Mandell, Douglas, and Bennett's
PRINCIPLES AND PRACTICE OF
INFECTIOUS DISEASES

Mandell, Douglas, and Bennett's
PRINCIPLES AND PRACTICE OF
INFECTIOUS DISEASES

seventh edition

Volume 2

GERALD L. MANDELL, MD, MACP
Professor of Medicine Emeritus
Owen R. Cheatham Professor of the Sciences Emeritus
Chief of Infectious Diseases Emeritus
University of Virginia Health Center
Charlottesville, Virginia

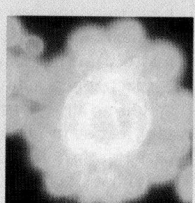

JOHN E. BENNETT, MD, MACP
Adjunct Professor of Medicine
Uniformed Services University of the Health Sciences
F. Edward Hébert School of Medicine
Bethesda, Maryland

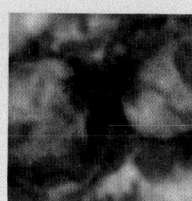

RAPHAEL DOLIN, MD
Maxwell Finland Professor of Medicine (Microbiology and Molecular Genetics)
Harvard Medical School
Attending Physician
Beth Israel Deaconess Medical Center
Brigham and Women's Hospital
Boston, Massachusetts

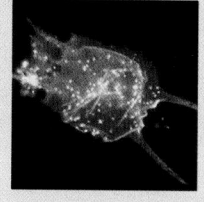

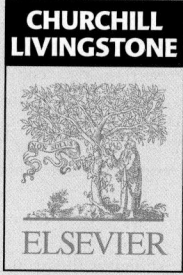

CHURCHILL
LIVINGSTONE

ELSEVIER

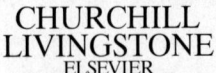

CHURCHILL
LIVINGSTONE
ELSEVIER

1600 John F. Kennedy Blvd.
Suite 1800
Philadelphia, PA 19103

MANDELL, DOUGLAS, AND BENNETT'S
PRINCIPLES AND PRACTICE OF INFECTIOUS DISEASES
Seventh Edition

Set ISBN: 978-0-4430-6839-3
Volume 1: Part no. 9996058433
Volume 2: Part no. 9996058492

Notices

Knowledge and best practice in this field are constantly changing. As new research and experience broaden our understanding, changes in research methods, professional practices, or medical treatment may become necessary.

Practitioners and researchers must always rely on their own experience and knowledge in evaluating and using any information, methods, compounds, or experiments described herein. In using such information or methods they should be mindful of their own safety and the safety of others, including parties for whom they have a professional responsibility.

With respect to any drug or pharmaceutical products identified, readers are advised to check the most current information provided (i) on procedures featured or (ii) by the manufacturer of each product to be administered, to verify the recommended dose or formula, the method and duration of administration, and contraindications. It is the responsibility of practitioners, relying on their own experience and knowledge of their patients, to make diagnoses, to determine dosages and the best treatment for each individual patient, and to take all appropriate safety precautions.

To the fullest extent of the law, neither the Publisher nor the authors, contributors, or editors assume any liability for any injury and/or damage to persons or property as a matter of product liability, negligence or otherwise, or from any use or operation of any methods, products, instructions, or ideas contained in the material herein.

Library of Congress Cataloging-in-Publication Data

Mandell, Douglas, and Bennett's principles and practice of infectious diseases / [edited by] Gerald L. Mandell, John E. Bennett, Raphael Dolin.—7th ed.
        p. ; cm.
    Includes bibliographical references and index.
    ISBN 978-0-4430-6839-3
  1. Communicable diseases.   I. Mandell, Gerald L.   II. Bennett, John E. (John Eugene).   III. Dolin, Raphael.   IV. Title: Principles and practice of infectious diseases.
    [DNLM: 1. Communicable Diseases. WC 100 M2713 2010]
    RC111.P78 2010
    616.9—dc22   2009022686

Executive Publisher: Natasha Andjelkovic
Senior Developmental Editor: Heather Krehling
Editorial Assistants: Brad McIlwain, Taylor Ball
Publishing Services Manager: Frank Polizzano
Senior Project Managers: Robin Hayward, Lee Ann Draud
Project Management Assistance: Joan Sinclair, Tina Rebane, Linda Van Pelt,
    Jeff Gunning, Rachel Miller, Pete Faber, Mary Ann Folcher, Peggy M. Gordon
Marketing Manager: Courtney Ingram
Multimedia Producer: Dan Martinez
Design Direction: Ellen Zanolle

Printed in the United States.

Last digit is the print number: 9 8 7 6 5 4 3 2 1

CONTRIBUTORS

N. Franklin Adkinson, Jr., MD
Professor of Medicine and Senior Laboratory Investigator, Johns Hopkins University School of Medicine, Baltimore, Maryland
β-Lactam Allergy

David M. Allen, MD
Partner, ID Specialists, Dallas, Texas
Acinetobacter Species

Ban Mishu Allos, MD
Assistant Professor of Medicine and Preventive Medicine, Vanderbilt University School of Medicine, Nashville, Tennessee
Campylobacter jejuni and Related Species

Guy W. Amsden, PharmD
Director, Department of Pharmaceutical Care Services, Bassett Healthcare, Cooperstown, New York
Pharmacokinetics and Pharmacodynamics of Anti-infective Agents; Tables of Antimicrobial Agent Pharmacology

David A. Anderson, PhD
Associate Professor, Deputy Director, and National Health and Medical Research Council Senior Research Fellow, Macfarlane Burnet Institute for Medical Research and Public Health, Melbourne, Victoria, Australia
Hepatitis E Virus

David R. Andes, MD
Associate Professor, University of Wisconsin School of Medicine and Public Health, Madison, Wisconsin
Cephalosporins

Fred Y. Aoki, MD
Professor, Departments of Medicine, Medical Microbiology, Pharmacology, and Therapeutics, University of Manitoba Faculty of Medicine; Health Sciences Centre, Winnipeg, Manitoba, Canada
Antiviral Drugs (Other than Antiretrovirals)

Petra M. Apfalter, MD, DTMH
Associate Professor, Medical University of Vienna, Vienna; Attending Physician, Elisabethinen Hospital Linz, Linz, Austria
Chlamydophila (Chlamydia) pneumoniae

Michael A. Apicella, MD
Professor and Head, Department of Microbiology, University of Iowa Carver College of Medicine, Iowa City, Iowa
Neisseria meningitidis

Cesar A. Arias, MD, MSc, PhD
Assistant Professor of Medicine, University of Texas Medical School at Houston, Houston, Texas; Director, Molecular Genetics and Antimicrobial Resistance Unit, Universidad El Bosque, Bogotá, Colombia
Enterococcus Species, *Streptococcus bovis* Group, and *Leuconostoc* Species

Michael H. Augenbraun, MD
Professor of Medicine, State University of New York Downstate College of Medicine; Director, Sexually Transmitted Diseases Clinic, Kings County Hospital Center, Brooklyn, New York
Genital Skin and Mucous Membrane Lesions

Dimitri T. Azar, MD
Professor of Ophthalmology, University of Illinois College of Medicine at Chicago; Professor and Head, Department of Ophthalmology and Visual Sciences, University of Illinois at Chicago Medical Center, Chicago, Illinois
Microbial Conjunctivitis; Microbial Keratitis

Larry M. Baddour, MD
Professor of Medicine, Mayo Clinic College of Medicine; Consultant, Infectious Diseases, Mayo Clinic, Rochester, Minnesota
Prosthetic Valve Endocarditis; Infections of Nonvalvular Cardiovascular Devices

Lindsey R. Baden, MD
Assistant Professor of Medicine, Harvard Medical School; Associate Physician, Director of Clinical Research (Division of Infectious Diseases), and Director of Transplant Infectious Diseases, Brigham and Women's Hospital; Director of Infectious Diseases, Dana-Farber Cancer Institute, Boston, Massachusetts
Vaccines for Human Immunodeficiency Virus-1 Infection

Carol J. Baker, MD
Professor of Pediatrics, Molecular Virology, and Microbiology, Department of Pediatrics, Section of Infectious Diseases, Baylor College of Medicine; Attending Physician, Texas Children's Hospital, Houston, Texas
Streptococcus agalactiae (Group B Streptococcus)

Ronald C. Ballard, PhD
Branch Chief, Laboratory Reference and Research Branch, Division of Sexually Transmitted Diseases Prevention, Centers for Disease Control and Prevention, Atlanta, Georgia
Klebsiella granulomatis (Donovanosis, Granuloma Inguinale)

Charles H. Ballow, PharmD
Director, Buffalo Clinical Research Center, Buffalo, New York
Pharmacokinetics and Pharmacodynamics of Anti-infective Agents

Scott D. Barnes, MD
Chief, Warfighter Refractive Eye Surgery Clinic, Womack Army Medical Center, Fort Bragg, North Carolina
Microbial Conjunctivitis; Microbial Keratitis

Miriam J. Baron, MD
Assistant Professor, Department of Medicine, Harvard Medical School; Associate Physician, Brigham and Women's Hospital, Boston, Massachusetts
Pancreatic Infection

Dan H. Barouch, MD, PhD
Associate Professor of Medicine, Harvard Medical School; Chief, Division of Vaccine Research, and Staff Physician, Beth Israel Deaconess Medical Center; Associate Physician, Brigham and Women's Hospital, Boston, Massachusetts
Vaccines for Human Immunodeficiency Virus-1 Infection; Adenoviruses

Alan Barrett, PhD
Professor, Department of Pathology, University of Texas Medical Branch, Galveston, Texas
Flaviviruses (Yellow Fever, Dengue, Dengue Hemorrhagic Fever, Japanese Encephalitis, West Nile Encephalitis, St. Louis Encephalitis, Tick-Borne Encephalitis)

Sarice L. Bassin, MD
Assistant Professor of Neurology, Northwestern University Feinberg
School of Medicine; Fellowship Director, Neurocritical Care,
Northwestern Memorial Hospital, McGaw Medical Center, Chicago,
Illinois
    Rhabdoviruses

Byron E. Batteiger, MD
Professor, Department of Medicine, Division of Infectious
Diseases, and Department of Microbiology and Immunology,
Indiana University School of Medicine, Indianapolis,
Indiana
    Introduction to *Chlamydia* and *Chlamydophila*; *Chlamydia
    trachomatis* (Trachoma, Perinatal Infections, Lymphogranuloma
    Venereum, and Other Genital Infections)

Stephen G. Baum, MD
Professor of Medicine and Professor of Microbiology and
Immunology, Albert Einstein College of Medicine of Yeshiva
University; Attending Physician, North Bronx Healthcare Network,
Bronx, New York
    Mumps Virus; Introduction to *Mycoplasma* and *Ureaplasma*;
    Mycoplasma pneumoniae and Atypical Pneumonia

Arnold S. Bayer, MD
Professor of Medicine, Department of Internal Medicine, David
Geffen School of Medicine at UCLA, Los Angeles; Associate Chief,
Adult Infectious Diseases, Department of Internal Medicine,
Harbor-UCLA Medical Center; Senior Investigator, St. John's
Cardiovascular Research Center, Los Angeles Biomedical Research
Institute, Torrance, California
    Endocarditis and Intravascular Infections

J. David Beckham, MD
Assistant Professor of Medicine, Division of Infectious Diseases,
University of Colorado Denver School of Medicine; Assistant
Professor of Medicine, University of Colorado Hospital, Aurora,
Colorado
    Encephalitis

Susan E. Beekmann, RN, MPH
University of Iowa Carver College of Medicine, Iowa
City, Iowa
    Infections Caused by Percutaneous Intravascular Devices

Beth P. Bell, MD, MPH
Associate Director for Epidemiologic Science, National Center for
Immunization and Respiratory Diseases, Centers for Disease Control
and Prevention, Atlanta, Georgia
    Hepatitis A Virus

John E. Bennett, MD
Adjunct Professor of Medicine, Uniformed Services University of the
Health Sciences F. Edward Hébert School of Medicine, Bethesda,
Maryland
    Chronic Meningitis; Introduction to Mycoses

Elie F. Berbari, MD
Associate Professor, Division of Infectious Diseases, Mayo Clinic
College of Medicine; Attending Physician, Mayo Clinic, Rochester,
Minnesota
    Osteomyelitis

Jonathan D. Berman, MD, PhD
Senior Vice President for Clinical Affairs, Fast-Track Drugs and
Biologics, LLC, North Potomac, Maryland
    Alternative Medicines for Infectious Diseases

Joseph S. Bertino, Jr., PharmD
Associate Professor of Pharmacology, Columbia University College
of Physicians and Surgeons, New York; Bertino Consulting,
Schenectady, New York
    Pharmacokinetics and Pharmacodynamics of Anti-infective Agents

Holly H. Birdsall, MD, PhD
Professor of Otolaryngology and Immunology, Baylor College of
Medicine; Associate Chief of Staff for Research, Michael E. DeBakey
Veterans Affairs Medical Center, Houston, Texas
    Antibodies

Alan L. Bisno, MD
Professor Emeritus, Department of Medicine, University of Miami
Miller School of Medicine; Staff Physician, Miami Veterans Affairs
Medical Center, Miami, Florida
    Classification of Streptococci; *Streptococcus pyogenes*;
    Nonsuppurative Poststreptococcal Sequelae: Rheumatic Fever and
    Glomerulonephritis

Hope H. Biswas, ScM
Staff Scientist, Blood Systems Research Institute, San Francisco,
California
    Human T-Cell Lymphotropic Virus Types I and II

Brian G. Blackburn, MD
Clinical Assistant Professor and Co-Director of Clinical Services,
Division of Infectious Diseases and Geographic Medicine, Stanford
University School of Medicine; Attending Physician, Department
of Internal Medicine, Division of Infectious Diseases and
Geographic Medicine, Stanford Hospital and Clinics, Stanford,
California
    Free-Living Amebas

Martin J. Blaser, MD
Frederick H. King Professor of Internal Medicine; Chair,
Department of Medicine; and Professor of Microbiology, New York
University School of Medicine; Chief, Medical Services, Bellevue
Hospital Center; Chief, Medical Services, New York University
Langone Medical Center; Staff Physician, Department of Medical
Services, New York Harbor Veterans Affairs Medical Center,
New York, New York
    Introduction to Bacteria and Bacterial Diseases; *Campylobacter
    jejuni* and Related Species; *Helicobacter pylori* and Other Gastric
    Helicobacter Species

David L. Blazes, MD, MPH
Chief, Global Emerging Infections System Operations, Armed Forces
Health Surveillance Center, Silver Spring, Maryland
    Outbreak Investigation

Thomas P. Bleck, MD
Assistant Dean and Professor of Neurological Sciences,
Neurosurgery, Medicine, and Anesthesiology, Rush Medical College
of Rush University; Associate Chief Medical Officer (Critical Care),
Rush University Medical Center, Chicago, Illinois
    Rhabdoviruses; *Clostridium tetani* (Tetanus); *Clostridium botulinum*
    (Botulism); Botulinum Toxin as a Biological Weapon

Nicole M. A. Blijlevens, MD, PhD
Consultant and Lecturer, Department of Haematology, Radboud
University Nijmegen Medical Centre, Nijmegen, The Netherlands
    Infections in the Immunocompromised Host: General Principles

David A. Bobak, MD
Associate Professor of Medicine, Division of Infectious Diseases and HIV Medicine, Case Western Reserve University School of Medicine; Associate Chair for Clinical Affairs, Division of Infectious Diseases and HIV Medicine; Director, Traveler's Healthcare Center; Chair, Health System Medication Safety and Therapeutics Committee; and Staff Physician, Transplant Infectious Diseases Clinic, University Hospitals of Cleveland–Case Medical Center, Cleveland, Ohio
  Nausea, Vomiting, and Noninflammatory Diarrhea

William Bonnez, MD
Associate Professor of Medicine, University of Rochester School of Medicine and Dentistry; Attending Physician, University of Rochester Medical Center, Rochester, New York
  Papillomaviruses

John C. Boothroyd, PhD
Professor of Microbiology and Immunology, Stanford University School of Medicine, Stanford, California
  Toxoplasma gondii

Luciana Borio, MD
Assistant Professor of Medicine, University of Pittsburgh School of Medicine; Senior Associate, Center for Biosecurity of the University of Pittsburgh Medical Center, Pittsburgh, Pennsylvania
  Bioterrorism: An Overview; Plague as a Bioterrorism Weapon

Patrick J. Bosque, MD
Associate Professor, Department of Neurology, University of Colorado Denver School of Medicine, Aurora; Attending Physician, Neurology Division, Department of Medicine, Denver Health Medical Center, Denver, Colorado
  Prions and Prion Diseases of the Central Nervous System (Transmissible Neurodegenerative Diseases)

Richard C. Boucher, Jr., MD
William Rand Kenan Professor of Medicine, Cystic Fibrosis Research and Treatment Center, University of North Carolina at Chapel Hill School of Medicine, Chapel Hill, North Carolina
  Cystic Fibrosis

Barry D. Brause, MD
Professor of Clinical Medicine, Weill Cornell Medical College; Attending Physician and Director of Infectious Diseases, Hospital for Special Surgery; Attending Physician, New York–Presbyterian Hospital, New York, New York
  Infections with Prostheses in Bones and Joints

Kevin E. Brown, MD
Consultant Medical Virologist, Virus Reference Department, Centre for Infections, Health Protection Agency, London, United Kingdom
  Human Parvoviruses, Including Parvovirus B19 and Human Bocavirus

Patricia D. Brown, MD
Associate Professor of Medicine, Wayne State University School of Medicine; Chief of Medicine, Detroit Receiving Hospital, Detroit, Michigan
  Infections in Injection Drug Users

Barbara A. Brown-Elliott, MS, MT(ASCP)SM
Assistant Professor of Microbiology and Supervisor, *Mycobacteria/ Nocardia* Laboratory, University of Texas Health Science Center, Tyler, Texas
  Infections Due to Nontuberculous Mycobacteria Other than *Mycobacterium avium-intracellulare*

Eileen M. Burd, PhD
Associate Professor, Emory University School of Medicine; Director, Clinical Microbiology, Emory University Hospital, Atlanta, Georgia
  Other Gram-Negative and Gram-Variable Bacilli

James E. Burns, MD, MBA
Clinical Assistant Professor, Department of Pediatrics, University of Virginia School of Medicine, Charlottesville; Deputy Commissioner, Virginia Department of Health, Richmond, Virginia
  Epiglottitis

Larry M. Bush, MD
Clinical Associate Professor of Medicine, University of Miami Miller School of Medicine, Miami; Clinical Associate Professor of Medicine, Florida Atlantic University School of Biomedical Science, Boca Raton; Chief, Infectious Diseases, John F. Kennedy Medical Center, Atlantis, Florida
  Peritonitis and Intraperitoneal Abscesses

David P. Calfee, MD, MS
Associate Professor of Medicine, Mount Sinai School of Medicine; Hospital Epidemiologist, Mount Sinai Hospital, New York, New York
  Rifamycins

Ellis S. Caplan, MD
Clinical Professor of Medicine, Division of Infectious Diseases, University of Maryland School of Medicine; Chief, Infectious Diseases, R. Adams Cowley Shock Trauma Center, Baltimore, Maryland
  Hyperbaric Oxygen

Michel Caraël, PhD
Professor Emeritus, Free University of Brussels, Brussels, Belgium; Manager, HIV and AIDS Data HUB, UNICEF and UNAIDS, Asia Pacific, Bangkok, Thailand
  Global Perspectives on Human Immunodeficiency Virus Infection and Acquired Immunodeficiency Syndrome

Charles C. J. Carpenter, MD
Professor of Medicine, Warren Alpert Medical School of Brown University; Director, Lifespan/Tufts/Brown Center for AIDS Research; Attending Physician, Division of Infectious Diseases, Miriam Hospital, Providence, Rhode Island
  Other Pathogenic Vibrios

Mary T. Caserta, MD
Associate Professor of Pediatrics, University of Rochester School of Medicine and Dentistry; Attending Physician, Golisano Children's Hospital at Strong, University of Rochester Medical Center, Rochester, New York
  Pharyngitis; Acute Laryngitis

Elio Castagnola, MD, PhD
Chief, Section for Infections in the Immunocompromised Host, Infectious Diseases Unit, Department of Hematology and Oncology, G. Gaslini Children's Hospital, Genoa, Italy
  Prophylaxis and Empirical Therapy of Infection in Cancer Patients

Richard E. Chaisson, MD
Professor of Medicine, Epidemiology, and International Health, Johns Hopkins University School of Medicine, Baltimore, Maryland
  General Clinical Manifestations of Human Immunodeficiency Virus Infection (Including the Acute Retroviral Syndrome and Oral, Cutaneous, Renal, Ocular, Metabolic, and Cardiac Diseases)

Henry F. Chambers, MD
Professor of Medicine, University of California, San Francisco, School of Medicine; Chief, Infectious Diseases, San Francisco General Hospital, San Francisco, California
  Penicillins and β-Lactam Inhibitors; Carbapenems and Monobactams

Stanley W. Chapman, MD
Professor of Medicine and Associate Professor of Microbiology, University of Mississippi School of Medicine; Division of Infectious Diseases, University of Mississippi Medical Center, Jackson, Mississippi
Blastomyces dermatitidis

James D. Chappell, MD, PhD
Assistant Professor of Pathology and Pediatrics, Vanderbilt University School of Medicine; Director, Clinical Diagnostic Virology Laboratory, Vanderbilt University Medical Center, Nashville, Tennessee
Introduction to Viruses and Viral Diseases

Sharon C-A. Chen, PhD, MB BS
Clinical Senior Lecturer, University of Sydney Faculty of Medicine, Sydney; Senior Staff Specialist, Centre for Infectious Diseases and Microbiology, Westmead Hospital, Westmead, New South Wales, Australia
Nocardia Species

Sanjiv Chopra, MD
Professor of Medicine, Harvard Medical School; Senior Consultant in Hepatology, Beth Israel Deaconess Medical Center, Boston, Massachusetts
Acute Viral Hepatitis

Anthony W. Chow, MD
Professor Emeritus, Department of Medicine, Division of Infectious Diseases, University of British Columbia Faculty of Medicine; Honorary Staff, Department of Medicine, Division of Infectious Disease, Vancouver Hospital Health Sciences Center, Vancouver, British Columbia, Canada
Infections of the Oral Cavity, Neck, and Head

Alexandra Chroneou, MD
University of Athens Medical School; Attending Physician, Sotiria Hospital for Chest Diseases, Athens, Greece
Nosocomial Pneumonia

Nicholas P. Cianciotto, PhD
Professor of Microbiology-Immunology, Northwestern University Feinberg School of Medicine, Chicago, Illinois
Legionella

Rebecca A. Clark, MD, PhD
Professor of Medicine, Louisiana State University Health Sciences Center; Clinical Medical Director, HIV Outpatient Program, Interim LSU Public Hospital, New Orleans, Louisiana
Human Immunodeficiency Virus Infection in Women

Robert A. Clark, MD
Professor of Medicine and Associate Chair for Research, Assistant Vice President for Clinical Research, and Director of the Institute for Integration of Medicine and Science, University of Texas Health Science Center at San Antonio; Staff Physician, University Health System and South Texas Veterans Health Care System, San Antonio, Texas
Granulocytic Phagocytes

Jeffrey I. Cohen, MD
Chief, Medical Virology Section, Laboratory of Clinical Infectious Diseases, National Institute of Allergy and Infectious Diseases, National Institutes of Health, Bethesda, Maryland
Introduction to Herpesviridae; Human Herpesvirus Types 6 and 7; Herpes B Virus

Myron S. Cohen, MD
Professor of Medicine, University of North Carolina at Chapel Hill School of Medicine; Chief, Division of Infectious Diseases, University of North Carolina Health Care, Chapel Hill, North Carolina
The Acutely Ill Patient with Fever and Rash

Ronit Cohen-Poradosu, MD
Research Associate, Channing Laboratory, Brigham and Women's Hospital and Harvard Medical School, Boston, Massachusetts
Anaerobic Infections: General Concepts

Susan E. Cohn, MD, MPH
Professor of Medicine, Division of Infectious Diseases, University of Rochester School of Medicine and Dentistry; Attending Physician, Strong Memorial Hospital, Rochester, New York
Human Immunodeficiency Virus Infection in Women

Mark Connors, MD
Chief, HIV-Specific Immunity Section, Laboratory of Immunoregulation, National Institute of Allergy and Infectious Diseases, National Institutes of Health, Bethesda, Maryland
The Immunology of Human Immunodeficiency Virus Infection

Joanne Cono, MD, ScM
Senior Advisor for Science and Global Health, Office of the Director, Coordinating Center for Infectious Diseases, Centers for Disease Control and Prevention, Atlanta, Georgia
Smallpox as an Agent of Bioterrorism

Lawrence Corey, MD
Head, Virology Division, and Professor of Medicine and Laboratory Medicine, University of Washington School of Medicine; Senior Vice President and Co-Director, Vaccine and Infectious Disease Institute, and Head, Program in Infectious Disease, Fred Hutchinson Cancer Research Center, Seattle, Washington
Herpes Simplex Virus

Patricia A. Cornett, MD
Health Science Clinical Professor, University of California, San Francisco, School of Medicine; Chief, Hematology/Oncology, San Francisco Veterans Affairs Medical Center, San Francisco, California
Malignant Diseases in Human Immunodeficiency Virus Infection

Heather L. Cox, PharmD
Assistant Professor of Medicine and Infectious Diseases, Department of Internal Medicine, University of Virginia School of Medicine; Clinical Specialist, Infectious Diseases, Department of Pharmacy Services, University of Virginia Health System, Charlottesville, Virginia
Linezolid and Other Oxazolidinones

William A. Craig, MD
Professor, University of Wisconsin School of Medicine and Public Health, Madison, Wisconsin
Cephalosporins

Donald E. Craven, MD
Professor of Medicine, Tufts University School of Medicine, Boston; Chairman, Department of Infectious Diseases, Lahey Clinic Medical Center, Burlington, Massachusetts
Nosocomial Pneumonia

Kent B. Crossley, MD
Professor of Medicine, University of Minnesota Medical School; Associate Chief of Staff for Education, Minneapolis Veterans Affairs Medical Center, Minneapolis, Minnesota
Infections in the Elderly

John A. Crump, MB ChB, DTM&H
Associate Professor of Medicine, Division of Infectious Diseases and International Health, Duke University School of Medicine; Director, Duke Tanzania Operations, Duke Global Health Institute, Durham, North Carolina
  Enteric Fever and Other Causes of Abdominal Symptoms with Fever

Clyde S. CrumpackerII, MD
Professor of Medicine, Harvard Medical School; Attending Physician, Division of Infectious Diseases, Beth Israel Deaconess Medical Center, Boston, Massachusetts
  Cytomegalovirus

James W. Curran, MD, MPH
Dean and Professor of Epidemiology, Rollins School of Public Health, Emory University; Co-Director, Emory Center for AIDS Research, Atlanta, Georgia
  Epidemiology and Prevention of Acquired Immunodeficiency Syndrome and Human Immunodeficiency Virus Infection

Bart J. Currie, FRACP, DTM&H
Professor in Medicine, Tropical and Emerging Infectious Diseases Division, Menzies School of Health Research and Northern Territory Clinical School; Infectious Diseases Physician, Royal Darwin Hospital, Darwin, Northern Territory, Australia
  Burkholderia pseudomallei and *Burkholderia mallei: Melioidosis* and *Glanders*

Michael P. Curry, MD
Assistant Professor of Medicine, Harvard Medical School; Medical Director, Liver Transplantation, Beth Israel Deaconess Medical Center, Boston, Massachusetts
  Acute Viral Hepatitis

Inger K. Damon, MD, PhD
Adjunct Clinical Faculty, Department of Medicine, Emory University School of Medicine; Chief, Poxvirus and Rabies Branch, Centers for Disease Control and Prevention, Atlanta, Georgia
  Orthopoxviruses: Vaccinia (Smallpox Vaccine), Variola (Smallpox), Monkeypox, and Cowpox; Other Poxviruses That Infect Humans: Parapoxviruses, Molluscum Contagiosum, and Yatapoxviruses; Smallpox as an Agent of Bioterrorism

Rabih O. Darouiche, MD
Professor of Medicine and Physical Medicine and Rehabilitation and Director, Center for Prostheses Infection, Baylor College of Medicine; Veterans Affairs Distinguished Service Professor, Michael E. DeBakey Veterans Affairs Medical Center, Houston, Texas
  Infections in Patients with Spinal Cord Injury

Roberta L. DeBiasi, MD
Associate Professor of Pediatrics, George Washington University School of Medicine and Health Sciences; Attending Physician, Division of Pediatric Infectious Diseases, Children's National Medical Center, Washington, DC
  Orthoreoviruses and Orbiviruses; Coltiviruses and Seadornaviruses

George S. Deepe, Jr., MD
Morgan Professor of Medicine, University of Cincinnati College of Medicine; Professor, Division of Infectious Diseases, University Hospital and Veterans Affairs Cincinnati Medical Center, Cincinnati, Ohio
  Histoplasma capsulatum

Carlos del Rio, MD
Professor and Chair, Hubert Department of Global Health, Rollins School of Public Health, Emory University; Co-Director, Emory Center for AIDS Research, Atlanta, Georgia
  Epidemiology and Prevention of Acquired Immunodeficiency Syndrome and Human Immunodeficiency Virus Infection

Gregory P. DeMuri, MD
Associate Professor, University of Wisconsin School of Medicine and Public Health; Attending Physician, American Family Children's Hospital, Madison, Wisconsin
  Sinusitis

David T. Dennis, MD, MPH
Faculty Affiliate, Department of Microbiology, Immunology, and Pathology, Colorado State University College of Veterinary Medicine and Biomedical Sciences, Fort Collins, Colorado; Medical Epidemiologist, Division of Influenza, Centers for Disease Control and Prevention, Atlanta, Georgia
  Yersinia Species, Including Plague

Peter Densen, MD
Executive Dean, University of Iowa Carver College of Medicine, Iowa City, Iowa
  Complement

Ben E. De Pauw, MD, PhD
Professor, Blood Transfusion and Transplantation Immunology, Radboud University Nijmegen Medical Centre, Nijmegen, The Netherlands
  Infections in the Immunocompromised Host: General Principles

Terence S. Dermody, MD
Dorothy Overall Wells Professor of Pediatrics and Professor of Microbiology and Immunology, Vanderbilt University School of Medicine; Director, Division of Pediatric Infectious Diseases, Monroe Carell Jr. Children's Hospital at Vanderbilt, Nashville, Tennessee
  Introduction to Viruses and Viral Diseases

Robin Dewar, PhD
Principal Scientist, SAIC–Frederick, National Cancer Institute–Frederick, Frederick, Maryland
  Diagnosis of Human Immunodeficiency Virus Infection

James H. Diaz, MD, MPH and TM, PhD
Professor of Public Health and Preventive Medicine and Head, Environmental and Occupational Health Sciences, School of Public Health; Professor of Anesthesiology, School of Medicine, Louisiana State University Health Sciences Center, New Orleans, Louisiana
  Introduction to Ectoparasitic Diseases; Lice (Pediculosis); Scabies; Myiasis and Tungiasis; Mites, Including Chiggers; Ticks, Including Tick Paralysis

Carl W. Dieffenbach, PhD
Director, Division of AIDS, National Institute of Allergy and Infectious Diseases, National Institutes of Health, Bethesda, Maryland
  Innate (General or Nonspecific) Host Defense Mechanisms

Jules L. Dienstag, MD
Carl W. Walter Professor of Medicine and Dean for Medical Education, Harvard Medical School; Attending Physician, Massachusetts General Hospital, Boston, Massachusetts
  Chronic Viral Hepatitis

Raphael Dolin, MD
Maxwell Finland Professor of Medicine (Microbiology and Molecular Genetics), Harvard Medical School; Attending Physician, Beth Israel Deaconess Medical Center and Brigham and Women's Hospital, Boston, Massachusetts
> Antiviral Drugs (Other than Antiretrovirals); Vaccines for Human Immunodeficiency Virus-1 Infection; Zoonotic Paramyxoviruses: Nipah, Hendra, and Menangle Viruses; Noroviruses and Other Caliciviruses; Astroviruses and Picobirnaviruses

Scott H. Donaldson, MD
Associate Professor of Medicine, Division of Pulmonary and Critical Care Medicine, University of North Carolina at Chapel Hill School of Medicine, Chapel Hill, North Carolina
> Cystic Fibrosis

J. Peter Donnelly, PhD
Coordinator of Studies in Supportive Care, Department of Haematology, Radboud University Nijmegen Medical Centre, Nijmegen, The Netherlands
> Infections in the Immunocompromised Host: General Principles

Michael S. Donnenberg, MD
Professor of Medicine and Professor of Microbiology and Immunology, University of Maryland School of Medicine, Baltimore, Maryland
> Enterobacteriaceae

Gerald R. Donowitz, MD
Edward W. Hook Professor of Medicine and Infectious Diseases, University of Virginia School of Medicine; Vice-Chair for Education, Department of Medicine, University of Virginia Health System, Charlottesville, Virginia
> Linezolid and Other Oxazolidinones; Acute Pneumonia

Philip R. Dormitzer, MD, PhD
Senior Director and Senior Project Leader, Viral Vaccine Research, Novartis Vaccines and Diagnostics, Cambridge, Massachusetts
> Rotaviruses

James M. Drake, MB BCh, MSc
Professor of Surgery, University of Toronto Faculty of Medicine; Neurosurgeon in Chief and Harold Hoffman Shopper's Drug Mart Chair in Pediatric Neurosurgery, Division of Neurosurgery, Hospital for Sick Children, Toronto, Ontario, Canada
> Cerebrospinal Fluid Shunt Infections

J. Stephen Dumler, MD
Professor, Department of Pathology, Division of Medical Microbiology, Johns Hopkins University School of Medicine; Professor, Department of Molecular Microbiology and Immunology, Johns Hopkins Bloomberg School of Public Health; Associate Director, Medical Microbiology, Department of Pathology, Johns Hopkins Hospital, Baltimore, Maryland
> *Rickettsia typhi* (Murine Typhus); *Ehrlichia chaffeensis* (Human Monocytotropic Ehrlichiosis), *Anaplasma phagocytophilum* (Human Granulocytotropic Anaplasmosis), and Other Anaplasmataceae

J. Stephen Dummer, MD
Professor of Medicine and Surgery and Chief, Transplant Infectious Diseases, Vanderbilt University School of Medicine, Nashville, Tennessee
> Risk Factors and Approaches to Infections in Transplant Recipients; Infections in Solid Organ Transplant Recipients

Herbert L. DuPont, MD
Professor of Epidemiology and Director, Center for Infectious Diseases, University of Texas School of Public Health; Vice Chairman, Department of Medicine, Baylor College of Medicine; Chief, Internal Medicine Service, St. Luke's Episcopal Hospital, Houston, Texas
> *Shigella* Species (Bacillary Dysentery)

David T. Durack, MB, DPhil
Consulting Professor of Medicine, Duke University School of Medicine, Durham, North Carolina; Senior Vice President, Beckton, Dickinson and Company, Franklin Lakes, New Jersey
> Fever of Unknown Origin; Prevention of Infective Endocarditis

Marlene L. Durand, MD
Assistant Professor, Harvard Medical School; Director, Infectious Disease Service, Massachusetts Eye and Ear Infirmary; Physician, Infectious Disease Unit, Massachusetts General Hospital, Boston, Massachusetts
> Endophthalmitis; Infectious Causes of Uveitis; Periocular Infections

Paul H. Edelstein, MD
Professor of Pathology and Laboratory Medicine, University of Pennsylvania School of Medicine; Director of Clinical Microbiology, Hospital of the University of Pennsylvania, Philadelphia, Pennsylvania
> *Legionella*

Michael B. Edmond, MD, MPH, MPA
Professor of Internal Medicine, Epidemiology, and Community Health and Chair, Division of Infectious Diseases, Virginia Commonwealth University School of Medicine; Hospital Epidemiologist, Virginia Commonwealth University Medical Center, Richmond, Virginia
> Organization for Infection Control; Isolation

John E. Edwards, Jr., MD
Professor of Medicine, David Geffen School of Medicine at UCLA, Los Angeles; Chief, Division of Infectious Diseases, Harbor-UCLA Medical Center, Torrance, California
> *Candida* Species

Morven S. Edwards, MD
Professor of Pediatrics, Section of Infectious Diseases, Baylor College of Medicine; Attending Physician, Texas Children's Hospital, Houston, Texas
> *Streptococcus agalactiae* (Group B Streptococcus)

George M. Eliopoulos, MD
Professor of Medicine, Harvard Medical School; Staff Physician, Division of Infectious Diseases, Beth Israel Deaconess Medical Center, Boston, Massachusetts
> Principles of Anti-infective Therapy

N. Cary Engleberg, MD
Professor, Department of Microbiology and Immunology, University of Michigan Medical School, Ann Arbor, Michigan
> Chronic Fatigue Syndrome

Joel D. Ernst, MD
Professor, Departments of Medicine, Pathology, and Microbiology, and Director, Division of Infectious Diseases, New York University School of Medicine, New York, New York
> *Mycobacterium leprae*

Rick M. Fairhurst, MD, PhD
Chief, Malaria Pathogenesis and Human Immunity Unit, Laboratory of Malaria and Vector Research, National Institute of Allergy and Infectious Diseases, National Institutes of Health, Bethesda, Maryland
  Plasmodium Species (Malaria)

Jessica K. Fairley, MD
Fellow, Division of Infectious Diseases and HIV Medicine, Case Western Reserve University School of Medicine, Cleveland, Ohio
  Cestodes (Tapeworms)

Stanley Falkow, PhD
Robert W. and Vivian K. Cahill Professor of Microbiology and Immunology and Professor of Medicine, Stanford University School of Medicine, Stanford, California
  A Molecular Perspective of Microbial Pathogenicity

Ann R. Falsey, MD
Professor of Medicine, University of Rochester School of Medicine and Dentistry; Attending Physician, Rochester General Hospital, Rochester, New York
  Human Metapneumovirus

Anthony S. Fauci, MD
Director, National Institute of Allergy and Infectious Diseases, National Institutes of Health, Bethesda, Maryland
  The Immunology of Human Immunodeficiency Virus Infection

Stephen M. Feinstone, MD
Chief, Laboratory of Hepatitis Viruses, Center for Biologics Evaluation and Research, U.S. Food and Drug Administration, Bethesda, Maryland
  Hepatitis A Virus

Thomas Fekete, MD
Professor of Medicine and Chief, Section of Infectious Diseases, Temple University School of Medicine, Philadelphia, Pennsylvania
  Bacillus Species and Related Genera Other than *Bacillus anthracis*

Paul D. Fey, PhD
Associate Professor, Department of Pathology and Microbiology, University of Nebraska Medical Center College of Medicine, Omaha, Nebraska
  Staphylococcus epidermidis and Other Coagulase-Negative Staphylococci

Steven M. Fine, MD, PhD
Assistant Professor of Medicine, University of Rochester School of Medicine and Dentistry; Attending Physician, Division of Infectious Diseases, University of Rochester Medical Center, Rochester, New York
  Vesicular Stomatitis Virus and Related Vesiculoviruses

Sydney M. Finegold, MD
Emeritus Professor of Medicine and Emeritus Professor of Microbiology, Immunology, and Molecular Genetics, David Geffen School of Medicine at UCLA; Staff Physician, Infectious Diseases Section, West Los Angeles Veterans Affairs Medical Center, Los Angeles, California
  Anaerobic Cocci

Neil O. Fishman, MD
Associate Professor of Medicine, University of Pennsylvania School of Medicine; Director, Department of Healthcare Epidemiology and Infection Prevention and Control, Hospital of the University of Pennsylvania, Philadelphia, Pennsylvania
  Antimicrobial Stewardship

Daniel W. Fitzgerald, MD
Associate Professor of Medicine, Weill Cornell Medical College, New York, New York
  Mycobacterium tuberculosis

Anthony R. Flores, MD, PhD, MPH
Postdoctoral Fellow, Pediatric Infectious Diseases, Baylor College of Medicine, Houston, Texas
  Pharyngitis

Vance G. Fowler, Jr., MD, MHS
Associate Professor of Medicine, Division of Infectious Diseases, Duke University School of Medicine, Durham, North Carolina
  Endocarditis and Intravascular Infections

David O. Freedman, MD
Professor of Medicine and Epidemiology, Gorgas Center for Geographic Medicine, Division of Infectious Diseases, University of Alabama at Birmingham School of Medicine; Director, University of Alabama at Birmingham Travelers Health Clinic, University of Alabama at Birmingham Health System, Birmingham, Alabama
  Protection of Travelers; Infections in Returning Travelers

Arthur M. Friedlander, MD
Adjunct Professor of Medicine, Uniformed Services University of the Health Sciences F. Edward Hébert School of Medicine, Bethesda; Senior Scientist, U.S. Army Medical Research Institute of Infectious Diseases, Frederick, Maryland
  Bacillus anthracis (Anthrax); Anthrax as an Agent of Bioterrorism

John N. Galgiani, MD
Professor, University of Arizona College of Medicine; Director, University of Arizona Valley Fever Center for Excellence; Chief Medical Officer, Valley Fever Solutions, Inc., Tucson, Arizona
  Coccidioides Species

John I. Gallin, MD
Director, Clinical Center, National Institutes of Health; Senior Investigator, Laboratory of Host Defenses, National Institutes of Health, Bethesda, Maryland
  Evaluation of the Patient with Suspected Immunodeficiency

Robert C. Gallo, MD
Director, Institute of Human Virology, and Professor, Department of Medicine, University of Maryland School of Medicine, Baltimore, Maryland
  Human Immunodeficiency Viruses

Wendy S. Garrett, MD, PhD
Instructor in Medicine, Harvard Medical School and Harvard School of Public Health; Dana-Farber Cancer Institute and Brigham and Women's Hospital, Boston, Massachusetts
  Gas Gangrene and Other *Clostridium*-Associated Diseases; *Bacteroides, Prevotella, Porphyromonas,* and *Fusobacterium* Species (and Other Medically Important Anaerobic Gram-Negative Bacilli)

Jeffrey A. Gelfand, MD
Clinical Professor of Medicine, Harvard Medical School; Attending Physician, Infectious Diseases Division, Massachusetts General Hospital, Boston, Massachusetts
  Babesia Species

Steven P. Gelone, PharmD
Associate Professor of Community Medicine and Preventive Health, Drexel University College of Medicine, Philadelphia; Vice President, Clinical Development, Virolharma Inc., Exton, Pennsylvania
  Topical Antibacterials

Anne A. Gershon, MD
Professor of Pediatrics and Director, Division of Pediatric Infectious Diseases, Columbia University College of Physicians and Surgeons, New York, New York
Rubella Virus (German Measles); Measles Virus (Rubeola)

David N. Gilbert, MD
Professor of Medicine, Oregon Health & Science University School of Medicine; Chief, Infectious Diseases, Providence Portland Medical Center, Portland, Oregon
Aminoglycosides

Peter H. Gilligan, PhD
Professor of Microbiology, Immunology and Pathology, and Laboratory Medicine, University of North Carolina at Chapel Hill School of Medicine, Chapel Hill, North Carolina
Cystic Fibrosis

Michael S. Glickman, MD
Associate Member, Division of Infectious Diseases, Immunology Program, Memorial Sloan-Kettering Cancer Center, New York, New York
Cell-Mediated Defense against Infection

Ulf B. Göbel, MD, PhD
Professor of Clinical Microbiology, Humboldt University of Berlin; Director, Institut für Mikrobiologie und Hygiene, Charité Universitätsmedizin Berlin, Berlin, Germany
Stenotrophomonas maltophilia and *Burkholderia cepacia* Complex

Deborah Goldstein, MD
Fellow, Division of Infectious Diseases, Department of Medicine, Georgetown University Hospital, Washington DC
Diagnosis of Human Immunodeficiency Virus Infection

Ellie J. C. Goldstein, MD
Clinical Professor of Medicine, David Geffen School of Medicine at UCLA; Director, Infection Control, Kindred Hospital–Los Angeles, Los Angeles; Director, R. M. Alden Research Laboratory, Santa Monica, California
Bites

Fred M. Gordin, MD
Professor of Medicine, George Washington University School of Medicine and Health Sciences; Chief, Infectious Diseases, Veterans Affairs Medical Center, Washington, DC
Mycobacterium avium Complex

Eduardo Gotuzzo, MD
Professor of Medicine and Principal Investigator, Alexander von Humboldt Tropical Medicine Institute, Cayetano Heredia University; Chief, Department of Infectious Diseases and Tropical Medicine, National Hospital Cayetano Heredia, Lima Peru
Vibrio cholerae

Paul S. Graman, MD
Professor of Medicine, University of Rochester School of Medicine and Dentistry; Attending Physician and Clinical Director, Infectious Diseases Division, Strong Memorial Hospital, Rochester, New York
Esophagitis

Margot Graves, BS
Public Health Microbiologist and Supervisor, Microbial Diseases Laboratory, Center for Infectious Disease, California Department of Public Health, Richmond, California
Capnocytophaga

Patricia M. Griffin, MD
Chief, Enteric Diseases Epidemiology Branch, Division of Foodborne, Bacterial, and Mycotic Diseases, National Center for Zoonotic, Vectorborne, and Enteric Diseases, Centers for Disease Control and Prevention, Atlanta, Georgia
Foodborne Disease

David E. Griffith, MD
Professor of Medicine and William A. and Elizabeth B. Moncrief Distinguished Professor, University of Texas Health Science Center at Tyler, Tyler, Texas
Antimycobacterial Agents

Richard L. Guerrant, MD
Thomas H. Hunter Professor of International Medicine; Director, Center for Global Health, Division of Infectious Diseases and International Health, University of Virginia School of Medicine, Charlottesville, Virginia
Principles and Syndromes of Enteric Infection; Nausea, Vomiting, and Noninflammatory Diarrhea; Inflammatory Enteritides; Enteric Fever and Other Causes of Abdominal Symptoms with Fever

David A. Haake, MD
Professor of Medicine in Residence, David Geffen School of Medicine at UCLA; Staff Physician, Veterans Affairs Greater Los Angeles Healthcare System, Los Angeles, California
Leptospira Species (Leptospirosis)

David W. Haas, MD
Associate Professor, Departments of Medicine, Microbiology, and Immunology, Vanderbilt University School of Medicine, Nashville, Tennessee
Mycobacterium tuberculosis

Caroline Breese Hall, MD
Professor of Pediatrics and Medicine, University of Rochester School of Medicine and Dentistry, Rochester, New York
Acute Laryngotracheobronchitis (Croup); Bronchiolitis; Respiratory Syncytial Virus

Scott Halperin, MD
Professor, Departments of Pediatrics and Microbiology and Immunology, Dalhousie University Faculty of Medicine; Head, Division of Pediatric Infectious Diseases, Dalhousie University and IWK Health Centre, Halifax, Nova Scotia, Canada
Bordetella pertussis

Margaret R. Hammerschlag, MD
Professor of Pediatrics and Medicine, State University of New York Downstate College of Medicine; Director, Division of Pediatric Infectious Diseases, State University of New York Downstate Medical Center, Brooklyn, New York
Chlamydophila (Chlamydia) pneumoniae

H. Hunter Handsfield, MD
Senior Research Leader, Battelle Centers for Public Health Research and Evaluation; Clinical Professor of Medicine, University of Washington Center for AIDS and Sexually Transmitted Diseases, Seattle, Washington
Neisseria gonorrhoeae

Rashidul Haque, MD, PhD
International Scientist, Laboratory Sciences Division, International Centre for Diarrheal Diseases Research, Dhaka, Bangladesh
Entamoeba Species, Including Amebiasis

Barry J. Hartman, MD
Clinical Professor of Medicine, Weill Cornell Medical College;
Attending Physician, New York–Presbyterian Hospital, New York,
New York
Acinetobacter Species

Roderick J. Hay, DM
Honorary Professor, Clinical Research Unit, London School of
Hygiene and Tropical Medicine, London; Emeritus Professor,
Queens University, Belfast, United Kingdom
Dermatophytosis and Other Superficial Mycoses

Frederick G. Hayden, MD
Stuart S. Richardson Professor of Clinical Virology and Professor of
Internal Medicine and Pathology, University of Virginia School of
Medicine, Charlottesville, Virginia
Antiviral Drugs (Other than Antiretrovirals)

Craig W. Hedberg, PhD
Division of Environmental Health Sciences, University of Minnesota
School of Public Health, Minneapolis, Minnesota
Epidemiologic Principles

David K. Henderson, MD
Deputy Director for Clinical Care, Clinical Center, National
Institutes of Health, Bethesda, Maryland
Hospital Preparedness for Emerging and Highly Contagious
Infectious Diseases: Getting Ready for the Next Epidemic or
Pandemic; Infections Caused by Percutaneous Intravascular
Devices; Human Immunodeficiency Virus in Health Care Settings;
Nosocomial Herpesvirus Infections

Donald A. Henderson, MD, MPH
21st Century Professor of Medicine, University of Pittsburgh School
of Medicine; Professor of Infectious Diseases and Microbiology,
University of Pittsburgh School of Public Health, Pittsburgh,
Pennsylvania; Distinguished Scholar, Center for Biosecurity of the
University of Pittsburgh Medical Center, Baltimore, Maryland
Bioterrorism: An Overview

J. Owen Hendley, MD
Professor of Pediatrics, University of Virginia School of Medicine.;
Attending Physician, Division of Pediatric Infectious Diseases,
University of Virginia Health System, Charlottesville, Virginia
Epiglottitis

Erik L. Hewlett, MD
Professor of Medicine and Pharmacology, Department of Medicine,
Division of Infectious Diseases and International Health, University
of Virginia School of Medicine, Charlottesville, Virginia
Toxins

Kevin P. High, MD, MS
Professor of Medicine and Chief, Section on Infectious Diseases,
Wake Forest University School of Medicine, Winston-Salem, North
Carolina
Nutrition, Immunity, and Infection

Adrian V. S. Hill, DPhil, DM
Professor of Human Genetics, Wellcome Trust Centre for Human
Genetics, University of Oxford, Oxford, United Kingdom
Human Genetics and Infection

David R. Hill, MD, DTM&H
Honorary Professor, London School of Hygiene and Tropical
Medicine; Director, National Travel Health Network and Centre,
University College London Hospitals National Health Service
Foundation Trust, London, United Kingdom
Giardia lamblia

Alan R. Hinman, MD, MPH
Adjunct Professor of Epidemiology and Global Health, Rollins
School of Public Health, Emory University, Atlanta; Senior Public
Health Scientist, Task Force for Global Health, Decatur, Georgia
Immunization

Martin S. Hirsch
Professor of Medicine, Harvard Medical School; Infectious Diseases
Unit, Massachusetts General Hospital, Boston, Massachusetts
Antiretroviral Therapy for Human Immunodeficiency Virus Infection

Lisa S. Hodges, MD
Assistant Professor of Medicine/Pediatrics, Louisiana State University
Health Sciences Center in Shreveport School of Medicine,
Shreveport, Louisiana
Francisella tularensis (Tularemia) as an Agent of Bioterrorism

Steven M. Holland, MD
Chief, Laboratory of Clinical Infectious Diseases, National Institute
of Allergy and Infectious Diseases, National Institutes of Health,
Bethesda, Maryland
Evaluation of the Patient with Suspected Immunodeficiency

Edward W. Hook III, MD
Professor of Medicine, Epidemiology and Microbiology, University
of Alabama at Birmingham School of Medicine and University of
Alabama at Birmingham School of Public Health, Birmingham,
Alabama
Endemic Treponematoses

David C. Hooper, MD
Professor of Medicine, Harvard Medical School; Chief, Infection
Control Unit, and Associate Chief, Division of Infectious Diseases,
Massachusetts General Hospital, Boston, Massachusetts
Quinolones; Urinary Tract Agents: Nitrofurantoin and Methenamine

Thomas M. Hooton, MD
Professor of Clinical Medicine and Director, Institute for Women's
Health, University of Miami Miller School of Medicine, Miami,
Florida
Nosocomial Urinary Tract Infections

C. Robert Horsburgh, Jr., MD, MUS
Professor of Epidemiology, Biostatistics, and Medicine and
Chairman, Department of Epidemiology, Boston University School
of Public Health; Attending Physician, Boston Medical Center,
Boston, Massachusetts
Mycobacterium avium Complex

Duane R. Hospenthal, MD, PhD
Professor of Medicine, Uniformed Services University of the Health
Sciences F. Edward Hébert School of Medicine, Bethesda, Maryland;
Chief, Infectious Disease Service, San Antonio Military Medical
Center and Brooke Army Medical Center, Fort Sam Houston, Texas
Agents of Chromoblastomycosis; Agents of Mycetoma; Uncommon
Fungi and *Prototheca*

James M. Hughes, MD
Professor of Medicine (Infectious Diseases), Emory University
School of Medicine; Professor of Public Health (Global Health),
Rollins School of Public Health, Emory University, Atlanta, Georgia
Emerging and Reemerging Infectious Disease Threats; Foodborne
Disease

Molly A. Hughes, MD, PhD
Assistant Professor of Medicine, Division of Infectious Diseases and
International Health, University of Virginia School of Medicine,
Charlottesville, Virginia
Toxins

Christopher D. Huston, MD
Assistant Professor, Division of Infectious Diseases, University of Vermont College of Medicine; Attending Physician, Fletcher Allen Health Care, Burlington, Vermont
  Microbial Adherence

Noreen A. Hynes, MD, MPH, DTM&H
Associate Professor of Medicine, Johns Hopkins University School of Medicine; Associate Professor of Public Health, Johns Hopkins Bloomberg School of Public Health, Baltimore, Maryland
  Bioterrorism: An Overview; Plague as a Bioterrorism Weapon

Jonathan R. Iredell, MB BS, PhD
Associate Professor, University of Sydney Faculty of Medicine, Sydney; Senior Staff Specialist, Centre for Infectious Diseases and Microbiology, Westmead Hospital, Westmead, New South Wales, Australia
  Nocardia Species

J. Michael Janda, PhD
Chief, Microbial Diseases Laboratory, Center for Infectious Disease, Division of Communicable Disease Control, California Department of Public Health, Richmond, California
  Capnocytophaga

Eric C. Johannsen, MD
Assistant Professor of Medicine, Harvard Medical School; Associate Physician, Division of Infectious Diseases, Brigham and Women's Hospital, Boston, Massachusetts
  Epstein-Barr Virus (Infectious Mononucleosis, Epstein-Barr Virus–Associated Malignant Diseases, and Other Diseases)

Warren D. Johnson, Jr., MD
B. H. Kean Professor of Tropical Medicine and Director, Center for Global Health, Weill Cornell Medical College; Attending Physician, New York–Presbyterian Hospital and Weill Cornell Medical Center, New York, New York
  Borrelia Species (Relapsing Fever)

Angela D. M. Kashuba, PharmD
Associate Professor, Eshelman School of Pharmacy; Director, Clinical Pharmacology and Analytical Chemistry Core, Center for AIDS Research, University of North Carolina at Chapel Hill, Chapel Hill, North Carolina
  Pharmacokinetics and Pharmacodynamics of Anti-infective Agents

Dennis L. Kasper, MD
Professor of Microbiology and Molecular Genetics, Harvard Medical School; William Ellery Channing Professor of Medicine, Brigham and Women's Hospital, Boston, Massachusetts
  Anaerobic Infections: General Concepts

Donald Kaye, MD
Professor of Medicine, Drexel University College of Medicine, Philadelphia, Pennsylvania
  Polymyxins (Polymyxin B and Colistin); Urinary Tract Infections

Keith S. Kaye, MD, MPH
Professor of Medicine, Wayne State University School of Medicine; Corporate Director, Hospital Epidemiology and Antimicrobial Stewardship, Detroit Medical Center, Detroit, Michigan
  Polymyxins (Polymyxin B and Colistin)

Kenneth M. Kaye, MD
Associate Professor, Department of Medicine, Harvard Medical School; Attending Physician, Division of Infectious Diseases, Brigham and Women's Hospital, Boston, Massachusetts
  Epstein-Barr Virus (Infectious Mononucleosis, Epstein-Barr Virus–Associated Malignant Diseases, and Other Diseases); Kaposi's Sarcoma–Associated Herpesvirus (Human Herpesvirus Type 8)

James W. Kazura, MD
Professor of International Health, Medicine, and Pathology, Case Western Reserve University School of Medicine; Attending Physician, University Hospitals Case Medical Center, Cleveland, Ohio
  Tissue Nematodes, Including Trichinellosis, Dracunculiasis, and the Filariases

George E. Kenny, PhD
Professor Emeritus, Department of Global Health, University of Washington School of Public Health, Seattle, Washington
  Genital Mycoplasmas: *Mycoplasma genitalium, Mycoplasma hominis,* and *Ureaplasma* Species

Jay S. Keystone, MD, MSc
Professor of Medicine, University of Toronto Faculty of Medicine; Tropical Disease Unit, Toronto General Hospital; Medisys Travel Health, Toronto, Ontario, Canada
  Cyclospora cayetanensis, Isospora belli, Sarcocystis Species, *Balantidium coli,* and *Blastocystis hominis*

Rima F. Khabbaz, MD
Director, National Center for Preparedness, Detection, and Control of Infectious Diseases, Centers for Disease Control and Prevention, Atlanta, Georgia
  Emerging and Reemerging Infectious Disease Threats

Charles H. King, MD, MS
Professor of International Health, Case Western Reserve University School of Medicine, Cleveland, Ohio
  Cestodes (Tapeworms)

Louis V. Kirchhoff, MD, MPH
Professor, Departments of Internal Medicine (Infectious Diseases) and Epidemiology, University of Iowa Carver College of Medicine; Staff Physician, Medical Service, Department of Veterans Affairs Medical Center, Iowa City, Iowa
  Trypanosoma Species (America Trypanosomiasis, Chagas' Disease): Biology of Trypanosomes; Agents of African Trypanosomiasis (Sleeping Sickness)

Jerome O. Klein, MD
Professor of Pediatrics, Boston University School of Medicine; Consultant in Pediatrics, Maxwell Finland Laboratory for Infectious Diseases, Boston Medical Center, Boston, Massachusetts
  Otitis Externa, Otitis Media, and Mastoiditis

Bettina M. Knoll, MD, PhD
Infectious Diseases Fellow, Mayo Clinic, Rochester, Minnesota
  Prosthetic Valve Endocarditis

Kirk U. Knowlton, MD
Professor of Medicine and Chief, Division of Cardiology, University of California, San Diego, School of Medicine, La Jolla, California
  Myocarditis and Pericarditis

Stephan A. Kohlhoff, MD
Assistant Professor of Pediatrics and Medicine, State University of New York Downstate College of Medicine; Co-Director, Division of Pediatric Infectious Diseases, State University of New York Downstate Medical Center, Brooklyn, New York
  Chlamydophila (Chlamydia) pneumoniae

Eija Könönen, PPS, PhD
Professor, Institute of Dentistry, University of Turku, Turku; Department of Infectious Disease Surveillance and Control, National Institute for Health and Welfare, Helsinki, Finland
  Anaerobic Gram-Positive Nonsporulating Bacilli

Dimitrios P. Kontoyiannis, MD
Adjunct Professor, Baylor College of Medicine; Professor, Department of Infectious Diseases, University of Texas M. D. Anderson Cancer Center, Houston, Texas
Agents of Mucormycosis and Entomophthoramycosis

Igor J. Koralnik, MD
Associate Professor of Neurology, Harvard Medical School; Director, Human Immunodeficiency Virus/Neurology Center, Beth Israel Deaconess Medical Center, Boston, Massachusetts
Neurologic Diseases Caused by Human Immunodeficiency Virus Type 1 and Opportunistic Infections; JC, BK, and Other Polyomaviruses: Progressive Multifocal Leukoencephalopathy

Anita A. Koshy, MD
Postdoctoral Fellow, Departments of Internal Medicine and of Microbiology and Immunology, Division of Infectious Diseases, Stanford University School of Medicine; Clinical Instructor, Department of Neurology, Stanford University Hospital, Stanford, California
Free-Living Amebas

Camille Nelson Kotton, MD
Assistant Professor, Harvard Medical School; Clinical Director, Transplant and Immunocompromised Host Infectious Diseases, Infectious Diseases Division, Massachusetts General Hospital, Boston, Massachusetts
Zoonoses

Joseph A. Kovacs, MD
Head, Acquired Immunodeficiency Syndrome Section, Critical Care Medicine Department, Clinical Center, National Institutes of Health, Bethesda, Maryland
Toxoplasma gondii

Phyllis Kozarsky, MD
Professor of Medicine/Infectious Diseases and Co-Director, Travel and Tropical Medicine, Emory University School of Medicine; Expert Consultant, Division of Global Migration and Quarantine, Centers for Disease Control and Prevention, Atlanta, Georgia
Cyclospora cayetanensis, Isospora belli, Sarcocystis Species, Balantidium coli, and Blastocystis hominis

Margaret James Koziel, MD
Associate Professor of Medicine, Harvard Medical School; Attending Physician, Beth Israel Deaconess Medical Center, Boston, Massachusetts
Hepatitis B Virus and Hepatitis Delta Virus

John N. Krieger, MD
Professor of Urology, University of Washington School of Medicine; Chief of Urology, Veterans Affairs Puget Sound Health Care System; Attending Urologist, University of Washington Medical Center, Harborview Medical Center, and Seattle Children's Hospital, Seattle, Washington
Prostatitis, Epididymitis, and Orchitis

Matthew J. Kuehnert, MD
Director, Office of Blood, Organ, and Other Tissue Safety, Division of Healthcare Quality Promotion, Centers for Disease Control and Prevention, Atlanta, Georgia
Nosocomial Hepatitis and Other Transfusion- and Transplantation-Transmitted Infections

James W. LeDuc, PhD
Professor, University of Texas Medical Branch School of Medicine; Deputy Director, Galveston National Laboratory, University of Texas Medical Branch, Galveston, Texas
Emerging and Reemerging Infectious Disease Threats

Laura M. Lee, BSN, RN
Special Assistant to the Deputy Director for Clinical Care, Clinical Center, National Institutes of Health, Bethesda, Maryland
Hospital Preparedness for Emerging and Highly Contagious Infectious Diseases: Getting Ready for the Next Epidemic or Pandemic

James E. Leggett, MD
Associate Professor of Medicine, Oregon Health & Science University School of Medicine; Assistant Director, Medical Education, Providence Portland Medical Center, Portland, Oregon
Aminoglycosides

Andres G. Lescano, PhD
Director, Public Health Training, Naval Medical Research Center Detachment, Lima, Peru
Outbreak Investigation

Paul N. Levett, PhD
Assistant Clinical Director, Saskatchewan Disease Control Laboratory, Regina, Saskatchewan, Canada
Leptospira Species (Leptospirosis)

Donald P. Levine, MD
Professor of Medicine, Wayne State University School of Medicine; Vice-Chief of Medicine, Detroit Receiving Hospital, Detroit, Michigan
Infections in Injection Drug Users

Matthew E. Levison, MD
Professor of Public Health, Drexel University School of Public Health; Adjunct Professor of Medicine, Drexel University College of Medicine, Philadelphia, Pennsylvania
Peritonitis and Intraperitoneal Abscesses

Russell E. Lewis, PharmD
Associate Professor, University of Houston College of Pharmacy; Adjunct Assistant Professor, University of Texas M. D. Anderson Cancer Center, Houston, Texas
Agents of Mucormycosis and Entomophthoramycosis

W. Conrad Liles, MD, PhD
Vice-Chair and Professor of Medicine and Canada Research Chair in Infectious Diseases and Inflammation, University of Toronto Faculty of Medicine; Director, Division of Infectious Diseases; Senior Scientist, McLaughlin-Rotman Centre for Global Health; and Senior Scientist, Toronto General Research Institute, University Health Network, Toronto, Ontario, Canada
Immunomodulators

Aldo A. M. Lima, MD, PhD
Professor, Federal University of Ceará School of Medicine, Fortaleza, Ceará, Brazil
Inflammatory Enteritides

Nathan Litman, MD
Professor of Pediatrics, Albert Einstein College of Medicine of Yeshiva University; Director of Pediatrics and Pediatric Infectious Diseases, Children's Hospital at Montefiore, Bronx, New York
Mumps Virus

Bennett Lorber, MD
Thomas M. Durant Professor of Medicine and Professor of Microbiology and Immunology, Temple University School of Medicine, Philadelphia, Pennsylvania
Bacterial Lung Abscess; Listeria monocytogenes

Larry I. Lutwick, MD
Professor of Medicine, Division of Infectious Diseases, State University of New York Downstate Medical Center College of Medicine; Director, Division of Infectious Diseases, Department of Medicine, Veterans Affairs New York Harbor Healthcare System—Brooklyn Campus, Brooklyn, New York
Infections in Asplenic Patients

Rob Roy MacGregor, MD
Professor of Medicine, Division of Infectious Diseases, University of Pennsylvania School of Medicine; Attending Physician, Hospital of the University of Pennsylvania, Philadelphia, Pennsylvania
Corynebacterium diphtheriae

Philip A. Mackowiak, MD, MBA
Professor and Vice Chairman, Department of Medicine, University of Maryland School of Medicine; Chief, Medical Care Clinical Center, Veterans Affairs Maryland Health Care System, Baltimore, Maryland
Temperature Regulation and the Pathogenesis of Fever; Fever of Unknown Origin

Lawrence C. Madoff, MD
Professor of Medicine, University of Massachusetts Medical School; Director, Division of Epidemiology and Immunization, Massachusetts Department of Public Health and University of Massachusetts Memorial Medical Center, Division of Infectious Disease and Immunology, Worcester, Massachusetts
Infections of the Liver and Biliary System; Pancreatic Infection; Splenic Abscess; Appendicitis; Diverticulitis and Typhlitis

Alan J. Magill, MD
Associate Professor of Preventive Medicine and Biometrics and Associate Professor of Medicine, Uniformed Services University of the Health Sciences F. Edward Hébert School of Medicine, Bethesda; Director, Division of Experimental Therapeutic, Walter Reed Army Institute of Research, Silver Spring, Maryland
Leishmania Species: Visceral (Kala-Azar), Cutaneous, and Mucosal Leishmaniasis

James H. Maguire, MD, MPH
Professor of Medicine, Harvard Medical School; Senior Physician, Division of Infectious Disease, Brigham and Women's Hospital, Boston, Massachusetts
Introduction to Helminth Infections; Intestinal Nematodes (Roundworms); Trematodes (Schistosomes and Other Flukes)

Frank Maldarelli, MD, PhD
Staff Clinician, Host-Virus Interaction Branch, and Head, In Vivo Biology Group, HIV Drug Resistance Program, National Cancer Institute, National Institutes of Health, Bethesda, Maryland
Diagnosis of Human Immunodeficiency Virus Infection

Lionel A. Mandell, MD
Professor of Medicine, McMaster University Faculty of Health Sciences; Attending Physician, Hamilton Health Sciences, Hamilton, Ontario, Canada
Fusidic Acid; Novel Antibiotics

Barbara J. Mann, PhD
Associate Professor of Medicine and Microbiology, University of Virginia School of Medicine, Charlottesville, Virginia
Microbial Adherence

Lewis Markoff, MD
Chief, Laboratory of Vector-Borne Virus Diseases, Office of Vaccines, Center for Biologics Evaluation and Research, U.S. Food and Drug Administration, Bethesda, Maryland
Alphaviruses

Jeanne M. Marrazzo, MD, MPH
Associate Professor of Medicine, Division of Allergy and Infectious Diseases, University of Washington School of Medicine, Seattle, Washington
Neisseria gonorrhoeae

Thomas J. Marrie, MD
Dean, Dalhousie University Faculty of Medicine, Halifax, Nova Scotia, Canada
Coxiella burnetii (Q Fever)

Thomas Marth, MD
Chief, Division of Internal Medicine, Krankenhaus Maria Hilf, Daun, Germany
Whipple's Disease

Gregory J. Martin, MD
Associate Professor of Medicine and Associate Professor of Preventive Medicine, Uniformed Services University of the Health Sciences F. Edward Hébert School of Medicine; Attending Physician, National Naval Medical Center, Bethesda, Maryland
Bacillus anthracis (Anthrax); Anthrax as an Agent of Bioterrorism

Georg Maschmeyer, MD, PhD
Academic Clinical Instructor, Charité University of Medicine, Berlin; Director, Department of Hematology and Oncology, Klinikum Ernst von Bergmann, Potsdam, Germany
Stenotrophomonas maltophilia and Burkholderia cepacia Complex

Henry Masur, MD
Chief, Critical Care Medicine Department, Clinical Center, National Institutes of Health, Bethesda, Maryland
Management of Opportunistic Infections Associated with Human Immunodeficiency Virus Infection

Alison Mawle, PhD
Associate Director for Laboratory Science, National Center for Immunization and Respiratory Diseases, Centers for Disease Control and Prevention, Atlanta, Georgia
Immunization

Kenneth H. Mayer, MD
Professor of Medicine and Community Health and Director, Brown University AIDS Program, Warren Alpert Medical School of Brown University; Attending Physician, Miriam Hospital, Providence, Rhode Island
Sulfonamides and Trimethoprim

John T. McBride, MD
Professor of Pediatrics, Northeastern Ohio Universities Colleges of Medicine and Pharmacy, Rootstown; Vice Chair, Department of Pediatrics, Akron Children's Hospital, Akron, Ohio
Acute Laryngotracheobronchitis (Croup); Bronchiolitis

William M. McCormack, MD
Distinguished Teaching Professor of Medicine and of Obstetrics and Gynecology, State University of New York Downstate Medical Center College of Medicine; Chief, Infectious Diseases Division, State University of New York Downstate Medical Center, Brooklyn, New York
Urethritis; Vulvovaginitis and Cervicitis

Kenneth McIntosh, MD
Professor of Pediatrics, Harvard Medical School; Professor, Department of Immunology and Infectious Diseases, Harvard School of Public Health; Emeritus Chief, Division of Infectious Diseases, Children's Hospital Boston, Boston, Massachusetts
Coronaviruses, Including Severe Acute Respiratory Syndrome (SARS)–Associated Coronavirus

Paul S. Mead, MD, MPH
Chief, Epidemiology and Surveillance Activity, Bacterial Disease Branch, National Center for Zoonotic, Vector-Borne, and Enteric Diseases, Centers for Disease Control and Prevention, Fort Collins, Colorado
   Yersinia Species, Including Plague

Daniel K. Meyer, MD
Assistant Professor of Medicine, University of Medicine and Dentistry of New Jersey—Robert Wood Johnson Medical School; Program Director, Division of Infectious Diseases, Cooper University Hospital, Camden, New Jersey
   Other Coryneform Bacteria and Rhodococci

Burt R. Meyers, MD
Clinical Professor, Department of Medicine/Infectious Diseases, Mount Sinai School of Medicine, New York; Attending Physician, New York Medical College, Valhalla, New York
   Tetracyclines and Chloramphenicol; Metronidazole

Mark A. Miller, MD
Associate Professor, McGill University Faculty of Medicine; Staff Physician, Jewish General Hospital, Montreal, Quebec, Canada
   Prebiotics, Probiotics, and Synbiotics

Samuel I. Miller, MD
Professor, Department of Immunology, University of Washington School of Medicine, Seattle, Washington
   Salmonella Species, Including *Salmonella* Typhi

David H. Mitchell, MB BS
Clinical Senior Lecturer, Department of Infectious Diseases, University of Sydney Faculty of Medicine, Sydney; Senior Staff Specialist, Centre for Infectious Diseases and Microbiology, Westmead Hospital, Westmead, New South Wales, Australia
   Nocardia Species

John F. Modlin, MD
Chair, Department of Pediatrics, Dartmouth-Hitchcock Medical Center; Infectious Disease and International Health, Children's Hospital at Dartmouth, Lebanon, New Hampshire
   Introduction to the Enteroviruses and Parechoviruses; Poliovirus; Coxsackieviruses, Echoviruses, Newer Enteroviruses, and Parechoviruses

Robert C. Moellering, Jr., MD
Shields Warren-Mallinckrodt Professor of Medical Research, Harvard Medical School; Staff Physician, Division of Infectious Diseases, Beth Israel Deaconess Medical Center, Boston, Massachusetts
   Principles of Anti-infective Therapy

Susan Moir, PhD
Staff Scientist, National Institute of Allergy and Infectious Diseases, National Institutes of Health, Bethesda, Maryland
   The Immunology of Human Immunodeficiency Virus Infection

Joel M. Montgomery, PhD
Epidemiologist, Influenza Division, Centers for Disease Control and Prevention, Atlanta, Georgia
   Outbreak Investigation

José G. Montoya, MD
Associate Professor of Medicine, Division of Infectious Diseases and Geographic Medicine, Stanford University School of Medicine; Attending Physician, Stanford University Medical Center; Director, Toxoplasma Serology Laboratory, Palo Alto Medical Foundation, Stanford, California
   Toxoplasma gondii

Thomas A. Moore, MD
Clinical Professor, Department of Medicine, University of Kansas School of Medicine–Wichita Campus, Wichita, Kansas
   Agents Active against Parasites and *Pneumocystis*

Philippe Moreillon, MD, PhD
Professor and Vice-Rector for Research, and Director of the Department of Fundamental Microbiology, University of Lausanne, Lausanne, Switzerland
   Staphylococcus aureus (Including Staphylococcal Toxic Shock)

Dean S. Morrell, MD
Clinical Associate Professor, University of North Carolina at Chapel Hill School of Medicine; Director of Residency Training Program, Pediatric Dermatology, University of North Carolina Health Care, Chapel Hill, North Carolina
   The Acutely Ill Patient with Fever and Rash

J. Glenn Morris, Jr., MD, MPHTM
Professor of Medicine, Division of Infectious Diseases, University of Florida College of Medicine; Director, University of Florida Emerging Pathogens Institute, Gainesville, Florida
   Human Illness Associated with Harmful Algal Blooms

Caryn Gee Morse, MD, MPH
Assistant Clinical Investigator, Laboratory of Immunoregulation, Clinical Research Section, National Institute of Allergy and Infectious Diseases, National Institutes of Health, Bethesda, Maryland
   Nutrition, Immunity, and Infection

Robin Moseley, MAT
Associate Director for Program Integration, National Center for Preparedness, Detection, and Control of Infectious Diseases, Centers for Disease Control and Prevention, Atlanta, Georgia
   Emerging and Reemerging Infectious Disease Threats

Robert R. Muder, MD
Professor of Medicine, University of Pittsburgh School of Medicine; Chief, Infectious Disease Section, Veterans Affairs Pittsburgh Healthcare System, Pittsburgh, Pennsylvania
   Other *Legionella* Species

Robert S. Munford, MD
Senior Clinician, Laboratory of Clinical Infectious Diseases, National Institute of Allergy and Infectious Diseases, National Institutes of Health, Bethesda, Maryland
   Sepsis, Severe Sepsis, and Septic Shock

Edward L. Murphy, MD, MPH
Professor, Departments of Laboratory Medicine and Epidemiology/Biostatistics, University of California, San Francisco, School of Medicine; Senior Investigator, Blood Systems Research Institute, San Francisco, California
   Human T-Cell Lymphotropic Virus Types I and II

Timothy F. Murphy, MD
University of Buffalo Distinguished Professor, Departments of Medicine and Microbiology, and Chief, Infectious Diseases, State University of New York at Buffalo School of Medicine and Biomedical Sciences, Buffalo, New York
   Moraxella catarrhalis, Kingella, and Other Gram-Negative Cocci; *Haemophilus* Species (Including *H. influenzae* and Chancroid)

Barbara E. Murray, MD
J. Ralph Meadows Professor of Medicine and Director, Division of Infectious Diseases, University of Texas Medical School at Houston, Houston, Texas
  Glycopeptides (Vancomycin and Teicoplanin), Streptogramins (Quinupristin-Dalfopristin), and Lipopeptides (Daptomycin); *Enterococcus* Species, *Streptococcus bovis* Group, and *Leuconostoc* Species

Clinton K. Murray, MD
Associate Professor, Uniformed Services University of the Health Sciences, Bethesda, Maryland; Clinical Associate Professor, University of Texas Health Science Center at San Antonio; Program Director, Infectious Disease Fellowships, San Antonio Uniformed Services Health Education Consortium, San Antonio, Texas
  Burns

Patrick R. Murray, PhD
Chief, Microbiology Service, Clinical Center, National Institutes of Health, Bethesda, Maryland
  The Clinician and the Microbiology Laboratory

Daniel M. Musher, MD
Professor of Medicine, Baylor College of Medicine; Chief, Infectious Disease, Michael E. DeBakey Veterans Affairs Medical Center, Houston, Texas
  Streptococcus pneumoniae

Esteban C. Nannini, MD
Assistant Professor, Division of Infectious Diseases, Facultad de Ciencias Médicas, Universidad Nacional de Rosario; Attending Physician, Sanatorio Parque, Rosario, Argentina
  Glycopeptides (Vancomycin and Teicoplanin), Streptogramins (Quinupristin-Dalfopristin), and Lipopeptides (Daptomycin)

Theodore E. Nash, MD
Head, Gastrointestinal Parasites Section, Laboratory of Parasitic Diseases, National Institute of Allergy and Infectious Diseases, National Institutes of Health, Bethesda, Maryland
  Giardia lamblia; Visceral Larva Migrans and Other Unusual Helminth Infections

William M. Nauseef, MD
Professor of Medicine and of Microbiology, Department of Medicine, University of Iowa Carver College of Medicine; Attending Physician, Iowa City Veterans Affairs Medical Center, Iowa City, Iowa
  Granulocytic Phagocytes

Marguerite A. Neill, MD
Associate Professor of Medicine, Warren Alpert Medical School of Brown University, Providence; Attending Physician, Division of Infectious Disease, Memorial Hospital of Rhode Island, Pawtucket, Rhode Island
  Other Pathogenic Vibrios

Judith A. O'Donnell, MD
Professor of Clinical Medicine, Division of Infectious Diseases, University of Pennsylvania School of Medicine; Hospital Epidemiologist and Director, Department of Infection Prevention and Control, Penn Presbyterian Medical Center, Philadelphia, Pennsylvania
  Topical Antibacterials

Christopher A. Ohl, MD
Associate Professor of Medicine, Wake Forest University School of Medicine; Medical Director, Center for Antimicrobial Utilization, Stewardship, and Epidemiology, Wake Forest University Baptist Medical Center, Winston-Salem, North Carolina
  Infectious Arthritis of Native Joints

Pablo C. Okhuysen, MD
Professor of Medicine, Division of Infectious Diseases, University of Texas Medical School at Houston; Medical Staff, Memorial Hermann Hospital–Texas Medical Center; Medical Staff, Lyndon B. Johnson General Hospital, Houston, Texas
  Sporothrix schenckii

Andrew B. Onderdonk, PhD
Professor of Pathology, Harvard Medical School; Director, Clinical Microbiology, Brigham and Women's Hospital, Boston, Massachusetts
  Gas Gangrene and Other *Clostridium*-Associated Diseases; *Bacteroides, Prevotella, Porphyromonas,* and *Fusobacterium* Species (and Other Medically Important Anaerobic Gram-Negative Bacilli)

Steven M. Opal, MD
Professor of Medicine, Warren Alpert Medical School of Brown University, Providence; Chief, Division of Infectious Diseases, Memorial Hospital of Rhode Island, Pawtucket, Rhode Island
  Molecular Mechanisms of Antibiotic Resistance in Bacteria

Walter A. Orenstein, MD
Deputy Director for Vaccine-Preventable Diseases, Integrated Health Solutions Development, Global Health Program, Bill and Melinda Gates Foundation, Seattle, Washington
  Immunization

Douglas R. Osman, MD, MPH
Associate Professor, Division of Infectious Diseases, Mayo Clinic College of Medicine; Consultant, Mayo Clinic, Rochester, Minnesota
  Osteomyelitis

Michael T. Osterholm, PhD, MPH
Professor, Division of Environmental Health Sciences, University of Minnesota School of Public Health; Adjunct Professor, University of Minnesota Medical School, Minneapolis, Minnesota
  Epidemiologic Principles

Stephen M. Ostroff, MD
Director, Bureau of Epidemiology, and Acting Physician General, Pennsylvania Department of Health, Harrisburg, Pennsylvania
  Emerging and Reemerging Infectious Disease Threats

Michael N. Oxman, MD
Professor of Medicine and Pathology, University of California, San Diego, School of Medicine, La Jolla; Staff Physician (Infectious Diseases), Veterans Affairs San Diego Healthcare System, San Diego, California
  Myocarditis and Pericarditis

Andrea V. Page, MD
Clinician-Scientist Training Program, Department of Medicine, University of Toronto Faculty of Medicine; Clinical Associate, Divisions of Internal Medicine and Infectious Diseases, University Health Network, Toronto, Ontario, Canada
  Immunomodulators

Tara N. Palmore, MD
Deputy Hospital Epidemiologist, Clinical Center, National Institutes of Health, Bethesda, Maryland
  Nosocomial Herpesvirus Infections

Eric G. Pamer, MD
Professor of Medicine, Weill Cornell Medical College; Chief, Infectious Diseases, Memorial Hospital, Memorial Sloan-Kettering Cancer Center, New York, New York
  Cell-Mediated Defense against Infection

Peter G. Pappas, MD
Professor of Medicine and Tinsley Harrison Clinical Scholar,
University of Alabama at Birmingham School of Medicine,
Birmingham, Alabama
  Chronic Pneumonia

Mark S. Pasternack, MD
Associate Professor of Pediatrics, Harvard Medical School; Chief,
Pediatric Infectious Disease Unit, Massachusetts General Hospital,
Boston, Massachusetts
  Cellulitis, Necrotizing Fasciitis, and Subcutaneous Tissue Infections;
  Myositis and Myonecrosis; Lymphadenitis and Lymphangitis

Thomas F. Patterson, MD
Chief, Division of Infectious Diseases; Professor of Medicine; and
Director, San Antonio Center for Medical Mycology, University of
Texas Health Science Center at San Antonio; Attending Physician,
South Texas Veterans Health Care System, San Antonio, Texas
  Aspergillus Species

Deborah Pavan-Langston, MD
Professor of Ophthalmology, Harvard Medical School; Attending
Physician, Massachusetts Eye and Ear Infirmary, Boston,
Massachusetts
  Microbial Conjunctivitis; Microbial Keratitis

David A. Pegues, MD
Professor of Clinical Medicine, David Geffen School of Medicine at
UCLA; Hospital Epidemiologist and Attending Physician, Ronald
Reagan UCLA Medical Center, Los Angeles, California
  Salmonella Species, Including *Salmonella* Typhi

Robert L. Penn, MD
Professor of Medicine, Louisiana State University Health Sciences
Center in Shreveport School of Medicine; Chief, Section of
Infectious Diseases, Louisiana State Health Sciences Center–
University Hospital, Shreveport, Louisiana
  Francisella tularensis (Tularemia); *Francisella tularensis* (Tularemia)
  as an Agent of Bioterrorism

John R. Perfect, MD
Professor of Medicine, Duke University School of Medicine and
Duke University Medical Center, Durham, North Carolina
  Cryptococcus neoformans

Stanley Perlman, MD, PhD
Professor of Microbiology and Pediatrics, University of Iowa Carver
College of Medicine, Iowa City, Iowa
  Coronaviruses, Including Severe Acute Respiratory Syndrome
  (SARS)–Associated Coronavirus

C. J. Peters, MD
Professor, Department of Microbiology and Immunology; Professor,
Department of Pathology; and John Sealy Distinguished University
Chair in Tropical and Emerging Virology, University of Texas
Medical Branch, Galveston; Adjunct Graduate Faculty, Texas A&M
University, College Station, Texas
  Marburg and Ebola Virus Hemorrhagic Fevers; California
  Encephalitis, Hantavirus Pulmonary Syndrome, and Bunyavirid
  Hemorrhagic Fevers; Lymphocytic Choriomeningitis Virus, Lassa
  Virus, and the South American Hemorrhagic Fevers; Viral
  Hemorrhagic Fevers as Agents of Bioterrorism

Phillip K. Peterson, MD
Professor of Medicine; Director, Division of Infectious Diseases and
International Medicine; and Co-Director, Center for Infectious
Diseases and Microbiology Translational Research, University of
Minnesota Medical School, Minneapolis, Minnesota
  Infections in the Elderly

William A. Petri, Jr., MD, PhD
Wade Hampton Frost Professor of Epidemiology; Professor of
Medicine, Microbiology, and Pathology; and Chief, Division of
Infectious Diseases and International Health, University of Virginia
School of Medicine; Attending Physician, University of Virginia
Health System, Charlottesville, Virginia
  Microbial Adherence; Introduction to Protozoal Diseases;
  Entamoeba Species, Including Amebiasis

Cathy A. Petti, MD
Associate Professor of Pathology and Medicine, University of Utah
School of Medicine, Salt Lake City, Utah
  Streptococcus anginosus Group

Larry K. Pickering, MD
Professor of Pediatrics, Emory University School of Medicine;
Executive Secretary, Advisory Committee on Immunization Practices
(ACIP), and Senior Adviser to the Director, National Center for
Immunization and Respiratory Diseases, Centers for Disease Control
and Prevention, Atlanta, Georgia
  Immunization

Gerald B. Pier, PhD
Professor of Medicine (Microbiology and Molecular Genetics),
Harvard Medical School; Microbiologist, Brigham and Women's
Hospital, Boston, Massachusetts
  Pseudomonas aeruginosa

Satish K. Pillai, MD
Instructor in Medicine, Harvard Medical School; Staff Physician,
Division of Infectious Diseases, Beth Israel Deaconess Medical
Center, Boston, Massachusetts
  Principles of Anti-infective Therapy

Peter Piot, MD, PhD
Professor of Global Health and Director, Institute for Global Health,
Imperial College London, London, United Kingdom
  Global Perspectives on Human Immunodeficiency Virus Infection
  and Acquired Immunodeficiency Syndrome

Susan F. Plaeger, PhD
Director, Basic Sciences Program, National Institute of Allergy and
Infectious Diseases, National Institutes of Health, Bethesda,
Maryland
  Innate (General or Nonspecific) Host Defense Mechanisms

Ronald E. Polk, PharmD
Professor of Pharmacy and Medicine, Virginia Commonwealth
University School of Pharmacy, Richmond, Virginia
  Antimicrobial Stewardship

Aurora Pop-Vicas, MD
Assistant Professor of Medicine, Warren Alpert Medical School of
Brown University, Providence; Infectious Disease Physician,
Memorial Hospital of Rhode Island, Pawtucket, Rhode Island
  Molecular Mechanisms of Antibiotic Resistance in Bacteria

John H. Powers, MD
Assistant Clinical Professor of Medicine, George Washington
University School of Medicine, Washington, DC; Assistant Clinical
Professor of Medicine, University of Maryland School of Medicine,
Baltimore; Senior Medical Scientist, National Institute of Allergy and
Infectious Diseases, National Institutes of Health, Bethesda,
Maryland
  Interpreting the Results of Clinical Trials of Antimicrobial Agents

Antonello Punturieri, MD, PhD
Program Director, Division of Lung Diseases, National Heart, Lung, and Blood Institute, National Institutes of Health, Bethesda, Maryland
  Chronic Obstructive Pulmonary Disease and Acute Exacerbations

Yok-ai Que, MD, PhD
Instructor and Researcher, University of Lausanne School of Medicine; Attending Physician, Department of Critical Care Medicine, Centre Hospitalier Universitaire Vaudois Lausanne, Lausanne, Switzerland
  Staphylococcus aureus (Including Staphylococcal Toxic Shock)

Ronald P. Rabinowitz, MD
Assistant Professor of Medicine, Division of Infectious Diseases, University of Maryland School of Medicine; Attending Physician, R. Adams Cowley Shock Trauma Center, Baltimore, Maryland
  Hyperbaric Oxygen

Shervin Rabizadeh, MD, MBA
Instructor, David Geffen School of Medicine at UCLA; Staff Physician, Department of Pediatrics, Cedars-Sinai Medical Center, Los Angeles, California
  Prebiotics, Probiotics, and Synbiotics

Reuben Ramphal, MD
Professor of Medicine, Division of Infectious Diseases, University of Florida College of Medicine, Gainesville, Florida
  Pseudomonas aeruginosa

Didier Raoult, MD, PhD
Professor and President, Marseille School of Medicine; Director, Clinical Microbiology Laboratory for the University Hospitals; Founder, WHO Collaborative Center; President, Université de la Méditerranée in Marseille, Marseille, France
  Introduction to Rickettsioses, Ehrlichioses, and Anaplasmosis; *Rickettsia akari* (Rickettsialpox); *Coxiella burnetii* (Q Fever); *Rickettsia prowazekii* (Epidemic or Louse-Borne Typhus); *Orientia tsutsugamushi* (Scrub Typhus)

Jonathan I. Ravdin, MD
Dean and Executive Vice President, Medical College of Wisconsin, Milwaukee, Wisconsin
  Introduction to Protozoal Diseases

Stuart C. Ray, MD
Associate Professor of Medicine, Johns Hopkins University School of Medicine, Baltimore, Maryland
  Hepatitis C

Annette C. Reboli, MD
Professor of Medicine, University of Medicine and Dentistry of New Jersey—Robert Wood Johnson Medical School; Deputy Chief of Medicine for Administration, Head of Infectious Diseases Division, and Hospital Epidemiologist, Cooper University Hospital, Camden, New Jersey
  Other Coryneform Bacteria and Rhodococci; *Erysipelothrix rhusiopathiae*

Pavani Reddy, MD
Assistant Professor, Division of Infectious Diseases, Northwestern University Feinberg School of Medicine; Director of Antimicrobial Stewardship, Northwestern Memorial Hospital, Chicago, Illinois
  Clostridium tetani (Tetanus); *Clostridium botulinum* (Botulism); Botulinum Toxin as a Biological Weapon

Richard C. Reichman, MD
Emeritus Professor of Medicine, University of Rochester School of Medicine and Dentistry; Attending Physician, University of Rochester Medical Center, Rochester, New York
  Papillomaviruses

Marvin S. Reitz, Jr., PhD
Professor, Institute of Human Virology and Department of Medicine, University of Maryland School of Medicine, Baltimore, Maryland
  Human Immunodeficiency Viruses

David A. Relman, MD
Professor of Medicine and Professor of Microbiology and Immunology, Stanford University School of Medicine, Stanford; Chief, Infectious Diseases, Veterans Affairs Palo Alto Health Care System, Palo Alto, California
  A Molecular Perspective of Microbial Pathogenicity

Cybèle A. Renault, MD, DTM&H
Clinical Assistant Professor, Department of Internal Medicine, Division of Infectious Diseases, Stanford University School of Medicine, Stanford; Attending Physician, Veterans Affairs Palo Alto Health Care System, Palo Alto, California
  Mycobacterium leprae

Angela Restrepo, PhD
Senior Researcher and Scientific Director, Corporación para Investigaciones Biológicas, Medellin, Colombia
  Paracoccidioides brasiliensis

John H. Rex, MD
Adjunct Professor of Medicine, University of Texas Medical School at Houston, Houston, Texas; Infection Clinical Vice President, AstraZeneca Pharmaceuticals, Macclesfield, United Kingdom
  Systemic Antifungal Agents; *Sporothrix schenckii*

Herbert Y. Reynolds, MD
Emeritus Professor of Medicine, Penn State University College of Medicine, Milton S. Hershey Medical Center, Hershey, Pennsylvania; Adjunct Professor of Medicine, Uniformed Services University of the Health Sciences F. Edward Hébert School of Medicine; Medical Officer, Division of Lung Diseases, National Heart, Lung and Blood Institute, National Institutes of Health, Bethesda, Maryland
  Chronic Obstructive Pulmonary Disease and Acute Exacerbations

Elizabeth G. Rhee, MD
Fellow, Department of Medicine, Harvard Medical School; Division of Viral Pathogenesis, Department of Medicine, Beth Israel Deaconess Medical Center; Attending Physician, Division of Infectious Diseases, Department of Medicine, Brigham and Women's Hospital, Boston, Massachusetts
  Adenoviruses

Kyu Y. Rhee, MD, PhD
Assistant Professor of Medicine, Microbiology, and Immunology and William Randolph Hearst Foundation Clinical Scholar in Microbiology and Infectious Diseases, Weill Cornell Medical College; Assistant Attending Physician, New York–Presbyterian Hospital and Weill Cornell Medical Center, New York, New York
  Borrelia Species (Relapsing Fever)

Lisa D. Rotz, MD
Director, Division of Bioterrorism Preparedness and Response, National Center for Preparedness, Detection, and Control of Infectious Diseases, Centers for Disease Control and Prevention, Atlanta, Georgia
  Smallpox as an Agent of Bioterrorism

Kathryn L. Ruoff, PhD
Associate Professor, Dartmouth Medical School, Hanover; Associate Director, Clinical Microbiology Laboratory, Dartmouth-Hitchcock Medical Center, Lebanon, New Hampshire
Classification of Streptococci

Mark E. Rupp, MD
Professor, Department of Internal Medicine, Division of Infectious Diseases, University of Nebraska Medical Center College of Medicine; Director, Department of Healthcare Epidemiology, Nebraska Medical Center, Omaha, Nebraska
Mediastinitis; *Staphylococcus epidermidis* and Other Coagulase-Negative Staphylococci

Charles E. Rupprecht, VMD, PhD
Section Lead, Rabies, Centers for Disease Control and Prevention, Atlanta, Georgia
Rhabdoviruses

Thomas A. Russo, MD
Professor of Medicine and Microbiology, Division of Infectious Diseases, State University of New York at Buffalo School of Medicine and Biomedical Sciences; Staff Physician, Veterans Affairs Western New York Health Care System, Buffalo, New York
Agents of Actinomycosis

William A. Rutala, PhD, MPH
Professor of Medicine and Director, Statewide Program in Infection Control and Epidemiology, University of North Carolina at Chapel Hill School of Medicine; Director, Hospital Epidemiology, Occupational Health and Safety Program, University of North Carolina Health Care System, Chapel Hill, North Carolina
The Acutely Ill Patient with Fever and Rash; Disinfection, Sterilization, and Control of Hospital Waste

Mirella Salvatore, MD
Assistant Professor, Department of Public Health, and Assistant Professor, Department of Medicine/Infectious Diseases, Weill Cornell Medical College; Assistant Attending Physician, New York–Presbyterian Hospital, New York, New York
Tetracyclines and Chloramphenicol; Metronidazole

Frank T. Saulsbury
Professor, Department of Pediatrics, Division of Immunology and Rheumatology, University of Virginia School of Medicine, Charlottesville, Virginia
Kawasaki Syndrome

Maria C. Savoia, MD
Vice Dean for Medical Education and Professor of Medicine, University of California, San Diego, School of Medicine, La Jolla, California
Myocarditis and Pericarditis

Paul E. Sax, MD
Associate Professor of Medicine, Harvard Medical School; Clinical Director, Division of Infectious Diseases and Human Immunodeficiency Virus Program, Brigham and Women's Hospital, Boston, Massachusetts
Pulmonary Manifestations of Human Immunodeficiency Virus Infection

W. Michael Scheld, MD
Gerald L. Mandell–Bayer Professor of Infectious Diseases and Professor of Medicine, University of Virginia School of Medicine; Clinical Professor of Neurosurgery and Director, Pfizer Initiative in International Health, University of Virginia Health System, Charlottesville, Virginia
Endocarditis and Intravascular Infections; Acute Meningitis

Joshua T. Schiffer, MD, MS
Senior Fellow, University of Washington School of Medicine and Fred Hutchinson Cancer Research Center, Seattle, Washington
Herpes Simplex Virus

David Schlossberg, MD
Professor of Medicine, Temple University School of Medicine; Adjunct Professor of Medicine, University of Pennsylvania School of Medicine; Medical Director, Tuberculosis Control Program, Philadelphia Department of Public Health, Philadelphia, Pennsylvania
Chlamydophila (Chlamydia) psittaci (Psittacosis)

Thomas Schneider, MD, PhD
Professor of Infectious Diseases, Charité University Hospital, Benjamin Franklin Campus, Berlin, Germany
Whipple's Disease

Jane R. Schwebke, MD
Professor of Medicine, University of Alabama at Birmingham School of Medicine, Birmingham, Alabama
Trichomonas vaginalis

Cynthia L. Sears, MD
Professor of Medicine, Divisions of Infectious Diseases and Gastroenterology, Johns Hopkins University School of Medicine, Baltimore, Maryland
Prebiotics, Probiotics, and Synbiotics

Carlos Seas, MD
Associate Professor of Medicine and Principal Investigator, Alexander von Humboldt Tropical Medicine Institute, Cayetano Heredia University; Attending Physician, National Hospital Cayetano Heredia, Lima, Peru
Vibrio cholerae

Kent A. Sepkowitz, MD
Professor of Medicine, Weill Cornell Medical College; Vice-Chairman of Medicine and Director, Hospital Infection Control, Memorial Sloan-Kettering Cancer Center, New York, New York
Nosocomial Hepatitis and Other Transfusion- and Transplantation-Transmitted Infections

Edward J. Septimus, MD
Affiliate Professor and Distinguished Senior Fellow, School of Public Policy, George Mason University, Fairfax, Virginia; Medical Director, Infection Prevention, HCA Healthcare System, Nashville, Tennessee
Pleural Effusion and Empyema

George K. Siberry, MD, MPH
Medical Officer, Pediatric, Adolescent, and Maternal Acquired Immunodeficiency Syndrome Branch, Eunice Kennedy Shriver National Institute of Child Health and Human Development, National Institutes of Health, Bethesda, Maryland
Pediatric Human Immunodeficiency Virus Infection

Costi D. Sifri, MD
Assistant Professor of Medicine, Division of Infectious Diseases and International Health, University of Virginia School of Medicine; Attending Physician, Department of Medicine, University of Virginia Health System, Charlottesville, Virginia
Infections of the Liver and Biliary System; Appendicitis; Diverticulitis and Typhlitis

Nina Singh, MD
Associate Professor of Medicine, University of Pittsburgh School of Medicine; Chief, Transplant Infectious Diseases, Veterans Affairs Pittsburgh Healthcare System, Pittsburgh, Pennsylvania
Infections in Solid Organ Transplant Recipients

Upinder Singh, MD
Assistant Professor, Department of Internal Medicine, Division of Infectious Diseases, Stanford University School of Medicine, Stanford, California
  Free-Living Amebas

Scott W. Sinner, MD
Clinical Assistant Professor of Medicine, University of Medicine and Dentistry of New Jersey–Robert Wood Johnson Medical School, New Brunswick; Physician in Private Practice, Hillsborough, New Jersey
  Viridans Streptococci, Groups C and G Streptococci, and *Gemella* Species

Sumathi Sivapalasingam, MD
Assistant Professor, Department of Medicine, Division of Infectious Diseases and Immunology, New York University School of Medicine, New York, New York
  Macrolides, Clindamycin, and Ketolides

Leonard N. Slater, MD
Professor of Medicine, Division of Infectious Diseases, University of Oklahoma College of Medicine; Chief, Section of Infectious Diseases, and Chairman, Infection Control Committee, Oklahoma City Veterans Affairs Medical Center; Medical Director, Employee Health Service, Oklahoma University Medical Center, Oklahoma City, Oklahoma
  Bartonella, Including Cat-Scratch Disease

A. George Smulian, MB BCh
Associate Professor, University of Cincinnati College of Medicine; Chief, Infectious Disease Section, Veterans Affairs Cincinnati Medical Center, Cincinnati, Ohio
  Pneumocystis Species

Jack D. Sobel, MD
Professor of Medicine, Wayne State University School of Medicine; Chief, Division of Infectious Diseases, Detroit Medical Center, Detroit, Michigan
  Urinary Tract Infections

Samir V. Sodha, MD, MPH
Medical Epidemiologist, Enteric Diseases Epidemiology Branch, Division of Foodborne, Bacterial, and Mycotic Diseases, National Center for Zoonotic, Vectorborne, and Enteric Diseases, Centers for Disease Control and Prevention, Atlanta, Georgia
  Foodborne Disease

M. Rizwan Sohail, MD
Assistant Professor of Medicine, Mayo Clinic College of Medicine; Consultant, Infectious Diseases, Mayo Clinic, Rochester, Minnesota
  Infections of Nonvalvular Cardiovascular Devices

Tom Solomon, BM, BCh, PhD, DTM&H
Head, Brain Infections Group, and Chair, Division of Neurological Science, University of Liverpool Faculty of Medicine, Liverpool, United Kingdom
  Flaviviruses (Yellow Fever, Dengue, Dengue Hemorrhagic Fever, Japanese Encephalitis, West Nile Encephalitis, St. Louis Encephalitis, Tick-Borne Encephalitis)

Yuli Song, PhD
Senior Scientist, Procter and Gamble Healthcare Research, Mason, Ohio
  Anaerobic Cocci

David E. Soper, MD
Professor, Departments of Obstetrics and Gynecology, Division of Infectious Diseases, Department of Medicine, Medical University of South Carolina, Charleston, South Carolina
  Infections of the Female Pelvis

Tania C. Sorrell, MB BS, MD
Professor of Clinical Infectious Diseases and Director, Centre for Infectious Diseases and Microbiology, University of Sydney Faculty of Medicine, Sydney; Director of Infectious Diseases, Sydney West Area Health Service, Westmead Hospital, Westmead, New South Wales, Australia
  Nocardia Species

P. Frederick Sparling, MD
Professor of Medicine, Microbiology and Immunology, University of North Carolina School of Medicine, Chapel Hill, North Carolina
  Neisseria gonorrhoeae

Walter E. Stamm, MD
Professor of Medicine, Division of Allergy and Infectious Diseases, University of Washington School of Medicine, Seattle, Washington
  Introduction to *Chlamydia* and *Chlamydophila*; *Chlamydia trachomatis* (Trachoma, Perinatal Infections, Lymphogranuloma Venereum, and Other Genital Infections)

James M. Steckelberg, MD
Professor, Division of Infectious Diseases, Mayo Clinic College of Medicine; Consultant, Mayo Clinic, Rochester, Minnesota
  Osteomyelitis

Allen C. Steere, MD
Professor of Medicine, Harvard Medical School; Director of Clinical and Translational Research, Department of Rheumatology, Massachusetts General Hospital, Boston, Massachusetts
  Borrelia burgdorferi (Lyme Disease, Lyme Borreliosis)

Neal H. Steigbigel, MD
Professor of Medicine, Division of Infectious Diseases and Immunology, New York University School of Medicine; Staff Physician, Medical Service, Infectious Diseases Section, New York Veterans Affairs Medical Center, New York, New York
  Macrolides, Clindamycin, and Ketolides

James P. Steinberg, MD
Professor of Medicine, Division of Infectious Diseases, Emory University School of Medicine; Chief Medical Officer, Emory University Hospital Midtown, Atlanta, Georgia
  Other Gram-Negative and Gram-Variable Bacilli

Theodore S. Steiner, MD
Associate Professor of Medicine, University of British Columbia Faculty of Medicine, Vancouver, British Columbia, Canada
  Principles and Syndromes of Enteric Infection

Timothy R. Sterling, MD
Professor of Medicine, Division of Infectious Diseases, Vanderbilt University School of Medicine; Nashville Metro Public Health Department Tuberculosis Clinic, Nashville, Tennessee
  General Clinical Manifestations of Human Immunodeficiency Virus Infection (Including the Acute Retroviral Syndrome and Oral, Cutaneous, Renal, Ocular, Metabolic, and Cardiac Diseases); *Mycobacterium tuberculosis*

David A. Stevens, MD
Professor of Medicine, Stanford University School of Medicine, Stanford; Chief, Division of Infectious Diseases, Department of Medicine, and Hospital Epidemiologist, Santa Clara Valley Medical Center; President and Principal Investigator, Infectious Disease Research Laboratory, California Institute for Medical Research, San Jose, California
 Systemic Antifungal Agents

Dennis L. Stevens, PhD, MD
Professor of Medicine, University of Washington School of Medicine, Seattle, Washington; Chief, Infectious Diseases, Boise Veterans Affairs Medical Center, Boise, Idaho
 Streptococcus pyogenes

Jacob Strahilevitz, MD
Senior Lecturer in Clinical Microbiology, Hebrew University; Staff Physician, Department of Clinical Microbiology and Infectious Diseases, Hadassah Medical Center, Jerusalem, Israel
 Quinolones

Charles W. Stratton IV, MD
Associate Professor of Pathology and Medicine, Vanderbilt University School of Medicine; Director, Clinical Microbiology Laboratory, Vanderbilt University Medical Center, Nashville, Tennessee
 Streptococcus anginosus Group

Anthony F. Suffredini, MD
Senior Investigator, Critical Care Medicine Department, Clinical Center, National Institutes of Health, Bethesda, Maryland
 Sepsis, Severe Sepsis, and Septic Shock

Kathryn N. Suh, MD
Assistant Professor of Medicine and Pediatrics, University of Ottawa Faculty of Medicine; Attending Physician, Division of Infectious Diseases, Ottawa Hospital, Ottawa, Ontario, Canada
 Cyclospora cayetanensis, Isospora belli, Sarcocystis Species, *Balantidium coli,* and *Blastocystis hominis*

Mark S. Sulkowski, MD
Associate Professor of Medicine and Medical Director, Viral Hepatitis Center, Johns Hopkins University School of Medicine, Baltimore; Johns Hopkins Rockland Physicians Practice and Research Group at Greenspring Station, Lutherville, Maryland
 Gastrointestinal and Hepatobiliary Manifestations of Human Immunodeficiency Virus Infection

Donna C. Sullivan, PhD
Professor of Medicine and Associate Professor of Microbiology, University of Mississippi School of Medicine; Division of Infectious Diseases, University of Mississippi Medical Center, Jackson, Mississippi
 Blastomyces dermatitidis

Morton N. Swartz, MD
Professor of Medicine, Harvard Medical School; Associate Firm Chief, Massachusetts General Hospital, Boston, Massachusetts
 Cellulitis, Necrotizing Fasciitis, and Subcutaneous Tissue Infections; Myositis and Myonecrosis; Lymphadenitis and Lymphangitis

Thomas R. Talbot, MD, MPH
Assistant Professor of Medicine and Preventive Medicine, Vanderbilt University School of Medicine; Chief Hospital Epidemiologist, Vanderbilt Medical Center, Nashville, Tennessee
 Surgical Site Infections and Antimicrobial Prophylaxis

C. Sabrina Tan, MD
Instructor in Medicine, Harvard Medical School; Staff Physician, Beth Israel Deaconess Medical Center, Boston, Massachusetts
 JC, BK, and Other Polyomaviruses: Progressive Multifocal Leukoencephalopathy

Nathan M. Thielman, MD, MPH
Associate Professor of Medicine, Division of Infectious Diseases and International Health, Duke University School of Medicine; Director, Duke Global Health Residency Program, Duke University Medical Center, Durham, North Carolina
 Antibiotic-Associated Colitis; Enteric Fever and Other Causes of Abdominal Symptoms with Fever

Chloe Lynn Thio, MD
Associate Professor of Medicine, Johns Hopkins University School of Medicine, Baltimore, Maryland
 Hepatitis B Virus and Hepatitis Delta Virus

David L. Thomas, MD, MPH
Professor of Medicine and Chief, Infectious Diseases, Johns Hopkins University School of Medicine, Baltimore, Maryland
 Hepatitis C

Lora D. Thomas, MD, MPH
Assistant Professor of Medicine, Vanderbilt University School of Medicine; Chief, Division of Infectious Diseases, Nashville Veterans Affairs Medical Center, Nashville, Tennessee
 Risk Factors and Approaches to Infections in Transplant Recipients

Anna R. Thorner, MD
Instructor, Department of Medicine, Harvard Medical School; Associate Physician, Division of Infectious Diseases, Brigham and Women's Hospital, Boston, Massachusetts
 Zoonotic Paramyxoviruses: Nipah, Hendra, and Menangle Viruses

Alan D. Tice, MD
Assistant Professor, John A. Burns School of Medicine, University of Hawaii at Manoa, Honolulu, Hawaii
 Outpatient Parenteral Antimicrobial Therapy

Angela María Tobón, MD
Director, Chronic Infectious Diseases Unit, Corporación para Investigaciones Biológicas, Medellin, Colombia
 Paracoccidioides brasiliensis

Edmund C. Tramont, MD
Associate Director, Special Projects, Division of Clinical Research, National Institute of Allergy and Infectious Diseases, National Institutes of Health, Bethesda, Maryland
 Innate (General or Nonspecific) Host Defense Mechanisms; *Treponema pallidum* (Syphilis)

John J. Treanor, MD
Professor of Medicine, Microbiology, and Immunology, University of Rochester School of Medicine and Dentistry; Attending Physician, Strong Memorial Hospital; Chief, Division of Infectious Diseases, Department of Medicine, University of Rochester Medical Center, Rochester, New York
 Influenza Viruses, Including Avian Influenza and Swine Influenza; Noroviruses and Other Caliciviruses; Astroviruses and Picobirnaviruses

Athe M. N. Tsibris, MD
Instructor in Medicine, Harvard Medical School; Clinical Assistant in Medicine, Massachusetts General Hospital, Boston, Massachusetts
 Antiretroviral Therapy for Human Immunodeficiency Virus Infection

Allan R. Tunkel, MD, PhD
Professor of Medicine, Drexel University College of Medicine, Philadelphia, Pennsylvania; Chair, Department of Medicine, Monmouth Medical Center, Long Branch, New Jersey
  Approach to the Patient with Central Nervous System Infection; Acute Meningitis; Cerebrospinal Fluid Shunt Infections; Brain Abscess; Subdural Empyema, Epidural Abscess, and Suppurative Intracranial Thrombophlebitis; Viridans Streptococci, Groups C and G Streptococci, and *Gemella* Species

Ronald B. Turner, MD
Professor of Pediatrics, University of Virginia School of Medicine, Charlottesville, Virginia
  The Common Cold; Rhinovirus

Kenneth L. Tyler, MD
Reuler-Lewin Family Professor of Neurology and Professor of Medicine and Microbiology, University of Colorado Denver School of Medicine, Aurora; Chief, Neurology Service, Denver Veterans Affairs Medical Center, Denver, Colorado
  Encephalitis; Orthoreoviruses and Orbiviruses; Coltiviruses and Seadornaviruses; Prions and Prion Diseases of the Central Nervous System (Transmissible Neurodegenerative Diseases)

Diederik van de Beek, MD, PhD
Neurologist, Center of Infection and Immunity Amsterdam (CINIMA), University of Amsterdam, Academic Medical Center, Amsterdam, The Netherlands
  Acute Meningitis

Edouard G. Vannier, PharmD, PhD
Assistant Professor of Medicine, Tufts University School of Medicine; Department of Medicine, Division of Geographic Medicine and Infectious Diseases, Tufts Medical Center, Boston, Massachusetts
  Babesia Species

Trevor C. Van Schooneveld, MD
Assistant Professor, Department of Internal Medicine, Division of Infectious Diseases, University of Nebraska Medical Center College of Medicine; Director, Antimicrobial Stewardship Program, Nebraska Medical Center, Omaha, Nebraska
  Mediastinitis

David W. Vaughn, MD, MPH
Director, Global Clinical Research and Development, GlaxoSmithKline Biologicals, King of Prussia, Pennsylvania
  Flaviviruses (Yellow Fever, Dengue, Dengue Hemorrhagic Fever, Japanese Encephalitis, West Nile Encephalitis, St. Louis Encephalitis, Tick-Borne Encephalitis)

Claudio Viscoli
Professor of Infectious Disease, University of Genoa Faculty of Medicine; Chief, Infectious Diseases Unit, San Martino University Hospital, Genoa, Italy
  Prophylaxis and Empirical Therapy of Infection in Cancer Patients

Paul A. Volberding, MD
Professor of Medicine, University of California, San Francisco, School of Medicine; Vice Chair, Department of Medicine, University of California, San Francisco, Medical Center; Chief, Medical Service, San Francisco Veterans Affairs Medical Center, San Francisco, California
  Malignant Diseases in Human Immunodeficiency Virus Infection

Ellen R. Wald, MD
Alfred Dorrance Daniels Professor on Diseases of Children, University of Wisconsin School of Medicine and Public Health; Pediatrician-in-Chief, American Family Children's Hospital, Madison, Wisconsin
  Sinusitis

David H. Walker, MD
Professor and Chairman, Department of Pathology, University of Texas Medical Branch School of Medicine; The Carmage and Martha Walls Distinguished University Chair in Tropical Diseases; Executive Director of the Center for Biodefense and Emerging Infectious Diseases; and Director of the WHO Collaborating Center for Tropical Diseases, University of Texas Medical Branch, Galveston, Texas
  Rickettsia rickettsii and Other Spotted Fever Group Rickettsiae (Rocky Mountain Spotted Fever and Other Spotted Fevers); *Rickettsia prowazekii* (Epidemic or Louse-Borne Typhus); *Rickettsia typhi* (Murine Typhus); *Ehrlichia chaffeensis* (Human Monocytotropic Ehrlichiosis), *Anaplasma phagocytophilum* (Human Granulocytotropic Anaplasmosis), and Other Anaplasmataceae

Richard J. Wallace, Jr., MD
Professor of Medicine and Chairman, Department of Microbiology, University of Texas Health Science Center at Tyler, Tyler, Texas
  Antimycobacterial Agents; Infectious Due to Nontuberculous Mycobacteria Other than *Mycobacterium avium-intracellulare*

Edward E. Walsh, MD
Professor of Medicine, University of Rochester School of Medicine and Dentistry; Attending Physician, Rochester General Hospital, Rochester, New York
  Acute Bronchitis

Peter D. Walzer, MD, MSc
Professor of Medicine, University of Cincinnati College of Medicine; Associate Chief of Staff for Research, Veterans Affairs Cincinnati Medical Center, Cincinnati, Ohio
  Pneumocystis Species

Christine A. Wanke, MD
Professor of Medicine and Public Health, Tufts University School of Medicine; Infectious Diseases Physician, Tufts Medical Center, Boston, Massachusetts
  Tropical Sprue: Enteropathy

Ronald G. Washburn, MD
Professor of Medicine, Section of Infectious Diseases, Louisiana State University Health Sciences Center in Shreveport School of Medicine; Associate Chief of Staff for Research and Development and Chief, Section of Infectious Diseases, Shreveport Veterans Affairs Medical Center, Shreveport, Louisiana
  Rat-Bite Fever: *Streptobacillus moniliformis* and *Spirillum minus*

Annemarie Wasley, ScD
Senior Research Epidemiologist, Global Immunization Division, National Center for Immunization and Respiratory Diseases, Centers for Disease Control and Prevention, Atlanta, Georgia
  Hepatitis A Virus

Valerie Waters, MD, MSc
Assistant Professor, Department of Pediatrics, University of Toronto Faculty of Medicine; Assistant Professor, Department of Pediatrics, Division of Infectious Diseases, Hospital for Sick Children, Toronto, Ontario, Canada
  Bordetella pertussis

David J. Weber, MD, MPH
Professor of Medicine, Pediatrics, and Epidemiology, University of North Carolina at Chapel Hill School of Medicine; Associate Chief of Staff and Medical Director, Hospital Epidemiology and Occupational Health, University of North Carolina Health Care, Chapel Hill, North Carolina
  The Acutely Ill Patient with Fever and Rash; Disinfection, Sterilization, and Control of Hospital Waste

Arnold N. Weinberg, MD
Professor of Medicine, Harvard Medical School; Attending
Physician, Infectious Disease Unit, Massachusetts General Hospital,
Boston, Massachusetts
  Zoonoses

Geoffrey A. Weinberg, MD
Professor of Pediatrics, University of Rochester School of Medicine
and Dentistry; Director, Pediatric Human Immunodeficiency Virus
Program, Golisano Children's Hospital, University of Rochester
Medical Center, Rochester, New York
  Pediatric Human Immunodeficiency Virus Infection

Gail G. Weinmann, MD
Deputy Director, Division of Lung Diseases, National Heart, Lung,
and Blood Institute, National Institutes of Health, Bethesda,
Maryland
  Chronic Obstructive Pulmonary Disease and Acute Exacerbations

Daniel J. Weisdorf, MD
Professor of Medicine, Division of Hematology, Oncology, and
Transplantation, and Director, Adult Blood and Marrow Transplant
Program, University of Minnesota Medical School, Minneapolis,
Minnesota
  Infections in Recipients of Hematopoietic Cell Transplantation

Louis M. Weiss, MD, MPH
Professor of Pathology, Division of Parasitology and Tropical
Medicine, and Professor of Medicine, Division of Infectious
Diseases, Albert Einstein College of Medicine of Yeshiva University;
Attending Physician, Weiler Hospital–Montefiore Medical Center
and Jacobi Medical Center, Bronx, New York
  Microsporidiosis

Michael E. Weiss, MD
Clinical Professor of Medicine, University of Washington School of
Medicine, Seattle, Washington
  β-Lactam Allergy

David F. Welch, PhD
Associate Clinical Professor of Pathology, University of Texas
Southwestern Medical School; President, Medical Microbiology
Consulting, LLC, Dallas, Texas
  Bartonella, Including Cat-Scratch Disease

Thomas E. Wellems, MD, PhD
Chief, Laboratory of Malaria and Vector Research, National Institute
of Allergy and Infectious Diseases, National Institutes of Health,
Bethesda, Maryland
  Plasmodium Species (Malaria)

Richard P. Wenzel, MD, MSc
William Branch Porter Professor and Chair, Department of Internal
Medicine, Virginia Commonwealth University School of Medicine,
Richmond, Virginia
  Organization for Infection Control; Isolation

Melinda Wharton, MD, MPH
Deputy Director, National Center for Immunization and Respiratory
Diseases, Centers for Disease Control and Prevention, Atlanta,
Georgia
  Immunization

A. Clinton White, Jr., MD
Paul R. Stalnaker, MD, Distinguished Professor of Internal
Medicine and Director, Infectious Disease Division, Department of
Internal Medicine, University of Texas Medical Branch, Galveston,
Texas
  Cryptosporidium Species

Richard J. Whitley, MD
Distinguished Professor of Pediatrics and Professor of Microbiology,
Medicine, and Neurosurgery, University of Alabama at Birmingham
School of Medicine; Loeb Eminent Scholar Chair in Pediatrics; Vice
Chairman, Department of Pediatrics; and Co-Director, Division of
Infectious Diseases, University of Birmingham at Alabama Health
System, Birmingham, Alabama
  Varicella-Zoster Virus

Kenneth H. Wilson, MD
Professor of Medicine, Division of Infectious Diseases and
International Health, Duke University School of Medicine;
Attending Physician, Durham Veterans Affairs Medical Center,
Durham, North Carolina
  Antibiotic-Associated Colitis

Walter R. Wilson, MD
Professor of Medicine and Assistant Professor of Microbiology,
Mayo Clinic College of Medicine; Consultant, Infectious Diseases,
Mayo Clinic, Rochester, Minnesota
  Prosthetic Valve Endocarditis; Infections of Nonvalvular
  Cardiovascular Devices

Frank G. Witebsky, MD
Assistant Chief, Microbiology Service, Department of Laboratory
Medicine, National Institutes of Health Clinical Center, National
Institutes of Health, Bethesda, Maryland
  The Clinician and the Microbiology Laboratory

Matthew C. Wolfgang, PhD
Assistant Professor, Department of Microbiology and Immunology,
University of North Carolina at Chapel Hill School of Medicine,
Chapel Hill, North Carolina
  Cystic Fibrosis

Peter F. Wright, MD
Professor of Pediatrics, Dartmouth Medical School, Hanover, New
Hampshire
  Parainfluenza Viruses

Edward J. Young, MD
Professor of Medicine, Molecular Virology, and Microbiology,
Baylor College of Medicine; Chief, Infection Control, Michael E.
DeBakey Veterans Affairs Medical Center, Houston, Texas
  Brucella Species

Jo-Anne H. Young, MD
Associate Professor of Medicine, Division of Infectious Disease, and
Director, Transplant Infectious Disease Program, University of
Minnesota Medical School, Minneapolis, Minnesota
  Infections in Recipients of Hematopoietic Cell Transplantation

Jie Lin Zhang, MD
Assistant Professor of Medicine, Harvard Medical School; Attending
Physician, Division of Infectious Diseases, Beth Israel Deaconess
Medical Center, Boston, Massachusetts
  Cytomegalovirus

Stephen H. Zinner, MD
Charles S. Davidson Professor of Medicine, Harvard Medical School,
Boston; Chair, Department of Medicine, Mount Auburn Hospital,
Cambridge, Massachusetts
  Sulfonamides and Trimethoprim

John J. Zurlo, MD
Professor of Medicine, Penn State University College of Medicine,
Milton S. Hershey Medical Center, Hershey, Pennsylvania
  Pasteurella Species

PREFACE TO THE FIRST EDITION

Infectious diseases traverse the usual boundaries established by medical specialists. All organ systems may be involved, and all physicians caring for patients may have to deal with infected patients. The format of this book was chosen with the intent that it would contain the necessary information to aid the practitioner in the understanding, diagnosis, and treatment of infectious diseases. Thus, internists, family or general practitioners, pediatricians, surgeons, obstetrician-gynecologists, urologists, residents and fellows in training, medical students, hospital infection control personnel, and clinical microbiologists should find the book a valuable reference.

In planning this book, the editors considered several different patterns of organization. The system adopted allows the reader to approach an infected patient three different ways: (a) by major clinical syndrome, (b) by specific etiologic organisms, and (c) by host characteristics for patients who are compromised.

Principles and Practice of Infectious Diseases consists of four major parts. The book may be perused as whole, or individual chapters may be examined when the reader is concerned with a specific problem. Part I covers the basic principles necessary for a clear understanding of the concepts of diagnosis and management of infectious disease. Chapters dealing with microbial virulence factors, host defense mechanisms, the epidemiology of infectious diseases, and the clinician and microbiology laboratory are included. In addition, there is a comprehensive discussion of anti-infective chemotherapy.

Part II considers major clinical syndromes. The syndromes are described, followed by a discussion of the potential etiologic agents, evaluation of differential diagnostic possibilities, and an outline of presumptive therapy. All major infectious diseases are discussed in this part of the book.

Part III describes all important pathogenic microbes for man and the diseases they cause. The pathogen is classified and described, the epidemiology is discussed, clinical manifestations are listed, and specific information on therapy and prevention is presented. The most comprehensive discussion of a disease entity can be found by reading about both the etiologic agent and the clinical syndrome. Thus, a comprehensive treatment of pneumococcal pneumonia could be found in reading the appropriate sections of the chapters on acute pneumonia and *Streptococcus pneumoniae*. We attempted to make the chapters dealing with etiologic agents and those dealing with syndromes complete. Therefore some repetition was unavoidable.

The final section, Part IV, covers special problems in infectious diseases including nosocomial infections, infections in impaired hosts, immunizations, and protection of travelers.

The editors are grateful to our expert contributors. These physicians are the world's leaders in their fields, and they diligently prepared carefully written, well-referenced "state of the art" chapters. Our secretaries were skillful and meticulous in their attention to the complexities of assembling *Principles and Practice of Infectious Diseases*. John de Carville, executive editor of John Wiley & Sons, encouraged, cajoled, and advised us from the formative steps all the way through to completion. Lastly, and perhaps most important, we are grateful to our wives and children for putting up with interminable editorial work and meetings.

GERALD L. MANDELL, MD

R. GORDON DOUGLAS, JR., MD

JOHN E. BENNETT, MD

PREFACE TO THE SEVENTH EDITION

It is interesting to compare the first edition with the new, seventh edition of *Principles and Practice of Infectious Diseases*. Since 1979, when the first edition was published, there have been scores of new antimicrobial agents and newly recognized diseases and pathogens, such as Legionnaires' disease, Lyme disease, Kaposi's sarcoma, human immunodeficiency virus (HIV)/acquired immunodeficiency syndrome (AIDS), multidrug-resistant tuberculosis, *Clostridium difficile* colitis, progressive multifocal leukoencephalopathy, severe acute respiratory syndrome (SARS), and the new H1N1 flu, to mention just a few. A comparison with the sixth edition, published in 2004, reveals a further increase in our knowledge of newly recognized diseases, microbes, and therapeutic agents. The developments in basic sciences have been astounding, with advances in genomics leading to rapid diagnoses and breakthrough therapies.

Principles and Practice of Infectious Diseases differs from other sources of information, such as many web-based resources, in that it is carefully edited and the content put into perspective by infectious diseases experts. The new edition combines the knowledge and experience of the world's authorities with the careful review of all chapters by all three editors.

This edition has been planned and designed for physicians (infectious diseases specialists, internists, family practitioners, travel medicine specialists, HIV/AIDS researchers), pharmacologists, public health experts, microbiologists, and basic scientists. Readers consulting the volumes can quickly find key clinical information to help in diagnosing and treating their patients. The text contains up-to-date information and includes numerous 2009 references. New chapters have been added, and all other chapters have been revised extensively, with tables, figures, and references updated.

Among the 330 chapters is excellent coverage of such topics as microbial pathogenesis, infections in cancer patients, emerging infections, new antimicrobial agents, antibiotic resistance, travel medicine, vaccines, infections related to exotic pets, and important aspects of agents of bioterrorism.

The online version of the book contains fully searchable text on the dedicated Expert Consult website. It will also allow us to present new developments in the field and advances in therapy via regular content updates. The website contains other added-value features such as a downloadable image library and drug database.

We could not have edited this book without the assistance and stoic patience of our wives, Judy Mandell, Shirley Bennett, and Kelly Dolin, who endured the many long hours their husbands spent at home, uncommunicative, laboring over yet another edition of this treatise. Our thanks also go to Janet Morgan for her invaluable assistance to Dr. Dolin.

GERALD L. MANDELL, MD

JOHN E. BENNETT, MD

RAPHAEL DOLIN, MD

CONTENTS

VOLUME 1

 PART I Basic Principles in the Diagnosis and Management of Infectious Diseases

SECTION A
MICROBIAL PATHOGENESIS

1 A Molecular Perspective of Microbial Pathogenicity 3
DAVID A. RELMAN | STANLEY FALKOW

2 Microbial Adherence 15
WILLIAM A. PETRI, JR. | BARBARA J. MANN | CHRISTOPHER D. HUSTON

3 Toxins 27
ERIK L. HEWLETT | MOLLY A. HUGHES

SECTION B
HOST DEFENSE MECHANISMS

4 Innate (General or Nonspecific) Host Defense Mechanisms 37
CARL W. DIEFFENBACH | EDMUND C. TRAMONT | SUSAN F. PLAEGER

5 Human Genetics and Infection 49
ADRIAN V. S. HILL

6 Antibodies 59
HOLLY H. BIRDSALL

7 Complement 77
PETER DENSEN

8 Granulocytic Phagocytes 99
WILLIAM M. NAUSEEF | ROBERT A. CLARK

9 Cell-Mediated Defense against Infection 129
MICHAEL S. GLICKMAN | ERIC G. PAMER

10 Nutrition, Immunity, and Infection 151
CARYN GEE MORSE | KEVIN P. HIGH

11 Prebiotics, Probiotics, and Synbiotics 161
SHERVIN RABIZADEH | MARK A. MILLER | CYNTHIA L. SEARS

12 Evaluation of the Patient with Suspected Immunodeficiency 167
STEVEN M. HOLLAND | JOHN I. GALLIN

SECTION C
EPIDEMIOLOGY OF INFECTIOUS DISEASES

13 Epidemiologic Principles 179
MICHAEL T. OSTERHOLM | CRAIG W. HEDBERG

14 Outbreak Investigation 193
ANDRES G. LESCANO | JOEL M. MONTGOMERY | DAVID L. BLAZES

15 Emerging and Reemerging Infectious Disease Threats 199
RIMA F. KHABBAZ | STEPHEN M. OSTROFF | JAMES W. LeDUC | ROBIN MOSELEY | JAMES M. HUGHES

16 Hospital Preparedness for Emerging and Highly Contagious Infectious Diseases: Getting Ready for the Next Epidemic or Pandemic 221
LAURA M. LEE | DAVID K. HENDERSON

SECTION D
CLINICAL MICROBIOLOGY

17 The Clinician and the Microbiology Laboratory 233
PATRICK R. MURRAY | FRANK G. WITEBSKY

SECTION E
ANTI-INFECTIVE THERAPY

18 Principles of Anti-infective Therapy 267
SATISH K. PILLAI | GEORGE M. ELIOPOULOS | ROBERT C. MOELLERING, JR.

19 Molecular Mechanisms of Antibiotic Resistance in Bacteria 279
STEVEN M. OPAL | AURORA POP-VICAS

20 Pharmacokinetics and Pharmacodynamics of Anti-infective Agents 297
GUY W. AMSDEN | CHARLES H. BALLOW | JOSEPH S. BERTINO, JR. | ANGELA D. M. KASHUBA

21 Penicillins and β-Lactam Inhibitors 309
HENRY F. CHAMBERS

22 Cephalosporins 323
DAVID R. ANDES | WILLIAM A. CRAIG

23 Carbapenems and Monobactams 341
HENRY F. CHAMBERS

24 β-Lactam Allergy 347
MICHAEL E. WEISS | N. FRANKLIN ADKINSON, JR.

25 Fusidic Acid 355
LIONEL A. MANDELL

26 Aminoglycosides 359
DAVID N. GILBERT | JAMES E. LEGGETT

27 Tetracyclines and Chloramphenicol 385
MIRELLA SALVATORE | BURT R. MEYERS

28 Rifamycins 403
DAVID P. CALFEE

29 Metronidazole 419
MIRELLA SALVATORE | BURT R. MEYERS

30 Macrolides, Clindamycin, and Ketolides 427
SUMATHI SIVAPALASINGAM | NEAL H. STEIGBIGEL

31 Glycopeptides (Vancomycin and Teicoplanin), Streptogramins (Quinupristin-Dalfopristin), and Lipopeptides (Daptomycin) 449
BARBARA E. MURRAY | ESTEBAN C. NANNINI

32 Polymyxins (Polymyxin B and Colistin) 469
KEITH S. KAYE | DONALD KAYE

33 Linezolid and Other Oxazolidinones 471
GERALD R. DONOWITZ | HEATHER L. COX

34 Sulfonamides and Trimethoprim 475
STEPHEN H. ZINNER | KENNETH H. MAYER

35 Quinolones 487
DAVID C. HOOPER | JACOB STRAHILEVITZ

36 Novel Antibiotics 511
LIONEL A. MANDELL

37 Urinary Tract Agents: Nitrofurantoin and Methenamine 515
DAVID C. HOOPER

38 Topical Antibacterials 521
JUDITH A. O'DONNELL | STEVEN P. GELONE

39 Antimycobacterial Agents 533
RICHARD J. WALLACE, JR. | DAVID E. GRIFFITH

40 Systemic Antifungal Agents 549
JOHN H. REX | DAVID A. STEVENS

41 Antiviral Drugs (Other Than Antiretrovirals) 565
FRED Y. AOKI | FREDERICK G. HAYDEN | RAPHAEL DOLIN

42 Immunomodulators 611
ANDREA V. PAGE | W. CONRAD LILES

43 Hyperbaric Oxygen 625
RONALD P. RABINOWITZ | ELLIS S. CAPLAN

44 Agents Active against Parasites and *Pneumocystis* 631
THOMAS A. MOORE

45 Alternative Medicines for Infectious Diseases 669
JONATHAN D. BERMAN

46 Antimicrobial Stewardship 677
RONALD E. POLK | NEIL O. FISHMAN

47 Interpreting the Results of Clinical Trials of Antimicrobial Agents 687
JOHN H. POWERS

48 Outpatient Parenteral Antimicrobial Therapy 699
ALAN D. TICE

49 Tables of Antimicrobial Agent Pharmacology 705
GUY W. AMSDEN

 PART II Major Clinical Syndromes

SECTION A
FEVER

50 Temperature Regulation and the Pathogenesis of Fever 765
PHILIP A. MACKOWIAK

51 Fever of Unknown Origin 779
PHILIP A. MACKOWIAK | DAVID T. DURACK

52 The Acutely Ill Patient with Fever and Rash 791
DAVID J. WEBER | MYRON S. COHEN | DEAN S. MORRELL | WILLIAM A. RUTALA

SECTION B
UPPER RESPIRATORY TRACT INFECTIONS

53 The Common Cold 809
RONALD B. TURNER

54 Pharyngitis 815
MARY T. CASERTA | ANTHONY R. FLORES

55 Acute Laryngitis 823
MARY T. CASERTA

56 Acute Laryngotracheobronchitis (Croup) 825
CAROLINE BREESE HALL | JOHN T. McBRIDE

57 Otitis Externa, Otitis Media, and Mastoiditis 831
JEROME O. KLEIN

58 Sinusitis 839
GREGORY P. DeMURI | ELLEN R. WALD

59 Epiglottitis 851
JAMES E. BURNS | J. OWEN HENDLEY

60 Infections of the Oral Cavity, Neck, and Head 855
ANTHONY W. CHOW

SECTION C
PLEUROPULMONARY AND BRONCHIAL INFECTIONS

61 Acute Bronchitis 873
EDWARD E. WALSH

62 Chronic Obstructive Pulmonary Disease and Acute Exacerbations 877
ANTONELLO PUNTURIERI | GAIL G. WEINMANN | HERBERT Y. REYNOLDS

63 Bronchiolitis 885
CAROLINE BREESE HALL | JOHN T. McBRIDE

64 Acute Pneumonia 891
GERALD R. DONOWITZ

65 Pleural Effusion and Empyema 917
EDWARD J. SEPTIMUS

66 Bacterial Lung Abscess 925
BENNETT LORBER

67 Chronic Pneumonia 931
PETER G. PAPPAS

68 Cystic Fibrosis 947
SCOTT H. DONALDSON | MATTHEW C. WOLFGANG | PETER H. GILLIGAN | RICHARD C. BOUCHER, JR.

SECTION D
URINARY TRACT INFECTIONS

69 Urinary Tract Infections 957
JACK D. SOBEL | DONALD KAYE

SECTION E
SEPSIS

70 Sepsis, Severe Sepsis, and Septic Shock 987
ROBERT S. MUNFORD | ANTHONY F. SUFFREDINI

SECTION F
INTRA-ABDOMINAL INFECTION

71 Peritonitis and Intraperitoneal Abscesses 1011
MATTHEW E. LEVISON | LARRY M. BUSH

72 Infections of the Liver and Biliary System 1035
COSTI D. SIFRI | LAWRENCE C. MADOFF

73 Pancreatic Infection 1045
MIRIAM J. BARON | LAWRENCE C. MADOFF

74 Splenic Abscess 1055
LAWRENCE C. MADOFF

75 Appendicitis 1059
COSTI D. SIFRI | LAWRENCE C. MADOFF

76 Diverticulitis and Typhlitis 1063
COSTI D. SIFRI | LAWRENCE C. MADOFF

SECTION G
CARDIOVASCULAR INFECTIONS

77 Endocarditis and Intravascular Infections 1067
VANCE G. FOWLER, JR. | W. MICHAEL SCHELD | ARNOLD S. BAYER

78 Prosthetic Valve Endocarditis 1113
BETTINA M. KNOLL | LARRY M. BADDOUR | WALTER R. WILSON

79 Infections of Nonvalvular Cardiovascular Devices 1127
M. RIZWAN SOHAIL | WALTER R. WILSON | LARRY M. BADDOUR

80 Prevention of Infective Endocarditis 1143
DAVID T. DURACK

81 Myocarditis and Pericarditis 1153
KIRK U. KNOWLTON | MARIA C. SAVOIA | MICHAEL N. OXMAN

82 Mediastinitis 1173
TREVOR C. VAN SCHOONEVELD | MARK E. RUPP

SECTION H
CENTRAL NERVOUS SYSTEM INFECTIONS

83 Approach to the Patient with Central Nervous System Infection 1183
ALLAN R. TUNKEL

84 Acute Meningitis 1189
ALLAN R. TUNKEL | DIEDERIK VAN DE BEEK | W. MICHAEL SCHELD

85 Cerebrospinal Fluid Shunt Infections 1231
ALLAN R. TUNKEL | JAMES M. DRAKE

86 Chronic Meningitis 1237
JOHN E. BENNETT

87 Encephalitis 1243
J. DAVID BECKHAM | KENNETH L. TYLER

88 Brain Abscess 1265
ALLAN R. TUNKEL

89 Subdural Empyema, Epidural Abscess, and Suppurative Intracranial Thrombophlebitis 1279
ALLAN R. TUNKEL

SECTION I
SKIN AND SOFT TISSUE INFECTIONS

90 Cellulitis, Necrotizing Fasciitis, and Subcutaneous Tissue Infections 1289
MARK S. PASTERNACK | MORTON N. SWARTZ

91 Myositis and Myonecrosis 1313
MARK S. PASTERNACK | MORTON N. SWARTZ

92 Lymphadenitis and Lymphangitis 1323
MARK S. PASTERNACK | MORTON N. SWARTZ

SECTION J
GASTROINTESTINAL INFECTIONS AND FOOD POISONING

93 Principles and Syndromes of Enteric Infection 1335
THEODORE S. STEINER | RICHARD L. GUERRANT

94 Esophagitis 1353
PAUL S. GRAMAN

95 Nausea, Vomiting, and Noninflammatory Diarrhea 1359
DAVID A. BOBAK | RICHARD L. GUERRANT

96 Antibiotic-Associated Colitis 1375
NATHAN M. THIELMAN | KENNETH H. WILSON

97 Inflammatory Enteritides 1389
ALDO A. M. LIMA | RICHARD L. GUERRANT

98 Enteric Fever and Other Causes of Abdominal Symptoms with Fever 1399
NATHAN M. THIELMAN | JOHN A. CRUMP | RICHARD L. GUERRANT

99 Foodborne Disease 1413
SAMIR V. SODHA | PATRICIA M. GRIFFIN | JAMES M. HUGHES

100 Tropical Sprue: Enteropathy 1429
CHRISTINE A. WANKE

101 Whipple's Disease 1435
THOMAS MARTH | THOMAS SCHNEIDER

SECTION K
BONE AND JOINT INFECTIONS

102 Infectious Arthritis of Native Joints 1443
CHRISTOPHER A. OHL

103 Osteomyelitis 1457
ELIE F. BERBARI | JAMES M. STECKELBERG | DOUGLAS R. OSMON

104 Infections with Prostheses in Bones and Joints 1469
BARRY D. BRAUSE

SECTION L
DISEASES OF THE REPRODUCTIVE ORGANS AND SEXUALLY TRANSMITTED DISEASES

105 Genital Skin and Mucous Membrane Lesions 1475
MICHAEL H. AUGENBRAUN

106 Urethritis   1485
WILLIAM M. McCORMACK

107 Vulvovaginitis and Cervicitis   1495
WILLIAM M. McCORMACK

108 Infections of the Female Pelvis   1511
DAVID E. SOPER

109 Prostatitis, Epididymitis, and Orchitis   1521
JOHN N. KRIEGER

SECTION M
EYE INFECTIONS

110 Microbial Conjunctivitis   1529
SCOTT D. BARNES | DEBORAH PAVAN-LANGSTON | DIMITRI T. AZAR

111 Microbial Keratitis   1539
SCOTT D. BARNES | DEBORAH PAVAN-LANGSTON | DIMITRI T. AZAR

112 Endophthalmitis   1553
MARLENE L. DURAND

113 Infectious Causes of Uveitis   1561
MARLENE L. DURAND

114 Periocular Infections   1569
MARLENE L. DURAND

SECTION N
HEPATITIS

115 Acute Viral Hepatitis   1577
MICHAEL P. CURRY | SANJIV CHOPRA

116 Chronic Viral Hepatitis   1593
JULES L. DIENSTAG

SECTION O
ACQUIRED IMMUNODEFICIENCY SYNDROME

117 Global Perspectives on Human Immunodeficiency
Virus Infection and Acquired Immunodeficiency
Syndrome   1619
PETER PIOT | MICHEL CARAEL

118 Epidemiology and Prevention of Acquired
Immunodeficiency Syndrome and Human
Immunodeficiency Virus Infection   1635
CARLOS DEL RIO | JAMES W. CURRAN

119 Diagnosis of Human Immunodeficiency Virus
Infection   1663
ROBIN DEWAR | DEBORAH GOLDSTEIN | FRANK MALDARELLI

120 The Immunology of Human Immunodeficiency Virus
Infection   1687
SUSAN MOIR | MARK CONNORS | ANTHONY S. FAUCI

121 General Clinical Manifestations of Human
Immunodeficiency Virus Infection (Including the
Acute Retroviral Syndrome and Oral, Cutaneous,
Renal, Ocular, Metabolic, and Cardiac
Diseases)   1705
TIMOTHY R. STERLING | RICHARD E. CHAISSON

122 Pulmonary Manifestations of Human
Immunodeficiency Virus Infection   1727
PAUL E. SAX

123 Gastrointestinal and Hepatobiliary
Manifestations of Human Immunodeficiency Virus
Infection   1737
MARK S. SULKOWSKI

124 Neurologic Diseases Caused by Human
Immunodeficiency Virus Type 1 and Opportunistic
Infections   1745
IGOR J. KORALNIK

125 Malignant Diseases in Human Immunodeficiency Virus
Infection   1765
PATRICIA A. CORNETT | PAUL A. VOLBERDING

126 Human Immunodeficiency Virus Infection
in Women   1781
SUSAN E. COHN | REBECCA A. CLARK

127 Pediatric Human Immunodeficiency Virus
Infection   1809
GEOFFREY A. WEINBERG | GEORGE K. SIBERRY

128 Antiretroviral Therapy for Human Immunodeficiency
Virus Infection   1833
ATHE M. N. TSIBRIS | MARTIN S. HIRSCH

129 Management of Opportunistic Infections
Associated with Human Immunodeficiency Virus
Infection   1855
HENRY MASUR

130 Vaccines for Human Immunodeficiency Virus-1
Infection   1887
DAN H. BAROUCH | LINDSEY R. BADEN | RAPHAEL DOLIN

SECTION P
MISCELLANEOUS SYNDROMES

131 Chronic Fatigue Syndrome   1897
N. CARY ENGLEBERG

Index   i

VOLUME 2

PART III Infectious Diseases and Their Etiologic Agents

SECTION A
VIRAL DISEASES

132 Introduction to Viruses and Viral Diseases   1907
JAMES D. CHAPPELL | TERENCE S. DERMODY

133 Orthopoxviruses: Vaccinia (Smallpox Vaccine), Variola (Smallpox), Monkeypox, and Cowpox   1923
INGER K. DAMON

134 Other Poxviruses That Infect Humans: Parapoxviruses, Molluscum Contagiosum, and Yatapoxviruses   1933
INGER K. DAMON

135 Introduction to Herpesviridae   1937
JEFFREY I. COHEN

136 Herpes Simplex Virus   1943
JOSHUA T. SCHIFFER | LAWRENCE COREY

137 Varicella-Zoster Virus   1963
RICHARD J. WHITLEY

138 Cytomegalovirus   1971
CLYDE S. CRUMPACKER II | JIE LIN ZHANG

139 Epstein-Barr Virus (Infectious Mononucleosis, Epstein-Barr Virus–Associated Malignant Diseases, and Other Diseases)   1989
ERIC C. JOHANNSEN | KENNETH M. KAYE

140 Human Herpesvirus Types 6 and 7   2011
JEFFREY I. COHEN

141 Kaposi's Sarcoma–Associated Herpesvirus (Human Herpesvirus Type 8)   2017
KENNETH M. KAYE

142 Herpes B Virus   2023
JEFFREY I. COHEN

143 Adenoviruses   2027
ELIZABETH G. RHEE | DAN H. BAROUCH

144 Papillomaviruses   2035
WILLIAM BONNEZ | RICHARD C. REICHMAN

145 JC, BK, and Other Polyomaviruses: Progressive Multifocal Leukoencephalopathy   2051
C. SABRINA TAN | IGOR J. KORALNIK

146 Hepatitis B Virus and Hepatitis Delta Virus   2059
MARGARET JAMES KOZIEL | CHLOE LYNN THIO

147 Human Parvoviruses, Including Parvovirus B19 and Human Bocavirus   2087
KEVIN E. BROWN

148 Orthoreoviruses and Orbiviruses   2097
ROBERTA L. DeBIASI | KENNETH L. TYLER

149 Coltiviruses and Seadornaviruses   2101
ROBERTA L. DeBIASI | KENNETH L. TYLER

150 Rotaviruses   2105
PHILIP R. DORMITZER

151 Alphaviruses   2117
LEWIS MARKOFF

152 Rubella Virus (German Measles)   2127
ANNE A. GERSHON

153 Flaviviruses (Yellow Fever, Dengue, Dengue Hemorrhagic Fever, Japanese Encephalitis, West Nile Encephalitis, St. Louis Encephalitis, Tick-Borne Encephalitis)   2133
DAVID W. VAUGHN | ALAN BARRETT | TOM SOLOMON

154 Hepatitis C   2157
STUART C. RAY | DAVID L. THOMAS

155 Coronaviruses, Including Severe Acute Respiratory Syndrome (SARS)–Associated Coronavirus   2187
KENNETH McINTOSH | STANLEY PERLMAN

156 Parainfluenza Viruses   2195
PETER F. WRIGHT

157 Mumps Virus   2201
NATHAN LITMAN | STEPHEN G. BAUM

158 Respiratory Syncytial Virus   2207
CAROLINE BREESE HALL

159 Human Metapneumovirus   2223
ANN R. FALSEY

160 Measles Virus (Rubeola)   2229
ANNE A. GERSHON

161 Zoonotic Paramyxoviruses: Nipah, Hendra, and Menangle Viruses   2237
ANNA R. THORNER | RAPHAEL DOLIN

162 Vesicular Stomatitis Virus and Related Vesiculoviruses   2245
STEVEN M. FINE

163 Rhabdoviruses   2249
SARICE L. BASSIN | CHARLES E. RUPPRECHT | THOMAS P. BLECK

164 Marburg and Ebola Virus Hemorrhagic Fevers   2259
C. J. PETERS

165 Influenza Viruses, Including Avian Influenza and Swine Influenza   2265
JOHN J. TREANOR

166 California Encephalitis, Hantavirus Pulmonary Syndrome, and Bunyavirid Hemorrhagic Fevers   2289
C. J. PETERS

167 Lymphocytic Choriomeningitis Virus, Lassa Virus, and the South American Hemorrhagic Fevers   2295
C. J. PETERS

168 Human T-Cell Lymphotropic Virus Types I and II   2303
EDWARD L. MURPHY | HOPE H. BISWAS

169 Human Immunodeficiency Viruses   2323
MARVIN S. REITZ, JR. | ROBERT C. GALLO

170 Introduction to the Enteroviruses and
    Parechoviruses   2337
    JOHN F. MODLIN

171 Poliovirus   2345
    JOHN F. MODLIN

172 Coxsackieviruses, Echoviruses, Newer Enteroviruses,
    and Parechoviruses   2353
    JOHN F. MODLIN

173 Hepatitis A Virus   2367
    ANNEMARIE WASLEY | STEPHEN M. FEINSTONE | BETH P. BELL

174 Rhinovirus   2389
    RONALD B. TURNER

175 Noroviruses and Other Caliciviruses   2399
    RAPHAEL DOLIN | JOHN J. TREANOR

176 Astroviruses and Picobirnaviruses   2407
    RAPHAEL DOLIN | JOHN J. TREANOR

177 Hepatitis E Virus   2411
    DAVID A. ANDERSON

SECTION B
PRION DISEASES

178 Prions and Prion Diseases of the Central Nervous
    System (Transmissible Neurodegenerative
    Diseases)   2423
    PATRICK J. BOSQUE | KENNETH L. TYLER

SECTION C
CHLAMYDIAL DISEASES

179 Introduction to *Chlamydia* and
    Chlamydophila   2439
    WALTER E. STAMM | BYRON E. BATTEIGER

180 *Chlamydia trachomatis* (Trachoma, Perinatal
    Infections, Lymphogranuloma Venereum, and Other
    Genital Infections)   2443
    WALTER E. STAMM | BYRON E. BATTEIGER

181 *Chlamydophila (Chlamydia) psittaci*
    (Psittacosis)   2463
    DAVID SCHLOSSBERG

182 *Chlamydophila (Chlamydia) pneumoniae*   2467
    MARGARET R. HAMMERSCHLAG | STEPHAN A. KOHLHOFF |
    PETRA M. APFALTER

SECTION D
MYCOPLASMA DISEASES

183 Introduction to *Mycoplasma* and *Ureaplasma*   2477
    STEPHEN G. BAUM

184 *Mycoplasma pneumoniae* and Atypical
    Pneumonia   2481
    STEPHEN G. BAUM

185 Genital Mycoplasmas: *Mycoplasma genitalium,*
    Mycoplasma hominis, and *Ureaplasma* Species   2491
    GEORGE E. KENNY

SECTION E
RICKETTSIOSES, EHRLICHIOSES, AND ANAPLASMOSIS

186 Introduction to Rickettsioses, Ehrlichioses, and
    Anaplasmosis   2495
    DIDIER RAOULT

187 *Rickettsia rickettsii* and Other Spotted Fever Group
    Rickettsiae (Rocky Mountain Spotted Fever and
    Other Spotted Fevers)   2499
    DAVID H. WALKER

188 *Rickettsia akari* (Rickettsialpox)   2509
    DIDIER RAOULT

189 *Coxiella burnetii* (Q Fever)   2511
    THOMAS J. MARRIE | DIDIER RAOULT

190 *Rickettsia prowazekii* (Epidemic or Louse-Borne
    Typhus)   2521
    DAVID H. WALKER | DIDIER RAOULT

191 *Rickettsia typhi* (Murine Typhus)   2525
    J. STEPHEN DUMLER | DAVID H. WALKER

192 *Orientia tsutsugamushi* (Scrub Typhus)   2529
    DIDIER RAOULT

193 *Ehrlichia chaffeensis* (Human Monocytotropic
    Ehrlichiosis), *Anaplasma phagocytophilum* (Human
    Granulocytotropic Anaplasmosis), and Other
    Anaplasmataceae   2531
    J. STEPHEN DUMLER | DAVID H. WALKER

SECTION F
BACTERIAL DISEASES

194 Introduction to Bacteria and Bacterial Diseases   2539
    MARTIN J. BLASER

195 *Staphylococcus aureus* (Including Staphylococcal
    Toxic Shock)   2543
    YOK-AI QUE | PHILIPPE MOREILLON

196 *Staphylococcus epidermidis* and Other
    Coagulase-Negative Staphylococci   2579
    MARK E. RUPP | PAUL D. FEY

197 Classification of Streptococci   2591
    KATHRYN L. RUOFF | ALAN L. BISNO

198 *Streptococcus pyogenes*   2593
    ALAN L. BISNO | DENNIS L. STEVENS

199 Nonsuppurative Poststreptococcal Sequelae:
    Rheumatic Fever and Glomerulonephritis   2611
    ALAN L. BISNO

200 *Streptococcus pneumoniae*   2623
    DANIEL M. MUSHER

201 *Enterococcus* Species, *Streptococcus bovis* Group,
    and *Leuconostoc* Species   2643
    CESAR A. ARIAS | BARBARA E. MURRAY

202 *Streptococcus agalactiae* (Group B
    Streptococcus)   2655
    MORVEN S. EDWARDS | CAROL J. BAKER

203 Viridans Streptococci, Groups C and G Streptococci,
    and *Gemella* Species   2667
    SCOTT W. SINNER | ALLAN R. TUNKEL

204 *Streptococcus anginosus* Group   2681
CATHY A. PETTI | CHARLES W. STRATTON IV

205 *Corynebacterium diphtheriae*   2687
ROB ROY MacGREGOR

206 Other Coryneform Bacteria and Rhodococci   2695
DANIEL K. MEYER | ANNETTE C. REBOLI

207 *Listeria monocytogenes*   2707
BENNETT LORBER

208 *Bacillus anthracis* (Anthrax)   2715
GREGORY J. MARTIN | ARTHUR M. FRIEDLANDER

209 *Bacillus* Species and Related Genera Other than *Bacillus anthracis*   2727
THOMAS FEKETE

210 *Erysipelothrix rhusiopathiae*   2733
ANNETTE C. REBOLI

211 *Neisseria meningitidis*   2737
MICHAEL A. APICELLA

212 *Neisseria gonorrhoeae*   2753
JEANNE M. MARRAZZO | H. HUNTER HANDSFIELD | P. FREDERICK SPARLING

213 *Moraxella catarrhalis*, *Kingella*, and Other Gram-Negative Cocci   2771
TIMOTHY F. MURPHY

214 *Vibrio cholerae*   2777
CARLOS SEAS | EDUARDO GOTUZZO

215 Other Pathogenic Vibrios   2787
MARGUERITE A. NEILL | CHARLES C. J. CARPENTER

216 *Campylobacter jejuni* and Related Species   2793
BAN MISHU ALLOS | MARTIN J. BLASER

217 *Helicobacter pylori* and Other Gastric *Helicobacter* Species   2803
MARTIN J. BLASER

218 Enterobacteriaceae   2815
MICHAEL S. DONNENBERG

219 *Pseudomonas aeruginosa*   2835
GERALD B. PIER | REUBEN RAMPHAL

220 *Stenotrophomonas maltophilia* and *Burkholderia cepacia* Complex   2861
GEORG MASCHMEYER | ULF B. GÖBEL

221 *Burkholderia pseudomallei* and *Burkholderia mallei*: Melioidosis and Glanders   2869
BART J. CURRIE

222 *Acinetobacter* Species   2881
DAVID M. ALLEN | BARRY J. HARTMAN

223 *Salmonella* Species, Including *Salmonella* Typhi   2887
DAVID A. PEGUES | SAMUEL I. MILLER

224 *Shigella* Species (Bacillary Dysentery)   2905
HERBERT L. DuPONT

225 *Haemophilus* Species (Including *H. influenzae* and Chancroid)   2911
TIMOTHY F. MURPHY

226 *Brucella* Species   2921
EDWARD J. YOUNG

227 *Francisella tularensis* (Tularemia)   2927
ROBERT L. PENN

228 *Pasteurella* Species   2939
JOHN J. ZURLO

229 *Yersinia* Species, Including Plague   2943
DAVID T. DENNIS | PAUL S. MEAD

230 *Bordetella pertussis*   2955
VALERIE WATERS | SCOTT HALPERIN

231 Rat-Bite Fever: *Streptobacillus moniliformis* and *Spirillum minus*   2965
RONALD G. WASHBURN

232 *Legionella*   2969
PAUL H. EDELSTEIN | NICHOLAS P. CIANCIOTTO

233 Other *Legionella* Species   2985
ROBERT R. MUDER

234 *Capnocytophaga*   2991
J. MICHAEL JANDA | MARGOT GRAVES

235 *Bartonella*, Including Cat-Scratch Disease   2995
LEONARD N. SLATER | DAVID F. WELCH

236 *Klebsiella granulomatis* (Donovanosis, Granuloma Inguinale)   3011
RONALD C. BALLARD

237 Other Gram-Negative and Gram-Variable Bacilli   3015
JAMES P. STEINBERG | EILEEN M. BURD

238 *Treponema pallidum* (Syphilis)   3035
EDMUND C. TRAMONT

239 Endemic Treponematoses   3055
EDWARD W. HOOK III

240 *Leptospira* Species (Leptospirosis)   3059
PAUL N. LEVETT | DAVID A. HAAKE

241 *Borrelia* Species (Relapsing Fever)   3067
KYU Y. RHEE | WARREN D. JOHNSON, JR.

242 *Borrelia burgdorferi* (Lyme Disease, Lyme Borreliosis)   3071
ALLEN C. STEERE

243 Anaerobic Infections: General Concepts   3083
RONIT COHEN-PORADOSU | DENNIS L. KASPER

244 *Clostridium tetani* (Tetanus)   3091
PAVANI REDDY | THOMAS P. BLECK

245 *Clostridium botulinum* (Botulism)   3097
PAVANI REDDY | THOMAS P. BLECK

246 Gas Gangrene and Other *Clostridium*-Associated Diseases   3103
ANDREW B. ONDERDONK | WENDY S. GARRETT

247 *Bacteroides*, *Prevotella*, *Porphyromonas*, and *Fusobacterium* Species (and Other Medically Important Anaerobic Gram-Negative Bacilli)   3111
WENDY S. GARRETT | ANDREW B. ONDERDONK

248 Anaerobic Cocci   3121
SYDNEY M. FINEGOLD | YULI SONG

249 Anaerobic Gram-Positive Nonsporulating Bacilli   3125
EIJA KÖNÖNEN

250   *Mycobacterium tuberculosis*   3129
DANIEL W. FITZGERALD | TIMOTHY R. STERLING | DAVID W. HAAS

251   *Mycobacterium leprae*   3165
CYBÈLE A. RENAULT | JOEL D. ERNST

252   *Mycobacterium avium* Complex   3177
FRED M. GORDIN | C. ROBERT HORSBURGH, JR.

253   Infections Due to Nontuberculous Mycobacteria Other than *Mycobacterium avium-intracellulare*   3191
BARBARA A. BROWN-ELLIOTT | RICHARD J. WALLACE, JR.

254   *Nocardia* Species   3199
TANIA C. SORRELL | DAVID H. MITCHELL | JONATHAN R. IREDELL | SHARON C-A. CHEN

255   Agents of Actinomycosis   3209
THOMAS A. RUSSO

SECTION G
MYCOSES

256   Introduction to Mycoses   3221
JOHN E. BENNETT

257   *Candida* Species   3225
JOHN E. EDWARDS, JR.

258   *Aspergillus* Species   3241
THOMAS F. PATTERSON

259   Agents of Mucormycosis and Entomophthoramycosis   3257
DIMITRIOS P. KONTOYIANNIS | RUSSELL E. LEWIS

260   *Sporothrix schenckii*   3271
JOHN H. REX | PABLO C. OKHUYSEN

261   Agents of Chromoblastomycosis   3277
DUANE R. HOSPENTHAL

262   Agents of Mycetoma   3281
DUANE R. HOSPENTHAL

263   *Cryptococcus neoformans*   3287
JOHN R. PERFECT

264   *Histoplasma capsulatum*   3305
GEORGE S. DEEPE, JR.

265   *Blastomyces dermatitidis*   3319
STANLEY W. CHAPMAN | DONNA C. SULLIVAN

266   *Coccidioides* Species   3333
JOHN N. GALGIANI

267   Dermatophytosis and Other Superficial Mycoses   3345
RODERICK J. HAY

268   *Paracoccidioides brasiliensis*   3357
ANGELA RESTREPO | ANGELA MARÍA TOBÓN

269   Uncommon Fungi and *Prototheca*   3365
DUANE R. HOSPENTHAL

270   *Pneumocystis* Species   3377
PETER D. WALZER | A. GEORGE SMULIAN

271   Microsporidiosis   3391
LOUIS M. WEISS

SECTION H
PROTOZOAL DISEASES

272   Introduction to Protozoal Diseases   3409
JONATHAN I. RAVDIN | WILLIAM A. PETRI, JR.

273   *Entamoeba* Species, Including Amebiasis   3411
WILLIAM A. PETRI, JR. | RASHIDUL HAQUE

274   Free-Living Amebas   3427
ANITA A. KOSHY | BRIAN G. BLACKBURN | UPINDER SINGH

275   *Plasmodium* Species (Malaria)   3437
RICK M. FAIRHURST | THOMAS E. WELLEMS

276   *Leishmania* Species: Visceral (Kala-Azar), Cutaneous, and Mucosal Leishmaniasis   3463
ALAN J. MAGILL

277   *Trypanosoma* Species (American Trypanosomiasis, Chagas' Disease): Biology of Trypanosomes   3481
LOUIS V. KIRCHHOFF

278   Agents of African Trypanosomiasis (Sleeping Sickness)   3489
LOUIS V. KIRCHHOFF

279   *Toxoplasma gondii*   3495
JOSÉ G. MONTOYA | JOHN C. BOOTHROYD | JOSEPH A. KOVACS

280   *Giardia lamblia*   3527
DAVID R. HILL | THEODORE E. NASH

281   *Trichomonas vaginalis*   3535
JANE R. SCHWEBKE

282   *Babesia* Species   3539
JEFFREY A. GELFAND | EDOUARD G. VANNIER

283   *Cryptosporidium* Species   3547
A. CLINTON WHITE, JR.

284   *Cyclospora cayetanensis, Isospora belli, Sarcocystis* Species, *Balantidium coli,* and *Blastocystis hominis*   3561
KATHRYN N. SUH | PHYLLIS KOZARSKY | JAY S. KEYSTONE

SECTION I
DISEASES DUE TO TOXIC ALGAE

285   Human Illness Associated with Harmful Algal Blooms   3569
J. GLENN MORRIS, JR.

SECTION J
DISEASES DUE TO HELMINTHS

286   Introduction to Helminth Infections   3573
JAMES H. MAGUIRE

287   Intestinal Nematodes (Roundworms)   3577
JAMES H. MAGUIRE

288   Tissue Nematodes, Including Trichinellosis, Dracunculiasis, and the Filariases   3587
JAMES W. KAZURA

289   Trematodes (Schistosomes and Other Flukes)   3595
JAMES H. MAGUIRE

290 Cestodes (Tapeworms) 3607
CHARLES H. KING | JESSICA K. FAIRLEY

291 Visceral Larva Migrans and Other Unusual Helminth Infections 3617
THEODORE E. NASH

SECTION K
ECTOPARASITIC DISEASES

292 Introduction to Ectoparasitic Diseases 3625
JAMES H. DIAZ

293 Lice (Pediculosis) 3629
JAMES H. DIAZ

294 Scabies 3633
JAMES H. DIAZ

295 Myiasis and Tungiasis 3637
JAMES H. DIAZ

296 Mites, Including Chiggers 3643
JAMES H. DIAZ

297 Ticks, Including Tick Paralysis 3649
JAMES H. DIAZ

SECTION L
DISEASES OF UNKNOWN ETIOLOGY

298 Kawasaki Syndrome 3663
FRANK T. SAULSBURY

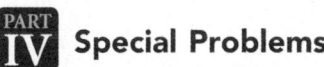

PART IV Special Problems

SECTION A
NOSOCOMIAL INFECTIONS

299 Organization for Infection Control 3669
MICHAEL B. EDMOND | RICHARD P. WENZEL

300 Isolation 3673
MICHAEL B. EDMOND | RICHARD P. WENZEL

301 Disinfection, Sterilization, and Control of Hospital Waste 3677
WILLIAM A. RUTALA | DAVID J. WEBER

302 Infections Caused by Percutaneous Intravascular Devices 3697
SUSAN E. BEEKMANN | DAVID K. HENDERSON

303 Nosocomial Pneumonia 3717
DONALD E. CRAVEN | ALEXANDRA CHRONEOU

304 Nosocomial Urinary Tract Infections 3725
THOMAS M. HOOTON

305 Nosocomial Hepatitis and Other Transfusion- and Transplantation-Transmitted Infections 3739
KENT A. SEPKOWITZ | MATTHEW J. KUEHNERT

306 Human Immunodeficiency Virus in Health Care Settings 3753
DAVID K. HENDERSON

307 Nosocomial Herpesvirus Infections 3771
TARA N. PALMORE | DAVID K. HENDERSON

SECTION B
INFECTIONS IN SPECIAL HOSTS

308 Infections in the Immunocompromised Host: General Principles 3781
J. PETER DONNELLY | NICOLE M. A. BLIJLEVENS | BEN E. DE PAUW

309 Prophylaxis and Empirical Therapy of Infection in Cancer Patients 3793
CLAUDIO VISCOLI | ELIO CASTAGNOLA

310 Risk Factors and Approaches to Infections in Transplant Recipients 3809
J. STEPHEN DUMMER | LORA D. THOMAS

311 Infections in Recipients of Hematopoietic Cell Transplantation 3821
JO-ANNE H. YOUNG | DANIEL J. WEISDORF

312 Infections in Solid Organ Transplant Recipients 3839
J. STEPHEN DUMMER | NINA SINGH

313 Infections in Patients with Spinal Cord Injury 3851
RABIH O. DAROUICHE

314 Infections in the Elderly 3857
KENT B. CROSSLEY | PHILLIP K. PETERSON

315 Infections in Asplenic Patients 3865
LARRY I. LUTWICK

316 Infections in Injection Drug Users 3875
DONALD P. LEVINE | PATRICIA D. BROWN

SECTION C
SURGICAL AND TRAUMA-RELATED INFECTIONS

317 Surgical Site Infections and Antimicrobial Prophylaxis 3891
THOMAS R. TALBOT

318 Burns 3905
CLINTON K. MURRAY

319 Bites 3911
ELLIE J. C. GOLDSTEIN

SECTION D
IMMUNIZATION

320 Immunization 3917
WALTER A. ORENSTEIN | LARRY K. PICKERING | ALISON MAWLE | ALAN R. HINMAN | MELINDA WHARTON

SECTION E
BIODEFENSE

321 Bioterrorism: An Overview 3951
LUCIANA BORIO | NOREEN A. HYNES | DONALD A. HENDERSON

322 Plague as a Bioterrorism Weapon 3965
LUCIANA BORIO | NOREEN A. HYNES

323 *Francisella tularensis* (Tularemia) as an Agent of Bioterrorism 3971
LISA S. HODGES | ROBERT L. PENN

324 Smallpox as an Agent of Bioterrorism 3977
LISA D. ROTZ | JOANNE CONO | INGER K. DAMON

325 **Anthrax as an Agent of Bioterrorism** 3983
GREGORY J. MARTIN | ARTHUR M. FRIEDLANDER

326 **Botulinum Toxin as a Biological Weapon** 3993
PAVANI REDDY | THOMAS P. BLECK

327 **Viral Hemorrhagic Fevers as Agents of Bioterrorism** 3995
C. J. PETERS

SECTION F
ZOONOSES

328 **Zoonoses** 3999
CAMILLE NELSON KOTTON | ARNOLD N. WEINBERG

SECTION G
PROTECTION OF TRAVELERS

329 **Protection of Travelers** 4009
DAVID O. FREEDMAN

330 **Infections in Returning Travelers** 4019
DAVID O. FREEDMAN

Index i

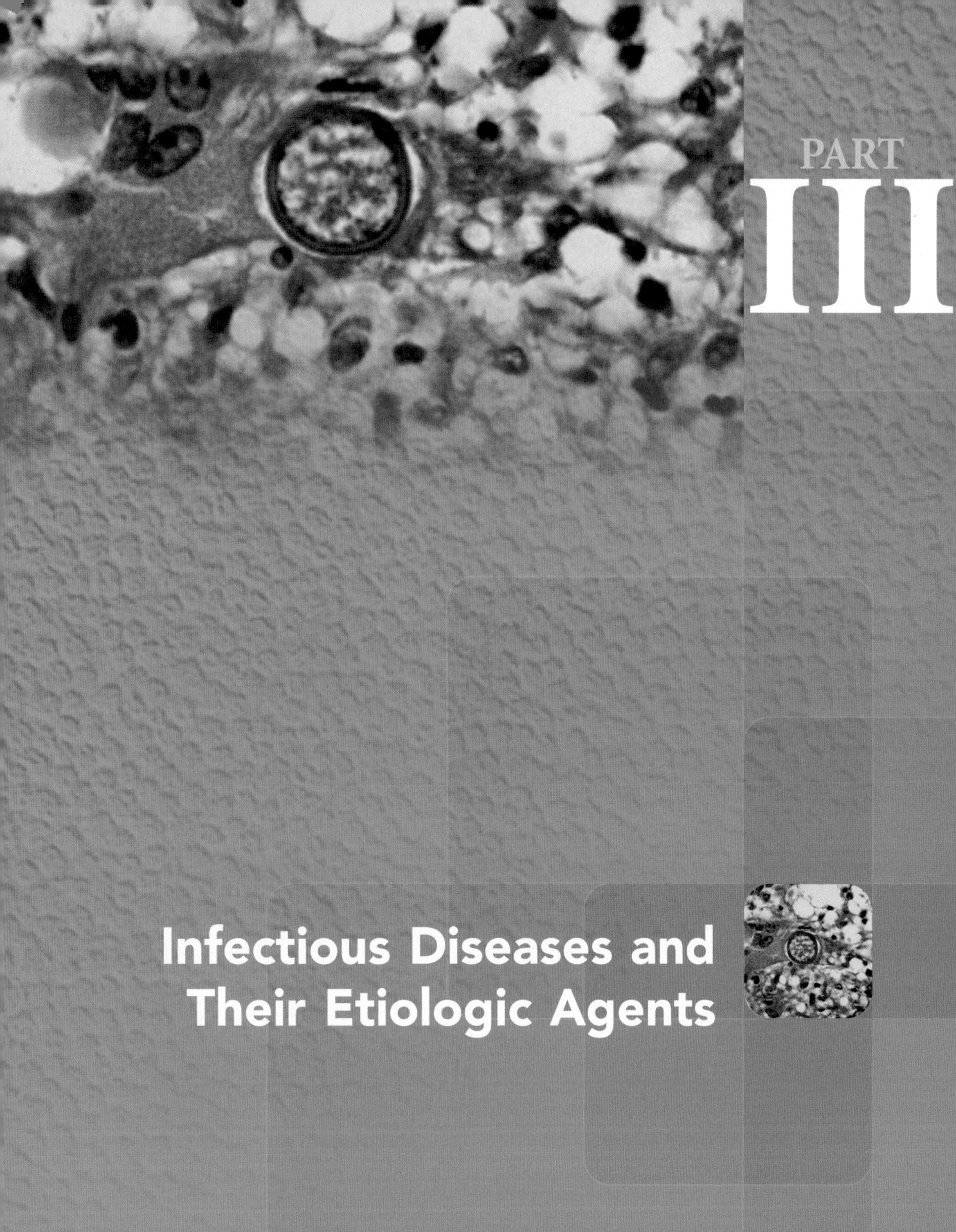

Infectious Diseases and Their Etiologic Agents

III

132

Introduction to Viruses and Viral Diseases

JAMES D. CHAPPELL | TERENCE S. DERMODY

History

Viruses exact an enormous toll on the human population and are the single most important cause of infectious disease morbidity and mortality worldwide. Viral diseases in humans were first noted in ancient times and have played a major role in social and ecologic history. Scientific approaches to the study of viruses and viral disease began in the 19th century and led to the identification of specific disease entities caused by viruses. Careful clinical observations enabled the identification of many viral illnesses and allowed several viral diseases to be differentiated (e.g., smallpox vs. chickenpox and measles vs. rubella). Progress in an understanding of disease at the level of cells and tissues, exemplified by the pioneering work of Virchow, allowed the pathology of many viral diseases to be defined. Finally, the work of Pasteur ushered in the systematic use of laboratory animals for studies of the pathogenesis of infectious diseases, including those caused by viruses.

The first viruses were identified as the 19th century ended. Ivanovsky and Beijerinck identified tobacco mosaic virus, and Loeffler and Frosch discovered foot-and-mouth disease virus. These observations were quickly followed by the discovery of yellow fever virus and the seminal research on the pathogenesis of yellow fever by Walter Reed and the U. S. Army Yellow Fever Commission.[1] By the end of the 1930s, tumor viruses, bacteriophages, influenza virus, mumps virus, and many arthropod-borne viruses had been identified. This process of discovery has continued with growing momentum to the present, with the zoonotic paramyxoviruses, Hendra and Nipah,[2,3] the skin cancer–associated Merkel cell polyomavirus,[4] and a newly identified parvovirus associated with respiratory tract disease, human bocavirus,[5] being the most recent additions to the catalogue of human disease–causing viruses.

In the 1940s, Delbruck, Luria, and others used bacteriophages as models to establish many basic principles of microbial genetics and molecular biology and identified key steps in viral replication.[6,7] The pioneering experiments of Avery and associates on the transformation of pneumococci established DNA as the genetic material[8] and set the stage for experiments by Hershey and Chase.[9] In the late 1940s, Enders and colleagues cultivated poliovirus in tissue culture.[10] This accomplishment led to the development of both formalin-inactivated (Salk)[11] and and live-attenuated (Sabin)[12] vaccines for polio and ushered in the modern era of experimental and clinical virology.

In recent years, x-ray crystallography has allowed visualization of virus structures at an atomic level of resolution. Nucleotide sequences of entire genomes of most human viruses are known, and functional domains of many viral structural and enzymatic proteins have been defined. This information is being applied to the development of new strategies to diagnose viral illnesses and design effective antiviral therapies. Techniques to detect viral genomes, such as the polymerase chain reaction (PCR) and its derivatives, have proven superior to conventional serologic assays and culture techniques for the diagnosis of many viral diseases. Nucleic acid–based strategies are now used routinely in the diagnosis of infections caused by enteroviruses, hepatitis B virus (HBV), hepatitis C virus (HCV), herpesviruses, human immunodeficiency virus (HIV) and, with increasing frequency, respiratory viral pathogens.

Perhaps an even more exciting development is the means to introduce new genetic material into viral genomes. Strategies now exist whereby specific mutations or even entire genes can be inserted into the genomes of many viruses. Such approaches can be exploited in the rational design of vaccines and the development of viral vectors for use in gene delivery. Furthermore, these powerful new techniques are leading to breakthroughs in foundational problems in viral pathogenesis, such as the nature of virus-cell interactions that produce disease, immunoprotective and immunopathologic host responses to infection, and viral and host determinants of contagion. Improved understanding of these aspects of viral infection will facilitate new approaches to the prevention, diagnosis, and treatment of viral diseases.

Virus Structure and Classification

The first classification of viruses as a group distinct from other microorganisms was based on their ability to pass through filters of a small pore size (filterable agents). Initial subclassifications were based primarily on pathologic properties such as specific organ tropism (e.g., hepatitis viruses) or common epidemiologic features such as transmission by arthropod vectors (e.g., arboviruses). Current classification systems are based on the following: (1) the type and structure of the viral nucleic acid and the strategy used in its replication; (2) the type of symmetry of the virus capsid (helical vs. icosahedral); and (3) the presence or absence of a lipid envelope (Table 132-1).

Virus particles—virions—can be schematically represented as a delivery system that surrounds a payload (Fig. 132-1). The delivery system consists of structural components used by the virus to survive in the environment and bind to host cells. The payload contains the viral genome and often includes enzymes required for the initial steps in viral replication. In almost all cases, the delivery system must be removed from the virion to allow viral replication to commence.

In addition to mediating attachment to host cells, the delivery system also plays a crucial role in determining the mode of transmission between hosts. Viruses containing lipid envelopes are sensitive to desiccation in the environment and, for the most part, are transmitted by the respiratory, parenteral, and sexual routes. Nonenveloped viruses are stable to harsh environmental conditions and often are transmitted by the fecal-oral route.

Viral genomes exist in a variety of forms and sizes and consist of RNA or DNA (see Table 132-1). Animal virus genomes range in size from 3 kb, encoding only three or four proteins in small viruses such as the hepadnaviruses, to more than 300 kb, encoding several hundred proteins in large viruses such as the poxviruses. Viral genomes are single- or double-stranded and circular or linear. RNA genomes are comprised of a single molecule of nucleic acid or multiple discrete segments, which can vary in number from as few as two in the arenaviruses up to 12 in some members of the Reoviridae. Viral nucleic acid is packaged in a protein coat, or capsid, that consists of multiple protein subunits. The combination of the viral nucleic acid and the surrounding protein capsid is referred to as the nucleocapsid (Fig. 132-2).

Structural details of many viruses have now been defined at an atomic level of resolution (Fig. 132-3). General features of virus structure can be gained from examination of electron micrographs of

TABLE 132-1	Classification of Viruses					
Family	*Example*	*Type of Nucleic Acid*	*Genome Size (kb or kb pair)*	*Envelope*	*Capsid Symmetry*	
RNA-Containing Viruses						
Picornaviridae	Poliovirus	SS (+) RNA	7-9	No	I	
Astroviridae	Astrovirus	SS (+) RNA	6-7	No	I	
Caliciviridae	Norwalk virus	SS (+) RNA	7-8	No	I	
Togaviridae	Rubella virus	SS (+) RNA	10-12	Yes	I	
Flaviviridae	Yellow fever virus	SS (+) RNA	10-12	Yes	S	
Coronaviridae	Coronavirus	SS (+) RNA	28-31	Yes	H	
Rhabdoviridae	Rabies virus	SS (−) RNA	11-15	Yes	H	
Paramyxoviridae	Measles virus	SS (−) RNA	13-18	Yes	H	
Filoviridae	Ebola virus	SS (−) RNA	19	Yes	H	
Arenaviridae	Lymphocytic choriomeningitis virus	2 SS (ambisense) RNA segments	11	Yes	S	
Bunyaviridae	California encephalitis virus	3 SS (ambisense) RNA segments	11-19	Yes	H	
Orthomyxoviridae	Influenza virus	6–8 SS (−) RNA segments*	10-15	Yes	H	
Reoviridae	Rotavirus	10-12 DS RNA segments*	19-32	No	I	
Retroviridae	HIV	2 identical SS (+) RNA segments	7-13	Yes	S	
DNA-Containing Viruses						
Hepadnaviridae	Hepatitis B virus	Circular DS DNA with SS portions	3-4	Yes	I	
Parvoviridae	Human parvovirus B-19	SS (+) or (−) DNA	4-6	No	I	
Polyomaviridae	JC virus	Circular DS DNA	5	No	I	
Papillomaviridae	Human papillomavirus	Circular DS DNA	7-8	No	I	
Adenoviridae	Adenovirus	Linear DS DNA	26-45	No	I	
Herpesviridae	Herpes simplex virus	Linear DS DNA	125-240	Yes	I	
Poxviridae	Vaccinia virus	Linear DS DNA	130-375	Yes	Complex	

*Reovirus and orbivirus: 10 segments; rotavirus: 11 segments; Colorado tick fever virus; 12 segments.
(+), message sense; (−), complement of message sense; DS, double-stranded; H, helical; I, icosahedral; S, spherical; SS, single-stranded.
Data from Condit RC. Principles of virology. In: Knipe DM, Howley PM, eds. *Fields Virology*. 5th ed. Philadelphia, Lippincott Raven Press, 2007:25-57.

negatively stained virions and thin-section electron micrographs of virus-infected tissues and cultured cells. These techniques allow rapid identification of viral size, shape, symmetry, and surface features, presence or absence of an envelope, and intracellular site of viral assembly. Cryoelectron microscopy and computer image processing techniques are used to determine the three-dimensional structures of spherical viruses at a level of resolution far superior to that of negatively stained electron micrographs. A major advantage of cryoelectron microscopy is that it allows structural studies of viruses to be performed under conditions that do not alter native virion structure. Moreover, recent advances in cryoelectron microscopy have extended the achievable resolution of particle-associated proteins to near-atomic levels, sufficient to recognize characteristic features of secondary structural elements.[13] Image reconstructions of cryoelectron micrographs, sometimes in combination with x-ray crystallography, also can be used to investigate structural aspects of various virus functions, including receptor binding[14-16] and interaction with antibodies.[17,18] Identification

of key motifs, such as receptor binding sites or immunodominant domains, provides the framework for understanding the structural basis of virus-cell interactions.

A number of general principles have emerged from studies of virus structure. In almost all cases, the capsid is composed of a repeating series of structurally similar subunits, each of which in turn is composed of only a few different proteins. The parsimonious use of structural proteins in a repetitive motif minimizes the amount of genetic information required to encode the viral capsid and leads to structural arrangements with symmetric features. All but the most complex viruses exhibit either helical or icosahedral symmetry (see Table 132-1). Viruses with helical symmetry contain repeating protein subunits bound at regular intervals along a spiral formed by the viral nucleic acid. Interestingly, all known animal viruses that show this type of symmetry have RNA genomes. Viruses with icosahedral symmetry display twofold, threefold, and fivefold axes of rotational symmetry, and viral nucleic acid is intimately associated with specific capsid proteins in an ordered packing arrangement.

The use of repeating subunits with symmetrical protein-protein interactions facilitates the assembly of the viral capsid. In most cases, viral assembly appears to be a spontaneous process that occurs under the appropriate physiologic conditions and often can be reproduced when recombinant viral proteins are expressed in the absence of viral replication.[19,20] For many viruses, assembly of the capsid proceeds through a series of intermediates, each of which nucleates the addition of subsequent components in the assembly sequence.

One of the most poorly understood aspects of viral assembly is the process that ensures that the viral nucleic acid is correctly packaged into the capsid. In the case of viruses with helical symmetry, there may be an initiation site on the nucleic acid to which the initial capsid protein subunit binds, triggering the addition of subsequent subunits. The genomes of most DNA-containing viruses are inserted into preassembled capsid intermediates (procapsids) through ATP-driven mechanisms.[21] In preparations of many icosahedral viruses, empty capsids (i.e., capsids lacking nucleic acid) are frequently observed,

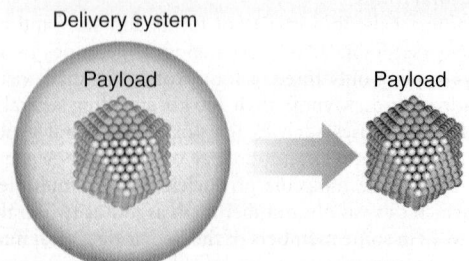

Delivery system

Payload   Payload

Figure 132-1 **Schematic diagram of a virus particle.** Viruses are simple structures consisting of a delivery system and a payload. The delivery system of a virus protects it against degradation in the environment and contains structures used to bind susceptible cells in the host. The payload of a virus contains the genome and enzymes necessary to initiate the first steps in viral replication.

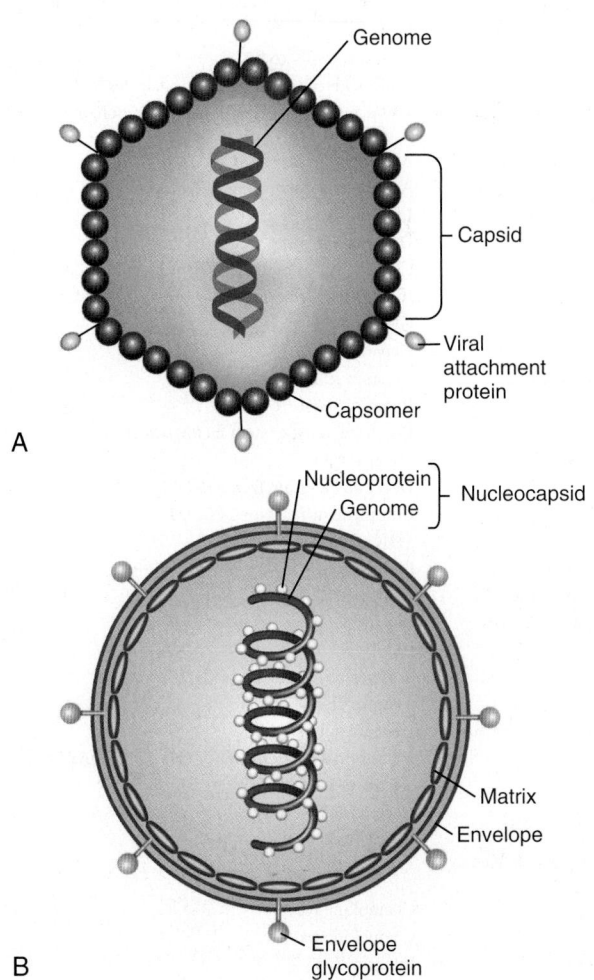

Figure 132-2 Nucleocapsid—combination of a viral nucleic acid and surrounding protein capsid. These schematic diagrams illustrate the structure of a nonenveloped icosahedral virus **(A)** and an enveloped helical virus **(B)**.

indicating that assembly may proceed to completion without a requirement for the viral genome.

In some viruses, the nucleocapsid is surrounded by a lipid envelope acquired as the virus particle buds from the host cell cytoplasmic, nuclear, or endoplasmic reticular membrane (see Fig. 132-2). Inserted into this lipid bilayer are virus-encoded proteins (e.g., the hemagglutinin [HA] and neuraminidase proteins of influenza virus and gp41 and gp120 of HIV), which are exposed on the surface of the virus particle. These viral proteins usually contain a glycosylated hydrophilic external portion and internal hydrophobic domains that span the lipid membrane and anchor the protein into the viral envelope. In some cases, another viral protein, often termed a *matrix protein*, associates with the internal (cytoplasmic) surface of the lipid envelope, where it can interact with the cytoplasmic domains of the envelope glycoproteins. Matrix proteins may play roles in stabilizing the interaction between viral glycoproteins and the lipid envelope, directing the viral genome to intracellular sites of viral assembly, or facilitating viral budding. Matrix proteins also can influence a diverse set of cellular functions, such as inhibition of host cell-transcription[22,23] and evasion of the cellular innate antiviral response.[24]

Virus-Cell Interactions

Viruses require an intact cell to replicate and can direct the synthesis of hundreds to thousands of progeny viruses during a single cycle of infection. In contrast to other microorganisms, viruses do not replicate by binary fission. Instead, the infecting particle must disassemble in order to direct synthesis of viral progeny.

ATTACHMENT

Viral replication occurs through an ordered series of steps (Table 132-2). The interaction between a virus and its host cell begins with attachment of the virus particle to specific receptors on the cell surface. Viral proteins that mediate the attachment function (viral attachment proteins) include the following: single-capsid components that extend from the virion surface, such as the attachment proteins of adenovirus,[25] reovirus,[26] and rotavirus[27,28]; surface glycoproteins of enveloped viruses, such as influenza virus[29,30] (Fig. 132-4) and HIV[31,32]; viral capsid proteins that form binding pockets that engage cellular receptors, such as the canyon formed by the capsid proteins of poliovirus[33] and rhinovirus[34]; and viral capsid proteins that contain extended loops capable of binding receptors, such as foot-and-mouth disease virus.[35] Studies of the attachment of several diverse virus groups, including adenoviruses, coronaviruses, herpesviruses, lentiviruses, and reoviruses, indicate that multiple interactions between virus and cell occur during the attachment step. These observations indicate that a specific

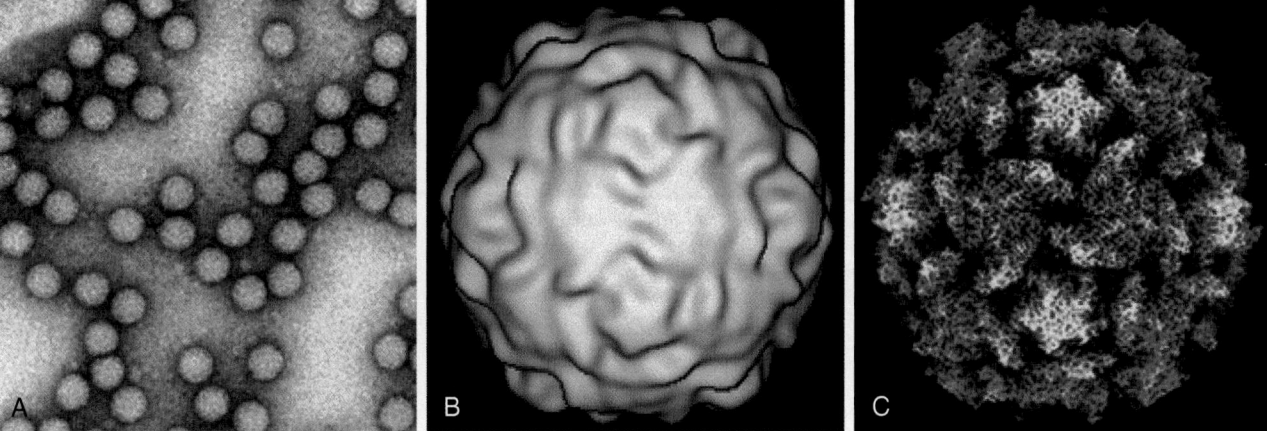

Figure 132-3   Structural studies of poliovirus. A, Negative-stained electron micrograph. **B,** Three-dimensional image reconstruction of cryoelectron micrographs. **C,** Structure determined by x-ray crystallography. *(Courtesy of Dr. James Hogle, Harvard University.)*

TABLE 132-2	Stages in Virus-Cell Interaction
1	Attachment
2	Penetration
3	Disassembly
4	Transcription
5	Translation
6	Replication
7	Assembly
8	Release

sequence of binding events between virus and cell optimizes specificity and contributes significant stability to the association.[36]

One of the most dynamic areas of virology concerns the identification of virus receptors on host cells. This interest stems in part from the critical importance of the attachment step as a determinant of target cell selection by many viruses. Several virus receptors have now been identified (Table 132-3), and three important principles have emerged from studies of these receptors. First, viruses have adapted to use cell surface molecules designed to facilitate a variety of normal cellular functions. Virus receptors may be highly specialized proteins with limited tissue distribution, such as complement receptors, growth factor receptors, or neurotransmitter receptors, or more ubiquitous components of cellular membranes, such as integrins and other intercellular adhesion molecules, glycosaminoglycans, or sialic acid–containing oligosaccharides. Second, many viruses use more than a single receptor to mediate multistep attachment and internalization. For example, adenovirus binds coxsackievirus and adenovirus receptor (CAR)[37] and the integrins αvβ3 or αvβ5[38]; herpes simplex virus (HSV) binds heparan sulfate[39-41] and herpesvirus entry mediator (HVEM/

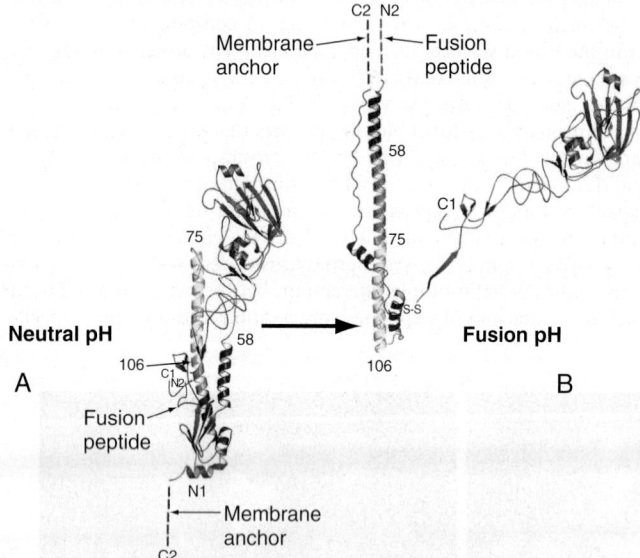

Figure 132-4 The folded structure of the influenza virus HA and its rearrangement when exposed to low pH. **A,** The HA monomer. HA1 is blue and HA2 is multicolored. The receptor-binding pocket resides in the virion-distal portion of HA1. The viral membrane would be at the bottom of this figure. **B,** Conformational change in HA induced by exposure to low pH. Note the dramatic structural rearrangement in HA2, in which amino acid residues 40-105 become a continuous alpha helix. Dashed lines indicate regions of undetermined structure. This model of HA in its fusion conformation is a composite of the HA1 domain structure and the low-pH HA2 structure. *(Adapted from Russell RJ, Kerry PS, Stevens DJ, et al. Structure of influenza hemagglutinin in complex with an inhibitor of membrane fusion. Proc Natl Acad Sci U S A. 2008;105:17736-17741, with permission.)*

TABLE 132-3	Receptors and Entry Mediators Used by Selected Human Viruses
Virus	**Receptor**
Adenovirus	Coxsackievirus and adenovirus receptor (CAR)[37,237]
	CD46[238,239]
	Integrins αvβ3, αvβ5[38]
	Sialic acid–containing oligosaccharides[240]
Coronavirus	9-O-acetylated sialic acid–containing oligosaccharides (HCoV-OC43)[241]
	Aminopeptidase N (HCoV-229E)[242,243]
	Angiotensin-converting enzyme 2 (SARS-CoV)[244]
Coxsackievirus	Integrin αvβ3[245]
	Decay accelerating factor (CD55)[246,247]
	Coxsackievirus and adenovirus receptor (CAR)[37]
	Intercellular adhesion molecule-1 (ICAM-1)[248]
	GRP78/BiP[249]
	Heparan sulfate[250]
Cytomegalovirus	Heparan sulfate[251,252]
	Integrins α2β1, α6β1, αvβ3[253]
	Platelet-derived growth factor-α receptor[254]
Echovirus	Integrin α2β1[255]
	Decay accelerating factor (CD55)[256,257]
Epstein-Barr virus	Complement receptor 2 (CD21)[258,259]
	MHC class II protein[66]
Hantaviruses	β3 Integrins[260]
Henipaviruses	Ephrin-B2[261,262]
Hepatitis A virus	Mucin-like protein TIM-1[263]
Hepatitis C virus	CD81[264,265]
	Scavenger receptor B1 (SRB1)[266,267]
	Claudin[268]
Herpes simplex virus	Heparan sulfate[39-41]
	Herpesvirus entry mediator (HVEM/HveA)[42]
	Nectin 1 (PRR1/HveC)[43]
	Nectin 2 (PRR2/HveB)[44]
Human immunodeficiency virus	CD4[45,46]
	Chemokine receptor CXCR4[47,48]
	Chemokine receptor CCR5[49-51]
Human metapneumovirus	Integrin αvβ1[269]
Human T cell leukemia virus	Glucose transporter GLUT-1[270]
Influenza virus	Sialic acid–containing oligosaccharides[30,271]
Kaposi's sarcoma herpesvirus	Integrin α3β1[272]
Lassa fever virus	α-Dystroglycan[273]
Measles virus	CD46[274,275]
	Signaling lymphocyte-activation molecule (SLAM)[276]
Parvovirus	Erythrocyte P antigen (globoside)[277]
Poliovirus	Poliovirus receptor (PVR, CD155)[163]
Polyomavirus JC	Serotonin receptor 5HT2A[278]
Rabies virus	Neural cell adhesion molecule (CD56)[279]
	Nerve growth factor receptor (p75NTR)[280]
Reovirus	Sialic acid–containing oligosaccharides[281,282]
	Junctional adhesion molecule-A (JAM-A)[53]
	β1 Integrins[283]
Rhinovirus	Intercellular adhesion molecule-1 (ICAM-1)[284-286]
	Low-density lipoprotein receptor[287]
Rotavirus	Sialic acid–containing oligosaccharides[288,289]
	Integrins α2β1, α4β1, αvβ3, αxβ2[290,291]

HveA),[42] nectin 1 (PRR1/HveC),[43] or nectin 2 (PRR2/HveB)[44]; and HIV binds CD4[45,46] and chemokine receptors CXCR4[47,48] or CCR5.[49-51] Third, in many cases, receptor expression is not the sole determinant of viral tropism for particular cells and tissues in the host. Therefore, although receptor binding is the first step in the interaction between virus and cell, subsequent events in the viral replication cycle also must be supported for productive viral infection to occur.

Several viruses bind receptors expressed at regions of cell-cell contact.[52] Junctional adhesion molecule-A (JAM-A), which serves as a receptor for reovirus[53] and feline calicivirus,[54] and CAR, which serves as a receptor for some coxsackieviruses and adenoviruses,[37] are expressed at tight junctions[55,56] and adherens junctions.[57,58] Junctional regions are sites of enhanced membrane recycling, endocytic uptake, and intracellular signaling.[59] Therefore, it is possible that viruses have selected junction-associated proteins as receptors to usurp the physiologic functions of these molecules. In this regard, interactions of coxsackievirus with decay-accelerating factor elicits a tyrosine kinase–based signaling cascade that mediates subsequent interactions of the virus with CAR in tight junctions.[60] Structures of viral proteins or whole viral particles in complex with sialic acid have been determined for some viruses, including the influenza virus HA[30,61] (see Fig. 132-4), polyomavirus,[62,63] and foot-and-mouth disease virus.[64] Sialic acid binding in each of these cases occurs in a shallow groove at the surface of the viral protein. However, the architectures of the binding sites differ. Structures of complexes of viral proteins or viral particles and cell surface protein receptors also have been determined. These include adenovirus fiber knob and CAR,[65] Epstein-Barr virus (EBV) gp42 and major histocompatibility complex (MHC) class II protein,[66] HSV glycoprotein D and HVEM/HveA,[67] HIV gp120 and CD4,[32] reovirus σ1 and JAM-A,[68] and rhinovirus and ICAM-1.[69] In several of these cases, the viral attachment proteins engage precisely the same domains used by their cognate receptors to bind natural ligands.

PENETRATION AND DISASSEMBLY

Once attachment has occurred, the virus must penetrate the cell membrane and the capsid must undergo a series of disassembly steps (uncoating) that prepare the virus for the next steps in viral replication. Enveloped viruses such as the paramyxoviruses and retroviruses enter cells by fusion of the viral envelope with the cell membrane (Fig. 132-5). Attachment of these viruses to the cell surface induces changes in viral envelope proteins required for membrane fusion. For example,

the binding of CD4 and certain chemokine receptors by HIV envelope glycoprotein gp120 induces a series of conformational changes in gp120 that lead to the exposure of transmembrane protein gp41.[70,71] Fusion of viral and cellular membranes proceeds through subsequent interactions of the hydrophobic gp41 fusion peptide with the cell membrane.[72-75]

Other viruses enter cells by receptor-mediated endocytosis (see Fig. 132-5). After receptor binding, virus-receptor complexes induce formation of clathrin-coated pits that invaginate from the cell membrane to form coated vesicles. These vesicles are rapidly uncoated and fuse with early endosomes, which sort internalized proteins for recycling to the cell surface or other cellular compartments, such as late endosomes or lysosomes.[76] Enveloped viruses such as dengue virus,[77] influenza virus,[78] and Semliki Forest virus[79] exploit the acidic environment of the endocytic compartment to induce conformational changes in surface glycoproteins required for membrane fusion. High-resolution structures at acidic pH of the influenza virus HA demonstrate the dramatic alterations in the conformation of viral attachment proteins required for membrane fusion[78] (see Fig. 132-4).

Endocytic uptake and acidification also are required for entry of some nonenveloped viruses such as adenovirus,[80,81] parvovirus,[82] and reovirus.[83,84] In these cases, acidic pH may facilitate disassembly of the viral capsid to enable subsequent penetration of endosomal membranes. In addition to acidic pH, endocytic cathepsin proteases are required for disassembly of several viruses, including Ebola virus,[85] Hendra virus,[86] reovirus,[87] and severe acute respiratory syndrome (SARS) coronavirus.[88]

In contrast to enveloped viruses, nonenveloped viruses cross cell membranes using mechanisms that do not involve membrane fusion. This group of viruses includes several human pathogens, with adenoviruses, picornaviruses, and rotaviruses serving as prominent examples. Despite differences in genome and capsid composition, each of these viruses must penetrate cell membranes to deliver the genetic payload to the interior of the cell. Capsid rearrangements triggered by receptor binding,[89,90] acidic pH,[80,81] or proteolysis[91,92] serve essential functions in membrane penetration by some nonenveloped viruses. Although a precise understanding of the biochemical mechanisms that underlie viral membrane penetration is generally lacking, small-capsid proteins of several nonenveloped viruses, such as adenovirus,[93] poliovirus,[94] and reovirus,[95] are required for membrane penetration, perhaps by forming pores in host cell membranes.

GENOME REPLICATION

Once a virus has entered a target cell, it must replicate its genome and proteins. Replication strategies used by single-stranded RNA-containing viruses depend on whether the genome can be used as mRNA. Translation-competent genomes, which include those of the coronaviruses, flaviviruses, picornaviruses, and togaviruses, are termed *plus* (+) *sense* and are translated by cellular ribosomes immediately following entry of the genome into the cytoplasm. For most viruses containing (+) sense RNA genomes, translation results in the synthesis of a large polyprotein that is cleaved into several smaller proteins through the action of viral proteases. One of these proteins is an RNA-dependent RNA polymerase (RdRp), which replicates the viral RNA. Genome replication of (+) sense RNA-containing viruses requires synthesis of a minus (−) sense RNA intermediate, which serves as template for production of (+) sense genomic RNA.

A different strategy is used by viruses containing (−) sense RNA genomes. The genomes of these viruses, which include the filoviruses, orthomyxoviruses, paramyxoviruses, and rhabdoviruses, cannot serve directly as mRNA. Therefore, viral particles must contain a previously generated RdRp to transcribe (+) sense mRNAs using the (−) sense genomic RNA as template. Genome replication of (−) sense RNA-containing viruses requires synthesis of a (+) sense RNA intermediate, which serves as template for production of (−) sense genomic RNA. Mechanisms that determine whether (+) sense RNAs are used as templates for translation or genome replication are not well understood.

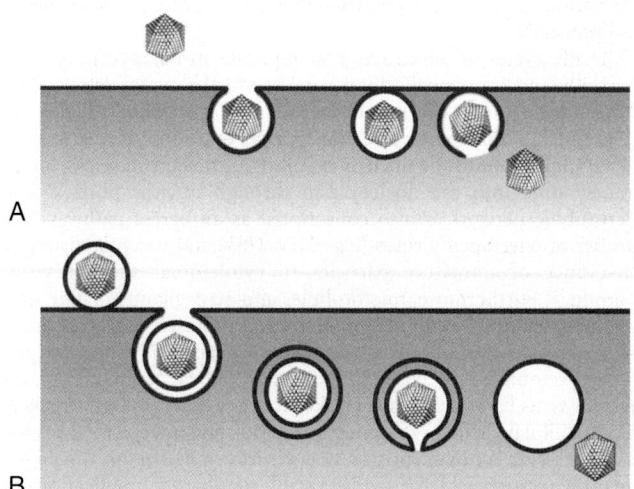

Figure 132-5 **Mechanisms of viral entry into cells. A,** Viral penetration at the cell surface. **B,** Viral internalization by receptor-mediated endocytosis.

RNA-containing viruses belonging to the family Reoviridae have segmented double-stranded (ds) RNA genomes. The innermost protein shell of these viruses (termed a *single-shelled particle* or *core*) contains an RdRp that catalyzes the synthesis of (+) sense mRNA using as a template the (−) sense strand of each dsRNA segment. The mRNAs of these viruses are capped at their 5′-termini by virus-encoded enzymes and then extruded into the cytoplasm through channels in the single-shelled particle.[96] The (+) sense mRNAs also serve as a template for replication of dsRNA gene segments. Viral genome replication is thus completely conservative; neither strand of parental dsRNA is present in newly formed genomic segments.

The retroviruses are RNA-containing viruses that replicate using a DNA intermediate. The viral genomic RNA is (+) sense and single-stranded; however, it does not serve as mRNA following viral entry. Instead, the retrovirus RNA genome is a template for synthesis of a double-stranded DNA copy, termed the *provirus*. Synthesis of the provirus is mediated by a virus-encoded RNA-dependent DNA polymerase or reverse transcriptase, so-named because of the reversal of genetic information from RNA to DNA. The provirus translocates to the nucleus and integrates into host DNA. Expression of this integrated DNA is regulated for the most part by cellular transcriptional machinery. However, the human retroviruses HIV and human T-cell leukemia virus (HTLV) encode proteins that augment transcription of viral genes. Intracellular signaling pathways are capable of activating retroviral gene expression and play important roles in inducing high levels of viral replication in response to certain stimuli.[97] Transcription of the provirus yields mRNAs that encode viral proteins and genome-length RNAs that are packaged into progeny virions. Such a replication strategy results in persistent infection in the host because the viral genome is maintained in the host cell genome and replicated with each cell division.

With the exception of the poxviruses, viruses containing DNA genomes replicate in the nucleus and for the most part use cellular enzymes for transcription and replication of their genomes. Transcription of most DNA-containing viruses is tightly regulated and results in the synthesis of early and late mRNA transcripts. The early transcripts encode regulatory proteins and proteins required for DNA replication, whereas the late transcripts encode structural proteins. Several DNA-containing viruses, such as adenovirus and human papillomavirus (HPV), induce cells to express host proteins required for viral DNA replication by stimulating cell-cycle progression. For example, the HPV E7 protein binds the retinoblastoma gene product pRB and liberates transcription factor E2F, which induces the cell cycle.[98,99] To prevent programmed cell death in response to E7-mediated unscheduled cell cycle progression, the HPV E6 protein mediates the ubiquitination and degradation of tumor suppressor protein p53.[100-102] Some DNA-containing viruses, such as the herpesviruses, can establish latent infections in the host. Unlike the retroviruses, genomes of the herpesviruses do not integrate into host chromosomes but instead exist as plasmid-like episomes. Mechanisms that govern establishment of latency and subsequent reactivation of replication are not well understood. However, microRNAs encoded by cytomegalovirus (CMV) may promote persistence by targeting viral and cellular mRNAs that control viral gene expression and replication and innate immune responses to viral infection.[103,104]

A fascinating aspect of virus-cell interactions is the replication microenvironments established in infected cells. Viral replication is a sophisticated interplay of transcription, translation, nucleic acid amplification, and particle assembly. Furthermore, infection must proceed under sensitive pathogen surveillance systems trained on virus-associated molecular patterns (e.g., unmethylated CpG dinucleotides in DNA viral genomes) and replicative intermediates (e.g., dsRNA generated during RNA virus replication) that may impose impassable blocks to infection.[105] Partitioning of the viral replication machinery from the surrounding intracellular milieu satisfies a logistic requirement to concentrate viral proteins and nucleic acid for efficient genome amplification and encapsidation while simultaneously shielding viral products from cellular sensors that provoke antiviral innate immune responses. Hence, as a rule, viral replication is a localized process, occurring within morphologically discrete cytoplasmic or nuclear structures variously termed *viral inclusions* (or *inclusion bodies*), *virosomes*, *viral factories*, or *viroplasm*. These entities are novel, metabolically active organelles formed by contributions from both virus and cell. Many highly recognizable features of viral cytopathic effect observed using light microscopy, such as dense nuclear inclusions or refractile cytoplasmic densities, represent locally concentrated regions of viral nucleic acid and protein.

Membrane-associated replicase complexes appropriated by (+) sense RNA viruses are perhaps the most conspicuous examples of compartmentalized viral replication. In cells infected by these viruses, intracellular membranes originating from the endoplasmic reticulum (ER; e.g., picornaviruses[106,107]), ER-Golgi intermediate compartment and *trans*-Golgi network (e.g., flaviviruses[108]), endolysosomal vesicles (e.g., alphaviruses[109]), and autophagic vacuoles (e.g., poliovirus[110]) are reduplicated and reorganized by viral proteins into platforms that anchor viral replication complexes consisting of the RdRp and other RNA-modifying enzymes necessary for RNA synthesis. Curiously, dsRNA viruses generate nonmembranous intracytoplasmic replication factories, even though their life cycles pass through a (+) polarity RNA intermediate. However, in an interesting functional parallel with (+) sense RNA viruses, the assembly pathway of rotavirus, a dsRNA virus, involves budding of immature particles into the ER, where a lipid envelope is transiently acquired and subsequently replaced by the outermost protein shell.[111] Perhaps additional roles for cellular membranes in nonmembrane-bound viral replication complexes await discovery.

The tight relationship of RNA virus replication to cellular membranes is less predictable for DNA viruses. For example, in distinction to the supporting role of autophagy in the replication of some RNA viruses, autophagosomes (stress-induced, double-membraned vesicles that remove noxious cytoplasmic materials to lysosomes for degradation) defend against infection by HSV-1, which encodes a protein that inhibits induction of autophagy and accentuates viral virulence.[112,113] The replication and assembly complexes of many DNA viruses, including adenoviruses, herpesviruses, papillomaviruses, polyomaviruses, and parvoviruses, are associated with promyelocytic leukemia (PML) nuclear bodies,[114,115] which have been ascribed functions in diverse nuclear processes encompassing gene regulation, tumor suppression, apoptosis, and removal of aggregated or foreign proteins.[116] It appears that DNA viruses exploit PML bodies in a variety of ways, which include consolidation and disposal of misfolded viral proteins, sequestration of host-cell stress response factors that block infection, and segregation of interfering cellular DNA repair proteins from sites of viral replication.[117]

The life cycles of all viruses that replicate in eukaryotic cells are physically and functionally intertwined with the cytoskeleton. Many viruses with nuclear replication programs, such as adenovirus, HSV, and influenza virus, are transported by motor proteins along microtubules toward the nucleus, resulting ultimately in release of the viral genome into the nucleoplasm through nuclear pores.[118] The microtubule network is also conscripted as an egress pathway by a number of enveloped viruses (e.g., HIV, HSV, and vaccinia virus) for conveyance of immature particles to cytolemmal sites of virion budding.[119] Furthermore, microtubules and actin filaments may serve as anchorage points for nucleoprotein complexes that coordinate genome expression or replication with cytoplasmic replication programs, exemplified by parainfluenza virus (PIV),[120] reovirus,[121] and vaccinia virus.[122] Because the cytoskeleton is a decentralized organelle linking cellular structural elements to the metabolic and transport machineries, it is not surprising that viruses capitalize on this highly integrative system, which provides a stable platform for replication and enables purposeful movement of virions or subviral components within cells to facilitate the requisite partitioning of viral assembly and disassembly.

CELL KILLING

Viral infection can compromise numerous cellular processes, such as nucleic acid and protein synthesis, maintenance of cytoskeletal architecture, and preservation of membrane integrity.[123] Many viruses also are capable of inducing the genetically programmed mechanism of cell death that leads to apoptosis of host cells.[124,125] Apoptotic cell death is characterized by cell shrinkage, membrane blebbing, condensation of nuclear chromatin, and activation of an endogenous endonuclease, which results in cleavage of cellular DNA into oligonucleosome-length DNA fragments.[126] These changes occur according to predetermined developmental programs or in response to certain environmental stimuli. In some cases, apoptosis may serve as an antiviral defense mechanism to limit viral replication by destruction of virus-infected cells or reduction of potentially harmful inflammatory responses elicited by viral infection.[127] In other cases, apoptosis may result from viral induction of cellular factors required for efficient viral replication.[124,125] Generally, RNA-containing viruses, including influenza virus, measles virus, poliovirus, reovirus, and Sindbis virus, induce apoptosis of host cells, whereas DNA-containing viruses, including adenovirus, CMV, EBV, HPV, and the poxviruses, encode proteins that block apoptosis. For some viruses, the duration of the viral infectious cycle may determine whether apoptosis is induced or inhibited. Viruses capable of completing an infectious cycle before induction of apoptosis would not require a means to inhibit this cellular response to viral infection. Interestingly, several viruses that cause encephalitis are capable of inducing apoptosis of infected neurons[128-130] (Fig. 132-6).

ANTIVIRAL DRUGS

Knowledge of viral replication strategies has provided insights into critical steps in the viral life cycle that can serve as potential targets for antiviral therapy. For example, drugs can be designed to interfere with virus binding to target cells or prevent penetration and disassembly once receptor engagement has occurred. Steps involved in the replication of the viral genome are also obvious targets for antiviral therapy. A number of antiviral agents inhibit viral polymerases, including those active against herpesviruses (e.g., acyclovir), HIV (e.g., zidovudine), and HBV (e.g., entecavir). Drugs that inhibit viral proteases have been developed, and several are now used to treat HIV infection. These drugs block the processing of the Gag and Gag-Pol polyproteins and serve as potent inhibitors of HIV replication.[131] Other viral enzymes also serve as targets for antiviral therapy. The influenza virus neuraminidase is required for the release of progeny influenza virus particles from infected cells. Oseltamivir and zanamivir bind the neuraminidase catalytic site and are potent inhibitors of the enzyme.[132] These drugs have been used in the prophylaxis and treatment of influenza virus infection.[133]

Better understanding of viral replication strategies and mechanisms of virus-induced cell killing is paving the way for the rational design of novel antiviral therapeutics. One of the most exciting approaches to the development of antiviral agents is the use of high-resolution x-ray crystallography to optimize interactions between these inhibitory molecules and their target viral proteins. Such structure-based drug design has led to the development of synthetic peptides (e.g., enfuvirtide) that inhibit HIV entry by blocking gp41-mediated membrane fusion.[134] Other vulnerable steps in HIV replication are targets of new drugs currently in clinical trials or recently approved for patient treatment. These include entry inhibitors that interfere with gp120 binding to CCR5,[135] agents that prevent proviral integration into cellular DNA through inhibition of viral integrase activity,[136] and "maturase" inhibitors that block the final events of viral capsid proteolytic processing required for HIV infectivity.[137] Several inhibitors of the HCV protease and polymerase also are in clinical development.[138]

Despite promising advances in rational antiviral drug design, current therapeutic approaches to some viral infections rely heavily on compounds with less specific mechanisms of action. One such agent, interferon (IFN)-α, efficiently inhibits a broad spectrum of viruses and

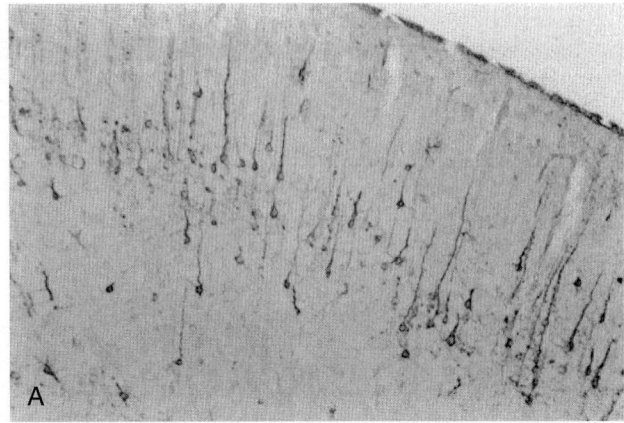
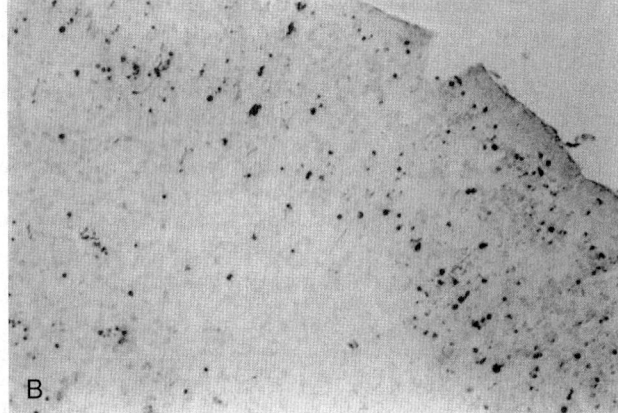

Figure 132-6 Reovirus-induced apoptosis in the murine central nervous system. Cells staining positive for (**A**) reovirus antigen and (**B**) fragmented DNA using terminal deoxy-UTP nick-end labeling (TUNEL) in consecutive sections of cerebral cortex obtained from a newborn mouse 6 days following intracranial inoculation with reovirus strain type 3 Dearing. Reovirus antigen–positive cells contain a dark precipitate in the cytoplasm, including neuronal processes. TUNEL-positive cells contain a dark precipitate in the nucleus (original magnification, ×25). *(Adapted from Oberhaus SM, Smith RL, Clayton GH, et al. Reovirus infection and tissue injury in the mouse central nervous system are associated with apoptosis. J Virol. 1997;71:2100-2106, with permission.)*

is secreted by diverse cell types as part of the host innate immune response. Recombinant IFN-α is presently used to treat HBV and HCV infections. Ribavirin, a synthetic guanosine analogue, inhibits the replication of many RNA- and DNA-containing viruses through complex mechanisms involving inhibition of viral RNA synthesis and disturbances in intracellular pools of GTP.[139,140] This drug is routinely used in combination with IFN-α to treat HCV infection and is sometimes administered in aerosolized form to treat respiratory syncytial virus (RSV) lower respiratory tract infection in severely ill and immunocompromised patients. Ribavirin therapy reduces the mortality associated with certain viral hemorrhagic fevers, such as that caused by Lassa virus.[141] Broader spectrum therapies exemplified by IFN-α and ribavirin remain part of the first-line defense against emerging pathogens and other susceptible viruses for which biochemical and structural information is insufficient to design high-potency agent-specific drugs.

Virus-Host Interaction

One of the most formidable challenges in virology is to apply knowledge gained from studies of virus-cell interactions in tissue culture systems to an understanding of how viruses interact with living hosts to produce disease. Virus-host interactions are often described in

TABLE 132-4	Stages in Virus-Host Interaction
1	Entry into the host
2	Primary replication
3	Spread
4	Cell and tissue tropism
5	Secondary replication
6	Cell injury or persistence
7	Host immune response

terms of pathogenesis and virulence. Pathogenesis is the process whereby a virus interacts with its host in a discrete series of stages to produce disease (Table 132-4). Virulence is the ability of a virus to produce disease in a susceptible host. Virulence is often measured in terms of the quantity of virus required to produce illness or death in 50% of a cohort of experimental animals infected with the virus. Virulence is dependent on viral and host factors and must be measured using carefully defined conditions (e.g., virus strain, dose, and route of inoculation, and host species, age, and immune status). In many cases, it has been possible to identify roles played by individual viral and host proteins at specific stages in viral pathogenesis and to define the importance of these proteins in viral virulence.

ENTRY

The first step in the process of virus-host interaction is the exposure of a susceptible host to viable virus under conditions that promote infection (Fig. 132-7). Infectious virus may be present in respiratory droplets or aerosols, in fecally contaminated food or water, or in a body fluid or tissue (e.g., blood, saliva, urine, semen, or a transplanted organ) to which the susceptible host is exposed. In some cases, the virus is inoculated directly into the host through the bite of an animal vector or through the use of a contaminated needle.

Infection also can be transmitted from mother to infant through virus that has infected the placenta or birth canal or by virus in breast milk. In some cases, acute viral infections result from the reactivation of endogenous latent virus (e.g., reactivation of HSV giving rise to herpes labialis) rather than de novo exposure to exogenous virus.

Exposure of respiratory mucosa to virus by direct inoculation or inhalation is an important route of viral entry into the host. A simple cough can generate up to 10,000 small, potentially infectious aerosol particles, and a sneeze can produce nearly 2 million. The distribution of these particles depends on a variety of environmental factors, the most important of which are temperature, humidity, and air currents. In addition to these factors, particle size is an important determinant of particle distribution. In general, smaller particles remain airborne longer than larger ones. Particle size also contributes to particle fate after inhalation. Larger particles (>6 μm) are generally trapped in the nasal turbinates, whereas smaller particles may ultimately travel to the alveolar spaces of the lower respiratory tract.

Fecal-oral spread represents an additional important route of viral entry into the host. Food, water, or hands contaminated by infected fecal material can facilitate the entry of a virus via the mouth into the gastrointestinal tract, the environment of which requires viruses that infect by this route to have certain physical properties. Viruses capable of enteric transmission must be acid-stable and resistant to bile salts. Because conditions in the stomach and intestine are destructive to lipids contained in viral envelopes, most viruses that spread by the fecal-oral route are nonenveloped. Interestingly, many viruses that enter the host via the gastrointestinal tract require proteolysis of certain capsid components to infect intestinal cells productively. Treatment of mice with inhibitors of intestinal proteases blocks infection by reovirus[142] and rotavirus,[143] which demonstrates the critical importance of proteolysis in the initiation of enteric infection by these viruses.

To produce systemic disease, a virus must cross the mucosal barrier that separates the luminal compartments of the respiratory, gastrointestinal, and genitourinary tracts from the host's parenchymal tissues. Studies with reovirus illustrate one strategy used by viruses to cross mucosal surfaces to invade the host after entry into the gastrointestinal tract.[144,145] After oral inoculation of mice, reovirus adheres to the surface of intestinal microfold cells (M cells) that overlie collections of intestinal lymphoid tissue (Peyer's patches). In electron micrographs, reovirus virions can be followed sequentially as they are transported within vesicles from the luminal to the subluminal surface of M cells. Virions subsequently appear within Peyer's patches and then spread to regional lymph nodes and extraintestinal lymphoid organs such as the spleen. A similar pathway of spread has been described for poliovirus[146] and HIV,[147] suggesting that M cells represent an important portal for viral invasion of the host after entry into the gastrointestinal tract.

SPREAD

Once a virus has entered the host, it can replicate locally or spread from the site of entry to distant organs to produce systemic disease

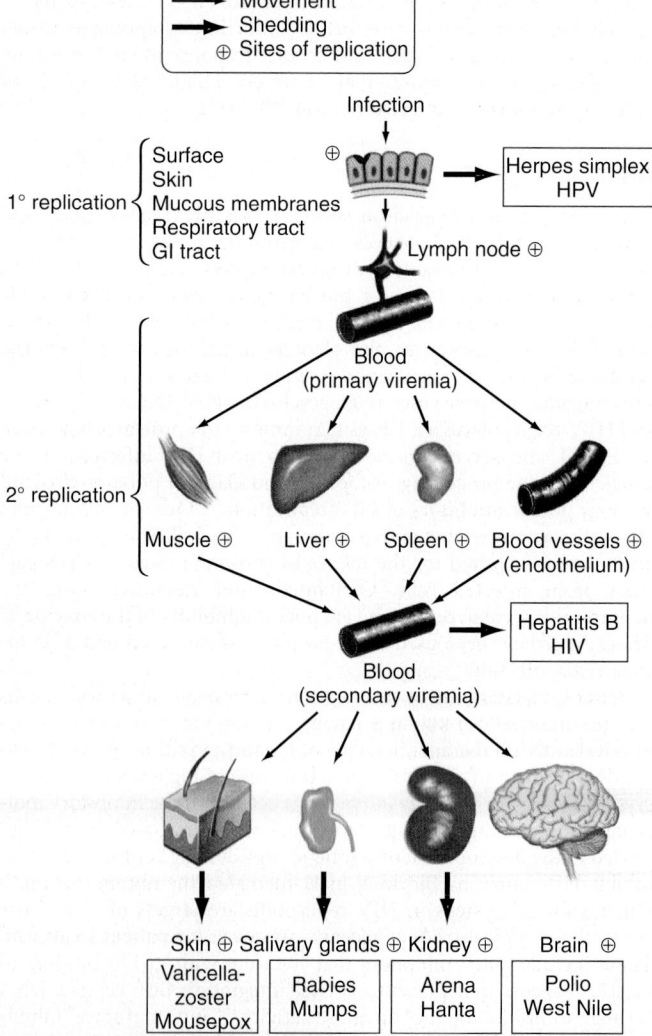

Figure 132-7   Entry and spread of viruses in human hosts. Some major steps in the viral spread and invasion of target organs are shown. Neural spread is not illustrated. GI, gastrointestinal; HIV, human immunodeficiency virus; HPV, human papillomavirus. (*Adapted from Nathanson N, Tyler KL. Entry, dissemination, shedding, and transmission of viruses. In: Nathanson N, eds.* Viral Pathogenesis. *Philadelphia: Lippincott-Raven; 1997:13-33, with permission.*)

(see Fig. 132-7). Examples of localized infections in which viral entry and replication occur at the same anatomic site include respiratory infections caused by influenza virus, RSV, and rhinovirus; enteric infections produced by astrovirus, calicivirus, and rotavirus; and dermatologic infections caused by HPV (warts) and paravaccinia virus (milker's nodules). Other viruses spread to distant sites in the host after primary replication at sites of entry. For example, poliovirus spreads from the gastrointestinal tract to the central nervous system (CNS) to produce meningitis, encephalitis, or poliomyelitis. Measles virus and varicella-zoster virus (VZV) enter the host through the respiratory tract and then spread to lymph nodes, skin, and viscera.

Release of some viruses occurs preferentially from the apical or basolateral surface of polarized cells, such as epithelial cells. In the case of enveloped viruses, polarized release is frequently determined by preferential sorting of envelope glycoproteins to sites of viral budding. Specific amino acid sequences in these viral proteins direct their transport to a particular aspect of the cell surface.[148,149] Polarized release of virus at apical surfaces may facilitate local spread of infection, whereas release at basolateral surfaces may facilitate systemic invasion by providing virus access to subepithelial lymphoid, neural, or vascular tissues.

Many viruses use the bloodstream to spread in the host from sites of primary replication to distant target tissues (see Fig. 132-7). In some cases, viruses may enter the bloodstream directly, such as during a blood transfusion or via an arthropod bite. More commonly, viruses enter the bloodstream after replication at some primary site. Important sites of primary replication preceding hematogenous spread of viruses include Peyer's patches and mesenteric lymph nodes for enteric viruses, bronchoalveolar cells for respiratory viruses, and subcutaneous tissue and skeletal muscle for alphaviruses and flaviviruses. In the case of reovirus, infection of endothelial cells leads to hematogenous dissemination in the host.[150]

Classic studies by Fenner with mousepox (ectromelia) virus have suggested that an initial low-titer viremia (primary viremia) serves to seed virus to a variety of intermediate organs, where a period of further replication leads to a high-titer viremia (secondary viremia) that disseminates virus to the ultimate target organs[151] (Fig. 132-8). It is often difficult to identify primary and secondary viremias in naturally occurring viral infections. However, replication of many viruses in reticuloendothelial organs (e.g., liver, spleen, lymph nodes, bone marrow), muscle, fat, and even vascular endothelial cells can play an important role in maintaining viremia.

Viruses that reach the bloodstream may travel free in plasma (e.g., enteroviruses and togaviruses) or in association with specific blood cells.[152] A number of viruses are spread hematogenously by macrophages (e.g., CMV, HIV, measles virus) or lymphocytes (e.g., CMV, EBV, HIV, HTLV, measles virus). Although many viruses have the ability to agglutinate erythrocytes in vitro (a process called hemagglutination), only in exceptional cases (e.g., Colorado tick fever virus) have erythrocytes been shown to transport virus in the bloodstream.

The maintenance of viremia depends on the interplay among factors that promote virus production and those that favor viral clearance. A number of variables have been identified that can affect the efficiency of virus removal from plasma. In general, the larger the viral particle, the more efficiently it is cleared. Viruses that induce high titers of neutralizing antibodies are more efficiently cleared than those that do not induce humoral immune responses. Finally, phagocytosis of virus by cells in the host reticuloendothelial system can contribute to viral clearance.

A major pathway used by viruses to spread from sites of primary replication to the nervous system is through nerves. Numerous diverse viruses, including Borna disease virus, coronavirus, HSV, poliovirus, rabies virus, reovirus, and Venezuelan equine encephalitis virus (VEE), are capable of neural spread. Several of these viruses accumulate at the neuromuscular junction after primary replication in skeletal muscle.[153,154] HSV appears to enter nerve cells via receptors that are located primarily at synaptic endings rather than on the nerve cell body.[155] Spread to the CNS of both rabies virus[153,154] and HSV[156] can

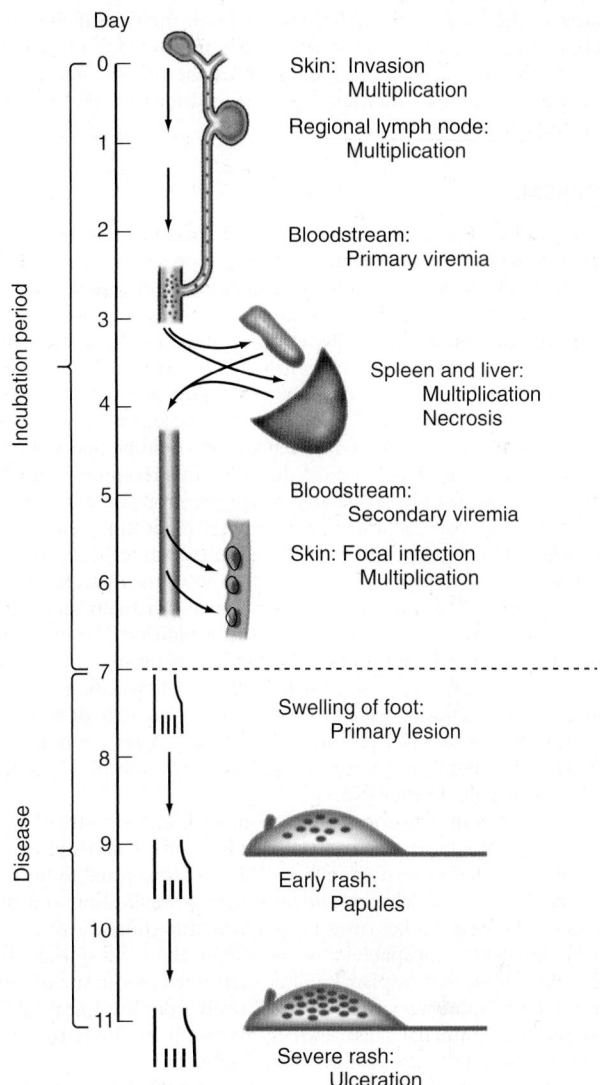

Day

Incubation period

Skin: Invasion
Multiplication

Regional lymph node:
Multiplication

Bloodstream:
Primary viremia

Spleen and liver:
Multiplication
Necrosis

Bloodstream:
Secondary viremia

Skin: Focal infection
Multiplication

Disease

Swelling of foot:
Primary lesion

Early rash:
Papules

Severe rash:
Ulceration

Figure 132-8 **Pathogenesis of mousepox virus infection.** Successive waves of viremia are shown to seed the spleen and liver and then the skin. *(From Fenner F. Mousepox [infectious ectromelia of mice]: a review. J Immunol. 1949;63:341-373, with permission.)*

be interrupted by scission of the appropriate nerves or by chemical agents that inhibit axonal transport. Neural spread of some of these viruses occurs by the microtubule-based system of fast axonal transport.[157]

Viruses are not limited to a single route of spread. VZV, for example, enters the host by the respiratory route and then spreads from respiratory epithelium to the reticuloendothelial system and skin via the bloodstream. Infection of the skin produces the characteristic exanthem of chickenpox. The virus subsequently enters distal terminals of sensory neurons and travels to dorsal root ganglia, where it establishes latent infection. Reactivation of VZV from latency results in transport of the virus in sensory nerves to skin, where it gives rise to vesicular lesions in a dermatomal distribution characteristic of zoster or shingles.

Poliovirus also is capable of spreading by hematogenous and neural routes. Poliovirus is generally thought to spread from the gastrointestinal tract to the CNS via the bloodstream, although it has been suggested that the virus may spread via autonomic nerves in the intestine to the brain stem and spinal cord.[158,159] This hypothesis is supported by experiments using transgenic mice expressing the human poliovirus receptor.[160] When these mice are inoculated with poliovirus intramuscularly in the hind limb, virus does not reach the CNS if the sciatic nerve ipsilateral to the site of inoculation is transected.[161] Once poliovirus reaches the CNS, axonal transport is the major route of viral dissemination. Similar mechanisms of spread may be used by other enteroviruses.

TROPISM

The capability of a virus to infect a distinct group of cells in the host is referred to as *tropism*. For many viruses, tropism is determined by the availability of virus receptors on the surface of a host cell. This concept was first appreciated in studies of poliovirus when it was recognized that the ability of the virus to infect specific tissues paralleled its capacity to bind homogenates of the susceptible tissues in vitro.[162] The importance of receptor expression as a determinant of poliovirus tropism was conclusively demonstrated by showing that cells not permissive for poliovirus replication could be made permissive by recombinant expression of the poliovirus receptor.[163] In addition to the availability of virus receptors, tropism also can be determined by postattachment steps in viral replication, such as the regulation of viral gene expression. For example, some viruses contain genetic elements, termed *enhancers*, that act to stimulate transcription of viral genes.[164,165] Some enhancers are active in virtually all types of cells, whereas others show exquisite tissue specificity. The promoter-enhancer region of JC polyomavirus is active in cultured human glial cells but not in HeLa cervical epithelial cells.[166] Cell-specific expression of the JC virus genome correlates well with the capacity of this virus in immunocompromised persons to produce progressive multifocal leukoencephalopathy, a disease in which JC virus infection is limited to oligodendroglia in the CNS.

Specific steps in virus-host interaction, such as the route of entry and pathway of spread, also can strongly influence viral tropism. For example, encephalitis viruses such as VEE are transmitted to humans by insect bites. These viruses undergo primary replication and then spread to the CNS by hematogenous and neural routes.[167] After oral inoculation, VEE is incapable of primary replication and spread to the CNS, illustrating that tropism can be determined by the site of entry into the host. Influenza virus buds exclusively from the apical surface of respiratory epithelial cells,[168] which may limit its ability to spread within the host and infect cells at distant sites.

A wide variety of host factors can influence viral tropism. These include age, nutritional status, and immune responsiveness as well as certain genetic polymorphisms that affect susceptibility to viral infection. Age-related susceptibility to infection is observed for many viruses, including reovirus,[169,170] RSV,[171-173] and rotavirus.[174,175] The increased susceptibility in young children to these viruses may in part be due to immaturity of the immune response but also may be related to intrinsic age-specific factors that enhance host susceptibility to infection. Nutritional status is a critical determinant of the tropism and virulence of many viruses. For example, persons with vitamin A deficiency have enhanced susceptibility to measles virus infection.[176,177] Similarly, the outcome of most viral infections is strongly linked to the immune competence of the host.

The genetic basis of host susceptibility to viral infections is complex. Studies with inbred strains of mice indicate that genetic variation can alter susceptibility to viral disease by a variety of mechanisms.[178] These can involve differences in immune responses, variability in the ability to induce antiviral mediators such as interferon, and differential expression of functional virus receptors. Polymorphisms in the expression of chemokine receptor CCR5, which serves as a coreceptor for HIV,[49-51] are associated with alterations in susceptibility to HIV infection in humans.[179,180]

PERSISTENT INFECTIONS

Many viruses are capable of establishing persistent infections, of which two types are recognized: chronic and latent. *Chronic viral infections*

are characterized by continuous shedding of virus for prolonged periods of time. Congenital infections with rubella virus and CMV and persistent infections with HBV and HCV are examples of chronic viral infections. *Latent viral infections* are characterized by maintenance of the viral genome in host cells in the absence of viral replication. Herpesviruses and retroviruses can establish latent infections. The distinction between chronic and latent infections is not readily apparent for some viruses, such as HIV, which can establish both chronic and latent infections in the host.[181-183] Viruses capable of establishing persistent infections must have a means of evading the host immune response and a mechanism of attenuating their virulence. Lentiviruses such as equine infectious anemia virus[184] and HIV[185-187] are capable of extensive antigenic variation resulting in escape from neutralizing antibody responses of the host. Several viruses encode proteins that directly attenuate the host immune response; for example, the adenovirus E3/19K protein and CMV US11 gene product block cell-surface expression of MHC class I proteins, resulting in diminished presentation of viral antigens to cytotoxic T lymphocytes (CTLs).[188,189] The poxviruses encode a variety of immunomodulatory molecules including CrmA, which blocks T-cell–mediated apoptosis of virus-infected cells.[190] In some cases (e.g., the CNS), preferential sites for persistent viral infections are not readily accessible by the immune system,[191] which may favor establishment of persistence.

VIRUSES AND CANCER

Several viruses produce disease by promoting malignant transformation of host cells. Work by Peyton Rous with an avian retrovirus was the first to demonstrate that viral infections can cause cancer.[192] Rous sarcoma virus encodes an oncogene, *v-src*, which is a homologue of a cellular proto-oncogene, *c-src*.[193,194] Cells infected with Rous sarcoma virus become transformed.[195-199] Several viruses are associated with malignancies in humans. EBV is associated with many neoplasms, including Burkitt's lymphoma, Hodgkin's disease, large B-cell lymphoma, leiomyosarcoma, and nasopharyngeal carcinoma. HBV and HCV are associated with hepatocellular carcinoma. HPV is associated with cervical cancer and a variety of anogenital neoplasms. Kaposi's sarcoma herpesvirus is associated with Kaposi's sarcoma and primary effusion lymphoma in persons with HIV infection.

Often, the linkage of a virus to a particular neoplasm can be attributed to transforming properties of the virus itself. For example, EBV encodes several latency-associated proteins that are responsible for immortalization of B cells; these proteins likely play crucial roles in the pathogenesis of EBV-associated malignancies.[200] Similarly, HPV encodes the E6 and E7 proteins that block apoptosis[100-102] and induce cell cycle progression,[98,99] respectively. It is hypothesized that unregulated expression of these proteins induced by the aberrant integration of the HPV genome into host DNA is responsible for malignant transformation.[201] The tumorigenicity of polyomaviruses, which are oncogenic in rodent species, is mediated by a family of viral proteins known as tumor (T) antigens. Reminiscent of the HPV E6 and E7 proteins, T antigens induce cell cycling and block the ensuing cellular apoptotic response to unscheduled cell division.[202] The normally episomal polyomavirus genome becomes integrated into cellular DNA during neoplastic transformation of nonpermissive cells unable to support the entire viral replication program, which would culminate in cell death. Recent discovery of a new human polyomavirus clonally integrated into cells of an aggressive form of skin cancer, Merkel cell carcinoma,[4] substantiates the long-standing suspicion that polyomaviruses can also promote neoplasia in humans.

In other cases, mechanisms of malignancy triggered by viral infection are less clear. HCV is an RNA-containing virus that lacks reverse transcriptase and a means of viral genome integration. However, chronic infection with HCV is strongly associated with hepatocellular cancer.[203] It is possible that increased cell turnover and inflammatory mediators elicited by chronic HCV infection increase the risk of genetic damage, which results in malignant transformation. Some HCV proteins also may play a contributory role in neoplasia. For example, the HCV core protein can protect cells against apoptosis induced by a variety of stimuli, including tumor necrosis factor-α (TNF-α).[204]

VIRAL VIRULENCE DETERMINANTS

Viral surface proteins involved in attachment and entry influence the virulence of diverse groups of viruses. For example, polymorphisms in the attachment proteins of influenza virus,[205,206] polyomavirus,[207] reovirus,[208] rotavirus,[209] and VEE[210] are strongly linked to virulence and can be accurately termed *virulence determinants*. Viral attachment proteins can serve this function by altering the affinity of virus-receptor interactions or modulating the kinetics of viral disassembly. Importantly, sequences in viral genomes that do not encode protein also can influence viral virulence. Mutations that contribute to the attenuated virulence of the Sabin strains of poliovirus are located in the 5′ nontranslated region of the viral genome.[211] These mutations attenuate poliovirus virulence by altering the efficiency of viral protein synthesis.

A number of viruses encode proteins that enhance virulence by modulation of host immune responses. In many cases, these proteins are dispensable for viral replication in cultured cells. In this way, immunomodulatory viral virulence determinants resemble classic bacterial virulence factors such as various types of secreted toxins.

HOST RESPONSES TO INFECTION

The immune response to viral infection involves complex interactions among leukocytes, nonhematopoietic cells, signaling proteins, soluble proinflammatory mediators, antigen-presenting molecules, and antibodies. These cells and molecules collaborate in a highly regulated fashion to limit viral replication and dissemination through recognition of broadly conserved molecular signatures, followed by virus-specific adaptive responses that further control infection and establish antigen-selective immunologic memory. The innate antiviral response is a local, transient, antigen-independent perimeter defense strategically focused at the site of virus incursion into an organ or tissue. Mediated by ancient families of membrane-associated and cytosolic molecules known as pattern recognition receptors (PRRs), the innate immune system detects pathogen-associated molecular patterns (PAMPs), which are basic structural components of microbial products including nucleic acids, carbohydrates, and lipids.[212] Viral PAMPs in the form of ssRNA, dsRNA, and DNA evoke the innate immune response through two groups of PRRs, the transmembrane Toll-like receptors (TLRs) and the cytosolic nucleic acid sensors. The latter include retinoic acid inducible gene-I (RIG-I), melanoma differentiation-associated gene 5 (Mda-5), and DNA-dependent activator of IFN-regulatory factors (DAI).[213,214] Nucleic acid binding by PRRs activates signaling pathways leading to the production and extracellular release of IFN-α and IFN-β. Through engagement of the cell-surface IFN-α/β receptor, these molecules mediate the upregulated expression of hundreds of gene products that corporately suppress viral replication and establish an intracellular antiviral state in neighboring uninfected cells. Well-described IFN-inducible gene products include the latent enzymes dsRNA-dependent protein kinase (PKR) and 2′,5′-oligoadenylate synthetase (OAS), both of which are activated by dsRNA.[215] PKR inhibits the initiation of protein synthesis through phosphorylation of translation initiation factor eIF2α. The 2′,5′-oligoandenylates generated by OAS bind and activate endoribonuclease RNAse L, which degrades viral mRNA. In addition to mediating the intracellular antiviral state, IFN-α/β also stimulates the antigen-independent destruction of virus-infected cells by a specialized population of lymphocytes known as natural killer (NK) cells.[216] Importantly, IFNs bridge innate and adaptive antiviral immune responses through multiple modes of action, which include enhancing viral antigen presentation by class I MHC proteins,[217] promoting the proliferation of MHC class I–restricted CD8+ CTLs,[218] and facilitating the functional maturation of dendritic cells.[219]

The adaptive immune response confers systemic and enduring pathogen-selective immunity through expansion and functional differentiation of viral antigen-specific T and B lymphocytes. Having both regulatory and effector roles, T lymphocytes are centrally positioned in the scheme of adaptive immunity. The primary cell type involved in the resolution of acute viral infection is the CD8+ CTL, which induces lethal proapoptotic signaling in virus-infected cells upon recognition of endogenously produced viral protein fragments presented by cell surface MHC class I molecules. Uncommonly, CD4+ T cells, which recognize MHC class II–associated viral oligopeptides processed from exogenously acquired proteins, also demonstrate cytotoxicity against viral antigen–presenting cells.[220] The usual function of CD4+ T lymphocytes is to orchestrate and balance cell-mediated (CTL) and humoral (B lymphocyte) responses to infection. Four principal classes of CD4+ helper T-cell subsets—Th1, Th2, Th17, and Treg (regulatory T)—have been defined based on characteristic patterns of cytokine secretion and effector activities.[221] Th1 and Th2 lymphocytes are usually associated with the development of cell-mediated and humoral responses, respectively, to viral infection. More recently described, Th17 and Treg CD4+ subsets are important for control of immune responses and prevention of autoimmunity, but their precise roles in viral disease and antiviral immunity are not clear. For certain persistent viral infections, such as those caused by HIV and HSV, Treg cells might exacerbate disease through suppression of CTLs or, paradoxically, ameliorate illness by attenuating immune-mediated cell and tissue injury.[222]

The primacy of cell-mediated immune responses in combating viral infections is revealed by the extreme vulnerability of individuals to chronic and life-threatening viral disease when cellular immunity is dysfunctional. Those with acquired immune deficiency syndrome (AIDS) exemplify the catastrophic consequences of collapsing cell-mediated immunity; progressive multifocal leukoencephalopathy caused by JC polyomavirus, along with severe mucocutaneous and disseminated CMV, HSV, and VZV infections, are frequent complications of vanishing CD4+ T cells. Similarly, iatrogenic cellular immunodeficiency associated with hematopoietic stem cell and solid organ transplantation or antineoplastic treatment regimens predisposes to severe, potentially fatal, infections with herpesviruses and respiratory viral pathogens such as adenovirus, PIV, and RSV,[223] all of which normally produce self-limited illness in immunocompetent hosts. Prevention and management of serious viral respiratory infections are significant challenges in myelosuppression units because of the communicability of respiratory viruses and paucity of effective drugs to combat these ubiquitous agents. Individuals with significantly impaired cell-mediated immunity also are at increased risk for enhanced viral replication and systemic disease following immunization with live, attenuated viral vaccines (e.g., measles-mumps-rubella (MMR) and VZV vaccines). Hence, live viral vaccines are generally contraindicated for immunocompromised persons.

In contrast to cell-mediated immune mechanisms, humoral responses usually are not a determinative factor in the resolution of primary viral infections. (One notable exception is a syndrome of chronic enteroviral meningitis in the setting of agammaglobulinemia.[224]) However, for most human viral pathogens, the presence of antibody is associated with protection against initial infection in vaccinees or reinfection in hosts with a history of natural infection.[225] Longitudinal studies indicate that levels of protective serum antibodies (induced by natural infection or immunization) to common viruses, including EBV, measles, mumps, and rubella, are remarkably stable, with calculated antibody half-lives ranging from several decades to thousands of years.[226] The protective role of antibodies on secondary exposure is frequently explained as interruption of viremic spread where a hematogenous phase is involved, such as occurs with measles, mumps, and rubella viruses; poliovirus, VZV; and most arboviruses. Nevertheless, most human viruses, excluding insect-transmitted agents, enter their hosts by transgression of a mucosal barrier, frequently undergoing primary replication in mucosal epithelium or adjacent lymphoid tissues. Neutralizing IgA exuded onto mucosal epithelial surfaces may protect against primary infection at this portal of viral entry. A classic example is gut mucosal immunity induced by orally administered Sabin poliovirus vaccine containing live-attenuated virus. Secretory IgA against poliovirus blocks infection at the site of primary replication and consequently interrupts the chain of viral transmission, although fully virulent revertant viruses arise at regular frequency in vaccine recipients, who may develop disease and also transmit revertant strains to nonimmune individuals. Clinical and experimental studies of immunity to HIV have led to the recognition that resident neutralizing antibodies probably are critical components of host resistance to primary HIV infection at the mucosal interface, and achievement of potent mucosal immunity is emerging as a guiding principle for the design of candidate HIV vaccines.[227] Despite the appearance of serum neutralizing antibodies to HIV several weeks after infection, viral eradication is thwarted by selection of neutralization-resistant variant strains from a mutant pool, which is perpetually replenished because of extreme plasticity within neutralization determinants on the viral envelope glycoproteins.[228]

Protection against viral infection by serum immunoglobulins is often correlated with antibody-mediated neutralization of viral infectivity in cultured cells. Antibodies interrupt the viral life cycle at early steps, which may include cross-linking virion particles into noninfectious aggregates, steric hindrance of receptor engagement, and interference with viral disassembly.[229] It is presumed that virus neutralization in cell culture by human serum is reflective of antibody activity in the intact host, but the mechanistic basis of infection blockade and disease prevention by antibodies in vivo is difficult to define precisely. For example, exclusively in vivo functions of the humoral antiviral response include Fc-mediated virion phagocytosis[230,231] and antibody-dependent cell-mediated cytotoxicity (ADCC). Although formally a branch of innate immunity, ADCC responses require effectors from both the innate and adaptive systems, NK cells, and antibodies, respectively.[232] The basis of ADCC is FcγRIIIa receptor-dependent recognition by NK cells of virus-specific IgG bound to antigens expressed on the surface of infected cells, leading to release of perforin and granzymes from NK cells that eventuate in target cell apoptosis. Neutrophils, lymphocytes, and macrophages also possess Fc receptors and may participate in ADCC.

REFERENCES

1. Reed W. Recent researches concerning the etiology, propagation and prevention of Yellow Fever by the United States Army Commission. *J Hyg*. 1902;2:101-109.
2. Murray K, Selleck P, Hooper P, et al. A morbillivirus that caused fatal disease in horses and humans. *Science*. 1995;268:94-97.
3. Chua KB, Bellini WJ, Rota PA, et al. Nipah virus: A recently emergent deadly paramyxovirus. *Science*. 2000;288:1432-1435.
4. Feng H, Shuda M, Chang Y, et al. Clonal integration of a polyomavirus in human Merkel cell carcinoma. *Science*. 2008; 319:1096-1100.
5. Allander T, Tammi MT, Eriksson M, et al. Cloning of a human parvovirus by molecular screening of respiratory tract samples. *Proc Natl Acad Sci U S A*. 2005;102:12891-12896.
6. Delbruck M. The growth of bacteriophage and lysis of the host. *J Gen Physiol*. 1940;23:643.
7. Luria SE. Bacteriophage: An essay on virus reproduction. *Science*. 1950;111:507-511.
8. Avery OT, MacLeod CM, McCarty M. Studies on the chemical nature of the substance inducing transformation of pneumococcal types. Induction of transformation by a desoxyribonucleic acid fraction isolated from pneumococcus type III. *J Exp Med*. 1944;79:137-158.
9. Hershey AD, Chase M. Independent functions of viral protein and nucleic acid in the growth of bacteriophage. *J Gen Physiol*. 1952;36:39-56.
10. Enders JF, Weller TH, Robbins FC. Cultivation of the Lansing strain of poliomyelitis virus in cultures of various human embryonic tissues. *Science*. 1949;109:85-87.
11. Salk JE. Studies in human subjects on active immunization against poliomyelitis. I. A preliminary report of experiments in progress. *JAMA*. 1953;151:1081-1098.
12. Sabin AB, Boulger LR. History of Sabin attenuated poliovirus oral live vaccine strains. *J Biol Stand*. 1973;1:115-118.
13. Zhang X, Settembre E, Xu C, et al. Near-atomic resolution using electron cryomicroscopy and single-particle reconstruction. *Proc Natl Acad Sci U S A*. 2008;105:1867-1872.
14. Chiu CY, Mathias P, Nemerow GR, et al. Structure of adenovirus complexed with its internalization receptor, αvβ5 integrin. *J Virol*. 1999;73:6759-6768.
15. He Y, Bowman VD, Mueller S, et al. Interaction of the poliovirus receptor with poliovirus. *Proc Natl Acad Sci U S A*. 2000;97:79-84.
16. Xiao C, Bator CM, Bowman VD, et al. Interaction of coxsackievirus A21 with its cellular receptor, ICAM-1. *J Virol*. 2001;75:2444-2451.
17. Che Z, Olson NH, Leippe D, et al. Antibody-mediated neutralization of human rhinovirus 14 explored by means of cryoelectron microscopy and X-ray crystallography of virus-Fab complexes. *J Virol*. 1998;72:4610-4622.
18. Nason EL, Wetzel JD, Mukherjee SK, et al. A monoclonal antibody specific for reovirus outer-capsid protein sigma3 inhibits sigma1-mediated hemagglutination by steric hindrance. *J Virol*. 2001;75:6625-6634.
19. Bertolotti-Ciarlet A, White LJ, Chen R, et al. Structural requirements for the assembly of Norwalk virus-like particles. *J Virol*. 2002;76:4044-4055.
20. Biemelt S, Sonnewald U, Galmbacher P, et al. Production of human papillomavirus type 16 virus-like particles in transgenic plants. *J Virol*. 2003;77:9211-9220.
21. Guo P, Lee TJ. Viral nanomotors for packaging of dsDNA and dsRNA. *Mol Microbiol*. 2007;64:886-903.
22. Ahmed M, Lyles DS. Effect of vesicular stomatitis virus matrix protein on transcription directed by host RNA polymerases I, II, and III. *J Virol*. 1998;72:8413-8419.
23. Ahmed M, McKenzie MO, Puckett S, et al. Ability of the matrix protein of vesicular stomatitis virus to suppress beta interferon gene expression is genetically correlated with the inhibition of host RNA and protein synthesis. *J Virol*. 2003;77:4646-4657.
24. Stojdl DF, Lichty BD, tenOever BR, et al. VSV strains with defects in their ability to shutdown innate immunity are potent systemic anti-cancer agents. *Cancer Cell*. 2003;4:263-275.
25. van Raaij MJ, Mitraki A, Lavigne G, et al. A triple β-spiral in the adenovirus fibre shaft reveals a new structural motif for a fibrous protein. *Nature*. 1999;401:935-938.
26. Chappell JD, Prota A, Dermody TS, et al. Crystal structure of reovirus attachment protein σ1 reveals evolutionary relationship to adenovirus fiber. *EMBO J*. 2002;21:1-11.
27. Shaw AL, Rothnagel R, Chen D, et al. Three-dimensional visualization of the rotavirus hemagglutinin structure. *Cell*. 1993;74:693-701.
28. Dormitzer PR, Sun ZY, Wagner G, et al. The rhesus rotavirus VP4 sialic acid binding domain has a galectin fold with a novel carbohydrate binding site. *EMBO J*. 2002;21:885-897.
29. Wilson IA, Skehel JJ, Wiley DC. Structure of the hemagglutinin membrane glycoprotein of influenza virus at 3-Å resolution. *Nature*. 1981;289:366-373.
30. Weis W, Brown JH, Cusack S, et al. Structure of the influenza virus haemagglutinin complexed with its receptor, sialic acid. *Nature*. 1988;333:426-431.
31. Lasky LA, Nakamura G, Smith DH, et al. Delineation of a region of the human immunodeficiency virus type 1 gp120 glycoprotein critical for interaction with the CD4 receptor. *Cell*. 1987;50:975-985.
32. Kwong PD, Wyatt R, Robinson J, et al. Structure of an HIV gp120 envelope glycoprotein in complex with the CD4 receptor and a neutralizing antibody. *Nature*. 1998;393:648-659.
33. Hogle JM, Chow M, Filman DJ. Three-dimensional structure of poliovirus at 2.9-Å resolution. *Science*. 1985;229:1358-1365.
34. Rossmann MG, Arnold E, Erickson JW, et al. Structure of a human common cold virus and functional relationship to other picornaviruses. *Nature*. 1985;317:145-153.
35. Acharya R, Fry E, Stuart D, et al. The three-dimensional structure of foot-and-mouth disease virus at 2.9-Å resolution. *Nature*. 1989;327:709-716.
36. Haywood AM. Virus receptors: Binding, adhesion strengthening, and changes in viral structure. *J Virol*. 1994;68:1-5.
37. Bergelson JM, Cunningham JA, Droguett G, et al. Isolation of a common receptor for Coxsackie B viruses and adenoviruses 2 and 5. *Science*. 1997;275:1320-1323.
38. Wickham TJ, Mathias P, Cheresh DA, et al. Integrins $\alpha_v\beta_3$ and $\alpha_v\beta_5$ promote adenovirus internalization but not virus attachment. *Cell*. 1993;73:309-319.
39. WuDunn D, Spear PG. Initial interaction of herpes simplex virus with cells is binding to heparan sulfate. *J Virol*. 1989;63:52-58.
40. Lycke E, Johansson M, Svennerholm B, et al. Binding of herpes simplex virus to cellular heparan sulphate; An initial step in the adsorption process. *J Gen Virol*. 1991;72:1131-1137.
41. Shieh MT, WuDunn D, Montgomery RI, et al. Cell surface receptors for herpes simplex virus are heparan sulfate proteoglycans. *J Cell Biol*. 1992;116:1273-1281.
42. Montgomery RI, Warner MS, Lum BJ, et al. Herpes simplex virus-1 entry into cells mediated by a novel member of the TNF/NGF receptor family. *Cell*. 1996;87:427-436.
43. Geraghty RJ, Krummenacher C, Cohen GH, et al. Entry of alphaherpesviruses mediated by poliovirus receptor-related protein 1 and poliovirus receptor. *Science*. 1998;280:1618-1620.
44. Warner MS, Geraghty RJ, Martinez WM, et al. A cell surface protein with herpesvirus entry activity (HveB) confers susceptibility to infection by mutants of herpes simplex virus type 1, herpes simplex virus type 2, and pseudorabies virus. *Virology*. 1998;246:179-189.
45. Dalgleish AG, Beverley PCL, Clapham PR, et al. The CD4 (T4) antigen is an essential component of the receptor for the AIDS retrovirus. *Nature*. 1984;312:763-767.
46. Maddon PJ, Dalgleish AG, McDougal JS, et al. The T4 gene encodes the AIDS virus receptor and is expressed in the immune system and the brain. *Cell*. 1986;47:333-348.
47. Feng Y, Broder CC, Kennedy PE, et al. HIV-1 entry cofactor: functional cDNA cloning of a seven-transmembrane, G protein-coupled receptor. *Science*. 1996;272:872-877.
48. Oberlin E, Amara A, Bachelerie F, et al. The CXC chemokine SDF-1 is the ligand for LESTR/fusin and prevents infection by T-cell-line-adapted HIV-1. *Nature*. 1996;382:833-835.
49. Deng H, Liu R, Ellmeier W, et al. Identification of a major co-receptor for primary isolates of HIV-1. *Nature*. 1996;381:661-666.
50. Dragic T, Litwin V, Allaway GP, et al. HIV-1 entry into CD4+ cells is mediated by the chemokine receptor CC-CKR-5. *Nature*. 1996;381:667-673.
51. Alkhatib G, Combadiere C, Broder CC, et al. CC CKR5: A RANTES, MIP-1alpha, MIP-1beta receptor as a fusion cofactor for macrophage-tropic HIV-1. *Science*. 1996;272:1955-1958.
52. Spear PG. Viral interactions with receptors in cell junctions and effects on junctional stability. *Dev Cell*. 2002;3:462-464.
53. Barton ES, Forrest JC, Connolly JL, et al. Junction adhesion molecule is a receptor for reovirus. *Cell*. 2001;104:441-451.
54. Makino A, Shimojima M, Miyazawa T, et al. Junctional adhesion molecule 1 is a functional receptor for feline calicivirus. *J Virol*. 2006;80:4482-4490.
55. Martin-Padura I, Lostaglio S, Schneemann M, et al. Junctional adhesion molecule, a novel member of the immunoglobulin superfamily that distributes at intercellular junctions and modulates monocyte transmigration. *J Cell Biol*. 1998;142:117-127.
56. Cohen CJ, Shieh JT, Pickles RJ, et al. The coxsackievirus and adenovirus receptor is a transmembrane component of the tight junction. *Proc Natl Acad Sci U S A*. 2001;98:15191-15196.
57. Takahashi K, Nakanishi H, Miyahara M, et al. Nectin/PRR: An immunoglobulin-like cell adhesion molecule recruited to cadherin-based adherens junctions through interaction with Afadin, a PDZ domain-containing protein. *J Cell Biol*. 1999;145:539-549.
58. Yoon M, Spear PG. Disruption of adherens junctions liberates nectin-1 to serve as receptor for herpes simplex virus and pseudorabies virus entry. *J Virol*. 2002;76:7203-7208.
59. Zahraoui A, Louvard D, Galli T. Tight junction, a platform for trafficking and signaling protein complexes. *J Cell Biol*. 2000;151:F31-F36.
60. Coyne CB, Bergelson JM. Virus-induced Abl and Fyn kinase signals permit coxsackievirus entry through epithelial tight junctions. *Cell*. 2006;124:119-131.
61. Eisen MB, Sabesan S, Skehel JJ, et al. Binding of the influenza A virus to cell-surface receptors: Structures of five hemagglutinin-sialyloligosaccharide complexes determined by X-ray crystallography. *Virology*. 1997;232:19-31.
62. Stehle T, Yan Y, Benjamin TL, et al. Structure of murine polyomavirus complexed with an oligosaccharide receptor fragment. *Nature*. 1994;369:160-163.
63. Stehle T, Harrison SC. High-resolution structure of a polyomavirus VP1-oligosaccharide complex: Implications for assembly and receptor binding. *EMBO J*. 1997;16:5139-5148.
64. Fry EE, Lea SM, Jackson T, et al. The structure and function of a foot-and-mouth disease virus-oligosaccharide receptor complex. *EMBO J*. 1999;18:543-554.

65. Bewley MC, Springer K, Zhang YB, et al. Structural analysis of the mechanism of adenovirus binding to its human cellular receptor, CAR. *Science*. 1999;286:1579-1583.
66. Mullen MM, Haan KM, Longnecker R, et al. Structure of the Epstein-Barr virus gp42 protein bound to the MHC class II receptor HLA-DR1. *Mol Cell*. 2002;9:375-385.
67. Carfi A, Willis SH, Whitbeck JC, et al. Herpes simplex virus glycoprotein D bound to the human receptor HveA. *Mol Cell*. 2001;8:169-179.
68. Kirchner E, Guglielmi KM, Strauss HM, et al. Structure of reovirus σ1 in complex with its receptor junctional adhesion molecule-A. *PLoS Pathog*. 2008;4:e1000235.
69. Kolatkar PR, Bella J, Olson NH, et al. Structural studies of two rhinovirus serotypes complexed with fragments of their cellular receptor. *EMBO J*. 1999;18:6249-6259.
70. Doranz BJ, Berson JF, Rucker J, et al. Chemokine receptors as fusion cofactors for human immunodeficiency virus type 1 (HIV-1). *Immunol Res*. 1997;16:15-28.
71. Moore JP, Trkola A, Dragic T. Co-receptors for HIV-1 entry. *Curr Opin Immunol*. 1997;9:551-562.
72. Kowalski M, Potz J, Basiripour L, et al. Functional regions of the envelope glycoprotein of human immunodeficiency virus type 1. *Science*. 1988;237:1351-1355.
73. Sattentau QJ. CD4 activation of HIV fusion. *Int J Cell Clon*. 1992;10:323-332.
74. Weissenhorn W, Dessen A, Harrison SC, et al. Atomic structure of the ectodomain from HIV-1 gp41. *Nature*. 1997;387:426-430.
75. Dutch RE, Jardetzky TS, Lamb RA. Virus membrane fusion proteins: Biological machines that undergo a metamorphosis. *Biosci Rep*. 2000;20:597-612.
76. Trowbridge IS, Collawn JE, Hopkins CR. Signal-dependent membrane protein trafficking in the endocytic pathway. *Annu Rev Cell Biol*. 1993;9:129-161.
77. Modis Y, Ogata S, Clements D, et al. Structure of the dengue virus envelope protein after membrane fusion. *Nature*. 2004;427:313-319.
78. Bullough PA, Hughson FM, Skehel JJ, et al. Structure of influenza haemagglutinin at the pH of membrane fusion. *Nature*. 1994;371:37-43.
79. Gibbons DL, Vaney MC, Roussel A, et al. Conformational change and protein-protein interactions of the fusion protein of Semliki Forest virus. *Nature*. 2004;427:320-325.
80. Varga MJ, Weibull C, Everitt E. Infectious entry pathway of adenovirus type 2. *J Virol*. 1991;65:6061-6070.
81. Greber UF, Willetts M, Webster P, et al. Stepwise dismantling of adenovirus 2 during entry into cells. *Cell*. 1993;75:477-486.
82. Basak S, Turner H. Infectious entry pathway for canine parvovirus. *Virology*. 1992;186:368-376.
83. Maratos-Flier E, Goodman MJ, Murray AH, et al. Ammonium inhibits processing and cytotoxicity of reovirus, a nonenveloped virus. *J Clin Invest*. 1986;78:1003-1007.
84. Sturzenbecker LJ, Nibert ML, Furlong DB, et al. Intracellular digestion of reovirus particles requires a low pH and is an essential step in the viral infectious cycle. *J Virol*. 1987;61:2351-2361.
85. Chandran K, Sullivan NJ, Felbor U, et al. Endosomal proteolysis of the Ebola virus glycoprotein is necessary for infection. *Science*. 2005;308:1643-1645.
86. Pager CT, Dutch RE. Cathepsin L is involved in proteolytic processing of the Hendra virus fusion protein. *J Virol*. 2005;79:12714-12720.
87. Ebert DH, Deussing J, Peters C, et al. Cathepsin L and cathepsin B mediate reovirus disassembly in murine fibroblast cells. *J Biol Chem*. 2002;277:24609-24617.
88. Huang I-C, Bosch BJ, Li F, et al. SARS coronavirus, but not human coronavirus NL63, utilizes cathepsin L to infect ACE2-expressing cells. *J Biol Chem*. 2006;281:3198-3203.
89. Fricks CE, Hogle JM. Cell-induced conformational change in poliovirus: Externalization of the amino terminus of VP1 is responsible for liposome binding. *J Virol*. 1990;64:1934-1945.
90. Greve JM, Forte CP, Marlor CW, et al. Mechanisms of receptor-mediated rhinovirus neutralization defined by two soluble forms of ICAM-1. *J Virol*. 1991;65:6015-6023.
91. Odegard AL, Chandran K, Zhang X, et al. Putative autocleavage of outer capsid protein μ1, allowing release of myristoylated peptide μ1N during particle uncoating, is critical for cell entry by reovirus. *J Virol*. 2004;78:8732-8745.
92. Dormitzer PR, Nason EB, Prasad BV, et al. Structural rearrangements in the membrane penetration protein of a non-enveloped virus. *Nature*. 2004;430:1053-1058.
93. Wiethoff CM, Wodrich H, Gerace L, et al. Adenovirus protein VI mediates membrane disruption following capsid disassembly. *J Virol*. 2005;79:1992-2000.
94. Danthi P, Tosteson M, Li QH, et al. Genome delivery and ion channel properties are altered in VP4 mutants of poliovirus. *J Virol*. 2003;77:5266-5274.
95. Agosto MA, Ivanovic T, Nibert ML. Mammalian reovirus, a nonfusogenic nonenveloped virus, forms size-selective pores in a model membrane. *Proc Natl Acad Sci U S A*. 2006;103:16496-16501.
96. Lawton JA, Estes MK, Prasad BVV. Three-dimensional visualization of mRNA release from actively transcribing rotavirus particles. *Nature Struct Biol*. 1997;4:118-121.
97. Nabel GJ. The role of cellular transcription factors in the regulation of human immunodeficiency virus gene expression. In: Cullen BR, eds. *Human Retroviruses*. Oxford: IRL Press; 1993:49-73.
98. Dyson N, Howley PM, Munger K, et al. The human papilloma virus-16 E7 oncoprotein is able to bind to the retinoblastoma gene product. *Science*. 1989;243:934-937.
99. Dyson N, Guida P, Munger K, et al. Homologous sequences in adenovirus E1A and human papillomavirus E7 proteins mediate interaction with the same set of cellular proteins. *J Virol*. 1992;66:6893-6902.
100. Scheffner M, Werness BA, Huibregtse JM, et al. The E6 oncoprotein encoded by human papillomavirus types 16 and 18 promotes the degradation of p53. *Cell*. 1990;63:1129-1136.
101. Werness BA, Levine AJ, Howley PM. Association of human papillomavirus types 16 and 18 E6 proteins with p53. *Science*. 1990;248:76-79.
102. Scheffner M, Huibregtse JM, Vierstra RD, et al. The HPV-16 E6 and E6-AP complex functions as a ubiquitin-protein ligase in the ubiquitination of p53. *Cell*. 1993;75:495-505.
103. Grey F, Meyers H, White EA, et al. A human cytomegalovirus-encoded microRNA regulates expression of multiple viral genes involved in replication. *PLoS Pathog*. 2007;3:e163.
104. Stern-Ginossar N, Elefant N, Zimmermann A, et al. Host immune system gene targeting by a viral miRNA. *Science*. 2007;317:376-381.
105. Randall RE, Goodbourn S. Interferons and viruses: An interplay between induction, signalling, antiviral responses and virus countermeasures. *J Gen Virol*. 2008;89:1-47.
106. Bienz K, Egger D, Pasamontes L. Association of polioviral proteins of the P2 genomic region with the viral replication complex and virus-induced membrane synthesis as visualized by electron microscopic immunocytochemistry and autoradiography. *Virology*. 1987;160:220-226.
107. Schlegel A, Giddings TH Jr, Ladinsky MS, et al. Cellular origin and ultrastructure of membranes induced during poliovirus infection. *J Virol*. 1996;70:6576-6588.
108. Mackenzie J. Wrapping things up about virus RNA replication. *Traffic*. 2005;6:967-977.
109. Froshauer S, Kartenbeck J, Helenius A. Alphavirus RNA replicase is located on the cytoplasmic surface of endosomes and lysosomes. *J Cell Biol*. 1988;107:2075-2086.
110. Jackson WT, Giddings TH Jr, Taylor MP, et al. Subversion of cellular autophagosomal machinery by RNA viruses. *PLoS Biol*. 2005;3:e156.
111. Estes MK, Kapikian AZ. Rotaviruses. In: Knipe DM, Howley PM, eds. *Fields Virology*. 5th ed. Philadelphia: Lippincott Williams & Wilkins; 2007:1917-1974.
112. Talloczy Z, Virgin HWt, Levine B. PKR-dependent autophagic degradation of herpes simplex virus type 1. *Autophagy*. 2006;2:24-29.
113. Orvedahl A, Alexander D, Talloczy Z, et al. HSV-1 ICP34.5 confers neurovirulence by targeting the Beclin 1 autophagy protein. *Cell Host Microbe*. 2007;1:23-35.
114. Everett RD. Interactions between DNA viruses, ND10 and the DNA damage response. *Cell Microbiol*. 2006;8:365-374.
115. Netherton C, Moffat K, Brooks E, et al. A guide to viral inclusions, membrane rearrangements, factories, and viroplasm produced during virus replication. *Adv Virus Res*. 2007;70:101-182.
116. Bernardi R, Pandolfi PP. Structure, dynamics and functions of promyelocytic leukaemia nuclear bodies. *Nat Rev Mol Cell Biol*. 2007;8:1006-1016.
117. Wileman T. Aggresomes and pericentriolar sites of virus assembly: Cellular defense or viral design? *Annu Rev Microbiol*. 2007;61:149-167.
118. Radtke K, Dohner K, Sodeik B. Viral interactions with the cytoskeleton: A hitchhiker's guide to the cell. *Cell Microbiol*. 2006;8:387-400.
119. Dohner K, Nagel CH, Sodeik B. Viral stop-and-go along microtubules: Taking a ride with dynein and kinesins. *Trends Microbiol*. 2005;13:320-327.
120. Gupta S, De BP, Drazba JA, et al. Involvement of actin microfilaments in the replication of human parainfluenza virus type 3. *J Virol*. 1998;72:2655-2662.
121. Parker JS, Broering TJ, Kim J, et al. Reovirus core protein μ2 determines the filamentous morphology of viral inclusion bodies by interacting with and stabilizing microtubules. *J Virol*. 2002;76:4483-4496.
122. Mallardo M, Schleich S, Krijnse Locker J. Microtubule-dependent organization of vaccinia virus core–derived early mRNAs into distinct cytoplasmic structures. *Mol Biol Cell*. 2001;12:3875-3891.
123. Wagner RR. Cytopathic effects of viruses: A general survey. In: Fraenkel-Conrat H, Wagner RR, eds. *Comprehensive Virology*. New York: Plenum Press; 1984:1-63.
124. O'Brien V. Viruses and apoptosis. *J Gen Virol*. 1998;79:1833-1845.
125. Roulston A, Marcellus RC, Branton PE. Viruses and apoptosis. *Ann Rev Microbiol*. 1999;53:577-628.
126. Wyllie AH, Kerr JFR, Currie AR. Cell death: The significance of apoptosis. *Int Rev Cytol*. 1980;68:251-306.
127. Everett H, McFadden G. Apoptosis: An innate immune response to virus infection. *Trends Microbiol*. 1999;7:160-165.
128. Lewis J, Wesselingh SL, Griffin DE, et al. Alphavirus-induced apoptosis in mouse brains correlates with neurovirulence. *J Virol*. 1996;70:1828-1835.
129. Jackson AC, Rossiter JP. Apoptosis plays an important role in experimental rabies virus infection. *J Virol*. 1997;71:5603-5607.
130. Oberhaus SM, Smith RL, Clayton GH, et al. Reovirus infection and tissue injury in the mouse central nervous system are associated with apoptosis. *J Virol*. 1997;71:2100-2106.
131. McQuade TK, Tomasselli AG, Liu L, et al. HIV-1 protease inhibitor with antiviral activity arrest HIV-like particle maturation. *Science*. 1990;247:454-456.
132. Woods JM, Bethell RC, Coates JA, et al. 4-Guanidino-2,4-dideoxy-2,3-dehydro-*N*-acetylneuraminic acid is a highly effective inhibitor both of the sialidase (neuraminidase) and of growth of a wide range of influenza A and B viruses *in vitro*. *Antimicrob Agents Chemother*. 1993;37:1473-1479.
133. Stiver G. The treatment of influenza with antiviral drugs. *CMAJ*. 2003;168:49-56.
134. Kilby JM, Eron JJ. Novel therapies based on mechanisms of HIV-1 cell entry. *N Engl J Med*. 2003;348:2228-2238.
135. MacArthur RD, Novak RM. Reviews of anti-infective agents: Maraviroc: The first of a new class of antiretroviral agents. *Clin Infect Dis*. 2008;47:236-241.
136. Pace P, Rowley M. Integrase inhibitors for the treatment of HIV infection. *Curr Opin Drug Discov Devel*. 2008;11:471-479.
137. Salzwedel K, Martin DE, Sakalian M. Maturation inhibitors: A new therapeutic class targets the virus structure. *AIDS Rev*. 2007;9:162-172.
138. Stauber RE, Kessler HH. Drugs in development for hepatitis C. *Drugs*. 2008;68:1347-1359.
139. Crotty S, Maag D, Arnold JJ, et al. The broad-spectrum antiviral ribonucleoside ribavirin is an RNA virus mutagen. *Nat Med*. 2000;6:1375-1379.
140. Leyssen P, Balzarini J, De Clercq E, et al. The predominant mechanism by which ribavirin exerts its antiviral activity *in vitro* against flaviviruses and paramyxoviruses is mediated by inhibition of IMP dehydrogenase. *J Virol*. 2005;79:1943-1947.
141. McCormick JB, King IJ, Webb PA, et al. Lassa fever. Effective therapy with ribavirin. *N Engl J Med*. 1986;314:20-26.
142. Bass DM, Bodkin D, Dambrauskas R, et al. Intraluminal proteolytic activation plays an important role in replication of type 1 reovirus in the intestines of neonatal mice. *J Virol*. 1990;64:1830-1833.
143. Vonderfecht SL, Miskuff RL, Wee S, et al. Protease inhibitors suppress the *in vitro* and *in vivo* replication of rotaviruses. *J Clin Invest*. 1988;82:2011-2016.
144. Wolf JL, Rubin DH, Finberg R, et al. Intestinal M cells: A pathway of entry of reovirus into the host. *Science*. 1981;212:471-472.
145. Wolf JL, Kauffman RS, Finberg R, et al. Determinants of reovirus interaction with the intestinal M cells and absorptive cells of murine intestine. *Gastroenterology*. 1983;85:291-300.
146. Sicinski P, Rowinski J, Warchol JB, et al. Poliovirus type 1 enters the human host through intestinal M cells. *Gastroenterology*. 1990;98:56-58.
147. Amerongen HM, Weltzin R, Farnet CM, et al. Transepithelial transport of HIV-1 by intestinal M cells: A mechanism for transmission of AIDS. *J AIDS*. 1991;4:760-765.
148. Ball JM, Mulligan MJ, Compans RW. Basolateral sorting of the HIV type 2 and SIV enveloope glycoproteins in polarized epithelial cells: Role of the cytoplasmic domain. *AIDS Res Hum Retrovir*. 1997;13:665-675.
149. Huang XF, Compans RW, Chen S, et al. Polarized apical targeting directed by the signal/anchor region of simian virus 5 hemagglutinin-neuraminidase. *J Biol Chem*. 1997;272:27598-27604.
150. Antar AAR, Konopka JL, Campbell JA, et al. Junctional adhesion molecule-A is required for hematogenous dissemination of reovirus. *Cell Host Microbe*. 2009;5:59-71.
151. Fenner F. The pathogenesis of acute exanthems. *Lancet*. 1948;2:915.
152. Tyler KL, Nathanson N. Pathogenesis of viral infections. In: Knipe DM, Howley PM, eds. *Fields Virology*. 4th ed. Philadelphia: Lippincott-Raven Press; 2001:199-243.
153. Tsiang H. Evidence for intraaxonal transport of fixed and street rabies virus. *J Neuropathol Exp Neurol*. 1979;38:286-297.
154. Lycke E, Tsiang H. Rabies virus infection of cultured rat sensory neurons. *J Virol*. 1987;61:2733-2741.
155. Ziegler RJ, Herman RE. Peripheral infection in culture of rat sensory neurons by herpes simplex virus. *Infect Immun*. 1980;28:620-623.
156. Kristensson K, Lycke E, Sjostrand J. Spread of herpes simplex virus in peripheral nerves. *Acta Neuropathology (Berlin)*. 1971;17:44-53.
157. Smith GA, Gross SP, Enquist LW. Herpesviruses use bidirectional fast-axonal transport to spread in sensory neurons. *Proc Natl Acad Sci U S A*. 2001;98:3466-3470.
158. Bodian D. Poliomyelitis: Pathogenesis and histopathology. In: Rivers TM, Horsfall FL, eds. *Viral and Rickettsial Infections of Man*. 3rd ed. Philadelphia: Lippincott; 1959:479-518.
159. Sabin AB. Paralytic poliomyelitis: old dogmas and new perspectives. *Rev Infect Dis*. 1981;3:543-564.
160. Ren R, Costantini FC, Gorgacz EJ, et al. Transgenic mice expressing a human poliovirus receptor: A new model for poliomyelitis. *Cell*. 1990;63:353-362.
161. Ren R, Racaniello VR. Poliovirus spreads from muscle to central nervous system by neural pathways. *J Infect Dis*. 1992;166:747-752.

162. Holland JJ. Receptor affinities as major determinants of enterovirus tissue tropisms in humans. *Virology*. 1961;15:312-326.
163. Mendelsohn CL, Wimmer E, Racaniello VR. Cellular receptor for poliovirus: Molecular cloning, nucleotide sequence, and expression of a new member of the immunoglobulin superfamily. *Cell*. 1989;56:855-865.
164. McKnight S, Tijan R. Transcriptional selectivity of viral genes in mammalian cells. *Cell*. 1986;46:795-805.
165. Maniatis T, Goodbourn S, Fischer JA. Regulation of inducible and tissue-specific gene expression. *Science*. 1987;236:1237-1245.
166. Kenney S, Natarajan V, Strike D, et al. JC virus enhancer-promoter active in human brain cells. *Science*. 1984;226:1337-1339.
167. Davis NL, Grieder FB, Smith JF, et al. A molecular genetic approach to the study of Venezuelan equine encephalitis virus pathogenesis. *Arch Virol* Supp. 1994;9:99-109.
168. Tucker SP, Compans RW. Virus infection of polarized epithelial cells. *Adv Virus Res*. 1993;42:187-247.
169. Tardieu M, Powers ML, Weiner HL. Age-dependent susceptibility to reovirus type 3 encephalitis: Role of viral and host factors. *Ann Neurol*. 1983;13:602-607.
170. Mann MA, Knipe DM, Fischbach GD, et al. Type 3 reovirus neuroinvasion after intramuscular inoculation: Direct invasion of nerve terminals and age-dependent pathogenesis. *Virology*. 2002;303:222-231.
171. Hall CB, Hall WJ, Speers DM. Clinical and physiologic manifestations of bronchiolitis and pneumonia: Outcome of respiratory syncytial virus. *Am J Dis Child*. 1979;133:798-802.
172. Henderson FW, Collier AM, Clyde WA, et al. Respiratory-syncytial-virus infections, reinfections and immunity. A prospective, longitudinal study in young children. *N Engl J Med*. 1979;300:530-534.
173. Glezen WP, Taber LH, Frank AL, et al. Risk of primary infection and reinfection with respiratory syncytial virus. *Amer J Dis Child*. 1986;140:543-546.
174. Rodriguez WJ, Kim HW, Brandt CD, et al. Rotavirus gastroenteritis in the Washington, D.C. area. Incidence of cases resulting in admission to the hospital. *Am J Dis Child*. 1980;134:777-779.
175. Bishop RF. Natural history of human rotavirus infections. In: Kapikian AZ, eds. *Viral Infections of the Gastrointestinal Tract*. New York: Marcel Dekker; 1994:131-168.
176. Barclay AJG, Foster A, Sommer A. Vitamin A supplements and mortality related to measles: A randomised clinical trial. *BMJ*. 1987;294:294-296.
177. Hussey GD, Klein M. Routine high-dose vitamin A therapy for children hospitalized with measles. *J Trop Pediatr*. 1993;39:342-345.
178. Rosenstreich DL, Weinblatt AC, O'Brien AD. Genetic control of resistance to infection in mice. *CRC Crit Rev Immunol*. 1982;3:263-300.
179. Dean M, Carrington M, Winkler C, et al. Genetic restriction of HIV-1 infection and progression to AIDS by a deletion allele of the CKR5 structural gene. *Science*. 1996;273:1856-1862.
180. Hoffman TL, MacGregor RR, Burger H, et al. CCR5 genotypes in sexually active couples discordant for human immunodeficiency virus type 1 infection status. *J Infect Dis*. 1997;176:1093-1096.
181. Ho DD, Neumann AU, Perelson AS, et al. Rapid turnover of plasma virions and CD4 lymphocytes in HIV-1 infection. *Nature*. 1995;373:123-126.
182. Wong JK, Hezareh M, Gunthard HF, et al. Recovery of replication-competent HIV despite prolonged suppression of plasma viremia. *Science*. 1997;278:1291-1295.
183. Finzi D, Hermankova M, Pierson T, et al. Identification of a reservoir for HIV-1 in patients on highly active antiretroviral therapy. *Science*. 1997;278:1295-1300.
184. Montelaro RC, Parekh B, Orrego A, et al. Antigenic variation during persistent infection by equine infectious anemia virus, a retrovirus. *J Biol Chem*. 1984;259:10539-10544.
185. Robert-Guroff M, Brown M, Gallo RC. HTLV-III-neutralizing antibodies in patients with AIDS and AIDS-related complex. *Nature*. 1985;316:72-74.
186. Weiss RA, Clapham PR, Cheingsong-Popou R, et al. Neutralization of human T lymphotropic virus type III by sera of AIDS and AIDS-risk patients. *Nature*. 1985;316:69-72.
187. Fauci A. Immunopathogenesis of HIV infection. *AIDS*. 1993;6:655-662.
188. Burgert H, Maryanski J, Kvist S. "E3/19K" protein of adenovirus type 2 inhibits lysis of cytolytic T lymphocytes by blocking cell-surface expression of histocompatibility class I antigens. *Proc Natl Acad Sci U S A*. 1987;84:1356-1360.
189. Wiertz E, Jones T, Sun L, et al. The human cytomegalovirus US11 gene product dislocates MHC class I heavy chains from the endoplasmic reticulum to the cytosol. *Cell*. 1996;84:769-779.
190. Tewari M, Telford WG, Miller RA, et al. CrmA, a poxvirus-encoded serpin, inhibits cytotoxic T-lymphocyte-mediated apoptosis. *J Biol Chem*. 1995;270:22705-22708.
191. Stevenson PG, Hawke S, Sloan DJ, et al. The immunogenicity of intracerebral virus infection depends on anatomical site. *J Virol*. 1997;71:145-151.
192. Rous P. A transmissible avian neoplasm: Sarcoma of the common fowl. *J Exp Med*. 1910;12:696-705.
193. Stehelin D, Varmus HE, Bishop JM, et al. DNA related to the transforming gene(s) of avian sarcoma viruses is present in normal avian DNA. *Nature*. 1976;260:170-173.
194. Takeya T, Hanafusa H. Nucleotide sequences of *c-src*. *Cell*. 1983;32:881-890.
195. Manaker RA, Groupe V. Discrete foci of altered chicken embryo cells associated with Rous sarcoma virus in tissue culture. *Virology*. 1956;2:838-840.
196. Temin HM, Rubin H. Characteristics of an assay for Rous sarcoma virus and Rous sarcoma cells in tissue culture. *Virology*. 1958;6:669-688.
197. Toyoshima K, Vogt PK. Temperature-sensitive mutants of an avian sarcoma virus. *Virology*. 1969;39:930-931.
198. Martin GS. Rous sarcoma virus: A function required for the maintenance of the transformed state. *Nature*. 1970;227:1021-1023.
199. Cooper JA, Howell B. The when and how of Src regulation. *Cell*. 1993;73:1051-1054.
200. Dolcetti R, Masucci MG. Epstein-Barr virus: Induction and control of cell transformation. *J Cell Physiol*. 2003;196:207-218.
201. Wentzensen N, Ridder R, Klaes R, et al. Characterization of viral-cellular fusion transcripts in a large series of HPV16 and 18 positive anogenital lesions. *Oncogene*. 2002;21:419-426.
202. Sullivan CS, Pipas JM. T antigens of simian virus 40: Molecular chaperones for viral replication and tumorigenesis. *Microbiol Mol Biol Rev*. 2002;66:179-202.
203. Tsukuma H, Hiyana T, Tanka S, et al. Risk factors for hepatocellular carcinoma among patients with chronic liver disease. *N Engl J Med*. 1993;328:1797-1801.
204. Marusawa H, Hijikata M, Chiba T, et al. Hepatitis C virus core protein inhibits Fas- and tumor necrosis factor alpha-mediated apoptosis via NF-kappaB activation. *J Virol*. 1999;73:4713-4720.
205. Nestorowicz A, Kawaoka Y, Bean WJ, et al. Molecular analysis of the hemagglutinin genes of Australian H7N7 influenza viruses: Role of passerine birds in maintenance or transmission? *Virology*. 1987;11:400-418.
206. Horimoto T, Kawaoka Y. Reverse genetics provides direct evidence for a correlation of hemagglutinin cleavability and virulence of an avian influenza A virus. *J Virol*. 1994;68:3120-3128.
207. Chen MH, Benjamin T. Roles of N-glycans with alpha2,6 as well as alpha2,3 linked sialic acid in infection by polyoma virus. *Virology*. 1997;233:440-442.
208. Bassel-Duby R, Spriggs DR, Tyler KL, et al. Identification of attenuating mutations on the reovirus type 3 S1 double-stranded RNA segment with a rapid sequencing technique. *J Virol*. 1986;60:64-67.
209. Offit PA, Blavat G, Greenberg HB, et al. Molecular basis of rotavirus virulence: Role of gene segment 4. *J Virol*. 1986;57:46-49.
210. Grieder FB, Davis NL, Aronson JF, et al. Specific restrictions in the progression of Venezuelan equine encephalitis virus–induced disease resulting from single amino acid changes in the glycoproteins. *Virology*. 1995;206:994-1006.
211. Brown F, Lewis BP. Poliovirus attenuation: Molecular mechanisms and practical aspects. *Dev Biol Stand*. 1993;78:1-187.
212. Kumagai Y, Takeuchi O, Akira S. Pathogen recognition by innate receptors. *J Infect Chemother*. 2008;14:86-92.
213. Takaoka A, Wang Z, Choi MK, et al. DAI (DLM-1/ZBP1) is a cytosolic DNA sensor and an activator of innate immune response. *Nature*. 2007;448:501-505.
214. Saito T, Gale M Jr. Principles of intracellular viral recognition. *Curr Opin Immunol*. 2007;19:17-23.
215. Sadler AJ, Williams BR. Interferon-inducible antiviral effectors. *Nat Rev Immunol*. 2008;8:559-568.
216. Biron CA, Nguyen KB, Pien GC, et al. Natural killer cells in antiviral defense: Function and regulation by innate cytokines. *Annu Rev Immunol*. 1999;17:189-220.
217. Samuel CE. Antiviral actions of interferons. *Clin Microbiol Rev*. 2001;14:778-809.
218. Le Bon A, Durand V, Kamphuis E, et al. Direct stimulation of T cells by type I IFN enhances the CD8+ T cell response during cross-priming. *J Immunol*. 2006;176:4682-4689.
219. Le Bon A, Tough DF. Links between innate and adaptive immunity via type I interferon. *Curr Opin Immunol*. 2002;14:432-436.
220. van de Berg PJ, van Leeuwen EM, ten Berge IJ, et al. Cytotoxic human CD4(+) T cells. *Curr Opin Immunol*. 2008;20:339-343.
221. Zhu J, Paul WE. CD4 T cells: Fates, functions, and faults. *Blood*. 2008;112:1557-1569.
222. Rouse BT, Sarangi PP, Suvas S. Regulatory T cells in virus infections. *Immunol Rev*. 2006;212:272-286.
223. Ison MG, Hayden FG. Viral infections in immunocompromised patients: What's new with respiratory viruses? *Curr Opin Infect Dis*. 2002;15:355-367.
224. McKinney RE Jr, Katz SL, Wilfert CM. Chronic enteroviral meningoencephalitis in agammaglobulinemic patients. *Rev Infect Dis*. 1987;9:334-356.
225. Slifka MK, Ahmed R. Long-term humoral immunity against viruses: Revisiting the issue of plasma cell longevity. *Trends Microbiol*. 1996;4:394-400.
226. Amanna IJ, Carlson NE, Slifka MK. Duration of humoral immunity to common viral and vaccine antigens. *N Engl J Med*. 2007;357:1903-1915.
227. Haynes BF, Shattock RJ. Critical issues in mucosal immunity for HIV-1 vaccine development. *J Allergy Clin Immunol*. 2008;122:3-9.
228. McMichael AJ. HIV vaccines. *Annu Rev Immunol*. 2006;24:227-255.
229. Parren PW, Burton DR. The antiviral activity of antibodies in vitro and in vivo. *Adv Immunol*. 2001;77:195-262.
230. Huber SA, Lodge PA. Coxsackievirus B-3 myocarditis in Balb/c mice. Evidence for autoimmunity to myocyte antigens. *Am J Pathol*. 1984;116:21-29.
231. McCullough KC, De Simone F, Brocchi E, et al. Protective immune response against foot-and-mouth disease. *J Virol*. 1992;66:1835-1840.
232. Trinchieri G. Biology of natural killer cells. *Adv Immunol*. 1989;47:187-376.
233. Russell RJ, Kerry PS, Stevens DJ, et al. Structure of influenza hemagglutinin in complex with an inhibitor of membrane fusion. *Proc Natl Acad Sci U S A*. 2008;105:17736-17741.
234. Nathanson N, Tyler KL. Entry, dissemination, shedding, and transmission of viruses. In: Nathanson N, ed. *Viral Pathogenesis*. Philadelphia: Lippincott-Raven; 1997:13-33.
235. Fenner F. Mousepox (infectious ectromelia of mice): A review. *J Immunol*. 1949;63:341-373.
236. Condit RC. Principles of virology. In: Knipe DM, Howley PM, eds. *Fields Virology*. 5th ed. Philadelphia: Lippincott Williams & Wilkins; 2007:25-57.
237. Tomko RP, Xu R, Philipson L. HCAR and MCAR: The human and mouse cellular receptors for subgroup C adenoviruses and group B coxsackieviruses. *Proc Natl Acad Sci U S A*. 1997;94:3352-3356.
238. Segerman A, Atkinson JP, Marttila M, et al. Adenovirus type 11 uses CD46 as a cellular receptor. *J Virol*. 2003;77:9183-9191.
239. Gaggar A, Shayakhmetov DM, Lieber A. CD46 is a cellular receptor for group B adenoviruses. *Nat Med*. 2003;9:1408-1412.
240. Arnberg N, Edlund K, Kidd AH, et al. Adenovirus type 37 uses sialic acid as a cellular receptor. *J Virol*. 2000;74:42-48.
241. Vlasak R, Luytjes W, Spaan W, et al. Human and bovine coronaviruses recognize sialic acid-containing receptors similar to those of influenza C viruses. *Proc Natl Acad Sci U S A*. 1988;85:4526-4529.
242. Delmas B, Gelfi J, L'Haridon R, et al. Aminopeptidase N is a major receptor for the entero-pathogenic coronavirus TGEV. *Nature*. 1992;357:417-420.
243. Yeager CL, Ashmun RA, Williams RK, et al. Human aminopeptidase N is a receptor for human coronavirus 229E. *Nature*. 1992;357:420-422.
244. Li W, Moore MJ, Vasilieva N, et al. Angiotensin-converting enzyme 2 is a functional receptor for the SARS coronavirus. *Nature*. 2003;426:450-454.
245. Roivainen M, Piirainen L, Hovi T, et al. Entry of coxsackievirus A9 into host cells: Specific interactions with $\alpha v\beta 3$ integrin, the vitronectin receptor. *Virology*. 1994;203:357-365.
246. Bergelson JM, Mohoanty JG, Crowell RL, et al. Coxsackievirus B3 adapted to growth in RD cells binds to decay-accelerating factor (CD55). *J Virol*. 1995;69:1903-1906.
247. Shafren DR, Bates RC, Agrez MV, et al. Coxsackieviruses B1, B3, and B5 use decay accelerating factor as a receptor for cell attachment. *J Virol*. 1995;69:3873-3877.
248. Shafren DR, Dorahy DJ, Ingham RA, et al. Coxsackievirus A21 binds to decay-accelerating factor but requires intercellular adhesion molecule 1 for cell entry. *J Virol*. 1997;71:4736-4743.
249. Triantafilou K, Fradelizi D, Wilson K, et al. GRP78, a coreceptor for coxsackievirus A9, interacts with major histocompatibility complex class I molecules which mediate virus internalization. *J Virol*. 2002;76:633-643.
250. Zautner AE, Korner U, Henke A, et al. Heparan sulfates and coxsackievirus-adenovirus receptor: Each one mediates coxsackievirus B3 PD infection. *J Virol*. 2003;77:10071-10077.
251. Neyts J, Snoeck R, Schols D, et al. Sulfated polymers inhibit the interaction of human cytomegalovirus with cell surface heparan sulfate. *Virology*. 1992;189:48-58.
252. Compton T, Nowlin DM, Cooper NR. Initiation of human cytomegalovirus infection requires initial interaction with cell surface heparan sulfate. *Virology*. 1993;193:834-841.
253. Feire AL, Koss H, Compton T. Cellular integrins function as entry receptors for human cytomegalovirus via a highly conserved disintegrin-like domain. *Proc Natl Acad Sci U S A*. 2004;101:15470-15475.
254. Soroceanu L, Akhavan A, Cobbs CS. Platelet-derived growth factor-α receptor activation is required for human cytomegalovirus infection. *Nature*. 2008;455:391-395.
255. Bergelson JM, Shepley MP, Chan BM, et al. Identification of the integrin VLA-2 as a receptor for echovirus 1. *Science*. 1992;255:1718-1720.
256. Bergelson JM, Chan M, Solomon KR, et al. Decay-accelerating factor (CD55), a glycosylphosphatidylinositol-anchored complement regulatory protein, is a receptor for several echoviruses. *Proc Natl Acad Sci U S A*. 1994;91:6245-6249.
257. Ward T, Pipkin PA, Clarkson NA, et al. Decay-accelerating factor CD55 is identified as the receptor for echovirus 7 using CELICS, a rapid immuno-focal cloning method. *EMBO J*. 1994;13:5070-5074.
258. Fingeroth JD, Weis JJ, Tedder TF, et al. Epstein-Barr virus receptor of human B lymphocytes is the C3d receptor CR2. *Proc Natl Acad Sci U S A*. 1984;81:4510-4514.

259. Frade R, Barel M, Ehlin-Henriksson B, et al. gp140, the C3d receptor of human B lymphocytes, is also the Epstein-Barr virus receptor. *Proc Natl Acad Sci U S A.* 1985;82:1490-1493.

260. Gavrilovskaya IN, Shepley M, Shaw R, et al. β3 integrins mediate the cellular entry of hantaviruses that cause respiratory failure. *Proc Natl Acad Sci U S A.* 1998;95:7074-7079.

261. Bonaparte MI, Dimitrov AS, Bossart KN, et al. Ephrin-B2 ligand is a functional receptor for Hendra virus and Nipah virus. *Proc Natl Acad Sci U S A.* 2005;102:10652-10657.

262. Negrete OA, Levroney EL, Aguilar HC, et al. EphrinB2 is the entry receptor for Nipah virus, an emergent deadly paramyxovirus. *Nature.* 2005;436:401-405.

263. Kaplan G, Totsuka A, Thompson P, et al. Identification of a surface glycoprotein on African green monkey kidney cells as a receptor for hepatitis A virus. *EMBO J.* 1996;15:4282-4296.

264. Pileri P, Uematsu Y, Campagnoli S, et al. Binding of hepatitis C virus to CD81. *Science.* 1998;282:938-941.

265. Lindenbach BD, Evans MJ, Syder AJ, et al. Complete replication of hepatitis C virus in cell culture. *Science.* 2005;309: 623-626.

266. Scarselli E, Ansuini H, Cerino R, et al. The human scavenger receptor class B type I is a novel candidate receptor for the hepatitis C virus. *EMBO J.* 2002;21:5017-5025.

267. Bartosch B, Vitelli A, Granier C, et al. Cell entry of hepatitis C virus requires a set of co-receptors that include the CD81 tetraspanin and the SR-B1 scavenger receptor. *J Biol Chem.* 2003;278:41624-41630.

268. Evans MJ, von Hahn T, Tscherne DM, et al. Claudin-1 is a hepatitis C virus co-receptor required for a late step in entry. *Nature.* 2007;446:801-805.

269. Cseke G, Maginnis MS, Cox RG, et al. Integrin αvβ1 promotes infection by human metapneumovirus. *Proc Natl Acad Sci U S A.* 2009;106:1566-1571.

270. Manel N, Kim FJ, Kinet S, et al. The ubiquitous glucose transporter GLUT-1 is a receptor for HTLV. *Cell.* 2003;115: 449-459.

271. Higa HH, Rogers GN, Paulson JC. Influenza virus hemagglutinins differentiate between receptor determinants bearing N-acetyl-, N-glycollyl-, and N,O-diacetylneuraminic acid groups. *Virology.* 1985;144:279-282.

272. Akula SM, Pramod NP, Wang FZ, et al. Integrin α3β1 (CD 49c/29) is a cellular receptor for Kaposi's sarcoma-associated herpesvirus (KSHV/HHV-8) entry into the target cells. *Cell.* 2002;108:407-419.

273. Cao W, Henry MD, Borrow P, et al. Identification of alpha-dystroglycan as a receptor for lymphocytic choriomeningitis virus and Lassa fever virus. *Science.* 1998;282:2079-2081.

274. Dörig RE, Marcil A, Chopra A, et al. The human CD46 molecule is a receptor for measles virus (Edmonston strain). *Cell.* 1993;75:295-305.

275. Naniche D, Varior-Krishnan G, Cervoni F, et al. Human membrane cofactor protein (CD46) acts as a cellular receptor for measles virus. *J Virol.* 1993;67:6025-6032.

276. Tatsuo H, Ono N, Tanaka K, et al. SLAM (CDw150) is a cellular receptor for measles virus. *Nature.* 2000;406:893-897.

277. Brown KE, Anderson SM, Young NS. Erythrocyte P antigen: Cellular receptor for B19 parvovirus. *Science.* 1993;262: 114-117.

278. Elphick GF, Querbes W, Jordan JA, et al. The human polyomavirus, JCV, uses serotonin receptors to infect cells. *Science.* 2004;306:1380-1383.

279. Thoulouze MI, Lafage M, Schachner M, et al. The neural cell adhesion molecule is a receptor for rabies virus. *J Virol.* 1998;72:7181-7190.

280. Tuffereau C, Benejean J, Blondel D, et al. Low-affinity nerve-growth factor receptor (P75NTR) can serve as a receptor for rabies virus. *EMBO J.* 1998;17:7250-7259.

281. Gentsch JR, Pacitti AF. Effect of neuraminidase treatment of cells and effect of soluble glycoproteins on type 3 reovirus attachment to murine L cells. *J Virol.* 1985;56:356-364.

282. Paul RW, Choi AH, Lee PWK. The α-anomeric form of sialic acid is the minimal receptor determinant recognized by reovirus. *Virology.* 1989;172:382-385.

283. Maginnis MS, Forrest JC, Kopecky-Bromberg SA, et al. β1 integrin mediates internalization of mammalian reovirus. *J Virol.* 2006;80:2760-2770.

284. Greve JM, Davis G, Meyer AM, et al. The major human rhinovirus receptor is ICAM-1. *Cell.* 1989;56:839-847.

285. Staunton DE, Merluzzi VJ, Rothlein R, et al. A cell adhesion molecule, ICAM-1, is the major surface receptor for rhinoviruses. *Cell.* 1989;56:849-853.

286. Tomassini JE, Graham D, DeWitt CM, et al. cDNA cloning reveals that the major group rhinovirus receptor on HeLa cells is intercellular adhesion molecule 1. *Proc Natl Acad Sci U S A.* 1989;86:4907-4911.

287. Hofer F, Gruenberger M, Kowalski H, et al. Members of the low-density lipoprotein receptor family mediate cell entry of a minor-group common cold virus. *Proc Natl Acad Sci U S A.* 1994;91:1839-1842.

288. Fukudome K, Yoshie O, Konno T. Comparison of human, simian, and bovine rotaviruses for requirement of sialic acid in hemagglutination and cell adsorption. *Virology.* 1989;172: 196-205.

289. Willoughby RE, Yolken RH, Schnaar RL. Rotaviruses specifically bind to the neutral glycosphingolipid asialo-GM1. *J Virol.* 1990;64:4830-4835.

290. Hewish MJ, Takada Y, Coulson BS. Integrins α2β1 and α4β1 can mediate SA11 rotavirus attachment and entry into cells. *J Virol.* 2000;74:228-236.

291. Graham KL, Halasz P, Tan Y, et al. Integrin-using rotaviruses bind α2β1 integrin α2 I domain via VP4 DGE sequence and recognize αXβ2 and αVβ3 by using VP7 during cell entry. *J Virol.* 2003;77:9969-9978.

133

Orthopoxviruses: Vaccinia (Smallpox Vaccine), Variola (Smallpox), Monkeypox, and Cowpox

INGER K. DAMON*

Background

The genus *Orthopoxvirus* belongs to the family of Poxviridae, a group of large complex double-stranded DNA viruses that replicate in the cytoplasm of the host cell and are defined by their genomic, structural, and antigenic similarities.[1,2] Humans can be infected by members of multiple poxvirus genera, but they are usually accidental hosts. Most human infections are zoonotic, and animal exposure and geographic location give clues to the etiologic agent. The orthopoxvirus, variola, however, is a selective human pathogen. Variola is the causative agent of smallpox, which in 1980 was declared by the World Health Organization (WHO) to be eradicated worldwide. Other orthopoxviruses known to infect humans are cowpox, vaccinia, and monkeypox. Species of poxvirus genera that infect humans, other than within the *Orthopoxvirus* genus, are discussed in Chapter 134. Recent comprehensive book chapter reviews and monographs on poxvirus virology have been published.[3-5]

The ability of sera raised against one orthopoxvirus species to cross neutralize another species is one of the fundamental reasons for cross protection provided with vaccination. Vaccinia virus is the orthopoxvirus species now characterized as the constituent of smallpox vaccine. In part because of the concern that variola could be used as an agent of bioterrorism or as a bioweapon (see Chapter 324), increased interest and research on orthopoxviruses and poxviruses has been seen. Significant new research on vaccinia is targeting both fundamental viral properties and use of the virus as a (vaccine) vector. The emergence in 2003 of human clinical illness caused by monkeypox in the United States and ongoing disease in Central Africa, the continued recurrence of human vaccinia infections in Brazil and the Indian subcontinent, and cowpox infections in Eurasia have also increased the need for knowledge of these viral pathogens. The orthopoxviruses, monkeypox virus, camelpox virus, and variola virus are all considered select agents by the Department of Health and Human Services (DHHS) or the U.S. Department of Agriculture (USDA); these considerations impose additional restrictions on use in research laboratories and on reporting on discovery of these agents in clinical specimens.[6]

Morphology and Chemical Structure

The poxviruses described in these chapters belong to the family Poxviridae, subfamily Chordopoxviridae.[1] The eight genera of vertebrate poxviruses are: *Orthopoxvirus, Parapoxvirus, Avipoxvirus, Capripoxvirus, Leporipoxvirus, Suipoxvirus, Molluscipoxvirus,* and *Yatapoxvirus.* Only species of *Orthopoxvirus, Parapoxvirus, Molluscipoxvirus,* and *Yatapoxvirus* are known to infect humans. The last three are discussed in Chapter 134. Orthopoxvirus virions are large and brick-shaped (as are the virions of yatapoxvirus and molluscipoxvirus). Poxvirus virions range in length from 220 to 450 nm and in width and depth from 140 to 260 nm.[7,8] The electron microscopic appearance of virions varies

somewhat with sample preparation.[3] On cryoelectron microscopy of unstained unfixed vitrified specimens, vaccinia and other orthopoxviruses appear as smooth rounded rectangles; a uniform core is surrounded by a 30-nm membrane. In conventional thin sections, the core appears dumbbell-shaped and is surrounded by a complex series of membranes. On negative stain, most virions have short surface tubules 10 nm in diameter and are referred to as M (mulberry) forms; a minority of virions, slightly larger and electron dense, appears to have a thick (20-nm to 25-nm) membrane or capsule (C form; Figure 133-1). Poxvirus particles contain about half of the approximately 200 potential virus genome-encoded proteins; virions are comprised of structural proteins and enzymes, including a virtually complete RNA polymerase system for primary transcription of viral genes.[3] The genome, which is within a nucleoprotein complex (nucleosome) inside the core, consists of a single linear molecule of double-stranded DNA that is composed, depending on the strain, of about 130 to 375 kilobase pairs of DNA and that is covalently closed at each end; the ends are hairpin-like telomeres. Complete genome DNA sequences have been reported for several different species of the orthopoxviruses described in this chapter; GenBank entries are compiled at a dedicated website (www.poxvirus.org).

During virus replication,[3,9,10] virion morphogenesis begins in the cytoplasm. Thin-section electron microscopic observations of cells early after infection show crescent-shaped membrane structures that progress to circular structures, called immature virions, which enclose a dense nucleoprotein complex. Primary transcription precedes the production of the crescents (cup shaped in three dimensions) and the immature virions. The bilayer surface membrane of the immature virion differentiates, with one layer becoming the outer membrane and the other becoming the core membrane, thereby forming an intracellular mature virion (MV). A small portion of MVs may be further processed to acquire a bilayer envelope of Golgi intermediate compartment membrane that contains specific viral proteins. The intracellular enveloped MV (IEV) then moves along cellular microtubules to the cell surface, where actin polymerizes behind IEV. IEVs exit the cell through distinctive microvilli by fusing the outermost lipoprotein layer with the plasma membrane, thereby releasing the MV within the inner lipoprotein layer. The released particle is the extracellular enveloped virion (EEV); enveloped virions (EVs) that stay attached to the outer surface of the cell are termed cell-associated EVs (CEVs). MVs and EVs are mature infectious particles, each with distinct surface antigenic properties. Enveloped and nonenveloped forms are believed to have different attachment sites on the cell[3]; however, the common result is fusion of the MV membrane with the plasma membrane, followed by entry and uncoating of the particle, release of viral contents into the cell, and initiation of virus-controlled transcription of early, intermediate, and late class proteins.[3] Fusion and entry processes have been recently reviewed.[5,11] Secretion or expression of viral proteins modulate the host immune response or intracellular signaling to permit the subsequent assembly, morphogenesis, release, and infectivity of progeny virions.

The dissemination of naturally released virions (EVs) is an important aspect of pathogenesis, and genes have been identified (e.g., *B5R*)

---

*All material in this chapter is in the public domain, with the exception of any borrowed figures or tables.

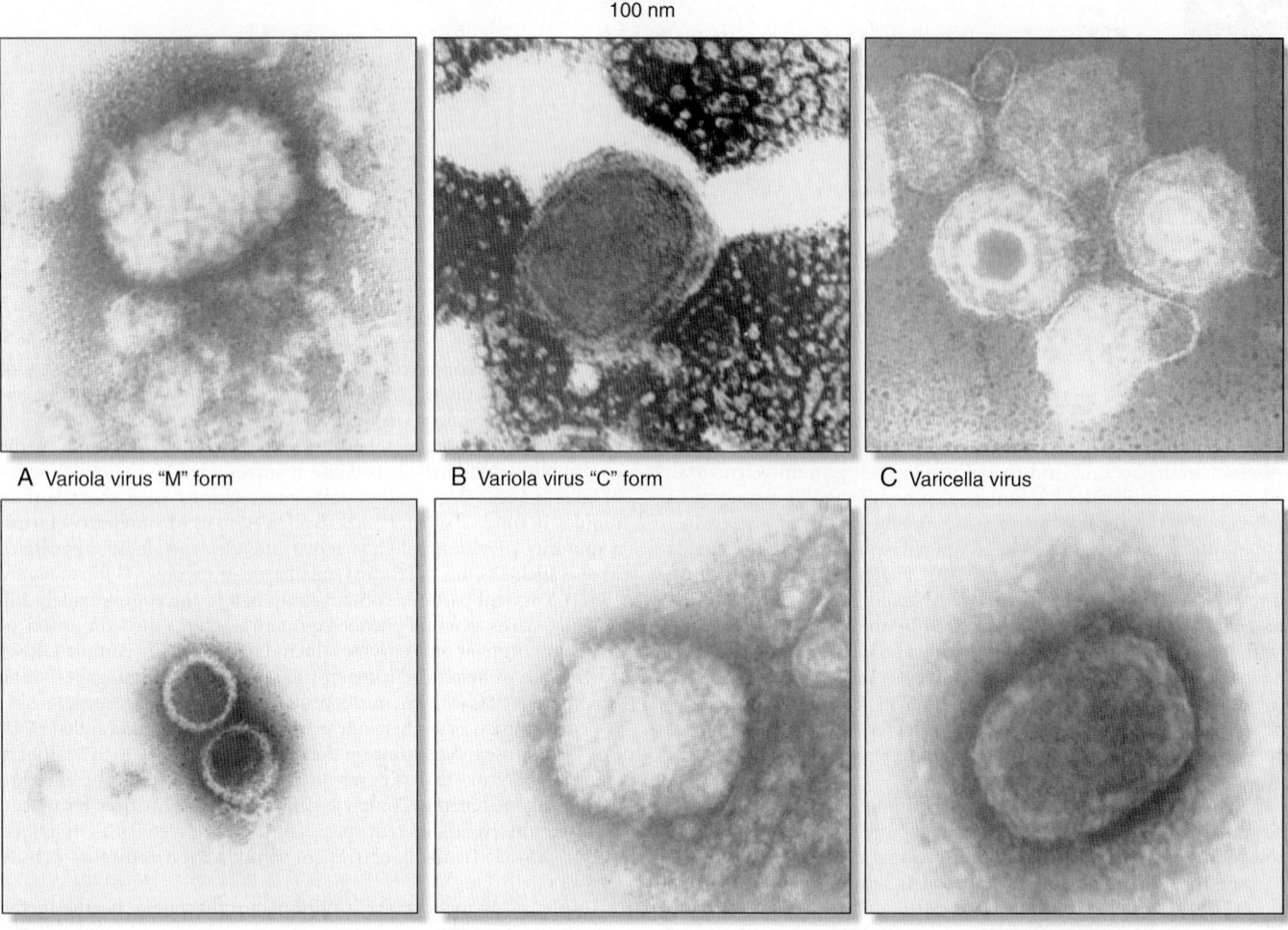

100 nm

A Variola virus "M" form   B Variola virus "C" form   C Varicella virus

D Varicella virus core   E Vaccinia virus "M" form   F Vaccinia virus "C" form

Figure 133-1   Electron micrographs of variola, varicella, and vaccinia virions. *(From the US CDC Public Health Information Library [PHIL] at http://phil.cdc.gov/phil/default.asp. Image ID 5 2426. Electron micrograph taken in 1975 by Dr James Nakano, CDC. This image is in the public domain and thus free of any copyright restrictions.)*

that code for proteins necessary for the proper development of EEVs and expression of virulence. Host cell factors are also involved in EEV dissemination.[9,10,12]

Pathogenesis

Poxvirus infections evolve either as a localized (skin) fairly benign infection or as a systemic infection. Systemic infection results in viral dissemination, with the formation of generalized skin lesions, and usually involves some degree of morbidity and mortality. The pathogenesis of human systemic orthopoxvirus infections is largely extrapolated and modeled from studies of the pathogenesis of the related orthopoxvirus infections in animals: mousepox (ectromelia) in mice, rabbitpox in rabbits, and monkeypox in nonhuman primates.[13-17] In addition, extensive literature exists on animal models used to examine the role of virally encoded proteins predicted to be involved in viral pathogenesis or used to examine the effect of therapeutic methods, or both.[18-20] The general paradigm for systemic orthopoxvirus pathogenesis is that the virus enters the host, through a respiratory route, a mucosal surface, or a break in the skin, and replicates locally. The virus then spreads through local lymphatics, causing a primary viremia, and subsequently spreads to the reticuloendothelial system. Replication in these organs results in the secondary viremia, usually associated with fever. The virus then ultimately seeds skin, causing a characteristic "pock" rash.

The host immune response probably involves all arms of the immune system. Complement, interferon, natural killer cells, and inflammatory cells are implicated in the early innate response; pox-specific antibodies (including neutralizing antibodies) are subsequent components of the humoral response, and pox-specific cytotoxic lymphocytes are involved in cellular clearance of infection.[21-26] Within their large genomes, poxviruses encode a number of proteins predicted to modulate the host's immune response, which affect both viral survival and disease pathogenesis. Various poxvirus-encoded proteins are predicted to bind and interfere with the function of host cytokines, chemokines, interferon, and complement. Other poxvirus-encoded proteins may interfere with apoptosis. Articles on immunomodulatory properties of poxviruses review specific properties of these virally encoded gene products.[5,27-29]

Vaccinia: Vaccine and Vaccine Adverse Events

Vaccinia is an orthopoxvirus and is the most studied of all poxviruses. At some point, it replaced cowpox as the smallpox "vaccine." The origin of vaccinia virus is uncertain.[30] A single strain of the virus, derived from the New York City Board of Health (NYCBOH) strain, is used for smallpox vaccine in the United States. Other strains have been used outside the United States.

Smallpox vaccine is administered with a special bifurcated needle designed to hold a small standardized inoculum of a live virus suspension between its prongs. The skin over the deltoid or triceps is pierced several times with the needle with enough vigor to allow a trace of blood to appear after several seconds. Within 2 to 5 days of inoculation, a papule forms at the vaccination site. This papule evolves into a vesicle and then a pustule, reaching its maximum size (about 1 cm in diameter) by 8 to 10 days after vaccination, after which it dries to a scab, which usually separates by day 14 to 21.[31,32] An areola may encircle the site as the lesion evolves. Low-grade fever is sometimes observed in children but rarely in adults. Regional lymphadenopathy may also occur. A scar at the inoculation site often provides lifelong evidence of successful vaccination, although a scar's presence may not guarantee a history of successful smallpox vaccination because it may have resulted from bacterial superinfection or vaccination with Calmette-Guérin bacillus.

IMMUNITY RESULTING FROM VACCINATION

Vaccinia immunization is cross protective against other orthopoxvirus infections, including variola. Preexposure vaccine efficacy is estimated to be as high as 100% for 1 to 3 years after vaccination,[33] and reports from the smallpox eradication efforts noted that "smallpox rarely occurs during the 4 or 5 years following successful vaccination in infancy."[34] Complete protection against smallpox after vaccination is not lifelong, although data suggest that substantial protection may persist for up to 15 to 20 years.[34-36] Experiences with monkeypox in the United States in 2003 suggest that immunity is not completely protective against systemic orthopoxvirus disease acquisition for more than 20 years after vaccination.[37,38] Protection against death from the disease may persist even longer than protection against disease.[39,40]

Likely because of the relatively long asymptomatic incubation period of systemic orthopoxvirus diseases (10 to 14 days), vaccinia is also effective as a postexposure prophylaxis when given to contacts of patients with smallpox. Vaccination should be performed as soon as possible after exposure; interpretation of data from the eradication program suggests that vaccination may not be as effective if given more than 3 days after the exposure.[41-44] Effectiveness was greater for those vaccinated previously.

Despite recent advances, the correlates of immunity against smallpox are poorly understood. Humoral responses, including neutralizing antibody, correlate with protection in both animal[45] and human[46-48] studies. Cell-mediated and T-cell responses are also believed to be critical for successful vaccination.[49] T-cell responses have been documented up to 35 years after vaccination.[50-52] Neutralizing antibody responses are also long lived.[51,53,54]

COMPLICATIONS RESULTING FROM VACCINATION

Of all vaccines used today, the smallpox vaccine has one of the highest rates of adverse events (http://www.cdc.gov/mmwr/preview/mmwrhtml/rr5204a1.htm).[31,55-59] Major complications include progressive vaccinia, eczema vaccinatum, generalized vaccinia, accidental infection, postvaccinial encephalitis, and carditis.

Progressive vaccinia, previously called vaccinia necrosum or vaccinia gangrenosum, is a rare and often fatal vaccine complication in persons with severe deficiencies of cellular immunity.[55] In 1 year (1968) in the United States, five cases among 6 million primary vaccinations and six cases among 8.6 million revaccinations were found.[57] Four of these 11 patients died. Progressive vaccinia is characterized by progressive often painless growth and spread of the vaccine virus beyond the inoculation site, often leading to necrosis, sometimes with metastases to other body sites.[60] This diagnosis should be considered if the vaccination site lesion continues to progress and expand without apparent healing more than 15 days after vaccination.[61] Initially, limited or no inflammation is present at the site, and histopathologic examination shows an absence of inflammatory cells.[62] Management of progressive vaccinia has historically included aggressive therapy with vaccinia immune globulin (VIG), methisazone, débridement, and whole blood transfusions from previously vaccinated individuals. The last procedure, designed to bolster cell-mediated immunity, often resulted in a graft-versus-host reaction.[60] Methisazone is now regarded as ineffective therapy. Supportive measures and attention to prevention of secondary bacterial infections are beneficial, and newer therapeutic agents such as cidofovir may also have a role, although its efficacy is unproven.[31,55] VIG is available from the Centers for Disease Control and Prevention (CDC) as an intravenous formulation.

Eczema vaccinatum can occur in people with a history of atopic dermatitis (eczema) irrespective of disease severity or activity. This complication is the clinical result of local spread or dissemination from the primary vaccination site in such persons or the result of inadvertent contact of another's unscabbed vaccination site with a susceptible atopic individual's skin.[63,64] A localized or generalized papular, vesicular, or pustular rash anywhere on the body or localized to previous eczematous lesions is the clinical presentation. Systemic illness with fever, malaise, and lymphadenopathy may occur. In the 1968 national survey, 66 cases (no deaths) among 14.5 million vaccinations (4.6 cases per million) and 60 cases (one death) among several million contacts were found. Treatment of eczema vaccinatum included the administration of VIG (0.6 mL/kg IM per 24 hours, repeated until no further lesions arise),[33] hemodynamic support with fluid replacement and electrolyte monitoring, and skin care.[31] In one study, early VIG administration reduced the mortality rate from 30% to 40% to 7%.[65] In 2007, a severe case of eczema vaccinatum was successfully treated with a combination of multiple doses of VIG IV, a single dose of cidofovir, a multiple day course of a compound under investigational study (ST-246, discussed in the section on therapy), intensive skin care management, and skin grafting.[66]

Generalized vaccinia is a nonspecific term that is used to describe a vesicular rash that develops after vaccination. Excluding dissemination associated with eczema vaccinatum and progressive vaccinia, documentation of virus in these vesicular rash lesions has been extremely rare[67]; true generalized vaccinia is believed to represent the end product of viremic spread of virus. No predisposing factors have been identified. Treatment is generally not necessary because the generalized rash is self-limited. The lesions evolve and resolve more quickly than the primary vaccination site, presumably because of a developing immune response to the virus. This complication is estimated to occur in about 242 of every 1 million primary vaccinations (http://www.bt.cdc.gov/agent/smallpox/vaccination/reactions-vacc-clinic.asp). In general, this complication of vaccination does not necessitate the administration of VIG unless it is severe and the patient is systemically ill or the patient has an underlying immunocompromising condition. Treatment with nonsteroidal anti-inflammatory agents or oral antipruritics may provide symptomatic relief.[31]

Postvaccination encephalomyelitis (PVEM) is a rare but serious complication that usually occurs only in primary vaccinees. The frequency of its occurrence differs widely from country to country and with the strain of vaccinia virus used in the vaccine. In the survey conducted in the United State in 1968, the frequency was 2.9 to 12.3 per million first-time vaccinees.[31] The incidence of PVEM was lower with the NYCBOH vaccinia virus strain than with the strain used in other countries.[68] No predisposing factors are known, although host factors are believed to be important; the pathophysiology is not well understood. Cases have variably displayed clinical and diagnostic features suggestive of a postimmunization demyelinating encephalomyelitis/acute demyelinating encephalomyelitis (ADEM) or direct viral invasion of the nervous system. This postvaccination reaction typically occurs 11 to 15 days after vaccination. Symptoms of PVEM include fever, headache, vomiting, confusion, delirium, disorientation, restlessness, drowsiness or lethargy, seizures, and coma. The cerebrospinal fluid can have an elevated pressure but generally has a normal cell count and chemistry profile.[69-71]

Infants younger than 2 years can also have a rare postvaccination encephalopathy (PVE) similar to PVEM develop. Acute onset of PVE occurs earlier in the postvaccination period (6 to 10 days after vaccination), involves the same symptoms as PVEM, and may also include hemiplegia and aphasia.[4,31]

The diagnosis of PVE or PVEM is one of exclusion because no specific tests are available to confirm the diagnosis of this complication and many other infectious and toxic etiologies can result in a similar clinical picture. Recent cases have shown the presence of orthopoxvirus-reactive antibodies in the cerebrospinal fluid (CSF).[72,73] The role of antiviral medications is unclear; VIG, although effective prophylactically, has not shown clear benefit after symptom onset. A few recent cases have responded to some combination of IVIG, steroids, and VIG.[72] A review of the pathogenesis of ADEM, and suggested therapies, is available (also see Chapter 87).[74]

Accidental infection occurs when virus from the vaccination site is transferred to another site or to another person through intimate skin contact. It usually occurs in primary vaccinees rather than revaccinees. Accidental self inoculation, which most commonly occurs on the face, mouth, lips, or genitalia, is usually not serious and requires no specific treatment. Inoculation of the conjunctiva, cornea, or eyelid is more serious and can be sight-threatening if not evaluated and treated appropriately. In the 5 years between 1963 and 1968, ocular vaccinia was observed in 348 persons: 259 vaccinees and 66 contacts. Of these, 22 had evidence of corneal involvement and 11 had permanent defects.[75] No controlled trials of therapeutics exist; current topical optic antivirals (trifluorothymidine, vidarabine)[76] have in vitro activity against vaccinia, and their off-label use for this purpose has been recommended by some ophthalmologists.[31]

Cardiac adverse events are rare and had not been reported before 2003 in any person vaccinated with the NYCBOH strain. Myocarditis had been reported after vaccination with the vaccine strains used in Europe and Australia,[77,78] and in the U.S. military population, myopericarditis was documented in 18 of 230,734 primary vaccinees immunized with the NYCBOH strain between 2002 and 2003.[79] Arrhythmias and myocardial ischemia have also been described, but the association with vaccination is not as clear.[80-84]

Vaccination programs designed to help civilian public health preparedness and military preparedness for the possible use of smallpox as a weapon of bioterrorism, implemented in 2002 through 2003, have documented lower adverse event rates than previously seen, in part because of stringent criteria and education programs to screen persons at risk for complications (http://www.bt.cdc.gov/agent/smallpox/vaccination/index.asp).[80,85,86] Nonetheless, instances of generalized rash, which may arise 10 to 14 days after vaccination, continued to be reported. On a clinical basis alone, distinguishing among generalized vaccinia is often difficult, which represents virus presumably spread hematogenously, a form of erythema multiforme, or erythematous urticaria eruptions that may be immunologically mediated. Laboratory identification of virus within the disseminated rash may differentiate these conditions. Studies of recent vaccination efforts have also identified focal and generalized folliculitis associated with vaccination.[87]

The 2001 recommendations of the Advisory Committee on Immunization Practices (ACIP) on vaccinia vaccination are available at http://www.cdc.gov/mmwr/preview/mmwrhtml/rr5010a1.htm. The ACIP recommends vaccination as a safeguard for laboratory and health care workers who are at high risk for orthopoxvirus infection. In the United States, the CDC Drug Service provides the vaccine after CDC approval of a formal request for this purpose by the administering physician. Vaccinia immunoglobulin is available to treat possible postvaccination complications, which can be severe. Supplemental recommendations of the ACIP were published in 2003 and constitute advice on vaccination of persons designated by public health authorities to conduct investigation and follow-up of initial smallpox cases that might necessitate direct contact with the patient. These recommendations are available at http://www.cdc.gov/mmwr/preview/mmwrhtml/rr5207a1.htm.[88] Recently, in the United States, the use of a cell-culture–grown clonal derivative of the NYCBOH/Dryvax (Wyeth Pharmaceuticals, Collegeville, PA) smallpox vaccine has replaced use of Dryvax. Studies and development of this new vaccine, ACAM2000, have been recently reviewed.[89]

VACCINIA VIRUS AS A ZOONOSIS

Vaccinia virus infections are not generally regarded as naturally occurring, although vaccinee-to-cattle and cattle-to-human transmissions occurred on farms during the smallpox eradication campaign. Sporadic outbreaks of infection caused by the vaccinia virus subspecies buffalopox virus that involve transmission between milking buffalo, cattle, and people have been reported, mainly in India but also in Egypt, Bangladesh, Pakistan, and Indonesia. Vaccinia-like lesions have been observed on the animals' teats and the milkers' hands. Biologic data and limited DNA analyses of isolates from an outbreak in India in 1985 suggest that buffalopox virus may be derived from vaccinia virus strains transmitted from humans to livestock during the smallpox vaccination era.[90-92] A vaccinia virus possibly related to the vaccine strain used during smallpox eradication in Brazil was found in cattle and farm worker handlers in rural Rio de Janeiro.[93,94] Subsequent reports and surveillance efforts indicate that these vaccinia virus infections are ongoing and that at least two clades or subgroups of vaccinia are circulating in Brazil, likely representing low-level endemic disease.[95-97] The ecologic factors that support the persistence of vaccinia in this region of the world remain unknown and are a topic of study.[98,99] In addition, at least one instance was found of human infection with a vaccinia-vector recombinant rabies virus vaccine in a bait dispersed to control rabies in wildlife; the bait was carried home by the family dog.[100]

VARIOLA

In 1980, the WHO General Assembly declared that smallpox had been eradicated; destruction of the remaining virus stocks, scheduled for 1999 and then 2002, has been delayed in an effort to permit research for improved preparedness in the event smallpox recurs as the result of the malevolent use of variola virus. The virus has a strict human host range and no animal reservoir. Variola major strains produced a disease with a severe prodrome, fever, and prostration. The virus was most often transmitted between humans via large-droplet respiratory particles inhaled by susceptible persons who had prolonged close face-to-face contact with an infectious person; it was spread less commonly via aerosol or direct contact with the rash lesion or sloughed crust material from the scab.[101] A toxemia or other form of systemic shock led to case-fatality rates of up to 30%. Secondary attack rates among unvaccinated contacts within households ranged from 30% to 80%. Variola minor strains (alastrim, amass, or Kaffir viruses) produced less severe infection and case-fatality rates of less than 1%, although secondary attack rates among unvaccinated contacts within households also ranged from 30% to 80%. The last naturally occurring smallpox case was in Somalia in October 1977, although a fatal laboratory-associated infection with variola major virus occurred at the University of Birmingham, England, in August 1978.[101]

Naturally acquired variola virus infection caused a systemic febrile rash illness. For ordinary smallpox, the most common clinical presentation, after an asymptomatic incubation period of 10 to 14 days (range, 7 to 17 days), was fever, with the temperature quickly rising to about 103° F, sometimes with dermal petechiae. Associated constitutional symptoms included backache, headache, vomiting, and prostration. Within a day or two after incubation, a systemic rash appeared that was characteristically centrifugally distributed (i.e., lesions were present in greater numbers on the oral mucosa, face, and extremities than on the trunk). Lesions were commonly manifested on the palms and soles (Figs. 133-2 and 133-3). Initially, the rash lesions appeared macular, then papular, enlarging and progressing to a vesicle by days 4 to 5 and a pustule by day 7; lesions were encrusted and scabby by day 14 and sloughed off (Fig. 133-4). Skin lesions were deep seated and in the same stage of development in any one area of the body. Milder and more severe forms of the rash were also documented. Less severe manifestations (modified smallpox or variola sine eruptione) occurred in some vaccinated individuals, whereas hemorrhagic or flat-pox types of smallpox are thought to have developed as a result of impaired immune response of patients.

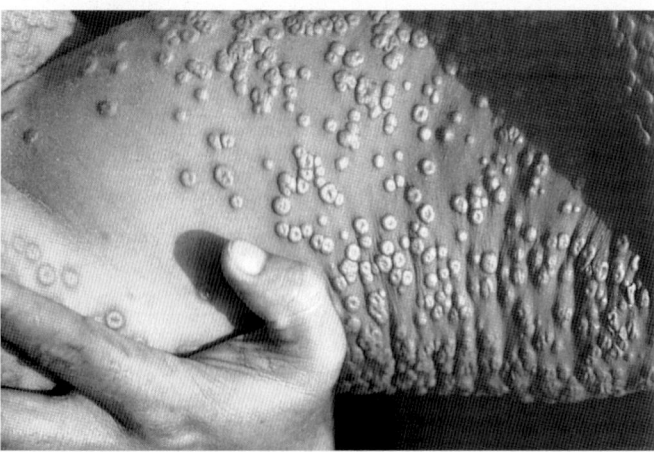

Figure 133-2   Smallpox lesions on skin of trunk. *(From the US CDC PHIL at http://phil.cdc.gov/phil/default.asp. Image ID 5 284. Photograph taken in 1973 by James Hicks, CDC. This image is in the public domain and thus free of any copyright restrictions.)*

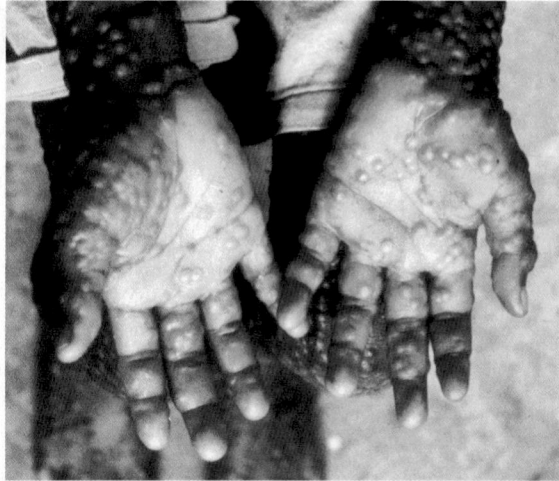

Figure 133-3   This child was infected with the smallpox virus and on day 8 of the rash shows the typical lesions on his palms. *(From the US CDC PHIL at http://phil.cdc.gov/phil/default.asp. Image ID 5 3303. Photograph taken in 1972 by Dr Paul B. Dean, CDC. This image is in the public domain and thus free of any copyright restrictions.)*

Variola major smallpox was differentiated into the following four main clinical types:

1. Ordinary smallpox (90% of cases) produced viremia, fever, prostration, and rash; mortality rates were generally proportionate to the extent of rash. With the WHO classification, mortality rates ranged from less than 10% for "ordinary discrete" smallpox to 50% to 75% for the rarer "ordinary confluent" presentation.
2. (Vaccine)-modified smallpox (5% of cases) produced a mild prodrome with few skin lesions in previously vaccinated people and a mortality rate well under 10%.
3. Flat smallpox (5% of cases) produced slowly developing focal lesions with generalized infection and an approximate 50% fatality rate.
4. Hemorrhagic smallpox (<1% of cases) induced bleeding into the skin and the mucous membranes and was invariably fatal within a week of onset.

A discrete type of the ordinary form, with a typical febrile prodrome and rash, resulted from alastrim variola minor infection.[101] The WHO established a classification system for smallpox case types based on disease presentation and rash burden. The hemorrhagic and flat types have already been briefly described. The ordinary type was subgrouped into three categories on the basis of the extent of rash on the face and the body. In the ordinary confluent category, no area of skin was visible between vesiculopustular rash lesions on the trunk or the face. Patches of normal skin were visible between rash lesions on the trunk in ordinary semiconfluent disease and on the face in ordinary discrete disease. (Vaccine)-modified disease arose with sparse numbers of lesions. Infection conferred lifelong immunity.[101,102]

Before its eradication, smallpox as a clinical entity was relatively easy to recognize, but other exanthematous illnesses were mistaken for this disease.[101-103] For example, the rash of severe chickenpox, caused by varicella-zoster virus, was often misdiagnosed as that of smallpox. However, chickenpox produces a centripetally distributed rash and rarely appears on the palms and soles. In addition, in the case of chickenpox, prodromal fever and systemic manifestations are mild, if manifest at all; the lesions are superficial in nature; and lesions in different developmental stages may be present in the same area of the body. Other diseases confused with vesicular-stage smallpox included monkeypox, generalized vaccinia, disseminated herpes zoster, disseminated herpes simplex virus infection, drug reactions (eruptions), erythema multiforme, enteroviral infections, scabies, insect bites, impetigo, and molluscum contagiosum. Diseases confused with hemorrhagic smallpox included acute leukemia, meningococcemia, and idiopathic thrombocytopenic purpura. The CDC, in collaboration with numerous professional organizations, has developed an algorithm for evaluation of patients with smallpox. The algorithm assists in differential diagnoses of the vesiculopustular stage of rash. The algorithm and additional laboratory testing information are available at http://emergency.cdc.gov/agent/smallpox/diagnosis/#diagnosis. The differential diagnosis of febrile vesicular pustular rash illnesses is presented in Table 133-1.

Monkeypox

Monkeypox virus was so named because it was first detected in captive Asiatic monkeys; however, the virus has been found naturally only in Africa (although it emerged in the United States as a result of global

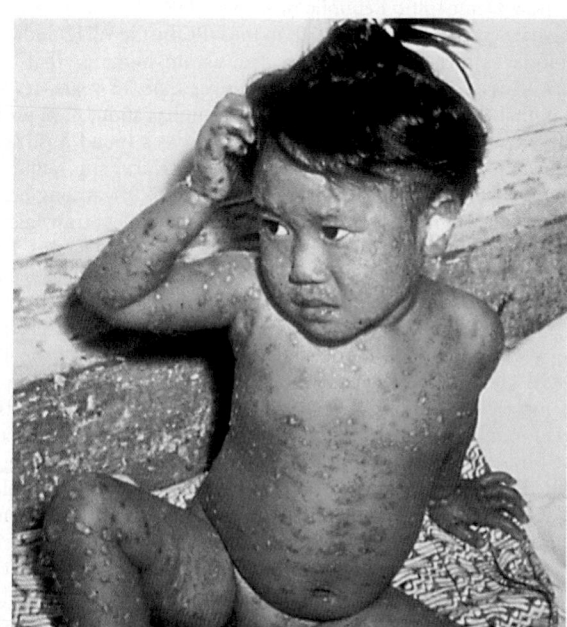

Figure 133-4   Smallpox lesions at day 17 of rash on a 5-year-old convalescing Indonesian child. *(From the US CDC PHIL at http://phil.cdc.gov/phil/default.asp. Image ID 5 2041. Photograph taken in 1963 by J. D. Millar, CDC. This image is in the public domain and thus free of any copyright restrictions.)*

TABLE 133-1	Differential Diagnosis of Febrile Vesicular Pustular Rash Illnesses That May Be Confused with Smallpox
Disease	**Clues**
Varicella	Most common in children younger than 10 years; children do not usually have a viral prodrome.
Disseminated herpes zoster	Immunocompromised or elderly persons; rash looks like varicella, usually begins or erupts in dermatomal pattern.
Impetigo (*Streptococcus pyogenes, Staphylococcus aureus*)	Honey-colored crusted plaques with bullae are classic but may begin as vesicles.
Drug eruptions	Exposure to medications.
Erythema multiforme minor	Target or bull's-eye lesions; often follows systemic viral infections such as herpes simplex; may include palms and soles.
Erythema multiforme (including Stevens-Johnson)	Involves conjunctivae and mucous membranes.
Enteroviral infections (especially hand, foot, and mouth disease)	Seasonal—summer and fall.
Disseminated herpes simplex	Similar to varicella.
Scabies and insect bites	Pruritus; patient not febrile.
Molluscum contagiosum	May disseminate in immunosuppressed individuals.
Generalized vaccinia	History of vaccination with smallpox vaccine or contact with vaccinated individual.
Monkeypox	Travel to endemic area; animal exposure.

Adapted from Evaluating Patients for Smallpox: Acute Generalized Vesicular or Pustular Rash Illness Protocol, at http://www.bt.cdc.gov/agent/smallpox/diagnosis/pdf/spox-poster-full.pdf.

commerce), and evidence points to rodents as important reservoir hosts. Reviews of human monkeypox infection are available.[104,105]

Monkeypox was first recognized by Von Magnus in Copenhagen in 1958 as an exanthema of primates in captivity. Later, the disease was seen in other captive animals, including primates in zoos and animal import centers. Particular attention was focused on it in 1970 when smallpox surveillance activities in Africa revealed cases of human monkeypox, clinically indistinguishable from smallpox, particularly in Zaire (now Democratic Republic of Congo [DRC]). Serosurveys and virologic investigations in the 1980s in the DRC by the WHO indicated that monkeys are sporadically infected, as are humans; that three fourths of cases, mainly in children younger than 15 years, resulted from animal contact; that vaccinia vaccination has about 85% protective efficacy; that monkeypox virus probably has a broad host range, including squirrels (*Funisciurus* spp. and *Heliosciurus* spp.); and that human monkeypox has a secondary attack rate of 9% among unvaccinated contacts within households (i.e., it is much less transmissible than smallpox). Since 1970, the disease has been seen in the DRC, Liberia, Ivory Coast, Sierra Leone, Nigeria, Benin, Cameroon, and Gabon; most cases have been in the DRC, which in 1980 had a population of about 30 million (338 cases were discovered prospectively during WHO-intensified monkeypox surveillance in Zaire from 1981 to 1986). Human monkeypox has recently been reported from the DRC, mainly in children younger than 15 years. On the basis of reported monkeypox onset dates in a largely retrospective study complicated by a concurrent outbreak of chickenpox, about 250 serosubstantiated cases of monkeypox occurred among 0.5 million people in 78 villages from February 1996 to October 1997. About three fourths of the cases appeared to result from human-to-human transmission; however, the secondary attack rate of 8% among unvaccinated contacts within households appeared to be about the same as in the 1981 to 1986 surveillance.[104,106]

Sporadic outbreaks continue to occur and cause concern,[104,107] but the most detailed clinical, epidemiologic, and ecologic information about virologic laboratory–confirmed disease in Africa was obtained before 1988. Initial animal surveys in Zaire detected monkeypox-specific antibodies in 85 of 347 squirrels (25%) sampled but from none

of 233 terrestrial rodents. Monkeypox-specific antibody has been detected in very few monkeys, which, like humans, are probably only occasional hosts.[108] Subsequent work[106] in the DRC found evidence of orthopoxvirus seroreactivity in some small terrestrial mammals tested, including Gambian rats (*Cricetomys emini*) and elephant shrews (*Petrodromus tetradactylus*). Studies in the 1980s that used direct virus sampling of trapped animals revealed virus in only one *Funisciurus* species.

In 2003, monkeypox infection of humans was identified in the United States as a result of exposure to ill prairie dogs, probably infected after exposure to infected West African small mammals imported as exotic pets.[109] From that work, a Gambian rat (*Cricetomys gambianus*), rope squirrel (*Funisciurus* sp.), and dormouse (*Graphiurus* sp.) from the affected African shipment of exotic species, originating in Ghana and implicated in the U.S. monkeypox outbreak, were found to be infected with monkeypox with viral isolation and nucleic acid detection (polymerase chain reaction).[109]

PATHOGENESIS

The pathogenesis of human monkeypox is surmised to be similar to that of smallpox: an acute febrile exanthema with an incubation period of about 12 days. During the incubation period, the virus is distributed initially to internal organs and then to the skin.[101,105] The main differences are a greater degree of lymphadenopathy and a lower capacity for human case-to-case spread. The major concerns are the source of infection and the mode of transmission.

CLINICAL FEATURES

In general, the clinical features of disease as seen in central Africa are those of a classic or modified case of smallpox. The most obvious difference is the pronounced lymphadenopathy, which involves the submandibular, cervical, and sublingual regions.

Most cases occur in unvaccinated children. In Zaire from 1981 to 1986, 291 cases (86%) occurred in children younger than 10 years and only 12 of them (4%) had vaccination scars. The illness lasts 2 to 4 weeks. Of 292 unvaccinated patients, 22 (7.5%) had a mild illness with less than 25 skin lesions and were not incapacitated; 55 (19%) had 25 to 99 lesions, were incapable of most physical activity, and needed nursing; and 218 (75%) had more than 100 lesions, were totally incapacitated, and needed intensive nursing. Complications occurred in about 40% of patients; the most common were bacterial skin infections (16%), respiratory (12%) and gastrointestinal (5%) disorders, and keratitis (3.8%). The overall mortality rate was approximately 10%; however, all the deaths occurred in unvaccinated children, in whom the group mortality rate is about 15%.[105] In the United States, disease in the 2003 outbreak appears to have been milder, and only three of the 37 laboratory-confirmed cases had complications or serious disease: keratitis, encephalopathy (with diffuse cortical, thalamic, and brainstem edema, meningeal enhancement, and left thalamic and right parietal signal abnormality on magnetic resonance imaging [MRI]),[109] and upper respiratory tract lymphadenitis with dysphagia and airway compromise.[110] No deaths were observed. Although routes of exposure and host factors may have been significantly different in the African and U.S. outbreaks, evidence of differences between DRC/Congo Basin and U.S./West African viral strains/clades is also evident.[111-113] Additional animal and human studies are beginning to define some of the viral genetic differences that may contribute to the differences in pathogenicity and apparent interhuman transmissibility of the two viral clades.[114,115] The skin lesions of monkeypox are illustrated in Figure 133-5.

DIAGNOSIS

Until 2003, human monkeypox had not been detected outside Africa. Clinical diagnosis may present a problem because fewer physicians now have experience with smallpox, which human monkeypox closely

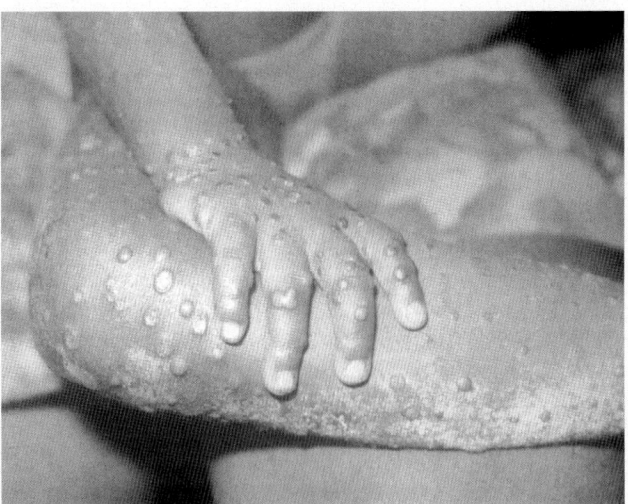

Figure 133-5 Monkeypox skin lesions.

resembles. In vaccinated individuals, the rash may be more pleomorphic and not in a uniform stage of development.[105] Access to a virus diagnostic laboratory should permit detection of the virus with electron microscopy and molecular methods, and this detection provides a diagnosis. In some circumstances, distinguishing between monkeypox and tanapox may be important. In the past, differentiation between monkeypox and variola was essential and could be done with examination of the pock appearance (hemorrhagic or not) and presence of pocks produced on chorioallantoic membrane at 39° C, a temperature that inhibits smallpox. Currently, an array of nucleic acid diagnostic techniques permits the speciation of these viruses.[116-121]

The close serologic relationships among orthopoxviruses make detection of monkeypox-specific antigens difficult, but methods are available and being refined that may be of value, particularly for epidemiologic studies of monkeypox virus in its natural reservoirs.[7,108] An immunoglobulin M (IgM) capture assay was shown to be sensitive and specific in identification of monkeypox cases 4 to 56 days after rash onset; this assay may have similar utility in the identification of human smallpox cases.[122]

EPIDEMIOLOGY AND CONTROL

Management of individual cases has been supportive, with case-to-case spread reduced with isolation and, if available, the use of smallpox vaccine for contacts. Potential use of newer therapeutics is discussed at the end of this chapter. Human cases in Africa occur in villages in the rain forests, where a variety of animals are captured for food. Infection of children might be explained by their playing or working with carcasses. The results of the comprehensive surveys carried out in the 1980s indicated that those infected were principally unvaccinated children and that case-to-case spread was unusual. Control measures are based on interposing a buffer zone of cleared land between the arboreal reservoir and cultivated land, the development of animal husbandry as a source of meat, and education in the handling of wildlife, with emphasis on any trapping done by those previously vaccinated; continued vaccination was not thought necessary.[105,108]

Only occasional human cases were reported from central Africa after cessation of routine surveillance activities after smallpox eradication, but a resurgence occurred in 1996 to 1997 that has not yet been fully explained. Increased political unrest leads to population displacement and breakdown of routine control measures, and the levels of vaccine-induced immunity decline with time. A potentially serious finding that requires clarification is the observation that human case-to-case transmission appears to have occurred more frequently from 1996 to 1997 than earlier.[107] More recently, a study of an outbreak in the Republic of Congo showed that the virus was transmitted quite

efficiently between successive generations of human transmission associated with a hospital compound; six generations of uninterrupted interhuman transmission were identified and supported with laboratory studies.[123] Human monkeypox continues to be reported in the Congo Basin, and mildly symptomatic monkeypox, or other orthopoxvirus infections, may also coexist in the area.[124-126] Comparison of the genomes of smallpox virus and monkeypox virus strains isolated up to 1986 suggested that they have evolved discretely,[127] and the results of complete genome analysis[128] confirm this observation. Laboratory workers studying monkeypox virus should be vaccinated with vaccinia and handle the virus in certified biosafety cabinets. Biosafety level 2 (BSL-2) containment, according to the *Biosafety in Microbiological and Biomedical Laboratories* definition, should be the minimum containment used. BSL-3 laboratory practices provide additional biosafety protection. As mentioned previously, additional select agent requirements apply to use of this virus.

Cowpox

COWPOX VIRUS

Cowpox sometimes occurs as a rare occupational infection of humans and can be acquired by contact with infected cows; more often, other animals (e.g., infected rats, pet cats, and zoo and circus elephants) have been sources of the disease. Phylogenies show that cowpox virus is a rather diverse species and is geographically restricted; it has been isolated from humans and a variety of animals in Europe and adjoining regions of Asia.[129-131] A serosurvey of wild animals in Great Britain found orthopoxvirus antibodies in a portion of bank and field voles and wood mice that were collected, which is consistent with small rodents being reservoir hosts for cowpox virus.[132]

CLINICAL

Most information is available from a detailed analysis of 54 human cases investigated from 1969 to 1993.[130] Lesions are generally restricted to the hands and face, and most patients (72%) have only one lesion. Multiple lesions may be caused by multiple primary inoculations, autoinoculation, and occasionally by lymphatic or viremic spread. Lesions in humans occur mainly on the fingers, with reddening and swelling; autoinoculation of other parts of the body may occur, and systemic severe infections have been reported, often in individuals with immunosuppression conditions.[133] Skin lesions are initially likened to those of a primary vaccinia virus vaccination; the site becomes papular, and in 4 to 5 days a vesicle develops. The lesion passes through macular, papular, vesicular, and pustular stages before forming a hard black crust. The lesion is usually painful, and erythema and edema are common at the late vesicular and pustular stages. Usually, lymphadenitis, fever, and general malaise occur, often referred to as influenza-like. These features are usually severe in children; 16 of 54 patients (30%) were hospitalized. Most cases take 6 to 8 weeks for recovery; in some cases, recovery can take more than 12 weeks. Scarring is usually permanent.

ORTHOPOXVIRUS LABORATORY DIAGNOSTICS

Electron microscopy of vesicle fluid or extracts of crusts is particularly valuable because it distinguishes between parapoxvirus, herpes virus, and other presumptive orthopoxvirus infections. Of 24 cases of cowpox in which adequate material was available, electron microscopy was successful in 23. Similar sensitivity was achieved in the diagnosis of smallpox.[8] Many protein-based diagnostic approaches have also been used[5,7] and further developed.[134] Nucleic acid–based diagnostics[117-119] are now commonly used to diagnose orthopoxvirus infections and to speciate them. Within currently defined species, not all strains of cowpox are identical, and genome analysis may show differences of epidemiologic value. As well, although the phylogenetic differences are not as great within the monkeypox virus and vaccinia virus species, diagnostic techniques have been developed to differentiate monkeypox virus clades and vaccinia strains.

Virus may be isolated on the chorioallantoic membrane, where the production of characteristic hemorrhagic pocks is diagnostic. A cytopathic effect occurs in many cell lines (Vero, MRC-5, RK13), and detection of A-type inclusions is usually diagnostic for human cowpox virus infections, as it would be if found in biopsy material.

■ Therapy: Orthopoxviruses

An active area of research involves the development and evaluation of therapeutics for orthopoxvirus infections. Currently, no antiviral drugs are licensed for use in the treatment of orthopoxvirus or other poxviral illnesses. Comprehensive reviews of the history and latest developments in poxvirus antivirals and therapeutics have been published.[5,76,135] In addition, such compounds are being tested on experimental models of variola-infected nonhuman primates[136] and on other animal models of orthopoxvirus infections.[19,20,137] Cidofovir, an antiviral in use for treatment of cytomegalovirus infections in patients with immunosuppression, appears to show promise as an antiviral for treatment of some poxvirus infections. The use of VIG is best described for treatment of certain complications of vaccinia (smallpox) vaccine administration,[31] but it may have utility in treatment of certain other orthopoxvirus infections. No clear benefit has been shown for this product alone in treatment of smallpox.[101]

The earliest drug compounds shown to have activity against orthopoxviruses, including vaccinia, were thiosemicarbazone derivatives. Initial case studies and case series suggested that they were effective in prophylaxis of smallpox and in treatment of progressive vaccinia and eczema vaccinatum.[138,139] However, subsequent double-blind controlled trials of smallpox prophylaxis revealed no benefit.[140]

A number of different classes of therapeutics have been tested for potential systemic or topical use against orthopoxviruses. These include compounds predicted to interfere with specific viral enzymes and cellular targets.[141] In vitro studies have usually focused on compounds currently licensed or under phase I or II study, although some novel compounds have also been studied. Promising candidates have then been studied in small animal models (mouse, rabbit, and others) and in nonhuman primates. Because monkeypox and smallpox both cause human illness, with mortality rates that range from 10% to 40% in nonvaccinated individuals, models have been designed to evaluate drug efficacy in systemic lethal disease created by intranasal, aerosol, or (historically) intracerebral virus challenge. Intravenous challenges classically have been designed to evaluate the effect of drug on rash development or illness progression, although higher challenge doses of virus have been used for a lethal model.[142] The primary animal models currently used involve a challenge of aerosolized or intranasal virus, which results in pulmonary disease and lethality. Models of localized rash lesions have involved scarification of animal skin. Treatment models of keratitis involve scarification of corneal tissue. Work evaluating the potential use of antivirals for treatment of systemic complications of vaccination (progressive vaccinia and eczema vaccinatum) has used immunodeficient mouse populations.

The most studied compounds are inhibitors of DNA polymerase. Some nucleoside analogue compounds with activity against herpesviruses, most notably acyclovir and its derivatives, do not have activity against poxviruses. Other compounds with antiherpesvirus activity do show in vitro and in vivo activity against poxviruses, specifically 5-iodo-2′-deoxyuridine, adenine arabinoside, and trifluorothymidine.[143-146] Because of their systemic toxicity, these compounds have also been used topically for treatment of orthopoxvirus (and herpes) ocular infections. Of the three compounds, trifluorothymidine appears to be most widely available. Many phosphonate-nucleoside analogues, for example, cidofovir, have antiorthopoxviral activity. In vitro, cidofovir has been shown to be active against the orthopoxviruses cowpox, vaccinia, monkeypox, and variola.[20,147,148] In in vivo studies, cidofovir has successfully protected challenged animals when given prophylactically or early in the evolution of disease, often before the onset of overt symptoms. Cidofovir has known renal toxicity and is administered with hydration and probenecid. It has a long intracellular half-life but is not orally bioavailable; the alkoxyalkyl ester analogue of cidofovir, 1-O-hexadecyloxypropyl cidofovir (HDP-CDV), is orally bioavailable, and a preliminary report of the protective effect of HDP-CDV (CMX-001) in mice challenged with aerosolized cowpox has been noted; as has its protective effect in a lethal model of mousepox infection.[148,149] Other nucleoside analogues are under study.[150,151]

ST-246 is a novel orally bioavailable compound with antiorthopoxvirus activity, characterized to inhibit orthopoxvirus release. Genetic characterization of viral mutants resistant to ST-246 indicate the viral target is the orthopoxvirus homologue of the vaccinia F13 protein, which is needed for wrapping of the virus before its release as an enveloped viral particle.[152] The drug has been shown to be active against multiple orthopoxvirus species, including monkeypox and variola virus.[153,154] ST-246 has been shown in a variety of small animal models, used prophylactically before the onset of symptoms or therapeutically after the onset of symptoms, to be effective in prevention of disease or to significantly mitigate illness severity and mortality.[155-157] As mentioned in the section on vaccinia virus, it has been used, in combination with other therapeutic methods, in the successful treatment of a severe human case of eczema vaccinatum. Recent animal studies have shown the drug has synergistic benefit when combined with CMX-001.[158]

Other antivirals tested against orthopoxviruses have predicted cellular targets. Ribavirin, an inosine monophosphate dehydrogenase inhibitor, shows *in vitro* activity against a number of orthopoxviruses[159] and has shown antiorthopoxviral activity in animal models of vaccinia-induced keratitis[160] and mouse tail pock lesions.[161] Case reports are seen of the use of ribavirin and VIG in the treatment of progressive vaccinia.[162] Initial therapy with ribavirin alone was ineffective at stemming new lesions; however, with the addition of VIG, new lesion development was stopped.

Additional studies of compounds targeting cellular kinases are of interest as another potential antiorthopoxvirus therapeutic strategy. Various cellular kinases (abl, src, and others) have been shown to be involved in the egress of virus, and blocking their function provides a different "antiviral" therapeutic mechanism of action.[163,164] Studies of an erbB kinase inhibitor (CI-1033) showed benefit in treatment of vaccinia-infected mice; its benefit was augmented with the use of a monoclonal antibody that neutralizes MV viral particles. In vitro, CI-1033 appeared to inhibit the local release of virus from an infected cell, so as to impede the ability of the virus to subsequently infect other surrounding (uninfected) cells.[165]

Recent comprehensive summaries of antiorthopoxvirus therapeutic development are available,[5,141,142,166,167,168] and this is an area of active research.

REFERENCES

1. Moyer RW, Arif BM, Black DN, et al. Poxviridae. In: van Regenmortel MHV, Fauquet CM, Bishop DHL, et al, eds. *Virus Taxonomy: Seventh Report of the International Committee on Taxonomy of Viruses*. San Diego: Academic Press; 2000:137-157.
2. Fenner F, Wittek R, Dumbell KR. *The Orthopoxviruses*. Boston: Academic Press; 1989:6.
3. Moss B. Poxviridae: The viruses and their replication. In: Fields BN, Knipe DM, Howley PM, et al, eds. *Fields' Virology*. 5th ed. Philadelphia: Lippincott Williams & Wilkins; 2007:2905-2947.
4. Damon IK. Poxviruses. In: Fields BN, Knipe DM, Howley PM, et al, eds. *Fields' Virology*. 5th ed. Philadelphia: Lippincott Williams & Wilkins; 2007:2947-2976.
5. Mercer AA, Schmidt A, Weber O, eds. *Poxviruses Advances in Infectious Diseases*. Boston: Birkhauser; 2007.
6. Centers for Disease Control and Prevention (CDC), Department of Health and Human Services (HHS). Possession, use, and transfer of select agents and toxins. Final rule. *Fed Regist*. 2008;73:61363-61366.
7. Damon IK. Poxviruses. In: Murray PR, Baron EJ, Jorgensen JH, et al, eds. *Manual of Clinical Microbiology*. 9th ed. Washington, DC: ASM Press; 2007:1631-1640.
8. Nakano JH. Poxviruses. In: Lennette EH, Schmidt NJ, eds. *Diagnostic Procedures for Viral, Rickettsial, and Chlamydial Infections*. 5th ed. Washington, DC: American Public Health Association; 1979:257-308.

9. Smith GL, Vanderplasschen A, Law M. The formation and function of extracellular enveloped vaccinia virus. *J Gen Virol.* 2002;83:2915-2931.
10. Smith GL. Vaccinia virus morphogenesis and dissemination. *Trends Microbiol.* 2008;16:472-479.
11. Moss B. Poxvirus entry and membrane fusion. *Virology.* 2006;344:48-54.
12. Payne LG. Significance of extracellular enveloped virus in the in vitro and in vivo dissemination of vaccinia virus. *J Gen Virol.* 1980;50:89-100.
13. Fenner F, Wittek R, Dumbell KR. *The Pathogenesis, Pathology, and Immunology of Orthopoxvirus Infections. The Orthopoxviruses.* Boston: Academic Press; 1989:85-141.
14. Roberts JA. Histopathogenesis of mousepox. I. Respiratory infection. *Br J Exp Pathol.* 1962;43:451-461.
15. Bedson HS, Duckworth MJ. Rabbitpox: An experimental study of the pathways of infection in rabbits. *J Pathol Bacteriol.* 1963;85:1-20.
16. Buller RM, Palumbo GJ. Poxvirus pathogenesis. *Microbiol Rev.* 1991;55:80-122.
17. Zaucha GM, Jahrling PB, Geisbert TW, et al. The pathology of experimental aerosolized monkeypox virus infection in cynomolgus monkeys (*Macaca fascicularis*). *Lab Invest.* 2001;81:1581-1600.
18. Smith S, Kotwal GJ. Immune response to poxvirus infections in various animals. *Crit Rev Microbiol.* 2002;28:149-185.
19. Martinez MJ, Bray M, Huggins JW. A mouse model of aerosol-transmitted orthopoxviral disease. *Arch Pathol Lab Med.* 2000;124:362-377.
20. Bray M, Martinez M, Smee DF, et al. Cidofovir protects mice against lethal aerosol or intranasal cowpox virus challenge. *J Infect Dis.* 2000;181:10-19.
21. Karupiah G, Fredrickson TN, Holmes KL, et al. Importance of interferons in recovery from mousepox. *J Virol.* 1993;63:4214-4226.
22. Wakamiya N, Okada N, Wang YL, et al. Tumor cells treated with vaccinia virus can activate the alternate pathway of mouse complement. *Jpn J Cancer Res.* 1989;80:765-770.
23. West BC, Eschete ML, Cox ME, et al. Neutrophil uptake of vaccinia virus in vitro. *J Infect Dis.* 1987;156:597-606.
24. Jones JF. Interactions between human neutrophils and vaccinia virus: Induction of oxidative metabolism and virus inactivation. *Pediatr Res.* 1982;16:525-529.
25. Doherty PC, Korngold R. Characteristics of poxvirus-induced meningitis: Virus specific and non-specific cytotoxic effectors in the inflammatory exudates. *Scand J Immunol.* 1983;18:1-7.
26. Blanden RV, Gardner ID. The cell-mediated response to ectromelia virus infection. I. Kinetics and characteristics of the primary effector T cell response in vivo. *Cell Immunol.* 1976;22:271-282.
27. Seet BT, Johnston JB, Brunetti CR, et al. Poxviruses and immune evasion. *Annu Rev Immunol.* 2003;21:377-423.
28. Smith GL, Symons JA, Khanna A, et al. Vaccinia virus immune evasion. *Immunol Rev.* 1997;159:137-154.
29. Johnston JB, MacFadden G. Poxvirus immunomodulatory strategies: Current perspectives. *J Virol.* 2003;77:6093-6100.
30. Baxby D. *Jenner's Smallpox Vaccine: The Riddle of Vaccinia Virus and Its Origin.* London: Heinemann Educational; 1981:1-214.
31. Cono J, Casey CG, Bell D. Smallpox vaccination and adverse reactions: Guidance for clinicians. *MMWR Recomm Rep.* 2003;52:1-28.
32. Arenstein AW, Rubins K, Relman DA. Smallpox vaccination. *N Engl J Med.* 2003;348:1925.
33. Neff JM. Vaccinia virus (cowpox). In: Mandell GL, Bennett JE, Dolin R, eds. *Principles and Practice of Infectious Diseases.* New York: Churchill Livingstone; 2000:1553-1555.
34. World Health Organization Expert Committee on Smallpox Eradication. Second report. *WHO Tech Rep Ser.* 1972;493:35.
35. Hammarlund E, Lewis MW, Hansen SG, et al. Duration of antiviral immunity after smallpox vaccination. *Nat Med.* 2003;9:1131-1137.
36. Taub DD, Ershler WB, Janowski M, et al. Immunity from smallpox vaccine persists for decades: A longitudinal study. *Am J Med.* 2008;121:1058-1064.
37. Karem KL, Reynolds M, Hughes C, et al. Monkeypox-induced immunity and failure of childhood smallpox vaccination to provide complete protection. *Clin Vaccine Immunol.* 2007;14:1318-1327.
38. Croft DR, Sotir MJ, Williams CJ, et al. Occupational risks during a monkeypox outbreak, Wisconsin, 2003. *Emerg Infect Dis.* 2007;13:1150-1157.
39. Mack TM. Smallpox in Europe, 1950-1971. *J Infect Dis.* 1972;125:161-169.
40. Hanna W, Baxby B. Studies in small-pox and vaccination. 1913. *Rev Med Virol.* 2002;12:201-209.
41. Massoudi MS, Barker L, Schwartz B. Effectiveness of postexposure vaccination for the prevention of smallpox: Results of a Delphi analysis. *J Infect Dis.* 2003;188:973-976.
42. Rao AR, Jacob ES, Kamalakshi S, et al. Epidemiological studies in smallpox: A study of intrafamilial transmission in a series of 254 infected families. *Indian J Med Res.* 1968;56:1826-1854.
43. Heiner GG, Fatima N, McCrumb FR. A study of intrafamilial transmission of smallpox. *Am J Epidemiol.* 1974;99:316-326.
44. Sommer A. The 1972 smallpox outbreak in Khulna Municipality, Bangladesh. II. Effectiveness of surveillance and containment in urban epidemic control. *Am J Epidemiol.* 1974;99:303-313.
45. Fenner F. Studies in mousepox: Infectious ectromelia of mice. IV. Quantitative investigations on the spread of virus through the host in actively and passively immunized animals. *Aust J Exp Biol Med.* 1947;27:1-18.
46. Mack TM, Noble J Jr, Thomas DB. A prospective study of serum antibody and protection against smallpox. *Am J Trop Med Hyg.* 1972;21:214-218.
47. Sarkar JK, Mitra AC, Mukherjee MK. The minimum protective levels of antibodies in smallpox. *Bull World Health Organ.* 1975;52:307-311.
48. McClain DJ, Harrison S, Yeager CL, et al. Immunologic responses to vaccinia vaccines administered by different parenteral routes. *J Infect Dis.* 1997;175:756-763.
49. Ennis FA, Cruz J, Demkowicz WE Jr, et al. Primary induction of human C^{D8+} cytotoxic T lymphocytes and interferon-γ–producing T cells after smallpox vaccination. *J Infect Dis.* 2002;185:1657-1659.
50. Demkowicz WE Jr, Littaua RA, Wang J, et al. Human cytotoxic T-cell memory: Long lived responses to vaccinia virus. *J Virol.* 1996;70:2627-2631.
51. Hammersland E, Lewis MW, Hansen SG, et al. Duration of antiviral immunity after smallpox vaccination. *Nat Med.* 2003;9:1131-1137.
52. Hsieh SM, Pan SC, Chen SY, et al. Age distribution for T cell reactivity to vaccinia virus in a healthy population. *Clin Infect Dis.* 2003;38:86-89.
53. Baruch E, Roth Y, Winder A, et al. The persistence of neutralizing antibodies after revaccination against smallpox. *J Infect Dis.* 1990;161:446-448.
54. Frey SE, Newman FK, Yan L, et al. Response to smallpox vaccine in persons immunized in the distant past. *JAMA.* 2003;289:3295-3296.
55. Bray M, Wright M. Progressive vaccinia. *Clin Infect Dis.* 2003;36:766-774.
56. Neff JM, Lane MM, Pert J, et al. Complications of smallpox vaccination. I. National survey in the United States, 1963. *N Engl J Med.* 1967;276:125-132.
57. Lane JM, Ruben FL, Beff JM, et al. Complications of smallpox vaccination, 1968: National surveillance in the United States. *N Engl J Med.* 1969;281:1201-1208.
58. Lane JM, Ruben F, Neff JM, et al. Complications of smallpox vaccination, 1968: Results of ten statewide surveys. *J Infect Dis.* 1970;122:303-309.
59. Feery BJ. Adverse reactions after smallpox vaccination. *Med J Aust.* 1977;2:41-42.
60. Fulginetti V, Kempe C, Hathaway W, et al. Progressive vaccinia in immunologically deficient individuals. *Birth Defects Orig Artic Ser.* 1968;4:129-145.
61. Goldstein J, Neff J, Lane J, et al. Smallpox vaccination reactions, prophylaxis and therapy of complications. *Pediatrics.* 1975;55:342-347.
62. Keidan SE, McCarthy K, Haworth JC. Fatal generalized vaccinia with failure of antibody production and absence of serum gamma globulin. *Arch Dis Child.* 1953;28:110-116.
63. Copeman PWM, Wallace HJ. Eczema vaccinatum. *BMJ.* 1964;5414:906-908.
64. Rachelefsky GS, Opelz G, Mickey R. Defective T cell function in atopic dermatitis. *J Allergy Clin Immunol.* 1976;57:569-576.
65. Kempe CH. Studies on smallpox and complications of smallpox vaccination. *Pediatrics.* 1960;26:176-189.
66. Vora S, Damon I, Fulginiti V, et al. Severe eczema vaccinatum in a household contact of a smallpox vaccinee. *Clin Infect Dis.* 2008;46:1555-1561.
67. Miller JR, Cirino NM, Philbin EF. Generalized vaccinia 2 days after smallpox revaccination. *Emerg Infect Dis.* 2003;12:1649-1650.
68. Fenner F, Henderson DA, Arita I, et al. *Smallpox and Its Eradication.* Geneva: World Health Organization; 1988:307.
69. De Vries E. *Postvaccinial Perivenous Encephalitis.* Amsterdam: Elsevier; 1960.
70. Tenembaum S, Nestor C, Fejerman N. Acute disseminated encephalomyelitis: A long term follow-up study of 84 pediatric patients. *Neurology.* 2002;59:1224-1231.
71. Gurvich E, Viseova I. Vaccinia virus in postvaccinial encephalitis. *Acta Virol.* 1983;27:154-159.
72. Van Dam CN, Syed S, Eron JJ, et al. Severe postvaccinia encephalitis with acute disseminated encephalomyelitis: Recovery with early intravenous immunoglobulin, high-dose steroids, and vaccinia immunoglobulin. *Clin Infect Dis.* 2009. Epub ahead of print.
73. Melekhin VV, Karem KL, Damon IK, et al. Encephalitis after secondary smallpox vaccination. *Clin Infect Dis.* 2009;48:e1-e2.
74. Miravalle A, Roos KL. Encephalitis complicating smallpox vaccination. *Arch Neurol.* 2003;60:925-928.
75. Ruben FL, Lane JM. Ocular vaccinia: An epidemiologic analysis of 348 cases. *Arch Ophthalmol.* 1970;84:45-48.
76. Kern E. *In vitro* activity of potential anti-poxvirus agents. *Antivir Res.* 2003;57:35-40.
77. Karjalainen J, Heikkila J, Nieminen MS, et al. Etiology of mild acute infectious myocarditis. *Acta Med Scand.* 1983;213:65-73.
78. Helle EJ, Koskenvuo K, Heikkila J, et al. Myocardial complications of immunisations. *Ann Clin Res.* 1978;10:280-287.
79. Halsell JS, Riddle JR, Atwood JE, et al. Myopericarditis following smallpox vaccination among vaccinia-naïve U.S. military personnel. *JAMA.* 2003;289:3283-3289.
80. Grabenstein JD, Winkenwerder W. U.S. military smallpox vaccination program experience. *JAMA.* 2003;289:3278-3282.
81. Supplemental recommendations on adverse events following smallpox vaccine in the pre-event vaccination program: Recommendations of the Advisory Committee on Immunization Practices. *MMWR Morb Mortal Wkly Rep.* 2003;52:282-284. <http://www.cdc.gov/mmwr/preview/mmwrhtml/mm5213a5.htm>
82. Cardiac adverse events following smallpox vaccination—United States, 2003. *MMWR Morb Mortal Wkly Rep.* 2003;52:248-250.
83. Macadam DB, Whitaker W. Cardiac complication after vaccination for smallpox. *BMJ.* 1962;5312:1099-1100.
84. Ahlborg B, Linroth K, Nordgren B. ECG—changes without subjective symptoms after smallpox vaccination of military personnel. *Acta Med Scand.* 1966;S464:127-134.
85. Update: Adverse events following civilian smallpox vaccination—United States, 2003. *MMWR Morb Mortal Wkly Rep.* 2003;52:819-820.
86. Update on cardiac and other adverse events following civilian smallpox vaccination—United States, 2003. *MMWR Morb Mortal Wkly Rep.* 2003;52:639-642.
87. Talbot TR, Bredenberg HK, Smith M, et al. Focal and generalized folliculitis following smallpox vaccination among vaccinia-naïve recipients. *JAMA.* 2003;289:3290-3294.
88. Wharton M, Strikas RA, Harpaz R, et al. Recommendations for using smallpox vaccine in a pre-event vaccination program. *MMWR Recomm Rep.* 2003;52:1-16.
89. Greenberg RN, Kennedy JS. ACAM2000: a newly licensed cell culture-based live vaccinia smallpox vaccine. *Expert Opin Investig Drugs.* 2008;17:555-564.
90. Dumbell KR, Richardson M. Virological investigations of specimens from buffaloes affected by buffalopox in Maharashtra State, India between 1985 and 1987. *Arch Virol.* 1993;128:257-267.
91. Mathew T. *Advances in Medical and Veterinary Virology, Immunology and Epidemiology: Cultivation and Immunological Studies on Pox Groups of Viruses with Special Reference to Buffalo Pox Virus.* New Delhi, India: Thajema Publishers; 1987.
92. Zafar A, Swanepoel R, Hewson R, et al. Nosocomial buffalopoxvirus infection, Karachi, Pakistan. *Emerg Infect Dis.* 2007;13:902-904.
93. Damaso CRA, Esposito JJ, Condit RC, et al. An emergent poxvirus from humans and cattle in Rio de Janeiro state: Cantagalo virus may derive from Brazilian smallpox vaccine. *Virology.* 2000;277:439-449.
94. Schatzmayr HG, Sampaio de Lemos ER, Mazur C, et al. Detection of poxvirus in cattle associated with human cases in the state of Rio de Janeiro: Preliminary report. *Mem Inst Oswaldo Cruz.* 2000;95:625-627.
95. Trindade GS, Guedes MI, Drumond BP, et al. Zoonotic vaccinia virus: Clinical and immunological characteristics in a naturally infected patient. *Clin Infect Dis.* 2009;48:e37-e40.
96. Trindade GS, Lobato ZI, Drumond BP, et al. Short report: Isolation of two vaccinia virus strains from a single bovine vaccinia outbreak in rural area from Brazil: Implications on the emergence of zoonotic orthopoxviruses. *Am J Trop Med Hyg.* 2006;75:486-490.
97. Leite JA, Drumond BP, Trindade GS, et al. Passatempo virus, a vaccinia virus strain, Brazil. *Emerg Infect Dis.* 2005;11:1935-1938.
98. Trindade GS, Emerson GL, Carroll DS, et al. Brazilian vaccinia viruses and their origins. *Emerg Infect Dis.* 2007;13:965-972.
99. da Fonseca FG, Trindade GS, Silva RL, et al. Characterization of a vaccinia-like virus isolated in a Brazilian forest. *J Gen Virol.* 2002;83:223-228.
100. Rupprecht CE, Blass L, Smith K, et al. Human infection due to recombinant vaccinia-rabies glycoprotein virus *N Engl J Med.* 2001;345:582-586.
101. Fenner F, Henderson DA, Arita I, et al. *Smallpox and Its Eradication.* Geneva: World Health Organization; 1988.
102. Breman JA, Henderson DA. Diagnosis and management of smallpox. *N Engl J Med.* 2002;346:1300-1308.
103. Dixon CW. *Differential Diagnosis Laboratory Diagnosis Post-mortem Appearance in Smallpox.* London: Churchill; 1962:67-91.
104. Bremen JG. Monkeypox: An emerging infection for humans? In: Scheld WM, Craig WA, Hughes JM, eds. *Emerging Infections 4.* Washington, DC: ASM Press; 2000:45-67.
105. Jezek Z, Fenner F. Human monkeypox. *Monogr Virol.* 1988;17:1-140.
106. Hutin YJF, Williams RJ, Malfait P, et al. Outbreak of human monkeypox in the Democratic Republic of Congo, 1996-1997. *Emerg Infect Dis.* 2000;7:434-438.
107. Heymann DL, Szczeniowski M, Esteves K. Re-emergence of monkeypox in Africa: A review of the past six years. *Br Med Bull.* 1998;54:693-702.
108. Khodacevich L, Jezek Z, Messinger D. Monkeypox virus: Ecology and public health significance. *Bull World Health Organ.* 1988;66:747-752.
109. Update: Multistate outbreak of monkeypox—Illinois, Indiana, Kansas, Missouri, Ohio, and Wisconsin, 2003. *MMWR Morb Mortal Wkly Rep.* 2003;52:642-646.
110. Anderson M, Frenkel LD, Homann S, et al. A case of severe monkeypox virus disease in an American child: Emerging infections and changing professional values. *Pediatr Infect Dis J.* 2003;22:1093-1096.
111. Reed KD, Melski JW, Graham MB, et al. The detection of monkeypox in humans in the western hemisphere. *N Engl J Med.* 2004;350:342-350.

112. Reynolds MG, Davidson WB, Curns AT, et al. Spectrum of infection and risk factors for human monkeypox, United States, 2003. *Emerg Infect Dis.* 2007;13:1332-1339.

113. Likos AM, Sammons SA, Olson VA, et al. A tale of two clades: Monkeypox viruses. *J Gen Virol.* 2005;86:2661-2672.

114. Chen N, Li G, Liszewski MK, et al. Virulence differences between monkeypox virus isolates from West Africa and the Congo basin. *Virology.* 2005;340:46-63.

115. Olson VA, Carroll DS, Abel JA, et al. A prairie dog animal model of systemic orthopoxvirus disease using West African and Congo Basin strains of monkeypox virus. *J Gen Virol.* 2009;90:323-333.

116. Ibrahim MS, Kulesh D, Saleh SS, et al. Real-time PCR assay to detect smallpox virus. *J Clin Microbiol.* 2003;41:3385-3389.

117. Meyer H, Ropp SL, Esposito JJ. Gene for A-type inclusion body protein is useful for a polymerase chain reaction assay to differentiate orthopoxviruses. *J Virol Methods.* 1997;64:217-222.

118. Meyer H, Ropp SL, Esposito JJ. Poxviruses. In: Warnes A, Stephenson J, eds. *Methods in Molecular Biology: Diagnostic Virology Protocols, 1998.* Totowa, NJ: Humana Press; 1998:199-211.

119. Ropp SL, Jin Q, Knight JC, et al. PCR strategy for identification and differentiation of smallpox and other orthopoxviruses. *J Clin Microbiol.* 1995;33:2069-2076.

120. Loparev VN, Massung RF, Esposito JJ, et al. Detection and differentiation of Old World orthopoxviruses: Restriction length polymorphism of the crmB gene region. *J Clin Microbiol.* 2001;39:94-100.

121. Li Y, Olson VA, Laue T, et al. Detection of monkeypox virus with real-time PCR assays. *J Clin Virol.* 2006;36:194-203.

122. Karem KL, Reynolds M, Braden Z, et al. Characterization of acute-phase humoral immunity to monkeypox: Use of immunoglobulin M enzyme-linked immunosorbent assay for detection of monkeypox infection during the 2003 North American outbreak. *Clin Diagn Lab Immunol.* 2005;12:867-872.

123. Learned LA, Reynolds MG, Wassa DW, et al. Extended interhuman transmission of monkeypox in a hospital community in the Republic of the Congo, 2003. *Am J Trop Med Hyg.* 2005;73:428-434.

124. Meyer H, Perrichot M, Stemmler P, et al. Outbreaks of disease suspected of being due to human monkeypox virus infection in the Democratic Republic of Congo in 2001. *J Clin Microbiol.* 2002;40:2919-2921.

125. Rimoin AW, Kisalu N, Kebela-Ilunga B, et al. Endemic human monkeypox, Democratic Republic of Congo, 2001-2004. *Emerg Infect Dis.* 2007;13:934-937.

126. Lederman ER, Reynolds MG, Karem K, et al. Prevalence of antibodies against orthopoxviruses among residents of Likouala region, Republic of Congo: Evidence for monkeypox virus exposure. *Am J Trop Med Hyg.* 2007;77:1150-1156.

127. Douglas NJ, Dumbell KR. Independent evolution of monkeypox and variola viruses. *J Virol.* 1992;66:7565-7567.

128. Shchelkunov SN, Totmenin AV, Safronov PF, et al. Analysis of the monkeypox genome. *Virology.* 2002;297:172-194.

129. Baxby D. Poxvirus infections in domestic animals. In: Darai G, ed. *Virus Diseases in Laboratory and Captive Animals.* Boston: Nijhoff; 1988:17-35.

130. Baxby D, Bennett M, Getty B. Human cowpox 1969-93: A review based on 54 cases. *Br J Dermatol.* 1994;131:598-607.

131. Bennett M, Gaskell CJ, Baxby D, et al. Feline cowpox infection. *J Small Anim Pract.* 1990;31:167-173.

132. Bennett M, Crouch AJ, Begon M, et al. Cowpox in British voles and mice. *J Comp Pathol.* 1997;116:35-44.

133. Pelkonen PM, Tarvainen K, Hynninen A, et al. Cowpox with severe generalized eruption, Finland. *Emerg Infect Dis.* 2003;9:1458-1461.

134. Dubois ME, Slifka MK. Retrospective analysis of monkeypox infection. *Emerg Infect Dis.* 2008;14:592-599.

135. Neyts J, De Clerq E. Therapy and short term prophylaxis of poxvirus infections: Historical background and perspectives. *Antivir Res.* 2003;57:25-33.

136. LeDuc J, Damon I, Meegan J, et al. Smallpox research activities: U.S. interagency collaboration. *Emerg Infect Dis.* 2002;8:742-745.

137. Keith KA, Hitchcock MJ, Lee WA, et al. Evaluation of nucleoside phosphonates and their analogs and prodrugs for inhibition of orthopoxvirus replication. *Antimicrob Agents Chemother.* 2003;47:2193-2198.

138. Bauer DJ. The antiviral and synergistic actions of isatin thiosemicarbazone and certain phenoxypyrimidines in vaccinia infection in mice. *Br J Exp Pathol.* 1955;36:105-114.

139. Rao M, McFadzean J, Squires S. The laboratory and clinical assessment of an iso-thiazole thiosemicarbazone (M&B 7714) against pox viruses. *Ann N Y Acad Sci.* 1965;130:118-127.

140. Heiner GG, Fatima N, Russell PK, et al. Field trials of methisazone as a prophylactic agent against smallpox. *Am J Epidemiol.* 1971;94:435-449.

141. Neyts J, De Clerq ED. Therapy and short term prophylaxis of poxvirus infections: Historical background and perspectives. *Antivir Res.* 2003;57:25-33.

142. Smee DF, Sidwell RW. A review of compounds exhibiting anti-orthopoxvirus activity in animal models. *Antivir Res.* 2003;57:41-52.

143. Neyts J, Verbeken E, De Clerq E. Effect of 5-iodo-2′-deoxyuridine on vaccinia virus (orthopoxvirus) infections in mice. *Antimicrob Agents Chemother.* 2002;46:2842-2847.

144. Hyndiuk R, Seideman S, Leibsohn JM. Treatment of vaccinial dermatitis with trifluorothymidine. *Arch Ophthalmol.* 1976;94:1785-1786.

145. Hyndiuk R, Okumoto M, Damiano R, et al. Treatment of vaccinial keratitis with vidarabine. *Arch Ophthalmol.* 1976;94:1363-1364.

146. Kaufman H, Nesburn A, Maloney E. Cure of vaccinia infection by 5-iodo-2-deoxyuridine. *Virology.* 1962;18:567-569.

147. Quenelle DC, Collins DJ, Kern ER. Efficacy of multiple or single dose cidofovir against vaccinia and cowpox virus infections in mice. *Antimicrob Agents Chemother.* 2003;47:3275-3280.

148. Winegarden KL, Ciesla SL, Aldern KA, et al. Oral pharmacokinetics and preliminary toxicology of 1-O-hexadecyloxypropyl-cidofovir in mice. Abstracts of the 15th International Conference on Antiviral Research, Prague, Czech Republic, March 17-21, 2002. *Antiviral Res.* 2002;53:A67.

149. Parker S, Touchette E, Oberle C, et al. Efficacy of therapeutic intervention with an oral ether-lipid analogue of cidofovir (CMX001) in a lethal mousepox model. *Antiviral Res.* 2008;77:39-49.

150. Smee D, Bailey K, Sidwell R. Treatment of lethal cowpox virus respiratory infections in mice with 2-amino-7-[(1,3-dihydroxy-2-propoxy)methyl]purine and its orally active diacetate ester prodrug. *Antiviral Res.* 2002;54:113-120.

151. Neyts J, De Clerq E. Efficacy of 2-amino-7-(1,3-dihydroxy-2-propoxymethyl) purine for treatment of vaccinia virus (orthopoxvirus) infections in mice. *Antimicrob Agents Chemother.* 2002;45:84-87.

152. Yang G, Pevear DC, Davies MH, et al. An orally bioavailable antipoxvirus compound (ST-246) inhibits extracellular virus formation and protects mice from lethal orthopoxvirus challenge. *J Virol.* 2005;79:13139-13149.

153. Smith SK, Olson VA, Karem KL, et al. ST246 in vitro efficacy against smallpox and monkeypox. *Antimicrob Agents Chemother.* 2008. [Epub ahead of print]

154. Duraffour S, Snoeck R, de Vos R, et al. Activity of the anti-orthopoxvirus compound ST-246 against vaccinia, cowpox and camelpox viruses in cell monolayers and organotypic raft cultures. *Antivir Ther.* 2007;12:1205-1216.

155. Nalca A, Hatkin JM, Garza NL, et al. Evaluation of orally delivered ST-246 as postexposure prophylactic and antiviral therapeutic in an aerosolized rabbitpox rabbit model. *Antiviral Res.* 2008;79:121-127.

156. Sbrana E, Jordan R, Hruby DE, et al. Efficacy of the antipoxvirus compound ST-246 for treatment of severe orthopoxvirus infection. *Am J Trop Med Hyg.* 2007;76:768-773.

157. Quenelle DC, Buller RM, Parker S, et al. Efficacy of delayed treatment with ST-246 given orally against systemic orthopoxvirus infections in mice. *Antimicrob Agents Chemother.* 2007;51:689-695.

158. Quenelle DC, Prichard MN, Keith KA, et al. Synergistic efficacy of the combination of ST-246 with CMX001 against orthopoxviruses. *Antimicrob Agents Chemother.* 2007;51:4118-4124.

159. Baker RO, Bray M, Huggins JW. Potential antiviral therapeutics for smallpox, monkeypox and other orthopoxvirus infections. *Antiviral Res.* 2003;57:13-23.

160. Sidwell R, Allen L, Khare G, et al. Effect of 1-beta-D-ribofuranosyl-1,2,4-triazole-3-carboxamide (Virazole, ICN 1229) on herpes and vaccinia keratitis and encephalitis in laboratory animals. *Antimicrob Agents Chemother.* 1973;3:242-246.

161. De Clerq E, Luczak M, Shugar D, et al. Effect of cytosine arabinoside, iododeoxyuridine, ethyldeoxyuridine, thiocyanatodeoxyuridine, and ribavirin on tail lesion formation in mice infected with vaccinia virus. *Proc Soc Exp Biol Med.* 1976;151:487-490.

162. Kesson A, Ferguson J, Rawlinson W, et al. Progressive vaccinia treated with ribavirin and vaccinia immune globulin. *Clin Infect Dis.* 1997;25:911-914.

163. Newsome TP, Weisswange I, Frischknecht F, et al. Abl collaborates with Src family kinases to stimulate actin-based motility of vaccinia virus. *Cell Microbiol.* 2006;8:233-241.

164. Reeves PM, Bommarius B, Lebeis S, et al. Disabling poxvirus pathogenesis by inhibition of Abl-family tyrosine kinases. *Nat Med.* 2005;11:731-739. Epub 2005 Jun 26. Erratum: 1361.

165. Yang H, Kim SK, Kim M, et al. Antiviral chemotherapy facilitates control of poxvirus infections through inhibition of cellular signal transduction. *J Clin Invest.* 2005;115:379-387.

166. Bray M. Pathogenesis and potential antiviral therapy of complications of smallpox vaccination. *Antiviral Res.* 2003;58:101-114.

167. Progress in the discovery of compounds inhibiting orthopoxviruses in animal models. *Antivir Chem Chemother.* 2008;19:115-124.

168. De Clercq E. Emerging antiviral drugs. *Expert Opin Emerg Drugs.* 2008;13:393-416.

134

Other Poxviruses That Infect Humans: Parapoxviruses, Molluscum Contagiosum, and Yatapoxviruses

INGER K. DAMON*

Parapoxviruses

Parapoxviruses, which are found worldwide, are common pathogens of sheep, goats, and cattle. Human infection, characterized by localized epithelial lesions, is an occupational hazard for those who handle infected animals. Parapoxvirus infection in sheep and goats is usually referred to as *sore mouth, scabby mouth, contagious pustular dermatitis/ ecthyma* or *orf*, and the corresponding human infection as *orf*. Taxonomically, the relevant parapoxvirus species is referred to as *Orf virus* (ORFV; synonym, contagious pustular dermatitis virus, and contagious ecthyma virus). Parapoxvirus infection of dairy cattle is usually referred to as *paravaccinia, pseudocowpox,* or *ring sores*, and the human equivalent as *paravaccinia, pseudocowpox,* or *milker's nodes*. The virus species is referred to as *Pseudocowpox virus* (PCPV). Parapoxvirus infection of beef cattle is referred to as *stomatitis papulosa*. The parapoxvirus species associated with beef cattle is referred to as *Bovine papular stomatitis virus* (BPSV). Other zoonotic infections, caused by tentative members of the parapoxvirus genus, shown to infect humans are derived from camel exposure (*contagious ecthyma* or *Ausdyk disease*) or, less often, from seals (*sealpox*).[1,2] The *Parapoxvirus of red deer in New Zealand* (PCNZ) is another parapoxvirus species. Lesions in animals are found on the skin, in the oropharyngeal mucosa, and on external surfaces. Other parapoxviruses documented to cause ungulate, pinniped, or other nonhuman animal infections may also cause human illness. Detailed reviews of members of this genus of poxviridae are available.[3-6]

MORPHOLOGY AND COMPOSITION OF THE AGENT

The parapoxviruses have a unique appearance among poxviruses, as revealed with negative-stain transmission electron microscopy. Most poxvirus virions are brick-shaped, but parapoxvirus particles are oblong, rounded, or ovoid. In addition, members of the *Parapoxvirus* genus have a characteristic M form that can be observed with negative-stain electron microscopy: one long spicule wraps the particle, giving a crisscross effect.[7] The stability of the virus in scabs is correlated with possible transmission of the virus through fomites.

The parapoxvirus genome consists of a linear double-stranded DNA of about 135 kilobase pairs (kbp) with covalently closed terminal hairpins; the genome is relatively high in G+C content and is smaller than other poxvirus genomes. Complete genome sequences of ORFV and BPSV have been reported.[8] Several proteins described to have potential roles in viral pathogenesis include a chemokine-binding protein,[9] an interleukin (IL)-10 homologue,[10] a vascular endothelial growth factor homologue,[11] an interferon resistance gene,[12] and a cytokine-binding protein.[13]

PATHOGENESIS AND IMMUNE RESPONSE

Infection, which occurs via cuts and scratches, usually remains localized in the epithelium or oral mucosa. Human lesions of orf are produced by hypertrophy and proliferation of epidermal cells, which is often marked and perhaps related to the endothelial growth factor homologue encoded by the virus and to leukocyte infiltration. Histologic examination of human lesions shows many small multilocular vesicles within the dermis; true macrovesicles rarely occur.[14,15] Generalized symptoms of lymphadenopathy, malaise, and disseminated lesions are uncommon, and the immune response is not protective against disease recurrence on a lifelong basis.[15,16] Second attacks occur in 8% to 12% of individuals.[15,17]

CLINICAL FEATURES

Detailed descriptions of human disease progression are available,[14-16] as are illustrations.[18,19] In brief, infection manifests as localized lesions at the site of inoculation by a diseased animal. The portal of entry is usually a break in the skin. Six stages of clinical disease are described. After a brief incubation period of 3 to 5 days, lesions begin as (pruritic) erythematous macules, then raise to form papules, often with a target appearance (days 7 to 14). Lesions become nodular or vesicular, and orf lesions often ulcerate after 14 to 21 days; this ulceration has been referred to as the acute stage. Complete healing can take up to 4 to 6 weeks and is characterized by a regenerative papilloma and regressive stages where normal epithelium once again is seen.[15] Very large granulomatous lesions occur, more frequently in individuals with immunocompromise, and these may need surgical removal; other less-invasive therapeutic methods may now be feasible and are discussed later in this chapter.[20] Milker's node lesions may have a more nodular appearance, without ulceration. Parapoxvirus infections reported in handlers of reindeer and musk-oxen in Norway are more granulomatous and persist for months.[21] Erythema multiforme and Stevens-Johnson syndrome have been associated with parapoxvirus infections.

DIAGNOSIS

Polymerase chain reaction diagnostic tests generic for parapoxvirus[22,23] and orf[23,24] have been reported; however, the infection is usually clinically diagnosed on the basis of exposure history and the presence of a characteristic lesion. Negative-stain transmission microscopy of lesion material examined by a skilled observer can be diagnostic if the characteristic structure is observed. Virus isolation in tissue culture usually requires primary ovine or bovine cells and may be difficult to attain.[25] The development of immunologic sera specific for parapoxviruses is another source for diagnostic reagents.[26]

EPIDEMIOLOGY

Infection with parapoxvirus is an occupational hazard of farm workers, abattoir workers, veterinarians, students, and others with frequent exposure to sheep, cattle, or goats. Human orf infection is most common in the spring, a time when the bottle-feeding of lambs may predispose humans to exposure risks, and in the fall, when slaughtering and shearing occur.[15] Of 191 cases of orf or milker's nodule with a known source surveyed from 1978 to 1995, 84% had an ovine source and 16% were transmitted by cattle. An additional 32 cases occurred

---

*All material in this chapter is in the public domain, with the exception of any borrowed figures or tables.

in abattoir workers.[27] A recent study evaluated a cluster of cases in children in the midwest United States and found that facial contact with infected animals often led to disease acquisition in children.[23] Most workers at risk are infected at some point in their career, and reinfection is not uncommon. Infected individuals should take care not to further infect themselves with autoinoculation or to spread infection to contacts, including animals. The vaccine used to control orf in sheep is fully virulent and has caused human infection.

TREATMENT

In most cases, the disease is self-limited. Anecdotal reports of the use of 3% cidofovir topical cream[28,29] have described apparent beneficial effects; however, no controlled trials are available. Recently, the use of the Toll-like receptor/interferon modulating compound, imiquimod, showed benefit in topical treatment of a giant orf lesion, after topical and intralesional cidofovir had been unsuccessful.[30]

Molluscum Contagiosum

Molluscum contagiosum, a disease that causes a benign self-limited skin "tumor" or papular eruption, occurs worldwide and is regarded as a specific human infection.[31] Although no evidence exists of disease transmission between humans and other animals, lesions that resemble molluscum and contain pox virions have been detected in species other than humans (e.g., horses and chimpanzees).

DESCRIPTION OF THE AGENT

Four subtypes, characterized by restriction endonuclease digests, have been described.[32] Disease presentation by all subtypes appears to be similar. The genome of molluscum contagiosum virus (MCV) subtype I has been sequenced.[33] This genome encodes several novel gene products involved in its pathogenesis and in evasion of the immune system, including an IL-18–binding protein[34] and apoptosis inhibitors,[35] among others.

PATHOGENESIS AND PATHOLOGY

Molluscum contagiosum lesions have long been known to have a distinctive pathology. In 1841, the first description of characteristic molluscum bodies—Henderson-Paterson bodies—was provided by Henderson and Paterson. Onset of infection occurs when the virus begins replication in the lower layers of the epidermis[36] and then extends upward. The incubation period is quite variable and can be lengthy (2 to 7 weeks; as long as 6 months has been suggested). The epidermis hypertrophies and extends down into the underlying dermal strata. Characteristic inclusions (Henderson-Paterson bodies, or molluscum bodies) are formed in the prickle cell layer and gradually enlarge as cells age and migrate to the surface. These cells are replaced by hyperplasia of the basal cell layer. The structure of the basement membrane remains intact; the hypertrophied epidermal cells, with their cytoplasm occupied by a large acidophilic granular mass (the molluscum body), project above the skin to appear as a tumor.[37] Little to no inflammatory infiltrate is seen until late in disease, just before natural resolution of the lesion occurs.[38]

CLINICAL FEATURES

Infection occurs after breakage of the skin. The characteristic lesion begins as a small papule and, when mature, is a discrete, 2-mm to 5-mm in diameter, smooth, dome-shaped, pearly or flesh-colored nodule that is often umbilicated (Fig. 134-1). A cheesy off-white, sometimes yellowish, material is easily expressed from lesions. Usually, 1 to 20 lesions occur, but occasionally, hundreds may be seen. Because of multiple simultaneous infections, or mechanical spread, these lesions may become confluent along the line of a scratch, and satellite lesions are occasionally seen.

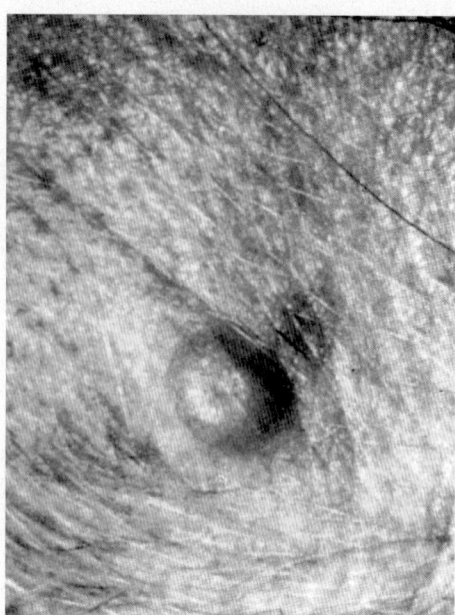

Figure 134-1   Molluscum contagiosum. *(Reprinted with permission from Wood MJ. Skin and soft tissue infection. In: Farrar WE, Wood MJ, Innes JA, et al, eds. Infectious Diseases Text and Color Atlas. Hong Kong: Gower Medical Publishing; 1992:11.17, Fig. 11.69. By permission of Mosby International Ltd.)*

In children, lesions occur mainly on the trunk and proximal extremities. In adults, they tend to occur on the trunk, pubic area, and thighs, but in all cases, infection may be transmitted to other parts with autoinoculation.[38] In patients with human immunodeficiency virus (HIV) , molluscum infections occur along the beard line in males; with facial involvement, reports of ocular involvement, such as lesions on the bulbar conjunctiva, have been found.[39] Individual lesions last for about 2 months, but the disease usually persists for 6 to 9 months.[40] Severe and prolonged infection tends to occur in individuals with impaired cell-mediated immunity, including persons with HIV infection.[31,41]

DIAGNOSIS

The clinical appearance of lesions is generally sufficiently characteristic to permit clinical diagnosis. Brick-shaped virions can usually be seen in large numbers if the cheesy material expressed from the lesion is examined with transmission negative-stain electron microscopy. The virus has not been cultured in standard tissue culture systems. The characteristic histopathology of these lesions is diagnostic; polymerase chain reaction (PCR) methods have been described.[42,43] On occasion, similar-appearing umbilicated lesions have been seen in patients with acquired immunodeficiency syndrome (AIDS) with disseminated cryptococcosis.

EPIDEMIOLOGY AND CONTROL

The virus occurs worldwide, and reports of increasing disease have paralleled reports of AIDS. Traditional modes of transmission are associated with mild skin trauma and in some cases fomites (shared towels); however, evidence is increasing that the disease is sexually transmitted and that genital lesions are common.[31] This disease presents a significant concern for individuals whose children are in daycare or school situations, where concerns about potential transmission to other children may exist. Covering of lesions and hand hygiene after contact with lesions should prevent transmission in these situations.

THERAPEUTICS

Infection is benign and recovery is usually spontaneous, but treatment may be sought for cosmetic reasons, particularly for facial or multiple lesions. Various treatments have been tried.[31] Cryotherapy,[44] mechanical curettage,[44,45] and chemical treatments include podophyllin/podofilox, cantharidin, iodine, and tretinoin.[45-47] Irritation is an adverse effect of many of the chemical methods of treatment. Topical application of an antiviral 3% cidofovir cream or suspension[48,49] has been reported to be beneficial, as has potentially immune-modulating cimetidine[50] or topical imiquimod therapy.[51] The absence of well-controlled trials makes assessment of the efficacy of various therapeutic regimens difficult for the clinician. For individuals with AIDS and molluscum, the use of highly active antiretroviral therapy, with improved CD4 counts, appears to be efficacious.

▣ Yatapoxviruses

The genus *Yatopoxvirus* includes tanapoxvirus and Yaba monkey tumor virus.

TANAPOX

Human infection with tanapox virus, which was first recognized in the Tana River basin area of Kenya in 1957, was best characterized during post–smallpox eradication surveillance efforts. An account of 264 laboratory-confirmed cases from Zaire (Democratic Republic of Congo), with color illustrations, is available,[52] as is information on the virus itself.[53] The genome of the virus has been sequenced.[54] Yaba-like disease virus of monkeys is a variant of the species of virus that causes tanapox in humans.[6,55] Recent anecdotal reports of human disease outside Africa have been published and illustrate the need to consider poxvirus causes of illness in travelers returning from and emigrants from areas where the virus is endemic.[56-58]

Pathophysiology and Clinical Features

Tanapox infection begins with a short febrile illness of 2 to 4 days with temperatures of 38°C to 39°C that is sometimes accompanied by headache, backache, or prostration. The eruption of a lesion is often heralded by pruritus at the site. The lesion appears as a hyperpigmented macule, often with central elevation. The macule then evolves to a papule, with palpable induration. Fever and systemic symptoms wane as the lesion manifests. The papule then becomes more "pock-like" but contains no fluid; umbilication or the formation of a pseudocrust has been reported at this stage. Typically, the papule evolves into a firm, deep-seated, elevated nodule. At the end of the first week, the lesion is surrounded by erythema and by indurated skin. Regional adenopathy is common at this stage. After this stage, lesions either ulcerate or became larger nodules, up to 2 cm in diameter. In the African series, maximum size was usually reached within 2 weeks, then the local inflammatory response began to wane and the lesion began to granulate. Resolution of lesions occurred within 6 weeks.[52]

Most cases (78% in one series[47]) involve a solitary nodule; however, as many as 10 lesions on one individual have been described. The most common location for lesions (72%) is the lower extremities, and the least common locations are the face and parts of the body that are normally covered by clothing.[52] Infection appears to confer lifelong immunity.

Diagnosis

For diagnosis of tanapox, the limited geographic distribution should be considered, as should travel history. Unique clinical features that allow the differentiation of tanapox from other orthopoxvirus infections include the nodular nature of the rash lesion, the local adenopathy, the paucity of lesions, the benign disease course, and the protracted course of rash resolution. As well, the solid nodular/ulcerated lesions are larger and develop more slowly than those of monkeypox, but they are smaller and develop more rapidly than do tropical ulcers.

Tanapox virus can be detected with electron microscopy, and the virions usually appear enveloped.[59] This finding does not exclude the possibility of infection with other morphologically similar brick-shaped poxviruses; nucleic acid testing[56,57] on-lesion extract could be used for that purpose. Tanapox virus grows in a number of cell lines (e.g., owl monkey kidney, Vero, MRC-5, BSC-1) but not on CAM.

Epidemiology and Control

Tanapox virus is restricted to Africa, principally to Kenya and the Democratic Republic of the Congo, and likely has a simian reservoir.[55] Cases of direct primate-to-human transmission, via a break in skin, have been described in animal handlers, although such cases appear to be extremely rare.[60,61] Several factors have led to speculation that an insect or arthropod intermediary may be involved in transmission of tanapox virus to humans: persons confirmed to have tanapox infection have denied contact with nonhuman primates but have reported arthropod and culcine mosquito bites before infection, and in patients in whom multiple lesions developed, no evidence was found that the virus had been spread mechanically.[52] Furthermore, the seasonal variation of human tanapox infections follows the activity of local arthropod populations. No human-to-human transmission has been reported. With the exception of vaccination, measures for the prevention of monkeypox are applicable to tanapox.

YABA MONKEY TUMOR VIRUS

Yaba monkey tumor virus (YMTV) is a distinct species of Yatapoxvirus. It was originally isolated as the cause of a cutaneous tumor on a rhesus monkey (*Mucaca mulatta*). In Asiatic monkeys, the virus causes benign histiocytomas that resolve in 1 to 2 months.[62] Serosurveys have suggested that African green monkeys are the natural host of YMTV.[63]

Clinical

Accidental needle stick infections of human animal handlers, and deliberate infections of human volunteers, show that humans have localized skin lesions develop at the site of inoculation.[64] Human infections have not been recently reported.

REFERENCES

1. Becher P, Konig M, Muller G, et al. Characterization of sealpox, a separate member of the parapoxviruses. *Arch Virol.* 2002; 147:113-114.
2. Nollens HH, Gulland FM, Jacobson ER, et al. Parapoxviruses of seals and sea lions make up a distinct subclade within the genus Parapoxvirus. *Virology.* 2006;349:316-324.
3. Haig DM, Mercer AA. Ovine diseases: Orf. *Vet Res.* 1998;29:311-326.
4. Mercer A, Fleming S, Robinson A, et al. Molecular genetic analyses of parapoxviruses pathogenic for humans. *Arch Virol Suppl.* 1997;13:25-34.
5. Robinson AJ, Lyttle DJ. Parapoxviruses: Their biology and potential as recombinant vaccines. In: Binns MM, Smith GL, eds. *Recombinant Poxviruses.* Boca Raton, FL: CRC Press; 1992:285-327.
6. Mercer AA, Schmidt A, Weber O, eds. *Poxviruses Advances in Infectious Diseases.* Boston: Birkhauser; 2007.
7. Nakano JH. Poxviruses. In: Lennette EH, Schmidt NJ, eds. *Diagnostic Procedures for Viral, Rickettsial, and Chlamydial Infections.* 5th ed. Washington, DC: American Public Health Association, Inc; 1979:257-308.
8. Delhon G, Tulman ER, Alfonso CL. Genomes of parapoxviruses, orf virus, and bovine papular stomatitis virus. *J Virol.* 2004;78:168-177.
9. Seet BT, McCaughan CA, Handel TM, et al. Analysis of an orf virus chemokine-binding protein: Shifting ligand specificities among a family of poxvirus viroceptors. *PNAS.* 2003;100:15137-15142.
10. Fleming SB, Haig DM, Nettleton P, et al. Sequence and functional analysis of a homolog of interleukin-10 encoded by the parapoxvirus orf virus. *Virus Genes.* 2000;21:85-95.
11. Savory LJ, Stacker SA, Fleming SB, et al. Viral vascular endothelial growth factor plays a critical role in orf virus infection. *J Virol.* 2000;74:10699-10706.
12. Haig DM, McInnes CJ, Thompson J, et al. The orf virus OV20.0L gene product is involved in interferon resistance and inhibits an interferon-inducible, double-stranded RNA-dependent kinase. *Immunology.* 1998;93:335-340.
13. Deane D, McInnes CJ, Percival A, et al. Orf virus encodes a novel secreted protein inhibitor of granulocyte-macrophage colony-stimulating factor and interleukin-2. *J Virol.* 2000;74:1313-1320.
14. Johannesen JV, Krogh HK, Solberg I, et al. Human orf. *J Cutan Pathol.* 1975;2:265-283.
15. Yirrell DL, Vestey JP. Human orf infections. *J Eur Acad Dermatol Venereol.* 1994;3:451-459.
16. Leavell UW, McNamara MJ, Muelling R, et al. Orf: Report of 19 human cases with clinical and pathological observations. *JAMA.* 1968;204:657-664.
17. Robinson AJ, Peterson GV. Orf virus infection of workers in the meat industry. *N Z Med J.* 1983;96:81-85.

18. Baxby D, Bennett M, Getty B. Human cowpox 1969-93: A review based on 54 cases. *Br J Dermatol*. 1994;131:598-607.

19. Diven DG. An overview of poxviruses. *J Am Acad Dermatol*. 2001;44:1-16.

20. Pether JVS, Guerrier CJW, Jones SM, et al. Giant orf in a normal individual. *Br J Dermatol*. 1986;115:497-499.

21. Falk ES. Parapoxvirus infections of reindeer and musk ox associated with unusual human infections. *Br J Dermatol*. 1978;99:647-654.

22. Inoshima Y, Morooka A, Sentsui H. Detection and diagnosis of parapoxvirus by the polymerase chain reaction. *J Virol Methods*. 2000;84:201-208.

23. Lederman ER, Austin C, Trevino I, et al. ORF virus infection in children: Clinical characteristics, transmission, diagnostic methods, and future therapeutics. *Pediatr Infect Dis J*. 2007;26:740-744.

24. Torafson EG, Gunadottir S. Polymerase chain reaction for laboratory diagnosis of cirus infections. *J Clin Virol*. 2002;24:79-84.

25. Fenner F, Nakano JH. Poxviridae: The poxviruses. In: Lennette EH, Halonen P, Murpy FA, eds. *The Laboratory Diagnoses of Infectious Diseases: Principles and Practices, v II. Viral, Rickettsial, and Chlamydial Diseases*. New York: Springer Verlag; 1988:177-210.

26. Czerny CP, Waldmann R, Scheubeck T. Identification of three distinct antigenic sites in parapoxviruses. *Arch Virol*. 1997; 142:807-821.

27. Baxby D, Bennett M. Poxvirus zoonoses. *J Med Microbiol*. 1997;46:17-20.

28. Geerinck K, Lukito G, Snoeck G, et al. A case of human orf in an immunocompromised patient treated successfully with cidofovir cream. *J Med Virol*. 2001;75:1205-1210.

29. McCabe D, Weston B, Storch G. Treatment of orf poxvirus lesion with cidofovir cream. *Pediatr Infect Dis J*. 2003;22:1027-1028.

30. Lederman ER, Green GM, DeGroot HE, et al. Progressive ORF virus infection in a patient with lymphoma: Successful treatment using imiquimod. *Clin Infect Dis*. 2007;44:e100-e103.

31. Birthistle K, Carrington D. Molluscum contagiosum virus. *J Infect*. 1997;34:21-28.

32. Nakamura J, Muraki Y, Yamada M, et al. Analysis of molluscum contagiosum genomes isolated in Japan. *J Med Virol*. 1995;46:339-348.

33. Senkevich TG, Bugert JJ, Sisler JJ, et al. Genome sequence of a human tumorigenic poxvirus: Prediction of specific host response evasion genes. *Science*. 1996;273:813-816.

34. Xiang Y, Moss B. IL-18 binding and inhibition of interferon gamma induction by human poxvirus-encoding proteins. *Proc Natl Acad Sci U S A*. 1999;96:11537-11542.

35. Bertin J, Armstrong RC, Ottilie S, et al. Death effector domain-containing herpesvirus and poxvirus proteins inhibit both Fas- and TNFR1-induced apoptosis. *Proc Natl Acad Sci U S A*. 1997;94:1172-1176.

36. Pierard-Franchimont C, Legrain A, Pierard GE. Growth and regression of molluscum contagiosum. *J Am Acad Dermatol*. 1983;9:669-672.

37. Shelly WB, Burmeister V. Demonstration of a unique viral structure: The molluscum viral colony sac. *Br J Dermatol*. 1986;115:557-562.

38. Brown S, Nalley JF, Kraus SJ. Molluscum contagiosum. *Sex Transm Dis*. 1981;8:227-234.

39. Pepose JS, Esposito JJ. Molluscum contagiosum, orf and vaccinia ocular infections in humans. In: Pepose JS, Holland GN, Wilhelmus KR, eds. *Ocular Infection and Immunity*. St Louis: Mosby; 1996:846-856.

40. Steffen C, Markman J. Spontaneous disappearance of molluscum contagiosum. *Arch Dermatol*. 1989;116:923-924.

41. Gottlieb SL, Myskowski PL. Molluscum contagiosum. *Int J Dermatol*. 1994;33:453-461.

42. Nunez A, Funes JM, Agromayor M, et al. Detection and typing of molluscum contagiosum virus in skin lesions using a simple lysis method and polymerase chain reaction. *J Med Virol*. 1996;50:342-349.

43. Thompson CH. Identification and typing of molluscum contagiosum virus in clinical specimens by polymerase chain reaction. *J Med Virol*. 1997;53:205-211.

44. Janniger CK, Schwartz RA. Molluscum contagiosum in children. *Cutis*. 1993;52:194-196.

45. Valentine CL, Diven DG. Treatment modalities for molluscum contagiosum. *Dermatol Ther*. 2000;13:285-289.

46. Silverburg NB, Sidbury R, Mancini AJ. Childhood molluscum contagiosum: Experience with cantharidin therapy in 300 patients. *J Am Acad Dermatol*. 2000;43:503-507.

47. Ohkuma M. Molluscum contagiosum treated with iodine solution and salicylic plaster. *Int J Dermatol*. 1990;29:443-445.

48. Calista D. Topical cidofovir for severe cutaneous human papillomavirus and molluscum contagiosum infection in patient with HIV/AIDS. A pilot study. *J Eur Acad Dermatol Venereol*. 2000;14:484.

49. Zabawaski EJ Jr, Cockerell CJ. Topical cidofovir for molluscum contagiosum in children. *Pediatr Dermatol*. 1999;16:414-415.

50. Dohil M, Prendiville JS. Treatment of molluscum contagiosum with oral cimetidine: Clinical experience on 13 patients. *Pediatr Dermatol*. 1996;13:310-312.

51. Hengge UR, Esser S, Schultewolter T, et al. Self administered topical 5% imiquod for the treatment of common warts and molluscum contagiosum. *Br J Dermatol*. 2000;143:1026-1031.

52. Jezek Z, Arita I, Szczeniowski M, et al. Human tanapox in Zaire: Clinical and epidemiological observations on cases confirmed by laboratory studies. *Bull World Health Organ*. 1985;63:1027-1035.

53. Knight JC, Novembre FJ, Brown DR, et al. Studies on tanapox virus. *Virology*. 1989;172:116-124.

54. Lee HJ, Essani K, Smith GL. The genome sequence of Yaba-like disease virus, a yatapoxvirus. *Virology*. 2001;281:170-192.

55. Downie A, Espana C. Comparison of tanapox and yaba-like viruses causing epidemic diseases in monkeys. *J Hyg Camb*. 1972;70:23-33.

56. Croitoru AG, Birge MB, Rudikoff D, et al. Tanapox virus infection. *Skin Med*. 2002;1:56.

57. Stich A, Meyer H, Kohler B, et al. Tanapox: First report in a European traveller and identification by PCR. *Trans R Soc Trop Med Hyg*. 2002;96:178-179.

58. Dhar AD, Werchniak AE, Li Y, et al. Tanapox infection in a college student. *N Engl J Med*. 2004;350:361-366.

59. Fenner F, Nakano JH. Poxviridae: The poxviruses. In: Lennette EH, Halonen P, Murphy FA, eds. *The Laboratory Diagnosis of Infectious Diseases: Principles and Practice, v II. Viral, Rickettsial, and Chlamydial Diseases*. New York: Springer Verlag; 1988:177-210.

60. McNulty WPJ, Lobitz WCJ, Hu F, et al. A pox disease in monkeys transmitted to man: Clinical and histological features. *Arch Dermatol*. 1968;97:286-293.

61. Hall AS, McNulty WP Jr. A contagious pox disease in monkeys. *J Am Vet Med Assoc*. 1967;151:833-838.

62. Bearcroft WG, Jamieson MF. An outbreak of subcutaneous tumors in rhesus monkeys. *Nature*. 1958;182:195-196.

63. Tsuchiya Y, Tagaya I. Sero-epidemiological survey on Yaba and 1211 virus infections among several species of monkeys. *J Hyg (Lond)*. 1971;69:445-451.

64. Grace JT Jr, Mirand EA. Yaba virus infection in humans. *Exp Med Surg*. 1965;23:213-216.

135

Introduction to Herpesviridae

JEFFREY I. COHEN*

Although there are hundreds of herpesviruses that infect nearly all animals, eight herpesviruses naturally infect humans (Table 135-1). A ninth herpesvirus, herpes B virus, which naturally infects macaques, can cause fatal encephalitis in humans. This chapter is an overview of herpesviruses that infect humans, and the subsequent chapters (Chapters 136 to 142) discuss the individual herpesviruses themselves.

Classification

Members of the herpesvirus family are distinguished from other virus families by their structure and genome. Herpesviruses contain a double-stranded DNA surrounded by an icosahedral nucleocapsid, which is wrapped inside a tegument consisting of several proteins and then surrounded by an envelope studded with viral glycoproteins (Fig. 135-1).[1] The envelope is derived from host cell membranes. Herpesviruses range in size from 120 to 260 nm in diameter. Virions contain a characteristic set of viral proteins as well as some host cell proteins.

Human herpesviruses are subdivided into three subfamilies (see Table 135-1). The Alphaherpesviruses include herpes simplex virus (HSV) types 1 and 2, varicella-zoster virus (VZV), and herpes B virus. These viruses are latent in neurons of sensory ganglia, and infection of cultured cells leads to rapid destruction of the cells. They cause mucocutaneous infections in healthy individuals. The Betaherpesviruses include cytomegalovirus (CMV), human herpesvirus 6 (HHV-6), and human herpesvirus 7 (HHV-7). These viruses have a more limited host range, replicate slowly in cell culture, and establish latency in mononuclear cells. Gammaherpesviruses include Epstein-Barr virus (EBV) and Kaposi's sarcoma–associated herpesvirus (KSHV, also known as HHV-8). These viruses establish latency in lymphoid cells and cause lytic infection in epithelial cells or fibroblasts. Beta- and Gammaherpesviruses can cause lymphoproliferation with mononucleosis.

EBV and HHV-6 are present as one of two types, referred to as types A and B. EBV types can differ depending on the geographic location of the infected individual. Although HSV-1 and HSV-2 share 50% or more sequence identity, different types of EBV and HHV-6 are much more closely related.

Genome Structure and Proteins

The human herpesviruses consist of 125,000 to 229,000 base pairs of double-stranded DNA (see Table 135-1), and their overall guanosine and cytosine content varies from 36% (for HHV-7) to 70% (for HSV-2). The genomes consist of long unique regions and short repeated regions. These repeats, as well as single nucleotide polymorphisms, are often useful for molecular epidemiologic studies because restriction endonuclease digestion results in different-sized fragments that can help to indicate whether different persons are infected with different strains of virus. Thus, after transplantation, the sizes of the repeated regions can help to indicate whether the viruses originate from the donor or the recipient.[2] EBV has terminal repeats at the ends of its genome. The number of terminal repeats is fixed in cells that were infected with the same clone of virus, but varies in number if the cells were infected with different viral clones.[3] The viral genome is linear inside the virion, but circularizes in infected cells. Portions of many herpesvirus genes overlap in the genome; most herpesvirus genes are not spliced.

HHVs encode 71 to 166 genes. Herpesviruses encode a core set of approximately 40 proteins that are conserved among all the herpesvirus species and include proteins involved in nucleic acid synthesis (e.g., viral DNA polymerase), nucleic acid metabolism (e.g., ribonucleotide reductase), protein modification (e.g., protein kinases), and virion structure (major capsid protein, glycoproteins B, H, and L). In addition, the Alpha-, Beta-, and Gammaherpesviruses each contain a conserved set of genes unique to each subfamily such as genes encoding proteins important for virus entry. Herpesviruses have a lytic phase of replication that results in cell death, and a latent phase of replication in which no or a very limited set of viral proteins are made.

Virus Replication

Herpesviruses use at least two principal methods to enter cells.[4] Virus can enter cells by endocytosis and subsequent fusion of the virion envelope to the endocytic membrane, which allows entry of the nucleocapsid into the cytoplasm. Alternatively, the virion envelope can fuse to the cell membrane on the cell surface to deliver the nucleocapsid directly to the cytoplasm. Viral glycoproteins bind to receptors on the cell membrane, which allows entry into the cell. Herpesviruses often have more than one cell surface receptor (see Table 135-1). The viral nucleocapsid is transported from the cytoplasm to the nucleus where the linear viral DNA circularizes, and DNA replication can begin. Replication proceeds in an orderly pattern of viral gene expression. The immediate-early genes are initially expressed that encode proteins that regulate viral gene expression. This is followed by the early viral proteins, many of which encode enzymes important for viral DNA replication or protein phosphorylation. Last, the late proteins are made, many of which encode structural proteins including the viral glycoproteins and nucleocapsid proteins. Viral genes are transcribed in the nucleus, and the proteins are synthesized in the cytoplasm. Herpesvirus nucleocapsids are assembled in the nucleus and undergo envelopment at the inner nuclear membrane, de-envelopment at the outer nuclear membrane, and re-envelopment at the cytoplasmic membrane, and then exit the cell. Lytic replication of herpesviruses inhibits host cell RNA and protein synthesis.

Virus Latency and Reactivation

The mechanisms by which herpesviruses establish and maintain latency are not well understood. Some viruses, such as HSV, express one family of latency associated transcripts that do not encode proteins, but may be important to prevent apoptosis.[5] Other viruses express proteins during latency. VZV expresses the IE63 protein, which inhibits the activity of interferon-α,[6] and EBV expresses the EBV nuclear antigen 1 protein, which allows viral episomes to partition to dividing latently infected B cells.[7] EBV and KSHV encode a number of latency proteins expressed in different types of virus-associated malignancies. Herpesvirus genomes exist in a circular, episomal form during latency.

Several mechanisms have recently been proposed for maintaining latency in herpesviruses. These include expression of viral micro RNAs during latency that inhibit expression of immediate-early viral genes,[8,9] and methylation of histone proteins associated with lytic genes, which results in compaction of chromatin and silencing of the lytic genes.[10,11] In addition, certain viral and cellular proteins, which are normally in the nucleus of cells undergoing herpesvirus replication, may be sequestered to the cytoplasm during latency so that the viral proteins cannot activate gene expression.[12,13]

---

*All material in this chapter is in the public domain, with the exception of any borrowed figures or tables.

TABLE 135-1	Biologic Features of Herpesviruses That Infect Humans				
		Genome			
Virus	*Subfamily*	*Size (kbp)*	*Receptor(s)*	*Sites of Latency*	
Human Virus					
HSV-1 (HHV-1)	α	152	Nectin-1, nectin-2 TNFRSF14, 3-OS-HS	Sensory and cranial nerve ganglia	
HSV-2 (HHV-2)	α	152	Nectin-1, nectin-2 TNFRSF14	Sensory and cranial nerve ganglia	
Varicella-zoster virus (HHV-3)	α	125	IDE	Sensory and cranial nerve ganglia	
Cytomegalovirus (HHV-5)	β	229	PDGFRα, EGFR? $\alpha_2\beta_1$, $\alpha_6\beta_1$, $\alpha_v\beta_3$	Monocytes, macrophages CD34+ cells	
HHV-6	β	165	CD46	CD34+ cells, monocytes, macrophages	
HHV-7	β	145	CD4?	CD4 cells	
Epstein-Barr virus (HHV-4)	γ	172	CD21, MHC class II	Memory B cells	
Kaposi's sarcoma–associated herpesvirus (HHV-8)	γ	165	Integrin $\alpha_3\beta_1$ XCT, DC-SIGN	B cells	
Simian Virus					
Herpes B virus (cercopithecine herpesvirus 1)	α	150	Unknown	Sensory and cranial nerve ganglia	

DC-SIGN, dendritic cell-specific ICAM-3 grabbing nonintegrin; EGFR, epidermal growth factor receptor; HHV, human herpesvirus; HSV, herpes simplex virus; IDE, insulin degrading enzyme; MHC, major histocompatibility complex; PDGFR, platelet-derived growth factor receptor; 3-O-S-HS, 3-O-sulfotransferases; TNFRSFI4, tumor necrosis factor receptor superfamily, member 14; XCT, light chain of the human cystine/glutamate transporter system.

Adapted from Straus SE. Introduction to Herpesviridae. In: Mandell GL, Bennett JE, Dolin R, eds. *Principles and Practice of Infectious Diseases*, 6th ed. Philadelphia: Elsevier, Churchill Livingstone; 2005:1756-1762.

Latent viral genomes can reactivate to produce infectious virus. Reactivation can be stimulated in some virus-infected cells by radiation, trauma to nerves (in the case of Alphaherpesviruses), hyperthermia,[14] or hypoxia.[15] Reactivation is more common in immunosuppressed or immunocompromised hosts that have impaired T-cell immunity. Reactivation allows the virus to be transmitted to other individuals, thereby perpetuating virus infection over time to other generations.

Pathogenesis

Many herpesviruses, such as HSV, EBV, CMV, HHV-6, and HHV-7, are shed from the oral mucosa without symptoms, and it is during asymptomatic shedding, rather than during symptomatic disease, that most viruses are transmitted from person to person. In contrast, VZV is only transmitted when patients have varicella or zoster.

Symptomatic disease due to some herpesviruses is associated with lytic virus replication resulting in skin lesions due to HSV or VZV or visceral lesions due to HSV, VZV, or CMV. Other diseases, such as erythema multiforme associated with HSV or hemolytic anemia associated with CMV or EBV, are due to the immune response to the virus. Most symptoms from infectious mononucleosis associated with EBV are due to the proliferation of T cells that respond to the infection rather than to lytic destruction of virus-infected B cells.

Most human encounters with herpesviruses are asymptomatic or induce very mild symptoms. Many persons infected with HSV-1 or HSV-2 are asymptomatic, and young children and infants infected with CMV and EBV are usually asymptomatic. In contrast, most

persons infected with VZV present with chickenpox and most with HHV-6 have fever. Infections are rarely fatal except in highly immunocompromised persons. It is in the best interest of the virus for the host to survive so that the infection can be transmitted to others. Although some herpesviruses (e.g., HSV, VZV, CMV, HHV-6) infect a wide range of cells in the body, others (e.g., EBV, HHV-7, KSHV) have a more narrow host range.

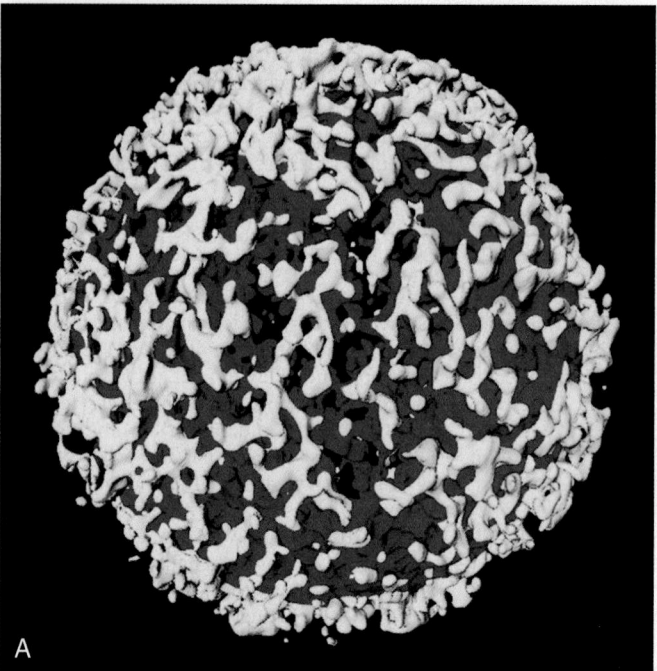

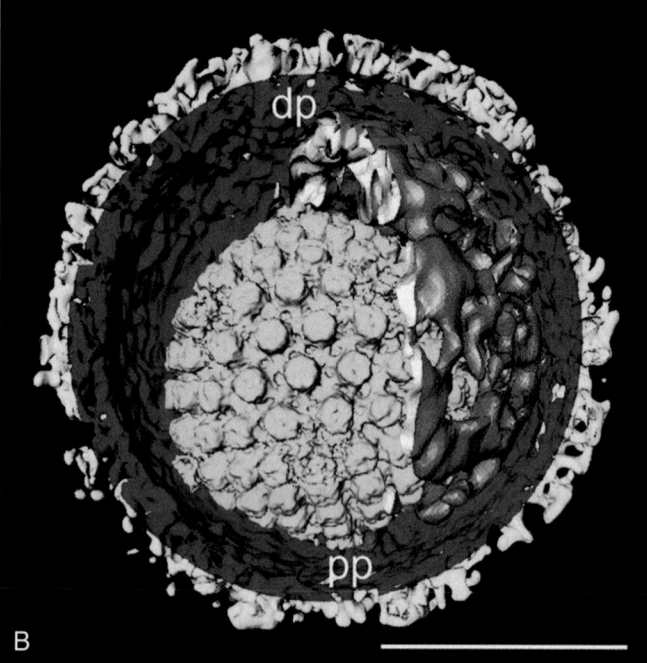

Figure 135-1 **Structure of a herpes simplex virus virion based on cryoelectron tomography. A,** The outer surface of the virion shows viral glycoproteins (*yellow*) embedded in the viral membrane (*blue*). **B,** The interior of the virion shows the viral nucleocapsid (*light blue*) surrounded by the protein tegument (*orange*), which is inside the viral envelope (*blue and yellow*). pp, proximal pole; dp, distal pole; scale bar, 100 nm. (*From Grünewald K, Desai P, Winkler DC, et al. Three-dimensional structure of herpes simplex virus from cryo-electron tomography.* Science. *2003;302:1396-1398, with permission.*)

Epidemiology

Nearly all adults are infected with HSV-1, VZV, EBV, HHV-6, and HHV-7 (Table 135-2). Approximately 20% to 50% of adults in the United States are infected with HSV-2, 40% to 70% are infected with CMV, and less than 5% are infected with KSHV. Rates of HSV-1, HSV-2, CMV, EBV, and KSHV are higher in developing countries than in the United States.

Herpesviruses are usually spread by direct contact because the enveloped viruses do not survive long in the environment; VZV is the exception and is spread by airborne transmission. HSV, EBV, CMV, and HHV-6 are spread by infected saliva; HHV-7 and KSHV are also likely spread by saliva. Sexual contact results in spread of HSV, CMV, KSHV, and perhaps EBV. Intrauterine infection with HSV, VZV, and CMV can occur; most infants infected with HSV acquire the infection at the time of delivery. CMV, EBV, and KSHV have been transmitted by organ transplantation, and CMV and EBV have been spread by blood transfusion.

Clinical Syndromes

Several herpesviruses cause similar clinical syndromes including vesicular skin lesions, retinitis, hepatitis, encephalitis, and mononucleosis; virus-specific diagnostic tests are needed to distinguish the virus that causes a particular syndrome (Tables 135-2 and 135-3).

Herpesviruses cause more severe disease in persons with impaired cellular, but not with impaired humoral immunity (see Table 135-2). Patients with impaired T-cell immunity, such as organ transplant recipients receiving immunosuppression therapy, hematopoietic cell transplant recipients, patients with acquired immunodeficiency syndrome, or patients with congenital T- or natural killer–cell deficiencies, have more severe herpesvirus infections.[16] Patients with HIV and low CD4 cell counts often have severe herpesvirus infections. Persistent erosive mucocutaneous oral or anogenital HSV infections may occur, and

resistance to acyclovir is not uncommon. VZV can cause verrucous skin lesions or small vessel central nervous system vasculitis or radiculopathy in patients with AIDS. CMV can cause encephalitis, retinitis, colitis, or radiculopathy; however, pneumonitis is rare in patients with acquired immunodeficiency syndrome. EBV is associated with central nervous system lymphomas or non-Hodgkin's lymphoma, whereas KSHV is associated with Kaposi's sarcoma, primary effusion lymphoma, and Castleman's disease in patients with acquired immunodeficiency syndrome. Interestingly, HHV-6 and HHV-7 rarely cause disease in patients with acquired immunodeficiency syndrome. Infection with HSV-2 increases the rate of transmission and infection with HIV.[17]

Immunity

Humoral immunity contributes to protection from primary infection with herpesviruses. Antibody acquired transplacentally protects neonates from HSV, VZV, and CMV; infection of neonates when mothers develop primary infection and lack virus-specific antibody near the time of birth can cause severe disease in the neonate. VZV and CMV infection during fetal development is associated with intrauterine growth retardation and birth defects. Antibody to VZV (varicella-zoster immunoglobulin) or CMV (CMV hyperimmunoglobulin) reduces the severity of primary disease in immunocompromised persons. Most herpesviruses spread in the body from cell to cell rather than as free virions, and therefore the effect of antibody is limited once infection is well established.

The observation that patients with hypogammaglobulinemia are not at risk of developing severe herpesvirus infections, whereas those with impaired cellular immunity can have life-threatening disease indicates the important role of cellular immunity in controlling the severity of herpesvirus disease. Numerous virus epitopes are recognized by CD4+ and CD8+ T cells, and few appear to be dominant in HSV and CMV infection.[18,19] Patients with mutations in genes in the innate immunity pathway such as TLR3[20] and UNC-393[21] are prone to develop HSV

TABLE 135-2	Features of Herpesvirus Infections and Seroepidemiology				
				Seroprevalence (%)	
			Healthy Children	Healthy Adults	
Virus	Primary Infection in Healthy Persons	Infection in Immunocompromised Persons		United States	Developing World
Herpes simplex virus 1	Gingivostomatitis Keratoconjunctivitis Cutaneous herpes Genital herpes	Gingivostomatitis Keratoconjunctivitis Cutaneous herpes Visceral infections	20-40	50-70	50-90
Herpes simplex virus 2	Genital herpes Cutaneous herpes Gingivostomatitis Aseptic meningitis Neonatal herpes	Genital herpes Cutaneous herpes Disseminated infection	0-5	20-50	20-60
Varicella-zoster virus	Varicella	Disseminated infection	50-75	85-95	50-80
Cytomegalovirus	Mononucleosis Hepatitis Congenital cytomegalic inclusion disease	Hepatitis Retinitis Other visceral infections	10-30	40-70	40-80
Epstein-Barr virus	Mononucleosis Hepatitis Encephalitis	Polyclonal and monoclonal lymphoproliferative syndromes Oral hairy leukoplakia	10-30	80-95	90-100
Human herpesvirus 6	Exanthem subitum, infantile fever and seizures, encephalitis	Fever and rash Encephalitis Bone marrow suppression	80-100	60-100	60-100
Human herpesvirus 7	Exanthem subitum, childhood fever and seizures, encephalitis	Encephalitis?	40-80	60-100	40-100
Kaposi's sarcoma–associated herpesvirus	Febrile exanthem Mononucleosis?	Kaposi's sarcoma, Castleman's disease, primary effusion lymphoma	<3	<3	10-60
Herpes B virus	Mucocutaneous lesions Encephalitis	?	0	<<1	<<1

Adapted from Straus SE. Introduction to Herpesviridae. In: Mandell GL, Bennett EJ, Dolin R, eds. *Principles and Practice of Infectious Diseases*, 6th ed. Philadelphia: Elsevier, Churchill Livingstone; 2005:1756-1762.

TABLE 135-3 Clinical Syndromes Associated with Human Herpesviruses

Syndrome	HSV-1	HSV-2	VZV	CMV	EBV	HHV-6	HHV-7	KSHV	Herpes B Virus
Gingivostomatitis	+	+	–	–	–	–	–	–	–
Genital lesions	+	+	–	–	–	–	–	–	–
Keratoconjunctivitis	+	+	+	–	–	–	–	–	–
Cutaneous lesions	+	+	+	–	–	–	–	+	+
Neonatal infection	+	+	+	+	–	–	–	–	–
Retinitis	+	+	+	+	–	–	–	–	–
Esophagitis	+	+	+	+	–	–	–	–	–
Pneumonitis	+	+	+	+	+	+	–	–	–
Hepatitis	+	+	+	+	+	+	–	–	–
Meningitis	–	+	+	–	–	+	–	–	–
Encephalitis	+	+	+	+	+	+	–	–	+
Myelitis	+	+	+	+	–	–	–	–	+
Mononucleosis	–	–	–	+	+	+	–	+?	–
Hemolytic anemia	–	–	+	+	+	+	–	–	–
Leukopenia	–	–	+	+	+	+	–	–	–
Thrombocytopenia	–	–	+	+	+	+	–	–	–

CMV, cytomegalovirus; EBV, Epstein-Barr virus; HHV, human herpesvirus; HSV, herpes simplex virus; KSHV, Kaposi's sarcoma–associated herpes virus; VZV, varicella-zoster virus..
Adapted from Straus SE. Introduction to Herpesviridae, In: Mandell GL, Bennett JE, Dolin R, eds. *Principles and Practice of Infectious Diseases*, 6th ed. Philadelphia: Elsevier, Churchill Livingstone; 2005:1756-1762.

encephalitis. Mutations in SLAM-associated protein[22] and XIAP[23] can result in severe EBV disease. Polymorphisms in HLA genes are associated with symptomatic HSV[24] or EBV infection,[25] whereas polymorphisms in TLR2[26] or interleukin-10[27] are associated with increased severity of HSV or EBV infection, respectively.

Herpesviruses encode numerous genes that inhibit cellular immune mechanisms.[28,29] EBV and KSHV encode homologues of the antiapoptotic protein bcl-2, whereas HSV, CMV, and HHV-6 encode other proteins that inhibit apoptosis. Many herpesviruses encode proteins that inhibit recognition of infected cells by $CD4^+$ and $CD8^+$ T and natural killer cells. HSV and CMV encode proteins that inhibit the TAP protein that is required for processing major histocompatibility complex class I molecules, and KSHV encodes proteins that enhance endocytosis of major histocompatibility complex class I molecules from the cell surface. HSV and CMV also encode proteins that inhibit major histocompatibility complex class II, and CMV and KSHV encode proteins that inhibit natural killer cells. HSV, VZV, EBV, CMV, and KHSV encode proteins that inhibit interferon. HSV encodes a glycoprotein (gE) that inhibits the activity of antibody, whereas HSV and KSHV encode proteins that inhibit complement. EBV and CMV encode interleukin-10 homologues, and KSHV encodes an interleukin-6 homologue. HHV-6 and HHV-8 encode chemokines, and CMV, EBV, HHV-6, HHV-7, and KSHV encode chemokine receptor homologues.[30] These proteins allow the virus to avoid destruction by the host immune system.

Oncogenesis

Two human herpesvirus, EBV and KSHV, are oncogenic in humans, whereas the other human herpesviruses are not associated with cancer.[31] Oncogenic viruses must be maintained in cells and be transmitted to progeny cells. Oncogenic viruses express a limited set of viral proteins during latency to avoid detection by the immune system and to provide functions needed to immortalize the cell. EBV and KSHV encode proteins that activate cellular gene expression and B-cell signaling pathways. EBV LMP-1 functions as an oncogene and mimics the activity of CD40 to activate nuclear factor kappa B and signal transducers and activators of transcription (STATs), whereas KSHV encodes several proteins (e.g., K1, K12, ORF74) with transforming activity. EBV is associated with Hodgkin's disease, non-Hodgkin's lymphoma, Burkitt's lymphoma, T-cell lymphoma, and nasopharyngeal carcinoma, and KSHV is associated with Kaposi's sarcoma, primary effusion lymphoma, and Castleman's disease.

Diagnosis

Most primary herpesvirus infections such as herpes gingivitis, genital herpes, varicella, and roseola are diagnosed by their clinical symptoms. Serology is useful for confirming acute or previous infection. Type-specific serologies are available for HSV-1 and HSV-2, either of which can cause oral or genital disease.

Polymerase chain reaction is the standard test for detection of HSV, VZV, EBV, CMV, or HHV-6 encephalitis; culture of virus from the cerebrospinal fluid is much less likely to be positive.[32] Polymerase chain reaction of cerebrospinal fluid is also useful for the diagnosis of HSV meningitis and can be an important clue for EBV central nervous system lymphoma in highly immunocompromised patients. Quantification of CMV and EBV DNA in the blood is useful for monitoring the risk of disease due to these viruses and for response to therapy in transplant recipients. Culture of herpesviruses is much less sensitive than polymerase chain reaction, but is useful for analysis of drug-resistant virus. Because asymptomatic shedding is common for most herpesviruses, a positive culture does not necessarily indicate that the virus is causing disease. Direct fluorescent antibody testing is useful for detection of VZV in skin lesions.

Lytic replication of herpesviruses causes characteristic intranuclear inclusions in tissues. CMV and HHV-6 cause both intranuclear and cytoplasmic inclusions, whereas HSV and VZV result in only intranuclear inclusions (Fig. 135-2). Immunohistochemistry with monoclonal antibodies can be used to identify specific viruses in tissues.

Treatment

Currently all FDA approved oral or intravenous antiviral agents for herpesvirus infections act at the same step of virus replication; they inhibit the viral DNA polymerase.[33] Some antiviral agents are phosphorylated by the HSV or VZV thymidine kinase (acyclovir, penciclovir) or CMV UL97 protein kinase (ganciclovir), whereas other antiviral drugs do not require phosphorylation (foscarnet, cidofovir). In general, foscarnet and cidofovir are more toxic to cells because they are active in both infected and uninfected cells. Valacyclovir, valganciclovir, and famciclovir are prodrugs that are converted to their active form (acyclovir, ganciclovir, penciclovir, respectively) by cellular enzymes. New drugs under development, such as marabavir, act at a different step of virus replication such as inhibiting viral protein kinases (see also Chapter 41).

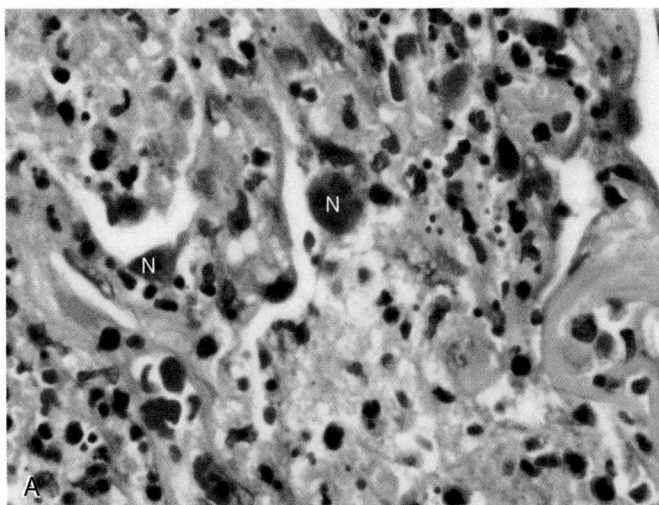

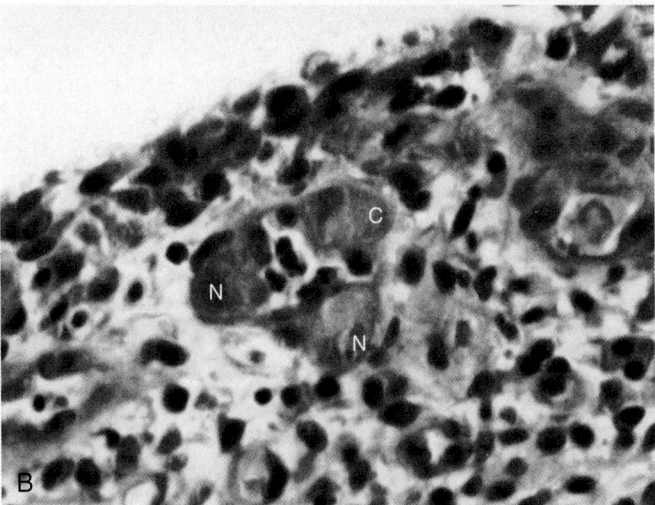

Figure 135-2 **Intranuclear inclusions in cells infected with herpes simplex virus (A) and intranuclear and cytoplasmic inclusions in cells infected with cytomegalovirus (B).** N, intranuclear; C, cytoplasmic. *(Courtesy of David Kleiner, Laboratory of Pathology, National Cancer Institute, National Institutes of Health, Bethesda, MD.)*

Resistance of HSV, VZV, or CMV to antiviral drugs usually only occurs in highly immunocompromised persons and is usually due to mutations in the HSV or VZV thymidine kinase or CMV protein kinase; foscarnet or, less often, cidofovir, is used to treat drug-resistant HSV, VZV, or CMV. Resistance to the latter two agents can occur due to mutations in the viral DNA polymerase. Antiviral therapy has not been proven to be clinically effective for HHV-6, HHV-7, and KSHV. Antiviral therapy is not beneficial for reducing symptoms of EBV disease, with the exception of oral hairy leukoplakia. Corticosteroids are occasionally used to treat severe manifestations of EBV, which are due to the T-cell proliferative response to the virus rather than to lytic replication in B cells.

Currently available antivirals inhibit lytic replication, not latent replication, and therefore do not affect the latent reservoir of viral DNA. One approach that has been suggested to reduce the latent reservoir of herpesvirus DNA is to activate lytic replication in latently infected cells (e.g., using a histone deacetylase inhibitor) and then treat with an inhibitor of lytic replication (acyclovir or ganciclovir). This approach has been used in vitro[34] and in patients with EBV-positive lymphomas.[35] Another approach is to infuse HLA-matched cytotoxic T cells to destroy latently infected cells. This has been successful for EBV and CMV disease.[36]

Prevention

Varicella immunoglobulin is used to decrease the severity of disease in immunocompromised persons exposed to chickenpox or shingles and CMV immunoglobulin to decrease disease in organ transplant recipients at high risk of CMV disease. Acyclovir reduces recurrences of HSV, and severity of varicella in uninfected immunocompromised persons exposed to VZV; ganciclovir reduces the risk of CMV disease in transplant recipients who often have virus reactivation.

Currently licensed vaccines are only available for VZV to prevent varicella and zoster.[37] These are live attenuated vaccines and differ only in the titer of the vaccine virus used; the shingles vaccine is approximately 14 times the titer of the varicella vaccine. Both vaccines induce humoral and cellular immunity. Live attenuated vaccines are not likely options for EBV and KSHV, which contain oncogenes and other genes that induce lymphocyte proliferation. Candidate vaccines for herpesviruses that are farthest along in clinical trials are subunit vaccines. A glycoprotein D vaccine for HSV-2,[38] glycoprotein B vaccine for CMV,[39] and glycoprotein gp350 for EBV[40] have all undergone clinical trials and continue to be tested in humans and are discussed further in the following chapters that discuss individual herpesviruses.

REFERENCES

1. Pellett PE, Roizman B. The family Herpesviridae: a brief introduction. In: Knipe DM, Howley PM, eds. *Fields Virology*. 5th ed. Philadelphia: Lippincott Williams & Wilkins; 2007;2479-2499.
2. Walker A, Petheram SJ, Ballard L, et al. Characterization of human cytomegalovirus strains by analysis of short tandem repeat polymorphisms. *J Clin Microbiol*. 2001;39:2219-2226.
3. Katz BZ, Raab-Traub N, Miller G. Latent and replicating forms of Epstein-Barr virus DNA in lymphomas and lymphoproliferative diseases. *J Infect Dis*. 1989;160:589-598.
4. Heldwein EE, Krummenacher C. Entry of herpesviruses into mammalian cells. *Cell Mol Life Sci*. 2008;65:1653-1668.
5. Perng GC, Jones C, Ciacci-Zanella J, et al. Virus-induced neuronal apoptosis blocked by the herpes simplex virus latency-associated transcript. *Science*. 2000;287:1500-1503.
6. Ambagala AP, Cohen JI. Varicella-zoster virus IE63, a major viral latency protein, is required to inhibit the alpha interferon-induced antiviral response. *J Virol*. 2007;81:7844-7851.
7. Hochberg D, Middeldorp JM, Catalina M, et al. Demonstration of the Burkitt's lymphoma Epstein-Barr virus phenotype in dividing latently infected memory cells in vivo. *Proc Natl Acad Sci U S A*. 2004;101:239-244.
8. Umbach JL, Kramer MF, Jurak I, et al. MicroRNAs expressed by herpes simplex virus 1 during latent infection regulate viral mRNAs. *Nature*. 2008;454:780-783.
9. Murphy E, Vanícek J, Robins H, et al. Suppression of immediate-early viral gene expression by herpesvirus-coded microRNAs: implications for latency. *Proc Natl Acad Sci U S A*. 2008;105:5453-5458.
10. Gary L, Gilden DH, Cohrs RJ. Epigenetic regulation of varicella-zoster virus open reading frames 62 and 63 in latently infected human trigeminal ganglia. *J Virol*. 2006;80:4921-4926.
11. Knipe DM, Cliffe A. Chromatin control of herpes simplex virus lytic and latent infection. *Nat Rev Microbiol*. 2008;6:211-221.
12. Kristie TM, Vogel JL, Sears AE. Nuclear localization of the C1 factor (host cell factor) in sensory neurons correlates with reactivation of herpes simplex virus from latency. *Proc Natl Acad Sci U S A*. 1999;96:1229-1233.
13. Lungu O, Panagiotidis CA, Annunziato PW, et al. Aberrant intracellular localization of Varicella-Zoster virus regulatory proteins during latency. *Proc Natl Acad Sci U S A*. 1998;95:7080-7085.
14. Sawtell NM, Thompson RL. Rapid in vivo reactivation of herpes simplex virus in latently infected murine ganglionic neurons after transient hyperthermia. *J Virol*. 1992;66:2150-2156.
15. Davis DA, Rinderknecht AS, Zoeteweij JP, et al. Hypoxia induces lytic replication of Kaposi sarcoma-associated herpesvirus. *Blood*. 2001;97:3244-3250.
16. Orange JS. Human natural killer cell deficiencies. *Curr Opin Allergy Clin Immunol*. 2006;6:399-409.
17. Corey L, Wald A, Celum CL, et al. The effects of herpes simplex virus-2 on HIV acquisition and transmission: a review of two overlapping epidemics. *J Acquir Immune Defic Syndr*. 2004;35:435-445.
18. Sylwester AW, Mitchell BL, Edgar JB, et al. Broadly targeted human cytomegalovirus-specific CD4+ and CD8+ T cells dominate the memory compartments of exposed subjects. *J Exp Med*. 2005;202:673-685.
19. Hosken N, McGowan P, Meier A, et al. Diversity of the CD8+ T-cell response to herpes simplex virus type 2 proteins among persons with genital herpes. *J Virol*. 2006;80:5509-5515.
20. Zhang SY, Jouanguy E, Ugolini S, et al. TLR3 deficiency in patients with herpes simplex encephalitis. *Science*. 2007;317:1522-1527.
21. Casrouge A, Zhang SY, Eidenschenk C, et al. Herpes simplex virus encephalitis in human UNC-93B deficiency. *Science*. 2006;314:308-312.
22. Sayos J, Wu C, Morra M, et al. The X-linked lymphoproliferative-disease gene product SAP regulates signals induced through the co-receptor SLAM. *Nature*. 1998;395:462-469.
23. Rigaud S, Fondanèche MC, Lambert N, et al. XIAP deficiency in humans causes an X-linked lymphoproliferative syndrome. *Nature*. 2006;444:110-114.
24. Lekstrom-Himes JA, Hohman P, Warren T, et al. Association of major histocompatibility complex determinants with the development of symptomatic and asymptomatic genital herpes simplex virus type 2 infections. *J Infect Dis*. 1999;179:1077-1085.
25. McAulay KA, Higins CD, Macween KF, et al. HLA class I polymorphisms are associated with development of infectious mononucleosis upon primary EBV infection. *J Clin Invest*. 2007;117:3042-3048.
26. Bochurd PY, Magaret AS, Koelle DM, et al. Polymorphisms in TLR2 are associated with increased viral shedding and lesional rate in patients with genital herpes simplex virus type 2 infection. *J Infect Dis*. 2007;196:505-509.

27. Helminen M, Lahdenpohja N, Hume M. Polymorphism of the interleukin-10 gene is associated with susceptibility to Epstein-Barr virus infection. *J Infect Dis.* 1999;180:496-499.
28. Tortorella D, Gewurz BE, Furman MH, et al. Viral subversion of the immune system. *Annu Rev Immunol.* 2000;18:861-926.
29. Powers C, DeFilippis V, Malouli D, et al. Cytomegalovirus immune evasion. *Curr Top Microbiol Immunol.* 2008;325:333-359.
30. Nicholas J. Human gammaherpesvirus cytokines and chemokine receptors. *Interferon Cytokine Res.* 2005;25:373-383.
31. Cohen JI. Herpesviruses. In: Kufe DW, Bast RC, Hait WN, et al. eds. *Cancer Medicine.* 7th ed. Hamilton: BC Decker; 2006;310-317.
32. DeBiasi RL, Kleinschmidt-DeMasters BK, Weinberg AM, et al. Use of PER for the diagnosis of herpesvirus infections of the central nervous system. *J Clin Virol.* 2002;25(Suppl 1):S5-S11.
33. Naesens L, De Clercq E. Recent developments in herpesvirus therapy. *Herpes.* 2001;8:12-16.
34. Feng WH, Hong G, Delecluse HJ, et al. Lytic induction therapy for Epstein-Barr virus-positive B-cell lymphomas. *J Virol.* 2004;78:1893-1902.
35. Perrine, SP, Hermine, O, Small, T et al. A phase 1/2 trial of arginine butyrate and ganciclovir in patients with Epstein-Barr virus-associated lymphoid malignancies. *Blood.* 2007;109:2571-2578.
36. Leen AM, Myers GD, Sili U, et al. Monoculture-derived T lymphocytes specific for multiple viruses expand and produce clinically relevant effects in immunocompromised individuals. *Nat Med.* 2006;12:1160-1166.
37. Oxman MN, Levin MJ, Johnson GR, et al. A vaccine to prevent herpes zoster and postherpetic neuralgia in older adults. *N Engl J Med.* 2005;352:2271-2284.
38. Stanberry LR, Spruance SL, Cunningham AL, et al. Glycoprotein-D-adjuvant vaccine to prevent genital herpes. *N Engl J Med.* 2002;347:1652-1661.
39. Zhang C, Buchanan H, Andrews W, et al. Detection of cytomegalovirus infection during a vaccine clinical trial in healthy young women: seroconversion and viral shedding. *J Clin Virol.* 2006;35:338-342.
40. Sokal EM, Hoppenbrouwers K, Vandermeulen C, et al. Recombinant gp350 vaccine for infectious mononucleosis: a phase 2, randomized, double-blind, placebo-controlled trial to evaluate the safety, immunogenicity, and efficacy of an Epstein-Barr virus vaccine in healthy young adults. *J Infect Dis.* 2007;196:1749-1753.

136

Herpes Simplex Virus

JOSHUA T. SCHIFFER | LAWRENCE COREY

Herpes simplex virus types 1 and 2 (HSV-1 and HSV-2) produce a wide variety of illnesses, including mucocutaneous infections, infections of the central nervous system (CNS), and an occasional infection of visceral organs; some of these conditions may be life threatening. The advent of effective chemotherapy for HSV infection has made their prompt recognition of clinical importance.

The word herpes (from the Greek, "to creep") has been used in medicine since antiquity. Cold sores (herpes febrilis) were described by the Roman physician Herodotus in AD 100.[1] Genital herpes was first described by John Astruc, physician to the king of France in 1736: the first English translation appeared in his treatise on venereal disease in 1754.[2,3] Infection in orolabial lesions was transmitted to other humans in the late 19th century. The disease was successfully transferred to rabbits in the early 20th century, and HSV was grown in vitro in 1925.[4,5] In the 1960s, Nahmias and Dowdle[6] reported two antigenic types of HSV with different sites of viral recovery.

Description of the Agent

The eight known human herpesviruses (HHVs) are divided by genomic and biologic behavior into three groups: the alphaherpesviruses (HSV-1, HSV-2, and varicella-zoster), the betaherpesviruses (HHV-6, HHV-7, and cytomegalovirus), and the gammaherpesviruses (Epstein-Barr virus, Kaposi's sarcoma-associated herpesvirus, and HHV-8) (see Chapter 135). Herpesviruses are morphologically similar, possessing an internal core containing double-stranded DNA, an icosahedral capsid with 162 capsomers, an amorphous material surrounding the capsid called a tegument, and a lipid envelope containing viral glycoproteins on its surface. Their overall diameter is approximately 160 nm.[7] Despite common morphologic features, the biologic and epidemiologic features of each of the herpesviruses are different. Although HSV-1 and HSV-2 are the two most closely related herpesviruses, the two agents are serologically and genetically distinct.[6]

The genome of HSV is a linear, double-stranded DNA molecule (molecular weight approximately 100×10^6) that encodes approximately 90 transcriptional units, 84 of which appear to encode proteins. The genetic organization has sequences from both terminal ends of the genome repeated in an inverted fashion. This divides the genome into two unique components.[8] The overall sequence homology between HSV-1 and HSV-2 is approximately 50%.[9] The homologous sequences are distributed over the entire genome map, and most of the polypeptides specified by one viral type are antigenically related to polypeptides of the other viral type. Many type-specific regions unique to HSV-1 and HSV-2 proteins do exist, however, and many of these regions appear to be important in host immunity.

HSV is genomically stable and restriction endonuclease or sequence analysis of viral DNA can be used to distinguish between the two subtypes and among strains of each subtype.[10,11] The variability of nucleotide sequences from clinical strains of HSV-1 and HSV-2 is such that HSV isolates obtained from two individuals can be easily differentiated.[12] Isolates from epidemiologically related sources, such as sexual partners, mother-infant pairs, and victims of a common-source outbreak, are identical.[13-15]

Viral replication has nuclear and cytoplasmic phases. The initial steps of replication include attachment and fusion between the viral envelope and cell membrane to liberate the nucleocapsid into the cytoplasm of the cell. Several cellular receptors and viral envelope glycoproteins are required for viral attachment. The initial attachment to the cell membrane involves the interactions of viral glycoproteins C and B with cellular heparin sulfate.[16] Subsequently, viral glycoprotein D binds to cellular co-receptors that belong to the tumor necrosis factor receptor family of proteins, the immunoglobulin superfamily (nectin family), or both.[17,18] The ubiquity of these receptors underscores the wide host range of herpesviruses, and their presence on sensory neurons implicates their role in the development of neuronal infection and, therefore, latency.[19-21]

After attachment, the de-enveloped tegument capsid structure is transported to nuclear pores, where viral DNA is released into the nucleus. After fusion of the virion envelope with the host cell membrane, the virions release several functional proteins. The virion host shutoff protein shuts off synthesis (by increasing cellular RNA degradation), whereas VP16 turns on transcription of immediate early genes of HSV replication.[22] Some of these immediate early gene products (designated α genes) are important determinants of neurovirulenece in animal models, whereas others are required for synthesis of a subsequent polypeptide group, the β or early polypeptides. Many β proteins are regulatory proteins and enzymes required for DNA replication. Most current antiviral drugs interfere with β proteins, such as the viral DNA polymerase enzyme. Transcription of the viral genome, replication of viral DNA, and assembly of capsids take place in the nucleus.[23] Moreover, the late (γ) class of HSV genes requires viral DNA replication for expression. These late proteins are structural and assist with viral egress. DNA replication takes place in a "rolling circle" pattern like a roll of toilet paper. Specific viral genes "clip" the end of the viral DNA into the procapsid.

After nucleocapsids are assembled in the nucleus, envelopment occurs as the nucleocapsids bud through the inner nuclear membrane into the perinuclear space. In some cells, viral replication in the nucleus forms two types of inclusion bodies: type A basophilic Feulgen-positive bodies that contain viral DNA and eosinophilic inclusion bodies that are devoid of viral nucleic acid or protein and represent a "scar" of infection. Virions are then transported through the endoplasmic reticulum and Golgi apparatus to the cell surface. The entire replication cycle takes 16 to 20 hours. HSV is cytopathic to cells that harbor the full cycle of HSV replication.[24]

HSV infection of some neuronal cells does not result in cell death. Instead, viral genomes are maintained by the cell in a repressed state compatible with survival and normal activities of the cell, called latency.[25,26] Latency is associated with transcription of only a limited number of virus-encoded RNAs.[27-29] Subsequent activation of the viral genome may occur, resulting in the normal pattern of regulated viral gene expression, replication, and release of HSV, although without apparent damage to the infected neuron. The release of virions from the neuron follows a complex process of anterograde transport down the length of neuronal axons.[30] Subsequent viral entry into epithelial cells can result in viral replication: this process is termed reactivation.[31,32]

Although infectious virus typically cannot be cultured from sensory or autonomic nervous system ganglia dissected from cadavers, maintenance and growth of the neural cells in tissue culture result in production of infectious virions (explantation) and in subsequent permissive infection of susceptible cells (cocultivation).[33] The fact that HSV replication was first detected in neurons during reactivation in vitro suggested that the neuron harbors latent virus in vivo.[27] Viral DNA and RNA have since been found in neural tissue at times when infectious virus cannot be isolated.[29,34] Documentation of individual neurons infected with multiple strains of drug-susceptible and drug-resistant virus has been shown in severely immunosuppressed patients, suggesting that the ganglia can be reseeded with HSV repeatedly during chronic infection.[35] Whether this is a common occurrence among immunocompetent persons is, as yet, unclear.

Three noncoding RNA latency-associated transcripts (LATs) are the only transcripts in abundance in the nuclei of latently infected neurons.[27,36,37] Deletion mutants of the genomic region that can become latent have been made, and the efficiency of their later reactivation is reduced.[36,38] In addition, substitution of HSV-1 LAT for HSV-2 LAT induces an HSV-1 reactivation pattern.[37] Thus, LATs appear to maintain, rather than establish, latency. HSV-1 LATs promote the survival of acutely infected neurons, perhaps by inhibiting apoptotic pathways.[39,40] Highly expressed during latency, LAT-derived micro RNA appears to silence expression of the key neurovirulence factor infected cell protein (ICP)34.5[41] and to bind in an antisense configuration to ICP0 messenger RNA to prevent expression of this immediate early protein that is vital to HSV reactivation. Recent work employing microdissection plus real-time polymerase chain reaction (PCR) of individual neurons from cadaveric trigeminal ganglia explants revealed that many more neurons (2% to 10%) harbor HSV than would be predicted by in situ hybridization studies for LAT and that copy number is similar in LAT positive and negative neurons.[42,43] This adds uncertainty to the role that LATs play in preventing reactivation. At present, the molecular mechanisms of HSV latency are not completely understood, and strategies to interrupt or maintain latency in neurons are not available.[44,45]

Epidemiology

Herpes simplex viruses have a worldwide distribution and are found in the most remote human populations. There are no known animal vectors for HSV, and although experimental animals are easily infected, humans appear to be the only natural reservoir. Herpes infection is the predominant cause of genital ulcers throughout the world. This is due to an overall decrease in *Treponema pallidum* and chancroid infections in most populations, increased use of HSV PCR for detection of HSV infection,[46] and the frequent reactivation of HSV-2 among persons infected with the human immunodeficiency virus (HIV).[47]

Infection with HSV-1 is acquired more frequently and earlier than infection with HSV-2.[48] More than 90% of adults have antibodies to HSV-1 by the fifth decade of life. Prevalence of antibody to HSV-1 increases with age and demonstrates an inverse correlation with socioeconomic status. In much of Asia and Africa, HSV-1 infection is nearly universal and is acquired early in childhood. However, in post–World War II era Western populations, 80% to 100% of middle-aged adults of lower socioeconomic status had antibodies to HSV-1 compared with only 30% to 50% of adults in higher socioeconomic groups.[49,50] Serosurveys continue to show a decrease in the age-specific prevalence rates for HSV-1 in both the United States and most of Europe, although socioeconomic class distinctions remain.[51] A decrease in HSV-1 acquisition in childhood accounts for the increased frequency of sexually acquired HSV-1 infections in adolescents and the increased proportion of neonatal HSV cases that are due to HSV-1.[48,50,52,53]

Antibodies to HSV-2 start to appear during puberty and correlate with initiation of sexual activity.[51,54] Widespread use of serologic testing has provided a detailed characterization of a worldwide HSV-2 pandemic over the past two decades (Table 136-1).[51,55-57] Most African surveys indicate very high levels of infection. Seroprevalence is lower in Europe, Australia, Latin America, and Asia, although it remains highly dependent on the risk of the group being evaluated. In the United States, nationwide surveys showed an increase in HSV-2 seroprevalence from 16.4% to 21.7% in adults between 1979 and 1991, with a decrease to 17% from 1999 to 2004.[51,55,58] The cumulative lifetime incidence of HSV-2 reaches 25% in white women, 20% in white men, 80% in black women, and 60% in black men. The higher rates of HSV-2 among African Americans may reflect patterns of sexual networking rather than high-risk individual behavior.

HSV-2 prevalence in a population is defined by geographic region, gender, sexual habits, and study population. There is consistently a higher prevalence of HSV-2 in women than in men.[49,50,52,56] The frequency of HSV-2 antibody is higher among HIV-infected persons, persons recruited from sexually transmitted disease (STD) clinics, and among homosexual men.[56,57,59] HSV-2 antibody levels are closely related to the lifetime number of sexual partners, age at initiation of sexual activity, and a history of other sexually acquired diseases.[60,61]

Incidence rates of HSV-2 infection are difficult to estimate due to the common nature of asymptomatic seroconversion, attenuation of symptoms due to previous HSV-1 infection, location of lesions in nonvisible locations (perianal), and differential access to health care and diagnostics. For instance, among HSV-seronegative women in the control arm of an HSV-2 vaccine trial, only half of seroconversions were clinically symptomatic.[62] Nevertheless, data are accumulating and vary among populations based on risk characteristics and geography. Vaccine and condom prevention studies conducted in serodiscordant couples document HSV-2 seroincidence levels between 6.7 and 8.6 infections per 100 person-years for women, and 1.5 to 3.7 per 100 person-years for men.[63-65] Seroincidence in several high-risk urban youth cohorts was 11.7 cases per 100 person-years.[66] In high-risk men who have sex with men (MSM), the seroincidence rate for HSV-2 was lower at 1.9 cases per 100 person-years, but the seroprevalence of HSV-2 was already 20% and the HSV-2 incidence was identical to that of HIV type 1 (HIV-1).[67] In African populations characterized by a high preexisting HSV-2 seroprevalence, the seroincidence was 1.8 to 12.9 per 100 person-years, with higher acquisition rates among persons with HIV-1 and among seronegative women in a monogamous relationship with a seropositive man.[68-70]

Cofactors for risk of genital HSV-2 acquisition in an individual are well defined from prospective trials. Women are at higher risk of HSV-2 acquisition than men.[62,63] Possible explanations include greater mucosal surface area as well as a higher likelihood of asymptomatic ulcers in men, which may facilitate transmission. It is uncertain whether past HSV-1 infection reduces the risk of infection with HSV-2. However, persons with previous HSV-1 are three times as likely to acquire HSV-2 subclinically.[62] In contrast with bacterial STDs, HSV-2 is commonly transmitted within long-term couples rather than casual sexual relationships. Longitudinal studies of such couples showed transmission rates varying from 3% to 12% per year.[63,65,71] The median time to transmission within discordant couples is 3 months, with a median number of only 24 sex acts before transmission.[65] Moreover, one third of source partners in serodiscordant couples deny a history of genital lesions.[72] Therefore, prevention efforts are essential. Knowledge of a long-term partner's HSV-2–positive status decreases transmission incidence by 50%, highlighting the importance of formal diagnosis and disclosure of infection.[65,73] Consistent condom use decreases HSV acquisition among women, and chemoprophylaxis of the source partner also decreases transmission.[65,71] Circumcision, which decreases HIV-1 acquisition, may have less effect on risk of HSV-2 acquisition.[74]

Transmission of Herpes Simplex Virus Infection

In 1921, Lipschutz[5] inoculated material from genital herpetic lesions into the skin of humans, eliciting clinical infection within 48 to 72 hours in six persons and within 24 days in one case. Transmission of HSV infections most frequently occurs through close contact with a person who is shedding virus at a peripheral site, at a mucosal surface, or in genital or oral secretions.[75,76] Infection occurs by inoculation of virus onto susceptible mucosal surfaces (e.g., the oropharynx, cervix, conjunctivae) or through small cracks in the skin. Because HSV is readily inactivated at room temperature and by drying, aerosol and fomitic spread are unusual means of transmission.[77] Transmission of HSV-1 from orogenital contact is increasingly recognized, perhaps because of a decrease in the age-specific prevalence of HSV-1 at the time that sexual activity starts.[78] Spread of HSV-1 infection from oral secretions to other skin areas is a hazard of certain occupations (e.g.,

TABLE 136-1	Herpes Simplex Virus Type 2 Seroprevalence in Selected Populations	
Population		Frequency of HSV-2 Infection (%)
United States		
General population		22
Women		26
Men		18
Women's clinic, Albuquerque, NM		31
Women in STD clinic, Birmingham, AL		64
HIV-1–negative MSM, Seattle, WA		26
San Francisco neighborhood survey		
Women		41
Men		25
Europe		
Blood donors, Germany		13
STD clinic, France		55
STD clinic, Milan, Italy		25
MSM, Italy		55
Ob/Gyn clinic, Italy		18
Blood donors, London, UK		8
General population, Helsinki, Finland		16
STD clinic, London, UK		
Women		25
Men		17
Randomly selected German population, 1996		13
STD clinic, The Netherlands		32
STD clinic, Sweden		17
Obstetric clinic, Sweden		33
Obstetric clinic, Estonia		24
Africa		
Rural adults, Rakai, Uganda		
Women		74
Men		57
Urban adults, Kisumu, Kenya		
Women		68
Men		35
Urban adults, Cotonou, Benin		
Women		30
Men		12
Urban adults, Yaounde, Cameroon		
Women		51
Men		27
Urban adults, Kinshasa, Zaire		41
Male factory workers, Zimbabwe		45
STD clinics, South African male		60
Commercial sex workers, Zaire		90
Latin America/South America		
Women seeking HIV-1 testing, Mexico City		29
Household survey of women, Costa Rica		39
Pregnant women, Sao Paulo, Brazil		39
MSM, Peru		52
STD clinic, Peru		83
Women in Brazil		42
Asia		
Married women, Bangladesh		12
Pregnant women, Japan		7
Commercial sex workers, Thailand		76
Women, Philippines		9
Antenatal clinic, India		14
Antenatal clinic, Sri Lanka		21
Australia		
Pregnant women		15
STD clinic		
Women		55
Men		35
STD clinic, Auckland, New Zealand		26

HIV-1, human immunodeficiency virus type 1; HSV-2, herpes simplex virus type 2; MSM, men who have sex with men; Ob/Gyn, obstetrics and gynecology; STD, sexually transmitted disease.

Adapted from Corey L, Wald A, Celum C, Quinn TC. The effects of HSV-2 on HIV-1 acquisition and transmission: a review of two overlapping epidemics. *J Acquir Immune Defic Syndr.* 2004;35:435-445.

dentists, respiratory care unit personnel), and laboratory-acquired and nosocomial outbreaks in hospital or nursery personnel have been reported.[77] Outbreaks among wrestlers are well recognized.[79] Transmission of HSV can occur in infants born to mothers excreting HSV at delivery.[80] Anal and perianal infections with HSV-1 or HSV-2 are common among sexually active MSM populations.[81] The majority of cases occur within 5 days of contact, highlighting the short incubation period of primary infection.

Precise virologic determinants of transmission likelihood are poorly understood. For HIV infection, a clear relationship between genital and plasma HIV viral load and per coital risk of HIV transmission is established.[82] However, because genital HSV-2 levels fluctuate rapidly over time, the degree to which source partner viral load during sex affects the likelihood of transmission is unknown.[83] Subclinical or asymptomatic shedding of HSV in oral and genital secretions is common, even in immunocompetent persons, and transmission occurs more commonly during asymptomatic shedding.[75,84] Frequency of detectable shedding is markedly heterogeneous among those seropositive for HSV-2, suggesting that per coital transmission may be highly dependent on the source partner.[84] A modeling study predicted that a core group of "super spreaders" with high reactivation rates may account for a disproportionately large percentage of new infections.[85] However, the frequency of symptomatic recurrences was a poor predictor of the likelihood of transmission in the valacyclovir prevention study.[86] DNA polymerase inhibitors that decrease the frequency of asymptomatic shedding as well as peak HSV-2 titers during recurrence decrease transmission within serodiscordant couples.[71]

Pathogenesis

Exposure to HSV at mucosal surfaces or abraded skin sites permits entry of the virus and initiation of its replication in cells of the epidermis and dermis.[87] Initial HSV infection is often subclinical, without apparent lesions. In animal models and human subjects, both clinical acquisition and subclinical acquisition are associated with sufficient viral replication to permit infection of either sensory or autonomic nerve endings.[29,87,88] After traversing the neuroepithelial gap and entering the neuronal cell, the virus or, more likely, the nucleocapsid is transported intra-axonally to the nerve cell bodies in ganglia.[89] For HSV-1 infection, trigeminal ganglia are most commonly infected, although extension to the inferior and superior cervical ganglia also occurs.[25,26] With genital infection, sacral nerve root ganglia (S2 to S5) are most commonly affected.[31] In humans, the interval from inoculation of virus in peripheral tissue to spread to the ganglia is unknown.

Viral replication occurs in ganglia and contiguous neural tissue during primary infection only.[87,88] After initial inoculation of the neural ganglion, virus spreads to other mucosal skin surfaces by centrifugal migration of infectious virions through peripheral sensory nerves. This mode of spread explains the characteristic development of new lesions distant from the initial crop of vesicles in patients with primary genital or orolabial HSV infection, the large surface area over which these vesicles may be visualized, and the recovery of virus from neural tissue distant from neurons innervating the inoculation site.[90] Contiguous spread of virus may also take place via autoinoculation and allow further extension of disease. Viremia is present during approximately 25% of primary HSV-2 infections, and its presence may affect the natural history of HSV-2 disease in terms of site, severity, and frequency of reactivation.[91]

After resolution of primary disease, infectious HSV can no longer be cultured from the ganglia. However, viral DNA is present in 2% to 11% of ganglion cells in the anatomic region of initial infection.[42] Therefore, many neurons may contribute to reactivation. The mechanism of reactivation is unknown. Recent studies indicate that host T-cell responses both at the ganglion and peripheral mucosal level influence the frequency and severity of HSV reactivation.[32,33] Recently, HSV-specific T cells have been recovered from peripheral nerve root ganglia. Resident CD8+ lymphocytes and lymphocyte-derived cytokines appear to be important in preventing infectious virions from being transported down the length of the axon for release in the basal layer of the epidermis.[92-94] CD8+ T cells juxtapose to HSV-1 latently infected neurons in the trigeminal ganglia[95] and can block reactivation with both interferon-γ release[96] and granzyme B degradation of immediate early protein, infected cell protein 4.[97] In addition, there appears to be a latent viral load in the ganglia that correlates positively with the number of neurons infected and the rate of reactivation, but inversely with the number of CD8+ cells present.[98,99] Yet, it is not known whether reactivating stimuli transiently suppress these immune cells, independently upregulate transcription of lytic genes, or both. However, once virus reaches the dermal-epidermal junction, there are two possible outcomes: subclinical shedding or recurrence defined clinically by a skin blister and ulceration (Fig. 136-1). Histologically, herpetic lesions involve a thin-walled vesicle or ulceration in the basal region, multinucleated cells that may include intranuclear inclusion, necrosis, and an acute inflammatory infection. Re-epithelialization occurs once viral replication is restricted, almost always in the absence of a scar. It is not known whether excess inflammation is present during brief asymptomatic shedding events.

Recent studies suggest that the rate of reactivation is far more frequent and dynamic than previously recognized[84,100] (Fig. 136-2). The use of daily anogenital PCR swabs showed that the median shedding rate of the 95% of patients with a positive HSV-2 antibody who shed virus is 25% of days, with a wide range of interpatient variability (range, 2% to 75%).[101] In addition, in a study with sampling performed every 6 hours, it was noted that 49% of genital reactivation episodes last less than 12 hours and 29% last less than 6 hours.[84] However, even these short bursts of reactivation were associated with copy numbers high enough to cause transmission. The conclusion from these recent studies was that ganglionic immunity is considerably less tight than previously believed, which, in turn, raises the possibility that peripheral immune control might dictate the likelihood and severity of recurrences as well as the frequency of subclinical shedding. There is a strong association between the magnitude of CD8+ lymphocyte response and clearance of virus from genital lesions.[102,103] The lack of this response, rather than low CD4+ lymphocyte count, also predicts frequent and severe HSV-2 recurrences in untreated, as well as treated, HIV-1–infected patients.[104,105] HSV-2 CD8+ and CD4+ T cells appear to persist for prolonged time periods (2 to 4 months) in genital skin previously involved in an HSV-2 reactivation. The location, effectiveness, and longevity of the T lymphocytes and perhaps other immune effector cells may be an important factor in the expression of disease and the likelihood of transmission over time.

Among immunocompetent persons who acquire HSV-1 orally and genitally, HSV-1 reactivates more frequently in the oral than in the genital region. Similarly, for HSV-2, reactivation in the genital region is 8 to 10 times more frequent than oral reactivation of HSV-2.[106,107] In experimental animal systems, both sacral and trigeminal ganglia contain latent virus, but reactivation differs according to the anatomic site of infection.[108] When the region containing the latency-associated transcripts of HSV-2 was inserted in an HSV-1 virus, increasing reactivation in sacral nerve root ganglia occurred, indicating that viral factors influence site of reactivation.[37]

Clinical studies demonstrate that host factors also influence reactivation. Immunocompromised patients have more severe disease.[109-111] Agammaglobulinemic patients appear to handle HSV infection normally. Neonatal HSV is more likely to occur in vaginally delivered infants when the mother has primary rather than recurrent infection because placental antibodies are generated after primary infection and increase in avidity over time.[112-114] Widespread local extension and dissemination can occur in patients with inadequate cell-mediated immunity, including infants, organ transplant recipients, and HIV-infected persons.[115] Viremic spread to visceral organs can lead to life-threatening disease.[109] Severe, even fatal, infections can also develop in individuals with innate immunity defects in natural killer cells and plasmacytoid dendritic cells.[116,117]

Multiple cell populations, including natural killer cells, macrophages, a variety of T lymphocytes, and lymphokines generated by these cells, play a role in host defense against HSV infection.[115,118] Experimental ablation of lymphocytes indicated that T cells play a major role in viral containment and prevention of lethal disseminated disease, although antibodies also help reduce viral titer in neural tissue.[119] In animals, passive transfer of primed lymphocytes confers protection against rechallenge.[118] Maximal protection usually requires the activation of multiple T-cell subpopulations, including cytotoxic T cells and T cells responsible for delayed hypersensitivity.[120,121] T cells may confer protection by the antigen-stimulated release of lymphokines (e.g., interferons), which have a direct antiviral effect, or may activate other nonspecific effector cells.[122,123]

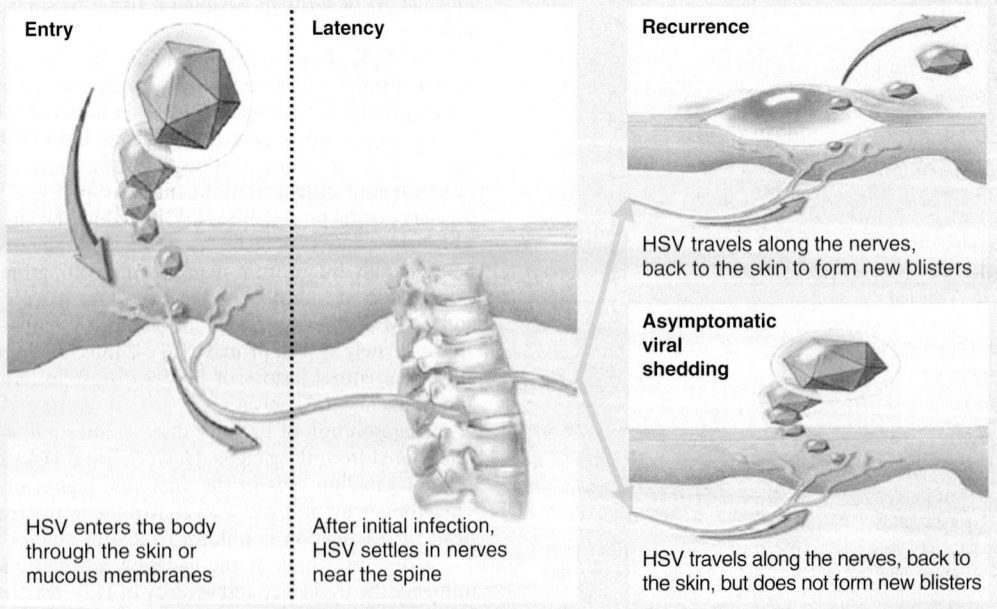

Entry

Latency

Recurrence

HSV travels along the nerves, back to the skin to form new blisters

Asymptomatic viral shedding

HSV enters the body through the skin or mucous membranes

After initial infection, HSV settles in nerves near the spine

HSV travels along the nerves, back to the skin, but does not form new blisters

Figure 136-1 **Schemata of herpes simplex virus (HSV) recurrence and asymptomatic viral shedding.**

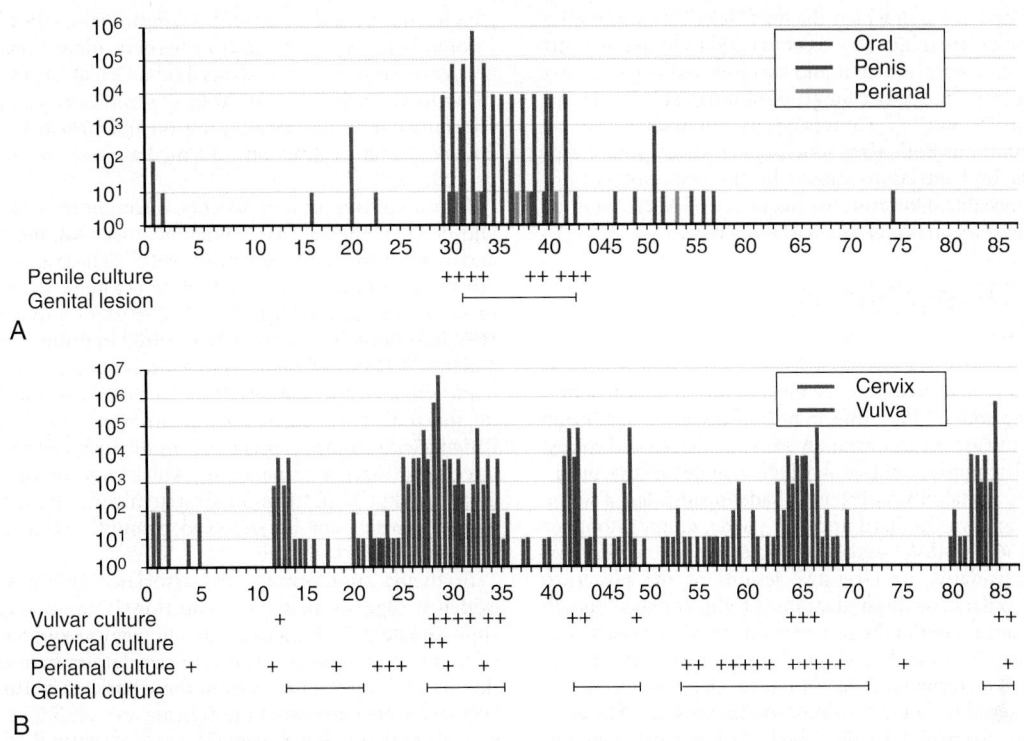

A

B

Figure 136-2 **Clinical and virologic shedding pattern as detected by viral culture and herpes simplex virus (HSV) DNA polymerase chain reaction in a man (A) and a woman (B).** The man began obtaining daily viral cultures around day 30 after acquisition of genital HSV type 2 infection. The woman was within 6 months of genital HSV type 2 acquisition when she was enrolled in the study.

There is an evolving appreciation that the cellular immune response to HSV-2 infection is highly compartmentalized and that responses in the neural ganglia, CNS, and mucosal sites may all play different roles.[94,124] Biopsies of herpetic lesions show that the predominant infiltrating cell is initially the CD4+ lymphocyte.[125,126] These lesion-infiltrating cells display activation markers such as interleukin-2 receptor, DR+, and ICAM-1+ and also secrete large amounts of interferon-γ.[127] Within 2 to 4 days, lesions are infiltrated with CD8+ T cells. Clearance of HSV-2 from genital lesions is associated with the infiltration of HSV-specific CD8+ T cells, and these cells are disproportionately represented in the mucosa in comparison with the serum.[102,128] CD8+ cells in the ganglia, conversely, control the rate of reactivation.[99]

The surface viral glycoproteins necessary for attachment also participate as antigens that are recognized by antibodies mediating neutralization and immune-mediated cytolysis (antibody-dependent cell-mediated cytotoxicity).[129] Monoclonal antibodies specific for each of the known viral glycoproteins have conferred experimental protection against subsequent neurologic disease or ganglionic latency.[130] In an ex vivo model of human reactivation, adequate neutralizing antibody concentrations prevented the successful transmission of HSV from dorsal root ganglion neurons to keratinocytes, despite successful antegrade transport of fully assembled particles down the length of the sensory neuron.[131] Antibodies are broadly generated against tegument, capsid and other nonessential viral glycoproteins, although the importance of antibody response magnitude, breadth, tissue compartment specificity, and subclass is not defined for HSV infection.[101]

Finally, innate immunity mechanisms appear to have a direct antiviral role. Plasma dendritic cells express Toll-like receptors and produce interferon-α,[132,133] defects in interferon receptors in mice promote enhanced infection,[134] Toll-like receptor 2 polymorphisms are associated with increased shedding and recurrence rate,[135] and a topically applied Toll-like receptor 7 and 8 agonist decreased shedding in a recent randomized trial.[136] However, the role of the innate immune response often is not neatly differentiated from acquired immunity: interferons that are produced by innate cells (plasmacytoid dendritic

cells, natural killer T cells, and natural killer cells) may influence the balance of Th1/Th2 response to HSV-2 and trigger similar transcription pathways in innate and acquired immune cells.[101,133]

The family of herpesviruses is evolutionarily ancient, infects a broad range of primitive and sophisticated hosts, and has developed complex mechanisms to evade sophisticated immune systems. Both HSV-1 and HSV-2 encode proteins that are directed at subverting innate and acquired responses.[137,138] ICP47 interacts with the transporter activity protein to prevent the interaction between HSV-specific peptides and HLA class I molecules. This interaction downregulates certain HSV peptides with HLA class I antigen on the cell surface and subverts the host CD8+ cytotoxic T-cell response to HSV.[138,139] The VHS protein shuts down host cell RNA and subsequent host defenses.[140] gJ protein inhibits cellular mechanisms of apoptosis and hence increases viral replication.[141,142] HSV γ34.5 ICP0 and US11 are virally derived proteins that counteract the antiviral effect of interferon-α.[143,144] UNC-93B is involved in Toll-like receptor signaling, and functional mutations in this gene were detected in a consanguineous cohort of patients with fatal HSV encephalitis.[145]

Some aspects of HSV disease may be related to immunopathologic events. In experimental animals, stromal keratitis associated with HSV-1 infection is precipitated by HSV-specific T cells.[146] Molecular cross-reactivity between the HSV proteins and cellular proteins seems to play a role in this phenomenon.[147]

Spectrum of Diseases Caused by Herpes Simplex Virus

HSV has been isolated from nearly all visceral and mucocutaneous sites. The clinical manifestations and course of HSV infection depend on the anatomic site involved, the age and immune status of the host, and the antigenic type of the virus. Presentations vary from subclinical mucosal shedding to overwhelming sepsis or encephalitis. First episodes of HSV disease, especially primary infections (first infections with either HSV-1 or HSV-2 in which the host lacks HSV antibodies in acute-phase serum), are frequently accompanied by systemic signs and symptoms, involve both mucosal and extramucosal sites, have a higher complication rate, and have a longer duration of symptoms and viral shedding from lesions.[148,149] Conversely, asymptomatic primary infection is also common. Both viral subtypes can cause genital and orofacial infections, and infections caused by the two subtypes are clinically indistinguishable. However, the frequency of reactivation of infection is influenced by anatomic site and virus type.[150]

Orofacial Herpes Simplex Virus Infection

Gingivostomatitis and pharyngitis are the most frequent clinical manifestations of first-episode HSV-1 infection,[151,152] usually result from primary infection, and are most commonly seen in children and young adults.[153,154] Clinical symptoms and signs, which include malaise, myalgias, inability to eat, irritability, and cervical adenopathy, last 3 to 14 days. Lesions may involve the hard and soft palate, gingiva, tongue, lip, and face (Fig. 136-3). HSV-1 and HSV-2 infection of the pharynx usually results in exudative or ulcerative lesions of the posterior pharynx, tonsillar pillars, or both. Lesions of the tongue, buccal mucosa, or gingiva occur later in the course in one third of cases. Fever lasts 2 to 7 days. It can be difficult to clinically differentiate HSV pharyngitis from bacterial pharyngitis, *Mycoplasma pneumoniae* infections, and pharyngeal ulcerations of noninfectious causes (e.g., Stevens-Johnson syndrome). Recurrent herpes labialis is the most frequent clinical manifestation of reactivation. No substantial evidence suggests that reactivation of orolabial HSV infection is associated with symptomatic recurrent pharyngitis.[155] Release of HSV from the trigeminal

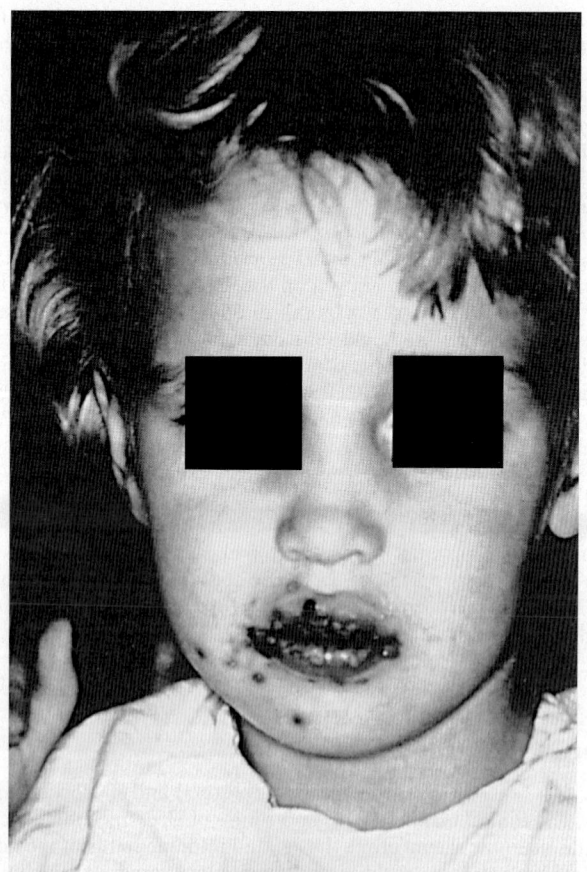

Figure 136-3 Primary herpes simplex virus gingivostomatitis in a child, extending to involve the cheek, chin, and periocular skin.

ganglia may be associated with asymptomatic salivary virus excretion, intraoral mucosal ulcerations, or herpetic ulcerations on the vermilion border of the lip or external facial skin. Orolabial HSV disease develops in approximately 50% to 70% of seropositive patients undergoing trigeminal nerve root decompression and 10% to 15% of those undergoing dental extraction a median of 3 days after these procedures.[155,156]

In immunosuppressed patients, infection may extend into mucosal and deep cutaneous layers. Friability, necrosis, bleeding, severe pain, and inability to eat or drink may result.[157] The lesions of HSV mucositis are similar to oral lesions caused by cytotoxic drug therapy, trauma, or fungal or bacterial infection.[158] Persistent and disabling ulcerative HSV infections are common in acquired immunodeficiency syndrome patients.[159] HSV and *Candida* infections often occur concurrently. Systemic acyclovir therapy speeds the rate of healing and relieves the pain of mucosal HSV infections in immunosuppressed patients.[157,158] Patients with atopic eczema or burns may acquire severe orofacial HSV infections (eczema herpeticum), which may rapidly involve extensive areas of skin with occasional systemic dissemination.[160] Extensive eczema herpeticum has resolved promptly with administration of intravenous acyclovir.[161]

Erythema multiforme is also associated with HSV infections, and evidence suggests that HSV infection is the precipitating event in approximately 75% of cases of cutaneous erythema multiforme.[162] HSV antigen was demonstrated in circulatory immune complexes and skin lesion biopsy samples from these patients.[163] Patients with severe HSV-associated erythema multiforme are candidates for chronic suppressive oral antiviral therapy.[164]

HSV-1 and varicella-zoster virus are implicated as common causes of Bell's palsy (facial paralysis of the mandibular portion of the facial nerve).[165] HSV DNA was found in ganglionic fluid in a high percentage of persons undergoing decompressive surgery for this entity, suggesting recent reactivation as the cause of disease.[166] These findings were corroborated by a trial that showed faster and more frequent resolution of facial paralyses with the prompt use of antiviral therapy directed at HSV-1 or varicella-zoster. It should be noted, however, that data on the results on antiviral therapy for Bell's palsy are conflicting, perhaps related to the timing of initiation of therapy.[167,168] As such, there is no consensus on the use of antivirals versus steroids versus both modalities for the treatment of Bell's palsy.

Genital Infection

First-episode primary genital herpes is associated with prolonged duration of symptoms, lesions (10 to 12 days), and viral shedding. This is particularly true for primary infection (i.e., HSV-1 and HSV-2 antibody negative), which is the case for approximately half of first-episode cases.[148] Approximately 25% of patients with their first clinical episode of symptomatic genital herpes have an HSV-2 antibody. Therefore, their acquisition likely occurred in the past and was asymptomatic.[169] First episodes of genital herpes caused by HSV-2 in patients who had previous HSV-1 infection are associated with less frequent systemic symptoms and faster healing than primary genital herpes, although rates of recurrence are the same.[148-150] The clinical courses of first-episode genital herpes among patients with HSV-1 and HSV-2 infections are similar; however, the 12-month recurrence rates among patients with first-episode HSV-2 and HSV-1 infections are 90% and 55%, respectively.[106,150] Genital HSV-1 infection is usually primary infection because HSV-1 acquisition is rare after HSV-2 infection.[170] Previous oral HSV-1 infection may protect against genital HSV-1 infection, although the degree of protection is unknown.

In 70% of women and 40% of men, first-episode genital herpes is accompanied by fever, headache, malaise, and myalgias. Pain, itching, dysuria, vaginal and urethral discharge, and tender inguinal lymphadenopathy are the predominant local symptoms and persist for several days after systemic symptoms. Local symptoms often peak between days 7 and 11 of detectable shedding, whereas inguinal tenderness can persist for several weeks. Widely spaced bilateral lesions

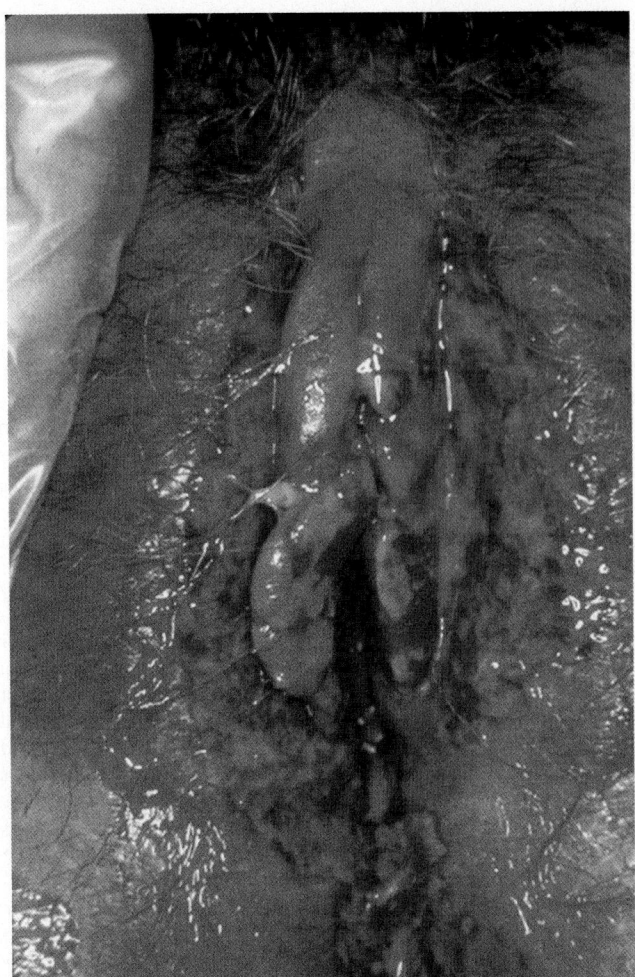

Figure 136-4 Primary genital herpes simplex virus type 2 infection of the vulva.

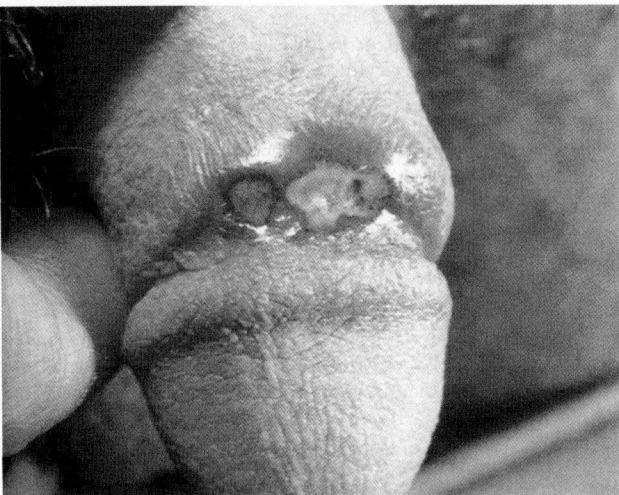

Figure 136-5 Chancroidal herpes simplex virus lesion on the penis. *(From Handsfield HH. Color Atlas and Synopsis of Sexually Transmitted Diseases, 2nd ed. New York: McGraw-Hill, 2001.)*

rectal intercourse.[177,178] Symptoms include anorectal pain, anorectal discharge, tenesmus, and constipation. Sigmoidoscopy reveals ulcerative lesions of the distal 10 cm of the rectal mucosa. Rectal biopsies show mucosal ulceration, necrosis, polymorphonuclear and lymphocytic infiltration of the lamina propria, and, occasionally, multinucleated intranuclear inclusion-bearing cells. External perianal lesions are

of the external genitalia are characteristic on examination (Figs. 136-4 and 136-5). Lesions may be present in varying stages, including vesicles, pustules, painful erythematous ulcers, crusting (dry surfaces), or re-epithelialization (mucosal surfaces). Multiple small lesions often coalesce into one larger ulcer. If untreated, formation of new ulcers between days 4 and 10 of infection is common. The mean time from the onset of a primary genital HSV lesion to complete healing is 19.5 days for women and 16.5 days for men.[148,149]

A clear mucoid discharge and dysuria are present in first-episode HSV in 83% of women and 44% of men. The severity of dysuria is often out of proportion with the urethral discharge seen on examination and the mild inflammation detected on urinalysis. HSV-2 cervicitis, when symptomatic, is notable for purulent or bloody vaginal discharge and can be difficult to differentiate from *Chlamydia trachomatis* and *Neisseria gonorrhoeae* infection. When present on speculum examination, cervical ulceration or necrosis is specific for HSV-2 infection. HSV-2 is present on the cervix and urethra in more than 80% of women with first-episode infections and 20% of women with recurrent lesions (Fig. 136-6).[171,172] Traditional colposcopy and Papanicolaou smear lack sensitivity for cervical HSV infection.[173] Moreover, HSV can be isolated from the urethra and urine of men and women without external genital lesions and from the urethra of 5% of women with the dysuria-frequency syndrome.[172-174] On occasion, HSV genital tract disease is manifested by endometritis and salpingitis in women and prostatitis in men.[175,176]

Both HSV-1 and HSV-2 can cause symptomatic or asymptomatic rectal and perianal infections. HSV proctitis is usually associated with

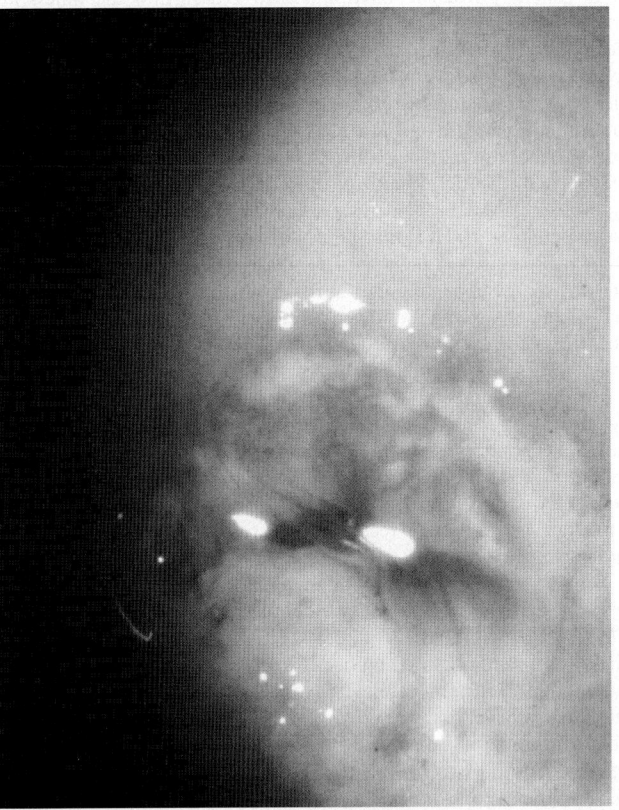

Figure 136-6 Herpes simplex virus cervicitis. *(From Corey L. Herpes simplex virus infections. In: Mandell GL, series ed. Atlas of Infectious Diseases, Volume V, Sexually Transmitted Diseases. Rein MF, ed. Philadelphia: Churchill Livingstone/Current Medicine; 1996, Fig. 15-21B.)*

present in approximately one half of cases.[177] Antiviral therapy speeds healing.[177-179] Perianal herpetic lesions also are found in immunosuppressed patients receiving cytotoxic therapy. Extensive perianal herpetic lesions, HSV proctitis, or both are common among HIV-infected patients.[159] Subclinical perianal shedding of HSV is detected both in heterosexual men and in women who report no rectal intercourse.[179,180] This phenomenon is due to the establishment of latency in the sacral dermatome from previous genital tract infection, with subsequent reactivation in epithelial cells in the perianal region.

Complications of Genital Herpes

The complications of genital herpes are related to local extension, spread to extragenital sites, or both.[80,181] Complications occur more frequently in women than in men.[148]

ASEPTIC MENINGITIS/TRANSVERSE MYELITIS/SACRAL RADICULOPATHY

Both HSV-1 and HSV-2 have been isolated from cerebrospinal fluid (CSF), although overt viral meningitis is much more common with HSV-2.[182,183] In one series, 36% of women and 13% of men with primary genital HSV-2 infection had stiff neck, headache, and photophobia on two consecutive examinations.[148] Hospitalization was necessary for 6.4% of women and 1.6% of men for aseptic meningitis in these patients. There was also a high frequency of CSF pleocytosis in patients without overt clinical evidence of meningeal irritation in a study of primary genital herpes in the early 1900s, suggesting that meningeal involvement may be quite common with primary genital herpes.[184]

Fever, headache, vomiting, photophobia, and nuchal rigidity are the predominant symptoms of HSV aseptic meningitis. Meningeal symptoms usually start 3 to 12 days after the onset of genital lesions. Symptoms generally reach a maximum 2 to 4 days into the illness and gradually recede without sequelae over 2 to 3 days. The CSF is usually clear, and opening pressures may be somewhat elevated. White blood cell counts in the CSF usually range from 10 to 1000 cells/mm³. The pleocytosis is predominantly lymphocytic in adults, although early in the course of disease and in neonates, a predominantly polymorphonuclear response may be seen. The CSF glucose level is usually more than 50% of the blood glucose, although hypoglycorrhachia has been reported.[185] The CSF protein is usually slightly elevated. In cases of aseptic meningitis, HSV may be isolated from the CSF, although HSV DNA PCR assay is a more sensitive diagnostic test.[183] The differential diagnosis of aseptic meningitis is broad, but the presence of both neurologic involvement and genital ulcerations narrows the possibilities to include sacral herpes zoster, Behçet's syndrome, collagen vascular disease, inflammatory bowel disease, and porphyria. Rarely, aseptic meningitis is the sole presenting sign of new HSV-2 acquisition. Use of systemic antiviral chemotherapy early in the course of primary genital herpes decreases subsequent development of aseptic meningitis. Controlled trials of intravenous acyclovir for established HSV meningitis have not been conducted. However, intravenous acyclovir 5 mg/kg every 8 hours is recommended for hospitalized symptomatic patients.

Benign recurrent lymphocytic meningitis, or Mollaret's meningitis, is characterized by recurrent episodes of meningitis lasting 3 to 7 days and resolving without neurologic sequelae.[186] Although the differential diagnosis for chronic meningitis is broad, HSV-2 is responsible for the majority of recurrent cases.[187] In one small series of patients with meningitis during first-episode genital HSV-2 infection, 27% had possible symptomatic evidence of recurrent meningitis, and 10% had documentation of recurrent disease by demonstration of HSV DNA in the CSF.[188] Prophylactic doses of DNA polymerase inhibitors often are encouraged for patients with frequent recurrent meningitis.

Autonomic nervous system dysfunction can occur in association with genital HSV infection.[189,190] Manifestations include hyperesthesia or anesthesia of the perineum, lower back, or sacral regions as well as

urinary retention and constipation. This complication occurs more frequently among women than men but is sometimes present in men with HSV proctitis. Physical examination reveals a large bladder, decreased sacral sensation, and poor rectal and perineal sphincter tone. Impotence and absent bulbocavernous reflexes have been noted in men. CSF pleocytosis may be present in some patients. Electromyography usually reveals slowed nerve conduction velocities and fibrillation potentials in the affected area, and urinary cystometric examination shows a large atonic bladder. Resolution occurs in most cases in 4 to 8 weeks.

Transverse myelitis has also been reported in association with primary genital HSV infection.[191] Decreased deep tendon reflexes and muscle strength in the lower extremities, as well as the previously described autonomic nervous system signs and symptoms, are present. Residual neurologic dysfunction may occur. Whether autonomic nervous system and spinal cord dysfunction results from viral invasion of the CNS or an unusual immunologic response to infection is unknown.

EXTRAGENITAL LESIONS

Extragenital lesions commonly develop during the course of primary genital herpes and are more common in women than in men. Extragenital lesions are most frequently located in the buttock, groin, or thigh area, although the finger and eye can also be involved. Among patients with primary HSV-2, extragenital lesions develop in 9%, most commonly on the buttocks. Among patients with primary genital HSV-1, 25% acquire extragenital lesions, most commonly in or around the mouth.[170] The distribution of lesions on the extremities or areas near the genital lesions, and their typical occurrence 2 weeks into the course of disease suggests that the majority of extragenital lesions develop by autoinoculation of virus or by viral reactivation in another part of the affected dermatome rather than viremic spread.[148,170] However, the common demonstration of plasma viremia during the course of primary HSV infection suggests that viremic spread may also be a factor.[91,192] Both HSV-1 and HSV-2 have been shown to be rare causes of pelvic inflammatory disease. Although this may represent dual infection with other sexually transmitted pathogens such as N. gonorrhoeae and C. trachomatis, extension of HSV infection into the uterine cavity with laparoscopic evidence of HSV-positive vesicular lesions on the fallopian tube has been reported.[175]

DISSEMINATED INFECTION

Blood-borne dissemination as manifested by multiple vesicles over widespread areas of the thorax and extremities occurs rarely in persons with primary mucocutaneous herpes.[193,194] Cutaneous dissemination usually occurs early in the disease and is often associated with aseptic meningitis, hepatitis, or pneumonitis. Other complications of primary genital HSV-2 infection include monoarticular arthritis,[195] thrombocytopenia,[196] adrenal necrosis,[197] and myoglobinuria.[198] Pregnancy may predispose to severe visceral dissemination of primary genital HSV disease.[199,200] Reactivation of genital HSV in immunosuppressed patients, especially those with impaired cellular immune responses, can be associated with interstitial pneumonia, hepatitis, and meningitis, similar to the manifestations of disseminated infection of the neonate.[201,202] Disseminated visceral infections in immunosuppressed and pregnant patients are associated with high mortality and should be treated with systemic antiviral chemotherapy.

SUPERINFECTION

Bacterial superinfection of genital herpes in immunocompetent patients is a rare complication. Pelvic cellulitis appears as an advancing erythema and swelling of the perineal area: such patients should receive systemic antimicrobial therapy. Fungal vaginitis is frequently encountered toward the end of genital herpes–associated symptoms and often leads to recurrence of pruritus and increased discharge;

concurrent yeast infection occurs more frequently in women with genital herpes.[148] Bacterial vaginosis also appears to be more common in women seropositive for HSV-2.[203]

Recurrent Mucocutaneous Herpes Simplex Virus Infections

In contrast to first episodes of genital infection, the symptoms, signs, and anatomic sites of infection of recurrent genital or orolabial herpes are usually localized to a defined mucocutaneous site.[204,205] Local symptoms such as pain and itching are mild to moderate compared with first episodes of infection, and the duration of the episode is shorter. Lesions are usually confined to one side, and the involved area is on average one tenth that of the primary infection.[206,207] Recurrent orolabial HSV tends to be of shorter duration than genital HSV. Orolabial lesions usually pass through clinical stages of infection more rapidly, and the median time from onset of tingling to healing averages 5 days.[151]

Both oral and genital HSV reactivations are frequently associated with prodromal symptoms that occur in the absence of lesions in 20% of episodes.[204] Prodromal symptoms vary from a mild tingling sensation, occurring 0.5 to 48 hours before eruption, to shooting pains in the buttocks, legs, or hips 1 to 5 days before eruption. In many patients, the prodromal symptoms are the most bothersome part of the episode. HSV is present on mucosal surfaces more frequently during the prodrome, suggesting that viral reactivation is associated with these symptoms.[180,207] The severity and mean duration of pain is longer in women (5.9 days) than in men (3.9 days), as is the likelihood of dysuria (27% vs. 9%), although dysuria is normally external and isolation of HSV from the urethra is considerably less common than during the first episode of HSV-2 infection. The mean duration of shedding (~4 days in both genders) is shorter than during primary infection but highly variable both between and within persons over time.[208]

The diverse clinical spectrum of recurrent HSV is increasingly recognized. First, subclinical reactivation of virus on mucosal surfaces is common.[180] In addition, studies of both orolabial and genital ulcerative lesions have found a surprisingly high frequency of HSV isolated from atypical clinical syndromes (~33%), including linear fissures or serpiginous ulcers without an erythematous base (see Fig. 136-5).[174] Even among experienced clinicians, false-positive and false-negative clinical diagnoses of genital herpes are common.[62,209,210] Therefore, we recommend that all ulcerative lesions on the oral and genital mucosa be sampled for HSV.[211] A definitive etiologic diagnosis is best established by demonstration of viral nucleic acid or isolation of virus from the affected area. The detection of HSV-2 does not rule out coinfection with *T. pallidum* or *Haemophilus ducreyi*, which should be considered in the appropriate clinical and epidemiologic context.[210,212]

Importantly, the vast majority of HSV-2–seropositive persons who deny having genital lesions are not truly asymptomatic, but have genital lesions that they do not recognize as herpetic. In several studies, seropositive women and men who were previously unaware of their diagnosis were educated regarding signs and symptoms of genital herpes. During follow-up periods of just a few months, classic recurrent lesions developed in 48% to 62% of these subjects.[75,205,213] In one study, localized genital symptoms developed in an additional 25%.[75] The rate of subclinical shedding was the same among men and women with recognized and unrecognized genital HSV, although recurrences were more likely and longer in those with previously recognized disease.

Frequency of Reactivation and Recurrence

The major morbidity of genital HSV-2 infection is a result of the high frequency of reactivation.[214] Ninety percent of persons who present with symptomatic first-episode genital HSV-2 experience clinical reac-

tivation of infection, and 98% experience subclinical HSV-2 shedding in genital mucosa.[215-218] The median recurrence rate is between 4 and 5 episodes per year, although there is great heterogeneity among patients: 20% of patients report more than 10 recurrences during the year after primary infection.[150] Studies of clinical reactivation of HSV-2 infection show a steady but gradual decrease in recurrence rates over time. In one study, annual recurrences of genital herpes decreased from an average of 5 to 2 per year over a 5- to 8-year period. The decrease most commonly occurred 3 to 5 years after acquisition. However, there was again great variability, with 20% of patients reporting increased recurrences over time.[219] Both recurrence and shedding persist at high levels even 10 years after initial infection (W. Phipps, personal communication).

HSV-2 recurs much more frequently in the genital tract than HSV-1. Less than 5% of people with primary HSV-1 infection of the genital tract will have more than four recurrences during their lifetime.[106] Men have slightly more recurrences than women. Prolonged duration of primary infection (>35 days) is also a predictor of early and frequent recurrence.[150] There are likely to be genetic determinants of frequency and severity of reactivation, but these remain unidentified.

Subclinical or asymptomatic viral shedding is a critical concept for understanding the epidemiologic and transmission features of genital and orolabial HSV infections.[72,220-222] Previous studies indicated that two thirds of mucosal HSV-1 or HSV-2 shedding episodes are subclinical.[180,217,222-224] New studies with frequent swabbing for HSV-2 in the anogenital tract detect a high number of previously missed shedding episodes that last less than 6 hours, which implies that the percentage of episodes that are not symptomatic is likely to be even higher (see Fig. 136-2).[84] Subclinical episodes of HSV may last less than 2 hours to several days, often involve more than one anatomic site, and, like clinical recurrences, occur most frequently after acquisition and then gradually decline to stable levels over a 2- to 3-year period. In women, the anatomic sites of asymptomatic shedding include the cervix, vulva, anus, and urethra.[180] In men, shedding occurs from the penile skin, urethra, anus, and occasionally semen.[218] Among MSM, perianal shedding is more common, whereas the converse is true for men who acquire HSV via heterosexual contact, suggesting that site of initial inoculation and latency influences the subsequent pattern of reactivation. Similar patterns of subclinical reactivation occur in the oropharynx where frequent shedding correlates with frequent recurrence.

HSV can be cultured from the lower genitourinary tract of women and men in the absence of genital ulcerations or other lesions. Detection of HSV DNA by PCR assays demonstrates HSV on mucosal surfaces three to four times more frequently than viral isolation.[211] Studies of antiviral therapy have shown that long-term daily therapy reduces viral excretion by 70% to 95% (from 28% to 8% of days), indicating that HSV DNA as detected by PCR on mucosal surfaces represents the replicating form of the virus and, hence, is likely infectious.[217] Most sexual and maternal-fetal transmissions occur during episodes of subclinical shedding. Similarly, subclinical shedding can cause primary genital HSV-1 infections through orogenital sexual activity. Counseling of patients with genital herpes therefore needs to emphasize the potential for infectivity regardless of symptomatology and to provide appropriate strategies to decrease the risk to patients' sexual partners.

Herpetic Whitlow

Herpetic whitlow (HSV infection of the finger) may occur as a complication of primary oral or genital herpes by inoculation of virus through a break in the epidermal surface or by direct introduction of virus into the hand through occupational or some other type of exposure.[225] Before the increased use of gloves in health care settings, HSV-1 was most commonly isolated from herpetic infections of the hand. However, one survey found HSV-2 as the predominant causative agent.[170] Clinical signs and symptoms of herpetic whitlow include the abrupt onset of edema, erythema, and localized tenderness of the infected finger. Vesicular or pustular lesions of the fingertip can be difficult to distinguish from lesions of pyogenic bacterial infection. Fever, lymphadenitis, and epitrochlear and axillary lymphadenopathy are common. The infection may recur. Prompt diagnosis (to avoid unnecessary and potentially exacerbating surgical therapy or transmission) is essential. Antiviral chemotherapy to speed the healing of the process is recommended.

Herpes Gladiatorum

HSV may infect almost any area of skin. Mucocutaneous HSV infections of the thorax, ears, face, and hands occur in outbreaks among wrestlers (herpes gladiatorium). Transmission of these infections is facilitated by trauma to the skin sustained during matches. Prompt diagnosis and therapy are required to contain the spread of this infection.[226]

Eye Infections

HSV infection of the eye is the most frequent cause of corneal blindness in the United States.[227,228] HSV keratitis arises with an acute onset of pain, blurring of vision, chemosis, conjunctivitis, and characteristic dendritic lesions of the cornea (Fig. 136-7). Use of topical glucocorticoids may exacerbate symptoms and lead to involvement of deep structures of the eye.[229] Débridement, topical antiviral treatment, interferon therapy, or a combination of these methods hastens healing. Primary disease is often self-limited but recurrences are common, and the deeper structures of the eye may sustain irreversible scarring due to immunopathologic injury. Both eyes are involved in approximately 5% of cases. HSV-1 blepharitis and conjunctivitis are distinguishable from other self-limited viral conjunctivitis cases by the presence of vesicles on the eyelid margin. Chorioretinitis occurs in neonates or in patients with HIV infection who have disseminated infection.[230] HSV and varicella-zoster virus also can cause acute necrotizing retinitis, a devastating condition that leads to painless vision loss and affects both eyes approximately 25% of the time. This entity can be seen both in immunocompetent persons, pregnant women, and in persons with HIV-1 infection. Retinal necrosis is rapid, and prompt systemic antiviral chemotherapy, systemic steroids to reduce inflammation, vitreal biopsy with PCR, and laser retinopexy are indicated. Residual blindness is common.[228,231,232]

Herpes Simplex Virus Encephalitis

HSV is the most commonly identified cause of acute, sporadic viral encephalitis in the United States, accounting for 10% to 20% of all cases.[233] The estimated incidence is approximately 2.3 cases per million

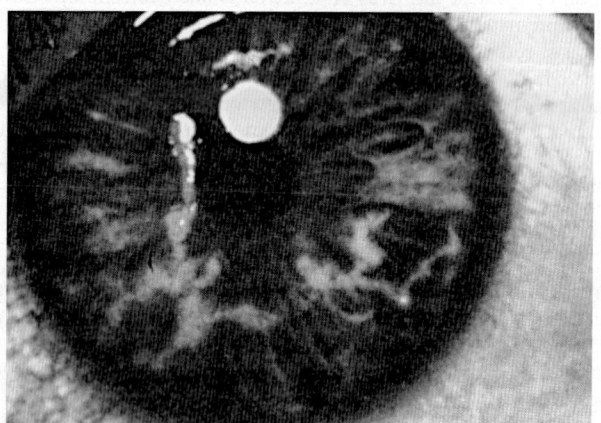

Figure 136-7 **Herpes simplex virus type 1 dendritic keratitis.** (From Pavan-Langston D, ed. Ocular Viral Disease, Volume 15. Boston: Little, Brown; 1975:19-36.)

persons per year. Unlike enteroviral infections, cases are distributed throughout the year, and the age distribution appears to be biphasic, with peaks at ages 5 to 30 years and more than 50 years of age.[234] HSV-1 causes more than 95% of cases.[235,236]

The pathogenesis of HSV encephalitis varies. In children and young adults, primary HSV infection may result in encephalitis; presumably, exogenously acquired virus enters the CNS by neurotropic spread from the periphery through the olfactory bulb. Most adults with HSV encephalitis have clinical or serologic evidence of mucocutaneous HSV-1 infection before the onset of symptoms.[236] However, in approximately 25% of patients examined, the HSV-1 strains from the oropharynx and brain tissue of the same patient differ; thus, some cases may result from reinfection with another strain of HSV-1 that reaches the CNS.[237] Reactivation of latent HSV-1 infection in trigeminal or autonomic nerve roots may be associated with extension of virus into the CNS through nerves innervating the middle cranial fossa. HSV DNA has been demonstrated by DNA hybridization in brain tissue obtained at autopsy from healthy adults.[236] Therefore, reactivation of long-standing latent CNS infection is a final possible mechanism for the development of HSV encephalitis.

The clinical hallmark of HSV encephalitis is acute onset of fever and focal neurologic (especially temporal lobe) symptoms. Differentiation of HSV encephalitis from other viral encephalitides, focal infections, and noninfectious processes is difficult.[238] The most sensitive noninvasive method for early diagnosis of HSV encephalitis is demonstration of HSV DNA in CSF by PCR, although uncommonly PCR may become positive only a few days after onset. Although titers of CSF and serum antibodies to HSV increase in most cases of HSV encephalitis, they rarely do so earlier than 10 days into the illness and, as such, are generally not helpful in establishing an early clinical diagnosis.[239-241]

Magnetic resonance imaging is the neuroimaging technique of choice for the detection of abnormalities associated with HSV encephalitis, and frequently gadolinium-enhanced lesions are seen in the temporal lobe. Brain biopsy was used extensively in the past to make the diagnosis of HSV encephalitis and has a low complication rate; demonstration of HSV antigen, HSV DNA, or HSV replication in brain tissue obtained by biopsy is highly sensitive. Brain biopsy is infrequently used now, but it provides the best opportunity to identify alternative, potentially treatable causes of encephalitis and may be considered when the clinical presentation is atypical or the diagnosis remains unclear.[238]

Most authorities recommend empirical use of intravenous acyclovir in patients with presumed HSV encephalitis until the diagnosis is confirmed or an alternative diagnosis is made. All confirmed cases should be treated with intravenous acyclovir at a dose of 30 mg/kg/day in three divided doses for 14 to 21 days.[242] Cases of clinical recurrence of encephalitis have been reported after therapy stopped that required more treatment. For this reason, some authorities prefer to treat initially for 21 days, and many continue therapy until HSV DNA has been eliminated from the CSF. Even with therapy, neurologic sequelae are frequent, especially in persons older than 35.

Visceral Infections

HSV infection of visceral organs usually results from viremia, and multiple-organ involvement is common. Occasionally, the clinical manifestations of HSV infection involve only the esophagus, lung, or liver. HSV esophagitis may result from direct extension of oropharyngeal HSV infection into the esophagus or by reactivation and spread of HSV to the esophageal mucosa through the vagus nerve.[243,244] It is a well-known complication in patients with acquired immunodeficiency syndrome and should be differentiated from Candida and cytomegalovirus infections and aphthous ulcers by histologic examination. The predominant symptoms of HSV esophagitis are odynophagia, dysphagia, substernal pain, and weight loss. The distal esophagus is most commonly involved with multiple oval ulcerations on an erythematous base, with or without a patchy white pseudomembrane. With extensive disease, diffuse friability may involve the entire esophagus. Neither endoscopic nor barium examination differentiates HSV esophagitis from esophageal ulcerations related to *Candida,* thermal injury, radiation, or corrosives. Endoscopically obtained secretions for cytologic examination and culture provide the most useful diagnostic material. Systemic antiviral chemotherapy usually reduces symptoms and heals ulcerations.

HSV pneumonitis is uncommon except in severely immunosuppressed patients and may result from extension of herpetic tracheobronchitis into lung parenchyma.[245-247] Because oral shedding of HSV can lead to contamination, a positive HSV culture from a respiratory specimen should be interpreted with caution in an unlikely host or in the absence of radiologic evidence of disease. However, demonstration of virus from lower respiratory tract specimens should be evaluated promptly as to whether there is evidence of tracheobronchitis or true parenchymal lung disease. HSV-1 pneumonia usually presents as a focal necrotizing pneumonitis. Hematogenous dissemination of virus from sites of oral or genital mucocutaneous disease may also occur and produce bilateral interstitial pneumonitis. Bacterial, fungal, and parasitic copathogens are commonly present, and the mortality rate from untreated HSV pneumonia in immunosuppressed patients is high (>80%).[245,246] HSV has also been observed in association with acute respiratory disease syndrome.[248,249] Most authorities believe that the presence of HSV in tracheal aspirates in such settings is due to reactivation of HSV in the tracheal region and localized tracheitis in persons with long-standing intubation. Such patients should be evaluated for the potential extension of HSV infection into lung parenchyma. Controlled trials evaluating the role that antiviral agents for HSV play in acute respiratory distress syndrome morbidity and mortality have not been conducted.

HSV is an uncommon cause of hepatitis in immunocompetent patients. HSV infection of the liver is associated with fever, abrupt elevations of bilirubin and serum aminotransferase levels, and leukopenia (<4000 white blood cells/μL). Disseminated intravascular coagulation may also develop.[197]

Interactions between Genital Herpes Simplex Virus Infection and Human Immunodeficiency Virus Infection

Persistent HSV infection is a common clinical presentation of HIV infection.[159] HSV-2 is also of primary importance in driving the HIV-1 epidemic based on both increased HIV-1 acquisition and transmission in the context of HSV-2 coinfection. Throughout the world, HSV-2 infection is common in those infected with HIV-1 and those at high risk of acquiring HIV-1. A majority of homosexual men with HIV infection have antibodies to HSV,[250] and one fourth of HIV-1–negative MSM are also seropositive for HSV-2.[59] In discordant HIV-1 heterosexual partners, both in the developed and developing world, HSV-2 infection is common among potential transmitters (70% and 95%, respectively) and those at risk of HIV-1 infection.[251]

HSV reactivation, especially perianal shedding in men and subclinical vulvar shedding in women, is more frequent in HIV-positive persons than HIV-negative control subjects. As with the HIV-negative population, mucosal HSV-2 reactivation rates vary considerably between patients.[179,252] For example, HSV DNA was detected on 30% to 80% of days in two cohorts of HIV-positive persons.[252,253] Low CD4 counts and high HIV viral loads are associated with an increased frequency of HSV shedding.[104,179,254] Highly active antiretroviral therapy seems to reduce the frequency of genital lesions substantially, but decreases the frequency of subclinical shedding only modestly.[104]

HSV-2 infection has important effects on the global epidemiology of HIV. Case-control and cohort studies have shown that previous HSV-2 infection is associated with an increased risk of acquiring HIV.[255-259] Per-contact probability of HIV-1 acquisition is affected equally by HSV-2 serostatus and HIV-1 plasma viral load in the source partner (Table 136-2). One review estimated a population-attributable

TABLE 136-2 Per-Contact Probability of Human Immunodeficiency Virus Type 1 Acquisition Stratified by Plasma Human Immunodeficiency Virus Type 1 RNA in Human Immunodeficiency Virus Type 1 Seropositive Partner and Herpes Simplex Virus Serostatus in the Susceptible Partner

HIV-1 Plasma RNA in Source Partner (Copies/mL)	Per-Contact Probability in the HIV-1–Susceptible Partner	
	HSV-2 Positive	HSV-2 Negative
<1,700	0.0001	0.00004
1,700-12,499	0.0023	0.0005
12,500-38,499	0.0018	0.0002
>38,499	0.0036	0.0007

HIV-1, human immunodeficiency virus type 1; HSV-2, herpes simplex virus type 2.
Adapted from Quinn T, Wawer M, Sewankambo N, et al. Viral load and heterosexual transmission of human immunodeficiency virus type 1. Rakai Project Study Group. *N Engl J Med.* 2000;342:921-929.

risk of 20% in populations with moderate HSV-2 prevalence, such as the United States, and 45% in populations with a very high HSV-2 seroprevalence.[260] A meta-analysis performed of all available prospectively conducted studies estimated an age-adjusted relative risk of 3.1 for HIV-1 acquisition in persons with HSV-2 infection.[251] The elevated risk was present in MSM and heterosexual men and women, but not in high-risk women. A mathematical model of coinfection predicted that approximately one fourth of infections in a high-prevalence city in Africa were directly attributable to HSV-2 and that HSV-2 facilitated spread of HIV into low-risk populations via stable long-term relationships.[261] Unfortunately, two large randomized, controlled trials showed no decrease in HIV-1 acquisition when acyclovir was given twice daily to high-risk HSV-2–seropositive women in Africa as well as high-risk MSM in Peru and the United States.[262,263] Recent studies indicate that HSV appears to imprint a focal inflammatory response of HIV-susceptible cells that is unaffected by antiviral therapy. Detailed in situ studies of posthealing biopsies indicate that despite clinical healing and the appearance of normal skin, an inflammatory focus of chemokine (C-C motif) receptor 5 (CCR-5)-expressing CD4$^+$ T cells, as well as dendritic cell-specific intercellular adhesion molecule-3-grabbing non-integrin (DC-SIGN)-expressing dendritic cells, persist in the region.[264] This residual focus of inflammatory cells provides increased potential for HIV to encounter susceptible cells through epithelial tears associated with intercourse or through epithelial cell transcytosis.

The risk of HIV transmission attributable to HSV-2 was examined in one study of discordant couples in Africa that estimated a higher per coital rate of transmission from patients with a reported history of genital ulcer disease.[82] Because HSV-2 is the most common genital ulcer disease in Africa, this suggests that HSV-2 might affect sexual HIV-1 transmission. Initial evidence also suggests that HSV-2 may enhance maternal-fetal HIV transmission.[265,266] Plasma HIV viral load is an important determinant of sexual transmission.[267] Therefore, the discovery of an approximate 30% increase in plasma and genital HIV-1 viral load in HSV-2–infected patients during and for several weeks after HSV-2 clinical and subclinical recurrence adds plausibility to the concept of enhanced HIV transmission.[253,257,268,269] Frequency of HSV-2 shedding correlates with HIV plasma viral load: twice-daily valacyclovir lowered the HIV-1 plasma viral load by approximately 0.2 to 0.5 log and decreased the frequency and mean quantity of HIV-1 shed in the genital tract.[270,271] The reductions in HIV plasma RNA take 6 to 12 weeks to demonstrate and are not seen with episodic use of these agents. It was initially hypothesized that HSV-2 DNA polymerase inhibitors decrease HIV-1 viral load indirectly by decreasing the overall level of T-cell activation relating to HSV-2 recrudescence. However, recent in vitro studies indicate that acyclovir may act directly on HIV-1 reverse transcriptase and might even predispose to the development of clinically important HIV-1 reverse transcriptase mutations.[272] Acyclovir requires HSV thymidine kinase for its initial phosphorylation step; therefore, in vivo, one would expect that its anti-HIV activity would require coinfection of a significant number of cells with both HIV-1 and HSV-2 for such an effect to be seen. A randomized trial is under way to evaluate whether treating the HSV-2/HIV-1–positive partner in a serodiscordant couple with prolonged acyclovir will decrease HIV-1 transmission[273] and whether such treatment induces important mutations in the HIV-1–infected person.

Laboratory studies support the idea that HSV may be an important cofactor in influencing the titer and frequency of mucosal HIV infection. The HSV regulatory proteins ICP0 and ICP4 can upregulate the rate of HIV replication in vitro[274-276]; herpetic lesions are also associated with an influx of activated CD4-bearing lymphocytes,[126] which may result in increased expression of HIV on mucosal surfaces in HSV-positive patients and greater surface area of HIV target cells in HSV-negative patients. Finally, in vivo, HSV-2 and HIV coinfection of epithelial cells results in a higher copy number of HSV virions.[275] HIV virions can be detected in genital herpes lesions and higher HIV-1 titers are found in genital secretions during episodes of subclinical HSV-2 reactivation.[277,278]

Herpes Simplex Virus Infections in Immunocompromised Hosts Not Infected with Human Immunodeficiency Virus

Organ transplant recipients, patients undergoing cancer chemotherapy, or those compromised by malnutrition or disorders of skin integrity such as burns or eczema are at risk of the development of severe HSV infections.[279-281] Besides causing extensive mucocutaneous infections, HSV may disseminate to visceral organs such as adrenal glands, liver, bone marrow, and the gastrointestinal tract in such persons. Most kidney, liver, and bone marrow transplant recipients excrete HSV-1 in saliva during the first 2 to 3 weeks after grafting.[280] Although these reactivations are often asymptomatic, extensive mucocutaneous ulcerations may occur (Fig. 136-8) and, if persistent, extend to the esophagus or lung. Because of the difficulty in distinguishing HSV from chemotherapy-related mucositis, most oncology centers use routine prophylaxis against HSV during the initial period after transplantation or initiation of chemotherapy to shorten the course or prevent mucocutaneous HSV infection. Prophylactic acyclovir reduced bacteremia with oral pathogens in patients after chemotherapy in a single trial.[282] The importance of adoptive T-cell immunity in controlling HSV resolution has been demonstrated. HSV-1–seropositive persons who received a bone marrow transplant from an HSV-seronegative donor were at higher risk of recurrence and acyclovir-resistant strains of HSV were more likely to develop than those who received marrow from HSV-1–positive donors.[283]

Neonatal Herpes

Infants acquire infection through contact with HSV-infected secretions, usually at the time of delivery.[112,113,230,284] Ninety percent of neonatal herpes is perinatally acquired, 5% to 8% is congenital, and a few cases are acquired postnatally.[230] Of the 70% of neonatal HSV infections caused by HSV-2, almost all result from contact with infected genital secretions during delivery. Although congenitally infected infants have been reported, these infants almost invariably are born to mothers who had primary HSV-1 or HSV-2 infection during pregnancy.[285,286] Features included microcephaly, hydrocephalus, and chorioretinitis. Neonatal HSV-1 infections also may be acquired through postnatal contact with health care workers or immediate family members who have symptomatic or asymptomatic orolabial HSV-1 infection.

Neonates (infants younger than 6 weeks) have the highest frequency of visceral or CNS infection, or both, of any HSV-infected population. If not treated, neonatal herpes undergoes dissemination or develops into CNS infection in more than 70% of cases. Without therapy, the overall rate of death from neonatal herpes is 65%; less than 20% of neonates with CNS infection develop normally.[230,287] CNS morbidity is less severe with HSV-1 than with HSV-2 infection.[288] Although skin lesions are the most commonly recognized features of disease, many infants do not acquire visible lesions until well into the course of disease.[289] Cutaneous involvement alone is not associated with mortality. High-dose (60 mg/kg/day) intravenous acyclovir divided in three daily doses for 21 days (14 days for cutaneous involvement only) reduces mortality and morbidity, but long-term disabilities are still common, especially in infants with HSV-2 infection involving the CNS.[290]

Infants born by cesarean section to women before the rupture of membranes or by vaginal delivery to women with no evidence of recent HSV infection are at minimal risk of the development of HSV infection, and most hospitals do not recommend segregating the infant from the rest of the newborn nursery. If a more cautious approach is desired, the infant can be put into an Isolette incubator to make hospital personnel aware of the necessity to use wound and skin precautions and proper hand-washing techniques. Infants born to women with active lesions should be placed in isolation. Viral cultures, liver function studies, and CSF examinations should be performed, and the infant should be observed closely for the first month of life. Any symptoms of neonatal disease (e.g., poor feeding, fever, hypothermia, skin lesions, lethargy, seizures) should be investigated expeditiously for evidence of neonatal HSV infection.

Management of contact between infant and mother should be handled on an individual basis. In women who acquire primary genital herpes late in pregnancy, the high incidence of extragenital lesions suggests that separation of mother and infant is warranted until therapy has produced a clinical and virologic response. Because recurrent maternal genital herpes is rarely associated with dissemination of disease or the development of extragenital lesions in exposed extremities, protection of the infant from exposure to infected genital secretions is adequate. When handling the infant in the hospital, the mother should wear a gown and observe proper hand-washing techniques. Orolabial herpes presents a greater risk of postnatal acquisition of HSV infections to the newborn than genital herpes.[13] Thus, nursery personnel and other adults with external lesions caused by HSV should not engage in intimate contact with the newborn.

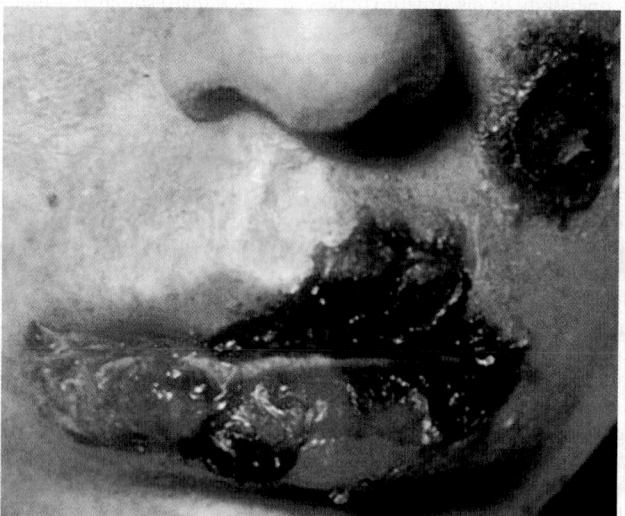

Figure 136-8 Severe mucocutaneous herpes simplex virus type 1 infection in a bone marrow transplant recipient. *(From Corey L. Herpes simplex virus infections. In: Mandell GL, series ed. Atlas of Infectious Diseases, Volume V, Sexually Transmitted Diseases. Rein MF, ed. Philadelphia: Churchill Livingstone/Current Medicine; 1996, Fig. 15-47B.)*

Herpes Simplex Virus in Pregnancy

Incidence data for neonatal HSV are similar to HIV infection before the advent of routine antiretroviral use in pregnancy and are higher

TABLE 136-3	Transmission Rates of Neonatal Herpes Simplex Virus by Maternal Herpes Simplex Virus Serologic Status among Women Who Delivered at the University of Washington and Madigan Army Hospitals	
Maternal HSV Serostatus	No./Total (%) of Infants with Neonatal HSV	Rate per 100,000 Live Births (95% Confidence Interval)
HSV seronegative	6/11,115 (0.054)	54 (19.8-118)
HSV-1 seropositive only	6/23,480 (0.026)	26 (9.3-56)
All HSV-2 seropositive	3/13,795 (0.022)	22 (4.4-64)
HSV-2 only	2/5,761 (0.035)	35 (4.2-126)
HSV-1 and HSV-2	1/8,034 (0.012)	12 (0.3-7.0)

HSV, herpes simplex virus; HSV-1, herpes simplex virus type 1; HSV-2, herpes simplex virus type 2.

Adapted from Brown ZA, Ashley RL, Selka S, et al. Effect of serologic status and cesarean delivery on transmission rates of herpes simplex virus from mother to infant. *JAMA.* 2003;289:203.

than congenital syphilis, toxoplasmosis, and congenital rubella during endemic years.[80] The prevalence of genital HSV infection during pregnancy, as well as the incidence of neonatal HSV infection, is influenced by socioeconomic status, age, and past sexual activity of the population of patients being examined.[291] In the United States, 22% of all pregnant women and 55% of non-Hispanic black pregnant women are HSV-2 seropositive.[292] However, the highest risk of transmitting HSV in the perinatal period occurs during the acquisition of HSV near the time of labor.[80,113,223] Table 136-3 depicts the frequency of neonatal infection in relation to maternal serologic states.

Clinical Course of Genital Herpes in Pregnancy

The clinical manifestations of recurrent genital herpes, including the frequency of subclinical versus clinical infection, duration of lesions, pain, and constitutional symptoms, are similar in pregnant and nonpregnant women. Recurrences increase in frequency over the course of pregnancy.[293,294] However, among women who are HSV-2 seropositive entering pregnancy, there is no effect on neonatal outcome, including birth weight and gestational age.[295] First-episode infections in pregnancy have more severe consequences for mother and infant.[223,285,296,297] Maternal visceral dissemination during the third trimester, as well as prematurity or intrauterine growth retardation, occasionally occur. The acquisition of primary disease in pregnancy, whether related to HSV-1 or HSV-2, carries the risk of potential transplacental transmission of virus to the neonate and can result in spontaneous abortion, although this is relatively uncommon.[298] We recommend antiviral treatment of newly acquired genital HSV during pregnancy with 7 to 10 days of acyclovir 400 mg three times daily or valacyclovir 500-1000 mg twice daily, although the effect of this intervention on transmission is unknown.

Criteria for laboratory screening and surveillance, as well as delivery procedures for women with recurrent genital HSV infections, are the questions frequently encountered by physicians caring for pregnant women.[299,300] The high HSV-2 prevalence rate in pregnancy and low incidence of neonatal disease (1/6000 to 20,000 live births) indicate that only a few infants are at risk of acquiring HSV (see Table 136-3).[301] Cesarean section is therefore not warranted for all women with recurrent genital disease.[302] Because intrapartum transmission of infection accounts for the majority of cases, only women who shed HSV at delivery need be considered for abdominal delivery.[112,302] Several studies showed no correlation between recurrence of viral shedding before delivery and the presence of viral shedding at term.[284,302,303] Hence, weekly virologic monitoring and amniocentesis are not recommended.

The frequency of transmission from mother to infant is markedly higher among women who acquire HSV near term (30% to 50%) than

among those who reactivate HSV-2 at delivery (<1%).[112] Although maternal HSV-2 antibody is protective, HSV-1 antibody offers little or no protection against neonatal HSV-2 infection.[304] Primary HSV-1 genital infection leads to a particularly high risk of transmission and accounts for an increasing proportion of neonatal HSV cases.[112,114] Moreover, during reactivation, HSV-1 appears more transmissible to the neonate than HSV-2.[304] Only 2% of women who are HSV-2 seropositive have HSV-2 isolated from cervical secretions at delivery, and only 1% of infants exposed in this manner develop infection, presumably because of the protective effects of maternally transferred antibodies and perhaps lower viral titers during reactivation.[112,223] Despite the low frequency of transmission of HSV in this setting, 30% to 50% of infants with neonatal HSV are born to mothers with established genital herpes.

Isolation of HSV by cervicovaginal swab at the time of delivery is the greatest risk factor for intrapartum HSV transmission (relative risk = 346); however, culture-negative, PCR-positive cases of intrapartum transmission are well described. New acquisition of HSV (odds ratio = 49), isolation of HSV-1 versus HSV-2 (odds ratio = 35), cervical versus vulvar HSV detection (odds ratio = 15), use of fetal scalp electrodes (odds ratio = 3.5), and young age confer further risk of transmission, whereas abdominal delivery is protective (odds ratio = 0.14).[112] Physical examination poorly predicts the absence of shedding,[305] and PCR far exceeds culture in terms of sensitivity and speed. Therefore, PCR detection at the onset of labor should be used to aid clinical decision making for women with an HSV-2 antibody. Because cesarean section appears to be an effective means of reducing maternal-fetal transmission, patients with recurrent genital herpes should be encouraged to come to the hospital early at the time of delivery for careful examination of the external genitalia and cervix, plus swab for viral isolation. Women who have no evidence of lesions should have a vaginal delivery. The presence of active lesions on the cervix or external genitalia is an indication for abdominal delivery.

This policy results in the exposure of some infants to episodes of asymptomatic cervical or vulvar shedding, or both.[305] The identification of HSV-exposed infants provides important information to the attending pediatrician. If first-episode exposure has occurred (e.g., if HSV serologies show that the mother is seronegative or if the mother is HSV-1 seropositive and the isolate at delivery is HSV-2), many authorities would initiate antiviral therapy of the infant with intravenous acyclovir.[306,307] At a minimum, viral cultures and PCR should be obtained from the throat, nasopharynx, eyes, and rectum of these infants immediately and at 5- to 10-day intervals. Lethargy, skin lesions, or fever should be evaluated promptly. All infants from whom HSV is isolated 24 hours after delivery should be treated with intravenous acyclovir at recommended treatment doses.

The relationship between the duration of ruptured membranes in the woman with clinically apparent lesions and transmission of HSV to the infant is not well defined.[303] Delivery of infants by cesarean section, even in women with intact membranes, occasionally results in neonatal herpes. Prolonged contact with infected secretions may increase the risk of acquisition. Many authorities recommend that if membranes are ruptured for more than 4 to 6 hours, cesarean section should no longer be considered protective against HSV transmission. However, transmission can occur from exposure to external genital lesions alone. Thus, in women with recurrent genital herpes who have active external genital lesions during labor, we still recommend abdominal delivery.

Prevention of Herpes Simplex Virus Acquisition in Pregnancy by Use of Antivirals

Controversy exists regarding the use of antiviral therapy during pregnancy. Antiviral therapy given after 36 weeks' gestation reduces, but does not totally eliminate, HSV-2 recurrence at delivery.[307,308] Systematic reviews suggest that the frequency of cesarean delivery can also be reduced.[309,310] Although mathematical models suggest that such an approach may be cost-effective in reducing cesarean deliveries, there are no data supporting the ability of this approach to reduce neonatal infection. Because the risk of neonatal transmission is low among HSV-2–seropositive women, the routine use of antiviral therapy among HSV-2–positive pregnant women would result in many women treated with few cases of neonatal HSV prevented, even if the effects on reducing maternal-fetal transmission are high. As such, we do not believe that routine use of antiviral therapy at the end of gestation should be recommended until better information on efficacy and potential neonatal safety is assessed. A more logical approach, described previously, that requires further study would be to screen low-risk seropositive mothers at delivery with rapid PCR and follow infants with HSV-2 exposure intensively after birth.

More effective screening programs would target HSV-2–seronegative women; 2% of women in one survey seroconverted during pregnancy and one third of these seroconversions occurred during the third trimester. Potential approaches range from counseling for routine abstinence in all women after 34 weeks' gestation to the use of routine serologic screening to identify HSV-susceptible women. Such women then would be counseled about the importance of engaging in only protected coitus during the latter part of pregnancy. Of particular interest are the 20% of women who are in a serodiscordant relationship and are at high risk of primary infection (3.5% for HSV-1, 20% for HSV-2).[311]

A third possible type of screening program could be to identify and treat the HSV-2–positive sex partners of seronegative pregnant women with antiviral therapy and follow them serially for seroconversion, although the expense would be substantial.[312] Clinical and demographic data do not differentiate women at high versus low risk of transmitting HSV to their infants.[313] Pregnancy also may enhance HSV acquisition, making standard prophylactic measures such as condoms potentially less effective.[314] Because nearly 30% of neonatal HSV is due to HSV-1, attention to reducing HSV-1 acquisition through orogenital sex is also of importance.

Diagnosis

Clinical criteria are essential for entertaining the diagnosis of HSV infections. Nevertheless, given the gravity of diagnosing a lifelong viral STD, we believe that appropriate management of the patient should always include laboratory confirmation. A clinical diagnosis often can be inferred when characteristic multiple vesicular lesions appear on an erythematous base. In this situation, given the prolonged morbidity of first-episode genital HSV infection and the ability of antiviral agents to mitigate systemic symptoms and prevent development of new ulcers, it is appropriate to initiate oral antiviral treatment while awaiting laboratory confirmation. It is increasingly recognized that herpetic lesions may resemble skin ulcerations of other causes.[60,209] Mucosal HSV infection can appear as urethritis or pharyngitis without cutaneous lesions. When there is clinical uncertainty, laboratory diagnosis is essential to guide therapy.[62]

HSV infection is best confirmed by isolation of virus in tissue culture or demonstration of HSV DNA in lesion scrapings.[209,211] HSV causes a discernible cytopathic effect in a variety of cell culture systems, generally within 48 to 96 hours after inoculation. Spin-amplified culture with subsequent staining for HSV antigen shortens the time needed to identify HSV to less than 24 hours. The sensitivity of viral isolation is higher in vesicular lesions than ulcerative lesions during the first rather than recurrent episodes of disease and in samples from immunosuppressed rather than immunocompetent patients. HSV DNA detection is three to four times more sensitive than viral isolation; is less affected by variation in specimen transport; is the preferred diagnostic method, if available; and is cost-effective compared with culture.[211] Laboratory confirmation permits subtyping of the virus, which may help predict frequency of reactivation after first-episode oral or genital HSV infection, site of CNS infection, and likelihood of drug resistance.[315] Staining of scrapings from the base of the lesions

with Wright, Giemsa (Tzanck preparation), or Papanicolaou stain demonstrates characteristic giant cells or intranuclear inclusions of HSV infection. These cytologic techniques are useful as quick office procedures to confirm the diagnosis. The limitations are that they do not differentiate between HSV and varicella-zoster virus infections, they are relatively insensitive, and correct identification of giant cells requires experience.

Evaluation of the seroprevalence of HSV-1 and HSV-2 has been markedly enhanced by the development of type-specific serologic assays.[316-318] These assays allow for detection of HSV-2 in the presence of HSV-1 antibodies and vice versa. Most commercially available assays measure antibodies to purified HSV-1 or HSV-2-specific proteins such as glycoproteins gG1 and gG2, which are antigenically distinct between the two subtypes. gG1 and gG2 assays are accurate for defining persons with long-standing HSV infections regardless of clinical symptoms and are adequate for clinical use, although some are not as sensitive for incident HSV-1 infection.[316,319-321] Another assay using an immunoblot format that identifies several type-specific antibodies, for example, gG2 and ICP-35 complex, was also developed.[319] The Western blot assay is the most accurate available test and has a sensitivity and specificity of greater than 98% for distinguishing HSV-1– and HSV-2–specific antibodies.[322,323] Assays that use whole viral extracts or antigens are inaccurate and should not be used for any stage of clinical diagnosis or epidemiologic studies.[324,325] Unfortunately, these assays have not been taken off the market and are in widespread use in many laboratories.

Acute- and convalescent-phase serum can be useful in demonstrating seroconversion during primary HSV-1 or HSV-2 infection. Only 5% of patients with recurrent orogenital HSV infections have a fourfold or greater increase in HSV antibody titer in the interval between collection of two samples. A specific but only partially sensitive immunoglobulin M assay to IgG2 was developed but is not commercially available.[326]

Treatment

The advent of antiviral drugs for HSV-1 and HSV-2 infections has made management of these infections a part of standard clinical practice (see Chapter 41). For mucocutaneous and visceral HSV infections, acyclovir and its related compounds famciclovir and valacyclovir are the mainstay of therapy. Several antiviral agents are available for topical use in HSV eye infections: idoxuridine, trifluorothymidine, topical vidarabine, and cidofovir. For HSV encephalitis and neonatal herpes, intravenous acyclovir is the treatment of choice. Acyclovir-resistant virus can be encountered in immunocompromised hosts and is treated with foscarnet or cidofovir.

Acyclovir was the first antiviral drug clearly demonstrated to be effective against HSV infections. It is an acyclic nucleoside analogue that is a substrate for HSV-specified thymidine kinase and is selectively phosphorylated by HSV-infected cells to acyclovir monophosphate.[327,328] Cellular enzymes then phosphorylate acyclovir monophosphate to acyclovir triphosphate, a competitive inhibitor of viral DNA polymerase. Acyclovir triphosphate is incorporated into the growing DNA chain of the virus and causes chain termination. Acyclovir has potent in vitro activity against both HSV-1 and HSV-2.[329]

Numerous trials of acyclovir in mucocutaneous HSV infections of the immunocompetent and immunosuppressed host have been conducted.[330-335] Famciclovir, the oral formulation of penciclovir, is also clinically effective in the treatment of a variety of HSV-1 and HSV-2 infections.[336-339] Valacyclovir is a valyl ester of acyclovir that has greater bioavailability than acyclovir.[340-342] The high blood levels of acyclovir achieved make valacyclovir useful for once-daily suppressive therapy and for short-course, 1- or 2-day treatment of orogenital HSV-1 infection.[343,344] Ganciclovir has activity against both HSV-1 and HSV-2, but because it is more toxic than acyclovir, valacyclovir, and famciclovir, it is generally not recommended for treatment of HSV infections.[345] Table 136-4 outlines a variety of treatment options for the use of these compounds.

TABLE 136-4	Antiviral Chemotherapy for Herpes Simplex Virus Infection

Mucocutaneous HSV Infections

Infections in Immunosuppressed Patients

Acute symptomatic first or recurrent episodes: Acyclovir 5 mg/kg IV q8h, acyclovir 400 mg PO qid, famciclovir 500 mg PO tid, or valacyclovir 500 mg PO bid for 7 to 10 days is effective. Treatment duration may vary from 7 to 14 days.

Suppression of reactivation disease: Acyclovir 5 mg/kg IV q8h, valacyclovir 500 mg PO bid, or acyclovir 400 to 800 mg PO three to five times daily prevents recurrences during the immediate 30-day post-transplantation period. Longer term suppression is often used for persons with continued immunosuppression. In bone marrow and renal transplant recipients, valacyclovir 2 g PO three to four times daily is also effective in preventing CMV infection. However, valacyclovir 2 g PO four times daily has been associated with TTP after extended use in HIV-positive persons. In HIV-infected persons, famciclovir 500 mg PO bid is effective in reducing clinical and subclinical reactivations of HSV-1 and -2.

Genital Herpes

First episodes: Acyclovir 200 mg PO five times daily (I) or 400 mg PO tid (V) for 7 to 10 days. Valacyclovir 1000 mg PO bid for 7 to 10 days (I). Famciclovir 250 mg PO tid for 7 to 10 days (I). Acyclovir 5 mg/kg IV q8h for 5 days is given for severe disease or neurologic complications such as aseptic meningitis. Treatment might be extended if healing is incomplete after ten days of therapy.

Symptomatic recurrent genital herpes: Acyclovir 200 mg PO five times daily for 5 days, 400 mg PO tid for 5 days (V), **800 mg PO tid for 2 days** or bid for 5 days (II). **Valacyclovir 500 mg PO bid for 3-5 days (I)** or 1 g/day PO for 5 days (I) or **1 g PO bid for 1 day (II)**. **Famciclovir** 125 mg PO bid for 5 days (I), 500 mg PO bid for 5 days (II), **1 g PO bid for 1 day (I), or 500 mg once and then 250 mg PO bid for three doses (I)**. All these therapies are effective in shortening lesion duration. Short-course options (1, 2, or 3 days of therapy) should be considered based on increased convenience, likelihood of adherence, and reduced cost and are shown in bold. Given the brief period of viral replication and rapid evolution of lesions, patients should be given drugs for self-administration when prodromal symptoms occur.

Suppression of recurrent genital herpes: Acyclovir 400 mg PO bid (I) or 400 to 800 mg PO bid to tid (I). Valacyclovir 500 mg/day PO (I) or 1000 mg/day PO (I) or 250 to 500 mg PO bid (I) prevents symptomatic reactivation. Persons with frequent reactivation (fewer than nine episodes per year) can take valacyclovir 500 mg/day PO; those with more than nine episodes per year should take valacyclovir 1000 mg/day PO or 500 mg PO bid. Consider suppression with valacyclovir for patients with frequent (more than six episodes) or severe recurrences, in immunocompromised patients, or as an adjunct to prevent transmission. Famciclovir 250 mg PO bid (I) or 500 mg PO bid (II).

Orolabial HSV Infections

First episode: Acyclovir 15 mg/kg PO (up to 200 mg) five times daily (II) or 400 mg PO tid (V) for 7 days. Famciclovir 500 mg PO bid (V). Valacyclovir 1000 mg PO bid (V) for 7 days.

Recurrent episodes: Acyclovir 400 mg PO five times daily for 5 days (II). **Valacyclovir 2000 mg PO bid for 1 day (I). Famciclovir 1500 mg PO once (I).** Self-initiated therapy with topical 1% penciclovir cream q2h during waking hours (I); topical acyclovir cream 5% five times daily for 4 days (I). Short-course options should be considered based on increased convenience and likelihood of adherence and are shown in bold. Given the brief period of viral replication and rapid evolution of lesions, patients should be given drugs for self-administration when prodromal symptoms occur.

Suppression of reactivation of orolabial HSV: Acyclovir 400 mg PO bid (II) or valacyclovir 500 mg/day or 1000 mg/day PO (II) or famciclovir 500 mg PO bid (V). Consider for patients with frequent (more than six episodes) or severe recurrences, in immunocompromised patients, or as an adjunct to prevent transmission.

Herpetic Whitlow

Acyclovir 200 mg PO five times daily for 7 to 10 days

HSV Proctitis

Acyclovir 400 mg PO five times daily is useful in shortening the course of infection. In immunosuppressed patients or in patients with severe infection, acyclovir 5 mg/kg IV q8h may be useful.

Herpetic Eye Infections

In acute keratitis, topical trifluorothymidine, vidarabine, idoxuridine, acyclovir, penciclovir, and interferon are all beneficial. Débridement may be required; topical steroids may worsen disease (see Chapter 111).

CNS HSV Infections

HSV encephalitis: Acyclovir 10 mg/kg IV q8h (30 mg/kg/day) for 14 to 21 days

HSV aseptic meningitis: No studies of systemic antiviral chemotherapy exist. Generally, acyclovir 5 mg/kg q8h IV should be used.

Autonomic radiculopathy: No studies are available.

Neonatal HSV Infections

Acyclovir 60 mg/kg/day IV (divided into three doses) for 21 days. Monitoring for relapse should be undertaken, and some authorities recommend continued suppression with oral acyclovir suspension for 3 to 4 months.

Visceral HSV Infections

HSV esophagitis: Acyclovir 15 mg/kg/day IV. In some patients with milder forms of immunosuppression, oral therapy with valacyclovir or famciclovir is effective.

HSV pneumonitis: No controlled studies exist. Acyclovir 15 mg/kg/day IV should be considered.

Disseminated HSV Infections

No controlled studies exist. Acyclovir 10 mg/kg IV q8h nevertheless should be given. No definite evidence indicates that therapy decreases the risk of death.

Erythema Multiforme–Associated HSV

Anecdotal observations suggest that acyclovir 400 mg PO bid or tid or valacyclovir 500 mg PO bid suppresses erythema multiforme.

Surgical Prophylaxis

Several surgical procedures such as laser skin resurfacing, trigeminal nerve root decompression, and lumbar disk surgery have been associated with HSV reactivation. Acyclovir 3 mg/kg IV and acyclovir 800 mg PO bid, valacyclovir 500 mg PO bid, or famciclovir 250 mg PO bid is effective in reducing reactivation. Therapy should be initiated 48 hours before surgery and continued for 3 to 7 days.

Infections with Acyclovir-Resistant HSV

Foscarnet 40 mg/kg IV q8h should be given until lesions heal. The optimal duration of therapy and the usefulness of its continuation to suppress lesions are unclear. Some patients may benefit from cutaneous application of trifluorothymidine or 5% cidofovir gel.

CMV, cytomegalovirus; CNS, central nervous system; HIV, human immunodeficiency virus; HSV, herpes simplex virus; TTP, thrombotic thrombocytopenic purpura. I, II, III, IV, and V represent level of evidence.

Adapted in part from Cernik C, Gallina K, Brodell RT. The treatment of herpes simplex infections: an evidence-based review. *Arch Intern Med*. 2008;168:1137-1144; and Spruance S, Aoki FY, Tyring S, et al. Short-course therapy for recurrent genital herpes and herpes labialis: entering an era of greater convenience, better treatment adherence, and reduced cost. *J Fam Pract*. 2007;56:30-36.

Increasingly, shorter courses of therapy are being used for treatment of recurrent mucocutaneous HSV-1 or HSV-2 in immunocompetent patients. One-day courses of famciclovir and valacyclovir are clinically effective, more convenient, and generally less costly than longer courses of therapy.[335,337,346-349]

Intravenous acyclovir (30 mg/kg/day, given as a 10-mg/kg infusion over 1 hour at 8-hour intervals) is effective in reducing the morbidity and mortality associated with HSV encephalitis.[242] Early initiation of therapy is a critical factor in outcome. The major side effect is transient renal insufficiency, usually caused by crystallization of the compound in the renal parenchyma. This adverse reaction can be avoided if the medication is given slowly over 1 hour, and the patient is well hydrated. Because CSF levels of acyclovir average only 30% to 50% of plasma levels, the dose of acyclovir used for treatment of CNS infection (30 mg/kg/day) is double that used for the treatment of mucocutaneous or visceral disease (15 mg/kg/day). For disseminated neonatal HSV, high-dose intravenous therapy is recommended (60 mg/kg/day in three divided doses) for 21 days.[290] In immunosuppressed patients, intravenous acyclovir or oral valacyclovir is used to prevent HSV reactivations during transplantation or chemotherapy; high doses of valacyclovir also prevent cytomegalovirus reactivations.[345]

Acyclovir-resistant strains of HSV are well described.[350-352] Almost all clinically significant acyclovir resistance is seen in immunocompromised patients, especially in HIV-infected persons. Although resistant strains are generated in local mucosal replicating sites in immunocompetent hosts receiving therapy, these strains are not archived in the latent pool and do not have an effect on treatment outcome.[353] Most acyclovir-resistant strains of HSV have a deficiency in thymidine kinase, the enzyme that phosphorylates acyclovir.[354,355] Thus, cross-resistance to famciclovir is usually found (see Chapter 41). Occasionally, an isolate with altered thymidine kinase specificity arises and is sensitive to famciclovir but not to acyclovir. In some patients infected with thymidine kinase–deficient virus, higher doses of acyclovir are associated with clearing of lesions.[356] In others, clinical disease progresses. Isolation of HSV from persisting lesions despite adequate doses and blood levels of acyclovir should raise the suspicion of resistance. Therapy with foscarnet should be initiated and is usually successful, although side effects from foscarnet are common and include renal insufficiency, electrolyte wasting, nausea, paresthesias, and seizures.[357,358] Because of its toxicity and cost, intravenous foscarnet is usually reserved for patients with extensive mucocutaneous infections and laboratory-confirmed resistance. Cidofovir is a nucleotide analogue and exists as a phosphonate or monophosphate form. Most thymidine kinase–deficient strains of HSV are sensitive to cidofovir, which can be used topically or given intravenously on a weekly basis. Cidofovir ointment speeds healing of acyclovir-resistant lesions,[359,360] but the drug itself also can cause mucocutaneous ulcer-

ations. The intravenous form very commonly causes renal failure, neutropenia, rash, and gastrointestinal distress due to concurrent probenecid dosing. Trifluridine ointment is useful for ophthalmic HSV infection and has been reported anecdotally to be useful for resistant mucosal HSV in AIDS patients.[361] Resiquimod, a topical Toll-like receptor-7 and -8 agonist, decreased shedding and recurrence rates of anogenital HSV-2, but further commercial development of this agent has ceased.[136]

Counseling and Prevention

Many patients with first-episode genital HSV experience substantial morbidity and, as a result, miss work or school. Yet, a significant proportion, particularly men, do not seek health care advice.[362] Many patients report feelings of depression and fear of rejection and discovery. These negative feelings tend to subside over time, although not completely.[363] Therefore, during acute illness, it is best to ensure symptomatic palliation by recommending antiviral therapy, anti-inflammatory pain medicines, sitz baths, and local drying of the lesions. The patient usually should be taught about the chronicity of infection and natural history of recurrence and asymptomatic reactivation on later visits. Women's concerns regarding issues relating to pregnancy and childbirth should be addressed as well. Some asymptomatic primary care patients, pregnant women, or sexually transmitted disease clinic patients will have their infection diagnosed by serology rather than symptoms. This is also likely to be a source of distress for patients, and similar strategies should be used. Particular emphasis should be placed on recognition of subtle genital ulcers.

Finally, strategies for the prevention of HSV-2 transmission should be emphasized to patients, particularly those in serodiscordant relationships. Partially effective strategies include full disclosure to the susceptible partner, condom use, abstinence during symptomatic lesions, and antiviral therapy.[71,73,364] Valacyclovir (500 mg/day) reduced transmission of genital herpes by 50% by suppression of episodes of subclinical shedding and is a primary, albeit imperfect, prevention strategy in serodiscordant relationships.[71] Development of an effective HSV vaccine would be the best approach for the prevention of HSV. To date, no licensed vaccine is available. Clinical trials of a vaccine consisting of HSV-2 gD2 protein in a unique monophosphoryl lipid A (MPL)-like adjuvant showed partial efficacy against HSV-2 infection (75% decrease in clinical disease and 40% decrease in seroconversion) in women seronegative for HSV-1; the vaccine is still undergoing clinical evaluation. Unfortunately, this vaccine did not show efficacy in phase 2 trials in men or HSV-1–seropositive women,[63] limiting its potential use globally. Other vaccine products and spermicides to prevent HSV acquisition are in early clinical stages of development.

REFERENCES

1. Wildy P. Herpes history and classification. In: Kaplan A, ed. *The Herpes Viruses*. New York: Academic Press; 1973:1-25.
2. Astruc J. *De Morbis Venereis Libri Sex*. Paris; 1736.
3. Hutfield D. History of herpes genitalis. *Br J Vener Dis*. 1996;42:263.
4. Parker F, Nye R. Studies on filterable viruses: II. Cultivation of herpes virus. *Am J Pathol*. 1925;1:337.
5. Lipschutz B. Untersuchungen uber die Aetiologie der Krankheiten der Herpes Gruppe (herpes zoster, herpes genitalis, herpes febrilis). *Arch Dermatol Symp (Berl)*. 1921;136:428.
6. Nahmias AJ, Dowdle WR. Antigenic and biologic differences in herpesvirus hominis. *Prog Med Virol*. 1968;10:110-159.
7. Roizman B. The structure and isomerization of herpes simplex virus genomes. *Cell*. 1979;16:481-494.
8. Dolan A, Jamieson FE, Cunningham C, et al. The genome sequence of herpes simplex virus type 2. *J Virol*. 1998;72:2010-2021.
9. Gentry GA, Lowe M, Alford G, et al. Sequence analyses of herpesviral enzymes suggest an ancient origin for human sexual behavior. *Proc Natl Acad Sci U S A*. 1988;85:2658-2661.
10. Buchman TG, Roizman B, Adams G, et al. Restriction endonuclease fingerprinting of herpes simplex virus DNA: a novel epidemiological tool applied to a nosocomial outbreak. *J Infect Dis*. 1978;138:488-498.
11. Schmidt OW, Fife KH, Corey L. Reinfection is an uncommon occurrence in patients with symptomatic recurrent genital herpes. *J Infect Dis*. 1984;149:645-646.
12. Buchman TG, Roizman B, Nahmias AJ. Demonstration of exogenous genital reinfection with herpes simplex virus type 2 by restriction endonuclease fingerprinting of viral DNA. *J Infect Dis*. 1979;140:295-304.
13. Douglas J, Schmidt O, Corey L. Acquisition of neonatal HSV-1 infection from a paternal source contact. *J Pediatr*. 1983;103:908-910.
14. Hammer SM, Buchman TG, D'Angelo LJ, et al. Temporal cluster of herpes simplex encephalitis: investigation by restriction endonuclease cleavage of viral DNA. *J Infect Dis*. 1980;141:436-440.
15. Lakeman AD, Nahmias AJ, Whitley RJ. Analysis of DNA from recurrent genital herpes simplex virus isolates by restriction endonuclease digestion. *Sex Transm Dis*. 1986;13:61-66.
16. Spear PG, Longnecker R. Herpesvirus entry: an update. *J Virol*. 2003;77:10179-10185.
17. Montgomery RI, Warner MS, Lum BJ, et al. Herpes simplex virus-1 entry into cells mediated by a novel member of the TNF/NGF receptor family. *Cell*. 1996;87:427-436.
18. Krummenacher C, Nicola AV, Whitbeck JC, et al. Herpes simplex virus glycoprotein D can bind to poliovirus receptor-related protein 1 or herpesvirus entry mediator, two structurally unrelated mediators of virus entry. *J Virol*. 1998;72:7064-7074.
19. Struyf F, Posavad CM, Keyaerts E, et al. Search for polymorphisms in the genes for herpesvirus entry mediator, nectin-1, and nectin-2 in immune seronegative individuals. *J Infect Dis*. 2002;185:36-44.
20. Haarr L, Shukla D, Rødahl E, et al. Transcription from the gene encoding the herpesvirus entry receptor nectin-1 (HveC) in nervous tissue of adult mouse. *Virology*. 2001;287:301-309.
21. Mata M, Zhang M, Hu X, et al. HveC (nectin-1) is expressed at high levels in sensory neurons, but not in motor neurons, of the rat peripheral nervous system. *J Neurovirol*. 2001;7:476-480.
22. Zelus BD, Stewart RS, Ross J. The virion host shutoff protein of herpes simplex virus type 1: messenger ribonucleolytic activity in vitro. *J Virol*. 1996;70:2411-2419.
23. Homa FL, Brown JC. Capsid assembly and DNA packaging in herpes simplex virus. *Rev Med Virol*. 1997;7:107-122.
24. Roizman B, Knipe DM. Herpes simplex viruses and their replication. In: Knipe DM, Howley PM, Griffin DE, et al, eds. *Field's Virology*. 5th ed. Philadelphia: Lippincott Williams & Wilkins; 2007.
25. Cushing H. Surgical aspects of major neuralgia of trigeminal nerve: report of 20 cases of operation upon the gasserian gan-

glion with anatomic and physiologic notes on the consequences of its removal. *JAMA*. 1905;44:773-779.
26. Stevens JG, Cook ML. Latent herpes simplex virus in spinal ganglia of mice. *Science*. 1971;173:843-845.
27. Stevens JG, Haarr L, Porter DD, et al. Prominence of the herpes simplex virus latency-associated transcript in trigeminal ganglia from seropositive humans. *J Infect Dis*. 1988;158:117-123.
28. Mehta A, Maggioncalda J, Bagasra O, et al. In situ DNA PCR and RNA hybridization detection of herpes simplex virus sequences in trigeminal ganglia of latently infected mice. *Virology*. 1995;206:633-640.
29. Burke RL, Hartog K, Croen KD, et al. Detection and characterization of latent HSV RNA by in situ and northern blot hybridization in guinea pigs. *Virology*. 1991;181:793-797.
30. Saksena MM, Wakisaka H, Tijono B, et al. Herpes simplex virus type 1 accumulation, envelopment, and exit in growth cones and varicosities in mid-distal regions of axons. *J Virol*. 2006; 80:3592-3606.
31. Baringer JR. Recovery of herpes simplex virus from human sacral ganglions. *N Engl J Med*. 1974;291:828-830.
32. Sawtell NM, Thompson RL. Rapid in vivo reactivation of herpes simplex virus in latently infected murine ganglionic neurons after transient hyperthermia. *J Virol*. 1992;66:2150-2156.
33. Sawtell NM, Thompson RL. Herpes simplex virus type 1 latency-associated transcription unit promotes anatomical site-dependent establishment and reactivation from latency. *J Virol*. 1992;66:2157-2169.
34. Carton CA, Kilbourne ED. Activation of latent herpes simplex by trigeminal sensory-root section. *N Engl J Med*. 1952;246: 172.
35. Wang K, Mahalingam G, Hoover S, et al. Diverse herpes simplex virus type 1 thymidine kinase mutants in individual human neurons and ganglia. *J Virol*. 2007;81:6817-6826.
36. Javier RT, Stevens JG, Dissette VB, et al. A herpes simplex virus transcript abundant in latently infected neurons is dispensable for establishment of the latent state. *Virology*. 1988;166:254-257.
37. Yoshikawa T, Hill JM, Stanberry LR, et al. The characteristic site-specific reactivation phenotypes of HSV-1 and HSV-2 depend upon latency-associated transcript region. *J Exp Med*. 1996;184:659.
38. Krause PR, Stanberry LR, Bourne N, et al. Expression of the herpes simplex virus type 2 latency-associated transcript enhances spontaneous reactivation of genital herpes in latently infected guinea pigs. *J Exp Med*. 1995;181:297-306.
39. Thompson RL, Sawtell NM. Herpes simplex virus type 1 latency-associated transcript gene promotes neuronal survival. *J Virol*. 2001;75:6660-6675.
40. Perng GC, Jones C, Ciacci-Zanella J, et al. Virus-induced neuronal apoptosis blocked by the herpes simplex virus latency-associated transcript. *Science*. 2000;287:1500-1503.
41. Tang S, Bertke AS, Patel A, et al. An acutely and latently expressed herpes simplex virus 2 viral microRNA inhibits expression of ICP34.5, a viral neurovirulence factor. *Proc Natl Acad Sci U S A*. 2008;105:10931-10936.
42. Wang K, Lau T, Morales M, et al. Laser-capture microdissection: refining estimates of the quantity and distribution of latent herpes simplex virus 1 and varicella-zoster virus DNA in human trigeminal ganglia at the single-cell level. *J Virol*. 2005;79: 14079-14087.
43. Chen X, Mata M, Kelley M, et al. The relationship of herpes simplex virus latency associated transcript expression to genome copy number: a quantitative study using laser capture microdissection. *J Neurovirol*. 2002;8:204-210.
44. Perng GC, Thompson RL, Sawtell NM, et al. An avirulent ICP34.5 deletion mutant of herpes simplex virus type 1 is capable of in vivo spontaneous reactivation. *J Virol*. 1995;69: 3033-3041.
45. Coen DM, Kosz-Vnenchak M, Jacobson JG, et al. Thymidine kinase-negative herpes simplex virus mutants establish latency in mouse trigeminal ganglia but do not reactivate. *Proc Natl Acad Sci U S A*. 1989;86:4736-4740.
46. Mertz KJ, Trees D, Levine WC, et al. Etiology of genital ulcers and prevalence of human immunodeficiency virus coinfection in 10 US cities. The Genital Ulcer Disease Surveillance Group. *J Infect Dis*. 1998;178:1795-1798.
47. Cowan FM, Johnson AM, Ashley R, et al. Relationship between antibodies to herpes simplex virus (HSV) and symptoms of HSV infection. *J Infect Dis*. 1996;174:470-475.
48. Cowan FM, Copas A, Johnson AM, et al. Herpes simplex virus type 1 infection: a sexually transmitted infection of adolescence? *Sex Transm Infect*. 2002;78:346-348.
49. Malkin JE, Morand P, Malvy D, et al. Seroprevalence of HSV-1 and HSV-2 infection in the general French population. *Sex Transm Infect*. 2002;78:201-203.
50. Tunback P, Bergstrom T, Andersson AS, et al. Prevalence of herpes simplex virus antibodies in childhood and adolescence: a cross-sectional study. *Scand J Infect Dis*. 2003;35:498-502.
51. Xu F, Sternberg M, Kottiri B, et al. Trends in herpes simplex virus type 1 and type 2 seroprevalence in the United States. *JAMA*. 2006;296:964-973.
52. Vyse AJ, Gay NJ, Slomka MJ, et al. The burden of infection with HSV-1 and HSV-2 in England and Wales: implications for the changing epidemiology of genital herpes. *Sex Transm Infect*. 2000;76:183-187.
53. Kropp R, Wong T, Cormier L, et al. Neonatal herpes simplex virus infections in Canada: results of a 3-year national prospective study. *Pediatrics*. 2006;117:1955-1962.
54. Cowan FM, Johnson AM, Ashley R, et al. Antibody to herpes simplex virus type 2 as serological marker of sexual lifestyle in populations. *Br Med J*. 1994;309:1325-1329.
55. Fleming D, McQuillan G, Johnson R, et al. Herpes simplex virus type 2 in the United States, 1976 to 1994. *N Engl J Med*. 1997;337:1105-1111.
56. Weiss H. Epidemiology of herpes simplex virus type 2 infection in the developing world. *Herpes*. 2004;11(Suppl 1):24A-35A.
57. Malkin JE. Epidemiology of genital herpes simplex virus infection in developed countries. *Herpes*. 2004;11(Suppl 1): 2A-23A.
58. Johnson RE, Nahmias AJ, Magder LS, et al. A seroepidemiologic survey of the prevalence of herpes simplex virus type 2 infection in the United States. *N Engl J Med*. 1989;321:7-12.
59. Corey L, Wald A, Celum C, et al. The effects of herpes simplex virus-2 on HIV-1 acquisition and transmission: a review of two overlapping epidemics. *J Acquir Immune Defic Syndr*. 2004; 35:435-445.
60. Koutsky LA, Ashley RL, Holmes KK, et al. The frequency of unrecognized type 2 herpes simplex virus infection among women: implications for the control of genital herpes. *Sex Transm Dis*. 1990;17:90-94.
61. Cherpes TL, Meyn LA, Krohn MA, et al. Risk factors for infection with herpes simplex virus type 2: role of smoking, douching, uncircumcised males, and vaginal flora. *Sex Transm Dis*. 2003;30:405-410.
62. Langenberg AG, Corey L, Ashley RL, et al. A prospective study of new infections with herpes simplex virus type 1 and type 2. Chiron HSV Vaccine Study Group. *N Engl J Med*. 1999;341: 1432-1438.
63. Stanberry LR, Spruance SL, Cunningham AL, et al. Glycoprotein-D-adjuvant vaccine to prevent genital herpes. *N Engl J Med*. 2002;347:1652-1661.
64. Corey L, Langenberg AG, Ashley R, et al. Recombinant glycoprotein vaccine for the prevention of genital HSV-2 infection: two randomized controlled trials. Chiron HSV Vaccine Study Group. *JAMA*. 1999;282:331-340.
65. Wald A, Langenberg A, Link K, et al. Effect of condoms on reducing the transmission of herpes simplex virus type 2 from men to women. *JAMA*. 2001;285:3100-3106.
66. Gottlieb SL, Douglas JM Jr, Foster M, et al. Incidence of herpes simplex virus type 2 infection in 5 sexually transmitted disease (STD) clinics and the effect of HIV/STD risk-reduction counseling. *J Infect Dis*. 2004;190:1059-1067.
67. Brown E, Wald A, Hughes J, et al. High risk of human immunodeficiency virus in men who have sex with men with herpes simplex virus type 2 in the EXPLORE study. *Am J Epidemiol*. 2006;164:733-741.
68. Kebede Y, Dorigo-Zetsma W, Mengistu Y, et al. Transmission of herpes simplex virus type 2 among factory workers in Ethiopia. *J Infect Dis*. 2004;190:365-372.
69. Kamali A, Nunn A, Mulder D, et al. Seroprevalence and incidence of genital ulcer infections in a rural Ugandan population. *Sex Transm Infect*. 1999;75:98-102.
70. McFarland W, Gwanzura L, Bassett M, et al. Prevalence and incidence of herpes simplex virus type 2 infection among male Zimbabwean factory workers. *J Infect Dis*. 1999;180:1459-1465.
71. Corey L, Wald A, Patel R, et al. Once-daily valacyclovir to reduce the risk of transmission of genital herpes. *N Engl J Med*. 2004;350:11-20.
72. Mertz GJ, Schmidt O, Jourden JL, et al. Frequency of acquisition of first-episode genital infection with herpes simplex virus from symptomatic and asymptomatic source contacts. *Sex Transm Dis*. 1985;12:33-39.
73. Wald A, Krantz E, Selke S, et al. Knowledge of partners' genital herpes protects against herpes simplex virus type 2 acquisition. *J Infect Dis*. 2006;194:42-52.
74. Weiss H, Thomas S, Munabi S, et al. Male circumcision and risk of syphilis, chancroid, and genital herpes: a systematic review and meta-analysis. *Sex Transm Infect*. 2006;82:101-110.
75. Wald A, Zeh J, Selke S, et al. Reactivation of genital herpes simplex virus type 2 infection in asymptomatic seropositive persons. *N Engl J Med*. 2000;342:844-850.
76. Blank H, Haines HG. Experimental human reinfection with herpes simplex virus. *J Invest Dermatol*. 1973;61:223-225.
77. Perl TM, Haugen TH, Pfaller MA, et al. Transmission of herpes simplex virus type 1 infection in an intensive care unit. *Ann Intern Med*. 1992;117:584-586.
78. Cherpes TL, Meyn LA, Hillier SL. Cunnilingus and vaginal intercourse are risk factors for herpes simplex virus type 1 acquisition in women. *Sex Transm Dis*. 2005;32:84-89.
79. Belongia EA, Goodman JL, Holland EJ, et al. An outbreak of herpes gladiatorum at a high-school wrestling camp. *N Engl J Med*. 1991;325:906-910.
80. Brown ZA, Selke S, Zeh J, et al. The acquisition of herpes simplex virus during pregnancy. *N Engl J Med*. 1997;337:509-515.
81. Quinn TC, Corey L, Chaffee RG, et al. The etiology of anorectal infections in homosexual men. *Am J Med*. 1981;71:395-406.
82. Gray R, Wawer M, Brookmeyer R, et al. Probability of HIV-1 transmission per coital act in monogamous, heterosexual, HIV-1-discordant couples in Rakai, Uganda. *Lancet*. 2001;357:1149-1153.
83. Sacks SL, Griffiths PD, Corey L, et al. Introduction: is viral shedding a surrogate marker for transmission of genital herpes? *Antiviral Res*. 2004;63(Suppl 1):S3-S9.
84. Mark KE, Wald A, Margaret AS, et al. Rapidly cleared episodes of herpes simplex virus reactivation in immunocompetent adults. *J Infect Dis*. 2008;198:1141-1149.
85. Blower S, Wald A, Gershengorn H, et al. Targeting virological core groups: a new paradigm for controlling herpes simplex virus type 2 epidemics. *J Infect Dis*. 2004;190:1610-1617.
86. Kim H, Wald A, Harris J, et al. Does frequency of genital herpes recurrences predict risk of transmission? Further analysis of the valacyclovir transmission study. *Sex Transm Dis*. 2008;35:124-128.
87. Stanberry LR, Kern ER, Richards JT, et al. Genital herpes in guinea pigs: pathogenesis of the primary infection and description of recurrent disease. *J Infect Dis*. 1982;146:397-404.
88. Sawtell NM. Quantitative analysis of herpes simplex virus reactivation in vivo demonstrates that reactivation in the nervous system is not inhibited at early times postinoculation. *J Virol*. 2003;77:4127-4138.
89. Rock DL, Fraser NW. Detection of HSV-1 genome in central nervous system of latently infected mice. *Nature*. 1983;302: 523-525.
90. Corey L, Spear PG. Infections with herpes simplex viruses (1). *N Engl J Med*. 1986;314:686-691.
91. Johnston C, Magaret A, Selke S, et al. Herpes simplex virus viremia during primary genital infection. *J Infect Dis*. 2008; 198:31-34.
92. Chen S, Garber D, Schaffer P, et al. Persistent elevated expression of cytokine transcripts in ganglia latently infected with herpes simplex virus in the absence of ganglionic replication or reactivation. *Virology*. 2000;278:207-216.
93. Liu T, Khanna K, Carriere B, et al. Gamma interferon can prevent herpes simplex virus type 1 reactivation from latency in sensory neurons. *J Virol*. 2001;75:11178-11184.
94. Liu T, Khanna K, Chen X, et al. CD8(+) T cells can block herpes simplex virus type 1 (HSV-1) reactivation from latency in sensory neurons. *J Exp Med*. 2000;191:1459-1466.
95. Verjans GM, Hintzen RQ, van Dun JM, et al. Selective retention of herpes simplex virus-specific T cells in latently infected human trigeminal ganglia. *Proc Natl Acad Sci U S A*. 2007;104: 3496-3501.
96. Decman V, Kinchington PR, Harvey SA, et al. Gamma interferon can block herpes simplex virus type 1 reactivation from latency, even in the presence of late gene expression. *J Virol*. 2005;79:10339-10347.
97. Knickelbein JE, Khanna KM, Yee MB, et al. Noncytotoxic lytic granule-mediated $CD8^+$ T cell inhibition of HSV-1 reactivation from neuronal latency. *Science*. 2008;322:268-271.
98. Hoshino Y, Qin J, Follmann D, et al. The number of herpes simplex virus-infected neurons and the number of viral genome copies per neuron correlate with the latent viral load in ganglia. *Virology*. 2008;372:56-63.
99. Hoshino Y, Pesnicak L, Cohen JI, et al. Rates of reactivation of latent herpes simplex virus from mouse trigeminal ganglia ex vivo correlate directly with viral load and inversely with number of infiltrating CD8+ T cells. *J Virol*. 2007;81:8157-8164.
100. Crespi C, Cumberland W, Wald A, et al. Longitudinal study of herpes simplex virus type 2 infection using viral dynamic modelling. *Sex Transm Infect*. 2007;83:359-364.
101. Koelle D, Corey L. Herpes simplex: insights on pathogenesis and possible vaccines. *Annu Rev Med*. 2008;59:381-395.
102. Koelle D, Posavad C, Barnum G, et al. Clearance of HSV-2 from recurrent genital lesions correlates with infiltration of HSV-specific cytotoxic T lymphocytes. *J Clin Invest*. 1998;101:1500-1508.
103. Koelle DM, Liu Z, McClurkan CM, et al. Expression of cutaneous lymphocyte-associated antigen by CD8(+) T cells specific for a skin-tropic virus. *J Clin Invest*. 2002;110:537-548.
104. Posavad C, Wald A, Kuntz S, et al. Frequent reactivation of herpes simplex virus among HIV-1-infected patients treated with highly active antiretroviral therapy. *J Infect Dis*. 2004;190: 693-696.
105. Posavad CM, Koelle DM, Shaughnessy MF, et al. Severe genital herpes infections in HIV-infected individuals with impaired herpes simplex virus-specific $CD8^+$ cytotoxic T lymphocyte responses. *Proc Natl Acad Sci U S A*. 1997;94:10289-10294.
106. Engelberg R, Carrell D, Krantz E, et al. Natural history of genital herpes simplex virus type 1 infection. *Sex Transm Dis*. 2003;30: 174-177.
107. Lafferty WE, Coombs RW, Benedetti J, et al. Recurrences after oral and genital herpes simplex virus infection: influence of site of infection and viral type. *N Engl J Med*. 1987;316:1444-1449.
108. Landry ML, Zibello TA. Ability of herpes simplex virus (HSV) types 1 and 2 to induce clinical disease and establish latency following previous genital infection with the heterologous HSV type. *J Infect Dis*. 1988;158:1220-1226.
109. Kusne S, Schwartz M, Breinig MK, et al. Herpes simplex virus hepatitis after solid organ transplantation in adults. *J Infect Dis*. 1991;163:1001-1007.
110. Modiano P, Salloum E, Gillet-Terver MN, et al. Acyclovir-resistant chronic cutaneous herpes simplex in Wiskott-Aldrich syndrome. *Br J Dermatol*. 1995;133:475-478.
111. Johnson JR, Egaas S, Gleaves CA, et al. Hepatitis due to herpes simplex virus in marrow-transplant recipients. *Clin Infect Dis*. 1992;14:38-45.
112. Brown Z, Wald A, Morrow R, et al. Effect of serologic status and cesarean delivery on transmission rates of herpes simplex virus from mother to infant. *JAMA*. 2003;289:203-209.

113. Prober CG, Sullender WM, Yasukawa LL, et al. Low risk of herpes simplex virus infections in neonates exposed to the virus at the time of vaginal delivery to mothers with recurrent genital herpes simplex virus infections. *N Engl J Med*. 1987;316: 240-244.
114. Brown EL, Morrow R, Krantz EM, et al. Maternal herpes simplex virus antibody avidity and risk of neonatal herpes. *Am J Obstet Gynecol*. 2006;195:115-120.
115. Koelle DM, Corey L. Recent progress in herpes simplex virus immunobiology and vaccine research. *Clin Microbiol Rev*. 2003;16:96-113.
116. Abbo L, Vincek V, Dickinson G, et al. Selective defect in plasmacytoid dendritic cell function in a patient with AIDS-associated atypical genital herpes simplex vegetans treated with imiquimod. *Clin Infect Dis*. 2007;44:e25-e27.
117. Dalloul A, Oksenhendler E, Chosidow O, et al. Severe herpes virus (HSV-2) infection in two patients with myelodysplasia and undetectable NK cells and plasmacytoid dendritic cells in the blood. *J Clin Virol*. 2004;30:329-336.
118. Manickan E, Rouse BT. Roles of different T-cell subsets in control of herpes simplex virus infection determined by using T-cell-deficient mouse-models. *J Virol*. 1995;69:8178-8179.
119. Kapoor AK, Nash AA, Wildy P, et al. Pathogenesis of herpes simplex virus in congenitally athymic mice: the relative roles of cell-mediated and humoral immunity. *J Gen Virol*. 1982;60: 225-233.
120. Smith CM, Belz GT, Wilson NS, et al. Cutting edge: conventional CD8 alpha+ dendritic cells are preferentially involved in CTL priming after footpad infection with herpes simplex virus-1. *J Immunol*. 2003;170:4437-4440.
121. Khanna KM, Bonneau RH, Kinchington PR, et al. Herpes simplex virus-specific memory CD8+ T cells are selectively activated and retained in latently infected sensory ganglia. *Immunity*. 2003;18:593-603.
122. Ashkar AA, Bauer S, Mitchell WJ, et al. Local delivery of CpG oligodeoxynucleotides induces rapid changes in the genital mucosa and inhibits replication, but not entry, of herpes simplex virus type 2. *J Virol*. 2003;77:8948-8956.
123. Kobelt D, Lechmann M, Steinkasserer A. The interaction between dendritic cells and herpes simplex virus-1. *Curr Top Microbiol Immunol*. 2003;276:145-161.
124. Zhu J, Koelle D, Cao J, et al. Virus-specific CD8+ T cells accumulate near sensory nerve endings in genital skin during subclinical HSV-2 reactivation. *J Exp Med*. 2007;204:595-603.
125. Cunningham AL, Turner RR, Miller AC, et al. Evolution of recurrent herpes simplex lesions: an immunohistologic study. *J Clin Invest*. 1985;75:226-233.
126. Koelle DM, Abbo H, Peck A, et al. Direct recovery of herpes simplex virus (HSV)-specific T lymphocyte clones from recurrent genital HSV-2 lesions. *J Infect Dis*. 1994;169:956-961.
127. Cunningham AL, Merigan TC. gamma Interferon production appears to predict time of recurrence of herpes labialis. *J Immunol*. 1983;130:2397-2400.
128. Posavad C, Koelle D, Shaughnessy M, et al. Severe genital herpes infections in HIV-infected individuals with impaired herpes simplex virus-specific CD8+ cytotoxic T lymphocyte responses. *Proc Natl Acad Sci U S A*. 1997;94:10289-10294.
129. Dubin G, Fishman NO, Eisenberg RJ, et al. The role of herpes simplex virus glycoproteins in immune evasion. *Curr Top Microbiol Immunol*. 1992;179:111-120.
130. Balachandran N, Bacchetti S, Rawls WE. Protection against lethal challenge of BALB/c mice by passive transfer of monoclonal antibodies to five glycoproteins of herpes simplex virus type 2. *Infect Immun*. 1982;37:1132-1137.
131. Mikloska Z, Sanna P, Cunningham A. Neutralizing antibodies inhibit axonal spread of herpes simplex virus type 1 to epidermal cells in vitro. *J Virol*. 1999;73:5934-5944.
132. Siegal FP, Kadowaki N, Shodell M, et al. The nature of the principal type 1 interferon-producing cells in human blood. *Science*. 1999;284:1835-1837.
133. Lund JM, Linehan MM, Iijima N, et al. Cutting edge: plasmacytoid dendritic cells provide innate immune protection against mucosal viral infection in situ. *J Immunol*. 2006;177:7510-7514.
134. Leib DA. Counteraction of interferon-induced antiviral responses by herpes simplex viruses. *Curr Top Microbiol Immunol*. 2002;269:171-185.
135. Bochud PY, Magaret AS, Koelle DM, et al. Polymorphisms in TLR2 are associated with increased viral shedding and lesional rate in patients with genital herpes simplex virus type 2 infection. *J Infect Dis*. 2007;196:505-509.
136. Mark K, Corey L, Meng T, et al. Topical resiquimod 0.01% gel decreases herpes simplex virus type 2 genital shedding: a randomized, controlled trial. *J Infect Dis*. 2007;195:1324-1331.
137. Jerome KR, Fox R, Chen Z, et al. Inhibition of apoptosis by primary isolates of herpes simplex virus. *Arch Virol*. 2001;146:2219-2225.
138. York IA, Roop C, Andrews DW, et al. A cytosolic herpes simplex virus protein inhibits antigen presentation to CD8+ T lymphocytes. *Cell*. 1994;77:525-535.
139. Tigges MA, Koelle D, Hartog K, et al. Human CD8+ herpes simplex virus-specific cytotoxic T-lymphocyte clones recognize diverse virion protein antigens. *J Virol*. 1992;66:1622-1634.
140. Murphy JA, Duerst RJ, Smith TJ, et al. Herpes simplex virus type 2 virion host shutoff protein regulates alpha/beta interferon but not adaptive immune responses during primary infection in vivo. *J Virol*. 2003;77:9337-9345.
141. Barcy S, Corey L. Herpes simplex inhibits the capacity of lymphoblastoid B cell lines to stimulate CD4+ T cells. *J Immunol*. 2001;166:6242-6249.
142. Jerome KR, Chen Z, Lang R, et al. HSV and glycoprotein J inhibit caspase activation and apoptosis induced by granzyme B or Fas. *J Immunol*. 2001;167:3928-3935.
143. Lin R, Noyce RS, Collins SE, et al. The herpes simplex virus ICP0 RING finger domain inhibits IRF3- and IRF7-mediated activation of interferon-stimulated genes. *J Virol*. 2004;78:1675-1684.
144. Sanchez R, Mohr I. Inhibition of cellular 2′-5′ oligoadenylate synthetase by the herpes simplex virus type 1 Us11 protein. *J Virol*. 2007;81:3455-3464.
145. Casrouge A, Zhang SY, Eidenschenk C, et al. Herpes simplex virus encephalitis in human UNC-93B deficiency. *Science*. 2006;314:308-312.
146. Thomas J, Rouse BT. Immunopathogenesis of herpetic ocular disease. *Immunol Res*. 1997;16:375-386.
147. Zhao ZS, Granucci F, Yeh L, et al. Molecular mimicry by herpes simplex virus-type 1: autoimmune disease after viral infection. *Science*. 1998;279:1344-1347.
148. Corey L, Adams HG, Brown ZA, et al. Genital herpes simplex virus infections: clinical manifestations, course, and complications. *Ann Intern Med*. 1983;98:958-972.
149. Reeves WC, Corey L, Adams HG, et al. Risk of recurrence after first episodes of genital herpes: relation to HSV type and antibody response. *N Engl J Med*. 1981;305:315-319.
150. Benedetti J, Corey L, Ashley R. Recurrence rates in genital herpes after symptomatic first-episode infection. *Ann Intern Med*. 1994;121:847-854.
151. Bader C, Crumpacker CS, Schnipper LE, et al. The natural history of recurrent facial-oral infection with herpes simplex virus. *J Infect Dis*. 1978;138:897-905.
152. Glezen WP, Fernald GW, Lohr JA. Acute respiratory disease of university students with special reference to the etiologic role of herpesvirus hominis. *Am J Epidemiol*. 1975;101:111-121.
153. Schmitt DL, Johnson DW, Henderson FW. Herpes simplex type 1 infections in group day care. *Pediatr Infect Dis J*. 1991;10: 729-734.
154. Amir J, Harel L, Smetana Z, et al. The natural history of primary herpes simplex type 1 gingivostomatitis in children. *Pediatr Dermatol*. 1999;16:259-263.
155. Openshaw H, Bennett HE. Recurrence of herpes simplex virus after dental extraction. *J Infect Dis*. 1982;146:707.
156. Pazin GJ, Armstrong JA, Lam MT, et al. Prevention of reactivated herpes simplex infection by human leukocyte interferon after operation on the trigeminal root. *N Engl J Med*. 1979;301: 225-230.
157. Straus SE, Smith HA, Brickman C, et al. Acyclovir for chronic mucocutaneous herpes simplex virus infection in immunosuppressed patients. *Ann Intern Med*. 1982;96:270-277.
158. Eisen D, Essell J, Broun ER, et al. Clinical utility of oral valacyclovir compared with oral acyclovir for the prevention of herpes simplex virus mucositis following autologous bone marrow transplantation or stem cell rescue therapy. *Bone Marrow Transplant*. 2003;31:51-55.
159. Siegal FP, Lopez C, Hammer GS, et al. Severe acquired immunodeficiency in male homosexuals, manifested by chronic perianal ulcerative herpes simplex lesions. *N Engl J Med*. 1981;305: 1439-1444.
160. Foley FD, Greenawald KA, Nash G, et al. Herpesvirus infection in burned patients. *N Engl J Med*. 1970;282:652-656.
161. Garland SM, Hill PJ. Eczema herpeticum in pregnancy successfully treated with acyclovir. *Aust N Z J Obstet Gynaecol*. 1994;34:214-215.
162. Shelley W. Herpes simplex virus as a cause of erythema multiforme. *JAMA*. 1967;210:153.
163. Orton PW, Huff JC, Tonnesen MG, et al. Detection of a herpes simplex viral antigen in skin lesions of erythema multiforme. *Ann Intern Med*. 1984;101:48-50.
164. Green JA, Spruance SL, Wenerstrom G, et al. Post-herpetic erythema multiforme prevented with prophylactic oral acyclovir. *Ann Intern Med*. 1985;102:632-633.
165. Vahlne A, Edstrom S, Arstila P, et al. Bell's palsy and herpes simplex virus. *Arch Otolaryngol*. 1981;107:79-81.
166. Furuta Y, Fukuda S, Chida E, et al. Reactivation of herpes simplex virus type 1 in patients with Bell's palsy. *J Med Virol*. 1998;54:162-166.
167. Sullivan FM, Swan IR, Donnan PT, et al. Early treatment with prednisolone or acyclovir in Bell's palsy. *N Engl J Med*. 2007; 357:1598-1607.
168. Hato N, Yamada H, Kohno H, et al. Valacyclovir and prednisolone treatment for Bell's palsy: a multicenter, randomized, placebo-controlled study. *Otol Neurotol*. 2007;28:408-413.
169. Bernstein D, Lovett M, Bryson Y. Serologic analysis of first-episode nonprimary genital herpes simplex virus infection: presence of type 2 antibody in acute serum samples. *Am J Med*. 1984;77:1055-1060.
170. Benedetti JK, Zeh J, Selke S, et al. Frequency and reactivation of nongenital lesions among patients with genital herpes simplex virus. *Am J Med*. 1995;98:237-242.
171. Bryson YJ, Dillon M, Lovett M, et al. Treatment of first episodes of genital herpes simplex virus infection with oral acyclovir: a randomized double-blind controlled trial in normal subjects. *N Engl J Med*. 1983;308:916-921.
172. Corey L, Fife KH, Benedetti JK, et al. Intravenous acyclovir for the treatment of primary genital herpes. *Ann Intern Med*. 1983; 98:914-921.
173. Stamm WE, Wagner KF, Amsel R, et al. Causes of the acute urethral syndrome in women. *N Engl J Med*. 1980;303:409-415.
174. Koutsky LA, Stevens CE, Holmes KK, et al. Underdiagnosis of genital herpes by current clinical and viral-isolation procedures. *N Engl J Med*. 1992;326:1533-1539.
175. Lehtinen M, Rantala I, Teisala K, et al. Detection of herpes simplex virus in women with acute pelvic inflammatory disease. *J Infect Dis*. 1985;152:78-82.
176. Morrisseau PM, Phillips CA, Leadbetter GW Jr. Viral prostatitis. *J Urol*. 1970;103:767-769.
177. Goodell SE, Quinn TC, Mkrtichian E, et al. Herpes simplex virus proctitis in homosexual men: clinical, sigmoidoscopic, and histopathological features. *N Engl J Med*. 1983;308:868-871.
178. Rompalo AM, Mertz GJ, Davis LG, et al. Oral acyclovir for treatment of first-episode herpes simplex virus proctitis. *JAMA*. 1988;259:2879-2881.
179. Schacker T, Hu HL, Koelle DM, et al. Famciclovir for the suppression of symptomatic and asymptomatic herpes simplex virus reactivation in HIV-infected persons: a double-blind, placebo-controlled trial. *Ann Intern Med*. 1998;128:21-28.
180. Wald A, Zeh J, Selke S, et al. Virologic characteristics of subclinical and symptomatic genital herpes infections. *N Engl J Med*. 1995;333:770-775.
181. Whitley R, Barton N, Collins E, et al. Mucocutaneous herpes simplex virus infections in immunocompromised patients: a model for evaluation of topical antiviral agents. *Am J Med*. 1982;73:236-240.
182. Skoldenberg B, Jeansson S, Wolontis S. Herpes simplex virus type 2 and acute aseptic meningitis: clinical features of cases with isolation of herpes simplex virus from cerebrospinal fluids. *Scand J Infect Dis*. 1975;7:227-232.
183. Schlesinger Y, Tebas P, Gaudreault-Keener M, et al. Herpes simplex virus type 2 meningitis in the absence of genital lesions: improved recognition with use of the polymerase chain reaction. *Clin Infect Dis*. 1995;20:842-848.
184. Ravaut P, Darré M. Les reactions nerveuses au cours de herpes genitaux. *Ann Dermatol Syphiligr*. 1904;5:481.
185. Brenton DW. Hypoglycorrhachia in herpes simplex type 2 meningitis. *Arch Neurol*. 1980;37:317.
186. Bruyn GW, Straathof LJ, Raymakers GM. Mollaret's meningitis: differential diagnosis and diagnostic pitfalls. *Neurology*. 1962; 12:745-753.
187. Tedder DG, Ashley R, Tyler KL, et al. Herpes simplex virus infection as a cause of benign recurrent lymphocytic meningitis. *Ann Intern Med*. 1994;121:334-338.
188. Bergstrom T, Vahlne A, Alestig K, et al. Primary and recurrent herpes simplex virus type 2-induced meningitis. *J Infect Dis*. 1990;162:322-330.
189. Riehle RA Jr, Williams JJ. Transient neuropathic bladder following herpes simplex genitalis. *J Urol*. 1979;122:263-264.
190. Goldmeier D, Bateman JR, Rodin P. Urinary retention and intestinal obstruction associated with ano-rectal herpes simplex virus infection. *Br Med J*. 1975;2:425.
191. Shturman-Ellstein R, Borkowsky W, Fish I, et al. Myelitis associated with genital herpes in a child. *J Pediatr*. 1976;88:523.
192. Diamond C, Mohan K, Hobson A, et al. Viremia in neonatal herpes simplex virus infections. *Pediatr Infect Dis J*. 1999;18: 487-489.
193. Frederick DM, Bland D, Gollin Y. Fatal disseminated herpes simplex virus infection in a previously healthy pregnant woman: a case report. *J Reprod Med*. 2002;47:591-596.
194. Moedy JL, Lerman SJ, White RJ. Fatal disseminated herpes simplex virus infection in a healthy child. *Am J Dis Child*. 1981; 135:45-47.
195. Friedman HM, Pincus T, Gibilisco P, et al. Acute monoarticular arthritis caused by herpes simplex virus and cytomegalovirus. *Am J Med*. 1980;69:241-247.
196. Whitaker JA 3rd, Hardison JE. Severe thrombocytopenia after generalized herpes simplex virus-2 (HSV-2) infection. *South Med J*. 1978;71:864-865.
197. Flewett TH, Parker RG, Philip WM. Acute hepatitis due to herpes simplex virus in an adult. *J Clin Pathol*. 1969;22:60-66.
198. Schlesinger JJ, Gandara D, Bensch KG. Myoglobinuria associated with herpes-group viral infections. *Arch Intern Med*. 1978;138:422-424.
199. Goyette RE, Donowho EM Jr, Hieger LR, et al. Fulminant herpesvirus hominis hepatitis during pregnancy. *Obstet Gynecol*. 1974;43:191-195.
200. Kobbermann T, Clark L, Griffin WT. Maternal death secondary to disseminated herpesvirus hominis. *Am J Obstet Gynecol*. 1980;137:742-743.
201. Nahmias AJ. Disseminated herpes-simplex-virus infections. *N Engl J Med*. 1970;282:684-685.
202. Sutton AL, Smithwick EM, Seligman SJ, et al. Fatal disseminated herpesvirus hominis type 2 infection in an adult with associated thymic dysplasia. *Am J Med*. 1974;56:545-553.
203. Kaul R, Nagelkerke N, Kimani J, et al. Prevalent herpes simplex virus type 2 infection is associated with altered vaginal flora and an increased susceptibility to multiple sexually transmitted infections. *J Infect Dis*. 2007;196:1692-1697.
204. Sacks SL. Frequency and duration of patient-observed recurrent genital herpes simplex virus infection: characterization of the nonlesional prodrome. *J Infect Dis*. 1984;150:873-877.

205. Frenkel LM, Garratty EM, Shen JP, et al. Clinical reactivation of herpes simplex virus type 2 infection in seropositive pregnant women with no history of genital herpes. *Ann Intern Med.* 1993;118:414-418.
206. Corey L, Holmes KK. Genital herpes simplex virus infections: current concepts in diagnosis, therapy, and prevention. *Ann Intern Med.* 1983;98:973-983.
207. Diaz-Mitoma F, Ruben M, Sacks S, et al. Detection of viral DNA to evaluate outcome of antiviral treatment of patients with recurrent genital herpes. *J Clin Microbiol.* 1996;34:657-663.
208. Sacks SL, Varner TL, Davies KS, et al. Randomized, double-blind, placebo-controlled, patient-initiated study of topical high- and low-dose interferon-alpha with nonoxynol-9 in the treatment of recurrent genital herpes. *J Infect Dis.* 1990;161:692-698.
209. Morse SA, Trees DL, Htun Y, et al. Comparison of clinical diagnosis and standard laboratory and molecular methods for the diagnosis of genital ulcer disease in Lesotho: association with human immunodeficiency virus infection. *J Infect Dis.* 1997;175:583-589.
210. Fast MV, D'Costa LJ, Nsanze H, et al. The clinical diagnosis of genital ulcer disease in men in the tropics. *Sex Transm Dis.* 1984;11:72-76.
211. Wald A, Huang ML, Carrell D, et al. Polymerase chain reaction for detection of herpes simplex virus (HSV) DNA on mucosal surfaces: comparison with HSV isolation in cell culture. *J Infect Dis.* 2003;188:1345-1351.
212. Chapel TA, Jeffries CD, Brown WJ. Simultaneous infection with *Treponema pallidum* and herpes simplex virus. *Cutis.* 1979;24:191-192.
213. Langenberg A, Benedetti J, Jenkins J, et al. Development of clinically recognizable genital lesions among women previously identified as having "asymptomatic" herpes simplex virus type 2 infection. *Ann Intern Med.* 1989;110:882-887.
214. Rand KH, Hoon EF, Massey JK, et al. Daily stress and recurrence of genital herpes simplex. *Arch Intern Med.* 1990;150:1889-1893.
215. Cone RW, Hobson AC, Brown Z, et al. Frequent reactivation of genital herpes simplex viruses among pregnant women. *JAMA.* 1994;272:792-796.
216. Krone MR, Tabet SR, Paradise M, et al. Herpes simplex virus shedding among human immunodeficiency virus-negative men who have sex with men: site and frequency of shedding. *J Infect Dis.* 1998;178:978-982.
217. Wald A, Corey L, Cone R, et al. Frequent genital herpes simplex virus 2 shedding in immunocompetent women: effect of acyclovir treatment. *J Clin Invest.* 1997;99:1092-1097.
218. Wald A, Zeh J, Selke S, et al. Genital shedding of herpes simplex virus among men. *J Infect Dis.* 2002;186(Suppl 1):S34-S39.
219. Benedetti JK, Zeh J, Corey L. Clinical reactivation of genital herpes simplex virus infection decreases in frequency over time. *Ann Intern Med.* 1999;131:14-20.
220. Bryson Y, Dillon M, Bernstein DI, et al. Risk of acquisition of genital herpes simplex virus type 2 in sex partners of persons with genital herpes: a prospective couple study. *J Infect Dis.* 1993;167:942-946.
221. Mertz GJ, Coombs RW, Ashley R, et al. Transmission of genital herpes in couples with one symptomatic and one asymptomatic partner: a prospective study. *J Infect Dis.* 1988;157:1169-1177.
222. Rooney JF, Felser JM, Ostrove JM, et al. Acquisition of genital herpes from an asymptomatic sexual partner. *N Engl J Med.* 1986;314:1561-1564.
223. Brown ZA, Benedetti J, Ashley R, et al. Neonatal herpes simplex virus infection in relation to asymptomatic maternal infection at the time of labor. *N Engl J Med.* 1991;324:1247-1252.
224. Mertz GJ, Benedetti J, Ashley R, et al. Risk factors for the sexual transmission of genital herpes. *Ann Intern Med.* 1992;116:197-202.
225. Gill MJ, Arlette J, Buchan K. Herpes simplex virus infection of the hand: a profile of 79 cases. *Am J Med.* 1988;84:89-93.
226. Anderson BJ. The epidemiology and clinical analysis of several outbreaks of herpes gladiatorum. *Med Sci Sports Exerc.* 2003;35:1809-1814.
227. Liesegang TJ, Melton LJ 3rd, Daly PJ, et al. Epidemiology of ocular herpes simplex: incidence in Rochester, Minn, 1950 through 1982. *Arch Ophthalmol.* 1989;107:1155-1159.
228. Cook SD. Herpes simplex virus in the eye. *Br J Ophthalmol.* 1992;76:365-366.
229. Benz MS, Glaser JS, Davis JL. Progressive outer retinal necrosis in immunocompetent patients treated initially for optic neuropathy with systemic corticosteroids. *Am J Ophthalmol.* 2003;135:551-553.
230. Whitley RJ, Nahmias AJ, Visintine AM, et al. The natural history of herpes simplex virus infection of mother and newborn. *Pediatrics.* 1980;66:489-494.
231. Culbertson WW, Blumenkranz MS, Haines H, et al. The acute retinal necrosis syndrome. Part 2: histopathology and etiology. *Ophthalmology.* 1982;89:1317-1325.
232. Holland GN. Acquired immunodeficiency syndrome and ophthalmology: the first decade. *Am J Ophthalmol.* 1992;114:86-95.
233. Olson LC, Buescher EL, Artenstein MS, et al. Herpesvirus infections of the human central nervous system. *N Engl J Med.* 1967;277:1271-1277.
234. Whitley RJ, Lakeman F. Herpes simplex virus infections of the central nervous system: therapeutic and diagnostic considerations. *Clin Infect Dis.* 1995;20:414-420.
235. Whitley RJ, Soong SJ, Hirsch MS, et al. Herpes simplex encephalitis: vidarabine therapy and diagnostic problems. *N Engl J Med.* 1981;304:313-318.
236. Fraser NW, Lawrence WC, Wroblewska Z, et al. Herpes simplex type 1 DNA in human brain tissue. *Proc Natl Acad Sci U S A.* 1981;78:6461-6465.
237. Whitley R, Lakeman AD, Nahmias A, et al. DNA restriction-enzyme analysis of herpes simplex virus isolates obtained from patients with encephalitis. *N Engl J Med.* 1982;307:1060-1062.
238. Whitley RJ, Cobbs CG, Alford CA Jr, et al. Diseases that mimic herpes simplex encephalitis: diagnosis, presentation, and outcome. NIAD Collaborative Antiviral Study Group. *JAMA.* 1989;262:234-239.
239. Aurelius E, Johansson B, Skoldenberg B, et al. Encephalitis in immunocompetent patients due to herpes simplex virus type 1 or 2 as determined by type-specific polymerase chain reaction and antibody assays of cerebrospinal fluid. *J Med Virol.* 1993;39:179-186.
240. Lakeman FD, Whitley RJ. Diagnosis of herpes simplex encephalitis: application of polymerase chain reaction to cerebrospinal fluid from brain-biopsied patients and correlation with disease. National Institute of Allergy and Infectious Diseases Collaborative Antiviral Study Group. *J Infect Dis.* 1995;171:857-863.
241. Rowley AH, Whitley RJ, Lakeman FD, et al. Rapid detection of herpes-simplex-virus DNA in cerebrospinal fluid of patients with herpes simplex encephalitis. *Lancet.* 1990;335:440-441.
242. Whitley RJ, Alford CA, Hirsch MS, et al. Vidarabine versus acyclovir therapy in herpes simplex encephalitis. *N Engl J Med.* 1986;314:144-149.
243. McBane RD, Gross JB Jr. Herpes esophagitis: clinical syndrome, endoscopic appearance, and diagnosis in 23 patients. *Gastrointest Endosc.* 1991;37:600-603.
244. McDonald GB, Sharma P, Hackman RC, et al. Esophageal infections in immunosuppressed patients after marrow transplantation. *Gastroenterology.* 1985;88:1111-1117.
245. Ramsey PG, Fife KH, Hackman RC, et al. Herpes simplex virus pneumonia: clinical, virologic, and pathologic features in 20 patients. *Ann Intern Med.* 1982;97:813-820.
246. Cook CH, Yenchar JK, Kraner TO, et al. Occult herpes family viruses may increase mortality in critically ill surgical patients. *Am J Surg.* 1998;176:357-360.
247. Graham BS, Snell JD Jr. Herpes simplex virus infection of the adult lower respiratory tract. *Medicine (Baltimore).* 1983;62:384-393.
248. Camps K, Jorens PG, Demey HE, et al. Clinical significance of herpes simplex virus in the lower respiratory tract of critically ill patients. *Eur J Clin Microbiol Infect Dis.* 2002;21:758-759.
249. Prellner T, Flamholc L, Haidl S, et al. Herpes simplex virus—the most frequently isolated pathogen in the lungs of patients with severe respiratory distress. *Scand J Infect Dis.* 1992;24:283-292.
250. Siegel D, Golden E, Washington AE, et al. Prevalence and correlates of herpes simplex infections: the population-based AIDS in Multiethnic Neighborhoods Study. *JAMA.* 1992;268:1702-1708.
251. Freeman E, Weiss H, Glynn J, et al. Herpes simplex virus 2 infection increases HIV acquisition in men and women: systematic review and meta-analysis of longitudinal studies. *AIDS.* 2006;20:73-83.
252. Augenbraun M, Feldman J, Chirgwin K, et al. Increased genital shedding of herpes simplex virus type 2 in HIV-seropositive women. *Ann Intern Med.* 1995;123:845-847.
253. Schacker T, Zeh J, Hu H, et al. Changes in plasma human immunodeficiency virus type 1 RNA associated with herpes simplex virus reactivation and suppression. *J Infect Dis.* 2002;186:1718-1725.
254. McClelland RS, Wang CC, Overbaugh J, et al. Association between cervical shedding of herpes simplex virus and HIV-1. *AIDS.* 2002;16:2425-2430.
255. Holmberg S, Stewart J, Gerber A, et al. Prior herpes simplex virus type 2 infection as a risk factor for HIV infection. *JAMA.* 1988;259:1048-1050.
256. Hook EW 3rd, Cannon RO, Nahmias AJ, et al. Herpes simplex virus infection as a risk factor for human immunodeficiency virus infection in heterosexuals. *J Infect Dis.* 1992;165:251-255.
257. Serwadda D, Gray R, Sewankambo N, et al. Human immunodeficiency virus acquisition associated with genital ulcer disease and herpes simplex virus type 2 infection: a nested case-control study in Rakai, Uganda. *J Infect Dis.* 2003;188:1492-1497.
258. Stamm W, Handsfield H, Rompalo A, et al. The association between genital ulcer disease and acquisition of HIV infection in homosexual men. *JAMA.* 1988;260:1429-1433.
259. Brown J, Wald A, Hubbard A, et al. Incident and prevalent herpes simplex virus type 2 infection increases risk of HIV acquisition among women in Uganda and Zimbabwe. *AIDS.* 2007;21:1515-1523.
260. Wald A, Link K. Risk of human immunodeficiency virus infection in herpes simplex virus type 2-seropositive persons: a meta-analysis. *J Infect Dis.* 2002;185:45-52.
261. Abu-Raddad L, Magaret A, Celum C, et al. Genital herpes has played a more important role than any other sexually transmitted infection in driving HIV prevalence in Africa. *PLoS ONE.* 2008;3:e2230.
262. Celum C, Wald A, Hughes J, et al. Effect of aciclovir on HIV-1 acquisition in herpes simplex virus 2 seropositive women and men who have sex with men: a randomised, double-blind, placebo-controlled trial. *Lancet.* 2008;371:2109-2119.
263. Watson-Jones D, Weiss HA, Rusizoka M, et al. Effect of herpes simplex suppression on incidence of HIV among women in Tanzania. *N Engl J Med.* 2008;358:1560-1571.
264. Zhu J, Hladik F, Woodward A, et al. Persistence of HIV-1 receptor-positive cells after HSV-2 reactivation: a potential mechanism for increased HIV-1 acquistion. *Nat Med.* 2009 (in press).
265. Chen KT, Segu M, Lumey LH, et al. Genital herpes simplex virus infection and perinatal transmission of human immunodeficiency virus. *Obstet Gynecol.* 2005;106:1341-1348.
266. Drake A, John-Stewart G, Wald A, et al. Herpes simplex virus type 2 and risk of intrapartum human immunodeficiency virus transmission. *Obstet Gynecol.* 2007;109:403-409.
267. Quinn T, Wawer M, Sewankambo N, et al. Viral load and heterosexual transmission of human immunodeficiency virus type 1. Rakai Project Study Group. *N Engl J Med.* 2000;342:921-929.
268. Mole L, Ripich S, Margolis D, et al. The impact of active herpes simplex virus infection on human immunodeficiency virus load. *J Infect Dis.* 1997;176:766-770.
269. Nagot N, Ouedraogo A, Konate I, et al. Roles of clinical and subclinical reactivated herpes simplex virus type 2 infection and human immunodeficiency virus type 1 (HIV-1)-induced immunosuppression on genital and plasma HIV-1 levels. *J Infect Dis.* 2008;198:241-249.
270. Nagot N, Ouédraogo A, Foulongne V, et al. Reduction of HIV-1 RNA levels with therapy to suppress herpes simplex virus. *N Engl J Med.* 2007;356:790-799.
271. Zuckerman R, Lucchetti A, Whittington W, et al. Herpes simplex virus (HSV) suppression with valacyclovir reduces rectal and blood plasma HIV-1 levels in HIV-1/HSV-2-seropositive men: a randomized, double-blind, placebo-controlled crossover trial. *J Infect Dis.* 2007;196:1500-1508.
272. McMahon MA, Siliciano JD, Lai J, et al. The anti-herpetic drug acyclovir inhibits HIV replication and selects the V75i reverse transcriptase multi-drug resistance mutation. *J Biol Chem.* 2008;283:31289-31293.
273. Lingappa JR, Celum C. Clinical and therapeutic issues for herpes simplex virus-2 and HIV co-infection. *Drugs.* 2007;67:155-174.
274. Albrecht MA, DeLuca NA, Byrn RA, et al. The herpes simplex virus immediate-early protein, ICP4, is required to potentiate replication of human immunodeficiency virus in CD4+ lymphocytes. *J Virol.* 1989;63:1861-1868.
275. Kucera LS, Leake E, Iyer N, et al. Human immunodeficiency virus type 1 (HIV-1) and herpes simplex virus type 2 (HSV-2) can coinfect and simultaneously replicate in the same human CD4+ cell: effect of coinfection on infectious HSV-2 and HIV-1 replication. *AIDS Res Hum Retroviruses.* 1990;6:641-647.
276. Margolis D, Rabson A, Straus S, et al. Transactivation of the HIV-1 LTR by HSV-1 immediate-early genes. *Virology.* 1992;186:788-791.
277. Mbopi Keou F, Grésenguet G, Mayaud P, et al. Genital herpes simplex virus type 2 shedding is increased in HIV-infected women in Africa. *AIDS.* 1999;13:536-537.
278. Schacker T, Ryncarz A, Goddard J, et al. Frequent recovery of HIV-1 from genital herpes simplex virus lesions in HIV-1-infected men. *JAMA.* 1998;280:61-66.
279. Straus SE, Seidlin M, Takiff H, et al. Oral acyclovir to suppress recurring herpes simplex virus infections in immunodeficient patients. *Ann Intern Med.* 1984;100:522-524.
280. Wade JC, Newton B, McLaren C, et al. Intravenous acyclovir to treat mucocutaneous herpes simplex virus infection after marrow transplantation: a double-blind trial. *Ann Intern Med.* 1982;96:265-269.
281. Meyers JD, Flournoy N, Thomas ED. Infection with herpes simplex virus and cell-mediated immunity after marrow transplant. *J Infect Dis.* 1980;142:338-346.
282. Ringden O, Heimdahl A, Lonnqvist B, et al. Decreased incidence of viridans streptococcal septicaemia in allogeneic bone marrow transplant recipients after the introduction of acyclovir. *Lancet.* 1984;1:744.
283. Nichols WG, Boeckh M, Carter RA, et al. Transferred herpes simplex virus immunity after stem-cell transplantation: clinical implications. *J Infect Dis.* 2003;187:801-808.
284. Arvin AM, Hensleigh PA, Prober CG, et al. Failure of antepartum maternal cultures to predict the infant's risk of exposure to herpes simplex virus at delivery. *N Engl J Med.* 1986;315:796-800.
285. Florman AL, Gershon AA, Blackett PR, et al. Intrauterine infection with herpes simplex virus: resultant congenital malformations. *JAMA.* 1973;225:129-132.
286. Kimura H, Futamura M, Kito H, et al. Detection of viral DNA in neonatal herpes simplex virus infections: frequent and prolonged presence in serum and cerebrospinal fluid. *J Infect Dis.* 1991;164:289-293.
287. Whitley R, Arvin A, Prober C, et al. Predictors of morbidity and mortality in neonates with herpes simplex virus infections. The National Institute of Allergy and Infectious Diseases Collaborative Antiviral Study Group. *N Engl J Med.* 1991;324:450-454.
288. Corey L, Whitley RJ, Stone EF, et al. Difference in neurologic outcome after antiviral therapy of neonatal central nervous system herpes simplex virus type 1 versus herpes simplex virus type 2 infection. *Lancet.* 1988;2:1-4.
289. Arvin AM, Yeager AS, Bruhn FW, et al. Neonatal herpes simplex infection in the absence of mucocutaneous lesions. *J Pediatr.* 1982;100:715-721.
290. Kimberlin DW, Lin CY, Jacobs RF, et al. Safety and efficacy of high-dose intravenous acyclovir in the management of

neonatal herpes simplex virus infections. *Pediatrics.* 2001;108:230-238.

291. Forsgren M, Skoog E, Jeansson S, et al. Prevalence of antibodies to herpes simplex virus in pregnant women in Stockholm in 1969, 1983 and 1989: implications for STD epidemiology. *Int J STD AIDS.* 1994;5:113-116.
292. Xu F, Markowitz LE, Gottlieb SL, et al. Seroprevalence of herpes simplex virus types 1 and 2 in pregnant women in the United States. *Am J Obstet Gynecol.* 2007;196(Suppl):e1-e6.
293. Brown ZA, Vontver LA, Benedetti J, et al. Genital herpes in pregnancy: risk factors associated with recurrences and asymptomatic viral shedding. *Am J Obstet Gynecol.* 1985;153:24-30.
294. Vontver LA, Hickok DE, Brown Z, et al. Recurrent genital herpes simplex virus infection in pregnancy: infant outcome and frequency of asymptomatic recurrences. *Am J Obstet Gynecol.* 1982;143:75-84.
295. Brown ZA, Benedetti J, Selke S, et al. Asymptomatic maternal shedding of herpes simplex virus at the onset of labor: relationship to preterm labor. *Obstet Gynecol.* 1996;87:483-488.
296. Chalhub EG, Baenziger J, Feigen RD, et al. Congenital herpes simplex type II infection with extensive hepatic calcification, bone lesions and cataracts: complete postmortem examination. *Dev Med Child Neurol.* 1977;19:527-534.
297. Hain J, Doshi N, Harger JH. Ascending transcervical herpes simplex infection with intact fetal membranes. *Obstet Gynecol.* 1980;56:106-109.
298. Abrams C. Isolation of herpes simplex from a mother and aborted fetus. *Ghana Med J.* 1966;5:41.
299. Kulhanjian JA, Soroush V, Au DS, et al. Identification of women at unsuspected risk of primary infection with herpes simplex virus type 2 during pregnancy. *N Engl J Med.* 1992;326:916-920.
300. Prober CG, Corey L, Brown ZA, et al. The management of pregnancies complicated by genital infections with herpes simplex virus. *Clin Infect Dis.* 1992;15:1031-1038.
301. Kropp RY, Wong T, Cormier L, et al. Neonatal herpes simplex virus infections in Canada: results of a 3-year national prospective study. *Pediatrics.* 2006;117:1955-1962.
302. Gibbs RS, Mead PB. Preventing neonatal herpes—current strategies. *N Engl J Med.* 1992;326:946-947.
303. Rouse DJ, Stringer JS. Cesarean delivery and risk of herpes simplex virus infection. *JAMA.* 2003;289:2208; author reply, 2209.
304. Brown EL, Gardella C, Malm G, et al. Effect of maternal herpes simplex virus (HSV) serostatus and HSV type on risk of neonatal herpes. *Acta Obstet Gynecol Scand.* 2007;86:523-529.
305. Gardella C, Brown Z, Wald A, et al. Poor correlation between genital lesions and detection of herpes simplex virus in women in labor. *Obstet Gynecol.* 2005;106:268-274.
306. Frenkel LM, Brown ZA, Bryson YJ, et al. Pharmacokinetics of acyclovir in the term human pregnancy and neonate. *Am J Obstet Gynecol.* 1991;164:569-576.
307. Watts DH, Brown Z, Money D, et al. A double-blind, randomized, placebo-controlled trial of acyclovir in late pregnancy for reduction of herpes simplex virus shedding and cesarean section. *Am J Obstet Gynecol.* 2003;188:836-843.
308. Sheffield J, Hill J, Hollier L, et al. Valacyclovir prophylaxis to prevent recurrent herpes at delivery: a randomized clinical trial. *Obstet Gynecol.* 2006;108:141-147.
309. Hollier L, Wendel G. Third trimester antiviral prophylaxis for preventing maternal genital herpes simplex virus (HSV) recurrences and neonatal infection. *Cochrane Database Syst Rev.* 2008:CD004946.
310. Scott L, Alexander J. Cost-effectiveness of acyclovir suppression to prevent recurrent genital herpes in term pregnancy. *Am J Perinatol.* 1998;15:57-62.
311. Gardella C, Brown Z, Wald A, et al. Risk factors for herpes simplex virus transmission to pregnant women: a couples study. *Am J Obstet Gynecol.* 2005;193:1891-1899.
312. Barnabas R, Carabin H, Garnett G. The potential role of suppressive therapy for sex partners in the prevention of neonatal herpes: a health economic analysis. *Sex Transm Infect.* 2002;78:425-429.
313. Mark KE, Kim HN, Wald A, et al. Targeted prenatal herpes simplex virus testing: can we identify women at risk of transmission to the neonate? *Am J Obstet Gynecol.* 2006;194:408-414.
314. Kaushic C, Ashkar AA, Reid LA, et al. Progesterone increases susceptibility and decreases immune responses to genital herpes infection. *J Virol.* 2003;77:4558-4565.
315. Corey L, Huang ML, Selke S, et al. Differentiation of herpes simplex virus types 1 and 2 in clinical samples by a real-time taqman PCR assay. *J Med Virol.* 2005;76:350-355.
316. Cowan FM, French RS, Mayaud P, et al. Seroepidemiological study of herpes simplex virus types 1 and 2 in Brazil, Estonia, India, Morocco, and Sri Lanka. *Sex Transm Infect.* 2003;79:286-290.
317. Lee FK, Coleman RM, Pereira L, et al. Detection of herpes simplex virus type 2-specific antibody with glycoprotein G. *J Clin Microbiol.* 1985;22:641-644.
318. Ashley RL, Wu L, Pickering JW, et al. Premarket evaluation of a commercial glycoprotein G-based enzyme immunoassay for herpes simplex virus type-specific antibodies. *J Clin Microbiol.* 1998;36:294-295.
319. Ashley RL, Militoni J, Lee F, et al. Comparison of Western blot (immunoblot) and glycoprotein G-specific immunodot enzyme assay for detecting antibodies to herpes simplex virus types 1 and 2 in human sera. *J Clin Microbiol.* 1988;26:662-667.
320. Morrow R, Friedrich D, Meier A, et al. Use of "biokit HSV-2 Rapid Assay" to improve the positive predictive value of Focus HerpeSelect HSV-2 ELISA. *BMC Infect Dis.* 2005;5:84.
321. Ngo T, Laeyendecker O, La H, et al. Use of commercial enzyme immunoassays to detect antibodies to the herpes simplex virus type 2 glycoprotein G in a low-risk population in Hanoi, Vietnam. *Clin Vaccine Immunol.* 2008;15:382-384.
322. Martins TB, Woolstenhulme RD, Jaskowski TD, et al. Comparison of four enzyme immunoassays with a Western blot assay for the determination of type-specific antibodies to herpes simplex virus. *Am J Clin Pathol.* 2001;115:272-277.
323. Turner KR, Wong EH, Kent CK, et al. Serologic herpes testing in the real world: validation of new type-specific serologic herpes simplex virus tests in a public health laboratory. *Sex Transm Dis.* 2002;29:422-425.
324. Ashley R, Cent A, Maggs V, et al. Inability of enzyme immunoassays to discriminate between infections with herpes simplex virus types 1 and 2. *Ann Intern Med.* 1991;115:520-526.
325. Morrow RA, Friedrich D. Inaccuracy of certain commercial enzyme immunoassays in diagnosing genital infections with herpes simplex virus types 1 or 2. *Am J Clin Pathol.* 2003;120:839-844.
326. Page J, Taylor J, Tideman RL, et al. Is HSV serology useful for the management of first episode genital herpes? *Sex Transm Infect.* 2003;79:276-279.
327. Dorsky DI, Crumpacker CS. Drugs five years later: acyclovir. *Ann Intern Med.* 1987;107:859-874.
328. Schaeffer HJ, Beauchamp L, de Miranda P, et al. 9-(2-hydroxyethoxymethyl) guanine activity against viruses of the herpes group. *Nature.* 1978;272:583-585.
329. Crumpacker CS, Schnipper LE, Zaia JA, et al. Growth inhibition by acycloguanosine of herpesviruses isolated from human infections. *Antimicrob Agents Chemother.* 1979;15:642-645.
330. Douglas JM, Critchlow C, Benedetti J, et al. A double-blind study of oral acyclovir for suppression of recurrences of genital herpes simplex virus infection. *N Engl J Med.* 1984;310:1551-1556.
331. Mindel A, Faherty A, Carney O, et al. Dosage and safety of long-term suppressive acyclovir therapy for recurrent genital herpes. *Lancet.* 1988;1:926-928.
332. Raborn GW, McGaw WT, Grace M, et al. Treatment of herpes labialis with acyclovir: review of three clinical trials. *Am J Med.* 1988;85:39-42.
333. Reichman RC, Badger GJ, Mertz GJ, et al. Treatment of recurrent genital herpes simplex infections with oral acyclovir: a controlled trial. *JAMA.* 1984;251:2103-2107.
334. Rooney JF, Straus SE, Mannix ML, et al. Oral acyclovir to suppress frequently recurrent herpes labialis: a double-blind, placebo-controlled trial. *Ann Intern Med.* 1993;118:268-272.
335. Wald A, Carrell D, Remington M, et al. Two-day regimen of acyclovir for treatment of recurrent genital herpes simplex virus type 2 infection. *Clin Infect Dis.* 2002;34:944-948.
336. Bartlett BL, Tyring SK, Fife K, et al. Famciclovir treatment options for patients with frequent outbreaks of recurrent genital herpes: the RELIEF trial. *J Clin Virol.* 2008;43:190-195.
337. Bodsworth N, Bloch M, McNulty A, et al. 2-day versus 5-day famciclovir as treatment of recurrences of genital herpes: results of the FaST study. *Sex Health.* 2008;5:219-225.
338. Sacks SL, Aoki FY. Famciclovir for the management of genital herpes simplex in patients with inadequate response to aciclovir or valaciclovir. *Clin Drug Investig.* 2005;25:803-809.
339. Sacks SL, Aoki FY, Diaz-Mitoma F, et al. Patient-initiated, twice-daily oral famciclovir for early recurrent genital herpes: a randomized, double-blind multicenter trial. Canadian Famciclovir Study Group. *JAMA.* 1996;276:44-49.
340. Laiskonis A, Thune T, Neldam S, et al. Valacyclovir in the treatment of facial herpes simplex virus infection. *J Infect Dis.* 2002;186(Suppl 1):S66-S70.
341. Reitano M, Tyring S, Lang W, et al. Valaciclovir for the suppression of recurrent genital herpes simplex virus infection: a large-scale dose range-finding study. International Valaciclovir HSV Study Group. *J Infect Dis.* 1998;178:603-610.
342. Soul-Lawton J, Seaber E, On N, et al. Absolute bioavailability and metabolic disposition of valaciclovir, the L-valyl ester of acyclovir, following oral administration to humans. *Antimicrob Agents Chemother.* 1995;39:2759-2764.
343. Strand A, Patel R, Wulf HC, et al. Aborted genital herpes simplex virus lesions: findings from a randomised controlled trial with valaciclovir. *Sex Transm Infect.* 2002;78:435-439.
344. Romanowski B, Marina RB, Roberts JN. Patients' preference of valacyclovir once-daily suppressive therapy versus twice-daily episodic therapy for recurrent genital herpes: a randomized study. *Sex Transm Dis.* 2003;30:226-231.
345. Burns LJ, Miller W, Kandaswamy C, et al. Randomized clinical trial of ganciclovir vs acyclovir for prevention of cytomegalovirus antigenemia after allogeneic transplantation. *Bone Marrow Transplant.* 2002;30:945-951.
346. Bavaro J, Drolette L, Koelle D, et al. One-day regimen of valacyclovir for treatment of recurrent genital herpes simplex virus 2 infection. *Sex Transm Dis.* 2008;35:383-386.
347. Spruance SL, Jones TM, Blatter MM, et al. High-dose, short-duration, early valacyclovir therapy for episodic treatment of cold sores: results of two randomized, placebo-controlled, multicenter studies. *Antimicrob Agents Chemother.* 2003;47:1072-1080.
348. Spruance S, Aoki FY, Tyring S, et al. Short-course therapy for recurrent genital herpes and herpes labialis. *J Fam Pract.* 2007;56:30-36.
349. Abudalu M, Tyring S, Koltun W, et al. Single-day, patient-initiated famciclovir therapy versus 3-day valacyclovir regimen for recurrent genital herpes: a randomized, double-blind, comparative trial. *Clin Infect Dis.* 2008;47:651-658.
350. Sacks SL, Wanklin RJ, Reece DE, et al. Progressive esophagitis from acyclovir-resistant herpes simplex: clinical roles for DNA polymerase mutants and viral heterogeneity? *Ann Intern Med.* 1989;111:893-899.
351. Erlich KS, Mills J, Chatis P, et al. Acyclovir-resistant herpes simplex virus infections in patients with the acquired immunodeficiency syndrome. *N Engl J Med.* 1989;320:293-296.
352. Englund JA, Zimmerman ME, Swierkosz EM, et al. Herpes simplex virus resistant to acyclovir: a study in a tertiary care center. *Ann Intern Med.* 1990;112:416-422.
353. Gupta R, Hill E, McClernon D, et al. Acyclovir sensitivity of sequential herpes simplex virus type 2 isolates from the genital mucosa of immunocompetent women. *J Infect Dis.* 2005;192:1102-1107.
354. Chibo D, Mijch A, Doherty R, et al. Novel mutations in the thymidine kinase and DNA polymerase genes of acyclovir and foscarnet resistant herpes simplex viruses infecting an immunocompromised patient. *J Clin Virol.* 2002;25:165-170.
355. McLaren C, Corey L, Dekket C, et al. In vitro sensitivity to acyclovir in genital herpes simplex viruses from acyclovir-treated patients. *J Infect Dis.* 1983;148:868-875.
356. Lehrman SN, Douglas JM, Corey L, et al. Recurrent genital herpes and suppressive oral acyclovir therapy: relation between clinical outcome and in-vitro drug sensitivity. *Ann Intern Med.* 1986;104:786-790.
357. Safrin S, Elbeik T, Phan L, et al. Correlation between response to acyclovir and foscarnet therapy and in vitro susceptibility result for isolates of herpes simplex virus from human immunodeficiency virus-infected patients. *Antimicrob Agents Chemother.* 1994;38:1246-1250.
358. Safrin S, Crumpacker C, Chatis P, et al. A controlled trial comparing foscarnet with vidarabine for acyclovir-resistant mucocutaneous herpes simplex in the acquired immunodeficiency syndrome. The AIDS Clinical Trials Group. *N Engl J Med.* 1991;325:551-555.
359. Lalezari J, Schacker T, Feinberg J, et al. A randomized, double-blind, placebo-controlled trial of cidofovir gel for the treatment of acyclovir-unresponsive mucocutaneous herpes simplex virus infection in patients with AIDS. *J Infect Dis.* 1997;176:892-898.
360. Mendel DB, Barkhimer DB, Chen MS. Biochemical basis for increased susceptibility to cidofovir of herpes simplex viruses with altered or deficient thymidine kinase activity. *Antimicrob Agents Chemother.* 1995;39:2120-2122.
361. Snoeck R, Andrei G, Gerard M, et al. Successful treatment of progressive mucocutaneous infection due to acyclovir- and foscarnet-resistant herpes simplex virus with (S)-1-(3-hydroxy-2-phosphonylmethoxypropyl)cytosine (HPMPC). *Clin Infect Dis.* 1994;18:570-578.
362. Richards J, Krantz E, Selke S, et al. Healthcare seeking and sexual behavior among patients with symptomatic newly acquired genital herpes. *Sex Transm Dis.* 2008;35:1015-1021.
363. Catotti DN, Clarke P, Catoe KE. Herpes revisited: still a cause of concern. *Sex Transm Dis.* 1993;20:77-80.
364. Wald A, Langenberg A, Krantz E, et al. The relationship between condom use and herpes simplex virus acquisition. *Ann Intern Med.* 2005;143:707-713.

137

Varicella-Zoster Virus

RICHARD J. WHITLEY

Varicella-zoster virus (VZV) causes two distinct clinical diseases. Varicella, more commonly called chickenpox, is the primary infection and results from exposure of a person susceptible to the virus. Chickenpox is ubiquitous and extremely contagious, but for the most part, it is a benign illness characterized by a generalized exanthematous rash. It occurs seasonally and in epidemics. Recurrence of infection results in the more localized phenomenon known as *herpes zoster*, often referred to as *shingles*, a common infection among the elderly. Two live, attenuated vaccines for the prevention of chickenpox and herpes zoster are available in the United States. Vaccination is recommended for use in healthy children and in susceptible adults to prevent chickenpox (see Chapter 320). Similarly, the herpes zoster vaccine is recommended for adults over 60 years of age to decrease the burden of illness and the overall incidence of shingles. The incidence of chickenpox was that of the annual birth rate but has been tremendously reduced with widespread vaccination. Surveillance for varicella in three counties in California, Texas, and Pennsylvania from 1995 to 2000 showed reductions in cases of varicella from 71% to 84% by years 1999 and 2000[1] with only 500 cases occuring in 2004.[2] It is estimated that there are approximately 1,000,000 cases of herpes zoster yearly in the United States, which result in over 2 million physician visits per year. Likely, this approximation is a gross underestimation of disease occurrence. Many of these individuals require long-term follow-up medical care for postherpetic neuralgia (PHN).

Historical Overview

Shingles has been recognized since ancient times as a unique clinical entity because of the dermatomal vesicular rash; however, chickenpox was often confused with smallpox.[3] In 1875, Steiner successfully transmitted VZV by inoculation of the vesicular fluid from a person suffering from chickenpox to "volunteers."[4] The infectious nature of VZV was further defined by von Bokay,[5,6] who observed chickenpox in persons who had close contact with others suffering from herpes zoster. He correctly described the mean incubation period for the development of chickenpox in susceptible patients as well as the average range in days. Kundratitz in 1925[7] showed that the inoculation of vesicular fluid from patients with herpes zoster into susceptible persons resulted in chickenpox. Similar observations were reported by Brunsgaard[8] and others,[9] and in 1943 Garland[10] suggested that herpes zoster was the consequence of the reactivation of latent VZV.

Since early in the 20th century, similarities in the histopathologic features of skin lesions and in epidemiologic and immunologic studies indicated that varicella and herpes zoster were caused by the same agent.[11,12] Tyzzer[13] described the histopathologic features of skin lesions resulting from VZV infections and noted the appearance of intranuclear inclusions and multinucleated giant cells. These descriptions came from histologic studies performed on serial skin biopsy specimens that were obtained during the first week of illness. The histopathologic descriptions were amplified by Lipschutz in 1921[14] for herpes zoster.

Isolation of VZV in 1958 permitted a definition of the biology of this virus.[12] Viral isolates from patients with either chickenpox or herpes zoster demonstrated similar changes in tissue culture, specifically the appearance of eosinophilic intranuclear inclusions and multinucleated giant cells. These findings are virtually identical to those present on clinically available biopsy material. Taken together, these data provided a universal acceptance that both diseases were caused

by VZV. By 1958, Weller and colleagues[12,15-17] established that there were neither biologic nor immunologic differences between the viral agents isolated from patients with these two clinical entities. Later studies provided their identity by rigorous biochemical methods.[18] Viral DNA from a patient with chickenpox who subsequently developed herpes zoster was examined by restriction endonuclease analysis, and the molecular identity of these two viruses was verified.[19,20]

The Pathogen and Its Replication

VZV is a member of the Herpesviridae family and shares structural characteristics with other members of the family. The virus has icosapentahedral symmetry and contains centrally located double-stranded DNA with a surrounding envelope. The size of the virus is approximately 150 to 200 nm, and it has a lipid-containing envelope with glycoprotein spikes.[19] The naked capsid has a diameter of approximately 90 to 95 nm.[21-23] The DNA contains 125,000 base pairs, or approximately 80 megadaltons, and encodes about 75 proteins. The organization of the viral genome is similar to that of other herpesviruses. There are unique long (105-kb) and unique short (5.2-kb) regions of the viral genome. Each unique sequence contains terminal repeat sequences. With replication, the unique short (U_s) region can invert upon itself and result in two isomeric forms.[24-26]

Five families of VZV glycoproteins (gp) have been identified: gpI, gpII, gpIII, gpIV, and gpV. The herpes simplex virus (HSV) homologues are gE, gB, gH, U_s7, and gC, respectively. Viral infectivity can be neutralized by monoclonal antibodies directed against gpI, gpII, and gpIII. These glycoproteins have been the subject of intense investigative interest because they represent the primary markers for both humoral and cell-mediated immune responses.

Only enveloped virions are infectious; this may account for the lability of VZV. Furthermore, the envelope is sensitive to detergent, ether, and air drying. VZV is highly cell associated and spreads from cell to cell by direct contact. Virus can be isolated in a variety of continuous and discontinuous cell culture systems of human and simian origin. Approximately 8 to 10 hours after infection, virus-specific immunofluorescence can be detected in the cells immediately adjacent to the initial focus of infection. This parallels the microscopic observation of the radial spread of the cytopathologic process.[27,28] Electron microscopic studies demonstrate the appearance of immature viral particles within 12 hours of the onset of infection. As with HSV, the naked capsids acquire their envelope at the nuclear membrane, being released into the perinuclear space where large vacuoles are formed.[21,29] Infectious virus is then spread to adjacent cells after fusion of plasma membranes.

Epidemiology of Varicella-Zoster Virus Infections

CHICKENPOX

Humans are the only known reservoir for VZV. Chickenpox follows exposure of the susceptible or seronegative person to VZV and represents the primary form of infection. Although it is assumed that the virus is spread by the respiratory route and replicates in the nasopharynx or upper respiratory tract, retrieval of virus from persons incubating VZV has been uncommon. However, the application of polymerase chain reaction (PCR) techniques to nasopharyngeal secretions of exposed and susceptible persons has detected VZV DNA and supports this hypothesis. Chickenpox was a common infection of childhood and affects both genders equally and people of all races. To a certain extent, the virus is endemic in the population at large; however, it becomes epidemic among susceptible persons during seasonal periods of late winter and early spring.[30] Intimate contact appears to be the key determinant for transmission.

Overall, chickenpox is a disease of childhood, because 90% of cases occur in children younger than 13 years. Typically, the virus is introduced into the susceptible school-aged or preschool child. In a study by Wells and Holla,[31] 61 of 67 susceptible children in kindergarten through the fourth grade contracted chickenpox. Approximately 10% of persons older than 15 years are considered susceptible to VZV infection. The incubation period of chickenpox (i.e., the time interval between exposure of a susceptible person to the time the vesicular rash develops in an index case) is generally regarded to be 14 to 15 days, but disease can appear within a range of 10 to 20 days.[32,33] Secondary attack rates among susceptible siblings within a household are between 70% and 90%.[34] Patients are infectious for a period of approximately 48 hours before the period of vesicle formation and generally for 4 to 5 days thereafter until all vesicles are crusted.

Although chickenpox exists worldwide among children, it occurs more frequently in adults who reside in tropical regions than in those who reside in other geographic areas. Stokes noted a higher incidence of chickenpox among soldiers serving abroad during World War II, in whom the incidence was 1.41 to 2.27 per 1000 persons annually. These rates contrast with those in the United States, which were approximately half those reported among the soldiers.[35]

HERPES ZOSTER

The epidemiology of herpes zoster is somewhat different. VZV characteristically becomes latent after primary infection within the dorsal root ganglia. Reactivation leads to herpes zoster, a sporadic disease. Histopathologic examination of the nerve root after infection with VZV demonstrates characteristics indicative of VZV infection. In persons who die after recent herpes zoster infection, an examination of the dorsal root ganglia reveals satellitosis, lymphocytic infiltration in the nerve root, and degeneration of the ganglia cells.[36,37] Intranuclear inclusions can be found within the ganglia cells. Although it is possible to demonstrate the presence of VZV by electron microscopy, it has not been possible to isolate this virus in cultures, usually from explants of dorsal root ganglia, as has been done after HSV infection. The biologic mechanism by which VZV establishes latency remains unknown.

Herpes zoster is a disease that occurs at all ages, but it afflicts about 20% or more of the population overall, mainly the elderly.[38,39] Herpes zoster, known also as shingles, occurs in persons who are seropositive for VZV or, more specifically, in those who have had chickenpox. Reactivation appears to be dependent on a balance between virus and host factors. Most patients who develop herpes zoster have no history of exposure to other persons with VZV infection at the time of the appearance of lesions. The highest incidence of disease varies between 5 and 10 cases per 1000 for persons older than 60 years.[15] Approximately 4% of patients experience a second episode of herpes zoster; however, recurrences of dermatomal lesions are usually caused by HSV. In a 7-year study performed by McGregor,[40] the annualized rate of herpes zoster was 4.8 cases per 1000 patients and three fourths of those patients were older than 45 years. Persons who are immunocompromised have a higher incidence of both chickenpox and shingles.[41-44] Herpes zoster occurs within the first 2 years of life in children born to women who have had chickenpox during pregnancy. These cases probably reflect in utero chickenpox with reactivation early in life.

Pathogenesis

Chickenpox occurs in susceptible persons who are exposed to virus after close personal contact. Histopathologic findings in human VZV infections, whether chickenpox or herpes zoster, are virtually identical.

The vesicles involve the corium, or dermis. As viral replication progresses, the epithelial cells undergo degenerative changes characterized by ballooning, with the subsequent appearance of multinucleated giant cells and prominent eosinophilic intranuclear inclusions. Under unusual circumstances, necrosis and hemorrhage may appear in the upper portion of the dermis. As the vesicle evolves, the fluid becomes cloudy as a consequence of the appearance of polymorphonuclear leukocytes, degenerated cells, and fibrin. Ultimately, either the vesicles rupture and release infectious fluid, or the fluid gradually becomes reabsorbed.

Transmission is likely by the respiratory route, followed by localized replication at an undefined site, which leads to seeding of the reticuloendothelial system and, ultimately, viremia. The occurrence of viremia in patients with chickenpox is supported by the diffuse and scattered nature of the skin lesions and can be verified in selected cases by the recovery of virus from the blood.[45] The mechanism of VZV reactivation that results in herpes zoster is unknown.

Clinical Manifestations

CHICKENPOX

Chickenpox is generally a benign, self-limited disease in immunocompetent children, whose incidence is markedly decreasing as the varicella vaccine becomes more widely used. There are fewer than 50 deaths per year in the United States.[46,47] For the normal unimmunized child, chickenpox-associated mortality is less than 2 per 100,000 cases. This risk increases by more than 15-fold for adults. The presenting manifestations of chickenpox are a rash, low-grade fever, and malaise. A prodrome of symptoms may occur 1 to 2 days before the onset of the exanthem in a few patients. For the most part, chickenpox in the immunocompetent child is associated with lassitude and a temperature of 100° to 103° F of 3 to 5 days' duration. Subsequent constitutional symptoms include malaise, pruritus, anorexia, and listlessness; these symptoms gradually resolve as the illness abates. The skin manifestations, which are the hallmark of infection, consist of maculopapules, vesicles, and scabs in varying stages of evolution. The lesions initially contain clear vesicular fluid, but over a very short period of time they pustulate and scab. Most lesions are small, having an erythematous base with a diameter of 5 mm to as large as 12 to 13 mm. The lesions can be round or oval; central umbilication occurs as healing progresses. The lesions have often been referred to as "dew-drop-like" during the early stages of formation. If they do not rupture within a few hours, the contents rapidly become purulent in appearance. The lesions appear on the trunk and face, and rapidly spread centrifugally to involve other areas of the body. Successive crops of lesions generally appear over a period of 2 to 4 days. Thus, early in the disease, the hallmark of the infection is the appearance of lesions at all stages, as noted previously. The lesions can also be found on the mucosa of the oropharynx and even the vagina; however, these sites are less commonly involved. The crusts completely fall off within 1 to 2 weeks after the onset of infection and leave a slightly depressed area of skin.

Immunocompromised children, particularly those with leukemia, have more numerous lesions, often with a hemorrhagic base. Healing takes nearly three times longer in this population.[41] These children are at greater risk for visceral complications, which occur in 30% to 50% of cases and can be fatal in as many as 15% of cases in the absence of therapy. A notable complication of cutaneous lesions is secondary bacterial infection, often in association with gram-positive organisms. Streptococcal toxic shock is a rare but potentially lethal complication of varicella. Infection in the neutropenic host can be systemic.

The most frequent noncutaneous site of involvement after chickenpox is the central nervous system (CNS); the neurologic abnormalities are manifested as acute cerebellar ataxia or encephalitis.[30,48-50] Cerebellar ataxia has been estimated to occur in 1 in 4000 cases among children younger than 15 years. Cerebellar ataxia can appear as late as 21 days after the onset of rash. It is more common, however, for acute cerebellar ataxia to present within 1 week of the onset of the exanthem. An extensive review by Underwood[50] of 120 cases demonstrated that ataxia, vomiting, altered speech, fever, vertigo, and tremor all were common on physical examination. Cerebrospinal fluid (CSF) from these patients often demonstrates lymphocytosis and elevated levels of protein. This is usually a benign complication in children, and resolution occurs within 2 to 4 weeks. PCR techniques can detect VZV DNA in the CSF.[51]

A more serious CNS complication is encephalitis, which can be life threatening in adults. Encephalitis is reported to occur in 0.1% to 0.2% of persons with the disease.[49] Underwood's review[50] reveals this illness to be characterized by depression in the level of consciousness with progressive headaches, vomiting, altered thought patterns, fever, and frequent seizures. The duration of disease in these patients is at least 2 weeks. Some patients experience progressive neurologic deterioration that leads to death. Mortality in patients who develop encephalitis has been estimated to range between 5% and 20%, and neurologic sequelae occur in as many as 15% of survivors.

A neurologic complication of note is the late appearance of cerebral angiitis after herpes zoster ophthalmicus. This problem has been noted in several patients and defined as being progressive, with a high mortality rate. Other nervous system manifestations of chickenpox include meningitis, transverse myelitis, and Reye's syndrome.

A serious and life-threatening complication is the appearance of varicella pneumonitis, a complication that occurs more commonly in adults and in immunocompromised persons.[30,48,52] Among adults, it is estimated to occur in 1 in 400 cases of infection and, not infrequently, in the absence of clinical symptoms, it appears 3 to 5 days into the course of illness and is associated with tachypnea, cough, dyspnea, and fever. Chest radiographs usually reveal nodular or interstitial pneumonitis. Varicella pneumonitis can be life threatening when it occurs in pregnant women during the second or third trimester.

In a prospective study of male military personnel, radiographic abnormalities were detected in nearly 16% of enlisted men who developed varicella, yet only one fourth of these persons had evidence of cough.[52] Only 10% of those with radiographic abnormalities developed evidence of tachypnea, indicating that asymptomatic pneumonitis may exist more commonly than was initially predicted. Other manifestations of noncutaneous and non-neurologic involvement include the appearance of myocarditis, nephritis, bleeding diatheses, and hepatitis.

Perinatal varicella is associated with a high death rate when maternal disease develops 5 days before delivery or up to 48 hours postpartum.[53,54] In large part, this is the consequence of the newborn failing to receive protective transplacental antibodies as well as the immaturity of the neonatal immune system. Under such circumstances, mortality has been reported to be as high as 30%. Affected children have progressive disease involving visceral organs, especially the lung. The outcome in these children was summarized by Brunell.[55] Congenital varicella, while uncommon, is characterized by skin scarring, hypoplastic extremities, eye abnormalities, and evidence of CNS impairment.[56]

Varicella has been associated epidemiologically with the development of Reye's syndrome and coadministration of aspirin. Therefore, the administration of aspirin is contraindicated in persons with varicella. Cutaneous complications of concern are the development of secondary skin infections, especially those caused by *Staphylococcus aureus*.

Chickenpox in the Immunocompromised Patient

Chickenpox in the immunocompromised child or adult is a cause of significant morbidity and mortality. As noted previously, the duration of healing of cutaneous lesions can be extended by a minimum of threefold. However, a more important problem is the progressive involvement of visceral organs. Data from a variety of immunocompromised patient populations indicate a broad spectrum of disease in persons with lymphoproliferative malignancies and solid tumors versus bone marrow transplant recipients. Approximately one third of children develop progressive disease with involvement of multiple organs, including the lungs, liver, and CNS.[41] Most of these children developed pneumonitis within the first week after the onset of infection, as do 20% of all those who acquire chickenpox. Mortality in this patient population has approximated 15% to 18%.[41,57,58] Patients with lymphoproliferative malignancies who require continuous chemotherapy appear to be at greatest risk for visceral involvement.

In persons undergoing human hematopoietic cell transplantation, the incidence of VZV infections over the first year has been estimated to be 30% by 1 year after transplantation. Eighty percent of these infections occurred within the first 9 months after transplantation, and 45% of these patients had cutaneous or visceral dissemination (see Chapter 311). Overall, 23 deaths occurred in one prospective series.[43] Risk factors identified for the acquisition of VZV infection included an age between 10 and 29 years, a diagnosis other than chronic myelogenous leukemia, the post-transplant use of antithymocyte globulin, allogeneic transplant, and acute or chronic graft-versus-host disease. Notably, graft-versus-host disease increases the probability of visceral dissemination significantly.

HERPES ZOSTER

Herpes zoster, or shingles, is characterized by a unilateral vesicular eruption with a dermatomal distribution. Thoracic and lumbar dermatomes are most commonly involved (Fig. 137-1). Herpes zoster may involve the eyelids when the first or second branch of the fifth cranial nerve is affected, but herpes zoster ophthalmicus is a sight-threatening condition. Although lesions on the tip of the nose are said to presage corneal lesions, absence of such skin lesions does not guarantee corneal sparing. Keratitis may be followed by severe iridocyclitis, secondary glaucoma, or neuroparalytic keratitis. Ophthalmologic consultation should be requested for any patient with suspected herpes zoster ophthalmicus. Generally, the onset of disease is heralded by pain within the dermatome that precedes the lesions by 48 to 72 hours. Early in the disease course, erythematous, maculopapular lesions appear that rapidly evolve into a vesicular rash. Vesicles may coalesce to form bullous lesions. In the normal host, these lesions continue to form over a period of 3 to 5 days, with the total duration of disease being 10 to 15 days. However, it may take as long as 1 month before the skin returns to normal.

Unusual cutaneous manifestations of herpes zoster, in addition to herpes zoster ophthalmicus, include the involvement of the maxillary or mandibular branch of the trigeminal nerve, which results in intra-oral involvement with lesions on the palate, tonsillar fossa, floor of the mouth, and tongue. When the geniculate ganglion is involved, the Ramsay Hunt syndrome may occur, with pain and vesicles in the external auditory meatus, loss of taste on the anterior two thirds of the tongue, and ipsilateral facial palsy.

No known factors are responsible for the precipitation of the episodes of herpes zoster. If herpes zoster occurs in children, the course is generally benign and not associated with progressive pain or discom-

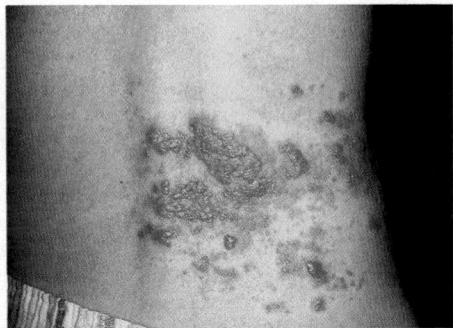

Figure 137-1 **Herpes zoster involving the lumbar dermatome.**

fort. In adults, systemic manifestations are mainly those associated with pain, as noted in the following paragraphs.

The most significant clinical manifestations of herpes zoster are the associated acute neuritis and, later, PHN. Modeling of pain attributed to herpes zoster defines three phases of disease: acute, subacute, and chronic.[59] Historically, the latter two make up PHN. As identified later, the impact of therapy on each phase can be defined. PHN, although uncommon in young people, may occur in as many as 25% to 50% of patients older than 50 years.[60-62] As many as 50% of persons older than 50 years have debilitating pain that persists for more than 1 month. PHN may cause constant pain in the involved dermatome or consist of intermittent stabbing pain. Pain may be worse at night or on exposure to temperature changes, and at its worst, the neuralgia can be incapacitating.[63]

Extracutaneous sites of involvement include the CNS, as manifested by meningoencephalitis or encephalitis. The clinical manifestations are similar to those of other viral infections of the brain. However, a rare manifestation of CNS involvement by herpes zoster is granulomatous cerebral angiitis, which usually follows zoster ophthalmicus. Involvement of the CNS with cutaneous herpes zoster probably is more common than recognized clinically. Frequently, patients who undergo CSF examination for other reasons during episodes of shingles are found to have evidence of pleocytosis without elevated protein levels. These patients are without signs of meningeal irritation and infrequently complain of headaches.

Classically, VZV infection involves sensory ganglia; however, motor paralysis can occur as a consequence of the involvement of the anterior horn cells, in a manner similar to that encountered with polio. Patients with involvement of the anterior horn cells are particularly likely to have excruciating pain. Other neuromuscular disorders associated with herpes zoster include Guillain-Barré syndrome, transverse myelitis,[64] and myositis.[65,66] Herpes zoster in the immunocompromised patient is more severe than in the normal person. Lesion formation continues for up to 2 weeks, and scabbing may not take place until 3 to 4 weeks into the disease course.[44] Patients with lymphoproliferative malignancies are at risk for cutaneous dissemination and visceral involvement, including varicella pneumonitis, hepatitis, and meningoencephalitis. However, even in the immunocompromised patient, disseminated herpes zoster is rarely fatal.

Herpes zoster has been recognized as a frequent infection in persons with human immunodeficiency virus (HIV) infection, occurring in 8% to 11% of patients. Although the occurrence of cutaneous dissemination is infrequent, complications such as VZV retinitis, acute retinal necrosis, and chronic progressive encephalitis have been reported.[67] Recently, the use of anti-TNF-α monoclonal antibodies has been associated with an increased incidence of herpes zoster.

Chronic herpes zoster may also occur in immunocompromised patients, particularly those with HIV infection. Patients have experienced new lesion formation with an absence of healing of the existing lesions. These syndromes can be particularly debilitating and, of interest, have been associated with the isolation of VZV isolates resistant to acyclovir.

Diagnosis

The diagnosis of both chickenpox and shingles is usually made by history and physical examination. In the first part of the 21st century, the differential diagnosis of varicella and herpes zoster is less confusing than it was 20 to 30 years ago. Smallpox or disseminated vaccinia was confused with varicella because of the similar appearance of the cutaneous lesions, and it could again pose a problem in the era of bioterrorism. With the worldwide eradication of smallpox, these disease entities only serve to confound the diagnosis if used by a bioterrorist or as a complication of vaccination. The characteristic skin rash of chickenpox with lesions in all stages of development provides the basis for the clinical diagnosis of infection. The presence of pruritus, pain, and low-grade fever also helps establish the diagnosis of chickenpox. The localization and distribution of a vesicular rash make the diagnosis

of herpes zoster highly likely; however, other viral exanthemas can occasionally be confused with this disease.

Impetigo and varicella can also be confused clinically. Impetigo is usually caused by group A β-hemolytic streptococci, often follows an abrasion of the skin or inoculation of bacteria at the site of the skin break, and can be associated with the formation of small vesicles in the surrounding area. Systemic signs of disease may be present if progressive cellulitis or secondary bacteremia develops. Unroofing lesions and careful Gram staining of the scraping of the base of the lesion should reveal gram-positive cocci in chains, suggestive of streptococci, or gram-positive cocci in clusters, suggestive of staphylococci, another cause of vesicular skin lesions, or both organisms. Treatment for these latter infections is distinctly different from that for chickenpox and requires administration of an appropriate antibiotic.

In a smaller number of cases, disseminated vesicular lesions can be caused by HSV. In these cases, disseminated HSV infection is usually a consequence of an underlying skin disease such as atopic dermatitis or eczema. An unequivocal diagnosis can be made only by isolation of the virus in tissue culture.

Disseminated enteroviral infections, particularly those caused by group A coxsackieviruses, have been reported to cause widespread distal vesicular lesions. These rashes are more commonly morbilliform in nature, with a hemorrhagic component rather than a vesicular or vesiculopustular appearance. Generally, these infections occur during the enterovirus season in late summer and early fall and are associated with lesions of the oropharynx, palms, and soles. This latter finding is helpful in distinguishing enteroviral disease from chickenpox.

Unilateral vesicular lesions in the dermatomal pattern should immediately lead the clinician to suspect a diagnosis of shingles. HSV and coxsackievirus infections can also cause dermatomal vesicular lesions. In such situations, diagnostic viral cultures remain the best method of establishing the cause of infection. Confirmation of the diagnosis is possible through the isolation of VZV in susceptible tissue culture cell lines or by the demonstration of either seroconversion or serologic rises using standard antibody assays of acute and convalescent serum specimens. A Tzanck smear, performed by scraping the base of the lesion, can demonstrate multinucleated giant cells; however, the sensitivity of this test is no better than 60%. Commercially available reagents are useful for direct fluorescent antibody staining of smears obtained from scraping vesicular lesions. With atypical skin lesions, such smears have adequate sensitivity and specificity to guide early management decisions. In research laboratories, PCR is a useful diagnostic tool; however, its expense and lack of uniform performance standards preclude routine diagnostic use. Useful antibody assays include immune adherence hemagglutination assay, fluorescence antibody to membrane antigen (FAMA) assay, and enzyme-linked immunosorbent assay (ELISA).[68] The application of PCR to the CSF can be used to detect VZV DNA and, therefore, infections of the CNS.

Therapy

The medical management of chickenpox and shingles in the normal host is directed toward reduction of complications. For chickenpox, hygiene is important, including bathing, astringent soaks, and closely cropped fingernails to avoid a source for secondary bacterial infection associated with scratching of the pruritic skin lesions. Pruritus can be decreased with topical dressing or the administration of antipruritic drugs. Soaks with aluminum acetate, or Burow's solution, in the management of herpes zoster can be both soothing and cleansing.[69] Acetaminophen should be used to reduce fever in patients with chickenpox because of the association between aspirin and Reye's syndrome.

Acyclovir is approved in the United States for the treatment of both chickenpox and herpes zoster in the normal host. Oral acyclovir therapy in normal children, adolescents, and adults shortens the duration of lesion formation by about 1 day, reduces the total number of new lesions by approximately 25%, and diminishes constitutional symptoms in one third of patients.[69-72] The American Academy of

Pediatrics recommends therapy for adolescents and adults as well as for high-risk groups of patients (e.g., premature infants, children with bronchopulmonary dysplasia) within 24 hours of onset of disease. In children 2 to 16 years old, the oral dosage is 20 mg/kg 4 times daily for 5 days (maximum of 800 mg daily). Adolescents and adults can receive up to 800 mg 5 times a day. Oral therapy of herpes zoster in the normal host accelerates cutaneous healing and reduces acute neuritis.

Acyclovir has been evaluated in controlled studies for all herpesvirus infections. Acyclovir is a guanine derivative that has a high degree of selectivity for the inhibition of VZV replication because of its selected phosphorylation and activation by the virus-coded thymidine kinase and its subsequent selective inhibition of the viral DNA polymerase. It is estimated that the concentration of acyclovir required to inhibit VZV replication in vitro is between 2.1 and 6.3 μM, which concentration is easily achieved after intravenous administration of acyclovir.[73] However, such concentrations are not easily achieved even after administration of high-dose oral acyclovir as summarized.[74] The recommended dosage for acyclovir is 5 to 10 mg/kg administered intravenously every 8 hours or, as suggested by some, 500 mg/m^2 intravenously every 8 hours, especially for children.

The prodrugs of acyclovir and penciclovir, namely, valaciclovir and famciclovir, respectively, have been licensed for therapy of herpes zoster.[75,76] The use of valaciclovir results in enhanced oral bioavailability, approximately 60%, compared with acyclovir. Famciclovir's oral bioavailability is approximately 80%. Both drugs appear superior to acyclovir for acceleration of cutaneous healing and are at least equally, if not more, efficacious for resolution of pain. Valaciclovir is administered at 1 g 3 times daily for 7 to 10 days.[75] Famciclovir is given at 500 mg 3 times daily for 7 to 10 days.[75] Both medications are well tolerated. These medications primarily affect the acute and subacute phases of disease, as noted earlier.

The concomitant administration of corticosteroids and an antiviral remains controversial. In one study, such regimens failed to affect PHN, although resolution of acute neuritis was accelerated.[77] This study was not placebo controlled. A placebo-controlled trial, using a 2 × 2 factorial design, demonstrated significant improvement in quality of life.[78] Patients older than 50 years who received acyclovir (800 mg 5 times daily for 3 weeks) and tapering doses of prednisone (60 mg daily for 7 days, 30 mg daily for 7 days, and 15 mg daily for 7 days) experienced resolution of acute neuritis, were able to sleep uninterrupted, and returned to their usual activity levels more promptly than did controls and also had lower analgesic requirements. Complications were not encountered; however, patients at risk for complications of high-dose steroid therapy were excluded.

Management of varicella pneumonitis and other complications requires excellent supportive nursing care in addition to evaluation, on an individual basis, of the potential need for antiviral therapy. The management of acute neuritis and PHN can be particularly problematic. It requires the judicious use of analgesics ranging from nonnarcotic to narcotic derivatives and may include the deployment of such drugs as amitriptyline hydrochloride, fluphenazine hydrochloride, lidocaine patches, gabapentin, and pregabalin.[79-82] Further, intrathecal administration of narcotics has been reported to be of value.[83]

Prevention

In the normal host, prophylaxis of chickenpox is achieved via vaccination. The potential for transmission of VZV within the hospital to immunosuppressed patients, particularly children, is a serious problem, which is discussed in detail in Chapter 307. Patients who require hospitalization because of varicella are a source of nosocomial infection within the hospital environment. Because approximately 10% of adults are seronegative, the risks in the medical care environment can be high. Those most likely to become infected are nurses and other medical personnel providing care to infected persons. Airflow can be a means of transmission of infection from one area to another in the hospital environment.

In the immunocompromised person who has not been previously exposed to chickenpox, the administration of varicella-zoster immune globulin (VZIG) (VariZig; see Chapter 320) has been shown to be useful for both prevention and amelioration of symptomatic chickenpox in high-risk persons.[84-87] VZIG should be administered to the immunodeficient patient younger than 15 years who has a negative or unknown history of chickenpox, who has not been vaccinated against VZV, or who has had contact in the household with a playmate or in a shared hospital room for more than 1 hour. Recent guidelines also recommend administration of VZIG to a pregnant woman who is known to be seronegative and who has had a significant exposure. VZIG should also be administered to a newborn infant whose mother had onset of chickenpox less than 5 days before delivery or up to 48 hours postpartum. The use of VZIG for susceptible immunocompetent persons older than 15 years must be evaluated on an individual basis.

A vaccine is licensed for the prevention of chickenpox in immunocompetent persons.[88-94] Studies performed to date indicate excellent protection after vaccination. The Oka strain of VZV was developed by Takahashi and colleagues in Japan and studied as a vaccine extensively in both healthy and leukemic children. In immunocompromised children, serologic evidence of host response after vaccination has been achieved in between 89% and 100% of vaccinated individuals. Vaccine-induced rash, however, is not uncommon and occurs in variable percentages of patients from approximately 6% to as high as 47%. The factor most predictive of the appearance of rash is the degree of immunosuppression. Specifically, for children with acute lymphoblastic leukemia, the likelihood of rash can be as high as 40% to 50%. The subsequent occurrence of natural varicella after community exposure is decreased in the larger control studies and averages 8% to 16%. Vaccination did not appear to increase the likelihood of subsequent herpes zoster during the period of follow-up.

The Advisory Committee on Immunization Practices (ACIP) recommends routine childhood vaccination.[95] In clinical trials, the development of antibody responses was higher than in the immunocompromised host and varied between 94% and 100%. Vaccine-induced rash was far less common in these individuals and occurred at a frequency of 0.5% to approximately 19% overall, with the rate for subsequent appearance of varicella after community exposure averaging between 1% and 5%. The impact of this vaccine is now being appreciated as documented in sentinel cities where the incidence of chickenpox has fallen dramatically.[1,96] Recently, the ACIP has recommended a second dose of vaccine at school entry in the light of small outbreaks[97] (see also Chapter 320).

The Oka vaccine was also evaluated in adults to prevent shingles, but a higher titer of live attenuated virus was required to elicit significant and durable increases in cell-mediated immune (CMI) responses. Thus, Zostavax was developed specifically for protection against herpes zoster. The zoster vaccine contains, on average, 19,400 plaque-forming units (PFU) per dose,[98] whereas the chickenpox vaccines contain either approximately 9800 PFU per dose (quadrivalent measles, mumps, rubella, and varicella vaccine)[99] or 1350 PFU per dose (monovalent varicella vaccine; Varivax).[100] A zoster vaccine, to be effective, should boost an older person's CMI responses and, therefore, mimic immunologic benefit of exposure of VZV-immune adults to chickenpox.[101] Indeed, several dose-ranging studies of vaccine defined a boost in waning CMI responses in older individuals.[102-104] The Shingles Prevention Study evaluated the high-titer, live attenuated zoster vaccine[105] in nearly 40,000 subjects over 60 years of age with a mean follow-up of 3 years. Benefit was defined in three specific areas. First, the incidence of herpes zoster was 50% lower in the vaccine group than in placebo recipients (5.4 cases per 1000 person-years vs. 11.1 cases per 1000 person-years, $P < 0.001$). For those patients who developed herpes zoster while on the study, vaccine virus was not detected by PCR. Second, the incidence of PHN was 67% lower among vaccine recipients (0.5 cases per 1000 person-years vs. 1.4 cases per 1000 person-years, $P < 0.001$). In addition, the median duration of pain among subjects in whom herpes zoster developed was shorter in the vaccine group, albeit of marginal clinical value (21 vs. 24 days, $P = 0.003$).

Third, vaccination significantly decreased the burden of illness overall for patients who developed zoster (as assessed by an area under the curve evaluation, $P = 0.008$). When patients were analyzed according to two age groups, the younger elderly (60 to 69 years old) and older elderly (>70 years of age), differences in vaccine efficacy were noted. Vaccination was more effective in preventing herpes zoster among the younger versus the older elderly. However, it prevented PHN and burden of illness to a similar extent in both groups. Notably, the risk of subsequent development of herpes zoster does not appear to be increased in vaccine recipients.[106]

In 2006, the U.S. Food and Drug Administration approved the zoster vaccine for the prevention of herpes zoster in persons 60 years of age or older.[98,105] This vaccine is not indicated for the treatment of PHN or herpes zoster.

The inactivated Oka vaccine is being evaluated for prevention of herpes zoster after human stem cell transplantation.[107]

REFERENCES

1. Seward JF, Watson BM, Peterson CL, et al. Varicella disease after introduction of varicella vaccine in the United States, 1995-2000. *JAMA.* 2002;287:606-611.
2. Seward JF, Marin M, Vazquez M. Varicella vaccine effectiveness in the US vaccination program: A review. *J Infect Dis.* 2008;197(suppl 2):S82-89.
3. Gordon JE, Meader FM. The period of infectivity and serum prevention of chickenpox. *JAMA.* 1929;93:2013-2015.
4. Steiner P. Zur inokulation der varicellen. *Wien Med Wochenschr.* 1875;25:306.
5. von Bokay J. Das auftreten der schafblattern unter besonderen umstanden. *Ungar Arch Med.* 1892;1:159.
6. von Bokay J. Uber den atiologischen zusammenhang der varizellen mit ewissen fallen von herpes zoster. *Wien Klin Wochemscher.* 1909;22:1323.
7. Kundratiz K. Experimentelle ubertragungen von herpes zoster auf menschen und die beziehungen von herpes zoster zu varicellen. *A Kinderheilkd.* 1925;39:379.
8. Brunsgaard E. The mutual relation between zoster and varicella. *Br J Dermatol Syph.* 1932;44:1.
9. School Epidemics Committee of Great Britain, Medical Research Council, Special Report Series. His Majesty's Stationery Office, 1938.
10. Garland J. Varicella following exposure to herpes zoster. *N Engl J Med.* 1943;228:336.
11. Seiler H. A study of herpes zoster particularly in its relationship to chicken pox. *J Hyg.* 1949;47:253-262.
12. Weller TH, Witton HM. The etiologic agents of varicella and herpes zoster: serologic studies with the viruses as propagated in vitro. *J Exp Med.* 1958;108:869-890.
13. Tyzzer EE. The histology of the skin lesions in varicella. *Philipp J Sci.* 1906:349.
14. Lipschutz B. Untersuchungen uber die atiologie der krankheiten der herpesgruppe (herpes zoster, herpes genitalis, and herpes febrilis). *Arch Dermatol Syph.* 1921;136:428-482.
15. Weller TH. Serial propagation in vitro of agents producing inclusion bodies derived from varicella and herpes zoster. *Proc Soc Exp Biol Med.* 1953;83:340.
16. Weller TH, Coons AH. Fluorescent antibody studies with agents of varicella and herpes zoster propagated in vitro. *Proc Soc Exp Biol Med.* 1954;86:789.
17. Weller TH, Stoddard MB. Intranuclear inclusion bodies in cultures of human tissue inoculated with varicella vesicle fluid. *J Immunol.* 1952;68:311-319.
18. Davison AJ, Scott JE. The complete DNA sequence of varicella-zoster virus. *J Gen Virol.* 1986;67:1759-1816.
19. Sawyer MH, Ostrove JM, Felser JM, et al. Mapping of the varicella zoster virus deoxypyrimidine kinase gene and preliminary identification of its transcript. *Virology.* 1986;149:1-9.
20. Dumas AM, Geelen JL, Mares W, et al. Infectivity and molecular weight of varicella-zoster virus DNA. *J Gen Virol.* 1980; 47:233-235.
21. Achong BC, Meurisse EV. Observation on the fine structure and replication of varicella virus in cultivated human amnion cells. *J Gen Virol.* 1968;3:305.
22. Almeida JD, Howatson AF, Williams MG. Morphology of varicella (chickenpox) virus. *Virology.* 1962;16:353.
23. Tournier P, Cathala F, Bernhard W. [Ultrastructure and intracellular development of varicella virus observed with electron microscope.]. *Presse Med.* 1957;65(52):1229-1234.
24. Straus SE, Ostrove JM, Inchauspe G, et al. NIH conference. Varicella-zoster virus infections: biology, natural history, treatment, and prevention. *Ann Intern Med.* 1988;108:221-237.
25. Gelb LD. Varicella-zoster virus. In: Fields BN, Knipe DM, eds. *Fields Virology.* New York: Raven Press; 1990:2011-2054.
26. Arvin A. Varicella-zoster virus. In: Fields BN, Knipe DM, Howley PM, eds. *Fields Virology.* Philadelphia: Lippincott-Raven; 1996:2547.
27. Rapp F, Vanderslice D. Spread of zoster virus in human embryonic lung cells and the inhibitory effect of iododeoxyuridine. *Virology.* 1964;22:321.
28. Vaczi L, Geder L, Koller M, et al. Influence of temperature on the multiplication of varicella virus. *Acta Microbiol Acad Sci Hung.* 1963;10:109.
29. Grose C, Perrotta DM, Brunell PA, et al. Cell-free varicella-zoster virus in cultured human melanoma cells. *J Gen Virol.* 1979;43:15-27.
30. Preblud SR. Varicella: complications and cost. *Pediatrics.* 1986;78:728-735.
31. Wells MW, Holla WA. Ventilation in the flow of measles and chickenpox through a community. *JAMA.* 1950;142:1337-1344.
32. Preblud SR, Orenstein WA, Bart KJ. Varicella: Clinical manifestations, epidemiology and health impact in children. *Pediatr Infect Dis.* 1984;3:505-509.
33. Hope-Simpson RE. Infectiousness of communicable diseases in the household (measles, chickenpox, and mumps). *Lancet.* 1952;2:549-554.
34. Ross AH. Modification of chickenpox in family contacts by administration of gamma globulin. *N Engl J Med.* 1962; 267:369-376.
35. Stokes J Jr, ed. Chickenpox: communicable diseases transmitted chiefly through respiratory and alimentary tracts. Preventive Medicine in World War II, Vol. IV. Washington, DC; Office of the Surgeon General, Department of the Army; 1958:55-56.
36. Bastian FO, Rabson AS, Yee CL, et al. Herpes virus varicella isolated from human dorsal root ganglia. *Arch Pathol.* 1974;97:331-336.
37. Esiri MM, Tomlinson AH. Herpes zoster: demonstration of virus in trigeminal nerve and ganglion by immunofluorescence and electron microscopy. *J Neurol Sci.* 1972;15:35-48.
38. Ragozzino MW, Melton LJ 3rd, Kurland LT, et al. Population-based study of herpes zoster and its sequelae. *Medicine.* 1982;61:310-316.
39. Hope-Simpson RE. The nature of herpes zoster: a long-term study and a new hypothesis. *Proc R Soc Med.* 1965;58:9-20.
40. McGregor RM. Herpes zoster, chickenpox, and cancer in general practice. *Br Med J.* 1957;1:84-87.
41. Feldman S, Hughes WT, Daniel CB. Varicella in children with cancer: seventy-seven cases. *Pediatrics.* 1975;56:388-399.
42. Arvin AM, Pollard RB, Rasmussen LE, et al. Cellular and humoral immunity in the pathogenesis of recurrent herpes viral infection in patients with lymphoma. *J Clin Invest.* 1980; 65:869-878.
43. Locksley RM, Flournoy N, Sullivan KM, et al. Infection with varicella-zoster virus after marrow transplantation. *J Infect Dis.* 1985;152:1172-1181.
44. Whitley RJ. Varicella-zoster virus infections. In: Galasso GJ, Merigan TC, Buchanan RA, eds. *Antiviral Agents and Viral Diseases of Man.* New York: Raven Press; 1984:517-541.
45. Asano Y, Itakura N, Hiroishi Y, et al. Viremia is present in incubation period in nonimmunocompromised children with varicella. *J Pediatr.* 1985;106:69-71.
46. Reynolds MA, Watson BM, Plott-Adams KK, et al. Epidemiology of varicella hospitalizations in the United States, 1995-2005. *J Infect Dis.* 2008;197(Suppl 2):S120-126.
47. Zhou F, Harpaz R, Jumaan AO, et al. Impact of varicella vaccination on health care utilization. *JAMA.* 2005;294: 797-802.
48. Fleisher G, Henry W, McSorley M, et al. Life threatening complications of varicella. *Am J Dis Child.* 1981;135:896-899.
49. Johnson R, Milbourn PE. Central nervous system manifestations of chickenpox. *Can Med Assoc J.* 1970;102:831-836.
50. Underwood EA. The neurological complications of varicella: a clinical and epidemiological study. *Br J Child Dis.* 1935; 32:376-378.
51. Burke DG, Kalayjian RC, Vann VR, et al. Polymerase chain reaction detection and clinical significance of varicella-zoster virus in cerebrospinal fluid from human immunodeficiency virus-infected patients. *J Infect Dis.* 1997;176:1080-1084.
52. Triebwasser J, Harris RE, Bryant RE, et al. Varicella pneumonia in adults: Report of seven cases and review of the literature. *Medicine.* 1967;46:409-420.
53. Brunell PA. Fetal and neonatal varicella-zoster infections. *Semin Perinatol.* 1983;7:47-56.
54. Preblud SR, Bregman DJ, Vernon LL. Deaths from varicella in infants. *Pediatr Infect Dis.* 1985;4:503-507.
55. Brunell PA. Placental transfer of varicella zoster antibody. *Pediatrics.* 1966;38:1034-1038.
56. Paryani SG, Arvin AM. Intrauterine infection with varicella-zoster virus after maternal varicella. *N Engl J Med.* 1986; 314:1542-1546.
57. Arvin AM, Kushner JH, Feldman S, et al. Human leukocyte interferon for treatment of varicella in children with cancer. *N Engl J Med.* 1982;306:761-767.
58. Whitley RJ, Soong SJ, Dolin R, et al. Early vidarabine therapy to control the complications of herpes zoster in immunosuppressed patients. *N Engl J Med.* 1982;307:971-975.
59. Arani RB, Soong SJ, Weiss HL, et al. Phase specific analysis of herpes zoster associated pain data: a new statistical approach. *Stat Med.* 2001;20:2429-2439.
60. De Moragas JM, Kierland RR. The outcome of patients with herpes zoster. *AMA Arch Derm.* 1957;75:193-196.
61. Watson PN, Evans RJ. Postherpetic neuralgia: A review. *Arch Neurol.* 1986;43:836-840.
62. Esmann V, Geil JP, Kroon S, et al. Prednisolone does not prevent post-herpetic neuralgia. *Lancet.* 1987;2:126-129.
63. Kost RG, Straus SE. Postherpetic neuralgia—pathogenesis, treatment, and prevention. *N Engl J Med.* 1996;335:32-42.
64. Hogan EL, Krigman MR. Herpes zoster myelitis. *Arch Neurol.* 1973;29:309-313.
65. Rubin D, Fusfeld RD. Muscle paralysis in herpes zoster. *Calif Med.* 1965;103:261-266.
66. Norris FH Jr, Dramov B, Calder CD, et al. Virus-like particles in myositis accompanying herpes zoster. *Arch Neurol.* 1969;21:25-31.
67. Gnann JW, Whitley RJ. Natural history and treatment of varicella-zoster in high risk populations. *J Hosp Infect.* 1991;18:317-329.
68. Forghani B, Schmidt NJ, Dennis J. Antibody assays for varicella-zoster virus: comparison of enzyme immunoassay with neutralization, immune adherence hemagglutination, and complement fixation. *J Clin Microbiol.* 1978;8:545-552.
69. Balfour HH Jr, Kelly JM, Suarez CS, et al. Acyclovir treatment of varicella in otherwise healthy children. *J Pediatr.* 1990; 116:633-639.
70. Dunkle LM, Arvin AM, Whitley RJ, et al. A controlled trial of acyclovir for chickenpox in normal children. *N Engl J Med.* 1991;325:1539-1544.
71. Balfour HH Jr, Rotbart HA, Feldman S, et al. Acyclovir treatment of varicella in otherwise healthy adolescents. The Collaborative Acyclovir Varicella Study Group. *J Pediatr.* 1992; 120:627-633.
72. Wallace MR, Bowler WA, Murray NB, et al. Treatment of adult varicella with oral acyclovir: a randomized, placebo-controlled trial. *Ann Intern Med.* 1992;117:358-363.
73. Huff JC, Bean B, Balfour HH Jr, et al. Therapy of herpes zoster with oral acyclovir. *Am J Med.* 1988;85:84-89.
74. Whitley RJ, Gnann J. Acyclovir: A decade later. *N Engl J Med.* 1992;327:782-789.
75. Beutner KR, Friedman DJ, Forszpaniak C, et al. Valacyclovir compared with acyclovir for improved therapy for herpes zoster in immunocompetent adults. *Antimicrob Agents Chemother.* 1995;39:1546-1553.
76. Tyring S, Barbarash RA, Nahlik JE, et al. Famciclovir for the treatment of acute herpes zoster: Effects on acute disease and postherpetic neuralgia: a randomized, double-blind, placebo-controlled trial. *Ann Intern Med.* 1995;123:89-96.
77. Wood MJ, Johnson RW, McKendrick MW, et al. A randomized trial of acyclovir for 7 days or 21 days with and without prednisolone for treatment of acute herpes zoster. *N Engl J Med.* 1994;330:896-900.
78. Whitley RJ, et al. Acyclovir with and without prednisone for the treatment of herpes zoster: a randomized, placebo-controlled trial. The National Institute of Allergy and Infectious Diseases Collaborative Antiviral Study Group. *Ann Intern Med.* 1996;125:376-383.
79. Dworkin RH, Johnson RW, Breuer J, et al. Recommendations for the management of herpes zoster. *Clin Infect Dis.* 2007;44(Suppl 1):S1-26.
80. Galer BS, Jensen MP, Ma T, et al. The lidocaine patch 5% effectively treats all neuropathic pain qualities: results of a randomized, double-blind, vehicle-controlled, 3-week efficacy study with use of the neuropathic pain scale. *Clin J Pain.* 2002;18:297-301.
81. Rowbotham M, Harden N, Stacey B, et al. Gabapentin for the treatment of postherpetic neuralgia: a randomized controlled trial. *JAMA.* 1998;280:1837-1842.
82. Dworkin RH, Schmader KE. Treatment and prevention of postherpetic neuralgia. *Clin Infect Dis.* 2003;36:877-882.
83. Gnann JW, Whitley RJ. Herpes zoster. *N Engl J Med.* 2002;347:340-346.
84. Brunell PA, Ross A, Miller LH, et al. Prevention of varicella by zoster immune globulin. *N Engl J Med.* 1969;280:1191-1194.
85. Gershon AA, Steinberg S, Brunell PA. Zoster immune globulin: A further assessment. *N Engl J Med.* 1974;290:243-245.
86. Zaia JA, Levin MJ, Preblud SR. Evaluation of varicella-zoster immune globulin: protection of immunosuppressed children after household exposure to varicella. *J Infect Dis.* 1983;147:737-743.
87. Centers for Disease Control and Prevention. Varicella zoster immune globulin for the prevention of chickenpox: recommendations of the immunization practices advisory committee. *Ann Intern Med.* 1984;100:859-865.

88. Takahashi M, Otsuka T, Okuno Y, et al. Live vaccine used to prevent the spread of varicella in children in hospitals. *Lancet.* 1974;2:1288-1290.

89. Gershon AA, Steinberg SP, Gelb L. Live attenuated varicella vaccine use in immunocompromised children and adults. *Pediatrics.* 1986;78:757-762.

90. Takahashi M. Clinical overview of varicella vaccine: development and early studies. *Pediatrics.* 1986;78:736-741.

91. Yabuuchi H, Baba K, Tsuda N, et al. A live varicella vaccine in a pediatric community. *Biken J.* 1984;27:43-49.

92. Horiuchi K. Chickenpox vaccination of healthy children: Immunological and clinical responses and protective effect in 1978-1982. *Biken J.* 1984;27:37-38.

93. Weibel RE, Neff BJ, Kuter BJ, et al. Live attenuated varicella virus vaccine: efficacy trial in healthy children. *N Engl J Med.* 1984;310:1409-1415.

94. Asano Y, Nagai T, Ito S, et al. Long-term protective immunity of recipients of the OKA strain of life varicella vaccine. *Pediatrics.* 1985;75:667-671.

95. Straus SE, Ostrove JM, Inchauspe G, et al. NIH Conference. Varicella-zoster virus infections: biology, natural history, treatment, and prevention. *Ann Intern Med.* 1988;108:221-237.

96. Prevention of varicella. Update recommendations of the Advisory Committee on Immunization Practices (ACIP). *MMWR Recomm Rep.* 1999;48(RR-6):1-5.

97. Chaves SS, Gargiullo P, Zhang JX, et al. Loss of vaccine-induced immunity to varicella over time. *N Engl J Med.* 2007;356(11):1121-1129.

98. Zostavax. Whitehouse Station, NJ: Merck & Co.; 2006 (package insert). Available at: http://www.fda.gov/cber/label/zostavaxLBf.pdf. Accessed 5/30/09.

99. ProQuad. Whitehouse Station, NJ: Merck & Co.; 2005 (package insert). Available at: http://www.fda.gov/cber/label/proquadLB2.pdf. Accessed 5/30/09.

100. Varivax. Whitehouse Station, NJ: Merck & Co.; 2005 (package insert). Available at: http://www.fda.gov/cber/label/varivaxfrozenLB.pdf. Accessed 5/30/09.

101. Levin MJ, Murray M, Zerbe GO, et al. Immune responses of elderly persons 4 years after receiving a live attenuated varicella vaccine. *J Infect Dis.* 1994;170:522-526.

102. Levin MJ, Barber D, Goldblatt E, et al. Use of a live attenuated varicella vaccine to boost varicella-specific immune responses in seropositive people 55 years of age and older: duration of booster effect. *J Infect Dis.* 1998;178(Suppl 1):S109-112.

103. Oxman MN. Immunization to reduce the frequency and severity of herpes zoster and its complications. *Neurology.* 1995;45(12 Suppl 8):S41-46.

104. Trannoy E, Berger R, Hollander G, et al. Vaccination of immunocompetent elderly subjects with a live attenuated Oka strain of varicella zoster virus: a randomized, controlled, dose-response trial. *Vaccine.* 2000;18:1700-1706.

105. Oxman MN, Levin MJ, Johnson GR, et al. Shingles Prevention Study Group. A vaccine to prevent herpes zoster and postherpetic neuralgia in older adults. *N Engl J Med.* 2005;352:2271-2284.

106. Lawrence R, Gershon AA, Holzman R, et al. The risk of zoster after vaccination in children with leukemia. *N Engl J Med.* 1988;318:543-548.

107. Hata A, Asanuma H, Rinki M, et al. Use of an inactivated varicella vaccine in recipients of hematopoietic-cell transplants. *N Engl J Med.* 2002;347:26-34.

138

Cytomegalovirus

CLYDE S. CRUMPACKER II | JIE LIN ZHANG

*H*uman cytomegalovirus (HCMV), a β herpes virus (see Chapter 135), is the largest virus to infect humans. Its genome is sufficient to encode 230 proteins, many of which play a significant role in downregulation of the immune response. Infection is common in all human populations and reaches 60% to 70% in U.S. cities[1] and nearly 100% in some parts of Africa. Disease is varied in humans infected with cytomegalovirus (CMV), from no disease in healthy hosts and congenital CMV syndrome in neonates, which is frequently fatal, to infectious mononucleosis syndrome in young adults. In the patient with immunocompromise, CMV produces its most significant and severe disease syndromes in lung, liver, kidney, and heart transplant recipients. CMV is the most common opportunistic pathogen detected in those settings and causes significant mortality and morbidity.[2] In bone marrow transplant recipients, CMV pneumonia is the most common life-threatening infectious complication after transplantation.[3] In patients with acquired immunodeficiency syndrome (AIDS), CMV is the most common viral pathogen, and CMV retinitis is the most frequent sight-threatening infection, even in the era of highly active antiretroviral therapy.[4] Fortunately, effective therapies for the treatment and prevention of serious CMV disease in patients with immunocompromise are being established, and principles for the use of these therapies are becoming more clear.[5]

As with all herpes viruses, CMV establishes latent infection in the host after recovery from acute infection. The exact mechanisms that control latency are unclear, but polymorphonuclear cells, T lymphocytes, endothelial vascular tissue, renal epithelial cells, and salivary glands may all harbor the virus in a nonreplicating or slowly replicating form. Activation from this latent state can occur after immunosuppression, other illness, or the use of chemotherapeutic agents.[6]

Both primary and secondary infection with CMV can occur. *Primary infection* occurs in patients who are seronegative and have never been infected with CMV. *Secondary infection* represents activation of a latent infection or reinfection in a person with seropositive immunity. Both infants and adults can be infected with multiple strains. Several different strains of CMV have been found at the same time in the urine of patients with AIDS.[7] Clinical CMV disease can result from either primary or secondary infection; in primary infection, virus usually replicates to a higher level and disease is more severe. Congenital infection of the neonate is almost always the result of primary infection of the mother during pregnancy.[8]

The emphasis in this chapter is on the clinical manifestations of CMV disease and the mechanisms of pathogenesis. Treatment and prevention with antiviral drugs have greatly changed the management of CMV disease in the patient with immunocompromise; this development is highlighted. Limitations of antiviral therapy, such as resistance to antiviral drugs, are discussed.

Description of the Pathogen

The era of modern virology of CMV began with the isolation of murine CMV.[9] Shortly after this time, the isolation of human CMV was reported by three independent groups led by Smith, Weller, Rowe, and colleagues.[10-12] Human CMV was isolated from the human salivary gland, and the term *cytomegalovirus* was first used to replace the term *salivary gland virus* or *cytomegalic inclusion disease virus*.[13] The first description of recognizable CMV disease in a healthy adult was documented in 1965.[14] A syndrome of CMV mononucleosis was found to occur sporadically or after transfusion with blood[15] or leukocyte products.[16]

Human CMV (HCMV) is the largest member of the human herpes virus group and is the largest known virus to infect humans. The CMV genome is a linear, double-stranded DNA molecule (230 Kbp) that has been completely sequenced[17] and contains nonoverlapping open reading frames for 230 proteins. Not all of the proteins have been identified, and the functions of many of the proteins are not known. The laboratory strain AD169 has been the best studied and was the first strain to have its nucleotide sequence determined. AD169 has a shorter genome than do many clinical isolates, and the Toledo strain of HCMV contains an additional 15 kilobase (kb) of DNA that is not present in strain AD169.[18] This large block of duplex DNA contains 19 genes that encode viral glycoproteins and other specialized functions. The large block of CMV genes in this region is designed to mimic and interact with cellular functions. The UL144 open reading frame (ORF) exhibits a great diversity of genetic polymorphism among clinical isolates. UL144 has strong nucleotide sequence homology with the human tumor necrosis factor-α (TNF-α) receptor family.[19] The UL146 ORF has a strong CXC cytokine homology.[19a] The regulation and function of many of these ORFs are still being determined. The structure of the HCMV genome makes it a member of the β group of human herpes viruses because it contains terminal repeat sequences that are complementary to each other. The HCMV genome contains a single origin of replication, and like all human herpes viruses, it encodes a DNA polymerase gene and a complete package of genes needed for its own DNA replication. Viral DNA polymerase is an important target for antiviral drugs, and all current therapies for CMV disease inhibit viral DNA polymerase as the final target.[5] CMV DNA polymerase is encoded by a CMV ORF designated UL54. CMV DNA polymerase is highly conserved with only a 4% occurrence of polymorphic nucleotide variation noted in clinical isolates[20] and has an important accessory protein, UL44, that enhances the processivity of DNA polymerase.[21] The UL54 and UL44 proteins form the functional complex of complete DNA polymerase in infected cells.

The CMV genome also encodes a protein phosphotransferase enzyme, the product of UL97, whose role in CMV DNA replication is not well understood.[22] This UL97 protein is able to phosphorylate ganciclovir to form ganciclovir monophosphate; this activation step is needed for ganciclovir to inhibit CMV DNA replication.[5,23,24] The role of UL97 in CMV replication is still being defined, but it has been shown to phosphorylate serine residues.[25] The UL97 protein may phosphorylate other proteins involved in DNA replication, and it can phosphorylate CMV UL144. The CMV UL97 protein phosphorylates and inactivates the cellular retinoblastoma tumor suppressor.[26]

Cytomegalovirus also contains many genes that encode proteins directly involved in downregulating the host immune system. One of the most important of these CMV proteins prevents cellular HLA-1 molecules from reaching the cell surface.[27] Thus, HLA-1 and CMV glycoproteins cannot form complexes on the cell surface to trigger recognition and destruction by CD8+ T lymphocytes, which enables the CMV genome to remain in infected cells and avoid immune destruction.

In the infectious virion, CMV double-stranded DNA is wrapped in a nucleoprotein core that is surrounded by matrix proteins and the pp65 antigen of CMV. The latter is important for diagnosis of CMV because it can be readily detected in the infected cells with immunofluorescence, immunoperoxidase, and other antigen detection methods.[28] A lipid envelope that surrounds the matrix and inner core contains viral glycoproteins that are involved in viral entry.

The cellular protein that serves as the specific receptor for CMV entry has not been identified, but CMV infects cells by a process of endocytosis. The CMV genome is uncoated within the cell, and the DNA protein core is transported to the nucleus of the cell. After synthesis of viral DNA polymerase, CMV replication occurs in the nuclei of infected cells and forms the large nuclear inclusions that are the hallmark of CMV infection in tissue culture and in infected cells, which represent aggregates of replicating CMV nucleoprotein cores. Recognition of these CMV nuclear inclusions is valuable in diagnosis of CMV infection.[29]

The ability of CMV to remain latent after infection contributes a great deal to serious CMV disease. Evidence for persistent CMV genomes and antigens exists in many tissues after initial infection, and CMV has been found in circulating mononuclear cells and in polymorphonuclear neutrophils.[30] CMV antigens have been detected in vascular endothelial cells; this site has been suggested as a cause of vascular inflammation and development of atherosclerosis. Detection of CMV intranuclear inclusions in renal epithelial cells and in pulmonary secretions provides evidence that CMV may persist in these tissues as well. The mechanisms that control latency are not known, but the ability of CMV to evade immune destruction of infected cells through downregulation of cell surface markers, such as HLA-1, may contribute to the capacity of the virus to remain undetected.[27] When immune suppression occurs in patients through HIV infection or immunosuppressive therapy, such as anti-lymphocyte antibody (OKT3) infusion,[31] CMV can reactivate and grow to high titers, producing end-organ disease.

In humans, a broad range of cell types are infected by HCMV, including epithelial cells, endothelial cells, neuronal cells, smooth muscle cells, and fibroblast monocytes and macrophages.[32] Recent work with endothelial cells has mapped a primary determinant of HCMV cell tropism to the UL131-128 locus.[33] Two messenger RNAs (mRNAs) are encoded by this locus, and they contain three ORFs: UL128, UL130 and UL131.[34] A mutation in any one of these three ORFs abolishes endothelial cell tropism.[33] Laboratory-adapted strains that do not efficiently infect endothelial cells consistently contain mutations in this region. The AD169 laboratory strain contains a single nucleotide change in the UL131 exon, and the Towne strain has a frame shift mutation in the carboxyl terminal region of UL130.[32,35] Neither of these laboratory strains is able to infect human umbilical vein endothelial cells (HUVECs), and when clinical strains are passaged in fibroblasts, as little as three passages can be sufficient to select for mutations in the UL131-128 locus.[33] These HCMV genes (UL131-128) are indispensable for growth in endothelial cells. HCMV-infected vascular endothelial cells have also been shown to be the source of HCMV infection of neutrophils.[36] When polymorphonuclear leukocytes pass through vascular tissue to reach the site of an infection, they become infected with HCMV present in the vascular endothelial cells.[36] Intact genes UL131-128 are necessary for this transfer to polymorphonuclear leukocytes.[33] Repair of the UL131 in AD169 allows CMV to infect endothelial and epithelial cells.[35]

Previous claims that CMV had oncogenic properties are now regarded with great skepticism. CMV is not associated with immortalization of cells in culture or with enhanced proliferation of cell DNA; rather, CMV infection may be associated with cellular arrest or decreased growth. CMV is not closely linked to any tumor in patients with immunocompromise and is distinguished from the oncogenic association of viruses such as Epstein-Barr virus (see Chapter 139).

Laboratory Diagnosis

The laboratory diagnosis of CMV infection depends on growth of the virus from urine or other body fluids or on demonstration of virion components such as viral antigens or viral DNA. Diagnosis almost always depends on laboratory confirmation and cannot be made on clinical grounds alone. The first useful laboratory test relied on the detection of large nuclear inclusion–bearing cells in the urine sediment.[29] This test was particularly useful for the newborn period, and

the associated disease was called *cytomegalic inclusion disease of infancy*. Growth of virus in human fibroblast cultures (MRC-5 cells) was laborious, and several weeks were needed for cell cultures to grow the virus. The culture technique could be greatly accelerated with the use of "shell vials" of cultured cells in which immediate early antigens were detected through the use of monoclonal antibodies.[28,37]

Direct detection of antigens in neutrophils with a monoclonal antibody against the CMV matrix protein pp65 has proved particularly useful.[38] This test provides a direct measure of the presence of CMV and can detect CMV antigen in the spinal fluid of patients with CMV polyradiculopathy syndrome and in the peripheral blood of patients with immunocompromise. Other methods for detection of CMV DNA or RNA have used labeled viral nucleic acid probes and nucleic acid hybridization in body fluids or tissue specimens.[1,39,40]

Polymerase chain reaction (PCR), which uses primers in the gene that encodes CMV immediate early antigen[41] or in the CMV DNA polymerase,[42] has provided a very sensitive technique for detection of CMV. PCR can detect small amounts of CMV DNA in many body fluids. It has been useful for the detection of CMV DNA in the cerebrospinal fluid of patients with CMV encephalitis or CMV polyradiculopathy syndrome.[43,44]

Three important papers have described the use of PCR for detection of CMV DNA in the blood of patients with AIDS; these findings reveal that the presence of CMV DNA could predict the development of CMV retinitis several months later.[45-47] Although all three studies used different PCR techniques, they showed remarkable agreement, with a positive predictive value of approximately 60% in correlation of the presence of CMV DNA with the subsequent development of clinical disease. Quantitative PCR has also been used to show that a high quantitative number of CMV DNA copies per milliliter of plasma was correlated with CMV disease activity in patients with AIDS.[48] The PCR assay for CMV DNA is also revolutionizing the approach to the management of CMV disease in liver, kidney, and bone marrow transplant recipients (see subsequent discussion).[49] With the availability of effective antiviral therapy, one goal of management is prevention of CMV disease through the use of the PCR assay to detect CMV DNA in plasma before end-organ disease has developed. Antiviral therapy can then be used to lower CMV DNA levels and prevent the development of CMV end-organ disease. This approach has been labeled *preemptive therapy*.[50] CMV antigen detection in cerebrospinal fluid cells and cerebrospinal fluid DNA levels determined with PCR have provided comparable information on the course of antiviral therapy for CMV infection of the central nervous system (CNS).[51] Another study has suggested that prophylactic treatment with ganciclovir may be better than CMV antigen-guided preemptive therapy in prevention of CMV pneumonia during the first 100 days after transplantation.[52] Additional comparative studies on the use of assays in plasma and in neutrophils are needed to assess their relative merits in different clinical conditions.

Clinical laboratories are rapidly adopting kit-based molecular technology for diagnosis of active CMV disease. Kits are based on PCR or on a solution hybridization capture assay.[53] Technology based on nucleic acid sequence-based amplification (NASBA), although promising,[16] is not widely used at the present time.

A research kit-based assay that uses PCR technology is the COBAS Amplicor CMV Monitor (Roche Molecular Diagnostics, Pleasanton, Calif). This assay uses plasma and is based on the coamplification of a 365-base pair sequence in the amino terminus of the CMV DNA polymerase gene and on a quantitation standard of a known concentration. The assay detects a range of 400 and 100,000 copies per milliliter. Several studies in a variety of populations susceptible to CMV infection have shown high sensitivity and specificity of this assay in detection of the presence of CMV DNA levels in blood.[54-57]

The Hybrid Capture CMV DNA Assay version 2.0 (Digene, Gaithersburg, MD) is a rapid signal-amplified solution hybridization assay that uses RNA probes for CMV DNA present in leukocytes and antibodies to capture the resulting RNA-DNA hybrids and expresses results as picograms per milliliter. As with the COBAS Amplicor, several studies have shown high sensitivity and specificity of this assay in detection of blood levels of CMV DNA in a variety of patient groups.[58,59]

Although data are accumulating to support the usefulness of these assays for the early detection of CMV disease, it is still not clear whether these tests are equally effective in predicting disease or response to therapy.[60-65] Two studies that compared the properties of the Digene Hybrid Capture Assay (2.0) with those of the quantitative COBAS Amplicor in a cohort of renal transplant recipients noted a correlation between the results with each assay. However, 8% to 9% discordance between results was observed within each group independently. Both studies noted a lower detection limit with the Digene 2.0. Tong and associates[60] observed that discordance was more likely to occur at the beginning or toward the end of infection. In this population, a CMV DNA cutoff of more than 40,000 copies/mL was estimated as specific for CMV disease. The sensitivity for this cutoff is only 29.4% (COBAS Amplicor) and 41.2% (Digene), but it may be increased to 76.5% and 82.4%, respectively, if the cutoff to predict disease is decreased to more than 1000 copies/mL. Because this cutoff was found to be associated with a low positive predictive value (46.2% [COBAS Amplicor] and 56% [Digene]), the authors suggest that this value should be used only to rule out CMV disease for this specific population.[66]

In a study that involved specimens from allogeneic stem cell transplant recipients, the Digene Hybrid Capture Assay was compared with the Roche CMV polymerase PCR assay and a Qiagen real time light cycler PCR assay on plasma specimens and whole virus standards. The authors concluded that the PCR assays showed better speed, sensitivity, and specificity. One study,[62] which prospectively analyzed the clinical use of weekly COBAS Amplicor assays and the pp65 antigenemia assay for prediction of the development of active CMV disease in 97 consecutive liver transplant recipients, found that CMV viral loads were highly correlated with levels of CMV antigenemia. Twenty-one patients were found to have active CMV disease. The optimal cutoff for CMV copy load to predict disease was determined to be in the range of 2000 to 5000 copies/mL; at more than 5000 copies/mL, 18 of 21 of cases of CMV would have been predicted. This cutoff was associated with a sensitivity of 85.7%, a specificity of 86.8%, a positive predictive value (PPV) of 64.3%, and a negative predictive value (NPV) of 95.7%. The optimal cutoff for antigenemia was determined to be in the range of four to six positive cells per slide (PPV, 50% to 60.7%; NPV, 96.6% to 94.2%). A second independent study observed that high peak viral loads (>10,000 copies/mL) were consistently associated with donor positive/recipient negative (D+/R–) patients after liver transplantation with active CMV infection.[63] Peak viral loads varied in symptomatic infections of D+/R+ and D–/R+ patients. Because peak viral loads of asymptomatic, non-treated D+/R+ patients did not exceed 5500 copies/mL, the optimal cutoff for this particular population was suggested to be 5000 copies/mL. A study of 51 allogeneic stem cell transplant recipients indicated that quantitative PCR detection occurred earlier than pp65 antigenemia and was useful clinically.[67] In a prospective study that compared a quantitative CMV PCR (COBAS) in plasma and pp65 antigenemia in patients after allogeneic stem cell transplantation (SCT), low levels of CMV viral load were found to be frequently detected after allogeneic SCT. In a prospective longitudinal study of 38 patients who were at risk for CMV infection after SCT, 534 blood samples were obtained with weekly monitoring for CMV infection for 100 days after SCT with simultaneous analysis of pp65 Ag and PCR. That study found that 74% of patients had active CMV infection within 100 days from SCT with use of those assays to detect CMV viral load in blood samples. Three patients (7.9%) had CMV gastrointestinal (GI) disease develop. The study concluded that plasma CMV DNA PCR (COBAS) and pp65 Ag assays were effective in detection of CMV infection, but discordance between both methods was frequently observed. The authors concluded that plasma CMV DNA PCR and pp65 Ag assays were complimentary for diagnosis and management of CMV infection.[68]

Additional comparative studies on the use of these assays in plasma and neutrophils are needed to assess their relative merits in different clinical conditions.[69-71] As new study findings become available, rapid laboratory diagnosis and its correlation with clinical conditions and outcomes will significantly change the clinical management of multiple aspects of CMV disease.

Cultivation of Cytomegalovirus

Human CMV has been cultured in human cells only, and previous claims that CMV could be grown in other animal cells have not been substantiated.[72] Although CMV can be readily cultured in human fibroblast cells, growth is characteristically slow. One to 4 weeks of growth may be necessary for the development of typical cytopathic changes in tissue culture. CMV produces characteristic infected cells, which are large and rounded and contain "ground-glass"–appearing inclusions in the cytoplasm. These infected cells, the hallmark of CMV, indicate the presence of CMV in the sample.[29]

Cytomegalovirus can be readily isolated from urine, mouth swabs, buffy coat, cervical tissue, and tissues obtained with biopsy or at post-mortem examination. Virus is demonstrable even in the presence of neutralizing antibody.

Cytomegalovirus is not usually cultured from healthy adults and may be difficult to culture from blood, even in patients with immunocompromise. Virus may be cultured from the cervix in healthy women[73] and from semen in healthy homosexual men.[74]

The growth of CMV from throat, urine, or blood is an abnormal finding, but only culture from blood is highly suggestive of a pathogenic CMV infection because CMV in throat or urine is frequently associated with asymptomatic infection. Patients who recover from acute CMV mononucleosis may shed CMV in the urine and throat for several weeks. Patients with immunosuppression may also shed CMV in throat washings or bronchoalveolar lavage. In the latter cases, histologic changes, such as intranuclear inclusions, are needed for the establishment of a diagnosis of CMV pneumonitis.[29]

Cytomegalovirus Mononucleosis

Primary infection with CMV in a young adult can produce an infectious *mononucleosis* syndrome with fever, lymphadenopathy, and relative lymphocytosis. Seventy-nine percent of infectious mononucleosis is estimated to be caused by the Epstein-Barr virus (EBV; see Chapter 139); most of the other 21% is caused by acute CMV infection.[75] Heterophil agglutinin test results are negative in CMV mononucleosis and usually positive in EBV mononucleosis. Another distinguishing feature of diseases caused by these two viruses is a sore throat with enlarged exudate-covered tonsils, which is more common with EBV infection. CMV-induced infectious mononucleosis syndrome has been called *typhoidal* because symptoms may be systemic in nature, fever may predominate, and few signs of enlarged lymph nodes or splenomegaly may be noted.[75]

The hematologic hallmark of infectious mononucleosis syndrome is a relative lymphocytosis, in which more than 50% of the peripheral white blood cell differential is composed of lymphocytes. Of these, 10% or more should comprise atypical lymphocytes that possess abnormal nuclei and exhibit rosetting around red blood cells.

The landmark study that defined the clinical features of infectious mononucleosis was an 8-year prospective study of 494 patients by investigators from Finland.[75] In that study, 79% of patients had positive heterophil agglutinin results and acute EBV infection; 73 patients older than 15 years of age had a negative heterophil response, and 33 of these patients (45%) had CMV infection. The first serum, which was taken 3 to 20 days after the onset of disease, showed that 11 of 19 patients were seronegative (titer, ≤1:4) and had a rise in complement-fixing antibodies. The peak titer was reached 4 to 7 weeks after the onset of disease. The presence of CMV in the urine was documented in 10 of 12 patients tested. This analysis led to the conclusion that CMV mononucleosis represents a primary infection in persons who were previously seronegative. The age range of infected patients was 18 to 66 years, with a median age of 29 years (higher than in the group with EBV-induced mononucleosis). Fever was common in all patients and persisted for 9 to 35 days (mean, 19 days). Lymphocytosis in these patients ranged from 55% to 86%; 12% to 55% of total leukocytes were atypical lymphocytes. In the patients with CMV infection, pharyngitis and tonsillitis were rare. Enlargement of both lymph nodes and spleen was not a prominent feature of CMV mononucleosis, although this can occur. Low-level liver function abnormalities are regular features of CMV mononucleosis and can be an important clue to diagnosis. The occurrence of severe hepatitis or jaundice is rare.

Cytomegalovirus mononucleosis may occur without a clear source, but "kissing" and direct transfer of infected lymphocytes and polymorphonuclear cells is sometimes identified as a source. Other forms of intimate sexual contact are also important in the transmission of CMV.

The most clearly identified source for transmission of CMV and EBV is blood transfusion. CMV is also readily transmitted with transfusion of leukocytes alone.[76] The greater the number of units of transfused blood a patient receives, the greater is the risk of infection from this source. When large amounts of blood have been transfused, CMV should be considered as a potential cause of postoperative fever. The risk of transmission of CMV from blood has been greatly reduced with the screening of blood for the presence of antibodies and with elimination of units from seropositive donors.[73,77]

In both CMV-induced and EBV-induced mononucleosis, laboratory abnormalities or transient immunologic aberrations can occur. These abnormalities include cold agglutinins, rheumatoid factor, mixed cryoglobulinemia, antinuclear antibodies, and anticomplementary activity.[75]

A study of 124 patients used elevated CMV immunoglobulin M (IgM) levels (>300 U/mL) as a measure of acute CMV infection; patients presented with fever, malaise, jaundice, hepatitis, sweats, or a mononucleosis-like illness, and a detailed analysis of symptoms was provided. The specificity of the CMV IgM assay was confirmed in every case with the use of a CMV immunoglobulin G (IgG) avidity assay. The authors were careful to include patients who exhibited the absence of EBV infection, hepatitis A, antibody to hepatitis B core antigen, *Toxoplasma gondii*, IgM antibodies, and rheumatoid factor. The study examined samples obtained from 7630 patients in the United Kingdom from December 1998 to June 2001 and found 106 patients with CMV infection who were treated by general practitioners and 18 who were hospitalized. In this group, the most frequent symptoms were malaise (67%), fever (46%), and sweats (46%). The most frequent laboratory finding was abnormal liver function test results (69%). Relapsing illness was observed in 12% of patients; symptoms persisted for up to 32 weeks, with a mean duration of symptoms of 7.8 weeks. No significant differences were seen between patients who were treated by general practitioners and those who were hospitalized, except that the same symptoms were more severe in those who were hospitalized. Four patients were pregnant at the time of acute CMV infection. Three delivered healthy children, but one child had severe intrauterine growth retardation and a severe hearing impairment. This study expands the range of clinical symptoms associated with laboratory-documented acute CMV infection.[78]

Associated Complications

A series of associated findings can occur with CMV infection; these may be the initial manifestation of disease even in the healthy host. The following sections describe these complications.

INTERSTITIAL PNEUMONIA

Interstitial pneumonia is the most severe complication of CMV disease in the patient with hematopoietic stem cell transplantation (HSCT), and it may also occur uncommonly in CMV-induced mononucleosis in the healthy host. In the large series from Finland,[75] CMV pneumonitis occurred in two of 33 patients. The main finding is one of interstitial infiltrates on chest radiography that eventually clear (Fig. 138-1), which is in sharp distinction to the finding of CMV pneumonitis in

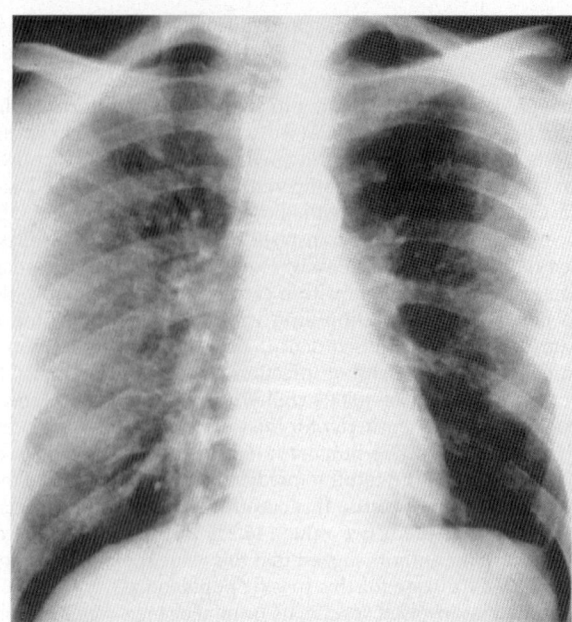

Figure 138-1 Bilateral interstitial pneumonitis caused by cytomegalovirus in bone marrow transplant recipient.

HSCT recipients, in whom CMV pneumonitis has a high mortality rate even with aggressive antiviral therapy. CMV pneumonitis that occurs with CMV mononucleosis is usually mild, and no treatment is necessary.

HEPATITIS

Hepatitis is commonly associated with CMV mononucleosis, but it is usually mild and is rarely symptomatic in the patient with immunocompetence. A 21-year-old patient with immunocompetence has been described in whom infectious hepatitis was suspected and who had a large and tender liver but no atypical lymphocytes. CMV was isolated from the urine, and a significant rise in complement-fixing antibodies was observed, which confirmed the diagnosis of acute CMV infection.[79] Granulomatous hepatitis may also be an initial manifestation of CMV infection that accompanies mononucleosis.[80] In these patients, fever, vomiting, and a profound atypical lymphocytosis of nearly 50% are noted. CMV is isolated from the throat, and a diagnostic rise in complement-fixing antibodies is seen. Liver biopsy in these patients reveals a resolving hepatitis with mononuclear cells infiltrating portal areas, along with microscopic granulomas with giant cells. In the setting of acute CMV infection, hepatitis usually resolves fully. When scattered microscopic granulomas are found on liver biopsy, CMV infection should be considered.

GUILLAIN-BARRÉ SYNDROME

The association of *Guillain-Barré syndrome* with CMV mononucleosis was initially described in 1971 when nine patients with acute CMV mononucleosis presented with polyneuritis that was characterized by sensory and motor weakness in the extremities. Cranial nerve involvement was also common, and four patients were treated in the respiratory unit.[81] Return of sensation was followed by motor improvement, and complete recovery occurred in about 3 months for most patients.

In a large series of 94 cases of Guillian-Barré syndrome, acute CMV infection was documented in 10 patients.[82] In nine of these patients, a high IgM immunofluorescent antibody titer was found on the initial specimen and showed a decline that was diagnostic for acute CMV infection by the time of discharge. The complement fixation antibody titer was already elevated in these patients, and no further rises were observed. All patients had atypical lymphocytes in a blood smear, and all recovered.

The strongest evidence that CMV may be a direct cause of polyradiculopathy and myopathy has been observed in patients with AIDS, in whom CMV inclusions have been shown in the nuclei of Schwann cells in association with a syndrome of motor weakness that leads to loss of bowel and bladder control (see subsequent discussion).[83]

MENINGOENCEPHALITIS

In association with CMV-induced infectious mononucleosis, *meningoencephalitis* has been infrequently reported in patients with immunocompetence.[84] Such patients may also have motor and sensory weakness similar to polyradiculopathy. Severe headache, photophobia, lethargy, and pyramidal tract findings are features that are more indicative of meningoencephalitis. The spinal fluid usually shows a moderate number of lymphocytes. In both CMV meningoencephalitis and CMV polyradiculopathy, the presence of CMV DNA detected with PCR can be helpful to the clinician in diagnosis.[43,44]

MYOCARDITIS

Complications of CMV-induced mononucleosis can include myocardial involvement or *myocarditis*. In three of eight cases, inversion of T waves was noted.[85] One patient was a 14-year-old boy who died with serologic evidence of acute CMV infection, hepatitis, myocarditis, and consumptive coagulopathy. Another report described a 43-year-old woman with immunocompetence with acquired myocarditis, heart failure, encephalitis, hepatitis, and adrenal insufficiency.[86] At autopsy, CMV was cultured from the adrenal glands. In children with congenital CMV infection, myocardial involvement is rarely reported.

THROMBOCYTOPENIA AND HEMOLYTIC ANEMIA

Thrombocytopenia and *hemolytic anemia* occur regularly in children with congenital CMV disease and occasionally as a complication of CMV mononucleosis in healthy adults. A 33-year-old man with serologic evidence of acute CMV infection and viruria had a profound decrease in platelet count to 500/mm³, a hemolytic anemia and hemoglobin of 3.6 g/dL, and a reticulocyte count of 12%.[87] The patient had generalized purpura and bleeding gums and recovered completely with prednisone treatment. In a 26-year-old man with acute CMV infection who presented with thrombocytopenia and purpura, decreased red cell survival and elevated reticulocyte count were seen.[88]

SKIN ERUPTIONS

Maculopapular and *rubelliform rashes* may also occur in the setting of CMV mononucleosis. These rashes may develop after administration of ampicillin[89] and are thought to result from immunologic reactions to cellular antigens that are uncovered or expressed in association with

the acute CMV infection. In an unusual report, a 40-year-old man with acute CMV viremia and viruria acquired epidermolysis 8 weeks after the onset of hepatitis.[90] Thus, the skin manifestations of acute CMV infection are usually mild but can occasionally be severe.

■ Cytomegalovirus Infection in Patients with Acquired Immunodeficiency Syndrome

The profound immunodeficiency caused by infection with human immunodeficiency virus–1 (HIV-1) results in defects in cellular immunity to many common infectious agents, including CMV. Coinfection with CMV has been noted in more than 90% of homosexual men with HIV-1 infection by serologic status.[91] A high percentage of homosexual men also have CMV that is detected in the urine, even in the absence of HIV-1 infection.[92] Patients who are infected with HIV-1 in whom CD4 cells are decreased to fewer than 100 cells/mm³ have a significantly increased risk for the development of serious CMV disease.

Cytomegalovirus is the most common viral opportunistic infection in patients with AIDS; it has been estimated that 21% to 44% of patients with AIDS acquired CMV disease in the era before the availability of highly active antiretroviral therapy (HAART).[4] CMV retinitis, by far the most common form of CMV disease, usually occurs when the CD4 cell count falls to less than 50 cells/mm³.[93] Autopsy studies have shown that up to 81% of patients with HIV had clinical or pathologic evidence of CMV disease by the time they died and 32% had CMV retinitis.[94] Retinal disease as a result of CMV occurs only rarely in patients with bone marrow or solid organ transplantation. CMV retinitis causes a complete-thickness infection through the retinal cells and results in progressive retinal destruction that leads to blindness within 4 to 6 months. Now that HAART is able to suppress HIV, the incidence of CMV end-organ disease has decreased by more than 80%,[95] which has greatly changed the management of CMV retinitis, discussed in detail in Chapter 129.[4] The most likely reason for the reduction in CMV disease is the improvement in CMV-specific immune responses that results from HAART.[96]

Cytomegalovirus retinitis is diagnosed predominantly on the basis of its clinical appearance. The characteristic appearance is a white fluffy retinal infiltrate that occurs with several areas of hemorrhage (Fig. 138-2). It can also appear as a granular white area without hemorrhage. This form must be distinguished from cotton wool spots, which are seen on the retinal tissue of patients with AIDS and are unrelated to CMV.

Initially, treatment of CMV retinitis included intravenous ganciclovir for 3 weeks at a dose of 7.5 to 15 mg/kg/d in three divided doses for 14 to 21 days, followed by a maintenance regimen of 5 to 6 mg/kg/d for 5 to 7 days per week[97] to prevent relapse. Oral ganciclovir, despite its low oral bioavailability (8%),[98] administered at a dose of 1000 mg taken three times a day, was found to be nearly equivalent to intravenous ganciclovir in prevention of progression and preservation

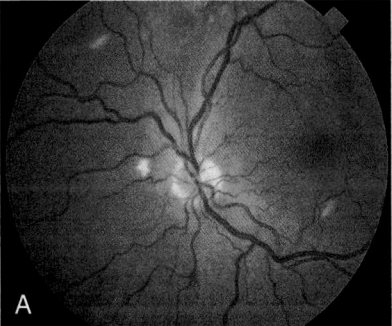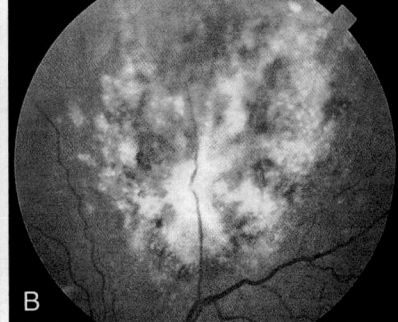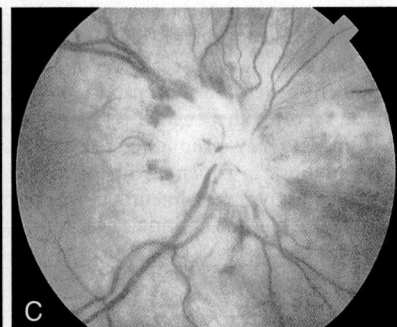

Figure 138-2 Cytomegalovirus (CMV) retinitis. A, Early disease with retinal involvement along blood vessels. **B,** Extensive retinal damage and retinal hemorrhages. **C,** CMV retinitis with papillitis.

of vision, particularly if the initial CMV retinitis was not sight-threatening.[99] Valganciclovir has supplanted oral ganciclovir for the treatment of CMV infection (see subsequent discussion).

A sustained-release ganciclovir implant device plus oral ganciclovir (4.5 g/d) to prevent infection in the other eye has significant advantages when used as therapy for CMV retinitis. This device is implanted surgically in the eye and does not interfere with vision. The implant releases a high intravitreal concentration of ganciclovir that maintains adequate levels of drug for 8 to 10 months.[99] New implants that can release ganciclovir for up to 2 years are now in use. The ganciclovir implant plus oral ganciclovir was able to prevent relapse of CMV retinitis for about 270 days in 25% of patients.[100] This outcome was far superior to that seen in patients on intravenous ganciclovir alone and compared favorably with that in patients who received implant and intravenous ganciclovir. The incidence rate of severe complications of ganciclovir toxicity, namely, marrow suppression leading to neutropenia and thrombocytopenia, was also decreased by approximately 40% in patients receiving oral ganciclovir.[99] However, in patients who received oral ganciclovir at a dose of 4.5 g/d, a higher rate of neutropenia was seen than in those who received either intravenous ganciclovir or placebo, limiting this effective dose for some patients.[101] Another important benefit among patients who received oral ganciclovir at a dose of 4.5 g/d along with the ganciclovir implant was a statistically significant decrease in the occurrence of Kaposi's sarcoma associated with AIDS.[101] Kaposi's sarcoma is closely linked with human herpes virus 8 (see Chapter 141), and this virus is sensitive to ganciclovir in vitro.

CENTRAL NERVOUS SYSTEM

In patients with AIDS, the most common CNS infection caused by CMV is polyradiculopathy.[83] This syndrome has a characteristic onset of ascending weakness in the lower extremities associated with a loss of deep tendon reflexes and ultimately loss of bowel and bladder control. The syndrome frequently begins as low back pain with a radicular or perianal radiation, followed in 1 to 6 weeks by a progressive flaccid paralysis. Marked pathologic changes are found in the cauda equina and the lumbosacral nerve roots with distinct mononuclear cell infiltrate destruction of axons, along with CMV inclusion in Schwann cells and epithelial cells.[83] Lumbar puncture reveals a characteristic picture of polymorphonuclear cells, mildly elevated protein, and modest lowering of cerebrospinal fluid sugar levels. The findings are frequently mistaken for those of bacterial meningitis, but bacterial culture results are negative. The diagnosis is usually made with detection of CMV DNA with PCR in the spinal fluid[43,44] or with culture of CMV from the spinal fluid.

Treatment with ganciclovir has improved weakness and polyradiculopathy in a few patients who were treated with ganciclovir alone or with ganciclovir and foscarnet early in the disease,[102,103] but treatment with ganciclovir alone generally has been disappointing.[104] Some of the poor treatment results may be because only about one third of the plasma concentration of intravenous ganciclovir is found in the cerebrospinal fluid; the CNS may represent a privileged site where only low concentrations of ganciclovir penetrate.[105]

The current favored treatment for CMV polyradiculopathy is early therapy with ganciclovir and foscarnet, although no vigorous clinical trials to document benefit have been published. Anecdotal observations have been reported that suggest that CMV meningoencephalitis in patients with AIDS may respond to ganciclovir and foscarnet.[106]

Other CNS findings in patients with AIDS include mononeuritis multiplex and painful peripheral neuropathy, which have been attributed to CMV.[107] The benefits of antiviral therapy for these conditions are uncertain.

GASTROINTESTINAL TRACT

Infection of the gastrointestinal tract with CMV had been frequent in patients with AIDS before the era of HAART. CMV can cause ulcers in the esophagus, and patients present with pain and difficulty swallowing. Through endoscopic examination, shallow ulcers are seen. The diagnosis of CMV esophagitis is made with demonstration of intranuclear inclusions on biopsy specimens of the ulcers or with culture of CMV from biopsy tissue.

Patients with AIDS may present with explosive watery diarrhea as a result of CMV colitis. Fever is common with CMV colitis, and occasionally, bloody diarrhea may be present. The diagnosis is made with sigmoidoscopy, which reveals plaque-like pseudomembranes, numerous erosions, and serpiginous ulcers.[108]

Cytomegalovirus colitis may be seen as a mass lesion that produces partial obstruction or as lesions that resemble Kaposi's sarcoma.[109] CMV may be present in the colon with other pathogens such as *Mycobacterium avium* complex and *Cryptosporidium*. With severe CMV colitis, perforation and gangrene have been described, although CMV infection alone may not be the only condition found in association with these findings. Diagnosis of CMV colitis is made with biopsy, which shows typical CMV inclusion bodies, or with culture of CMV from biopsy material. CMV inclusion bodies are usually seen in the mucosal epithelium[108] or in mucosal crypts.[109] The first report of successful treatment of CMV colitis described the use of ganciclovir in 1986[110]; this was followed by a placebo-controlled study with intravenous ganciclovir at a dose of 5 mg/kg for 14 days, in which a reduction was observed in the frequency of CMV-infected colonic and urinary cultures in the ganciclovir treatment group compared with the placebo group ($P = .03$ and $P < .001$, respectively). Colonoscopy scores improved more frequently in those who received ganciclovir (23% of patients) than in the placebo group (9%; $P = .03$).[111] However, diarrhea persisted at the end of treatment in both groups. These results suggest that treatment for 14 days may be inadequate for the colon to heal and diarrhea to resolve. In another study of bone marrow transplantation patients with CMV colitis, ganciclovir had no apparent clinical benefit.[112] Cultures became negative with ganciclovir treatment, but gastrointestinal symptoms improved in both the ganciclovir-treated and placebo-treated groups. No evidence has been found that maintenance therapy with ganciclovir is useful in prevention of relapse of CMV colitis.

Other parts of the digestive system can be infected with CMV. Patients with AIDS may acquire acute CMV pancreatitis.[113] Cholecystitis has been associated with the presence of CMV in the bile duct, gallbladder, and biliary tree,[113] including acalculous cholecystitis, papillary stenosis, and sclerosing cholingitis.[114]

Antiviral Therapy

Three antiviral drugs that act to inhibit the viral DNA polymerase have been shown to be effective in the treatment of CMV end-organ disease and have been approved for use in the United States: ganciclovir, foscarnet, and cidofovir (see Chapters 41 and 129). Another drug, valacyclovir, appears to delay the time to retinitis progression in patients with CMV retinitis.[115] An antisense inhibitor of CMV, fomivirsen, can be used for direct injection into intravitreal fluid for the treatment of CMV retinitis and has also been approved by the U.S. Food and Drug Administration (FDA).[116] These drugs have been used to treat many forms of CMV disease in patients with AIDS and in other patients with immunocompromise, for example, recipients of bone marrow transplants or solid organ transplants. Individual drugs that have been useful in the treatment of CMV-associated disease are discussed in the following sections.

GANCICLOVIR

Ganciclovir, a nucleoside analogue of guanosine and a homologue of acyclovir, was the first antiviral drug shown to be effective in the treatment of CMV disease in humans.[5,117-119] It inhibits all the herpes viruses and blocks transformation of normal cord blood lymphocytes by EBV.[120,121]

For antiviral activity, ganciclovir requires phosphorylation by a virus-specific enzyme, but CMV does not have a thymidine kinase enzyme homologue to the herpes simplex virus thymidine kinase. The phosphotransferase product of the UL97 gene of CMV converts ganciclovir to ganciclovir monophosphate. Monophosphate is then phosphorylated by cellular enzymes to triphosphate. Ganciclovir triphosphate, a potent inhibitor of the CMV DNA polymerase enzyme, is a competitive inhibitor of the incorporation of deoxyguanosine triphosphate into elongating viral DNA. After cleavage of the pyrophosphate, ganciclovir monophosphate is incorporated into the end of the growing chain of viral DNA, greatly slowing replication.[122] Ganciclovir is not an absolute chain terminator, and short fragments of CMV DNA continue to be synthesized.[123,124] All of the drug's antiviral effects are as result of its ability to inhibit the synthesis of CMV DNA and CMV replication by slowing the elongation of viral DNA.[5]

The half-life of ganciclovir triphosphate in CMV-infected cells is 16.5 hours, compared with only 2.5 hours for acyclovir triphosphate.[125] Although ganciclovir triphosphate is not as effective an inhibitor of CMV DNA polymerase as is acyclovir triphosphate, this concentration of ganciclovir triphosphate in CMV-infected cells is 10 times the concentration of acyclovir triphosphate.[125] The high level of ganciclovir triphosphate and its prolonged intracellular half-life make ganciclovir a more effective inhibitor than acyclovir of CMV replication in vivo.

VALGANCICLOVIR

Valganciclovir is the valine ester of ganciclovir; it has a much greater oral bioavailability than does ganciclovir (about 68% is absorbed compared with 6% to 8% for oral ganciclovir). A valine esterase in the human intestinal mucosa cleaves the valine, and ganciclovir enters the blood stream. Two 450-mg tablets orally (PO) result in blood levels that are equivalent to those attained with intravenous ganciclovir at a dose of 5 mg/kg/d. In a treatment study of CMV retinitis in patients with HIV, valganciclovir was found to be equivalent to intravenous ganciclovir for the treatment and maintenance of CMV retinitis in patients on HAART. The adverse effects of valganciclovir are similar to those of ganciclovir: mainly, neutropenia and thrombocytopenia.[126] Valganciclovir has supplanted oral ganciclovir because of its improved bioavailability and convenience.

Resistance to Ganciclovir
The major mechanism of CMV resistance to ganciclovir is the selection of mutants that are unable to phosphorylate ganciclovir. These viruses have mutations in two main regions of the UL97 protein. These are point mutations at codon 460 and point mutations or deletions around codons 590 to 596.[127,128] A mutation at codon 520 also confers an inability to phosphorylate ganciclovir.[129] Ganciclovir-resistant viruses that have mutations or deletions in regions of the UL97 protein that affect nucleotide binding and phosphate transfer have also been described.

Cytomegalovirus clinical isolates that were resistant to ganciclovir were first reported in 1989.[130] These isolates were taken from three patients with immunocompromise with CMV disease who had disease progression and died despite therapy and in whom all viral culture results remained positive. In a subsequent study of 72 patients with CMV retinitis who were receiving maintenance ganciclovir therapy, 80% became culture-negative after 3 months of treatment.[131] Among those who remained culture-positive, resistant CMV was isolated in 38% (with an overall incidence rate of 8%), and resistance was clearly associated with disease progression. Nine resistant strains of CMV were obtained from these 72 patients, and all failed to phosphorylate ganciclovir (Fig. 138-3).[132] All strains remained sensitive to foscarnet, a drug that acts directly on the viral DNA polymerase (see subsequent discussion).

Another mechanism of resistance to ganciclovir involves mutations that occur in the CMV DNA polymerase gene.[133] These have been identified in clinical isolates and are less common than mutations in

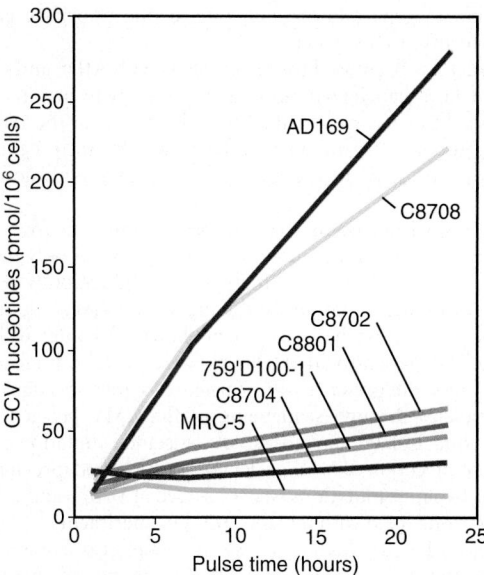

Figure 138-3 Intracellular phosphorylation by clinical isolates. *(From Stanat SC, Reardon JE, Erice A, et al. Ganciclovir-resistant cytomegalovirus clinical isolates: Modes of resistance to ganciclovir. Antimicrob Agents Chemother. 1991;35:2191-2197.)*

the UL97 gene.[134] CMV strains with mutations in both the UL97 gene and the CMV DNA polymerase gene have also been reported.[135] These exhibit a high degree of resistance with a 50% inhibiting concentration (IC_{50}) greater than 30 µmol/L. The inhibitory concentration of CMV clinical isolates that are sensitive to ganciclovir is 6.0 µmol/L or less.[135] Some clinical isolates reveal an intermediate sensitivity between 6 and 12 µmol/L. In a study undertaken to correlate mutations in either the UL97 gene or the DNA polymerase gene with resistance, the presence of a mutation in either gene was associated with an IC_{50} greater than 7 µmol/L.[134] In an analysis of variability in the DNA polymerase gene of CMV, among 40 clinical isolates that were all sensitive to ganciclovir and foscarnet, less than 4% variability was found. No mutations were found in highly conserved regions of the viral DNA polymerase in wild-type isolates, which indicates that mutations that occur in these highly conserved regions are more likely to be a result of selection by antiviral drugs.[136]

Of patients treated with ganciclovir for CMV retinitis over a prolonged period, 27% showed evidence of ganciclovir resistance after 9 months.[137] The detection of cytomegalovirus resistant to ganciclovir in the blood or urine of a patient with CMV retinitis was associated with an increased risk of adverse ocular outcomes.[138]

In the era of HAART, the incidence rate of drug-resistant CMV in the setting of AIDS has decreased to 5% per year because of more effective control of CMV with combination antiretroviral therapy.[139] In solid organ transplant recipients, the highest rate of drug resistance occurs when a CMV seronegative recipient receives a donor organ from a CMV seropositive donor (D+/R−). Resistance is more common after lung or kidney-pancreas transplantation.[139-142]

FOSCARNET

Foscarnet, a pyrophosphate analogue that binds directly to the DNA polymerase of CMV and other herpes viruses (see Chapter 41), is a reversible competitive inhibitor that does not become incorporated into elongating viral DNA. Foscarnet must be present in high concentrations inside the cell to remain in contact with the DNA polymerase enzyme and inhibit DNA polymerase activity. When the intracellular concentration of foscarnet decreases, foscarnet no longer binds to the DNA polymerase and viral DNA synthesis resumes.[143] Ganciclovir-resistant strains of CMV that have a mutation or a deletion in the UL97 protein kinase gene and are not able to phosphorylate ganciclovir remain sensitive to foscarnet.

Foscarnet has been used to treat patients with AIDS and CMV retinitis who have ganciclovir-resistant virus or who are intolerant of ganciclovir[144]; its use has resulted in stabilization of the retinitis and healing. Patients must be on long-term maintenance regimens with intravenous foscarnet to prevent the relapse or progression of CMV retinitis.

Cytomegalovirus strains that exhibit resistance to foscarnet have been reported, with mutations within the CMV DNA polymerase gene at codons 711 and 714[145] in the highly conserved region II of the polymerase. Additional mutations in the highly conserved regions VI and III of the polymerase have also been shown to confer resistance to foscarnet.[146] In patients with AIDS who were treated with foscarnet for CMV retinitis, the presence of foscarnet resistance was detected in 30 clinical isolates through sequencing of the CMV *pol* gene in these isolates. Nine isolates had foscarnet resistance mutations; seven of these were at codon V781L or V715M, which had previously been reported. Two new mutations were observed at V787L and E756Q, and these were confirmed with marker transfer experiments.[146] The clinical significance of CMV foscarnet resistance was also assessed in these patients with CMV retinitis and AIDS. The phenotypic plaque reduction assay (PRA) with IC_{50} more than 400 mmol/L was found to correlate with genotypic resistance, whereas the DNA hybridization assay (DHA) for resistance showed that an IC_{50} more than 600 mmol/L correlated with the presence of resistance mutations. Sixteen of 18 isolates showed a concordant plaque reduction assay and DNA hybridization assay phenotype. In 44 patients treated with foscarnet, resistance to foscarnet increased the risk of retinitis progression (odds ratio, 148; *P* = .016). The incidence of foscarnet resistance after 6 months was 13%; after 12 months of therapy, it was 37%.[147] To date, the resistance mutations in the CMV DNA polymerase that confer resistance to foscarnet do not usually occur in regions of the polymerase that confer resistance to ganciclovir. One report described a clinical isolate that had a mutation in CMV DNA polymerase region III and exhibited resistance to foscarnet and ganciclovir.[148]

Foscarnet 90 mg/kg/d given intravenously in two divided doses had been shown to be equivalent to ganciclovir for the initial treatment of CMV retinitis,[149] but mortality among patients with AIDS was improved in those who received foscarnet. In a subsequent study of CMV retinitis in patients with AIDS, the survival benefit was not confirmed,[150] but the combination of ganciclovir and foscarnet was superior for the treatment of retinitis.

Foscarnet is associated with significant nephrotoxicity and metabolic toxicity.[130] Renal failure, hypocalcemia, hypomagnesemia, and hypophosphatemia are serious consequences of foscarnet therapy that can be effectively managed through close monitoring of serum creatinine levels and replacement of magnesium, calcium, and phosphate losses with oral supplements.

CIDOFOVIR

Cidofovir ([S]-1[3-hydroxy-2(phosphorylmethoxy) propyl] cytokine) is a nucleotide analogue of cytosine that has significant antiviral activity against CMV in vitro (see Chapter 41). The IC_{50} for cidofovir against CMV clinical isolates is 2.0 µmol/L.[151] Cidofovir contains a phosphonate group and does not need to be phosphorylated by a viral enzyme. It is therefore active against thymidine kinase–deficient herpes simplex virus[152] and cytomegalovirus, in which mutations in the UL97 gene confer resistance to ganciclovir. Cidofovir is converted by cellular enzymes to cidofovir triphosphate, which is the active inhibitor of the viral DNA polymerase. Cidofovir triphosphate has a long intracellular half-life and needs to be given only once weekly. The maximal tolerated dose is 5 mg/kg weekly given intravenously.[153] This dose is given weekly for 2 weeks for induction and then is given once every 2 weeks. The drug has been approved for treatment only for CMV retinitis in patients with AIDS. Cidofovir must be administered with oral probenecid (2 g) before each intravenous dose. The major toxicity of cidofovir

results from its uptake by the proximal convoluted renal tubular cells, which produces degeneration and necrosis of these cells that may be irreversible.[154] Patients with irreversible nephrotoxicity from cidofovir given without probenecid have needed dialysis. Probenecid prevents the uptake of cidofovir and spares the renal tubular cells from degenerative damage.

CROSS-RESISTANCE TO ANTIVIRAL DRUGS IN CYTOMEGALOVIRUS CLINICAL ISOLATES

All clinically approved systemic antiviral drugs act to inhibit the viral DNA polymerase as a final target. The possibility for cross resistance among all drugs that act on the viral DNA polymerase exists, but at present, distinct patterns appear to be emerging. An early study showed that resistance to ganciclovir in the viral DNA polymerase of herpes simplex virus could be overcome by an analogue of foscarnet, phosphonoactive acid, which suggests that drugs that act on the viral polymerase can act synergistically[155] to overcome resistance to drugs that act on the DNA polymerase. Synergistic activity of ganciclovir and foscarnet against CMV has been shown in vitro.[156] If a clinical isolate of CMV is highly resistant to ganciclovir (IC_{50} = 30 µmol/L) and contains mutations in both the UL97 and DNA polymerase genes, cross resistance to cidofovir may also be observed.[157,158] These isolates still remain sensitive to foscarnet. Cross resistance between ganciclovir and foscarnet has not been observed with one exception,[148] which may reflect the fact that ganciclovir and foscarnet bind to different regions of the viral DNA polymerase. Resistance mutations to antiviral drugs against CMV appear to cluster in three distinct regions on the DNA polymerase; significant overlap has not been observed (Fig. 138-4).[158]

MARIBAVIR

The UL97 protein is also the target of the antiviral drug *maribavir,* an L-ribofuranosyl nucleoside, which is a potent inhibitor of CMV replication by inhibition of DNA synthesis and egress of nucleocapsids from the nucleus of infected cells.[159] Maribavir strongly inhibits the kinase activity of the viral UL97. Maribavir is a competitive inhibitor with ATP for binding to the UL97.[160,161] Maribavir also inhibits phosphorylation and accumulation of EBV early antigen D, which is an essential cofactor in EBV replication.[162]

A phase II trial of maribavir in bone marrow transplant patients showed that maribavir prophylaxis after transplant was effective in preventing CMV disease and greatly decreased CMV infection compared with placebo.[163] This study of maribavir prophylaxis to prevent CMV infection in allogeneic stem cell transplant recipients was a randomized double-blind placebo controlled dose ranging study. Twenty-

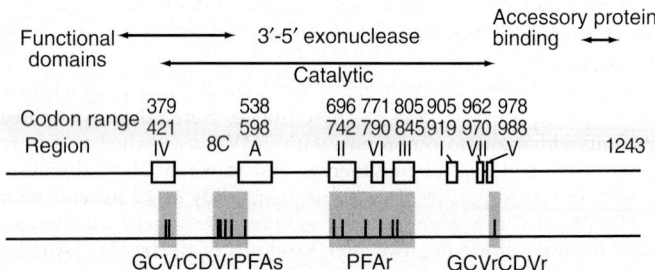

Figure 138-4 Map of the cytomegalovirus (CMV) DNA polymerase. CMV DNA polymerase shows functional domains and highly conserved regions of DNA nucleotide sequences (I to VII). *Shaded areas* are regions associated with drug-resistance phenotypes. Codons mapped to drug resistance in clinical isolates are shown as *bars.* CDV, Cidofovir; GCV, ganciclovir; PFA, foscarnet. (*Adapted from Chou S, Lurain NS, Weinberg A, et al. Interstrain variation in the human cytomegalovirus DNA polymerase sequence and its effect on genotype diagnosis of antiviral drug resistance. Antimicrob Agents Chemother. 1999;43:1500-1502.*)

eight patients received placebo, and 111 patients were randomized to receive maribavir at 100 mg twice daily, 400 mg once daily, or 400 mg twice daily. Within the first 100 days after transplantation, the incidence rate of CMV infection as determined with CMV pp65 antigen detection was lowered in each of the maribavir groups (15%, 19%, and 15%, respectively) compared with the placebo group (39%). The incidence rate of CMV infection based on plasma CMV DNA was lower in each of the maribavir groups (7%, 11%, and 19%, respectively) compared with the placebo group (45%). Three cases of CMV disease were found in placebo control subjects, and none in any maribavir patients. Maribavir was well tolerated, and the main side effects were a taste disturbance, nausea, and vomiting. Maribavir had no adverse effects on neutrophil or platelet counts, in contrast to ganciclovir treatment in the stem cell transplant population.[163] These results suggested that maribavir treatment may avoid the myelosuppression seen with ganciclovir. Large scale phase III trials of prophylaxis with maribavir in stem cell transplant recipients are under way.

When CMV develops resistance to maribavir, mutations are found in the UL97 protein but in regions that are distinct from mutations that confer ganciclovir resistance. Passage of laboratory strains of HCMV in the presence of maribavir resulted in a mutation L397R in UL97, which was associated with high-level MBV resistance.[164] Recently, passage of two clinical HCMV isolates in the presence of maribavir, beginning at 0.3 μmol/L and increasing to 1.5 μmol/L, resulted in resistant viruses with mutations at T409M and V353A of UL97 and a 20-fold increase in IC_{50} concentration needed to inhibit CMV replication.[161] When the T409M and V353A mutations were transferred to a CMV laboratory strain, the recombinant viruses also showed 15-fold and 80-fold increases, respectively, in maribavir resistance. Experiments with an error-prone strain of CMV resulted in confirmation of a new maribavir mutation at codon 411 (H411L or H411N). V353A and T409M are the most commonly selected UL97 mutations in vitro.[160] Combinations of UL97 mutations at codon 353 with those at codons 409 or 411 result in very high levels of maribavir resistance (>150-fold increased IC_{50}), which is similar to that observed with L397R alone.[160]

The known maribavir resistance mutations (codons 353, 397, 409, and 411) are located in the vicinity of the kinase ATP binding domain and are upstream of known ganciclovir (GCV) resistance mutations.[161] Structural models of UL97 kinase strongly suggest that maribavir is an ATP competitive kinase inhibitor.[160] The mutation at L397R has been suggested to affect maribavir binding either by affecting a contact point or by altering spacing between residues 353 and 409-411.[160] A lack of cross resistance between GCV-resistant isolates of CMV and those that are resistant to maribavir is generally reported. Recently identified maribavir resistant UL97 mutants have been tested against GCV and found to be susceptible to GCV.[159,160]

Prevention of Cytomegalovirus Disease

One of the most significant advances in the field was the demonstration that serious CMV disease could be prevented after bone marrow and solid organ transplantation with antiviral therapy. Prevention of life-threatening CMV pneumonia or other CMV-associated disease in recipients of bone marrow, heart, and liver transplants with administration of ganciclovir was clearly shown in four independent studies from 1991 to 1995. In bone marrow transplantation in particular, the development of interstitial pneumonia up to 120 days after the transplantation procedure is most frequently caused by CMV and has a very high mortality. In one of the studies from 1991, positive CMV culture results from any site at any time after bone marrow transplantation were used as an indication of when intravenous ganciclovir therapy should be started.[165] This was found to be more effective in the prevention of CMV pneumonia or death (97% efficacy) than was screening for CMV by means of bronchoalveolar lavage at day 35 (75% efficacy)[166] and gave a reliable indication of when ganciclovir should be

started. In a study in which CMV was detected with bronchoalveolar lavage in 20 patients who then received a full course of ganciclovir treatment, CMV pneumonia did not develop in any patient.[166] This strategy of prevention of CMV pneumonia was quickly confirmed in heart transplant recipients who were seropositive for CMV and received ganciclovir or placebo for 28 days after transplantation.[167] Among patients who received ganciclovir, the incidence rate of CMV disease at 120 days after transplantation was reduced from 46% to 9%. The incidence rate of CMV infection at day 60 was 56% in the placebo group and only 19% in the ganciclovir group.[167] Among 250 patients who received ganciclovir or acyclovir intravenously after liver transplantation, ganciclovir almost completely prevented CMV disease during a follow-up period of 120 days, whereas CMV infection occurred in 38% of acyclovir recipients.[168]

Oral ganciclovir was first shown to be effective in prevention of CMV disease in patients with AIDS who had fewer than 100 CD4 cells/mm^3 of blood. In a study that compared oral ganciclovir at a dose of 1000 mg every 8 hours with placebo in 725 patients, only 14% of patients in the ganciclovir group acquired CMV disease compared with 26% of those in the placebo group.[169] A trend toward longer survival time was noted in the ganciclovir group. Patients who received ganciclovir also had significantly fewer positive urine culture results for CMV than did those who received placebo, thus providing a virologic correlation with clinical benefit. Analysis of plasma CMV DNA in patients who acquired CMV disease showed that oral ganciclovir primarily benefitted those with very low plasma CMV DNA at baseline, and it was effective in prevention of CMV retinitis among those with a low copy number of CMV DNA at baseline.[48] If a high copy number of CMV DNA was present at baseline, little evidence indicated that oral ganciclovir would prevent CMV disease.[170] Because oral ganciclovir has a low oral bioavailability (6% to 8%), the maximum serum concentration is 1.2 μg/mL.[98] This concentration is probably too low to be active against high copy numbers of actively replicating CMV.

Oral ganciclovir has also been shown to be effective in the prevention of CMV disease among liver transplant recipients and in the reduction of mortality from CMV infection.[98,171] In kidney transplantation patients, oral ganciclovir has been effective in the prevention of CMV disease and in the reduction of CMV DNA levels in plasma. In patients who have received oral ganciclovir, the level of CMV DNA in plasma may be reduced to undetectable levels, but rejection of transplanted kidney still occurs. This suggests that CMV disease may not be the only reason for rejection of kidney transplants; rigorous control of CMV replication does not eliminate renal graft rejection.[172]

Valganciclovir represents a significant advance in the prevention of CMV disease and has replaced oral ganciclovir. The significant increase in oral bioavailability provided by valganciclovir over oral ganciclovir results in a dramatic antiviral effect. In a study that compared valganciclovir at 900 mg/d with oral ganciclovir at 1000 mg three times a day in 364 CMV D+/R− solid organ transplant patients, the patients who received valganciclovir had an incidence rate of CMV viremia above the limit of quantitative (400 copies/mL) of 2.5% versus 10.4% for oral ganciclovir (P = .001).[173] Valganciclovir was also associated with a longer duration of time to development of viremia and a lower peak CMV load in plasma. The main reason for this superior viral suppression with valganciclovir is the higher exposure compared with oral ganciclovir.

The ganciclovir area under the curve (AUC, 0 to 24 h = 46.3 mg/h/mL) after 900 mg daily in this study was comparable with intravenous (IV) ganciclovir at 5 mg/kg/d in liver transplant patients.[173] Another measure of the enhanced suppression of viremia observed with valganciclovir was a decrease in ganciclovir resistance. At 1 year after transplant, no ganciclovir-resistant mutants were associated with valganciclovir treatment compared with the low incidence rate of ganciclovir mutants of 1.9% in patients who received oral ganciclovir for 100 day prophylaxis. In patients in whom CMV disease developed after oral ganciclovir treatment, 6.1% had ganciclovir-resistant virus. The enhanced antiviral suppression achieved with valganciclovir did not translate into a reduced overall long-term incidence of CMV disease compared with oral ganciclovir. At 6 months, 12.1% of valganciclovir recipients and 15.2% of ganciclovir recipients had CMV disease develop.[173] By 12 months, the incidence rate of CMV disease was 17.2% in the valganciclovir group and 18.4% in the ganciclovir group. The two groups were comparable in the incidence of CMV disease and in all signs, symptoms, and laboratory criteria.

Interesting differences were seen in the incidence rates of CMV disease by type of organ transplant in the valganciclovir and ganciclovir groups, with 8% and 23% for kidney, 6% and 10% for heart, 0% and 17% for pancreas-kidney, and 19% and 12% for liver transplants, respectively.[173]

Cytomegalovirus Infection in Transplantation Patients

After HSCT and solid organ transplantation, the severe immunosuppressive regimens that are used to prevent rejection of the transplant make the recipient prone to severe CMV disease (see also Chapters 311 and 312). In each form of transplantation, the occurrence of CMV disease is different. The severity of the end-organ disease caused by CMV is related to the degree of immune suppression. The more severe the immune suppression, such as that necessary after HSCT, the more severe is the disease that occurs. Therefore, CMV pneumonia during the first 120 days after HSCT is much more severe and life-threatening than it is in a patient after renal transplantation. All major transplantations (kidney, liver, heart, heart-lung, and HSCT marrow) are associated with an increased risk of CMV infection. In a summary of 16 studies of 1276 patients, the rate of infection after renal transplantation as measured with a serologic rise in antibody to CMV or isolation of virus from blood, urine, or throat was found to range from 59% to 70%, with a median rate of 70%.[73] The infection rate was significantly higher among recipients who were seropositive before organ transplantation (84%), and it was lower in seronegative recipients (52%). Primary infections can occur in which a patient is infected from exposure to blood in a dialysis center or intensive care unit; however, this is uncommon now because of the use of filtered blood. Although CMV may be acquired from a transplanted organ, most CMV-associated disease represents reactivation of virus in the recipient.[73]

CYTOMEGALOVIRUS INFECTION ACQUIRED FROM DONATED ORGANS

Although attempts to isolate infectious CMV from organs of healthy hosts are usually unsuccessful, the presence of CMV antigen in major visceral organs has been reported. This makes it likely that CMV is activated after transplantation. In the case of kidney transplant recipients, two studies have reported the development of primary infection in 83% of seronegative recipients who received kidneys from seropositive donors.[174,175] The development of CMV infection in those who received kidneys from seronegative donors was rare. CMV infection is also common among seronegative recipients who receive liver transplants from seropositive donors; in these cases, as many as 50% to 70% of recipients acquire CMV disease. The CMV seropositive recipient is also at risk of development of CMV infection after transplant of an organ from a seropositive donor. In a study of 486 renal transplant recipients, CMV antigenemia occurred most commonly in seronegative recipients of kidney transplants from seropositive donors (D+/R−), but donor status also had a significant effect on CMV antigenemia in seropositive recipients (D+/R+; P = .006; odds ratio [OR], 2.2). Thus, the authors concluded that donor status played a significant role in determination of CMV in the seropositive recipient.[176] In a trial that compared oral ganciclovir at 3 g/d with placebo for the prevention of CMV disease, 44% of seronegative placebo recipients who received a liver transplant from a seropositive donor acquired CMV disease.[171] Evidence that the donor organ is a source of CMV is provided by the demonstration that identical CMV strains were found in two organ recipients who acquired CMV disease and shared a common organ donor.[73]

IMMUNOSUPPRESSIVE THERAPY

Immunosuppressive drugs play a major role in reactivation of CMV.[177] Cytologic drugs such as cyclophosphamide and azathioprine are sufficient in themselves to reactivate CMV.[178] Corticosteroids alone are not able to enhance CMV infection but act synergistically with other agents. The use of high doses of corticosteroids plus azathioprine has been associated with a very high incidence of CMV reactivation.[179]

Cyclosporine has been widely used as a primary immunosuppressive agent, and its potency has contributed to the success of transplants. The use of cyclosporine by itself does not increase CMV disease. A controlled trial in kidney transplantation patients that compared azathioprine and prednisone with cyclosporine and prednisone showed that infection and severity of CMV disease were comparable in both groups of patients.[180] The other mainstay of immunosuppression, tacrolimus, does not enhance CMV infection, although CMV-associated disease is not eliminated by it.[181] Some novel immunosuppressive regimens, however, increase the frequency of severe CMV disease; the most notable of these is the OKT3 antiserum infusion that is used to treat rejection in liver transplantation patients.[31] The use of OKT3 is associated with an increase in CMV hepatitis and dissemination of CMV in such patients. The type of organ that is transplanted is an important determinant of the morbidity of CMV disease, as is discussed in the following sections.

HEMATOPOIETIC STEM CELL TRANSPLANTATION

The most common life-threatening infectious complication of allogeneic HSCT is interstitial pneumonia from CMV, which usually occurs within the first 120 days after transplantation. This pneumonitis usually shows an interstitial pattern rather than alveolar disease, but nodules may also be present on chest radiographic films. CMV pneumonia is usually rapid in onset with respiratory symptoms of less than 2 weeks in duration. Fever, nonproductive cough, and dyspnea that progresses to hypoxia are common in severe cases. Hypoxia frequently necessitates assisted ventilation. In HSCT patients, CMV pneumonia has a very high mortality rate (in one large series, 84%).[3] Part of the severity of CMV pneumonia noted in HSCT patients may be the result of a graft-versus-host reaction in the lung. Graft-versus-host disease has been reported more commonly in those with CMV pneumonia (82%) than in those without CMV pneumonia (27%).[3]

In kidney transplant recipients, pneumonia from CMV is less severe than that seen in bone marrow transplantation patients, and ganciclovir treatment has been lifesaving. In HSCT recipients, however, the severe interstitial pneumonia has been difficult to treat with any single therapy. Attempts to treat with ganciclovir, acyclovir, vidarabine, human leukocyte interferon, and lymphoblastoid interferon plus acyclovir have had only limited success.[110,182,183] Among 10 bone marrow transplant recipients treated with ganciclovir for CMV pneumonia, only one patient survived, although CMV was promptly cleared from the urine and pulmonary secretions of all 10.[182] Among another 20 HSCT recipients with CMV pneumonia, only 38% survived after treatment with ganciclovir. Four of these survivors also received high-titer CMV immune globulin.[183] In three uncontrolled trials, survival rates among HSCT patients treated with intravenous ganciclovir and high-dose intravenous CMV immune globulin ranged from 52% to 69%.[184-186] Although these trials were uncontrolled, the combination of ganciclovir and high-titer CMV immune globulin is the currently recommended therapy for CMV pneumonia in HSCT patients.

Results from European studies have not supported the favorable results observed in these three studies.[187] A retrospective study of 49 allogeneic HSCT recipients treated with ganciclovir and intravenous immune globulin showed that only 35% had response to treatment. At 1 month after diagnosis, the mortality rate of the combined treatment was 69%. The American patients studied may not be comparable with the European patients who received this treatment because of differences in immunosuppressive regimens used in the two locations.

Antiviral prophylaxis and preventive therapy are both effective in decreasing the incidence of CMV disease among transplant patients. Ganciclovir has been the most frequently used anti-CMV drug; it effectively prevents CMV disease during the first 3 months after allogeneic HSCT when administered during engraftment for pp65 antigenemia or detection of CMV DNA with PCR.[188-190] The use of ganciclovir also improves survival in selected patients at high risk.[190-192]

Valacyclovir was compared with IV ganciclovir for prevention of CMV disease in 168 patients after allogeneic HSCT. Study patients received acyclovir after transplant, until the time of neutrophil engraftment; they then were randomly assigned to receive either oral valacyclovir or IV ganciclovir for 100 days. No significant difference was observed between the study arms for the incidence of CMV disease or the median time to onset of CMV disease. In this study, valacyclovir and ganciclovir were equivalent, and the authors concluded that oral valacyclovir may provide an alternative for patients who cannot tolerate ganciclovir because of neutropenia.[193]

The report of a phase II trial of maribavir to prevent CMV disease after bone marrow transplantation offers promising results, in that maribavir prophylaxis after transplant is effective in preventing CMV disease and greatly decreasing CMV infection compared with placebo. In the first 100 days after transplantation, the incidence of CMV pp65 antigen detection and plasma CMV DNA was reduced with maribavir treatment. No CMV disease occurred in the maribavir patients.[163] Maribavir was well tolerated and had no adverse effect on neutrophil or platelet counts.

The use of strategies to prevent CMV disease results in a syndrome called *late-onset CMV disease*, which in many cases involves infection with ganciclovir-resistant viruses.[193,194] Ganciclovir therapy and graft-versus-host disease and its treatment can delay recovery of CMV-specific T-cell immunity after HSCT. This CMV-specific immunodeficiency can persist after ganciclovir therapy is stopped. The continued detection of CMV pp65 antigen or CMV DNA in plasma or peripheral blood leukocytes and the presence of lymphopenia after 3 months of ganciclovir preventive therapy are strong predictors of late CMV disease and death.[193] Late CMV disease developed at a median of 146 days after bone marrow transplantation in 18% of 146 patients, with a mortality rate of 46%. Preventive measures against late CMV disease should be directed at patients in whom CMV became reactivated during the first 3 months after transplantation and in patients with poor CMV-specific immunity and low CD4 cell counts.

LIVER TRANSPLANTATION

Cytomegalovirus remains the pathogen most commonly isolated after solid organ transplantation, including liver transplantation.[195,196] CMV hepatitis, an important problem that occurs after transplantation in adults, children, and infants, is more common after primary CMV infection. CMV disease, a leading cause of morbidity during the first 14 weeks after transplantation, increases costs and length of hospital stay.[197] The incidence of CMV hepatitis is greatest after transplantation from a CMV-seropositive donor. All cases of CMV hepatitis are characterized by prolonged fever, elevated bilirubinemia, and elevated liver enzyme concentrations. CMV hepatitis can also lead to liver failure that necessitates repeat transplantation. Management may be difficult because the signs of severe CMV hepatitis can be difficult to distinguish from graft rejection. Liver biopsy is the only reliable way to distinguish rejection from CMV hepatitis.[198] The clinician must distinguish between these two possibilities because rejection is treated with an increase in immunosuppression whereas CMV infection is treated with a decrease in immunosuppression and initiation of antiviral therapy. CMV predisposes to other opportunistic infections[199] and increases the risk for allograft rejection.[200] Attempts to prevent CMV disease in liver transplant recipients through administration of CMV immune globulin[201] or oral acyclovir[202,203] or a combination of the two[204] have had little effect on the incidence of CMV disease in seronegative recipients. The best results of prophylaxis for CMV disease in liver transplant recipients have been achieved with prolonged courses of intravenous ganciclovir.[167] Among 250 patients randomly assigned to receive ganciclovir or acyclovir intravenously after liver transplantation, ganciclovir recipients had an incidence rate of CMV disease of 0.8% during a follow-up period of 120 days, whereas CMV disease occurred in 38% of acyclovir recipients. Intravenous ganciclovir reduced the incidence of CMV infection in patients who were positive for CMV antigen and in those who were CMV antigen–negative. The striking decrease in CMV disease included decreases in pneumonia, gastrointestinal disease, hepatitis, retinitis, encephalitis, and CMV syndrome (see subsequent discussion).

A long course of oral ganciclovir, 1000 mg three times a day, was compared with matching placebo in liver transplant recipients.[171] The drug was begun no later than 10 days after transplantation and was continued until the day 98 after transplantation. Oral ganciclovir reduced the incidence of CMV disease in all subgroups when compared with placebo. The 6-month incidence rate of CMV disease was 18.9% in the placebo group and 4.8% (7 of 150) in the ganciclovir group ($P < .001$). In the high-risk group of seronegative recipients of seropositive livers (D+/R–), the incidence rate of CMV disease was 44% in the placebo group and 14.8% in the ganciclovir group. A benefit was also seen among those who received antilymphocyte globulin, in whom the frequency of CMV disease was 32.9% in the placebo group and 4.6% in the ganciclovir group. The study showed that oral ganciclovir prophylaxis was still effective despite the intense immunosuppression of antilymphocyte antibodies. Oral ganciclovir for prophylaxis was still not as effective as intravenous ganciclovir, which was associated with an incidence rate of 0.8% of CMV disease compared with 4.8% among oral ganciclovir recipients.[171]

The usual dose-limiting toxicity of ganciclovir is myelosuppression, which is less common in solid organ transplant recipients[167] than in HSCT patients[165] or in patients with AIDS.[169] In the study of oral ganciclovir for liver transplant recipients, no associated significant myelotoxicity was observed. A trend toward a higher serum creatinine concentration was noted in ganciclovir recipients, which reflects the mild nephrotoxic effects of ganciclovir.[167]

Valganciclovir has supplanted the use of oral ganciclovir among these patients. In the first clinical trial in transplant populations, valganciclovir was as clinically effective as oral ganciclovir in prevention of CMV disease in organ transplants. In liver transplant recipients, however, 19% of valganciclovir patients had CMV disease compared with 12% in those who received oral ganciclovir at 1000 mg/d. This result differed from kidney transplants where 8% of valganciclovir patients had CMV disease compared with 23% for ganciclovir. This difference is not explained.[173]

KIDNEY TRANSPLANTATION

Morbidity from CMV is lowest among kidney transplant recipients, but primary infection from a seropositive donor to a seronegative recipient can occur and is significantly more symptomatic than is secondary infection. Two studies[174,175] reported the clinical and laboratory findings from a total of 154 renal transplantation patients with CMV infection. In one of the series, 13 of 18 primary infections were associated with at least two of the following symptoms: fever, leukopenia, atypical lymphocytes, lymphocytosis, hepatosplenomegaly, myalgia, and arthralgia. This constellation of findings has been called the *CMV syndrome*, which is now defined as CMV infection accompanied by an otherwise unexplained fever of longer than 48 hours, malaise, and a fall in neutrophil count for three consecutive days.[171] This most common manifestation of CMV-associated illness in kidney transplant recipients contrasts with the appearance of secondary CMV infections, of which only 19% have been associated with fever.

Clinically significant CMV hepatitis is a rare occurrence among patients after renal transplantation,[205] but elevated hepatic enzyme (aspartate aminotransferase) levels were seen in 10 of 16 cases (63%) of primary CMV infection in kidney transplant recipients.[175] Five cases of CMV interstitial pneumonia were found in this group. Rejection of the transplanted kidney was also observed in four of 16 patients with primary infection. In this study, 24 seronegative patients who received kidneys from seronegative donors and remained seronegative did not undergo rejection. This study is one of the few that reached the conclusion that CMV infection may increase the likelihood of rejection of the transplanted organ.[175] In a large series of 126 kidney transplantation patients, hepatic dysfunction was observed in 22%.[206] Severe hepatitis was observed in seven, and CMV was isolated from the bodily fluids of all seven. At autopsy, five of these patients had evidence of CMV in the liver.

In a small series of kidney transplantation patients in whom CMV pneumonia developed, a mortality rate of 48% was noted.[207] This rate is much less than that observed among bone marrow transplantation patients in whom mortality rates as high as 84% have been reported.[3] In kidney transplant recipients who acquire CMV pneumonia, ganciclovir alone has been effective therapy for severe interstitial pneumonia, as was previously noted.[208]

Kidney transplant recipients have also been extensively studied in attempts to prevent CMV disease. In a study of CMV infection, hyperimmune globulin was administered to 24 seronegative kidney transplant recipients within 72 hours of transplantation and was continued for 16 weeks. The rate of CMV infection was 71% compared with 77% in 35 control subjects, but the rate of symptomatic disease decreased from 60% to 21%.[209] This study reported one death from CMV in the treated group and five deaths in the control group; the higher rates of CMV disease and death may have been related to the widespread use of antithymocyte globulin. Prophylaxis with immunoglobulin was not shown to be effective in primary CMV disease after other solid organ transplants, such as liver transplants.[210] CMV antigen detection has been used at the start of ganciclovir as preemptive therapy in CMV antibody–positive kidney transplantation patients and has met with success in the prevention of CMV disease.[211] Oral ganciclovir therapy has also been successful in lowering CMV DNA levels and in preventing CMV disease after renal transplantation.

Valganciclovir is now used widely used after kidney transplantation.[172] In the original study in which valganciclovir was compared with oral ganciclovir to prevent CMV disease in kidney transplant patients, 8% of valganciclovir patients had CMV disease develop compared with 23% of ganciclovir patients.[173]

DRUG RESISTANCE IN SOLID ORGAN RECIPIENTS

Estimates are that more than 67% of solid organ transplant recipients who are CMV seronegative (R−) or who receive an organ from a seropositive donor (D+) have evidence of CMV infection. Only a small subgroup of these patients actually has CMV end-organ disease develop. Primary infection with CMV that occurs in CMV-seronegative recipients of solid organ transplants from seropositive donors (D+/R−) is associated with the greatest increase in risk of disease. A long-term study of a large number of solid organ transplant recipients focused on the virologic characteristics related to drug resistance.[142] This study found that (D+/R−) serostatus was the only clear-cut predictor of drug resistance among patients in the Chicago and Cleveland cohorts. In the Cleveland cohort, high peak virus load was significantly associated with drug-resistant CMV. Ganciclovir was used for prophylaxis and treatment of all recipients; most of those in whom ganciclovir resistance developed received multiple courses of ganciclovir therapy. Two important host factors were strongly associated with the detection of ganciclovir-resistant CMV strains: lung transplantation and (D+/R−) CMV serostatus.[142] Among all transplant groups, 28 of the 30 transplant recipients with resistant CMV strains were D+/R−. This finding is similar to a finding by Limaye and colleagues.[141] Drug-resistant CMV was documented phenotypically and genotypically most frequently in lung transplant recipients in 2.2% of 228 Cleveland lung transplant recipients and in 4.6% of 325 Chicago lung transplant recipients during a 7-year period from 1994 to 2001. When the D+/R− subgroup of recipients was examined, drug resistance in CMV isolates rose to 10.5% for the Cleveland cohort and 18.3% for the

Chicago lung transplant recipients. This study also used direct genotypic drug resistance assays, which use DNA extracts of clinical specimens as templates for direct PCR amplification and sequencing to detect known drug resistance mutations. This greatly shortens the time needed to detect resistance, eliminates the need for cultures, and enables detection of all known mutations in either of the CMV genes UL97 and UL54, which indicate resistance of CMV to ganciclovir. This can make resistance testing available in 3 days and allows the clinician to use resistance assays when making patient management decisions. This study shows that drug resistance is an important aspect of CMV pathogenesis in solid organ transplant recipients. All patients with drug-resistant strains had CMV-related disease, and at least 50% died as a result of the infection.[142]

Cytomegalovirus Infection and Cardiovascular Diseases

The role of CMV as a potential factor in the development of cardiovascular (CV) disease has been the object of substantial epidemiologic, clinical, and laboratory studies.[20,212-233] Epidemiologic studies have generally used the detection of CMV IgG antibody to determine the presence of CMV infection. In a number of these studies, the correlation of CMV infection with CV disease is statistically significant ($P <$ .05), with a 95% confidence interval (CI) and a study size of patients from 40 to 3168 with a median age from 49 to 65.4 years.[212-218] Studies have detected CMV genomic DNA in the plasma, in coronary atherectomy, at myocardial autopsy, and in donor heart valves of patients with CV disease PCR and in situ hybridization tests were both used.[215-219]

One of these clinical trial studies is the Heart Outcomes Prevention Evaluation (HOPE) study, which is a prospective, multicenter, randomized clinical trial that defined factors for the prevention of CV events among 9541 patients with previous coronary artery disease, stroke, peripheral vascular disease, or high-risk diabetes.[212] The baseline enrollment blood samples from 3168 Canadian patients in the HOPE study were analyzed to measure the relation between serostatus and 494 adjudicated trial outcomes of myocardial infarction (MI), stroke, or CV death over 4.5 years of follow-up. Patients had a mean age of 65.4 years, and 77.6% were men. CMV IgG antibody was present in 2220 of 3153 patients (70.4%). CMV serostatus was associated with an excess of CV events (log rank test, 0.03), with an unadjusted hazards ratio (HR) of 1.26 (95% CI, 1.03, 1.54; $P = .02$) and an adjusted HR of 1.24 (1.01, 1.53; $P = .04$). CMV was associated with the outcomes of MI alone and with the primary events combined with revascularization. CMV was also associated with the primary outcome of CV disease with adjusted HR of 1.05 (95% CI, 0.59, 1.88; $P = .86$) for women and 1.28 (95% CI, 1.03, 1.59; $P = .03$) for men. The authors concluded that the presence of CMV was associated with a subsequent MI, stroke, or CV death in patients of the HOPE study.[212]

Animal model experiments have shown that murine cytomegalovirus (MCMV) or rat cytomegalovirus (RCMV) infection markedly increases the expression of proinflammatory cytokines such TNF-α, interferon-γ (INF-γ), and interleukin-10 (IL-10) and results in atherosclerotic lesions in vessel walls of the experimental animals.[220-222] Studies in mice have shown that persistent infection of vascular cells by MCMV alone causes a significant increase of arterial blood pressure.[249] In addition, the ultraviolet (UV)-inactivated MCMV significantly increases the mean of atherosclerotic lesion areas and the infiltration of T cells, which suggests that MCMV-associated cardiovascular lesions do not require active virus replication in cardiovascular cells.[223] Moreover, gene therapy with DNA encoding subtypes of INF significantly reduces the infiltration of CD8+ T cells into myocardium in mice, which suggests that the autoimmune responses induced by chronic MCMV infection may play an important role in pathogenesis of MCMV myocarditis.[224]

In vitro cell culture and molecular biology analyses have shown that CMV can infect cardiovascular endothelial cells (ECs) and vessel smooth muscle cells (SMCs) in a chronic or persistent manner.[225-233] CMV infection of EC and SMC activates several signal transduction pathways, including p53, NFκB, and IκB kinase-related pathways in host cells. Furthermore, CMV infection increases expression of proinflammatory cytokines and vascular adhesion factors, such TNF-α, IL-1, IL-6, MCP-1, leukotrienes (LTs), vascular endothelial growth factor (VEGF), and vascular cell adhesion molecule–1 (VCAM-1).[225-233] CMV infection induced expression of proinflammatory cytokines may also sequentially upregulate expression of intercellular adhesion molecules on the noninfected neighboring cells through paracrine action.[229-233]

The potential role of CMV in the pathogenesis of CV disease continues to be a subject of active research interest. Carefully designed and controlled studies that use anti-CMV therapy are needed to ultimately assess the contribution of CMV infection to the development and risks of CV disease.[222a]

Congenital Cytomegalovirus Infection

Intrauterine CMV infections occur in 0.5% to 22% of all live births.[234] This mode of infection is less frequent than perinatal infection but is associated with the most serious CMV disease that occurs during the neonatal period. The diagnosis of congenital infection is best found with viruria within the first week of life. The presence of IgM antibodies against CMV in cord serum is suggestive but not completely specific for congenital infection. Clinically significant congenital infection occurs most often in infants born to primiparous mothers with a primary infection during pregnancy.[73] Such infection is diagnosed in the mother through a change in antibody titer from negative to positive or with detection of IgM antibody.

In a group of 3712 pregnant women from upper and lower socioeconomic groups in Alabama, 21 primary infections were found in 1382 seronegative mothers.[235] Among this group of 21 mothers, 11 congenital infections occurred; three were symptomatic. This finding indicates that the intrauterine infection rate of infants after primary CMV infection is high (55%). The rate of primary infection (0.52%) did not vary with socioeconomic status or immune status of the population. The rate of intrauterine CMV infection (24 in 8416 pregnancies) from primary infection was 0.3%; 25% of the cases were symptomatic. These data indicate that primary infection at any stage of pregnancy presents a risk for intrauterine infection; the risk is highest during the first half of pregnancy.[236]

Congenital infection was observed in 20 babies from 2330 mothers (0.5%) who were seropositive.[235] This type of congenital infection occurs more frequently among mothers from lower socioeconomic groups with a high prevalence of past infection. None of the 20 babies had symptoms of congenital infection.[235] Other reports have claimed that symptomatic infection may rarely result from infection in an immune mother.[237] These results indicate that the neonate who acquires CMV disease generally acquires infection from a mother who is not immune. When mothers are immune, most infections among babies are asymptomatic. A small number of infections develop from transplacental infection. Perinatal infection occurs when CMV is carried in the cervix during late stages of pregnancy and when CMV is carried in breast milk.

Symptoms that occur in children who are infected congenitally from nonimmune mothers involve fulminant cytomegalic inclusion disease, which consists of jaundice, hepatosplenomegaly, petechial rash, and multiple organ involvement. CNS findings of microcephaly, motor disability, chorioretinitis, and cerebral calcifications are present.[238] At birth or shortly thereafter, onset of lethargy, respiratory distress, and seizures occurs. The child may die in days or a few weeks. Jaundice and hepatosplenomegaly may subside, but neurologic sequelae, microcephaly, and mental retardation persist. Many extraneural defects, including hearing disorders, have been associated with congenital infection, and most disease manifestations are the result of inflammation from virus invasion.[238] Interference with organ development (such as occurs with rubella) is not seen with CMV infection.

Infections that occur in babies postnatally are different from congenital infections; diffuse visceral and CNS diseases do not occur. The

clinical picture may resemble CMV mononucleosis in some respects, although the full mononucleosis syndrome is usually absent. CMV mononucleosis may occur rarely in young children,[14] and much more severe CMV-associated disease can occur as the result of exchange transfusions.[239]

Although perinatal infections are completely asymptomatic and cause no obvious long-term abnormalities, subtle effects on hearing and intelligence have been reported. In a study of 8644 neonates from middle-class socioeconomic families, 53 were identified with IgM antibodies against CMV in cord blood (0.6%).[240] Forty-four of these children were evaluated at 3.5 to 7.0 years of age. The mean intelligence quotient (IQ) for the group was 103, which was lower than that of a matched control group. The school failure rate of this group was 2.7 times that of matched controls of the same socioeconomic status. Thirteen percent of these children (5 of 40) had severe bilateral hearing loss, and three had profound deafness. Inapparent CMV infection during the perinatal period is being invoked as a cause of the 1-in-1000 incidence rate of profound deafness in American children. Another report described the incidence of sensorineural hearing loss among those with neonatal CMV infection. In this study, 59 patients had congenital intrauterine infection, and eight had symptoms at birth.[241] Twenty-one children had perinatal CMV infection, and none had hearing loss. Late-onset hearing loss developed in 17% of those with symptomatic congenital infection and in 14% of those with asymptomatic congenital CMV infection. In this study, histopathology showed virus in the cells of the organ of Corti and in neurons of the spira ganglia.[241] Rare typical nuclear inclusions were seen in cells of the cochlea. The problem of hearing loss associated with CMV cannot be predicted with severity of infection or IgM level at birth. This problem of hearing loss from CMV has been cited as a major stimulus for vaccine development and for research into other preventive measures for CMV infection.

Cytomegalovirus Infection in Pregnant Women

Possible sources of sexual transmission of CMV include virus in the uterine cervix and in semen. About 1% to 2% of women in the United States who undergo a routine medical examination in a private practice setting are found to carry the virus in the cervix.[73] In Taiwan, 18% of a group with infrequent sexual relations had CMV isolated from the cervix.[242] A study of 134 women who attended a sexually transmitted diseases clinic in Seattle revealed that 34% of women older than 21 years of age had shed CMV in the cervix and that many of these women had evidence of shedding of multiple strains of CMV.[243] Frequency of colonization correlated with the number of sexual partners and age of first sexual intercourse, although no direct evidence has confirmed that CMV in the cervix comes from sexual intercourse or that it is transmitted via sexual intercourse. CMV is also found in high titers in the semen of both homosexual and heterosexual men.[74]

An increased rate of cervical infection occurs during the late stages of pregnancy. CMV in the uterine cervix is a source of infection transmitted to the neonate during passage through the birth canal. Three studies of 987 pregnant women showed an increasing prevalence rate of infection that progressed from first (0 to 2%), second (6% to 10%), and third trimesters (11% to 28%; Table 138-1).[244-246] These three studies examined distinct populations. The study from Japan[244] included a nonpromiscuous middle-class population that was 85% CMV seropositive. The study from Alabama in the United States included a young sexually promiscuous group with a 10% rate of gonorrhea and a CMV-seropositive status of 89%.[245] The third study included 71 Native American Navajo and 125 middle-class white and black pregnant women.[246]

High cervical CMV excretion during the third trimester of pregnancy presents a risk of infection for the neonate during the birth process, but this risk may not be as important as that associated with transmission of perinatal infection from infected milk. In a study of 50 babies born to mothers who were nonsecretors, only two (4%) became infected, but 12.5% of babies born to mothers who secreted

TABLE 138-1   Cervical Cytomegalovirus Infection during Pregnancy

Source	First Trimester	Second Trimester	Third Trimester	Overall Infection
Numazaki et al[244]	0/30 (0)*	6/62 (9.7%)	17/61 (27.9%)	23/153 (15.0%)
Montgomery et al[246]	1/43 (2%)	6/83 (7.2%)	6/49 (12.2%)	13/175 (7.4%)
Stagno et al[245]	3/183 (1.6%)†	22/359 (6.1%)	42/371 (11.3%)	63/659 (9.6%)
Total infected/tested	4/256	34/504	65/481	99/987
Percentage infected	1.6	6.7	13.5	10.0

*Represents number of patients with positive results per number of patients tested.
†Number infected per number of specimens tested.
From Ho M. Cytomegalovirus. In Mandell GL, Bennett JE, Dolin R, editors. *Principles and Practice of Infectious Diseases*, 4th ed. New York: Churchill Livingstone; 1995:1351.

CMV from the cervix during the first or second trimester became infected and 37% of babies born to mothers who secreted during the third trimester became infected. The infection rate of babies whose mothers shed virus postpartum and who were presumably shedding at birth rose to 57%.[247] During pregnancy, primary infection in the mother may manifest as a mild mononucleosis syndrome, but it is usually asymptomatic and is associated with CMV viruria for 4 to 7 days. The former belief was that recurrent infections during pregnancy were largely asymptomatic. Boppana and coworkers[248] showed that reinfection with a different strain of CMV during pregnancy can lead to intrauterine transmission and symptomatic congenital infection. This conclusion was based on the appearance of antibodies directed against new strain-specific epitopes of CMV glycoprotein H not present in maternal blood before the current pregnancy. To promote our understanding of the true frequency and clinical importance of congenital CMV infection caused by recurrent maternal infections, further investigation with larger, long-term prospective studies is needed.[248]

REFERENCES

1. Zhang LJ, Hanpf P, Rutherford C, et al. Detection of cytomegalovirus, DNA, RNA, and antibody in normal donor blood. *J Infect Dis.* 1995;171:1002-1006.
2. Patel R, Surydman DR, Rubin RH, et al. Cytomegalovirus prophylaxis in solid organ transplant recipients. *Transplantation.* 1996;61:1279-1289.
3. Myers JD, Flournoy N, Thomas ED. Risk factors for cytomegalovirus infection after human marrow transplantation. *J Infect Dis.* 1986;153:478-488.
4. Masur H, Whitcup SM, Cartwright C, et al. Advances in the management of AIDS-related CMV retinitis. *Ann Intern Med.* 1996;125:126-136.
5. Crumpacker CS. Ganciclovir. *N Engl J Med.* 1996;335:721-729.
6. Ho M. Cytomegalovirus. In: Mandell GM, Bennett JE, Dolin R, eds. *Principles and Practice of Infectious Diseases.* 4th ed. New York: Churchill Livingstone; 1995.
7. Spector SA, Hirata KK, Neumann TR. Identification of multiple cytomegalovirus strains in homosexual men with acquired immunodeficiency syndrome. *J Infect Dis.* 1984;6:953-956.
8. Griffiths PD, Stagno S, Pass RF, et al. Infection with cytomegalovirus during pregnancy: Specific IgM antibodies as a marker of recent primary infection. *J Infect Dis.* 1982;145:647-653.
9. Smith MG. Propagation of salivary gland virus of the mouse in tissue cultures. *Proc Soc Exp Biol Med.* 1954;86:435-440.
10. Smith MG. Propagation in tissue cultures of a cytopathogenic virus from human salivary gland virus (SGV) disease. *Proc Soc Exp Biol Med.* 1956;92:424-430.
11. Weller TH, Macauley JC, Craig JM, et al. Isolation of intranuclear inclusion producing agents from infants with illnesses resembling cytomegalic inclusion disease. *Proc Soc Exp Biol Med.* 1957;94:4-12.
12. Rowe WP, Hartley JW, Waterman S, et al. Cytopathogenic agent resembling human salivary gland virus recovered from tissue cultures of human adenoids. *Proc Soc Exp Biol Med.* 1956;92:418-424.
13. Weller TH, Hanshaw JB, Scott DE. Serologic differentiation of viruses responsible for cytomegalic inclusion disease. *Virology.* 1960;12:130-132.
14. Klemola E, Kaarianen L. Cytomegalovirus as a possible cause of a disease resembling infectious mononucleosis. *Br Med J.* 1965;1099:102.
15. Kaarianen L, Klemola E, Paloheimo J. Rise of cytomegalovirus antibodies in an infectious-mononucleosis-like syndrome after transfusion. *Br Med J.* 1966;2:1270-1272.
16. Winston DJ, Ho WG, Howell CL, et al. Cytomegalovirus infections associated with leukocyte transfusions. *Ann Intern Med.* 1980;93:671-675.
17. Chee MS, Bankier AT, Becks S, et al. Analysis of the protein-coding content of the sequence of human cytomegalovirus strain—AD 169. *Curr Top Microbiol Immunol.* 1990;154:125-169.
18. Cha T, Tom S, Kemble GW, et al. Human cytomegalovirus clinical isolates carry at least 19 genes not found in laboratory strains. *J Virol.* 1996;70:78-83.
19. Lurain NS, Kapell KS, Huang DD, et al. Human cytomegalovirus UL144 open reading frame: sequence hypervariability in low-passage clinical isolates. *J Virol.* 1999;73:10040-10050.
19a. Penfold ME, Dairaghi DJ, Duke GM, et al. Cytomegalovirus encodes a potent alpha chemokine. *Proc Natl Acad Sci U S A.* 1999;96:9839-9844.
20. Zhou YF, Shou M, Harrell RF, et al. Chronic non-vascular cytomegalovirus infection: effects on the neointimal response to experimental vascular injury. *Cardiovasc Res.* 2000;45:1019-1025.
21. Rul PF, Powell KL. Physical and functional interaction of human cytomegalovirus DNA polymerase and its accessory protein (ZCP36) expressed in insect cells. *J Virol.* 1992;66:4126-4133.
22. Chee MS, Lawrence GL, Barell BG. Alpha-, beta- and gamma-herpesviruses encode a putative phosphotransferase. *J Gen Virol.* 1989;70:1151-1160.
23. Sullivan V, Talarico CL, Stanat SC, et al. A protein kinase homologue controls phosphorylation of ganciclovir in human cytomegalovirus infected cells. *Nature.* 1992;358:162-164. [Errata. *Nature.* 1992;359:85 and. 1993;366:756.]
24. Littler E, Stuart AD, Chee MS. Human cytomegalovirus UL 97 open reading frame encodes a protein that phosphorylates the antiviral nucleoside analogue ganciclovir. *Nature.* 1992;358:160-162.
25. He Z, He YS, Kim Y, et al. The human cytomegalovirus UL97 protein is a protein kinase that autophosphorylates on serines and threonines. *J Virol.* 1997;71:405-411.
26. Hume AJ, Finkel JS, Kamil JP, et al. Phosphorylation of retinoblastoma protein by viral protein with cyclin-dependent kinase function. *Science.* 2008;320:797-799.
27. Beersma MF, Bizlemaker MJ, Ploegh HL. Human cytomegalovirus down regulates HLA class I expression by reducing the stability of class I H chains. *J Immunol.* 1993;151:4455-4464.
28. Schuster EA, Bencke JS, Tegtmeier GE, et al. Monoclonal antibody for rapid laboratory detection of cytomegalovirus infections: Characterization and diagnostic application. *Mayo Clin Proc.* 1985;60:577-585.
29. Fetterman GH. A new laboratory aid in the clinical diagnosis of inclusion disease of infancy. *Am J Clin Pathol.* 1952;22:424-425.
30. Rinaldo CR, Black PH, Hirsch MS. Interactions of cytomegalovirus with leukocytes from patients with mononucleosis due to cytomegalovirus. *J Infect Dis.* 1977;136:667-678.
31. Singh N, Dummer JS, Ho M, et al. Infections with cytomegalovirus and other herpesviruses in 121 liver transplant recipients: Transmission by donated organ and the effect of OKT3 antibodies. *J Infect Dis.* 1988;158:124-131.
32. Plachter B, Sinzger C, Jahn G. Cell types involved in replication and distribution of human cytomegalovirus. *Adv Virus Res.* 1996;46:195-261.
33. Hahn G, Revello MG, Patrone M, et al. Human cytomegalovirus UL131-128 genes are indispensable for virus growth in endothelial cells and virus transfer to leukocytes. *J Virol.* 2004;78:10023-10033.
34. Akter P, Cunningham C, McSharry BP, et al. Two novel spliced genes in human cytomegalovirus. *J Gen Virol.* 2003;84:1117-1122.
35. Wang D, Shenk T. Human cytomegalovirus UL131 open reading frame is required for epithelial cell tropism. *J Virol.* 2005;79:10330-10338.
36. Grundy JE, Lawson KM, MacCormac LP, et al. Cytomegalovirus-infected endothelial cells recruit neutrophils by the secretion of C-X-C chemokines and transmit virus by direct neutrophil-endothelial cell contact and during neutrophil transendothelial migration. *J Infect Dis.* 1998;177:1465-1474.
37. Martin WJ, Smith TJ. Rapid detection of cytomegalovirus in bronchoalveolar lavage specimens by a monoclonal antibody method. *J Clin Microbiol.* 1986;23:1006-1008.
38. van der Bij W, Schirm J, Torensma R, et al. Comparison between viremia and antigenemia for detection of cytomegalovirus in blood. *J Clin Microbiol.* 1988;26:2531-2535.
39. Chou S, Merigan TC. Rapid detection and quantitation of human cytomegalovirus in urine through DNA hybridization. *N Engl J Med.* 1983;308:921-925.
40. Churchill MA, Zaia JA, Forman SJ, et al. Quantitation of human cytomegalovirus DNA in lungs from bone marrow transplant recipients with interstitial pneumonia. *J Infect Dis.* 1987;155:501-509.
41. Stanier P, Kitchen AD, Taylor DL, et al. Detection of human cytomegalovirus in peripheral mononuclear cells and urine samples using PCR. *Mol Cell Probes.* 1992;6:51-58.
42. Gerna G, Zipeto D, Parea M, et al. Monitoring of human cytomegalovirus infections and ganciclovir treatment in heart transplant recipients by determination of viremia, antigenemia, and DNAemia. *J Infect Dis.* 1991;164:488-498.
43. Wolf DG, Spector SA. Diagnosis of human cytomegalovirus central nervous system disease in AIDS patients by DNA amplification from cerebrospinal fluid. *J Infect Dis.* 1992;166:1412-1415.
44. Fox JD, Brink NS, Zuckerman MA, et al. Detection of herpesvirus DNA by nested polymerase chain reaction in cerebrospinal fluid of human immunodeficiency virus-infected persons with neurologic disease: A prospective evaluation. *J Infect Dis.* 1995;172:1087-1090.
45. Bowen F, Sabiwca Wilson P, et al. Cytomegalovirus (CMV) viraemia detected by polymerase chain reaction identifiers. A group at high risk of CMV disease. *AIDS.* 1997;11:889-893.
46. Shinkai M, Boizette SA, Powderly W, et al. Utility of urine and leukocyte cultures and plasma DNA PCR for identification of AIDS patients at risk for developing human cytomegalovirus disease. *J Infect Dis.* 1997;175:302-332.
47. Dodt KK, Jacobsen PH, Hofman B, et al. Development of cytomegalovirus (CMV) disease can be predicted in HIV infected patients by CMV polymerase chain reaction and antigenemia test. *AIDS.* 1997;11F:21-28.
48. Spector SA, Wong R, Hiza K, et al. Plasma cytomegalovirus (CMV) DNA load predicts CMV disease and survival in AIDS patients. *J Clin Invest.* 1998;101:497-502.
49. Imbert-Marcille BM, Cantarovich D, Ferre-Aubineau V, et al. Usefulness of DNA viral load quantification for cytomegalovirus disease monitoring in renal and pancreas/renal transplant recipients. *Transplantation.* 1997;63:1476-1481.
50. Singh N, Yu VL, Mieles L, et al. High-dose acyclovir compared with short-course preemptive ganciclovir therapy to prevent cytomegalovirus disease in liver transplant recipients: A randomized trial. *Ann Intern Med.* 1994;120:375-381.
51. Flood J, Drew WL, Miner R, et al. Diagnosis of cytomegalovirus (CMV) polyradiculopathy and documentation of in vivo anti-CMV activity in cerebrospinal fluid by using branched DNA signal amplification and antigen assays. *J Infect Dis.* 1997;176:348-352.
52. Boeckl M, Gooley TA, Myerson D, et al. Cytomegalovirus pp65 antigenemia guided early treatment with ganciclovir marrow transplantation: A randomized double blind study. *Blood.* 1997;88:4063-4071.
53. Avery RK, Adal KA, Longworth DL, et al. A survey of allogeneic bone marrow transplant programs in the United States regarding cytomegalovirus prophylaxis and pre-emptive therapy. *Bone Marrow Transplant.* 2000;26:763-767.
54. Schulenburg A, Watkins-Riedel T, Greinix HT, et al. CMV monitoring after peripheral blood stem cell and bone marrow transplantation by pp65 antigen and quantitative PCR. *Bone Marrow Transplant.* 2001;28:765-768.
55. Boivin G, Belanger R, Delage R, et al. Quantitative analysis of cytomegalovirus (CMV) viremia using the pp65 antigenemia assay and the COBAS AMPLICOR CMV MONITOR PCR test after blood and marrow allogeneic transplantation. *J Clin Microbiol.* 2000;38:4356-4360.
56. Masaoka T, Hiraoka A, Ohta K, et al. Evaluation of the AMPLICOR CMV, COBAS AMPLICOR CMV monitor and antigenemia assay for cytomegalovirus disease. *Jpn J Infect Dis.* 2001;54:12-16.

57. Sia IG, Wilson JA, Smith TF, et al. Evaluation of the COBAS AMPLICOR CMV MONITOR test for detection of viral DNA in specimens taken from patients after liver transplantation. *J Clin Microbiol.* 2000;38:600-606.
58. Ho SK, Li FK, Lai KN, et al. Comparison of the CMV brite turbo assay and the digene hybrid capture CMV DNA (Version 2.0) assay for quantitation of cytomegalovirus in renal transplant recipients. *J Clin Microbiol.* 2000;38:3743-3745.
59. Mazzulli T, Drew LW, Yen-Lieberman B, et al. Multicenter comparison of the digene hybrid capture CMV DNA assay (Version 2.0), the pp65 antigenemia assay, and cell culture for detection of cytomegalovirus viremia. *J Clin Microbiol.* 1999;37:958-963.
60. Tong CY, Cuevas LE, Williams H, et al. Comparison of two commercial methods for measurement of cytomegalovirus load in blood samples after renal transplantation. *J Clin Microbiol.* 2000;38:1209-1213.
61. Siennicka J, Rechnio M, Durlik M, et al. Quantitative detection of CMV DNA by PCR and hybridization methods in renal transplant recipients. *Acta Microbiol Pol.* 2000;49:261-264.
62. Humar A, Gregson D, Caliendo AM, et al. Clinical utility of quantitative cytomegalovirus viral load determination for predicting cytomegalovirus disease in liver transplant recipients. *Transplantation.* 1999;68:1305-1311.
63. Piiparinen H, Hockerstedt K, Lappalainen M, et al. Monitoring of viral load by quantitative plasma PCR during active cytomegalovirus infection of individual liver transplant patients. *J Clin Microbiol.* 2002;40:2945-2952.
64. Flexman J, Kay I, Fonte R, et al. Differences between the quantitative antigenemia assay and the cobas amplicor monitor quantitative PCR assay for detecting CMV viraemia in bone marrow and solid organ transplant patients. *J Med Virol.* 2001;64:275-282.
65. Caliendo AM, St George K, Allega J, et al. Distinguishing cytomegalovirus (CMV) infection and disease with CMV nucleic acid assays. *J Clin Microbiol.* 2002;40:1581-1586.
66. Erice A, Tierney C, Hirsch M, et al. Cytomegalovirus (CMV) and human immunodeficiency virus (HIV) burden, CMV end-organ disease, and survival in subjects with advanced HIV infection (AIDS Clinical Trials Group Protocol 360). *Clin Infect Dis.* 2003;37:567-578.
67. Corez KJ, Fischer SH, Fahle GA, et al. Clinical trial of quantitative real-time polymerase chain reaction for detection of cytomegalovirus in peripheral blood of allogeneic hematopoietic stem-cell transplant recipients. *J Infect Dis.* 2003;188:967-972.
68. Gentile G, Picardi A, Capobianchi A, et al. A prospective study comparing quantitative cytomegalovirus (CMV) polymerase chain reaction in plasma and PP65 antigenemia assay in monitoring patients after allogeneic stem cell transplantation. *BMC Infect Dis.* 2006;6:167.
69. Razonable RR, Brown RA, Wilson J, et al. The clinical use of various blood compartments for cytomegalovirus (CMV) DNA quantitation in transplant recipients with CMV disease. *Transplantation.* 2002;73:968-973.
70. Gerna G, Baldanti F, Lilleri D, et al. Human cytomegalovirus pp67 mRNAemia versus pp65 antigenemia for guiding preemptive therapy in heart and lung transplant recipients: A prospective, randomized, controlled, open-label trial. *Transplantation.* 2003;75:1012-1019.
71. Weinberg A, Schissel D, Giller R. Molecular methods for cytomegalovirus surveillance in bone marrow transplant recipients. *J Clin Microbiol.* 2002;40:4203-4206.
72. Dunkel EC, Scheer DI, Zhu Q, et al. A rabbit model for human cytomegalovirus-induced chorioretinal disease (retraction). *J Infect Dis.* 1998;177:1778.
73. Ho M. *Cytomegalovirus: Biology and Infection.* 2nd ed. New York: Plenum; 1991:440.
74. Lang DJ, Kummer JF. Demonstration of cytomegalovirus in semen. *N Engl J Med.* 1972;287:756-758.
75. Klemola E, von Essen R, Henle G, et al. Infectious-mononucleosis-like disease with negative heterophil agglutination test. Clinical features in relation to Epstein-Barr virus and cytomegalovirus and antibodies. *J Infect Dis.* 1970;121:608-614.
76. Chou S, Kim DY, Norman DJ. Transmission of cytomegalovirus by pretransplant leukocyte transfusions in renal transplant candidates. *J Infect Dis.* 1987;155:565-567.
77. Bowden RA, Sayers M, Flourney N, et al. Cytomegalovirus immune globulin and seronegative blood products to prevent primary cytomegalovirus infection after marrow transplantation. *N Engl J Med.* 1986;314:1006-1010.
78. Wreghitt TG, Teare EL, Sule O, et al. Cytomegalovirus infection in immunocompetent patients. *Clin Infect Dis.* 2003;37:1603-1606.
79. Carter AR. Cytomegalovirus disease presenting as hepatitis. *Br Med J.* 1968;3:786.
80. Bonkowsky HL, Lee RV, Klatskin G. Acute granulomatous hepatitis: Occurrence in cytomegalovirus mononucleosis. *JAMA.* 1984;37:1284-1288.
81. Leonard JC, Tobin JOH. Polyneuritis associated with cytomegalovirus infections. *Q J Med.* 1971;40:435-442.
82. Schmitz H, Enders G. Cytomegalovirus as a frequent cause of Guillain-Barre syndrome. *J Med Virol.* 1977;1:21-27.
83. Eidelberg D, Sotrel A, Vogel H, et al. Progressive polyradiculopathy in acquired immune deficiency syndrome. *Neurology.* 1986;36:912-916.
84. Klemola E, Kaariainen L, von Essen R, et al. Further studies on cytomegalovirus mononucleosis in previously healthy individuals. *Acta Med Scand.* 1967;182:311-322.
85. Tiula E, Leinikki P. Fatal cytomegalovirus infection in a previously healthy boy with myocarditis and consumption coagulopathy as presenting signs. *Scand J Infect Dis.* 1972;4:57-60.
86. Waris E, Rasanen P, Kreus KE, et al. Fatal cytomegalovirus disease in a previously healthy adult. *Scand J Infect Dis.* 1972;4:61-67.
87. Chanarin I, Walford DM. Thrombocytopenic purpura in cytomegalovirus mononucleosis. *Lancet.* 1973;1:238-239.
88. Harris AI, Meyer RJ, Brody EA. Cytomegalovirus-induced thrombocytopenia and hemolysis in an adult. *Ann Intern Med.* 1975;83:670-671.
89. Klemola E. Hypersensitivity reactions to ampicillin in cytomegalovirus mononucleosis. *Scand J Infect Dis.* 1970;2:29-31.
90. Muller-Stamou A, Senn HJ, Emody G. Epidermolysis in a case of severe cytomegalovirus infection. *Br Med J.* 1974;3:609-610.
91. Collier AC, Meyers JD, Corey L, et al. Cytomegalovirus infection in homosexual men. *Am J Med.* 1987;82:493-600.
92. Drew WL, Mills J, Levy J, et al. Cytomegalovirus infection and abnormal T-leukocyte subset ratios in homosexual men. *Ann Intern Med.* 1985;103:61-63.
93. Gallant JE, Moore RD, Richman DP, et al. Incidence and natural history of cytomegalovirus disease in patients with advanced human immunodeficiency virus disease treated with zidovudine. *J Infect Dis.* 1992;166:1223-1227.
94. McKenzie R, Travis WD, Dolan SA, et al. The causes of death in patients with human immunodeficiency virus infection: A clinical and pathologic study with emphasis on the role of pulmonary diseases. *Medicine (Baltimore).* 1991;70:326-343.
95. Hammer SM, Squires KE, Hughes MD, et al. A controlled trial of two nucleosides analogues plus indinavir in persons with immunodeficiency virus infection and CD4 cell counts of 200 per cubic millimeter or less. *N Engl J Med.* 1997;337:725-732.
96. Autran B, Carcelain G, Li TS, et al. Positive effects of combined antiretroviral therapy on CD4 T-cell homeostasis and function in advanced HIV disease. *Science.* 1997;277:112-116.
97. Mills J, Jacobsen MA, O'Donnell JJ, et al. Treatment of cytomegalovirus retinitis in patients with AIDS. *Rev Infect Dis.* 1988;3:S522-S531.
98. Anderson RD, Griffy KG, Jung D, et al. Ganiciclovir absolute bioavailability and steady state pharmacokinetics after oral administration of two 3000-mg/d dosing regimens in human immunodeficiency virus- and cytomegalovirus-seropositive patients. *Clin Ther.* 1995;17:425-432.
99. Drew WI, Ives D, Lalezari JP, et al. Oral ganciclovir as maintenance treatment for cytomegalovirus retinitis in patients with AIDS. *N Engl J Med.* 1995;333:615-620.
100. Martin DF, Parks DJ, Mellow SD, et al. Treatment of cytomegalovirus retinitis with an intraocular sustained release ganciclovir implant: A randomized controlled clinical trial. *Arch Ophthamol.* 1994;112:1531-1539.
101. Martin DF, Kuppermann BD, Wolitz RA, et al, for the Roche Ganciclovir Study Group. Oral ganciclovir for patients with cytomegalovirus retinitis treated with a ganciclovir implant. *N Engl J Med.* 1999;340:1063-1070.
102. Miller RG, Storcy JR, Greco CM. Ganciclovir in the treatment of progressive AIDS-related polyradiculopathy. *Neurology.* 1990;40:569-574.
103. Fuller GN, Gill SK, Guiloff RJ, et al. Ganciclovir for lumbosacral polyradiculopathy in AIDS. *Lancet.* 1990;335:48-49.
104. Jacobson MA, Mills J, Rush J, et al. Failure of antiviral therapy for acquired immunodeficiency syndrome-related cytomegalovirus myelitis. *Arch Neurol.* 1988;45:1090-1092.
105. Fletcher CV, Balfour HH. Evaluation of ganciclovir for cytomegalovirus disease. *DICP.* 1989;23:5-12.
106. Enting R, de Gans J, Reiss P, et al. Ganciclovir/foscarnet for cytomegalovirus meningoencephalitis in AIDS. *Lancet.* 1992;340:559-560.
107. Fuller GN. Cytomegalovirus and the peripheral nervous system in AIDS. *J Acquir Immune Defic Syndr.* 1992;5:S33-S36.
108. Knapp AB, Horst DA, Eliopoulos G, et al. Widespread cytomegalovirus gastroenterocolitis in a patient with acquired immunodeficiency syndrome. *Gastroenterology.* 1983;85:1399-1402.
109. Meiselman MS, Cello JP, Margaretten W. Cytomegalovirus colitis. Report of the clinical, endoscopic, and pathologic findings in two patients with acquired immune deficiency syndrome. *Gastroenterology.* 1985;88:171-175.
110. Collaborative DHPG Treatment Study Group. Treatment of serious cytomegalovirus infections with 9-(1,3-dihydroxy-2-propoxymethyl)guanine in patients with AIDS and other immunodeficiencies. *N Engl J Med.* 1986;314:801-805.
111. Dieterich DT, Kotler DP, Busch DF, et al. Ganciclovir treatment of cytomegalovirus colitis in AIDS: A randomized, double-blind, placebo-controlled multicenter study. *J Infect Dis.* 1992;167:278-282.
112. Reed EC, Bowden RA, Dandliker PS, et al. Treatment of cytomegalovirus pneumonia with ganciclovir and intravenous cytomegalovirus immunoglobulin in patients with bone marrow transplants. *Ann Intern Med.* 1988;109:783-788.
113. Texidor HS, Honig CL, Norsoph E, et al. Cytomegalovirus infection of the alimentary canal: Radiologic findings with pathologic correlation. *Radiology.* 1987;163:317-323.
114. Blumberg RS, Kelsey P, Perrone T, et al. Cytomegalovirus- and cryptosporidium-associated acalculous gangrenous cholecystitis. *Am J Med.* 1984;76:1118-1123.
115. Feinberg JE, Hurwitz S, Cooper D, et al. A randomized double-blind trial of valaciclovir prophylates for cytomegalovirus disease in patients with advanced human immunodeficiency virus infection. *J Infect Dis.* 1998;177:48-56.
116. Goudrield J, Khardori N. Cytomegalovirus: The taming of the beast? *Lancet.* 1997;350:1718-1719.
117. Martin JC, Dvorak CA, Smee DF, et al. 9-[(1,3-Dihydroxy-2-propoxy)methyl] guanine: A new potent and selective antiherpes agent. *J Med Chem.* 1983;26:759-761.
118. Ashton WT, Karkas JD, Field AK, et al. Activation by thymidine kinase and potent antiherpetic activity of 2′-nor-2′-deoxyguanosine (2′NDG). *Biochem Biophys Res Commun.* 1982;108:1716-1721.
119. Ogilvie UK, Cheriyan UD, Radatus OX, et al. Biologically active acyclonucleoside analogues. II. The synthesis of 9-(2-hydroxy-1-[hydroxymethyl, ethoxymethyl]guanine) BIOLF-62. *Can J Chem.* 1982;60:3005-3010.
120. Cheng YC, Huang ES, Lin JC, et al. Unique spectrum of activity of 9-[(1,3-dihydroxy-2-propoxy)methyl]-guanine against herpesviruses in vitro and its mode of action against herpes simplex virus type 1. *Proc Natl Acad Sci U S A.* 1983;80:2767-2770.
121. Field AK, Davies ME, DeWitt C, et al. 9[{2-Hydroxy-1-(hydroxymethyl) ethoxy}methyl]guanine: A selective inhibitor of herpes group virus replication. *Proc Natl Acad Sci U S A.* 1983;80:4139-4143.
122. Cheng YC, Grill SP, Dutschman GE, et al. Metabolism of 9-(1,3-dihydroxy-2-propoxymethyl)guanine, a new anti-herpes virus compound, in herpes simplex virus-infected cells. *J Biol Chem.* 1983;258:12460-12464.
123. Hamzeh FM, Lietman PS. Intranuclear accumulation of subgenomic noninfectious human cytomegalovirus DNA in infected cells in the presence of ganciclovir. *Antimicrob Agents Chemother.* 1991;35:1818-1823.
124. Hamzeh FM, Lietman PS, Gibson W, et al. Identification of the lytic origin of DNA replication in human cytomegalovirus by a novel approach utilizing ganciclovir-induced chain termination. *J Virol.* 1990;64:6184-6195.
125. Biron KK, Stanat SC, Sorrell JB, et al. Metabolic activation of the nucleoside analog 9-[{hydroxy-1-(hydroxymethyl)ethoxy} methyl]guanine in human diploid fibrolasts infected with human cytomegalovirus. *Proc Natl Acad Sci U S A.* 1985;82:2473-2477.
126. Martin DF, Sierra-Madero J, Walmsley S, et al. A controlled trial of valganciclovir as induction therapy for cytomegalovirus retinitis. *N Engl J Med.* 2002;346:1119-1126.
127. Chou S, Erice A, Jordan MC, et al. Analysis of the UL97 phosphotransferase coding sequence in clinical cytomegalovirus isolates and identification of mutations conferring ganciclovir resistance. *J Infect Dis.* 1995;171:576-583.
128. Lurain NS, Spatford LE, Thompson KD. Mutation in the UL97 open reading frame of human cytomegalovirus strains resistant to ganciclovir. *J Virol.* 1994;68:4427-4431.
129. Erice A, Gil-Roda C, Perez JL, et al. Antiviral susceptibilities and analysis of UL97 and DNA polymerase sequences of clinical cytomegalovirus isolates from immunocompromised patients. *J Infect Dis.* 1997;175:1087-1092.
130. Erice A, Chou S, Biron KK, et al. Progressive disease due to ganciclovir-resistant cytomegalovirus in immunocompromised patients. *N Engl J Med.* 1989;320:289-293.
131. Drew WL, Miner RC, Busch DF, et al. Prevalence of resistance in patients receiving ganciclovir for serious cytomegalovirus infection. *J Infect Dis.* 1991;163:716-719.
132. Stanat SC, Reardon JE, Erice A, et al. Ganciclovir resistant cytomegalovirus clinical isolates: Mode of resistance to ganciclovir. *Antimicrob Agents Chemother.* 1991;35:2191-2197.
133. Lurain NS, Thompson KD, Holmes EW, et al. Point mutations in the DNA polymerase gene of human cytomegalovirus that result in resistance to antiviral agents. *J Virol.* 1992;66:7146-7152.
134. Chou S, Guentzel S, Michels KR, et al. Frequency of UL97 phosphotransferase mutations related to ganciclovir resistance in clinical cytomegalovirus isolates. *J Infect Dis.* 1995;172:239-242.
135. Sullivan V, Biron KK, Talarico C, et al. A point mutation in the human cytomegalovirus DNA polymerase gene confers resistance to ganciclovir and phosphonylmethoxyalkyl derivatives. *Antimicrob Agents Chemother.* 1993;37:19-25.
136. Chou S, Lurain NS, Weinberg A, et al. Interstrain variation in the human cytomegalovirus DNA polymerase sequence and its effect on genotype diagnosis of antiviral drug resistance. *Antimicrob Agents Chemother.* 1999;43:1500-1502.
137. Jabs DA, Enger C, Dunn JP, et al, for the CMV Retinitis and Viral Resistance Study Group. Cytomegalovirus retinitis and viral resistance: Ganciclovir resistance. *J Infect Dis.* 1998;177:770-773.
138. Jabs DA, Martin BK, Forman MS, et al. Cytomegalovirus resistance to ganciclovir and clinical outcomes of patients with cytomegalovirus retinitis. *Am J Ophthalmol.* 2003;135:26-34.
139. Martin BK, Ricks MO, Forman MS, et al. Change over time in incidence of ganciclovir resistance in patients with cytomegalovirus retinitis. *Clin Infect Dis.* 2007;44:1001-1008.
140. Singh N, Wannstedt C, Keyes L, et al. Impact of evolving trends in recipient and donor characteristics on cytomegalovirus infec-

tion in liver transplant recipients. *Transplantation.* 2004;77:106-110.

141. Limaye AP, Corey L, Koelle DM, et al. Emergence of ganciclovir-resistant cytomegalovirus disease among recipients of solid-organ transplants. *Lancet.* 2000;356:645-649.
142. Lurain NS, Bhorade SM, Pursell KJ, et al. Analysis and characterization of antiviral drug-resistant cytomegalovirus isolates from solid organ transplant recipients. *J Infect Dis.* 2002;186:760-768.
143. Crumpacker CS. Mechanism of action of foscarnet against viral polymerases. *Am J Med.* 1992;92:2A3S-2A7S.
144. Jacobson MA, Wulfsohn M, Feinberg JE, et al. Phase II dose-ranging trial of foscarnet salvage therapy for cytomegalovirus retinitis in AIDS patients intolerant of or resistant to ganciclovir (ACTG protocol 093). *AIDS.* 1994;8:451-459.
145. Baldanti F, Underwood MR, Stanat SC, et al. Single amino acid changes in the DNA polymerase confer foscarnet resistance and slow growth phenotype, while mutation in the UL 97-encoded phosphotransferase confers ganciclovir resistance in the double-resistant human cytomegalovirus strains removed from patients with AIDS. *J Virol.* 1996;70:1390-1395.
146. Chou S, Marousek G, Parenti DM, et al. Mutation in region III of the DNA polymerase gene conferring foscarnet resistance in cytomegalovirus isolates from 3 subjects receiving prolonged antiviral therapy. *J Infect Dis.* 1998;178:526-530.
147. Weinberg A, Jabs DA, Chou S, et al. Mutations conferring foscarnet resistance in a cohort of patients with acquired immunodeficiency syndrome and cytomegalovirus retinitis. *J Infect Dis.* 2003;187:777-784.
148. Chou S, Marousek GI, Van Wechel LC, et al. Growth and drug resistance phenotypes resulting from cytomegalovirus DNA polymerase region III mutations observed in clinical specimens. *Antimicrob Agents Chemother.* 2007;51:4160-4162.
149. Studies of Ocular Complications of AIDS Research Group, AIDS Clinical Trials Group. Mortality in patients with the acquired immunodeficiency syndrome treated with either foscarnet or ganciclovir for cytomegalovirus retinitis. *N Engl J Med.* 1992;326:213-220. [Erratum, N Engl J Med. 1992;326:1172.]
150. Studies of Ocular Complications of AIDS Research Group, AIDS Clinical Trials Group. Combination foscarnet and ganciclovir therapy vs. monotherapy for the treatment of relapsed cytomegalovirus retinitis in patients with AIDS: The Cytomegalovirus Retreatment Trial. *Arch Ophthalmol.* 1996;114:23-33.
151. Ho HT, Woods KL, Bronson JJ, et al. Intercellular metabolism of the antiherpes agent (S)-1-{3-hydroxy-2-(phosphonylmethoxy)propyl}cytosine. *Mol Pharmacol.* 1992;41:197-202.
152. Lalezari JP, Jaffe HS, Stagg RG, et al. Randomized controlled study of the safety and efficacy of intravenous cidofovir for the treatment of relapsing cytomegalovirus retinitis in patients with AIDS. *J AIDS.* 1998;17:339-344.
153. Polis MA, Spooner KM, Baird BF, et al. Anticytomegaloviral activity and safety of ganciclovir in patients with human immunodeficiency virus infection and cytomegaloviruses. *Antimicrob Agents Chemother.* 1995;39:882-886.
154. Lalezari JP, Stagg RJ, Kupperman BD, et al. Intravenous ganciclovir for peripheral cytomegalovirus retinitis in patients with AIDS. *Ann Intern Med.* 1997;126:257-263.
155. Crumpacker CS, Kowalsky PN, Oliver SA, et al. Resistance of herpes simplex virus to 9-{[2-hydroxy-1-(hydroxymethyl) ethoxy]methyl}guanine: Physical mapping of drug synergism within the viral DNA polymerase locus. *Proc Natl Acad Sci U S A.* 1984;81:1556-1560.
156. Manischevitz JF, Quinnan GV, Lane HC, et al. Synergistic effect of ganciclovir and foscarnet on cytomegalovirus replication in vitro. *Antimicrob Agents Chemother.* 1990;34:373-375.
157. Cherrington JM, Fuller MD, Lamy PD, et al. In vitro antiviral susceptibilities of isolates from CMV retinitis patients receiving first or second line cidofovir therapy, relationship to clinical outcome. *J Infect Dis.* 1998;178:1821-1825.
158. Chilar T, Fuller MD, Cherrington JM. Characterization of drug resistance associated mutations in the human cytomegalovirus DNA polymerase gene by using recombinant mutant viruses generated from overlapping DNA fragments. *J Virol.* 1998;72;5927-5936.
159. Biron KK, Harvey RJ, Chamberlain SC, et al. Potent and selective inhibition of human cytomegalovirus replication by 1263W94, a benzimidazole L-riboside with a unique mode of action. *Antimicrob Agents Chemother.* 2002;46:2365-2372.
160. Chou S. Cytomegalovirus UL97 mutations in the era of ganciclovir and maribavir. *Rev Med Virol.* 2008;18:233-246.
161. Chou S, Marousek GI. Accelerated evolution of maribavir resistance in a cytomegalovirus exonuclease domain II mutant. *J Virol.* 2008;82:246-253.
162. Gershburg E, Pagano JS. Phosphorylation of the Epstein-Barr virus (EBV) DNA polymerase processivity factor EA-D by the EBV-encoded protein kinase and effects of the L-riboside benzimidazole 1263W94. *J Virol.* 2002;76:998-1003.
163. Winston DJ, Young JA, Pullarkat V, et al. Maribavir prophylaxis for prevention of cytomegalovirus infection in allogeneic stem cell transplant recipients: a multicenter, randomized, double-blind, placebo-controlled, dose-ranging study. *Blood.* 2008;111:5403-5410.
164. Chou S, Wechel LC, Marousek GI. Cytomegalovirus UL97 kinase mutations that confer maribavir resistance. *J Infect Dis.* 2007;196:91-94.
165. Goodrich JM, Mori M, Gleaves CA, et al. Early treatment with ganciclovir to prevent cytomegalovirus disease after allogeneic bone marrow transplantation. *N Engl J Med.* 1991;325:1601-1607.
166. Schmidt GM, Horack DA, Niland JC, et al. A randomized, controlled trial of prophylactic ganciclovir for cytomegalovirus pulmonary infection in recipients of allogeneic bone marrow transplants. *N Engl J Med.* 1991;324:1005-1011.
167. Merigan TC, Renlund DG, Keay S, et al. A controlled trial of ganciclovir to prevent cytomegalovirus disease after heart transplantation. *N Engl J Med.* 1992;326:1182-1186.
168. Winston DJ, Wirin D, Shaked A, et al. Randomized comparison of ganciclovir and high-dose acyclovir for long-term cytomegalovirus prophylaxis in liver-transplant recipients. *Lancet.* 1995;346:69-74.
169. Spector SA, McKinley GF, Lalezari JP, et al. Oral ganciclovir for the prevention of cytomegalovirus disease in persons with AIDS. *N Engl J Med.* 1996;334:1491-1497.
170. Spector SA, Wong R, Hiza K, et al. Plasma cytomegalovirus (CMV) DNA load predicts CMV disease and survival in AIDS patients. *J Clin Invest.* 1998;101:497-502.
171. Gane E, Salida F, Valdecasas GJC, et al. Randomized trial of efficacy and safety of oral ganciclovir in the prevention of cytomegalovirus disease in liver transplant recipients. *Lancet.* 1997;350:1729-1733.
172. Brennan D, Garlick K, Singer G, et al. Prophylactic oral ganciclovir compared to deferred therapy for control of cytomegalovirus disease in renal transplant patients. *Transplantation.* 1997;64:1843-1846.
173. Chou S, Wechel LC, Marousek GI. Cytomegalovirus UL97 kinase mutations that confer maribavir resistance. *J Infect Dis.* 2007;196:91-94.
174. Ho M, Suwansirikul S, Dowling JN, et al. The transplanted kidney as a source of cytomegalovirus infection. *N Engl J Med.* 1975;293:1109-1112.
175. Betts RF, Freeman RB, Douglas RG Jr, et al. Transmission of cytomegalovirus infection with renal allograft. *Kidney Int.* 1975;8:387-394.
176. Paya C, Humar A, Dominguez E, et al. Efficacy and safety of valganciclovir vs. oral ganciclovir for prevention of cytomegalovirus disease in solid organ transplant recipients. *Am J Transplant.* 2004;4:611-620.
177. Ho M. Virus infections after transplantation in man. *Arch Virol.* 1977;55:1-24.
178. Dowling JN, Saslow AR, Ho M, et al. Cytomegalovirus infection in patients receiving immunosuppressive therapy for rheumatologic disorders. *J Infect Dis.* 1976;133:399-408.
179. Rubin RH. Infection in the renal transplant patient. In: Rubin RH, Young LS, eds. *Clinical Approach to Infection in the Compromised Host.* New York: Plenum; 1981:553-605.
180. Dummer JS, Hardy A, Poorsatter A, et al. Early infections in kidney, heart and liver transplant recipients on cyclosporine. *Transplantation.* 1983;36:259-267.
181. Thomason AW. FK-506—How much potential? *Immunol Today.* 1990;11:6-9.
182. Shepp DH, Dandliker PS, de Miranda P, et al. Activity of 9-[2-hydroxy-1-(hydroxymethyl)ethoxymethyl]guanine in the treatment of cytomegalovirus pneumonia. *Ann Intern Med.* 1985;103:368-373.
183. Crumpacker CS, Marlowe S, Zhang JL, et al. Ganciclovir Bone Marrow Transplant Treatment Group. Treatment of cytomegalovirus pneumonia. *Rev Infect Dis.* 1988;10:S538-S546.
184. Emmanuel D, Cunningham I, Jules-Elysee K, et al. Cytomegalovirus pneumonia after bone marrow transplantation successfully treated with the combination of ganciclovir and high-dose intravenous immune globulin. *Ann Intern Med.* 1988;109:783-788.
185. Reed EC, Bowden RA, Dandliker PS, et al. Treatment of cytomegalovirus pneumonia with ganciclovir and intravenous cytomegalovirus immunoglobulin in patients with bone marrow transplants. *Ann Intern Med.* 1988;109:783-788.
186. Schmidt GM, Kovacs A, Zaia JA, et al. Ganciclovir/immunoglobulin combination therapy for the treatment of human cytomegalovirus-associated interstitial pneumonia in bone marrow allograft recipients. *Transplantation.* 1988;46:905-907.
187. Ljungman P, Engelhard D, Link H. Treatment of interstitial pneumonitis due to cytomegalovirus with ganciclovir and intravenous immune globulin: Experience of European bone marrow transplantation. *Clin Infect Dis.* 1992;14:831-835.
188. Winston DJ, Ho WG, Bartoni K, et al. Ganciclovir prophylaxis of cytomegalovirus infection and disease in allogeneic bone marrow transplant recipients. Results of a placebo-controlled, double-blind trial. *Ann Intern Med.* 1993;118:179-184.
189. Boeckh M, Gooley TA, Myerson D, et al. Cytomegalovirus pp65 antigenemia-guided early treatment with ganciclovir versus ganciclovir at engraftment after allogeneic marrow transplantation: A randomized double-blind study. *Blood.* 1996;88:4063-4071.
190. Einsele H, Ehninger G, Hebart H, et al. Polymerase chain reaction monitoring reduces the incidence of cytomegalovirus disease and the duration and side effects of antiviral therapy after bone marrow transplantation. *Blood.* 1995;86:2815-2820.
191. Ljungman P, Aschan J, Lewensohn-Fuchs I, et al. Results of different strategies for reducing cytomegalovirus-associated mortality in allogeneic stem cell transplant recipients. *Transplantation.* 1998;66:1330-1334.
192. Boeckh M, Leisenring W, Riddell SR, et al. Late cytomegalovirus disease and mortality in recipients of allogeneic hematopoietic stem cell transplants: Importance of viral load and T-cell immunity. *Blood.* 2003;101:407-414.
193. Winston DJ, Yeager AM, Chandrasekar PH, et al. Randomized comparison of oral valacyclovir and intravenous ganciclovir for prevention of cytomegalovirus disease after allogeneic bone marrow transplantation. *Clin Infect Dis.* 2003;36:749-758.
194. Krause H, Hebart H, Jahn G, et al. Screening for CMV-specific T cell proliferation to identify patients at risk of developing late onset CMV disease. *Bone Marrow Transplant.* 1997;19:1111-1116.
195. Patel R, Snydman DR, Rubin RH, et al. Cytomegalovirus prophylaxis in solid organ transplant recipients. *Transplantation.* 1996;61:1279-1289.
196. Stratta RJ, Shaeffer MS, Markin RS, et al. Clinical patterns of cytomegalovirus disease after liver transplantation. *Arch Surg.* 1989;124:1443-1450.
197. McCarthy JM, Karim MA, Keown PA. The cost impact of cytomegalovirus disease in renal transplant recipients. *Transplantation.* 1993;55:1277-1282.
198. Demetris AJ, Lasky S, Van Thiel DH, et al. Pathology of hepatic transplantation. *Am J Pathol.* 1985;116:151-161.
199. Paya CV, Weisner RH, Hermans PE, et al. Risk factors for cytomegalovirus and severe bacterial infections following liver transplantation: A prospective multivariate time-dependent analysis. *J Hepatol.* 1993;18:185-195.
200. O'Grady JG, Alexander GJ, Sutherland S, et al. CMV infection and donor/recipient HLA antigens: Interdependent co-factors in the pathogenesis of vanishing bile duct syndrome after liver transplantation. *Lancet.* 1988;2:302-305.
201. Snydman DR, Werner BG, Dougherty NN, et al, for the Boston Center for Liver Transplantation CMVIG Study Group. Cytomegalovirus immune globulin prophylaxis in liver transplantation. A randomized, double-blind, placebo-controlled trial. *Ann Intern Med.* 1993;119:984-991.
202. Singh N, Yu VL, Mieles L, et al. High-dose acyclovir compared with short-course preemptive ganciclovir therapy to prevent cytomegalovirus disease in liver transplant recipients. *Ann Intern Med.* 1994;120:375-381.
203. Martin M, Manez R, Linden P, et al. A prospective randomized trial comparing sequential ganciclovir-high dose acyclovir to high dose acyclovir for prevention of cytomegalovirus disease in adult liver transplant recipients. *Transplantation.* 1994;58:779-785.
204. Stratta RJ, Shaefer MS, Cushing KA, et al. A randomized prospective trial of acyclovir and immune globulin prophylaxis in liver transplant recipients receiving OKT3 therapy. *Arch Surg.* 1992;127:55-64.
205. Ho M. Cytomegalovirus. In: Mandell J, Bennett J, Dolin R, eds. *Principles of Infectious Disease.* Philadelphia: Saunders; 1996.
206. Aldrete JS, Sterling WA, Hathaway BM, et al. Gastrointestinal and hepatic complications affecting patients with renal allografts. *Am J Surg.* 1975;129:115-124.
207. Petersen PK, Balfour HH Jr, Marker SC, et al. Cytomegalovirus disease in renal allograft recipients: A prospective study of the clinical features, risk factors and impact on renal transplantation. *Medicine (Baltimore).* 1980;59:283-300.
208. Hecht DW, Snydman DR, Crumpacker CS, et al, for the Boston Renal Transplant CMV Study Group. Ganciclovir for treatment of renal transplant-associated primary cytomegalovirus pneumonia. *J Infect Dis.* 1988;157:187-190.
209. Snydman DR, Werner BG, Heinze-Lacey B, et al. Use of cytomegalovirus immune globulin to prevent cytomegalovirus disease in renal-transplant recipients. *N Engl J Med.* 1987;317:1049-1054.
210. Snydman DR, Werner BG, Dougherty NN, et al. Cytomegalovirus prophylaxis in liver transplantation. *Ann Intern Med.* 1993;119:984-991.
211. Hibberd PL, Tolkoff-Rubin NE, Conti D, et al. Preemptive ganciclovir therapy to prevent cytomegalovirus disease in cytomegalovirus antibody-positive renal transplant recipients: A randomized controlled trial. *Ann Intern Med.* 1995;123:18-26.
212. Smieja M, Gnarpe J, Lonn E, et al. Multiple infections and subsequent cardiovascular events in the Heart Outcomes Prevention Evaluation (HOPE) Study. *Circulation.* 2003;107:251-257.
213. Muhlestein JB, Horne BD, Carlquist JF, et al. Cytomegalovirus seropositivity and C-reactive protein have independent and combined predictive value for mortality in patients with angiographically demonstrated coronary artery disease. *Circulation.* 2000;102:1917-1923.
214. Ziemann M, Sedemund-Adib B, Reiland P, et al. Increased mortality in long-term intensive care patients with active cytomegalovirus infection. *Crit Care Med.* 2008;36:3145-3150.
215. Guech-Ongey M, Brenner H, Twardella D, et al. Role of cytomegalovirus sero-status in the development of secondary cardiovascular events in patients with coronary heart disease under special consideration of diabetes. *Int J Cardiol.* 2006;111:98-103.
216. Schlitt A, Blankenberg S, Weise K, et al. Herpesvirus DNA (Epstein-Barr virus, herpes simplex virus, cytomegalovirus) in circulating monocytes of patients with coronary artery disease. *Acta Cardiol.* 2005;60:605-610.
217. Gredmark S, Jonasson L, Van Gosliga D, et al. Active cytomegalovirus replication in patients with coronary disease. *Scand Cardiovasc J.* 2007;41:230-234.

218. Kyto V, Vuorinen T, Saukko P, et al. Cytomegalovirus infection of the heart is common in patients with fatal myocarditis. *Clin Infect Dis.* 2005;40:683-688.

219. Donoso Mantke O, Meyer R, et al. Frequent detection of viral nucleic acids in heart valve tissue. *J Clin Microbiol.* 2004; 42:2298-2300.

220. Tang-Feldman YJ, Wojtowicz A, Lochhead GR, et al. Use of quantitative real-time PCR (qRT-PCR) to measure cytokine transcription and viral load in murine cytomegalovirus infection. *J Virol Methods.* 2006;131:122-129.

221. Vliegen I, Duijvestijn A, Grauls G, et al. Cytomegalovirus infection aggravates atherogenesis in apoE knockout mice by both local and systemic immune activation. *Microbes Infect.* 2004;6:17-24.

222. Rott D, Zhu J, Zhou YF, et al. IL-6 is produced by splenocytes derived from CMV-infected mice in response to CMV antigens, and induces MCP-1 production by endothelial cells: a new mechanistic paradigm for infection-induced atherogenesis. *Atherosclerosis.* 2003;170:223-228.

222a. Cheng J, Ke Q, Jin Z, et al. Cytomegalovirus infection causes an increase of arterial blood pressure. *PLoS Pathog.* 2009; 5:e1000427.

223. Vliegen I, Herngreen SB, Grauls GE, et al. Mouse cytomegalovirus antigenic immune stimulation is sufficient to aggravate atherosclerosis in hypercholesterolemic mice. *Atherosclerosis* 2005;181:39-44.

224. Bartlett EJ, Lenzo JC, Sivamoorthy S, et al. Type I IFN-beta gene therapy suppresses cardiac CD8+ T-cell infiltration during autoimmune myocarditis. *Immunol Cell Biol.* 2004;82:119-126.

225. Speir E, Modali R, Huang ES, et al. Potential role of human cytomegalovirus and p53 interaction in coronary restenosis. *Science.* 1994;265:391-394.

226. Gravel SP, Servant MJ. Roles of an IkappaB kinase-related pathway in human cytomegalovirus-infected vascular smooth muscle cells: a molecular link in pathogen-induced proatherosclerotic conditions. *J Biol Chem.* 2005;280:7477-7486.

227. Villacres MC, Longmate J, Auge C, et al. Predominant type 1 CMV-specific memory T-helper response in humans: evidence for gender differences in cytokine secretion. *Hum Immunol.* 2004;65:476-485.

228. Soderberg-Naucler C. HCMV microinfections in inflammatory diseases and cancer. *J Clin Virol.* 2008;41:218-223.

229. Bolovan-Fritts CA, Trout RN, Spector SA. Human cytomegalovirus-specific CD4+-T-cell cytokine response induces fractalkine in endothelial cells. *J Virol.* 2004;78:13173-13181.

230. Lunardi C, Bason C, Corrocher R, et al. Induction of endothelial cell damage by hCMV molecular mimicry. *Trends Immunol.* 2005;26:19-24.

231. Woodroffe SB, Garnett HM, Danis VA. Interleukin-1 production and cell-activation response to cytomegalovirus infection of vascular endothelial cells. *Arch Virol.* 1993;133:295-308.

232. Dengler TJ, Raftery MJ, Werle M, et al. Cytomegalovirus infection of vascular cells induces expression of pro-inflammatory adhesion molecules by paracrine action of secreted interleukin-1beta. *Transplantation.* 2000;69:1160-1168.

233. Reinhardt B, Schaarschmidt P, Bossert A, et al. Upregulation of functionally active vascular endothelial growth factor by human cytomegalovirus. *J Gen Virol.* 2005;86:23-30.

234. Stagno S, Pass RF, Dworsky ME, et al. Congenital and perinatal cytomegalovirus infections. *Semin Perinatol.* 1983;7:31-42.

235. Stagno S, Pass RF, Dworsky ME, et al. Congenital cytomegalovirus infection: The relative importance of primary and recurrent maternal infection. *N Engl J Med.* 1982;306:945-949.

236. Stagno S, Whitley RJ. Herpesvirus infections of pregnancy. Part I: Cytomegalovirus and Epstein-Barr virus infection. *N Engl J Med.* 1985;313:1270-1274.

237. Ahlfors K, Harris S, Ivarsson S, et al. Secondary maternal cytomegalovirus infection causing symptomatic congenital infection. *N Engl J Med.* 1981;305:284.

238. Hanshaw JB. Developmental abnormalities associated with congenital cytomegalovirus infection. In: Wollam DHM, ed. *Advances in Teratology. v. 4.* New York: Academic Press; 1970:64.

239. Yeager AS, Grumet FC, Hafleigh EB, et al. Prevention of transfusion-acquired cytomegalovirus infection in newborn infants. *J Pediatr.* 1981;98:281-287.

240. Hanshaw JB, Scheiner AP, Moxley AW, et al. School failure and deafness after "silent" congenital cytomegalovirus infection. *N Engl J Med.* 1976;295:468-470.

241. Stagno S, Reynolds DW, Amos CS, et al. Auditory and visual defects resulting from symptomatic and subclinical congenital cytomegaloviral and *Toxoplasma* infections. *Pediatrics.* 1977;59:669-678.

242. Alexander ER. Maternal and neonatal infection with cytomegalovirus in Taiwan [abstract]. *Pediatr Res.* 1967;1:210.

243. Chandler SH, Handsfield HH, McDougall JK. Isolation of multiple strains of cytomegalovirus from women attending a clinic for sexually transmitted diseases. *J Infect Dis.* 1987;155:655-660.

244. Numazaki Y, Yano N, Morizuka T, et al. Primary infection with human cytomegalovirus: Virus isolation from healthy infants and pregnant women. *Am J Epidemiol.* 1970;91:410-417.

245. Stagno S, Reynolds D, Tsiantos A, et al. Cervical cytomegalovirus excretion in pregnant and non-pregnant women: Suppressions in early gestation. *J Infect Dis.* 1975;131:522-527.

246. Montgomery RL, Youngblood LA, Medearis DN Jr. Recovery of cytomegalovirus from the cervix in pregnancy. *Pediatrics.* 1972;49:524-531.

247. Reynolds DW, Stagno S, Hosty TS, et al. Maternal cytomegalovirus excretion and perinatal infection. *N Engl J Med.* 1973;289:1-5.

248. Boppana SB, Rivera LB, Fowler KB, et al. Intrauterine transmission of cytomegalovirus to infants of women with preconceptional immunity. *N Engl J Med.* 2001;344:1366-1371.

139

Epstein-Barr Virus (Infectious Mononucleosis, Epstein-Barr Virus–Associated Malignant Diseases, and Other Diseases)

ERIC C. JOHANNSEN | KENNETH M. KAYE

Epstein-Barr virus (EBV) is a ubiquitous human herpes virus. Infection with EBV is common, worldwide in distribution, and largely subclinical in early childhood. EBV has been established as the causative agent of heterophile-positive infectious mononucleosis, which occurs most frequently in late adolescence or early adulthood. In addition, EBV is causally associated with the development of malignant diseases, including Burkitt's lymphoma, lymphoproliferative disease, Hodgkin's lymphoma, primary central nervous system (CNS) lymphomas in acquired immunodeficiency syndrome (AIDS), and nasopharyngeal carcinoma based on seroepidemiologic data and the detection of EBV genomes in these tumors. Some epidemiologic studies describe an association between EBV and autoimmune diseases, particularly multiple sclerosis; however, a causal relationship is not established.

History

Historical accounts of infectious mononucleosis often attribute the initial description of the disease to Filatov or Pfeiffer, who nearly simultaneously at the end of the 19th century described an illness characterized by malaise, fever, hepatosplenomegaly, lymphadenopathy, and abdominal discomfort.[1,2] This illness came to be known as Drusenfieber (glandular fever) and occurred in family outbreaks. However, without specific techniques with which to establish the diagnosis, the concept of Drusenfieber as a clinical entity fell into disrepute. Between 1910 and 1920, a number of observers reported cases of apparent spontaneous remission of leukemia, with a clinical course that is consistent with the spontaneous resolution of infectious mononucleosis.[3,4] The establishment of infectious mononucleosis as a clinical entity is credited to Sprunt and Evans,[5] who in 1920 described six cases of fever, lymphadenopathy, and prostration that occurred in previously healthy young adults. The authors pointed out the mononuclear lymphocytosis that developed in each of the patients and contrasted the pathologic appearance of these lymphocytes with the uniform lymphocyte morphology observed in children with other infections. Two years later, Downey and McKinlay[6] described additional cases of infectious mononucleosis and provided a more detailed morphologic description of the atypical lymphocyte. The recognition of atypical lymphocytosis as a hematologic marker for the disease led to more accurate descriptions of the clinical manifestations of this illness.

A major advance occurred in 1932, when Paul and Bunnell,[7] investigating immunologic mechanisms in serum sickness, unexpectedly encountered high titers of spontaneously occurring sheep red blood cell agglutinins in the sera of patients with infectious mononucleosis. Davidsohn[8] later enhanced the specificity of detection of this heterophile antibody with differential absorption of serum with guinea pig kidney and beef erythrocytes.

During the 1940s and 1950s, substantial efforts were made to detect a causative agent for infectious mononucleosis. Attempts to culture etiologically related bacteria and viruses from patients with infectious mononucleosis proved unsuccessful. The disease could not be transmitted to animals. Interpretation of experimental attempts to transmit the disease to humans was hindered by the failure to appreciate the widespread occurrence of asymptomatic infection in preadolescents and the absence of a serologic marker of immunity.[9-11]

The identification of EBV followed the description by Burkitt[12] in 1958 of an unusual lymphoma with a predilection for the head and neck. The geographic distribution of this tumor paralleled that of certain mosquito-borne diseases in Africa, and a search for an etiologically related arbovirus was undertaken. Epstein and associates[13] in 1964 described the presence of particles that resembled herpes viruses in tissue cultures of biopsy specimens from patients with Burkitt's lymphoma. However, attempts to propagate the virus in conventional tissue cultures were unsuccessful. An indirect immunofluorescent antibody technique to this virus, now called Epstein-Barr virus, was developed by Werner and Gertrude Henle,[14] and high titers of this antibody were detected in patients with Burkitt's lymphoma. Additional studies revealed that 90% of American adults had demonstrable EBV antibodies as well.[14] The development of infectious mononucleosis in a technician in the Henles' laboratory on whom sequentially obtained sera were analyzed for EBV antibody suggested that acute EBV infection may be associated with this illness.[15] Large-scale epidemiologic studies[16-19] showed that heterophile-positive infectious mononucleosis occurred in patients without preexisting EBV antibody and, conversely, heterophile-positive infectious mononucleosis was always accompanied by acquisition of EBV antibodies. These epidemiologic studies indicated that subclinical EBV infection also occurred. With specific antibody tests for EBV, it became apparent that 10% to 20% of the cases of mononucleosis, of which most were heterophile negative, were caused by other agents, the most frequent of which was cytomegalovirus (CMV). This chapter deals primarily with EBV-induced infectious mononucleosis.

Description of Epstein-Barr Virus

PHYSICAL PROPERTIES

Epstein-Barr virus (EBV), or human herpes virus 4, is a gamma-1 herpes virus. Like the other members of the Herpesviridae family, EBV has a double-stranded DNA genome encased in an icosahedral protein nucleocapsid surrounded by a lipid envelope embedded with viral glycoproteins. Herpes viruses also have an amorphous protein layer, the tegument, which lies between the capsid and envelope. The B95-8 laboratory strain of EBV, the first herpes virus genome sequenced, was found to have a 12-kilobase (kb) deletion, and the wild-type EBV genome is now known to be approximately 184 kb in size and to encode almost 100 proteins.[20,21]

TABLE 139-1	Frequency of Epstein-Barr Virus Shedding	
Population Description	**Oropharyngeal Shedding Rate (Range)**	**Reference**
EBV-seronegative individuals	0	82
Seropositive healthy adults	12%-25%	82-87
Solid tumor patients	27%	86, 87
HIV-1–infected individuals	50%	88
Renal transplant recipients	56%-70%	85, 87
Infectious mononucleosis patients	50%-100%	82-84, 325
Critically ill leukemia or lymphoma patients	74%-92%	86, 87

LIFE CYCLE

Primary infection with EBV results from exposure to the oral secretions of seropositive individuals through kissing, sharing of food, or other intimate contact. The long-accepted concept that EBV infection spreads to B lymphocytes after initial productive (lytic) infection of oral epithelial cells[22,23] has been challenged. Tonsillar biopsies from patients with primary EBV infection did not reveal any infected epithelial cells, but infected lymphocytes were readily seen.[24,25] EBV undoubtedly has clinically significant tropism for epithelial cells as is seen in nasopharyngeal carcinoma and oral hairy leukoplakia. It remains possible that significant infection of oral epithelial cells occurs in nontonsillar sites or that an initial round of lytic replication precedes spread to the B-cell compartment and the onset of symptoms.[26,27] Infected B lymphocytes incite an intense cytotoxic T-cell response, and these T cells constitute the atypical lymphocytosis characteristic of primary EBV infection.[28,29] In healthy individuals, most infected B lymphocytes are cleared through immune surveillance, but between one and 50 B cells per million remain quiescently infected and serve as the reservoir for lifelong infection of the individual.[30,31] Thus, EBV shares the properties of lifelong latency and persistence with other members of the herpes virus family. In contrast to that of alpha herpes viruses (herpes simplex virus and varicella-zoster virus), shedding of infectious EBV particles into the saliva from periodic reactivation of latently infected cells is entirely asymptomatic. This shedding occurs in otherwise healthy persons but is more frequent in immunosuppressed hosts (Table 139-1).

The host range of the virus is limited. In vitro cultivation of the virus has been described primarily in B lymphocytes and also in nasopharyngeal epithelial cells of humans and certain nonhuman primates.[32] EBV binds to its receptor, the CD21 molecule, through an interaction with its major envelope glycoprotein, gp350. CD21 is a 145-kDa glycoprotein that is also the receptor for the d region of the third component of complement and is also termed the C3d receptor or CR2.[33,34] This receptor is demonstrable on B lymphocytes and nasopharyngeal epithelial cells of humans and certain nonhuman primates and on a small proportion of complement receptor–bearing, non-B, non-T lymphocytes.[35-39] Another EBV glycoprotein, gp42, binds major histocompatibility complex (MHC) class II molecules, which serve as co-receptors for infection of B cells.[40-44]

LATENT INFECTION AND GROWTH TRANSFORMATION

After infection with EBV, B lymphocytes enter the cell cycle and proliferate continuously in a process termed *transformation* or *immortalization;* these cells can be propagated in vitro indefinitely.[45] This ability of EBV to convert peripheral blood B cells into immortalized lymphoblastoid cell lines (LCLs) is widely used in genomic studies as a means of preserving DNA samples from volunteer donors for future use.[46] In vivo EBV-driven B-cell proliferation is observed during infectious mononucleosis, in which it probably serves to expand rapidly the pool of infected B lymphocytes. These B lymphocytes are usually rapidly cleared from the circulation.[47-50] However, in the absence of an intact immune response, EBV infection can result in life-threatening lymphoproliferative disease (LPD).[51,52] The growth-transforming properties of EBV can act in concert with genetic and environmental cofactors to cause malignant diseases in immunocompetent hosts as well.[53,54]

Epstein-Barr virus infection of B lymphocytes is characterized by a state of viral latency, in which the genome circularizes in the nucleus and is replicated as an episome in concert with host chromosomes by cell enzymes. The infection is latent in the sense that viral particles are not being produced, but it is anything but quiescent. Limited viral gene expression persists, and these genes exert effects on the infected cell. In vitro latent infection of B lymphocytes with EBV is characterized by the expression of latent infection membrane proteins 1 and 2 (LMP1 and LMP2), six EBV nuclear antigens (EBNAs), and two small, nuclear, noncoding RNAs (EBV-encoded RNAs [EBERs]) that are transcribed by RNA polymerase III (Table 139-2).[55] Additional EBV transcripts have been detected in latent infection and are termed complementary strand transcripts (CSTs) or BamH1 A rightward transcripts (BARTs). Translation of these transcripts into proteins has not been shown, but they appear to serve as precursors for two of three clusters of EBV-encoded microRNAs (miRNAs) whose role in EBV biology remains unclear.[56,57] Recombinant reverse genetic analysis has determined that only *LMP1, EBNA1, EBNA2, EBNA3A, EBNA3C,* and *EBNALP* are critical for B-cell growth transformation.[55] The mechanisms by which these EBV genes promote B-lymphocyte growth have been the subject of intense investigation.

After the virus gains entry to susceptible B lymphocytes, EBNA2 and EBNALP are the first proteins expressed. *EBNA2* is an acidic transac-

TABLE 139-2	Patterns of Epstein-Barr Virus (EBV) Latent Gene Expression							
				EBV-Associated Malignant Diseases				
		Acute Infection	**Healthy Carrier**	**Latency III**		**Latency II**		**Latency I**
EBV Gene	**Function**	**IM**	**PBB**	**LPD**	**PCNSL**	**HL**	**NPC**	**BL**
EBNA1	EBV genome maintenance	+	?	+	+	+	+	+
EBNA2	Activate expression of EBV/host genes	+	−	+	+	−	−	−
EBNA3s*	Unknown	+	−	+	+	−	−	−
EBNALP	Coactivates with EBNA2	+	−	+	+	−	−	−
LMP1	Mimics CD40 signaling	+	−	+	+	+	+	−
LMP2	Mimics BCR signaling	+	+	+	+	+	+	−
EBERs	Noncoding, highly expressed RNAs	+	+	+	+	+	+	+

*Includes EBNA3A, EBNA3B, and EBNA3C.
BL, Burkitt's lymphoma; HL, Hodgkin's lymphoma; IM, infectious mononucleosis; NPC, nasopharyngeal carcinoma; PBB, peripheral blood B cell; PCNSL, primary central nervous system lymphoma.

tivator that acts as the major switch to turn on latent virus gene expression and several B-cell gene products (including CD21, CD23, and c-fgr). It has no intrinsic sequence-specific DNA binding capacity but rather is targeted to promoters by binding to a host DNA binding protein RBP-Jκ (also called CBF1 or CSL), a downstream component of the Notch signaling pathway.[58,59] By an incompletely understood mechanism, EBNALP cooperates with EBNA2 to activate expression of the remaining nuclear proteins and LMP1 and LMP2.[60] *LMP1* is the major EBV-encoded oncogene, and its expression in transgenic mice results in B-cell lymphomas.[61,62] It constitutively activates signaling pathways that mimic the growth and survival signals given to B cells by CD4+ T lymphocytes through the CD40 surface glycoprotein. LMP1 sends this signal through its cytoplasmic tail, which binds a set of second messenger proteins similar but not identical to those used by CD40.[63,64] Unlike CD40, LMP1 does not require the presence of ligand to form patches in the cell membrane but self associates constitutively, approximating its cytoplasmic tails to activate signaling.[65] This results in the activation of nuclear factor κB (NF-κB), c-jun, upregulation of adhesion molecules (intercellular adhesion molecule 1, LFA-1, and LFA-3), cytokine production, B-cell proliferation, and induction of an antiapoptotic state.[47,54] A second EBV latent membrane protein, LMP2, mimics another signal necessary for B-cell survival.[66] By interacting with signaling molecules of the B-cell receptor (BCR), LMP2 mimics BCR engagement by constitutive patching in the membrane in a manner analogous to LMP1. LMP2 probably also interferes with normal signaling through the BCR by antigenic stimulation to inhibit activation of lytic viral replication (discussed subsequently). Interestingly, LMP2 is not necessary for EBV-mediated outgrowth of B cells in vitro but is probably a critical component of the viral strategy in vivo. The nuclear protein EBNA1 acts to promote the replication of the viral genome by the host machinery when the virus is in the latent, episomal state and to ensure proper segregation of the EBV genome to both daughter cells. The EBNA3 proteins are of uncertain function but are known to interact with the same DNA binding protein as EBNA2 (RBP-Jκ) and may modulate virus and cell gene expression. The function of the highly expressed, noncoding EBV RNAs (EBERs) is incompletely understood.

Epstein-Barr virus–associated malignant diseases are exclusively associated with latent infection and latent gene expression. Three general patterns of expression of EBV-encoded proteins have been observed in association with latency (see Table 139-2).[47,48] Expression of all latent genes is seen in LPD in immunosuppressed hosts, in primary CNS lymphoma of patients with AIDS, and during primary EBV infection (infectious mononucleosis), and this program of gene expression is often referred to as latency III.[53] EBV-associated nasopharyngeal carcinomas, Hodgkin's lymphoma, and T-cell lymphomas exhibit a more restricted pattern of EBV gene expression (latency II) that includes LMP1, LMP2, EBNA1, and the EBERs and EBNA1.[67-69] In Burkitt's lymphoma (latency I) only EBERs and EBNA1 are expressed.[53] The more restricted patterns of latent gene expression in some tumors are probably in part the result of the intense immune response against viral proteins.

LYTIC INFECTION

Latent infection can be activated to lytic infection by stimulation of host B cells by certain chemicals, calcium ionophores, or antibodies to surface immunoglobulin.[70] The physiologic signals that reactivate EBV lytic replication are unknown, but signaling through the B-cell receptor after antigenic stimulation is a possible scenario. After this inciting event, two EBV-encoded transcriptional activators are expressed: BZLF1 and BRLF1. Expression of these immediate early genes leads to a cascade of events that culminate in the production of early EBV gene (early antigen [EA]) products responsible for viral replication (e.g., thymidine kinase and DNA polymerase) and late (structural) genes of the virus including viral capsid antigens (VCAs).[71] Lytic infection produces EBV virions and can cause host cell death.

Epidemiology

SERUM ANTIBODY PREVALENCE

Antibodies to EBV have been found in all population groups studied, and most studies have shown no predilection for either gender. Antibodies are acquired earlier in life in developing countries than in industrialized countries, but by adulthood, 90% to 95% of most populations have demonstrable EBV antibodies.[72,73] In the United States and in Great Britain, EBV seroconversion occurs before the age of 5 years in about 50% of the population.[73-75] A second wave of seroconversion occurs midway through the second decade of life. EBV seroconversion may occur at a younger average age in the southern United States than in other areas of that country.[76] Lower socioeconomic groups have a higher EBV antibody prevalence than more affluent age-matched control groups.

Two strains of EBV have been defined on the basis of viral gene sequences expressed during latency and their ability to transform B lymphocytes.[70] The strains (type 1 [A] or 2 [B]) are not distinguishable serologically, but they express unique epitopes that are identified by cytotoxic T lymphocytes (CTLs). Although the initial thought was that specific geographic distributions existed for these two strains of EBV, it is now clear that both are widely distributed and that individuals can be coinfected with both strains.

INCIDENCE OF INFECTION

Clinically apparent infectious mononucleosis is more common in populations in which primary EBV exposure is delayed until after the first decade of life. The disease is diagnosed most frequently among adolescents of higher socioeconomic groups in industrialized countries.[77] The incidence of infectious mononucleosis in a large epidemiologic study in the United States was 45.2 cases per 100,000 per year and was highest in the 15-year-old to 24-year-old age group.[78] The incidence was the same for women as for men, but the peak age-specific incidence occurred 2 years earlier in women. Infectious mononucleosis is 30 times more frequent in whites than in blacks. The infrequency of infectious mononucleosis among blacks, noted as early as 1940, is probably a reflection of earlier primary EBV infection and the higher frequency of subclinical infections in children.[79-81] No clear seasonal incidence has been noted.

METHODS OF SPREAD

Low titers of EBV are present in throat washings of persons with infectious mononucleosis.[82-84] Susceptible roommates of students with infectious mononucleosis or with inapparent EBV infection have EBV seroconversion no more frequently than the general susceptible college population.[18,76] Only 6% of those with infectious mononucleosis cite previous contact with another case of infectious mononucleosis.[78] The virus persists in the B-cell compartment for the life of the infected host and can be cultured from throat washings from 10% to 20% of healthy adults, from 50% of kidney transplant recipients, and from greater proportions of those critically ill with leukemia or lymphoma (see Table 139-1).[85-87] Approximately 50% of men with human immunodeficiency virus type–1 (HIV-1) infection who have sex with men shed EBV in oropharyngeal secretions.[88] EBV DNA or protein, or both, have also been identified in parotid duct and uterine cervical epithelia, although the implications of this distribution are unclear with respect to viral transmission.[89,90]

Epstein-Barr virus, like other herpes viruses, is relatively labile in the laboratory, and the virus has not been recovered from environmental sources, including fomites. These data suggest that EBV is a widespread agent that is not particularly contagious and that most cases of infectious mononucleosis are probably contracted by intimate contact between susceptible individuals and asymptomatic shedders of EBV. Among young adults, spread of the virus may be facilitated by the transfer of saliva with kissing.[91,92] Serologic evidence suggests that the virus may also be spread among susceptible individuals within families.[93,94] EBV has also been spread via blood transfusion and after open heart surgery as the postpump perfusion syndrome.[95] Most postpump perfusion infectious mononucleosis is, however, heterophile negative and attributable to CMV.

Although several apparent epidemics of infectious mononucleosis have been described, these reports have not been substantiated with EBV serologic data and have lacked rigorous epidemiologic, clinical, or laboratory support. Some of these have resulted from errors in the performance of Monospot tests.[96] On the basis of the previously discussed information, true epidemics of infectious mononucleosis are unlikely to occur.

PUBLIC HEALTH IMPACT

College and military populations experience the highest morbidity from infectious mononucleosis, although cases occur in other groups as well. Infectious mononucleosis accounted for 5% of all hospitalizations of University of Wisconsin students, with an incidence rate of 450 admissions per 100,000 students per year. Other American universities have reported similar incidence rates.[97,98] Approximately 12% of susceptible college students undergo EBV seroconversion yearly.[18,19] Many of these infections are subclinical (see subsequent discussion).[18,76] Although primary EBV infection may be clinically apparent in only about 10% of military cases, infectious mononucleosis ranked fourth as the cause of days lost because of illness in army personnel.[99,100] Detailed information about the impact of infectious mononucleosis on the general population is not available because infectious mononucleosis is not a reportable disease in most states. However, morbidity from infectious mononucleosis likely is generally underestimated because a specific diagnosis may not be made and the nonspecific illness can be attributed to a variety of other causes.

Pathogenesis

HOST IMMUNE RESPONSE

Epstein-Barr virus presents a formidable challenge to the immune system. At the height of acute infection, up to 20% of peripheral blood B lymphocytes may express EBNA, and 0.005% to 0.5% of circulating mononuclear cells are capable of forming continuous cell lines if cultured in vitro.[101,102] The immune response to EBV-infected transformed lymphocytes is complex and involves both humoral and cell-mediated immune mechanisms.[28] An intact immune response is critical to prevention of the unchecked proliferation of these cells as seen in LPD but is also responsible for most of the symptoms of infectious mononucleosis. The increase in prevalence in symptomatic acute EBV infection with age of seroconversion is probably the result of differences in the immune responses of different age groups.

The cellular immune response to EBV is complex and well integrated and includes CD8+ and CD4+ CTLs and natural killer (NK) cells.[29,103-106] The massive atypical lymphocytosis of infectious mononucleosis is composed primarily of antigen-stimulated CD8+ cytotoxic T cells. In one study, 40% of circulating CD8+ T cells were reactive against a single EBV epitope.[107] These lymphocytes probably produce most of the signs and symptoms of infectious mononucleosis through the abundant production of cytokines, including tumor necrosis factor, interleukin-1 (IL-1), and IL-6.[108] During acute infection, CD8+ T cells specific for lytic antigens predominate, but with convalescence, a shift occurs toward cells that recognize latent proteins, particularly the EBNA3 proteins.[28,107,109] T cells reactive against EBV latent proteins are sufficiently numerous that unselected mononuclear cells from EBV-immune adults suppress the outgrowth of autologous EBV-infected B lymphocytes in vitro.[106] An expansion of EBV-specific CD4+ lymphocytes has also been described in infectious mononucleosis but is small in magnitude, and its significance in containing acute EBV infection is unclear.[110,111]

The humoral immune response to EBV has been extensively studied, primarily as a means to diagnose EBV infection (see Laboratory Diag-

nosis section for detailed discussion). In general, specific antibodies directed against EBV lytic antigens (VCA and EA) are demonstrable in most patients with infectious mononucleosis. By contrast, antibody responses to the latency-associated EBV nuclear antigens (EBNA1, EBNA2, EBNA3s, and EBNALP) do not develop until convalescence.[28] The significance of any of these antibody responses to containment of EBV infection is not established; however, antibodies to EBV surface glycoproteins have been shown to prevent experimental EBV infection.[112-114]

For unclear reasons, primary EBV infection is associated with the synthesis of large amounts of antibodies reactive against antigens found on sheep, horse, and beef red cells. These so-called heterophile antibodies are a heterogeneous group of predominantly immunoglobulin M (IgM) antibodies that do not react with specific EBV proteins.[115] Detection of these antibodies in sera of patients with mononucleosis syndromes predicts acute EBV infection with high sensitivity and specificity and is discussed in the section Laboratory Diagnosis. No good correlation is found between the heterophile titer and the severity of the illness, and no clearly defined role exists for heterophile antibodies in the pathogenesis of EBV disease or in immune clearance of the virus.

Epstein-Barr virus has evolved multiple strategies to elude this aggressive immune response. The EBV BCRF1 protein shares 70% homology with the cytokine IL-10. This EBV protein is functional and is thought to mimic IL-10 inhibition of interferon-γ synthesis by mononuclear cells in the peripheral blood. Thus, BCRF1 expression during lytic infection is expected to promote a shift toward Th2 differentiated CD4+ effectors that can provide B-cell help but do not promote the CD8+ responses needed to kill EBV-infected cells.[116,117] Another EBV protein, BARF1, can function as a soluble receptor for colony-stimulating factor 1 and may interfere with the ability of this cytokine to enhance expression of interferon-α from monocytes.[118] EBV also encodes a bcl2 homologue that is expressed during lytic replication and may act to prevent apoptosis of the host cell.[119] Finally, the virus has evolved a strategy for ensuring its persistence in the memory B cell compartment. After acute infection resolves, most latent proteins are no longer expressed to circumvent the strong immune pressure exerted against EBV. However, in any cycling cell, EBV must express EBNA1 to ensure that its genome is replicated. To prevent targeting of this key protein, EBNA1 contains a sequence of expanded glycine-alanine repeats, not necessary for its function in genome maintenance, capable of inhibiting proteasomal processing of the protein.[120] Without this processing, EBNA1 peptides cannot be presented on class I MHC molecules, and cells that express EBNA1 may elude immune surveillance.

HISTOPATHOLOGIC FINDINGS

Because biopsies are rarely obtained in patients with uncomplicated infectious mononucleosis, most data come from pathologic examination of tissues obtained from fatal cases or from cases with atypical features in which biopsy specimens were obtained for diagnostic evaluation. During the acute phase of the illness, lymph nodes throughout the body are moderately enlarged. Individual nodes reveal increased numbers of enlarged, moderately active lymphoid follicles. Germinal centers are also enlarged, with cores that contain blast cells, histiocytes, and lymphocytes. Although the reticulin framework remains intact, invasion by the hyperplastic pulp makes its borders less distinct.[121] In studies of spleens obtained at autopsy or at surgery after rupture, the organ is usually two to three times its normal weight.[122] The splenic capsule and trabeculae are edematous, thinned, and invaded by lymphoid cells. Most of the increased splenic size is the result of hyperplasia of the red pulp. Throughout the red pulp, pleomorphic blast cells are evident. The spleen is often congested with focal, particularly subcapsular, hemorrhages. The white pulp is relatively normal. Tonsillar biopsy specimens obtained during the course of mononucleosis reveal intense proliferation with numerous mitoses.[123] Bone marrow aspirate and biopsy specimens are often strikingly normal when compared with the florid changes noted in peripheral blood. Biopsy specimens are usually normocellular to mildly hypercellular. Small granulomas may be present, but these are not specific for mononucleosis and have no prognostic significance.[124,125]

Changes in hepatic histologic features are usually mild. Hepatocytes show minimal swelling and vacuolization. Pleomorphic lymphocytic and monocytic portal infiltration is usually evident. Bile ducts may be minimally swollen, but frank biliary stasis is rare.[126,127] A number of histopathologic changes have been reported in the nervous system in fatal cases of infectious mononucleosis.[123,128,129] These changes include neuronal degeneration, perivascular cuffing, perivascular hemorrhage, and astrocytic hyperplasia. Little mononuclear infiltration may be present despite demonstrable degenerative changes in the neurons of the cortex, basal ganglia, cerebellum, or spinal cord.

Clinical Manifestations

INFECTIOUS MONONUCLEOSIS (PRIMARY INFECTION)

Spectrum of Illness
Epstein-Barr virus induces a broad spectrum of illness in humans. Classic or typical infectious mononucleosis is an acute illness characterized clinically by sore throat, fever, and lymphadenopathy; serologically by the transient appearance of heterophile antibodies; and hematologically by a mononuclear leukocytosis that consists, in part, of atypical lymphocytes (Table 139-3). An individual case may have most but not necessarily all the aforementioned characteristics. Specific serologic tests for EBV infection indicate that infection results in a spectrum of clinical manifestations. Attempts to exclude cases that fail to meet the classic criteria for infectious mononucleosis result in artificial and often misleading distinctions.

The age of the patient has a profound influence on the clinical expression of EBV infection. In children, primary EBV infection is often asymptomatic. Young children may be more likely to exhibit rashes, neutropenia, or pneumonia than individuals with primary EBV infection at an older age.[130] Clinically apparent infections in very young children are heterophile negative in about one half of the cases.[131] The proportions of clinically apparent disease and of heterophile-positive cases increase with age. By 4 years of age, 80% of children with primary EBV infection are heterophile antibody positive.[132] During the course of the illness, 90% of the adolescents with clinically apparent infectious mononucleosis should be heterophile positive.

In patients of college age, the ratio of clinically apparent to inapparent EBV infection ranges from 1:3 to 3:1.[18,76] In military recruits, this ratio has been as low as 1:10.[100] Because of previously existing immunity, the disease is less common in older patients. When it does occur, however, clinical and serologic manifestations are similar to those found in adolescents.[133] In general, EBV infection is inapparent or is a self-limited illness that lasts 2 or 3 weeks. In rare cases, the disease can

be devastating and can be accompanied by severe prostration, major complications, and even death,[134] as discussed subsequently.

Symptoms
Most cases of infectious mononucleosis consist of the clinical triad of sore throat, fever, and lymphadenopathy (Table 139-4). Epidemiologic studies suggest that the incubation period of acute infectious mononucleosis is 30 to 50 days, but this has not yet been confirmed with molecular epidemiologic techniques.[83,138] Thus, the incubation period of the illness is somewhat speculative. The onset may be abrupt, but often several days of prodromal symptoms can be elicited, including chills, sweats, feverish sensations, anorexia, and malaise. Loss of taste for cigarettes is common early in the illness but is not specific for infectious mononucleosis. Retroorbital headaches, myalgias, and feelings of abdominal fullness are other common prodromal symptoms. The most frequent symptom is sore throat, which may be the most severe the patient has experienced.[135,136] Other patients seek medical attention because of prolonged fever or malaise and less frequently because of incidentally encountered lymphadenopathy. Rarely, the first manifestation of illness is one of the complications of infectious mononucleosis described subsequently.

Signs
The signs of infectious mononucleosis are summarized in Table 139-5. Fever is present in more than 90% of patients with infectious mononucleosis. The fever usually peaks in the afternoon with temperatures of 38°C to 39°C, although a temperature as high as 40°C is not uncommon. In most cases, fever resolves over a 10-day to 14-day period. A rash, which may be macular, petechial, scarlatiniform, urticarial, or erythema multiforme–like, is present in about 5% of patients. The administration of ampicillin or amoxicillin produces a pruritic, maculopapular eruption in 90% to 100% of the patients (Fig. 139-1), and this rash may appear after cessation of treatment with the drug.[140,141] The ampicillin-related rash does not necessarily predict future intoler-

TABLE 139-4	Symptoms of Infectious Mononucleosis[97,135-137]		
Symptom	Rate	Percentage	Range (%)
Sore throat	409/502	82	70-88
Malaise	243/426	57	43-76
Headache	216/426	51	37-55
Anorexia	117/546	21	10-27
Myalgias	66/326	20	12-22
Chills	54/326	16	9-18
Nausea	18/156	12	2-17
Abdominal discomfort	37/426	9	2-14
Cough	3/56	5	5
Vomiting	3/56	5	5
Arthralgias	1/56	2	2

TABLE 139-3	Manifestations of Epstein-Barr Virus–Induced Infectious Mononucleosis
Clinical	
Fever	
Sore throat	
Lymphadenopathy	
Hematologic	
More than 50% mononuclear cells	
More than 10% atypical lymphocytes	
Serologic	
Transient appearance of heterophile antibodies	
Permanent emergence of antibodies to EBV	

TABLE 139-5	Signs of Infectious Mononucleosis[135-137,139]		
Sign	Rate	Percentage	Range (%)
Lymphadenopathy	495/526	94	93-100
Pharyngitis	444/526	84	69-91
Fever	399/526	76	63-100
Splenomegaly	244/470	52	50-63
Hepatomegaly	34/370	12	6-14
Palatal enanthem	18/156	11	5-13
Jaundice	37/426	9	4-10
Rash	49/470	10	0-15

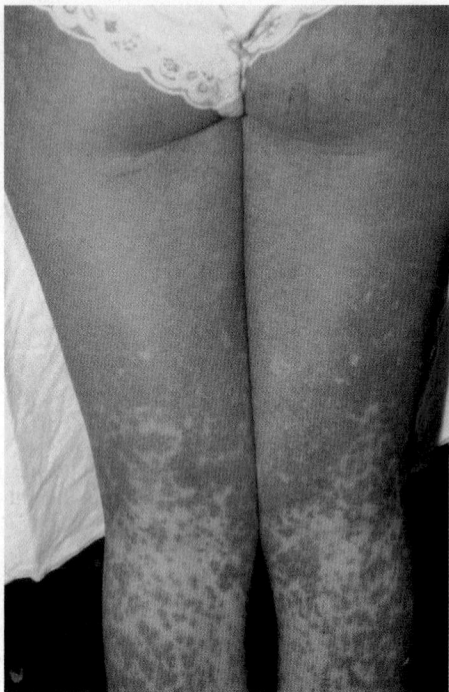

Figure 139-1 **Patient with infectious mononucleosis and ampicillin-induced rash.** Maculopapular rash extends over the trunk and extremities. Rash frequently has a violaceous hue and is often accompanied by pruritus. *(Courtesy of Dr. Stephen Gellis.)*

ance to ampicillin or amoxicillin.[142,143] Periorbital edema has been reported in up to one third of cases in some series,[136] but it has been observed less frequently in others.[137] Tonsillar enlargement is usually present, occasionally with tonsils meeting at the midline. The pharynx is erythematous with an exudate in about one third of cases. Palatal petechiae may be seen in 25% to 60% of cases but are not diagnostic of infectious mononucleosis. The petechiae are usually multiple, are 1 to 2 mm in diameter, occur in crops that last 3 to 4 days, and are usually seen at the junction of the hard and soft palate.[144] Cervical adenopathy, usually symmetrical, is present in 80% to 90% of patients. Posterior adenopathy is most common, but submandibular and anterior adenopathies are quite frequent as well, and axillary and inguinal adenopathies also occur. Individual nodes are freely movable, are not spontaneously painful, and are only mildly tender to palpation. The results of examination of the lungs and heart are usually normal. Abdominal examination may detect hepatomegaly in 10% to 15% of cases, although mild tenderness to fist percussion over the liver is present somewhat more frequently.[135,137] Jaundice is present in approximately 5% of cases.[136] Splenomegaly is present in about one half of cases if sought carefully over the course of the illness. The splenomegaly is usually maximal at the beginning of the second week of illness and regresses over the next 7 to 10 days. The results of neurologic examination are generally normal, although occasional complications may occur (see subsequent discussion).

Complications
Most patients with infectious mononucleosis recover uneventfully. Complications that occasionally occur have been extensively reported in the literature. Even these complications have generally resolved fully, although rare fatalities have been reported.

Hematologic. Autoimmune hemolytic anemia occurs in 0.5% to 3% of the patients with infectious mononucleosis.[145,146] Cold agglutinins, almost always of the IgM class, are present in 70% to 80% of cases.[147] Anti-i specificity has been reported in 20% to 70% of cases.[148,149] Most

but not all cases of autoimmune hemolytic anemia in infectious mononucleosis are mediated by antibodies of this specificity.[150-153] The hemolysis usually becomes clinically apparent during the second or third week of illness and subsides over a 1-month to 2-month period.[154] Corticosteroids may hasten recovery in some cases. Hemophagocytic syndrome, a rare complication of EBV infection, is discussed subsequently in a separate section.

Mild thrombocytopenia is common in infectious mononucleosis. Platelet counts less than 140,000/mm^3 were noted in 50% of patients with uncomplicated infectious mononucleosis in one series.[155] Profound thrombocytopenia with bleeding occurs rarely,[156] but platelet counts less than 1000/mm^3 and deaths from intracerebral bleeding have been reported.[157,158] The mechanism for the thrombocytopenia is not known. The presence of normal or increased numbers of megakaryocytes in the marrow coupled with reports of antiplatelet antibodies suggests that peripheral destruction of platelets may occur, possibly on an autoimmune basis.[148,152,159] Corticosteroids have been reported to be beneficial for the thrombocytopenia in some but not all cases.[156-158,160] For refractory cases, splenectomy may be indicated.[159] Neutropenia is seen rather frequently in uncomplicated infectious mononucleosis. The neutropenia is usually mild and self limiting, although deaths associated with bacterial sepsis or pneumonia, or both, have been reported.[161-168] Anaerobic sepsis without associated granulocytopenia, presumably of pharyngeal origin, has also been reported.[169]

Splenic Rupture. Splenic rupture is a rare but dramatic complication of infectious mononucleosis. Lymphocytic infiltration of the capsule, trabeculae, and vascular walls coupled with rapid splenic enlargement predisposes the organ to rupture. The incidence of rupture is highest in the second or third week of illness but may be the first sign of infectious mononucleosis. Abdominal pain is uncommon in infectious mononucleosis,[170] and splenic rupture must be strongly considered whenever abdominal pain occurs. The onset of this pain may be insidious or abrupt. Pathologic examination of some ruptured spleens has revealed subcapsular hematomas that suggest that rupture may be preceded by intermittent subcapsular bleeding. The pain, usually in the left upper quadrant, may radiate to the left scapular area. Left upper quadrant tenderness to palpation, with or without rebound tenderness, is usually present along with peritoneal signs or shifting dullness. In rare cases, splenic rupture is unaccompanied by pain and is manifested as shock. Laboratory findings include a falling hematocrit and, in some cases, an elevated left hemidiaphragm. The abdominal catastrophe may reverse the usual differential count of infectious mononucleosis and evoke a neutrophilia. Confirmatory findings should not be awaited if splenic rupture is suspected. Prompt splenectomy is the treatment of choice, although nonoperative observation and splenorrhaphy have a role in the management of selected patients with subcapsular splenic hematoma.[171,172] Because a history of trauma may be elicited in about one half the cases of splenic rupture,[173] elimination of contact sports, attention to constipation, and caution in splenic palpation are prudent measures for at least the first month after diagnosis (see Treatment section).

Neurologic. Neurologic complications, which occur in less than 1% of the cases, can dominate the clinical presentation (Table 139-6).[174-189] On occasion, these neurologic signs can be the first or only manifesta-

TABLE 139-6	Neurologic Complications of Infectious Mononucleosis	
Encephalitis[175-179]	Brachial plexus neuropathy[184]
Meningitis[175]	Seizures[175,179]
Guillain-Barré syndrome[179]	Subacute sclerosing panencephalitis[185]
Optic neuritis[181]	Transverse myelitis[186]
Retrobulbar neuritis[182]	Psychosis[187]
Cranial nerve palsies[179]	Demyelination[188]
Mononeuritis multiplex[183]	Hemiplegia[189]

tion of infectious mononucleosis. In many cases, the heterophile antibody determination is negative, atypical lymphocytes may be low in number or delayed in appearance, and the diagnosis must be made by changes in EBV-specific antibodies.[174,175,180] The encephalitis seen with infectious mononucleosis may be acute in onset and rapidly progressive and severe but is usually associated with complete recovery. The encephalitis is commonly manifested as a cerebellitis but may also be global.[176-178] The clinical presentation may also resemble that of aseptic meningitis. In both encephalitis and meningitis, changes in the spinal fluid are mild. The opening pressure is normal or slightly elevated. A predominantly mononuclear pleocytosis may be present, with most cell counts much less than 200/mm³. Atypical lymphocytes have been seen in the cerebrospinal fluid (CSF) in a number of cases. The protein level is usually normal to mildly elevated, and the glucose concentration is usually normal. Low titers of EBV VCA can be found in the CSF.[179] Cases of Guillain-Barré syndrome, Bell's palsy, and transverse myelitis have been reported in primary EBV infection.[180] Although neurologic complications are the most frequent cause of death in infectious mononucleosis, the benign outcome of most of these episodes should be emphasized.[190] Eighty-five percent of the patients with neurologic complications recover completely.[174]

Hepatic. Hepatic manifestations consist largely of self-limited elevations of hepatocellular enzyme levels, which are present in 80% to 90% of the cases of infectious mononucleosis.[191] Reported cases of infectious mononucleosis leading to cirrhosis or other chronic sequelae are poorly documented.

Renal. Abnormal urinary sediment is common in acute infectious mononucleosis.[192,193] Microscopic hematuria and proteinuria are the most frequently noted abnormalities.[194] Overt renal dysfunction is, however, extremely rare, although sporadic cases of acute renal failure in association with infectious mononucleosis have been reported.[195] The renal manifestations of infectious mononucleosis have been hypothesized as usually attributable to interstitial nephritis from renal infiltration by activated T lymphocytes.[195] Renal dysfunction in association with EBV-associated rhabdomyolysis has also been reported, although not all cases of rhabdomyolysis are accompanied by renal dysfunction.[196]

Cardiac. Clinically significant cardiac disease is uncommon. Electrocardiographic abnormalities, usually confined to ST-T wave abnormalities, were reported in 6% of the cases in one series.[197] Pericarditis and fatal myocarditis have also been observed.[198,199]

Pulmonary. Pulmonary manifestations of infectious mononucleosis are rare.[200-203] Early studies reported the presence of interstitial infiltrates in 3% to 5% of the cases. However, systematic examination for other causes of nonbacterial pneumonias, for example, *Mycoplasma*, was not carried out in these studies, and whether these infiltrates were related to EBV infection is not clear. Pneumonia has, however, been reported, and in at least one instance, EBERs were found in pulmonary tissue.[204,205] The attribution of pulmonary lesions to EBV infection should be made only after other pathogens have been carefully excluded.

Death. Death from infectious mononucleosis is rare.[190,206] Death may occur either as a result of overwhelming EBV infection or from complications of the disease. Neurologic complications of the illness, splenic rupture, and upper airway obstruction are the most frequent causes of death from infectious mononucleosis in previously healthy persons. Deaths from complications associated with granulocytopenia, thrombocytopenia, hepatic failure, and myocarditis have also been reported.[153,166,190,199,207,208]

Clinical Course

Most cases of infectious mononucleosis resolve spontaneously over a 2-week to 3-week period. The sore throat is usually maximal for 3 to 5 days and then gradually resolves over the course of a week to 10 days.

Patients remain febrile for 10 to 14 days, but in the last 5 to 7 days, the fever is usually low grade and associated with little morbidity. The prostration associated with infectious mononucleosis is generally more gradual in its resolution. As the illness resolves, patients often have days of relative well being that alternate with recrudescence of symptoms.

X-LINKED LYMPHOPROLIFERATIVE DISEASE

An X-linked syndrome has been described in which boys, without other evidence of immunodeficiency, develop overwhelming primary EBV infection with demonstrable virus in lymph nodes, spleen, thymus, and other organs.[209,210] This syndrome has been designated *X-linked lymphoproliferative syndrome* and is sometimes referred to as Purtilo's syndrome or Duncan's disease. Affected boys develop a large proliferation of polyclonal B and T cells in response to primary EBV infection that frequently results in fulminant hepatitis and hemophagocytic syndrome (discussed subsequently). Patients who survive primary EBV infection frequently develop progressive agammaglobulinemia, or they may develop lymphoma within several years after initial infection.[211-216] This disorder was linked to mutations in the signaling lymphocyte activation molecule (SLAM)–associated protein (SAP) gene in 1998.[217] SAP is thought to be an important mediator of signal transduction in T and NK cells; however, why mutations in SAP confer a specific susceptibility to EBV infection remains to be explained.[218,219]

CHRONIC ACTIVE EPSTEIN-BARR VIRUS INFECTION

Persistent EBV infection has been suggested as a frequent cause of fatigue and malaise in young and middle-aged adults.[220-223] This speculation has arisen from reports of a syndrome characterized by fatigue, sore throat, mild cognitive dysfunction, and myalgias initially noted in association with an apparent increase in antibody titers to the EBV EA complex[220,221] (see Laboratory Diagnosis section). These reports have included primarily young adults, usually with a female preponderance, who report a nonspecific symptom complex more reminiscent of the prodrome of infectious mononucleosis than of the syndrome itself (often known as *chronic mononucleosis syndrome* or *chronic fatigue syndrome*). These patients have been noted either sporadically[220,221,224] or in epidemic clusters.[223] The initial suggestion that the syndrome is attributable to EBV has become untenable on the basis of serologic and epidemiologic observations.[224,225] Investigation of the syndrome has been hampered by the vagueness of the symptoms and the absence of objective laboratory diagnostic criteria. A consensus case definition has emerged that focuses on fatigue rather than on EBV as the central feature of the syndrome.[226,227] The chronic fatigue syndrome is discussed in more detail in Chapter 131.

In contrast to the nonspecific syndrome just noted, patients have been identified in whom EBV appears to play a direct role in ongoing objective organ system dysfunction.[228-231] These cases have been termed *chronic active EBV* (CAEBV) infection and are extremely rare in the United States. CAEBV is more frequent in Asia and South America where, in striking contrast to other EBV lymphoproliferative diseases, it has been associated with EBV infection of NK or T cells.[232-234] To distinguish CAEBV from other nonspecific syndromes, diagnostic criteria have been proposed.[235-237] First, patients have severe illness that lasts more than 6 months, began as primary EBV infection, and is associated with markedly elevated titers to EBV lytic antigens (VCA immunoglobulin G [IgG] ≥ 1:640 or EA IgG ≥ 1:160) or EBV DNA level in the blood (>300 copies/µg DNA). Second, histologic evidence of major organ involvement is present such as interstitial pneumonia, hemophagocytosis, uveitis, lymphadenitis, or persistent hepatitis. Third, affected tissues should contain elevated amounts of EBV DNA, RNA, or proteins by in situ hybridization or immunohistochemical staining. The prognosis for these patients is poor, with most dying of progressive pancytopenia and hypogammaglobulinemia or NK/T-cell nasal lymphoma within a few years, although survival for more than

10 years after diagnosis has been observed.[231] Presentation before age 8 years, without thrombocytopenia, or with an NK cell phenotype is associated with an improved prognosis.[238] Antiviral therapy with acyclovir or ganciclovir is of no proven benefit, but case reports of adoptive immunotherapy and bone marrow transplantation for patients with CAEBV have been found.[230,239-243] The pathogenesis of CAEBV is not well understood but is probably the result of an immune defect that permits the proliferation of EBV infected T or NK cells.[244] The limited number of cases of CAEBV diagnosed in the United States often include disease associated with EBV infection of B cells.[243] Whether B cell CAEBV represents a distinct clinicopathologic entity is an intriguing but academic question because the prognosis is similarly poor and treatment options are no different than NK or T-cell CAEBV.

EPSTEIN-BARR VIRUS–ASSOCIATED HEMOPHAGOCYTIC LYMPHOHISTIOCYTOSIS

The hemophagocytic syndrome is characterized by excessive lymphocyte and macrophage (histiocyte) activation and infiltration of bone marrow, lymph nodes, spleen, and liver with prominent phagocytosis of erythrocytes and nucleated cells.[245] Although the hemophagocytic syndrome can occur as a consequence of X-linked lymphoproliferative syndrome (XLP) or CAEBV, it can present as a distinct clinical entity in the absence of these diseases and has been called *hemophagocytic lymphohistiocytosis* (HLH). Children are primarily affected, usually before the age of 3 years, with high fevers, pancytopenia, liver dysfunction, and coagulopathy.[245,246] HLH usually develops as the sequelae of a viral infection, most commonly primary EBV infection. Most, if not all, cases of HLH are associated with a monoclonal proliferation of T cells that are usually CD8+.[246-248] In EBV-associated HLH, most infiltrating T lymphocytes are monoclonally infected with EBV.[249-251] These unregulated proliferating T cells are thought to account for the markedly elevated levels of tumor necrosis factor (TNF)–α, interferon gamma, M-CSF, IL-6, IL-10, IL-18, and sIL-2R that typify HLH and drive macrophage activation.[252,253] Familial forms of HLH have revealed that this is an autosomal recessive disorder characterized by impaired NK cell activity and have linked the disease to mutations in PRF1 (perforin), MUNC13-4, and UNC13D.[246] These latter two genes are believed to be essential for release of perforin-containing cytotoxic granules from NK and CD8+ T cells. In one study, five of 20 sporadic (nonfamilial) cases of HLH were also associated with mutations in the PRF1 gene. Interestingly, PRF1 mutations were not seen in any of the six cases linked to EBV; however, MUNC13-4 and UNC13D were not evaluated.[254] Untreated, the prognosis of EBV-associated HLH is poor. However, treatment with the etoposide, dexamethasone, cyclosporine-based HLH-94 protocol has been associated with survival rates of approximately 75%.[255]

ORAL HAIRY LEUKOPLAKIA

As previously stated, reactivation of lytic EBV replication with viral shedding in the saliva is usually entirely asymptomatic. An important exception to this rule is *oral hairy leukoplakia* (OHL), which arises as a corrugated or "hairy" white lesion usually on the lateral surface of the tongue but sometimes elsewhere. This nonmalignant lesion is seen in AIDS and other states of immunosuppression and is caused by unchecked lytic replication of EBV.[256,257] The diagnosis of OHL is based on the typical appearance of the lesions in the appropriate clinical setting. The differential diagnosis includes oral candidiasis, which, unlike OHL, can be removed with gentle scraping of the tongue. Alternatively, thrush may be diagnosed with a KOH wet mount or should respond to an empirical trial of antifungal therapy. Biopsy for histology and in situ hybridization or immunofluorescence staining for EBV is rarely necessary but confirms the diagnosis. Polymerase chain reaction (PCR) detection of EBV in "oral scrapes" is neither sensitive nor specific for OHL.[258]

EPSTEIN-BARR VIRUS–ASSOCIATED MALIGNANT DISEASES

Epstein-Barr virus is an extremely well-adapted parasite that establishes lifelong latent infection without lasting adverse effects in about 95% of the human population. However, in immunosuppressed hosts, the growth-transforming properties of EBV can result in malignant disease. EBV in conjunction with environmental or genetic factors, or both, can rarely result in malignant disease in immunocompetent hosts (Table 139-7).

Lymphoproliferative Disease

In the absence of effective immune surveillance, uncontrolled proliferation of EBV-infected B lymphocytes may occur. This disorder is referred to as *lymphoproliferative disease* and represents the in vivo equivalent of the immortalized B-cell lines seen with EBV infection in vitro. Proliferating B cells in LPD express all EBV latent proteins (latency III), including the EBNA3 proteins that are normally strong targets for CD8+ cytotoxic T cells (see Table 139-2).[28,55] Patients with LPD typically present with symptoms similar to those of infectious mononucleosis or with fever and lymphomatous infiltration of lymph nodes, spleen, liver, bone marrow, kidney, lung, CNS, or intestine (Fig. 139-2). The frequency of this disease in solid organ and bone marrow transplant recipients has led to the designation *post-transplantation lymphoproliferative disease* (PTLD), but it can be seen in any patient receiving high-dose immune suppression or in those with inherited disorders that affect T-cell immunity. Patients with more severe cellular immune impairment, such as those receiving T cell–depleted bone marrow transplants or antithymocyte globulin, are at increased risk for PTLD, as are those with primary EBV infection after transplantation.[51,52] Notably, the timing of risk for PTLD differs in stem cell versus solid organ transplant recipients because of differences in immune suppression. In stem cell transplants, the overall risk is 1%, and this risk is greatest within the first 5 months after transplantation when the immune suppression is severe and before immune reconstitution.[259] In solid organ transplantation, the risk is more prolonged because of the need for long-term immunosuppression. PTLD is most

TABLE 139-7	Epstein-Barr Virus (EBV)–Associated Malignant Diseases		
Malignant Disease	*EBV Association*	*Population at Risk*	*Cofactors*
Lymphoproliferative disease	~90%	Transplantation patients	Immunosuppression
Primary CNS lymphoma	100%	AIDS with very low CD4+ count	Immunosuppression
Hodgkin's lymphoma	~50%, depending on histologic subtype	Children (developing countries) Young adults (western countries)	Unknown
Nasopharyngeal carcinoma	100% undifferentiated 30%-100% squamous	Southern Chinese, Inuit	Genetic predisposition and dietary factors
Burkitt's lymphoma	>95% endemic ~20% sporadic ~40% HIV associated	African children Independent of CD4+ count	C-myc translocations (all) Malaria (endemic only)

Adapted from Kieff E, Rickinson AB. Epstein-Barr virus and its replication. In: Knipe D, Howley P, Griffin D, et al, eds. *Fields Virology*. 5th ed. Philadelphia: Lippincott Williams & Wilkins; 2007:2603-2654.

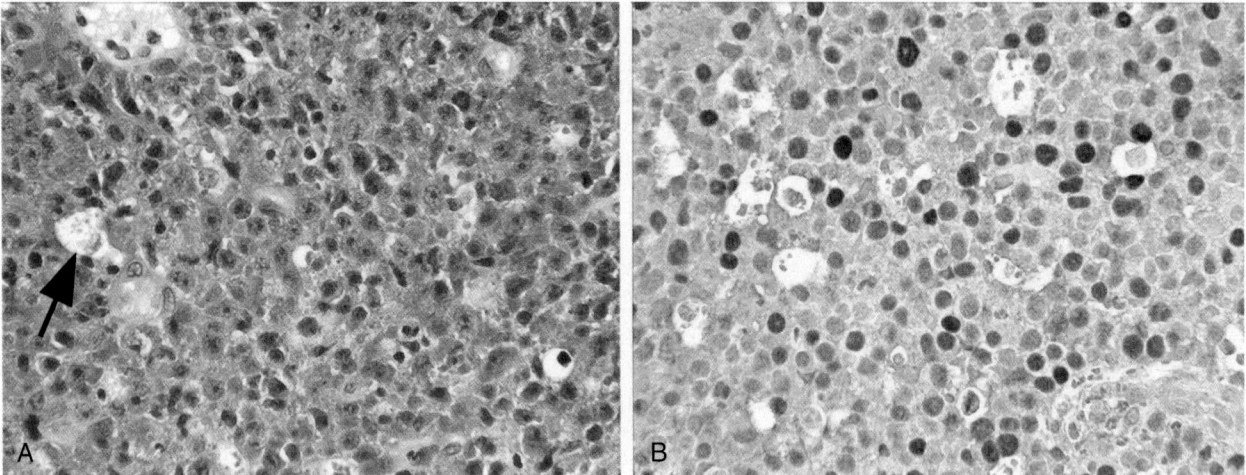

Figure 139-2 **Posttransplantation lymphoproliferative disease involving the colon. A,** Tumor is composed of large, atypical lymphoid cells (hematoxylin and eosin). Scattered macrophages (*arrow*) are seen, producing "starry-sky" appearance. **B,** In situ hybridization for Epstein-Barr virus (EBV)–encoded RNA (EBER; *brown*) shows variably intense nuclear staining in most tumor cells, indicating EBV infection. (Original magnification, ×400.) *(Courtesy of Dr. Jeffery Kutok.)*

common in multivisceral transplantation (up to 33%), least common in renal and liver transplantation (~1% to 2%), and intermediate in heart or lung (2% to 9%) or intestinal (~10%) transplantation.[260,261] Up to half of PTLDs occur in the setting of primary EBV infection. These may arise early after transplantation and often occur in children, who are more likely to be EBV seronegative.[262] Diffuse large cell lymphoma, a B-cell lymphoma seen in patients with HIV, bears a striking resemblance to PTLD. As with PTLD, it occurs in the setting of profound immunosuppression; those with the lowest CD4 counts for the longest time are at greatest risk. Presentation as primary CNS lymphoma is frequent, and essentially all CNS lymphomas are EBV positive, whereas about two thirds of AIDS-associated diffuse large cell lymphomas outside the CNS are EBV positive.[263]

Burkitt's Lymphoma

Burkitt's lymphoma is a high-grade lymphoma with characteristic small, noncleaved B cells and is endemic in equatorial Africa. Endemic Burkitt's lymphoma is geographically associated with *Plasmodium falciparum* malaria and usually arises as a tumor of the jaw. Although the fact that more than 90% of Burkitt's lymphomas are EBV associated has been long appreciated, the role of the virus in its pathogenesis is unclear because most of the EBV transforming genes are not expressed. In fact, viral gene expression is restricted to EBNA1 and the EBERs (latency I; see Table 139-2).[48,53,54] It is unlikely that EBV is merely a passenger because terminal repeat analysis of EBV genomes has confirmed that the viral infection occurred before expansion of the tumor.[264] Also, persons in endemic regions with elevated titers to EBV lytic antigens are at high risk for Burkitt's lymphoma.[265] In addition to EBV association, virtually all Burkitt's lymphomas contain a chromosomal translocation that involves the c-myc oncogene and an immunoglobulin heavy or light chain locus. The unregulated expression of this potent oncogene probably supplants the need for expression of many of the EBV transforming genes that otherwise would serve as targets for immune surveillance. In addition to the endemic form of the disease, sporadic Burkitt-like lymphomas are seen that typically arise as abdominal masses. These lymphomas also contain c-*myc* translocations but are less consistently associated with EBV (only about 25% of cases).[263] Persons with HIV are at increased risk for Burkitt-like lymphoma, independent of degree of immunodeficiency.[266]

Hodgkin's Lymphoma

Hodgkin's lymphoma is an unusual malignant disease in that the malignant Hodgkin and Reed-Sternberg (HRS) cells constitute as little as 1% of the tumor. The balance of the tumor mass is composed of an infiltrate of reactive mononuclear and stromal cells. An infectious etiology for Hodgkin's lymphoma was proposed as early as 1966 on the basis of the epidemiology of the disease, but definitive evidence was slow to evolve because of technical difficulties presented by the scarcity of the HRS cells.[267-269] Subsequently, EBV DNA and protein expression were shown in HRS cells from some forms of Hodgkin's lymphoma.[270,271] The strongest associations are with the mixed cellularity (Fig. 139-3) and lymphocyte-depleted histologic subtypes.[67] No association with the lymphocyte predominant subtype could be proved, and this is now considered a distinct, non–EBV-associated entity. Even in classic Hodgkin's lymphoma, considerable variation is found in the strength of the association with EBV, which depends on other factors such as age, gender, ethnicity, and country of residence. There is, however, general agreement that in EBV-associated Hodgkin's lymphoma, the malignant HRS cells represent postgerminal center B cells that express a latency II EBV gene pattern (LMP1, LMP2, EBNA1, and EBERs; see Table 139-2). EBV genomes, when present in HRS cells, are monoclonal with terminal repeat analysis, which suggests that EBV infection preceded the development of the malignant disease.[271] Many HRS contain "crippling mutations" in their immunoglobulin genes or fail to express surface immunoglobulins and thus lack a critical antiapoptotic signal normally transmitted by the B cell receptor (BCR). Expression of EBV LMP2A can serve as a surrogate BCR signal and may allow the survival of cells otherwise destined to undergo apoptosis from failure to express functional immunoglobulin.[272] Activation of NF-κB signaling is also typical of HRS cells, which suggests activation of this pathway by LMP1.[273] In some EBV-negative HRS cells, IκBα gene mutations have been reported that could serve as an alternative means of constitutively activating the NF-κB pathway.[274] Speculation is tempting that EBV gene expression can serve as one step in the malignant transformation of HRS cells that is circumvented by other mutational events in EBV-negative forms of the disease.

Nasopharyngeal Carcinoma

Nasopharyngeal carcinoma is a rare disease in most western countries, but its prevalence rate approaches 50 per 100,000 in southern China

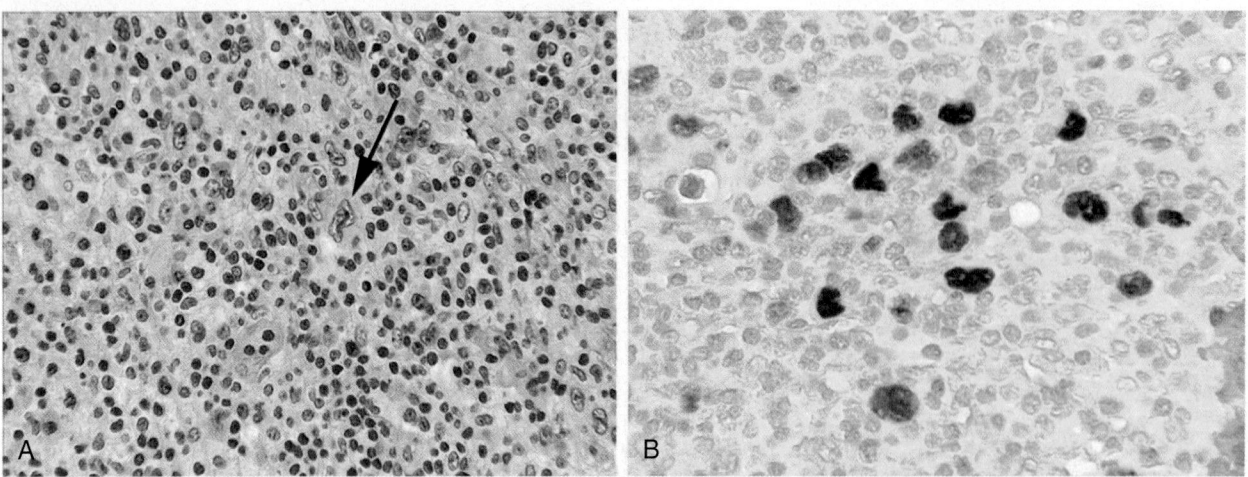

Figure 139-3   **Mixed cellularity classic Hodgkin's lymphoma. A,** Lymph node architecture is effaced by infiltrate comprised of small lymphocytes, epithelioid histiocytes, plasma cells, eosinophils, and Hodgkin and Reed-Sternberg cells *(arrow;* hematoxylin and eosin). **B,** In situ hybridization for Epstein-Barr virus (EBV)–encoded RNA (EBER; *brown)* shows EBV infection in malignant Hodgkin and Reed-Sternberg cells. (Original magnification, ×400.) *(Courtesy of Dr. Jeffery Kutok.)*

and among the Inuit in Alaska.[275] An association between EBV and nasopharyngeal carcinoma was first suggested with the observation that patients with this malignant disease had elevated IgG and immunoglobulin A (IgA) titers to EBV lytic antigens (VCA and EA).[276] The undifferentiated form (Fig. 139-4) is EBV associated in nearly 100% of cases, whereas squamous nasopharyngeal carcinomas are inconsistently EBV associated, particularly outside endemic regions. The undifferentiated form bears some resemblance to Hodgkin's lymphoma in that the tumor consists of EBV-positive cells (of epithelial origin in this case) that express a latency II gene pattern infiltrated with reactive, nonmalignant lymphoid cells.[68,277,278] Terminal repeat assays have confirmed that these epithelial cells contain monoclonal EBV genomes, placing EBV infection early in the genesis of the malignant disease as seen in EBV-associated B-cell neoplasia.[279] In addition to EBV, evidence indicates that genetic and environmental factors may have roles in tumor development.[280-282]

Other Malignant Diseases
Nasal NK and *T-cell lymphomas* are angiocentric lymphomas that typically present as a midline facial destructive disease (lethal midline

granuloma) but can also arise at other extranodal sites.[283] They are highly associated with EBV, and, like nasopharyngeal carcinoma (NPC) and Hodgkin's lymphoma (HL), malignant cells typically express a latency II gene pattern.[284] As discussed previously, persons with CAEBV are at high risk of development of this subtype of peripheral T-cell lymphoma.[285,286] A similar angiocentric malignant disease, *lymphomatoid granulomatosis* (LG), is now known to be a distinct clinical entity caused by EBV-infected proliferating B lymphocytes with an exuberant reactive T-cell infiltrate. Patients with LG typically present with pulmonary lesions and synchronous brain, skin, kidney, or liver lesions that can be easily mistaken for disseminated fungal infections.[287] An EBV association has been reported in some gastric cancers, breast cancer, hepatocellular cancers, and smooth muscle tumors, but the contribution of EBV to the pathogenesis of these malignant diseases remains to be established.[288-290]

In addition to the Burkitt-like lymphomas and diffuse large cell lymphomas, persons with HIV (or other immunosuppression) are at increased risk for an unusual EBV-associated lymphoma, *primary effusion lymphoma* (PEL).[291,292] These human herpesvirus 8 (Kaposi's sarcoma–associated herpesvirus)–related lymphomas are often

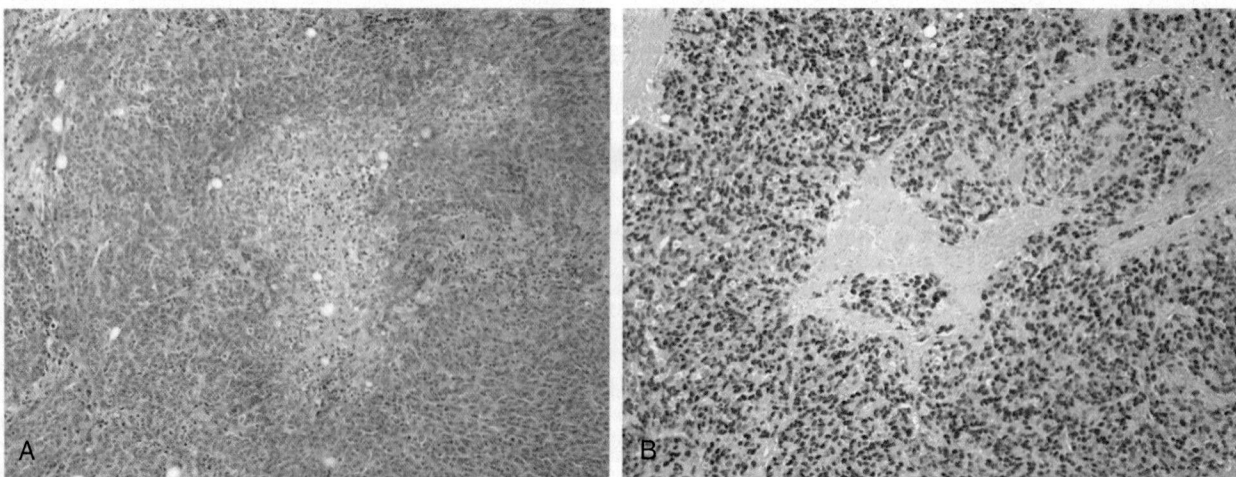

Figure 139-4   **Nasopharyngeal carcinoma. A,** Nests of metastatic undifferentiated nasopharyngeal carcinoma in a fibrous stroma in lymph node (hematoxylin and eosin). Metastases often lack infiltrating lymphocytes. **B,** In situ hybridization for Epstein-Barr virus (EBV)–encoded RNA (EBER; *brown)* shows EBV infection in most cells in the same area of tissue. (Magnification, ×100.) *(Courtesy of Dr. Miguel Rivera.)*

coinfected with EBV. PELs derived their name from a tendency to arise within potential body cavities such as the pleural, pericardial, or peritoneal spaces and frequently follow an aggressive clinical course. *Pyothorax-associated lymphoma* (PAL) is sometimes confused with PEL but differs in that it is strictly EBV (not Kaposi's sarcoma-associated herpesvirus) associated, forms an identifiable mass lesion, arises in patients with long-standing pleural-based inflammation, and is seen in patients without HIV.[293] In pediatric patients with AIDS, EBV has been reported in leiomyosarcoma biopsy specimens as well.[294]

MULTIPLE SCLEROSIS AND OTHER AUTOIMMUNE DISEASES

Viruses have long been suspected as environmental triggers for autoimmune diseases in genetically predisposed individuals. EBV has been a candidate on the basis of seroepidemiologic studies that link it to systemic lupus erythematosus, rheumatoid arthritis, and *multiple sclerosis* (MS).[295-297] Although definitive proof is lacking, patients with MS are more likely to be EBV seropositive than age-matched control subjects.[297] This difference is most notable in pediatric patients in whom the rate of EBV seropositivity of control subjects is much lower.[298] Patients with MS have higher titers to EBV antigens, while elevated titers are not observed in other viruses, including CMV, varicella-zoster virus (VZV), and herpes simplex virus (HSV).[298-302] Furthermore, prospective studies have shown that antibody titers, particularly to EBNA1, are elevated more than 10 years before the onset of MS symptoms.[303-305] In addition, a history of symptomatic infectious mononucleosis is associated with a two-fold increased risk of development of MS relative to asymptomatic primary EBV infection.[306] Finally, the presence of oligoclonal IgG in the CSF is a well-established hallmark of MS. Cepok and associates[307] determined that the two most frequent MS-specific reactivities in CSF recognized peptides found in the EBV proteins EBNA1 and BRRF2. Thus, a body of data supports an association of EBV infection with MS. Whether or not these observed differences in immune responses to EBV cause MS or are merely an epiphenomenon that results from the same immunologic dysregulation that causes MS remains to be seen.

Laboratory Diagnosis

INFECTIOUS MONONUCLEOSIS

Hematologic Findings

The central hematologic manifestation of the illness is a circulating lymphocytosis. At presentation, a relative and absolute mononuclear lymphocytosis is found in about 70% of the cases. The lymphocytosis peaks during the second or third week of illness, and monocytes and lymphocytes account for 60% to 70% of the total white cell counts of 12,000 to 18,000/mm³. However, higher white cell counts are not uncommon, and occasional patients manifest 30,000 to 50,000 leukocytes/mm³. Atypical lymphocytes are the hematologic hallmark of infectious mononucleosis and account for about 30% of the differential count at their zenith.[136,137] The wide range in the atypical lymphocytosis is well recognized, and some cases show none or only a few atypical lymphocytes, whereas 90% or more of the circulating lymphocytes may be atypical in other cases. These atypical lymphocytes are composed largely of reactive CD8⁺ cytotoxic T cells and are not pathognomonic for infectious mononucleosis (Table 139-8). They are also noted in other syndromes, including CMV infection, primary HIV infection, viral hepatitis, toxoplasmosis, rubella, mumps, and roseola, and in drug reactions.[308,309] The atypical lymphocyte is generally larger than the mature lymphocyte encountered in peripheral blood. The cytoplasm is often vacuolated and basophilic, and its edges have a rolled-up appearance with a tendency to flow around adjacent red blood cells (RBCs) on a peripheral smear. Nuclei are often lobulated and are eccentrically placed. Although the cells may appear quite immature, the heterogeneity of morphologic and tinctorial character-

TABLE 139-8	Differential Diagnosis of Atypical Lymphocytosis
Epstein-Barr virus primary infection (infectious mononucleosis)	
Cytomegalovirus primary infection (heterophile-negative mononucleosis)*	
Human herpes virus 6 primary infection (roseola)	
Primary HIV infection	
Toxoplasmosis	
Acute viral hepatitis	
Rubella, mumps	
Drug reactions (e.g., phenytoin, sulfa)	

*CMV is the most common cause of heterophile-negative mononucleosis.

istics of such cells helps to distinguish atypical lymphocytes from the more uniform lymphoblasts of acute lymphocytic leukemia.[6,308]

A relative and absolute neutropenia is evident in 60% to 90% of the cases, and neutrophils that remain in circulation exhibit a mild left shift.[162,163] In most cases, the neutropenia is mild, with total granulocyte counts of 2000 to 3000/mm³, although profound granulocytopenia has also been reported.[161,164-168,212,310] The neutropenia is usually self limited, and counts rise gradually toward normal by a month after presentation.[162]

Thrombocytopenia is also common, and 50% of the patients in one series manifested platelet counts of less than 140,000/mm³.[155] Although cases of profound thrombocytopenia with bleeding have been reported,[156-160] these cases are rare and contrast markedly with the generally benign course of the common mild thrombocytopenia.

Heterophile Antibodies

Heterophile antibodies, originally described by Paul and Bunnell[7] as sheep erythrocyte agglutinins, are present in about 90% of cases at some point during the illness. Beef erythrocyte hemolysins and agglutinating antibodies to horse, goat, and camel erythrocytes are also demonstrable in infectious mononucleosis. The classic heterophile antibody titer is reported as the highest serum dilution at which sheep erythrocytes are agglutinated after absorption of the test serum by guinea pig kidney (Table 139-9). The differential absorption permits a distinction between naturally occurring Forssman antibodies, the antibodies of serum sickness, and heterophile antibodies of infectious mononucleosis. Beef red cell hemolysins do not need differential absorption for interpretation. Although titers may vary depending on laboratory techniques, a titer of 40 or greater after guinea pig absorption along with a compatible clinical presentation is strong evidence for infectious mononucleosis.

Heterophile antibodies may be seen at the onset of illness or may appear later in the course of the illness. A delayed appearance of heterophile antibodies may be associated with a more prolonged convalescence.[311] Horse red cell agglutination is more sensitive than tests for sheep red cell agglutination or beef red cell hemolysis. Horse red cell agglutinins persist for a year after diagnosis in 75% of the cases,[312] whereas sheep cell agglutinins fall to titers of less than 40 by a year in 70% of cases. False-positive titers greater than 40 of sheep and horse erythrocyte agglutinins have been found in 12% and 6.7% of sera, respectively.[313] Commercial spot kits are available and are generally specific and sensitive for heterophile antibodies. The correlation

TABLE 139-9	Heterophile Antibodies: Effect of Absorption		
		After Absorption with	
Source of Serum	*Unabsorbed*	*Guinea Pig Kidney*	*Beef Red Cells*
Infectious mononucleosis	++++	+++	0
Serum sickness	+++	0	0
Normal serum (Forssman antibody)	+	0	+

between the results obtained with the use of these kits and results of the classic tube heterophile method is quite good, although the sensitivity of the spot and slide tests is slightly greater than that of the classic tube heterophile test. Occasional false-positive Monospot test responses have been reported in patients with lymphoma or hepatitis, but the rarity of this event makes confirmation of a positive Monospot test result with EBV-specific serology unnecessary.[314-316] Three cases of false-positive Monospot tests in the setting of primary HIV infection have been reported.[317] One study of 132 patients with positive Monospot test results found no instances of primary HIV infection.[318] However, the exact rate of false-positive Monospot test results among patients with primary HIV infection is not known.

Epstein-Barr Virus–Specific Antibodies

In addition to the transient heterophile antibodies, infection with EBV results in the development of virus-specific antibodies. Antibodies are formed to structural proteins or VCAs, nonstructural proteins expressed early in the lytic cycle or EAs, and nuclear proteins expressed during latent infections or EBNAs. A determination of EBV-specific antibodies is rarely necessary for the diagnosis of infectious mononucleosis because 90% of the cases are heterophile positive and few false-positive results are obtained if the test is properly performed (see previous discussion). For heterophile-negative cases and for diagnosis in atypical cases, a determination of EBV antibodies may help to establish a cause (Table 139-10).[319]

Antibodies to VCA as measured with immunofluorescence arise early in the course of the illness and are seen at presentation in most cases. IgG antibodies to VCA are usually present at titers of 80 or greater on the first visit to a physician. Because these initially detected levels are close to peak VCA titers, a fourfold rise in titer is seen in only 10% to 20% of the cases. After recovery, detectable titers of VCA IgG antibody are maintained for life. Thus, IgG VCA antibody titers may be of little help in the diagnosis of infectious mononucleosis. Conversely, IgM antibodies to VCA are sensitive and specific for infectious mononucleosis. IgM antibody titers greater than 5 as measured with indirect immunofluorescence are seen in 90% of cases early in the illness. Titers fall rapidly thereafter, and in only 10% of the cases are titers greater than 5 retained by 4 months after diagnosis.[312,320] IgM VCA antibodies are not seen in the general population; thus, their presence is virtually diagnostic of acute EBV infection.

Serum antibodies to EAs are also seen with indirect immunofluorescence, and two distinct patterns of fluorescence emerge.[319,320] Certain sera stain both nuclei and cytoplasm diffusely (anti-EA-D), whereas the staining of other sera is restricted (anti-EA-R) to cytoplasmic aggregates. Anti-EA-D antibody is found in about 70% of patients with acute infectious mononucleosis (see Table 139-10). Anti-EA-D titers arise later in the course of illness than those to VCA and disappear after recovery. Anti-EA-D antibodies may be found in the sera of patients with advanced nasopharyngeal carcinoma but are absent from the general population. The appearance of anti-EA-D antibodies in a patient with IgG VCA antibodies suggests recent EBV infection. Unfortunately, only 70% of EBV-induced cases manifest anti-EA-D antibodies. The presence and titer of anti-EA-D antibodies correlate with the duration and severity of clinical illness.[320] Anti-EA-R antibodies are only occasionally seen in infectious mononucleosis (see Table 139-10). They are present more often in protracted or atypical cases, arise after the anti-EA-D antibodies peak, and remain detectable for up to 2 years.[321] Anti-EA-R antibodies are also present in higher titers in patients with African Burkitt's lymphoma and occasionally in healthy persons who also have high VCA titers.[322]

Antibodies to EBNA appear late in the course of all cases of infectious mononucleosis and persist for life.[323] The appearance of EBNA antibodies in a patient who was previously VCA positive and EBNA negative is strong evidence of recent EBV infection. These antibodies may be reactive against any of the six nuclear proteins expressed during latent infection. Neutralizing antibodies to EBV also appear late in the course of infectious mononucleosis and reach maximal levels 6 to 7 weeks after the onset of illness.[324] Neutralizing antibodies persist at stable titers (mean, 40) for life. The appearance or a rise in titer of neutralizing antibodies to EBV also indicates recent EBV infection. Neutralizing antibodies are, however, difficult to measure, and tests for them are not routinely available.

Detection of Epstein-Barr Virus

Epstein-Barr virus may be cultured from oropharyngeal washings or from circulating lymphocytes of 80% to 90% of patients with infectious mononucleosis.[83,84,91,101,325] Cultivation of the virus is, however, not routinely available in most diagnostic virology laboratories. This, coupled with the ubiquity of virus shedding in both healthy persons and in those with unrelated illnesses, renders cultivation of the virus of little clinical use (see Table 139-1). Rapid diagnostic techniques based on DNA hybridization or monoclonal antibody techniques have also been developed but for similar reasons are not helpful in the diagnosis of mononucleosis.[326-328] Interestingly, up to 50% of memory B cells are infected with EBV during infectious mononucleosis, compared with 1 in 10^4 to 1 in 10^6 memory B cells that contain virus in healthy individuals.[329,330] Virus DNA can be detected in the plasma early in the course of infectious mononucleosis, in addition to in lymphocytes. Detection of EBV DNA in plasma is otherwise infrequent in healthy individuals.[331] EBV viral load in blood is initially high in mononucleosis but then rapidly declines (see subsequent discussion of EBV viral load).[332]

TABLE 139-10	Antibodies to Epstein-Barr Virus (EBV)			
Antibody Specificity	Time of Appearance in Infectious Mononucleosis	Percentage of EBV-Induced Mononucleosis Cases with Antibody	Persistence	Comments
Viral Capsid Antigens (VCAs)				
IgM VCA	At clinical presentation	100	4-8 wk	Highly sensitive and specific; major diagnostic utility
IgG VCA	At clinical presentation	100	Lifelong	High titer at presentation and lifelong persistence make IgG VCA more useful as epidemiologic tool than as diagnostic tool in individual cases
Early Antigens				
Anti-EA-D	Peaks at 3-4 wk after onset	70	3-6 mo	Correlated with severe disease; also seen in nasopharyngeal carcinoma
Anti-EA-R	2 wk to several months after onset	Low	2 mo to >3 y	Occasionally seen with unusually severe or protracted illness; also seen in African Burkitt's lymphoma
EBV nuclear antigen	3-4 wk after onset	100	Lifelong	Late appearance helpful in diagnosis of heterophile-negative cases

Other Laboratory Abnormalities

Liver function test results are abnormal in almost all cases of infectious mononucleosis.[191,333,334] Levels of the hepatocellular enzymes aspartate aminotransferase, alanine aminotransferase, and lactate dehydrogenase are most commonly elevated, and one of the three is abnormal in about 90% of the cases. Elevations are usually mild, with individual values in the range of two to three times the upper limit of normal. Elevation to more than 10 times the upper limit of normal necessitates a search for another diagnosis.[191] The alkaline phosphatase level is elevated in about 60% of the cases.[333,334] Mild elevation of the bilirubin level is noted in approximately 45% of cases, although frank jaundice occurs in only about 5%. Elevations are maximal in the second week of illness and decline gradually over a 3-week to 4-week period.

Cryoproteins are present in modest amounts in 90% to 95% of patients.[149,335] The cryoproteins are generally mixed cryoglobulins of IgG and IgM classes. When the cryoglobulins are dissociated, antibody of anti-i or anti-I or both specificities is usually seen.[335,336]

EPSTEIN-BARR VIRUS VIRAL LOAD

The detection of EBV DNA from blood has become increasingly used for a number of EBV-associated diseases. In its most modern form, DNA is quantitated with real time PCR to determine a specific copy number. Although the use of EBV loads holds much promise, the technique is currently hampered by a lack of standardization across different centers. For instance, the units of measurement vary across studies, such as number of virus DNA copies per milliliter of blood or per microgram of total DNA. In addition, different sample types are used to assay viral loads and can include whole blood, plasma, or peripheral blood mononuclear cells. EBV is a cell-associated virus and therefore typically is found in the peripheral blood mononuclear cell component of blood; but in certain disease states, notably nasopharyngeal carcinoma, it can be found in high levels in plasma, likely because of cell death and release of episomal DNA into the circulation. Further, extensive variability in quantitation can be found as a result of a lack of standardization among different laboratories because of differing DNA extraction techniques and different gene amplification targets.[337,338] Taken together, these factors have resulted in a lack of validated data from multicenter trials. Thus, individual centers often have their own protocols for monitoring viral load and decision points for intervention. This situation differs greatly from other pathogens such as HIV or hepatitis B or C, which have regulatory requirements for assay calibration, largely from needs for blood donor screening.[338-342] Notably, although interlaboratory variation on the same samples is quite high, intralaboratory variation tends to be very low, which indicates accuracy within each system and suggests that quantitative tracking of individual patients in any one laboratory permits accurate assessment of trends.[337,338]

▪ Post-transplant Lymphoproliferative Disease (PTLD)

Perhaps the disease in which EBV loads have been most intensively studied is *post-transplant lymphoproliferative disease* (PTLD). Although standard protocols are not available and controlled trials have not been performed, a number of studies report that the EBV viral load can be predictive of PTLD, especially in the setting of T-cell depleted stem cell transplants.[262,331,343-345] Many transplantation centers therefore now monitor EBV loads and view elevated values as evidence for increased risk of PTLD in stem cell transplantation. Some centers now routinely treat high EBV loads with rituximab, an anti-CD20 antibody that kills B cells and rapidly lowers EBV load, or with other approaches (discussed subsequently).[346,347] Rituximab lowered the rate of PTLD compared with historical controls in one study.[348]

The use of EBV viral loads is less clear after PTLD in solid organ transplantation, and large studies are needed to define protocols. After solid organ transplantation, EBV viral loads tend to remain consistently high, without a clear risk for development of PTLD.[349-352] A rapid increase in viral loads may be of concern for development of PTLD. EBV load monitoring is particularly important after transplantation in individuals who are EBV seronegative, especially if the donor is EBV positive, because these patients are at higher risk for PTLD after primary infection.[262]

NASOPHARYNGEAL CARCINOMA

Nasopharyngeal carcinoma is difficult to diagnose in its early stages; therefore, patients typically present with advanced disease. The most common initial presenting symptom is a neck mass (Fig. 139-5). Diagnosis requires endoscopy to visualize the nasopharynx and histologic examination of biopsy tissue.[353] Radiologic studies are helpful in revealing the extent of disease (Fig. 139-6). Patients with nasopharyngeal carcinoma have elevated levels of serum IgA directed against EBV VCA and EA.[354-356] The elevation of the IgA antibodies may occur several years before the onset of nasopharyngeal carcinoma. In light of this finding, a program of screening individuals for elevated EBV IgA VCA and EA titers has been instituted in southern China, where nasopharyngeal carcinoma is one of the leading malignant diseases. Individuals with elevated IgA titers are then observed closely for the development of disease. This screening program enhanced the diagnosis of nasopharyngeal carcinoma in earlier as opposed to more advanced stages of disease.

Detection of EBV DNA in nasopharyngeal brush biopsies has also been proposed in one study as a possible screening mechanism in high-risk populations. This study detected EBV DNA in 19 of 21 brush biopsies from patients with recently diagnosed nasopharyngeal carcinoma but only in 1.3% of control subjects.[357]

Cell-free EBV DNA in plasma is commonly detected in patients with nasopharyngeal carcinoma.[353] Cell-free EBV DNA is postulated to be released into the circulation on tumor cell death. In two studies by the same authors[358,359] of patients with nasopharyngeal carcinoma, quantitative analysis of the concentration of DNA in plasma was useful in monitoring patients for recurrence of disease. Further, patients with nasopharyngeal carcinoma presenting with higher plasma level viral loads have poorer outcomes and higher rates of early recurrence or metastasis after radiotherapy.[360,361]

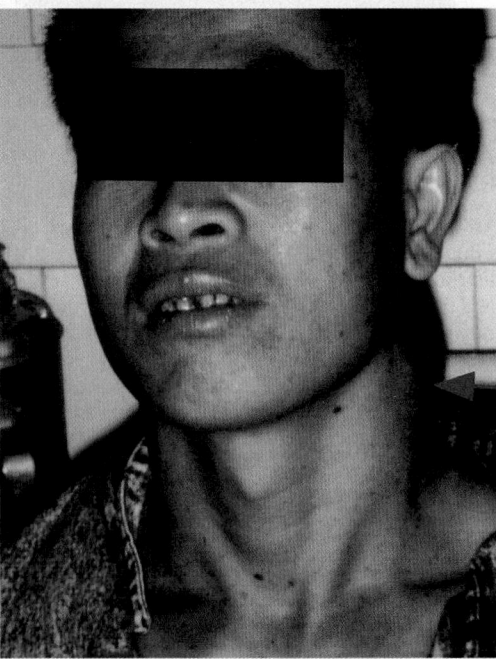

Figure 139-5 **Patient with nasopharyngeal carcinoma and neck mass** *(arrow).*

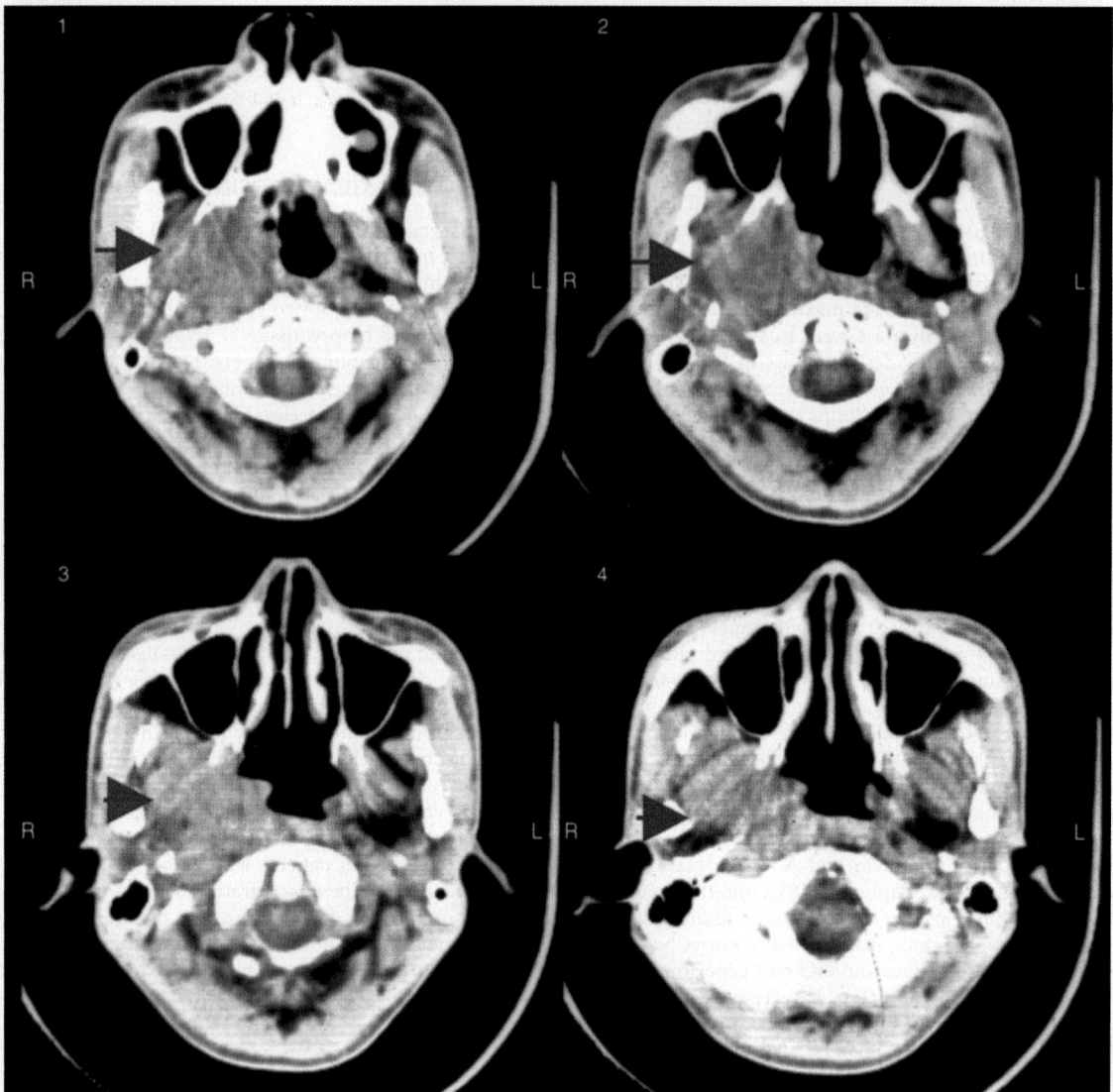

Figure 139-6   Computed tomographic scan images of 25-year-old man with nasopharyngeal carcinoma *(arrow).* Tumor involves right parapharyngeal space. *(Courtesy of Dr. Yi Zeng.)*

CENTRAL NERVOUS SYSTEM LYMPHOMA IN ACQUIRED IMMUNODEFICIENCY SYNDROME

Polymerase chain reaction detection of EBV DNA in CSF has been useful in the diagnosis of CNS lymphoma in patients with HIV.[362-365] Nearly all primary CNS lymphomas in HIV disease are EBV associated, as discussed previously. Whereas patients with HIV without CNS lymphoma rarely have detectable EBV DNA in CSF, EBV DNA is frequently detected when CNS lymphoma is present. Therefore, CSF PCR for EBV used in conjunction with radiologic studies may reduce the need for brain biopsy in certain instances. Quantification of EBV DNA in CSF may also be useful for monitoring the effects of CNS lymphoma therapy.[366]

Differential Diagnosis of Infectious Mononucleosis

In most cases, the diagnosis of infectious mononucleosis is straightforward. The clinical manifestations of sore throat, fever, lymphadenopathy, and malaise coupled with atypical lymphocytosis and a positive heterophile test result establish the diagnosis of EBV-induced infectious mononucleosis. Difficulties arise, however, when the clinical manifestations are less striking, particularly when the heterophile test results are negative.

Heterophile-negative infectious mononucleosis may be caused by several different agents. Attention to the clinical manifestations of the illness and proper use of the laboratory provide an etiologic diagnosis in 85% to 90% of all cases of infectious mononucleosis. The frequency with which heterophile-negative infectious mononucleosis is seen depends largely on three factors: (1) age of the population of patients (EBV-induced infectious mononucleosis tends to be a milder illness and is more often heterophile negative in pediatric populations than in young adults); (2) sensitivity of the heterophile test (heterophile antibodies are more often demonstrable with horse red cell agglutination than with beef red-cell hemolysis or with sheep red-cell agglutination); and (3) diligence with which heterophile antibodies are sought (typical cases of infectious mononucleosis may be heterophile negative on presentation but, if retested later in the course of the illness, may become heterophile positive).

The most frequent cause of heterophile-negative infectious mononucleosis in most populations is CMV.[367] Although differentiation of individual cases of EBV-induced versus CMV-induced infectious mononucleosis may be difficult, certain features are more common in CMV infections. CMV more frequently follows transfusion and is more often manifested as a typhoid-like syndrome without sore throat and lymphadenopathy. Splenomegaly may be slightly more prominent with CMV-induced disease, whereas the atypical lymphocytosis is usually less intense in CMV-induced infectious mononucleosis. In age-matched control subjects, the results of liver function tests are less elevated when the agent is CMV. Cryoglobulins are seen in both EBV-induced and CMV-induced disease, but anti-i specificity is not seen in CMV-induced mononucleosis.[336] The illness may be attributed to CMV with serologic evidence of acute CMV infection and no evidence of acute EBV infection.

Heterophile-negative infectious mononucleosis may also be caused by EBV. As previously noted, this is not uncommon in the pediatric age group.[131,132] The diagnosis rests on the demonstration of appropriate changes in specific EBV serologic tests (see Table 139-10).

Viral hepatitis may result in fever, lymphadenopathy, malaise, and an atypical lymphocytosis. Generally, the atypical lymphocytosis is of lesser magnitude, and accounts for less than 10% of the leukocytes. In viral hepatitis, hepatocellular enzyme levels are usually markedly elevated at the initial visit, whereas in infectious mononucleosis, the results of liver function tests are only mildly elevated initially and rise gradually over a 1-week to 2-week period. In addition, specific serologic tests are currently available for the detection of infection with hepatitis A, B, and C viruses.

Acute toxoplasmosis may also give rise to an infectious mononucleosis–like illness. Usually the degree of the lymphocytosis is mild, and a diagnosis can be made with serologic tests for *Toxoplasma*. Rubella may also occasionally be manifested by fever, lymphadenopathy, and a mild atypical lymphocytosis, but the appearance of the exanthem and the clinical course of the illness are generally not confused with those of infectious mononucleosis. A serologic diagnosis of recent rubella infection can be obtained if the diagnosis remains in doubt. Infectious lymphocytosis of childhood is a disease of uncertain cause that is characterized by fever, lymphadenopathy, occasionally diarrhea, and a lymphocytosis that consists almost exclusively of small mature lymphocytes. The disease is most common in the pediatric age group, may occur in epidemics, and is not associated with EBV infection.[368]

A streptococcal sore throat may also mimic infectious mononucleosis clinically. Adenopathy is generally submandibular and anterior cervical, and splenomegaly is absent in streptococcal sore throat. Culture of group A β-hemolytic streptococci from the throat is supportive but not conclusive evidence for this diagnosis because colonization with the organism is common in this population of patients. Serologic tests for recent infection with group A streptococci may help to establish the cause.

Patients with primary HIV infection may also present with fever, lymphadenopathy, and pharyngitis.[369-371] Such patients may also have a maculopapular rash and signs of aseptic meningitis. Patients with primary HIV infection are typically heterophile negative; however, rare cases of heterophile-positive primary HIV infection have been reported.[317] Thus, serum or plasma should be sent for HIV RNA (viral load) as part of the evaluation of heterophile-negative infectious mononucleosis and may even be appropriate in heterophile-positive patients at high risk (see Chapter 121). Patients with primary HIV infection typically have negative or indeterminate HIV serology.

▣ Treatment

INFECTIOUS MONONUCLEOSIS

Supportive

Treatment of infectious mononucleosis is largely supportive because more than 95% of the patients recover uneventfully without specific therapy. The level of activity is generally tailored to what the individual patient can tolerate comfortably. To avoid trauma to the spleen, contact sports or heavy lifting should be avoided during the first month of illness and until any splenomegaly has resolved. Ultrasound scan examination can be used to monitor spleen size. If constipation is present, it should be treated with a gentle laxative. Acetaminophen

or nonsteroidal antiinflammatory agents can be helpful in relieving the sore throat and in suppressing the fever. Sore throat may be further alleviated with gargling with warm salt water.

Antiviral Agents

Acyclovir, ganciclovir, and foscarnet inhibit EBV replication in vitro.[372-374] However, these agents target the viral DNA polymerase, which is expressed only during lytic infection. Because EBV infection is predominantly latent, that these agents are ineffective in treatment of infectious mononucleosis is not surprising. Further, the clinical symptoms and signs of infectious mononucleosis are largely the result of the vigorous immune response directed against EBV. A meta-analysis of five randomized, controlled trials showed no significant benefit of acyclovir in the treatment of infectious mononucleosis. These trials included patients with mild, moderate, and severe mononucleosis. As expected, viral shedding from the oropharynx, where lytic replication commonly occurs, was reduced, but inhibition of shedding was lost 3 weeks after withdrawal of the antiviral agent.[375-379]

Corticosteroids

Corticosteroids should not generally be used in uncomplicated infectious mononucleosis. A double-blind, placebo-controlled trial showed that the combination of acyclovir and prednisolone did not reduce the duration of symptoms or result in an earlier return to work.[378] Other studies with corticosteroids have indicated that corticosteroids decrease the period of febrility and hasten the resolution of tonsillopharyngeal symptoms but do not reproducibly affect lymphadenopathy or liver and spleen involvement.[380-384] One particular reason to avoid corticosteroids in uncomplicated disease is that they have rarely been linked with complications such as encephalitis and myocarditis.[47,384] In addition, there is a theoretical risk that corticosteroids may inhibit the host immune response, resulting in a larger reservoir of latently infected cells that could potentially put patients at risk for EBV-associated malignant disease.

Corticosteroids may be helpful in cases of complicated infectious mononucleosis.[384-386] Tonsillar enlargement that causes airway compromise may respond rapidly to corticosteroids, eliminating the need for tracheostomy. Corticosteroids may also be helpful in autoimmune hemolytic anemia, severe thrombocytopenia, and aplastic anemia. Some investigators also advocate the use of corticosteroids for CNS involvement, myocarditis, or pericarditis. In selected cases of severe or prolonged prostration, corticosteroids may be of benefit. If corticosteroids are administered in these situations, treatment should be initiated in doses equivalent to 60 to 80 mg of prednisone per day given in a split daily regimen. The response is usually rapid, and the dosage can be tapered over a 1-week to 2-week period.

LYMPHOPROLIFERATIVE DISEASE

The overall mortality rate remains high, at about 50%, for LPD. Outcome appears to be enhanced with early diagnosis and treatment.[387] Multiple methods are used in the treatment of LPD, but large trials are still needed to determine the best approaches.[51,52,262,388] The approach to therapy differs depending on whether LPD arises in hematopoietic stem cell or solid organ transplantation. The mainstay of LPD therapy in solid organ transplantation is reduction of immune suppression. This strategy is logical because LPD most likely results from ineffective immune surveillance of EBV-infected B cells. Reduction of immune suppression leads to regression of tumors in up to 50% of cases. However, this approach is usually ineffective in stem cell transplantation because these patients receive high-dose chemotherapy and radiation to ablate the immune system and are dependent on engraftment of donor immune cells.[387] Reduction of immunosuppression can increase the risk of graft rejection. Surgical resection and radiotherapy are often used in localized LPD and can be combined with reduction of immune suppression in solid organ transplant recipients with good results. Interferon-α produces antiviral effects and boosts immune function and is used for LPD treatment but risks graft rejection. Accurate assessment of the efficacy of interferon-α is difficult because it is usually combined with other treatment methods.

Antiviral therapy with agents such as acyclovir or ganciclovir is commonly used to treat LPD, with or without immunoglobulin.[51,52,388] Most LPD cells are latently infected by EBV and therefore do not express the EBV DNA polymerase. Because acyclovir and ganciclovir are directed against the EBV DNA polymerase, the latently infected tumor cells should not be susceptible to these agents. Acyclovir or ganciclovir may prevent expansion of the overall pool of EBV-infected B cells by preventing cell-to-cell spread through inhibition of lytic replication that otherwise occurs in a small percentage of cells. Immune globulin may possibly neutralize released EBV virus or exert antibody-dependent cell-mediated toxicity on tumor cells. One experimental approach has been to induce lytic infection (and therefore induce expression of the EBV DNA polymerase) in LPD cells with treatment with arginine butyrate followed by ganciclovir.[389] Initial results have been promising. Cytotoxic chemotherapy, usually with regimens used for non-Hodgkin's lymphoma, is often used after other initial approaches have failed but tends to be associated with high mortality rates.

Treatment and prophylaxis of LPD with antibodies targeted against B cells is often used in hematopoietic stem cell transplantation.[51,52,388] Rituximab is a monoclonal antibody directed against the CD20 B-cell antigen. Binding of this antibody to B cells produces cell death through complement fixation or antibody-dependent cell-mediated cytoxicity (ADCC). Response rates range from approximately 70% to 100% with rituximab in different studies, and these differences may be a result of the timeliness of diagnosis.[387] Rituximab causes profound B-cell depletion for up to 8 months, so prophylaxis should be reserved for patients believed to be at particularly high risk for LPD. Rituximab has also been used as ancillary therapy in solid organ transplantation in patients who do not respond well to reduction of immunosuppression.

Adoptive immunotherapy is another approach to LPD treatment. It is particularly useful in allogeneic stem cell recipients where LPD usually arises from donor cells and the donor is often available to harvest CTLs. This strategy is based on reconstitution of a cellular immune response against EBV to treat the infected tumor cells. Allogeneic stem cell recipients with LPD have been treated with unselected, donor mononuclear cells.[390,391] This approach results in response rates of up to 90% but also results in a high rate of graft-versus-host disease (GVHD) because of the presence of the infused alloreactive T cells. To avoid GVHD, another approach has been to infuse selected, donor-derived, EBV-specific CTLs.[392,393] Marking of transferred T cells has shown that they persist up to 18 months. This approach has also been used with success as prophylaxis for LPD in hematopoietic stem cell transplant recipients. Of note, a patient died of PTLD despite receiving adoptive immunotherapy. Analysis of the patient's tumor showed a deletion in EBNA-3B, a gene that is not necessary for B-cell growth transformation. Because the infused CTLs were largely directed against EBNA-3B, they selected for the mutated EBV. This report raises concern about escape mutants with CTL therapy.[394]

Adoptive immunotherapy can also be used in solid organ transplant recipients. The organ recipient's CTLs can be expanded in vitro and then infused back into the patient.[395] The infused CTLs do not expand as robustly as in hematopoietic stem cell transplantation and only exhibit transient persistence, perhaps at least partially because of continued immunosuppression.[387] A limitation to this method occurs in primary EBV infection, in which rapid onset LPD may not allow time to generate EBV-specific CTLs. Another approach in solid organ transplants has been to use closely matched, allogeneic CTLs. A bank of about 100 CTLs from healthy donors has been used on a best possible human leukocyte antigen (HLA) match basis to treat LPD.[396] In a phase II multicenter trial, 33 patients with LPD who had failure with conventional therapy were treated with these allogeneic CTLs.[397] A response rate of 52% was seen at 6 months, and 14 patients achieved complete remission.

Measurement of the EBV DNA load in the blood may be helpful for prediction of response to treatment of LPD. In one study, a decrease in the EBV DNA load within 72 hours correlated with response to therapy in seven responders, and all nonresponders had an increased EBV load at 72 hours.[398] Of note, however, after treatment with rituximab, peripheral blood mononuclear cell EBV DNA levels can fall even in the setting of tumor progression.[399]

EPSTEIN-BARR VIRUS TARGETED THERAPY IN ASSOCIATED MALIGNANT DISEASES

A comprehensive discussion of multimodality therapy for all EBV-associated malignant diseases is beyond the scope of this chapter. The success of EBV immunotherapy in LPD has prompted its investigation in other EBV-associated malignant diseases. These malignant diseases, however, present challenges for immunotherapy that LPD does not. First, EBV gene expression is more limited in other tumors, and unlike LPD, they do not express the immunodominant EBNA3 proteins. Second, because other EBV-associated malignant diseases arise in the setting of an apparently intact immune response, that immunotherapy should work is not obvious. Several small clinical trials have evaluated the safety and efficacy of CTL infusions for EBV-positive Hodgkin's lymphoma, and more recently nasopharyngeal carcinoma. In one study, 14 patients with relapsed Hodgkin's lymphoma were given infusions of autologous CTLs that had been expanded in vitro with antigenic stimulation with EBV transformed LCLs.[400] After 40 months of follow-up, results were five complete responses, one partial response, five patients with stable disease, and three with no response. Infused CTLs were shown to home to tumor sites and persist for at least 12 months and were well tolerated. A second study examined the effect of autologous EBV-specific CTLs that were enriched for LMP2A-specific reactivity.[401] With this therapy, two of three patients with active Hodgkin's lymphoma achieved a complete response; the other had no response, and five of five patients without active disease remained in remission after treatment. The use of allogeneic EBV-specific CTLs has also been examined for Hodgkin's lymphoma in a single study of six patients.[402] Three patients who received only CTL infusions had a partial response, two of three patients who received fludarabine followed by CTL infusion achieved a partial response, and the third had stable disease.

At least three studies have examined the use of autologous EBV-specific CTLs in nasopharyngeal carcinoma. One study reported a decrease in EBV viral load in three of four treated patients with stage IV or V disease but did not detect any clinical responses.[403] A second study of six patients with refractory stage III or IV nasopharyngeal carcinoma observed two complete and one partial response; one patient had stable disease, and two had nonresponses.[404] Four other patients in remission treated with CTL infusions remained in remission with a minimum follow-up of 19 months. A third study evaluated EBV-specific CTL infusions in 10 patients with refractory stage IV disease.[405] This treatment resulted in two partial responses, four patients with stable disease, and four patients with progression despite therapy. A second approach to immunotherapy used in nasopharyngeal carcinoma is use of vaccines to induce responses against EBV antigens. Among 16 patients with recurrent or metastatic nasopharyngeal carcinoma who were vaccinated with dendritic cells pulsed with LMP2A peptides, only two patients had a partial response, although nine were seen to have increased epitope-specific cytotoxicity.[406] Another vaccine with a vaccinia strain modified vaccinia Ankara (MVA) to express a hybrid EBNA1-LMP2A protein appears to be safe in patients with nasopharyngeal carcinoma and is currently in clinical trials.[407] In summary, limited data suggest that EBV immunotherapy in patients with advanced EBV-positive Hodgkin's lymphoma or nasopharyngeal carcinoma is well tolerated and may be beneficial. By contrast, antiviral drugs have no established role in the treatment of EBV malignant diseases.

ORAL HAIRY LEUKOPLAKIA

Oral hairy leukoplakia differs from most EBV-related diseases in that the EBV infection is predominantly lytic rather than latent.

In this setting of active lytic infection, agents such as acyclovir, ganciclovir, and foscarnet are effective in therapy.[408-411] Topical therapy, such as use of podophyllum resin, has also been shown to have efficacy against OHL.[412,413] In the setting of HIV-related OHL, oral lesions usually regress with the institution of effective antiretroviral therapy.

▪ Prevention

PUBLIC HEALTH MEASURES

Because the spread of virus requires intimate contact, isolation of patients with infectious mononucleosis is not necessary. Elevated viremia is seen for several months after recovery, so consideration should be given to postponement of blood donation by patients with infectious mononucleosis for at least 6 months after the onset of illness.

VACCINE

Epstein-Barr virus vaccine development has been an elusive goal for many years. Because EBV infection does not cause severe disease in most instances, a vaccine must be particularly safe.[49] The only herpes virus vaccine currently licensed by the Food and Drug Administration is a live attenuated varicella-zoster vaccine. Because of EBV's associations with malignant diseases, acceptance of a live attenuated vaccine is highly unlikely.

The goals of an EBV vaccine are not yet clearly defined[262] and likely will be determined based on the levels of protection provided by different vaccine formulations. Complete protection from infection, at first glance, appears to be the primary goal, but its attainment may be limited by the biology of the virus (see subsequent discussion). Another potential goal is prevention of symptomatic infection of infectious mononucleosis, without necessarily prevention of lifelong latent viral infection. In such a case, determination is critical of whether the vaccine also provides any protection against complications of EBV, such as malignancy disease or fulminant primary infection in X-linked lymphoproliferative disease. Another possibility might be a vaccine that prevents EBV-associated malignant diseases but without prevention of latent infection or even symptoms of mononucleosis.

Two major approaches have been taken to EBV vaccine development. One approach is to induce EBV neutralizing antibody directed against the viral glycoprotein gp350, which binds to the EBV cellular receptor.[414] Immunization with gp350 protects against EBV-induced lymphomas in an animal model.[415] Interestingly, despite initial expectations, cell-mediated immunity appears to play an important role in the gp350 vaccination prevention of lymphoma in this model.[416] A small trial in China with recombinant vaccinia virus expressing gp350 protected six of nine children from EBV infection at 16 months compared with none of 10 control subjects.[417] However, the use of live vaccinia-based vaccines is unlikely to become widespread.[262] Phase I and II studies of a gp350 vaccine have recently shown protection from symptoms of infectious mononucleosis but did not prevent asymptomatic infection with EBV. Of note, one initially EBV seropositive participant experienced an oligoarthritis reaction, which may have been related to the vaccine.[418-420] Symptomatic mononucleosis has been suggested to lead to a long-term deficit in T-cell responsiveness, so this vaccine could possibly have benefits in addition to prevention of symptomatic illness with its accompanying loss of productivity.[418,421]

The second approach has been to develop a vaccine with known EBV MHC class I restricted CTL epitopes.[422-424] Although such a vaccine would not necessarily be designed to prevent primary infection, it is expected to ameliorate the symptoms of mononucleosis.[422] Another important potential use of such a vaccine would be to boost the CTL response to avoid development of, or possibly treat, EBV-associated malignant diseases. A significant number of EBV epitopes recognized by CTLs have now been identified. A phase I trial has been completed in Australia with a single EBNA3 EBV epitope. In this trial, in which two placebo recipients who became EBV infected, one had symptomatic mononucleosis; none of four vaccine recipients who acquired EBV infection were symptomatic.[425] To generate a broad-based CTL response, a vaccine containing multiple EBV epitopes is necessary. In addition, because CTLs from individuals with different human leukocyte antigen alleles recognize different EBV epitopes, inclusion of relevant epitopes in a vaccine is important. Therefore, current efforts have fused multiple peptide epitopes together for use in vaccines.[49,422]

REFERENCES

1. Filatov NF. *Lektuse ob ostrikh infektsion Nikh Lolieznyak (Lectures on Acute Infectious Disease of children)*. Moscow: U. Deitel; 1885.
2. Pfeiffer E. Drusenfieber. *Jahrb Kinderheilkd*. 1889;29:257.
3. Türk W. Septische Erkrankungen bei Verkümmerung des Granulozytensystems. *Wien Klin Wochenschr*. 1907;20:157.
4. Hall AJ. A case resembling acute lymphatic leukaemia, ending in complete recovery. *Proc R Soc Med*. 1915;8:15-19.
5. Sprunt TP, Evans FA. Mononuclear leukocytosis in reaction to acute infections ("infectious mononucleosis"). *Johns Hopkins Hosp Bull*. 1920;31:410.
6. Downey H, McKinlay CA. Acute lymphadenosis compared with acute lymphatic leukemia. *Arch Intern Med*. 1923;32:82-112.
7. Paul JR, Bunnell W. The presence of heterophile antibodies in infectious mononucleosis. *Am J Med Sci*. 1932;183:90-104.
8. Davidsohn I. Serologic diagnosis of infectious mononucleosis. *JAMA*. 1937;108:289-295.
9. Evans AS. Experimental attempts to transmit infectious mononucleosis to man. *Yale J Biol Med*. 1947;20:19-26.
10. Evans AS. Further experimental attempts to transmit infectious mononucleosis to man. *J Clin Invest*. 1950;29:508-512.
11. Niederman JC, Scott RB. Studies on infectious mononucleosis: Attempts to transmit the disease to human volunteers. *Yale J Biol Med*. 1965;38:1-10.
12. Burkitt D. A sarcoma involving the jaws in African children. *Br J Surg*. 1958;46:218-223.
13. Epstein MA, Achong BA, Barr YM. Virus particles in cultured lymphoblasts from Burkitt's lymphoma. *Lancet*. 1964;1:702-703.
14. Henle G, Henle W. Immunofluorescence in cells derived from Burkitt lymphoma. *J Bacteriol*. 1966;91:1248-1256.
15. Henle G, Henle W, Diehl V. Relation of Burkitt's tumor associated herpes-type virus to infectious mononucleosis. *Proc Natl Acad Sci U S A*. 1968;59:94-101.

16. Niederman JC, McCollum RW, Henle G, et al. Infectious mononucleosis: Clinical manifestations in relation to EB virus antibodies. *JAMA*. 1968;203:205-209.
17. Evans AS, Niederman JC, McCollum RW. Seroepidemiologic studies of infectious mononucleosis with EB virus. *N Engl J Med*. 1968;279:1121-1127.
18. Sawyer RN, Evans AS, Niederman JC, et al. Prospective studies of a group of Yale University freshmen. I. Occurrence of infectious mononucleosis. *J Infect Dis*. 1971;123:263-270.
19. University Health Physicians and PHLS Laboratories. A joint investigation of infectious mononucleosis and its relationship to EB virus antibody. *Br Med J*. 1971;4:643-646.
20. Baer R, Bankier AT, Biggin MD, et al. DNA sequence and expression of the B95-8 Epstein-Barr virus genome. *Nature*. 1984;310:207-211.
21. Parker BD, Bankier A, Satchwell S, et al. Sequence and transcription of Raji Epstein-Barr virus DNA spanning the B95-8 deletion region. *Virology*. 1990;179:339-346.
22. Allday MJ, Crawford DH. Role of epithelium in EBV persistence and pathogenesis of B-cell tumours. *Lancet*. 1988;1:855-857.
23. Sixbey JW, Nedrud JG, Raab-Traub N, et al. Epstein-Barr virus replication in oropharyngeal epithelial cells. *N Engl J Med*. 1984;310:1225-1230.
24. Anagnostopoulos I, Hummel M, Kreschel C, et al. Morphology, immunophenotype, and distribution of latently and/or productively Epstein-Barr virus–infected cells in acute infectious mononucleosis: Implications for the interindividual infection route of Epstein-Barr virus. *Blood*. 1995;85:744-750.
25. Niedobitek G, Agathanggelou A, Herbst H, et al. Epstein-Barr virus (EBV) infection in infectious mononucleosis: Virus latency, replication and phenotype of EBV-infected cells. *J Pathol*. 1997;182:151-159.

26. Borza CM, Hutt-Fletcher LM. Alternate replication in B cells and epithelial cells switches tropism of Epstein-Barr virus. *Nat Med*. 2002;8:594-599.
27. Farrell PJ. Cell-switching and kissing. *Nat Med*. 2002;8:559-560.
28. Moss DJ, Burrows SR, Silins SL, et al. The immunology of Epstein-Barr virus infection. *Philos Trans R Soc Lond B Biol Sci*. 2001;356:475-488.
29. Rickinson AB, Moss DJ. Human cytotoxic T lymphocyte responses to Epstein-Barr virus infection. *Annu Rev Immunol*. 1997;15:405-431.
30. Babcock GJ, Decker LL, Volk M, et al. EBV persistence in memory B cells in vivo. *Immunity*. 1998;9:395-404.
31. Wagner HJ, Bein G, Bitsch A, et al. Detection and quantification of latently infected B lymphocytes in Epstein-Barr virus–seropositive, healthy individuals by polymerase chain reaction. *J Clin Microbiol*. 1992;30:2826-2829.
32. Sixbey JW, Vesterinen EH, Nedrud JG, et al. Replication of Epstein-Barr virus in human epithelial cells infected in vitro. *Nature*. 1983;306:480-483.
33. Fingeroth JD, Weiss JJ, Tedder TF, et al. Epstein-Barr virus receptor of human B lymphocytes is the C3d receptor CR2. *Proc Natl Acad Sci U S A*. 1984;81:4510-4514.
34. Frade R, Barel M, Ehlin-Eriksson B, et al. gp140, the C3d receptor of human B lymphocytes, is also the Epstein-Barr virus receptor. *Proc Natl Acad Sci U S A*. 1985;82:1490-1493.
35. Young LS, Sixbey JW, Clark D, et al. Epstein-Barr virus receptor on human pharyngeal epithelia. *Lancet*. 1986;1:240-242.
36. Sixbey JW, Davis DS, Young LS, et al. Human epithelial cell expression of an Epstein-Barr virus receptor. *J Gen Virol*. 1987;68:805-811.
37. Jondal M, Klein G. Surface markers on human B and T lymphocytes. II. Presence of Epstein-Barr virus receptors on B lymphocytes. *J Exp Med*. 1973;138:1365-1378.

38. Yefenof E, Bakacs T, Einhorn L, et al. Epstein-Barr virus receptors, complement receptors and EBV infectibility of different lymphocyte fractions of human peripheral blood. I. Complement receptor distribution and complement binding by separated lymphocyte subpopulations. *Cell Immunol.* 1978;35:34-42.
39. Einhorn L, Steinitz M, Yefenof E, et al. Epstein-Barr virus receptors, complement receptors and EBV infectibility of different lymphocyte fractions of human peripheral blood. II. Epstein-Barr virus studies. *Cell Immunol.* 1978;35:43-58.
40. Haan KM, Kwok WW, Longnecker R, et al. Epstein-Barr virus entry utilizing HLA-DP or HLA-DQ as a coreceptor. *J Virol.* 2000;74:2451-2454.
41. Li Q, Spriggs MK, Kovats S, et al. Epstein-Barr virus uses HLA class II as a cofactor for infection of B lymphocytes. *J Virol.* 1997;71:4657-4662.
42. McShane MP, Mullen MM, Haan KM, et al. Mutational analysis of the HLA class II interaction with Epstein-Barr virus glycoprotein 42. *J Virol.* 2003;77:7655-7662.
43. Mullen MM, Haan KM, Longnecker R, et al. Structure of the Epstein-Barr virus gp42 protein bound to the MHC class II receptor HLA-DR1. *Mol Cell.* 2002;9:375-385.
44. Wang X, Hutt-Fletcher LM. Epstein-Barr virus lacking glycoprotein gp42 can bind to B cells but is not able to infect. *J Virol.* 1998;72:158-163.
45. Pope JH, Horne MK, Scott W. Transformation of foetal human leukocytes in vitro by filtrates of a human leukaemic cell line containing herpes-like virus. *Int J Cancer.* 1968;3:857-866.
46. Steinberg K, Beck J, Nickerson D, et al. DNA banking for epidemiologic studies: A review of current practices. *Epidemiology.* 2002;13:246-254.
47. Cohen JI. Epstein-Barr virus infection. *N Engl J Med.* 2000;343:481-492.
48. Crawford DH. Biology and disease associations of Epstein-Barr virus. *Philos Trans R Soc Lond B Biol Sci.* 2001;356:461-473.
49. Macsween KF, Crawford DH. Epstein-Barr virus: Recent advances. *Lancet Infect Dis.* 2003;3:131-140.
50. Thorley-Lawson DA. Epstein-Barr virus: Exploiting the immune system. *Nat Rev Immunol.* 2001;1:75-82.
51. Andreone P, Gramenzi A, Lorenzini S, et al. Posttransplantation lymphoproliferative disorders. *Arch Intern Med.* 2003;163:1997-2004.
52. Loren AW, Porter DL, Stadtmauer EA, et al. Post-transplant lymphoproliferative disorder: A review. *Bone Marrow Transplant.* 2003;31:145-155.
53. Kuppers R. B cells under influence: Transformation of B cells by Epstein-Barr virus. *Nat Rev Immunol.* 2003;3:801-812.
54. Young LS, Murray PG. Epstein-Barr virus and oncogenesis: From latent genes to tumours. *Oncogene.* 2003;22:5108-5121.
55. Kieff E, Rickinson AB. Epstein-Barr virus and its replication. In: Knipe D, Howley P, Griffin D, et al, eds. *Fields Virology*. Philadelphia: Lippincott Williams & Wilkins; 2007:2603-2654.
56. Smith P. Epstein-Barr virus complementary strand transcripts (CSTs/BARTs) and cancer. *Semin Cancer Biol.* 2001;11:469-476.
57. Edwards RH, Marquitz AR, Raab-Traub N. Epstein-Barr virus BART microRNAs are produced from a large intron prior to splicing. *J Virol.* 2008;82:9094-9106.
58. Grossman SR, Johannsen E, Tong X, et al. The Epstein-Barr virus nuclear antigen 2 transactivator is directed to response elements by the J kappa recombination signal binding protein. *Proc Natl Acad Sci U S A.* 1994;91:7568-7572.
59. Henkel T, Ling PD, Hayward SD, et al. Mediation of Epstein-Barr virus EBNA2 transactivation by recombination signal-binding protein J kappa. *Science.* 1994;265:92-95.
60. Harada S, Kieff E. Epstein-Barr virus nuclear protein LP stimulates EBNA-2 acidic domain–mediated transcriptional activation. *J Virol.* 1997;71:6611-6618.
61. Kulwichit W, Edwards RH, Davenport EM, et al. Expression of the Epstein-Barr virus latent membrane protein 1 induces B cell lymphoma in transgenic mice. *Proc Natl Acad Sci U S A.* 1998;95:11963-11968.
62. Wang D, Liebowitz D, Kieff E. An EBV membrane protein expressed in immortalized lymphocytes transforms established rodent cells. *Cell.* 1985;43:831-840.
63. Mosialos G, Birkenbach M, Yalamanchili R, et al. The Epstein-Barr virus transforming protein LMP1 engages signaling proteins for the tumor necrosis factor receptor family. *Cell.* 1995;80:389-399.
64. Uchida J, Yasui T, Takaoka-Shichijo Y, et al. Mimicry of CD40 signals by Epstein-Barr virus LMP1 in B lymphocyte responses. *Science.* 1999;286:300-303.
65. Gires O, Zimber-Strobl U, Gonnella R, et al. Latent membrane protein 1 of Epstein-Barr virus mimics a constitutively active receptor molecule. *EMBO J.* 1997;16:6131-6140.
66. Merchant M, Swart R, Katzman RB, et al. The effects of the Epstein-Barr virus latent membrane protein 2A on B cell function. *Int Rev Immunol.* 2001;20:805-835.
67. Flavell KJ, Murray PG. Hodgkin's disease and the Epstein-Barr virus. *Mol Pathol.* 2000;53:262-269.
68. Raab-Traub N. Epstein-Barr virus in the pathogenesis of NPC. *Semin Cancer Biol.* 2002;12:431-441.
69. Su IJ. Epstein-Barr virus and T-cell lymphoma. *EBV Rep.* 1996;3:1-6.
70. Straus SE, Cohen JI, Tosato G, et al. Epstein-Barr virus infections: Biology, pathogenesis and management. *Ann Intern Med.* 1992;118:45-58.
71. Ragoczy T, Heston L, Miller G. The Epstein-Barr virus Rta protein activates lytic cycle genes and can disrupt latency in B lymphocytes. *J Virol.* 1998;72:7978-7984.
72. Henle G, Henle W, Clifford P, et al. Antibodies to Epstein-Barr virus in Burkitt's lymphoma and control groups. *J Natl Cancer Inst.* 1969;43:1147-1154.
73. Pereira MS, Blake JM, Macrae AD. EB virus antibody at different ages. *Br Med J.* 1969;4:526-527.
74. Porter DD, Wimberly I, Benyesh-Melnick M. Prevalence of antibodies to EB virus and other herpesviruses. *JAMA.* 1969;208:1675-1679.
75. Gerber P, Birch SM, Rosenblum EN. The incidence of complement fixing antibodies in sera of human and non-human primates to viral antigens derived from Burkitt's lymphocyte cells. *Proc Natl Acad Sci U S A.* 1967;58:478-484.
76. Hallee TJ, Evans AS, Niederman JC, et al. Infectious mononucleosis at the United States Military Academy. A prospective study of a single class over 4 years. *Yale J Biol Med.* 1974;47:182-195.
77. Nye FJ. Social class and infectious mononucleosis. *J Hyg (Lond).* 1973;71:145-149.
78. Heath CW Jr, Brodsky AL, Potolsky AI. Infectious mononucleosis in a general population. *Am J Epidemiol.* 1972;95:46-52.
79. Bernstein A. Infectious mononucleosis. *Medicine (Baltimore).* 1940;19:85-159.
80. Henle G, Henle W. Observations on childhood infections with the Epstein-Barr virus. *J Infect Dis.* 1970;121:303-310.
81. Tamir D, Benderly A, Levy J, et al. Infectious mononucleosis and Epstein-Barr virus in childhood. *Pediatrics.* 1974;53:330-335.
82. Gerber P, Nonoyama M, Lucas S, et al. Oral excretion of Epstein Barr virus by healthy subjects and patients with infectious mononucleosis. *Lancet.* 1972;2:988-989.
83. Chang RS, Golden HD. Transformation of human leukocytes from throat washings from infectious mononucleosis patients. *Nature.* 1971;234:359-360.
84. Niederman JC, Miller G, Pearson HA, et al. Infectious mononucleosis: Epstein Barr virus shedding in saliva and the oropharynx. *N Engl J Med.* 1976;294:1355-1359.
85. Strauch B, Siegel N, Andrews LL, et al. Oropharyngeal excretion of Epstein Barr virus by renal transplant recipients and other patients treated with immunosuppressive drugs. *Lancet.* 1974;1:234-237.
86. Chang RS, Lewis JP, Abildgaard CF. Prevalence of oropharyngeal excreters of leukocyte transforming agents among a human population. *N Engl J Med.* 1973;289:1325-1329.
87. Chang RS, Lewis JS, Reynolds RD, et al. Oropharyngeal excretion of Epstein Barr virus by patients with lymphoproliferative disorders and by recipients of renal homografts. *Ann Intern Med.* 1978;88:34-40.
88. Ferbas J, Rahman MA, Kingsley LA, et al. Frequent oropharyngeal shedding of Epstein-Barr virus in homosexual men during early HIV infection. *AIDS.* 1992;6:1273-1278.
89. Wolf H, Haus M, Wilmer E. Persistence of Epstein Barr virus in the parotid gland. *J Virol.* 1984;51:795-798.
90. Sixbey JW, Lemon SM, Pagano JS. A second site for Epstein-Barr virus shedding: The uterine cervix. *Lancet* 1986;2:122-124.
91. Lipman M, Andrews L, Niederman J, et al. Direct visualization of enveloped Epstein-Barr herpesvirus in throat washing with leukocyte transforming activity. *J Infect Dis.* 1975;132:520-523.
92. Hoagland RS. The transmission of infectious mononucleosis. *Am J Med Sci.* 1955;229:262-272.
93. Fleisher GR, Pasquariello PS, Warren WS, et al. Intrafamilial transmission of Epstein-Barr virus infections. *J Pediatr.* 1981;98:16-19.
94. Larsson BO, Linde A. Intrafamilial transmission of Epstein-Barr virus infection among six adult members of one adult family. *Scand J Infect Dis.* 1990;22:363-366.
95. Gerber P, Walsh JH, Rosenblum EN, et al. Association of EB virus infection with the post perfusion syndrome. *Lancet.* 1969;1:593-595.
96. Herbert JT, Feorino P, Caldwell GG. False-positive epidemic infectious mononucleosis. *Am Fam Physician.* 1977;115:119-121.
97. Evans AS. Infectious mononucleosis in University of Wisconsin students. Report of a 5 year investigation. *Am J Hyg.* 1960;71:342-362.
98. Evans AS. Epidemiology and pathogenesis of infectious mononucleosis. In: *Proceedings of the International Infectious Mononucleosis Symposium*. Evanston, Ill: American College Health Association; 1967:40.
99. Evans AS. Infectious mononucleosis in the Armed Forces. *Mil Med.* 1970;135:300-304.
100. Lehane DE. A seroepidemiologic study of infectious mononucleosis. The development of EB virus antibody in a military population. *JAMA.* 1970;212:2240-2242.
101. Rocchi G, DeFelici A, Ragona G, et al. Quantitative evaluation of Epstein-Barr virus infected mononuclear peripheral blood leukocytes in infectious mononucleosis. *N Engl J Med.* 1977;296:132-134.
102. Robinson JE, Smith D, Niederman J. Plasmacytic differentiation of circulating Epstein-Barr virus infected B-lymphocytes during acute infectious mononucleosis. *J Exp Med.* 1981;153:235-244.
103. Blazar B, Patarroyo M, Klein E, et al. Increased sensitivity of human lymphoid lines to natural killer cells after induction of the Epstein-Barr viral cycle by superinfection or sodium butyrate. *J Exp Med.* 1980;151:614-627.
104. Rickinson AB, Crawford D, Epstein MA. Inhibition of the in vitro outgrowth of Epstein-Barr virus transformed lymphocytes by thymus dependent lymphocytes from infectious mononucleosis patients. *Clin Exp Immunol.* 1977;28:72-79.
105. Thorley-Lawson DA, Chess L, Strominger JA. Suppression of in vitro Epstein Barr virus infection: A new role for the adult human T lymphocyte. *J Exp Med.* 1977;146:495-508.
106. Schooley RT, Haynes BF, Payling-Wright CR, et al. Development of suppressor T-lymphocytes for Epstein-Barr virus induced B-lymphocyte outgrowth: Assessment by two quantitative systems. *Blood.* 1981;57:510-517.
107. Callan MF, Tan L, Annels N, et al. Direct visualization of antigen-specific CD8+ T cells during the primary immune response to Epstein-Barr virus in vivo. *J Exp Med.* 1998;187:1395-1402.
108. Foss HD, Herbst H, Hummel M, et al. Patterns of cytokine gene expression in infectious mononucleosis. *Blood.* 1994;83:707-712.
109. Catalina MD, Sullivan JL, Bak KR, et al. Differential evolution and stability of epitope-specific $CD8^+$ T cell responses in EBV infection. *J Immunol.* 2001;167:4450-4457.
110. Amyes E, Hatton C, Montamat-Sicotte D, et al. Characterization of the CD4+ T cell response to Epstein-Barr virus during primary and persistent infection. *J Exp Med.* 2003;198:903-911.
111. Precopio ML, Sullivan JL, Willard C, et al. Differential kinetics and specificity of EBV-specific CD4+ and CD8+ T cells during primary infection. *J Immunol.* 2003;170:2590-2598.
112. Hoffman GJ, Lazarowitz SG, Hayward SD. Monoclonal antibody against a 250,000-dalton glycoprotein of Epstein-Barr virus identifies a membrane antigen and a neutralizing antigen. *Proc Natl Acad Sci U S A.* 1980;77:2979-2983.
113. Qualtiere LF, Chase R, Pearson GR. Purification and biologic characterization of a major Epstein Barr virus–induced membrane glycoprotein. *J Immunol.* 1982;129:814-818.
114. Thorley-Lawson DA, Geilinger K. Monoclonal antibodies against the major glycoprotein (gp350/220) of Epstein-Barr virus neutralize infectivity. *Proc Natl Acad Sci U S A.* 1980;77:5307-5311.
115. Henle W, Henle G, Hewetson J, et al. Failure to detect heterophile antigens in Epstein Barr virus infected cells and to demonstrate interaction of heterophile antibodies with Epstein Barr virus. *Clin Exp Immunol.* 1974;17:281-286.
116. Hsu DH, de Waal Malefyt R, Fiorentino DF, et al. Expression of interleukin-10 activity by Epstein-Barr virus protein BCRF1. *Science.* 1990;250:830-832.
117. Moore KW, Vieira P, Fiorentino DF, et al. Homology of cytokine synthesis inhibitory factor (IL-10) to the Epstein-Barr virus gene *BCRFI*. *Science.* 1990;248:1230-1234.
118. Cohen JI, Lekstrom K. Epstein-Barr virus BARF1 protein is dispensable for B-cell transformation and inhibits alpha interferon secretion from mononuclear cells. *J Virol.* 1999;73:7627-7632.
119. Henderson S, Huen D, Rowe M, et al. Epstein-Barr virus–coded BHRF1 protein, a viral homologue of Bcl-2, protects human B cells from programmed cell death. *Proc Natl Acad Sci U S A.* 1993;90:8479-8483.
120. Levitskaya J, Coram M, Levitsky V, et al. Inhibition of antigen processing by the internal repeat region of the Epstein-Barr virus nuclear antigen-1. *Nature.* 1995;375:685-688.
121. Downey H, Stasney J. The pathology of the lymph nodes in infectious mononucleosis. *Folia Haematol (Leipz).* 1936;54:417-438.
122. Smith EB, Custer RP. Rupture of spleen in infectious mononucleosis: Clinicopathologic report of 7 cases. *Blood.* 1946;1:317-333.
123. Custer RP, Smith EB. The pathology of infectious mononucleosis. *Blood.* 1948;3:830-857.
124. Hovde RF, Sundberg RD. Granulomatous lesions in the bone marrow in infectious mononucleosis. *Blood.* 1950;5:209-232.
125. Pease GL. Granulomatous lesions in bone marrow. *Blood.* 1956;11:720-734.
126. Nelson RS, Darragh JH. Infectious mononucleosis hepatitis. A clinicopathologic study. *Am J Med.* 1956;21:26-33.
127. Sullivan BH, Irey NS, Pieggi VJ, et al. The liver in infectious mononucleosis. *Am J Dig Dis.* 1957;2:210-223.
128. Bergin JD. Fatal encephalopathy in glandular fever. *J Neurol Neurosurg Psychiatry.* 1960;23:69-73.
129. Ambler M, Stoll J, Tzamaloukas A, et al. Focal encephalomyelitis in infectious mononucleosis. A report with pathologic description. *Ann Intern Med.* 1971;75:579-583.
130. Sumaya CV, Ench Y. Epstein-Barr virus infectious mononucleosis in children. I. Clinical and general laboratory findings. *Pediatrics.* 1985;75:1003-1010.
131. Schmitz H, Volz D, Krainick-Riechert CH, et al. Acute Epstein-Barr virus infections in children. *Med Microbiol Immunol.* 1972;158:58-63.
132. Sumaya CV, Ench Y. Epstein-Barr virus infectious mononucleosis in children. II. Heterophil antibody and viral-specific responses. *Pediatrics.* 1985;75:1011-1019.
133. Horwitz CA, Henle W, Henle G, et al. Clinical and laboratory evaluation of elderly patients with heterophile antibody positive infectious mononucleosis. Report of seven patients ages 40 to 78. *Am J Med.* 1976;61:333-339.
134. Britton S, Andersson-Anvret M, Gergely P, et al. Epstein Barr virus immunity and tissue distribution in a fatal case of infectious mononucleosis. *N Engl J Med.* 1978;298:89-92.

135. Cameron D, MacBear LM. *A Clinical Study of Infectious Mononucleosis and Toxoplasmosis*. Baltimore: Williams & Wilkins; 1973:8.
136. Hoagland RJ. Infectious mononucleosis. *Am J Med*. 1952;13:158-171.
137. Mason WR Jr, Adams EK. Infectious mononucleosis. An analysis of 100 cases with particular attention to diagnosis, liver function tests, and treatment of selected cases with prednisone. *Am J Med Sci*. 1958;236:447-459.
138. Hoagland RJ. The incubation period of infectious mononucleosis. *Am J Public Health Nations Health*. 1964;54:1699-1705.
139. Joncas J, Chaisson JP, Turcotte J, et al. Studies on infectious mononucleosis. III. Clinical data, serologic and epidemiologic findings. *Can Med Assoc J*. 1968;98:848-854.
140. Pullen H, Wright N, Murdock J McC. Hypersensitivity reactions to antibacterial drugs in infectious mononucleosis. *Lancet*. 1967;2:1176-1178.
141. Patel BM. Skin rash with infectious mononucleosis and ampicillin. *Pediatrics*. 1967;40:910-911.
142. Bierman CW, Pierson WE, Zeitz SJ, et al. Reactions associated with ampicillin therapy. *JAMA*. 1972;220:1098-1100.
143. Nazareth I, Mortimer P, McKendrick GD. Ampicillin sensitivity in infectious mononucleosis: Temporary or permanent? *Scand J Infect Dis*. 1972;4:229-230.
144. Caird FI, Holt PR. The enanthem of glandular fever. *Br Med J*. 1958;1:85-87.
145. Karzon DT. Infectious mononucleosis. *Adv Pediatr*. 1976;22:231-265.
146. Hoagland RJ. *Infectious Mononucleosis*. New York: Grune & Stratton; 1967:64.
147. Horwitz CA, Moulds J, Henle W, et al. Cold agglutinins in infectious mononucleosis and heterophile antibody negative mononucleosis like syndromes. *Blood*. 1977;50:195-202.
148. Jenkins WJ, Koster HG, Marsh WL, et al. Infectious mononucleosis: An unsuspected source of anti-i. *Br J Haematol*. 1965;11:480-483.
149. Capra JD, Dowling P, Cook S, et al. An incomplete cold reactive γG antibody with i specificity in infectious mononucleosis. *Vox Sang*. 1969;16:10-17.
150. Bowman HS, Marsh WL, Schumacher HR, et al. Auto anti-N immunohemolytic anemia in infectious mononucleosis. *Am J Clin Pathol*. 1974;61:465-472.
151. Troxel DB, Innella F, Cohen RJ. Infectious mononucleosis complicated by hemolytic anemia due to anti-i. *Am J Clin Pathol*. 1966;46:625-631.
152. Wilkinson LS, Petz LD, Garraty G. Reappraisal of the role of anti-i in haemolytic anemia in infectious mononucleosis. *Br J Haematol*. 1973;25:715-722.
153. Rosenfield RE, Schmidt PJ, Calvo RC, et al. Anti-i, a frequent cold agglutinin in infectious mononucleosis. *Vox Sang*. 1965;10:631-634.
154. Worlledge SM, Dacie JV. Hemolytic and other anemias in infectious mononucleosis. In: Carter RL, Penman HG, eds. *Infectious Mononucleosis*. Oxford: Blackwell Scientific; 1969:82-120.
155. Carter RL. Platelet levels in infectious mononucleosis. *Blood*. 1965;25:817-821.
156. Clark BF, Davies SH. Severe thrombocytopenia in infectious mononucleosis. *Am J Med Sci*. 1964;248:703-708.
157. Radel EG, Schorr JB. Thrombocytopenic purpura with infectious mononucleosis. *J Pediatr*. 1963;63:46-60.
158. Goldstein E, Porter DY. Fatal thrombocytopenia with cerebral hemorrhage in mononucleosis. *Arch Neurol*. 1969;20:533-535.
159. Ellman L, Carvalho A, Jacobson BM, et al. Platelet autoantibody in a case of infectious mononucleosis presenting as thrombocytopenic purpura. *Am J Med*. 1973;55:723-726.
160. Grossman LA, Wolff SM. Acute thrombocytopenic purpura in infectious mononucleosis. *JAMA*. 1959;171:2208-2210.
161. Schooley RT, Densen P, Harmon D, et al. Antineutrophil antibodies in infectious mononucleosis. *Am J Med*. 1984;76:85-90.
162. Carter RL. Granulocyte changes in infectious mononucleosis. *J Clin Pathol*. 1966;19:279-283.
163. Cantow EK, Kostinas JE. Studies on infectious mononucleosis. IV. Changes in the granulocytic series. *Am J Clin Pathol*. 1966;46:43-47.
164. Wulff HR. Acute agranulocytosis following infectious mononucleosis. Report of a case. *Scand J Haematol*. 1965;2:180-182.
165. Habib MA, Babka JC, Burningham RA. Case report. Profound granulocytopenia associated with infectious mononucleosis. *Am J Med Sci*. 1973;265:339-346.
166. Neel EU. Infectious mononucleosis. Death due to agranulocytosis and pneumonia. *JAMA*. 1976;236:1493-1494.
167. Eriksson KF, Holmberg L, Gustafbergstrand C. Infectious mononucleosis and agranulocytosis. *Scand J Infect Dis*. 1979;11:307-309.
168. Hammond WP, Harlan JM, Steinberg SE. Severe neutropenia in infectious mononucleosis. *West J Med*. 1979;131:92-97.
169. Dagan R, Powell KR. Postanginal sepsis following infectious mononucleosis. *Arch Intern Med*. 1987;147:1581-1583.
170. Hoagland RJ, Henson HM. Splenic rupture in infectious mononucleosis. *Ann Intern Med*. 1957;46:1184-1191.
171. Peters RM, Gordon LA, Nonsurgical treatment or splenic hemorrhage in an adult with infectious mononucleosis. *Am J Med*. 1986;80:123-125.
172. McLean ER, Diehl W, Edoga JK, et al. Failure of conservative management of splenic rupture in a patient with mononucleosis. *J Pediatr Surg*. 1987;22:1034-1035.
173. Smith EB. The anatomic pathology of infectious mononucleosis and its complications. In: *Proceedings of the International Infectious Mononucleosis Symposium*. Washington, DC: American College Health Association; 1967:109.
174. Bernstein TC, Wolff HG. Involvement of the nervous system in infectious mononucleosis. *Ann Intern Med*. 1950;33:1120-1138.
175. Silverstein A, Steinberg S, Nathanson M. Nervous system involvement in infectious mononucleosis. The heralding and/or major manifestation. *Arch Neurol*. 1972;26:353-358.
176. Bennett DR, Peters HA. Acute cerebellar syndrome secondary to infectious mononucleosis in a 52 year old man. *Ann Intern Med*. 1961;55:147-149.
177. Gilbert JW, Culebras A. Cerebellitis in infectious mononucleosis. *JAMA*. 1972;220:727.
178. Bejada S. Cerebellitis in glandular fever. *Med J Aust*. 1976;1:153-156.
179. Joncas JH, Chicoine L, Thivierge R, et al. Epstein-Barr virus antibodies in the cerebrospinal fluid. *Am J Dis Child*. 1974;127:282-285.
180. Grose C, Henle W, Henle G, et al. Primary Epstein Barr virus infections in acute neurologic diseases. *N Engl J Med*. 1975;292:392-395.
181. Tanner OR. Ocular manifestations of infectious mononucleosis. *Arch Ophthalmol*. 1954;51:229-241.
182. Shechter FR, Lipsius EI, Rasansky HN. Retrobulbar neuritis. *Am J Dis Child*. 1955;89:58-61.
183. Gautier-Smith PC. Neurological complications of glandular fever (infectious mononucleosis). *Brain*. 1965;88:323-324.
184. Watson P, Ashby P. Brachial plexus neuropathy associated with infectious mononucleosis. *Can Med Assoc J*. 1976;114:758-767.
185. Forino PM, Humphrey D, Hochberg F, et al. Mononucleosis associated subacute sclerosing panencephalitis. *Lancet*. 1975;2:530-532.
186. Cotton PB, Webb-Peploe MM. Acute transverse myelitis as a complication of glandular fever. *Br Med J*. 1966;654-655.
187. Raymond RW, Williams RL. Infectious mononucleosis with psychosis. Report of a case. *N Engl J Med*. 1948;239:542-544.
188. Bray PF, Culp KW, McFarlin DE, et al. Demyelinating disease after neurologically complicated primary Epstein-Barr virus infection. *Neurology*. 1992;42:278-282.
189. Adamson DJ, Gordon PM. Hemiplegia: A rare complication of acute Epstein-Barr virus (EBV) infection. *Scand J Infect Dis*. 1992;24:379-380.
190. Penman HG. Fatal infectious mononucleosis: A critical review. *J Clin Pathol*. 1970;23:765-771.
191. Finkel M, Parker GW, Fanselau HA. The hepatitis of infectious mononucleosis: Experience with 235 cases. *Mil Med*. 1964;129:533-538.
192. Hoagland RJ. The clinical manifestations of infectious mononucleosis: A report of two hundred cases. *Am J Med Sci*. 1960;240:21-29.
193. Stevens JE. Infectious mononucleosis: A clinical analysis of 210 sporadic cases. *Va Med Mon*. 1952;79:74-80.
194. Lee S, Kjellstrand CM. Renal disease in infectious mononucleosis. *Clin Nephrol*. 1978;9:236-240.
195. Mayer HB, Wanke CA, Williams M, et al. Epstein-Barr virus–induced infectious mononucleosis complicated by acute renal failure: Case report and review. *Clin Infect Dis*. 1996;22:1009-1018.
196. Osmah H, Finkelstein R, Brook JG. Rhabdomyolysis complicating acute Epstein-Barr virus infection. *Infection*. 1995;23:119-120.
197. Hoagland RJ. Mononucleosis and heart disease. *Am J Med Sci*. 1964;248:1-6.
198. Shapiro SC, Dimich I, Steier M. Pericarditis as the only manifestation of infectious mononucleosis. *Am J Dis Child*. 1973;126:662-663.
199. Frishman W, Kraus ME, Zabkar J, et al. Infectious mononucleosis and fatal myocarditis. *Chest*. 1977;72:535-538.
200. Mundy GR. Infectious mononucleosis with pulmonary parenchymal involvement. *Br Med J*. 1972;1:219-220.
201. Offit PA, Fleisher GR, Koven NI, et al. Severe Epstein-Barr virus pulmonary involvement. *J Adolesc Health Care*. 1981;2:121-125.
202. Andiman WA, McCarthy P, Markowitz RI, et al. Clinical, virologic, and serologic evidence of Epstein-Barr virus infection in association with childhood pneumonia. *J Pediatr*. 1981;99:880-886.
203. Barbera JA, Hayashi S, Hegele RG, et al. Detection of Epstein-Barr virus in lymphocytic interstitial pneumonia by *in situ* hybridization. *Am Rev Respir Dis*. 1992;145:940-946.
204. Sriskandan S, Labrecque LG, Schofield J. Diffuse pneumonia associated with infectious mononucleosis: Detection of Epstein-Barr virus in lung tissue by *in situ* hybridization. *Clin Infect Dis*. 1996;22:578-579.
205. Haller A, von Segesser L, Baumann PC, et al. Severe respiratory insufficiency complicating Epstein-Barr virus infection: Case report and review. *Clin Infect Dis*. 1995;21:206-209.
206. Lukes RJ, Cox FH. Clinical and morphologic findings in 30 fatal cases of infectious mononucleosis. *Am J Pathol*. 1958;34:586.
207. Allen UR, Bass BH. Fatal hepatic necrosis in glandular fever. *J Clin Pathol*. 1963;16:337-341.
208. Dorman JM, Glick TH, Shannon DC, et al. Complications of infectious mononucleosis: A fatal case in a 2-year-old child. *Am J Dis Child*. 1974;128:239-243.
209. Purtilo DT, Cassel CK, Yang JPS, et al. X-linked recessive progressive combined variable immunodeficiency (Duncan's disease). *Lancet*. 1975;1:935-940.
210. Purtilo DT, Cassel CK, Yang JPS. Fatal infectious mononucleosis in familial lymphohistiocytosis. *N Engl J Med*. 1974;291:736.
211. Purtilo DT, Bhawan J, Hutt LM, et al. Epstein-Barr virus infections in the X-linked recessive lymphoproliferative syndrome. *Lancet*. 1978;1:798-801.
212. Provisor AJ, Iacuone JJ, Chilcote RR, et al. Acquired agammaglobulinemia after a life-threatening illness with clinical and laboratory features of infectious mononucleosis in three related male children. *N Engl J Med*. 1975;293:62-65.
213. Purtilo DT, Yang JP, Cassel CK, et al. X-linked recessive progressive combined variable immunodeficiency. *Lancet*. 1975;1:935-940.
214. Hamilton JK, Paquin L, Sullivan J, et al. X-linked lymphoproliferative syndrome registry report. *J Pediatr*. 1980;96:669-673.
215. Purtilo DT, DeFloria D Jr, Hutt L, et al. Variable phenotypic expression of an X-linked expressive lymphoproliferative syndrome. *N Engl J Med*. 1977;297:1077-1080.
216. Sullivan JL, Byron KS, Brewster FE, et al. X-linked lymphoproliferative syndromes: Natural history of the immunodeficiency. *J Clin Invest*. 1983;71:1765-1778.
217. Sayos J, Wu C, Morra M, et al. The X-linked lymphoproliferative-disease gene product SAP regulates signals induced through the co-receptor SLAM. *Nature*. 1998;395:462-469.
218. Latour S, Veillette A. Molecular and immunological basis of X-linked lymphoproliferative disease. *Immunol Rev*. 2003;192:212-224.
219. Schwartzberg PL, Mueller KL, Qi H, et al. SLAM receptors and SAP influence lymphocyte interactions, development and function. *Nat Rev Immunol*. 2009;9:39-46.
220. Jones JF, Ray CG, Minnich LL, et al. Evidence for active Epstein Barr virus infection in patients with persistent, unexplained illnesses: Elevated anti-early antigen antibodies. *Ann Intern Med*. 1985;102:1-7.
221. Straus SE, Tosato G, Armstrong G, et al. Persisting illness and fatigue in adults with evidence of Epstein-Barr virus infection. *Ann Intern Med*. 1985;102:7-16.
222. Straus SE. The chronic mononucleosis syndrome. *J Infect Dis*. 1988;157:405-412.
223. Holmes GP, Kaplan JE, Stewart JA, et al. A cluster of patients with a chronic mononucleosis-like syndrome. *JAMA*. 1987;257:2297-3302.
224. Buchwald D, Sullivan JL, Komaroff AL. Frequency of "chronic active Epstein-Barr virus infection" in a general medical practice. *JAMA*. 1987;257:2303-2307.
225. Horwitz CA, Henle W, Henle G, et al. Long-term serological follow-up of patients for Epstein-Barr virus after recovery from infectious mononucleosis. *J Infect Dis*. 1985;151:1150-1153.
226. Holmes GP, Kaplan JE, Gantz NM, et al. Chronic fatigue syndrome: A working case definition. *Ann Intern Med*. 1988;108:387-389.
227. Holmes GP. Defining the chronic fatigue syndrome. *Rev Infect Dis*. 1991;13: S54-S55.
228. Virelizier J-L, Lenoir G, Griscelli C. Persistent Epstein-Barr virus infection in a child with hypergammaglobulinaemia and immunoblastic proliferation associated with a selective defect in immune interferon secretion. *Lancet*. 1978;2:231-234.
229. Katano H, Ali MA, Patera AC, et al. Chronic active Epstein-Barr virus infection associated with mutations in perforin that impair its maturation. *Blood*. 2004;103:1244-1252.
230. Savoldo B, Huls MH, Liu Z, et al. Autologous Epstein-Barr virus (EBV)-specific cytotoxic T cells for the treatment of persistent active EBV infection. *Blood*. 2002;100:4059-4066.
231. Kimura H, Hoshino Y, Kanegane H, et al. Clinical and virologic characteristics of chronic active Epstein-Barr virus infection. *Blood*. 2001;98:280-286.
232. Jones JF, Shurin S, Abramowsky C, et al. T-cell lymphomas containing Epstein-Barr viral DNA in patients with chronic Epstein-Barr virus infections. *N Engl J Med*. 1988;318:733-741.
233. Quintanilla-Martinez L, Kumar S, Fend F, et al. Fulminant EBV^+ T-cell lymphoproliferative disorder following acute/chronic EBV infection: A distinct clinicopathologic syndrome. *Blood*. 2000;96:443-451.
234. Kasahara Y, Yachie A. Cell type specific infection of Epstein-Barr virus (EBV) in EBV-associated hemophagocytic lymphohistiocytosis and chronic active EBV infection. *Crit Rev Oncol Hematol*. 2002;44:283-294.
235. Ohshima K, Kimura H, Yoshino T, et al. Proposed categorization of pathological states of EBV-associated T/natural killer-cell lymphoproliferative disorder (LPD) in children and young adults: Overlap with chronic active EBV infection and infantile fulminant EBV T-LPD. *Pathol Int*. 2008;58:209-217.
236. Okano M, Kawa K, Kimura H, et al. Proposed guidelines for diagnosing chronic active Epstein-Barr virus infection. *Am J Hematol*. 2005;80:64-69.
237. Straus SE. Acute progressive Epstein-Barr virus infections. *Annu Rev Med*. 1992;43:437-449.
238. Kimura H, Morishima T, Kanegane H, et al. Prognostic factors for chronic active Epstein-Barr virus infection. *J Infect Dis*. 2003;187:527-533.
239. Kawa K, Okamura T, Yasui M, et al. Allogeneic hematopoietic stem cell transplantation for Epstein-Barr virus–associated T/NK-cell lymphoproliferative disease. *Crit Rev Oncol Hematol*. 2002;44:251-257.

240. Kuzushima K, Yamamoto M, Kimura H, et al. Establishment of anti–Epstein-Barr virus (EBV) cellular immunity by adoptive transfer of virus-specific cytotoxic T lymphocytes from an HLA-matched sibling to a patient with severe chronic active EBV infection. *Clin Exp Immunol.* 1996;103:192-198.
241. Okano M. Therapeutic approaches for severe Epstein-Barr virus infection. *Pediatr Hematol Oncol.* 1997;14:109-119.
242. Gotoh K, Ito Y, Shibata-Watanabe Y, et al. Clinical and virological characteristics of 15 patients with chronic active Epstein-Barr virus infection treated with hematopoietic stem cell transplantation. *Clin Infect Dis.* 2008;46:1525-1534.
243. Cohen JI. Optimal treatment for chronic active Epstein-Barr virus disease. *Pediatr Transplant.* 2009;13:393-396.
244. Kimura H. Pathogenesis of chronic active Epstein-Barr virus infection: is this an infectious disease, lymphoproliferative disorder, or immunodeficiency? *Rev Med Virol.* 2006;16:251-261.
245. Janka G, Imashuku S, Elinder G, et al. Infection- and malignancy-associated hemophagocytic syndromes. Secondary hemophagocytic lymphohistiocytosis. *Hematol Oncol Clin North Am.* 1998;12:435-444.
246. Ishii E, Ohga S, Imashuku S, et al. Review of hemophagocytic lymphohistiocytosis (HLH) in children with focus on Japanese experiences. *Crit Rev Oncol Hematol.* 2005;53:209-223.
247. Kawaguchi H, Miyashita T, Herbst H, et al. Epstein-Barr virus-infected T lymphocytes in Epstein-Barr virus-associated hemophagocytic syndrome. *J Clin Invest.* 1993;92:1444-1450.
248. Noma T, Kou K, Yoshizawa I, et al. Monoclonal proliferation of Epstein-Barr virus-infected T-cells in a patient with virus-associated haemophagocytic syndrome. *Eur J Pediatr.* 1994;153:734-738.
249. Imashuku S, Hibi S, Tabata Y, et al. Outcome of clonal hemophagocytic lymphohistiocytosis: analysis of 32 cases. *Leuk Lymphoma.* 2000;37:577-584.
250. Kikuta H, Sakiyama Y, Matsumoto S, et al. Fatal Epstein-Barr virus-associated hemophagocytic syndrome. *Blood.* 1993;82:3259-3264.
251. Su IJ, Chen RL, Lin DT, et al. Epstein-Barr virus (EBV) infects T lymphocytes in childhood EBV-associated hemophagocytic syndrome in Taiwan. *Am J Pathol.* 1994;144:1219-1225.
252. Imashuku S. Clinical features and treatment strategies of Epstein-Barr virus-associated hemophagocytic lymphohistiocytosis. *Crit Rev Oncol Hematol.* 2002;44:259-272.
253. Kikuta H. Epstein-Barr virus-associated hemophagocytic syndrome. *Leuk Lymphoma.* 1995;16:425-429.
254. Ueda I, Morimoto A, Inaba T, et al. Characteristic perforin gene mutations of haemophagocytic lymphohistiocytosis patients in Japan. *Br J Haematol.* 2003;121:503-510.
255. Imashuku S, Teramura T, Tauchi H, et al. Longitudinal follow-up of patients with Epstein-Barr virus-associated hemophagocytic lymphohistiocytosis. *Haematologica.* 2004;89:183-188.
256. Greenspan JS, Greenspan D, Lennette ET, et al. Replication of Epstein-Barr virus within the epithelial cells of oral "hairy" leukoplakia, an AIDS-associated lesion. *N Engl J Med.* 1985;313:1564-1571.
257. Triantos D, Porter SR, Scully C, Teo CG. Oral hairy leukoplakia: Clinicopathologic features, pathogenesis, diagnosis, and clinical significance. *Clin Infect Dis.* 1997;25:1392-1396.
258. Scully C, Porter SR, Di Alberti L, et al. Detection of Epstein-Barr virus in oral scrapes in HIV infection, in hairy leukoplakia, and in healthy non–HIV-infected people. *J Oral Pathol Med.* 1998;27:480-482.
259. Curtis RE, Travis LB, Rowlings PA, et al. Risk of lymphoproliferative disorders after bone marrow transplantation: a multi-institutional study. *Blood.* 1999;94:2208-2216.
260. Cockfield SM. Identifying the patient at risk for post-transplant lymphoproliferative disorder. *Transpl Infect Dis.* 2001;3:70-78.
261. Preiksaitis JK. New developments in the diagnosis and management of posttransplantation lymphoproliferative disorders in solid organ transplant recipients. *Clin Infect Dis.* 2004;39:1016-1023.
262. Williams H, Crawford DH. Epstein-Barr virus: the impact of scientific advances on clinical practice. *Blood.* 2006;107:862-869.
263. Hamilton-Dutoit SJ, Raphael M, Audouin J, et al. In situ demonstration of Epstein-Barr virus small RNAs (EBER 1) in acquired immunodeficiency syndrome–related lymphomas: Correlation with tumor morphology and primary site. *Blood.* 1993;82:619-624.
264. Neri A, Barriga F, Inghirami G, et al. Epstein-Barr virus infection precedes clonal expansion in Burkitt's and acquired immunodeficiency syndrome–associated lymphoma. *Blood.* 1991;77:1092-1095.
265. de-The G, Geser A, Day NE, et al. Epidemiological evidence for causal relationship between Epstein-Barr virus and Burkitt's lymphoma from Ugandan prospective study. *Nature.* 1978;274:756-761.
266. Levine AM. Acquired immunodeficiency syndrome–related lymphoma: Clinical aspects. *Semin Oncol.* 2000;27:442-453.
267. Gutensohn N, Cole P. Epidemiology of Hodgkin's disease. *Semin Oncol.* 1980;7:92-102.
268. MacMahon B. Epidemiology of Hodgkin's disease. *Cancer Res.* 1966;26:1189-1201.
269. Mueller N, Evans A, Harris NL, et al. Hodgkin's disease and Epstein-Barr virus. Altered antibody pattern before diagnosis. *N Engl J Med.* 1989;320:689-695.
270. Pallesen G, Hamilton-Dutoit SJ, Rowe M, et al. Expression of Epstein-Barr virus latent gene products in tumour cells of Hodgkin's disease. *Lancet.* 1991;337:320-322.
271. Weiss LM, Movahed LA, Warnke RA, et al. Detection of Epstein-Barr viral genomes in Reed-Sternberg cells of Hodgkin's disease. *N Engl J Med.* 1989;320:502-506.
272. Ambinder RF. Epstein-barr virus and hodgkin lymphoma. *Hematology Am Soc Hematol Educ Program.* 2007;204-209.
273. Bargou RC, Leng C, Krappmann D, et al. High-level nuclear NF-kappa B and Oct-2 is a common feature of cultured Hodgkin/Reed-Sternberg cells. *Blood.* 1996;87:4340-4347.
274. Jungnickel B, Staratschek-Jox A, Brauninger A, et al. Clonal deleterious mutations in the IkappaBalpha gene in the malignant cells in Hodgkin's lymphoma. *J Exp Med.* 2000;191:395-402.
275. Zeng Y, Zhang LG, Li HY, et al. Serological mass survey for early detection of nasopharyngeal carcinoma in Wuzhou City, China. *Int J Cancer.* 1982;29:139-141.
276. Henle G, Henle W. Epstein-Barr virus–specific IgA serum antibodies as an outstanding feature of nasopharyngeal carcinoma. *Int J Cancer.* 1976;17:1-7.
277. Chan AT, Teo PM, Johnson PJ. Nasopharyngeal carcinoma. *Ann Oncol.* 2002;13:1007-1015.
278. Niedobitek G. Epstein-Barr virus infection in the pathogenesis of nasopharyngeal carcinoma. *Mol Pathol.* 2000;53:248-254.
279. Raab-Traub N, Flynn K. The structure of the termini of the Epstein-Barr virus as a marker of clonal cellular proliferation. *Cell.* 1986;47:883-889.
280. Farrow DC, Vaughan TL, Berwick M, et al. Diet and nasopharyngeal cancer in a low-risk population. *Int J Cancer.* 1998;78:675-679.
281. Liebowitz D. Nasopharyngeal carcinoma: The Epstein-Barr virus association. *Semin Oncol.* 1994;21:376-381.
282. Yuan JM, Wang XL, Xiang YB, et al. Preserved foods in relation to risk of nasopharyngeal carcinoma in Shanghai, China. *Int J Cancer.* 2000;85:358-363.
283. Jaffe ES, Chan JK, Su IJ, et al. Report of the Workshop on Nasal and Related Extranodal Angiocentric T/Natural Killer Cell Lymphomas. Definitions, differential diagnosis, and epidemiology. *Am J Surg Pathol.* 1996;20:103-111.
284. Chiang AK, Tao Q, Srivastava G, et al. Nasal NK- and T-cell lymphomas share the same type of Epstein-Barr virus latency as nasopharyngeal carcinoma and Hodgkin's disease. *Int J Cancer.* 1996;68:285-290.
285. Kanegane H, Nomura K, Miyawaki T, Tosato G. Biological aspects of Epstein-Barr virus (EBV)–infected lymphocytes in chronic active EBV infection and associated malignancies. *Crit Rev Oncol Hematol.* 2002;44:239-249.
286. Kawa K. Diagnosis and treatment of Epstein-Barr virus–associated natural killer cell lymphoproliferative disease. *Int J Hematol.* 2003;78:24-31.
287. Jaffe ES, Wilson WH. Lymphomatoid granulomatosis: pathogenesis, pathology and clinical implications. *Cancer Surv.* 1997;30:233-248.
288. Herrmann K, Niedobitek G. Epstein-Barr virus–associated carcinomas: Facts and fiction. *J Pathol.* 2003;199:140-145.
289. Lee ES, Locker J, Nalesnik M, et al. The association of Epstein-Barr virus with smooth-muscle tumors occurring after organ transplantation. *N Engl J Med.* 1995;332:19-25.
290. Takada K. Epstein-Barr virus and gastric carcinoma. *Mol Pathol.* 2000;53:255-261.
291. Cesarman E, Chang Y, Moore PS, et al. Kaposi's sarcoma–associated herpesvirus-like DNA sequences in AIDS-related body-cavity-based lymphomas. *N Engl J Med.* 1995;332:1186-1191.
292. Cesarman E, Nador RG, Aozasa K, et al. Kaposi's sarcoma–associated herpesvirus in non-AIDS related lymphomas occurring in body cavities. *Am J Pathol.* 1996;149:53-57.
293. Aozasa K. Pyothorax-associated lymphoma. *J Clin Exp Hematop.* 2006;46:5-10.
294. McClain KL, Leach CT, Jenson HB, et al. Association of Epstein-Barr virus with leiomyosarcomas in children with AIDS. *N Engl J Med.* 1995;332:12-18.
295. Alspaugh MA, Henle G, Lennette ET, et al. Elevated levels of antibodies to Epstein-Barr virus antigens in sera and synovial fluids of patients with rheumatoid arthritis. *J Clin Invest.* 1981;67:1134-1140.
296. Evans AS, Rothfield NF, Niederman JC. Raised antibody titres to E.B. virus in systemic lupus erythematosus. *Lancet.* 1971;1:167-168.
297. Sumaya CV, Myers LW, Ellison GW. Epstein-Barr virus antibodies in multiple sclerosis. *Arch Neurol.* 1980;37:94-96.
298. Alotaibi S, Kennedy J, Tellier R, et al. Epstein-Barr virus in pediatric multiple sclerosis. *JAMA.* 2004;291:1875-1879.
299. Bray PF, Bloomer LC, Salmon VC, et al. Epstein-Barr virus infection and antibody synthesis in patients with multiple sclerosis. *Arch Neurol.* 1983;40:406-408.
300. Myhr KM, Riise T, Barrett-Connor E, et al. Altered antibody pattern to Epstein-Barr virus but not to other herpesviruses in multiple sclerosis: a population based case-control study from western Norway. *J Neurol Neurosurg Psychiatry.* 1998;64:539-542.
301. Sundstrom P, Juto P, Wadell G, et al. An altered immune response to Epstein-Barr virus in multiple sclerosis: a prospective study. *Neurology.* 2004;62:2277-2282.
302. Wandinger K, Jabs W, Siekhaus A, et al. Association between clinical disease activity and Epstein-Barr virus reactivation in MS. *Neurology.* 2000;55:178-184.
303. Ascherio A, Munger KL, Lennette ET, et al. Epstein-Barr virus antibodies and risk of multiple sclerosis: a prospective study. *JAMA.* 2001;286:3083-3088.
304. DeLorenze GN, Munger KL, Lennette ET, et al. Epstein-Barr virus and multiple sclerosis: evidence of association from a prospective study with long-term follow-up. *Arch Neurol.* 2006;63:839-844.
305. Levin LI, Munger KL, Rubertone MV, et al. Temporal relationship between elevation of Epstein-Barr virus antibody titers and initial onset of neurological symptoms in multiple sclerosis. *JAMA.* 2005;293:2496-2500.
306. Nielsen TR, Rostgaard K, Nielsen NM, et al. Multiple sclerosis after infectious mononucleosis. *Arch Neurol.* 2007;64:72-75.
307. Cepok S, Zhou D, Srivastava R, et al. Identification of Epstein-Barr virus proteins as putative targets of the immune response in multiple sclerosis. *J Clin Invest.* 2005;115:1352-1360.
308. Wood TA, Frenkel EP. The atypical lymphocyte. *Am J Med.* 1967;42:923-936.
309. Chin TDY. Diagnosis of infectious mononucleosis. *South Med J.* 1976;69:654-658.
310. Penman HG. Extreme neutropenia in glandular fever. *J Clin Pathol.* 1968;21:48-49.
311. Chretien JH, Esswein JG, Holland WG, et al. Predictors of the duration of infectious mononucleosis. *South Med J.* 1977;70:437-439.
312. Evans AS, Niederman JC, Cenabre LC, et al. A prospective evaluation of heterophile and Epstein Barr virus specific IgM antibody tests in clinical and subclinical infectious mononucleosis. Specificity and sensitivity of the tests and persistence of antibody. *J Infect Dis.* 1975;132:546-554.
313. Hochberg FG, Miller G, Schooley RT, et al. Central nervous system lymphoma related to Epstein-Barr virus. *N Engl J Med.* 1983;309:745-748.
314. Basson V, Sharp AA. Monospot: A differential slide test for infectious mononucleosis. *J Clin Pathol.* 1969;22:324-325.
315. Seitanidis B. A comparison of the Monospot with the Paul-Bunnell test in infectious mononucleosis and other diseases. *J Clin Pathol.* 1969;22:321-323.
316. Wolf P, Dorfman R, McClenahan J, et al. False-positive infectious mononucleosis spot test in lymphoma. *Cancer.* 1970;25:626-628.
317. Vidrih JA, Walensky RP, Sax PE, et al. Positive Epstein-Barr virus heterophile antibody tests in patients with primary human immunodeficiency virus infection. *Am J Med.* 2001;111:192-194.
318. Walensky RP, Rosenberg ES, Ferraro MJ, et al. Investigation of primary human immunodeficiency virus infection in patients who test positive for heterophile antibody. *Clin Infect Dis.* 2001;33:570-572.
319. Henle W, Henle G, Horwitz CA. Epstein-Barr virus specific diagnostic tests in infectious mononucleosis. *Hum Pathol.* 1974;5:551-565.
320. Henle W, Henle G, Niederman JC, et al. Antibodies to early antigens induced by Epstein Barr virus in infectious mononucleosis. *J Infect Dis.* 1971;124:58-67.
321. Horwitz CA, Henle W, Henel G, et al. Clinical evaluation of patients with infectious mononucleosis and development of antibodies to the R component of the Epstein-Barr virus induced early antigen complex. *Am J Med.* 1975;58:330-338.
322. Reedman BM, Klein G. Cellular localization of an Epstein Barr virus associated complement fixing antigen in producer and nonproducer lymphoblastoid cell lines. *Int J Cancer.* 1973;11:499-520.
323. Henle G, Henle W, Horwitz CA. Antibodies to Epstein Barr virus associated nuclear antigen in infectious mononucleosis. *J Infect Dis.* 1974;130:231-239.
324. Hewetson JF, Rocchi S, Henle W, et al. Neutralizing antibodies to Epstein Barr virus in healthy populations and patients with infectious mononucleosis. *J Infect Dis.* 1973;128:283-289.
325. Miller G, Niederman JC, Andrews LL. Prolonged oropharyngeal excretion of Epstein Barr virus after infectious mononucleosis. *N Engl J Med.* 1973;288:229-232.
326. Yamamoto M, Kimura H, Hironaka T, et al. Detection and quantification of virus DNA in plasma of patients with Epstein-Barr virus–associated diseases. *J Clin Microbiol.* 1995;33:1765-1768.
327. Jones JF, Shurin S, Abramowsky C, et al. T cell lymphomas containing Epstein-Barr viral DNA in patients with chronic Epstein-Barr virus infections. *N Engl J Med.* 1988;318:733-741.
328. Diaz-Mitoma F, Preiksaitis JK, Leung WC, et al. DNA-DNA dot hybridization to detect Epstein-Barr virus in throat washings. *J Infect Dis.* 1987;155:297-303.
329. Babcock GJ, Decker LL, Volk M, et al. EBV persistence in memory B cells in vivo. *Immunity.* 1998;9:395-404.
330. Hochberg D, Souza T, Catalina M, et al. Acute infection with Epstein-Barr virus targets and overwhelms the peripheral memory B-cell compartment with resting, latently infected cells. *J Virol.* 2004;78:5194-5204.
331. Kimura H, Ito Y, Suzuki R, Nishiyama Y. Measuring Epstein-Barr virus (EBV) load: the significance and application for each EBV-associated disease. *Rev Med Virol.* 2008;18:305-319.
332. Balfour HH Jr, Holman CJ, Hokanson KM, et al. A prospective clinical study of Epstein-Barr virus and host interactions during acute infectious mononucleosis. *J Infect Dis.* 2005;192:1505-1512.
333. Baron DN, Bell JL, Demmett WN. Biochemical studies on hepatic involvement in infectious mononucleosis. *J Clin Pathol.* 1965;18:209-211.

334. Rosalki SB, Jones TG, Verney AF. Transaminase and liver function studies in infectious mononucleosis. *Br Med J*. 1960;1: 929-932.
335. Kaplan ME. Cryoglobulinemia in infectious mononucleosis: Quantitation and characterization of the cryoproteins. *J Lab Clin Med*. 1968;71:754-765.
336. Horwitz CA, Moulds J, Henle W, et al. Cold agglutinins in infectious mononucleosis and heterophil-antibody-negative mononucleosis-like syndromes. *Blood*. 1977;50:195-202.
337. Hayden RT, Hokanson KM, Pounds SB, et al. Multicenter comparison of different real-time PCR assays for quantitative detection of Epstein-Barr virus. *J Clin Microbiol*. 2008;46:157-163.
338. Preiksaitis JK, Pang XL, Fox JD, et al. Interlaboratory comparison of Epstein-Barr virus viral load assays. *Am J Transplant*. 2009;9:269-279.
339. Pisani G, Cristiano K, Saldanha J, et al. External quality assessment for the detection of blood-borne viruses in plasma by nucleic acid amplification technology: the first human immunodeficiency virus and hepatitis B virus studies (HIV EQA/1 and HBV EQA/1) and the fifth hepatitis C virus study (HCV EQA/5). *Vox Sang*. 2004;87:91-95.
340. Saldanha J, Gerlich W, Lelie N, et al. An international collaborative study to establish a World Health Organization international standard for hepatitis B virus DNA nucleic acid amplification techniques. *Vox Sang*. 2001;80:63-71.
341. Saldanha J, Heath A, Aberham C, et al. World Health Organization collaborative study to establish a replacement WHO international standard for hepatitis C virus RNA nucleic acid amplification technology assays. *Vox Sang*. 2005;88:202-204.
342. Saldanha J, Lelie N, Heath A. Establishment of the first international standard for nucleic acid amplification technology (NAT) assays for HCV RNA. WHO Collaborative Study Group. *Vox Sang*. 1999;76:149-158.
343. Baiocchi OC, Colleoni GW, Caballero OL, et al. Quantification of Epstein-Barr viral load and determination of a cut-off value to predict the risk of post-transplant lymphoproliferative disease in a renal transplant cohort. *Haematologica*. 2004;89:366-368.
344. Riddler SA, Breinig MC, McKnight JL. Increased levels of circulating Epstein-Barr virus (EBV)-infected lymphocytes and decreased EBV nuclear antigen antibody responses are associated with the development of posttransplant lymphoproliferative disease in solid-organ transplant recipients. *Blood*. 1994;84:972-984.
345. van Esser JW, van der Holt B, Meijer E, et al. Epstein-Barr virus (EBV) reactivation is a frequent event after allogeneic stem cell transplantation (SCT) and quantitatively predicts EBV-lymphoproliferative disease following T-cell–depleted SCT. *Blood*. 2001;98:972-978.
346. Meerbach A, Wutzler P, Hafer R, et al. Monitoring of Epstein-Barr virus load after hematopoietic stem cell transplantation for early intervention in post-transplant lymphoproliferative disease. *J Med Virol*. 2008;80:441-454.
347. Wagner HJ, Cheng YC, Huls MH, et al. Prompt versus preemptive intervention for EBV lymphoproliferative disease. *Blood*. 2004;103:3979-3981.
348. van Esser JW, Niesters HG, van der Holt B, et al. Prevention of Epstein-Barr virus-lymphoproliferative disease by molecular monitoring and preemptive rituximab in high-risk patients after allogeneic stem cell transplantation. *Blood*. 2002;99:4364-4369.
349. Carpentier L, Tapiero B, Alvarez F, et al. Epstein-Barr virus (EBV) early-antigen serologic testing in conjunction with peripheral blood EBV DNA load as a marker for risk of posttransplantation lymphoproliferative disease. *J Infect Dis*. 2003;188:1853-1864.
350. Doesch AO, Konstandin M, Celik S, et al. Epstein-Barr virus load in whole blood is associated with immunosuppression, but not with post-transplant lymphoproliferative disease in stable adult heart transplant patients. *Transpl Int*. 2008;21:963-971.
351. Hopwood PA, Brooks L, Parratt R, et al. Persistent Epstein-Barr virus infection: unrestricted latent and lytic viral gene expression in healthy immunosuppressed transplant recipients. *Transplantation*. 2002;74:194-202.
352. Sato T, Fujieda M, Tanaka E, et al. Monitoring of Epstein-Barr virus load and antibody in pediatric renal transplant patients. *Pediatr Int*. 2008;50:454-458.
353. Chan KC, Lo YM. Circulating EBV DNA as a tumor marker for nasopharyngeal carcinoma. *Semin Cancer Biol*. 2002;12: 489-496.
354. de The G, Zeng Y. Population screening for EBV markers: toward improvement of nasopharyngeal carcinoma control. In: Epstein MA, Achong BG, eds. *The Epstein-Barr Virus: Recent Advances*. New York: Wiley; 1986:237-249.
355. Zeng Y. Seroepidemiological studies on nasopharyngeal carcinoma in China. *Adv Cancer Res*. 1985;44:121-138.
356. Zeng Y, Deng H, Zhong J, et al. A 10 year prospective study on nasopharyngeal carcinoma in Wuzhou city and Zangwu county, Guangxi, China. In: Tursz T, Ablashi DV, de The G, et al, eds. *The Epstein-Barr Virus and Associated Diseases*. Paris: Colloque INSERM/John Libbey Eurotext; 1993:735-741.
357. Tune CE, Liavaag PG, Freeman JL, et al. Nasopharyngeal brush biopsies and detection of nasopharyngeal cancer in a high-risk population. *J Natl Cancer Inst*. 1999;91:796-800.
358. Lo YM, Chan LY, Chan AT, et al. Quantitative and temporal correlation between circulating cell-free Epstein-Barr virus DNA and tumor recurrence in nasopharyngeal carcinoma. *Cancer Res*. 1999;59:5452-5455.
359. Lo YM, Chan LY, Lo KW, et al. Quantitative analysis of cell-free Epstein-Barr virus DNA in plasma of patients with nasopharyngeal carcinoma. *Cancer Res*. 1999;59:1188-1191.
360. Lin JC, Wang WY, Chen KY, et al. Quantification of plasma Epstein-Barr virus DNA in patients with advanced nasopharyngeal carcinoma. *N Engl J Med*. 2004;350:2461-2470.
361. Lo YM, Chan AT, Chan LY, et al. Molecular prognostication of nasopharyngeal carcinoma by quantitative analysis of circulating Epstein-Barr virus DNA. *Cancer Res*. 2000;60:6878-6881.
362. Antinori A, Ammassari A, De Luca A, et al. Diagnosis of AIDS-related focal brain lesions: A decision-making analysis based on clinical and neuroradiologic characteristics combined with polymerase chain reaction assays in CSF. *Neurology*. 1997;48:687-694.
363. Arribas JR, Clifford DB, Fichtenbaum CJ, et al. Detection of Epstein-Barr virus DNA in cerebrospinal fluid for diagnosis of AIDS-related central nervous system lymphoma. *J Clin Microbiol*. 1995;33:1580-1583.
364. De Luca A, Antinori A, Cingolani A, et al. Evaluation of cerebrospinal fluid EBV-DNA and IL-10 as markers for in vivo diagnosis of AIDS-related primary central nervous system lymphoma. *Br J Haematol*. 1995;90:844-849.
365. Lechowicz MJ, Lin L, Ambinder RF. Epstein-Barr virus DNA in body fluids. *Curr Opin Oncol*. 2002;14:533-537.
366. Antinori A, Cingolani A, De Luca A, et al. Epstein-Barr virus in monitoring the response to therapy of acquired immunodeficiency syndrome–related primary central nervous system lymphoma. *Ann Neurol*. 1999;45:259-261.
367. Horwitz CA, Henle W, Henle G, et al. Heterophile negative infectious mononucleosis and mononucleosis-like illness. Laboratory confirmation of 43 cases. *Am J Med*. 1977;63:947-957.
368. Blacklow NR, Kapikian AZ. Serological studies with EB virus in infectious lymphocytosis. *Nature*. 1970;226:647.
369. Ho DD, Sarngadharan MG, Resnick L, et al. Primary human T-lymphotropic virus type III infection. *Ann Intern Med*. 1985;103:880-883.
370. Cooper DA, Gold J, MacLean P, et al. Acute AIDS retrovirus infection: Definition of a clinical illness associated with seroconversion. *Lancet*. 1985;1:537-540.
371. Goudsmit J, de Wolf F, Paul DA, et al. Expression of human immunodeficiency virus antigen (HIV-Ag) in serum and cerebrospinal fluid during acute and chronic infection. *Lancet*. 1986;2:177-180.
372. Summers WC, Klein G. Inhibition of Epstein-Barr virus DNA synthesis and late gene expression by phosphonoacetic acid. *J Virol*. 1976;18:151-155.
373. Colby BM, Shaw JE, Elion GB, et al. Effect of acyclovir [9-(2-hydroxyethoxymethyl)guanine] on Epstein-Barr virus DNA replication. *J Virol*. 1980;34:560-568.
374. Lin JC, Smith MC, Pagano JS. Prolonged inhibitory effect of 9-(1,3-dihydroxy-2-propoxymethyl)guanine against replication of Epstein-Barr virus. *J Virol*. 1984;50:50-55.
375. Andersson J, Skoldenberg B, Henle W, et al. Acyclovir treatment in infectious mononucleosis: A clinical and virological study. *Infection*. 1987;15:14-20.
376. Andersson J, Britton S, Ernberg I, et al. Effect of acyclovir on infectious mononucleosis: A double-blind, placebo-controlled study. *J Infect Dis*. 1986;153:283-290.
377. van der Horst C, Joncas J, Aronheim G, et al. Lack of effect of peroral acyclovir for the treatment of infectious mononucleosis. *J Infect Dis*. 1991;164:788-792.
378. Tynell E, Aurelius E, Brandell A, et al. Acyclovir and prednisolone treatment of acute infectious mononucleosis: A multicenter, double-blind, placebo-controlled study. *J Infect Dis* 1996;174:324-331.
379. Torre D, Tambini R. Acyclovir for treatment of infectious mononucleosis: A meta-analysis. *Scand J Infect Dis*. 1999;31: 543-547.
380. Schumacher HR, Jacobson WA, Bemiller CR. Treatment of infectious mononucleosis. *Ann Intern Med*. 1963;58:217-228.
381. Bender CE. The value of corticosteroids in the treatment of infectious mononucleosis. *JAMA*. 1967;15:529-531.
382. Klein EM, Cochran JF, Buck RL. The effects of short-term corticosteroid therapy on the symptoms of infectious mononucleosis pharyngotonsillitis: A double blind study. *J Am Coll Health Assoc*. 1969;17:446-452.
383. Collins M, Fleischer G, Kreisberg J, et al. Role of steroids in the treatment of infectious mononucleosis in the ambulatory college student. *J Am Coll Health Assoc*. 1984;33:101-105.
384. Straus SE, Cohen JI, Tosato G, et al. NIH conference. Epstein-Barr virus infections: Biology, pathogenesis, and management. *Ann Intern Med*. 1993;118:45-58.
385. Papesch M, Watkins R. Epstein-Barr virus infectious mononucleosis. *Clin Otolaryngol*. 2001;26:3-8.
386. McGowan JE Jr, Chesney PJ, Crossley KB, et al. Guidelines for the use of systemic glucocorticosteroids in the management of selected infections. Working Group on Steroid Use, Antimicrobial Agents Committee, Infectious Diseases Society of America. *J Infect Dis*. 1992;165:1-13.
387. Gottschalk S, Rooney CM, Heslop HE. Post-transplant lymphoproliferative disorders. *Annu Rev Med*. 2005;56:29-44.
388. Preiksaitis JK, Keay S. Diagnosis and management of posttransplant lymphoproliferative disorder in solid-organ transplant recipients. *Clin Infect Dis*. 2001;33:S38-S46.
389. Faller DV, Mentzer SJ, Perrine SP. Induction of the Epstein-Barr virus thymidine kinase gene with concomitant nucleoside antivirals as a therapeutic strategy for Epstein-Barr virus–associated malignancies. *Curr Opin Oncol*. 2001;13:360-367.
390. Papadopoulos EB, Ladanyi M, Emanuel D, et al. Infusions of donor leukocytes to treat Epstein-Barr virus–associated lymphoproliferative disorders after allogeneic bone marrow transplantation. *N Engl J Med*. 1994;330:1185-1191.
391. Porter DL, Orloff GJ, Antin JH. Donor mononuclear cell infusions as therapy for B-cell lymphoproliferative disorder following allogeneic bone marrow transplant. *Transplant Sci*. 1994;4:12-14; discussion 14-16.
392. Rooney CM, Smith CA, Ng CY, et al. Use of gene-modified virus-specific T lymphocytes to control Epstein-Barr-virus–related lymphoproliferation. *Lancet*. 1995;345:9-13.
393. Rooney CM, Smith CA, Ng CY, et al. Infusion of cytotoxic T cells for the prevention and treatment of Epstein-Barr virus–induced lymphoma in allogeneic transplant recipients. *Blood*. 1998;92:1549-1555.
394. Gottschalk S, Ng CY, Perez M, et al. An Epstein-Barr virus deletion mutant associated with fatal lymphoproliferative disease unresponsive to therapy with virus-specific CTLs. *Blood*. 2001;97:835-843.
395. Nalesnik MA, Rao AS, Zeevi A, et al. Autologous lymphokine-activated killer cell therapy of lymphoproliferative disorders arising in organ transplant recipients. *Transplant Proc*. 1997;29:1905-1906.
396. Wilkie GM, Taylor C, Jones MM, et al. Establishment and characterization of a bank of cytotoxic T lymphocytes for immunotherapy of epstein-barr virus-associated diseases. *J Immunother*. 2004;27:309-316.
397. Haque T, Wilkie GM, Jones MM, et al. Allogeneic cytotoxic T-cell therapy for EBV-positive posttransplantation lymphoproliferative disease: results of a phase 2 multicenter clinical trial. *Blood*. 2007;110:1123-1131.
398. van Esser JW, Niesters HG, Thijsen SF, et al. Molecular quantification of viral load in plasma allows for fast and accurate prediction of response to therapy of Epstein-Barr virus–associated lymphoproliferative disease after allogeneic stem cell transplantation. *Br J Haematol*. 2001;113:814-821.
399. Yang J, Tao Q, Flinn IW, et al. Characterization of Epstein-Barr virus–infected B cells in patients with posttransplantation lymphoproliferative disease: Disappearance after rituximab therapy does not predict clinical response. *Blood*. 2000;96:4055-4063.
400. Bollard CM, Aguilar L, Straathof KC, et al. Cytotoxic T lymphocyte therapy for Epstein-Barr virus+ Hodgkin's disease. *J Exp Med*. 2004;200:1623-1633.
401. Bollard CM, Gottschalk S, Leen AM, et al. Complete responses of relapsed lymphoma following genetic modification of tumor-antigen presenting cells and T-lymphocyte transfer. *Blood*. 2007;110:2838-2845.
402. Lucas KG, Salzman D, Garcia A, Sun Q. Adoptive immunotherapy with allogeneic Epstein-Barr virus (EBV)-specific cytotoxic T-lymphocytes for recurrent, EBV-positive Hodgkin disease. *Cancer*. 2004;100:1892-1901.
403. Chua D, Huang J, Zheng B, et al. Adoptive transfer of autologous Epstein-Barr virus-specific cytotoxic T cells for nasopharyngeal carcinoma. *Int J Cancer*. 2001;94:73-80.
404. Straathof KC, Bollard CM, Popat U, et al. Treatment of nasopharyngeal carcinoma with Epstein-Barr virus–specific T lymphocytes. *Blood*. 2005;105:1898-1904.
405. Comoli P, Pedrazzoli P, Maccario R, et al. Cell therapy of stage IV nasopharyngeal carcinoma with autologous Epstein-Barr virus-targeted cytotoxic T lymphocytes. *J Clin Oncol*. 2005;23: 8942-8949.
406. Lin CL, Lo WF, Lee TH, et al. Immunization with Epstein-Barr Virus (EBV) peptide-pulsed dendritic cells induces functional CD8+ T-cell immunity and may lead to tumor regression in patients with EBV-positive nasopharyngeal carcinoma. *Cancer Res*. 2002;62:6952-6958.
407. Hui EP, Ma BB, Chan SL, et al. Therapeutic vaccination with modified vaccinia Ankara (MVA) encoding Epstein-Barr virus (EBV) target antigens in EBV+ nasopharyngeal carcinoma (NPC). *J Clin Oncol*. 2008;26, abstr 3052.
408. Albrecht H, Stellbrink HJ, Brewster D, et al. Resolution of oral hairy leukoplakia during treatment with foscarnet. *AIDS*. 1994;8:1014-1016.
409. Greenspan D, De Souza YG, Conant MA, et al. Efficacy of desciclovir in the treatment of Epstein-Barr virus infection in oral hairy leukoplakia. *J Acquir Immune Defic Syndr*. 1990;3: 571-578.
410. Newman C, Polk BF. Resolution of oral hairy leukoplakia during therapy with 9-(1,3-dihydroxy-2-propoxymethyl)guanine (DHPG). *Ann Intern Med*. 1987;107:348-350.
411. Resnick L, Herbst JS, Ablashi DV, et al. Regression of oral hairy leukoplakia after orally administered acyclovir therapy. *JAMA*. 1988;259:384-388.
412. Gowdey G, Lee RK, Carpenter WM. Treatment of HIV-related hairy leukoplakia with podophyllum resin 25% solution. *Oral Surg Oral Med Oral Pathol Oral Radiol Endod*. 1995;79:64-67.
413. Lozada-Nur F, Costa C. Retrospective findings of the clinical benefits of podophyllum resin 25% sol on hairy leukoplakia. Clinical results in nine patients. *Oral Surg Oral Med Oral Pathol*. 1992;73:555-558.
414. Thorley-Lawson DA, Poodry CA. Identification and isolation of the main component (gp350-gp220) of Epstein-Barr virus responsible for generating neutralizing antibodies in vivo. *J Virol*. 1982;43:730-736.

415. Morgan AJ. Epstein-Barr virus vaccines. *Vaccine*. 1992;10:563-571.

416. Wilson AD, Lovgren-Bengtsson K, Villacres-Ericsson M, et al. The major Epstein-Barr virus (EBV) envelope glycoprotein gp340 when incorporated into Iscoms primes cytotoxic T-cell responses directed against EBV lymphoblastoid cell lines. *Vaccine*. 1999;17:1282-1290.

417. Gu SY, Huang TM, Ruan L, et al. First EBV vaccine trial in humans using recombinant vaccinia virus expressing the major membrane antigen. *Dev Biol Stand*. 1995;84:171-177.

418. Balfour HH Jr. Epstein-Barr virus vaccine for the prevention of infectious mononucleosis: and what else? *J Infect Dis*. 2007;196:1724-1726.

419. Moutschen M, Leonard P, Sokal EM, et al. Phase I/II studies to evaluate safety and immunogenicity of a recombinant gp350 Epstein-Barr virus vaccine in healthy adults. *Vaccine*. 2007;25:4697-4705.

420. Sokal EM, Hoppenbrouwers K, Vandermeulen C, et al. Recombinant gp350 vaccine for infectious mononucleosis: a phase 2, randomized, double-blind, placebo-controlled trial to evaluate the safety, immunogenicity, and efficacy of an Epstein-Barr virus vaccine in healthy young adults. *J Infect Dis*. 2007;196:1749-1753.

421. Sauce D, Larsen M, Curnow SJ, et al. EBV-associated mononucleosis leads to long-term global deficit in T-cell responsiveness to IL-15. *Blood*. 2006;108:11-18.

422. Bharadwaj M, Moss DJ. Epstein-Barr virus vaccine: A cytotoxic T-cell-based approach. *Expert Rev Vaccines*. 2002;1:467-476.

423. Khanna R, Sherritt M, Burrows SR. EBV structural antigens, gp350 and gp85, as targets for ex vivo virus-specific CTL during acute infectious mononucleosis: Potential use of gp350/gp85 CTL epitopes for vaccine design. *J Immunol*. 1999;162:3063-3069.

424. Moss DJ, Schmidt C, Elliott S, et al. Strategies involved in developing an effective vaccine for EBV-associated diseases. *Adv Cancer Res*. 1996;69:213-245.

425. Elliott SL, Suhrbier A, Miles JJ, et al. Phase I trial of a CD8+ T-cell peptide epitope-based vaccine for infectious mononucleosis. *J Virol*. 2008;82:1448-1457.

140

Human Herpesvirus Types 6 and 7

JEFFREY I. COHEN*

Human herpesviruses 6 and 7 (HHV-6 and HHV-7) are both members of the β-herpesvirus subfamily. Both viruses infect T cells, are present ubiquitously, and can cause exanthema subitum (or roseola infantum). In addition, both viruses frequently reactivate in highly immunocompromised patients but rarely cause serious disease in these patients.

Human Herpesvirus Type 6

HISTORY

HHV-6 was discovered by Salahuddin and colleagues in 1986 in patients with lymphoproliferative disorders and HIV.[1] Subsequently, two variants of HHV-6 were described, HHV-6A and HHV-6B.[2] HHV-6B was shown to be an etiologic agent of exanthema subitum,[3] whereas HHV-6A has rarely been associated with disease.

DESCRIPTION OF THE VIRUS

HHV-6 is a member of the *Roseolovirus* genus of β-herpesviruses and shares a number of features with cytomegalovirus including numerous homologous viral proteins and similar genomic structures.[4] HHV-6A and HHV-6B, which share 90% nucleotide sequence identity, are sufficiently different in their sequences and in their cell tropism that they could be classified as separate species of herpesviruses. The receptor for HHV-6 is CD46, which interacts with a complex consisting of viral glycoproteins gH, gL, gQ1, and gQ2. The HHV-6 genome contains about 165 kilobase pairs of DNA.

EPIDEMIOLOGY

Over 95% of adults are seropositive for HHV-6. Maternal antibody to HHV-6 declines during the first 5 months of life. About 40% to 50% of children are infected by 1 year of age, and 77% to 82% are infected by 2 years of age (Fig. 140-1).[5,6] The peak of infection occurs at 9 to 21 months. Approximately 90% of infections in children are symptomatic; in one study 40% of infants with HHV-6 were seen by a physician.[5] There is no seasonal peak for primary HHV-6 infection.[5] HHV-6 is usually transmitted horizontally, presumably by infected saliva from close contacts to children. Outbreaks of HHV-6 infection have been reported at daycare centers.

HHV-6 infects peripheral blood mononuclear cells (PBMCs) and cells in the liver, salivary glands, endothelial cells, and central nervous system. HHV-6 DNA was detected in PBMCs from 22%, and in cervical swabs from 7.5%, of pregnant women.[7] HHV-6 was also detected in about 1% of cord blood samples and in fetal blood, indicating a potential for fetal disease. Congenital infection with HHV-6 is most often due to chromosomally integrated virus passed in the germline DNA. In one study, 86% of congenital infections were from chromosomally integrated viral DNA, and 14% were due to transplacental infection.[8] These infants have 10^5 or 10^6 copies of HHV-6 DNA per microgram of cellular DNA. HHV-6 DNA persists in the blood intermittently after primary infection in most children, and can reactivate in healthy children without apparent illness.[9] HHV-6 has been transmitted by organ transplantation[10] and has been transmitted to hema-topoietic cell transplant recipients by virus integrated into the chromosome of the donor cells.[11]

HHV-6 frequently reactivates in immunocompromised patients. About 50% of hematopoietic cell and about 33% of solid organ transplant recipients reactivate HHV-6 as defined by detection of viral DNA in the peripheral blood.[12,13] Over 95% of HHV-6 reactivations in hematopoietic cell transplant recipients are due to HHV-6B. Reactivation of the virus usually occurs within the first month of transplant, and reactivation is increased with reduced cellular immunity, particularly in patients receiving anti-CD3 antibody or corticosteroids, and in those who have undergone allogeneic or cord blood transplants.[13,14] Reactivation has also been reported in 54% of critically ill patients who are not otherwise immunocompromised.[15]

PATHOGENESIS

In addition to infecting its primary target, CD4+ T cells, HHV-6 infects other T cells, B cells, NK cells, monocytes, macrophages, epithelial cells, and neural cells. HHV-6A has a greater predilection to infect neural cells than does HHV-6B, whereas HHV-6B is more commonly detected in PBMCs than HHV-6A. Infection of lymphocytes with HHV-6 results in ballooning of the cells with intranuclear inclusions, followed by cell death. HHV-6 establishes a latent infection in CD34+ hematopoietic stem cells, monocytes, and/or macrophages, and a persistent infection in salivary glands. HHV-6 is detected in saliva, but at a much lower frequency than HHV-7. Cellular immunity is more important than humoral immunity for controlling HHV-6 infection.

HHV-6 induces expression of CD4 on the surface of T cells, which can increase susceptibility to HIV infection. However, infection of cells with HHV-6 results in reduced expression of the HIV coreceptor CXCR4 on the surface of cells and increased expression of the RANTES chemokine, which can inhibit replication of CCR5 tropic HIV strains in HHV-6-infected cells. HHV-6A inhibits expression of MHC class I on dendritic cells.

CLINICAL MANIFESTATIONS

Infantile Fever and Seizures

The incubation time for HHV-6 infection is estimated to be 1 to 2 weeks. Infantile fever is the most common manifestation of HHV-6 infection. More than 90% of children infected with HHV-6 have symptoms, including fussiness, rhinorrhea, and fever in over half of patients; cough, diarrhea, and rash occur in about one third of patients (Table 140-1).[5] It is estimated that 5% to 25% of visits to emergency rooms for fever in infants are due to HHV-6. Children older than 6 months of age are more likely to have fever than are younger children.[5] Of children under 3 years of age who present to emergency rooms with fever, 10% had primary infection with HHV-6; this number increased to 20% for children 6 to 12 months old (Fig. 140-2).[16] The mean age of primary HHV-6 infection was 9.4 months, the median duration of illness was 6 days, and the mean temperature was 39.6°C. In another study of 243 children presenting to the emergency room with HHV-6, over 50% had fever of 40°C or higher, malaise, otitis, and nasal congestion.[17]

HHV-6 is a responsible for about one third of febrile seizures in children up to 2 years of age.[16] Of 160 children presenting with acute HHV-6 infections, 13% had seizures and the median age of children with HHV-6 and seizures was 14 months. Primary infection with HHV-6 is more frequently associated with severe seizures, long sei-

*All material in this chapter is in the public domain, with the exception of any borrowed figures or tables.

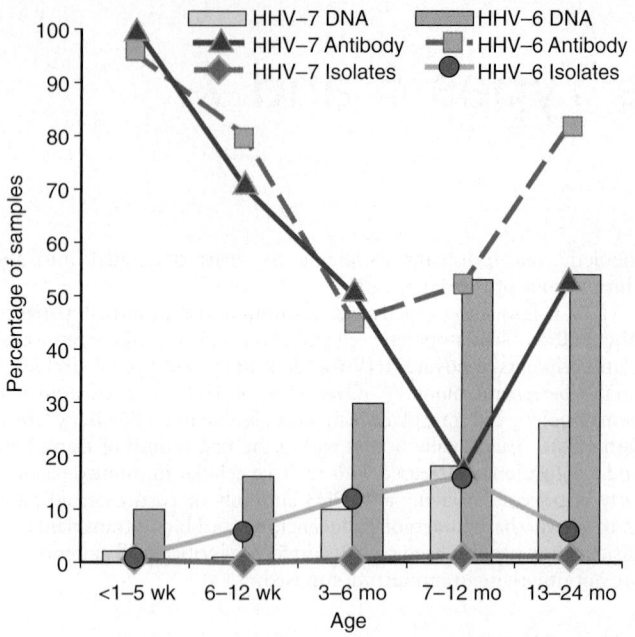

Figure 140-1 Percentages of blood samples from children 2 years of age or younger with antibody, virus culture, and virus PCR for **HHV-6 and HHV-7.** *(From Hall CB, Caserta MT, Schnabel KC, et al. Characteristics and acquisition of human herpesvirus (HHV) 7 infections in relation to infection with HHV-6. J Infect Dis. 2006;193:1063-1069).*

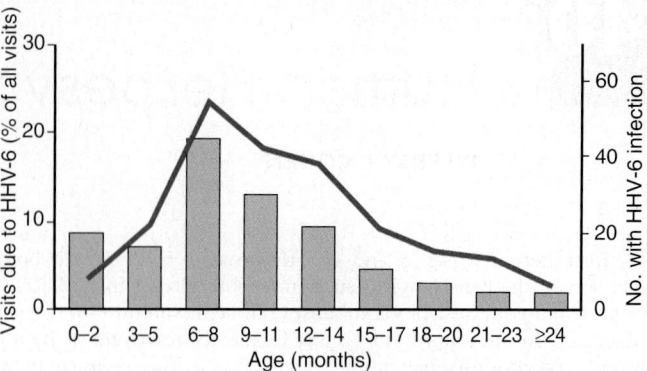

Figure 140-2 Percentage of visits to the emergency department for febrile illnesses associated with HHV-6 (*line*) and the number of children with primary HHV-6 infection (*bars*). *(From Hall CB, Long CE, Schnabel KC, et al. Human herpesvirus-6 infection in children: A prospective study of complications and reactivation. N Engl J Med. 1994;331:432-438.)*

(red papules on the soft palate or base of the uvula). The median duration of symptoms is 9 days. Rare complications include febrile seizures, meningitis, and encephalitis. Patients often have leukocytosis during the first day, followed by leukopenia with a relative lymphocytosis and in some cases thrombocytopenia.

Other Neurologic Symptoms Associated with HHV-6

HHV-6 is a rare cause of meningitis; the virus also can cause encephalitis in otherwise healthy children who present with an altered level of consciousness, seizures, psychosis, or cranial nerve deficits.[20] These children usually present with a panencephalitis and can have persistent neurologic sequelae. Eight percent (13/156) of young children hospitalized in Britain and Ireland with encephalitis or fever and seizures were found to have acute HHV-6 infection.[21] HHV-6 DNA was

zures, and recurrent seizures than seizures not associated with HHV-6.[18]

Exanthem Subitum (Roseola Infantum or Sixth Disease)

Exanthem subitum is caused by either HHV-6B or HHV-7. Approximately 25% of patients with HHV-6 infection in the United States present with exanthem subitum;[5] in contrast, in Japan about 75% of primary HHV-6 infections result in exanthem subitum.[19] The disease begins with a high fever that usually lasts for 3 to 4 days.[5,19] At the time of defervescence, patients develop a macular or maculopapular rash that begins on the neck or the trunk, spreads to the extremities, and persists for a few hours to 2 days (Fig. 140-3). The disease may be accompanied by cough, cervical and occipital lymphadenopathy, erythema of the tympanic membranes, conjunctivitis, eyelid edema, bulging fontanelles, lymphadenopathy, diarrhea, or Nagayama spots

TABLE 140-1	Incidence of Symptoms and Visits to a Physician among Children with Primary HHV-6 Infection and Age-Matched Controls without HHV-6 Infection		
Variable	*HHV-6-Positive* (N = 80)	*HHV-6-Negative* (N = 80)	*P-Value*
	% (95% CI)*		
Any symptom	94 (88-99)	71 (61-81)	0.004
Fever	58 (47-68)	14 (6-21)	<0.001
Fussiness	70 (60-80)	46 (35-57)	0.009
Rhinorrhea	66 (56-77)	46 (35-57)	0.02
Cough	34 (23-44)	33 (22-43)	0.87
Vomiting	8 (2-13)	5 (0-10)	0.53
Diarrhea	26 (17-36)	11 (4-18)	0.05
Rash	31 (21-41)	8 (2-13)	0.002
Roseola	24 (14-33)	3 (0-6)	0.003
Seizure	0 (0-2)	0 (0-2)	—
Visit to physician	39 (28-49)	19 (10-27)	0.009

*CI, confidence interval.
From Zerr DM, Meier AS, Selke SS, et al. A population-based study of primary human herpesvirus 6 infection. *N Engl J Med.* 2005;352:768-776.

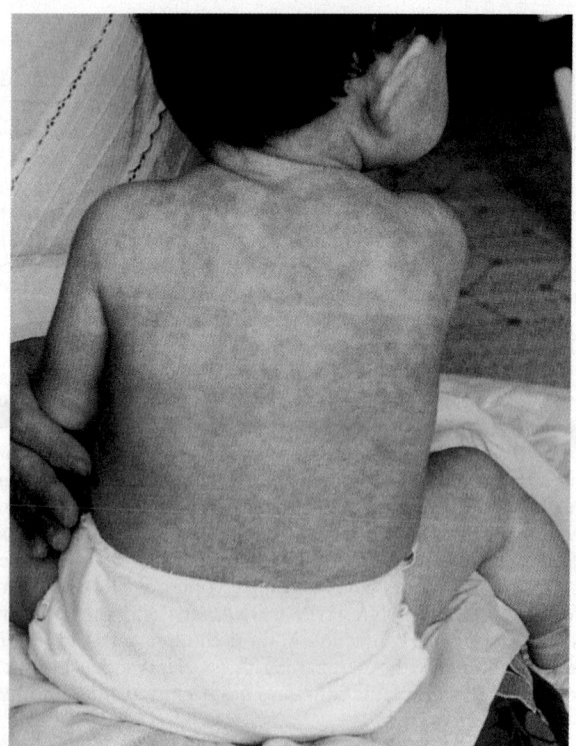

Figure 140-3 A child with exanthem subitum. *(Courtesy of Professor K. Yaminishi, Osaka University Medical School, Osaka, Japan.)*

detected in the cerebrospinal fluid (CSF) of 7% (9/138) patients with encephalitis with a lymphocytic pleocytosis, but no specific differences were noted in patients with encephalitis attributed to HHV-6 versus those due to other causes.[22] HHV-6 DNA was detected in the CSF of 0.4% (4/1000) of persons in the California Encephalitis Project study.[23]

HHV-6 has been associated with multiple sclerosis based on detection of DNA in CSF and DNA and viral antigens in the brain; however, viral DNA and proteins have also been detected in the brain of controls[24,25] and the role of HHV-6 in multiple sclerosis is controversial.[26] HHV-6 antigen was detected in astrocytes cultured from the brain of patients with mesial temporal lobe epilepsy.[27]

Infectious Mononucleosis

Older patients who develop primary infection with HHV-6 may present with infectious mononucleosis with fever, lymphadenopathy, generalized rash, and atypical lymphocytes.[28] Lymph node biopsies show intranuclear and cytoplasmic inclusions with HHV-6 antigens (Fig. 140-4).[29]

Other Complications in Healthy Persons

HHV-6 has been associated with chronic or fulminant hepatitis,[30] thrombocytopenic purpura, myocarditis, and hemophagocytic syndrome in case reports. While HHV-6 DNA has been found in some

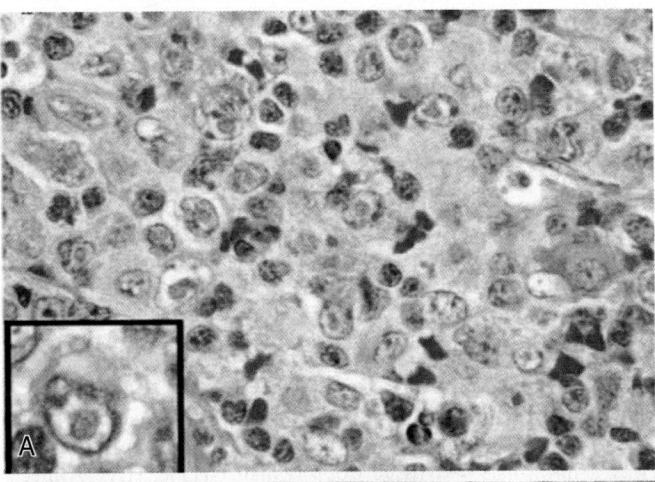

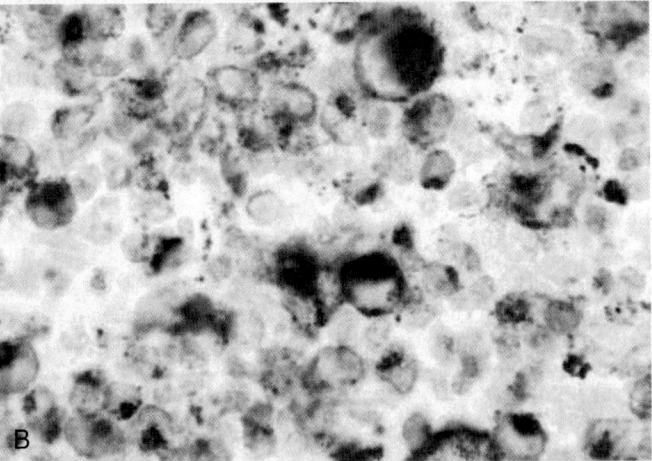

Figure 140-4 **Eosinophilic intranuclear and cytoplasmic inclusions with hematoxylin and eosin stain (A) and immunohistochemical staining with antibody to HHV-6 envelope glycoprotein gp60 in viral inclusions (B) in a lymph node from a patient with HHV-6 infectious mononucleosis.** *(From Maric I, Bryant R, Abu-Asab M, et al. Human herpesvirus-6-associated acute lymphadenitis in immunocompetent adults.* Mod Pathol. *2004;17:1427-1433.)*

lymphomas, there is no compelling evidence that HHV-6 is associated with malignancy. HHV-6 is not a cause of chronic fatigue syndrome.

Congenital Infection

HHV-6 congenital infections (defined by detection of virus in cord blood) occurred in 1% (57/5638) of births and, unlike infections later in life, were asymptomatic.[31]

Infection in the Immunocompromised Host

Since a large proportion of hematopoietic cell and organ transplant recipients reactivate HHV-6 with viral DNA in the peripheral blood (see Epidemiology, above), it is often difficult to confirm that symptoms in transplant recipients are due to HHV-6.

HHV-6 is frequently associated with fever and rash early after transplant.[13,32] The virus has also been associated with delayed monocyte and platelet engraftment in hematopoietic cell transplant recipients.[33] One study showed that high levels of HHV-6 DNA in the blood correlated with delayed platelet engraftment after transplant.[34] HHV-6 infects hematopoietic progenitor cells inhibiting colony formation in vitro[35] and has been associated with bone marrow suppression and delayed engraftment in some[12] but not other[36] studies. The association of HHV-6 reactivation with cytomegalovirus (CMV) infection and graft-versus-host disease may make it difficult to confirm HHV-6 as a primary cause of marrow suppression or graft rejection.

One of best documented manifestations of HHV-6 in immunosuppressed patients is encephalitis.[37] About 50 cases have been reported in the literature, and most were diagnosed by detection of HHV-6 in the CSF;[38] HHV-6 antigen in the brain is more specific for diagnosis. Patients often present 2 to 6 weeks after hematopoietic cell transplant with headache and confusion and a nonfocal neurologic examination that may progress to seizures, psychosis, and cranial nerve deficits. While the CT scan is usually unremarkable initially, the MRI shows abnormalities in 75% of patients with changes in the gray matter of the temporal lobes, especially the medial aspect of these lobes. The CSF shows an elevated protein in two thirds of cases with a mild lymphocytic pleocytosis in the minority of patients. Limbic encephalitis, presenting with short-term memory loss and insomnia, with HHV-6 proteins or RNA in the hippocampus and amygdala, has been reported in hematopoietic cell transplant recipients.[37,39,40] Nine transplant patients were reported to have limbic encephalitis with MRI changes involving the amygdala and hippocampus, inappropriate diuretic hormone secretion, and anterograde amnesia.[41]

Although HHV-6 DNA was detected at high levels in the lungs of bone marrow transplant patients with idiopathic pneumonia compared with lower levels in the lungs of control immunocompetent patients,[42] other studies have not confirmed these findings.[36] The high frequency of virus reactivation in these patients emphasizes the importance of detecting viral proteins in tissues (see Diagnosis, below).

Case reports have described HHV-6 associated with giant cell hepatitis,[10] other forms of hepatitis, colitis, and gastroduodenitis in transplant recipients. HHV-6 antigen was detected in PBMCs infiltrating biopsies of gastroduodenal mucosa in 23% of liver transplant recipients, but also in 19% of immunocompetent patients with upper gastrointestinal symptoms; the number of HHV-6 positive cells tended to be higher in the transplant patients than in the immunocompetent patients.[43] HHV-6 proteins have been detected in tubular epithelia of kidneys undergoing rejection after transplantation.

HHV-6 has less commonly been associated with encephalitis and pneumonitis in AIDS patients. HHV-6 has generally not been shown to influence the rate of progression of HIV to AIDS.

LABORATORY DIAGNOSIS

Healthy Persons

The diagnosis of exanthem subitum is usually made clinically. The most frequently used diagnostic test for acute HHV-6 disease in children is comparison of acute and convalescent serum for seroconversion to HHV-6.[44] The observation of asymptomatic reactivations of

HHV-6 in healthy persons indicates that detection of a 4-fold or greater rise in titer alone may not be diagnostic of acute infection. HHV-6 IgG is usually present 1 week after infection, peaks in the second week, and persists for life. An alternative diagnostic test for acute disease in children is detection of HHV-6 DNA in sera or plasma at a time when antibody to the virus is absent, reflecting the transient viremia that occurs before the onset of antibody; however, this test is less specific than seroconversion.[44] Currently used serologic tests include immunofluorescent antibody, enzyme-linked immunosorbent assay (ELISA), and immunoblot assays. These tests cannot distinguish HHV-6A from HHV-6B, and there can be cross-reactivity of HHV-6 with HHV-7. HHV-6 IgM is present early in infection and persists for a few weeks; however, virus-specific IgM may not be detectable in some children, and this antibody has been detected in some adults, suggesting virus reactivation.

Culture of HHV-6 from PBMCs, serum, or plasma of patients with exanthem subitum during the febrile period is considered diagnostic[3] but is available only in research laboratories. Detection of HHV-6 DNA in plasma in children under 2 years is not considered sufficiently specific to differentiate infants with acute HHV-6 infection from those with serious bacterial infections.[45]

Immunocompromised Persons
Diagnosis of HHV-6 as the cause of symptoms in immunocompromised patients is often difficult. Since HHV-6 frequently reactivates in a large proportion of these patients, it is important to distinguish latent infections that are not associated with disease from productive HHV-6 infections that may cause disease. A high or a rising level of viral DNA, or detection of viral RNA (available only as a research test), in the blood is more likely to distinguish productive infection associated with HHV-6 disease from latent viral DNA. In a study of hematopoietic cell transplant recipients, the presence of over 10^3 copies of HHV-6 DNA per 10^6 PBMCs was statistically associated with myelosuppression, pneumonitis, fever, and rash.[12] Detection of viral DNA in the serum or plasma may also be more predictive of disease than finding HHV-6 in PBMCs. Detection of HHV-6 RNA, and especially viral proteins, in tissues is more specific for active disease than is detection of viral DNA. In addition to a rising level of HHV-6 in the blood, and preferably detection of HHV-6 in tissue, other potential causes of disease (including CMV, which is often associated with HHV-6) must be excluded before HHV-6 can be considered to have a causative role in disease.

Detection of HHV-6 in the CSF is strongly suggestive of central nervous system (CNS) disease but is not absolutely diagnostic, as some patients with HHV-6 in the CSF have had other CNS diseases documented at autopsy, and HHV-6 has been detected in the CSF of children years after acute infection.[46] In one study, HHV-6 DNA was detected in the CSF of 8/11 (73%) patients with neurologic dysfunction and 3/11 (27%) of asymptomatic hematopoietic cell transplant recipients.[47] While another study reported HHV-6 in the CSF of 23% of transplant recipients with encephalitis, compared with only 1% of transplant recipients without encephalitis, controls were not well matched for the level of immunosuppression.[48] Thus, other causes of encephalitis must be ruled out before diagnosis of HHV-6 encephalitis is accepted based on CSF findings. Detection of HHV-6 proteins in the brain is more specific than detection of DNA, as viral DNA has been detected by polymerase chain reaction (PCR) in the brain of about one third of healthy persons.[49]

The use of PCR for diagnosis of HHV-6 is complicated by the finding that HHV-6 is integrated into chromosomal DNA in 0.7% to 1.5% of persons.[50] Stem cells containing integrated copies of HHV-6 have transmitted viral DNA to recipients.[11] Therefore, HHV-6 integration into host chromosomes, in addition to HHV-6 productive infection, must be considered when a diagnosis is based on detection of HHV-6 in leukocytes or in CSF that may contain leukocytes.

TREATMENT
HHV-6 is sensitive to ganciclovir, foscarnet, and cidofovir in vitro; the latter two agents are more active in cell culture. HHV-6, like CMV, is

not sensitive to acyclovir. HHV-6 U69 is a protein kinase that phosphorylates ganciclovir. HHV-6 DNA levels in the CSF and serum declined with ganciclovir or foscarnet therapy in one series; however, without a control group it is unknown whether this was treatment related.[47] Antiviral therapy has been used in some immunocompromised patients, but no controlled studies have shown that these drugs are effective. Some anecdotal reports suggest that patients with HHV-6 encephalitis may have responded to a 7-day course of ganciclovir or foscarnet. Ganciclovir-resistant HHV-6, due to a mutation in the viral U69 protein kinase, has been isolated from a patient with AIDS.[51] Prophylaxis with ganciclovir has been reported to reduce HHV-6 reactivation,[52,53] but this is not recommended owing to the toxicity of the drug and the low incidence of disease in immunocompromised patients.

Human Herpesvirus Type 7
HISTORY
HHV-7 was discovered by Frenkel and colleagues in 1990 in a healthy person[54] and was shown to be a cause of exanthem subitum.[55]

DESCRIPTION OF THE VIRUS
HHV-7, like HHV-6, is a member of the *Roseolovirus* genus and shares 20% to 75% amino acid identity with HHV-6 in many of their viral proteins.[4] The HHV-7 genome contains about 145 kilobase pairs of DNA.

EPIDEMIOLOGY
HHV-7 infections occur at a later age than HHV-6 infections (see Fig. 140-1).[6] About 18% of children are infected with HHV-7 by 1 year of age and 53% by 2 years. Most children are infected between ages 2 and 5 presumably from infected saliva of parents and siblings.[56] HHV-7 DNA was detected in PBMCs from 67%, and in cervical swabs from 3%, of pregnant women.[7] About 50% of hematopoietic cell and 20% of solid organ transplant recipients reactivate HHV-7 as indicated by viral DNA in the peripheral blood.[13,57]

PATHOGENESIS
HHV-7 has a narrower tissue tropism than HHV-6. HHV-7 infects $CD4^+$ T cells, epithelial cells in the salivary glands, and cells in the lungs and skin. HHV-7 is frequently shed in saliva at high levels throughout life in most adults and children.[58] The virus has been detected in breast milk and establishes latency in $CD4^+$ cells. HHV-7 induces degradation of major histocompatibility complex (MHC) class I molecules.

CLINICAL MANIFESTATIONS
Primary HHV-7 infection may be asymptomatic or associated with fever or febrile seizures. In a study of 30 children with HHV-7 viremia, the most common clinical presentation was seizures, which occurred at 12 to 63 months of age; 10 of 12 patients had febrile seizures.[6] The second most common presentation of HHV-7 viremia was nonspecific fever with a mean temperature of 40.1°C. Less common symptoms were upper respiratory tract disease, vomiting, and diarrhea. Leukopenia was frequently noted. In a study of 496 children presenting to the emergency room, children with HHV-7 had a similar level of fever, rash, and gastrointestinal symptoms but were older and more likely to have seizures than those with HHV-6.[59]

HHV-7 is also a cause of exanthem subitum, although most cases are due to HHV-6. HHV-7 has been less frequently associated with CNS disease than HHV-6, but two cases of hemiplegia associated with HHV-7 have been described. HHV-7 has been associated with encephalitis in immunocompetent[60] and immunosuppressed[61] patients. Ten percent (15/156) of young children hospitalized in Britain and Ireland with encephalitis or fever and seizures were found to have an acute HHV-7 infection.[44] HHV-7 was not reported to cause congenital infection (defined as viral DNA in cord blood) in over 5600 births.[31]

LABORATORY DIAGNOSIS

Like HHV-6, the most common diagnostic test for HHV-7 in children is seroconversion based on detection of antibody by indirect immunofluorescence assay or ELISA.[44] Detection of HHV-7 in serum or plasma is much less common than for HHV-6; therefore, the presence of HHV-7 DNA in blood in the absence of antibody is more likely to be indicative of acute infection. HHV-7 has been cultured from PBMCs of patients with exanthem subitum, but this is done only in research laboratories.

Unlike HHV-6, levels of HHV-7 in the blood did not correlate with disease in immunocompromised patients.[12] Since HHV-7 DNA has been detected in the brain by PCR in 37% of adults,[62] detection of HHV-7 protein is more specific than viral DNA for the diagnosis of encephalitis.

TREATMENT

Like HHV-6, HHV-7 is most susceptible to foscarnet and cidofovir in vitro, although virus replication is also inhibited by ganciclovir. There are insufficient clinical reports to indicate whether these drugs are effective in vivo.

REFERENCES

1. Salahuddin SZ, Ablashi DV, Markham PD, et al. Isolation of a new virus, HBLV, in patients with lymphoproliferative disorders. *Science.* 1986;234:596-601.
2. Schirmer EC, Wyatt LS, Yamanishi K, et al. Differentiation between two distinct classes of viruses now classified as human herpesvirus 6. *Proc Natl Acad Sci U S A.* 1991;88:5922-5926.
3. Yamanishi K, Okuno T, Shiraki K, et al. Identification of human herpesvirus-6 as a causal agent for exanthem subitum. *Lancet.* 1988;1(8594):1065-1067.
4. Yamanishi K, Mori Y, Pellett PE. Human herpesviruses 6 and 7. In: Knipe DM, Howley PM, et al. eds. *Fields Virology 2006.* 5th ed. Philadelphia: Wolters Kluwer, Lippincott Williams & Wilkins; 2007:2819-2845.
5. Zerr DM, Meier AS, Selke SS, et al. A population-based study of primary human herpesvirus 6 infection. *N Engl J Med.* 2005;352:768-776.
6. Hall CB, Caserta MT, Schnabel KC, et al. Characteristics and acquisition of human herpesvirus (HHV) 7 infections in relation to infection with HHV-6. *J Infect Dis.* 2006;193:1063-1069.
7. Caserta MT, Hall CB, Schnabel K, et al. Human herpesvirus (HHV)-6 and HHV-7 infections in pregnant women. *J Infect Dis.* 2007;196:1296-1303.
8. Hall CB, Caserta MT, Schnabel K, et al. Chromosomal integration of human herpesvirus 6 is the major mode of congenital human herpesvirus 6 infection. *Pediatrics.* 2008;122:513-520.
9. Caserta MT, McDermott MP, Dewhurst S, et al. Human herpesvirus 6 (HHV6) DNA persistence and reactivation in healthy children. *J Pediatr.* 2004;145:478-484.
10. Potenza L, Luppi M, Barozzi P, et al. HHV-6A in syncytial giant-cell hepatitis. *N Engl J Med.* 2008;359:593-602.
11. Clark, DA, Nacheva EP, Leong HN, et al. Transmission of integrated human herpesvirus 6 through stem cell transplantation: Implications for laboratory diagnosis. *J Infect Dis.* 2006;193:912-916.
12. Boutolleau D, Fernandez C, André E, et al. Human herpesvirus (HHV)-6 and HHV-7: two closely related viruses with different infection profiles in stem cell transplantation recipients. *J Infect Dis.* 2003;187:179-186.
13. Dockrell DH, Paya CV. Human herpesvirus-6 and -7 in transplantation. *Rev Med Virol.* 2001;11:23-36.
14. Sashihara J, Tanaka-Taya K, Tanaka S, et al. High incidence of human herpesvirus 6 infection with a high viral load in cord blood stem cell transplant recipients. *Blood.* 2002;100:2005-2011.
15. Razonable RR, Fanning C, Brown RA, et al. Selective reactivation of human herpesvirus 6 variant a occurs in critically ill immunocompetent hosts. *J Infect Dis.* 2002;185:110-113.
16. Hall CB, Long CE, Schnabel KC, et al. Human herpesvirus-6 infection in children: a prospective study of complications and reactivation. *N Engl J Med.* 1994;331:432-438.
17. Pruksananonda P, Hall CB, Insel RA, et al. Primary human herpesvirus 6 infection in young children. *N Engl J Med.* 1992;326:1445-1450.
18. Suga S, Suzuki K, Ihira M, et al. Clinical characteristics of febrile convulsions during primary HHV-6 infection. *Arch Dis Child.* 2000;82:62-66.
19. Asano Y, Yoshikawa T, Suga S, et al. Clinical features of infants with primary human herpesvirus 6 infection (exanthem subitum, roseola infantum). *Pediatrics.* 1994;93:104-108.
20. Suga S, Yoshikawa T, Asano Y, et al. Clinical and virological analyses of 21 infants with exanthem subitum (roseola infantum) and central nervous system complications. *Ann Neurol.* 1993;33:597-603.
21. Ward KN, Andrews NJ, Verity CM, et al. Human herpesviruses-6 and -7 each cause significant neurological morbidity in Britain and Ireland. *Arch Dis Child.* 2005;90:619-623.

22. McCullers JA, Lakeman FD, Whitley RJ. Human herpesvirus 6 is associated with focal encephalitis. *Clin Infect Dis.* 1995;21:571-576.
23. Isaacson E, Glaser CA, Forghani B, et al. Evidence of human herpesvirus 6 infection in 4 immunocompetent patients with encephalitis. *Clin Infect Dis.* 2005;40:890-893.
24. Cermelli C, Berti R, Soldan SS, et al. High frequency of human herpesvirus 6 DNA in multiple sclerosis plaques isolated by laser microdissection. *J Infect Dis.* 2003;187:1377-1387.
25. Goodman AD, Mock DJ, Powers JM, et al. Human herpesvirus 6 genome and antigen in acute multiple sclerosis lesions. *J Infect Dis.* 2003;187:1365-1376.
26. Clark D. Human herpesvirus type 6 and multiple sclerosis. *Herpes.* 2004;11(Suppl 2):112A-119A.
27. Fotheringham J, Donati D, Akhyani N, et al. Association of human herpesvirus-6B with mesial temporal lobe epilepsy. *PLoS Med.* 2007;4(5):e180.
28. Akashi K, Eizuru Y, Sumiyoshi Y, et al. Brief report: Severe infectious mononucleosis-like syndrome and primary human herpesvirus 6 infection in an adult. *N Engl J Med.* 1993;329:168-171.
29. Maric I, Bryant R, Abu-Asab M, et al. Human herpesvirus-6-associated acute lymphadenitis in immunocompetent adults. *Mod Pathol.* 2004;17:1427-1433.
30. Härmä M, Höckerstedt K, Lautenschlager I. Human herpesvirus-6 and acute liver failure. *Transplantation.* 2003;76:536-539.
31. Hall CB, Caserta MT, Schnabel KC, et al. Congenital infections with human herpesvirus 6 (HHV6) and human herpesvirus 7 (HHV7). *J Pediatr.* 2004;145:472-477.
32. Chang FY, Singh N, Gayowski T, et al. Fever in liver transplant recipients: Changing spectrum of etiologic agents. *Clin Infect Dis.* 1998;26:59-65.
33. Zerr DM, Corey L, Kim HW, et al. Clinical outcomes of human herpesvirus 6 reactivation after hematopoietic stem cell transplantation. *Clin Infect Dis.* 2005;40:932-940.
34. Ljungman P, Wang FZ, Clark DA, et al. High levels of human herpesvirus 6 DNA in peripheral blood leucocytes are correlated to platelet engraftment and disease in allogeneic stem cell transplant patients. *Br J Haematol.* 2000;111:774-781.
35. Isomura H, Yamada M, Yoshida M, et al. Suppressive effects of human herpesvirus 6 on in vitro colony formation of hematopoietic progenitor cells. *J Med Virol.* 1997;52:406-412.
36. Yoshikawa T, Asano Y, Ihira M, et al. Human herpesvirus 6 viremia in bone marrow transplant recipients: clinical features and risk factors. *J Infect Dis.* 2002;185:847-853.
37. Drobyski WR, Knox KK, Majewski D, et al. Brief report: Fatal encephalitis due to variant B human herpesvirus-6 infection in a bone marrow-transplant recipient. *N Engl J Med.* 1994;330:1356-1360.
38. Zerr DM. Human herpesvirus 6 and central nervous system disease in hematopoietic cell transplantation. *J Clin Virol.* 2006;37(Suppl 1):S52-56.
39. Fotheringham J, Akhyani N, Vortmeyer A, et al. Detection of active human herpesvirus-6 infection in the brain: correlation with polymerase chain reaction detection in cerebrospinal fluid. *J Infect Dis.* 2007;195:450-454.
40. Wainwright MS, Martin PL, Morse RP, et al. Human herpesvirus 6 limbic encephalitis after stem cell transplantation. *Ann Neurol.* 2001;50:612-619.
41. Seeley WW. Post-transplant acute limbic encephalitis. *Neurology.* 2007;69:156-165.
42. Cone RW, Hackman RC, Huang ML, et al. Human herpesvirus 6 in lung tissue from patients with pneumonitis after bone marrow transplantation. *N Engl J Med.* 1993;329:156-161.
43. Halme L, Arola J, Höckerstedt K, et al. Human herpesvirus 6 infection of the gastroduodenal mucosa. *Clin Infect Dis.* 2008;46:434-439.

44. Ward KN. The natural history and laboratory diagnosis of human herpesviruses-6 and -7 infections in the immunocompetent host. *J Clin Virol.* 2005;32:183-193.
45. Zerr DM, Frenkel LM, Huang ML, et al. Polymerase chain reaction diagnosis of primary human herpesvirus-6 infection in the acute care setting. *J Pediatr.* 2006;149:480-485.
46. Caserta MT, Hall CB, Schnabel K, et al. Neuroinvasion and persistence of human herpesvirus 6 in children. *J Infect Dis.* 1994;170:1586-1589.
47. Zerr DM, Gupta D, Huang ML, et al. Effect of antivirals on human herpesvirus 6 replication in hematopoietic stem cell transplant recipients. *Clin Infect Dis.* 2002;34:309-317.
48. Wang FZ, Linde A, Hägglund H, et al. Human herpesvirus 6 DNA in cerebrospinal fluid specimens from allogeneic bone marrow transplant patients: does it have clinical significance? *Clin Infect Dis.* 1999;28:562-568.
49. Cuomo L, Trivedi P, Cardillo MR, et al. Human herpesvirus 6 infection in neoplastic and normal brain tissue. *J Med Virol.* 2001;63:45-51.
50. Leong HN, Tuke PW, Tedder RS, et al. 2007. The prevalence of chromosomally integrated human herpesvirus 6 genomes in the blood of UK blood donors. *J Med Virol.* 79:45-51.
51. Manichanh C, Olivier-Aubron C, Lagarde JP, et al. Selection of the same mutation in the U69 protein kinase gene of human herpesvirus-6 after prolonged exposure to ganciclovir in vitro and in vivo. *J Gen Virol.* 2001;82:2767-2776.
52. Tokimasa S, Hara J, Osugi Y, et al. Ganciclovir is effective for prophylaxis and treatment of human herpesvirus-6 in allogeneic stem cell transplantation. *Bone Marrow Transplant.* 2002;29:595-598.
53. Rapaport D, Engelhard D, Tagger G, et al. Antiviral prophylaxis may prevent human herpesvirus 6 reactivation in bone marrow transplant recipients. *Transpl Infect Dis.* 2002;4:10-16.
54. Frenkel N, Schirmer EC, Wyatt LS, et al. Isolation of a new herpesvirus from human CD4+ T cells. *Proc Natl Acad Sci U S A.* 1990;87:748-752.
55. Tanaka K, Kondo T, Torigoe S, et al. Human herpesvirus 7: Another causal agent for roseola (exanthem subitum). *J Pediatr.* 1994;125:1-5.
56. Wyatt LS, Rodriguez WJ, Balachandran N, et al. Human herpesvirus 7: antigenic properties and prevalence in children and adults. *J Virol.* 1991;65:6260-6265.
57. Chan PKS, Li CK, Chik KW, et al. Risk factors and clinical consequences of human herpesvirus 7 infection in pediatric hematopoietic stem cell transplant recipients. *J Med Virol.* 2004;72:668-674.
58. Ihira M, Yoshikawa T, Ohashi M, et al. Variation of human herpesvirus 7 shedding in saliva. *J Infect Dis.* 2003;188:1352-1354.
59. Caserta MT, Hall CB, Schnabel K, et al. Primary human herpesvirus 7 infection: a comparison of human herpesvirus 7 and human herpesvirus 6 infections in children. *J Pediatr.* 1998;133:386-389.
60. Ward KN, Kalima P, MacLeod KM, et al. Neuroinvasion during delayed primary HHV-7 infection in an immunocompetent adult with encephalitis and flaccid paralysis. *J Med Virol.* 2002;67:538-541.
61. Chan PKS, Chik KW, To KF, et al. Case report: Human herpesvirus 7 associated fatal encephalitis in a peripheral blood stem cell transplant recipient. *J Med Virol.* 2002;66:493-496.
62. Chan PKS, Ng HK, Cheung JLK, et al. Prevalence and distribution of human herpesvirus 7 in normal brain. *J Med Virol.* 2000;62:345-348.

141

Kaposi's Sarcoma–Associated Herpesvirus (Human Herpesvirus Type 8)

KENNETH M. KAYE

Kaposi's sarcoma (KS)–associated herpesvirus (KSHV or HHV-8) is the eighth, and most recently discovered, human herpesvirus. KSHV was discovered as a result of its connection with KS and is also linked with primary effusion lymphoma (PEL) and multicentric Castleman's disease. The role of KSHV in malignancy has generated much interest in this virus.

History

Kaposi's sarcoma was first described in 1872 by Moritz Kaposi, a prominent Hungarian dermatologist.[1] Kaposi described findings in five men of "idiopathic multiple pigmented sarcoma of the skin."[2] He noted aggressive disease and emphasized that the syndrome was incurable and rapidly lethal.[3] In fact, three of the men reported by Kaposi were dead within 16 months of presentation, and autopsy demonstrated disseminated disease. Despite the aggressive nature of the disease Kaposi described, KS subsequently came to be regarded as an indolent disease in elderly men of Mediterranean and eastern European descent. It is not clear what accounted for the evolution in the defining features of KS from the aggressive, rapidly fatal disorder described by Kaposi to a relatively mild one. During the 1950s, KS was recognized as an important disease in areas of sub-Saharan Africa.[4] Then, in 1981, Alvin Friedman-Kein reported on 50 young men who had had sex with men with KS of the skin, lymph nodes, mucosa, and viscera.[5] This report heralded the AIDS epidemic. The similarity of the original syndrome described by Kaposi and that seen in human immunodeficiency virus (HIV) infection is striking and raises the question of whether AIDS-like immune suppression was present in the men initially described.[3]

KSHV was identified in 1994 in KS lesions by Chang and Moore and colleagues using a polymerase chain reaction (PCR)–based technique termed *representational difference analysis*.[6] This technique searches for DNA, such as from a virus, that is present in diseased tissue and absent in normal tissue.[7] These investigations were based on epidemiologic observations suggesting that an infectious agent may have an etiologic role in KS. KS occurred at a 20-fold higher rate in men who had had sex with men who had AIDS compared with those who contracted AIDS by other means, such as by a blood-borne route. Subsequent to this seminal discovery, work by many groups worldwide has elucidated much about this virus.

Classification and Biology

KSHV is the only known human rhadinovirus (gamma-2 herpesvirus) and is related to other rhadinoviruses, including those that infect New (South American) and Old (African) World monkeys and rodents (murine gamma herpesvirus 68).[8-12] Two Old World monkey rhadinoviruses (RFHVMm and RFHVMn) are found in retroperitoneal fibromatosis. This entity has histologic similarities to KS. Herpesvirus saimiri (HVS), a New World virus, can cause T-cell lymphoma when infecting New World monkeys that are not its natural host.[13] Epstein-Barr virus, a gamma-1 herpesvirus, is KSHV's closest human relative.

KSHV is an enveloped virus that measures 140 nm in diameter, and its appearance by electron microscopy is indistinguishable from that of other herpesviruses.[14,15] KSHV attaches to cells prior to entry by binding to cell surface heparin sulfate and the integrin $\alpha_3\beta_1$.[16] The KSHV genome contains approximately 140 kb of unique sequence,[8,17] which encodes approximately 100 open reading frames (ORFs). The nomenclature of the ORFs is based on that of HVS due to high sequence and positional homology with those of HVS and the fact that HVS was the only fully sequenced gamma-2 herpesvirus prior to KSHV. ORFs without homology to those in HVS are numbered sequentially with K prefixes. A number of KSHV genes are homologues of human genes that were presumably "pirated" from mammalian cells during the evolution of the virus. The unique KSHV sequence is flanked by approximately 40 copies[18] of 0.8-kb guanine and cytosine-rich terminal repeat elements.

KSHV is capable of both latent and lytic infection.[9,19,20] Due to its capacity for latent infection, KSHV persistence in its human host is lifelong, similar to other herpesviruses. During lytic infection, many encapsidated viral progeny are produced in a cell and then released as the infected cell dies. Almost all of the nearly 100 KSHV genes are devoted to, and only expressed during, lytic infection. These genes encode proteins responsible for replication of the viral DNA and packaging the DNA into capsids. The viral genome is linear, with terminal repeats on each end when packaged in viral capsids. In addition to genes involved in virus replication, some genes expressed during lytic infection are involved in immune evasion, preventing the host from properly responding to and targeting the infected cells.[21-23]

Latent KSHV infection sharply contrasts with lytic infection.[19,20,24] Latent infection predominates over lytic infection in KSHV-infected tumors and cell lines, with only a small fraction of infected cells undergoing lytic infection. In latently infected cells, the viral genome circularizes by fusing at its terminal repeat ends and persists as a multiple-copy (ranging in number from 10 to 50 copies) extrachromosomal episome (plasmid) within the nucleus. Only approximately five KSHV genes are expressed during latent infection. Rather than causing cell death, these genes encourage cell survival. Because promotion of cell survival is also a prominent feature of malignancy, it is not surprising that KSHV is associated with certain tumors.[25]

Genes expressed in latent infection have important roles in tumorigenesis.[19,20,24,26] To persist in latent infection in proliferating cells such as tumor cells, KSHV episomes must replicate and efficiently segregate to progeny nuclei. The viral latency-associated nuclear antigen (LANA or ORF73) gene mediates KSHV DNA replication and then tethers episomes to chromosomes during mitosis to ensure efficient segregation to daughter cells. LANA also exerts effects on transcriptional regulation and cell growth. Viral cyclin D (ORF72) is a homologue of cell cyclin D and stimulates the G1-to-S transition of the cell cycle. The viral cyclin D is resistant to the multiple inhibitors that normally inhibit cell cyclin D, resulting in unchecked cell growth. The KSHV viral FLICE-inhibitory protein (vFLIP or K13) activates nuclear factor kappa B and inhibits apoptosis (or cell suicide), thereby preventing the cell from eliminating itself once it "knows" it is infected. The kaposin locus encodes overlapping ORFs, and this transcript and its protein products are induced in lytic infection. Kaposin A (K12) exerts transforming effects and kaposin B acts to increase the expression of cytokines. Latency-associated membrane protein (LAMP or K15) interacts with growth control proteins. LANA2 (vIRF3) is expressed in B cells, not KS tissue, and inhibits apoptosis.

Although only a small percentage (~1%) of cells within tumors undergo lytic infection, these cells may also have an important role in tumorigenesis. For instance, in lytic infection, a G protein–coupled receptor homologue (ORF74) is expressed that is constitutively active and has paracrine effects.[27] Therefore, although the cell with lytic infection will die, it can produce factors that have growth effects on nearby cells. In fact, transgenic mice expressing this viral protein have KS-like lesions.[28,29]

Cell culture and transformation models of KSHV remain rather limited. Primary bone marrow endothelial cells can be infected and transformed, but only approximately 5% of the cells are infected, with paracrine effects stimulating growth in the other cells.[30] Due to a lack of a cell line permissive for KSHV lytic replication, the mainstay of KSHV production is from cell lines derived from KSHV primary effusion lymphomas. The vast majority of cells in these lines are latently infected, but lytic infection (and virions) can be induced by several methods such as incubation with phorbol esters. However, this method produces relatively low titers of virus. The most tractable models so far used to study the effects of KSHV virus infection are in dermal microvascular cells.[20] KSHV induces phenotypic changes in these cells, such as spindle formation, but does not immortalize or fully transform them.

Pathogenesis

KSHV has an etiologic role in KS, PEL, and multicentric Castleman's disease. Overall, KSHV is well adapted to its human host and usually does not cause disease. Such a situation is ideal from the virus's point of view because a commensal existence without harm to its host enhances its long-term survival. Suppression of the immune system appears to disturb the delicate balance between KSHV and its human host and can lead to KSHV-associated malignancy. However, other poorly understood factors also contribute to tumorigenesis. For instance, the cause of the more frequent occurrence of KS in men rather than in women, despite a similar prevalence of KSHV infection in many instances, is not clear. Furthermore, prior to the HIV epidemic, KS occurred relatively frequently in Uganda and Cameroon but not in Botswana and the Gambia, despite KSHV infection being common to all these countries.[31] These findings argue for as yet unknown factors interacting with KSHV to induce KS.

Epidemiology

Assays to identify KSHV-infected individuals are still evolving.[9,20,32-34] Serologic assays for antibodies against specific KSHV antigens expressed during the latent or lytic phases of infection have been most commonly used. The assays differ in sensitivity and specificity, resulting in some that likely overestimate and others that underestimate seropositivity. With these limitations in mind, certain general conclusions regarding prevalence of KSHV infection can be made. Detection of KSHV DNA by PCR of blood is less sensitive than the serologic assays, reflecting highly variable levels of viremia occurring in both those with and those without KSHV-induced disease.

KSHV differs from other herpesviruses in that it does not cause worldwide ubiquitous infection.[9,20,32] Instead, the prevalence of infection in the general population varies significantly in different areas of the world. Sub-Saharan Africa has the highest rate of infection, with approximately 50% of the population infected. Seroprevalence is approximately 10% in the Mediterranean region, although in certain areas of Italy, it approaches 30%. Seroprevalence in the United States and northern Europe is approximately 5%, but only 0.2% of individuals in Japan are positive. Despite the low prevalence of KSHV in the general population in the United States, approximately 15% to 20% of HIV-negative and approximately 40% of HIV-positive men who have sex with men are KSHV seropositive.[35] In contrast to the general population, approximately 90% to 100% of individuals with KS are seropositive, consistent with KSHV's etiologic role in this disease.

There are several patterns of KSHV transmission. In the United States, KSHV is spread predominantly through sexual contact among men who have sex with men. Among men who have sex with men, KSHV seropositivity is associated with high numbers of sexual part-

ners, a history of sexually transmitted diseases, and the use of amyl nitrates.[35,36] In contrast to the well-documented sexual transmission among men who have sex with men, the evidence for heterosexual KSHV transmission is conflicting.[37-41] In areas of the world where KSHV infection is more prevalent, nonsexual transmission also occurs, and KSHV infection occurs among children before they are sexually active.[42,43] Intrafamilial clustering has also been documented as further evidence of nonsexual transmission.[44] Saliva is likely a unifying vehicle of both sexual and nonsexual KSHV transmission. Relatively high titers of KSHV DNA can be found in the saliva of infected individuals, whereas high levels of virus are not found at other sites. In one study of 50 KSHV-infected men who had sex with men without KS, 30% of oropharyngeal samples compared to 1% of anal and genital samples were positive for KSHV. KSHV from the oral cavity was 2.5 logs higher than the titer at other sites.[35] Interestingly, deep ("French") kissing was a risk factor for KSHV transmission among men who have sex with men.[35] HLA alleles may influence the degree of KSHV shedding in saliva.[45] Solid organ transplantation from a seropositive donor to a seronegative recipient has also been shown to transmit KSHV.[46] Vertical transmission from mother to infant can occur but appears to be rare.[47] Transmission by blood transfusion can also occur, and the risk is greatest in regions of high KSHV seroprevalence. Whether or not the blood supply should be screened in the United States, where the seroprevalence is low, remains controversial. However, there is currently no Food and Drug Administration–approved diagnostic test for KSHV infection, limiting potential strategies to screen blood products for KSHV infection.[48-50]

Clinical Manifestations

PRIMARY INFECTION

A primary infection syndrome for KSHV has not been clearly described, and most infections are probably asymptomatic or unrecognized. In a prospective Egyptian study, 86 children 1 to 4 years of age presenting to the emergency department with fever of unclear origin were evaluated for KSHV infection. Six of the children likely had primary KSHV infection because they were seronegative but had KSHV DNA detected in saliva. In three of these subjects, follow-up serology was obtained, and all three seroconverted to KSHV. All but one of the six had a maculopapular rash that began on the face and gradually spread downward over the trunk and extremities. Five of the six also had associated upper respiratory tract symptoms. Fever persisted for a median of 10 days.[51] Primary KSHV infection was associated with mild symptoms of diarrhea, fatigue, localized rash (ankle and face), and lymphadenopathy (cervical and submental) in four of five HIV-negative men.[52] A 43-year-old HIV-infected man developed fever, athralgia, cervical lymphadenopathy, and splenomegaly 5 weeks after KSHV seroconversion, and his illness spontaneously resolved within 10 weeks. Biopsies showed angiolymphoid hyperplasia and foci of KS. Neither lesions nor clinical symptoms had recurred after 8 years of follow-up (on highly active antiretroviral therapy [HAART]).[53] Four months after transplantation, two renal allograft recipients developed primary KSHV infection from the same KSHV-positive donor. One recipient developed disseminated KS and the other a syndrome of fever, splenomegaly, cytopenia, and marrow failure with plasmacytosis. KSHV infection of immature progenitor cells from the aplastic bone marrow was noted for the patient with marrow failure.[54] Although these data are very limited, it appears that primary infection in immunocompetent hosts is self-limited, whereas primary infection in immunosuppressed hosts can be severe and have significant consequences.

KAPOSI'S SARCOMA

KS typically involves the skin and manifests as lesions that enlarge from patches to plaques to nodules.[55,56] The lesions often begin as violaceous and later evolve into a brown color due to hemosiderin deposition (Fig. 141-1). KS lesions are composed of vascular spaces,

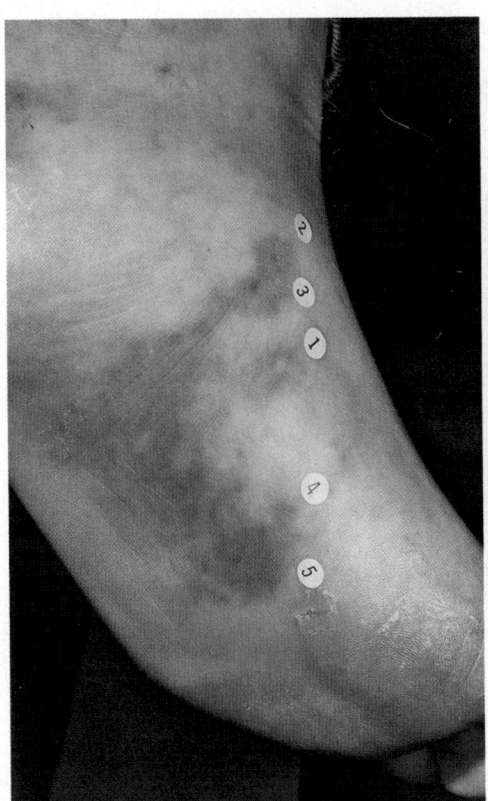 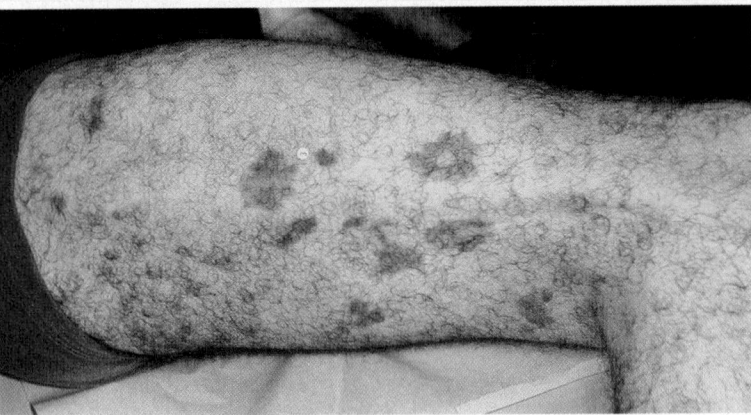

Figure 141-1   Kaposi's sarcoma of the foot (left) and leg (right) in two HIV-positive patients. Lesions are highly vascular and often occur on the lower extremities. Newer KS lesions are typically violaceous (foot) and evolve to a brownish color (leg) over time due to hemosiderin deposition. Labels are present as part of a clinical treatment trial. *(Courtesy of Bruce Dezube, MD.)*

extravasated erythrocytes, and several different types of cells (Fig. 141-2). These include the malignant spindle cells and infiltrating mononuclear cells, such as hemosiderin-laden macrophages. The highly vascular nature of KS gives it its purple color. In the nodular stage, nearly all spindle cells are KSHV infected (see Fig. 141-2).

Four variants of KS occur that differ epidemiologically and clinically.[9,20,57,58] The occurrence of KS largely reflects the seroprevalence of the population, with KS more common in areas with high KSHV seropositivity. Classical KS occurs in elderly men of Mediterranean or eastern European descent, predominantly involves the skin of the lower extremities, and is indolent. Endemic KS occurs in certain sub-Saharan African countries. At least two forms of endemic KS occurred prior to the HIV epidemic. In adults, cutaneous KS occurred in an approximately 20:1 ratio of men to women; it clinically resembled classical KS in adults. However, in children younger than 10 years, KS caused an aggressive, multifocal, lymphadenopathic form, often without cutaneous lesions, that was frequently fatal.[55,56,59] Epidemic KS, which refers to KS in HIV-infected individuals, tends to be aggressive, commonly involving the skin, gastrointestinal tract, and respiratory tract. In contrast to classical KS, lesions commonly involve the face (often the nose), genitalia, and oral cavity (palatal and gingival), in addition to the lower extremities.[60] This form is most common in the United States, where it predominantly affects men who have sex with men. However, KS largely occurs in heterosexual HIV-infected individuals in Africa. Since the start of the HIV epidemic in Africa, the ratio of men to women with KS has dropped 10-fold to approximately 2:1. The number of childhood cases of KS has also significantly increased in Africa with the AIDS epidemic.[61,62] For instance, in Zambia in the early 1980s, KS accounted for 0% to 2% of childhood malignancies, but by 1992 it accounted for approximately 25% of childhood malignancies.[62-64] Iatrogenic KS occurs in individuals who are immunosuppressed such as from organ transplantation and tends to be aggressive. Kidney allograft recipients appear to be at higher risk for

developing KS compared to other transplant recipients.[65] KS regressed in renal transplant patients with KS who were switched from cyclosporine to rapamycin (sirolimus) immunosuppression. Therefore, rapamycin (or one of its analogues) immunosuppression should be considered in transplant recipients with KS.[66,67] Interestingly, reduction of immune suppression can lead to KS remission, highlighting the critical role of immune response in this infection. Similarly, epidemic KS often responds to boosting of the immune response with HAART.[56,68] The incidence of KS in HIV infection has decreased significantly in developed countries since the introduction of HAART, but the standardized incidence rate remains highest for KS compared to other cancers in HIV infection.[69,70]

Although KS can often be recognized by a trained observer, the diagnosis is easily confirmed by biopsy.[56,60] Early stages of KS can be more difficult to recognize. The differential diagnosis of KS includes bacillary angiomatosis, which is caused by *Bartonella* species. Skin lesions of bacillary angiomatosis are very vascular and may mimic those of KS.[56]

The measurement of KSHV viral loads has been performed on peripheral blood of patients with KS. Viral loads are performed by PCR of viral DNA either in plasma or in peripheral blood mononuclear cells (PBMCs), and studies vary as to which blood component is used. One study showed that detection of KSHV DNA in PBMCs of HIV-infected individuals without KS predicted the development of KS lesions.[71] Plasma KSHV DNA levels were greater in more advanced KS disease compared to less advanced disease; they were also greater in AIDS KS compared to classical KS.[72,73] KSHV levels were higher in PBMCs in patients with active KS compared to those with KS in remission,[73] and KSHV levels in buffy coat cells were higher in those patients with higher rates of eruptions of KS lesions.[74] A study comparing plasma and PBMC KSHV load in patients with KS found that there was generally a linear relationship between the two,[72] although there was significant variation in the correlation for many individuals. Despite the

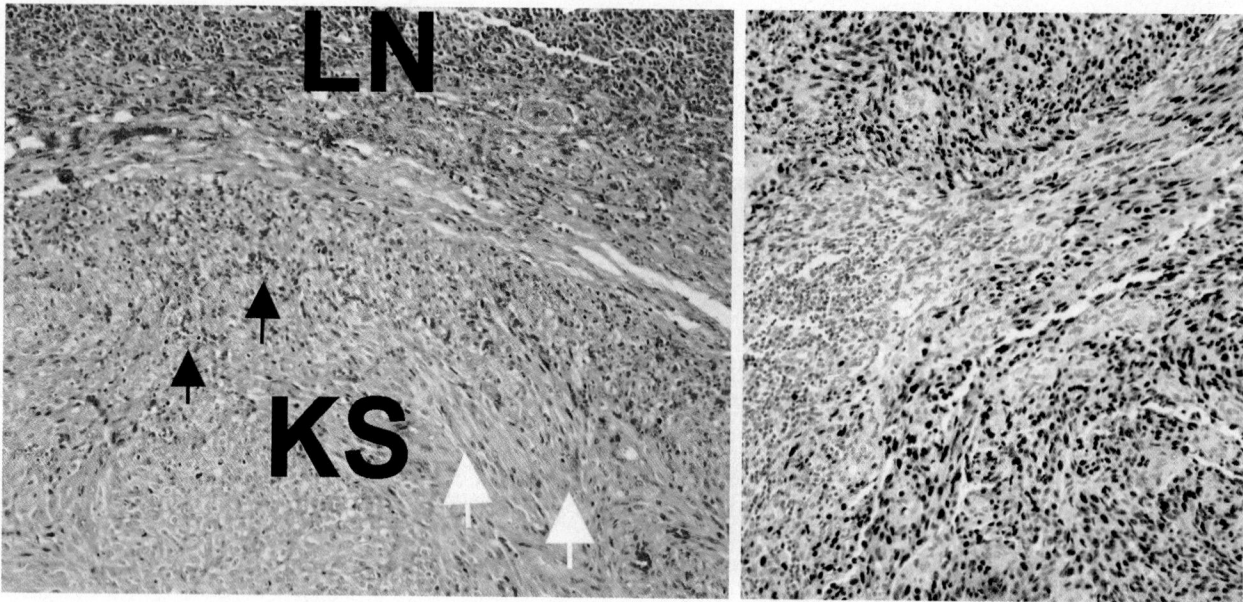

Figure 141-2 **Kaposi's sarcoma involving a lymph node. Left,** A spindle cell proliferation *(white arrows)* containing poorly formed vascular spaces with entrapped red blood cells *(black arrows)*. Areas of uninvolved lymph node (LN) are seen at the top (hematoxylin and eosin). **Right,** Immunohistochemical detection of KSHV LANA *(brown)* in the nuclei of many spindle cells indicates KSHV infection (×200). *(Courtesy of Dan Jones, MD, PhD.)*

detection of KSHV in the blood of KS patients and apparent correlation with KSHV load and disease activity, the clinical use of viral loads for monitoring KS activity or as a guide for therapy is limited by the relatively low levels of KSHV viremia.[73] In contrast, the levels of KSHV viremia are significantly higher in multicentric Castleman's disease.

Treatment of KS in HIV infection is palliative and not curative.[56,60,66,68] Depending on the severity of disease, treatment options may include observation, topical therapy, or systemic therapy (see Chapter 125). Local therapy may include chemotherapeutic agents, laser treatment, cryotherapy, and irradiation. Systemic therapy is reserved for more severe disease and includes liposomal anthracyclines, paclitaxel, and vinorelbine.

PRIMARY EFFUSION LYMPHOMA

PEL was first described in 1989 in HIV-infected patients.[75] It occurs in the potential body spaces of the pleural, pericardial, and peritoneal cavities.[9,76] Lymphoma cells (Fig. 141-3) grow in suspension with little or no contiguous solid mass component. Cells contain clonal immunoglobulin gene arrangements, indicating a B-cell origin, despite lacking most typical B-cell antigens. The malignant cells are infected with KSHV, and Epstein-Barr virus often coinfects the cells. PEL is rare, accounting for approximately 3% of AIDS-related lymphomas and only an estimated 0.4% of non–AIDS-associated large cell non-Hodgkin's lymphoma.[77] The prognosis is poor, with death often occurring within months of diagnosis. Patients with PEL tend to have higher levels of KSHV viremia than those with KS but lower levels than those with multicentric Castleman's disease.[73,78]

MULTICENTRIC CASTLEMAN'S DISEASE

Castleman's disease is a rare lymphoproliferative disorder first described in 1956[79] that occurs in two forms. Localized Castleman's disease (hyaline vascular variant) is not associated with KSHV and has an indolent clinical course. Multicentric Castleman's disease (plasma cell variant), first described in 1978,[80] is associated with KSHV and has a much more aggressive clinical course, frequently resulting in death. Multicentric Castleman's disease is often associated with fever, hepatosplenomegaly, and generalized lymphadenopathy.

Complications include infection (often a cause of death) and the development of either lymphoma or KS.[81] KSHV is almost always linked to multicentric Castleman's disease in HIV-infected individuals, and KSHV infection is linked to approximately 50% of cases in individuals without HIV infection.[82,83] Interleukin-6 (IL-6), which induces B-cell differentiation, is expressed at high levels in the germinal centers of affected lymph nodes and may be responsible for the high numbers of plasma cells present (Fig. 141-4A). Interestingly, KSHV encodes a homologue of IL-6 that is expressed in lytic infection and may have a role in disease.[84,85] KSHV-infected plasmablasts are typically seen in the mantle zone of affected lymph nodes (Fig. 141-4B).[86] Although the optimal therapy for multicentric Castleman's disease is not clearly defined, treatment modalities include steroids and chemotherapy.[81,87]

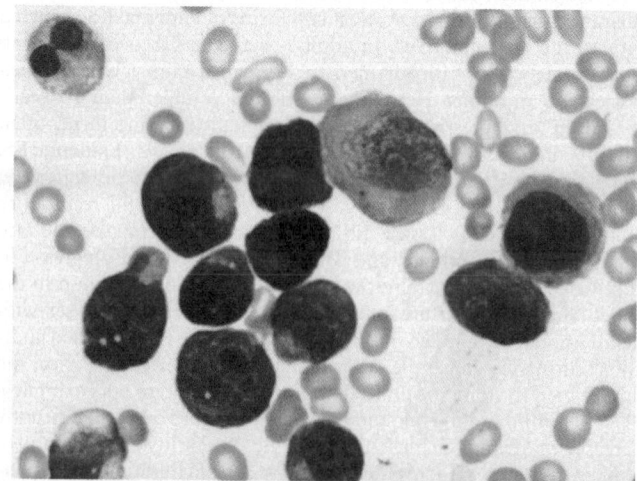

Figure 141-3 **KSHV-infected primary effusion lymphoma cells from this pleural effusion have plasmacytoid features and deeply basophilic cytoplasm.** Red blood cells are interspersed among the lymphoma cells. (Wright Giemsa, ×1000.) *(Courtesy of Dan Jones, MD, PhD.)*

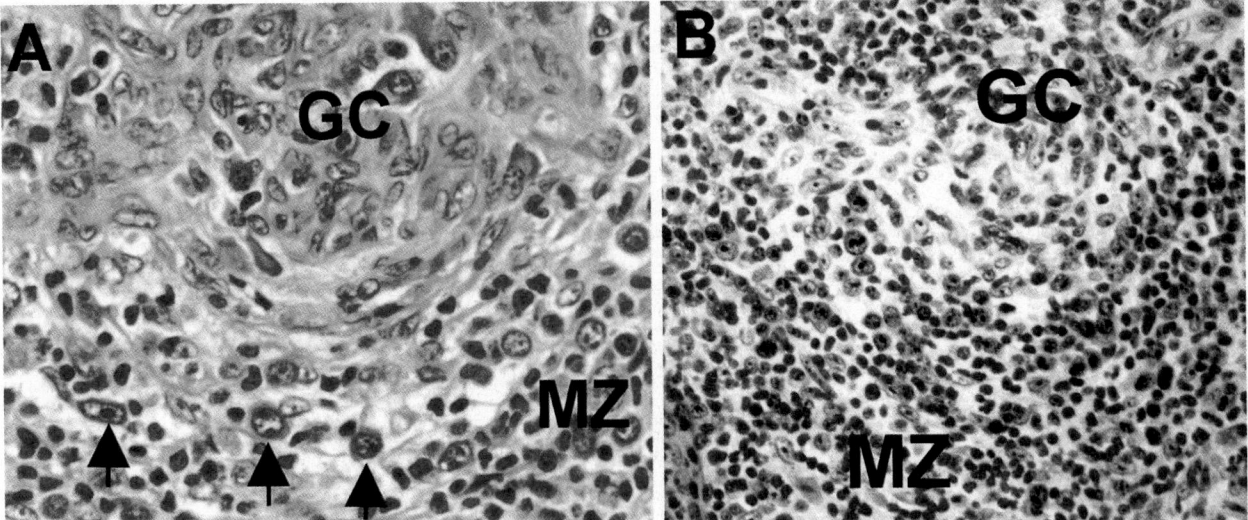

Figure 141-4 Multicentric Castleman's disease in a lymph node of an HIV-negative patient. A, Regressed germinal center (GC) has atypical plasmablasts *(arrows)* concentrated in the follicle mantle zone (MZ) (hematoxylin and eosin, ×600). **B,** Immunohistochemical detection of KSHV LANA *(brown)* in the nuclei of plasmablasts indicates KSHV-infected cells (×400). *(Courtesy of Dan Jones, MD, PhD.)*

Interestingly, KSHV viral loads in peripheral blood are relatively high in multicentric Castleman's disease (ranging up to 4 or 5 logs). High KSHV levels can be found in both PBMCs and plasma.[78] Furthermore, the presence of symptoms or active disease has been associated with higher levels of KSHV in PBMCs compared to in the absence of symptoms or when disease is in remission.[73,88] For this reason, KSHV viral loads may be useful for monitoring activity of disease during treatment of patients with multicentric Castleman's disease.[73] It is unclear why there are higher levels of KSHV DNA in multicentric Castleman's disease compared with KS. It is possible that there may be increased levels of lytic replication occurring in patients with multicentric Castleman's disease,[73,89] but this question remains open.

OTHER SYNDROMES

A number of syndromes have been linked to KSHV infection but are either disputed in the literature or have not been confirmed. These include the skin diseases pemphigus and bullous pemphigoid, sarcoid, Kikuchi's disease, multiple myeloma, hemophagocytic syndrome, and primary pulmonary hypertension.[9,90] An intriguing link between KSHV and ketosis-prone diabetes has been observed.[91]

Treatment and Prevention

Several agents have activity against KSHV lytic replication, but none have established roles in KSHV-associated diseases. Ganciclovir, foscarnet, cidofovir, and adefovir, but not acyclovir, inhibit KSHV lytic replication.[92-95] A likely reason for a lack of efficacy of these agents in KSHV-associated diseases is that they target lytic, rather than latent, replication of KSHV. The vast majority of KSHV-infected cells in KS, PEL, and multicentric Castleman's disease are latently, not lytically, infected. Development of agents that target latent infection would therefore likely result in a major advance in treatment of KSHV-associated diseases.

Lytic KSHV infection has a role in the biology and transmission of KSHV. Notably, a study investigating CMV retinitis in AIDS showed that ganciclovir reduced the incidence of KS.[96] Also, a randomized study showed that oral valganciclovir reduced oropharyngeal KSHV shedding,[97] indicating that interference with lytic infection might reduce rates of KSHV transmission. However, although valganciclovir was well tolerated in this study, the adverse effects of ganciclovir or valganciclovir would mitigate against either being used widely for the prevention of KSHV transmission or disease.

REFERENCES

1. Kaposi M. Idiopathisches multiples Pigmentsarkom der Haut. *Archiv Dermatol Syphilis.* 1872;3:265-273.
2. Sternbach G, Moritz VJ. Kaposi: idiopathic pigmented sarcoma of the skin. *J Emerg Med.* 1995;13:671-674.
3. Breimer L. Original description of Kaposi's sarcoma. *BMJ.* 1994;308:1303-1304.
4. Antman K, Chang Y. Kaposi's sarcoma. *N Engl J Med.* 2000;342:1027-1038.
5. Kaposi's sarcoma and Pneumocystis pneumonia among homosexual men—New York City and California. *MMWR Morb Mortal Wkly Rep.* 1981;30:305-308.
6. Chang Y, Cesarman E, Pessin MS, et al. Identification of herpesvirus-like DNA sequences in AIDS-associated Kaposi's sarcoma. *Science.* 1994;266:1865-1869.
7. Lisitsyn N, Wigler M. Cloning the differences between two complex genomes. *Science.* 1993;259:946-951.
8. Russo JJ, Bohenzky RA, Chien M-C, et al. Nucleotide sequence of the Kaposi sarcoma-associated herpesvirus (HHV8). *Proc Natl Acad Sci U S A.* 1996;93:14862-14887.
9. Ablashi DV, Chatlynne LG, Whitman JE Jr, et al. Spectrum of Kaposi's sarcoma-associated herpesvirus, or human herpesvirus 8, diseases. *Clin Microbiol Rev.* 2002;15:439-464.
10. Greensill J, Sheldon JA, Renwick NM, et al. Two distinct gamma-2 herpesviruses in African green monkeys: a second gamma-2 herpesvirus lineage among old world primates? *J Virol.* 2000;74:1572-1577.
11. Davison AJ. Evolution of the herpesviruses. *Vet Microbiol.* 2002;86:69-88.
12. Virgin HW, Latreille P, Wamsley P, et al. Complete sequence and genomic analysis of murine gammaherpesvirus 68. *J Virol.* 1997;71:5894-5904.
13. Jung JU, Trimble JJ, King NW, et al. Identification of transforming genes of subgroup A and C strains of *Herpesvirus saimiri. Proc Natl Acad Sci U S A.* 1991;88:7051-7055.
14. Wu L, Lo P, Yu X, et al. Three-dimensional structure of the human herpesvirus 8 capsid. *J Virol.* 2000;74:9646-9654.
15. Trus BL, Heymann JB, Nealon K, et al. Capsid structure of Kaposi's sarcoma-associated herpesvirus, a gammaherpesvirus, compared to those of an alphaherpesvirus, herpes simplex virus type 1, and a betaherpesvirus, cytomegalovirus. *J Virol.* 2001; 75:2879-2890.
16. Akula SM, Pramod NP, Wang FZ, et al. Integrin alpha3beta1 (CD 49c/29) is a cellular receptor for Kaposi's sarcoma-associated herpesvirus (KSHV/HHV-8) entry into the target cells. *Cell.* 2002;108:407-419.
17. Neipel F, Albrecht JC, Fleckenstein B. Cell-homologous genes in the Kaposi's sarcoma-associated rhadinovirus human herpesvirus 8: determinants of its pathogenicity? *J Virol.* 1997; 71:4187-4192.
18. Lagunoff M, Ganem D. The structure and coding organization of the genomic termini of Kaposi's sarcoma-associated herpesvirus (human herpesvirus 8). *Virology.* 1997;236:147-154.
19. Verma SC, Robertson ES. Molecular biology and pathogenesis of Kaposi sarcoma-associated herpesvirus. *FEMS Microbiol Lett.* 2003;222:155-163.
20. Dourmishev LA, Dourmishev AL, Palmeri D, et al. Molecular genetics of Kaposi's sarcoma-associated herpesvirus (human herpesvirus-8) epidemiology and pathogenesis. *Microbiol Mol Biol Rev.* 2003;67:175-212.
21. Moore PS, Chang Y. Kaposi's sarcoma-associated herpesvirus immunoevasion and tumorigenesis: two sides of the same coin? *Annu Rev Microbiol.* 2003;57:609-639.
22. Means RE, Choi JK, Nakamura H, et al. Immune evasion strategies of Kaposi's sarcoma-associated herpesvirus. *Curr Top Microbiol Immunol.* 2002;269:187-201.
23. Liang C, Lee JS, Jung JU. Immune evasion in Kaposi's sarcoma-associated herpes virus associated oncogenesis. *Semin Cancer Biol.* 2008;18:423-436.
24. Schulz TF. Kaposi's sarcoma-associated herpesvirus (human herpesvirus-8). *J Gen Virol.* 1998;79:1573-1591.
25. Cesarman E. Kaposi's sarcoma-associated herpesvirus—The high cost of viral survival. *N Engl J Med.* 2003;349:1107-1109.
26. Ganem D. KSHV infection and the pathogenesis of Kaposi's sarcoma. *Annu Rev Pathol.* 2006;1:273-296.
27. Bais C, Santomasso B, Coso O, et al. G-protein-coupled receptor of Kaposi's sarcoma-associated herpesvirus is a viral oncogene and angiogenesis activator. *Nature.* 1998;391:86-89.

28. Holst PJ, Rosenkilde MM, Manfra D, et al. Tumorigenesis induced by the HHV8-encoded chemokine receptor requires ligand modulation of high constitutive activity. *J Clin Invest.* 2001;108:1789-1796.
29. Yang TY, Chen SC, Leach MW, et al. Transgenic expression of the chemokine receptor encoded by human herpesvirus 8 induces an angioproliferative disease resembling Kaposi's sarcoma. *J Exp Med.* 2000;191:445-454.
30. Flore O, Rafii S, Ely S, et al. Transformation of primary human endothelial cells by Kaposi's sarcoma-associated herpesvirus. *Nature.* 1998;394:588-592.
31. Dedicoat M, Newton R. Review of the distribution of Kaposi's sarcoma-associated herpesvirus (KSHV) in Africa in relation to the incidence of Kaposi's sarcoma. *Br J Cancer.* 2003;88:1-3.
32. Chatlynne LG, Ablashi DV. Seroepidemiology of Kaposi's sarcoma-associated herpesvirus (KSHV). *Semin Cancer Biol.* 1999;9:175-185.
33. Hudnall SD. Crazy 8: unraveling human herpesvirus 8 seroprevalence. *Clin Infect Dis.* 2004;39:1059-1061.
34. Hudnall SD, Chen T, Rady P, et al. Human herpesvirus 8 seroprevalence and viral load in healthy adult blood donors. *Transfusion.* 2003;43:85-90.
35. Pauk J, Huang ML, Brodie SJ, et al. Mucosal shedding of human herpesvirus 8 in men. *N Engl J Med.* 2000;343:1369-1377.
36. Martin JN, Ganem DE, Osmond DH, et al. Sexual transmission and the natural history of human herpesvirus 8 infection. *N Engl J Med.* 1998;338:948-954.
37. Malope BI, MacPhail P, Mbisa G, et al. No evidence of sexual transmission of Kaposi's sarcoma herpes virus in a heterosexual South African population. *AIDS.* 2008;22:519-526.
38. Engels EA, Atkinson JO, Graubard BI, et al. Risk factors for human herpesvirus 8 infection among adults in the United States and evidence for sexual transmission. *J Infect Dis.* 2007;196:199-207.
39. Smith NA, Sabin CA, Gopal R, et al. Serologic evidence of human herpesvirus 8 transmission by homosexual but not heterosexual sex. *J Infect Dis.* 1999;180:600-606.
40. Kedes DH, Operskalski E, Busch M, et al. The seroepidemiology of human herpesvirus 8 (Kaposi's sarcoma-associated herpesvirus): distribution of infection in KS risk groups and evidence for sexual transmission [published erratum appears in *Nat Med.* 1996;2:1041]. *Nat Med.* 1996;2:918-924.
41. Cannon MJ, Dollard SC, Smith DK, et al. Blood-borne and sexual transmission of human herpesvirus 8 in women with or at risk for human immunodeficiency virus infection. *N Engl J Med.* 2001;344:637-643.
42. Gessain A, Mauclere P, van Beveren M, et al. Human herpesvirus 8 primary infection occurs during childhood in Cameroon, Central Africa. *Int J Cancer.* 1999;81:189-192.
43. Andreoni M, El-Sawaf G, Rezza G, et al. High seroprevalence of antibodies to human herpesvirus-8 in Egyptian children: evidence of nonsexual transmission. *J Natl Cancer Inst.* 1999;91:465-469.
44. Angeloni A, Heston L, Uccini S, et al. High prevalence of antibodies to human herpesvirus 8 in relatives of patients with classic Kaposi's sarcoma from Sardinia. *J Infect Dis.* 1998;177:1715-1718.
45. Alkharsah KR, Dedicoat M, Blasczyk R, et al. Influence of HLA alleles on shedding of Kaposi sarcoma-associated herpesvirus in saliva in an African population. *J Infect Dis.* 2007;195:809-816.
46. Munoz P, Alvarez P, de Ory F, et al. Incidence and clinical characteristics of Kaposi sarcoma after solid organ transplantation in Spain: importance of seroconversion against HHV-8. *Medicine (Baltimore).* 2002;81:293-304.
47. Brayfield BP, Phiri S, Kankasa C, et al. Postnatal human herpesvirus 8 and human immunodeficiency virus type 1 infection in mothers and infants from Zambia. *J Infect Dis.* 2003;187:559-568.
48. Blajchman MA, Vamvakas EC. The continuing risk of transfusion-transmitted infections. *N Engl J Med.* 2006;355:1303-1305.
49. Moore PS, Chang Y, Jaffe HW. Transmission of human herpesvirus 8 by blood transfusion. *N Engl J Med.* 2007;356:88-89.
50. Hladik W, Dollard SC, Mermin J, et al. Transmission of human herpesvirus 8 by blood transfusion. *N Engl J Med.* 2006;355:1331-1338.
51. Andreoni M, Sarmati L, Nicastri E, et al. Primary human herpesvirus 8 infection in immunocompetent children. *JAMA.* 2002;287:1295-1300.
52. Wang QJ, Jenkins FJ, Jacobson LP, et al. Primary human herpesvirus 8 infection generates a broadly specific CD8(+) T-cell response to viral lytic cycle proteins. *Blood.* 2001;97:2366-2373.
53. Oksenhendler E, Cazals-Hatem D, Schulz TF, et al. Transient angiolymphoid hyperplasia and Kaposi's sarcoma after primary infection with human herpesvirus 8 in a patient with human immunodeficiency virus infection. *N Engl J Med.* 1998;338:1585-1590.
54. Luppi M, Barozzi P, Schulz TF, et al. Bone marrow failure associated with human herpesvirus 8 infection after transplantation. *N Engl J Med.* 2000;343:1378-1385.
55. Habif TP. *Clinical Dermatology*, 3rd ed. St. Louis: Mosby-Year Book; 1996.
56. Hengge UR, Ruzicka T, Tyring SK, et al. Update on Kaposi's sarcoma and other HHV8 associated diseases. Part 1: Epidemiology, environmental predispositions, clinical manifestations, and therapy. *Lancet Infect Dis.* 2002;2:281-292.
57. Friedman-Kien AE, Saltzman BR. Clinical manifestations of classical, endemic African, and epidemic AIDS-associated Kaposi's sarcoma. *J Am Acad Dermatol.* 1990;22:1237-1250.
58. Sarid R, Klepfish A, Schattner A. Virology, pathogenetic mechanisms, and associated diseases of Kaposi sarcoma-associated herpesvirus (human herpesvirus 8). *Mayo Clin Proc.* 2002;77:941-949.
59. Wabinga HR, Parkin DM, Wabwire-Mangen F, et al. Trends in cancer incidence in Kyadondo County, Uganda, 1960-1997. *Br J Cancer.* 2000;82:1585-1592.
60. Dezube BJ, Groopman JE. AIDS-related Kaposi's sarcoma: clinical features and treatment. Available at www.uptodate.com; 2003. Accessed November 12.
61. Wabinga HR, Parkin DM, Wabwire-Mangen F, et al. Cancer in Kampala, Uganda, in 1989-91: changes in incidence in the era of AIDS. *Int J Cancer.* 1993;54:26-36.
62. Bayley AC. Occurrence, clinical behaviour and management of Kaposi's sarcoma in Zambia. *Cancer Surv.* 1991;10:53-71.
63. Patil PS, Elem B, Gwavava NJ, et al. The pattern of paediatric malignancy in Zambia (1980-1989): a hospital-based histopathological study. *J Trop Med Hyg.* 1992;95:124-127.
64. Chintu C, Athale UH, Patil PS. Childhood cancers in Zambia before and after the HIV epidemic. *Arch Dis Child.* 1995;73:100-105.
65. Iscovich J, Boffetta P, Franceschi S, et al. Classic Kaposi sarcoma: epidemiology and risk factors. *Cancer.* 2000;88:500-517.
66. Sullivan RJ, Pantanowitz L, Casper C, et al. HIV/AIDS: epidemiology, pathophysiology, and treatment of Kaposi sarcoma-associated herpesvirus disease: Kaposi sarcoma, primary effusion lymphoma, and multicentric Castleman disease. *Clin Infect Dis.* 2008;47:1209-1215.
67. Stallone G, Schena A, Infante B, et al. Sirolimus for Kaposi's sarcoma in renal-transplant recipients. *N Engl J Med.* 2005;352:1317-1323.
68. Scadden DT. AIDS-related malignancies. *Annu Rev Med.* 2003;54:285-303.
69. Patel P, Hanson DL, Sullivan PS, et al. Incidence of types of cancer among HIV-infected persons compared with the general population in the United States, 1992-2003. *Ann Intern Med.* 2008;148:728-736.
70. Engels EA, Biggar RJ, Hall HI, et al. Cancer risk in people infected with human immunodeficiency virus in the United States. *Int J Cancer.* 2008;123:187-194.
71. Whitby D, Howard MR, Tenant-Flowers M, et al. Detection of Kaposi sarcoma associated herpesvirus in peripheral blood of HIV-infected individuals and progression to Kaposi's sarcoma. *Lancet.* 1995;346:799-802.
72. Campbell TB, Borok M, White IE, et al. Relationship of Kaposi sarcoma (KS)-associated herpesvirus viremia and KS disease in Zimbabwe. *Clin Infect Dis.* 2003;36:1144-1151.
73. Marcelin AG, Motol J, Guihot A, et al. Relationship between the quantity of Kaposi sarcoma-associated herpesvirus (KSHV) in peripheral blood and effusion fluid samples and KSHV-associated disease. *J Infect Dis.* 2007;196:1163-1166.
74. Nsubuga MM, Biggar RJ, Combs S, et al. Human herpesvirus 8 load and progression of AIDS-related Kaposi sarcoma lesions. *Cancer Lett.* 2008;263:182-188.
75. Knowles DM, Inghirami G, Ubriaco A, et al. Molecular genetic analysis of three AIDS-associated neoplasms of uncertain lineage demonstrates their B-cell derivation and the possible pathogenetic role of the Epstein-Barr virus. *Blood.* 1989;73:792-799.
76. Hengge UR, Ruzicka T, Tyring SK, et al. Update on Kaposi's sarcoma and other HHV8 associated diseases. Part 2: Pathogenesis, Castleman's disease, and pleural effusion lymphoma. *Lancet Infect Dis.* 2002;2:344-352.
77. Carbone A, Gloghini A, Vaccher E, et al. Kaposi's sarcoma-associated herpesvirus DNA sequences in AIDS-related and AIDS-unrelated lymphomatous effusions. *Br J Haematol.* 1996;94:533-543.
78. Tedeschi R, Marus A, Bidoli E, et al. Human herpesvirus 8 DNA quantification in matched plasma and PBMCs samples of patients with HHV8-related lymphoproliferative diseases. *J Clin Virol.* 2008;43:255-259.
79. Castleman B, Iverson L, Menendez VP. Localized mediastinal lymph node hyperplasia resembling thymoma. *Cancer.* 1956;9:822-830.
80. Gaba AR, Stein RS, Sweet DL, et al. Multicentric giant lymph node hyperplasia. *Am J Clin Pathol.* 1978;69:86-90.
81. Herrada J, Cabanillas F, Rice L, et al. The clinical behavior of localized and multicentric Castleman disease. *Ann Intern Med.* 1998;128:657-662.
82. Soulier J, Grollet L, Oksenhendler E, et al. Kaposi's sarcoma-associated herpesvirus-like DNA sequences in multicentric Castleman's disease. *Blood.* 1995;86:1276-1280.
83. Gessain A, Sudaka A, Briere J, et al. Kaposi sarcoma-associated herpes-like virus (human herpesvirus type 8) DNA sequences in multicentric Castleman's disease: is there any relevant association in non-human immunodeficiency virus-infected patients? *Blood.* 1996;87:414-416.
84. Moore PS, Boshoff C, Weiss RA, et al. Molecular mimicry of human cytokine and cytokine response pathway genes by KSHV. *Science.* 1996;274:1739-1744.
85. Parravinci C, Corbellino M, Paulli M, et al. Expression of a virus-derived cytokine, KSHV vIL-6, in HIV-seronegative Castleman's disease. *Am J Pathol.* 1997;151:1517-1522.
86. Dupin N, Fisher C, Kellam P, et al. Distribution of human herpesvirus-8 latently infected cells in Kaposi's sarcoma, multicentric Castleman's disease, and primary effusion lymphoma. *Proc Natl Acad Sci U S A.* 1999;96:4546-4551.
87. Brown JR, Harris NL, Freedman AS. Castleman's disease. Available at www.uptodate.com; 2003. Accessed November 19.
88. Oksenhendler E, Carcelain G, Aoki Y, et al. High levels of human herpesvirus 8 viral load, human interleukin-6, interleukin-10, and C reactive protein correlate with exacerbation of multicentric Castleman disease in HIV-infected patients. *Blood.* 2000;96:2069-2073.
89. Parravicini C, Chandran B, Corbellino M, et al. Differential viral protein expression in Kaposi's sarcoma-associated herpesvirus-infected diseases: Kaposi's sarcoma, primary effusion lymphoma, and multicentric Castleman's disease. *Am J Pathol.* 2000;156:743-749.
90. Cool CD, Rai PR, Yeager ME, et al. Expression of human herpesvirus 8 in primary pulmonary hypertension. *N Engl J Med.* 2003;349:1113-1122.
91. Sobngwi E, Choukem SP, Agbalika F, et al. Ketosis-prone type 2 diabetes mellitus and human herpesvirus 8 infection in sub-Saharan Africans. *JAMA.* 2008;299:2770-2776.
92. Kedes DH, Ganem D. Sensitivity of Kaposi's sarcoma-associated herpesvirus replication to antiviral drugs: implications for potential therapy. *J Clin Invest.* 1997;99:2082-2086.
93. Medveczky MM, Horvath E, Lund T, et al. In vitro antiviral drug sensitivity of the Kaposi's sarcoma-associated herpesvirus. *AIDS.* 1997;11:1327-1332.
94. Neyts J, De Clercq E. Antiviral drug susceptibility of human herpesvirus 8. *Antimicrob Agents Chemother.* 1997;41:2754-2756.
95. Flore O, Gao SJ. Effect of DNA synthesis inhibitors on Kaposi's sarcoma-associated herpesvirus cyclin and major capsid protein gene expression. *AIDS Res Hum Retroviruses.* 1997;13:1229-1233.
96. Martin DR, Kuppermann BD, Wolitz RA, et al. Oral ganciclovir for patients with CMV retinitis treated with a ganciclovir impant. *N Engl J Med.* 1999;340:1063-1070.
97. Casper C, Krantz EM, Corey L, et al. Valganciclovir for suppression of human herpesvirus-8 replication: a randomized, double-blind, placebo-controlled, crossover trial. *J Infect Dis.* 2008;198:23-30.

142

Herpes B Virus

JEFFREY I. COHEN*

Herpes B virus (cercopithecine herpesvirus 1, herpesvirus simiae) causes a disease in macaque monkeys that is similar to that seen with herpes simplex virus (HSV) type 1 in humans; however, infection of immunocompetent humans with herpes B virus can result in a fatal encephalitis. Persons who are scratched, bitten, or have splashes to mucosal surfaces with material from macaque monkeys should be evaluated for possible herpes B virus infection, and when appropriate, they should receive postexposure prophylaxis or treatment.

History

Herpes B virus was first described in 1933[1] in a researcher who died after being bitten by a macaque. Sabin and Wright[2] isolated the virus and named it B virus after the patient's last name. About 50 cases of herpes B virus in humans have been reported in the literature, with 26 well-documented cases.[3]

Description of the Virus

Herpes B virus is an alphaherpesvirus, in the same subfamily as HSV. The complete sequence of herpes B virus[4] shows that it is closely related to HSV with a conserved genomic structure, and the viral glycoproteins show about 50% amino acid identity between the two viruses.

Epidemiology

Herpes B virus is endemic in old world macaques, and most macaques in captivity (unless separated from their parents at birth and reared apart from other animals) should be considered as possibly infected. Most macaques are infected during adolescence, and nearly 100% of adult ($\geq$2.5 years old) macaques bred in captivity or in the wild are infected.[5] The virus naturally infects all types of old world macaques including rhesus macaques (*Macaca mulatta*), cynomolgus monkeys (*Macaca fascicularis*), and pig-tailed macaques (*Macaca nemestrina*). The virus has also been isolated from bonnet, Japanese, stumptail, and other macaques, but no other old or new world monkeys are naturally infected.[6] Herpes B virus has also been detected in free-ranging monkeys in Bali and other sites in Southeast Asia.[7]

Humans are inadvertent hosts. Humans have been infected by bites and scratches from macaques. Other exposures that have transmitted the virus are a needlestick injury from a needle that was exposed to tissue around the eye of a macaque or a needle that was thought to be used to inject monkeys, contamination of wounds with macaque saliva, lacerations from bottles containing macaque cell cultures, scratches from cages, exposure to monkey nervous tissue at autopsy, and possible aerosol exposures.[3] One case was reported due to a splash to the eye from material from a caged macaque.[8] A single case of human-to-human transmission of herpes B virus was reported in a woman who became infected after applying hydrocortisone cream to her contact dermatitis lesions and her husband's herpes B virus skin lesions.[9] Herpes B virus was reported in a primate worker who had not cared for primates for over 10 years. The disease was presumed to be due to reactivation of the virus from latency in the worker;[10] however, this case is considered controversial and the patient may have had an unrecognized exposure to herpes B virus more recently. All cases of herpes B virus, except for the patient with mucosal splash, have been due to percutaneous exposure. While a large number of animal bites and scratches occur each year, cases of herpes B virus are rare; nonetheless the potential for fatalities requires that each of these exposures be evaluated.

Pathogenesis

Animals are infected through the mucosa or skin from oral or genital secretions of other animals. Herpes B virus rarely causes disease in macaques, although oral lesions can occur (Fig. 142-1). The virus is latent in the sensory ganglia of the animals and can reactivate with shedding. Sites of shedding include the genital tract and oral and conjunctival mucosa. On a given day, about 2% of herpes B virus–seropositive healthy adult monkeys shed virus.[11] Shedding is more common in animals that are ill, immunocompromised, stressed, or breeding. Like herpes simplex virus in humans, latently infected macaques shed virus intermittently and often in the absence of lesions. Peripheral blood of macaques has been reported to contain herpes B virus in animals that are ill;[12] and viremia rarely, if ever, occurs in healthy macaques.[13]

Humans are infected from monkey oral, genital, or ocular secretions or monkey nervous system tissues, with a usual incubation period of 5 days to 3 weeks (range, 2 days to 5 weeks). The virus replicates at the site of infection and then ascends the peripheral nervous system in retrograde fashion before advancing to the central nervous system (CNS). Antibody to HSV does not protect humans from herpes B virus infection.

Clinical Manifestations

Asymptomatic infection (i.e., seropositivity without disease) of human primate workers with herpes B virus, including most of those who had histories of bites and scratches, has not been detected.[14,15] Most human infections have been reported from animals without any symptoms. Infection of humans with herpes B virus can initially manifest in three different forms. First, patients may present with nonspecific flu-like symptoms including fever, chills, myalgias, and malaise before presenting with CNS symptoms. Second, patients may present with symptoms at the site of herpes B virus inoculation, which can include itching, tingling, numbness, or pain. Some patients have a vesicular rash at the inoculation site and may have lymphadenopathy in the draining lymph nodes. Third, patients may present directly with peripheral or CNS symptoms. Patients with the first two presentations may develop weakness or paresthesias involving the nerve at the site of infection before developing CNS symptoms. These symptoms include headache, nuchal rigidity, nausea, vomiting, confusion, dysphagia, dysarthria, ataxia, urinary retention, and cranial nerve palsies. The disease progresses from the upper spinal cord to the brainstem and then results in a global encephalitis manifested by seizures, ascending paralysis, hemiplegia, coma, and respiratory failure. Additional symptoms can include sinusitis, conjunctivitis, hiccups, and abdominal pain. The mortality rate in untreated humans is estimated at 70%[6] and is considerably lower in persons treated at an early stage of the disease.

Laboratory Diagnosis After Exposure

Some authorities recommend obtaining baseline serum at the time of exposure in order to simultaneously test it with serum obtained about 3 to 6 weeks later to document seroconversion or a four-fold rise in titer.

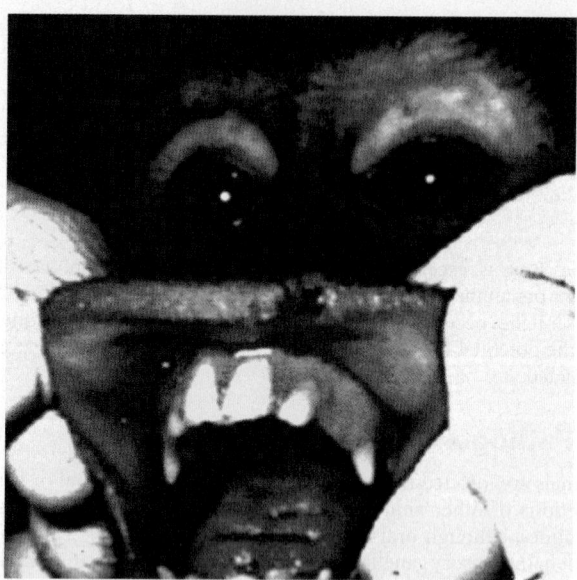

Figure 142-1   **Macaque with a lesion on the upper lip due to herpes B virus infection.** (*Courtesy of J. Hilliard, Georgia State University, Atlanta, Georgia.*)

Persons receiving acyclovir may have delayed seroconversion; serum might be obtained from patients receiving postexposure prophylaxis 3 to 6 weeks after the exposure and at 12 weeks. Since asymptomatic infection has never been reported, other authorities do not recommend testing serum, except to confirm a diagnosis in persons with symptoms compatible with herpes B virus disease. Positive serologies are confirmed using competition ELISA or Western blotting.[14]

Cultures of the wound or exposed mucosa should be obtained only after cleansing is performed, so as not to delay first aid or removal of virus from the site. Some authorities feel that cultures are not especially helpful, since decisions must be made regarding postexposure prophylaxis before the results return. While a negative culture is not helpful (since sampling error may have occurred), a positive culture indicates a true exposure, although not necessarily an infection. Any patient who has a positive culture for herpes B virus needs subsequent follow-up cultures to be certain that they are not shedding virus.

Polymerase chain reaction (PCR) for herpes B virus DNA can be performed on lesion swabs,[16] spinal fluid,[17] and other sites; a positive PCR in the setting of symptoms consistent with herpes B virus is considered diagnostic of infection.

Some authorities recommend testing the primate with which the patient was in contact for herpes B virus by culture or serologic test. However, the monkeys can be in the process of seroconverting at the time of the exposure, and a positive serologic test in a monkey does not indicate that it is actively shedding virus. Herpes B virus cultures may be negative owing to sampling error, and obtaining these cultures can result in a risk of herpes B virus infection to the person collecting the specimens.

Culture, serologic testing, and PCR testing of humans and primates in the United States is performed by the National B Virus Resource Center in Atlanta, Georgia; the virus should be isolated only in a BL-3 laboratory. Their Web site (http://www.gsu.edu/~wwwvir/index.html) offers useful information on collecting and shipping specimens. Similar testing is performed in the United Kingdom by the Health Protection Agency at the Center for Infections (http://www.hpa.org.uk/srmtests/).

Postexposure Evaluation and Prophylaxis

First aid, with prompt, thorough irrigation of wounds and exposed mucosal tissues is essential to reduce the likelihood of infection.

Mucous membranes should be flushed with saline, and wounds irrigated with detergent (e.g., chlorhexidine or povidone-iodine) for 15 minutes.[3] A health care professional should evaluate the inoculation site and thoroughness of cleansing, document the type of exposure (including whether it involved a macaque), consider obtaining baseline serum samples, consider culturing the wound, educate the patient regarding signs and symptoms of herpes B virus, identify a local medical consultant if the need arises, and consider postexposure prophylaxis. The medical history of the monkey should be evaluated, including whether it is ill or immunocompromised or has lesions compatible with herpes B virus infection. All these factors increase the risk that the animal is actively shedding herpes B virus.

Postexposure prophylaxis with oral acyclovir or ganciclovir has been shown to be effective in a rabbit model of herpes B virus infection[18,19] but has not formally been shown to be effective in humans. Nonetheless, although postexposure prophylaxis with antiviral therapy has been recommended only since 1995,[6] no cases of herpes B virus have been reported to date in persons receiving postexposure prophylaxis within 3 days of exposure.[3]

A working group convened by the Centers for Disease Control and Prevention (CDC) prepared a series of recommendations for postexposure prophylaxis of herpes B virus in 2002.[3] Certain types of exposure to macaques were considered to impart a much higher risk of herpes B virus infection in humans. These include inadequately cleansed wounds, deep puncture wounds (which are difficult to clean), bites to the head and face (in which virus can quickly travel to the CNS), exposures involving materials known or highly likely to be infected with herpes B virus, and exposures involving ill or immunocompromised macaques or those with lesions consistent with herpes B virus disease. Recommendations concerning which patients should receive postexposure prophylaxis are described in Table 142-1. Postexposure prophylaxis is given as early as possible and within 5 days of the exposure, since animals given antiviral medication have benefited as late as 5 days after inoculation.[18,19] Postexposure prophylaxis is not

TABLE 142-1	Recommendations for Postexposure Prophylaxis for Persons Exposed to Herpes B Virus

Prophylaxis Recommended

Skin exposure* (with loss of skin integrity) or mucosal exposure (with or without injury) to a high-risk source (e.g., a macaque that is ill, immunocompromised, or known to be shedding virus or that has lesions compatible with herpes B virus disease)

Inadequately cleaned skin exposure (with loss of skin integrity) or mucosal exposure (with or without injury)

Laceration of the head, neck, or torso

Deep puncture bite

Needlestick associated with tissue or fluid from the nervous system, lesions suspicious for herpes B virus, eyelids, or mucosa

Puncture or laceration after exposure to objects (a) contaminated either with fluid from monkey oral or genital lesions or with nervous system tissues, or (b) known to contain herpes B virus

A post-cleansing culture is positive for herpes B virus

Prophylaxis Considered

Mucosal splash that has been adequately cleaned

Laceration (with loss of skin integrity) that has been adequately cleaned

Needlestick involving blood from an ill or immunocompromised macaque

Puncture or laceration occurring after exposure to (a) objects contaminated with body fluid (other than that from a lesion), or (b) potentially infected cell culture

Prophylaxis Not Recommended

Skin exposure in which the skin remains intact

Exposure associated with non-macaque species of nonhuman primates

*Exposures include macaque bites or scratches, or contact with ocular, oral, or genital secretions, nervous system tissues, or materials contaminated by macaques (e.g., cages or equipment).

From Cohen JI, Davenport DS, Stewart JA, et al. Recommendations for prevention and therapy of persons exposed to B virus (Cercopithecine herpesvirus 1). *Clin Infect Dis.* 2002;35:1191-1203.

a substitute for prompt and thorough cleansing of the infected site. Most authorities recommend either valacyclovir 1 g three times daily or acyclovir 800 mg five times daily for 14 days, although these medications are not approved for this use by the U.S. Food and Drug Administration. High doses of the oral drugs are used, since the dose needed to inhibit virus replication by 50% (IC_{50}) for herpes B virus is 18 μg/mL,[19] which is about 10 times higher than that for herpes simplex virus. Valacyclovir is the drug of choice owing to the higher levels of acyclovir achieved than with oral acyclovir. Since rabbit studies have been performed with acyclovir, either valacyclovir or acyclovir rather than penciclovir or famciclovir is recommended. If symptoms compatible with herpes B virus disease occur while patients are receiving postexposure prophylaxis, treatment for herpes B virus should be started; thus, it is important to follow up patients with a potential herpes B virus exposure whether or not they receive postexposure prophylaxis.

Diagnosis of Herpes B Virus Disease

A physical examination of the lesion site (looking for vesicles) and a complete neurologic examination should be performed in persons with herpes B virus disease. Cultures of conjunctiva, oropharynx, and the exposure site are recommended, along with obtaining serum for herpes B virus serologic testing. An MRI of the brain should be performed, and CSF should be sent for PCR.[6,17,20,21] Electroencephalography may help differentiate herpes B virus, which initiates with upper spinal cord and brainstem involvement and results in a diffuse encephalitis, from HSV encephalitis, which usually involves one of the temporal lobes. Somatosensory evoked potentials can help identify early lesions in the brain or spinal cord.

PCR for herpes B virus has been reported using primers for glycoprotein G (gG), which differs from gG in HSV-1 and HSV-2.[21] Real-time PCR was as specific, but twice as sensitive, as culture to detect herpes B virus in human and monkey specimens.

Treatment

Intravenous treatment rather than oral prophylaxis should be initiated in any patient with signs or symptoms of herpes B virus, or a positive culture or PCR (not including a post-cleansing culture or PCR from the wound) if the patient has had a documented exposure to a macaque. In the absence of CNS symptoms, either acyclovir 12.5 to 15 mg/kg intravenously every 8 hours or ganciclovir 5 mg/kg intravenously every 12 hours is recommended until symptoms resolve and two cultures over a 2-week period are negative for herpes B virus.[3] Since animal models show that herpes B virus is more sensitive to ganciclovir than acyclovir,[19] most experts recommend ganciclovir for patients with CNS symptoms.

If herpes B virus can establish latency and reactivate in humans, then discontinuation of antiviral therapy could allow reactivation to occur. Therefore, many authorities recommend that persons who survive herpes B virus infection be maintained on oral acyclovir or valacyclovir, initially at doses used for postexposure prophylaxis and later at suppressive doses, for a prolonged time after intravenous therapy is stopped.[3,6] Repeated cultures for herpes B virus are often recommended after intravenous therapy has been changed to oral therapy to confirm that herpes B virus shedding is not occurring, or when antiviral therapy is discontinued.

Prior to antiviral therapy, about 80% of persons with herpes B virus infection died; with antiviral therapy, it is estimated that 80% of patients survive.[22] Although there have been relatively few cases of documented herpes B virus infection treated in the era of antiviral therapy, five patients with laboratory-confirmed infection with herpes B virus (some of whom had CNS symptoms) who were treated with intravenous acyclovir or ganciclovir had their symptoms resolve within 2 to 3 weeks of therapy.[9,15,23,24] Like HSV encephalitis, therapy for herpes B virus encephalitis is likely to be more effective when given earlier.

Prevention

A vaccine for herpes B virus does not yet exist. Prevention of herpes B virus requires strict precautions when working with nonhuman primates. In view of a fatal case of herpes B virus occurring in a woman who received a splash to her eyes, primate workers exposed to macaques should wear goggles or glasses with side shields and a mask, or a chin-length face shield and a mask to prevent infection of the eyes and oral mucosa.[3] While only a single case of person-to-person transmission of herpes B virus has been reported,[9] persons infected with the virus can shed infectious virus for over 1 week, even while receiving intravenous acyclovir;[3] therefore, body fluids should be considered potentially infectious. Oral and genital secretions from persons who have been exposed to herpes B virus, when it is not yet known whether they are infected, should be considered potentially infectious to others. If the incubation period for herpes B virus (generally 5 weeks in untreated persons) has passed and the person is asymptomatic and/or serologies are persistently negative (at least 12 weeks after exposure in patients given antiviral prophylaxis), then the likelihood of infection and virus transmission is exceedingly low.

It is essential that persons exposed to macaques be educated regarding the importance of first aid and the need for rapid cleansing of wounds or mucosal exposures, the need to see health care personnel regarding evaluation for postexposure prophylaxis, and the signs and symptoms of herpes B virus disease so that early therapy can be initiated.

REFERENCES

1. Gay FP, Holden M. Isolation of herpes virus from several cases of epidemic encephalitis. *Proc Soc Exp Biol Med.* 1933;30:1051-1053.
2. Sabin AB, Wright AM. Acute ascending myelitis following a monkey bite, with the isolation of a virus capable of reproducing the disease. *J Exp Med.* 1934;59:115-136.
3. Cohen JI, Davenport DS, Stewart JA, et al. Recommendations for prevention and therapy of persons exposed to B virus (Cercopithecine herpesvirus 1). *Clin Infect Dis.* 2002;35:1191-1203.
4. Perelygina L, Zhu L, Zurkuhlen H, et al. Complete sequence and comparative analysis of the genome of herpes B virus (Cercopithecine herpesvirus 1) from a rhesus monkey. *J Virol.* 2003;77:6167-6177.
5. Weigler BJ, Roberts JA, Hird DW, et al. A cross sectional survey for B virus antibody in a colony of group housed rhesus macaques. *Lab Anim Sci.* 1990;40:257-261.
6. Holmes GP, Chapman LE, Stewart JA, et al. Guidelines for the prevention and treatment of B-virus infections in exposed persons: the B virus Working Group. *Clin Infect Dis.* 1995;20:421-439.
7. Engel GA, Jones-Engel L, Schillaci MA, et al. Human exposure to herpesvirus B-seropositive macaques, Bali, Indonesia. *Emerg Infect Dis.* 2002;8:789-795.
8. Centers for Disease Control and Prevention. Fatal Cercopithecine herpesvirus 1 (B virus) infection following a mucocutaneous exposure and interim recommendations for worker protection. *MMWR Morb Mortal Wkly Rep.* 1998;47:1073-1076, 1083.
9. Holmes GP, Hilliard JK, Klontz KC, et al. B virus (Herpesvirus simiae) infection in humans: epidemiologic investigation of a cluster. *Ann Intern Med.* 1990;112:833-839.
10. Fierer J, Bazeley P, Braude AI. Herpes B virus encephalomyelitis presenting as ophthalmic zoster: a possible latent infection reactivated. *Ann Intern Med.* 1973;79:225-228.
11. Keeble SA, Christofinis GJ, Wood W. Natural B virus infection in rhesus monkeys. *J Pathol Bacteriol.* 1958;76:189-199.
12. Simon MA, Daniel MD, Lee-Parritz D, et al. Disseminated Herpes B virus infection in a cynomolgus monkey. *Lab Anim Sci.* 1993;43:545-550.
13. Keeble SA. B virus infection in monkeys. *Ann N Y Acad Sci.* 1960;85:960-969.
14. Freifeld AG, Hilliard J, Southers J, et al. A controlled sero-prevalence survey of primate handlers for evidence of asymptomatic herpes B virus infection. *J Infect Dis.* 1995;171:1031-1034.
15. Davenport DS, Johnson DR, Holmes GP, et al. Diagnosis and management of human B virus (Herpesvirus simiae) infections in Michigan. *Clin Infect Dis.* 1994;19:33-41.
16. Scinicariello F, Eberle R, Hilliard JK. Rapid detection of B virus (herpesvirus simiae) DNA by polymerase chain reaction. *J Infect Dis.* 1993;168:747-750.
17. Scinicariello F, English WJ, Hilliard JK. Identification by PCR of meningitis caused by herpes B virus. *Lancet.* 1993;341:1660-1661.
18. Boulter EA, Thornton D, Bauer DJ, et al. Successful treatment of experimental B virus (Herpesvirus simiae) infection with acyclovir. *Br Med J.* 1980;280:681-683.
19. Zwartouw HT, Humphreys CR, Collins P. Oral chemotherapy of fatal B virus (herpesvirus simiae) infection. *Antiviral Res.* 1989;11:275-283.
20. Slomka MJ, Brown DW, Clewley JP, et al. Polymerase chain reaction for detection of herpesvirus simiae (B virus) in clinical specimens. *Arch Virol.* 1993;131:89.
21. Perelygina L, Patrusheva I, Manes N, et al. Quantitative real-time PCR for detection of monkey B virus (Cercopithecine herpesvirus 1) in clinical samples. *J Virol Methods.* 2003;109:245-251.
22. Whitley RJ, Hilliard J. Cercopithecine herpes virus 1 (B virus). In: Knipe DM, Howley PM, et al, eds. *Fields Virology 2007.* 5th ed. Philadelphia: Wolters Kluwer, Lippincott Williams & Wilkins; 2007:2889-2903.
23. Centers for Disease Control. B virus infections in humans—Michigan. *MMWR Morb Mortal Wkly Rep.* 1989;38:453-454.
24. Artenstein AW, Hicks CB, Goodwin BS Jr, et al. Human infection with B virus following a needlestick injury. *Rev Infect Dis.* 1991;13:288-291.

143

Adenoviruses

ELIZABETH G. RHEE | DAN H. BAROUCH

In 1953, Rowe and colleagues isolated a novel cytopathic agent from surgical human adenoid samples undergoing spontaneous degeneration in tissue culture.[1] Soon after, Hilleman and Werner recovered similar viral agents from cases of acute respiratory disease (ARD) in military personnel.[2] To denote their origin, these agents were designated adenoviruses. Subsequently, links to clinical disease were established by studies in which rising anti-adenovirus antibody titers were detected in historic serum samples from World War II military personnel and from patients with ARD, exudative tonsillitis, and atypical pneumonia.[3] In 1955, adenovirus serotype 8 was identified as a cause of epidemic keratoconjunctivitis.[4]

In the 20 years following the discovery of adenoviruses by Rowe and associates, more than 30 different serotypes were identified and were shown to cause several clinical syndromes, including upper and lower respiratory tract infections, keratoconjunctivitis, and infantile gastroenteritis.[5] Epidemiologic studies in the 1960s and 1970s established that adenovirus infections are very common, causing 5% to 10% of all febrile illnesses in infants and young children.[6] Although clinically evident adenovirus infections are typically mild and self-limiting in immunocompetent patients, outbreaks of severe respiratory disease associated with significant morbidity and occasional deaths have been observed in neonates and military recruits[7-9] and, more recently, in civilian populations.[7,10] Adenoviruses have also emerged as serious opportunistic pathogens in immunocompromised patients who have undergone hematopoietic stem cell or solid organ transplantation.[11,12] With the advent of molecular diagnostics, 51 human adenovirus serotypes have been identified to date. Although several serotypes have not been linked to clinical disease, many have been shown to cause a broad range of clinical syndromes, including hepatitis, hemorrhagic cystitis, nephritis, myocarditis, and meningoencephalitis.[13]

In 1962, adenovirus serotype 12 was shown to cause tumors in rodent cells.[14] This was the first description of a human virus that could induce malignant tumors in animals, and certain adenoviruses became model systems for studying oncogenesis. However, the oncogenic potential of adenoviruses has not been associated with any malignancies in humans. Adenoviruses also provided an important model system for studying viral and cellular gene expression and regulation, cell cycle control, and DNA replication.[15] Recently, intense interest has focused on utilizing modified adenoviruses as vectors for gene therapy and vaccines for infectious diseases and cancers.

Description of the Pathogen

Adenoviruses are nonenveloped, lytic DNA viruses. Mature virions are 70 to 90 nm in diameter and contain a linear 36-kb double-stranded DNA core complex encased in an icosahedral capsid (Fig. 143-1). The adenovirus capsid is composed primarily of three major capsid proteins called *hexon*, *penton*, and *fiber* (Fig. 143-2). There are 252 subunits called *capsomeres*, including 240 hexon proteins and 12 penton proteins that form the 20 surfaces and 12 vertices of the capsid. At each vertex a penton protein is located at the base from which a fiber protein protrudes. The fiber protein interacts with primary cellular receptors and consists of a distal–globular knob, a central shaft, and a tail that anchors the wandlike fiber to its penton base.[15,16] Less well-characterized are several minor proteins, including IIIa, VI, VIII, and IX, that contribute to stabilization of the capsid structure. Most of the epitopes recognized by group- and serotype-specific antibodies are present on the hexon and fiber proteins. Hexon proteins contain seven short hypervariable regions that are located on the solvent-exposed surface and that represent serotype-specific targets of dominant neutralizing antibodies. Fiber proteins also contain certain serotype-specific antigenic determinants that are responsible for in vitro hemagglutination characteristics.[17]

More than 100 adenoviruses have been isolated from vertebrates, ranging from reptiles to humans. Nonhuman adenoviruses have not been demonstrated to cause clinical disease in humans. Human adenoviruses belong to the genera *mastadenovirus* (encompassing all mammalian adenoviruses) and are further divided into six subgroups (A through F) based on their hemagglutination characteristics (Table 143-1). Further characterization into 51 serotypes has been determined by their resistance to neutralization by antibodies to other known adenoviruses.[18] Adenoviruses have also been classified by their oncogenic properties (including their ability to transform cells in cultures and cause tumors in animals) and by the percentage of guanine and cytosine in adenovirus DNA; these classification schemes are outlined elsewhere.[15]

▣ Interactions with the Host

Adenoviruses can cause a broad range of clinical syndromes, but it is not well understood why specific adenovirus serotypes are often associated with particular syndromes. The portal of viral entry often appears to determine the primary site of disease, as seen in the spread of ARD by respiratory droplets or of infantile diarrhea by fecal-oral transmission, whereas other organ-limited diseases such as hemorrhagic cystitis likely result from a viremic phase of infection. Tissue tropism varies between different adenovirus groups; group C, E, and some B viruses typically infect the respiratory tract; group D viruses can cause ocular and gastrointestinal infections; and group A and F viruses target the gastrointestinal tract. Viral tropism may be partially determined by differences in virus binding and host cell entry, which is typically initiated by binding of the fiber knob to a high-affinity receptor on the cell surface. Internalization of the virus particle is then mediated by association of the penton base with cell surface integrins.[19]

The primary cellular receptor for the majority of adenoviruses, including groups A, C, E, and F adenoviruses, is the coxsackie B virus–adenovirus receptor (CAR), a transmembrane protein belonging to the immunoglobulin superfamily. CAR is a component of epithelial cell tight junctions and is abundantly expressed in heart, pancreas, the central and peripheral nervous systems, prostate, testis, lung, liver, and intestine.[20] In contrast, several group B and group D adenoviruses bind the transmembrane protein CD46, which is also widely expressed.[21] In addition, a number of other receptors, including CD80 and CD86,[22] sialic acid,[23] and heparan sulfate proteoglycans,[24] have been shown to contribute to attachment and internalization of specific adenovirus serotypes into host cells. It has also been demonstrated that coagulation factor X mediates binding of the adenovirus serotype 5 hexon protein to hepatocytes, providing a rationale for the hepatic tropism of this serotype.[25]

After internalization into endosomes, the virus capsid undergoes conformational changes and is released into the cytoplasm. The virion is then transported by microtubules to the nucleopore, where the adenovirus genome is transferred into the nucleus. Activation of viral transcription leads to expression of early proteins that result in deregulation of the cell cycle and modulation of host antiviral immune responses. These early regulatory proteins are under the control of early region 1A (E1A) genes, which in turn control expression from

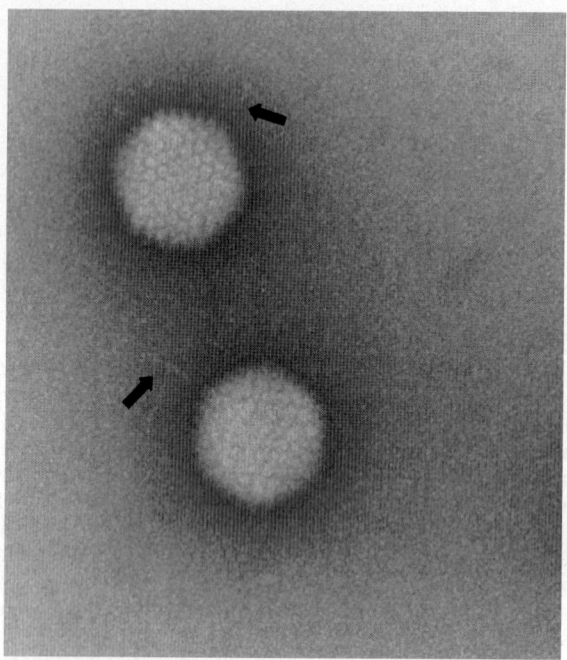

Figure 143-1 **Electron micrograph of adenovirus particles.** Arrows indicate fibers.

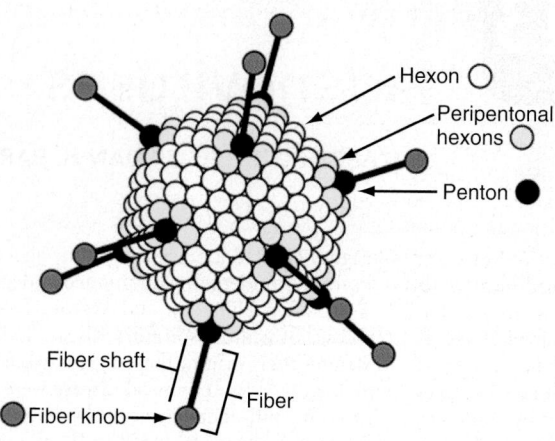

Figure 143-2 **Schematic of an adenovirus capsid.**

other early genes (E1B, E2, E3, and E4). The E3 genes encode several proteins that modulate host immune responses, including inhibition of major histocompatibility complex class I expression and antigen presentation and downregulation of Fas, tumor necrosis factor (TNF), and TNF-related apoptosis-inducing ligand (TRAIL) receptors that lead to inhibition of apoptosis. Within several hours of infection, viral DNA synthesis is initiated, followed by production of viral structural proteins encoded by late genes. New virions are assembled in the nucleus of infected cells and are released by cell lysis.[15]

There is evidence that adenovirus can persist as a latent infection for years after an acute initial infection. Intermittent fecal excretion of group C adenoviruses has been demonstrated to persist for months after an initial acute respiratory infection.[6,26,27] Persistent adenovirus secretion into tears has been documented up to 10 years following conjunctivitis.[28] T lymphocytes in tonsils and adenoids are the most likely potential reservoirs of adenovirus because they have been demonstrated to harbor adenovirus DNA for several years in the absence of infectious particles.[29] Although latency has been well described, the mechanisms for this phase of infection are not established.

Epidemiology

Adenovirus infections are ubiquitous. Most individuals have serologic evidence of prior adenovirus infection by age 10 years, often having experienced infection by several adenovirus serotypes during early childhood.[5] Approximately 50% of all adenovirus infections result in

subclinical disease, and most symptomatic infections are mild and self-resolving.[26] Therefore, the majority of adenovirus infections remain undocumented, and epidemiologic data are derived from several surveillance studies and investigations of sporadic outbreaks. Epidemiologic studies conducted in the United States in the 1960s and 1970s demonstrated that 5% to 10% of all febrile illnesses in infants and young children are attributable to adenovirus infections, typically involving the respiratory tract and commonly caused by serotypes 1, 2, 3, and 5.[6,26] According to a survey from the United Kingdom, 61% of documented adenovirus infections were present in children younger than 5 years of age.[30] Although serotypes that cause respiratory illness may be transmitted through aerosolized droplets, prolonged secretion after acute infection occurs through the gastrointestinal tract, such that fecal-oral transmission may account for a substantial number of infections in young children.[26] Sporadic outbreaks of pediatric infections have been documented in day care centers, summer camps, and public swimming pools.[31]

In contrast, acute adenovirus infections are less common in immunocompetent adults, with the notable exception of military recruits. In this population, several epidemics of ARD caused by adenoviruses have been well documented and have led to significant morbidity.[32] Initial studies in military personnel demonstrated that these epidemics were most commonly due to adenovirus serotypes 4 and 7, leading to the development of a live oral vaccine that was administered to the military until 1999.[33,34] After discontinuation of this vaccine, outbreaks of adenovirus-related respiratory infections reemerged.[9,35] In subsequent studies of military personnel, investigators have demonstrated that serotypes 3, 4, and 21 are the most common adenovirus infections[10] and that several group B adenoviruses, including serotypes 3, 7, 14, and 21, have caused ARD outbreaks.[10,35-37]

Severe or fatal adenovirus infections in immunocompetent adults are rare, but in 2006 and 2007 several clusters of severe ARD were caused by a virulent strain of adenovirus serotype 14 that affected military personnel, infants, and immunocompetent adults. The major-

TABLE 143-1	Classification of Adenoviruses			
Group	**Hemagglutination Groups**		**Serotypes**	**Common Sites of Infection**
A	IV (little or no agglutination)		12, 18, 31	GI tract, respiratory tract
B	I (complete agglutination of monkey erythrocytes)		3, 7, 11, 14, 16, 21, 34, 35, 50	Respiratory tract, GU tract
C	III (partial agglutination of rat erythrocytes)		1, 2, 5, 6	Respiratory tract, liver
D	II (complete agglutination of rat erythrocytes)		8-10, 13, 15, 17, 19, 20, 22-30, 32, 33, 36-39, 42-49, 51	Eye, GI tract
E	III		4	Respiratory tract
F	III		40, 41	GI tract

GI, gastrointestinal; GU, genitourinary.

ity of hospitalized patients in these outbreaks were admitted to the intensive care unit, and several patients died, including previously healthy young adults.[7,36]

Transmission of adenovirus infections typically occurs through respiratory droplets or the fecal-oral route from individuals with acute infection or asymptomatic viral shedding postinfection. Rare cases of transmission through cervical secretions have been documented in neonates.[8,38] Infections can also be spread by contact with contaminated fomites because adenoviruses can survive for extended periods on environmental surfaces. In one study, an isolate responsible for epidemic keratoconjunctivitis (EKC) remained viable for 35 days on an inanimate surface.[39] Nosocomially acquired adenovirus infections have been documented in outbreaks of keratoconjunctivitis[40] and respiratory disease[41] on hospital wards.

Clinical Syndromes

Most adenovirus infections are self-limiting, although fatal infections can occur in immunocompromised hosts, neonates, and, occasionally, healthy children and adults. Severe disease is also associated with certain serotypes, including adenovirus 5, 7, 14, and 21. A broad spectrum of clinical adenovirus-associated disease exists, presumably as a result of the diverse serotypes and tissue tropisms of adenoviruses (Table 143-2).

RESPIRATORY TRACT DISEASE

In children, adenoviruses cause approximately 5% of upper respiratory tract infections and 10% of pneumonias.[42] Most commonly, upper respiratory tract disease presents as mild pharyngitis or tracheitis accompanied by coryza. The common serotypes that cause these syndromes are adenovirus 1, 2, 5, and 6 and occasionally 3 and 7. Other systemic manifestations, including fever, malaise, headache, myalgia, and abdominal pain, are common.[43-45] Exudative tonsillitis and cervical adenopathy may be present and can be clinically indistinguishable

TABLE 143-2	Clinical Diseases Caused by Adenovirus Infection	
Clinical Disease	**Populations at Risk**	**Causal Adenovirus Serotypes**
Pharyngitis	Infants, children	1-7
Pharyngoconjunctival fever	Children	3, 7
Pertussis-like syndrome	Children	5
Pneumonia	Infants, children	1-3, 21
	Military recruits	4, 7, 14
Acute respiratory disease	Military recruits	3, 4, 7, 14, 21
Conjunctivitis	Children	1-4, 7
Epidemic keratoconjunctivitis	Adults, children	8, 11, 19, 37
Gastroenteritis	Infants	31, 40, 41
	Children	2, 3, 5
Intussusception	Children	1, 2, 4, 5
Hemorrhagic cystitis	Children	7, 11, 21
	HSCT recipients, renal transplant recipients	34, 35
Meningoencephalitis	Children, immunocompromised hosts	2, 6, 7, 12, 32
Hepatitis	Pediatric liver transplant recipients	1-3, 5, 7
Nephritis	Renal transplant recipients	11, 34, 35
Myocarditis	Children	7, 21
Urethritis	Adults	2, 19, 37
Disseminated disease	Neonates, immunocompromised hosts	1, 2, 5, 11, 31, 34, 35, 40

HSCT, hematopoietic stem cell transplant.

from group A streptococcal infection.[43] In children younger than 1 year, otitis media can also be a common presentation.[44,45] Adenoviruses have also been associated with a pertussis-like syndrome in cases in which the bacteria were never cultured.[46,47] Several adenovirus serotypes, including 1 through 5, 7, 14, and 21, can cause pneumonia in children and may occasionally result in sequelae such as bronchiectasis. Certain subgroup B adenoviruses (3, 7, 14, and 21) have been associated with severe and complicated pneumonias, particularly in infants. In retrospective studies from South America, adenovirus serotype 7 infection resulted in substantial mortality rates in infants with pneumonia,[48,49] and in an outbreak of adenovirus serotype 30 infections in neonatal patients in the United States, pneumonia was associated with increased mortality.[50]

Several outbreaks of ARD have been documented in military recruits, most commonly caused by serotypes 4, 7, 14, and 21. The clinical syndrome is characterized by fever, sore throat, cough, hoarseness, and rhinorrhea and may progress to involve the lower respiratory tract. Symptoms usually last 3 to 5 days, and on examination, pharyngitis, rales, and rhonchi may be present. On chest radiographs, bilateral patchy ground-glass opacities are consistent with the appearance of viral pneumonia. Rare extrapulmonary complications have been reported, including meningoencephalitis, hepatitis, myocarditis, nephritis, neutropenia, and disseminated intravascular coagulopathy.[51,52]

OCULAR DISEASE

Pharyngoconjunctival fever is a common syndrome consisting of benign follicular conjunctivitis, fever, pharyngitis, and cervical adenitis, commonly caused by adenovirus serotypes 3 and 7. Palpebral and bulbar conjunctivitis may be the sole finding and is typically bilateral. It is a common sporadic illness in children and has also been associated with outbreaks in children's summer camps, swimming pools, and lakes. The illness is usually mild and self-limited.[53]

In contrast, EKC is a more serious illness. Patients present with unilateral or bilateral follicular conjunctivitis followed by corneal subepithelial infiltrates that are painful and can cause blurry vision. Prominent preauricular lymphadenopathy is common. The incubation period typically lasts 8 to 10 days, and virus can be isolated for up to 9 days after the onset of symptoms.[54] Adenovirus serotypes 8, 19, and 37 have all been documented to cause outbreaks. Although usually self-limited, EKC can take up to 1 month to resolve and is associated with significant patient morbidity. Corneal opacities may persist for several months to years after infection.[55,56] EKC is highly contagious, and outbreaks have been documented in schools, military bases, and hospital wards. Transmission by instruments, eye drops, and skin has been documented in ophthalmic practices.[39,57]

GASTROINTESTINAL TRACT DISEASE

The detection of adenovirus isolates from the stool of patients with and without clinical disease confounded initial attempts to attribute diarrheal illnesses to adenoviruses. Subclinical infections, confirmed by positive stool cultures and antibody responses, appeared to account for the majority of infections. Furthermore, positive stool cultures without gastrointestinal symptoms were often observed for weeks to months following respiratory adenoviral disease. Subsequently, the identification of "noncultivatable" adenoviruses on electron microscopy examination of symptomatic patients' stools led to the discovery of enteric adenovirus serotypes 40 and 41, which have been closely associated with infantile diarrhea. These viruses can be detected readily by polymerase chain reaction (PCR) and antigen detection assays, and they can be grown in special cell lines. Acute infantile gastroenteritis results in a watery diarrhea that lasts 8 to 12 days on average, accompanied by fever and vomiting.[58,59] In young children, approximately 2% to 5% of acute diarrheal illnesses are caused by adenoviruses 40 and 41.[60] Although cases are generally acquired in the community, nosocomial infections have been reported as well. In addition to adenovirus serotypes 40 and 41, serotypes 2, 3, 8, and 31 have been associated with infantile diarrhea in some reports.[61]

Lower serotype adenoviruses (1, 2, 5, and 6), but not adenoviruses 40 or 41, are associated with mesenteric adenitis, which can clinically mimic appendicitis and have been shown on occasion to cause intussusception. In these cases, adenoviruses have been isolated from stool cultures and lymph nodes. In several studies of children with intussusception, evidence of adenovirus infection ranged from 22% to 61%.[62,63]

GENITOURINARY TRACT DISEASE

In children, adenoviruses can cause acute hemorrhagic cystitis, which is a benign, self-limited illness. Patients present with gross hematuria lasting 3 days on average, without fever or hemodynamic instability. Microscopic hematuria and dysuria may persist for several more days, but tests for renal function remain normal. Boys are two or three times more commonly affected than girls. In Japan, several case series of hemorrhagic cystitis have attributed up to 70% of infections to adenovirus. In the United States, only 20% of hemorrhagic cystitis cases can be linked to acute adenovirus infection. Adenovirus serotypes 11 and 21 are most commonly isolated, although adenovirus serotype 7 has also been detected.[64,65]

Cases of hemorrhagic cystitis and tubulointerstitial nephritis, either as isolated syndromes or as part of disseminated disease, have been reported in renal transplant and stem cell transplant recipients caused by adenovirus serotypes 11, 34, and 35. In immunocompetent adult males, rare cases of nongonococcal urethritis have been associated with adenovirus serotypes 19 and 37.[66,67]

CENTRAL NERVOUS SYSTEM DISEASE

Adenoviruses have been associated with sporadic cases of meningitis and meningoencephalitis, either as a primary manifestation or as a complication of systemic or respiratory infection. In rare cases, adenovirus has been cultured only from cerebrospinal fluid (CSF) in immunocompetent patients[68] and patients undergoing chemotherapy for lymphoma.[69] More commonly, meningoencephalitis has been reported as a complication of severe pneumonia, seen primarily with serotype 7 infection, although also reported with serotypes 1, 6, and 12.[51] Spinal fluid cell counts and chemistries are variable in these cases.

OTHER CLINICAL SYNDROMES

Myocarditis caused by adenovirus has been described in several case series of acute myocarditis in children, based on detection of virus in myocardial tissue by PCR.[70,71] In one large study that included neonates and adults, adenovirus PCR of cardiac tissue was positive in 23% of patients with myocarditis, 12% of patient with dilated cardiomyopathy, and in none of the control patients, suggesting that adenovirus may be a common cause of myocarditis.[71]

Rare cases of myositis associated with rhabdomyolysis,[72] arthritis,[73] and pancreatitis[74] caused by adenovirus have been reported. Disseminated adenoviral disease has been best described in pediatric and immunocompromised patients, particularly in neonates, infants, and stem cell transplant recipients. Several serotypes, including adenovirus 3, 7, 21, and 30, have been isolated in these cases.[75,76]

▪ Infections in Immunocompromised Patients

Adenoviruses have emerged as important opportunistic pathogens in immunocompromised hosts. Infections can range from asymptomatic shedding of virus to disseminated and potentially life-threatening disease. The majority of clinically significant adenovirus infections occur in hematopoietic stem cell transplant (HSCT) and solid organ transplant (SOT) recipients. The incidence of adenovirus infections in these populations has increased in the past 20 years due to improvements in diagnostic methods, more aggressive conditioning regimens, and the institution of surveillance for adenoviral infection by PCR at some centers.[11,12] These populations are also more likely to have coinfection with more than one serotype.[10]

HEMATOPOIETIC STEM CELL TRANSPLANT RECIPIENTS

The rates of adenovirus disease in HSCT recipients are difficult to assess due to variations in diagnostics and study inclusion criteria, but mortality rates with adenovirus disease in this population are significant, ranging from 6% to 70% in different case series.[11] In a study of 1050 HSCT recipients, 4.8% of patients were found to shed adenovirus asymptomatically and 0.9% had invasive disease.[77] Pediatric HSCT recipients have a threefold higher risk of adenovirus infections and are more likely to have severe disease.[78,79] The increased risk of clinical disease in children is likely due to an increased risk of acquiring primary infection, although reactivation of latent infection or reactivation of infection in the transplanted cells may also occur. In addition to younger age, other risk factors for infection include unrelated donor, graft-versus-host disease, T-cell depletion of the graft, cord transplants, aggressive immunosuppression, total body irradiation, and low T-lymphocyte counts after transplantation.[80] Adenovirus is usually detected within the first 100 days post-transplant, with a mean at day 58 and ranging up to day 333 in one study.[81] The presence of adenovirus DNA in blood, a greater degree of immunosuppression, lymphocytopenia, and a rising viral load all increase the risk for serious adenovirus-related clinical disease.[82] In the pediatric HSCT population, the most common adenoviral disease is diarrhea or gastroenteritis.[83] Cases of pneumonia, hemorrhagic cystitis, pneumonitis, tubulointerstitial nephritis, hepatitis, cholangiohepatitis, encephalitis, and disseminated disease have been reported as well.[11]

Surveillance of blood samples by adenovirus PCR to assess risk of infection has become a common practice in some pediatric HSCT centers.[84,85] This practice is based on studies that have shown that adenovirus can be detected in blood 2 or 3 weeks before the development of clinical symptoms.[84] Studies have also shown that increasing viral load measurements have been associated with increased mortality once clinical disease is established. However, the potential use of preemptive therapy in these situations is unclear.[86-88]

SOLID ORGAN TRANSPLANT RECIPIENTS

In SOT recipients, the transplanted organ is typically the primary site of disease. Clinical adenovirus disease may be due to a primary infection or reactivation of latent virus in the transplanted organ because infections are more common in children and in patients with donor-positive/recipient-negative adenovirus status. Severe disease, which may include dissemination, is more common in the pediatric transplant population, particularly liver and lung recipients, and in patients who receive antilymphocyte antibodies.[11] In adults, adenovirus infection may be less severe. In one prospective study that included adult liver, heart, and kidney recipients, viremia was documented by PCR in 7% of cases, and more than half of the patients remained asymptomatic and were able to clear the infection spontaneously.[89]

Adenovirus hepatitis has been well described in pediatric liver transplant recipients. In a case series, rates of hepatitis ranged from 3% to 10% and frequently led to graft loss and death, with mortality rates up to 53%.[81] Most commonly, hepatitis is caused by adenovirus serotype 5, but cases caused by adenovirus serotypes 1 and 2 have also been documented. Lung transplant recipients may develop adenovirus pneumonia in the early post-transplant period. One study of adults and children documented a 1.3% prevalence in this population, and subsequent graft failure, death, or bronchiolitis obliterans has been reported.[90,91] Renal transplant recipients can develop acute hemorrhagic cystitis, sometimes complicated by tubulointerstitial nephritis. Adenovirus serotypes 11, 34, and 35 have been detected in these cases. In general, adenovirus infections are less common and less serious in renal transplant recipients, although cases of pneumonia and rare cases of fatal disseminated infections have been reported.[89,92] Adenovirus infections involving the grafted organ have also been reported in cardiac transplant and small bowel transplant recipients.[11]

HIV/AIDS PATIENTS

Most observations regarding adenovirus infections in HIV-positive patients were made prior to the availability of highly active antiretroviral therapy. In these studies, the risk of adenovirus infection was 28% in patients with AIDS and 17% in patients with CD4 counts greater than 200 cells/μL.[93] Although adenovirus can be isolated frequently from the stool and urine of patients with AIDS, no causative link with diarrhea, hematuria, or other clinical syndromes has been established. Several novel adenovirus serotypes have been detected in the stool of AIDS patients, including many of the group D serotypes and the last nine adenovirus serotypes.[13,94] If symptoms are present, they are usually attributed to other opportunistic infections. Rare cases of fatal hepatic necrosis, fatal pneumonia, encephalitis, nephritis, and systemic infection caused by adenoviruses have been reported, but adenovirus infections in AIDS patients are an uncommon cause of morbidity or mortality.[95-97]

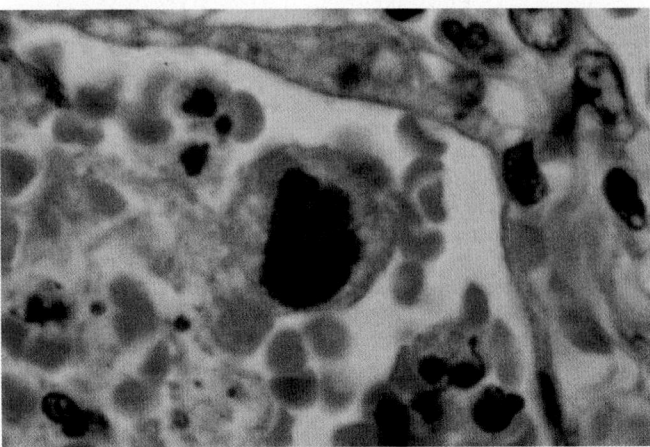

Figure 143-3 Lung biopsy specimen from a patient with adenovirus pneumonia showing a characteristic "smudge cell" (hematoxylin-eosin stain. ×400). *(Courtesy of Franz C. Lichtenberg, MD, Department of Pathology, Brigham and Women's Hospital, Boston, MA.)*

Diagnosis

Because most adenovirus infections in immunocompetent patients are mild and self-limited, diagnosis is not routinely pursued. However, establishing a diagnosis may be useful in the setting of outbreaks or for individuals who are immunosuppressed or seriously ill. Traditional methods of determining adenovirus infection include viral culture, antigen-specific assays, and serologies. Recently, detection by PCR has become widespread due to greater sensitivity and specificity and also rapid turnaround.

With the exception of serotypes 40 and 41, adenoviruses are detectable by routine tissue culture. They grow well in human epithelial cell lines, producing a typical cytopathic effect within 2 to 7 days, although some group D serotypes can take up to 4 weeks to isolate. Viruses may be recovered from nasopharyngeal swabs or aspirates, throat swabs, conjunctival swabs or scrapings, stool or rectal swabs, urine, CSF, and tissue. Viral excretion is detectable in the first 1 to 3 days in patients with pharyngitis, 3 to 5 days in patients with pharyngoconjunctival fever, and up to 2 weeks in patients with keratoconjunctivitis.[98] If culture is not available, direct antigen detection provides rapid diagnosis. The immunofluorescence assay (IFA) is useful for respiratory samples and tissue, and enzyme-linked immunosorbent assay is the test of choice to detect adenoviruses 40 and 41 in stool.[99] The sensitivity of virus detection by IFA of respiratory samples is 40% to 60% lower compared with culture.[100] Adenovirus infection may also be established by detecting a fourfold or greater rise in adenovirus-specific antibody titers in paired acute and convalescent sera. Serotype analysis of viral isolates is not routine but can be determined in a reference virology lab by determining hemagglutination patterns and performing serum neutralization assays against a panel of type-specific sera.

Detection of adenoviral DNA by PCR has become increasingly attractive for diagnosis, identification of serotype, and quantification of virus from a variety of clinical specimens, including fixed tissues, serum, and blood. Primers may be directed against conserved hexon or fiber genes, but more specific typing can be done by a multiplex PCR format followed by sequencing to detect and identify all 51 serotypes.[101,102] Real-time PCR has also permitted quantification of virus, which is sometimes employed in monitoring viral loads in peripheral blood samples from immunocompromised patients, particularly pediatric HSCT patients. The specificity of PCR in asymptomatic, immunocompetent adults is high, ranging from 96% to 100% in studies of urine, throat swabs, and peripheral blood.[11,103]

When obtained, tissue should be sent for culture and pathologic examination. Histopathologic findings in the lung include diffuse interstitial pneumonitis, necrotizing bronchitis, bronchiolitis, and pneumonia with mononuclear cell infiltration and hyaline membrane formation.[104] Early postinfection, infected cells may display small eosinophilic inclusions. During late infection, basophilic intranuclear inclusions surrounded by a thin, clear halo emerge and eventually enlarge to obscure the nuclear membrane. This produces "smudge cells," which are characteristic of adenovirus infections (Fig. 143-3). In contrast with cytomegalovirus, there are no intracytoplasmic inclusions or multinucleated giant cells. Further study by electron microscopy, adenovirus-specific immunohistochemical assays, and in situ DNA hybridization can be performed to make the diagnosis.

Treatment

There are currently no approved antiviral agents for the treatment of adenovirus infections. Clearance of adenovirus infection in HSCT and SOT patients is typically associated with immune reconstitution, particularly with improved absolute lymphocyte counts and CD4 T-cell counts.[105,106] There are no prospective, controlled trials of antiviral drugs for adenovirus infections, and thus clinical experience is limited to retrospective case series and case reports, primarily in immunosuppressed patients. Cidofovir has good in vitro activity against adenovirus and has been reported to be useful in certain animal models of ocular adenovirus infections.[107] However, a large, multicenter trial to evaluate the potential efficacy of topical cidofovir for EKC was discontinued due to toxicity.[108] In several case series and case reports involving pediatric and adult HSCT recipients, with a variety of clinical adenovirus syndromes, treatment with cidofovir appeared to be associated with clinical improvement in a subset of patients, although fatalities still occurred and significant nephrotoxicity was noted.[79,109-111] Moreover, it was not clear if the clinical improvement in these individuals was due to the drug. Ribavirin use has been reported in several cases of adenovirus infection in HSCT recipients, but results in case series have been mixed[112,113] and may be explained in part by the observation that in vitro activity of ribavirin appears restricted to group C serotypes.[114] Vidarabine and ganciclovir are reported to possess in vitro activity against adenovirus, but there are scant clinical data for these agents.[115] In some centers, preemptive therapy has been proposed to treat patients who are at risk for adenovirus infection. In a study of 58 pediatric HSCT recipients in which patients were prospectively screened weekly for evidence of infection and then treated with cidofovir, symptoms and viremia resolved in the majority of recipients.[109] It is clear that larger prospective studies are needed to determine if any of these antiviral agents have clinical efficacy and whether their use is warranted in particular clinical settings.

Immunotherapy by adoptive T-cell therapy is being pursued by some groups but remains an investigative approach. One group reported the induction of effective T-cell responses after infusion of adenovirus-specific donor CD4 and CD8 T cells into pediatric HSCT patients.[116-118] Intravenous immunoglobulin has also been used in immunocompromised patients with mixed results.[119,120]

Prevention

Because of the morbidity seen with respiratory adenovirus infections in military recruits, successful live oral vaccines for serotypes 4 and 7 were developed and administered in the military starting in 1971. The vaccine was packaged in enteric capsules that ensured that replication would occur in the gastrointestinal tract and not the airways, resulting in subclinical infection and good neutralizing antibody responses. The sole manufacturer discontinued vaccine production in 1996, and vaccination stopped in 1999 when the supply was exhausted.[34] Since then, ARD has recurred in military recruits at rates similar to those of the prevaccination era, with several outbreaks affecting up to 80% of recruits, resulting in hospitalization rates ranging from 11% to 20% and producing occasional fatalities.[37,121] Due to the reemergence of ARD, a vaccine against adenoviruses 4 and 7 has been redeveloped and is currently advancing through clinical trials.[122]

Adenoviruses as Vectors for Gene Therapy and Vaccination

There has been intense investigation during the past two decades into the capacity of adenoviruses to serve as a vector platform for delivery of genes for both gene therapy and vaccination. Typically, adenoviruses are rendered replication incompetent by deletion of the E1 gene, which allows the insertion of a transgene expression cassette that encodes a gene of interest. Scores of human clinical trials utilizing adenovirus vectors have been conducted, and others are currently in progress or are planned. Adenovirus vectors have been well studied and have several advantages over other available vectors, including their ability to be produced at high titers, to infect several cell types including both dividing and nondividing cells, and to accommodate gene inserts stably.

Applications for gene therapy have primarily focused on delivery of a functional gene to replace a dysfunctional or absent gene product for diseases such as cystic fibrosis, ornithine transcarbamylase deficiency, hemophilia, and bilirubin UDP glucuronosyl transferase deficiency. Although promising in several animal models, early human gene therapy studies have proven disappointing due to inefficient gene delivery.[123] Initial studies also demonstrated that adenovirus vectors at high doses elicit early innate immune responses, including production of proinflammatory cytokines that can lead to systemic toxicity and resulted in the death of a volunteer in a clinical trial.[124,125] Vector-specific immune responses also develop rapidly and limit the utility of repeat vector administration. Several strategies to minimize vector-specific immunity have been developed, including using different human adenovirus serotypes, nonhuman adenoviruses, and structurally modified adenoviruses to create novel vectors.

Adenovirus vectors are also being developed as vaccines for both infectious diseases and cancer, primarily due to their ability to elicit robust cellular immune responses against encoded transgenes. These vectors contain genes encoding pathogen-specific antigens and elicit robust CD8+ T-lymphocyte responses. Adenovirus vector-based vaccine candidates are currently being explored for a variety of infectious diseases, including malaria, herpes simplex virus, tuberculosis, and HIV-1,[126] although a phase IIB efficacy study using an adenovirus serotype 5 vector for HIV-1 has failed. Clinical trials for adenovirus vectors are also being conducted in the tumor vaccine field. Strategies include directly delivering genes that control cell growth, apoptosis, and angiogenesis or genes that express cytokines to induce antitumor responses. Another approach has been to modify adenovirus vectors to replicate and induce lysis in tumor cells but not normal cells. Adenovirus vectors utilizing these strategies have advanced into phase II and III clinical trials for treatment of head and neck cancers.[127,128]

REFERENCES

1. Rowe WP, Huebner RJ, Gilmore LK, et al. Isolation of a cytopathogenic agent from human adenoids undergoing spontaneous degeneration in tissue culture. *Proc Soc Exp Biol Med.* 1953;84:570-573.
2. Hilleman MR, Werner JH. Recovery of new agent from patients with acute respiratory illness. *Proc Soc Exp Biol Med.* 1954;85:183-188.
3. Ginsberg HS, Gold E, Jordan WS Jr, et al. Relation of the new respiratory agents to acute respiratory diseases. *Am J Public Health Nation's Health.* 1955;45:915-922.
4. Jawetz E, Kimura S, Nicholas AN, et al. New type of APC virus from epidemic keratoconjunctivitis. *Science.* 1955;122:1190-1191.
5. Knight V, Kasel JA. Adenoviruses. In: Knight V, ed. *Viral and Mycoplasmal Infections of the Respiratory Tract.* Philadelphia: Lea & Febiger; 1973:65-86.
6. Fox JP, Hall CE, Cooney MK. The Seattle Virus Watch. VII. Observations of adenovirus infections. *Am J Epidemiol.* 1977;105:362-386.
7. Centers for Disease Control and Prevention. Acute respiratory disease associated with adenovirus serotype 14—four states, 2006-2007. *MMWR Morb Mortal Wkly Rep.* 2007;56:1181-1184.
8. Pinto A, Beck R, Jadavji T. Fatal neonatal pneumonia caused by adenovirus type 35: report of one case and review of the literature. *Arch Pathol Lab Med.* 1992;116:95-99.
9. Ryan MA, Gray GC, Smith B, et al. Large epidemic of respiratory illness due to adenovirus types 7 and 3 in healthy young adults. *Clin Infect Dis.* 2002;34:577-582.
10. Gray GC, McCarthy T, Lebeck MG, et al. Genotype prevalence and risk factors for severe clinical adenovirus infection, United States 2004-2006. *Clin Infect Dis.* 2007;45:1120-1131.
11. Echavarria M. Adenoviruses in immunocompromised hosts. *Clin Microbiol Rev.* 2008;21:704-715.
12. Ison MG. Adenovirus infections in transplant recipients. *Clin Infect Dis.* 2006;43:331-339.
13. De Jong JC, Wermenbol AG, Verweij-Uijterwaal MW, et al. Adenoviruses from human immunodeficiency virus-infected individuals, including two strains that represent new candidate serotypes Ad50 and Ad51 of species B1 and D, respectively. *J Clin Microbiol.* 1999;37:3940-3945.
14. Trentin JJ, Yabe Y, Taylor G. The quest for human cancer viruses. *Science.* 1962;137:835-841.

15. Berk AJ. Adenoviridae: the viruses and their replication. In: Knipe DM, Howley PM, eds. *Fields Virology.* 5th ed. Philadelphia: Lippincott Williams & Wilkins; 2007:2355-2394.
16. Valentine RC, Pereira HG. Antigens and structure of the adenovirus. *J Mol Biol.* 1965;13:13-20.
17. Russell WC, Kemp GD. Role of adenovirus structural components in the regulation of adenovirus infection. *Curr Top Microbiol Immunol.* 1995;199:81-98.
18. Hierholzer JC, Adrian T, Anderson LJ, et al. Analysis of antigenically intermediate strains of subgenus B and D adenoviruses from AIDS patients. *Arch Virol.* 1988;103:99-115.
19. Wickham TJ, Mathias P, Cheresh DA, et al. Integrins alpha v beta 3 and alpha v beta 5 promote adenovirus internalization but not virus attachment. *Cell.* 1993;73:309-319.
20. Meier O, Greber UF. Adenovirus endocytosis. *J Gene Med.* 2004;6:S152-S163.
21. Gaggar A, Shayakhmetov DM, Lieber A. CD46 is a cellular receptor for group B adenoviruses. *Nature Med.* 2003;9:1408-1412.
22. Short JJ, Pereboev AV, Kawakami Y, et al. Adenovirus serotype 3 utilizes CD80 (B7.1) and CD86 (B7.2) as cellular attachment receptors. *Virology.* 2004;322:349-359.
23. Arnberg N, Edlund K, Kidd AH, et al. Adenovirus type 37 uses sialic acid as a cellular receptor. *J Virol.* 2000;74:42-48.
24. Dechecchi MC, Melotti P, Bonizzato A, et al. Heparan sulfate glycosaminoglycans are receptors sufficient to mediate the initial binding of adenovirus types 2 and 5. *J Virol.* 2001;75:8772-8780.
25. Waddington SN, McVey JH, Bhella D, et al. Adenovirus serotype 5 hexon mediates liver gene transfer. *Cell.* 2008;132:397-409.
26. Fox JP, Brandt CD, Wassermann FE, et al. The virus watch program: a continuing surveillance of viral infections in metropolitan New York families. VI. Observations of adenovirus infections: virus excretion patterns, antibody response, efficiency of surveillance, patterns of infections, and relation to illness. *Am J Epidemiol.* 1969;89:25-50.
27. Adrian T, Schafer G, Cooney MK, et al. Persistent enteral infections with adenovirus types 1 and 2 in infants: no evidence of reinfection. *Epidemiol Infect.* 1988;101:503-509.
28. Kaye SB, Lloyd M, Williams H, et al. Evidence for persistence of adenovirus in the tear film a decade following conjunctivitis. *J Med Virol.* 2005;77:227-231.

29. Garnett CT, Erdman D, Xu W, et al. Prevalence and quantitation of species C adenovirus DNA in human mucosal lymphocytes. *J Virol.* 2002;76:10608-10616.
30. Cooper RJ, Hallett R, Tullo AB, et al. The epidemiology of adenovirus infections in Greater Manchester, UK 1982-96. *Epidemiol Infect.* 2000;125:333-345.
31. Foy HM, Cooney MK, Hatlen JB. Adenovirus type 3 epidemic associated with intermittent chlorination of a swimming pool. *Arch Environ Health.* 1968;17:795-802.
32. Hilleman MR. Efficacy of and indications for use of adenovirus vaccine. *Am J Public Health Nation's Health.* 1958;48:153-158.
33. Top Jr FH, Dudding BA, Russell PK, et al. Control of respiratory disease in recruits with types 4 and 7 adenovirus vaccines. *Am J Epidemiol.* 1971;94:142-146.
34. Gaydos CA, Gaydos JC. Adenovirus vaccines in the U.S. military. *Milit Med.* 1995;160:300-304.
35. Russell KL, Broderick MP, Franklin SE, et al. Transmission dynamics and prospective environmental sampling of adenovirus in a military recruit setting. *J Infect Dis.* 2006;194:877-885.
36. Binn LN, Sanchez JL, Gaydos JC. Emergence of adenovirus type 14 in US military recruits—a new challenge. *J Infect Dis.* 2007;196:1436-1437.
37. Metzgar D, Osuna M, Kajon AE, et al. Abrupt emergence of diverse species B adenoviruses at US military recruit training centers. *J Infect Dis.* 2007;196:1465-1473.
38. Montone KT, Furth EE, Pietra GG, et al. Neonatal adenovirus infection: a case report with in situ hybridization confirmation of ascending intrauterine infection. *Diagn Cytopathol.* 1995;12:341-344.
39. Azar MJ, Dhaliwal DK, Bower KS, et al. Possible consequences of shaking hands with your patients with epidemic keratoconjunctivitis. *Am J Ophthalmol.* 1996;121:711-712.
40. Birenbaum E, Linder N, Varsano N, et al. Adenovirus type 8 conjunctivitis outbreak in a neonatal intensive care unit. *Arch Dis Child.* 1993;68:610-611.
41. Gerber SI, Erdman DD, Pur SL, et al. Outbreak of adenovirus genome type 7d2 infection in a pediatric chronic-care facility and tertiary-care hospital. *Clin Infect Dis.* 2001;32:694-700.
42. Brandt CD, Kim HW, Vargosko AJ, et al. Infections in 18,000 infants and children in a controlled study of respiratory tract

disease. I. Adenovirus pathogenicity in relation to serologic type and illness syndrome. *Am J Epidemiol.* 1969;90:484-500.
43. Dominguez O, Rojo P, de Las Heras S, et al. Clinical presentation and characteristics of pharyngeal adenovirus infections. *Pediatr Infect Dis J.* 2005;24:733-734.
44. Edwards KM, Thompson J, Paolini J, et al. Adenovirus infections in young children. *Pediatrics.* 1985;76:420-424.
45. Pacini DL, Collier AM, Henderson FW. Adenovirus infections and respiratory illnesses in children in group day care. *J Infect Dis.* 1987;156:920-927.
46. Nelson KE, Gavitt F, Batt MD, et al. The role of adenoviruses in the pertussis syndrome. *J Pediatr.* 1975;86:335-341.
47. Ferrer A, Calico I, Manresa JM, et al. Microorganisms isolated in cases of pertussis-like syndrome. *Enfermedades Infecciosas Microbiol Clin.* 2000;18:433-438.
48. Murtagh P, Cerqueiro C, Halac A, et al. Adenovirus type 7h respiratory infections: a report of 29 cases of acute lower respiratory disease. *Acta Paediatr.* 1993;82:557-561.
49. Frabasile S, Vitureira N, Perez G, et al. Genotyping of Uruguayan human adenovirus isolates collected between 1994 and 1998. *Acta Virol.* 2005;49:129-132.
50. Faden H, Wynn RJ, Campagna L, et al. Outbreak of adenovirus type 30 in a neonatal intensive care unit. *J Pediatr.* 2005;146:523-527.
51. Simila S, Jouppila R, Salmi A, et al. Encephaloningitis in children associated with an adenovirus type 7 epidemic. *Acta Paediatr Scand.* 1970;59:310-316.
52. Wadell G, Varsanyi TM, Lord A, et al. Epidemic outbreaks of adenovirus 7 with special reference to the pathogenicity of adenovirus genome type 7b. *Am J Epidemiol.* 1980;112:619-628.
53. Bell JA, Rowe WP, Engler JI, et al. Pharyngoconjunctival fever: epidemiological studies of a recently recognized disease entity. *J Am Med Assoc.* 1955;157:1083-1092.
54. Koc J, Wigand R, Weil M. The efficiency of various laboratory methods for the diagnosis of adenovirus conjunctivitis. *Zentralbl Bakteriol Mikrobiol Hygiene.* 1987;263:607-615.
55. Dawson C, Darrell R. Infections due to adenovirus type 8 in the United States. I. An outbreak of epidemic keratoconjunctivitis originating in a physician's office. *N Engl J Med.* 1963;268:1031-1034.
56. Dawson C, Darrell R, Hanna L, et al. Infections due to adenovirus type 8 in the United States. II. Community-wide infection with adenovirus type 8. *N Engl J Med.* 1963;268:1034-1037.
57. Jernigan JA, Lowry BS, Hayden FG, et al. Adenovirus type 8 epidemic keratoconjunctivitis in an eye clinic: risk factors and control. *J Infect Dis.* 1993;167:1307-1313.
58. Van R, Wun CC, O'Ryan ML, et al. Outbreaks of human enteric adenovirus types 40 and 41 in Houston day care centers. *J Pediatr.* 1992;120:516-521.
59. Uhnoo I, Wadell G, Svensson L, et al. Importance of enteric adenoviruses 40 and 41 in acute gastroenteritis in infants and young children. *J Clin Microbiol.* 1984;20:365-372.
60. de Jong JC, Wigand R, Kidd AH, et al. Candidate adenoviruses 40 and 41: fastidious adenoviruses from human infant stool. *J Med Virol.* 1983;11:215-231.
61. Krajden M, Brown M, Petrasek A, et al. Clinical features of adenovirus enteritis: a review of 127 cases. *Pediatr Infect Dis J.* 1990;9:636-641.
62. Bines JE, Liem NT, Justice FA, et al. Risk factors for intussusception in infants in Vietnam and Australia: adenovirus implicated, but not rotavirus. *J Pediatr.* 2006;149:452-460.
63. Montgomery EA, Popek EJ. Intussusception, adenovirus, and children: a brief reaffirmation. *Hum Pathol.* 1994;25:169-174.
64. Lee HJ, Pyo JW, Choi EH, et al. Isolation of adenovirus type 7 from the urine of children with acute hemorrhagic cystitis. *Pediatr Infect Dis J.* 1996;15:633-634.
65. Mufson MA, Belshe RB. A review of adenoviruses in the etiology of acute hemorrhagic cystitis. *J Urol.* 1976;115:191-194.
66. Harnett GB, Phillips PA, Gollow MM. Association of genital adenovirus infection with urethritis in men. *Med J Aust.* 1984;141:337-338.
67. Swenson PD, Lowens MS, Celum CL, et al. Adenovirus types 2, 8, and 37 associated with genital infections in patients attending a sexually transmitted disease clinic. *J Clin Microbiol.* 1995;33:2728-2731.
68. Soeur M, Wouters A, de Saint-Georges A, et al. Meningoencephalitis and meningitis due to an adenovirus type 5 in two immunocompetent adults. *Acta Neurol Belg.* 1991;91:141-150.
69. Fianchi L, Scardocci A, Cattani P, et al. Adenovirus meningoencephalitis in a patient with large B-cell lymphoma. *Ann Hematol.* 2003;82:313-315.
70. Martin AB, Webber S, Fricker FJ, et al. Acute myocarditis: rapid diagnosis by PCR in children. *Circulation.* 1994;90:330-339.
71. Bowles NE, Ni J, Kearney DL, et al. Detection of viruses in myocardial tissues by polymerase chain reaction: evidence of adenovirus as a common cause of myocarditis in children and adults. *J Am Coll Cardiol.* 2003;42:466-472.
72. Sakata H, Taketazu G, Nagaya K, et al. Outbreak of severe infection due to adenovirus type 7 in a paediatric ward in Japan. *J Hosp Infect.* 1998;39:207-211.
73. Fraser KJ, Clarris BJ, Muirden KD, et al. A persistent adenovirus type 1 infection in synovial tissue from an immunodeficient patient with chronic, rheumatoid-like polyarthritis. *Arthritis Rheum.* 1985;28:455-458.
74. Niemann TH, Trigg ME, Winick N, et al. Disseminated adenoviral infection presenting as acute pancreatitis. *Hum Pathol.* 1993;24:1145-1148.
75. Munoz FM, Piedra PA, Demmler GJ. Disseminated adenovirus disease in immunocompromised and immunocompetent children. *Clin Infect Dis.* 1998;27:1194-1200.
76. Abzug MJ, Levin MJ. Neonatal adenovirus infection: four patients and review of the literature. *Pediatrics.* 1991;87:890-896.
77. Shields AF, Hackman RC, Fife KH, et al. Adenovirus infections in patients undergoing bone-marrow transplantation. *N Engl J Med.* 1985;312:529-533.
78. Howard DS, Phillips IG, Reece DE, et al. Adenovirus infections in hematopoietic stem cell transplant recipients. *Clin Infect Dis.* 1999;29:1494-1501.
79. Muller WJ, Levin MJ, Shin YK, et al. Clinical and in vitro evaluation of cidofovir for treatment of adenovirus infection in pediatric hematopoietic stem cell transplant recipients. *Clin Infect Dis.* 2005;41:1812-1816.
80. van Tol MJ, Kroes AC, Schinkel J, et al. Adenovirus infection in paediatric stem cell transplant recipients: increased risk in young children with a delayed immune recovery. *Bone Marrow Transpl.* 2005;36:39-50.
81. Kojaoghlanian T, Flomenberg P, Horwitz MS. The impact of adenovirus infection on the immunocompromised host. *Rev Med Virol.* 2003;13:155-171.
82. van Tol MJ, Claas EC, Heemskerk B, et al. Adenovirus infection in children after allogeneic stem cell transplantation: diagnosis, treatment and immunity. *Bone Marrow Transpl.* 2005;35:S73-S76.
83. de Mezerville MH, Tellier R, Richardson S, et al. Adenoviral infections in pediatric transplant recipients: a hospital-based study. *Pediatr Infect Dis J.* 2006;25:815-818.
84. Lion T, Baumgartinger R, Watzinger F, et al. Molecular monitoring of adenovirus in peripheral blood after allogeneic bone marrow transplantation permits early diagnosis of disseminated disease. *Blood.* 2003;102:1114-1120.
85. Sivaprakasam P, Carr TF, Coussons M, et al. Improved outcome from invasive adenovirus infection in pediatric patients after hemopoietic stem cell transplantation using intensive clinical surveillance and early intervention. *J Pediatr Hematol Oncol.* 2007;29:81-85.
86. Schilham MW, Claas EC, van Zaane W, et al. High levels of adenovirus DNA in serum correlate with fatal outcome of adenovirus infection in children after allogeneic stem-cell transplantation. *Clin Infect Dis.* 2002;35:526-532.
87. Echavarria M, Forman M, van Tol MJ, et al. Prediction of severe disseminated adenovirus infection by serum PCR. *Lancet.* 2001;358:384-385.
88. Leruez-Ville M, Minard V, Lacaille F, et al. Real-time blood plasma polymerase chain reaction for management of disseminated adenovirus infection. *Clin Infect Dis.* 2004;38:45-52.
89. Humar A, Kumar D, Mazzulli T, et al. A surveillance study of adenovirus infection in adult solid organ transplant recipients. *Am J Transplant.* 2005;5:2555-2559.
90. Ohori NP, Michaels MG, Jaffe R, et al. Adenovirus pneumonia in lung transplant recipients. *Hum Pathol.* 1995;26:1073-1079.
91. Doan ML, Mallory GB, Kaplan SL, et al. Treatment of adenovirus pneumonia with cidofovir in pediatric lung transplant recipients. *J Heart Lung Transplant.* 2007;26:883-889.
92. Stalder H, Hierholzer JC, Oxman MN. New human adenovirus (candidate adenovirus type 35) causing fatal disseminated infection in a renal transplant recipient. *J Clin Microbiol.* 1977;6:257-265.
93. Khoo SH, Bailey AS, de Jong JC, et al. Adenovirus infections in human immunodeficiency virus-positive patients: clinical features and molecular epidemiology. *J Infect Dis.* 1995;172:629-637.
94. Hierholzer JC, Wigand R, Anderson LJ, et al. Adenoviruses from patients with AIDS: a plethora of serotypes and a description of five new serotypes of subgenus D (types 43-47). *J Infect Dis.* 1988;158:804-813.
95. Krilov LR, Rubin LG, Frogel M, et al. Disseminated adenovirus infection with hepatic necrosis in patients with human immunodeficiency virus infection and other immunodeficiency states. *Rev Infect Dis.* 1990;12:303-307.
96. Anders KH, Park CS, Cornford ME, et al. Adenovirus encephalitis and widespread ependymitis in a child with AIDS. *Pediatr Neurosurg.* 1990;16:316-320.
97. Shintaku M, Nasu K, Ito M. Necrotizing tubulo-interstitial nephritis induced by adenovirus in an AIDS patient. *Histopathology.* 1993;23:588-590.
98. Wold WSM, Horwitz MS. Adenoviruses. In: Knipe DM, Howley PM, eds. *Fields Virology.* 5th ed. Philadelphia: Lippincott Williams & Wilkins; 2007:2395-2436.
99. Gleaves CA, Militoni J, Ashley RL. An enzyme immunoassay for the direct detection of adenovirus in clinical specimens. *Diagn Microbiol Infect Dis.* 1993;17:57-59.
100. Shetty AK, Treynor E, Hill DW, et al. Comparison of conventional viral cultures with direct fluorescent antibody stains for diagnosis of community-acquired respiratory virus infections in hospitalized children. *Pediatr Infect Dis J.* 2003;22:789-794.
101. Ebner K, Suda M, Watzinger F, et al. Molecular detection and quantitative analysis of the entire spectrum of human adenoviruses by a two-reaction real-time PCR assay. *J Clin Microbiol.* 2005;43:3049-3053.
102. Casas I, Avellon A, Mosquera M, et al. Molecular identification of adenoviruses in clinical samples by analyzing a partial hexon genomic region. *J Clin Microbiol.* 2005;43:6176-6182.
103. Echavarria M, Sanchez JL, Kolavic-Gray SA, et al. Rapid detection of adenovirus in throat swab specimens by PCR during respiratory disease outbreaks among military recruits. *J Clin Microbiol.* 2003;41:810-812.
104. Becroft DM. Histopathology of fatal adenovirus infection of the respiratory tract in young children. *J Clin Pathol.* 1967;20:561-569.
105. Chakrabarti S, Mautner V, Osman H, et al. Adenovirus infections following allogeneic stem cell transplantation: incidence and outcome in relation to graft manipulation, immunosuppression, and immune recovery. *Blood.* 2002;100:1619-1627.
106. Heemskerk B, Veltrop-Duits LA, van Vreeswijk T, et al. Extensive cross-reactivity of $CD4^+$ adenovirus-specific T cells: implications for immunotherapy and gene therapy. *J Virol.* 2003;77:6562-6566.
107. de Oliveira CB, Stevenson D, LaBree L, et al. Evaluation of cidofovir (HPMPC, GS-504) against adenovirus type 5 infection in vitro and in a New Zealand rabbit ocular model. *Antiviral Res.* 1996;31:165-172.
108. Kinchington PR, Romanowski EG , Jerold Gordon Y. Prospects for adenovirus antivirals. *J Antimicrob Chemother.* 2005;55:424-429.
109. Yusuf U, Hale GA, Carr J, et al. Cidofovir for the treatment of adenoviral infection in pediatric hematopoietic stem cell transplant patients. *Transplantation.* 2006;81:1398-1404.
110. Ljungman P, Ribaud P, Eyrich M, et al. Cidofovir for adenovirus infections after allogeneic hematopoietic stem cell transplantation: a survey by the Infectious Diseases Working Party of the European Group for Blood and Marrow Transplantation. *Bone Marrow Transpl.* 2003;31:481-486.
111. Nagafuji K, Aoki K, Henzan H, et al. Cidofovir for treating adenoviral hemorrhagic cystitis in hematopoietic stem cell transplant recipients. *Bone Marrow Transpl.* 2004;34:909-914.
112. Hromas R, Clark C, Blanke C, et al. Failure of ribavirin to clear adenovirus infections in T cell-depleted allogeneic bone marrow transplantation. *Bone Marrow Transpl.* 1994;14:663-664.
113. Lankester AC, Heemskerk B, Claas EC, et al. Effect of ribavirin on the plasma viral DNA load in patients with disseminating adenovirus infection. *Clin Infect Dis.* 2004;38:1521-1525.
114. Morfin F, Dupuis-Girod S, Mundweiler S, et al. In vitro susceptibility of adenovirus to antiviral drugs is species-dependent. *Antiviral Ther.* 2005;10:225-229.
115. Kitabayashi A, Hirokawa M, Kuroki J, et al. Successful vidarabine therapy for adenovirus type 11-associated acute hemorrhagic cystitis after allogeneic bone marrow transplantation. *Bone Marrow Transpl.* 1994;14:853-854.
116. Feuchtinger T, Matthes-Martin S, Richard C, et al. Safe adoptive transfer of virus-specific T-cell immunity for the treatment of systemic adenovirus infection after allogeneic stem cell transplantation. *Br J Haematol.* 2006;134:64-76.
117. Feuchtinger T, Richard C, Joachim S, et al. Clinical grade generation of hexon-specific T cells for adoptive T-cell transfer as a treatment of adenovirus infection after allogeneic stem cell transplantation. *J Immunother.* 2008;31:199-206.
118. Leen AM, Myers GD, Bollard CM, et al. T-cell immunotherapy for adenoviral infections of stem-cell transplant recipients. *Ann N Y Acad Sci.* 2005;1062:104-115.
119. Crooks BN, Taylor CE, Turner AJ, et al. Respiratory viral infections in primary immune deficiencies: significance and relevance to clinical outcome in a single BMT unit. *Bone Marrow Transpl.* 2000;26:1097-1102.
120. Dagan R, Schwartz RH, Insel RA, et al. Severe diffuse adenovirus 7a pneumonia in a child with combined immunodeficiency: possible therapeutic effect of human immune serum globulin containing specific neutralizing antibody. *Pediatr Infect Dis.* 1984;3:246-251.
121. Kolavic-Gray SA, Binn LN, Sanchez JL, et al. Large epidemic of adenovirus type 4 infection among military trainees: epidemiological, clinical, and laboratory studies. *Clin Infect Dis.* 2002;35:808-818.
122. Lyons A, Longfield J, Kuschner R, et al. A double-blind, placebo-controlled study of the safety and immunogenicity of live, oral type 4 and type 7 adenovirus vaccines in adults. *Vaccine.* 2008;26:2890-2898.
123. Grubb BR, Pickles RJ, Ye H, et al. Inefficient gene transfer by adenovirus vector to cystic fibrosis airway epithelia of mice and humans. *Nature.* 1994;371:802-806.
124. Schnell MA, Zhang Y, Tazelaar J, et al. Activation of innate immunity in nonhuman primates following intraportal administration of adenoviral vectors. *Mol Ther.* 2001;3:708-722.
125. Raper SE, Chirmule N, Lee FS, et al. Fatal systemic inflammatory response syndrome in an ornithine transcarbamylase deficient patient following adenoviral gene transfer. *Mol Genet Metab.* 2003;80:148-158.
126. Barouch DH. Challenges in the development of an HIV-1 vaccine. *Nature.* 2008;455:613-619.
127. Roth JA. Adenovirus p53 gene therapy. *Expert Opin Biol Ther.* 2006;6:55-61.
128. Nemunaitis J, Khuri F, Ganly I, et al. Phase II trial of intratumoral administration of ONYX-015, a replication-selective adenovirus, in patients with refractory head and neck cancer. *J Clin Oncol.* 2001;19:289-298.

144

Papillomaviruses

WILLIAM BONNEZ | RICHARD C. REICHMAN

Papillomaviruses have been detected in a variety of higher vertebrates. *Human papillomaviruses* (HPVs) are widespread throughout the population, produce epithelial tumors of the skin and mucous membranes, and have been closely associated with genital tract malignant diseases. HPVs are strictly species specific, and cross-species infections do not occur even in experimental conditions. The infectious nature of human warts was initially seen in the late 19th century when human wart extracts were shown to produce warts with injection into humans. Ciuffo[1] suggested that the infectious agent of warts was a virus after he was able to transmit the infection through cell-free filtrates in 1907. Despite these early observations, HPVs have not been studied with standard virologic techniques because they have not been propagated successfully in tissue culture or in standard laboratory animals. For this reason, much of our knowledge of the biology of HPVs and the diseases with which they are associated has depended on the use of molecular biologic techniques and, more recently, of organotypic cultures and complex animal models. These techniques have led to an understanding of the genomic organization of these viruses, the functions of different viral genes, and the multiplicity of HPV types. Detailed reviews of these subjects are available.[2-6]

Virology

Papillomaviruses constitute the *Papillomavirus* genus of the Papillomaviridae family. They are nonenveloped viruses that are 55 nm in diameter and have an icosahedral capsid composed of 72 capsomeres that enclose a double-stranded circular DNA genome. Virion particles contain at least two capsid proteins. The major capsid protein constitutes 80% of the virion by weight and has a molecular weight of about 56,000 daltons. The minor capsid protein has a molecular weight of approximately 76,000 daltons.

The HPV genome consists of approximately 7900 base pairs. All putative coding sequences (open reading frames [ORFs]) are arranged on one DNA strand, and all papillomaviruses share the same genomic organization.[5-7] Specific protein products are derived from these ORFs. However, analyses of viral messenger RNA (mRNA) transcripts suggest that most viral proteins derive from splicing of more than one ORF-specific mRNA. The genome is divided functionally into three regions. A noncoding upstream regulatory region contributes to the control of DNA replication and transcription of eight to nine ORFs that are divided into early (E1 to E7) and late (L1 and L2) regions.[5-7] E1 is involved in viral plasmid replication.[8] The E2 product is an important modulator of viral transcription and also plays a role in viral replication.[8] E4 proteins form filamentous cytoplasmic networks and share the same cellular distribution as cytokeratin intermediate filaments, with which they may interact. The E5 protein is located in the cellular membrane and prevents the acidification of endosomes.[2,9] It stimulates the transforming activity of the epidermal growth factor receptor and contributes to the oncogenicity of HPV.[7,8,10] The gene products of E6 and E7 of oncogenic HPV types have major transforming properties through the binding of various cellular factors and key tumor suppressor proteins.[2-4,6,7] The E6 protein binds to the p53 tumor suppressor gene product and abrogates its activity by accelerating its degradation. The E7 protein also binds to a tumor suppressor gene product, the retinoblastoma protein, and to related proteins, thus inhibiting their functions. Both E6 and E7 proteins can impede apoptosis. The L1 and L2 ORFs encode the major and minor capsid proteins, respectively.[6,7]

Although the genomes of several papillomaviruses can transform certain cell lines in tissue culture, only recently have both replication and propagation of HPV been possible in vitro, with use of organotypic culture systems.[7,11] In addition, HPV types 6, 11, 16, 40, and 59 have been propagated successfully in human skin grafted in the athymic (nude) mouse or the mouse with severe combined immunodeficiency.[12] HPV-infected grafts recovered from these animals can maintain viral particle production in vitro.

Virions of most HPV types cannot be purified from naturally occurring lesions in significant quantities, and well-characterized type-specific antigens have not been available until recently.[13] Therefore, types are determined according to the degree of nucleic acid sequence homology rather than with serologic techniques. Distinct HPV types share less than 90% of DNA sequences in the L1 ORF, and subtypes share between 90% and 98%.[14] HPVs belong to five of the 18 Papillomaviridae genera: alpha, beta, gamma, mu, and nu. A genus may be further divided into species. For example, HPV-16 is the representative type of species 9, which also includes types 31, 33, 35, 52, and 67. At least 111 HPV types have now been characterized, and many others have been recognized. HPVs are host-specific, and each type is, to a large extent, associated with a distinct histopathologic process (Table 144-1).

A broadly cross-reactive genus-specific antigenic determinant, located in the middle of the major capsid protein,[15] can be prepared with denaturation of viral particles, typically from bovine papillomavirus, with detergents and reducing agents. Antisera prepared against this papillomavirus common antigen have been used in the immunocytochemical diagnosis of HPV infections (see Diagnosis section).[16] The antigenic characteristics of native viral particles can also be studied with the use of virus-like particles (VLPs). These are obtained with the expression in eukaryotic systems of the L1 or L1 and L2 ORFs (see Prevention section). A close correlation appears to exist between genotype and serotype.[13]

Epidemiology

INCIDENCE AND PREVALENCE

Although clinical HPV infections are the most recognizable and most important for the patient and practitioner, subclinical and asymptomatic latent infections are probably most common, and past HPV infections represent an even larger group.[17-19] The study of these different types of infection poses different technical problems, and their respective interrelated epidemiologies are not equally well understood.

As Table 144-1 illustrates, HPV infections can also be divided according to predominant anatomic location. Thus, the genital or mucosal infections are recognized as distinct from the nongenital infections, which include the cutaneous infections.

Three types of cutaneous HPV infections are widespread throughout the general population.[20] Common warts, which represent up to 71% of all cutaneous warts, occur frequently among school-aged children, with prevalence rates of 4% to 20%.[21,22] Although less common (34% of cutaneous warts), plantar warts are observed frequently among adolescents and young adults. Juvenile or flat warts are the least common of the three types (4%) and occur predominantly in children. Other groups at high risk for the development of cutaneous warts include butchers, meat packers, and fish handlers.[23] Epidermodysplasia

TABLE 144-1	Human Papillomavirus Types and Their Disease Association	
	HPV Types*	
Disease	**Frequent Association**	**Less Frequent Association**
Plantar warts	1, 2	4, 63
Common warts	2, 1, 4	26,[†] 27, 29, 41,[‡] 57, 65, 77[‡]
Common warts of meat, poultry, and fish handlers	7, 2	1, 3, 4, 10, 28
Flat and intermediate warts	3, 10	26, 27,[†] 28, 38, 41,[‡] 49,[†] 75, 76
Epidermodysplasia verruciformis	5,[‡] 8,[‡] 9, 12, 14,[‡] 15, 17[‡]	19, 20,[‡§] 21, 22, 23, 24, 25, 36, 37, 38,[‡] 47,[‡] 49, 50, 93
Condylomata acuminata	6, 11	16,[‡] 18,[‡] 31,[‡] 33,[‡] 35,[‡] 40, 42, 43, 44, 45,[‡] 51,[‡] 52,[‡] 53,[‡] 54, 55, 56,[‡] 58,[‡] 59,[‡] 66, 68,[‡] 70
Intraepithelial neoplasia, unspecified		26,[‡] 30,[‡] 34, 39,[‡] 40, 53,[‡] 57, 59,[‡] 61, 62, 67,[‡] 68,[‡] 69, 71, 81, 83
Low-grade	6, 11	16,[‡] 18,[‡] 31,[‡] 33,[‡] 35,[‡] 42, 43, 44,[§] 45,[‡] 51,[‡] 52,[‡] 54, 61, 70, 72, 74[†]
High-grade	16,[‡] 18[‡]	6, 11, 31,[‡] 34,[‡] 33,[‡] 35,[‡] 39,[‡] 42, 44, 45,[‡] 51,[‡] 52,[‡] 56,[‡] 58,[‡] 66,[‡] 67[‡]
Cervical carcinoma	16,[‡] 18[‡]	31,[‡] 33,[‡] 35,[‡] 39,[‡] 45,[‡] 51,[‡] 52,[‡] 56,[‡] 58,[‡] 59,[‡] 66,[‡] 67,[‡] 68,[‡] 73,[†‡] 82[‡]
Recurrent respiratory papillomatosis	6, 11	16,[‡] 18,[‡] 31,[‡] 33,[‡] 35,[‡] 39[‡]
Focal epithelial hyperplasia of Heck	13, 32	18,[‡] 33,[‡] 45[‡]
Conjunctival papillomas and carcinomas	6, 11, 16[‡]	
Other cutaneous lesions[¶]		36, 37, 38,[‡] 41,[‡] 48,[†‡] 60, 72,[†] 88, 92, 93, 94, 95, 96, 107, 110, 111
Other genital lesions		30,[‡] 84,[‡] 85, 86,[‡] 87, 89, 90, 91, 97, 101, 102, 103, 106

*The distinction between frequent and less frequent association is arbitrary in many instances. Large descriptive statistics of HPV type distribution by disease are not available for most HPV types. Moreover, many HPV types have been looked for or identified only once.

[†]Types first recovered from patients with immunosuppression or immunodeficiency.

[‡]Types with high malignant potential or isolated in only one or a few lesions that were malignant.

[§]HPV-46 was found to be HPV-20, HPV-64 is a variant of HPV-34, and HPV-55 is HPV-44.

[¶]Includes epidermoid cysts, keratoacanthoma, laryngeal carcinoma, and malignant melanoma.

Information on HPV DNA sequences is available in GenBank and EMBL databases. In addition, older but extensive data are available on the World Wide Web at http://hpv-web.lanl.gov/HTML_FILES/HPVcompintro4.html. Note that the sequence information on some of the newer genotypes is not yet available.

verruciformis is a rare, typically autosomal recessive condition characterized by the appearance early in life of disseminated cutaneous warts and frequent malignant transformation.[24]

An estimated 6.2 million genital HPV infections occurred in the age group 15 years to 44 years in the United States in 2000.[25] These infections are the most commonly acquired viral sexually transmitted infections (STIs). Accordingly, 20 million Americans are likely infected and contagious. More accurate assessments come from direct surveys of the U.S. population. In a sample of 1921 females aged 14 to 59 years, the overall prevalence rate of cervical HPV DNA was 27%. Three fifths of these were high-risk types for cervical neoplasms.[26] Most of the sexually active population is likely to be infected in a lifetime.[17]

The prevalence rate of condyloma acuminatum (plural, condylomata acuminata), or anogenital warts (venereal warts), in the general population is approximately 1%.[17] In a U.S. survey of 18-year-olds to 59-year-olds, 5.6% reported having had genital warts.[27] The incidence of the disease has risen. The annual number of initial visits to physicians' offices for genital warts almost doubled between 2000 and 2006, from 220,000 to 422,000.[28] Smaller studies in better-defined populations of patients have also shown dramatic increases in the prevalence of this disease.[29] Approximately 500,000 persons each year are estimated to acquire symptomatic genital warts.[30] HPV infection of the cervix gives rise to the most common cause of squamous cell abnormalities on Papanicolaou (Pap) smears.[31]

The incidence rate of recurrent respiratory papillomatosis, which is primarily a disease of the larynx, is estimated to be 4.3 per 100,000/year for the juvenile-onset form of the disease and 1.8 per 100,000/year for the adult-onset form.[32] Prevalence rates are about 2-fold to 9-fold more.[32]

TRANSMISSION

Close personal contact is assumed to be important for the transmission of most cutaneous warts, although strong epidemiologic evidence for this assumption is lacking.[23,33] Minor trauma at the site of inoculation may also be important, as suggested by the high frequency of disease among meat handlers.[23]

Evidence that anogenital warts are sexually transmitted includes the observations that the age of onset is similar to that in other sexually transmitted diseases (STDs) and that the disease develops in approximately two thirds of sexual contacts of patients with anogenital warts.[34,35] In addition, patients with anogenital warts often have other concomitant STDs or a history of such infections. Also, as outlined in Table 144-1, particular HPV types are associated with these lesions. These types are rarely found at other sites. Finally, a large number of sexual partners is associated with greater risk of condylomata acuminata or HPV infection of the cervix.[17,36,37] Despite these observations in adults, young children may acquire genital warts from hand contact with nongenital lesions.[38] Approximately one fifth of prepubertal children with condyloma acuminatum have HPV type 1 or 2 in the lesions.[39-41] Conversely, HPV-6 DNA has been identified in cutaneous warts of family contacts of children with anogenital warts.[40]

In adults, estimates of the rate of HPV transmission (expressed as number of events per 100 person months) are 4.9 from penis to cervix and 17.4 from cervix to penis.[42]

Recurrent respiratory papillomatosis in young children is thought to be acquired via passage through an infected birth canal.[32] This hypothesis is based on the observations that similar HPV types are associated with both respiratory papillomatosis and anogenital warts and that a large percentage of the mothers of these children have a history of genital tract HPV disease.[32] In addition, neonates are more likely to harbor HPV DNA in the oral cavity if the cervix of the mother contains HPV DNA.[32] Many children with recurrent respiratory papillomatosis are first-born babies who were delivered vaginally to young (often teenaged) mothers. Although the median age of onset of recurrent respiratory papillomatosis is 3 years, cases have been documented at birth, even after cesarean section.[32] This observation suggests that the disease may be acquired in utero, probably via ascending infection from the mother's genital tract. The role of cesarean section, if any, in prevention of transmission is unknown, and the procedure is not recommended for that purpose.[32] Family members and others with close personal contact with these patients are not at risk for development of the disease. In the adult-onset form, recurrent respiratory papillomatosis is associated with a higher than expected number of lifetime sexual partners and with oral-genital contact.[32]

The role of fomites in the transmission of HPV infection is uncertain. However, nosocomial transmission appears possible because infectious virus can be recovered from the fumes released from lesions during treatment with carbon dioxide laser or electrocoagulation.[43] In addition, HPVs are resistant to heat, and use of an autoclave is probably necessary for sterilization of contaminated instruments.[44,45]

ASSOCIATION BETWEEN HUMAN PAPILLOMAVIRUS AND MALIGNANT DISEASES

The oncogenic potential of animal papillomaviruses was shown many years ago.[46] Observations of patients with epidermodysplasia verruciformis provided the initial evidence that suggested that HPVs might also be carcinogenic. In these patients, characteristic skin lesions induced by specific HPV types frequently undergo malignant transformation, particularly when they occur in sun-exposed areas.[24] Most research investigating the oncogenic potential of HPVs has focused on genital tract malignant diseases.

The low prevalence of cancer of the uterine cervix among Catholic nuns,[47] the direct association of risk with number of sexual partners, and the increased risk of malignant disease that is associated with a male sexual partner whose previous consort had cervical cancer have been observations consistent with a sexually transmitted agent playing a role in the pathogenesis of cervical cancer.[48-50] Among several agents, herpes simplex virus type 2 (HSV-2) was once strongly suspected. However, over the past 30 years, a large and coherent body of biologic and epidemiologic observations has shown that HPV infection is the necessary, if not sufficient, cause of cervical cancer.[51] This evidence can be summarized as follows:

1. The association between those HPV types called high-risk oncogenic (see Table 144-1) and cervical cancer is strong, with odds ratios that range from 50 to 100 fold. For the most oncogenic of these viruses, HPV-16 for squamous cell carcinoma (SCC) and HPV-18 for adenocarcinoma, the odds ratios range from 100 to 900. In a worldwide survey, HPV DNA was found in 99.7% of cervical cancer samples.[52]
2. The association has been consistent through many studies done in different countries and populations.
3. The association has been specific, so that among the approximately 40 HPV types associated with the genitalia, or more broadly, the mucosal surfaces, only a subset of the types (at least 15) are oncogenic for the cervix. In addition, the same HPV types, with sometimes slightly different frequencies, are found in other SCCs. Forty percent of carcinomas of the vulva, vagina, and penis are associated with HPV.[53] This association is much higher if only warty and basaloid histologic variants of these tumors are considered. HPV is found in 90% of anal SCCs. Moreover, up to 60% of oropharyngeal cancers might be attributed to high-risk HPV, with 95% HPV-16 or HPV-18.[54]

   HPV-16 has been found in some SCCs of the conjunctiva and of the nail bed.

   The HPV types found in the SCCs of patients with epidermodysplasia verruciformis have also been found in about a third of SCCs and basal cell carcinomas in immunocompetent hosts and in up to 80% of immunosuppressed hosts. Nevertheless, the biologic basis of this association is still uncertain.[55]
4. The development of cervical abnormalities and cancer is preceded by HPV infection. Most HPV infections are transient and last a mean of 13.5 months for high-risk HPVs and 4.8 months for low-risk types. However, between 15% and 30% of women with normal cervical cytology, but high-risk HPV infection, have cervical intraepithelial neoplasia (CIN) grades 2 or 3 develop in the following 4 years. Conversely, CIN 2 or 3 is unlikely to develop in women with milder cytologic squamous abnormalities who are negative for high-risk HPV. Although clearance of HPV DNA appears to precede clearance of cervical lesions, persistence of HPV DNA after treatment for CIN 2 or 3 is a predictor of relapse.

   The temporal association between HPV and cervical premalignant lesions has proven to be useful for prevention strategies. Hence, HPV testing is more sensitive than repeated cervical cytology in identification of women with atypical squamous cells of unknown significance (ASC-US) than those with CIN 2 or 3.

   The number of sexual partners, the age of first sexual intercourse, and the sexual behavior of the husband are risk factors for HPV infections and also for cervical cancer, which occurs later in life. This temporal sequence is consistent with a causal link between infection and cancer.
5. In some studies, a direct association is found between viral load and the risk of cancer, which is consistent with a biologic gradient.
6. Several lines of biologic evidence support an oncogenic role for HPV. Virtually all neoplastic cells in cervical cancer tissue contain HPV DNA, including metastases. The E6 and E7 genes are expressed at higher levels in neoplasms than in benign lesions. When the E6 or E7 genes of high-risk HPV types are introduced in normal cells, they cause malignant transformation in cell culture. Transgenic animals carrying these genes have SCCs develop. The role of E6 and E7 genes proteins is further discussed in the Pathogenesis section.
7. Papillomaviruses can cause cancer in animal experimental models, such as the cottontail rabbit papillomavirus (CRPV) in the domestic rabbit and bovine papillomaviruses in the cow. Moreover, human neonatal foreskin grafts infected with HPV-16 and placed in severe combined immunodeficiency (SCID) mice develop intraepithelial neoplasias.[56]
8. Other alternative risk factors for cervical cancer, such as the use of oral contraceptives, high parity, tobacco smoking, nutrition (vitamins C and E, carotenoids, xanthophylls), immunosuppression, prior HSV-2 or *Chlamydia trachomatis* infection, have not reached the strength and coherence of the evidence gathered for HPV. Their contribution may be only secondary to the primary role played by HPV infection.
9. Finally, the clinical trials of the HPV vaccine (see Prevention section) have amply shown that immunization against HPV types 6, 11, 16, and 18 confers protection not only against subsequent infection but also against disease (warts and intraepithelial neoplasias of all grades) caused by the homologous genotype in the cervix, vagina, and vulva and in the external male genitalia, although for warts only at that site.

⬛ Pathogenesis

The pathogenesis of HPV disease has been reviewed by several authors.[2-4,6-10,57-59] The incubation period was established experimentally with inoculation of human subjects with extracts of cutaneous warts.[1,60] Most often, warts developed within 3 to 4 months, although lesions occasionally grew as early as 6 weeks or as long as 2 years after inoculation. A similar incubation period was observed for genital warts among wives of American soldiers returning from the Korean War.[61] All types of squamous epithelium may be infected by HPV, but with the exception of the cervical glandular epithelium, other tissues appear to be resistant to productive infection. Gross histologic appearances of individual lesions vary with the site of infection and the virus type. Figure 144-1 is a schematic diagram of a typical exophytic cutaneous wart.

Although little is known about the first stage of HPV infection, the virus replicative cycle is assumed to begin with the entry of particles into the stratum germinativum (basale) because viral DNA is detected in the nuclei of the basal cells.[58,59] As the basal cells differentiate and progress to the surface of the epithelium, HPV DNA replicates and is transcribed, and viral particles are assembled in the nucleus. Ultimately, complete virions are released, probably still tightly associated with the remnants of the shed dead keratinocyte shell.[62] In a wart or condyloma, viral replication is associated with excessive proliferation of all of the epidermal layers except the basal layer. This process produces acanthosis, parakeratosis, and hyperkeratosis. A deepening of the rete ridges, where normally present, produces the typical papillomatous cytoarchitecture. Some infected cells undergo the characteristic transformation of koilocytosis. With histology, koilocytes (from the Greek *koilos*, "cavity") are large, usually polygonal, squamous cells with a shrunken nucleus lodged inside a large cytoplasmic vacuole. Cytoplasmic keratohyalin inclusion bodies may also be observed. Excessive proliferation of the basal-like cells (basaloid proliferation)

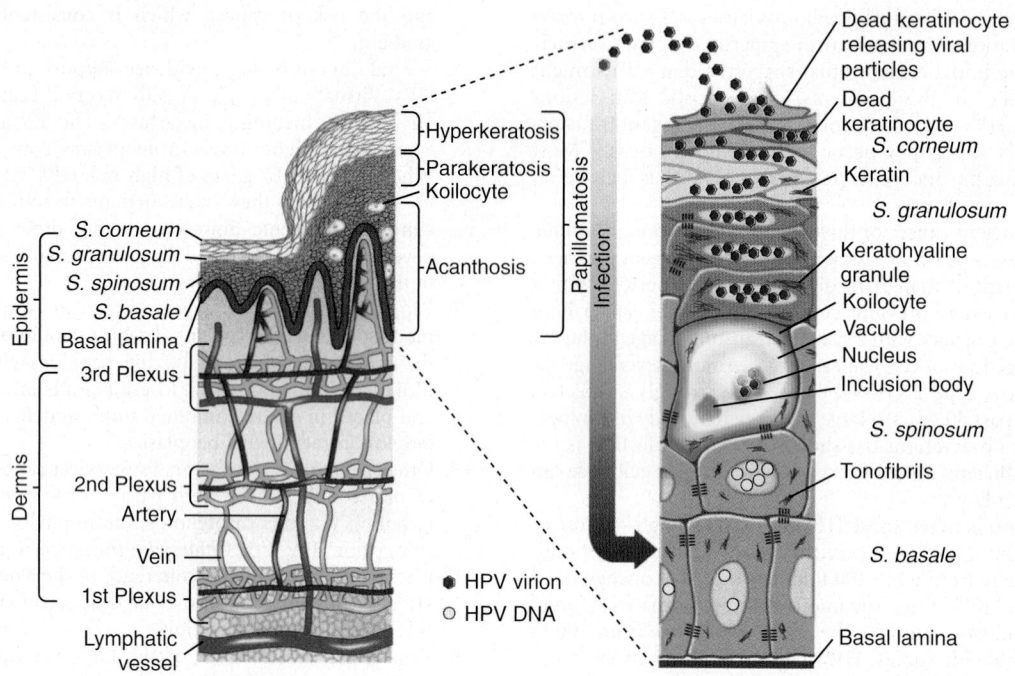

Figure 144-1 Exophytic cutaneous wart: human papillomavirus (HPV) pathogenesis. **A,** Histologic features. **B,** Cytologic features (see text for details). *S.,* Stratum.

with a high nuclear/cytoplasmic ratio, accompanied by a high number of mitoses, some abnormal (dyskaryosis), is a feature of incipient and malignant HPV disease.

Normal-appearing epithelium may contain HPV DNA,[63,64] and the presence of residual DNA after the treatment of warts may lead to recurrent disease. In benign lesions caused by HPV, viral DNA is located extrachromosomally in the nuclei of infected cells. However, when HPV DNA is detected in high-grade intraepithelial neoplasias and cancers, it is generally integrated.[4,7,59] Integration of HPV DNA may occur at preferential sites in host cell chromosomes,[3] and it specifically disrupts the E2 ORF. Interruption of E2 probably plays a role in the pathogenesis of malignant disease because expression of this ORF normally leads to downregulation of E6 and E7, whose products interfere with the p53 and retinoblastoma tumor suppressor proteins (see Virology section).[2-4,7,10,57] Nevertheless, the frequency of viral integration varies with the HPV genotype and does not appear to be necessary for oncogenesis.[57] Other events are also important, including hypermethylation of viral and cellular DNA; inhibition of apoptosis and telomerase activation, which both confer immortality; and cooperation with activated cellular oncogenes. The development of chromosomal instability and deletions (6p, 3p, 4p, 6q, 10p, and ultimately 11q) occur as the lesion becomes a high-grade intraepithelial neoplasia.[4,7,59]

Host defense responses to HPV infection are poorly understood. Nevertheless, several clinical observations suggest that an effective immune system is important in the resolution of HPV infection. HPV diseases occur frequently and are often severe in patients with both primary and secondary immunodeficiencies (e.g., Wiskott-Aldrich syndrome, common variable immunodeficiency).[65] Severe frequent HPV disease is also seen in patients with lymphoproliferative disorders and in those with human immunodeficiency virus (HIV) infections.[66-69] The range of HPV-related diseases in HIV infection includes cutaneous warts, anogenital warts, CIN in women, and anal intraepithelial neoplasia and cancer in men who have sex with men (MSM).[66,70,71] HIV infection increases by 4-fold to 40-fold the inci-

dence and prevalence rates of genital warts and CIN.[70] The prevalence of these conditions is greater with low counts of CD4+ T lymphocytes and high HIV-1 RNA levels. Compared with subjects with HIV seronegativity, patients with AIDS have an increased risk for the development of in situ or invasive squamous cell carcinomas of the cervix, vulva-vagina, anus (both genders), and penis.[72] Contrary to the expectation that led to the inclusion of cervical cancer as an AIDS-defining illness, the progression to AIDS does not appear to augment the risk of cervical cancer.[72-74] This could reflect better appreciation among health care providers for disease in women and earlier detection of more easily treated lesions.[74] However, the same observation has been made with anal cancer for which preventive measures appear less likely to have had a large impact.[74] Immunosuppressive therapy, notably in renal allograft recipients, has also been associated with high rates of extensive HPV infection.[68,69] Another indication of the role of the immune system comes from the observation that the regression of a wart may be promptly followed by the spontaneous regression of others.[75,76] Although the relative immunosuppression of pregnancy appears to be associated with an increased incidence and severity of HPV disease,[35,77] rates of HPV infection are not clearly found to be substantially higher in this population than in nonpregnant women.[78-80]

The frequency, severity, and persistence of HPV infections and diseases in patients with immunocompromise strongly argue for a determinant role of the immune system, especially its cellular arm.[74,81] Unfortunately, our understanding of the immune system in HPV infections is limited.[80a] Epidermodysplasia verruciformis is a genodermatosis that results from the inactivation of two genes, *EVER1/TMC6* and *EVER2/TMC8*, that code for endoplasmic transporter proteins. Mutations that affect the CXCR4 chemokine receptor or the Janus kinase-3 genes have been described in patients with extensive verrucosis. Evidence also shows that HPV-16 E6 and E7 proteins may inhibit the toll-like receptor (TLR) 9, a component of innate immunity.

The cell proliferation induced by HPV is also associated with increased leukocyte trafficking and angiogenesis, which is the result of the production of numerous cytokines and chemokines, including tumor necrosis factor-α (TNF-α); monocyte chemotactic protein-1 (MCP-1); chemokine CCL27; vascular endothelial cell growth factor (VEGF); interferons α, β, and γ; interferon-γ-inducible protein 10 (IP-10), CXCL10; retinoic acid; and tumor growth factor-β.[2,4,7]

These molecular changes highlight the importance of the adaptive and native immune system in controlling HPV disease. Concomitantly, at the histologic level, an alteration is seen in the number and function of the natural killer and helper T cells and cutaneous Langerhans cells.[82,83] These cells contribute to the local and systemic immune response, which becomes more apparent in regressing warts, as they show a clear lymphomononuclear cell infiltrate.[84]

A humoral and cellular immune response does develop after HPV infection, but its laboratory correlates are not necessarily uniform or constant. The E7 and L1 proteins are the strongest antigens.[85-87] The enhancement after immunization of antibody formation against the L1 native protein has been exploited to produce the first currently available vaccine (see Prevention section).

The ability of HPV infections and diseases to persist and progress can be explained in part by the ability of the E5, E6, and E7 proteins to suppress the immune system at different levels.[88] Immunogenetic factors are also important. In a large case-control study of the association of human leukocyte antigen (HLA) classes A, B, and C, DRB1, and DQB1 alleles and cervical SCC, several low-magnitude (about two-fold or less) associations were observed.[89] For example, HLA class I allele A*0301 increased the risk, and B*1501 decreased it. Similarly, HLA class II allele DQB1*0301 was a risk, and DRB1*1302 was protective. A particular combination of alleles, B*4402-DRB1*1101-DQB1*1302 increased the risk 10-fold. The same immunogenetic risk factors were noted with cervical adenocarcinoma and vulvar SCC. These results confirm the important role that helper and cytotoxic cell responses play in the development of HPV-associated genital cancer.

Clinical Manifestations

CUTANEOUS WARTS

Cutaneous warts include deep plantar warts, common warts, and plane or flat warts.[90,91]

Deep plantar warts (verrucae plantaris), also called *myrmecia* (from the Greek, meaning "ant hill"), affect mostly adolescents and young adults. The lesions characteristically look like raised bundles of soft keratotic fibers 2 mm to 1 cm in diameter; shaving reveals punctate, bleeding blood vessels. These lesions are often painful and may also be located on the palms of the hands.

Common warts (verrucae vulgaris) appear as well-demarcated, exophytic, hyperkeratotic papules with a rough surface. They may occur on the dorsum of the hand, between the fingers, around the nails (periungual warts), on the palms or soles, or rarely on mucous membranes. Warts may coalesce and reach a diameter of 1 cm. Morphologic variants of common warts include mosaic warts, which appear as cobblestone-like patches of aggregated warts several square centimeters in diameter and barely rising above an indurated base. Filiform warts on the head and vegetating, hyperproliferative warts on the hands of butchers, fish handlers, and meat packers also occur.[23]

Plane warts (verrucae planae) are commonly found on children and appear as multiple, slightly elevated papules with an irregular contour and distribution and a smooth surface. They occur on the face, neck, and hands. When more protuberant, these lesions are called *intermediate warts.*

Cutaneous warts are usually asymptomatic, although they may bleed and can be painful when located over weight-bearing surfaces or points of friction. Rarely, cutaneous warts may degenerate into verrucous carcinomas.[92] The natural history of cutaneous warts is poorly characterized. Spontaneous resolution appears to occur in 50% and 90% of children within 1 and 5 years, respectively.[20] In a given patient, two thirds of the warts that resolve spontaneously do so within 2 months.[93]

EPIDERMODYSPLASIA VERRUCIFORMIS

Epidermodysplasia verruciformis is an autosomal recessive genodermatosis linked to gene loci on chromosome 17.[81] The lesions are associated with a large array of HPV types (see Table 144-1), most of which are specific for epidermodysplasia verruciformis.[24,81] These warts have several morphologic variants. They may resemble flat warts but more commonly resemble lesions of pityriasis versicolor, which cover the torso and upper extremities. Over extensor surfaces, these warts may become hypertrophic and coalescent. In most patients, warts appear in the first decade of life. Beginning in young adulthood, in about one third of patients, the lesions undergo malignant transformation into invasive squamous cell carcinomas, particularly in sun-exposed areas. Although these patients may have depressed cellular immunity,[81] they appear to have normal resistance to other pathogens. Epidermodysplasia verruciformis does not appear to be contagious to healthy contacts. Of interest, lesions that resemble epidermodysplasia verruciformis are observed in solid organ allograft recipients.[19]

ANOGENITAL WARTS

Anogenital warts are flesh-colored to gray-colored, hyperkeratotic, exophytic papules, either sessile on the skin or, more frequently, attached by a short, broad peduncle (Fig. 144-2). Lesions range from smooth, pearly papules to more jagged, acuminate growths. They vary in size from less than a millimeter in diameter to several square centimeters when they merge into plaques. In uncircumcised men, the preputial cavity is involved in 85% to 90% of cases.[35,94] In the United States, where about 85% of the male population is circumcised, the penile shaft is the most common site of lesions. The urethral meatus

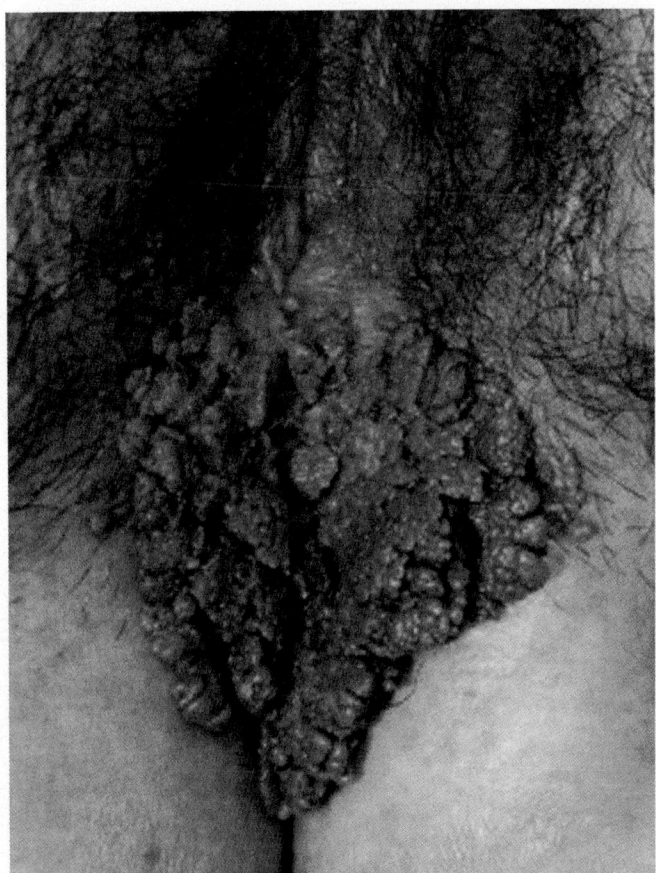

Figure 144-2 **Vulvar condylomata acuminata.** *(From Gagné H. Colposcopy of the vagina and vulva. Obstet Gynecol Clin North Am. 2008;35:659-669.)*

is also involved in 1% to 25% of patients.[95] Urethral warts are clearly visible with eversion of the meatus or with the use of a pediatric nasal speculum. They are mostly confined to the fossa navicularis or, less frequently, to the distal 3 cm of the urethra. Involvement of the bladder or proximal urethra is exceptional.[95] Involvement of the perianal area varies according to sexual practice, from very high among MSM (about 10%, and double with HIV seropositivity) to low among heterosexual men.[96,97] Lesions are only occasionally observed on the scrotum, perineum, groin, or pubic area.

In women, most lesions are distributed over the posterior introitus and, to a lesser degree, over the labia majora and minora and the clitoris (see Fig. 144-2). In order of decreasing frequency, the perineum, vagina, anus, cervix, and urethra each represent less than one quarter of the sites of involvement.[35]

The use of the colposcope and prior soaking of examined tissues with 3% to 5% acetic acid has expanded the clinical spectrum of anogenital warts, particularly those caused by HPV types 16 and 18, which can be small acetowhite papules.[98] This technique was initially used to show the existence of flat condylomas on the uterine cervix. Typically, these lesions are shiny white patches with poorly defined borders and an irregular surface that contains characteristic capillary loops.[99,100] The presence of external genital warts may indicate the existence of cervical HPV squamous epithelial lesions, including CIN.[101,102] Morphologic differentiation among the grades of cervical squamous epithelial lesions is not sufficiently reliable, and biopsy is strongly recommended for diagnosis.[103,104]

In the vagina, in addition to flat condylomas, small white nodosities centered on a capillary loop, called *spiked condylomas*, have been described.[105] The vulvar introitus may display prominent, sometimes painful, papillae whose relation to HPV infection is unlikely but controversial.[106,107] HPV infection of the vulva may also appear as white patches revealed or accentuated with the application of acetic acid, but acetowhitening lacks specificity.[108]

In men, acetic acid soaking or examination with a colposcope has shown HPV-infected papules and macules to be up to two times more common than exophytic condylomas, particularly on the prepuce and scrotum.[98,109] With a range in size from minuscule to 1 cm in diameter, round sessile papules with brown to slate blue pigmentation are encountered on both male (Fig. 144-3) and female external genitalia. These lesions, and similarly colored macules, are important to recognize because they may represent either HPV-6 or HPV-11 infected benign condylomas,[110,111] seborrheic keratoses,[112] or intraepithelial neoplasias associated with HPV type 16 or 18 infection.[111-113]

About three quarters of patients with anogenital warts are asymptomatic. However, itching and burning, pain, and tenderness are encountered frequently. In addition, the disease can have serious psy-

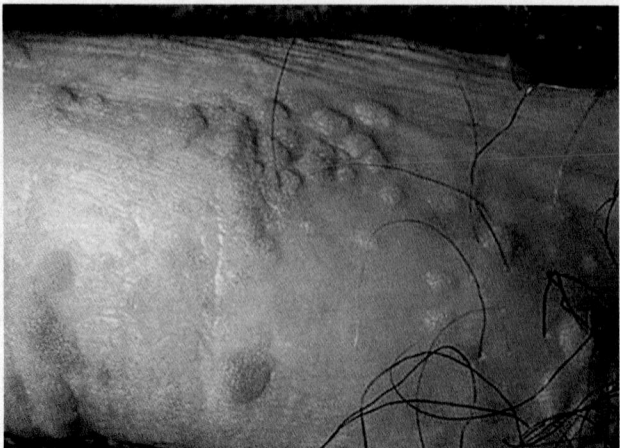

Figure 144-3 Pigmented penile warts mimicking bowenoid papulosis. *(From Habit TP, ed. Clinical Dermatology, 4th ed. London, Mosby, 2004.)*

chologic effects.[114] The natural history of genital warts, particularly of subclinical HPV disease, is poorly understood, but spontaneous remission may occur, as shown by the results of randomized, placebo-controlled therapeutic trials that indicate up to 10% to 20% spontaneous remission rates in untreated lesions over a 3-month to 4-month period.[115-119]

Exophytic genital warts may rarely transform into invasive squamous cell carcinomas, including verrucous carcinoma. They may also reach considerable size, particularly during pregnancy or immunosuppression.[120] When large condylomas reveal histologic features of local destructive invasion without metastases, they may be called *Buschke-Löwenstein tumors*, a term that regroups verrucous carcinomas and giant condylomas.[121-123] A related lesion, condylomatous (warty) carcinoma, may metastasize.[123] Genital HPV infections may also belong to the spectrum of penile, anal, vulvar, vaginal, and cervical intraepithelial neoplasias (PIN, AIN, VIN, VAIN, and CIN, respectively).[124,125] For historical reasons, some variants of intraepithelial neoplasias are further recognized. Histologically, pigmented papules of the external genitalia may show condylomatous cytoarchitecture with evidence of intraepithelial neoplasia.[111] This clinicopathologic entity is called *bowenoid papulosis* (see Fig. 144-3).[126] *Bowenoid papulosis* can evolve to *Bowen's disease*, which manifests as a flat red-to-brown plaque with well-demarcated borders and a scaly irregular surface.[127] On the glans penis, the lesion is known as *erythroplasia of Queyrat*. Histologically, carcinoma in situ is present. HPV-16 and HPV-18 have been recovered from both *bowenoid papulosis* and *Bowen's disease*.[128] The natural history of intraepithelial neoplasias is best understood in cervical lesions.[129] Clearly, the outcome (regression, no change, or progression) is highly variable and depends on the histologic grade of the tumor, the HPV type, and the method of diagnosis (conization, punch biopsy, or scraping). CIN grade 1 lesions have an approximate probability of 60% to regress, 30% to remain unchanged, 10% to progress to CIN 3, and 1% to progress to invasive cancer.[129] For CIN 2, the figures are 40%, 40%, 20%, and 5%, respectively. The risk of progression to cancer is the highest with CIN 3 at 12%; only a third of these lesions disappear spontaneously.

Perianal warts are common among homosexual men, and up to two thirds of patients with external anal warts also have internal lesions.[130] Consequently, the presence of perianal warts or anal symptoms in association with a history of anal sexual play or intercourse should prompt a digital rectal examination and an anoscopic evaluation. After the malignant transformation of anal condylomas was described,[131] the association between anorectal dysplasia or cancer and HPV infection was recognized in MSM.[132,133] Passive anal intercourse carries a risk of anal cancer in MSM, and heterosexual men and women with a history of anogenital warts have a 30-fold increased risk of disease compared with control populations.[134] The anus and the cervix have a different biology respective to HPV. HPV infections in women with and without HIV are 79% and 43% prevalent in the anus, respectively, but only 53% and 25% in the cervix.[135] In the general population, a history of anal warts increases by about 10 times the risk of anal cancer.[136] During pregnancy, HPV shedding may increase and condylomas may become so large as to impair normal delivery mechanically.[80,120,137] Anogenital warts in children should always raise the possibility of sexual abuse, but in very young children, nongenital or possibly perinatal transmission may be the predominant mode of acquisition.[138-140]

RECURRENT RESPIRATORY PAPILLOMATOSIS

Recurrent respiratory papillomatosis has been described by several authors.[32] Patients present with hoarseness or, in infants, with an altered cry. Sometimes these symptoms are accompanied by respiratory distress or stridor. The disease may spread to the trachea and lungs and lead to obstruction, infection, and respiratory failure. In young children, rapid growth of lesions often threatens the upper respiratory tract and frequently necessitates surgical excision to avoid asphyxiation. In adults, the course of the disease is usually less aggressive. Lesions may, however, undergo malignant transformation, particularly in patients who have received radiation therapy or in cases with lung involvement.

OTHER HUMAN PAPILLOMAVIRUS INFECTIONS

Oral squamous cell papillomas (or squamous papillomas) are the most common HPV-related oral lesions. A closely related entity, with slightly different histologic features, is oral condyloma acuminatum. Both types of lesions are caused by mucosal HPV (mostly HPV-6, HPV-11, and HPV-16). Oral verrucae vulgaris are rarer and can be differentiated reliably only with histology. They are caused by cutaneous HPVs (HPV-2, HPV-4, HPV-57).[141] Focal epithelial hyperplasia of the oral cavity (Heck's disease) is caused predominantly by HPV-3 and HPV-13 and tends to regress spontaneously.[142] Other HPV infections may also occur in the oral cavity.[142] Conjunctival HPV-related papillomas and SCCs, and periungual SCCs, have been described.[51] HPV DNA has also been identified in other skin lesions, such as epidermoid cysts, seborrheic keratoses (especially vulvar), skin squamous cell and basal carcinomas,[19] and aerodigestive carcinomas. The prevalence of HPV in these different lesions varies, which makes a causative link difficult to establish.

▣ Diagnosis

The diagnosis of warts is usually made clinically with physical examination. Exophytic warts have a characteristic appearance. Deep plantar warts may be confused with calluses, but paring usually reveals typical punctate, thrombosed capillaries. Nevi, seborrheic keratoses, acrochordons, acanthomas, molluscum contagiosum, lichen planus, syringomas, and dermofibromas may be confused with cutaneous warts. Lesions of epidermodysplasia verruciformis may be similar to those of flat warts or pityriasis versicolor, but the patient's history should clarify the diagnosis.

Condyloma acuminatum of the external anogenital tract should rarely be confused with other STDs such as condyloma latum of syphilis, nodular scabies, genital herpes, lymphogranuloma venereum, chancroid, or granuloma inguinale. Nevertheless, molluscum contagiosum, particularly in its more atypical presentations, may be difficult to distinguish from anogenital warts. In contrast to those of condyloma acuminatum, the lesions of molluscum contagiosum tend to predominate over the pubis and are rarely pedunculated but rather appear as smooth, sessile domes, the color of the skin or lighter, with a depressed center from which cheesy material can be expressed. In men, a normal anatomic variant of the corona, hirsutoid papillomatosis (pearly coronal papules, papillae corona glandis), can be difficult to differentiate from small warts. A similar anatomic presentation exists in the vulvar introitus, where lesions may appear identical to those of HPV-related vulvar papillomatosis. On the keratinized vulva, hidradenoma papilliferum may be confused with a large wart. On the scrotum, epidermoid cysts and angiokeratomas should be easy to identify. Small and flat HPV lesions may sometimes be difficult to distinguish from lichen planus, lichen sclerosus et atrophicus, lichen nitidus, or syringomas, even with the help of the colposcope and acetic acid application. Finally, pigmented HPV lesions may be confused with nevi or seborrheic keratoses (see Fig. 144-3).

Although initially designed for the evaluation of the female internal genital tract, the colposcope, with prior application for 3 to 5 minutes of a 3% to 5% acetic acid solution, has become an important diagnostic tool for other HPV infections as well.[143] In studies of male partners of women with either cervical condylomas or dysplasias, biopsy-proven genital condylomas were detected in 65% to 88% of the patients, respectively. More significantly, 43% to 73% of the lesions were seen only with a colposcope, whereas acetowhitening alone was used for the diagnosis in 22% of patients.[98,144,145] The same technique applied to the vulva revealed subclinical papillomavirus infection in 96% of women with vulvar warts and 80% of women who were partners of men with penile warts.[146] In the oral cavity, 83% of HPV lesions are seen only with the colposcope.[147] The clinical significance of lesions that are detectable with acetowhitening only is unknown, and aceto-

whitening lacks specificity for the diagnosis of HPV infection, particularly for external anogenital warts.[112,148,149]

Lesions of the external genitalia that are pigmented (see Fig. 144-3), appear as plaques, bleed, or are large should have biopsies to establish the diagnosis and rule out malignancy.[111] Biopsy is also indicated to confirm the diagnosis of epidermodysplasia verruciformis and to determine the cause of lesions of the oral cavity and upper airways.

Anoscopic examination should be considered in patients with perianal warts, anal symptoms, or a history of receptive anal intercourse. Most intraanal lesions are below the pectinate line, and sigmoidoscopy is not routinely indicated.[150,151] The oral cavity should be examined in all patients with anogenital warts because of the possibility of concomitant oral warts.[147]

Evaluation of the vagina and cervix, when appropriate, should include colposcopy and acetic acid application and should seek to rule out invasive cancer.[143] An international colposcopic terminology has now been developed, which should improve diagnostic accuracy and reliability.[100] Women with a history of anogenital HPV disease, or whose sexual partners have had anogenital HPV disease, should have a cytologic examination of a cervical smear (Pap smear), at least as part of regular screening (see Prevention section). Koilocytes on a cytologic smear are the hallmark of HPV infection.[152] More important, diagnoses of dysplasia and cancer can also be made from the smear.[153] Depending on the patient's age and the location and nature of the HPV infection, the sensitivity of the Pap smear in detection of HPV infection ranges from 30% to 90%.[154]

The use of the colposcope during the anoscopic examination (high-resolution anoscopy [HRA]) combined with anal cytology has been applied with success to the diagnosis of intraanal HPV infections.[155] It can be a screening tool for anal intraepithelial neoplasias in homosexual or bisexual males or in the female with HIV.[135,156-158] So far, only New York State recommends anal cytology and HRA for the management of women with HIV with high-grade intraepithelial neoplasia and of any patient with HIV with abnormal anal physical findings (http://www.hivguidelines.org). Nevertheless, this approach has yet to be validated with randomized, blinded, long-term studies of outcomes and costs.

A development in cervical cytology has been the introduction of a liquid-based collection technology.[153,159,160] Now that HPV DNA testing is part of the screening strategy, this technology allows the performance of both cytology and HPV DNA testing on the same sample.[159-161]

Cervical cytology has benefited from the development of the Bethesda system, last revised in 2001. This interpretation scheme addresses the adequacy of the specimen, classifies its pathologic features, and provides guidelines for management and follow-up, updated in 2006 (http://www.asccp.org/consensus.shtml).[160-162] HPV-related squamous cell abnormalities are regrouped in four categories: 1, atypical squamous cells (a) of undetermined significance (ASC-US) or (b) for which a high-grade squamous intraepithelial lesion (ASC-H) cannot be excluded; 2, low-grade squamous intraepithelial lesion (LSIL), a diagnosis that regroups the previous cytologic and histologic diagnoses of koilocytic or condylomatous atypia, mild dysplasia, and CIN 1; 3, high-grade squamous intraepithelial lesion (HSIL), previously including moderate and severe dysplasia, CIN 2 and CIN 3, and carcinoma in situ (CIS); and 4, squamous cell carcinoma (SCC).

The general histopathologic features of HPV infection are usually characteristic (see Pathogenesis section). Therefore, biopsy can be used to confirm most diagnoses. In addition, histologic examination can identify the presence of intraepithelial neoplasia or invasive cancer. Although histology is the gold standard, like cytology it suffers from lack of accuracy and reliability where disease grades are concerned.[153,163]

To enhance the sensitivity and specificity of cytohistopathology, several techniques are available, mostly in research settings.[164] These techniques rely on demonstration of either papillomavirus antigens or nucleic acids in biopsy specimens. The papillomavirus common antigen is usually detected with peroxidase-antiperoxidase immunocytochemical staining. It is present in about half of HPV lesions, although less frequently with HPV-16 or HPV-18 infections.[16]

Two HPV DNA detection tests, the Hybrid Capture II (Digene Corporation) and the Cervista HPV HR and HPV 16/18 (Hologic Inc.)

assays, are approved by the U.S. Food and Drug Administration (FDA) for the triage of ASC-US Pap smears and for the primary screening of cervical cancer in combination with cytology. The Hybrid Capture II assay is based on a liquid hybridization reaction performed in a 96-well microplate. The sample DNA is reacted with RNA probes targeted to genital high-risk HPVs (types 16, 18, 31, 33, 35, 39, 45, 51, 52, 56, 58, 59, and 68). This assay is rapid and, unlike the polymerase chain reaction (PCR)–based assays, not susceptible to cross contamination. It is also only slightly less sensitive than PCR assays.[164] The Cervista assays were approved in March 2009. The HPV HR version detects the same high-risk genotypes as the Hybrid Capture II, as well as type 66. The HPV 16/18 version is limited to those two types. The technology is based on type-specific oligonucleotide overlapping probes, a cleavase enzyme, and a fluorescent signal amplification.

Many other new screening technologies have been developed, which, in addition to HPV genotyping, rely on various other approaches such as HPV mRNA detection, HPV viral load, HPV integration, methylation profile, p16 protein detection, and proliferation or cell cycle markers.[5,164] None are yet FDA-approved.

Virus cultivation techniques are not available for the clinical diagnosis of HPV infections. HPV infection may elicit a serologic response. In patients with cutaneous warts, condyloma acuminatum, or recurrent respiratory papillomatosis, antibodies directed against the viral capsid have been detected.[165-167] Recombinant virus-like particles (VLP) based on the L1 or L1 and L2 proteins offer the same antigenic properties as viral capsids.[168] They have been used extensively to show with enzyme-linked immunosorbent assay that about one half to almost 90% of patients with HPV infection have capsid antibodies.[86] Anti-HPV antibodies tend to disappear with disease resolution but can persist for several years in asymptomatic patients.[86] A fraction of the antibodies produced in response to HPV infection are neutralizing, but probably not in amounts sufficient to offer significant protection.[169] No commercial assays are available for the serologic diagnosis of HPV infections because of insufficient sensitivity and clinical specificity. Such assays have been used for seroepidemiologic surveys. Moreover, assays that measure binding and neutralizing activity against the viral capsid have been useful in assessment of the immune response after HPV vaccination (see Prevention section).

Treatment

Highly effective and safe treatments for HPV diseases are not yet available, and the current therapies are not designed to eradicate HPV infection. Rather, their purpose is to decrease or, if possible, eliminate clinical manifestations. The current therapeutic armamentarium has been largely developed empirically over decades and too often relies on the physical or chemical destruction of lesions. Newer approaches are directed at molecular viral targets and immunomodulation.[170,171]

CUTANEOUS WARTS

The choice of treatments for cutaneous warts is complicated by the existence of weak and confusing evidence.[172,173] Nevertheless, the most common approach, the topical application of preparations that contain salicylic acid, a keratolytic agent, is effective for the treatment of common warts.[172,173] A meta-analysis of six placebo-controlled clinical trials revealed a complete response rate of 75% (144 of 191) in the cases, compared with 48% (89 of 185) in the control groups.[172] A widely available over-the-counter preparation for self treatment is a salicylic acid and lactic acid paint (salicylic acid, lactic acid, collodion, 1:1:4 [SAL]) that is typically applied daily for up to 12 weeks. The cornified layer that typically covers skin warts may need to be removed. This removal is done with a hot water soak, followed by abrasion with a pumice stone, sand paper, or an emery board. Occlusive bandages seem to increase treatment effectiveness. Mosaic warts tend to be more resistant to treatment than myrmecia.

Cryotherapy is a popular treatment, but it requires a health practitioner. It is typically accomplished with cotton wool buds dipped in liquid nitrogen and applied to the lesion or with spraying of liquid nitrogen.[174] Randomized, placebo-controlled studies have been inconclusive on the efficacy of cryotherapy, but, when compared with salicylic acid preparations, cryotherapy appears to be equivalent.[172] Variations in technique may account for these confusing results. However, aggressive cryotherapy, a 10-second sustained freeze, is more effective than briefer traditional cryotherapy, despite a higher incidence of pain and blisters.[175] More than one treatment is often needed. A 2-week interval offers the best balance between the occurrence of side effects and brevity of treatment.[176] Treatment beyond 3 months, or about four cryotherapies, presents little advantage.[177]

A randomized study with blind evaluation compared cryotherapy with duct tape application, an occlusive treatment that has long been in the medical lore, for the treatment of common warts.[178] Complete clearance of the warts occurred in 85% (22 of 26) of the patients who received occlusive therapy but in only 60% (15 of 25) of the patients treated with cryotherapy. However, this trial had limitations with blinding and follow-up. Two subsequent placebo-controlled trials of duct tape application produced negative results.[179,180]

Other treatment methods that are less often used include glutaraldehyde, formaldehyde, podofilox, and cantharidin. Their use is empirical. Intralesional bleomycin has been better studied, but when it is compared with placebo, the results are inconclusive.[172] It is usually reserved for the treatment of periungual warts.

Allergic sensitization with dinitrochlorobenzene (DNCB) followed by direct application of DNCB on the lesions has been found to be twice as effective as placebo.[172,181] However, the use of DNCB is risky, and other sensitizing agents, such as 2,3-diphenylcyclopropenone, squaric acid dibutyl ester, and 10% masoprocol cream (Actinex, Schwarz Pharmaceuticals, Mequon, WI), appear to be safer and as effective.[181,182]

Imiquimod is an immunomodulator that is approved by the FDA for the topical treatment of genital warts (see subsequent section). When used off label in an open study, imiquimod 5% cream applied once a day, 5 days per week, for up to 16 weeks on varied common warts resulted in a complete response.[183]

Cimetidine, an H_2 blocker that has immunomodulatory properties, has been widely publicized as an effective treatment for cutaneous warts on the basis of uncontrolled studies. Yet several placebo-controlled, double-blind studies have failed to confirm that claim.[181]

Electrosurgery and laser surgery are used, but they can be expensive and have not been rigorously evaluated.[172,181,184-186] Electrosurgery is relatively contraindicated for the treatment of plantar warts because of the risk of permanent and painful scarring. Laser surgery is also not scar-free, but it may be useful for the treatment of periungual and subungual warts.

Photodynamic therapy, which relies on laser light to activate locally the cytotoxicity of a compound administered systemically or applied topically, is superior to placebo for the treatment of cutaneous warts.[172] However, the technique is costly and not widely available.

Suggestion, hypnosis, homeopathy, and distant healing are among alternative approaches that have been proposed for the treatment of cutaneous warts.[187-191] More rigorous evaluations of these interventions showed little, if any, promise.

Particular treatment methods have been proposed for some specific types of warts. For example, flat warts rarely need treatment, but when they do, cryotherapy or electrosurgery (electrodesiccation) is used. Cryotherapy may also be used for the treatment of eyelid and periungual warts, and electrodesiccation is useful to remove flat or filiform warts.

ANOGENITAL WARTS

The treatment methods for condyloma acuminatum are numerous yet unsatisfactory, but guidelines that attempt to optimize the therapeutic approach have been published.[119,192-196] Because no or scant evidence shows that treatment directly affects eradication of HPV, or transmission of infection, or prevents the uncommon development of neoplasms, the rationale for treatment is restricted.[63,197,198] It includes cosmesis, relief of local symptoms, alleviation of the adverse psychologic impact caused by the presence of anogenital warts,[114] and restoration of normal physiologic function (e.g., debulking of lesions that obstruct the birth canal). Before treatment is initiated, the goals of therapy, alternatives, costs, and potential side effects should be discussed with patients. Also, within 3 to 4 months, approximately 10% to 20% of patients have spontaneous resolution of the disease.[115-119] Independent of treatment, patient counseling is part of management.[199]

None of the available treatment methods is dramatically superior to the others, but each may have its particular advantages. Because convenience is one of the greatest advantages, the availability over the past few years of patient-applied therapies, podofilox and imiquimod, has been of considerable interest.

Podofilox (podophyllotoxin) is a derivative of podophyllin, which was long the mainstay of genital wart treatment by practitioners. Podophyllin, a resin extract from the rhizome of *Podophyllum peltatum* (podophyllum resin [USP]) or *Podophyllum emodi*, has been the principal mode of therapy for many years.[200,201] The active molecules are lignans, particularly podophyllotoxin. Although podophyllin is a mitotic poison, its mode of action in warts is unknown. The compound is usually applied as a 10% to 25% solution in benzoin, directly on the wart, once weekly. Washing of lesions within 12 hours is recommended to minimize local reactions. Lack of regression after four applications suggests the need for alternative therapy. Podophyllin has never been compared with a placebo. Its effectiveness has been evaluated in a series of randomized controlled trials against other treatment methods; complete clearance rates ranged from 20% to 40%, with accounting for the frequent recurrences.[94,200] Side effects are both local and systemic.[200,201] Chemical burns are seen in one third to one half of the patients. Transient pseudoneoplastic histopathologic changes have also been reported. Neurologic, hematologic, and febrile complications, sometimes leading to death, and allergic sensitization have been associated with administration of topical podophyllin. Therefore, areas larger than 10 cm^2 should not be treated. The drug is contraindicated in pregnancy.

Podophyllotoxin is available in the United States under the generic name podofilox. It offers distinct advantages over podophyllin. It is chemically uniform and of standardized potency. Podofilox is also more efficacious and less toxic than podophyllin.[94,201-203] Finally, it does not need to be washed off. Randomized controlled studies have shown that 0.5% podofilox solution applied twice daily for 3 consecutive days every week for up to 4 weeks results in rates of complete response from 45% to 58%.[119,196,203-206] A gel formulation is easier to apply without spillover. Side effects are mostly mild and similar in nature to those of podophyllin. As with podophyllin, relapses are common and occur in 33% to 91% of patients.[119,196,203-206] Application of podofilox to prevent recurrences is effective and well tolerated, but the long-term outcome after cessation of treatment is unknown.[207] In addition to podofilox 0.5% (Condylox, Watson, Corona, CA) solution, a 0.5% gel is now available. It yielded a 45% (81 of 181) complete clearance rate after 8 weeks in a large randomized controlled trial, as opposed to 4% (5 of 93) for the vehicle only.[208]

Imiquimod is an imidazoquinolineamine that induces the production of interferon-α and other cytokines. It appears to exert its unique antitumor and antiviral action by binding to the toll-like receptors 7 and possibly 8 of dendritic cells.[209] It is available as a 5% cream (Aldara, 3M Pharmaceuticals, St. Paul, MN) for the self treatment of condyloma acuminatum.[210] This preparation was compared with vehicle alone in a randomized double-blind trial and was given three times a week, on alternate days, for up to 8 weeks.[211] At the end of the treatment period, 108 patients were evaluable and the complete response rate was 37% in the imiquimod group compared with nil in the control group ($P < .001$). Nineteen percent of the patients had a recurrence during the 10 weeks of follow-up. In a similar study, the treatment duration was extended up to 16 weeks, and imiquimod 5% cream was compared with a 1% cream and with vehicle.[212] At the end of treatment, the complete response rates were 50%, 21%, and 14% in the three respective groups. Imiquimod 5% cream was significantly superior to either of the two other preparations ($P < .001$). In the 5% imiquimod group, 72% of women had a complete response, compared with 33% of the men. During the 12 weeks of follow-up, recurrences were noted in 13%, 0, and 10% of the subjects in the three groups, respectively. The adverse reactions were local and included itching and burning sensations, erythema, erosions, and swelling; they were well tolerated. The daily administration of imiquimod 5% cream offers some enhancement of efficacy, mostly in men, but a substantially higher incidence of side effects.[213] Therefore, Aldara is approved for thrice-weekly use only. Additional clinical trials have complemented and supported the results of these pivotal studies.[195,214,215] Imiquimod also appears to be useful for the treatment of other possibly HPV-related conditions, such as actinic keratoses, basal cell carcinomas, and squamous cell carcinomas in situ.[183]

A new preparation, polyphenon E, that contains green tea catechins was approved in 2008 by the FDA as a 15% ointment, Veregen (Doak, Fairfield, NJ).[216] These compounds have some antiviral and anticarcinogenic activities. The product is self applied three times a day on the lesions until complete disappearance, but for no more than 16 weeks. Three randomized controlled clinical studies have been conducted in men and women with genital warts, with a total of more than 300 subjects in the 15% ointment arm. In the aggregate, the complete clearance rate was 58% with the active compound and 34% in the placebo arm. Efficacy was better in women than men. The side effects were local and included erythema (18%), pruritus (14%), pain (14%), and ulceration (12%). The drug is contraindicated in pregnancy. The red stain of the substance and its frequency of administration are potential drawbacks.

Various provider-applied therapies are available. They can be divided into nonsurgical and surgical treatments, which are as follows.

Podophyllin resin (see previous discussion) is still used widely where cost is an issue, although podofilox 0.5% solution or gel is more effective and safer to use.[201]

Trichloracetic acid and, to a lesser extent, bichloracetic acid have been favored by gynecologists for the treatment of genital warts.[217] They can both be used during pregnancy. Trichloracetic acid in a 10% to 90% solution is used topically at weekly intervals. The application is painful and can cause ulcers. The unreacted acid should be removed with talcum powder or bicarbonate of soda. In one comparative trial, trichloracetic acid therapy appeared to be equivalent to cryotherapy, with complete response and relapse rates of 81% and 36%, respectively.[218] Another study was also unable to detect any differences, with complete response rates of 64% for cryotherapy and 70% for trichloracetic acid.[219] Trichloracetic acid at 50% does not add to the effects of podophyllin alone and is ineffective in the treatment of vaginal and cervical warts.[220,221]

Cryotherapy is administered with liquid nitrogen or cryoprobe. Lesions are frozen every 1 or 2 weeks. Cryotherapy is regarded as an effective treatment, with cure rates in the 50% to 100% range, and it is safe even during pregnancy.[218,222] One comparative study suggested that cryotherapy is more effective than podophyllin but probably less effective than electrosurgery.[223-225] Side effects are tolerable and include burning, which resolves within a few hours, and ulceration, which heals in 7 to 10 days with little or no scarring.

Other surgical techniques are available for the treatment of anogenital warts.[194-196] Conventional surgery with scissors offers the advantage of immediate eradication of visible lesions. This technique has been reserved mainly for the treatment of perianal warts, but it can be advantageously applied to other genital warts if they are limited in number. Up to one third of patients have recurrences, and scarring, typically limited to some skin discoloration, is the most common complication.[226-229] Electrosurgical techniques have often been applied for the treatment of external genital warts, with results probably superior to those of cryotherapy, but scarring may occur.[224,225] Complete response rates of 80% to 90% have been reported with carbon dioxide laser therapy.[230-232] In a comparative assessment, however, laser therapy was not deemed to be superior to conventional surgery,[227] and subsequent better-designed studies indicated a long-term complete response rate of 19% to 39%.[233,234] Laser therapy is expensive, may require general anesthesia, and is frequently accompanied by pain and scarring.

The availability of lidocaine-prilocaine (EMLA) cream, which should be applied about 1 hour before the procedure, has facilitated local anesthesia before cryotherapy and laser surgery.[235-238]

Two treatments that are now rarely used but still deserve mention are 5-fluorouracil and intralesional interferon. 5-Fluorouracil, used topically as a 5% cream applied daily, has been reported to have cure rates of 30% to 95%; the best results have been obtained with intra-urethral warts.[94,239,240] In a comparative trial in men, 5-fluorouracil appeared to be equivalent in efficacy to podophyllin.[241] In addition, prophylactic activity of 5-fluorouracil has been reported for vulvar warts.[242] This drug is not widely used because it often produces substantial pain, ulceration, and, if applied in the urethra, dysuria.[94] Like other antimetabolites, 5-fluorouracil is contraindicated during pregnancy.

Interferons have antiviral, immunomodulatory, and antiproliferative properties.[243,244] Encouraging in vitro and preliminary clinical studies were confirmed by four randomized, double-blind trials that showed the efficacy of intralesionally administered interferon-α and interferon-β compared with placebo.[75,245-247] Parenterally administered interferons have also been evaluated for treatment of condyloma acuminatum but have generally been ineffective.[115-117,248] Interferon, in the doses used, has been generally well tolerated. Side effects (influenza-like symptoms, neutropenia, and thrombocytopenia) are usually mild and are seen more frequently with higher doses. Imiquimod, an interferon-α inducer, is a more practical and cheaper substitute for interferon. No published experience is found with pegylated interferons.

Cidofovir is an acyclic nucleotide that is a potent inhibitor of the DNA polymerase of cytomegalovirus and other herpes viruses and is licensed for the intravenous treatment of cytomegalovirus retinitis. Although HPVs do not possess a DNA polymerase, this compound triggers the apoptosis of HPV-infected cells.[249] In a randomized, vehicle-controlled trial of a compounded 1% gel applied daily to genital warts for 5 consecutive days every other week, at 12 weeks, the treated group had 47% (9 of 19) complete clearance compared with 0 (0 of 11) in the vehicle group ($P = .006$).[250] Pain, pruritus, rash, erosions, and ulcerations were frequently noted, but equally in both groups. The cost, the risk of carcinogenesis associated with cidofovir, and the absence of long-term data are reservations about this non–FDA-approved treatment.

Although guidelines are helpful, firm recommendations on the proper treatment strategy for condyloma acuminatum are not always possible. The divergent results of several cost-benefit analyses reinforce this point.[251-253] Costs may vary widely for a given therapy, recurrences are common yet long-term outcomes are not well studied, and the significance of the antecedent genital wart history and treatment is poorly known. Furthermore, the importance of factors such as gender, wart location, size, and number is largely unknown with respect to each treatment. Nevertheless, the duration of lesions (>1 year), their number (>10), and their location on dry rather than moist skin are adverse predictors of treatment response.[195,254,255] Treatment response may improve with the discontinuation of oral contraceptive use, pubic hair shaving, and tobacco smoking.[256,257]

In practice, availability, convenience, adverse reactions, location of lesions, and characteristics of the patient are determinant in the treatment choice. Patient-applied therapies should receive preference. Warts of the urinary meatus can be treated with careful application of podophyllin, podofilox,[94] or cryotherapy.[258] 5-Fluorouracil cream may also be used.[94,259] Laser surgery and instillations of interferon-α can also be used with intraurethral warts.[109,260] Perianal and anal warts may be treated with scalpel removal,[226-228] cryotherapy,[261] laser surgery,[262] trichloracetic or bichloracetic acid,[194] or even, as adjunctive therapy, with imiquimod-soaked anal tampons.[263]

For vaginal warts, cryotherapy (sprays), trichloracetic acid, and podophyllin are simple options[264]; laser therapy[265,266] and cryotherapy[267]

have the advantage of being relatively safe during pregnancy, and they may be used for treatment of cervical warts as well. Although intralesional interferon may be indicated for the treatment of single, very large warts, laser therapy seems to be better suited for large, extensive lesions.

The genital warts of patients with immunocompromise, including those with HIV, seem relatively refractory to treatment.[268] Thus, podophyllin, podofilox, intralesional interferon, and imiquimod alone have been largely ineffective.[269-273] Combination therapy appears more successful, such as electrosurgery plus cold-blade excision[269,274] or plus intralesional interferon for anal warts.[275] Imiquimod may also be used as adjunctive therapy.[276] Nevertheless, single therapy, especially for small (<1 cm^2) intraanal lesions, may be effective, as shown with trichloracetic acid, liquid nitrogen, or the use of an infrared coagulator.[158,277] Lesion healing is generally not a problem after surgery.[278] Further recommendations for the management of HIV patients with HPV infections are available from the Centers for Disease Control and Prevention (CDC; http://www.cdc.gov/mmwr/preview/mmwrhtml/rr5315a1.htm and http://www.cdc.gov/mmwr/preview/mmwrhtml/rr5804a1.htm?s_cid=rr5804a1_e) and the New York State Department of Health (http://www.hivguidelines.org). The effects of highly active antiretroviral therapy (HAART) on HPV diseases are still debated. HAART appears to increase the incidence of genital and oral warts, does not affect AIN, and may help the regression of CIN.[279-281]

Because internal genital warts are often associated with genital dysplasias and malignant diseases and because of the special skills and technical resources necessary for proper diagnosis and management, patients with internal lesions should be referred to a qualified specialist.

OTHER WARTS

The lesions of epidermodysplasia verruciformis should be carefully observed, and any malignant changes should be treated with surgical techniques (cold blade or laser), cryotherapy, or 5-fluorouracil ointments.[24] Retinoids in combination with intralesional interferon or calciferol help with the management of the lesions of epidermodysplasia verruciformis.[24,282]

The management of recurrent respiratory papillomatosis is complex.[32,283,284] For the primary debulking of lesions, most surgeons use the CO_2 laser. Mechanical devices such as a microresector are also used. Photodynamic laser therapy is gaining acceptance. The recurrent nature of the disease requires a careful balance between the risks and benefits of the surgery, which can be achieved only by experienced and skilled operators. Tracheostomy should be avoided because the papillomatosis could then extend to the tracheostomy site and further down the respiratory tree. Radiotherapy is contraindicated because of the known risk of malignant transformation. Different adjuvant therapies are available. Parenteral interferon-α may yield long-term complete responses in a quarter of patients. Over the past 5 years, the interest has moved to the intralesional injection of cidofovir.[285] The enthusiasm generated by the results of the early case series has precluded the completion of a properly designed study. Because of the small size of the case series, the long-term risks, including those of malignant disease, are not well understood. Indole-3-carbinol (I3C) and its main active metabolite, diindolyl methane (DIM), are derivatives of cruciferous vegetables (e.g., broccoli, cabbage, cauliflower) that are widely used by patients with recurrent respiratory papillomatosis. By increasing the 2-hydroxylation of estradiol, these compounds favor the formation of 2-hydroxyestrone, a nonestrogenic, antiproliferative, antiangiogenic, and apoptotic molecule, instead of 16α-hydroxyestrone. A randomized, placebo-controlled clinical trial has shown the ability of I3C to induce regression of biopsy-proven CIN 2 or 3.[286] A similar trial has not been conducted for recurrent respiratory papillomatosis.

Oral warts (squamous papillomas, condylomata acuminata, and verruca vulgaris) can be treated with surgical excision, cryotherapy, laser surgery, or podophyllin application.[287] Because of its benign natural history, focal epithelial hyperplasia should not be treated.

Prevention

At present, no effective methods of prevention for cutaneous warts are available, other than avoiding contact with infectious lesions. In the case of plantar warts, this avoidance is achieved effectively in swimming pools with wearing of protective foot equipment (verruca socks).[33]

Male condoms offer an imperfect protection against female acquisition of HPV infection. However, a prospective study of 82 college-aged women, virgin at enrollment, showed protection against HPV cervical infection in direct relationship with frequency of condom use during intercourse.[288] Two randomized trials make a more dramatic argument in favor of condoms by showing that male condom use for at least 3 months promoted regression of CIN and clearance of HPV DNA in the female sexual partners and regression of HPV-associated penile lesions in the patient.[289,290] This occurred only in couples with concordant HPV types.[291] Therefore, reinfection is clinically important.

Although the U.S. Centers for Disease Control and Prevention state that the evaluation of partners is unnecessary for the management of genital warts, examination of the partners provides an opportunity to educate, counsel, and screen for HPV disease and other STDs.[194,199]

The Pap smear is an essential tool for the screening and prevention of cervical cancer.[292] The American Cancer Society, in 2002, and the U.S. Preventive Services Task Force and the American College of Obstetricians and Gynecologists, in 2003, released their latest guidelines for the screening of cervical cancer.[293-295] These guidelines are summarized in Table 144-2. Consensus guidelines for the management of the cytologic and histologic abnormalities have been issued by the American Society for Colposcopy and Cervical Pathology.[159,163] Additional sources provide further guidance on the use of HPV DNA testing.[160,161] In the female with HIV, the Pap smear should be obtained twice the first year after the diagnosis of HIV infection and, if the results are normal, annually thereafter.[194] No clinically validated guidelines can be provided at the moment for the screening of anal cancer with anal cytology in the patient with HIV. However, the rising incidence of anal cancer in the HIV population has led New York State to recommend this approach (http://www.hivguidelines.org). Recurrent respiratory papillomatosis of children may be acquired by the infant during passage through the birth canal, as discussed previously. Cesarean section has probably only a limited role, if any, in the prevention of respiratory papillomatosis.[32]

A major development in the field of HPV diseases has been the availability since June 2006 of an FDA-approved vaccine for the prevention of several genital HPV diseases, including cervical cancer. This quadrivalent vaccine, Gardasil (Merck, West Point, PA), is directed against HPV types 6, 11, 16, and 18, thus aiming at 80% to 90% of the agents of genital warts and 70% of the agents of cervical cancer.[296] It is made with the expression in baker's yeast of the L1 gene of these genotypes. The major capsid protein made spontaneously folds into capsomeres and then into properly conformed capsids devoid of any infectious nucleic acid; they are called virus-like particles (VLP). A similar L1 VLP vaccine, directed against only HPV-16 and HPV-18 (Cervarix, GlaxoSmithKline, London, UK) and made in insect cells, is only available outside the United States currently (June 2009).[297] Although Gardasil is adjuvanted with a proprietary amorphous aluminum hydrophosphate sulfate, Cervarix has an AS04 adjuvant that contains a mixture of monophosphoryl lipid A adsorbed on hydrated aluminum hydroxide.

Virions and VLPs are capable of inducing the formation of neutralizing antibodies in high titers that are sufficient to protect the vaccine recipient.[298] Protection is not dependent on a cellular immune response.

The protective effectiveness of the HPV vaccine was shown in a randomized, placebo-controlled trial in which women, ages 16 to 23 years, free of HPV infection and abnormal cervical cytology, were given an intramuscular HPV-16 VLP vaccine at months 0, 2, and 6 or the adjuvant alone as a placebo.[299] None of the women who received the vaccine (0 of 768) had HPV infection develop, whereas 5.4% (41 of 765) in the placebo group did ($P < .001$). As a secondary end point, none of the HPV-16 vaccine recipients had HPV-16–associated CIN develop, but nine of 41 HPV-16–infected placebo recipients (22%)

did. In that study, 290 women were also followed for a mean of 8.5 years. None of the vaccine-recipients and 5 of the placebo-recipients developed HPV-16–associated CIN, a favorable indication of the longevity of the protection.[299a] Several phase III trials that used prevention of disease, especially high-grade intraepithelial neoplasia, instead of infection as the primary endpoint led to the vaccine approval.[296,298]

TABLE 144-2	Summary of Cervical Cancer Screening Guidelines
When to Begin Pap Test Screening	
USPSTF and ACS	Approximately 3 years after a woman begins having sexual intercourse but no later than 21 years old.
How Often?	
USPSTF	Every 3 years (regardless of the cervical cytology technique used).
ACS	1. Annually with conventional cytology. *or* 2. At or after age 30 years, women who have had three consecutive, technically satisfactory normal-negative cytology results may be screened every 2 to 3 years. UNLESS a. They have a history of in utero diethylstilbestrol (DES) exposure. b. They are HIV-positive. c. They have immunocompromise from organ transplantation, chemotherapy, or chronic corticosteroid treatment.
When to Discontinue Screening	
USPSTF	At age 65 years in women who have had normal results previously and who are not otherwise at high risk for cervical cancer.
ACS	At age 70 years or older in women with an intact cervix and who have had three or more documented, consecutive, technically satisfactory, normal-negative cervical cytology tests and no abnormal-positive cytology tests within the 10-year period before age 70 years. EXCEPTIONS: a. Women who have not been previously screened. b. Women for whom information about previous screening is unavailable. c. Women for whom past screening is unlikely. d. Women with a history of (i) cervical cancer, (ii) in utero exposure to DES. e. Women with immunocompromise (e.g., because of organ transplantation, HIV infection, chemotherapy, or chronic corticosteroid treatment). f. Women who have tested positive for HPV DNA.
Screening after Hysterectomy	
USPSTF and ACS	Not necessary if (total) hysterectomy was for benign disease.
Screening with HPV DNA Testing (Hybrid Capture II Test for High-Risk HPV)	
USPSTF	Not recommended.
ACS	It should be used, with cytology, only at age 30 years or older and not more frequently than every 3 years.
Additional Guidelines	
ACS	Regular health care visits, including gynecologic care (including pelvic examination) and STD screening and prevention, should be done. Counseling and education related to HPV infection is critical if HPV DNA testing is done.
ACOG	Yearly testing using cytology alone remains an acceptable screening plan.
CDC	Women who have external genital warts do not need to have Pap tests more frequently than women who do not have warts, unless otherwise indicated. In women with HIV, a cervical cytology should be obtained twice in the first year after diagnosis of HIV infection and, if the results are normal, annually thereafter.

USPSTF, US Preventive Services Task Force; *ACS*, American Cancer Society; *ACOG*, American College of Obstetrics and Gynecology.
American Cancer Society (ACS)[293]: http://caonline.amcancersoc.org/cgi/content/short/52/6/342.
US Preventive Services Task Force (USPSTF)[294]: http://www.ahrq.gov/clinic/uspstf/uspscerv.htm.
American College of Obstetrics and Gynecology (ACOG).[295]
Centers for Disease Control and Prevention (CDC)[163]: http://www.cdc.gov/std/treatment.

These trials totaled 17,000 females, ages 16 to 26 years, who were seronegative and HPV DNA–negative for the vaccine types at entry. The per-protocol analysis showed a 100% efficacy after 3 years of follow-up at prevention of CIN of any grade, adenocarcinoma in situ (AIS), VIN 1 and VAIN 1, external genital warts caused by any of the vaccine types, and VIN 2 or 3 and VAIN 2 or 3 caused by HPV types 16 or 18. When the subjects who did not receive the full immunization series, had minor protocol violations, or had an abnormal Pap smear at entry were included, the vaccine efficacy for these different conditions ranged from 82% to 98%. When women who were seropositive or HPV DNA positive for the vaccine types were included, the efficacy decreased to 44% for CIN 2/3 and AIS and to 76% for genital warts.[300] The same figures were 18% and 51%, respectively, if diseases of any HPV types, not just vaccine types, were included. However, these efficacy results actually do improve with more follow-up time, as the rates of disease acquisition diverge further between vaccine and placebo recipients. To show that the vaccine is likely effective if administered to children aged 9 to 15 years who otherwise are difficult to study because of their low rate of HPV disease, the neutralizing antibody levels were used as substitute and were shown to be higher in boys and girls than in the women.[296,298] Clinical trials have indicated that Gardasil is also effective in older women (ages 24 to 45 years) and in males for the prevention of genital warts (data available online at http://www.cdc.gov/vaccines/recs/acip/slides.htm).[300a] Evidence also shows that the vaccine offers some cross protection against CIN 2 or 3 and AIS caused by types 31 (related to type 16) and 45 (related to type 45). Immunization of males is under consideration because it might result in increased herd immunity and also because of the rising incidence of HPV-related anal and oropharyngeal cancers.

Gardasil is indicated for the prevention of SCC and AIS of the cervix; CIN 1, 2, and 3; VAIN 2 and 3; VIN 2 and 3; and external genital warts in women from ages 9 through 26 years. The Advisory Committee on Immunization Practices (ACIP) has recommended vaccination for girls aged 11 through 12 years and a catch-up immunization for 13-year-olds to 26-year-olds.[299] The vaccine is given as an intramuscular injection (0.5 mL) at months 0, 2, and 6. To date, no booster is necessary, and data show that protection lasts for at least 5 years.[169] Because syncope may occur after the immunization, observation of the subject for 15 minutes after the injection is recommended. The other significant adverse reactions from the immunization are pain at the injection site (85%) and swelling (26%). Fever was reported with

13.5% of the vaccine immunizations compared with 10.2% with the placebo. The vaccine otherwise appears to be safe. A great deal of concern, so far unsubstantiated, has been generated by this immunization and the risk of Guillain-Barré syndrome, multiple sclerosis, and other autoimmune disorders. Several monitoring tools have been put in place by the CDC and the Nordic countries to examine any possible relationship to the vaccine (see the ACIP October 2008 session, available online at http://www.cdc.gov/vaccines/recs/acip/slides.htm).

No prior testing for the presence of cervical HPV DNA, cytologic abnormalities, or antibodies to HPV is necessary because they are not contraindications for vaccination. Only a small percentage of subjects would have a present or past infection to all HPV types included in the vaccine, and protection against the HPV types for which the subject is naive is not altered by prior or current infections by other vaccine types.

The vaccine is contraindicated in subjects allergic to yeast (*Saccharomyces cerevisae*) or who have had a prior allergic reaction to the vaccine or its components. No data exist on the presence of the vaccine antigens or of the antibodies induced by the vaccine in breast milk. Pregnancy is a contraindication. Should the series of three immunizations be interrupted, one should complete the series whenever possible. Oral contraceptives do not alter the immunogenicity of the vaccine. Because this is an inert, noninfectious vaccine, it is not contraindicated for patients with immunodeficiency or immunosuppression. However, no data are available at present on the vaccine efficacy in these populations. The need for patients to continue cervical cancer screening per standard of care must be communicated.

In the primary target population, ages 11 to 12 years, two other vaccines are on the immunization calendar: tetanus, diphtheria, and acellular pertussis (Tdap) and the quadrivalent meningococcal vaccine (see Chapter 320). Although not formally studied, the administration of these vaccines (at different anatomic sites) along with Gardasil has been approved by ACIP and the American Academy of Pediatrics.[301,302] The coadministration of Gardasil with the hepatitis B vaccine (Recombivax HB, Merck) showed no interaction in the immune response to each vaccine.[303] The manufacturer charges $120 per dose, but the actual cost to the patient varies a great deal and can be considerably higher. Most major health care insurers reimburse the vaccine up to age 18 years. The Vaccine for Children program is a federal program administered by the states that covers the costs of vaccination for disadvantaged children.

REFERENCES

1. Ciuffo G. Imnesto positivo con filtrato di verruca volgare. *G Ital Mal Venere.* 1907;48:12-17.
2. Hebner CM, Laimins LA. Human papillomaviruses: basic mechanisms of pathogenesis and oncogenicity. *Rev Med Virol.* 2006;16:83-97.
3. Zheng ZM, Baker CC. Papillomavirus genome structure, expression, and post-transcriptional regulation. *Front Bios.* 2006;11:2286-2302.
4. Snijders PJ, Steenbergen RD, Heideman DA, et al. HPV-mediated cervical carcinogenesis: concepts and clinical implications. *J Pathol.* 2006;208:152-164.
5. Bonnez W. *Guide to Genital HPV Diseases and Prevention.* New York: Informa Healthcare Publishers; 2009.
6. Bonnez W. Papillomavirus. In: Richman RD, Whitley RJ, Hayden FG, eds. *Clinical Virology.* 3rd ed. Washington, DC: American Society for Microbiology; 2009:603-644.
7. Garcea RL, DiMaio D. *The Papillomaviruses.* New York: Springer; 2007.
8. Kadaja M, Silla T, Ustav E, et al. Papillomavirus DNA replication: from initiation to genomic instability. *Virology.* 2009;384:360-368.
9. Talbert-Slagle K, DiMaio D. The bovine papillomavirus E5 protein and the PDGF beta receptor: it takes two to tango. *Virology.* 2009;384:345-351.
10. Howie HL, Katzenellenbogen RA, Galloway DA. Papillomavirus E6 proteins. *Virology.* 2009;384:324-334.
11. Wang HK, Duffy AA, Broker TR, Chow LT. Robust production and passaging of infectious HPV in squamous epithelium of primary human keratinocytes. *Genes Dev.* 2009;23:181-194.
12. Bonnez W. Murine models of human papillomavirus-infected human xenografts. *Papillomavirus Rep.* 1998;9:27-38.
13. Giroglou T, Sapp M, Lane C, et al. Immunological analyses of human papillomavirus capsids. *Vaccine.* 2001;19:1783-1793.
14. Bernard HU. The clinical importance of the nomenclature, evolution and taxonomy of human papillomaviruses. *J Clin Virol.* 2005;32:S1-S6.
15. Strike DG, Bonnez W, Rose RC, et al. Expression in *Escherichia coli* of seven DNA segments comprising the complete L1 and L2 open reading frames of human papillomavirus type 6b and the location of the "common antigen." *J Gen Virol.* 1989;70:543-555.
16. Jenson AB, Kurman RJ, Lancaster WD. Detection of papillomavirus common antigens in lesions of skin and mucosa. *Clin Dermatol.* 1985;3:56-63.
17. Trottier H, Franco EL. The epidemiology of genital human papillomavirus infection. *Vaccine.* 2006;24:S1-S15.
18. Antonsson A, Forslund O, Ekberg H, et al. The ubiquity and impressive genomic diversity of human skin papillomaviruses suggest a commensalic nature of these viruses. *J Virol.* 2000;74:11636-11641.
19. Sterling JC. Human papillomavirus and skin cancer. *J Clin Virol.* 2005;32:S67-S71.
20. Massing AM, Epstein WL. Natural history of warts. A two year study. *Arch Dermatol.* 1963;87:306-310.
21. Williams HC, Pottier A, Strachan D. The descriptive epidemiology of warts in British schoolchildren. *Br J Dermatol.* 1993;128:504-511.
22. Larsson PA, Liden S. Prevalence of skin diseases among adolescents 12-16 years of age. *Acta Derm Venereol.* 1980;60:415-423.
23. Bonnez W. A comment on "Butcher's warts: Dermatological heritage or testable misinformation?" *Arch Dermatol.* 2002;138:411.
24. Gewirtzman A, Bartlett B, Tyring S. Epidermodysplasia verruciformis and human papilloma virus. *Curr Opin Infect Dis.* 2008;21:141-146.
25. Weinstock H, Berman S, Cates W Jr. Sexually transmitted diseases among American youth: incidence and prevalence estimates, 2000. *Perspect Sex Reprod Health.* 2004;36:6-10.
26. Dunne EF, Unger ER, Sternberg M, et al. Prevalence of HPV infection among females in the United States. *JAMA.* 2007;297:813-819.
27. Dinh TH, Sternberg M, Dunne EF, Markowitz LE. Genital warts among 18- to 59-year-olds in the United States, national health and nutrition examination survey, 1999-2004. *Sex Transm Dis.* 2008;35:357-360.
28. Centers for Disease Control and Prevention. *Sexually Transmitted Disease Surveillance, 2006.* Atlanta: Department of Health and Human Services; 2007.
29. Koshiol JE, Laurent SA, Pimenta JM. Rate and predictors of new genital warts claims and genital warts-related healthcare utilization among privately insured patients in the United States. *Sex Trans Dis.* 2004;31:748-752.
30. Chesson HW, Blandford JM, Gift TL, et al. The estimated direct medical cost of sexually transmitted diseases among American youth, 2000. *Perspect Sex Reprod Health.* 2004;36:11-19.
31. Stoler MH. Advances in cervical screening technology. *Modern Pathology.* 2000;13:275-284.
32. Derkay CS, Darrow DH. Recurrent respiratory papillomatosis. *Ann Otol Rhinol Laryngol.* 2006;115:1-11.
33. Bunney MH. Prevention of plantar warts by the use of protective footwear in swimming pool. *Commun Med.* 1972;127:127-129.
34. Barrett TJ, Silbar JD, McGinley JP. Genital warts: A venereal disease. *JAMA.* 1954;154:333-334.
35. Oriel JD. Natural history of genital warts. *Br J Vener Dis.* 1971;47:1-13.
36. Habel LA, van den Eeden SK, Sherman KJ, et al. Risk factors for incident and recurrent condylomata acuminata among women. A population-based study. *Sex Transm Dis.* 1998;25:285-292.

37. van den Eeden SK, Habel LA, Sherman KJ, et al. Risk factors for incident and recurrent condylomata acuminata among men. A population-based study. *Sex Transm Dis.* 1998;25:278-284.

38. Fairley CK, Gay NJ, Forbes A, et al. Hand-genital transmission of genital warts? An analysis of prevalence data. *Epidemiol Infect.* 1995;115:169-176.

39. Obalek S, Jablonska S, Favre M, et al. Condylomata acuminata in children: Frequent association with human papillomaviruses responsible for cutaneous warts. *J Am Acad Dermatol.* 1990;23:205-213.

40. Cohen BA, Honig P, Androphy E. Anogenital warts in children: Clinical and virologic evaluation for sexual abuse. *Arch Dermatol.* 1990;126:1575-1580.

41. Gutman LT, Herman-Giddens ME, Phelps WC. Transmission of human genital papillomavirus disease: Comparison of data from adults and children. *Pediatrics.* 1993;91:31-38.

42. Hernandez BY, Wilkens LR, Zhu X, et al. Transmission of human papillomavirus in heterosexual couples. *Emerg Infect Dis.* 2008;14:888-894.

43. Sawchuk WS, Weber PJ, Lowy DR, et al. Infectious papillomavirus in the vapor of warts treated with carbon dioxide laser or electrocoagulation: Detection and protection. *J Am Acad Dermatol.* 1989;21:41-49.

44. Bonnez W, Rose RC, Borkhuis C, et al. Evaluation of the temperature sensitivity of human papillomavirus (HPV) type 11 using the human xenograft severe combined immunodeficiency (SCID) mouse model. *J Clin Microbiol.* 1994;32:1575-1577.

45. Roden RB, Lowy DR, Schiller JT. Papillomavirus is resistant to desiccation. *J Infect Dis.* 1997;176:1076-1079.

46. Campo MS. Animal models of papillomavirus pathogenesis. *Virus Res.* 2002;89:249-261.

47. Fraumeni JF Jr, Lloyd JW, Smith EM, et al. Cancer mortality among nuns: Role of marital status in etiology of neoplastic disease in women. *J Natl Cancer Inst.* 1969;42:455-468.

48. Human papillomaviruses. *IARC Monogr Eval Carcinog Risks Hum.* 1995;94:1-379.

49. Morris M, Tortolero-Luna G, Malpica A, et al. Cervical intraepithelial neoplasia and cervical cancer. *Obstet Gynecol Clin North Am.* 1996;23:347-410.

50. Franco EL. Epidemiology of anogenital warts and cancer. *Obstet Gynecol Clin North Am.* 1996;23:597-623.

51. Bosch FX, Lorincz A, Munoz N, et al. The causal relation between human papillomavirus and cervical cancer. *J Clin Pathol.* 2002;55:244-265.

52. Munoz N, Bosch FX, Castellsague X, et al. Against which human papillomavirus types shall we vaccinate and screen? The international perspective. *Int J Cancer.* 2004;111:278-285.

53. Parkin DM, Bray F. Chapter 2: The burden of HPV-related cancers. *Vaccine.* 2006;24:S11-S25.

54. D'Souza G, Kreimer AR, Viscidi R, et al. Case-control study of human papillomavirus and oropharyngeal cancer. *N Engl J Med.* 2007;356:1944-1956.

55. Sterling JC. Human papillomaviruses and skin cancer. *J Clin Virol.* 2005;32:S67-S71.

56. Bonnez W, DaRin C, Borkhuis C, et al. Isolation and propagation of human papillomavirus type 16 in human xenografts implanted in the severe combined immunodeficiency mouse. *J Virol.* 1998;72:5256-5261.

57. McLaughlin-Drubin ME, Munger K. The human papillomavirus E7 oncoprotein. *Virology.* 2009;384:335-344.

58. Doorbar J. The papillomavirus life cycle. *J Clin Virol.* 2005;32:S7-S15.

59. Woodman CB, Collins SI, Young LS. The natural history of cervical HPV infection: unresolved issues. *Nature Rev Cancer.* 2007;7:11-22.

60. Goldschmidt H, Klingman AM. Experimental inoculation of humans with ectodermotropic viruses. *J Invest Dermatol.* 1958;31:175-182.

61. Barrett TJ, Silbar JD, McGinley JP. Genital warts: A venereal disease. *JAMA.* 1954;154:333-334.

62. Lehr E, Jarnik M, Brown DR. Human papillomavirus type 11 alters the transcription and expression of loricrin, the major cell envelope protein. *Virology.* 2002;298:240-247.

63. Ferenczy A, Mitao M, Nagai N, et al. Latent papillomavirus and recurring warts. *N Engl J Med.* 1985;313:784-788.

64. Steinberg BM, Gallagher T, Stoler M, et al. Persistence and expression of human papillomavirus during interferon therapy. *Arch Otolaryngol Head Neck Surg.* 1988;114:27-32.

65. Kirchner H. Immunobiology of human papillomavirus infection. *Prog Med Virol.* 1986;33:1-41.

66. Garman ME, Tyring SK. The cutaneous manifestations of HIV infection. *Dermatol Clin.* 2002;20:193-208.

67. Peto J. Cancer epidemiology in the last century and the next decade. *Nature.* 2001;411:390-395.

68. Leigh IM, Buchanan JA, Harwood CA, et al. Role of human papillomaviruses in cutaneous and oral manifestations of immunosuppression. *J Acquir Immune Defic Syndr.* 1999;21:S49-S57.

69. Penn I. Cancers in renal transplant recipients. *Adv Ren Replace Ther.* 2000;7:147-156.

70. Palefsky JM, Gillison ML, Strickler HD. Chapter 16: HPV vaccines in immunocompromised women and men. *Vaccine.* 2006;24:S140-S146.

71. Kojic EM, Cu-Uvin S. Update: human papillomavirus infection remains highly prevalent and persistent among HIV-infected individuals. *Curr Opin Oncol.* 2007;19:464-469.

72. Frisch M, Biggar RJ, Goedert JJ. Human papillomavirus-associated cancers in patients with human immunodeficiency virus infection and acquired immunodeficiency syndrome. *J Natl Cancer Inst.* 2000;92:1500-1510.

73. Centers for Disease Control and Prevention. 1993 revised classification system for HIV infection and expanded surveillance case definition for AIDS among adolescents and adults. *MMWR Morb Mortal Wkly Rep.* 1992;41:1-19.

74. Biggar RJ, Chaturvedi AK, Goedert JJ, et al. AIDS-related cancer and severity of immunosuppression in persons with AIDS. *J Natl Cancer Inst.* 2007;99:962-972.

75. Reichman RC, Oakes D, Bonnez W, et al. Treatment of condyloma acuminatum with three different interferons administered intralesionally: A double-blind, placebo-controlled trial. *Ann Intern Med.* 1988;108:675-679.

76. Tagami H. Regression phenomenon of numerous flat warts: An experiment on the nature of tumor immunity in man. *Int J Dermatol.* 1983;22:570-571.

77. Arena S, Marconi M, Ubertosi M, et al. HPV and pregnancy: Diagnostic methods, transmission and evolution. *Minerva Ginecol.* 2002;54:225-237.

78. Kemp EA, Hakenewerth AM, Laurent SL, et al. Human papillomavirus prevalence in pregnancy. *Obstet Gynecol.* 1992;79:649-656.

79. Morrison EA, Gammon MD, Goldberg GL, et al. Pregnancy and cervical infection with human papillomaviruses. *Int J Gynaecol Obstet.* 1996;54:125-130.

80. Nobbenhuis MA, Helmerhorst TJ, van den Brule AJ, et al. High-risk human papillomavirus clearance in pregnant women: Trends for lower clearance during pregnancy with a catch-up postpartum. *Br J Cancer.* 2002;87:75-80.

80a. Einstein MH, Schiller JT, Viscidi RP, et al. Clinician's guide to human papillomavirus immunology: knowns and unknowns. *Lancet Infect Dis.* 2009;9:347-356.

81. Orth G. Genetics of epidermodysplasia verruciformis: Insights into host defense against papillomaviruses. *Semin Immunol.* 2006;18:362-374.

82. Stanley M. Immune responses to human papillomavirus. *Vaccine.* 2006;24:S16-S22.

83. Hong K, Greer CE, Ketter N, et al. Isolation and characterization of human papillomavirus type 6–specific T cells infiltrating genital warts. *J Virol.* 1997;71:6427-6432.

84. Oguchi M, Komura J, Tagami H, et al. Ultrastructural studies of spontaneously regressing plane warts. Macrophages attack verruca-epidermal cells. *Arch Dermatol Res.* 1981;270:403-411.

85. Bonnez W, DaRin C, Rose RC, et al. Use of human papillomavirus type 11 virions in an ELISA to detect specific antibodies in humans with condylomata acuminata. *J Gen Virol.* 1991;72:1343-1347.

86. Dillner J. The serological response to papillomaviruses. *Semin Cancer Biol.* 1999;9:423-430.

87. Konya J, Dillner J. Immunity to oncogenic human papillomaviruses. *Adv Cancer Res.* 2001;82:205-238.

88. Kanodia S, Fahey LM, Kast WM. Mechanisms used by human papillomaviruses to escape the host immune response. *Current Cancer Drug Targets.* 2007;7:79-89.

89. Madeleine MM, Johnson LG, Smith AG, et al. Comprehensive analysis of HLA-A, HLA-B, HLA-C, HLA-DRB1, and HLA-DQB1 loci and squamous cell cervical cancer risk. *Cancer Res.* 2008;68:3532-3539.

90. Grussendorf-Conen E-I. Papillomavirus-induced tumors of the skin: Cutaneous warts and epidermodysplasia verruciformis. In: Syrjänen K, Gissmann L, Koss LG, eds. *Papillomaviruses and Human Disease.* New York: Springer Verlag; 1987:158-181.

91. Jablonska S, Orth G, Obalek S, et al. Cutaneous warts. Clinical, histologic, and virologic correlations. *Clin Dermatol.* 1985;3:71-82.

92. Schwartz RA. Verrucous carcinoma of the skin and mucosa. *J Am Acad Dermatol.* 1995;32:1-21.

93. Allington HV. Review of the psychotherapy of warts. *AMA Arch Derm Syphilol.* 1952;66:316-326.

94. von Krogh G. Podophyllotoxin for condylomata acuminata eradication. Clinical and experimental comparative studies on *Podophyllum lignans*, colchicine and 5-fluorouracil. *Acta Derm Venereol Suppl (Stockh).* 1981;98:1-48.

95. Kaplinsky RS, Pranikoff K, Chasan S, et al. Indications for urethroscopy in male patients with penile condylomata. *J Urol.* 1995;153:1120-1121.

96. Goorney BP, Waugh MA, Clarke J. Anal warts in heterosexual men. *Genitourin Med.* 1987;63:216.

97. Oriel JD. Anal warts and anal coitus. *Br J Vener Dis.* 1971;47:373-376.

98. Barrasso R, De Brux J, Croissant O, et al. High prevalence of papillomavirus-associated penile intraepithelial neoplasia in sexual partners of women with cervical intraepithelial neoplasia. *N Engl J Med.* 1987;317:916-923.

99. Reid R, Laverty CR, Coppleson M, et al. Noncondylomatous cervical wart virus infection. *Obstet Gynecol.* 1980;55:476-483.

100. Walker P, Dexeus S, De Palo G, et al. International terminology of colposcopy: An updated report from the International Federation for Cervical Pathology and Colposcopy. *Obstet Gynecol.* 2003;101:175-177.

101. Walker PG, Colley NV, Grubb C, et al. Abnormalities of the uterine cervix in women with vulvar warts. *Br J Vener Dis.* 1983;59:120-123.

102. Schwebke JR, Zajackowski ME. Effect of concurrent lower genital tract infections on cervical cancer screening. *Genitourin Med.* 1997;73:383-386.

103. Väyrynen M, Syrjänen H, Castrén O, et al. Colposcopy in women with papillomavirus lesions of the uterine cervix. *Obstet Gynecol.* 1985;65:409-415.

104. Dexeus S, Cararach M, Dexeus D. The role of colposcopy in modern gynecology. *Eur J Gynaecol Oncol.* 2002;23:269-277.

105. Roy M, Meisels A, Fortier M, et al. Vaginal condylomata: A human papillomavirus infection. *Clin Obstet Gynecol.* 1981;24:461-483.

106. Strand A, Wilander E, Zehbe I, et al. Vulvar papillomatosis, aceto-white lesions, and normal-looking vulvar mucosa evaluated by microscopy and human papillomavirus analysis. *Gynecol Obstet Invest.* 1995;40:265-270.

107. Gentile G, Formelli G, Pelusi G, et al. Is vestibular micropapillomatosis associated with human papillomavirus infection? *Eur J Gynaecol Oncol.* 1997;18:523-525.

108. Strand A, Rylander E. Human papillomavirus. Subclinical and atypical manifestations. *Dermatol Clin.* 1998;16:817-822.

109. Rosemberg SK, Jacobs H, Fuller T. Some guidelines in the treatment of urethral condylomata with carbon dioxide laser. *J Urol.* 1982;127:906-908.

110. Campion MJ. Clinical manifestations and natural history of genital human papillomavirus infection. *Obstet Gynecol Clin North Am.* 1987;14:363-388.

111. Demeter LM, Stoler MH, Bonnez W, et al. Penile intraepithelial neoplasia: Clinical presentation and an analysis of the physical state of human papillomavirus DNA. *J Infect Dis.* 1993;168:38-46.

112. Gross G, Ikenberg H, Gissmann L, et al. Papillomavirus infection of the anogenital region: Correlation between histology, clinical picture, and virus type. Proposal of a new nomenclature. *J Invest Dermatol.* 1985;85:147-152.

113. Löwhagen G-B, Bolmstedt A, Ryd W, et al. The prevalence of "high-risk" HPV types in penile condyloma-like lesions: Correlation between HPV type and morphology. *Genitourin Med.* 1993;69:87-90.

114. Maw RD, Reitano M, Roy M. An international survey of patients with genital warts: Perceptions regarding treatment and impact on lifestyle. *Int J STD AIDS.* 1998;9:571-578.

115. Schonfeld A, Nitke S, Schattner A, et al. Intramuscular human interferon-β injections in treatment of condylomata acuminata. *Lancet.* 1984;1:1038-1042.

116. Reichman RC, Oakes D, Bonnez W, et al. Treatment of condyloma acuminatum with three different alpha interferon preparations administered parenterally: A double-blind, placebo-controlled trial. *J Infect Dis.* 1990;162:1270-1276.

117. Condylomata International Collaborative Study Group. Recurrent condylomata acuminata treated with recombinant interferon alfa-2a. A multicenter double-blind placebo-controlled clinical trial. *JAMA.* 1991;265:2684-2687.

118. Schiffman MH. Latest HPV findings: Some clinical implications. *Contemp OB/GYN.* 1993;38:27-40.

119. Beutner KR, Wiley DJ, Douglas JM, et al. Genital warts and their treatment. *Clin Infect Dis.* 1998;28:S37-S56.

120. Osborne NG, Adelson MD. Herpes simplex and human papillomavirus genital infections: Controversies around obstetric management. *Clin Obstet Gynecol.* 1990;33:801-811.

121. Becker FT, Walder HJ, Larson DM. Giant condylomata acuminata. Buschke-Lowenstein tumor. *Arch Dermatol.* 1969;100:184-186.

122. Kibrite A, Zeitouni NC, Cloutier R. Aggressive giant condyloma acuminatum associated with oncogenic human papilloma virus: A case report. *Can J Surg.* 1997;40:143-145.

123. Cubilla AL, Velazques EF, Reuter VE, et al. Warty (condylomatous) squamous cell carcinoma of the penis: A report of 11 cases and proposed classification of 'verruciform' penile tumors. *Am J Surg Pathol.* 2000;24:505-512.

124. Anderson MC, Brown CL, Buckley CH, et al. Current views on cervical intraepithelial neoplasia. *J Clin Pathol.* 1991;44:969-978.

125. Okagaki T. Impact of human papillomavirus research on the histopathologic concepts of genital neoplasms. *Curr Top Pathol.* 1992;85:273-307.

126. Wade TR, Kopf AW, Ackerman AB. Bowenoid papulosis of the penis. *Cancer.* 1978;42:1890-1903.

127. De Villez RL, Stevens CS. Bowenoid papules of the genitalia. A case progressing to Bowen's disease. *J Am Acad Dermatol.* 1980;3:149-152.

128. Ikenberg H, Gissmann L, Gross G, et al. Human papillomavirus type 16–related DNA in genital Bowen's disease and in bowenoid papulosis. *Int J Cancer.* 1983;32:563-565.

129. Östör AG. Natural history of cervical intraepithelial neoplasia: A critical review. *Int J Gynecol Pathol.* 1993;12:186-192.

130. Schlappner OLA, Schaffer EA. Anorectal condylomata acuminata: A missed part of the condyloma spectrum. *Can Med Assoc J.* 1978;118:172-173.

131. Prassad ML, Abcarian H. Malignant potential of perianal condyloma acuminatum. *Dis Colon Rectum.* 1980;23:191-197.

132. Metcalf AM, Dean T. Risk of dysplasia in anal condyloma. *Surgery.* 1995;118:724-726.

133. Koblin BA, Hessol NA, Zauber AG, et al. Increased incidence of cancer among homosexual men, New York City and San Francisco, 1978-1990. *Am J Epidemiol.* 1996;144:916-923.

134. Daling JR, Weiss NS, Hislop TG, et al. Sexual practices, sexually transmitted diseases, and the incidence of anal cancer. *N Engl J Med.* 1987;317:973-977.

135. Bratcher J, Palefsky J. Anogenital human papillomavirus coinfection and associated neoplasia in HIV-positive men and women. *PRN Notebook*. 2008;13:1-8; available at http://www.prn.org/index.php/coinfections/article/anogenital_hpv_neoplasia_hiv_positive_502.

136. Frisch M, Glimelius B, van den Brule AJ, et al. Sexually transmitted infection as a cause of anal cancer. *N Engl J Med*. 1997;337:1350-1358.

137. Ziegler A, Kastner C, Chang-Claude J. Analysis of pregnancy and other factors on detection of human papilloma virus (HPV) infection using weighted estimating equations for follow-up data. *Stat Med*. 2003;22:2217-2233.

138. Watts DH, Koutsky LA, Holmes KK, et al. Low risk of perinatal transmission of human papillomavirus: Results from a prospective cohort study. *Am J Obstet Gynecol*. 1998;178:365-373.

139. Armstrong DK, Handley JM. Anogenital warts in prepubertal children: Pathogenesis, HPV typing and management. *Int J STD AIDS*. 1997;8:78-81.

140. Hammerschlag MR. Sexually transmitted diseases in sexually abused children: Medical and legal implications. *Sex Transm Dis*. 1998;74:167-174.

141. Bonnez WA. Issues with HIV and oral human papillomavirus infections. *AIDS Reader*. 2002;12:174-176.

142. Syrjänen S. Human papillomavirus infections and oral tumors. *Med Microbiol Immunol (Berl)*. 2003;192:123-128.

143. Sellors JW, Sankaranarayanan R. *Colposcopy and Treatment of Cervical Intraepithelial Neoplasia: A Beginners' Manual*. Lyon: International Agency for Research on Cancer; 2003; available at http://whqlibdoc.who.int/publications/2003/9283204123_eng.pdf.

144. Sedlacek TV, Cunnane M, Carpiniello V. Colposcopy in the diagnosis of penile condyloma. *Am J Obstet Gynecol*. 1986;154:494-496.

145. Krebs H-B, Schneider V. Human papillomavirus-associated lesions of the penis: Colposcopy, cytology, and histology. *Obstet Gynecol*. 1987;70:299-304.

146. Singer A, Campion MJ, Clarkson PK, et al. Recognition of subclinical human papillomavirus infection of the vulva. *J Reprod Med*. 1986;31:985-986.

147. Panici PB, Scambia G, Perrone L, et al. Oral condyloma lesions in patients with extensive genital human papillomavirus infection. *Am J Obstet Gynecol*. 1992;167:451-458.

148. Reid R, Greenberg M, Jenson AB, et al. Sexually transmitted papillomaviral infections: I. The anatomic distribution and pathologic grade of neoplastic lesions associated with different viral types. *Am J Obstet Gynecol*. 1987;156:212-222.

149. Jonsson M, Karlsson R, Evander M, et al. Acetowhitening of the cervix and vulva as a predictor of subclinical human papillomavirus infection: Sensitivity and specificity in a population-based study. *Obstet Gynecol*. 1997;90:744-747.

150. McMillan A. Sigmoidoscopy: A necessary procedure in the routine investigation of homosexual men? *Genitourin Med*. 1987;63:44-46.

151. Parker BJ, Cossart YE, Thompson H, et al. The clinical management and laboratory assessment of anal warts. *Med J Aust*. 1987;147:59-63.

152. Sidawy MK. Cytology in gynecological disorders. *Curr Top Pathol*. 1992;85:233-272.

153. Sherman ME. Chapter 11: Future directions in cervical pathology. *J Natl Cancer Inst Monogr*. 2003;31:72-79.

154. Nanda K, McCrory DC, Myers ER, et al. Accuracy of the Papanicolaou test in screening for and follow-up of cervical cytologic abnormalities: A systematic review. *Ann Intern Med*. 2000;132:810-819.

155. Palefsky JM, Holly EA, Hogeboom CJ, et al. Anal cytology as a screening tool for anal squamous intraepithelial lesions. *J Acquir Immune Defic Syndr Hum Retrovirol*. 1997;14:415-422.

156. Goldie SJ, Kuntz KM, Weinstein MC, et al. The clinical effectiveness and cost-effectiveness of screening for anal squamous intraepithelial lesions in homosexual and bisexual HIV-positive men. *JAMA*. 1999;281:1822-1829.

157. Palefsky JM, Holly EA, Ralston ML, et al. Anal squamous intraepithelial lesions in HIV-positive and HIV-negative homosexual and bisexual men: Prevalence and risk factors. *J Acquir Immune Defic Syndr Hum Retrovirol*. 1998;17:320-326.

158. Chin-Hong PV, Palefsky JM. Natural history and clinical management of anal human papillomavirus disease in men and women infected with human immunodeficiency virus. *Clin Infect Dis*. 2002;35:1127-1134.

159. Russell J, Crothers BA, Kaplan KJ, et al. Current cervical screening technology considerations: liquid-based cytology and automated screening. *Clin Obstet Gynecol*. 2005;48:108-119.

160. Wright TC Jr, Massad LS, Dunton CJ, et al. 2006 consensus guidelines for the management of women with abnormal cervical cancer screening tests. *Am J Obstet Gynecol*. 2007;197:346-355.

161. Wright TC Jr, Massad LS, Dunton CJ, et al. 2006 consensus guidelines for the management of women with cervical intraepithelial neoplasia or adenocarcinoma in situ. *Am J Obstet Gynecol*. 2007;197:340-350.

162. Solomon D, Davey D, Kurman R, et al. The 2001 Bethesda System: Terminology for reporting results of cervical cytology. *JAMA*. 2002;287:2114-2119.

163. Stoler MH, Schiffman M. Interobserver reproducibility of cervical cytologic and histologic interpretations. Realistic estimates from the ASCUS-LSIL Triage Study. *JAMA*. 2001;285:1500-1505.

164. Gravitt PE, Coutlee F, Iftner T, et al. New technologies in cervical cancer screening. *Vaccine*. 2008;26:K42-K52.

165. Kienzler JL, Lemoine MT, Orth G, et al. Humoral and cell-mediated immunity to human papillomavirus type 1 (HPV-1) in human warts. *Br J Dermatol*. 1983;108:665-672.

166. Bonnez W, DaRin C, Rose RC, et al. Use of human papillomavirus type 11 virions in an ELISA to detect specific antibodies in humans with condylomata acuminata. *J Gen Virol*. 1991;72:1343-1347.

167. Bonnez W, Kashima HK, Leventhal B, et al. Antibody response to human papillomavirus (HPV) type 11 in children with juvenile-onset recurrent respiratory papillomatosis. *Virology*. 1992;188:384-387.

168. Rose RC, Reichman RC, Bonnez W. Human papillomavirus type 11 (HPV-11) recombinant virus-like particles (VLPs) induce the formation of neutralizing antibodies and detect HPV-specific antibodies in human sera. *J Gen Virol*. 1994;75:2075-2079.

169. Olsson SE, Villa LL, Costa RL, et al. Induction of immune memory following administration of a prophylactic quadrivalent human papillomavirus (HPV) types 6/11/16/18 L1 virus-like particle (VLP) vaccine. *Vaccine*. 2007;25:4931-4939.

170. Underwood MR, Shewchuk LM, Hassell AM, et al. Searching for antiviral drugs for human papillomaviruses. *Antiviral Ther*. 2000;5:229-242.

171. Snoeck R. Papillomavirus and treatment. *Antiviral Res*. 2006;71:181-191.

172. Gibbs S, Harvey I, Sterling J, et al. Local treatments for cutaneous warts: Systematic review. *BMJ*. 2002;325:461.

173. Luk NM, Tang YM. Warts (non-genital). *BMJ Clin Evid*. 2007;12:1-18.

174. Jackson AD. Cryosurgery: A guide for GPs. *Practitioner*. 1999;243:131-136.

175. Connolly M, Bazmi K, O'Connell M, et al. Cryotherapy of viral warts: A sustained 10-s freeze is more effective than the traditional method. *Br J Dermatol*. 2001;145:554-557.

176. Bourke JF, Berth-Jones J, Hutchinson PE. Cryotherapy of common viral warts at intervals of 1, 2 and 3 weeks. *Br J Dermatol*. 1995;132:433-436.

177. Berth-Jones J, Hutchinson PE. Modern treatment of warts: Cure rates at 3 and 6 months. *Br J Dermatol*. 1992;127:262-265.

178. Focht DR III, Spicer C, Fairchok MP. The efficacy of duct tape vs cryotherapy in the treatment of verruca vulgaris (the common wart). *Arch Pediatr Adolesc Med*. 2002;156:971-974.

179. de Haen M, Spigt MG, van Uden CJ, et al. Efficacy of duct tape vs placebo in the treatment of verruca vulgaris (warts) in primary school children. *Arch Ped Adolesc Med*. 2006;160:1121-1125.

180. Wenner R, Askari SK, Cham PM, et al. Duct tape for the treatment of common warts in adults: a double-blind randomized controlled trial. *Arch Dermatol*. 2007;143:309-313.

181. Torrelo A. What's new in the treatment of viral warts in children. *Pediatr Dermatol*. 2002;19:191-199.

182. Buckley DA, Du Vivier AW. The therapeutic use of topical contact sensitizers in benign dermatoses. *Br J Dermatol*. 2001;145:385-405.

183. Najarian DJ, English JC III. Imiquimod cream: A new multipurpose topical therapy for dermatology. *P&T*. 2003;28:122-126.

184. Benton EC. Therapy of cutaneous warts. *Clin Dermatol*. 1997;15:449-455.

185. Tanzi EL, Lupton JR, Alster TS. Lasers in dermatology: Four decades of progress. *J Am Acad Dermatol*. 2003;49:1-31; quiz 31-34.

186. Odell RC. Electrosurgery: Principles and safety issues. *Clin Obstet Gynecol*. 1995;38:610-620.

187. Shenefelt PD. Hypnosis in dermatology. *Arch Dermatol*. 2000;136:393-399.

188. Johnson RFQ, Barber TX. Hypnosis, suggestion, and warts: An experimental investigation implicating the importance of "believed-in efficacy." *Am J Clin Hypn*. 1978;20:165-174.

189. Spanos NP, Stenstrom RJ, Johnston JC. Hypnosis, placebo, and suggestion in the treatment of warts. *Psychosom Med*. 1988;50:245-260.

190. Smolle J, Prause G, Kerl H. A double-blind, controlled clinical trial of homeopathy and an analysis of lunar phases and postoperative outcome. *Arch Dermatol*. 1998;134:1368-1370.

191. Harkness EF, Abbot NC, Ernst E. A randomized trial of distant healing for skin warts. *Am J Med*. 2000;108:448-452.

192. Beutner KR, Reitano MV, Richwald GA, et al. External genital warts: Report of the American Medical Association Consensus Conference. *Clin Infect Dis*. 1998;27:796-806.

193. von Krogh G. Management of anogenital warts (condylomata acuminata). *Eur J Dermatol*. 2001;11:598-603; quiz 604.

194. Workowski KA, Berman SM. Centers for Disease Control and Prevention sexually transmitted diseases treatment guidelines. *Clin Infect Dis*. 2007;44:S73-S76.

195. Wiley DJ, Douglas J, Beutner K, et al. External genital warts: Diagnosis, treatment, and prevention. *Clin Infect Dis*. 2002;35:S210-S224.

196. Buck HW Jr. Warts (genital). *BMJ Clin Evid*. 2007;12:1-20.

197. Krebs H-B, Helmkamp BF. Does the treatment of genital condylomata in men decrease the treatment failure rate of cervical dysplasia in the female sexual partner? *Obstet Gynecol*. 1990;76:660-663.

198. Sigurgeirsson B, Lindelöf B, Eklund G. Condylomata acuminata and risk of cancer: An epidemiological study. *BMJ*. 1991;303:341-344.

199. Gilbert LK, Alexander L, Grosshans JF, et al. Answering frequently asked questions about HPV. *Sex Transm Dis*. 2003;30:193-194.

200. Miller RA. Podophyllin. *Int J Dermatol*. 1985;24:491-498.

201. von Krogh G, Longstaff E. Podophyllin office therapy against condyloma should be abandoned. *Sex Transm Infect*. 2001;77:409-412.

202. Beutner KR. Podophyllotoxin in the treatment of genital human papillomavirus infection: A review. *Semin Dermatol*. 1987;6:10-18.

203. Lacey CJ, Goodall RL, Tennvall GR, et al. Randomised controlled trial and economic evaluation of podophyllotoxin solution, podophyllotoxin cream, and podophyllin in the treatment of genital warts. *Sex Transm Infect*. 2003;79:270-275.

204. Beutner KR, Friedman-Kien AE, Artman NN, et al. Patient-applied podofilox for treatment of genital warts. *Lancet*. 1989;1:831-834.

205. Kirby P, Dunne A, King DH, et al. Double-blind randomized clinical trial of self-administered podofilox solution versus vehicle in the treatment of genital warts. *Am J Med*. 1990;88:465-469.

206. Greenberg MD, Rutledge LH, Reid R, et al. A double-blind, randomized trial of 0.5% Podofilox and placebo for the treatment of genital warts in women. *Obstet Gynecol*. 1991;77:735-739.

207. Bonnez W, Elswick RK Jr, Bailey-Farchione A, et al. Efficacy and safety of 0.5% podofilox solution in the treatment and suppression of anogenital warts. *Am J Med*. 1994;96:420-425.

208. Tyring S, Edwards L, Cherry LK, et al. Safety and efficacy of 0.5-percent podofilox gel in the treatment of anogenital warts. *Arch Dermatol*. 1998;134:33-38.

209. Hurwitz DJ, Pincus L, Kupper TS. Imiquimod: A topically applied link between innate and acquired immunity. *Arch Dermatol*. 2003;139:1347-1350.

210. Slade HB, Owens ML, Tomai MA, et al. Imiquimod 5% cream (Aldara(tm)). *Exp Opin Invest Drugs*. 1998;7:437-449.

211. Beutner KR, Spruance SL, Hougham AJ, et al. Treatment of genital warts with an immune-response modifier (imiquimod). *J Am Acad Dermatol*. 1998;38:230-239.

212. Edwards L, Ferenczy A, Eron L, et al. Self-administered topical 5% imiquimod cream for external anogenital warts. *Arch Dermatol*. 1998;134:25-30.

213. Beutner KR, Tyring SK, Trofatter KF Jr, et al. Imiquimod, a patient-applied immune-response modifier for treatment of external genital warts. *Antimicrob Agents Chemother*. 1998;42:789-794.

214. Moore RA, Edwards JE, Hopwood J, et al. Imiquimod for the treatment of genital warts: A quantitative systematic review. *BMC Infect Dis*. 2001;1:3.

215. Garland SM, Sellors JW, Wikstrom A, et al. Imiquimod 5% cream is a safe and effective self-applied treatment for anogenital warts: Results of an open-label, multicentre phase IIIB trial. *Int J STD AIDS*. 2001;12:722-729.

216. Meltzer SM, Monk BJ, Tewari KS. Green tea catechins for treatment of external genital warts. *Am J Obstet Gynecol*. 2009;200:233.e7.

217. Richart RM, Kaufman RM, Woodruff JD. Advances in managing condylomas. *Contemp OB/GYN*. 1982;20:164-171, 175, 177, 180, 182, 187, 188, 190-192, 194.

218. Godley MJ, Bradbeer CS, Gellan M, et al. Cryotherapy compared with trichloracetic acid in treating genital warts. *Genitourin Med*. 1987;63:390-392.

219. Abdullah AN, Walzman M, Wade A. Treatment of external genital warts comparing cryotherapy (liquid nitrogen) and trichloracetic acid. *Sex Transm Dis*. 1993;20:344-345.

220. Gabriel G, Thin RNT. Treatment of anogenital warts: Comparison of trichloracetic acid and podophyllin versus podophyllin alone. *Br J Vener Dis*. 1983;59:124-126.

221. Boothby RA, Carlson JA, Rubin M, et al. Single application treatment of human papillomavirus infection of the cervix and vagina with trichloracetic acid: A randomized trial. *Obstet Gynecol*. 1990;76:278-280.

222. Stone KM. Human papillomavirus infection and genital warts: Update on epidemiology and treatment. *Clin Infect Dis*. 1995;20:S91-S97.

223. Bashi SA. Cryotherapy versus podophyllin in the treatment of genital warts. *Int J Dermatol*. 1985;24:535-536.

224. Stone KM, Becker TM, Hadgu A, et al. Treatment of external genital warts: A randomised clinical trial comparing podophyllin, cryotherapy, and electrodesiccation. *Genitourin Med*. 1990;66:16-19.

225. Simmons PD, Langlet F, Thin RNT. Cryotherapy versus electrocautery in the treatment of genital warts. *Br J Vener Dis*. 1981;57:273-274.

226. Jensen SL. Comparison of podophyllin application with simple surgical excision in clearance and recurrence of perianal condylomata acuminata. *Lancet*. 1985;2:1146-1148.

227. Duus BR, Philipsen T, Christensen JD, et al. Refractory condylomata acuminata: A controlled clinical trial of carbon dioxide laser versus conventional surgical treatment. *Genitourin Med*. 1985;61:59-61.

228. McMillan A, Scott GR. Outpatient treatment of perianal warts by scissor excision. *Genitourin Med*. 1987;63:114-115.

229. Bonnez W, Oakes D, Choi A, et al. Therapeutic efficacy and complications of excisional biopsy of condyloma acuminatum. *Sex Transm Dis*. 1996;23:273-276.

230. Baggish MS. Improved laser techniques for the elimination of genital and extragenital warts. *Am J Obstet Gynecol.* 1985;153:545-550.
231. Reid R. Physical and surgical principles governing expertise with the carbon dioxide laser. *Obstet Gynecol Clin North Am.* 1987;14:513-535.
232. Bar-Am A, Shilon M, Peyser MR, et al. Treatment of male genital condylomatous lesions by carbon dioxide laser after failure of previous nonlaser methods. *J Am Acad Dermatol.* 1991;24:87-89.
233. Petersen CS, Bjerring P, Larsen J, et al. Systemic interferon alpha-2b increases the cure rate in laser treated patients with multiple persistent genital warts: A placebo-controlled study. *Genitourin Med.* 1991;67:99-102.
234. Condylomata International Collaborative Study Group. Randomized placebo-controlled double-blind combined therapy with laser surgery and systemic interferon-alpha 2a in the treatment of anogenital condylomata acuminatum. *J Infect Dis.* 1993;167:824-829.
235. Lassus A, Kartamaa M, Happonen H-P. A comparative study of topical analgesia with a lidocaine/prilocaine cream (EMLA(r)) and infiltration anesthesia for laser surgery of genital warts in men. *Sex Transm Dis.* 1990;17:130-132.
236. Rylander E, Sjoberg I, Lillieborg S, et al. Local anesthesia of the genital mucosa with a lidocaine/prilocaine cream (EMLA) for laser treatment of condylomata acuminata: A placebo-controlled study. *Obstet Gynecol.* 1990;75:302-306.
237. Mansell-Gregory M, Romanowski B. Randomised double blind trial of EMLA for the control of pain related to cryotherapy in the treatment of genital HPV lesions. *Sex Transm Infect.* 1998; 74:274-275.
238. Gupta AK, Koren G, Shear NH. A double-blind, randomized, placebo-controlled trial of eutectic lidocaine/prilocaine cream 5% (EMLA) for analgesia prior to cryotherapy of warts in children and adults. *Pediatr Dermatol.* 1998;15:129-133.
239. de Benedictis JT, Marmar JL, Praiss DE. Intraurethral condylomata acuminata: Management and a review of the literature. *J Urol.* 1977;118:767-769.
240. Dretler SP, Klein LA. The eradication of intraurethral condyloma acuminata with 5 per cent 5-fluorouracil cream. *J Urol.* 1975;113:195-198.
241. Wallin J. 5-Fluorouracil in the treatment of penile and urethral condylomata acuminata. *Br J Vener Dis.* 1977;53:240-243.
242. Krebs H-B. Prophylactic topical 5-fluorouracil following treatment of human papillomavirus-associated lesions of the vulva and vagina. *Obstet Gynecol.* 1986;68:837-841.
243. Edwards L. The interferons. *Dermatol Clin.* 2001;19:139-146, ix.
244. Parmar S, Platanias LC. Interferons: Mechanisms of action and clinical applications. *Curr Opin Oncol.* 2003;15:431-439.
245. Eron LJ, Judson F, Tucker S, et al. Interferon therapy for condylomata acuminata. *N Engl J Med.* 1986;315:1059-1064.
246. Friedman-Kien A, Eron LJ, Conant M, et al. Natural interferon alfa for treatment of condylomata acuminata. *JAMA.* 1988;259: 533-538.
247. Vance JC, Bart BJ, Hansen RC, et al. Intralesional recombinant alpha-2 interferon for the treatment of patients with condyloma acuminatum or verruca plantaris. *Arch Dermatol.* 1986;122: 272-277.
248. Condylomata International Collaborative Study Group. A comparison of interferon alfa-2a and podophyllin in the treatment of primary condylomata acuminata. *Genitourin Med.* 1991;67: 394-399.
249. Johnson JA, Gangemi JD. Selective inhibition of human papillomavirus-induced cell proliferation by (*S*)-1-[3-hydroxy-2-(phosphonylmethoxy)propyl]cytosine. *Antimicrob Agents Chemother.* 1999;43:1198-1205.
250. Snoeck R, Bossens M, Parent D, et al. Phase II double-blind, placebo-controlled study of the safety and efficacy of cidofovir topical gel for the treatment of patients with human papillomavirus infection. *Clin Infect Dis.* 2001;33:597-602.
251. Strauss MJ, Khanna V, Koenig JD, et al. The cost of treating genital warts. *Int J Dermatol.* 1996;35:340-348.
252. Langley PC, Tyring SK, Smith MH. The cost effectiveness of patient-applied versus provider-administered intervention strategies for the treatment of external genital warts. *Am J Manag Care.* 1999;5:69-77.
253. Alam M, Stiller M. Direct medical costs for surgical and medical treatment of condylomata acuminata. *Arch Dermatol.* 2001;137:337-341.
254. Bonnez W, Oakes D, Bailey-Farchione A, et al. A randomized, double-blind, placebo-controlled trial of systemically administered alpha-, beta-, or gamma-interferon in combination with cryotherapy for the treatment of condyloma acuminatum. *J Infect Dis.* 1995;171:1081-1089.
255. Wilson JD, Brown CB, Walker PP. Factors involved in clearance of genital warts. *Int J STD AIDS.* 2001;12:789-792.
256. Ross JD. Is oral contraceptive associated with genital warts? *Genitourin Med.* 1996;72:330-333.
257. Feldman JG, Chirgwin K, Dehovitz JA, et al. The association of smoking and risk of condyloma acuminatum in women. *Obstet Gynecol.* 1997;89:346-350.
258. Sand PK, Shen W, Bowen LW, et al. Cryotherapy for the treatment of proximal urethral condyloma acuminatum. *J Urol.* 1987;137:874-876.
259. Ng N, Vuignier BI, Hart LL. Fluorouracil in condyloma acuminatum. *Drug Intel Clin Pharm.* 1987;21:175-176.
260. Levine LA, Elterman L, Rukstalis DB. Treatment of subclinical intraurethral human papilloma virus infection with interferon alfa-2b. *Urology.* 1996;47:553-557.
261. Dodi G, Infantino A, Moretti R, et al. Cryotherapy of anorectal warts and condylomata. *Cryosurgery.* 1982;19:287-288.
262. Bullingham RP, Lewis RG. Laser versus electrical cautery in the treatment of condylomata acuminata of the anus. *Surg Gynecol Obstet.* 1982;155:865-867.
263. Kaspari M, Gutzmer R, Kaspari T, et al. Application of imiquimod by suppositories (anal tampons) efficiently prevents recurrences after ablation of anal canal condyloma. *Br J Dermatol.* 2002;147:757-759.
264. Centers for Disease Control and Prevention. 1998 guidelines for the treatment of sexually transmitted diseases. *MMWR Morb Mortal Wkly Rep.* 1998;47:1-116.
265. Ferenczy A. Treating genital condyloma during pregnancy with the carbon dioxide laser. *Am J Obstet Gynecol.* 1984;148:9-12.
266. Wertheimer A. Indirect colposcopy and laser vaporization in the management of vaginal condylomata. *J Reprod Med.* 1986;31: 39-42.
267. Matsunaga J, Bergman A, Bhatia NN. Genital condylomata acuminata in pregnancy: Effectiveness, safety and pregnancy outcome following cryotherapy. *Br J Obstet Gynaecol.* 1987;94: 168-172.
268. Bonnez W. Sexually transmitted human papillomavirus infection. In: Dolin R, Masur H, Saag M, eds. *AIDS Therapy.* 3rd ed. Philadelphia: Saunders; 2008.
269. Beck DE, Jaso RG, Zajac RA. Surgical management of anal condylomata in the HIV-positive patient. *Dis Colon Rectum.* 1990;33:180-183.
270. Orkin BA, Smith LE. Perineal manifestations of HIV infection. *Dis Colon Rectum.* 1992;35:310-314.
271. Kilewo CD, Urassa WK, Pallangyo K, et al. Response to podophyllotoxin treatment of genital warts in relation to HIV-1 infection among patients in Dar es Salaam, Tanzania. *Int J STD AIDS.* 1995;6:114-116.
272. Douglas JM, Rogers M, Judson FN. The effect of asymptomatic infection with HTLV-III on the response of anogenital warts in intralesional treatment with recombinant alpha-2 interferon. *J Infect Dis.* 1986;154:331-334.
273. Gilson RJ, Shupack JL, Friedman-Kien AE, et al. A randomized, controlled, safety study using imiquimod for the topical treatment of anogenital warts in HIV-infected patients. Imiquimod Study Group. *AIDS.* 1999;13:2397-2404.
274. Miles AJG, Mellor CH, Gazzard B, et al. Surgical management of anorectal disease in HIV-positive homosexuals. *Br J Surg.* 1990;77:869-871.
275. Fleshner PR, Freilich MI. Adjuvant interferon for anal condyloma: A prospective, randomized trial. *Dis Colon Rectum.* 1994;37:1255-1259.
276. Conant MA. Immunomodulatory therapy in the management of viral infections in patients with HIV infection. *J Am Acad Dermatol.* 2000;43:S27-S30.
277. Stier EA, Goldstone SE, Berry JM, et al. Infrared coagulator treatment of high-grade anal dysplasia in HIV-infected individuals: an AIDS malignancy consortium pilot study. *J Acquir Immune Defic Syndr.* 2008;47:56-61.
278. Lord RVN. Anorectal surgery in patients infected with human immunodeficiency virus: Factors associated with delayed wound healing. *Ann Surg.* 1997;226:92-99.
279. O'Brien ME, Clayton JL, Clark R, et al. Association between antiretroviral therapy and condyloma acuminatum. 39th Meeting of the Infectious Disease Society of America, San Francisco, 2001:659.
280. Greenspan D, Canchola AJ, MacPhail LA, et al. Effect of highly active antiretroviral therapy on frequency of oral warts. *Lancet.* 2001;357:1411-1412.
281. Heard I, Palefsky JM, Kazatchkine M. The impact of HIV antiviral therapy on human papillomavirus (HPV) infections and HPV-related diseases. *Antivir Ther.* 2004;9:13-22.
282. Majewski S, Skopinska M, Bollag W, et al. Combination of isotretinoin and calcitriol for precancerous and cancerous skin lesions. *Lancet.* 1994;344:1510-1511.
283. Auborn KJ. Therapy for recurrent respiratory papillomatosis. *Antivir Ther.* 2002;7:1-9.
284. Kimberlin DW. Pharmacotherapy of recurrent respiratory papillomatosis. *Expert Opin Pharmacother.* 2002;3:1091-1099.
285. Pransky SM, Albright JT, Magit AE. Long-term follow-up of pediatric recurrent respiratory papillomatosis managed with intralesional cidofovir. *Laryngoscope.* 2003;113:1583-1587.
286. Bell MC, Crowley-Nowick P, Bradlow HL, et al. Placebo-controlled trial of indole-3-carbinol in the treatment of CIN. *Gynecol Oncol.* 2000;78:123-129.
287. Dilley DC, Siegel MA, Budnick S. Diagnosing and treating common oral pathologies. *Pediatr Clin North Am.* 1991;38: 1227-1264.
288. Winer RL, Hughes JP, Feng Q, et al. Condom use and the risk of genital human papillomavirus infection in young women. *N Engl J Med.* 2006;354:2645-2654.
289. Hogewoning CJ, Bleeker MC, van den Brule AJ, et al. Condom use promotes regression of cervical intraepithelial neoplasia and clearance of human papillomavirus: A randomized clinical trial. *Int J Cancer.* 2003;107:811-816.
290. Bleeker MC, Hogewoning CJ, Voorhorst FJ, et al. Condom use promotes regression of human papillomavirus-associated penile lesions in male sexual partners of women with cervical intraepithelial neoplasia. *Int J Cancer.* 2003;107:804-810.
291. Bleeker MC, Hogewoning CJ, Berkhof J, et al. Concordance of specific human papillomavirus types in sex partners is more prevalent than would be expected by chance and is associated with increased viral loads. *Clin Infect Dis.* 2005;41:612-620.
292. Monsonego J, Bosch FX, Coursaget P, et al. Cervical cancer control, priorities and new directions. *Int J Cancer.* 2004;108: 329-333.
293. Saslow D, Runowicz CD, Solomon D, et al. American Cancer Society guideline for the early detection of cervical neoplasia and cancer. *CA Cancer J Clin.* 2002;52:342-362.
294. U.S. Preventive Services Task Force. *Screening for Cervical Cancer.* AHRQ Publication No. 03-515A, January 2003. Rockville, Md: Agency for Healthcare Research and Quality; 2003.
295. ACOG Practice Bulletin. Cervical cytology screening. Number 45, August 2003. *Int J Gynaecol Obstet.* 2003;83:237-247.
296. Barr E, Sings HL. Prophylactic HPV vaccines: new interventions for cancer control. *Vaccine.* 2008;26:6244-6257.
297. Keam SJ, Harper DM. Human papillomavirus types 16 and 18 vaccine (recombinant, AS04 adjuvanted, adsorbed) [Cervarix]. *Drugs.* 2008;68:359-372.
298. Bonnez W. Human papillomavirus vaccine-recent results and future developments. *Current Opin Pharmacol.* 2007;7:1-8.
299. Koutsky LA, Ault KA, Wheeler CM, et al. A controlled trial of a human papillomavirus type 16 vaccine. *N Engl J Med.* 2002;347:1645-1651.
299a. Rowhani-Rahbar A, Mao C, Alvarez FB, et al. Long-term efficacy of a prophylactic human papillomavirus type 16 vaccine. *25th International Papillomavirus Conference.* May 8-14, 2009. Malmö, Sweden. Abstract O-01.03.
300. Barr E, Gause CK, Bautista OM, et al. Impact of a prophylactic quadrivalent human papillomavirus (types 6, 11, 16, 18) L1 virus-like particle vaccine in a sexually active population of North American women. *Am J Obstet Gynecol.* 2008;198:261. e1-261.e11.
300a. Munoz N, Manalastas R Jr, Pitisuttithum P, et al. Safety, immunogenicity, and efficacy of quadrivalent human papillomavirus (types 6, 11, 16, 18) recombinant vaccine in women aged 24-45 years: a randomized, double-blind trial. *Lancet.* 2009; 373:1949-1957.
301. Markowitz LE, Dunne EF, Saraiya M, et al. Quadrivalent Human Papillomavirus Vaccine: Recommendations of the Advisory Committee on Immunization Practices (ACIP). *MMWR—Morbidity and Mortality Weekly Report.* 2007;56: 1-24.
302. American Academy of Pediatrics Committee on Infectious Diseases. Recommended immunization schedules for children and adolescents: United States, 2007. *Pediatrics.* 2007;119: 207-208.
303. Wheeler CM, Bautista OM, Tomassini JE, et al. Safety and immunogenicity of co-administered quadrivalent human papillomavirus (HPV)-6/11/16/18 L1 virus-like particle (VLP) and hepatitis B (HBV) vaccines. *Vaccine.* 2008;26:686-696.

145

JC, BK, and Other Polyomaviruses: Progressive Multifocal Leukoencephalopathy

C. SABRINA TAN | IGOR J. KORALNIK

The human polyomaviruses, *JC virus* (JCV) and *BK virus* (BKV), are ubiquitous in most human populations throughout the world and do not cause disease in individuals with immunocompetence. As much as 90% and 86% of the general adult population are seropositive for BKV and JCV, respectively.[1,2] In individuals with immunosuppression, JCV is the etiologic agent of a demyelinating disease of the central nervous system, progressive multifocal leukoencephalopathy (PML), whereas BKV causes nephropathy, hemorrhagic cystitis, and ureteral stenosis. PML is an AIDS-defining opportunistic infection.[3] BKV nephropathy is a cause of allograft loss in kidney transplant recipients. Recently, three new human polyomaviruses have been characterized. This chapter describes features of the human polyomaviruses and their associated diseases.

Virology

HISTORY

Polyomaviruses are small (45-nm) nonenveloped viruses that are comprised of 72 capsomeres with icosahedral symmetry, harbor a circular double-stranded DNA, and belong to the Papovaviridae family. The other member of the Papovaviridae family is the *Papillomavirus* genus. The polyoma genus was named after the murine polyoma virus that caused numerous tumors in newborn mice.[4] The polyomaviruses are ubiquitous in nature and are species-specific, including humans (JCV, BKV), monkeys (simian virus 40 [SV40]), and mice (mouse polyomavirus). In humans, JCV was first isolated from the brain of a patient with PML whose initials were J.C.[5] Similarly, B.K. were the initials of a kidney transplant patient in whom BKV-associated ureteral stenosis was first described.[6] The newest members of the polyomaviruses are WU (Washington University) and KI (Karolinska Institute), both recently isolated from human respiratory tract secretions and named according to the institutions at which they were discovered, and Merkel cell carcinoma virus (MCV), named because it was detected in Merkel cell carcinoma tissues.[7-9]

EPIDEMIOLOGY

Both JCV and BKV have worldwide distribution, including geographically isolated populations with little exposure to other infections.[10] Although seroprevalence for both BKV and JCV increases rapidly with age,[11] primary infection of each virus occurs independently.[12] After primary infection, BKV and JCV can be detected in renal tubular epithelial cells, where they may remain latent. Although JC viruria occurs independent of the host's immune status, JC viremia is usually only detected in individuals with immunosuppression. Indeed, JCV is found in the urine of 20% to 30% of healthy and immunosuppressed individuals alike, with or without PML.[13,14] However, JCV viremia has been only detected in 20% to 40% of individuals who are HIV-positive without PML and in 60% to 80% of patients with PML.[15,16] Conversely, BK viruria occurs in 0 to 20% of asymptomatic individuals with immunocompetence,[1] but viral shedding in the urine is higher in individuals with immunosuppression (10% to 60%),[17-19] which correlates with the degrees of immunosuppression.[20] Specifically, in the urine of patients who are HIV-positive, BK viral load increases with decreased CD4+ T-cell counts.[21,22] Although BKV is usually not detected in the peripheral blood of individuals with either immunocompetence or immunosuppression, the detection of BKV DNA in the plasma of renal transplant patients is an indication of development of BKV-induced nephropathy.[17,23]

GENOME

Polyomaviruses have a circular double-stranded genomic DNA of approximately 5 kb. The genomes of BKV and JCV have been used extensively in human population migration studies because of their extremely conserved coding regions. JCV and BKV share approximately 70% genome homology,[24] and all polyomaviruses maintain the feature of coding DNA from both strands. The early proteins, large T and small t, are transcribed counterclockwise from one strand, whereas the late proteins, VP1, VP2, VP3, and agnoprotein, are transcribed clockwise from the opposite strand (Fig. 145-1). The genome can be divided into three distinct areas: 1, the early genes region, which includes the large T and small t antigens, regulatory proteins responsible for viral transformation, replication, and regulation of gene expression; 2, the late genes region, which encodes the capsid proteins VP1, VP2, and VP3 and the agnoprotein; and 3, the noncoding regulatory region. The agnoprotein is important both in regulation of JCV transcription and translation and in dysregulation of host cell cycle and DNA repairs.[25,26] Similar to the origin of DNA replication, the noncoding regulatory region also contains several binding sites for nuclear factors, which play important roles in JCV transcription. Deletions, insertions, and rearrangements in the regulatory region are associated with tissue tropism and virulence. The archetype regulatory region is mainly found in JCV isolated from kidney cells and consequently from urine. It is thought to be the type from which all other JCV regulatory region sequences have evolved. The rearranged type of regulatory region of JCV is principally detected in the brain and cerebrospinal fluid (CSF) of patients with PML. Whereas the rearranged type of regulatory region is found in the peripheral blood of patients with PML, a mixture of both types is present in the bone marrow.[15,27] Which type of regulatory region is associated with primary infection is not known.

RECEPTORS AND CELL ENTRY

JC Virus

Data suggested that N-linked glycoprotein containing an alpha (2,6)-linked sialic acid may act as a JCV receptor. In addition, evidence from cultured cell lines showed that JCV uses the serotonergic 5HT2a receptors for cell entry.[28] Pharmacologic blockade of the serotonergic receptors restricts JCV infection in vitro. The 5HT2a receptor is present on glial cells and astrocytes and on B lymphocytes, platelets, and kidney epithelial cells. JCV also uses clarithrin-coated pits on cell surfaces after binding and adsorption, mediated by the capsid protein, VP1. Cell

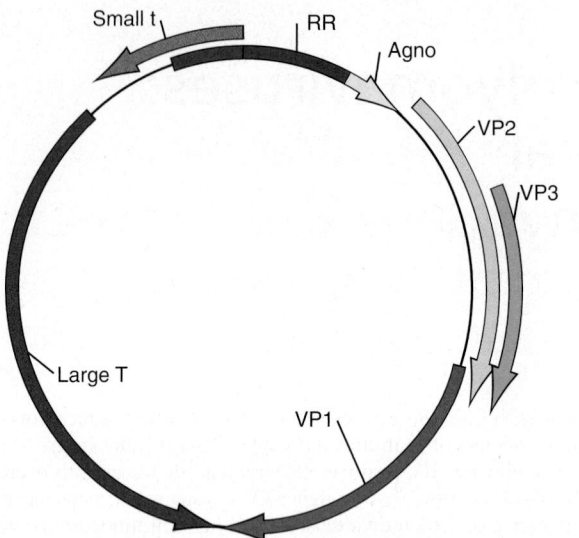

Figure 145-1   Polyomavirus genomic map (~5 kb). RR, regulatory region. *(Courtesy of Dr. Yiping Chen.)*

entry occurs via endocytosis and results in fusion of virus-carrying vesicle with the nuclear membrane.[29]

BK Virus

BK virus uses an N-linked glycoprotein containing an alpha (2,3)-linked sialic acid as a receptor. Entry into the cell occurs via caveolae-mediated endocytosis.[30]

NEW HUMAN POLYOMAVIRUSES

In 2007, two new viruses were discovered; phylogenetic analyses have placed them in the polyomavirus genus. The KI and WU polyomaviruses were first isolated from respiratory samples with high-throughput screens.[7,8] Subsequently, molecular evidence indicated a worldwide distribution for both viruses in the respiratory secretions of children, with incidence rates as high as 2.5% in Australia[31] for KI and 7% in South Korea[32] for WU. A study analyzing nasopharyngeal aspirates in the United Kingdom showed a bimodal age distribution of KI virus and detection of the WU virus in samples from patients younger than 15 years old.[33] Both KI and WU share significant genomic and protein similarities with BKV and JCV. Although the DNA of these viruses is convincingly present in the respiratory tracts of patients with respiratory diseases, as yet, no reported serologic assay or isolation of mature viral particles exists. Therefore, the proof of their existence as bona fide infectious agents remains to be established.

The Merkel cell polyomavirus (MCV) was discovered in 2008 in up to 80% of tissues with Merkel cell carcinoma, an aggressive and deadly neuroectodermal tumor that principally affects patients with immunosuppression.[9] Molecular studies indicate that MCV shares a similar genome with the other human polyomaviruses and that integration of MCV into the tumor genome most likely takes place before clonal expansion of tumor cells. Unlike KI and WU, MCV is most similar to the African green monkey lymphotropic polyomavirus. Interestingly, all three newly discovered polyomaviruses differ from all other human polyomaviruses by not containing a gene that encodes the agnoprotein. The agnoprotein was initially named because its function was unknown. However, this protein appears to have important regulatory functions of both the polyomaviruses and the host cells. The significance of the agnoprotein deletion in these three most recently discovered polyomaviruses remains to be determined.

Progressive Multifocal Leukoencephalopathy and Other JC Virus–Associated Syndromes

EPIDEMIOLOGY

Progressive multifocal leukoencephalopathy was initially described in 1958.[34] The disease was estimated to occur in 0.07% of individuals with hematologic malignant diseases,[35] such as leukemia and lymphoma, or in rare patients with solid organ cancer or in organ transplant recipients. Since the 1980s, in the era of HIV infection, PML has been recognized as a major opportunistic infection that affects up to 5% of patients with AIDS.[3] Currently, 80% of patients with PML have AIDS, 13% have hematologic malignant diseases, 5% are either solid organ or bone marrow transplant recipients, and 2% have chronic inflammatory diseases.[36] Lastly, a new group of patients with PML has emerged among patients treated with immunomodulatory medications for malignant diseases or autoimmune diseases, such as patients treated with natalizumab for multiple sclerosis or Crohn's disease,[37-39] rituximab for lymphoma[40,41] or lupus,[42] and efalizumab for psoriasis.[43]

PATHOGENESIS

Primary infection of JCV is asymptomatic, after which the virus becomes clinically latent. JCV DNA is detected with polymerase chain reaction (PCR) in the tonsillar tissues of 39% of healthy individuals, which suggests a possible oral or respiratory route of infection.[44,45] Detection of JCV in urine of healthy adults indicates that the kidney is a site of latency. Immunohistochemical staining shows viral proteins in the kidney tubular epithelial cells. Detection of JCV DNA in the bone marrow[44a] and brain of patients without PML suggests these are also possible additional sites of latency.

In patients with PML, JCV infects oligodendrocytes and astrocytes in the brain and rarely the spinal cord, which causes a lytic infection that results in the destruction of the myelin sheath. Pathologic examinations of PML lesions show extensive demyelination of the affected areas.

CLINICAL MANIFESTATIONS

Classic Progressive Multifocal Leukoencephalopathy

Because PML causes multifocal demyelination of the white matter of the central nervous system (CNS), the resulting neurologic deficits correspond to the location of the lesions. Although initial symptoms of PML can vary greatly from patient to patient, the predominant symptoms include coordination difficulties, gait imbalance, cognitive dysfunction, visual problems, and limb paresis. The optic nerves and the spinal cord of the central nervous system are usually spared, but incidental postmortem findings of PML lesions have been discovered in the spinal cord of a patient who was HIV-positive with hemispheric PML.[46] Furthermore, although PML lesions are generally located in the white matter, seizures, which are usually considered to be of cortical origin, can be seen in up to 18% of patients with PML and are associated with the localization of demyelinated lesions immediately adjacent to the cortex (Table 145-1).[47]

Progressive Multifocal Leukoencephalopathy–Immune Reconstitution Inflammatory Syndrome

Inflammatory PML has been frequently detected when the immune response is rapidly restored with highly active antiretroviral therapy (HAART) treatment in patients with HIV. Patients usually have an increasing $CD4^+$ count and a decreasing plasma HIV viral load. Unlike classic PML, the PML–immune reconstitution inflammatory syndrome (IRIS) lesions display contrast enhancement on magnetic resonance imaging (MRI), which indicates a breakdown of the blood-brain barrier, along with worsening of the initial presenting symptoms. Conditions may stabilize after the initial worsening of symptoms, but fatal outcome has been reported.[48,49]

TABLE 145-1	JC Virus–Associated Diseases			
Clinical Presentation	*Classic PML*	*PML-IRIS*	*JCV GCN*	*JCV E*
Onset	Subacute	Immune recovery	Chronic	Subacute
MRI	Asymmetric, well-demarcated, nonenhancing subcortical white matter lesions; hyperintense in T2 and FLAIR; hypointense in T1	Contrast-enhancing lesions and possible mass effect	Cerebellar atrophy	Cortical lesions
Neurologic symptoms	Based on location	Based on location and inflammation	Cerebellar syndrome	Encephalopathy
Histology	Demyelinating lesions often at gray/white junction; JCV detected in enlarged oligodendrocytes, bizarre astrocytes; presence of CD8+ T cells near JCV-infected cells	Demyelination similar to classic PML but with marked inflammatory infiltrates	Focal areas of cell loss in granule cell layer of cerebellum; JCV detected in enlarged granule cell neurons	Focal areas of cell loss in hemispheric cortex; JCV detected in enlarged pyramidal neurons

E, encephalopathy; FLAIR, fluid attenuated inversion recovery; GCN, granule cell neuropathy; IRIS, immune reconstitution inflammatory syndrome; JCV, JC virus; MRI, magnetic resonance imaging; PML, progressive multifocal leukoencephalopathy.

In autopsy samples of patients with PML-IRIS, mainly CD8+ lymphocytes were detected in the lesions with a paucity of CD4+ lymphocytes.[49-51] The reported time of onset of PML-IRIS ranged from 4 to 108 weeks after start of HAART.[48,49] In some cases, HAART was started as treatment for PML,[48-54] and in others, PML was diagnosed at the time of IRIS presentation.[48,55]

JC Virus Granule Cell Neuronopathy

Demyelination of white matter in the cerebellum is well described in patients with PML. In addition to oligodendrocytes and astrocytes, JCV can also infect and destroy cerebellar granule cell neurons. This neuronal infection can result in a novel syndrome characterized by cerebellar atrophy, gait ataxia, and incoordination, without associated demyelination.[56] This novel syndrome, distinct from PML, is called JCV granule cell neuronopathy (GCN).[57,58] JCV GCN appears to be caused by a JCV variant harboring a 10-bp deletion in the C terminus of the VP1 gene.[59] A recent histologic survey indicated that infection of granule cell neurons may be found in up to half of patients with PML.[60]

JC Virus Encephalopathy

JC virus can also infect hemispheric cortical pyramidal neurons. The clinical presentation differs from both classic PML and JCV GCN. Brain lesions are initially restricted to the gray matter on MRI, and the patient presents with a global cognitive decline and aphasia, rather than with focal neurologic deficits such as sensory or motor dysfunction.[61]

JC Virus Meningitis

Although JCV is not routinely tested for in the CSF of patients with meningeal symptoms, several studies have documented JCV as the only pathogen present in the CSF of patients with typical meningitis symptoms, including neck stiffness and diplopia.[62-64] Whether these cases result from JCV primary infection or reactivation is unclear. Because JCV PCR is not routinely performed in the CSF of patients with meningitis who do not have CNS lesions, the exact incidence of JCV meningitis is unknown.

DIAGNOSIS

Imaging

Radiographically, PML brain lesions typically appear as multiple white matter lesions, usually sparing the cortex, that do not conform to particular vascular territories. No associated mass effect or contrast enhancement is generally seen. Both computer tomography (CT) scan imaging and MRI can be used in the diagnosis of PML. Lesions appear in the white matter as hypodense or patchy on CT scan, and on MRI, as areas of hyperintense (bright) signal on T2-weighted and fluid attenuated inversion recovery (FLAIR) images, and as hypointense (dark) signal on T1-weighted images. MRI is more sensitive than CT scan and is the imaging method of choice for diagnosis of PML. As the name PML suggests, multiple lesions are usually present; they are often located in the subcortical white matter or in the cerebellar peduncles.[65,66] Lesions may also be found in gray matter structures such as the basal ganglia or thalamus, which also contain myelinated fibers. Although features of MRI appearance are not linked to survival time, the rare detection of mass effect predicts poor prognosis.[67] Lastly, atypical PML lesions, including ones with contrast enhancement, are seen in inflammatory PML that results from IRIS (Fig. 145-2).[48]

Brain Biopsy

Brain biopsy is the gold standard for the diagnosis of PML. This test has a sensitivity that ranges from 64% to 96% and a specificity of 100%. Histologic examination shows demyelinated areas, with reactive gliosis and enlarged and bizarre astrocytes, and macrophages that contain phagocytosed myelin and cellular debris. These lesions are located in both cortical and subcortical regions of the brain.[68] JCV can be detected in infected oligodendrocytes with enlarged amphophilic nuclei located at the periphery of the lesions. Intraparenchymal and perivascular infiltrates by CD8+ T cells are usually present in PML-IRIS (Fig. 145-3).[49]

Cerebrospinal Fluid Polymerase Chain Reaction

Brain biopsy may not be feasible in some patients, depending on the location of the lesions and the disability of the patient. In addition, biopsy carries an inherent morbidity and mortality risk. Therefore, spinal fluid examination is more commonly used as an alternative method of diagnosis. Patients with PML generally have a nonspecific CSF profile, including mild pleocytosis, with slightly elevated protein, and normal glucose. The detection of JCV with PCR of CSF had a sensitivity of 72% to 92% and a specificity of 92% to 100%[69] before extensive availability of HAART. However, in the post-HAART era, the sensitivity of PCR detection of CSF has decreased significantly to 58% with no changes in the specificity in patients with HIV presenting with PML while on HAART.[70]

PROGNOSIS

Progressive multifocal leukoencephalopathy is a fatal disease in most cases. Before the HAART era, only 10% of patients who were HIV-positive with PML lived longer than a year after diagnosis.[71,72] After the extensive use of HAART, the 1-year survival rate has increased to 50%.[72] A number of studies have delineated several prognostic markers that include: patients who present with a lower JCV CSF burden,[73] detectable JCV-specific immune response in blood and CSF,[74-77] and development of inflammatory immune response in the CNS.[78,79] Because positive JCV serology is detected in most individuals, including those with PML, the humoral immune response alone is not able to prevent viral reactivation. However, cellular immune response to JCV has been detected in patients with PML, and a strong response is associated with better prognosis. Studies have documented the presence of cytotoxic T lymphocytes that recognize two human leukocyte antigen A*0201-restricted epitopes of the major capsid protein VP1 in

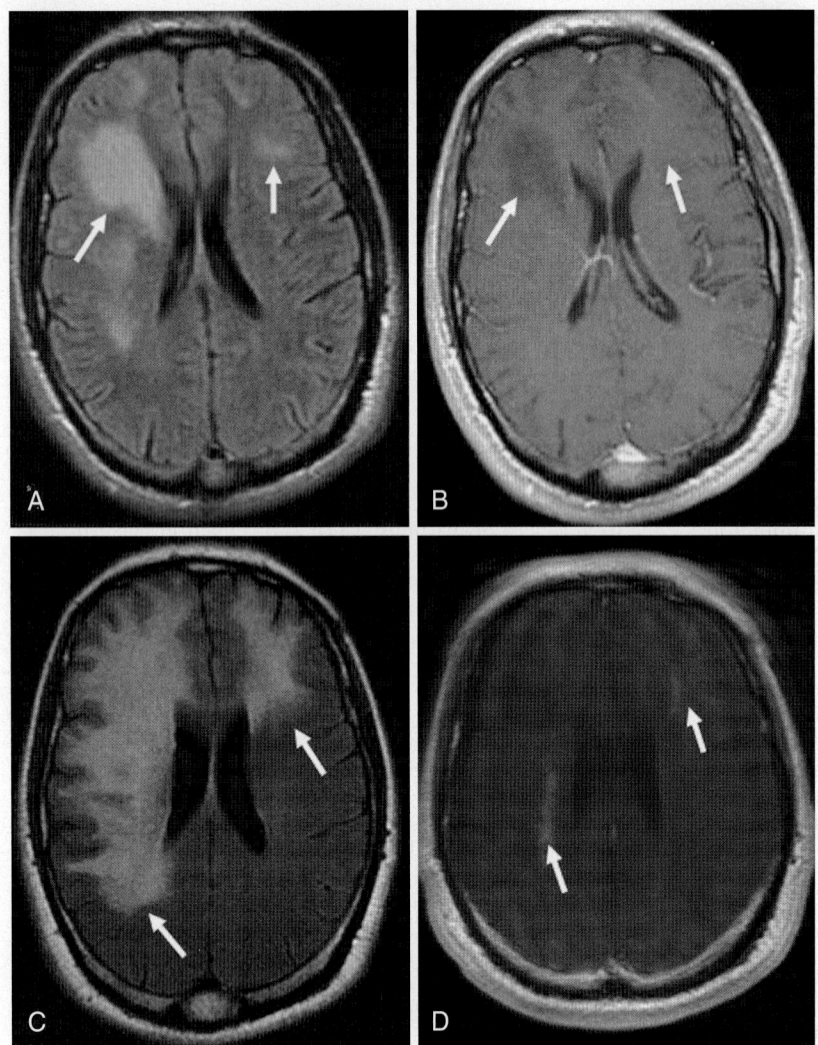

Figure 145-2 Magnetic resonance image of patient with human immunodeficiency virus infection with classic progressive multifocal leukoencephalopathy at presentation. A, Fluid attenuated inversion recovery (FLAIR) images show lesions in right and left frontal lobes *(arrows)*, which do not enhance after gadolinium injection on T1-weighted images in **B.** Magnetic resonance image of same patient shows progressive multifocal leukoencephalopathy–immune reconstitution inflammatory syndrome (PML-IRIS) after treatment with highly active antiretroviral therapy (HAART), displaying progression of lesions in both hemispheres in FLAIR images in **C.** Peripheral enhancement can be seen, in T1-weighted images, **D,** after gadolinium *(arrows)*.

patients with PML who survived more than 1 year.[75,80-82] Furthermore, elevation of myoinositol, a marker of inflammation detected with magnetic resonance spectroscopy in PML lesions, was associated with a better prognosis.[79,83]

TREATMENT

No specific treatment exists for PML. However, in patients with HIV, initiation or optimization of HAART has been associated with an increase in PML survival rate at 1 year from 10% to 50%.[72] For patients who are HIV negative, improvement of the immune status through reduction of immunosuppression may allows for the adaptive immune system to take control of the infection. Because a strong cellular immunity against JCV has been associated with a better clinical outcome, immunotherapies aimed at boosting this immune response may become a treatment option for PML.[84] Cytarabine has shown an in vitro effect in controlling JCV replication and multiplication.[85] One randomized controlled clinical trial with patients who were HIV positive with PML did not show efficacy,[86] but one small retrospective study did show stabilization after intravenous treatment with cytarabine[87] in seven of 19 HIV-negative patients (37%) with PML who had leukemia or lymphoma. Cidofovir is another potent antiviral agent that has shown in vitro activities against murine polyomavirus and SV40, but it has not been tested against JCV or BKV. However, multiple studies in different centers with cidofovir in patients both with and without HIV have not shown a significant effect in changing the disease course.[72,88-90] Lastly, because in vitro studies revealed that JCV infects cells via the serotonin

receptor 5HT2a, mirtazapine, a serotonin receptor blocker, has been considered as a potential candidate for containment of JCV infection.[28] However, clinical improvement of PML with mirtazapine remains anecdotal so far.[91] Recently, a large pharmacologic screening study suggested that mefloquine, an antimalarial medication, has the ability to inhibit JCV replication in cell culture.[92] Thus, a multicenter study is currently examining the role of mefloquine in the treatment of PML.

In treatment of patients with inflammatory PML, where brain swelling and mass effect can be present, a short course of corticosteroids including prednisone, dexamethasone, and methylprednisolone may be used sparingly for mitigation of the inflammation surrounding the lesion, especially with a risk of brain herniation. However, the use of these medications in PML-IRIS cases remains a matter of debate.[93,94] In patients with HIV, no evidence exists that interruption of HAART during corticosteroid treatment is beneficial. In published case studies, most clinicians chose to continue HAART therapy after the diagnosis of PML-IRIS. Short-term interruption of HAART can be used to temporarily reduce the uncontrolled immune reaction. However, clinicians need to be aware that disruptions in HAART have been associated with higher HIV viral load rebound and lower CD4 counts.[95,96] Furthermore, whether a recurrence of IRIS may develop upon restarting HAART is also unclear. Corticosteroids, including dexamethasone, prednisone, and hydrocortisone, have been used anecdotally for their anti-inflammatory and immunosuppressive effects.[97] However, no clear guidelines exist for corticosteroid treatments of patients with PML-IRIS. Therefore, these medications should only be used in cases with clear clinical or radiologic worsening attributable to IRIS, includ-

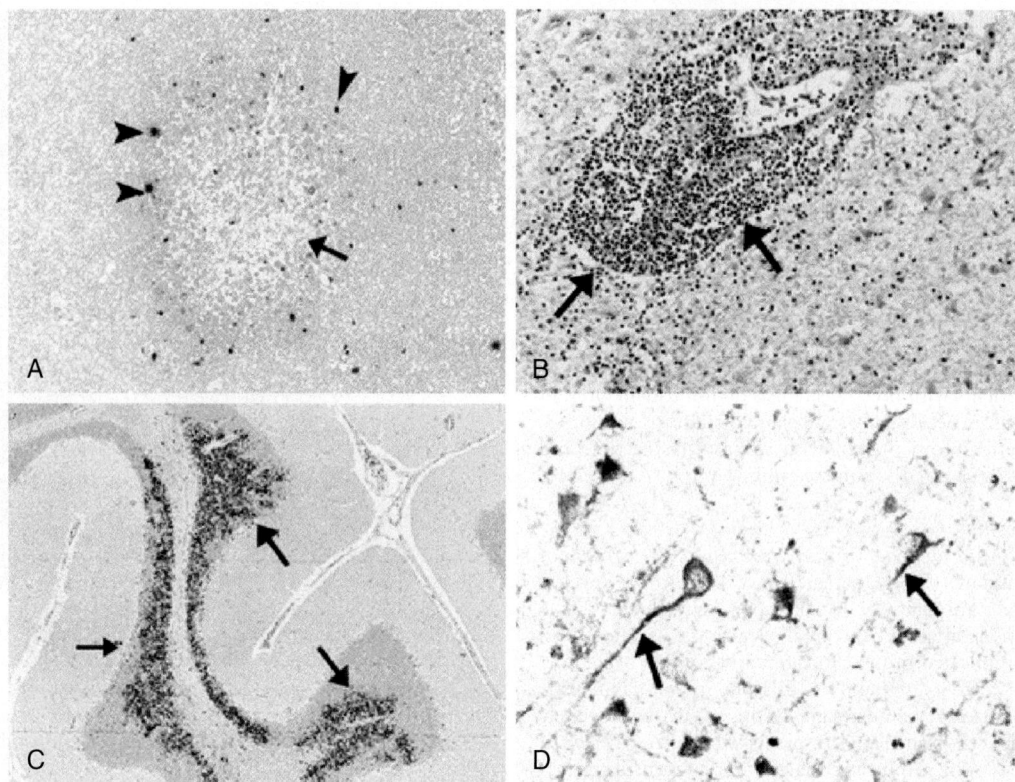

Figure 145-3   **Histologic features of JC virus (JCV) infection in the central nervous system. A,** Classic progressive multifocal leukoencephalopathy (PML), with demyelinating lesion in white matter *(arrow)* surrounded by multiple JCV-infected glial cells *(dark blue, arrowheads).* **B,** Progressive multifocal leukoencephalopathy–immune response inflammatory syndrome (PML-IRIS), with marked lymphocytic perivascular infiltrates *(arrows).* **C,** JCV granule cell neuronopathy in a patient with human immunodeficiency virus infection with focal JCV infection of granule cell neurons *(dark blue, arrows).* **D,** JCV encephalopathy with hemispheric cortical neurons *(brown)* infected with JCV *(blue, arrows).* **(A, C,** and **D** *courtesy of Dr. Christian Wühtrich.* **B** *courtesy of Dr. Françoise Gray.)*

ing life-threatening situations associated with cerebral edema and impending brain herniation.

Nephropathy and Other BK Virus–Associated Diseases

EPIDEMIOLOGY

Although BKV-induced nephropathy rarely occurs in a native kidney,[98,99] the prevalence rate of this condition in kidney transplant recipients ranges from 1% to 10%.[100,101] Diagnosis is made on average 44 weeks after transplantation with a peak around 24 weeks.[17] With the availability of potent immunosuppressive medications, such as tacrolimus and mycophenolate, a trend has been seen toward increasing prevalence of BKV-induced nephropathy in renal transplant patients.[102] Incidences of BK viremia and viruria decrease significantly 1 year after transplantation, diminishing the risk of BKV reactivation.[103] In addition, the incidence rate of BKV-induced ureteral stenosis in renal transplant patients is estimated to be 3%[104]; it occurs in 0.5% to 6% of the general transplant population.[105] Lastly, hemorrhagic cystitis is the most prevalent BKV-associated complication and occurs in 10% to 25% of bone marrow transplant recipients.[106]

BK VIRUS PATHOGENESIS

BK virus primary infection occurs in childhood and is asymptomatic. Thereafter, the virus remains latent in the kidney. Most cases of asymptomatic BK viruria are not associated with nephropathy or hemorrhagic cystitis. Therefore, BKV pathogenesis is the result of several factors, which include: host predisposition, target organ damage, and

immunosuppression. During the initial posttransplant period, severe therapeutic immunosuppressive conditioning regimens are a trigger for reactivation of BKV in renal cells. Such reactivation may lead to productive infection and lysis of kidney tubular epithelial cells. Although the ability of the host to mount a BKV-specific immunity can be limited by immunosuppressive medications, the resulting cell lysis and necrosis mediated by the immune cells may trigger further renal dysfunction. In the host, BKV seropositivity, older age, and high anti-BKV immunoglobulin G (IgG) levels before transplant have been associated with increased risk of BKV reactivation.[107] Furthermore, in the late engraftment period, the recovery of immune function may produce additional injury from inflammation caused by immune reconstitution, resulting in hemorrhagic cystitis.[108] Lastly, alloimmune dysregulation may play an important role because BKV-induced hemorrhagic cystitis is rarely detected in autologous transplant recipients who received similar conditioning regimens.[109]

CLINICAL MANIFESTATIONS

Nephropathy

BK virus has a tropism for cells of the genitourinary tract. Infection with BKV in patients with immunocompromise can result in asymptomatic hematuria, both hemorrhagic and nonhemorrhagic cystitis, and ureteral stenosis. Furthermore, BKV can induce interstitial nephritis in patients with HIV or renal transplantation. However, in patients with a renal allograft, BKV-induced renal tubular epithelial infection results in nephropathy, which is not associated with any specific immunosuppressive medication. BK viruria and viremia usually precede nephropathy. The factors associated with detection of BKV in urine and blood include high donor BK antibody titer and, possibly, absence of the human leukocyte antigen (HLA)-C7 class I allele in both donor and recipient.[110] In addition, a higher risk of development of BKV nephropathy is associated with older age, male gender, comorbidity of diabetes mellitus, and White ethnicity.[101] Onset of BKV nephropathy after transplant ranges from 6 days to 5 years, with a mean time of 10 to 13 months.[111,112] Clinical manifestation of BKV nephropathy is similar to graft rejection, with slowly increasing serum creatinine levels without symptoms. Hematuria and fever can be detected in some patients.[113,114] Laboratory findings suggest renal insufficiency and urinary abnormalities. A rise in quantitative BKV serology can be seen with reactivation of the virus; however, this increase does not prevent progression of disease.[110]

Ureteral Stenosis
Renal transplant patients with ureteral stenosis do not usually present with pain or discomfort because the transplanted kidney is not innervated. However, patients can present with urinary obstruction and laboratory findings of elevated serum creatinine levels.

Hemorrhagic Cystitis
Because of BKV tropism for renal urinary tract cells, close to 50% of bone marrow transplant (BMT) patients have BK viruria develop within 2 months of transplant,[24,106] usually after engraftment.[115] The rate of BK viruria is no different between allogeneic versus autologous grafts,[116] and it is implicated in the clinical manifestations of hemorrhagic cystitis (10% to 25%), ureteral stenosis, and interstitial nephritis. However, most cases of hemorrhagic cystitis occur in allogeneic hematopoietic stem cell transplant recipients who also have graft versus host disease,[109] which indicates that immune reconstitution is part of the pathogenesis. Diagnosis of BKV-induced hemorrhagic cystitis is considered when postengraftment BMT patients present with hematuria, dysuria, urgency, frequency, or suprapubic pain. With severe bleeding and clot formation, complications can include urinary tract obstruction and renal failure.

DIAGNOSIS

Urine Polymerase Chain Reaction
In the appropriate clinical setting, detection of BK viruria and renal insufficiency is diagnostic of BKV-induced nephropathy. Urine cytology containing decoy cell (enlarged nucleus with a single large basophilic intranuclear inclusion) is an indication of viral infection but not specific to BKV infection because these cells are also associated with JCV and adenovirus infections.[117,118] Although detection of BKV DNA with PCR in the urine of patients with hemorrhagic cystitis is sensitive, it is nonspecific because asymptomatic BK viruria is common. However, an increased BK viral load in urine along with hematuria can aid in the diagnosis.

Renal Biopsy
Renal biopsy is often used in the diagnosis of nephropathy. Histologic examination of renal biopsy shows viral replication in the tubular epithelium cells with large intranuclear inclusions and cell detachment (Fig. 145-4).[119] These cytopathic changes are initially localized to the medulla and distal tubules, with progression to the proximal tubules. However, renal biopsy is associated with a false-negative rate up to 30% because of the focal nature of the disease.

Blood Polymerase Chain Reaction
BK virus DNA can be detected in the plasma of kidney transplant recipients. However, this test is more useful in ruling out BKV nephropathy than in diagnosing it. BKV PCR in blood has a negative predictive value of 100% but only a positive predictive value of 50% for BKV nephropathy.[24] One study, however, indicated that plasma BK viral load above 10^4 copies per mL has a sensitivity and specificity of 93% in prediction of histologic manifestations of nephropathy.[120] Unlike in nephropathy, BK virus is usually not detected in the blood of patients with hemorrhagic cystitis or ureteral stenosis.

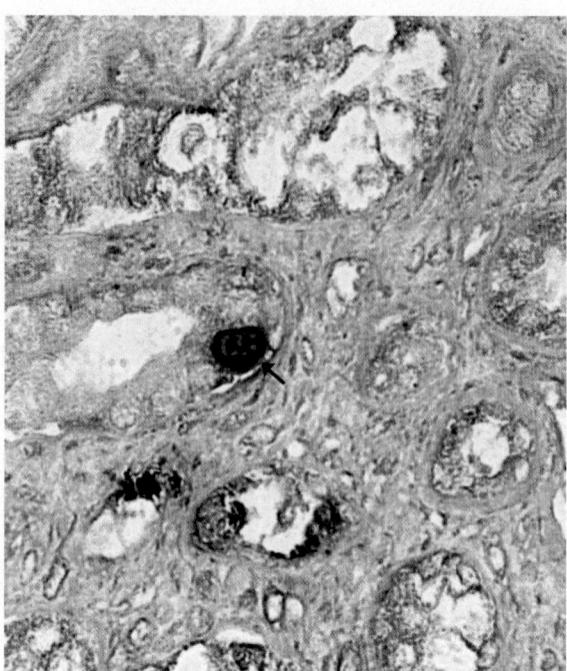

Figure 145-4 Histology of BKV nephropathy. BK virus–infected cell (*arrow*) in renal tubular epithelium. (*Courtesy of Department of Pathology, Beth Israel Deaconess Medical Center, Boston MA.*)

PROGNOSIS

BK virus–induced nephropathy is associated with irreversible graft failure in 1% to 10% of cases.[44] Histologic findings of mild viral cytopathic changes with minimum inflammatory infiltrates or fibrosis correlated with better prognosis for allograft outcome.[120] Studies have shown decreased incidence of nephropathy with early screening for BK viruria and viremia and subsequent reduction of immunosuppressives.[23,121-123] In post–renal transplant patients with BKV nephropathy, a robust BKV-specific cellular immune response correlates with decreased viruria and viremia, whereas the humoral immune response correlated with decreased viremia only.[124]

TREATMENT

Nephropathy
Treatment for BK virus–induced nephropathy is reduction of immunosuppression. Multiple antiviral agents, including cidofovir, leflunomide, quinolones, and intravenous immunoglobulin, have shown varying success in small clinical studies.[125-128] However, patients in these studies also had concomitant decrease of immunosuppressive medications. Because no specific antiviral therapy exists for BKV, reduction of immunosuppression is the therapy of choice[123] and has to be balanced with the increase in risk of graft rejection. The clearance of BK virus from plasma is a surrogate marker for resolving renal tissue pathology.

Ureteral Stenosis
Post–renal transplant patients with the occurrence of BKV-associated ureteral stenosis can benefit from reduced immune suppression. Further treatments primarily involve surgical interventions that relieve the obstruction.

Hemorrhagic Cystitis
Treatment of hemorrhagic cystitis is symptomatic and includes continuous bladder irrigations, analgesia, hyperhydration, forced diuresis, and transfusion to maintain platelet levels above 50,000 and hematocrit values greater than 25%.

REFERENCES

1. Knowles WA. Discovery and epidemiology of the human polyomaviruses BK virus (BKV) and JC virus (JCV). *Adv Exp Med Biol.* 2006;577:19-45.
2. Weber T, Trebst C, Frye S, et al. Analysis of the systemic and intrathecal humoral immune response in progressive multifocal leukoencephalopathy. *J Infect Dis.* 1997;176:250-254.
3. Berger JR, Kaszovitz B, Post MJ, et al. Progressive multifocal leukoencephalopathy associated with human immunodeficiency virus infection. A review of the literature with a report of sixteen cases. *Ann Intern Med.* 1987;107:78-87.
4. Gross L. A filterable agent, recovered from Ak leukemic extracts, causing salivary gland carcinomas in C3H mice. *Proc Soc Exp Biol Med.* 1953;83:414-421.
5. Padgett BL, Walker DL, ZuRhein GM, et al. Cultivation of papova-like virus from human brain with progressive multifocal leucoencephalopathy. *Lancet.* 1971;1:1257-1260.
6. Gardner SD, Field AM, Coleman DV, et al. New human papovavirus (B.K.) isolated from urine after renal transplantation. *Lancet.* 1971;1:1253-1257.
7. Allander T, Andreasson K, Gupta S, et al. Identification of a third human polyomavirus. *J Virol.* 2007;81:4130-4136.
8. Gaynor AM, Nissen MD, Whiley DM, et al. Identification of a novel polyomavirus from patients with acute respiratory tract infections. *PLoS Pathog.* 2007;3:e64.
9. Feng H, Shuda M, Chang Y, et al. Clonal integration of a polyomavirus in human Merkel cell carcinoma. *Science.* 2008;319:1096-1100.
10. Brown P, Tsai T, Gajdusek DC. Seroepidemiology of human papovaviruses. Discovery of virgin populations and some unusual patterns of antibody prevalence among remote peoples of the world. *Am J Epidemiol.* 1975;102:331-340.
11. Knowles WA, Pipkin P, Andrews N, et al. Population-based study of antibody to the human polyomaviruses BKV and JCV and the simian polyomavirus SV40. *J Med Virol.* 2003;71:115-123.
12. Shah KV, Daniel RW, Warszawski RM. High prevalence of antibodies to BK virus, an SV40-related papovavirus, in residents of Maryland. *J Infect Dis.* 1973;128:784-787.
13. Doerries K. Human polyomavirus JC and BK persistent infection. *Adv Exp Med Biol.* 2006;577:102-116.
14. Kitamura T, Aso Y, Kuniyoshi N, et al. High incidence of urinary JC virus excretion in nonimmunosuppressed older patients. *J Infect Dis.* 1990;161:1128-1133.
15. Koralnik IJ, Schmitz JE, Lifton MA, et al. Detection of JC virus DNA in peripheral blood cell subpopulations of HIV-1-infected individuals. *J Neurovirol.* 1999;5:430-435.
16. Tornatore C, Berger JR, Houff SA, et al. Detection of JC virus DNA in peripheral lymphocytes from patients with and without progressive multifocal leukoencephalopathy. *Ann Neurol.* 1992;31:454-462.
17. Nickeleit V, Klimkait T, Binet IF, et al. Testing for polyomavirus type BK DNA in plasma to identify renal-allograft recipients with viral nephropathy. *N Engl J Med.* 2000;342:1309-1315.
18. Howell DN, Smith SR, Butterly DW, et al. Diagnosis and management of BK polyomavirus interstitial nephritis in renal transplant recipients. *Transplantation.* 1999;68:1279-1288.
19. Bressollette-Bodin C, Coste-Burel M, Hourmant M, et al. A prospective longitudinal study of BK virus infection in 104 renal transplant recipients. *Am J Transplant.* 2005;5:1926-1933.
20. Ahsan N, Shah KV. Polyomaviruses and human diseases. *Adv Exp Med Biol.* 2006;577:1-18.
21. Knowles WA, Pillay D, Johnson MA, et al. Prevalence of long-term BK and JC excretion in HIV-infected adults and lack of correlation with serological markers. *J Med Virol.* 1999;59:474-479.
22. Gluck TA, Knowles WA, Johnson MA, et al. BK virus-associated haemorrhagic cystitis in an HIV-infected man. *AIDS.* 1994;8:391-392.
23. Hirsch HH, Knowles W, Dickenmann M, et al. Prospective study of polyomavirus type BK replication and nephropathy in renal-transplant recipients. *N Engl J Med.* 2002;347:488-496.
24. Hirsch HH, Steiger J. Polyomavirus BK. *Lancet Infect Dis.* 2003;3:611-623.
25. Safak M, Barrucco R, Darbinyan A, et al. Interaction of JC virus agno protein with T antigen modulates transcription and replication of the viral genome in glial cells. *J Virol.* 2001;75:1476-1486.
26. Khalili K, White MK, Sawa H, et al. The agnoprotein of polyomaviruses: a multifunctional auxiliary protein. *J Cell Physiol.* 2005;204:1-7.
27. Marzocchetti A, Wuthrich C, Tan CS, et al. Rearrangement of the JC virus regulatory region sequence in the bone marrow of a patient with rheumatoid arthritis and progressive multifocal leukoencephalopathy. *J Neurovirol.* 2008;14:455-458.
28. Elphick GF, Querbes W, Jordan JA, et al. The human polyomavirus, JCV, uses serotonin receptors to infect cells. *Science.* 2004;306:1380-1383.
29. Eash S, Manley K, Gasparovic M, et al. The human polyomaviruses. *Cell Mol Life Sci.* 2006;63:865-876.
30. Dugan AS, Eash S, Atwood WJ. Update on BK virus entry and intracellular trafficking. *Transpl Infect Dis.* 2006;8:62-67.
31. Bialasiewicz S, Whiley DM, Lambert SB, et al. A newly reported human polyomavirus, KI virus, is present in the respiratory tract of Australian children. *J Clin Virol.* 2007;40:15-18.
32. Han TH, Chung JY, Koo JW, et al. WU polyomavirus in children with acute lower respiratory tract infections, South Korea. *Emerg Infect Dis.* 2007;13:1766-1768.
33. Abedi Kiasari B, Vallely PJ, Corless CE, et al. Age-related pattern of KI and WU polyomavirus infection. *J Clin Virol.* 2008;43:123-125.
34. Astrom KE, Mancall EL, Richardson EP. Progressive multifocal leukoencephalopathy. *Brain.* 1958;81:93-127.
35. Power C, Gladden JG, Halliday W, et al. AIDS- and non-AIDS-related PML association with distinct p53 polymorphism. *Neurology.* 2000;54:743-746.
36. Koralnik IJ, Schellingerhout D, Frosch MP. Case records of the Massachusetts General Hospital. Weekly clinicopathological exercises. Case 14-2004. A 66-year-old man with progressive neurologic deficits. *N Engl J Med.* 2004;350:1882-1893.
37. Langer-Gould A, Atlas SW, Green AJ, et al. Progressive multifocal leukoencephalopathy in a patient treated with natalizumab. *N Engl J Med.* 2005;353:375-381.
38. Kleinschmidt-DeMasters BK, Tyler KL. Progressive multifocal leukoencephalopathy complicating treatment with natalizumab and interferon beta-1a for multiple sclerosis. *N Engl J Med.* 2005;353:369-374.
39. Van Assche G, Van Ranst M, Sciot R, et al. Progressive multifocal leukoencephalopathy after natalizumab therapy for Crohn's disease. *N Engl J Med.* 2005;353:362-368.
40. Rey J, Belmecheri N, Bouayed N, et al. JC papovavirus leukoencephalopathy after first line treatment with CHOP and rituximab. *Haematologica.* 2007;92:e101.
41. Bonavita S, Conforti R, Russo A, et al. Infratentorial progressive multifocal leukoencephalopathy in a patient treated with fludarabine and rituximab. *Neurol Sci.* 2008;29:37-39.
42. Harris HE. Progressive multifocal leucoencephalopathy in a patient with systemic lupus erythematosus treated with rituximab. *Rheumatology (Oxford).* 2008;47:224-225.
43. Genetech: Important safety information. Accessed 2008. Available at <http://www.gene.com/gene/products/information/pdf/raptiva_dhcp.pdf>.
44. Monaco MC, Jensen PN, Hou J, et al. Detection of JC virus DNA in human tonsil tissue: evidence for site of initial viral infection. *J Virol.* 1998;72:9918-9923.
44a. Tan CS, Dezube BJ, Bhargava P, et al. Detection of JC virus DNA and proteins in the bone marrow of HIV-positive and HIV-negative patients: implications for viral latency and neurotropic transformation. *J Infect Dis.* 2009;199:881-888.
45. Goudsmit J, Wertheim-van Dillen P, van Strien A, et al. The role of BK virus in acute respiratory tract disease and the presence of BKV DNA in tonsils. *J Med Virol.* 1982;10:91-99.
46. Bernal-Cano F, Joseph JT, Koralnik IJ. Spinal cord lesions of progressive multifocal leukoencephalopathy in an acquired immunodeficiency syndrome patient. *J Neurovirol.* 2007;13:474-476.
47. Lima MA, Drislane FW, Koralnik IJ. Seizures and their outcome in progressive multifocal leukoencephalopathy. *Neurology.* 2006;66:262-264.
48. Du Pasquier RA, Koralnik IJ. Inflammatory reaction in progressive multifocal leukoencephalopathy: harmful or beneficial? *J Neurovirol.* 2003;9:25-31.
49. Vendrely A, Bienvenu B, Gasnault J, et al. Fulminant inflammatory leukoencephalopathy associated with HAART-induced immune restoration in AIDS-related progressive multifocal leukoencephalopathy. *Acta Neuropathol (Berl).* 2005;109:449-455.
50. Venkataramana A, Pardo CA, McArthur JC, et al. Immune reconstitution inflammatory syndrome in the CNS of HIV-infected patients. *Neurology.* 2006;67:383-388.
51. D'Amico R, Sarkar S, Yusuff J, et al. Immune reconstitution after potent antiretroviral therapy in AIDS patients with progressive multifocal leukoencephalopathy. *Scand J Infect Dis.* 2007;39:347-350.
52. Martinez JV, Mazziotti JV, Efron ED, et al. Immune reconstitution inflammatory syndrome associated with PML in AIDS: a treatable disorder. *Neurology.* 2006;67:1692-1694.
53. Rushing EJ, Liappis A, Smirniotopoulos JD, et al. Immune reconstitution inflammatory syndrome of the brain: case illustrations of a challenging entity. *J Neuropathol Exp Neurol.* 2008;67:819-827.
54. Kastrup O, Wanke I, Esser S, et al. Evolution of purely infratentorial PML under HAART: negative outcome under rapid immune reconstitution. *Clin Neurol Neurosurg.* 2005;107:509-513.
55. Hoffmann C, Horst HA, Albrecht H, et al. Progressive multifocal leucoencephalopathy with unusual inflammatory response during antiretroviral treatment. *J Neurol Neurosurg Psychiatry.* 2003;74:1142-1144.
56. Hecht JH, Glenn OA, Wara DW, et al. JC virus granule cell neuronopathy in a child with CD40 ligand deficiency. *Pediatr Neurol.* 2007;36:186-189.
57. Du Pasquier RA, Corey S, Margolin DH, et al. Productive infection of cerebellar granule cell neurons by JC virus in an HIV+ individual. *Neurology.* 2003;61:775-782.
58. Koralnik IJ, Wuthrich C, Dang X, et al. JC virus granule cell neuronopathy: A novel clinical syndrome distinct from progressive multifocal leukoencephalopathy. *Ann Neurol.* 2005;57:576-580.
59. Dang X, Koralnik IJ. A granule cell neuron-associated JC virus variant has a unique deletion in the VP1 gene. *J Gen Virol.* 2006;87:2533-2537.
60. Wuthrich C, Cheng YM, Joseph JT, et al. Frequent infection of cerebellar granule cell neurons by polyomavirus JC in progressive multifocal leukoencephalopathy. *J Neuropathol Exp Neurol.* 2009;68:15-25.
61. Wüthrich C, Dang X, Westmoreland S, et al. Fulminant JC virus encephalopathy with productive infection of cortical pyramidal neurons. *Ann Neurol.* In press.
62. Viallard JF, Ellie E, Lazaro E, et al. JC virus meningitis in a patient with systemic lupus erythematosus. *Lupus.* 2005;14:964-966.
63. Blake K, Pillay D, Knowles W, et al. JC virus associated meningoencephalitis in an immunocompetent girl. *Arch Dis Child.* 1992;67:956-957.
64. Behzad-Behbahani A, Klapper PE, Vallely PJ, et al. BKV-DNA and JCV-DNA in CSF of patients with suspected meningitis or encephalitis. *Infection.* 2003;31:374-378.
65. Skiest DJ. Focal neurological disease in patients with acquired immunodeficiency syndrome. *Clin Infect Dis.* 2002;34:103-115.
66. Whiteman ML, Post MJ, Berger JR, et al. Progressive multifocal leukoencephalopathy in 47 HIV-seropositive patients: neuroimaging with clinical and pathologic correlation. *Radiology.* 1993;187:233-240.
67. Post MJ, Yiannoutsos C, Simpson D, et al. Progressive multifocal leukoencephalopathy in AIDS: are there any MR findings useful to patient management and predictive of patient survival? AIDS Clinical Trials Group, 243 Team. *AJNR Am J Neuroradiol.* 1999;20:1896-1906.
68. Moll NM, Rietsch AM, Ransohoff AJ, et al. Cortical demyelination in PML and MS: Similarities and differences. *Neurology.* 2007.
69. Cinque P, Scarpellini P, Vago L, et al. Diagnosis of central nervous system complications in HIV-infected patients: cerebrospinal fluid analysis by the polymerase chain reaction. *AIDS.* 1997;11:1-17.
70. Marzocchetti A, Di Giambenedetto S, Cingolani A, et al. Reduced rate of diagnostic positive detection of JC virus DNA in cerebrospinal fluid in cases of suspected progressive multifocal leukoencephalopathy in the era of potent antiretroviral therapy. *J Clin Microbiol.* 2005;43:4175-4177.
71. Berger JR, Pall L, Lanska D, et al. Progressive multifocal leukoencephalopathy in patients with HIV infection. *J Neurovirol.* 1998;4:59-68.
72. Antinori A, Cingolani A, Lorenzini P, et al. Clinical epidemiology and survival of progressive multifocal leukoencephalopathy in the era of highly active antiretroviral therapy: data from the Italian Registry Investigative Neuro AIDS (IRINA). *J Neurovirol.* 2003;9:47-53.
73. Yiannoutsos CT, Major EO, Curfman B, et al. Relation of JC virus DNA in the cerebrospinal fluid to survival in acquired immunodeficiency syndrome patients with biopsy-proven progressive multifocal leukoencephalopathy. *Ann Neurol.* 1999;45:816-821.
74. Koralnik IJ. Overview of the cellular immunity against JC virus in progressive multifocal leukoencephalopathy. *J Neurovirol.* 2002;8:59-65.
75. Du Pasquier RA, Kuroda MJ, Schmitz JE, et al. Low frequency of cytotoxic T lymphocytes against the novel HLA-A*0201-restricted JC virus epitope VP1(p36) in patients with proven or possible progressive multifocal leukoencephalopathy. *J Virol.* 2003;77:11918-11926.
76. Lima MA, Marzocchetti A, Autissier P, et al. Frequency and phenotype of JC virus-specific CD8+ T lymphocytes in the peripheral blood of patients with progressive multifocal leukoencephalopathy. *J Virol.* 2007;81:3361-3368.
77. Du Pasquier RA, Autissier P, Zheng Y, et al. Presence of JC virus-specific CTL in the cerebrospinal fluid of PML patients: rationale for immune-based therapeutic strategies. *AIDS.* 2005;19:2069-2076.
78. Berger JR, Levy RM, Flomenhoft D, et al. Predictive factors for prolonged survival in acquired immunodeficiency syndrome-associated progressive multifocal leukoencephalopathy. *Ann Neurol.* 1998;44:341-349.
79. Katz-Brull R, Lenkinski RE, Du Pasquier RA, et al. Elevation of myoinositol is associated with disease containment in progressive multifocal leukoencephalopathy. *Neurology.* 2004;63:897-900.
80. Koralnik IJ, Du Pasquier RA, Letvin NL. JC virus-specific cytotoxic T lymphocytes in individuals with progressive multifocal leukoencephalopathy. *J Virol.* 2001;75:3483-3487.
81. Koralnik IJ, Du Pasquier RA, Kuroda MJ, et al. Association of prolonged survival in HLA-A2+ progressive multifocal leukoencephalopathy patients with a CTL response specific for a commonly recognized JC virus epitope. *J Immunol.* 2002;168:499-504.
82. Du Pasquier RA, Kuroda MJ, Zheng Y, et al. A prospective study demonstrates an association between JC virus-specific cytotoxic T lymphocytes and the early control of progressive multifocal leukoencephalopathy. *Brain.* 2004;127:1970-1978.
83. Chang L, Ernst T, Tornatore C, et al. Metabolite abnormalities in progressive multifocal leukoencephalopathy by proton

magnetic resonance spectroscopy. *Neurology.* 1997;48:836-845.

84. Marzocchetti A, Lima M, Tompkins T, et al. Efficient in vitro expansion of JC virus-specific CD8(+) T-cell responses by JCV peptide-stimulated dendritic cells from patients with progressive multifocal leukoencephalopathy. *Virology.* 2009;383:173-177.

85. Hou J, Major EO. The efficacy of nucleoside analogs against JC virus multiplication in a persistently infected human fetal brain cell line. *J Neurovirol.* 1998;4:451-456.

86. Hall CD, Dafni U, Simpson D, et al. Failure of cytarabine in progressive multifocal leukoencephalopathy associated with human immunodeficiency virus infection. AIDS Clinical Trials Group 243 Team [see comments]. *N Engl J Med.* 1998;338:1345-1351.

87. Aksamit AJ. Treatment of non-AIDS progressive multifocal leukoencephalopathy with cytosine arabinoside. *J Neurovirol.* 2001;7:386-390.

88. Marra CM, Rajicic N, Barker DE, et al. A pilot study of cidofovir for progressive multifocal leukoencephalopathy in AIDS. *AIDS.* 2002;16:1791-1797.

89. Osorio S, de la Camara R, Golbano N, et al. Progressive multifocal leukoencephalopathy after stem cell transplantation, unsuccessfully treated with cidofovir. *Bone Marrow Transplant.* 2002;30:963-966.

90. Herrlinger U, Schwarzler F, Beck R, et al. Progressive multifocal leukoencephalopathy: cidofovir therapy in three patients with underlying hematological disease. *J Neurol.* 2003;250:612-614.

91. Verma S, Cikurel K, Koralnik IJ, et al. Mirtazapine in progressive multifocal leukoencephalopathy associated with polycythemia vera. *J Infect Dis.* 2007;196:709-711.

92. Brickelmaier M, Lugovskoy A, Kartikeyan R, et al. Identification and characterization of mefloquine efficacy against JC virus in vitro. *Antimicrob Agents Chemother.* 2009;53:1840-1849.

93. Tan K, Roda R, Ostrow L, et al. PML-IRIS in patients with HIV infection. Clinical manifestations and treatment with steroids. *Neurology.* 2009;72:1458-1464.

94. Berger JR. Steroids for PML-IRIS. A double-edged sword? *Neurology.* 2009;72:1454-1455.

95. Li X, Margolick JB, Conover CS, et al. Interruption and discontinuation of highly active antiretroviral therapy in the multicenter AIDS cohort study. *J Acquir Immune Defic Syndr.* 2005;38:320-328.

96. Steingrover R, Pogany K, Fernandez Garcia E, et al. HIV-1 viral rebound dynamics after a single treatment interruption depends on time of initiation of highly active antiretroviral therapy. *AIDS.* 2008;22:1583-1588.

97. Czock D, Keller F, Rasche FM, et al. Pharmacokinetics and pharmacodynamics of systemically administered glucocorticoids. *Clin Pharmacokinet.* 2005;44:61-98.

98. Limaye AP, Smith KD, Cook L, et al. Polyomavirus nephropathy in native kidneys of non-renal transplant recipients. *Am J Transplant.* 2005;5:614-620.

99. Barber CE, Hewlett TJ, Geldenhuys L, et al. BK virus nephropathy in a heart transplant recipient: case report and review of the literature. *Transpl Infect Dis.* 2006;8:113-121.

100. Nickeleit V, Hirsch HH, Zeiler M, et al. BK-virus nephropathy in renal transplants-tubular necrosis, MHC-class II expression and rejection in a puzzling game. *Nephrol Dial Transplant.* 2000;15:324-332.

101. Hirsch HH, Brennan DC, Drachenberg CB, et al. Polyomavirus-associated nephropathy in renal transplantation: interdisciplinary analyses and recommendations. *Transplantation.* 2005;79:1277-1286.

102. Ramos E, Drachenberg CB, Portocarrero M, et al. BK virus nephropathy diagnosis and treatment: experience at the University of Maryland Renal Transplant Program. *Clin Transpl.* 2002;143-153.

103. Koukoulaki M, Grispou E, Pistolas D, et al. Prospective monitoring of BK virus replication in renal transplant recipients. *Transpl Infect Dis.* 2009;11:1-10.

104. Coleman DV, Mackenzie EF, Gardner SD, et al. Human polyomavirus (BK) infection and ureteric stenosis in renal allograft recipients. *J Clin Pathol.* 1978;31:338-347.

105. Karam G, Hetet JF, Maillet F, et al. Late ureteral stenosis following renal transplantation: risk factors and impact on patient and graft survival. *Am J Transplant.* 2006;6:352-356.

106. Arthur RR, Shah KV, Baust SJ, et al. Association of BK viruria with hemorrhagic cystitis in recipients of bone marrow transplants. *N Engl J Med.* 1986;315:230-234.

107. Wong AS, Chan KH, Cheng VC, et al. Relationship of pretransplantation polyoma BK virus serologic findings and BK viral reactivation after hematopoietic stem cell transplantation. *Clin Infect Dis.* 2007;44:830-837.

108. Leung AY, Yuen KY, Kwong YL. Polyoma BK virus and haemorrhagic cystitis in haematopoietic stem cell transplantation: a changing paradigm. *Bone Marrow Transplant.* 2005;36:929-937.

109. Leung AY, Yuen KY, Cheng VC, et al. Clinical characteristics of and risk factors for herpes zoster after hematopoietic stem cell transplantation. *Haematologica.* 2002;87:444-446.

110. Bohl DL, Storch GA, Ryschkewitsch C, et al. Donor origin of BK virus in renal transplantation and role of HLA C7 in susceptibility to sustained BK viremia. *Am J Transplant.* 2005;5:2213-2221.

111. Randhawa PS, Finkelstein S, Scantlebury V, et al. Human polyoma virus-associated interstitial nephritis in the allograft kidney. *Transplantation.* 1999;67:103-109.

112. Ramos E, Drachenberg CB, Papadimitriou JC, et al. Clinical course of polyoma virus nephropathy in 67 renal transplant patients. *J Am Soc Nephrol.* 2002;13:2145-2151.

113. Vasudev B, Hariharan S, Hussain SA, et al. BK virus nephritis: risk factors, timing, and outcome in renal transplant recipients. *Kidney Int.* 2005;68:1834-1839.

114. Dall A, Hariharan S. BK virus nephritis after renal transplantation. *Clin J Am Soc Nephrol.* 2008;3:S68-75.

115. Bedi A, Miller CB, Hanson JL, et al. Association of BK virus with failure of prophylaxis against hemorrhagic cystitis following bone marrow transplantation. *J Clin Oncol.* 1995;13:1103-1109.

116. Azzi A, Cesaro S, Laszlo D, et al. Human polyomavirus BK (BKV) load and haemorrhagic cystitis in bone marrow transplantation patients. *J Clin Virol.* 1999;14:79-86.

117. Kahan AV, Coleman DV, Koss LG. Activation of human polyomavirus infection-detection by cytologic technics. *Am J Clin Pathol.* 1980;74:326-332.

118. Traystman MD, Gupta PK, Shah KV, et al. Identification of viruses in the urine of renal transplant recipients by cytomorphology. *Acta Cytol.* 1980;24:501-510.

119. Drachenberg RC, Drachenberg CB, Papadimitriou JC, et al. Morphological spectrum of polyoma virus disease in renal allografts: diagnostic accuracy of urine cytology. *Am J Transplant.* 2001;1:373-381.

120. Drachenberg CB, Papadimitriou JC, Hirsch HH, et al. Histological patterns of polyomavirus nephropathy: correlation with graft outcome and viral load. *Am J Transplant.* 2004;4:2082-2092.

121. Burgos D, Lopez V, Cabello M, et al. Polyomavirus BK nephropathy: the effect of an early diagnosis on renal function or graft loss. *Transplant Proc.* 2006;38:2409-2411.

122. Almeras C, Foulongne V, Garrigue V, et al. Does reduction in immunosuppression in viremic patients prevent BK virus nephropathy in de novo renal transplant recipients? A prospective study. *Transplantation.* 2008;85:1099-1104.

123. Brennan DC, Agha I, Bohl DL, et al. Incidence of BK with tacrolimus versus cyclosporine and impact of preemptive immunosuppression reduction. *Am J Transplant.* 2005;5:582-594.

124. Chen Y, Trofe J, Gordon J, et al. Interplay of cellular and humoral immune responses against BK virus in kidney transplant recipients with polyomavirus nephropathy. *J Virol.* 2006;80:3495-3505.

125. Leung AY, Chan MT, Yuen KY, et al. Ciprofloxacin decreased polyoma BK virus load in patients who underwent allogeneic hematopoietic stem cell transplantation. *Clin Infect Dis.* 2005;40:528-537.

126. Williams JW, Javaid B, Kadambi PV, et al. Leflunomide for polyomavirus type BK nephropathy. *N Engl J Med.* 2005;352:1157-1158.

127. Sener A, House AA, Jevnikar AM, et al. Intravenous immunoglobulin as a treatment for BK virus associated nephropathy: one-year follow-up of renal allograft recipients. *Transplantation.* 2006;81:117-120.

128. Randhawa PS. Anti-BK virus activity of ciprofloxacin and related antibiotics. *Clin Infect Dis.* 2005;41:1366-1367; author reply 1367.

Hepatitis B Virus and Hepatitis Delta Virus

MARGARET JAMES KOZIEL | CHLOE LYNNE THIO

Introduction

Hepatitis B virus (HBV) infects more than 500 million people worldwide. It is the leading cause of chronic hepatitis, cirrhosis, and hepatocellular carcinoma (HCC), and these sequelae of chronic infection account for more than one million deaths annually. The outcome of infection and spectrum of illness varies widely. During the acute phase, infections range from asymptomatic hepatitis to icteric hepatitis, including fulminant hepatitis. Once chronic infection is established, the spectrum of illness ranges from the asymptomatic, healthy carrier state to progressive liver disease that results in the sequelae of end-stage liver disease, including cirrhosis and HCC. Even though HBV cannot be cultured, enough is known about the viral life cycle that specific antivirals are available to control viral replication in patients. Moreover, the identification of the correlates of protective immunity has facilitated the widespread use of a highly effective vaccine, which by preventing chronic carriage of the virus and the subsequent development of HCC represents the first true cancer vaccine.

HISTORICAL BACKGROUND AND CLASSIFICATION

Hippocrates recognized the spread of jaundice by infectious agents as early as 4000 BC. The early cases of HBV infection were linked to the use of conventional viral vaccines, which were prepared from or contained human serum. In 1885, Lurman described the appearance of jaundice in 15% of 1289 shipyard workers who received smallpox vaccine prepared from human lymph.[1] Epidemics of hepatitis were also recorded following the administration of yellow fever vaccine, which was stabilized with human serum.[2] In the early part of the 20th century, the increasing use of contaminated syringes and needles by diabetics on insulin, and by patients treated for syphilis at venereal disease clinics, elevated the importance of serum hepatitis.[3,4] This led to the association of hepatitis B with blood and blood products, and to its distinction from infectious hepatitis, caused by hepatitis A virus, a member of the *Picornaviridae* family.[5] The first hint of viral etiology came from the studies of Blumberg, who reported the discovery of a human antigen in Australian Aborigines termed Australian (Au) antigen.[6] Subsequently, the Au antigen came to be known as hepatitis B surface antigen (HBsAg), and its association with acute hepatitis was established. For this discovery, Dr. Baruch Blumberg received the Nobel Prize in Physiology and Medicine in 1976. In 1971, Dane, an electron microscopist, visualized the presence of 22-nm HBsAg subviral particles along with the complete 42-nm virus particles in the blood of hepatitis B patients (Fig. 146-1).[7]

Due to their unique biologic and molecular characteristics, and their liver tropism, HBV and HBV-like animal viruses were given the status of a new family designated *Hepadnaviridae* (*hepa*totropic *DNA viruses*).[8] HBV, the human pathogen, and other mammalian hepatitis viruses with sequence homology and similar genome organization are grouped in the genus *Orthohepadnavirus*. The genus *Avihepadnavirus* includes viruses that infect ducks, geese, and heron. The *Hepadnavirus* animal models, which include duck hepatitis virus (DHBV),[9] woodchuck hepatitis virus (WHV), and ground squirrel hepatitis virus, have been extensively studied and have contributed to the current knowledge of the molecular biology of HBV infection and replication. However, these viral genomes are considerably divergent from human HBV, and there are limited tools to study the immune reaction to the

virus in these animals. The primary host for HBV is human, but other primates such as chimpanzees, gibbons, orangutans, African green monkeys, and squirrel monkeys have been found positive for HBsAg. However, the use of these animals for the study of pathogenesis is both difficult and expensive. Thus, a convenient animal model or an efficient tissue culture system for HBV remains unavailable. HBV was molecularly cloned from patients' sera in 1979 and its complete DNA sequence determined.[10-12] These advances led to a surge of investigations on the molecular aspects of HBV molecular biology, chief among which are the regulatory schemes of gene expression and replication.

BIOLOGY

HBV is a small DNA virus, whose 3200 kilobases (kb) partially double-stranded DNA genome is maintained in a circular conformation.[13] Partially duplex DNA molecules represent incomplete synthesis of the viral DNA during morphogenesis (Fig. 146-2).[14] One of the unique features of HBV infection is the production of large quantities of subviral spherical and filamentous HBsAg particles in addition to complete virus particles. Under electron microscopy, these are distinguished by a diameter of 42 nm for complete virus (Dane) particles, and 22-nm spherical and filamentous structures for subviral particles (see Fig. 146-1).[7] HBsAg is expressed on the exterior of all these particles. HBsAg subviral particles reach a titer of 10^{13}/mL, whereas viral particles range in titer from 10^4/mL to 10^9/mL. All of these particles circulate in blood and permit convenient diagnosis of viral antigen by enzyme-linked immunosorbent assay (ELISA) or radioimmunoassay (RIA).[15] HBsAg forms the viral component of the lipoprotein envelope, which encloses a core shell containing the viral DNA genome and the virus-encoded polymerase protein. The nucleocapsid or core is composed of a 21 kDa basic phosphoprotein commonly known as hepatitis B core antigen (HBcAg).[16] A cell-derived kinase activity has been shown to be associated with the virion particles,[17] but the functional significance of this enzyme is not understood.

The 20-nm HBsAg particles and filaments are composed of three forms of surface antigen polypeptides, and lipids derived from hepatocyte membranes. The lipid content is approximately 30% by weight and includes phospholipids, cholesterol, cholesterol esters, and triglycerides.[18,19] These particles are devoid of HBV DNA genome and hence are noninfectious. Because of their high immunogenicity, purified HBsAg particles can be used as an HBV vaccine. HBsAg elicits neutralizing antibodies, which offer protection from reinfection.[20,21] The high titers of HBsAg in patients during natural infection can potentially serve to adsorb neutralizing antibody and thus protect the virus from host defenses.

ATTACHMENT, ENTRY, AND HEPATOTROPISM

HBV primarily infects hepatocytes. It enters hepatocytes via an unidentified liver cell–specific receptor, consistent with the strict hepatotropism exhibited by this and other members of *Hepadnaviridae*. Candidate receptor molecules include endonexin, carboxypeptidase, and serum apolipoproteins, but none appear to fulfill the criteria for a liver cell–specific receptor that confers hepatotropism to HBV and other related hepatitis viruses. There is evidence that hepatocyte entry may be a multistep process involving binding to heparan sulfate proteoglycans, which are found on a variety of cells, followed by a highly

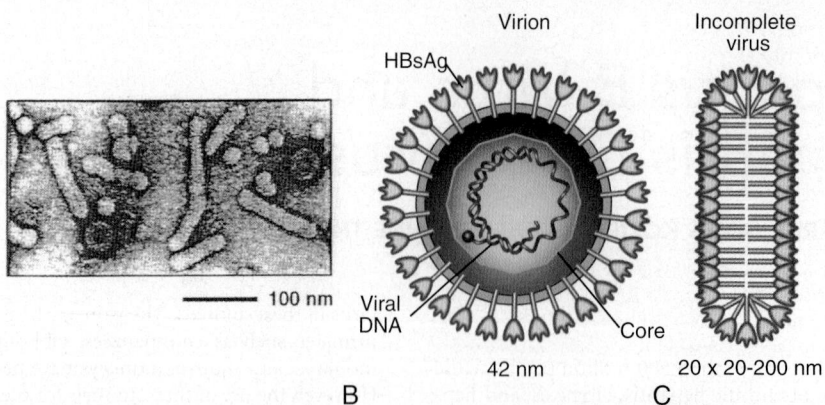

Figure 146-1   **Structure of hepatitis B virus (HBV) and hepatitis B surface antigen (HBsAg) particles. A,** Electron micrograph of negatively stained HBV. **B,** Diagram of 42-nm HBV showing partially duplex DNA genome with a covalently linked protein at the 5' end of the complete minus strand. **C,** Diagram of 22-nm HBsAg filament. *(Adapted from Flint SJ, Enquist LW, Racaniello VR, et al. Principles of Virology, 2nd ed. Washington, DC: ASM Press; 2004, p 808.)*

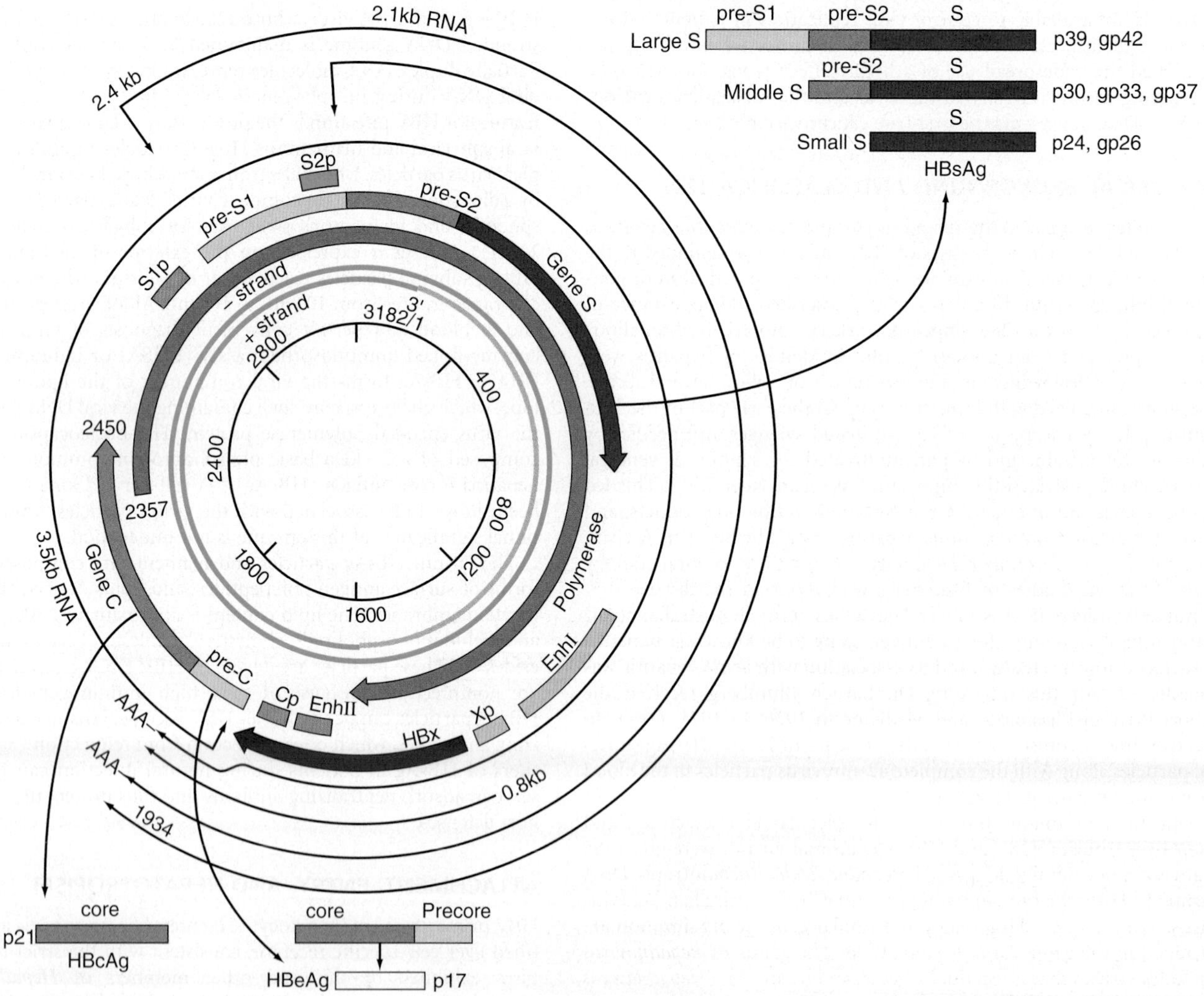

Figure 146-2   **Hepatitis B virus (HBV) genome organization, map of viral transcripts, and proteins.** The partially double-stranded 3.2-kb viral DNA is shown in the inner circle. The single-stranded (ss) region is indicated in yellow-orange. The extent of the ss region varies from molecule to molecule. HBV-encoded overlapping genes are indicated in the outer circles in various colors. Four promoter regions preceding a corresponding gene are indicated as S1p, S2p, Cp, and Xp. Two enhancer elements (I and II) are also shown. Viral transcripts are indicated in the outermost circles *(thin lines).* The three forms of HBsAg, HBcAg, and HBeAg (surface, core, and early antigen) polypeptides are also shown. *(Adapted from Hepatitis viruses. In Murray PA, Rosenthal KS, Kobayashi GS, et al, eds: Medical Microbiology, 4th ed. St. Louis, MO, Mosby; 2002, pp 591-605.)*

HBV-specific step.[22] Bound virions deliver core particles into the cytoplasm, which make their way into the nucleus through the nuclear pore complex.[23] In the nucleus, the virion DNA, which is partially duplex is matured into a covalently closed circular (CCC) DNA form (Fig. 146-3).[24] Liver specificity is also displayed at the level of viral gene expression, which is controlled largely by the promoters and enhancers (see Fig. 146-2).[25]

The liver appears to be the major but may not be the only site of viral infection. The presence of HBV DNA in other cell types, especially lymphocytes, has been described.[26] Clear and coherent evidence for viral DNA replication, transcription, and translation in all of these cells has not been clearly demonstrated. However, infectious WHV can be found in lymphocytes following mitogenic stimulation, implicating lymphocytes as a second reservoir for HBV.[27,28]

VIRAL GENOME

HBV uses unique transcriptional and translational strategies to maximize the limited coding capacity of its genome. The HBV DNA genome is a partially double-stranded molecule within the virions (see Fig.

146-1).[29] The complete (negative) strand contains a protein covalently linked to its 5′ terminus.[30] The incomplete (plus) strand displays variable length and bears a 5′ capped oligoribonucleotide at its 5′ end (see Fig. 146-2).[31] The asymmetry of the DNA strands reflects the incomplete synthesis of DNA during maturation of viral particles. HBV DNA codes for four overlapping open reading frames (ORFs): S, for the surface antigen or envelope gene (HBsAg); C, for the nucleocapsid (core) and "e" antigen gene (HBcAg, HBeAg); P, for the polymerase gene; and X, for the HBx gene (see Fig. 146-2). The surface antigen ORF contains three in-frame initiator codons from which small or major (S), middle (M), and large kDa (L) HBsAg polypeptides are synthesized, respectively. These polypeptides are variably glycosylated to yield several species: S, p24/gp26, M, p30/gp33/gp37, and L, p39/gp42 kDa HBsAg polypeptides, respectively. L and M HBsAg contain characteristic preS-1 and preS-2 domains and hence these proteins are also referred to as preS-1 and preS-2 proteins, respectively. The 22-nm subviral particles are composed of mostly S and lesser amounts of M polypeptides and few or no L polypeptides. The 42-nm Dane particles, which represent the complete virus, contain all three HBsAg forms. The L polypeptide carries the receptor recognition domain,[32] so it is

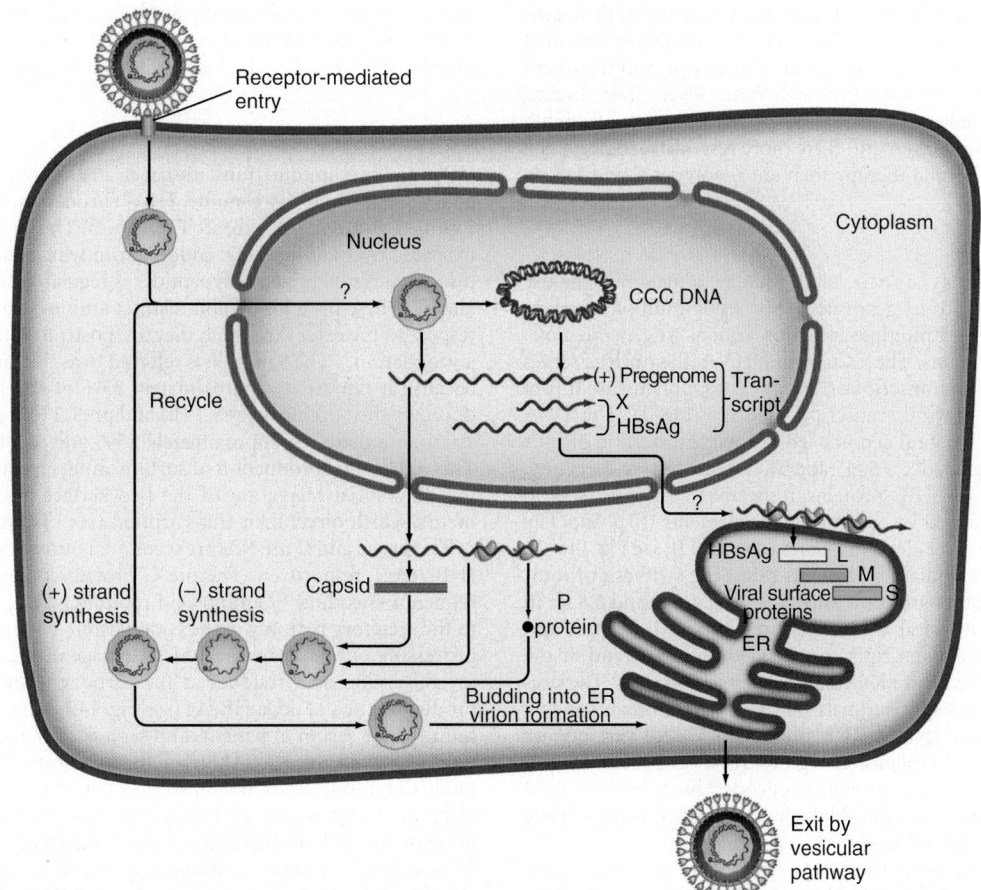

Figure 146-3 **Hepatitis B virus (HBV) life cycle.** The virion attaches to a susceptible hepatocyte through recognition of a cell surface receptor that has yet to be identified. The mechanism of virus uptake is unknown, and repair of the gapped (+) DNA strand is accomplished by as yet unidentified enzymes. The DNA is translocated to the nucleus, where it is found in a covalently closed circular form called CCC DNA. The (−) strand of such CCC DNA is the template for transcription by cellular RNA polymerase II of a longer-than-genome-length RNA called the pregenome and shorter, subgenomic transcripts. Viral messenger RNAs (mRNAs) are transported from the nucleus. The hepatitis B surface antigens encoding viral mRNAs are translated by ribosomes bound to the endoplasmic reticulum (ER), and the proteins enter the secretory pathway. The pregenome RNA is translated at low efficiency to produce a 90-kDa polymerase protein, P, which possesses reverse transcriptase activity. This protein then binds to a specific site at the 5′ end of its own transcript, where viral DNA synthesis is eventually initiated. The pregenomic RNA also serves as mRNA for the capsid protein. Concurrently with capsid formation, the RNA-P protein complex is packaged and reverse transcription begins with synthesis of (−) strand DNA followed by (+) strand DNA synthesis. Before the completion of +−strand synthesis, core particles mature and these structures acquire envelopes by budding into the ER, where viral morphogenesis is completed. Progeny-enveloped virions are released from the cell by exocytosis or are recycled to the nucleus, where the process is repeated. (*Adapted from Flint SJ, Enquist LW, Racaniello VR, et al. Principles of Virology, 2nd ed. Washington, DC: ASM Press; 2004, p 809.*)

necessary for binding the unidentified hepatocyte receptor.[33] Thus, the meager amounts or absence of L protein in the 22-nm particles prevents these abundant forms from competing with virions for cell surface receptors.

The C region or the core ORF contains two in-frame initiator codons with the first ATG responsible for e antigen polypeptide synthesis (HBeAg) (see Fig. 146-2). The second ATG serves as an initiation codon for the HBcAg polypeptide. HBeAg is secreted from cells and accumulates in serum as an immunologically distinct soluble antigen and serves as a marker of ongoing viral replication.[34] Both gene products (core and e polypeptides) are made from the same reading frame. The P and X ORFs encode the polymerase and the HBx proteins, respectively.

Prior to the advent of current molecular methods, HBV was divided into serotypes based on the antibody response to HBsAg. However, HBV is now divided into eight genotypes (A-H) based on genetic diversity of at least 8% in the HBV genome.[35,36] Within these genotypes are subgenotypes, which differ by a minimum of 4%. These genotypes and subgenotypes are distributed geographically with genotypes A in North America, Europe, and parts of Africa; genotypes B and C in Asia; genotype D in India, the Middle East, the Mediterranean region, and parts of Africa; gentotype E in Africa; and genotype F in South America. Genotypes G and H have been identified more recently, so their geographic distribution is less clear. There are accumulating data that these genotypic differences are associated with disease and treatment outcomes. Genotype C is associated with more severe liver disease, slower HBeAg seroconversion compared to genotype B, and higher rates of HCC.[37-39] Genotypes A and B are more responsive to pegylated (PEG) interferon (IFN) alfa therapy than are genotypes C and D.[40]

TRANSCRIPTION

The HBV genome displays a remarkable strategy to maximize the use of the limited capacity of its genomic size by using multiple overlapping reading frames and multiple initiation codons to generate antigenically different proteins. The CCC viral DNA in the nucleus serves as the substrate for viral transcription and uses host polymerase II (pol II) in the synthesis of viral transcripts (see Fig. 146-3). The DNA sequence analysis of the viral genome led to the identification of four different genes designated C, S, P, and X, which encode HBc/eAg, HBsAg, polymerase, and HBx proteins, respectively.[15] The expression of these genes is regulated by four promoter elements (S1p, S2p, Cp, and Xp) and two enhancer elements (enhancer I and II; see Fig. 146-2). These transcriptional regulatory elements direct the synthesis of multiple viral transcripts that are approximately 3.5, 2.4/2.1, and 0.8 kb in length, respectively. All viral transcripts are unspliced, capped, and polyadenylated. All the transcripts are encoded on one strand of the DNA and co-terminate at an identical polyadenylation site.[41] The pregenomic RNA contains splice signals that allow the human splicing mechanism to produce spliced RNA transcripts. Splice variants are common in vivo with prevalence as high as 96%.[42] A protein known as the HBV splice-generated protein is encoded by a singly spliced pregenomic RNA[43]; however, the biologic significance of this splice protein has not been determined.

The preS-1 (S1p) promoter directs the synthesis of the 2.4-kb transcripts, which code for the large envelope (L HBsAg) polypeptide. This promoter contains binding sites for two liver-enriched transcription factors, HNF-3 and HNF-1, which are primarily responsible for the liver-specific activity of this promoter.[44] The preS-2 or S (S2p) promoter directs the transcription of multiple species of messenger RNAs (mRNAs) coding for preS-2/M and S HBsAg polypeptides. Collectively these RNA species are approximately 2.1 kb in length with 5′ heterogeneous ends. The mRNAs, which initiate downstream of the preS-2 initiator ATG, code for the S, or the major polypeptide. The S2p promoter also displays liver specificity and is controlled by the enhancer II element located about 2000 bp away (see Fig. 146-2).[45] The S2p promoter is stronger than the S1p promoter, which results in the synthesis of an excess of the major S over the L (preS-1) and M (preS-

2) forms of the HBsAg. This regulation is especially critical for synthesizing the appropriate levels of the three forms of surface proteins within the cell. The basis for the differential regulation of these promoters is governed by mechanisms that involve both positive and negative cis-acting elements and the trans-acting transcriptional factors.[15,46]

The core/pregenomic promoter (Cp) governs the expression of two longer-than-genome-length transcripts (3.5 kb) designated precore (pre-C) and core (C) RNAs. The slightly longer precore RNA directs the translation of HBeAg polypeptide. The shorter C RNA is used for the translation of core and polymerase proteins. The ATG for the polymerase (reverse transcriptase) is located several hundred nucleotides from the 5′ end (see Fig. 146-2). The C RNA, after its translation into core polypeptides, packages its own RNA, which then functions as a pregenome RNA (pregenomic RNA). The Cp promoter contains binding sites for several liver-enriched and ubiquitous transcription factors.[47] Immediately juxtaposed to this lies enhancer II, which in concert with enhancer I plays a regulatory role in the overall HBV gene expression. A complex scheme of transcriptional regulation appears to operate within these control elements.[48]

The X promoter (Xp) is located immediately downstream of enhancer I and regulates the synthesis of the low abundance 0.8-kb X transcripts that correlate with similar levels of HBx protein synthesis in infected cells.[49,50] Both ubiquitous and liver-enriched factors binding to enhancer I regulate the biosynthesis of X transcripts.

TRANSLATION

HBV also uses unique translational strategies to maximize the limited coding capacity of its genome. HBV encodes three major viral transcripts (2.4/2.1, 3.5, 0.9 kb; see Fig. 146-2). The S region contains three in-frame translational start codons from which the synthesis of three distinct surface antigen polypeptides is regulated (L/preS-1, M/preS-2, and S). These proteins exhibit distinct amino-termini and differ with respect to the extent in which they are posttranslationally modified by glycosylation.[51] The S protein is referred to as the major surface antigen because it represents approximately 85% of the HBsAg that is produced by the virus. The preS-1 (L) and preS-2 (M) proteins are present at an abundance of approximately 15% and 1% to 2%, respectively. This differential production of surface antigen proteins correlates with the differential regulation of the two surface antigen promoter elements, which direct their transcription (see "Transcription").

The pre-C and C mRNAs are translated into e and core polypeptides (HBc/eAg), respectively. The pre-C protein contains a signal peptide sequence encoding 19 amino acid residues, which targets this protein to the secretory pathway in the endoplasmic reticulum (ER).[52] Further processing of the protein includes cleavage of the signal peptide, and several amino acid residues at the carboxy-terminus leading to the production of a 17-kDa HBeAg (see Fig. 146-2). HBeAg is secreted and found in the serum of patients and serves as a marker of active replication in chronic hepatitis. Although the function of HBeAg is not clearly understood, one study demonstrated that it downregulated Toll-like receptor 2 expression on hepatocytes and monocytes leading to a decrease in cytokine expression.[53] These data suggest a role for HBeAg in modifying the innate immune response to HBV. HBeAg is dispensable for replication, as nonsense or frameshift mutations in the pre-C are found in nature. In HBV carriers, mutant viruses with defects in the pre-C region arise spontaneously and are both infectious and pathogenic.[54,55] The C RNA initiates downstream of the pre-C ATG and translates into HBcAg and less frequently into polymerase. Because polymerase ATG is located several hundred nucleotides downstream of the 5′ end (see Fig. 146-2), the ribosomes must access this initiator codon by a mechanism different from ribosome scanning. As this process is inefficient, one polymerase protein is translated for every 200 to 300 molecules of core polypeptides.

HBV polymerase protein consists of 832 aa and is composed of four domains: terminal protein (TP), spacer, reverse transcriptase (RT), and ribonuclease H (RNaseH) (Fig. 146-4).[15] The TP domain repre-

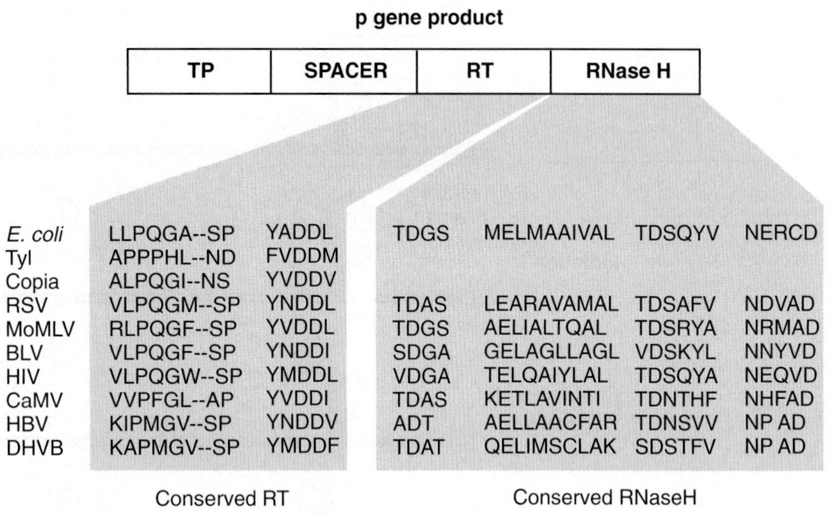

p gene product

| TP | SPACER | RT | RNase H |

	Conserved RT		Conserved RNaseH			
E. coli	LLPQGA--SP	YADDL	TDGS	MELMAAIVAL	TDSQYV	NERCD
Tyl	APPPHL--ND	FVDDM				
Copia	ALPQGI--NS	YVDDV				
RSV	VLPQGM--SP	YNDDL	TDAS	LEARAVAMAL	TDSAFV	NDVAD
MoMLV	RLPQGF--SP	YVDDL	TDGS	AELIALTQAL	TDSRYA	NRMAD
BLV	VLPQGF--SP	YNDDI	SDGA	GELAGLLAGL	VDSKYL	NNYVD
HIV	VLPQGW--SP	YMDDL	VDGA	TELQAIYLAL	TDSQYA	NEQVD
CaMV	VVPFGL--AP	YVDDI	TDAS	KETLAVINTI	TDNTHF	NHFAD
HBV	KIPMGV--SP	YNDDV	ADT	AELLAACFAR	TDNSVV	NP AD
DHVB	KAPMGV--SP	YMDDF	TDAT	QELIMSCLAK	SDSTFV	NP AD

Figure 146-4 Domain structure of the hepadnaviral polymerase protein. Top, Schematic depiction of the functional domains of P protein. TP, terminal protein; RT, reverse transcriptase; RNaseH, ribonuclease H. **Bottom,** Amino acid sequence alignments with other RNA-dependent DNA polymerases; these homologies form the basis of the assignment of the RT and RNaseH domains. (*Adapted from Ganem DE, Schneider RI. Hepadnaviridae: the viruses and their replication. In Knipe D, Howley P, eds.* Fundamental Virology, *4th ed. Philadelphia: Lippincott Williams and Wilkins; 2001, pp 1285-1331.*)

sents the portion of the polymerase protein that is covalently bound to minus-strand DNA. The spacer domain or tether region connects the TP domain to the RT, which contains the catalytic domain for the polymerase. The RT domain contains the characteristic YMDD consensus sequence, the catalytic site for RT and is a major focus of current drug development in HBV (see Fig. 146-4 and "Nucleoside and Nucleotide Therapies"). The RT domain is followed by an RNaseH domain, which functions to hydrolyze the pregenomic RNA template after reverse transcription within the nucleocapsid.[56,57]

REPLICATION

Although HBV is a DNA-containing virus, the replication occurs via an RNA intermediate, a characteristic that places hepadnaviruses close to retroviruses. Much of our understanding of HBV replication strategy comes from the classic experiments of Summers and Mason,[58] which demonstrated that HBV amplifies via reverse transcription of an RNA intermediate and that these events occur within the subviral core particles in the cytoplasm. The complex mechanisms by which pregenomic RNA is converted to partially double-stranded virion DNA has been studied in considerable detail (Fig. 146-5).[59] HBV replication begins with the encapsidation of pregenomic RNA by the core polypeptide along with the polymerase.[60,61] The pregenomic RNA contains terminally redundant 200 nucleotide sequences, which include an epsilon (ε) stem-loop structure and a short sequence of 11 to 12 nucleotides termed DR1 (see Fig. 146-5). The HBV polymerase binds pregenomic RNA preferentially at the 5′ copy of the ε stem-loop structure on its own molecule. The interaction between the ε signal of the pregenomic RNA and the polymerase and the core leads to the formation of a ribonucleoprotein complex. The HBV capsid or core assembles into a replication-competent particle.[15] The sequence of events and the mechanism of assembly remain to be characterized. The TP domain of the polymerase protein functions as a protein primer for the initiation of reverse transcription in a process called *nucleotide priming* or *protein-primed reverse transcription* (see Fig. 146-4).[62] The positive strand is extended to variable lengths to yield mature HBV DNA. The cessation of the positive strand synthesis at various stages of its synthesis coincides with the maturation of the core particles and their entry into the ER leading to the packaging of partially duplex genomic DNA found in hepatitis B (HB) virions (see Fig. 146-3).[63] This entry prevents access to cytoplasmic deoxynucleotide pools needed for completion of DNA synthesis. Matured core particles face two options at this stage: either they enter the ER, undergo virion packaging with HBsAg polypeptides, and bud from the membrane as 42-nm Dane particles, or they enter the nucleus and deliver the partially duplex DNA and repeat the cycle of replication (see Fig. 146-3). In the nucleus,

virion DNA is repaired to produce CCC DNA molecules. About 5 to 50 copies of CCC DNA accumulate in the nucleus of an infected hepatocyte. CCC DNA serves as a substrate of viral mRNA synthesis; it is the stable form of HBV DNA that is most resistant to antiviral treatment and the host immune response.[64] In summary, the salient features of HBV replication are the use of viral RNA as a template for reverse transcription; protein-priming in which both the TP and the RT domains of the viral polymerase participate; and incomplete plus-strand synthesis that results in a partially duplex DNA genome found within the hepatitis B virion particles.

HBx

HBx is a regulatory protein that is required for the viral life cycle, but its precise role is not clearly understood.[65] This protein acts as a regulator of both viral and cellular gene expression. It does not directly bind DNA but appears to interact with host factors that bind DNA,[66] including transcription factors and components of basal transcriptional machinery.[15] The cellular targets are numerous and the list of the cellular functions HBx has been shown to modulate continues to grow.[15] Overall, the functions of HBx are characterized as transcriptional transactivators. NF-kB was one of the first HBx-responsive elements identified.[67] Because the NF-kB site does not exist within the HBV genome, it is believed that the trans-activating potential of HBx extends to cellular target genes involved in inflammation. Other HBx-responsive transcription factors include ATF-2/CREB, AP-1, STAT-3, and NF-AT.[68,69] Within the cytoplasm, it also localizes to the mitochondria and induces oxidative stress via calcium signaling.[70,71] These activities may mediate mitochondria-mediated liver injury. HBx has also been shown to modulate cellular signal transduction pathways.[72,73] It was shown to activate Src kinase and stimulate the Ras-Raf-MAP kinase signal transduction pathway.[74] The physiologic significance of any of these observations remains to be established in the context of human infections. HBx is not known to be directly oncogenic, but based on its role in activation of transcription factors, elevation of reactive oxygen species, and inhibition of apoptosis,[75] it is considered a potential contributor to the processes of liver oncogenesis.[15]

MORPHOGENESIS AND ASSEMBLY

Envelopment of the nucleocapsid occurs in the ER or ER-Golgi intermediate compartments.[15] All three forms of the surface proteins are synthesized in the ER as integral transmembrane proteins and are involved in the virion morphogenesis.[76] The overall ratio of these proteins is approximately 1000:10:1. Viral assembly begins with the translation of C RNA into core and polymerase proteins. After its

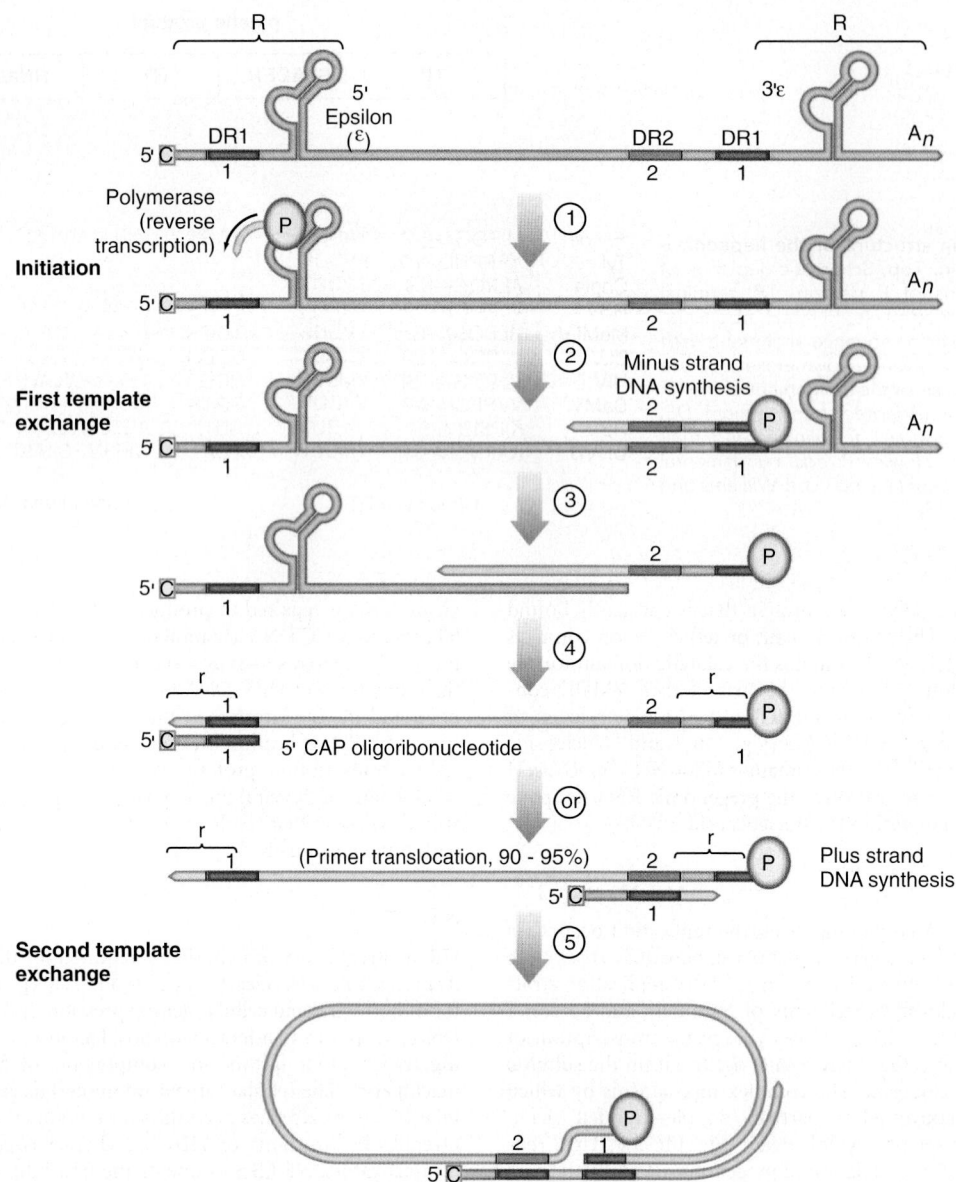

Figure 146-5 **Hepatitis B virus (HBV) replication pathway.** The terminally redundant pregenomic RNA (*top line*) is capped and polyadenylated. Boxes 1 and 2 represent DR1 and DR2, respectively. The horizontal bracket labeled R represents the terminally redundant region of the RNA. The epsilon (ε) stem-loops are indicated at the termini. Pregenome RNA packaging into cores is initiated by the interaction of polymerase (P) protein with the 5' copy of ε. Minus-strand DNA synthesis is initiated at the 5'ε of the RNA and is primed by P protein. After the first template exchange (step 2), DNA synthesis continues, using the 3' copy of DR1 as the template (step 3). As synthesis proceeds, the newly copied RNA template is degraded by the associated ribonuclease H activity of the polymerase (step 4). Elongation of (–) strand DNA is finished on complete copying of the pregenomic RNA template. The product is a terminally redundant complete (–) strand DNA species. The redundancies (8 to 10 nucleotides) are labeled r. At this time, the primer for (+) strand synthesis is generated from the 5'-terminal 15 to 18 nucleotides of the pregenomic RNA. The primer is capped and includes the sequence to the 3' end of DR1. Elongation of the (+) strand results in a duplex linear genome. In the majority of cases, the primer is translocated to base pair with the DR2 sequence near the 5' end of (–) strand DNA (step 5). The (+) strand synthesis is initiated, and then elongation begins. On reaching the 5' end of (–) strand DNA, an intramolecular template exchange occurs, resulting in a circular DNA genome (step 5). This exchange is facilitated by the short terminal redundancy in (–) strand DNA. The (+) strand DNA synthesis then continues for a variable distance, resulting in the relaxed circular partially duplex form of the genome found in mature virions. (*Adapted from Tavis JE. The replication strategy of the hepadnaviruses. Viral Hepatitis Rev. 1996;2:205-218.*)

translation, the polymerase protein apparently binds to the ε signal on the same molecule that now functions as a pregenome, forming a preassembly complex that triggers core protein association. Core protein monomers rapidly dimerize and provide a pool of assembly intermediates. Virion formation initiates by specific interactions between core particles and after budding, the virions are secreted via vesicular transport through the remaining compartments of the secre-

tory pathways and are eventually released into the bloodstream. M protein is not important for morphogenesis but is required for infectivity. L protein is required for virion morphogenesis,[77] and its retention in an early compartment of the secretory pathway leads to the efficiency of the assembly process. During chronic hepatitis, accumulation of the L surface protein-containing particles has been associated with the pathologic phenotype of ground-glass hepatocytes.[15]

Hepatitis Delta Virus

Delta agent was identified by Mario Rizzetto in 1977 as a nuclear antigen distinct from HBsAg, HBcAg, and HBeAg in hepatocytes of some HBsAg carriers in Italy (Fig. 146-6). It soon became clear that this passenger virus, termed hepatitis D virus (HDV) accompanied HBV infection. This unique RNA genome resembles plant pathogens including viroids and virusoids.[78] HDV is the only member of the genus *Deltavirus*.[79] In nature, HDV is only found in patients who are also infected with HBV. The regions of highest prevalence include the Mediterranean basin, North Africa, and South America.[80] In the United States, the prevalence is low in the general population but high in drug users. Globally, about 10% of HBV-infected individuals are coinfected with HDV. HDV infection of chronic carriers is frequently associated with severe sequelae of chronic hepatitis and accounts for cases of fulminant hepatitis. There are seven known genotypes (I to VII).[81] Genotype I is the most common worldwide and associated with severe pathogenicity. Genotype II is found in Asia and HDV associated with this genotype is of milder forms. Genotype III is found in South America and is associated with the most severe form of HDV.[82] Genotype IV is found in Taiwan and genotypes V through VII are found in west and central Africa.

HDV is an enveloped virus of 36 nm that is distinct from 22-nm HBsAg or 42-nm HBV particles (see Fig. 146-6).[83] The HDV genome is a small single-stranded, circular RNA genome that is enclosed by hepatitis delta antigen, which functions as a nucleocapsid for the viral genome.[84,85] The viral envelope consists of the three forms (L, M, and S) of HBsAg. Because the HBsAg envelope is derived from the HBV-infected cells, HDV cannot be propagated without HBV.

HEPATITIS DELTA ANTIGEN

The nucleocapsid or the hepatitis delta (HD) antigen consists of two species: small S-HDAg (24 kDa) and large L-HDAg (27 kDa) (Fig. 146-7). Both are initiated from the same ATG codon and have similar N-terminal sequences but differ in the use of termination codons.[86] Each is translated from a distinct species of RNA. The L-HDAg transcript is produced by a unique RNA editing event, which results in the

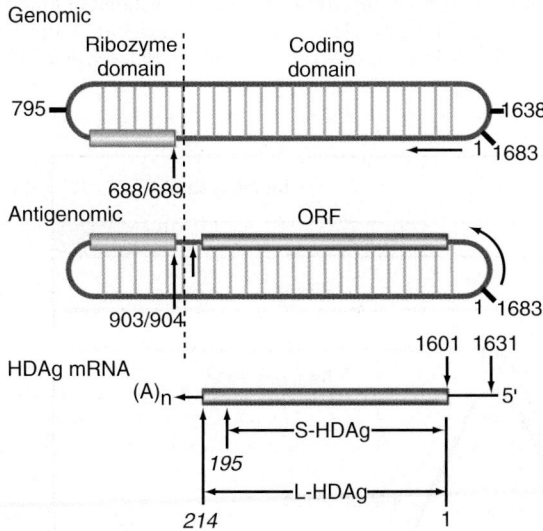

Figure 146-6   Schematic structures of hepatitis D virus genomic and antigenomic RNA and hepatitis D antigen (HDAg)-encoding messenger RNA (mRNA). The minimum ribozymes are indicated by light boxes. The italicized numbers for HDAg are amino acid residues. All other numbers are nucleotide positions on the genomic-sense RNA. ORF, open reading frame. *(Adapted from Macnaughton TB, Lai MC. The molecular biology of hepatitis delta virus. In Ou JE, ed. Hepatitis Viruses. Norwell, MA: Kluwer; 2002, pp 109-128.)*

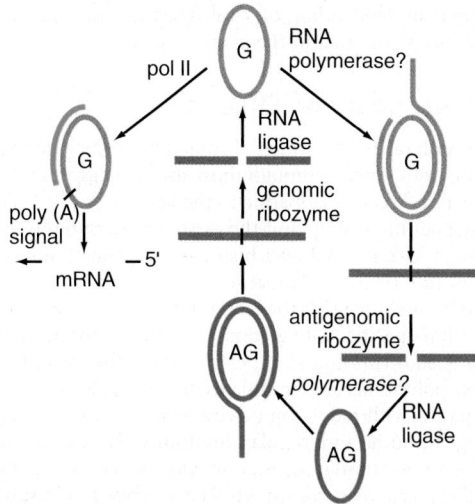

Figure 146-7   Proposed model of hepatitis D virus RNA replication. The hepatitis D antigen-encoding messenger RNA is synthesized by polymerase II (pol II) from the genomic RNA template independently of RNA replication. The enzymes for genomic and antigenomic RNA replication are not yet known. AG, antigenomic strand; G, genomic strand. *(Adapted from Macnaughton TB, Lai MC. The molecular biology of hepatitis delta virus. In Ou JE, ed. Hepatitis Viruses. Norwell, MA: Kluwer; 2002, pp 109-128.)*

addition of 19 amino acid residues at its N-terminus.[87] Both L- and S-HDAgs are phosphorylated, contain nuclear localization signal, and are localized to the nucleus.[88,89] They multimerize with each other through antiparallel coiled-coils.[90] L-HDAg is a clathrin adaptor-like protein that binds to the host clathrin heavy chain, facilitating HDV assembly of new particles.[91] It also acts as a dominant-negative inhibitor of replication. S-HDAg is involved in the initiation of RNA replication and is believed to have RNA chaperone activity.[92]

HEPATITIS D VIRUS RNA GENOME AND REPLICATION

The HDV RNA genome is 1.7 kb but does not encode protein. Instead, the complementary antigenomic HDV RNA codes for HDAg and contains a sequence of approximately 85 nucleotides with an intrinsic ribozyme activity (see Fig. 146-7).[93,94] The HDV ribozyme activity is absolutely required for RNA replication.[95] It is estimated that about 100,000 copies of genomic RNAs can be found in an infected hepatocyte. S-HDAg is believed to be involved in RNA replication and may serve as an RNA chaperone.[96] Because HDV does not encode a polymerase it recruits the host RNA pol II for this activity.[92,97] HDV interacts with the clamp of RNA pol II, a structure that holds RNA and DNA in place. HDAg loosens the clamp, which facilitates forward translocation of RNA pol II while sacrificing fidelity.[98] HDV envelopment follows the scheme of virion assembly similar to HBV. Because HDV assembly can also occur in an L protein–independent fashion,[99] noninfectious HDV virions can be produced in abundance (about 90%). These particles are noninfectious because of the absence of preS-1 domain, which is required for infectivity.

HDV infects only hepatocytes with no evidence of extrahepatic sites of its replication. The mechanism of HDV entry is similar to HBV, as it requires L HBsAg for entry through an unidentified, liver cell–specific receptor. Like HBV, there is no culture system for HDV. The host range of HDV is limited to those species that can support the replication of hepadnaviruses and supply in trans the HBsAg envelope. For instance, HDV can infect woodchucks and can be packaged with HBsAg derived from WHV.[100] Chimpanzees are susceptible to HDV infection and the infection is similar to that in humans.[80] Chimpanzees, therefore, have served as an experimental model and contributed to the current understanding of viral infection. In chimpanzees, the HDV infection is confined to the liver.

Pathogenesis of Disease

The exact mechanisms by which chronic liver injury occurs in HBV infection are not known, although most studies suggest that the hepatitis virus is not directly cytopathic to the hepatocyte.[101,102] There is no robust tissue culture system, but the existence of asymptomatic hepatitis B carriers with normal liver histology and function suggests that the virus is not directly cytopathic. Extensive human and animal studies have now shown that the liver injury mediated by HBV is initiated by a viral-specific cellular and humoral immune response. In more than 95% of immunocompetent adults, the immune response is vigorous, polyclonal, and multispecific and results in acute, self-limited hepatitis with reduction of viral load and the development of long-lasting humoral and cellular immunity. Persistent infection is associated with necroinflammatory activity, which eventually leads to cirrhosis. The mechanism for this viral persistence and immune-mediated liver injury is not known.

ACUTE HEPATITIS B

Natural recovery from acute HBV probably depends on multiple components of cellular immune responses, including natural killer (NK) cells, natural killer T (NK T) cells, and virus-specific CD4+ T cells and CD8+ cytotoxic T lymphocytes (CTL). Both NK and NK T cells contribute to clearance through production of IFN-α/β, which mediates noncytopathic control of viral replication.[103] Acute HBV infection is also accompanied by a strong and transient expansion of CD4+ T cells directed against multiple epitopes within the HBV. HBc is the dominant antigen recognized by CD4+ T cells in most cases of acute, resolving HBV infection.[104] These HBc-specific CD4+ T cells provide help for the production of antibody to HBsAg and are also associated with the development of a vigorous and polyclonal cytotoxic CTL capable of recognizing different epitopes within the HBV genome.[105] Individuals who successfully clear HBV infection, either spontaneously or after IFN therapy, maintain these broad and strong peripheral CTL responses.[106] CD4+ and CTL memory in the presence of low levels of persisting HBV DNA has been shown to persist up to 23 years after infection despite markers of serologic recovery. Both virus-specific CD4+ and CTL contribute to control of HBV replication through both direct cytolysis of infected cells but, more importantly, through pro-

duction of cytokines that control viral replication.[107] Analysis of the NK, CTL, and CD4+ T-cell responses in the incubation phase has demonstrated that CTL response increases in parallel with alanine aminotransferase (ALT), consistent with the previously observed notions that CTL activity is responsible for liver injury, and peak about the time that the HBV DNA titers begin to fall.[108]

HBcAg is extremely immunogenic during HBV infection and after immunization. IgM anti-HBc is the first antibody to be detected, usually appearing within 1 month of the appearance of HBsAg and 1 to 2 weeks before the rise in ALT (Fig. 146-8). During convalescence, the titer of IgM anti-HBc declines while the titers of IgG anti-HBc increase. Although IgM anti-HBc is frequently considered to be associated with acute infection, it can persist for up to 2 years in 20% of individuals, and low titers may be found in chronically infected individuals, which rise during acute flares in HBV.

The development of surface antibody (anti-HBs) follows the disappearance of surface antigen and marks recovery from HBV infection. Anti-HBs is sufficient for protection against HBV infection, as demonstrated by the success of the current HBV vaccines, even if it is not the sole operative mechanism clearing acute infection. The "a" determinant is the predominant B-cell epitope common to all HBV subtypes. Antibodies against this epitope confer immunity to all HBV subtypes. Coexistence of HBsAg and anti-HBs is reported in up to 24% of chronically infected individuals, in which case the anti-HBs is directed against one of the subtypic determinants and a mutation preventing neutralization of the virus has occurred. Other surface antigens that stimulate antibody responses include the preS-1 and preS-2 antigens. Antibody to these develops during recovery and can be detected before anti-HBs; however, routine serologic assays are not readily available. Mutation in the S gene usually occurs in the a determinant, which allows the virus to escape antibody neutralization. This may occur following the use of hepatitis B immunoglobulin for passive immunization of newborns and transplant recipients.

CHRONIC HEPATITIS B

Persistent HBV infection may result because of the failure of initial innate and adaptive immune responses. Among infants who become infected at birth, both viral and host factors play a role in the development of chronic infection. The presence of HBeAg and the viral titer in the mother are both directly related to the likelihood of infant infection. In animal models, HBeAg may be toleragenic,[109] and because HBeAg and HBcAg are cross-reactive at the T-cell level, deletion of the

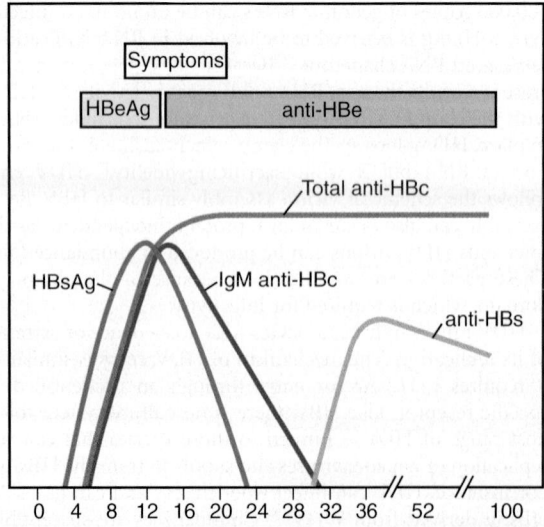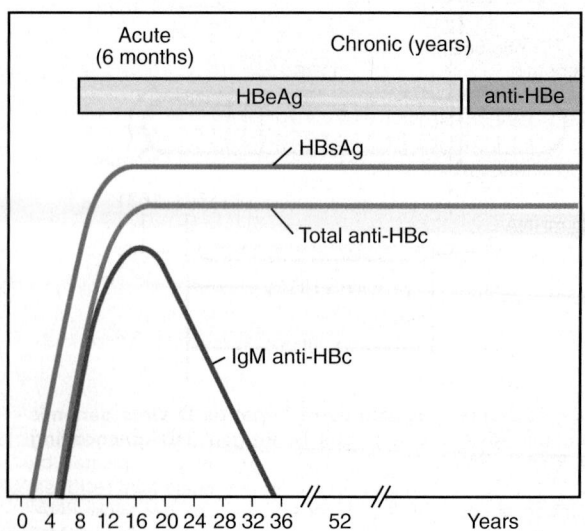

Figure 146-8 **Typical course of hepatitis B. Left,** Typical course of acute hepatitis B. **Right,** Chronic hepatitis B. HBc, hepatitis B core; HBe, hepatitis B early; HBsAg, hepatitis B surface antigen; IgM, immunoglobulin M.

CD4+ HBc-specific T-cell responses results in ineffective CTL responses to HBcAg.

Adult immunocompetent individuals who fail to clear acute HBV infection also have less vigorous CD4+ T-cell and CTL responses. In contrast to acute resolving infection, peripheral CD4+ T-cell and CTL responses in those individuals who develop chronic infection are weak and more narrowly focused.[110] The mechanisms by which HBV evades the immune response and results in chronic infection in these adults remain obscure. In part this is determined by host genetic factors, as persons with certain human leukocyte antigen (HLA) alleles appear to be more susceptible to chronic infection.[111-114] It has also been suggested that the size of initial viral inoculum and viral kinetics may be such that the immune system is overwhelmed by the virus and becomes "exhausted."[115] Despite the weak and narrowly focused response of the peripheral blood CTL, HBV-specific CD4+ and CD8+ T cells can be isolated from the livers of chronic HBV patients that are capable of ex vivo, class-I-restricted cytolytic activity in response to envelope and core peptides. The cytotoxicity mediated by these cells appears to be sufficiently strong to cause liver injury but not strong enough to eradicate virus from all hepatocytes.[116,117] In addition to the virus-specific cells, the inflamed liver contains other cells that may participate in hepatocyte damage.[118]

HEPATITIS D VIRUS

HDAg is the only viral protein known to be expressed during HDV infection. Detection of antibody is the usual method for diagnosis of acute infection. During HDV infection, IgM and IgG antibodies can be detected in the serum of infected individuals. A high titer of IgM anti-HDV is strongly associated with elevated hepatitis D viremia and the severity of liver injury, whereas a more favorable course to HDV infection is found in individuals with IgG-anti HDV. Although these antibody responses are present during acute and chronic infection, there is no convincing evidence of a protective role of anti-HDV antibodies.[119] Woodchucks immunized with recombinant HDAg are only partially protected from subsequent challenge with HDV, which suggests that other mechanisms are responsible for immunity.[120]

The mechanisms of liver damage in HDV infection are unclear. In contrast to HBV, the hepatocyte injury resulting from HDV infection may be caused by a direct viral cytopathic effect rather than immune-mediated damage.[121] The presence of HDV-specific, T-cell responses correlates with lower ALT levels, suggesting that immune control of viral replication leads to lesser degrees of liver injury.[118,119] However, histologic assessment demonstrates that the degree of cellular infiltration in the portal tracts and lobules correlates with the degree of staining for HDAg in the liver, suggesting that the immune response contributes to hepatocellular injury.[122]

HEPATOCELLULAR CARCINOMA

Although epidemiologic evidence supports the role of HBV as a causal agent of liver cancer (see "Epidemiology of Hepatitis B"),[123,124] the molecular mechanisms addressing the link between the viral infection and the development of HCC have been highly debated.[125] Despite a large body of work on this subject, a clear view of how HBV infection triggers events that lead to liver oncogenesis remains elusive. HCC development, like other cancers, proceeds in multiple steps that correlate with specific lesions associated with livers of patients with HCC. These include altered hepatic foci, dysplastic (neoplastic) nodules, and low- and high-grade HCCs. These lesions are characterized as exhibiting different levels of cell differentiation. Similar to other well-characterized human cancers, HCC progresses through these individual stages. The molecular switches associated with each step of HCC development still need to be identified. Although the WHV model has been valuable in the study of hepadnavirus pathogenesis, there are important differences. Compared to HBV, the WHV is a more potent hepatocarcinogen. Nearly 100% of woodchucks infected with WHV develop HCC at about 18 to 24 months of age.[126] Similarly, in humans, HCC

is mostly associated with cirrhosis but in woodchucks, this association is uncommon.

HBV-related HCCs are derived from the clonal expansion of a single transformed cell or cancerous cells.[123] Whereas 80% of HBV-associated HCC tumors contain integrated viral DNA, most of the HBV genes are either truncated or transcriptionally inactivated.[15] As opposed to retroviral replication, HBV DNA integration is not an obligatory part of the viral life cycle but may instead serve as an insertional mutagen.[127] Following integration into the host chromosomes, the HBV DNA control elements such as enhancers or promoters can act in cis to activate a cellular oncogene. HBV integrates randomly at multiple sites in the host chromosomes and molecular analyses of the HBV integration junction sites have not revealed specific integration adjacent to or neighboring cellular oncogenes.[128] In the case of WHV, however, the integration next to the cellular N-myc2 gene was observed in 40% to 50% of woodchuck HCC tumors.[99] Efforts to document a similar case for insertional activation by HBV have been largely unsuccessful. Alternatively, integration of viral DNA could have far-reaching consequences rather than merely activating or repressing neighboring genes. Unstable integration events might frequently lead to genomic instability by causing chromosomal aberrations such as amplifications, translocations, and deletions, all of which have the potential for initiating events that lead to liver neoplasia. Indeed, in HBV-associated liver tumors, the HBV DNA integrants are highly rearranged with deletions, inversions, and sequence reiterations.[129]

The pleiotropic functions of HBx in HCC have been implicated in the processes of liver oncogenesis and have been the subject of multiple investigations.[130] Prominent among these are the ability of HBx to activate transcription factors by direct physical interaction or modulate cellular signal transduction pathways, or both, thereby modifying the host gene expression profile. Other functions include its effects on DNA repair processes and potential to cause direct oxidative damage to host DNA by elevating the intracellular levels of reactive oxidant species (ROS) in cells.[15,65,100] These and other properties of HBx have been implicated in contributing to the genesis of HCC. Because most of the HBV genes are extinguished in advanced tumors, the viral role in the development of HCC is most likely to be at the stage(s) of initiation or promotion of hepatocarcinogenesis, or both. This would preclude the presence of HBx in maintaining the transformed phenotype.

Finally, HBV-associated HCC may be due to the repeated cellular division associated with the inflammatory response.[15,131] HCC associated with HBV nearly always arises in the context of cirrhosis, although a few cases of HCC without cirrhosis have been reported.[132] Cirrhosis is the result of years of inflammation and associated repair processes, during which there is considerable cell killing and repeated hepatocyte regeneration. In all types of liver damage, there is evidence of enhanced production of free radicals or significant decrease of antioxidant defense, or both.[133] Oxidative stress over a long period may give rise to high mutation rates in infected hepatocytes. Mutations, which confer in a cell a proliferative advantage and provide opportunities for achieving a transformed phenotype, are perpetuated. Therefore, according to this model, the role of HBV, if any, is merely to induce liver injury and the subsequent events are all secondary to the host immune response.

Epidemiology of Hepatitis B

The prevalence of HBV carriage varies widely, and is inversely proportional to the age of acquisition of infection. The prevalence rates range from the low-prevalence areas of 0.1% to 2% (United States, Canada, Western Europe, Australia, and New Zealand), to areas with intermediate prevalence of 2% to 7% (Japan, central Asia, Israel, Eastern and Southern Europe, Central America, and South America), to areas of greater than 8% seroprevalence (Southeast Asia, China, Middle East except Israel, Haiti and Dominican Republic, and Africa; Fig. 146-9 and Table 146-1). In areas of high seroprevalence, HBV is more likely to be acquired perinatally, with an attendant high risk of chronic infection of 90%. For infections acquired in later childhood, between the

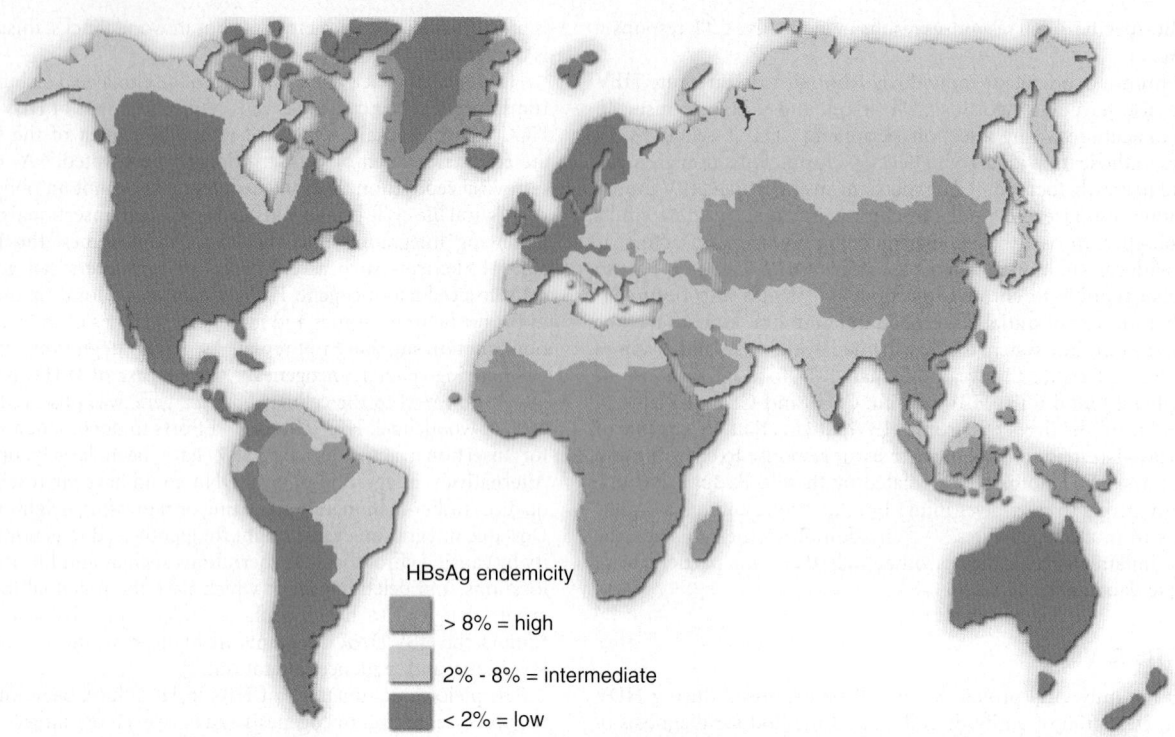

HBsAg endemicity

> 8% = high

2% - 8% = intermediate

< 2% = low

Figure 146-9 **Global prevalence of hepatitis B surface antigenemia.** *(From World Health Organization. Introduction of Hepatitis B Vaccine into Childhood Immunization Services. Geneva: WHO; 2001. WHO/V and B/01.31. Available at http://www.who.int/csr/disease/hepatitis/whocdscrlyo20022.)*

ages of 1 and 5 years, the risk of chronic infection is between 10% and 20%, and for infections acquired by immunocompetent adults the risk is approximately 5%. This leads to a vicious cycle whereby the infected infant is likely to acquire HBV and in turn pass it on to playmates, future sexual partners, and, in the case of infected women, infants.

The epidemiology of HBV is changing with the advent of universal vaccination programs adopted by many countries. For example, in the United States the estimated number of new infections per year was more than 275,000 in the mid 1980s, whereas following the adoption of universal vaccination for infants and "catch-up" vaccination for older children in 1991 there were estimated to be 46,000 new cases in 2006 (Fig. 146-10).[134] The highest rates are among males between the ages of 25 and 44 years.[135] However, there are still estimated to be between 750,000 and 1 million HBV carriers in the United States, of whom 20% to 40% will develop serious sequelae during their lifetime, and 5000 will die annually due to complications of chronic liver disease including HCC. Worldwide, the number of chronic carriers is estimated to be more than 400 million.

Despite an increasing incidence of HCC associated with HCV infection in Japan and the Western hemisphere, chronic HBV infection remains the most important cause of HCC worldwide.[136] The classic epidemiologic studies conducted in Taiwan among HBV carriers established the absolute link between HBV infection and HCC.[137,138] These studies suggest that the interval between acquisition of infection and development of HCC spans several decades (average 30 years). HCC is the fifth most common cancer worldwide with an estimated half a million new cases diagnosed annually.[139] The lifetime risk for HBV chronic carriers is currently estimated to be about 20% to 40%.[136] The incidence of HCC varies geographically and among different ethnic groups. It occurs commonly in HBV-endemic areas, which

TABLE 146-1	Global Seroprevalence Rates and Modes of Transmission of Hepatitis B		
Characteristic	*High*	*Intermediate*	*Low*
Carrier rate (%)	>8	2-7	<2
Distribution	Southeast Asia, China, Alaskan Eskimos, sub-Saharan Africa, Middle East except Israel, Haiti, Dominican Republic	Eastern and southern, Europe, western Mediterranean, central Asia, Latin and South America, Israel	United States, Canada, western Europe, Australia, New Zealand
Age at infection	Perinatal and early childhood	Childhood	Adult
Mode of transmission	Maternal and perinatal	Percutaneous	Sexual, percutaneous

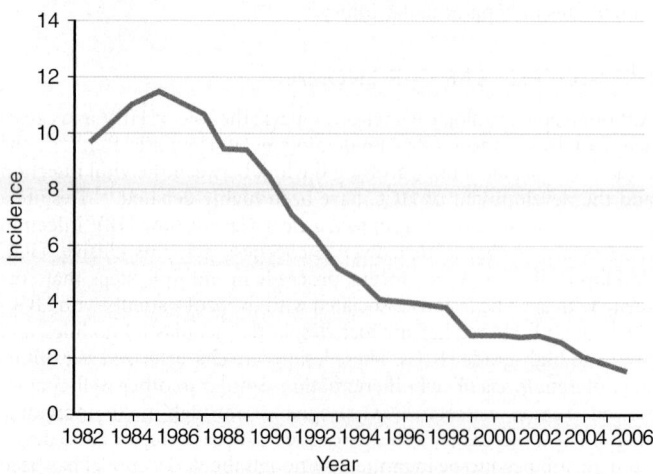

Figure 146-10 **Incidence of acute hepatitis B per 100,000 population by year—United States, 1982 to 2006.** *(Adapted from Surveillance Summaries: Surveillance for Acute Viral Hepatitis—United States, 2006. MMWR Morb Mortal Wkly Rep. 2008;57[SS02]:1-24.)*

include sub-Saharan Africa and Southeast Asia. In parts of sub-Saharan Africa and Asia, HBV-related HCC is one of the leading causes of cancer and HBV carriers have a 100-fold relative risk of HCC compared to noncarriers.[140] In Western Europe and North America, HCC is rare and reflects a 0.1% to 0.5% rate of chronic hepatitis. A report from Taiwan indicates a dramatic reduction of the incidence of HCC in the population coinciding with mass vaccination against HBV (see "Active Immunization").[141] In Asia, HCC has been associated with higher body mass index, higher HBV DNA levels, and genotype C.[142-144]

EPIDEMIOLOGY OF DELTA HEPATITIS

Infection with HDV has a worldwide distribution, although there are considerable geographic differences that do not entirely mirror the prevalence of HBV infection. In northern Europe and in the United States, where HDV is not endemic, the infection is mainly confined to intravenous drug users,[145] whereas it has virtually disappeared in multiply transfused subjects and hemophiliacs as a result of universal blood screening for HBsAg and HBV vaccination campaigns.[146] In areas where HDV is endemic in the general population, such as the Mediterranean basin, most cases of HDV transmission are due to inapparent parenteral exposure.[147]

Routes of Transmission

Hepatitis B replicates to high titer in the blood (10^8 to 10^{10} virions/mL), especially during the acute phase of illness. Any parenteral or mucosal exposure to infected blood thus represents a potential risk for acquisition of hepatitis B, and accounts for the 100 times more efficient transmission of HBV compared to HIV after needlestick exposure.[148] HBV is also found in other body fluids to a variable degree, including semen, saliva, cervical secretions, and leukocytes, and can survive for long periods on environmental surfaces. Thus, exposure to even minute amounts of blood or contaminated secretions may transmit virus, and infection can occur in settings of prolonged, close personal contact, such as occurs between children, or among residents of institutions for the developmentally disabled, probably due to inapparent contact of infected secretions with nonintact skin. The typical mode of transmission of HBV varies in part with the prevalence of infection (see Table 146-1). Perinatal infection is the predominant mode of transmission in high-prevalence areas, whereas horizontal transmission, particularly in early childhood, accounts for most cases of chronic HBV infection in intermediate prevalence areas. Unprotected sexual intercourse and intravenous drug use in adults are the major routes of spread in low-prevalence areas. Persons at increased risk of acquiring HBV infection include members of the following groups: parenteral drug users, heterosexual men and women and homosexual men with multiple partners, household contacts and sexual partners of HBV carriers, infants born to HBV-infected mothers, patients and staff in custodial institutions for the developmentally disabled, recipients of certain plasma-derived products (including patients with congenital coagulation defects), hemodialysis patients, health and public safety workers who have contact with blood, and persons born in areas of high HBV endemicity and their children (Table 146-2). Persons at risk of exposure to HBV should be screened for markers of HBV infection and receive hepatitis B vaccine if seronegative (see "Prevention of Hepatitis B Infection").

Clinical Manifestations and Prognosis

The spectrum of clinical manifestations of HBV infection varies in both acute and chronic infection. During the acute phase, manifestations range from subclinical or anicteric hepatitis to icteric hepatitis and, in some cases, fulminant hepatitis. During the chronic phase, manifestations range from an asymptomatic carrier state to the signs and symptoms of cirrhosis and HCC. Extrahepatic manifestations also can occur with both acute and chronic infection.

TABLE 146-2	Prevalence of Hepatitis B in Selected Populations	
	HBV Marker (%)	
Population	*Prevalence HBsAg⁺*	*Any Marker*
Residents in endemic areas	10-20	70-85
Alaskan natives	5-15	40-70
Residents of institutions for mentally disabled	10-20	35-38
Parenteral drug users	5-10	60-80
Men who have sex with men	4-8	35-80
Household contacts of HBsAg⁺	3-6	30-60
Hemodialysis patients	3-10	20-80
Prison inmates	1-8	10-80
Heterosexuals with multiple sex partners	0.5	5-20
Health care workers	0.5	3-10
General U.S. population	0.2	4.8
Blacks	0.85	13
Whites	0.19	3

HBsAg, hepatitis B surface antigen; HBV, hepatitis B virus.

ACUTE HEPATITIS B

After exposure to HBV, there is an incubation period of 1 to 4 months.[149] Acute hepatitis B is a clinical syndrome indistinguishable from other acute hepatidites, and often consists of a flulike syndrome with malaise, fatigue, anorexia, nausea, vomiting, and right upper quadrant discomfort. Serum sickness-like manifestations may be present prior to the onset of jaundice. Physical signs include jaundice and tender hepatomegaly. The likelihood of developing icteric illness is inversely proportional to age. Symptomatic hepatitis rarely develops in children less than 1 year, in 10% of children less than 5 years, and between 30% to 80% of adults.[150] Most reported cases of HBV are the result of icteric illness, but it is believed that there are a far larger number of infections that either result in subclinical illness or illness only diagnosed in retrospect. The acute illness may be more severe in the setting of other coinfections, such as simultaneous acquisition of hepatitis D, or with underlying liver disease such as alcoholic liver disease. The symptoms and jaundice generally disappear after 1 to 3 months, but some patients have prolonged fatigue even after resolution of the elevated serum aminotransferases. (See Fig. 146-8 for an illustration of a typical clinical and laboratory course of acute hepatitis B compared to that of chronic hepatitis B.)

LABORATORY FINDINGS

Laboratory testing during the acute phase reveals elevations in the concentration of ALT and aspartate aminotransferase (AST) levels; values up to 1000 to 2000 IU/L are typically seen during the acute phase with ALT being higher than AST. The serum bilirubin concentration may be normal in patients with anicteric hepatitis. The prothrombin time (PT) is the best indicator of prognosis, with a high PT indicative of fulminant liver failure.[151] Among patients who recover, normalization of serum aminotransferases usually occurs within 1 to 4 months. Persistent elevation of serum ALT for more than 6 months indicates progression to chronic hepatitis. During the acute phase, there is development of IgM against the core antigen, followed by the development of IgG anti-HBc (see "Making a Viral Diagnosis"). Markers of viral replication, such as HBs antigenemia and HBV DNA in the serum, will be present at the same time as anti-HBc.

Most adult immunocompetent patients clear the infection, but chronic hepatitis (defined by persistent elevation in serum aminotransferases for more than 6 months or HBsAg in serum) develops in less than 5% of adults, 10% to 25% of young children, and 80% to 90% of infants.[150] Rates are similar whether or not there is symptomatic acute disease. Loss of HBV DNA, HBeAg, HBsAg, and IgM anti-HBc and the development of anti-HBe and anti-HBs characterize immunity. An individual who has acquired natural immunity through infection will develop both anti-HBs and anti-HBc. Patients who recover from acute hepatitis B are probably not truly cured of infection, as a significant number of patients will have HBV DNA detectable by polymerase chain reaction (PCR) many years after clinical recovery.[152] They generally have lifelong protection from disease unless there is significant immunosuppression with loss of protective immune responses, such as in the setting of human immunodeficiency virus (HIV) or bone marrow transplant.[153,154]

FULMINANT HEPATITIS

Fulminant hepatitis B is rare, occurring in only 0.1% to 0.5% of patients, and causes less than 10% of fulminant liver failure in the United States.[155,156] Patients typically present with rapidly progressive acute hepatitis, with less than 28 days from the time of symptom onset, accompanied by signs of liver failure such as coagulopathy, encephalopathy, and cerebral edema. Poor prognostic factors for transplant-free survival include a lower mean arterial pressure on admission and low platelet count.[155] Laboratory testing may not reveal HBsAg due to early clearance, but will have IgM anti-HBc and a positive HBV DNA.

The pathogenesis of fulminant hepatic failure is not clear, but may be related to massive immune responses against the virus. Staining of the liver in fulminant HBV often reveals few copies of HBV, suggesting that it is the exuberant immune response that is primarily responsible for the pathogenesis.[157] Fulminant hepatitis is also more common in the setting of coinfection with hepatitis D[158] and withdrawal of immunosuppressant therapy, such as may occur following transplantation.[159] In addition to host factors relating to immune status, several variants of HBV have also been implicated in several outbreaks of fulminant HBV.[160] At least some of the variants lead to premature termination of e antigen (the pre-C mutants), and so there will be detection of core antigen in the blood without detection of HBeAg. Because HBeAg may serve as a tolerogen,[161] the postulated mechanism is that there is enhancement of the immune response. However, careful epidemiologic studies have raised questions about whether these mutants and other mutations within the core are truly more common in fulminant disease,[162,163] and the relatively low levels of virus and robust immune response may be due to other, as yet undefined, viral and host factors.

CHRONIC HEPATITIS B

Chronic hepatitis is defined by at least 6 months of persistent HBV disease. Many patients with chronic hepatitis B are not diagnosed as a result of follow-up after a case of icteric illness or due to specific symptoms, but rather as a result of incidental elevations in serum aminotransferases or due to membership in a specific risk category. Symptoms, if present, can be as nonspecific as fatigue, unless cirrhosis or HCC are present. Other less common symptoms include nausea, right upper quadrant tenderness, anorexia, myalgias, and arthralgias. Symptoms often do not correlate with severity of disease, levels of serum aminotransferases, or hepatic injury on liver biopsy. The physical examination may be normal, or there may be an enlarged liver. The presence of jaundice, splenomegaly, ascites, encephalopathy, or pedal edema suggests cirrhosis.

LABORATORY TESTING IN CHRONIC HEPATITIS B

Laboratory findings in chronic hepatitis B are as variable as the clinical manifestations. Serum aminotransferases may be normal, although most patients with chronic active hepatitis have at least mild-to-moderate elevations. Patients will have markers of viral replication including HBsAg and often HBeAg or HBV DNA as well. During flares of disease activity or just prior to seroconversion to anti-HBe status, there may be marked elevations in the serum aminotransferases to more than 20 times normal. Flares of disease activity may be due to changes in the level of baseline HBV replication, followed by an immune

response against the virus. In some patients, this results in repopulation of the viral species with a new variant.[164] Patients with flares of disease activity should be followed for the development of anti-HBe, which signals control of viral replication.[165] The spontaneous rate of seroconversion varies by age, but in otherwise healthy adults is estimated at 10% to 20% per year.[166] Cirrhosis should be suspected if there is evidence of hypersplenism, manifest as decreased platelet count, or impaired hepatic synthetic function, indicated by hypoalbuminemia, hyperbilirubinemia, or decreased albumin. Similar to the range of findings observed in other laboratory tests, findings on liver biopsy range from minimal inflammation to cirrhosis.

There are no characteristic findings that can distinguish hepatitis B from other forms of viral hepatitis, although liver biopsies can be stained for the presence of HBsAg and HBcAg. The most characteristic feature of chronic HBV is the ground-glass hepatocyte, which is thought to be due to accumulation of HBsAg within the ER.[167] Differentiation from alcoholic liver disease can be made by characteristic patterns of steatosis, Mallory bodies, and micronodular cirrhosis, whereas chronic HCV is marked by steatosis and characteristic lymphoid follicles within portal tracts. Immunosuppressed hosts may have a variant of HBV known as fibrosing cholestatic hepatitis, which reveals periportal fibrosis, hepatocyte ballooning, bile stasis, and mild or absent inflammation.[168]

NATURAL HISTORY OF CHRONIC HEPATITIS B

The natural history of hepatitis B can be viewed as three phases that are the result of the interplay between the virus and the host.[169] Viral factors include the level of replication, and host factors include gender, alcohol consumption, infection with other hepatitis viruses such as hepatitis C virus (HCV), and the extent of immunosuppression. The first phase is the immunotolerant phase, in which there is circulating HBsAg, HBeAg, and high levels of HBV DNA. There is very little immune response against the virus, and so there are minimal elevations of serum aminotransferases and minimal inflammation in the liver. In cases of perinatal infection, this phase may last for decades during which there are very low rates of spontaneous seroconversion to anti-HBe. The cumulative rate of spontaneous HBeAg clearance is estimated to be approximately 2% during the first 3 years of life and only 15% after 20 years of infection in cases of perinatal infection.[170,171] In contrast, among immunocompetent adults this phase is typically present only during the incubation period.

During the second phase of the infection, there is a reduction in HBV DNA levels and an increase in immunity, accompanied by increased aminotransferases and inflammation in the liver. This is thought to be the period in which there is augmentation of both innate and acquired HBV immunity, leading to cytolytic destruction of hepatocytes, as the peak of the immune response coincides with the aminotransferase elevations.[172] In adults, this is usually the period of symptomatic acute hepatitis B, although this phase of infection can last for decades if the immune reaction is not sufficiently vigorous to lead to viral clearance.

The third phase heralds the conversion from HBe antigenemia to anti-HBe, usually followed by a decrease in viral replication and reduction in aminotransferases. This seroconversion event is often, but not always, accompanied by increase in aminotransferases above baseline, suggesting that there is immune control of the virus.[165] However, both HBsAg and low levels of HBV DNA persist, and hence this stage is referred to as the inactive carrier state. Seroconversion may be clinically silent or accompanied by dramatic elevations in aminotransferases, suggesting fulminant hepatitis. As IgM anti-HBc may increase during these flares, this may lead to the erroneous diagnosis of acute hepatitis.[173] Not every acute exacerbation leads to anti-HBe seroconversion, and repeated episodes of these flares are a risk factor for HCC.

In perinatally acquired infection, this period usually occurs in the second to third decade of life, and seroconversion rates may approach 10% to 20% per year.[137,170] Similar rates are observed in adults with chronic infection. In a study of 1536 Alaskan natives who acquired

HBV as adults, more than 70% of subjects cleared HbeAg during the first 10 years of follow-up.[174] The likelihood of seroconversion is inversely related to the serum aminotransferase. In children with normal ALT, the seroconversion rate is less than 2% during the first 3 years of life and 4% to 5% in older children. Spontaneous seroconversion occurs in 50% of those with serum aminotransferases greater than five times the upper limit of normal compared to less than 10% in those with lower aminotransferases.[175] Spontaneous seroconversion is marked by the appearance of HBcAg-specific CD4+ and CD8+ T cells,[176] but the precise factors that lead up to this event are unknown, and cannot be linked to specific viral mutants, as was previously believed.[177] Males and older individuals are also more likely to have spontaneous seroconversion, and viral genotype may play a role.[38] Trials of anti-HBV therapy should account for this rate of spontaneous seroconversion, as a therapeutic agent may not offer increased rates of HBe seroconversion above the spontaneous seroconversion rate observed in a given cohort.

After the development of anti-HBe, patients are in the third phase of illness, the nonreplicative phase. Termination of virus replication is associated in most patients with biochemical and histologic regression of inflammatory activity.[178] Some individuals will also clear HBsAg, although this is unusual, occurring in less than 1% of patients per year in adults and 0.05% to 0.8% in infection acquired in infancy or childhood.[174,179] In the absence of cirrhosis the prognosis of healthy carriers is generally good, although these patients can have reactivation of replication if immunosuppressed.[180]

PRECORE OR HBe-NEGATIVE MUTANTS

Early reports described patients in whom HBeAg was absent, although HBV DNA continued to be present at a high level, typically in association with severe liver disease.[181-184] This is due to the development of HBV mutants that cannot produce HBeAg due to mutations in the pre-C or core promoter (see "Translation").[185] The most frequent pre-C mutation is a G to A change at nucleotide 1986, which creates a premature stop codon in the pre-C region and abolishes production of HBeAg.[186] However, other variants are reported in both the pre-C and core promoter regions. All these mutations abrogate HBeAg synthesis without affecting the replication of the virus. Most of these pre-C mutations exhibit enhanced levels of HBV replication.[187] Other mutations, for example, in the signal peptide, lead to diminished levels of HBeAg expression.[188,189] Pre-C HBV mutants often become dominant viral quasispecies in the viral populations within an individual.

Originally, this was thought to be predominately a geographic phenomenon, as HBeAg negative hepatitis is more prevalent in certain parts of the world, especially Asia and the Mediterranean. However, more recent studies suggest that the likelihood of HBeAg negative chronic HBV is related to duration of infection, as suggested by the older age at presentation,[190] which would make it appear to be of higher prevalence in areas where perinatal transmission predominates. HBeAg negative disease is also more frequent with genotypes B, C, and D than with genotype A infection.[191] A recent prospective study demonstrated that HBeAg negative chronic hepatitis accumulates over time after anti-HBe seroconversion, with a cumulative incidence of 25% at 16 years of follow-up.[192] Patients with HBeAg negative but HBV DNA positive hepatitis tend to have more severe inflammation and a higher likelihood of cirrhosis, and 29% to 38% are cirrhotic at the time of initial presentation.[190,193] These patients have very low rates of spontaneous seroconversion of less than 0.5% per year[192] and are more difficult to treat.[182]

PROGNOSIS OF CHRONIC HEPATITIS B

The likelihood of morbidity and mortality in chronic hepatitis B is directly related to the development of cirrhosis. For persons who clear HBsAg, the prognosis is good although perhaps surprisingly is not entirely benign. In one study of 189 patients who were noncirrhotic at the time of HBsAg clearance, three (1.6%) developed cirrhosis, two (1.1%) developed HCC, and one died of HCC. These complications all

developed in patients with concurrent HCV or HDV infection, however.[194] In the absence of cirrhosis, the long-term prognosis even of HBsAg-positive patients is good. In a 16-year follow-up study of 317 HBsAg-positive blood donors from Montreal, for example, only three died from HBV-related cirrhosis and none developed HCC.[195] Higher rates of mortality are reported in other cohorts and may be related to disease duration. In one study of HBsAg-positive patients in England and Wales, during a mean 22 years of follow-up, 17.4% of deaths in the cohort of HBsAg-positive subjects were due to HCC or liver disease.[196] The risk of developing cirrhosis in chronic HBsAg-positive patients ranges from 1 to 5.4 per 100 person-years, with a 5-year cumulative probability of progression ranging from 8% to 20%.[190,197,198]

Multiple variables account for the wide estimates of risk. A recent study from Taiwan of 3582 people with chronic hepatitis B followed for 11 years found that the strongest predictor of progression to cirrhosis was the HBV DNA level, which was independent of the HBeAg status and inflammation as represented by ALT values.[199] Individuals with greater than 10^6 copies/mL of HBV DNA had a 36.2% cumulative incidence of cirrhosis compared to 4.5% in those with less than 300 copies/mL. Most of the people in this study acquired HBV in infancy or early childhood; thus, this study may not be applicable to adult-acquired HBV. The rate of progression to cirrhosis may be higher in patients who are HBeAg negative compared to those who are HBeAg positive,[182] although these findings may be confounded by a longer duration of disease in HBeAg-negative patients. Patients with more severe inflammation and fibrosis at the time of presentation are also more likely to progress to cirrhosis. Fattovich and colleagues found that 30% of patients with moderate, chronic active hepatitis developed cirrhosis on histology after 6 years, whereas 50% of patients with severe, chronic active hepatitis (bridging necrosis) developed cirrhosis on histology after 4 years.[175] Similarly, in one study the severity of the fibrosis was 0%, 6%, and 17%, respectively, of individuals with no, mild, or moderate degrees of fibrosis present on the initial biopsy.[200] Consumption of alcohol also increases both the risk of cirrhosis and HCC.[201] Infection with hepatitis C, when accompanied by active replication of both viruses, also increases the rate of progression to cirrhosis,[202,203] as does delta hepatitis.[204]

For patients with compensated cirrhosis, survival is 84% at 5 years and 68% at 10 years.[205] Once cirrhosis develops, the risk of decompensation is 20% to 25% per year.[175,206] The prognosis is very poor after the development of decompensation, with estimated survival rates of only 55% to 70% at 1 year and 14% to 35% at 5 years.[197,207] In one study of European patients with biopsy-proven cirrhosis, during a 6-year period of follow-up, HCC developed in 32 (9%) of the 349 patients, and decompensation was observed in 88 (28%) of 317 tumor-free patients. After the first episode of decompensation, the probability of survival was only 35% at 5 years.[197]

Another major cause of mortality in chronic HBV is HCC, which has a poor prognosis unless caught in a small, surgically resectable stage. The risk of HCC in persons with cirrhosis is estimated to be 6% to 15%.[193,197,208] For example, in one study, the likelihood of developing HCC over a 5-year time period is 9% in persons with Child's A cirrhosis with an incidence per 100 person-years of 2.2.[205] Risk factors for the development of HCC are male sex, age, alcohol, the presence of HBeAg, and higher levels of HBV DNA. In one study of over 11,000 men, the incidence rate of HCC was 1169 cases per 100,000 person-years among men who were positive for both HBsAg and HBeAg, 324 per 100,000 person-years for those who were positive for HBsAg only, and 39 per 100,000 person-years for those who were negative for both.[209] The relative risk of HCC was 9.6 (95% confidence interval [CI], 6.0 to 15.2) among men who were positive for HBsAg alone and 60.2 (95% CI, 35.5 to 102.1) among those who were positive for both HBsAg and HBeAg, as compared with men who were negative for both.[209] In one case-control study, the relative risk of HCC was 4.5 for alcohol use alone, 12.6 for HBsAg alone, and 53.9 for patients with both viral hepatitis and alcohol use.[210] Levels of HBV DNA are also a risk factor, with levels above 105 copies/mL being strongly linked to the development of HCC.[142] Clearance of HBsAg by the age of 50 appears to decrease the risk of HCC.[211] Men are between 2 and 4 times more likely than women to develop HCC,[212] which may be due to the presence of other cofactors, such as alcohol, or a direct effect of testosterone on HBV replication.[213]

HEPATITIS D

HDV is spread by blood, blood products, and bodily secretions similar to HBV.[214] Following exposure, there is a short incubation period of 3 to 7 weeks. As HDV requires a helper function from HBV, disease may occur as an acute coinfection with HBV or as a superinfection of a chronic HBV infection. As with hepatitis B, the clinical presentation and natural history are highly variable. The incubation period during coinfection may display a biphasic pattern of ALT levels due to different titers of the virus, as the incubation period is inversely proportional to the dose of the virus. Usually the first episode is due to hepatitis B replication and immune response, followed by that of hepatitis D. Superinfection of chronic carriers with HDV generally results in severe hepatitis with a relatively short incubation period followed by chronic hepatitis D in most of the cases. Superinfection with HDV is also associated with fulminant hepatitis and chronic active hepatitis with cirrhosis. Fulminant hepatitis, a severe form of acute hepatitis, is 10 times more common in coinfection. The diagnosis of HDV may be established using PCR, which is more sensitive than hybridization assays,[215] as well as both IgM and IgG anti-HDAg.

Most simultaneous acute infections in adults are cleared along with hepatitis B. Of acute coinfections, 1% to 3% become chronic, and 70% to 80% of superinfections develop into chronic hepatitis D. Once chronic infection is established, the clinical course of hepatitis is accelerated. Cirrhosis occurs in 60% to 80% of chronic hepatitis D patients, and the risk of HCC is about threefold.[216] Superinfection progresses to chronicity in over 90% of cases. These patients have more severe liver disease, with a 60% to 80% chance of cirrhosis, and an increased risk of HCC.[217-219] In one study where the seroprevalence rate for HDV was 6%, the relative risk of cirrhosis and HCC was 2.58 and 2.87, respectively, in patients with both infections compared to those with HBV alone.[217] The high risk of HCC may reflect the higher rate of cirrhosis.

EXTRAHEPATIC MANIFESTATIONS OF HEPATITIS B

Extrahepatic manifestations, which are thought to be mediated by circulating immune complexes, can be seen in both acute and chronic HBV. Acute hepatitis may be manifest in 10% to 20% of patients as a serum-sickness–like illness with fever, skin rash, arthralgias, and polyarthritis, typically occurring just prior to the onset and subsiding with the development of jaundice. The skin rash can be of virtually any type, including erythematous, macular, maculopapular, urticarial, or petechial. Polyarteritis nodosa (PAN) is a rare complication of HBV. It is a vasculitis of small-to-medium-size arteries, and typically presents with fever, rash, hypertension, eosinophilia, abdominal pain, renal disease, and polyarthritis. A variable proportion of patients with PAN are HBV positive, and some of those may benefit from antiviral treatment.[220] Steroids may improve the manifestations but may worsen the hepatitis B. Both nucleosides and IFN alfa have been used.[221,222] There is also a rare but distinctive manifestation in children, papular acrodermatitis (Gianotti-Crosti syndrome), which consists of 2- to 3-mm, flat, erythematous, and papular eruptions localized to the face and extremities, along with generalized lymphadenopathy in the setting of acute hepatitis B.[223-225] Glomerular disease also occurs as a manifestation of HBV infection. Nephrotic syndrome secondary to membranous or membranoproliferative glomerulonephritis is a rare complication of HBV infection occurring predominantly in children with active viral replication. The typical presentation is with nephrotic range proteinuria. Approximately 30% to 60% of children with HBV-related membranous nephropathy undergo spontaneous remission, usually in association with HBeAg to anti-HBe seroconversion.[226] Progression to renal failure can occur, particularly in adults. Its prognosis

is variable, but in adults it may lead to progressive renal insufficiency.[227] It can be successfully treated with IFN alfa.[228]

Clinical Manifestations and Natural History in Special Hosts

INDIVIDUALS WITH HUMAN IMMUNODEFICIENCY VIRUS INFECTION

Because of common parenteral routes of transmission, HBV and HIV are frequently seen in concert. In a study of 16,248 HIV-infected patients receiving care, the incidence of acute HBV was 12.2 cases per 1000 person-years, which was lower in those taking either antiretroviral therapy (ART) with lamivudine, ART without lamivudine, or with one or more doses of HBV vaccine.[229] Current estimates are that 65% of individuals who are HIV seropositive in the United States are positive for some marker of past HBV infection, and 6% to 14% are HBsAg positive.[230] In the regions with high HBV endemicity, up to 20% of HIV-infected persons are coinfected with chronic HBV.[231] Patients with HIV and AIDS are more likely to have chronic HBV infection, have increased replication manifest as higher HBV DNA burdens, and are more likely to be HBeAg positive.[232] Despite lower serum aminotransferases, patients with HIV/HBV coinfection are more likely to have cirrhosis on biopsy.[233] This translates into a higher observed liver-related mortality for patients with coinfection compared to those with either virus alone.[234] In coinfected individuals, the liver-related mortality rate was highest with lower nadir CD4+ T-cell counts and was twice as high after 1996, when effective ART was introduced, which may be confounded by the longer duration of HBV infection in those surviving into the ART era. Loss of CD4+ T cells in persons with HIV can be accompanied by reactivation of disease in previously healthy carriers[235] and rapidly progressive, fibrosing cholestatic hepatitis in others.[236] Isolated anti-HBc is found in approximately 20% of HIV-infected patients,[237] but rates of occult hepatitis B in this group are variable ranging from less than 5% up to 90%.[237-241]

HEPATITIS B AFTER LIVER TRANSPLANTATION

In the absence of specific therapy, most patients with hepatitis B will have reinfection of the allograft. In some patients, rapidly progressive liver failure develops marked by a histologic variant known as fibrosing cholestatic hepatitis.[168] Hepatitis B hyperimmune globulin (HBIg) can prevent reinfection of the allograft, but it is expensive and must be continued indefinitely to prevent reinfection. Lamivudine may also be used to treat and prevent recurrent HBV infection, although its long-term effectiveness is limited by lamivudine resistance (see "Nucleoside and Nucleotide Therapies").[242] The long-term survival following liver transplantation for hepatitis B is generally very good when HBIg and antivirals are combined. In one large study conducted between 1988 and 2002, the 1-, 5-, and 10-year patient survival rates were 91%, 81%, and 73%,[243] respectively, which is comparable to other conditions leading to transplantation.

HEPATITIS B AFTER OTHER TYPES OF TRANSPLANTATION

Due to the frequent need for blood products in some groups of patients, patients with other types of transplantation are also at risk for HBV infection, followed by progressive hepatitis during the period of immunosuppression. In the past, large numbers of patients in chronic hemodialysis became infected through contaminated dialysis equipment and blood transfusions due to chronic anemia. With better appreciation of appropriate infection control measures and vaccination of patients, the incidence of hepatitis B among patients with chronic renal disease has decreased. Renal transplantation is associated with reduced survival in HBsAg-positive hemodialysis patients, compared to improved survival in HCV-seropositive patients.[244] Similarly, recipients of bone marrow transplants are also at risk of recurrent hepatitis B, which may present as a severe flare at the time of withdrawal of immunosuppression[245] or as progressive chronic liver disease.[246] T-cell-depleted recipients appear to be at particular risk.[247] Interestingly, however, there have also been case reports of cure of hepatitis B after bone marrow transplantation due to the transfer of HBV-specific immune cells in the graft.[248,249]

COINFECTION WITH HEPATITIS C

Coinfection with HCV and active replication of both viruses is unusual, although 10% to 20% of patients with evidence of HBV may carry some marker of both infections.[175,250] Coinfection with hepatitis C often seems to result in suppression of HBV replication and these patients are often negative for HBeAg.[251,252] However, when both viruses are replicating, the liver disease is usually more severe than in patients infected by HBV alone.[219,253] Patients with dual HBV and HCV infection may also have a higher rate of HCC compared to patients infected by either virus alone.[254] Patients with occult hepatitis B (HBV DNA by PCR only) may have a reduced response rate to IFN alfa monotherapy of hepatitis C,[255] but the response rate to combined IFN and ribavirin appears equal to those with HCV alone.[256]

Making a Viral Diagnosis

Infection with HBV is associated with characteristic patterns of hepatitis B antigens and antibodies. In addition to confirming the stage of HBV infection, proper interpretation of the available tests will aid in the monitoring of patients and selection for antiviral therapy.

ACUTE HEPATITIS

The diagnosis of acute hepatitis B is based on the detection of HBsAg and IgM anti-HBc (Table 146-3 and see Fig. 146-8). During the replicative phase of infection, HBeAg and HBV DNA are also present. Recovery is accompanied by the disappearance of markers of HBV replication and the appearance of antibodies to these proteins.

HBsAg is the serologic hallmark of HBV infection. It can be detected by RIAs or ELISAs. HBsAg appears in serum 1 to 10 weeks after an acute exposure to HBV, prior to the onset of symptoms or elevation of serum ALT. In patients who subsequently recover, HBsAg usually becomes undetectable after 4 to 6 months. Persistence of HBsAg for more than 6 months generally defines chronic infection, although in rare cases HBsAg may persist for as long as 1 year.[150] HBeAg is a secretory protein that is processed from the pre-C protein, and is a marker of HBV replication and infectivity.[34] During recovery from acute infection, anti-HBe appears first followed by anti-HBs. In most patients who recover, anti-HBs persists for life, thereby conferring long-term immunity.

HBcAg is an intracellular antigen that is not detectable in serum. Anti-HBc can be detected throughout the course of HBV infection, and its presence signifies natural infection. During acute infection, anti-HBc is predominantly IgM class and can be the sole marker of HBV infection during the window period between the disappearance of HBsAg and the appearance of anti-HBs. The detection of IgM anti-HBc is usually regarded as an indication of acute HBV infection. However, IgM anti-HBc may remain detectable up to 2 years after the acute infection. IgG anti-HBc persists even in individuals with HBs antigenemia, indicating that the presence of this antibody does not confer protection against viral replication.

PAST HEPATITIS B INFECTION

Previous HBV infection is characterized by the presence of anti-HBs and IgG anti-HBc. Immunity to HBV infection after vaccination is indicated by the presence of anti-HBs only.

CHRONIC HEPATITIS B INFECTION

The diagnosis of chronic HBV infection is based on the persistence of HBsAg for more than 6 months. Additional tests for HBV replication—HBeAg and serum HBV DNA—should be performed in those with chronic hepatitis B. The presence of HBe antigenemia signifies increased infectivity and higher HBV DNA leading to higher rates of vertical and nosocomial transmission.[34] In adults, if HBeAg is negative, HBV DNA is undetectable and serum aminotransferases are normal, the patient is likely a healthy carrier and does not need further evaluation, although most experts recommend periodic (every 6 to 12 months) evaluation of aminotransferases and HBV DNA to detect the rare instances of reactivation. The annual rate of flares of ALT is about 4%, with pre-C mutations, male sex, and age over 30 being predictors of flares.[257] Patients with perinatal HBV infection, in particular, may have normal or minimally elevated serum aminotransferases due to immune tolerance, but they are distinguished from the healthy carrier by high HBV DNA levels.[258]

Those with progressive liver disease can be either HBeAg negative or positive, have detectable HBV DNA, and usually have elevated serum ALT concentrations. The HBV DNA level in HBeAg-positive, chronic hepatitis B patients tends to be higher than those with HBeAg-negative chronic hepatitis B. HBeAg-negative patients have a stop codon mutation in the pre-C region that prevents the production of HBeAg (see "Precore or HBe-Negative Mutants"),[181] and so HBV DNA is the measurement of viral replication.

In HBeAg-positive patients, development of anti-HBe can occur at any point during chronic HBV infection; it occurs spontaneously in a small percent of patients per year. It is often accompanied by an increase in serum aminotransferases, followed by a disappearance of HBeAg and HBV DNA from the serum and improvement in liver inflammation. However, some patients continue to have active liver disease and detectable HBV DNA in serum after HBeAg seroconversion.[259]

TABLE 146-3	Interpretation of Serologic Tests in Hepatitis B				
Test	*Acute Hepatitis B*	*Immunity through Infection**	*Immunity through Vaccination*	*Chronic Hepatitis B†*	*Healthy Carrier*
HBsAg	+	−	−	+	+
Anti-HBs	−	+	+	−	−
HBeAg	+	−	−	+/−	−
Anti-HBe	−	+/−	−	+/−	+
Anti-HBc	+	+	−	+	+
IgM anti-HBc	+	−	−	−	−
HBV DNA‡	+	−	−	+	+ (low)
ALT	Elevated	Normal	Normal	Elevated	Normal

*Occasionally individuals with past infection have isolated anti-HBc only. The presence of an isolated IgG anti-HBc may indicate a window period during acute infection or remote prior infection with loss of HBsAg or anti-HBs. In such cases, an HBV DNA test may prove useful.
†Chronic hepatitis B with a pre-core mutant is HBeAg− and anti-HBe+.
‡Presence of HBV DNA depends on the sensitivity of the test used.
ALT, alanine aminotransferase; HBc, hepatitis B core; HBe, hepatitis B early; HBsAg, hepatitis B surface antigen; HBV, hepatitis B virus; IgM, immunoglobulin M.

Patients with chronic hepatitis B should have HBV DNA quantified as well as be tested for other conditions such as hepatitis C, HIV, and immunity to hepatitis A. If they are nonimmune to hepatitis A, they should be vaccinated as fulminant hepatitis A, although rare, can occur in patients with chronic hepatitis B.

MEASURES OF HEPATITIS B REPLICATION

PCR-based assays are the standard way to quantify HBV replication. Several real-time PCR assays are available now and have lower limits of sensitivity of approximately 10 IU/mL and upper limits of 4×10^9 IU/mL. The older hybridization assays are less sensitive; therefore, they are not recommended. A study from Taiwan with 3653 participants with chronic hepatitis B demonstrated that HBV DNA levels correlate with the risk of developing either cirrhosis or HCC.[142,199] There was a dose-response relationship between the HBV DNA level and the risk for these outcomes. The major role of HBV DNA assays is to evaluate patients with either HBeAg-positive or -negative chronic hepatitis B to assess candidacy for treatment. In those who are treated, following HBV DNA is essential to monitor the treatment response. There are several circumstances in which HBV DNA is useful. The first is distinguishing the window period of acute infection from chronic infection in those patients who are IgG anti-HBc only. HBV DNA is also useful in cases of fulminant hepatitis, where there may be undetectable levels of HBsAg on presentation. HBV DNA testing is also indicated in patients with biochemical or histologic evidence of viral replication but negative HBeAg testing. These individuals are likely to have pre-C mutants. The major role of HBV DNA assays, however, is in patients with chronic HBV to assess both candidacy and response to antiviral therapy. Patients with high pretreatment levels of HBV DNA are less likely to respond to IFN, although responses to nucleoside agents appear not to be affected by the level of pretreatment HBV DNA.[260-262] Clearance of serum HBV DNA may be used as one of the end points in assessing response to antiviral treatment.

The enhanced sensitivity of the newer tests, especially PCR-based methods, has also raised questions about the significance of low-level viremia. Recovery from acute infection was formerly thought to be accompanied by complete clearance of HBV from serum. However, use of PCR-based methods has demonstrated that some individuals may have very low level replication in the absence of any biochemical or histologic markers of liver injury.[263] The significance of this is not known, although some studies have suggested that such "occult" hepatitis B is associated with progressive liver disease. The threshold level that is associated with a risk of progression of chronic liver disease is not known. An arbitrary value of greater than 20,000 IU/mL or 10^5 copies/mL has been suggested as a diagnostic criterion for chronic hepatitis,[263] but lower levels may be seen in patients with ongoing liver injury, especially in HBeAg-negative patients. Because levels of HBV DNA may fluctuate over time in a given individual, the use of HBV DNA testing as a sole determination of future prognosis is not recommended.[264]

ISOLATED ANTI-HBc

The isolated presence of anti-HBc alone is not uncommon, being present in 0.4% to 1.7% of blood donors in low-prevalence areas[265] and in 10% to 20% of the population in endemic countries.[266] Isolated anti-HBc can be found in patients during the window period of acute hepatitis, many years after resolution of acute hepatitis, due to a decline of anti-HBs to undetectable titers; or, rarely, after years of chronic infection with decline of HBsAg to titers below the limit of detection. Individuals with anti-HBc alone should have repeat testing done to exclude false-positive results; IgM anti-HBc to exclude acute hepatitis; and HBV DNA testing. Isolated anti-HBc is more common in people coinfected with either chronic hepatitis C or HIV. The clinical significance of isolated anti-HBc with or without a low-level positive HBV DNA test is not clear; however, such patients should be considered potentially infectious, as transmission of HBV from blood and organ donors with anti-HBc alone has been reported.[267,268]

Management of Hepatitis B

ACUTE HEPATITIS B

Treatment in acute hepatitis B is generally supportive. Medication lists should be reviewed, and patients should be reminded to avoid medications metabolized by the liver if possible or limit the doses. This is particularly true for agents such as acetaminophen, which patients may be taking to minimize discomfort and fever. Treatment of fulminant hepatitis is also supportive, including liver transplantation for those patients who do not appear to have spontaneous recovery. Treatment with antiviral agents is not indicated for acute hepatitis B;[269] however, there is some evidence of benefit for cases of acute fulminant HBV.[270,271]

CHRONIC HEPATITIS B

The goals of antiviral therapy in hepatitis B are reduction of the morbidity and mortality due to liver disease. There are a variety of end points that have been used to define response to treatment in clinical trials, including normalization of serum aminotransferases (biochemical response), improvement in liver histology (histologic responses), improvement in the level of HBV DNA or achieving undetectable HBV DNA in the serum (virologic response), and loss of HBeAg with or without anti-HBe (serologic response).[264,272] Elimination of HBsAg is rare but important, as the risk of liver cancer continues to be elevated above baseline among patients with persistent HBs antigenemia.[211]

Because long-term studies have demonstrated that either seroconversion to anti-HBe or durable suppression of HBV DNA is associated with reduction in cirrhosis,[273,274] an improvement in survival,[275-278] and reduction of the rates of HCC,[279] these are the most common surrogate markers used in both clinical practice and clinical trials to monitor the efficacy of therapy. For HBeAg-positive patients who achieve seroconversion to anti-HBe, therapy is usually continued for 6 to 12 months after seroconversion to achieve a durable response.[280-282] For those who do not seroconvert on treatment or who are HBeAg negative, therapy with a nucleoside/tide is generally continued indefinitely; unless resistance develops, therapy is usually effective for long periods of time.[283-288]

SELECTION OF PATIENTS FOR TREATMENT
(See also Chapter 116)

The currently available treatments all have limited short- and long-term efficacy, as well as substantial costs, both in terms of side effects (e.g., as in the case of IFN) and financial considerations. Thus, not all patients warrant treatment. Current recommendations are to treat patients with evidence of viral replication (either HBeAg positive with a nonamplified HBV DNA of >20,000 IU/mL, or, in the case of HBeAg-negative disease, with HBV DNA > 2000 IU/mL) and serum aminotransferases greater than two times the upper limit of normal, or with evidence of moderate-to-severe necroinflammation on biopsy (Table 146-4).[272] However, strict interpretation of these guidelines may miss host and viral factors (e.g., pre-C mutations) that are predictive of long-term adverse outcomes;[289] thus, therapy can also be guided by age of the patient and histologic findings. The choice of therapy, particularly of initial nucleoside/tide treatment, is undergoing substantial evaluation and in part is governed by patient considerations of tolerability and limited data about the optimal strategy to prevent the development of antiviral resistance over the long term.

INTERFERON

IFN alfa is the recombinant version of one or more proteins that are naturally produced by the body in response to viral infection. These proteins have antiviral, antiproliferative, immunomodulatory, and

TABLE 146-4	Selection of Patients for Treatment in Chronic Hepatitis B		
HBeAg	HBV DNA*	ALT†	*Treatment Strategy*
+	>20,000 IIU/mL	<2 × ULN	Observe patient Consider liver biopsy if age > 40, ALT > 1 but <2 × ULN, family history HCC, HIV+; treat if moderate-to-severe inflammation or fibrosis
+	>20,000 IIU/mL	>2 × ULN	Observe 3-6 mos for spontaneous HBe seroconversion Treatment with PEG IFN (48 wk) or NUC (at least 1 yr; minimum 6 mo after HBe seroconversion)
−	>20,000 IIU/mL	>2 × ULN	Treatment with PEG IFN (48 wk) or NUC (end point not defined; likely indefinite)
−	>2000 IIU/mL	1 to <2 × ULN	Consider liver biopsy and treatment if moderate-to-severe inflammation or fibrosis (PEG IFN or NUC)
−	>2000 IIU/mL	<ULN	Observe; treat if HBV DNA or ALT increase
+/−	+	Cirrhosis	Compensated: Treat with NUC if HBV DNA > 2000 IU/mL; if HBV DNA < 2000 IU/mL consider treatment if ALT > ULN Decompensated: NUC; consider liver transplantation
+/−	−	Cirrhosis	Compensated: Observe Decompensated: Consider liver transplantation

*Conversion factor to copies/mL = 5.6 (20,000 IU/mL is approximately 10^5 copies/mL).

†Also use moderate-to-severe necroinflammation on liver biopsy as guide.

ALT, alanine aminotransferase; HBeAg, hepatitis B early antigen; HBV, hepatitis B virus; IFN, interferon alfa; NUC, nucleoside or nucleotide; ULN, upper limit of normal.

Adapted from Lok AS, McMahon BJ. Chronic hepatitis B. *Hepatology.* 2007;45:507-539.

antifibrotic effects. The mechanism by which it is effective has not been established, although IFN alfa has been used in the treatment of hepatitis B for more than 25 years.[261] Most recently, PEG IFN alfa, given as a once-a-week injection of 180 µg, has supplanted standard IFN alfa for treatment of hepatitis B. The efficacy of IFN alfa depends on the patient.[290,291] Factors predictive of a high response to PEG IFN alfa in HbeAg-negative disease are low HBV DNA, age, female sex, and genotype B or C (compared to genotype D).[292] Treatment of patients with normal ALT, whether adults or children, results in response rates of less than 10%,[293] suggesting the importance of the immune response in IFN-based therapy.

In HBeAg-positive patients, therapy is usually given for 48 weeks, irrespective of the time to seroconversion. One-year rates of seroconversion are 27%;[40,294] the durability of the response is improved if PEG IFN alfa is continued for at least 24 weeks after seroconversion. Loss of HBeAg and HBsAg were maintained in 37% and 11%, respectively, for 3 years after treatment with PEG IFN alfa.[295] In HBeAg-negative patients, the end point of therapy is usually normalization of ALT and loss of serum HBV DNA. The rate of sustained undetectable HBV DNA, measured 24 weeks after 48 weeks of treatment, is approximately 19% in HBeAg-negative disease. Given the toxicity of IFN alfa, most providers do not use it in HBeAg-negative disease as the tolerability of long-term nucleosides/tides is better. Nevertheless, sustained responses can be achieved in 15% to 25% of patients and long-term follow-up showed that 15% to 30% of sustained responders cleared HBsAg.[291,296] In addition, long-term responders appear to have reduced risks of HCC and liver-related deaths. PEG IFN alfa, along with ribavirin, may also be used in the setting of dual infection with HBV and HCV.[297]

PEG IFN alfa is administered as subcutaneous injections. Patients should be treated for at least 12 months, but it is not clear if longer duration of treatment will increase the rate of sustained response.[298] IFN alfa therapy causes many side effects, including flulike illness, fever, myalgias, headache, and fatigue. Many of these acute side effects improve after the first days to weeks of dosing, although they can linger in individual patients for the full duration of therapy. Other side effects seen after prolonged dosing include leukopenia and thrombocytopenia, hair loss, and changes in mood, including irritability, sleep disorders, and depression, which can be severe. IFN therapy can also lead to the development of auto-antibodies, such as antithyroid antibodies, and worsening of other autoimmune disorders.[299]

IFN alfa is contraindicated in decompensated cirrhosis, as it may precipate flares of disease activity with subsequent decompensation.[300,301] However, IFN alfa is safe and may be effective in patients with compensated cirrhosis. In clinical trials of patients with HBeAg-positive, chronic hepatitis, up to 60% of patients included had histologic cirrhosis, and less than 1% of patients who received standard doses of IFN alfa developed hepatic decompensation.[301]

NUCLEOSIDE AND NUCLEOTIDE THERAPIES

Recognition that HBV, like HIV, has an RT step in its life cycle had led to the testing of many nucleoside agents (Table 146-5). Because these agents are better tolerated than IFN alfa, this has led to long-term use of these agents for the purpose of both viral suppression and improvement in histologic disease. Unlike IFN alfa, nucleoside/tide agents can be used in the setting of hepatic decompensation[302] and may even prevent or delay the need for transplantation in this setting.[303] However, resistance to these agents develops over time. The rapidity of HBV DNA suppression is predictive of the virologic, serologic, biochemical, and histologic benefit of therapy; moreover, the degree of suppression is inversely related to the likelihood of resistance.[260]

LAMIVUDINE

Lamivudine is the negative enantiomer of 2′ to 3′ dideoxy-3′-thiacytidine (see Chapter 41). It is phosphorylated by host enzymes, and it is the incorporation of the triphosphate form into DNA that results in premature chain termination. Lamivudine is administered at 100 mg/day and, unlike IFN, is well tolerated, with side effects no different than placebo in most series. The recommended dose for children is 3 mg/kg/day with a maximum dose of 100 mg/day. Dose reduction is necessary for patients with renal insufficiency (creatinine clearance <50 mL/min). Several large, randomized clinical trials in patients with HBeAg-positive HBV and elevated aminotransferases have demonstrated HBeAg seroconversion rates of 16% to 18% compared to 4% to 6% of controls.[304,305] In addition to virologic improvement, histologic improvement (defined as a reduction in necroinflammatory score greater than 2 points) was observed in 49% to 56% of treated patients and in 23% to 25% of controls. These benefits increased over time. A multinational study of Asian patients showed that seroconversion rates increased over time from 17% to 27% at 2 years, 40% at 3 years, 47% at 4 years, and 50% by 5 years.[283,284] An important predictor of response is the pretreatment aminotransferase level. At 1 year, HBeAg seroconversion was seen in 5% of patients with ALT less than two times the upper limit of normal, 26% of those with ALT two to five times the upper limit of normal, and 64% of those with ALT greater than five times the upper limit of normal.[306] Conversely, those with normal aminotransferases have less than a 10% chance of seroconversion.[262] Patients with HBeAg-negative hepatitis appear to have similar response rates,[286,307,308] as do patients who have previously failed IFN alfa therapy.[309] Genotype, as with all the oral agents, is not a known predictor of response. Unlike IFN alfa, lamivudine can be given in both compensated and decompensated cirrhosis, although the likelihood of HBeAg seroconversion is small in these groups.[302,310]

One of the major issues with lamivudine treatment is the duration and the durability of response, as resistance develops rapidly during

TABLE 146-5	Approved Agents for Treatment of Chronic Hepatitis B*					
	PEG IFN alfa	*Lamivudine*	*Adefovir*	*Entecavir*	*Telbivudine*	*Tenofovir*
Route	Subcutaneous	Oral	Oral	Oral	Oral	Oral
Dose	180 μg/wk	100 mg/day[†]	10 mg/day[†]	0.5 mg/day[†] (1.0 if Lam resistant)	600 mg/day[†]	300 mg/day[†]
Duration (wk)	48	48 to ≥52	≥48	≥48	≥52	≥48
Tolerability	Flulike symptoms	Good	Follow renal function	Good	Good	Follow renal function
HBe seroconversion	27%	16%-21%	12%	21%	22%	21%
Undetectable HBV DNA	25%-63%	60%-73%	51%-64%	67%-90%	60%-88%	80%-95%
ALT normalization	39%	41%-75%	48%-61%	68%	60%	77%
HBeAg loss	3%	<1%	0%	2%	<1%	3%
Viral resistance	None	15%-30%	Minimal	None[‡]	6%	0%

*All data are for 1 year unless otherwise noted.
[†]Dose adjust for creatinine clearance.
[‡]None; otherwise, 7% if preexisting lamivudine resistance.
ALT, alanine aminotransferase; HBeAg, hepatitis B early antigen; HBV, hepatitis B virus; IFN, interferon alfa; NUC, nucleoside or nucleotide; ULN, upper limit of normal.
Adapted from Lok AS, McMahon BJ. Chronic hepatitis B. *Hepatology.* 2007;45:507-539; Dienstag JL. Hepatitis B infection. *N Engl J Med.* 2008;359:1486-1500.

monotherapy (see "Viral Resistance"). Lamivudine can suppress HBV replication, but cannot eliminate CCC DNA, which leads to prompt relapse of viremia once therapy is discontinued in the majority of patients who do not achieve HBeAg seroconversion. For those patients with HBeAg-positive HBV who do have HBeAg seroconversion, current recommendations are to treat for 1 year and then discontinue therapy.[311] Due to the risk of relapse, therapy should not be discontinued prior to 1 year even if seroconversion occurs rapidly. If patients do not have HBeAg seroconversion but have suppressed HBV DNA replication, then therapy may be continued, as there is evidence of progressive enhancement of the HBeAg seroconversion rate with longer duration of treatment, and patients may continue to derive histologic benefit.[273] Once HBeAg seroconversion has occurred, the rate of durable response ranges from 30% to 80%.[312] The duration of additional lamivudine therapy after HBeAg seroconversion and pretreatment serum HBV DNA levels are independent predictors for posttreatment relapse.[309]

ADEFOVIR

Adefovir dipivoxil is the oral prodrug of adefovir, a phosphonate nucleotide analogue of adenosine monophosphate (see Chapter 41). It inhibits HBV DNA polymerase at much lower doses than those that inhibit human DNA polymerase. Phase I and II clinical trials showed that adefovir decreased serum HBV DNA levels by 2 to 4 $\log_{10}$;[313] however, it is the least potent of the oral agents. Two large multicenter trials have demonstrated the efficacy of adefovir in chronic HBV, which led to its approval in the United States. In a study of 515 patients with HBeAg-positive HBV, 21% of patients treated with adefovir at 10 mg/day had suppression of HBV DNA to undetectable levels compared to 0% of controls, and 53% of treated patients had improvement in histology compared to 25% of controls.[314] Of the adefovir group, 12% had HBeAg seroconversion compared to 6% of controls. Similarly, in HBeAg-negative, chronic HBV, after 48 weeks of adefovir at 10 mg/day, 51% of treated patients had suppression of HBV compared to 0% of untreated controls, and 64% had histologic improvement compared to 33% of controls.[315] Initially it was believed that resistance did not develop, at least up to 60 weeks of treatment,[316] although a recent report describes the development of a novel asparagine-to-threonine mutation at residue rtN236T in domain D of the HBV polymerase, with increased serum HBV DNA and reduced susceptibility to adefovir in vitro.[317] After 240 weeks of treatment, the cumulative probability of resistance was 29%, but virologic resistance and biochemical relapse was only noted in 11% of patients.[287,288]

In clinical trials, headache and abdominal pain are the most common side effects. Although adefovir used in higher doses (120 mg/day) as used previously for HIV leads to substantial degrees of Fanconi-like renal toxicity, adefovir at the low doses used to treat HBV does not appear to lead to such renal toxicity.[315] In vitro and preliminary clinical data showed that adefovir is effective in suppressing the replication of lamivudine-resistant HBV mutants[313,318]; thus, adefovir may be useful for treatment of individuals already resistant to lamivudine.

ENTECAVIR

Entecavir is a guanosine analogue that inhibits all three functions of the HBV polymerase: priming, negative-strand reverse transcription, and synthesis of the positive-strand HBV DNA. It received FDA approval for the treatment of HBeAg-negative and -positive chronic hepatitis B in 2005. In a double-blind controlled trial of 709 HBeAg-positive patients, the 354 who received 48 weeks of entecavir had a decline in HBV DNA of 6.9 log copies/mL, which was superior to the 5.4 log copies/mL in the 355 who received lamivudine.[319] The dose of entecavir was 0.5 mg/day for those who were lamivudine naïve and 1.0 mg/day in those who had taken lamivudine previously. Furthermore, 67% in the entecavir group compared to 36% in the lamivudine group achieved HBV DNA that was less than 300 copies/mL, and histologic improvement occurred in 72% and 62% in the entecavir and lamivudine groups, respectively. However, HBeAg seroconversion was similar between the groups. Results after 96 weeks of treatment showed similar efficacy rates.[320] Entecavir results in a greater log fold change from baseline in HBV DNA after treatment, compared to adefovir (-6.23 $\log_{10}$ copies/mL vs. -4.42 $\log_{10}$ copies/mL at week 12);[321] and both mean HBV DNA and the percent with undetectable serum HBV DNA are greater in the entecavir group. Similarly, in the HBeAg-negative patients, 70% of the 331 in the entecavir group had histologic improvement compared to 61% of the 317 in the lamivudine group. An undetectable HBV DNA was achieved in 90% in the entecavir group, compared to 72% in the lamivudine group. Side effects include headache, abdominal pain, and diarrhea.

Entecavir inhibits HIV-1 replication and can select for the lamivudine-resistant HIV mutation M184V when given as monotherapy;[322] thus, HIV status should be checked prior to initiating therapy for chronic hepatitis B with entecavir. Furthermore, it should not be given to an HIV coinfected patient without a suppressive highly active ART (HAART) regimen.

TELBIVUDINE

Telbivudine is an L-nucleoside analogue that is structurally related to lamivudine (see Chapter 41) and thus has overlapping resistance patterns at the rtM204 position. Unlike lamivudine, it is not known to inhibit HIV-1 replication. The GLOBE trial was the registration trial for telbivudine and was an international study randomizing patients to 600 mg of telbivudine daily (n = 680) or to 100 mg of lamivudine (n = 687).[323] This study included both HBeAg-positive and -negative patients with HBV DNA greater than 6 $\log_{10}$ copies/mL and elevated ALT. At 52 weeks, the decrease in HBV DNA in the HBeAg-positive patients was significantly greater in the telbivudine group, at 6.5 $\log_{10}$ copies/mL compared to 5.5 $\log_{10}$ copies/mL in the lamivudine group.

The proportion with undetectable HBV DNA (<300 copies/mL) was greater in the telbivudine than the lamivudine group (60% vs. 40%, respectively), but HBeAg seroconversions, as with other nucleoside analogues, were similar between the groups at 22% and 21%, respectively. At week 104, telbivudine continued to be superior, but the decrease in HBV DNA from baseline in the telbivudine group decreased to 5.7 $\log_{10}$ copies/mL, and the proportion with undetectable HBV DNA decreased to 56%. These changes were due to development of resistance at the rtM204I, which reached 25% at week 104. Results of the HBeAg-negative group also showed superiority of telbivudine over lamivudine, and demonstrated poor durability of response due to development of resistance, which occurred in 8.6% of the telbivudine group. The lower rate of resistance in HBeAg-negative patients is due to the lower HBV DNA levels at the start of therapy. Individuals were divided into groups based on their week 24 HBV DNA: undetectable, detectable but less than 3 $\log_{10}$ copies/mL, 3 to 4 $\log_{10}$ copies/mL, and greater than 4 $\log_{10}$ copies/mL. At week 24, those who were in the undetectable group had the greatest proportion (77%) of individuals with undetectable HBV DNA, and those in the greater than 4 $\log_{10}$ copies/mL group had the smallest proportion (12%) in the undetectable group. One side effect from telbivudine that is notable is the increased risk of creatinine kinase elevations (seven times normal), which occurred in 7.5% of the telbivudine and 3.1% of the lamivudine group. About 70% of these decreased to less than two times normal by the next visit without a change in therapy. The creatinine kinase elevations did not correlate with clinical symptoms. One patient had creatinine kinase elevation and muscle pain, which resolved over 9 to 12 months after discontinuation of the telbivudine.[324]

TENOFOVIR DISOPROXIL FUMARATE

Tenofovir disoproxil fumarate (DF) was approved for treatment of hepatitis B in 2008 and is also approved for treatment of HIV-1 (see Chapter 41). In two phase III trials comparing tenofovir to adefovir, a significantly higher proportion of patients receiving tenofovir DF than those receiving adefovir dipivoxil had reached the primary end point of HBV DNA at less than 400 copies/mL by week 48.[325] Viral suppression occurred in more HBeAg-negative patients receiving tenofovir DF than patients receiving adefovir dipivoxil (93% vs. 63%, $P < 0.001$), and in more HBeAg-positive patients receiving tenofovir DF than patients receiving adefovir dipivoxil (76% vs. 13%, $P < 0.001$). Significantly, more HBeAg-positive patients treated with tenofovir DF than those treated with adefovir dipivoxil had normalized ALT levels (68% vs. 54%, $P = 0.03$) and loss of HBsAg (3% vs. 0%, $P = 0.02$). At week 48, amino acid substitutions within HBV DNA polymerase associated with phenotypic resistance to tenofovir DF or to other drugs used to treat HBV infection had not developed in any of the patients. Tenofovir DF produced a similar HBV DNA response in patients regardless of prior lamivudine use. After 48 weeks, those receiving adefovir were switched to tenofovir DF in the open-label phase of the study. After 96 weeks, 91% of the HBeAg-negative patients in the original tenofovir DF group had HBV DNA at less than 400 copies/mL, and 89% in the adefovir-to-tenofovir DF group achieved this goal. In an intent-to-treat analysis of the HBeAg-positive group, 78% in both groups had HBV DNA at less than 400 copies/mL after 96 weeks. HBeAg seroconversion occurred in 26% in the continuous tenofovir DF group and 24% in the adefovir-to-tenofovir DF group. The major side effect of tenofovir DF that has been noted in HIV-infected patients is possible renal insufficiency with increases in serum creatinine. In these two registration trials of HBV-monoinfected patients, none of the patients developed a creatinine clearance less than 50 mL/min.

VIRAL RESISTANCE

The major limitation in the use of oral agents for hepatitis B is the development of resistance, which has been observed with the use of all approved agents, albeit at different times and frequencies. Genotypic resistance to lamivudine develops rapidly, with between 14% and 32%

of patients having evidence of mutations after 1 year of treatment.[304,305] Cumulative resistance increases over time, with one study demonstrating cumulative rates of 15%, 38%, 55%, 67%, and 69%, at 1, 2, 3, 4, and 5 years, respectively.[283] The most common mutation affects the rtM204V/I position of the HBV DNA polymerase, which is essential for polymerase activity, and leads to substitution of isoleucine (I) or valine (V) for methionine at position 204 of the DNA polymerase.[283,326] Due to variations within genotypes, previous numbering systems have noted this amino acid as position 552, 550, 539, or 549.[327] HBV mutants with the rtM204V/I appear to have reduced replication capacity in vitro and in vivo compared to wild-type HBV.[328] However, the rtM204V/I variant is frequently accompanied by a leucine-to-methionine substitution in an upstream region (L180M; previously 528, 526, 515, or 525). The combined M204I/V/L180M double mutation restores replication capacity, at least in vitro.[328] Recently another novel mutation (Met –> Ser change at rt204; M204S), which confers lamivudine resistance in vivo and in vitro, leading to virologic breakthrough and ALT increases, was described.[329] The rates of lamivudine resistance in patients treated for HBeAg-negative chronic hepatitis B appear to be more variable (0% to 27% at 1 year and 10% to 56% at 2 years).[308,330] Even in the presence of documented rtM204V/I mutants, however, continuation of lamivudine appears to result in improvement in histologic injury.[273]

Although the rates of resistance to telbivudine are lower than to those of lamivudine (11% vs. 26% at 2 years), resistance may preclude its widespread use.[331] Telbivudine was not active against HBV strains bearing lamivudine mutations L180M/M204V/I, but remained active against the M204V single mutant in vitro, potentially explaining the difference in resistance profiles between telbivudine and lamivudine. Against HBV genomes with known telbivudine-resistance mutations, rtM204I and rtL80I/M204I, telbivudine, lamivudine, and entecavir lost 353- to greater than 1000-fold activity, whereas adefovir and tenofovir exhibited no more than three- to fivefold change. Conversely, against HBV cell lines expressing adefovir resistance mutations rtN236T and rtA181V, or the rtA194T mutant associated with resistance to tenofovir, telbivudine remained active as shown by respective fold changes of 0.5 (rtN236T) and 1.0 (rtA181V and rtA194T).[332]

Entecavir has a high genetic barrier to resistance as it requires the presence of multiple mutations including the rtM204V and the rtL180M along with either the rtT184S/A/I/L or rtC202G/C. In addition, it has the most potent and rapid suppression of HBV DNA, suggesting that resistance may develop less frequently in clinical practice. In patients who are treatment naïve and do not have a preexisting rtM204V or rtL180M, the rates of resistance are less than 1% per year with a 5-year cumulative rate of 1.2%.[333] However, in patients with the characteristic lamivudine mutations rtM204V and rtL180M, the cumulative incidence is 51% after 5 years.

Resistance to adefovir is rare through week 60 in treatment-naïve patients;[287,288,316] however, resistance rises to 22% in those with preexisting lamivudine resistance.[334] The signature mutations are rtN236T and rtA181T/V. Tenofovir DF resistance rates appear low, but precise mutations with confirmed resistance to tenofovir DF have not been fully characterized. The adefovir-resistance mutations rtA181T/V and rtN236T confer decreased sensitivity to tenofovir DF. In one retrospective study, patients with these mutations were less likely to achieve HBV DNA less than 400 copies/mL on tenofovir DF than those without the mutations.[335]

Assays for genotypic or phenotypic resistance are not yet widely available, but resistance is clinically manifest as reappearance of HBV DNA, with a greater than one $\log_{10}$ change or reappearance of detectable HBV DNA. Serum aminotransferases may or may not become elevated, and there are rare instances of acute exacerbations and hepatic decompensation.[336] However, most patients appear to have somewhat lower aminotransferase and HBV DNA levels compared to pretreatment levels. The impact of this emergence on disease activity is unpredictable. Although continued disease suppression or even HBeAg seroconversion occurs in some patients, in others, hepatitis may relapse, and liver failure has been reported despite continuation of nucleoside/tide. Because the mutations that confer resistance may diminish viral fitness in vitro and in vivo, most experts currently recommend adding an additional agent with a nonoverlapping resistance pattern (e.g., adding tenofovir to lamivudine) rather than switching agents.[337] In general, the nucleosides (lamivudine, telbivudine, and entecavir) are not cross-resistant with the nucleotides (adefovir, tenofovir). Addition of adefovir or tenofovir in patients with lamivudine resistance resulted in durable prevention of breakthrough, with 80% maintaining undetectable HBV DNA and 100% without clinical or virologic breakthrough.[338-341]

Given the overlapping reading frames, mutations in the HBV polymerase can lead to changes in the surface antigen including in the immunogenic a determinant. One study demonstrated that a triple mutant that occurs on lamivudine monotherapy (rtV173L/rtL180M/rtM204V) leads to the surface changes sE164D/I195M. These changes in the surface antigen lead to reduced binding of anti-HBs in vitro, and thus the virus behaves as a vaccine escape mutant.[342]

OTHER AGENTS AND COMBINATION THERAPY

The other agent that is approved for HIV treatment but is also active against HBV is emtricitabine. Emtricitabine is similar to lamivudine, but it has a longer half-life. Mutations that confer resistance to lamivudine also confer resistance to emtricitabine. Clevudine is also in development for treatment of HBV (see Chapter 41).[343]

Combination therapy for hepatitis B is attractive as it may increase potency and decrease the rates for developing resistance; however, these concepts have not been clearly demonstrated to date. The combination of PEG IFN alfa and lamivudine had greater HBV DNA decline compared to monotherapy with either one alone at the end of 48 weeks of treatment. However, the relapse rate in the combination group was higher, so 24 weeks after the end of treatment, there was no difference between the PEG IFN group alone or with lamivudine regardless of HBeAg status.[40,344] Given the expansion in the number of oral agents available, it is desirable to consider combining these as is done in HIV therapy. The anti-HBV drugs all target the same part of the HBV life cycle; thus, the situation is not entirely analogous to HIV in which drugs target different aspects of the viral life cycle. In a WHV model, combination therapy with adefovir or tenofovir along with lamivudine or emtricitabine was superior to any of these drugs as monotherapy.[345] A study in humans demonstrated that adefovir plus lamivudine for 104 weeks had larger declines in HBV DNA (−5.2 versus −3.4 log$_{10}$ copies/mL) and decreased development of drug-resistant HBV (15% vs. 43%) compared to lamivudine monotherapy.[346] This advantage in the combination, however, was only seen after the first 52 weeks of therapy and was primarily due to the difference in emergence of resistance rather than the increased potency of the combination. A study of adefovir with emtricitabine compared with adefovir monotherapy for 96 weeks demonstrated that the HBV DNA decline in the combination group was greater than in the monotherapy group (5.30 vs. 3.98 log$_{10}$ copies/mL).[347] In this study, the differences were noted in the first 4 weeks of treatment, suggesting that there was increased potency. Alternatively, the combination of telbivudine and lamivudine was not superior to telbivudine alone, which may be related to the similar mechanism of action and cross-resistance of these drugs.[348] Thus, there is potential advantage for combination therapy, but further work is needed to define the optimal combination.

▨ Management in Special Populations

LIVER TRANSPLANTATION

Historically, rates of recurrence of HBV were high (90%), and the consequences of reinfection were devastating, such that HBV was considered a relative contraindication to liver transplantation. Treatment of HBV-related liver disease in transplant patients is difficult for several reasons, including the high levels of HBV replication and the ongoing immunosuppressive treatment. HBIg was introduced in the early 1980s and nucleosides in the early 1990s, with progressive reduction in likelihood of recurrence with each intervention. U.S. transplantation centers typically use a fixed dose schedule of HBIg, with monthly infusions of 10,000 IU, whereas European centers typically vary the dose of HBIg to maintain the trough anti-HBs at greater than 100 IU/mL. Using HBIg alone, recurrence rates are 20% to 25%, depending on the schedule and trough anti-HBs titer. Mutations in the HBs a determinant are associated with recurrence of hepatitis B.[349] Due to the significant expense of HBIg, lamivudine monotherapy was also attempted, with recurrence rates of 10% to 32% at 1 year and 40% to 50% at 3 years.[350]

Thus, the current standard of care typically uses lamivudine plus HBIg, with rates of reinfection as low as 10%.[351,352] Recent studies demonstrate that the use of lamivudine both pre- and postoperatively may allow a reduction in the dose of HBIg, resulting in considerable cost savings.[353] Two-year patient survival increased from 85% in 1988 to 1993, prior to the availability of antivirals, to 94% since 1997, after which patients received a combination of hepatitis B immune globulin and lamivudine (p < 0.05). The 2-year recurrence rates in these two periods were 42% and 8% (p < 0.05). In summary, with currently available combination therapy, survival is excellent in patients undergoing liver transplantation for HBV disease, even in those with active viral replication pretransplantation.

Monotherapy with lamivudine has resulted in the emergence of HBV variants that are resistant to these compounds as discussed previously. Molecular analysis of these mutations has shown changes in the gene for the viral DNA polymerase. Because of the overlapping nature of the HBV ORFs, nucleotide changes in the polymerase may result in amino acid changes not only in the polymerase protein, but also in the surface protein, which could in turn theoretically alter binding of HBIg.[354] Lamivudine resistance post-transplantation has on occasion been associated with severe and even fatal post-transplantation disease in patients receiving combination therapy with lamivudine plus hepatitis B immune globulin.[355] However, this is not universal and patients may derive benefit from continuing lamivudine.[242,356] Antiviral therapy failure is not a predictor of either transplantation failure or death pretransplant.[357]

Fortunately, the availability of new hepatitis B antivirals such as adefovir has resulted in viral suppression of lamivudine-resistant variants[313] and even resolution of graft failure in these patients who have them.[358] A recent small study of 34 patients showed that adefovir in combination with lamivudine provided equivalent protection to HBIg plus lamivudine,[359] although the long-term durability and side effects are not known.

HUMAN IMMUNODEFICIENCY VIRUS

Treatment of individuals with HIV is complicated by the dual activity of some agents against both HIV and HBV leading to the potential of developing resistance in both viruses. Given these issues, if HIV treatment is indicated, then it is recommended to simultaneously treat HBV regardless of its disease stage. Tenofovir DF and emtricitabine are a recommended backbone of HIV treatment, and both drugs are efficacious against HBV in HIV-infected individuals.[360] If only HBV needs treatment, then the drugs that are active against HBV and do not lead to HIV drug resistance are telbivudine, adefovir, and PEG IFN. Entecavir was previously thought not to affect HIV replication, but it was shown to inhibit HIV replication both in vivo and in vitro. Furthermore, entecavir can select for the HIV drug-resistant virus M184V.[322] Telbivudine is not ideal given its high rates of resistance in HBV monotherapy and unknown rates in HIV coinfection. Early HAART has also been advocated in this group as controlling HIV may also slow down liver disease progression.

The efficacy of the nucleoside/tide agents does not seem to be compromised by coinfection with HIV.[361] However, with lamivudine monotherapy, drug resistance develops more rapidly than in HBV monoinfection,[362] but it is not known if this is true for other, newer anti-HBV agents. The efficacy of PEG IFN in HIV coinfection is not known. Lamivudine-resistant HBV is common in HIV coinfection as it has been a backbone agent for HIV therapy for years. Due to cross-resistance with other drugs, the best treatment option against lamivu-dine-resistant HBV is to add tenofovir DF to lamivudine. Adding tenofovir DF instead of switching may delay the development of teno-fovir-resistant HBV, as has been demonstrated with a related drug, adefovir.

RECIPIENTS OF CYTOTOXIC CHEMOTHERAPY

Several reports have demonstrated the risk of reactivation of HBV even in the presence of anti-HBs, although reactivation is most common in those who are HBsAg positive.[363-365] For example, in 244 HBsAg-positive patients undergong chemotherapy, 3% experienced reactivation of disease.[366] Use of nucleoside therapy prior to the institution of che-motherapy has been demonstrated to decrease the risk.[367,368] A recent meta-analysis demonstrated benefit for prophylactic lamivudine prior to chemotherapy in patients who are HBsAg positive.[352] The optimal duration of prophylactic therapy is unknown but most recommend continuing treatment for a minimum of 6 months after stopping chemotherapy.[272,369]

HEPATITIS DELTA

Lamivudine is ineffective at controlling HDV replication[370]; thus, IFN alfa is the only approved option for treatment. However, the efficacy of IFN alfa in the treatment of HDV is limited unless high doses (9 million units three times a week) are used.[371] Of note, IFN alfa appears to affect the biochemical and histologic improvement, but does not affect HDV DNA levels.[372] If HDV replication is controlled and there is normalization of serum aminotransferases, the effect appears to be very durable. Improvement in liver histology was maintained 10 years posttreatment among the patients who received high-dose IFN alfa.[372]

▣ Other Management Issues in Chronic Hepatitis B

Patients with chronic hepatitis B should be counseled about disease-modifying factors as well as means to prevent spread of HBV to other persons. For example, patients should be counseled about the means of spread of delta hepatitis and hepatitis C to avoid superinfec-tion with these viruses. Patients should also be counseled to consume minimal if any alcohol in the absence of data regarding safe levels of consumption, and because consumption of large amounts of alcohol is clearly a risk factor for more rapid progression to cirrhosis. Other major issues in the management of patients with chronic HBV include prevention of hepatitis A, prevention of spread of HBV, and surveil-lance for HCC.

HEPATITIS A VACCINATION

The official recommendation of the Advisory Committee for Immu-nization Practices (ACIP) in the United States is that all persons with chronic liver disease be vaccinated against hepatitis A virus (HAV).[373] The data supporting this recommendation are not strong,[374] as at least one study revealed that the risk of fulminant HAV is significantly increased only in patients with underlying hepatitis C and not hepatitis B.[375] However, the guidelines of the American Association for the Study of Liver Disease call for immunization of all patients with chronic HBV against HAV.[311]

SCREENING AND VACCINATION OF CONTACTS

Sexual and household contacts of persons with HBV are at increased risk of infection. All sexual partners and household contacts should be tested for HBV and vaccinated if seronegative. Until the immunization series is complete, sexual partners should use barrier methods. Both

patients and contacts should be counseled regarding the modes of transmission, and advised on methods to prevent household transmis-sion, including avoiding sharing of items that might be contaminated with small amounts of blood, such as toothbrushes, and the need to cover open wounds. Pregnant women or women who wish to become pregnant and are infected with HBV should also be counseled on the risk of transmission to the newborn and the method to prevent such transmission. The combination of HBIg and concurrent hepatitis B vaccine have been shown to be 95% efficacious in the prevention of perinatal transmission of HBV[135] (see Chapter 320).

Recommendations for the health care worker infected with HBV vary from country to country. Although there is general agreement that individuals with HBeAg or HBV DNA greater than 5×10^4 copies/mL pose the greatest risk of transmission,[376] there have been docu-mented cases of transmission from health care workers in the absence of HBeAg and during "low-risk" procedures.[377,378] In the United States, the Centers for Disease Control and Prevention (CDC) recommend that invasive procedures not be performed without expert guidance and review of procedures to be performed by the health care worker.[379,380] In other countries, HBsAg-positive carriers are specifi-cally forbidden to perform invasive procedures in which there is risk of inadvertent exposure of the patient to the provider's blood (e.g., deep surgical procedures in which there is limited visibility into the surgical wound).[381,382]

SURVEILLANCE FOR HEPATOCELLULAR CARCINOMA

In multiple longitudinal studies, carriers of HBsAg have been shown to be at increased risk of developing HCC.[209] The goal of HCC screen-ing is to detect small, surgically resectable tumors because the progno-sis for more advanced lesions is poor. Current recommendations are for periodic screening in HBsAg-positive persons at high risk for HCC, such as men over the age of 45 years, patients with cirrhosis, and patients with a positive family history.[383] In general, the longer the duration of disease in HBsAg-positive patients, the greater is the risk for HCC. The combination of serum-α-fetoprotein (AFP) and ultra-sound repeated every 6 months appears to offer the best sensitivity and specificity, although lower risk individuals may be screened with AFP alone.

▣ Prevention of Hepatitis B Virus Infection

Successful vaccination is not only effective in preventing HBV infec-tion but it also prevents the sequelae of chronic HBV infection, and thus is the first example that cancer can be prevented by vaccination.[141] In Taiwan, which was an early adopter of universal HBV vaccination in children, the average annual incidence of HCC in 6- to 14-year-olds declined from 0.70 per 100,000 children before widespread vaccination to 0.36 after initiation of widespread vaccination (P < .01). The cor-responding rates of mortality from HCC also decreased. The incidence of HCC in children 6 to 9 years of age declined from 0.52 for those born between 1974 and 1984 to 0.13 for those born between 1984 and 1986.[384] Currently available vaccines are both safe and effective, with seroconversion rates of more than 90% in healthy adults and children. The major obstacles to true universal vaccination have been the cost in developing nations, failure to reach high-risk groups, and failure to convince potential recipients that vaccines are necessary.

POSTEXPOSURE IMMUNOPROPHYLAXIS

Postexposure prophylaxis with HBIg and vaccine is recommended for all nonimmune individuals who have percutaneous, sexual contact, ocular, or mucous membrane exposure to blood, including human bites that penetrate the skin (see Chapter 320). The first dose of 0.06 mL/kg (or 5 mL for adults) should be administered as soon as possible, preferably within 12 hours, although there is a window period of up to 24 hours.[385] The first vaccine dose should be given at the same time although in a different site, followed by the remainder of the series. For individuals who are vaccinated but who do not have documentation of adequate titers of anti-HBs, recommendations are to administer both HBIg and vaccine pending documentation of adequate anti-HBs. Individuals who have failed to respond to a vaccine series require two doses of HBIg 1 month part.[135]

ACTIVE IMMUNIZATION

Both plasma-derived and recombinant forms of vaccine are available. Both are comparable in terms of efficacy and durability. Plasma-derived vaccine was developed first, and is no longer available in North America and Europe, but is still widely used in parts of Asia and India. More than 200 million doses of plasma-derived vaccines have been distributed globally, and they are both safe and effective. They are cheaper to produce than recombinant preparations, especially in areas of high seroprevalence of HBs antigenemia. However, concerns about the use of any plasma-derived product have led to the widespread adoption of recombinant vaccines in developed countries. Because anti-HBs alone is sufficient to confer protective immunity, most recombinant vaccines have expressed HBsAg only. Two thimerosal free vaccines that express HBsAg (Engerix-B and Recombivax-HB) are widely available (see Chapter 320). These vaccines are approved for use in all age groups. A combination vaccine (Twinrix), which expresses both HBsAg and hepatitis A, is also available and is approved for use in adults in the United States and Europe. This vaccine is typically used for convenience when protection against both viruses is needed.

INDICATIONS FOR VACCINATION

All persons at high risk of acquiring HBV (see "Routes of Transmission") should be offered vaccination if nonimmune. Recent CDC guidelines recommend that persons born in areas of high and intermediate HBV endemicity, infants not vaccinated but born to mothers from a high HBV endemic area, and persons in high-risk HBV groups should be tested for HBV markers and vaccinated if there is ongoing risk for HBV acquisition.[386] Many countries have now moved to universal vaccination of all infants and incorporation of hepatitis B vaccines into routine childhood immunization programs. Universal vaccination of all neonates with catch-up vaccination of older children began in 1991 in the United States. Countries that adopted universal vaccination programs in the 1980s have already begun to see declines in the rate of chronic HCV infection and subsequent HCC.

DOSE REGIMEN

Two recombinant hepatitis B vaccines have been licensed in the United States: Engerix-B and Recombivax-HB. Engerix-B is formulated to contain 20 μg HBsAg/mL, and Recombivax-HB contains 10 μg HBsAg/mL (Table 146-6). The recommendation for adults is to administer Engerix-B 20 μg or Recombivax-HB 10 μg in three doses at months 0, 1 to 2, and then at 6 to 12 months. In infants, three doses of 0.5 mL vaccine are required to complete the course, the timing of which depends on the clinical setting.[135] For adolescents (11 to 19 years old), three doses of 0.5 mL of Recombivax-HB or 1.0 mL of Engerix-B are recommended. Either vaccine can be interchanged during the series of injections. An optional two-dose regimen of Recombivax-HB has also been approved for adolescents aged 11 to 15 years (1.0 mL containing 10 μg of HBsAg with a second dose given 4 to 6 months after the first dose).[387]

Vaccines should be administered intramuscularly as deposition of the vaccine into adipose tissue results in a lower seroconversion rate.[388] Adverse reactions are uncommon, and most consist of soreness at the injection site. Low-grade fever, malaise, headache, and myalgias are seen in less than 1% of vaccinees. The vaccine can be administered during pregnancy. There were case reports of neurologic sequelae after vaccination, including demyelinating disease,[389] raising concerns that hepatitis B immunization was linked to multiple sclerosis. However, numerous studies failed to confirm an association of multiple sclerosis with vaccination.[390,391]

PREVENTION OF PERINATAL TRANSMISSION

The risk of maternal-infant transmission is related to the HBV replicative status of the mother. The risk is 85% to 90% to infants born to HBeAg-positive mothers and 32% to infants born to HBeAg-negative mothers.[392,393] Maternal serum HBV DNA levels also correlate with the risk of transmission.[394] Maternal-infant transmission may occur in utero, at the time of birth, or after birth. The high protective efficacy (95%) of neonatal vaccination suggests that infection occurs predominantly at or after birth. There is no evidence that cesarean section prevents maternal-infant transmission, and thus routine cesarean section is not recommended. Neither breast-feeding nor amniocentesis appears to increase the risk of transmission.[395]

The current recommendation is to provide passive-active immunization to newborns of carrier mothers. Infants should receive both HBIg (0.06 mL/kg) and vaccine, and the first dose of vaccine should be given within 12 hours of birth, and the second and third doses at 1 and at 6 to 12 months, respectively. This regimen has a protective

TABLE 146-6	Doses and Schedules of Licensed Hepatitis B Vaccines*				
Hepatitis B Vaccines	Age	Dose		Volume	Schedule
Engerix-B	<20 yr	10 μg		10 μg/0.5 mL	Infants†: birth, 1-4, 6-18 mo; Older children: 0, 1-2, 4 mo
	>20 yr	20 μg		20 μg/1.0 mL	0, 1, 6 mo
	Dialysis	40 μg		2-20 μg/1.0 mL doses	0, 1, 2, 6 mo
Recombivax HB	<20 yr	5 μg		5 μg/0.5 mL	Infants†: birth, 1-4, 6-18 mo; Older children: 0, 1-2, 4 mos
	11-15 yr	10 μg		10 μg/1.0 mL	0, 4-6 mo
	>20 yr	10 μg		10 μg/1.0 mL	0, 1, 6 mo
	Dialysis	40 μg‡		40 μg/1.0 mL	0, 1, 6 mo
Combination Vaccines	Age§	Antigen		Volume	Schedule
Comvax	6 wk-4 yr	PedvaxHIB‖ and Recombivax		0.5 mL	2, 4, 12-15 mo
Pediarix	6 wk-6 yr	Engerix B, Infarix (DTaP), and IPV		0.5 mL	2, 4, 6 mo
Twinrix	>18 yr	Havrix (HAV) and Engerix B (20 μg)		1.0 mL	0, 1, 6 mo

*All vaccines should be administered intramuscularly in the deltoid.
†Infants born to hepatitis B surface antigen (HBsAg)-positive mothers should have hepatitis B immune globulin (HBIG) within 12 hours of delivery, along with vaccine at a separate site. If mother's HBsAg status is unknown, administer vaccine within 12 hours and test mother. If mother is HBsAg positive, administer HBIG within 1 week.
‡Special formulation.
§Birth dose should be monovalent vaccine only; subsequent doses can be combination.
‖PedvaxHIB, licensed Haemophilus influenzae type B vaccine; Infarix, licensed diphtheria, tetanus, and acellular pertussis vaccine (DTaP); Havrix, licensed hepatitis A virus (HAV) vaccine.

efficacy of 95%.[392,393] One study of lamivudine given to HBsAg-positive mothers with high HBV DNA showed a trend in favor of lamivudine prophylaxis, but it was not statistically significant.[396]

EFFICACY

A protective level of immune response after vaccination is defined as a titer of anti-HBs of greater than 10 IU/L. Although this was somewhat arbitrary, clinical studies suggest that a decrease in titer below this level is associated with a risk of infection. In a 5-year follow-up study of 773 homosexual men vaccinated in 1980, the acute infection rate increased seven times when the anti-HBs titer decreased below the level of 10 IU/L.[397] Long-term data from Taiwan indicate that the vaccine provides long-term protection up to 20 years; at this time, booster doses are not recommended.[398]

Using the definition of greater than 10 IU/L anti-HBs as a positive response, the overall seroconversion rate is about 95% in healthy adults. Factors that may reduce the immunogenicity of the vaccine include age over 40 years, weight, genetics, smoking, HIV or any form of immunosuppression, improper administrations (e.g., administration into the buttock or subcutaneous injection), and freezing of the vaccine. In patients on chronic hemodialysis, the response rate to recombinant vaccines is 50% to 60%.[399] In patients with HIV, response rates are 40% to 70% and are not necessarily tightly correlated with CD4+ counts.[400,401] Because the response rate in otherwise healthy individuals is so high, routine postvaccination testing is not recommended, except for health care workers and others who are at high risk of repeated exposure to HBV, such as intravenous drug users and homosexual men. Testing should be performed 1 to 2 months after the vaccine series, except in infants born to HBsAg-positive mothers, in which testing should be performed at age 9 to 15 months.

In individuals with hemodialysis or chronic renal failure, several approaches have been used to increase vaccine efficacy. One approach was intradermal injection, which although successful was technically difficult.[402] Most individuals now receive an increased dose, which should be administered prior to the onset of dialysis if possible (see Table 146-6). For individuals with HIV, transient increases in the CD4+ T-cell counts through administration of interleukin-2 or granulocyte-macrophage colony-stimulating factor (GM-CSF) did not increase postvaccination titers.[403] It is not clear whether individuals who were vaccinated prior to a decline in CD4+ T-cell counts retain immunity, or whether vaccinations above a threshold CD4+ count are more likely to result in protective immunity. Finally, there are other individuals for whom nonresponse is genetically determined by the presence of HLA haplotypes.[404]

DURABILITY OF RESPONSE

The current recommendation for otherwise healthy individuals who have no or inadequate anti-HBs titers after a primary series is to administer one or more doses of vaccine. After one to two doses, up to 25% of previously non- or hyporesponders may have adequate

titers, and with three doses up to 50% may have adequate titers.[135] Individuals who still have inadequate titers are not protected from HBV infection and should receive HBIg on exposure.

There is excellent durability of response after a successful primary series. Of infants and young children who have received hepatitis B vaccine 50% to 85% continue to have protective titers of anti-HBsAg 9 to 15 years after immunization. In addition, even if titers of anti-HBs fall to less than the commonly defined protective level (10 IU), most of these infants and young children will continue to be protected against HBV 9 to 15 years after immunization.[405-408] In a 5-year follow-up of 773 men who have sex with men vaccinated in 1980, the HBV infection rate was significantly lower in the vaccinated group (2.9% vs. 21%) despite the observation that at 5 years, 15% of the vaccinees had undetectable anti-HBs and another 27% had anti-HBs titers below 10 IU/L.[397] The risk of late infection with hepatitis B in those with an initially adequate vaccine response increased markedly when antibody levels decreased below 10 IU, but only 1 of 34 late infections resulted in viremia and liver inflammation.[397] Thus, the CDC does not currently recommend that otherwise healthy individuals who were vaccinated as adults or children have routine booster doses of vaccine. The only group in whom routine boosters are recommended are patients on hemodialysis, in whom antibody levels should be checked yearly, and a booster dose of vaccine given if the anti-HBs is below 10 IU/mL.[409] Revaccination at this level should also be considered in HIV-infected persons if they have ongoing risk for exposure.[410]

HEPATITIS B SURFACE ANTIGEN ESCAPE MUTANTS

HBs mutants have been described in infants infected with HBV following passive-active vaccination,[411] as well as in liver transplant recipients who have received prolonged courses of HBIg to prevent recurrence in the allograft.[349,412] The most common mutation is a glycine-to-arginine substitution at codon 145 (G145R) in the a determinant of HBsAg. This mutation decreases binding of HBsAg to anti-HBs and may explain why these infants develop "escape" infection. The G145R mutation has also been observed in liver transplant recipients who developed recurrent HBV infection despite HBIg prophylaxis. The prevalence of these escape mutants is increasing over time,[413,414] but the clinical and epidemiologic importance and the impact on current vaccination strategies is unclear. However, in a chimpanzee model of infection, the current vaccines appear to protect against the spread of HBs mutants.[415] Due to the overlapping ORFs in HBV, the catalytic domain of HBV Pol overlaps with the immunogenic a determinant of the HBsAg. A triple mutant that is selected for by lamivudine (rtV173L/rtL180M/rtM204V) leads to the envelope mutations sE164D/I195M. These envelope mutations behave as a vaccine escape mutant in vitro.[416]

ACKNOWLEDGMENTS

We wish to thank Aleem Siddiqui for his contributions to this chapter in the Sixth Edition of this book.

REFERENCES

1. Lurman A. Eine icterus Epidemic. *Berlin Klinische Wochenschrift.* 1885;22:20-23.
2. Findlay G, MacCallum F. Note on acute hepatitis and yellow fever immunization. *Trans Soc Trop Med Hyg.* 1937;31:297.
3. Bigger J, Dubi S. Jaundice in syphilitics under treatment. *Lancet.* 1943;1:457.
4. Flaum A, Malmros H, Persson E. Eine nosocomiale icterus epidemic. *Acta Med Scand Suppl.* 1926;16:544.
5. Feinstone S, Kapikian A, Purcell R, et al. Transfusion associated hepatitis not due to viral hepatitis type A or B. *N Engl J Med.* 1975;282:767.
6. Blumberg B, Alter H, Visnich S. A "new" antigen in leukemia sera. *JAMA.* 1965;191:541-546.
7. Dane DS, Cameron C, Briggs M. Virus-like particles in serum of patients with Australia antigen associated hepatitis. *Lancet.* 1970;2:695-698.
8. Robinson W, Marion P, Feitelson M, et al. *The Hepadnavirus Group: Hepatitis B and Related Viruses.* Philadelphia: Franklin Institute Press; 1982.

9. Mason WS, Seal G, Summers J. Virus of Pekin ducks with structural and biological relatedness to human hepatitis B virus. *J Virol.* 1980;36(3):829-836.
10. Sninsky JJ, Siddiqui A, Robinson WS, et al. Cloning and endonuclease mapping of the hepatitis B viral genome. *Nature.* 1979;279(5711):346-348.
11. Galibert F, Mandart E, Fitoussi F, et al. Nucleotide sequence of the hepatitis B virus genome (subtype ayw) cloned in *E. coli. Nature.* 1979;281(5733):646-650.
12. Valenzuela P, Gray P, Quiroga M, et al. Nucleotide sequence of the gene coding for the major protein of hepatitis B virus surface antigen. *Nature.* 1979;280(5725):815-819.
13. Landers TA, Greenberg HB, Robinson WS. Structure of hepatitis B Dane particle DNA and nature of the endogenous DNA polymerase reaction. *J Virol.* 1977;23(2):368-376.
14. Robinson WS, Clayton DA, Greenman RL. DNA of a human hepatitis B virus candidate. *J Virol.* 1974;14(2):384-391.
15. Ganem D, Schneider RJ. The molecular biology of the hepatitis B viruses. In: Howley PM, Knipe DM, eds. *Fields Virology.* 4th ed. New York: Lippincott; 2001.

16. Roossinck MJ, Siddiqui A. In vivo phosphorylation and protein analysis of hepatitis B virus core antigen. *J Virol.* 1987;61(4):955-961.
17. Albin C, Robinson WS. Protein kinase activity in hepatitis B virus. *J Virol.* 1980;34(1):297-302.
18. Gavilanes F, Gonzalez-Ros JM, Peterson DL. Structure of hepatitis B surface antigen: characterization of the lipid components and their association with the viral proteins. *J Biol Chem.* 1982;257(13):7770-7777.
19. Peterson DL. Isolation and characterization of the major protein and glycoprotein of hepatitis B surface antigen. *J Biol Chem.* 1981;256(13):6975-6983.
20. Gerin JL, Alexander H, Shih JW, et al. Chemically synthesized peptides of hepatitis B surface antigen duplicate the d/y specificities and induce subtype-specific antibodies in chimpanzees. *Proc Natl Acad Sci U S A.* 1983;80(8):2365-2369.
21. Thornton G, Moriarty A, Milich D, et al. Protection of chimpanzees from hepatitis B virus infection after immunization with synthetic peptides. In: Brown F, Channock T, Ginsberg H,

Lerner R, eds. *Vaccines 89*. Cold Spring Harbor, NY: Cold Spring Harbor Laboratory, 1989:467.
22. Schulze A, Gripon P, Urban S. Hepatitis B virus infection initiates with a large surface protein-dependent binding to heparan sulfate proteoglycans. *Hepatology*. 2007;46(6):1759-1768.
23. Rabe B, Vlachou A, Pante N, et al. Nuclear import of hepatitis B virus capsids and release of the viral genome. *Proc Natl Acad Sci U S A*. 2003;100(17):9849-9854.
24. Mason WS, Seal G, Summers J. Virus of Pekin ducks with structural and biological relatedness to human hepatitis B virus. *J Virol*. 1983;36(3):829-836.
25. Kosovsky M, Qadri I, Siddiqui A. *The Regulation of Hepatitis B Virus Gene Expression: An Overview of the CIS- and Trans-acting Components*. London: Imperial College Press; 1998.
26. Romet-Lemonne JL, McLane MF, Elfassi E, et al. Hepatitis B virus infection in cultured human lymphoblastoid cells. *Science*. 1983;221(4611):667-669.
27. Korba BE, Cote PJ, Shapiro M, et al. In vitro production of infectious woodchuck hepatitis virus by lipopolysaccharide-stimulated peripheral blood lymphocytes. *J Infect Dis*. 1989; 160(4):572-576.
28. Michalak TI, Pardoe IU, Coffin CS, et al. Occult lifelong persistence of infectious hepadnavirus and residual liver inflammation in woodchucks convalescent from acute viral hepatitis. *Hepatology*. 1999;29(3):928-938.
29. Hruska JF, Clayton DA, Rubenstein JL, et al. Structure of hepatitis B Dane particle DNA before and after the Dane particle DNA polymerase reaction. *J Virol*. 1977;21(2):666-672.
30. Gerlich WH, Robinson WS. Hepatitis B virus contains protein attached to the 5′ terminus of its complete DNA strand. *Cell*. 1980;21(3):801-809.
31. Lien JM, Aldrich CE, Mason WS. Evidence that a capped oligoribonucleotide is the primer for duck hepatitis B virus plus-strand DNA synthesis. *J Virol*. 1986;57(1):229-236.
32. Neurath AR, Kent SB, Strick N, et al. Identification and chemical synthesis of a host cell receptor binding site on hepatitis B virus. *Cell*. 1986;46(3):429-436.
33. Gripon P, Cannie I, Urban S. Efficient inhibition of hepatitis B virus infection by acylated peptides derived from the large viral surface protein. *J Virol*. 2005;79(3):1613-1622.
34. Baraldini M, Facchini A, Miglio F, et al. Radioimmunoassay for hepatitis B "e" antigen and antibody: correlations with viral replication and prognostic value. *Vox Sang*. 1981;41(3):139-145.
35. Okamoto H, Tsuda F, Sakugawa H, et al. Typing hepatitis B virus by homology in nucleotide sequence: comparison of surface antigen subtypes. *J Gen Virol*. 1988;69(Pt 10):2575-2583.
36. Allain JP. Epidemiology of hepatitis B virus and genotype. *J Clin Virol*. 2006;36 (Suppl 1):S12-S17.
37. Kao JH, Chen PJ, Lai MY, et al. Hepatitis B genotypes correlate with clinical outcomes in patients with chronic hepatitis B. *Gastroenterology*. 2000;118(3):554-559.
38. Chu CJ, Hussain M, Lok AS. Hepatitis B virus genotype B is associated with earlier HBeAg seroconversion compared with hepatitis B virus genotype C. *Gastroenterology*. 2002;122(7): 1756-1762.
39. Sumi H, Yokosuka O, Seki N, et al. Influence of hepatitis B virus genotypes on the progression of chronic type B liver disease. *Hepatology*. 2003;37(1):19-26.
40. Lau GK, Piratvisuth T, Luo KX, et al. Peginterferon Alfa-2a, lamivudine, and the combination for HBeAg-positive chronic hepatitis B. *N Engl J Med*. 2005;352(26):2682-2695.
41. Russnak R, Ganem D. Sequences 5′ to the polyadenylation signal mediate differential poly(A) site use in hepatitis B viruses. *Genes Dev*. 1990;4(5):764-776.
42. Rosmorduc O, Petit MA, Pol S, et al. In vivo and in vitro expression of defective hepatitis B virus particles generated by spliced hepatitis B virus RNA. *Hepatology*. 1995;22(1):10-19.
43. Soussan P, Tuveri R, Nalpas B, et al. The expression of hepatitis B spliced protein (HBSP) encoded by a spliced hepatitis B virus RNA is associated with viral replication and liver fibrosis. *J Hepatol*. 2003;38(3):343-348.
44. Raney AK, Milich DR, McLachlan A. Characterization of hepatitis B virus major surface antigen gene transcriptional regulatory elements in differentiated hepatoma cell lines. *J Virol*. 1989;63(9):3919-3925.
45. Zhou DX, Yen TS. Differential regulation of the hepatitis B virus surface gene promoters by a second viral enhancer. *J Biol Chem*. 1990;265(34):20731-20734.
46. Bulla GA, Siddiqui A. The hepatitis B virus enhancer modulates transcription of the hepatitis B virus surface antigen gene from an internal location. *J Virol*. 1988;62(4):1437-1441.
47. Lopez-Cabrera M, Letovsky J, Hu KQ, et al. Multiple liver-specific factors bind to the hepatitis B virus core/pregenomic promoter: trans-activation and repression by CCAAT/enhancer binding protein. *Proc Natl Acad Sci U S A*. 1990;87(13):5069-5073.
48. Guo W, Chen M, Yen TS, et al. Hepatocyte-specific expression of the hepatitis B virus core promoter depends on both positive and negative regulation. *Mol Cell Biol*. 1993;13(1):443-448.
49. Siddiqui A, Jameel S, Mapoles J. Expression of hepatitis B virus X gene in mammalian cells. *Proc Natl Acad Sci U S A*. 1987;84(8):2513-2517.
50. Treinin M, Laub O. Identification of a promoter element located upstream from the hepatitis B virus X gene. *Mol Cell Biol*. 1987;7(1):545-548.
51. Heermann K-H GW. Surface proteins of hepatitis B viruses. In: McLachlan A, ed. *Molecular Biology of the Hepatitis B Virus*. LaJolla, Calif: CRC Press; 1991:109-144.
52. Ou JH, Laub O, Rutter WJ. Hepatitis B virus gene function: the precore region targets the core antigen to cellular membranes and causes the secretion of the e antigen. *Proc Natl Acad Sci U S A*. 1986;83(6):1578-1582.
53. Visvanathan K, Skinner NA, Thompson AJ, et al. Regulation of Toll-like receptor-2 expression in chronic hepatitis B by the precore protein. *Hepatology*. 2007;45(1):102-110.
54. Bonino F, Brunetto MR, Rizzetto M, et al. Hepatitis B virus unable to secrete e antigen. *Gastroenterology*. 1991;100(4):1138-1141.
55. Gunther S, Meisel H, Reip A, et al. Frequent and rapid emergence of mutated pre-C sequences in HBV from e-antigen positive carriers who seroconvert to anti-HBe during interferon treatment. *Virology*. 1992;187(1):271-279.
56. Schodel F, Weimer T, Will H, et al. Amino acid sequence similarity between retroviral and *E. coli* RNase H and hepadnaviral gene products. *AIDS Res Hum Retroviruses*. 1988;4(6): ix-xi.
57. Radziwill G, Tucker W, Schaller H. Mutational analysis of the hepatitis B virus P gene product: domain structure and RNase H activity. *J Virol*. 1990;64(2):613-620.
58. Summers J, Mason WS. Replication of the genome of a hepatitis B–like virus by reverse transcription of an RNA intermediate. *Cell*. 1982;29(2):403-415.
59. Seeger C, Mason WS. Hepatitis B virus biology. *Microbiol Mol Biol Rev*. 2000;64(1):51-68.
60. Pollack JR, Ganem D. An RNA stem-loop structure directs hepatitis B virus genomic RNA encapsidation. *J Virol*. 1993; 67(6):3254-3263.
61. Wang GH, Zoulim F, Leber EH, et al. Role of RNA in enzymatic activity of the reverse transcriptase of hepatitis B viruses. *J Virol*. 1994;68(12):8437-8442.
62. Wang GH, Seeger C. The reverse transcriptase of hepatitis B virus acts as a protein primer for viral DNA synthesis. *Cell*. 1992;71(4):663-670.
63. Lutwick LI, Robinson WS. DNA synthesized in the hepatitis B Dane particle DNA polymerase reaction. *J Virol*. 1977;21(1): 96-104.
64. Le Mire MF, Miller DS, Foster WK, et al. Covalently closed circular DNA is the predominant form of duck hepatitis B virus DNA that persists following transient infection. *J Virol*. 2005; 79(19):12242-12252.
65. Zoulim F, Saputelli J, Seeger C. Woodchuck hepatitis virus X protein is required for viral infection in vivo. *J Virol*. 1994; 68(3):2026-2030.
66. Maguire HF, Hoeffler JP, Siddiqui A. HBV X protein alters the DNA binding specificity of CREB and ATF-2 by protein-protein interactions. *Science*. 1991;252(5007):842-844.
67. Siddiqui A, Gaynor R, Srivivasan A, et al. Trans-activation of viral enhancers including long terminal repeat of the human immunodeficiency virus by the hepatitis B virus X protein. *Virology*. 1989;169(2):479-484.
68. Benn J, Su F, Doria M, et al. Hepatitis B virus HBx protein induces transcription factor AP-1 by activation of extracellular signal-regulated and c-Jun N-terminal mitogen-activated protein kinases. *J Virol*. 1996;70(8):4978-4985.
69. Waris G, Siddiqui A. Interaction between STAT-3 and HNF-3 leads to the activation of liver-specific hepatitis B virus enhancer 1 function. *J Virol*. 2002;76(6):2721-2729.
70. Rahmani Z, Huh KW, Lasher R, et al. Hepatitis B virus X protein colocalizes to mitochondria with a human voltage-dependent anion channel, HVDAC3, and alters its transmembrane potential. *J Virol*. 2000;74(6):2840-2846.
71. Shirakata Y, Koike K. Hepatitis B virus X protein induces cell death by causing loss of mitochondrial membrane potential. *J Biol Chem*. 2003;278(24):22071-22078.
72. Cross JC, Wen P, Rutter WJ. Transactivation by hepatitis B virus X protein is promiscuous and dependent on mitogen-activated cellular serine/threonine kinases. *Proc Natl Acad Sci U S A*. 1993; 90(17):8078-8082.
73. Kekule AS, Lauer U, Weiss L, et al. Hepatitis B virus transactivator HBx uses a tumour promoter signalling pathway. *Nature*. 1993;361(6414):742-745.
74. Benn J, Schneider RJ. Hepatitis B virus HBx protein activates Ras-GTP complex formation and establishes a Ras, Raf, MAP kinase signaling cascade. *Proc Natl Acad Sci U S A*. 1994;91(22): 10350-10354.
75. Elmore LW, Hancock AR, Chang SF, et al. Hepatitis B virus X protein and p53 tumor suppressor interactions in the modulation of apoptosis. *Proc Natl Acad Sci U S A*. 1997;94(26):14707-14712.
76. Huovila AP, Eder AM, Fuller SD. Hepatitis B surface antigen assembles in a post-ER, pre-Golgi compartment. *J Cell Biol*. 1992;118(6):1305-1320.
77. Bruss V, Ganem D. The role of envelope proteins in hepatitis B virus assembly. *Proc Natl Acad Sci U S A*. 1991;88(3):1059-1063.
78. Gerin JL. Animal models of hepatitis delta virus infection and disease. *Ilar J*. 2001;42(2):103-106.
79. van Regenmortel M, Fauquet C, Bishop D, et al. Virus taxonomy: the classification and nomenclature of viruses. In: *The Seventh Report of the International Committee on Taxonomy of Viruses; 2000*. San Diego, Calif: Academic Press; 2000.
80. Rizzetto M, Canese MG, Gerin JL, et al. Transmission of the hepatitis B virus–associated delta antigen to chimpanzees. *J Infect Dis*. 1980;141(5):590-602.
81. Deny P. Hepatitis delta virus genetic variability: from genotypes I, II, III to eight major clades? *Curr Top Microbiol Immunol*. 2006;307:151-171.
82. Casey JL, Brown TL, Colan EJ, et al. A genotype of hepatitis D virus that occurs in northern South America. *Proc Natl Acad Sci U S A*. 1993;90(19):9016-9020.
83. Rizzetto M, Purcell RH, Gerin JL. Epidemiology of HBV-associated delta agent: geographical distribution of anti-delta and prevalence in polytransfused HBsAg carriers. *Lancet*. 1980; 1(8180):1215-1218.
84. Gerin JL, Casey JL, Purcell RH. Hepatitis delta virus. In: Knipe DM, Howley PM, eds. *Fields Virology*. New York: Lippincott; 2001:3037-3050.
85. MacNaughton TB, Lai MM. Genomic but not antigenomic hepatitis delta virus RNA is preferentially exported from the nucleus immediately after synthesis and processing. *J Virol*. 2002;76(8):3928-3935.
86. Weiner AJ, Choo QL, Wang KS, et al. A single antigenomic open reading frame of the hepatitis delta virus encodes the epitope(s) of both hepatitis delta antigen polypeptides p24 delta and p27 delta. *J Virol*. 1988;62(2):594-599.
87. Luo GX, Chao M, Hsieh SY, et al. A specific base transition occurs on replicating hepatitis delta virus RNA. *J Virol*. 1990; 64(3):1021-1027.
88. Chang MF, Chang SC, Chang CI, et al. Nuclear localization signals, but not putative leucine zipper motifs, are essential for nuclear transport of hepatitis delta antigen. *J Virol*. 1992; 66(10):6019-6027.
89. Xia YP, Lai MM. Oligomerization of hepatitis delta antigen is required for both the trans-activating and trans-dominant inhibitory activities of the delta antigen. *J Virol*. 1992;66(11): 6641-6648.
90. Wang JG, Lemon SM. Hepatitis delta virus antigen forms dimers and multimeric complexes in vivo. *J Virol*. 1993;67(1):446-454.
91. Huang C, Chang SC, Yu IC, et al. Large hepatitis delta antigen is a novel clathrin adaptor-like protein. *J Virol*. 2007:81(11):5985-5994. Epub 2007 Mar 21.
92. Lai MM. The molecular biology of hepatitis delta virus. *Annu Rev Biochem*. 1995;64:259-286.
93. Sharmeen L, Kuo MY, Dinter-Gottlieb G, et al. Antigenomic RNA of human hepatitis delta virus can undergo self-cleavage. *J Virol*. 1988;62(8):2674-2679.
94. Wu HN, Lin YJ, Lin FP, et al. Human hepatitis delta virus RNA subfragments contain an autocleavage activity. *Proc Natl Acad Sci U S A*. 1989;86(6):1831-1835.
95. Macnaughton TB, Wang YJ, Lai MM. Replication of hepatitis delta virus RNA: effect of mutations of the autocatalytic cleavage sites. *J Virol*. 1993;67(4):2228-2234.
96. Huang YH, Wu JC, Chau GY, et al. Detection of serum hepatitis B, C, and D viral nucleic acids and its implications in hepatocellular carcinoma patients. *J Gastroenterol*. 1998;33(4):512-516.
97. Taylor J. Replication of human hepatitis delta virus: recent developments. *Trends Microbiol*. 2003;11(4):185-190.
98. Yamaguchi Y, Mura T, Chanarat S, et al. Hepatitis delta antigen binds to the clamp of RNA polymerase II and affects transcriptional fidelity. *Genes Cells*. 2007;12(7):863-875.
99. Nassal M. Hepatitis B virus morphogenesis. *Curr Top Microbiol Immunol*. 1996;214:297-337.
100. Ponzetto A, Cote PJ, Popper H, et al. Transmission of the hepatitis B virus–associated delta agent to the eastern woodchuck. *Proc Natl Acad Sci U S A*. 1984;81(7):2208-2212.
101. Ferrari C, Missale G, Boni C, et al. Immunopathogenesis of hepatitis B. *J Hepatol*. 2003;39(Suppl 1):S36-S42.
102. Chang JJ, Lewin SR. Immunopathogenesis of hepatitis B virus infection. *Immunol Cell Biol*. 2007;85(1):16-23.
103. Baron JL, Gardiner L, Nishimura S, et al. Activation of a non-classical NKT cell subset in a transgenic mouse model of hepatitis B virus infection. *Immunity*. 2002;16(4):583-594.
104. Ferrari C, Bertoletti A, Penna A, et al. Identification of immunodominant T cell epitopes of the hepatitis B virus nucleocapsid antigen. *J Clin Invest*. 1991;88(1):214-222.
105. Penna A, Chisari FV, Bertoletti A, et al. Cytotoxic T lymphocytes recognize an HLA-A2-restricted epitope within the hepatitis B virus nucleocapsid antigen. *J Exper Med*. 1991;174(6):1565-1570.
106. Penna A, Artini M, Cavalli A, et al. Long-lasting memory T cell responses following self-limited acute hepatitis B. *J Clin Invest*. 1996;98(5):1185-1194.
107. Guidotti LG, Chisari FV. Noncytolytic control of viral infections by the innate and adaptive immune response. *Annu Rev Immunol*. 2001;19:65-91.
108. Guidotti LG, Chisari FV. Cytokine-induced viral purging—role in viral pathogenesis. *Curr Opin Microbiol*. 1999;2(4):388-391.
109. Milich DR, Schodel F, Peterson DL, et al. Characterization of self-reactive T cells that evade tolerance in hepatitis B e antigen transgenic mice. *Eur J Immunol*. 1995;25(6):1663-1672.
110. Bertoletti A, Sette A, Chisari FV, et al. Natural variants of cytotoxic epitopes are T-cell receptor antagonists for antiviral cytotoxic T cells. *Nature*. 1994;369(6479):407-410.

111. Thursz MR, Kwiatkowski D, Allsopp CE, et al. Association between an MHC class II allele and clearance of hepatitis B virus in the Gambia. *N Engl J Med*. 1995;332(16):1065-1069.
112. Frodsham AJ. Host genetics and the outcome of hepatitis B viral infection. *Transpl Immunol*. 2005;14(3-4):183-186.
113. Thio CL, Mosbruger T, Astemborski J, et al. Mannose binding lectin genotypes influence recovery from hepatitis B virus infection. *J Virol*. 2005;79(14):9192-9196.
114. Thio CL, Astemborski J, Thomas R, et al. Interaction between RANTES promoter variant and CCR5Delta32 favors recovery from hepatitis B. *J Immunol*. 2008;181(11):7944-7947.
115. Chisari FV. Rous-Whipple Award Lecture. Viruses, immunity, and cancer: lessons from hepatitis B. *Am J Pathol*. 2000; 156(4):1117-1132.
116. Barnaba V, Franco A, Alberti A, et al. Recognition of hepatitis B virus envelope proteins by liver-infiltrating lymphocytes in chronic HBV infection. *J Immunol*. 1989;143(8):2650-2655.
117. Barnaba V, Franco A, Alberti A, et al. Selective killing of hepatitis B envelope antigen-specific B cells by class I-restricted, exogenous antigen-specific T lymphocytes. *Nature*. 1990;345: 258-260.
118. Maini MK, Boni C, Lee CK, et al. The role of virus-specific CD8(+) cells in liver damage and viral control during persistent hepatitis B virus infection. *J Exp Med*. 2000;191(8):1269-1280.
119. Nisini R, Paroli M, Accapezzato D, et al. Human CD4+ T-cell response to hepatitis delta virus: identification of multiple epitopes and characterization of T-helper cytokine profiles. *J Virol*. 1997;71(3):2241-2251.
120. Karayiannis P, Saldanha J, Jackson AM, et al. Partial control of hepatitis delta virus superinfection by immunisation of woodchucks (*Marmota monax*) with hepatitis delta antigen expressed by a recombinant vaccinia or baculovirus. *J Med Virol*. 1993; 41(3):210-214.
121. Cole SM, Gowans EJ, Macnaughton TB, et al. Direct evidence for cytotoxicity associated with expression of hepatitis delta virus antigen. *Hepatology*. 1991;13(5):845-851.
122. Negro F, Rizzetto M. Pathobiology of hepatitis delta virus. *J Hepatol*. 1993;17(Suppl 3):S149-S153.
123. Beasley RP, Hwang LY, Lin CC, et al. Hepatocellular carcinoma and hepatitis B virus: a prospective study of 22,707 men in Taiwan. *Lancet*. 1981;2(8256):1129-1133.
124. Williams R. Global challenges in liver disease. *Hepatology*. 2006;44(3):521-526.
125. Cougot D, Neuveut C, Buendia MA. HBV induced carcinogenesis. *J Clin Virol*. 2005;34(Suppl 1):S75-S78.
126. Popper H, Roth L, Purcell RH, et al. Hepatocarcinogenicity of the woodchuck hepatitis virus. *Proc Natl Acad Sci U S A*. 1987; 84(3):866-870.
127. Brechot C, Pourcel C, Louise A, et al. Presence of integrated hepatitis B virus DNA sequences in cellular DNA of human hepatocellular carcinoma. *Nature*. 1980;286(5772):533-535.
128. Koike K, Kobayashi M, Gondo M, et al. Hepatitis B virus DNA is frequently found in liver biopsy samples from hepatitis C virus–infected chronic hepatitis patients. *J Med Virol*. 1998; 54(4):249-255.
129. Buendia MA. Hepatitis B viruses and cancerogenesis. *Biomed Pharmacother*. 1998;52(1):34-43.
130. Caselmann W, Koshy R. *Transactivators of HBV, Signal Transduction and Tumorigenesis*. London: Imperial College Press; 1998.
131. Brunetto MR, Giarin MM, Oliveri F, et al. Wild-type and e antigen-minus hepatitis B viruses and course of chronic hepatitis. *Proc Natl Acad Sci U S A*. 1991;88(10):4186-4190.
132. Yu MW, Yang YC, Yang SY, et al. Hormonal markers and hepatitis B virus–related hepatocellular carcinoma risk: a nested case-control study among men. *J Natl Cancer Inst*. 2001;93(21): 1644-1651.
133. Hussain S, Hofseth L, Harris C. Radical causes of cancer. *Nat Rev*. 2003;3:276-285.
134. McNabb SJ, Jajosky RA, Hall-Baker PA, et al. Summary of notifiable diseases—United States, 2006. *MMWR Morb Mortal Wkly Rep*. 2008;55(53):1-92.
135. Hepatitis B virus: a comprehensive strategy for eliminating transmission in the United States through universal childhood vaccination. Recommendations of the Immunization Practices Advisory Committee (ACIP). *MMWR Recomm Rep*. 1991; 40(RR-13):1-25.
136. Chen CJ, Chen DS. Interaction of hepatitis B virus, chemical carcinogen, and genetic susceptibility: multistage hepatocarcinogenesis with multifactorial etiology. *Hepatology*. 2002;36(5): 1046-1049.
137. Liaw YF, Chu CM, Lin DY, et al. Age-specific prevalence and significance of hepatitis B e antigen and antibody in chronic hepatitis B virus infection in Taiwan: a comparison among asymptomatic carriers, chronic hepatitis, liver cirrhosis, and hepatocellular carcinoma. *J Med Virol*. 1984;13(4):385-391.
138. Lai MY, Chen DS, Chen PJ, et al. Status of hepatitis B virus DNA in hepatocellular carcinoma: a study based on paired tumor and nontumor liver tissues. *J Med Virol*. 1988;25(3):249-258.
139. Pisani P, Parkin DM, Bray F, et al. Estimates of the worldwide mortality from 25 cancers in 1990. *Int J Cancer*. 1999;83:18-29.
140. Beasley RP. Hepatitis B virus. The major etiology of hepatocellular carcinoma. *Cancer*. 1988;61(10):1942-1956.
141. Chang MH, Chen CJ, Lai MS, et al. Universal hepatitis B vaccination in Taiwan and the incidence of hepatocellular carcinoma in children. Taiwan Childhood Hepatoma Study Group. *N Engl J Med*. 1997;336(26):1855-1859.
142. Chen CJ, Yang HI, Su J, et al. Risk of hepatocellular carcinoma across a biological gradient of serum hepatitis B virus DNA level. *JAMA*. 2006;295(1):65-73.
143. Huang Y, Wang Z, An S, et al. Role of hepatitis B virus genotypes and quantitative HBV DNA in metastasis and recurrence of hepatocellular carcinoma. *J Med Virol*. 2008;80(4):591-597.
144. Yu MW, Shih WL, Lin CL, et al. Body-mass index and progression of hepatitis B: a population-based cohort study in men. *J Clin Oncol*. 2008;26(34):5576-5582.
145. Novick DM, Farci P, Croxson TS, et al. Hepatitis D virus and human immunodeficiency virus antibodies in parental drug abusers who are hepatitis B surface antigen positive. *J Infect Dis*. 1988;158:795-803.
146. Rosina F, Saracco G, Rizzetto M. Risk of post-transfusion infection with the hepatitis delta virus: a multicenter study. *N Engl J Med*. 1985;321:1488-1491.
147. Liaw YF, Chiu KW, Chu CM, et al. Heterosexual transmission of hepatitis delta virus in the general population of an area endemic for hepatitis B virus infection: a prospective study. *J Infect Dis*. 1990;162:1170-1172.
148. Gerberding JL. Incidence and prevalence of human immunodeficiency virus, hepatitis B virus, hepatitis C virus, and cytomegalovirus among health care personnel at risk for blood exposure: final report from a longitudinal study. *J Infect Dis*. 1994;170(6): 1410-1417.
149. Hoofnagle JH. Type B hepatitis: virology, serology and clinical course. *Semin Liver Dis*. 1981;1(1):7-14.
150. McMahon BJ, Alward WL, Hall DB, et al. Acute hepatitis B virus infection: relation of age to the clinical expression of disease and subsequent development of the carrier state. *J Infect Dis*. 1985; 151(4):599-603.
151. Lee WM. Medical progress: hepatitis B virus infection. *N Engl J Med*. 1997;337(24):1733-1745.
152. Rehermann B, Ferrari C, Pasquinelli C, et al. The hepatitis B virus persists for decades after patients' recovery from acute viral hepatitis despite active maintenance of a cytotoxic T lymphocyte response. *Nat Med*. 1996;2:1104-1108.
153. Al-Taie OH, Mork H, Gassel AM, et al. Prevention of hepatitis B flare-up during chemotherapy using lamivudine: case report and review of the literature. *Ann Hematol*. 1999;78(5): 247-249.
154. Bessesen M, Ives D, Condreay L, et al. Chronic active hepatitis B exacerbations in human immunodeficiency virus–infected patients following development of resistance to or withdrawal of lamivudine. *Clin Infect Dis*. 1999;28(5):1032-1035.
155. Schiodt FV, Atillasoy E, Shakil AO, et al. Etiology and outcome for 295 patients with acute liver failure in the United States. *Liver Transpl Surg*. 1999;5(1):29-34.
156. Wai CT, Fontana RJ, Polson J, et al. Clinical outcome and virological characteristics of hepatitis B–related acute liver failure in the United States. *J Viral Hepat*. 2005;12(2):192-198.
157. Wright TL, Mamish D, Combs C, et al. Hepatitis B virus and apparent fulminant non-A, non-B hepatitis. *Lancet*. 1992; 339(8799):952-955.
158. Wu JC, Chen CL, Hou MC, et al. Multiple viral infection as the most common cause of fulminant and subfulminant viral hepatitis in an area endemic for hepatitis B: application and limitations of the polymerase chain reaction. *Hepatology*. 1994;19(4): 836-840.
159. Vento S, Cainelli F, Mirandola F, et al. Fulminant hepatitis on withdrawal of chemotherapy in carriers of hepatitis C virus. *Lancet*. 1996;347(8994):92-93.
160. Liang TJ, Hasegawa K, Munoz SJ, et al. Hepatitis B virus precore mutation and fulminant hepatitis in the United States: a polymerase chain reaction–based assay for the detection of specific mutation. *J Clin Invest*. 1994;93(2):550-555.
161. Milich DR, Jones JE, Hughes JL, et al. Is a function of the secreted hepatitis B e antigen to induce immunologic tolerance in utero? *Proc Natl Acad Sci U S A*. 1990;87(17):6599-6603.
162. Sterneck M, Kalinina T, Gunther S, et al. Functional analysis of HBV genomes from patients with fulminant hepatitis. *Hepatology*. 1998;28(5):1390-1397.
163. Bartholomeusz A, Locarnini S. Hepatitis B virus mutants and fulminant hepatitis B: fitness plus phenotype. *Hepatology*. 2001; 34(2):432-435.
164. Liu CJ, Chen PJ, Lai MY, et al. A prospective study characterizing full-length hepatitis B virus genomes during acute exacerbation. *Gastroenterology*. 2003;124(1):80-90.
165. Perrillo RP. Acute flares in chronic hepatitis B: the natural and unnatural history of an immunologically mediated liver disease. *Gastroenterology*. 2001;120(4):1009-1022.
166. Wong JB, Koff RS, Tine F, et al. Cost-effectiveness of interferon-alpha 2b treatment for hepatitis B e antigen-positive chronic hepatitis B. *Ann Intern Med*. 1995;122(9):664-675.
167. Gerber MA, Hadziyannis S, Vissoulis C, et al. Electron microscopy and immunoelectronmicroscopy of cytoplasmic hepatitis B antigen in hepatocytes. *Am J Pathol*. 1974;75(3):489-502.
168. Harrison RF, Davies MH, Goldin RD, et al. Recurrent hepatitis B in liver allografts: a distinctive form of rapidly developing cirrhosis. *Histopathology*. 1993;23(1):21-28.
169. Fattovich G, Bortolotti F, Donato F. Natural history of chronic hepatitis B: special emphasis on disease progression and prognostic factors. *J Hepatol*. 2008;48(2):335-352.
170. Lok AS, Lai CL, Wu PC, et al. Spontaneous hepatitis B e antigen to antibody seroconversion and reversion in Chinese patients with chronic hepatitis B virus infection. *Gastroenterology*. 1987; 92(6):1839-1843.
171. Chang MH, Hsu HY, Hsu HC, et al. The significance of spontaneous hepatitis B e antigen seroconversion in childhood: with special emphasis on the clearance of hepatitis B e antigen before 3 years of age. *Hepatology*. 1995;22(5):1387-1392.
172. Yang PL, Althage A, Chung J, et al. Hydrodynamic injection of viral DNA: a mouse model of acute hepatitis B virus infection. *Proc Natl Acad Sci U S A*. 2002;99(21):13825-13830.
173. Liaw YF, Chu CM, Huang MJ, et al. Determinants for hepatitis B e antigen clearance in chronic type B hepatitis. *Liver*. 1984; 4(5):301-306.
174. McMahon BJ, Holck P, Bulkow L, et al. Serologic and clinical outcomes of 1536 Alaska Natives chronically infected with hepatitis B virus. *Ann Intern Med*. 2001;135(9):759-768.
175. Fattovich G, Brollo L, Giustina G, et al. Natural history and prognostic factors for chronic hepatitis type B. *Gut*. 1991; 32(3):294-298.
176. Tsai SL, Chen PJ, Lai MY, et al. Acute exacerbations of chronic type B hepatitis are accompanied by increased T cell responses to hepatitis B core and e antigens: implications for hepatitis B e antigen seroconversion. *J Clin Invest*. 1992;89(1):87-96.
177. Schulte-Frohlinde E, Foster GR. Spontaneous seroconversion in chronic hepatitis B: role of mutations in the precore/core gene. *Dig Dis Sci*. 1998;43(8):1714-1718.
178. Fattovich G, Rugge M, Brollo L, et al. Clinical, virologic and histologic outcome following seroconversion from HBeAg to anti-HBe in chronic hepatitis type B. *Hepatology*. 1986;6(2): 167-172.
179. Liaw YF, Lin SM, Sheen IS, et al. Acute hepatitis C virus superinfection followed by spontaneous HBeAg seroconversion and HBsAg elimination. *Infection*. 1991;19(4):250-251.
180. Kawatani T, Suou T, Tajima F, et al. Incidence of hepatitis virus infection and severe liver dysfunction in patients receiving chemotherapy for hematologic malignancies. *Eur J Haematol*. 2001;67(1):45-50.
181. Carman WF, Jacyna MR, Hadziyannis S, et al. Mutation preventing formation of hepatitis B e antigen in patients with chronic hepatitis B infection. *Lancet*. 1989;2(8663):588-591.
182. Fattovich G, Brollo L, Alberti A, et al. Long-term follow-up of anti-HBe-positive chronic active hepatitis B. *Hepatology*. 1988; 8(6):1651-1654.
183. Gunther S, Sommer G, Von Breunig F, et al. Amplification of full-length hepatitis B virus genomes from samples from patients with low levels of viremia: frequency and functional consequences of PCR-introduced mutations. *J Clin Microbiol*. 1998;36(2):531-538.
184. Hawkins AE, Gilson RJ, Bickerton EA, et al. Conservation of precore and core sequences of hepatitis B virus in chronic viral carriers. *J Med Virol*. 1994;43(1):5-12.
185. Tong SP, Li JS, Vitvitski L, et al. Evidence for a base-paired region of hepatitis B virus pregenome encapsidation signal which influences the patterns of precore mutations abolishing HBe protein expression. *J Virol*. 1993;67(9):5651-5655.
186. Hadziyannis SJ, Vassilopoulos D. Immunopathogenesis of hepatitis B e antigen negative chronic hepatitis B infection. *Antiviral Res*. 2001;52(2):91-98.
187. Tong SP, Li JS, Vitvitski L, et al. Active hepatitis B virus replication in the presence of anti-HBe is associated with viral variants containing an inactive pre-C region. *Virology*. 1990;176(2): 596-603.
188. Lok AS, Akarca U, Greene S. Mutations in the pre-core region of hepatitis B virus serve to enhance the stability of the secondary structure of the pre-genome encapsidation signal. *Proc Natl Acad Sci U S A*. 1994;91(9):4077-4081.
189. Volz T, Lutgehetmann M, Wachtler P, et al. Impaired intrahepatic hepatitis B virus productivity contributes to low viremia in most HBeAg-negative patients. *Gastroenterology*. 2007;133(3): 843-852.
190. Zarski JP, Marcellin P, Cohard M, et al. Comparison of anti-HBe-positive and HBe-antigen-positive chronic hepatitis B in France. French Multicentre Group. *J Hepatol*. 1994;20(5):636-640.
191. Chan HL, Hussain M, Lok AS. Different hepatitis B virus genotypes are associated with different mutations in the core promoter and precore regions during hepatitis B e antigen seroconversion. *Hepatology*. 1999;29(3):976-984.
192. Hsu YS, Chien RN, Yeh CT, et al. Long-term outcome after spontaneous HBeAg seroconversion in patients with chronic hepatitis B. *Hepatology*. 2002;35(6):1522-1527.
193. Di Marco V, Lo Iacono O, Camma C, et al. The long-term course of chronic hepatitis B. *Hepatology*. 1999;30(1):257-264.
194. Chen YC, Sheen IS, Chu CM, et al. Prognosis following spontaneous HBsAg seroclearance in chronic hepatitis B patients with or without concurrent infection. *Gastroenterology*. 2002;123(4): 1084-1089.
195. Villeneuve JP, Desrochers M, Infante-Rivard C, et al. A long-term follow-up study of asymptomatic hepatitis B surface antigen-positive carriers in Montreal. *Gastroenterology*. 1994; 106(4):1000-1005.
196. Crook PD, Jones ME, Hall AJ. Mortality of hepatitis B surface antigen-positive blood donors in England and Wales. *Int J Epidemiol*. 2003;32(1):118-124.
197. Fattovich G, Giustina G, Schalm SW, et al. Occurrence of hepatocellular carcinoma and decompensation in western European patients with cirrhosis type B. The EUROHEP Study

Group on Hepatitis B Virus and Cirrhosis. *Hepatology.* 1995;21(1):77-82.

198. Moreno-Otero R, Garcia-Monzon C, Garcia-Sanchez A, et al. Development of cirrhosis after chronic type B hepatitis: a clinicopathologic and follow-up study of 46 HBeAg-positive asymptomatic patients. *Am J Gastroenterol.* 1991;86(5):560-564.

199. Iloeje UH, Yang HI, Su J, et al. Predicting cirrhosis risk based on the level of circulating hepatitis B viral load. *Gastroenterology.* 2006;130(3):678-686.

200. Ikeda K, Saitoh S, Suzuki Y, et al. Disease progression and hepatocellular carcinogenesis in patients with chronic viral hepatitis: a prospective observation of 2215 patients. *J Hepatol.* 1998;28(6):930-938.

201. Donato F, Tagger A, Gelatti U, et al. Alcohol and hepatocellular carcinoma: the effect of lifetime intake and hepatitis virus infections in men and women. *Am J Epidemiol.* 2002;155(4):323-331.

202. Liaw YF. Hepatitis C virus superinfection in patients with chronic hepatitis B virus infection. *J Gastroenterol.* 2002;37 (Suppl 13):S65-S68.

203. Crespo J, Lozano JL, de la Cruz F, et al. Prevalence and significance of hepatitis C viremia in chronic active hepatitis B. *Am J Gastroenterol.* 1994;89(8):1147-1151.

204. Fattovich G, Boscaro S, Noventa F, et al. Influence of hepatitis delta virus infection on progression to cirrhosis in chronic hepatitis type B. *J Infect Dis.* 1987;155(5):931-935.

205. Realdi G, Fattovich G, Hadziyannis S, et al. Survival and prognostic factors in 366 patients with compensated cirrhosis type B: a multicenter study. The Investigators of the European Concerted Action on Viral Hepatitis (EUROHEP). *J Hepatol.* 1994;21(4):656-666.

206. Liaw YF, Lin DY, Chen TJ, et al. Natural course after the development of cirrhosis in patients with chronic type B hepatitis: a prospective study. *Liver.* 1989;9(4):235-241.

207. de Jongh FE, Janssen HL, de Man RA, et al. Survival and prognostic indicators in hepatitis B surface antigen-positive cirrhosis of the liver. *Gastroenterology.* 1992;103(5):1630-1635.

208. Fattovich G. Progression of hepatitis B and C to hepatocellular carcinoma in Western countries. *Hepatogastroenterology.* 1998;45(Suppl 3):S1206-S1213.

209. Yang HI, Lu SN, Liaw YF, et al. Hepatitis B e antigen and the risk of hepatocellular carcinoma. *N Engl J Med.* 2002;347(3):168-174.

210. Hassan MM, Hwang LY, Hatten CJ, et al. Risk factors for hepatocellular carcinoma: synergism of alcohol with viral hepatitis and diabetes mellitus. *Hepatology.* 2002;36(5):1206-1213.

211. Yuen MF, Wong DK, Fung J, et al. HBsAg seroclearance in chronic hepatitis B in Asian patients: replicative level and risk of hepatocellular carcinoma. *Gastroenterology.* 2008;135(4):1192-1199.

212. Chen CJ, Yu MW, Liaw YF. Epidemiological characteristics and risk factors of hepatocellular carcinoma. *J Gastroenterol Hepatol.* 1997;12(9-10):S294-S308.

213. Farza H, Salmon AM, Hadchouel M, et al. Hepatitis B surface antigen gene expression is regulated by sex steroids and glucocorticoids in transgenic mice. *Proc Natl Acad Sci U S A.* 1987;84(5):1187-1191.

214. Ponzetto A, Forzani B, Parravicini PP, et al. Epidemiology of hepatitis delta virus (HDV) infection. *Eur J Epidemiol.* 1985;1(4):257-263.

215. Jardi R, Buti M, Cotrina M, et al. Determination of hepatitis delta virus RNA by polymerase chain reaction in acute and chronic delta infection. *Hepatology.* 1995;21(1):25-29.

216. Beral V, Blum H, Ma B. Hepatitis D virus. *IARC Monographs on the Evaluation of Carcinogenic Risks to Humans.* 1994;59:223-253.

217. Tamura I, Kurimura O, Koda T, et al. Risk of liver cirrhosis and hepatocellular carcinoma in subjects with hepatitis B and delta virus infection: a study from Kure, Japan. *J Gastroenterol Hepatol.* 1993;8(5):433-436.

218. Lozano JL, Crespo J, de la Cruz F, et al. Correlation between hepatitis B viremia and the clinical and histological activity of chronic delta hepatitis. *Med Microbiol Immunol (Berl).* 1994;183(3):159-167.

219. Weltman MD, Brotodihardjo A, Crewe EB, et al. Coinfection with hepatitis B and C or B, C and delta viruses results in severe chronic liver disease and responds poorly to interferon-alpha treatment. *J Viral Hepat.* 1995;2(1):39-45.

220. Guillevin L, Lhote F, Cohen P, et al. Polyarteritis nodosa related to hepatitis B virus: a prospective study with long-term observation of 41 patients. *Medicine (Baltimore).* 1995;74(5):238-253.

221. Avsar E, Savas B, Tozun N, et al. Successful treatment of polyarteritis nodosa related to hepatitis B virus with interferon alpha as first-line therapy. *J Hepatol.* 1998;28(3):525-526.

222. Simsek H, Telatar H. Successful treatment of hepatitis B virus-associated polyarteritis nodosa by interferon alpha alone. *J Clin Gastroenterol.* 1995;20(3):263-265.

223. Boeck K, Mempel M, Schmidt T, et al. Gianotti-Crosti syndrome: clinical, serologic, and therapeutic data from nine children. *Cutis.* 1998;62(6):271-274; quiz 86.

224. De Gaspari G, Bardare M, Costantino D. AU antigen in Crosti-Gianotti acrodermatitis. *Lancet.* 1970;1(7656):1116-1117.

225. Fergin P. Gianotti-Crosti syndrome: non-parenterally acquired hepatitis B with a distinctive exanthem. *Med J (Aust).* 1983;1(4):175-176.

226. Gilbert RD, Wiggelinkhuizen J. The clinical course of hepatitis B virus–associated nephropathy. *Pediatr Nephrol.* 1994;8(1):11-14.

227. Lhotta K. Beyond hepatorenal syndrome: glomerulonephritis in patients with liver disease. *Semin Nephrol.* 2002;22(4):302-308.

228. Conjeevaram HS, Hoofnagle JH, Austin HA, et al. Long-term outcome of hepatitis B virus–related glomerulonephritis after therapy with interferon alfa. *Gastroenterology.* 1995;109(2):540-546.

229. Kellerman SE, Hanson DL, McNaghten AD, et al. Prevalence of chronic hepatitis B and incidence of acute hepatitis B infection in human immunodeficiency virus–infected subjects. *J Infect Dis.* 2003;188(4):571-577.

230. Alter MJ. Epidemiology of viral hepatitis and HIV coinfection. *J Hepatol.* 2006;44(Suppl 1):S6-S9.

231. Nyirenda M, Beadsworth MB, Stephany P, et al. Prevalence of infection with hepatitis B and C virus and coinfection with HIV in medical inpatients in Malawi. *J Infect.* 2008;57(1):72-77.

232. Gilson RJ, Hawkins AE, Beecham MR, et al. Interactions between HIV and hepatitis B virus in homosexual men: effects on the natural history of infection. *AIDS.* 1997;11(5):597-606.

233. Colin JF, Cazals-Hatem D, Loriot MA, et al. Influence of human immunodeficiency virus infection on chronic hepatitis B in homosexual men. *Hepatology.* 1999;29(4):1306-1310.

234. Thio CL, Seaberg EC, Skolasky R Jr, et al. HIV-1, hepatitis B virus, and risk of liver-related mortality in the Multicenter Cohort Study (MACS). *Lancet.* 2002;360(9349):1921-1926.

235. Altfeld M, Rockstroh JK, Addo M, et al. Reactivation of hepatitis B in a long-term anti-HBs-positive patient with AIDS following lamivudine withdrawal. *J Hepatol.* 1998;29(2):306-309.

236. Fang JW, Tung FY, Davis GL, et al. Fibrosing cholestatic hepatitis in a transplant recipient with hepatitis B virus precore mutant. *Gastroenterology.* 1993;105(3):901-904.

237. Neau D, Winnock M, Galperine T, et al. Isolated antibodies against the core antigen of hepatitis B virus in HIV-infected patients. *HIV Med.* 2004;5(3):171-173.

238. Santos EA, Yoshida CF, Rolla VC, et al. Frequent occult hepatitis B virus infection in patients infected with human immunodeficiency virus type 1. *Eur J Clin Microbiol Infect Dis.* 2003;22(2):92-98.

239. Sherman KE, Shire N, Rouster S, et al. Prevelance of occult hepatitis B infections in HIV patients: analysis of a geographically distributed ACTG cohort. In 10th Conference on Retroviruses and Opportunistic Infections; 2003; Boston, 2003.

240. Tsui JI, French AL, Seaberg EC, et al. Prevalence and long-term effects of occult hepatitis B virus infection in HIV-infected women. *Clin Infect Dis.* 2007;45(6):736-740.

241. Shire NJ, Rouster SD, Stanford SD, et al. The prevalence and significance of occult hepatitis B virus in a prospective cohort of HIV-infected patients. *J Acquir Immune Defic Syndr.* 2007;44(3):309-314.

242. Terrault NA. Treatment of recurrent hepatitis B infection in liver transplant recipients. *Liver Transpl.* 2002;8(10 Suppl 1):S74-S81.

243. Steinmuller T, Seehofer D, Rayes N, et al. Increasing applicability of liver transplantation for patients with hepatitis B–related liver disease. *Hepatology.* 2002;35(6):1528-1535.

244. Gane E, Pilmore H. Management of chronic viral hepatitis before and after renal transplantation. *Transplantation.* 2002;74(4):427-437.

245. Bird GL, Smith H, Portmann B, et al. Acute liver decompensation on withdrawal of cytotoxic chemotherapy and immunosuppressive therapy in hepatitis B carriers. *Q J Med.* 1989;73(270):895-902.

246. Locasciulli A, Alberti A, Bandini G, et al. Allogeneic bone marrow transplantation from HBsAg⁺ donors: a multicenter study from the Gruppo Italiano Trapianto di Midollo Osseo (GITMO). *Blood.* 1995;86(8):3236-3240.

247. Mertens T, Kock J, Hampl W, et al. Reactivated fulminant hepatitis B virus replication after bone marrow transplantation: clinical course and possible treatment with ganciclovir. *J Hepatol.* 1996;25(6):968-971.

248. Ilan Y, Nagler A, Adler R, et al. Ablation of persistent hepatitis B by bone marrow transplantation from a hepatitis B-immune donor. *Gastroenterology.* 1993;104(6):1818-1821.

249. Lau GK, Suri D, Liang R, et al. Resolution of chronic hepatitis B and anti-HBs seroconversion in humans by adoptive transfer of immunity to hepatitis B core antigen. *Gastroenterology.* 2002;122(3):614-624.

250. Fong TL, Di Bisceglie AM, Waggoner JG, et al. The significance of antibody to hepatitis C virus in patients with chronic hepatitis B. *Hepatology.* 1991;14(1):64-67.

251. Shih CM, Lo SJ, Miyamura T, et al. Suppression of hepatitis B virus expression and replication by hepatitis C virus core protein in HuH-7 cells. *J Virol.* 1993;67(10):5823-5832.

252. Sagnelli E, Coppola N, Scolastico C, et al. Virologic and clinical expressions of reciprocal inhibitory effect of hepatitis B, C, and delta viruses in patients with chronic hepatitis. *Hepatology.* 2000;32(5):1106-1110.

253. Zarski JP, Bohn B, Bastie A, et al. Characteristics of patients with dual infection by hepatitis B and C viruses. *J Hepatol.* 1998;28(1):27-33.

254. Sun CA, Farzadegan H, You SL, et al. Mutual confounding and interactive effects between hepatitis C and hepatitis B viral infections in hepatocellular carcinogenesis: a population-based case-control study in Taiwan. *Cancer Epidemiol Biomarkers Prev.* 1996;5(3):173-178.

255. Zignego AL, Fontana R, Puliti S, et al. Impaired response to alpha interferon in patients with an inapparent hepatitis B and hepatitis C virus coinfection. *Arch Virol.* 1997;142(3):535-544.

256. Liu CJ, Chen PJ, Lai MY, et al. Ribavirin and interferon is effective for hepatitis C virus clearance in hepatitis B and C dually infected patients. *Hepatology.* 2003;37(3):568-576.

257. Kumar M, Chauhan R, Gupta N, et al. Spontaneous increases in alanine aminotransferase levels in asymptomatic chronic hepatitis B virus–infected patients. *Gastroenterology.* 2009;136(4):1272-1280. Epub 2009 Jan 16.

258. Bortolotti F. Chronic viral hepatitis in childhood. *Baillieres Clin Gastroenterol.* 1996;10(2):185-206.

259. Bonino F, Rosina F, Rizzetto M, et al. Chronic hepatitis in HBsAg carriers with serum HBV-DNA and anti-HBe. *Gastroenterology.* 1986;90(5 Pt 1):1268-1273.

260. Yuen MF, Sablon E, Hui CK, et al. Factors associated with hepatitis B virus DNA breakthrough in patients receiving prolonged lamivudine therapy. *Hepatology.* 2001;34(4 Pt 1):785-791.

261. Manns MP. Current state of interferon therapy in the treatment of chronic hepatitis B. *Semin Liver Dis.* 2002;22(Suppl 1):7-13.

262. Perrillo RP, Lai CL, Liaw YF, et al. Predictors of HBeAg loss after lamivudine treatment for chronic hepatitis B. *Hepatology.* 2002;36(1):186-194.

263. Pawlotsky JM. Molecular diagnosis of viral hepatitis. *Gastroenterology.* 2002;122(6):1554-1568.

264. Lok AS, Heathcote EJ, Hoofnagle JH. Management of hepatitis B: 2000—Summary of a workshop. *Gastroenterology.* 2001;120(7):1828-1853.

265. Hadler SC, Murphy BL, Schable CA, et al. Epidemiological analysis of the significance of low-positive test results for antibody to hepatitis B surface and core antigens. *J Clin Microbiol.* 1984;19(4):521-525.

266. Lok AS, Lai CL, Wu PC. Prevalence of isolated antibody to hepatitis B core antigen in an area endemic for hepatitis B virus infection: implications in hepatitis B vaccination programs. *Hepatology.* 1988;8(4):766-770.

267. Hoofnagle JH, Seefe LB, Bales ZB, et al. Type B hepatitis after transfusion with blood containing antibody to hepatitis B core antigen. *N Engl J Med.* 1978;298(25):1379-1383.

268. Dickson RC, Everhart JE, Lake JR, et al. Transmission of hepatitis B by transplantation of livers from donors positive for antibody to hepatitis B core antigen. The National Institute of Diabetes and Digestive and Kidney Diseases Liver Transplantation Database. *Gastroenterology.* 1997;113(5):1668-1674.

269. Kumar M, Satapathy S, Monga R, et al. A randomized controlled trial of lamivudine to treat acute hepatitis B. *Hepatology.* 2007;45(1):97-101.

270. Lisotti A, Azzaroli F, Buonfiglioli F, et al. Lamivudine treatment for severe acute HBV hepatitis. *Int J Med Sci.* 2008;5(6):309-312.

271. Tillmann HL, Hadem J, Leifeld L, et al. Safety and efficacy of lamivudine in patients with severe acute or fulminant hepatitis B, a multicenter experience. *J Viral Hepat.* 2006;13(4):256-263.

272. Lok AS, McMahon BJ. Chronic hepatitis B. *Hepatology.* 2007;45(2):507-539.

273. Dienstag JL, Goldin RD, Heathcote EJ, et al. Histological outcome during long-term lamivudine therapy. *Gastroenterology.* 2003;124(1):105-117.

274. Malekzadeh R, Mohamadnejad M, Rakhshani N, et al. Reversibility of cirrhosis in chronic hepatitis B. *Clin Gastroenterol Hepatol.* 2004;2(4):344-347.

275. van Zonneveld M, Honkoop P, Hansen BE, et al. Long-term follow-up of alpha-interferon treatment of patients with chronic hepatitis B. *Hepatology.* 2004;39(3):804-810.

276. Papatheodoridis GV, Dimou E, Dimakopoulos K, et al. Outcome of hepatitis B e antigen-negative chronic hepatitis B on long-term nucleos(t)ide analog therapy starting with lamivudine. *Hepatology.* 2005;42(1):121-129.

277. Papatheodoridis GV, Manesis E, Hadziyannis SJ. The long-term outcome of interferon-alpha treated and untreated patients with HBeAg-negative chronic hepatitis B. *J Hepatol.* 2001;34(2):306-313.

278. Niederau C, Heintges T, Lange S, et al. Long-term follow-up of HBeAg-positive patients treated with interferon alfa for chronic hepatitis B. *N Engl J Med.* 1996;334(22):1422-1427.

279. Liaw YF, Sung JJ, Chow WC, et al. Lamivudine for patients with chronic hepatitis B and advanced liver disease. *N Engl J Med.* 2004;351(15):1521-1531.

280. Dienstag JL, Cianciara J, Karayalcin S, et al. Durability of serologic response after lamivudine treatment of chronic hepatitis B. *Hepatology.* 2003;37(4):748-755.

281. Dienstag JL, Schiff ER, Mitchell M, et al. Extended lamivudine retreatment for chronic hepatitis B: maintenance of viral suppression after discontinuation of therapy. *Hepatology.* 1999;30(4):1082-1087.

282. Ryu SH, Chung YH, Choi MH, et al. Long-term additional lamivudine therapy enhances durability of lamivudine-induced HBeAg loss: a prospective study. *J Hepatol.* 2003;39(4):614-619.

283. Liaw YF, Leung NW, Chang TT, et al. Effects of extended lamivudine therapy in Asian patients with chronic hepatitis B. Asia Hepatitis Lamivudine Study Group. *Gastroenterology.* 2000;119(1):172-180.

284. Leung NW, Lai CL, Chang TT, et al. Extended lamivudine treatment in patients with chronic hepatitis B enhances hepatitis B e

antigen seroconversion rates: results after 3 years of therapy. *Hepatology*. 2001;33(6):1527-1532.
285. Rizzetto M, Tassopoulos NC, Goldin RD, et al. Extended lamivudine treatment in patients with HBeAg-negative chronic hepatitis B. *J Hepatol*. 2005;42(2):173-179.
286. Hadziyannis SJ, Papatheodoridis GV, Dimou E, et al. Efficacy of long-term lamivudine monotherapy in patients with hepatitis B e antigen-negative chronic hepatitis B. *Hepatology*. 2000;32 (4 Pt 1):847-851.
287. Hadziyannis SJ, Tassopoulos NC, Heathcote EJ, et al. Long-term therapy with adefovir dipivoxil for HBeAg-negative chronic hepatitis B. *N Engl J Med*. 2005;352(26):2673-2681.
288. Hadziyannis SJ, Tassopoulos NC, Heathcote EJ, et al. Long-term therapy with adefovir dipivoxil for HBeAg-negative chronic hepatitis B for up to 5 years. *Gastroenterology*. 2006;131(6): 1743-1751.
289. Tong MJ, Hsien C, Hsu L, et al. Treatment recommendations for chronic hepatitis B: an evaluation of current guidelines based on a natural history study in the United States. *Hepatology*. 2008;48(4):1070-1078.
290. Heathcote J. Treatment of HBe antigen-positive chronic hepatitis B. *Semin Liver Dis*. 2003;23(1):69-80.
291. Hadziyannis SJ, Papatheodoridis GV, Vassilopoulos D. Treatment of HBeAg-negative chronic hepatitis B. *Semin Liver Dis*. 2003;23(1):81-88.
292. Bonino F, Marcellin P, Lau GK, et al. Predicting response to peginterferon alpha-2a, lamivudine and the two combined for HBeAg-negative chronic hepatitis B. *Gut*. 2007;56(5):699-705.
293. Torre D, Tambini R. Interferon-alpha therapy for chronic hepatitis B in children: a meta-analysis. *Clin Infect Dis*. 1996; 23(1):131-137.
294. Janssen HL, van Zonneveld M, Senturk H, et al. Pegylated interferon alfa-2b alone or in combination with lamivudine for HBeAg-positive chronic hepatitis B: a randomised trial. *Lancet*. 2005;365(9454):123-129.
295. Buster EH, Hansen BE, Buti M, et al. Peginterferon alpha-2b is safe and effective in HBeAg-positive chronic hepatitis B patients with advanced fibrosis. *Hepatology*. 2007;46(2):388-394.
296. Marcellin P, Bonino F, Lau GK, et al. Sustained response of hepatitis B e antigen-negative patients 3 years after treatment with peginterferon alfa-2a. *Gastroenterology*. 2009;136:2169-2179.
297. Liu CJ, Chuang WL, Lee CM, et al. Peginterferon alfa-2a plus ribavirin for the treatment of dual chronic infection with hepatitis B and C viruses. *Gastroenterology*. 2009;136(2):496-504.
298. Lampertico P, Del Ninno E, Vigano M, et al. Long-term suppression of hepatitis B e antigen-negative chronic hepatitis B by 24-month interferon therapy. *Hepatology*. 2003;37(4):756-763.
299. Deutsch M, Dourakis S, Manesis EK, et al. Thyroid abnormalities in chronic viral hepatitis and their relationship to interferon alfa therapy. *Hepatology*. 1997;26(1):206-210.
300. Hoofnagle JH, Di Bisceglie AM, Waggoner JG, et al. Interferon alfa for patients with clinically apparent cirrhosis due to chronic hepatitis B. *Gastroenterology*. 1993;104(4):1116-1121.
301. Perillo R, Schiff E, Davis G, et al. A Randomized, controlled trial of interferon alfa-2b alone and after prednisone withdrawal for the treatment of chronic hepatitis B. *N Engl J Med*. 1990;323: 295-301.
302. Villeneuve JP, Condreay LD, Willems B, et al. Lamivudine treatment for decompensated cirrhosis resulting from chronic hepatitis B. *Hepatology*. 2000;31(1):207-210.
303. Fontana RJ, Keeffe EB, Carey W, et al. Effect of lamivudine treatment on survival of 309 North American patients awaiting liver transplantation for chronic hepatitis B. *Liver Transpl*. 2002;8(5):433-439.
304. Dienstag JL, Schiff ER, Wright TL, et al. Lamivudine as initial treatment for chronic hepatitis B in the United States. *N Engl J Med*. 1999;341(17):1256-1263.
305. Lai C-L, Chien R-N, Leung NWY, et al. A one-year trial of lamivudine for chronic hepatitis B. *N Engl J Med*. 1998; 339(2):61-68.
306. Chien RN, Liaw YF, Atkins M. Pretherapy alanine transaminase level as a determinant for hepatitis B e antigen seroconversion during lamivudine therapy in patients with chronic hepatitis B. Asian Hepatitis Lamivudine Trial Group. *Hepatology*. 1999; 30(3):770-774.
307. Lau DT, Khokhar MF, Doo E, et al. Long-term therapy of chronic hepatitis B with lamivudine. *Hepatology*. 2000;32(4 Pt 1):828-834.
308. Tassopoulos NC, Volpes R, Pastore G, et al. Efficacy of lamivudine in patients with hepatitis B e antigen-negative/hepatitis B virus DNA-positive (precore mutant) chronic hepatitis B. Lamivudine Precore Mutant Study Group. *Hepatology*. 1999;29(3): 889-896.
309. Schiff ER. Lamivudine for hepatitis B in clinical practice. *J Med Virol*. 2000;61(3):386-391.
310. Yao FY, Bass NM. Lamivudine treatment in patients with severely decompensated cirrhosis due to replicating hepatitis B infection. *J Hepatol*. 2000;33(2):301-307.
311. Lok AS, McMahon BJ. Chronic hepatitis B. *Hepatology*. 2001;34(6):1225-1241.
312. Lee KM, Cho SW, Kim SW, et al. Effect of virological response on post-treatment durability of lamivudine-induced HBeAg seroconversion. *J Viral Hepat*. 2002;9(3):208-212.
313. Perrillo R, Schiff E, Yoshida E, et al. Adefovir dipivoxil for the treatment of lamivudine-resistant hepatitis B mutants. *Hepatology*. 2000;32(1):129-134.
314. Marcellin P, Chang TT, Lim SG, et al. Adefovir dipivoxil for the treatment of hepatitis B e antigen-positive chronic hepatitis B. *N Engl J Med*. 2003;348(9):808-816.
315. Hadziyannis SJ, Tassopoulos NC, Heathcote EJ, et al. Adefovir dipivoxil for the treatment of hepatitis B e antigen-negative chronic hepatitis B. *N Engl J Med*. 2003;348(9):800-807.
316. Yang H, Westland CE, Delaney WE, et al. Resistance surveillance in chronic hepatitis B patients treated with adefovir dipivoxil for up to 60 weeks. *Hepatology*. 2002;36(2):464-473.
317. Angus P, Vaughan R, Xiong S, et al. Resistance to adefovir dipivoxil therapy associated with the selection of a novel mutation in the HBV polymerase. *Gastroenterology*. 2003;125(2):292-297.
318. Xiong X, Flores C, Yang H, et al. Mutations in hepatitis B DNA polymerase associated with resistance to lamivudine do not confer resistance to adefovir in vitro. *Hepatology*. 1998;28(6): 1669-1673.
319. Chang TT, Gish RG, de Man R, et al. A comparison of entecavir and lamivudine for HBeAg-positive chronic hepatitis B. *N Engl J Med*. 2006;354(10):1001-1010.
320. Gish RG, Lok AS, Chang TT, et al. Entecavir therapy for up to 96 weeks in patients with HBeAg-positive chronic hepatitis B. *Gastroenterology*. 2007;133(5):1437-1444.
321. Leung N, Peng CY, Hann HW, et al. Early hepatitis B virus DNA reduction in hepatitis B e antigen-positive patients with chronic hepatitis B: a randomized international study of entecavir versus adefovir. *Hepatology*. 2009;49(1):72-79.
322. McMahon MA, Jilek BL, Brennan TP, et al. The HBV drug entecavir—effects on HIV-1 replication and resistance. *N Engl J Med*. 2007;356(25):2614-2621.
323. Lai CL, Gane E, Liaw YF, et al. Telbivudine versus lamivudine in patients with chronic hepatitis B. *N Engl J Med*. 2007; 357(25):2576-2588.
324. Lai CL, Gane E, Liaw YF, et al. Globe Study Group. Telbivudine versus lamivudine in patients with chronic hepatitis B. *N Engl J Med*. 2007;357:2576-2588.
325. Marcellin P, Heathcote EJ, Buti M, et al. Tenofovir disoproxil fumarate versus adefovir dipivoxil for chronic hepatitis B. *N Engl J Med*. 2008;359(23):2442-2455.
326. Das K, Xiong X, Yang H, et al. Molecular modeling and biochemical characterization reveal the mechanism of hepatitis B virus polymerase resistance to lamivudine (3TC) and emtricitabine (FTC). *J Virol*. 2001;75(10):4771-4779.
327. Stuyver LJ, Locarnini SA, Lok A, et al. Nomenclature for antiviral-resistant human hepatitis B virus mutations in the polymerase region. *Hepatology*. 2001;33(3):751-757.
328. Ono SK, Kato N, Shiratori Y, et al. The polymerase L528M mutation cooperates with nucleotide binding-site mutations, increasing hepatitis B virus replication and drug resistance. *J Clin Invest*. 2001;107(4):449-455.
329. Bozdayi AM, Uzunalimoglu O, Turkyilmaz AR, et al. YSDD: a novel mutation in HBV DNA polymerase confers clinical resistance to lamivudine. *J Viral Hepat*. 2003;10(4):256-265.
330. Lok AS, Hussain M, Cursano C, et al. Evolution of hepatitis B virus polymerase gene mutations in hepatitis B e antigen-negative patients receiving lamivudine therapy. *Hepatology*. 2000;32(5):1145-1153.
331. Liaw YF, Gane E, Leung N, et al. 2-Year GLOBE trial results: telbivudine is superior to lamivudine in patients with chronic hepatitis B. *Gastroenterology*. 2009;136(2):486-495.
332. Seifer M, Patty A, Serra I, et al. Telbivudine, a nucleoside analog inhibitor of HBV polymerase, has a different in vitro cross-resistance profile than the nucleotide analog inhibitors adefovir and tenofovir. *Antiviral Res*. 2009;81(2):147-155.
333. Tenney DJ, Rose RE, Baldick CJ, et al. Long-term monitoring shows hepatitis B virus resistance to entecavir in nucleoside-naive patients is rare through 5 years of therapy. *Hepatology*. 2009;49:1503-1514.
334. Chen CH, Wang JH, Lee CM, et al. Virological response and incidence of adefovir resistance in lamivudine-resistant patients treated with adefovir dipivoxil. *Antivir Ther*. 2006;11(6):771-778.
335. Villet S, Pichoud C, Billioud G, et al. Impact of hepatitis B virus rtA181V/T mutants on hepatitis B treatment failure. *J Hepatol*. 2008;48(5):747-755.
336. Liaw YF. Acute exacerbation and superinfection in patients with chronic viral hepatitis. *J Formos Med Assoc*. 1995;94(9):521-528.
337. Yim HJ, Hussain M, Liu Y, et al. Evolution of multi-drug resistant hepatitis B virus during sequential therapy. *Hepatology*. 2006;44(3):703-712.
338. Kuo A, Dienstag JL, Chung RT. Tenofovir disoproxil fumarate for the treatment of lamivudine-resistant hepatitis B. *Clin Gastroenterol Hepatol*. 2004;2(3):266-272.
339. Yatsuji H, Suzuki F, Sezaki H, et al. Low risk of adefovir resistance in lamivudine-resistant chronic hepatitis B patients treated with adefovir plus lamivudine combination therapy: two-year follow-up. *J Hepatol*. 2008;48(6):923-931.
340. Lampertico P, Vigano M, Manenti E, et al. Low resistance to adefovir combined with lamivudine: a 3-year study of 145 lamivudine-resistant hepatitis B patients. *Gastroenterology*. 2007;133(5):1445-1451.
341. van Bommel F, Zollner B, Sarrazin C, et al. Tenofovir for patients with lamivudine-resistant hepatitis B virus (HBV) infection and high HBV DNA level during adefovir therapy. *Hepatology*. 2006;44(2):318-325.
342. Torresi J, Earnest Silveira L, Deliyannis G, et al. Reduced antigenicity of the hepatitis B virus HBsAg protein arising as a consequence of sequence changes in the overlapping polymerase gene that are selected by lamivudine therapy. *Virology*. 2005; 293(2):305-313.
343. Yoo BC, Kim JH, Kim TH, et al. Clevudine is highly efficacious in hepatitis B e antigen-negative chronic hepatitis B with durable off-therapy viral suppression. *Hepatology*. 2007;46(4):1041-1048.
344. Marcellin P, Lau GK, Bonino F, et al. Peginterferon alfa-2a alone, lamivudine alone, and the two in combination in patients with HBeAg-negative chronic hepatitis B. *N Engl J Med*. 2004; 351(12):1206-1217.
345. Menne S, Butler SD, George AL, et al. Antiviral effects of lamivudine, emtricitabine, adefovir dipivoxil, and tenofovir disoproxil fumarate administered orally alone and in combination to woodchucks with chronic woodchuck hepatitis virus infection. *Antimicrob Agents Chemother*. 2008;52(10):3617-3632.
346. Sung JJ, Lai JY, Zeuzem S, et al. Lamivudine compared with lamivudine and adefovir dipivoxil for the treatment of HBeAg-positive chronic hepatitis B. *J Hepatol*. 2008;48(5): 728-735.
347. Hui CK, Zhang HY, Bowden S, et al. 96 weeks combination of adefovir dipivoxil plus emtricitabine vs. adefovir dipivoxil monotherapy in the treatment of chronic hepatitis B. *J Hepatol*. 2008;48(5):714-720.
348. Lai CL, Leung N, Teo EK, et al. A 1-year trial of telbivudine, lamivudine, and the combination in patients with hepatitis B e antigen-positive chronic hepatitis B. *Gastroenterology*. 2005; 129(2):528-536.
349. Ghany MG, Ayola B, Villamil FG, et al. Hepatitis B virus S mutants in liver transplant recipients who were reinfected despite hepatitis B immune globulin prophylaxis. *Hepatology*. 1998;27(1):213-222.
350. Perrillo RP, Wright T, Rakela J, et al. A multicenter United States-Canadian trial to assess lamivudine monotherapy before and after liver transplantation for chronic hepatitis B. *Hepatology*. 2001;33(2):424-432.
351. Lok AS. Prevention of recurrent hepatitis B post-liver transplantation. *Liver Transpl*. 2002;8(10 Suppl 1):S67-S73.
352. Loomba R, Rowley AK, Wesley R, et al. Hepatitis B immunoglobulin and lamivudine improve hepatitis B–related outcomes after liver transplantation: meta-analysis. *Clin Gastroenterol Hepatol*. 2008;6(6):696-700.
353. Gane EJ, Angus PW, Strasser S, et al. Lamivudine plus low-dose hepatitis B immunoglobulin to prevent recurrent hepatitis B following liver transplantation. *Gastroenterology*. 2007;132(3): 931-937.
354. Locarnini S, McMillan J, Bartholomeusz A. The hepatitis B virus and common mutants. *Semin Liver Dis*. 2003;23(1):5-20.
355. Bock CT, Tillmann HL, Torresi J, et al. Selection of hepatitis B virus polymerase mutants with enhanced replication by lamivudine treatment after liver transplantation. *Gastroenterology*. 2002;122(2):264-273.
356. Seehofer D, Rayes N, Steinmuller T, et al. Occurrence and clinical outcome of lamivudine-resistant hepatitis B infection after liver transplantation. *Liver Transpl*. 2001;7(11):976-982.
357. Osborn MK, Han SH, Regev A, et al. Outcomes of patients with hepatitis B who developed antiviral resistance while on the liver transplant waiting list. *Clin Gastroenterol Hepatol*. 2007;5(12): 1454-1461.
358. Mutimer D, Feraz-Neto BH, Harrison R, et al. Acute liver graft failure due to emergence of lamivudine resistant hepatitis B virus: rapid resolution during treatment with adefovir. *Gut*. 2001;49(6):860-863.
359. Angus PW, Patterson SJ, Strasser SI, et al. A randomized study of adefovir dipivoxil in place of HBIG in combination with lamivudine as post-liver transplantation hepatitis B prophylaxis. *Hepatology*. 2008;48(5):1460-1466.
360. Matthews GV, Avihingsanon A, Lewin SR, et al. A randomized trial of combination hepatitis B therapy in HIV/HBV coinfected antiretroviral naive individuals in Thailand. *Hepatology*. 2008; 48(4):1062-1069.
361. Peters MG, Andersen J, Lynch P, et al. Randomized controlled study of tenofovir and adefovir in chronic hepatitis B virus and HIV infection: ACTG A5127. *Hepatology*. 2006;44(5):1110-1116.
362. Matthews GV, Bartholomeusz A, Locarnini S, et al. Characteristics of drug resistant HBV in an international collaborative study of HIV-HBV-infected individuals on extended lamivudine therapy. *AIDS*. 2006;20(6):863-870.
363. Yeo W, Chan PK, Zhong S, et al. Frequency of hepatitis B virus reactivation in cancer patients undergoing cytotoxic chemotherapy: a prospective study of 626 patients with identification of risk factors. *J Med Virol*. 2000;62(3):299-307.
364. Yeo W, Chan PK, Chan HL, et al. Hepatitis B virus reactivation during cytotoxic chemotherapy-enhanced viral replication precedes overt hepatitis. *J Med Virol*. 2001;65(3):473-477.
365. Hui CK, Cheung WW, Zhang HY, et al. Kinetics and risk of de novo hepatitis B infection in HBsAg-negative patients undergoing cytotoxic chemotherapy. *Gastroenterology*. 2006;131(1): 59-68.
366. Hui CK, Cheung WW, Zhang HY, et al. Kinetics and risk of de novo hepatitis B infection in HBsAg-negative patients undergo-

ing cytotoxic chemotherapy. *Gastroenterology.* 2006;131(1): 59-68.

367. Idilkerman R, Arat M, Soydan E, et al. Lamivudine prophylaxis for prevention of chemotherapy-induced hepatitis B virus reactivation in hepatitis B virus carriers with malignancies. *J Viral Hepat.* 2004;11(2):141-147.

368. Shibolet O, Ilan Y, Gillis S, et al. Lamivudine therapy for prevention of immunosuppressive-induced hepatitis B virus reactivation in hepatitis B surface antigen carriers. *Blood.* 2002;100(2): 391-396.

369. Hui CK, Cheung WW, Au WY, et al. Hepatitis B reactivation after withdrawal of pre-emptive lamivudine in patients with haematological malignancy on completion of cytotoxic chemotherapy. *Gut.* 2005;54(11):1597-1603.

370. Lau DT, Doo E, Park Y, et al. Lamivudine for chronic delta hepatitis. *Hepatology.* 1999;30(2):546-549.

371. Villa E, Grottola A, Buttafoco P, et al. High doses of alpha-interferon are required in chronic hepatitis due to coinfection with hepatitis B virus and hepatitis C virus: long term results of a prospective randomized trial. *Am J Gastroenterol.* 2001;96(10): 2973-2977.

372. Farci P, Mandas A, Coiana A, et al. Treatment of chronic hepatitis D with interferon alfa-2a. *N Engl J Med.* 1994;330(2):88-94.

373. Prevention of hepatitis A through active or passive immunization: recommendations of the Advisory Committee on Immunization Practices (ACIP). *MMWR Recomm Rep.* 1996; 45(RR-15):1-30.

374. Keeffe EB. Is hepatitis A more severe in patients with chronic hepatitis B and other chronic liver diseases? *Am J Gastroenterol.* 1995;90(2):201-205.

375. Vento S, Garofano T, Renzini C, et al. Fulminant hepatitis associated with hepatitis A virus superinfection in patients with chronic hepatitis C. *N Engl J Med.* 1998;338(5):286-290.

376. Corden S, Ballard AL, Ijaz S, et al. HBV DNA levels and transmission of hepatitis B by health care workers. *J Clin Virol.* 2003;27(1):52-58.

377. Transmission of hepatitis B to patients from four infected surgeons without hepatitis B e antigen. The Incident Investigation Teams and others. *N Engl J Med.* 1997;336(3):178-184.

378. Spijkerman IJ, van Doorn LJ, Janssen MH, et al. Transmission of hepatitis B virus from a surgeon to his patients during high-risk and low-risk surgical procedures during 4 years. *Infect Control Hosp Epidemiol.* 2002;23(6):306-312.

379. Leads from the MMWR. Update: universal precautions for prevention of transmission of human immunodeficiency virus, hepatitis B virus, and other bloodborne pathogens in health-care settings. *JAMA.* 1988;260(4):462-465.

380. Management of healthcare workers infected with hepatitis B virus, hepatitis C virus, human immunodeficiency virus, or other bloodborne pathogens. AIDS/TB Committee of the Society for Healthcare Epidemiology of America. *Infect Control Hosp Epidemiol.* 1997;18(5):349-363.

381. Proceedings of the Consensus Conference on Infected Health Care Worker Risk for transmission of bloodborne pathogens. *Can Commun Dis Rep.* 1998;24(Suppl 4):i-iii, 1-25; i-iii, 1-28.

382. Mele A, Ippolito G, Craxi A, et al. Risk management of HBsAg or anti-HCV positive healthcare workers in hospital. *Dig Liver Dis.* 2001;33(9):795-802.

383. Bruix J, Sherman M. Management of hepatocellular carcinoma. *Hepatology.* 2005;42(5):1208-1236.

384. Chang MH, Chen CJ, Lai MS, et al. Universal hepatitis B vaccination in Taiwan and the incidence of hepatocellular carcinoma in children. Taiwan Childhood Hepatoma Study Group. *N Engl J Med.* 1997;336(26):1855-1859.

385. Recommendation of the Immunization Practices Advisory Committee (ACIP) post-exposure prophylaxis of hepatitis B. *MMWR Morb Mortal Wkly Rep.* 1984;33(21):285-290.

386. Implementation of newborn hepatitis B vaccination—worldwide, 2006. *MMWR Morb Mortal Wkly Rep.* 2008;57(46): 1249-1252.

387. Alternate two dose hepatitis B vaccination schedule for adolescents aged 11 to 15 years. *MMWR Morb Mortal Wkly Rep.* 2000;49:261.

388. Lindsay KL, Herbert DA, Gitnick GL. Hepatitis B vaccine: low postvaccination immunity in hospital personnel given gluteal injections. *Hepatology.* 1985;5(6):1088-1090.

389. Herroelen L, de Keyser J, Ebinger G. Central-nervous-system demyelination after immunisation with recombinant hepatitis B vaccine. *Lancet.* 1991;338(8776):1174-1175.

390. Ascherio A, Zhang SM, Hernan MA, et al. Hepatitis B vaccination and the risk of multiple sclerosis. *N Engl J Med.* 2001;344(5):327-332.

391. DeStefano F, Verstraeten T, Jackson LA, et al. Vaccinations and risk of central nervous system demyelinating diseases in adults. *Arch Neurol.* 2003;60(4):504-509.

392. Stevens CE, Taylor PE, Tong MJ, et al. Yeast-recombinant hepatitis B vaccine: efficacy with hepatitis B immune globulin in prevention of perinatal hepatitis B virus transmission. *JAMA.* 1987;257(19):2612-2616.

393. Stevens CE, Toy PT, Tong MJ, et al. Perinatal hepatitis B virus transmission in the United States: prevention by passive-active immunization. *JAMA.* 1985;253(12):1740-1745.

394. Wong VC, Ip HM, Reesink HW, et al. Prevention of the HBsAg carrier state in newborn infants of mothers who are chronic carriers of HBsAg and HBeAg by administration of hepatitis-B vaccine and hepatitis-B immunoglobulin: double-blind randomised placebo-controlled study. *Lancet.* 1984;1(8383):921-926.

395. Beasley RP, Stevens CE, Shiao IS, et al. Evidence against breastfeeding as a mechanism for vertical transmission of hepatitis B. *Lancet.* 1975;2(7938):740-741.

396. van Zonneveld M, van Nunen AB, Niesters HG, et al. Lamivudine treatment during pregnancy to prevent perinatal transmission of hepatitis B virus infection. *J Viral Hepat.* 2003;10(4): 294-297.

397. Hadler SC, Francis DP, Maynard JE, et al. Long-term immunogenicity and efficacy of hepatitis B vaccine in homosexual men. *N Engl J Med.* 1986;315(4):209-214.

398. Ni YH, Huang LM, Chang MH, et al. Two decades of universal hepatitis B vaccination in Taiwan: impact and implication for future strategies. *Gastroenterology.* 2007;132(4):1287-1293.

399. Propst T, Propst A, Lhotta K, et al. Reinforced intradermal hepatitis B vaccination in hemodialysis patients is superior in antibody response to intramuscular or subcutaneous vaccination. *Am J Kidney Dis.* 1998;32(6):1041-1045.

400. Wong EK, Bodsworth NJ, Slade MA, et al. Response to hepatitis B vaccination in a primary care setting: influence of HIV infection, CD4+ lymphocyte count and vaccination schedule. *Int J STD AIDS.* 1996;7(7):490-494.

401. Collier AC, Corey L, Murphy VL, et al. Antibody to human immunodeficiency virus (HIV) and suboptimal response to hepatitis B vaccination. *Ann Intern Med.* 1988;109(2):101-105.

402. Waite NM, Thomson LG, Goldstein MB. Successful vaccination with intradermal hepatitis B vaccine in hemodialysis patients previously nonresponsive to intramuscular hepatitis B vaccine. *J Am Soc Nephrol.* 1995;5(11):1930-1934.

403. Valdez H, Mitsuyasu R, Landay A, et al. Interleukin-2 increases CD4+ lymphocyte numbers but does not enhance responses to immunization: results of A5046s. *J Infect Dis.* 2003;187(2): 320-325.

404. Alper CA, Kruskall MS, Marcus-Bagley D, et al. Genetic prediction of nonresponse to hepatitis B vaccine. *N Engl J Med.* 1989;321(11):708-712.

405. Ding L, Zhang M, Wang Y, et al. A 9-year follow-up study of the immunogenicity and long-term efficacy of plasma-derived hepatitis B vaccine in high-risk Chinese neonates. *Clin Infect Dis.* 1993;17(3):475-479.

406. Da Villa G, Peluso F, Picciotto L, et al. Persistence of anti-HBs in children vaccinated against viral hepatitis B in the first year of life: follow-up at 5 and 10 years. *Vaccine.* 1996;14(16):1503-1505.

407. Wu JS, Hwang LY, Goodman KJ, et al. Hepatitis B vaccination in high-risk infants: 10-year follow-up. *J Infect Dis.* 1999; 179(6):1319-1325.

408. Williams IT, Goldstein ST, Tufa J, et al. Long-term antibody response to hepatitis B vaccination beginning at birth and to subsequent booster vaccination. *Pediatr Infect Dis J.* 2003; 22(2):157-163.

409. Saab S, Weston SR, Ly D, et al. Comparison of the cost and effectiveness of two strategies for maintaining hepatitis B immunity in hemodialysis patients. *Vaccine.* 2002;20(25-26):3230-3235.

410. Workowski KA, Berman SM. Sexually transmitted diseases treatment guidelines, 2006. *MMWR Recomm Rep.* 2006; 55(RR-11):1-94.

411. Carman WF, Zanetti AR, Karayiannis P, et al. Vaccine-induced escape mutant of hepatitis B virus. *Lancet.* 1990;336(8711):325-329.

412. Carman WF, Trautwein C, van Deursen FJ, et al. Hepatitis B virus envelope variation after transplantation with and without hepatitis B immune globulin prophylaxis. *Hepatology.* 1996; 24(3):489-493.

413. Hsu HY, Chang MH, Liaw SH, et al. Changes of hepatitis B surface antigen variants in carrier children before and after universal vaccination in Taiwan. *Hepatology.* 1999;30(5):1312-1317.

414. He C, Nomura F, Itoga S, et al. Prevalence of vaccine-induced escape mutants of hepatitis B virus in the adult population in China: a prospective study in 176 restaurant employees. *J Gastroenterol Hepatol.* 2001;16(12):1373-1377.

415. Ogata N, Cote PJ, Zanetti AR, et al. Licensed recombinant hepatitis B vaccines protect chimpanzees against infection with the prototype surface gene mutant of hepatitis B virus. *Hepatology.* 1999;30(3):779-786.

416. Torresi J, Earnest-Silveira L, Deliyannis G, et al. Reduced antigenicity of the hepatitis B virus HBsAg protein arising as a consequence of sequence changes in the overlapping polymerase gene that are selected by lamivudine therapy. *Virology.* 2002; 293(2):305-313.

147

Human Parvoviruses, Including Parvovirus B19 and Human Bocavirus

KEVIN E. BROWN

Parvum is Latin for small, and Parvoviridae are among the smallest known DNA-containing viruses that infect mammalian cells. The virions are nonenveloped particles about 22 nm in diameter with icosahedral symmetry. The Parvoviridae are divided into two subfamilies, Parvovirinae and Densovirinae, on the basis of their ability to infect vertebrate or invertebrate cells, respectively. The Parvovirinae are further subdivided into five genera on the basis of their transcription map, their ability to replicate efficiently either autonomously or with helper virus, and their sequence homology. The five genera are: *Parvovirus, Dependovirus, Erythrovirus, Bocavirus,* and *Amdovirus.*[1]

At least four different parvoviruses are known to infect humans. Parvovirus B19 (B19V) is the best characterized, and is classified as a member of the *Erythrovirus* genus, of which it is the type species. The other human viruses are the human adeno-associated viruses (AAVs, or dependoviruses), human bocavirus (HBoV), and human parvovirus 4. The last two viruses have not officially been classified yet, but HBoV is clearly a member of the *Bocavirus* genus, whereas human parvovirus 4 is markedly different from all other known viruses, and will probably become part of a new genus.

Parvovirus B19 (B19V)

B19V was discovered in 1974 during evaluations of assays for hepatitis B surface antigen using panels of serum samples.[2] Sample 19 in panel B (hence B19) gave an anomalous result, a "false positive" in the relatively insensitive counterimmunoelectrophoresis assay, and when the precipitin line was excised, electron microscopy showed the presence of 23-nm particles resembling parvoviruses. Although originally labeled serum parvovirus-like particle or human parvovirus, in 1985 the virus was officially recognized as a member of the Parvoviridae, and the International Committee on Taxonomy of Viruses recommended the name B19V to prevent confusion with other viruses.

An association of B19V with significant clinical disease was not made until 1981, but it is now known that B19V infection has a wide variety of disease manifestations dependent on the immunologic and hematologic status of the host (Table 147-1). In normal immunocompetent children, B19V is the cause of erythema infectiosum (EI), also called fifth disease or "slapped cheek" disease, which is an innocuous illness with rash. Occasionally, especially in women, fifth disease leads to an acute symmetrical polyarthropathy, which can mimic rheumatoid arthritis. In persons with underlying hemolytic disorders or increased erythropoiesis, or both, infection leads to a temporary failure of red blood cell production and transient aplastic crisis (TAC). In the immunocompromised host, persistent B19V viremia manifests as pure red cell aplasia (PRCA) and chronic anemia, and in the fetus, in which the immune response is immature, infection may lead to fetal death in utero, hydrops fetalis, or rarely the development of congenital anemia.

The Virus

By electron microscopy, B19V particles have the typical parvovirus morphology (Fig. 147-1). Mature infectious particles have a molecular weight of 5.6×10^6 and a buoyant density in cesium chloride gradients of 1.41 g/mL. As a consequence of the lack of envelope and limited DNA content, B19V is resistant to physical inactivation. Although the virus can be inactivated by heat in low concentrations of protein,[3] the virus resists inactivation at 56° C for more than 60 minutes, and at high viral concentrations, it resists 80° C for 72 hours in clotting factor concentrates.[4] B19V is stable in lipid solvents such as ether and chloroform but can be inactivated by formalin, β-propiolactone, oxidizing agents, and γ-irradiation.

The B19V genome size is limited, consisting of a single strand of DNA of approximately 5600 nucleotides, with identical inverted, 365-nucleotide-long terminal repeat sequences at each end. The transcription map of B19V distinguishes it from other Parvovirinae. There is a single strong promoter at the far left side of the genome and unusual polyadenylation signals in the middle of the genome.[5] The three major viral proteins, one nonstructural protein and two capsid proteins, are produced by alternative splicing from the promoter and its accompanying leader sequence. The relative quantities of the major and minor capsid proteins are in part regulated by the presence of multiple upstream AUG codons situated before the authentic transcription initiation codon.[6] In addition, there are transcripts for several smaller proteins of 7.5 and 11 kD. Although the 11-kD protein is known to be required for producing infectious virus, the role of the 7.5-kD protein is unknown.[7]

The only unspliced transcript encodes the nonstructural protein, a 78-kD phosphoprotein.[8] Consistent with its role in viral propagation, the protein has DNA-binding properties and adenosine and guanosine triphosphatase activity.[9] Expression of the nonstructural protein causes host cell death through induction of apoptosis.[10]

The B19V virion is an icosahedron consisting of 60 copies of the capsid proteins. Most of the capsid is VP2, a 58-kD protein, with 5% or less of the larger 84-kD, VP1 protein. VP1 protein differs from VP2 by an additional 227 amino acids at the amino terminus. Using genetic engineering techniques, the capsid proteins can be expressed in a variety of mammalian,[11] insect,[12,13] and yeast[14] cell lines. Capsid proteins self-assemble in the absence of B19V DNA, and in these systems protein expression leads to formation of recombinant empty capsids; VP1 is not required for capsid formation.

The atomic structure of both B19V VP2 empty capsids and infectious virus has been resolved.[15,16] The virion surface has a major depression encompassing the fivefold axis, similar to the canyon structure found in RNA-containing icosahedral viruses. In B19V capsids, there is also a hollow cylindrical structure around the fivefold axes that appears to penetrate to the inside of the virion. The structural distribution of VP1 in the B19V capsid structure cannot be inferred from the crystallographic structures, but on the basis of antibody-binding and structural studies, in infectious B19V the VP1 unique region appears to be exposed on the viral surface adjacent to the fivefold axis cylinder.[16] It has been shown that the VP1 unique region of all parvoviruses, including B19V, has a phospholipase A_2 motif.[17] Infection studies with B19V (and other parvoviruses) show that this motif is required for viral infectivity.[17,18]

It is now recognized that there are three different genotypes, with approximately 10% variability at the DNA level between them.[19] Most of the B19V identified is genotype 1,[20] the original B19V genotype, and is distributed worldwide. Genotype 3 seems to be the predominant B19V genotype in Ghana, representing more than 90% of the sequences identified.[21] Genotype 2 has been primarily identified in tissues of older

TABLE 147-1	Disease Manifestations and Persistence of Parvovirus B19 Infection in Different Host Populations	
Disease	*Acute or Chronic*	*Host*
Fifth disease	Acute	Normal children
Polyarthropathy syndrome	Acute or chronic	Normal adults
Transient aplastic crisis	Acute	Patients with increased erythropoiesis
Hydrops fetalis or congenital anemia	Acute or chronic	Fetus (<20 wk)
Persistent anemia	Chronic	Immunodeficient or immunocompromised patients

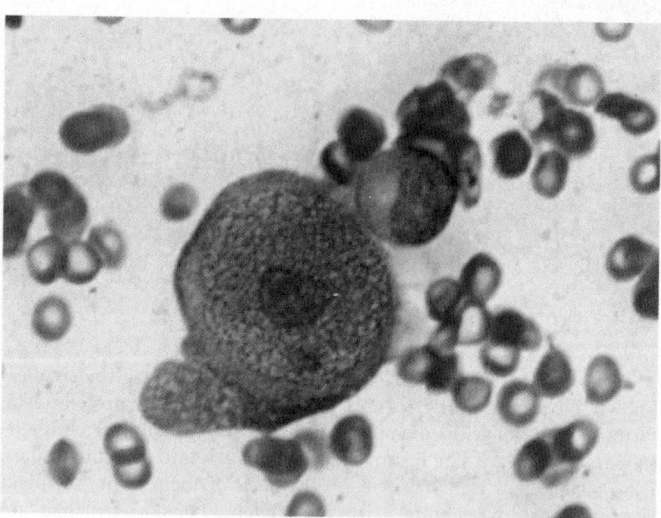

Figure 147-2 Giant pronormoblast in patient with B19 infection.

patients (born before 1973), suggesting that it may have circulated more frequently prior to the 1970s.[22] However, blood samples or donations containing high-titer genotype 2 are occasionally identified,[23] and genotype 2 and 3 sequences have been identified in blood and tissues from many different parts of the world,[24-27] suggesting a more widespread distribution than originally assumed. However, the true prevalence of these different genotypes is currently unknown.

Despite the differences in the DNA sequences, the capsid protein sequence is conserved between the different genotypes, and there is evidence for both serologic and cross-neutralization.[23,28,29]

Pathogenesis

Parvovirus B19, like the other autonomous parvoviruses, is dependent on mitotically active cells for replication. However, B19V has a very narrow target cell range and can be propagated efficiently only in human erythroid progenitor cells. The virus cannot be easily cultivated in the laboratory, apart from in primary erythroblasts.[30] Humans are the only known host of parvovirus B19; all primates tested are resistant to B19V infection, although primates have their own related erythroviruses.[31]

In human erythroid cells derived from bone marrow, susceptibility to parvovirus B19 increases with differentiation; the pluripotent stem cell appears to be spared, and the main target cells are erythroid progenitors (cells capable of giving rise to erythroid colonies in vitro) and CD 36-positive erythroblasts.[31,32] Infection with parvovirus B19 is cytotoxic[33] because of expression of the nonstructural protein in infected cells.[34] Infected cultures are characterized by the presence of giant

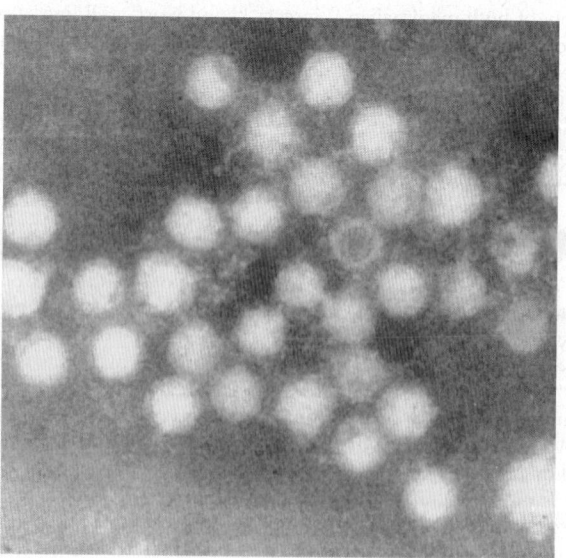

Figure 147-1 Electron micrograph of parvovirus B19 particles showing icosahedral symmetry. *(Electron micrograph courtesy of Dr. Anne Field.)*

pronormoblasts, 25 to 32 μm in diameter, with cytoplasmic vacuolization, immature chromatin, and large eosinophilic nuclear inclusion bodies (Fig. 147-2). By electron microscopy, virus particles are seen in the nucleus and cytoplasmic membrane lining, and infected cells show marginated chromatin, pseudopod formation, and cytoplasmic vacuolation,[34] all of which are typical of cells undergoing apoptosis.

Erythroid specificity of parvovirus B19 is, in part, due to the tissue distribution of the virus's cellular receptor globoside, also known as blood group P antigen.[34] P antigen is found on erythroid progenitors, erythroblasts, and megakaryocytes.[35] It is also present on endothelial cells, which may be targets of viral infection involved in the pathogenesis of transplacental transmission, possibly vasculitis, and the rash of fifth disease and on fetal myocardial cells. Rare individuals who genetically lack P antigen on erythrocytes are resistant to B19V infection, and their bone marrow cannot be infected with B19V in vitro.[36] However, although P antigen is required for infection, it is not sufficient for viral entry, and additional B19V receptors have been proposed as putative cellular receptors.[37,38] In addition, the erythroid specificity may also be modulated by specific erythroid cell transcription factors.

Studies in healthy volunteers showed that B19V infection led to an acute but self-limited (4 to 8 days) cessation of red cell production and a corresponding decline in hemoglobin level.[39] In patients with normal erythroid turnover, this short interruption of red cell production does not lead to anemia, but in patients with high red cell turnover related to hemolysis, blood loss, or other causes, the temporary failure of erythropoiesis can precipitate an aplastic crisis. The anemia improves as the immune response develops. In patients who are immunocompromised, infection may persist and produce chronic PRCA.

The infected fetus may suffer severe effects because red blood cell turnover is high and the immune response deficient. During the second trimester there is a great increase in red cell mass. Parvovirus particles can be detected by electron microscopy within the hematopoietic tissues of the liver and thymus.[40] B19V DNA and capsid antigen have been detected in the myocardium of infected fetuses,[41] and there is evidence that the fetus may develop myocarditis,[42] compounding the severe anemia and secondary cardiac failure. By the third trimester, a more effective fetal immune response to the virus probably accounts for the decrease in fetal loss at this stage of pregnancy.

The pathogenesis of the rash in EI and polyarthropathy is almost certainly immune complex mediated (Fig. 147-3). In volunteer studies, these appeared when high-titer viremia was no longer detectable and coincident with a detectable immune response.[39] Similar findings have been reported in chronically infected individuals who received immunoglobulin therapy.[43] However, in vitro studies have shown that the

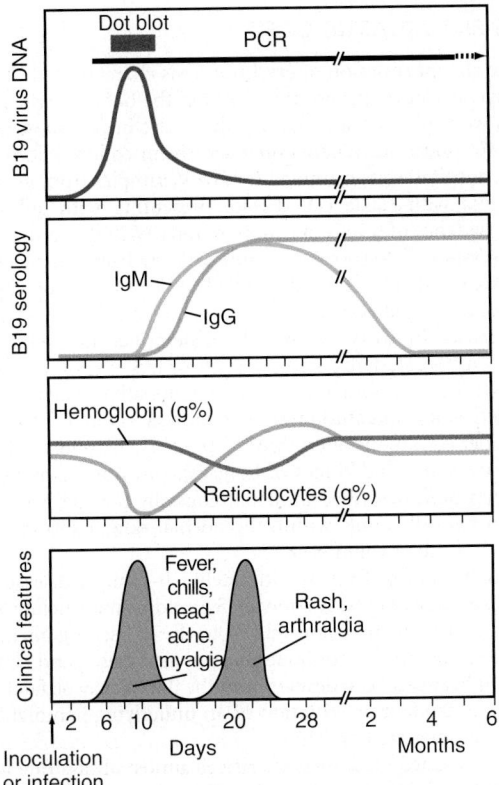

Figure 147-3 **Virologic, immunologic, and clinical courses after acute B19 infection in a healthy individual.** IgG, immunoglobulin G; PCR, polymerase chain reaction. *(From Anderson MJ, Higgins PG, Davis LR, et al. Experimental parvoviral infection in humans. J Infect Dis. 1985;152:257-265; Patou G, Pillay D, Myint S, Pattison J. Characterization of a nested polymerase chain reaction assay for detection of parvovirus B19. J Clin Microbiol. 1993;31:540-546.)*

B19V nonstructural protein not only induces apoptosis in host cells but also induces activation of interleukin-6,[41] and the phospholipase motif in the VP1u region is functional[44]; both of these findings could contribute in vivo to the B19-induced arthropathy.

Epidemiology

PREVALENCE AND INCIDENCE

Parvovirus B19 infection is common in childhood, and by age 15 years approximately 50% of children have detectable immunoglobulin G (IgG) against B19V. Infection also occurs in adult life, and more than 80% of elderly people have detectable antibody.[45] Women of childbearing age in the United States and Europe have an annual seroconversion rate of approximately 1%.[46,47] Studies in different countries (France, Germany, Japan, the United Kingdom, and the United States) show similar patterns, with a slightly higher prevalence in children from countries such as Africa and Brazil. Some isolated tribal populations have a much lower prevalence: 2% on Rodriguez Island, Africa,[48] and 4% to 10% among the tribes around Belem, Brazil.[49]

Although antibody is prevalent in the general population, high-titer viremia (>10⁹ genome copies/mL) is rare: approximately 1 per 20,000 to 1 per 40,000 units of blood during epidemic seasons contains high-titer B19V.[46] However, estimates of the prevalence of lower levels of B19V DNA vary widely depending on the sensitivity of the method used,[50] with approximately 1% of donations having detectable B19V DNA by sensitive polymerase chain reaction (PCR).[51] The significance of these low levels of B19V DNA in blood samples is unknown.[50]

MECHANISM AND ROUTES OF TRANSMISSION

Parvovirus B19 infections in temperate climates are more common in the late winter, spring, and early summer months.[52] Rates of infection may also increase every 3 to 4 years, as reflected by corresponding increases in the major clinical manifestations of B19V infection, TACs, and EI.[53,54]

B19V DNA has been found in the respiratory secretions of patients at the time of viremia,[55] suggesting that infection is generally spread by a respiratory route of transmission. The virus can be readily transmitted by close contact, and the secondary attack rate has been calculated in various settings; in one study, the rate of secondary attack from symptomatic TAC or EI patients to susceptible (IgG-negative) household contacts was approximately 50%.[55] For school outbreaks, serologic studies are generally not available, but 10% to 60% of students may develop a rash consistent with B19V infection.[56,57] The highest secondary attack rates and annual seroconversion rates, even in the absence of known community outbreaks, are for workers in close contact with affected children, such as daycare providers and school personnel.[58] Nosocomial transmission in hospital situations has been described[59] but is probably infrequent, especially from patients with chronic infection. Nevertheless, patients with TAC or persistent disease should be considered infectious and appropriate precautions taken to limit interaction with other patients and susceptible staff.

The virus can be found in serum, and infection can be transmitted by blood and blood products[60] including albumin and plasma.[61,62] As described previously, parvoviruses, including B19V, are very heat resistant, and they can withstand the usual thermal treatment aimed at infectious agents in blood products. In addition, solvent-detergent methods, which inactivate only lipid-enveloped viruses, are ineffective. B19V infection has been transmitted by steam-treated, dry-heated, and solvent-detergent-treated factors, although hemophiliacs who received heat-treated factor VIII alone had a lower prevalence of B19V antibody and lower rates of seroconversion than those receiving non-heat-treated factor.[63]

Clinical Manifestations

ERYTHEMA INFECTIOSUM

Manifestations of parvovirus B19 infection vary, even in the normal host, from asymptomatic or subclinical infection (most people with B19V specific antibody have no recollection of any specific symptoms) to a biphasic illness with symptoms during the viremic and immune complex-mediated stages of the disease, but EI is the major manifestation. EI was well characterized clinically before the discovery of B19V.[64] This exanthematous rash illness of childhood was probably first described by Robert Willan in 1799 and illustrated in his 1808 textbook. The disease was rediscovered in Germany, where in 1899 Sticker termed it *erythema infectiosum*, and 6 years later Cheinisse classified it as the "fifth rash disease" of the six classic exanthems of childhood.[65] Often the epidemiologic data suggested "a common-source exposure to a highly effective transmitter," and an atypical rubella virus or echovirus was thought to be responsible. However, neither virus could be reproducibly isolated from patients with fifth disease. In 1983, after an outbreak of EI in London, all 31 affected children or adolescents had anti-B19-specific IgM.[66] Similar results were obtained in other epidemics of fifth disease, and parvovirus B19 is now recognized as the etiologic agent.

Clinical symptoms begin with a nonspecific prodromal illness, which often goes unrecognized; there may be symptoms of fever, coryza, headache, and mild gastrointestinal distress, including nausea and diarrhea. In 2 to 5 days, the classic "slapped cheek" rash appears, a fiery red eruption on the cheek, accompanied by relative circumoral pallor (Fig. 147-4). There may be a second-stage rash within a few days, and an erythematous maculopapular exanthem on the trunk and limbs; as this eruption fades, it produces a typical lacy appearance. There is great variation in the dermatologic symptoms: the classic

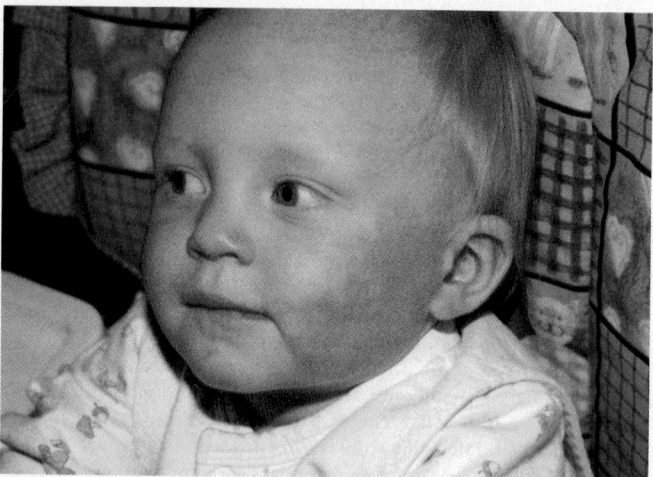

Figure 147-4 Slapped-cheek appearance of a child with fifth disease.

slapped cheek is much more common in children than adults; the second-stage eruption may vary from a very faint, barely perceptible erythema to a florid exanthem; and the rash may be transient or recurrent for weeks. Rarely, other dermatologic presentations are seen: vesicopustular rash,[67] papular-purpuric glove and sock syndrome,[68] other purpuric rashes with or without Koplik spots,[69,70] and erythema multiforme.[71] Pruritus, especially on the soles of the feet, can be the dominant symptom.[72]

ARTHROPATHY

Although B19V infection in children is usually mild and of short duration, a large proportion of adults, especially women, suffer arthralgia or frank arthritis, with painful joints often accompanied by swelling and stiffness.[57] The arthralgia is usually symmetrical, with mainly the small joints of hands and feet involved, and generally lasts for 1 to 3 weeks, although it may persist or recur for months or even years. In the absence of a history of rash, the symptoms may be mistaken for those of acute rheumatoid arthritis, especially because prolonged symptoms do not correlate with serologic studies, such as the duration of B19V IgM response, or persistent viremia. In addition, B19V infection can be associated with transient rheumatoid factor production.[73] In one large study of patients attending an "early synovitis" clinic in England, 12% had evidence of recent infection with B19V.[74] Three patients would have fulfilled the American Rheumatism Association's diagnostic criteria for definite rheumatoid arthritis. B19V infection should be considered as part of the differential diagnosis in any patient presenting with acute arthritis.

It has been postulated that B19V is involved in the initiation and perpetuation of rheumatoid arthritis leading to joint lesions,[75] but these results have not been reproducible by other groups. In contrast, parvoviral B19V DNA is frequently found in synovial tissue of patients with rheumatoid arthritis, chronic arthropathy, and control subjects. In one carefully performed controlled study, although B19V DNA was indeed detected in synovial tissue of 28% of individuals with chronic arthritis, it was also found in 48% of nonarthropathy controls,[76] indicating that PCR-detectable DNA may persist in synovial tissues for months or years. In addition, in one study with long-term follow-up, none of the 54 patients with B19-associated arthralgia reported persistence of joint swelling or restricted motion, and no evidence of inflammatory joint disease was found.[77] Therefore, it seems unlikely that B19V plays a role in classic erosive rheumatoid arthritis. The association of B19V and juvenile rheumatic disease is more convincing,[78] but whether it is the cause of the disease or one of many potential triggers is less clear.

TRANSIENT APLASTIC CRISIS

TAC, the abrupt cessation of erythropoiesis characterized by reticulocytopenia, absent erythroid precursors in the bone marrow, and precipitous worsening of anemia, was the first clinical illness associated with B19V infection. When stored sera from children admitted to a London hospital were examined for B19V, samples from six Jamaican immigrants with sickle cell disease presenting with aplastic crisis showed evidence of recent infection with B19V (either antigenemia or seroconversion).[79] Retrospective studies of sera from Jamaican patients with sickle cell disease showed that 86% of TACs were associated with recent parvovirus infection.[80]

TAC caused by B19V has now been described in a wide range of patients with underlying hemolytic disorders, including hereditary spherocytosis, thalassemia, red cell enzymopathies such as pyruvate kinase deficiency, and autoimmune hemolytic anemia.[81] TAC can also occur under conditions of erythroid "stress," such as hemorrhage, iron deficiency anemia, and kidney or bone marrow transplantation. Acute anemia has been described in hematologically normal persons,[82] and a drop in red cell count (within the normal range) and reticulocytes was seen in healthy volunteers.[39]

Although suffering from an ultimately self-limiting disease, patients with aplastic crisis can be severely ill. Symptoms may include dyspnea, lassitude, and even confusion related to the worsening anemia. Congestive heart failure, severe bone marrow necrosis,[83] and cerebrovascular complications[84] can develop, and the illness may be fatal. Aplastic crisis can be the first presentation of an underlying hemolytic disease in a well-compensated patient.

Community-acquired aplastic crisis is almost always due to parvovirus B19,[85] and B19V infection should be the presumptive diagnosis in any patient with anemia related to abrupt cessation of erythropoiesis as documented by reduced reticulocytes and bone marrow appearance. In contrast to patients with EI, patients with TAC are often viremic at the time of presentation, with concentrations of virus as high as 10^{14} genome copies/mL (iU/mL); thus, the diagnosis is readily made by detection of B19V DNA in the serum. As B19V DNA levels fall in serum, B19V-specific IgM becomes detectable. TAC is easily treated by blood transfusion. After acute infection, immunity is lifelong.

TAC and B19V infection in hematologically normal patients are often associated with changes in other blood lineages, varying degrees of neutropenia,[86] and thrombocytopenia.[87] Some cases of idiopathic thrombocytopenic purpura and Henoch-Schönlein purpura[88] have been reported to follow parvovirus B19 infection. Transient pancytopenia after parvovirus infection is rare. Although some cases of chronic neutropenia of childhood have also been ascribed to parvovirus B19 infection,[89] other studies have not confirmed an association.[90]

Parvovirus B19 does not appear to be the cause of true (chronic) aplastic anemia[91] or transient erythroblastopenia of childhood (TEC),[92] the temporary failure of red cell production in normal children. Sporadic cases of TEC with thrombocytopenia with evidence of recent B19V infection have been described, whereas "classic" TEC is associated with *high* platelet counts.

PURE RED CELL APLASIA

Persistent B19V infection that results in PRCA has been reported in a wide variety of immunosuppressed patients, including patients with congenital immunodeficiency, acquired immunodeficiency syndrome (AIDS), and lymphoproliferative disorders and transplant recipients.[93] The stereotypical presentation is with persistent anemia rather than immune-mediated symptoms of rash or arthropathy. Patients have absent or low levels of B19V-specific antibody and persistent or recurrent parvoviremia as detected by B19V DNA in the serum. Bone marrow examination generally reveals the presence of scattered giant pronormoblasts. Administration of immunoglobulin can be beneficial and ameliorative, if not curative.[94]

The prevalence of B19-induced anemia in human immunodeficiency virus (HIV)-seropositive patients is probably higher than that recognized. In one early study of 50 patients with AIDS, no patients with B19V viremia were identified. In a larger cohort study, B19V DNA was found in only 1 of 191 (0.5%) HIV-seropositive homosexuals. However, B19V DNA was found in 5 of 30 (17%) transfusion-dependent HIV-seropositive homosexuals, and when a hematocrit of less than 20 mL/dL was used as a criterion, 4 of 13 (31%) were positive.[95] In contrast to the earlier studies, the marrow morphology need not be suggestive of PRCA, and giant pronormoblasts may not be present.

In less severely immunosuppressed patients (e.g., patients with systemic lupus erythematosus receiving steroid therapy), prolonged anemia after B19V infection has also been described.[96] However, in these patients there was a spontaneous, albeit delayed, development of antibodies, and viremia resolved without therapy. Such patients represent one end of the spectrum of disease manifestations of B19V in patients with a compromised immune system.

VIRUS-ASSOCIATED HEMOPHAGOCYTIC SYNDROME

Virus-associated hemophagocytic syndrome (VAHS) is characterized by histiocytic hyperplasia, marked hemophagocytosis, and cytopenia in association with a systemic viral illness.[97] In contrast to malignant histiocytosis, VAHS is usually a benign, self-limiting illness in which histiocytic proliferation is reversible. Hemophagocytosis is not uncommon and occurs in the setting of a wide range of infections, not only viral but also bacterial, rickettsial, fungal, and parasitic.[98] However, in many patients there is underlying immunosuppression, usually iatrogenic, so that the role of the incriminated pathogen as an etiologic agent or coincidental opportunistic infection remains unclear.

Parvovirus B19 infection has been detected in 15 cases of hemophagocytosis syndrome among children and adults.[99] The majority of patients were previously healthy, but four patients were immunosuppressed by drug therapies. In all but one case, there was a favorable outcome (one immunosuppressed patient died of fulminant aspergillosis). Further studies are required to determine whether parvovirus B19 is a major cause of VAHS as well as the rate of VAHS in otherwise uncomplicated parvovirus B19 infection.

FETAL INFECTION (HYDROPS FETALIS AND MISCARRIAGE)

Parvovirus B19 causes 10% to 15% of all cases of nonimmune hydrops fetalis.[100] Nonimmune hydrops fetalis is rare (1 per 3000 births), and in approximately 15% of cases the etiology is unknown. In a study of 63 cases, 8 were due to parvovirus B19 infection. When pathologic studies have been undertaken, B19-infected fetuses showed evidence of leukoerythroblastic reaction in the liver and large pale cells with eosinophilic inclusion bodies and peripheral condensation or margination of the nuclear chromatin. Parvovirus B19 DNA can be detected by PCR and in situ hybridization, and viral particles by electron microscopy.

Even in the absence of treatment, an adverse fetal outcome is not typical after maternal B19V infection. In a prospective British study of more than 400 women with serologically confirmed B19V during pregnancy, the excess rate of fetal loss was confined to the first 20 weeks of pregnancy and averaged only 9%.[101] No abnormalities were found at birth in the surviving infants, even when there was evidence of intrauterine infection by the presence of B19V IgM in the umbilical cord blood, and there were no long-term sequelae in the 129 children observed for more than 7 years. Similar findings have been found in studies in other countries.[102,103]

No systematic studies have shown evidence for congenital abnormalities after B19V infection,[101,104] although there are case reports of congenital ocular and neurologic abnormalities after maternal B19V infection. Rare cases of congenital anemia after a history of maternal B19V exposure have been reported.[105,106] In these cases, the virus load is generally low, and the anemia does not respond to immu-

noglobulin therapy. The B19V infection may mimic Diamond-Blackfan anemia,[107] and the role of in utero B19V infection inducing constitutional bone marrow failure such as that in Diamond-Blackfan anemia is still not clear.

OTHER DISEASE MANIFESTATIONS

B19V infection has been associated with a range of other disease manifestations including neurologic disease, myocarditis, kidney disease, hepatitis, and vasculitis. However, most of these are case reports or limited PCR-based studies with poorly documented controls. Determining the role of B19V in these diseases is often difficult; the diseases are rare, and B19V may not be the only cause. In addition, with sensitive PCR-based assays, B19V DNA can be detected in many tissues including bone marrow, synovial, and other tissues from healthy individuals probably lifelong after infection.[22,108] If the disease is rare, large multicenter trials may be required to substantiate or disprove the causal relationship.

Encephalitis and more often aseptic meningitis have been described in serologically confirmed B19V infection[109] and detection of B19V DNA in cerebrospinal fluid. The long-term outcome of infection was generally favorable, and only rarely did long-term sequelae occur. Brachial plexus neuropathy with weakness and sensory loss has also been described in patients with B19V infection,[110] and in one study, 50% of patients with classic fifth disease (confirmed serologically) experienced neurologic symptoms (tingling and numbness in the fingers or toes).[111]

There have been several case reports of myocarditis associated with B19V infection in both children and adults.[112,113] In many of the case reports, the diagnosis of B19V as the cause is made simply on the detection of the B19V DNA genome, and given the known persistence of B19V DNA in tissues, this may be erroneous. However, the putative role of B19V in the pathogenesis of myocarditis warrants further investigation, particularly because P antigen is found on fetal myocardial cells, and B19V appears to cause myocarditis in the fetus.[41,42]

Similarly, a number of case reports have described an association of parvovirus B19 infection and glomerulonephritis in both children and adults.[114]

The role of parvovirus B19 in both hepatitis and vasculitis remains unclear. Although transient elevation of liver transaminases is not uncommon in B19V infection, frank hepatitis associated with B19V infection has rarely been reported.[115] Parvovirus B19 has been suggested as a possible causative agent of fulminant liver failure and associated aplastic anemia on the basis of PCR studies.[116] However, the detection of B19V DNA in control liver tissue is not uncommon, and with appropriate controls we have been unable to confirm this putative relationship.[24,117]

Several case reports have described positive B19V serology in patients with vasculitis or polyarteritis nodosum, systemic necrotizing vasculitis, and Kawasaki disease, a multisystem vasculitis of early childhood. However, other studies have failed to confirm a relationship between B19V and vasculitis[118] or Kawasaki disease.[119]

▣ Immune Response

Both virus-specific IgM and IgG antibodies are made after experimental[39] and natural parvovirus B19 infection (see Fig. 147-3). After intranasal inoculation of volunteers, virus can be detected first at days 5 to 6, and levels peak at days 8 to 9. IgM antibody to virus appears about 10 to 12 days after experimental inoculation, and IgG antibody appears at about 2 weeks (see Fig. 147-3). The time course is similar in natural infections. In patients with TAC, 10^8 to 10^{14} genome copies per milliliter of viral DNA may circulate. IgM antibody may be present in patients with TAC at the time of reticulocyte nadir and during the subsequent 10 days; IgG usually appears during the period of hematopoietic recovery. High-titer viremia is not detectable in patients with clinical fifth disease (the manifestations are secondary to immune complex formation).

IgM antibody may be found in serum samples for several months after exposure.[120] IgG persists for life, and levels rise with reexposure.[39] Measurable IgA antibodies specific to B19V may play a role in protection against infection by the nasopharyngeal route.[121]

In immunocompetent individuals, the early antibody response is to the major capsid protein VP2, but as the immune response matures reactivity to the minor capsid protein VP1 dominates. Sera from patients with persistent B19V infection typically contain antibody to VP2 but not to VP1.[122] The importance of an immune response to VP1 for protective immunity has been confirmed in animal experiments using recombinant capsids. Rabbits immunized with capsids containing only VP2 produced a strong antibody response, as measured by enzyme-linked immunosorbent assay (ELISA), but the sera had low neutralization titers. In contrast, rabbits immunized with capsids containing VP1 produced antibody with neutralizing titers comparable to those produced in humans after acute B19V infection.[123] In addition, the importance of the humoral arm of the immune response is shown by recovery from infection with the appearance of circulating specific antivirus antibody, and administration of commercial immunoglobulins can cure or ameliorate persistent parvovirus infection in immunodeficient patients.

The role of the cellular immune response in limiting parvovirus B19 infection has been studied less intensively. Using a combination of recombinant capsids and peptides from the NS and capsid proteins, it is now clear that B19V infection induces profound CD8[+124] and CD4[+125-127] responses, both of which are required for viral clearance.

Persistent B19V infection is the result of failure to produce effective neutralizing antibodies by the immunocompromised host. Perhaps because of the limited numbers of epitopes presented to the immune system by parvovirus B19, the congenital immunodeficiency states associated with persistent infection may be clinically subtle, with susceptibility largely restricted to parvovirus, although multiple immune system defects are apparent when direct testing of T- and B-cell function is performed.

Diagnosis

There is no suitable method for virus isolation from clinical specimens, and the detection of virus relies on the detection of B19V DNA. High-titer B19V DNA can be detected in serum at the time of TAC using dot-blot hybridization (sensitivity level > 10^6 genome copies/mL) or quantitative PCR, and in situ hybridization has been used to identify B19V DNA in bone marrow and other cells. In immunocompetent individuals, B19V DNA is detectable at high titer for only 2 to 4 days (see Fig. 147-3), and the diagnosis of acute B19V infection is therefore based on IgM assays, ideally performed by the capture technique.[128] In an ELISA, antibody can be detected in more than 90% of cases by the third day of TAC or at the time of rash in EI. IgM antibody remains detectable for 2 to 3 months after infection.

B19V IgG can be detected by capture assay or indirect assay. IgG is usually present by the seventh day of illness and is probably present for life thereafter. As more than 50% of the population has IgG antibody to B19V infection, this test is not helpful for the diagnosis of acute infection. Immunocompromised or immunodeficient patients with chronic infection typically do not mount an immune response to the virus, and testing for B19V antigens or more usually for viral DNA is necessary to document recent infection.

The sensitivity level of detection of B19V has greatly increased with the use of PCR, but at the risk of possible contamination and false-positive results, confusing interpretation. Even in immunocompetent persons, low levels of B19V DNA may be detectable by PCR for more than 4 months in serum after acute infection,[129,130] and for years in bone marrow, synovium, liver, heart, and other tissues.[22,108] As noted ealier in this chapter, detection of B19V DNA in tissues does not prove that the disease is due to B19V infection. In general, the diagnosis of acute or chronic infection can be made on the basis of quantitative (real-time) PCR in combination with serologic assays for B19-specific IgG or IgM, or both.[131]

Investigation of B19V fetal or congenital infection should be accompanied by serologic studies of the maternal serum. At the time of fetal infection, the mother should have evidence of recent B19V infection with detectable IgG and possibly IgM. If the IgM titer is low or absent, recent infection can be documented using IgG avidity studies, or measuring B19V DNA levels.[132] Fetal infection can be confirmed by amniotic fluid sampling, by fetal blood sampling, or from postmortem tissue.

Treatment

In the overwhelming majority of children and adults, B19V infection is a benign and self-limiting infection that results in lifelong immunity and requires no treatment other than symptomatic relief. Patients with arthralgia and arthritis usually respond to nonsteroidal anti-inflammatory drugs, although in some patients symptoms can persist for months and even years.[74] In patients with hematologic disease or persistent infection, specific treatment may be necessary.

Immunocompetent patients with TAC have a self-limiting illness, and typical TAC is readily treated by blood transfusion and supportive therapy alone. In one study of sickle cell patients with aplastic crisis, 87% required blood transfusions and 61% required hospitalization for their symptoms. One death occurred before transfusion could be given,[133] which underscores the importance of prompt medical intervention.

In immunosuppressed patients with documented, persistent B19V infection, temporary cessation of immunosuppression may be sufficient to allow the host to mount an immune response and resolve the B19V infection, and no additional treatment is required.[134] In cases in which cessation of immunosuppression is not feasible or is ineffective, administration of immunoglobulin can be beneficial.[43,94] The usual regimen is IV IgG at a dose of 0.4 g/kg for 5 days. Patients often respond with a marked reduction in the level of B19V viremia, reticulocytosis, and resolution of the anemia within 1 to 2 weeks of treatment. However, monitoring for relapse is important, by observation of the reticulocyte counts and quantitative assays for B19V DNA when indicated. If relapse occurs less than 6 months after the initial treatment, especially in HIV-positive patients, an empirical maintenance treatment with a single-day infusion of 0.4 g/kg IgG every 4 weeks may control the B19V viremia.

The role of intrauterine blood transfusions in the treatment of hydrops fetalis related to maternal parvovirus B19 has been shown to be beneficial.[135,136] However, intrauterine blood transfusions have risks, and B19-associated hydrops is known to resolve spontaneously and the fetus can be normal at delivery. In addition there remains the theoretical risk that treatment may be confounded by an increased incidence of antibody-enhanced infection and damage, especially to myocardial cells and the immune system.[105]

Prevention and Vaccination

The only measures currently available to prevent B19V infection are those designed to interrupt virus transmission. However, because patients are viremic and infectious before the symptoms of EI, isolation of patients with fifth disease is not rational. Patients with TAC and PRCA are both viremic and infectious and should be appropriately separated from high-risk contacts. The Centers for Disease Control and Prevention recommend that patients with TAC have droplet isolation precautions for 7 days, and for patients with chronic infection, isolation should be continued for the duration of their hospitalization.[137]

The humoral immune response plays the major role in the normal immune response to parvovirus. Although antibodies appear protective in both passive and active immunizations, insufficient data are available to assess the efficacy of immunoprophylaxis.[138,139]

Prospects for vaccination are favorable, with a B19V empty capsid vaccine currently under development. The presence of VP1 protein in the capsid immunogen appears critical for the production of antibodies that neutralize virus activity in vitro, and capsids with supranormal VP1 content are even more efficient in inducing neutralizing activity in immunized animals. Phase I trials of a VP1-enhanced baculovirus-produced B19V vaccine looked promising,[140] and phase II trials are in progress. However, the target populations for such a vaccine remain to be determined. Should only those at high risk for severe or life-threatening disease, such as sickle cell patients, be protected? Or, in view of the wide variety of disease manifestations affecting all strata of the population, should a universal vaccine policy be pursued?

Other Human Parvoviruses

HUMAN DEPENDOVIRUSES

To date at least nine different primate dependoviruses have been described,[141] and AAVs 1, 2, 3, 8, and 9 are common agents of human infections.[141] Although AAV DNA has been detected in a wide range of tissues, including some fetal abortion tissues, none of the dependoviruses have been definitively linked with disease in either humans or animals. This lack of pathogenicity, plus the ability of the genome to infect both dividing and nondividing cells and to integrate into the human genome, has made the dependoviruses popular choices to modify and use as gene therapy vectors in a number of different clinical settings.[142]

HUMAN BOCAVIRUS

Bocaviruses are parvoviruses that infect the respiratory and gastrointestinal tracts of young animals. Recently, sequences of a human bocavirus (HBoV) were identified in respiratory samples of Swedish children with lower respiratory tract infections using a molecular screening method.[143] The nucleotide sequences of HBoV have been determined and have 42% to 43% amino acid identity to animal parvoviruses, the minute virus of canines, and the bovine parvovirus. The genomic organization of HBoV is also similar to animal parvoviruses.[143] Currently, HBoV can be detected only by PCR techniques,

and sequences have been detected in respiratory secretions, in blood, and in feces.[144-146] HBoV-specific antibodies have been detected using binding assays with viral capsid proteins.[147] Subsequent studies have identified HBoV DNA sequences in children in many different parts of the world, but other pathogenic viruses are often present in the samples. Seroepidemiology studies indicate that bocavirus is a common infection of early childhood, with most acquiring antibodies in the first 4 years of life.[148] Despite the observation that it is often found with other pathogens, there is increasing evidence that the virus itself is pathogenic and especially associated with wheezing and respiratory disease in young children.[149] HBoV has been detected worldwide and has been observed in 1.5% to 19% of respiratory secretions in prevalence studies primarily from children with acute respiratory disease.[144] Several studies have reported that HBoV is more frequent in patients with respiratory tract symptoms than in asymptomatic individuals.[150-153] A variety of respiratory diseases have been implicated in HBoV infection including lower and upper respiratory tract illnesses,[147] primarily in young children. HBoV infections in otherwise normal adults with respiratory illnesses appear to be uncommon, but have been reported mainly from immunocompromised individuals.[153-155] The association of HBoV infection with respiratory illness is confounded by the frequent coinfection with other respiratory viruses, and the apparently long period of HBoV shedding after infections.[144] Additional information on the pathogenetic significance of HBoV infection will emerge from ongoing studies. Currently there is no known treatment.

HUMAN PARVOVIRUS 4 (PARV4)

Using similar methods to those used to identify HBoV, a fourth group of parvoviruses, Parv4,[156] has also recently been found, with three different genotypes of Parv4 identified to date.[157] The viral sequences are commonly found in pooled serum samples,[158] and in bone marrow and lymphoid tissue of IDUs and hemophiliacs.[159] However, whether the virus is itself pathogenic is unknown. The virus has not been grown in culture, but preliminary studies of the transcription map suggest that Parv4 does not group with any of the other parvovirus genera.

REFERENCES

1. Tattersall P, Bergoin M, Bloom ME, et al. Parvoviridae. In Fauquet CM, Mayo MA, Maniloff J, et al, eds. *Virus Taxonomy: Classification and Nomenclature of Viruses: Eighth Report of the International Committee on Taxonomy of Viruses.* New York: Elsevier Academic Press; 2005:353-369.
2. Cossart YE, Field AM, Cant B, et al. Parvovirus-like particles in human sera. *Lancet.* 1975;1:72-73.
3. Yunoki M, Tsujikawa M, Urayama T, et al. Heat sensitivity of human parvovirus B19. *Vox Sang.* 2003;85:67-68.
4. Bartolomei Corsi O, Azzi A, Morfini M, et al. Human parvovirus infection in haemophiliacs first infused with treated clotting factor concentrates. *J Med Virol.* 1988;25:165-170.
5. Ozawa K, Ayub J, Hao YS, et al. Novel transcription map for the B19 (human) pathogenic parvovirus. *J Virol.* 1987;61:2395-2406.
6. Ozawa K, Ayub J, Young N. Translational regulation of B19 parvovirus capsid protein production by multiple upstream AUG triplets. *J Biol Chem.* 1988;263:10922-10926.
7. Zhi N, Mills IP, Lu J, et al. Molecular and functional analyses of a human parvovirus B19 infectious clone demonstrates essential roles for NS1, VP1, and the 11-kilodalton protein in virus replication and infectivity. *J Virol.* 2006;80:5941-5950.
8. Ozawa K, Young N. Characterization of capsid and noncapsid proteins of B19 parvovirus propagated in human erythroid bone marrow cell cultures. *J Virol.* 1987;61:2627-2630.
9. Momoeda M, Wong S, Kawase M, et al. A putative nucleoside triphosphate-binding domain in the nonstructural protein of B19 parvovirus is required for cytotoxicity. *J Virol.* 1994;68:8443-8446.
10. Moffatt S, Yaegashi N, Tada K, et al. Human parvovirus B19 nonstructural (NS1) protein induces apoptosis in erythroid lineage cells. *J Virol.* 1998;72:3018-3028.
11. Kajigaya S, Frickhofen N, Kurtzman G, et al. A genetically engineered cell line that produces empty capsids of human parvovirus B19. *Vaccines.* 1990;90:63-68.
12. Kajigaya S, Fujii H, Field A, et al. Self-assembled B19 parvovirus capsids, produced in a baculovirus system, are antigenically and

immunogenically similar to native virions. *Proc Natl Acad Sci U S A.* 1991;88:4646-4650.
13. Brown CS, Van Lent JW, Vlak JM, et al. Assembly of empty capsids by using baculovirus recombinants expressing human parvovirus B19 structural proteins. *J Virol.* 1991;65:2702-2706.
14. Lowin T, Raab U, Schroeder J, et al. Parvovirus B19 VP2-proteins produced in *Saccharomyces cerevisiae:* comparison with VP2-particles produced by baculovirus-derived vectors. *J Vet Med B Infect Dis Vet Public Health.* 2005;52:348-352.
15. Kaufmann B, Simpson AA, Rossmann MG. The structure of human parvovirus B19. *Proc Natl Acad Sci U S A.* 10-8-2004;101:11628-11633.
16. Kaufmann B, Chipman PR, Kostyuchenko VA, et al. Visualization of the externalized VP2 N termini of infectious human parvovirus B19. *J Virol.* 2008;82:7306-7312.
17. Zadori Z, Szelei J, Lacoste MC, et al. A viral phospholipase A2 is required for parvovirus infectivity. *Dev Cell.* 2001;1:291-302.
18. Filippone C, Zhi N, Wong S, et al. VP1u phospholipase activity is critical for infectivity of full-length parvovirus B19 genomic clones. *Virology.* 2008;374:444-452.
19. Servant A, Laperche S, Lallemand F, et al. Genetic diversity within human erythroviruses: identification of three genotypes. *J Virol.* 2002;76:9124-9134.
20. Nguyen QT, Wong S, Heegaard ED, et al. Identification and characterization of a second novel human erythrovirus variant, A6. *Virology.* 2002;301:374-380.
21. Candotti D, Etiz N, Parsyan A, et al. Identification and characterization of persistent human erythrovirus infection in blood donor samples. *J Virol.* 2004;78:12169-12178.
22. Norja P, Hokynar K, Aaltonen LM, et al. Bioportfolio: lifelong persistence of variant and prototypic erythrovirus DNA genomes in human tissue. *Proc Natl Acad Sci U S A.* 2006;103:7450-7453.
23. Blumel J, Eis-Hubinger AM, Stuhler A, et al. Characterization of Parvovirus B19 genotype 2 in KU812Ep6 cells. *J Virol.* 2005;79:14197-14206.

24. Wong S, Young NS, Brown KE. Prevalence of parvovirus B19 in liver tissue: no association with fulminant hepatitis or hepatitis-associated aplastic anemia. *J Infect Dis.* 2003;187:1581-1586.
25. Cohen BJ, Gandhi J, Clewley JP. Genetic variants of parvovirus B19 identified in the United Kingdom: implications for diagnostic testing. *J Clin Virol.* 2006;36:152-155.
26. Sanabani S, Neto WK, Pereira J, et al. Sequence variability of human erythroviruses present in bone marrow of Brazilian patients with various parvovirus B19-related hematological symptoms. *J Clin Microbiol.* 2006;44:604-606.
27. Freitas RB, Melo FL, Oliveira DS, et al. Molecular characterization of human erythrovirus B19 strains obtained from patients with several clinical presentations in the Amazon region of Brazil. *J Clin Virol.* 2008;43:60-65.
28. Corcoran A, Doyle S, Allain JP, et al. Evidence of serological cross-reactivity between genotype 1 and genotype 3 erythrovirus infections. *J Virol.* 2005;79:5238-5239.
29. Ekman A, Hokynar K, Kakkola L, et al. Biological and immunological relations among human parvovirus B19 genotypes 1 to 3. *J Virol.* 2007;81:6927-6935.
30. Wong S, Zhi N, Filippone C, et al. Ex vivo-generated CD36+ erythroid progenitors are highly permissive to human parvovirus B19 replication. *J Virol.* 2008;82:2470-2476.
31. Brown KE, Young NS. The simian parvoviruses. *Rev Med Virol.* 1997;7:211-218.
32. Takahashi T, Ozawa K, Takahashi K, et al. Susceptibility of human erythropoietic cells to B19 parvovirus in vitro increases with differentiation. *Blood.* 1990;75:603-610.
33. Yaegashi N, Niinuma T, Chisaka H, et al. Parvovirus B19 infection induces apoptosis of erythroid cells in vitro and in vivo. *J Infect.* 1999;39:68-76.
34. Morey AL, Ferguson DJ, Fleming KA. Ultrastructural features of fetal erythroid precursors infected with parvovirus B19 in vitro: evidence of cell death by apoptosis. *J Pathol.* 1993;169:213-220.
35. Rouger P, Gane P, Salmon C. Tissue distribution of H, Lewis and P antigens as shown by a panel of 18 monoclonal antibodies. *Rev Fr Transfus Immunohematol.* 1987;30:699-708.

36. Brown KE, Hibbs JR, Gallinella G, et al. Resistance to parvovirus B19 infection due to lack of virus receptor (erythrocyte P antigen). N Engl J Med. 1994;330:1192-1196.

37. Weigel-Kelley KA, Yoder MC, Srivastava A. Alpha5beta1 integrin as a cellular coreceptor for human parvovirus B19: requirement of functional activation of beta1 integrin for viral entry. Blood. 2003;102:3927-3933.

38. Munakata Y, Saito-Ito T, Kumura-Ishii K, et al. Ku80 autoantigen as a cellular coreceptor for human parvovirus B19 infection. Blood. 2005;106:3449-3456.

39. Anderson MJ, Higgins PG, Davis LR, et al. Experimental parvoviral infection in humans. J Infect Dis. 1985;152:257-265.

40. Field AM, Cohen BJ, Brown KE, et al. Detection of B19 parvovirus in human fetal tissues by electron microscopy. J Med Virol. 1991;35:85-95.

41. Morey AL, Keeling JW, Porter HJ, et al. Clinical and histopathological features of parvovirus B19 infection in the human fetus. Br J Obstet Gynaecol. 1992;99:566-574.

42. Naides SJ, Weiner CP. Antenatal diagnosis and palliative treatment of non-immune hydrops fetalis secondary to fetal parvovirus B19 infection. Prenat Diagn. 1989;9:105-114.

43. Frickhofen N, Abkowitz JL, Safford M, et al. Persistent B19 parvovirus infection in patients infected with human immunodeficiency virus type 1 (HIV-1): a treatable cause of anemia in AIDS. Ann Intern Med. 1990;113:926-933.

44. Lu J, Zhi N, Wong S, et al. Activation of synoviocytes by the secreted phospholipase A2 motif in the VP1-unique region of parvovirus B19 minor capsid protein. J Infect Dis. 2006;193:582-590.

45. Rohrer C, Gartner B, Sauerbrei A, et al. Seroprevalence of parvovirus B19 in the German population. Epidemiol Infect. 2008;1-12.

46. Koch WC, Adler SP. Human parvovirus B19 infections in women of childbearing age and within families. Pediatr Infect Dis J. 1989;8:83-87.

47. Mossong J, Hens N, Friederichs V, et al. Parvovirus B19 infection in five European countries: seroepidemiology, force of infection and maternal risk of infection. Epidemiol Infect. 2008;136:1059-1068.

48. Schwarz TF, Gürtler LG, Zoulek G, et al. Seroprevalence of human parvovirus B19 infection in Sao Tomé and Principe, Malawi and Mascarene Islands. Int J Med Microbiol. 1989;271:231-236.

49. de Freitas RB, Wong D, Boswell F, et al. Prevalence of human parvovirus (B19) and rubella virus infections in urban and remote rural areas in northern Brazil. J Med Virol. 1990;32:203-208.

50. Brown KE, Simmonds P. Parvoviruses and blood transfusion. Transfusion. 2007;47:1745-1750.

51. Kleinman SH, Glynn SA, Lee TH, et al. Prevalence and quantitation of parvovirus B19 DNA levels in blood donors with a sensitive polymerase chain reaction screening assay. Transfusion. 2007;47:1756-1764.

52. Anderson MJ, Cohen BJ. Human parvovirus B19 infections in United Kingdom 1984-86 [letter]. Lancet. 1987;1:738-739.

53. Kelly HA, Siebert D, Hammond R, et al. The age-specific prevalence of human parvovirus immunity in Victoria, Australia compared with other parts of the world. Epidemiol Infect. 2000;124:449-457.

54. Serjeant GR, Serjeant BE, Thomas PE, et al. Human parvovirus infection in homozygous sickle cell disease. Lancet. 1993;341:1237-1240.

55. Chorba T, Coccia P, Holman RC, et al. The role of parvovirus B19 in aplastic crisis and erythema infectiosum (fifth disease). J Infect Dis. 1986;154:383-393.

56. Gillespie SM, Cartter ML, Asch S, et al. Occupational risk of human parvovirus B19 infection for school and day-care personnel during an outbreak of erythema infectiosum. J Am Med Assoc. 1990;263:2061-2065.

57. Woolf AD, Campion GV, Chishick A, et al. Clinical manifestations of human parvovirus B19 in adults. Arch Intern Med. 1989;149:1153-1156.

58. Adler SP, Manganello AM, Koch WC, et al. Risk of human parvovirus B19 infections among school and hospital employees during endemic periods. J Infect Dis. 1993;168:361-368.

59. Seng C, Watkins P, Morse D, et al. Parvovirus B19 outbreak on an adult ward. Epidemiol Infect. 1994;113:345-353.

60. Azzi A, Morfini M, Mannucci PM. The transfusion-associated transmission of parvovirus B19. Transfus Med Rev. 1999; 13:194-204.

61. Brown KE, Young NS, Alving BM, et al. Parvovirus B19: implications for transfusion medicine: summary of a workshop. Transfusion. 2001;41:130-135.

62. Koenigbauer UF, Eastlund T, Day JW. Clinical illness due to parvovirus B19 infection after infusion of solvent/detergent-treated pooled plasma. Transfusion. 2000;40:1203-1206.

63. Williams MD, Cohen BJ, Beddall AC, et al. Transmission of human parvovirus B19 by coagulation factor concentrates. Vox Sang. 1990;58:177-181.

64. Balfour HH. Erythema infectiosum (fifth disease): clinical review and description of 91 cases seen in an epidemic. Clin Pediatr (Phila). 1969;8:721-727.

65. Cheinisse L. Une cinquième maladie éruptive: le mégal-érythème épidémique. Sem Med. 1905;25:205-207.

66. Anderson MJ, Jones SE, Fisher-Hoch SP, et al. Human parvovirus, the cause of erythema infectiosum (fifth disease)? [letter]. Lancet. 1983;1:1378.

67. Naides SJ, Piette W, Veach LA, et al. Human parvovirus B19-induced vesiculopustular skin eruption. Am J Med. 1988;84:968-972.

68. Smith PT, Landry ML, Carey H, et al. Papular-purpuric gloves and socks syndrome associated with acute parvovirus B19 infection: case report and review. Clin Infect Dis. 1998;27:164-168.

69. Shiraishi H, Umetsu K, Yamamoto H, et al. Human parvovirus (HPV/B19) infection with purpura. Microbiol Immunol. 1989; 33:369-372.

70. Evans LM, Grossman ME, Gregory N. Koplik spots and a pur-puric eruption associated with parvovirus B19 infection. J Am Acad Dermatol. 1992;27:466-467.

71. Lobkowicz F, Ring J, Schwarz TF, et al. Erythema multiforme in a patient with acute human parvovirus B19 infection. J Am Acad Dermatol. 1989;20:849-850.

72. Jacks TA. Pruritus in parvovirus infection. J R Coll Gen Pract. 1987;37:210-211.

73. Luzzi GA, Kurtz JB, Chapel H. Human parvovirus arthropathy and rheumatoid factor [letter]. Lancet. 1985;1:1218.

74. White DG, Woolf AD, Mortimer PP, et al. Human parvovirus arthropathy. Lancet. 1985;1:419-421.

75. Takahashi Y, Murai C, Shibata S, et al. Human parvovirus B19 as a causative agent for rheumatoid arthritis. Proc Natl Acad Sci U S A. 1998;95:8227-8232.

76. Soderlund M, von Essen R, Haapasaari J, et al. Persistence of parvovirus B19 DNA in synovial membranes of young patients with and without chronic arthropathy. Lancet. 1997;349:1063-1065.

77. Speyer I, Breedveld FC, Dijkmans BA. Human parvovirus B19 infection is not followed by inflammatory joint disease during long term follow-up: a retrospective study of 54 patients. Clin Exp Rheumatol. 1998;16:576-578.

78. Lehmann HW, Knoll A, Kuster RM, et al. Frequent infection with a viral pathogen, parvovirus B19, in rheumatic diseases of childhood. Arthritis Rheum. 2003;48:1631-1638.

79. Pattison JR, Jones SE, Hodgson J, et al. Parvovirus infections and hypoplastic crisis in sickle-cell anaemia. Lancet. 1981; 1:664-665.

80. Serjeant GR, Topley JM, Mason K, et al. Outbreak of aplastic crisis in sickle cell anaemia associated with parvovirus-like agent. Lancet. 1981;2:595-597.

81. Young NS. Hematologic manifestations and diagnosis of parvovirus B19 infections. Clin Adv Hematol Oncol. 2006;4: 908-910.

82. Hamon MD, Newland AC, Anderson MJ. Severe aplastic anaemia after parvovirus infection in the absence of underlying haemolytic anaemia [letter]. J Clin Pathol. 1988;41:1242.

83. Conrad ME, Studdard H, Anderson LJ. Aplastic crisis in sickle cell disorders: bone marrow necrosis and human parvovirus infection. Am J Med Sci. 1988;295:212-215.

84. Wierenga KJ, Serjeant BE, Serjeant GR. Cerebrovascular complications and parvovirus infection in homozygous sickle cell disease. J Pediatr. 2001;139:438-442.

85. Anderson MJ, Davis LR, Hodgson J, et al. Occurrence of infection with a parvovirus-like agent in children with sickle cell anaemia during a two-year period. J Clin Pathol. 1982;35: 744-749.

86. Saunders PW, Reid MM, Cohen BJ. Human parvovirus induced cytopenias: a report of five cases [letter]. Br J Haematol. 1986;63:407-410.

87. Inoue S, Kinra NK, Mukkamala SR, et al. Parvovirus B-19 infection: aplastic crisis, erythema infectiosum and idiopathic thrombocytopenic purpura. Pediatr Infect Dis J. 1991;10:251-253.

88. Lefrère JJ, Couroucé AM, Muller JY, et al. Human parvovirus and purpura [letter]. Lancet. 1985;2:730.

89. McClain K, Estrov Z, Chen H, et al. Chronic neutropenia of childhood: frequent association with parvovirus infection and correlations with bone marrow culture studies. Br J Haematol. 1993;85:57-62.

90. Hartman KR, Brown KE, Green SW, et al. Lack of evidence for parvovirus B19 viraemia in children with chronic neutropenia [letter]. Br J Haematol. 1994;84:895-896.

91. Hsu HC, Lee YM, Su WJ, et al. Bone marrow samples from patients with aplastic anemia are not infected with parvovirus B19 and Mycobacterium tuberculosis. Am J Clin Pathol. 2002;117:36-40.

92. Skeppner G, Kreuger A, Elinder G. Transient erythroblastopenia of childhood: prospective study of 10 patients with special reference to viral infections. J Pediatr Hematol Oncol. 2002;24: 294-298.

93. Frickhofen N, Young NS. Persistent parvovirus B19 infections in humans. Microb Pathog. 1989;7:319-327.

94. Kurtzman GJ, Cohen B, Meyers P, et al. Persistent B19 parvovirus infection as a cause of severe chronic anaemia in children with acute lymphocytic leukaemia. Lancet. 1988;2:1159-1162.

95. Abkowitz JL, Brown KE, Wood RW, et al. Human parvovirus B19 (HPV B19) is not a rare cause of anemia in HIV-seropositive individuals [abstract]. Clin Res. 1993;41:393A.

96. Koch WC, Massey G, Russell CE, et al. Manifestations and treatment of human parvovirus B19 infection in immunocompromised patients. J Pediatr. 1990;116:355-359.

97. Risdall RJ, McKenna RW, Nesbit ME, et al. Virus-associated hemophagocytic syndrome. Cancer. 1979;44:993-1002.

98. Reiner AP, Spivak JL. Hematophagic histiocytosis: a report of 23 new patients and a review of the literature. Medicine (Baltimore). 1988;67:369-388.

99. Shirono K, Tsuda H. Parvovirus B19-associated haemophagocytic syndrome in healthy adults. Br J Haematol. 1995;89:923-926.

100. Ismail KM, Martin WL, Ghosh S, et al. Etiology and outcome of hydrops fetalis. J Matern Fetal Med. 2001;10:175-181.

101. Miller E, Fairley CK, Cohen BJ, et al. Immediate and long term outcome of human parvovirus B19 infection in pregnancy. Br J Obstet Gynaecol. 1998;105:174-178.

102. Enders M, Weidner A, Zoellner I, et al. Fetal morbidity and mortality after acute human parvovirus B19 infection in pregnancy: prospective evaluation of 1018 cases. Prenat Diagn. 2004;24:513-518.

103. Yaegashi N, Niinuma T, Chisaka H, et al. Serologic study of human parvovirus B19 infection in pregnancy in Japan. J Infect. 1999;38:30-35.

104. Rodis JF, Rodner C, Hansen AA, et al. Long-term outcome of children following maternal human parvovirus B19 infection. Obstet Gynecol. 1998;91:125-128.

105. Brown KE, Green SW, Antunez de Mayolo J, et al. Congenital anaemia after transplacental B19 parvovirus infection. Lancet. 1994;343:895-896.

106. Heegaard ED, Hasle H, Skibsted L, et al. Congenital anemia caused by parvovirus B19 infection. Pediatr Infect Dis J. 2000;19:1216-1218.

107. Heegaard ED, Hasle H, Clausen N, et al. Parvovirus B19 infection and Diamond-Blackfan anaemia. Acta Paediatr. 1996;85:299-302.

108. Soderlund-Venermo M, Hokynar K, Nieminen J, et al. Persistence of human parvovirus B19 in human tissues. Pathol Biol (Paris). 2002;50:307-316.

109. Tabak F, Mert A, Ozturk R, et al. Prolonged fever caused by parvovirus B19-induced meningitis: case report and review. Clin Infect Dis. 1999;29:446-447.

110. Walsh KJ, Armstrong RD, Turner AM. Brachial plexus neuropathy associated with human parvovirus infection. Br Med J. 1988;296:896.

111. Faden H, Gary GW Jr, Korman M. Numbness and tingling of fingers associated with parvovirus B19 infection [letter]. J Infect Dis. 1990;161:354-355.

112. Enders G, Dotsch J, Bauer J, et al. Life-threatening parvovirus B19-associated myocarditis and cardiac transplantation as possible therapy: two case reports. Clin Infect Dis. 1998;26:355-358.

113. Chia JK, Jackson B. Myopericarditis due to parvovirus B19 in an adult. Clin Infect Dis. 1996;23:200-201.

114. Waldman M, Kopp JB. Parvovirus B19 and the kidney. Clin J Am Soc Nephrol. 2007;2(Suppl 1):S47-S56.

115. Yoto Y, Kudoh T, Haseyama K, et al. Human parvovirus B19 infection associated with acute hepatitis. Lancet. 1996;347:868-869.

116. Langnas AN, Markin RS, Cattral MS, et al. Parvovirus B19 as a possible causative agent of fulminant liver failure and associated aplastic anemia. Hepatology. 1995;22:1661-1665.

117. Lee WM, Brown KE, Young NS, et al. Brief report: no evidence for parvovirus B19 or hepatitis E virus as a cause of acute liver failure. Dig Dis Sci. 2006;51:1712-1715.

118. Eden A, Mahr A, Servant A, et al. Lack of association between B19 or V9 erythrovirus infection and ANCA-positive vasculitides: a case-control study. Rheumatology (Oxford). 2003;42:660-664.

119. Chua PK, Nerurkar VR, Yu Q, et al. Lack of association between Kawasaki syndrome and infection with parvovirus B19, human herpesvirus 8, TT virus, GB virus C/hepatitis G virus or Chlamydia pneumoniae. Pediatr Infect Dis J. 2000;19:477-479.

120. Anderson LJ, Tsou C, Parker RA, et al. Detection of antibodies and antigens of human parvovirus B19 by enzyme-linked immunosorbent assay. J Clin Microbiol. 1986;24:522-526.

121. Erdman DD, Usher MJ, Tsou C, et al. Human parvovirus B19 specific IgG, IgA, and IgM antibodies and DNA in serum specimens from persons with erythema infectiosum. J Med Virol. 1991;35:110-115.

122. Kurtzman GJ, Cohen BJ, Field AM, et al. Immune response to B19 parvovirus and an antibody defect in persistent viral infection. J Clin Invest. 1989;84:1114-1123.

123. Rosenfeld SJ, Young NS, Alling D, et al. Subunit interaction in B19 parvovirus empty capsids. Arch Virol. 1994;136:9-18.

124. Isa A, Kasprowicz V, Norbeck O, et al. Prolonged activation of virus-specific CD8+ cells after acute B19 infection. PLoS Med. 2005;2:e343.

125. von Poblotzki A, Gerdes C, Reischl U, et al. Lymphoproliferative responses after infection with human parvovirus B19. J Virol. 1996;70:7327-7330.

126. Lindner J, Barabas S, Saar K, et al. CD4+ T-cell responses against the VP1-unique region in individuals with recent and persistent parvovirus B19 infection. J Vet Med B Infect Dis Vet Public Health. 2005;52:356-361.

127. Kasprowicz V, Isa A, Tolfvenstam T, et al. Tracking of peptide-specific CD4+ T-cell responses after an acute resolving viral infection: a study of parvovirus B19. J Virol. 2006;80:11209-11217.

128. Anderson MJ, Davis LR, Jones SE, et al. The development and use of an antibody capture radioimmunoassay for specific IgM to a human parvovirus-like agent. J Hyg (Lond). 1982; 88:309-324.

129. Patou G, Pillay D, Myint S, et al. Characterization of a nested polymerase chain reaction assay for detection of parvovirus B19. J Clin Microbiol. 1993;31:540-546.

130. Musiani M, Zerbini M, Gentilomi G, et al. Persistent B19 parvovirus infections in haemophilic HIV-1 infected patients. *J Med Virol.* 1995;46:103-108.
131. Gallinella G, Zuffi E, Gentilomi G, et al. Relevance of B19 markers in serum samples for a diagnosis of parvovirus B19-correlated diseases. *J Med Virol.* 2003;71:135-139.
132. Enders M, Weidner A, Rosenthal T, et al. Improved diagnosis of gestational parvovirus B19 infection at the time of nonimmune fetal hydrops. *J Infect Dis.* 2008;197:58-62.
133. Goldstein AR, Anderson MJ, Serjeant GR. Parvovirus associated aplastic crisis in homozygous sickle cell disease. *Arch Dis Child.* 1987;62:585-588.
134. Smith MA, Shah NR, Lobel JS, et al. Severe anemia caused by human parvovirus in a leukemia patient on maintenance chemotherapy. *Clin Pediatr (Phila).* 1988;27:383-386.
135. Fairley CK, Smoleniec JS, Caul OE, et al. Observational study of effect of intrauterine transfusions on outcome of fetal hydrops after parvovirus B19 infection. *Lancet.* 1995;346:1335-1337.
136. Rodis JF, Borgida AF, Wilson M, et al. Management of parvovirus infection in pregnancy and outcomes of hydrops: a survey of members of the Society of Perinatal Obstetricians. *Am J Obstet Gynecol.* 1998;179:985-988.
137. Bolyard EA, Tablan OC, Williams WW, et al. Guideline for infection control in health care personnel, 1998. Hospital Infection Control Practices Advisory Committee. *Infect Control Hosp Epidemiol.* 1998;19:407-463.
138. Pillay D, Patou G, Hurt S, et al. Parvovirus B19 outbreak in a children's ward. *Lancet.* 1992;339:107-109.
139. Torok TJ, Pavia AT, Anderson LJ. Efficacy of immune globulin for prevention of human parvovirus B19 infection [abstract]. Montpellier, France: Sixth Parvovirus Workshop; 1995:P6 #8.
140. Ballou WR, Reed JL, Noble W, et al. Safety and immunogenicity of a recombinant parvovirus B19 vaccine formulated with MF59C.1. *J Infect Dis.* 2003;187:675-678.
141. Gao G, Vandenberghe LH, Alvira MR, et al. Clades of Adeno-associated viruses are widely disseminated in human tissues. *J Virol.* 2004;78:6381-6388.
142. Daya S, Berns KI. Gene therapy using adeno-associated virus vectors. *Clin Microbiol Rev.* 2008;21:583-593.
143. Allander T, Tammi MT, Eriksson M, et al. Cloning of a human parvovirus by molecular screening of respiratory tract samples. *Proc Natl Acad Sci U S A.* 2005;102:12891-12896.
144. Allander T. Human bocavirus. *J Clin Virol.* 2008;41:29-33.
145. Vicente D, Cilla G, Montes M, et al. Human bocavirus, a respiratory and enteric virus. *Emerg Infect Dis.* 2007;13:636-637.
146. Lau SK, Yip CC, Que TL, et al. Clinical and molecular epidemiology of human bocavirus in respiratory and fecal samples from children in Hong Kong. *J Infect Dis.* 2007;196:986-993.
147. Lindner J, Karalar L, Schimanski S, et al. Clinical and epidemiological aspects of human bocavirus infection. *J Clin Virol.* 2008;43:391-395.
148. Kahn JS, Kesebir D, Cotmore SF, et al. Seroepidemiology of human bocavirus defined using recombinant virus-like particles. *J Infect Dis.* 2008;198:41-50.
149. Allander T, Jartti T, Gupta S, et al. Human bocavirus and acute wheezing in children. *Clin Infect Dis.* 2007;44:904-910.
150. Kesebir D, Vazquez M, Weibel C, et al. Human bocavirus infection in young children in the United States: molecular epidemiological profile and clinical characteristics of a newly emerging respiratory virus. *J Infect Dis.* 2006;194:1276-1282.
151. Allander T, Jartti T, Gupta S, et al. Human bocavirus and acute wheezing in children. *Clin Infect Dis.* 2007;44:904-910.
152. Fry AM, Lu X, Chittaganpitch M, et al. Human bocavirus: a novel parvovirus epidemiologically associated with pneumonia requiring hospitalization in Thailand. *J Infect Dis.* 2007;195:1038-1045.
153. Maggi F, Andreoli E, Pifferi M, et al. Human bocavirus in Italian patients with respiratory diseases. *J Clin Virol.* 2007;38:321-325.
154. Manning A, Russell V, Eastick K, et al. Epidemiological profile and clinical associations of human bocavirus and other human parvoviruses. *J Infect Dis.* 2006;194:1283-1290.
155. Kupfer B, Vehreschild J, Cornely O, et al. Severe pneumonia and human bocavirus in adults. *Emerg Infect Dis.* 2006;12:1614-1616.
156. Jones MS, Kapoor A, Lukashov VV, et al. New DNA viruses identified in patients with acute viral infection syndrome. *J Virol.* 2005;79:8230-8236.
157. Simmonds P, Douglas J, Bestetti G, et al. A third genotype of the human parvovirus PARV4 in sub-Saharan Africa. *J Gen Virol.* 2008;89:2299-2302.
158. Fryer JF, Delwart E, Hecht FM, et al. Frequent detection of the parvoviruses, PARV4 and PARV5, in plasma from blood donors and symptomatic individuals. *Transfusion.* 2007;47:1054-1061.
159. Manning A, Willey SJ, Bell JE, et al. Comparison of tissue distribution, persistence, and molecular epidemiology of parvovirus B19 and novel human parvoviruses PARV4 and human bocavirus. *J Infect Dis.* 2007;195:1345-1352.

148

Orthoreoviruses and Orbiviruses

ROBERTA L. DeBIASI | KENNETH L. TYLER

The Reoviridae family of viruses consists of nine genera, whose members have a widely varied host range, including plants and invertebrate (insects, crustaceans) and vertebrate (mammalian, reptilian, avian) animals. Five genera have been etiologically linked with diseases of humans: *Orthoreovirus, Orbivirus, Rotavirus, Coltivirus,* and *Seadornavirus.* The genome of all Reoviridae consists of linear double-stranded RNA surrounded by a nonenveloped icosahedral capsid 60 to 80 nm in diameter. Genomic material is organized into 10 to 12 segments, which are capable of reassortment and resultant generation of novel viruses.[1] This chapter summarizes clinically relevant information pertaining to human infection due to orthoreoviruses and orbiviruses. Rotaviruses, coltiviruses, and seadornaviruses are discussed in Chapters 149 and 150.

Orthoreoviruses

BACKGROUND AND EPIDEMIOLOGY

Reoviruses were first discovered in the 1950s after isolation from human enteric specimens, and they were subsequently documented to infect a wide range of hosts. Reovirus serotypes 1, 2, and 3 are found ubiquitously in the environment, and their sources include stagnant and river water and untreated sewage. The term *reovirus* is an acronym for *respiratory enteric orphan virus,* which emphasizes the anatomic site from which these viruses were initially isolated as well as the fact that infection of humans, although common, is only rarely associated with significant disease. Human infection primarily results in either asymptomatic infection or mild, self-limited symptoms such as upper respiratory illness and gastroenteritis.[2,3] Rarely, reoviruses have been identified as the causative agent in human cases of meningitis, encephalitis, pneumonia, and myocarditis and are potentially associated with biliary atresia and choledochal cysts (discussed later).[2-4] Serologic studies of reovirus prevalence have documented steady increases from infancy (5% to 10% seropositivity at 1 year of age; 30% at 2 years of age; 50% at 5 years of age) through adulthood (50% at 20 to 30 years of age; >80% by 60 years of age),[4,5] reflecting immunity acquired as a consequence of natural infection. Despite this, it has been difficult to provide convincing evidence linking reoviruses to specific human diseases. Transmission occurs by the fecal-oral and airborne routes in humans. Reovirus infection serves as an important experimental animal model of viral encephalitis and myocarditis, which are beyond the scope of this discussion but are reviewed in Chapters 81 and 87.[6]

CLINICAL DISEASE

Respiratory

Mild upper respiratory illness consisting primarily of rhinorrhea and pharyngitis accompanied by low-grade fever, headache, and malaise (35% to 80%), with or without mild diarrhea (15% to 65%), has been described in children during outbreaks and was produced in experimental reovirus infections of adult volunteers.[7,8] In children, a maculopapular (and in one case vesicular) exanthem has been described,[4] as has otitis media. Rarer reports of lower respiratory tract disease have included interstitial or confluent pneumonia, one of which was fatal.[9] A novel reassortant reovirus designated as BYD1 strain was isolated in 2003 from five patients with severe acute respiratory syndrome (SARS) who were coinfected with SARS-associated coronavirus (SARS-CoV). Subsequent characterization in animal experimental models has

suggested a possible copathogenic role for this virus in SARS.[10,11] More recently, two new and closely related reoviruses (Melaka and Kampar viruses) have been identified and characterized from six adult and pediatric Malaysian patients with acute respiratory infection.[12,13] Both viruses are presumably of bat origin with transmission to humans by bat droppings or contaminated fruits. Index adult cases suffered from high fever, chills and rigors, sore throat, headache, and myalgia. Human-to-human transmission has been substantiated by serologic analysis of secondary cases, including children.

Gastrointestinal and Hepatobiliary

A 20-year study of children with diarrhea implicated reoviruses in only 0.1% of cases, and those occurred mainly in infants younger than 1 year.[2] A role for reovirus infection in the pathogenesis of extrahepatic biliary atresia (EHBA) and choledochal cysts (CDCs) has long been proposed based on similarities between pathologic changes observed in pediatric patients suffering from these diseases and reovirus-infected mice.[14] However, results from serology-based, as well as more recent molecular-based, studies are conflicting.[14,15] In one study, reovirus RNA was detected in hepatic or biliary tissues from 55% of patients with EHBA and 78% of patients with CDCs, compared with 21% of patients with other hepatobiliary diseases and 12% of autopsy cases.[14] However, a subsequent study failed to detect reovirus genome in hepatobiliary tissues taken from 26 patients with EHBA and 28 patients with congenital dilation of the bile duct.[15] No convincing data exist to support an etiologic role for reovirus infection in the setting of idiopathic cholestatic liver diseases in adults.

Central Nervous System

Reovirus types 1, 2, and 3 have been isolated from cerebrospinal fluid of infants with meningitis, systemic illness, or both. Reovirus type 1 was isolated from a previously healthy 3-month-old with symptoms of meningitis, diarrhea, vomiting, and fever.[16] Reovirus type 2 (subsequently identified as a new mammalian reovirus type 2 Winnepeg) was isolated from the cerebrospinal fluid of an 8-week-old presenting with active varicella-zoster virus, *Escherichia coli* sepsis, intermittent fever, diarrhea, and feeding intolerance.[17,18] A novel serotype 3 reovirus (T3C/96) was isolated from a 6-week-old with meningitis and was subsequently shown to be capable of producing lethal encephalitis in newborn mice.[19] These reports illustrate the rare but possible neuroinvasive potential of reoviruses in the human host.

Reovirus as an Oncolytic Agent

Reoviruses induce apoptosis in multiple cell types.[6] Reoviruses replicate preferentially in cells with the activated gene of *ras* family or *ras*-signaling pathway, which is the case in as many as 60% to 80% of human malignancies and 90% of metastatic disease.[20] A wide range of preclinical studies have demonstrated the potential application of reoviruses as an anticancer oncolytic agent.[21] Multiple tumor types have been shown to be susceptible to reovirus infection in vitro as a novel antitumor agent, including breast, ovarian, brain (glioma, medulloblastoma), colon, melanoma, bladder, pancreatic, prostate, and lung cancers; childhood sarcoma; and head and neck tumors.[22,23] Human clinical trials with mammalian reovirus serotype 3 Dearing (Reolysin, Oncolytics Biotech Inc., Calgary, Alberta, Canada) began in 2002. To date, more than 230 patients have been treated in 12 trials (in the United States, Canada, and the United Kingdom), using Reolysin intratumorally or intravenously, alone or in combination with other chemotherapeutic agents or radiation therapy.[24,25] Results of a phase I trial for reovirus as treatment for recurrent malignant glioma in 12 adult patients have recently been reported.[26] Stereotactic intratumoral administration of the genetically unmodified reovirus was well tolerated in these patients: 10 patients had tumor progression, 1 had stabilization, and 1 patient was not evaluable for response. Characterization of immune responses to intravenous Reolysin have also been reported.[27] Phase II trials evaluating systemic Reolysin as monotherapy are in progress for sarcoma, melanoma, and ovarian cancers. A pivotal phase II/III randomized trial using systemic Reolysin in combination with paclitaxel/carboplatin for patients with refractory head and neck cancers is planned.

Orbiviruses

BACKGROUND AND EPIDEMIOLOGY

The genus *Orbivirus* contains more than 100 subspecies classified within 14 serogroups, infecting a broad range of arthropod and vertebrate hosts. Orbiviruses are named based on their characteristic doughnut-shaped capsomers. The bulk of disease due to orbiviruses occurs in nonhuman vertebrates; the most frequently identified are bluetongue virus (sheep, cattle, goats, and wild ungulates), African horse sickness virus (horses, donkeys, and dogs), and epizootic hemorrhagic disease virus (deer). Disease in humans has been reported infrequently (fewer than 100 cases reported in the literature worldwide). However, infection can occur in humans who serve as an incidental host during the maintenance cycle of vector-borne transmission between nonhuman vertebrate hosts. Vectors for disease include mosquitoes, midges, gnats, sandflies, and ticks.[28,29]

CLINICAL DISEASE

Only four orbivirus serogroups have been linked to disease in humans; these are the viruses belonging to the Kemerovo antigenic complex, including Kemerovo, Lipovnik, and Tribec viruses (Russia and eastern Europe), Orungo virus (sub-Saharan Africa), Lebombo virus (South Africa and Nigeria), and Changuinola virus (Central America).[29] The spectrum of reported human disease includes neurologic infection (encephalitis, meningitis, meningoencephalitis, polyradiculitis) as well as acute febrile illnesses. Many orbiviruses preferentially infect vascular endothelial cells; thus, clinical and laboratory manifestations can mimic those seen in the setting of rickettsial illnesses. No deaths have been reported due to human orbivirus infection, and patients generally recover without long-term sequelae of infection. All age groups may be infected; however, the pediatric population is overrepresented in seroprevalence studies. In animals, orbivirus infection has been linked to congenital abnormalities such as hydranencephaly, arthrogryposis, and deafness, but this has not been reported in humans.[29]

Clinical Features of Specific Agents

Kemerovo Virus Antigenic Complex. Viruses of the Kemerovo complex (Kemerovo, Tribec, and Lipovnik) are transmitted by *Ixodes* sp. ticks in Russian and Eastern Europe and were first isolated in 1963 from ticks and patients with meningitis and meningoencephalitis. Meningoencephalitis and polyradiculitis have been linked to Lipovnik virus in former Czechoslovakia. Seroprevalence studies in healthy residents of the former Czech Republic indicate up to 18% seropositivity; additional serologic evaluation of neurologic patients from Central Europe with tick-borne encephalitis virus demonstrated the presence of concurrent Lipovnik virus antibodies in more than 50% of patients.[30]

Oklahoma Tick Fever. In the United States, cases of acute febrile illness, subsequently designated as Oklahoma tick fever, have been reported in Oklahoma and Texas and attributed to orbivirus infection, likely a Kemerovo-related virus. Clinical features of these reports included myalgia, vomiting, and severe abdominal pain. Laboratory features include transient leukopenia, thrombocytopenia, and anemia, suggesting possible rickettsial disease; however, serologic analysis for Rocky Mountain spotted fever, Colorado tick fever, and Powassan virus was negative.[28] Diagnosis was based on positive serology for Kemerovo group-related orbiviruses (Sixgun City and Lipovnik viruses). Viremia was not present in these patients; therefore, a specific viral etiology was not confirmed in these cases. Transmission of Kemerovo-related viruses in rabbit and large animal populations has been documented in Midwestern states, but no human cases have been reported to date.

Orungo Virus. Orungo virus is transmitted primarily by *Aedes* sp. but also by *Culex* and *Anopheles* spp. mosquitoes in regions of sub-Saharan Africa. Seroprevalence studies in that region are as high as 24% to 34%.[31] Acute febrile illness, including fever, headache, and myalgia has been reported, as has one case of encephalitis in a child with convulsions and flaccid paralysis.[32,33] Coinfection with yellow fever virus has been documented.[34]

Lebombo Virus. Transmission of Lebombo virus occurs from *Aedes* and *Mansonia* spp. mosquitoes in South Africa and Nigeria. A case of nonspecific acute febrile illness has been reported in a Nigerian child.[32]

Changuinola Virus. Acute febrile illness due to Changuinola virus has been reported in a single human case from Panama. Seroprevalence studies indicate high rates of seropositivity in parts of South America, but the infection-to-disease ratio is unknown. Transmission has been proposed by *Phlebotomus* sp. flies.

African Horse Sickness Virus. Naturally occurring infection of humans with African horse sickness virus has not been reported. However, four workers in a South African veterinary office were infected in 1989 with accidentally aerosolized freeze-dried virus present in a vaccine containing attenuated viral strains. Illness was severe in all exposed workers: three developed frontotemporal encephalitis, and all four developed uveochorioretinitis. Diagnosis was confirmed serologically.[35]

Diagnosis

Laboratory diagnosis of orbivirus infection is made serologically by a fourfold rise in acute and convalescent serum antibody response, or virus isolation from serum or cerebrospinal fluid by inoculation of suckling mice or cell cultures (Vero or BHK021). Virus-specific immunoglobulin M testing is available at reference laboratories, including the Centers for Disease Control and Prevention and the United States Army Medical Research Institute for Infectious Diseases. No specific therapy is available.

REFERENCES

1. Schiff LA, Nibert ML, Tyler KL. Orthoreoviruses and their replication. In: Knipe DM, Roizman B, Howley PM, et al, eds. *Fields Virology*. Philadelphia: Lippincott Williams & Wilkins; 2007.
2. Giordano MO, Martinez LC, Isa MB, et al. Twenty year study of the occurrence of reovirus infection in hospitalized children with acute gastroenteritis in Argentina. *Pediatr Infect Dis J*. 2002; 21:880-882.
3. El-Rai FM, Evans AS. Reovirus infections in children and young adults. *Arch Environ Health*. 1963;7:700-704.
4. Lerner AM, Cherry JD, Klein JO, et al. Infections with reoviruses. *N Engl J Med*. 1962;267:947-952.
5. Tai, JH, Williams JV, Edwards KM, et al. Prevalence of reovirus-specific antibodies in young children in Nashville, Tennessee. *J Infect Dis*. 2005;191:1221-1224.
6. Clarke P, DeBiasi RL, Goody R, et al. Mechanisms of reovirus-induced cell death and tissue injury: role of apoptosis and virus-induced perturbation of host-cell signaling and transcription factor activation. *Viral Immunol*. 2005;18:89-115.
7. Rosen L, Evans HE, Spickard A. Reovirus infections in human volunteers. *Am J Hyg*. 1963;77:29-37.
8. Rosen L, Hovis JF, Mastrota FM, et al. Observations on a newly recognized virus (Abney) of the reovirus family. *Am J Hyg*. 1960;71:258-265.
9. Tillotson JR, Lerner AM. Reovirus type 3 associated with fatal pneumonia. *N Engl J Med*. 1967;276:1060-1063.
10. Song L, Zhou Y, He J, et al. Comparative sequence analyses of a new mammalian reovirus genome and the mammalian reovirus S1 genes from six new serotype 2 human isolates. *Virus Genes*. 2008;37:392-399.
11. He C, Yang Q, Lei M, et al. Diffuse alveolar lesion in BALB/c mice induced with human reovirus BYD1 strain and its potential relation with SARS. *Exp Anim*. 2006;55:439-447.
12. Chua KB, Crameri G, Hyatt A, et al. A previously unknown reovirus of bat origin is associated with an acute respiratory disease in humans. *Proc Natl Acad Sci U S A*. 2007;104:11424-11429.

13. Chua KB, Voon K, Crameri G, et al. Identification and characterization of a new orthoreovirus from patients with acute respiratory infections. *PLoS ONE.* 2008;3:e3803.

14. Tyler KL, Sokol RJ, Oberhaus SM, et al. Detection of reovirus RNA in hepatobiliary tissues from patients with extrahepatic biliary atresia and choledochal cysts. *Hepatology.* 1998;27: 1475-1482.

15. Saito T, Shinozaki K, Matsunaga T, et al. Lack of evidence for reovirus infection in tissues from patients with biliary atresia and congenital dilatation of the bile duct. *J Hepatol.* 2004; 40:203-211.

16. Johansson PJ, Sveger T, Ahlfors K, et al. Reovirus type 1 associated with meningitis. *Scand J Infect Dis.* 1996;28:117-120.

17. Hermann L, Embree J, Hazelton P, et al. Reovirus type 2 isolated from cerebrospinal fluid. *Pediatr Infect Dis J.* 2004;23:373-375.

18. Jiang J, Hermann L, Coombs KM. Genetic characterization of a new mammalian reovirus, type 2 Winnipeg (T2W). *Virus Genes.* 2006;33:193-204.

19. Tyler KL, Barton ES, Ibach ML, et al. Isolation and molecular characterization of a novel type 3 reovirus from a child with meningitis. *J Infect Dis.* 2004;189:1664-1675.

20. Figova K, Hrabeta J, Eckschlager T. Reovirus—possible therapy of cancer. *Neoplasma.* 2006;53:457-462.

21. Kim M, Chung YH, Johnston RN. Reovirus and tumor oncolysis. *J Microbiol.* 2007;45:187-192.

22. Comins C, Heinemann L, Harrington K, et al. Reovirus: viral therapy for cancer 'as nature intended'. *Clin Oncol (R Coll Radiol).* 2008;20:548-554.

23. Yap TA, Brunetto A, Pandha H, et al. Reovirus therapy in cancer: has the orphan virus found a home? *Expert Opin Investig Drugs.* 2008;17:1925-1935.

24. Stoeckel J, Hay JG. Drug evaluation: Reolysin–wild-type reovirus as a cancer therapeutic. *Curr Opin Mol Ther.* 2006;8:249-260.

25. Liu TC, Kirn D. Systemic efficacy with oncolytic virus therapeutics: clinical proof-of-concept and future directions. *Cancer Res.* 2007;67:429-432.

26. Forsyth P, Roldan G, George D, et al. A phase I trial of intratumoral administration of reovirus in patients with histologically confirmed recurrent malignant gliomas. *Mol Ther.* 2008;16: 627-632.

27. White CL, Twigger KR, Vidal L, et al. Characterization of the adaptive and innate immune response to intravenous oncolytic reovirus (Dearing type 3) during a phase I clinical trial. *Gene Ther.* 2008;15:911-920.

28. Tsai TF. Arboviral infections in the United States. *Infect Dis Clin North Am.* 1991;5:73-102.

29. Tsai TF. Orbiviruses and coltiviruses. In: Feigen RD, Cherry J, eds. *Textbook of Pediatric Infectious Diseases.* Philadelphia: WB Saunders; 2004:1897-1901.

30. Libikova H, Heinz F, Ujhazyova D, et al. Orbiviruses of the Kemerovo complex and neurological diseases. *Med Microbiol Immunol.* 1978;166:255-263.

31. Tomori O, Fabiyi A. Neutralizing antibodies to Orungo virus in man and animals in Nigeria. *Trop Geogr Med.* 1976;28: 233-238.

32. Moore DL, Causey OR, Carey DE, et al. Arthropod-borne viral infections of man in Nigeria, 1964-1970. *Ann Trop Med Parasitol.* 1975;69:49-64.

33. Familusi JB, Moore DL, Fomufod AK, et al. Virus isolates from children with febrile convulsions in Nigeria. A correlation study of clinical and laboratory observations. *Clin Pediatr (Phila).* 1972;11:272-276.

34. Monath TP, Craven RB, Adjukiewicz A, et al. Yellow fever in the Gambia, 1978–1979: epidemiologic aspects with observations on the occurrence of orungo virus infections. *Am J Trop Med Hyg.* 1980;29:912-928.

35. Swanepoel R, Erasmus BJ, Williams R, et al. Encephalitis and chorioretinitis associated with neurotropic African horsesickness virus infection in laboratory workers. Part III. Virological and serological investigations. *S Afr Med J.* 1992;81: 458-461.

149

Coltiviruses and Seadornaviruses

ROBERTA L. DeBIASI | KENNETH L. TYLER

Coltivirus and *Seadornavirus* are two of five genera of the Reoviridae virus family that have been documented to cause human disease; *Orthoreovirus*, *Orbivirus*, and *Rotavirus* are discussed in Chapters 148 and 150. Like all Reoviridae, coltiviruses and seadornaviruses are non-enveloped double-stranded RNA viruses with a segmented genome. Coltiviruses have 12 gene segments enclosed within two capsids. Coltiviruses were classified within the *Orbivirus* genus until 1991, at which time their distinct molecular identity was established, and a unique genus was proposed.[1-4] Coltiviruses were initially subclassified into the tick-borne subgroup A (North American and European distribution) and mosquito-borne subgroup B (Asian distribution) viruses. In the year 2000, subgroup B coltiviruses were reclassified into the newly designated genus *Seadornavirus* (an acronym for *Southeast Asian dodeca RNA virus*) based on sequence data and antigenic properties. Coltiviruses associated with human disease include the type-specific Colorado tick fever virus (CTFV; North America), Eyach virus (EYAV; France, Germany, Czech Republic), and Salmon River virus (SRV; North America). The only Seadornavirus implicated in human disease to date is Banna virus (BAV; Indonesia and China). However, Seadornavirus infection is considered an emerging infectious disease, and the full spectrum of human disease is likely underrecognized.[3,5-7] Although not yet isolated from humans, the seadornaviruses Kadipiro and Liao ning have been isolated from mosquitoes and replicate well in mice,[3,8] suggesting the potential for human infection.

Coltiviruses

COLORADO TICK FEVER VIRUS

Epidemiology

A recent comprehensive review of CTFV indicates that up to 400 cases are reported in the United States each year, making it the second most commonly identified arboviral infection in the United States, after West Nile virus.[9] Ticks are the principal vectors of coltiviruses but have also been isolated from mosquitoes, rodents, and humans.[6,10] Coltiviruses exhibit a high frequency of RNA segment reassortment in tick vectors.[11] CTFV is maintained in an epizootic cycle between the principal vector, *Dermacentor andersoni*, and small mammals such as porcupines, ground squirrels, and chipmunks. Humans are infected by the bite of adult ticks.[9,12] The geographic distribution of the type-specific CTFV includes China, Europe, and North America. In the United States, the distribution of CTFV coincides with the range of the principal vector, *D. andersoni*. The virus has been isolated in 11 states, primarily within the Rocky Mountain region (California, Colorado, Idaho, Montana, Nevada, New Mexico, Oregon, South Dakota, Utah, Washington, and Wyoming) as well as southwestern Canada.[9] Most cases occur in Colorado, Montana, Utah, and Wyoming.[9] Elevations of 4000 to 10,000 feet and rocky outcroppings are especially suited to CTFV.[9,12,13] Transmission coincides with the seasonal activity of *D. andersoni* ticks, with most cases occurring between April and July.[9] Disease transmission can occur even as a consequence of brief tick attachment, in contrast with the requirement for prolonged tick attachment for transmission of *Borrelia burgdorferi* or *Rickettsia rickettsii*.[9] Ninety percent of patients report tick exposure, but only 48% recall tick attachment.[14] Half of reported cases occur in patients between 20 and 49 years of age, with an additional 25% occurring in patients younger than 20 years.[9,14] Transfusion-related symptomatic infection has been reported.[15] CTFV patients should not be allowed to serve as blood product or hematopoietic stem cell donors until infection has fully resolved, and reverse transcriptase–polymerase chain reaction (RT-PCR) assays on blood are negative, a process that may take 4 months or longer (see later). Intrauterine transmission during human pregnancy has resulted in the birth of healthy infants but also has been potentially associated with spontaneous abortion and other congenital anomalies.[16] Laboratory transmission cases have also been reported.

Clinical Features

CTFV has been isolated from patients with acute febrile syndromes, meningitis, and encephalitis in North America. The first published clinical descriptions of CTFV appeared as early as 1855 with identification of the virus in 1946 after isolation from human serum.[9,17] At least 22 strains of CTFV have been described,[18] many of which cause disease in humans. Onset of symptoms usually occurs after an incubation of 3 to 5 days (range, 0 to 14 days).[9,14,19] Symptoms classically include abrupt onset of fever, chills, and headache, which may be accompanied by retroorbital pain, photophobia, conjunctivitis, myalgia, generalized weakness, or lethargy.[9,14,19] Other reported clinical findings include pharyngitis (20% of patients), palatal enanthem, nausea, vomiting, diarrhea, abdominal pain, and splenomegaly.[9,14,19] Rash occurs in a minority (5% to 12%) of patients and has been described as macular, maculopapular, or petechial.[9] Fever typically lasts 2 to 3 days and either resolves completely or, in 50% of cases, recurs after a period of 1 to 3 days of fever remittance (although malaise may continue), described as the *saddleback fever pattern*. This second phase of febrile illness lasts about 2 days.[14,19] Full resolution of symptoms typically occurs within 1 week. Older patients (>30 years or age) may have fatigue, persisting for weeks to months.[9] Neurologic complications (aseptic meningitis, meningoencephaltis, or encephalitis) are more common in the pediatric population, occurring in up to 10% of symptomatic children.[9] Other rarely reported complications include myocarditis, pericarditis, pneumonitis, hepatitis, and epididymo-orchitis.[6,9,18] Severity of illness is sufficient to necessitate hospitalization in up to 20% of CTFV patients.[6] Mortality has not been reported in adults and is rare in children, with deaths reported in the pediatric population secondary to hemorrhagic shock, disseminated intravascular coagulation, or meningoencephalitis.[9,14,19]

Laboratory and Diagnostic Findings

Leukopenia (900 to 4000 cells/mm³) is common (65% of patients),[6] with a nadir typically occurring 6 days after symptom onset.[20] A relative lymphocytosis is common, although atypical lymphocytes and neutrophils with toxic granules have also been reported. Moderate thrombocytopenia (20,000 to 97,000/μL) may also be present.[20] Bone marrow aspiration shows reduction in mature granulocytes and megakaryocytes and increase in immature forms.[18] In patients with meningitis, meningoencephalitis, or encephalitis, cerebrospinal fluid (CSF) may demonstrate a lymphocytic pleocytosis of up to 300 white blood cells/mm³, mild elevations of protein, and normal to slightly decreased glucose concentration, none of which are distinguishable from other causes of meningoencephalitis.[9,19]

The virus can be isolated from blood and CSF. CTF viremia is prolonged, persisting up to 4 months after onset of illness in 50% of cases, related to infection of hematopoietic progenitor cells and persistence through erythrocyte maturation.[6,21,22] A quantitative real-time RT-PCR assay for the detection of CTF viral RNA in human clinical samples, including serum, has recently been described.[23,24] The sensitivity of this assay has been shown to be greater than that of isolation of virus in Vero cells. The assay may be particularly useful for diagnosis during the first 5 to 6 days of illness.[23]

A variety of methods for serologic diagnosis have been used.[25] An immunofluorescence assay allows rapid detection of anti-CTFV antibodies. A plaque reduction neutralization assay can detect neutralizing antibodies that appear 14 to 21 days after onset of disease. An enzyme-linked immunosorbent assay (ELISA) detects immunoglobulin M (IgM) and IgG antibodies that appear concurrently or several days after neutralizing antibodies. IgM titers for CTFV peak 30 to 40 days after infection, then rapidly fall after day 45. ELISA based on recombinant VP7 and Western blot based on synthetic VP12 also show good sensitivity.[26] The complement-fixation test is insensitive; complement-fixing antibodies are detectable only late in infection for 75% of patients and are not detectable in 25% of patients.

The differential diagnosis of CTFV includes rickettsial diseases (Rocky Mountain spotted fever, ehrlichiosis), tularemia, relapsing fever, and Lyme disease as well as other causes of viral meningitis and encephalitis.

Treatment

No specific antiviral therapy is available, and treatment is supportive. Aspirin should be avoided because it may exacerbate the potential for hemorrhage associated with thrombocytopenia.[9] Animal models show increased survival with ribavirin, but no human data support efficacy or safety in treatment of CTFV of humans.[9] Tick prevention strategies are most important in limiting disease in humans. Infection with CTFV is thought to provide long-lasting immunity against reinfection.

SALMON RIVER VIRUS

SRV (CTFV-Ca) is considered a serotype of CTFV and has been associated with human disease. It was isolated from a viremic patient with a CTFV-like illness and named for the area where infection was likely acquired: at the middle fork of Idaho's Salmon River. Some experts have postulated that SRV may be the cause of most CTFV-like illnesses in Idaho and Montana. Many small and large mammals are infected naturally with the virus, but only humans develop clinical illness.[27]

EYACH VIRUS

EYAV is an antigenically related but distinct virus from CTFV that was first isolated from *Ixodes* sp. ticks in France and Germany.[6,10,18,28,29] EYAV has subsequently been implicated in febrile illness and neuro-logic syndromes (encephalitis and polyradiculoneuritis) in patients from the former Czech Republic.[30] Antibodies to EYAV were detected in sera and CSF from 12% of Czech patients, most of whom had clinical presentations suggestive of tick-borne encephalitis virus infection. EYAV was not isolated from these patients. The natural cycle of the virus is still not fully known. The reservoir is thought to be the European rabbit, and serologic surveys demonstrated EYAV antibodies in deer, ovines, and caprines.[1] Virus isolation and propagation are not feasible in cell culture and typically require intracranial injection of suckling mice. Complement fixation and neutralization assays for EYAV are not widely available. A highly sensitive and specific ELISA directed at recombinant VP6 protein of EYAV is available, which effectively distinguishes between CTFV and EYAV.[31] In an evaluation of 340 sera from French blood donors, specificity for this ELISA was 100%, and no cross-reactivity was detected with antibody to CTFV. PCR has also been used for diagnosis.[4]

Seadornaviruses

BANNA VIRUS

Epidemiology and Clinical Features

Seadornaviruses are mosquito-borne arboviruses endemic to Southeast Asia, particularly Indonesia and China. The epidemiology of seadornaviruses remains poorly documented. BAV, the type species of the genus, is the only seadornavirus that has been isolated from humans and associated with human disease.[3,6,7,32] BAV has been isolated from multiple mosquito species (*Anopheles*, *Culex*, and *Aedes* spp.), pigs, and cattle, as well as humans, suggesting widespread distribution throughout Southeast Asia.[5,6] BAV was first isolated in 1987 from CSF and sera from encephalitis patients in southern China (Yunnan province) and has subsequently been detected in up to 24% of patients with unexplained fever or encephalitis in other parts of China.[6,7,33] Patients infected with BAV exhibit influenza-like symptoms, myalgia, arthralgia, fever, and encephalitis.[6] Infection with BAV may be underreported because it circulates in regions with a high incidence of Japanese encephalitis and could be misdiagnosed as this disease.[10] Two other seadornaviruses, Kadipiro and Liao ning, have been isolated only from mosquitoes but may be emerging human pathogens.[6,8]

Serologic diagnostic assays have been developed based on the outer coat proteins responsible for cell attachment and neutralization.[7,26,31,34] Molecular diagnostics have been designed for detection of BAV, including RT-PCR.[25,35] No specific therapy exists; treatment is symptomatic for fever and pain relief. Strong and long-lasting immunologic responses have been documented in patients infected with BAV.[6]

REFERENCES

1. Attoui H, Jaafar FM, Biagini P, et al. Genus *Coltivirus* (family Reoviridae): genomic and morphologic characterization of Old World and New World viruses. *Arch Virol.* 2002;147:533-561.
2. Attoui H., Billoir F, Biagini P, et al. Sequence determination and analysis of the full-length genome of Colorado tick fever virus, the type species of genus *Coltivirus* (family Reoviridae). *Biochem Biophys Res Commun.* 2000;273:1121-1125.
3. Attoui H, Billoir F, Biagini P, et al. Complete sequence determination and genetic analysis of Banna virus and Kadipiro virus: proposal for assignment to a new genus (*Seadornavirus*) within the family Reoviridae. *J Gen Virol.* 2000;81:1507-1515.
4. Attoui H, Charrel RN, Billoir F, et al. Comparative sequence analysis of American, European and Asian isolates of viruses in the genus Coltivirus. *J Gen Virol.* 1998;79(Pt 10):2481-2489.
5. Nabeshima T, Nga PT, Posadas G, et al. Isolation and molecular characterization of Banna virus from mosquitoes, Vietnam. *Emerg Infect Dis.* 2008;14:1276-1279.
6. Attoui H, Mohd Jaafar F, de Micco P, et al. Coltiviruses and seadornaviruses in North America, Europe, and Asia. *Emerg Infect Dis.* 2005;11:1673-1679.
7. Tao SJ, Chen BQ. Studies of coltivirus in China. *Chin Med J (Engl).* 2005;118:581-586.
8. Attoui H, Mohd Jaafar F, Belhouchet M, et al. Liao ning virus, a new Chinese seadornavirus that replicates in transformed and embryonic mammalian cells. *J Gen Virol.* 2006;87:199-208.
9. Romero JR, Simonsen KA. Powassan encephalitis and Colorado tick fever. *Infect Dis Clin North Am.* 2008;22:545-559, x.
10. Charrel RN, Attoui H, Butenko AM, et al. Tick-borne virus diseases of human interest in Europe. *Clin Microbiol Infect.* 2004;10:1040-1055.
11. Brown SE, Miller BR, McLean RG, et al. Co-circulation of multiple Colorado tick fever virus genotypes. *Am J Trop Med Hyg.* 1989;40:94-101.
12. McLean RG, Shriner RB, Pokorny KS, et al. The ecology of Colorado tick fever in Rocky Mountain National Park in 1974. III. Habitats supporting the virus. *Am J Trop Med Hyg.* 1989;40:86-93.
13. Emmons RW. Ecology of Colorado tick fever. *Annu Rev Microbiol.* 1988;42:49-64.
14. Goodpasture HC, Poland JD, Francy DB, et al. Colorado tick fever: clinical, epidemiologic, and laboratory aspects of 228 cases in Colorado in 1973-1974. *Ann Intern Med.* 1978;88:303-310.
15. Leiby DA, Gill JE. Transfusion-transmitted tick-borne infections: a cornucopia of threats. *Transfus Med Rev.* 2004;18:293-306.
16. Parsonson IM, Della-Porta AJ, Snowdon WA. Developmental disorders of the fetus in some arthropod-borne virus infections. *Am J Trop Med Hyg.* 1981;30:660-673.
17. Florio L, Miller MS, Mugrage ER. Colorado tick fever: isolation of the virus from Dermacentor andersoni in nature and a laboratory study of the transmission of the virus in the tick. *J Immunol.* 1950;64:257-263.
18. Klasco R, Colorado tick fever. *Med Clin North Am.* 2002;86:435-440, ix.
19. Spruance SL, Bailey A. Colorado tick fever. A review of 115 laboratory confirmed cases. *Arch Intern Med.* 1973;131:288-293.
20. Andersen RD, Entringer MA, Robinson WA. Virus-induced leukopenia: Colorado tick fever as a human model. *J Infect Dis.* 1985;151:449-453.
21. Philipp CS, Callaway C, Chu MC, et al. Replication of Colorado tick fever virus within human hematopoietic progenitor cells. *J Virol.* 1993;67:2389-2395.
22. Hughes LE, Casper EA, Clifford CM. Persistence of Colorado tick fever virus in red blood cells. *Am J Trop Med Hyg.* 1974;23:530-532.
23. Lambert AJ, Kosoy O, Velez JO, et al. Detection of Colorado Tick Fever viral RNA in acute human serum samples by a quantitative real-time RT-PCR assay. *J Virol Methods.* 2007;140:43-48.
24. Johnson AJ, Karabatsos N, Lanciotti RS. Detection of Colorado tick fever virus by using reverse transcriptase PCR and application of the technique in laboratory diagnosis. *J Clin Microbiol.* 1997;35:1203-1208.

25. Attoui H, Billoir F, Bruey, JM, et al. Serologic and molecular diagnosis of Colorado tick fever viral infections. *Am J Trop Med Hyg*. 1998;59:763-768.

26. Mohd Jaafar F, Attoui H, Gallian P, et al. Recombinant VP7-based enzyme-linked immunosorbent assay for detection of immunoglobulin G antibodies to Colorado tick fever virus. *J Clin Microbiol*. 2003;41:2102-2105.

27. Tsai T. Orbiviruses and coltiviruses. In: Feigen RD, Cherry J, eds. *Textbook of Pediatric Infectious Diseases*. Philadelphia: WB Saunders; 2004:1897-1901.

28. Chastel C. Erve and Eyach: two viruses isolated in France, neuropathogenic for man and widely distributed in Western Europe. *Bull Acad Natl Med*. 1998;182:801-809; discussion 809-810.

29. Rehse-Kupper B, Casals J, Rehse E, et al. Eyach: An arthropod-borne virus related to Colorado tick fever virus in the Federal Republic of Germany. *Acta Virol*. 1976;20:339-342.

30. Malkova D, Holubova J, Kolman JM, et al. Antibodies against some arboviruses in persons with various neuropathies. *Acta Virol*. 1980;24:298.

31. Mohd Jaafar F, Attoui H, De Micco P, et al. Recombinant VP6-based enzyme-linked immunosorbent assay for detection of immunoglobulin G antibodies to Eyach virus (genus Coltivirus). *J Clin Virol*. 2004;30:248-253.

32. Mohd Jaafar F, Attoui H, Mertens PP, et al. Structural organization of an encephalitic human isolate of Banna virus (genus Seadornavirus, family Reoviridae). *J Gen Virol*. 2005;86:1147-1157.

33. Xu P, Wang Y, Zuo J, et al. New orbiviruses isolated from patients with unknown fever and encephalitis in Yunnan province. *Chinese J Virol*. 1990;6:27-33.

34. Mohd Jaafar F, Attoui H, Gallian P, et al. Recombinant VP9-based enzyme-linked immunosorbent assay for detection of immunoglobulin G antibodies to Banna virus (genus *Seadornavirus*). *J Virol Methods*. 2004;116:55-61.

35. Billoir F, Attoui H, Simon S, et al. Molecular diagnosis of group B coltiviruses infections. *J Virol Methods*. 1999;81:39-45.

150

Rotaviruses

PHILIP R. DORMITZER

History and Overview

Rotaviruses constitute a genus within the Reoviridae, a family of non-enveloped, icosahedral animal viruses with double-stranded, segmented RNA genomes. The family Reoviridae also includes the reoviruses, which have occasionally been isolated from patients with respiratory illnesses but have not been established as a cause of human disease (see Chapter 148), and the coltiviruses and seadornaviruses, which cause disease in humans (see Chapter 149). Rotavirus is the most important cause of severe, dehydrating gastroenteritis in children younger than 5 years in all socioeconomic groups and in all regions of the world.[1] It is responsible for approximately 611,000 infant and childhood deaths annually, with these deaths occurring primarily in the developing world.[1] In temperate climates, rotavirus causes the annual peak in pediatric hospitalizations for dehydration related to gastroenteritis during the cooler months of the year.[2]

Before the association of rotaviruses with human disease, etiologic agents were not identified in most cases of childhood gastroenteritis. In 1973, electron microscopic examination of duodenal biopsy specimens from six of nine children with acute gastroenteritis revealed similar viral particles, which were approximately 70 nm in diameter.[3] Morphologically, these particles were indistinguishable from viruses previously identified in specimens from mice and cows with diarrhea,[4,5] and were designated rotaviruses because of their appearance in electron micrographs as wheels with spokes (Fig. 150-1). The antigenic similarity between the human and bovine agents was confirmed when an exchange of matched liquid stool and convalescent-phase sera between a veterinary and a medical laboratory showed that antibodies in the sera of children and calves agglutinated the rotavirus particles in the stools of both species.[6] The human sera also neutralized the infectivity of the bovine agent, which had been adapted to growth in cell culture.[6]

Since the discovery of the agent, understanding of rotavirus replication, pathogenesis, and immunity has relied on the study of strains that grow well in cell culture and on large and small animal models for rotavirus infection and disease. The ability to "mate" rotavirus strains by coinfecting cells to achieve reassortment of the 11 genome segments has allowed classic genetic studies. Extensive global epidemiology has relied on an elaborate serology, now supplemented by nucleic acid-based diagnostics. This scientific background enabled the recent introduction of live-attenuated vaccines for human use. These vaccines have started to change the epidemiology and clinical impact of rotaviruses in the regions where they are being introduced.[7] Extension of effective immunization to the most severely affected populations in developing countries is the next important challenge. The application of molecular and structural biology promises to provide the scientific basis for the next generation of vaccines.

Viral Structure

The rotavirus virion is a nonenveloped icosahedral particle, which is approximately 770 Å in diameter, excluding the VP4 spikes (Fig. 150-2).[8] It consists of three concentric protein layers, which encapsidate 11 segments of tightly packed, double-stranded RNA, together with polymerase and capping enzyme complexes. Each genome segment contains one or, in the case of genome segment 11, two open reading frames. These segments encode six structural proteins (VP1 to VP4, VP6, and VP7) and six nonstructural proteins (NSP1 to NSP6).

The innermost protein shell consists of 120 copies of VP2, arranged in an icosahedral lattice (T = 1 with two VP2 molecules making up each icosahedral asymmetrical unit).[8] The VP1 polymerase and VP3 capping enzyme are anchored inside the VP2 shell adjacent to pores at the icosahedral fivefold vertices. The middle layer consists of 780 copies of VP6, which form thick trimeric pillars in an icosahedral lattice (T = 13 *levo*). Although not exposed on the virus surface, VP6 is the target of the most abundant antibodies elicited by rotavirus infection. The genome, VP1, VP3, and the inner two protein layers make up the transcriptionally active, double-layered subviral particle (DLP).

The thin outermost layer consists of 780 copies of a coat glycoprotein, VP7, and 60 VP4 spikes, which protrude from the virion.[8] One hundred and thirty-two aqueous holes perforate the outer and middle layers. VP4 and VP7 translocate the DLP across a host membrane and into the cytoplasm. Both outer layer proteins are neutralization antigens.[9] VP4 is the major cell attachment protein as well as a determinant of virulence and growth restriction in cell culture.[10,11] VP7 forms the icosahedral lattice (T = 13 *levo*) of the outermost layer, which is in register with the VP6 lattice of the middle layer. VP4 and VP7 are shed from the virion during entry. In vitro, chelation of calcium from the virion causes dissociation of VP7 trimers,[12] leading to virus uncoating and activation of the viral polymerase.[13]

The rotavirus particle is physically hardy and resists inactivation by treatment with fluorocarbons, ether, and concentrations of chlorine typically used to treat sewage effluent and drinking water.[14] However, the particle is inactivated by calcium chelators and by antiseptic agents that contain relatively high concentrations of alcohols (>40%), free chlorine (>20,000 ppm), or iodophores (>10,000 ppm iodine).[15] A commonly used hand-sanitizing agent (Purell), which contains 62% ethanol, substantially reduces viable rotavirus carriage on fingertips[16] and a disinfectant spray (Lysol), which contains 79% ethanol and 0.1% *o*-phenylphenol, prevents the experimental transmission of rotavirus from fomites to human volunteers.[17] Rotavirus survival in the environment is significantly decreased at high relative humidity.[14]

Viral Replication

Efficient rotavirus infectivity requires priming of the virus by intestinal trypsin, which cleaves the spike protein, VP4, into an amino-terminal fragment, VP8*, and a carboxy-terminal fragment, VP5*. The VP8* fragment contains a hemagglutination domain, which forms the spike "heads," and the VP5* fragment contains a membrane interaction domain, which forms the spike "body" (see Fig. 150-2).[18,19] Cleavage into VP5* and VP8* triggers an initial rearrangement of VP4 that increases the rigidity of the spikes.[20]

The rotavirus cell entry pathway involves virus interactions with several cell surface molecules.[21] Some rotavirus strains, including many that cause disease in nonhuman animals, attach to cells when the VP8* heads of the VP4 spikes bind neuraminidase-sensitive sialosides on cell membrane glycoproteins or glycolipids.[18,22] Most strains that cause human disease bind an alternative receptor, possibly an integrin, using the VP5* fragment of VP4.[21,23] During entry, the VP5* fragment of VP4 undergoes a dramatic fold-back rearrangement, translocating its hydrophobic apex from one end of the molecule to the other.[19] This motion resembles the fold-back rearrangments of enveloped virus-fusion proteins, which mediate fusion between a virus envelope and a

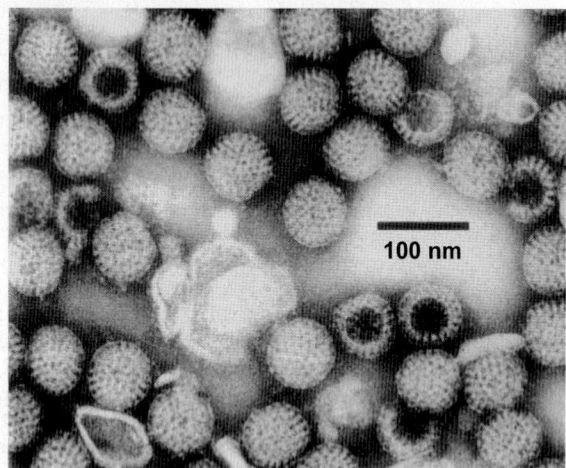

Figure 150-1   Electron micrograph of negatively stained rotavirus virions in a stool filtrate from a child with gastroenteritis. The outer capsid appears as a thin rim surrounding stubby protrusions made up of VP6 trimers. "Empty" particles with dark centers lack genomic RNA. *(From Kapikian AZ, Kim HW, Wyatt RG, et al. Reoviruslike agent in stools: association with infantile diarrhea and development of serologic tests. Science. 1974;185:1049-1053.)*

cellular membrane. By analogy, it is likely that the "jackknifing" of VP5* helps nonenveloped rotavirus particles breach a cellular membrane during entry. The membrane breach must be substantial. Because naked rotavirus double-stranded RNA genome segments are not infectious, the entire transcriptionally active 710-Å DLP must be translocated into the cytoplasm to initiate infection.

Dependence of rotavirus entry on dynamin function suggests, but does not prove, that rotavirus enter cells through endosomes.[24] Endo-

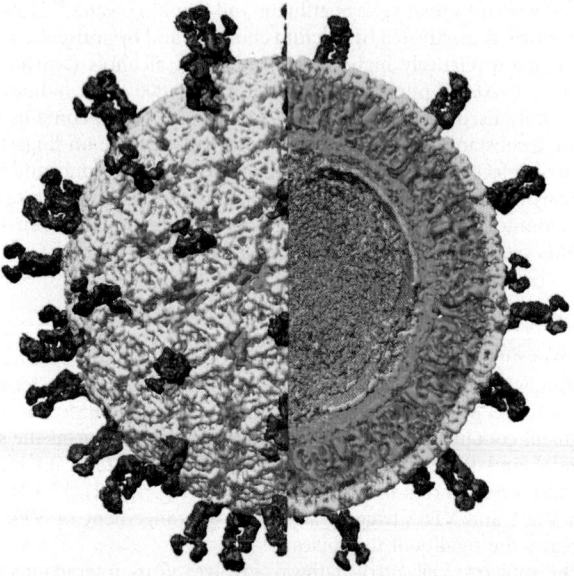

Figure 150-2   Electron cryomicroscopy image reconstruction of the rotavirus (strain SA11-4F) triple-layered particle at 9.5 Å resolution. VP2, the innermost icosahedral layer protein, is green. VP6, the middle icosahedral layer protein, is blue. VP7, the outermost icosahedral layer protein, is yellow. VP4, the spike protein, is red, and a layer of the particle interior, which is filled with genomic RNA, the polymerase, and the capping enzyme, is orange. The virions used to create this reconstruction were produced in the presence of trypsin, so that VP4 has been cleaved into VP5* and VP8*. *(From Li Z, Baker ML, Jiang W, et al. Rotavirus architecture at subnanometer resolution. J Virol. 2008, Epub ahead of print, by permission.)*

somal acidification and clathrin function do not seem to be required for entry, as they are for many other viruses, suggesting unique aspects of the rotavirus pathway.[24] Falling endosomal calcium concentration is probably required for rotavirus entry.[25] Because rotavirus virions uncoat when calcium concentrations fall,[13] low endosomal calcium concentrations could trigger a series of linked molecular rearrangements leading to membrane permeabilization and entry.

Once in the cytoplasm, the rotavirus DLP functions as a self-contained transcriptase, extruding capped, nonpolyadenylated messenger RNA (mRNA) through channels at its fivefold icosahedral vertices.[13,26] The genome remains encapsidated throughout transcription. The translation of viral mRNAs is enhanced by circularization, mediated by the specific binding of the rotavirus nonstructural protein NSP3 to the 3′ end of viral mRNA and to the cellular cap-binding protein eIF4G.[27,28] Thus, NSP3 substitutes for a cellular polyadenylic acid-binding protein to favor the translation of the nonpolyadenylated viral mRNAs over polyadenylated host mRNAs.

Rotavirus genome replication must overcome two major challenges: one copy of each of 11 different RNAs must be selected for packaging, and the newly synthesized double-stranded RNA must be sequestered so that it does not induce an interferon response. The mechanism of selective packaging remains obscure; the mechanism of genome sequestration is better understood.[29] The polymerase, VP1, specifically binds rotavirus mRNAs by recognizing a consensus sequence (UGUG) near their 3′ ends but holds the mRNAs in an inactive complex.[30] The mRNA shifts to a position that permits negative strand synthesis only when the polymerase binds a decamer of the inner shell protein, VP2.[29] The dependence of negative-strand synthesis on VP1-mRNA complexes binding to the inner shell protein ensures that double-stranded genomic RNA is synthesized within a nascent particle.

Several viral nonstructural proteins are involved in genome replication and the assembly of precursor particles.[29] DLPs are assembled in viral "factories," termed *viroplasms*, which form through the interaction of rotavirus nonstructural proteins NSP2 and NSP5.[31] NSP2 is an octomeric doughnut-shaped structure with RNA-binding, helix-destabilizing, nucleoside triphosphatase, and nucleoside diphosphate kinase-like activities.[32] Activities proposed for NSP2 include acting as a molecular motor to drive replicating mRNA into the nascent particles and maintaining nucleotide pools in viroplasms during replication.[32,33] NSP5 is a phosphoprotein with an autokinase activity.[34] It probably has a regulatory role, competing with single-stranded RNA to bind in grooves of the NSP2 octamer.[35] Once VP6 binds the nascent particle, the newly formed DLP can transcribe mRNA, amplifying virus yield.

Newly transcribed rotavirus mRNA enters two pools: mRNA that remains sequestered within viroplasms is replicated and packaged; mRNA that escapes viroplasms is translated.[36] Despite the barrier imposed by the need to introduce recombinant mRNA into viroplasms for replication, recombinant genes have been incorporated into infectious rotavirus genomes.[37] The reverse genetics system entails transfecting cells with a plasmid bearing a T7 promoter-controlled recombinant gene, infecting with a vaccinia virus expressing T7 polymerase, coinfecting with a helper rotavirus, and selecting against wild-type helper virus progeny with neutralizing antibodies. In this way, a recombinant rotavirus with a chimeric VP4 that is an antigenic mosaic of P genotypes has been produced.[38] As reverse genetics are made more efficient, the technique promises accelerated basic discovery and, potentially, rationally attenuated vaccine strains.

Following genome replication and DLP assembly, the outer capsid is added through an unusual maturation process. The DLP binds the cytoplasmic tail of NSP4, a rotavirus nonstructural protein that is resident in the membranes of the endoplasmic reticulum (ER) and viroplasm-associated vesicles, and buds into the ER lumen, transiently acquiring an envelope.[39,40] VP7, also resident in the ER, mediates removal of the transient envelope and binds the DLP, locking the VP4 spike protein in place.[41,42] Thus, rotavirus penetrates membranes twice. During entry, rotavirus penetrates a cellular membrane through a mechanism involving rearrangements of cleaved VP4 as the outer capsid disassembles; during maturation, rotavirus penetrates an envelope derived from the ER through a mechanism that involves VP7 and possibly NSP4 as the outer capsid assembles. Rotavirus egress from infected enterocytes is accomplished by release from the apical surface after vesicular transport from the ER by a pathway that bypasses the Golgi apparatus.[43]

Clinical Features

Infants and young children with diarrhea caused by rotavirus are more likely to have severe symptoms and become dehydrated than patients with diarrhea related to other common enteric pathogens.[44,45] The clinical features of rotavirus gastroenteritis in humans have been studied in experimental infections in adults. In one such study, 4 of 18 adult volunteers developed vomiting 1 to 3 days after oral administration of a virulent rotavirus strain.[46] This was followed by diarrhea lasting 1 to 4 days and associated with anorexia, crampy abdominal pain, and low-grade fever. Viral shedding in stool was detected for 6 to 10 or more days. Two thirds of the adult volunteers developed serologic evidence of infection without disease. Similarly, most natural rotavirus infections of adults are asymptomatic, manifested only by a rise in antibody titer.[47] However, natural rotavirus infection of adults can also cause severe and even fatal disease.[48]

Observational studies of children in North America hospitalized with rotavirus gastroenteritis reveal a similar, although more severe, pattern of disease.[44,45,49] Rotavirus gastroenteritis in children generally begins with vomiting and fever, which lasts 2 to 3 days, and progresses to profuse watery diarrhea, which continues for 4 to 5 days. Vomiting is more common and prolonged with rotavirus gastroenteritis than with pediatric gastroenteritis caused by most other agents.[45]

Laboratory findings in children hospitalized with rotavirus gastroenteritis reflect isotonic dehydration and include a high, urine-specific gravity and metabolic acidosis.[44,49] Rotavirus gastroenteritis is not generally associated with leukocytosis but is sometimes accompanied by a mild elevation in transaminases and uric acid levels.[44,49] Liquid stools from children with rotavirus diarrhea usually do not contain blood or fecal leukocytes,[44,59] although the presence of fecal leukocytes does not exclude rotavirus as an etiology.[45] Typically, virus is detected in stools of children by antigenic assays for 4 to 10 days after the onset of symptoms.[44] When a sensitive reverse transcriptase-polymerase chain reaction (RT-PCR) assay is used, shedding of viral RNA can be detected for up to 57 days from immunocompetent children, although this does not necessarily indicate shedding of infectious particles.[50]

Dehydration and severe electrolyte abnormalities leading to cardiovascular failure are the most common proximate causes of death from rotavirus gastroenteritis.[51] Seizures and aspiration of vomitus may also lead to death.[51] In a case series from Toronto, parents of 16 of 21 infants and young children who died from rotavirus gastroenteritis had made contact with a physician during the course of the illness. Nevertheless, after a median 2 days of illness, 20 of the 21 ultimately presented to the hospital either dead or moribund. In a number of cases, communication barriers between physician and parent related to language or culture may have contributed to the fatal outcomes.[51]

The spectrum of illness after rotavirus infection of infants and children also includes mild gastroenteritis and asymptomatic infection. In some newborn nurseries, difficult-to-eradicate endemic rotavirus strains asymptomatically infect neonates year round.[52,53] A common VP4 type (P[6]) and genetic stability over time suggest that these nursery strains may be less virulent than most circulating strains,[52] although maternally transmitted immunity or maturational resistance may also protect the neonates from disease. Because outbreaks of rotavirus diarrhea in neonatal nurseries also occur, any component of maturational resistance cannot be absolute.[54]

Rotavirus also has extraintestinal manifestations. Viremia, which is common in symptomatic and asymptomatic rotavirus infection, has unknown clinical significance in immunocompetent children.[55] In immunocompromised children, rotavirus infection has been associated with chronic diarrhea and extraintestinal infection. Conditions associated with chronic rotavirus infection include severe combined immunodeficiency (SCID), X-linked agammaglobulinemia, cartilage hair hypoplasia, acquired immunodeficiency syndrome (AIDS), and DiGeorge syndrome.[56-59] Rotavirus shed from chronically infected children often has altered genome segments.[57,59] Immunohistochemical staining for rotavirus structural and nonstructural proteins in autopsy specimens has demonstrated rotavirus replication in the hepatocytes and renal tubular cells of immunodeficient children with chronic rotavirus infection at the time of death.[56] Relatively severe rotavirus gastroenteritis has been noted in adult inpatients with immunosuppression related to bone marrow or renal transplantation.[60,61] Rotavirus is associated with diarrhea in adults with AIDS and very low CD4 counts but is not one of the more common causes of diarrhea in this population.[62]

Rotavirus has been detected in association with a number of syndromes other than gastroenteritis, including respiratory infections,[63] necrotizing enterocolitis,[64] pneumatosis intestinalis,[65] hepatic abscess,[66] myocarditis,[67] seizures,[68] and meningoencephalitis.[68] As rotavirus infection is universal, these associations may be coincidental rather than causative, and an etiologic association has not been established. Although intestinal intussusception has been temporally associated with immunization with Rotashield, a live-attenuated rotavirus vaccine no longer on the market (see "Immunization"), intestinal intussuception does not appear to be associated with natural rotavirus infection.[69]

Links between rotavirus infection and the subsequent development of autoimmune disease have been proposed. Although some strains of rotavirus can cause biliary atresia in mouse models, and group C rotavirus has been detected in liver tissue from biliary atresia patients, rotavirus has not been convincingly demonstrated to cause this condition in humans.[70-72] Similarly, depending on timing, rotavirus infection can either accelerate or delay the onset of diabetes in nonobese diabetic (NOD) mice,[73] but rotavirus infection has not been significantly associated with the development of type I diabetes in humans.[74] Serologic evidence of more frequent rotavirus infection has been associated with the development of celiac disease in predisposed children.[75] The introduction of effective rotavirus immunization will clarify whether symptomatic infection with group A rotaviruses is a trigger for such distinctive clinical syndromes.

Pathogenesis

The pathogenesis of rotavirus diarrhea is complex and incompletely understood, with potential roles for a viral enterotoxin, malabsorption related to mucosal damage and depression of disaccharidases, and secretion mediated by the enteric nervous system (ENS). Postmortem examination of the gastrointestinal tract of gnotobiotic pigs with diarrhea after experimental infection with a virulent human rotavirus strain demonstrated that virus replicates primarily in the villous epithelium of the small intestine.[76] This pattern is consistent with the patchy villous epithelial distribution of rotavirus antigen noted after immunofluorescent staining of duodenal biopsy specimens from children with severe gastroenteritis.[77] Light microscopic examination of such duodenal biopsy specimens reveals shortened and blunted villi with a cuboidal epithelium, crypt hypertrophy, and mononuclear cell infiltration of the lamina propria.[3,78]

The severity of diarrhea in children with rotavirus gastroenteritis correlates with the degree of mucosal damage, which suggests that malabsorption related to loss of absorptive cells may contribute to rotavirus diarrhea late in infection.[78] However, in experimentally infected gnotobiotic pigs, diarrhea precedes villous atrophy.[76] Similarly, small intestinal biopsies from children with relatively mild rotavirus gastroenteritis do not consistently display histologic changes, probably reflecting patchy epithelial injury.[79] These observations indicate that potentially absorptive villous epithelial cells remain despite net fluid losses and that factors other than destruction of the intestinal epithelium are also important in the pathogenesis of rotavirus gastroenteritis.

In several animal models, rotavirus infection induces a net secretion of fluid, sodium, and chloride from intestinal segments.[80] Glucose cotransport of electrolytes is inhibited,[81] although the degree of inhibition in humans does not prevent the use of oral rehydration solutions. Furthermore, decreased disaccharidase activity makes less glucose available for cotransport.[3,81] Changes in the molecular weight distribution of absorbed polyethylene glycol in children with rotavirus gastroenteritis indicate an increase in paracellular permeability.[82] Experiments in cell culture suggest that disruption of tight junctions by VP8* or NSP4 may mediate this increased permeability.[83,84]

In some animal models, the rotavirus nonstructural glycoprotein NSP4 acts as an enterotoxin to induce a secretory state.[86] Although most NSP4 is resident in the ER membrane, a portion traffics to the plasma membrane by a Golgi-independent route and releases a peptide corresponding to residues 112-175.[39,86] This region contains an enterotoxin with a tetrameric coiled-coil structure.[87] The enterotoxin, applied extracellularly, inhibits glucose-coupled sodium transport and stimulates phospholipase C to produce inositol 1,4,5 triphosphate, which leads to calcium influx and release of calcium from intracellular stores.[88,89] The resulting elevated intracellular calcium level leads to a secretory state by activating an anion channel, distinct from the cystic fibrosis transmembrane regulator.[90] Although orally administered antibodies against NSP4 protect mice from rotavirus diarrhea, actively acquired anti-NSP4 antibody fails to protect gnotobiotic piglets from challenge, and the role of an extracellular enterotoxin in human rotavirus gastroenteritis is not yet established.[85,91]

The ENS has a role in the pathogenesis of rotavirus gastroenteritis. Treatment of rotavirus-infected mice with lidocaine (a sodium channel-blocking anesthetic), granisetron (a serotonin receptor antagonist), or a VIP receptor antagonist attenuates diarrhea.[92,93] The ability of racecadotril, an enkephalinase inhibitor, to attenuate rotavirus diarrhea in children confirms that ENS-mediated secretion contributes to the pathogenesis of diarrhea in humans and is a target for therapeutic intervention (see "Treatment").[94] As diarrhea induced by bacterial toxins can also be ameliorated by inhibition of the ENS, roles for an enterotoxin and the ENS in the pathogenesis of rotavirus diarrhea are not mutually exclusive.

Serologic Classification

The diversity of rotaviruses, their ability to exchange genome segments encoding antigenic determinants, and changing diagnostic technology have led to evolving serology and classification systems. Rotavirus strains are classified by serogroup, subgroup, G serotype, and P serotype as well as by genetic groupings, such as electropherotype, G genotype, P genotype, and genogroup.

The broadest serologic designation is the serogroup. The seven serogroups, A through G, are defined by the cross-recognition of particles by serum antibody obtained from parenterally hyperimmunized animals.[95] Serogroup determinants are predominantly located on VP2 and VP6 (the innermost and middle layer proteins). Genetic exchange has not been observed between members of different serogroups. Serogroups A, B, and C cause disease in humans and other animals, whereas groups D through G have been described only in nonhuman animals. Serogroup A is the most important clinically, as group A viruses cause the endemic gastroenteritis of children; groups B and C have been associated with epidemics of gastroenteritis affecting all ages. Group B includes the strain ADRV (adult diarrhea rotavirus), which has been associated with large outbreaks of severe diarrhea in adults in China.[96] Group C viruses have been associated with less severe gastroenteritis in both children and adults.[97,98] Serogroup A is subdivided into subgroups I, II, I+II, and non-I non-II on the basis of monoclonal antibody recognition of antigenic determinants on VP6.[11]

Within group A, rotavirus serotypes are defined on the basis of reciprocal cross-neutralization by antibody. Initially, rotavirus serotypes were designated by a unitary system, which primarily reflected neutralizing antibodies directed against VP7. This system did not fully explain cross-neutralization patterns because VP4 also contains neutralization determinants.[99-101] Group A rotaviruses are now classified into serotypes with a binomial nomenclature, in which neutralization by antibodies against VP7 defines "G" serotype (for glycoprotein antigen) and neutralization by antibodies against VP4 defines "P" serotype (for protease-sensitive antigen). Further complicating the serology, VP7 and VP4 are each targets both of homotypic antibodies that neutralize only within serotype and of heterotypic antibodies that neutralize several serotypes.[102,103] In the case of VP4, serotype-specific epitopes are predominantly found on the variable VP8* hemagglutination domain, at the tips of the spikes, and heterotypic epitopes are predominantly found on the more conserved membrane interaction domain, within the body of the spikes.[18,19,102]

To date, at least 15 G serotypes (G1 to G15) have been identified, of which five (G1-4 and G9) commonly infect humans, and six more (G5-6, G8, and G10-12) have been detected less frequently.[95,104] The sequence of the genome segment encoding VP7 accurately predicts G serotype,[105] so genotyping provides a practical surrogate for G serotype determination. Serotype G2 viruses predominate in outbreaks of group A rotavirus gastroenteritis among adults, which suggests that heterotypic immunity after natural infection may protect less effectively against G2 viruses or that G2 viruses may be particularly virulent in adults.[106]

To date, 14 P serotypes (with serotypes 1, 2, and 5 each divided into subtypes A and B) have been identified.[95,104] Immunologic reagents for determining P serotype are limited, and P serotyping is complicated by cross-reactivity between P serotypes. Therefore, P genotyping is more commonly used for classification. At least 27 P genotypes (P1 to P27) have been identified thus far.[95,104] Unlike G serotypes, which have a one-to-one correspondence with G genotypes, some P serotypes include more than one P genotype. In strain descriptions, the genotype is enclosed in brackets after the serotype designation. Thus, G2P1B[4] refers to a virus of G serotype 2, P serotype 1B, and P genotype 4. The P types known to infect humans include P1A[8], P1B[4], P2A[6], P3[9], P4[10], P5A[3], P7[5], P8[11], P11[14], P12[19], and P[25].[95,104]

A limited number of serotypic combinations cause the majority of symptomatic infections of humans. Rotaviruses with four such combinations (G1P[8], G2P[4], G3P[8], and G4P[8]) caused 88.5% of pediatric rotavirus gastorenteritis cases, worldwide over the three decades from 1973 to 2003.[95] However, there is substantial geographic and temporal variation in strain distribution. For example, G1P[8] causes over 70% of rotavirus infections in North America and Europe but only 23% in Africa.[95] Serotypic and genotypic diversity is greater in Africa, Asia, and South America than in North America, Europe, and Australia.[95]

The emergence of G9 rotavirus strains emphasizes the fluidity of rotavirus evolution. G9 strains were first known to have infected humans in 1980. They were then detected in the United States and Japan through the mid-1980s, disappeared for about a decade, and then reemerged in the mid-1990s in three lineages and in association with a variety of P types to become the fifth most common G type causing human disease worldwide.[107,108] In another example, although P[6] strains were initially detected in association with asymptomatic nursery infections, they have now become prevalent causes of diarrhea in South America, Africa, and the Indian subcontinent.[52,53,95] Reassortment between human and animal rotavirus strains, antigenic drift, and the occasional introduction of animal rotaviruses into the pool of viruses circulating among humans provide a continuous introduction of genetic diversity, necessitating ongoing surveillance to determine whether rotavirus vaccines will require strain changes in the future for continued efficacy.[109]

Alternative genetic classification methods correlate to varying degrees with serologic classification. RNA electropherotype distinguishes group A strains as "long," "short," and "supershort" on the basis of the electrophoretic mobility of genome segments 10 and 11. In general, subgroup I rotaviruses have a short electropherotype, and subgroup II rotaviruses have a long electropherotype.[110] Human rotavirus strains have been classified in three genogroups on the basis of overall genome sequence similarity.[111] Full genome analysis, designating genotypes for each of the 11 genome segments, indicates that the two main genogroups of human rotaviruses share origins with the rotaviruses of domesticated animals: the Wa-like genogroup with porcine rotavirues and the DS-1-like genogroup with bovine rotaviruses.[112]

Epidemiology

Rotavirus infection is universal, and almost all children acquire serum antibody against the virus in the first 2 or 3 years of life.[113] Severe gastroenteritis caused by rotavirus most commonly affects infants and children between 6 months and 2 years of age,[114] although in poorer populations the peak of illness may be somewhat earlier.[114-116] The age of greatest susceptibility to severe disease may be bracketed by the waning of maternally transferred passive immunity and the maturation of the gastrointestinal tract at about 6 months, and by the acquisition of active immunity related to natural infection later in childhood.

Rotavirus is the most common cause of severe dehydrating diarrhea leading to the hospitalization of infants and children in both the developed and developing world. Analyses of published studies indicate that rotavirus causes approximately 139 million cases of gastroenteritis and 611,000 childhood deaths each year worldwide.[1,117] Whereas the incidence of rotavirus gastroenteritis is similar in developed and developing countries, mortality is concentrated in poorer nations (Fig. 150-3).[1] The causes of higher mortality rates from rotavirus in the developing world may include the greater prevalence of malnutrition, less access to treatment, larger inoculum size, and synergy with other intestinal flora or pathogens.[115] Although rotavirus vaccines are not yet widely used in regions where rotavirus deaths are common, global mortality rates from rotavirus infection are thought to have fallen by approximately 30% since 1985.[1] Improved access to treatment, particularly increased use of oral rehydration solutions, probably plays a role in the lower mortality rates, although better nutrition and a lower incidence of comorbidities may also contribute.

The physical hardiness of the rotavirus particle, the high particle concentration in stool (up to 10^{11} particles/mL),[118] and the small minimum infectious dose ($ID_{50} = 10$ focus-forming units)[119] account for the weak association between the incidence of rotavirus gastroenteritis and the level of economic development or hygiene. In developed countries, rotavirus is a major cause of morbidity and health care costs. Although about 75% of children in the United States experience rotavirus gastroenteritis in the first 5 years of life, only about 20 to 40 die each year as a result.[120] In the United States, approximately 3 million cases of childhood rotavirus gastroenteritis are responsible for approximately 735,000 physician visits and 27,000 hospitalizations annually.[120,121] This disease burden results in approximately $319 million in direct health care costs and $893 million in total economic costs to society.[120]

Rotavirus gastroenteritis has a marked seasonality in temperate climates, with a peak of cases in the cooler months each year (Fig. 150-4A).[2,114,122] In North America, annual rotavirus epidemics have begun in the fall in the southwest, spreading north and east, reaching the eastern seaboard by late winter, and tapering off in the spring.[122] In the tropics, although the seasonality is less pronounced, infection is most common in the cooler and drier times of the year.[123] Because the rotavirus particle is inactivated more quickly in conditions of relatively high humidity, dry weather may promote transmission.[14] During a rotavirus season, multiple strains, representing several P and G types, usually circulate. In a single region, the dominant strains differ from year to year; in the same year, the dominant strains differ regionally.[124]

The best documented mode of rotavirus transmission is fecal-oral.[119] However, winter seasonality and universal infection early in life are more typical of pathogens with respiratory spread. Experiments on the transmission of rotavirus gastroenteritis (epizootic diarrhea of infant mice) between cages of mice support the possibility of airborne spread.[125] Although rotavirus can be foodborne, it is not a major cause of foodborne illness.[126] Transmission by contaminated water has also been documented. For example, a large outbreak of group B rotavirus gastroenteritis in China was attributed to fecal contamination of water supplies.[96]

Attendance at daycare is a risk factor for pediatric hospitalization due to rotavirus gastroenteritis.[127] The illness can spread in families, and may cause gastroenteritis in the adult caregivers for small children.[128,129] It is likely that the large viral inoculum ingested by these caregivers is, in part, responsible for illness despite some level of acquired immunity. Rotavirus outbreaks have occurred in nursing home populations and sometimes have resulted in fatalities.[48,106] Rotavirus is an important cause of nosocomial infection; in addition to the asymptomatic infections associated with rotavirus endemics in newborn nurseries, rotavirus causes symptomatic hospital-acquired outbreaks associated with circulation of rotavirus in the community.[130] Rotavirus also can cause traveler's diarrhea.[131]

Rotavirus is a major veterinary pathogen, causing disease in infant cattle, sheep, swine, and camels as well as in adult chickens and turkeys and in domestic pets such as cats and dogs. Some strains that circulate and cause disease in humans are more closely related to animal rotavirus strains than to other human rotavirus strains, and strains that currently circulate in domestic animals occasionally cause human disease.[132,133] In addition, some human rotaviruses have individual

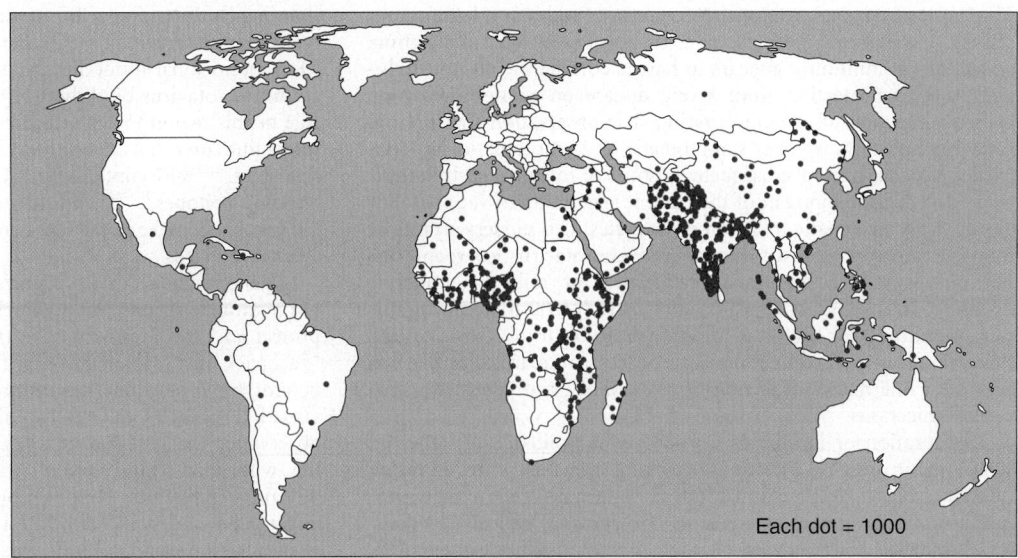

Figure 150-3 **Estimated global distribution of annual rotavirus-related deaths.** *(Adapted from Parashar UD, Gibson CJ, Bresee JS, et al. Rotavirus and severe childhood diarrhea. Emerg Infect Dis. 2006;12:304-306.)*

Each dot = 1000

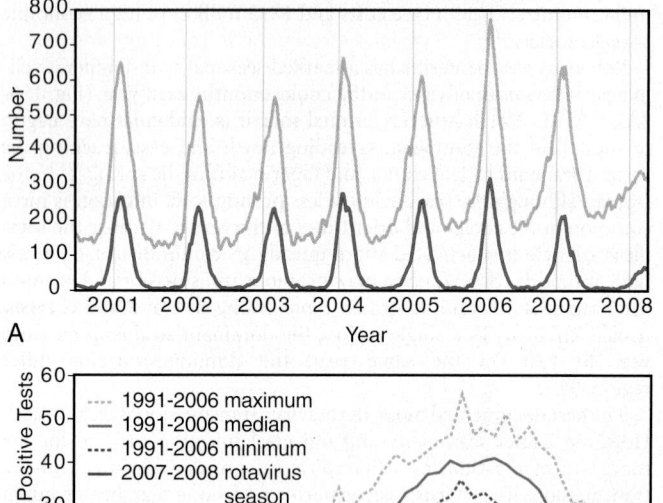

Figure 150-4   Seasonality of rotavirus infection and decreased incidence with the introduction of immunization in the United States. A, Total number of rotavirus tests and positive test results from laboratories of the National Respiratory and Enteric Virus Surveillance System, July 2, 2000 to May 3, 2008. **B,** Percentage of rotavirus tests with positive results from participating laboratories. *(Adapted from Centers for Disease Control and Prevention. Delayed onset and diminished magnitude of rotavirus activity—United States, November 2007-May 2008. MMWR. 2008;57:697-700.)*

genome segments that are closely related to those of animal rotaviruses, suggesting reassortment between viruses with different primary hosts.[132,134] Nevertheless, in non-native hosts most rotavirus strains are attenuated and do not spread efficiently. No major rotavirus gastroenteritis outbreaks have been directly linked to contact with infected animals.

Immunity

The immune response to rotavirus is complex and redundant: innate, cellular, and humoral mechanisms contribute to clearance of infection, and humoral immunity appears to have a dominant (but not exclusive) role in protection from severe disease on reinfection or on primary infection after immunization. The observation that natural rotavirus infection, whether symptomatic or asymptomatic, provides partial protection from subsequent episodes of rotavirus gastroenteritis guided the development of the current generation of vaccines. For example, asymptomatic infection of neonates with nursery strains of rotavirus protects against subsequent severe rotavirus gastroenteritis but not against asymptomatic reinfection or mild to moderate disease.[135] In a prospective observational study, 200 Mexican infants were monitored for rotavirus infection from birth to 2 years of age. Protection from subsequent moderate or severe rotavirus diarrhea was 87% after one natural infection of any severity and 100% after two natural infections.[113]

The duration of immunity to rotavirus is limited, with repeated symptomatic rotavirus infections occurring (generally with decreasing severity) in both children and adults.[106,113,136] In isolated human communities with limited prior exposure to rotaviruses, explosive epidemics of rotavirus diarrhea with high attack rates in adults are seen.[48,137]

Although some experimental animals, including mice, show maturational resistance to rotavirus disease,[125,138] these clinical observations suggest that maturational resistance is less significant in humans and does not fully account for the lower incidence of severe disease in older children and adults. Rather, repeated asymptomatic or mildly symptomatic episodes of rotavirus gastroenteritis throughout life appear to be important for maintaining immunity.[47,139]

In experimental studies of passively transferred immunity to rotavirus in mice, circulating neutralizing antibody does not protect against disease; however, the presence of sufficient levels of neutralizing monoclonal or colostrum-derived antibody in the gut does protect.[140,141] In immunized mice, the appearance of immunoglobulin A (IgA) in the gut correlates with clearance of infection.[142] Passive infusion of neutralizing antibodies into monkeys protects from experimental challenge and, at high dose, results in detectable antibody in stool.[143] These experimental results corroborate the observation that, in naturally exposed children, preexisting rotavirus-specific serum IgA and fecal IgA, which reflect duodenal IgA, are associated with protection from disease.[128,139,144] Virus-specific serum antibody may correlate with protection in children because it signifies previous infection without necessarily being a primary effector of protection.[116,145]

The evidence that breast-feeding protects human infants from rotavirus diarrhea is mixed. In Bangladesh, hospitalized children with rotavirus diarrhea are more likely to be breast-fed than patients with diarrhea from other causes, which suggests that breast-feeding prevents rotavirus gastroenteritis less effectively than it prevents gastroenteritis caused by other agents.[146] Nevertheless, in some clinical studies of rotavirus gastroenteritis, breast-feeding is associated with reduced frequency of vomiting, less severe dehydration, or (for infants less than 6 months of age) a lower risk of hospitalization.[127,147,148]

Serotype influences but does not determine the degree of protection from challenge. Protection after natural infection or immunization appears to be somewhat more reliable against viruses of the same serotype (G type) as the immunizing strain.[113,136,149-152] On the other hand, cross-protection between serotypes clearly also occurs, particularly after multiple infections.[113,149,153] This finding correlates with the primarily homotypic neutralizing antibody response to primary infection and the increasingly heterotypic responses to reinfection with the same or other serotypes.[154,155]

The mechanisms of rotavirus neutralization by antibodies have been examined in detail. Neutralizing monoclonal antibodies that recognize the VP8* fragment of VP4 block the attachment of sialic acid–dependent rotaviruses to cells or trigger virus uncoating;[156,157] antibodies that recognize the VP5* fragment of VP4 block a postbinding entry event;[156] and antibodies against the VP7 coat protein block virion uncoating.[158] Although VP8*, which has high sequence variability, contains predominantly P-type specific neutralization epitopes, VP5*, which is relatively conserved, contains heterotypic neutralizing epitopes.[102,159] Most monoclonal antibodies that recognize VP4 and neutralize human strains of rotavirus bind the VP5* fragment,[159] possibly reflecting the role of this region in cell attachment for strains (including most that infect humans) that do not bind neuraminidase-sensitive cell surface sialosides.[22,23] VP7 contains both G-type specific and heterotypic neutralizing epitopes.[103] Therefore, antibodies that recognize VP5* and VP7 probably make important contributions to heterotypic protection against rotavirus.

IgA monoclonals that recognize the middle layer protein, VP6, do not neutralize virions, but do block transcription by DLPs in vitro and protect mice from rotavirus infection when secreted into the serum by "backpack" hybridoma tumors.[160,161] Host J-chains are required for heterotypic protection after immunization of mice with recombinant virus-like particles (VLPs) containing only VP2 and VP6.[162] These observations suggest that anti-VP6 IgA can block infection by interfering with viral transcription while being transcytosed across the intestinal epithelium. However, protection is not provided by immunogens that lack VP4 and VP7 in all animal models. For example, immunization of gnotobiotic pigs with VP2/6 VLPs boosts protective responses elicited by immunization with live virus, but primary immunization with these VLPs does not protect gnotobiotic pigs from diarrhea on challenge with a virulent human rotavirus strain.[163] Llama single-chain antibody fragments that recognize VP6 can neutralize virions across serotypes and subgroups and, administered intragastrically, passively protect mice from challenge, suggesting a novel approach to orally administered antibody prophylaxis.[164] Potentially, the small antigen combining sites of the fragments, which lack light chains, could access VP6 through gaps in the VP7 shell.

The role of innate and cellular immunity in clearing and preventing rotavirus infection has been studied in an adult mouse model of rotavirus infection (but not diarrhea). Although some rotavirus-inoculated SCID mice persistently shed virus, 40% of SCID mice on a C57BL/6 background do clear the infection.[165] This observation indicates that innate immune mechanisms can resolve rotavirus infections but are unreliable. Indeed, rotavirus antagonizes innate immunity through the action of nonstructural protein NSP1, which degrades several interferon response factors, thus blocking type I interferon expression.[166] Mice that are T-cell deficient on the basis of an αβ/γδ T-cell receptor knockout clear primary infection shortly after immunocompetent mice, mount a modest IgA response (primarily against VP6), and are resistant to reinfection on challenge.[165] Most B cell-deficient mice (J$_H$D knockouts) with intact CD8$^+$ T cells also clear primary rotavirus infections but can be reinfected.[167] Thus, although cell-mediated or humoral immunity effectively clears primary infection, humoral immunity is more effective at protecting mice from infectious challenge.

Diagnosis

Rotavirus gastroenteritis is not clearly distinguished from other causes of acute gastroenteritis on clinical grounds alone. Because the standard treatment for rotavirus gastroenteritis is rehydration and supportive care, a specific microbiologic diagnosis is not required in most cases. However, with prolonged diarrhea, in complicated cases, in immunocompromised hosts, when alternative diagnoses are considered, or when epidemiologic or infection control data are needed, it may be desirable to establish rotavirus as the etiologic agent. Definitively diagnosing rotavirus gastroenteritis may also the prevent unnecessary and potentially harmful use of antibiotics.

Rotavirus can be detected by numerous techniques, including a variety of commercial antigenic assays, RT-PCR, electron microscopy, immune electron microscopy, polyacrylamide gel electrophoresis (PAGE) for viral genomic RNA, and viral culture. Detection of viral antigen in stool or rectal swabs, most commonly using enzyme-linked immunosorbent assay (ELISA) or latex agglutination formats, forms the basis for practical, commercially available, and widely used diagnostic kits.[168] Latex agglutination is particularly suitable for use in areas with limited resources, although a confirmatory technique is desirable to evaluate indeterminate results because of the limited sensitivity of the test.[168,169] Commercial antigenic assays primarily detect the VP2 and VP6 proteins of the subviral double-layered particle and detect only group A rotaviruses. Serotype-specific ELISAs, based on recognition of VP7 or VP4, allow determination of serotype without the need to perform neutralization assays.[100] Although there are various techniques for measuring serum, fecal, and salivary antibodies against rotavirus, the acute and generally self-limited nature of rotavirus infections limits the usefulness of these techniques for clinical decision making.

Multiplexed RT-PCR has become a major diagnostic technique used in epidemiologic studies. RT-PCR allows determination of P and G types and permits finer definition of strain differences.[170,171] Real-time RT-PCR provides greater sensitivity and speed than conventional or nested PCR diagnosis.[172] DNA oligonucleotide microarray methods now being introduced offer greater robustness to sequence drift (which can prevent PCR amplification if a primer binding site is affected) and greater ability to distinguish a mixed infection from a single strain infection.[173]

Both electron microscopy and PAGE can detect unusual strains of rotavirus (such as non–group A rotaviruses) that might be missed by standard antigenic or nucleic acid-based assays. Electron microscopy of stool specimens negatively stained with phosphotungstic acid is rapid and, despite only moderate sensitivity, has high specificity because of the distinctive appearance of rotavirus particles (Fig. 150-1).[174] Electrophoresis of simply prepared stool suspensions on polyacrylamide gels followed by silver staining for the pattern of 11 segments of genomic double-stranded RNA allows both diagnosis and tracking of rotavirus strains in molecular epidemiologic investigations.[175] Rotavirus can be detected, although with relatively low sensitivity, by growth in cell culture. Human rotavirus strains have proved more difficult to culture routinely than most animal rotavirus strains but in many cases can be propagated in MA104 cells or primary green monkey kidney cells grown in roller tubes with the addition of trypsin to the cell culture medium.[118,176]

Treatment

Recommendations for treatment are summarized in a guideline from the Centers for Disease Control and Prevention (CDC).[177] As rotavirus gastroenteritis is generally self-limited, and dehydration is the primary cause of morbidity and mortality, rehydration and restoration of electrolyte balance are the primary therapies. Oral rehydration solutions (ORSs) are effective in treating dehydration related to rotavirus gastroenteritis, even in the presence of moderate vomiting, and are preferred over IV rehydration in cases of mild or moderate dehydration.[177,178] The principle on which these solutions are based is the solute-coupled cotransport of sodium by enterocytes, which continues to operate even in the damaged gut.[179] Effective solutes include glucose, amino acids, and short oligopeptides.

In 2002, the World Health Organization (WHO) revised the recommended standard oral rehydation formula to a low osmolarity (245 mOsm/L) solution, which is associated with less vomiting, lower stool output, and a reduced need for intravenous (IV) infusions. The low osmolarity formulation is 75 mM Na$^+$, 20 mM K$^+$, 65 mM Cl$^-$, 10 mM citrate, and 75 mM glucose (see reference for acceptable variations).[180] When oral hydration cannot be maintained because of severe vomiting, depressed level of consciousness, or intestinal ileus, and in cases of severe dehydration (with loss of more than 9% of body weight), IV hydration with lactated Ringer's solution, normal saline, or a similar solution is recommended.[177] However, when the patient has been resuscitated and is able to take oral fluids, oral rehydration should be instituted. Despite the depressed disaccharidase levels associated with rotavirus gastroenteritis, it is recommended that nursing infants continue to breastfeed during rehydration and that children resume a diet as soon as they can tolerate feeding. The early reinstitution of an age-appropriate diet, avoiding foods high in simple sugars, has nutritional benefits and shortens the duration of diarrhea by about half a day.[177,181]

Randomized controlled trials in developing countries have demonstrated that short courses of zinc supplementation for 10 to 14 days can significantly decrease the prevalence of diarrheal disease in the following 2 to 3 months (odds ratio = 0.66) and that zinc supplementation during an episode of acute diarrhea can decrease duration of illness (15% reduced probability of continued diarrhea on any given day).[182,183] On this basis, the WHO has recommended zinc supplementation (10-14 days of 10 mg/day for infants under 6 months and 20 mg/day for older infants) together with oral rehydration therapy.[184] Because the benefits of zinc supplementation in well-nourished populations have not been established, this intervention is not currently recommended by the CDC for infants and children in the United States.[177]

Racecadotril (no commercial preparations currently available in the United States) is an enkephalinase inhibitor that inhibits intestinal hypersecretion and has been evaluated as an adjunct to ORS in a placebo-controlled trial in Peru. Racecadotril combined with ORS cut total stool output and the duration of diarrhea by about half compared with the use of ORS alone for treatment of rotavirus gastroenteritis.[94] Although these results are promising, the clinical role of racecadotril is not yet clearly established.[177]

Oral administration of immunoglobulins is not indicated for routine use, but may have a role in treating chronic rotavirus diarrhea and may merit further evaluation for prophylaxis in high-risk settings in which vaccination has not yet been shown to be efficacious. In case reports, feeding human serum immune globulin to children with chronic rotavirus diarrhea has been followed by resolution of diarrhea and viral shedding.[185] When given prophylactically to low-birth-weight infants, oral gamma globulin reduced the severity of diarrhea associated with neonatal rotavirus infections.[186]

Because of complications including ileus and respiratory depression, antimotility agents such as loperamide have no role in the treatment of childhood gastroenteritis.[177] Bismuth subsalicylate (Pepto-Bismol) has been shown to decrease the duration of diarrhea and the intake of ORS in children with gastroenteritis,[187] but the modest benefits observed and a theoretical possibility of Reye's syndrome related to salicylate absorption argue against routine use of this agent.[177] Although its mechanism of action is unclear, probiotic treatment of childhood gastroenteritis, including rotavirus gastroenteritis, by oral administration of lactobacilli appears to shorten the duration of diarrhea by about 0.7 days, based on a meta-analysis of randomized, blinded, controlled trials.[188]

Immunization

Because lack of access to treatment is one of the major causes of childhood mortality from rotavirus, and improved sanitation has limited impact on rotavirus prevalence, prevention by immunization is a critical approach to decreasing the impact of this infection. In 1998, the first human rotavirus vaccine, RotaShield (Wyeth Lederle Vaccines) was approved by the U.S. Food and Drug Administration (FDA) and was recommended for infants by the Advisory Committee on Immunization Practices (ACIP). This quadrivalent, reassortant vaccine was based on a modified "Jennerian" approach, using a live animal virus to immunize humans. To broaden the serotype specificity of the immune response, VP7 from each of the G types 1 to 4 was presented on the genetic background of a simian rotavirus strain (RRV), which is attenuated for humans on the basis of host range restriction and passage in cell culture. In phase III trials, RotaShield proved safe and highly effective against moderate to severe diarrhea in both developed (United States and Finland) and developing (Venezuela) countries.[149,189,190]

In 1999, after more than 1 million doses of RotaShield had been administered, an association between immunization and intestinal intussusception (telescoping of the intestine) led the manufacturer to voluntarily withdraw the vaccine from the market.[191] A case-control study revealed a significantly increased incidence of intestinal intussusception in vaccinees in the 3 to 14 days after administration of the first dose (odds ratio = 21.7) and a smaller increase after the second dose (odds ratio = 3.3).[192] The relative risk of intussusception shortly after immunization increased with increasing age of receiving a first dose of RotaShield.[193] Reanalysis of the case-control study database and a study of overall rates of hospitalization for intussusception following vaccine introduction suggested that a compensatory decrease in intussusception may have followed the brief period of increased risk immediately after immunization, yielding no overall increased risk of intussusception in vaccinees.[194]

The unknown mechanism of the temporal association between intussusception and immunization combined with the failure to observe this complication in pre-licensure clinical trials of RotaShield increased the size of the phase III trials required for licensure of subsequent live-attenuated rotavirus vaccines in most nations. Nevertheless, two other live-attenuated rotavirus vaccines, RotaRix (GlaxoSmithKline) and Rotateq (Merck), have achieved licensure with no observed association with intestinal intussusception in clinical trials.[151,195]

Rotarix, an oral, live-attenuated vaccine, is derived from a human rotavirus isolate (strain 89-12; P[8]G1) that has been attenuated by serial passage in cell culture.[151] Because Rotarix is monovalent, breadth of coverage relies on cross-protection between serotypes, as has been observed following natural rotavirus infection.[113] In a phase III trial carried out in Finland and in middle-income Latin American populations, Rotarix proved efficacious (84.7%) against severe gastorenteritis from any rotavirus serotype. The vaccine was 87.3% effective against severe gastroenteritis caused by strains that shared the P[8] VP4 type with the vaccine and 91.8% effective against strains that shared both VP4 type and VP7 type (G1) with the vaccine.[151] Although efficacy criteria were not met for doubly mismatched G2P[4] strains in the initial phase III trial or after a second year of monitoring a subset of infants from that trial, Rotarix achieved 85.5% protection against severe diarrhea caused by G2P[4] strains in a placebo controlled, double-blind study in European infants.[151,153,196] Since Rotarix was first licensed in Mexico and the Dominican Republic in 2004, approvals have followed in more than 90 nations, including the European Union in February 2006 and the United States in April 2008. The ACIP has recommended immunization with Rotarix at 2 and 4 months of age, the first dose to be given before 15 weeks of age.[197]

RotaTeq is a multivalent, orally administered, modified Jennerian vaccine. The five strains in Rotateq are reassortants with a bovine rotavirus (strain WC3) background. Each has a VP7 from one of four prevalent human rotavirus G serotypes (G1, G2, G3, and G4) or a bovine G serotype (G6) combined with a VP4 from the common human rotavirus P genotye, P[8], or a bovine rotavirus P genotype, P[7].[198] In a phase III trial, RotaTeq was highly efficacious (>98% protection) against severe rotavirus gastroenteritis and efficacia against any diarrhea caused by G1 or G2 rotaviruses (74.9% and 63.4% protection, respectively).[195] RotaTeq was licensed in the United States and the European Union in 2006. The ACIP has recommended RotaTeq for routine use in the United States, with doses given at 2, 4, and 6 months of age, the first dose to be given before 13 weeks of age.[199] Subsequent recommendations increase the maximum age of first immunization to less than 15 weeks of age.[197] Early data from the 2007-2008 rotavirus season, the first full season of RotaTeq use, indicate that the onset of rotavirus disease activity in the United States was delayed by 2 to 4 months and decreased in magnitude by more than 50% relative to previous years (Fig. 150-4B).[7] Based on estimated rates of vaccine coverage, it appears that Rotateq not only provided substantial protection to vaccinees but also elicited a degree of herd immunity.[7] As of September 2007, with more than 100,000 doses of Rotateq administered, post-licensure monitoring has not revealed any significant association between Rotateq administration and intestinal intussusception.[200]

Ongoing monitoring will assess how circulating rotavirus strains evolve in response to the new immune pressure imposed by rotavirus immunization. The largest potential impact of rotavirus vaccines on mortality is in impoverished populations of Asia and Africa, among whom live-attenuated oral approaches to immunzation against rotavirus and other agents have proven less efficacious than in more affluent settings.[201] Rotarix and Rotateq are now being tested in such populations.[202] The introduction of locally developed and produced vaccines, such as a human neonatal strain 116E vaccine candidate under investigation in India, could help overcome economic barriers to widespread immunization.[152] In fact, in 2000, the Lanzhou lamb vaccine, a monovalent ovine rotavirus (P[12]G10), was licensed in China as a live-attenuated oral vaccine. More than 5 million infants and children have been immunized with this vaccine, but it was not tested in a placebo-controlled phase III trial, and limited data are available on its efficacy and safety.[203] Parenteral vaccines, such as recombinant, noninfectious, virus-like particles[204] or inactivated rotavirus particles,[201] could potentially prove stable without a cold chain and could be more easily integrated into childhood immunization programs than the live-attenuated vaccines, lowering practical barriers to universal immunization in the most challenging settings.

ACKNOWLEDGMENTS

I thank Albert Z. Kapikian for providing electron micrographs of rotavirus particles; Umesh D. Parashar for providing epidemiologic data and artwork; and B.V. Venkataram Prasad and Matthew L. Baker for providing an electron cryomicroscopy image reconstruction of a rotavirus virion.

REFERENCES

1. Parashar UD, Gibson CJ, Bresee JS, et al. Rotavirus and severe childhood diarrhea. *Emerg Infect Dis.* 2006;12:304-306.
2. Cook SM, Glass RI, LeBaron CW, et al. Global seasonality of rotavirus infections. *Bull World Health Organ.* 1990;68: 171-177.
3. Bishop RF, Davidson GP, Holmes IH, et al. Virus particles in epithelial cells of duodenal mucosa from children with acute non-bacterial gastroenteritis. *Lancet.* 1973;2:1281-1283.
4. Adams WR, Kraft LM. Epizootic diarrhea of infant mice: identification of the etiologic agent. *Science.* 1963;141:359-360.
5. Mebus CA, Underdahl NR, Rhodes MB, et al. Calf diarrhea (scours): reproduced with a virus from a field outbreak. *Univ Nebr Res Bull.* 1969;233.
6. Flewett TH, Bryden AS, Davies H, et al. Relation between viruses from acute gastroenteritis of children and newborn calves. *Lancet.* 1974;2:61-63.
7. Centers for Disease Control and Prevention. Delayed onset and diminished magnitude of rotavirus activity—United States, November 2007-May 2008. *MMWR.* 2008;57:697-700.
8. Li Z, Baker ML, Jiang W, et al. Rotavirus architecture at subnanometer resolution. *J Virol.* 2009;83:1754-1766.
9. Greenberg HB, Valdesuso J, van Wyke K, et al. Production and preliminary characterization of monoclonal antibodies directed at two surface proteins of rhesus rotavirus. *J Virol.* 1983;47: 267-275.
10. Offit PA, Blavat G, Greenberg HB, et al. Molecular basis of rotavirus virulence: role of gene segment 4. *J Virol.* 1986;57: 46-49.
11. Greenberg HB, Flores J, Kalica AR, et al. Gene coding assignments for growth restriction, neutralization and subgroup specificities of the W and DS-1 strains of human rotavirus. *J Gen Virol.* 1983;64:313-320.
12. Dormitzer PR, Greenberg HB, Harrison SC. Purified recombinant rotavirus VP7 forms soluble, calcium-dependent trimers. *Virology.* 2000;277:420-428.
13. Cohen J, Laporte J, Charpilienne A, et al. Activation of rotavirus RNA polymerase by calcium chelation. *Arch Virol.* 1979;60: 177-186.
14. Ansari SA, Springthorpe VS, Sattar SA. Survival and vehicular spread of human rotaviruses: possible relation to seasonality of outbreaks. *Rev Infect Dis.* 1991;13:448-461.
15. Lloyd-Evans N, Springthorpe VS, Sattar SA. Chemical disinfection of human rotavirus-contaminated inanimate surfaces. *J Hyg (Lond).* 1986;97:163-173.
16. Macinga DR, Sattar SA, Jaykus L-A, et al. Improved inactivation of nonenveloped enteric viruses and their surrogates by a novel alcohol-based hand sanitizer. *Appl Env Microbiol.* 2008;74: 5047-5052.
17. Ward RL, Bernstein DI, Knowlton DR, et al. Prevention of surface-to-human transmission of rotaviruses by treatment with disinfectant spray. *J Clin Microbiol.* 1991;29:1991-1996.
18. Dormitzer PR, Sun ZY, Wagner G, et al. The rhesus rotavirus VP4 sialic acid binding domain has a galectin fold with a novel carbohydrate binding site. *EMBO J.* 2002;21:885-897.
19. Dormitzer PR, Nason EB, Prasad BV, et al. Structural rearrangements in the membrane penetration protein of a non-enveloped virus. *Nature.* 2004;430:1053-1058.
20. Crawford SE, Mukherjee SK, Estes MK, et al. Trypsin cleavage stabilizes the rotavirus VP4 spike. *J Virol.* 2001;75:6052-6061.
21. Lopez S, Arias CF. Early steps in rotavirus cell entry. *Curr Top Microbiol Immunol.* 2006;309:39-66.
22. Ciarlet M, Ludert JE, Iturriza-Gomara M, et al. Initial interaction of rotavirus strains with N-acetylneuraminic (sialic) acid residues on the cell surface correlates with VP4 genotype, not species of origin. *J Virol.* 2002;76:4087-4095.
23. Zarate S, Espinosa R, Romero P, et al. The VP5 domain of VP4 can mediate attachment of rotaviruses to cells. *J Virol.* 2000; 74:593-599.
24. Sanchez-San Martin C, Lopez T, Arias CF. Characterization of rotavirus cell entry. *J Virol.* 2004;78:2310-2318.
25. Chemello ME, Aristimuno OC, Michelangeli F, et al. Requirement for vacuolar H^+-ATPase activity and Ca^{2+} gradient during entry of rotavirus into MA104 cells. *J Virol.* 2002;76: 13083-13087.
26. Lawton JA, Estes MK, Prasad BV. Three-dimensional visualization of mRNA release from actively transcribing rotavirus particles. *Nat Struct Biol.* 1997;4:118-121.
27. Groft CM, Burley SK. Recognition of eIF4G by rotavirus NSP3 reveals a basis for mRNA circularization. *Mol Cell.* 2002;9: 1273-1283.
28. Vende P, Piron M, Castagne N, et al. Efficient translation of rotavirus mRNA requires simultaneous interaction of NSP3 with the eukaryotic translation intiation factor EIF4G and the mRNA 3' end. *J Virol.* 2000;74:7064-7071.
29. Patton JT, Vasquez-Del Carpio R, Tortorici MA, et al. Coupling of rotavirus genome replication and capsid assembly. *Adv Virus Res.* 2007;69:167-201.
30. Lu X, McDonald SM, Tortorici MA, et al. Mechanism for coordinated RNA packaging and genome replication by rotavirus polymerase VP1. *Structure.* 2008;16:1678-1688.
31. Fabbretti E, Afrikanaova I, Vascotto F. Two non-structural rotavirus proteins, NSP2 and NSP5, form viroplasm-like structures in vivo. *J Gen Virol.* 1999;80:333-339.
32. Kumar M, Jayaram H, Vasquez-Del Carpio R, et al. Crystallographic and biochemical analysis of rotavirus NSP2 with nucleotides reveals a nucleoside disphosphate kinase-like activity. *J Virol.* 2007;81:12272-12284.
33. Schuck P, Taraporewala Z, McPhie P, et al. Rotavirus nonstructural protein NSP2 self-assembles into octamers that undergo ligand-induced conformational changes. *J Biol Chem.* 2001;276:9679-9687.
34. Bar-Magen, T, Spencer E, Patton JT. An ATPase activity associated with the rotavirus phosphoprotein NSP5. *Virology.* 2007;369:89-99.
35. Jiang X, Jayaram H, Kumar M, et al. Cryoelectron microscopy structures of rotavirus NSP2-NSP5 and NSP2-RNA complexes: implications for genome replication. *J Virol.* 2006;80:10829-10835.
36. Silvestri LS, Taraporewala ZF, Patton JT. Rotavirus replication: plus-sense templates for double-stranded RNA synthesis are made in viroplasms. *J Virol.* 2004;78:7763-7774.
37. Komoto S, Sasaki J, Taniguchi K. Reverse genetics system for introduction of site-specific mutations into the double-stranded RNA genome of infectious rotavirus. *PNAS.* 2006;103: 4646-4651.
38. Komoto S, Kugita M, Sasaki J, et al. Generation of recombinant rotavirus with an antigenic mosaic of cross-reactive neutralization epitopes on VP4. *J Virol.* 2008;82:6753-6757.
39. Berkova Z, Crawford SE, Trugnan G, et al. Rotavirus NSP4 induces a novel vesicular compartment regulated by calcium and associated with viroplasms. *J Virol.* 2005;80:6061-6071.
40. O'Brien JA, Taylor JA, Bellamy AR. Probing the structure of rotavirus NSP4: a short sequence at the extreme C terminus mediates binding to the inner capsid particle. *J Virol.* 2000;74:5388-5394.
41. Lopez T, Camacho M, Zayas M, et al. Silencing the morphogenesis of rotavirus. *J Virol.* 2005;79:184-192.
42. Trask SD, Dormitzer PR. Assembly of highly infectious rotavirus particles recoated with recombinant outer capsid proteins. *J Virol.* 2006;80:11293-11304.
43. Jourdan N, Maurice M, Delautier D, et al. Rotavirus is released from the apical surface of cultured human intestinal cells through nonconventional vesicular transport that bypasses the Golgi apparatus. *J Virol.* 1997;71:8268-8278.
44. Kovacs A, Chan L, Hotrakitya C, et al. Rotavirus gastroenteritis: clinical and laboratory features and use of the Rotazyme test. *Am J Dis Child.* 1987;141:161-166.
45. Rodriguez WJ, Kim HW, Arrobio JO, et al. Clinical features of acute gastroenteritis associated with human reovirus-like agent in infants and young children. *J Pediatr.* 1977;91: 188-193.
46. Kapikian AZ, Wyatt RG, Levine MM, et al. Oral administration of human rotavirus to volunteers: induction of illness and correlates of resistance. *J Infect Dis.* 1983;147:95-106.
47. Kim HW, Brandt CD, Kapikian AZ, et al. Human reovirus-like agent infection: occurrence in adult contacts of pediatric patients with gastroenteritis. *JAMA.* 1977;238:404-407.
48. Hrdy DB. Epidemiology of rotaviral infection in adults. *Rev Infect Dis.* 1987;9:461-469.
49. Tallett S, MacKenzie C, Middleton P, et al. Clinical, laboratory, and epidemiologic features of a viral gastroenteritis in infants and children. *Pediatrics.* 1977;60:217-222.
50. Richardson S, Grimwood K, Gorrell R, et al. Extended excretion of rotavirus after severe diarrhoea in young children. *Lancet.* 1998;351:1844-1848.
51. Carlson JA, Middleton PJ, Szymanski MT, et al. Fatal rotavirus gastroenteritis: an analysis of 21 cases. *Am J Dis Child.* 1978;132:477-479.
52. Rodger SM, Bishop RF, Birch C, et al. Molecular epidemiology of human rotaviruses in Melbourne, Australia, from 1973 to 1979, as determined by electrophoresis of genome ribonucleic acid. *J Clin Microbiol.* 1981;13:272-278.
53. Gorziglia M, Green K, Nishikawa K, et al. Sequence of the fourth gene of human rotaviruses recovered from asymptomatic or symptomatic infections. *J Virol.* 1988;62:2978-2984.
54. Widdowson MA, van Doornum GJ, van der Poel WH, et al. An outbreak of diarrhea in a neonatal medium care unit caused by a novel strain of rotavirus: investigation using both epidemiologic and microbiological methods. *Infect Control Hosp Epidemiol.* 2002;23:665-670.
55. Blutt SE, Matson DO, Crawford SE, et al. Rotavirus antigenemia is associated with viremia. *PLoS Med.* 2007;4:e121.
56. Gilger MA, Matson DO, Conner ME, et al. Extraintestinal rotavirus infections in children with immunodeficiency. *J Pediat.* 1992;120:912-917.
57. Wood DJ, David TJ, Chrystie IL, et al. Chronic enteric virus infection in two T-cell immunodeficient children. *J Med Virol.* 1988;24:435-444.
58. Saulsbury FT, Winkelstein JA, Yolken RH. Chronic rotavirus infection in immunodeficiency. *J Pediatr.* 1980;97:61-65.
59. Oishi I, Kimura T, Murakami T, et al. Serial observations of chronic rotavirus infection in an immunodeficient child. *Microbiol Immunol.* 1991;35:953-961.
60. Yolken RH, Bishop CA, Townsend TR, et al. Infectious gastroenteritis in bone-marrow-transplant recipients. *N Engl J Med.* 1982;306:1010-1012.
61. Peigue-Lafeuille H, Henquell C, Chambon M, et al. Nosocomial rotavirus infections in adult renal transplant recipients. *J Hosp Infect.* 1991;18:67-70.
62. Thomas PD, Pollok RCG, Gazzard BG. Enteric viral infections as a cause of diarrhea in the acquired immunodeficiency syndrome. *HIV Med.* 1999;1:19-24.
63. Zheng BJ, Chang RX, Ma GZ, et al. Rotavirus infection of the oropharynx and respiratory tract in young children. *J Med Virol.* 1991;34:29-37.
64. Rotbart HA, Nelson WL, Glode MP, et al. Neonatal rotavirus-associated necrotizing enterocolitis: case control study and prospective surveillance during an outbreak. *J Pediatr.* 1988; 112:87-93.
65. Capitanio MA, Greenberg SB. Pneumatosis intestinalis in two infants with rotavirus gastroenteritis. *Pediatr Radiol.* 1991;21: 361-362.
66. Grunow JE, Dunton SF, Waner JL. Human rotavirus-like particles in a hepatic abscess. *J Pediatr.* 1985;106:73-76.
67. Cioc AM, Nuovo GJ. Histologic and in situ viral findings in the myocardium in cases of sudden, unexpected death. *Mod Pathol.* 2002;15:914-922.
68. Lynch M, Lee B, Azimi P, et al. Rotavirus and central nervous system symptoms: cause or contaminant? Case reports and review. *Clin Infect Dis.* 2001;33:932-938.
69. Bines JE, Liem NT, Justice FA, et al. Risk factors for intussusception in infants in Vietnam and Australia: adenovirus implicated, but not rotavirus. *J Pediatr.* 2006;149:452-460.
70. Riepenhoff-Talty M, Gouvea V, Evans MJ, et al. Detection of group C rotavirus in infants with extrahepatic biliary atresia. *J Infect Dis.* 1996;174:8-15.
71. Allen SR, Jafri M, Donnelly B, et al. Effect of rotavirus strain in the murine model of biliary atresia. *J Virol.* 2007;81: 1671-1679.
72. Rauschenfels S, Krassmann M, Al-Masri AN, et al. Incidence of hepatotropic viruses in biliary atresia. *Eur J Pediatr.* 2009;168: 469-476.
73. Graham KL, Sanders N, Tan Y, et al. Rotavirus infection accelerates type 1 diabetes in mice with established insulitis. *J Virol.* 2008;82:6139-6149.
74. Makela M, Oling V, Marttila J, et al. Rotavirus-specific T cell responses and cytokine mRNA expression in children with diabetes-associated autoantibodies and type 1 diabetes. *Clin Exp Immunol.* 2006;145:261-270.
75. Stene LC, Honeyman MC, Hoffenberg EJ, et al. Rotavirus infection frequency and risk of celiac disease autoimmunity in early childhood: a longitudinal study. *Am J Gastoenterol.* 2006;101: 2333-2340.
76. Ward LA, Rosen BI, Yuan L, et al. Pathogenesis of an attenuated and a virulent strain of group A human rotavirus in neonatal gnotobiotic pigs. *J Gen Virol.* 1996;77:1431-1441.
77. Davidson GP, Goller I, Bishop RF, et al. Immunofluorescence in duodenal mucosa of children with acute enteritis due to a new virus. *J Clin Pathol.* 1975;28:263-266.
78. Davidson GP, Barnes GL. Structural and functional abnormalities of the small intestine in infants and young children with rotavirus enteritis. *Acta Paediatr Scand.* 1979;68:181-186.
79. Kohler T, Erben U, Wiedersberg H, et al. [Histological findings of the small intestinal mucosa in rotavirus infections in infants and young children]. *Kinderarztl Prax.* 1990;58:323-327.
80. Lundgren O, Svensson L. Pathogenesis of rotavirus diarrhea. *Microbes Infect.* 2001;3:1145-1156.
81. Davidson GP, Gall DG, Petric M, et al. Human rotavirus enteritis induced in conventional piglets: intestinal structure and transport. *J Clin Invest.* 1977;60:1402-1409.
82. Stintzing G, Johansen K, Magnusson KE, et al. Intestinal permeability in small children during and after rotavirus diarrhoea

assessed with different-size polyethyleneglycols (PEG 400 and PEG 1000). *Acta Paediatr Scand.* 1986;75:1005-1009.
83. Tafazoli F, Zeng CQ, Estes MK, et al. NSP4 enterotoxin of rotavirus induces paracellular leakage in polarized epithelial cells. *J Virol.* 2001;75:1540-1546.
84. Nava P, Loperz S, Arias CF, et al. The rotavirus surface protein VP8 modulates the gate and fence function of tight junctions in epithelial cells. *J Cell Sci.* 2004;117:5509-5519.
85. Ball JM, Tian P, Zeng CQ, et al. Age-dependent diarrhea induced by a rotaviral nonstructural glycoprotein. *Science.* 1996;272:101-104.
86. Zhang M, Zeng CQ, Morris AP, et al. A functional NSP4 enterotoxin peptide secreted from rotavirus-infected cells. *J Virol.* 2000;74:11663-11670.
87. Bowman GD, Nodelman IM, Levy O, et al. Crystal structure of the oligomerization domain of NSP4 from rotavirus reveals a core metal-binding site. *J Mol Biol.* 2000;304:861-871.
88. Halaihel N, Lievin V, Ball JM, et al. Direct inhibitory effect of rotavirus NSP4(114-135) peptide on the Na^+-D-glucose symporter of rabbit intestinal brush border membrane. *J Virol.* 2000;74:9464-9470.
89. Dong Y, Zeng CQ, Ball JM, et al. The rotavirus enterotoxin NSP4 mobilizes intracellular calcium in human intestinal cells by stimulating phospholipase C-mediated inositol 1,4,5-trisphosphate production. *PNAS.* 1997;94:3960-3965.
90. Morris AP, Scott JK, Ball JM, et al. NSP4 elicits age-dependent diarrhea and Ca^{2+} mediated I^- influx into intestinal crypts of CF mice. *Am J Physiol.* 1999;277:G431-444.
91. Yuan L, Honma S, Ishida S, et al. Species-specific but not genotype-specific primary and secondary isotype-specific NSP4 antibody responses in gnotobiotic calves and piglets infected with homologous host bovine (NSP4[A]) or porcine (NSP4[B]) rotavirus. *Virology.* 2004;330:92-104.
92. Lundgren O, Peregrin AT, Persson K, et al. Role of the enteric nervous system in the fluid and electrolyte secretion of rotavirus diarrhea. *Science.* 2000;287:491-495.
93. Kordasti S, Sjovall H, Lundgren O, et al. Serotonin and vasoactive intestional peptide antagonists attenuate rotavirus diarrhea. *Gut.* 2004;53:952-957.
94. Salazar-Lindo E, Santisteban-Ponce J, Chea-Woo E, et al. Racecadotril in the treatment of acute watery diarrhea in children. *N Engl J Med.* 2000;343:463-467.
95. Santos N, Hoshino Y. Global distribution of rotavirus serotypes/genotypes and its implication for the development and implementation of an effective rotavirus vaccine. *Rev Med Virol.* 2005;15:29-56.
96. Hung T, Chen GM, Wang CG, et al. Waterborne outbreak of rotavirus diarrhoea in adults in China caused by a novel rotavirus. *Lancet.* 1984;1:1139-1142.
97. Nilsson M, Svenungsson B, Hedlund KO, et al. Incidence and genetic diversity of group C rotavirus among adults. *J Infect Dis.* 2000;182:678-684.
98. Jiang B, Dennehy PH, Spangenberger S, et al. First detection of group C rotavirus in fecal specimens of children with diarrhea in the United States. *J Infect Dis.* 1995;172:45-50.
99. Hoshino Y, Sereno MM, Midthun K, et al. Independent segregation of two antigenic specificities (VP3 and VP7) involved in neutralization of rotavirus infectivity. *PNAS.* 1985;82:8701-8704.
100. Coulson BS. VP4 and VP7 typing using monoclonal antibodies. *Arch Virol Suppl.* 1996;12:113-118.
101. Ward RL, McNeal MM, Sander DS, et al. Immunodominance of the VP4 neutralization protein of rotavirus in protective natural infections of young children. *J Virol.* 1993;67:464-468.
102. Mackow ER, Shaw RD, Matsui SM, et al. The rhesus rotavirus gene encoding protein VP3: location of amino acids involved in homologous and heterologous rotavirus neutralization and identification of a putative fusion region. *PNAS.* 1988;85:645-649.
103. Mackow ER, Shaw RD, Matsui SM, et al. Characterization of homotypic and heterotypic VP7 neutralization sites of rhesus rotavirus. *Virology.* 1988;165:511-517.
104. Santos N, Honma S, Timenetsky M do C, et al. Development of a microtiter plate hybridization-based PCR-enzyme-linked immunosorbent assay for identification of clinically relevant human group A rotavirus G and P genotypes. *J Clin Micro.* 2008;46:462-469.
105. Green KY, Sears JF, Taniguchi K, et al. Prediction of human rotavirus serotype by nucleotide sequence analysis of the VP7 protein gene. *J Virol.* 1988;62:1819-1823.
106. Griffin DD, Fletcher M, Levy ME, et al. Outbreaks of adult gastroenteritis traced to a single genotype of rotavirus. *J Infect Dis.* 2002;185:1502-1505.
107. Hoshino Y, Honma S, Jones RW, et al. A porcine G9 rotavirus strain shares neutralization and VP7 phylogenetic sequence lineage 3 characteristics with contemporary G9 rotavirus strains. *Virology.* 2005;332:177-188.
108. Cao D, Santos N, Jones RW, et al. The VP7 genes of two G9 rotaviruses isolated in 1980 from diarrheal stool samples collected in Washington, DC, are unique molecularly and serotypically. *J Virol.* 2008;82:4175-4179.
109. Gentsch JR, Laird AR, Biefelt B, et al. Serotype diversity and reassortment between human and animal rotavirus strains: implications for rotavirus vaccine programs. *J Infect Dis.* 2005;192:S146-S159.
110. Hoshino Y, Kapikian AZ. Classification of rotavirus VP4 and VP7 serotypes. *Arch Virol Suppl.* 1996;12:99-111.
111. Heiman EM, McDonald SM, Barro M, et al. Group A human rotavirus genomics: evidence that gene constellations are influenced by protein-protein interactions. *J Virol.* 2008;82:11106-11116.
112. Matthijnssens J, Ciarlet M, Heiman E, et al. Full genome-based classification of rotaviruses reveals a common origin between human Wa-like and porcine rotavirus strains and human DS-1-like and bovine rotavirus strains. *J Virol.* 2008;82:3204-3219.
113. Velazquez FR, Matson DO, Calva JJ, et al. Rotavirus infections in infants as protection against subsequent infections. *N Engl J Med.* 1996;335:1022-1028.
114. Brandt CD, Kim HW, Rodriguez WJ, et al. Pediatric viral gastroenteritis during eight years of study. *J Clin Microbiol.* 1983;18:71-78.
115. Dagan R, Bar-David Y, Sarov B, et al. Rotavirus diarrhea in Jewish and Bedouin children in the Negev region of Israel: epidemiology, clinical aspects and possible role of malnutrition in severity of illness. *Pediatr Infect Dis J.* 1990;9:314-321.
116. Velazquez FR, Matson DO, Guerrero ML, et al. Serum antibody as a marker of protection against natural rotavirus infection and disease. *J Infect Dis.* 2000;182:1602-1609.
117. Parashar UD, Hummelman EG, Bresee JS, et al. Global illness and deaths caused by rotavirus disease in children. *Emerg Infect Dis.* 2003;9:565-572.
118. Ward RL, Knowlton DR, Pierce MJ. Efficiency of human rotavirus propagation in cell culture. *J Clin Microbiol.* 1984;19:748-753.
119. Ward RL, Bernstein DI, Young EC, et al. Human rotavirus studies in volunteers: determination of infectious dose and serological response to infection. *J Infect Dis.* 1986;154:871-880.
120. Widdowson M-A, Meltzer MI, Zhang X, et al. Cost-effectiveness and potential impact of rotavirus vaccination in the United States. *Pediatrics.* 2007;119:684-697.
121. Payne DC, Staat MA, Edwards KM, et al. Active, population-based surveillance for severe rotavirus gastroenteritis in children in the United States. *Pediatrics.* 2008;122:1235-1243.
122. Laboratory-based surveillance for rotavirus—United States, July 1996-June 1997. *MMWR.* 1997;46:1092-1094.
123. Levy K, Hubbard AE, Eisenberg JNS. Seasonality of rotavirus disease in the tropics: a systematic review and meta-analysis. *Int J Epidemiol.* 2008; Epub ahead of print.
124. Desselberger U, Iturriza-Gomara M, Gray JJ. Rotavirus epidemiology and surveillance. *Novartis Found Symp.* 2001;238:125-127.
125. Kraft LM. Studies on the etiology and transmission of epidemic diarrhea of infant mice. *J Exp Med.* 1957;106:743-755.
126. Mead PS, Slutsker L, Dietz V, et al. Food-related illness and death in the United States. *Emerg Infect Dis.* 1999;5:607-625.
127. Dennehy PH, Cortese MM, Begue RE, et al. A case-control study to determine risk factors for hospitalization for rotavirus gastroenteritis. *Pediatr Infect Dis J.* 2006;25:1123-1131.
128. Matson DO, O'Ryan ML, Herrera I, et al. Fecal antibody responses to symptomatic and asymptomatic rotavirus infections. *J Infect Dis.* 1993;167:577-583.
129. Rodriguez WJ, Kim HW, Brandt CD, et al. Common exposure outbreak of gastroenteritis due to type 2 rotavirus with high secondary attack rate within families. *J Infect Dis.* 1979;140:353-357.
130. Chandran AC, Heinzen RR, Santosham M, et al. Nosocomial rotavirus infections: a systematic review. *J Pediatr* 2006:149:448-451.
131. Black RE. Epidemiology of travelers' diarrhea and relative importance of various pathogens. *Rev Infect Dis.* 1990;12:S73-79.
132. Nakagomi O, Nakagomi T. Interspecies transmission of rotaviruses studied from the perspective of genogroup. *Microbiol Immunol.* 1993;37:337-348.
133. De Grazia S, Martella V, Giammanco GM, et al. Canine-origin G3P[3] rotavirus strain in child with acute gastroenteritis. *Emerg Infect Dis.* 2007;13:1091-1093.
134. Browning GF, Snodgrass DR, Nakagomi O, et al. Human and bovine serotype G8 rotaviruses may be derived by reassortment. *Arch Virol.* 1992;125:121-128.
135. Bishop RF, Barnes GL, Cipriani E, et al. Clinical immunity after neonatal rotavirus infection: a prospective longitudinal study in young children. *N Engl J Med.* 1983;309:72-76.
136. Chiba S, Yokoyama T, Nakata S, et al. Protective effect of naturally acquired homotypic and heterotypic rotavirus antibodies. *Lancet.* 1986;2:417-421.
137. Linhares AC, Pinheiro FP, Freitas RB, et al. An outbreak of rotavirus diarrhea among a nonimmune, isolated South American Indian community. *Am J Epidemiol.* 1981;113:703-710.
138. Bass DM, Baylor M, Broome R, et al. Molecular basis of age-dependent gastric inactivation of rhesus rotavirus in the mouse. *J Clin Invest.* 1992;89:1741-1745.
139. Coulson BS, Grimwood K, Hudson IL, et al. Role of coproantibody in clinical protection of children during reinfection with rotavirus. *J Clin Microbiol.* 1992;30:1678-1684.
140. Offit PA, Clark HF. Protection against rotavirus-induced gastroenteritis in a murine model by passively acquired gastrointestinal but not circulating antibodies. *J Virol.* 1985;54:58-64.
141. Offit PA, Shaw RD, Greenberg HB. Passive protection against rotavirus-induced diarrhea by monoclonal antibodies to surface proteins VP3 and VP7. *J Virol.* 1986;58:700-703.
142. Burns JW, Krishnaney AA, Vo PT, et al. Analyses of homologous rotavirus infection in the mouse model. *Virology.* 1995;207:143-153.
143. Westerman LE, McClure HM, Jiang B, et al. Serum IgG mediates mucosal immunity against rotavirus infection. *PNAS.* 2005;102:7268-7273.
144. Gonzalez R, Franco M, Sarmiento L, et al. Serum IgA levels induced by rotavirus natural infection, but not following vaccine (Rotashield), correlate with protection. *J Med Virol.* 2005;76:608-612.
145. Ward RL, Clemens JD, Knowlton DR, et al. Evidence that protection against rotavirus diarrhea after natural infection is not dependent on serotype-specific neutralizing antibody. *J Infect Dis.* 1992;166:1251-1257.
146. Glass RI, Stoll BJ, Wyatt RG, et al. Observations questioning a protective role for breast-feeding in severe rotavirus diarrhea. *Acta Paediatr Scand.* 1986;75:713-718.
147. Weinberg RJ, Tipton G, Klish WJ, et al. Effect of breast-feeding on morbidity in rotavirus gastroenteritis. *Pediatrics.* 1984;74:250-253.
148. Duffy LC, Byers TE, Riepenhoff-Talty M, et al. The effects of infant feeding on rotavirus-induced gastroenteritis: a prospective study. *Am J Public Health.* 1986;76:259-263.
149. Rennels MB, Glass RI, Dennehy PH, et al. Safety and efficacy of high-dose rhesus-human reassortant rotavirus vaccines: report of the National Multicenter Trial. United States Rotavirus Vaccine Efficacy Group. *Pediatrics.* 1996;97:7-13.
150. Bernstein DI, Glass RI, Rodgers G, et al. Evaluation of rhesus rotavirus monovalent and tetravalent reassortant vaccines in US children. US Rotavirus Vaccine Efficacy Group. *JAMA.* 1995;273:1191-1196.
151. Ruiz-Palacios GM, Perez-Schael I, Velazquez FR, et al. Safety and efficacy of an attenuated vaccine against severe rotavirus gastroenteritis. *N Engl J Med.* 2006;354:11-22.
152. Bhandari N, Sharma P, Glass RI. Safety and immunogenicity of two live attenuated human rotavirus vaccine candidates, 116E and I321, in infants: results of a randomised controlled trial. *Vaccine.* 2006;24:5817-5823.
153. Vesikari T, Karvonen A, Prymula R, et al. Efficacy of human rotavirus vaccine against rotavirus gastorenteritis during the first 2 years of life in European infants: randomised, double-blind controlled study. *Lancet.* 2007;370:1757-1763.
154. Ward RL, Sander DS, Schiff GM, et al. Effect of vaccination on serotype-specific antibody responses in infants administered WC3 bovine rotavirus before or after a natural rotavirus infection. *J Infect Dis.* 1990;162:1298-1303.
155. Green KY, Taniguchi K, Mackow ER, et al. Homotypic and heterotypic epitope-specific antibody responses in adult and infant rotavirus vaccinees: Implications for vaccine development. *J Infect Dis.* 1990;161:667-679.
156. Ruggeri FM, Greenberg HB. Antibodies to the trypsin cleavage peptide VP8 neutralize rotavirus by inhibiting binding of virions to target cells in culture. *J Virol.* 1991;65:2211-2219.
157. Zhou YJ, Burns JW, Morita Y, et al. Localization of rotavirus VP4 neutralization epitopes involved in antibody-induced conformational changes of virus structure. *J Virol.* 1994;68:3955-3964.
158. Ludert JE, Ruiz MC, Hidalgo C, et al. Antibodies to rotavirus outer capsid glycoprotein VP7 neutralize infectivity by inhibiting virion decapsidation. *J Virol.* 2002;76:6643-6651.
159. Kobayashi N, Taniguchi K, Urasawa S. Identification of operationally overlapping and independent cross-reactive neutralization regions on human rotavirus VP4. *J Gen Virol.* 1990;71:2615-2623.
160. Feng N, Lawton JA, Gilbert J, et al. Inhibition of rotavirus replication by a non-neutralizing, rotavirus VP6-specific IgA mAb. *J Clin Invest.* 2002;109:1203-1213.
161. Burns JW, Siadat-Pajouh M, Krishnaney AA, et al. Protective effect of rotavirus VP6-specific IgA monoclonal antibodies that lack neutralizing activity. *Science.* 1996;272:104-107.
162. Schwartz-Cornil I, Benureau Y, Greenberg H, et al. Heterologous protection induced by the inner capsid proteins of rotavirus requires transcytosis of mucosal immunoglobulins. *J Virol.* 2002;76:8110-8117.
163. Gonzalez AM, Nguyen TV, Azevedo MS, et al. Antibody responses to human rotavirus (HRV) in gnotobiotic pigs following a new prime/boost vaccine strategy using oral attenuated HRV priming and intranasal VP2/6 rotavirus-like particle (VLP) boosting with ISCOM. *Clin Exp Immunol.* 2004;135:361-367.
164. Garaicoechea L, Olichon A, Marcoppido G, et al. Llama-derived single-chain antibody fragments directed to rotavirus VP6 protein possess broad neutralizing activity in vitro and confer protection against diarrhea in mice. *J Virol.* 2008;82:9753-9764.
165. Franco MA, Greenberg HB. Immunity to rotavirus in T cell deficient mice. *Virology.* 1997;238:169-179.
166. Barro M, Patton JT. Rotavirus NSP1 inhibits expression of type I interferon by antagonizing the function of interferon regulatory factors IRF3, IRF5, and IRF7. *J Virol.* 2007;81:4473-4481.
167. Franco MA, Greenberg HB. Role of B cells and cytotoxic T lymphocytes in clearance of and immunity to rotavirus infection in mice. *J Virol.* 1995;69:7800-7806.
168. Doern GV, Herrmann JE, Henderson P, et al. Detection of rotavirus with a new polyclonal antibody enzyme immunoassay (Rotazyme II) and a commercial latex agglutination test (Rotalex): comparison with a monoclonal antibody enzyme immunoassay. *J Clin Microbiol.* 1986;23:226-229.

169. Raboni SM, Nogueira MB, Hakim VM, et al. Comparison of latex agglutination with enzyme immunoassay for detection of rotavirus in fecal specimens. *Am J Clin Pathol*. 2002;117: 392-394.

170. Gouvea V, Glass RI, Woods P, et al. Polymerase chain reaction amplification and typing of rotavirus nucleic acid from stool specimens. *J Clin Microbiol*. 1990;28:276-282.

171. Gentsch JR, Glass RI, Woods P, et al. Identification of group A rotavirus gene 4 types by polymerase chain reaction. *J Clin Microbiol*. 1992;30:1365-1373.

172. Pang XL, Lee B, Boroumand N, et al. Increased detection of rotavirus using a real time reverse transcription-polymerase chain reaction (RT-PCR) assay in stool specimens from children with diarrhea. *J Med Virol*. 2004;72:496-501.

173. Honma S, Chizhikov V, Santos N, et al. Development and validation of DNA microarray for genotyping group A rotavirus VP4 (P[4], P[6], P[8], P[9], and P[14]) and VP7 (G1 to G6, G8 to G10, and G12) genes. *J Clin Microbiol*. 2007;45:2641-2648.

174. Brandt CD, Kim HW, Rodriguez WJ, et al. Comparison of direct electron microscopy, immune electron microscopy, and rotavirus enzyme-linked immunosorbent assay for detection of gastroenteritis viruses in children. *J Clin Microbiol*. 1981;13: 976-981.

175. Dolan KT, Twist EM, Horton-Slight P, et al. Epidemiology of rotavirus electropherotypes determined by a simplified diagnostic technique with RNA analysis. *J Clin Microbiol*. 1985;21: 753-758.

176. Sato K, Inaba Y, Shinozaki T, et al. Isolation of human rotavirus in cell cultures: Brief report. *Arch Virol*. 1981;69:155-160.

177. King CK, Glass R, Breese JS, et al. Managing acute gastroenteritis among children: oral rehydration, maintenance, and nutritional therapy. *MMWR*. 2003;52:1-16.

178. Santosham M, Daum RS, Dillman L, et al. Oral rehydration therapy of infantile diarrhea: a controlled study of well-nourished children hospitalized in the United States and Panama. *N Engl J Med*. 1982;306:1070-1076.

179. Schedl HP, Clifton JA. Solute and water absorption by human small intestine. *Nature*. 1963;199:1264-1267.

180. World Health Organization. *Reduced Osmolarity Oral Rehydration Salts (ORS) Formulation*. WHO/FCH/CAH/01.22. Geneva, Switzerland. 2002.

181. Brown KH, Gastanaduy AS, Saavedra JM, et al. Effect of continued oral feeding on clinical and nutritional outcomes of acute diarrhea in children. *J Pediatr*. 1988;112:191-200.

182. Bhutta ZA, Black RE, Brown KH, et al. Prevention of diarrhea and pneumonia by zinc supplementation in children in developing countries: pooled analysis of randomized controlled trials. *J Peds*. 1999;135:689-697.

183. Bhutta ZA, Bird SM, Black RE, et al. Therapeutic effects of zinc in actue and persistent diarrhea in developing countries: pooled analysis of randomized controlled trials. *Am J Clin Nutr*. 2000;72:1516-1522.

184. World Health Organization/United Nations Childrens Fund Joint Statement. *Clinical Management of Acute Diarrhoea*. Geneva, Switzerland. 2004.

185. Guarino A, Guandalini S, Albano F, et al. Enteral immunoglobulins for treatment of protracted rotaviral diarrhea. *Pediatr Infect Dis J*. 1991;10:612-614.

186. Barnes GL, Doyle LW, Hewson PH, et al. A randomised trial of oral gammaglobulin in low-birth-weight infants infected with rotavirus. *Lancet*. 1982;1:1371-1373.

187. Figueroa-Quintanilla D, Salazar-Lindo E, Sack RB, et al. A controlled trial of bismuth subsalicylate in infants with acute watery diarrheal disease. *N Engl J Med*. 1993;328:1653-1658.

188. Van Niel CW, Feudtner C, Garrison MM, et al. Lactobacillus therapy for acute infectious diarrhea in children: a meta-analysis. *Pediatrics*. 2002;109:678-684.

189. Joensuu J, Koskenniemi E, Vesikari T. Prolonged efficacy of rhesus-human reassortant rotavirus vaccine. *Pediatr Infect Dis J*. 1998;17:427-429.

190. Perez-Schael I, Guntinas MJ, Perez M, et al. Efficacy of the rhesus rotavirus-based quadrivalent vaccine in infants and young children in Venezuela. *N Engl J Med*. 1997;337: 1181-1187.

191. Intussusception among recipients of rotavirus vaccine—United States, 1998-1999. *MMWR*. 1999;48:577-581.

192. Murphy TV, Gargiullo PM, Massoudi MS, et al. Intussusception among infants given an oral rotavirus vaccine. *N Engl J Med*. 2001;344:564-572.

193. Simonsen L, Viboud C, Elixhauser A, et al. More on RotaShield and intussusception: the role of age at the time of vaccination. *J Infect Dis*. 2005;192:S36-S43.

194. Murphy BR, Morens DM, Simonsen L, et al. Reappraisal of the association of intussusception with the licensed live rotavirus vaccine challenges initial conclusions. *J Infect Dis*. 2003; 187:1301-1308.

195. Vesikari T, Matson DO, Dennehy P, et al. Safety and efficacy of a pentavalent human-bovine (WC3) reassortant rotavirus vaccine. *New Engl J Med*. 2006;354:23-33.

196. Bernstein DI, Sack DA, Reisinger K, et al. Second-year follow-up evaluation of live, attenuated human rotavirus vaccine 89-12 in healthy infants. *J Infect Dis*. 2002;186:1487-1489.

197. Cortese MM, Parashar UD. Centers for Disease Control and Prevention. Prevention of rotavirus gastroenteritis among infants and children: recommendations of the Advisory Committee on Immunization Practices (ACIP). *MMWR Recomm Rep*. 2009;58:1-25.

198. Clark HF, Offit PA, Ellis RW, et al. The development of multivalent bovine rotavirus (strain WC3) reassortant vaccine for infants. *J Infect Dis*. 1996;174:S73-S80.

199. Parashar UD, Alexander JP, Glass RI. Prevention of rotavirus gastroenteritis among infants and children: recommendation of the Advisory Committee on Immunization Practices (ACIP). *MMWR*. 2006;55:1-13.

200. Haber P, Patel M, Izurieta HS, et al. Postlicensure monitoring of intussusception after RotaTeq vaccination in the United States, February 2006, to September 25, 2007. *Pediatrics*. 2008;121:1206-1212.

201. Jiang B, Gentsch JR, Glass RI. Inactivated rotavirus vaccines: a priority for accelerated vaccine development. *Vaccine*. 2008;26:6754-6758.

202. World Health Organization. Evaluating clinical trial data and guiding future research for rotavirus vaccines. *Weekly Epidem Rec*. 2008;83:385-392.

203. Fu C, Wang M, Liang J, et al. Effectiveness of Lanzhou lamb rotavirus vaccine against rotavirus requiring hospitalization: a matched case-control study. *Vaccine*. 2007;25:8756-8761.

204. Istrate C, Hinkula J, Charpilienne A, et al. Parenteral adminstration of RF8-2/6/7 rotavirus-like particles in a one dose regimen induce protective immunity in mice. *Vaccine*. 2008;26: 4594-4601.

151

Alphaviruses

LEWIS MARKOFF

All the medically important alphaviruses are arthropod vector borne. Most have hosts in nature other than humans and vectors that are crucial to the virus life cycle. Three mosquito-borne alphaviruses currently cause human disease in the United States: eastern equine encephalitis (EEE), western equine encephalitis (WEE), and Venezuelan equine encephalitis (VEE) viruses. These are among the "New World" alphaviruses, defined by their antigenic and nucleotide sequence relatedness as well as by their geographic distribution. "Old World" alphavirus species of major importance include Chikungunya (CHIK) (in Africa and Asia), O'nyong-nyong (Africa), Mayaro (South America), Ross River (Australia, Oceania), Sindbis (Africa, Scandinavia, the countries of the former Soviet Union, Asia), and Barmah Forest virus (Australia). The Old World alphaviruses primarily cause fever, rash, and arthropathy. Relevant information on medically important alphaviruses and some related species is presented in Table 151-1.

History

WEE and EEE viruses were initially recovered from the brains of horses with encephalitis in California (1930) and New Jersey (1933), respectively. By 1938, both of these agents had been established as causes of encephalitis in humans.[1] Similarly, the VEE virus was first isolated from the brains of horses in Venezuela during an epidemic of encephalitis in 1938.[2] The first reports of VEE infection of humans were from laboratories where equine isolates were being studied in 1943. Apparently, this outbreak was caused by the aerosol spread of infectious virus to laboratory workers. Naturally acquired VEE virus in humans was first reported from Colombia in 1952 in association with an epizootic disease in equines.[3] The first reports of VEE virus infection of humans in the United States were published in 1968.[4] Retrospective analysis of historical accounts suggests that CHIK virus caused epidemics of fever, rash, and arthralgia in Indonesia (1779), East Africa (1823, 1870), India (1824, 1871, 1901, 1923), the Far East (1901), West Africa (1925), and the Southeastern United States (1827). The virus was first isolated during an epidemic in Tanzania in 1952 and 1953.[5] An epidemic of CHIK that originated in Africa, and then spread to islands in the Indian Ocean, India, and elsewhere in Asia, Africa, and Europe, is currently ongoing (2004 to the present).[6]

Pathogens

The alphaviruses constitute a genus in the family Togaviridae.[7] The genus contains at least 30 different viruses classified into 7 serocomplexes.[8] These are lipid-enveloped virions with a diameter of 50 to 60 nm. The alphavirus genome is an 11- to 12-kilobase bicistronic positive-strand (or message sense) RNA. In virus particles, genomic RNA is complexed with the virus-coded core protein in an icosahedral nucleocapsid structure. Two glycoproteins, E1 and E2, are inserted in the lipid membrane surrounding the nucleocapsid and project outward from the membrane. E1 and E2 appear to form both hetero- and homodimers in the course of virion morphogenesis.[9] An additional small viral structural protein, the 6K protein,[10] and a second protein, derived from the 6K gene segment by ribosomal frame-shifting (TF protein),[11] are also associated with membranes. 6K protein enhances membrane permeability by inducing pore formation,[12] and 6K expression in cultured cells induces caspase-dependent apoptosis.[13] E2 appears primarily responsible for attachment of virus to the cell surface. E2 antibodies, but not generally E1 antibodies, can neutralize virus infectivity. E1 has hemagglutinin activity and contains alphavirus cross-reactive epitopes.

Alphaviruses enter cells by receptor-mediated endocytosis. After the E2 envelope protein binds to the cellular receptor, the virus particle is engulfed in an endocytic vesicle, and a low pH–dependent fusion reaction mediated by the E1 envelope protein results in the release of virus particle contents into the cytoplasm. Four viral nonstructural proteins are then derived by translation of the 5′-terminal two thirds of genomic RNA and sequential cleavage of the resulting polyprotein. Partial cleavage products of the nonstructural polyprotein initiate negative-strand RNA synthesis after infection. Complete processing of the nonstructural precursor is necessary for subsequent plus-strand RNA synthesis and for evasion of the cellular antiviral response, which is mediated by nsp2.[14] Viral structural proteins are encoded by a subgenomic (26S) messenger RNA colinear with the 3′-terminal one third of the genome. Initial products of translation of the 26S messenger RNA include a 62-kDa E2 precursor polypeptide, PE2 or "p62"; E1; and the hydrophobic 6K protein. PE2 and E1 form a stable heterodimer in the endoplasmic reticulum that is transported to the plasma membrane through the secretory pathway. PE2 is cleaved by cellular enzymes in acidic transport vesicles to produce E2, and the E2/E1 heterodimer is acquired on nascent particles by budding at the plasma membrane. The cleavage of PE2 destabilizes the heterodimer with E1 such that it is more readily dissociated by low pH, which activates the fusion process for mature virions.[9,15-17]

Complement fixation, hemagglutination inhibition (HI), and the plaque reduction-neutralization test define seven distinct alphavirus antigenic complexes and distinguish among virus species within a complex. EEE, VEE, and WEE are prototype viruses for each of three antigenic complexes.[18] The WEE genome and those of WEE-like viruses, except for Aura virus (see later), are intragenic recombinants: the nonstructural and core protein genes are derived from an EEE-like ancestral genome, whereas the structural glycoproteins E1 and E2 are derived from the genome of a Sindbis-like virus.[19] Results of complement fixation, HI, and plaque reduction neutralization test assays are largely dependent on antigenicity of E2. Therefore, some of the Old World alphaviruses, Sindbis virus and Sindbis-like viruses, group with WEE and related New World viruses. CHIK, O'nyong-nyong, Mayaro, and Ross River viruses are grouped with Semliki Forest virus in a fourth complex. Middelburg, Nduma, and Barmah Forest viruses, respectively, constitute the single species in each of the three additional alphavirus serogroups (see Table 151-1).

Partial and complete nucleotide sequencing of alphavirus genomes has permitted the phylogenetic subgrouping of the alphaviruses. When 3′-terminal sequences for more than two dozen different alphaviruses were compared, genetically distinct clades appeared to coincide with each of the seven complexes as defined by antigenic distinctions, with only minor discrepancies between the two methods.[8] Within each clade or complex, there are viruses that exist in regions of the world that are geographically distant from one another yet share medically important characteristics in addition to their genetic and antigenic relatedness. For example, despite their nonoverlapping geographic distribution, members of the EEE and VEE complexes share encephalitic potential in equines and humans, and the Semliki Forest virus complex of Mayaro (limited to Latin America) and O'nyong-nyong (limited to Africa) viruses produce identical fever-rash-arthralgia syndromes. The WEE complex includes viruses that produce either arthralgic (Sindbis virus–like subgroup) or encephalitic (WEE and Highlands J virus subgroup) syndromes, regardless of their respective geographic distribu-

TABLE 151-1	Medically Important Alphaviruses and Some Related Alphavirus Species				
Antigenic Complex	Virus	Geographic Distribution	Animal Reservoir	Human Vector*	Human Disease (Animals Affected)
EEE	EEE	NA, SA, Caribbean	Birds	Aedes	Encephalitis (horses, birds)
WEE	WEE	NA, SA	Birds, horses	Culex tarsalis	Fever, encephalitis (horses, birds [especially emus])
	Aura	SA	Birds		
	Fort Morgan	Colorado	Birds		
	Highlands J	Eastern U.S.	Birds	Culex, Aedes	(Encephalitis in turkeys, pheasants, partridges, ducks, emus, horses)
	Kyzylagach	Azerbaijan	Birds		
	Sindbis	AUS, AFR, EUR, Asia Minor	Birds	Aedes	Fever, arthritis, rash
	Whataroa	AUS, NZ	Birds		
VEE	VEE	NA, SA	Horses and others	Psorophora, Aedes	Fever, encephalitis (horses)
	Cabassou	SA			
	Everglades	Florida	Mammals	Ochlerotatus	Encephalitis
	Pixuna	Brazil	Mammals		
SF	Semliki Forest	AFR	Mammals	Aedes	Fever, arthritis, rash? (rare)
	Bebaru	Asia			
	Chikungunya	ADR, Southeast Asia, Philippines	Primates	Culex, Aedes	Fever, arthritis, rash
	Getah	Asia	Mammals	Culex, Aedes	Fever? (horses)
	Mayaro	SA		Haemagogus, Aedes	Fever, arthritis, rash
	O'nyong-nyong	AFR		Anopheles	Fever, arthritis, rash
	Ross River	AUS, South Pacific	Mammals	Aedes, Culex	Fever, arthritis, rash
BF	Barmah Forest	AUS	Birds	Aedes	Fever, arthritis, rash

*The mosquito vector genus or species required for epizootic transmission of infection is shown. No epizootic vector is listed for viruses that rarely cause disease or for which there are no reports of disease.

AFR, Africa; AUS, Australia; EEE, eastern equine encephalitis; EUR, Europe; NA, North America; NZ, New Zealand; SA, South America; U.S., United States; VEE, Venezuelan equine encephalitis; WEE, western equine encephalitis.

tions. The encephalitic potential of the latter viruses probably reflects the genetic contribution of the EEE-like ancestral virus core and nonstructural genes rather than that of the Sindbis-like *E1* and *E2* genes.

Within the EEE antigenic complex, there are North American and South American subtypes based on HI testing. A phylogenetic analysis suggested that the North American subtypes constitute a single lineage and that there are three distinct lineages among South American subtypes. Each of the four lineages seemed also to be antigenically distinct according to results of plaque reduction neutralization tests.[20] This finding has significance in relation to EEE virus vaccine development. As mentioned, the WEE antigenic complex includes the New World viruses WEE, Buggy Creek, Highlands J, Fort Morgan, and Aura and the Old World viruses Sindbis and the Sindbis subtypes Babanki (Africa), Ockelbo (Northern Europe), Kyzylagach (Azerbaijan, China), and Whataroa (New Zealand). Five subtypes of VEE are recognized. Subtype I occurs in tropical America and is medically most important. Four geographic variants of subtype I are distinguishable. Variants IAB and IC were associated with equine epizootics and human epidemics that occurred between the 1920s and the early 1970s. Variants ID and IE and subtype II (Everglades virus) are less virulent and are associated with enzootic disease. A phylogenetic study of alphaviruses, using both whole genome sequences and predicted total protein sequences[21] (Fig. 151-1) essentially confirmed the classifications cited previously. Using the Rubella virus genome (family: Togaviridae; genus: Rubivirus) as a comparator, all the medically important alphaviruses were grouped into two clades, the Semliki Forest clade, including CHIK, O'nyong-nyong, and Ross River viruses, and the Sindbis-equine encephalitis clade, including Sindbis, VEE, WEE, and EEE viruses.

Epidemiology

ENCEPHALITIS-CAUSING ALPHAVIRUSES

Alphaviruses are limited in their geographic distribution by the range of their respective arthropod vectors. EEE virus infection occurs focally

along the eastern and Gulf coasts of the United States, and documented cases have occurred as far north as southern Canada and as far south as northern areas of South America and the Caribbean.[22] EEE is a summertime disease, occurring most frequently in children and elderly people. A few human cases occur each year. Although relatively rare, an outbreak is usually noteworthy because of the high case-fatality rate (50% to 70%). The incidence of equine cases greatly exceeds that in humans, and outbreaks resulting in the deaths of hundreds of horses have been reported in the Northeastern United States and Florida.[22] In horses, the infection may involve multiple organ systems, including the heart, spleen, urinary tract, and gastrointestinal tract as well as the entire central nervous system (CNS).[23]

In North America, the principal enzootic vector for EEE is the mosquito *Culiseta melanura*, which breeds in freshwater swamps and feeds on passerine birds. Infection of avian species may result in death in some cases and may be without apparent consequence in others. In either case, it results in viremia of sufficient magnitude and frequency to maintain a reservoir of infected mosquitoes.[24] Transmission from birds to horses and humans is mediated by mosquitoes other than *C. melanura*, which is highly ornithophilic. Possible vectors include *Aedes* and *Coquillettidia* spp.[25] Horses and humans develop only low or undetectable levels of viremia. Therefore, these hosts do not serve as reservoirs for further virus spread. In summary, conditions for EEE epizootics include the presence of *C. melanura* and susceptible bird populations coincident with vector mosquitoes capable of feeding on both birds and the horses or humans in the vicinity. In temperate climates, maintenance of epizootics is theoretically interdicted by winter and may account for the relative rarity of these epidemics. However, EEE virus can be isolated from the same endemic foci in successive years, and nucleotide sequencing of the genomes of 42 EEE viruses isolated along the east coast of the United States suggested that the virus does persist or "overwinter" in cold climates. The same data set also suggested that EEE virus strains migrate from south to north along the east coast of the United States.[26] As for VEE (see previously) and other alphaviruses, mosquito transmission is not the only mode

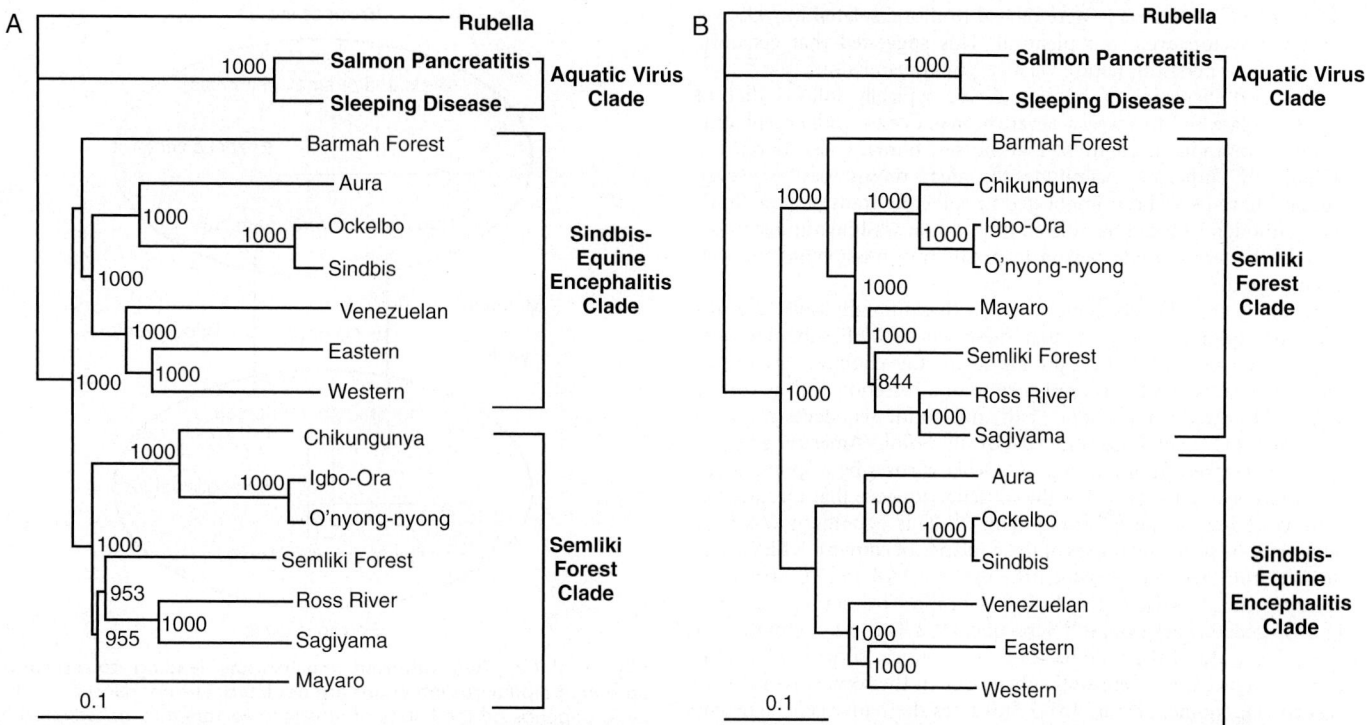

Figure 151-1 **Phylograms examining the complete genomes of the alphaviruses.** These trees were generated using Clustal X and neighbor joining analysis. Each of the alphavirus clades are identified in bold. Rubella, Salmon Pancreatitis, and Sleeping Disease viruses are in bold to denote their placement as outgroups. **A,** Whole complementary DNA alphaviral genomic sequences. **B,** Whole amino acid alphaviral genomic sequences. *(Reprinted with permission from Luers AJ, Adams SD, Smalley JV, et al. A phylogenetic study of the genus Alphavirus employing whole genome comparison. Comp Func Genom. 2005;6:217-227.).*

of spread for EEE virus. The virus is also highly infectious by the aerosol route.[27] However, this mode of infection poses a risk associated only with handling of infected birds or with laboratory exposure.

EEE is a rare disease in South America, with only two case reports, but strains of EEE virus that are genetically distinct from EEE viruses isolated in North America do persist there.[28] A recent serosurvey in a Peruvian population exposed to EEE virus showed that infections occur without subsequent illness, suggesting that South American strains are relatively avirulent in humans.[29] This difference in virulence between North and South American isolates may be due to differences in replication efficiency in neuronal cells and in interferon (IFN) sensitivity, and is probably multigenic in origin.[30]

The WEE viruses are distributed primarily in the Americas. A subtype of WEE, isolated in Argentina, is presumed to be representative of endemic strains in South America.[31] In North America, WEE is a summertime disease of horses and humans in states west of the Mississippi River and in corresponding Canadian provinces. The vector is *Culex tarsalis*. Risk factors for infection include rural residence, outdoor employment in farming (because the vector favors irrigated areas), and male sex. During an epidemic, a very high percentage of the adult population seroconverts, but the case-to-infection ratio ranges from less than 1:1000 in older adults to nearly 1:1 in infants. Thus, encephalitis is most frequent in infants younger than 1 year. However, encephalitis is most severe in older adults. Case-fatality rates are 3% to 4%. In contrast, EEE infection rates are low in an epidemic, but the case-to-infection ratio is higher than that for WEE and is highest in the young.[32] In a laboratory-based study of WEE virus virulence, eight individual strains of WEE virus displayed either high or low virulence phenotypes in mice. The eight strains segregated into one of two genotypes that correlated with their pathogenicity.[33]

Between 1964 and 2000, 640 total cases of WEE and 182 total cases of EEE were reported to the Centers for Disease Control and Prevention. WEE cases all occurred before 1996 and occurred most com-

monly in Colorado (173 cases), Texas (94 cases), North Dakota (78 cases), and California (53 cases), with additional significant numbers of cases in Missouri, South Dakota, and Kansas. EEE occurred most commonly in Florida (53 cases), Georgia (22 cases), and Massachusetts (21 cases) as well as in New Jersey, North Carolina, and Louisiana. The fact that there were no case reports of WEE between 1996 and 2000 and also between 2000 and 2007 suggests that control efforts and other natural variables have had a dramatic negative effect on the disease incidence.[34] In contrast, 31 of the 182 cases of EEE reported between 1964 and 2000 occurred in 1996 or later, and cases continued to be reported at a rate of less than 10 per year between 2000 and 2007.[35] EEE cases in Massachusetts are reported to cluster in cycles lasting 2 to 3 years that recur every 10 to 20 years.[34-36] Currently, EEE is estimated to cause about 1% of all cases of viral encephalitis in the United States.[36]

Epizootic strains of VEE virus (1D, 1E, and II subtypes) have the special capacity to cause disease in horses and humans. VEE virus infections in South America and Central America have been associated with tens of thousands of both equine and human cases.[37] For epizootic viruses, equines play an important role in maintenance because they develop high-titer viremia and are thus likely to transmit infection to mosquitoes. At least 10 mosquito species, including *Culex, Aedes, Mansonia, Psorophora,* and *Deinocerites,* have been identified as probable epidemic vectors.[38] Epizootics have been documented in Venezuela, Colombia, Ecuador, and Peru at intervals of 10 years or less since the 1930s. Typically, epizootics begin in areas of tropical forest during the rainy season. In the center of an epizootic, transmission usually continues until all horses are dead or immune. Spread may be to contiguous areas or may be sporadic. Major Venezuelan outbreaks occurred in 1962, 1973, and 1995, the last outbreak involving as many as 100,000 human cases.[39] Nearly all viruses isolated during the 1995 outbreak were closely related to the 1C subtype viruses that had been isolated in 1973. Five years later, viruses isolated from a few scattered cases of VEE in Venezuela were related to those isolated in 1995, yet epizootic vectors were not plentiful. This suggested that epizootic viruses could persist in nature via a cryptic transmission cycle.[40]

Increased incidence of human disease typically follows that of equine disease by 1 to 2 weeks. Severe human disease with encephalitis is most common in children. Like horses, humans also develop a viremia of sufficient magnitude to infect mosquitoes. However, humans have never been implicated in epidemic transmission. Similarly, although VEE can be isolated from throat washings and is infectious by the aerosol route, person-to-person transmission has not been documented.[41]

Studies comparing epizootic strains with commonly isolated enzootic ones originally suggests that these sets of VEE subtypes were highly unrelated. In fact, *Culex taeniopus*, the common vector for enzootic strains of VEE, is refractory to oral infection with epizootic virus.[42] However, comparisons of the nucleotide sequences of newly emerging (1C-like) epizootic viruses in South America suggests that they evolved from a group of 1D-like viruses by a spontaneous mutation or mutations within the *E2* gene sequence that increase the positive charge of the E2 ectodomain.[43,44] This hypothesis was later supported by studies in horses of the virulence of chimeric VEE viruses derived from genomes in which the subtype 1AB and 1C structural glycoprotein genes had been substituted for those of a subtype 1D virus in a 1D genetic background.[45] Subsequently, a Thr to Lys mutation at amino acid 213 of the subtype 1D E2 protein was shown to be sufficient to induce the 1C epizootic phenotype in the context of a closely related 1D genome.[46] Figure 151-2 illustrates alternative general mechanisms by which viruses like EEE virus, WEE virus, and VEE virus might transition from an enzootic to an epizootic cycle.

Horses are not amplifying hosts for enzootic strains of VEE. These viruses are principally maintained by their mosquito vector and rodents that thrive in tropical and subtropical swamps and forests. Humans living in these areas manifest a high prevalence of antibody. These viruses cause encephalitis sporadically in Central America (subtypes ID and IE) and Florida (subtype II).

ALPHAVIRUSES CAUSING FEVER, RASH, AND POLYARTHRITIS

Chikungunya Virus
Chikungunya means "to walk bent over," in reference to the crippling arthritic manifestations of the disease. *Aedes* mosquitoes of the subgenus *Stegomyia* are the principal vectors in Africa, and the virus seems to be maintained by transmission to nonhuman primates. Humans with appropriate concentrations also provide a reservoir for the infection of mosquitoes. A major epidemic of CHIK virus apparently started in Kenya in 2004, causing an estimated 500,000 cases in Africa, and spread initially in 2006 to the island of Reunion in the Indian Ocean. On Reunion, approximately 265,000 of 770,000 inhabitants reported symptoms of disease in 2006, with 237 deaths.[47] The outbreak subsequently spread to the southeast coast of India, the islands of Mauritius, Seychelles, and Mayotte and to Madagascar and Italy. An outbreak of CHIK fever, believed to originate directly from Africa, also occurred in 2006 in Malaysia.[6] At least 1,400,000 cases of CHIK fever were reported in 2006 to 2007 in India. The major vector involved in the outbreak on Reunion and in Italy was *Aedes albopictus*, whereas *Aedes aegypti* is implicated as a vector in urban epidemics in India and elsewhere in Asia. A single mutation in the E1 envelope glycoprotein is associated with adaptation of African CHIK virus strains to *Aedes albopictus* mosquitoes.[48] In 2005 to 2006, 12 cases of CHIK fever were diagnosed among travelers returning to the United States from these endemic or epidemic areas.[49] Cases occurring in northeastern Italy seem to have originated with a man visiting Italy from India.[50]

Serologic survey of native populations using the HI assay suggests that epidemics occur periodically when the youngest group of inhabitants of an endemic area are susceptible. Twenty percent to more than 90% of the population of tropical and subtropical Africa show serologic evidence of past infection. The following factors suggest the

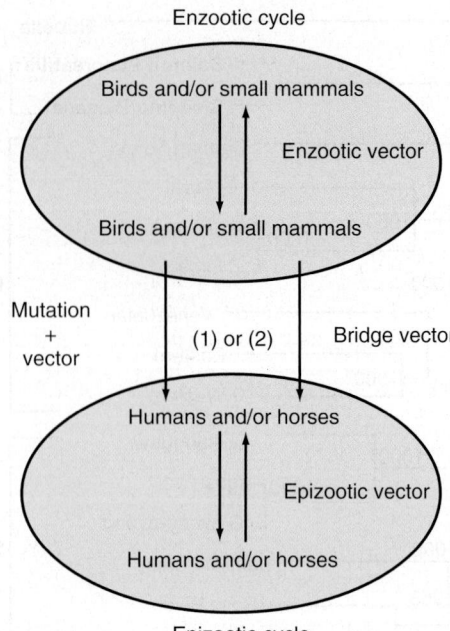

Figure 151-2 Two different mechanisms leading to epizootic spread of alphavirus infections are depicted. The normal enzootic life cycle depends on the habits of mosquito vectors that are adapted to feed on the required small animal hosts, including birds and rodents. Virus infection spreads to horses or humans, or both, when either (1) a mutation occurs in the viral genome adapting it to replication in large animals and in vector mosquitoes that are adapted to feed on them, or (2) a "bridging" vector transmits virus directly from animals involved in the enzootic cycle to humans or horses. Once the epizootic cycle is initiated, virus is spread by a different vector or set of vectors adapted to the large animal host. Venezuelan equine encephalitis virus is an example of an alphavirus that requires a mutation to initiate epizootic spread (mechanism 1). Eastern equine encephalitis virus is an example of an alphavirus that can spread to humans and horses by the action of a bridging vector mosquito (mechanism 2).

potential for future major CHIK fever epidemics, especially in the Western hemisphere: (1) the increasing prevalence of *Aedes* species, especially *albopictus*, in North and South America and Europe,[47] (2) the increasing mobility of populations residing in endemic or currently epidemic areas (3) the lack of a requirement for an animal host, other than humans to support the CHIK virus life cycle, and (4) the presence of large populations of immunologically naïve individuals in the West.[5,6]

O'nyong-nyong Virus
O'nyong-nyong virus is closely related to CHIK virus, both antigenically and genetically. It initially appeared in Uganda in the form of an epidemic that involved 2 million people in its final extent by the middle-to-late 1960s. The virus then disappeared until 1996, when it reappeared in the context of a second epidemic in southern Uganda. The reemerging virus was shown by nucleotide sequence analysis to be closely related to the 1959 strain.[51] During the fall of 2003, there was a third outbreak of O'nyong-nyong fever in the Ivory Coast that was initially mistaken for measles.[52] Both O'nyong-nyong virus and CHIK virus are closely related to a third virus, Igbo-Aura, also found in Africa. Risk factors for O'nyong-nyong fever include residence in rural villages where the vector *Anopheles* mosquitoes congregate. A nonhuman primate reservoir of infection has not been identified.

Sindbis Virus
Sindbis virus is transmitted among birds by *Culex* mosquitoes. Studies in South Africa show that extensive human disease occurs in parallel with years of abundant rainfall in association with flooding of usually

arid regions. Thus, infected mosquitoes and susceptible humans are presumably brought into proximity. Infection rates may approach 15% during a major transmission season. Sindbis virus and the flavivirus West Nile virus share the avian-*Culex* mosquito hosts (see Chapter 153). In South Africa, the Nile Valley of Egypt, and Israel, individuals with antibodies to Sindbis virus frequently also have antibodies to West Nile virus. In northern Europe, symptomatic infection is called Pogosta disease and is recognized in the region between 60° and 65° north latitude in Sweden, Finland, and the Commonwealth of Independent States. Pogosta disease is characterized by arthritis, pruritic rash, fatigue, mild fever, headache, and muscle pain. It is a disease of adults who work or vacation in forested areas. Between 1981 and 1996, 2183 cases of Pogosta disease were serologically confirmed in Finland, for an annual average of 136 cases, but the disease peaks in 7-year cycles.[53] The virus has been isolated from *Culiseta*, *Aedes*, and *Culex* mosquitoes. A recent serosurvey among migratory birds in Finland suggests that the grouse is the major avian host of Sindbis virus in that locale.[54]

Ross River Virus

Ross River virus is a cause of epidemic polyarthritis, myalgia, and fatigue, in humid northern tropical areas of Australia. It is the most common and most widespread arboviral disease in Australia. Joint symptoms are especially intense and may last as long as 3 years after fever and rash have abated.[55] Spread to the Pacific Islands has been documented. The facts that this virus has been isolated from mosquitoes and that human disease is seasonal are clues to its dependence on vector transmission. A second alphavirus, Barmah Forest disease virus, is also found in northern Australia. Disease caused by Barmah Forest disease virus is increasing; 1895 cases were reported in 2005 to 2006. Barmah Forest disease virus causes, in general, a less severe arthritis that is shorter in duration than that caused by Ross River virus.[56]

Mayaro Virus

Mayaro virus was first isolated in the Caribbean in the 1950s in association with an epidemic of febrile illness with rash and occasional arthropathy. It has since been documented to have caused epidemics in Brazil and Bolivia. The virus has been isolated from *Haemagogus* mosquitoes and from marmosets as well as other nonhuman primates.[57] These may provide a reservoir for virus in the natural setting.

A long list of alphaviruses, including Bebaru, Cabassou, Getah, Kyzylagach, Middelburg, Nduma, Pixuna, Sagiyama, Semliki Forest, Una, and Whataroa viruses, either are not known to cause human disease or disease is of the fever-arthropathy type and is rare.

▥ Pathogenesis

The locus of alphavirus replication in the mosquito is the midgut epithelium, which is targeted after the mosquito has taken a blood meal from a viremic host. In the mosquito, the infection is generally thought to be a lifelong, persistent, productive one, although there may be associated necrotic changes in the midgut.[58] Alphavirus infections of humans are initiated by the bite of an infected mosquito, which results in the deposition of virus in subcutaneous and possibly cutaneous tissues. The initial phase of infection is marked by viremia and a febrile response, signaling the replication of virus in non-neural tissues. The earliest measurable VEE immune response is antibody directed against a virion surface component that is non-neutralizing but mediates viral clearance. This is followed by the advent of neutralizing antibodies with E2 specificity. Before CNS invasion in experimental animals, VEE replicates in lymphoid tissues, resulting in necrotic changes, and in bone marrow, resulting in lymphopenia. Lymphoid infection in mice is followed by high-titer viremia, during which the peripheral CNS is seeded, mainly through the olfactory system.[59] VEE also replicates in the pancreas and salivary glands of experimental animals but does not seem to have a diabetogenic effect in humans who have survived encephalitis. Infection of neurons by VEE in animals leads to an acute encephalitis with necrosis, mild to moderate neutrophilic infiltrate, gliosis, and perivascular cuffing with involvement of Purkinje cells.[60] Susceptibility of mice to VEE and death is enhanced in mice lacking IFN regulatory factors (IRF-1 and IRF-2), IFN receptors, or type I IFN itself.[61,62] In addition, inducible nitric oxide synthase gene function is associated with recovery from VEE in mice. VEE-induced neuronal cell death is by apoptosis.[63]

EEE causes lesions throughout the brain and spinal cord, most severely involving the cerebral cortex and basal ganglia. WEE causes focal necrosis in the striatum, globus pallidus, cerebral cortex, thalamus, pons, and meninges. Transplacental spread of VEE and WEE may affect the fetus, resulting in massive cerebral necrosis.[37,64]

Although it does not commonly invade the human CNS, Sindbis virus causes a fatal encephalitis in mice that serves as a model for study of alphavirus encephalitis in humans. Neurovirulence is directly related to previous mouse-brain adaptation of the virus, route of administration, and genetic differences among mouse strains; it is inversely related to age.[65] The initial event appears to be infection of capillary endothelial cells, allowing virus to reach neuronal cells through the microvasculature or through transport across vessel walls into the brain parenchyma.[66] Once infected, mature neurons are more resistant to apoptotic cell death caused by Sindbis virus than immature neurons, which may account for the increased susceptibility of very young mice to Sindbis encephalitis.[67] Apoptosis is triggered by the fusion event that occurs during virus entry. Fusion-associated conformational changes in sphingomyelin activate the enzyme sphingomyelinase, resulting in an increase in ceramide, a proapoptotic substance.[68] Despite the role of sphingomyelinases in triggering apoptosis, young mice deficient in this enzyme exhibit an increased susceptibility to virus dissemination and encephalitis with apoptotic cell death.[69] To explain this finding, alphaviruses can trigger apoptotic cell death by a variety of other mechanisms. For example, the 6K protein induces apoptosis in conjunction with its function as a viroporin.[13] The outcome of infection at the cellular level seems related to the neuronal response to produce mediators of apoptosis (e.g., BAX) versus antagonists of apoptosis (e.g., BCL-2, Beclin-1, and certain protease inhibitors).[67]

In adult mice infected with neuro-adapted Sindbis virus, Sindbis virus–infected and neighboring uninfected neurons die by the necrotic pathway and secondary to inflammation, respectively, as well as by apoptosis.[70] Murine cortical neurons in culture were protected specifically from necrotic and inflammatory cell death by antagonists of a subclass of glutamate receptors (AMPA receptor antagonists).[71,72] Further evaluation of the mechanism of protection revealed that the inflammatory response was markedly diminished in the brains of treated mice; lymphocytes were not activated and failed to proliferate. Viral clearance was also delayed in treated mice, despite the protective efficacy of the drug.[71]

The humoral immune response is primarily responsible for clearance of Sindbis virus from the CNS, not only by direct neutralization of virus infectivity but also by antibody-dependent, complement-mediated cytolysis of infected cells.[73] In addition, certain Sindbis virus–specific monoclonal antibodies can induce virus clearance from the CNS by restricting viral gene expression in neurons. Despite this effect of extracellular antibody, viral RNA could be shown to persist in infected neurons for several months. Removal of antibody resulted in recrudescence of infection.[74] This phenomenon was completely independent of a cell-mediated immune response and suggested a mechanism for persistence of alphavirus infections in the CNS. Although neurologic symptoms may be among the sequelae of human infection with the neurotropic flaviviruses, long-term persistence of infectious alphaviruses in the CNS has not been documented. However, there is some suggestion that alphaviruses that cause the fever/rash/arthritis syndrome may persist for weeks or months in affected joints (see later).

T cells seem to be required primarily for late clearance of viral RNA from neurons.[75] However, they may also be involved in clearance of infectious virus, at least in specialized situations. For example, mice immunized with the Sindbis nonstructural protein nsp-2 do not develop a protective humoral immune response but do recover from paralysis caused by Sindbis virus replication in the CNS. Presumably protection is T cell mediated,[76] but possibly mice were protected because anti-nsp2 antibodies interfere with the role of endogenous nsp2 in suppressing IFNs.[77] IFN-γ–secreting T cells were required for noncytolytic clearance of virus from spinal cord and brain stem neurons but were not effective in clearance of virus from cortical neurons.[78] In addition, consistent with the results of studies using AMPA antagonists,[72] T cells may also contribute to the damaging inflammatory response associated with fatal acute viral encephalomyelitis through production of IFN-γ.[79]

The mechanisms by which alphaviruses cause rash and arthritis are less well studied. During self-limited infection with a non-neurotropic alphavirus, such as CHIK virus, the level of viremia closely parallels the fever curve. As viremia fades and fever subsides, HI and neutralizing antibody titers start to increase, suggesting that these immune responses curtail infection. Biopsy of the maculopapular to macular rash in CHIK infection shows lymphocytic perivascular cuffing and extravasation of erythrocytes from superficial capillaries.[80] Arthralgia may accompany early symptoms of fever and malaise (CHIK virus) or may be slightly delayed and quite severe, leading to frank arthritis (Ross River virus). The disease caused by these viruses is believed to be initiated by viral replication, which induces host inflammatory responses in the affected tissues. This is based on the detection of Ross River virus RNA and antigen in joint tissues, as well as the presence of inflammatory cellular infiltrates, consisting primarily of monocytes and virus-infected macrophages within synovial effusions.[81,82] Similarly, CHIK virus antigens have been detected in muscle-biopsy specimens exhibiting severe myositis with inflammatory macrophages, T lymphocytes, and myofibril pathology.[83] The severity of Ross River virus disease was markedly reduced in mice that were depleted of macrophages. Treated mice also had decreased concentrations of the inflammatory cytokines tumor necrosis factor-α, IFN-γ, and macrophage chemoattractant protein 1.[84] Complement receptor 3 also promotes inflammation at sites of Ross River virus infection in the mouse model.[85] Concomitant with these findings, sulfasalazine, which blocks nuclear factor-κB, ameliorated inflammatory disease in human subjects.[84] A general scheme for the time course of the pathogenesis of acute alphavirus diseases is shown in Figure 151-3.

Clinical Manifestations

ALPHAVIRUSES CAUSING ENCEPHALITIS

EEE is heralded by a 5- to 10-day prodrome of headache, high fever, chills, nausea, and vomiting or diarrhea. In patients in whom CNS involvement develops, initial symptoms are followed by mental confusion and somnolence often accompanied by photophobia. Seizures or convulsions occur most often in younger patients. Seizures are usually tonic-clonic, but may also be of the partial-complex type. Progression to frank coma can occur rapidly. Physical examination may reveal nuchal rigidity, depressed or hyperactive reflexes, tremors, muscle twitching, spastic paralysis, bilateral papilledema, and cranial nerve palsies, which can be secondary to increased cerebrospinal fluid (CSF) pressure or directly related to inflammation. Cranial nerves VI, VII, and XII are most often affected. Infants may develop bulging fontanelles. Other occasional findings include cyanosis secondary to depressed respiratory drive and facial, periorbital, or generalized edema.[36,86]

Laboratory findings in acute EEE are as follows.[36,86] A polymorphonuclear leukocytosis is present in most cases to levels of 15,000 cells/mm³ or higher. Hyponatremia, when noted, may be due to the syndrome of inappropriate antidiuretic hormone. CSF protein is increased, and 500 to 2000 cells/mm³ are present, mostly lymphocytes. Red blood cells are occasionally noted as well. Hypoglycorrhachia is not present. Serologic tests are positive for antibodies to EEE virus (see later).

Neurologic sequelae include mental retardation, behavioral changes, convulsive disorders, and paralysis. These may occur in 70% of those recovering from EEE infection. Negative prognostic signs in EEE are

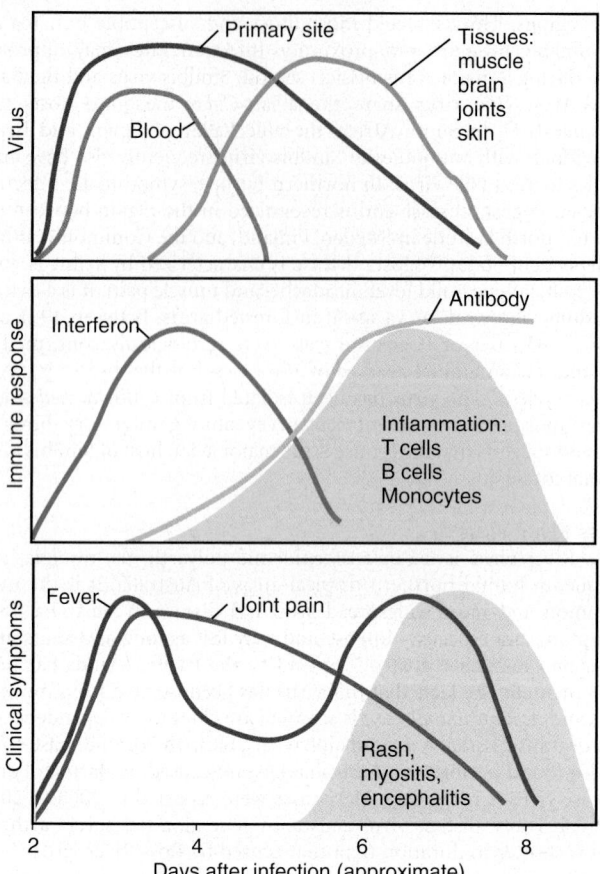

Figure 151-3 Schematic diagram of the pathogenesis of alphavirus-induced disease. Viremia may be accompanied by production of interferon, other proinflammatory cytokines, and fever. Virus then spreads through the blood to other target tissues. As the immune response is induced, the viremia is terminated, but fever is renewed with the appearance of a mononuclear inflammatory response in the infected tissues. In infections that lead to rash and arthritis, joint pain usually appears early after infection and before the appearance of the rash. *(From Griffin D. The alphaviruses. In: Knipe DM, Howley PM, eds. Fields Virology. 5th ed. Philadelphia: Lippincott Williams & Wilkins; 2007:1031.)*

age older than 40, rapid progression to coma, severe hyponatremia, and CSF cell counts higher than 500/mm³.[36,86] Among patients who recover, sequelae are less frequent in adults.

WEE infection is also heralded by a short prodromal phase lasting 1 to 4 days. Signs and symptoms during this period are very similar to those described for EEE. In adults, the prodromal phase may subside spontaneously with no neurologic complications. In subjects who do progress, the course of encephalitis resembles that of EEE as well, except that focal neurologic abnormalities may be less common.[36,87] Laboratory studies usually reveal a polymorphonuclear leukocytosis, but counts are significantly lower than those noted for EEE. The CSF protein is usually increased, and lymphocytes and red blood cells are present. Cell counts are lower than those noted for EEE. Glucose is normal. Neurologic sequelae occur in 30% of young patients and are similar to those noted for EEE.[87] Parkinsonism is an occasional late sequela of WEE encephalitis in adults.

The most common clinical manifestation of epizootic VEE infection is a febrile illness with malaise after an incubation period of 1 to 6 days. Chills, myalgia, and headache with or without photophobia, hyperesthesia, and vomiting are common. Occasionally patients report a sore throat. Fever may remit in a short time, with recrudescence the next day. Approximately 4% of children and less than 1% of adults progress to severe encephalitis, which usually occurs after a few days to a week of the prodromal illness.[38] Features of encephalitis include nuchal rigidity, ataxia, convulsions, coma, and paralysis, in ascending order of severity. Laboratory studies characteristically reveal lymphopenia, sometimes accompanied by neutropenia and mild thrombocytopenia within a day or two of onset. Serum glutamic oxaloacetic transaminase (aspartate aminotransferase) and lactate dehydrogenase enzymes are typically increased. CSF examination reveals a few hundred lymphocytes. The overall case-fatality rate is less than 1%, but approaches 20% in those who progress to encephalitis. Nearly all individuals in endemic areas contract enzootic VEE infection, as suggested by the results of serologic surveys.[38] Most seem to have experienced the influenza-like prodromal illness or to have had asymptomatic infection.

ALPHAVIRUSES CAUSING FEVER, RASH, AND POLYARTHRITIS

CHIK fever is taken as the prototype of the diseases caused by this large group of alphaviruses. This is an acute viral infection characterized by a rapid transition from a state of good health to illness that includes severe arthralgia and fever.[88] The incubation period ranges from 1 to 12 days. Body temperature increases abruptly to as high as 40°C and is often accompanied by shaking chills. After a few days, fever may abate and recrudesce, giving rise to a "saddleback" fever curve (see Fig. 151-3). Arthralgia is polyarticular, favoring the small joints and sites of previous injuries, and is most intense on arising. Patients typically avoid movement as much as possible. Joints may swell without significant fluid accumulation. These symptoms may last from 1 week to several months and are accompanied by myalgia. The rash characteristically appears on the first day of illness, but onset may be delayed. It usually arises as a flush over the face and neck, which evolves to a maculopapular or macular form that may be pruritic. The latter lesions appear on the trunk, limbs, face, palms, and soles, in that order of frequency. Petechial skin lesions have also been noted. Headache, photophobia, retro-orbital pain, sore throat with objective signs of pharyngitis, nausea, and vomiting also occur in this setting. Laboratory test results may reveal a mild leukopenia with relative lymphocytosis. The erythrocyte sedimentation rate is usually markedly elevated, and the C-reactive protein is positive.[89] Severe arthritic involvement is most commonly seen in adults, whereas children occasionally present with symptoms referable to the CNS, including seizures and convulsions. Long-term joint involvement has been reported in association with human leukocyte antigen B27.[64]

As a result of the recent CHIK epidemic, additional clinical aspects of the disease have been documented. In 88 patients on Reunion Island who were assessed a median of 18 months after onset of disease, 56 reported persistent arthralgia, and half of those reported a resulting reduction in their ability to carry out daily activities. All had polyarticular involvement, and pain was continuous in more than half of those who reported arthralgia. Approximately 40% of the total had persisting CHIK-specific immunoglobulin (Ig) M antibodies.[90] Transient ocular involvement was described among adult patients in South India, with the main manifestations including anterior uveitis, optic neuritis, retrobulbar neuritis, and dendritic lesions.[91] In another study emanating from Reunion Island, atypical cases of CHIK were defined as those in which patients developed symptoms other than fever and arthralgia. A total of 610 such cases were studied, among which 222 were graded as severe. Of these, 65 patients died. Atypical manifestations included meningoencephalitis, hepatitis, bullous dermatitis, pneumonia, and diabetes.[92] According to a report from another hospital on Reunion Island, serious acute CHIK virus infection resulted in encephalitis (14 cases), myocarditis, hepatitis, and Guillain-Barré syndrome among 33 patients who were admitted to an intensive care unit. There was a 48% fatality rate in this severely ill group.[93]

Mother-to-child transmission of CHIK virus infection was demonstrated in a retrospective study of neonates. Clinical signs seen in 38 infants included fever (79%), rash (82%), pain (100%), and peripheral edema (58%). Laboratory abnormalities included thrombocytopenia, lymphopenia, decreased prothrombin, and elevation of alanine aminotransferase. Virus was detected in the CSF of 22 of 24 infants evaluated by polymerase chain reaction; 14 of these subjects had abnormal findings on brain magnetic resonance imaging with white matter lesions or intraparenchymal hemorrhages. Myocardial hypertrophy, ventricular dysfunction, pericarditis, and coronary artery dilatation were documented in a minority of this group, and one neonate died of necrotizing enterocolitis.[94] Among all patients, the case-fatality rate on Reunion Island was estimated at 1/1000. Higher rates were calculated for Mauritius and parts of India.

Cases of CHIK fever among travelers returning to their home countries from the epidemic areas have been characterized. In one study from Germany, CHIK infection was documented in 20 of 69 patients who initially reported CHIK-like symptoms, including fever and arthralgia. Two thirds of the patients had persistent arthralgia for longer than 2 months, and 13% had it for longer than 6 months. Active viremia was reported in all patients who reported to clinic within the first week of illness.[95] In a 14-month prospective report from France, 47 patients were diagnosed and followed. Nearly all had fever, rash, and arthritis, and 38 of 47 had rheumatism persisting longer than 2 weeks, characterized by severe joint pain, tenosynovitis, and significant loss of ability to function.[96]

Diagnosis

The epidemiology of each of the disease entities caused by alphaviruses is highly specific and provides a major clue to diagnosis. Thus, knowledge of the recent travel or outdoor exposure history of the patient is of vital importance. In certain locales, during epidemic spread of a disease, the diagnosis is obvious. In the United States, the initial signs and symptoms of EEE or WEE infection may mimic those of enteroviruses. Encephalitis caused by the flaviviruses West Nile virus and St. Louis encephalitis virus may occur in the same setting as encephalitis caused by WEE, although clinical disease related to St. Louis encephalitis is more common in elderly people than in infants. Similarly, West Nile-virus encephalitis should be considered in the differential diagnosis of a viral encephalitis in areas of the United States where EEE traditionally occurs. Centers for Disease Control and Prevention criteria for the diagnosis of an arboviral encephalitis require the presence of an acute febrile illness with encephalitis during a time when virus transmission is likely plus one of the following criteria: (1) greater than fourfold increase in viral antibody titer between acute and convalescent sera; (2) virus isolation from CSF, blood, or tissue; or (3) IgM positive to the virus in CSF.

For EEE, the virus can sometimes be isolated from serum during the prodrome,[36] but historically most cases are diagnosed by testing paired sera in HI tests or in a neutralization assay because only low-level viremia occurs in human subjects. Convalescing patients may manifest high complement fixation antibody titers, and IgM antibodies can be detected by enzyme-linked immunosorbent assay (ELISA).[97] Magnetic resonance imaging with specialized imaging techniques such as fluid-attenuated inversion recovery and T_2 weighting is of value for both diagnosis and following the clinical course of encephalitis.[98] EEE caused focal radiographic changes involving the basal ganglia, thalamus, and brainstem, in descending order of frequency, in one study of 36 cases.[86]

Diagnostic testing for WEE follows a similar pattern except that viremia is usually not detectable. The presence of WEE in a specimen may be documented by inoculating suckling mice or embryonated eggs. In contrast, sera taken from patients with VEE infection within 48 hours of onset are usually positive for virus. However, sera from patients with full-blown encephalitis are usually negative, and the diagnosis may be made by complement fixation testing. ELISA for VEE-specific IgM in sera and CSF is available. IgM and IgG ELISAs using attenuated VEE as antigen are the most sensitive diagnostic tests but should be followed up with the plaque reduction neutralization assay to prove specificity.[99]

Sensitive nucleic acid amplification assays using the reverse-transcriptase polymerase chain reaction are under development for rapid diagnosis of EEE, WEE, VEE, and West Nile virus infections.[100] Most recently, ELISA and reverse-transcriptase polymerase chain reaction have been combined in a single, rapid-detection system that uses biotinylated oligonucleotide probes complementary to unique amplified nucleotide sequences in the WEE, EEE, VEE, and Mayaro virus genomes.[101] Human monoclonal antibodies directed against epizootic VEE viruses have been expressed in bacteriophage and are being used for rapid diagnostic assays.[102] Where and when these assays are available, they constitute a very rapid substitute for actual culturing of virus from a clinical specimen.

CHIK fever may be clinically indistinguishable from disease caused by Mayaro, O'nyong-nyong, Ross River, or Sindbis virus. In addition, parvovirus infection, the prodrome of hepatitis B, juvenile rheumatoid arthritis, dengue fever, and rubella, may also be confused with CHIK fever or with the other alphavirus infections. Patients with CHIK fever are usually viremic for the first 48 hours, and the virus is easily isolated by in vivo or in vitro methods. Viremia may be so intense (titer >10^7 plaque-forming units/mL of blood) as to yield measurable amounts of hemagglutinating activity from sera.[103] Consequently, virus in sera can also often be detected by ELISA directly.[104] As previously mentioned, the decrease in levels of viremia parallels a rapid increase in titers of HI and neutralizing antibodies. ELISA testing for virus-binding antibodies may detect cross-reactive immune responses to other alphaviruses. The recent CHIK epidemics in Africa and Asia have stimulated the development of rapid diagnostic tests based on variations of the real-time reverse-transcriptase polymerase chain reaction, with particular emphasis on their ability to distinguish dengue from CHIK.[104,105]

Treatment and Prevention

There is no specific treatment for any of the diseases caused by alphaviruses. For encephalitis, supportive measures and intensive nursing care are indicated. Ribavirin and other nucleoside analogues have some in vitro activity against these viruses in tissue culture but are not in use clinically. Intravenous immunoglobulin was apparently effective in promoting recovery of at least one patient with acute EEE infection who had full-blown encephalitis and coma.[98]

Prevention of WEE and EEE depends primarily on control of vector mosquito populations. During outbreaks, susceptible individuals engaged in high-risk activities should be advised to avoid exposure as much as is practicable by using effective mosquito repellents and netting, wearing full-length trousers and long-sleeved shirts, and avoiding outdoor activities at least during periods of maximal mosquito activity. Inactivated vaccines against EEE and WEE are available for limited human use. Similar veterinary vaccines are used against EEE in horses and birds and against WEE in horses. The inactivated EEE vaccine is derived from a North American virus isolate and may not be efficacious in the prevention of disease caused by the South American antigenic variant of EEE virus.[106]

Both formalin-inactivated and live, attenuated vaccines to prevent VEE infection are limited use in humans. Efficacy of the formalin-inactivated vaccine was greatly enhanced in mice when antigens were microencapsulated in biodegradable microspheres.[107] The live, attenuated VEE vaccine strain TC-83 is used in the diagnostic ELISA, and large-scale vaccination of horses with this strain is the major approach to the prevention of VEE epizootics. A live, attenuated vaccine to prevent CHIK fever (strain TSI-GSD-218) has been shown to be safe in volunteers at the level of phase II clinical trials.[108] One study in which the experimental live, attenuated VEE and CHIK fever vaccines were sequentially administered to human volunteers indicated that preexisting alphavirus immunity interferes with a subsequent neutralizing antibody response to a heterologous vaccine virus.[109]

The live VEE and CHIK vaccine candidates mentioned previously were derived several years ago by serial passage of virulent human isolates in tissue culture, and neither one is licensed by any regulatory authority. Newer approaches to alphavirus vaccine development, both live and DNA types, have involved the use of recombinant DNA technology. Attenuated mutant-VEE viruses have been developed with a goal to both prevent VEE and use VEE as a vector for presentation of foreign antigens, because of the propensity of VEE virus to target dendritic cells. One viable mutant virus derived from VEE infectious DNA, which contains mutations affecting cleavage of the viral structural proteins, was avirulent in mice, produced solid mucosal immunity against VEE, and currently shows promise primarily as a vaccine for horses.[110,111] This genetic backbone provided the basis for a number of VEE DNA-based vaccines designed to induce immunity to foreign viral and nonviral antigens,[112-114] especially when mucosal immune responses are considered to be of crucial importance for protection,[114] but progress has slowed in recent years with regard to vaccines for human use.

Novel vaccines to prevent EEE and CHIK are based on a Sindbis virus infectious DNA; in each case, the Sindbis structural protein genes were replaced by those of EEE virus or CHIK virus, in the context of a Sindbis infectious DNA.[115,116] Each of these vaccines was immunogenic and protective in mice. Neither of these candidates has entered clinical trials. Vaccinology is a rapidly changing field, and the reader is advised to search the literature for up-to-date information on alphavirus vaccines and the therapeutic use of recombinant DNA–derived vaccines based on alphavirus genomes.

REFERENCES

1. Fothergill LD, Dingle JH, Farber S, et al. Human encephalitis caused by a virus of eastern variety of equine encephalitis. *N Engl J Med.* 1983;219:411.
2. Beck CG, Wyckof RWG. Venezuelan equine encephalitis. *Science.* 1938;88:530.
3. San Martin-Barberi C, Groot H, Osborn-Mesa E. Human epidemic in Colombia caused by the Venezuelan equine encephalitis virus. *Am J Trop Med Hyg.* 1954;3:283.
4. Ehrenkranz NJ, Ventura AK. Venezuelan equine encephalitis virus infection in man. *Annu Rev Med.* 1974;25:9-14.
5. Peters CJ, Dalrymple JM. Alphaviruses. In: Fields BN, Knipe DM, eds. *Virology.* 2nd ed. New York: Raven Press; 1990: 713-761.
6. Pialoux G, Gauzere BA, Jaureguiberry S, et al. Chikungunya, an epidemic arbovirosis. *Lancet Infect Dis.* 2007;7:319-327.
7. Francki RIB, Fauquet CM, Knudson DL, et al. Classification and nomenclature of viruses. *Arch Virol.* 1991;2(Suppl):223.
8. Powers AM, Brault AC, Shirako Y, et al. Evolutionary relationships and systematics of the alphaviruses. *J Virol.* 2001;75: 10118-10131.
9. Strauss JH, Strauss EG. Virus evolution: how does an enveloped virus make a regular structure. *Cell.* 2001;105:5-8.
10. Gaedigk-Nitschko K, Schlesinger MJ. The Sindbis virus 6K protein can be detected in virions and is acylated with fatty acids. *Virology.* 1990;175:274-281.
11. Firth AE, Chung BY, Fleeton MN, et al. Discovery of frameshifting in alphavirus 6K resolves a 20-year enigma. *Virol J.* 2008;5:108.

12. Sanz MA, Perez L, Carrasco L. Semliki Forest virus 6K protein modifies membrane permeability after inducible expression in *Escherichia coli* cells. *J Biol Chem.* 1994;269:12106-12110.
13. Madan V, Castello A, Carrasco L. Viroporins from RNA viruses induce caspase-dependent apoptosis. *Cell Microbiol.* 2008;10: 437-451.
14. Gorchakov R, Frolova E, Sawicki S, et al. A new role for ns polyprotein cleavage in Sindbis virus replication. *J Virol.* 2008;82:6218-6231.
15. Smit JM, Klimstra WB, Ryman KD, et al. PE2 cleavage mutants of Sindbis virus: Correlation between virus infectivity and pH-dependent membrane fusion activation of the spike heterodimer. *J Virol.* 2001;75:11196-11204.
16. Zhang X, Fugere M, Day R, et al. Furin processing and proteolytic activation of Semliki Forest virus. *J Virol.* 2003;77: 2981-2989.
17. Mukhopadyay S, Zhang W, Gabler S, et al. Mapping the structure and function of the E1 and E2 glycoproteins in alphaviruses. *Structure.* 2006;14:63-73.
18. Calisher CH, Shope RE, Brandt WE, et al. Proposed antigenic classification of registered arboviruses. I. Togaviridae. *Alphavirus Intervirol.* 1980;14:229-232.
19. Weaver SC, Kang W, Shirako Y, et al. Recombinational history and molecular evolution of Western equine encephalitis complex alphaviruses. *J Virol.* 1997;71:613-623.
20. Brault AC, Powers AM, Chavez CL, et al. Genetic and antigenic diversity among eastern equine encephalitis viruses from

North, Central, and South America. *Am J Trop Med Hyg.* 1999;61:579-586.
21. Luers AJ, Adams SD, Smalley JV, et al. A phylogenetic study of the genus Alphavirus employing whole genome comparison. *Comp Func Genom.* 2005;6:217-227.
22. Monath TP. Arthropod-borne encephalitides in the Americas. *Bull World Health Organ.* 1979;57:513-533.
23. Del Piero F, Wilkins PA, Dubovi EJ, et al. Clinical, pathologic, immunohistochemical, and virologic findings of eastern equine encephalitis in two horses. *Vet Pathol.* 2001;38:451-456.
24. Shope RE, de Andrade AHP, Bensabeth G, et al. The epidemiology of EEE, WEE, SLE, and Tralock viruses. *Am J Epidemiol.* 1966;84:467-477.
25. Chamberlain RW. Vector relationship of the arthropod-borne encephalitides in North America. *Ann N Y Acad Sci.* 1958; 70:312-319.
26. Young DS, Kramer LD, Maffel JG, et al. Molecular epidemiology of eastern equine encephalitis virus, New York. *Emerg Infect Dis.* 2008;14:454-460.
27. Reed DS, Lackemeyer MG, Garza NL, et al. Severe encephalitis in cynomolgus macaques exposed to aerosolized eastern equine encephalitis virus. *J Infect Dis.* 2007;196: 441-450.
28. Kondig JP, Turrell MJ, Lee JS, et al. Genetic analysis of South American eastern equine encephalitis viruses isolated from mosquitoes collected in the Amazon Basin region of Peru. *Am J Trop Med Hyg.* 2007;76:408-416.

29. Aguilar PV, Robich RM, Turell MJ, et al. Endemic eastern equine encephalitis in the Amazon region of Peru. *Am J Trop Med Hyg*. 2007;76:293-298.
30. Aguilar PV, Adams AP, Wang E, et al. Structural and nonstructural protein genome regions of eastern equine encephalitis virus are determinants of interferon sensitivity and murine neurovirulence. *J Virol*. 2008;82:4920-4930.
31. Reisen WK, Monath TP. Western equine encephalomyelitis. In: Monath TP, ed. *The Arboviruses: Epidemiology and Ecology*. Vol. 5. Boca Raton, FL: CRC Press; 1989:90-137.
32. Feemster RF. Equine encephalitis in Massachusetts. *N Engl J Med*. 1957;257:701-704.
33. Nagata LP, Hu WG, Parker M, et al. Infectivity variation and genetic diversity among strains of Western equine encephalitis virus. *J Gen Virol*. 2006;87:2353-2361.
34. Centers for Disease Control and Prevention. <www.cdc.gov>.
35. <http://www.infectiousdiseasenews.com/200605/equine.asp>
36. Hirsch MS, DeMaria A, Schaefer PW, et al. Case 22-2008: a 52-year-old woman with fever and confusion. *N Engl J Med*. 2008;359:294-303.
37. Groot H. The health and economic impact of Venezuelan equine encephalitis. In: *Venezuelan Encephalitis, Proceedings of the Workshop-Symposium on Venezuelan Encephalitis Virus*. Washington, DC: Pan American Health Organization; 1972:244.
38. Johnson KM, Martin DH. Venezuelan equine encephalitis. *Adv Vet Sci Comp Med*. 1974;18:79.
39. Weaver SC, Salas R, Rico-Hesse R, et al. Re-emergence of epidemic Venezuelan equine encephalitis in South America. VEE Study Group. *Lancet*. 1996;348:436-440.
40. Navarro JC, Medina G, Vazquez C, et al. Postepizootic persistence of Venezuelan equine encephalitis virus, Venezuela. *Emerg Infect Dis*. 2005;11:1907-1915.
41. Bowen GS, Fashinell TR, Dean PB, et al. Clinical aspects of human Venezuelan equine encephalitis in Texas. *Bull Pan Am Health Org*. 1976;10:46-57.
42. Scherer WF, Cupp EW, Dziem GM, et al. Mesenteronal infection threshold of an epizootic strain of Venezuelan equine encephalitis virus in *Culex* (*Melanoconion*) *taeniopus* mosquitoes and its implication to the apparent disappearance of this virus from an enzootic habitat in Guatemala. *Am J Trop Med Hyg*. 1982;31:1030-1037.
43. Powers AM, Oberste MS, Brault AC, et al. Repeated emergence of epidemic/epizootic Venezuelan equine encephalitis from a single genotype of enzootic subtype 1D virus. *J Virol*. 1997;71: 6697-6705.
44. Brault AC, Powers AM, Holmes EC, et al. Positively charged amino acid substitutions in the E2 envelope glycoprotein are associated with the emergence of Venezuelan equine encephalitis virus. *J Virol*. 2002;76:1718-1730.
45. Greene IP, Paessler S, Austgen L, et al. Envelope glycoprotein mutations mediate equine amplification and virulence of epizootic Venezuelan equine encephalitis virus. *J Virol*. 2005;79:9128-9133.
46. Anishchenko M, Bowen RA, Paessler S, et al. Venezuelan encephalitis emergence mediated by a phylogenetically predicted viral mutation. *Proc Natl Acad Sci U S A*. 2006;103: 4994-4999.
47. Charrel, RN, Lamballerie X, Raoult D. Chikungunya outbreaks—the globalization of vector-borne diseases. *N Engl J Med*. 2007;356:769-771.
48. Kumar NP, Joseph R, Kamaraj T, et al. A 226V mutation in virus during the 2007 chikungunya outbreak in Kerala, India. *J Gen Virol*. 2008;89:1945-1948.
49. Centers for Disease Control and Prevention. Update: chikungunya fever diagnosed among international travelers—United States, 2006. *MMWR Morb Mortal Wkly Rep*. 2007;56:276-277.
50. Rezza G, Nicoletti L, Angelini R, et al. Infection with chikungunya in Italy: An outbreak in a temperate region. *Lancet*. 2007; 370:1840-1846.
51. Lanciotti RS, Ludwig ML, Rwaguma EB, et al. Emergence of epidemic O'nyong-nyong fever in Uganda after a 35-year absence: genetic characterization of the virus. *Virology*. 1998;252:258-268.
52. Posey DL, O'Rourke T, Roehrig JT, et al. Short report: O'nyong-nyong fever in West Africa. *Am J Trop Med Hyg*. 2005;73: 32.
53. Brummer-Korventkontio M, Vapalahti O, Kuusisto P, et al. Epidemiology of Sindbis virus infections in Finland 1981-96: possible factors explaining a peculiar disease pattern. *Epidemiol Infect*. 2002;129:335-345.
54. Kurkela S, Ratti O, Huhtamo E, et al. Sindbis virus infection in resident birds, migratory birds, and humans, Finland. *Emerg Infect Dis*. 2008;14:41-47.
55. Mudge PR. Clinical features of epidemic polyarthritis. *Arbovirus Res Aust*. 1982:158-166.
56. Jacups SP, Whelan PI, Currie BJ. Ross River virus and Barmah Forest virus infections: a review of history, ecology, and predictive models, with implications for northern Australia. *Vector Borne Zoonotic Dis*. 2008;8:283-297.
57. Pinheiro FP, LeDuc JW. Mayaro virus disease. In: Monath TP, ed. *The Arboviruses: Epidemiology and Ecology*. Boca Raton, FL: CRC Press; 1988:137-150.
58. Weaver SC, Lorenz LH, Scott TW. Pathologic changes in the midgut of *Culex tarsalis* following infection with Western equine encephalomyelitis virus. *Am J Trop Med Hyg*. 1992;47:691-701.
59. Charles PC, Walters E, Margolis F, et al. Mechanism of neuroinvasion of Venezuelan equine encephalitis virus in the mouse. *Virology*. 1995;208:662-671.
60. Gorelkin L. Venezuelan equine encephalitis in an adult animal host. *Am J Pathol*. 1973;73:425-432.
61. Grieder FB, Vogel SN. Role of interferon and interferon regulatory factors in early protection against Venezuelan equine encephalitis virus infection. *Virology*. 1999;257:106-118.
62. Schoneboom BA, Lee JS, Grieder FB. Early expression of IFN alpha/beta and iNOS in the brains of Venezuelan equine encephalitis virus-infected mice. *J Interferon Cytokine Res*. 2000;20:205-215.
63. Jackson AC, Rossiter JP. Apoptotic cell death is an important cause of neuronal cell injury in Venezuelan equine encephalitis virus infection of mice. *Acta Neuropathol (Berl)*. 1997;93: 349-353.
64. Tsai TF, Monath TP. Viral diseases in North America transmitted by arthropods or from vertebrate reservoirs. In: Feigin RD, Cherry JD, eds. *Textbook of Pediatric Infectious Diseases*. 2nd ed. Philadelphia: WB Saunders; 1988:1417.
65. Thach DC, Kimura T, Griffin DE. Differences between C57Bl/6 and BALB/c mice in mortality and virus replication after intranasal infection with neuroadapted Sindbis virus. *J Virol*. 2000;74:6156-6161.
66. Dropulic B, Masters CL. Entry of neurotropic arboviruses into the central nervous system: an in vitro study using mouse brain endothelium. *J Infect Dis*. 1990;161:685-691.
67. Griffin DE. Neuronal cell death in alphavirus encephalitis. *Curr Top Microbiol Immunol*. 2005;289:57-77.
68. Jan JT, Chatterjee S, Griffin DE. Sindbis virus entry into cells triggers apoptosis by activating sphingomyelinase, leading to release of ceramide. *J Virol*. 2000;74:6425-6432.
69. Ng CG, Griffin DE. Acid sphingomyelinase deficiency increases susceptibility to fatal alphavirus encephalomyelitis. *J Virol*. 2006;80:10989-10999.
70. Havert MB, Schonfeld B, Griffin DE, et al. Divergent neuronal cell death pathways activated in different target cell populations during neuroadapted Sindbis virus infection of mice. *J Virol*. 2000;74:5352-5356.
71. Nargi-Aizenman JL, Griffin DE. Sindbis virus-induced neuronal death is both necrotic and apoptotic and is ameliorated by *N*-methyl-D-aspartate receptor antagonists. *J Virol*. 2001;75: 7114-7121.
72. Greene IP, Lee EY, Prow N, et al. Protection from fatal viral encephalomyelitis: AMPA receptor antagonists have a direct effect on the inflammatory response to infection. *Proc Natl Acad Sci U S A*. 2008;105:3575-3580.
73. Grosfeld H, Lustig S, Gozes Y, et al. Divergent envelope E2 alphavirus sequences spanning amino acids 297 to 352 induce in mice virus-specific immunity and antibodies with complemented-mediated cytolytic activity. *Virology*. 1992;66: 1084-1090.
74. Levine B, Griffin DE. Persistence of viral RNA in mouse brains after recovery from acute alphavirus encephalitis. *J Virol*. 1992;66:6429-6435.
75. Kimura T, Griffin DE. The role of $CD8^+$ T cells and major histocompatibility complex class I expression in the central nervous system of mice infected with neurovirulent Sindbis virus. *J Virol*. 2000;74:6117-6125.
76. Gorrell MD, Lemm JA, Rice CM, et al. Immunization with nonstructural proteins promotes functional recovery of alphavirus-infected neurons. *J Virol*. 1997;71:3415-3419.
77. Breakwell L, Dosenovic P, Karlsson Hedestam GB, et al. Semliki Forest virus nonstructural protein 2 is involved in suppression of the type I interferon response. *J Virol*. 2007;81:8677-8684.
78. Binder GK, Griffin DE. Interferon-γ-mediated site-specific clearance of alphavirus from CNS neurons. *Science*. 2000; 293:303-306.
79. Rowell JF, Griffin DE. Contribution of T cells to mortality in neurovirulent Sindbis virus encephalomyelitis. *J Neuroimmunol*. 2002;127:106-114.
80. Fourie ED, Morrison JGL. Rheumatoid arthritis syndrome after chikungunya fever. *S Afr Med J*. 1979;56:130-132.
81. Soden M, Vasudevan H, Roberts B, et al. Detection of viral ribonucleic acid and histologic analysis of inflamed synovium in Ross River virus infection. *Arthritis Rheum*. 2000;43: 365-369.
82. Suhrbier A, La Linn M. Clinical and pathologic aspects of arthritis due to Ross River virus and other alphaviruses. *Curr Opin Rheumatol*. 2004;16:374-379.
83. Ozden S, Huerre M, Riviere JP, et al. Human muscle satellite cells as targets of chikungunya virus infection. *PLoS ONE*. 2007;2:e527.
84. Lidbury BA, Rulli NE, Suhrbier A. Macrophage-derived proinflammatory factors contribute to the development of arthritis and myositis after infection with arthrogenic alphavirus. *J Infect Dis*. 2008;197:1585-1593.
85. Morrison TE, Simmons JD, Heise MT. Complement receptor 3 promotes severe Ross River virus-induced disease. *J Virol*. 2008;82:11263-11272.
86. Deresiewicz RL, Thaler SJ, Zamani AA. Clinical and neuroradiographic manifestations of eastern equine encephalitis. *N Engl J Med*. 1997;336:1867-1874.
87. Nandalur M, Urban AW. Western equine encephalitis. 2002; <www.emedicine.com/ med/topic3155.htm>.
88. Deller JJ, Russell PK. Chikungunya disease. *Am J Trop Med Hyg*. 1968;17:1007-1011.
89. Kennedy AC, Fleming J, Solomon L. Chikungunya viral arthropathy: a clinical description. *J Rheumatol*. 1980;7: 231-236.
90. Borgherini G, Poubeau P, Jossaume A, et al. Persistent arthralgia associated with chikungunya virus: a study of 88 adult patients on Reunion Island. *Clin Infect Dis*. 2008;47:469-475.
91. Lalitha P, Rathinam S, Banushree K, et al. Ocular involvement associated with an epidemic outbreak of chikungunya virus infection. *Am J Ophthalmol*. 2007;144:552-556.
92. Economopoulou A, Dominguez M, Helnyk B, et al. Atypical chikungunya virus infections: clinical manifestations, mortality, and risk factors for severe disease during the 2005-2006 outbreak in Reunion. *Epidemiol Infect*. 2008;11:1-8.
93. Lemant J, Boisson V, Winer A, et al. Serious acute chikungunya virus infection requiring intensive care during the Reunion Island outbreak in 2005-2006. *Crit Care Med*. 2008;36: 2536-2541.
94. Ramful D, Carbonnier M, Pasquet M, et al. Mother-to-child transmission of chikungunya virus infection. *Pediatr Infect Dis*. 2007;26:811-815.
95. Taubitz W, Cramer JP, Kapaun A, et al. Chikungunya fever in travelers: clinical presentation and course. *Clin Infect Dis*. 2007;45:e1-e4.
96. Simon F, Parola P, Grandadam M, et al. Chikungunya infection: an emerging rheumatism among travelers returned from Indian Ocean islands: Report of 47 cases. *Medicine (Baltimore)*. 2007;86:123-137.
97. Calisher CH, El-Kafrawi AO, Al-Deen Mahmud MI, et al. Complex-specific immunoglobulin M antibody patterns in humans infected with alphaviruses. *J Clin Microbiol*. 1986;23:155-159.
98. Golomb MR, Durand ML, Schaefer PW, et al. A case of immunotherapy-responsive eastern equine encephalitis with diffusion-weighted imaging. *Neurology*. 2001;56:420-421.
99. Coates DM, Makh SR, Jones N, et al. Assessment of assays for the serodiagnosis of Venezuelan equine encephalitis. *J Infect Dis*. 1992;25:279-289.
100. Lambert AJ, Martin DA, Lanciotti RS. Detection of North American eastern and western equine encephalitis viruses by nucleic acid amplification assays. *J Clin Microbiol*. 2003;41: 379-385.
101. Wang E, Paessler S, Aguilar PV, et al. An RT-PCR-ELISA for rapid detection and differentiation of alphavirus infections. *J Clin Microbiol*. 2006;44:4000-4008.
102. Kirsch MI, Hulseweh B, Nacke C, et al. Development of human antibody fragments using antibody phage display for the detection and diagnosis of Venezuelan equine encephalitis virus. *BMC Biotechnol*. 2008;8:66.
103. Carey DE, Myers RM, DeRanitz CM, et al. The 1964 chikungunya epidemic at Vellore, South India, including observations about concurrent dengue. *Trans R Soc Trop Med Hyg*. 1969;63:434-435.
104. Edwards CJ, Welch SR, Chamberlain J, et al. Molecular diagnosis and analysis of chikungunya virus. *J Clin Virol*. 2007; 39:271-275.
105. Dash PK, Parida M, Santhosh SR, et al. Development and evaluation of a 1-step duplex reverse transcription polymerase chain reaction for differential diagnosis of chikungunya and dengue infection. *Diagn Microbiol Infect Dis*. 2008;62:52-57.
106. Strizki JM, Repik PM. Differential reactivity of immune sera from human vaccinees with field strains of equine encephalitis virus. *Am J Trop Med Hyg*. 1995;53:564-570.
107. Greenway TE, Eldridge JH, Ludwig G, et al. Enhancement of protective immune responses to Venezuelan equine encephalitis virus with micro-encapsulated vaccine. *Vaccine*. 1995;13: 1411-1420.
108. Edelman R, Tacket CO, Wasserman SS, et al. Phase II safety and immunogenicity study of live chikungunya virus vaccine TSI-GSD-218. *Am J Trop Med Hyg*. 2000;62:681-685.
109. McClain DJ, Pittman PR, Ramsburg HH, et al. Immunologic interference from sequential administration of live attenuated alphavirus vaccines. *J Infect Dis*. 1998;177:634-641.
110. Fine DL, Roberts BA, Teehee ML, et al. Venezuelan equine encephalitis virus vaccine candidate (V3526) safety, immunogenicity and efficacy in horses. *Vaccine*. 2007;25:1868-1875.
111. Charles PC, Brown KW, Davis NL, et al. Mucosal immunity induced by immunization with a live attenuated Venezuelan equine encephalitis vaccine candidate. *Virology*. 1997;228: 153-160.
112. Davis NL, Brown KW, Johnston RE. A viral vaccine vector that expresses foreign genes in lymph nodes and protects against mucosal challenge. *J Virol*. 1996;70:3781-3787.
113. Pushko P, Parker M, Ludwig GV, et al. Replicon-helper systems from attenuated Venezuelan equine encephalitis virus: expression of heterologous genes in vitro and immunization against heterologous pathogens in vivo. *Virology*. 1997;239:389-401.
114. Carey IJ, Betts MR, Irlbeck DM, et al. Humoral, mucosal, and cellular immunity in response to a human immunodeficiency virus type 1 immunogen expressed by a Venezuelan equine encephalitis virus vaccine vector. *J Virol*. 1997;71:3031-3038.
115. Wang E, Volkova E, Adams AP, et al. Chimeric alphavirus vaccine candidates for chikungunya. *Vaccine*. 2008;26:5030-5039.
116. Wang E, Petrakova O, Adams AP, et al. Chimeric Sindbis/eastern equine encephalitis vaccine candidates are highly attenuated and immunogenic in mice. *Vaccine*. 2007;25:7573-7581.

Rubella Virus (German Measles)

ANNE A. GERSHON

Rubella (German measles) is an acute exanthematous viral infection of children and adults. The clinical illness is characterized by rash, fever, and lymphadenopathy and resembles a mild case of measles (rubeola). Although many infections with the agent are subclinical, this virus has the potential to cause fetal infection, with resultant birth defects, and (uncommonly but especially in adults) various forms of arthritis.

Rubella virus was first isolated in 1962 by Parkman and colleagues[1] and by Weller and Neva.[2] Rubella virus is classified in the Togaviridae family[3,4] on the basis of its single-stranded positive-sense polyadenylated RNA genome, replication strategy, icosahedral capsid, and lipoprotein envelope. Rubella virus is closely related to the alphaviruses, but in contrast to alphaviruses, no vector is required for its transmission, and it is serologically distinct from alphaviruses.[4] Therefore, rubella virus alone has been placed in a separate genus, *Rubivirus*. There are 2 clades, and as many as 13 genotypes.[5] On electron microscopy, rubella virus is roughly spherical. Its envelope, which has short surface projections, has a diameter of about 60 nm. The envelope surrounds the 20-sided nucleocapsid, which has a diameter of about 30 nm and is composed of a helix of protein and RNA. Rubella virus matures by budding from the cell membrane.[6]

Three structural polypeptides associated with rubella virus are termed *E1*, *E2*, and *C*. There are also two nonstructural proteins that are related to replication and transcription. E1 and E2 are transmembrane glycoproteins, and C is the capsid protein that surrounds the RNA of the virion. Hemagglutinin and complement-fixing antigens are composed of varying proportions and mixtures of E1, E2, and C.[7,8] E1 is important in attachment, fusion, hemagglutination, and neutralization.

Rubella virus is relatively unstable. It is inactivated by lipid solvents, trypsin, formalin, ultraviolet light, and extremes of pH and heat, and it is inhibited by amantadine.[9] Cytopathic effects may not be noted in all cell lines in which rubella virus replicates. However, cytopathic effects are readily observed in the rabbit kidney cell line RK-13 and in primary African green monkey cells.[7]

Epidemiology

Rubella was not distinguished clinically from certain other exanthematous infections until the late 19th century. It was at one time termed *third disease*, when measles and scarlet fever were called *first disease* and *second disease*, respectively.[10] Because postnatal rubella is such a mild illness, the disease was considered to be of only minor importance for many years. However, in 1941, when Gregg[11] recognized the link between maternal rubella and certain congenital defects, a more complete picture of disease due to rubella virus began to emerge.

Before widespread vaccine use, the incidence of clinical cases of postnatal rubella was highest in the spring, and it was traditionally recognized to be most common in children 5 to 9 years of age.[12] Rubella is only a moderately contagious illness, in contrast to measles. Therefore, in the prevaccine era, only 80% to 90% of adults were immune to rubella, whereas 98% were immune to measles.[13]

Epidemics of rubella of minor proportions occurred in the prevaccine era every 6 to 9 years, and large-scale epidemics occurred at intervals of up to 30 years. The most recent major epidemic in the United States occurred in 1964, during which some 12,500,000 persons were infected.[14] Since the licensure of a live-attenuated rubella vaccine in 1969, there have been no large rubella epidemics in countries where the vaccine is widely used. However, limited outbreaks continued to occur in settings such as workplaces, schools, and military camps, where groups of susceptible individuals had close contact with each other.[13,15] In 2001, only 23 cases of postnatal rubella and 3 confirmed cases of congenital rubella syndrome were reported to the Centers for Disease Control and Prevention (CDC).[16] An increase in susceptibility to rubella was noted among Hispanic young adults for some years, and there were increasing efforts to identify rubella-susceptible women before they became pregnant.[16,17]

Importantly, in 2005, rubella was declared no longer endemic in the United States.[5,18-20] Since 2001, there were fewer than 25 annual postnatal cases and only rare cases of the congenital rubella syndrome. Ninety-five percent of school-aged children were vaccinated, more than 90% of the population had immunity, there was adequate surveillance to detect outbreaks, and there was molecular evidence that there are no circulating American genotypes of rubella virus; rubella was considered eliminated from the United States.[21] This was a major advance in public health and occurred at a similar time to when measles was no longer endemic in the United States, also as a result of widespread immunization. Similarly to measles, isolated cases of rubella may be imported into the United States from another country, but only with the possibility of limited spread of rubella. Mathematical models indicate that transmission of rubella ceases at 90% immunization levels, which has been achieved in the United States.[5,22] Global efforts are underway to decrease the global burden of rubella and congenital rubella syndrome.[23]

Transmission of Rubella

Rubella virus is spread in droplets that are shed from respiratory secretions of infected persons. Patients are most contagious while the rash is erupting, but they may shed virus from the throat from 10 days before until 15 days after the onset of the rash. Patients with subclinical cases of illness may also transmit the infection to others.[9]

Infants with congenital rubella shed large quantities of virus from body secretions for many months and therefore may transmit the infection to those who care for them. These babies continue to excrete rubella virus despite high titers of neutralizing antibody, a puzzling phenomenon that has yet to be explained.[24] The possibility of immune tolerance due to fetal infection has been raised.[8] Infants of recent immigrants from developing countries who have congenital rubella may infect susceptible persons if the diagnosis is not made and contacts are not immunized.

Persons who receive rubella vaccine do not transmit rubella to others, although the virus may be transiently isolated from the pharynx. It may be that the quantity of virus shed is too small to be infectious.[17]

Maintenance of Immunity to Rubella

After an attack of rubella, lifelong protection against the disease develops in most persons. However, the factors responsible for this protection are not precisely understood. Antibody titers to rubella virus develop, but the significance of the decline of antibody titers with time remains unclear. Cell-mediated immunity to rubella virus associated with CD4$^+$ and CD8$^+$ T lymphocytes has also been detected by in vitro assays[7,25] months to years after an attack of rubella. The long-term persistence of humoral and cellular immunity to rubella in a group of cloistered nuns who had no opportunity for reexposure to rubella virus has been documented.[26] The persistence of specific antibody for as long as 14 years after immunization has also been demonstrated.[27,28]

Nevertheless, despite the presence of specific immunity to rubella virus, it appears that reinfection with rubella virus can occur. This had been long suspected on clinical grounds alone.[29,30] Rubella reinfections have been documented by detection of a significant boost in rubella antibody titers in naturally immune persons after reexposure to the virus. Most reinfections are asymptomatic.[31] It is likely that the virus can multiply locally in the upper respiratory tract but that viremia occurs infrequently because the host's immune response eradicates the virus before it can invade the blood. However, in rare instances, patients have been reported to have proven rubella reinfection occurring years after naturally acquired rubella, with symptoms indicative of viremia (e.g., arthritis, rash).[32]

Rubella reinfection occurring months or years after the receipt of rubella vaccine has also been observed. Several investigators have documented reinfections in up to 80% of persons who had received rubella vaccine previously and were subsequently exposed to rubella during an epidemic.[31,33] Most of these reinfections were not characterized by clinical illness but were identified only by a rise in antibody titer. Viremia is probably extremely rare in such cases,[33-35] although rubella virus has been recovered from throat secretions in reinfections.[31,34] In one study of eight seronegative adult vaccinees who were experimentally challenged with wild-type rubella virus, replication in the respiratory tract was found in seven subjects, and viremia was present in two.[36] However, these subjects also experienced only a mild illness or remained asymptomatic.[36]

Reinfections are more common among vaccinees than among persons who have experienced natural rubella, and they are most common among persons with hemagglutination inhibition (HAI) antibody titers of 1:64 or less.[31,33,34] It has been suggested that there may also be qualitative differences in antibody between persons with vaccine-induced immunity and those with natural immunity because in one study, even with similar HAI titers, vaccinees were 10 times more likely to be reinfected than were those with natural immunity to rubella.[31]

Whether rubella reinfection that occurs during pregnancy can result in transmission of the virus to the fetus has been the subject of much debate. Several case reports in the older literature that ascribed fetal defects to maternal rubella reinfection actually involved primary maternal infections in all likelihood.[37,38] Viremia was documented in one woman with detectable rubella antibody before immunization.[39] Boué and colleagues[40] studied a small number of women with documented subclinical cases of rubella reinfection during pregnancy who carried their babies to term; all of the babies were found to be normal. In a number of other case reports of rubella reinfection during pregnancy, babies born (at term) to the affected mothers had symptoms suggestive of congenital rubella.[41-46] Most of these reinfections occurred years after natural infection, although some occurred years after immunization.[45,46] However, these transmissions are acknowledged to be extremely rare events, particularly considering the exceedingly low incidence of congenital rubella in the United States today.

In summary, it appears that persons who are immune to rubella, by virtue either of having had the natural infection or of having received rubella vaccine, may be reinfected when reexposed. However, this reinfection is usually asymptomatic and detectable only by serologic means. Viremia in reinfection appears to be a rare event.

The presence of large numbers of immune people in a community appears to be able to prevent rubella epidemics from occurring; this effect is termed *herd immunity*. Although it has been documented that herd immunity does not entirely eliminate the spread of rubella, it probably plays a major role in control of this infection, which is now rare in the United States.[5]

Pathogenesis

The incubation period for rubella ranges from 12 to 23 days (average, 18 days). As in measles (see Chapter 160), a primary and a secondary viremia are believed to accompany rubella. Rubella virus has been detected in leukocytes of patients as early as 1 week before the onset of symptoms.[47] Also as in measles, the rubella rash appears as immunity develops and the virus disappears from the blood,[7] suggesting that the rash is immunologically mediated. Although circulating immune complexes are detectable during rubella, they do not appear to contribute to the development of rash.[7,48] Rubella virus has been isolated from involved skin,[49] but this does not preclude the possibility that the rash is secondary to an immune response to the virus.

Clinical Manifestations

Age is the most important determinant of the severity of rubella. Postnatally acquired rubella is usually an innocuous infection, and, as is true for many viral illnesses, children have milder disease than adults. In contrast, the fetus is at high risk for development of severe rubella, with serious sequelae if infected transplacentally in early pregnancy because of maternal rubella.

POSTNATAL RUBELLA

Many, if not most, cases of postnatal rubella are subclinical.[14,50] Among those patients who are symptomatic, children do not experience a prodromal phase, but adults may have a prodrome of malaise, fever, and anorexia for several days. The major clinical manifestations of postnatal rubella are adenopathy, which may last several weeks, and rash. The lymph nodes involved include the posterior auricular, posterior cervical, and suboccipital chains. On occasion, splenomegaly also occurs.[51] These symptoms are not specific for rubella, and clinically the disease may resemble measles, toxoplasmosis, scarlet fever, roseola, parvovirus B19 infection, and certain enterovirus infections.

The rash of rubella begins on the face and moves down the body. It is maculopapular but not confluent, may desquamate during convalescence, and may be absent in some cases. An enanthem consisting of petechial lesions on the soft palate (Forschheimer's spots) has been described for rubella, but this enanthem is not diagnostic for rubella (unlike Koplik's spots in measles). The rash may be accompanied by mild coryza and conjunctivitis. Usually the rash lasts 3 to 5 days. Fever, if present, rarely lasts beyond the first day of rash.

COMPLICATIONS OF POSTNATAL RUBELLA

The complications of postnatal rubella, in contrast to those of measles, are uncommon. Bacterial superinfections after rubella are rare.

Arthritis or arthralgia has been reported in as many as one third of women with rubella; this complication is less common in children and in men.[52] The arthritis tends to involve the fingers, wrists, and knees, and it occurs either as the rash is appearing or soon afterward. It can be rather slow to resolve, as long as 1 month. Rarely does chronic arthritis develop.

The pathogenesis of rubella arthritis is not entirely understood. The frequency of detection and the quantity of circulating immune complexes are higher in rubella vaccinees who report joint complaints than in those with no joint involvement.[48,53] Rubella virus has been isolated from joint effusions in patients with acute or recurrent rubella arthritis associated with either previous natural infection or vaccination.[54-63] Rubella virus has been isolated from peripheral blood mononuclear cells in patients with chronic arthritis.[61,64] A persistent rubella virus infection of human synovial cells cultured *in vitro* was reported, and this was advanced as an explanation for the pathogenesis of chronic forms of rubella arthritis.[65]

Hemorrhagic manifestations occur as a complication in about 1 of every 3000 cases of rubella.[51,66] In contrast to other complications of rubella, hemorrhagic manifestations occur more often in children than in adults. This complication may be secondary to both thrombocytopenia and vascular damage, and it is probably immunologically mediated.[66] Some investigators have proposed that mild thrombocytopenia often goes undetected in apparently uncomplicated rubella.[67] Thrombocytopenia may last from weeks to months and may cause serious problems if bleeding into vital areas (e.g., brain, kidney, eye) occurs.[51] Thrombocytopenic purpura as the single clinical manifestation of rubella in children has also been reported.[66]

Encephalitis is an extremely uncommon complication of rubella; its incidence during an epidemic was reported to be 1 in 5000 cases. It occurs more frequently in adults than in children, and it is associated with a mortality rate of 20% to 50%.[51,68,69] Survivors usually have no sequelae.[7] A fatal case of rubella encephalitis in a 2-month-old child whose mother had rubella in the last week of pregnancy has been reported.[70]

Mild hepatitis has been described as an unusual complication of rubella.[71]

CONGENITAL RUBELLA SYNDROME

Rubella can be a disastrous disease in early gestation and can lead to fetal death, premature delivery, and an array of congenital defects. The incidence of congenital rubella in a given population is quite variable, depending on the number of susceptible individuals, the circulation of virus in the community, and, in recent times, the use of rubella vaccine. The rubella epidemic of 1964 left 30,000 affected infants in its wake. Between 1969 and 1979, however, an average of 39 cases per year were reported to the CDC.[72-74] Since the advent of the 21st century, congenital rubella has been essentially eliminated from the United States.[16,21]

The effects of rubella virus on the fetus are, to a large extent, dependent on the time of infection; in general, the younger the fetus when infected, the more severe the illness. During the first 2 months of gestation, the fetus has a 65% to 85% chance of being affected, with an outcome of multiple congenital defects or spontaneous abortion, or both.[7] Rubella during the third month of fetal life has been associated with a 30% to 35% chance of developing a single defect, such as deafness or congenital heart disease. Fetal infection during the fourth month carries a 10% risk for a single congenital defect. Occasionally, fetal damage (deafness alone) is seen if rubella occurs up to the 20th week of gestation.[75]

The specific signs and symptoms of congenital rubella may be classified as temporary (e.g., low birth weight), permanent (e.g., deafness), and developmental (e.g., myopia).[72] The most common manifestations are deafness, cataract or glaucoma, congenital heart disease, and mental retardation; a list of the major clinical manifestations is presented in Table 152-1.[72]

Prospective studies of the congenital rubella syndrome suggest that it should not be considered a static disease. Some children whose mothers had rubella during pregnancy and who, at birth, were considered normal were found to have manifestations of congenital rubella when they reached school age.[76,77] Diabetes mellitus in late childhood has also been observed 50 times more frequently in children who had congenital rubella than in normal children.[7,78] Insulin-dependent diabetes has been reported in 40% of adult survivors of congenital rubella from the 1942 epidemic.[79] Of interest, in a follow-up study of 242 children who had congenital rubella, rubella virus–induced diabetes had genetic and immunologic features similar to those observed in other forms of insulin-dependent diabetes: the frequency of the human leukocyte antigen allele HLA-DR3 was increased, and that of HLA-DR2 was decreased.[80] Antibodies to pancreatic islet cells or cytotoxic surface antibodies were present in 80% of the patients with abnormalities in serum glucose concentration.[80] At autopsy of congenital rubella patients, the virus was isolated from the pancreas, which was noted to have a subnormal number of glandular cells.[80] Progressive encephalopathy resembling subacute sclerosing panencephalitis was observed in children with congenital rubella.[81,82] In 1991, a group of 40 adults born with the congenital rubella syndrome between 1939 and 1943 were reexamined. Although they had multiple defects involving

TABLE 152-1	Congenital Rubella: Transient (T), Permanent (P), and Developmental (D) Manifestations	
Common	*Uncommon or Rare*
Low birth weight (T)	Jaundice (T)
Thrombocytopenic purpura (T)	Dermatoglyphic "abnormality" (P)
Hepatosplenomegaly (T)	Glaucoma (P)
Bone "lesions" (T)	Cloudy cornea (T)
Large anterior fontanelle (T)	Severe myopia (P, D)
Meningoencephalitis (T)	Myocardial abnormalities (P)
Hearing loss (P, D)	Hepatitis (T)
Cataract (and microphthalmia) (P)	Generalized lymphadenopathy (T)
Retinopathy (P)	Hemolytic anemia (T)
Patent ductus arteriosus (P)	Rubella pneumonitis (T)
Pulmonic stenosis (P, D)	Diabetes mellitus (P, D)
Mental retardation (P, D)	Thyroid disorders (P, D)
Behavior disorders (P, D)	Seizure disorders (D)
Central language disorders (P, D)	Precocious puberty (D)
Cryptorchidism (P)	Degenerative brain disease (D)
Inguinal hernia (P)	
Spastic diplegia (P)	
Microcephaly (P)	

From Cooper LZ. Congenital rubella in the United States. In: Krugman S, Gershon A, eds. *Infections of the Fetus and Newborn Infant.* New York: Alan R. Liss; 1975:1. Reprinted with permission of John Wiley & Sons, Inc. Copyright © 1975. This material is used by permission of Wiley-Liss, Inc., a subsidiary of John Wiley & Sons, Inc.

hearing, diabetes, growth retardation, and eye and heart abnormalities, most were well adjusted socially. There was no increased incidence of malignant disease in these 50-year-old survivors.[83]

Infants with congenital rubella develop high titers of neutralizing antibody that may persist for years.[84] However, these children may eventually lose detectable antibody.[85] Reinfection with rubella has also been documented in some of these children.[86] Impairment of cell-mediated immunity to rubella antigen was found in some children with congenital rubella.[87]

A number of pathologic mechanisms have been proposed to explain certain manifestations of congenital rubella. It has been suggested that persistent infection with rubella virus leads to a mitotic arrest of cells, which in turn causes inhibition of cellular growth and, consequently, retarded organ growth.[88] Additional hypotheses put forth to explain the growth retardation associated with congenital rubella are that infection leads to angiopathy with placental and fetal vasculitis, which compromises growth,[89] and that tissue necrosis without inflammation or fibrotic damage leads to cellular damage.[90] Another possible explanation is that infection of various types of cells during gestation interferes with the normal balance of growth and differentiation, which leads to defects in organogenesis.[7] Human fibroblasts infected with rubella virus in vitro were found to produce a growth inhibitor, which might also account for fetal growth retardation.[91] An increased frequency of chromosomal breakage was found in cultured cells from children with congenital rubella, compared with cells from healthy children.[92] Molecular evidence of cell cycle arrest caused by rubella virus has been obtained.[93] It has been postulated that lymphocyte abnormalities in patients with the congenital rubella syndrome may predispose them to organ-specific autoimmunity.[94]

Diagnosis

Because rubella is usually a mild disease with nonspecific symptoms, it is often difficult to diagnose clinically. The disease has been confused with other infections such as scarlet fever, mild measles, infectious mononucleosis, toxoplasmosis, roseola, erythema infectiosum, and certain enteroviral infections.[95,96] Routine laboratory studies are not helpful for diagnosis because they may reveal only leukopenia and atypical lymphocytes; more specific laboratory diagnostic techniques are usually necessary.

Virus isolation from throat swabs, urine, synovial fluid, or other body secretions is an acceptable method for diagnosis. However, this technique is time-consuming and expensive, so it is usually reserved for special circumstances, such as investigation of arthritis and other conditions presumed to represent complications of postnatal rubella, and for the diagnosis of congenital rubella.[7,9] The diagnosis of congenital rubella infection has been made by isolation of virus from amniotic fluid.[97] Today, molecular methods such as reverse transcriptase–polymerase chain reaction (RT-PCR) are preferred to virus isolation.[8]

The laboratory diagnosis of postnatal rubella is most conveniently made serologically. At one time, HAI was the preferred means of measuring rubella antibody titers, but this technique has been supplanted by simpler, more accurate methods of similar sensitivity.[9,96,98-104]

These include enzyme-linked immunosorbent assay (ELISA), passive latex agglutination test, and radial hemolysis test. These tests are variable in their sensitivity. Most of these tests may be used to measure either immunoglobulin G (IgG) or IgM antibodies. A demonstration of specific IgG on one serum sample is evidence of immunity to rubella. Acute rubella infection may be diagnosed either by a demonstration of specific IgM in one serum sample or by a fourfold or greater increase in rubella antibody titer in acute and convalescent specimens assayed in the same test.[8,105] Positive rubella IgM antibody tests have been associated not only with primary infection but also with reinfection with rubella virus.[106] This phenomenon may explain, at least in part, why apparent false-positive results on IgM-rubella ELISA testing in pregnant women have been reported.[107] Results of many of these serologic tests are available within a matter of minutes or hours and yield prompt, useful information.

For a serologic diagnosis of congenital rubella in the neonatal period, antibody to rubella virus should be measured in both infant and maternal sera. It may be necessary to perform several antibody determinations on serum from the infant to detect whether the titer of rubella antibody is falling, which indicates passively acquired maternal antibody, or rising, which suggests rubella infection. If rubella IgM is detected in a newborn infant's serum, then transplacental rubella infection has occurred. Congenital rubella infection has been diagnosed by the following tests or procedures: placental biopsy at 12 weeks, demonstration of rubella antigen with monoclonal antibody, cordocentesis and detection of RNA by in situ hybridization,[108] and PCR.[109] It may also be diagnosed by the presence of specific IgM in fetal blood, but this may not be detectable until as late as 22 weeks of gestation.[110,111]

Treatment

Because postnatal rubella is such a mild infection in most instances, no treatment is indicated. There is no specific therapy, but for patients with fever and arthritis or arthralgia, the treatment of symptoms is indicated. At one time, immune globulin (IG) was advocated for the prevention or modification of rubella in susceptible pregnant women who were exposed to the infection. However, it was discovered that, although IG might suppress symptoms, it would not necessarily prevent viremia.[112] Therefore, indications for the use of IG for rubella prophylaxis are few. Possibly, IG may be given to a susceptible pregnant woman who is exposed to rubella and for whom abortion is not an option if she should develop the disease. With the advent of rubella vaccine, it is now possible to immunize susceptible women of childbearing age against rubella before they become pregnant.

Vaccination against Rubella

Rubella virus was isolated in 1962[1,2] and attenuated in 1966[113]; the live-attenuated vaccine was licensed for use in the United States in 1969. The rationale for use of the vaccine is to prevent congenital rubella by control of postnatal rubella (see Chapter 320). In the United States, the first strategy was to vaccinate prepubertal children so as to minimize exposure of susceptible pregnant women to rubella. More recently, there has been an emphasis on immunization of rubella-susceptible women of childbearing age who are not pregnant. Often, this is done just after delivery of an infant; nursing mothers who are vaccinated do not cause harm to their infants. In some other countries, the approach has been to vaccinate girls against rubella as they approach puberty.

Immunization programs in the United States have dramatically reduced the transmission of rubella in young children and prevented major epidemics of rubella. There have been no such epidemics for the past 40 years, a phenomenon never previously observed in the United States. A distressing miniepidemic of congenital rubella in 21 infants occurred in 1990 in southern California. More than 55% of their mothers had a total of 22 missed opportunities for vaccination at the time of marriage or after previous delivery of a child; therefore, more than half of these cases of congenital rubella were preventable.[114]

The incidence of postnatal rubella fell to an all-time low in 1988, but by 1991, it had increased threefold. There was a concomitant increase in cases of congenital rubella syndrome during the same period, although there was still a decline of more than 98% in cases of rubella compared with the prevaccine era. The observed increase in cases was attributed to failure to immunize rather than vaccine failure.[73] With improvements in vaccine delivery since 1991, the incidence of rubella in the United States fell. Fewer than 300 cases were reported in 1995 and in 1996,[115] and only 23 postnatal cases were reported in 2001.[16] As noted previously, endemic rubella has been eliminated from the United States. There remains, however, a continued need to emphasize the importance of immunization of susceptible women of childbearing age who are not pregnant and of hospital employees, as well as infants and children.[113,114,116,117]

At present, the only rubella vaccine available in the United States is RA 27/3. This vaccine has been widely used in Europe and is more immunogenic than the previously used vaccines, HPV 77 DE5 and Cendehill, with fewer side effects. RA 27/3 vaccine also stimulates the production of secretory as well as humoral IgA, which may account for its increased immunogenic potency.[118-120]

COMPLICATIONS OF VACCINATION

Rubella vaccine may cause viremia,[121,122] and therefore the main complications are fever, adenopathy, arthritis, and arthralgia. All the complications are more common in adults than in children, and they are most common in women older than 25 years of age.[123-125] In one study, up to 40% of such vaccinees developed joint complications[124]; however, all reactions were transient. It is uncommon for children to develop complications. In general, the incidence of joint complications, even in adults, is lower after vaccination than after natural rubella.[13,122] In 1991, a committee of the Institute of Medicine examined the issue of chronic arthritis after administration of RA 27/3 rubella vaccine and concluded that there is a rare causal relationship.[126] The risk for arthritis is increased in persons with HLA alleles DR1, DR4, and DR6.[127] Evidence in vitro indicates that wild-type strains of rubella virus can be propagated more efficiently in joint tissues than can vaccine strains.[128]

EFFICACY OF VACCINATION

Since the introduction of rubella vaccine, the number of reported cases of clinical rubella has declined progressively. The vaccines available today, when properly administered, produce a seroconversion rate of about 95% after one dose.[13] Seroconversion in response to rubella vaccine is not impaired in children with upper respiratory tract infections.[129] Because antibody titers are lower after vaccination than after natural disease, the question has been raised as to whether the antibody titer, years after vaccination, will remain high enough to prevent clinical rubella. Only time and continued surveillance will provide an answer to this question, but at present there is little evidence of waning immunity,[27,28] as reflected by the low incidence of rubella in the United States. Booster injections of rubella vaccine therefore are not routinely indicated.

EFFECTS OF RUBELLA VACCINE ON THE FETUS

Since rubella vaccine was licensed in 1969, the CDC has monitored the outcome in babies born to women who were reported to have been inadvertently immunized against rubella during early pregnancy. As of late 1987, 812 such women who carried their infants to term had been included in the CDC study, with no cases of the congenital rubella syndrome attributed to rubella vaccine.[130] The observed risk for congenital rubella after immunization therefore is reported as zero; however, the theoretical maximal risk could be as high as 1% to 2%. This is in contrast to a 20% or greater risk after maternal rubella in the first trimester.[130] Of interest, the vaccine-type virus can cross the placenta, and rubella virus has been isolated from both decidua and fetal tissue at abortion after inadvertent vaccination of pregnant women.[130-134] Rubella virus was isolated from the fetus of a woman given rubella vaccine 7 weeks before conception.[135] A single case of persistent infection of a fetus whose mother was inadvertently immunized in early pregnancy has been recorded; the infant had no signs or symptoms of the congenital rubella syndrome.[136]

Based on an analysis of 293 normal infants born to rubella-susceptible mothers vaccinated 1 to 2 weeks before or 4 to 6 weeks after conception, for whom the theoretical risk to the fetus is 1.3%, the CDC recommends that women avoid pregnancy for 28 days after rubella vaccination.[137] Although it is not recommended that rubella vaccine be administered to women who are pregnant, the currently recognized minimal theoretical fetal risk does not mandate automatic termination of a pregnancy. Many, if not most, of such vaccinated women may wish to carry their baby to term.

REFERENCES

1. Parkman PD, Buescher EC, Artenstein MS. Recovery of rubella virus from army recruits. *Proc Soc Exp Biol Med.* 1962;111:225.
2. Weller TH, Neva FA. Propagation in tissue culture of cytopathic agents from patients with rubella-like illness. *Proc Soc Exp Biol Med.* 1962;111:215.
3. Andrewes CH. Generic names of viruses of vertebrates. *Virology.* 1970;40:1070.
4. Horzinek M, Maess J, Laufs R. Studies on the substructure of togaviruses. II. Analysis of equine arteritis, rubella, bovine viral diarrhea, and hog cholera viruses. *Arch Gesamte Virusforsch.* 1971;33:306.
5. Icenogle JP, Frey TK, Abernathy E, et al. Genetic analysis of rubella viruses found in the United States between 1966 and 2004: evidence that indigenous rubella viruses have been eliminated. *Clin Infect Dis* 2006;43(Suppl 3):S133-S140.
6. Murphy FA, Halomen PE, Harrison AK. Electron microscopy of the development of rubella virus in BHK-21 cells. *J Virol.* 1968;2:1223.
7. Chandler J, Wolinsky JS, Tingle A. Rubella. In: Fields BM, Knipe DM, Chanock RM, et al, eds. *Virology*. 4th ed. New York: Raven Press, 2001;963-990.
8. Bellini WJ, Icenogle J. Measles and rubella virus. In: Murray PR, Baron EJ, Jorgenson JH, et al. *Manual of Clinical Microbiology.* Washington, DC: ASM Press; 2003:1389-1403.
9. Beor J, O'Shea S. Rubella virus. In: Lennette EH, Lennette DA, Lennette ET, eds. *Diagnostic Procedures for Viral and Rickettsial Infections.* 7th ed. New York: American Public Health Association; 1995:583-600.
10. Shapiro L. The numbered diseases: First through sixth. *JAMA.* 1971;194:680.
11. Gregg NM. Congenital cataract following German measles in the mother. *Trans Ophthalmol Soc Aust.* 1941;3:35.
12. Witte JJ, Karchmer AW, Case G, et al. Epidemiology of rubella. *Am J Dis Child.* 1969;118:107.
13. Krugman S. Present status of measles and rubella immunization in the United States: A medical progress report. *J Pediatr.* 1977;90:1.
14. Horstmann DM. Rubella: The challenge of its control. *J Infect Dis.* 1971;123:640.
15. Danovaro-Holliday MC, LeBaron CW, Allenworth C, et al. A large rubella outbreak with spread from the workplace to the community. *JAMA.* 2000;284:2733-2739.
16. Reef SE, Frey TK, Theall K, et al. The changing epidemiology of rubella in the 1990s: on the verge of elimination and new challenges for control and prevention. *JAMA.* 2002;287:464-472.
17. Sheridan E, Aitken C, Jeffries D, et al. Congenital rubella syndrome: A risk in immigrant populations. *Lancet.* 2002;359:674-675.
18. Plotkin SA. The history of rubella and rubella vaccination leading to elimination. *Clin Infect Dis.* 2006;43(Suppl 3):S164-168.
19. Reef SE, Cochi SL. The evidence for the elimination of rubella and congenital rubella syndrome in the United States: a public health achievement. *Clin Infect Dis.* 2006;43(Suppl 3):S123-S125.
20. Reef SE, Redd SB, Abernathy E, et al. The epidemiological profile of rubella and congenital rubella syndrome in the United States, 1998-2004: the evidence for absence of endemic transmission. *Clin Infect Dis.* Nov 1 2006;43(Suppl 3):S126-132.
21. Centers for Disease Control and Prevention. Elimination of rubella and congenital rubella syndrome: United States, 1969-2004. *MMWR Morb Mortal Wkly Rep.* 2005;54:279-282.
22. Bloom S, Smith P, Stanwyck C, et al. Has the United States population been adequately vaccinated to achieve rubella elimination? *Clin Infect Dis.* 2006;43(Suppl 3):S141-145.
23. Best JM, Castillo-Solorzano C, Spika JS, et al. Reducing the global burden of congenital rubella syndrome: report of the World Health Organization Steering Committee On Research Related To Measles and Rubella Vaccines and Vaccination, June 2004. *J Infect Dis.* 2005;192:1890-1897.
24. Cooper LZ, Green RH, Krugman S, et al. Neonatal thrombocytopenic purpura and other manifestations of rubella contracted in vitro. *Am J Dis Child.* 1965;110:416.
25. Steele RW, Hensen SA, Vincent MM, et al. A ^{51}Cr microassay technique for cell-mediated immunity to viruses. *J Immunol.* 1973;110:1502.
26. Rossier E, Phipps PH, Weber JM, et al. Persistence of humoral and cell-mediated immunity to rubella virus in cloistered nuns and in schoolteachers. *J Infect Dis.* 1981;144:137-141.
27. Horstmann D, Schluederberg A, Emmons JE, et al. Persistence of vaccine-induced immune responses to rubella: Comparison with natural infection. *Rev Infect Dis.* 1985;7(Suppl):80-85.
28. Plotkin S, Buser F. History of RA27/3 rubella vaccine. *Rev Infect Dis.* 1985;7(Suppl):77-78.
29. Hillenbrand FKM. Rubella in a remote community. *Lancet.* 1956;2:64.
30. Fry J, Dillane JB, Fry L. Rubella 1962. *Br Med J.* 1962;2:833.
31. Horstmann DM, Liebhaber H, Le Bouvier GL, et al. Rubella: Reinfection of vaccinated and naturally immune persons exposed in an epidemic. *N Engl J Med.* 1970;283:771.
32. Wilkins J, Leedom JM, Salvotore MA, et al. Clinical rubella with arthritis resulting from reinfection. *Ann Intern Med.* 1972;77:930.
33. Davis WJ, Larson HE, Simsarian JP, et al. A study of rubella immunity and resistance to infection. *JAMA.* 1971;215:600.
34. Wilkins J, Leidom JM, Portnoy B, et al. Reinfection with rubella virus despite live vaccine-induced immunity. *Am J Dis Child.* 1969;118:275.
35. Forrest JM, Menser MA, Honeyman MC, et al. Clinical rubella eleven months after vaccination. *Lancet.* 1972;2:399.
36. Schiff G, Young B, Stefanovic GM, et al. Challenge with rubella virus after loss of detectable vaccine-induced immunity. *Rev Infect Dis.* 1985;7(Suppl):156-163.
37. Northrop RL, Gardner WM, Guttmann WF. Rubella reinfection during early pregnancy: A case report. *Obstet Gynecol.* 1972;39:524.
38. Biano S, Cochran W, Herrmann KL, et al. Rubella reinfection during pregnancy. *Am J Dis Child.* 1975;129:1353.
39. Balfour HH, Groth KE, Edelman CK. Rubella viraemia and antibody responses after rubella vaccination and reimmunization. *Lancet.* 1981;1:1078.
40. Boué A, Nicolas A, Montagron B. Reinfection with rubella in pregnant women. *Lancet.* 1971;1:2151.
41. Eilard T, Strannegard O. Rubella reinfection in pregnancy followed by transmission to the fetus. *J Infect Dis.* 1974;129:594.
42. Levine JB, Berkowitz CD, St Geme JW. Rubella virus reinfection during pregnancy leading to late-onset congenital rubella syndrome. *J Pediatr.* 1982;100:589.
43. Fosgren M, Carlson G, Strongert K. Case of congenital rubella after maternal reinfection. *Scand J Infect Dis.* 1979;11:81-93.
44. Partridge JW, Flewett TH, Whitehead JEM. Congenital rubella affecting an infant whose mother had rubella antibodies before conception. *Br Med J.* 1981;282:187-188.
45. Bott LM, Eizenberg DH. Congenital rubella after successful vaccination. *Med J Aust.* 1982;1:514-515.
46. Robinson J, Lemay M, Vaudry WL. Congenital rubella after anticipated maternal immunity: Two cases and a review of the literature. *Pediatr Infect Dis J.* 1994;13:812-815.
47. Heggie AD, Robbins FC. Rubella in naval recruits. *N Engl J Med.* 1964;271:231.
48. Coyle PK, Wolinsky JS, Buimovici-Klein E, et al. Rubella-specific immune complexes after congenital infection and vaccination. *Infect Immun.* 1982;36:498-503.
49. Heggie AD. Pathogenesis of rubella exanthem. Isolation of rubella virus from skin. *N Engl J Med.* 1971;285:664.
50. Buescher EL. Behavior of rubella virus in adult populations. *Arch Gesamte Virusforsch.* 1965;16:470.
51. Heggie AD, Robbins FC. Natural rubella acquired after birth. *Am J Dis Child.* 1969;118:12.
52. Johnson RE, Hall AP. Rubella arthritis. *N Engl J Med.* 1958;258:743.
53. Vergani D, Morgan-Capner P, Davies ET, et al. Joint symptoms, immune complexes and rubella. *Lancet.* 1980;1:321-322.
54. Hildebrandt HM, Maasab HF. Rubella synovitis in a one-year-old patient. *N Engl J Med.* 1966;274:1428.
55. Phillips CA, Behbehani AM, Johnson LW, et al. Isolation of rubella virus: An epidemic characterized by rash and arthritis. *JAMA.* 1965;191:615.
56. Ogra PL, Herd JK. Arthritis associated with induced rubella infection. *J Immunol.* 1971;107:810-813.
57. Smith CA, Petty RE, Tingle AJ. Rubella virus and arthritis. *Rheum Dis Clin North Am.* 1987;13:265-274.
58. Grahame R, Armstrong R, Simmons NA, et al. Isolation of rubella virus from synovial fluid in five cases of seronegative arthritis. *Lancet.* 1981;2:649-651.
59. Grahame R, Armstrong R, Simmons NA, et al. Chronic arthritis associated with the presence of intrasynovial rubella virus. *Ann Rheum Dis.* 1983;42:2-13.
60. Fraser JR, Cunningham AL, Hayes K, et al. Rubella arthritis in adults: Isolation of virus, cytology, and other aspects of synovial infection. *Clin Exp Rheumatol.* 1983;1:287-293.
61. Chantler JK, Tingle AJ, Petty RE. Persistent rubella virus infection associated with chronic arthritis in children. *N Engl J Med.* 1985;313:1117-1123.
62. Chantler JK, da Roza DM, Bonnie ME, et al. Sequential studies on synovial lymphocyte stimulation by rubella antigen, and rubella virus isolation in an adult with persistent arthritis. *Ann Rheum Dis.* 1985;44:564-568.
63. Bosma TJ, Etherington J, O'Shea S, et al. Rubella virus and chronic joint disease: is there an association? *J Clin Microbiol* 1998;36:3524-3526
64. Chantler JK, Ford DK, Tingle AJ. Persistent rubella infection and rubella-associated arthritis. *Lancet.* 1982;1:1323-1325.
65. Cunningham AL, Fraser JRE. Persistent rubella virus infection of human synovial cells cultured in vitro. *J Infect Dis.* 1985;151:638-645.
66. Ozsoyla S, Kanra G, Savas G. Thrombocytopenic purpura related to rubella infection. *Pediatrics.* 1978;62:567.
67. Boyer WL, Sherman FE, Michaels RH, et al. Purpura in congenital and acquired rubella. *N Engl J Med.* 1965;273:1362.
68. Steen E, Torp KH. Encephalitis and thrombocytopenic purpura after rubella. *Arch Dis Child.* 1956;31:470.
69. Sherman FE, Michaels RH, Kenny FM. Acute encephalopathy (encephalitis) complicating rubella. *JAMA.* 1965;192:675.
70. Sheinis M, Sarov I, Maor E, et al. Severe neonatal rubella following maternal infection. *Pediatr Infect Dis J.* 1985;4:202-203.
71. Zeldis JB, Miller JG, Dienstag JL. Hepatitis in an adult with rubella. *Am J Med.* 1985;79:515-516.
72. Cooper LZ. Congenital rubella in the United States. In: Krugman S, Gershon A, eds. *Infections of the Fetus and the Newborn Infant.* New York: Alan R. Liss; 1975:1.
73. Centers for Disease Control and Prevention. Increase in rubella and congenital rubella—United States. *MMWR Morb Mortal Wkly Rep.* 1991;40:93-99.
74. Centers for Disease Control and Prevention. Control and prevention of rubella: Evaluation and management of suspected outbreaks, rubella in pregnant women, and surveillance for

congenital rubella syndrome. *MMWR Morb Mortal Wkly Rep.* 2001;50(Suppl):1-22.

75. Marshall WC. Rubella: Current problems and recent developments. *Br J Clin Pract.* 1976;30:56.

76. Menser MA, Forrest JM. Rubella: High incidence of defects in children considered normal at birth. *Med J Aust.* 1974;1:123.

77. Peckham CS. Clinical and laboratory study of children exposed in utero to maternal rubella. *Arch Dis Child.* 1972;47:571.

78. Norris JM, Dorman JS, Rewers M, et al. The epidemiology and genetics of insulin-dependent diabetes mellitus. *Arch Pathol Lab Med.* 1987;111:905-909.

79. Menser MA, Forrest JM, Honeyman MC, et al. Diabetes, HLA antigens and congenital rubella. *Lancet.* 1974;2:1508-1509.

80. Ginsberg-Felner F, Witt ME, Fedun B, et al. Diabetes mellitus and auto-immunity in patients with the congenital rubella syndrome. *Rev Infect Dis.* 1985;7(Suppl):170-176.

81. Townsend JJ, Baringer JR, Wolinsky JS, et al. Progressive rubella panencephalitis: Late onset after congenital rubella. *N Engl J Med.* 1975;292:990.

82. Weil MC, Itabashi HH, Cremer NE, et al. Chronic progressive panencephalitis due to rubella virus simulating subacute sclerosing panencephalitis. *N Engl J Med.* 1975;292:994.

83. McIntosh ED, Menser MA. A fifty-year follow-up of congenital rubella. *Lancet.* 1992;340:414-415.

84. Alford CA, Neva FA, Weller TH. Virologic and serologic studies on human products of conception after maternal rubella. *N Engl J Med.* 1964;271:1275.

85. Hardy JB, Sever JL, Gilkeson MR. Declining antibody titers in children with congenital rubella. *J Pediatr.* 1969;75:213.

86. Doege TC, Kim KK. Studies of rubella and its prevention with gamma globulin. *JAMA.* 1967;200:584.

87. Fuccillo DA, Steele RW, Hensen SA, et al. Impaired cellular immunity to rubella virus in congenital rubella. *Infect Immun.* 1974;9:81.

88. Naeye RL, Blanc W. Pathogenesis of congenital rubella. *JAMA.* 1965;194:1277.

89. Driscoll SG. Histopathology of gestational rubella. *Am J Dis Child.* 1969;118:49.

90. Tondury G, Smith DW. Fetal rubella pathology. *J Pediatr.* 1966;68:867.

91. Plotkin SA, Vaheri A. Human fibroblasts infected with rubella virus produce a growth inhibitor. *Science.* 1967;154:659.

92. Nusbacher J, Hirschhorn K, Cooper LZ. Chromosomal abnormalities in congenital rubella. *N Engl J Med.* 1967;276:1409.

93. Atreya CD, Mohan KV, Kulkarni S. Rubella virus and birth defects: molecular insights into the viral teratogenesis at the cellular level. *Birth Defects Res A Clin Mol Teratol* 2004;70:431-437.

94. Rabinowe SL, George KL, Loughlin R, et al. Congenital rubella: Monoclonal antibody-defined T cell abnormalities in young adults. *Am J Med.* 1986;81:779-782.

95. Bell EF, Ross CA, Grist NR. ECHO 9 infection in pregnant women with suspected rubella. *J Clin Pathol.* 1975;28:267.

96. Black JB, Durigon E, Kite-Powell K, et al. Seroconversion to human herpesvirus 6 and human herpesvirus 7 among Brazilian children with clinical diagnoses of measles or rubella. *Clin Infect Dis.* 1996;23:1156-1158.

97. Levin MJ, Oxman MN, Moore MG, et al. Diagnosis of congenital rubella in utero. *N Engl J Med.* 1974;290:1187.

98. Chernesky M, Wyman L, Mahoney J, et al. Clinical evaluation of the sensitivity and specificity of a commercially available enzyme immunoassay for detection of rubella virus-specific immunoglobulin M. *J Clin Microbiol.* 1984;20:400-404.

99. Field PR, Gong CM. Diagnosis of postnatally acquired rubella by use of three enzyme-linked immunoadsorbent assays for specific immunoglobulins G and M and single radial hemolysis for specific immunoglobulin G. *J Clin Microbiol.* 1944;20:951-958.

100. Wittenburg RA, Roberts M, Elliott L, et al. Comparative evaluation of commercial rubella virus antibody kits. *J Clin Microbiol.* 1985;21:161-163.

101. Hedman K, Salonen E, Keski-Oja J, et al. Single-serum radial hemolysis to detect recent rubella infection. *J Infect Dis.* 1986;154:1018-1023.

102. Ferraro MJ, Kallas WM, Welch KP, et al. Comparison of a new, rapid enzyme immunoassay with a latex agglutination test for qualitative detection of rubella antibodies. *J Clin Microbiol.* 1987;25:1722-1724.

103. Mubareka S, Richards H, Gray M, et al. Evaluation of commercial rubella immunoglobulin G avidity assays. *J Clin Microbiol* 2007;45:231-233.

104. Tipples GA, Hamkar R, Mohktari-Azad T, et al. Evaluation of rubella IgM enzyme immunoassays. *J Clin Virol* 2004;30:233-238.

105. Best JM, O'Shea S, Tipples G, et al. Interpretation of rubella serology in pregnancy: Pitfalls and problems. *BMJ.* 2002;325:147-148.

106. Morgan-Capner P, Hodgson J, Hambling MH, et al. Detection of rubella-specific IgM in subclinical reinfection in pregnancy. *Lancet.* 1985;1:244-246.

107. Belin E, Safyer S, Braslow C. False positive IgM-rubella enzyme-linked immunoassay in three first trimester pregnant patients. *Pediatr Infect Dis J.* 1990;9:671-672.

108. Terry GM, Ho TL, Warren RC, et al. First trimester prenatal diagnosis of congenital rubella: A laboratory investigation. *BMJ.* 1986;292:930-933.

109. Bosma TJ, Corbett KM, Eckstein MB, et al. Use of PCR for prenatal and postnatal diagnosis of congenital rubella. *J Clin Microbiol.* 1995;33:2881-2887.

110. Daffos F, Forestier F, Grangeot-Keros L, et al. Prenatal diagnosis of congenital rubella. *Lancet.* 1984;2:1-3.

111. Grose C, Itani O, Weiner C. Prenatal diagnosis of fetal infection: Advances from amniocentesis to cordocentesis—Congenital toxoplasmosis, rubella, cytomegalovirus, varicella virus, parvovirus and human immunodeficiency virus. *Pediatr Infect Dis J.* 1989;8:459-460.

112. Schiff GM. Titered lots of immune globulin: Efficacy in the prevention of rubella. *Am J Dis Child.* 1969;118:322.

113. Parkman PD, Meyer HM, Kirschstein RL, et al. Attenuated rubella virus. I. Development and laboratory characterization. *N Engl J Med.* 1966;275:569.

114. Ewert DP, Frederick PD, Moscola L. Resurgence of congenital rubella syndrome in the 1990s: Report on missed opportunities and failed prevention policies among women of childbearing age. *JAMA.* 1992;267:2616-2620.

115. Watson JC, Hadler SC, Dykewicz CA, et al. Measles, mumps, and rubella: Vaccine use and strategies for elimination of measles, rubella, and congenital rubella syndrome and control of mumps. Recommendations of the Advisory Committee on Immunization Practices (ACIP). *MMWR Morb Mortal Wkly Rep.* 1998;47(RR-8):1-57.

116. Mellinger AK, Cragan JD, Atkinson WL, et al. High incidence of congenital rubella syndrome after a rubella outbreak. *Pediatr Infect Dis J.* 1995;14:573-578.

117. Robinson JL, Lee BE, Preiksaitis JK, et al. Prevention of congenital rubella syndrome: What makes sense in 2006? *Epidemiol Rev* 2006;28:81-87.

118. Plotkin SA, Farquhar JD, Katz M, et al. Attenuation of RA 27/3 rubella virus in W1-38 human diploid cells. *Am J Dis Child.* 1969;118:178.

119. LeBouvier GL, Plotkin SA. Precepitin responses to rubella vaccine RA 27/3. *J Infect Dis.* 1971;123:220.

120. Ogra PL, Kerr-Grant D, Umana G, et al. Antibody response in serum and nasopharynx after naturally acquired and vaccine-induced infection with rubella virus. *N Engl J Med.* 1971;285:1333.

121. Modlin JF, Brandling-Bennett AD, Witte JJ, et al. A review of 5 years' experience with rubella vaccine in the United States. *Pediatrics.* 1975;55:20.

122. Tingle AJ, Chantler JK, Pot KH, et al. Postpartum rubella immunization: Association with development of prolonged arthritis, neurological sequelae, and chronic rubella viremia. *J Infect Dis.* 1985;152:606-612.

123. Horstmann DM, Liebheber H, Kohorn EI. Postpartum vaccination of rubella-susceptible women. *Lancet.* 1970;2:1003.

124. Lerman ST, Nankervis GA, Heggie AD, et al. Immunologic response, virus excretion and joint reactions with rubella vaccine: A study of adolescent girls and young women given live attenuated virus vaccine (HPV-77 DE5). *Ann Intern Med.* 1971;74:67.

125. Weibel RE, Benor DE. Chronic arthropathy and musculoskeletal symptoms associated with rubella vaccines: A review of 124 claims submitted to the National Vaccine Injury Compensation Program. *Arthritis Rheum.* 1996;39:1529-1534.

126. Howson CP, Katz M, Johnston RB Jr, et al. Chronic arthritis after rubella vaccination. *Clin Infect Dis.* 1992;15:307-312.

127. Mitchell LA, Tingle AJ, MacWilliam L, et al. HLA-DR class II associations with rubella vaccine-induced joint manifestations. *J Infect Dis.* 1998;177:5-12.

128. Miki NPH, Chantler JK. Differential ability of wild-type and vaccine strains of rubella virus to replicate and persist in human joint tissue. *Clin Exp Rheumatol.* 1992;10:3-12.

129. Dennehy PH, Saracen CL, Peter G. Seroconversion rates to combined measles-mumps-rubella-varicella vaccine of children with upper respiratory infection. *Pediatrics.* 1994;94:514-516.

130. Centers for Disease Control and Prevention. Rubella vaccination during pregnancy 1971-1986. *MMWR Morb Mortal Wkly Rep.* 1987;36:457-461.

131. Phillips CA, Maeck JVS, Rogers WA, et al. Intrauterine rubella infection following immunization with rubella vaccine. *JAMA.* 1970;213:624.

132. Vahieri A, Vesikari T, Oker-Blum N, et al. Isolation of attenuated rubella-vaccine virus from human products of conception and uterine cervix. *N Engl J Med.* 1972;286:1071.

133. Wyll SA, Herrmann K. Inadvertent rubella vaccination of pregnant women: Fetal risk in 215 cases. *JAMA.* 1973;225:1472.

134. Modlin JF, Herrmann K, Brandling-Bennett AD, et al. Risk of congenital abnormality after inadvertent rubella vaccination of pregnant women. *N Engl J Med.* 1976;294:972.

135. Fleet WF, Benz EW, Karzon DT, et al. Fetal consequences of maternal rubella immunization. *JAMA.* 1974;227:621.

136. Hofmann J, Kortung M, Pustowoit B, et al. Persistent fetal rubella vaccine virus infection following inadvertent vaccination during early pregnancy. *J Med Virol.* 2000;61:155-158.

137. Centers for Disease Control and Prevention. Notice to readers: Revised ACIP recommendation for avoiding pregnancy after receiving a rubella-containing vaccine. *MMWR Morb Mortal Wkly Rep.* 2001;50:1117.

153

Flaviviruses (Yellow Fever, Dengue, Dengue Hemorrhagic Fever, Japanese Encephalitis, West Nile Encephalitis, St. Louis Encephalitis, Tick-Borne Encephalitis)

DAVID W. VAUGHN | ALAN BARRETT | TOM SOLOMON

The *Flavivirus* genus consists of more than 60 species, most of which are arthropod-transmitted or zoonotic viruses, including some 30 known to cause human disease.[1] Many of the remainder have an unknown pathogenic potential but have been implicated in laboratory disease infections, and several are veterinary pathogens. The agents are classified in the family Flaviviridae (from *flavus*, Latin for "yellow" and for *yellow fever virus*, the type species), together with viruses in the *Pestivirus* genus (which are of veterinary importance) and those in the genus *Hepacivirus* (hepatitis C–like viruses) on the basis of similar morphologic characteristics and genomic structures.[1] However, there are no antigenic relationships between viruses in the respective genera.

From a global perspective, the public health burdens of flavivirus infections such as dengue, yellow fever (YF), Japanese encephalitis (JE), and tick-borne encephalitis (TBE) have been of sufficient magnitude to stimulate, at an early stage, the development of vaccines to control the diseases.[2-4] The licensure and distribution of effective vaccines for YF for more than 70 years, JE for more than 50 years, and TBE for more than 30 years have led to significant reductions in incidence and, in some locations, the effective disappearance of cases; dengue vaccines are under active development.[5] Many of the other flaviviruses cause considerable morbidity, but their appearances as individual cases or outbreaks are infrequent or are too local in impact to have stimulated a concerted approach to prevention and control.

Flavivirus infections are important considerations in the differential diagnosis of central nervous system (CNS) infection, hemorrhagic fever, and acute febrile illnesses with arthropathy or rash, especially in returned travelers.[6,7] By evaluating the epidemiologic history, including the places and dates of travel, activities, and immunizations, in conjunction with clinical features of the illnesses and their incubation periods, the clinician can obtain important clues to pursue or exclude a diagnosis. The diseases of chief importance in this group are described later in this chapter.

History

YELLOW FEVER

Although the historical record and molecular taxonomic studies of viral strains have indicated an African origin of YF, the disease was first recognized in an outbreak that occurred in the New World in 1648 (Fig. 153-1A).[8] The virus probably was introduced by *Aedes aegypti*–infested slave-trading vessels from West Africa. Through the next two centuries, similar outbreaks spread by saltation to port cities in the New World and in Europe. The resulting calamities were illustrated by the 1793 Philadelphia epidemic, in which one tenth of the city's population died, and by the 1878 Mississippi Valley epidemic of 100,000 cases, the cost of which equaled the national budget. Sanitary measures, especially the introduction of piped water, inadvertently served to diminish transmission of the disease, although its mosquito-

borne route of spread was not demonstrated until 1900 and its viral cause not until after 1928. Theiler's development of the attenuated 17D vaccine strain in the 1930s was recognized by a Nobel Prize, but more than 60 years later, vaccine implementation (Expanded Program of Immunization) in areas with endemic transmission remains incomplete, and outbreaks recur periodically.[9]

DENGUE

Because of dengue fever's nonspecific clinical features, the interpretation of historical records for evidence of past epidemics is open to speculation.[10] However, Benjamin Rush's description of a 1780 Philadelphia epidemic was the earliest description in English of so-called break-bone fever. Subsequently, sporadic outbreaks were reported throughout the tropics and subtropics. Outbreaks were common in the continental United States through the early decades of the 20th century, the last large ones occurring in Florida in 1934 and in New Orleans in 1945. Clinical descriptions of dengue complicated by hemorrhages, shock, and death were reported in outbreaks in Australia in 1897, in Greece in 1928, and in Formosa in 1931. Mosquito-borne transmission of the infection by *A. aegypti* was demonstrated in 1903, and its viral etiology in 1906. While isolating the virus in 1944, Sabin demonstrated the failure of two viral strains to cross-protect humans, thus establishing the existence of dengue viral serotypes. Hammon characterized two more serotypes in 1956. After World War II, the start of a pandemic with intensified transmission of multiple viral serotypes began in Southeast Asia, leading to outbreaks of dengue hemorrhagic fever (DHF). In the past 30 years, a similar pattern of intensified viral transmission and increased DHF incidence has been established in Southwest Asia, the Americas, and Oceania, fueled by secular changes toward urbanization, population growth, and increased mobility.

JAPANESE ENCEPHALITIS

JE virus was isolated from a patient in a fatal case in Japan in 1934, but summertime encephalitis outbreaks leading to thousands of cases were described before that year and were called *Japanese B encephalitis*, to differentiate the disease from von Economo's encephalitis lethargica, which was known as *type A encephalitis* (the qualifying *B* has fallen into disuse). Mosquito-borne transmission of the virus was established in 1938. The burden of annual epidemics led to the introduction in the 1960s of vaccines that effectively eliminated the disease in Japan, Korea, and Taiwan and reduced its annual incidence in China by 10-fold, from 160,000 cases in 1966 to 16,000 in 1996. Since the 1970s, the incidence of the disease has increased in countries of Southeast Asia, India, Nepal, and Sri Lanka, probably owing in part to changes in agricultural productivity and increased recognition (see Fig. 153-1B). An estimated 35,000 to 50,000 cases and 10,000 to 15,000 deaths

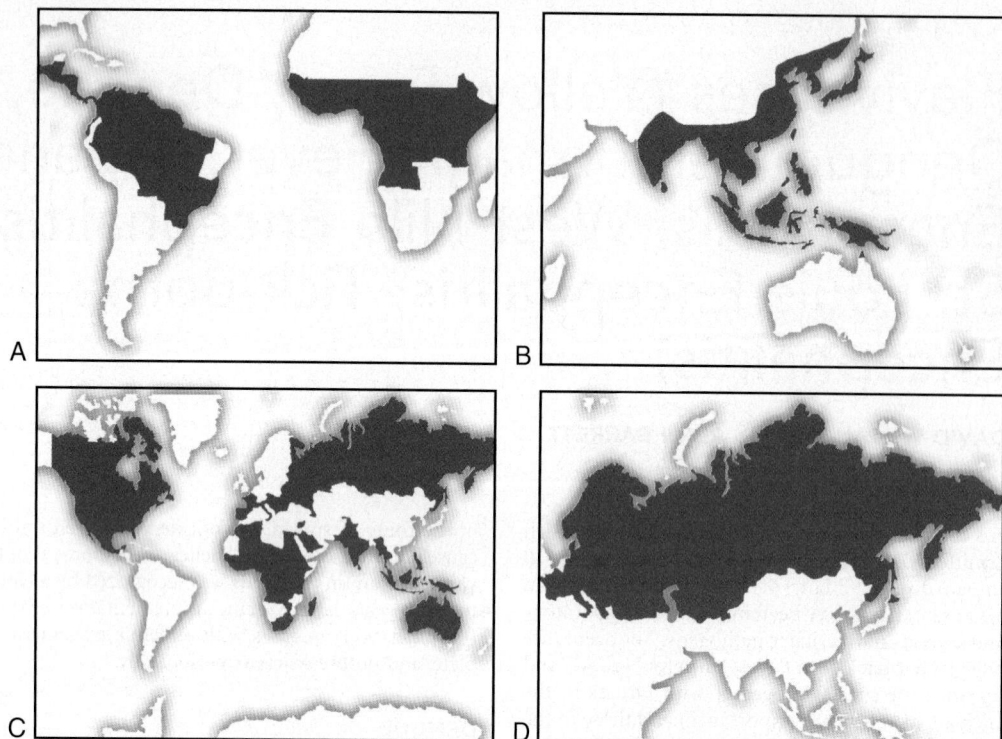

Figure 153-1 **Geographic distribution of medically important flaviviruses. A,** Regions with yellow fever viral transmission. **B,** Regions with Japanese encephalitis viral transmission. **C,** Countries with West Nile virus transmission. **D,** Countries with tick-borne encephalitis transmission.

are reported annually, making the JE virus the most important cause of epidemic viral encephalitis worldwide. In addition, novel introductions to northern Australia in 1995 and 1998, and twice to western Pacific islands, have underscored the ability of this virus to spread. Childhood immunization programs have been established in Thailand and areas of Vietnam, India, and Sri Lanka, but a great deal more remains to be done.

WEST NILE ENCEPHALITIS

West Nile (WN) virus was isolated from the blood of a febrile woman in the West Nile region of Uganda in 1937, and mosquito transmission between vertebrate hosts (especially birds) was demonstrated soon afterward. Although not associated with neurologic disease at that time, the virus was shown by serologic cross-reactivity to be closely related to the then recently identified neurotropic viruses, JE virus and St. Louis encephalitis (SLE) virus. Later, sporadic cases and larger outbreaks of febrile disease (WN fever) were reported in the Middle East and Africa, in some instances in association with arthralgia and a rash. In the 1950s, meningeal irritation and meningoencephalitis were noted in a few patients in Israel. Outbreaks of equine and human meningoencephalitis occurred in southern France during the 1960s, and a subtype of WN virus (Kunjin virus) was isolated in Australasia. Since the 1990s, the epidemiology of WN virus has changed, with increasing frequency and severity of outbreaks in southern Europe, Russia, and the Middle East, and spread of the virus to the Americas (see Fig. 153-1C). The first outbreak in the Western Hemisphere occurred in the northeastern United States in 1999. The virus rapidly spread across the continent, reaching the Pacific Coast in 2002. During 2002 and again in 2003, more than 2000 cases of CNS disease and 200 deaths were reported from the United States, with additional cases in Canada and enzootic transmission reported in the Carribean and Central America. Since 2003, the number of cases reported in the United States has decreased, but there are still more than 1000 neurologic cases per year. WN virus activity has not been reported in tropical

South America, but there was an outbreak in Argentina in equines in 2003.[11]

ST. LOUIS ENCEPHALITIS

SLE was first reported as an epidemic of unknown cause in St. Louis, Missouri, in 1933, although outbreaks compatible with SLE had been described from the 1920s. A U.S. Public Health Service investigation identified the viral cause and, on the basis of epidemiologic features, surmised a mosquito-borne mode of transmission, which subsequently was proved by viral isolations from *Culex* sp. mosquitoes in outbreaks in the Yakima Valley, Washington. With the occurrence of more than 10,000 cases in more than 50 outbreaks through 1990, the disease was the most important cause of epidemic viral encephalitis in the United States until WN virus became established. In 1975, there were 2900 cases of SLE in 31 states, and more than 200 cases occurred during an epidemic in Florida in 1990. SLE continues to be seen in the United States, particularly among elderly people in the southern states.[12] Interestingly, there is evidence that WN virus is displacing SLE virus in its ecosystem in California and Texas.[13,14]

TICK-BORNE ENCEPHALITIS

Descriptions of a disease compatible with TBE appeared in Austria in the early 1930s, although isolation of the virus responsible for this disease (then known as *Central European encephalitis*—CEE) was not reported until 1948. However, investigation of similar cases in the far eastern part of Russia in 1932 had led to descriptions of so-called Russian spring-summer encephalitis (RSSE), and in 1937, the virus was isolated from the blood of patients and from *Ixodes* sp. tick vectors. It is now recognized that three closely related subtypes of TBE virus exist, whose names reflect the geographic areas that they principally affect: European, Siberian, and Far Eastern (see Fig. 153-1D). However, across this vast geographic area, the disease has been given a range of different names, including CEE, RSSE, Far Eastern encephalitis, and biphasic milk fever. This last name reflects the transmission of TBE virus through ingestion of unpasteurized milk from infected livestock, first confirmed during a common source epidemic leading to 660 cases in Czechoslovakia in 1951.

The disease arises in a large geographic area. During the past two decades, both new endemic foci and an increase in cases have been reported in many European countries.[15] The incidence of TBE varies according to location and year. After the collapse of the former Soviet Union and reduced use of pesticides and vaccine against TBE, the annual incidence rose to more than 10,000 cases. In Austria, where there had been several hundred cases annually, a formalin-inactivated vaccine was introduced in the 1970s. Administration of a purified form of the vaccine in mass campaigns since the 1980s has led to a dramatic reduction in the number of cases. The TBE group serocomplex also includes viruses that are rare causes of human neurologic disease (such as Powassan virus, first isolated from a fatal case in Ontario, Canada, in 1958, and louping ill virus, first isolated from a sheep in Scotland in 1930) and viruses that produce a hemorrhagic fever syndrome (such as the Omsk hemorrhagic fever and Kyasanur Forest disease viruses).

Pathogens

Flaviviruses are icosahedral, are about 50 nm in diameter, and consist of a lipid envelope covered densely with surface projections consisting of 180 copies of the M (membrane) and 180 copies of the E (envelope) glycoproteins.[16,17] The latter are organized as dimers, paired horizontally head to tail, on the virion surface. The viruses are unstable in the environment and are sensitive to heat, ultraviolet radiation, disinfectants (including alcohol and iodine), and acid pH. The nucleocapsid joins the capsid (C) protein to a single strand of positive-sense RNA of 11 kilobases, which includes a 10-kilobase open reading frame that is translated as a single polyprotein precursor, which is co- and posttranslationally processed to yield 10 proteins. The order of protein gene products from the 5′ end is C, premembrane (preM, a precursor of the mature M protein), E, and a series of seven nonstructural proteins needed in the viral replicative process: NS1, NS2A, NS2B, NS3, NS4A, NS4B, NS5. The genome is flanked by a short (about 100 nucleotide) 5′ noncoding region and a 3′ noncoding region that is variable in length (100 to 700 nucleotides).

The E protein exhibits important biologic properties, including attachment to host cell receptors, endosomal membrane fusion, and display of sites mediating hemagglutination and viral neutralization.[16] Its carboxyl terminus provides a membrane anchor, and the ectodomain is folded into three structural and corresponding antigenic domains (domains I, II, and III).[18] Domain II is involved in fusion, and domain III is involved in receptor binding. Viral neutralizing epitopes are found in all three domains; because the protein is folded, they are nonlinear and conformationally dependent. PreM protein chaperones the E protein in the cell secretory pathway, preventing its misfolding, before it is cleaved to its M form in the mature virion. NS1 is expressed on the surface of infected cells and is also excreted as a complement-fixing antigen. Although antibodies to NS1 do not neutralize the virus, they contribute to protective immunity, probably by antibody-dependent cellular cytotoxicity and cell-mediated responses against infected cells.[19] Aside from their replicative functions, NS1, NS2A, NS3, and NS5 display epitopes mediating viral serotype and flavivirus cross-reactive human leukocyte antigen (HLA)–restricted lymphocytic responses.[20,21] Studies suggest that NS4B and NS5 are involved in interferon (IFN) antagonism.[22,23]

Viral attachment to unidentified cellular receptors is followed by endocytic uptake of virus-containing vesicles. Acidic-induced changes of the viral envelope lead to fusion activity, uncoating of the nucleocapsid, and viral RNA release into the cytoplasm. Glycosaminoglycans and proteoglycans have been implicated as co-receptors in some studies, but proteinaceous receptors are thought also to be involved, and viral binding evidently varies with cell type.[24,25] The viral polyprotein is co- and post-translationally processed by passage through the rough endoplasmic reticulum, providing the replicative complex for further viral RNA and protein synthesis and the assembly of nascent virions that mature through the Golgi and trans-Golgi network. Immature virions collect in the highly proliferated endoplasmic reticulum and secretory vesicles before release, although intracellular nucleocapsid accumulations have been observed in some virus cell systems.

Flaviviruses are adapted to grow in a wide variety of insect, tick, and vertebrate cells and at temperatures spanning the normal temperatures of their arthropod, reptilian, mammalian, and avian hosts. Cytopathologic changes and plaque formation develop in Vero, LLCMK2, BHK-21, PS, and primary chick and duck embryo cells, whereas infection of mosquito cell lines (e.g., C6/36, AP61) is typically nondestructive and may persist.

A wide range of vertebrates, including mammals, birds, and reptiles, are naturally infected as amplifying hosts in the transmission cycle of alternating arthropod and vertebrate infection.[1] These infections are usually asymptomatic, but individual viruses may be pathogenic for domesticated or wild animals; for example, several neurotropic flaviviruses, including JE, SLE, WN, Kunjin, TBE, and Powassan viruses, produce encephalitis in horses, and certain TBE viral strains are neurotropic for dogs, sheep, and goats. JE virus is an important cause of swine abortion; louping ill is a manifestation of encephalitis in sheep; and YF and Kyasanur Forest disease are lethal in some monkey species. Laboratory rodents are generally susceptible to neurotropic infection, with sensitivity inversely related to age.

With few exceptions, the flaviviruses can be classified by cross-neutralization assays into eight antigenic groups, of which the most important are the JE complex, consisting of JE, SLE, WN, and Murray Valley encephalitis viruses; the dengue complex of dengue 1 through 4 viruses; the mammalian tick-borne virus complex, including TBE, louping ill, Powassan, Kyasanur Forest disease, and Omsk hemorrhagic fever viruses; YF virus; and a complex of non–vector-borne rodent- and bat-associated viruses.[1,26] Genetic studies largely support the antigenic classification and suggest the evolution of flaviviruses from viruses found only in insects to mosquito-borne viruses and subsequently non–vector-borne flaviviruses and tick-borne viruses.[27] Genomic sequencing studies of specific viruses have facilitated evolution studies, and the tracking of viral movements historically and in epidemics. For example, YF viral strains have been divided into seven genotypes: three in East and Central Africa, two in West Africa, and two in South America, with a close relationship between West African and South American viruses supporting the hypothesis that YF virus was introduced to the Western Hemisphere from Africa.[28] Genotypic markers have been of particular help in understanding the emergence of dengue and JE epidemics in the wake of viral introductions from other regions.[29,30] Genotypes also have been correlated with viral biologic characteristics that underlie their transmission patterns. For example, SLE viral genotypes from the eastern and western United States exhibit distinct neurovirulence and transmission characteristics that are consistent with epidemiologic observations.[31,32] On a clinical level, structural distinctions between strains associated with classic dengue and with DHF have been described, providing potential clues to molecular determinants of dengue viral virulence.[32]

Epidemiology

YELLOW FEVER

YF is transmitted in areas of sub-Saharan Africa and South America (see Fig. 153-1A). The disease has never been documented in Asia, but, in principle, anthroponotic (vector-borne person-to-person) transmission of the virus could occur there and in other A. aegypti–infested locations, including the southern United States.[3,33,34] Epidemic ("urban") YF is transmitted by A. aegypti mosquitoes; the mosquitoes are infected after feeding on viremic humans and then spread the infection in subsequent feeding attempts. The threat of epidemic transmission arises when a person with a forest-acquired infection travels to an A. aegypti–infested location while viremic.

The fluctuating incidence of YF has been dominated by epidemics in Africa; 90% of annual 200,000 cases are in Africa, and there were 34 outbreaks between 1985 and 2005. However, official reports considerably underestimate the true magnitude of those epidemics, which field studies estimated as 50-fold greater.[34-36] Epidemic attack rates ranged as high as 30 in 1000 persons, with case-fatality ratios of 20% to 50%. Since 2000, outbreaks in West Africa have produced more than 2000 reported cases in Burkina Faso, Cote d'Ivoire, Guinea, Ghana, Sudan, Cameroon, Togo, and Liberia. The variable size and frequency of epidemics in recent years may reflect cyclic changes in viral activity and human immunity, acquired in recent epidemics and through vaccination in emergency campaigns and the World Health Organization (WHO) Expanded Program of Immunization.

In South America, an annual mean of about 100 cases has been reported in the past 25 years, reflecting the occurrence of forest-acquired infections in the greater Magdalena, Orinoco, and Amazon River basins.[37,38] In its *jungle cycle,* the virus is transmitted from tree-hole *Haemagogus* and *Sabethes* spp. mosquitoes to forest monkeys in wandering epizootics that follow movements of the animals and of the virus to susceptible populations. Cases in humans predominate between January and March among men 15 to 45 years of age who are bitten incidentally by infected mosquitoes while employed as agricultural and forestry workers, soldiers, and settlers. Recent outbreaks frequently have occurred among nonimmune migrants from their coastal or Andean homes to at-risk locations in the tropical zone. An intensification of enzootic viral transmission frequently produces clusters of monkey deaths, indicating an increased transmission risk to humans. The last urban outbreak in the Western Hemisphere took place in Paraguay in 2008 following a period of 54 years since the last urban outbreak in Trinidad in 1954. The growth of urban areas and their reinfestation by *A. aegypti* have renewed concern for the emergence of epidemics, especially in cities that border forested areas, and has been exemplified by the situation in Paraguay in 2008. Since 1995, several patients with jungle-acquired disease have been hospitalized in Brazilian cities and in Santa Cruz, Bolivia—fortunately, without urban spread. The imminent threat of epidemic transmission continues to prompt mass vaccination campaigns and other control measures.[37-39]

In the moist savanna of Africa, a variety of tree-hole–breeding mosquitoes transmit infections among humans and monkeys during the end of the rainy season, leading to early infections in children and sporadic cases that are typically unrecognized. Annual infections in the range of 1% are estimated in areas of West Africa, suggesting that more than 200,000 endemic cases may occur annually.[34,40] Infections are spread readily by migration, with the potential for involvement of *A. aegypti* in urban areas and in dry locations where stored water provides breeding sites. During the dry season, the virus survives in infected mosquito eggs that are resistant to desiccation.

DENGUE AND DENGUE HEMORRHAGIC FEVER

Four serotypes of dengue are recognized and correspond to four distinct virus species (dengue-1 to dengue-4) based on antigenic and genetic characteristics. They are transmitted in the tropics, in an area roughly between 35 degrees north and 35 degrees south latitude, corresponding to the distribution of *A. aegypti*, the principal mosquito vector (Fig. 153-2).[41] *Aedes albopictus, Aedes polynesiensis,* and other species can transmit the virus in specific circumstances. Although enzootic transmission among forest monkeys in Asia and Africa has been described, anthroponotic viral transmission is sufficient to maintain the virus, and these animal infections could represent either epiphenomena or potentially a vestigial sylvatic cycle.[42] The intensification of dengue transmission in tropical cities, where growing populations live under crowded conditions, can be understood in view of the close relationship of *A. aegypti* to humans.[43,44] After the female mosquito feeds on a viremic person, viral replication in the mosquito over 1 to 2 weeks (extrinsic incubation period) occurs before it can transmit the virus on subsequent feeding attempts. Feeding attempts may occur several times a day over the insect's lifetime of 1 to 4 weeks. Mechanical transmission, without extrinsic incubation, has also been suggested. *A. aegypti* is adapted to breed around human dwellings, where the insects oviposit in uncovered water storage containers as well as miscellaneous containers holding water, such as vases, flower dishes, cans, automobile tires, and other discarded objects. Adult mosquitoes shelter indoors and bite during 1- to 2-hour intervals in the morning and late afternoon. In areas with endemic transmission, 1 of every 20 houses may contain an infected mosquito.[45] Cases often cluster in households, and human movements and the mosquito's peregrinations within a range of 800 m rapidly spread the infection.[46,47] In tropical areas, transmission is maintained throughout the year and intensifies at the start of the rainy season, when infected vector mosquitoes are more abundant as higher humidity lengthens their life span and increased temperatures shorten the extrinsic incubation period.

When the virus is introduced into susceptible populations, usually by viremic travelers, epidemic attack rates may reach 50% to 70%. Because cross-protective immunity among the serotypes is limited, epidemic transmission recurs with the introduction of novel virus types. Furthermore, because secondary infections predispose to DHF (see later discussion), the concurrent transmission of multiple viral

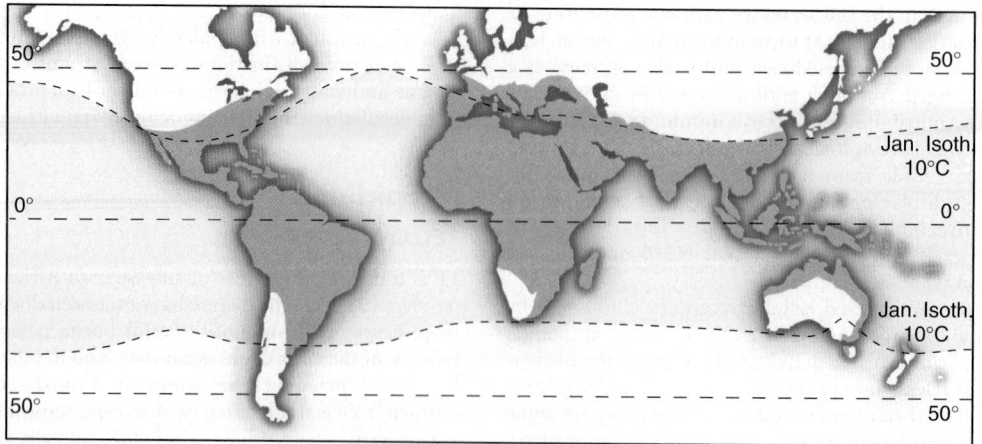

Figure 153-2 **Approximate actual and potential distribution of *Aedes aegypti*.** The band between the 10°C isotherms represents potential distribution. *(From World Health Organization. Technical Guide for Diagnosis, Treatment, Surveillance, Prevention, and Control of Dengue Haemorrhagic Fever, 2nd ed. Geneva: World Health Organization; 1997.)*

serotypes establishes the necessary conditions for endemic DHF. Under these circumstances, virtually all DHF cases occur in individuals with secondary infections, primarily children, with a relative risk for developing DHF in secondary compared with primary infection being as high as 100.[48-51] The central role of prior immunity for at least some virus types is illuminated by the phenomenon of DHF in infants, born to immune mothers, who are infected for the first time before 1 year of age. In these cases, the age distribution of disease onset parallels the expected decline of passively acquired maternal antibodies.[52-54] Outbreaks in Cuba in 1981 and 1997, in which DHF cases occurred only in the age cohort exposed during the last epidemic period (older than 3 years and older than 17 years, respectively), further underscored secondary infection as a critical precondition for DHF, at least for some serotypes.[55-57] However, anecdotal DHF cases in persons with primary infections have been reported, pointing to the contributory roles of viral strain and host factors.[58,59] Race and specific HLA haplotypes have been implicated in the risk for acquiring DHF, and a variable predominance of severe cases has been observed in girls and in children with good nutrition, indicating the contributions of both genetic and acquired host factors to susceptibility to the syndrome.[60-62]

Intensified dengue transmission in Asia after World War II evolved in the previously described pattern, resulting in novel epidemics of DHF beginning in the 1950s. Dengue infection rates in Southeast Asian areas with hyperendemic transmission are now in the range of 5% to 10%, with DHF incidence rates of 10 to 300 per 100,000 persons.[44,63] In Thailand, dengue accounts for one third of acute febrile illnesses in children seeking medical attention.[48,64] Although DHF still is principally a disease of children younger than 15 years of age in hyperendemic areas, the peak age of risk has risen as dengue virus transmission has declined in some hyperendemic areas due to increased use of screens and air-conditioning. Dengue occurs in all age groups when new to an area and, in the case of secondary infections with some dengue virus serotypes, may occur only in previously immunologically primed adults.[56]

The most dramatic ascendance of dengue and DHF has occurred in the Caribbean and in Latin America, where *A. aegypti* has become widely reestablished since its near-eradication as part of YF-control efforts ending in the 1970s.[44,65-67] Before 1977, only dengue-2 and dengue-3 viruses were transmitted in the Western Hemisphere, and DHF was virtually nonexistent. Introductions of dengue-1 virus in 1977 (in Cuba and elsewhere) and dengue-4 four years later were followed by their rapid spread broadly in the region. The introduction to Cuba in 1981 of a novel dengue-2 viral strain from Southeast Asia produced the first major DHF epidemic in the hemisphere, resulting in 116,143 hospitalizations, including 10,000 for shock. Santiago de Cuba escaped the 1981 dengue-2 outbreak until a resurgence in 1997, at which time only adults infected during the 1977-1979 dengue-1 outbreak became ill.[56] A partial explanation for increasing disease frequency is the apparent superior replication capacity of some viruses from Southeast Asia in vector mosquitoes.[68] Since 1989, recurrent DHF outbreaks have been reported in most of Central and South America resulting in several thousand DHF cases each year.[8,67,69] With the reintroduction of a novel dengue-3 strain to Central America in 1994, all four dengue virus serotypes now circulate in the Americas, increasing dengue incidence and severity in the region.[70,71]

The dissemination of dengue viruses by viremic travelers has been facilitated by the increased mobility of people living within endemic areas and internationally by burgeoning air travel. Between 1997 and 2000, a total of 390 anecdotal dengue cases were confirmed among travelers returning to the United States.[72] Incidence rates among American soldiers during World War II were as high as 300 per 1000 persons per month in the Pacific.[73] More recently, rates for those assigned temporarily to Somalia and Haiti were in the range of 1 in 1000 per month.[74] In several studies, dengue virus infection was documented in 7% to 45% of febrile returned travelers.[75,76] Small numbers of autochthonous cases acquired in Texas towns bordering Mexico were recognized in 1980, 1986, 1995, and 2005.[77,78]

Infection can be transmitted by accidental needlestick.[79] The high incidence of infection in endemic areas suggests that transfusion-associated cases could occur frequently, but in these same populations, immunity in recipients is also high, and differentiating a transfusion-transmitted case from a natural infection would be difficult.

JAPANESE ENCEPHALITIS

JE is transmitted in Asia over an area spanning one third of the world's circumference, from Pakistan at the westernmost edge to far eastern Russia (see Fig. 153-1B) (Table 153-1). The disease is endemic and periodically epidemic in Southeast Asia, China, and the Asian subcontinent.[80] During 2005-2006, there were large outbreaks in Northern India causing several thousand deaths.[81] Sporadic cases are reported in tropical Asia, including the Indonesian and Philippine archipelagoes, but field studies suggest a higher incidence.[82,83] Twice, in 1947 and 1990, the virus was introduced to the western Pacific, resulting in outbreaks on Guam and Saipan. The virus invaded the Torres Strait islands of Australia in 1995 and the Australian mainland in 1998.[30,84]

Worldwide, 160,000 cases of JE were reported to the WHO in 1966 and 16,000 cases in 1996, the 10-fold decline reflecting widespread childhood immunization in China, Japan, Korea, and Taiwan as well as regional economic development and the declining emphasis on agriculture. In the latter three countries, few cases are reported currently, although enzootic viral transmission persists. In areas with endemic transmission, an annual incidence of 2.5 per 10,000 children younger than 15 years is estimated, with a case-fatality rate of 25% and disability in 45% of surviving patients.[3,80] Extrapolating this incidence to the population of 700 million children younger than 15 years in the region, an estimated 175,000 JE cases, 45,000 deaths, and 78,000 cases of newly disabled children would occur annually in the absence of immunization.[82] Allowing for the countries where there is immunization, the expected number of cases annually is greater than 125,000. The fact that only one fifth of these are officially recorded probably reflects the lack of reporting from many countries where no surveillance currently exists.[82] In an era in which polio has declined to the point of eradication, JE is now preeminent among causes of pediatric CNS infections in the region. The introduction of new WHO Surveillance guidelines in many Asian countries should improve detection.[85,86]

Within temperate areas, JE is transmitted sporadically from July to September, at a relatively low incidence and with periodic seasonal epidemics. In subtropical Asia, viral transmission extends from March to October in a hyperendemic pattern, resulting in cases throughout the year and the absence of easily detected seasonal epidemics. The geographic distribution of different JE virus genotypes was postulated to explain the differences in clinical epidemiology,[84] but it is now thought to be best explained by the virus's evolution in the Indonesia-Malaysia region and its subsequent spread as more recently evolved genotypes.[87]

The virus is transmitted by *Culex tritaeniorhynchus* and related ground-pool–breeding mosquitoes to pigs and aquatic birds, which are the principal viral-amplifying hosts.[88] Viremic adult pigs are asymptomatic, but infected pregnant sows abort or deliver stillbirths. Infected horses and humans are symptomatic but incidental hosts. Because rice paddies provide favorable breeding habitats for vector mosquitoes, the risk for infection is highest in rural areas. However, both pigs and rice paddies are found at the edges of some Asian cities, resulting in isolated cases and, rarely, urban outbreaks. The mosquito vectors chiefly feed outdoors, in the evenings, and prefer animal to human hosts.

More than 99% of infections with JE virus are subclinical; consequently, in areas with endemic transmission, infections acquired naturally at an early age result in immunity in more than 80% of young adults. Cases occur chiefly in children between 2 and 10 years of age, with a slight predominance of boys. In Japan, Korea, and Taiwan, children are protected by immunizations, and cases occur principally

TABLE 153-1   Estimated Risk for Japanese Encephalitis by Country and Season*

Country	Affected Areas	Transmission Season	Comments
Australia[†]	Islands of Torres Strait	February-April peak; year-round transmission risk	Localized outbreak in Torres Strait in 1995 and sporadic cases in 1998 in Torres Strait and on mainland Australia at Cape York Peninsula
Bangladesh	Few data, but probably widespread	Possibly July-December, as in northern India	Outbreak reported from Tangail District, Dacca Division; sporadic cases in Rajshahi Division
Bhutan	No data	No data	—
Brunei	Presumed to be sporadic-endemic, as in Malaysia	Presumed year-round transmission	—
Cambodia	Endemic-hyperendemic countrywide	Presumed to be May-October	Cases in refugee camps on Thai border and from Phnom Penh
Democratic Republic of Korea	Presumed to be countrywide in rural areas <800 m altitude	July-October	Epidemics in 1970s; few recent data
India	Reported cases from all states except Arunachal, Dadra, Daman, Diu, Gujarat, Himachal, Jammu, Kashmir, Lakshadweep, Meghalaya, Nagar Haveli, Orissa, Punjab, Rajasthan, and Sikkim	South India: May-October in Goa, October-January in Tamil Nadu, August-December in Karnataka Second peak: April-June in Mandya District Andrha Pradesh: September-December[†] North India: July-December	Outbreaks in West Bengal, Bihar, Karnataka, Tamil Nadu, Andhra Pradesh, Kerala, Assam, Uttar Pradesh, Manipure, and Goa; urban cases reported (e.g., in Luchnow)
Indonesia	Kalimantan, Bali, Nusa, Tenggara, Sulawesi, Mollucas, Irian Jaya, and Lombok	Probably year-round risk; varies by island; peak risks associated with rainfall, rice cultivation, and presence of pigs Peak periods of risk: November-March, June and July in some years	Endemic on Bali, Java, and possibly in Lombok; sporadic cases recognized elsewhere
Japan[†]	Rare; sporadic cases on all islands except Hokkaido	June-September, except April-December on Ryuku Islands (Okinawa)	Vaccination not routinely recommended for travel to Tokyo and other major cities; enzootic transmission without human cases observed on Hokkaido
Laos	Presumed to be endemic-hyperendemic countrywide	Presumed to be May-October	—
Malaysia	Sporadic-endemic in all states of Peninsula, Sarawak, and probably Sabah	Year-round transmission; October-February in Sarawak	Most cases from Penang, Perak, Salangor, Johore, and Sarawak
Myanmar	Presumed to be endemic-hyperendemic countrywide	Presumed to be May-October	Repeated outbreaks in Shan State in Chiang Mai valley
Nepal	Hyperendemic in southern lowlands (Terai); sporadic cases in Kathmandu valley	July-December	Vaccination not recommended for travelers visiting only high-altitude areas
Pakistan	May be transmitted in central deltas	Presumed to be June-January	Cases reported near Karachi; endemic areas overlap those for West Nile virus; lower Indus Valley might be an endemic area
Papua New Guinea	Normanby Islands and Western Province	Probably year-round risk	Localized sporadic cases
People's Republic of China[†]	Cases in all provinces except Xizang (Tibet), Xinjiang, Qinghai Temperate areas: endemic to periodically epidemic Southern China: hyperendemic Hong Kong: rare cases in new territories	Northern China: May-September Southern China: April-October (Guangxi, Yunnan, Guangdong, and southern Fujian; Sichuan, Guizhou, Hunan, and Jiangxi provinces) Hong Kong: April-October	Vaccination not routinely recommended for travelers to urban areas only
Philippines	Presumed to be endemic on all islands	Uncertain; speculations based on locations and agroecosystems West Luzon, Mindoro, Negros, Palawan: April-November Elsewhere: year-round, with greatest risk April-January	Outbreaks described in Nueva Ecija, Luzon (including January 2004), and Manila
Republic of Korea[†]	Sporadic-endemic with occasional outbreaks	July-October	Last major outbreaks were 1982-1983
Russia	Far eastern maritime areas south of Khabarousk	Peak period July-September	Sporadic transmission in rural and sylvatic cycles
Singapore	Higher rates of enzootic transmission in western rural areas of island	Year-round transmission with April peak	Vaccination not routinely recommended; two sporadic cases in 2001
Sri Lanka	Endemic in all but mountainous areas; periodically epidemic in northern and central provinces	October-January; secondary peak of enzootic transmission in May-June	Outbreaks in central (Anuradhapura) and northwestern provinces
Taiwan[†]	Endemic, sporadic cases island-wide	April-October; June peak	Cases reported in and around Taipei and the Kao-hsiung–Pingtung river basins
Thailand[†]	Hyperendemic in north; sporadic-endemic in south	May-October	Annual outbreaks in Chiang Mai Valley; sporadic cases in Bangkok suburbs
Vietnam[†]	Endemic-hyperendemic in all provinces	May-October in the North, year-round in the South	Highest rates in and near Hanoi
Western Pacific	Two epidemics reported in Guam and Saipan since 1947	Uncertain; possibly September-January	Enzootic cycle may not be sustainable; epidemics have occurred after introductions of virus

*Assessments are based on publications, surveillance reports, and personal communications. Extrapolations have been made from available data. Transmission patterns may change.
[†]Locally reported incidence rates may not reflect risks to nonimmune visitors because high immunization rates in local populations may obscure ongoing enzootic transmission.
Modified from references 2 and 90, and updated from ProMed Mail (http://www.promedmail.org/), and following the Global Alliance for Vaccines and Immunizations, Southeast Asia and Western Pacific Regional Working Group's Japanese Encephalitis Meeting: Setting the Global Agenda on Public Health Solutions and National Needs, Bangkok, Thailand, 2002.

in elderly people, reflecting waning immunity or other biologic factors associated with senescence.[89]

Expatriate and traveler cases have been recognized since 1932, and outbreaks among American, British, and Australian soldiers in World War II, Korea, and Vietnam were considered militarily important. Travelers of all ages without naturally acquired protective antibodies are at risk for acquisition of the illness. The risk is slight, estimated to be 1 in 150,000 person-months of exposure, reflecting low vector mosquito infection rates (0.5%) and the small case-to-infection ratio (0.3%).[90] However, cases of JE among travelers even on short trips to southeast Asia serve as a reminder of the unpredictable risk for acquiring this disease.[91-93]

WEST NILE ENCEPHALITIS

WN virus is one of the most widely distributed arboviruses, being found across much of Africa, southern Europe, the Middle East, Asia, Australia (Kunjin subtype), and more recently, the Americas.[94,95] Recent outbreaks have included almost 400 confirmed cases in Romania in 1996, almost 200 cases in the Volgograd region of Russia in 1999, and more than 200 cases in Israel in 2000 (Table 153-2).[95] In 1999, the virus appeared in North America for the first time in the New York area, with 62 confirmed human cases and 25 equine cases. The virus rapidly established itself in North America with a peak in 2003 of nearly 10,000 clinical cases, including 286 cases of neurologic disease. Since 2004, the number of cases has decreased, but there are still 1000 to 1500 neurologic cases per year, and there has been a consistent mortality rate of 10% among neurologic cases. Like JE, many of the survivors of WN neurologic infection suffer from neuropsychiatric impairment that may last as long as 3 to 4 years. Surprisingly, there are few reports of human disease south of the United States, with a few cases reported in Argentina.

WN virus is transmitted in an enzootic cycle between birds, by mosquitoes (Fig. 153-3). Recent studies in the United States have demonstrated infection in at least 300 different bird species and 62 mosquito species. In addition, at least 30 vertebrate species are infected, but they have insufficient viremia to infect a feeding mosquito and are considered "dead-end" hosts. Some, however, may have clinical infection (e.g., in humans). Members of the order Passeriformes (jays, blackbirds, finches, warblers, sparrows, and crows) appear to be important in transmission of the virus in nature; the family Corvidae (crows and blue jays) is particularly susceptible. In some areas, arrival of the virus was heralded by dying birds falling from the sky. The lack of resistance and fatal infection of avian intermediary hosts provided evidence for the novel introduction of the virus to the ecosystem of the Western hemisphere, unlike the asymptomatic infection of autochthonous birds by the closely related SLE virus. Of the many mosquito species from which WN virus has been isolated, *Culex* sp. appears to be important in the enzootic cycle, although the species varies by geographic location. Transovarial transmission of the virus in mosquitoes probably provides for viral overwintering. During the 2002 outbreak in the United States, it became clear that on rare occasions viral transmission can occur by transplantation of infected organs, from infected blood products, transplacentally, and, possibly, through breast milk.[96,97] During the height of the 2002 epidemic, the risk for infection by transfusion was estimated to be as high as 21 per 10,000 donations,[96,97] and blood screening using real-time polymerase chain reaction (PCR) has been instituted and has dramatically decreased the risk for contaminated blood (see Chapter 305).

The means by which WN virus is introduced to new areas are not completely understood. Migratory birds are thought to be important for movement of the virus from Africa into southern Europe. They may have been involved in its introduction into North America, although importation of viremic exotic birds or amphibians and inadvertent transport of mosquitoes are alternative explanations.[98] Molecular genetic evidence suggests a single introduction into the United States of a strain, possibly from the Middle East.[99]

Most human infections with WN virus are asymptomatic. Epidemiologic surveys taken after the 1999 outbreak in New York suggested that about 1 in 5 people infected with WN virus develops fever and that only about 1 in 150 develops CNS disease.[96,97] These rates are similar to the attack rates for the Romanian 1997 outbreak,[100] but they appear to be much higher than those reported from Egypt and South Africa,[101,102] most likely because of preexisting antibodies in people in Africa. In New York, Romania, and Israel, the risk for neurologic disease increased with age, which may explain, in part, the different

TABLE 153-2	Outbreaks of West Nile Virus Infection*					
Year of Outbreak	Country	No. of Suspected Cases	No. of Cases Investigated	No. of Confirmed Cases	No. of Deaths	Notes
1957	Israel	419	247	About 180	4	Included first naturally occurring encephalitis cases (12 patients)
1974	South Africa	18,000	558	307	0	Estimated 18,000 cases of WN fever
1962-1966	France (Camargue)	—	—	14	1	Many horses also affected
1994	Algeria	50	18	17	8	—
1996	Romania	835	509	393	17	Continuing cases in 1997-1999
1997	Tunisia	173	129	111	8	—
1998	Democratic Republic of Congo	35	35	23	0	Military personnel newly arrived in this area
1999	USA (New York)	719	719	62	7	—
1999	Russia (Volgograd Region)	826	318	183	40	—
2000	Israel	—	—	233	33	91 nonhospitalized patients with WN fever also identified
2000-2001	USA	—	—	85	24	—
2002	USA	—	—	4156	284	2956 with CNS disease
2003	USA	—	—	9862	264	2866 with CNS disease
2004	USA	—	—	2539	100	1142 with CNS disease
2005	USA	—	—	3000	119	1294 with CNS disease
2006	USA	—	—	4269	177	1459 with CNS disease
2007	USA	—	—	3630	124	1217 with CNS disease

*Only details of selected outbreaks are shown. Criteria for hospitalization, case definitions, and diagnostic methods varied among outbreaks, and some numbers are approximations.
CNS, central nervous system; WN, West Nile.

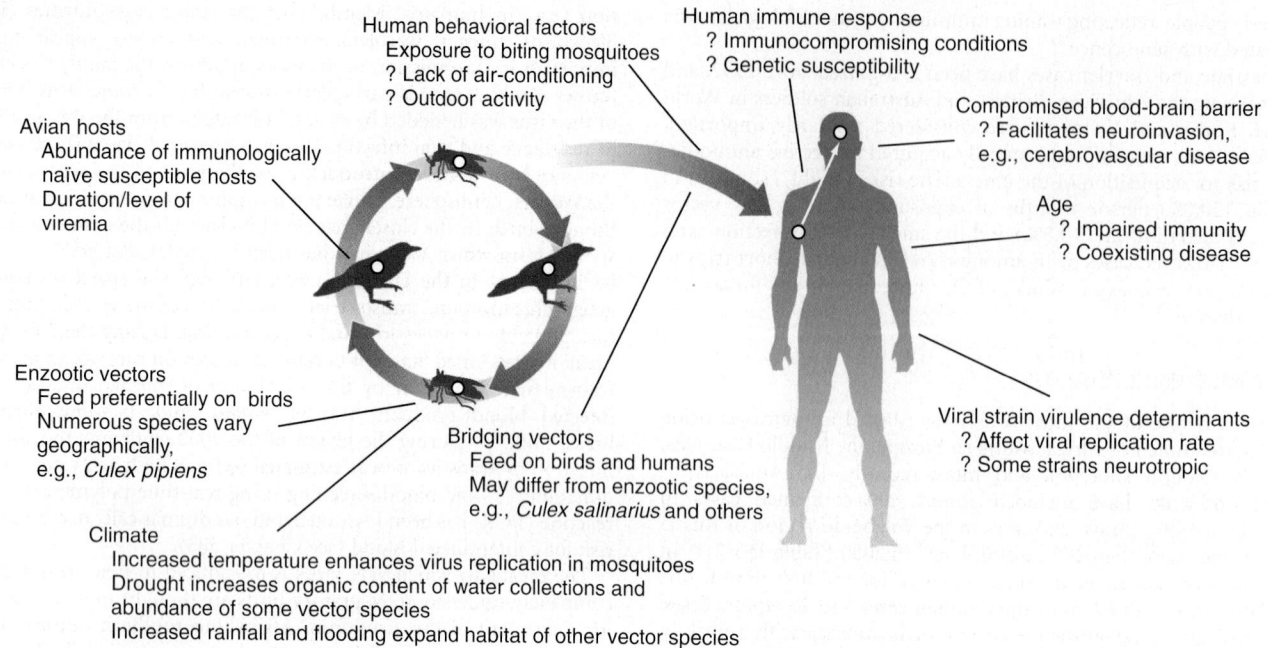

Figure 153-3 West Nile virus transmission cycle and examples of modifying climatologic, vertebrate, mosquito, and human factors on infection and illness.

epidemiologic patterns seen in parts of Africa. In Egypt, most of the population is infected during childhood, and neurologic disease is rare.[101] In South Africa, a large outbreak affected an estimated 18,000 people of all ages, yet only a single West Nile encephalitis (WNE) case was reported.[102]

ST. LOUIS ENCEPHALITIS

Outbreak-associated cases of SLE have been reported from virtually all U.S. states, the provinces of Ontario and Manitoba in Canada, and Sonora State in Mexico, whereas only sporadic cases have been reported from Argentina, Brazil, Panama, Trinidad, French Guiana, Surinam, Curacao, Jamaica, and the Dominican Republic. Enzootic viral transmission has also been recognized in Alberta and British Columbia in Canada and in Ecuador, Guatemala, and Haiti and may occur elsewhere in the hemisphere.[103,104]

In the United States, the virus is transmitted to birds in three distinct cycles overlapping those of WN virus: by *Culex pipiens* and *Culex quinquefasciatus* in the midwestern and eastern states, by *Culex nigripalpus* in Florida, and by *Culex tarsalis* in the Great Plains and farther west. Humans are infected incidentally from the enzootic cycle and, as with WN infection, humans are dead-end hosts. Characteristics of the vectors and their respective transmission cycles define epidemiologic features in each location.

In the eastern states, SLE is transmitted periodically in localized and regional outbreaks at lengthy intervals without significant transmission in intervening years. Outbreaks in the late summer and fall occur in urban areas, often in older neighborhoods, where polluted wastewater provides breeding habitat for *C. pipiens* and *C. quinquefasciatus*, the northern and southern house mosquitoes, respectively. More than 50 epidemics, ranging in the hundreds of cases, have been recognized in small towns or cities, including Houston, Dallas, Memphis, New Orleans, Chicago, and Detroit. The largest epidemic, in 1976, led to more than 3000 cases of neurologic infection nationally, similar in scale and geographic location to recent WNE outbreaks. In three outbreaks since 1991, disproportionate risk was reported among homeless persons infected with the human immunodeficiency virus (HIV), probably reflecting their increased vulnerability to mosquito bites in the evening, when the vectors are most active.[105] Between 1992 and

2000, much smaller outbreaks and sporadic cases occurred (median, 14 cases; range, 2 to 26 cases annually). The 2001 outbreak in Louisiana produced 71 cases and was a reminder of the continued enzootic transmission and epidemic potential of this virus.[106]

Outbreaks in Florida occur more diffusely in suburban and urban locations, where swales and ground pools provide breeding sites for *C. nigripalpus*.[107] In the western states, SLE is transmitted perennially and at a low level in rural areas, frequently in association with irrigated farms and pastures. Forty years ago, outbreaks in agricultural areas occurred at regular intervals; more recently, cases have been more sporadic and frequently have involved vocational exposures or have occurred in proximity to cities. Small urban outbreaks have also occurred. The decline in cases has been attributed to secular changes in land use, air-conditioning of residences, and other factors leading to reduced exposure. Diminished exposure to infection has been confirmed in rural California populations, in whom seroprevalence rates now range from 0.1 to 11%.[104]

The risk for illness is associated most strongly with advanced age, but a slightly elevated risk is also seen in infants. The importance of age is reflected in the declining ratio of asymptomatic to symptomatic infection, which ranges from 800 : 1 in children to 85 : 1 in adults older than 60 years (Fig. 153-4).[108] Between 1999 and 2007, 75% of all patients were older than 40 years, with an increased risk in males and in blacks.[12]

TICK-BORNE ENCEPHALITIS

TBE virus is classified as one species within the mammalian group of tick-borne flaviviruses and is further subdivided into three subtypes: Far Eastern (previously RSSE), Siberian (previously west-Siberian), and European (previously CEE). In this chapter, this latest classification is followed, although many of the older references use the earlier names for virus subtypes.

The three subtypes of TBE virus, as well as other related tick-borne flaviviruses, are transmitted across the Holarctic, with some evidence for their dissemination from an Asian source.[27,109] The Far Eastern subtype is transmitted in eastern Russia, Korea, China, and parts of Japan; the European subtype and related viral strains are found in Scandinavia, Europe, and eastern states of the former Soviet Union;

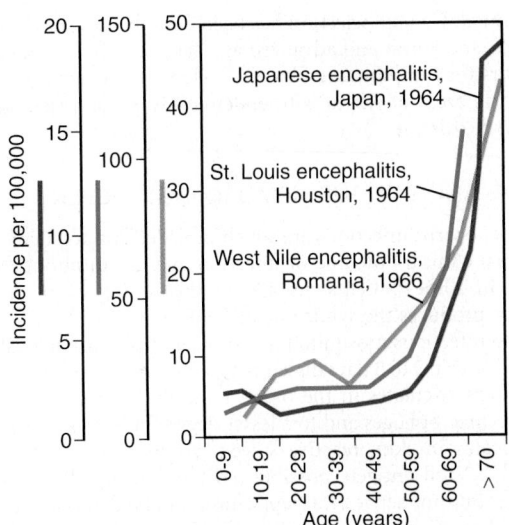

Figure 153-4 Age-specific incidence of St. Louis encephalitis, West Nile encephalitis, and Japanese encephalitis.

and the Siberian subtype is found in western Siberia (see Fig. 153-1D). The geographic distributions overlap in eastern Europe, where both Siberian and Far Eastern subtypes may be isolated.[15] Louping ill virus is found in the British Isles, and Powassan virus in North America and northern Asia. Closely related tick-borne flaviviruses include Turkish and Spanish sheep encephalitis viruses, which are found in southern Europe,[110] and two viruses that cause hemorrhagic fever—Kyasanur Forest disease virus in India and Omsk hemorrhagic fever virus in Siberia.

TBE has been recognized throughout Europe, except in Portugal and the Benelux countries, but endemic transmission is most intense in Austria, areas of Germany, Poland, Hungary, the former Yugoslavia, Czechoslovakia, and the Baltic states and western Russia. In these countries, incidence rates in unvaccinated populations have approached 50 in 100,000 persons, but the risk is highly focal. In Austria, national vaccination programs have reduced the incidence of disease to fewer than 1 in 1,000,000.[111] Sporadic cases are reported from France, Liechtenstein, Sweden, Switzerland, Italy, and Greece. In the Far East, TBE cases occur principally among people working or living in sylvatic locations in Russia, Korea, northern China, and Hokkaido Island, Japan. New models based on environmental factors and satellite data suggest that climate change is partially responsible for the increased incidence in Europe.[112] Longitudinal studies show the virus now circulates at greater altitudes in the Czech Republic.

The viruses are transmitted horizontally between ticks and vertebrates and through the winter by vertical transmission in the ticks and latent infections in hibernating animals. The virus passes transovarially and transtadially, from egg to larva, nymph, and adult, so all stages of the tick and both male and female ticks transmit infections to animals and humans. In addition, it appears that virus may be transmitted between ticks, as they feed on the skin of the same host, through infected host reticuloendothelial and inflammatory cells, without the need for host viremia.[113] Larval and nymphal ticks feed principally on birds and small mammals, and adult ticks on larger mammals such as roe deer, deer, domestic goats, sheep, cows, dogs, cats, and humans. Human infections are incidental to the transmission cycle. Animal movements can spread ticks and the virus to new foci.

Within the ranges of *Ixodes ricinus* and *Ixodes persulcatus*, the principal tick vectors of the European and Far Eastern subtypes, respectively, the ticks are distributed focally in sheltered microhabitats with high humidity and moderate temperatures, limited to elevations lower than 1000 m. Landscape ecology studies have characterized forest ecotones to fields or meadows, and low stands of deciduous trees and

brush with a thick canopy, as high-risk biotopes that correlate with foci of human cases.[114] Transmission foci tend to be highly stable but are subject to human environmental modifications and possibly climate change.[115] In central Europe, cases occur from April until November, peaking in June and July, with a secondary rise in October.

Cases occur mainly in adults, 20 to 50 years of age, with a male predominance, reflecting occupational exposure in forestry and farming. But children at outdoor play and persons with vocational exposure while hiking, berry picking, or mushroom gathering also may be at risk, depending on the location and season. However, the risk for most persons with short-term exposures is low. Among American soldiers stationed in central Europe, no cases and a low rate of seroconversion (0.1% to 0.4%) have been reported.[116] Louping ill is principally an occupational disease of veterinarians, sheepherders, and butchers.[117]

TBE virus is stable at acid pH, and consumption of unpasteurized milk or milk products from infected goats, sheep, or cows previously accounted for 10% to 20% of cases in some parts of central Europe. The possibility that Powassan virus can be transmitted from raw milk products in the United States has been suggested.[118] Slaughter or butchering of infected animals or meat is a principal mode of transmission for louping ill virus to humans and also has been reported in TBE and in outbreaks of Alkhurma virus (see later discussion).[119] Infection has also been acquired from infected ticks carried to households on fomites.

In addition to TBE virus, *I. ricinus* also transmits several *Borrelia* spp. responsible for Lyme disease (as well as *Anaplasma phagocytophilum*, *Babesia microti*, and several species of rickettsia), and dual infections of ticks and humans are observed. However, in at-risk areas, Lyme disease is far more common than the other diseases. This difference reflects the low proportion of virus-infected ticks (0.1% to 5%) and the 10-fold higher borrelial infection rates of ticks in the same location. This distinction may result from the brevity of viremia in animal hosts, which provides an opportunity for tick infection of only a few days; in contrast, persistent borrelial infections of rodents offer a higher likelihood of tick infection during feeding. An analogous situation occurs in the United States, where *Ixodes scapularis* transmits Lyme disease, babesiosis, human anaplasmosis, and a genotype of Powassan virus represented by deer tick virus.[120] However, *Ixodes cookei* ticks (the principal vector of Powassan virus) and *I. scapularis* differ somewhat in their host range, which may further limit opportunities for the viral and borrelial transmission cycles to intersect.

Pathogenesis

YELLOW FEVER

Early stages of YF infection can be inferred from human vaccine studies and from experimental wild-type viral infections of primates. Two days after inoculation of the attenuated 17D vaccine, levels of tumor necrosis factor-α (TNF-α), interleukin-1 receptor antagonist (IL-1RA), and to a lesser extent, interleukin-6 (IL-6) increase, with a secondary TNF-α peak 7 days later.[3,33,121,122] The cytokines are synthesized in response to local spread of the vaccine and again as a response to viremia, which peaks between days 3 and 6.[3,33,123] TNF-α elevations correspond to declines in the lymphocyte count. After wild-type viral infection, the grippe phase of early YF presumably is associated with a similarly timed elaboration of cytokines. In experimentally inoculated rhesus monkeys, the virus replicates initially in local lymph nodes, followed rapidly by blood-borne infection of fixed macrophages, especially Kupffer cells in the liver, and further spread and replication in liver, lung, kidney, and adrenal glands, and most prolifically in regional lymph tissue, spleen, and bone marrow.[3,33] Infection by mosquito feeding, which introduces cytokines from the insect's saliva, is believed to differ from experimental needle inoculation in the outcome of local viral replication and distribution, but the importance of these factors in modulating human flavivirus infections is unknown.

Pathologic changes are most pronounced in the liver and kidneys, but widespread hemorrhages are found on mucosal surfaces, in the skin, and within various organs. Numerous petechial hemorrhages and erosion of the gastric mucosa contribute to the hematemesis that typically introduces the illness. Hepatocellular damage is characterized by a patchy mid-zonal distribution, sparing cells around the central vein and portal triad. The extent of lobular necrosis is variable, with an average of 60%, but even with confluent lobular necrosis, the reticular architecture is preserved. The preservation of the reticulin network, minimal inflammatory changes, and the morphology of degenerating hepatocytes are consistent with apoptosis as the principal pathway of cell death. Early changes in infected hepatocytes consist of glycogen depletion and cloudy swelling, followed by accumulations of fat and of ceroid pigment. Necrotic cells finally undergo coagulation, with the formation of characteristic eosinophilic Councilman bodies, which correspond to apoptotic cells. Viral antigen is identified initially in Kupffer cells and appears later in hepatocytes, Councilman bodies, and endothelial cells.[124-126] Healing occurs without fibrosis.

Albuminuria and renal insufficiency reflect prerenal factors, including vomiting and myocarditis, as well as parenchymal invasion and, in advanced illness, acute tubular necrosis.[33,127] Viral antigen can be identified in the kidney and also in the heart, in which degenerative fatty infiltration of the myocardium and of the conduction system contributes to decreased output and arrhythmias.[126] Neurologic findings probably reflect metabolic disturbances, cerebral edema, and hemorrhages rather than encephalitis. The cause of the bleeding diathesis is ill defined but probably represents a combination of reduced hepatic synthesis of clotting factors, intravascular coagulation, thrombocytopenia, and endothelial and platelet dysfunction. A combination of direct parenchymal damage and a systemic inflammatory response–like syndrome appears to contribute to shock and a fatal outcome. Neutralizing antibodies elaborated within the first week of illness clear the virus, and recovery is followed by lifelong immunity.

Heterologous flavivirus immunity (e.g., previous dengue) is believed to provide partial protection against infection, which may contribute to the absence of YF in Asia.[128] However, in contrast to the situation with DHF, there is no evidence of antibody-mediated immune enhancement. Genetic selection has been described in survivors of YF epidemics, and youth and advanced age have both been implicated as risk factors for symptomatic illness.[3,129] Hepatitis B carriage, which is prevalent in areas of Africa with endemic YF, is not a risk factor for symptomatic disease.[130]

DENGUE AND DENGUE HEMORRHAGIC FEVER

Most dengue virus infections are subclinical. Self-limited dengue fever is the usual clinical outcome of infection, but an immunopathologic response in some patients, usually in the setting of heterologous immunity, produces the syndrome of DHF (Fig. 153-5).[131-133]

After an infectious mosquito bite, the virus replicates in local lymph nodes and within 2 to 3 days disseminates through the blood to various tissues. Virus circulates in the blood typically for 5 days in infected monocyte-macrophages and to a lesser degree in B cells and T cells. It also replicates in skin, reactive spleen lymphoid cells, and macrophages.[134,135] Viral antigen, possibly reflecting an uptake of immune complexes, but not active viral replication, can be demonstrated more widely in liver Kupffer cells and endothelia, renal tubular cells, and alveolar macrophages and endothelia. Almost all patients are viremic at the point of clinical presentation with fever and clear the virus from the blood within days after defervescence.[136,137] The malaise and influenza-like symptoms that typify dengue probably reflect patients' cytokine response; however, myalgia, a cardinal feature of the illness, may also indicate pathologic changes in muscle, typified by a moderate perivascular mononuclear infiltrate with lipid accumulation.[138] Musculoskeletal pain (break-bone fever) conceivably could reflect viral infection of bone marrow elements, including mobile macrophages and dendritic cells (CD11b/CD18 [MAC-1]-positive) and relatively nonmotile adventitial reticular cells (nerve growth factor receptor–positive).[135] Local suppression of erythrocytic, myelocytic, and thrombocytic poiesis within 4 to 5 days is reflected in peripheral cytopenia. Histopathologic examination of skin from patients with rash discloses a minor degree of lymphocytic dermal vasculitis and, variably, viral antigen.[134,136] Elevated hepatic transaminase concentrations have been reported in most cases of dengue, with the aspartate aminotransferase (AST) level initially higher than that of alanine aminotransferase

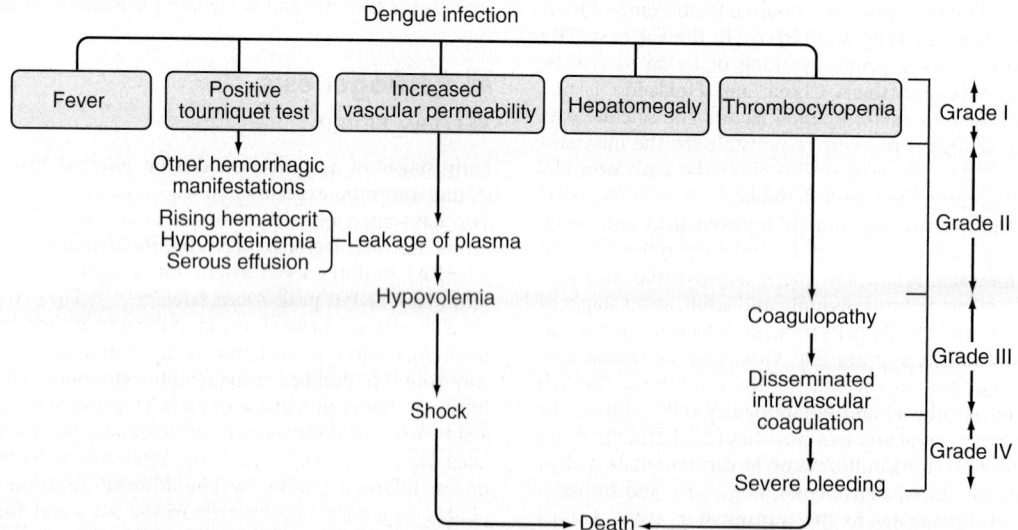

Figure 153-5 **Clinical spectrum, pathophysiology, and classification of dengue hemorrhagic fever.** At the top are key clinical findings; in the center, pathophysiologic mechanisms; and on the side, the World Health Organization classification of cases: *Grade 1:* Fever accompanied by nonspecific constitutional symptoms; the only hemorrhagic manifestations are a positive tourniquet test result, easy bruising, or both. *Grade 2:* Spontaneous bleeding in addition to the manifestations of grade 1, usually in the form of skin hemorrhages or other hemorrhages. *Grade 3:* Circulatory failure manifested by a rapid, weak pulse and narrowing of pulse pressure or hypotension, with the presence of cold, clammy skin and restlessness. *Grade 4:* Profound shock with undetectable blood pressure or pulse. *(From World Health Organization. Technical Guide for Diagnosis, Treatment, Surveillance, Prevention, and Control of Dengue Haemorrhagic Fever, 2nd ed. Geneva: World Health Organization; 1997.)*

(ALT), and with levels higher in DHF compared with dengue fever.[64,139] In fatal cases, histopathologic findings resemble those of early mild YF, with hypertrophy of Kupffer cells, focal ballooning, and necrosis of hepatocytes in a mid-zonal distribution, with occasional Councilman body formation, mild fatty changes, and a scant periportal mononuclear cell response.[140] Viral antigen has been demonstrated in hepatocytes, Kupffer cells, and endothelia.[135] Neurologic complications have been attributed chiefly to metabolic alterations and to focal and sometimes massive intracranial hemorrhages, but anecdotal cases and limited case series have indicated the possibility of viral CNS invasion and encephalitis.[141-144]

Shock in dengue shock syndrome (DSS) occurs after the sudden extravasation of plasma into extravascular sites, including the pleural and abdominal cavities, usually with the defervescence of fever.[132,145] The extensive increase in vascular permeability is associated with immune activation, as manifested by increased levels of plasma-soluble tumor necrosis factor receptor (sTNFR/75), IL-8, IFN-γ, and other mediators and local endothelial production of IL-8 RANTES with apoptotic endothelial cell death.[146-153] In addition, immune complex formation activates the complement system, with increases in C3a and C5a.[154] Levels of IL-6 and intercellular adhesion molecule-1 are depressed in parallel with hypoalbuminemia and the general loss of serum proteins. The rapid, predictable reversibility of the syndrome within 48 hours and the paucity of histopathologic correlates—usually perivascular edema with diapedesis of red cells and widespread focal hemorrhages—suggest that the inflammatory response produces a vasculopathy. Reduced cardiac output may contribute further to shock.[155] The hemorrhagic diathesis is complex and not well understood, reflecting a combination of cytokine action and vascular injury, viral antibodies binding to platelets or cross-reacting with plasminogen and other clotting factors, reduced platelet function and survival, and a mild consumptive coagulopathy.[156-159]

The increased frequency of DHF in secondary dengue virus infections has suggested a role for heterologous antibodies in enhancing viral uptake and replication in Fc receptor–bearing cells (antibody-mediated immune enhancement).[160,161] Simultaneously, levels of TNF-α, soluble CD8, and soluble IL-2 that are higher in patients with DHF than in those with dengue fever indicate an activation of cross-reactive memory CD4+ and CD8+ T cells in response to a second infection.[146] The resulting production of IL-2, IFN-γ, and other lymphokines is reinforced by the increased abundance of infected target cells resulting from IFN-γ–mediated upregulation of Fc receptors and flavivirus-induced expression of major histocompatibility complex type I and II molecules that further activate T lymphocytes.[162,163] Activated infected monocytes and endothelia produce and release with their lysis TNF-α, IL-1, platelet-activating factor (PAF), IL-8, and RANTES, which act in synergy with lymphokines, histamine, and viral immune complex–induced C3a and C5a to produce the temporary vascular endothelial dysfunction that leads to plasma leakage. Paralleling the pathogenetic role of secondary enhancing antibodies in DHF, memory cellular responses to heterologous antigens also may contribute to immunopathology. While activated cells responding to cross-reactive antigens predominate over primary responses to the infecting virus, following the paradigm of original antigenic sin, they are marked for apoptosis and are ineffective in viral clearance, and they may be a source of cytokines with a negative clinical effect.[146]

Although infection with any of the serotypes can produce DHF, there is some indication for a greater propensity after second infections with certain serotypes or with specific strains of putatively greater virulence in a given partially immune population.[57,164,165] Trends toward an increased or fluctuating severity of illness during prolonged outbreaks have been attributed to the evolution of viral quasispecies.[166]

The rise of levels of serum neutralizing antibodies is correlated with the clearance of viremia, but immunity is associated with both humoral and cellular immune responses.[136,153] The latter are mediated by CD4+ and CD8+ cells that recognize serotype-specific, dengue serotype–cross-reactive epitopes, and flavivirus–cross-reactive epitopes.[20,167-169] The stimulation of cross-protective immunity from infection with one dengue viral serotype must be limited and brief because infection with a second type during the same transmission season is not uncommon. Illness after infection with two serotypes (i.e., a third bout of dengue) occurs infrequently, and illness after three infections, virtually never. Repeated episodes of DHF have been recognized rarely, presumably because immune factors that promote immunopathologic responses are outweighed by immune responses that clear the infection.[170]

FLAVIVIRUS ENCEPHALITIS

The variable and potentially lengthy incubation period of 4 to 21 days (usually 1 week) may reflect the interval for viral replication in the skin Langerhans cells and local lymph nodes, with a subsequent brief viremia before the virus invades the CNS.[171] Virus can rarely be recovered from blood, usually less than 1 week after the onset of illness and before the onset of neurologic symptoms, but sometimes later in an immunosuppressed patient; for WN virus, detection by real-time PCR is more common.[172] The large proportion of infections that are asymptomatic, about 300 times the number of symptomatic cases, is striking and remarkably consistent among SLE, JE, and WNE. Subclinical infection presumably reflects the peripheral clearance of virus before neuroinvasion.

Innate responses are thought to be critical to this clearance. For example, during WN virus infection, the host response limits viral spread through the activation of the IFN regulatory factor 3 pathway.[173] A Toll-like receptor 3–dependent inflammatory response is thought to be involved in brain penetration of the virus and neuronal injury in animal models.[174] CNS expression of the chemokine receptor CCR5 and its ligand CCL5 are prominently upregulated by WN virus, associated with CNS infiltration of CD4+, CD8+ T cells, NK1.1+ cells, and macrophages that express CCR5.

A range of host genetic polymorphisms in cytokine genes, and their promoters, have been shown to be important in a number of inflammatory and infectious conditions. In mouse models of flavivirus encephalitis, polymorphisms in the IFN-induced gene 2-5-oligoadenylate synthetase-1 (OAS-1) are associated with different outcomes following infection.[174,175] Other genetic polymorphisms may be relevant in protecting neurons against oxidative damage, or by restricting disease progression, perhaps by acting at the level of leukocyte trafficking to the brain. For example, in one recent study of humans with WN virus infection, a defective allele in the chemokines receptor CCR5 (CCR5Δ32), found predominantly in whites, was found to be highly significantly associated with symptomatic WN virus infection in two independent populations in the United States. A similar polymorphism is associated with severe disease in TBE.[175] Impaired function of helper T cells to nonstructural protein 3 has been associated with severity of outcome following infection with JE virus.[176]

In animal models of arboviral encephalitis, virus enters the CNS by crossing the vascular endothelium or through the olfactory epithelium, where the blood-brain barrier is impaired. However, in humans, the evidence suggests transmission across the vascular endothelium, either by passive transfer or by replication in endothelial cells.[177] For JE, endothelial cell function may be disrupted.[172]

Within the brain, virions spread from cell to cell. Pathologic changes consist of meningeal congestion and inflammation, brain edema, and widespread encephalitis with a predilection for the hippocampus and temporal cortex, thalamus, substantia nigra, cerebellum, periventricular areas of the brain stem, and anterior spinal cord. Destruction of lower motor neuron nuclei in the brain stem and the anterior horns of the cervical and upper lumbar cord is frequently seen in TBE, more so in the Far Eastern form of the disease and less often in JE, SLE, and WNE. Focal neuronal degeneration and necrosis with neuronophagia evolve to the formation of glial nodules and, with healing, spongiform changes. Viral antigen appears in neuronal bodies and their processes and later in phagocytic cells.[178] Perivascular inflammatory infiltrates consist of activated CD4+ and CD8+ T cells, macrophages, and B cells.

In one pathologic study of TBE, viral antigen was identified predominantly in large neurons; there was a poor topographic relation between inflammatory infiltrates, mainly T cells and macrophages, and distribution of antigen, suggesting an immune-mediated neuronal cell death rather than direct viral lysis.[179]

Within the cerebrospinal fluid (CSF), T cells predominate above their proportion in serum, with a correspondingly lower ratio of B and natural killer cells. T-cell activation is evidenced by the expression of HLA-DR followed by CD25 (IL-2 receptor) and CD71 (transferrin receptor) and increased CSF levels of neopterin and β_2-microglobulin.[180,181] A variety of processes may contribute to neuronal cell death, including apoptosis, cytoplasmic swelling, vacuolation, and membrane breakdown.

The rare recovery of virus from CSF, usually in patients with fulminant and fatal disease, is associated with the absence of intrathecal antibodies, indicating an important role of viral neutralization in recovery.[182] CD4+ and CD8+ cellular responses to JE viral N53 and N53-induced IFN-γ correlated with protection from illness and with prognosis, indicating a key role of this instructional protein in helping to stimulate an anamnestic antibody response, as well as in viral clearance of established CNS infection.[176] On the other hand, intrathecal immune-complex formation and antineurofilament and antimyelin basic protein antibodies have also been reported in association with a poor outcome, suggesting immunopathologic injury.[183,184] Immunopathology is implicated in some animal models of flavivirus encephalitis[185] and is supported by the observation that in some immunocompromised patients infected with WN virus, there is a delayed onset of clinical features despite high levels of viremia.[186]

The biphasic and relatively prolonged course of illness in TBE is reflected in CSF neopterin, β_2-microglobulin, and intrathecal immunoglobulin G (IgG) synthesis that remains elevated for 6 weeks and pleocytosis that persists considerably longer than in other CNS infections, consistent with a protracted inflammatory reaction.[187] Although this time course alludes to a postinfectious process, pathologic changes with viral antigen in neurons, focal and perivascular infiltrates, and the recovery of virus from patients with fatal cases are consistent with a primary encephalitis.[188] In some studies of chronic, progressive TBE, mutations in the virus NS1 gene and defective T-cell responses have been reported.[189,190]

Delayed CNS clearance of JE virus has also been suggested by the presence of infectious virus, antigen, or IgM antibodies in CSF several weeks after the onset of illness. JE viral antigen has been detected in peripheral blood mononuclear cells months after clinical recovery.[191,192] Clinically, subacute and progressive paralysis of the limb musculature and chronic epilepsy are well-known features of TBE,[193,194] and CNS viral persistence has been demonstrated.[195] Similar chronic symptomatic infections have been modeled in TBE virus– and WN virus–infected monkeys.

Advanced age is preeminent among the risk factors for development of neurologic infection. In susceptible populations, illness rates rise steeply with age, although infections uniformly attack persons of all ages, indicating age-related host factors rather than increased exposure as the risk factor (see Fig. 153-4).[1,37,100,108] The biologic basis for the age-related susceptibility is ill defined. Studies in mice indicate a critical role of the early antibody response in containing viral replication and limiting dissemination in the CNS. Although the age-related risk may simply reflect immunosenescence, other observations indicate roles for functional or structural CNS changes that facilitate neuroinvasion. As examples, in some studies, neurocysticercosis was more prevalent in patients with fatal cases of JE than in patients dying of other conditions; and in one study, hypertension was associated with an increased incidence of fatal SLE.[196] The interaction of concurrent viral, bacterial, or parasitic infections has been reported to alter expected outcomes of TBE and JE, related to either facilitated neuroinvasion or immune factors.[197,198] Heterologous dengue immunity has been associated with a better outcome in SLE and JE.[199-201]

Clinical Features

YELLOW FEVER

YF illness ranges in severity from an undifferentiated, self-limited grippe to hemorrhagic fever that is fatal in 50% of cases.[3,33,127] In addition, between 5% and 50% of infections are inapparent. After an incubation period of 3 to 6 days, fever, headache, and myalgias begin abruptly, accompanied by few physical findings except conjunctival injection, facial flushing, a relative bradycardia (Faget's sign), and on laboratory examination, leukopenia. In most cases, resolution of this *period of infection* concludes the illness, but in others, the remission of fever for a few hours to several days is followed by renewed symptoms, including high fever, headache, lumbosacral back pain, nausea, vomiting, abdominal pain, and somnolence (*period of intoxication*). Profound weakness and prostration ensue, compounded by poor oral intake and protracted vomiting, but the severe multisystemic illness is dominated by icteric hepatitis and a hemorrhagic diathesis with prominent gastrointestinal bleeding and hematemesis, epistaxis, gum bleeding, and petechial and purpuric hemorrhages. Albuminuria is a constant feature that aids in the differentiation of YF from other causes of viral hepatitis. Deepening jaundice and elevations in transaminase levels continue for several days, at the same time that azotemia and progressive oliguria ensue. Whereas direct bilirubin levels rise to 5 to 10 mg/dL, alkaline phosphatase levels are only slightly raised; not infrequently, AST may be elevated above ALT because of myocardial damage.[202] Ultimately, hypotension, shock, and metabolic acidosis develop, compounded by myocardial dysfunction and arrhythmias as late events and acute tubular necrosis in some patients. Confusion, seizures, and coma distinguish the late stages of illness, but CSF examination discloses an increased protein level without pleocytosis, consistent with cerebral edema or encephalopathy. Death usually occurs within 7 to 10 days after onset. If the patient survives the critical period of illness, secondary bacterial infections resulting in pneumonia or sepsis are common complications. Recovery has not been followed by chronic hepatitis.

Clinically, severe YF resembles other viral hemorrhagic fevers occurring in Africa and South America, so laboratory confirmation is required to make the diagnosis. Early exclusion of other causes with the potential for person-to-person spread is important to prevent nosocomial transmission. Other forms of viral hepatitis, particularly hepatitis E (which frequently appears in outbreaks), leptospirosis, malaria, typhoid, typhus, relapsing fever, acute fatty liver of pregnancy, and toxin-related hepatitis, are alternative diagnoses.

DENGUE FEVER AND DENGUE HEMORRHAGIC FEVER

Classic dengue fever is an acute febrile disease with headaches, musculoskeletal pain, and rash, but the severity of illness and clinical manifestations vary with age and virus type. Infection is often asymptomatic or nonspecific, consisting of fever, malaise, pharyngeal injection, upper respiratory symptoms, and rash—particularly in children.[8,203,204] Dengue virus types 2 and 4 may be more likely to cause inapparent infections in flavivirus-naïve persons.[137] Disease severity may be increased among infants and elderly people.[205] After an incubation period of 4 to 7 days, fever—often with chills, severe frontal headache, and retro-orbital pain—develops abruptly with a rapid progression to prostration, severe musculoskeletal and lumbar back pain, and abdominal tenderness. Anorexia, nausea, vomiting, hyperesthesia of the skin, and dysgeusia are common complaints. Initially, the skin appears flushed, but within 3 to 4 days and with the lysis of fever, an indistinct macular and sometimes scarlatiniform rash develops, sparing the palms and soles. As the rash fades or desquamates, localized clusters of petechiae on the extensor surfaces of the limbs may remain. A second episode of fever and symptoms may ensue ("saddle-back" pattern). Recovery may be followed by a prolonged period of listlessness, easy fatigability, and even depression.

Although virtually all cases are uncomplicated, minor bleeding from mucosal surfaces (usually epistaxis, bleeding from the gums, hematuria, and metrorrhagia) is not uncommon, and gastrointestinal hemorrhage and hemoptysis can occur (see Fig. 153-5).[206] In patients with preexisting peptic ulcer disease, severe, even fatal, gastric bleeding can be precipitated.[207] Subcapsular splenic bleeding and rupture, uterine hemorrhage resulting in spontaneous abortion, and severe postpartum bleeding have also been reported.[208,209] It is important to differentiate these phenomena from the bleeding diathesis that accompanies the life-threatening syndrome of hypotension and circulatory failure in DHF-DSS.

Hepatitis frequently complicates dengue fever.[64,139,210] In Taiwan, transaminase levels raised 10-fold above normal were observed in 11% of cases, with rare deaths due to hepatic failure. Neurologic symptoms associated with dengue fever have been reported sporadically and attributed to hemorrhages or cerebral edema, but recovery of virus from the CSF, intrathecal viral-specific IgM, and immunohistochemical evidence of infection in the brain indicate the possibility of primary dengue encephalitis in some cases.[141-143,211] Myositis with rhabdomyolysis has also been reported.

Vertical transmission of dengue virus to neonates whose mothers had an onset of primary or secondary dengue fever up to 5 weeks before delivery has resulted in acute neonatal dengue manifesting as fever, cyanosis, apnea, mottling, hepatomegaly, and reduced platelet counts as low as 11,000/mm^3.[203,212] One baby died of intracerebral hemorrhage, but others, although ill, did not have other signs of DHF, and they recovered without incident. Dengue virus was isolated from the neonates in some cases. The outcome of infection acquired earlier in pregnancy has not been addressed satisfactorily. Anecdotal reports have described spontaneous abortion (see earlier discussion) and a variety of birth defects and, in a postepidemic investigation, an increase in neural tube defects.[213] Other investigations have found no increases in abnormal pregnancy outcomes.[212,214,215] In a study of cord blood samples from infants delivered 5 to 9 months after an outbreak, 4 of 59 samples had viral-specific IgM, but all the infants appeared normal.[216]

The central clinical features of DHF-DSS are hemorrhagic phenomena and hypovolemic shock caused by increased vascular permeability and plasma leakage.[145,217,218] The early clinical features in children who ultimately develop DHF-DSS are indistinguishable from those of ordinary dengue fever, namely, fever, malaise, headache, musculoskeletal pain, facial flushing, anorexia, nausea, and vomiting. However, with the defervescence of fever 2 to 7 days later, reduced perfusion and early signs of shock are manifested by central cyanosis, restlessness, diaphoresis, and cool, clammy skin and extremities. Abdominal pain is a common complaint. In cases with a benign course of illness, blood pressure and pulse may be maintained, but a rapid and weak pulse, narrowing of the pulse pressure to less than 20 mm Hg, and in the most extreme cases, an unobtainable blood pressure establish the shock syndrome. The platelet count declines, and petechiae appear in widespread distribution with spontaneous ecchymoses. Bleeding occurs at mucosal surfaces from the gastrointestinal tract and at venipuncture sites. The liver is palpably enlarged in up to 75% of patients, with variable splenomegaly. Increased amylase levels and sonographic evidence of pancreatic enlargement are found in up to 40% of patients. Pleural effusions can be detected in more than 80% of cases if a decubitus film is taken; in combination with an elevated hematocrit and hypoalbuminemia, reflecting hemoconcentration, these studies provide objective measures of plasma loss. However, ultrasonography has been more sensitive in detecting pleural effusions, ascites, and gallbladder edema in more than 95% of severe cases, and pararenal and perirenal effusions in 77%, as well as hepatic and splenic subcapsular and pericardial effusions.[219,220] The presence of pleural and peritoneal effusions is associated with severe disease. Acute respiratory distress syndrome (ARDS) may develop with capillary-alveolar leakage.[221] In untreated patients, hypoperfusion complicated by myocardial dysfunction and reduced ejection fraction results in metabolic acidosis and organ failure. With support through the critical period of

illness, spontaneous resolution of vasculopathy and circulatory failure usually can be expected within 2 to 3 days, with complete recovery afterward. The duration of illness ranges from 7 to 10 days in most cases. Fatality rates have reached 50% in underserved populations, but in experienced centers, fewer than 1% of cases are fatal. Encephalopathy, prolonged shock, and hepatic or renal failure infrequently complicate the illness but are associated with a poor prognosis. As would be expected in areas where dengue infects 10% of children each year, concurrent infection with bacteria, parasites, and other viral pathogens occurs frequently. Dual infections, principally gram-negative sepsis, have been reported in 1 of 200 children hospitalized with dengue, resulting in prolonged fever and hospitalization.[222]

Attempts to differentiate dengue fever clinically from other acute febrile illnesses are unlikely to be successful, although the diagnosis is aided if laboratory examination indicates leukopenia, neutropenia, thrombocytopenia, or mildly elevated AST levels.[7,64,166] Even when facial flushing was included as a selective criterion in a study that also included DHF patients, the only differentiating symptoms were anorexia, nausea, and vomiting. A positive tourniquet test, a requirement in the DHF case definition, is obtained more often than in children with other febrile illnesses, but its specificity is low. In comparison with chikungunya, another epidemic A. aegypti–borne infection, dengue patients are less likely to have conjunctivitis, rash, and musculoskeletal pain.[223] The difficulty of differentiating dengue from rubella, measles, and even influenza has been underscored by the early misrecognition of entire epidemics. The clinical differentiation of DHF from YF and other viral hemorrhagic fevers is also difficult, and diagnosis requires laboratory confirmation.

Clinical or laboratory differentiation, at the time of first presentation, of children destined to develop DHF would facilitate intervention before the sudden onset of shock.[224] In one study, AST elevations greater than 60 U/mL, leukocyte counts less than 5000/mm^3, and absolute neutrophil counts less than 3000/mm^3 had higher predictive values than the tourniquet test in differentiating dengue from other febrile illnesses.[64,166] In another study, an elevated sTNFR/75 level had a sensitivity of 93% and a negative predictive value of 95% in foretelling shock.[151] Several other cytokines are being evaluated as markers predicting mild or severe disease, although there are few prospective studies, results vary, and implementation of useful measures at the point of care may be a challenge.[153,225]

JAPANESE ENCEPHALITIS

Infection is symptomatic in fewer than 1% of cases of JE, but the illness is usually a severe encephalitis, leading frequently to coma and to a fatal outcome in 25% of cases. The spectrum of clinical illness is probably broader than is appreciated from an evaluation of hospitalized patients. JE cases are found among hospitalized children with acute pyrexia of undetermined origin, and undoubtedly, many patients with febrile illnesses and headache or aseptic meningitis do not present to a hospital. Studies have drawn attention to patients presenting with spinal paralysis without encephalitic signs, initially misdiagnosed as poliomyelitis cases, and conversely, acute behavioral changes mimicking psychosis without motor signs.[1,2,177,226,227] The earliest symptoms are lethargy and fever and, frequently, headache, abdominal pain, nausea, and vomiting. Lethargy increases over several days, when uncharacteristic behaviors associated with an agitated delirium, unsteadiness, and abnormal motor movements may develop, advancing to progressive somnolence and coma. Although the prodrome may evolve over several days to 1 week, some children present with a sudden convulsion after a brief febrile illness.

The chief findings are high fever and altered consciousness, ranging from mild disorientation or a subtle personality change to a severe state of confusion, delirium, and coma.[1,2,177] Mutism has been a presentation in some cases. Nuchal rigidity is a variable finding, present in one third to two thirds of the cases. Cranial nerve palsies resulting in facial paralysis and disconjugate gaze are detected in one third of the cases. Muscular weakness can be associated with decreased or increased tone and can be generalized or asymmetrical, with hemiparesis or unusual distributions of flaccid and spastic paralysis. Hyperreflexia, ankle clonus, and other abnormal reflexes may be elicited. Disordered movements such as nonstereotypical flailing, ataxia, or tremor may be present initially. Not uncommonly, choreoathetosis, rigidity, masked facies, and other extrapyramidal signs appear later in the illness. Focal or generalized seizures develop in up to 85% of children and 10% of adults.[228] Multiple seizures and status epilepticus are associated with a poor outcome. Subtle motor status epilepticus, in which the only clinical manifestation might be the twitching of a finger or eyebrow, may also occur but is easily overlooked.[228]

Signs of increased intracranial pressure, such as papilledema and hypertension, are detected in a minority of patients, although some fatal cases show evidence of uncal or tentorial herniation, and clinical signs consistent with brain stem herniation syndromes are not uncommon.[228] More than one third of patients in coma need ventilatory support. Fulminant cases may be rapidly fatal. More typically, improvement can be expected after 1 week with the defervescence of fever. Neurologic function is regained gradually over several weeks, with further recovery after hospital discharge over intervals of months to years.[229,230] Infections from stasis ulcers, urinary tract infection, pneumonia, and bacteremia frequently complicate the lengthy recovery from coma and paralysis and may be secondary causes of death. The virulence of the infection is underscored by contemporary fatality rates of 25% in locations with intensive care facilities. Neurologic abnormalities such as seizure disorders, motor and cranial nerve paresis, cortical blindness, and movement disorders persist in up to one third of patients after 5 years. A greater proportion, perhaps even 75% of recovered children, exhibit behavioral and psychological abnormalities. Anecdotal cases of clinical relapse weeks after hospital discharge with recovery of virus from peripheral blood have alluded to delayed viral clearance or persistence, but the significance of these observations is uncertain.[192] In illness acquired during the first or second trimesters of pregnancy, the virus can infect the fetal-placental unit and precipitate abortion.[231] Cases acquired in the third trimester have not been reported to interrupt pregnancy. Congenital infections have been reported only when the virus was newly introduced to a susceptible adult population because almost all women in endemic areas have acquired immunity. Nonimmune travelers may have an increased risk.

Laboratory studies disclose peripheral leukocytosis, as high as 30,000/mm³ with a left shift, and hyponatremia. The CSF opening pressure is elevated in about 50% of patients.[228] Pleocytosis ranges from less than 10 to several thousand cells per cubic millimeter, with a median of several hundred cells of a predominantly lymphocytic composition. CSF protein may be normal or elevated up to 100 mg/dL. The electroencephalogram discloses a pattern of diffuse slow waves (theta or delta) with superimposed seizure activity, including periodic lateralized epileptiform discharges (PLEDS).[228,232] Brain imaging reveals diffuse white matter edema and abnormal signals mainly in the thalamus (often with evidence of hemorrhage), basal ganglia, cerebellum, midbrain, pons, and spinal cord.[233,234] Electromyography shows changes of chronic partial denervation consistent with anterior horn cell destruction.

In rural Asia, tuberculous, cerebral malaria, and bacterial meningitis (especially partially treated) are the principal alternative diagnoses.[7,82,235,236] Typhoid fever with tremors and ataxia, dengue infection with encephalopathy, lead poisoning, heat stroke, and enterovirus 71 encephalitis have all been confused with JE. In JE-endemic areas, any encephalitis outbreak is initially assumed to be JE, but the outbreak of the previously unknown Nipah virus in Malaysia in 1999 (see Chapter 161) and outbreaks of Chandipura virus infection in India since 2003 showed how easy it is to be misled.[237] WN and JE virus infections in particular may be mutually misrecognized because the viruses overlap in their distribution in Southwest Asia and can produce clinically indistinguishable illnesses in contemporaneous outbreaks and because differentiation in laboratory tests may be difficult.

WEST NILE ENCEPHALITIS

Most infections are asymptomatic; when symptoms do occur, they develop after an incubation period that typically lasts 2 to 6 days but may extend to 14 days, or even longer in immunosuppressed persons. In recent outbreaks, the syndrome of WN fever occurred in about 20% of infected individuals, who developed a sudden onset of an acute, nonspecific, influenza-like illness lasting 3 to 6 days, with high fever and chills, malaise, headache, backache, arthralgia, myalgia, and retroorbital pain, without overt neurologic signs.[94,95,177] Other nonspecific features include anorexia, nausea, vomiting, diarrhea, cough, and sore throat. In some epidemics, a flushed face, conjunctival injection, and generalized lymphadenopathy were common, and a maculopapular or pale roseolar rash was reported in about 50% of patients, more frequently in children. In one outbreak, 20% of patients with WN fever were reported to have hepatomegaly, and 10% had splenomegaly.[238] Myocarditis, pancreatitis, and hepatitis have also been described occasionally in severe WN virus infection.

Neurologic disease occurs in fewer than 1% of infected individuals. Patients typically have a febrile prodrome of 1 to 7 days, which may be biphasic, before developing neurologic symptoms (Fig. 153-6). Although in most cases, the prodrome is nonspecific, 15% to 20% of patients have features suggestive of WN fever, including eye pain, facial congestion, or a rash; fewer than 5% have lymphadenopathy.[239] In recent outbreaks, approximately two thirds of hospitalized patients had encephalitis (with or without signs of meningeal irritation), and one third had meningitis.[100,240,241] Acute flaccid paralysis caused by virus infection of the anterior horn of the spinal cord (myelitis) has been recognized in recent outbreaks.[242-244] The clinical picture suggests poliomyelitis; paralysis is frequently asymmetrical and may or may not be associated with meningoencephalitis. Once paralysis is established, little long-term improvement has been described. Although convulsions occurred in about 30% of patients in the early descriptions of

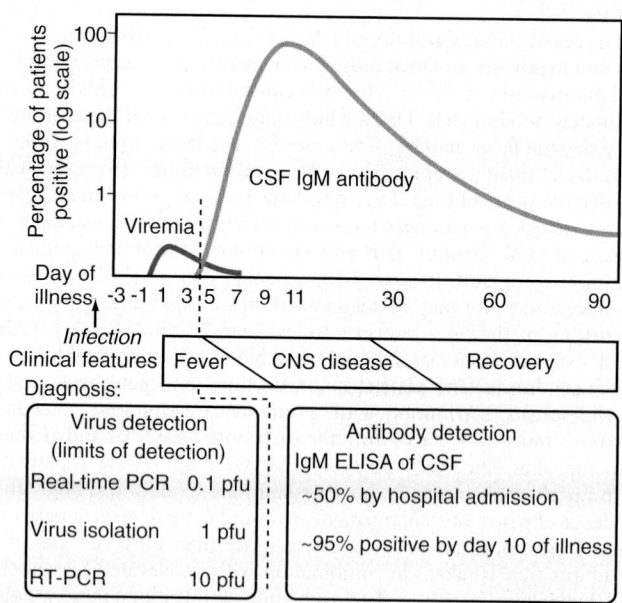

Figure 153-6 Schematic representation of the clinical course of West Nile encephalitis. Schematic includes viremia, development of antibody, and implications for diagnosis (as approximate percentage of patients). Limits of virus detection are expressed as plaque-forming units (pfu) per 100 μL; human viremia is thought to be less than 10 pfu/100 μL. The first day of fever is taken as the first day of illness; most patients are not admitted to hospital until day 3 to 5 of illness. CSF, cerebrospinal fluid; CNS, central nervous system; ELISA, enzyme-linked immunosorbent assay; IgM, immunoglobulin M; PCR, polymerase chain reaction; RT, reverse transcriptase. *(From Solomon T, Ooi MH. West Nile encephalitis. BMJ. 2003;326:865-869.)*

WNE, they did not appear to be an important feature in the more recent outbreaks.[241,245] Other neurologic features include cranial neuropathies, optic neuritis, and ataxia. Stiffness, rigidity, spasms, bradykinesia, and tremors, associated with basal ganglia damage, have also recently been recognized in WNE.[245,246]

In recent outbreaks, overall case-fatality rates for hospitalized patients ranged from 4% to 14% but were higher in older patients.[240,241,245] Other risk factors for death include the presence of profound weakness, deep coma, failure to produce IgM antibody, impaired immunity, and coexisting illness such as hypertension or diabetes mellitus.[241,247] Neurologic sequelae are common among survivors. In one study, half of hospitalized patients still had a functional deficit at discharge,[248] and only one third had recovered fully by 1 year.

About 50% of patients have a peripheral leukocytosis, and 15% have leukopenia.[241,248] Hyponatremia sometimes occurs in patients with encephalitis. Examination of the CSF typically shows a moderate lymphocytic pleocytosis, although sometimes there are no cells, or neutrophils may predominate. The protein is moderately elevated, and the glucose ratio is typically normal. Magnetic resonance imaging may show high signal intensities in the thalamus in T_2-weighted images and diffusion-weighted images in some patients, although this is a late finding and occurs in the more severely ill patients (Fig. 153-7).[245,246] Electroencephalograms show diffuse slowing and, in some cases, focal seizure activity. Nerve conduction studies typically show the reduced motor axonal amplitudes consistent with anterior horn cell damage, although there may also be some slowing of conduction velocities and some changes to sensory nerves.[177]

ST. LOUIS ENCEPHALITIS

SLE has been classified into three syndromes, characterized respectively by constitutional symptoms and headache (febrile headache), aseptic meningitis, and fatal encephalitis.[1,103,108] The proportion of cases in each category is age dependent, with increasing proportions of encephalitis and fatal cases in adults, especially in elderly people. The illness usually begins with a febrile prodrome of malaise, fever, headache, and myalgias, sometimes with upper respiratory or abdominal symptoms, that evolves over several days to more than 1 week with progressive lethargy, periods of confusion, and the onset of tremors, clumsiness, and ataxia. Vomiting and diarrhea are common, and some patients complain of dysuria, urgency, and incontinence.

Altered consciousness, marked by confusion, delirium, or somnolence, is the predominant presenting feature, and generalized motor weakness is more usual than are focal signs. Indications of meningeal irritation are inconstant and are elicited more often in children. Mental clouding may be subtle and manifested only by slight disorientation.

Most patients do not progress to deep coma. Tremulousness involving the eyelids, tongue, lips, and extremities is usual, and cerebellar and cranial nerve signs are common.[106,249] Various abnormal movements may be present, including myoclonic jerks and nystagmus. Convulsions are infrequent and signal a poor prognosis, except in children; subtle motor seizures also have been reported. Most patients improve over several days; however, pneumonia, thrombophlebitis and pulmonary embolism, stroke, gastrointestinal hemorrhage, and nosocomial infection can complicate recovery. The mortality rate is 8% overall and 20% among patients older than 60 years of age. In recovered adults, asthenia, emotional lability, anxiety, irritability, forgetfulness, tremor, dizziness, and unsteadiness may persist for months, accompanied by tremor, asymmetrical deep tendon reflexes, and visual disturbances.[250] No cases of clinical relapse or progressive illness have been described. Infants and young children frequently exhibit significant neurologic sequelae when discharged, but psychomotor function is usually recovered on later follow-up.[251] Little is known of the risk or outcome of congenital infection. Pregnancy and delivery progressed normally in one case in which infection was acquired during the third trimester (T. F. Tsai, unpublished observation). HIV-positive individuals appear to be at greater risk for acquisition of SLE, but whether this is related to their immune status or to other factors (e.g., increased risk for exposure due to homelessness) is not clear.[105]

The peripheral white cell count may be slightly elevated. In some patients, microscopic hematuria, proteinuria, and pyuria have been reported. Hyponatremia due to syndrome of inappropriate secretion of antidiuretic hormone (SIADH) occurs in more than one third of patients, and the concentrations of ALT and creatine phosphokinase may be slightly elevated. One third of patients have an increased CSF opening pressure, and there is typically a moderate mononuclear pleocytosis, with an elevated protein concentration. The electroencephalogram shows diffuse slowing and seizure activity, including PLEDs. Magnetic resonance imaging may show high signal intensity in the substantia nigra.[252] The diagnosis should be suspected if the case is one of a cluster in the summer or early fall, especially if the patient is an elderly or homeless person. A cerebral ischemic event, heat stroke, medication or drug toxicity, or other cause of delirium or encephalopathy has frequently been the initial diagnosis in confirmed cases. Other infectious causes of aseptic meningitis or acute encephalitis, including WNE, which can be transmitted contemporaneously, cannot easily be distinguished on a clinical basis.

TICK-BORNE ENCEPHALITIS

Infection leads to symptoms of TBE in only 1 in 250 persons. Three quarters of patients are able to recall a tick bite occurring a median of

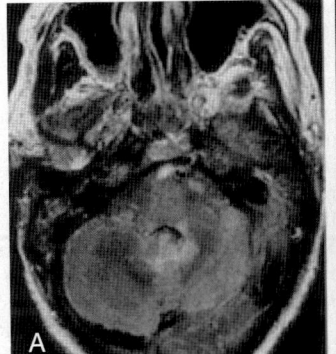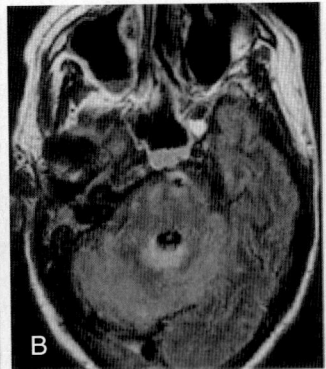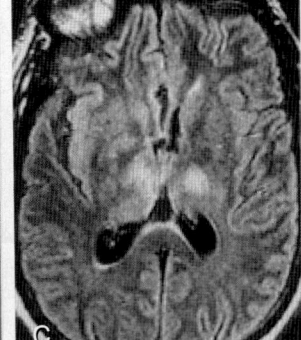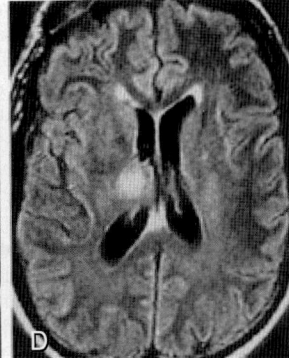

Figure 153-7 Magnetic resonance imaging changes in West Nile encephalitis. Fluid-attenuated inversion recovery images for a patient with West Nile encephalitis on day 10 of hospitalization, showing increased signal intensity in the periventricular gray matter of the fourth ventricle at the vermis of the cerebellum (**A** and **B**) and increased signal intensity in both thalami and the right caudate nucleus (**C** and **D**). *(From Solomon T, Dung NM, Kneen R, et al. Seizures and raised intracranial pressure in Vietnamese patients with Japanese encephalitis. Brain. 2002;125:1084-1093. By permission of the Oxford University Press.)*

8 days (range, 4 to 28 days) before symptoms developed.[187,253,254] The illness usually begins with a nonspecific grippe of fever, malaise, headache, nausea, vomiting, and myalgias that may be accompanied by fasciculation. Within 1 week, these symptoms resolve spontaneously. In most patients who have the "febrile form" of the disease, there are no further symptoms,[109] but in others who progress to more severe illness, the remission of symptoms is temporary, usually 2 to 8 days (range, 1 to 20 days), before high fever, headache, and vomiting resume. The second phase may be limited to a "meningeal form" with aseptic meningitis (commonly in children), or it may manifest as a "meningoencephalitis form," a "poliomyelitic form" with poliomyelitis-like flaccid paralysis, or a "polyradiculoneuritic form" with a Guillain-Barré–like paralysis, which usually resolves spontaneously. In one series, almost 50% of hospitalized patients had meningitis, 40% had meningoencephalitis, and 10% had meningoencephalomyelitis.[255] Neurologic infections usually are benign in children, whereas severe disease occurs more often in elderly persons. The Far Eastern form of TBE is reported as more severe, with fatalities occurring in 20% of hospitalized patients and residual neurologic sequelae in up to 60% of recovered patients.[193] Although differences in hospital admission rates may have confounded some of these observations, intrinsic differences in the neurovirulence of different TBE viral subtypes have been shown in experimental animal infections.

Early prodromal symptoms may be undetected in children, whose illness in more than two thirds of cases consists of aseptic meningitis. Altered consciousness, ataxia, tremor, paresthesias, focal signs, and less often, seizures characterize the presentation with encephalitis. Limb weakness and paralysis usually represent lower motor neuron lesions caused by myelitis or radicular neuritis; paresis may be transient, or it may evolve to permanent weakness and muscular atrophy. The shoulder girdle and upper limb musculature are affected most frequently, and urinary bladder continence and other autonomic functions can also be disturbed. Involvement of cranial nerves III, VII, IX, X, and XI produces gaze and peripheral facial paralysis and dysphagia. The outcome generally is good, especially in children, but the prognosis varies with age. A hemorrhagic syndrome has been reported in some cases and also in a laboratory-acquired louping ill infection.[256]

About 1% of cases are fatal, most often in elderly people. Sequelae are reported in up to 40% to 60% of patients, most frequently consisting of psychological disturbances such as asthenia, headache, memory loss and decreased concentration, anxiety, and emotional lability. Residual motor abnormalities include ataxia and incoordination, tremor, dysphasia, and in fewer than 5% of cases, specific cranial or spinal muscular paralysis.[187,257] Progressive motor weakness and epilepsia partialis continua (Kozhevnikov's epilepsy) are specific syndromes that may reflect a chronic encephalitic process. Pneumonia, heart failure, and other complications associated with prolonged hospitalization have been reported.

Powassan encephalitis is a severe encephalitis with a case-fatality rate of about 10%. Focal features have occurred in more than 50% of reported cases; in one patient, the clinical presentation with olfactory hallucinations and temporal lobe seizures mimicked herpes encephalitis.[258] Significant residua of hemiplegia, quadriplegia, or aphasia may result, and spinal paralysis with residual muscular wasting is similar to the myelitis associated with TBE.

Examination of the peripheral blood in TBE discloses leukopenia in the initial phase of illness, and leukocytosis up to 20,000/mm^3 during the second phase, with a transition to leukopenia again before recovery. Thrombocytopenia can also occur in the initial viremic phase.[259] An elevated erythrocyte sedimentation rate and C-reactive protein concentration are common by the time patients present with neurologic disease, and elevated ALT and AST levels and electrocardiographic abnormalities have been reported anecdotally.[253] There is a moderate lymphocytic CSF pleocytosis (average, <100 leukocytes/mm^3). The CSF protein level, although normal at the onset of neurologic symptoms, rises during the next 6 weeks, with an increase in the IgG index, indicating intrathecal synthesis. The albumin CSF-to-serum ratio, indicating disturbed blood-brain barrier permeability,

can remain abnormal for as long as 1 year.[187] The number and distribution of CSF lymphocytes and their cell markers differ in TBE and neuroborreliosis, a fact that may have diagnostic value in rapidly identifying patients for antibiotic treatment.[181] Abnormal magnetic resonance imaging signals are found most consistently in the thalami and basal ganglia.[260] Electroencephalograms show diffuse slowing in 90% of patients with encephalitis, with or without focal abnormalities.[253]

Although a history of tick bite is not given in all cases, exposure to an endemic focus during the transmission season should trigger suspicion. TBE is transmitted under the same circumstances as *Borrelia burgdorferi*, and clinically, their radicular and aseptic meningitis syndromes can overlap. Anecdotal observations suggest that neurologic symptoms of Lyme disease may occur more often in the context of concurrent TBE, and, conversely, that TBE may be more severe in a dual infection.[197,198] TBE results in a more prolonged course of illness and hospitalization than do the other acute encephalitides of presumed viral origin; this pattern and the presence of spinal paralysis may aid in making the diagnosis.

Laboratory Diagnosis

Viral isolation is relevant to the diagnosis of suspected YF and dengue because patients may present while still viremic and viral infectivity titers in blood are sufficiently high that attempts may be successful. However, real-time reverse transcriptase–PCR (RT-PCR) has become the technique of choice to detect viremia. Identifying the infective dengue viral serotype is important chiefly for public health reasons, but an individual patient also may benefit because future exposure to other serotypes places the patient at higher risk for DHF. Neurotropic flaviviruses can occasionally be isolated from blood taken within the first week of illness and before the onset of neurologic symptoms, or later if patients are immunosuppressed. In general, viral recovery from blood is successful only before an antibody response develops. Contrary to expectation, the isolation of neurotropic viruses from the CSF is usually unsuccessful except in the early stages of fulminant illness.

Tissue samples, whether from biopsy or autopsy, ideally should be divided into aliquots that are frozen at −70° C for viral isolation and fixed in buffered formalin and glutaraldehyde for light and electron microscopy. Viscerotomy liver samples are frequently taken after death as a means of postmortem YF diagnosis, but because pathologic changes are not pathognomonic, a purely histologic diagnosis should be considered presumptive and should be supplemented with immunohistochemical staining using viral-specific antibodies. Liver biopsy should never be attempted from patients with suspected YF, because they are at risk for fatal hemorrhage. SLE, WN, TBE, and JE viruses have been isolated from brain, lung, liver, spleen, and kidney with varied success, depending on the duration of illness and the day of death. Diverse areas of the brain and spinal cord should be sampled. JE virus is rarely cultured from peripheral blood using conventional techniques, but culture of virus from white blood cells separated from blood clots may be positive.[261] SLE virus was also isolated from vitreous humor in one case. Suckling mice and C6/36 or AP61 mosquito cell cultures are the most sensitive systems for viral isolation, but Vero, LLCMK$_2$, PS, and other continuous vertebrate cell lines are also used.[262]

Multiplex PCR assays in various formats that simultaneously identify the presence of dengue virus and its serotype in serum samples are used only in specialized laboratories in the United States and several Asian, African, and South American countries.[263] YF virus genomic sequences have also been detected in blood, but clinical experience is limited. In patients with flavivirus encephalitis, RT-PCR of the CSF has not proved very useful, although it may have a role in the detection of TBE virus in acute serum. However, real-time (TaqMan) PCR has proved sensitive in detecting WN virus in the CSF and serum and has been used for screening of blood products.[97,263]

Laboratory diagnosis of most cases, especially in travelers who come to clinical attention after viremia has cleared, depends principally on the serologic testing of serum and, in the case of neurologic infections, the CSF.[264] IgM detection by antibody capture enzyme-linked immunosorbent assay (ELISA) is the preferred technique for a specific diagnosis, although some laboratories successfully detect IgM and IgG antibodies by indirect immunofluorescence assay. The assay is more than 95% sensitive when serum specimens obtained between 7 and 10 days after the onset are tested. In secondary flavivirus infections, a combination of IgM and IgG ELISA is 100% sensitive as early as 4 to 5 days after the onset of illness. Both CSF and serum should be examined in cases of flavivirus encephalitis because IgM may appear earlier in the CSF. If both specimens are tested, positive results are obtained in almost all patients by 10 days after the onset of illness, with, in general, a 10% increase in cumulative positivity per day (see Fig. 153-6). However, some patients die without making an antibody response.[177] Serum IgM in dengue infection declines to undetectable levels within 60 days, but antibodies persist for up to 9 months in recovered SLE and TBE patients and for longer than 16 months in some WNE patients,[265] potentially limiting the specificity of tests (see later discussion).

Heterologous reactions with other flaviviruses are problematic where numerous flaviviruses cocirculate due to extensive serologic cross-reactivity between flaviviruses, but in tropical Asia, where only JE and dengue viruses infect humans, the infections are easily distinguished. Circumstances are more complex in Africa and even in Australia, where more flaviviruses cocirculate. Recent vaccination against JE or YF, or recent infection with dengue or SLE virus, may cause a false-positive WN virus IgM antibody test result; neutralization assays such as the plaque reduction neutralization test and ELISA that detect antibody to NS5 are more specific.[266] Fractionation of IgM before hemagglutination inhibition testing and competitive epitope-blocking ELISA improve specificity. However, among sera from African patients, all serologic approaches frequently fail to resolve previous and recent infections. Heterologous flavivirus antibodies have become an issue even among specimens submitted in the United States for arboviral diagnosis. Previous dengue virus infection, reflecting prior exposures in persons who have resided abroad, is now a frequent finding that can interfere with interpretation of the serologic diagnosis of a recent flavivirus infection. These heterologous dengue antibodies frequently pose difficulties in the interpretation of tests for SLE, WNE, and Powassan encephalitis. Although neutralization tests provide the greatest specificity, they are time-consuming, are expensive to perform, are offered only in specialized laboratories, and require control reference sera to obtain reliable results. Hemagglutination inhibition and complement fixation tests are now used infrequently, but they still have utility under some circumstances. Complement fixation antibodies, which recognize NS1 protein, are relatively specific in distinguishing between antigenic complexes, and because they rise rather late (often 4 to 6 weeks after the onset) and decline with a half-life of 3 years, positive reactions indicate infection in the intermediate period after the disappearance of IgM antibodies. Recent studies have shown that NS1 protein is present early in dengue virus infection and offers a new technique to diagnose a dengue virus infection based on NS1 antigen capture ELISA.[267] Hemagglutination inhibition and neutralizing antibodies can persist for decades after infection. Rapid immunochromatographic tests formatted as small folders to detect dengue and JE IgM and IgG have demonstrated high sensitivity and specificity in field evaluations (100% and 90%, respectively, for the dengue test) and should facilitate laboratory confirmation of cases in clinical facilities.[268]

In a patient with a compatible illness, a case is confirmed by a fourfold change in the serum antibody titer or, alternatively, in encephalitis patients, by the demonstration of viral-specific IgM in CSF, reflecting intrathecal immune response. An elevated serum IgM antibody level alone is considered presumptive evidence of recent infection if high IgM prevalence rates in the population prevail because of frequent asymptomatic infections and because antibodies may persist beyond a single transmission season.

Serologic testing for SLE, WN, dengue, and other selected arboviruses is performed at several private laboratories, most state laboratories, the Centers for Disease Control and Prevention, the U.S. Army Medical Research Institute for Infectious Diseases, and other reference laboratories. In addition, an indirect immunofluorescence assay kit for the domestic arboviruses that includes an SLE antigen can be purchased in the United States, and a TBE ELISA kit can be obtained in Europe. Dengue immunochromatographic folders and ELISA kits are sold in Asia and Australia.[269]

Prevention and Therapy

YELLOW FEVER

Hospitalization in an intensive care facility where the patient can be sequestered from mosquitoes is recommended to provide close clinical monitoring and supportive care and to prevent anthroponotic transmission. Blood in the acute phase of illness is potentially infectious. No antiviral therapy is available, and specific supportive interventions have not been evaluated. General support with oxygen, fluids, and pressors is indicated to treat and prevent hypotension and metabolic acidosis. Histamine-2 (H2) receptor antagonists and sucralfate may be of value in preventing or ameliorating gastric bleeding. Avoidance of sedatives and drugs dependent on hepatic metabolism is prudent, and the medication-dosing intervals should be adjusted with reduced renal function. Encephalopathy should be investigated for treatable metabolic causes, particularly hypoglycemia. Fresh-frozen plasma and vitamin K have been administered to replenish clotting factors. The effect of heparin therapy is unproved. Secondary infections should be pursued and treated.

YF is vaccine preventable with the attenuated 17D vaccine, which produces immunity in more than 95% of recipients and long-term (at least 10 years and possibly lifelong) protection with a single 0.5-mL subcutaneous dose.[3] Vaccination has been associated with anaphylaxis in 1 of every 116,000 doses, but the relative roles of hypersensitivity to chicken eggs and gelatin are unclear because the vaccine is produced in chick embryos, and gelatin, which is added as a vaccine stabilizer, has been implicated in other hypersensitivity events.[270] Equally serious, however, are rare but potentially fatal cases of vaccine-associated CNS infection or systemic illness, mimicking wild-type infection, which have been reported from multiple countries. To date, a total of 41 cases of yellow fever vaccine–associated viscerotropic disease (YEL-AVD) have been reported. All known cases are primary vaccinees and range in age from 4 to 79 years, with a mean age of about 50 years. Clinical signs of high fever, arthralgia, myalgia, headache, and vomiting usually occur with 2 to 5 days after immunization and are followed by elevated liver enzymes and bilirubin, and thrombocytopenia and lymphocytopenia. Subsequently, combinations of fulminant hepatitis, shock, renal failure, and disturbances of coagulation, all consistent with YF, have been observed. When laboratory tests for virus have been undertaken, large quantities of vaccine virus are detected in tissues or blood. The clinical and laboratory picture, plus the histology and immunohistochemistry at autopsy, are similar to those seen with wild-type YF infection. The case-fatality rate is about 60%. There have been 39 cases of YEL-AND, but only 2 have been fatal. The age range is 1 to 78 years, with a mean of about 43 years of age. Clinical signs of headache and fever (>101.5°F), focal neurologic dysfunction, and altered mental state are first seen from 2 to 30 days after immunization and are accompanied by CSF pleocytosis or elevated protein.[271-273]

The rate of YEL-AVD is 0.3 to 0.4 per 100,000 doses administered, which has resulted in no change in vaccine recommendations for travelers. However, providers are admonished to ensure that the traveler's destination is an endemic area because two cases of vaccine-associated systemic illness have occurred in persons traveling to areas free of YF. Because of the well-established risk for vaccine-associated encephalitis in infants, YF vaccine is contraindicated in infants younger than 4 months of age and is recommended for 4- to 9- month-old infants only under situations of high risk. YF and measles vaccines are coadministered at the 9-month Expanded Program of Immunization visit under WHO–United Nations Children's Fund recommendations in 35 African countries; however, compliance is low. The vaccine's risk in pregnancy has not been established. Cord blood IgM viral antibodies indicating congenital infection were reported in one case without evidence of birth defects.[274,275] In small studies, the vaccine was less immunogenic in pregnant women and was asymptomatic HIV-infected adults (77% antibody response) and HIV-infected infants (17% antibody response). No adverse events were reported in the latter two studies, but a fatal CNS infection has been reported in one HIV-infected vaccinee.[274-279]

Travelers to at-risk South American and African countries should receive the vaccine at 10-year intervals to meet international requirements. The vaccine can be given concurrently with measles, oral polio, hepatitis A or B, meningococcal polysaccharide, oral or intramuscular typhoid, or oral cholera vaccines; chloroquine; or immune serum globulin.

Prevention of epidemic *A. aegypti*–borne YF follows the approach for dengue control, with the reduction of peridomestic breeding sites. In dry savanna and urban locations where drinking water frequently must be stored, the simple expedient of covering the containers or reservoirs eliminates a principal source of breeding. Surveillance of viral activity by monitoring of viral infection rates in sylvatic mosquitoes has been proposed as an early warning system for West and Central Africa, where outbreaks frequently emerge in a region-wide distribution. The discovery of intensified viral activity, even in a small number of sentinel sites, may be a sufficiently sensitive predictor of viral activity in a broader area to trigger timely and effective mass immunization. In South America, surveys to detect dead monkeys on the forest floor are conducted to monitor viral transmission and risk for its spillover to humans.

DENGUE AND DENGUE HEMORRHAGIC FEVER

Antipyretics may help to relieve the symptoms of dengue fever, but to avert Reye's syndrome and hemostatic complications, aspirin should not be used. Oral rehydration is indicated to replace losses from vomiting and high fever. Attentive clinical monitoring of patients with suspected DHF-DSS and anticipatory and supportive care are lifesaving and have reduced fatality rates by 50- to 100-fold. Treatment algorithms and protocols to monitor patients by clinical and laboratory markers based on the practice at the Queen Sirikit National Institute of Child Health (formerly Bangkok Children's Hospital) have been published.[280] The critical activities are monitoring of circulation and vascular leakage by serial clinical assessments of pulse, blood pressure, skin perfusion, urine output, and hematocrit, to trigger intravenous fluid therapy. An increase in hematocrit of greater than 20% (e.g., from 35% to 42%) indicates a significant loss of intravascular volume and the urgent need for fluid resuscitation. Normal saline is administered to maintain circulation and, under continued monitoring, for recurrent shock. Shock necessitates rapid intervention with isotonic crystalloid or colloid solutions, or, if needed, plasma or whole-blood transfusions.[281] Anecdotal reports suggest that desmopressin may reduce the need for intravenous fluids and improve hemostasis; however, no controlled trials have been performed.[282] Because vascular integrity is usually restored spontaneously in 48 hours, overhydration resulting in pulmonary edema is a risk, and positive-pressure ventilation with positive end-expiratory pressure may be needed. As a result of the danger of ARDS due to capillary leakage and excessive fluid administration, DHF-DSS has been reported to be the third most common cause of ARDS in hospitalized children in Malaysia.[221] Whole-blood, platelet, and fresh-frozen plasma transfusions may be needed if there is significant hemorrhage, but caution is indicated in the administration of heparin except in patients with clear signs of disseminated intravascular coagulopathy.[283] Preventive transfusions may be harmful and should be avoided, and invasive procedures should be minimized to avoid hemorrhagic complications. Treatment to end virus replication could be beneficial, although viremia levels usually are already decreasing dramatically at the time of presentation to health care providers.[284] In some locations, intravenous immune globulin has been used empirically, but no benefit has been established

in a controlled evaluation. Neither high-dose methylprednisolone (30 mg/kg) nor AC-17 (carbazochrome sodium sulfonate), which is believed to reduce vascular permeability, was beneficial in controlled trials.[285,286] Treatment with anti-TNF antibody and antioxidants is being evaluated in mouse models of dengue.[287,288] Secondary and concurrent infections should be investigated and treated.

Dengue prevention currently relies on public health and community-based *A. aegypti* control programs to remove and destroy mosquito-breeding sites.[46] The ubiquity of containers that potentially provide breeding habitats in urban neighborhoods and individual houses makes this a formidable challenge. Although a combination of vector surveillance, area treatment, and monitoring can be effective, it has rarely been successful for prolonged periods. Insecticidal fogging is considered unhelpful, but in sealed houses, indoor insecticidal sprays should be effectual.[289] Several approaches to vaccine development are being pursued. The most advanced approach is a tetravalent combination of traditionally attenuated dengue strains, although approaches using molecular attenuation and chimeric viruses are undergoing clinical evaluation.[8] Travelers are well advised to protect themselves by using repellents and insecticidal sprays indoors.

FLAVIVIRUS ENCEPHALITIS

No specific therapy for flavivirus encephalitis has been developed. Anecdotal use of IFN-α in the prophylaxis and treatment of JE and SLE cases has been reported, but a phase III randomized double-blind, placebo-controlled trial of interferon-α-2a in children with JE showed that it did not improve the outcome at hospital discharge or at 3 months' follow-up.[290] A mixture of JE-virus–neutralizing monoclonal antibodies was reportedly beneficial in a clinical trial in China, but considerable experience with TBE immune globulin therapy has highlighted the potential hazards of immunotherapy.[291,292] Passive immunization appears to have been associated with exacerbation of the disease, and its use, even within the recommended interval of 96 hours after a tick bite, should be undertaken with due caution. However, there were no reports of such deterioration in uncontrolled trials of immune globulin in WNE,[293] and a multicenter controlled trial of intravenous immune globulin in the treatment of WNE is underway in the United States. Humanized monoclonal antibodies against WN virus envelope protein have shown efficacy in mice and hamsters, even when given as a single dose on day 5 after infection, and when the virus has reached the CNS system.[294,295]

Corticosteroid therapy for TBE resulted in a more rapid reduction of fever but prolonged hospitalization, whereas in JE a small trial of corticosteroid treatment failed to show benefit or harm.[296] In a small controlled study, tetracycline administered as an immunomodulator was shown to reduce elaboration of proinflammatory cytokines and to hasten recovery from TBE.[297] Antisense oligomers that inhibit WN virus replication in vitro have been reported,[298] and an RNA interference screen approach has examined in detail virus and human host cell interactions, identifying potential targets for antiviral treatments.[299] In addition, cell-based high-throughput assays have been developed to screen compound libraries for agents effective against WN virus and other flaviviruses.[300]

Supportive care should focus on controlling seizures, providing ventilatory support in respiratory failure, and monitoring and reducing cerebral edema. In many parts of Asia, mannitol, corticosteroids, or both are given to patients with severe JE. Fluid and electrolyte administration should balance circulatory needs, the avoidance of cerebral edema, and SIADH. Secondary infections should be anticipated and treated, and careful nursing attention should be paid to minimize complications such as bed sores and contractures.

There are currently three JE vaccines licensed and others in various stages of development. An inactivated mouse brain–derived vaccine produced in Japan, Korea, Taiwan, Thailand, and Vietnam is administered in early childhood in two primary doses, with four to six additional boosters at various intervals until 15 years of age.[201] The efficacy in field trials was 91%. The Japanese and Korean vaccines have been distributed internationally to military personnel and travelers in three 1-mL doses, administered subcutaneously, on days 0, 7, and 30. Angioedema and generalized urticaria with onset up to 3 days after vaccination have occurred in about 0.3% of vaccinees; therefore, in travelers, the series should be completed 1 week before departure.[301] Anecdotal cases of acute disseminated encephalomyelitis temporally related to vaccination have been reported.[2] Because of vaccine side effects and the slight risk for acquiring the disease during travel, vaccination is not recommended routinely and is reserved for expatriates in Asia, persons with a high risk for exposure, and travelers spending more than 30 days during the transmission season in an endemic area (see Table 153-1). However, because individual cases have occurred in travelers with exposures as brief as a few days, more liberal use of vaccine may be appropriate in some circumstances.[91,92]

Because of the issues described previously, the mouse brain–derived vaccines are being phased out. Production of JE-VAX by the Biken laboratories in Japan has ceased, but newer vaccines are in development (Table 153-3).[302] These include tissue culture–derived inactivated vaccines, based on Beijing-1 and P3 strains of virus, which are produced in Japan and China for local use.

A live-attenuated vaccine (SA-14-14-2) developed by Chinese researchers has been used extensively in China, and since issues over the cells used in its production have been resolved, it has also been used in South Korea, Nepal, India, and Sri Lanka.[303] Two doses are administered during spring campaigns to children older than 1 year. The live vaccine, however, is highly efficacious after even one dose.[2,303,304] The vaccine has an extensive history of safe use, with respective efficacies of 98%. More than 9 million children were vaccinated in India in the summer of 2006.[305]

The structural genes from this vaccine have been inserted into the backbone genome of the YF 17D vaccine to make a live chimeric vaccine that is now in advanced development.[306] The SA14-14-2 attenuated virus was also used to make the new inactivated Vero-cell–derived vaccine, which proved safe and immunogenic in a noninferiority comparison with the Biken vaccine.[307] With the phasing out of the Biken vaccines, this vaccine is being considered as an alternative for travelers. The recommendations for JE vaccination in travelers are being reviewed by the Advisory Committee on Immunization Practices (ACIP). Whatever the vaccine availability and recommendations, to minimize the risk for acquiring infection, travelers should avoid outdoor exposure at dusk and should use mosquito repellents and mosquito-excluding bed nets.

No human vaccines against WN or SLE viruses are licensed; however, formalin-inactivated and canarypox-vectored WN virus vaccines for horses are commercially available in the United States. A live-attenuated chimeric WN/YF 17D vaccine is under clinical evaluation.[306,308] Chimeric vaccines of WN virus combined with dengue virus 2 or 4 have also been developed and provide complete protection against WN virus in challenge experiments.[309]

Two inactivated TBE vaccines, derived from chick embryo cells infected with European subtype TBE virus, are licensed in Europe and distributed with considerable uptake rates in areas that have a high transmission risk.[111] Mass vaccination has been practiced in Austria since the 1990s. Administration in three doses over a period of 1 year, with an additional booster 3 years later, has been highly effective in reducing rates of disease. An abbreviated 0-, 7-, and 21- or 28-day immunization schedule also is immunogenic.[310] Cross-protection against the Far Eastern subtype of TBE virus has been shown in animals, but clinical efficacy against the disease has not been reported. Chiefly mild adverse events (fever and local reactions) are reported; however, neurologic adverse events including Guillain-Barré syndrome have been noted, albeit without a proven causal association, in about 1 of every 1 million vaccinees. Although no formal cost benefit analysis has been done, the immunization campaign in Austria had an estimated yearly benefit in the 1990s that was equivalent to $80 million, on the basis of morbidity prevented, without taking into account the vaccination costs.[311]

The vaccine is not licensed in the United States and no longer is held as an investigational new drug by the U.S. Army. For most travelers, the risk for acquiring the disease is extremely low, and personal protective measures (e.g., avoidance of risky habitats, wearing protective clothing, using repellents) are appropriate. Expatriates may choose to be immunized abroad, and for the exceptional short-term traveler with high-risk activities, preexposure prophylaxis with TBE immune globulin (0.05 mL/kg intramuscularly) is an alternative, although its efficacy is unproved, and breakthrough cases and enhanced disease have been reported. Live-attenuated and naked DNA vaccines are under development.

Vector control is impractical as a means of JE prevention because of the extensive areas that must be treated. Pig immunization effec-

TABLE 153-3	Summary of Vaccines against Japanese Encephalitis			
Description	Virus Strain	Common Name	Manufacturer or Developer	Notes
Inactivated Vaccines				
Mouse brain	Nakayama	BIKEN	Japan, BIKEN	Manufactured for international distribution; production now discontinued
Mouse brain	Nakayama	Green Cross	Korea, Green Cross	Some available internationally through Green Cross partnership; distribution by India by Shanta Biotech
Mouse brain	Beijing-1		Japan	Manufactured for the domestic market
Primary hamster kidney	P3		China	Previously China's principal vaccine
Vero cell	P3		China	Recently licensed in China
Live Attenuated Vaccines				
Primary hamster kidney	SA14-14-2		China	Widely used in China, also in trials in Nepal and South Korea
Primary hamster kidney	SA14-5-3		China	Abandoned after clinical trials due to poor immunogenicity
Inactivated Vaccines in Advanced Development and Clinical Trials				
Vero cell	Beijing-1	BK-VJE	Japan, BIKEN	Targeted for Japanese market
Vero cell	Beijing-1	Kaketsuken	Japan, Kaketsuken	Targeted for Japanese market
Vero cell	SA14-14-2	JE-PIV/IC51	WRAIR, Intercell	Marketing and distribution agreement with Novartis for United States, Europe, and some Asian and Latin American markets
Live, Attenuated Chimeric Vaccines in Advanced Development and Clinical Trials				
Yellow fever 17D vectored	SA14-14-2	ChimeriVax-Je	Acambis	Marketing and distribution agreements with Sanofi Pasteur and Bharat Biotech International Ltd. (Indian subcontinent)

From Beasley DW, Lewthwaite P, Solomon T. Current use and development of vaccines for Japanese encephalitis. *Expert Opin Biol Ther.* 2008;8:95-106.

tively prevents abortions in sows and can modulate the transmission of disease to humans, but wide-scale implementation is impractical. Emergency truck-mounted or aerial applications of adulticides are routinely administered in response to SLE and WNE epidemics, usually in conjunction with programs of avian or mosquito surveillance that provide early warning of increased viral transmission. Public health warnings to avoid outdoor activities in the evening and rescheduling of evening high school football games and Halloween trick-or-treat activities to daylight hours were demonstrated to reduce the risk for acquiring SLE in central Florida. In the absence of effective therapies or prophylaxis, public health interventions are the only available preventive measures. Control of TBE in defined locations by the area-wide application of acaricides has been effective in reducing vector ticks, but widespread implementation is impractical.

Other Flavivirus Infections

MURRAY VALLEY ENCEPHALITIS

Murray Valley encephalitis virus is a member of the antigenic complex of JE, SLE, and WNE viruses, and, like them, it is transmitted in a mosquito-avian cycle, chiefly by *Culex annulirostris*. Foci of perennial viral transmission are maintained in western Australia, where sporadic cases and small outbreaks occur. Most sporadic cases occur in aboriginal children living in areas where they are exposed to the virus, but cases have also occurred among travelers to these areas,[312,313] including a visitor from Europe.[314] At infrequent intervals since the initial recognition of the disease in 1917, the virus has spread to the heavily populated southeastern river valleys, where it has produced larger outbreaks, most recently in 1981. Sporadic cases also have been recognized in Papua New Guinea. About 350 cases have been reported in total, with a case-fatality rate of 20% in the most recent outbreak. The onset of encephalitis is preceded by a prodrome of headache, nausea, vomiting, photophobia, and neck stiffness, followed within 2 to 5 days by changes in sensorium, stupor, and motor signs. Coma, limb paralysis, and respiratory depression necessitating ventilatory support

develop in severe cases. Recovery is followed by motor paralysis in severe cases and by milder motor disturbances and emotional and psychological symptoms in a higher proportion of survivors. Serologic diagnosis is potentially encumbered by cross-reactive antibodies to Kunjin, Kokobera, JE, Edge Hill, Alfuy, Sepik, dengue, and other flaviviruses in the region. Supportive treatment has reduced mortality and morbidity. Regional surveillance of sentinel chicken infections is maintained as an early warning system.

ROCIO ENCEPHALITIS

Rocio encephalitis was recognized to be the novel cause of a series of encephalitis outbreaks that occurred from 1975 to 1977 in the Ribiera Valley and Santista lowlands in coastal São Paulo and Paraná States, Brazil.[315] More than 1000 cases were identified, chiefly in fishermen and others with outdoor occupations. The virus was isolated from human brain, and its relationship to SLE virus was shown antigenically and, later, by genomic sequencing. The virus is transmitted from *Psorophora* sp. mosquitoes to birds, and human infections are incidental. Sporadic asymptomatic infections have been detected in field studies, but outbreaks have not recurred. In 1996, serologic evidence of infection was reported in Bahia State, far to the north, but the virus has not been isolated outside the original focus. A prodrome of fever, headache, malaise, vomiting, and conjunctivitis precedes the onset of altered consciousness, motor weakness, and frequently, cerebellar signs. Neurologic infection progresses to coma in one third of cases and death in 10%. Neurologic and psychological sequelae have been reported in 20% of survivors. Supportive treatment is potentially life-saving. Emergency applications of insecticides have been implemented in outbreak control.

KYASANUR FOREST DISEASE

The report of an outbreak of monkey deaths and hemorrhagic fever with jaundice in 1957 in the Kyasanur Forest of Mysore (now Karnataka) State, India, triggered an investigation of what was suspected to

TABLE 153-4	Less Commonly Recognized Flaviviral Infections			
Virus	**Clinical Syndrome**	**Geographic Distribution**	**Transmission Cycle**	**Mode of Transmission**
Alkhurma[119]	Hemorrhagic fever, encephalitis	Saudi Arabia	Presumably tick-borne	DC, ?V
Alma-Arasan[320]	Febrile illness, meningitis	Kazakhstan	*Ixodes persulcatus*–?	V
Apoi[323]	Encephalitis	Japan	Rodent–?	L
Banzi[324]	Nonspecific febrile illness	South and East Africa	*Culex rubinotus*–rodent	V
Bussuquara[325]	Fever, arthralgias	Brazil, Colombia, Panama	*Culex melaconion* spp.–rodent	V
Edge Hill[326]	Fever, polyarthritis	Australia	*Aedes vigilax*–marsupial	V
Ilhéus[325,327]	Fever, myalgia, encephalitis	Argentina, Brazil, Colombia, Guatemala, Panama, Trinidad	*Psorophora ferox*–bird	V, E
Karshi[320]	Nonspecific febrile illness	Uzbekistan	Various ticks–rodent	V
Kokobera[328]	Fever, polyarthralgia	Australia, Papua New Guinea	*Culex annulirostris*–? Marsupial	V
Koutango[1]	Fever, rash, arthralgia	West and Central Africa	Tick–rodent	L
Kunjin[95]	Fever, polyarthralgia, encephalitis	Australia, Malaysia, Thailand	*Culex annulirostris*–bird	V
Langat[329]	Fever, encephalitis	Malaysia, Thailand, Russia	*Ixodes* tick–rodent	V
Modoc[330]	Aseptic meningitis	Western United States, Canada	Rodent–rodent	Z
Negishi[323]	Encephalitis	Japan, China, Russia	Tick–unknown	L, V
Rio Bravo[331]	Nonspecific febrile illness, meningitis	Western United States, Canada	Bat–bat	Z, L
Sepik[332]	Nonspecific febrile illness	Papua New Guinea	*Mansonia* spp.–?	V
SPH 16111–related viruses[333]	Pneumonia, encephalitis, lymphadenopathy, rash	São Paulo, Brazil	Unknown	U
Spondweni[334]	Fever, arthralgia, rash	South and West Africa	*Aedes* spp.–?	L, V
Usutu[335]	Fever, rash	South and Central Africa	*Culex* spp.–bird	V
Wesselsbron[336]	Fever, arthralgia, rash, encephalitis	Sub-Saharan Africa, Thailand	*Aedes* spp.–?	V, L, DC
Zika[337]	Fever, rash, arthralgia	West, East, and Central Africa; Indonesia, Malaysia	*Aedes* spp.–monkey	V

DC, contact with infected sheep; E, experimental infection; L, laboratory-acquired infection; U, unknown; V, vector-borne; Z, zoonotic infection.

be the much-feared introduction of YF to Asia.[316-319] The virus, isolated from dead langur monkeys and *Haemaphysalis* sp. ticks, was shown to be a novel member of the antigenic complex of tick-borne flaviviruses that was transmitted between various ixodid ticks and forest rodents, insectivores, and monkeys. That epidemic and subsequent sporadic cases and outbreaks occurred during the dry season among peasants clearing forests for pasture, and the endemic area gradually spread and enlarged in connection with those activities. Serologic evidence of infection has also been reported in northwestern India and from the Andaman Islands. Despite the local availability of vaccine, from January 1999 through January 2005, an increasing number of cases were detected in Kamataka State of India. The incubation period is 3 to 8 days, after which illness begins abruptly with fever, headache, chills, vomiting, myalgia, photophobia, and conjunctival suffusion. Facial and conjunctival hyperemia, lymphadenopathy, hepatosplenomegaly, and petechiae are found on examination. Diffuse hemorrhages from the nares, gums, and gastrointestinal tract develop, with hemorrhagic pulmonary edema in 40% of cases and renal failure in severe cases. After defervescence and a remission of symptoms for as long as 1 to 3 weeks, a second phase of illness develops, with neurologic symptoms in 15% to 50% of patients. Laboratory findings are similar to those of DHF, with leukopenia, thrombocytopenia, an elevated hematocrit reflecting hemoconcentration, and elevated hepatic transaminase levels. Patients have detectable viremias up to 12 days after the onset of illness. Between 5% and 10% of cases are fatal, and iridokeratitis has been reported in survivors. A genotypic variant of Kyasanur Forest disease virus, Alkhurma haemorrhagic fever virus, has been recently identified in Saudi Arabia and shares 89% nucleotide homology with Kyasanur Forest disease virus.

OMSK HEMORRHAGIC FEVER

Omsk hemorrhagic fever virus is transmitted between *Dermacentor* sp. ticks and small mammals in forest-steppe zones of the Omsk, Novosibirsk, Kurgan, and Tjumen regions of western Siberia, but the disease emerged in significant form only after muskrats were introduced to the region to establish a fur industry.[320-322] Outbreaks between 1945 and 1958 led to muskrat epizootics and 1500 human cases, chiefly among trappers, their family members, and laboratory workers. Infection is transmitted directly from infected animal tissues or by tick bite, with a peak in spring or early summer and another peak in autumn. The illness resembles Kyasanur Forest disease, but neuropsychiatric sequelae have been reported more often. The case-fatality rate is less than 3%. Inactivated TBE vaccine (produced in Russia) has been reported to offer cross-protection against the disease.

LESS COMMONLY RECOGNIZED FLAVIVIRUS INFECTIONS

Small numbers or even single cases of the diseases listed in Table 153-4 have been reported. In some instances, experimental human infection (evaluated as cancer therapy) provides the only knowledge of their pathogenicity.

REFERENCES

1. Lindenbach BD, Thiel HJ, Rice CM. Flaviviruses. In: Knipe DM, Howley PM, eds. *Field's Virology*. 5th ed. Philadelphia: Lippincott Williams-Wilkins; 2007:1103-1113.
2. Halstead SB, Tsai TF. Japanese encephalitis vaccines. In: Plotkin SA, Orenstein WA, eds. *Vaccines*. 4th ed. Philadelphia: WB Saunders; 2004:919-958.
3. Monath TP. Yellow fever vaccine. In: Plotkin SA, Orenstein WA, eds. *Vaccines*. 4th ed. Philadelphia: WB Saunders; 2004:815-880.
4. Barrett PN, Dorner F, Plotkin SA. Tick-borne encephalitis vaccine. In: Plotkin SA, Orenstein WA, eds. *Vaccines*. 4th ed. Philadelphia: WB Saunders; 2004:767-780.
5. Halstead S, Vaughn DW. Dengue fever vaccine. In: Jong EC, Zuckerman JN, eds. *Travelers' Vaccines*. Hamilton, Ontario: BC Decker Inc; 2004:298-310.
6. Freedman DO, Weld LH, Kozarsky PE, et al. Spectrum of disease and relation to place of exposure among ill returned travelers. *N Engl J Med*. 2006;354:119-130.
7. Tsai TF, Niklasson B. Arboviruses and zoonotic viruses. In: DuPont HL, Steffen R, eds. *Textbook of Travel Medicine and Health*. 2nd ed. Hamilton, Ontario: BC Decker; 2001:290-312.
8. Bryant JE, Holmes EC, Barrett AD. Out of Africa: a molecular perspective on the introduction of yellow fever virus into the Americas. *PLoS Pathog*. 2007;3:e75.
9. Barrett AD, Higgs S. Yellow fever: a disease that has yet to be conquered. *Annu Rev Entomol*. 2007;52:209-229.
10. Vaughn DW, Whitehead SS, Durbin AP. Dengue. In: Barret AD, Stanberry L, eds. *Vaccines for Biodefense and Emerging and Neglected Diseases*. Philadelphia: Elsevier; 2009:285-321.
11. Morales MA, Barrandeguy M, Fabbri C, et al. West Nile virus isolation from equines in Argentina, 2006. *Emerg Infect Dis*. 2006;12:1559-1561.
12. Reimann CA, Hayes EB, Diguiseppi C, et al. Epidemiology of neuroinvasive arboviral disease in the United States, 1999-2007. *Am J Trop Med Hyg*. 2008;79:974-979.
13. May FJ, Li L, Zhang S, et al. Genetic variation of St. Louis encephalitis virus. *J Gen Virol*. 2008;89:1901-1910.
14. Reisen WK, Lothrop HD, Wheeler SS, et al. Persistent West Nile virus transmission and the apparent displacement St. Louis encephalitis virus in southeastern California, 2003-2006. *J Med Entomol*. 2008;45:494-508.
15. Suss J. Epidemiology and ecology of TBE relevant to the production of effective vaccines. *Vaccine*. 2003;21(Suppl 1):S19-S35.
16. Heinz FX, Allison SL. Flavivirus structure and membrane fusion. *Adv Virus Res*. 2003;59:63-97.
17. Kuhn RJ, Zhang W, Rossmann MG, et al. Structure of dengue virus: Implications for flavivirus organization, maturation, and fusion. *Cell*. 2002;108:717-725.
18. Rey FA, Heinz FX, Mandl C, et al. Nature: The envelope glycoprotein from tick-borne encephalitis virus at 2 A resolution. *Nature*. 1995;375:291-298.
19. Co MD, Terajima M, Cruz J, et al. Human cytotoxic T lymphocyte responses to live attenuated 17D yellow fever vaccine: Iden-

tification of HLA-B35-restricted CTL epitopes on nonstructural proteins NS1, NS2b, NS3, and the structural protein E. *Virology*. 2002;293:151-163.
20. Brinton M, Perelygen AA. Genetic resistance to flaviviruses. *Adv Virus Res*. 2003;60:43-85.
21. Stephens HA, Klaythong R, Sirikong M, et al. HLA-A and -B allele associations with secondary dengue virus infections correlate with disease severity and the infecting viral serotype in ethnic Thais. *Tissue Antigens*. 2002;60:309-318.
22. Muñoz-Jordan JL, Sánchez-Burgos GG, Laurent-Rolle M, et al. Inhibition of interferon signaling by dengue virus. *Proc Natl Acad Sci U S A*. 2003;100:14333-14338.
23. Best SM, Morris KL, Shannon JG, et al. Inhibition of interferon-stimulated JAK-STAT signaling by a tick-borne flavivirus and identification of NS5 as an interferon antagonist. *J Virol*. 2005;79:12828-12839.
24. Wei HY, Jiang LF, Fang DY, et al. Dengue virus type 2 infects human endothelial cells through binding of the viral envelope glycoprotein to cell surface polypeptides. *J Gen Virol*. 2003;84:3095-3098.
25. Hilgard P, Stockert R. Heparan sulfate proteoglycans initiate dengue virus infection of hepatocytes. *Hepatology*. 2000;32:1069-1077.
26. Van Regenmortel M, Fauquet CM, Bishop DH. Flaviviruses. In: *Virus Taxonomy. Seventh Report of the International Committee on Taxonomy of Viruses*. San Diego: Academic Press; 2000:859-878.
27. Cook S, Holmes EC. A multigene analysis of the phylogenetic relationships among the flaviviruses (family: Flaviviridae) and the evolution of vector transmission. *Arch Virol*. 1998;151:309-325.
28. Chang GJ, Cropp BC, Kinney RM, et al. Nucleotide sequence variation of the envelope protein gene identifies two distinct genotypes of yellow fever virus. *J Virol*. 1995;69:5773.
29. Rico-Hesse R, Harrison LM, Salas RA, et al. Origins of dengue type 2 viruses associated with increased pathogenicity in the Americas. *Virology*. 1997;230:244.
30. Hanna JN, Ritchie SA, Phillips DA, et al. An outbreak of Japanese encephalitis in the Torres Strait, Australia, 1995. *Med J Aust*. 1996;165:256.
31. Trent DW, Monath TP, Bown GS, et al. Variation among strains of St Louis encephalitis virus: Basis for genetic, pathogenic and epidemiologic classification. *Ann N Y Acad Sci*. 1980;354:219.
32. Rico-Hesse R. Microevolution and virulence of dengue viruses. *Adv Virus Res*. 2003;59:315-341.
33. Monath TP. Yellow fever: An update. *Lancet Infect Dis*. 2001;1:11-20.
34. Barrett AD, Monath TP. Epidemiology and ecology of yellow fever virus. *Adv Virus Res*. 2003;61:291-315.
35. Robertson SE, Hull BP, Tomori O, et al. Yellow fever: A decade of reemergence. *JAMA*. 1996;276:1157.

36. Monath TP. Yellow fever: Victor, Victoria? Conqueror, conquest? Epidemics and research in the last forty years and prospects for the future. *Am J Trop Med Hyg*. 1991;45:1-43.
37. de Filippis AM, Nogueira RM, Schatzmayr HG, et al. Outbreak of jaundice and hemorrhagic fever in the southeast of Brazil in 2001: Detection and molecular characterization of yellow fever virus. *J Med Virol*. 2002;68:620-627.
38. Vasconcelos PF, Costa ZG, Travassos Da Rosa ES, et al. Epidemic of jungle yellow fever in Brazil, 2000: Implications of climatic alterations in disease spread. *J Med Virol*. 2001;65:598-604.
39. Van der Stuyft P, Gianella A, Pirard M, et al. Urbanisation of yellow fever in Santa Cruz, Bolivia. *Lancet*. 1999;353:1558-1562.
40. Monath TP, Nasidi A. Should yellow fever vaccine be included in the expanded program of immunization in Africa? A cost-effectiveness analysis for Nigeria. *Am J Trop Med Hyg*. 1993;48:274.
41. World Health Organization. *Technical Guide for Diagnosis, Treatment, Surveillance, Prevention, and Control of Dengue Haemorrhagic Fever*. 2nd ed. Geneva: World Health Organization; 1997.
42. Wang E, Ni H, Xu R, et al. Evolutionary relationships of endemic/epidemic and sylvatic dengue viruses. *J Virol*. 2000;74:3227-3234.
43. Reiter P, Lathrop S, Bunning M, et al. Texas lifestyle limits transmission of dengue virus. *Emerg Infect Dis*. 2003;9:86-89.
44. Gubler DJ. Dengue and dengue hemorrhagic fever. *Clin Microbiol Rev*. 1998;11:480-496.
45. Kuno G. Factors influencing the transmission of dengue viruses. In: Gubler DJ, Kuno G, eds. *Dengue and Dengue Hemorrhagic Fever*. New York: CAB International; 1997:61-88.
46. Reiter P, Gubler DJ. Surveillance and control of urban dengue vectors. In: Gubler DJ, Kuno G, eds. *Dengue and Dengue Hemorrhagic Fever*. New York: CAB International; 1997:425-462.
47. De Benedictis J, Chow-Shaffer E, Costero A, et al. Identification of the people from whom engorged *Aedes aegypti* took blood meals in Florida, Puerto Rico, using polymerase chain reaction-based DNA profiling. *Am J Trop Med Hyg*. 2003;68:437-446.
48. Burke DS, Nisalak A, Johnson DE, et al. A prospective study of dengue infections in Bangkok. *Am J Trop Med Hyg*. 1988;38:172-180.
49. Sangkawhibha N, Rohanasuphor S, Ahandrik S, et al. Risk factors in dengue shock syndrome: A prospective study in Rayong, Thailand. I. The 1980 outbreak. *Am J Epidemiol*. 1984;120:653-669.
50. Thein S, Aung MM, Shwe TN, et al. Risk factors in dengue shock syndrome. *Am J Trop Med Hyg*. 1997;56:566-572.
51. Halstead SB. Dengue and hemorrhagic fevers of Southeast Asia. *Yale J Biol Med*. 1965;37:434-454.
52. Nguyen TH, Lei HY, Nguyen TL, et al. Dengue hemorrhagic fever in infants. *J Infect Dis*. 2004;189:221-232.

53. Watanaveeradej V, Endy TP, Samakoses R, et al. Transplacentally transferred maternal-infant antibodies to dengue virus. *Am J Trop Med Hyg.* 2003;69:123-128.
54. Halstead SB, Lan NT, Myint TT, et al. Dengue hemorrhagic fever in infants: research opportunities ignored. *Emerg Infect Dis.* 2002;8:1474-1479.
55. Kouri GP, Guzman MG, Bravo JR, et al. Dengue haemorrhagic fever/dengue shock syndrome: Lessons from the Cuban epidemic. *Bull World Health Organ.* 1989;67:375-380.
56. Guzman MG, Kouri G, Valdes L, et al. Epidemiologic studies on Dengue in Santiago de Cuba, 1997. *Am J Epidemiol.* 2000;152:793-799.
57. Vaughn DW. Invited commentary: Dengue lessons from Cuba. *Am J Epidemiol.* 2000;152:800-803.
58. Scott RM, Nimmanitya S, Bancroft WH, et al. Shock syndrome in primary dengue infections. *Am J Trop Med Hyg.* 1976;25:866-874.
59. Rosen L. Comments on the epidemiology, pathogenesis and control of dengue. *Med Trop (Mars).* 1999;59:495-498.
60. Bravo JR, Guzman MG, Louri GP. Why dengue hemorrhagic fever in Cuba? I. Individual risk factors for dengue hemorrhagic fever/dengue shock syndrome. *Trans R Soc Trop Med Hyg.* 1987;81:816-820.
61. Thisyakorn U, Nimmanitya S. Nutritional status of children with dengue hemorrhagic fever. *Clin Infect Dis.* 1993;16:295-297.
62. Chiewslip P, Scott RM, Bhamarapravati N. Histocompatibility antigens and dengue hemorrhagic fever. *Am J Trop Med Hyg.* 1981;30:1100-1105.
63. Halstead SB. The XXth century dengue pandemic: Need for surveillance and research. *World Health Stat Q.* 1992;45:292-298.
64. Kalayanarooj S, Vaughn DW, Nimmannitya S, et al. Early clinical and laboratory indicators of acute dengue illness. *J Infect Dis.* 1997;176:313-321.
65. Castleberry JS, Mahon CR. Dengue fever in the Western Hemisphere. *Clin Lab Sci.* 2003;16:34-38.
66. Ramirez-Ronda CH, Garcia CD. Dengue in the Western Hemisphere. *Infect Dis Clin North Am.* 1994;8:107-128.
67. Thomas SJ, Strickman D, Vaughn DW. Dengue epidemiology: Virus epidemiology, ecology, and emergence. *Adv Virus Res.* 2003;61:235-289.
68. Anderson JR, Rico-Hesse R. Aedes aegypti vectorial capacity is determined by the infecting genotype of dengue virus. *Am J Trop Med Hyg.* 2006;75:886-892.
69. Guzman MG, Kouri G. Dengue and dengue hemorrhagic fever in the Americas: Lessons and challenges. *J Clin Virol.* 2003;27:1-13.
70. Guzman MG, Vazquez S, Martinez E, et al. Dengue in Nicaragua, 1994: Reintroduction of serotype 3 in the Americas. *Bol Oficina Sanit Panam.* 1996;12: 102-110.
71. Uzcategui NY, Comach G, Camacho D, et al. Molecular epidemiology of dengue virus type 3 in Venezuela. *J Gen Virol.* 2003;84:1569-1575.
72. Imported dengue—United States, 1999-2000. *MMWR Morb Mortal Wkly Rep.* 2002;51:281-283.
73. McCoy OR, Sabin AB. Dengue. In: Coates JB, Hoff EC, Hoff PM, eds. *Preventive medicine in World War II: Communicable disease. VII. Arthropodborne Diseases Other Than Malaria.* Washington, DC: Office of the Surgeon General; 1946: 29-62.
74. Trofa AF, DeFraites RF, Smoak BL, et al. Dengue in US military personnel in Haiti. *JAMA.* 1997;277:1546-1548.
75. Jelinek T, Muhlberger N, Harms G, et al. Epidemiology and clinical features of imported dengue fever in Europe: Sentinel surveillance data from TropNetEurop. *Clin Infect Dis.* 2002;35:1047-1052.
76. Wichmann O, Gascon J, Schunk M, et al. Severe dengue virus infection in travelers: risk factors and laboratory indicators. *J Infect Dis.* 2007;195:1089-1096.
77. Rawlings JA, Hendricks KA, Burgess CR, et al. Dengue surveillance in Texas, 1995. *Am J Trop Med Hyg.* 1998;59:95.
78. Dengue hemorrhagic fever: U.S.-Mexico border, 2005. *MMWR Morb Mortal Wkly Rep.* 2007;56:785-789.
79. Langgartner J, Audebert F, Scholmerich J, et al. Dengue virus infection transmitted by needle stick injury. *J Infect.* 2002;44:269-270.
80. Endy TP, Nisalak A. Japanese encephalitis virus: Ecology and epidemiology. *Curr Top Microbiol Immunol.* 2002;267:11-48.
81. Mudur G. Japanese encephalitis outbreak kills 1300 children in India. *BMJ.* 2005;331(7528):1288.
82. Tsai TF. New initiatives for the control of Japanese encephalitis by vaccination. Minutes of a WHO/CVI meeting, Bangkok, Thailand, 13-15 October 1998. *Vaccine.* 2000;18(Suppl):21-25.
83. Kari K, Liu W, Gautama K, et al. A hospital-based surveillance for Japanese encephalitis in Bali, Indonesia. *BMC Med.* 2006;4:8.
84. Paul WS, Moore PS, Karabatsos N, et al. Outbreak of Japanese encephalitis on the island of Saipan, 1990. *J Infect Dis.* 1993;167:1053-1058.
85. Solomon T, Thao TT, Lewthwaite P, et al. A cohort study to assess the new WHO Japanese encephalitis surveillance standards. *Bull World Health Organ.* 2008;86:178-186.
86. World Health Organization. Japanese encephalitis surveillance standards—Field Test Version. http://www.who.int/vaccines-documents/DocsPDF06/843.pdf; accessed online 7/8/2009.
87. Solomon T, Ni H, Beasley DW, et al. Origin and evolution of Japanese encephalitis virus in Southeast Asia. *J Virol.* 2003;77:3091-3098.
88. Rosen L. The natural history of Japanese encephalitis virus. *Ann Revu Microbiol.* 1986;40:395.
89. Kitaoka M. Shift of age distribution of cases of Japanese encephalitis in Japan during the period 1950 to 1967. In: Hammon WM, Kitaoka M, Downs WG, eds. *Immunization for Japanese Encephalitis.* Tokyo: Igaku-Shoin; 1972:287-291.
90. Tsai TF. Immunization Practices Advisory Committee (ACIP). Inactivated Japanese encephalitis virus vaccine: Recommendations of the ACIP. *MMWR Morb Mortal Wkly Rep.* 1993; 42(RR-1):1-15.
91. Buhl MR, Black FT, Andersen PL, et al. Fatal Japanese encephalitis in a Danish tourist visiting Bali for 12 days. *Scand J Infect Dis.* 1996;28:189.
92. Shlim DR, Solomon T. Japanese encephalitis vaccine for travelers: Exploring the limits of risk. *Clin Infect Dis.* 2002;35:183-188.
93. Lehtinen VA, Huhtamo E, Siikamäki H, et al. Japanese encephalitis in a Finnish traveler on a two-week holiday in Thailand. *J Clin Virol.* 2008;43:93-95.
94. Campbell GL, Marfin AA, Lanciotti RS, et al. West Nile virus. *Lancet Infect Dis.* 2002;9:519-529.
95. Solomon T, Ooi MH. West Nile encephalitis. *BMJ.* 2003; 326:865-869.
96. Pealer LN, Marfin AA, Petersen LR, et al. Transmission of West Nile virus through blood transfusion in the United States in 2002. *N Engl J Med.* 2003;349:1236-1245.
97. Ravindra KV, Freifeld AG, Kalil AC, et al. West Nile virus–associated encephalitis in recipients of renal and pancreatic transplants: Case series and literature review. *Clin Infect Dis.* 2004;38:1257-1260.
98. Rappole JH, Derrickson SR, Hubalek Z. Migratory birds and spread of West Nile virus in the Western Hemisphere. *Emerg Infect Dis.* 2000;6:319-328.
99. Lanciotti RS, Roehrig JT, Deubel V, et al. Origin of the West Nile virus responsible for an outbreak of encephalitis in the northeastern United States. *Science.* 1999;286:2333-2337.
100. Tsai TF, Popovici F, Cernescu C, et al. West Nile encephalitis epidemic in southeastern Romania. *Lancet.* 1998;352:767-771.
101. Taylor R, Work T, Rizk F, et al. A study of the ecology of West Nile virus in Egypt. *Am J Trop Med Hyg.* 1956;5:579-620.
102. McIntosh BM, Jupp PG. Epidemics of West Nile and Sindbis viruses in South Africa with *Culex (culex) univittatus* Theobold as vector. *S Afr J Sci.* 1976;72:295-300.
103. Monath TP, Tsai TF. St Louis encephalitis: Lessons from the last decade. *Am J Med Hyg.* 1987;37:40S.
104. Reisen WK. Epidemiology of St. Louis encephalitis virus. *Adv Virus Res.* 2003;61:139-183.
105. Okhuysen PC, Crane JK, Pappas J. St. Louis encephalitis in patients with human immunodeficiency virus infection. *Clin Infect Dis.* 1993;17:140-141.
106. Jones SC, Morris J, Hill G, et al. St. Louis encephalitis outbreak in Louisiana in 2001. *J La State Med Soc.* 2002;154:303-306.
107. Meehan PJ, Wells DL, Paul W, et al. Epidemiological features of and public health response to a St. Louis encephalitis epidemic in Florida, 1990-1991. *Epidemiol Infect.* 2000;125:181-188.
108. Luby JP, Miller G, Gardner P, et al. The epidemiology of St Louis encephalitis in Houston, Texas, 1964. *Am J Epidemiol.* 1967;86:584-597.
109. Gritsun TS, Lashkevich VA, Gould EA. Tick-borne encephalitis. *Antiviral Res.* 2003;57:129-146.
110. Heinz FX. Molecular aspects of TBE virus research. *Vaccine.* 2003;21(Suppl 1):S3-S10.
111. Kunz C. TBE vaccination and the Austrian experience. *Vaccine.* 2003;21(Suppl 1):S50-S55.
112. Randolph E, Rogers DJ. Fragile transmission cycles of tick-borne encephalitis virus may be disrupted by predicted climate change. *Proc R Soc Lond B Biol Sci.* 2000;267:1741-1744.
113. Nuttall PA, Labuda M. Dynamics of infection in tick vectors and at the tick-host interface. *Adv Virus Res.* 2003;60:233-272.
114. Daniel M, Kolar J, Zeman P, et al. Predictive map of *Ixodes ricinus* high-incidence habitats and a tick-borne encephalitis risk assessment using satellite data. *Exp Appl Acarol.* 1998; 22:417-433.
115. Daniel M, Danielova V, Kriz B, et al. Shift of the tick *Ixodes ricinus* and tick-borne encephalitis to higher altitudes in central Europe. *Eur J Clin Microbiol Infect Dis.* 2003;22:327-328.
116. McNeil JG, Lednar WM, Stansfield SK, et al. Central European tick-borne encephalitis: Assessment of risk for persons in the armed services and vacationers. *J Infect Dis.* 1985;152:650-651.
117. Davidson MM, Williams H, MacLoed JA. Louping ill in man: A forgotten disease. *J Infect.* 1991;23:241-249.
118. Woodall JP, Roz A. Experimental milk-borne transmission of Powassan virus in the goat. *Am J Trop Med Hyg.* 1977;26: 190-192.
119. Charrel RN, de Lamballerie X. The Alkhurma virus (family Flaviviridae, genus *Flavivirus*): An emerging pathogen responsible for hemorrhage fever in the Middle East. *Med Trop (Mars).* 2003;63:296-299.
120. Kuno G, Artsob H, Karabatsos N, et al. Genomic sequencing of deer tick virus and phylogeny of Powassan-related viruses of North America. *Am J Trop Med Hyg.* 2001;65:671-676.
121. Hacker UT, Jelinek T, Erhardt S, et al. In vivo synthesis of tumor necrosis factor-α in healthy humans after live yellow fever vaccination. *J Infect Dis.* 1998;177:774-778.
122. Bonnevie-Nielsen V, Heron I, Monath TP, et al. Lymphocytic 2′,5′-oligoadenylate synthetase activity increases prior to the appearance of neutralizing antibodies and immunoglobulin M and immunoglobulin G antibodies after primary and secondary immunization with yellow fever vaccine. *Clin Diagn Lab Immunol.* 1995;2:302-306.
123. Wheelock EF, Sibley WA. Circulating virus, interferon and antibody after vaccination with the 17-D strain of yellow fever virus. *N Engl J Med.* 1965;273:194-198.
124. Monath TP, Ballinger ME, Miller BR, et al. Detection of yellow fever viral RNA by nucleic acid hybridization and viral antigen by immunocytochemistry in fixed human liver. *Am J Trop Med Hyg.* 1989;40:663-668.
125. Deubel V, Huerre M, Cathomas G, et al. Molecular detection and characterization of yellow fever virus in blood and liver specimens of a non-vaccinated fatal human case. *J Med Virol.* 1997;53:212-217.
126. DeBrito T, Sigueira SAC, Santos RTM, et al. Human fatal yellow fever: Immunohistochemical detection of viral antigens in the liver, kidney and heart. *Pathol Res Pract.* 1992;188:177.
127. Monath TP. Yellow fever: A medically neglected disease. *Rev Infect Dis.* 1987;9:165-175.
128. Monath TP. The absence of yellow fever in Asia: Hypotheses. A cause for concern? *Virus Inform Exch Newslett.* 1989;6:106-107.
129. DeVries RRP, Meera Khan P, Bernini LF, et al. Genetic control of survival in epidemics. *J Immunogenet.* 1979;6:271-287.
130. Monath TP, Hadler SC. Type B hepatitis and yellow fever infections in West Africa. *Trans R Soc Trop Med Hyg.* 1987; 18:172-173.
131. Halstead SB, Shotwell H, Casals J. Studies on the pathogenesis of dengue infection in monkeys. II. Clinical laboratory responses to heterologous infection. *J Infect Dis.* 1973;128:15-22.
132. Halstead SB. Antibody, macrophages, dengue virus infection, shock and hemorrhage: A pathogenetic cascade. *Rev Infect Dis.* 1989;11:S830-S839.
133. Halstead SB. Pathogenesis of dengue: Challenges to molecular biology. *Science.* 1988;239:476-481.
134. Wu SJ, Grouard-Vogel G, Sun W, et al. Human skin Langerhans cells are targets of dengue virus infection. *Nat Med.* 2000;6:816-820.
135. Jessie K, Fong MY, Devi S, et al. Localization of dengue virus in naturally infected human tissues by immunohistochemistry and in situ hybridization. *J Infect Dis.* 2004;189:1411-1418.
136. Vaughn DW, Green S, Kalayanarooj S, et al. Dengue in the early febrile phase: Viremia and antibody responses. *J Infect Dis.* 1997;176:322-330.
137. Vaughn DW, Green S, Kalayanarooj S, et al. Dengue viremia titer, antibody response pattern, and virus serotype correlate with disease severity. *J Infect Dis.* 2000;181:2-9.
138. Malheiros SMF, Oliveira ASB, Schmidt B, et al. Dengue: Muscle biopsy findings in 15 patients. *Arq Neuropsiquiatr.* 1993;51: 159.
139. Kuo C-H, Tai D-I, Chang-Chien C-S, et al. Liver biochemical tests and dengue fever. *Am J Trop Med Hyg.* 1992;47:265-270.
140. Bhamarapravati N, Toochinda P, Boonyapaknavik V. Pathology of Thailand hemorrhagic fever. V. A study of 100 autopsy cases. *Ann Trop Med Parasitol.* 1967;61:500-510.
141. Lum LCS, Lam SK, Choy YS, et al. Dengue encephalitis: A true entity? *Am J Trop Med Hyg.* 1996;54:256-259.
142. Hommel D, Talarmin A, Deubel V, et al. Dengue encephalitis in French Guinea. *Res Virol.* 1998;149:235-238.
143. Solomon T, Dung NM, Vaughn DW, et al. Neurological manifestations of dengue infection. *Lancet.* 2000;355:1053-1059.
144. Wasay M, Channa R, Jumani M, et al. Encephalitis and myelitis associated with dengue viral infection clinical and neuroimaging features. *Clin Neurol Neurosurg.* 2008;110:635-640.
145. Monath TP. Early indicators in acute dengue infection. *Lancet.* 1997;350:1719-1720.
146. Mongkolsapaya J, Dejnirattisai W, Xu XN, et al. Original antigenic sin and apoptosis in the pathogenesis of dengue hemorrhagic fever. *Nat Med.* 2003;9:921-927.
147. Espina LM, Valero NJ, Hernandez JM, et al. Increased apoptosis and expression of tumor necrosis factor-alpha caused by infection of cultured human monocytes with dengue virus. *Am J Trop Med Hyg.* 2003;68:48-53.
148. Gagnon SJ, Mori M, Kurane I, et al. Cytokine gene expression and protein production in peripheral blood mononuclear cells of children with acute dengue virus infections. *J Med Virol.* 2002;67:41-46.
149. Green S, Vaughn DW, Kalayanarooj S, et al. Elevated plasma interleukin-10 levels in acute dengue correlate with disease severity. *J Med Virol.* 1999;59:329-334.
150. Green S, Rothman A. Immunopathological mechanisms in dengue and dengue hemorrhagic fever. *Curr Opin Infect Dis.* 2006;19:429-436.
151. Bethell DB, Flobbe K, Phuong CXT, et al. Pathophysiologic and prognostic role of cytokines in dengue hemorrhagic fever. *J Infect Dis.* 1998;177:778.
152. Avirutnan P, Malasit P, Seliger B, et al. Dengue virus infection of human endothelial cells leads to chemokine production, complement activation, and apoptosis. *J Immunol.* 1998;161: 6338-6346.
153. Rothman AL. Immunology and immunopathogenesis of dengue disease. *Adv Virus Res.* 2003;60:397-419.
154. Bokisch VA, Top FH Jr, Russell PK, et al. The potential pathogenic role of complement in dengue hemorrhagic shock syndrome. *N Engl J Med.* 1973;289:996-1000.

155. Kabra SK, Juneja R, Madhulika, et al. Myocardial dysfunction in children with dengue haemorrhagic fever. *Natl Med J India*. 1998;11:59-61.
156. Huang YH, Lei HY, Liu HS, et al. Tissue plasminogen activator induced by dengue virus infection of human endothelial cells. *J Med Virol*. 2003;70:610-616.
157. Krishnamurti C, Kalayanarooj S, Cutting MA, et al. Mechanisms of hemorrhage in dengue without circulatory collapse. *Am J Trop Med Hyg*. 2001;65:840-847.
158. Mairuhu AT, MacGillavry MR, Setiati TE, et al. Is clinical outcome of dengue-virus infections influenced by coagulation and fibrinolysis? A critical review of the evidence. *Lancet Infect Dis*. 2003;3:33-41.
159. Falconar AKI. The dengue virus nonstructural-1 protein (NS1) generates antibodies to common epitopes on human blood clotting, integrin/adhesin proteins and binds to human endothelial cells: Potential implications in haemorrhagic fever pathogenesis. *Arch Virol*. 1997;142:897.
160. Kliks SC, Nisalak A, Brandt WE, et al. Antibody dependent enhancement of dengue virus growth in human monocytes as a risk factor for dengue hemorrhagic fever. *Am J Trop Med Hyg*. 1989;40:444.
161. Halsted SB. Neutralization of antibody-dependent enhancement of dengue virus. *Adv Virus Res*. 2003;60:421-467.
162. Mullbacher A, Lobigs M. Up-regulation of MHC class I by flavivirus-induced peptide translocation into the endoplasmic reticulum. *Immunity*. 1995;3:207.
163 Mathew A, Rothman AL. Understanding the contribution of cellular immunity to dengue disease pathogenesis. *Immunol Rev*. 2008;225:300-313.
164. Watts DM, Porter KR, Putvatana P, et al. Failure of secondary infection with American genotype dengue 2 to cause dengue haemorrhagic fever. *Lancet*. 1999;354:1431-1434.
165. Kochel TJ, Watts DM, Halstead SB, et al. Effect of dengue-1 antibodies on American dengue-2 viral infection and dengue haemorrhagic fever. *Lancet*. 2002;360:310-312.
166. Deparis X, Murgue B, Roche C, et al. Changing clinical and biological manifestations of dengue during the dengue-2 epidemic in French Polynesia in 1996/97: Description and analysis in a prospective study. *Trop Med Int Health*. 1998;3:859-865.
167. Mathew A, Kurane I, Green S, et al. Predominance of HLA-restricted cytotoxic T-lymphocyte responses to serotype-cross-reactive epitopes on nonstructural proteins following natural secondary dengue virus infection. *J Virol*. 1998;72:3999-4004.
168. Kurane I, Zeng L, Brinton MA, et al. Definition of an epitope on NS3 recognized by human $CD4^+$ cytotoxic T lymphocyte clones cross-reactive for dengue virus types 2, 3, and 4. *Virology*. 1998;240:169-174.
169. Mangada MM, Endy TP, Nisalak A, et al. Dengue-specific T cell responses in peripheral blood mononuclear cells obtained prior to secondary dengue virus infections in Thai schoolchildren. *J Infect Dis*. 2002;185:1697-1703.
170. Gibbons RV, Kalanarooj S, Jarman RG, et al. Analysis of repeat hospital admissions for dengue to estimate the frequency of third or fourth dengue infections resulting in admissions and dengue hemorrhagic fever, and serotype sequences. *Am J Trop Med Hyg*. 2007;77:910-913.
171. Chambers TJ, Diamond MS. Pathogenesis of flavivirus encephalitis. *Adv Virus Res*. 2003;60:273-342.
172. Lanciotti RS, Kerst AJ, Nasci RS, et al. Rapid detection of West Nile virus from human clinical specimens, field-collected mosquitoes, and avian samples by a TaqMan reverse transcriptase-PCR assay. *J Clin Microbiol*. 2000;38:4066-4071.
173. Fredericksen BL, Smith M, Katze MG, et al. The host response to West Nile virus infection limits viral spread through the activation of the interferon regulatory factor 3 pathway, *J Virol*. 2004;78:7737-7747.
174. Wang T, Town T, Alexopoulou L, et al. Toll-like receptor 3 mediates West Nile virus entry into the brain causing lethal encephalitis. *Nat Med*. 2004;10:1366-1373.
175. Kindberg E, Mickiene A, Ax C, et al. A deletion in the chemokine receptor 5 (CCR5) gene is associated with tickborne encephalitis. *J Infect Dis*. 2008;197:266-269.
176. Kumar P, Sulochana P, Nirmala G, et al. Impaired T helper 1 function of nonstructural protein 3-specific T cells in Japanese patients with encephalitis with neurological sequelae. *J Infect Dis*. 2004;189:880-891.
177. Solomon T, Vaughn DW. Pathogenesis and clinical features of Japanese encephalitis and West Nile virus infections. *Curr Top Microbiol Immunol*. 2002;267:171-194.
178. Desai A, Shankar SK, Ravi V, et al. Japanese encephalitis virus antigen in the human brain and its topographic distribution. *Acta Neuropathol*. 1995;89:368.
179. Gelpi E, Preusser M, Garzuly F, et al. Visualization of Central European tick-borne encephalitis in fatal human cases. *J Neuropathol Exp Neurol*. 2005;64:506-512.
180. Johnson RT, Intralawan P, Puapanwatton S. Japanese encephalitis: Identification of inflammatory cells in cerebrospinal fluid. *Ann Neurol*. 1986;20:691.
181. Tomazic J, Ihan A. Flow cytometric analysis of lymphocytes in cerebrospinal fluid in patients with tick-borne encephalitis. *Acta Neurol Scand*. 1997;95:29.
182. Leake CJ, Burke DS, Nisalak A, et al. Isolation of Japanese encephalitis virus from clinical specimens using a continuous mosquito cell line. *Am J Trop Med Hyg*. 1986;35:1045-1050.
183. Desai A, Ravi V, Guru SC, et al. Detection of autoantibodies to neural antigens in the CSF of Japanese encephalitis patients and correlation of findings with the outcome. *J Neurol Sci*. 1994;122:109-116.
184. Desai A, Ravi V, Chandramuki A, et al. Proliferative response of human peripheral blood mononuclear cells to Japanese encephalitis virus. *Microbiol Immunol*. 1995;39:269.
185. Leyssen P, Paeshuyse J, Charlier N, et al. Impact of direct virus-induced neuronal dysfunction and immunological damage on the progression of flavivirus (Modoc) encephalitis in a murine model. *J Neurovirol*. 2003;9:69-78.
186. Iwamoto M, Jernigan DB, Guasch A, et al. Transmission of West Nile virus from an organ donor to four transplant recipients. *N Engl J Med*. 2003;348:2196-2203.
187. Gunther G, Haglund M, Lindquist L, et al. Tick-borne encephalitis in Sweden in relation to aseptic meningo-encephalitis of other etiology: A prospective study of clinical course and outcome. *J Neurol*. 1997;244:230.
188. Tomazic J, Poljak M, Popovi M, et al. Tick-borne encephalitis: Possibly a fatal disease in its acute stage. PCR amplification of TBE RNA from postmortem brain tissue (Case report). *Infection*. 1997;25:41-43.
189. Gritsun TS, Frolova TV, Zhankov AI, et al. Characterization of a Siberian virus isolated from a patient with progressive chronic tick-borne encephalitis, *J Virol*. 2003;77:25-36.
190. Naslednikova IO, Ryazantseva NV, Novitskii VV, et al. Chronic tick-borne encephalitis virus antigenemia: possible pathogenesis pathways. *Bull Exp Biol Med*. 2005;139:451-454.
191. Ravi V, Desai AS, Shenoy PK, et al. Persistence of Japanese encephalitis virus in the human nervous system. *J Med Virol*. 1993;40:326-329.
192. Sharma S, Mathur A, Prakash R, et al. Japanese encephalitis virus latency in peripheral blood lymphocytes and recurrence of infection in children. *Clin Exp Immunol*. 1991;85:85-89.
193. Silber LA, Soloviev VD. Far Eastern tick-borne spring-summer (spring) encephalitis. In: Davis BD, Fisher SH, eds. *American Review of Soviet Medicine*. New York: America-Soviet Medical Society; 1946:1.
194. Ogawa M, Okubo H, Tsuji Y, et al. Chronic progressive encephalitis occurring 13 years after Russian spring-summer encephalitis. *J Neurol Sci*. 1973;19:363.
195. Gritsun TS, Frolova TV, Zhankov AI, et al. Characterization of a Siberian virus isolated from a patient with progressive chronic tick-borne encephalitis. *J Virol*. 2003;77:25-36.
196. Broun GO. Relationship of hypertensive vascular disease to mortality in cases of St Louis encephalitis. *Med Bull St. Louis Univ*. 1952;4:32.
197. Cimperman J, Maraspin V, Lotri-Furlan S, et al. Double infection with tick-borne encephalitis virus and *Borrelia burgdorferi sensu laou*. *Wien Klin Wochenschr*. 2002;114:620-622.
198. Oksi J, Viljanen MK, Kalimo H, et al. Fatal encephalitis caused by concomitant infection with tick-borne encephalitis virus and *Borrelia burgdorferi*. *Clin Infect Dis*. 1993;16:392-396.
199. Edelman R, Schneider RJ, Chieowanich P, et al. The effect of dengue virus infection on the clinical sequelae of Japanese encephalitis: A one year follow-up study in Thailand. *Southeast Asian J Trop Med Public Health*. 1975;6:308-315.
200. Bond JO, Hammon WM. Epidemiologic studies of possible cross protection between dengue and St Louis encephalitis arboviruses in Florida. *Am J Epidemiol*. 1970;92:321-329.
201. Hoke CH, Nisalak A, Singawhipa N, et al. Protection against Japanese encephalitis by inactivated vaccines. *N Engl J Med*. 1988;319:608-614.
202. Francis TI, Moore DL, Edington GM, et al. A clinicopathological study of human yellow fever. *Bull World Health Organ*. 1972;46:659-667.
203. Endy TP, Chunsuttiwat S, Nisalak A, et al. Epidemiology of inapparent and symptomatic acute dengue virus infection: A prospective study of primary school children in Kamphaeng Phet, Thailand. *Am J Epidemiol*. 2002;156:40-51.
204. Hanafusa S, Chanyasanha C, Sujirarat D, et al. Clinical features and differences between child and adult dengue infections in Rayong Province, southeast Thailand. *Southeast Asian J Trop Med Public Health*. 2008;39:252-259.
205. Garcia-Rivera EJ, Rigau-Perez JG. Dengue severity in the elderly in Puerto Rico. *Rev Panam Salud Publica*. 2003;13:362-368.
206. Thisyakorn U, Thisyakorn C. Dengue infections with unusual manifestations. *J Med Assoc Thai*. 1994;77:410-413.
207. Tsai JC, Juo CH, Chen PC. Upper gastrointestinal bleeding in dengue fever. *Am J Gastroenterol*. 1991;86:33-35.
208. Imbert P, Sordet D, Hovette P, et al. Spleen rupture in a patient with dengue fever. *Trop Med Parasitol*. 1993;44:327-328.
209. Chye JK, Lim CT, Ng KB, et al. Vertical transmission of dengue. *Clin Infect Dis*. 1997;25:1374-1377.
210. Innis BL, Mhint KSA. Acute liver failure is one important cause of fatal dengue infection. *Southeast Asian J Trop Med Public Health*. 1990;21:658-662.
211. Ramos C, Sanchez G, Pando RH, et al. Dengue virus in the brain of a fatal case of hemorrhagic dengue fever. *J Neurovirol*. 1998;4:465-468.
212. Phongsamart W, Yoksan S, Vanaprapa N, et al. Dengue virus infection in late pregnancy and transmission to the infants. *Pediatr Infect Dis J*. 2008;27:500-504.
213. Sharma JB, Gulati N. Potential relationships between dengue fever and neural tube defects in a northern district of India. *Int J Gynecol Obstet*. 1992;39:291-295.
214. Mirovsky J, Holub J, Nguyen BC. Influence de la dengue sur la grossesse et le foetus. *Gynecol Obstet (Paris)*. 1965;65:673.
215. Tan PC, Rajasingam G, Devi S, et al. Dengue infection in pregnancy: prevalence, vertical transmission, and pregnancy outcome. *Obstet Gynecol*. 2008;111:1111-1117.
216. Fernandez R, Rodriguez T, Borbonet F, et al: Study of the relationship dengue- pregnancy in a group of Cuban mothers (in Spanish). *Rev Cubana Med Trop*. 1994;46:76-78.
217. Cohen SN, Halstead SB. Shock associated with dengue infection. I. The clinical and physiologic manifestations of dengue hemorrhagic fever in Thailand, 1964. *J Pediatr*. 1966;68:448-456.
218. Kautner I, Robinson MJ, Kuhnle U. Dengue virus infection: Epidemiology, pathogenesis, clinical presentation, diagnosis and prevention. *J Pediatr*. 1997;131:516-524.
219. Setiawan MW, Samsi TK, Wulur H, et al. Dengue haemorrhagic fever: Ultrasound as an aid to predict the severity of the disease. *Pediatr Radiol*. 1998;28:1-4.
220 Statler J, Mammen M, Lyons A, et al. Sonographic findings of healthy volunteers infected with dengue virus. *J Clin Ultrasound*. 2008;36:413-417.
221. Lum LCS, Thong MK, Cheah YK, et al. Dengue-associated adult respiratory distress syndrome. *Ann Trop Paediatr*. 1995;15:335.
222. Pancharoen C, Thisyakorn U. Coinfections in dengue patients. *Pediatr Infect Dis J*. 1998;17:81-82.
223. Halstead SB, Nimmannitya S, Margiotta MR. Dengue and chikungunya virus infection in man in Thailand. II. Observations on disease in outpatients. *Am J Trop Med Hyg*. 1969;18:972-983.
224. Halstead SB. Dengue. *Lancet*. 2007;370:1644-1652.
225. Bozza FA, Cruz OG, Zagne SM, et al. Multiplex cytokine profile from dengue patients: MIP-1beta and IFN-gamma as predictive factors for severity. *BMC Infect Dis*. 2008;8:86.
226. Solomon T, Kneen R, Dung NM, et al. Poliomyelitis-like illness due to Japanese encephalitis virus. *Lancet*. 1998;351:1094-1097.
227. Dickerson RB, Newton JR, Hansen JE. Diagnosis and immediate prognosis of Japanese B encephalitis. *Am J Med*. 1952;12:227.
228. Solomon T, Dung NM, Kneen R, et al. Seizures and raised intracranial pressure in Vietnamese patients with Japanese encephalitis. *Brain*. 2002;125:1084-1093.
229. Ooi MH, Lewthwaite P, Lai BF, et al. The epidemiology, clinical features, and long-term prognosis of Japanese encephalitis in central Sarawak, Malaysia, 1997-2005. *Clin Infect Dis*. 2008;47:458-468.
230. Ding D, Hong Z, Zhao SJ, et al. Long-term disability from acute childhood Japanese encephalitis in Shanghai, China. *Am J Trop Med Hyg*. 2007;77:528-533.
231. Chaturvedi UC, Mathur A, Chandra A, et al. Transplacental infection with Japanese encephalitis virus. *J Infect Dis*. 1980;141:712-715.
232. Misra UK, Kalita J, Jain SK, et al. Radiological and neurophysiological changes in Japanese encephalitis. *J Neurol Neurosurg Psychiatry*. 1994;57:1484-1487.
233. Singh P, Kalra N, Ratho RK, et al. Coexistent neurocysticercosis and Japanese B encephalitis: MR imaging correlation. Am J *Neuroradiol*. 2001;22:1131-1136.
234. Kalita J, Misra UK, Pandey S, et al. A comparison of clinical and radiological findings in adults and children with Japanese encephalitis. *Arch Neurol*. 2003;60:1760-1764.
235. Srey VH, Sadones H, Ong S, et al. Etiology of encephalitis syndrome among hospitalized children and adults in Takeo, Cambodia, 1999-2000. *Am J Trop Med Hyg*. 2002;66:200-207.
236. Kumar A. Movement disorders in the tropics. *Parkinsonism Relat Disord*. 2002;9:69-75.
237. Chadha MS, Arankalle VA, Jadi RS, et al. An outbreak of Chandipura virus encephalitis in the eastern districts of Gujarat state, India. *Am J Trop Med Hyg*. 2005;73(3):566-570.
238. Goldblum N, Sterk VV, Paderski B. West Nile fever: The clinical features of the disease and the isolation of West Nile virus from the blood of nine human cases. *Am J Hyg*. 1954;59:89-103.
239. Asnis DS, Conetta R, Teixeira AA, et al. The West Nile Virus outbreak of 1999 in New York: The Flushing Hospital experience. *Clin Infect Dis*. 2000;30:413-418; erratum in Clin Infect Dis. 2000;30:841.
240. Chowers MY, Lang R, Nassar F, et al. Clinical characteristics of the West Nile fever outbreak, Israel, 2000. *Emerg Infect Dis*. 2001;7:675-678.
241. Nash D, Mostashari F, Fine A, et al. The outbreak of West Nile virus infection in the New York City area in 1999. *N Engl J Med*. 2001;344:1807-1814.
242. Gadoth N, Weitzman S, Lehmann EE. Acute anterior myelitis complicating West Nile fever. *Arch Neurol*. 1979;36:172-173.
243. Leis AA, Stokic DS, Webb RM, et al. Clinical spectrum of muscle weakness in human West Nile virus infection. *Muscle Nerve*. 2003;28:302-308.
244. Sejvar JJ, Leis AA, Stokic DS, et al. Acute flaccid paralysis and West Nile virus infection. *Emerg Infect Dis*. 2003;9:788-793.
245. Sejvar JJ, Haddad MB, Tierney BC, et al. Neurologic manifestations and outcome of West Nile virus infection. *JAMA*. 2003;290:511-515.
246 Solomon T, Fisher AF, Beasley DW, et al. Natural and nosocomial infection in a patient with West Nile encephalitis and extrapyramidal movement disorders. *Clin Infect Dis*. 2003;36:E140-E145.
247. Cernescu C, Ruta SM, Tardei G, et al. A high number of severe neurologic clinical forms during an epidemic of West Nile virus infection. *Rom J Virol*. 1997;48:13-25.
248 Weiss D, Carr D, Kellachan J, et al. Clinical findings of West Nile virus infection in hospitalized patients, New York and New Jersey, 2000. *Emerg Infect Dis*. 2001;7:654-658.

249. Wasay M, Diaz-Arrastia R, Suss RA, et al. St Louis encephalitis: A review of 11 cases in a 1995 Dallas, Tex, epidemic. *Arch Neurol.* 2000;57:114-118.
250. Azar GJ, Bond JO, Chappell GL, et al. Follow-up studies of St Louis encephalitis in Florida: Sensorimotor findings. *Am J Public Health.* 1966;56:1074-1081.
251. Palmer RJ, Finley KH. Sequelae of encephalitis: Report of a study after the California epidemic. *Calif Med.* 1956;84:98-100.
252. Cerna F, Mehrad B, Luby JP, et al. St. Louis encephalitis and the substantia nigra: MR imaging evaluation. *Am J Neuroradiol.* 1999;20:1281-1283.
253. Kaiser R. The clinical and epidemiological profile of tick-borne encephalitis in southern Germany 1994-1998: A prospective study of 656 patients. *Brain.* 1999;122:2067-2078.
254. Mickiene A, Laiskonis A, Gunther G, et al. Tickborne encephalitis in an area of high endemicity in Lithuania: Disease severity and long-term prognosis. *Clin Infect Dis.* 2002;35:650-658.
255. Cizman M, Rakar R, Zakotnik B, et al. Severe forms of tick-borne encephalitis in children. *Wien Klin Wochenschr.* 1999;111:484-487.
256. Ternovoi VA, Kurzhukov GP, Sokolov YV, et al. Tick-borne encephalitis with hemorrhagic syndrome, Novosibirsk region, Russia, 1999. *Emerg Infect Dis.* 2003;9:743-746.
257. Haglund M, Forsgren M, Lindh G, et al. A 10-year follow-up study of tick-borne encephalitis in the Stockholm area and a review of the literature: Need for a vaccination strategy. *Scand J Infect Dis.* 1996;28:217-224.
258. Conway D, Rossier E, Spence L, et al. Powassan virus encephalitis with shoulder girdle involvement. *Can Dis Weekly Rep.* 1976;85:2.
259. Lotric-Furlan S, Strle F. Thrombocytopenia: A common finding in the initial phase of tick-borne encephalitis. *Infection.* 1995;23:203-206.
260. Alkadhi H, Kollias SS. MRI in tick-borne encephalitis. *Neuroradiology.* 2000;42:753-755.
261. Sapkal GN, Wairagkar NS, Ayachit VM, et al. Detection and isolation of Japanese encephalitis virus from blood clots collected during the acute phase of infection. *Am J Trop Med Hyg.* 2007;77(6):1139-1145.
262. Tsai TF, Chandler LJ. Arboviruses. In: Murray PR, Baron EJ, Jorensen J, et al, eds. *Manual of Clinical Microbiology.* 8th ed. Washington, DC: American Society of Microbiology; 2003: 1553-1569.
263. Lanciotti R. Molecular amplification assays for the detection of flaviviruses. *Adv Virus Res.* 2003;61:67-99.
264. Kuno G. Serodiagnosis of flaviviral infections and vaccinations in humans. *Adv Virus Res.* 2003;61:3-65.
265. Roehrig JT, Nash D, Maldin B, et al. Persistence of virus-reactive serum immunoglobulin M antibody in confirmed West Nile virus encephalitis cases. *Emerg Infect Dis.* 2003;9:376-379.
266. Shi PY, Wong SJ. Serologic diagnosis of West Nile virus infection. *Expert Rev Mol Diagn.* 2003;3:733-741.
267. Bessoff K, Delorey M, Sun W, et al. Comparison of two commercially available dengue virus (DENV) NS1 capture enzyme-linked immunosorbent assays using a single clinical sample for diagnosis of acute DENV infection. *Clin Vaccine Immunol.* 2008;15(10):1513-1518.
268. Cuzzubbo AJ, Vaughn DW, Nisalak A, et al. Comparison of PanBio Dengue Duo IgM and IgG Capture ELISA and Venture Technologies Dengue IgM and IgG Dot Blot. *J Clin Virol.* 2000;16:135-144
269. Blacksell SD, Bell D, Kelley J, et al. Prospective study to determine accuracy of rapid serological assays for diagnosis of acute dengue virus infection in Laos. *Clin Vaccine Immunol.* 2007;14:1458-1464.
270. Kelso JM, Mootrey GT, Tsai TF. Anaphylaxis from yellow fever vaccine. *J Allergy Clin Immunol.* 1999;103:698-701.
271. Barrett AD, Monath TP, Barban V, et al. 17D yellow fever vaccines: new insights. A report of a workshop held during the World Congress on medicine and health in the tropics, Marseille, France, Monday 12 September 2005. *Vaccine.* 2007;25:2758-2765.
272. Lindsey NP, Schroeder BA, Miller ER, et al. Adverse event reports following yellow fever vaccination. *Vaccine.* 2008;26: 6077-6082.
273. Hayes EB. Acute viscerotropic disease following vaccination against yellow fever. *Trans R Soc Trop Med Hyg.* 2007;101: 967-971.
274. Advisory Committee on Immunization Practices. Yellow fever vaccine. Recommendations of the ACIP, 2002. *MMWR Morb Mortal Wkly Rep.* 2002;RR-17:1-11.
275. Tsai TF, Paul R, Lynberg MC, et al. Congenital yellow fever virus infection after immunization in pregnancy. *J Infect Dis.* 1993;168:1520-1523.
276. Kengsakul K, Sathirapongsasuti K, Punyagupta S. Fatal myeloencephalitis following yellow fever vaccination in a case with HIV infection. *J Med Assoc Thai.* 2002;85:131-134.
277. Nasidi A, Monath TP, Vandenberg J, et al. Yellow fever vaccine and pregnancy: A four year prospective study. *Trans R Soc Trop Med Hyg.* 1993;87:337.
278. Goujon C, Tohr M, Feuillie V, et al. Good tolerance and efficacy of yellow fever vaccine among subjects who are carriers of human immunodeficiency virus (Abstract). Fourth International Conference on Travel Medicine, Acapulco, Mexico, April 23-27, 1995:63.
279. Sibailly TS, Wiktor SZ, Tsai TF, et al. Poor antibody response to yellow fever vaccination in children infected with human immunodeficiency virus type 1. *Pediatr Infect Dis J.* 1997; 16:1177-1179.
280. *Dengue Haemorrhagic Fever: Diagnosis, Treatment, Prevention and Control.* 2nd ed. Geneva, World Health Organization; 1997.
281. Ngo NT, Cao XT, Kneen R, et al. Acute management of dengue shock syndrome: A randomized double-blind comparison of 4 intravenous fluid regimens in the first hour. *Clin Infect Dis.* 2001;32:204-213.
282. Pea L, Roda L, Moll F. Desmopressin treatment for a case of dengue hemorrhagic fever/dengue shock syndrome. *Clin Infect Dis.* 2001;33:1611-1612.
283. Lum LC, Abdel-Latif-Yel A, Goh AY, et al. Preventive transfusion in dengue shock syndrome—is it necessary? *J Pediatr.* 2003;143:682-684.
284. Diamond MS, Roberts TG, Edgil D, et al. Modulation of Dengue virus infection in human cells by alpha, beta, and gamma interferons. *J Virol.* 2000;74:4957-4966.
285. Tassniyom S, Vasanawathana S, Dhiensiri T, et al. Failure of carbazochrome sodium sulfonate (AC-17) to prevent dengue vascular permeability or shock: A randomized, controlled trial. *J Pediatr.* 1997;131:525-528.
286. Tassniyom S, Vasanawathana S, Chirawatkul A, et al. Failure of high-dose methylprednisolone in established dengue shock syndrome: A placebo-controlled, double-blind study. *Pediatrics.* 1993;92:111-115.
287. Atrasheuskaya A, Petzelbauer P, Fredeking TM, et al. Anti-TNF antibody treatment reduces mortality in experimental dengue virus infection. *FEMS Immunol Med Microbiol.* 2003;35:33-42.
288. Yen YT, Chen HC, Lin YD, et al. TNF-α enhancing dengue virus-induced endothelium production of reactive nitrogen and oxygen species is key to hemorrhage development. *J Virol.* 2008;82:12312-12324.
289. Kyle JL, Harris E. Global spread and persistence of dengue. *Annu Rev Microbiol.* 2008;62:71-92.
290. Solomon T, Dung NM, Wills B, et al. Interferon alfa-2a in Japanese encephalitis: A randomised double-blind placebo-controlled trial. *Lancet.* 2003;361:821-826.
291. Arras C, Fescharek R, Gregersen JP. Do specific hyperimmunoglobulins aggravate clinical course of tick-borne encephalitis? *Lancet.* 1996;347:1331.
292. Kluger G, Schottler A, Waldvogel K, et al. Tickborne encephalitis despite specific immunoglobulin prophylaxis. *Lancet.* 1995;346:1502.
293. Shimoni Z, Niven MJ, Pitlick S, et al. Treatment of West Nile virus encephalitis with intravenous immunoglobulin. *Emerg Infect Dis.* 2001;7:759.
294. Oliphant T, Engle M, Nybakken G, et al. Development of a humanized monoclonal antibody with therapeutic potential against West Nile virus. *Nat Med.* 2005;11:522-530.
295. Morrey JD, Siddharthan V, Olsen AL, et al. Defining limits of humanized neutralizing monoclonal antibody treatment for West Nile virus neurological infection in a hamster model. *Antimicrob Agents Chemother.* 2007;51:2396-2402.
296. Hoke CH Jr, Vaughn DW, Nisalak A, et al. Effect of high-dose dexamethasone on the outcome of acute encephalitis due to Japanese encephalitis virus. *J Infect Dis.* 1992;165:631.
297. Atrasheuskaya AV, Fredeking TM, Ignatyev GM. Changes in immune parameters and their correction in human cases of tick-borne encephalitis. *Clin Exp Immunol.* 2003;131:148-154.
298. Deas TS, Binduga-Gajewska I, Tilgner M, et al. Inhibition of flavivirus infections by antisense oligomers specifically suppressing viral translation and RNA replication. *J Virol.* 2005;79:4599-5509.
299. Krishnan MN, Ng A, Sukumaran B, et al. RNA interference screen for human genes associated with West Nile virus infection. *Nature.* 2008;455:242-245.
300. Puig-Basagoiti F, Tilgner M, Forshey B, et al. Triaryl pyrazoline compound inhibits flavivirus RNA replication. *Antimicrob Agents Chemother.* 2006;50:1320-1329.
301. Plesner AM. Allergic reactions to Japanese encephalitis vaccine. *Immunol Allergy Clin North Am.* 2003;23:665-697.
302. Beasley DW, Lewthwaite P, Solomon T. Current use and development of vaccines for Japanese encephalitis. *Expert Opin Biol Ther.* 2008;8:95-106.
303. Bista MB, Banerjee MK, Shin SH, et al. Efficacy of single-dose SA 14-14-2 vaccine against Japanese encephalitis: A case control study. *Lancet.* 2001;358:791-795.
304. Hennessy S, Liu Z, Tsai TF, et al. Effectiveness of live-attenuated Japanese encephalitis vaccine (SA14-14-2): A case-control study. *Lancet.* 1996;347:1583-1586.
305. World Health Organization. Safety of Japanese encephalitis vaccination in India. *Weekly Epidemiological Record.* 2007;82:23.
306. Monath TP, Guirakhoo F, Nichols R, et al. Chimeric live, attenuated vaccine against Japanese encephalitis (ChimeriVax-JE): Phase 2 clinical trials for safety and immunogenicity, effect of vaccine dose and schedule, and memory response to challenge with inactivated Japanese encephalitis antigen. *J Infect Dis.* 2003;188:1213-1230.
307. Tauber E, Kollaritsch H, Korinek M, et al. Safety and immunogenicity of a Vero-cell-derived, inactivated Japanese encephalitis vaccine: a non-inferiority, phase III, randomised controlled trial. *Lancet.* 2007;370:1847-1853.
308. Hall RA, Khromykh AA. ChimeriVax-West Nile vaccine. *Curr Opin Mol Ther.* 2007;9:498-504.
309. Pletnev AG, Putnak R, Speicher J, et al. West Nile virus/dengue type 4 virus chimeras that are reduced in neurovirulence and peripheral virulence without loss of immunogenicity or protective efficacy. *Proc Natl Acad Sci U S A.* 2002;99:3036-3041.
310. Zent O, Jilg W, Plentz A, et al. Kinetics of the immune response after primary and booster immunization against tick-borne encephalitis (TBE) in adults using the rapid immunization schedule. *Vaccine.* 2003;21:4655-4660.
311. Lindquist L, Vapalahti O. Tick-borne encephalitis. *Lancet.* 2008;371:1861-1871.
312. Bennett NM. Murray Valley encephalitis, 1974: Clinical features. *Med J Aust.* 1976;2:446-450.
313. Burrow JN, Whelan PI, Kilburn CJ, et al. Australian encephalitis in the Northern Territory: clinical and epidemiological features, 1987-1996. *Aust N Z J Med.* 1998;28:590-596.
314. Douglas MW, Stephens DP, Burrow JN, et al. Murray Valley encephalitis in an adult traveller complicated by long-term flaccid paralysis: case report and review of the literature. *Trans R Soc Trop Med Hyg.* 2007;101(3):284-288.
315. Lopes O, Sacchetta L de A, Coimbra TLM, et al. Emergence of a new arbovirus disease in Brazil. II. Epidemiologic studies on 1975 epidemic. *Am J Epidemiol.* 1978;108:394.
316. Pavri K. Clinical, clinicopathologic, and hematologic features of Kyasanur Forest disease. *Rev Infect Dis Suppl.* 1989;4S:854.
317. Prabha A, Prabhu MG, Raghuvcer CV, et al. Clinical study of 100 cases of Kyasanur Forest disease with clinicopathological correlation. *Indian J Med Sci.* 1993;47:124.
318. Pattnaik P. Kyasanur forest disease: an epidemiological view in India. *Rev Med Virol.* 2006;16:151-165.
319. Lehrer AT, Holbrook MR. Tick-borne encephalitis. In: Barret AD, Stanberry L, eds. *Vaccines for Biodefense and Emerging and Neglected Diseases.* Philadelphia: Elsevier; 2008:713-734.
320. Lvov DK. Arboviral zoonoses of northern Eurasia (Eastern Europe and The Commonwealth of Independent States). In: Beran GW, ed. *Handbook of Zoonoses.* 2nd ed. Boca Raton, Fla: CRC; 1994:237.
321. Charrel RN, Attoui H, Butenko AM, et al. Tick-borne virus diseases of human interest in Europe. *Clin Microbiol Infect.* 2004;10:1040-1055.
322. Grard G, Moureau G, Charrel RN, et al. Genetic characterization of tick-borne flaviviruses: new insights into evolution, pathogenetic determinants and taxonomy. *Virology.* 2007;361: 80-92.
323. Kurane I, Takasaki T, Yamada K. Trends in flavivirus infections in Japan. *Emerg Infect Dis.* 2000;6:569-571.
324. Smithburn KC, Paterson HE, Heymann CS, et al. An agent related to Uganda S virus from man and mosquitoes in South Africa. *S Afr Med J.* 1959;33:959.
325. Figueiredo LT. The Brazilian flaviviruses. *Microbes Infect.* 2000;2:1643-1649.
326. Aaskov JG, Phillips DA, Wiemers MA. Possible clinical infection with Edge Hill virus. *Trans R Soc Trop Med Hyg.* 1993;87: 452-453.
327. Southam CM, Moore AE. West Nile, Ilheus, and Bunyamwera infections in man. *Am J Trop Med.* 1951;31:724-741.
328. Boughton CR, Hawkes RA, Naim HM. Illness caused by a Kokobera-like virus in southeastern Australia. *Med J Aust.* 1986;145:90-92.
329. Webb HE. Leukaemia and neoplastic processes treated with Langat and Kyasanur Forest disease viruses: A clinical and laboratory study of 28 patients. *BMJ.* 1966;5482:258-266.
330. Reeves WC. *Epidemiology and Control of Mosquito-Borne Arboviruses in California, 1943-1987.* Sacramento, Calif: California Mosquito Vector Control Association; 1990.
331. Sulkin SE, Burns KF, Shelton DF, et al. Bat salivary gland virus: Infections of man and monkey. *Tex Rep Biol Med.* 1962;20:113-127.
332. Woodroofe GM, Marshall ID. Arboviruses from the Sepik district of New Guinea. In: *John Curtin School of Medical Research Annual Report.* Canberra, Australia: Australian National University; 1971:90.
333. Nassar ES, Coimbra TL, Rocco IM, et al. Human disease caused by an arbovirus closely related to Ilheus virus: Report of five cases. *Intervirology.* 1997;40:247-252.
334. Wolfe MS, Calisher CH, McGuire K. Spondweni virus infection in a foreign resident of Upper Volta. *Lancet.* 1982;2:1306.
335. *Rapport Annuel du Centre Collaborateur OMS de Reference et de Recherche pours les Arbovirus.* Dakar: Institut Pasteur; 1983.
336. Heymann CS, Kokernot RH, De Meillon B. Wesselsbron virus infections in man. *S Afr Med J.* 1958;32:543-545.
337. Digoutte J-P, Salaun J-J, Robin Y, et al. Les arboviroses mineures en Afrique centrale et occidentale. *Med Trop (Mars).* 1980; 40:523-533.

154

Hepatitis C

STUART C. RAY | DAVID L. THOMAS

Non-A, Non-B Viral Hepatitis and Hepatitis C

When serologic tests for hepatitis A virus (HAV) and hepatitis B virus (HBV) were developed during the 1970s, it became evident that most cases of transfusion-associated hepatitis must be caused by yet another agent, leading to the term *non-A, non-B hepatitis* (NANB).[1,2] Studies in chimpanzees confirmed that blood-borne NANB hepatitis was transmissible and due to a relatively small, lipid-enveloped virus.[3,4] In the late 1980s, Michael Houghton's laboratory at Chiron Corporation, working with Daniel Bradley's laboratory at the Centers for Disease Control and Prevention (CDC), identified a virally encoded antigen associated with NANB hepatitis and called the agent "hepatitis C virus" (HCV).[5] This finding rapidly led to the molecular cloning of the complete viral genome[6] and other major discoveries, including the proclivity of this virus to establish persistent infection, and its strong association with chronic hepatitis, cirrhosis, and hepatocellular carcinoma.

Hepatitis C Virus

VIRION PROPERTIES AND CLASSIFICATION

HCV is a roughly spherical, enveloped, positive-strand RNA virus approximately 55 nm in diameter (Fig. 154-1).[7-10] Its structure, genomic organization, and replication cycle support classification as a member of the family *Flaviviridae*, yet it is sufficiently distinct to merit classification within a separate genus, *Hepacivirus*. Related genera include the genus *Flavivirus* (e.g., yellow fever virus and dengue viruses) and the genus *Pestivirus* (e.g., bovine viral diarrhea virus and classical swine fever virus). Several "GB" viruses are also in the Flaviviridae family,[11,12] although they have not yet been assigned to a particular genus. These include GB virus C (GBV-C), which was previously inappropriately considered to be a "hepatitis" virus (i.e., "hepatitis G virus"), and GB virus B (GBV-B), which is a true primate hepatitis virus and has the highest level of genetic relatedness to HCV of any animal virus.[13] Sucrose-gradient studies of infectious plasma and sera suggest that HCV may associate with low-density lipoproteins and, in some samples, with antibody in high-density complexes that are less infectious for chimpanzees.[14-17]

ORGANIZATION OF THE HCV GENOME

The genome of HCV is a positive-sense, single-stranded RNA molecule approximately 9.6 kb in length. Unlike a typical eukaryotic messenger RNA (mRNA), the HCV genomic RNA is neither 5′ capped nor polyadenylated, and contains a large open reading frame (ORF) encoding a single large polyprotein (~3010 aa). A frame-shifting event occurring near the 5′ end of the ORF has been suggested to shift some translating ribosomes into an alternative, truncated reading frame, giving rise to a putative "F" protein that, if it exists, is of uncertain function in the viral life cycle. The large ORF is flanked by highly conserved 5′ and 3′ untranslated regions (UTRs) that function in both translation and viral RNA replication (Fig. 154-2).[6]

Nontranslated RNA Segments

The HCV 5′UTR is approximately 341 nucleotides in length, demonstrates extensive secondary and tertiary RNA structure (see Fig. 154-2), and contains two overlapping functional regions. The 5′ 125 nucleotides are essential for viral RNA replication, probably for recognition of the RNA by the viral replicase, whereas the remainder of the 5′UTR appears to play an accessory role in this process.[18] An overlapping, approximately 300-nucleotide segment acts as an "internal ribosomal entry site" (IRES), directing the cap-independent translation of the viral ORF.[18-23] The HCV IRES and the closely related IRES elements of pestiviruses are unique among eukaryotic RNAs in that they are capable of binding directly to the 40S ribosome subunit in the absence of any protein translation initiation factor.[24-26] The binary complex formed by the 5′UTR RNA and the 40S subunit appears to involve specific macromolecular interactions around the initiator AUG codon of HCV.[27] Thus, HCV initiates translation of its proteins via a unique prokaryotic-like mechanism that may prove to be a useful target for future antiviral drug development.

The 3′UTR consists of a relatively variable 30 to 60 nucleotide segment downstream of the termination codon that is followed by a highly variable poly-U/UC tract of 50 to 100 nucleotides. Downstream of the poly-U/UC tract there is a highly conserved 98-base sequence (the "3′-X" region).[28-30] This highly structured 3′ terminal 98-base sequence is the most conserved segment of the HCV genome. Experiments in vitro indicate that "kissing loop" interactions between RNA structures in the 3′-X region and NS5B coding region, as well as 33 consecutive U residues in the poly-U/UC tract, are absolutely required for viral RNA replication.[31-33] Recent work indicates that the poly-U/UC tract is the principal pathogen-associated molecular pattern (PAMP) of HCV sensed by the human cytoplasmic pattern recognition receptor (PRR) RIG-I (see "Mechanisms of Persistence").[34] A highly unusual feature of HCV replication that involves the UTRs is the presence of complementary sequences for liver-specific microRNA 122 (miR122), an interaction that has been found to be necessary for HCV replication, potentially contributes to the liver tropism of HCV, and may represent a therapeutic target.[35]

Polyprotein

The approximately 9.0-kb ORF encodes a polyprotein that is cotranslationally processed into at least 10 proteins. These include three "structural" proteins: the nucleocapsid protein, core (C), and two envelope proteins (E1 and E2); two proteins that are essential for virion production but are not required for viral RNA replication (p7 and NS2); and five nonstructural proteins that form the viral RNA replicase complex (NS3, NS4A, NS4B, NS5A, and NS5B; see Fig. 154-2). Processing of the polyprotein is directed by both cellular and viral proteases. Four distinct signal sequences within the amino third of the polyprotein direct the translocation of the nascent protein into the ER, with the result that signal peptidase cleaves the polyprotein at the C/E1, E1/E2, E2/p7, and p7/NS2 junctions. The nascent NS2/NS3 protein is a cysteine protease that acts only *in cis* to cleave the NS2/NS3 junction, whereas the NS3 protein contains a second (serine) protease activity that catalyzes the remaining *in trans* polyprotein cleavages among the nonstructural proteins. Full expression of NS3 protease activity requires formation of a complex with the NS4A protein.

Structural Proteins

The 191 aa segment at the amino terminus of the HCV polyprotein is cleaved from the nascent polypeptide by signal peptidase, forming the highly basic core protein which has RNA-binding activity.[36-39] A further cleavage occurs just upstream of the signal peptide sequence, within

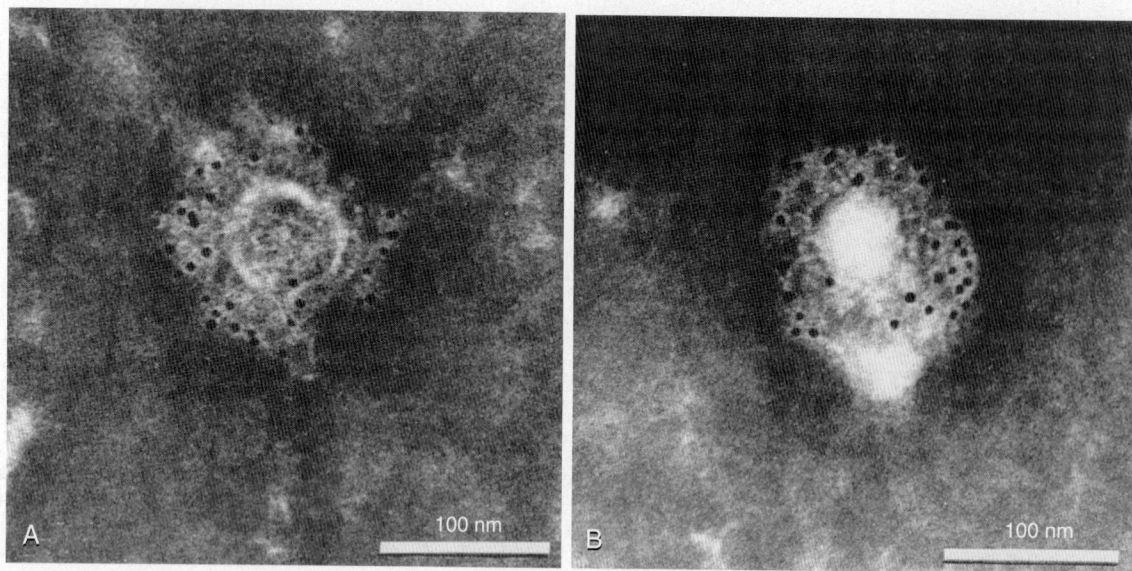

Figure 154-1 **A and B, Electron microscopic images of hepatitis C virus (HCV) virions concentrated from human plasma by high-speed centrifugation.** The virions are identified by staining with gold-labeled antibodies to the HCV envelope proteins. *(From Kaito M, Watanabe S, Tsukiyama-Koham K, et al. Hepatitis C virus particle detected by immunoelectron microscopic study. J Gen Virol. 1994;75:1755-1760.)*

the membranes of the endoplasmic reticulum (ER) and is directed by signal peptide peptidase.[40] This releases a mature core protein of about 171 amino acids into the cytoplasm of the cell, where it is associated with the surface of lipid droplets in a membranous compartment.[41]

A number of biologic activities have been associated with the core protein, including suppression of HBV replication, alterations in regulation of the cell cycle and transcription of cellular proto-oncogenes, either induction or suppression of apoptosis, and transformation of rat embryo fibroblasts.[42-52] The core protein has also been suggested to interfere with anti-HCV immune responses through a variety of mechanisms, including NK cell inhibition via upregulation of MHC class I expression, inhibition of T-cell proliferation via interaction with complement receptor gC1qR, and interaction with the cytoplasmic tail of several cellular receptors belonging to the tumor necrosis factor (TNF) receptor family.[48,49,51,53,54] However, these data are derived largely from studies in which core has been overexpressed from recombinant cDNA. It is not clear whether core exerts any of these biologic effects when expressed by replicating virus within the liver, and in many cases contradictory in vitro evidence against such effects can be found in the literature. The core protein is immunogenic; both core protein and antibody to it are typically present in the serum of infected individuals.

Yellow fever virus and other members of the genus *Flavivirus* have a single major envelope protein and a glycosylated, cell-associated NS-1 protein that can elicit neutralizing antibodies. However, HCV has two major envelope glycoproteins (E1 and E2) and no comparable NS-1 protein. Signal peptidases direct cleavage of the HCV polyprotein at amino acid residues 383 and 746 (numbering based on the prototype strain H77), producing the E1 and E2 proteins, respectively (see Fig. 154-2).[37] These are secreted into the ER as type 1 membrane proteins, remaining anchored to the membrane by a hydrophobic C-terminal anchor sequence (Fig. 154-3). The E1 and E2 proteins are heavily glycosylated, with sugar moieties representing about 50% of the mature mass of each. The two major envelope proteins associate with each other as a noncovalent heterodimeric complex; covalently linked complexes have also been identified, but are thought to arise from misfolded forms of the proteins.[55] In HCV cell culture, E1 and E2 are localized to the ER compartment, perhaps due to ER-retention signals located in the transmembrane domain.[41,56-58] This suggests that, like other members of the *Flaviviridae*, HCV particles assemble and exit the cell by budding into intracytoplasmic vesicles, and then follow the secretory pathway for release.

A highly variable segment approximately 30 amino acid residues in length near the amino terminus of E2 has been called the hypervariable region 1 (HVR-1).[59-61] It is the most genetically variable segment of the

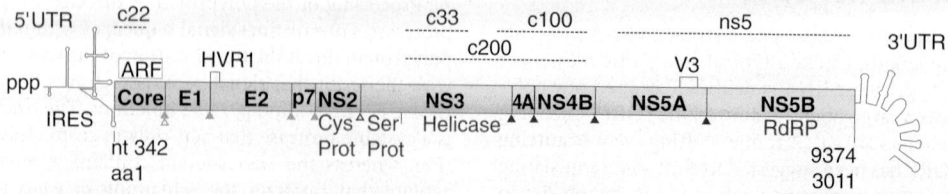

Figure 154-2 **Organization of the hepatitis C virus (HCV) genome and viral polyprotein.** The 5' and 3' untranslated region (UTR) RNA structures *(curves)* flank the major open reading frame (ORF). Unlike eukaryotic mRNA, the viral RNA genome has 5' triphosphate ("ppp") and no 3' polyadenylation. The 5'UTR contains an internal ribosomal entry site (IRES). Triangles indicate sites of cleavage by host cellular signal peptidase *(brown, open indicating additional processing by signal peptide peptidase)* and viral proteases *(red, open indicating cleavage by the NS2/NS3 cysteine protease)*. Putative structural *(purple)* and nonstructural *(blue)* mature proteins *(boxes)* generated by these cleavage events are labeled, below which in red are viral enzymatic functions NS2/NS3 cysteine protease (Cys Prot), NS3 serine protease (Ser Prot), NS3 helicase, and the NS5B RNA-dependent RNA polymerase (RdRP). Positions of the first and last nucleotides (nt) and amino acids (aa) of the polyprotein ORF are shown, based on reference genome H77 (GenBank accession number AF009606). Above the ORF are positions of the alternate reading frame (ARF) protein, variable regions HVR-1 and V3, and *(dashed lines)* the antigens included in the EIA and RIBA serologic assays. See "Organization of the HCV Genome."

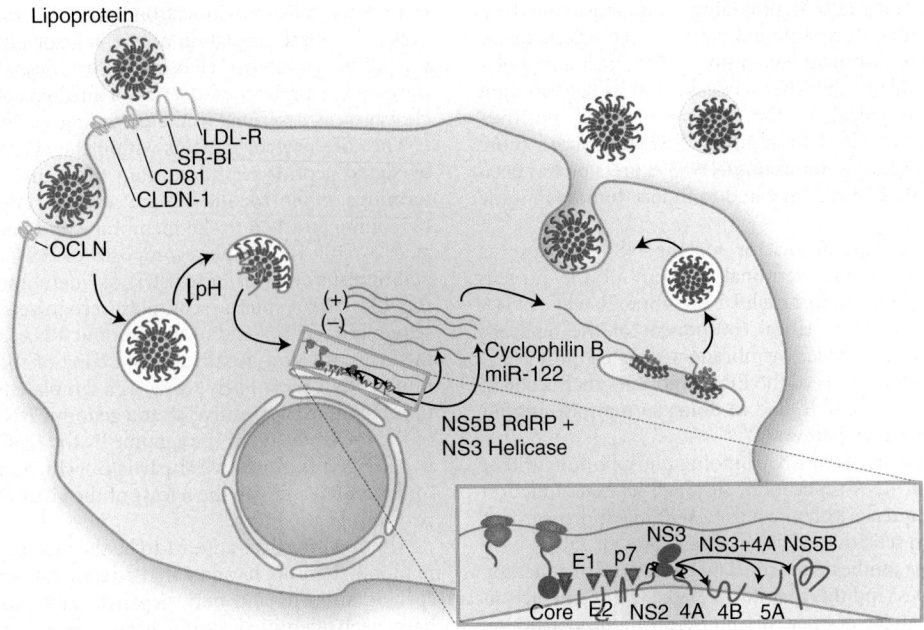

Figure 154-3 **Putative major events in the replication of hepatitis C virus (HCV).** Specific steps include: attachment and penetration of the virion into the hepatocyte via a receptor complex that has not been fully characterized; pH-dependent membrane fusion and release of viral RNA (*solid green line*) into cytoplasm; cap-independent translation directed by the internal ribosomal entry site (IRES), and processing of the viral polyprotein (*triangles*) resulting in production of the viral proteins (*blue*) core, envelope proteins E1 and E2, putative viroporin p7, and 5 nonstructural proteins that are essential for RNA replication that form the replicase complex; assembly of a "membranous web" from ER structures (mediated by NS4B) and the replicase complex at the 3' end of the virion RNA; synthesis of a minus-strand replicative intermediate RNA ("−"); synthesis of multiple positive-strand copies ("+") of the RNA; assembly of virus particles in late ER, early Golgi compartments; and release of progeny virus from the cell. Many of these details have yet to be confirmed by direct experimental evidence. See "Replication." (*Graphic art by Jocelyn Ray.*)

envelope proteins and is assumed to exist as a polypeptide loop on the surface of the virion. Infected persons frequently have antibodies that react with synthetic peptides representing the HVR-1 sequences of the virus with which they are infected. The appearance of such antibodies seems to alter the quasispecies, selecting variants with HVR-1 sequences that are less reactive. Available evidence suggests that the HVR-1 harbors one or more neutralization epitopes, and that it is a site of mutations causing immune escape during acute and chronic infection.[62-65] Such mutations may occur at little cost to the virus, as the extent of sequence heterogeneity within the HVR-1 indicates that there are few sequence-related constraints on its function; however, some constraints have been observed (see "Humoral Immunity").[66-68] It has been suggested that the HVR-1 may function as an immunologic decoy during infection by masking a deeper, more highly conserved structure within the envelope, such as a recognition site for the cellular receptor.[69] Importantly, deletion of this region does not eliminate the ability of the virus to infect chimpanzees, suggesting that it is not critical for viral entry or release.[70]

p7 and NS2 Proteins
These two proteins may play roles in viral particle assembly or egress from the cell, but neither is required for viral RNA replication.[71] A signal peptidase cleavage near the carboxyl-terminus of E2 generates the p7 (formerly NS2A) protein (see Fig. 154-2). This is a small, 63 aa hydrophobic polypeptide that appears capable of forming a voltage-gated ion channel in a manner that suggests it may be a viroporin. This activity is essential for production of infectious virions, and inhibited in vitro by amantadine and long-alkyl-chain iminosugar derivatives, thereby representing a possible therapeutic target.[71-74]

The NS2 (formerly NS2B) protein is a membrane-associated dimeric cysteine protease with two composite active sites that mediate cleavage at the NS2/NS3 junction.[75-77] The transmembrane and protease domain

structures of NS2 are essential for production of infectious virions in cell culture, whereas the protease activity is not.[71,78] The precise role of the NS2 transmembrane and protease domains in virion assembly remains unknown, though structural analysis and in vitro study of cultured intergenotype chimeric viruses suggests that NS2 may interact directly with p7 and NS3.[77,79]

Nonstructural Proteins Involved in RNA Replication
Proteins spanning the region within the polyprotein from NS3 to NS5B (see Fig. 154-2) are required for RNA replication, which occurs in a membrane-associated replicase complex within the cytoplasm. The NS3 protein possesses serine protease activity localized to its amino terminal third, and an RNA helicase with NTPase activity in its carboxy-terminal domain. The mature, fully active NS3 protease requires the noncovalent association of NS3 with the NS4A protein, which becomes an integral part of the protease structure.[80-83] Atomic-level resolution structures of these domains have been solved separately and together, and these have been explored as targets for antiviral drug discovery efforts (see "Specific Small Antivirals for Hepatitis C").[80,84,85] The NS3 serine protease is active *in trans*, is dependent on zinc, and is responsible for the NS3/NS4A *cis* cleavage, as well as the NS4A/NS4B, NS4B/NS5A, and NS5A/NS5B cleavages that follow in the processing of the polyprotein. The carboxy-terminal 465 amino acids of NS3 contain the NTPase and RNA helicase activities, which are likely to direct the unwinding of duplex RNA molecules at some point during the replication of the viral genome. There is evidence that the helicase has 3' to 5' directionality and binds to the 3' poly-U/UC sequence.[86,87] No cleavage site has been identified between the NS3 protease and helicase, and functional studies suggest that these domains are interdependent.[88]

NS3 protease activity has been shown to interfere with interferon-mediated signaling by blocking the virus-activated phosphorylation of interferon regulatory factor 3 (IRF3), providing a mechanism by which HCV might evade innate cellular antiviral defenses (see "Mechanisms of Persistence").[89] The multifunctional nature of NS3, including polyprotein processing, its role in the RNA replicase, and its contribution to immune evasion, is typical for the proteins of small, positive-stranded RNA viruses like HCV. In addition, NS3 may play a more direct role in viral pathogenesis; for example, NS3 expression has been shown to transform NIH 3T3 cell lines and to induce tumors in nude mice.[90]

The NS4A protein acts as a cofactor for the NS3 protease, as described previously. An amino terminal segment of the protein anchors the NS3/4A complex to intracellular membranes, while NS4A also interacts with NS5A as a critical component of the replicase complex. NS4B is a hydrophobic, membrane-associated protein. It appears to mediate modifications of the ER membranes that occur in association with replicase assembly, and in doing so may also inhibit normal ER-to-Golgi secretory pathways.[91,92]

NS5A is a membrane-anchored RNA-binding phosphoprotein that appears to play a role in RNA replication, although its exact function remains obscure.[93-95] Sequence polymorphisms within a short segment of NS5A (the interferon sensitivity determining region, or ISDR) have been correlated in some studies with resistance to interferon therapy for some HCV genotypes, and this may be mediated by the interaction of NS5A with the catalytic domain of interferon-induced dsRNA-activated protein kinase R (PKR).[96-99] Inactivation of PKR by NS5A could mitigate both the antiviral and antiproliferative activities of interferon, though this remains unproven. In addition, NS5A may induce expression of IL-8, which antagonizes expression of interferon-stimulated genes.[100]

The NS5B is a membrane-bound protein that contains a Gly-Asp-Asp motif characteristic of RNA-dependent RNA polymerases and is considered to be the catalytic core of the replicase complex. The RNA-binding activity of NS5B is stimulated by cyclophilin B and inhibited by cyclosporine A.[101,102] As with the enzymatic activities of the NS3 protein, the NS5B RNA polymerase has proven to be a useful target for antiviral drug development with nucleoside analogues and non-nucleoside small molecule inhibitors, as well as cyclosporine A analogues, now in the development pipeline (see "Specific Small Molecule Antivirals for Hepatitis C").

In addition to the polyprotein described above, ribosomal frame-shifting may generate the F (frame shift) or ARF (alternate reading frame) protein from a short ORF found within the core region of some genotype 1 isolates.[103-105] Some subjects with HCV infection, but not those with HBV, have been found to have serum antibody and T-cell reactivity to in vitro synthesized F protein, suggesting that the protein can be expressed in vivo. The role of the F protein remains speculative, and recent evidence suggests that a related RNA element, rather than the ARF protein itself, is required for infection in vitro and in vivo.[106]

REPLICATION

Details of the viral life cycle were initially examined using replication-competent subgenomic RNA replicons in cultured cells, and then more recently with a cell culture system that completes the viral life cycle from cell entry to release of infectious virions. These studies and reasonable analogies with other positive-strand RNA viruses suggest the following scenario (see Fig. 154-3). The virus is likely to enter the cell through interaction with more than one specific cell surface receptor molecule; suggested receptor molecules include CD81, the LDL receptor, DC-SIGN, L-SIGN, human scavenger receptor SR-B1, and the tight junction protein claudin-1.[107-113] Following attachment, penetration, and uptake into a cellular endosome, local pH changes may alter the conformation of the envelope proteins, resulting in fusion with the endosomal membrane. The viral RNA is released into the cytoplasm, where it acts as mRNA directing the cap-independent translation of the viral polyprotein. The ability to rescue infectious virus by intrahepatic inoculation of synthetic, genome-length RNA in chimpanzees, as well as the replication competence of viral RNA in

transfected cells, provides strong proof for this step in the replication cycle.[114,115] Viral translation occurs in association with the rough ER by the process of internal ribosome entry (described previously), and the polyprotein undergoes a series of further cotranslational proteolytic cleavages, as described in the preceding section.

The core protein remains within the cytoplasm following cleavage by signal peptide peptidase from the signal sequence at its carboxy-terminus, while E1 and E2 are secreted into the lumen of the ER, remaining attached to the membrane and becoming heavily glycosylated. A replicase complex, composed of NS3, NS4A, NS4B, NS5A, and NS5B forms cytoplasmic clusters of "membranous webs" derived from the ER. This replicase complex recognizes specific structures and sequences at the 3' end of the genomic RNA, and subsequently directs the synthesis of a negative-strand copy of the genome. The resulting duplex RNA most likely serves as a template for the synthesis of multiple copies of the positive-strand genomic RNA, following recognition of the opposite end of the genome by the replicase. The genomic RNA is packaged into new viral particles, which are likely to be extruded into the ER leading to the release of the virus via the vesicular secretory pathway.

Although the liver appears to be the primary source of virus present in blood, there are few data that directly support this conjecture. HCV-specific antigens and both negative- and positive-strand HCV RNA have been identified within hepatocytes, indicating that replication occurs in this cell type via a negative-strand intermediate as outlined previously.[116-118] However, additional data suggest that the virus may also replicate within peripheral mononuclear cells of lymphoid or perhaps bone marrow origin (see "Viral Tropism").[119,120]

Mathematical models of viral kinetics suggest a half-life of approximately 2.5 hours for virions in the bloodstream and that up to 1.0×10^{12} virions are produced each day in a chronically infected human.[121,122] This rate meets or exceeds comparable estimates of the production of human immunodeficiency virus (HIV).[123]

GENETIC DIVERSITY

Quasispecies Variation

The high level of virion turnover, the absence of proofreading by the NS5B RNA polymerase, and the "tolerance" of many genomic regions for multiple nucleotides results in the relatively rapid accumulation of viral mutations. Multiple HCV variants can be recovered from the plasma and liver of an infected individual at any time. As a result, like many RNA viruses, HCV exists in each infected person as a quasispecies, or "swarm" of closely related but distinct genetic sequences.[61,124] For example, up to 85% of cDNA clones obtained from viral RNAs in the blood of a recently infected individual may represent unique genetic variants.[125] During RNA replication, mutations most likely occur in a nearly random fashion throughout the genome, whereas fixation of a substitution within the quasispecies population depends on how that substitution influences viral "fitness" as related to its effect on functional protein/RNA structures, the capacity of the virus for replication, and the host-viral interaction.

Immunologic responses appear to be important selective forces. For example, viral RNAs containing spontaneous mutations within the HVR-1 segment of the E2 protein (discussed previously) may be favored for survival in the host when they reduce the binding of preexisting neutralizing antibodies to the viral envelope, and may be relatively neutral in terms of viral replication.[126-129] Significantly, agammaglobulinemic patients have slower evolution of amino acid sequence changes within HRV-1.[130,131] There is also evidence that cellular immune responses may drive the selection of specific quasispecies variants.[68,132,133] Thus, quasispecies variants recovered from blood reflect the balance of production and selective forces.

Although the nucleotide substitutions identified in circulating virus represent only a fraction of all mutations generated during viral replication, these mutations are estimated to occur at an overall rate of $0.9 - 1.92 \times 10^{-3}$ base substitutions per site per year during chronic infection.[134-136] Variation within an HCV quasispecies swarm can be described either in terms of the number of nucleotide differences between variants within a single blood sample (i.e., *genetic diversity*) or in terms of the number of distinct variants (i.e., *genetic complexity*). There is considerable interest in determining the clinical correlates of these parameters. Although much remains to be learned, it appears that genetic complexity is linked to the extent of disease and the duration of infection.[137,138] This is consistent with the hypothesis that immunologic responses affect both the extent of disease progression and the generation of sequence diversity. Thus, quasispecies variation results from the persistence of infection in the face of an active but less than completely effective immune response; it is not likely, however, to be the sole cause of persistence (see "Mechanisms of Persistence"). Differences in the HCV quasispecies present in the blood and liver (and possibly other tissues) have been described, suggesting that differences in tissue tropism may also influence genetic variation.[120,139,140]

The extent of genetic diversity varies markedly throughout the HCV genome, being highest in the segment that encodes the amino terminus of the second envelope protein, E2, within the so-called HVR-1, and lowest in the core gene and the 5′ and 3′ nontranslated segments of the genome.[126-129,141] High conservation at some loci suggests functional constraint (mutations may be lethal or sufficiently disadvantageous to replication to be undetectable among surviving virus populations).

HCV Genotypes

In addition to the impressive heterogeneity that often exists among HCV sequences present in a single infected individual (i.e., quasispecies variation), there is also remarkable genetic heterogeneity and divergence among HCV sequences recovered from different individuals (i.e., strain and genotype variation). Phylogenetic evaluation of HCV sequences recovered from multiple geographic regions suggests that there are at least six major genotypes or clades, with a provisional identification of a seventh genotype in a specimen originating from central Africa.[142,143] These genotypes are even more diverse than those

causing the worldwide HIV-1 pandemic (Fig. 154-4), in part due to a much longer epidemic history for HCV.[144] Depending on the genomic region evaluated, HCV sequences assigned to different genotypes may have less than 50% nucleotide sequence identity. Significantly, this level of nucleotide sequence divergence usually correlates with substantial serotypic differences among other RNA viruses (e.g., poliovirus type 1 vs. poliovirus type 2, which are not cross-neutralizable in assays of antibody-mediated neutralization). Little is known, however, of the extent of serotypic variation among HCV strains. Despite extensive study, there is little evidence that HCV genotypes differ in transmissibility, level of replication, or rate of progression of the resulting liver disease. There are genotype differences in response to interferon-based treatments and emerging data of differences in small molecule inhibitory activity (see "Treatment").

Within individual HCV genotypes, strains can be further grouped into subgenotypes (subtypes) that generally share 75% to 85% nucleotide sequence identity within the core-E1 and NS5B regions of the genome.[142,145] In contrast, the quasispecies variants that exist within a single person generally have 91% to 99% identity in these regions.[146] The phylogenetic grouping of HCV strains is largely independent of the segment of the genome that is analyzed.[142,147]

The geographic distribution of HCV genotypes is not fully characterized, but some trends are apparent. Within the United States, 60% to 70% of isolates are either of genotype 1a or 1b (Fig. 154-5).[148,149] In contrast, genotype 4 infections are prevalent throughout Africa and the Middle East.[150] For example, more than 90% of the viral sequences recovered in an Egyptian survey were of genotype 4.[151] Types 5 and 6 have been reported in South Africa and Southeast Asia.[152-154] Genotype 3 occurs in Asia, but has been linked in other geographic regions to illicit drug use.[155] Differences between early proposals for genotype nomenclature may cause some confusion in interpreting such studies; however, there is general acceptance of a revised nomenclature.[13,156]

VIRAL TROPISM

HCV replicates within the hepatocyte, and the liver-specific expression of miR122 may contribute to this specificity as noted previously. However, replication may also occur in other cell types. Some studies have suggested the presence of negative-strand (replicative intermediate) HCV RNA in T cells, B cells, and monocytes, especially in patients with chronic infection.[157-159] Others have suggested that this occurs rarely,[119] or not at all,[160,161] but, as already mentioned, differences in dominant quasispecies populations in these various compartments are supportive of extrahepatic infection. Substantial evidence also supports the ability of HCV to replicate at low levels in cultured human cells of T- and B-cell origin.[162]

HCV RNA also has been detected in cutaneous lesions of persons with HCV-related cryoglobulinemia and vasculitis,[163] in renal biopsies of patients with HCV-associated membranoproliferative glomerulonephritis,[164] and (with variable success) in various body fluids including saliva, semen, tears, urine, and ascitic fluid.[165-167] Unlike HBV, HCV replication does not produce DNA that can integrate its genetic information into chromosomal DNA. Because of this, the detection of HCV sequences in these tissues and fluids may indicate the presence of infectious virus, though transmission via these fluids appears to be rare (see "Transmission of HCV").

EXPERIMENTAL MODELS

Autonomously Replicating Viral Replicons and Genome-Length RNAs

Specially constructed subgenomic HCV RNAs ("replicons") and genome-length RNAs undergo autonomous replication in certain cultured cells. These model systems have provided important information regarding HCV RNA replication mechanisms and virus-host cell interactions. The first such replicons were dicistronic RNAs derived from molecularly cloned cDNA (Fig. 154-6A).[168] The expression of a selectable antibiotic marker, such as neomycin phosphotransferase (Neo),

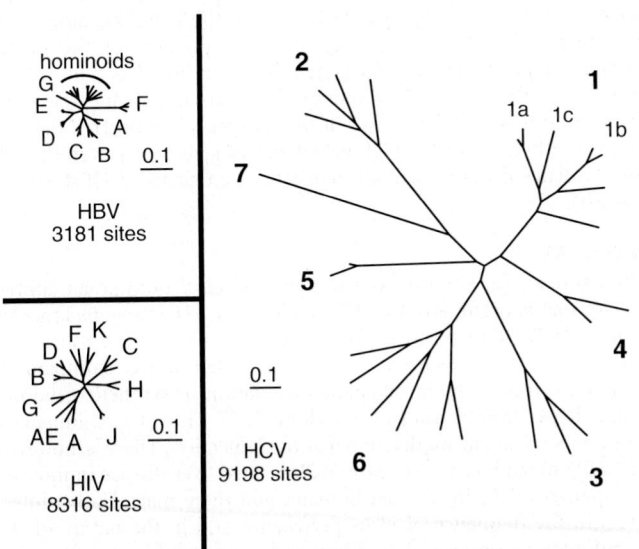

Figure 154-4 **Phylogenetic trees for hepatitis B virus (HBV), human immunodeficiency virus (HIV), and hepatitis C virus (HCV) shown to the same scale in terms of nucleotide genetic distance, based on full-length genome nucleotide sequences.** Sequences of representative strains for major genotypes were obtained from GenBank and aligned using ClustalX with minor manual adjustment, then sites containing gaps were removed resulting in an alignment of 3181 sites for HBV, 8316 sites for HIV, and 9198 sites for HCV. Maximum likelihood trees were inferred using PAUP* version 4b10, with the model (GTR+I+G in all three cases) and parameters selected by ModelTest 3.7 using the AIC criterion.

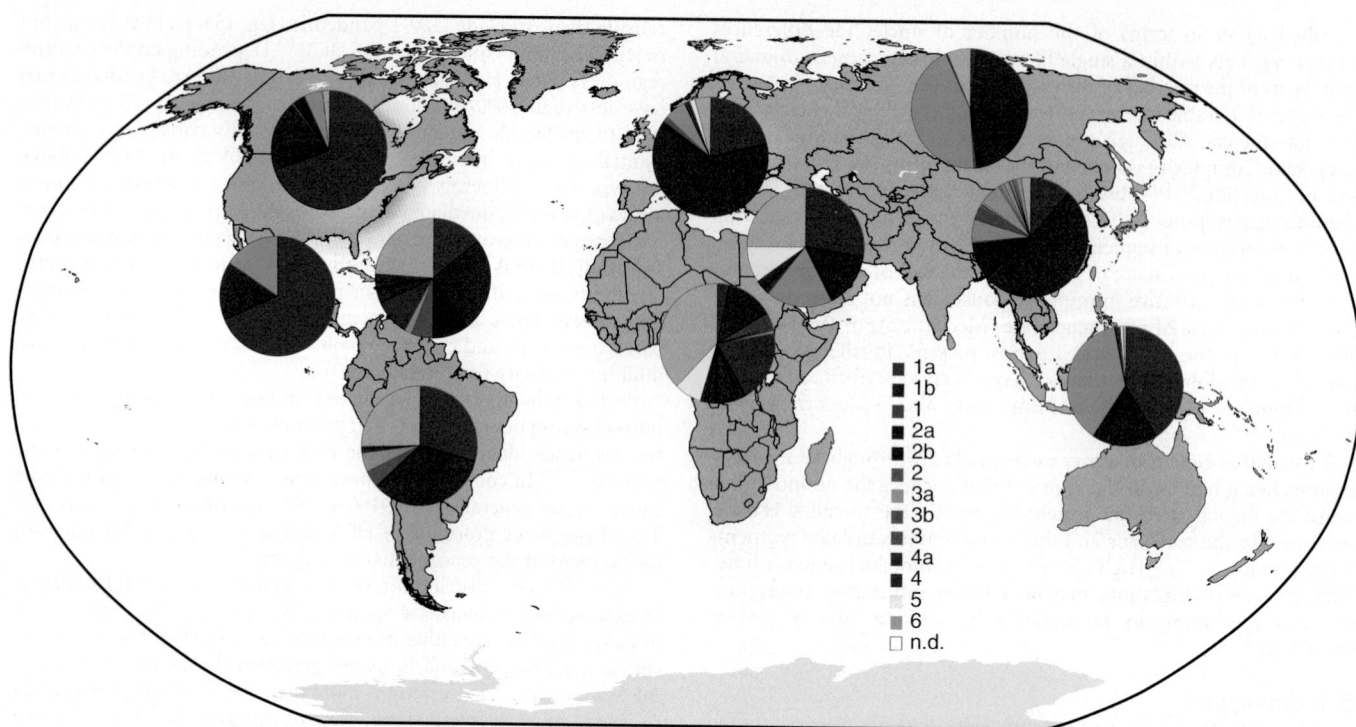

Figure 154-5 **Hepatitis C virus (HCV) subtype distribution worldwide, based on availability in online databases because population-based sampling is not consistently available.** Adapted from data generated using the interactive "Geography" tool at http://hcv.lanl.gov. Geographic information was available for 39,316 sequences, which were clustered by region: Africa, Asia, Caribbean, Central America, Europe, former USSR, Middle East, North America, Oceania, and South America. A putative 7th genotype has been proposed for virus found in Central Africa.

from the upstream cistron of these dicistronic RNAs under control of the natural HCV IRES allowed the selection of stable cell clones supporting replication of the RNA following its transfection into the cells. The downstream cistron, encoding either the NS2-NS5B or NS3-NS5B nonstructural proteins, was placed under the translational control of a picornaviral IRES. Such RNAs demonstrate a surprisingly robust replication phenotype in cultured human hepatoma cells (Huh7 cells), but typically only after the accumulation of adaptive mutations within the HCV sequence (often in the NS5A protein).[169] Interestingly, such mutations appear to attenuate substantially the ability of the virus to replicate in chimpanzees.[170] Some HCV RNAs have been further adapted to growth in HeLa cells and even cells of murine origin.[171]

As subgenomic replicon RNAs typically lack the sequence encoding the structural proteins (core and E1, E2, and p7), they are not capable of producing infectious particles. However, replication-competent, selectable dicistronic RNAs that encode all of the viral proteins also have been developed and also do not appear to produce infectious particles despite substantial replication in hepatoma cells.[172] The nature of the apparent block in virion production in these cells is not known, but it was recognized that many of the adaptive mutations that increased replicon efficiency (in terms of RNA production) impaired replication in vivo in the chimpanzee model. Although the first replicons were made from genotype 1b strains of HCV, RNAs from other genotypes (e.g., genotypes 1a and 2a) have been adapted to highly efficient replication in Huh7 cells. These subgenomic HCV replicons and genome-length RNAs appear to recapitulate the natural mechanisms of HCV RNA replication, and are useful for discerning differences in the susceptibility of different viral strains and genotypes to new candidate antiviral compounds and for studying mechanisms of resistance.

Propagation of Virus in Cell Cultures

The description in 2005 of a complete cell culture system for propagating HCV (designated HCVcc) opened a new era in HCV research,

enabling in vitro study of a complete viral life cycle.[10,173,174] Key aspects of this system were the recognition that the JFH-1 genomic RNA clone replicated efficiently without the need for adaptive mutations, and the isolation of highly permissive derivatives of the Huh7 hepatoma cell line, which may be defective in some components of the innate immune response. The HCVcc system has been broadened to include chimeras of the JFH-1 (HCV subtype 2a) strain that include portions of other strains, and derivatives of the subtype 1a strain H77 that are important because of the high prevalence of genotype 1 even though these isolates do not currently replicate as efficiently as JFH-1 (Fig. 154-6B).

Animal Models

The chimpanzee, *Pan troglodytes*, is the principal nonhuman animal species that is permissive for HCV replication. Percutaneous inoculation of HCV RNA-positive plasma, and in one instance saliva, has resulted in HCV infection.[175-177] Also, as noted above, chimpanzees have been infected by intrahepatic inoculation of synthetic genome-length RNA derived from cDNA clones.[114,115] Thus, the chimpanzee represents a valuable model for hepatitis C infection. There is, however, generally much less evidence for HCV-related liver disease in infected chimpanzees than in infected humans, and there may also be differences in the frequency of virus persistence and in the nature of the immunologic response.[177] As chimpanzees are an endangered species, the use of this animal model has been severely limited by costs, scarcity of the animals, and ethical concerns. Thus, it is of interest that GBV-B infection of nonendangered tamarins or marmosets shows substantial promise as a surrogate animal model for hepatitis C. GBV-B has greater sequence homology with HCV than any other animal virus, replicates within the liver of these animals, and can cause both acute and chronic hepatitis with many features resembling hepatitis C.[178]

Initially, mouse models of HCV infection were limited to transgenic mice that express transgenes encoding all or some HCV proteins under the control of liver-specific constitutive or inducible promoters.[179-181]

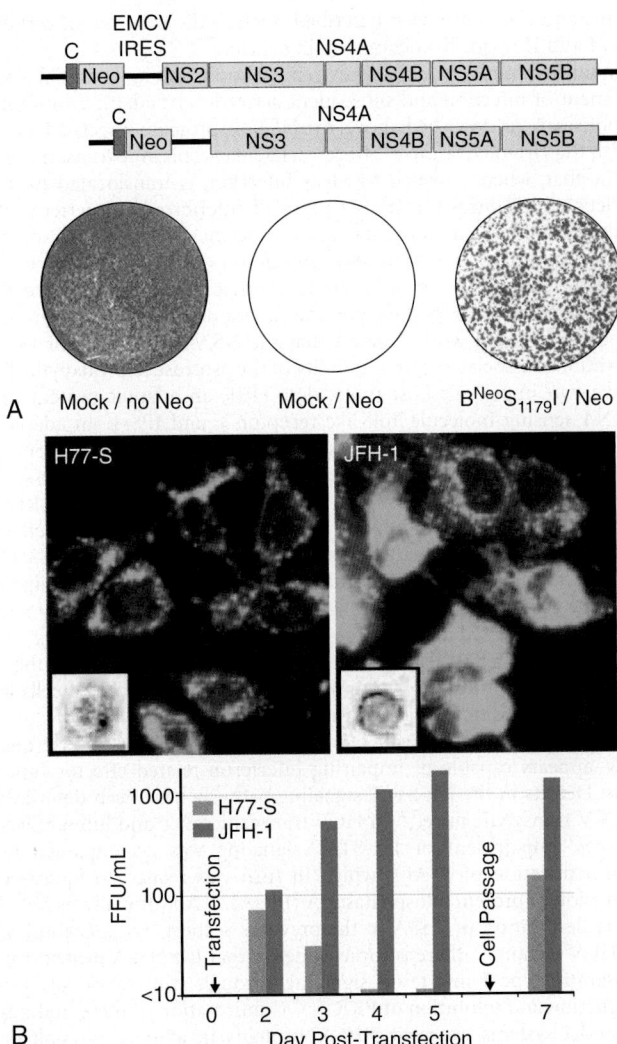

demonstrated broad neutralization of a heterologous viral swarm for some antibodies, but only at high titers.

Natural History and Pathogenesis

VIRAL PERSISTENCE

In experimentally infected chimpanzees and in humans, HCV RNA can be detected in plasma within days of exposure, often 1 to 4 weeks before liver enzyme levels rise.[175,184-188] Viremia peaks in the first 8 to 12 weeks of infection, then drops to lower levels and persists (Fig. 154-7).[189] In some instances, plasma HCV RNA becomes undetectable in the first few months and remains undetectable indefinitely (viral clearance); in other instances, viremia is inconsistently detected early and a stable pattern of recovery or persistence is not evident for more than 6 months.[175,187,190-193] Some instances of intermittent viremia may reflect reinfection, which has been observed in active injection drug users.[190] In other cases, rebounding viremia may represent escape from an initially successful immune response.[133,191,193,194] Overall, viremia persists in 50% to 85% of acutely infected persons (see "Treatment of Acute Hepatitis C").[187,190,195,196]

Because of limitations in experimental models and the infrequent recognition of natural acute infection, the mechanisms of viral clearance are poorly understood. There are clinical and epidemiologic clues that suggest host factors are critical. The role of the host in viral persistence is evident in common source outbreaks in which a large number of persons were accidentally infected with the same HCV inoculum and only some recovered.[197] In addition, HCV infection more often persists in African Americans than whites and in persons infected with HIV, compared to immunocompetent persons.[198,199] Persons also are more likely to clear HCV infection if they develop clinical symptoms (i.e., become jaundiced), which correlates with a more vigorous immune response.[190] Nonetheless, it has been difficult to define the immunologic mechanisms of HCV persistence and their genetic determinants.

Humoral Immunity

Within months of infection, antibodies are detectable in blood to multiple recombinant antigens that correspond to structural and non-

Figure 154-6 Organization of subgenomic hepatitis C virus (HCV) replicons, and selection of antibiotic-resistant human hepatoma cells following transfection with a neomycin phosphotransferase-expressing RNA replicon. A, The genetic organization of subgenomic replicons encoding the NS3-NS5B and NS2-NS5B segments of the viral polyprotein, as described by Lohmann et al.[168] is shown at top of figure. Below are photographs of cultures of human hepatoma (Huh7) cells that were either mock transfected or transfected with a subgenomic NS3-NS5B replicon RNA containing a cell-culture adaptation mutation within NS5A (B^NeoS_1179I). Following transfection, the cells in the two plates on the right were treated with G418 (neomycin). All cultures were stained with crystal violet approximately 3 weeks later. **B,** Hepatitis C virus cell culture (HCVcc) using the highly permissive Huh-7.5 cell line transfected with viral clones H77-S (*upper panel left*, at 96 hours) and JFH-1 (*upper panel right*, at 48 hours), then fixed and stained with a fluorescently tagged monoclonal antibody to the Core protein (upper panel insets are anti-E2 immunogold-labeled viral particles). Lower panel shows the time course of HCVcc infection, measured as focus-forming units (FFU) per mL. *(From Yi M, Villanueva RA, Thomas DL, et al. Production of infectious genotype 1a hepatitis C virus (Hutchinson strain) in cultured human hepatoma cells. PNAS (USA). 2006;103:2310-2315.)*

More recently, xenotransplantation of human hepatocytes to immunodeficient mice with chronic liver disease has resulted in a small-animal model that supports HCV replication.[182] For example, mice with severe combined immunodeficiency (SCID) transgenic for expression of plasminogen activator under control of the albumin promoter were transplanted with human hepatocytes and then used to test for protection in passive immunization using various monoclonal antibodies specific for HCV envelope genes.[183] These experiments

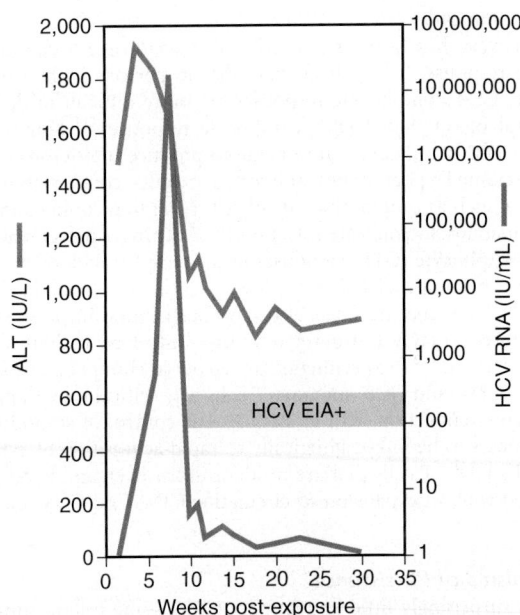

Figure 154-7 Acute hepatitis C virus (HCV) infection in a health care worker following a needlestick accident (time zero). *(From Sulkowski MS, Ray SC, Thomas DL. Needlestick transmission of hepatitis C. JAMA. 2002;287:2406-2413.)*

structural genes.[200] Emergence of HCV-specific antibodies does not correlate temporally with viral recovery. Indeed, although virtually all immunocompetent persons develop antibody responses to some HCV antigens, most infections persist. Viral recovery also has been described in persons with congenital agammaglobulinemia.[201] Alternately, humoral immune responses can neutralize individual variants. For example, there were fewer HCV infections in liver transplant recipients who received immune globulin prior to 1990, when it contained antibody to HCV.[202] Likewise, in a randomized controlled study, immune globulin administration was associated with a reduced incidence of sexual HCV transmission.[203] In the chimpanzee model, Farci and colleagues showed that antibodies could neutralize HCV infection in chimpanzees if those antibodies were directed at the HVR-1 sequence in the E2 protein, and that the same antibodies did not neutralize an inoculum collected later that had amino acid changes in the envelope sequence.[62,204] Krawczynski and coworkers have shown that postexposure immune globulin administration prolonged the incubation of HCV infection, and in later studies, was associated with early termination of infection.[205] Persons with reduced humoral immunity also accumulate fewer amino acid mutations in the E2 sequence.[131,206] In persons who recover from HCV infection, HCV antibody responses decline, sometimes below the level of detection by commercial assays.[177,190,207] In contrast, CD4+ lymphocyte responses often are maintained (see "Cellular Immunity").

Several functional expression systems have been described for the HCV envelope proteins, including the use of pseudotyped lentiviruses in cell-culture-based assays for neutralizing antibodies.[208-210] Application of this system to samples from one well-characterized individual suggested that HCV escapes continuously from neutralizing antibody responses in vivo.[65] Antibodies to HCV envelope proteins appear later and at lower titers compared to antibodies directed against nonstructural proteins, suggesting that neutralizing antibodies may play only a minor role in spontaneous resolution.[200,210] However, recent data from a common-source outbreak suggest that use of a much better-matched autologous envelope antigen reveals earlier appearance of neutralizing antibodies.[211] Collectively, the available data suggest that the humoral immune response can neutralize individual HCV variants and possibly limit the severity or even risk of recurrent infection, but are neither necessary nor sufficient for primary viral clearance.

Cellular Immunity

Viral recovery has been associated with a vigorous, broad cellular immune response.[191,212-214] It appears that in persons with persistent infection, CD4+ lymphocyte responses are more difficult to detect in peripheral blood than CD8+ lymphocyte responses.[215] Some HCV-specific CD8+ lymphocytes are unable to produce interferon-γ (a so-called "stunned" phenotype) and often express counter-regulatory molecules such as programmed death 1 (PD-1) that could contribute to their inability to eradicate infection.[216-218] Stronger polyclonal cytotoxic T lymphocyte (CTL) responses in the peripheral blood and liver also have been associated with lower levels of circulating HCV RNA.[219,220] HCV-specific CTLs also have been found in persons who were exposed to HCV but never were known to have had HCV antibody or viremia.[221,222] Experiments carried out in chimpanzees indicate that both CD4+ and CD8+ memory T cells play critical roles in protection against reinfection with HCV.[223,224] The control of second infections appears to be linked kinetically to rapid acquisition of cytolytic activity by CD8+ T cells that are resident in the liver, and is normally associated with an expansion of circulating CD4+ and CD8+ memory T cells.[224]

Mechanisms of Persistence

There is surprisingly little known about why some cellular immune responses are broad and vigorous and others ineffective. Coinfection with HIV or schistosomiasis has been associated with viral persistence, which corresponds with a diminished CD4+ lymphocyte response.[198,225,226] Host differences between persons whose infections

persist and clear have been described, such as the presence of certain class I and II major histocompatibility alleles.[227-230]

Innate immunity is probably extremely important in the initial containment of infection and subsequent activation of adaptive immune responses.[231] As described above, the NS3/4A protease directs a blockade of the virus activation of IRF3,[232] a latent cytoplasmic transcription factor that, when activated by virus infection, is translocated to the nucleus and induces the transcription of interferon-β. Interferon-β, through subsequent autocrine and paracrine mechanisms, subsequently stimulates the synthesis of interferon-α and a wide variety of other antiviral cytokines and chemokines that both inhibit viral replication and help to orchestrate the subsequent adaptive immune response.[89] Recent work suggests that the NS3/4A blockade of IRF3 activation is associated with the ability of the protease to proteolytically cleave two important host molecules: TRIF, an adapter protein for dsRNA sensing molecule Toll-like receptor 3; and IPS-1, an adaptor protein in the RIG-I signaling cascade.[233-235] When infected by sendai virus, hepatoma cells supporting HCV replicons transcribe less of NF-κB-regulated cytokines, like IL-6 and IL-12, as well as IRF3-regulated interferons and interferon-stimulated genes (ISGs), an effect that is blocked by treatment with small molecule inhibitors of NS3/4A protease.[233,235] Gene expression microarray studies have shown vigorous type 1 interferon responses within the livers of both acutely and chronically infected chimpanzees, indicating that these effects are incomplete.[236,237] Further research is needed to resolve whether these interferons are produced by uninfected cells, recently infected cells in which NS3/4A is not yet active, or another mechanism.

In addition to potentially blocking the induction of interferons, HCV appears capable of impairing interferon-related effector functions. Defects in the Jak-STAT signaling pathway have been described in HCV transgenic mice.[238] In HCV transgenic mice and human liver biopsies, impairment of Jak-STAT signaling was accompanied by hypomethylation of STAT1, which in turn was related to increased expression of protein phosphatase 2A (PP2A).[239] Additionally, as noted in the description of NS5A in the previous section "Organization of the HCV Genome," there is some evidence that the NS5A protein can antagonize type I interferon signaling through stimulation of IL-8 production and inhibition of PKR.[98,100] Confirmation of these findings in model systems expressing HCV proteins in a more physiologic context is needed before any firm conclusions can be drawn.

NK and NKT cells are abundant in liver and, through production of interferon-γ and other cytokines, prime cellular immune responses.[240] Thus, it is important that the binding of the E2 protein to CD81 has been associated with inhibition of NK cell activity.[241,242] Likewise, HLA Cw*04 and its related haplotypes, which reportedly bind to inhibitory killer immunoglobulin-like receptors on NK cells, have been associated with viral persistence.[227,243] Notably, the least inhibitory HLA-C-NKIR haplotypes are most strongly associated with recovery. HCV may interfere with NK cell activation of dendritic cells, which facilitate T-cell priming.[244] In some studies, but not others, HCV infection has been associated with measurable impairment of peripheral dendritic cell function.[245,246] This impairment is one possible mechanism that might explain the arrested development and then collapse of cellular immune response observed during the transition from acute to chronic infection.[247] Whether intrahepatic dendritic cells are infected with HCV is unknown. In addition, Crispe and others have pointed out that immune responses within the liver may inherently be biased toward tolerance because of the frequent exposure of the intrahepatic environment to antigenic material borne in food.[231]

Still other mechanisms have been suggested to reduce the susceptibility of infected cells to cytolytic attack by immune cells. The HCV core protein may bind to the cytoplasmic tail of the TNF-α receptor and the lymphotoxin-β receptor, based on ectopic expression studies.[48,49,51] This binding occurs immediately adjacent to the death domain, and may modulate signal transduction through the receptor. Although the biologic effects of this interaction remain controversial, it is possible that it protects the infected cell against TNF-α-mediated apoptotic cell death. Although this has not been observed in HCV transgenic mice, defects in Fas-mediated apoptosis have been documented in HCV-transgenic mice, both in vivo and in hepatocyte explant cultures ex vivo.[248]

The highly glycosylated nature of the viral envelope may protect it against antibody-mediated neutralization, analogous to the "glycan shield" hypothesis for HIV-1.[249] Furthermore, the envelope may have evolved a flexible structure (namely the HVR-1) that serves as an immunologic decoy and protects an otherwise vulnerable, conserved receptor-binding ligand from antibody attack.[69] In addition, the virus may downregulate replication to a level that is too low to disrupt cellular homeostasis, limiting the amounts of viral PAMPs and antigens produced.

Finally, HCV sequence variation and immune escape from both T and B cells may also contribute to viral persistence.[69,250] Mutation within the amino acid sequence of a critical epitope may allow a new quasispecies variant to evade a previously suppressive immune response, either cellular or humoral.[64,65,116] In several studies, acutely infected persons who developed persistent infection had a more complex quasispecies.[69,250] In agreement with that finding, viral escape in CTL epitopes has been reported frequently in persistently infected persons even when examined during acute infection.[133] Consistent with this notion, probable escape mutations within class I major histocompatibility complex-restricted epitopes were observed in chimpanzees that had an inadequate CD8+ memory T-cell response due to antibody depletion of CD4+ memory cells.[224] In summary, it appears likely that many factors contribute to HCV persistence, and that HCV may have evolved a variety of redundant and overlapping mechanisms of immune evasion to ensure its long-term persistence in the majority of immunologically normal persons who become infected. It is probable that additional mechanisms of viral immune evasion will be identified in the future.

DISEASE PROGRESSION

Although HCV infection leads to hepatic inflammation and steatosis, the major pathologic consequence of persistent HCV infection is the development of hepatic fibrosis, which may progress to life-threatening cirrhosis and a greatly increased risk of hepatocellular carcinoma. These long-term complications generally occur more than 20 years after the onset of infection, though more rapid progression has been reported.[251-253] There are wide estimates (5% to 25%) of the probability of cirrhosis occurring within 20 years of infection and very little information available on progression beyond 30 years (Fig. 154-8).[254,255] In two separate studies of women infected by contaminated Rh immune globulin, the incidence of cirrhosis during 15 to 20 years of follow-up was very low (<5%).[256-258] However, disease progression may have been limited in these cohorts by the relatively young

age and exclusive female gender of the infected persons, as well as possibly a lower than normal frequency of important cofactors like alcohol ingestion. In another cohort of 1667 HCV-infected injection drug users infected an estimated average of 14 years and followed an average of 8.8 years, the incidence of liver-related mortality was also low (3 per 1000 person years).[198] Liver biopsies were performed on a random sample of 210 HCV-infected members of this cohort, and only 10% had evidence of serious liver disease (Ishak modified fibrosis scores of 3 to 6) and there was little progression an average of 3 years later.[259,260]

In yet another study, Seeff and coworkers evaluated mortality and morbidity in a cohort of patients a mean of 18 years following posttransfusion hepatitis in comparison with control patients who were similarly transfused but had not developed recognizable hepatitis.[256,261] Overall mortality was high, reflecting the severity of underlying conditions, but not increased in HCV-infected patients. Liver-related mortality was slightly higher in patients with posttransfusion hepatitis (3%) than controls (1.5%), and it was estimated that approximately 10% of patients with posttransfusion hepatitis had cirrhosis 20 years later.[256] Other studies of posttransfusion hepatitis have reported a higher rate of cirrhosis.[251,253] In a community-based study, Alberti tested 4820 Italian Telecom employees for HCV infection, and evaluated liver disease in 78 of those who were infected.[262] Significant hepatic histologic abnormalities were detected in 40%.

Limited data concerning progression over periods greater than 30 years come from studies involving the retrospective identification of HCV-infected persons by testing of stored sera. Seeff and coworkers found 17 persons whose sera, stored since 1948 to 1954, contained HCV antibodies.[263] Seven had already died (one of liver disease), two could not be located, and eight were contacted. Five had no evidence of liver disease, two had biochemical evidence of cirrhosis but no symptoms, and one died before evaluation of a cancer of unknown primary that involved the liver. Once cirrhosis occurs, the rates of progression to liver failure (decompensated cirrhosis) and hepatocellular carcinoma are approximately 2% to 4% and 1% to 7% per year, respectively.[264-266]

This variability and uncertainty in the estimated frequency of life-threatening liver injury relates to limitations in basic research tools and the variable impact of environmental, host, and possibly viral factors for disease progression in different study cohorts (Table 154-1). Studies in tertiary care facilities generally predict higher rates of progression because they include a greater proportion of symptomatic subjects (referral bias). Assessment of disease is also difficult. Because HCV infection generally does not cause symptoms, it is difficult to assess the incremental progression of disease prior to clinical manifestation of cirrhosis or end-stage liver disease (ESLD; see "Clinical Manifestations of HCV Infection"). Liver fibrosis can be evaluated by biopsy (see "Liver Biopsy"). A comparison of biopsy scores with estimates of the duration of infection led Poynard and coworkers to advance the notion that fibrosis progresses linearly.[267] In their study of 2235 persons, the median estimated rate of fibrosis progression per year was 0.133 "fibrosis units" (95% confidence interval [CI] 0.125-0.143). Given that the factors that determine progression, such as alcohol use, vary over time, it is surprising that fairly consistent results have been reported from other studies, such as the prospective studies of Ghany and coworkers (0.12/year) and Wali and coworkers (0.15/year).[268,269] However, liver biopsies are not easily obtained, especially outside of referral centers, and can misrepresent the amount of disease due to variability in sampling and interpretation.[270-272]

The leading environmental determinant appears to be alcohol ingestion.[273-275] Whereas excessive alcohol ingestion and HCV infection independently may cause cirrhosis, combined exposure has a synergistic effect.[198,273,276] This is especially true with very heavy alcohol ingestion (more than 50 to 125 g/day), which in one study increased the risk of cirrhosis approximately 100-fold.[273] The mechanism underlying this synergy with an environmental toxin remains obscure, but both alcohol and HCV infection may cause microvesicular steatosis; this fact suggests a common pathway involving mitochondrial injury.[277,278]

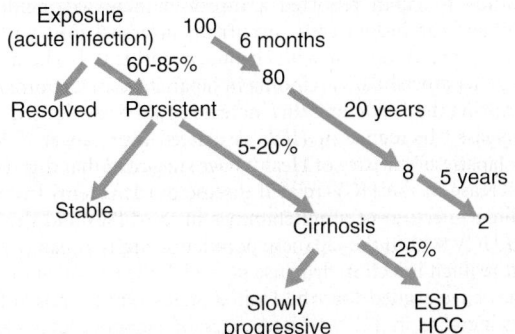

Figure 154-8 Natural history of hepatitis C virus (HCV) infection. Estimates of the most common outcomes of HCV infection are provided extrapolated to the hypothetical acute infection of 100 persons (100, 80, 8, 2). ESLD, end stage liver disease (e.g., esophageal varices, ascites, or hepatic encephalopathy); HCC, hepatocellular carcinoma. See "Disease Progression."

TABLE 154-1	Factors Associated with Cirrhosis in Persons with Hepatitis C Infection		
Factor	**Impact**	**Comment**	
Environmental			
Alcohol use	+4	The importance of minimal alcohol ingestion (<20 g daily) has not been established.	
Host			
HIV infection	+4	Increasingly important as HIV-related survival improves. May be masked by competing mortality.	
Age	+4	Strong effect; increases as low as 40 years. Hard to distinguish from infection duration.	
Duration of HCV infection	+3	Cirrhosis is rare before 10 years.	
HLA type	+1?	HLA B54 is correlated with increased risk of cirrhosis; DRB1*0301 with lack of cirrhosis.	
Viral			
Quasispecies complexity	+1	Cross-sectional studies cannot assess causality, and complexity may be confounded by duration of infection.	
HCV genotype 1	+1?	Genotype 1b in some but not other studies; could be confounded by longer duration of 1b infections.	
Quantitative measures of viremia (serum or plasma HCV RNA level)	+2	Not always detected or lost in multivariate analysis of age or HIV.	

Coinfection with HBV may also accelerate disease progression, but persistent GBV-C (so-called *hepatitis G virus*) infection does not appear to affect hepatitis C.[279-283] HIV infection increases the level of HCV viremia and is associated with more rapid progression of liver disease (see "HIV Coinfection").[284-288] Likewise, schistosomiasis coinfection is associated with much more rapid progression of HCV-related fibrosis in Egypt.[289] Increased progression of liver disease also has been reported in immunosuppression associated with agammaglobulinemia and transplantation.[290-292]

There is substantial evidence that disease progression is increased in persons infected at older ages, and this factor alone may explain much of the variability in studies, as those infected through transfusions appear to have the highest rates of progression to cirrhosis.[198,262,267] Although there are few studies detailing the natural history of HCV infection in children, the overall rate of disease progression appears quite slow, with few notable exceptions.[293-295] Strong associations between progression of fibrosis and both older age and various forms of immunosuppression remain largely unexplained.

Hepatic Fibrosis

Liver fibrosis is the net result of a complex, tightly regulated dynamic process in which collagen and other proteins are deposited and removed from a matrix in the subendothelial space between hepatocytes and the sinusoidal endothelium. Accumulation of liver fibrosis occurs in response to all forms of liver injury, and with viral hepatitis begins in the periportal zone and gradually extends as "septae" that may expand and "bridge" between portal tracts.[296] As the matrix expands and changes its composition, normal liver physiology can be disrupted and the architecture of the organ altered, although it is not clear whether this process is clinically evident prior to development of cirrhosis. The hepatic stellate cell (Ito cell) appears to be the chief architect of this matrix, responding to a variety of stimuli leading to various stages of activation (see Friedman's excellent review[297]).

Cytokines, reactive oxygen species, and other mediators of inflammation can initiate stellate cell activation, which can be perpetuated by autocrine and paracrine stimulation. Kupffer cells can play an important role in initiating and perpetuating fibrogenesis, through production of TGFβ, metalloproteinases, and reactive oxygen species.[298-300] CD8+ and CD4+ lymphocytes also appear to influence the pathogenesis of fibrosis, chiefly through stellate cell activation. In the CCl₄ mouse model, fibrogenesis is enhanced when Th1/CD8+ lymphocyte responses (in particular, interferon-γ) are depleted and by expression of Th2/CD4 lymphocyte-derived cytokines such as IL-4.[301] These data are interesting in light of the clinical observation of greater progression of fibrosis in persons coinfected with schistosomiasis in whom Th2-like responses predominated,[289] as well as extremely rapid fibrosis progression in persons with congenital agammaglobulinemia.[290] Similarly, recent evidence suggests that alcohol-related liver injury and fibrosis may be mediated in part by microbial translocation products including lipopolysaccharide, which may trigger TLR4 on stellate cells, resulting in recruitment of Kupffer cells and sensitization of stellate cells to the profibrotic action of TGFβ.[302]

Nonetheless, it remains unknown why only some immunocompetent persons with chronic hepatitis C develop cirrhosis. There is little reason to believe that certain HCV variants are more virulent than others or that the virus is cytopathic. In acute infection, the virus replicates at a high level for weeks with little or no evidence of liver damage. In a few studies, cirrhosis was associated with infection with genotype 1b virus, the presence of a greater complexity of HCV quasispecies, and higher levels of viremia.[137,303,304] However, there is less correlation between the level of viremia and disease progression than exists in HIV infection,[305,306] and the genotype and viral complexity findings have not been confirmed.

Host genetic factors probably play a role in determining why some infected persons develop cirrhosis. Wiley and coworkers have reported that African Americans have slower progression of fibrosis, compared to whites, a finding that appeared independent of other factors and which has also been noted by others.[307] Specific HLA alleles have been associated with differences in the progression of disease, as have polymorphisms in several genes believed to play a role in disease pathogenesis, including TGFβ.[308-310] With few exceptions, however, the link between these polymorphisms and the pathogenesis of disease remains unclear.

Hepatocellular Carcinoma

The risk of hepatocellular carcinoma is increased in HCV-infected persons, particularly in those with cirrhosis. In recent years there has been an increasing incidence of hepatocellular carcinoma in Western countries that has been attributed to prior increases in the prevalence of HCV infection.[311,312] Worldwide, there is considerable variation in the fraction of hepatocellular carcinoma attributed to HCV infection.[313-316] In Japan, Korea, and Southern Europe, 50% to 75% of hepatocellular carcinomas are associated with HCV infection.[317] In one Italian study, HCV infection was found in 71% of patients with liver cancer, and HBV infection in only 15%.[316]

One study in Japan reported a threefold increased incidence of hepatocellular carcinoma cases occurring in association with HCV infection compared to those with chronic hepatitis B.[317] The mortality rate due to hepatocellular carcinoma in Japan increased approximately twofold during the 1980s, and this increase could be attributed entirely to an increased incidence of HCV-associated liver cancer.[318] Reports from the Japanese Ministry of Health have suggested that this relatively recent increase in the HCV-related disease burden stems from widespread illicit injection of amphetamines in the 1950s and the related spread of HCV within the Japanese population approximately 25 to 30 years before illicit injection drug use peaked in the United States. Some authorities have argued that the United States should thus anticipate a similar increase in HCV-related cases of hepatocellular cancer, a phenomenon that is perhaps already being seen. Recent studies in the United States indicate that approximately one quarter of persons with hepatocellular carcinoma have HCV infection.[319,320] Interestingly, however, whereas cases of life-threatening cirrhosis appear to greatly outnumber cases of liver cancer related to HCV infection in the United States, the opposite appears to be the case at present in Japan.

As with cirrhosis, several cofactors have been proposed in the development of HCV-associated hepatocellular carcinoma. HBV coinfection appears to increase the risk of hepatocellular carcinoma in HCV-infected persons.[280,321] Infection with genotype 1b virus also has been associated with hepatocellular carcinoma, but this may reflect longer duration of infection.[315,319,322] Alcohol and tobacco use, older age, and male gender are associated with hepatocellular carcinoma among HCV-infected persons.[280,315]

Relatively little is known about how chronic HCV infection leads to cancer. The HCV genome is not reverse-transcribed to DNA, and thus cannot integrate into host cell chromosomes. Transforming activities have been associated with the core and NS3 proteins.[47,90] Strong evidence in favor of a direct or indirect transforming action of the core protein comes from studies of transgenic mice that develop such tumors in the absence of an immune response.[180,323] In addition, it is possible that NS5A promotes the development of tumors by repressing the antitumor activity of PKR.[98] However, in humans, chronic HCV replication is not by itself sufficient to cause hepatocellular carcinoma, even when accompanied by inflammation, because it does not usually occur in the large number of persons with long-term HCV infection and no cirrhosis. Even in the transgenic mouse model, liver cancer probably occurs as a result of increased hepatocyte turnover, dysregulation of pro-apoptotic and anti-apoptotic cellular signaling pathways, and/or the generation of free hydroxyl radicals that are capable of damaging cellular DNA.[278,324]

Clinical Manifestations of HCV Infection

ACUTE HEPATITIS C

Although usually not associated with symptoms, acute HCV infection may cause malaise, nausea, and right upper quadrant pain, followed by dark urine and jaundice (see Chapter 115). Such infections are clinically indistinguishable in the individual patient from other types of acute viral hepatitis. HCV RNA can be detected in blood within days of exposure and is followed by elevations in serum levels of the liver-specific enzyme and alanine aminotransferase (ALT), aspartate aminotransferase (AST), and in some cases bilirubin.[187,190,325] The most detailed information of the time course of acute infection comes from studies of HCV-contaminated transfusion recipients. Mosley and coworkers performed a lookback study of 94 persons infected by transfusion.[188] In 67 sera collected between the fourth and eighth day post-transfusion, HCV RNA was detected in all but two, underscoring the rapid onset of viral replication. There was wide variation in incubation (time to elevated ALT or symptoms), which ranged from 6 to 112 days (median 46 days). Shorter incubation was associated with higher ALT and jaundice was only detected in 21%.

FULMINANT HEPATITIS C

The frequency with which HCV causes fulminant hepatitis is controversial. HCV infection has been associated with 40% to 60% of fulminant NANB in Japan, but it is a very uncommon cause of fulminant liver disease in Western countries.[326-328] This discordance might arise from variation either in host factors or viral strains, or both. There appears to be an increased likelihood of fulminant liver disease following acute HAV infection in persons with underlying chronic hepatitis C.[329]

CHRONIC HEPATITIS C

From 50% to 85% of persons with acute hepatitis C infection develop persistent infection with long-term viremia (described in the previous section "Viral Persistence"; see also Chapter 116 and Fig. 154-8). Thus, although only one in six cases of symptomatic acute viral hepatitis is due to HCV infection, HCV is the leading infectious cause of chronic

liver disease in the United States. Persistently infected individuals tend to have few symptoms that are clearly caused by HCV infection (e.g., fatigue or malaise), leading some to question if hepatitis C is of any consequence in the majority of patients who never develop cirrhosis.[330] Alternatively, many patients who suffer with chronic fatigue or other nonspecific symptoms will ask whether HCV infection is the cause (and if treatment will help). Many quality-of-life indices are reduced in HCV-infected patients, even in the absence of cirrhosis, and they improve with successful therapy.[331-333] It is challenging in individual patients to disentangle the degree to which symptoms are due to the infection, the related liver disease, the psychological impact of having a chronic disease, or underlying depression that can be linked to illicit drug use.

Once chronic, HCV infection usually persists for decades. Serum ALT levels typically fluctuate independent of symptoms, whereas serum HCV RNA levels remain fairly constant.[195,251,334,335] The degree of inflammation present within liver biopsies also varies over time.[252,336] Some individuals will develop fibrosis that typically begins in portal triads, but can bridge between triads or central veins and ultimately destroy the hepatic architecture, progressing to cirrhosis.[296] There is a poor correlation between necroinflammatory liver injury, serum ALT levels, serum HCV RNA levels, and the extent of fibrosis.[337] Once established, 10% to 20% of HCV-infected persons with cirrhosis will decompensate clinically within 5 years, as evidenced by esophageal varices, ascites, coagulopathy, encephalopathy, or hepatocellular carcinoma.[264-266] A recent study underscored the importance of hepatocellular carcinoma in cirrhotic patients.[338] Of 214 persons with chronic hepatitis C and compensated (Child's A) cirrhosis followed an average of 114 months, 32% developed hepatocellular carcinoma, which occurred at a rate of 3.9% per annum.

Chronic HCV infection is associated with metabolic disorders such as insulin resistance, type 2 diabetes mellitus, and steatosis.[277,339-341] Interestingly, there is strong evidence of a direct viral link between steatosis and genotype 3 chronic HCV infection. The prevalence of steatosis is increased in patients with genotype 3 HCV infection and steatosis improves with successful HCV treatment.[277,342] In patients with the more common genotype 1 HCV infection, there is also a correlation with insulin resistance and steatosis, which reduces the likelihood of responding to interferon-based HCV therapy.[340,341]

Liver histology remains the best indicator of disease stage (See "Liver Biopsy"). Hepatic histology can be especially helpful when the duration of infection is known. For example, patients infected more than 25 years with little inflammation and no more than mild portal fibrosis are unlikely to develop cirrhosis in the ensuing 5 years.[260] This information can be useful if there are relative contraindications to treatment or if serious adverse reactions occur. However, for many patients the duration of infection is unknown and liver histology shows intermediate amounts of fibrosis and inflammation. Too little is known about the natural history of disease for such patients to reliably predict the long-term prognosis (10 years or more) with only a single biopsy.

HEPATOCELLULAR CARCINOMA

Primary hepatocellular carcinoma is typically a late complication of chronic hepatitis C, usually occurring in patients with cirrhosis.[315,316] HCV-related liver cancer has been particularly evident in Japan and Italy and often follows two or more decades of infection. The incidence is also increasing in the United States, and it is the principal concern in the natural history of cirrhosis.[338,343] Clinical findings can include a sudden worsening of prior symptoms and signs of cirrhosis (fatigue, ascites, and jaundice), often in association with right upper quadrant pain. However, small, asymptomatic hepatocellular carcinomas are not uncommonly detected at the time of liver transplantation. Serum α-fetoprotein levels are often very high, but the utility of this test in screening has been questioned.[344] Ultrasonography or computed tomography reveals an intrahepatic mass, but a specific diagnosis requires liver biopsy.

EXTRAHEPATIC MANIFESTATIONS OF HCV INFECTION

HCV infection is strongly associated with essential mixed cryoglobulinemia, membranoproliferative glomerulonephritis, and porphyria cutanea tarda. Up to half of HCV-infected persons have circulating cryoglobulins. However, only a small percentage develop the vasculitic syndrome of essential cryoglobulinemia (type II or type III, with circulating polyclonal IgG and IgM immune complexes).[345,346] Membranoproliferative glomerulonephritis may occur in association with HCV-related cryoglobulinemia, generally in the absence of vasculitis.[164,346] There is some evidence that treatment of HCV infection stabilizes renal disease progression.[347] HCV infection is also associated with B-cell lymphoproliferative disorders.[348-350] Chronic HCV infection has also been found in 60% to 80% of persons with sporadic (but not familial) porphyria cutanea tarda.[351,352] To a lesser extent, HCV infection has been associated with Mooren corneal ulcers, Sjögren's syndrome, lichen planus, and idiopathic pulmonary fibrosis.[353] The pathogenesis of such conditions remains unknown. However, sialadenitis resembling that occurring in Sjögren's syndrome has been observed in transgenic mice expressing HCV envelope proteins.[354] Thyroid autoantibodies, Hashimoto's thyroiditis, and hypothyroidism have been associated with chronic hepatitis C in women.[355]

Laboratory Assessment of HCV Infection

SEROLOGY

The laboratory diagnosis of HCV infection is based principally on detection of antibodies to recombinant HCV polypeptides. There have been several "generations" of enzyme immunoassays (EIAs) that measure antibodies directed against NS4, core, NS3, and NS5 sequences.[356-358] The U.S. Food and Drug Administration (FDA) has approved two EIAs: Abbott HCV EIA 2.0 (Abbott Laboratories, Abbott Park, IL) and ORTHO HCV Version 3.0 ELISA (Ortho-Clinical Diagnostics, Raritan, NJ), as well as a chemiluminescence immunoassay VITROS Anti-HCV assay (Ortho-Clinical Diagnostics, Raritan, NJ). The sensitivity of the third-generation assay is estimated to be 97%, and it can detect HCV antibody within 6 to 8 weeks of exposure.[359,360] These assays are measures of HCV infection, not immunity. Surrogate neutralizing tests based on pseudotyped lentivirus particles have been previously described (see "Humoral Immunity"). Assays for IgM HCV antibodies are not clinically useful.

So-called confirmatory tests are commonly used to evaluate a positive EIA result. The FDA has licensed the recombinant immunoblot assay (RIBA) Chiron RIBA HCV 3.0 SIA (Chiron Corporation, Emeryville, CA) as a supplemental antibody test. The RIBA generally identifies the specific antigens to which antibodies are reacting in the EIA, and may be positive (two antigens), indeterminate (one antigen), or negative.[361,362] EIA- and RIBA-positive sera usually contain HCV RNA, as indicated by direct detection (see "Direct Detection") and by lookback studies of donations that caused infection after transfusion.[363,364] EIA-positive, RIBA-indeterminate sera may also contain HCV RNA, especially if the reactivity was to core or NS3 antigens (the c22-3 and c33-c bands), respectively.[365]

The EIA is configured to optimize sensitivity, as the primary use of the assay is for screening for HCV infection. As with all tests, the predictive value of the EIA is directly related to the prevalence of infection in the population screened. Among injection drug users, HCV RNA can be detected in approximately 85% of second-generation EIA-positive sera. More than 98% of EIA-positive, RNA-negative sera from these injection drug users are RIBA-positive, indicating that most EIA reactive samples among drug users are true positive results (D. Thomas, unpublished data). At the other extreme, up to 40% of all third-generation EIA-positive blood donations from otherwise healthy individuals do not have detectable HCV RNA or a positive RIBA.[365]

Use of high-signal/cutoff ratios has largely replaced RIBA testing to improve the specificity of EIA results. In clinical laboratories, EIA-reactive samples with high optical density (e.g., >3.8 for the previously mentioned Ortho and Abbott EIA tests) are nearly always RIBA positive or contain HCV RNA.[366] Thus, HCV testing recommendations generally call for EIA screening followed by RNA testing.[367]

DIRECT DETECTION

HCV RNA can be detected in plasma and serum by a variety of molecular techniques including reverse-transcription PCR (RT-PCR), real time PCR, transcription-mediated amplification (TMA), and branched DNA (bDNA) technologies. Initially, tests used to quantify the amount of virus were less sensitive than those used to detect HCV RNA and also did not precisely characterize HCV RNA in persons with levels estimated at more than six $_{log10}$ international units per milliliter (IU/mL). Accordingly, some tests are FDA approved specifically for detection and others for quantification. More recently developed real time PCR assays quantify virus across a wide range and have comparable sensitivity (10 to 50 IU/mL) to qualitative assays.[368-370]

In persistently infected persons not receiving treatment, HCV RNA levels tend to remain stable (within one-half log_{10}) over years.[371,372] A number of factors may affect the estimate of HCV quantity including the assay used, time to serum separation, storage temperature, collection tube, and testing laboratory.[370,373] To improve the comparability of HCV RNA results, clinicians should use the same assay and laboratory to monitor a patient on treatment and laboratories should report quantitative results in international units, which correspond to a standardized amount of HCV RNA rather than viral particles.[374] Algorithms have been published for the conversion of proprietary unit values provided by commercially available assays to international units.[375]

HCV core antigen may also be detected in sera by EIA (Ortho-Clinical Diagnostics, Raritan, NJ).[375] The HCV core antigen titer corresponds closely with the HCV RNA level but the test is not widely used in practice.[376]

Genotype

Determination of the viral genotype is useful in predicting the response to therapy (see "Genetic Diversity"). Several assays are commercially available to determine HCV genotypes based on direct evaluation of 5' noncoding sequence, Trugene 5'NC HCV Genotyping Kit (Bayer Healthcare Diagnostics Division, Tarrytown, NY); hybridization to genotype-specific 5' noncoding oligonucleotide probes, INNO-LiPa HCV II (Innogenetics, Ghent, Belgium) and Versant HCV Genotyping Assay 2.0 (Bayer Healthcare Diagnostics Division, Tarrytown, NY).[377] The line probe assay accurately identifies the genotype, which is generally sufficient for clinical decision making, but it occasionally misclassifies the subtype. A serologic method for establishing genotype (but not subtype) also has been developed but is not widely available.

CLINICAL APPLICATION OF TESTS FOR HCV

Diagnosis

Chronic HCV infection is usually diagnosed by testing for antibodies to HCV using a licensed EIA, then by testing EIA reactive sera for HCV RNA to assess if the infection is persistent. Because information on HCV RNA level is useful for predicting and monitoring treatment response, it is expedient to use a quantitative HCV RNA test to confirm the presence of viremia.[375] Ideally, the quantitative HCV RNA test should have a sensitivity limit of less than 50 IU/mL and a wide linear range so that the same assay can be used to monitor throughout treatment. A negative RNA test result (<50 IU/mL) in a person found to have HCV antibodies by EIA most likely indicates that HCV infection has resolved. Other interpretations include that the EIA is falsely positive, that the HCV RNA test is falsely negative, or rarely, that a person has intermittent or low-level viremia. The latter condition may occur transiently in the initial two years of infection, but is extremely rare with chronic hepatitis C.

Although the RIBA has limited usefulness in clinical practice, it can be valuable to ascertain if a positive EIA test in a person with nondetectable HCV RNA represents resolved prior infection or whether the EIA test represented a false-positive result (a negative immunoblot result). In the latter scenario, no further testing is needed, which makes the RIBA useful when there is a strong suspicion that the EIA is falsely positive (e.g., when there are no risk factors, as is often the case for blood donors or persons tested for insurance reasons). The specificity of a positive HCV EIA also varies with the optical density of the result and this information can be used instead of RIBA in clinical settings.[366] For example, for the Ortho and Abbott HCV EIA assays mentioned above, values greater than 3.8 times the cutoff are highly specific for HCV infection.[367] In acute HCV infection or in immunosuppressed states, a negative EIA does not exclude HCV infection. HCV RNA testing is helpful if seronegative acute HCV infection is suspected, as HCV RNA can be detected within 2 to 3 days after an exposure, whereas antibodies to HCV are detectable an average of 7 to 8 weeks later.[187,188] HCV RNA testing can also be used to screen for HCV infection in persons with negative HCV EIA results who are known to have conditions associated with diminished antibody production, such as HIV infection and hemodialysis.

Pretreatment Evaluation

After HCV infection is confirmed and appropriate counseling is provided to reduce the risk of transmission to others, to caution against alcohol intake, and to recommend HAV and HBV vaccines for those susceptible, it is appropriate to consider whether the patient is likely to benefit from specific treatment for hepatitis C (see "Selection of Patients"). When treatment is being considered, it is appropriate to quantify HCV RNA and to determine the HCV genotype. In addition, many authorities also recommend liver disease staging and screening for other underlying causes of liver disease (e.g., autoimmune liver disease, hemochromatosis, Wilson's disease, α_1-antitrypsin deficiency, and chronic hepatitis B), as well as for HIV infection if there are risk factors.[378,379]

LIVER BIOPSY

Liver biopsy remains the most definitive method for assessing the stage of liver injury associated with HCV infection. Biopsy may identify other causes of liver disease, such as alcohol use or hemochromatosis, and also provides important information on four distinct HCV-related processes: periportal necrosis (piecemeal necrosis), parenchymal injury, portal inflammation, and fibrosis.[296,336,380] Based on the sum of scores, a standardized grading system, the histologic activity index (HAI) or "Knodell score," provides a numeric representation of the extent of disease that ranges from 0 to 22 (Table 154-2).[380] However,

the extent of fibrosis is likely to be the most important finding in patients with chronic hepatitis C. Several alternate systems have been developed to "score" liver biopsies (see Table 154-2).[381,382]

Although biopsy is the best available method for determining the type and extent of liver injury, there are limitations. Although interobserver variance has been described, the main concern is with the insensitivity of the test (failing to detect significant fibrosis), which is a function of the size of the sample taken.[383-385] Tissue samples less than 15 mm long are especially likely to miss significant disease. Complications such as serious bleeding may also occur, although infrequently (<1%).[383,384] The histologic "snapshot" of the current state of inflammation and fibrosis also does not predict the future course of disease with the level of certainty expected for an invasive screening test. Contraindications to liver biopsy include uncorrectable coagulopathy and clinical evidence of decompensated cirrhosis.

NONINVASIVE MARKERS OF HEPATIC FIBROSIS

Given the limitations of the liver biopsy, there is substantial interest in developing noninvasive markers of hepatic fibrosis. A large number of serum fibrosis markers have been considered, ranging from liver-related enzymes like ALT, AST, and γ-glutamyl transferase (GGT), direct and indirect measurements of molecules made or processed by the liver, such as the prothrombin time; platelet count and levels of serum albumin, bilirubin, γ-globulin, and apolipoprotein A_1; and markers of inflammation, fibrinolysis, fibrogenesis, or stellate cell activation (YKL-40, hyaluronic acid, procollagen III N peptide, transforming growth factor-β [TGF-β], α-2-macroglobulin, α-2 globulin).

Liver enzymes are inexpensive, readily available, and the most studied.[260,268,386] Longitudinal trends in ALT and AST levels may improve their correlation with histologic disease.[259,260,268,387,388] In addition, a change in the ratio of AST to ALT has been reported to be a reliable indicator of development of cirrhosis.[389,390] Among other routine laboratory tests, decreased platelet count, reversal of AST/ALT ratio, and prolonged prothrombin time are the earliest indicators of cirrhosis.[391,392] However, in most instances these tests are not sufficiently sensitive or specific to play a major role in clinical decision making.

The European MULTIVIRC group found that in using a combination of markers (α-2-macroglobulin, haptoglobin, apolipoprotein A1, GGT, ALT, and total bilirubin), they could achieve relatively high negative and positive predictive values for significant liver fibrosis.[393] The related assay is commercially available in the United States (Fibro-SURE, Lab Corp). However, the high negative and positive predictive values required scores that only pertained to 12% and 34% of subjects, respectively. In addition, the test does not appear to predict future fibrosis progression as well as contemporaneous disease.[260] Other groups have reported variable success with other "multitest" fibrosis algorithms designed for detection of significant fibrosis (metavir 2 to

	Liver biopsy			Noninvasive		
Histologic Finding	Modified HAI[382]	METAVIR[381]	Knodell*[380]	Fibroscan[399]	Fibrotest[393]	APRI[394]
No fibrosis	0	0	0		<0.21	
Expansion of some portal zones	1	1	1			
Expansion of most portal zones	2	1	1	<7.1	0.27-0.31	≤0.5
Expansion of most portal zones and occasional bridging	3	2†		7.1-9.4	0.48-0.58	
Expansion of most portal zones and marked bridging	4	3‡	3	9.5-12.4	0.58-0.72	>1.5
Marked bridging and occasional nodules	5	3				
Cirrhosis	6	4	4	12.5	>0.74	

TABLE 154-2 Comparison of Systems Used to Grade Liver Fibrosis in HCV-Infected Persons

*HAI, histologic activity index; Fibroscan is a radiographic technique; Fibrotest is marketed as FibroSURE in the United States; APRI, AST to platelet-ratio index. Other thresholds have been used for some of these noninvasive tests. See "Noninvasive Markers of Hepatic Fibrosis."

†>1 septum.

‡Portal-central septae.

4) or cirrhosis (metavir 4) among persons with chronic hepatitis C, with or without HIV coinfection.[394-397] For example, in 192 subjects with chronic hepatitis C, significant fibrosis could be predicted accurately in 51% of patients by using the aspartate aminotransferase-to-platelet ratio index (APRI), which is calculated by dividing the AST level (upper level of normal) by the platelet count (10^9/L) and multiplying by 100.[394] Diagnostic accuracies of various marker panels vary across studies. However, when compared to the liver biopsy, the accuracy (area under a receiver operating curve) rarely exceeds 0.8 to 0.9. It is very likely that this "ceiling" reflects error in the biopsy reference standard as much as inaccuracy in the surrogate tests themselves.[398]

Significant liver disease can also be detected by hepatic imaging with ultrasound, computed tomography, and magnetic resonance imaging. These modalities may detect a small nodular liver, ascites, an enlarged spleen, intra-abdominal varices, and hepatocellular carcinoma. However, although potentially useful in the management of persons known to have cirrhosis (e.g., in screening for hepatocellular carcinoma), or for avoiding a biopsy when cirrhosis is strongly suspected clinically, such imaging methods usually offer little for initial staging of HCV infection. In contrast, transient elastography (Fibroscan) has been introduced as a noninvasive method of staging liver disease in persons with chronic hepatitis C.[399-401] Based on the premise that liver fibrosis can be predicted by measuring liver stiffness, this noninvasive test can discriminate metavir 0 to 1 fibrosis from more significant stages (metavir 2 to 4) and is especially sensitive for detection of cirrhosis.

In 2009 use of one or more liver staging methods is recommended for patients with chronic hepatitis C. Liver biopsy remains a preferred method for some, whereas others rely on noninvasive tests, and still others use both. As much of the value of staging relates to assessment of treatment urgency, liver biopsy is not typically recommended when the treatment decision is already clear, for example, in patients with a very high likelihood of a favorable outcome or conversely a treatment contraindication.[378] In such patients, staging should generally still be done with noninvasive tests to assess whether hepatocellular carcinoma screening is indicated (metavir 3 to 4).

Persons with chronic hepatitis C and bridging fibrosis or cirrhosis (metavir 3 to 4) should be screened for hepatocellular carcinoma.[344] Elevations in serum α-fetoprotein (AFP) may indicate the development of hepatocellular carcinoma in persons with HCV-related cirrhosis; however, AFP is neither sensitive nor specific and liver ultrasound testing every 6 to 12 months is the preferred method to screen for hepatocellular cancer in these patients.[344]

Epidemiology of Hepatitis C

HCV is most often transmitted by percutaneous exposure to blood. However, the predominant modes of transmission may change over time and differ between, and even within, countries. In economically developed countries, most new HCV infections are related to illicit injection drug use, though blood transfusions were once important sources of infection. HCV may also be transmitted between sexual partners and from a mother to her infant, though this is relatively uncommon compared to HBV. HCV can also be transmitted by percutaneous medical procedures, when there is a breach in infection control protocols. This transmission route is especially important in settings with insufficient resources to maintain infection control standards.

PREVALENCE OF HCV

HCV infection has been reported in virtually every country where it has been carefully evaluated, suggesting that HCV, unlike HIV, has a long-standing global distribution. Although there are only a few regions of the world where prevalence data are representative, it is estimated that more than 170 million persons are infected worldwide.[402] In developed nations, the HCV prevalence is typically 1% to 2% in the general population and less than 0.5% among blood donors. An estimate of hepatitis C prevalence in the United States is

available from the 1999 to 2002 National Health and Nutrition Examination Survey (NHANES).[403] Overall, the results of this survey indicate that there are approximately 4.1 million individuals who have been infected with HCV in the United States, or 1.6% of the general population. This is an underestimate of the total number of infected persons, however, as nearly 2 million incarcerated persons in the United States were not included in the NHANES survey yet have an extraordinarily high prevalence of infection, on the order of 20% to 40%.[404] The prevalence of HCV infection in the United States is higher among racial minorities than in white Americans, and greater in African Americans than in Mexican Americans. In addition, the prevalence is increased in persons of lower socioeconomic status, and those born between 1945 and 1964.

Although the prevalence of HCV is remarkably similar in many parts of the world, there are a few distinct geographic regions where infection is especially common. In Egypt, for example, HCV infection occurs in 10% to 30% of the general population.[405,406] Similarly high rates of infection have been found in certain regions of Japan, Taiwan, and Italy. In such areas, HCV infection is generally more prevalent among persons over 40 years of age, and uncommon under the age of 20.[407-410] This cohort effect suggests that transmission occurred through a practice that has been discontinued, such as traditional folk remedies or reuse of needles for injection.[407,411,412] It is likely that a national campaign to treat schistosomiasis infections was responsible for many infections in Egypt.[413] Injection therapy for schistosomiasis was administered to entire villages in the 1970s, and needles were frequently reused.

A high prevalence of HCV infection also has been reported in some urban areas of developed countries. In Baltimore, Maryland, HCV infection was found in 18% of patients attending an inner-city emergency department and in 15% of persons attending a nearby clinic for sexually transmitted diseases.[414,415] A very high prevalence of HCV infection has also been noted among incarcerated persons in California, Maryland, and Texas.[404] Undoubtedly, in these settings, prior illicit injection drug use is chiefly responsible.

INCIDENCE OF HCV INFECTION

In the 1980s, the annual incidence of HCV infection in the United States was approximately 15 out of 100,000, but since then it has declined significantly.[416] The CDC has estimated that at least two thirds of all community-acquired HCV infections are related to illicit injection drug use.

TRANSMISSION OF HCV

Biologic Basis of Transmission
HCV transmission requires that infectious virions contact susceptible cells that are permissive for replication. HCV RNA can be detected in blood (including serum and plasma), saliva, tears, seminal fluid, ascitic fluid, and cerebrospinal fluid.[166,167,417] HCV-RNA-containing blood is infectious when inoculated intravenously (e.g., by transfusion). In addition, a chimpanzee has been infected by intravenous inoculation of saliva.[176] However, there is very little information available regarding the potential infectivity of HCV-RNA-containing body fluids. Furthermore, it is not clear whether cells other than hepatocytes can be infected (and thus whether infection requires direct percutaneous inoculation into the bloodstream).

Percutaneous Transmission
Infection occurs in more than 90% of seronegative recipients who are transfused with blood from HCV-antibody–positive donors.[364,418] Prior to the introduction of nonspecific surrogate tests (serum ALT and antibody to HBV core protein) as well as specific EIAs for detection of HCV infection in blood donations, approximately 17% of HCV infections in the United States were caused by transfusion.[419] Use of the HCV EIA test to screen donations reduced the risk of transfusion-transmitted hepatitis C substantially, and that risk is less than 1 : 100,000

in areas (like the United States) where donations are also screened for HCV RNA.[420,421]

HCV also has been transmitted by intravenous administration of contaminated blood products including immune globulin.[422,423] In recent years, however, the risk of transmission by these products has been effectively eliminated by the introduction of solvent-detergent and other virus inactivation procedures. Transplantation of organs from HCV-infected donors almost always results in HCV infection in seronegative recipients,[424] and in seropositive recipients it may lead to superinfection with a second distinct viral strain.[425]

Contaminated needles and other paraphernalia associated with illicit drug use account for the majority of HCV infections in most developed countries. Since 1992, at least two thirds of new HCV infections in the United States have been associated with illicit drug use.[426] Worldwide, 50% to 95% of persons acknowledging drug use have HCV infection.[427-430] HCV infection generally occurs within months of initiating the illicit use of injected drugs. In one cohort, 80% of subjects acknowledging 2 or more years of injection use were infected with the virus, a prevalence that was higher than that of HIV or HBV infection.[427,431] Early acquisition of HCV is probably related to the practice of older (infected) intravenous drug users teaching new (uninfected) initiates by demonstrating on themselves and then on the new initiate.[432] In the United States, there appears to have been a significant reduction in the incidence of HCV associated with illicit drug use since the late 1980s.[426]

HCV may be transmitted by other percutaneous exposures that are not associated with drug use but which occur too infrequently to be detected in many studies. For example, tattooing has been associated with HCV infection in some studies.[433,434] Human bite and folk remedies such as acupuncture and scarification rituals may also be associated with HCV infection.[435]

Nosocomial Infection
Worldwide, unsafe medical practices might be the dominant route of HCV transmission. In countries where there are adequate resources to observe universal precautions, nosocomial transmission is uncommon and associated with breaches in infection control protocols.[436,437] Nonetheless, a recent report from Spain suggests that nosocomial spread may be one of the more preventable forms of HCV transmission.[438] The investigators considered 109 cases of acute hepatitis diagnosed between 1998 and 2005. In the 6-month period preceding the diagnosis of acute hepatitis C, hospital admission was recognized in 73 (67%) of cases, whereas intravenous drug use was only reported in 9 (8%) and sexual contact in 6 (5%). Among the 73 patients in whom hospital admission was the only risk factor, 33 underwent surgery and 24 were admitted to a medical emergency unit or a medical ward; the remaining 16 patients underwent an invasive diagnostic or therapeutic procedure. In some instances, the transmission vector is identified (e.g., multidose saline containers, heparin flush vials, or colonoscope).[439-442] In one example, 16 persons were infected from a single source patient through preparation of radiopharmaceutical injections.[443] The nosocomial transmission of HCV within hemodialysis units is a particular concern related to contamination of surfaces and failure to adhere to hand hygiene and glove use in dialysis units.[444-446]

In economically developing regions of the world, HCV transmission occurs from the widespread use (and reuse) of injections and other percutaneous practices in both traditional and unconventional medical settings. For example, one analysis estimated that the annual ratio of injections per person ranged from 1.7 to 11.3 and that reuse of equipment without sterilization was as high as 75% in some areas such as in Southeast Asia.[447] As mentioned above, widespread use of injections for schistosomiasis appears to explain the approximate 20% population prevalence of HCV in Egypt.[413]

Transmission of HCV to health care workers occurs after 1% to 2% of accidental needlestick exposures to HCV-infected patients.[448-450] Studies of such accidents indicate that the risk of HCV transmission is intermediate (~3% per documented exposure to susceptible host) between that of HIV (~0.3%) and HBV (~30%).[448,450,451] Although hollow-bore needlestick exposures account for most documented

instances of HCV transmission, HCV infection has also been reported from blood splashed on the conjunctiva, and from a solid bore needlestick.[452] Despite these risks, the prevalence of HCV infection among dental and medical health care workers is less than or similar to that of the general population.[453-455]

HCV also may be transmitted from health care providers to patients.[456,457] Performance of procedures in which percutaneous injuries can occur (e.g., intrathoracic surgery) are a common feature. In community-based studies in the United States, patients with acute HCV infection do not commonly report recent interaction with a health provider, and work restrictions are not routinely required for HCV-infected health care workers.[426] Thus, whereas nosocomial exposure is a leading cause of infection in developing countries, it is rare where resources permit adherence to universal precautions.

Sexual Transmission
Although transmission of HCV during sexual intercourse is difficult to prove, there is mounting circumstantial evidence that it occurs. HCV RNA has been detected in semen and saliva,[166,458] and persons with multiple sexual partners as well as commercial sex workers have a high HCV prevalence.[459,460] In multiple studies of families of HCV-infected patients carried out in Japan and in Europe, sexual partners generally have been the only household contacts at increased risk for infection with the same viral variant, a risk that increases with the duration of the relationship.[459,461-463] Although these observations are consistent with sexual transmission, other common exposures such as sharing razors or needles cannot be ruled out.

The association between sexual behavior and HCV infection is much weaker than for HBV or HIV infections. Studies of long-term sexual partners of HCV-infected hemophiliacs and transfusion recipients generally show little or no evidence for HCV transmission, even if there was unprotected sexual intercourse.[464-467] Vandelli and coworkers studied 895 monogamous sexual partners of persons with chronic hepatitis C for over 8000 person-years and found no convincing instances of HCV transmission, despite unprotected intercourse occurring an average of 1.8 times per week.[468] HCV prevalence among men who have sex with men also is generally lower than for other infections like HIV, HBV, and syphilis, for which sexual transmission is well established.[469,470] In one study, only 4.6% of a cohort of homosexual men were infected with HCV, whereas 81% had been infected with HBV.[471]

Thus, available data suggest that HCV may be transmitted during sexual intercourse, but that this occurs rarely. One conjecture is that sexual transmission occurs more often from persons with acute HCV infection than from those with chronic hepatitis C. This might explain the high prevalence in settings in which exposure to someone with acute hepatitis C is likely (e.g., partner of an injection drug user) and the relatively low transmission incidence in long-term sexual partners of those with chronic hepatitis C. Nonetheless, individuals in long-term monogamous relationships should be informed of the low risk of future transmission and, according to recent U.S. Public Health Service Guidelines, encouraged to discuss this risk and the use of barrier precautions with their sexual partners.[378,416]

Maternal-Infant Transmission
HCV is uncommonly transmitted from mother to infant. Estimates of the perinatal transmission frequency range from 0% to 4% in larger studies.[472-475] The timing of transmission is not known. However, HCV RNA has been detected within a month of birth in non-breast-fed infants delivered by cesarean section, suggesting that transmission occurs in utero in at least some instances.[474] Because of the passive transfer of maternal HCV antibodies, the diagnosis of infant HCV infection must be based on detection of viral RNA or the persistence of antibody after 18 months of age.

HCV RNA has been detected in breast milk.[476] However, in most studies, the risk of HCV transmission is similar in breast-fed and bottle-fed babies.[473,477,478] Neither the CDC nor the American Academy of Pediatrics recommends that HCV-infected mothers bottle-feed to prevent HCV transmission.[416,479] Likewise, although one study showed a reduction in perinatal HCV transmission in women who had elective cesarean sections, this measure is not routinely recommended for HCV-infected mothers.[416,480]

Transmission Cofactors
Risk factors for HCV transmission chiefly relate to the probability of virus reaching the recipient bloodstream. The donor HCV RNA level matters, especially at the extremes. In a review of 2022 parenteral, sexual, and perinatal HCV exposures, HCV was transmitted only by individuals with detectable viremia.[481] Moreover, nonparenteral (e.g., perinatal) transmission of HCV is very rare when the level of viremia is low.[482] Some but not all studies indicate that infection with HIV may be an important cofactor for both sexual and maternal-infant transmission,[473,483,484] possibly because HIV infection is also associated with higher HCV RNA levels.[285,286,485]

Treatment of Chronic Hepatitis C

There is intense interest in developing therapeutic regimens that are capable of inhibiting HCV replication, eradicating infection, and improving the natural history of the disease (see also Chapter 116). Treatment with interferon-α (typically recombinant interferon-α) is the best characterized and has undergone a series of incremental improvements by extending the duration of therapy, using interferon-α in combination with oral ribavirin, use of pegylated formulations of interferon-α (peginterferon-α) with ribavirin, and, most recently, adding small molecule inhibitors of HCV replication to that regimen. Major challenges remain, including the cost, adverse reactions, and efficacy of current treatments, as well as the limited penetration of treatment into the population with the highest infection prevalence, like injection drug users. Nonetheless, vigorous drug development is ongoing and major advances in HCV treatment are anticipated.

TREATMENT RESPONSES

Virologic Responses
The primary aim of treatment is to prevent complications of chronic hepatitis C by eradication of infection. Treatment can permanently eradicate HCV infection such that HCV RNA is no longer detectable in blood or liver, titers of antibodies to HCV decline, and HCV-related liver pathology remits or improves.[486,487] Accordingly, treatment responses chiefly are characterized by the results of HCV RNA testing at various milestones (Fig. 154-9). Virologic response is considered "rapid" (rapid virologic response, or RVR) when HCV RNA is undetectable (<50 IU/mL) 4 weeks after starting and "early" (early virologic response, or EVR) when the HCV RNA level drops by at least two logs (or becomes undetectable) 12 weeks after starting. Undetectable virus at the end of therapy is referred to as an end of treatment response (ETR). A sustained virologic response (SVR) is defined as the absence of HCV RNA in serum by a sensitive test at the end of treatment and 6 months later. A term *relapse* is used when HCV RNA is detected again in persons who achieved an ETR. Persons in whom HCV RNA levels fail to decline by at least two logs by 24 weeks are considered nonresponders, whereas those whose HCV RNA levels decline but never become undetectable are referred to as partial responders.

Histologic and Clinical Responses to Therapy
Liver histology (chiefly inflammation but in some cases fibrosis) may improve in patients receiving interferon-α or peginterferon-α in combination with ribavirin, particularly in those patients achieving an SVR.[488-492] One retrospective study considered outcomes of 479 persons with chronic hepatitis C a median of 2.1 years after they underwent interferon-α-based treatment. The risk of a clinical event (liver failure, liver cancer, or death) was substantially lower in the 30% who had achieved an SVR compared to the others.[493] It is difficult to assess if SVR prevented the clinical events in this study or if it was a marker of a lower pretreatment disease stage (which increases

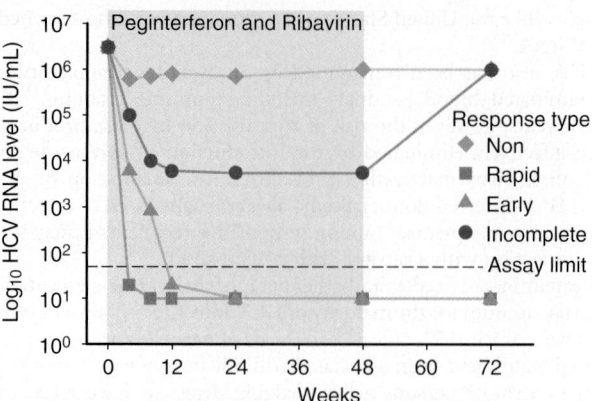

Figure 154-9 **Patterns of HCV RNA response to 48 weeks of interferon and ribavirin therapy for chronic hepatitis C.** Non (or null) response means less than 2 $\log_{10}$ IU/mL decline by 12 weeks; rapid virologic response means HCV RNA undetectable after 4 weeks; early virologic response means HCV undetectable or decline of greater than or equal to 2 $\log_{10}$ after 12 weeks; and incomplete means a response of more than 2 $\log_{10}$ IU/mL but not undetectable by 24 weeks, a circumstance that often is associated with relapse. Detection limit of many assays is 50 IU/mL.

SVR likelihood). In reports from Japan, interferon-α use is associated with a reduced incidence of hepatocellular carcinoma, observations that are difficult to generalize to other settings with lower hepatocellular incidences.[494-496] Thus, although there are emerging data demonstrating improvements in clinical outcomes associated with HCV treatment, additional prospective studies with longer follow-up are needed (and ongoing).

The clinical benefit of treatment appears largely limited to achieving a virologic response on treatment, compared to continued "maintenance" therapy in persons without initial viral suppression. In a large multicenter trial, 1050 persons with chronic hepatitis C and advanced fibrosis who failed to respond to previous peginterferon and ribavirin therapy were randomized to either peginterferon-α-2a (90 μg/week for 3.5 years) or no treatment. In the two groups, no difference was detected in the risk of death, hepatocellular carcinoma, hepatic decompensation, or, for those with bridging fibrosis at baseline, an increase in the Ishak fibrosis score of 2 or more points.[497] The percentage of patients with at least one serious adverse event was 38.6% in the treatment group and 31.8% in the control group.

TREATMENT

Interferon-α
The type 1 interferons (which include multiple types of interferon-α as well as interferon-β) comprise a heterogeneous group of cytokines that are expressed in response to viral infection. Interferons may alter the course of virus infections both directly and indirectly. With HCV, there is strong in vivo and in vitro evidence for a direct, interferon-mediated antiviral response, which in some cases the virus may be able to partially evade (see "Mechanisms of Persistence").[122,232] However, the exact effector mechanism(s) by which interferon-α exerts its antiviral effect against HCV are poorly understood. Two possibilities include the specific interruption of IRES-directed viral translation or the accelerated degradation of viral RNA. Interferon-α is also an immunomodulator, and among other effects, upregulates the level of expression of histocompatibility antigens on the surface of hepatocytes.

Serum levels of interferon-α peak approximately 6 hours after subcutaneous dosing and are undetectable by 16 hours. The drug is removed principally by renal catabolism, and has an estimated half-life of approximately 2 hours. The correlation between the serum level and the biologic activity is poorly understood. Decreases in the quantity of circulating HCV RNA can be detected within 8 hours of the initiation

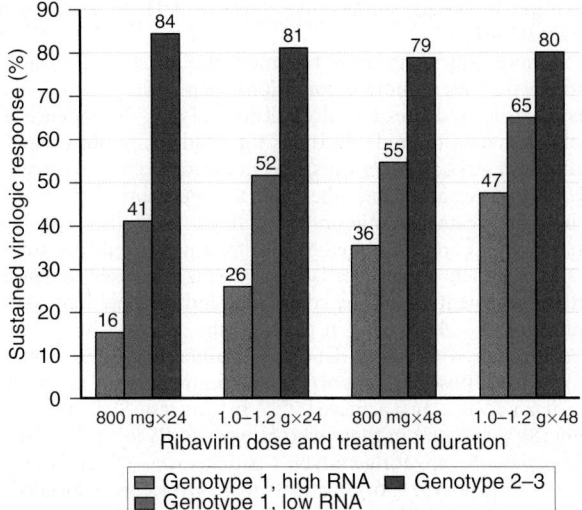

Figure 154-10 **Factors that predict response to treatment of hepatitis C virus (HCV) infection.** Sustained virologic response rates to standard interferon and ribavirin are provided for pairs of pretreatment factors. Although higher rates are achieved with peginterferon-α and ribavirin, similar differences are observed according to pretreatment factors. *(From Hadziyannis SJ, Sette H Jr, Morgan TR, et al. Peginterferon-alpha2a and ribavirin combination therapy in chronic hepatitis C: a randomized study of treatment duration and ribavirin dose. Ann Intern Med. 2004;140:346-355.)*

of therapy; an approximate 90% reduction in the level of viremia may be evident within 48 hours.[122] However, rebounds in viremia have been reported between doses given 48 hours apart, leading to development of longer acting formulations.

Recombinant interferon-α-2b, interferon-α-2a, and consensus interferon-α (acon-1) have been approved by the FDA for treatment of hepatitis C. The first large-scale clinical trials compared 3 million units of interferon-α-2b given subcutaneously three times a week for 6 months versus placebo and achieved SVR rates less than 15%.[498,499] Extension of the length of therapy to 12 to 18 months improved the SVR rates to 20% to 30%.[500] Overall, similar SVR rates have been reported with interferon-α-2a and acon-1.[501,502]

Peginterferon-α
By conjugating an inert polyethelene glycol molecule to interferon-α, the renal excretion is reduced and half-life is increased. Two such pegylated formulations of recombinant interferon-α have been approved for treatment of HCV infection in the United States, the 12-kd peginterferon-α-2b (Pegintron; Schering Plough) and the 40-kd peginterferon-α-2a (Pegasys; Hoffmann-La Roche). Because of their prolonged half-lives, they can be administered by subcutaneous injection once weekly. In large randomized, controlled trials, higher SVR rates have been achieved with the peginterferon-α products compared with standard interferon-α, and even higher rates when peginterferon-α was combined with oral ribavirin given twice daily.[503-506]

Combination Therapy with Ribavirin and Interferon-α
Ribavirin is a guanosine analogue with high oral bioavailability and is exceptionally broad although it is not particularly potent in antiviral activity. At least four different mechanisms of action have been proposed to explain its efficacy in the treatment of HCV infection: (1) ribavirin is a potent inhibitor of cellular inosine monophosphate dehydrogenase and thus may influence intracellular nucleoside pools; (2) it has been suggested that it may weakly inhibit the NS5B-encoded RNA-dependent RNA polymerase; (3) it has been shown to promote the mutagenicity of RNA viruses; and (4) ribavirin may possibly modulate the Th1/Th2 balance in the host immune response.[507-510] When administered alone, ribavirin therapy appears to reduce liver enzyme levels

in 21% to 43% of patients.[511-513] However, HCV RNA levels were significantly reduced in only a few percent of patients receiving ribavirin monotherapy. The use of orally administered ribavirin in combination with interferon-α and peginterferon-α significantly enhances the SVR rate by reducing relapse.[514-516] Interestingly, this "protection" against relapse appears to also occur when peginterferon is combined with a small molecule inhibitor like telaprevir.

Efficacy and Response Indicators
In early 2009, the combined use of peginterferon-α and ribavirin still represents the standard of care for treatment of HCV infection.[378,379,517] The dose for peginterferon-α-2a is 180 μg per week together with ribavirin using doses of 1000 mg for those weighing 75 kg or less and 1200 mg for those weighing more than 75 kg; the dose for peginterferon-α-2b is 1.5 μg/kg per week together with ribavirin using doses of 800 mg for those weighing less than 65 kg; 1000 mg for those weighing more than 65 to 85 kg; 1200 mg for those weighing more than 85 to 105 kg, and 1400 mg for those weighing more than 105 kg.[378] The optimal treatment duration of therapy and dose of ribavirin were investigated in a multicenter randomized, controlled trial in which all patients received peginterferon-α-2a at a dose of 180 μg, while patients in the four arms received either 24 or 48 weeks of ribavirin at either 800 mg or 1.0 to 1.2 g daily (Fig. 154-10).[518] Among patients with genotype 1, the SVR was highest in persons who received the higher ribavirin dose and who were treated for 48 weeks. Interestingly, in patients with genotypes 2 or 3, no differences were detected in SVR rates, suggesting that, for persons with genotype 2 or 3 infection, peginterferon-α should be given for only 24 weeks in combination with 800 mg of ribavirin. Additional studies have shown a modestly reduced efficacy of 16 versus 24 weeks of therapy for genotype 2 or 3 HCV infection.[519]

The response to peginterferon plus ribavirin varies substantially according to pretreatment characteristics, most importantly the HCV

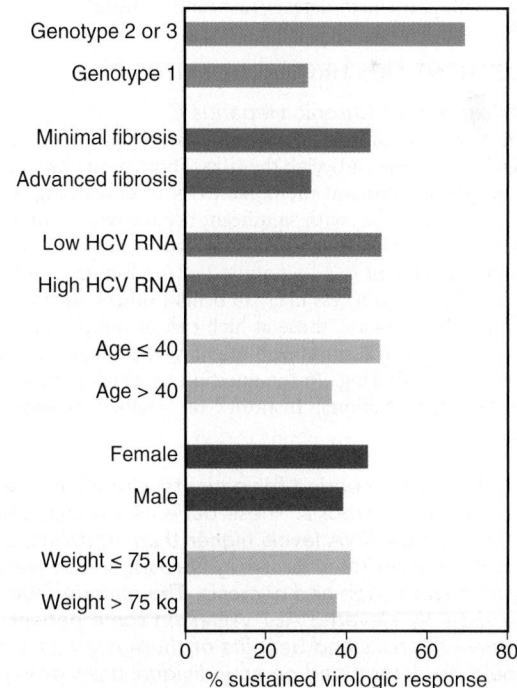

Figure 154-11 **Sustained virologic response rates in persons taking peginterferon and ribavirin according to duration of treatment and ribavirin dose, stratified by hepatitis C virus (HCV) genotype and HCV RNA level.** *(From Hadziyannis SJ, Sette H Jr, Morgan TR, et al. Peginterferon-alpha2a and ribavirin combination therapy in chronic hepatitis C: a randomized study of treatment duration and ribavirin dose. Ann Intern Med. 2004;140:346-355.)*

genotype (Fig. 154-11). The highest SVR rates are reported in patients who had genotype 2 or 3 HCV infections, lower pretreatment HCV RNA levels, younger ages, lower body weights, and an absence of bridging fibrosis, cirrhosis, and steatosis (or insulin resistance).[505,506,518] In the two large pivotal efficacy trials of pegylated interferon-α-2a and 2b, among patients with genotype 1 infections, SVRs were 42% to 46%, whereas the response rates in those with genotype 2 or 3 were 76% to 82%.[505,506] In the peginterferon-α-2a study, the data were analyzed further by combining genotype and viral load.[505] Persons with genotype 1 and a high viral load who received the combination of peginterferon-α-2a and ribavirin had an SVR of 41%, whereas the rate among those with genotype 1 and a low viral load treated with the same regimen was 56%. In contrast, among persons with genotypes 2 and 3 and a high viral load given peginterferon-α-2a and ribavirin, the SVR rate was 74%, compared with those with genotypes 2 and 3 and a low viral load who had an SVR of 81%. African Americans have a lower rate of response to interferon-α, which, as with the lower rates of spontaneous clearance, is unexplained.[520,521]

Adverse Reactions

Adverse reactions to interferon-α are common. Flu-like symptoms are experienced by most persons within 6 hours of the first dose, but generally diminish after 1 to 2 weeks. Fatigue, depression, and cognitive changes may occur and sometimes be unacceptable, although therapy can generally be continued with counseling and antidepressant administration. Hair thinning is a common late complication of therapy. Asymptomatic retinal abnormalities occur but their significance is not known.[522] Interferon-α also commonly causes mild-to-moderate transient bone marrow suppression, manifested by anemia, thrombocytopenia, and especially neutropenia. These hematologic reactions may require dose-reduction and/or administration of medications that stimulate blood cell production. Ribavirin causes a 1-5 g/dL reduction in hemoglobin (anemia) in 90% of persons; in one registration trial, 25% of persons had at least a 25% reduction in hemoglobin (see excellent review by Sulkowski[523]). Ribavirin use is also associated with gout, birth defects, rash, and sinusitis.

MANAGEMENT OF CHRONIC HEPATITIS C

Initial Treatment of Chronic Hepatitis C

It may be difficult in individual patients to ascertain whether the benefits of HCV treatment outweigh the risks. Those most likely to benefit from treatment are those at the highest risk of developing end-stage liver disease (ESLD) (i.e., with significant hepatic fibrosis or early cirrhosis; see "Natural History and Pathogenesis") and those most likely to respond to treatment (e.g., genotype 2 or 3 infection, or a low level of viremia). Treatment is less likely to benefit others, such as persons with minimal liver disease, those at high risk of complications, those unlikely to respond, and those who might have difficulty adhering to treatment and monitoring. To the question of which patients should be treated, a 2002 National Institutes of Health Consensus Panel concluded:

Treatment is recommended for patients with an increased risk of developing cirrhosis. These patients are characterized by detectable HCV RNA levels higher than 50 IU/mL, a liver biopsy with portal or bridging fibrosis, and at least moderate inflammation and necrosis. The majority also have persistently elevated ALT values. In some patient populations, the risks and benefits of therapy are less clear and should be determined on an individual basis or in the context of clinical trials.[517]

Seven years later, there has been little change in this guideline.[378,379] Many experts routinely provide treatment for all HCV-infected patients with genotype 2 or 3 infection, as response rates exceed 70% and treatment is for 6 rather than 12 months. This practice has also been supported in formal guidelines and will likely extend into treatment of genotype 1 infection as SVR rates improve with new treat-

ments and in certain subsets, like those with HCV levels less than 800,000 IU/mL.

It is more difficult to make treatment decisions for HCV-infected persons who have comorbid conditions such as HIV infection, renal disease, cirrhosis, depression, alcoholism, and drug dependence. There are also few data to guide decisions for children, persons with renal insufficiency, African Americans, injection drug users, those with fatty liver/insulin resistance, and other special populations.[517,524-529]

Virologic treatment milestones (defined previously) establish a probability for cure that, together with treatment need (disease severity) and treatment experience (adverse events), are used to determine whether treatment should be continued, and for how long. An SVR occurs rarely (~1% to 3%) in persons who fail to achieve an EVR, which together with recent data that "maintaining" treatment when an SVR is not possible, supports the recommendation to stop treatment if an EVR is not achieved.[378,379] In contrast, SVR occurs commonly (80% to 90%) in those who achieve an RVR.[505,530-533] Attempts to abbreviate therapy for genotype 1 patients who achieve an RVR to 24 weeks or genotype 2 or 3 patients to 16 weeks are associated with modestly reduced SVR expectations.[519,531] The duration of treatment for genotype 1 HCV infection should probably be longer than 48 weeks (e.g., 72 weeks) in persons with EVR but whose HCV RNA is not undetectable until 24 weeks after starting.[534]

Treatment of Acute Hepatitis C

Treatment of HCV infection within the first 6 months of infection with interferon-α usually results in an SVR.[535-539] In a German study, 60 patients with acute HCV (51 with symptomatic acute infection) were studied: 6 were given therapy immediately; of the remaining 54, 37 had at least one blood specimen in which HCV RNA could not be detected and 24 (44%) had durable recovery without treatment.[538] Ten patients were not treated, leaving 20 who were treated after a delay of 3 to 6 months after the onset of symptoms to see if there was spontaneous recovery. These 20 and the 6 treated immediately were given the "best available treatment," ranging from interferon-α (3 million units thrice weekly alone) to peginterferon-α and ribavirin; 21 (81%) of 26 had SVR. The authors concluded that the delayed treatment approach resulted in a 91% overall clearance rate (self-limited and treatment-related) and allowed 44% of patients to avoid unnecessary treatment. In another study from Japan, 13 of 15 persons randomized to start within 8 weeks had an SVR compared to 8 of 15 in whom treatment was delayed by 12 months.[540] Another study suggests that excellent results can be achieved up to 12 weeks after acute infection.[539] Thus, many recommend that treatment be withheld for 8 to 12 weeks to assess the natural outcome, especially in persons who are icteric, as they have the highest spontaneous clearance rates.[378]

Retreatment

Initial treatment can fail in three ways: there can be relapse, partial response, and nonresponse.[541] Persons who relapsed or had a partial response following standard interferon-α monotherapy can achieve an SVR with retreatment with a more potent regimen.[542,543] However, true nonresponders to interferon-α and ribavirin are much less likely to respond to a second course of therapy, even with peginterferon-α and ribavirin.[544] The likelihood of responding to a second course of treatment is also lower for persons with unfavorable response indicators, such as genotype 1 infection rather than genotype 2 or 3 infection, or for African Americans compared to whites. There is evidence that maintenance therapy (half-dose peginterferon) does not attenuate the progression of serious liver disease or cirrhosis in nonresponders (see "Histologic and Clinical Responses to Therapy").[497]

SPECIFIC SMALL MOLECULE ANTIVIRALS FOR HEPATITIS C

An improved understanding of HCV replication and atomic-level resolution structures of several critical viral enzymes have greatly accelerated the development of more potent and specific antiviral

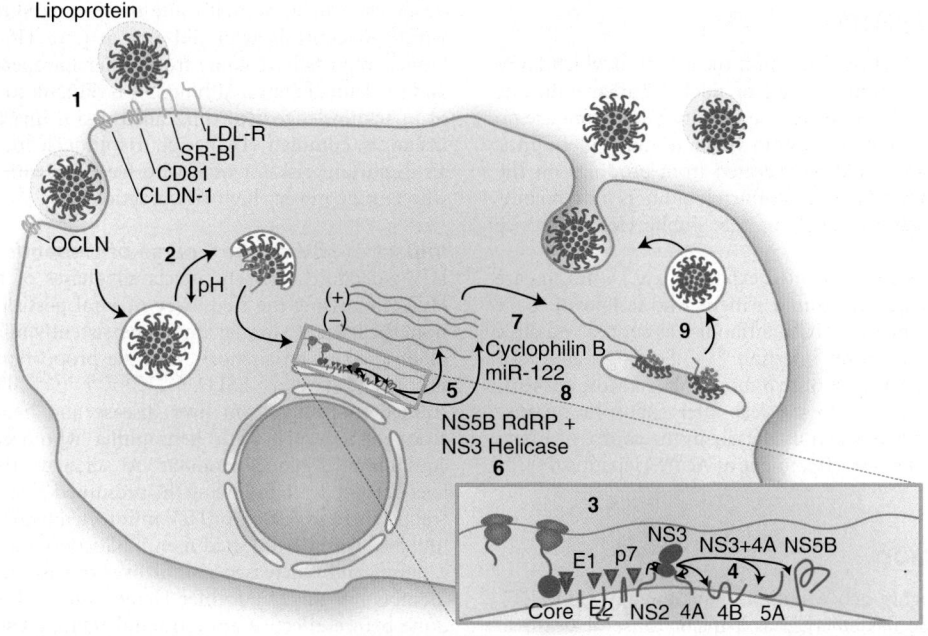

1. Entry
2. Uncoating
3. NS2/NS3 cysteine protease
4. NS3/NS4A serine protease
5. NS5B RdRP
6. NS3 Helicase
7. NS5B interaction with CypB
8. MicroRNA-122 requirement
9. Virion maturation and release

Figure 154-12 Enhanced understanding of hepatitis C virus (HCV) replication leads to new therapeutic targets. The life cycle (also shown in Fig. 154-3) has been labeled here with key steps for which therapeutic agents have been investigated. (*Graphic art by Jocelyn Ray.*)

agents (Fig. 154-12). In various stages of development are compounds that inhibit viral enzymes (e.g., NS3 serine protease or NS5B polymerase), immune activators (e.g., Toll cell receptor 7 agonists, T-cell vaccines, and monoclonal immune globulin), microRNAs that appear to inhibit replication by binding to the 5'-UTR, cyclosporin A, and the related cyclophilin inhibitors.[35,545-548] The first such compound that was characterized was an inhibitor of the NS3 serine protease.[545] In an initial phase I study, 31 patients with genotype 1 infection and minimal liver fibrosis were treated with BILN 2061 given orally twice daily for 2 days and reductions in HCV RNA level of 2 to 3 $\log_{10}$ copies/mL were noted. Although later phase testing of that compound was aborted due to toxicity, other potent protease inhibitors have been developed and, in early 2009, two are in phase III studies.

Telaprevir (VX-950) is a reversible, selective inhibitor of the HCV NS3/4A protease. When a dose of 750 mg every 8 hours for 14 days was administered, a median HCV RNA decline of 3.99 $\log_{10}$ (range −5.28 to −1.26) was reported; the same dose used with peginterferon-α-2a produced a median decline of −5.49 $\log_{10}$ (range, −6.54 to −4.30).[549] Boceprevir (SCH 503034) is another protease inhibitor that has advanced to phase III studies. Mean reduction of HCV RNA of 1.61 $\log_{10}$ was reported for a 400-mg dose.[550]

HCV replication can also be suppressed by nucleoside and non-nucleoside inhibitors of the HCV NS5B polymerase.[551] Through mechanisms that remain unclear, up to 3.6 $\log_{10}$ inhibition was reported to have occurred following a single dose of one compound by Nettles and colleagues at AASLD 2008.

The magnitude of inhibition of the NS3/4A protease and NS5B polymerase of HCV isolates varies with the respective RNA sequence. One implication is that the clinical effectiveness of these compounds can differ between genotypes and subtypes. Use of these compounds can rapidly select for variants within a subtype that are less inhibited.[552,553] In one study, HCV isolates were studied from 507 treatment-naïve persons with genotype 1 infection.[554] Collectively, 8.6% of the patients infected with genotype 1a and 1.4% of those infected with genotype 1b carried at least one mutation that conferred resistance to a protease or NS5B polymerase inhibitor. However, it appears that high-level protease-resistant isolates are not commonly dominant (~2%) in the pretreatment quasispecies.[554,555]

Prevention

PRE-EXPOSURE PREVENTION

The key to reducing the incidence of HCV infection is decreasing exposure to contaminated blood. The incidence of posttransfusion HCV infection has been reduced to very low levels by screening blood donations for HCV antibody as well as surrogate markers of HCV infection.[420,556] Although the impact is more difficult to measure, nosocomial HCV transmission in developing countries should decrease with worldwide adherence to universal precautions. There is some evidence that needle-exchange programs reduce HCV transmission among illicit drug users.[557] However, most studies have not found reduced HCV transmission associated with needle exchange, and more work is necessary to prevent transmission in this setting.

Efforts to develop an HCV vaccine are complicated by the extensive genetic and possibly antigenic diversity existing among different HCV genotypes, as well as the absence of solid immunity following natural infections, as discussed previously. Nonetheless, there is evidence that immunity can be acquired that protects against *persistent* HCV infection, both in chimpanzees and in humans. Chimpanzees that responded immunologically to an initial HCV infection, or that were immunized with an experimental vaccine, have been readily infected on subsequent experimental challenge with the virus.[558] Significantly, however, infection appears to be attenuated following prior infection or immunization, and rarely becomes persistent.[186,224,559-562] Lanford and coworkers have recently shown that such protection can even be achieved across HCV genotypes.[563] Likewise, injection drug users who recovered from an initial HCV infection were shown to be less likely to become viremic.[199] When viremia did occur, it often was at a low level and resolved. These data suggest that a vaccine might be capable of preventing viral persistence, and the significant pathologic consequences of HCV infection.

POSTEXPOSURE PREVENTION

Early studies provide conflicting data about the extent to which HCV infection is modified by administration of pooled human immune globulin.[205,564,565] However, because HCV seropositive donations are no longer included in the plasma pools from which immune globulin is manufactured, no benefit would be expected from products on the market today. Administration of immune globulin is not recommended following exposure to HCV in U.S. Public Health Service guidelines.[416]

An individual who has a documented exposure (e.g., a health care worker sustaining a needlestick from a patient who is known to be infected) should be screened for HCV antibodies as soon as possible after exposure to exclude prior infection.[189,416] Serology and ALT testing should be repeated at least once 6 months later. Most authorities also test for HCV RNA 2 to 4 weeks after exposure, because interferon-α is more effective when used early in the course of infection rather than years later (see "Treatment of Acute Hepatitis C").[537]

HIV Coinfection

Since the advent of highly active antiretroviral therapy (HAART), HCV-related liver disease has emerged as a major cause of death in HIV-infected persons.[566-568] In the large D:A:D study, 23,441 HIV-infected persons were followed from December 1999 through February 2004 and 1246 died.[568] The primary causes of death were AIDS (31.1%) and liver failure (14.5%). Among those who died of liver-related causes, 54.6% had achieved HIV RNA suppression (<400 c/mL) and half of liver-related deaths occurred in persons with CD4 lymphocyte counts greater than 200 cells/mm³. The relative contribution of liver-related mortality is likely to increase as HIV outcomes continue to improve with expanded use of better tolerated antiretroviral therapy. Accumulating population data show that liver disease will attenuate the remarkable long-term benefits of antiretroviral therapy in the subset coinfected with HCV (see also Chapters 116 and 123).[569,570]

EPIDEMIOLOGY AND NATURAL HISTORY

Epidemiology of Coinfection

Because of shared routes of transmission, HCV infection is found in persons with HIV much more frequently than in the general population. In the United States and Europe, 15% to 30% of HIV-infected persons are coinfected with HCV.[571,572] However, the prevalence of HIV/HCV coinfection varies markedly depending on the route of HIV infection, with 50% to 95% of HIV-infected injection drug users being coinfected, compared with less than 10% of HIV-infected homosexual men.[573]

HIV infection may enhance the transmissibility of HCV. The most conclusive data derive from studies comparing the rate of perinatal transmission of HCV from HIV/HCV coinfected mothers with those infected by HCV only.[473,480] It is unknown whether the association of HIV infection with higher HCV RNA levels is the reason for more frequent perinatal (and sexual) HCV transmission.[285,485] There are fewer studies investigating whether HIV/HCV coinfected persons are more likely to transmit HCV by sexual intercourse, but such persons appear to be much more likely to transmit HIV than HCV to their partners. In one study, HIV infection was detected in 13% of 162 female sexual partners of HIV/HCV coinfected hemophilia patients, whereas only 3% were HCV-infected.[483] The greater transmissibility of HIV by sexual intercourse, and related recommendations to prevent HIV transmission by using barrier precautions for every act of sexual intercourse, are more than satisfactory precautions to prevent spread of HCV to sexual partners.

Transmission of HCV among HIV infected men who have sex with men has also been reported, including several recent outbreaks.[574-576] In one recent outbreak, 60 HIV-infected men who acquired HCV had more high-risk sexual practices and were more likely to have shared drugs via a nasal or anal route in the preceding year in comparison with 130 controls who did not acquire HCV infection.[574,575,575,576] Similar reports have come from other European countries, Australia, and the United States. Although it is difficult to exclude the possibility of unacknowledged (or unrecalled) prior injection drug use in these instances, cumulatively the reports underscore that HCV infection is an important risk for men who have sex with men, especially those who engage in very high risk practices.

Impact of HIV on the Course of Hepatitis C Infection

HIV infection adversely affects all phases of the natural history of HCV, increasing the frequency of viral persistence after acute infection, the level of viremia among persistently infected persons, the rate of progression to cirrhosis, and the proportion of persons who will ultimately develop ESLD.[190,198,284,285,485,577-583] Darby and coworkers studied mortality from liver disease and hepatocellular carcinoma among 4865 men with hemophilia who were exposed to HCV-contaminated blood products. At all ages, the cumulative risk of liver-related death following the presumed exposure to HCV was 1.4% (range, 0.7% to 3.0%) for HIV uninfected men and 6.5% (range, 4.5% to 9.5%) for HIV-infected men.[577] Goedert and colleagues also found a significantly increased risk of liver disease in HIV/HCV coinfected members of the Multicenter Hemophilia Cohort Study.[584] In studies done before effective antiretroviral therapy use was widespread, the impact of liver disease on mortality in HIV/HCV coinfected persons was lower in injection drug users than in hemophilia patients. Thomas and colleagues did not detect more ESLD in HIV-infected members of a study of 1667 HCV-infected current and former injection drug users.[198] This apparent discrepancy was chiefly due to very high competing causes of mortality in the HIV-infected drug users. Overall, Graham and coworkers estimated that HIV infection increases the risk of cirrhosis twofold.[585]

Impact of HCV on the Course of HIV Infection

It remains unclear whether chronic hepatitis C affects the natural history of HIV disease. In the Swiss cohort study, Greub and colleagues reported that among 3111 patients receiving HAART, HCV-infected persons had a modestly increased risk of progression to a new AIDS-defining event or death, even among the subgroup with continuous suppression of HIV replication.[586] They also reported that the magnitude of the CD4 cell increase following effective anti-HIV therapy was significantly less than that observed in HCV uninfected persons, suggesting that HCV coinfection may blunt immune recovery.[586] Alternatively, among 1742 patients in a Baltimore HIV clinic, differences in the progression to AIDS or death chiefly appeared to be attributed to lower exposure to highly active antiretroviral therapy among the HCV-coinfected injection drug users.[587] Likewise, Chung and coworkers failed to detect a difference in immune restoration in HIV/HCV coinfected participants in a well-controlled AIDS Clinical Trial Group study, suggesting that the effect of HCV infection on progression of HIV is not large.[588]

HCV Infection and Antiretroviral Therapy

There is a complex relationship between antiretroviral therapy and liver disease progression in HIV-infected persons. On the one hand, antiretroviral therapy can itself be hepatotoxic. Hepatotoxicity occurs in about 10% of persons given a new antiretroviral regimen, more often if the person is HCV-coinfected.[589-591] In some cases, HAART-associated hepatotoxicity has been linked to liver failure and death.[592] However, in most cases it is manifested by an elevation in liver enzymes (often greater than fivefold normal) in the absence of symptoms. Although there is no reason to withhold HAART from HCV-infected persons, close monitoring is advisable if there is cirrhosis. Treatment of HCV infection also may reduce the incidence of antiretroviral therapy–related hepatotoxicity.[593]

On the other hand, antiretroviral therapy may protect against the adverse effects of HIV infection on liver disease.[581,594,595] In one recent prospective study, HAART exposure and effectiveness was compared in 184 HIV/HCV coinfected persons who had at least two liver biopsies between January 1998 and July 2006 and 41 (24%) had significant progression (≥2 point increase in Ishak scoring system).[596] Little difference was detected in this study in the rate of fibrosis progression according to antiretroviral use between biopsies. However, a number of factors can confound even prospective studies of this type as antiretroviral use and effectiveness is biased by factors that also affect liver fibrosis, like alcohol use.

PATHOGENESIS

The pathogenesis of HIV/HCV coinfection is poorly understood. HIV infection is likely to affect the adaptive immune response to HCV. Similar to experimental depletion of $CD4^+$ lymphocytes in the chimpanzee model, HIV infection of $CD4^+$ lymphocytes activated to combat HCV could diminish $CD8^+$ lymphocyte responses as well as maturation of humoral immunity.[224] Kim and coworkers have correlated the nadir of CD4 lymphocyte depletion with the magnitude of reduction in HCV-specific $CD8^+$ lymphocyte responses in HIV-infected persons (who interestingly do not have lower Epstein-Barr virus– or cytomegalovirus-specific $CD8^+$ T-cell responses).[226,597] Likewise, Netski found that HCV-specific humoral responses were indirectly correlated with $CD4^+$ lymphocyte suppression.[598] Thus, HIV-related CD4 lymphocyte depletion probably contributes to the clinical observation that HIV infection reduces the likelihood of spontaneous HCV clearance.[198]

Whether HIV replication in hepatocytes, Kupffer cells, and/or stellate cells occurs and directly affects HCV replication or fibrogenesis is largely unknown. Likewise, HCV replication in monocytes and lymphocytes has been inferred, but only at low levels and in a minority of cells.[160,588] Chung and coworkers have reported that HIV proteins like p24 and virus (produced from other cells) can enhance HCV replication in vitro and increase transforming growth factor β 1 expression and that these processes can be blocked by antibodies to the CCR5 or CXCR5 HIV coreceptors.[599] Increased STAT1 activation and Fas ligand expression in HIV-infected persons may lead to increased hepatocyte apoptosis, an effect that appears to be enhanced by both HCV and HIV envelope proteins.[600,601]

HIV infection may also enhance liver fibrosis by increasing translocation of microbial products from the gut. HIV infection of gut lymphoid tissues is associated with enhanced microbial translocation and these products are taken up near the portal vein by Kupffer cells.[602,603] As has been shown in an experimental model of alcohol-related liver disease, that process may lead to increased Toll cell 4 activation of stellate cells, especially if the Kupffer cell ability to take up bacterial products is diminished by HIV infection.[302] Cirrhosis itself, irrespective of the etiology, increases shunting of blood past the liver and might explain some of these findings.

The interaction between antiretroviral therapy and HCV infection is also poorly understood. Hepatoxicity in HIV/HCV coinfected persons could reflect decreased drug metabolism, HCV-specific immune reconstitution, or increased susceptibility to mitochondrial dysfunction.[278,604-607] Chung and coworkers demonstrated that HCV RNA levels in plasma actually increase in the first months after HAART and do so more in persons with low pretreatment CD4 lymphocyte counts.[588,608] Thus, the mechanisms by which these viruses interact and the pathogenesis of coinfection remain important research topics.

DIAGNOSIS AND TREATMENT OF HCV IN HIV-INFECTED PERSONS

Serologic Testing
According to U.S. Public Health Service Guidelines, all HIV-infected persons should be screened for HCV infection at entry into health care (http://AIDSinfo.nih.gov). HCV screening should be done as in persons without HIV infection (see "Clinical Application of Tests for HCV"). In HIV-infected persons, HCV antibody titers may decline

below the level of detection, especially in those with advanced immunodeficiency (CD4 cell count <100/mm³).[609-612] There are also case reports of HCV *seroreversion* occurring in association with immunosuppression and *seroconversion* associated with HAART therapy.[605,613] Thus, although uncommon in other settings,[614] HCV antibody-negative persons with HIV infection who have unexplained liver disease should be tested for HCV RNA to exclude the possibility of seronegative infection.[378,572]

Treatment of HCV Infection in HIV-Infected Persons
Treatment of HCV infection in HIV-infected persons is similar in many respects to persons without HIV. The current standard of care is also the combination of peginterferon-α and ribavirin.[615-618] In the largest published study (APRICOT), 868 persons were randomized to receive either standard interferon-α-2a (3 μU, thrice weekly) plus ribavirin (800 mg daily), peginterferon-α-2a 180 μg per week plus placebo, or peginterferon-α-2a 180 μg weekly plus ribavirin 800 mg daily; the SVR rates were 12%, 20%, and 40%, respectively.[616] As in HIV-uninfected persons, virologic response to peginterferon and ribavirin vary by genotype and pretreatment HCV RNA level.[615-618] In APRICOT, the peginterferon/ribavirin SVR rate was 29% for genotype-1-infected persons and 62% for those infected with genotype 2 or 3 infection; SVR rates were also greater than 60% in genotype-1-infected persons with pretreatment HCV RNA levels less than or equal to 800,000 IU/mL compared to 18% for genotype-1-infected persons with higher HCV RNA levels and the same treatment.[616] As in persons without HIV infection, those who took peginterferon and ribavirin but did not achieve EVR (85 of 289) almost never achieve an SVR (2 of 85).[615-618]

HIV-infected persons have a higher incidence of some serious adverse events. Ribavirin-associated anemia may be a greater problem in persons coinfected with HIV than in those with monoinfection, a problem that is compounded by concomitant zidovudine use.[619] Ribavirin also interacts with ddI, raising ddI levels and toxicity including fatal hyperlactatemia.[620] Although interferon-α therapy is associated with a dose-related reduction in white blood cell count and absolute CD4 count, the percentage of CD4 cells remains essentially unchanged and its use is not associated with the development of opportunistic infections.[615-618] Liver failure has also occurred in HIV/HCV coinfected persons on peginterferon-α and ribavirin therapy, especially when treatment is started in persons who already have Childs B cirrhosis.[621] Liver transplantation is the only treatment available for HIV/HCV coinfected persons with decompensated cirrhosis (i.e., Childs B or C cirrhosis).[622] However, the availability of liver transplant for HIV/HCV coinfected persons in most areas is low. Clearly, prevention of liver failure (and the need for transplantation) must remain the primary goal.

Selection of Patients
It is often difficult to decide whether to treat HCV infection in individual coinfected patients, as the increased risk of cirrhosis must be weighed against lower SVR rates and additional safety concerns. As for patients who are not infected with HIV, such decisions may be influenced by the results of liver biopsy, interpreted in light of other factors that might reduce the benefits of treatment (such as the stage of HIV infection or alcohol use) and comorbid conditions (such as depression) that might increase treatment toxicity.

If HIV treatment is indicated, antiretroviral therapy should be optimized before providing HCV treatment as it is reasonable to expect better results. Patients with decompensated liver disease (Childs B or C) are not treatment candidates and should be considered for liver transplantation, which remains experimental in HIV-infected persons but can be lifesaving.[622,623]

ACKNOWLEDGMENT

The authors thank Stanley Lemon for his extensive contributions to earlier versions of this chapter. Dr. Thomas' effort was funded in part by U.S. Public Health Service grants R01 DA013324m, R01 DA016078, and R01 DA013806, and Dr. Ray's effort was funded by R01 DA024565.

REFERENCES

1. Feinstone SM, Kapikian AZ, Purcell RH, et al. Transfusion-associated hepatitis not due to viral hepatitis type A or B. *N Engl J Med*. 1975;292:767-770.
2. Prince AM, Brotman B, Grady GF, et al. Long-incubation post-transfusion hepatitis without serological evidence of exposure to hepatitis-B virus. *Lancet*. 1974;2:241-246.
3. Tabor E, Gerety RJ, Drucker JA, et al. Transmission of non-A, non-B hepatitis from man to chimpanzee. *Lancet*. 1978;1:463-466.
4. Alter HJ, Purcell RH, Holland PV, et al. Transmissible agent in non-A, non-B hepatitis. *Lancet*. 1978;1:459-463.
5. Choo Q-L, Kuo G, Weiner AJ, et al. Isolation of a cDNA clone derived from a blood-borne non-A, non-B viral hepatitis genome. *Science*. 1989;244:359-364.
6. Choo QL, Richman KH, Han JH, et al. Genetic organization and diversity of the hepatitis C virus. *Proc Natl Acad Sci U S A*. 1991;88:2451-2455.
7. Shimizu YK, Feinstone SM, Kohara M, et al. Hepatitis C virus: detection of intracellular virus particles by electron microscopy. *Hepatology*. 1996;23:205-209.
8. Kaito M, Watanabe S, Tsukiyama-Kohara K, et al. Hepatitis C virus particle detected by immunoelectron microscopic study. *J Gen Virol*. 1994;75:1755-1760.
9. Wakita T, Pietschmann T, Kato T, et al. Production of infectious hepatitis C virus in tissue culture from a cloned viral genome. *Nat Med*. 2005;11:791-796.
10. Wakita T, Pietschmann T, Kato T, et al. Production of infectious hepatitis C virus in tissue culture from a cloned viral genome. *Nat Med*. 2005;11:791-796.
11. Simons JN, Leary TP, Dawson GJ, et al. Isolation of novel virus-like sequences associated with human hepatitis. *Nat Med*. 1995;1:564-569.
12. Theodore D, Lemon SM. GB virus C, hepatitis G virus, or human orphan flavivirus? *Hepatology*. 1997;25:1285-1286.
13. Robertson B, Myers G, Howard C, et al. Classification, nomenclature, and database development for hepatitis C virus (HCV) and related viruses: proposals for standardization. International Committee on Virus Taxonomy. *Arch Virol*. 1998;143:2493-2503.
14. Hijikata M, Shimizu YK, Kato H, et al. Equilibrium centrifugation studies of hepatitis C virus: evidence for circulating immune complexes. *J Virol*. 1993;67:1953-1958.
15. Kanto T, Hayashi N, Takehara T, et al. Buoyant density of hepatitis C virus recovered from infected hosts: Two different features in sucrose equilibrium density-gradient centrifugation related to degree of liver inflammation. *Hepatology*. 1994;19:296-302.
16. Choo SH, So HS, Cho JM, Ryu WS. Association of hepatitis C virus particles with immunoglobulin: A mechanism for persistent infection. *J Gen Virol*. 1995;76:2337-2341.
17. Miyamoto H, Okamoto H, Sato K, et al. Extraordinarily low density of hepatitis C virus estimated by sucrose density gradient centrifugation and the polymerase chain reaction. *J Gen Virol*. 1992;73:715-718.
18. Friebe P, Lohmann V, Krieger N, et al. Sequences in the 5′ nontranslated region of hepatitis C virus required for RNA replication. *J Virol*. 2001;75:12047-12057.
19. Brown EA, Zhang H, Ping LH, et al. Secondary structure of the 5′ nontranslated regions of hepatitis C virus and pestivirus genomic RNAs. *Nucleic Acids Res*. 1992;20:5041-5045.
20. Bukh J, Purcell RH, Miller RH. Sequence analysis of the 5′ noncoding region of hepatitis C virus. *Proc Natl Acad Sci U S A*. 1992;89:4942-4946.
21. Kamoshita N, Tsukiyama-Kohara K, Kohara M, et al. Genetic analysis of internal ribosomal entry site on hepatitis C virus RNA: Implication for involvement of the highly ordered structure and cell type-specific transacting factors. *Virology*. 1997;233:9-18.
22. Han JH, Shyamala V, Richman KH, et al. Characterization of the terminal regions of hepatitis C viral RNA: Identification of conserved sequences in the 5′ untranslated region and poly(A) tails at the 3′ end. *Proc Natl Acad Sci U S A*. 1991;88:1711-1715.
23. Honda M, Ping LH, Rijnbrand RC, et al. Structural requirements for initiation of translation by internal ribosome entry within genome-length hepatitis C virus RNA. *Virology*. 1996;222:31-42.
24. Pestova TV, Shatsky IN, Fletcher SP, et al. A prokaryotic-like mode of cytoplasmic eukaryotic ribosome binding to the initiation codon during internal translation initiation of hepatitis C and classical swine fever virus RNAs. *Genes Dev*. 1998;12:67-83.
25. Spahn CM, Kieft JS, Grassucci RA, et al. Hepatitis C virus IRES RNA-induced changes in the conformation of the 40s ribosomal subunit. *Science*. 2001;291:1959-1962.
26. Otto GA, Puglisi JD. The pathway of HCV IRES-mediated translation initiation. *Cell*. 2004;119:369-380.
27. Honda M, Brown EA, Lemon SM. Stability of a stem-loop involving the initiator AUG controls the efficiency of internal initiation of translation on hepatitis C virus RNA. *RNA*. 1996;2:955-968.
28. Yamada N, Tanihara K, Takada A, et al. Genetic organization and diversity of the 3′ noncoding region of the hepatitis C virus genome. *Virology*. 1996;223:255-261.
29. Kolykhalov AA, Feinstone SM, Rice CM. Identification of a highly conserved sequence element at the 3′ terminus of hepatitis C virus genome RNA. *J Virol*. 1996;70:3363-3371.
30. Tanaka T, Kato N, Cho MJ, et al. Structure of the 3′ terminus of the hepatitis C virus genome. *J Virol*. 1996;70:3307-3312.
31. Friebe P, Bartenschlager R. Genetic analysis of sequences in the 3′ nontranslated region of hepatitis C virus that are important for RNA replication. *J Virol*. 2002;76:5326-5338.
32. Yi M, Lemon SM. 3′ nontranslated RNA signals required for replication of hepatitis C virus RNA. *J Virol*. 2003;77:3557-3568.
33. You S, Rice CM. 3′ RNA elements in hepatitis C virus replication: Kissing partners and long poly(U). *J Virol*. 2008;82:184-195.
34. Saito T, Owen DM, Jiang F, et al. Innate immunity induced by composition-dependent RIG-I recognition of hepatitis C virus RNA. *Nature*. 2008;454:523-527.
35. Jopling CL, Yi M, Lancaster AM, et al. Modulation of hepatitis C virus RNA abundance by a liver-specific MicroRNA. *Science*. 2005;309:1577-1581.
36. Grakoui A, Wychowski C, Lin C, et al. Expression and identification of hepatitis C virus polyprotein cleavage products. *J Virol*. 1993;67:1385-1395.
37. Hijikata M, Kato N, Ootsuyama Y, et al. Gene mapping of the putative structural region of the hepatitis C virus genome by in vitro processing analysis. *Proc Natl Acad Sci U S A*. 1991;88:5547-5551.
38. Barba G, Harper F, Harada T, et al. Hepatitis C virus core protein shows a cytoplasmic localization and associates to cellular lipid storage droplets. *Proc Natl Acad Sci U S A*. 1997;94:1200-1205.
39. Yasui K, Wakita T, Tsukiyama-Kohara K, et al. The native form and maturation process of hepatitis C virus core protein. *J Virol*. 1998;72:6048-6055.
40. McLauchlan J, Lemberg MK, Hope G, et al. Intramembrane proteolysis promotes trafficking of hepatitis C virus core protein to lipid droplets. *EMBO J*. 2002;21:3980-3988.
41. Rouille Y, Helle F, Delgrange D, et al. Subcellular localization of hepatitis C virus structural proteins in a cell culture system that efficiently replicates the virus. *J Virol*. 2006;80:2832-2841.
42. Chen SY, Kao CF, Chen CM, et al. Mechanisms for inhibition of hepatitis B virus gene expression and replication by hepatitis C virus core protein. *J Biol Chem*. 2003;278:591-607.
43. Chang SC, Yen J-H, Kang H-Y, et al. Nuclear localization signals in the core protein of hepatitis C virus. *Biochem Biophys Res Commun*. 1994;205:1284-1290.
44. Santolini E, Migliaccio G, La Monica N. Biosynthesis and biochemical properties of the hepatitis C virus core protein. *J Virol*. 1994;68:3631-3641.
45. Suzuki R, Matsuura Y, Suzuki T, et al. Nuclear localization of the truncated hepatitis C virus core protein with its hydrophobic C terminus deleted. *J Gen Virol*. 1995;76:53-61.
46. Ray RB, Meyer K, Ray R. Suppression of apoptotic cell death by hepatitis C virus core protein. *Virology*. 1996;226:176-182.
47. Ray RB, Lagging LM, Meyer K, et al. Hepatitis C virus core protein cooperates with ras and transforms primary rat embryo fibroblasts to tumorigenic phenotype. *J Virol*. 1996;70:4438-4443.
48. Chen CM, You LR, Hwang LH, et al. Direct interaction of hepatitis C virus core protein with the cellular lymphotoxin-β receptor modulates the signal pathway of the lymphotoxin-β receptor. *J Virol*. 1997;71:9417-9426.
49. Matsumoto M, Hsieh TY, Zhu NL, et al. Hepatitis C virus core protein interacts with the cytoplasmic tail of lymphotoxin-β receptor. *J Virol*. 1997;71:1301-1309.
50. Ray RB, Steele R, Meyer K, et al. Transcriptional repression of p53 promoter by hepatitis C virus core protein. *J Biol Chem*. 1997;272:10983-10986.
51. Zhu NL, Khoshnan A, Schneider R, et al. Hepatitis C virus core protein binds to the cytoplasmic domain of tumor necrosis factor (TNF) receptor 1 and enhances TNF-induced apoptosis. *J Virol*. 1998;72:3691-3697.
52. Shrivastava A, Manna SK, Ray R, et al. Ectopic expression of hepatitis C virus core protein differentially regulates nuclear transcription factors. *J Virol*. 1998;72:9722-9728.
53. Herzer K, Falk CS, Encke J, et al. Upregulation of major histocompatibility complex class I on liver cells by hepatitis C virus core protein via p53 and TAP1 impairs natural killer cell cytotoxicity. *J Virol*. 2003;77:8299-8309.
54. Kittlesen DJ, Chianese-Bullock KA, Yao ZQ, et al. Interaction between complement receptor gC1qR and hepatitis C virus core protein inhibits T-lymphocyte proliferation. *J Clin Invest*. 2000;106:1239-1249.
55. Yi M, Kaneko S, Yu DY, et al. Hepatitis C virus envelope proteins bind lactoferrin. *J Virol*. 1997;71:5997-6002.
56. Op De Beeck A, Cocquerel L, Dubuisson J. Biogenesis of hepatitis C virus envelope glycoproteins. *J Gen Virol*. 2001;82:2589-2595.
57. Dubuisson J, Hsu HH, Cheung RC, et al. Formation and intracellular localization of hepatitis C virus envelope glycoprotein complexes expressed by recombinant vaccinia and Sindbis viruses. *J Virol*. 1994;68:6147-6160.
58. Ralston R, Thudium K, Berger K, et al. Characterization of hepatitis C virus envelope glycoprotein complexes expressed by recombinant vaccinia viruses. *J Virol*. 1993;67:6753-6761.
59. Weiner AJ, Brauer MJ, Rosenblatt J, et al. Variable and hypervariable domains are found in the regions of HCV corresponding to the flavivirus envelope and NS1 proteins and the pestivirus envelope glycoproteins. *Virology*. 1991;180:842-848.
60. Kato N, Ootsuyama Y, Ohkoshi S, et al. Characterization of hypervariable regions in the putative envelope protein of hepatitis C virus. *Biochem Biophys Res Commun*. 1992;189:119-127.
61. Kato N, Ootsuyama Y, Tanaka T, et al. Marked sequence diversity in the putative envelope proteins of hepatitis C viruses. *Virus Res*. 1992;22:107-123.
62. Farci P, Shimoda A, Wong D, et al. Prevention of hepatitis C virus infection in chimpanzees by hyperimmune serum against the hypervariable region 1 of the envelope 2 protein. *Proc Natl Acad Sci U S A*. 1996;93:15394-15399.
63. Kato N, Sekiya H, Ootsuyama Y, et al. Humoral immune response to hypervariable region 1 of the putative envelope glycoprotein (gp70) of hepatitis C virus. *J Virol*. 1993;67:3923-3930.
64. Weiner AJ, Geysen HM, Christopherson C, et al. Evidence for immune selection of hepatitis C virus (HCV) putative envelope glycoprotein variants: potential role in chronic HCV infections. *Proc Natl Acad Sci U S A*. 1992;89:3468-3472.
65. von Hahn T, Yoon JC, Alter H, et al. Hepatitis C virus continuously escapes from neutralizing antibody and T-cell responses during chronic infection in vivo. *Gastroenterology*. 2007;132:667-678.
66. McAllister J, Casino C, Davidson F, et al. Long-term evolution of the hypervariable region of hepatitis C virus in a common-source-infected cohort. *J Virol*. 1998;72:4893-4905.
67. Penin F, Combet C, Germanidis G, et al. Conservation of the conformation and positive charges of hepatitis C virus E2 envelope glycoprotein hypervariable region 1 points to a role in cell attachment. *J Virol*. 2001;75:5703-5710.
68. Ray SC, Fanning L, Wang XH, et al. Divergent and convergent evolution after a common-source outbreak of hepatitis C virus. *J Exp Med*. 2005;201:1753-1759.
69. Ray SC, Wang YM, Laeyendecker O, et al. Acute hepatitis C virus structural gene sequences as predictors of persistent viremia: hypervariable region 1 as decoy. *J Virol*. 1998;73:2938-2946.
70. Forns X, Thimme R, Govindarajan S, et al. Hepatitis C virus lacking the hypervariable region 1 of the second envelope protein is infectious and causes acute resolving or persistent infection in chimpanzees. *Proc Natl Acad Sci U S A*. 2000;97:13318-13323.
71. Jones CT, Murray CL, Eastman DK, et al. Hepatitis C virus p7 and NS2 proteins are essential for production of infectious virus. *J Virol*. 2007;81:8374-8383.
72. Lin C, Lindenbach BD, Pragai BM, et al. Processing in the hepatitis C virus E2-NS2 region: identification of p7 and two distinct E2-specific products with different C termini. *J Virol*. 1994;68:5063-5073.
73. Griffin SD, Beales LP, Clarke DS, et al. The p7 protein of hepatitis C virus forms an ion channel that is blocked by the antiviral drug amantadine. *FEBS Lett*. 2003;535:34-38.
74. Pavlovic D, Neville DC, Argaud O, et al. The hepatitis C virus p7 protein forms an ion channel that is inhibited by long-alkyl-chain iminosugar derivatives. *Proc Natl Acad Sci U S A*. 2003;100:6104-6108.
75. Grakoui A, McCourt DW, Wychowski C, et al. A second hepatitis C virus-encoded proteinase. *Proc Natl Acad Sci U S A*. 1993;90:10583-10587.
76. Santolini E, Pacini L, Fipaldini C, et al. The NS2 protein of hepatitis C virus is a transmembrane polypeptide. *J Virol*. 1995;69:7461-7471.
77. Lorenz IC, Marcotrigiano J, Dentzer TG, et al. Structure of the catalytic domain of the hepatitis C virus NS2-3 protease. *Nature*. 2006;442:831-835.
78. Jirasko V, Montserret R, Appel N, et al. Structural and functional characterization of nonstructural protein 2 for its role in hepatitis C virus assembly. *J Biol Chem*. 2008;283:28546-28562.
79. Yi M, Ma Y, Yates J, et al. Compensatory mutations in E1, p7, NS2, and NS3 enhance yields of cell culture-infectious intergenotypic chimeric hepatitis C virus. *J Virol*. 2007;81:629-638.
80. Kim JL, Morgenstern KA, Lin C, et al. Crystal structure of the hepatitis C virus NS3 protease domain complexed with a synthetic NS4A cofactor peptide. *Cell*. 1996;87:343-355.
81. Tanji Y, Hijikata M, Satoh S, et al. Hepatitis C virus-encoded nonstructural protein NS4A has versatile functions in viral protein processing. *J Virol*. 1995;69:1575-1581.
82. Failla C, Tomei L, De Francesco R. Both NS3 and NS4A are required for proteolytic processing of hepatitis C virus nonstructural proteins. *J Virol*. 1994;68:3753-3760.
83. Lin C, Pragai BM, Grakoui A, et al. Hepatitis C virus NS3 serine proteinase: Trans-cleavage requirements and processing kinetics. *J Virol*. 1994;68:8147-8157.
84. Yao NH, Hesson T, Cable M, et al. Structure of the hepatitis C virus RNA helicase domain. *Nat Struct Biol*. 1997;4:463-467.

85. Kim JL, Morgenstern KA, Griffith JP, et al. Hepatitis C virus NS3 RNA helicase domain with a bound oligonucleotide: the crystal structure provides insights into the mode of unwinding. *Structure.* 1998;6:89-100.
86. Tai CL, Chi WK, Chen DS, Hwang LH. The helicase activity associated with hepatitis C virus nonstructural protein 3 (NS3). *J Virol.* 1996;70:8477-8484.
87. Kim DW, Kim J, Gwack Y, et al. Mutational analysis of the hepatitis C virus RNA helicase. *J Virol.* 1997;71:9400-9409.
88. Beran RK, Pyle AM. Hepatitis C viral NS3-4A protease activity is enhanced by the NS3 helicase. *J Biol Chem.* 2008;283:29929-29937.
89. Gale M, Foy EM. Evasion of intracellular host defence by hepatitis C virus. *Nature.* 2005;436:939-945.
90. Sakamuro D, Furukawa T, Takegami T. Hepatitis C virus nonstructural protein NS3 transforms NIH 3T3 cells. *J Virol.* 1995;69:3893-3896.
91. Egger D, Wolk B, Gosert R, et al. Expression of hepatitis C virus proteins induces distinct membrane alterations including a candidate viral replication complex. *J Virol.* 2002;76:5974-5984.
92. Konan KV, Giddings TH Jr, Ikeda M, et al. Nonstructural protein precursor NS4A/B from hepatitis C virus alters function and ultrastructure of host secretory apparatus. *J Virol.* 2003;77:7843-7855.
93. Macdonald A, Harris M. Hepatitis C virus NS5A: tales of a promiscuous protein. *J Gen Virol.* 2004;85:2485-2502.
94. Tellinghuisen TL, Marcotrigiano J, Rice CM. Structure of the zinc-binding domain of an essential component of the hepatitis C virus replicase. *Nature.* 2005;435:374-379.
95. Huang L, Hwang J, Sharma SD, et al. Hepatitis C virus nonstructural protein 5A (NS5A) is an RNA-binding protein. *J Biol Chem.* 2005;280:36417-36428.
96. Witherell GW, Beineke P. Statistical analysis of combined substitutions in nonstructural 5A region of hepatitis C virus and interferon response. *J Med Virol.* 2001;63:8-16.
97. Enomoto N, Sakuma I, Asahina Y, et al. Mutations in the nonstructural protein 5A gene and response to interferon in patients with chronic hepatitis C virus 1b infection. *N Engl J Med.* 1996;334:77-81.
98. Gale MJJ, Korth MJ, Tang NM, et al. Evidence that hepatitis C virus resistance to interferon is mediated through repression of the PKR protein kinase by the nonstructural 5A protein. *Virology.* 1997;230:217-227.
99. Enomoto N, Sakuma I, Asahina Y, et al. Comparison of full-length sequences of interferon-sensitive and resistant hepatitis C virus 1b: sensitivity to interferon is conferred by amino acid substitutions in the NS5A region. *J Clin Invest.* 1995;96:224-230.
100. Polyak SJ, Khabar KS, Paschal DM, et al. Hepatitis C virus nonstructural 5A protein induces interleukin-8, leading to partial inhibition of the interferon-induced antiviral response. *J Virol.* 2001;75:6095-6106.
101. Nakagawa M, Sakamoto N, Enomoto N, et al. Specific inhibition of hepatitis C virus replication by cyclosporin A. *Biochem Biophys Res Commun.* 2004;313:42-47.
102. Watashi K, Ishii N, Hijikata M, et al. Cyclophilin B is a functional regulator of hepatitis C virus RNA polymerase. *Mol Cell.* 2005;19:111-122.
103. Xu Z, Choi J, Yen TS, et al. Synthesis of a novel hepatitis C virus protein by ribosomal frameshift. *EMBO J.* 2001;20:3840-3848.
104. Roussel J, Pillez A, Montpellier C, et al. Characterization of the expression of the hepatitis C virus F protein. *J Gen Virol.* 2003;84:1751-1759.
105. Branch AD, Stump DD, Gutierrez JA, et al. The hepatitis C virus alternate reading frame (ARF) and its family of novel products: the alternate reading frame protein/F-protein, the double-frameshift protein, and others. *Semin Liver Dis.* 2005;25:105-117.
106. McMullan LK, Grakoui A, Evans MJ, et al. Evidence for a functional RNA element in the hepatitis C virus core gene. Proc Natl Acad Sci U S A. 2007;104:2879-2884.
107. Agnello V, Abel G, Elfahal M, et al. Hepatitis C virus and other flaviviridae viruses enter cells via low density lipoprotein receptor. *Proc Natl Acad Sci U S A.* 1999;96:12766-12771.
108. Scarselli E, Ansuini H, Cerino R, et al. The human scavenger receptor class B type I is a novel candidate receptor for the hepatitis C virus. *EMBO J.* 2002;21:5017-5025.
109. Gardner JP, Durso RJ, Arrigale RR, et al. L-SIGN (CD 209L) is a liver-specific capture receptor for hepatitis C virus. *Proc Natl Acad Sci U S A.* 2003;100:4498-4503.
110. Lozach PY, Lortat-Jacob H, De Lavalette A De L, et al. DC-SIGN and L-SIGN are high affinity binding receptors for hepatitis C virus glycoprotein E2. *J Biol Chem.* 2003;278:20358-20366.
111. Pileri P, Uematsu Y, Campagnoli S, et al. Binding of hepatitis C virus to CD81. *Science.* 1998;282:938-941.
112. Evans MJ, von Hahn T, Tscherne DM, et al. Claudin-1 is a hepatitis C virus co-receptor required for a late step in entry. *Nature.* 2007;446:801-805.
113. Grove J, Huby T, Stamataki Z, et al. Scavenger receptor BI and BII expression levels modulate hepatitis C virus infectivity. *J Virol.* 2007;81:3162-3169.
114. Kolykhalov AA, Agapov EV, Blight KJ, et al. Transmission of hepatitis C by intrahepatic inoculation with transcribed RNA. *Science.* 1997;277:570-574.
115. Yanagi M, Purcell RH, Emerson SU, et al. Transcripts from a single full-length cDNA clone of hepatitis C virus are infectious when directly transfected into the liver of a chimpanzee. *Proc Natl Acad Sci U S A.* 1997;94:8738-8743.
116. Shimizu YK, Hijikata M, Iwamoto A, et al. Neutralizing antibodies against hepatitis C virus and the emergence of neutralization escape mutant viruses. *J Virol.* 1994;68:1494-1500.
117. Negro F, Pacchioni D, Shimizu Y, et al. Detection of intrahepatic replication of hepatitis C virus RNA by in situ hybridization and comparison with histopathology. *Proc Natl Acad Sci U S A.* 1992;89:2247-2251.
118. Krawczynski K, Beach MJ, Bradley DW, et al. Hepatitis C antigens in hepatocytes: immuno-morphologic detection and identification. *Gastroenterology.* 1992;103:622-629.
119. Lerat H, Berby F, Trabaud MA, et al. Specific detection of hepatitis C virus minus strand RNA in hematopoietic cells. *J Clin Invest.* 1996;97:845-851.
120. Shimizu YK, Igarashi H, Kanematu T, et al. Sequence analysis of the hepatitis C virus genome recovered from serum, liver, and peripheral blood mononuclear cells of infected chimpanzees. *J Virol.* 1997;71:5769-5773.
121. Lam NP, Neumann AU, Gretch DR, et al. Dose-dependent acute clearance of hepatitis C genotype 1 virus with interferon alfa. *Hepatology.* 1997;26:226-231.
122. Neumann AU, Lam NP, Dahari H, et al. Hepatitis C viral dynamics in vivo and the antiviral efficacy of interferon-alpha therapy. *Science.* 1998;282:103-107.
123. Ramratnam B, Bonhoeffer S, Binley J, et al. Rapid production and clearance of HIV-1 and hepatitis C virus assessed by large volume plasma apheresis. *Lancet.* 1999;354:1782-1785.
124. Martell M, Esteban JI, Quer J, et al. Hepatitis C virus (HCV) circulates as a population of different but closely related genomes: quasispecies nature of HCV genome distribution. *J Virol.* 1992;66:3225-3229.
125. Wang YM, Ray SC, Laeyendecker O, et al. Assessment of hepatitis C virus sequence complexity by electrophoretic mobilities of both single- and double-stranded DNAs. *J Clin Microbiol.* 1998;36:2982-2989.
126. Kurosaki M, Enomoto N, Marumo F, et al. Rapid sequence variation in the hypervariable region of hepatitis C virus during the course of chronic infection. *Hepatology.* 1993;18:1293-1299.
127. Kao J-H, Chen P-J, Lai M-Y, et al. Quasispecies of hepatitis C virus and genetic drift of the hypervariable region in chronic type C hepatitis. *J Infect Dis.* 1995;172:261-264.
128. Kato N, Ootsuyama Y, Sekiya H, et al. Genetic drift in hypervariable region 1 of the viral genome in persistent hepatitis C virus infection. *J Virol.* 1994;68:4776-4784.
129. Van Doorn L-J, Capriles I, Maertens G, et al. Sequence evolution of the hypervariable region in the putative envelope region E2/NS1 of hepatitis C virus is correlated with specific humoral immune responses. *J Virol.* 1995;69:773-778.
130. Odeberg J, Yun ZB, Sönnerborg A, et al. Variation of hepatitis C virus hypervariable region 1 in immunocompromised patients. *J Infect Dis.* 1997;175:938-943.
131. Booth JC, Kumar U, Webster D, et al. Comparison of the rate of sequence variation in the hypervariable region of E2/NS1 region of hepatitis C virus in normal and hypogammaglobulinemic patients. *Hepatology.* 1998;27:223-227.
132. Weiner A, Erickson AL, Kansopon J, et al. Persistent hepatitis C virus infection in a chimpanzee is associated with emergence of a cytotoxic T lymphocyte escape variant. *Proc Natl Acad Sci U S A.* 1995;92:2755-2759.
133. Cox AL, Mosbruger T, Mao Q, et al. Cellular immune selection with hepatitis C virus persistence in humans. *J Exp Med.* 2005;201:1741-1752.
134. Ogata N, Alter HJ, Miller RH, Purcell RH. Nucleotide sequence and mutation rate of the H strain of hepatitis C virus. *Proc Natl Acad Sci U S A.* 1991;88:3392-3396.
135. Abe K, Inchauspe G, Fujisawa K. Genomic characterization and mutation rate of hepatitis C virus isolated from a patient who contracted hepatitis during an epidemic of non-A, non-B hepatitis in Japan. *J Gen Virol.* 1992;73:2725-2729.
136. Okamoto H, Kojima M, Okada S, et al. Genetic drift of hepatitis C virus during an 8.2-year infection in a chimpanzee: variability and stability. *Virology.* 1992;190:894-899.
137. Honda M, Kaneko S, Sakai A, et al. Degree of diversity of hepatitis C virus quasispecies and progression of liver disease. *Hepatology.* 1994;20:1144-1151.
138. Wang XH, Netski DM, Astemborski J, et al. Progression of fibrosis during chronic hepatitis C is associated with rapid virus evolution. *J Virol.* 2007;81:6513-6522.
139. Cabot B, Esteban JI, Martell M, et al. Structure of replicating hepatitis C virus (HCV) quasispecies in the liver may not be reflected by analysis of circulating HCV virions. *J Virol.* 1997;71:1732-1734.
140. Maggi F, Fornai C, Vatteroni ML, et al. Differences in hepatitis C virus quasispecies composition between liver, peripheral blood mononuclear cells and plasma. *J Gen Virol.* 1997;78:1521-1525.
141. Rispeter K, Lu M, Behrens SE, et al. Hepatitis C virus variability: sequence analysis of an isolate after 10 years of chronic infection. *Virus Genes.* 2000;21:179-188.
142. Simmonds P, Holmes EC, Cha T-A, et al. Classification of hepatitis C virus into six major genotypes and a series of subtypes by phylogenetic analysis of the NS-5 region. *J Gen Virol.* 1993;74:2391-2399.
143. Murphy D, Chamberland J, Dandavino R, et al. A new genotype of hepatitis C virus originating from central Africa. *Hepatology.* 2007;46:623A.
144. Pybus OG, Charleston MA, Gupta S, et al. The epidemic behavior of the hepatitis C virus. *Science.* 2001;292:2323-2325.
145. Bukh J, Purcell RH, Miller RH. Sequence analysis of the core gene of 14 hepatitis C virus genotypes. *Proc Natl Acad Sci U S A.* 1994;91:8239-8243.
146. Bukh J, Miller RH, Purcell RH. Genetic heterogeneity of hepatitis C virus: quasispecies and genotypes. *Semin Liver Dis.* 1995;15:41-63.
147. Simmonds P, Smith DB, McOmish F, et al. Identification of genotypes of hepatitis C virus by sequence comparisons in the core, E1 and NS-5 regions. *J Gen Virol.* 1994;75:1053-1061.
148. Zein NN, Rakela J, Krawitt EL, et al. Hepatitis C virus genotypes in the United States: epidemiology, pathogenicity, and response to interferon therapy. *Ann Intern Med.* 1996;125:634-639.
149. Lau JYN, Davis GL, Prescott LE, et al. Distribution of hepatitis C virus genotypes determined by line probe assay in patients with chronic hepatitis C seen at tertiary referral centers in the United States. *Ann Intern Med.* 1996;124:868-876.
150. Dusheiko GM, Schmilovitz-Weiss H, Brown D, et al. Hepatitis C virus genotypes: an investigation of type-specific differences in geographic origin and disease. *Hepatology.* 1994;19:13-18.
151. Ray SC, Arthur RR, Carella A, et al. Genetic epidemiology of hepatitis C virus throughout Egypt. *J Infect Dis.* 2000;182:698-707.
152. Simmonds P. Variability of hepatitis C virus. *Hepatology.* 1995;21:570-583.
153. Mellor J, Walsh EA, Prescott LE, et al. Survey of type 6 group variants of hepatitis C virus in southeast Asia by using core based genotyping assay. *J Clin Microbiol.* 1996;34(2):417-423.
154. Simmonds P, Mellor J, Sakuldamrongpanich T, et al. Evolutionary analysis of variants of hepatitis C virus found in South-East Asia: comparison with classifications based upon sequence similarity. *J Gen Virol.* 1996;77:3013-3024.
155. Pawlotsky J-M, Tsakiris L, Roudot-Thoraval F, et al. Relationship between hepatitis C virus genotypes and sources of infection in patients with chronic hepatitis C. *J Infect Dis.* 1995;171:1607-1610.
156. Simmonds P, Bukh J, Combet C, et al. Consensus proposals for a unified system of nomenclature of hepatitis C virus genotypes. *Hepatology.* 2005;42:962-973.
157. Chang TT, Young KC, Yang YJ, et al. Hepatitis C virus RNA in peripheral blood mononuclear cells: comparing acute and chronic hepatitis C virus infection. *Hepatology.* 1996;23:977-981.
158. Navas S, Martín J, Quiroga JA, et al. Genetic diversity and tissue compartmentalization of the hepatitis C virus genome in blood mononuclear cells, liver, and serum from chronic hepatitis C patients. *J Virol.* 1998;72:1640-1646.
159. Zehender G, Meroni L, De Maddalena C, et al. Detection of hepatitis C virus RNA in CD19 peripheral blood mononuclear cells of chronically infected patients. *J Infect Dis.* 1997;176:1209-1214.
160. Lanford RE, Chavez D, Von Chisari F, et al. Lack of detection of negative-strand hepatitis C virus RNA in peripheral blood mononuclear cells and other extrahepatic tissues by the highly strand-specific rTth reverse transcriptase PCR. *J Virol.* 1995;69:8079-8083.
161. Laskus T, Radkowski M, Wang LF, et al. Hepatitis C virus negative strand RNA is not detected in peripheral blood mononuclear cells and viral sequences are identical to those in serum: a case against extrahepatic replication. *J Gen Virol.* 1997;78:2747-2750.
162. Sung VM, Shimodaira S, Doughty AL, et al. Establishment of B-cell lymphoma cell lines persistently infected with hepatitis C virus in vivo and in vitro: the apoptotic effects of virus infection. *J Virol.* 2003;77:2134-2146.
163. Agnello V, Abel G. Localization of hepatitis C virus in cutaneous vasculitic lesions in patients with type II cryoglobulinemia. *Arthritis Rheum.* 1997;40:2007-2015.
164. Johnson RJ, Gretch DR, Yamabe H, et al. Membranoproliferative glomerulonephritis associated with hepatitis C virus infection. *N Engl J Med.* 1993;328:465-470.
165. Chen M, Yun Z-B, Sällberg M, et al. Detection of hepatitis C virus RNA in the cell fraction of saliva before and after oral surgery. *J Med Virol.* 1995;45:223-226.
166. Fiore RJ, Potenza D, Monno L, et al. Detection of HCV RNA in serum and seminal fluid from HIV-1 co-infected intravenous drug addicts. *J Med Virol.* 1995;46:364-367.
167. Mendel I, Muraine M, Riachi G, et al. Detection and genotyping of the hepatitis C RNA in tear fluid from patients with chronic hepatitis C. *J Med Virol.* 1997;51:231-233.
168. Lohmann V, Korner F, Koch J, et al. Replication of subgenomic hepatitis C virus RNAs in a hepatoma cell line. *Science.* 1999;285:110-113.
169. Blight KJ, Kolykhalov AA, Rice CM. Efficient initiation of HCV RNA replication in cell culture. *Science.* 2000;290:1972-1974.
170. Bukh J, Pietschmann T, Lohmann V, et al. Mutations that permit efficient replication of hepatitis C virus RNA in Huh-7 cells prevent productive replication in chimpanzees. *Proc Natl Acad Sci U S A.* 2002;99:14416-14421.
171. Laras A, Zacharakis G, Hadziyannis SJ. Absence of the negative strand of GBV-C/HGV RNA from the liver. *J Hepatol.* 1999;30:383-388.

172. Ikeda M, Yi M, Li K, et al. Selectable subgenomic and genome-length dicistronic RNAs derived from an infectious molecular clone of the HCV-N strain of hepatitis C virus replicate efficiently in cultured Huh-7 cells. *J Virol.* 2002;76:2997-3006.

173. Yi M, Villanueva RA, Thomas DL, et al. Production of infectious genotype 1a hepatitis C virus (Hutchinson strain) in cultured human hepatoma cells. *Proc Natl Acad Sci U S A.* 2006;103:2310-2315.

174. Lindenbach BD, Evans MJ, Syder AJ, et al. Complete replication of hepatitis C virus in cell culture. *Science.* 2005;309:623-626.

175. Farci P, Alter HJ, Wong D, et al. A long-term study of hepatitis C virus replication in non-A, non-B hepatitis. *N Engl J Med.* 1991;325:98-104.

176. Abe K, Inchauspe G. Transmission of hepatitis C by saliva. *Lancet.* 1991;337:248.

177. Bassett SE, Brasky KM, Lanford RE. Analysis of hepatitis C virus-inoculated chimpanzees reveals unexpected clinical profiles. *J Virol.* 1998;72:2589-2599.

178. Martin A, Bodola F, Sangar DV, et al. Chronic hepatitis associated with GB virus B persistence in a tamarin after intrahepatic inoculation of synthetic viral RNA. *Proc Natl Acad Sci U S A.* 2003;100:9962-9967.

179. Kawamura T, Furusaka A, Koziel MJ, et al. Transgenic expression of hepatitis C virus structural proteins in the mouse. *Hepatology.* 1997;25:1014-1021.

180. Moriya K, Fujie H, Shintani Y, et al. The core protein of hepatitis C virus induces hepatocellular carcinoma in transgenic mice. *Nat Med.* 1998;4:1065-1067.

181. Wakita T, Taya C, Katsume A, et al. Efficient conditional transgene expression in hepatitis C virus cDNA transgenic mice mediated by the Cre/loxP system. *J Biol Chem.* 1998;273:9001-9006.

182. Mercer DF, Schiller DE, Elliott JF, et al. Hepatitis C virus replication in mice with chimeric human livers. *Nat Med.* 2001;7:927-933.

183. Law M, Maruyama T, Lewis J, et al. Broadly neutralizing antibodies protect against hepatitis C virus quasispecies challenge. *Nat Med.* 2008;14:25-27.

184. Shimizu YK, Weiner AJ, Rosenblatt J, et al. Early events in hepatitis C virus infection of chimpanzees. *Proc Natl Acad Sci U S A.* 1990;87:6441-6444.

185. Abe K, Inchauspe G, Shikata T, et al. Three different patterns of hepatitis C virus infection in chimpanzees. *Hepatology.* 1992;15:690-695.

186. Bassett SE, Guerra B, Brasky K, et al. Protective immune response to hepatitis C virus in chimpanzees rechallenged following clearance of primary infection. *Hepatology.* 2001;33:1479-1487.

187. Cox AL, Netski DM, Mosbruger T, et al. Prospective evaluation of community-acquired acute-phase hepatitis C virus infection. *Clin Infect Dis.* 2005;40:951-958.

188. Mosley JW, Operskalski EA, Tobler LH, et al. Viral and host factors in early hepatitis C virus infection. *Hepatology.* 2005;42:86-92.

189. Sulkowski MS, Ray SC, Thomas DL. Needlestick transmission of hepatitis C. *JAMA.* 2002;287:2406-2413.

190. Villano SA, Vlahov D, Nelson KE, et al. Persistence of viremia and the importance of long-term follow-up after acute hepatitis C infection. *Hepatology.* 1999;29:908-914.

191. Thimme R, Oldach D, Chang KM, et al. Determinants of viral clearance and persistence during acute hepatitis C virus infection. *J Exp Med.* 2001;194:1395-1406.

192. Prince AM, Brotman B, Inchauspe G, et al. Patterns and prevalence of hepatitis C virus infection in posttransfusion non-A, non-B hepatitis. *J Infect Dis.* 1993;167:1296-1301.

193. Mosley JW, Operskalski EA, Tobler LH, et al. The course of hepatitis C viraemia in transfusion recipients prior to availability of antiviral therapy. *J Viral Hepat.* 2008;15:120-128.

194. Erickson AL, Kimura Y, Igarashi S, et al. The outcome of hepatitis C virus infection is predicted by escape mutations in epitopes targeted by cytotoxic T lymphocytes. *Immunity.* 2001;15:883-895.

195. Alter MJ, Margolis HS, Krawczynski K, et al. The natural history of community acquired hepatitis C in the United States. *N Engl J Med.* 1992;327:1899-1905.

196. Barrera JM, Bruguera M, Ercilla MG, et al. Persistent hepatitis C viremia after acute self-limiting posttransfusion hepatitis C. *Hepatology.* 1995;21:639-644.

197. Kenny-Walsh E. Clinical outcomes after hepatitis C infection from contaminated anti-D immune globulin. Irish Hepatology Research Group. *N Engl J Med.* 1999;340:1228-1233.

198. Thomas DL, Astemborski J, Rai RM, et al. The natural history of hepatitis C virus infection: Host, viral, and environmental factors. *JAMA.* 2000;284:450-456.

199. Mehta SH, Cox A, Hoover DR, et al. Protection against persistence of hepatitis C. *Lancet.* 2002;359:1478-1483.

200. Netski DM, Mosbruger T, Depla E, et al. Humoral immune response in acute hepatitis C virus infection. *Clin Infect Dis.* 2005;41:667-675.

201. Adams G, Kuntz S, Rabalais G, et al. Natural recovery from acute hepatitis C virus infection by agammaglobulinemic twin children. *Pediatr Infect Dis J.* 1997;16:533-534.

202. Feray C, Gigou M, Samuel D, et al. Incidence of hepatitis C in patients receiving different preparations of hepatitis B immunoglobulins after liver transplantation. *Ann Intern Med.* 1998;128:810-816.

203. Piazza M, Sagliocca L, Tosone G, et al. Sexual transmission of the hepatitis C virus and efficacy of prophylaxis with intramuscular immune serum globulin—A randomized controlled trial. *Arch Intern Med.* 1997;157:1537-1544.

204. Farci P, Alter HJ, Wong DC, et al. Prevention of hepatitis C virus infection in chimpanzees after antibody-mediated in vitro neutralization. *Proc Natl Acad Sci U S A.* 1994;91:7792-7796.

205. Krawczynski K, Alter MJ, Tankersley DL, et al. Effect of immune globulin on the prevention of experimental hepatitis C virus infection. *J Infect Dis.* 1996;173:822-828.

206. Gaud U, Langer B, Petropoulou T, et al. Changes in hypervariable region 1 of the envelope 2 glycoprotein of hepatitis C virus in children and adults with humoral immune defects. *J Med Virol.* 2003;69:350-356.

207. Takaki A, Wiese M, Maertens G, et al. Cellular immune responses persist and humoral responses decrease two decades after recovery from a single-source outbreak of hepatitis C. *Nat Med.* 2000;6:578-582.

208. Bartosch B, Dubuisson J, Cosset FL. Infectious hepatitis C virus pseudo-particles containing functional E1-E2 envelope protein complexes. *J Exp Med.* 2003;197:633-642.

209. Roccasecca R, Ansuini H, Vitelli A, et al. Binding of the hepatitis C virus E2 glycoprotein to CD81 is strain specific and is modulated by a complex interplay between hypervariable regions 1 and 2. *J Virol.* 2003;77:1856-1867.

210. Logvinoff C, Major ME, Oldach D, et al. Neutralizing antibody response during acute and chronic hepatitis C virus infection. *Proc Natl Acad Sci U S A.* 2004;101:10149-10154.

211. Pestka JM, Zeisel MB, Blaser E, et al. Rapid induction of virus-neutralizing antibodies and viral clearance in a single-source outbreak of hepatitis C. *Proc Natl Acad Sci U S A.* 2007;104:6025-6030.

212. Missale G, Bertoni R, Lamonaca V, et al. Different clinical behaviors of acute hepatitis C virus infection are associated with different vigor of the anti-viral cell-mediated immune response. *J Clin Invest.* 1996;98:706-714.

213. Diepolder HM, Gerlach JT, Zachoval R, et al. Immunodominant CD4+ T-cell epitope within nonstructural protein 3 in acute hepatitis C virus infection. *J Virol.* 1997;71:6011-6019.

214. Gruner NH, Gerlach TJ, Jung MC, et al. Association of hepatitis C virus-specific CD8+ T cells with viral clearance in acute hepatitis C. *J Infect Dis.* 2000;181:1528-1536.

215. Chang KM, Thimme R, Melpolder JJ, et al. Differential CD4+ and CD8+ T-cell responsiveness in hepatitis C virus infection. *Hepatology.* 2001;33:267-276.

216. Gruener NH, Lechner F, Jung MC, et al. Sustained dysfunction of antiviral CD8+ T lymphocytes after infection with hepatitis C virus. *J Virol.* 2001;75:5550-5558.

217. Wedemeyer H, He XS, Nascimbeni M, et al. Impaired effector function of hepatitis C virus-specific CD8+ T cells in chronic hepatitis C virus infection. *J Immunol.* 2002;169:3447-3458.

218. Rutebemberwa A, Ray SC, Astemborski J, et al. High-programmed death-1 levels on hepatitis C virus-specific T cells during acute infection are associated with viral persistence and require preservation of cognate antigen during chronic infection. *J Immunol.* 2008;181:8215-8225.

219. Nelson DR, Marousis CG, Davis GL, et al. The role of hepatitis C virus-specific cytotoxic T lymphocytes in chronic hepatitis C. *J Immunol.* 1997;158:1473-1481.

220. Rehermann B, Chang KM, McHutchison JG, et al. Quantitative analysis of the peripheral blood cytotoxic T lymphocyte response in patients with chronic hepatitis C virus infection. *J Clin Invest.* 1996;98:1432-1440.

221. Bronowicki JP, Vetter D, Uhl G, et al. Lymphocyte reactivity to hepatitis C virus (HCV) antigens shows evidence for exposure to HCV in HCV-seronegative spouses of HCV-infected patients. *J Infect Dis.* 1997;176:518-522.

222. Koziel MJ, Wong DKH, Dudley D, et al. Hepatitis C virus-specific cytolytic T lymphocyte and T helper cell responses in seronegative persons. *J Infect Dis.* 1997;176:859-866.

223. Shoukry NH, Grakoui A, Houghton M, et al. Memory CD8+ T cells are required for protection from persistent hepatitis C virus infection. *J Exp Med.* 2003;197:1645-1655.

224. Grakoui A, Shoukry NH, Woollard DJ, et al. HCV persistence and immune evasion in the absence of memory T cell help. *Science.* 2003;302:659-662.

225. Kamal SM, Bianchi L, Al Tawil A, et al. Specific cellular immune response and cytokine patterns in patients coinfected with hepatitis C virus and *Schistosoma mansoni*. *J Infect Dis.* 2001;184:972-982.

226. Kim AY, Schulze zur WJ, Kuntzen T, et al. Impaired hepatitis C virus-specific T cell responses and recurrent hepatitis C virus in HIV coinfection. *PLoS Med.* 2006;3:e492.

227. Thio CL, Gao X, Goedert JJ, et al. HLA-Cw*04 and hepatitis C virus persistence. *J Virol.* 2002;76:4792-4797.

228. Thursz M, Yallop R, Goldin R, et al. Influence of MHC class II genotype on outcome of infection with hepatitis C virus. The HENCORE group. Hepatitis C European Network for Cooperative Research. *Lancet.* 1999;354:2119-2124.

229. Thio CL, Thomas DL, Goedert JJ, et al. Racial differences in HLA class II associations with hepatitis C virus outcomes. *J Infect Dis.* 2001;184:16-21.

230. Neumann-Haefelin C, McKiernan S, Ward S, et al. Dominant influence of an HLA-B27 restricted CD8+ T cell response in mediating HCV clearance and evolution. *Hepatology.* 2006;43:563-572.

231. Crispe IN. Hepatic T cells and liver tolerance. *Nat Rev Immunol.* 2003;3:51-62.

232. Foy E, Li K, Wang C, et al. Regulation of interferon regulatory factor-3 by the hepatitis C virus serine protease. *Science.* 2003;300:1145-1148.

233. Li K, Foy E, Ferreon JC, et al. Immune evasion by hepatitis C virus NS3/4A protease-mediated cleavage of the Toll-like receptor 3 adaptor protein TRIF. *Proc Natl Acad Sci U S A.* 2005;102:2992-2997.

234. Meylan E, Curran J, Hofmann K, et al. Cardif is an adaptor protein in the RIG-I antiviral pathway and is targeted by hepatitis C virus. *Nature.* 2005;437:1167-1172.

235. Loo YM, Owen DM, Li K, et al. Viral and therapeutic control of IFN-beta promoter stimulator 1 during hepatitis C virus infection. *Proc Natl Acad Sci U S A.* 2006;103:6001-6006.

236. Su AI, Pezacki JP, Wodicka L, et al. Genomic analysis of the host response to hepatitis C virus infection. *Proc Natl Acad Sci USA.* 2002;99:15669-15674.

237. Bigger CB, Brasky KM, Lanford RE. DNA microarray analysis of chimpanzee liver during acute resolving hepatitis C virus infection. *J Virol.* 2001;75:7059-7066.

238. Blindenbacher A, Duong FH, Hunziker L, et al. Expression of hepatitis C virus proteins inhibits interferon alpha signaling in the liver of transgenic mice. *Gastroenterology.* 2003;124:1465-1475.

239. Duong FHT, Filipowicz M, Tripodi M, et al. Hepatitis C virus inhibits interferon signaling through up-regulation of protein phosphatase 2A. *Gastroenterology.* 2004;126:263-277.

240. Liu ZX, Govindarajan S, Okamoto S, et al. NK cells cause liver injury and facilitate the induction of T cell-mediated immunity to a viral liver infection. *J Immunol.* 2000;164:6480-6486.

241. Tseng CT, Klimpel GR. Binding of the hepatitis C virus envelope protein E2 to CD81 inhibits natural killer cell functions. *J Exp Med.* 2002;195:43-49.

242. Crotta S, Stilla A, Wack A, et al. Inhibition of natural killer cells through engagement of CD81 by the major hepatitis C virus envelope protein. *J Exp Med.* 2002;195:35-41.

243. Khakoo SI, Thio CL, Martin MP, et al. HLA and NK cell inhibitory receptor genes in resolving hepatitis C virus infection. *Science.* 2004;305:872-874.

244. Jinushi M, Takehara T, Tatsumi T, et al. Negative regulation of NK cell activities by inhibitory receptor CD94/NKG2A leads to altered NK cell-induced modulation of dendritic cell functions in chronic hepatitis C virus infection. *J Immunol.* 2004;173:6072-6081.

245. Bain C, Fatmi A, Zoulim F, et al. Impaired allostimulatory function of dendritic cells in chronic hepatitis C infection. *Gastroenterology.* 2001;120:512-524.

246. Kanto T, Hayashi N, Takehara T, et al. Impaired allostimulatory capacity of peripheral blood dendritic cells recovered from hepatitis C virus-infected individuals. *J Immunol.* 1999;162:5584-5591.

247. Cox AL, Mosbruger T, Lauer GM, et al. Comprehensive analyses of CD8+ T cell responses during longitudinal study of acute human hepatitis C. *Hepatology.* 2005;42:104-112.

248. Disson O, Haouzi D, Desagher S, et al. Impaired clearance of virus-infected hepatocytes in transgenic mice expressing the hepatitis C virus polyprotein. *Gastroenterology.* 2004;126:859-872.

249. Wei X, Decker JM, Wang S, et al. Antibody neutralization and escape by HIV-1. *Nature.* 2003;422:307-312.

250. Farci P, Shimoda A, Coiana A, et al. The outcome of acute hepatitis C predicted by the evolution of the viral quasispecies. *Science.* 2000;288:339-344.

251. Tong MJ, El-Farra NS, Reikes AR, et al. Clinical outcomes after transfusion-associated hepatitis C. *N Engl J Med.* 1995;332:1463-1466.

252. Kiyosawa K, Sodeyama T, Tanaka E, et al. Interrelationship of blood transfusion, non-A, non-B hepatitis and hepatocellular carcinoma: Analysis by detection of antibody to hepatitis C virus. *Hepatology.* 1990;12:671-675.

253. Hopf U, Moller B, Kuther D, et al. Long-term follow-up of posttransfusion and sporadic chronic hepatitis non-A, non-B and frequency of circulating antibodies to hepatitis C virus (HCV). *J Hepatol.* 1990;10:69-76.

254. Di Bisceglie AM, Goodman ZD, Ishak KG, et al. Long-term clinical and histopathological follow-up of chronic posttransfusion hepatitis. *Hepatology.* 1991;14:969-974.

255. Tremolada F, Casarin C, Alberti A, et al. Long-term follow-up of non-A, non-B (type C) post-transfusion hepatitis. *J Hepatol.* 1992;16:273-281.

256. Seeff LB. Natural history of hepatitis C. *Hepatology.* 1997;26:21S-28S.

257. Power JP, Lawlor E, Davidson F, et al. Hepatitis C viraemia in recipients of Irish intravenous anti-D immunoglobulin. *Lancet.* 1994;344:1166-1167.

258. Wiese M, Berr F, Lafrenz M, et al. Low frequency of cirrhosis in a hepatitis C (genotype 1b) single-source outbreak in Germany: a 20-year multicenter study. *Hepatology.* 2000;32:91-96.

259. Rai R, Wilson LE, Astemborski J, et al. Severity and correlates of liver disease in hepatitis C virus-infected injection drug users. *Hepatology.* 2002;35:1247-1255.

260. Wilson LE, Torbenson M, Astemborski J, et al. Progression of liver fibrosis among injection drug users with chronic hepatitis C. *Hepatology.* 2006;43:788-795.

261. Seeff LB, Buskell-Bales ZB, Wright EC, et al. Long-term mortality after transfusion-associated non-A, non-B hepatitis. *N Engl J Med*. 1992;327:1906-1911.
262. Alberti A, Noventa F, Benvegnu L, et al. Prevalence of liver disease in a population of asymptomatic persons with hepatitis C virus infection. *Ann Intern Med*. 2002;137:961-964.
263. Seeff LB, Miller RN, Rabkin CS, et al. 45-year follow-up of hepatitis C virus infection in healthy young adults. *Ann Intern Med*. 2000;132:105-111.
264. Fattovich G, Giustina G, Degos F, et al. Morbidity and mortality in compensated cirrhosis C: a follow-up study of 384 patients. *Gastroenterology*. 1997;112:463-472.
265. Colombo M, De Franchis R, Del Ninno E, et al. Hepatocellular carcinoma in Italian patients with cirrhosis. *N Engl J Med*. 1991;325:675-680.
266. Tsukuma H, Hiyama T, Tanaka S, et al. Risk factors for hepatocellular carcinoma among patients with chronic liver disease. *N Engl J Med*. 1993;328:1797-1801.
267. Poynard T, Bedossa P, Opolon P. Natural history of liver fibrosis progression in patients with chronic hepatitis C. *Lancet*. 1997;349:825-832.
268. Ghany MG, Kleiner DE, Alter H, et al. Progression of fibrosis in chronic hepatitis C. *Gastroenterology*. 2003;124:97-104.
269. Wali M, Lewis S, Hubscher S, et al. Histological progression during short-term follow-up of patients with chronic hepatitis C virus infection. *J Viral Hepat*. 1999;6:445-452.
270. Intraobserver and interobserver variations in liver biopsy interpretation in patients with chronic hepatitis C. The French METAVIR Cooperative Study Group. *Hepatology*. 1994;20:15-20.
271. Feldmann G. Critical analysis of the methods used to morphologically quantify hepatic fibrosis. *J Hepatol*. 1995;22:49-54.
272. Westin J, Lagging LM, Wejstal R, et al. Interobserver study of liver histopathology using the Ishak score in patients with chronic hepatitis C virus infection. *Liver*. 1999;19:183-187.
273. Corrao G, Aricò S. Independent and combined action of hepatitis C virus infection and alcohol consumption on the risk of symptomatic liver cirrhosis. *Hepatology*. 1998;27:914-919.
274. Ostapowicz G, Watson KJR, Locarnini SA, et al. Role of alcohol in the progression of liver disease caused by hepatitis C virus infection. *Hepatology*. 1998;27:1730-1735.
275. Pessione F, Degos F, Marcellin P, et al. Effect of alcohol consumption on serum hepatitis C virus RNA and histological lesions in chronic hepatitis C. *Hepatology*. 1998;27:1717-1722.
276. Schiff ER. Hepatitis C and alcohol. *Hepatology*. 1997;26:39S-42S.
277. Monto A, Alonzo J, Watson JJ, et al. Steatosis in chronic hepatitis C: relative contributions of obesity, diabetes mellitus, and alcohol. *Hepatology*. 2002;36:729-736.
278. Okuda M, Li K, Beard MR, et al. Mitochondrial injury, oxidative stress, and antioxidant gene expression are induced by hepatitis C virus core protein. *Gastroenterology*. 2002;122:366-375.
279. Fong TL, Di Bisceglie AM, Waggoner JG, et al. The significance of antibody to hepatitis C virus in patients with chronic hepatitis B. *Hepatology*. 1991;14:64-67.
280. Chiba T, Matsuzaki Y, Abei M, et al. The role of previous hepatitis B virus infection and heavy smoking in hepatitis C virus–related hepatocellular carcinoma. *Am J Gastroenterol*. 1996;91:1195-1203.
281. Benvegnù L, Fattovich G, Noventa F, et al. Concurrent hepatitis B and C virus infection and risk of hepatocellular carcinoma in cirrhosis: a prospective study. *Cancer*. 1994;74:2442-2448.
282. Enomoto M, Nishiguchi S, Fukuda K, et al. Characteristics of patients with hepatitis C virus with and without GB virus C/hepatitis G virus co-infection and efficacy of interferon alfa. *Hepatology*. 1998;27:1388-1393.
283. Laskus T, Radkowski M, Wang LF, et al. Lack of evidence for hepatitis G virus replication in the livers of patients coinfected with hepatitis C and G viruses. *J Virol*. 1997;71:7804-7806.
284. Eyster ME, Diamondstone LS, Lien JM, et al. Natural history of hepatitis C virus infection in multitransfused hemophiliacs: effect of coinfection with human immunodeficiency virus. The Multicenter Hemophilia Cohort Study. *J Acquir Immune Defic Syndr*. 1993;6:602-610.
285. Thomas DL, Shih JW, Alter HJ, et al. Effect of human immunodeficiency virus on hepatitis C virus infection among injecting drug users. *J Infect Dis*. 1996;174:690-695.
286. Sherman KE, O'Brien J, Gutierrez AG, et al. Quantitative evaluation of hepatitis C virus RNA in patients with concurrent human immunodeficiency virus infections. *J Clin Microbiol*. 1993;31:2679-2682.
287. Bierhoff E, Fischer HP, Willsch E, et al. Liver histopathology in patients with concurrent chronic hepatitis C and HIV infection. *Virchows Arch Int J Pathol*. 1997;430:271-277.
288. Cribier B, Schmitt C, Rey D, et al. HIV increases hepatitis C viraemia irrespective of the hepatitis C virus genotype. *Res Virol*. 1997;148:267-271.
289. Kamal SM, Rasenack JW, Bianchi L, et al. Acute hepatitis C without and with schistosomiasis: correlation with hepatitis C-specific CD4(+) T-cell and cytokine response. *Gastroenterology*. 2001;121:646-656.
290. Bjoro K, Froland SS, Yun Z, et al. Hepatitis C infection in patients with primary hypogammaglobulinemia after treatment with contaminated immune globulin. *N Engl J Med*. 1994;331:1607-1611.
291. Gretch DR, Bacchi CE, Corey L, et al. Persistent hepatitis C virus infection after liver transplantation: clinical and virological features. *Hepatology*. 1995;22:1-9.
292. Collier J, Heathcote J. Hepatitis C viral infection in the immunosuppressed patient. *Hepatology*. 1998;27:2-6.
293. Vogt M, Lang T, Frosner G, et al. Prevalence and clinical outcome of hepatitis C infection in children who underwent cardiac surgery before the implementation of blood-donor screening. *N Engl J Med*. 1999;341:866-870.
294. Kage M, Fujisawa T, Shiraki K, et al. Pathology of chronic hepatitis C in children. Child Liver Study Group of Japan. *Hepatology*. 1997;26:771-775.
295. Ni YH, Chang MH, Lin KH, et al. Hepatitis C viral infection in thalassemic children: clinical and molecular studies. *Pediatr Res*. 1996;39:323-328.
296. Goodman ZD, Ishak KG. Histopathology of hepatitis C virus infection. *Semin Liver Dis*. 1995;15:70-81.
297. Friedman SL. Liver fibrosis—from bench to bedside. *J Hepatol*. 2003;38(Suppl 1):S38-S53.
298. Winwood PJ, Schuppan D, Iredale JP, et al. Kupffer cell-derived 95-kd type IV collagenase/gelatinase B: characterization and expression in cultured cells. *Hepatology*. 1995;22:304-315.
299. Paradis V, Scoazec JY, Kollinger M, et al. Cellular and subcellular localization of acetaldehyde-protein adducts in liver biopsies from alcoholic patients. *J Histochem Cytochem*. 1996;44:1051-1057.
300. Matsuoka M, Tsukamoto H. Stimulation of hepatic lipocyte collagen production by Kupffer cell–derived transforming growth factor beta: implication for a pathogenetic role in alcoholic liver fibrogenesis. *Hepatology*. 1990;11:599-605.
301. Shi Z, Wakil AE, Rockey DC. Strain-specific differences in mouse hepatic wound healing are mediated by divergent T helper cytokine responses. *Proc Natl Acad Sci U S A*. 1997;94:10663-10668.
302. Seki E, De Minicis S, Osterreicher CH, et al. TLR4 enhances TGF-beta signaling and hepatic fibrosis. *Nat Med*. 2007;13:1324-1332.
303. Nousbaum J-B, Pol S, Nalpas B, et al. Hepatitis C virus type 1b (II) infection in France and Italy. *Ann Intern Med*. 1995;122:161-168.
304. Gretch D, Corey L, Wilson J, et al. Assessment of hepatitis C virus RNA levels by quantitative competitive RNA polymerase chain reaction: high titer viremia correlates with advanced stage of disease. *J Infect Dis*. 1994;169:1219-1225.
305. Vlahov D, Graham N, Hoover D, et al. Prognostic indicators for AIDS and infectious disease death in HIV-infected injection drug users—Plasma viral load and CD4+ cell count. *JAMA*. 1998;279:35-40.
306. Mellors JW, Rinaldo CRJ, Gupta P, et al. Prognosis in HIV-1 infection predicted by the quantity of virus in plasma. *Science*. 1996;272:1167-1170.
307. Wiley TE, Brown J, Chan J. Hepatitis C infection in African Americans: its natural history and histological progression. *Am J Gastroenterol*. 2002;97:700-706.
308. Reynolds WF, Patel K, Pianko S, et al. A genotypic association implicates myeloperoxidase in the progression of hepatic fibrosis in chronic hepatitis C virus infection. *Genes Immun*. 2002;3:345-349.
309. Asti M, Martinetti M, Zavaglia C, et al. Human leukocyte antigen class II and III alleles and severity of hepatitis C virus–related chronic liver disease. *Hepatology*. 1999;29:1272-1279.
310. Powell EE, Edwards-Smith CJ, Hay JL, et al. Host genetic factors influence disease progression in chronic hepatitis C. *Hepatology*. 2000;31:828-833.
311. El Serag HB, Mason AC. Rising incidence of hepatocellular carcinoma in the United States. *N Engl J Med*. 1999;340:745-750.
312. Deuffic S, Poynard T, Valleron AJ. Correlation between hepatitis C virus prevalence and hepatocellular carcinoma mortality in Europe. *J Viral Hepat*. 1999;6:411-413.
313. Saito I, Miyamura T, Ohbayashi A, et al. Hepatitis C virus infection is associated with the development of hepatocellular carcinoma. *Proc Natl Acad Sci U S A*. 1990;87:6547-6549.
314. Bukh J, Miller RH, Kew MC, et al. Hepatitis C virus RNA in southern African blacks with hepatocellular carcinoma. *Proc Natl Acad Sci U S A*. 1993;90:1848-1851.
315. Bruno S, Silini E, Crosignani A, et al. Hepatitis C virus genotypes and risk of hepatocellular carcinoma in cirrhosis: a prospective study. *Hepatology*. 1997;25:754-758.
316. Simonetti RG, Camma C, Fiorello F, et al. Hepatitis C virus infection as a risk factor for hepatocellular carcinoma in patients with cirrhosis. *Ann Intern Med*. 1992;116:97-102.
317. Edamoto Y, Tani M, Kurata T, et al. Hepatitis C and B virus infections in hepatocellular carcinoma—Analysis of direct detection of viral genome in paraffin embedded tissues. *Cancer*. 1996;77:1787-1791.
318. Kiyosawa K, Furuta S. Hepatitis C virus and hepatocellular carcinoma. *Curr Stud Hematol Blood Transfus*. 1994;61:98-120.
319. Zein NN, Poterucha JJ, Gross JB Jr, et al. Increased risk of hepatocellular carcinoma in patients infected with hepatitis C genotype 1b. *Am J Gastroenterol*. 1996;91:2560-2562.
320. Yu MC, Yuan JM, Ross RK, et al. Presence of antibodies to the hepatitis B surface antigen is associated with an excess risk for hepatocellular carcinoma among non-Asians in Los Angeles county, California. *Hepatology*. 1997;25:226-228.
321. Kew MC, Yu MC, Kedda MA, et al. The relative roles of hepatitis B and C viruses in the etiology of hepatocellular carcinoma in southern African blacks. *Gastroenterology*. 1997;112:184-187.
322. Silini E, Bottelli R, Asti M, et al. Hepatitis C virus genotypes and risk of hepatocellular carcinoma in cirrhosis: a case-control study. *Gastroenterology*. 1996;111:199-205.
323. Lerat H, Honda M, Beard MR, et al. Steatosis and liver cancer in transgenic mice expressing the structural and nonstructural proteins of hepatitis C virus. *Gastroenterology*. 2002;122:352-365.
324. Nakamoto Y, Guidotti LG, Kuhlen CV, et al. Immune pathogenesis of hepatocellular carcinoma. *J Exp Med*. 1998;188:341-350.
325. Aach RD, Stevens CE, Hollinger FB, et al. Hepatitis C virus infection in post-transfusion hepatitis. *N Engl J Med*. 1991;325:1325-1329.
326. Yanagi M, Kaneko S, Unoura M, et al. Hepatitis C virus in fulminant hepatic failure. *N Engl J Med*. 1991;324:1895-1896.
327. Farci P, Alter HJ, Shimoda A, et al. Hepatitis C virus–associated fulminant hepatic failure. *N Engl J Med*. 1996;335:631-634.
328. Wright TL, Hsu H, Donegan E, et al. Hepatitis C virus not found in fulminant non-A, non-B hepatitis. *Ann Intern Med*. 1991;115:111-112.
329. Vento S, Garofano T, Renzini C, et al. Fulminant hepatitis associated with hepatitis A virus superinfection in patients with chronic hepatitis C. *N Engl J Med*. 1998;338:286-290.
330. Koretz RL, Abbey H, Coleman E, et al. Non-A, non-B post-transfusion hepatitis: looking back in the second decade. *Ann Intern Med*. 1993;119:110-115.
331. Foster GR, Goldin RD, Thomas HC. Chronic hepatitis C virus infection causes a significant reduction in quality of life in the absence of cirrhosis. *Hepatology*. 1998;27:209-212.
332. Bernstein D, Kleinman L, Barker CM, et al. Relationship of health-related quality of life to treatment adherence and sustained response in chronic hepatitis C patients. *Hepatology*. 2002;35:704-708.
333. Spiegel BMR, Younossi ZM, Hays RD, et al. Impact of hepatitis C on health-related quality of life: a systematic review and quantitative assessment. *Hepatology*. 2005;41:790-800.
334. Conry-Cantilena C, Vanraden MT, Gibble J, et al. Routes of infection, viremia, and liver disease in blood donors found to have hepatitis C virus infection. *N Engl J Med*. 1996;334:1691-1696.
335. Inglesby TV, Rai R, Astemborski J, et al. A prospective, community-based evaluation of liver enzymes in individuals with hepatitis C after drug use. *Hepatology*. 1999;29:590-596.
336. Perrillo RP. The role of liver biopsy in hepatitis C. *Hepatology*. 1997;26:57S-61S.
337. Shakil AO, Conry-Cantilena C, Alter HJ, et al. Volunteer blood donors with antibody to hepatitis C virus: clinical, biochemical, virologic, and histologic features. *Ann Intern Med*. 1995;123:330-337.
338. Sangiovanni A, Prati GM, Fasani P, et al. The natural history of compensated cirrhosis due to hepatitis C virus: a 17-year cohort study of 214 patients. *Hepatology*. 2006;43:1303-1310.
339. Mehta SH, Brancati FL, Sulkowski MS, et al. Prevalence of type 2 diabetes mellitus among persons with hepatitis C virus infection in the United States. *Hepatology*. 2001;33:1554.
340. Lonardo A, Adinolfi LE, Loria P, et al. Steatosis and hepatitis C virus: mechanisms and significance for hepatic and extrahepatic disease. *Gastroenterology*. 2004;126:586-597.
341. Shintani Y, Fujie H, Miyoshi H, et al. Hepatitis C virus infection and diabetes: direct involvement of the virus in the development of insulin resistance. *Gastroenterology*. 2004;126:840-848.
342. Poynard T, Ratziu V, McHutchison J, et al. Effect of treatment with peginterferon or interferon alfa-2b and ribavirin on steatosis in patients infected with hepatitis C. *Hepatology*. 2003;38:75-85.
343. Davila JA, Morgan RO, Shaib Y, et al. Hepatitis C infection and the increasing incidence of hepatocellular carcinoma: a population-based study. *Gastroenterology*. 2004;127:1372-1380.
344. Bruix J, Sherman M. Management of hepatocellular carcinoma. *Hepatology*. 2005;42:1208-1236.
345. Agnello V, Chung RT, Kaplan LM. A role for hepatitis C virus infection in Type II cryoglobulinemia. *N Engl J Med*. 1992;327:1490-1495.
346. Misiani R, Bellavita P, Fenili D, et al. Hepatitis C virus infection in patients with essential mixed cryoglobulinemia. *Ann Intern Med*. 1992;117:573-577.
347. Alric L, Plaisier E, Theault S, et al. Influence of antiviral therapy in hepatitis C virus–associated cryoglobulinemic MPGN. *Am J Kidney Dis*. 2004;43:617-623.
348. Rasul I, Shepherd FA, Kamel-Reid S, et al. Detection of occult low-grade B-cell non-Hodgkin's lymphoma in patients with chronic hepatitis C infection and mixed cryoglobulinemia. *Hepatology*. 1999;29:543-547.
349. Negri E, Little D, Boiocchi M, et al. B-cell non-Hodgkin's lymphoma and hepatitis C virus infection: a systematic review. *Int J Cancer*. 2004;111:1-8.
350. Matsuo K, Kusano A, Sugumar A, et al. Effect of hepatitis C virus infection on the risk of non-Hodgkin's lymphoma: a meta-analysis of epidemiological studies. *Cancer Sci*. 2004;95:745-752.
351. Herrero C, Vicente A, Bruguera M, et al. Is hepatitis C virus infection a trigger of porphyria cutanea tarda? *Lancet*. 1993;341:788-789.
352. DeCastro M, Sanchez J, Herrera JF, et al. Hepatitis C virus antibodies and liver disease in patients with porphyria cutanea tarda. *Hepatology*. 1993;17:551-557.

353. Gumber SC, Chopra S. Hepatitis C: a multifaceted disease—Review of extrahepatic manifestations. *Ann Intern Med.* 1995;123:615-620.
354. Koike K, Moriya K, Ishibashi K, et al. Sialadenitis histologically resembling Sjogren syndrome in mice transgenic for hepatitis C virus envelope genes. *Proc Natl Acad Sci U S A.* 1997;94:233-236.
355. Tran A, Quaranta JF, Benzaken S, et al. High prevalence of thyroid autoantibodies in a prospective series of patients with chronic hepatitis C before interferon therapy. *Hepatology.* 1993;18:253-257.
356. McHutchinson JG, Person JL, Govindarajan S, et al. Improved detection of hepatitis C virus antibodies in high-risk populations. *Hepatology.* 1992;15:19-25.
357. Nakatsuji Y, Matsumoto A, Tanaka E, et al. Detection of chronic hepatitis C virus infection by four diagnostic systems: first-generation and second-generation enzyme-linked immunosorbent assay, second-generation recombinant immunoblot assay and nested polymerase chain reaction analysis. *Hepatology.* 1992;16:300-305.
358. Chien DY, Choo QL, Tabrizi A, et al. Diagnosis of hepatitis C virus (HCV) infection using an immunodominant chimeric polyprotein to capture circulating antibodies: reevaluation of the role of HCV in liver disease. *Proc Natl Acad Sci U S A.* 1992;89:10011-10015.
359. Courouce A-M, Le Marrec N, Girault A, et al. Anti-hepatitis C virus (anti-HCV) seroconversion in patients undergoing hemodialysis: comparison of second- and third-generation anti-HCV assays. *Transfusion.* 1994;34:790-795.
360. Vallari DS, Jett BW, Alter HJ, et al. Serological markers of post-transfusion hepatitis C viral infection. *J Clin Microbiol.* 1992;30:552-556.
361. van der Poel CL, Cuypers HTM, Reesink HW, et al. Confirmation of hepatitis C virus infection by new four-antigen recombinant immunoblot assay. *Lancet.* 1991;337:317-319.
362. Buffet C, Charnaux N, Laurent-Puig P, et al. Enhanced detection of antibodies to hepatitis C virus by use of a third-generation recombinant immunoblot assay. *J Med Virol.* 1994;43:259-261.
363. McGuinness PH, Bishop GA, Lien A, et al. Detection of serum hepatitis C virus RNA in HCV antibody-seropositive volunteer blood donors. *Hepatology.* 1993;18:485-490.
364. Vrielink H, van der Poel CL, Reesink HW, et al. Look-back study of infectivity of anti-HCV ELISA-positive blood components. *Lancet.* 1995;345:95-96.
365. Damen M, Zaaijer HL, Cuypers HTM, et al. Reliability of the third-generation recombinant immunoblot assay for hepatitis C virus. *Transfusion.* 1995;35:745-749.
366. Pawlotsky JM, Lonjon I, Hezode C, et al. What strategy should be used for diagnosis of hepatitis C virus infection in clinical laboratories? *Hepatology.* 1998;27:1700-1702.
367. Alter MJ, Kuhnert WL, Finelli L. Guidelines for laboratory testing and result reporting of antibody to hepatitis C virus. Centers for Disease Control and Prevention. *MMWR Recomm Rep.* 2003;52:1-13, 15.
368. Lau JY, Davis GL, Kniffen J, et al. Significance of serum hepatitis C virus RNA levels in chronic hepatitis C. *Lancet.* 1993;341:1501-1504.
369. Sarrazin C, Hendricks DA, Sedarati F, et al. Assessment, by transcription-mediated amplification, of virologic response in patients with chronic hepatitis C virus treated with peginterferon alpha-2a. *J Clin Microbiol.* 2001;39:2850-2855.
370. Davis GL, Lau JYN, Urdea MS, et al. Quantitative detection of hepatitis C virus RNA with a solid-phase signal amplification method: definition of optimal conditions for specimen collection and clinical application in interferon-treated patients. *Hepatology.* 1994;19:1337-1341.
371. Gordon SC, Dailey PJ, Silverman AL, et al. Sequential serum hepatitis C viral RNA levels longitudinally assessed by branched DNA signal amplification. *Hepatology.* 1998;28:1702-1706.
372. Nguyen TT, Sedghi-Vaziri A, Wilkes LB, et al. Fluctuations in viral load (HCV RNA) are relatively insignificant in untreated patients with chronic HCV infection. *J Viral Hepat.* 1996;3:75-78.
373. Miskovsky EP, Carella AV, Gutekunst K, et al. Clinical characterization of a competitive PCR assay for quantitative testing of hepatitis C virus. *J Clin Microbiol.* 1996;34:1975-1979.
374. Saldanha J, Lelie N, Heath A. Establishment of the first international standard for nucleic acid amplification technology (NAT) assays for HCV RNA. WHO Collaborative Study Group. *Vox Sang.* 1999;76:149-158.
375. Pawlotsky JM. Use and interpretation of virological tests for hepatitis C. *Hepatology.* 2002;36:S65-S73.
376. Bouvier-Alias M, Patel K, Dahari H, et al. Clinical utility of total HCV core antigen quantification: a new indirect marker of HCV replication. *Hepatology.* 2002;36:211-218.
377. Stuyver L, Wyseur A, Van Arnhem W, et al. Second-generation line probe assay for hepatitis C virus genotyping. *J Clin Microbiol.* 1996;34:2259-2266.
378. Ghany MG, Strader DB, Thomas DL, et al. Diagnosis, management, and treatment of hepatitis C. *Hepatology.* 2009;49:1335-1374.
379. Dienstag JL, McHutchison JG. American Gastroenterological Association medical position statement on the management of hepatitis C. *Gastroenterology.* 2006;130:225-230.
380. Knodell RG, Ishak KG, Black WC, et al. Formulation and application of a numerical scoring system for assessing histological activity in asymptomatic chronic active hepatitis. *Hepatology.* 1981;1:431-435.
381. Bedossa P, Poynard T. An algorithm for the grading of activity in chronic hepatitis C. *Hepatology.* 1996;24:289-293.
382. Ishak K, Baptista A, Bianchi L, et al. Histological grading and staging of chronic hepatitis. *J Hepatol.* 1995;22:696-699.
383. Goldin RD, Goldin JG, Burt AD, et al. Intra-observer and inter-observer variation in the histopathological assessment of chronic viral hepatitis. *J Hepatol.* 1996;25:649-654.
384. McGill DB, Rakela J, Sinsmeister AR, et al. A 21-year experience with major hemorrhage after percutaneous liver biopsy. *Gastroenterology.* 1990;99:1392-1400.
385. Regev A, Berho M, Jeffers LJ, et al. Sampling error and intra-observer variation in liver biopsy in patients with chronic HCV infection. *Am J Gastroenterol.* 2002;97:2614-2618.
386. Gordon SC, Fang JW, Silverman AL, et al. The significance of baseline serum alanine aminotransferase on pretreatment disease characteristics and response to antiviral therapy in chronic hepatitis C. *Hepatology.* 2000;32:400-404.
387. Persico M, Persico E, Suozzo R, et al. Natural history of hepatitis C virus carriers with persistently normal aminotransferase levels. *Gastroenterology.* 2000;118:760-764.
388. Mathurin P, Moussalli J, Cadranel JF, et al. Slow progression rate of fibrosis in hepatitis C virus patients with persistently normal alanine transaminase activity. *Hepatology.* 1998;27:868-872.
389. Williams AL, Hoofnagle JH. Ratio of serum aspartate to alanine aminotransferase in chronic hepatitis. Relationship to cirrhosis. *Gastroenterology.* 1988;95:734-739.
390. Sheth SG, Flamm SL, Gordon FD, et al. AST/ALT ratio predicts cirrhosis in patients with chronic hepatitis C virus infection. *Am J Gastroenterol.* 1998;93:44-48.
391. Oberti F, Valsesia E, Pilette C, et al. Noninvasive diagnosis of hepatic fibrosis or cirrhosis. *Gastroenterology.* 1997;113:1609-1616.
392. Matsumura H, Moriyama M, Goto I, et al. Natural course of progression of liver fibrosis in Japanese patients with chronic liver disease type C—a study of 527 patients at one establishment. *J Viral Hepat.* 2000;7:268-275.
393. Imbert-Bismut F, Ratziu V, Pieroni L, et al. Biochemical markers of liver fibrosis in patients with hepatitis C virus infection: a prospective study. *Lancet.* 2001;357:1069-1075.
394. Wai CT, Greenson JK, Fontana RJ, et al. A simple noninvasive index can predict both significant fibrosis and cirrhosis in patients with chronic hepatitis C. *Hepatology.* 2003;38:518-526.
395. Forns X, Ampurdanes S, Llovet JM, et al. Identification of chronic hepatitis C patients without hepatic fibrosis by a simple predictive model. *Hepatology.* 2002;36:986-992.
396. Kelleher TB, Mehta SH, Bhaskar K, et al. Prediction of hepatic fibrosis in HIV/HCV co-infected patients using serum fibrosis markers: the SHASTA index. *J Hepatol.* 2005;43:78-84.
397. Sterling RK, Lissen E, Clumeck N, et al. Development of a simple noninvasive index to predict significant fibrosis in patients with HIV/HCV coinfection. *Hepatology.* 2006;43:1317-1325.
398. Mehta SH, Lau B, Afdhal NH, et al. Exceeding the limits of liver histology markers. *J Hepatol.* 2009;50:36-41.
399. Castera L, Vergniol J, Foucher J, et al. Prospective comparison of transient elastography, Fibrotest, APRI, and liver biopsy for the assessment of fibrosis in chronic hepatitis C. *Gastroenterology.* 2005;128:343-350.
400. de Lédinghen V, Douvin C, Kettaneh A, et al. Diagnosis of hepatic fibrosis and cirrhosis by transient elastography in HIV/hepatitis C virus–coinfected patients. *J Acquir Immune Defic Syndr.* 2006;41:175-179.
401. Foucher J, Chanteloup E, Vergniol J, et al. Diagnosis of cirrhosis by transient elastography (FibroScan): a prospective study. *Gut.* 2006;55:403-408.
402. World Health Organization. Hepatitis C: global prevalence. *Wkly Epidemiol Rec.* 1997;341-348.
403. Armstrong GL, Wasley A, Simard EP, et al. The prevalence of hepatitis C virus infection in the United States, 1999 through 2002. *Ann Intern Med.* 2006;144:705-714.
404. Baillargeon J, Wu H, Kelley MJ, et al. Hepatitis C seroprevalence among newly incarcerated inmates in the Texas correctional system. *Public Health.* 2003;117:43-48.
405. Abdel-Wahab MF, Zakaria S, Kamel M, et al. High seroprevalence of hepatitis C infection among risk groups in Egypt. *Am J Trop Med Hyg.* 1994;51:563-567.
406. Kamel MA, Ghaffar YA, Wasef MA, et al. High HCV prevalence in Egyptian blood donors. *Lancet.* 1992;340:427.
407. Osella AR, Misciagna G, Leone A, et al. Epidemiology of hepatitis C virus infection in an area of southern Italy. *J Hepatol.* 1997;27:30-35.
408. Chiaramonte M, Stroffolini T, Lorenzoni U, et al. Risk factors in community-acquired chronic hepatitis C virus infection: a case-control study in Italy. *J Hepatol.* 1996;24:129-134.
409. Nakashima K, Ikematsu H, Hayashi J, et al. Intrafamilial transmission of hepatitis C virus among the population of an endemic area of Japan. *JAMA.* 1995;274:1459-1461.
410. Guadagnino V, Stroffolini T, Rapicetta M, et al. Prevalence, risk factors, and genotype distribution of hepatitis C virus infection in the general population: a community-based survey in southern Italy. *Hepatology.* 1997;26:1006-1011.
411. Prati D, Capelli C, Silvani C, et al. The incidence and risk factors of community-acquired hepatitis C in a cohort of Italian blood donors. *Hepatology.* 1997;25:702-704.
412. Noguchi S, Sata M, Suzuki H, et al. Routes of transmission of hepatitis C virus in an endemic rural area of Japan—Molecular epidemiologic study of hepatitis C virus infection. *Scand J Infect Dis.* 1997;29:23-28.
413. Frank C, Mohamed MK, Strickland GT, et al. The role of parenteral antischistosomal therapy in the spread of hepatitis C virus in Egypt. *Lancet.* 2000;355:887-891.
414. Thomas DL, Cannon RO, Shapiro CN, et al. Hepatitis C, hepatitis B, and human immunodeficiency virus infections among non-intravenous drug-using patients attending clinics for sexually transmitted diseases. *J Infect Dis.* 1994;169:990-995.
415. Kelen GD, Green GB, Purcell RH, et al. Hepatitis B and hepatitis C in emergency department patients. *N Engl J Med.* 1992;326:1399-1404.
416. Centers for Disease Control and Prevention. Recommendations for prevention and control of hepatitis C virus (HCV) infection and HCV-related chronic disease. *MMWR.* 1998;47(No. RR-19):1-39.
417. Wang JT, Wang TH, Sheu JC, et al. Hepatitis C virus RNA in saliva of patients with posttransfusion hepatitis and low efficiency of transmission among spouses. *J Med Virol.* 1992;36:28-31.
418. Esteban JI, Lopez-Talavera JC, Genesca J, et al. High rate of infectivity and liver disease in blood donors with antibodies to hepatitis C virus. *Ann Intern Med.* 1991;115:443-449.
419. Centers for Disease Control and Prevention. Public Health Service interagency guidelines for screening blood, plasma, organs, tissue and semen for evidence of hepatitis B and C. *MMWR.* 1991;40:1-23.
420. Donahue JG, Munoz A, Ness PM, et al. The declining risk of post-transfusion hepatitis C virus infection. *N Engl J Med.* 1992;327:369-373.
421. Schreiber GB, Busch MP, Kleinman SH, et al. The risk of transfusion-transmitted viral infections. The Retrovirus Epidemiology Donor Study. *N Engl J Med.* 1996;334:1685-1690.
422. Blanchette V, Walker I, Gill P, et al. Hepatitis C infection in patients with hemophilia: results of a national survey. Canadian Hemophilia Clinic Directors Group. *Transfus Med Rev.* 1994;8:210-217.
423. Kinoshita T, Miyake K, Okamoto H, et al. Imported hepatitis C virus genotypes in Japanese hemophiliacs. *J Infect Dis.* 1993;168:249-250.
424. Pereira BJG, Milford EL, Kirkman RL, et al. Prevalence of hepatitis C virus RNA in organ donors positive for hepatitis C antibody and in the recipients of their organs. *N Engl J Med.* 1992;327:910-915.
425. Konig V, Bauditz J, Lobeck H, et al. Hepatitis C virus reinfection in allografts after orthotopic liver transplantation. *Hepatology.* 1992;16:1137-1143.
426. Alter MJ. Epidemiology of hepatitis C. *Hepatology.* 1997;26:62S-65S.
427. Thomas DL, Vlahov D, Solomon L, et al. Correlates of hepatitis C virus infections among injection drug users in Baltimore. *Medicine.* 1995;74:212-220.
428. Bolumar F, Hernandez-Aguado I, Ferrer L, et al. Prevalence of antibodies to hepatitis C in a population of intravenous drug users in Valencia, Spain, 1990-1992. *Int J Epidemiol.* 1996;25:204-209.
429. Van Ameijden EJ, van den Hoek JA, Mientjes GH, et al. A longitudinal study on the incidence and transmission patterns of HIV, HBV and HCV infection among drug users in Amsterdam. *Eur J Epidemiol.* 1993;9:255-262.
430. Patti AM, Santi AL, Pompa MG, et al. Viral hepatitis and drugs: a continuing problem. *Int J Epidemiol.* 1993;22:135-139.
431. Garfein RS, Vlahov D, Galai N, et al. Viral infections in short-term injection drug users: the prevalence of the hepatitis C, hepatitis B, human immunodeficiency, and human T-lymphotropic viruses. *Am J Public Health.* 1996;86:655-661.
432. Garfein RS, Doherty MC, Monterroso ER, et al. Prevalence and incidence of hepatitis C virus infection among young adult injection drug users. *J Acquir Immune Defic Syndr Hum Retrovirol.* 1998;18(Suppl 1):S11-S19.
433. Ko YC, Ho MS, Chiang TA, et al. Tattooing as a risk of hepatitis C virus infection. *J Med Virol.* 1992;38:288-291.
434. Sun DX, Zhang FG, Geng YQ, et al. Hepatitis C transmission by cosmetic tattooing in women. *Lancet.* 1996;347:541.
435. Dusheiko GM, Smith M, Scheuer PJ. Hepatitis C virus transmission by human bite. *Lancet.* 1990;336:503-504.
436. Thompson ND, Perz JF, Moorman AC, et al. Nonhospital health care–associated hepatitis B and C virus transmission: United States, 1998-2008. *Ann Intern Med.* 2009;150:33-39.
437. Acute hepatitis C virus infections attributed to unsafe injection practices at an endoscopy clinic—Nevada, 2007. *MMWR* 2008;57:513-517.
438. Martinez-Bauer E, Forns X, Armelles M, et al. Hospital admission is a relevant source of hepatitis C virus acquisition in Spain. *J Hepatol.* 2008;48:20-27.
439. Dumpis U, Kovalova Z, Jansons J, et al. An outbreak of HBV and HCV infection in a paediatric oncology ward: epidemiological investigations and prevention of further spread. *J Med Virol.* 2003;69:331-338.
440. Ross RS, Viazov S, Khudyakov YE, et al. Transmission of hepatitis C virus in an orthopedic hospital ward. *J Med Virol.* 2009;81:249-257.
441. Bronowicki JP, Venard V, Botté C, et al. Patient-to-patient transmission of hepatitis C virus during colonoscopy. *N Engl J Med.* 1997;337:237-240.

442. Allander T, Gruber A, Naghavi M, et al. Frequent patient-to-patient transmission of hepatitis C virus in a haematology ward. *Lancet*. 1995;345:603-607.
443. Patel PR, Larson AK, Castel AD, et al. Hepatitis C virus infections from a contaminated radiopharmaceutical used in myocardial perfusion studies. *JAMA*. 2006;296:2005-2011.
444. Girou E, Chevaliez S, Challine D, et al. Determinant roles of environmental contamination and noncompliance with standard precautions in the risk of hepatitis C virus transmission in a hemodialysis unit. *Clin Infect Dis*. 2008;47:627-633.
445. Schvarcz R, Johansson B, Nyström B, et al. Nosocomial transmission of hepatitis C virus. *Infection*. 1997;25:74-77.
446. Munro J, Biggs JD, McCruden EAB. Detection of a cluster of hepatitis C infections in a renal transplant unit by analysis of sequence variation of the NS5a gene. *J Infect Dis*. 1996;174:177-180.
447. Hutin YJ, Hauri AM, Armstrong GL. Use of injections in healthcare settings worldwide, 2000: literature review and regional estimates. *BMJ*. 2003;327:1075.
448. Kiyosawa K, Sodeyama T, Tanaka E, et al. Hepatitis C in hospital employees with needlestick injuries. *Ann Intern Med*. 1991;115:367-369.
449. Ridzon R, Gallagher K, Ciesielski C, et al. Simultaneous transmission of human immunodeficiency virus and hepatitis C virus from a needle-stick injury. *N Engl J Med*. 1997;336:919-922.
450. Mitsui T, Iwano K, Masuko K, et al. Hepatitis C virus infection in medical personnel after needlestick accident. *Hepatology*. 1992;16:1109-1114.
451. Seeff LB, Wright EC, Zimmerman HJ, et al. Type B hepatitis after needle-stick exposure: prevention with hepatitis B immune globulin. *Ann Intern Med*. 1978;88:285-293.
452. Sartori M, La Terra G, Aglietta M, et al. Transmission of hepatitis C via blood splash into conjunctiva. *Scand J Infect Dis*. 1993;25:270-271.
453. Thomas DL, Gruninger SE, Siew C, et al. Occupational risk of hepatitis C infections among general dentists and oral surgeons in North America. *Am J Med*. 1996;100:41-45.
454. Thomas DL, Factor S, Kelen G, et al. Hepatitis B and C in health care workers at the Johns Hopkins Hospital. *Arch Intern Med*. 1993;153:1705-1712.
455. Gerberding JL. Incidence and prevalence of human immunodeficiency virus, hepatitis B virus, hepatitis C virus, and cytomegalovirus among health care personnel at risk for blood exposure: final report from a longitudinal study. *J Infect Dis*. 1994;170:1410-1417.
456. Esteban JI, Gómez J, Martell M, et al. Transmission of hepatitis C virus by a cardiac surgeon. *N Engl J Med*. 1996;334:555-560.
457. Cardell K, Widell A, Fryden A, et al. Nosocomial hepatitis C in a thoracic surgery unit: retrospective findings generating a prospective study. *J Hosp Infect*. 2008;68:322-328.
458. Liou TC, Chang TT, Young KC, et al. Detection of HCV RNA in saliva, urine, seminal fluid, and ascites. *J Med Virol*. 1992;37:197-202.
459. Thomas DL, Zenilman JM, Alter HJ, et al. Sexual transmission of hepatitis C virus among patients attending sexually transmitted diseases clinics in Baltimore: an analysis of 309 sex partnerships. *J Infect Dis*. 1995;171:768-775.
460. van Doornum GJJ, Hooykaas C, Cuypers MT, et al. Prevalence of hepatitis C virus infections among heterosexuals with multiple partners. *J Med Virol*. 1991;35:22-27.
461. Akahane Y, Kojima M, Sugai Y, et al. Hepatitis C virus infection in spouses of patients with type C chronic liver disease. *Ann Intern Med*. 1994;120:748-752.
462. Chayama K, Kobayashi M, Tsubota A, et al. Molecular analysis of intraspousal transmission of hepatitis C virus. *J Hepatol*. 1995;22:431-439.
463. Kao JH, Chen PJ, Yang PM, et al. Intrafamilial transmission of hepatitis C virus: the important role of infections between spouses. *J Infect Dis*. 1992;166:900-903.
464. Bresters D, Mauser-Bunschoten ED, Reesink HW, et al. Sexual transmission of hepatitis C. *Lancet*. 1993;342:210-211.
465. Everhart JE, Di Bisceglie AM, Murray LM, et al. Risk for non-A, non-B (type C) hepatitis through sexual or household contact with chronic carriers. *Ann Intern Med*. 1990;112:544-545.
466. Brettler DB, Mannucci PM, Gringeri A, et al. The low risk of hepatitis C virus transmission among sexual partners of hepatitis C infected hemophilic males: an international, multicenter study. *Blood*. 1992;80:540-543.
467. Gordon SC, Patel AH, Kulesza GW, et al. Lack of evidence for the heterosexual transmission of hepatitis C. *Am J Gastroenterol*. 1992;87:1849-1851.
468. Vandelli C, Renzo F, Romano L, et al. Lack of evidence of sexual transmission of hepatitis C among monogamous couples: results of a 10-year prospective follow-up study. *Am J Gastroenterol*. 2004;99:855-859.
469. Osmond DH, Charlebois E, Sheppard HW, et al. Comparison of risk factors for hepatitis C and hepatitis B virus infection in homosexual men. *J Infect Dis*. 1993;167:66-71.
470. Bodsworth NJ, Cunningham P, Kaldor J, et al. Hepatitis C virus infection in a large cohort of homosexually active men: independent associations with HIV-1 infection and injecting drug use but not sexual behaviour. *Genitourin Med*. 1996;72:118-122.
471. Zaaijer HL, Cuypers HTM, Reesink HW, et al. Reliability of polymerase chain reaction for detection of hepatitis C virus. *Lancet*. 1993;341:722-724.
472. Ohto H, Terazawa S, Nobuhiko S, et al. Transmission of hepatitis C virus from mothers to infants. *N Engl J Med*. 1994;330:744-750.
473. Zanetti AR, Tanzi E, Paccagnini S, et al. Mother-to-infant transmission of hepatitis C virus. *Lancet*. 1995;345:289-291.
474. Resti M, Azzari C, Mannelli F, et al. Mother to child transmission of hepatitis C virus: prospective study of risk factors and timing of infection in children born to women seronegative for HIV-1. Tuscany Study Group on Hepatitis C Virus Infection. *BMJ*. 1998;317:437-441.
475. Mast EE, Hwang LY, Seto DS, et al. Risk factors for perinatal transmission of hepatitis C virus (HCV) and the natural history of HCV infection acquired in infancy. *J Infect Dis*. 2005;192:1880-1889.
476. Ogasawara S, Kage M, Kosai K, et al. Hepatitis C virus RNA in saliva and breastmilk of hepatitis C carrier mothers. *Lancet*. 1993;341:561.
477. Resti M, Azzari C, Lega L, et al. Mother-to-infant transmission of hepatitis C virus. *Acta Paediatr*. 1995;84:251-255.
478. Lin H-H, Kao J-H, Hsu H-Y, et al. Absence of infection in breast-fed infants born to hepatitis C virus–infected mothers. *J Pediatr*. 1995;126:589-591.
479. American Academy of Pediatrics. Committee on Infectious Diseases. Hepatitis C virus infection. *Pediatrics*. 1998;101:481-485.
480. Gibb DM, Goodall RL, Dunn DT, et al. Mother-to-child transmission of hepatitis C virus: evidence for preventable peripartum transmission. *Lancet*. 2000;356:904-907.
481. Dore GJ, Kaldor JM, McCaughan GW. Systematic review of role of polymerase chain reaction in defining infectiousness among people infected with hepatitis C virus. *BMJ* 1997;315:333-337.
482. Thomas DL, Villano SA, Riester KA, et al. Perinatal transmission of hepatitis C virus from human immunodeficiency virus type 1–infected mothers. *J Infect Dis*. 1998;177:1480-1488.
483. Eyster ME, Alter HJ, Aledort LM, et al. Heterosexual co-transmission of hepatitis C virus (HCV) and human immunodeficiency virus (HIV). *Ann Intern Med*. 1991;115:764-768.
484. Lam JPH, McOmish F, Burns SM, et al. Infrequent vertical transmission of hepatitis C virus. *J Infect Dis*. 1993;167:572-576.
485. Eyster ME, Fried MW, Di Bisceglie AM, et al. Increasing hepatitis C virus RNA levels in hemophiliacs: relationship to human immunodeficiency virus infection and liver disease. *Blood*. 1994;84:1020-1023.
486. Lau DT, Kleiner DE, Ghany MG, et al. 10-year follow-up after interferon-α therapy for chronic hepatitis C. *Hepatology*. 1998;28:1121-1127.
487. Marcellin P, Boyer N, Gervais A, et al. Long-term histologic improvement and loss of detectable intrahepatic HCV RNA in patients with chronic hepatitis C and sustained response to interferon-α therapy. *Ann Intern Med*. 1997;127:875-881.
488. Poynard T, McHutchison J, Manns M, et al. Impact of pegylated interferon alfa-2b and ribavirin on liver fibrosis in patients with chronic hepatitis C. *Gastroenterology*. 2002;122:1303-1313.
489. Shiffman ML, Hofmann CM, Contos MJ, et al. A randomized, controlled trial of maintenance interferon therapy for patients with chronic hepatitis C virus and persistent viremia. *Gastroenterology*. 1999;117:1164-1172.
490. Heathcote EJ, Keeffe EB, Lee SS, et al. Re-treatment of chronic hepatitis C with consensus interferon. *Hepatology*. 1998;27:1136-1143.
491. Serfaty L, Aumaître H, Chazouillères O, et al. Determinants of outcome of compensated hepatitis C virus–related cirrhosis. *Hepatology*. 1998;27:1435-1440.
492. Kaneko T, Tanji Y, Satoh S, et al. Production of two phosphoproteins from the NS5A region of the hepatitis C viral genome. *Biochem Biophys Res Commun*. 1994;205:320-326.
493. Veldt BJ, Heathcote EJ, Wedemeyer H, et al. Sustained virologic response and clinical outcomes in patients with chronic hepatitis C and advanced fibrosis. *Ann Intern Med*. 2007;147:677-684.
494. Nishiguchi S, Kuroki T, Nakatani S, et al. Randomised trial of effects of interferon-α on incidence of hepatocellular carcinoma in chronic active hepatitis C with cirrhosis. *Lancet*. 1995;346:1051-1055.
495. Shiratori Y, Imazeki F, Moriyama M, et al. Histologic improvement of fibrosis in patients with hepatitis C who have sustained response to interferon therapy. *Ann Intern Med*. 2000;132:517-524.
496. Shiratori Y, Ito Y, Yokosuka O, et al. Antiviral therapy for cirrhotic hepatitis C: association with reduced hepatocellular carcinoma development and improved survival. *Ann Intern Med*. 2005;142:105-114.
497. Di Bisceglie AM, Shiffman ML, Everson GT, et al. Prolonged therapy of advanced chronic hepatitis C with low-dose peginterferon. *N Engl J Med*. 2008;359:2429-2441.
498. Davis GL, Balart LA, Schiff ER, et al. Treatment of chronic hepatitis C with recombinant interferon alfa. *N Engl J Med*. 1989;321:1501-1506.
499. Di Bisceglie AM, Martin P, Kassianides C, et al. Recombinant interferon alfa therapy for chronic hepatitis C. *N Engl J Med*. 1989;321:1506-1510.
500. Poynard T, Bedossa P, Chevallier M, et al. A comparison of three interferon alfa-2b regimens for the long-term treatment of chronic non-A, non-B hepatitis. *N Engl J Med*. 1995;332:1457-1462.
501. Keeffe EB, Hollinger FB, Bailey R, et al. Therapy of hepatitis C: consensus interferon trials. *Hepatology*. 1997;26:101S-107S.
502. Lee WM. Therapy of hepatitis C: interferon alfa-2a trials. *Hepatology*. 1997;26:89S-95S.
503. Zeuzem S, Feinman SV, Rasenack J, et al. Peginterferon alfa-2a in patients with chronic hepatitis C. *N Engl J Med*. 2000;343:1666-1672.
504. Heathcote EJ, Shiffman ML, Cooksley WG, et al. Peginterferon alfa-2a in patients with chronic hepatitis C and cirrhosis. *N Engl J Med*. 2000;343:1673-1680.
505. Fried MW, Shiffman ML, Reddy KR, et al. Peginterferon alfa-2a plus ribavirin for chronic hepatitis C virus infection. *N Engl J Med*. 2002;347:975-982.
506. Manns MP, McHutchison JG, Gordon SC, et al. Peginterferon alfa-2b plus ribavirin compared with interferon alfa-2b plus ribavirin for initial treatment of chronic hepatitis C: a randomised trial. *Lancet*. 2001;358:958-965.
507. Crotty S, Cameron CE, Andino R. RNA virus error catastrophe: direct molecular test by using ribavirin. *Proc Natl Acad Sci U S A*. 2001;98:6895-6900.
508. Lanford RE, Guerra B, Lee H, et al. Antiviral effect and virus-host interactions in response to alpha interferon, gamma interferon, poly(i)-poly(c), tumor necrosis factor alpha, and ribavirin in hepatitis C virus subgenomic replicons. *J Virol*. 2003;77:1092-1104.
509. Patterson JL, Fernandez-Larson R. Molecular mechanisms of action of ribavirin. *Rev Infect Dis*. 1990;12:1139-1146.
510. Pawlotsky JM, Dahari H, Neumann AU, et al. Antiviral action of ribavirin in chronic hepatitis C. *Gastroenterology*. 2004;126:703-714.
511. Bodenheimer HCJ, Lindsay KL, Davis GL, et al. Tolerance and efficacy of oral ribavirin treatment of chronic hepatitis C: a multicenter trial. *Hepatology*. 1997;26:473-477.
512. Dusheiko G, Main J, Thomas H, et al. Ribavirin treatment for patients with chronic hepatitis C: results of a placebo-controlled study. *J Hepatol*. 1996;25:591-598.
513. Di Bisceglie AM, Conjeevaram HS, Fried MW, et al. Ribavirin as therapy for chronic hepatitis C—A randomized, double-blind, placebo-controlled trial. *Ann Intern Med*. 1995;123:897-903.
514. Davis GL, Esteban-Muir R, Rustgi VK, et al. Interferon alfa-2b alone or in combination with ribavirin for the treatment of relapse of chronic hepatitis C. *N Engl J Med*. 1998;339:1493-1499.
515. McHutchison JG, Gordon SC, Schiff ER, et al. Interferon alfa-2b alone or in combination with ribavirin as initial treatment for chronic hepatitis C. *N Engl J Med*. 1998;339:1485-1492.
516. Poynard T, Marcellin P, Lee SS, et al. Randomised trial of interferon α2b plus ribavirin for 48 weeks or for 24 weeks versus interferon α2b plus placebo for 48 weeks for treatment of chronic infection with hepatitis C virus. *Lancet*. 1998;352:1426-1432.
517. National Institutes of Health Consensus Development Conference Statement: Management of hepatitis C: 2002 (June 10-12, 2002). *Hepatology*. 2002;36:S3-S20.
518. Hadziyannis SJ, Sette H Jr, Morgan TR, et al. Peginterferon-alpha2a and ribavirin combination therapy in chronic hepatitis C: a randomized study of treatment duration and ribavirin dose. *Ann Intern Med*. 2004;140:346-355.
519. Shiffman ML, Suter F, Bacon BR, et al. Peginterferon alfa-2a and ribavirin for 16 or 24 weeks in HCV genotype 2 or 3. *N Engl J Med*. 2007;357:124-134.
520. Reddy KR, Hoofnagle JH, Tong MJ, et al. Racial differences in responses to therapy with interferon in chronic hepatitis C. *Hepatology*. 1999;30:787-793.
521. Theodore D, Shiffman ML, Sterling RK, et al. Intensive interferon therapy does not increase virological response rates in African Americans with chronic hepatitis C. *Dig Dis Sci*. 2003;48:140-145.
522. Manesis EK, Moschos M, Brouzas D, et al. Neurovisual impairment: a frequent complication of alpha-interferon treatment in chronic viral hepatitis. *Hepatology*. 1998;27:1421-1427.
523. Sulkowski MS. Anemia in the treatment of hepatitis C virus infection. *Clin Infect Dis*. 2003;37(Suppl 4):S315-S322.
524. Wright TL. Treatment of patients with hepatitis C and cirrhosis. *Hepatology*. 2002;36:S185-S194.
525. Edlin BR. Prevention and treatment of hepatitis C in injection drug users. *Hepatology*. 2002;36:S210-S219.
526. Jonas MM. Children with hepatitis C. *Hepatology*. 2002;36:S173-S178.
527. Sylvestre DL. Approaching treatment for hepatitis C virus infection in substance users. *Clin Infect Dis*. 2005;41(Suppl 1):S79-S82.
528. Muir AJ, Bornstein JD, Killenberg PG. Peginterferon alfa-2b and ribavirin for the treatment of chronic hepatitis C in blacks and non-Hispanic whites. *N Engl J Med*. 2004;350:2265-2271.
529. Romero-Gomez M, Del Mar Viloria M, Andrade RJ, et al. Insulin resistance impairs sustained response rate to peginterferon plus ribavirin in chronic hepatitis C patients. *Gastroenterology*. 2005;128:636-641.
530. Jensen DM, Morgan TR, Marcellin P, et al. Early identification of HCV genotype 1 patients responding to 24 weeks peginterferon alpha-2a (40 kd)/ribavirin therapy. *Hepatology*. 2006;43:954-960.
531. Yu ML, Dai CY, Huang JF, et al. Rapid virological response and treatment duration for chronic hepatitis C genotype 1 patients: a randomized trial. *Hepatology*. 2008;47:1884-1893.

532. Ferenci P, Laferl H, Scherzer TM, et al. Peginterferon alfa-2a and ribavirin for 24 weeks in hepatitis C type 1 and 4 patients with rapid virological response. *Gastroenterology*. 2008;135:451-458.
533. Davis GL. Monitoring of viral levels during therapy of hepatitis C. *Hepatology*. 2002;36:S145-S151.
534. Berg T, Von Wagner M, Nasser S, et al. Extended treatment duration for hepatitis C virus type 1: comparing 48 versus 72 weeks of peginterferon-alfa-2a plus ribavirin. *Gastroenterology*. 2006;130:1086-1097.
535. Vogel W, Graziadei I, Umlauft F, et al. High-dose interferon-α_{2b} treatment prevents chronicity in acute hepatitis C—A pilot study. *Dig Dis Sci*. 1996;41:81S-85S.
536. Gursoy M, Gur G, Arslan H, et al. Interferon therapy in haemodialysis patients with acute hepatitis C virus infection and factors that predict response to treatment. *J Viral Hepat*. 2001;8:70-77.
537. Jaeckel E, Cornberg M, Wedemeyer H, et al. Treatment of acute hepatitis C with interferon alfa-2b. *N Engl J Med*. 2001;345:1452-1457.
538. Gerlach JT, Diepolder HM, Zachoval R, et al. Acute hepatitis C: high rate of both spontaneous and treatment-induced viral clearance. *Gastroenterology*. 2003;125:80-88.
539. Kamal SM, Fouly AE, Kamel RR, et al. Peginterferon alfa-2b therapy in acute hepatitis C: impact of onset of therapy on sustained virologic response. *Gastroenterology*. 2006;130: 632-638.
540. Nomura H, Sou S, Tanimoto H, et al. Short-term interferon-alfa therapy for acute hepatitis C: a randomized controlled trial. *Hepatology*. 2004;39:1213-1219.
541. Shiffman ML. Retreatment of patients with chronic hepatitis C. *Hepatology*. 2002;36:S128-S134.
542. Cheng SJ, Bonis PA, Lau J, et al. Interferon and ribavirin for patients with chronic hepatitis C who did not respond to previous interferon therapy: a meta-analysis of controlled and uncontrolled trials. *Hepatology*. 2001;33:231-240.
543. Cummings KJ, Lee SM, West ES, et al. Interferon and ribavirin vs interferon alone in the re-treatment of chronic hepatitis C previously nonresponsive to interferon: a meta-analysis of randomized trials. *JAMA*. 2001;285:193-199.
544. Shiffman ML, Di Bisceglie AM, Lindsay KL, et al. Peginterferon alfa-2a and ribavirin in patients with chronic hepatitis C who have failed prior treatment. *Gastroenterology*. 2004;126:1015-1023.
545. Lamarre D, Anderson PC, Bailey M, et al. An NS3 protease inhibitor with antiviral effects in humans infected with hepatitis C virus. *Nature*. 2003;426:186-189.
546. Paeshuyse J, Kaul A, De Clercq E, et al. The non-immunosuppressive cyclosporin DEBIO-025 is a potent inhibitor of hepatitis C virus replication in vitro. *Hepatology*. 2006;43: 761-770.
547. Nakagawa M, Sakamoto N, Tanabe Y, et al. Suppression of hepatitis C virus replication by cyclosporin A is mediated by blockade of cyclophilins. *Gastroenterology*. 2005;129: 1031-1041.
548. Horsmans Y, Berg T, Desager JP, et al. Isatoribine, an agonist of TLR7, reduces plasma virus concentration in chronic hepatitis C infection. *Hepatology*. 2005;42:724-731.
549. Forestier N, Reesink HW, Weegink CJ, et al. Antiviral activity of telaprevir (VX-950) and peginterferon alfa-2a in patients with hepatitis C. *Hepatology*. 2007;46:640-648.
550. Sarrazin C, Rouzier R, Wagner F, et al. SCH 503034, a novel hepatitis C virus pro-tease inhibitor, plus pegylated interferon alpha-2b for genotype 1 nonresponders. *Gastroenterology*. 2007;132:1270-1278.
551. Sarrazin NM, Howe AY, Gao T, et al. HCV796: a selective nonstructural protein 5B polymerase inhibitor with potent antihepatitis C virus activity in vitro, in mice with chimeric human livers, and in humans infected with hepatitis C virus. *Hepatology*. 2009;49:745-752.
552. Zhou Y, Muh U, Hanzelka BL, et al. Phenotypic and structural analyses of hepatitis C virus NS3 protease Arg155 variants: sensitivity to telaprevir (VX-950) and interferon alpha. *J Biol Chem*. 2007;282:22619-22628.
553. Sarrazin C, Kieffer TL, Bartels D, et al. Dynamic hepatitis C virus genotypic and phenotypic changes in patients treated with the protease inhibitor telaprevir. *Gastroenterology*. 2007;132: 1767-1777.
554. Kuntzen T, Timm J, Berical A, et al. Naturally occurring dominant resistance mutations to hepatitis C virus protease and polymerase inhibitors in treatment-naive patients. *Hepatology*. 2008;48:1769-1778.
555. Bartels DJ, Zhou Y, Zhang EZ, et al. Natural prevalence of hepatitis C virus variants with decreased sensitivity to NS3.4A protease inhibitors in treatment-naive subjects. *J Infect Dis*. 2008;198:800-807.
556. Blajchman MA, Bull SB, Feinman SV. Post-transfusion hepatitis: impact of non-A, non-B hepatitis surrogate tests. *Lancet*. 1995;345:21-25.
557. Hagan H, Jarlais DCD, Friedman SR, et al. Reduced risk of hepatitis B and hepatitis C among injection drug users in the Tacoma syringe exchange program. *Am J Public Health*. 1995;85:1531-1537.
558. Farci P, Alter HJ, Govindarajan S, et al. Lack of protective immunity against reinfection with hepatitis C virus. *Science*. 1992;258:135-140.
559. Major ME, Mihalik K, Puig M, et al. Previously infected and recovered chimpanzees exhibit rapid responses that control hepatitis C virus replication upon rechallenge. *J Virol*. 2002;76:6586-6595.
560. Weiner AJ, Paliard X, Selby MJ, et al. Intrahepatic genetic inoculation of hepatitis C virus RNA confers cross-protective immunity. *J Virol*. 2001;75:7142-7148.
561. Forns X, Payette PJ, Ma X, et al. Vaccination of chimpanzees with plasmid DNA encoding the hepatitis C virus (HCV) envelope E2 protein modified the infection after challenge with homologous monoclonal HCV. *Hepatology*. 2000;32:618-625.
562. Choo QL, Kuo G, Ralston R, et al. Vaccination of chimpanzees against infection by the hepatitis C virus. *Proc Natl Acad Sci U S A*. 1994;91:1294-1298.
563. Lanford RE, Guerra B, Chavez D, et al. Cross-genotype immunity to hepatitis C virus. *J Virol*. 2004;78:1575-1581.
564. Seeff LB, Zimmerman JH, Wright EL, et al. A randomized double-blind controlled trial of the efficacy of immune serum globulin for the prevention of post-transfusion hepatitis. A Veterans Administration Cooperative Study. *Gastroenterology*. 1977;72:111-121.
565. Sanchez-Quijano A, Pineda JA, Lissen E, et al. Prevention of post-transfusion non-A, non-B hepatitis by nonspecific immunoglobulin in heart surgery patients. *Lancet*. 1988;i:1245-1249.
566. Bica I, McGovern B, Dhar R, et al. Increasing mortality due to end-stage liver disease in patients with human immunodeficiency virus infection. *Clin Infect Dis*. 2001;32:492-497.
567. Rosenthal E, Pialoux G, Bernard N, et al. Liver-related mortality in human-immunodeficiency-virus-infected patients between 1995 and 2003 in the French GERMIVIC Joint Study Group Network (MORTAVIC 2003 Study). *J Viral Hepat*. 2007;14:183-188.
568. Weber R, Sabin CA, Friis-Moller N, et al. Liver-related deaths in persons infected with the human immunodeficiency virus: the D:A:D study. *Arch Intern Med*. 2006;166:1632-1641.
569. Lohse N, Hansen AB, Pedersen G, et al. Survival of persons with and without HIV infection in Denmark, 1995-2005. *Ann Intern Med*. 2007;146:87-95.
570. Sackoff JE, Hanna DB, Pfeiffer MR, et al. Causes of death among persons with AIDS in the era of highly active antiretroviral therapy: New York City. *Ann Intern Med*. 2006;145:397-406.
571. Sherman KE, Rouster SD, Chung RT, et al. Hepatitis C virus prevalence among patients infected with human immunodeficiency virus: a cross-sectional analysis of the US adult AIDS Clinical Trials Group. *Clin Infect Dis*. 2002;34:831-837.
572. Alberti A, Clumeck N, Collins S, et al. Short statement of the first European consensus conference on the treatment of chronic hepatitis B and C in HIV co-infected patients. *J Hepatol*. 2005;42:615-624.
573. Sulkowski MS, Thomas DL. Hepatitis C in the HIV-infected person. *Ann Intern Med*. 2003;138:197-207.
574. Luetkemeyer A, Hare CB, Stansell J, et al. Clinical presentation and course of acute hepatitis C infection in HIV-infected patients. *J Acquir Immune Defic Syndr*. 2006;41:31-36.
575. Danta M, Brown D, Bhagani S, et al. Recent epidemic of acute hepatitis C virus in HIV-positive men who have sex with men linked to high-risk sexual behaviours. *AIDS*. 2007;21:983-991.
576. Fierer DS, Uriel AJ, Carriero DC, et al. Liver fibrosis during an outbreak of acute hepatitis C virus infection in HIV-infected men: a prospective cohort study. *J Infect Dis*. 2008; 198:683-686.
577. Darby SC, Ewart DW, Giangrande PL, et al. Mortality from liver cancer and liver disease in haemophilic men and boys in UK given blood products contaminated with hepatitis C. *Lancet*. 1997;350:1425-1431.
578. Soto B, Sánchez-Quijano A, Rodrigo L, et al. Human immunodeficiency virus infection modifies the natural history of chronic parenterally-acquired hepatitis C with an unusually rapid progression to cirrhosis. *J Hepatol*. 1997;26:1-5.
579. Garcia-Samaniego J, Rodriguez M, Berenguer J, et al. Hepatocellular carcinoma in HIV-infected patients with chronic hepatitis C. *Am J Gastroenterol*. 2001;96:179-183.
580. Kim WR, Gross JB, Poterucha JJ, et al. Outcome of hospital care of liver disease associated with hepatitis C in the United States. *Hepatology*. 2001;33:201-206.
581. Benhamou Y, Bochet M, Di Martino V, et al. Liver fibrosis progression in human immunodeficiency virus and hepatitis C virus coinfected patients. The MULTIVIRC Group. *Hepatology*. 1999;30:1054-1058.
582. Monga HK, Rodriguez-Barradas MC, Breaux K, et al. Hepatitis C virus infection–related morbidity and mortality among patients with human immunodeficiency virus infection. *Clin Infect Dis*. 2001;33:240-247.
583. Di Martino V, Rufat P, Boyer N, et al. The influence of human immunodeficiency virus coinfection on chronic hepatitis C in injection drug users: a long-term retrospective cohort study. *Hepatology*. 2001;34:1193-1199.
584. Goedert JJ, Eyster ME, Lederman MM, et al. End-stage liver disease in persons with hemophilia and transfusion-associated infections. *Blood*. 2002;100:1584-1589.
585. Graham CS, Baden LR, Yu E, et al. Influence of human immunodeficiency virus infection on the course of hepatitis C virus infection: a meta-analysis. *Clin Infect Dis*. 2001;33:562-569.
586. Greub G, Ledergerber B, Battegay M, et al. Clinical progression, survival, and immune recovery during antiretroviral therapy in patients with HIV-1 and hepatitis C virus coinfection: the Swiss HIV Cohort Study. *Lancet*. 2000;356:1800-1805.
587. Sulkowski MS, Moore RD, Mehta SH, et al. Hepatitis C and progression of HIV disease. *JAMA*. 2002;288:199-206.
588. Chung RT, Evans SR, Yang Y, et al. Immune recovery is associated with persistent rise in hepatitis C virus RNA, infrequent liver test flares, and is not impaired by hepatitis C virus in co-infected subjects. *AIDS*. 2002;16:1915-1923.
589. Martinez E, Blanco JL, Arnaiz JA, et al. Hepatotoxicity in HIV-1-infected patients receiving nevirapine-containing antiretroviral therapy. *AIDS*. 2001;15:1261-1268.
590. Sulkowski MS, Thomas DL, Chaisson RE, et al. Hepatotoxicity associated with antiretroviral therapy in adults infected with human immunodeficiency virus and the role of hepatitis C or B virus infection. *JAMA*. 2000;283:74-80.
591. den Brinker M, Wit FW, Wertheim-van Dillen PM, et al. Hepatitis B and C virus co-infection and the risk for hepatotoxicity of highly active antiretroviral therapy in HIV-1 infection. *AIDS*. 2000;14:2895-2902.
592. Cattelan AM, Erne E, Salatino A, et al. Severe hepatic failure related to nevirapine treatment. *Clin Infect Dis*. 1999;29:455-456.
593. Labarga P, Soriano V, Vispo ME, et al. Hepatotoxicity of antiretroviral drugs is reduced after successful treatment of chronic hepatitis C in HIV-infected patients. *J Infect Dis*. 2007;196:670-676.
594. Brau N, Salvatore M, Rios-Bedoya CF, et al. Slower fibrosis progression in HIV/HCV-coinfected patients with successful HIV suppression using antiretroviral therapy. *J Hepatol*. 2006;44:47-55.
595. Qurishi N, Kreuzberg C, Rockstroh JK, et al. Effect of antiretroviral therapy on liver-related mortality in patients with HIV and hepatitis C coinfection. *Lancet*. 2004;362:1708-1713.
596. Sulkowski MS, Mehta SH, Torbenson MS, et al. Rapid fibrosis progression among HIV/hepatitis C virus–co-infected adults. *AIDS*. 2007;21:2209-2216.
597. Kim AY, Lauer GM, Ouchi K, et al. The magnitude and breadth of hepatitis C virus–specific $CD8^+$ T cells depend on absolute $CD4^+$ T-cell count in individuals coinfected with HIV-1. *Blood*. 2005;105:1170-1178.
598. Netski DM, Mosbruger T, Astemborski J, et al. $CD4^+$ T cell–dependent reduction in hepatitis C virus–specific humoral immune responses after HIV infection. *J Infect Dis*. 2007;195:857-863.
599. Lin W, Weinberg EM, Tai AW, et al. HIV increases HCV replication in a TGF-beta1–dependent manner. *Gastroenterology*. 2008;134:803-811.
600. Balasubramanian A, Ganju RK, Groopman JE. Signal transducer and activator of transcription factor 1 mediates apoptosis induced by hepatitis C virus and HIV envelope proteins in hepatocytes. *J Infect Dis*. 2006;194:670-681.
601. Munshi N, Balasubramanian A, Koziel M, et al. Hepatitis C and human immunodeficiency virus envelope proteins cooperatively induce hepatocytic apoptosis via an innocent bystander mechanism. *J Infect Dis*. 2003;188:1192-1204.
602. Brenchley JM, Price DA, Schacker TW, et al. Microbial translocation is a cause of systemic immune activation in chronic HIV infection. *Nat Med*. 2006;12:1365-1371.
603. Balagopal A, Philp FH, Astemborski J, et al. Human immunodeficiency virus–related microbial translocation and progression of hepatitis C. *Gastroenterology*. 2008;135:226-233.
604. Veronese L, Rautaureau J, Sadler BM, et al. Single-dose pharmacokinetics of amprenavir, a human immunodeficiency virus type 1 protease inhibitor, in subjects with normal or impaired hepatic function. *Antimicrob Agents Chemother*. 2000;44: 821-826.
605. John M, Flexman J, French MAH. Hepatitis C virus–associated hepatitis following treatment of HIV-infected patients with HIV protease inhibitors: an immune restoration disease? *AIDS*. 1998;12:2289-2293.
606. Barbaro G, Di Lorenzo G, Asti A, et al. Hepatocellular mitochondrial alterations in patients with chronic hepatitis C: ultrastructural and biochemical findings. *Am J Gastroenterol*. 1999;94:2198-2205.
607. Soriano V, Sulkowski M, Bergin C, et al. Care of patients with chronic hepatitis C and HIV co-infection: recommendations from the HIV-HCV International Panel. *AIDS*. 2002; 16:813-828.
608. Contreras AM, Hiasa Y, He W, et al. Viral RNA mutations are region specific and increased by ribavirin in a full-length hepatitis C virus replication system. *J Virol*. 2002;76:8505-8517.
609. Ragni MV, Ndimbie OK, Rice EO, et al. The presence of hepatitis C virus (HCV) antibody in human immunodeficiency virus–positive hemophilic men undergoing HCV "seroreversion." *Blood*. 1993;82:1010-1015.
610. Marcellin P, Martinot-Peignoux M, Elias A, et al. Hepatitis C virus (HCV) viremia in human immunodeficiency virus-seronegative and -seropositive patients with indeterminate HCV recombinant immunoblot assay. *J Infect Dis*. 1994;170:433-435.
611. Chamot E, Hirschel B, Wintsch J, et al. Loss of antibodies against hepatitis C virus in HIV-seropositive intravenous drug users. *AIDS*. 1990;4:1275-1277.
612. George SL, Gebhardt J, Klinzman D, et al. Hepatitis C virus viremia in HIV-infected individuals with negative HCV antibody tests. *J Acquir Immune Defic Syndr*. 2002;31: 154-162.
613. Lefrère JJ, Guiramand S, Lefrère F, et al. Full or partial seroreversion in patients infected by hepatitis C virus. *J Infect Dis*. 1997;175:316-322.

614. Thio CL, Nolt KR, Astemborski J, et al. Screening for hepatitis C virus in human immunodeficiency virus–infected individuals. *J Clin Microbiol.* 2000;38:575-577.

615. Carrat F, Bani-Sadr F, Pol S, et al. Pegylated interferon alfa-2b vs standard interferon alfa-2b, plus ribavirin, for chronic hepatitis C in HIV-infected patients: a randomized controlled trial. *JAMA.* 2004;292:2839-2848.

616. Torriani FJ, Rodriguez-Torres M, Rockstroh JK, et al. Peginterferon alfa-2a plus ribavirin for chronic hepatitis C virus infection in HIV-infected patients. *N Engl J Med.* 2004;351:438-450.

617. Chung RT, Andersen J, Volberding P, et al. Peginterferon alfa-2a plus ribavirin versus interferon alfa-2a plus ribavirin for chronic hepatitis C in HIV-coinfected persons. *N Engl J Med.* 2004;351:451-459.

618. Laguno M, Murillas J, Blanco JL, et al. Peginterferon alfa-2b plus ribavirin compared with interferon alfa-2b plus ribavirin for treatment of HIV/HCV co-infected patients. *AIDS.* 2004;18:F27-F36.

619. Alvarez D, Dieterich DT, Brau N, et al. Zidovudine use but not weight-based ribavirin dosing impacts anaemia during HCV treatment in HIV-infected persons. *J Viral Hepat.* 2006;13:683-689.

620. Lafeuillade A, Hittinger G, Chadapaud S. Increased mitochondrial toxicity with ribavirin in HIV/HCV coinfection. *Lancet.* 2001;357:280-281.

621. Mauss S, Valenti W, Depamphilis J, et al. Risk factors for hepatic decompensation in patients with HIV/HCV coinfection and liver cirrhosis during interferon-based therapy. *AIDS.* 2004;18:F21-F25.

622. Neff GW, Bonham A, Tzakis AG, et al. Orthotopic liver transplantation in patients with human immunodeficiency virus and end-stage liver disease. *Liver Transpl.* 2003;9:239-247.

623. Roland ME, Havlir DV. Responding to organ failure in HIV-infected patients. *N Engl J Med.* 2003;348:2279-2281.

155

Coronaviruses, Including Severe Acute Respiratory Syndrome (SARS)–Associated Coronavirus

KENNETH McINTOSH | STANLEY PERLMAN

The family Coronaviridae contains two genera, the *Coronaviruses* and the *Toroviruses*. The two genera appear similar on electron microscopy, and they share similar strategies of replication (along with the other members of the order *Nidovirales*, including *Arterivirus*). They differ, however, in the size of their RNA genome and structural proteins, as well as the morphology of their nucleocapsids. Coronaviruses (CoVs) are primarily respiratory pathogens in humans and were until recently considered to cause upper respiratory tract illness and probably also some undetermined fraction of viral diarrhea. During the winter of 2002 to 2003, an alarming new disease appeared, severe acute respiratory syndrome, or SARS, and was quickly attributed to a new CoV, the SARS CoV. The outbreak originated in southern Peoples Republic of China, probably following transmission from a small mammal such as the palm civet (*Paguma larvata*) or raccoon dog (*Nyctereutes procyonoides*) to humans. These animals, kept in cages and slaughtered in market settings for exotic food, were probably themselves intermediate hosts for a virus originating in Chinese horseshoe bats.[1,2] Consistent with this, SARS CoV isolated from palm civets showed evidence of rapid adaptation to this intermediate host.[3] In retrospect, the emergence of SARS is consistent with what is known about CoVs as a group: they are important pathogens in animals causing a wide variety of diseases through a wide variety of pathogenic mechanisms, and they have been noted to mutate frequently and infect new species.[4] Toroviruses are, at least as currently known, exclusively enteric pathogens, both in animals and in humans.

History

RESPIRATORY CORONAVIRUSES AND SEVERE ACUTE RESPIRATORY SYNDROME

In 1965, Tyrrell and Bynoe[5] cultured a virus obtained from the respiratory tract of a boy with a common cold by passage in human embryonic tracheal organ cultures. The medium from these cultures consistently produced colds in volunteers. The agent was ether sensitive but not related to any known human virus. Subsequently, electron microscopy of fluids from infected organ cultures revealed particles that resembled infectious bronchitis virus of chickens.[6] At about the same time, Hamre and Procknow[7] recovered a cytopathic agent in tissue culture from medical students with colds. The prototype virus was named 229E and was found on electron microscopy to have a similar or identical morphology (Fig. 155-1).[6]

Using techniques similar to those used by Tyrrell and Bynoe, McIntosh and colleagues[8] reported the recovery of several infectious bronchitis-like agents from the human respiratory tract, the prototype of which was named OC43 (OC for organ culture). At much the same time, mouse hepatitis virus and transmissible gastroenteritis virus of swine were shown to have the same morphology on electron microscopy.[9,10] Very shortly thereafter, the name *coronavirus* (the prefix *corona* denoting the crownlike appearance of the surface projections) was chosen to signify this new genus.[11]

The number of animal CoVs quickly grew, including viruses causing diseases in rats, mice, chickens, turkeys, cattle, wild ruminants, dogs, cats, rabbits, and pigs, with manifestations in the respiratory and gastrointestinal tracts, central nervous system, liver, reproductive tract, and others. Through sequencing and antigenicity studies, the animal and human CoVs (HCoVs) were divided into three groups: group 1, which contained HCoV-229E as well as numerous animal viruses; group 2, which contained HCoV-OC43 plus the closely related animal viruses bovine CoV and mouse hepatitis virus; and group 3, which included only avian viruses related to infectious bronchitis virus (Fig. 155-2).

SARS was first identified in Guangdong Province of the Peoples Republic of China in November 2002[12] and spread from there first to Hong Kong, then to countries in Southeast Asia, to Europe, to North America, and finally throughout the world. A CoV was independently and almost simultaneously isolated from SARS patients by several laboratories and found by sequencing to be only distantly related to all previously characterized human or animal CoVs.[13-17] The SARS outbreak stimulated a rapid and intense public health response coordinated by the World Health Organization, and by July 2003, transmission had ceased throughout the world. Despite this heroic effort, however, there were more than 8000 cases, and more than 750 deaths were reported.[18] SARS CoV is considered to belong to CoV group 2, although it, along with the animal and bat viruses most closely related, is now labeled a group 2b virus, with the other group 2 viruses, including HCoV-OC43, in group 2a (see Fig. 155-2).[19]

With the emergence of SARS and the identification of the SARS CoV, the HCoV field became suddenly much more active. Sensitive molecular methods were developed to detect viruses identical or very closely related to HCoV-229E and HCoV-OC43 in the respiratory tract, and two new species were discovered, NL63 and HKU1.[20-22] HCoV-NL63 was found independently by three groups, two in the Netherlands and, somewhat later, the third in New Haven, Connecticut.[23] In all three cases, positive samples were from infants and children with respiratory disease. HCoV-HKU1 was found in Hong Kong in an adult with respiratory disease. These two new HCoV strains subsequently have been found worldwide and appear to have pathogenicity similar to that of HCoV-229E and HCoV-OC43, with the possible exception that NL63 is more frequently found in children with croup.[24,25]

GASTROINTESTINAL CORONAVIRUSES AND TOROVIRUSES

In view of the prominence of CoVs in animal enteric diseases, it is not surprising that CoV-like particles (CoVLPs) have also been described in human fecal matter. During the past 15 to 20 years, reports of such particles have been numerous, but these particles have been difficult to characterize further, in part, because they are difficult to grow in vitro.

Toroviruses were, like CoVs, first described in animals. They were first detected in the feces of cattle (Breda virus) and horses (Berne virus).[26,27] Shortly thereafter, Beards and colleagues[28] examined human fecal material and reported finding particles with a similar appearance that aggregated in the presence of antiserum to the bovine and equine viruses. Neither the human nor the bovine viruses grow in tissue culture.

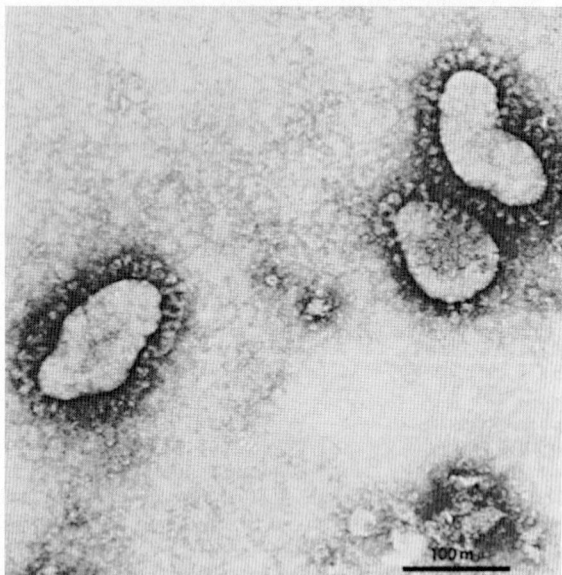

Figure 155-1 Coronavirus, strain HCoV-229E, harvested from infected WI-38 cells (phosphotungstic acid stain). *(From McIntosh K, Dees JH, Becker WB, et al. Recovery in tracheal organ cultures of novel viruses from patients with respiratory disease.* Proc Natl Acad Sci U S A. *1967;57:933-940.)*

Description of the Pathogens

CORONAVIRUSES

The CoV nucleic acid is RNA, approximately 30 kilobases in length, of positive sense, single stranded, polyadenylated, and infectious. The RNA, the largest known viral RNA (Fig. 155-3), codes for (in order from the 5′ end) a large polyprotein that is cleaved by virus-encoded proteases to form several nonstructural proteins including an RNA-dependent RNA polymerase and an adenosine triphosphatase helicase, followed by either four or five structural proteins intermingled with a variable number of nonstructural and minor structural proteins.[29] The first of the major structural proteins is a surface hemagglutinin-esterase protein, present on HCoVs OC43 and HKU1 and some group 2 animal CoVs, that may play some role in the attachment and/or release of the particle at the cell surface. This gene contains sequences similar to the hemagglutinin of influenza C virus, likely evidence of an interfamily recombinational event that occurred many years ago. The next gene encodes the surface glycoprotein that forms the petal-shaped surface projections and is responsible for attachment and the stimulation of neutralizing antibody. This is followed by a small envelope protein, a membrane glycoprotein, and a nucleocapsid protein that is complexed with the RNA. There are several other open reading frames whose coding functions are not clear. The strategy of replication of CoVs is similar to that of other nidoviruses, in that all messenger RNAs form a nested set with common polyadenylated 3′ ends, with only the unique portion of the 5′ end being translated.[4] As in other RNA viruses, mutations are common in nature, largely because the RNA-dependent RNA polymerase lacks proofreading capabilities. CoVs are also capable of genetic recombination if two viruses infect the same cell at the same time.

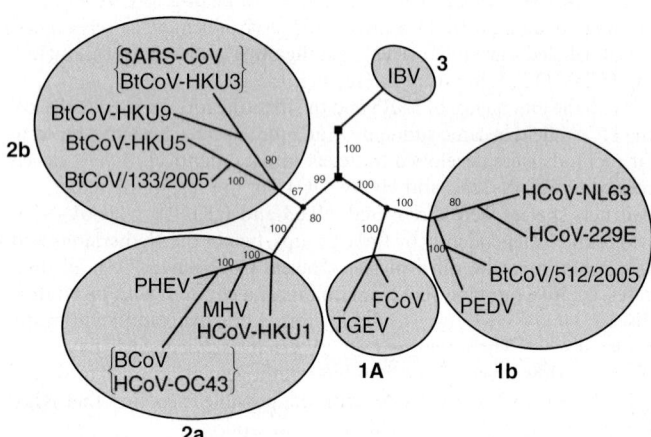

Figure 155-2 Coronavirus phylogeny. A tree showing evolutionary relationship between coronaviruses in different groups. Human coronaviruses are indicated in red. The unrooted maximum parsimonious tree was inferred by using multiple nucleotide alignments of the RNA-dependent RNA polymerase-helicase region of the indicated coronaviruses, using PAUPP* v.4.0b10 software. The viruses that were analyzed were HCoV-NL-63, 229E, HKU-1, OC43, SARS-CoV, porcine epidemic diarrhea virus (PEDV), bat coronaviruses (BtCoV) HKU3, HKU5, HKU9, 133, and 512, feline coronavirus (FCoV), transmissible gastroenteritis virus (TGEV), mouse hepatitis virus (MHV), bovine coronavirus (BCoV), porcine hemagglutinating encephalomyelitis virus (PHEV), and infectious bronchitis virus (IBV). BCoV and HCoV-OC43 are very closely related and are indicated on the same branch of this phylogenetic tree. *(Modified from Gorbalenya AE. Genomics and evolution of the nidovirales. In: Perlman S, Gallagher TM, Snijder EJ, eds. Nidoviruses. Washington, DC: ASM Press; 2008:15-28, Figure 2, with permission from ASM Press.)*

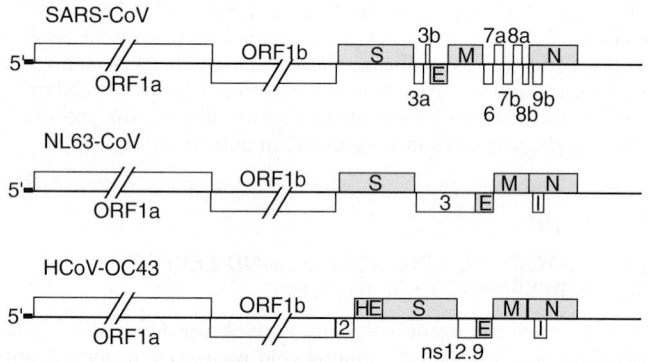

Figure 155-3 Genome organization of representative human coronaviruses. All coronavirus genomes have the same basic structure and mechanism of replication.[4] The 5′ end of each genome encodes a leader sequence, which is attached to each virus-specific messenger RNA transcript by a novel mechanism of discontinuous replication. The first two thirds of each genome encode replicase-associated genes. Gene 1 is translated as two large polyproteins, with the first expressed from ORF1a and the second from ORF1a/b following a −1 frameshift event. These polyproteins are then cleaved into individual proteins by two virus-encoded proteases. The major structural genes, the hemagglutinin-esterase (HE), surface (S), envelope (E), transmembrane (M), and nucleocapsid (N) proteins, are indicated in green. The nonreplicase, accessory genes located at the 3′ end of the genome are indicated with open boxes. The functions of these proteins are largely not known, and there is no sequence homology between accessory proteins of different coronaviruses. Some of these proteins are virion associated, but none are required for virus replication. The open reading frames encoding these proteins are numbered in order of appearance from the 5′ end of the genome, with the exception of ns12.9 of HCoV-OC43. I is an internal protein expressed from an alternative reading frame located within the N gene. It is equivalent to SARS CoV–specific protein 9b. ORF, open reading frame.

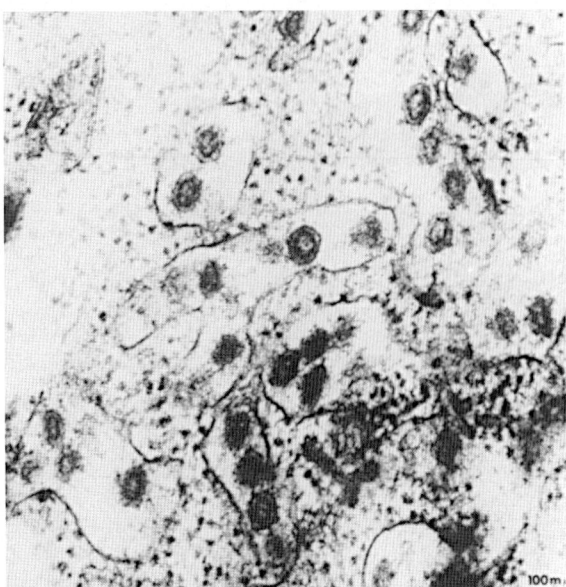

Figure 155-4   Coronavirus strain 229E in WI-38 cells. *(From Becker WB, McIntosh K, Dees JH, et al. Morphogenesis of avian infectious bronchitis virus and a related human virus (strain 229E). J Virol. 1967;1(5):1019-1027.)*

All CoVs develop exclusively in the cytoplasm of infected cells (Fig. 155-4). They bud into cytoplasmic vesicles from membranes of the pre-Golgi endoplasmic reticulum. These virus-filled vesicles are then extruded by the exocytic secretory pathway.[30] The resultant virus particles have a diameter of 70 to 80 nm on thin-section electron microscopy, and 60 to 220 nm on negative staining, and are pleomorphic, with widely spaced, petal-shaped projections 20 nm long (see Fig 155-1).

The cellular receptor for 229E and most other group 1 CoVs is aminopeptidase N.[31] Interestingly, NL63, the other known group 1 HCoV, uses as its cellular receptor angiotensin-converting enzyme II,[32] the same receptor as is used by the SARS CoV.[33] Mouse hepatitis virus, a group 2 CoV related to strain OC43, uses as its receptor a member of the carcinoembryonic antigen family.[34] HCoV-OC43 itself may use one of several cell surface molecules, including 9-O-acetylated neuraminic acid and the HLA-I molecule.[35]

All the respiratory HCoVs grow only with difficulty in tissue culture. Despite this, several of them, including 229E, NL63, and the SARS CoV, were discovered because they produced a detectable cytopathic effect, the first in human embryonic kidney,[7] the second in LLC-MK2,[20] and the third in Vero E6 cells.[14] HCoVs OC43 and HKU-1 have only been grown in tissue culture after laboratory adaptation.[36,37] Detection of all these viruses in clinical specimens is most conveniently and sensitively achieved using the polymerase chain reaction.

Likewise, the enteric CoVs have been difficult to cultivate in vitro. All but a few strains have been detected only by electron microscopy of human fecal material.[38-42] Some strains have been characterized by immune electron microscopy and found to be related to HCoV-OC43.[43] Two strains obtained from an outbreak of necrotizing enterocolitis in Texas and passaged in intestinal organ cultures were reported to contain four or five proteins with apparent molecular weights similar to those of other CoVs but not related antigenically to known strains.[44] The evidence favors the view that these isolates, as well as particles antigenically related to HCoV-OC43, are members of the family Coronaviridae, although their association with human disease is not yet proven. Other less well studied strains, called, for lack of a better name, CoVLPs, may also be CoVs, but the evidence is less compelling.

TOROVIRUSES

Toroviruses have a morphology, a genome organization, and a strategy of replication similar to those of CoVs.[19] They are membrane-coated viruses that are somewhat smaller and more pleomorphic than enteric CoVs (100-120 nm in their largest diameter), and their club-shaped surface projections are somewhat less distinct.[45,46] The nucleic acid–containing core of the virus assumes a doughnut shape (i.e., a torus) if viewed from a certain angle by electron microscopy.[27,46,47] The Berne virus was first isolated from horses with diarrhea in the 1970s and grows in equine cell tissue culture. The human toroviruses, like the bovine toroviruses, do not grow in tissue culture.

The surface glycoproteins on the surface of toroviruses have no significant sequence homology with the surface proteins of CoVs.[48] A second surface protein with hemagglutinin-esterase activity and sequence homology to the hemagglutinin-esterase proteins of both influenza C virus and mouse hepatitis virus has been found on the bovine Breda virus, but not on the equine Berne virus.[49] It is not known whether this molecule exists on human toroviruses, although human toroviruses do hemagglutinate rabbit erythrocytes.[46] There is also more than 90% identity in the 3′ end of the genome between human and animal toroviruses.[46,48] The toroviruses, like CoVs, contain membrane and nucleoproteins, but there is no significant sequence homology in the respective genes between the toroviruses and CoVs. In contrast, the toroviral replicase contains a sequence similar to that of CoVs, and the strategy of replication is similar, although not identical.[48,50]

Epidemiology

RESPIRATORY CORONAVIRUSES

Evidence of respiratory CoV infections has been found wherever in the world it has been sought. In temperate climates, respiratory CoV infections occur more often in the winter and spring than in the summer and fall. The contribution of CoV infections to the total number of upper respiratory illnesses may be as high as 35% during times of peak viral activity. Overall, the proportion of adult colds produced by CoVs may be reasonably estimated at 15%.

Early studies of HCoV-OC43 and 229E in the United States demonstrated periodicity, with large epidemics occurring at 2- to 3-year intervals.[51] Strain HCoV-229E tended to be epidemic throughout the United States, whereas strain HCoV-OC43 appeared in localized outbreaks. Similar studies of NL63 and HKU1 have not been done, but it seems from the available data that they also vary widely in incidence from year to year and place to place. Reinfection is common and may be due to the rapid diminution of antibody levels after infection.[52] Infection occurs at all ages but is most common in children. Approximately half of persons infected (as judged by an increase in antibody titer) become ill, and virus, detected by molecular methods, is found in both symptomatic and asymptomatic individuals.

SEVERE ACUTE RESPIRATORY SYNDROME

The SARS epidemic began in Guangdong Province in the Peoples Republic of China in mid-November 2002.[12] It came to worldwide attention in March 2003 when cases of severe, acute pneumonia were reported to the World Health Organization from Hong Kong, Hanoi, and Singapore. Disease spread in hospitals to health care workers, visitors, and patients, and among family members. Occasionally spread was also noted in other settings including hotels, apartment complexes, and markets. Worldwide spread was rapid, but focal (Fig 155-5). The largest numbers of cases were reported from the Peoples Republic of China, Hong Kong, Taiwan, Singapore, and Toronto, Canada. The overall case-fatality rates in these locations ranged from 7% to 17%, but persons with underlying medical conditions and those older than 65 years of age had mortality rates as high as 50%. There was no mortality in children younger than the age of 12 years.

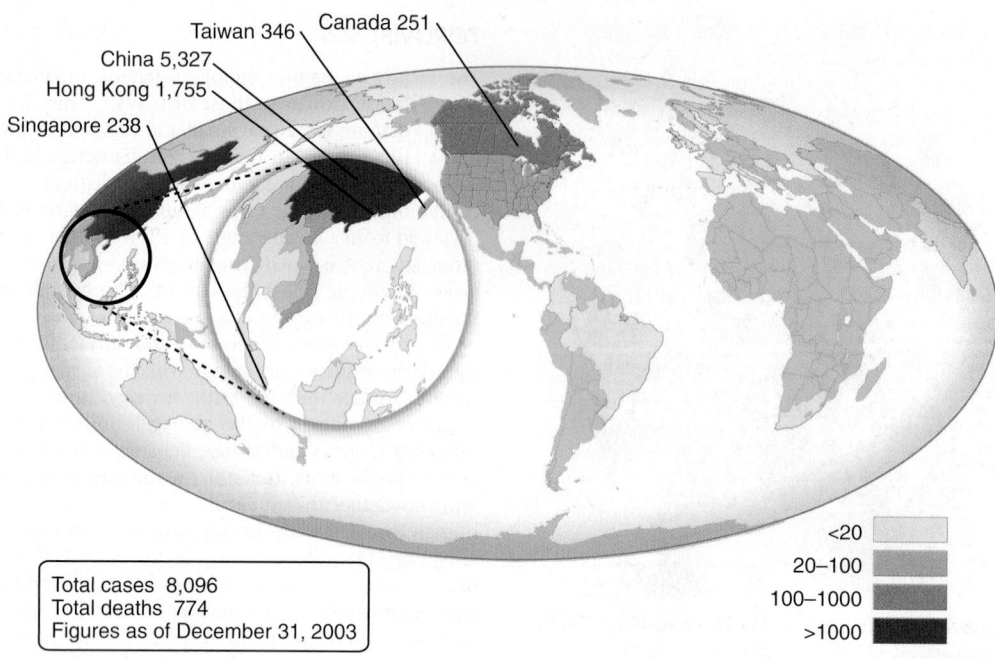

Figure 155-5 **World map of countries with severe acute respiratory syndrome and the number of cases as of December 31, 2003.** (*Source: World Health Organization.*)

In response to the global spread and associated severe disease, the World Health Organization coordinated a rapid and intense control program that included isolation of cases, careful attention to contact, droplet and airborne infection control procedures, quarantine of exposed persons in some settings, and efforts to control spread between countries through travel advisories and travel alerts. Presumably as a result of these efforts, global transmission ceased by July 2003.

A few subsequent cases of SARS have been detected, but all have been either a result of laboratory spread or individual cases related to contact with civet cats. There has been no, or very limited, human-to-human spread since the epidemic of 2002 to 2003.

Spread of SARS to humans is thought to have occurred primarily through droplet transmission and direct contact or fomite transmission. In most instances, an individual case transmitted to very few others. There were, however, several well-documented instances in which small-particle airborne transmission occurred, in one of which a single case infected 100 or more persons ("superspreading events").[53] Spread in hospital settings appeared to be surprisingly efficient, but it could be effectively suppressed with the enforcement of droplet and contact precautions.[54] On average, it was estimated that one infected person would infect approximately three others and that containment measures, including quarantine, would have a major effect on the course of the epidemic.[55,56] This proved to be the case. Containment measures were efficacious, in part, because patients were most contagious only after lower respiratory disease developed.[57] The chain of spread was finally broken in the Peoples Republic of China, the last country to experience endemic spread, in June 2003.

It now seems almost certain that the human epidemic began with the spread of SARS CoV from palm civets or other animals sold in live wild game markets to humans in Guangdong Province in the Peoples Republic of China, and that the virus adapted itself through mutation and possibly recombination, until it transmitted readily among humans. Variants of SARS CoV likely transmitted to animal handlers in the animal markets multiple times. However, the vast majority of these transmissions were abortive as evidenced by a high SARS CoV seroprevalence rate in animal handlers in these markets in the absence of SARS-like disease.[58] The virus that spread worldwide came largely from a single infected individual who traveled from Guangdong Province to Hong Kong and infected a large number of individuals in a superspreading event before succumbing to the disease. In contrast,

the virus that was epidemic in the Peoples Republic of China was more variable. The SARS CoV most likely did not originate in civets, and the prevailing consensus at present is that SARS-like viruses from horseshoe bats in southern Peoples Republic of China were the ultimate source.[2]

GASTROINTESTINAL CORONAVIRUSES

Enteric CoVs (or CoVLPs) have been most frequently associated with gastrointestinal disease in neonates and infants younger than 12 months. Particles have been found in the stools of adults with the acquired immunodeficiency syndrome.[59,60] Asymptomatic shedding is common, particularly in tropical climates[61] and in populations living in poor hygienic conditions.[62] The viruses can be detected for prolonged periods[39,41,63] and without any apparent seasonal pattern.[64]

Pathogenesis

RESPIRATORY CORONAVIRUSES

Respiratory CoVs replicate in ciliated epithelial cells of the nasopharynx, probably producing both direct degeneration of ciliated cells[65] and an outpouring of chemokines and interleukins, with a resultant common-cold symptom complex similar to that produced by rhinovirus infection.[66] The incubation period is, on average, 2 days, and the peak of respiratory symptoms, as well as viral shedding, is reached at approximately 3 or 4 days after inoculation.[67]

The pattern of virus replication of CoVs must be at least in part determined by virus-receptor interaction. The two best defined receptors for the respiratory CoVs are aminopeptidase N for strain HCoV-229E and angiotensin-converting enzyme II for NL63.

The pathogenicity of SARS is more complex and involves systemic spread. The route of infection of the SARS CoV is probably through the respiratory tract. After an incubation period that is usually 4 to 7 days, but can be as long as 10 to 14 days, the disease begins, starting usually with fever and other systemic (influenza-like) symptoms, with cough and dyspnea developing a few days to a week later.[68] Although the lung is the focus of the disease process, there are often signs of involvement in other organ systems, including diarrhea, leukopenia, thrombocytopenia, and, most notably, pan-lymphopenia.[69] Virus has been detected in respiratory secretions, blood, stool, and urine specimens and tissue from the lung and kidney. Based on polymerase chain reaction testing, virus titer is highest during the second week of illness[70] and can often be detected into the third week of illness and sometimes for as long as several months.[15,71] Pulmonary symptoms may worsen late in the course of the illness, with the development of adult respiratory distress syndrome.[70] There may also be late evidence of liver and kidney involvement.

The pulmonary pathology of infection by the SARS CoV has been described extensively,[14,72,73] but little has been published about the pathology in other organ systems.[73-75] The extrapulmonary pathologic changes found most consistently at autopsy are extensive necrosis of the white pulp of the spleen and a generalized small vessel arteritis.[73,74] In the lung, there is hyaline membrane formation, interstitial infiltration with lymphocytes and mononuclear cells, and desquamation of pneumocytes in the alveolar spaces. Giant cells are a constant finding and usually have macrophage markers. In bronchoalveolar lavage, biopsy, and autopsy specimens viral particles have been noted in type I and II pneumocytes.[18,76]

Clinical Manifestations

RESPIRATORY CORONAVIRUSES

Almost all the antigenically distinct respiratory CoV strains that were isolated in the 1960s have been administered to volunteers, and all these produce illness with similar characteristics.[5,67,77] A summary of these characteristics is given in Table 155-1, in which a comparison is made with colds produced by rhinoviruses in similarly inoculated volunteers. The incubation period of CoV colds was longer and their duration somewhat shorter, but the symptoms were very similar. Asymptomatic infection was sometimes seen and, indeed, has been a feature of serologic surveys of natural infection of children and adults.[78,79]

TABLE 155-1	Clinical Features of Colds Produced by Experimental Infection with Four Viruses			
	Coronaviruses		**Rhinoviruses**	
Feature	*229E*	*B814*	*Type 2 (HGP or PK)*	*DC*
No. of volunteers inoculated	26	75	213	251
No. (%) getting colds	13 (50)	34 (45)	78 (37)	77 (31)
Incubation period (days)				
Mean	3.3	3.2	2.1	2.1
Range	2-4	2-5	1-5	1-4
Duration (days)				
Mean	7	6	9	10
Range	3-18	2-17	3-19	2-26
Maximum no. of handkerchiefs used daily				
Mean	23	21	14	18
Range	8-105	8-120	3-38	33-60
Malaise (%)	46	47	28	25
Headache (%)	85	53	56	56
Chill (%)	31	18	28	15
Pyrexia (%)	23	21	14	18
Mucopurulent nasal discharge (%)	0	62	83	80
Sore throat (%)	54	79	87	73
Cough (%)	31	44	68	56
No. (%) of volunteers with colds of indicated severity				
Mild	10 (77)	24 (71)	63 (80)	36 (47)
Moderate	2 (15)	7 (20)	12 (15)	28 (36)
Severe	1 (8)	3 (9)	4 (5)	13 (17)

Data from Bradburne AF, Bynoe ML, Tyrrell DAJ. Effects of a "new" human respiratory virus in volunteers. *Br Med J.* 1967;3:767-769.

More serious respiratory tract illness is probably also caused by all four strains of non-SARS CoV. The evidence for this is not conclusive, but it seems likely that all strains can produce pneumonia and bronchiolitis in infants,[23,25,80,81] otitis and exacerbations of asthma in children and young adults,[82-84] pneumonia in healthy adults,[85] exacerbations of asthma and chronic bronchitis in adults,[86] both serious bronchitis and pneumonia in the elderly,[87,88] and pneumonia in the immunocompromised host.[89,90] HCoVs are found in asymptomatic individuals of all ages, and, when accompanied by illness, are also sometimes accompanied by infections with other potential respiratory pathogens. These characteristics (infection without disease, coinfection during disease) are features of many respiratory pathogens, including particularly rhinoviruses, adenoviruses, human metapneumovirus, human bocavirus, and parainfluenza viruses, but also (although less frequently) respiratory syncytial virus and influenza virus. Because infections with respiratory HCoVs are so common, however, it seems likely that they are responsible for a significant portion of these serious lower respiratory tract diseases, even though the basic pathogenicity of HCoVs (judging from volunteer studies) is similar to that of rhinoviruses, and clearly less than that of respiratory syncytial virus, influenza viruses, and certain adenovirus types. There is also some evidence that infection with NL63 in children is different from the other respiratory HCoVs in that several series have found an excess of children with croup.[24,25]

SEVERE ACUTE RESPIRATORY SYNDROME

The first symptom in most cases of SARS was fever, usually accompanied by headache, malaise, or myalgia. This was followed, usually in a few days, but as long as a week later, by a nonproductive cough and, in more severe cases, dyspnea. Approximately 25% of patients had diarrhea. Interestingly, upper respiratory symptoms such as rhinorrhea and sore throat usually did not occur.[68,70,91,92] The chest radiograph was frequently abnormal, showing scattered air-space opacification, usually in the periphery and lower zones of the lung.[93] Spiral computed tomography demonstrated both ground-glass opacification and consolidation, often in a subpleural distribution.[94-96]

Lymphopenia was common,[70,72,91] with normal or somewhat depressed neutrophils. Paradoxically, neutrophilia was associated with poor outcomes.[69] The decrease in lymphocytes in the blood was most marked for CD4 cells, but was seen in all T-cell phenotypes, including CD3 and CD8, as well as natural killer cells. Creatine kinase was often abnormal, as were lactic dehydrogenase and aspartate aminotransferase.

Approximately 25% of patients developed severe pulmonary disease that progressed to adult respiratory distress syndrome. Adult respiratory distress syndrome with SARS CoV infection was most likely to develop in patients older than 50 years or with underlying disease such as diabetes, cardiac disease, and chronic hepatitis.[70,91,92,97] The overall mortality rate was between 9% and 12%, with the highest rates in the elderly and adults with underlying liver disease. In some patients, clinical deterioration occurred during the second week of illness, as virus levels decreased, suggesting that disease was partly immune mediated.[70]

Pediatric disease was, interestingly, significantly less severe than adult disease, although the features were very similar.[98,99] Disease during pregnancy was very severe, with high mortality in both the mother and fetus.[100] Congenital transmission did not occur.

GASTROINTESTINAL CORONAVIRUSES AND TOROVIRUSES

The nature of the illness associated with enteric CoV infection is much less clear. One study found a significant association of gastroenteritis in infants 2 to 12 months of age with the presence of CoVLPs in the stool.[43] Another study, confined to infants in a neonatal intensive care unit, found highly significant associations between the presence of CoVLPs in the stool and the presence of water-loss stools, bloody stools, abdominal distention, and bilious gastric aspirates.[41] A further study of symptomatic infants shedding CoVLPs pointed to possible differences between CoVLP-associated diarrhea and rotavirus diarrhea: although fever and vomiting were of very similar incidence, stools were more often occult blood positive (18% in CoVLP-associated vs. 0% in rotavirus-associated disease), less often watery (66% vs. 92%), and more often mucoid (32% vs. 8%).[63] Finally, CoVs have been associated with at least three outbreaks of necrotizing enterocolitis in newborns,[40,41,44] and the best characterized strains[44] were isolated in infants with this illness.

The pathogenicity of human toroviruses is still in doubt, although the few controlled studies that have been done have shown a more consistent association with illness than those of enteric CoVs. Torovirus particles are found in the feces of both symptomatic and asymptomatic individuals, but there has been a clear excess in the former, implying a pathogenic role in diarrheal disease.[101,102]

In a study from Brazil, 20 of 91 fecal samples from children in the community with diarrhea contained torovirus antigen detectable by enzyme-linked immunosorbent assay, and toroviruses were significantly associated with both acute and chronic diarrhea ($P = .02$ for both).[102] In a study from Canada, symptomatic and asymptomatic hospitalized children were sampled for fecal viruses: toroviruses were found in 35% of the former and 14.5% of the latter. In comparison with those with stools containing either rotaviruses or astroviruses, torovirus-infected children were older (mean age, 4.0 years vs. 2.0 years), and their infections were more often acquired in hospital (57.6% vs. 31.3%). Vomiting was less frequent with torovirus infection, but occult blood was more frequent. A large proportion of symptomatic torovirus infections were in immunocompromised children.[101]

NEUROLOGIC SYNDROMES

Like many other viruses, CoVs have been sought as possible etiologic agents in multiple sclerosis. The search has been stimulated by the capacity of JHM, a well-studied strain of mouse hepatitis virus, to produce in mice and rats an immune-mediated chronic demyelinating encephalitis histologically similar to multiple sclerosis.[103,104] HCoV-OC43[105,106] and HCoV-229E[107] have been detected in brain tissue from multiple sclerosis patients using virus isolation,[105] in situ hybridization, immunohistology,[106] and polymerase chain reaction.[107] Moreover, T-cell lines established from patients with multiple sclerosis by stimulation with myelin basic protein or HCoV-229E were found to be cross-reactive with the opposite antigen, suggesting that molecular mimicry might be a possible pathogenic mechanism for the disease association.[108] Recently an adolescent boy with acute demyelinating encephalitis was reported to have HCoV-OC43 RNA in both the respiratory tract and the cerebrospinal fluid.[109] Despite these intriguing reports, compelling evidence is lacking to establish an etiologic or pathogenetic association of CoVs with central nervous system disease in humans.

Laboratory Diagnosis

RESPIRATORY CORONAVIRUSES

Although some human respiratory CoVs grow in tissue culture directly from clinical samples and although antigen detection systems have been developed for both HCoV-OC43 and HCoV-229E,[110,111] laboratory diagnosis of CoV respiratory infections is best accomplished by molecular methods. Reverse-transcriptase polymerase chain reaction systems have been developed using many different primers and detectors. From a clinical point of view, a single generic test for respiratory CoVs would be desirable, and such tests have been developed. However, when tested side-by-side with specific systems, the generic systems have a somewhat lower sensitivity.[81] Systems that combine primers and probes specific for several CoVs have also had considerable success.[112]

SEVERE ACUTE RESPIRATORY SYNDROME

Although SARS CoV was grown from respiratory tract specimens in Vero E6 and fetal rhesus monkey kidney cells, the more sensitive and rapid reverse-transcriptase polymerase chain reaction assays were most widely used to detect infection. Virus was detected by reverse-transcriptase polymerase chain reaction in upper and lower respiratory tract, blood, stool, and urine specimens. Early in the illness, specimens were found positive only in approximately one third of patients.[70] Use of samples from multiple sources increased the yield. Virus was detected most frequently during the second week of illness.[15,70,71]

Antibody tests have been developed using tissue culture grown virus and indirect immunofluorescence or enzyme-linked immunosorbent assay. Immunoglobulin M antibody can be detected in most patients for a limited period of time, and immunoglobulin G antibody appears first approximately 10 days after onset of fever and becomes essentially universal after 4 weeks.[70]

GASTROINTESTINAL CORONAVIRUSES AND TOROVIRUSES

Laboratory diagnosis of the gastrointestinal CoVs and of human toroviruses depends now entirely on electron microscopy of stool specimens and detection of characteristic particles in negatively stained specimens. Such testing is best performed in laboratories with extensive previous experience.

Treatment

Given the severity of SARS, clinicians throughout the world empirically treated most patients with corticosteroids and intravenous or oral ribavirin.[113] It is now known that ribavirin has little activity against SARS CoV in vitro, and there is no evidence that it was helpful in treating SARS cases. There is anecdotal and at least partially controlled evidence of the benefit of either corticosteroid or interferon-α treatment. Certain protease inhibitors, in particular lopinavir/ritonavir, have activity against the SARS CoV in vitro. Opinions differ on the efficacy of these treatments.[114] Nevertheless, one critical review concludes that nearly all reported studies were inconclusive and that none of the many treatments used during the epidemic had any beneficial effects.[115]

Prevention

Rigorous application of hospital infection control procedures, particularly those directed at contact and droplet spread, was shown to have a major beneficial effect on the spread of the SARS CoV.[54] The containment of the global SARS outbreak is a testament to the power of the cooperation and collaboration engendered by the World Health Organization to address a major public health threat.

Vaccines for animal CoVs have been developed and widely used with variable efficacy. In one instance, a vaccine for feline infectious peritonitis appeared to lead to enhanced disease with subsequent natural infection. If SARS does return, an effective vaccine would be extremely helpful in control efforts, and a variety of vaccination strategies, including inactivated, subunit, and live-attenuated vaccines, are being pursued.[114] In addition, hospitals have been advised on improvement of infection control procedures, so that in future epidemics of respiratory viruses, they will not be a major source of spread of infection, as occurred in the 2002 epidemic of SARS.

REFERENCES

1. Lau SK, Woo PC, Li KS, et al. Severe acute respiratory syndrome coronavirus-like virus in Chinese horseshoe bats. *Proc Natl Acad Sci U S A.* 2005;102:14040-14045.
2. Vijaykrishna D, Smith GJ, Zhang JX, et al. Evolutionary insights into the ecology of coronaviruses. *J Virol.* 2007;81:4012-4020.
3. Song HD, Tu CC, Zhang GW, et al. Cross-host evolution of severe acute respiratory syndrome coronavirus in palm civet and human. *Proc Natl Acad Sci U S A.* 2005;102:2430-2435.
4. Lai MM, Perlman S, Anderson LJ. Coronaviridae. In: Knipe DEA, ed. *Fields Virology.* 5th ed. Lippincott Williams & Wilkins; 2007.
5. Tyrrell DAJ, Bynoe ML. Cultivation of a novel type of common-cold virus in organ cultures. *Br Med J.* 1965;1:1467-1470.
6. Almeida JD, Tyrrell DAJ. The morphology of three previously uncharacterized human respiratory viruses that grow in organ culture. *J Gen Virol.* 1967;1:175-178.
7. Hamre D, Procknow JJ. A new virus isolated from the human respiratory tract. *Proc Soc Exp Biol Med.* 1966;121:190-193.
8. McIntosh K, Dees JH, Becker WB, et al. Recovery in tracheal organ cultures of novel viruses from patients with respiratory disease. *Proc Natl Acad Sci U S A.* 1967;57:933-940.
9. McIntosh K, Becker WB, Chanock RM. Growth in suckling-mouse brain of "IBV-like" viruses from patients with upper respiratory tract disease. *Proc Natl Acad Sci U S A.* 1967;58:2268-2273.
10. Witte KH, Tajima M, Easterday BC. Morphologic characteristics and nucleic acid type of transmissible gastroenteritis virus of pigs. *Arch Gesamte Virusforsch.* 1968;23:53-70.
11. Tyrrell DA, Almeida JD, Cunningham CH, et al. Coronaviridae. *Intervirology.* 1975;5:76-82.
12. Zhao Z, Zhang F, Xu M, et al. Description and clinical treatment of an early outbreak of severe acute respiratory syndrome (SARS) in Guangzhou, PR China. *J Med Microbiol.* 2003;52:715-720.
13. Peiris JS, Lai ST, Poon LL, et al. Coronavirus as a possible cause of severe acute respiratory syndrome. *Lancet.* 2003;361:1319-1325.
14. Ksiazek TG, Erdman D, Goldsmith CS, et al. A novel coronavirus associated with severe acute respiratory syndrome. *N Engl J Med.* 2003;348:1953-1966.
15. Drosten C, Gunther S, Preiser W, et al. Identification of a novel coronavirus in patients with severe acute respiratory syndrome. *N Engl J Med.* 2003;348:1967-1976.
16. Marra MA, Jones SJ, Astell CR, et al. The genome sequence of the SARS-associated coronavirus. *Science.* 2003;300:1399-1404.
17. Rota PA, Oberste MS, Monroe SS, et al. Characterization of a novel coronavirus associated with severe acute respiratory syndrome. *Science.* 2003;300:1394-1399.
18. Peiris JS, Guan Y, Yuen KY. Severe acute respiratory syndrome. *Nat Med.* 2004;10:S88-S97.
19. Gorbalenya AE. Genomics and evolution of the nidovirales. In: Perlman S, Gallagher TM, Snijder EJ, eds. *Nidoviruses.* Washington, DC: ASM Press; 2008:15-28.
20. van der Hoek L, Pyrc K, Jebbink MF, et al. Identification of a new human coronavirus. *Nat Med.* 2004;10:368-373.
21. Fouchier RA, Hartwig NG, Bestebroer TM, et al. A previously undescribed coronavirus associated with respiratory disease in humans. *Proc Natl Acad Sci U S A.* 2004;101:6212-6216.
22. Woo PC, Lau SK, Chu CM, et al. Characterization and complete genome sequence of a novel coronavirus, coronavirus HKU1, from patients with pneumonia. *J Virol.* 2005;79:884-895.
23. Esper F, Weibel C, Ferguson D, et al. Evidence of a novel human coronavirus that is associated with respiratory tract disease in infants and young children. *J Infect Dis.* 2005;191:492-498.
24. van der Hoek L, Sure K, Ihorst G, et al. Croup is associated with the novel coronavirus NL63. *PLoS Med.* 2005;2:e240.
25. Choi EH, Lee HJ, Kim SJ, et al. The association of newly identified respiratory viruses with lower respiratory tract infections in Korean children, 2000-2005. *Clin Infect Dis.* 2006;43:585-592.
26. Woode GN, Reed DE, Runnels PL, et al. Studies with an unclassified virus isolated from diarrheic calves. *Vet Microbiol.* 1982;7:221-240.
27. Weiss M, Steck F, Horzinek MC. Purification and partial characterization of a new enveloped RNA virus (Berne virus). *J Gen Virol.* 1983;64(Pt 9):1849-1858.
28. Beards GM, Hall C, Green J, et al. An enveloped virus in stools of children and adults with gastroenteritis that resembles the Breda virus of calves. *Lancet.* 1984;1:1050-1052.
29. Snijder EJ, Bredenbeek PJ, Dobbe JC, et al. Unique and conserved features of genome and proteome of SARS-coronavirus, an early split-off from the coronavirus group 2 lineage. *J Mol Biol.* 2003;331:991-1004.
30. Becker WB, McIntosh K, Dees JH, et al. Morphogenesis of avian infectious bronchitis virus and a related human virus (strain 229E). *J Virol.* 1967;1:1019-1027.
31. Yeager CL, Ashmun RA, Williams RK, et al. Human aminopeptidase N is a receptor for human coronavirus 229E. *Nature.* 1992;357:420-422.
32. Hofmann H, Pyrc K, van der Hoek L, et al. Human coronavirus NL63 employs the severe acute respiratory syndrome coronavirus receptor for cellular entry. *Proc Natl Acad Sci U S A.* 2005;102:7988-7993.

33. Li W, Moore MJ, Vasilieva N, et al. Angiotensin-converting enzyme 2 is a functional receptor for the SARS coronavirus. *Nature.* 2003;426:450-454.
34. Williams RK, Jiang GS, Holmes KV. Receptor for mouse hepatitis virus is a member of the carcinoembryonic antigen family of glycoproteins. *Proc Natl Acad Sci U S A.* 1991;88:5533-5536.
35. Collins AR. Human coronavirus OC43 interacts with major histocompatibility complex class I molecules at the cell surface to establish infection. *Immunol Invest.* 1994;23:313-321.
36. Bruckova M, McIntosh K, Kapikian AZ, et al. The adaptation of two human coronavirus strains (OC38 and OC43) to growth in cell monolayers. *Proc Soc Exp Biol Med.* 1970;135:431-435.
37. Vabret A, Dina J, Gouarin S, et al. Detection of the new human coronavirus HKU1: a report of 6 cases. *Clin Infect Dis.* 2006;42:634-639.
38. Mathan M, Mathan VI, Swaminathan SP, et al. Pleomorphic virus-like particles in human faeces. *Lancet.* 1975;1:1068-1069.
39. Baker SJ, Mathan M, Mathan VI, et al. Chronic enterocyte infection with coronavirus: one possible cause of the syndrome of tropical sprue? *Dig Dis Sci.* 1982;27:1039-1043.
40. Chany C, Moscovici O, Lebon P, et al. Association of coronavirus infection with neonatal necrotizing enterocolitis. *Pediatrics.* 1982;69:209-214.
41. Vaucher YE, Ray CG, Minnich LL, et al. Pleomorphic, enveloped, virus-like particles associated with gastrointestinal illness in neonates. *J Infect Dis.* 1982;145:27-36.
42. Maass G, Baumeister HG, Freitag N. [Viruses as causal agents of gastroenteritis in infants and young children (author's transl)]. *MMW Munch Med Wochenschr.* 1977;119:1029-1034.
43. Gerna G, Passarani N, Battaglia M, et al. Human enteric coronaviruses: antigenic relatedness to human coronavirus OC43 and possible etiologic role in viral gastroenteritis. *J Infect Dis.* 1985;151:796-803.
44. Resta S, Luby JP, Rosenfeld CR, et al. Isolation and propagation of a human enteric coronavirus. *Science.* 1985;229:978-981.
45. Weiss M, Horzinek MC. The proposed family Toroviridae: agents of enteric infections: brief review. *Arch Virol.* 1987;92:1-15.
46. Duckmanton L, Luan B, Devenish J, et al. Characterization of torovirus from human fecal specimens. *Virology.* 1997;239:158-168.
47. Beards GM, Brown DW, Green J, et al. Preliminary characterisation of torovirus-like particles of humans: comparison with Berne virus of horses and Breda virus of calves. *J Med Virol.* 1986;20:67-78.
48. Snijder EJ, Horzinek MC. Toroviruses: replication, evolution and comparison with other members of the coronavirus-like superfamily. *J Gen Virol.* 1993;74:2305-2316.
49. Cornelissen LA, Wierda CM, van der Meer FJ, et al. Hemagglutinin-esterase, a novel structural protein of torovirus. *J Virol.* 1997;71:5277-5286.
50. de Groot RJ. Molecular biology and evolution of toroviruses. In: Perlman S, Gallagher TM, Snijder EJ, eds. *Nidoviruses.* Washington, DC: ASM Press; 2008:133-146.
51. Monto AS. Medical reviews: coronaviruses. *Yale J Biol Med.* 1974;47:234-251.
52. Callow KA, Parry HF, Sergeant M, et al. The time course of the immune response to experimental coronavirus infection of man. *Epidemiol Infect.* 1990;105:435-446.
53. Severe acute respiratory syndrome—Singapore, 2003. *MMWR Morb Mortal Wkly Rep.* 2003;52:405-411.
54. Seto WH, Tsang D, Yung RW, et al. Effectiveness of precautions against droplets and contact in prevention of nosocomial transmission of severe acute respiratory syndrome (SARS). *Lancet.* 2003;361:1519-1520.
55. Lipsitch M, Cohen T, Cooper B, et al. Transmission dynamics and control of severe acute respiratory syndrome. *Science.* 2003;300:1966-1970.
56. Riley S, Fraser C, Donnelly CA, et al. Transmission dynamics of the etiological agent of SARS in Hong Kong: impact of public health interventions. *Science.* 2003;300:1961-1966.
57. Hung IF, Cheng VC, Wu AK, et al. Viral loads in clinical specimens and SARS manifestations. *Emerg Infect Dis.* 2004;10:1550-1557.
58. Guan Y, Zheng BJ, He YQ, et al. Isolation and characterization of viruses related to the SARS coronavirus from animals in southern China. *Science.* 2003;302:276-278.
59. Kern P, Muller G, Schmitz H, et al. Detection of coronavirus-like particles in homosexual men with acquired immunodeficiency and related lymphadenopathy syndrome. *Klin Wochenschr.* 1985;63:68-72.
60. Schmidt W, Schneider T, Heise W, et al. Stool viruses, coinfections, and diarrhea in HIV-infected patients. Berlin Diarrhea/Wasting Syndrome Study Group. *J Acquir Immune Defic Syndr Hum Retrovirol.* 1996;13:33-38.
61. Marshall JA, Birch CJ, Williamson HG, et al. Coronavirus-like particles and other agents in the faeces of children in Efate, Vanuatu. *J Trop Med Hyg.* 1982;85:213-215.
62. Marshall JA, Thompson WL, Gust ID. Coronavirus-like particles in adults in Melbourne, Australia. *J Med Virol.* 1989;29:238-243.
63. Mortensen ML, Ray CG, Payne CM, et al. Coronaviruslike particles in human gastrointestinal disease: epidemiologic, clinical,

and laboratory observations. *Am J Dis Child.* 1985;139:928-934.
64. Payne CM, Ray CG, Borduin V, et al. An eight-year study of the viral agents of acute gastroenteritis in humans: ultrastructural observations and seasonal distribution with a major emphasis on coronavirus-like particles. *Diagn Microbiol Infect Dis.* 1986;5:39-54.
65. Afzelius BA. Ultrastructure of human nasal epithelium during an episode of coronavirus infection. *Virchows Arch.* 1994;424:295-300.
66. Tyrrell DA, Cohen S, Schlarb JE. Signs and symptoms in common colds. *Epidemiol Infect.* 1993;111:143-156.
67. Bradburne AF, Bynoe ML, Tyrrell DA. Effects of a "new" human respiratory virus in volunteers. *Br Med J.* 1967;3:767-769.
68. Donnelly CA, Ghani AC, Leung GM, et al. Epidemiological determinants of spread of causal agent of severe acute respiratory syndrome in Hong Kong. *Lancet.* 2003;361:1761-1766.
69. Wong RS, Wu A, To KF, et al. Haematological manifestations in patients with severe acute respiratory syndrome: retrospective analysis. *Br Med J.* 2003;326:1358-1362.
70. Peiris JS, Chu CM, Cheng VC, et al. Clinical progression and viral load in a community outbreak of coronavirus-associated SARS pneumonia: a prospective study. *Lancet.* 2003;361:1767-1772.
71. Ren Y, Ding HG, Wu QF, et al. [Detection of SARS-CoV RNA in stool samples of SARS patients by nest RT-PCR and its clinical value]. *Zhongguo Yi Xue Ke Xue Yuan Xue Bao.* 2003;25:368-371.
72. Lee N, Hui D, Wu A, et al. A major outbreak of severe acute respiratory syndrome in Hong Kong. *N Engl J Med.* 2003;348:1986-1994.
73. Nicholls JM, Poon LL, Lee KC, et al. Lung pathology of fatal severe acute respiratory syndrome. *Lancet.* 2003;361:1773-1778.
74. Ding Y, Wang H, Shen H, et al. The clinical pathology of severe acute respiratory syndrome (SARS): a report from China. *J Pathol.* 2003;200:282-289.
75. Gu J, Gong E, Zhang B, et al. Multiple organ infection and the pathogenesis of SARS. *J Exp Med.* 2005;202:415-424.
76. Nicholls JM, Butany J, Poon LL, et al. Time course and cellular localization of SARS-CoV nucleoprotein and RNA in lungs from fatal cases of SARS. *PLoS Med.* 2006;3:e27.
77. Bradburne AF. Antigenic relationships amongst coronaviruses. *Arch Gesamte Virusforsch.* 1970;31:352-364.
78. van Gageldonk-Lafeber AB, Heijnen ML, Bartelds AI, et al. A case-control study of acute respiratory tract infection in general practice patients in The Netherlands. *Clin Infect Dis.* 2005;41:490-497.
79. Kusel MM, de Klerk NH, Holt PG, et al. Role of respiratory viruses in acute upper and lower respiratory tract illness in the first year of life: a birth cohort study. *Pediatr Infect Dis J.* 2006;25:680-686.
80. McIntosh K, Chao RK, Krause HE, et al. Coronavirus infection in acute lower respiratory tract disease of infants. *J Infect Dis.* 1974;130:502-507.
81. Gerna G, Campanini G, Rovida F, et al. Genetic variability of human coronavirus OC43-, 229E-, and NL63-like strains and their association with lower respiratory tract infections of hospitalized infants and immunocompromised patients. *J Med Virol.* 2006;78:938-949.
82. McIntosh K, Ellis EF, Hoffman LS, et al. The association of viral and bacterial respiratory infections with exacerbations of wheezing in young asthmatic children. *J Pediatr.* 1973;82:578-590.
83. Mertsola J, Ziegler T, Ruuskanen O, et al. Recurrent wheezy bronchitis and viral respiratory infections. *Arch Dis Child.* 1991;66:124-129.
84. Pitkaranta A, Virolainen A, Jero J, et al. Detection of rhinovirus, respiratory syncytial virus, and coronavirus infections in acute otitis media by reverse transcriptase polymerase chain reaction. *Pediatrics.* 1998;102:291-295.
85. Wenzel RP, Hendley JO, Davies JA, et al. Coronavirus infections in military recruits: three-year study with coronavirus strains OC43 and 229E. *Am Rev Respir Dis.* 1974;109:621-624.
86. Nicholson KG, Kent J, Ireland DC. Respiratory viruses and exacerbations of asthma in adults. *Br Med J.* 1993;307:982-986.
87. Falsey AR, Walsh EE, Hayden FG. Rhinovirus and coronavirus infection-associated hospitalizations among older adults. *J Infect Dis.* 2002;185:1338-1341.
88. Graat JM, Schouten EG, Heijnen ML, et al. A prospective, community-based study on virologic assessment among elderly people with and without symptoms of acute respiratory infection. *J Clin Epidemiol.* 2003;56:1218-1223.
89. Pene F, Merlat A, Vabret A, et al. Coronavirus 229E-related pneumonia in immunocompromised patients. *Clin Infect Dis.* 2003;37:929-932.
90. Kumar D, Erdman D, Keshavjee S, et al. Clinical impact of community-acquired respiratory viruses on bronchiolitis obliterans after lung transplant. *Am J Transplant.* 2005;5:2031-2036.
91. Booth CM, Matukas LM, Tomlinson GA, et al. Clinical features and short-term outcomes of 144 patients with SARS in the greater Toronto area. *JAMA.* 2003;289:2801-2809.

92. Lew TW, Kwek TK, Tai D, et al. Acute respiratory distress syndrome in critically ill patients with severe acute respiratory syndrome. *JAMA.* 2003;290:374-380.

93. Wong KT, Antonio GE, Hui DS, et al. Severe acute respiratory syndrome: radiographic appearances and pattern of progression in 138 patients. *Radiology.* 2003;228:401-406.

94. Antonio GE, Wong KT, Hui DS, et al. Imaging of severe acute respiratory syndrome in Hong Kong. *AJR Am J Roentgenol.* 2003;181:11-17.

95. Muller NL, Ooi GC, Khong PL, et al. Severe acute respiratory syndrome: radiographic and CT findings. *AJR Am J Roentgenol.* 2003;181:3-8.

96. Wong KT, Antonio GE, Hui DS, et al. Thin-section CT of severe acute respiratory syndrome: evaluation of 73 patients exposed to or with the disease. *Radiology.* 2003;228:395-400.

97. Fowler RA, Lapinsky SE, Hallett D, et al. Critically ill patients with severe acute respiratory syndrome. *JAMA.* 2003;290:367-373.

98. Chiu, WK, Cheung PC, Ng KL, et al. Severe acute respiratory syndrome in children: experience in a regional hospital in Hong Kong. *Pediatr Crit Care Med.* 2003;4:279-283.

99. Hon KL, Leung CW, Cheng WT, et al. Clinical presentations and outcome of severe acute respiratory syndrome in children. *Lancet.* 2003;361:1701-1703.

100. Wong SF, Chow KM, de Swiet M. Severe acute respiratory syndrome and pregnancy. *Br J Obstet Gynaecol.* 2003;110:641-642.

101. Jamieson FB, Wang EE, Bain C, et al. Human torovirus: a new nosocomial gastrointestinal pathogen. *J Infect Dis.* 1998;178:1263-1269.

102. Koopmans MP, Goosen ES, Lima AA, et al. Association of torovirus with acute and persistent diarrhea in children. *Pediatr Infect Dis J.* 1997;16:504-507.

103. Nagashima K, Wege H, Meyermann R, et al. Corona virus induced subacute demyelinating encephalomyelitis in rats: a morphological analysis. *Acta Neuropathol (Berl).* 1978;44:63-70.

104. Haring J, Perlman S. Mouse hepatitis virus. *Curr Opin Microbiol.* 2001;4:462-466.

105. Burks JS, DeVald BL, Jankovsky LD, et al. Two coronaviruses isolated from central nervous system tissue of two multiple sclerosis patients. *Science.* 1980;209:933-934.

106. Murray RS, Brown B, Brian D, et al. Detection of coronavirus RNA and antigen in multiple sclerosis brain. *Ann Neurol.* 1992;31:525-533.

107. Stewart JN, Mounir S, Talbot PJ. Human coronavirus gene expression in the brains of multiple sclerosis patients. *Virology.* 1992;191:502-505.

108. Boucher A, Desforges M, Duquette P, et al. Long-term human coronavirus-myelin cross-reactive T-cell clones derived from multiple sclerosis patients. *Clin Immunol.* 2007;123:258-267.

109. Yeh EA, Collins A, Cohen ME, et al. Detection of coronavirus in the central nervous system of a child with acute disseminated encephalomyelitis. *Pediatrics.* 2004;113:e73-e76.

110. McIntosh K, McQuillin J, Reed SE, et al. Diagnosis of human coronavirus infection by immunofluorescence: method and application to respiratory disease in hospitalized children. *J Med Virol.* 1978;2:341-346.

111. Lina B, Valette M, Foray S, et al. Surveillance of community-acquired viral infections due to respiratory viruses in Rhone-Alpes (France) during winter 1994 to 1995. *J Clin Microbiol.* 1996;34:3007-3011.

112. Kuypers J, Martin ET, Heugel J, et al. Clinical disease in children associated with newly described coronavirus subtypes. *Pediatrics.* 2007;119:e70-e76.

113. So LK, Lau AC, Yam LY, et al. Development of a standard treatment protocol for severe acute respiratory syndrome. *Lancet.* 2003;361:1615-1617.

114. Groneberg DA, Poutanen SM, Low DE, et al. Treatment and vaccines for severe acute respiratory syndrome. *Lancet Infect Dis.* 2005;5:147-155.

115. Stockman LJ, Bellamy R, Garner P. SARS: systematic review of treatment effects. *PLoS Med.* 2006;3:e343.

156

Parainfluenza Viruses

PETER F. WRIGHT

History

The three major parainfluenza viruses[1] were first isolated from humans among the flurry of new viruses identified in the late 1950s. Initially described in association with laryngotracheobronchitis (croup) in hospitalized children, parainfluenza viruses were characterized as viruses that had the property of hemadsorption of red blood cells. Subsequently, their important role in human respiratory disease in childhood and more recently in patients with immunocompromise has been well described. In the 1960s, mucosal immunoglobulin A (IgA) antibody was shown to have a protective role against parainfluenza viruses; these viruses remain the viruses for which mucosal immune protection has been most clearly shown. Advances in reverse genetics have led to characterization of the role of individual parainfluenza viral proteins and the rational design of vaccine candidates for prevention of human respiratory disease caused by these viruses.[2]

Description of Viruses

CLASSIFICATION AND STRUCTURE

Human parainfluenza viruses are classified as five types that belong to the Paramyxoviridae family[3,4] and are members of the genera *Respirovirus* (parainfluenza types 1 and 3) and *Rubulavirus* (parainfluenza types 2, 4A, and 4B). They have a lipid bilayer envelope derived from the host cell, are roughly spherical with a diameter of 150 to 200 nm, have glycoprotein spikes that extend from the envelope surface, and have a single-stranded, nonsegmented, negative-sense RNA genome. The human pathogens included in this family are the five parainfluenza viruses (designated parainfluenza types 1, 2, 3, 4A, and 4B), mumps, measles, Hendra and Nipah viruses (see Chapter 161),[5,6] human metapneumovirus (see Chapter 159),[7] and respiratory syncytial virus (see Chapter 158). Significant animal pathogens within the family include Sendai virus, simian virus type 5, Newcastle disease virus, canine distemper virus, and rinderpest.

REPLICATION

Parainfluenza viruses attach to sialic acid–containing cellular molecules via the hemagglutinin-neuraminidase (HN) protein.[3] Sialic acid–expressing cells are widespread, and thus, the specificity of attachment does not explain the respiratory tract tropism of parainfluenza viruses. The HN protein is coupled with the activated fusion (F) protein to allow cell entry of the virus.[8,9] Activation of the F protein is via proteolytic cleavage, which is mediated by cellular serine proteases. In the case of Sendai virus, F-protein cleavage may occur by a protease that is unique to a subset of respiratory cells called Clara cells.[10] The unique localization of the protease may be a factor in limiting the replication of parainfluenza viruses to the respiratory tract. Differences in tropism are striking between closely related viruses, as, for example, the respiratory localization of parainfluenza viruses contrasted to the preference of mumps for acinar tissue. Parainfluenza viruses do not appear to enter or unfold in the acid environment of the endosome, as occurs with influenza viruses. The nucleocapsid complex consists of the viral RNA and three internal proteins—nucleocapsid protein (NP), polymerase protein (L), and phosphorylated nucleocapsid–associated protein (P)—that initiate a primary transcription event to generate the messenger RNA from which viral proteins are translated. In addition, a full-length antigenome with positive-sense RNA is formed from which the genome is replicated. Diversity in expression of the P-gene–coded products leads to additional regulatory proteins whose functions are not fully defined, although some may inhibit the interferon pathway.[11] Virion assembly takes place within the cytoplasm in several steps. The new NP protein assembles with the genomic RNA to form a helical structure. The P-protein and L-protein complexes then join to form the nucleocapsid. After being synthesized in the endoplasmic reticulum and traveling a secretory pathway in the cell, the envelope proteins assemble at the cell surface with a polarity that favors the apical surface of the cell. The other major structural protein, matrix protein, plays a role in virus assembly and release from the cell surface by budding. The neuraminidase component of the HN protein may aid in release from the cell and prevention of virus aggregation by cleaving sialic acid residues to which the virus would otherwise reattach. The entire process is not efficient in that many incomplete noninfectious particles are formed that can interfere with the yield of infectious virus.

Pathogenesis

TROPISM

Parainfluenza viruses cause acute respiratory infections. The peak of illness is associated with peak virus shedding based on observations in children infected with a partially attenuated parainfluenza type 3 vaccine candidate.[12] Parainfluenza viruses replicate exclusively in cells of the respiratory epithelial layer.[4] The epithelial layer is a complex mixture of cell types that vary as one traverses to different depths of the upper and then lower respiratory tracts. Clinically, parainfluenza viruses most typically cause illness in the large airways of the lower respiratory tract manifested as laryngotracheobronchitis, or croup.[13] The reasons for this particular localization are not known. The best evidence is that parainfluenza viruses replicate in the ciliated epithelial cells that line much of the upper and lower respiratory tracts.[14] Not only do they grow in these superficial cells, but they are also released by budding only from the apical surface of the cell back into the mucin layer above the epithelium.[15]

As with influenza viruses, a surface protein of parainfluenza viruses, the fusion or F protein, is cleaved by a serine protease, a process necessary for replication of the virus. With Sendai virus, a murine virus closely related to parainfluenza virus type 1, mutations in the F protein that allow more ready cleavage lead to a mutant that replicates throughout the body.[16] Conversely, mutants of Sendai virus that are no longer cleaved by trypsin are highly attenuated.[17] In rodent models, a protease produced by the Clara cells of the respiratory tract has been identified that mediates this cleavage in Sendai and influenza viruses.[10] Clara cells are secretory cells that release this protease into the respiratory tract, where it presumably acts in a paracrine fashion to cleave virus in the extracellular environment or in the process of budding from cells. Early in Sendai infection, Clara cells secrete an abundance of tryptase Clara. The enzyme is found overlying the adjoining ciliated cells in which parainfluenza is replicating. The human counterpart of this protein has not been identified, but serine protease activity is seen in human secretions.[18]

Some of the parainfluenza viruses cause cell fusion and syncytia formation. The precise role of syncytia formation in disease is not known. It could potentially allow cell-to-cell spread without the virus

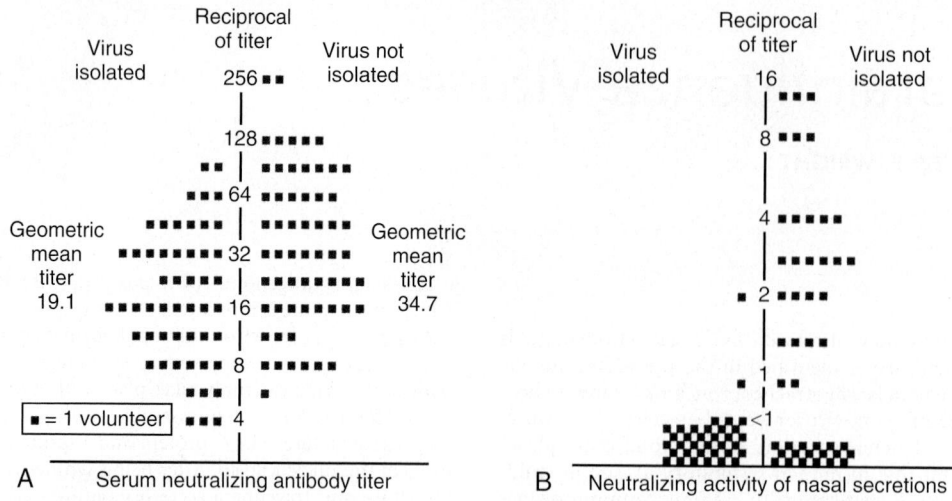

Figure 156-1 **A,** Serum neutralizing antibody titer before challenge with parainfluenza type 1 virus. **B,** Neutralizing activity of nasal secretions before challenge with parainfluenza type 1 virus. *(From Smith CB, Purcell RH, Bellanti JA, et al. Protective effect of antibody to parainfluenza type 1 virus. N Engl J Med. 1966:275:1145-1152. Copyright © 1996 Massachusetts Medical Society. All rights reserved.)*

being exposed to neutralizing antibody in the extracellular environment.

IMMUNE RESPONSE

Serum neutralizing antibodies and T-cell recognition are directed toward epitopes on the HN and F surface proteins of parainfluenza virus.[4] Monoclonal antibodies are preferentially formed to epitopes on the HN virus. In experimental animals, antibodies raised to an HN vaccinia construct were considerably more protective than antibodies to protein F.[19] After several infections, antibodies may develop that cross neutralize different parainfluenza strains.

In spite of these immunologic targets, children and adults are repeatedly infected with parainfluenza viruses over the course of a lifetime. Reinfection is more likely to solely involve the upper respiratory tract, with sparing of the lower respiratory tract after the first or second exposure in individuals with immunocompetence.[20] However, symptomatic disease with lower respiratory tract involvement can be seen after reinfection with parainfluenza type 3.[21]

Antigenic variation occurs, but it is not progressive.[22] Thus, reinfection probably reflects a waning of immunity over time rather than antigenic drift of the virus. This pattern is in obvious contrast to influenza virus, in which progressive antigenic drift is one of the major ways that the virus escapes immune surveillance.

Immunity to parainfluenza viruses, no matter how poorly sustained, can be readily seen. Prior infection in animal models blocks virus recovery on subsequent challenge. Experimental infection of adults with wild-type viruses is modulated by the level of immunity,[23] and infection of seropositive children with live-attenuated vaccines is more difficult than ready infection of immunologically naive children.[24] In both adults and children, recovery of virus is dramatically lowered by recent past exposure to the virus.

The most important component of resistance appears to be mucosal immunity. In animal models, greater protection is afforded with intranasal than with systemic administration of parainfluenza type 3 glycoproteins. In addition, passive IgA antibody delivered into the respiratory tract of mice provides greater protection than does immunoglobulin G (IgG). In adults, after an experimental parainfluenza type 1 challenge, reisolation of virus was inversely correlated with the detection of local neutralizing antibody in secretions and not with serum antibody (Fig. 156-1).[25] In children, prior natural infection blocks the replication of live-attenuated, intranasally administered virus vaccines, which replicate freely in naive children, including children in the first 6 months of life with passively acquired maternal

serum antibody. IgA antibody has the property of being transcytosed across epithelial cells from the basolateral surface to release at the apical surface into the respiratory tract. Antibody and virus have been proposed to potentially colocalize within cells and result in intracellular inhibition of virus assembly and release.[26]

In addition to prevention of reinfection, immunity is involved in termination of primary infection. In animal models, the role of CD8[+] T-cells is critical in virus clearance. Lymphoid cells, some of which are virus specific and some of which are bystanders, accumulate in the regional peribronchial lymph nodes during acute infection. The bystander lymphoid cells presumably contribute to the establishment of immunologic memory. The cells active in cytotoxic destruction of virally infected cells appear to accumulate in the airways and can be found in bronchoalveolar lavage fluid.[27] The severity of disease in individuals with T-cell deficits (see Clinical Manifestations section) suggests the importance of T-cell immunity in clearance of infection. Parainfluenza virus type 3 has been shown to downregulate granzyme B, one of the perforins that mediates cytotoxicity, thus suggesting a mechanism for immune modulation by parainfluenza viruses.[28]

Epidemiology

A number of studies have examined the impact of respiratory viral infections in pediatric practice.[21,29] Parainfluenza type 3 is the most frequently recovered of the parainfluenza virus types in longitudinal studies of respiratory illness in children. Roughly half as many parainfluenza type 1 isolates are found as parainfluenza type 3 isolates, and one quarter as many isolates of parainfluenza type 2 are found as type 3 (Table 156-1).[21] Parainfluenza viruses vary in their seasonal epidemiology by type. Parainfluenza type 3 virus is endemic, with isolation throughout the year; however, a distinct peak is seen in the spring months of April and May.[29] Parainfluenza virus types 1 and 2 cause annual fall epidemics of disease and often alternate in years, so an individual type may be seen only every 2 years. Parainfluenza virus types 4A and 4B are isolated so seldomly that their seasonality is not well described.[30]

In the unique environment of overwintering on the South Pole where 20 people were isolated for 6 months, parainfluenza virus types 1 and 3 were repeatedly isolated through the quarantine period, which suggests that persistent or repeated infection was spread in this small cohort.[31] In tissue culture cells, persistent parainfluenza virus type 3 infection can also be established.

The early age at which parainfluenza type 3 virus is first recovered is another trait that distinguishes it from types 1 and 2. Parainfluenza

TABLE 156-1	Diagnoses, Signs, and Symptoms in Patients from Whom Parainfluenza Viruses Were Isolated				
	Type				
Number of Isolates	*1 (n = 77)*	*2 (n = 33)*	*3 (n = 157)*	*Other (n = 19)*	*P**
Diagnosis					
Acute otitis	38†	30	52	32	.03
Croup	16	6	5	21	.01
Bronchiolitis	1	9	6	0	
Signs and Symptoms					
Cough	73	67	81	77	
Hoarseness	28	18	11	39	.001
Rales/rhonchi	6	15	15	11	
Wheezing	9	12	4	5	
Temperature, >38°C	33	16	38	6	.004
Irritability	47	30	54	72	.02

*Fisher's exact test for null hypothesis that all types are alike.
†Values are percentages of patients with the finding.
(Data from Reed G, Jewett PH, Thompson J, et al. Epidemiology and clinical impact of parainfluenza virus infections in otherwise healthy infants and young children <5 years old. *J Infect Dis.* 1997;175:807-813.)

type 3 virus, like respiratory syncytial virus, is commonly seen in the first 6 months of life, an age at which most viral infections are prevented or attenuated by maternal antibody. By age 5 years, almost all children have experienced infection with all three parainfluenza types. The impact of parainfluenza virus infections is best reflected by the peaks of hospitalization for croup that occur during biannual type 1 epidemics, which have been estimated to cause 18,000 hospitalizations nationwide.[32] In all croup cases from which virus can be isolated, about 60% of the isolates are parainfluenza.[33] The cost of a typical parainfluenza type 1 and 2 fall epidemic was estimated at $190 million for emergency department use and hospitalization.[34] Parainfluenza type 3 virus is more endemic and less associated with the distinctive clinical finding of croup, but it causes more hospitalizations for lower respiratory tract illness than do either parainfluenza type 1 or 2. Although the best studies are now more than 40 years old, the role of parainfluenza viruses as the second leading contributor to pediatric hospitalization for respiratory disease, after respiratory syncytial virus, is unlikely to have changed.[35] Nosocomial spread of parainfluenza viruses among hospitalized patients has been shown to occur.[36]

In adults, parainfluenza viruses have been implicated in about 10% of acute respiratory illnesses. Disease is also seen in the elderly, but without the impact of respiratory syncytial virus or influenza.[37] Definition of the role of parainfluenza viruses in the elderly may require sensitive assays such as polymerase chain reaction (PCR)[38] to detect the low-level shedding that typically accompanies viral infections in the elderly. Studies to date implicate parainfluenza viruses in less than 5% of acute respiratory infections in the elderly.[39] Nevertheless, a nursing home outbreak has been described.

Clinical Manifestations

Parainfluenza viruses cause a spectrum of respiratory illnesses. In healthy children, most illnesses are upper respiratory, although 30% to 50% are associated with otitis media[40] (see Table 156-1). In a 20-year epidemiologic study at Vanderbilt University, 15% of parainfluenza isolates were associated with lower respiratory tract disease.[21] Lower respiratory tract disease was manifested as either bronchiolitis, with types 2 and 3, or croup, with type 1.[21] Croup is characterized by a barking cough, a hoarse voice, and stridor. Radiographically, croup is distinguished by the "steeple sign" of progressive subglottic narrowing. As noted, among the virus isolates obtained from cases of croup, about 60% are parainfluenza. In some children, repeated episodes of spasmodic croup may occur. Whether these episodes are separate illnesses is unclear. In adults with immunocompetence, clinical manifestations are primarily those of an upper respiratory tract infection.

Parainfluenza infections cause severe disease in both adult and pediatric hematopoietic stem cell transplants (HSCT) and in solid organ transplant recipients.[41-43] In HSCT recipients at the University of Texas M. D. Anderson Cancer Center, 56% of 61 parainfluenza isolates were associated with uncomplicated upper respiratory illness; however, pneumonia developed in the remaining patients, with a mortality rate of 37%.[44] Other patients with immunosuppression can have prolonged shedding of parainfluenza viruses, particularly parainfluenza type 3.[45] Fatal pneumonias have been described in children with severe combined immunodeficiency syndrome.[46] In developed countries, parainfluenza virus infections do not appear to be more severe in children with HIV, although prolonged virus shedding occurs.[47] In developing countries, parainfluenza virus infections have been associated with increased morbidity and mortality.[48] Rarely, parainfluenza virus types 2 and 3 have been isolated from cerebrospinal fluid in association with aseptic meningitis. Parainfluenza viruses have not been strongly associated with asthma in adults.[49] However, childhood asthma continues to be linked with early respiratory viral infection.[50]

Diagnosis

As with many viruses, three approaches to the diagnosis of parainfluenza virus infection are currently used: viral culture, detection of viral antigen or nucleic acid, and serologic analysis. The gold standard remains the isolation of virus in tissue culture. Parainfluenza viruses are rarely isolated from healthy children, so the finding of a parainfluenza virus with an acute respiratory illness is strong proof of an association. The sensitivity of the method is greatest in primary infection, where 4 to 5 $\log_{10}$ of virus can be recovered per milliliter of nasal secretions for up to 10 days after the onset of illness.[51] In adults and older children undergoing repeated infections, the height and duration of virus shedding are much lower. In suspected lower respiratory tract disease in an immunocompromised host or transplant recipient, direct sampling of the lower respiratory tract with lung biopsy or lavage may be necessary to recover the agent. Nasal washings inoculated into shell vial cultures may be positive early (see Chapter 17) but may also remain positive for several weeks after initial shedding, which complicates their interpretation.

Sensitive cell lines for parainfluenza virus include primary rhesus or cynomolgus monkey kidney cells and a monkey kidney line, LLC-MK2. After primary isolation and identification with hemadsorption, the putative parainfluenza virus must be typed via immunofluorescence or hemadsorption inhibition. With parainfluenza type 2, hemadsorption cannot be relied on for identification of all isolates, and immunofluorescence must be used to detect growth. Critical to the success of isolating parainfluenza viruses is the way in which the specimen is collected (optimally with nasal wash or nasal aspiration), refrigerated (the specimen must be kept at 4°C), and transported (promptly to the laboratory). Rapid diagnosis does not have the sensitivity of tissue culture and entails direct immunofluorescence of exfoliated cells and enzyme-linked immunosorbent assay (ELISA) capture techniques. No commercial ELISA kits are currently available. Polymerase chain reaction amplification has been described that can detect parainfluenza types 1, 2, and 3 in a single multiplex assay[52] and has sensitivity of 95% to 100% and specificity of 97% to 100%.[53] PCR has been reported to increase the sensitivity of viral detection by 1.5 times compared with culture.[54] Serologic tests can be used to track the age-related acquisition of infection in infancy, and comparison of antibody titers in closely timed paired sera during and after an illness is a moderately sensitive and specific, although slow, method of diagnosis. An acute serum specimen should be obtained within 4 days of the onset of illness, and a convalescent serum specimen within 2 weeks of the illness.

Therapy

The effectiveness of specific antivirals for parainfluenza virus infection has not been established. The use of ribavirin as an aerosolized or intravenous preparation has been reported after heart and HSCT in anecdotal cases,[41] but controlled studies are lacking.

In children, the weight of opinion is that aerosolized steroids have an important role to play in the management of croup as a clinical illness.[55] One study compared nebulized budesonide with intramuscular dexamethasone and placebo in moderately severe croup in 144 children seen in the emergency department.[56] All patients received racemic epinephrine and cool mist. Viral cultures were done in 133 of the patients, with parainfluenza viruses recovered from 46 of the children, 29 of whom had parainfluenza type 1. Only seven viruses other than parainfluenza were identified. Seventy-one percent of the placebo group needed hospitalization versus 38% in the budesonide group and 23% in the dexamethasone group. The results in each group were significantly different from each other, and systemic steroids are the current treatment of choice. Nebulized epinephrine provides short-term relief, but return to the baseline obstruction occurs within 2 hours.[57] Its use in combination with either oral or intramuscular dexamethasone seems indicated. The value of cool mist has not been shown in small controlled trials, but the clinical impression is one of improvement of children in the shower or during a ride to the hospital with exposure to cool air.[58]

Prevention

An inactivated whole-virus trivalent parainfluenza vaccine was explored in the late 1960s. Although it was immunogenic, it was not protective.[59] This vaccine was evaluated in parallel with an inactivated respiratory syncytial virus (RSV) vaccine that resulted in enhanced illness on natural reexposure to RSV. Because the trivalent parainfluenza vaccine did not enhance illness, development of inactivated and subunit vaccines has continued. Several subunit vaccines have been developed, but none have entered clinical testing.

Two live-attenuated, intranasally administered parainfluenza type 3 vaccines are in development.[60] One is derived from a bovine parainfluenza type 3 virus. This vaccine protects against a challenge with human parainfluenza type 3 virus in chimpanzees. The bovine strain has been evaluated in phase I trials in adults, children, and infants.[61-63] It appears to be safe and immunogenic and is undergoing commercial development. In parallel, a cold-adapted parainfluenza type 3 virus vaccine was attenuated with multiple passages of a human strain in tissue culture.[64] After 45 passages in tissue culture cells, it was evaluated for protection in a chimpanzee challenge model and subsequently in stepwise studies in young children and infants.[65] The safety and immunogenicity profiles of the cold-passaged virus are comparable with those of the bovine strain, and it is undergoing further clinical evaluation. The potential for use of attenuated parainfluenza type 3 (PIV3) strains to generate parainfluenza type 1 and 2 vaccines on the same genetic background as the type 3 strains is now being explored. Finally, the bovine PIV3 has been used as a backbone into which the human PIV3 HN gene has been inserted as has the RSV F protein.[66] Critical questions that must still be answered are whether these vaccines can enable infants to mount an immune response, whether interference between strains occurs, and what degree of protection or amelioration of illness is provided by such vaccine approaches.[67]

REFERENCES

1. Chanock RM, Parrott RH, Cook K, et al. Newly recognized myxovirus in children with respiratory diseases. *N Engl J Med.* 1958;258:207-213.
2. Durbin AP, Hall SL, Siew JW, et al. Recovery of infectious human parainfluenza virus type 3 from cDNA. *Virology.* 1997;235:323-332.
3. Lamb RA, Parks GD. Paramyxoviridae: The viruses and their replication. In: Knipe DM, Howley PM, eds. *Fields Virology.* Philadelphia: Lippincott Williams and Wilkins; 2007:1449-1496.
4. Karron RA, Collins PL. Parainfluenza viruses. In: Knipe DM, Howley PM, eds. *Fields Virology.* Philadelphia: Williams and Wilkins; 2007:1497-1526.
5. Wang LF, Michelski WP, Yu M, et al. A novel P/V/C gene in the new member of the member of the Paramyxoviridae family, which causes lethal infection in humans, horses, and other animals. *J Virol.* 1998;72:1482-1490.
6. Wong KT, Shieh WJ, Zaki SR, Tan CT. Nipah virus infection; an emerging paramyxoviral zoonosis. *Springer Semin Immunopathol.* 2002;24:215-228.
7. van den Hoogen BG, de Jong JC, Groen J, et al. A newly discovered human pneumovirus isolated from young children with respiratory tract disease. *Nature Med.* 2001;7:719-724.
8. Yao Q, Hu X, Compans RW. Association of the parainfluenza virus fusion and hemagglutinin-neuraminidase glycoproteins on cell surfaces. *J Virol.* 1997;71:650-656.
9. Lamb RA. Paramyxovirus fusion: A hypothesis for changes. *Virology.* 1993;197:1-11.
10. Tashiro M, Yokogoshi Y, Tobita K, et al. Tryptase Clara, an activating protease for Sendai virus in rat lungs, is involved in pneumopathogenicity. *J Virol.* 1992;66:7211-7216.
11. He B, Paterson RG, Stock N, et al. Recovery of paramyxovirus simian virus 5 with a V protein lacking the conserved cysteine-rich domain: The multifunctional V protein blocks both interferon-beta induction and interferon signaling. *Virology.* 2002; 303:15-32.
12. Wright PF. Parainfluenza viruses 342-350. In: Belshe RB, ed. *Textbook of Human Virology.* 2nd ed. St Louis: Mosby; 1991.
13. Parrott RH, Vargosko AJ, Kim HW, et al. Clinical features of infection with hemadsorption viruses. *N Engl J Med.* 1959;260:731-738.
14. Massion PP, Funari P, Ikeda S, et al. Parainfluenza (Sendai) virus infects ciliated cells and secretory cells but not basal cells of rat tracheal epithelium. *Am J Respir Cell Mol Biol.* 1993;9:361-370.
15. Blau DM, Compans RW. Polarization of viral entry and release in epithelial cells. *Semin Virol.* 1996;7:245-253.
16. Tashiro M, Yokogoshi M, Tobita K, et al. Organ tropism of Sendai virus in mice; proteolytic activation of the fusion glycoprotein in mouse organs and budding site at the bronchial epithelium. *J Virol.* 1990;64:3627-3634.
17. Tashiro M, Seto JT, Choosakul S, et al. Changes in specific cleavability of the Sendai virus fusion protein: Implications for pathogenicity in mice. *J Virol.* 1992;73:1575-1579.
18. Morel-Barbey CL, Oeltmann TN, Edwards KM, et al. Role of respiratory tract protease in infectivity of influenza virus. *J Infect Dis.* 1987;155;667-672.
19. Spriggs MK, Murphy BR, Prince GA, et al. Expression of the F and HN glycoproteins of human parainfluenza virus type 3 by recombinant vaccinia viruses: Contribution of the individual proteins to host immunity. *J Virol.* 1987;61:3416-3423.
20. Glezen WP, Frank AL, Taber LH, et al. Parainfluenza virus type 3: Seasonality and risk of infection and reinfection in young children. *J Infect Dis.* 1984;150:851-857.
21. Reed G, Jewett PH, Thompson J, et al. Epidemiology and clinical impact of parainfluenza virus infections in otherwise healthy infants and young children < 5 years old. *J Infect Dis.* 1997;175: 807-813.
22. van Wyke Coelingh KL, Winter C, Murphy BR. Antigentic variation in the hemagglutinin-neuraminidase protein of human parainfluenza type 3 virus. *Virology.* 1985;143:569-582.
23. Kapikian AZ, Chanock RM, Reichelderfer TE, et al. Inoculation of human volunteers with parainfluenza virus type 3. *JAMA.* 1961;178:537-541.
24. Karron RA, Wright PF, Newman FK, et al. A live human parainfluenza type 3 virus is attenuated and immunogenic in healthy infants and children. *J Infect Dis.* 1995;172:1445-1450.
25. Smith CB, Purcell RH, Bellanti JA, et al. Protective effect of antibody to parainfluenza type 1 virus. *N Engl J Med.* 1966;275:1145-1152.
26. Mazanec MB, Coudret CL, Fletcher DR. Intracellular neutralization virus by immunoglobulin A anti-hemagglutination monoclonal antibodies. *J Virol.* 1995;69:1339-1343.
27. Hou S, Doherty PC. Clearance of Sendai virus CD8+ T cells requires direct targeting to virus-infected epithelium. *Eur J Immunol.* 1995;25:111.
28. Sieg S, Xia L, Huang Y, et al. Specific inhibition of granzyme B by parainfluenza virus type 3. *J Virol.* 1995;69:3538-3541.
29. Glezen WP, Loda FA, Clyde WA, et al. Epidemiologic patterns of acute lower respiratory disease of children in a pediatric group practice. *J Pediatr.* 1971;78:397-406.
30. Gardner SD. The isolation of parainfluenza 4 sub-types A and B in England and serological studies of their prevalence. *J Hyg (Lond).* 1969;67:540-545.
31. Muchmore HG, Parkinson AJ, Humphries JE, et al. Persistent parainfluenza virus shedding during isolation at the South Pole. *Nature.* 1981;289:187-189.
32. Marx A, Torok TJ, Holman RC, et al. Pediatric hospitalizations for croup (laryngotracheobronchitis): Biennial increases associated with human parainfluenza virus 1 epidemics. *J Infect Dis.* 1997;176:1423-1427.
33. Denny FW, Murphy TF, Clyde WA Jr, et al. Croup: An 11 year study in a pediatric practice. *Pediatrics.* 1983;71:871-876.
34. Hendrickson KJ, Kuhn SM, Savatski LL. Epidemiology and cost of infection with human parainfluenza virus types 1 and 2 in young children. *Clin Infect Dis.* 1994;18:770-779.
35. Chanock RM, Parrott RH. Acute respiratory disease in infancy and childhood: Present understanding and prospects for prevention. *J Pediatr.* 1965;36:21-30.
36. Karron RA, O'Brien KL, Froehlich JL, et al. Molecular epidemiology of parainfluenza type 3 virus outbreak on a pediatric ward. *J Infect Dis.* 1993;167:1441-1445.
37. Nicholson KG, Kent J, Hammersley V, et al. Acute viral infections of upper respiratory tract in elderly people living in the community: Comparative, prospective, population based study of disease burden. *BMJ.* 1997;315:1060-1064.
38. Echevarria JE, Erdman DD, Swierkosz EM, et al. Simultaneous detection and identification of human parainfluenza viruses 1, 2 and 3 from clinical samples by multiplex PCR. *J Clin Microbiol.* 1998;36:1388-1391.
39. Falsey AR, McCann RM, Hall WJ, et al. Acute respiratory tract infection in daycare centers for older persons. *J Am Geriatr Soc.* 1995;43:30-36.
40. Henderson FW, Collier AM, Sanyal MA, et al. A longitudinal study of respiratory viruses and bacteria in the etiology of acute otitis media with effusion. *N Engl J Med.* 1982;306:1377-1384.
41. Boeckh M. The challenge of respiratory virus infections in hematopoietic cell transplant recipients. *Br J Haematol.* 2008;143: 455-467.
42. Wendt CH, Weisdorf DJ, Jordan CM, et al. Parainfluenza virus respiratory infection after bone marrow transplantation. *N Engl J Med.* 1992;326:921-926.
43. Cortez KJ, Erdman DD, Peret TC, et al. Outbreak of human parainfluenza virus 3 infections in a hematopoietic stem cell transplant population. *J Infect Dis.* 2001;184:1093-1097.
44. Lewis VA, Champlin R, Englund J, et al. Respiratory disease due to parainfluenza virus in adult bone marrow transplant recipients. *J Clin Infect Dis.* 1996;23:1033-1037.
45. Scully RE, Mark EJ, McNeeley WF, et al. Case records of the Massachusetts General Hospital. *N Engl J Med.* 1996;335:1133-1140.
46. Jarvis WR, Middleton PJ, Gelfand EW. Parainfluenza pneumonia in severe combined immunodeficiency disease. *J Pediatr.* 1979;93:423-425.
47. King JC Jr, Burke AR, Clemens JD, et al. Respiratory syncytial virus illnesses in human immunodeficiency virus- and noninfected children. *Pediatr Infect Dis J.* 1993;12:733-739.
48. Madhi SA, Ramasamy N, Petersen K, et al. Severe lower respiratory tract infections associated with human parainfluenza viruses 1-3 in children infected and noninfected with HIV type 1. *Eur J Clin Microbiol Infect Dis.* 2002;21:499-505.
49. Sokhandan M, McFadden R, Huang YT, et al. The contribution of respiratory viruses to severe exacerbations of asthma in adults. *Chest.* 1995;107:1570-1575.
50. Wu P, Dupont WD, Griffin MR, et al. Evidence of a causal role of winter virus infection during infancy in early childhood asthma. *Am J Respir Crit Care Med.* 2008;178:1097-1098.
51. Frank AL, Taber LH, Wells CR, et al. Patterns of shedding of myxoviruses and paramyxoviruses in children. *J Infect Dis.* 1981;144:433-441.

52. Fan J, Hendrikson KJ, Savatski LL. Rapid simultaneous diagnosis of infections with respiratory syncytial viruses A and B, influenza viruses A and B, and human parainfluenza types 1,2, and 3 by multiplex quantitative reverse transcription-polymerase chain reaction-enzyme hybridization assay (Hexaplex). *Clin Infect Dis.* 1998;26:1397-1402.

53. Henrickson KJ. Parainfluenza viruses. *Clin Microbiol Rev.* 2003; 16:242-264.

54. Weinberg GA, Erdman DD, Edwards KM, et al. Superiority of reverse-transcriptase polymerase chain reaction to conventional viral culture in the diagnosis of acute respiratory tract infections in children. *J Infect Dis.* 2004;189:706-710.

55. Jaffee DM. The treatment of croup with glucocorticoids. *N Engl J Med.* 1998;339:553-555.

56. Johnson DA, Jacobson S, Edney PC, et al. A comparison of nebulized budesonide, intramuscular dexamethasone, and placebo for moderately severe croup. *N Engl J Med.* 1998;339: 498-503.

57. Skolnick NS. Treatment of croup: A critical review. *Am J Dis Child.* 1998;143:1045-1049.

58. Bourchier D, Dawson KP, Fergusson DM. Humidification in viral croup: A controlled trial. *Aust Paediatr J.* 1984;20:289-291.

59. Chin J, Magoffin RL, Shearer LA, et al. Field evaluation of a respiratory syncytial virus vaccine and a trivalent parainfluenza virus vaccine in a pediatric population. *Am J Epidemiol.* 1969;89:449-463.

60. Murphy BR, Collins PL. Current status of respiratory syncytial virus (RSV) and parainfluenza virus type 3 (PIV3) vaccine development: Memorandum from a joint WHO/NIAID meeting. *Bull World Health Organ.* 1997;75:307-313.

61. Clements ML, Belshe RB, King J, et al. Evaluation of bovine, cold-adapted human, and wild-type human parainfluenza type 3 viruses in adult volunteers and in chimpanzees. *J Clin Microbiol.* 1991;29:1175-1182.

62. Karron RA, Wright PF, Hall SL, et al. A live attenuated bovine parainfluenza virus type 3 vaccine is safe, infectious, immuno-genic, and phenotypically stable in infants and children. *J Infect Dis.* 1995;171:1107-1114.

63. Karron RA, Makene M, Gay K, et al. Evaluation of a live attenuated bovine parainfluenza type 3 vaccine in two- to six-month-old infants. *Pediatr Infect Dis J.* 1996;15:650-654.

64. Belshe RB, Hissom FK. Cold adaption of parainfluenza virus type 3: Induction of three phenotypic markers. *J Med Virol.* 1982;10: 235-242.

65. Karron RA, Belshe RB, Wright PF, et al. A live human parainfluenza type 3 virus vaccine is attenuated and immunogenic in young infants. *Pediatr Infect Dis.* 2003;22:394-405.

66. Tang RS, Spaete RR, Thompson MW, et al. Development of a PIV-vectored RSV vaccine: preclinical evaluation of safety, toxicity, and enhanced disease and initial clinical testing in healthy adults. *Vaccine.* 2008;26:6373-6382.

67. Sato M, Wright PF. Current status of vaccines for parainfluenza virus infections. *Pediatr Infect Dis J.* 2008;27:S123-S125. Review.

157

Mumps Virus

NATHAN LITMAN | STEPHEN G. BAUM

Mumps is an acute generalized viral infection that occurs primarily in school-aged children and adolescents. The most prominent manifestation of this disease is nonsuppurative swelling and tenderness of the salivary glands, with one or both parotid glands involved in most cases. The disease is benign and self-limited, with one third of affected persons having subclinical infection. Meningitis and epididymo-orchitis represent the two most important of the less frequent manifestations of this disease. As is characteristic of many viral infections, mumps is usually a more severe illness in persons past the age of puberty than in children and more commonly leads to extrasalivary gland involvement in these older patients. Although the use of effective vaccines has markedly reduced the incidence of mumps, the occurrence of outbreaks of mumps in the United Kingdom, Canada, United States, and elsewhere in recent years has raised concerns regarding the possible resurgence of the disease.

History

Hippocrates described mumps and its contagious characteristics in the fifth century BC. In the late 1700s, Hamilton emphasized the occurrence of orchitis as a manifestation of mumps. The experimental production of the disease in monkeys by Johnson and Goodpasture in 1934[1] provided the evidence that a filterable virus was present in the saliva of patients with mumps. In 1945, Habel reported the cultivation of mumps virus in the chick embryo.[2] Enders and colleagues described the skin test and development of complement-fixing antibodies after mumps in humans.[3] A killed virus vaccine used in the early 1950s on human subjects achieved limited success[4] and, in 1966, Buynak and Hilleman reported the development of an effective live virus vaccine.[5]

The etymology of the word *mumps* is unclear. It may arise from the English noun *mump*, meaning a lump, or from the English verb *to mump*, defined as "to be sulky"—a description of the characteristic facial expression. Alternatively, the term *mumps* has been ascribed to the mumbling speech pattern of the affected person. In the older literature, mumps may have been called "epidemic parotitis."

Virology

Mumps virus is a member of the Paramyxoviridae family, which includes the following genera: *Rubulavirus* (mumps virus, New Castle disease virus, human parainfluenza virus types 2, 4a, and 4b), *Paramyxovirus* (human parainfluenza virus types 1 and 3), *Morbillivirus* (measles), and *Pneumovirus* (human respiratory syncytial virus). The complete mumps virion has an irregular spherical shape, with a diameter ranging from 90 to 300 nm and averaging about 200 nm. The nucleocapsid is enclosed by an envelope that has three layers and is about 10 nm thick.[6] The external surface is regularly studded with glycoproteins possessing hemagglutinin, neuraminidase, and cell fusion activity. The middle component of the envelope is a lipid bilayer acquired from the host cell as the virus buds off the cytoplasmic membrane. The innermost surface of the envelope is a nonglycosylated membrane protein that maintains the outer structure of the virus. The genome of the virus is contained in a nucleocapsid that is a helical structure composed of a continuous linear molecule of single-stranded RNA genome surrounded by symmetrically repeating protein subunits. The genome codes for eight proteins—the hemagglutinin-neuraminidase protein (HN), the fusion protein (F), the nucleocapsid protein (NP), the phosphoprotein (P), the matrix protein (M), the hydrophobic protein (SH), and the L proteins.[7] The P protein contains two nonstructural proteins, V and I. F and HN proteins appear to be the most prominent determinants of immunity. Although only one serotype of mumps virus is known, there are 13 genotypes (A to M) that have been determined, based on sequencing of the SH protein, which is the most variable protein among mumps strains.[8-10]

Mumps virus is ether-sensitive by virtue of its lipid envelope. It is stable at 4°C for several days and at −65°C for months to years; however, repeated freezing and thawing may diminish viral activity.

The virus replicates in a variety of cell cultures as well as in embryonated hens' eggs.[11] For primary viral isolation, monkey kidney, human embryonic kidney, or HeLa cell cultures are used for primary isolation. Cytopathic effects such as the appearance of intracytoplasmic eosinophilic inclusions, rounding of cells, or the fusion of cells into giant multinucleate syncytia may be noted.[12] The presence of mumps virus is usually confirmed by the hemagglutination inhibition (HAI) test, which uses convalescent serum after mumps infection to inhibit the adsorption of chick erythrocytes added to mumps-infected epithelial cells.

Epidemiology

Mumps is endemic throughout the world. In the United States, before the licensing of live-attenuated mumps vaccine in 1967, epidemics occurred every 2 to 5 years.[13] Although the disease occurred throughout the year, the peak incidence was between January and May.[14] Epidemics have been reported in military populations and other closed communities such as prisons, boarding schools, ships, and remote islands.[15,16] Meyer demonstrated that mumps is spread throughout the community by children in schools, with secondary spread to family members.[17] There has been more than a 99% decline in the annual U.S. incidence of mumps since 1967, with an average of only 265 cases/year reported to the Centers for Disease Control and Prevention (CDC) from 2001 to 2005; the seasonal variation that was evident in earlier years is no longer apparent.[18] However, there have been outbreaks of mumps reported from various sites, including the Netherlands,[8] United Kingdom,[19] United States,[20] and Canada.[21] In the 2006 outbreak in the United States, 6584 cases of mumps were detected; 85% of patients were in Iowa and the seven contiguous states; the highest attack rate was for the age group of 18 to 24 years, which comprised 29% of all cases, and 83% of this group attended college.[20] The outbreak virus was of genotype G, the same virus genotype that had caused an outbreak in the United Kingdom during 2004 to 2006.[19] Surprisingly, for those patients with known vaccine status, only 13% had not received vaccine, and 63% had received two or more doses of mumps containing vaccine. The reasons for the outbreaks and the apparent vaccine failures are not clear, and may have been multiple.[21,22] These include possible waning immunity and exposure pressure from crowded conditions in dormitories, where susceptible individuals may have gathered. Genotypic differences between the vaccine Jeryl Lynn strain (A) and the circulating mumps strain in outbreaks in the United States and United Kingdom (G) were present. However, the genotype A viruses were apparently effective in controlling genotype G outbreaks, so the role of genotype differences in vaccine failure, if any, are unclear. The epidemic rapidly subsided, so that by 2008 there were only 376 cases of mumps reported to the CDC.

Mumps is uncommon in infants younger than 1 year. Resistance to infection in this age group is on the basis of passive immunity acquired by the placental transfer of maternal antibody. In the prevaccine era, more than 50% of cases occurred in the 5- to 9-year-old age group, and 90% of the cases occurred in children younger than 14 years. In 2001, 49% of infections were reported in persons older than 15 years. In the prevaccine era, 80% to 90% U.S. of adults older than 20 years were immune to mumps on the basis of natural infection. At present, in the United States, immunity to mumps in children and most young adults relies on prior vaccination. Men and women have the same frequency of development of parotitis with mumps infection.[23]

Humans are the only known natural host; however, monkeys and other laboratory animals have been experimentally infected.[1] Although persistent infections in cultured cells are commonly established by mumps virus,[24] a carrier state is not known to exist in humans.

Pathogenesis

The virus is naturally transmitted via direct contact, droplet nuclei, or fomites and enters through the nose or mouth. More intimate contact is needed to transmit mumps than for measles or varicella. The period of peak contagion is just before or at the onset of parotitis.

Experimental mumps infection has been produced in humans and monkeys by direct instillation of the virus into Stensen's duct.[1] However, the incubation period in this experimental model is shorter than in naturally occurring disease, and initial infection of the parotid gland does not explain the fact that meningitis or other manifestations of mumps infection may occur before the onset of parotitis. It has been suggested that during the incubation period, the virus proliferates in the upper respiratory tract epithelium and viremia ensues, with secondary dissemination and localization to glandular and neural tissue.[25,26]

Pathology

Salivary glands from patients infected with mumps are rarely available for pathologic examination because of the benign course in the great majority of the cases. When parotid glands have been examined, diffuse interstitial edema has been found, along with a serofibrinous exudate consisting primarily of mononuclear leukocytes. Neutrophils and necrotic debris accumulate within the ductal lumen, and the ductal epithelium shows degenerative changes. The glandular cells are relatively spared, but may also be involved with edema and overflow of the inflammatory reaction from the interstitial tissues. The multinucleate syncytia and intracytoplasmic eosinophilic inclusions that are occasionally seen in mumps-infected tissue culture are not present in vivo. When the pancreas or the testis is involved, the microscopic picture is similar to that seen in the salivary glands, except that interstitial hemorrhage and polymorphonuclear leukocytes are more frequently noted in orchitis. Local areas of infarction may occur because the vascular supply is compromised by increased pressure caused by edema within an inelastic tunica albuginea. When the process has been particularly severe, atrophy of the germinal epithelium may result, with accompanying hyalinization and fibrosis.

The description of brain involvement in mumps encephalitis has most often been that of a postinfectious encephalitis characterized by perivenous demyelinization, perivascular mononuclear cuffing, and a generalized increase in microglial cells, with relative sparing of neurons.[27] However, descriptions of what appears to be a primary mumps encephalitis have been reported that show widespread neuronolysis but no evidence of demyelinization.[28]

Clinical Manifestations

The incubation period of mumps averages 16 to 18 days, with a range of 2 to 4 weeks. Characteristically, the prodromal symptoms are non-specific and include low-grade fever, anorexia, malaise, and headache. Within 1 day, the nature of the illness becomes apparent when the patient complains of an earache, and tenderness can be elicited by palpation of the ipsilateral parotid. The involved gland is soon visibly enlarged and progresses to a maximum size over the next 2 to 3 days. The most severe pain accompanies the period of rapid enlargement. At its height, parotitis results in lifting of the ear lobe upward and outward. Lesser degrees of enlargement can more readily be appreciated by viewing the patient from behind. The enlarged parotid gland obscures the angle of the mandible, whereas cervical adenopathy does not hide this anatomic landmark. Usually, one parotid gland enlarges 1 or 2 days after the other; however, mumps results in unilateral parotitis alone in one quarter of patients with salivary gland involvement. The orifice of Stensen's duct is frequently edematous and erythematous. Trismus may result from the parotitis, and the patient may have difficulty with pronunciation and mastication. Ingestion of citrus fruits or juices typically exacerbates the pain. During the first 3 days of illness, the patient's temperature may range from normal to 40°C. After parotid swelling has reached its peak, pain, fever, and tenderness rapidly resolve, and the parotid gland returns to normal size within 1 week. Complications of parotitis are rare but are reported to include sialectasia resulting in recurrent acute and chronic sialadenitis.[29]

Involvement of the other salivary glands may occur in conjunction with parotitis in up to 10% of cases but is rare as the sole manifestation of mumps infection (Table 157-1). Submandibular gland involvement mimics signs of anterior cervical lymphadenopathy. The sublingual glands are the least frequently inflamed during mumps infection; when involvement occurs, it is usually bilateral and may be associated with swelling of the tongue. Presternal pitting edema develops in 6% of patients with mumps, most commonly in those who have submandibular adenitis.[30] The proposed mechanism for the involvement of the tongue and presternal area is obstruction of the lymphatic drainage of those regions by enlarged salivary glands.

Central nervous system involvement is the most common extrasalivary gland manifestation of mumps. As documentation of the remarkable neurotropism of this virus, Bang and Bang[31] reported the presence of cerebrospinal fluid (CSF) pleocytosis in 51% of 255 patients with mumps but without other evidence of meningitis. Clinical meningitis occurs in 1% to 10% of persons with mumps parotitis,[32] but on the other hand, only 40% to 50% of patients with mumps meningitis, confirmed by serology or viral isolation, have parotitis.[32-35] Meningeal symptoms, like any of the other manifestations of mumps infection, may occur before, during, after, or in the absence of parotitis. Its onset averages 4 days after the appearance of salivary gland involvement but may be as early as 1 week before or as late as 2 weeks after parotitis.[31-34] Men are afflicted three times as often as women,[32-35] but the age distribution is the same as for uncomplicated mumps. Ritter has noted that mumps meningitis with parotitis is most frequent in the spring, whereas meningitis without parotitis is most frequent in summer.[33]

TABLE 157-1	Frequency of Common Clinical Manifestations of Mumps
Manifestation	*Frequency (%)*
Glandular	
Parotitis	60-70
Submandibular and/or sublingual sialadenitis	10
Epididymo-orchitis*	25 (postpubertal men)
Oophoritis*	5 (postpubertal women)
Neural	
Cerebrospinal fluid pleocytosis	50
Meningitis	1-10
Encephalitis	0.1
Transient high-frequency deafness	4
Other	
Electrocardiographic abnormalities	5-15
Renal function abnormalities (mild)	>60

*Rare before puberty and usually unilateral.

The typical clinical features associated with viral meningitis are present—that is, headache, vomiting, fever, and nuchal rigidity. Lumbar puncture yields CSF containing 10 to 2000 white blood cells (WBC)/mm^3. The predominating cells are usually lymphocytes, but 20% to 25% of patients have a polymorphonuclear leukocyte predominance.[34] Protein levels are normal to mildly elevated, and 90% to 95% of patients have a CSF protein content lower than 70 mg/dL.[34,35] Hypoglycorrhachia (CSF glucose concentration lower than 40 mg/dL) is reported in 6% to 30% of the patients[34-36] and appears to be more common than in other viral meningitides. These CSF abnormalities may persist for 5 weeks or longer.[33,36] The finding of a depressed CSF sugar level with a moderate to marked pleocytosis may cause the physician to consider bacterial meningitis in the differential diagnosis, especially if neutrophils predominate, as they may early in the disease. As in other cases of meningitis, when mononuclear cells prevail in the CSF, tuberculous and fungal disorders should be considered.

Abatement of fever by lysis and resolution of symptoms generally occur 3 to 10 days after the onset of illness. The meningitis is benign, with complete recovery and an absence of sequelae. Before the introduction of the live-attenuated mumps vaccine in 1967, mumps accounted for approximately 10% of cases of aseptic meningitis in the United States. At present, aseptic meningitis is rarely attributed to mumps.

Encephalitis is reported to occur in from 1 in 6000[37] to 400[38] cases of mumps. The former ratio probably represents a more accurate estimate. There appears to be a bimodal distribution of cases according to the time of onset—an early group in which onset coincides with the presence of parotitis and a larger late group in which the condition develops 7 to 10 days after the onset of parotitis. As noted earlier ("Pathology"), early-onset encephalitis represents direct damage to neurons as a result of viral invasion, whereas late-onset disease is a postinfectious demyelinating process related to the host response to infection. These two processes probably represent the ends of a continuum of disease. Some patients die after the primary viral invasion of the brain, and some of those who survive produce antibodies to the virus or neural breakdown products and develop an "autoimmune" reaction. The clinical features are generally those of a nonfocal encephalitis; in addition to marked changes in the level of consciousness, neurologic findings may include convulsions, paresis, aphasia, and involuntary movements. CSF values are similar to those in uncomplicated meningitis. Fever is high, and characteristically temperatures of 40° to 41°C are present. Neurologic manifestations and fever gradually resolve over a period of 1 to 2 weeks. Sequelae such as psychomotor retardation and convulsive disorders are reported,[33-35] but their frequency cannot be determined from the available data. Death occurs in 1.4% of reported cases.[38]

Through the mid-1960s, mumps was the leading recognized cause of viral encephalitis in the United States, being responsible for 20% to 30% of cases. However, by 1981, it represented only 0.5% of cases of viral encephalitis nationwide and, by the 1990s, mumps encephalitis was rare. The major factor accounting for this change was an effective mumps immunization program.

The term *meningoencephalitis* is frequently used when describing patients with various degrees of CNS involvement.[28,32,33,36,39] This term should be eliminated in reference to mumps because it confuses a common and essentially benign condition (meningitis) with a relatively uncommon and serious illness (encephalitis) that might result in neurologic residua or death. Clearly, many patients with mumps meningitis may have lethargy, as may a large percentage of those with any viral infection such as influenza. However, the presence of profound changes in the level of consciousness or other findings suggestive of supratentorial involvement indicate the clear diagnosis of encephalitis as distinct from the ambiguous designation of meningoencephalitis. Although nuchal rigidity and CSF pleocytosis may be present in patients with encephalitis, the meningeal component is a trivial aspect of this illness.

Transient high-frequency-range deafness has been reported in 4.4% of cases of mumps in a military population.[40] Permanent unilateral deafness occurs in 1 in 20,000 cases of mumps.[41] The onset of otologic symptoms may be gradual or abrupt; vertigo is frequently present. On subsequent testing, vestibular function has been normal.

Other neurologic syndromes rarely associated with mumps include cerebellar ataxia,[42] facial palsy,[43] transverse myelitis,[44] ascending polyradiculitis (Guillain-Barré syndrome),[45] and a poliomyelitis-like syndrome.[46] There are now several well-documented cases of aqueductal stenosis and hydrocephalus developing after CNS infection caused by mumps.[47-49] Experimental and clinical reports have clearly implicated mumps as the probable causative agent of this disorder.[50-52]

Epididymo-orchitis is the most common extrasalivary gland manifestation in the adult. It develops in 20% to 30% of postpubertal male adolescents with mumps infection and is bilateral in one of six of those with testicular involvement.[53,54] Although it has been reported in infancy, it is rare before puberty. Two thirds of cases occur during the first week of parotitis, and another 25% arise during the second week.[53] However, gonadal involvement may precede parotitis or occur as the only manifestation of mumps. The onset is abrupt, with temperatures in the range of 39° to 41°C, chills, headache, vomiting, and testicular pain. Genital examination reveals warmth, swelling, and tenderness of the involved testicle and erythema of the scrotum. Epididymitis is present in 85% of cases and usually precedes the orchitis. The testis may be enlarged to three to four times its normal size. Constitutional complaints and fever generally parallel the severity of gonadal involvement. Fever resolves in 84% of patients in 5 days or less. Pain and swelling resolve shortly after defervescence. However, tenderness may persist for longer than 2 weeks in 20% of the cases.[53] Early in convalescence, a loss of turgor may be appreciated. When testes are examined months to years later, some degree of atrophy is noted in 50% of patients.

The anxiety engendered by mumps orchitis is difficult to allay. The psychological fears of sexual impotence and sterility far outweigh the potential debility from testicular atrophy. Clearly, most men who have unilateral orchitis need fear nothing other than a possible cosmetic imbalance. Even those with bilateral involvement should be assured that impotence (other than psychogenic) is not a sequela and that sterility is rare. In large surveys of infertile men, mumps is infrequently implicated as the causative disorder. Twenty-eight cases of testicular malignancy in men with atrophy of the testis due to mumps orchitis have been reported.[55]

Oophoritis develops in 5% of postpubertal women with mumps. Symptoms include fever, nausea, vomiting, and lower abdominal pain. Impaired fertility and premature menopause have been reported as a consequence of ovarian involvement but must be considered to be rare.[56]

Joint involvement during mumps is noted infrequently in adults and rarely in children.[57,58] Migratory polyarthritis is the most frequently described clinical form. Monoarticular arthritis and arthralgia have also been reported; both large and small joints are involved. Symptoms most commonly start 10 to 14 days after the onset of parotitis and may last up to 5 weeks. The process resolves spontaneously without residual joint damage.

Pancreatitis is manifested by severe epigastric pain and tenderness accompanied by fever, nausea, and vomiting. It is uncommon as a severe illness; however, many affected persons may complain of mild degrees of upper abdominal discomfort.

Electrocardiographic changes appear in up to 15% of patients with mumps; the most common abnormalities are depressed ST segments, flattened or inverted T waves, and prolonged P-R intervals.[59,60] Clinically manifested myocarditis is rare; however, deaths associated with myocarditis have been reported during the acute illness and after a chronically progressive deteriorating course.[59,60]

Utz and associates[61] have prospectively evaluated renal function in 20 young adult Navy servicemen admitted with mumps. These investigators discovered transient mild to moderate abnormalities of urinary concentration, creatinine clearance, and phenolsulfonphthalein excretion in most of this group. Hughes and co-workers have reported two deaths related to mumps-associated nephritis.[62]

A variety of other manifestations have accompanied mumps infection, but must be considered extremely rare; these include thyroiditis,[63] mastitis,[64] prostatitis,[65] hepatitis,[66] and thrombocytopenia.[67]

Complications

Gestational viral infections were extensively investigated in a controlled cohort study by Siegel and colleagues.[68-70] They observed excess fetal deaths when mumps developed during the first trimester; second- and third-trimester mumps infections were not associated with increased fetal mortality.[68] Low birth weight (less than 2500 g) was identified in 7.7% of infants born to mumps-infected mothers, compared with 3.3% of a control group; this is not, however, a statistically significant difference. Although the number of cases was small, when the data were analyzed with respect to the onset of infection, the effect on birth weight was greatest when mumps occurred in the first trimester.[69] A variety of congenital malformations have been described in pregnancies complicated by maternal mumps[71]; however, these anomalies are described in single case reports without comparison with an uninfected control population. As reported by Siegel and associates,[70] occurrence rates of major congenital defects were equal in both mumps and control newborn populations; even when the data were analyzed by trimester, no trends could be established. Similar results were obtained by a British team after reviewing 500 pregnancies complicated by maternal mumps.[72]

St. Geme and co-workers[73] have suggested an "embryopathic" relationship between intrauterine mumps infection and endocardial fibroelastosis (EFE) on the basis of the presence of skin test reactivity to mumps antigen in a high percentage of the EFE patients. Experimentally induced infection of the chick embryo has added histopathologic support to this association.[74] Although some observers have disputed that mumps plays a causative role,[75] studies using polymerase chain reaction (PCR) techniques have demonstrated mumps viral RNA in more than 70% of samples of myocardium from patients with autopsy-proven EFE.[76] There has been a marked decline in the incidence of EFE in the last 3 decades corresponding to the declining incidence of mumps.

A similar controversy exists over the possible role of mumps in the etiology of juvenile diabetes mellitus. Diabetes, transient or permanent, which developed soon after mumps, has been the subject of a number of case reports.[77,78] However, it is not clear whether this is simply coincidental. Epidemiologic studies have demonstrated a 7-year periodicity in the incidence of both mumps and childhood diabetes, with a 3- to 4-year lag time between their respective peaks.[79] Coxsackievirus B4 has also been epidemiologically linked to diabetes.[80] Although the frequency of EFE has declined in recent years, there has not been a decline in the frequency of juvenile diabetes mellitus coincident with the decreasing frequency of mumps after introduction of the mumps vaccine.

Immunology

After clinical or subclinical mumps infection, a variety of immunologic responses can be demonstrated. Complement-fixing antibodies directed against the NP protein (historically, S antigen) appear rapidly; sometimes they are present at the onset of clinically apparent illness. Antibody titers against the HN protein (historically, V antigen) rise more slowly and peak at about 2 to 4 weeks after the beginning of disease.[81] However, anti-NP antibody titers decline rapidly over a period of several months to undetectable levels, whereas anti-HN antibody titers drop more slowly and persist for years. This pattern of response provides the possibility of a serologic diagnosis of mumps from a single serum specimen. An acute-phase serum demonstrating a high anti-NP–low anti-HN titer or a high anti-NP–high anti-HN titer can be interpreted as evidence of current or recent infection, respectively. The presence in serum of only anti-HN antibodies would indicate a more remote infection with mumps. IgM antibodies to mumps are the earliest humoral responses and usually fall within 2 to

6 months. IgM anti-NP antibodies detected by capture or enzyme-linked immunosorbent assay (ELISA) are the most sensitive early serologic responses, and are used by the CDC to detect acute or recent infection (see later).

Neutralizing antibodies appear during convalescence, are directed against HN and F proteins, and detectable titers persist for years. Although assays for these antibodies constitute the most reliable test to determine whether a person is immune to mumps, such assays are cumbersome and not routinely performed. Assays for HAI antibodies, which also develop after the onset of mumps, are the simplest of the serologic studies, but results are unreliable because of potential cross-reaction with other paramyxoviruses. ELISAs for antibody to mumps have been developed[82,83] and are widely available.

Delayed hypersensitivity to an intradermally administered mumps skin test antigen develops between 3 weeks and 3 months after mumps.[3] The skin test was widely used as a measure of immunity to mumps and as a test for the competence of delayed hypersensitivity. The use of mumps skin test antigen to determine immunity to mumps has been abandoned because of the variability of lots of the skin test antigen and of the occurrence of false-positive and false-negative results.

Transplacental transfer of maternal mumps complement-fixing, HAI, and neutralizing antibodies has been demonstrated.[84] Titers in maternal and cord serum are almost identical. Neutralizing antibodies persist for several months and account for the rarity of mumps in young infants, as well as for the lack of response to immunization in this age group. One attack of mumps, whether inapparent or clinically manifested, confers lifelong immunity.

Diagnosis

Historically, the diagnosis of mumps has been made on the basis of a history of exposure and of parotid swelling and tenderness accompanied by mild to moderate constitutional symptoms.

The WBC and differential counts in mumps are normal, or there may be a mild leukopenia with a relative lymphocytosis. When meningitis, orchitis, or pancreatitis is present, leukocytosis with a shift to the left is most commonly encountered. The serum amylase level is elevated in the presence of parotitis and may remain abnormal for 2 to 3 weeks. Serum amylase levels may also be elevated in the absence of clinical salivary gland involvement. Mumps pancreatitis also increases amylase levels; differentiation from salivary gland amylase may be achieved by isoenzyme analysis or serum pancreatic lipase determinations.

The typical CSF findings in mumps meningitis have been described previously. Similar although less marked CSF abnormalities are present in half of patients with mumps parotitis but without apparent CNS involvement. In a patient with aseptic meningitis, an elevated serum amylase level should suggest mumps infection.

Laboratory confirmation of typical mumps is unnecessary. However, when parotitis is absent or recurrent, when extrasalivary gland manifestations are prominent, or when documentation of the presence of a specific viral disorder is desired, a variety of diagnostic aids can be used.

The definitive diagnosis of mumps depends on serologic studies, viral isolation, or PCR assay. The presence of IgM antibodies as determined by ELISA or a fourfold rise between acute and convalescent sera on complement fixation, HAI, ELISA, or neutralization testing confirms the diagnosis. The HAI test can be affected by heterologous antibody responses to parainfluenza virus infection. Because parotitis can be caused by parainfluenza 3 virus,[85] serologic testing and virus isolation studies for parainfluenza 3 virus should be undertaken if the HAI test is used in the diagnosis of mumps. Immunity to mumps is usually assessed by ELISA. This assay combines ease of performance with reliability. Reverse transcriptase (RT)–PCR assays have been developed that are highly sensitive and specific, and appear to be significantly more sensitive than tissue culture isolation methods.[7,86,87]

Virus is usually present in saliva for about 1 week, from 2 to 3 days before to 4 to 5 days after the onset of parotitis.[88] However, virus has been isolated from saliva as early as 6 days before and as late as 9 days after the first signs of salivary gland involvement. In addition, virus may be recovered from the saliva of persons with inapparent infection or those who manifest only extrasalivary gland signs.[89] A recent review of viral shedding data by the CDC, American Academy of Pediatrics (AAP), and Healthcare Infection Control Practices Advisory Committee (HICPAC) has concluded that virus shedding is relatively low by 5 days after onset of parotitis, and recommended that isolation of patients is not necessary for more than 5 days after clinical illness in the hospital or community setting.[90] The virus is frequently isolated from the CSF in patients with clinical meningitis during the first 3 days of meningeal symptoms[32] and is present as late as the sixth day of CNS disease. Viruria has been detected during the first 2 weeks of illness: in one study, 72% of urine specimens during the first 5 days of illness yielded a positive culture.[61] Viremia has rarely been detected and has been found only during the first 2 days of illness.[25,26] Mumps viral RNA has been detected by PCR assay in clinical specimens from patients with mumps infection and in throat swabs of healthy children following administration of mumps vaccine.[91-93]

Differential Diagnosis

A variety of entities may simulate mumps but can be easily differentiated from mumps on the basis of chronicity or associated symptoms. Infectious processes involving parotid glands are most likely to be confused with mumps because of their acute onset and associated fever. Parainfluenza 3 virus, coxsackieviruses, and influenza A viruses have been reported to cause acute parotitis.[85,94,95] These entities can be differentiated from mumps only by viral culture or serology. Bilateral parotid swelling is often seen in children with human immunodeficiency virus (HIV) infection. Suppurative parotitis, most often caused by *Staphylococcus aureus* or gram-negative organisms, usually occurs in the postoperative period, in premature newborns, or in debilitated patients with poor oral intake. The gland is warm, hard, and extremely tender; the overlying skin is erythematous. Massage of the parotid expresses purulent drainage from Stensen's duct.

Parotid enlargement caused by drugs or metabolic disorders is usually bilateral and asymptomatic. Phenylbutazone, thiouracil, iodides, and phenothiazines have been implicated in this condition.[65] Diabetes mellitus, malnutrition, cirrhosis, and uremia are among the metabolic disorders that can cause parotid swelling.[65]

Tumors, cysts, and obstruction caused by stones or structure are usually unilateral. Rare conditions that may mimic mumps include Mikulicz's syndrome, Parinaud's syndrome, uveoparotid fever of sarcoidosis, and Sjögren's syndrome.

Treatment

Therapy for mumps parotitis is symptomatic and supportive. Treatment with analgesic-antipyretics such as aspirin or acetaminophen relieves pain caused by salivary gland inflammation and reduces fever. Topical application of warm or cold packs to the parotid may also relieve discomfort. Intravenous fluid administration may be necessary for patients with meningitis or pancreatitis who have persistent vomiting. Lumbar puncture may relieve the headache associated with meningitis.

Management of orchitis is purely symptomatic. Bed rest, narcotic analgesics, support of the inflamed testis with a "bridge," and ice packs make the patient feel more comfortable. An anesthetic block of the spermatic cord with 1% procaine hydrochloride may alleviate severe pain.[96] There is no convincing evidence that the use of steroids or diethylstilbestrol or incision of the tunica albuginea produces more rapid resolution of the orchitis or prevents subsequent atrophy. Interferon-alfa 2b administered to four men with bilateral mumps orchitis resulted in prompt resolution of symptoms, with no evidence of testicular atrophy or oligospermia during follow-up study.[97] Further investigation to establish the efficacy of this treatment is needed.

Gellis and colleagues[98] have shown that 20 mL of mumps immune globulin administered intramuscularly to adult men with mumps reduces the incidence of orchitis from 27.4% to 7.8%. However, mumps immune globulin is no longer commercially available.

Prevention

As noted, recommendations for the management of patients with mumps include isolation for 5 days after the onset of parotid swelling to prevent the spread of infection to susceptible persons.[90] This measure may be of little value, particularly in closed populations such as schools or hospitals,[99] because virus is present in saliva days before parotitis develops and because those with clinically inapparent infection can shed virus.

Passive protection to exposed susceptible persons may have been afforded by mumps immune globulin, available in the past. However, Reed and associates[16] reported that use of mumps immune globulin during an epidemic in Alaska did not reduce clinical parotitis or inapparent infection rates and did not diminish the incidence of meningitis and orchitis.

Active immunization with the Jeryl Lynn strain of attenuated mumps virus vaccine has been available in the United States since December 1967. The vaccine is prepared in chick embryo cell culture.[5] A single subcutaneous immunization produces protective levels of mumps-neutralizing antibodies in more than 95% of vaccines.[5] Although the antibody levels produced are lower than after natural infection, adequate titers are maintained for at least 10.5 years.[100] Adverse reactions to the vaccine are uncommon; transient suppression of tuberculin-delayed hypersensitivity has been reported and parotitis and orchitis have been recognized rarely. Vaccine virus is not present in secretions of immunized children. In Japan, aseptic meningitis associated with mumps vaccine virus occurred in 0.05% to 0.3% of recipients of the Urabe AM 9 mumps vaccine; manifestations began 2 to 4 weeks after immunization.[101,102] U.S. studies did not reveal evidence of an increased risk of aseptic meningitis after administration of the Jeryl Lynn strain of mumps vaccine.[103]

All children older than 12 months should be immunized. Vaccination should take place at 12 to 15 months and again at 4 to 6 years of age, as part of immunization with the combined live measles-mumps-rubella (MMR) virus vaccine. Most states now require evidence of immunity to mumps (i.e., documented immunization, physician-diagnosed disease, or antibody studies) for school entrance and attendance (see Chapter 320). A two-dose immunization regimen is recommended for all adolescents and health care personnel without evidence of mumps immunity. Other adults should receive at least one dose of vaccine. Immunization after exposure may not provide protection from natural infection.

As with other live virus vaccines, mumps vaccine should not be administered to pregnant women, patients receiving immunosuppressive therapy, or those with severe febrile illnesses, advanced malignancies, or congenital or acquired immunodeficiencies. Serious reactions to the mumps component of MMR have not been reported in limited studies in HIV-infected patients. However, a fatal case of measles pneumonitis occurred in a 21-year-old man with advanced HIV disease who was vaccinated with MMR vaccine; therefore, it should not be administered to such patients [104] (see Chapter 320). Individuals with HIV infection who are not severely immunocompromised may be immunized with MMR vaccine.

REFERENCES

1. Johnson CD, Goodpasture EW. An investigation of the etiology of mumps. *J Exp Med.* 1934;59:1.
2. Habel K. Cultivation of mumps virus in the developing chick embryo and its application to the studies of immunity to mumps in man. *Publ Health Rep.* 1945;60:201.
3. Enders JF, Cohen S, Kane LW. Immunity in mumps. II. The development of complement fixing antibody and dermal hypersensitivity in human beings following mumps. *J Exp Med.* 1945;81:119.
4. Habel K. Vaccination of human beings against mumps; vaccine administered at the start of an epidemic. I. Incidence and severity of mumps in vaccinated and control groups. *Am J Hyg.* 1951;54:295.
5. Buynak EB, Hilleman MR. Live attenuated mumps virus vaccine. I. Vaccine development. *Proc Soc Exp Biol Med.* 1966;123:768.
6. Kleiman MB. Mumps virus. In: Lennette EH, ed. *Laboratory Diagnosis of Viral Infections.* 2nd ed. New York: Marcel Dekker; 1992;549-566.
7. Carbone KM, Rubin S. Mumps virus. In: Knipe DM, Howley PM, eds. *Fields Virology*, 5th ed, vol 1. Philadelphia: Lippincott Williams & Wilkins, 2007:1527-1550.
8. Kaaijk P, van der Zeijst BA, Boog MC, et al. Increased mumps incidence in the Netherlands: Review on the possible role of vaccine strain and genotype. *Eurosurveillance.* 2008;13:18914.
9. Santos CL, Ishida MA, Foster PG, et al. Detection of a new mumps virus genotype during parotitis epidemic of 2006-2007 in the state of Sao Paulo, Brazil. *J Med Virol.* 2008;80:323.
10. Cui A, Myers R, Xu W, et al. Analysis of the genetic variability of the mumps SH gene in viruses circulating in the UK between 1996 and 2005. *Infect Genet Evol.* 2009;9:71.
11. Deinhardt FW, Shramek GJ. Mumps virus. In: Lennette EH, Spaulding EH, Truant JP, eds. *Manual of Clinical Microbiology.* Washington DC: American Society for Microbiology; 1974:703-708.
12. Henle G, Deinhardt F, Girardi A. Cytolytic effects of mumps virus in tissue cultures of epithelial cells. *Proc Soc Exp Biol Med.* 1954;87:386.
13. Centers for Disease Control and Prevention. Mumps surveillance 1973. *MMWR Morb Mortal Wkly Rep.* 1974;23:431.
14. Centers for Disease Control and Prevention. Summary of notifiable diseases, United States, 1991. *MMWR Morb Mortal Wkly Rep.* 1991;40:3.
15. Philip RN, Reinhard KR, Lackman DB. Observations on a mumps epidemic in a "virgin" population. *Am J Hyg.* 1959;69: 91.
16. Reed D, Brown G, Merrick R, et al. A mumps epidemic on St. George Island, Alaska. *JAMA.* 1967;199:967.
17. Meyer MG. An epidemiologic study of mumps; its spread in schools and families. *Am J Hyg.* 1962;75:259.
18. Anderson LJ, Seward JF. Mumps epidemiology and immunity. *Pediatr Infect Dis J* 2008;27:S75.
19. Cohen C, White JM, Savage EJ, et al. Vaccine effectiveness estimates, 2004-2005 mumps outbreak, England. *Emerg Infect Dis.* 2007;13:12.
20. Dayan GH, Quinlisk MP, Parker AA, et al. Recent resurgence of mumps in the United States. *N Engl J Med.* 2008;358:1580.
21. Conly JM, Johnston BL. Is mumps making a comeback? *Can J Infect Dis Med Microbiol.* 2007;18:7.
22. Dayan GH, Rubin S. Mumps outbreaks in vaccinated populations: Are available mumps vaccines effective enough to prevent outbreaks? *Clin Infect Dis.* 2008;47:1458.
23. Centers for Disease Control and Prevention. Mumps surveillance, Report No. 1. January 1968.
24. Truant AL, Hullum JV. A persistent infection of baby hamster kidney—21 cells with mumps virus and the role of temperature sensitive variants. *J Med Virol.* 1977;1:49.
25. Kilham L. Isolation of mumps virus from the blood of a patient. *Proc Soc Exp Biol Med.* 1948;69:99.
26. Overman JR. Viremia in human mumps infection. *Arch Intern Med.* 1958;102:354.
27. Donohue WL, Playfair FD, Whitaker L. Mumps encephalitis. *J Pediatr.* 1955;47:395.
28. Taylor FB, Toreson WE. Primary mumps meningo-encephalitis. *Arch Intern Med.* 1963;112:216.
29. Travis LW, Hecht DW. Acute and chronic inflammatory diseases of the salivary glands, diagnosis and management. *Otolaryng Clin North Am.* 1977;10:329.
30. Gellis SS, Peters M. Mumps with presternal edema. *Bull Johns Hopkins Hosp.* 1944;75:241.
31. Bang HO, Bang J. Involvement of the central nervous system in mumps. *Acta Med Scand.* 1943;113:487.
32. McLean DM, Bach RD, Larke RPB, et al. Mumps meningoencephalitis, Toronto, 1963. *Can Med Assoc J.* 1964;90:458.
33. Ritter BS. Mumps meningoencephalitis in children. *J Pediatr.* 1958;52:424.
34. Levitt LP, Rich TA, Kinde SW, et al. Central nervous system mumps. *Neurology.* 1970;20:829.
35. Johnstone JA, Ross CAC, Dunn M. Meningitis and encephalitis associated with mumps infection. *Arch Dis Child.* 1972; 47:647.
36. Wilfert CM. Mumps meningoencephalitis with low cerebrospinal-fluid glucose, prolonged pleocytosis and elevation of protein. *N Engl J Med.* 1969;280:855.
37. Russell RR, Donald JC. The neurological complications of mumps. *Br Med J.* 1958;2:27.
38. Centers for Disease Control (CDC). Mumps surveillance, January 1977-December 1982. September 1984.
39. Azimi PH, Shaban S, Hilty MD, et al. Mumps meningoencephalitis-prolonged abnormality of cerebrospinal fluid. *JAMA.* 1975;234:1161.
40. Vuori M, Lahikainen EA, Peltonen T. Perceptive deafness in connection with mumps. *Acta Otolaryngol.* 1962;55:231.
41. Everberg G. Deafness following mumps. *Acta Otolaryngol.* 1957;48:397.
42. Cohen HA, Ashkenazi A, Nussinovitch M, et al. Mumps-associated acute cerebellar ataxia. *Am J Dis Child.* 1992;146:930.
43. Beardwell A. Facial palsy due to the mumps virus. *Br J Clin Pract.* 1969;23:37.
44. Nussinovitch M, Brand N, Frydman M, et al. Transverse myelitis following mumps in children. *Acta Paediatr.* 1992;81:183.
45. Ghosh S. Guillain-Barré syndrome complicating mumps. *Lancet.* 1967;1:895.
46. Lennette EH, Caplan GE, Magoffin RL. Mumps virus infection simulating paralytic poliomyelitis. *Pediatrics.* 1960;25:788.
47. Timmons GD, Johnson KP. Aqueductal stenosis and hydrocephalus after mumps encephalitis. *N Engl J Med.* 1970;283:1505.
48. Bray PF. Mumps: A cause of hydrocephalus? *Pediatrics.* 1972;49:446.
49. Oran B, Ceri A, Yilmaz H, et al. Hydrocephalus in mumps meningoencephalitis: Case report. *Pediatr Infect Dis J.* 1995;14:724.
50. Johnson RT, Johnson KP. Hydrocephalus following viral infection. The pathology of aqueductal stenosis developing after experimental mumps virus infection. *J Neuropathol Exp Neurol.* 1968;27:591.
51. Herndon RM, Johnson RT, Davis LE, et al. Ependymitis in mumps virus meningitis. *Arch Neurol.* 1974;30:475.
52. Uno M, Takano T, Yamano T, et al. Age-dependent susceptibility in mumps-associated hydrocephalus: Neuropathologic features and brain barriers. *Acta Neuropathol (Berl).* 1997;94:207.
53. Candel S. Epididymitis in mumps, including orchitis: Further clinical studies and comments. *Ann Intern Med.* 1951;34:20.
54. Lambert B. The frequency of mumps and of mumps orchitis. *Acta Genet Stat Med.* 1951;2(Suppl 1):1.
55. Kaufman JJ, Bruce PT. Testicular atrophy following mumps, a cause of testis tumour? *J Urol.* 1963;35:67.
56. Morrison JC, Givens JR, Wiser WL. Mumps oophoritis: A cause of premature menopause. *Fertil Steril.* 1975;26:655.
57. Appelbaum E, Kohn J, Steinman RE, et al. Mumps arthritis. *Arch Intern Med.* 1952;90:217.
58. Caranasos GJ, Felder JR. Mumps arthritis. *Arch intern Med.* 1967;119:394.
59. Kussy JC, Fatal mumps myocarditis. *Minn Med.* 1974;57:285.
60. Roberts WC, Fox SM. Mumps of the heart, clinical and pathologic features. *Circulation.* 1965;32:342.
61. Utz JP, Houk VN, Alling DW. Clinical and laboratory studies of mumps. IV. Viruria and abnormal renal function. *N Engl J Med.* 1964;270:1283.
62. Hughes WT, Steigman AJ, Delong HF. Some implications of fatal nephritis associated with mumps. *Am J Dis Child.* 1966;111:297.
63. Eylan E, Zmucky R, Sheba C. Mumps virus and subacute thyroiditis: Evidence of a causal association. *Lancet.* 1957;1: 1062.
64. Gershon AA. Mumps. In: Gershon AA, Hotez PJ, Katz SL, eds. *Krugman's Infectious Diseases in Children*, 11th ed. Philadelphia: Mosby, 2004:391-401.
65. Pomeroy C, Jordan MC. Mumps. In: Hoeprich PD, Jordan MC, eds. *Infectious Diseases.* 5th ed. Philadelphia: JB Lippincott; 1994:829-834.
66. Petersdorf RG, Bennett IL. Treatment of mumps orchitis with adrenal hormones: Report of 23 cases with a note on the hepatic involvement in mumps. *Arch Intern Med.* 1957;99:222.
67. Graham DY, Brown CH, Benrey J, et al. Thrombocytopenia: A complication of mumps. *JAMA.* 1974;227:1162.
68. Siegel M, Fuerst HT, Peress NS. Comparative fetal mortality in maternal virus diseases: A prospective study on rubella, measles, mumps, chickenpox and hepatitis. *N Engl J Med.* 1966;274: 768.
69. Siegel M, Fuerst HT. Low birth weight and maternal virus diseases: A prospective study of rubella, measles, mumps, chickenpox and hepatitis. *JAMA.* 1966;197:680.
70. Siegel MS. Congenital malformations following chickenpox, measles, mumps, and hepatitis. Results of a cohort study. *JAMA.* 1973;226:1521.
71. Gershon AA. Chickenpox, measles and mumps. In: Remington JS, Klein JO, eds. *Infectious Diseases of the Fetus and Newborn.* Philadelphia: WB Saunders: 1990:395-445.
72. Manson MM, Logan WPD, Loy RM. *Rubella and other virus infections in pregnancy. Reports on Public Health and Medical Subjects*, No. 101. London: Ministry of Health; 1960.
73. St Geme JW, Noren GR, Adams P. Proposed embryopathic relation between mumps virus and primary endocardial fibroelastosis. *N Engl J Med.* 1966;275:339.
74. St Geme JW, Peralta H, Farias E, et al. Experimental gestational mumps virus infection and endocardial fibroelastosis. *Pediatrics.* 1971;48:821.
75. Gersony WM, Katz SL, Nadas AS. Endocardial fibroelastosis and the mumps virus. *Pediatrics.* 1966;37:430.
76. Ni J, Bowles NE, Kim YH, et al. Viral infection of the endocardium in endocardial fibroelastosis. Molecular evidence for the role of mumps virus as an etiologic agent. *Circulation.* 1997;95:133.
77. Dacou-Voutetakis C, Constantinidis M, Moschos A, et al. Diabetes mellitus following mumps: Insulin reserve. *Am J Dis Child.* 1974;127:890.
78. Hinden E. Mumps followed by diabetes. *Lancet.* 1962;1:1138.
79. Sultz HA, Hart BA, Zielezny M, et al. Is mumps virus an etiologic factor in juvenile diabetes mellitus? *J Pediatr.* 1975;86:654.
80. Gamble DR, Kinsley ML, Fitzgerald MG, et al. Viral antibodies in diabetes mellitus. *Br Med J.* 1969;3:627.
81. Henle G, Harris S, Henle W. The reactivity of various human sera with mumps complement fixation antigens. *J Exp Med.* 1948;88:133.
82. Nigro G, Nanni F, Midulla M. Determination of vaccine-induced and naturally acquired class-specific antibodies by two indirect ELISAs. *J Virol Methods.* 1986;13:91.
83. Doern GV, Robbie L, St Amand R. Comparison of the Vidas and Bio-Whittaker enzyme immunoassays for detecting IgG reactive with varicella-zoster virus and mumps virus. *Diagn Microbiol Infect Dis.* 1997;28:31.
84. Hodes D, Brunell PA. Mumps antibody placental transfer and disappearance during the first year of life. *Pediatrics.* 1970; 45:99.
85. Zollar LM, Mufson MA. Acute parotitis associated with parainfluenza 3 virus infection. *Am J Dis Child.* 1970;119:147.
86. Cusi MG, Bianchi S, Valassina M, et al. Rapid detection and typing of circulating mumps virus by reverse transcription/polymerase chain reaction. *Res Virol.* 1996;147:227.
87. Poggio GP, Rodriguez C, Cisterna D, et al. Nested PCR for rapid detection of mumps virus in cerebrospinal fluid from patients with neurological diseases. *J Clin Microbiol.* 2000;38:274.
88. Polgreen PM, Bohnett LC, Cavanaugh JE, et al. The duration of mumps virus shedding after the onset of symptoms. *Clin Infect Dis.* 2008;46:1447.
89. Henle G, Henle W, Wendell KK, et al. Isolation of mumps virus from human beings with induced apparent or inapparent infections. *J Exp Med.* 1948;88:223.
90. Centers for Disease Control and Prevention. Updated recommendations for isolation of persons with mumps. *MMWR Morb Mortal Wkly Rep.* 2008;57:1103.
91. Boriskin YuS, Booth JC, Yamada A. Rapid detection of mumps virus by the polymerase chain reaction. *J Virol Methods.* 1993;42:23.
92. Hosoya M, Honzumi K, Sato M, et al. Application of PCR for various neurotropic viruses on the diagnosis of viral meningitis. *J Clin Virol.* 1998;11:117.
93. Nagai T, Nakayama T. Mumps vaccine virus genome is present in throat swabs obtained from uncomplicated healthy recipients. *Vaccine.* 2001;19:1353.
94. Howlett JG, Somlo F, Kalz F. A new syndrome of parotitis with herpangina caused by the coxsackie virus. *Can Med Assoc J.* 1957;77:5.
95. Brill SJ, Gilfillan RF. Acute parotitis associated with influenza type. A. *N Engl J Med.* 1977;296:1391.
96. Lyon RP, Bruyn HB. Mumps epididymo-orchitis: Treatment by anesthetic block of the spermatic cord. *JAMA.* 1966;196:736.
97. Erpenbach KH. Systemic treatment with interferon-alpha 2B: An effective method to prevent sterility after bilateral mumps orchitis. *J Urol.* 1991;146:54.
98. Gellis SS, McGuiness AC, Peters M. A study on the prevention of mumps orchitis with gamma globulin. *Am J Med Sci.* 1945;210:661.
99. Brunell PA, Brickman A, O'Hare D, et al. Ineffectiveness of isolation of patients as a method of preventing the spread of mumps. *N Engl J Med* 1968;279:1357.
100. Weibel RE, Buynak EB, McLean AA, et al. Persistence of antibody in human subjects following administration of combined liver attenuated measles, mumps, and rubella vaccines. *Proc Soc Exp Biol Med.* 1980;165:260.
101. Fuginaga T, Youichi M, Tamura H, et al. A prefecture-wide survey of mumps meningitis associated with measles, mumps and rubella vaccine. *Pediatr Infect Dis J.* 1991;10:204.
102. Sugiura A, Yamada A. Aseptic meningitis as a complication of mumps. *Pediatr Infect Dis J.* 1991;10:209.
103. Black S, Shinfeld H, Ray P, et al. Risk of hospitalization because of aseptic meningitis after measles-mumps-rubella vaccination in one to two year old children: An analysis of the Vaccine Safety Datalink (VSD) Project. *Pediatr Infect Dis J.* 1997;16:500.
104. Angel JA, Walpita P, Lerch RA, et al. Vaccine-associated measles pneumonitis in an adult with AIDS. *Ann Intern Med.* 1998;129:104.

158

Respiratory Syncytial Virus

CAROLINE BREESE HALL

Were we but able to explain
The fiefdom of the microbe—
Why one man is his serf,
Another is his lord
When all are his domain....
C.B.H.

Respiratory syncytial virus (RSV) is the major cause of lower respiratory tract illness in young children.[1,2] So effectively does RSV spread that essentially all persons have experienced RSV infection within the first few years of life. Immunity, however, is not complete, and reinfection is common. Although life-threatening infections most commonly occur during the first couple of years of life, RSV infections contribute an appreciable share of the morbidity caused by acute upper and lower respiratory tract infections among older children and adults. The health care costs associated with outpatient infections add appreciably to the estimated cost of $300 to $600 million for hospitalized infants with RSV infection.[2-4] Of concern and increasing recognition are the growing morbidity and costs associated with RSV infections in older adults.[5-7]

History

RSV was discovered in 1956, but was not initially associated with respiratory illness among infants. Indeed, when a group of 14 chimpanzees were noted to be suffering from colds and coryza, Morris and co-workers[8] isolated a new virus from one of the chimpanzees. They called this new agent *chimpanzee coryza agent* (CCA). Whether this agent was also able to infect humans was not then known, but cross-infection was suspected because one laboratory worker developed specific antibody to CCA. Subsequently, Chanock and colleagues[9] confirmed that the agent caused respiratory illness in humans when they obtained two isolates from children that were indistinguishable from CCA.[9] These isolates were recovered from the throat swabs of a child with bronchopneumonia (Long strain) and from a child with laryngotracheobronchitis (Snyder strain). Subsequently, specific neutralizing antibody to CCA was found to be present in most children by the time they reached school age. The "chimpanzee coryza agent" was then more appropriately renamed *respiratory syncytial virus* to denote its clinical and laboratory manifestations.

Description

CLASSIFICATION

RSV belongs to the order Mononegavirales, family Paramyxoviridae, and the subfamily Pneumovirinae. The two genera within the Pneumovirinae subfamily are *Metapneumovirus*, containing human metapneumovirus (hMPV), and *Pneumovirus*, which contains human RSV and the morphologically and biologically similar pneumonia virus of mice, bovine RSV, ovine RSV, and caprine RSV. Distinctive features of RSV include the number and order of genes and the lack of hemagglutinin and neuraminidase activity.

VIRAL STRUCTURE AND CHARACTERISTICS

RSV is an enveloped, medium-sized (120 to 300 nm) RNA virus with a nonsegmented, single-stranded, negative-sense genome that is asso-ciated with viral proteins throughout its length, which forms the nucleocapsid[4,10] (Figs. 158-1 and 158-2). The viral envelope has a bilipid layer derived from the plasma membrane of the host cells. Its surface has transmembrane surface glycoprotein spikes 11 to 12 nm in length and 6 to 10 nm apart, which on electron microscopy give it a thistle-like appearance[10] (Fig. 158-3).

The complete genome of RSV (A2 strain) has been sequenced[10] (see Fig. 158-2). The viral RNA consists of 15,222 nucleotides that are transcribed into 10 monocistronic polyadenylated messenger RNAs (mRNAs), each of which encodes for one of the major proteins, except for M2 mRNA, which possesses two overlapping open reading frames that encode for two separate proteins (M2-1, the transcription processivity factor, and M2-2, a regulatory protein). Four proteins, N (nucleoprotein), P (phosphoprotein), L (polymerase), and M2-1, are associated with the nucleocapsid. Associated with the envelope are three transmembrane surface proteins, F (fusion), G (attachment), and SH (small nonglycosylated hydrophobic protein). The M (matrix) protein accumulates at the inner surface of the envelope and is important in the virus's morphogenesis. Two proteins, NS1 and NS2, are small nonstructural accessory proteins that may have a role in modifying the immune response to RSV by inhibiting apoptosis and interferon production.[10,11]

The two major glycosylated surface proteins, F and G, are integral to the infectivity and pathogenicity of the virus. They are the major immunoprotective antigens and are the two targets for neutralization. The larger glycoprotein, G, is the primary mediator of attachment of the virus to host cells, although it possesses no hemagglutinin or neuraminidase, which are present in the attachment proteins of other paramyxoviruses. The F protein initiates viral penetration by fusing viral and host cellular membranes and promotes viral spread by melding infected cells to adjacent uninfected cells, thereby resulting in RSV's characteristic syncytia. Efficient fusion, however, appears to require the coexpression of all three of the surface glycoproteins, F, G, and SH.

LABORATORY PROPERTIES

RSV poorly withstands slow freezing and thawing and changes in pH and temperature. At 55°C, infectivity is rapidly diminished, and at 25°C, only 10% infectivity remains at 48 hours, and at 4°C, 1% remains after 7 days.[12] The optimal pH for RSV is 7.5. Inactivation occurs quickly with acidic media (pH < 5), ether, and chloroform and with detergents such as 0.1% sodium deoxycholate, sodium dodecyl sulfate, and Triton X-100.

The survival of RSV in the environment appears to depend in part on the drying time and dew point. At room temperature, RSV in the secretions of patients may survive on nonporous surfaces, such as countertops, for 3 to 30 hours.[13] On porous surfaces, such as cloth and paper tissue, survival is generally shorter, usually less than 1 hour. The infectivity of RSV on the hands is variable from person to person but is usually less than 1 hour.

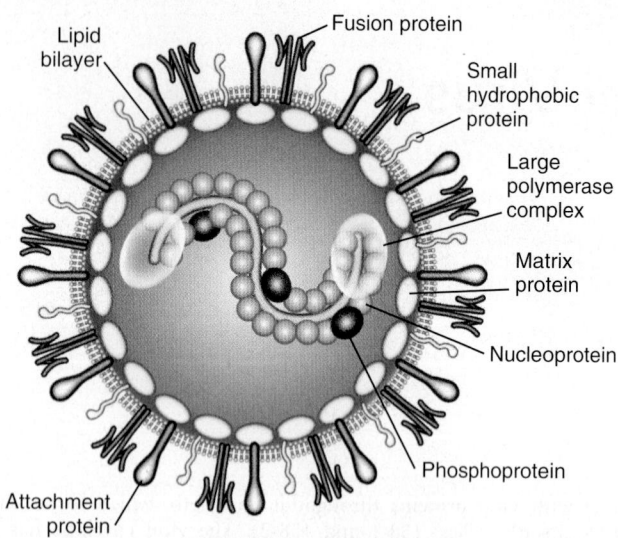

Figure 158-1 Structure of respiratory syncytial virus. *(Adapted from the Massachusetts Medical Society. Hall CB. Respiratory syncytial virus and parainfluenza virus. N Engl J Med. 2001;344:1917-1928.)*

Human heteroploid cell lines are usually preferred for primary isolation. Most commonly used are HEp-2, HeLa, and A549 cell lines. RSV may also be recovered in human kidney, amnion, diploid fibroblastic cells, and monkey kidney cells. Continual monitoring of these cell lines is required, and as with passage and laboratory conditions, their sensitivity may vary. RSV replication and syncytia formation require that the culture media contain calcium and glutamine. Serial propagation of RSV may change the growth characteristics, including diminishing the cytopathic effect (CPE) of syncytia formation and altering the susceptibility to neutralization, which may be related to the production of quasispecies.[14] With primary isolation in sensitive heteroploid cell cultures, characteristic CPE may be first detected after an average of 3 to 5 days. With laboratory-adapted strains, new infectious virus may first be detected 10 to 12 hours after inoculation. The typical syncytia develop about 10 to 24 hours later and progress until the cell sheet is completely destroyed, which is usually within 4 days.

The viral surface glycoproteins may be detected by immunofluorescence 7 to 10 hours after inoculation. Subsequently, cell-free virus may be demonstrated in the culture medium, but up to 90% of the virus remains cell-associated.[10] Release of cell-associated virus requires agitation or sonication. However, a large proportion of the virions released appear empty and noninfectious.

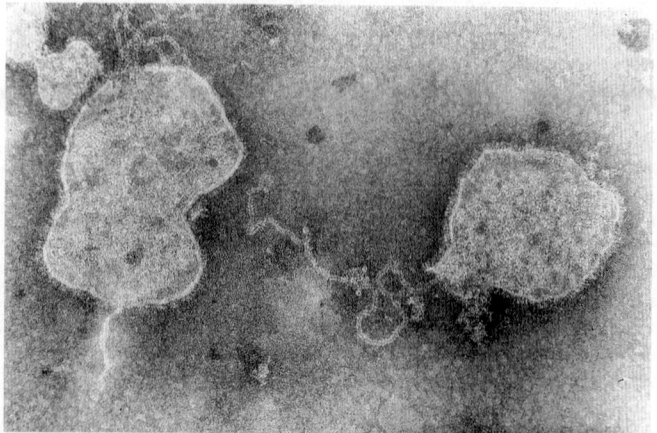

Figure 158-3 Negative contrast electron micrograph of respiratory syncytial virus.

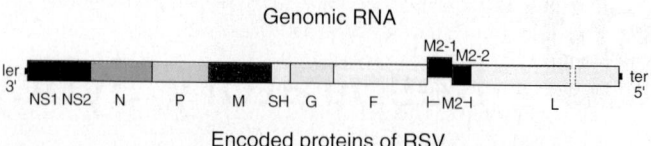

Figure 158-2 Simplified representation of the negative-sense RNA genome of respiratory syncytial virus (RSV) and the encoded proteins. The genome is shown 3′ with the leader extragenic region (ler) and with the 5′ trailer extragenic region (ter). The viral genes are depicted by the divided bars. Each viral gene transcribes a single mRNA encoding protein with the exception of M2 mRNA, which transcribes two proteins, M2-1 and M2-2.

INFECTION IN ANIMALS

The respiratory tract of a variety of animal species may be experimentally infected with RSV,[15] but natural symptomatic infection is limited mostly to humans and chimpanzees with human RSV strains, and to cows with bovine RSV (BRSV). BRSV is antigenically and genetically closely related to human RSV, and antibodies directed against the F, N, P, and M proteins of either virus recognize the heterologous virus. BRSV strains similarly consist of two major antigenic subgroups. Ovine and caprine strains of RSV also have been recovered, and genetic analysis suggests that caprine RSV is more closely related than ovine RSV to BRSV and human RSV.[10]

Although animal models develop upper respiratory tract infection, their lack of symptomatic lower respiratory tract disease comparable to that observed with infants is problematic. Closest is disease in chimpanzees because they readily acquire infection from infected contacts and shed moderate levels of RSV in their respiratory secretions.[10] Nevertheless, their disease is generally mild and without the degree of lower respiratory tract involvement observed in infants. Rodents are the most commonly used models, particularly cotton rats and mice, but replication of RSV is only semipermissive and highly variable, even among inbred strains of mice.[16]

Epidemiology

DISTRIBUTION

In every geographic area studied, RSV infections are ubiquitous and clinically similar in causing the most severe disease during infancy and repetitive infections throughout life.[4,17,18] The seasonal occurrence, however, varies according to geography and climate.

SEASONAL OCCURRENCE

RSV is singular in its ability to produce reliably a major burden of infections every year.[19,20] In temperate climates, the outbreaks occur primarily in the winter or spring and spread across the United States over a period of 20 or more weeks, generally from October to May. In warmer climates, RSV activity may be more prolonged or even present throughout the year.[18,21-23] What factors initiate and terminate the recurring patterns of RSV activity has been a subject of ongoing curiosity and investigation but remains a conundrum.[22,24,25] A complex, and currently incompletely understood, interaction of local meteorological conditions may explain part of the geographically variable epidemiologic patterns. Among these are the ambient temperature, humidity, and sunlight, and their effects on RSV's stability and infectivity. However, because the only source of RSV infection is an infected individual, human behavior is an indefinable factor integral to its transmission.[22,26]

ANTIGENIC VARIATION

Strain differences among RSV isolates may also affect the intensity, severity, and diversity of RSV outbreaks.[27] RSV isolates are divided into two antigenic groups, A and B, and into subtypes within each group.[10,28] The two strain groups have 81% nucleotide identity, but the proteins between the A and B strains vary appreciably. The major genetic diversity between groups A and B resides with the G protein, followed by M2-2 and SH proteins. This is reflected in the relative antigenic relatedness between the two groups of only 1% to 7% for the G proteins, in comparison to 50% for the F proteins. Nucleotide and amino acid sequence analysis within both A and B strain groups has further revealed subtypes of distinctive lineage or clades.[10]

Strains of both groups circulate simultaneously during outbreaks, but the proportions that are A and B vary, as do the subtypes.[27-29] Even in widely separated geographic areas, the cocirculating strains may have similar genotypes and parallel evolutionary lineages. Analyses of the proteins of strains collected over decades and from diverse areas suggest that the pressure of the population's immunity may result in a selective advantage for the dominance of strains that are most divergent from those that have recently circulated in the area. However, the relationship of the circulating strain groups and subtypes to the clinical severity and manifestations of the RSV infections among young children has been inconsistent and, thus, inconclusive.[29-31]

EPIDEMIOLOGIC MANIFESTATIONS

The characteristic epidemiologic ramifications of RSV's presence within a community are notable rises in the number of cases of bronchiolitis, pneumonia, and hospital admissions of young children, especially infants with acute lower respiratory tract disease.[2,32,33] RSV outbreaks may vary year to year in size and intensity, but these barometers of RSV's presence in a community generally remain. Severe lower respiratory tract illness from RSV in previously healthy children occurs most frequently in the first year of life and is almost always associated with primary infection. Essentially all children have experienced RSV infection within the first several years of life one or more times. Repeated infections are common not only among young children but also throughout life.[5,34-37]

PREVALENCE AND INCIDENCE

RSV is the most frequent cause of bronchiolitis and is estimated to cause 40% to 90% of bronchiolitis hospitalizations and up to 50% of pneumonia admissions among infants.[1,3,33] Ten to 30% of tracheobronchitis cases have been associated with RSV infection, but only 2% to 10% of croup cases. Bronchiolitis is the leading cause of all hospitalizations among infants in the United States, and the annual rate increased 2.4 times between 1980 and 1996.[1] RSV was estimated to account for 50% to 80% of the bronchiolitis cases. Overall, as many as 120,000 children each year have been reported to be hospitalized with RSV infection.[1,38]

The yearly rates of RSV hospitalizations estimated from national databases have been variable, ranging from about 2 to 44 per 1000 children within the first 2 to 5 years of life.[1,32,39-41] Children within the first year of life consistently had the highest rates of hospitalization for bronchiolitis and other RSV-associated illnesses, and the preponderance of admissions were among infants younger than 6 months. Recent population-based studies in the United States have indicated the current hospitalization rates are 17 per 1000 children younger than 6 months and 3 per 1000 children younger than 5 years.[2,33] These rates were more than 3 times the rates from parainfluenza or influenza viral infections over 4 years of surveillance among the same population of children.[42,43] The reported RSV hospitalization rates from European countries have been generally similar, ranging from 2.5 to 11 per 1000 children within the first 4 years of life and highest, among those less than 12 months of age, 19 to 22 per 1000 children.[3,44-46]

The rates of hospitalization among children, however, may vary according to the presence of risk factors. Many host, socioeconomic, and environmental factors have been associated with a greater likelihood of young children developing more severe RSV infection and

requiring hospitalization (see "Patients at High Risk for Severe Infection").

Little information has existed concerning the health care burden resulting from RSV illness among outpatients, especially among children cared for by office practices. However, population-based surveillance during 2000 to 2004, examining laboratory-proven RSV hospitalizations and emergency department and outpatient visits in the counties surrounding Rochester, Nashville, and Cincinnati indicated that outpatient visits constituted a major proportion of the health care burden attributable to RSV infection.[2] Of all visits for acute respiratory illnesses (ARI) among children within the first 5 years of life, RSV infection was documented among 20% of ARI hospitalizations, 18% of emergency department ARI visits, and 15% of office ARI visits. The estimated rates of ARI visits from RSV among children younger than 5 years in pediatric practices (80 per 1000 children) was about 3 times higher than that observed among emergency department patients and 26 times the rates among hospitalized children.

Even less information exists on the health care burden imposed by RSV infection among older children and adults. Recurrent RSV infections are common among school-aged children and adults who are exposed to RSV at school, home, work, or during military training.[37,40,47] In urban Rochester, 44% of the families followed with young children became infected with RSV during the winter months when RSV was prevalent in the community.[36] Of the exposed family members, 46% acquired RSV infection. Although the attack rate was highest among infants, 38% to 47% of older children and adults developed RSV infection. In the Houston family study in which children were followed from birth, the infection rate was 68.8 per 100 children in the first year of life, and during the second year, at least half were reinfected.[34]

More recently recognized is the frequency of RSV infections among older adults and the resulting appreciable clinical and economic impact.[5,48,49] RSV infection among older individuals is remarkably similar to influenza with respect to clinical manifestations and as a cause of hospitalization. In London, the rate of hospitalization attributable to RSV infection among the elderly has been estimated at 0.7 per 1000 adults 65 years or older, compared with 1.1 estimated for influenza.[50] In the United States, 2% to 9% of all lower respiratory tract–related hospitalizations among those 65 years or older have been associated with RSV infections, resulting in a cost estimated in 1999 of $150 million to $680 million each year.[7]

Pathogenesis

Infection with RSV is primarily acquired through close contact with an infected individual or direct inoculation into the eyes and nose of infectious secretions.[26,51,52] Large-particle aerosols engendered by coughs and sneezes of an ill person may transmit RSV to others within a radius of about 3 feet. Longer-distance spread by small-particle (droplet nuclei) aerosols appears to be much less likely.[26] However, infection occurring from touching objects that have been contaminated with infectious secretions, followed by self-inoculation into the eyes or nose, is an important mode of transmission.

Experimental infection occurs in adult volunteers after an incubation of 3 to 8 days, with an average of 5 days.[53-55] In naturally acquired infection, the average incubation period appears similar, with a range of 2 to 8 days. The mucosa of the nose and eye appear to be equally sensitive portals of entry, in contrast to the mouth.[55]

RSV replicates in respiratory epithelium, primarily involving the ciliated columnar cells, but additional cells, such as intraepithelial dendritic cells, may be involved.[56] During primary infection, lower respiratory tract infection usually is manifest by bronchiolitis, and the initial pathologic findings are a lymphocytic peribronchiolar infiltration, predominantly CD69+ monocytes, with edema of the walls and surrounding tissue.[56-58] Subsequently, the characteristic proliferation and necrosis of the epithelium of the bronchioles develop. The lumina of these small airways become obstructed from the sloughed epithelium and from the increased mucus secretion. The airway of the young infant is particularly vulnerable to any degree of inflammation and obstruction because resistance to the flow of air is related inversely to the cube of the radius. Impedance to the flow of air occurs during both inspiration and expiration but is greater in the latter when the lumen is narrowed further by the positive expiratory pressure. Hyperinflation, therefore, results from air trapping peripheral to the sites of partial occlusion. With complete obstruction, the trapped air eventually becomes absorbed, producing the characteristic multiple areas of atelectasis. Young infants are at increased risk for developing such areas of atelectasis because the collateral channels that maintain alveolar expansion in the presence of airway obstruction are not yet well developed. These changes result in an increase in lung volume and expiratory resistance.

Infants with lower respiratory tract disease from RSV often have pathologic evidence of both pneumonia and bronchiolitis. Patients with pneumonia demonstrate an interstitial infiltration of mononuclear cells that may be accompanied by edema and necrotic areas that lead to alveolar filling.[56,57] Some histologic evidence of recovery is present in most children with bronchiolitis within the first week of illness and is marked by the beginning regeneration of the bronchiolar epithelium. However, ciliated cells may not be present for weeks.

IMMUNITY AND PATHOGENESIS OF DISEASE

Diverse theories and supporting data have been offered to explain how RSV engenders these pathogenic findings. Much of our current knowledge regarding the immunologic responses to RSV is from studies in vitro and in animal models. In humans, the immune response cannot be separated from the confounding and poorly understood influence of genetics, environment, age, and antigenic experience.[59-61] Consensus exists that during primary infection, disease is both virally and immunologically mediated. RSV produces its most devastating illness when specific, maternally derived antibody is invariably and abundantly present. The severity of RSV infection in the young infant with high levels of specific antibody and the augmented disease induced by the inactivated RSV vaccine developed in the 1960s first suggested the putative singular role of the immune response in RSV's pathogenesis in infants.[62-64]

The potential importance of the host's immune response to the development of disease and the subsequent rowen of long-term complications has been further supported by the observation that RSV is not very invasive or cytopathogenic.[65] Viral loads do not correlate with the histopathology. Reducing viral replication during RSV with the administration of neutralizing antibody has not diminished the pulmonary pathology in rodent models or ameliorated clinical disease in infants.[66,67]

The relative contribution of the immune response to disease in infants, however, has been questioned by the observation that among children with bronchiolitis, those with RSV bronchiolitis produced a more robust response of proinflammatory cytokines in their nasal washes than did children with non-RSV bronchiolitis, but it was not associated with more severe disease and, indeed, appeared protective against hypoxia.[68] Furthermore, examination of fatal RSV cases has shown that RSV antigen was extensively present in the pulmonary tissue, indicating abundant viral replication.[69] Cytokine production on the other hand was nearly absent, and the expression of apoptosis was increased. These children with fatal RSV infection, therefore, appeared to have had an inadequate immune response and unabashed viral replication. Whether the innate or adaptive immune responses, or both, are enhanced or suppressed in association with more severe disease remains controversial, but most likely the pathogenicity of RSV infection results from varying and currently ill-defined combinations of the contributions of the virus and host.

Innate Immunity

The first barrier of defense against RSV infection in infants is the innate immune response, which is initiated by infection of the respiratory epithelium.[61,65,70,71] This early innate response does not evoke an immune memory. Infection of the respiratory epithelium, antigen-processing cells (dendrites), and macrophages produces multiple alterations in gene expression, which result in the production of cell surface markers and the release of cytokines and chemokines (Fig. 158-4). Inflammatory cells are recruited to the respiratory tract and consist of neutrophils as well as macrophages, mononuclear cells, T cells, NK cells, and eosinophils. Integral to the type of inflammatory cytokines and chemokines evoked and their polarization toward Th1 or Th2 cellular responses are the pattern recognition proteins, toll-like

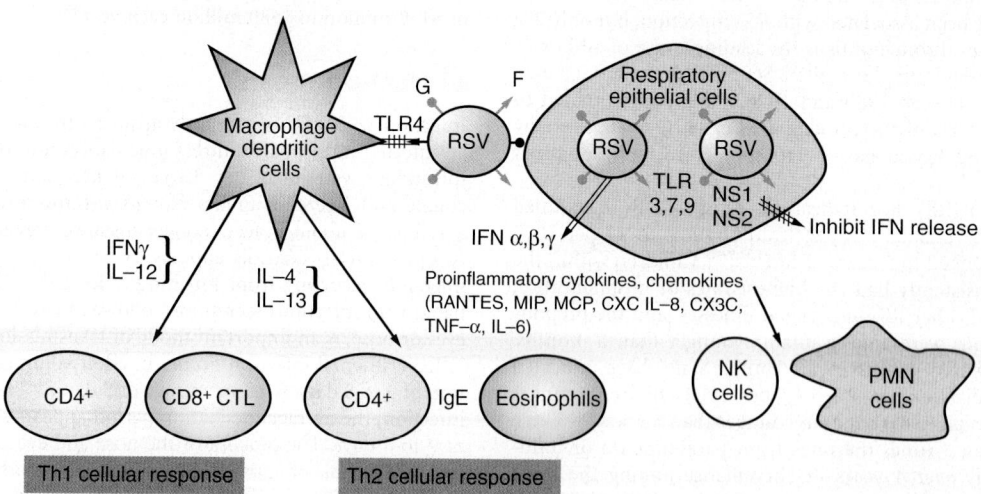

Figure 158-4 **Early innate and adaptive immunity response to respiratory syncytial virus (RSV).** RSV's envelope glycoprotein G attaches to the respiratory tract epithelial cells by glucosamine glycans expressed on the cell surface, and F interacts with antigen-presenting cells (macrophages, dendritic cells) through toll-like receptor 4 (TLR4) protein. This triggers the production and release of antiviral interferons (IFN-α, IFN-β, IFN-γ) and cascade of proinflammatory cytokines and chemokines. Two early nonstructural RSV gene products (NS1, NS2) antagonize interferon production. The chemokines recruit polymorphonuclear neutrophils (PMN cells), natural killer (NK) cells, and CD4+ and CD8+ T cells. A Th1-type cellular response becomes dominant under the influence of IFN-γ and interleukin-12 (IL-12), whereas under the influence of IL-4 and IL-13, the cellular response is skewed toward Th2 with the production of immunoglobulin E (IgE) and eosinophils. *(Adapted from Hall CB, Walsh EE. Respiratory Syncytial Virus. In: Feigin R, Cherry J, Demmler G, Kaplan S, eds. Textbook of Pediatric Infectious Diseases. 6th ed. Philadelphia: Elsevier Saunders; 2009:2462-2487.)*

receptors (TLRs).[70] The variability in the endowed innate defense and susceptibility of the host are also being increasingly correlated with polymorphisms in genes that are integral to various components of innate immunity.[70,72]

Adaptive Immunity

The relative contributions and interactions of different arms of the immune response to either a primary or recurrent exposure to RSV are not well defined. Their significance in the pathogenesis of natural disease or that seen after immunization is complex and unclear. However, considerable evidence suggests that an effective, nondetrimental immune response to RSV infection requires a fine balance of the multiple components of immunity, and that balance is determined by both host and viral factors.[59,65]

Serum neutralizing antibody provides some, but not complete, protection against RSV infection. Higher titers of antibody generally correlate with better resistance to infection, but no defined level of neutralizing antibody is predictive of the risk for infection, the severity of illness, or recovery in children or adults.[73,74] Higher levels of maternal antibody have been correlated with lower infection rates and with less severe illness in some studies, but not in others.[75,76] More recently, the trials of administration of RSV monoclonal antibody to high-risk infants have demonstrated protection against more severe RSV disease.[77]

Passively derived maternal antibody usually declines to undetectable levels by 6 months of age, but occasionally it may remain up to 9 to 12 months of age. During primary infection, serum immunoglobulin M (IgM) antibody appears within several days, but it is transient and detectable usually only for a few weeks.[65] During the second week, IgG antibody appears, usually peaks in the fourth week, and begins to decline after 1 to 2 months. The IgA serum antibody response is more variable in infants. An anamnestic response involving all three immunoglobulin classes occurs after reinfection, and after about three infections, the titers reach levels similar to those in adults.

Primary and subsequent infection produce antibody to many of the RSV proteins. However, the major immunoprotective antigens are two large surface glycoproteins, F and G.[10] Both contain neutralizing epitopes, but those on the F protein are conserved between the two strain groups, resulting in antibody to the F protein being cross-reactive between group A and B strains. In contrast, the response to the variable G protein is group and genotype specific.[78]

Although young children are able to produce neutralizing antibodies directed against both the F and G proteins, the neutralizing antibody responses, especially to the F protein, are blunted in infants younger than 6 months.[79] The G protein is heavily glycosylated and, therefore, is a poor immunogen in infants. Furthermore, maternal antibody appears to have more of a dampening effect on the antibody response to G than to F. In infants, the antibody response to the F and G proteins mainly involves the subclasses IgG_1 and IgG_3. However, adults respond to the G protein with antibodies in both the IgG_1 and the IgG_2 subclasses, and the adult response to the F protein is predominantly IgG_1. Antibodies after primary and recurrent infection usually decline substantially within months. Subsequent to natural infection, 75% of adults demonstrate a fourfold or greater drop in titer.[80] A protective role for local antibody in RSV infection has been suggested because RSV spreads from cell to cell, and in animal studies, circulating antibody does not prevent viral replication in the nasal passages.[73,81] RSV-specific IgA antibody, which is produced in nasal secretions during primary and subsequent infection, has been associated with protecting the upper respiratory tract from infection and has been correlated with clearance of viral shedding.[73] Serum-derived IgG, although present in the nasal secretions, is more protective against lower than upper respiratory tract infection. Children with RSV infection may also produce transient specific IgE antibody responses in the respiratory tract. Levels in the nasal secretions of both RSV-specific IgE antibodies and of cysteinyl leukotrienes have been correlated with increased risk for more severe acute infection with wheezing and with later episodes of recurrent wheezing.[82,83]

Cell-mediated immunity is likely to be pivotal in the clearance of virus and in recovery, but it has not been clearly shown to have a role in protection against reinfection and illness. The central role of the cellular immune response is supported by observations that adults and children with deficiencies of cellular immunity, as well as experimentally immunosuppressed animals, have more severe disease and prolonged shedding.[84,85] However, most of our information delineating the specific components of the cellular response induced by RSV are derived from rodent models and to a much lesser extent from humans.

Multiple suppressive effects on the cellular immune response are associated with RSV infection. Diminished in vitro lymphoproliferative responses during initial and repeated infections suggest impaired RSV-specific helper T-cell responses. Furthermore, RSV-infected dendrites have diminished ability to activate CD4+ T cells, and enhanced apoptosis of CD4+ and CD8+ lymphocytes is observed among infants with RSV bronchiolitis.[86-88]

RSV infection in both animals and humans engenders a spectrum of both Th1- and Th2-dominant responses (see Fig. 158-4). Th1-dominant responses, characterized by the production of CD8+ cytotoxic lymphocyte (CTL) and Th1 CD4+ cells secreting interleukin-2 (IL-2), interferon-γ (IFN-γ), and tumor necrosis factor-α (TNF-α) are associated with viral clearance and minimal pulmonary cytopathology. In contrast, Th2-dominant responses induce Th2 CD4+ cells, which stimulate IL-4, IL-5, IL-10, and IL-13 secretion. These Th2 cytokines affect CD8+ T-cell function and impair viral clearance.[16] IL-4 and IL-13 also augment isotype switching to IgE, and a Th2-biased response has been correlated with wheezing, more severe disease, and greater cellular inflammation and eosinophilia in the lung.[82,89]

Whether RSV evokes predominantly a Th1- or Th2-biased response has been shown to be influenced by the individual's genetic background, age, and previous RSV experience and the specific antigen. Infants within the first several months of life have been observed to have higher levels of Th2-type cytokines in nasal secretions than older infants.[90] Inactivated virus, as used in the initial formalin-inactivated vaccine and even in subunit vaccines, is more likely to induce a Th2-like response in experiments with unprimed animals than is live virus.[16] Antigenic stimulation with the F protein is associated with a predominantly Th1 response, whereas the G protein produces a Th2-biased response, possibly because its CX3C motif adversely affects the CD8+ T-cell response.[91]

The complexities and remaining conundrums of the immune response to RSV do not allow a definitive explanation that encompasses the widely divergent clinical and experimental observations gathered over the past 50 years. However, the wealth of data currently available indicate that mucosal antibodies offer first-line defense against infection of the upper respiratory tract, and serum neutralizing antibodies, once thought to be detrimental, provide limited protection against illness. The evoked T-cell responses are integral to efficient viral clearance and recovery, and their relative polarization toward Th1 or Th2 patterns appear to mold the clinical manifestations within the undefined genetic cast.

Clinical Manifestations

Clinical observations over the half century of RSV's recognition have confirmed the important immunologic correlates that naturally acquired immunity to RSV infection is incomplete, variable, and not durable. Repeated infections are common, but severe disease rarely occurs after the primary encounter. Lower respiratory tract involvement may occur with repeated infections, but it is generally confined to those at either end of the age spectrum.[34,35,73]

INFECTION AMONG YOUNG CHILDREN

Primary infections with RSV frequently involve the lower respiratory tract, particularly among infants within the first several months of life. Most commonly these present as bronchiolitis, followed by pneumonia and tracheobronchitis.[2,34,35] Croup is the least common form of clinical illness and usually accounts for less than 2% to 10% of the cases. Upper respiratory tract signs almost always accompany the lower respiratory tract disease, or the infection may be confined to the upper respiratory tract, which in young children is commonly associated with fever and otitis media (Fig. 158-5). Rarely is the first infection asymptomatic.[34-36,92] The risk for lower respiratory tract involvement occurring with the first infection is high. Pneumonia or bronchiolitis has been estimated to occur in 30% to 71%, depending on the age and population.[2,34,35,92,93] Among infants younger than 6 months, those with underlying cardiopulmonary disease, and those in close contact with other young children, such as those attending daycare, the proportion developing lower respiratory tract disease may be even higher.[35] Furthermore, the severity of illness among outpatient preschool-aged children is considerable, with two thirds manifesting wheezing and three fourths developing labored breathing (see Fig. 158-5).

RSV infection among young children and older individuals usually starts with an upper respiratory tract illness with nasal congestion and a cough. Hoarseness and laryngitis are not prominent features. A low-grade fever, lasting for 2 to 4 days, occurs in most young children early in the course of the illness. The height or duration of the fever does not correlate with the severity of the disease and is frequently absent in the presence of lower respiratory tract involvement and at the time of hospitalization. With progression of disease to the lower respiratory tract, the cough may become more prominent and productive, followed by an increased respiratory rate, dyspnea, and retractions of the intercostal muscles. With bronchiolitis, both expiratory and inspiratory obstruction may be evident. On auscultation, the infant may have crackles and wheezing. The rapid variability in the presence and intensity of these physical findings is characteristic of bronchiolitis. Repeated observations of the infant, therefore, are required for adequate assessment of clinical severity.[94]

Infants hospitalized with RSV lower respiratory tract infection commonly have some impairment of oxygenation.[94] This reflects diffuse viral involvement of the lung parenchyma, which causes an abnormally low ratio of ventilation to perfusion. Usually this is not clinically apparent, and mild degrees of desaturation may persist despite clinical improvement. A small proportion of hospitalized infants will develop alveolar hypoventilation and progressive hypercarbia and may require assisted ventilation. Hospitalization, if required, averages 3 days.[2] For most infants, however, the duration of the acute illness is 3 to 10 days, but respiratory signs, especially cough, may be present for 4 or more weeks.

The abnormalities observed on chest radiograph may be minimal irrespective of the severity of the child's illness. Hyperaeration has been shown to be especially indicative of RSV infection and may be associated with peribronchial thickening.[95,96] Most children exhibit only airway disease. Less than 10% of bronchiolitis cases have evidence of both airway and airspace disease, and only about 1% have parenchymal consolidation.[95] However, about 20% to 35% of children with RSV lower respiratory tract disease have opacities, which are commonly misdiagnosed as bacterial pneumonia. These most commonly are subsegmental in the right upper or middle lobe and result from atelectasis. Pleural fluid is rarely demonstrated.

OTITIS MEDIA

Acute otitis media is a common complication of RSV infection among young children.[97-100] Among children within the first 3 years of life who developed acute otitis media, as many as 74% have had RSV detected in their middle ear fluid. Acute otitis media usually develops about 5 days after the onset of the respiratory illness and is more common among children older than 1 year than in infants. Even among older children and previously healthy adults with RSV infection, otitis and earache are common complications.[36,47] RSV has been recovered from the middle ear fluid as the sole pathogen, with bacteria, or with another virus in up to 0% to 10% of cases.[97,99] The most frequent concurrent bacterial pathogens are those commonly found in the respiratory tract, especially *Streptococcus pneumoniae*, *Haemophilus influenzae*, and *Moraxella catarrhalis*.[100] RSV is detected slightly more often among children as the sole pathogen than in conjunction with bacteria.

Whether RSV primarily causes the frequently observed otitis media accompanying RSV infection by direct viral invasion or by augmentation of obstruction of the eustachian tube in conjunction with the bacterial infection, or both, is unclear. However, clinical and experimental evidence suggests that coinfection of RSV with a bacterial pathogen may prolong the duration and worsen the outcome of otitis media, resulting in a greater chance of treatment failure with antibiotics and persistent effusion.

INFECTIONS AMONG OLDER CHILDREN AND ADULTS

The frequency of RSV infections at all ages is well illustrated among families with young children and among those in contact with young children, as in schools and daycare facilities.[34-36] In these settings, repetitive RSV infections may occur in successive years. Among longitudinally followed children attending daycare facilities, almost all, 98%, have been shown to acquire RSV infection during their first year, and 75% and 65% during their second and third years, respectively.[35] Recurrent infections commonly are upper respiratory tract illnesses, but 20% to 50% of recurrent infections among preschool-aged children involve the lower respiratory tract.[34] Second episodes of lower respiratory tract illness among children are rarely as severe as the initial episode, and many are associated with wheezing.

Adults also may have repetitive RSV infection occurring within sequential years, especially those living or working with children or in confined military and university settings.[36,37,47,51,101,102] The lack of durable immunity evoked by natural infection is illustrated by a study of 15 healthy adults who became ill with a community-acquired RSV A strain and were subsequently challenged with an RSV A strain at repetitive intervals over 2 to 26 months.[73] Within 2 months of their natural infection, 47% became reinfected, and by 8 months, two thirds had been reinfected. However, successive infections, especially those occurring within close intervals, were associated with decreasing symptoms and shedding.

RSV infection among older adults has been recognized for some time, but the extent of the burden RSV places on the health care of this growing population has not been appreciated fully.[5,48,103] In long-term care facilities, 5% to 27% of respiratory infections have been reported to be caused by RSV. The attack rate generally has been estimated as 1% to 15%, the rate of pneumonia as 10% to 20%, and the mortality as 2% to 5%.[49] A retrospective cohort analysis estimated that among Tennessee nursing home patients, RSV was associated with 15

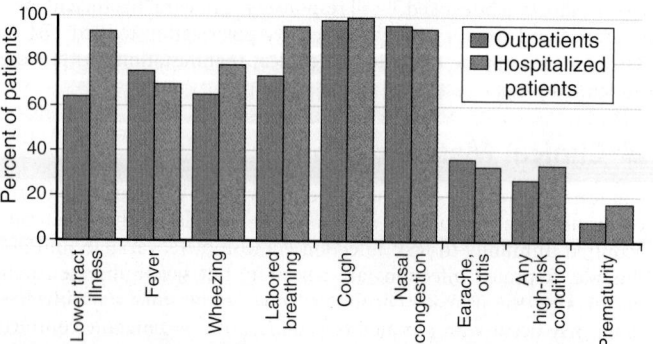

Figure 158-5 **Clinical characteristics of children younger than 5 years with respiratory syncytial virus (RSV) who were outpatients compared with those who were hospitalized.** RSV infection was laboratory confirmed during population-based surveillance of acute respiratory illnesses conducted in counties surrounding Nashville, TN, Rochester, NY, and Cincinnati, OH during 2000 to 2004. *(Data from Hall CB, Weinberg GA, Iwane MK, et al. The burden of respiratory syncytial virus infection in young children. N Engl J Med. 2009;360:588-598.)*

hospitalizations, 17 deaths, and 76 antibiotic courses per 1000 people, and 7% of hospitalizations and 9% of deaths from cardiopulmonary disease.[104] Among all older adults admitted with cardiopulmonary conditions, 10% had RSV infection, compared with 13% with influenza.[105] Illness was equally severe among the two groups: 18% required intensive care, and 10% of the RSV patients died, compared with 6% of the influenza patients. Similarly, among a prospectively studied population of older adults living in the community, RSV was identified as the cause of 7% and influenza as the cause of 9% of respiratory illnesses with identifiable pathogens.[106] The morbidity associated with the two viruses was also comparable: 82% of the RSV patients and 79% of the influenza patients developed lower respiratory tract disease. Among adults attending daycare facilities, 10% of acute respiratory infections were found to be caused by RSV, a rate similar to the rates for influenza and coronaviruses.[107]

A 4-year study of respiratory illnesses among two cohorts of prospectively followed elderly adults emphasizes the epidemiologic and clinical impact of RSV infection among this elderly population[5] (Table 158-1). Two cohorts of individuals 65 years or older were prospectively followed; 608 were healthy and living in the community, and 504 were high-risk elderly people with cardiopulmonary conditions. A third group of 1388 adults hospitalized with acute cardiopulmonary conditions was also evaluated. Using viral isolation, reverse transcriptase–polymerase chain reaction (RT-PCR), and serology, RSV infection was identified among 10% of those in each of the three groups studied. In comparison, influenza infection was identified among 4% of the individuals in the prospectively followed cohorts and among 11% of the hospitalized patients. Clinically the illnesses from RSV and influenza were remarkably similar. Among the healthy elderly outpatients, those with RSV infection and those with influenza were ill for an average 16

TABLE 158-2	Types of Acute Respiratory Infection in Adults Who Are Infected with Respiratory Syncytial Virus (RSV)		
Type of Acute Respiratory Illness	No. of Patients	Percentage of Patients with Symptomatic RSV Infection (n = 177)	Percentage of All Patients with RSV Infection (n = 211)
Asymptomatic	34	—	16
Symptomatic	177	—	84
Upper respiratory tract	131	74	62
With fever	52	29	25
Without fever	79	45	37
Lower respiratory tract	46	26	22
Tracheobronchitis	36	20	17
Wheezing	10	6	5

From Hall CB, Long CE, Schnabel KC. Respiratory syncytial virus infections in previously healthy working adults. *Clin Infect Dis.* 2001;33:792-796. Copyright 2001 with permission from the Infectious Diseases Society of America.

days. Of those with RSV infection, 39% were unable to perform their activities of daily living, which was not significantly different than the proportion (54%) with influenza. Among the hospitalized RSV patients, intensive care was required for 15%, and the mortality rate was 8%, compared with 12% and 7%, respectively, among influenza patients. Almost all RSV infections were symptomatic and frequently associated with appreciable functional impairment and use of health care services.

The increased morbidity associated with RSV infection observed among older adults is only partly explained by the presence of comorbid conditions and age-associated decline in pulmonary function.[108] Evidence is accumulating that among healthy older adults, age adversely affects the immune response to RSV infection. Humoral immunity to RSV among elderly people, however, is equal to or greater than that produced by young adults.[48,74] Age may have its greatest effect on the cellular adaptive response. Experiments with rodents have shown specific defects in the cellular response to RSV infection related to senescence, including the timing and type of the pulmonary cytokine response.[109,110]

RSV's burden among young healthy adults has been less well studied and thus generally unrecognized. Yet the studies that have examined RSV infections among this young population suggest that its impact may be considerable and also comparable to that from influenza.[36,47,101] Among working, healthy adults, RSV infection was symptomatic in 84%, and 22% had lower respiratory tract manifestations (Table 158-2). In comparison to influenza infection occurring in these same individuals, fever was less frequent, but earache and sinus pain and a persistent productive cough were significantly more common with RSV infection (Table 158-3). Thirty-eight percent of those with RSV infection missed work, and the average duration of illness was 9.5 days, which was significantly longer than that produced by influenza.

The frequency of RSV infections and their influenza-like manifestations have also been noted among university students and military recruits.[37,101,102] Wheezing was more frequently associated with RSV infection, and the proportion of military recruits with RSV infection requiring ward confinement was the same as for influenza. Among university students with cough persisting for 6 or more days, RSV was identified more often than the parainfluenza viruses, adenoviruses, pertussis, *Mycoplasma pneumoniae*, or *Chlamydophila pneumoniae*. In more than half of those with RSV infection, the clinical manifestations were indistinguishable from those of pertussis, and most were treated with a macrolide.[102]

TABLE 158-1	Respiratory Syncytial Virus (RSV) Compared with Influenza among Hospitalized Adults*	
Characteristics	RSV (N = 132)	Influenza A (N = 144)
Age (yr)	76 ± 13	76 ± 12
Female sex—N (%)	84 (64)	81 (56)
Chronic illness—N (%)		
Any cardiac disease	71 (54)	71 (49)
Congestive heart failure	39 (30)	33 (23)
Any lung disease	77 (58)	79 (55)
Any heart or lung disease	106 (80)	113 (78)
Diabetes mellitus	35 (27)	28 (19)
Residence in a long-term care facility—N (%)	16 (12)	15 (10)
Smoking (current or past)—N (%)	88 (67)	98 (68)
Influenza vaccination—N (%)	99 (75)	98 (68)
Katz ADL score—mean ± SD	1.2 ± 2.4	1.3 ± 3.0
IADL score—mean ± SD	4.1 ± 4.1	3.3 ± 4.0
Length of hospital stay—days	14 ± 41	8 ± 5
Findings on chest radiography— N (%)		
Infiltrate found	41 (31)	43 (30)
Congestive heart failure	17 (13)	15 (10)
Other	24 (18)	27 (19)
Admission to intensive care unit— N (%)	20 (15)	17 (12)
Use of mechanical ventilation— N (%)	17 (13)	15 (10)
Higher level of care at discharge than at admission—N (%)	7 (5)	8 (6)
Death—N (%)	10 (8)	10 (7)

*Plus-minus values are means plus or minus standard deviation. The Katz Activities of Daily Living (ADL) score and the Instrumental Activities of Daily Living (IADL) score are functional assessments based on a 12-point scale, with 0 representing total independence and 12 representing total dependence. Percentage may not sum to 100 because of rounding.
Modified from Falsey A, Hennessey PA, Formica MA, et al. Respiratory syncytial virus infection in elderly and high-risk adults. *N Engl J Med.* 2005;352:1749-1759.

■ Complications

PATIENTS AT HIGH RISK FOR SEVERE INFECTION

Children with underlying conditions affecting cardiopulmonary function or immunity are most likely to increase the risk for developing

TABLE 158-3	Clinical Characteristics of Illness Due to Influenza or Respiratory Syncytial Virus (RSV) among 211 Previously Healthy Adults		
	No. (%) of Adults with Illness Due to:		
Characteristic	*RSV (n = 177)*	*Influenza (n = 59)*	**P**
Sign or symptom			
Fever (temperature, >37.8°C)	50 (58)	43 (73)	<.001
Nasal congestion, rhinorrhea	157 (89)	46 (78)	<.04
Sore throat	102 (58)	32 (54)	.65
Ear pain	35 (20)	3 (5)	<.01
Headache	70 (40)	48 (81)	<.001
Sinus pain	55 (31)	8 (14)	<.01
Cough			
Nonproductive	150 (85)	47 (80)	.36
Productive	92 (52)	14 (24)	<.001
Lower respiratory tract signs, wheezing	28 (16)	5 (9)	.16
Work absence	67 (38)	39 (66)	<.001
Duration of illness, mean days (range)	9.5 (1–20)	6.8 (39–66)	<.001

From Hall CB, Long CE, Schnabel KC. Respiratory syncytial virus infections in previously healthy working adults. *Clin Infect Dis.* 2001;33:792-796. Copyright 2001 with permission from the Infectious Diseases Society of America.

complicated RSV infection among individuals of any age. Among young children, those most likely to require hospitalization are those who are premature and those with underlying chronic lung disease, cyanotic or complicated congenital heart disease, immunosuppressive conditions, or other chronic diseases that affect the handling of respiratory secretions such as neuromuscular disease.[2,77,111,112] About one third of children within the first 5 years of life hospitalized with RSV infection have one or more of these underlying conditions, and the proportion is greater among those older than 2 years.[2] Among children with RSV infection evaluated in pediatric practices and emergency departments, about one fourth have a preexisting chronic condition.

Preterm gestation, with or without associated chronic lung disease, is clearly a major risk factor for more severe RSV disease.[2,77,112] Hospitalization rates among infants with gestational ages of less than 36 weeks are three or more times higher than the rate for full-term infants. As the gestational age decreases below 32 weeks, the chance of admission with RSV infections rises, and the need for intensive care significantly increases. Recently recognized, however, is the disproportionate economic and clinical burden contributed by late preterm infants, those with gestational ages of 33 to 35 weeks, with RSV infections who represent about three fourths of all preterm infants.[77,113] These late preterm infants, compared with full-term infants, not only have significantly increased costs and risk for hospitalization but also have a significantly greater need for medical resources for at least the subsequent year.

Children with congenital heart disease have long been noted to have increased morbidity and mortality when infected with RSV. Congenital heart conditions have ranked among the top three major conditions among infants hospitalized with RSV infection, and about one fourth to one third require intensive care, and one fifth require mechanical ventilation.[114-117] Infants hospitalized in the first few months of life with uncorrected cyanotic congenital heart disease are at particular peril. However, the increased rate of hospitalization among children with congenital heart disease for RSV remains beyond infancy and appears greatest during the second year of life.[115,117] More complicated or serious illness has been associated with cyanotic congenital heart conditions and those accompanied by pulmonary hypertension. Nevertheless, all types of congenital cardiac abnormalities with functional impairment have been associated with increased risk for hospitalization with RSV infection, especially if needed surgical correction has not yet occurred. Recent advances in surgical and intensive care management of these children, including early correction, have appreciably reduced the mortality from RSV infection among infants with

congenital heart disease from 30% in the 1970s to less than 2% currently.

Multiple demographic and environmental factors also have been evaluated for augmenting the risk for more severe RSV infection.[2,118] Those most frequently associated with RSV disease requiring hospitalization among young children are male gender, crowded living conditions, lower socioeconomic status, exposure to other young children in the home or daycare, exposure to tobacco smoke, and lack of breastfeeding. However, the degree of risk these factors play in the expression of RSV disease in children has been difficult to quantify, and the reported data have been inconsistent and conflicting. The two independent risk factors that appear to be most important for hospitalization with RSV infection are prematurity and young age, especially within the first 3 months of life.[2,77]

Much evidence exists that the genetic background of an individual has important, but mostly undefined, effects on the susceptibility to RSV infection and more severe disease.[119] Groups of children with certain racial and ethnic backgrounds have notably increased rates of hospitalization and severe RSV infection, including Native American Indian and Alaskan Native infants, especially those living in the Yukon-Kuskokwim Delta region who have RSV hospitalization rates 3 to 4 times that observed for other U.S. infants.[77,120] The outcome of primary RSV infection also has been increasingly correlated with specific genetic polymorphisms. Children with more severe RSV disease have been shown to be more likely to have variations in certain genetic loci which affect the immune response.[59,61,72] Among these are loci involved in the expression of cytokines and inflammatory chemokines associated with the development of wheezing and reactive airway disease.

Immunocompromised Patients

Greater awareness of RSV as a cause of morbidity and mortality among immunocompromised patients has resulted from the increasing numbers of patients receiving solid organ and hematopoietic cell transplantation (HCT) with more intensive chemotherapy regimens and also from the greater availability of sensitive techniques for identification of RSV infection, such as PCR assays. The reported frequency of RSV infection among immunocompromised patients varies widely from about 5% to 50%, depending on the type of immunosuppression.[85,121-126] Recent retrospective case series suggest a mortality rate of about 9% to 18%.

RSV is usually introduced onto wards that house immunocompromised patients by medical staff or visitors who have a community-acquired RSV infection that may be mild or unrecognized.[124,125] Once introduced, however, the spread may be rapid and difficult to control and accompanied by appreciable morbidity and mortality.[85,121,123] The severity of the RSV infection among these patients is primarily related to the degree of immunosuppression[85,124,125,127]; severe combined immunodeficiency states and HCT recipients are particularly at risk for a poor outcome. Among transplant recipients, the source and timing of the transplant are major factors. More severe disease has been correlated with occurrence of RSV infection within 2 months of receiving the transplant and before engraftment, and with the presence of acute or chronic graft-versus-host disease. Lymphopenia significantly increases the chance of progression to severe lower respiratory tract disease. Among children, young age also is associated with a poorer prognosis.

RSV infection in these patients may clinically mimic other opportunistic agents and result in the correct etiology not being diagnosed or even suspected. The presence of upper respiratory tract signs, sinusitis, and wheezing may be more indicative of RSV infection than other pathogens.[126] Concurrent infections by other infectious agents, including community-acquired infections, may further confound or delay the diagnosis of RSV infection.[125,128] The manifestations of RSV infection range from asymptomatic to severe lower respiratory tract disease and respiratory failure. Among HCT patients, RSV infection within a year of transplantation was significantly associated with severe airflow decline.[129] With lower respiratory tract involvement, roentgenographic findings range from focal interstitial infiltrates, sometimes with hyperinflation or with lobar consolidation, to generalized alveolar and interstitial infiltrates, or even to a picture of acute respiratory distress syndrome.[123,126] With high-resolution computed tomography, the characteristic findings are airspace consolidation, small centrilobular nodules, ground-glass opacities, and thickening of the bronchial walls. These manifestations tend to have an asymmetrical but bilateral distribution.[130]

Among patients with human immunodeficiency virus (HIV) infection, RSV has been the most frequently identified cause of viral respiratory disease.[121] Although most of these RSV infections are community acquired, HIV patients also are at particular risk for nosocomial infection from RSV. The manifestations of RSV infection vary according to the stage and severity of the HIV infection. Most develop lower respiratory tract disease, but it generally is not as severe as that occurring among the more highly immunosuppressed transplant recipients.[131] HIV patients who have evidence of immunocompromise may shed RSV for prolonged periods, and the infection usually involves the lower respiratory tract. Confounding this, however, is the observation that children with HIV infection and concurrent viral respiratory infections also have a higher rate of bacterial coinfections.[131] Furthermore, the clinical outcome of respiratory viral infections has not been consistently different between children with and those without HIV infection.

No definitive guidelines are currently available for optimal therapy for immunocompromised patients with RSV infection. Determining the effectiveness of the various therapeutic regimens that have been used in highly compromised patients is hampered by limited data, lack of prospective controlled trials, and the diversity of the patient population. Furthermore, the efficacy of therapy among transplant recipients depends on the length of time between the post-transplantation onset of infection and the time at which therapy is initiated.[85,123]

The therapeutic and prophylactic agents used for RSV infection among highly immunocompromised patients have generally focused on intravenous immune globulin products, and more recently on the passive administration of humanized monoclonal antibody against the RSV F protein (palivizumab), with or without concurrent ribavirin therapy. The use of these alone or in combination has been evaluated primarily by observational and retrospective studies, and the results have been mixed, with some suggesting a trend toward diminished morbidity and progression to lower respiratory tract disease when used therapeutically.[123,124,127,132-134] However, consensus exists that these agents appear safe and well tolerated by highly immunosuppressed patients. Prophylactic administration of palivizumab to immunocompromised patients has not been adequately evaluated and is not recommended.[77] The American Academy of Pediatrics, nevertheless, states that children with severe immunodeficiencies may benefit from prophylaxis. Using a decision analysis model to evaluate the effect of palivizumab prophylaxis to prevent RSV mortality following bone marrow transplantation in children, the survival rate was estimated to increase by 10%, and that 12 children would need to be treated to prevent one fatal RSV infection.[135]

Most important in the management of immunocompromised patients is prevention of RSV infection by strict adherence to infection control policies. The Centers for Disease Control and Prevention guidelines for preventing opportunistic infections in hematopoietic stem cell transplant recipients provides evidence-based recommendations for control of RSV infection and transmission. These guidelines emphasize preventing the introduction of community respiratory viruses, including RSV, onto units with compromised patients and stress the importance of early diagnosis.[136,137]

ACUTE COMPLICATIONS

Apnea is one of the most frightening and striking of acute complications among young infants with RSV infection. Up to 20% of infants hospitalized with RSV infection have been admitted with apnea.[138,139] Among infants evaluated in the emergency department with unspecified bronchiolitis, 3% had a diagnosis of apnea. Most at risk for developing apnea are preterm infants with a gestational age of 32 weeks or less, those with a history of apnea of prematurity, and infants of young postnatal age, less than 44 weeks after conception. Characteristically, the apnea occurs at the onset of the RSV infection and may be the initial sign, before respiratory symptoms are noted.

The pathophysiology of apnea associated with RSV is not clear. In a model of RSV-infected weanling rats with capsaicin-induced apnea, apnea appeared to result from sensorineural stimulation occurring during RSV infection that involved the release of γ-aminobutyric acid and substance P.[140] Clinically, the apnea associated with RSV infection is nonobstructive. The prognosis is generally good following the acute RSV infection with no subsequent episodes, even with later acquired respiratory infections.

Infants admitted with RSV lower respiratory tract disease may be at increased risk for aspiration, which can appear clinically similar to bronchiolitis with airway hyperreactivity.[141,142] In one study of infants hospitalized with the diagnosis of RSV bronchiolitis and followed over a 12-month period, 83% developed reactive airway disease if they received neither ribavirin nor therapy for aspiration. However, the development of hyperreactive airways was reduced to 45% in infants who were given thickened feedings along with early ribavirin therapy. Furthermore, the decrease in episodes of reactive airway disease was greater in infants who received both ribavirin and thickened feedings than in infants who received either therapy alone.[142]

A complicating or coexistent bacterial infection is a frequent concern among those caring for young infants hospitalized with RSV lower respiratory tract disease. As a result, many children with RSV infection unnecessarily receive antibiotics. In part, this is because of their young age, the presence of fever, and, particularly, the relatively common appearance on the chest radiograph of opacities from viral infiltrates and atelectasis, which are commonly mistaken for consolidation of bacterial pneumonia. However, multiple studies in the United States have shown that a secondary bacterial infection is an unusual complication of RSV infection.[143-146] A 9-year prospective study of infants hospitalized with RSV lower respiratory tract disease identified secondary bacterial pneumonia in less than 1%.[143] Furthermore, antibiotic therapy has not been shown to improve the rate of recovery among infants with RSV lower respiratory tract disease.[147] More frequent is coinfection with another viral or bacterial agent, commonly acquired by this young age group. Most common of these coinfections are other respiratory viruses, such as adenoviruses, influenza, parainfluenza viruses, human metapneumovirus, and bocavirus.[148] Urinary tract infections are the most frequently identified concurrent bacterial infections.[149] In developing countries, however, complicating bacterial infections are more common and may contribute appreciably to the high mortality rate from RSV.

LONG-TERM COMPLICATIONS

Recurrent wheezing after RSV lower respiratory tract disease and bronchiolitis in infancy has long been recognized as a frequent sequela, but a direct link between the two remains unclear. About 30% to 50% of children hospitalized with RSV infection later develop repeated occurrences of wheezing.[61,150] For many children, the severity of the recurrent wheezing episodes decreases with age, although in some, pulmonary function abnormalities may persist without clinical manifestations.[151-153] Others may have persistent wheezing into adolescence, or have wheezing cease during childhood, but recur as adults. The frequency of this long-term sequela in the general population is confounded by most studies having focused on children with more severe illness, those hospitalized with RSV infection or bronchiolitis.[61,150] Similarities between the immune responses after RSV infection and the responses observed with reactive airway disease have been offered as a possible explanation for the immunopathogenesis of the putative link between RSV bronchiolitis and the long-term pulmonary sequelae that may persist clinically into adolescence and substantially contribute to the development of reactive airways in adulthood.

Epidemiologic evidence indicates that atopy in the child or family is not a major cause of this link. However, in a murine model of allergen-induced airway inflammation and remodeling, previous RSV infection could induce airway abnormalities in mice exposed to allergen through the airway, even though these mice had not been previously sensitized to the allergens.[154] This suggests that even without an atopic family background, RSV infection may provoke an allergic phenotype. In addition, RSV infection has been shown both in vitro and in children infected with RSV to produce an immunologic response similar to that observed with allergic sensitization, one with a predominantly Th2 T-cell profile and release of proinflammatory mediators, IgE, and neuropeptides[59,61,89,150,155,156] (see "Immunity and Pathogenesis of Disease"). A similar response, however, may be produced by viruses other than RSV.[150] The direct correlation between RSV lower respiratory tract disease and pulmonary sequelae likely remains elusive because the clinical syndrome of hyperreactive airways results from many different genetic, developmental, and environmental disorders.[61,157]

Diagnosis

RSV infection among young children is most often diagnosed clinically in the setting of the community's RSV season. Among adults, however, the findings are less specific, and RSV is commonly not suspected. A laboratory diagnosis may be made by viral isolation, using standard cell cultures or shell vials by one of the rapid diagnostic tests, or by serology.

Viral isolation, once the standard technique, mostly has been supplanted by one of the rapid antigen assays or by nucleic acid amplification, PCR. The sensitivity of viral isolation is highly dependent on the sensitivity of the cell lines, the specific laboratory's expertise, and the quality and handling of the specimen. RSV is a relatively labile virus and requires prompt inoculation without subjecting the specimen to major temperature changes during transportation. Nasopharyngeal washes or tracheal secretions are generally better than nasal swabs, although combined throat swab and swabs of both nares improve the rate of recovery over a single nasal swab.[158,159] Specific cytopathic changes usually appear within 2 to 5 days, but the range is 2 to 10 days. The major advantages of isolation in cell culture are having an isolate for further characterization for epidemiologic, research, sensitivity, diagnostic, and other potential research analyses, and, second, of identifying coinfecting viral agents.

Multiple rapid direct antigen detection tests are widely available and are used by most laboratories.[158] Direct and indirect immunofluorescent assays are both sensitive (93% to 98%) and specific (92% to 97%) but require several hours and skilled laboratory personnel. Most frequently used are the commercially available rapid detection tests using an enzyme immunoassay (EIA) method and to a lesser extent the optical immunoassay (OIA), which has a sensitivity of 88% to 95% and specificity of 97% to 100%. EIA tests have the advantages of rapidity, ease, and relatively low cost. Their disadvantage is their wide range of specificity (75% to 100%) and sensitivity (usually 60% to 70%, with ranges of about 50% to 90%).[158] The accuracy of these tests may vary according to the manufacturer and the viral strain but are highly dependent on the adequacy of the specimen and whether it was obtained during the peak of RSV activity in the community. The positive predictive value of these assays falls precipitously when the prevalence of RSV is low in the community. These tests also perform less well in immunocompromised and elderly populations.[49,158]

RT-PCR for the diagnosis of RSV infections has consistently demonstrated much higher rates of specificity and sensitivity than the rapid antigen diagnostic assays.[158] Among 496 specimens obtained from children with RSV infection determined by viral isolation or duplicate positive RT-PCR assays, about 50% were positive by both RT-PCR and culture, and 50% by RT-PCR alone. Less than 1% were positive only by viral isolation. The RT-PCR assays also allow the strain group of RSV to be concurrently determined. Rapidly evolving new technologies have allowed enhanced methods of detection with real-time monitoring (real-time RT-PCR). Other respiratory pathogens may be simultaneously identified, and with sensitive multiple-function systems, a limited number of agents may be detected with concurrent quantitative analyses. The rapidly expanding microassay technology allows the simultaneous highly sensitive detection of potentially innumerable agents.[160,161]

Serologic diagnosis of RSV infection is primarily useful for epidemiologic studies rather than for patient management, not only because of the delay required to obtain convalescent sera, but also because young infants, many older individuals, and immunocompromised patients may not produce a significant rise in antibody titer, depending on the assay used. Serologic diagnosis most frequently uses enzyme immunoassays and neutralization assays. These also allow detection of specific antibody classes. Earlier methods of serologic diagnosis by using assays that detect specific IgM antibodies are of limited usefulness because specific IgM antibodies are not consistently detectable in patients with proven RSV infection and may require 1 to 7 weeks to appear after the onset of illness. Secretory class-specific antibodies to RSV in nasopharyngeal secretions may also be detected by enzyme immunoassays. Because these secretory antibodies may be present earlier in infection than humoral antibodies, their detection has been used as an adjunct to diagnosis by antigen detection.

Treatment

Most children and adults with RSV infection require no more than the usual care given to ensure comfort, fever control, and adequate fluid intake. For bronchiolitis, the most commonly administered medications are those used for exacerbations of hyperreactive airway disease, primarily bronchodilators and corticosteroids, and also antibiotics.[94,162] Multiple studies and meta-analyses have shown these agents are not consistently effective for RSV disease or bronchiolitis of unspecified cause among previously healthy young children and, thus, are not routinely recommended (see Chapter 63).

Antibiotic therapy for children with RSV lower respiratory tract disease should be reserved for those with specific evidence of a coexisting bacterial infection.[94] Preemptive administration of antibiotics to children with RSV infection or bronchiolitis has not been associated with an improved outcome. Furthermore, complicating or secondary bacterial infections, other than otitis media among children with RSV infection in developed countries, is unusual.[143,144]

Ribavirin (1-β-D-ribofuranosyl-1,2,4-triazole-3-carboxamide), a synthetic nucleoside, is the only currently approved specific treatment for RSV lower respiratory tract disease in hospitalized infants (see Chapter 41). The drug, administered as a small-particle aerosol, has shown some clinical benefit and improved levels of oxygenation in some studies, but an improvement in the duration of hospitalization or short-term outcome has not been consistently demonstrated. An analysis of the studies examining the effect of ribavirin therapy among children with RSV lower respiratory tract disease included 11 relatively small randomized controlled trials. Of these, 7 showed clinical benefit, and 4 did not.[94] A Cochrane analysis of randomized placebo-controlled trials evaluating ribavirin for the therapy of children hospitalized with RSV lower respiratory tract disease found that ribavirin reduced the duration of mechanical ventilation and length of hospitalization.[163] Significant reduction in respiratory failure or deaths was not shown, but few children had either.

In view of the unclear degree of benefit relative to the considerable cost of aerosolized ribavirin, the American Academy of Pediatrics recommends that ribavirin should not be used routinely in the management of RSV lower respiratory tract infections.[77,94] Ribavirin therapy should be considered on an individual basis for children who have severe disease or who are at high-risk for developing complicated or severe disease.

Many new approaches are being investigated to develop therapies specific for RSV disease.[10,61,164] Among these are new inosine monophosphate dehydrogenase inhibitors, the class to which ribavirin belongs. Other approaches include the development of inhibitors of attachment and fusion, including small peptide fusion inhibitors, N protein, and RNA-dependent RNA polymerase inhibitors. Much interest and effort recently has been focused on developing oligonucleotides that interfere with viral RNA, antisense/siRNA inhibitors. Some of these have shown promise in clinical trails. An alternative approach has been to develop anti-inflammatory and immunomodulatory therapies.

Prevention

The viper's venom,
the serpent's spell
daunts not the tortoise
beneath his shell....
C.B.H.

INFECTION CONTROL

Prevention rather than treatment is the preferable, but yet unattained, goal for the control of RSV infection. Avoiding infection at home through interruption of the transmission of the virus is difficult and unlikely to be effective. However, general precautions may be useful against the spread of infectious secretions on hands and fomites. These include good hand hygiene, use of hand-rub antiseptic products, and care of contaminated tissues, toys, and other objects likely to be contaminated with secretions.[137]

On hospital wards, however, RSV poses a particular hazard for nosocomial spread.[51,123,165-167] Yearly outbreaks occur with widespread infection among both children and adults, including medical personnel who may continue to work despite upper respiratory tract signs. Furthermore, the lack of durable immunity to RSV results in a large, potentially susceptible population of patients of all ages. Considerable morbidity and mortality have been associated with nosocomial RSV infection among those with underlying conditions, especially prematurity and cardiopulmonary and immunocompromised conditions. Strict adherence to recommended guidelines, therefore, is essential and cost-effective.

RSV may be spread by close contact and by direct inoculation of large droplets from the secretions of an infected person, as well as by indirect spread from hands that touch infectious secretions in the environment.[51,166] Careful hand hygiene by all personnel, therefore, is integral to preventing nosocomial transmission (Table 158-4). Additional procedures aimed at preventing self-inoculation include the wearing of eye-nose goggles and gloves. Gloves enhance hand hygiene methods by diminishing the likelihood that personnel will touch their eyes or nose. Procedures aimed at reducing the risk for the introduction and spread of RSV to other personnel and patients include the wearing gowns for close contact with infected patients, isolation or cohorting of infected patients, and use of rapid diagnostic techniques. In addition, during the RSV season, staff with signs of respiratory illness should not care for high-risk patients, and visitors should be screened for respiratory illness. Of prime importance is that infection control procedures for RSV be reviewed yearly with all personnel, before and during the RSV season, to maintain compliance.[51]

PROPHYLAXIS

Prophylaxis using the passive administration of RSV-specific antibody currently is available primarily for those groups most at risk for developing severe or complicated RSV disease. High-risk children administered monthly doses of intravenous immune globulin containing high levels of RSV neutralizing antibody (RSV-IGIV) or intramuscular monoclonal antibody have shown reduced rates of hospitalization from RSV infection.[77] RSV-IGIV is no longer available and has been replaced by palivizumab, a humanized monoclonal antibody that has been estimated to be 50 to 100 times more effective than the intravenously administered polyclonal antibody. Palivizumab was developed from a mouse monoclonal antibody directed against a protective

TABLE 158-4	Infection Control Procedures, both Standard Precautions and Contact Precautions, for Prevention of Respiratory Syncytial Virus (RSV) Infection Recommended by Centers for Disease Control and Prevention
Recommendation Category, Procedure	**Comments**
Category 1-B Recommendations*	
Hand washing	Water with soap or antibacterial agent or waterless antiseptic hand rub
Wearing gloves	Combined with hand washing before and after each glove change; may diminish self-inoculation
Wearing gowns	When direct contact with patient or patient secretions is likely
Wearing masks plus eye protection	Eyes and nose are major sites for inoculation
Housing patient in private room or in a cohort isolated from other patients	Patients with documented infection can be grouped and isolated from other patients; beds should be separated by >0.9 m
Use of dedicated patient care equipment	Equipment, including toys, assigned to specific patients
Sometimes Recommended with Less or No Supporting Evidence	
Staff assigned according to patient's RSV status	Specific staff care only for patients with RSV infection
Visitor restrictions during RSV season	Some qualify by restricting young children only
Screening visitors for illness during RSV season	Visitor assessed by trained personnel or advised by use of an educational patient information list

*From Garner JS. Guidelines for isolation precautions in hospitals. *Infect Control Hosp Epidemiol.* 1996;17:53-80.

From Hall CB. Nosocomial respiratory syncytial virus infections: The "Cold War" has not ended. *Clin Infect Dis.* 2000;360:588-598.

epitope of the RSV fusion (F) protein. Only the antigen-recognition site was inserted into the spine of a human antibody. Immunoprophylaxis of five monthly intramuscular doses of 15 mg/kg initiated a month before the RSV season has been shown to reduce hospitalization rates by 34% to 82% among selected groups of high-risk infants.[77] Palivizumab administration does not prevent infection with RSV but is associated with diminished clinical severity, the risk for developing lower respiratory tract disease, and need for hospitalization.

Currently, palivizumab is recommended for selected children who are younger than 2 years and are considered to have a high risk for developing severe RSV disease. Included are those with prematurity (<32 weeks' gestation), chronic lung disease, functionally important cardiac disease, and chronic conditions that interfere with the handling of respiratory secretions.[77] Infants born between 32 and 35 weeks' gestation also have significantly greater risk for hospitalization and use of medical services for RSV disease than full-term infants.[77,168] However, considering that most premature infants are between 32 and 35 weeks' gestation and that palivizumab prophylaxis is very expensive, the American Academy of Pediatrics recommends that infants born from 32 to 35 weeks' gestation be considered for prophylaxis if they are younger than 3 months of age at the start of the RSV season and have additional risk factors.[77]

Controversy exists concerning the extent of the use of palivizumab prophylaxis based primarily on the concern of its considerable cost relative to its benefit. Economic analyses in general have not shown an overall savings in health care costs for prophylaxis of all infants less than 32 weeks' gestation and with underlying high-risk conditions, but the benefit relative to the cost among those at highest risk increases.[169,170] Palivizumab prophylaxis has not been shown to reduce the mortality from RSV, but currently in the United States, the mortality from RSV infection, even among high-risk infants, is very low. The effect of palivizumab on the long-term sequelae of RSV infection has not been adequately evaluated.[171]

Additional products are being evaluated for the prevention of RSV disease in high-risk individuals, including a newer humanized monoclonal antibody, motavizumab.[172] Motavizumab is derived from palivizumab and is also directed against the F protein. In vitro, it exhibits a 20-fold improvement in RSV neutralization. A recent multicenter study of more than 6000 high-risk infants showed that infants receiving motavizumab compared with those receiving palivizumab had a 26% relative reduction in RSV hospitalization and was superior to palivizumab in reducing RSV-related outpatient visits for lower respiratory tract disease.[173]

IMMUNIZATION

The optimal means of prophylaxis for RSV infection would be an effective vaccine. However, the challenges to achieve this are appreciable. Ideally, a vaccine should provide better protection than natural disease, which does not confer durable immunity. Also, concern still exists that an unpredictable abnormal response could occur in some vaccinees during their first maternal RSV infection, such as was observed during the trials with the initial formalin-inactivated RSV vaccine.[62] Furthermore, immunization would have to be initiated within the first weeks of life because most hospitalization for RSV occurs in the first several months of life. Additional considerations include that the populations potentially in need of immunization are diverse, and that no adequate animal model exists to judge the efficacy or safety of a vaccine before human trials. Even the response to a vaccine administered to adults and healthy older children may not predict the vaccine's safety or protection among very young infants.

The young age at initiation of immunization is of major anatomic and immunologic importance for the potential development of adverse effects. The physiologic consequences of any associated increase in respiratory secretions elicited by a live-attenuated vaccine are magnified in the infant in whom alveolar development is incomplete and the lumina of the small airways are highly susceptible to obstruction from increased production of mucus and secretions.[174]

The immunologic repertoire of young infants is also incomplete, and their immune response is variable. This may be compounded by the presence of specific maternal antibody. Among 0- to 24-month-old children hospitalized with RSV infection, 66% of infants younger than 6 months developed detectable levels of RSV neutralizing antibody.[175] The preinfection level of maternal antibody appeared to be more important than age in determining the infant's response. However, among infants administered a candidate live-attenuated RSV vaccine, all seronegative children older than 6 months developed at least a fourfold antibody response following a dose of vaccine, whereas only 44% of infants 2 to 4 months of age were able to do so after two doses.[176]

Cytotoxic T-cell responses have been shown to be impaired following RSV infection in rodent models,[177] and among young infants, the induction of a cytotoxic cellular response from RSV immunization appears variable.[176] Of the children given the live candidate RSV vaccine in the study cited earlier, less than 40% of those under 5 months of age produced a detectable, but transient, cytotoxic T-cell response to RSV, compared with 65% of those 6 to 24 months of age.

RSV immunization in early life is further complicated by the apparent bias toward a Th2-type immunologic response to RSV that exists during the first 3 months of life.[90] A vaccine given during this period, therefore, may result in an altered cytokine and inflammatory response to the vaccine and to subsequent encounters with wild RSV, which may contribute to airway dysfunction and allergic manifestations.[61,65] The possibility that sensitization to other concomitant antigens also may occur has been suggested by experiments in animal models.[178] This implies that any candidate RSV vaccine also should be evaluated when administered with other vaccines that are currently recommended for infants.

The efficacy of a candidate RSV vaccine may also relate to its ability to stimulate an adequate local antibody response in the respiratory tract, which may be the first line of defense.[10] Despite high levels of RSV antibodies in the serum, little reaches the respiratory secretions. Transudation of serum antibodies is poor, resulting in RSV antibody levels being 80 to 160 times less in the respiratory tract secretions or even less in the nasal secretions compared with the antibody levels in the serum. Nevertheless, a major potential advantage of a live-attenuated intranasal vaccine in comparison to a subunit vaccine is that it is more apt to mimic naturally evoked immunity and induce local respiratory tract antibodies.

Current candidate RSV vaccines have resulted from two main approaches: development of immunogenic subunit components of RSV or live-attenuated vaccines. Candidate vaccines have primarily aimed at eliciting responses to the two major surface glycoproteins of RSV, F and G, because both neutralize virus infectivity and induce both helper T and cytotoxic T lymphocytes. The nonprotective response of the initial formalin-inactivated vaccine and the clinical outcome of enhanced disease with subsequent natural infection likely resulted in part from the formalin disruption of epitopes of these surface glycoproteins.[179] The formalin-inactivated vaccine did induce a T-cell response, but it appears to have been unbalanced, skewed toward $CD4^+$ T-cell activation with a poor $CD8^+$ T-cell response.[180]

The subunit candidate vaccines have focused on F and G proteins, primarily using the F protein because of its considerable cross-reactivity between group A and B RSV strains. In contrast, the G protein exhibits limited cross-reactivity between the two strain groups. These purified F protein vaccines have been safe and variably immunogenic among individuals who are seropositive from previous natural RSV infection. Nevertheless, they may offer the possibility of boosting the immunity among some groups of older children and adults who have an increased risk for developing more severe RSV infection, and among pregnant women as a means of augmenting maternal antibody levels in the infant.[181] However, because of the aforementioned concerns about the initial experience with RSV being elicited by nonreplicating virus, live-attenuated vaccines have been judged a more appropriate approach for RSV-naïve infants. More immunogenic vaccines are being explored, including those consisting of synthetic viral peptides and vaccines using recombinant vectors and plasmids containing complementary DNA of the F and G genomes. Information on the safety and potential protection that these vaccines may offer awaits adequate evaluations in clinical trials.

The initial live-virus candidate vaccines were derived from serial passage of temperature-sensitive (ts) mutants of wild RSV strains at progressively lower temperatures. These cold passage (cp) strains were subsequently subjected to chemical mutagenesis and screened to identify mutants with suitable attenuation. Despite promising results in adult volunteers, subsequent studies proved these initial strains to be unsuitable in young children. They resulted in unacceptable degrees of illness, were overattenuated and not protective, or were genetically unstable, with reversion to wild-type virus that was then shed. New live-attenuated virus candidate vaccines have been improved by repeated rounds of chemical mutagenesis, producing mutants that are more attenuated and that provide improved stability and immunogenicity.[10]

The use of reverse genetics has resulted in generations of newly designed candidate strains from the cold-passage and temperature-sensitive vaccines, which contain mutations specifically chosen for their attenuating, immunogenic, and other advantageous characteristics.[182] These candidate "designer gene" vaccines are potentially safer, have increased breadth of antigenic expression, and allow combination vaccines with parainfluenza and other respiratory pathogens.[183] Recombinant genetic engineering methods offer considerable promise for developing multiple vaccines for the diverse groups of infants, older children, and adults who could benefit from diminished severity, if not complete protection, from the ubiquitous yearly outbreaks of RSV infection.

REFERENCES

1. Shay D, Holman R, Newman R, et al. Bronchiolitis-associated hospitalizations among US children, 1980-1996. *JAMA.* 1999;282:1440-1446.
2. Hall C, Weinberg G, Iwane M, et al. The burden of respiratory syncytial virus infection among healthy children. *N Engl J Med.* 2009;360:588-598.
3. Forster J, Ihorst G, Rieger C, et al. Prospective population-based study of viral lower respiratory tract infections in children under 3 years of age (the PRI.DE study). *Eur J Pediatr.* 2004;163:709-716.
4. Hall C. Respiratory syncytial virus and parainfluenza virus. *N Engl J Med.* 2001;344:1917-1928.
5. Falsey A, Hennessey P, Formica M, et al. Respiratory syncytial virus infection in elderly and high-risk adults. *N Engl J Med.* 2005;352:1749-1759.
6. Walsh E, Peterson D, Falsey A. Risk factors for severe respiratory syncytial virus infection in elderly persons. *J Infect Dis.* 2004;189:233-238.
7. Han L, Alexander J, Anderson L. Respiratory syncytial virus pneumonia among the elderly: an assessment of disease burden. *J Infect Dis.* 1999;179:25-30.
8. Morris J, Blount R, Savage R. Recovery of cytopathogenic agent from chimpanzees with coryza. *Proc Soc Exp Biol Med.* 1956;92:544-549.
9. Chanock R, Roizman B, Myers R. Recovery from infants with respiratory illness of a virus related to chimpanzee coryza agent (CCA): I. Isolation, properties and characterization. *Am J Hyg.* 1957;66:281-290.
10. Collins P, Crowe J Jr. Respiratory syncytial virus and metapneumovirus. In: Kinpe DM, Howley PM, Griffin DE, et al, eds. *Fields Virology.* 5th ed. Philadelphia, PA: Lippincott Williams & Wilkins; 2007;368:73-82.
11. Tran K, He B, Teng M. Replacement of the respiratory syncytial virus nonstructural proteins NS1 and NS2 by the V protein of parainfluenza virus 5. *Virology.* 2007.
12. Hambling M. Survival of the respiratory syncytial virus during storage under various conditions. *Br J Exp Pathol.* 1964;45:647-655.
13. Hall C, Douglas RJ, Geiman J. Possible transmission by fomites of respiratory syncytial virus. *J Infect Dis.* 1980;141:98-102.
14. Marsh R, Connor A, Gias E, et al. Increased susceptibility of human respiratory syncytial virus to neutralization by anti-fusion protein antibodies on adaptation to replication in cell culture. *J Med Virol.* 2007;79:829-837.
15. Domachowske J, Bonville C, Rosenberg H. Animal models for studying respiratory syncytial virus infection and its long term effects on lung function. *Pediatr Infect Dis J.* 2004;23:S228-S234.
16. Graham B, Rutigliano J, Johnson T. Respiratory syncytial virus immunobiology and pathogenesis. *Virology.* 2002;297:1-7.
17. Berman S. Epidemiology of acute respiratory infections in children of developing countries. *Rev Infect Dis.* 1991;13:S454-S462.
18. Shek L, Lee B. Epidemiology and seasonality of respiratory tract virus infections in the tropics. *Paediatr Respir Rev.* 2003;4:105-111.
19. Meissner C. Summary: Seasonal and geographic variation in respiratory syncytial virus outbreaks across the United States. *Pediatr Infect Dis J.* 2007;26:S60.
20. Centers for Disease Control. The National Respiratory and Enteric Virus Surveillance System (NREVSS). 2008. (Accessed November 14, 2008, at: http://www.cdc.gov/surveillance/nrevss/rsv/default.html)
21. Light M. Respiratory syncytial virus seasonality in southeast Florida: results from three area hospitals caring for children. *Pediatr Infect Dis J.* 2007;26:S55-S59.
22. Welliver R. Temperature, humidity, and ultraviolet b radiation predict community respiratory syncytial virus activity. *Pediatr Infect Dis J.* 2007;26:S29-S35.
23. Fergie J, Purcell K. Respiratory syncytial virus laboratory surveillance and hospitalization trends in south Texas. *Pediatr Infect Dis J.* 2007;26:S51-S54.
24. Donaldson G. Climate change and the end of the respiratory syncytial virus season. *Clin Infect Dis.* 2006;42:677-679.
25. Noyola D, Mandeville P. Effect of climatological factors on respiratory syncytial virus epidemics. *Epidemiol Infect.* 2008;136:1328-1332.
26. Hall C, Douglas RJ. Modes of transmission of respiratory syncytial virus. *J Pediatr.* 1981;99:100-103.
27. Peret T, Hall C, Hammond G, et al. Circulation patterns of group A and B human respiratory syncytial virus genotypes in 5 communities in North America. *J Infect Dis.* 2000;181:1891-1896.
28. Matheson J, Rich F, Cohet C, et al. Distinct patterns of evolution between respiratory syncytial virus subgroups A and B from New Zealand isolates collected over thirty-seven years. *J Med Virol.* 2006;78:1354-1364.
29. Hall C, Walsh E, Schnabel K, et al. Occurrence of groups A and B of respiratory syncytial virus over 15 years: associated epidemiologic and clinical characteristics in hospitalized and ambulatory children. *J Infect Dis.* 1990;162:1283-1290.
30. Papadopoulos N, Gourgiotis D, Javadyan A, et al. Does respiratory syncytial virus subtype influences the severity of acute bronchiolitis in hospitalized infants? *Respir Med.* 2004;98:879-882.
31. Brandenburg A, van Beek R, Moll H, et al. G protein variation in respiratory syncytial virus group A does not correlate with clinical severity. *J Clin Microbiol.* 2000;38:2849-2852.
32. Boyce T, Mellen B, Mitchel EJ, et al. Rates of hospitalization for respiratory syncytial virus infection among children in Medicaid. *J Pediatr.* 2000;137:865-870.
33. Iwane M, Edwards K, Szilagyi P, et al. Population-based surveillance for hospitalizations associated with respiratory syncytial virus, influenza virus, and parainfluenza viruses among young children. *Pediatrics.* 2004;113:1758-1764.
34. Glezen W, Taber L, Frank A, et al. Risk of primary infection and reinfection with respiratory syncytial virus. *Am J Dis Child.* 1986;140:543-546.
35. Henderson F, Collier A, Clyde W, et al. Respiratory syncytial virus infections, reinfections and immunity: A prospective, longitudinal study in young children. *N Engl J Med.* 1979;300:530-534.
36. Hall C, Geiman J, Biggar R, et al. Respiratory syncytial virus infections within families. *N Engl J Med.* 1976;294:414-419.
37. O'Shea M, Ryan M, Hawksworth A, et al. Symptomatic respiratory syncytial virus infection among previously healthy young adults living in a crowded military environment. *Clin Infect Dis.* 2005;41:311-317.
38. Pelletier A, Mansbach J, Camargo CJ. Direct medical costs of bronchiolitis hospitalizations in the United States. *Pediatrics.* 2006;118:2418-2423.
39. Leader S, Kohlhase K. Respiratory syncytial virus-coded pediatric hospitalizations, 1997-1999. *Pediatr Infect Dis J.* 2002;21:629-632.
40. Schanzer D, Langley J, Tam T. Hospitalization attributable to influenza and other viral respiratory illnesses in Canadian children. *Pediatr Infect Dis J.* 2006;25:795-800.
41. Howard T, Stang P. Burden of RSV Hospitalizations in the US. In: *ISPOR Fifth Annual International Meeting; Value in Health*; 2000:117.
42. Poehling K, Edwards K, Weinberg G, et al. The underrecognized burden of influenza in young children. *N Engl J Med.* 2006;355:31-40.
43. Weinberg G, Hall C, Iwane M, et al. Parainfluenza virus infections in children. *J Pediatr.* 2009;154:694-699.
44. Weigl J, Puppe W, Schmitt H. Incidence of respiratory syncytial virus-positive hospitalizations in Germany. *Eur J Clin Microbiol Infect Dis.* 2001;20:452-459.
45. Nicholson K, McNally T, Silverman M, et al. Rates of hospitalisation for influenza, respiratory syncytial virus and human metapneumovirus among infants and young children. *Vaccine.* 2006;24:102-108.
46. Fjaerli H, Farstad T, Bratlid D. Hospitalisations for respiratory syncytial virus bronchiolitis in Akershus, Norway, 1993-2000: a population-based retrospective study. *BMC Pediatr.* 2004;25:1-7.
47. Hall C. Respiratory syncytial virus infections in previously healthy working adults. *Clin Infect Dis.* 2001;33:792-796.
48. Murata Y. Respiratory syncytial virus infection in adults. *Curr Opin Pulm Med.* 2008;14:235-240.
49. Falsey A, Walsh E. Respiratory syncytial virus infection in elderly adults. *Drugs Aging.* 2005;22:577-587.
50. Mangtani P, Hajat S, Kovats S, et al. The association of respiratory syncytial virus infection and influenza with emergency admissions for respiratory disease in London: an analysis of routine surveillance data. *Clin Infect Dis.* 2006;42:640-646.
51. Hall C. Nosocomial respiratory syncytial virus infections: the "cold war" has not ended. *Clin Infect Dis.* 2000;31:590-596.
52. Hall C. Building Characteristics and the Spread of Infectious Diseases. In: *Green Schools: Attributes for Health and Learning.* Washington, DC: National Academies Press; 2007:105-119.
53. Johnson K, Chanock R, Rifkind D, et al. Respiratory syncytial virus. IV. Correlation of virus shedding, serologic response, and illness in adult volunteers. *JAMA.* 1961;176:663-667.
54. Kravetz H, Knight V, Chanock R, et al. Respiratory syncytial virus: III. Production of illness and clinical observations in adult volunteers. *JAMA.* 1961;176:657-663.
55. Hall C, Douglas RJ, Schnabel K, et al. Infectivity of respiratory syncytial virus by various routes of inoculation. *Infect Immun.* 1981;33:779-783.
56. Johnson J, Gonzales R, Olson S, et al. The histopathology of fatal untreated human respiratory syncytial virus infection. *Mod Pathol.* 2007;20:108-119.
57. Visscher D, Myers J. Bronchiolitis: the pathologist's perspective. *Proc Am Thorac Soc.* 2006;3:41-47.
58. Adams J, Imagawa D, Zike K. Epidemic bronchiolitis and pneumonia related to respiratory syncytial virus. *JAMA.* 1961;176:1037-1039.
59. Openshaw P, Tregoning J. Immune responses and disease enhancement during respiratory syncytial virus infection. *Clin Microbiol Rev.* 2005;18:541-555.
60. Peebles RJ, Graham B. Pathogenesis of respiratory syncytial virus infection in the murine model. *Proc Am Thorac Soc.* 2005;2:110-115.
61. Moore M, Peebles R Jr. Respiratory syncytial virus disease mechanisms implicated by human, animal model, and in vitro data facilitate vaccine strategies and new therapeutics. *Pharmacol Ther.* 2006;112:405-424.
62. Kim H, Canchola J, Brandt C, et al. Respiratory syncytial virus disease in infants despite prior administration of antigenic inactivated vaccine. *Am J Epidemiol.* 1969;89:422-434.
63. Fulginiti V, Eller J, Sieber O, et al. Respiratory virus immunization I. A field trial of two inactivated respiratory virus vaccines: an aqueous trivalent parainfluenza virus vaccine, and an alum-precipitated respiratory syncytial virus vaccine. *Am J Epidemiol.* 1969;89:435-448.
64. Kapikian A, Mitchell R, Chanock R, et al. An epidemiologic study of altered clinical reactivity to respiratory syncytial (RS) virus infection in children previously vaccinated with an inactivated RS virus vaccine. *Am J Epidemiol.* 1969;89:405-421.
65. Collins P, Graham B. Viral and host factors in human respiratory syncytial virus pathogenesis. *J Virol.* 2008;82:2040-2055.
66. Prince G, Mathews A, Curtis S, et al. Treatment of respiratory syncytial virus bronchiolitis and pneumonia in a cotton rat model with systemically administered monoclonal antibody (palivizumab) and glucocorticosteroid. *J Infect Dis.* 2000;182:1326-1330.
67. Malley R, DeVincenzo J, Ramilo O, et al. Reduction of respiratory syncytial virus (RSV) in tracheal aspirates in intubated infants by use of humanized monoclonal antibody to RSV F protein. *J Infect Dis.* 1998;178:1555-1561.
68. Bennett B, Garofalo R, Cron S, et al. Immunopathogenesis of respiratory syncytial virus bronchiolitis. *J Infect Dis.* 2007;195:1532-1540.
69. Welliver T, Reed J, Welliver R Sr. Respiratory syncytial virus and influenza virus infections: observations from tissues of fatal infant cases. *Pediatr Infect Dis J.* 2008;27:S92-S96.
70. Finberg R, Wang J, Kurt-Jones E. Toll like receptors and viruses. *Rev Med Virol.* 2007;17:35-43.
71. Crowe J, Williams J. Immunology of viral respiratory tract infection in infancy. *Paediatr Respir Rev.* 2003;4:112-119.
72. Hull J. Genetic susceptibility to RSV disease. In: Cane PA, ed. *Respiratory Syncytial Virus.* The Netherlands: Elsevier, Amsterdam; 2007:115-140.
73. Hall C, Walsh E, Long C, et al. Immunity to and frequency of reinfection with respiratory syncytial virus. *J Infect Dis.* 1991;163:693-698.
74. Walsh E, Falsey A. Age related differences in humoral immune response to respiratory syncytial virus infection in adults. *J Med Virol.* 2004;73:295-299.
75. Glezen W, Paredes A, Allison J, et al. Risk of respiratory syncytial virus infection for infants from low-income families in relationship to age, sex, ethnic group, and maternal antibody level. *J Pediatr.* 1981;98:708-715.
76. Parrott R, Kim H, Arrobio J, et al. Epidemiology of respiratory syncytial virus infection in Washington, DC II. Infection and disease with respect to age, immunologic status, race, and sex. *Am J Epidemiol.* 1973;98:289-300.
77. American Academy of Pediatrics. Respiratory syncytial virus. In: Pickering L, Baker C, Long S, eds. *Red Book: 2009 Report of the Committee on Infectious Diseases.* 28th ed. Elk Grove Village, IL: American Academy of Pediatrics; 2009: In press.
78. Scott P, Ochola R, Sande C, et al. Comparison of strain-specific antibody responses during primary and secondary infections with respiratory syncytial virus. *J Med Virol.* 2007;79:1943-19450.
79. Wright P, Gruber W, Peters M, et al. Illness severity, viral shedding, and antibody responses in infants hospitalized with bronchiolitis caused by respiratory syncytial virus. *J Infect Dis.* 2002;185:1011-1018.
80. Falsey A, Singh H, Walsh E. Serum antibody decay in adults following natural respiratory syncytial virus infection. *J Med Virol.* 2006;78:1493-1497.
81. Prince G, Horswood R, Chanock R. Quantitative aspects of passive immunity to respiratory syncytial virus infection in infant cotton rats. *J Virol.* 1985;55:517-520.
82. Welliver R, Wong D, Sun M, et al. The development of respiratory syncytial virus-specific IgE and the release of histamine in naso-pharyngeal secretions after infection. *N Engl J Med.* 1981;305:841-846.
83. Welliver R, Garofalo R, Ogra P. Beta-chemokines, but neither T helper type 1 nor T helper type 2 cytokines, correlate with severity of illness during respiratory syncytial virus infection. *Pediatr Infect Dis J.* 2002;21:457-561.
84. Hall C, Powell K, MacDonald N, et al. Respiratory syncytial virus infection in children with compromised immune function. *N Engl J Med.* 1986;315:77-81.
85. Kim Y, Boeckh M, Englund J. Community respiratory virus infections in immunocompromised patients: hematopoietic stem cell and solid organ transplant recipients, and individuals with human immunodeficiency virus infection. *Semin Respir Crit Care Med.* 2007;28:222-242.
86. Chi B, Dickensheets H, Spann K, et al. Alpha and lambda interferon together mediate suppression of CD4 T cells induced by respiratory syncytial virus. *J Virol.* 2006;80:5032-5040.
87. Guerrero-Plata A, Casola A, Suarez G, et al. Differential response of dendritic cells to human metapneumovirus and respiratory syncytial virus. *Am J Respir Cell Mol Biol.* 2006;34:320-329.

88. Roe M, Bloxham D, White D, et al. Lymphocyte apoptosis in acute respiratory syncytial virus bronchiolitis. *Clin Exp Immunol.* 2004;137:139-145.
89. Openshaw P. Antiviral immune responses and lung inflammation after respiratory syncytial virus infection. *Proc Am Thorac Soc.* 2005;2:121-125.
90. Kristjansson S, Bjarnarson S, Wennergren G, et al. Respiratory syncytial virus and other respiratory viruses during the first 3 months of life promote a local TH2-like response. *J Allergy Clin Immunol.* 2005;116:805-811.
91. Harcourt J, Alvarez R, Jones L, et al. Respiratory syncytial virus G protein and G protein CX3C motif adversely affect CX3CR1+ T cell responses. *J Immunol.* 2006;176:1600-1608.
92. Kim H, Arrobio J, Brandt C, et al. Epidemiology of respiratory syncytial virus infection in Washington, D.C. I. Importance of the virus in different respiratory tract disease syndromes and temporal distribution of infection. *Am J Epidemiol.* 1973;98:216-225.
93. Glezen W, Denny F. Epidemiology of acute lower respiratory disease in children. *N Engl J Med.* 1973;288:498-505.
94. American Academy of Pediatrics. Diagnosis and management of bronchiolitis. *Pediatrics.* 2006;118:1774-1793.
95. Schuh S, Lalani A, Allen U, et al. Evaluation of the utility of radiography in acute bronchiolitis. *J Pediatr.* 2007;150:429-433.
96. Friis B, Eiken M, Hornsleth A, et al. Chest x-ray appearances in pneumonia and bronchiolitis. *Acta Paediatr Scand.* 1990;79:219-225.
97. Chonmaitree T, Revai K, Grady J, et al. Viral upper respiratory tract infection and otitis media complication in young children. *Clin Infect Dis.* 2008;46:815-823.
98. Heikkinen T, Thint M, Chonmaitree T. Prevalence of various respiratory viruses in the middle ear during acute otitis media. *N Engl J Med.* 1999;340:260-264.
99. Patel J, Nguyen D, Revai K, et al. Role of respiratory syncytial virus in acute otitis media: implications for vaccine development. *Vaccine.* 2007;25:1683-1689.
100. Kleemola M, Nokso-Koivisto J, Herva E, et al. Is there any specific association between respiratory viruses and bacteria in acute otitis media of young children? *J Infect.* 2006;52:181-187.
101. Louie J, Hacker J, Gonzales R, et al. Characterization of viral agents causing acute respiratory infection in a San Francisco University Medical Center Clinic during the influenza season. *Clin Infect Dis.* 2005;41:822-828.
102. Harris J, Erdman D, Dhashemi S, et al. Respiratory syncytial virus (RSV) and persistent cough at a University Health Service. In: *39th Annual Meeting of the Infectious Diseases Society of America*; Oct. 25-28, 2001; San Francisco: 2001.
103. Walsh E, Peterson D, Falsey A. Is clinical recognition of respiratory syncytial virus infection in hospitalized elderly and high-risk adults possible? *J Infect Dis.* 2007;195:1046-1051.
104. Ellis J, Alvarez-Aguero A, Gregory V, et al. Influenza A/H1N2 viruses, United Kingdom, 2001-02 influenza season. *Emerg Infect Dis.* 2003;9:304-310.
105. Falsey A, Cunningham C, Barker W, et al. Respiratory syncytial virus and influenza A infections in the hospitalized elderly. *J Infect Dis.* 1995;172:389-394.
106. Nicholson K, Kent J, Hammersley V, et al. Acute viral infections of upper respiratory tract in elderly people living in the community: comparative, prospective, population based study of disease burden. *BMJ.* 1997;315:1060-1064.
107. Falsey A, McCann R, Hall W, et al. Acute respiratory tract infection in daycare centers for older persons. *J Am Geriatr Soc.* 1995;43:30-36.
108. Falsey A. Respiratory syncytial virus infection in adults. *Semin Respir Crit Care Med.* 2007;28:171-181.
109. Boukhvalova M, Yim K, Kuhn K, et al. Age-related differences in pulmonary cytokine response to respiratory syncytial virus infection: modulation by anti-inflammatory and antiviral treatment. *J Infect Dis.* 2007;195:511-518.
110. Liu B, Kimura Y. Local immune response to respiratory syncytial virus infection is diminished in senescence-accelerated mice. *J Gen Virol.* 2007;88:2552-2558.
111. Panitch H. Viral respiratory infections in children with technology dependence and neuromuscular disorders. *Pediatr Infect Dis J.* 2004;23:S222-S227.
112. Simon A, Ammann R, Wilkesmann A, et al. Respiratory syncytial virus infection in 406 hospitalized premature infants: results from a prospective German multicentre database. *Eur J Pediatr.* 2007;166:1273-1283.
113. McLaurin K, Hall C, Jackson E, et al. Persistence of morbidity and cost differences between late-preterm and term infants during the first year of life. *Pediatrics.* 2009;123:653-659.
114. Navas L, Wang E, de Carvalho V, et al. Improved outcome of respiratory syncytial virus infection in a high-risk hospitalized population of Canadian children. *J Pediatr.* 1992;121:348-354.
115. MacDonald N, Hall C, Suffin S, et al. Respiratory syncytial viral infection in infants with congenital heart disease. *N Engl J Med.* 1982;307:397-400.
116. Romero J. Palivizumab prophylaxis of respiratory syncytial virus disease from 1998 to 2002: results from four years of palivizumab usage. *Pediatr Infect Dis J.* 2003;22:S46-S54.
117. Altman C, Englund J, Demmler G, et al. Respiratory syncytial virus in patients with congenital heart disease: a contemporary look at epidemiology and success of preoperative screening. *Pediatr Cardiol.* 2000;21:433-438.
118. Simoes E. Environmental and demographic risk factors for respiratory syncytial virus lower respiratory tract disease. *J Pediatr.* 2003;143:S118-S126.
119. Grimwood K, Cohet C, Rich F, et al. Risk factors for respiratory syncytial virus bronchiolitis hospital admission in New Zealand. *Epidemiol Infect.* 2008;136:1333-1341.
120. Singleton R, Bruden D, Bulkow L. Respiratory syncytial virus season and hospitalizations in the Alaskan Yukon-Kuskokwim Delta. *Pediatr Infect Dis J.* 2007;26:S46-S50.
121. Mendoza Sanchez M, Ruiz-Contreras J, Vivanco J, et al. Respiratory virus infections in children with cancer or HIV infection. *J Pediatr Hematol Oncol.* 2006;28:154-159.
122. Raboni S, Nogueira M, Tsuchiya L, et al. Respiratory tract viral infections in bone marrow transplant patients. *Transplantation.* 2003;76:142-146.
123. Champlin R, Whimbey E. Community respiratory virus infections in bone marrow transplant recipients: the M.D. Anderson Cancer Center experience. *Biol Blood Marrow Transplant.* 2001;7:8s-10s.
124. Khanna N, Widmer A, Decker M, et al. Respiratory syncytial virus infection in patients with hematological diseases: single-center study and review of the literature. *Clin Infect Dis.* 2008;46:402-412.
125. El Saleeby C, Somes G, DeVincenzo J, et al. Risk factors for severe respiratory syncytial virus disease in children with cancer: the importance of lymphopenia and young age. *Pediatrics.* 2008;121:235-243.
126. Sable C, Hayden F. Orthomyxoviral and paramyxoviral infections in transplant patients. *Infect Dis Clin North Am.* 1995;9:987-1003.
127. Chemaly R, Ghosh S, Bodey G, et al. Respiratory viral infections in adults with hematologic malignancies and human stem cell transplantation recipients: a retrospective study at a major cancer center. *Medicine (Baltimore).* 2006;85:278-287.
128. Koskenvuo M, Mottonen M, Rahiala J, et al. Mixed bacterial-viral infections in septic children with leukemia. *Pediatr Infect Dis J.* 2007;26:1133-1136.
129. Erard V, Chien J, Kim H, et al. Airflow decline after myeloablative allogeneic hematopoietic cell transplantation: the role of community respiratory viruses. *J Infect Dis.* 2006;193:1619-1625.
130. Gasparetto E, Escuissato D, Marchiori E, et al. High-resolution CT findings of respiratory syncytial virus pneumonia after bone marrow transplantation. *AJR Am J Roentgenol.* 2004;182:1133-1137.
131. Madhi S, Venter M, Madhi A, et al. Differing manifestations of respiratory syncytial virus-associated severe lower respiratory tract infections in human immunodeficiency virus type 1-infected and uninfected children. *Pediatr Infect Dis J.* 2001;20:164-170.
132. de Fontbrune F, Robin M, Porcher R, et al. Palivizumab treatment of respiratory syncytial virus infection after allogeneic hematopoietic stem cell transplantation. *Clin Infect Dis.* 2007;45:1019-1024.
133. Chavez-Bueno S, Mejias A, Merryman R, et al. Intravenous palivizumab and ribavirin combination for respiratory syncytial virus disease in high-risk pediatric patients. *Pediatr Infect Dis J.* 2007;26:1089-1093.
134. Boeckh M, Englund J, Li Y, et al. Randomized controlled multicenter trial of aerosolized ribavirin for respiratory syncytial virus upper respiratory tract infection in hematopoietic cell transplant recipients. *Clin Infect Dis.* 2007;44:245-249.
135. Thomas N, Hollenbeak C, Ceneviva G, et al. Palivizumab prophylaxis to prevent respiratory syncytial virus mortality after pediatric bone marrow transplantation: a decision analysis model. *J Pediatr Hematol Oncol.* 2007;29:227-232.
136. Dykewicz C. Guidelines for preventing opportunistic infections among hematopoietic stem cell transplant recipients: focus on community respiratory virus infections. *Biol Blood Marrow Transplant.* 2001;7:19S-22S.
137. Centers for Disease Control. Guideline for Hand Hygiene in Health-Care Settings. Recommendations of the Healthcare Infections Control Practices Advisory Committee and the HICPAC/SHEA/APIC/IDSA Hand Hygiene Task Force. *MMWR Morb Mortal Wkly Rep.* 2002;51.
138. Church N, Anas N, Hall C, et al. Respiratory syncytial virus-related apnea in infants: Demographics and outcome. *Am J Dis Child.* 1984;138:247-250.
139. Willwerth B, Harper M, Greenes D. Identifying hospitalized infants who have bronchiolitis and are at high risk for apnea. *Ann Emerg Med.* 2006;48:441-447.
140. Sabogal C, Auais A, Napchan G, et al. Effect of respiratory syncytial virus on apnea in weanling rats. *Pediatr Res.* 2005;57:819-825.
141. Hernandez E, Khoshoo V, Thoppil D, et al. Aspiration: a factor in rapidly deteriorating bronchiolitis in previously healthy infants? *Pediatr Pulmonol.* 2002;33:30-31.
142. Khoshoo V, Ross G, Kelly B, et al. Benefits of thickened feeds in previously healthy infants with respiratory syncytial virus bronchiolitis. *Pediatr Pulmonol.* 2001;31:301-302.
143. Hall C, Powell K, Schnabel K, et al. Risk of secondary bacterial infection in infants hospitalized with respiratory syncytial viral infection. *J Pediatr.* 1988;113:266-271.
144. Purcell K, Fergie J. Concurrent serious bacterial infections in 2396 infants and children hospitalized with respiratory syncytial virus lower respiratory tract infections. *Arch Pediatr Adolesc Med.* 2002;156:322-324.
145. Purcell R, Fergie J. Concurrent serious bacterial infections (CSBIs) in 912 infants and young children hospitalized for treatment of respiratory syncytial virus (RSV) lower respiratory tract infection (LRT) at Driscoll Children's Hospital, 2000-2002. In: *Pediatric Academic Societies Annual Meeting*; May 3-6, 2003; Seattle, WA; 2003. abstract # 1906.
146. Oray-Schrom P, Phoenix C, St Martin D, et al. Sepsis workup in febrile infants 0-90 days of age with respiratory syncytial virus infection. *Pediatr Emerg Care.* 2003;19:314-319.
147. Kneyber MC, van Woensel J, Uijtendaal E, et al. Azithromycin does not improve disease course in hospitalized infants with respiratory syncytial virus (RSV) lower respiratory tract disease: A randomized equivalence trial. *Pediatr Pulmonol.* 2008;43:142-149.
148. Choi E, Lee H, Kim S, et al. The association of newly identified respiratory viruses with lower respiratory tract infections in Korean children, 2000-2005. *Clin Infect Dis.* 2006;43:585-592.
149. Purcell K, Fergie J. Lack of usefulness of an abnormal white blood cell count for predicting a concurrent serious bacterial infection in infants and young children hospitalized with respiratory syncytial virus lower respiratory tract infection. *Pediatr Infect Dis J.* 2007;26:311-315.
150. Gern J. Viral Respiratory infection and the link to asthma. *Pediatr Infect Dis J.* 2008;27:S97-S103.
151. Martinez F. Heterogeneity of the association between lower respiratory illness in infancy and subsequent asthma. *Proc Am Thorac Soc.* 2005;2:157-161.
152. Taussig L, Wright A, Holberg C, et al. Tucson Children's Respiratory Study: 1980 to present. *J Allergy Clin Immunol.* 2003;111:661-675.
153. Sigurs N. Respiratory syncytial virus lower respiratory tract illness in infancy and subsequent morbidity. *Acta Paediatr.* 2007;96:156-157.
154. Tourdot S, Mathie S, Hussell T, et al. Respiratory syncytial virus infection provokes airway remodelling in allergen-exposed mice in absence of prior allergen sensitization. *Clin Exp Allergy.* 2008;38:1016-1024.
155. Welliver R. Respiratory syncytial virus and other respiratory viruses. *Pediatr Infect Dis J.* 2003;22:s6-s12.
156. Piedimonte G. Contribution of neuroimmune mechanisms to airway inflammation and remodeling during and after respiratory syncytial virus infection. *Pediatr Infect Dis J.* 2003;22:S66-S75.
157. Patino C, Martinez F. Interactions between genes and environment in the development of asthma. *Allergy.* 2001;56:279-286.
158. Henrickson K, Hall C. Diagnostic assays for respiratory syncytial virus disease. *Pediatr Infect Dis J.* 2007;26:S36-S40.
159. Lambert S, Whiley D, O'Neill N, et al. Comparing nose-throat swabs and nasopharyngeal aspirates collected from children with symptoms for respiratory virus identification using real-time polymerase chain reaction. *Pediatrics.* 2008;122:e615-e620.
160. Chiu C, Urisman A, Greenhow T, et al. Utility of DNA microarrays for detection of viruses in acute respiratory tract infections in children. *J Pediatr.* 2008;153:76-83.
161. Takahashi H, Norman S, Mather E, et al. Evaluation of the NanoChip 400 system for detection of influenza A and B, respiratory syncytial, and parainfluenza viruses. *J Clin Microbiol.* 2008;46:1724-1727.
162. Behrendt C, Decker M, Burch D, et al. International variation in the management of infants hospitalized with respiratory syncytial virus. *Eur J Pediatr.* 1998;157:215-220.
163. Ventre K, Randolph A. Ribavirin for respiratory syncytial virus infection of the lower respiratory tract in infants and young children. Cochrane Database Syst Rev. 2007:CD000181.
164. Sidwell R, Barnard D. Respiratory syncytial virus infections: recent prospects for control. *Antiviral Res.* 2006;71:379-390.
165. Hall C, Douglas RJ, Geiman J, et al. Nosocomial respiratory syncytial virus infections. *N Engl J Med.* 1975;293:1343-1346.
166. Goldmann D. Epidemiology and prevention of pediatric viral respiratory infections in health-care institutions. *Emerg Infect Dis.* 2001;7:249-253.
167. Halasa N, Williams J, Wilson G, et al. Medical and economic impact of a respiratory syncytial virus outbreak in a neonatal intensive care unit. *Pediatr Infect Dis J.* 2005;24:1040-1044.
168. Carbonell-Estrany X, Bont L, Doering G, et al. Clinical relevance of prevention of respiratory syncytial virus lower respiratory tract infection in preterm infants born between 33 and 35 weeks gestational age. *Eur J Clin Microbiol Infect Dis.* 2008;27:891-899.
169. Elhassan N, Sorbero M, Hall C, et al. Cost-effectiveness analysis of palivizumab in premature infants without chronic lung disease. *Arch Pediatr Adolesc Med.* 2006;160:1070-1076.
170. Reeve C, Whitehall J, Buettner P, et al. Cost-effectiveness of respiratory syncytial virus prophylaxis with palivizumab. *J Paediatr Child Health.* 2006;42:248-252.
171. Simoes E, Groothuis J, Carbonell-Estrany X, et al. Palivizumab prophylaxis, respiratory syncytial virus, and subsequent recurrent wheezing. *J Pediatr.* 2007;151:34-42, e1.
172. Wu H, Pfarr D, Johnson S, et al. Development of motavizumab, an ultra-potent antibody for the prevention of respiratory syncytial virus infection in the upper and lower respiratory tract. *J Mol Biol.* 2007;368:652-665.
173. Carbonell-Estrany X, Genevieve L, Micki H, Edward C. Phase 3 Trial of Motavizumab (MEDI-524), an Enhanced Potency

Respiratory Syncytial Virus (RSV) Specific Monoclonal Antibody (Mab) for the Prevention of Serious RSV Disease in High Risk Infants. Pediatric Academic Societies Annual Meeting, 2007.

174. Welliver R. Review of epidemiology and clinical risk factors for severe respiratory syncytial virus (RSV) infection. *J Pediatr.* 2003;143:S112-S117.

175. Shinoff J, O'Brien K, Thumar B, et al. Young infants can develop protective levels of neutralizing antibody after infection with respiratory syncytial virus. *J Infect Dis.* 2008.

176. Karron R, Wright P, Belshe R, et al. Identification of a recombinant live attenuated respiratory syncytial virus vaccine candidate that is highly attenuated in infants. *J Infect Dis.* 2005; 191:1093-1104.

177. Vallbracht S, Unsold H, Ehl S. Functional impairment of cytotoxic T cells in the lung airways following respiratory virus infections. *Eur J Immunol.* 2006;36:1434-1442.

178. Peebles R, Hashimoto K, Collins R, et al. Immune interaction between respiratory syncytial virus infection and allergen sensitization critically depends on timing of challenges. *J Infect Dis.* 2001;184:1374-1379.

179. Murphy B, Prince G, Walsh E, et al. Dissociation between serum neutralizing antibody responses of infants and children who received inactivated respiratory syncytial virus vaccine. *J Clin Microbiol.* 1986;24:197-202.

180. Moghaddam A, Olszewska W, Wang B, et al. A potential molecular mechanism for hypersensitivity caused by formalin-inactivated vaccines. *Nat Med.* 2006;12:905-907.

181. Greenberg H, Piedra P. Immunization against viral respiratory disease: a review. *Pediatr Infect Dis J.* 2004;23:S254-S261.

182. Collins P, Murphy B. New generation live vaccines against human respiratory syncytial virus designed by reverse genetics. *Proc Am Thorac Soc.* 2005;2:166-173.

183. Hurwitz J. Development of Recombinant Sendai Virus Vaccines for Prevention of Human Parainfluenza and Respiratory Syncytial Virus Infections. *Pediatr Infect Dis J.* 2008;27:S126-S128.

Human Metapneumovirus

ANN R. FALSEY

Human metapneumovirus (hMPV) is a newly discovered respiratory pathogen first described by investigators in the Netherlands in 2001.[1] This previously unidentified virus was isolated from the nasopharyngeal secretions of 28 Dutch children with upper respiratory infections, and samples were collected over a 20-year period. The virus exhibited paramyxovirus-like morphology, and genetic analysis was most similar to the Pneumovirinae family of which respiratory syncytial virus (RSV) is the most prominent member. Serologic analyses indicate that infection with hMPV is nearly universal by age 5 years, and that the virus had been circulating undetected for at least 50 years. hMPV appears to account for a significant proportion of the respiratory illnesses that were not recognized as being caused by other viral pathogens.

Virus

hMPV is a nonsegmented, single-stranded, negative-sense RNA virus belonging to the order Mononegavirales, family Paramyxoviridae, subfamily Pneumovirinae, and genus *Metapneumovirus*.[1] Consistent with the morphology of a paramyxovirus, hMPV particles are pleomorphic, spherical, or filamentous with a lipid envelope and projections on the surface as imaged by electron microscopy (Fig. 159-1).[1,2] Within the subfamily Pneumovirinae are the genera *Pneumovirus* and *Metapneumovirus*. Members of the *Pneumovirus* genus include human RSV and a number of animal pathogens, such as bovine, ovine, and caprine RSVs, and pneumonia virus of mice. Until recently, the only member of the *Metapneumovirus* genus was avian pneumovirus (APV), also known as *turkey rhinotracheitis virus*.[3] APV causes upper respiratory tract infection of turkeys and other avian species and was first reported in the late 1970s in South Africa. Originally classified as a pneumovirus, APV was placed into a separate new genus, *Metapneumovirus*, because it had a different gene number and gene order and only 40% homology with mammalian pneumoviruses.

The original genetic analysis of hMPV by van den Hoogen and colleagues indicated a gene order of 3′-N-P-M-F-M2-SH-G-L-5′.[1] These eight genes encode for at least nine proteins and include nucleoprotein (N), phosphoprotein (P), matrix protein (M), fusion protein (F), transcription elongation factor (M2-1), RNA synthesis regulatory factor (M2-2), small hydrophobic protein (SH), attachment protein (G), and major polymerase subunit (L).[4] The F protein appears to be the major immunodominant protein and contains several features conserved among paramyxovirus F proteins including a putative cleavage site and fusion domains.[5] The G protein of hMPV is smaller than RSV G protein, but the predicted amino acid sequence suggests a similar structure and heavy glycosylation. The absence of the nonstructural interferon-inhibiting genes *NS1* and *NS2* is the most striking difference between hMPV and RSV and confirmed its classification in the *Metapneumovirus* genus (Fig. 159-2).[6]

Sequence homology of *N, P, M,* and *F* genes of hMPV indicate the highest identity with APV serotype C (APV-C), one of four avian pneumovirus types.[6] Given the close relationship between hMPV and APV-C, it is speculated that the human virus originated from birds. In view of human serologic data that indicate the presence of hMPV antibodies for at least 50 years, it is presumed that a zoonotic event must have taken place before 1958. Although current evidence links hMPV with APV, animal challenge studies indicate that hMPV is a primary human pathogen rather than an avian pathogen that incidentally affects humans.[1]

Genetic variation among hMPV isolates has been observed, and the sequences are found to cluster in two major genotypes (A and B) and four subgroups with two sublineages (A1, A2a, A2b, B1, and B2).[7,8] The two isolates representing each of the major genotypes have been completely sequenced, and amino acid identities between genotypes were 80% and 90%, respectively, similar to the differences found between RSV groups A and B. The greatest diversity is found in two of the surface glycoproteins, the small hydrophobic surface (SH) and attachment (G) proteins (59% and 37% identity, respectively), which is considerably greater than the diversity observed in the RSV groups.

Pathogenesis

Information regarding hMPV disease pathogenesis is derived primarily from animal models. The location of hMPV infection has been demonstrated to be type 2 alveolar and bronchiolar epithelial cells in cynomolgus macaques.[4] In rodent models, hMPV replicates efficiently in the upper and lower airways with peak viral titers between days 3 and 5. Lung infection is characterized by alveolar and interstitial inflammation.[4] Although hMPV and RSV are closely related viruses, cytokine profiles of hMPV- and RSV-infected mice are different. Stronger interferon-α (IFN-α) and IFN-γ responses and weaker induction of interleukin-1 (IL-1), IL-6, and tumor necrosis factor-α (TNF-α) are seen with hMPV compared with RSV. Greater interferon responses of hMPV may be in part due to the lack of the nonstructural proteins, which suppress type 1 IFN responses during RSV infection. In normal human volunteers, peripheral blood mononuclear cells stimulated with hMPV produce a stronger innate and weaker adaptive cytokine response than RSV.[9] In contrast, inflammatory cytokines measured in nasal secretions of babies infected with hMPV are less than infants infected with RSV.[10]

Limited human pathologic data indicate that bronchiolar epithelial cells are infected with hMPV, and prolonged inflammation may be observed. Bronchoalveolar lavage specimens from hMPV-infected children reveal epithelial degenerative changes, eosinophilic cytoplasmic inclusions, and multinucleated giant cells.[11] Lung biopsy samples obtained 1 month after initial diagnosis from hMPV-infected children exhibited chronic airway inflammation with foamy and hemosiderin-laden macrophages. Lung tissue from an 89-year-old woman who died during hMPV infection demonstrated diffuse alveolar damage and hyaline membranes with organization, fibrin thrombi, and peribronchial inflammation.[12] Immunohistochemical staining confirmed hMPV antigens in the cytoplasm of the bronchiolar epithelial cells.

Epidemiology

hMPV is a ubiquitous pathogen that affects all age groups.[1,13-15] Seroprevalence studies indicate that by age 5 years, most children have been infected with hMPV. Illness caused by both RSV and hMPV appears to be common in young children, but primary infection with hMPV occurs at a slightly older age.[16,17] Whereas nearly 100% of children are infected with RSV by age 2 years, data from the Netherlands show that about 50% are seropositive for hMPV by age 2 years and 100% by age 5 years.[1] hMPV accounts for about 1% to 5% of childhood upper respiratory infections (URI) and 10% to 15% of hospitalizations for lower respiratory tract infections (LRI); however, rates may vary depending on the specific age group and year of study.[14,16-21] As a cause of serious lower respiratory tract disease in children, hMPV ranks

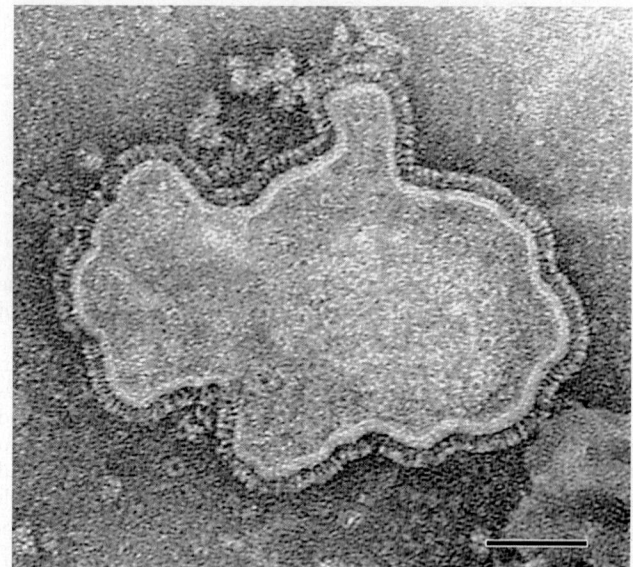

Figure 159-1 **Negative-stain electron micrograph of human meta-pneumovirus.** This pleomorphic form of the virus is stain-penetrated, thereby permitting visualization of portions of the virus envelope and nucleocapsid. A border composed of the surface projection proteins may also be seen around the virus periphery. Phosphotungstic acid negative stain, pH 6.5. *Bar marker represents 100 nm. (Courtesy of Charles Humphrey, PhD, research biologist, and Dean Erdman, PhD, Centers for Disease Control and Prevention.)*

second or third behind RSV and influenza.[16,17,20,22] A number of studies indicate that the peak age for hospitalization with hMPV is somewhat older than for hospitalization associated with RSV infection.[16,17] Reinfection occurs throughout life, and about 2% of acute respiratory illnesses in the general population are due to hMPV.[14,15]

Numerous epidemiologic studies have now documented worldwide hMPV circulation.[1,5,16,20,23,24] In temperate climates, the virus circulates predominantly in late winter and early spring months, frequently overlapping with other seasonal respiratory pathogens.[13,19,25] However, low levels of hMPV activity can occur during the summer months.[21,24] In the southern hemisphere, hMPV circulates in the summer, and in the subtropics, peak activity is in the spring and early summer.[16] Studies spanning multiple seasons indicate a fairly regular biannual pattern of alternating large and small outbreaks, which tend to be anticyclic with RSV activity.[26] In a 5-year study from Sweden, the average incidence of hMPV infection was 2.9% but ranged from 0.8% to 5.9% depending on the year.[19] Numerous studies from around the world confirm the

APV

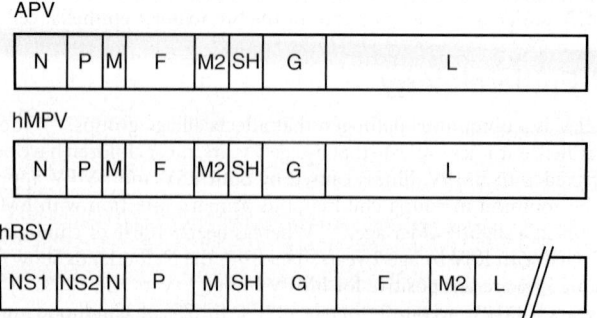

Figure 159-2 **Schematic representation of the gene order and sequence of avian pneumovirus (APV), human metapneumovirus (hMPV), and human respiratory syncytial virus (hRSV).** Gene lengths are not drawn to scale.

presence of two major genotypes of hMPV, which, like the RSV groups, often circulate concurrently within the same community.[20,25] The prevalence of genotypes and subgroups varies significantly each year, suggesting that immune pressure plays a roll in the dominant circulating genotype.

Clinical Manifestations

The clinical manifestations of hMPV infection are similar to those of RSV and range from mild URI to bronchiolitis and severe pneumonia requiring mechanical ventilation.[4,13] The spectrum of disease depends on the age and the health of the host. As with most respiratory viruses, the clinical syndrome is not distinct. Fever, cough, and coryza are the most common symptoms. The incubation period between exposure and onset of clinical symptoms is not precisely known, although cases of nosocomial transmission suggest an incubation period of about 5 to 6 days.[16]

CHILDREN

Most young children with hMPV infection exhibit fever, cough, and rhinorrhea (Table 159-1).[16,17,27] Fever appears to be more common with hMPV than with RSV, and febrile seizures were noted in 16% of patients with hMPV compared with 3.1% in RSV-infected children in one study.[16] Wheezing is also common, with rates ranging from 22% to 83% depending on the age group studied.[17,18] In children younger than 3 years, acute otitis media has been documented in up to 60% of hMPV-infected children, and hMPV RNA can be detected in middle ear fluid in some cases.[28,29] Conjunctivitis, pharyngitis, and laryngitis all occur with variable frequencies.[17,27,30] Less common symptoms include maculopapular truncal rash and diarrhea.[16] Notably, 2 of 26 French children with hMPV infection had diarrhea and high fever without respiratory symptoms.[30] Rarely, encephalitis has been attributed to hMPV infection.[31] Laboratory findings are relatively nonspecific, with lymphopenia and elevated hepatic transaminase values described.[16] Hypoxia and radiographic changes are common in hMPV-infected children, and abnormal chest radiographs have been found in 26% to 53% of hospitalized children.[16,27] Radiographic findings, which include peribronchial cuffing, perihilar infiltrates, patchy opacities, and hyperinflation, are similar to those in children with RSV infection (Fig. 159-3). Lobar consolidation has only rarely been described and may be due to bacterial complications.[23,32] Clinical diagnoses most frequently associated with hMPV hospitalization in children include bronchiolitis (in 47% to 84%), asthma (in 11% to 25%), and pneumonia (in 11% to 17%). The mean length of hospitalization for these children is 3 to 5 days.[16,17,27,30]

Viruses are commonly associated with exacerbations of childhood asthma. One of the first studies linking hMPV and asthma was from Finland, where hMPV was detected in 8% of children (10 of 132) admitted with wheezing during the winter months, and in seven cases hMPV was the sole pathogen identified.[33] The association of hMPV and asthma may in part depend on the age group studied. In a case-controlled study of 133 children hospitalized with acute wheezing, the

TABLE 159-1	Comparison of Signs and Symptoms in Children with hMPV, RSV, and Influenza A		
	hMPV (%)	*RSV (%)*	*Influenza A (%)*
Fever	52-80	47-57	78-81
Cough	90-100	99	96
Rhinorrhea	88-92	91	84
Retraction	65-92	95	82
Wheezing	22-83	23-65	5-57
Lacrimation	25	31	31
Diarrhea	8-17	17	9-27
Vomiting	10-25	8	10

hMPV, human metapneumovirus; RSV, respiratory syncytial virus.
Data compiled from references 17, 18, and 22.

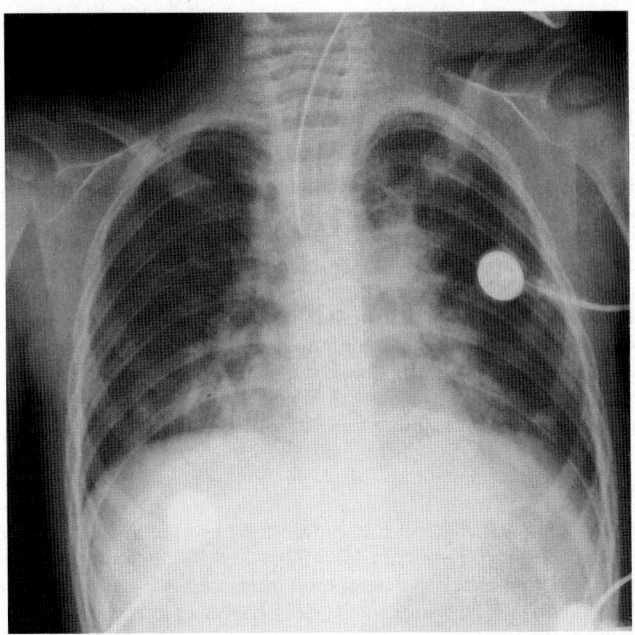

Figure 159-3 Chest radiograph of child with human metapneumo-virus (hMPV) infection. This 23-month-old child admitted to an intensive care unit required mechanical ventilation for 4 days. Nasal wash was positive for 5.5×10^6 copies/mL of hMPV by reverse transcriptase–polymerase chain reaction. The child recovered and was discharged to home off antibiotics on hospital day 6. Chest radiograph demonstrates patchy bilateral infiltrates. *(Courtesy of Janet A. Englund, MD, Professor of Pediatrics, Seattle Children's Hospital, University of Washington.)*

presence of hMPV was significant in children younger than 3 years, but not in older children.[34] In older children, the dominant pathogen associated with asthma exacerbations was rhinovirus.[35]

Although lower respiratory tract involvement appears common with hMPV infection, overall disease appears somewhat milder than that of RSV or influenza A. In a Canadian study of children younger than 3 years, none of the hMPV-infected children were admitted to an intensive care unit, whereas 15% of those with RSV and 16% of those with influenza A required intensive care.[17] In this study, about 25% of the hMPV-infected children had underlying medical conditions, compared with 7% of children infected with RSV. A high viral load in respiratory secretions has been correlated with lower respiratory tract involvement and hospitalization in young children infected with hMPV.[36] There are conflicting data regarding disease severity and the role of hMPV genotypes. Several studies suggest that severity or specific symptoms may vary with genotype.[37] However, the bulk of current evidence indicates that the severity of illness associated with hMPV A is similar to hMPV B infection.[25,36] Other risk factors for severe disease are similar to RSV and include prematurity, esophageal reflux, and underlying heart and lung disease.[24,32]

Because of the winter seasonality of hMPV, coinfection with other respiratory pathogens is common. Several investigators have noted that illness associated with dual hMPV and RSV infection is more severe than with either pathogen alone.[38,39] In a study of children younger than 2 years, coinfection with hMPV and RSV was associated with a 10-fold increased relative risk for mechanical ventilation.[38] A number of other studies have either not demonstrated the association of severity with dual infection or found low coinfection rates of hMPV and other respiratory pathogens.[4]

ADULTS

The clinical manifestations of hMPV infection in adults, like those in children, appear to depend on age and health status. Healthy adults

generally present with influenza-like illness and common cold syndromes.[13,15] In a 4-year prospective study of respiratory illnesses in New York, hMPV was detected by serology or reverse transcriptase–polymerase chain reaction (RT-PCR) in 2.2% to 10.5% of young, healthly elderly and high-risk adult cohorts, depending on the year.[15] Asymptomatic infection or very mild illness was common; about 40% of older adults and 70% of young adults with serologic evidence of infection each year reported no illnesses. Although mild infection in adults is common, it is unusual to find hMPV RNA in respiratory secretions in asymptomatic persons.[40] Symptoms in young adults are not distinctive from other respiratory viral illnesses, although in one study, hoarseness was more common among hMPV-infected patients than among those with RSV. In addition to respiratory illnesses, a mononucleosis-like syndrome due to hMPV has also been reported in healthly adults.[41] With increasing age, the impact of hMPV is greater. Healthy older adults with hMPV infection experience wheezing and dyspnea more often than do young adults, although more symptomatic, healthy older persons generally do not require medical attention. In contrast, adults with underlying cardiopulmonary conditions are at high risk for hospitalization. In a study of 1471 hospitalized patients during the winter, 118 (8.5%) illnesses were identified as hMPV related.[15] Similar to RSV and influenza, 85% of patients with hMPV requiring hospitalization had chronic heart or lung conditions. Common admission diagnoses were chronic obstructive pulmonary disease (COPD) exacerbation, pneumonia, and congestive heart failure. It is estimated that hMPV infection accounts for 4% to 12% of COPD, 7% of asthma, and 4% of community-acquired pneumonia admissions in adults.[42-44] Illnesses are characterized by severe cough and lack of fever. Chest radiographs revealing patchy, multilobar infiltrates associated with small pleural effusions are noted in 50% of cases.[43] Rates of respiratory failure and death of 12% and 7%, respectively, have been reported and are similar to influenza- and RSV-associated morbidity and mortality in this population.[15] Lastly, hMPV outbreaks have been reported in long-term care facilities and may result in high rates of pneumonia and death.[12] In one serologic study, hMPV was the most commonly identified respiratory viral infection among nursing home residents.[45]

IMMUNOCOMPROMISED HOSTS

As is found with other common respiratory viruses, hMPV infection is associated with severe illness and pneumonitis in immunocompromised patients.[46,47] Most fatalities described to date have involved patients receiving chemotherapy or recipients of hemopoetic stem cell transplantation (HSCT) or solid organ transplantation. Symptoms of infection typically begin with nasal congestion, fever, and cough and may evolve into diffuse pneumonia with respiratory failure. In one report of five hMPV-infected HSCT recipients, four developed rapidly progressive respiratory failure and had a septic shock–like picture with pulmonary hemorrhage.[46] Chest radiographs most often show bilateral airspace opacities, and computed tomography scan findings consist of patchy areas of ground-glass opacification and multiple nodules.[48] Along with diffuse alveolar damage, smudge cell formation has been found on histopathologic examination and is a distinctive finding compared with infection with other paramyxoviruses (Fig. 159-4).[49] Although severe hMPV illness is often observed in HSCT recipients, mild disease and even persistent asymptomatic shedding have also been described.[50] Bronchiolitis obliterans and allograft rejection in lung transplant recipients has been linked to hMPV infection.[47] Among HIV-infected children, hMPV has been associated with higher rates of bacterial complications and mortality compared with non–HIV-infected children.[23]

Diagnosis

The virus probably remained unidentified for many years because the clinical syndrome is not distinct and because isolation of the virus with standard cell culture techniques is difficult. hMPV replicates slowly in

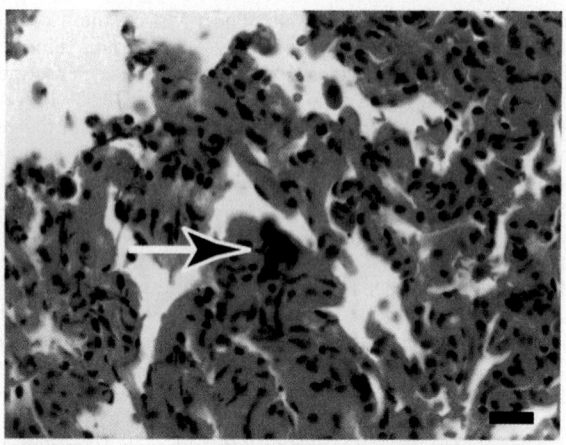

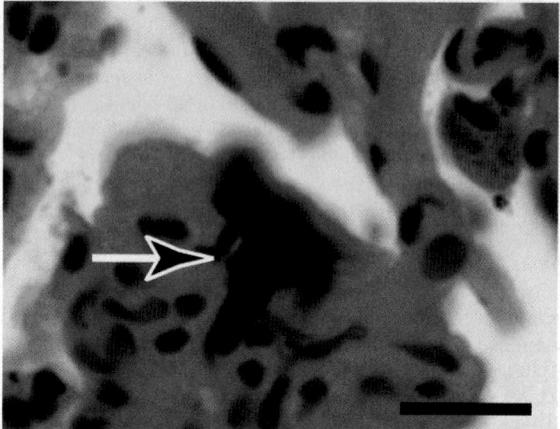

Figure 159-4 Photomicrograph of human metapneumovirus (hMPV) infection in lung tissue. Hematoxylin-eosin staining of transbronchial biopsy samples from a patient with hMPV infection. *Arrows* indicate smudge cells at low and high magnification. *Scale bars,* 20 μm. *(Courtesy of Micheal J. Holtzman, MD, Seldin Professor of Medicine and Cell Biology, Washington University School of Medicine, with permission from the* Journal of Infectious Disease.*)*

continuous cell lines traditionally used for viral isolation, does not display hemagglutinating activity, and appears to be relatively trypsin dependent.[1] Four methods of diagnosis are currently used: viral culture, immunofluorescence assay (IFA), RT-PCR, and serology.

VIRAL CULTURE

Isolation of hMPV requires inoculation of the sample on tertiary cynomolgus monkey kidney (tMK) cells or rhesus monkey kidney (LLC-MK2) cells in medium containing trypsin. Cultures should be observed for 21 days for cytopathic effect (CPE). The characteristic CPE in LLC-MK2 cells consists of small, round, granular, and refringent cells without large syncytia, and it is usually apparent after a mean of 17 days (range, 3 to 23 days) (Fig. 159-5).[2,13] Confirmation of hMPV infection requires either IFA with hMPV-specific antibodies or RT-PCR of the cell supernatant. The use of shell vial cultures may significantly speed time to identification of virus.[51]

IMMUNOFLUORESCENCE ASSAY

Virus-specific monoclonal antibodies are now commercially available for direct detection of hMPV in respiratory secretions using IFA.[52] In children, 85% of RT-PCR–positive specimens were IFA positive. Although this technique is less sensitive than RT-PCR, it may be a useful alternative in commercial microbiology laboratories that lack molecular diagnostic capabilities. Similar to RSV, rapid diagnosis by

IFA in adults may be insensitive owing to low viral load in secretions.

REVERSE TRANSCRIPTASE–POLYMERASE CHAIN REACTION

Because of difficulties with cell culture, molecular techniques for diagnosis of hMPV are favored. The conserved regions of several genes, including those of the F, N, M, and L proteins, have been used successfully in both nested and single-round PCR.[53] Real-time PCR using the *N* and *L* gene primers appear to be the most sensitive assays. Because there is no gold standard for the diagnosis of hMPV, the infection can be confirmed by amplification of two different gene products.[16] Detection of hMPV has been successfully incorporated into several commercially available multiplex PCR assays that simultaneously detect panels of common respiratory viruses.[54]

SEROLOGY

Because seropositivity is nearly universal by age 5 years, a definitive serologic diagnosis requires a fourfold rise in antibody titer or seroconversion. Serologic diagnosis is most often accomplished by enzyme immunoassay (EIA) using whole virus lysates of the representative strains of the two major genotypes or recombinant F or N proteins as antigen, or IFA using hMPV-infected cells fixed to slides.[4,15,55] Antibody responses are cross-reactive, and therefore distinguishing genotype by serology is not possible.[55]

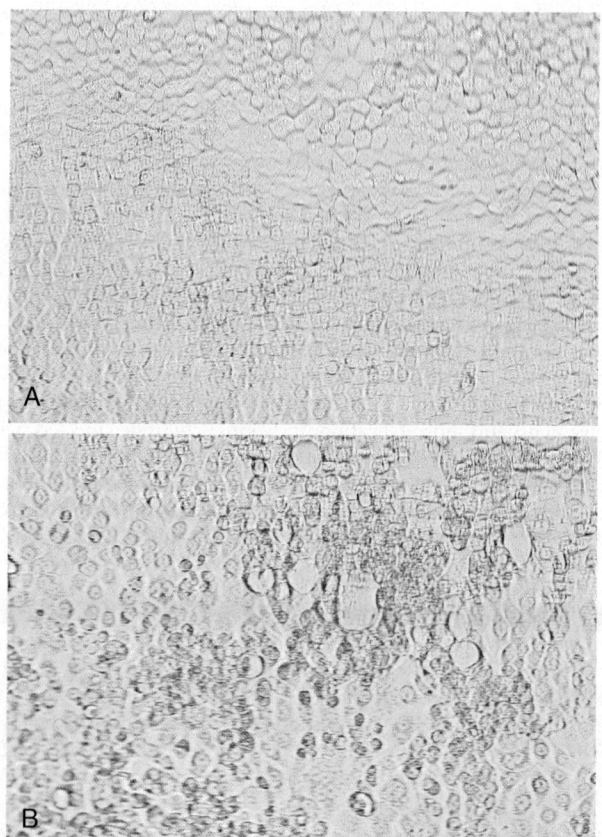

Figure 159-5 Photomicrograph of human metapneumovirus (hMPV) (CAN97-83) in LLC-MK2 cells. LLC-MK2 cells in a semiconfluent monolayer were infected with hMPV (provided by Dr. Guy Boivan) and allowed to grow for 11 days. **A,** Uninfected LLC-MK2 cells. **B,** Infected LLC-MK2 cells. Granular cytopathic effects, without syncytia formation, are evident.

Treatment and Prevention

Treatment of hMPV infection is supportive because therapeutic antivirals or antibody preparations for the treatment or prevention of hMPV infection are not available. Ribavirin, a nucleoside analogue with broad antiviral activity, is approved for the treatment of serious RSV infections in young children (see Chapter 41), and polyclonal intravenous immune globulin (IVIG) is approved for the prophylaxis of RSV infections in high-risk children (see Chapter 158). These two agents were tested by comparing their abilities to inhibit hMPV and RSV in tissue culture and found to have equivalent antiviral activity for both viruses.[56] In the mouse model, ribavirin combined with corticosteroid treatment was effective in reducing viral titers and histologic inflammation of the lung.[57] hMPV-specific fusion inhibitors are currently in development, and animal models indicate these agents may be useful for prophylaxis and preemptive treatment of hMPV infection.[58] Ribavirin and IVIG have been used in seriously ill immunocompromised patients; however, no recommendations for use of these agents can be made until data from controlled clinical trials are available.

The mode of transmission of hMPV is unknown, but given its close relationship with RSV, it is likely to have a similar mode of spread. Efficient transmission of RSV occurs as a result of direct contact with infected secretions through fomites or large-particle aerosols. Shedding of hMPV may occur for up to 3 weeks in children with primary infection.[24] Nosocomial transmission of hMPV has been documented in hospital settings and long-term care facilities among patients and health care workers.[12,16,30] Careful hand hygiene is of primary importance, and the use of gowns and gloves can be considered in outbreak situations.

No vaccine is currently available for the prevention of hMPV. Reinfection occurs throughout life despite the development of an antibody response.[21] Nevertheless, efforts to produce a vaccine for hMPV are ongoing.[59] Because of concerns that inactivated vaccines may produce enhanced disease similar to RSV in immunologically naïve persons, live-attenuated vaccines are favored for development in children. Vectored, recombinant, and chimeric vaccine candidates appear promising in small rodent and nonhuman primate models.

REFERENCES

1. van den Hoogen BG, de Jong JC, Groen J, et al. A newly discovered human pneumovirus isolated from young children with respiratory tract disease. *Nat Med.* 2001;7:719-724.
2. Peret TC, Boivin G, Li Y, et al. Characterization of human metapneumoviruses isolated from patients in North America. *J Infect Dis.* 2002;185:1660-1663.
3. Cook JKA, Cavanagh D. Detection and differentiation of avian pneumoviruses (metapneumoviruses). *Avian Pathol.* 2002;31:132.
4. Deffrasnes C, Hamelin ME, Boivin G. Human metapneumovirus. *Semin Respir Crit Care Med.* 2007;28:213-221.
5. Kahn JS. Epidemiology of human metapneumovirus. *Clin Microbiol Rev.* 2006;19:546-557.
6. van den Hoogen BG, Besterbroer TM, Osterhaus AD, et al. Analysis of the genomic sequence of a human metapneumovirus. *Virology.* 2002;295:119-132.
7. Biacchesi S, Skiadopoulos MH, Boivin G, et al. Genetic diversity between human metapneumovirus subgroups. *Virology.* 2003; 315:1-9.
8. Huck B, Scharf G, Neumann-Haefelin D, et al. Novel human metapneumovirus sublineage. *Emerg Infect Dis.* 2006;12: 147-150.
9. Douville RN, Bastien N, Li Y, et al. Human metapneumovirus elicits weak IFN-gamma memory responses compared with respiratory syncytial virus. *J Immunol.* 2006;176:5848-5855.
10. Laham FR, Israele V, Casellas JM, et al. Differential production of inflammatory cytokines in primary infection with human metapneumovirus and with other common respiratory viruses in infancy. *J Infect Dis.* 2004;189:2047-2056.
11. Vargas SO, Kozakewich HP, Perez-Atayde AR, et al. Pathology of human metapneumovirus infection: Insights into the pathogenesis of a newly identified respiratory virus. *Pediatr Dev Pathol.* 2004;7:478-486; discussion 421.
12. Boivin G, De Serres G, Hamelin ME, et al. An outbreak of severe respiratory tract infection due to human metapneumovirus in a long-term care facility. *Clin Infect Dis.* 2007;44:1152-1158.
13. Boivin G, Abed Y, Pelletier G, et al. Virological features and clinical manifestations associated with human metapneumovirus: A new paramyxovirus responsible for acute respiratory-tract infections in all age groups. *J Infect Dis.* 2002;186:1330-1334.
14. Gray GC, Capuano AW, Setterquist SF, et al. Multi-year study of human metapneumovirus infection at a large US Midwestern medical referral center. *J Clin Virol.* 2006;37:269-276.
15. Walsh EE, Peterson DR, Falsey AR. Human metapneumovirus infections in adults: Another piece of the puzzle. *Arch Intern Med.* 2008;168:2489-2496.
16. Peiris JSM, Tang W, Chan K, et al. Children with respiratory disease associated with metapneumovirus in Hong Kong. *Emerg Infect Dis.* 2003;9:628-633.
17. Boivin G, De Sarres G, Cote S, et al. Human metapneumovirus infections in hospitalized children. *Emerg Infect Dis.* 2003;9: 634-640.
18. Williams JV, Harris PA, Tollefson SJ, et al. Human metapneumovirus and lower respiratory tract disease in otherwise healthy infants and children. *N Engl J Med.* 2004;350:443-450.
19. Rafiefard F, Yun Z, Orvell C. Epidemiologic characteristics and seasonal distribution of human metapneumovirus infections in five epidemic seasons in Stockholm, Sweden, 2002-2006. *J Med Virol.* 2008;80:1631-1638.
20. Sloots TP, Mackay IM, Bialasiewicz S, et al. Human metapneumovirus, Australia, 2001-2004. *Emerg Infect Dis.* 2006;12: 1263-1266.
21. Williams JV, Wang CK, Yang CF, et al. The role of human metapneumovirus in upper respiratory tract infections in children: A 20-year experience. *J Infect Dis.* 2006;193:387-395.
22. Bosis S, Esposito S, Niesters HG, et al. Impact of human metapneumovirus in childhood: Comparison with respiratory syncytial virus and influenza viruses. *J Med Virol.* 2005;75:101-104.
23. Madhi SA, Ludewick H, Kuwanda L, et al. Pneumococcal coinfection with human metapneumovirus. *J Infect Dis.* 2006;193: 1236-1243.
24. Robinson JL, Lee BE, Bastien N, et al. Seasonality and clinical features of human metapneumovirus infection in children in northern Alberta. *J Med Virol.* 2005;76:98-105.
25. Agapov E, Sumino KC, Gaudreault-Keener M, et al. Genetic variability of human metapneumovirus infection: Evidence of a shift in viral genotype without a change in illness. *J Infect Dis.* 2006;193:396-403.
26. Mackay IM, Bialasiewicz S, Jacob KC, et al. Genetic diversity of human metapneumovirus over 4 consecutive years in Australia. *J Infect Dis.* 2006;193:1630-1633.
27. Esper F, Boucher D, Weibel C, et al. Human metapneumovirus infection in the United States: Clinical manifestations associated with a newly emerging respiratory infection in children. *Pediatrics.* 2003;111:1407-1410.
28. Heikkinen T, Osterback R, Peltola V, et al. Human metapneumovirus infections in children. *Emerg Infect Dis.* 2008;14: 101-106.
29. Williams JV, Tollefson SJ, Nair S, et al. Association of human metapneumovirus with acute otitis media. *Int J Pediatr Otorhinolaryngol.* 2006;70:1189-1193.
30. Freymuth F, Vabret A., Legrand L, et al. Presence of the new human metapneumovirus in French children with bronchiolitis. *Pediatr Infect Dis J.* 2003;22:92-94.
31. Schildgen O, Glatzel T, Geikowski T, et al. Human metapneumovirus RNA in encephalitis patient. *Emerg Infect Dis.* 2005; 11:467-470.
32. Wilkesmann A, Schildgen O, Eis-Hubinger AM, et al. Human metapneumovirus infections cause similar symptoms and clinical severity as respiratory syncytial virus infections. *Eur J Pediatr.* 2006;165:467-475.
33. Jartti T, van den Hoogen BG, Garofalo RP, et al. Metapneumovirus and acute wheezing in children. *Lancet.* 2003;360:1394.
34. Williams JV, Crowe JE Jr, Enriquez R, et al. Human metapneumovirus infection plays an etiologic role in acute asthma exacerbations requiring hospitalization in adults. *J Infect Dis.* 2005;192:1149-1153.
35. Khetsuriani N, Kazerouni NN, Erdman DD, et al. Prevalence of viral respiratory tract infections in children with asthma. *J Allergy Clin Immunol.* 2006;118:1199-1206.
36. Bosis S, Esposito S, Osterhaus AD, et al. Association between high nasopharyngeal viral load and disease severity in children with human metapneumovirus infection. *J Clin Virol.* 2008;42: 286-290.
37. Vicente D, Montes M, Cilla G, et al. Differences in clinical severity between genotype A and genotype B human metapneumovirus infection in children. *Clin Infect Dis.* 2006;42:e111-e113.
38. Semple MG, Cowell A, Dove W, et al. Dual infection of infants by human metapneumovirus and human respiratory syncytial virus is strongly associated with severe bronchiolitis. *J Infect Dis.* 2005;191:382-386.
39. Foulongne V, Guyon G, Rodiere M, et al. Human metapneumovirus infection in young children hospitalized with respiratory tract disease. *Pediatr Infect Dis J.* 2006;25:354-359.
40. Ostehaus A, Fouchier R. Human metapneumovirus in the community. *Lancet.* 2003;361:890-891.
41. Li IW, To KK, Tang BS, et al. Human metapneumovirus infection in an immunocompetent adult presenting as mononucleosis-like illness. *J Infect.* 2008;56:389-392.
42. Hamelin ME, Cote S, Laforge J, et al. Human metapneumovirus infection in adults with community-acquired pneumonia and exacerbation of chronic obstructive pulmonary disease. *Clin Infect Dis.* 2005;41:498-502.
43. Johnstone J, Majumdar SR, Fox JD, et al. Human metapneumovirus pneumonia in adults: Results of a prospective study. *Clin Infect Dis.* 2008;46:571-574.
44. Martinello RA, Esper F, Weibel C, et al. Human metapneumovirus and exacerbations of chronic obstructive pulmonary disease. *J Infect.* 2006;53:248-254.
45. Falsey AR, Dallal GE, Formica MA, et al. Long-term care facilities: A cornucopia of viral pathogens. *J Am Geriatr Soc.* 2008;56: 1281-1285.
46. Englund JA, Boeckh M, Kuypers J, et al. Brief communication: Fatal human metapneumovirus infection in stem-cell transplant recipients. *Ann Intern Med.* 2006;144:344-349.
47. Larcher C, Geltner C, Fischer H, et al. Human metapneumovirus infection in lung transplant recipients: Clinical presentation and epidemiology. *J Heart Lung Transplant.* 2005;24:1891-1901.
48. Franquet T, Rodriguez S, Martino R, et al. Human metapneumovirus infection in hematopoietic stem cell transplant recipients: High-resolution computed tomography findings. *J Comput Assist Tomogr.* 2005;29:223-227.
49. Sumino KC, Agapov E, Pierce RA, et al. Detection of severe human metapneumovirus infection by real-time polymerase chain reaction and histopathological assessment. *J Infect Dis.* 2005;192:1052-1060.
50. Debiaggi M, Canducci F, Sampaolo M, et al. Persistent symptomless human metapneumovirus infection in hematopoietic stem cell transplant recipients. *J Infect Dis.* 2006;194:474-478.
51. Reina J, Ferres F, Alcoceba E, et al. Comparison of different cell lines and incubation times in the isolation by the shell vial culture of human metapneumovirus from pediatric respiratory samples. *J Clin Virol.* 2007;40:46-49.
52. Landry ML, Cohen S, Ferguson D. Prospective study of human metapneumovirus detection in clinical samples by use of light diagnostics direct immunofluorescence reagent and real-time PCR. *J Clin Microbiol.* 2008;46:1098-1100.
53. Maertzdorf J, Wang CK, Brown JB, et al. Real-time reverse transcriptase PCR assay for detection of human metapneumoviruses from all known genetic lineages. *J Clin Microbiol.* 2004;42: 981-986.
54. Li H, McCormac MA, Estes RW, et al. Simultaneous detection and high-throughput identification of a panel of RNA viruses causing respiratory tract infections. *J Clin Microbiol.* 2007;45: 2105-2109.
55. Leung J, Esper F, Weibel C, et al. Seroepidemiology of human metapneumovirus (hMPV) on the basis of a novel enzyme-linked immunosorbent assay utilizing hMPV fusion protein expressed in recombinant vesicular stomatitis virus. *J Clin Microbiol.* 2005;43:1213-1219.
56. Wyde PR, Chetty SN, Jewell AM, et al. Comparison of the inhibition of human metapneumovirus and respiratory syncytial virus by ribavirin and immune serum globulin in vitro. *Antiviral Res.* 2003;60:51-59.
57. Hamelin ME, Prince GA, Boivin G. Effect of ribavirin and glucocorticoid treatment in a mouse model of human metapneumovirus infection. *Antimicrob Agents Chemother.* 2006;50:774-777.
58. Deffrasnes C, Hamelin ME, Prince GA, et al. Identification and evaluation of a highly effective fusion inhibitor for human metapneumovirus. *Antimicrob Agents Chemother.* 2008;52:279-287.
59. Herfst S, Fouchier RA. Vaccination approaches to combat human metapneumovirus lower respiratory tract infections. *J Clin Virol.* 2008;41:49-52.

160

Measles Virus (Rubeola)

ANNE A. GERSHON

Measles, an acute infection caused by rubeola virus, is highly contagious and usually seen in children. The illness is characterized by cough, coryza, fever, and a maculopapular rash that begins several days after the initial symptoms appear. There is a characteristic enanthem, Koplik's spots, that is specific for measles and that precedes the onset of rash. Recovery from measles is the rule, but serious complications of the respiratory tract and central nervous system (CNS) may occur. Measles in the United States has been largely controlled since the introduction of live-attenuated measles vaccine in 1963; it remains a serious problem in developing countries but successful efforts are now being carried out for improved control of the disease.[1]

Measles virus (MV) belongs to the genus *Morbillivirus* of the family Paramyxoviridae. It is closely related to the viruses causing canine and phocine distemper, rinderpest of cattle, peste des petits ruminants of goats and sheep, and morbilli of certain aquatic animals. Although these viruses are distinct agents, they share certain antigens.[2,3] Wild measles virus is pathogenic only for primates.

Description of the Pathogen

MV is an enveloped, nonsegmented, single-stranded, negative-sense RNA virus. It encodes for at least eight structural proteins.[3]

MORPHOLOGY

On electron microscopy, measles virions are pleomorphic spheres with a diameter of 100 to 250 nm. Virions consist of an inner nucleocapsid that is a coiled helix of protein and RNA, and an envelope that bears two types of short surface projections.[3,4] These projections include the hemagglutinin (H) and the fusion (F) proteins. The molecular weight of the single-stranded RNA is 4.5 kDa. Because the entire genome has been sequenced, it is possible to differentiate between wild measles virus and vaccine-type virus.

CHEMICAL AND ANTIGENIC COMPOSITION

Measles virus encodes at least eight structural proteins. These have letter names and include the following: F, C, H, L (large), M (matrix), N, P, and V. Three of them, the nucleoprotein (N), the phosphopolymerase protein (P), and the large protein (L), are complexed with RNA. C and V interact with cellular proteins and also play roles in the regulation of transcription and replication of the virus. Three are associated with the viral envelope: the M protein, a nonglycosylated protein, associated with the inner lipid bilayer, and the two glycoproteins H and F.[5] The H glycoprotein is involved in attachment of the virus to host cells and the F glycoprotein is involved in spread of the virus from one cell to another. The complement regulatory protein CD46, which is widely distributed in primate tissues, serves as a receptor for the measles virus,[3,6] as does signaling lymphocyte activation molecule (SLAM; CDw150).[7] It has been postulated that another receptor for measles virus exists on epithelial cells, but it remains to be exactly identified.[8] Multiple receptors probably enable MV to enter different types of cells during infection. The H glycoprotein constitutes the antigen that mediates hemagglutination. The hemagglutination inhibition (HI) test, using red blood cells from Old World monkeys, is an historically important serologic test for measuring antibody to measles virus. The F glycoprotein causes hemolysis. Unlike many other paramyxoviruses, neuraminidase is not found on the enve-

lope of measles virus.[9] Genetic and antigenic variations of measles virus are now recognized; the sequence of genes coding for H and N is the most variable.[10] Numerous genotypes have been described.[11,12] Measles virus antigens and their role in human disease[5,13] are discussed later.

GROWTH OF MEASLES VIRUS IN TISSUE CULTURE

Measles virus was first successfully isolated in the laboratory by Enders and Peebles in 1954.[14] The virus was initially propagated in primary human renal cells, but later was cultivated in cultured simian kidney cells. Wild measles virus is rather difficult to propagate in vitro because it is slow-growing and only a limited number of types of cell cultures are permissive for the virus.[12] Typically, cytopathic effects produced by measles virus in tissue cultures consist of stellate cells with increased refractility and, especially on passage, multinucleated syncytial giant cells containing intranuclear inclusions. In the absence of cytopathic effects, virus replication can also be detected by hemadsorption of rhesus monkey erythrocytes. Presumptive isolates of measles virus are identified by typing with monoclonal antibodies using immunofluorescence or plaque reduction tests.[3,15] Polymerase chain reaction (PCR) assays for measles virus are also available (see later).

HOST RANGE

Humans are the only natural host for wild measles virus, but monkeys may also be infected. In general, illness caused by measles virus is milder in monkeys than that in humans.[16] It has not been possible to infect small laboratory animals, such as rodents, with wild measles virus. However, newborn and suckling rodents may be infected with vaccine strains administered by the intracerebral route.[17,18]

Epidemiology

Measles has been recognized as a disease for some 2000 years, but its infectious nature was not recognized until about 150 years ago. In 1846, Panum[19] studied an epidemic of measles in the Faroe Islands and noted that the disease was contagious, that there was an incubation period of about 2 weeks, and that infection appeared to confer lifelong immunity. The next major advance in the understanding of measles occurred in 1954, when Enders and Peebles[14] successfully propagated wild measles virus in primary human renal tissue culture cells. This was a prerequisite for the development of a live attenuated measles vaccine, which was licensed for use in the United States in 1963.[20]

Measles is seen in every country in the world. Without a vaccine, epidemics of measles lasting 3 to 4 months could be predicted to occur every 2 to 5 years. Countries in which measles vaccine is widely used have experienced a marked decrease in the incidence of disease. For example, for many years, 200,000 to 500,000 cases of measles were reported annually in the United States. Since 1963, when the vaccine was licensed, the incidence of measles in the United States has decreased by almost 99%.[21,22] This decrease has been especially pronounced since the early 1980s, when state laws requiring proof of immunity to measles for school entry were enacted. The yearly incidence of measles in the United States reached a nadir in 1983, when 1,497 cases were reported to the Centers for Disease Control and Prevention (CDC) in Atlanta. In the late 1980s and early 1990s, however, there was an increase in the incidence of measles; this was brought under control by increasing the rate of immunization and by introducing a two-dose schedule of measles vaccine for all children.[23-25] In 1990, more than 25,000 cases of measles and 89 measles-associated deaths were reported to the CDC.[26] In 1991, however, the number of reported cases dropped significantly, to 9,643.[27] Between 1993 and 1996, fewer than 1,000 annual cases in the United States were reported to the CDC.[28] Between 2000 and 2007, an average of 63 annual cases were reported.[29] Using molecular techniques, it was demonstrated that transmission of indigenous measles largely ceased in the United States by 1993. Since that time, most cases of measles in the United States have resulted from international importation of measles virus.[11]

In the first 6 months of 2008, however, 131 measles cases were reported to the CDC; 13% were associated with importations from Europe, Asia, and the Middle East. Of these cases, 99 (76%) were epidemiologically or virologically linked to importations. Most of these patients were younger than 20 years, and 91% were unvaccinated or had an unknown vaccination status. Of the unvaccinated individuals, many of whom declined vaccination for philosophical and/or religious reasons, 85% were eligible for vaccination. When vaccination coverage fell to 80% to 85%, measles once again became endemic in the United Kingdom. Although current vaccine coverage in the United States, which is over 90%, is sufficient to prevent sustained outbreaks of measles, it is not sufficient to prevent imported cases, with resultant limited U.S. spread.

Measles continues to be a worldwide problem that primarily affects children in developing countries. In 2000, it was estimated that more than 750,000 deaths attributed to measles occurred globally. With the advent of World Health Organization (WHO)– and United Nations Children's Fund (UNICEF)–supported immunization programs, the estimated deaths globally have been reduced to 242,000 annually. The largest reduction in deaths was observed in Africa.[30] At present, there is minimal evidence that immunity induced by measles vaccine wanes significantly with time.[24,31-35] The major reasons why measles has not fully been eliminated from the United States are failure to immunize all persons who qualify for vaccination, primary vaccine failure, and importation of measles to the United States from other countries.[11,34-37]

SPREAD OF INFECTION

The measles virion is very labile; it is sensitive to acid, proteolytic enzymes, strong light, and drying.[3] The virus, however, remains infective in droplet form in air for several hours, especially under conditions of low relative humidity. This latter fact may account for the increased incidence of measles in winter.[38]

Measles is an airborne virus that is spread by direct contact with droplets from respiratory secretions of infected persons. It is one of the most communicable of the infectious diseases, most infectious during the late prodromal phase of the illness, when cough and coryza are at their peak[16]; however, the disease is probably contagious from several days before until several days after the onset of rash. Measles virus has been isolated from respiratory secretions of patients with measles only until up to 48 hours after the onset of rash.[39] Airborne spread of measles in physicians' offices[40,41] and in a sports complex[42] has been observed.

Diseases Associated with Measles Virus

Subacute sclerosing panencephalitis (SSPE) is a chronic degenerative fatal neurologic disease that occurs on average 7 years after an attack of measles, particularly in children who had measles before 2 years of age. Possibly it is an autoimmune disease.[12] A few children who received measles vaccine and who had no prior history of measles have been observed to develop SSPE. It is thought that these children may have had a subclinical case of measles before receiving vaccine. The

incidence of SSPE in the United States has declined dramatically since the introduction of measles vaccine.[21,43] It is almost invariably caused by wild-type virus; a single case of inclusion-body encephalitis caused by the vaccine strain was reported in 1999.[44] Based on the number of cases of measles in children during 1989 to 1991, and the number of cases of SSPE reported to the CDC following those years, it was estimated that the risk of SSPE after measles is 10 times greater than was originally thought, or 1 per 11,000 cases. Genotyping revealed that these SSPE cases were caused by the wild type measles circulating during those years. It appears therefore that vaccination can prevent significantly more cases of SSPE than was originally projected.[45]

Patients with SSPE have unusually high measles antibody titers, both in their serum and in their cerebrospinal fluid.[46] SSPE is caused by a persistent infection with a measles-related virus in the CNS that occurs despite a vigorous immune response on the part of the host. The pathogenesis of SSPE is extremely complex and has been ascribed to a combination of host factors and viral replicative phenomena. Although a measles-like virus has occasionally been isolated, using cocultivation techniques, from the brains of patients with SSPE at autopsy,[47,48] the infection is usually characterized by an inability to produce viral progeny.[49] This inability may be a result of defects in the formation of gene products arising from genomic mutations caused by errors of RNA replication. Originally, the inability to replicate was ascribed to failure of the infective virus to produce measles M protein.[50] Later, it was realized that this failure was related to mutations of the gene encoding this protein. Now it is recognized that defects in envelope gene products H and F also occur as a result of other genomic mutations of the causative virus. Host factors such as defective cellular immunity and the ability of specific antibodies to confine the virus to intracellular multiplication are also postulated to play a role in the pathogenesis of SSPE.[49-54] Measles virus RNA was demonstrated by an in situ reverse transcriptase–polymerase chain reaction (RT-PCR) assay in neurons, astrocytes, oligodendrocytes, and vascular endothelial cells in the brain of a patient who died from SSPE.[55]

The evidence that multiple sclerosis, Crohn's disease, and systemic lupus erythematosus are etiologically linked with measles virus is much weaker than that for SSPE,[56-58] and measles virus infection is probably unrelated to these diseases. A causative role for measles virus in Paget's disease of bone has been raised as a possibility but as yet is unproven.[59-62]

Pathogenesis

Measles virus (MV) was thought to infect by invasion of the respiratory epithelium from which it spreads to the local lymph nodes, blood, spleen, lymphatic tissue, lung, thymus, liver, and skin.[3,60,61] Recent studies in monkeys, however, have suggested that MV enters lymphoid cells of the upper respiratory tract using the SLAM receptor. After replication in lymphoid cells, MV then invades epithelial cells in organs such as the respiratory tract, intestine, bladder, and skin using a different as yet unidentified receptor. When MV infects epithelial cells, progeny is released into the airway and thus the virus can be transmitted to new individuals.[8] Studies on volunteers inoculated with live measles virus have indicated that infection may occur after instillation of virus at any point from the nose to the lower parts of the respiratory tract.[59]

Measles virus has been isolated from the leukocytes of patients with clinical measles.[63] The virus has also been propagated in vitro in human T and B lymphocytes and in monocytes.[64] The major infected cell in the blood is the monocyte.[3,65] Endothelial and epithelial cells are also infected. Infected tissues include the thymus, spleen, lymph nodes, liver, skin, conjunctiva, intestine, bladder, and lung.[3]

Infection of the entire respiratory mucosa accounts for the cough and coryza that are classic signs of measles. In addition, measles may directly cause croup, bronchiolitis, and pneumonia. Damage to the respiratory tract from edema and loss of cilia may predispose to secondary bacterial invasion, resulting in complications such as otitis media and pneumonia.[16]

Within a few days after generalized involvement of the respiratory tract has occurred, Koplik's spots appear and are followed by the development of a rash. Both manifestations are believed to result from similar pathologic mechanisms. On microscopic examination of skin and mucous membranes, multinucleate giant cells and other similar histologic changes are observed in the epidermis and oral epithelium.[66] The appearance of the measles rash coincides temporally with the appearance of serum antibody and the termination of communicability of the disease. Therefore, it has been postulated that the skin and mucous membrane manifestations of measles actually represent hypersensitivity of the host to the virus. MV antigen has been demonstrated in the involved skin and mucous membranes by immunofluorescence.[66-68] MV has also been isolated from the rash in its early stages.[61] If hypersensitivity is the actual cause of the rash, however, it is probably mediated by cellular rather than humoral immunity,[69] and therefore patients with agammaglobulinemia who contract measles develop a rash. Patients with deficiencies in cell-mediated immunity, on the other hand, may develop measles giant cell (Hecht's) pneumonia without a rash after an exposure to measles or if measles vaccine is given.[70,71]

Immunity

Immunity to measles after an attack of the disease appears to be lifelong. Similarly, after measles vaccination, immunity is of many years' duration and probably lifelong in most persons.[21] How measles antibody persists for years after infection is not understood. One possible explanation is that the virus becomes latent after acute infection and provides an immunologic stimulus to antibody formation. However, latent measles virus has not been demonstrated in humans or in experimental animals. An alternative explanation for the persistence of measles antibody is that reexposure to the virus results in persistent antigenic stimulation. Reinfection with measles can occur and is almost always asymptomatic even though a boost in antibody titer can be detected.[72] Cellular immunity to MV probably also plays a role in the prevention of recurrent measles, because patients with agammaglobulinemia do not have multiple attacks of measles. A cell-mediated response to measles antigen in the absence of detectable measles antibody was reported in two physicians in whom no disease developed, despite repeated exposures to measles.[73] Therefore, when humoral antibodies to measles are absent or of low titer, cellular immunity to the virus may protect against subsequent illness. Cellular immunity to MV in peripheral blood of persons with a history of measles has been shown by in vitro lymphocyte stimulation after exposure to measles antigen[74] and by demonstration of measles-specific class I and II cytotoxic T cells.[75-77] A complex interplay of cellular immunity and cytokines occurs before, during, and after measles infection in healthy persons.[78]

During infection, CD8 and CD4 T cells are activated and probably participate in the clearance of virus and the development of rash. During recovery, suppression of cell-mediated responses occurs, with elevation of suppressive cytokines such as interleukin-4, which may be responsible for depressed delayed-type hypersensitivity to tuberculin.[3,79] Effects of vaccine on the immune system that resemble the effects of naturally occurring measles have also been described.[80]

Clinical Manifestations

The incubation period of measles is 10 to 14 days; it is often somewhat longer in adults than in children. A prodromal phase lasting several days begins after the incubation period. It is manifested by malaise, fever, anorexia, conjunctivitis, and respiratory symptoms such as cough and coryza, and may resemble a severe upper respiratory tract infection. Toward the end of the prodrome, just before the appearance of the rash, Koplik's spots appear.

Koplik's spots are pathognomonic of measles. First noted by Koplik in 1896, they consist of bluish gray specks on a red base.[81] They have been likened to grains of sand and, without examination of the buccal

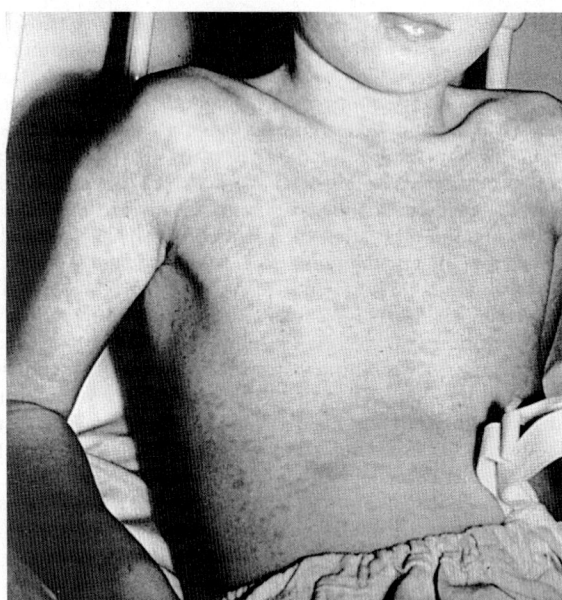

Figure 160-1 Typical rash on a patient with measles.

mucosa in good light, may be overlooked. Most often they appear on the mucosa opposite the second molars. However, in severe cases, the entire mucous membrane of the mouth may be involved. This enanthem persists for several days and begins to slough as the rash appears.

The rash of measles usually begins on the face and proceeds down the body to involve the extremities last, including the palms and soles (Fig. 160-1). During the healing phase, the involved areas (except palms and soles) may desquamate. The rash is erythematous and maculopapular; as it progresses, it becomes confluent, especially on the face and the neck. The rash usually lasts about 5 days and starts to clear first on the skin that was initially involved. The patient with measles is usually most ill during the first or second day of the rash. Several days after the appearance of the rash, the fever abates and the patient begins to feel better. The entire uncomplicated illness from late prodrome to resolution of the fever and rash lasts 7 to 10 days; cough may be the last symptom to disappear.

COMPLICATIONS

The most common complications of measles involve the respiratory tract and CNS. Involvement of the respiratory tract is part of the virus infection itself. In addition, bacterial superinfection may occur in any area of the respiratory tract, including the middle ear. Superinfection may be secondary to local tissue damage inflicted by the virus and depression of cellular immunity. Pneumonia accompanying measles may be caused by direct viral invasion of the lungs or by bacterial superinfection.[82] Roentgenographic evidence of pneumonia is common, even during apparently uncomplicated measles.[16] In infants who die of measles, pneumonia accounts for about 60% of deaths, whereas in children 10 to 14 years of age, death is more often observed to be from complications of acute encephalitis.[83,84]

Encephalitis after measles in normal hosts may be acute or chronic (e.g., SSPE). Acute measles encephalitis manifests with a resurgence of fever during convalescence and frequently with headaches, seizures, and changes in the state of consciousness. Up to 50% of patients with measles but no symptoms that suggest cerebral involvement may have abnormalities detected by electroencephalography,[85] so it is believed that viral invasion of the CNS is a common feature of measles. However, only 1 in 1000 to 2000 patients with measles develops clinical signs of encephalitis. Measles encephalitis ranges from mild to severe, and a high proportion of patients who recover are left with neurologic sequelae.

MV has been isolated from the brains of several persons dying of measles encephalitis.[86-89] However, virus isolation is uncommon and usually requires special virologic techniques such as cocultivation. It is hypothesized that acute measles encephalitis is caused by hypersensitivity to virus in brain tissue. Both viral and host antigens are present on the surface of measles-infected cells in vitro.[90] Therefore, hypersensitivity may be directed against viral and host (brain) antigens, which accounts for the encephalitic symptoms. Demyelination, vascular cuffing, gliosis, and infiltration of fat-laden macrophages near blood vessel walls are noted in brain tissue from patients with measles encephalitis.[3] In a laboratory study of serum and cerebrospinal fluid from 19 patients with postinfectious measles encephalitis, similarities between experimental allergic encephalomyelitis (e.g., immune responses to myelin basic protein, early destruction of myelin) were demonstrated in about 50%. There was no evidence of intrathecal synthesis of antibody against measles virus, which suggests that immunopathology, rather than viral multiplication, is involved in the pathogenesis of measles encephalitis.[91]

Transient hepatitis has also been reported during acute measles.[92]

SPECIAL CONSIDERATIONS

Modified Measles

An extremely mild form of measles has been observed in persons with some degree of passive immunity to the virus. This includes some babies younger than 1 year who have passively acquired maternal antibody to measles virus and some susceptible persons who received immune globulin after an exposure to measles. The symptoms of modified measles are variable, and certain classic symptoms such as the prodromal period, conjunctivitis, Koplik's spots, and rash may be absent. The incubation period may be prolonged. At times, the infection is subclinical and, with a great degree of passively acquired immunity, may be prevented completely.[72]

Atypical Measles

The syndrome of atypical measles has been described in persons who received killed measles vaccine (or killed vaccine followed soon afterward by live vaccine) and who, several years later, were exposed to wild measles virus.[93,94] Initially, these patients have an undetectable or a very low measles antibody titer. They then develop unusual manifestations of measles followed by the appearance of extremely high measles antibody titers (e.g., 1 : 100,000) in their serum.[95] After a prodrome of fever and pain for 1 to 2 days, the rash appears. Unlike classic measles, it begins peripherally and may be urticarial, maculopapular, hemorrhagic, vesicular, or some combination of these types. The disease may be misdiagnosed as varicella, Rocky Mountain spotted fever, Henoch-Schönlein purpura, drug eruption, or toxic shock syndrome. The patient has a high fever, edema of the extremities, interstitial pulmonary infiltrates, hepatitis and, on occasion, a pleural effusion. The disease tends to be severe with a somewhat more prolonged course than regular measles. At least one fatality has been reported. No specific therapy is available. Measles virus has not been isolated from these patients, and they do not appear to transmit measles to others.[94]

The pathogenesis of this syndrome is believed to be one of hypersensitivity to MV in a partially immune host. Whether cell-mediated or humoral immune mechanisms, or both, are involved remains controversial.[94,96,97] One hypothesis concerning pathogenesis is that killed measles vaccine lacks the antigen that stimulates the immunity that prevents entry of measles virus into cells, thereby allowing measles infection to occur, despite the partial immunity derived from killed vaccine.[98,99] In an animal model, the low avidity of measles antibodies induced by the inactivated vaccine fails to neutralize the wild-type virus, leading to deposition of immune complexes, vasculitis, and pneumonitis.[3]

Recurrences of atypical measles have not been reported. Therefore, those who received killed measles vaccine (or killed vaccine followed soon afterward by live vaccine) in the past may be reimmunized with live measles vaccine. It is important that persons who have received killed vaccine be made aware, however, that severe local reactions can follow an injection of live vaccine.[100,101] Usually, the reaction consists of tenderness and erythema around the injection site. However, severe local edema and high fever may also occur. Immunization with live vaccine should be strongly considered because the associated risk is lower than the risk of being exposed to the wild-type virus.[102]

Immunocompromised Patients

Severe measles may occur in those with compromised or deficient cellular immunity, such as those being treated for malignant disease, after transplantation, and in individuals with acquired immunodeficiency syndrome (AIDS) or any form of congenital immunodeficiency.[70,103-105] In a report of measles cases occurring in immunocompromised patients in 1989 to 1990, combined with some recorded in the literature, the case-fatality rate for severe measles in children and young adults was calculated to be 70% in 40 oncology patients and 40% in 11 patients infected with the human immunodeficiency virus (HIV).[106] Of the oncology patients, 40% had no rash, 58% had pneumonitis, and 20% had encephalitis. Of the HIV-infected patients, 27% had no rash, and 82% had pneumonia. Should immunocompromised patients be inadvertently exposed to measles, they may develop giant cell pneumonia without evidence of a rash.[70,103,106] In such cases, the clinical diagnosis of measles may be difficult or impossible to establish. Because these children may also have poor antibody responses, virus isolation from infected tissue (or identification of measles antigen by immunofluorescence) may be the only means of diagnosis. A chronic form of encephalitis resembling SSPE, often with a concomitant pneumonia, has also been reported in those with deficient cellular immunity.[51,52] This entity has been classified as subacute measles encephalitis and may be confirmed by the presence of measles RNA or infectious virus in brain tissue.[107] Even in the era of molecular diagnostic techniques, however, this diagnosis may be difficult to establish, particularly if the person had no history of clinical measles in the past.[108] Malnourished children, especially in developing countries, have also been reported to develop severe measles. This may be related to poor cell-mediated immune responses resulting from malnutrition.[109] Intense exposure to the virus because of crowding may also play a role in the severity of measles in developing countries.[110,111]

Immunocompromised patients with no history of clinical measles who are exposed to the infection should be passively immunized with immunoglobulin, even if they have previously been immunized (see later).

Pregnant Women and Their Offspring

Rubeola during pregnancy, in contrast to German measles (rubella), is not known to cause congenital anomalies of the fetus.[112] However, measles in pregnancy has been associated with spontaneous abortion and premature delivery.[16] Measles can be severe in pregnancy. From 1988 to 1991, when there was a resurgence of measles in the United States, a number of pregnant women developed measles. Of 13 such women hospitalized in Houston, 54% had respiratory complications requiring admission to the intensive care unit, and one died.[113] These women were thought to have primary measles pneumonia. Measles in the offspring of mothers with measles ranges from mild to severe.[114,115] It is therefore recommended that infants born to women with active measles be passively immunized with immunoglobulin at birth.

Persons with Tuberculosis

It has long been thought that tuberculosis is aggravated in persons who contract natural measles, presumably because of a depression of cell-mediated immunity by MV.[3] For example, the tuberculin test has been reported to become negative for about 1 month after measles or measles vaccination.[16] It seems prudent to defer measles vaccination in persons with known tuberculosis until antituberculosis therapy is underway. In geographic areas and populations where tuberculosis is rare, it is not mandatory to perform a tuberculin test on an infant before administering measles vaccine.[116]

Occurrence in Adults

Measles has long been regarded as an illness of childhood. When it occurs in adults, it is often a more severe illness. In a series of 3220 young adult military recruits with measles between 1976 and 1979, about 3% developed pneumonia requiring hospitalization. Bacterial superinfection of the respiratory tract occurred in 30%, and 17% had evidence of bronchospasm. In addition, 31% had laboratory evidence of hepatitis, 29% had otitis media, and 25% had sinusitis.[117] In patients with measles reported to the CDC in 1991, the incidence of complications was higher in those older than 20 years than in children.[26]

Diagnosis

Classic measles with cough, coryza, conjunctivitis, Koplik's spots, and a maculopapular rash beginning on the face is easily diagnosed clinically. Often, there is a striking leukopenia, perhaps related to the infection and death of leukocytes. A laboratory diagnosis of measles is helpful when the clinician is unfamiliar with the illness because of the decline in cases of clinical measles since the introduction of measles vaccine. A laboratory diagnosis may also be helpful in cases of possible atypical measles, or when unexplained pneumonia or encephalitis occurs in an immunocompromised patient. The differential diagnosis of measles includes rubella, Kawasaki syndrome, scarlet fever, roseola, infectious mononucleosis and rickettsial, enteroviral, and adenoviral infections.

Measles may be diagnosed in the laboratory by virus isolation, identification of measles antigen or RNA in infected tissues, or demonstration of a significant serologic response to MV. Virus isolation is technically difficult, and facilities for isolation are not always available. It is particularly useful, however, for patients with fatal pneumonia and patients with an immunodeficiency, in whom an antibody response may be minimal. Immunofluorescent examination of cells from nasal exudates or from urinary sediment for the presence of measles antigen may be useful for rapid diagnosis of measles.[112,118] A sensitive RT-PCR amplification method to demonstrate measles virus RNA is available, and nucleotide sequencing can be used for precise characterization of diagnostic specimens.[12,119]

A commonly used laboratory diagnostic method is the serologic response to the virus. A fourfold or greater increase in measles antibody titer in acute and convalescent serum specimens is considered diagnostic for measles. SSPE may be diagnosed by the demonstration of high measles antibody titers in serum and cerebrospinal fluid in the presence of a compatible illness.[118] A number of methods are available for measuring antibodies to measles, usually through hospital or state health department laboratories. Neutralization, which requires propagation of the virus in vitro, is technically difficult and infrequently used. Complement fixation lacks sensitivity and is rarely used. The HI test is not used frequently today because it has been supplanted by the enzyme-linked immunosorbent assay (ELISA), for which many diagnostic kits are commercially available.

The ELISA is sensitive and simple to perform, and is now widely used.[120,121] This assay can also be adapted to detect specific IgM antibody[122] and is therefore useful for the diagnosis of acute measles on one serum sample. Measles IgM persists for as long as 1 month after disease onset. Antibody tests that use capillary blood collected on filter paper from finger- or heel-stick specimens has been described and are used by some state health department laboratories.[123]

Prevention

Since the use of live measles vaccine, methods to prevent measles have changed dramatically. Prevention today is ideally carried out long before an anticipated exposure to measles by the administration of live vaccine during the early part of the second year of life. However, there are rare occasions when passive immunization against measles with immune globulin must be used.

Included in the group of persons for whom passive immunization is recommended are those who are at high risk for developing severe or fatal measles, are susceptible, and/or have been exposed to the infection. This includes children with malignant disease, particularly if they are receiving chemotherapy, radiotherapy, or both, and children with significant deficits in cell-mediated immunity, including patients with AIDS. Babies younger than 1 year (including newborns whose mothers have measles) are also at increased risk after an exposure to measles. Because measles has been reported even after vaccination in HIV-infected children, it has been recommended that they also be passively immunized with immunoglobulin after a recognized exposure.[105,106,116,124] To be effective, passive immunization must be given within 6 days after an exposure; administration after 6 days would not be expected to influence the course of the disease.

For a healthy infant younger than 1 year who has been exposed to measles, the modifying dose of immunoglobulin is 0.25 mL/kg IM. An infant passively immunized in this fashion should be given live measles vaccine at the age of 15 months.[116] For immunocompromised exposed children, a larger dose of immunoglobulin is required. These children should be given immunoglobulin, 0.5 mg/kg IM, with a maximum of 15 mL.

Active immunization against measles was developed in the early 1960s. Live and killed measles vaccines were licensed for use in the United States in 1963. Killed vaccine was withdrawn from the market in 1967, after the recognition of atypical measles in recipients of this vaccine. The first marketed live measles vaccine was the Edmonston B strain. This vaccine was associated with a fairly high incidence of moderately severe side reactions such as rash and fever, and it was therefore often administered along with a dose of immunoglobulin. Subsequently, more attenuated vaccines were developed from the Edmonston strain.[125] Because the incidence of vaccine reactions is low with these vaccines, immunoglobulin is no longer given along with measles vaccine.

In 1976, it was recommended that all healthy children be given live measles vaccine at 15 months. At present, it is recommended that children be immunized between the ages of 12 and 15 months (usually given as measles-mumps-rubella [MMR] vaccine or measles-mumps-rubella-varicella [MMRV] vaccine).[116] A second is recommended later in childhood.[102,116] Properly administered measles vaccine has been associated with persistence of immunity to measles for many years.[125-128] In one study, although measles HI antibodies were no longer detectable in some subjects, antibodies were demonstrated by neutralization, and revaccination was associated with a classic booster antibody response.[126] The estimated rate of secondary immune failure was calculated as less than 0.2%. In the general population, 95% of properly immunized children can be expected to respond serologically to measles vaccine. MMRV has been licensed for use in healthy children (not adults) in the United States and in many other countries. After two doses, this vaccine provides an adequate immune response to all four viral antigens with a single injection[129] (see Chapter 320).

Vaccination is not usually recommended for infants younger than 12 months because the induction of immunity may be suppressed by residual transplacentally acquired antibodies. In situations in which the incidence of natural measles before the age of 1 year is high, live measles vaccine may be given at 6 to 9 months of age but should be routinely followed by additional doses. Measles antibody titers are lower in women vaccinated as children than in women who have had natural measles, and the offspring of vaccinated women often lose transplacentally acquired measles antibodies before they are 1 year old.[130,131] Therefore, vaccination can be routinely given as early as 12 months of age, because most women in their childbearing years today were vaccinated as children. For individuals who were passively immunized after an exposure to measles, vaccination should not be performed for 5 months after a dose of 0.25 mL/kg or 6 months after a dose of 0.50 mL/kg.[116] Transient fever and rash develop about 1 week after vaccination in 5% to 15% of children. In a 1986 study of 1162 twins who were given either MMR or placebo, there were side effects (fever, irritability, drowsiness, conjunctivitis) in 0.5% to 4%.[132] Symptoms of CNS dysfunction after measles vaccine are exceedingly rare.[133] Because measles may be severe in adults, immunization of adults who were not vaccinated previously, who have no history of measles, and who were born after 1956 is recommended by the CDC.[102] A 1986 Chicago study of hospital employees, however, indicated that only 1 of 266 (0.03%) was susceptible to measles; about one third were born after 1957.[134]

A number of reasons for apparent primary vaccine failures of measles vaccine have been proposed.[21] These include improper storage of vaccine at temperatures exceeding 4°C, failure to use the proper diluent for the lyophilized vaccine, exposure of the vaccine to light or heat, and vaccination in the presence of low levels of passive antibody. The latter may occur if infants are immunized at 12 months of age or younger, if children are vaccinated 1 or 2 months after receiving an injection of immunoglobulin, if the more attenuated vaccines are given with immunoglobulin, or if live measles vaccine is administered soon after killed measles vaccine. No deleterious effects have been associated with measles revaccination. Although it is probably unusual, sustained transmission of measles has been reported in secondary schools, even when 95% of the students were immune and more than 99% were immunized.[135,136]

Live measles vaccine is contraindicated in persons with deficits in cell-mediated immunity and in pregnant women. Fatal measles in children with AIDS has been reported.[124,137] Although the potential risks of measles vaccine in these children are unknown, they are less than the disease itself. It is currently recommended that children with known asymptomatic HIV infection receive measles vaccine after the age of 12 months.[104,116] The use of measles vaccine should also be considered for children with known HIV infection who manifest symptoms if their CD4 T-cell levels are relatively well preserved, especially if they live in locations where there may be transmission of measles, such as certain inner city areas.[116] One case of fatal measles pneumonia resulting from vaccine virus in an HIV-infected vaccinated young adult has been described after a second dose of vaccine.[105,138] Children who have been treated for malignant disease may be given measles vaccine 3 months after they complete their course of therapy.[116] High-risk children such as those described may be given monovalent measles vaccine or MMR, but they should not be given MMRV vaccine, which contains a significantly higher dose of the varicella component. No safety data for MMRV in high-risk children are available.[139]

Serious hypersensitivity reactions to measles vaccine in persons allergic to egg protein have been reported. Persons with a history of anaphylactic reactions after the ingestion of eggs should be vaccinated only with extreme caution.[140,141]

Susceptible persons who are exposed to measles, with the exception of young infants, pregnant women, and immunocompromised persons, may be given live measles vaccine to prevent disease as an alternative to immunoglobulin. If the vaccine is given shortly after exposure, clinical cases of measles may be prevented because clinical manifestations associated with measles vaccine occur in about 7 days, compared with an incubation period of 10 days for clinical measles.[16]

An experimental measles vaccine, a derivative of the original Edmonston B vaccine strain termed *Edmonston-Zagreb vaccine*, administered at a dose 10 to 100 times higher than usual, proved to be immunogenic in 4- to 6-month-old infants.[142] Despite its short-term safety, however, the rate of mortality from causes other than measles in these vaccinees in Senegal was significantly higher than that in children who received standard vaccine.[143] Therefore, this vaccine is no longer in use.

The possibility that an abnormal immune reaction to vaccine-type measles virus in MMR vaccine might cause autism in young children was raised in 1998 by Wakefield and colleagues.[144] This idea was never accepted by the vast majority of the scientific community, and 10 of the original 13 authors of the paper eventually withdrew their names from the article in retraction of its content, in part because of conflict of interest by Wakefield.[145] After extensive review, numerous national committees, including the Institute of Medicine, concluded that there is no evidence to support this hypothesis.[146-148] A recent case-control study involving three independent laboratories failed to identify an association between autism and measles RNA in the gut or exposure to MMR vaccine.[149] Three other recent scientific studies have failed to identify an association between MMR vaccine and subsequent development of autism.[150-152]

Unfortunately, in the United Kingdom, where there has been extensive adverse publicity about MMR, the incidence of measles has recently increased as a result of suboptimal vaccination rates.[153]

Treatment

Patients with measles should be given supportive therapy such as antipyretics and fluids as indicated. Bacterial superinfection should be promptly treated with appropriate antimicrobials, but prophylactic antibiotics to prevent superinfection are of no known value and are therefore not recommended.

Vitamin A, 200,000 IU administered orally to children for 1 day, has been used successfully to decrease the severity of measles, especially in those with vitamin A deficiency (see Chapter 45).[154-156] (Children, 6 months to 1 year old, should receive 100,000 IU.) Side effects include transient vomiting and headache.[157] This treatment has also been recommended to be considered in the United States for children with measles who are hospitalized and are 6 months to 2 years of age or who are immunodeficient, have malabsorption, or are malnourished.[116] Administration of vitamin A has been reported to reduce seroconversion in vaccinees and should therefore be avoided at or after immunization.[158] The efficacy of ribavirin administered intravenously or by aerosol for treatment of severe measles is unproven.[113,124,159]

REFERENCES

1. Progress in global measles control and mortality reduction, 2000-2006. *MMWR Morb Mortal Wkly Rep.* 2007;56:1237.
2. Imagawa DT. Relationships among measles, canine distemper and rinderpest viruses. *Prog Med Virol.* 1968;10:160.
3. Griffin, DE. Measles Virus. In: Fields BN, ed. *Virology.* 5th ed. New York: Raven Press; 2007:1551-1585.
4. Waterson AP. Measles virus. *Arch Gesamte Virusforsch.* 1965;16:57.
5. Choppin PW, Richardson CD, Merz DC, et al. The functions and inhibition of the membrane glycoproteins of paramyxoviruses and myxoviruses and the role of the measles virus M protein in subacute sclerosing panencephalitis. *J Infect Dis.* 1981;143:352.
6. Naniche D, Varior-Krishnsnan G, Cervoni F, et al. Human membrane cofactor protein (CD46) acts as a cellular receptor for measles virus. *J Virol.* 1993;67:6025.
7. Tatsuo H, Ono N, Tanaka, K, et al. SLAM (CDw150) is a cellular receptor for measles virus. *Nature.* 2000;406:893.
8. Leonard VH, Sinn PL, Hodge G, et al. Measles virus blind to its epithelial cell receptor remains virulent in rhesus monkeys but cannot cross the airway epithelium and is not shed. *J Clin Invest.* 2008;118:2448.
9. Howe C, Schlueberg A. Neuraminidase associated with measles virus. *Biochem Biophys Res Commun.* 1970;40:606.
10. Rota JS, Rota PA, Redd SB, et al. Genetic analysis of measles viruses isolated in the United States, 1995-1996. *J Infect Dis.* 1998;177:204.
11. Rota PA, Liffick SL, Rota JS, et al. Molecular epidemiology of measles virus in the United States, 1997-2001. *Emerg Infect Dis.* 2002;8:902.
12. Bellini WJ, Icenogle J. Measles and rubella virus. In: Murray PR, Baron EJ, Jorgenson JH, et al, eds. *Manual of Clinical Microbiology.* 9th ed. Washington DC: ASM Press; 2007:1378-1391.
13. Hall WW, Choppin PW. Measles-virus proteins in the brain tissue of patients with subacute sclerosing panencephalitis: Absence of the M protein. *N Engl J Med.* 1981;304:1152.
14. Enders JF, Peebles TC. Propagation in tissue cultures of cytopathogenic agents from patients with measles. *Proc Soc Exp Biol Med.* 1954;86:277.
15. Enders JF. Measles virus, historical review, isolation and behavior in various systems. *Am J Dis Child.* 1962;103:282.
16. Kempe CH, Fulginiti VA. The pathogenesis of measles virus infection. *Arch Gesamte Virusforsch.* 1965;16:103.
17. Burnstein T, Frankel JW, Jensen JH. Adaptation of measles virus to suckling hamsters. *Fed Proc.* 1958;17:507.
18. Imagawa DT, Adams JM. Propagation of measles virus in suckling mice. *Proc Soc Exp Biol Med.* 1958;98:567.
19. Panum P. Observations made during the epidemic of measles on the Faroe Islands in the year 1846. *Med Classics.* 1938-1939;3:829.
20. Katz SL, Enders JF, Holloway A. The development and evaluation of an attenuated measles virus vaccine. *Am J Public Health.* 1962;52(Suppl):5.
21. Krugman S. Present status of measles and rubella immunization in the United States: A medical progress report. *J Pediatr.* 1977;90:1.
22. Atkinson WL, Hadler SC, Redd SB, et al. Measles surveillance—United States, 1991. *MMWR Morb Mortal Wkly Rep CDC Surveill Summ.* 1992;41:1.
23. Schlenker TL, Bain C, Baughman AL, et al. Measles herd immunity: Association of attack rates with immunization rates in preschool children. *JAMA.* 1992;267:823.
24. Frank J, Orenstein W, Bart K, et al. Major impediments to measles elimination. *Am J Dis Child.* 1985;139:881.
25. Hutchins S, Markowitz L, Atkinson W, et al. Measles outbreaks in the United States 1987 through 1990. *Pediatr Infect Dis J.* 1996;15:31.
26. Centers for Disease Control (CDC). Public-sector vaccination efforts in response to the resurgence of measles among preschool-aged children–United States, 1989-1991. *MMWR Morb Mortal Wkly Rep.* 1992;41:522.

27. Centers for Disease Control (CDC). Measles vaccination levels among selected groups of preschool-aged children—United States. *MMWR Morb Mortal Wkly Rep*. 1991;40:36.
28. Centers for Disease Control and Prevention. Measles: United States. *MMWR Morb Mortal Wkly Rep*. 1995;45:305.
29. Centers for Disease Control. Measles: United States, 2000. *MMWR Morb Mortal Wkly Rep*. 2002;51:120.
30. World Health Organization. Measles. Available at: http://www.who.int/mediacentre/factsheets/fs286/en/index.html; 2008.
31. Markowitz LE, Preblud SR, Fine PE, et al. Duration of live measles vaccine-induced immunity. *Pediatr Infect Dis J*. 1990;9:101.
32. Krugman S. Further-attenuated measles vaccine: Characteristics and use. *Rev Infect Dis*. 1983;5:477.
33. Mathias RG, Meekison WG, Arcand TA, et al. The role of secondary vaccine failures in measles outbreaks. *Am J Public Health*. 1989;79:475.
34. Gindler JS, Atkinson W, Markowitz LE, et al. Epidemiology of measles in the United States in 1989 and 1990. *Pediatr Infect Dis J*. 1992;841.
35. Anders JF, Jacobson RM, Poland G, et al. Secondary failure rates of measles vaccines: A meta-analysis of published studies. *Pediatr Infect Dis J*. 1996;15:62.
36. Frank JA, Orenstein WA, Bart KJ, et al. Major impediments to measles elimination. *Am J Dis Child*. 1985;39:881.
37. Bennish M, Arnow PM, Beem MO, et al. Epidemic measles in Chicago in 1983: Sustained transmission in the preschool population. *Am J Dis Child*. 1986;140:341.
38. De Jong JG. The survival of measles virus in air, in relation to the epidemiology of measles. *Arch Gesamte Virusforsch*. 1965; 16:97.
39. Ruckle G, Rogers KD. Studies with measles virus: II. Isolation of virus and immunologic studies in persons who have had the natural disease. *J Immunol*. 1957;78:341.
40. Bloch AB, Orenstein W, Ewing WM, et al. Measles outbreak in a pediatric practice: Airborne transmission in an office setting. *Pediatrics*. 1985;75:767.
41. Remington PL, Hall W, Davis IH, et al. Airborne transmission of measles in a physician's office. *JAMA*. 1985;253:1574.
42. Ehresmann KR, Hedberg CW, Grimm MB, et al. An outbreak of measles at an international sporting event with airborne transmission in a domed stadium. *J Infect Dis*. 1995;171: 679.
43. Modlin JF, Jabbour JT, Witte JJ, et al. Epidemiologic studies of measles, measles vaccine, and subacute sclerosing panencephalitis. *Pediatrics*. 1977;59:505.
44. Bitnun A, Shannon P, Durward A, et al. Measles inclusion-body encephalitis caused by the vaccine strain of measles virus. *Clin Infect Dis*. 1999;29:855.
45. Bellini WJ, Rota JS, Lowe LE, et al. Subacute sclerosing panencephalitis: More cases of this fatal disease are prevented by measles immunization than was previously recognized. *J Infect Dis*. 2005;192:1686.
46. Connolly JH, Allen IV, Hurwitz LJ, et al. Measles-virus antibody and antigen in subacute sclerosing panencephalitis. *Lancet*. 1967;1:542.
47. Barbosa LH, Fuccillo DA, Sever JL, et al. Subacute sclerosing panencephalitis: Isolation of measles virus from a brain biopsy. *Nature*. 1969;221:974.
48. Payne FE, Baublis JV, Itabashi HH. Isolation of measles virus from cell cultures of brain from a patient with subacute sclerosing panencephalitis. *N Engl J Med*. 1969;281:585.
49. Cattaneo R, Schmidt A, Billeter MA, et al. Multiple viral mutations rather than host factors cause defective measles virus gene expression in a subacute sclerosing panencephalitis line. *J Virol*. 1988;62:1388.
50. Hall WW, Lamb RA, Choppin PW. Measles and subacute sclerosing panencephalitis virus proteins: Lack of antibodies to the M protein in patients with subacute sclerosing panencephalitis. *Proc Soc Natl Acad Sci U S A*. 1979;76:2047.
51. Aicardi J, Goutieres F, Arsenio-Nunes ML, et al. Acute measles encephalitis in children with immunosuppression. *Pediatrics*. 1977;59:232.
52. Breitfeld V, Hashida Y, Sherman FE, et al. Fatal measles infection in children with leukemia. *Lab Invest*. 1973;28:279.
53. Gerson KL, Haslam HA. Subtle immunologic abnormalities in four boys with subacute sclerosing panencephalitis. *N Engl J Med*. 1971;285:78.
54. Sever JL. Persistent measles infection of the central nervous system: Subacute sclerosing panencephalitis. *Rev Infect Dis*. 1983;4:467.
55. Isaacson SH, Asher DM, Goded MS, et al. Widespread, restricted low-level measles virus infection of brain in a case of subacute sclerosing panencephalitis. *Acta Neuropathol*. 1996;91:135.
56. Adams JM, Imagawa DT. Measles antibodies in multiple sclerosis. *Proc Soc Exp Biol Med*. 1962;111:562.
57. Tannenbaum M, Hsu K, Buda J, et al. Electron microscopic virus-like material in systemic lupus erythematosus: With preliminary immunologic observations on presence of measles antigen. *J Urol*. 1971;105:615.
58. Feeney M, Winwood P, Snook J. A case-control study of measles vaccination and inflammatory bowel disease. *Lancet*. 1997;350: 764.
59. Kress S, Schluederberg AE, Hornick RB, et al. Studies with live attenuated measles-virus vaccine. *Am J Dis Child*. 1961;101:701.
60. Fenner F. The pathogenesis of the acute exanthems. *Lancet*. 1948;2:915.
61. Sergiev PS, Ryazantseva NE, Shroit IG. The dynamics of pathological processes in experimental measles in monkeys. *Acta Virol (Engl)*. 1960;4:265.
62. Siris ES. Seeking the elusive etiology of Paget disease: A progress report. *J Bone Miner Res*. 1996;11:1599.
63. Gresser I, Chany C. Isolation of measles virus from the washed leucocytic fraction of blood. *Proc Soc Exp Biol Med*. 1963;113:695.
64. Joseph BS, Lampert PW, Oldstone MBA. Replication and persistence of measles virus in defined subpopulations of human leukocytes. *J Virol*. 1975;16:1638.
65. Esolen IM, Ward BJ, Moench TR, et al. Infection of monocytes during measles. *J Infect Dis*. 1993;168:47.
66. Suringa DWR, Bank LJ, Ackerman AB. Role of measles virus in skin lesions and Koplik's spots. *N Engl J Med*. 1970;283:1139.
67. Kimura A, Tosaka K, Nakao T. Measles rash: I. Light and electron microscopic study of skin eruptions. *Arch Virol*. 1975;47:295.
68. Kimura A, Tosaka K, Nakao T. An immunofluorescent and electron microscopic study of measles skin eruptions. *Tohoku J Exp Med*. 1975;117:245.
69. Lackmann PJ. Immunopathology of measles. *Proc R Soc Med*. 1974;67:12.
70. Enders JF, McCarthy K, Mitus A, et al. Isolation of measles virus at autopsy in case of giant cell pneumonia without rash. *N Engl J Med*. 1959;261:875.
71. Mitus A, Holloway A, Evans AE, et al. Attenuated measles vaccine in children with acute leukemia. *Am J Dis Child*. 1962;103:413.
72. Krugman S, Giles JP, Friedman H, et al. Studies on immunity to measles. *J Pediatr*. 1965;66:471.
73. Ruckdeschel JC, Graziano KD, Mardiney MR. Additional evidence that the cell-associated immune system is the primary host defense against measles (rubeola). *Cell Immunol*. 1975; 17:11.
74. McFarland HF, Pedone CA, Mingioli ES, et al. The response of human lymphocyte subpopulations to measles, mumps, and vaccinia virus antigens. *J Immunol*. 1980;125:221.
75. Kreth HW, ter Mulen V, Eckert G. Demonstration of HLA restricted killer cells in patients with acute measles. *Med Microbiol Immunol*. 1979;165:203.
76. Lucas CJ, Biddison WE, Nelson ID, et al. Killing of measles virus infected cells by human cytotoxic T cells. *Infect Immunol*. 1982;38:226.
77. Jacobson S, Rose JW, Flerlage ML, et al. Induction of measles virus-specific human cytotoxic T cells by purified measles virus nucleocapsid and hemagglutinin polypeptides. *Viral Immunol*. 1987;1:153.
78. Griffin DE, Ward BJ, Jauregui E, et al. Immune activation in measles. *N Engl J Med*. 1989;320:1667.
79. Smithwick EM, Berkovich S. In vitro suppression of the lymphocyte response to tuberculin by live measles virus. *Proc Soc Exp Biol Med*. 1966;123:276.
80. Hussey GD, Goddard EA, Hughes J, et al. The effect of Edmonston-Zagreb and Schwartz measles vaccines on immune responses in infants. *J Infect Dis*. 1996;173:1320.
81. Koplik H. The diagnosis of the invasion of measles from a study of the exanthemata as it appears on the buccal mucous membranes. *Arch Pediatr*. 1896;13:918.
82. Quiambao BP, Gatchalian SR, Halonen P, et al. Coinfection is common in measles-associated pneumonia. *Pediatr Infect Dis J*. 1998;17:89.
83. Barkin RM. Measles mortality: A retrospective look at the vaccine era. *Am J Epidemiol*. 1975;102:341.
84. Barkin RM. Measles mortality. Analysis of the primary cause of death. *Am J Dis Child*. 1975;129:307.
85. Gibbs FA, Gibbs EL, Carpenter PR, et al. Electroencephalographic changes in "uncomplicated" childhood diseases. *JAMA*. 1959;171:1050.
86. McLean DM, Best JM, Smith PA, et al. Viral infections of Toronto children during 1965: II. Measles encephalitis and other complications. *Can Med Assoc J*. 1966;94:905.
87. Meulen VT, Müller D, Käckell Y, et al. Isolation of infectious measles virus in measles encephalitis. *Lancet*. 1972;2:1172.
88. Scott TF. Postinfectious and vaccinial encephalitis. *Med Clin North Am*. 1967;51:701.
89. Shaffer MF, Rake G, Hodes HL. Isolation of virus from a patient with fatal encephalitis complicating measles. *Am J Dis Child*. 1942;64:815.
90. Drzenick R, Rott R. Host-specific antigens of lipid-containing RNA viruses: Viruses as a carrier of cell-specific antigens. *Int Arch Allergy*. 1969;36(Suppl):146.
91. Johnson RT, Griffin D, Hirsch R, et al. Measles encephalomyelitis: Clinical and immunologic studies. *N Engl J Med*. 1984;310:137-141.
92. McLellan RK, Gleiner JA. Acute hepatitis in an adult with rubeola. *JAMA*. 1982;247:2000.
93. Rauh LW, Schmidt R. Measles immunization with killed virus vaccine. *Am J Dis Child*. 1965;109:232.
94. Fulginiti VA, Eller JJ, Downie AW, et al. Altered reactivity to measles virus. *JAMA*. 1967;202:1075.
95. Frey HM, Krugman S. Atypical measles syndrome: Unusual hepatic, pulmonary, and immunologic aspects. *Am J Med*. 1981;281:55.
96. Lennon RG, Isacson P, Rosales T, et al. Skin tests with measles and poliomyelitis vaccines in recipients of inactivated measles virus vaccine: Delayed dermal hypersensitivity. *JAMA*. 1967;200:275.
97. Bellanti JA, Sanga RL, Klutinis B, et al. Antibody responses in serum and nasal secretions of children immunized with inactivated and attenuated measles-virus vaccines. *N Engl J Med*. 1969;280:628.
98. Norrby E, Ruckle GE, Meulen VT. Differences in the appearance of antibodies to structural components of measles virus after immunization with inactivated and live virus. *J Infect Dis*. 1975;132:262.
99. Annunziato D, Kaplan M, Hall WW, et al. Atypical measles syndrome: Pathologic and serologic features. *Pediatrics*. 1982;70:203.
100. Scott TJ, Bonanno DE. Reactions to live-measles virus vaccine in children previously inoculated with killed-virus vaccine. *N Engl J Med*. 1967;277:248.
101. Stetler HC, Gens RD, Seastrom GR. Severe local reactions to live measles virus vaccine following an immunization program. *Am J Public Health*. 1983;73: 899-900.
102. Centers for Disease Control and Prevention (CDC). General recommendations on immunization: Recommendations of the Immunization Practices Advisory Committee (ACIP). *MMWR Morb Mortal Wkly Rep*. 1994;43(RR-1):1.
103. Mitus A, Enders JF, Craig JM, et al. Persistence of measles virus and depression of antibody formation in patients with giant cell pneumonia after measles. *N Engl J Med*. 1959;261:882.
104. Centers for Disease Control and Prevention (CDC). Recommendations of the Immunization Practices Advisory Committee: Immunization of children infected with human immunodeficiency virus: Supplementary ACIP statement. *MMWR Morb Mortal Wkly Rep*. 1988;37:1813.
105. Centers for Disease Control and Prevention (CDC). Measles pneumonitis following M-M-R vaccination of a patient with HIV infection. *MMWR Morb Mortal Wkly Rep*. 1996; 45:603.
106. Kaplan LJ, Daum RS, Smaron M, et al. Severe measles in immunocompromised patients. *JAMA*. 1992;267:1237.
107. Mustafa MM, Weitman SD, Winick NJ, et al. Subacute measles encephalitis in the young immunocompromised host: Report of two cases diagnosed by polymerase chain reaction and treated with ribavirin and review of the literature. *Clin Infect Dis*. 1993;16:654.
108. Turner A, Jeyaratnam D, Haworth F, et al. Measles-associated encephalopathy in children with renal transplants. *Am J Transplant*. 2006;6:1459.
109. Katz M, Stiehm ER. Host defense in malnutrition. *Pediatrics*. 1977;59:490.
110. Aaby P, Bukh J, Lisse IM, et al. Measles mortality, state of nutrition, and family structure: A community study for Guinea-Bissau. *J Infect Dis*. 1983;147:693.
111. Aaby P, Bukh J, Hoff G, et al. High measles mortality in infancy related to intensity of exposure. *J Pediatr*. 1986;109:40.
112. Gershon A, Young N. Chickenpox, measles, and mumps. In: Remington J, Klein J, eds. *Infectious Diseases of the Fetus and Newborn Infants*. Philadelphia: WB Saunders; 1994: 591-602.
113. Atmar RL, Englund JA, Hammill H. Complications of measles during pregnancy. *Clin Infect Dis*. 1992;14:217-226.
114. Bloch AB, Orenstein WA, Hinman AR. Comment. *J Infect Dis*. 1981;143:753.
115. Gazala E, Karplus M, Liberman JR, et al. The effect of maternal measles on the fetus. *Pediatr Infect Dis J*. 1985;4:203.
116. Committee on Infectious Diseases, American Academy of Pediatrics. *Red Book: 2006 Report of the Committee on Infectious Diseases*. 27th ed. Evanston, Ill: American Academy of Pediatrics; 2006.
117. Gremillion DH, Crawford GE. Measles pneumonia in young adults: An analysis of 106 cases. *Am J Med*. 1981;71:539.
118. Schiff GM. Measles (rubeola). In: Lennette EH, ed. *Laboratory Diagnosis of Viral Infections*. 2nd ed. New York: Marcel Dekker; 1992:535-547.
119. Matsuzono Y, Narita M, Ishiguro N, et al. Detection of measles virus from clinical samples using polymerase chain reaction. *Arch Pediatr Adolesc Med*. 1994;148:289.
120. Rice GPA, Casali P, Oldstone MBA. A new solid-phase enzyme-linked immunosorbent assay for specific antibodies to measles virus. *J Infect Dis*. 1983;147:1055.
121. Weigle K, Murphy D, Brunell P. Enzyme-linked immunosorbent assay for evaluation of immunity to measles virus. *J Clin Microbiol*. 1984;19:376.
122. Mayo DR, Brennan T, Cormier DP, et al. Evaluation of a commercial measles virus immunoglobulin M enzyme immunoassay. *J Clin Microbiol*. 1991;29:2865.
123. Wassilak S, Bernier R, Herrmann K, et al. Measles seroconfirmation using dried capillary blood specimens in filter paper. *Pediatr Infect Dis J*. 1984;3:117.
124. Krasinski K, Borkowsky W. Measles and measles immunity in children infected with human immunodeficiency virus. *JAMA*. 1989;261:2512.
125. Miller C. Live measles vaccine: A 21-year follow-up. *Br Med J*. 1987;295:22.
126. Krugman S. Further-attenuated measles vaccine: Characteristics and use. *Rev Infect Dis*. 1983;5:477.
127. Pederson IR, Mordhorst CH, Ewald T, et al. Long-term antibody response after measles vaccination in an isolated arctic society in Greenland. *Vaccine*. 1986;4:173.
128. Amanna IJ, Carlson NE, Slifka MK. Duration of humoral immunity to common viral and vaccine antigens. *N Engl J Med* 2007;357:1903.

129. Centers for Disease Control and Prevention (CDC). Prevention of varicella: Recommendations of the Advisory Committee on Immunization Practices (ACIP). *MMWR Morb Mortal Wkly Rep.* 2007;56:1.
130. Chui L, Marusyk RG, Pabst HF. Measles virus–specific antibody in infants in a highly vaccinated society. *J Med Virol.* 1991;33:199.
131. Johnson CE, Nalin DR, Chui LW, et al. Measles vaccine immunogenicity in 6- versus 15-month-old infants born to mothers in the measles vaccine era. *Pediatrics.* 1994;93:939.
132. Peltola H, Heinonen O. Frequency of true adverse reactions to measles-mumps-rubella vaccine. *Lancet.* 1986;1:939.
133. Weibel RE, Caserta V, Benor DE, et al. Acute encephalopathy followed by permanent brain injury or death associated with further attenuated measles vaccines: A review of claims submitted to the National Vaccine Injury Compensation Program. *Pediatrics.* 1998;101:383.
134. Chou T, Weil D, Arnow P. Prevalence of measles antibodies in hospital personnel. *Infect Control.* 1986;7:309.
135. Wassilak S, Orenstein W, Strickland P, et al. Continuing measles transmission in students despite a school-based outbreak control program. *Am J Epidemiol.* 1985;122:208.
136. Gustafson T, Lievens A, Brunell P, et al. Measles outbreak in a fully immunized secondary-school population. *N Engl J Med.* 1987;316:771.
137. Centers for Disease Control (CDC). Measles in HIV-infected children, United States. *MMWR Morb Mortal Wkly Rep.* 1988;37:183.
138. Angel JB, Walpita P, Lerch RA, et al. Vaccine-associated measles pneumonitis in an adult with AIDS. *Ann Intern Med.* 1998;129:104.
139. Centers for Disease Control (CDC). Guidelines for prevention and treatment of opportunistic infections among HIV-exposed and HIV-infected children. *MMWR Morb Mortal Wkly Rep.* 2009; available at http://aidsinfo.nih.gov/contentfiles/pediatric_OI.pdf.
140. Herman JJ, Radin R, Schneiderman R. Allergic reactions to measles (rubeola) vaccine in patients hypersensitive to egg protein. *J Pediatr.* 1983;102:196.
141. James JM, Burks AW, Robertson P, et al. Safe administration of the measles vaccine to children allergic to eggs. *N Engl J Med.* 1995;332:1262.
142. Whittle HC, Mann G, Eccles M, et al. Immunisation of 4-6 month old Gambian infants with Edmonston-Zagreb measles vaccine. *Lancet.* 1984;2:834.
143. Garenne M, Leroy O, Beau J-P, et al. Child mortality after high-titre measles vaccines: Prospective study in Senegal. *Lancet.* 1991;338:903.
144. Wakefield AJ, Murch SH, Anthony A, et al. Ileal-lymphoid-nodular hyperplasia, nonspecific colitis, and pervasive developmental disorder in children. *Lancet.* 1998;351:637.
145. Murch SH, Anthony A, Casson DH, et al. Retraction of an interpretation. *Lancet.* 2004;363:750.
146. Fombonne E, Chakrabarti S. No evidence for a new variant of MMR-induced autism. *Pediatrics.* 2001;108:E58.
147. Taylor B, Lingam R, Simmons A, et al. Autism and MMR vaccination in North London: No causal relationship. *Mol Psychiatry.* 2002;7(Suppl 2):S7
148. Taylor B, Miller E, Lingam R, et al. Measles, mumps, and rubella vaccination and bowel problems or developmental regression in children with autism: population study. *BMJ.* 2002; 324:393.
149. Hornig M, Briese T, Buie T, et al. Lack of association between measles virus vaccine and autism with enteropathy: A case-control study. *PLoS ONE.* 2008;3:e3140.
150. D'Souza Y, Fombonne E, Ward BJ. No evidence of persisting measles virus in peripheral blood mononuclear cells from children with autism spectrum disorder. *Pediatrics.* 2006;118:1664.
151. Afzal MA, Ozoemena LC, O'Hare A, et al. Absence of detectable measles virus genome sequence in blood of autistic children who have had their MMR vaccination during the routine childhood immunization schedule of UK. *J Med Virol.* 2006;78:623.
152. Baird G, Pickles A, Simonoff E, et al. Measles vaccination and antibody response in autism spectrum disorders. *Arch Dis Child.* 2008;93:832.
153. Coughlan S, Connell J, Cohen B, et al. Suboptimal measles-mumps-rubella vaccination coverage facilitates an imported measles outbreak in Ireland. *Clin Infect Dis.* 2002;35:84.
154. Arrieta C, Zaleska M, Stutman H, et al. Vitamin A levels in children with measles in Long Beach, California. *J Pediatr.* 1992;121:75.
155. Frieden TR, Sowell AL, Henning K, et al. Vitamin A levels and severity of measles. *Am J Dis Child.* 1992;146:182.
156. Hussey GD, Klein M. A randomized, controlled trial of vitamin A in children with severe measles. *N Engl J Med.* 1990; 323:160.
157. D'Souza RM, D'Souza R. Vitamin A for preventing secondary infections in children with measles: A systematic review. *J Trop Pediatr.* 2002;48:72.
158. Semba RD, Munasir Z, Beeler J, et al. Reduced seroconversion to measles in infants given vitamin A with measles vaccination. *Lancet.* 1995;345:1330.
159. Forni AL, Schluger NW, Roberts RB. Severe measles pneumonitis in adults: Evaluation of clinical characteristics and therapy with intravenous ribavirin. *Clin Infect Dis.* 1994;19:454.

161

Zoonotic Paramyxoviruses: Nipah, Hendra, and Menangle Viruses

ANNA R. THORNER | RAPHAEL DOLIN

Hendra and Nipah viruses are highly pathogenic zoonotic paramyxoviruses that emerged during the 1990s in Australia and Southeast Asia, respectively. In 1994, in Queensland, Australia, Hendra virus caused two outbreaks of fatal illness in horses and their human caretakers.[1,2] Additional outbreaks involving humans occurred in 2004 and 2008.[3,4] Nipah virus was first recognized when it caused an outbreak of severe encephalitis in pig farmers in Malaysia and abattoir workers in Singapore in 1998 and 1999.[5,6] Multiple outbreaks have occurred subsequently in Bangladesh and India.[7-14] In 1997, another zoonotic paramyxovirus, Menangle virus, caused decreased farrowing rates and stillbirths in pigs, as well as an influenza-like illness in two humans who had occupational exposure to infected pigs.[15,16] The *Pteropus* species of fruit bat, also known as the flying fox, was the reservoir of all three viruses.[8,17-19] Because Nipah and Hendra viruses are Biosafety Level 4 agents, research with these pathogens has been difficult to perform.[20,21] However, the development of pseudovirus and reverse genetics techniques has increased opportunities for their investigation.[20-22]

Virology

CLASSIFICATION

Nipah and Hendra viruses are members of the *Henipavirus* genus within the Paramyxovirinae subfamily of the Paramyxoviridae family.[23] In addition to the *Henipavirus* genus, the Paramyxovirinae subfamily also includes the genera *Respirovirus* (human parainfluenza virus types 1 and 3), *Rubulavirus* (mumps, Newcastle disease, human parainfluenza types 2, 4A, and 4B, and Menangle virus), *Morbillivirus* (measles), and *Avulavirus*.[24-26] Nipah and Hendra viruses are most similar to the viruses of the *Respirovirus* and *Morbillivirus* genera, but there is significantly less sequence homology between Nipah or Hendra virus and the members of either of these genera.[24] Nipah and Hendra viruses share a high degree of sequence homology and have similar genomic organization (Fig. 161-1).

STRUCTURE AND MOLECULAR BIOLOGY

Nipah and Hendra Viruses

Nipah and Hendra viruses have a single-stranded, nonsegmented, negative-sense RNA genome that is fully encapsidated by protein.[27] Nipah virus particles range in diameter from 120 to 500 nm,[24] and Hendra virus particles range from 40 to 600 nm.[28] The paramyxovirus envelope contains two transmembrane glycoproteins: an attachment protein or cell receptor-binding glycoprotein (G) and a fusion protein (F).[24] Thin-section electron microscopy (EM) of infected cells reveals filamentous nucleocapsids contained within cytoplasmic inclusions and incorporated into virions budding from the plasma membrane. Hendra virus has a double-fringed appearance caused by projections on the surface of the viral envelope, whereas Nipah virus has only a single layer of surface projections (Fig. 161-2).[24,29]

Henipaviruses cause the formation of syncytia in infected Vero cells.[29] An unusual feature of Nipah virus infection is that nucleocapsid aggregates form at the periphery of infected syncytial cells late in infection. In contrast, Hendra virus nucleocapsid aggregates form

randomly throughout the cytoplasm. Both Nipah and Hendra viruses have herringbone nucleocapsid structures.[24,28] Both viruses, but particularly Nipah virus, cause tubule-like structures to be present in the cytoplasm of infected cells.[29] These structures are unique to Hendra, Nipah, and Sendai viruses, a paramyxovirus that infects animals such as mice. The attachment proteins (G) of Hendra and Nipah viruses lack hemagglutinin and neuraminidase activity, which most other paramyxovirus attachment proteins possess.[27,30,31] The attachment proteins of Nipah and Hendra viruses use ephrin-B2 and -B3 as receptors, which are present in neurons and arterial endothelial cells.[32-35]

The genomes of the Henipaviruses have six transcription units that encode six major structural proteins.[27] The transcription units include the nucleocapsid (N), phosphoprotein (P), matrix protein (M), fusion protein (F), glycoprotein or attachment protein (G), and large protein or RNA polymerase (L). This genome arrangement is most similar to those of the *Respirovirus* and *Morbillivirus* genera. The mRNA of the P genes of Nipah and Hendra viruses are cotranscriptionally edited by the insertion of G residues at editing sites, which leads to the translation of multiple gene products; this is a characteristic shared by other members of the Paramyxovirinae subfamily.[36,37]

Hendra and Nipah viruses share 68% to 92% amino acid homology in the protein-coding regions and 40% to 67% nucleotide identity in the untranslated regions.[37-40] Both viruses are approximately 18.2 kb in length, whereas most of the other members of the Paramyxovirinae subfamily are substantially shorter, ranging from 15.1 to 15.9 kb,[27] with the exception of the recently described Beilong and J viruses.[41,41a] A Nipah virus strain isolated during an outbreak in Bangladesh was six nucleotides shorter than the strain isolated in Malaysia and shared 92% sequence homology with it.[42] The length of the genomes of the Henipaviruses is in multiples of six nucleotides, which is a property shared by the other members of the Paramyxovirinae subfamily and is important for efficient replication.[21,43]

Menangle Virus

Like the other paramyxoviruses, Menangle virus consists of an enveloped, nonsegmented, negative-sense RNA genome that is tightly associated with nucleocapsid proteins.[25] EM reveals that the morphology of Menangle virus is similar to that of other members of the Paramyxoviridae family.[16] The viral particles appear spherical or pleomorphic and range from 30 to 100 nm in diameter. Virus isolated from the lungs, brains, and hearts of affected piglets causes cytopathic effects, including vacuolation and syncytia formation, when grown in baby hamster kidney cells (BHK21). Menangle virus, like Nipah and Hendra viruses, contains herringbone nucleocapsids. It has an envelope with a single fringe of surface projections 17 ± 4 nm in length. Its genome encodes all six of the major structural proteins described previously for Hendra and Nipah viruses. Sequencing of the nucleoprotein (NP), P, M, F, and hemagglutinin-neuraminidase (HN) genes revealed that Menangle virus is a member of the *Rubulavirus* genus.[25] Ultrastructural analysis also supports this classification.[16] Unlike the other rubulaviruses, Menangle virus lacks hemagglutinin and neuraminidase activity.[25] The HN protein shares only 16% to 20% sequence homology with other Rubulavirus HN proteins. Menangle virus also lacks the hexapeptide NRKSCS, which is conserved in the other Rubulavirus

2237

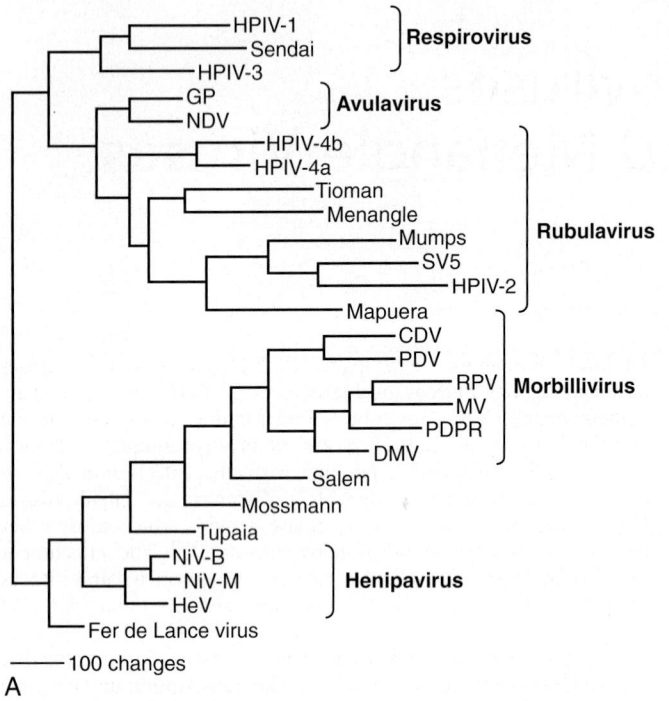

A

—— 100 changes

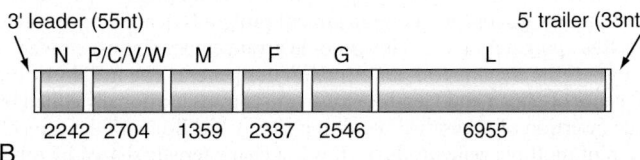

3' leader (55nt)   5' trailer (33nt)

N   P/C/V/W   M   F   G   L

2242   2704   1359   2337   2546   6955

B

Figure 161-1 **Phylogenetic tree of the subfamily Paramyxovirinae based on the nucleocapsid gene sequence (A) and schematic of the Nipah virus genome (B).** HPIV-1, human parainfluenza virus type 1; HPIV-3, human parainfluenza virus type 3; GP, goose paramyxovirus; NDV, Newcastle disease virus; HPIV-4b, human parainfluenza virus type 4b; HPIV-4a, human parainfluenza virus type 4a; SV5, simian virus 5; HPIV-2, human parainfluenza virus type 2; CDV, canine distemper virus; PDV, phocid distemper virus; RPV, rinderpest virus; MV, measles virus; PDPR, peste-des-petits-ruminants virus; DMV, dolphin morbillivirus; NiV-B, Nipah virus, Bangladesh strain; NiV-M, Nipah virus, Malaysia strain; HeV, Hendra virus. In **B**, *shaded sections* indicate viral gene coding regions, whereas the *unshaded sections* indicate noncoding regions of each gene. The numbers below each coding region indicate the nucleotide length of each gene. *(Reprinted from Lo MK, Rota PA. The emergence of Nipah virus, a highly pathogenic paramyxovirus. J Clin Virol. 2008;43:396-400.)*

and the Respirovirus HN proteins and is thought to be necessary for neuraminidase activity; only the last two amino acids in the sequence motif are conserved in the Menangle virus HN protein.

Nipah Virus

EPIDEMIOLOGY

An outbreak of severe encephalitis occurred in pig farmers in the Perak state of Malaysia in September 1998.[5,6,44] By December, the outbreak had spread to pig farmers in the Negeri Sembilan state. In March 1999, 11 abattoir workers in Singapore who came into contact with pigs that were imported from Malaysia developed an encephalitis syndrome with associated pneumonia.[45] The last cases occurred in May 1999 in the Selangor state of Malaysia.[46] There were a total of 276 cases of acute Nipah virus infection, 106 of which were fatal (case-fatality rate, 38%).[24,45,47] Of the cases in Malaysia, 70% occurred in individuals who

worked directly with pigs,[46] and a case-control study showed that exposure to sick pigs was a risk factor for Nipah virus infection.[45] The outbreak ended after more than 1 million pigs were culled.[48]

Nipah virus was isolated from the respiratory secretions and urine of 8 of 20 patients with acute infection in Malaysia.[49] Despite evidence of Nipah virus shedding from infected patients during the outbreaks in Malaysia and Singapore, serologic studies of exposed health care workers did not show evidence of nosocomial transmission.[50,51] However, there was a single case report of a nurse who cared for patients with Nipah virus encephalitis who developed the characteristic lesions of Nipah virus encephalitis on magnetic resonance imaging (MRI) despite having no signs or symptoms of infection.[52]

Subsequent outbreaks of Nipah virus encephalitis have occurred in Bangladesh nearly every year from 2001 to 2008, with the exception of the years 2002 and 2006.[8-14,53] Outbreaks also occurred in regions of India neighboring Bangladesh in 2001 and 2007 (Table 161-1).[7,53] All of the outbreaks occurred between January and May. Several epidemiologic features distinguished the outbreaks in Bangladesh and India from those that occurred in Malaysia and Singapore, including the absence of an intermediate host, evidence of person-to-person spread, and higher case-fatality rates in Bangladesh and India. Some of the outbreaks in Bangladesh and India involved multiple cases of person-to-person transmission and clustering of cases within households.[7,8,13,53-55] During the outbreak in India in 2001, 45 of 60 patients (75%) had a history of exposure to individuals infected with Nipah virus.[7] Many of the affected individuals were health care workers, sug-

TABLE 161-1	Nipah, Hendra, and Menangle Virus Outbreaks				
Year(s) of Outbreak	Country	Cases	Deaths	Case-Fatality Rate (%)	Mode of Acquisition
Nipah Virus					
1998-1999[5]	Malaysia	265	105	40	Exposure to sick pigs
1999[6]	Singapore	11	1	9	Exposure to sick pigs
Total		276	106	38	
2001[7]	India	66	49	74	Person-to-person, nosocomial
2001[8]	Bangladesh	13	9	69	Person-to-person, exposure to sick cow
2003[8,52]	Bangladesh	12	8	67	Person-to-person
2004[9,10,53]	Bangladesh	31	23	74	Climbing trees, person-to-person
2004[11]	Bangladesh	36	27	75	Person-to-person
2004-2005[12]	Bangladesh	12	11	92	Raw date palm sap exposure
2007[13]	Bangladesh	8	5	63	
2007[13]	Bangladesh	7	3	43	
2007[51]	India	30	5	17	Person-to-person
2008[14]	Bangladesh	9	8	89	
Total		224	148	66	
Hendra Virus					
1994[1]	Australia	1	1	100	Exposure to sick horse
1994[2]	Australia	1	1	100	Exposure to sick horse
2004[3]	Australia	1	0	0	Exposure to sick horse
2008[4]	Australia	2	1	50	Exposure to sick horse
Totals		5	3	60	
Menangle Virus					
1997[16]	Australia	2	0	0	Exposure to infected pigs

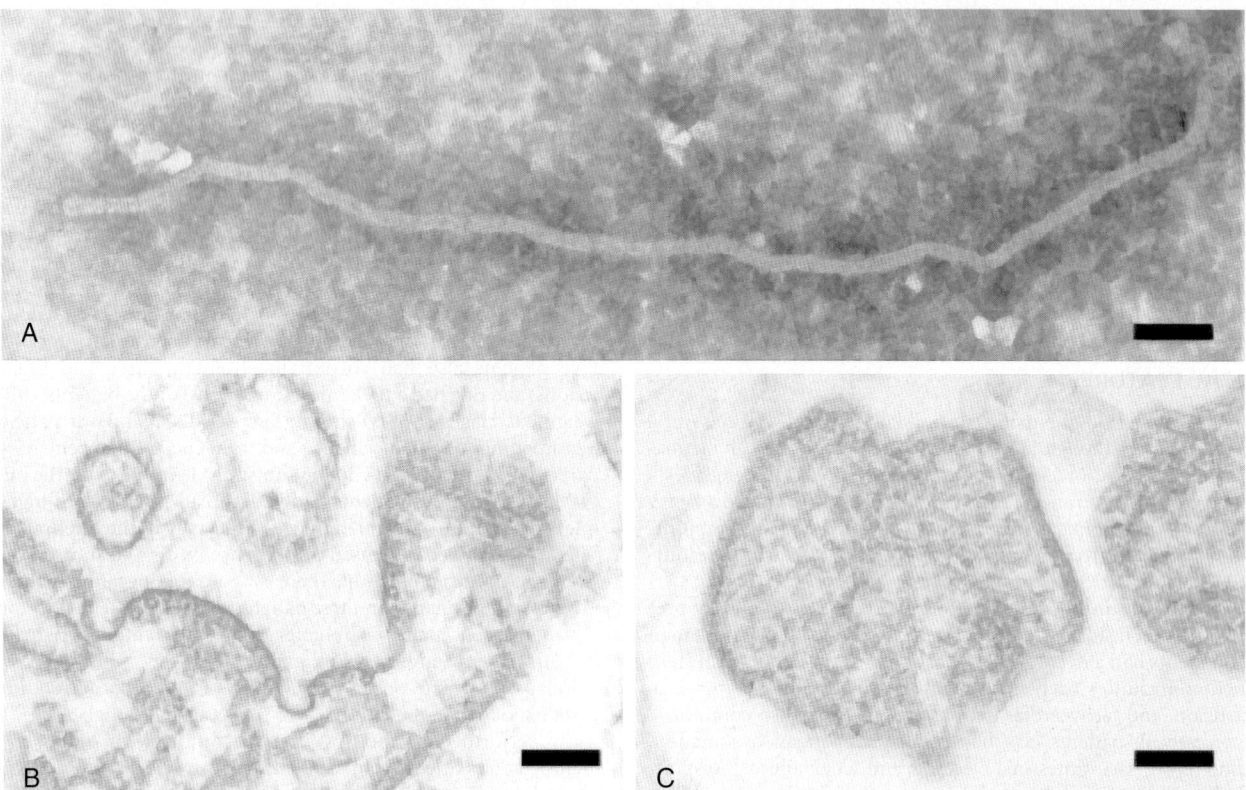

Figure 161-2 **Ultrastructural characteristics of Nipah virus isolate in cell culture as seen by negative stain (A) and thin-section (B and C) electron microscopy. A,** A single nucleocapsid with the typical herringbone appearance characteristic of the family Paramyxoviridae. **B,** Viral nucleocapsids, as seen in cross and longitudinal sections, aligned along the plasma membrane of Nipah virus-infected Vero E6 cells. **C,** Extracellular Nipah virus particle showing a curvilinear tangle of nucleocapsids enclosed within the viral envelope. Scale bars = 100 nm. *(Reprinted from Chua KB, Bellini WJ, Rota PA, et al. Nipah virus: a recently emergent deadly paramyxovirus. Science. 2000;288:1432-1435, with permission. Copyright 2000 American Association for the Advancement of Science. All rights reserved.)*

gesting that nosocomial transmission played an important role in the outbreak. Nipah virus was also identified on environmental surfaces in a hospital during an outbreak.[11] However, two other studies did not demonstrate evidence of nosocomial spread during outbreaks in Bangladesh, although in one of them, individuals who lived with or cared for patients with Nipah virus were more likely to acquire Nipah virus infection.[8,56] The increased incidence of person-to-person spread in Bangladesh and India compared with Malaysia and Singapore may have been due to the higher rates of respiratory involvement in patients in Bangladesh and India, which could have facilitated transmission.[10]

Other risk factors associated with the outbreaks in Bangladesh or India, or both, included exposure to sick cows,[8] consumption of contaminated raw date palm sap,[12] and climbing trees.[9] Fruit bats are known to feed from the pots that are used to collect date palm sap, which probably led to contamination of the sap that was later consumed by people.[12] Although most patients affected by Nipah virus were adults, in two outbreaks in Bangladesh, the median age of affected individuals was 12 years.[9,10] The lower median age and male predominance in one of these outbreaks were probably due to a behavior that increased the risk of infection, such as climbing trees.[9]

The case-fatality rate was substantially higher in the outbreaks in Bangladesh than in Malaysia and Singapore. In the largest published series, which included 92 patients from four of the outbreaks in Bangladesh, the case-fatality rate was 74% compared with 38% in the outbreak in Malaysia and Singapore.[10,24,45,47] The highest case-fatality rate that has been observed was 92% during an outbreak in Bangladesh in 2005 that involved 12 individuals.[12] The increased mortality observed in the outbreaks in Bangladesh and India may have been due to increased virulence of the Nipah virus strains involved, although other

factors, such as inadequate facilities for the care of critically ill patients and malnutrition, could have played a role.[10]

Although it was initially thought that Japanese encephalitis had caused the outbreak in Malaysia, researchers cultured a paramyxovirus from the cerebrospinal fluid (CSF) that caused syncytia formation in Vero cells from two of the first three patients who died from Nipah virus.[44] The virus stained with anti-Hendra virus antibodies by indirect immunofluorescence and an enzyme-linked immunosorbent assay (ELISA) for anti-Hendra immunoglobulin M (IgM) antibodies was positive in the CSF of all three patients. Given the epidemiologic and clinical differences between Hendra virus and the outbreak of encephalitis in Malaysia, it was proposed that a paramyxovirus that was related but distinct from Hendra virus had caused the outbreak.[44] It was named Nipah virus after the village in which the first patient from whom the virus was isolated resided.[44,46]

RESERVOIRS AND INTERMEDIATE HOSTS

Following the initial outbreak of Nipah virus in Malaysia, bats were screened for the presence of anti-Nipah antibodies because they were already known to be the reservoir of Hendra virus. Island flying foxes (*Pteropus hypomelanus*) and Malayan flying foxes (*Pteropus vampyrus*) were found to have neutralizing antibodies to Nipah virus.[19] Subsequently, viruses that caused Hendra virus-like cytopathic effect in Vero cells and stained strongly for Nipah and Hendra virus antibodies were identified from two urine samples from *P. hypomelanus* and from fruit that had been partially eaten by a fruit bat.[57] *Pteropus giganteus* is the reservoir of Nipah virus in Bangladesh[8] and is probably also the reservoir in India given that its natural habitat includes this region, although this has not been proven by serologic studies.[7] Anti-Nipah virus antibodies have been detected in *Pteropus* species of bats in other countries, such as Cambodia, Thailand, and Indonesia.[58-60] In addition, anti-Nipah virus antibodies or Nipah virus RNA, or both, have been found rarely in non-*Pteropus* species of bats in Malaysia and Thailand.[19,59]

The only animals that are known to have served as intermediate hosts of Nipah virus were pigs during the initial outbreak in Malaysia and Singapore.[5,6] Nipah virus infection has also been demonstrated serologically in cats, dogs, horses, and goats.[46,48] Of these less commonly infected species, only dogs have been shown to have clinical disease.[6]

CLINICAL FEATURES

The incubation period of Nipah virus in Malaysia ranged from several days to 2 months, although more than 90% of patients had an incubation period of 2 weeks or less.[61] In four of the outbreaks in Bangladesh, the incubation period ranged from 6 to 11 days, with a median of 9 days.[10] Although subclinical infection can occur, the ratio of symptomatic to subclinical infection was approximately 3:1 during the outbreak in Malaysia.[62]

In the outbreaks in Malaysia and Singapore, patients typically presented with fever, headache, dizziness, and vomiting.[46,61,63,64] More than 50% of patients had a decreased level of consciousness and brain stem dysfunction, including such signs as myoclonus, areflexia, hypotonia, hypertension, and tachycardia. Cerebellar signs were also common.[64] Some severely ill patients also had multisystem organ dysfunction, including sepsis, gastrointestinal bleeding, and renal failure.[61] Respiratory findings were uncommon in the outbreaks in Malaysia and Singapore, with only 14% of patients in Malaysia having a nonproductive cough[61] and 3 of 11 patients in Singapore having evidence of pneumonia.[45] In contrast, in a study of four of the outbreaks in Bangladesh, 62

of 92 patients (69%) had respiratory difficulty, and at least five patients had acute respiratory distress syndrome.[10]

In the most severely affected patients in the outbreak in Malaysia, electroencephalogram (EEG) revealed bilateral temporal periodic complexes of sharp and slow waves occurring every 1 or 2 seconds.[46] The typical MRI findings were multiple 2- to 7-mm lesions best visualized in the T_2-weighted images, without associated cerebral edema or mass effect; they were disseminated throughout the brain but were most commonly present in the subcortical and deep white matter of the cerebral hemispheres (Fig. 161-3A).[61,65] In a study of eight patients with Nipah virus encephalitis in Malaysia, all patients had multiple small bilateral foci of T_2 prolongation in the subcortical and deep white matter as well as in the periventricular areas and the corpus callosum.[66] Five patients also had cortical involvement, three had brain stem lesions, and one had a thalamic lesion. In five of the patients, diffusion-weighted images (DWIs) showed increased signal. Four patients had leptomeningeal enhancement, and four had enhancement of the parenchymal lesions. In a follow-up study 1 month after the outbreak in Malaysia, 5 of 12 patients had widespread small foci of high signal intensity on the T_1-weighted images, especially in the cerebral cortex.[67] The DWIs showed decreased prominence or disappearance over time. At the 6-month follow-up, there was no radiographic evidence of progression or relapse. In three patients who underwent MRI for acute Nipah virus encepahalitis in Bangladesh, confluent high-signal lesions in both the gray and the white matter were seen.[68]

Relapsed or late-onset encephalitis, or both, occurred in some patients following the outbreaks in Malaysia and Bangladesh.[61,65,69,70] A study performed 24 months after the outbreak in Malaysia, which included 160 patients who survived Nipah virus infection, found that 12 patients (7.5%) had developed a relapse of encephalitis.[69] Of 89 patients who initially had nonencephalitic disease or asymptomatic infection, 10 patients (11%) had late-onset encephalitis, with a mean time to neurologic findings of 8.4 months. Four of the 22 patients

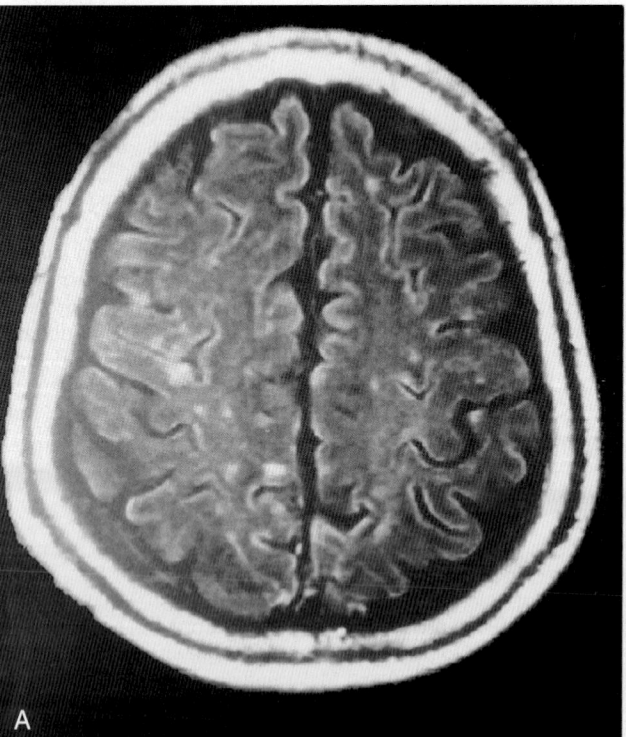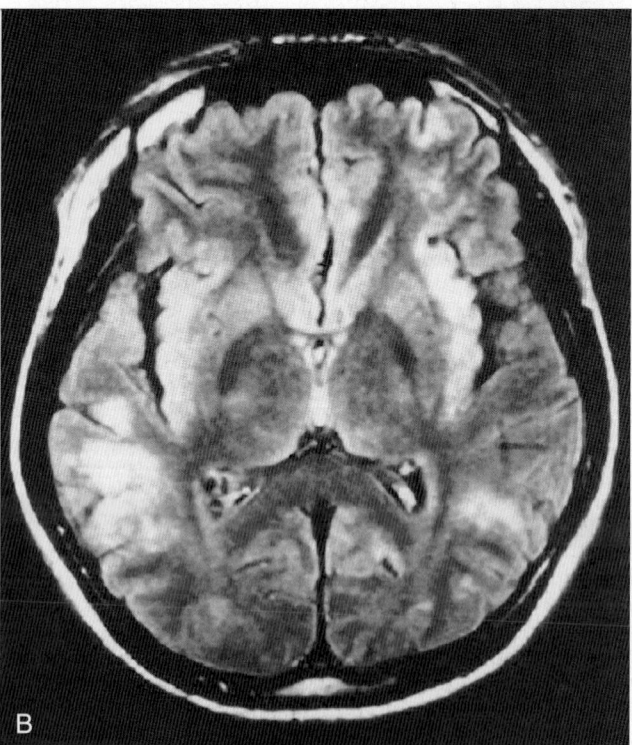

Figure 161-3 **Axial magnetic resonance imaging findings in patients with acute (A) and relapsed (B) Nipah virus encephalitis with use of fluid-attenuated inversion recovery. A,** Multiple discrete hyperintense lesions in the white and gray matter of a patient with acute Nipah virus encephalitis. **B,** Confluent lesions primarily involving the cortical gray matter in a patient with relapsed Nipah virus encephalitis. *(Reprinted from Goh KJ, Tan CT, Chew NK, et al. Clinical features of Nipah virus encephalitis among pig farmers in Malaysia. N Engl J Med. 2000;342:1229-1235, with permission. Copyright 2000, Massachusetts Medical Society. All rights reserved.)*

(18%) with relapsed or late-onset encephalitis died. Brain MRI in patients with relapsed disease usually showed patchy confluent cortical gray matter lesions (see Fig. 161-3B).[61,65,69]

In a study of long-term neurologic and functional outcomes that included 22 patients from Bangladesh who survived Nipah virus illness, 17 of whom had encephalitis and five of whom had febrile illness, all but one patient had disabling fatigue that lasted for a median of 5 months (range, 8 days to 8 months).[70] Seven of 17 patients (41%) with encephalitis, but none with febrile illness, had persistent neurologic deficits, including encephalopathy, ocular motor palsies, cervical dystonia, focal weakness, and facial paralysis. Four patients had late-onset neurologic abnormalities months following the acute illness.

LABORATORY ABNORMALITIES AND DIAGNOSTIC TESTS

Leukopenia (11%), thrombocytopenia (30%), and elevated levels of alanine aminotransferase (33%) and aspartate aminotransferase (42%) were the most common laboratory abnormalities in the outbreak in Malaysia.[61] The CSF was abnormal (elevated white blood cell [WBC] count or protein level, or both) in 75% of 92 patients evaluated; the mean CSF WBC count was 41 cells/µL (range, 0 to 842 cells/µL), and the mean protein level was 0.69 g/L (range, 0.12 to 2.15 g/L).[61] CSF glucose was normal in all patients. Unlike the outbreak in Malaysia, all 18 patients evaluated during an outbreak in India and 4 of 6 patients evaluated during outbreaks in Bangladesh had a normal CSF WBC count (≤5 cells/µL).[7,10] Among patients with acute Nipah virus infection in Malaysia, virus-specific antibodies were present in the serum in greater than 70% of samples but in less than one third of CSF samples.[46] Isolation of Nipah virus from the CSF was strongly associated with mortality.[71] Stored CSF samples from 84 patients with Nipah virus encephalitis (27 fatal and 57 nonfatal) were cultured for Nipah virus. The virus could be cultured from the CSF of 17 fatal cases and 1 nonfatal case.[71] Transmission EM of negative-stained CSF specimens can also be used to detect Nipah virus.[72] Other methods that have been developed for the detection of Nipah virus include polymerase chain reaction (PCR), serum neutralization tests, and monoclonal antibodies.[73-75]

PATHOLOGY

Nipah virus causes a multiorgan vasculitis with a predilection for the central nervous system.[76,77] On autopsy, patients with Nipah virus infection from the outbreak in Malaysia exhibited widespread endothelial involvement, characterized by vasculitis, thrombosis, ischemia, and parenchymal necrosis. This was most marked in the central nervous system, although the lungs, heart, and kidneys were also involved. Syncytial giant cell formation was present in affected vessels. Viral inclusions were detectable both by light microscopy and by EM. Immunohistochemistry revealed the presence of Nipah virus antigens in the endothelial and smooth muscle cells of blood vessels, as well as in neurons and other affected cells.

TREATMENT

The mainstay of therapy for Nipah virus infection is supportive care, including monitoring in the intensive care unit for patients with severe illness. In an open-label trial of oral or intravenous ribavirin in patients with Nipah virus encephalitis in Malaysia, 45 of 140 patients (32%) in the ribavirin group died, compared with 29 of 54 (54%) in the control group.[78] Although these observational data suggest that ribavirin is beneficial, it is not possible to draw conclusions about efficacy.

PREVENTION

No vaccine is available for the prevention of Nipah virus, although several have been studied in animal models, including vaccinia virus-expressed recombinant Nipah virus F and G proteins, recombinant

soluble Nipah and Hendra virus attachment proteins, and canarypox virus-based vaccine vectors carrying genes of Nipah virus F or G proteins.[21,79,80] Monoclonal antibodies have also been shown to neutralize Nipah and Hendra viruses in vitro.[81]

Hendra Virus

EPIDEMIOLOGY

In September 1994, an outbreak of an acute respiratory illness occurred in thoroughbred horses in Queensland, Australia.[1,82] Affected horses had fever, facial swelling, severe respiratory distress, ataxia, and copious frothy nasal discharge, which was sometimes blood-tinged. The index case was a pregnant mare at pasture, who died after a 2-day illness. During the next 2 weeks, 13 more horses at the same stable died or were euthanized. There were four nonfatal cases, two of which had mild neurologic sequelae. Three more horses were found to have seroconverted without having had signs of clinical illness. Within 1 week of the death of the equine index case, a horse trainer and a stablehand became ill with a severe influenza-like illness. The trainer died after developing respiratory and renal failure, whereas the stablehand recovered. Infection with Hendra virus was demonstrated in both human cases by viral culture, immunoelectron microscopy, serology, and PCR using primers derived from other paramyxoviruses.[1,28,82]

In October 1995, a second outbreak of Hendra virus was retrospectively discovered after the death of a thoroughbred stud owner who had developed a relapse of encephalitis 13 months following a mild and self-limited episode of meningitis.[2] It was subsequently determined that two horses had died in August 1994 on his farm in Mackay, in central Queensland, Australia, approximately 1000 km from the original outbreak. The first horse was a pregnant thoroughbred that had developed severe respiratory distress, ataxia, and swelling of the cheeks and supraorbital fossa during a 24-hour period. The second horse had licked the face of the dead mare through a fence. The second horse, a 2-year-old colt, died 11 days later, after a 24-hour clinical course of aimless pacing, muscle trembling, and hemorrhagic nasal discharge. The etiologic agent was originally called equine Morbillivirus, but the name was later changed to Hendra virus, after the suburb where the first outbreak was identified.[83]

In 2004, a veterinarian in Cairns, Queensland, developed a fever, dry cough, sore throat, cervical lymphadenopathy, myalgias, and malaise 1 week after performing an autopsy on a horse that was later found to have Hendra virus.[3] She was diagnosed with Hendra virus by convalescent serologies but recovered fully. An outbreak in five horses in Brisbane, Queensland, in July 2008 resulted in Hendra virus infection in two veterinary workers, one of whom died.[4]

A serologic survey of wildlife species that were present at the site of the outbreaks was performed.[17] A total of 168 animals from more than 16 species were tested, including rodents, marsupials, birds, amphibians, and insects, yet none were seropositive for Hendra virus. Nomadic birds and flying foxes (bats of the *Pteropus* genus) were then targeted as likely reservoirs, given their presence in the regions of both outbreaks and their ability to travel long distances. Anti-Hendra virus antibodies were found in several types of flying fox throughout Queensland. Hendra virus was subsequently isolated from the reproductive tract of a pregnant gray-headed flying fox that had become entangled on a wire fence and from tissue from aborted flying fox fetuses.[18] The bat isolates were identical to the isolate that infected the horses that died. Flying foxes are thought to have subclinical infection.[83-85]

CLINICAL FEATURES

Clinical features of Hendra virus infection range from a self-limited influenza-like syndrome to a fatal respiratory illness. The incubation period is approximately 5 to 8 days.[1,3,31,82] One patient had an influenza-like illness, characterized by fever, myalgias, headache, lethargy, and vertigo.[1] He was unwell for 6 weeks but then recovered. Another individual had a dry cough, sore throat, cervical lymphadenopathy, myalgias, fatigue, and fever that lasted for 4 days.[3] The illness lasted for a total of 8 days. Another patient presented with a similar syndrome but rapidly developed respiratory distress requiring mechanical ventilation.[1,28] He also had acidosis, dehydration, an arterial thrombosis in his right lower extremity, and cardiac irritability. He died 6 days after the onset of illness from asystolic cardiac arrest.

A relapse of encephalitis occurred in one patient 14 months after a horse that he had cared for died from Hendra virus.[2] He was a 35-year-old man who had aseptic meningitis in August 1994, after caring for two sick horses and assisting with their autopsies. He initially developed a sore throat, headache, drowsiness, vomiting, and neck stiffness, and he was found to have 560 WBC/μL in his CSF, with a polymorphonuclear predominance, and negative bacterial and viral cultures. He recovered fully, but 13 months later he developed irritability, low back pain, and a seizure. During the following week, he had a low-grade fever and recurrent seizures. By day 7 of hospitalization, he had a right hemiplegia, brain stem signs, and a decreased level of consciousness requiring intubation. He remained febrile and unconscious and was found by EEG to be having seizure activity despite control of clinically apparent seizures. He died 25 days after admission.

LABORATORY ABNORMALITIES AND DIAGNOSTIC TESTS

One of the patients who died from Hendra virus infection had thrombocytopenia and elevated levels of creatine kinase, lactate dehydrogenase, aspartate aminotransferase, alanine aminotransferase, and glutamyltransferase.[28] He also had signs of dehydration and acidosis. In contrast, a patient who survived had no laboratory abnormalities.[31]

Hendra virus forms syncytia when grown in Vero cells.[29] This cytopathic effect and the typical EM findings of the herringbone nucleocapsid and the double-fringed appearance of the surface projections of the viral envelope aid in its identification.[28,29] Other methods of detection include enzyme-linked immunosorbent assay (ELISA) for IgM and IgG in the serum or CSF and also a serum neutralization assay.[86]

PATHOLOGY

The autopsy of the horse trainer who died of acute Hendra virus infection revealed interstitial pneumonia characterized by lung congestion, edema, and hemorrhage.[28,82] Histologic examination revealed focal necrotizing alveolitis with giant cells, syncytia formation, and viral inclusions. He also had mild chronic myocarditis and regions of inflammation with necrosis in the kidney, as well as a pulmonary embolism.[82] Kidney tissue inoculated in cell culture caused syncytia formation, whereas lung, liver, and spleen tissue did not.[28,82]

The autopsy of the patient who died from relapsed encephalitis revealed a leptomeningitis with a cellular infiltrate that contained lymphocytes and plasma cells.[2] There were discrete foci of necrosis in the neocortex, basal ganglia, brain stem, and cerebellum, with sparing of the subcortical white matter. Rare multinucleated endothelial cells were detected in the brain, liver, spleen, and lungs. Immunohistochemistry of brain tissue was positive for Hendra virus. Electron microscopy revealed aggregates of nucleocapsids in cell remnants. Hendra virus could not be cultured from the brain.

TREATMENT

Because no specific antiviral therapies have been evaluated for the treatment of Hendra virus infection, treatment involves only supportive care, such as intravenous hydration and mechanical ventilation, when indicated. In vitro data indicate that ribavirin has activity against Hendra virus.[78] It penetrates the blood-brain barrier and reaches a mean CSF-to-plasma ratio of 0.7.[87]

Emergence of Henipaviruses

Phylogenetic analyses show that Nipah and Hendra viruses are old viruses,[28,88] which suggests that their recent emergence was due to ecologic factors rather than virus mutations.[83] Ecologic change that drew flying foxes closer to horses, pigs, and humans was probably the largest contributor to the emergence of Hendra and Nipah viruses. Deforestation has caused flying foxes to move into suburban and urban areas to use the trees in these regions for roosting. In fact, the pig farm that was the site of the large outbreak of Nipah virus infection in Malaysia is also an orchard, which meant that flying foxes were in close proximity to the pigs. The close quarters and transport of pigs throughout Malaysia and Singapore resulted in further spread of disease.

Menangle Virus

EPIDEMIOLOGY

From April to September 1997, the farrowing rate at a commercial piggery in New South Wales, Australia, decreased from 82% to 60%.[16] The number of live piglets declined, and the rate of mummified and stillborn piglets increased. Occasional abortions also occurred. The stillborn piglets had abnormalities that included severe degeneration of the brain and spinal cord, arthrogryposis, brachygnathia, and, rarely, fibrinous body cavity effusions and pulmonary hypoplasia. Of pigs at the affected piggery, 96% had neutralizing antibodies against the virus, whereas serum and plasma samples collected from pigs at the piggery prior to May 1997 were negative.[16,89]

A large colony of fruit bats was found to roost within 200 m of the affected piggery from October to April.[16] Given the proximity of the fruit bats to the piggery and the previous Hendra virus outbreak, fruit bats were immediate targets of the investigation. Forty-two (34%) of 125 serum samples from fruit bats in New South Wales and Queensland, Australia, were positive for neutralizing antibodies against Menangle virus. Antibodies were found in several species of fruit bat.[90] Other species in the area, including rodents, birds, cattle, sheep, cats, and a dog, were all seronegative.[16]

A total of 251 humans who had had potential exposures to infected pigs were tested serologically.[16] Only two of these individuals were found to have neutralizing antibodies, one of whom worked at the affected piggery and one of whom worked at a piggery that had received a shipment of pigs from the affected piggery. Both of these individuals had an influenza-like illness during the weeks after exposure to likely infectious material. They were also tested for a broad range of viruses, bacteria, and parasites that could have caused this illness, but none of the results suggested an alternative diagnosis.[15]

PATHOGENESIS

Respiratory spread has been proposed as the likely mode of transmission among pigs, but it is less clear how the virus spreads from pigs to humans.[15] Both of the humans who were infected had exposure to body fluids of infected pigs. The first individual helped to birth pigs, and he reported that splashes of amniotic fluid and blood often occurred. He also reported having frequent minor wounds of his hands and forearms. The second patient performed autopsies on pigs without wearing gloves or protective eye wear. Little is known about the pathogenesis and pathology of Menangle virus, but it is likely to have features in common with Hendra and Nipah viruses, its ability to leap from fruit bats to pigs to humans, and the phylogenetic relationship between Menangle virus and the Henipaviruses.

CLINICAL FEATURES AND DIAGNOSTIC TESTS

The first individual with Menangle virus reported that in early June 1997 he had the sudden onset of malaise and chills, followed by severe headache and myalgias.[15] He remained in bed for 10 days. Four days into the illness, he developed a spotty erythematous rash. His physician noted that in addition to the rash, he also had abdominal tenderness and lymphadenopathy. He returned to work after 2 weeks but continued to have fatigue. He lost 10 kg during the illness. An evaluation 2 months after the illness revealed mild right lower abdominal tenderness and an enlarged spleen on ultrasound. The liver was at the upper limit of normal. Urinalysis, complete blood count (CBC), blood chemistries, erythrocyte sedimentation rate (ESR), and C-reactive protein (CRP) were all normal.

The second patient also became ill in early June 1997 with fever, chills, rigors, sweats, malaise, back pain, severe frontal headache, and photophobia.[15] The headache lasted for 4 or 5 days. On the fourth day of illness, he noticed a spotty erythematous truncal rash, which lasted for 7 days. His acute illness lasted for approximately 10 days, during which time he lost 3 kg. Two months after the illness, he underwent a clinical evaluation. Urinalysis, CBC, ESR, and CRP were normal. Blood chemistries were normal, except for mildly elevated hepatic enzymes. However, he was found to have antibodies against hepatitis C, which could have explained these findings. Abdominal ultrasound revealed mild hepatomegaly and a spleen size at the upper limit of normal. Both patients had antibodies against Menangle virus, with titers of 1:128 and 1:512, respectively.

REFERENCES

1. Murray K, Rogers R, Selvey L, et al. A novel morbillivirus pneumonia of horses and its transmission to humans. *Emerg Infect Dis.* 1995;1:31-33.
2. O'Sullivan JD, Allworth AM, Paterson DL, et al. Fatal encephalitis due to novel paramyxovirus transmitted from horses. *Lancet.* 1997;349:93-95.
3. Hanna JN, McBride WJ, Brookes DL, et al. Hendra virus infection in a veterinarian. *Med J Aust.* 2006;185:562-564.
4. ProMED-mail. Hendra virus, human, equine—Australia (Queensland). ProMED mail. August 21, 2008;20080821.2606.
5. Outbreak of Hendra-like virus—Malaysia and Singapore, 1998-1999. *MMWR Morb Mortal Wkly Rep.* 1999;48:265-269.
6. Update: outbreak of Nipah virus—Malaysia and Singapore, 1999. *MMWR Morb Mortal Wkly Rep.* 1999;48:335-337.
7. Chadha MS, Comer JA, Lowe L, et al. Nipah virus-associated encephalitis outbreak, Siliguri, India. *Emerg Infect Dis.* 2006;12:235-240.
8. Hsu VP, Hossain MJ, Parashar UD, et al. Nipah virus encephalitis reemergence, Bangladesh. *Emerg Infect Dis.* 2004;10:2082-2087.
9. Montgomery JM, Hossain MJ, Carroll GD, et al. Risk factors for Nipah virus encephalitis in Bangladesh. *Emerg Infect Dis.* 2008;14:1526-1532.
10. Hossain MJ, Gurley ES, Montgomery JM, et al. Clinical presentation of Nipah virus infection in Bangladesh. *Clin Infect Dis.* 2008;46:977-984.
11. Gurley ES, Montgomery JM, Hossain MJ, et al. Person-to-person transmission of Nipah virus in a Bangladeshi community. *Emerg Infect Dis.* 2007;13:1031-1037.
12. Luby SP, Rahman M, Hossain MJ, et al. Foodborne transmission of Nipah virus, Bangladesh. *Emerg Infect Dis.* 2006;12:1888-1894.
13. ICDDR, B. Person-to-person transmission of Nipah infection in Bangladesh, 2007. *Health Sci Bull.* 2007;5:2-6.
14. ICDDR, B. Outbreaks of Nipah virus in Rajbari and Manikgonj, February 2008. *Health Sci Bull.* 2008;6:12-13.
15. Chant K, Chan R, Smith M, et al. Probable human infection with a newly described virus in the family Paramyxoviridae. The NSW Expert Group. *Emerg Infect Dis.* 1998;4:273-275.
16. Philbey AW, Kirkland PD, Ross AD, et al. An apparently new virus (family Paramyxoviridae) infectious for pigs, humans, and fruit bats. *Emerg Infect Dis.* 1998;4:269-271.
17. Young PL, Halpin K, Selleck PW, et al. Serologic evidence for the presence in *Pteropus* bats of a paramyxovirus related to equine morbillivirus. *Emerg Infect Dis.* 1996;2:239-240.
18. Halpin K, Young PL, Field HE, et al. Isolation of Hendra virus from pteropid bats: a natural reservoir of Hendra virus. *J Gen Virol.* 2000;81:1927-1932.
19. Yob JM, Field H, Rashdi AM, et al. Nipah virus infection in bats (order Chiroptera) in peninsular Malaysia. *Emerg Infect Dis.* 2001;7:439-441.
20. Eaton BT, Broder CC, Middleton D, et al. Hendra and Nipah viruses: different and dangerous. *Nat Rev Microbiol.* 2006; 4:23-35.
21. Halpin K, Mungall BA. Recent progress in henipavirus research. *Comp Immunol Microbiol Infect Dis.* 2007;30:287-307.
22. Yoneda M, Guillaume V, Ikeda F, et al. Establishment of a Nipah virus rescue system. *Proc Natl Acad Sci U S A.* 2006;103:16508-16513.
23. Mayo MA. A summary of taxonomic changes recently approved by ICTV. *Arch Virol.* 2002;147:1655-1663.
24. Chua KB, Bellini WJ, Rota PA, et al. Nipah virus: a recently emergent deadly paramyxovirus. *Science.* 2000;288:1432-1435.
25. Bowden TR, Westenberg M, Wang LF, et al. Molecular characterization of Menangle virus, a novel paramyxovirus which infects pigs, fruit bats, and humans. *Virology.* 2001;283:358-373.
26. Bowden TR, Boyle DB. Completion of the full-length genome sequence of Menangle virus: characterisation of the polymerase gene and genomic 5' trailer region. *Arch Virol.* 2005;150:2125-2137.
27. Wang L, Harcourt BH, Yu M, et al. Molecular biology of Hendra and Nipah viruses. *Microbes Infect.* 2001;3:279-287.
28. Murray K, Selleck P, Hooper P, et al. A morbillivirus that caused fatal disease in horses and humans. *Science.* 1995;268:94-97.
29. Hyatt AD, Zaki SR, Goldsmith CS, et al. Ultrastructure of Hendra virus and Nipah virus within cultured cells and host animals. *Microbes Infect.* 2001;3:297-306.
30. Yu M, Hansson E, Langedijk JP, et al. The attachment protein of Hendra virus has high structural similarity but limited primary sequence homology compared with viruses in the genus Paramyxovirus. *Virology.* 1998;251:227-233.
31. Rota PA, Ksiazek TG, Berlini WJ. Zoonotic paramyxoviruses. In: Richman DD, Whitley RJ, Hayden FG, eds. *Clinical Virology.* Washington, DC: American Society for Microbiology Press; 2009:889-903.
32. Bonaparte MI, Dimitrov AS, Bossart KN, et al. Ephrin-B2 ligand is a functional receptor for Hendra virus and Nipah virus. *Proc Natl Acad Sci U S A.* 2005;102:10652-10657.
33. Negrete OA, Levroney EL, Aguilar HC, et al. EphrinB2 is the entry receptor for Nipah virus, an emergent deadly paramyxovirus. *Nature.* 2005;436:401-405.
34. Negrete OA, Wolf MC, Aguilar HC, et al. Two key residues in ephrinB3 are critical for its use as an alternative receptor for Nipah virus. *PLoS Pathog.* 2006;2:e7.
35. Bowden TA, Aricescu AR, Gilbert RJ, et al. Structural basis of Nipah and Hendra virus attachment to their cell-surface receptor ephrin-B2. *Nat Struct Mol Biol.* 2008;15:567-572.
36. Lo MK, Rota PA. The emergence of Nipah virus, a highly pathogenic paramyxovirus. *J Clin Virol.* 2008;43:396-400.
37. Harcourt BH, Tamin A, Ksiazek TG, et al. Molecular characterization of Nipah virus, a newly emergent paramyxovirus. *Virology.* 2000;271:334-349.
38. Yu M, Hansson E, Shiell B, et al. Sequence analysis of the Hendra virus nucleoprotein gene: comparison with other members of the subfamily Paramyxovirinae. *J Gen Virol.* 1998;79:1775-1780.
39. Chan YP, Chua KB, Koh CL, et al. Complete nucleotide sequences of Nipah virus isolates from Malaysia. *J Gen Virol.* 2001;82:2151-2155.
40. Harcourt BH, Tamin A, Halpin K, et al. Molecular characterization of the polymerase gene and genomic termini of Nipah virus. *Virology.* 2001;287:192-201.
41. Li Z, Yu M, Zhang H, et al. Beilong virus, a novel paramyxovirus with the largest genome of non-segmented negative-stranded RNA viruses. *Virology.* 2006;346:219-228.

41a. Jack PJM, Boyle DB, Eaton BT, et al. The complete genome sequence of J virus reveals a unique genome structure in the family Paramyxoviridae. *J Virol.* 2005:79:10690-10700.

42. Harcourt BH, Lowe L, Tamin A, et al. Genetic characterization of Nipah virus, Bangladesh, 2004. *Emerg Infect Dis.* 2005;11:1594-1597.
43. Calain P, Roux L. The rule of six, a basic feature for efficient replication of Sendai virus defective interfering RNA. *J Virol.* 1993;67:4822-4830.
44. Chua KB, Goh KJ, Wong KT, et al. Fatal encephalitis due to Nipah virus among pig-farmers in Malaysia. *Lancet.* 1999;354:1257-1259.
45. Paton NI, Leo YS, Zaki SR, et al. Outbreak of Nipah-virus infection among abattoir workers in Singapore. *Lancet.* 1999;354:1253-1256.
46. Chua KB. Nipah virus outbreak in Malaysia. *J Clin Virol.* 2003;26:265-275.
47. Parashar UD, Sunn LM, Ong F, et al. Case-control study of risk factors for human infection with a new zoonotic paramyxovirus, Nipah virus, during a 1998-1999 outbreak of severe encephalitis in Malaysia. *J Infect Dis.* 2000;181:1755-1759.
48. Lam SK, Chua KB. Nipah virus encephalitis outbreak in Malaysia. *Clin Infect Dis.* 2002;34:S48-S51.
49. Chua KB, Lam SK, Goh KJ, et al. The presence of Nipah virus in respiratory secretions and urine of patients during an outbreak of Nipah virus encephalitis in Malaysia. *J Infect.* 2001;42:40-43.
50. Mounts AW, Kaur H, Parashar UD, et al. A cohort study of health care workers to assess nosocomial transmissibility of Nipah virus, Malaysia, 1999. *J Infect Dis.* 2001;183:810-813.
51. Chan KP, Rollin PE, Ksiazek TG, et al. A survey of Nipah virus infection among various risk groups in Singapore. *Epidemiol Infect.* 2002;128:93-98.
52. Tan CT, Tan KS. Nosocomial transmissibility of Nipah virus. *J Infect Dis.* 2001;184:1367.
53. World Health Organization. Nipah outbreak in India and Bangladesh. WHO Newsletter: available at <http://www.searo.who.int/en/Section10/Section372_13452.htm>.
54. ICDDR, B. Outbreaks of encephalitis due to Nipah/Hendra-like viruses, Western Bangladesh. *Health Sci Bull.* 2003;1:1-6.
55. ICDDR, B. Person-to-person transmission of Nipah virus during outbreak in Faridpur District, 2004. *Health Sci Bull.* 2004;2:5-9.
56. Gurley ES, Montgomery JM, Hossain MJ, et al. Risk of nosocomial transmission of Nipah virus in a Bangladesh hospital. *Infect Control Hosp Epidemiol.* 2007;28:740-742.
57. Chua KB, Koh CL, Hooi PS, et al. Isolation of Nipah virus from Malaysian Island flying-foxes. *Microbes Infect.* 2002;4:145-151.
58. Reynes JM, Counor D, Ong S, et al. Nipah virus in Lyle's flying foxes, Cambodia. *Emerg Infect Dis.* 2005;11:1042-1047.
59. Wacharapluesadee S, Lumlertdacha B, Boongird K, et al. Bat Nipah virus, Thailand. *Emerg Infect Dis.* 2005;11:1949-1951.
60. Sendow I, Field HE, Curran J, et al. Henipavirus *in Pteropus vampyrus* bats, Indonesia. *Emerg Infect Dis.* 2006;12:711-712.
61. Goh KJ, Tan CT, Chew NK, et al. Clinical features of Nipah virus encephalitis among pig farmers in Malaysia. *N Engl J Med.* 2000;342:1229-1235.
62. Tan CT, Chua KB. Nipah virus encephalitis. *Curr Infect Dis Rep.* 2008;10:315-320.
63. Chong HT, Kunjapan SR, Thayaparan T, et al. Nipah encephalitis outbreak in Malaysia; clinical features in patients from Seremban. *Can J Neurol Sci.* 2002;29:83-87.
64. Lee KE, Umapathi T, Tan CB, et al. The neurological manifestations of Nipah virus encephalitis, a novel paramyxovirus. *Ann Neurol.* 1999;46:428-432.
65. Sarji SA, Abdullah BJ, Goh KJ, et al. MR imaging features of Nipah encephalitis. *AJR Am J Roentgenol.* 2000;175:437-442.
66. Lim CC, Sitoh YY, Hui F, et al. Nipah viral encephalitis or Japanese encephalitis? MR findings in a new zoonotic disease. *AJNR Am J Neuroradiol.* 2000;21:455-461.
67. Lim CC, Lee KE, Lee WL, et al. Nipah virus encephalitis: serial MR study of an emerging disease. *Radiology.* 2002;222:219-226.
68. Quddus R, Alam S, Majumdar MA, et al. A report of 4 patients with Nipah encephalitis from Rajbari district, Bangladesh in the January 2004 outbreak. *Neurol Asia.* 2004;9:33-37.
69. Tan CT, Goh KJ, Wong KT, et al. Relapsed and late-onset Nipah encephalitis. *Ann Neurol.* 2002;51:703-708.
70. Sejvar JJ, Hossain J, Saha SK, et al. Long-term neurological and functional outcome in Nipah virus infection. *Ann Neurol.* 2007;62:235-242.
71. Chua KB, Lam SK, Tan CT, et al. High mortality in Nipah encephalitis is associated with presence of virus in cerebrospinal fluid. *Ann Neurol.* 2000;48:802-805.
72. Chow VT, Tambyah PA, Yeo WM, et al. Diagnosis of Nipah virus encephalitis by electron microscopy of cerebrospinal fluid. *J Clin Virol.* 2000;19:143-147.
73. Wacharapluesadee S, Hemachudha T. Duplex nested RT-PCR for detection of Nipah virus RNA from urine specimens of bats. *J Virol Methods.* 2007;141:97-101.
74. Bossart KN, McEachern JA, Hickey AC, et al. Neutralization assays for differential henipavirus serology using Bio-Plex protein array systems. *J Virol Methods.* 2007;142:29-40.
75. Zhu Z, Bossart KN, Bishop KA, et al. Exceptionally potent cross-reactive neutralization of Nipah and Hendra viruses by a human monoclonal antibody. *J Infect Dis.* 2008;197:846-853.
76. Hooper P, Zaki S, Daniels P, et al. Comparative pathology of the diseases caused by Hendra and Nipah viruses. *Microbes Infect.* 2001;3:315-322.
77. Wong KT, Shieh WJ, Kumar S, et al. Nipah virus infection: pathology and pathogenesis of an emerging paramyxoviral zoonosis. *Am J Pathol.* 2002;161:2153-2167.
78. Chong HT, Kamarulzaman A, Tan CT, et al. Treatment of acute Nipah encephalitis with ribavirin. *Ann Neurol.* 2001;49:810-813.

79. Guillaume V, Contamin H, Loth P, et al. Nipah virus: vaccination and passive protection studies in a hamster model. *J Virol.* 2004;78:834-840.

80. Weingartl HM, Berhane Y, Caswell JL, et al. Recombinant Nipah virus vaccines protect pigs against challenge. *J Virol.* 2006;80:7929-7938.

81. Zhu Z, Dimitrov AS, Bossart KN, et al. Potent neutralization of Hendra and Nipah viruses by human monoclonal antibodies. *J Virol.* 2006;80:891-899.

82. Selvey LA, Wells RM, McCormack JG, et al. Infection of humans and horses by a newly described morbillivirus. *Med J Aust.* 1995;162:642-645.

83. Field H, Young P, Yob JM, et al. The natural history of Hendra and Nipah viruses. *Microbes Infect.* 2001;3:307-314.

84. Williamson MM, Hooper PT, Selleck PW, et al. Experimental Hendra virus infection in pregnant guinea-pigs and fruit bats (*Pteropus poliocephalus*). *J Comp Pathol.* 2000;122:201-207.

85. Williamson MM, Hooper PT, Selleck PW, et al. Transmission studies of Hendra virus (equine morbillivirus) in fruit bats, horses and cats. *Aust Vet J.* 1998;76:813-818.

86. Daniels P, Ksiazek T, Eaton BT. Laboratory diagnosis of Nipah and Hendra virus infections. *Microbes Infect.* 2001;3:289-295.

87. Connor E, Morrison S, Lane J, et al. Safety, tolerance, and pharmacokinetics of systemic ribavirin in children with human immunodeficiency virus infection. *Antimicrob Agents Chemother.* 1993;37:532-539.

88. Gould AR. Comparison of the deduced matrix and fusion protein sequences of equine morbillivirus with cognate genes of the Paramyxoviridae. *Virus Res.* 1996;43:17-31.

89. Kirkland PD, Love RJ, Philbey AW, et al. Epidemiology and control of Menangle virus in pigs. *Aust Vet J.* 2001;79:199-206.

90. Philbey AW, Kirkland PD, Ross AD, et al. Infection with Menangle virus in flying foxes (*Pteropus* spp.) in Australia. *Aust Vet J.* 2008;86:449-454.

162

Vesicular Stomatitis Virus and Related Vesiculoviruses

STEVEN M. FINE

Vesicular stomatitis virus (VSV) most prominently causes a vesicular disease in domestic animals that resembles foot-and-mouth disease. Outbreaks within domestic animal herds decrease production and result in restrictions on the transport and sale of animals and animal products, which results in significant economic losses. VSV infects a high percentage of people who live in endemic areas; VSV-associated disease in humans is generally mild, although significant morbidity can occur. In addition, because the VSV-G protein can bind to numerous cell types, VSV has earned a major role in molecular biology research involving the transduction of genetic material into cells and as a vaccine vector.

Classification and Morphology

Vesicular stomatitis virus is enveloped and contains a single strand of negative-sense RNA that encodes five structural proteins: the glycoprotein (G), membrane (or matrix) protein (M), nucleoprotein (N), and two internal proteins (L and P).[1,2] It belongs to the family Rhabdoviridae, genus *Vesiculovirus*,[3] and it assumes the bullet morphology characteristic of the Rhabdoviridae. Approximately 1200 identical copies of the G protein cover its surface in an ordered, densely packed array of spikes, which present only one antigenic determinant accessible to neutralizing antibodies.[4,5] Of the nine confirmed and 22 tentative species of vesiculoviruses discovered thus far (Table 162-1), six cause animal or human disease: VS-New Jersey (VS-NJ), VS-Indiana (VS-I), VS-Alagoas, Chandipura, Isfahan, and Piry.[6-9]

Molecular Biology

The VSV-G protein binds to the surface of most cell types. Thus, molecular biologists often replace the envelope proteins in other viral vectors with VSV-G to expand the host range of the vector. Viruses produced in cell lines that express the VSV-G protein are thus *pseudotyped* with VSV-G on their surfaces. They can infect a large variety of cells and are therefore tremendously useful for gene transduction.[10,11] VSV is also used as an expression vector in candidate vaccines.[12,13] Live attenuated VSV vectors are being tested for use in vaccines for HIV,[14] Ebola,[15] malaria,[16] and avian influenza.[17]

Epidemiology

EPIZOOTIC

In North America, VSV disease caused by VS-NJ or VS-I appears in sporadic, epizootic outbreaks in domesticated horses and cattle, mainly in the central and southwestern United States and Canada and in Mexico. Outbreaks of VS-I occurred in 1942, 1956, 1964, 1965, 1997, and 1998[18] and of VS-NJ in 1944, 1949, 1957, 1963, 1982, 1985, 1995, 1997, and 2006.[19,20] Outbreaks typically begin in late spring, spread to adjacent or remote herds, and abate after heavy frost. The vector is not known, although insects are suspected. VSV was isolated from a mosquito during an epizootic outbreak in New Mexico[21] and from biting midges and black flies that may be responsible for long-distance transport of the virus.[22-24] The 1995 epizootic episode in the southwestern United States began in May, in horses in New Mexico, and by October had spread to 367 premises in Arizona, Colorado, New Mexico, Utah, and Wyoming. Seventy-eight percent of cases were in horses and 22% in cattle; one case was in a llama. Production losses, quarantines, and restrictions on livestock shows, auctions, and rodeos cost an estimated $50 to $100 million.[19]

ENZOOTIC

In parts of Central and South America and in the United States on Ossabaw Island, Georgia, outbreaks of disease from enzootic VS-NJ predictably appear near the beginning of the dry season (November) and last through March. Farms located near forests, and those with poultry, experience higher rates of attack.[25] One year in Costa Rica, 9% to 11% of cattle on affected farms had disease develop, which constituted 2.6% of cattle overall.[25,26] Lactation and a high acute VSV antibody titer increase the risk of disease for a given animal, but other diseases do not predispose to VSV disease.[25] The reservoirs and vectors for enzootic disease are not known, but phlebotomine sand flies harbor virus in enzootic areas.[6-8,27-29] They can transmit VSV to animals and transovarially to a new generation of sand flies in which it can then replicate.[28,30,31] Mosquitoes can also harbor VSV and can transmit infection to animals in a laboratory setting.[32] In addition, VSV-infected black flies feeding on uninfected mice can horizontally infect other black flies feeding on the same mouse.[24] The high prevalence rate of VS-NJ antibodies in cows in enzootic areas of Costa Rica (82% for VS-NJ and 17.7% for VS-I)[26] indicates a high lifetime probability of infection, and many of these infections are probably subclinical. Wild animals in enzootic areas also have VS-I and VS-NJ antibodies, with VS-I mainly in arboreal and semiarboreal species and VS-NJ in bats, Carnivora, some rodents, and white-tailed deer.[33,34] Animals with high titers of neutralizing antibodies can become reinfected with other strains.[25]

ANIMAL DISEASE

Vesicular stomatitis virus infection causes an acute vesicular disease in horses, cattle, swine, goats, llamas, and some wild animals.[19,35] Excess salivation, with fever and blisters or vesicles in and around the mouth, nose, hooves, or teats, appears after a 2-day to 8-day incubation period. Vesicles may burst, and the epithelium may slough, leaving large contiguous areas exposed and irritated. Secondary bacterial infection that leads to mastitis may complicate the course, and lameness from foot lesions can develop. A debilitating, nonvesicular manifestation with systemic symptoms, such as fever and weight loss, sometimes occurs. Most animals recover after 2 to 3 weeks,[25,36] but viral sequences may persist.[37]

HUMAN DISEASE

Humans usually contract VSV during close contact with infected animals.[38,39] Most human VSV infections go unrecognized, which indicates either mild or subclinical illness; however, infection is not always benign. Of eight animal handlers who contracted VS-I during a 1965 epizootic episode in cattle, seven reported an illness that included fever, malaise, myalgias, emesis, and pharyngitis, and two had oral vesicular lesions develop in 24 to 48 hours. Although most had mild

TABLE 162-1	Vesiculoviruses	
Species	*Location of Isolation*
VS-Indiana	United States
VS-New Jersey	United States
VS-Alagoas	Brazil[6]
VS-Carajas	Brazil[8]
Maraba	Brazil[8]
Piry	Brazil
Cocal	Trinidad[18]
Chandipura	India[64,65]
Isfahan	Iran[7]

Adapted from Travassos da Rosa AP, Tesh RB, Travassos da Rosa JF, et al. Carajas and Maraba viruses, two new vesiculoviruses isolated from phlebotomine sand flies in Brazil. *Am J Trop Med Hyg.* 1984;33:999-1006; and ICTV database 2002 of the 2002 International Committee on Taxonomy of Viruses. Available at http://www.ncbi.nlm.nih.gov/ICTVdb.

illness that quickly resolved, one otherwise healthy man had pharyngeal and buccal lesions, lymphadenopathy, and a 20-lb weight loss over 3 weeks.[36] In another case, 30 hours after self inoculation with VS-I, a laboratory worker had development of fever, chills, retroorbital pain, myalgias, nausea, emesis, and diarrhea, which resolved in 3 days.[40]

Vesicular stomatitis virus is neurotropic in baby mice,[41] and two cases of VSV meningoencephalitis have been reported in children. In one case, a 3-year-old boy from Panama infected with VS-I had fever, chills, emesis, and generalized tonic-clonic seizures and remained neurologically impaired at discharge.[9]

A related vesiculovirus, Chandipura, appears to infect humans more readily than VSV and has recently been implicated in outbreaks of encephalitis in parts of India. In 2003, an outbreak of encephalitis occurred in children in Andra Paresh, India, with a high fatality rate (183 of 329 cases, or 55%). Chandipura was detected in 28 of 51 cases (51%) with either presence of viral RNA, immunoglobulin M (IgM) antibodies, or both.[42] In 2004, an outbreak of encephalitis in children was noted in Eastern India and involved 26 cases, with a fatality rate of 78.3%. Laboratory studies in nine of 13 patients[43] revealed Chandipura RNA in serum specimens. Chandipura virus has been isolated from sand flies,[44] which were believed to be the likely vector of spread in the first outbreak but were not detected in a small number of sand fly samples in the second outbreak.

In an area of Iran enzootic for Isfahan, all residents older than 5 years were seropositive in one study,[7] and in a VS-Alagoas–endemic area of Colombia, 62% to 83% of people were seropositive,[6] indicating previous infection. This relatively high rate of seropositivity, which increases with age, also occurs with other serotypes in their respective enzootic areas.[27,33,39,45]

Diagnosis

Vesicular stomatitis virus causes lesions that look like those of the more dangerous foot-and-mouth disease; therefore, VSV outbreaks demand urgent diagnosis. Current diagnostic methods include complement fixation, serum neutralization, enzyme-linked immunosorbent assay (ELISA), or viral isolation in tissue culture.[19] Recently developed assays, with reverse transcription and the polymerase chain reaction, ease the collection of samples, can be used to identify viral RNA from lesions previously treated with toxic substances, and are being adapted for general use.[46]

Host Response and Treatment

Studies in mice showed that the presence of B cells and antibody responses was associated with recovery and the development of resistance to VSV; however, CD4+ cells also contribute to long-term survival, and secretion of interleukin-12 may be beneficial.[47-49] Antibody-mediated neutralization blocks virus-to-cell binding and requires 200 to 500 VSV-G-protein–specific immunoglobulin G molecules per virus particle.[2,4] Neutralizing antibodies bind to the same G-protein epitope and protect against infection with the same strain.[5,50] However, in endemic areas, up to 10% of cattle with high titers of neutralizing antibodies become infected each year with clinical symptoms, presumably from mutant strains.[25]

Human infections with VSV are usually mild and generally do not necessitate treatment. No specific treatments exist, and antiviral agents have not been evaluated in vivo. Interferon-α, interferon-β, and interferon-γ inhibit VSV growth in vitro[51-53] and protect newborn mice from lethal VSV infection.[54] Prostaglandins A_1 and A_2,[55,56] ribavirin,[57,58] and some experimental compounds[59-61] inhibit VSV in vitro. In animals, secondary bacterial infections of the mouth, teats, and hooves should be treated appropriately, and a mild antiseptic mouthwash may relieve pain from blisters.[62] Nutritional support may help animals that stop eating.

Prevention and Vaccination

Experimental vaccination with a recombinant vaccinia vector that expresses the VSV-G protein stimulated neutralizing antibody production and protected mice against lethal VSV disease after intravenous challenge. In cattle, protection was incomplete, but it correlated with high antibody titer.[63] The U.S. Department of Agriculture has approved a killed vaccine for animals, but its efficacy is unknown.[19]

REFERENCES

1. Banerjee AK, Barik S. Gene expression of vesicular stomatitis virus genome RNA. *Virology.* 1992;188:417-428.
2. Dietzschold B, Schneider LG, Cox JH. Serological characterization of the three major proteins of vesicular stomatitis virus. *J Virol.* 1974;14:1-7.
3. Knudson DL. Rhabdoviruses. *J Gen Virol.* 1973;20:105-130.
4. Kelley JM, Emerson SU, Wagner RR. The glycoprotein of vesicular stomatitis virus is the antigen that gives rise to and reacts with neutralizing antibody. *J Virol.* 1972;10:1231-1235.
5. Bachmann MF, Rohrer UH, Kundig TM, et al. The influence of antigen organization on B cell responsiveness. *Science.* 1993;262:1448-1451.
6. Tesh RB, Boshell J, Modi GB, et al. Natural infection of humans, animals, and phlebotomine sand flies with the Alagoas serotype of vesicular stomatitis virus in Colombia. *Am J Trop Med Hyg.* 1987;36:653-661.
7. Tesh R, Saidi S, Javadian E, et al. Isfahan virus, a new vesiculovirus infecting humans, gerbils, and sandflies in Iran. *Am J Trop Med Hyg.* 1977;26:299-306.
8. Travassos da Rosa AP, Tesh RB, Travassos da Rosa JF, et al. Carajas and Maraba viruses, two new vesiculoviruses isolated from phlebotomine sand flies in Brazil. *Am J Trop Med Hyg.* 1984;33:999-1006.
9. Quiroz E, Moreno N, Peralta PH, et al. A human case of encephalitis associated with vesicular stomatitis virus (Indiana serotype) infection. *Am J Trop Med Hyg.* 1988;39:312-314.
10. Arai T, Matsumoto K, Saitoh K, et al. A new system for stringent, high-titer vesicular stomatitis virus G protein-pseudotyped retrovirus vector induction by introduction of Cre recombinase into stable prepackaging cell lines. *J Virol.* 1998;72:1115-1121.
11. Yee JK, Friedmann T, Burns JC. Generation of high-titer pseudotyped retroviral vectors with very broad host range. *Methods Cell Biol.* 1994;43:99-112.
12. Lichty BD, Power AT, Stojdl DF, et al. Vesicular stomatitis virus: re-inventing the bullet. *Trends Mol Med.* 2004;10:210-216.
13. Liniger M, Zuniga A, Naim HY. Use of viral vectors for the development of vaccines. *Expert Rev Vaccines.* 2007;6:255-266.
14. Clarke DK, Cooper D, Egan MA, et al. Recombinant vesicular stomatitis virus as an HIV-1 vaccine vector. *Springer Semin Immunopathol.* 2006;28:239-253.
15. Geisbert TW, Daddario-Dicaprio KM, Lewis MG, et al. Vesicular stomatitis virus-based ebola vaccine is well-tolerated and protects immunocompromised nonhuman primates. *PLoS Pathog.* 2008;4:e1000225.
16. Li S, Locke E, Bruder J, et al. Viral vectors for malaria vaccine development. *Vaccine.* 2007;25:2567-2574.
17. Kalhoro NH, Veits J, Rautenschlein S, et al. A recombinant vesicular stomatitis virus replicon vaccine protects chickens from highly pathogenic avian influenza virus (H7N1). *Vaccine.* 2009;27:1174-1183.
18. Jonkers AH. The epizootiology of the vesicular stomatitis viruses: A reappraisal. *Am J Epidemiol.* 1967;86:286-291.
19. Bridges VE, McCluskey BJ, Salman MD, et al. Review of the 1995 vesicular stomatitis outbreak in the western United States. *J Am Vet Med Assoc.* 1997;211:556-560.
20. Rodriguez LL. Emergence and re-emergence of vesicular stomatitis in the United States. *Virus Res.* 2002;85:211-219.
21. Sudia WD, Fields BN, Calisher CH. The isolation of vesicular stomatitis virus (Indiana strain) and other viruses from mosquitoes in New Mexico, 1965. *Am J Epidemiol.* 1967;86:598-602.
22. Cupp EW, Mare CJ, Cupp MS, et al. Biological transmission of vesicular stomatitis virus (New Jersey) by *Simulium vittatum* (Diptera: Simuliidae). *J Med Entomol.* 1992;29:137-140.
23. Mead DG, Maré CJ, Ramberg FB. Bite transmission of vesicular stomatitis virus (New Jersey serotype) to laboratory mice by *Simulium vittatum* (Diptera: Simuliidae). *J Med Entomol.* 1999;36:410-413.
24. Mead DG, Ramberg FB, Besselsen DG, et al. Transmission of vesicular stomatitis virus (New Jersey serotype) between infected

and non-infected black flies co-feeding on non-viremic deer mice. *Science.* 2000;287:485-487.

25. Vanleeuwen JA, Rodriguez LL, Waltner-Toews D. Cow, farm, and ecologic risk factors of clinical vesicular stomatitis on Costa Rican dairy farms. *Am J Trop Med Hyg.* 1995;53:342-350.

26. Rodriguez LL, Vernon S, Morales AI, et al. Serological monitoring of vesicular stomatitis New Jersey virus in enzootic regions of Costa Rica. *Am J Trop Med Hyg.* 1990;42:272-281.

27. Shelokov A, Peralta PH. Vesicular stomatitis virus, Indiana type: An arbovirus infection of tropical sandflies and humans? *Am J Epidemiol.* 1967;86:149-157.

28. Comer JA, Tesh RB, Modi GB, et al. Vesicular stomatitis virus, New Jersey serotype: Replication in and transmission by *Lutzomyia shannoni* (Diptera: Psychodidae). *Am J Trop Med Hyg.* 1990;42:483-490.

29. Corn JL, Comer JA, Erickson GA, et al. Isolation of vesicular stomatitis virus New Jersey serotype from phlebotomine sand flies in Georgia. *Am J Trop Med Hyg.* 1990;42:476-482.

30. Tesh RB, Chaniotis BN, Johnson KM. Vesicular stomatitis virus, Indiana serotype: Multiplication in and transmission by experimentally infected phlebotomine sandflies (*Lutzomyia trapidoi*). *Am J Epidemiol.* 1971;93:491-495.

31. Tesh RB, Chaniotis BN. Transovarial transmission of viruses by phlebotomine sandflies. *Ann N Y Acad Sci.* 1975;266:125-134.

32. Calisher CH, Monath TP, Sabattini MS, et al. A newly recognized vesiculovirus, Calchaqui virus, and subtypes of Melao and Maguari viruses from Argentina, with serologic evidence for infections of humans and horses. *Am J Trop Med Hyg.* 1987;36:114-119.

33. Tesh RB, Peralta PH, Johnson KM. Ecologic studies of vesicular stomatitis virus. I. Prevalence of infection among animals and humans living in an area of endemic VSV activity. *Am J Epidemiol.* 1969;90:255-261.

34. Johnson KM, Tesh RB, Peralta PH. Epidemiology of vesicular stomatitis virus: Some new data and a hypothesis for transmission of the Indian serotype. *J Am Vet Med Assoc.* 1969;155:2133-2140.

35. Green SL. Vesicular stomatitis in the horse. *Vet Clin North Am Equine Pract.* 1993;9:349-353.

36. Fields BN, Hawkins K. Human infection with the virus of vesicular stomatitis during an epizootic. *N Engl J Med.* 1967;277:989-994.

37. Letchworth GJ, Barrera JC, Fishel JR, et al. Vesicular stomatitis New Jersey virus RNA persists in cattle following convalescence. *Virology.* 1996;219:480-484.

38. Reif JS, Webb PA, Monath TP, et al. Epizootic vesicular stomatitis in Colorado, 1982: Infection in occupational risk groups. *Am J Trop Med Hyg.* 1987;36:177-182.

39. Brody JA, Fischer GF, Peralta PH. Vesicular stomatitis virus in Panama. Human serologic patterns in a cattle raising area. *Am J Epidemiol.* 1967;86:158-161.

40. Johnson KM, Vogel JE, Peralta PH. Clinical and serological response to laboratory-acquired human infection by Indiana type vesicular stomatitis virus (VSV). *Am J Trop Med Hyg.* 1966;15:244-246.

41. Bi Z, Barna M, Komatsu T, et al. Vesicular stomatitis virus infection of the central nervous system activates both innate and acquired immunity. *J Virol.* 1995;69:6466-6472.

42. Rao BL, Basu A, Wairagkar NS, et al. A large outbreak of acute encephalitis with high fatality rate in children in Andhra Pradesh, India, in 2003, associated with Chandipura virus. *Lancet.* 2004;364:869-874.

43. Chadha MS, Arankalle VA, Jadi RS, et al. An Outbreak of Chandipura Virus Encephalitis in the Eastern Districts of Gujarat State, India. *AM J Trop Med Hyg.* 2005;73:566-570.

44. Basak S, Mondal A, Polley S, et al. Reviewing Chandipura: a vesiculovirus in human epidemics. *Biosci Rep.* 2007;27:275-298.

45. Cline BL. Ecological associations of vesicular stomatitis virus in rural Central America and Panama. *Am J Trop Med Hyg.* 1976;25:875-883.

46. Rodriguez LL, Fitch WM, Nichol ST. Ecological factors rather than temporal factors dominate the evolution of vesicular stomatitis virus. *Proc Natl Acad Sci U S A.* 1996;93:13030-13035.

47. Bachmann MF, Kalinke U, Althage A, et al. The role of antibody concentration and avidity in antiviral protection. *Science.* 1997;276:2024-2027.

48. Thomsen AR, Nansen A, Andersen C, et al. Cooperation of B cells and T cells is required for survival of mice infected with vesicular stomatitis virus. *Int Immunol.* 1997;9:1757-1766.

49. Komatsu T, Barna M, Reiss CS. Interleukin-12 promotes recovery from viral encephalitis. *Viral Immunol.* 1997;10:35-47.

50. Bachmann MF, Hengartner H, Zinkernagel RM. T helper cell-independent neutralizing B cell response against vesicular stomatitis virus: Role of antigen patterns in B cell induction? *Eur J Immunol.* 1995;25:3445-3451.

51. Witter F, Barouki F, Griffin D, et al. Biologic response (antiviral) to recombinant human interferon alpha 2a as a function of dose and route of administration in healthy volunteers. *Clin Pharmacol Ther.* 1987;42:567-575.

52. Maheshawari RK, Friedman RM. Interferon induced inhibition of enveloped viruses. *Prog Clin Biol Res.* 1985;202:297-305.

53. Baxt B, Sonnabend JA, Bablianian R. Effects of interferon on vesicular stomatitis virus transcription and translation. *J Gen Virol.* 1977;35:325-334.

54. DeClercq E, De Somer P. Protective effect of interferon and polyacrylic acid in newborn mice infected with a lethal dose of vesicular stomatitis virus. *Life Sci.* 1968;7:925-933.

55. Pica F, Rossi A, Santirocco N, et al. Effect of combined alpha IFN and prostaglandin A1 treatment on vesicular stomatitis virus replication and heat shock protein synthesis in epithelial cells. *Antiviral Res.* 1996;29:187-198.

56. Parker J, Ahrens PB, Ankel H. Antiviral effects of cyclopentenone prostaglandins on vesicular stomatitis virus replication. *Antiviral Res.* 1995;26:83-96.

57. Fernandez-Larsson R, O'Connell K, Koumans E, et al. Molecular analysis of the inhibitory effect of phosphorylated ribavirin on the vesicular stomatitis virus in vitro polymerase reaction. *Antimicrob Agents Chemother.* 1989;33:1668-1673.

58. Toltzis P, Huang AS. Effect of ribavirin on macromolecular synthesis in vesicular stomatitis virus-infected cells. *Antimicrob Agents Chemother.* 1986;29:1010-1016.

59. Shuto S, Obara T, Saito Y, et al. New neplanocin analogues: 6. Synthesis and potent antiviral activity of 6'-homoneplanocin A1. *J Med Chem.* 1996;39:2392-2399.

60. Spinu K, Vorozhbit V, Grushko T, et al. Antiviral activity of tomatoside from *Lycopersicon esculentum* Mill. *Adv Exp Med Biol.* 1996;404:505-509.

61. Muller-Decker K, Amtmann E, Sauer G. Inhibition of the phosphorylation of the regulatory non-structural protein of vesicular stomatitis virus by an antiviral xanthate compound. *J Gen Virol.* 1987;68:3045-3056.

62. Animal and Plant Health Inspection Service. *Precautions for Horses Diagnosed with Vesicular Stomatitis.* Lakewood, CO: Colorado Department of Agriculture Animal Industry Division; 1998.

63. Mackett M, Yilma T, Rose JK, et al. Vaccinia virus recombinants: Expression of VSV genes and protective immunization of mice and cattle. *Science.* 1985;227:433-435.

64. Fontenille D, Traore-Lamizana M, Trouillet J, et al. First isolations of arboviruses from phlebotomine sand flies in West Africa. *Am J Trop Med Hyg.* 1994;50:570-574.

65. Bhatt PN, Rodrigues FM. Chandipura: A new arbovirus isolated in India from patients with febrile illness. *Indian J Med Res.* 1967;55:1295-1305.

163

Rhabdoviruses

SARICE L. BASSIN | CHARLES E. RUPPRECHT | THOMAS P. BLECK

Rabies is a viral disease that produces an almost uniformly fatal encephalitis in humans and most other mammals. It has been present throughout recorded history, and literature, and likely predates the evolution of humans. Rabies remains one of the most common viral causes of mortality in the developing world. Exposure to the virus has profound medical and economic implications throughout the world, with as many as 10 million people annually receiving postexposure treatment (PET) to prevent rabies.[1] Although current technology can produce safe agents for PET, deviations from recommended PET regimens can lead to prophylaxis failure and fatal illness.

Rabies, Latin for "madness," derives from rabere, to rave, and is related to the Sanskrit word for violence, rabhas. The Greek term for rabies, lyssa, also means madness, and it provides the genus name (Lyssavirus). The Babylon Eshnuna code contains the first known mention of rabies in the 23rd century BC.[2] Democritus provided a clear description of animal rabies in about 500 BC. Wound cauterization was the preferred treatment in the 1st century AD and was recommended for the management of rabid animal bites until the mid 20th century.[2] This treatment remained the only real therapy until Pasteur introduced a vaccine based on attenuated rabies virus in 1885.

Rabies in the Western Hemisphere predated Columbus but remained rare because of low population density.[3] Bats spread the disease among cattle and humans in Central America in the early 16th century.[4] Rabies epizootics began in the northern and eastern United States in the 19th century, reflecting the importation of foxes for hunting.[5] Globally, 99% of all cases of human rabies result from transmission from dogs.[1]

Rabies was diagnosed clinically only until 1903, when Adelchi Negri described the cytoplasmic inclusions that bear his name.[6] These inclusions were the only pathologic marker before the development of the fluorescent antibody test in 1958.[7]

Virology

CLASSIFICATION

The Rhabdoviridae are rod-shaped, negative-sense, nonsegmented, single-stranded RNA viruses. Three genera infect animals (Lyssavirus, Vesiculovirus, and Ephemerovirus); one infects plants; and several other members are uncharacterized. Rabies (serotype 1) is the type species of the Lyssavirus genus,[5] vesicular stomatitis virus that of the Vesiculovirus genus, and bovine ephemeral fever that of the Ephemerovirus genus. Rabies is enzootic, and sometimes epizootic, in a variety of mammals. Australian bat lyssavirus (ABLV) is genetically distinct from rabies virus but causes rabies-like disease in Australian flying foxes and insectivorous bats. Two human deaths in Australia, both after a rabies-like illness, were from ABLV infection acquired from animals.[8] The five other members of the genus rarely cause human disease (Table 163-1). New putative lyssavirus species are still emerging in bats around the world.[9,10]

Vesiculoviruses share many of the virologic characteristics of the lyssaviruses. They infect a large number of animal and insect species; humans are occasionally infected via contact with animals, typically via respiratory secretions.[11] Seven vesiculoviruses are known to occasionally infect humans.[12] Another negative-sense single-stranded RNA virus, borna, produces central nervous system (CNS) infection in birds and primates, and some authors have suggested that it is related to human psychiatric disorders. In contrast to the rhabdoviruses, however, it replicates in the nucleus rather than in the cytoplasm. It is not a rhabdovirus, and its taxonomy remains uncertain.

COMPOSITION

Lyssaviruses are bullet-shaped, with an average length of 180 nm and an average diameter of 75 nm.[13] The complete virus includes a helical nucleocapsid with 30 and 35 coils between 4.2 and 4.6 nm in length.[14] This is enclosed in a lipoprotein envelope 7.5 to 10 nm thick, from which glycoprotein (G protein) spikes project 10 nm.[15] These spikes cover the surface of the virus except at the blunt end (Fig. 163-1).

The rabies genome is a single, negatively stranded RNA molecule that weighs 4.6×10^3 kd[16] and encodes five genes: N, NS (or M_1), M (or M_2), G, and L (Table 163-2).[17] Phosphorylation of the N nucleoprotein is necessary for efficient transcription replication of the viral RNA,[18,19] and the N nucleoprotein is potentially immunogenic.[20] It is probably needed to switch from the transcription of gene products to the production of a full-length positively stranded RNA.[21] The NS phosphoprotein (also called P in more recent studies) may control the L protein, an RNA-dependent RNA polymerase.[22,23] The M, or matrix, protein is located between the nucleocapsid and the lipoprotein envelope[24]; it, in concert with the G protein, is responsible for the assembly and budding of bullet-shaped particles.[25] This M protein determines the balance between transcription and replication[26] and affects RNA synthesis.[27]

The G protein is involved in cellular reception and is the antigen that induces neutralizing antibodies. Variability in this protein is responsible for serotypic differences among lyssaviruses,[28] and mutations at position 333 (with substitution of glutamine or isoleucine for arginine) disrupt virulence.[29] This arginine residue appears to be essential for fusion of the viral envelope with neurons.[30] Molecular modifications of the G protein can increase its antigenicity.[31]

REPLICATION STRATEGY

Neuronal attachment is probably mediated by more than one mechanism, including binding to a ganglioside[32] and independently to the neural cell adhesion molecule (CD56).[33] In muscle, the virus binds to the nicotinic acetylcholine receptor.[34] Once bound to the receptor, the virus is probably internalized with receptor-mediated endocytosis to form a coated pit, which then fuses with a lysosome, from which the nucleocapsid escapes into the cytosol.[35] The viral envelope forms from host membranes into which the G and M proteins are inserted.[36] The envelope includes small amounts of host proteins.[23]

The virus does not tolerate a pH level below 3 or above 11, and it is inactivated by ultraviolet light, sunlight, desiccation, formalin, phenol, ether, trypsin, β-propiolactone, and detergents.

Epidemiology

HUMAN RABIES

Rabies is currently distributed worldwide except for Antarctica and a few island nations. In 2007 (the last year for which global data are available), 103 nations reported the presence of rabies, and 42 reported its absence.[37] Worldwide, dogs account for 54% of animal rabies, terrestrial wildlife for 42%, and bats for 4%.

TABLE 163-1	Members of the Lyssavirus Genus	
Virus	*Serotype*	*Reservoir*
Rabies	1	Found worldwide except for a few island nations, Australia, and Antarctica.
Lagos bat	2	Probably enzootic in fruit bats; no reported human cases.
Mokola	3	Probably an insectivore or rodent species limited to parts of Africa; a few domestic animal and two human cases reported.
Duvenhage	4	Probably insectivorous bats; cases identified in South Africa, Zimbabwe, and Senegal.
European bat lyssavirus 1 (EBLV1)	5	European insectivorous bats (probably *Eptesicus serotinus*).
European bat lyssavirus 2 (EBLV2)	6	European insectivorous bats (probably *Myotis dasycneme*).
Australian bat lyssavirus	7	Flying foxes and insectivorous bats.

Adapted from Rupprecht CE, Smith JS, Fekadu M, Childs JE. The ascension of wildlife rabies: A cause for public health concern or intervention? *Emerg Infect Dis.* 1995;1:107-114.

The epidemiology of human rabies reflects that of local animal rabies.[38] In developing areas where canine rabies remains common, most human cases result from dog bites. In regions where dogs are immunized, most human cases follow exposure to rabid wild animals.

The World Health Organization (WHO) estimates that 55,000 humans die of rabies annually. These deaths probably represent an underestimate of the worldwide incidence rate of the disease, which may cause as many as 100,000 deaths annually.[5] A disproportionate number of those affected are children under the age of 15 years.[39] An estimated 10 million persons receive PET annually, with most treatments with types of vaccine that carry a risk of neurologic complications.[1,40]

In countries of low prevalence, an increasing percentage of cases are imported, occur after long incubation periods, or lack a known source of exposure.[41,42] In the United States, one to four cases were reported annually in the past decade (Fig. 163-2), and the sources of human cases have changed from predominantly domestic animals (1945 to 1965) to largely unknown sources (1976 to present). Three cases of human rabies were reported from Texas, Indiana, and California during 2006. The cases in Indiana and Texas were from bat rabies

variants. The case in California was from canine rabies acquired in the Philippines.[41] One human rabies case was reported during 2007. This fatality, from Minnesota, was believed to be from a bat exposure.[43]

In 2003, a 23-year-old man in Virginia died of raccoon strain of rabies; no history of animal exposure could be elicited from the patient's family or acquaintances.[44] To date, no other cases have been reported of human rabies infection from a raccoon variant.

ANIMAL RABIES

In the developing world, rabies is predominantly a problem of domestic and feral animals. In the United States, the major canine variants of the rabies virus in dogs, *Canis lupus*, were declared eliminated in 2006 as a result of aggressive oral vaccination programs.[43] As the developed nations have largely eliminated rabies from domestic animals, wild animals are left as the major affected group. Wild animals accounted for greater than 90% of the reported cases of rabies in the United States in 2007.[41] The incidence of wild animal rabies has been increasing during the past two decades (Fig. 163-3), and the number of cases reported in 2007 was up 6% from 2006.[41] A resurgence of

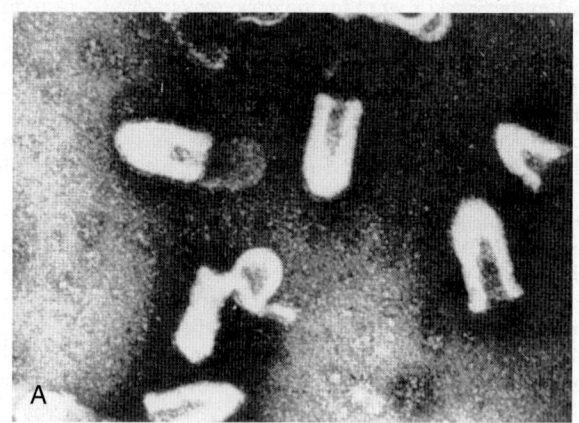

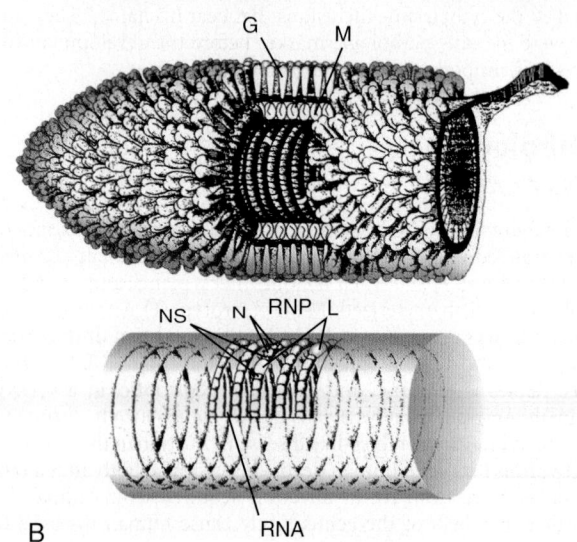

Figure 163-1 Rabies virus morphology. A, Electron micrograph of rabies virus. Original magnification, ×55,000. **B,** Schematic illustration of rabies virus *(top),* showing surface glycoprotein (G) projections extending from lipid envelope surrounding RNP and matrix protein (M) lining envelope. Helical ribonucleoprotein (RNP) *(bottom)* comprises single-stranded RNA genome, plus nucleoprotein (N), phosphoprotein (NS), and transcriptase (L). *(From Dietzschold B, Rupprecht CE, Fu ZF, Koprowski H. Rhabdoviruses. In: Fields BN, Knipe DM, Howley PM, et al, eds. Fields Virology. 3rd ed. Philadelphia: Lippincott Raven; 1996:1137-1159.)*

TABLE 163-2	Rhabdoviral Genes and Products		
Gene	*Synonyms*	*Size (kDa)*	*Function*
N (nucleocapsid)	—	50	—
NS (nonstructural)	M₁, P	40	Originally thought to encode a nonstructural protein but now known to produce a structural protein that is phosphorylated by kinases in the host cell and that joins with L.
M (matrix)	M₂	26	Responsible for the assembly and budding of bullet-shaped particles, in concert with the G protein.
G (glycoprotein)	—	65	Attachment to host cell receptors.
L (large)	—	160-190	RNA-dependent RNA polymerase; required for transcription of the negatively stranded viral RNA; appears to form a complex with NS.

Adapted from Rupprecht CE, Smith JS, Fekadu M, Childs JE. The ascension of wildlife rabies: A cause for public health concern or intervention? *Emerg Infect Dis.* 1995;1:107-114.

raccoon rabies in the United States began in 1977 near the Virginia–West Virginia border, and in the ensuing two decades, the territory expanded to involve most of the eastern states. More than 20,000 cases of raccoon rabies have been reported, with several thousand secondary cases in dogs and other animals.[45] Increases in cases of rabid raccoons during 2007 were reported by 11 of the 20 eastern states where raccoon rabies is enzootic.[43]

Bats are increasingly the source of human rabies in the United States.[46] The epizoology of bat rabies is changing from typical reservoirs (e.g., the common big brown bat) to include previously rarely affected species (e.g., the silver-haired bat).[47] Most of the human rabies cases known to have been contracted from bats in the United States since 1980 involve the silver-haired/eastern pipistrelle bat rabies virus variant.[48] Rabies is also increasing among previously rarely affected species in other parts of the United States, such as coyotes.[49] In rare wild animal species (e.g., spotted hyenas), rabies infection may not lead to clinically apparent disease.[50] In at least one bat species (*Eptesicus serotinus*), salivary samples may contain viral RNA without detectable RNA in concurrent brain samples.[51] The implications of this finding for screening wild animals after potentially infectious human contact remain to be determined.

Previously unidentified rabies variants from potential cross-species transmission are still emerging around the world.[42,52,53] Molecular epidemiologic evidence reinforces the importance of avoiding contact with downed bats or other wildlife.[54,55]

Pathogenesis

Rabies infection begins with centripetal spread of the virus via peripheral nerves to the CNS, proliferation within the CNS, and centrifugal spread via peripheral nerves to many tissues.[27,56] After the virus enters through a break in the skin, across a mucosal surface, or through the respiratory tract, it replicates in muscle cells and, in so doing, infects the muscle spindle. It then infects the nerve that innervates the spindle and moves centrally within the axons of these neurons. Replication occurs in peripheral neurons, but not usually in glia, either peripheral or central. Virus is present in dorsal root ganglia within 60 to 72 hours of inoculation and before its arrival in spinal cord neurons, which confirms its transport within sensory neurons.

Some studies suggest that the neuromuscular junction is also a major site of neuronal invasion[57] and blocking acetylcholine receptors inhibits viral attachment.[58] Partial sequence homology exists between rabies virus glycoprotein and several snake neurotoxins that bind to this receptor.[59] However, rabies virus can enter neurons that do not express acetylcholine receptors, albeit with less efficiency, which indicates the existence of other receptors.[60]

Natural rabies infection appears to require a period of local viral replication, perhaps to increase the inoculum, before nervous system infection occurs. Timely administration of antirabies immunoglobulin and active immunization can prevent spread of the virus into the nervous system, thereby preventing disease. Once the virus has entered peripheral nerves, current therapeutic techniques probably do not

readily prevent subsequent replication and spread, and the virus quickly moves centrally. Rabies virus ascends via fast axonal transport, probably involving an interaction between the cytoplasmic dynein light chain with the rabies virus NS phosphoprotein.[61] Herpes simplex virus and tetanus toxin also make use of the microtubular transport systems.[62] After reaching the spinal cord, the virus spreads throughout the CNS, following established patterns of synaptic connectivity.[63] Virtually every neuron is infected.[35]

After CNS infection, virus spreads to the rest of the body via peripheral nerves. The high concentration of virus in saliva results from viral shedding from sensory nerve endings in the oral mucosa[36] and also reflects replication in the salivary glands.

The mechanisms by which rabies damages the CNS are obscure because pathologic evidence of neuronal necrosis is frequently minimal or absent.[64] Rabies may interfere with neurotransmission[65] and with endogenous opioid systems,[66] and the almost 30-fold increase in local nitric oxide production[67] suggests an excitotoxic mechanism. An inverse relationship is found between the concentration of G protein produced and the pathogenicity of different viral strains, and a monotonic relationship is found between pathogenicity and the induction of neuronal apoptosis.[68] The infection is also capable of inducing apoptosis in T lymphocytes,[69] which may relate to the failure of the immune response to control the disease.

PATHOLOGY

The brain in furious rabies (see subsequent discussion) usually appears unremarkable grossly,[70] except for the vascular congestion. The microscopic pathology of rabies is typically encephalitis with Negri bodies (Fig. 163-4). However, not all autopsy specimens show the perivascular lymphocytic cuffing and necrosis that characterize encephalitis, and some cases look histologically like meningitis.[71] Negri bodies are concentrated in hippocampal pyramidal cells and less frequently in cortical neurons and cerebellar Purkinje cells.[70] They are round or oval, usually eosinophilic, cytoplasmic inclusions between 1 and 7 μm across, and they contain viral nucleocapsids.[72] The acidophilic lyssa body is ultrastructurally identical to the Negri body.[73] Negri bodies and lyssa bodies are detected in only a relatively small percentage of the cells that are infected (as determined with immunohistochemistry).[74]

Paralytic rabies affects primarily the spinal cord, with severe inflammation and necrosis.[75] The brain stem is involved to a lesser extent. A

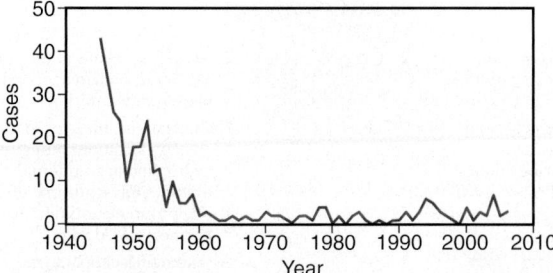

Figure 163-2 **Reported cases of human rabies in the United States by year, 1945-2006.** (*From McNabb SJN, Jajosky RA, Hall-Baker PA, et al. Summary of Notifiable Diseases: United States, 2006. Morb Mortal Wkly Rep. 2008;53:1-94.*)

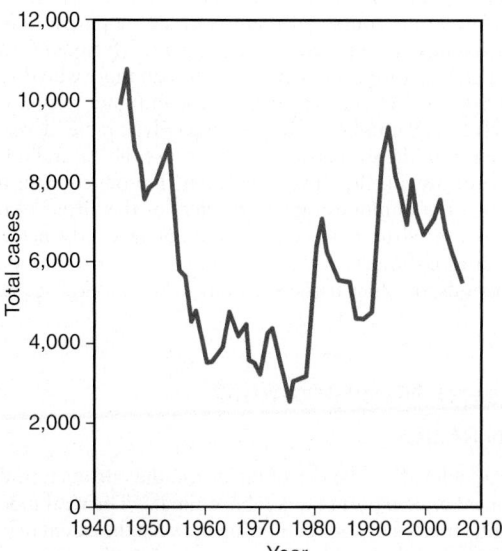

Figure 163-3 **Reported cases of animal rabies in the United States by year, 1945-2006.** (*From McNabb SJN, Jajosky RA, Hall-Baker PA, et al. Summary of Notifiable Diseases: United States, 2006. Morb Mortal Wkly Rep. 2008;53:1-94.*)

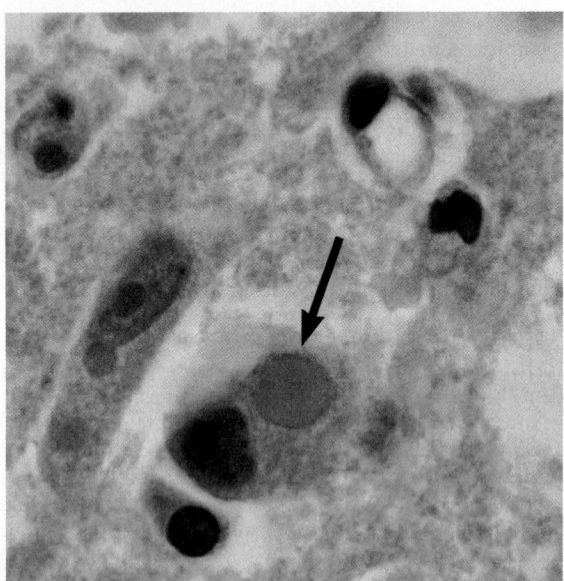

Figure 163-4 **Negri body** *(arrow).* Original magnification, ×400. *(Courtesy of Maria-Beatriz Lopes, MD, Division of Neuropathology, University of Virginia.)*

few patients have cortical Negri bodies. Segmental demyelination occurs in the peripheral nerves and resembles acute inflammatory polyneuropathy (Guillain-Barré syndrome).

Systemic pathology is most remarkable for the presence of myocarditis.[76] This cardiac disorder resembles the myocarditis that occurs in hypercatecholaminergic states such as pheochromocytoma, subarachnoid hemorrhage, and tetanus.[62] Negri bodies are found in the hearts of some patients, which suggests a direct viral role in this condition.[77] Atrial ganglioneuritis suggests that the virus reaches the myocardium via spread from the nervous system.[78]

IMMUNE RESPONSES

The immune response to natural rabies infection is insufficient to prevent disease. Rabies can produce immunosuppression,[79] and if unvaccinated patients have a measurable antibody response develop, it occurs late in the course.[80] Patients with development of a cellular immune response tend to have the encephalitic (furious) form rather than the paralytic form, and they die faster than those who do not have such a response.[81] Differences in the host immune response appear more likely to explain whether furious or paralytic rabies develops than do differences in the strains of virus that cause the natural infection.[82] Some investigators believe that interleukin-1 production in the CNS may explain the immunosuppressive effect of the virus.[83] One study suggests that the virus may persist in macrophages and emerge later to produce disease,[84] which may explain some cases with very long incubation periods, or other tissue locations in which viral sequestration occurs.

Clinical Manifestations

HUMAN RABIES

Several variables affect the risk of rabies and the rate of clinical disease development after exposure to a rabid animal.[85] The viral inoculum is important, reflected by the relationship between the extent of exposure to the saliva and the rapidity of progression. A bite with prominent salivary contamination (e.g., through exposed skin) is more likely to produce rabies than a bite through thick clothing that removes saliva from the animal's teeth. Multiple bites are more likely to transmit the disease than a single bite. The location of the bite also influences the

risk of rabies: bites on the face are more likely to result in disease than those on the extremities. Salivary contamination of a preexisting wound can transfer virus, as can exposure of mucous membranes or the respiratory tract to aerosolized virus.[86]

Transmission between humans has been documented in corneal transplantation.[87,88] One recipient received standard PET plus interferon and did not have rabies develop.[88] In 2004, rabies was confirmed as the cause of death of multiple organ transplant recipients. Two kidneys, one liver, and an iliac artery segment were transplanted from a man in Texas who had died of unknown encephalopathy, later determined to be rabies virus. A public health inquiry determined that the infected donor had reported being bitten by a bat.[89] Six patients received organ or tissue donation from a woman in Germany who had been infected with rabies from a dog bite during a trip to India. Three of six recipients subsequently died of rabies.[90] The three other recipients, all of whom received PET, did not have symptoms of rabies develop.

The reported incubation period for rabies varies from a few days to more than 19 years, although 75% of patients become ill in the first 90 days after exposure. The three solid organ transplant patients described previously all became ill within 1 month of transplantation. The shorter period of incubation in these patients is theorized to be related to their immunosuppressed state.[91]

The initial symptoms of rabies resemble those of other systemic viral infections, including fever, headache, malaise, and disorders of the upper respiratory and gastrointestinal tracts (Table 163-3).[92] Initial neurologic symptoms may include subtle changes in personality and cognition and paresthesias or pain near the exposure site. Rabies is rarely considered early in the differential diagnosis. In one series, physicians considered rabies in only three of 21 patients on the first visit, despite an exposure history in many.[92] The prodrome typically lasts about 4 days, but up to 10 days may elapse before more specific symptoms and signs supervene.[92] Myoedema (mounding of part of the muscle struck with a reflex hammer, which then disappears in a few seconds) is present during the prodrome and persists throughout the disease.[93]

Human rabies infections are divided into two forms: furious (or "encephalitic") and paralytic (or "dumb"). The furious form presents with the hydrophobia, delirium, and agitation that form the common picture of rabies. About a fifth of patients present with the paralytic form and have little clinical evidence of cerebral involvement until late in the course. The spinal cord and brain stem bear the brunt of the illness in the paralytic form. The pathogenetic distinction between the two types of rabies is unclear; it does not appear to be based on virologic or antigenic differences.[94] In either form, the symptomatic course

TABLE 163-3	Durations of Different Stages of Rabies	
Stage	**Duration (% of Cases)**	**Associated Findings**
Incubation period	<30 d (25%) 30-90 d (50%) 90 d to 1 y (20%) >1 y (5%)	None.
Prodrome and early symptoms	2-10 d	Paresthesias or pain at the wound site; fever; malaise; anorexia; nausea and vomiting.
Acute neurologic disease; Furious rabies (80% of cases)	2-7 d	Hallucinations; bizarre behavior; anxiety; agitation; biting; hydrophobia; autonomic dysfunction; syndrome of inappropriate antidiuretic hormone (SIADH).
Paralytic rabies (20% of cases)	2-7 d	Ascending flaccid paralysis.
Coma, death*	0-14 d	—

*Rare recoveries have been reported.
Data from Fishbein DB. Rabies in humans. In: Baer GM, ed. *The Natural History of Rabies.* 2nd ed. Boca Raton, Fla: CRC Press; 1991:519-549.

usually runs 2 to 14 days before coma supervenes. In one series of 32 patients, the median duration of illness was 19 days.[95] Some of the cases of human rabies reported in recent years have not fit into these classic forms of rabies. The diagnosis should be considered for any unexplained progressive encephalitis.

Furious Rabies

Hydrophobia is the symptom most identified with *furious rabies*. Sir William Gowers[96] provides a seminal depiction of hydrophobia and its sequelae, in which he described:

"... some discomfort about the throat, an occasional sense of choking, or a little difficulty in swallowing liquids ... The attempt to drink occasions some spasm in the pharynx, which increases in the course of a few hours, and spreads to the muscles of respiration, causing a short, quick inspiration, a "catch in the breath ..." This increases in severity to a strong inspiratory effort, in which the extraordinary muscles of respiration, sterno-mastoid, scaleni, etc., and even the facial muscles, take part; the shoulders are raised, and the angles of the mouth drawn outwards. As the intensity of the spasm increases, so does the readiness with which it is excited. It may be caused by the mere contact of water with the lips, and a state of cutaneous hyperæsthesia develops, so that various impressions, such as a draught of air, which normally excite a respiratory effort, bring on the spasm. The mere movement of air caused by raising the bedclothes may be sufficient. The patient is often unable to swallow the saliva, which is usually abundant and viscid, so that it hangs about the mouth and is expelled with difficulty ... Vomiting is common ... The attacks of spasm are very distressing to the patient; the mental state which they occasion increases the readiness with which they are produced; and in some cases the mere sight of water or the sound of dropping water will cause an attack. It may even be excited by visual impressions which cause a similar sensation, as the reflection from a looking glass, or even a strong light. The sufferer's horror and dread of these excitants becomes intense. Thus the disturbance in the act of swallowing liquids, which constitutes ... the first symptom and keynote of the disease, spreads, on the one hand, to mental disturbance, and on the other to extensive muscular spasm. In each of these directions further symptoms develop. The spasm, at first confined to the muscles of deglutition and respiration, spreads to the other muscles of the body, and the paroxysms, at first respiratory, afterwards become general, and assume a convulsive character, although still excited by the same causes. The convulsions may consist of general muscular rigidity, sometimes tetanoid in character, with actual opisthotonus ... Actual delusions occasionally supervene, and there may even be wild delirium. The mental derangement is most intense during the paroxysms of spasms, and the frenzied patient may spit his saliva at those about him, and often attempts to bite them with his teeth, making occasional strange sounds in his throat which have been thought to resemble the barking of a dog."

Hydrophobia represents an exaggerated irritant reflex of the respiratory tract, possibly arising from the nucleus ambiguus.[97] Other findings include episodic hyperactivity, seizures, and aerophobia. Hyperventilation is frequently present. Along with coma, evidence of pituitary dysfunction often develops, especially disordered water balance (either inappropriate antidiuresis or diabetes insipidus). Hyperventilation gives way to forms of periodic and ataxic respiration,[97] and eventually apnea supervenes. Cardiac arrhythmias are common, predominantly supraventricular tachycardias and bradycardias, and reflect either brain stem dysfunction or myocarditis.[98] Autonomic dysfunction is observed, including pupillary dilation, anisocoria, piloerection, markedly increased salivation and sweating, and rarely, priapism[99] or spontaneous ejaculation.[100] Two cases are reported of rabies-associated cerebral artery vasospasm that was treatable with drugs directed at the nitric oxide synthase pathway.[101] This vasospasm may relate to a deficiency of tetrahydrobioterin, and might be ameliorated by its replacement.[102]

With exceptions in some rare reports, patients entering coma generally die within 1 to 2 weeks despite maximal supportive care. Patients with furious rabies who receive maximal intensive care support and survive for a longer-than-expected period appear to pass through the paralytic phase before death.[94]

Paralytic (Dumb) Rabies

Patients with *paralytic rabies*, unlike those with the furious form, do not have hydrophobia, aerophobia, hyperactivity, or seizures. Their initial findings suggest an ascending paralysis, including hypophonia, resembling acute inflammatory polyneuropathy (Guillain-Barré syndrome), or a symmetric quadriparesis. Weakness may be more severe in the extremity where the virus was introduced. Meningeal signs (headache, neck stiffness) may be prominent despite a normal sensorium. As the disease progresses, the patient becomes confused and then declines into coma.

Nonneurologic Findings

In addition to the cardiac arrhythmias already mentioned, the systemic complications of rabies are similar to those of other critically ill patients. The virus disseminates to many organs,[103,104] but proof of its role in other organ dysfunction is lacking. Gastrointestinal disturbances include bleeding, vomiting, diarrhea, and ileus.[105] Death is usually from cerebral edema or myocarditis, with cardiac arrhythmia or congestive heart failure as mechanisms.[106]

ANIMAL RABIES

A complete description of the effects of rabies on behavior in all of the species that can be infected is beyond the scope of this text. WHO studies have established a crude ranking of rabies susceptibility, which is summarized in Table 163-4.[107] Descriptions of the behavioral changes of rabid animals are available elsewhere.[108,109]

Diagnosis

The diagnosis of rabies poses little difficulty in a nonimmunized patient with hydrophobia after a bite by a known rabid animal. The presentation in areas where domestic animals are immunized is seldom this straightforward. During the incubation period, no diagnostic studies in the patient are useful; recognition of an exposure to a potentially rabid animal should prompt prophylactic treatment. When symptoms begin, standard laboratory testing does not reliably distinguish rabies from other encephalitides. The cerebrospinal fluid (CSF) may be normal; however, pleocytosis, mild elevation of red blood cells, and modest increase in protein have been described.[110,111]

TABLE 163-4	Susceptibility of Various Animal Species to Rabies		
Very High	*High*	*Moderate*	*Low*
Wolves	Hamsters	Dogs	Opossums
Foxes	Skunks	Primates	
Coyotes	Raccoons		
Kangaroo rats	Domestic cats		
Cotton rats	Rabbits		
Jackals	Bats		
Voles	Cattle		

Data from World Health Organization. Sixth Report of the Expert Committee on Rabies: Technical Report Series 523. Geneva: World Health Organization; 1973.

Direct fluorescent antibody (DFA) staining of biopsy or necropsy (animal or human) tissue remains the standard for the diagnosis of rabies. In humans, the procedure of choice is DFA analysis of a skin biopsy obtained from the nape of the neck, above the hairline.[112] The virus tends to localize in hair follicles. During the first week of symptoms, about 50% of samples reveal rabies virus, with an increasing percentage thereafter.[113] The reverse transcriptase–polymerase chain reaction (RT-PCR) is another diagnostic procedure of choice in suspected human rabies.[114] This test can be performed on CSF or saliva of patients or on tissue. RT-PCR allows more specific determination of the geographic and host species origin of a particular rabies virus.[115,116] It can be successfully performed on decomposed brain material,[117] whereas older techniques failed with that material.[118] The older corneal impression test[119] is no longer in common use. Current recommendations for diagnostic testing in animals and humans, with instructions for sample collection and submission, are available at http://www.cdc.gov/rabies or by calling the rabies laboratory of the Centers for Disease Control and Prevention (CDC) at (404) 639-1050. In the United States, the state health department should be consulted whenever the diagnosis of rabies is suspected. The state rabies consultation contact phone numbers are also available at the CDC web site.

The rapid fluorescent focus inhibition test (RFFIT) is a serologic test for neutralizing antirabies antibody.[120] A few untreated patients have detectable antibody by day 6 of clinical illness, 50% by day 8, and usually 100% by day 15. Any CSF levels are diagnostically valuable, even in patients who have received PET. CSF may also be examined for the presence of specific oligoclonal bands not found in the serum as a method of confirmation of CNS infection.[121]

Computed tomographic scan results of the brain are usually normal early in the course,[88] unless hypoxia has supervened. Later, evidence of cerebral swelling may supervene if the patient receives prolonged critical care support (Fig. 163-5). Magnetic resonance (MR) images

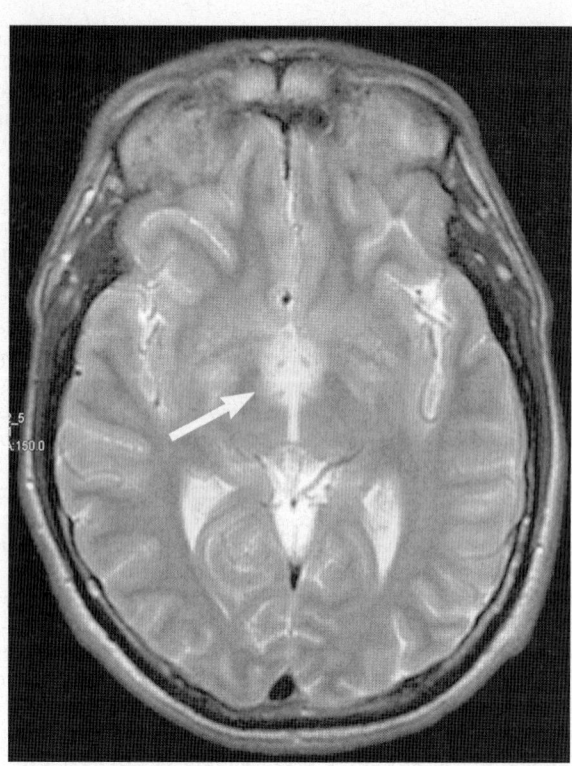

Figure 163-6   **T2-weighted MR image showing increased signal in diencephalon** *(arrow)*.

show areas of increased T_2 signal in the hippocampi, hypothalamus, brain stem, and sometimes other areas.[122] Figure 163-6 shows a T_2 image, with involvement of the thalamus and hypothalamus highlighted. Late in the course, gadolinium enhancement may occur in the most profoundly involved areas, indicating breakdown of the blood-brain barrier. In paralytic rabies, MR imaging of the spinal cord and nerve roots may be useful.[123] No imaging finding is pathomnemonic for rabies.

DIFFERENTIAL DIAGNOSIS

With furious rabies, the major differential consideration is another viral encephalitis. In the absence of exposure to a rabid animal, and if hydrophobia and hyperactivity are not prominent, distinguishing between the possibilities may be difficult.[124] Because the CSF and electroencephalographic (EEG) findings in rabies may mimic those of herpes simplex encephalitis, some patients receive empiric therapy with acyclovir while awaiting a more secure diagnosis (e.g., with PCR). Tetanus is occasionally confused with rabies because opisthotonic posturing may be seen in either.[62] However, the other symptoms of rabies, such as hydrophobia, are not seen in tetanus, and CSF and EEG results are normal in tetanus. Strychnine poisoning should be considered and can be excluded with laboratory testing.

Paralytic rabies may resemble acute inflammatory polyneuropathy, transverse myelitis, or poliomyelitis. Electromyographic studies may be useful in distinguishing rabies from polyneuropathy. In transverse myelitis, pain at the level of the lesion may be helpful, as may the finding of a high T_2 signal lesion. A sensory level is characteristic of transverse myelitis, whereas in rabies, sensory function is typically normal.[99] Fever usually precedes weakness in poliomyelitis, and the resolution of fever with the onset of neurologic findings favors this diagnosis. A history of poliomyelitis immunization should be sought.

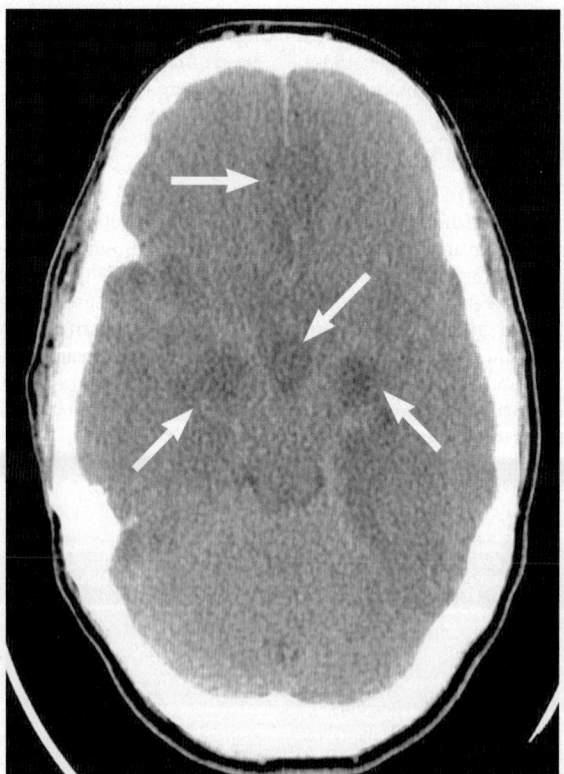

Figure 163-5   **Noncontrast computed tomographic scan showing areas of both severe cerebral edema** *(arrows)* **and more widespread swelling.**

The sometimes prolonged incubation period of rabies recalls the slow infections of the CNS caused by conventional viruses (e.g., progressive multifocal leukoencephalopathy).[125] However, rabies requires neither a defect in host immunity nor a mutation in the virus to produce disease, which distinguishes it from the agents in this group. Spongiform changes in brain tissue in rabies[126] may resemble those seen in the prion diseases.[127]

Although CNS reactions to the rabies vaccines available in developed countries are exceptionally rare, patients who receive older vaccine forms that contain myelin determinants occasionally have development of acute disseminated encephalomyelitis (ADEM; also called postvaccinial encephalomyelitis; see Prevention section). ADEM is a syndrome with many precipitants other than rabies vaccine. It resembles encephalitis, or occasionally, it presents as a mass lesion that resembles a brain abscess. It typically begins 10 to 14 days after vaccine exposure, which would constitute an unusually brief incubation period for rabies. In the absence of viral isolation, a high RFFIT titer in spinal fluid is evidence for rabies rather than ADEM, even in patients who have been immunized,[128] as are positive RT-PCR results. ADEM produces high-T_2 lesions visible with MR imaging.[129] However, differences in the distribution of the MR lesions in rabies and ADEM may aid in the differential diagnosis.[130]

Patients potentially exposed to rabies may have a psychologic reaction termed rabies hysteria.[131] They may refuse to drink water; in contrast, the patient with rabies attempts, at least initially, to drink but is halted by pharyngeal spasms.

▨ Prevention

PREEXPOSURE PROPHYLAXIS

Although control of animal rabies is central to prevention of human disease, few nations have eliminated it, and those that have been successful usually maintain quarantine procedures lest the disease reappear. Therefore, prophylactic procedures (for domestic animals and selected humans) and PET for humans remain essential. Prophylaxis for cats and dogs in many countries is required by law; in the United States, the use of 1-year or 3-year vaccines is permitted, although only the 3-year vaccines are recommended.[132] Vaccination should be performed or supervised by a veterinarian; improper administration can lead to lack of immunity.[133] Measurement of animal seroconversion rates may be considered to ensure protection,[134] and immunization of livestock is recommended in areas of increasing rabies prevalence.

Vaccination of wild animals is an effective public health measure.[135] The use of vaccines effective after ingestion allows immunization of wild animals.[136] An intensive 4-year campaign in Belgium nearly eliminated rabies from the fox population.[137] This approach may also be effective in dogs.[138] Veterinary vaccines cost about $0.50 per dose in the United States. In contrast, Semple-type (grown in sheep brain cultures) human vaccines cost about $5 per course, Vero cell vaccine in France about $160 per course, and human diploid cell rabies vaccine (HDCV) in the United States more than $500 per course.[139]

Preexposure prophylaxis is confined to people with a relatively high risk of rabies exposure, such as veterinarians, laboratory workers who use rabies virus, spelunkers, and people who plan to visit countries of high dog rabies prevalence where access to appropriate medical care is limited. Current recommendations for international travelers are available at the the CDC website (http://www.cdc.gov/rabies). A series of three intramuscular or intradermal injections (days 0, 7, and 21 or 28) is sufficient; antibody response determination is not required in normal hosts. Booster doses every 2 to 3 years are usually recommended for individuals frequently at risk of exposure. An adequate antibody response is generally considered to be complete neutralization at the 1:5 serum dilution level with the rapid fluorescent focus inhibition test, which is equivalent to the 0.5 IU/mL antibody titers suggested by the WHO.

POSTEXPOSURE TREATMENT

In New York State, the number of humans who received PET increased from 84 in 1989 to more than 1000 in 1992.[140] The median cost per patient in Massachusetts was $2376 in 1995, with estimates of the total cost to the state as high as $6.4 million.[141] Despite the relative high costs, the recent cost-effectiveness analysis of the Advisory Committee on Immunization Practices showed that it is always cost saving to administer PET if a patient is bitten by a rabid animal that has tested positive for rabies or if a patient is bitten by a reservoir vector species, even if the animal is not available for testing.[41]

The cornerstone of rabies prevention is wound care, which potentially reduces the risk of rabies by 90%.[142] Thorough washing with a 20% soap solution is as effective as the formerly recommended quaternary ammonium compounds.[143] Irrigation with a virucidal agent such as povidone-iodine is advisable.[144] After wound care, the clinician must decide whether to institute passive and active immunization. Prompt consultation with public health officials is advised because this decision is based on the current incidence of rabies in the animal species involved in the exposure.[145] The most recent report of the Immunization Practices Advisory Committee, is available at http://www.cdc.gov/rabies.[146]

In countries of low prevalence, a healthy dog or cat that has bitten, or otherwise transferred saliva to, a human is observed for 10 days. If the animal's behavior remains normal, the patient need not receive PET beyond proper wound care. If the animal's behavior changes, it should undergo immediate pathologic examination for evidence of rabies infection. If infection is confirmed, there is adequate time to institute PET. Wild mammal exposure, especially if the animal exhibits uncharacteristic behavior, warrants PET in most circumstances. If the animal is available for pathologic examination, and if pathologic examination of the brain does not indicate the presence of rabies virus, PET may be discontinued (Fig. 163-7). Discovery of a bat in a room with an infant or a child who cannot report the occurrence of a bite reliably, and on whom no bite is found, raises the issue of PET. If the bat is captured and tests positive for rabies, PET is indicated. If the bat is not captured, the decision about PET must be individualized. PET appears to be safe in pregnant women and should not be withheld when an indication exists.[147]

Postexposure treatment should always include administration of both passive antibody and vaccine for both bite and nonbite exposures in persons with no previous vaccination for rabies. Rabies immune globulin is available in human (HRIG) and equine forms (pooled antiserum of equine origin [ARS] and purified antirabies serum of equine origin [ERIG]). These immunoglobulins are purified from the sera of hyperimmunized donors. Two HRIG preparations are available in the United States: Imogam Rabies-HT (Pasteur Merieux) and BayRab (Bayer). HRIG is given only once in a dose of 20 IU/kg, and is applicable to all age groups, including children. The most recent WHO and CDC recommendations call for the entire dose to be infiltrated into the wound if anatomically feasible.[1,146] Any remaining volume should be administered intramuscularly (IM) at an anatomic site distant from that used for the active vaccine. The recommended dose of ERIG is 40 IU/kg. Failure to infiltrate wounds with rabies immune globulin, or surgical closure of wounds before immune globulin infiltration, has been associated with the development of rabies in patients despite otherwise proper PET.[148] If HRIG is not administered when active vaccination is begun, it can be administered through day 7 of the postexposure prophylaxis series.[146] The successful experimental administration of antirabies monoclonal antibodies raises the possibility that HRIG and ERIG might be replaced by a more easily produced and safer product.[149]

Many different forms of rabies vaccine have been produced since Pasteur's original success in 1882. In some developing nations, Semple-type vaccine is still used, but it carries a risk of central and peripheral neurologic complications in the range of 1 per 200 to 1600 vaccinees.[92] Production of vaccine in sheep CNS, a common method of Semple-type vaccine production, also carries the theoretic risk of

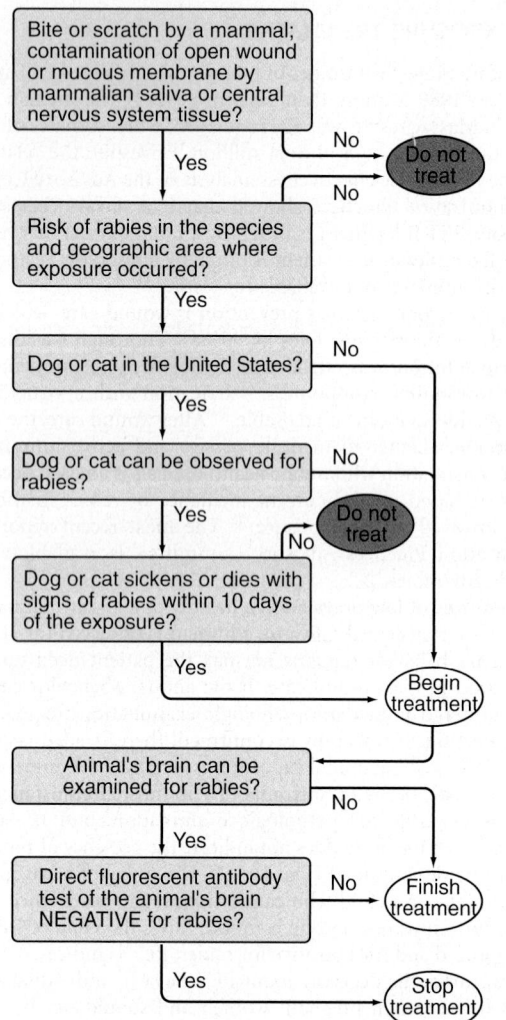

Figure 163-7 Algorithm for human rabies postexposure prophylaxis. In highly suspect animals, treatment should be started immediately and discontinued if fluorescent antibody test results of the animal brain are negative. In some cases with low risk, treatment may be delayed for up to 48 hours pending the result of fluorescent antibody testing.

transmitting the scrapie prion.[150] Suckling mouse brain vaccine is effective and safer, with a neurologic complication rate of approximately 1:8000.

The currently available vaccines licensed for human use in the United States include human diploid cell vaccine (HDCV; Imovax) and purified chick embryo cell vaccine (PCECV; RabAvert). Both are inactivated virus vaccines that are remarkably safe and immunogenic. Local reactions (pain, swelling, or induration) are common, but systemic symptoms (fever, headache, malaise, nausea, abdominal pain, or adenopathy) occur in only a minority of patients. Serious reactions have been exceedingly rare, with the Guillain-Barré syndrome reported rarely.[151] To report a vaccine reaction, call the appropriate number (for HDCV, Sanofi Pasteur at 800-822-2463; for PCECV, Novartis Vaccines at 800-244-7668). Corticosteroids should be given only to patients with a life-threatening vaccine reaction because they interfere with the development of immunity. Patients with immunocompromise may not respond adequately to vaccination, and antibody titers should be measured 2 to 4 weeks after immunization.[146]

In other countries, other PET vaccines (e.g., vaccines grown in chick embryos or Vero cell cultures)[152] and regimens are often used. Consultation with the rabies officer of the state health department may be helpful for the management of patients in whom PET has been initiated with a vaccine not approved for use in the United States.

Cross-protection is provided by rabies HDCV to ABLV.[153] Protocols for potential exposure to ABLV encourage thorough cleaning of the wound, use of the same vaccine doses and schedules as recommended for rabies, and testing the bat if possible for ABLV. Protocols differ in the specific recommendations regarding the influence of both bat testing and type of exposure on PET.[154]

The usual dose of HDCV for postexposure prophylaxis is 1.0 mL IM on the day of exposure (or as soon as possible thereafter), and repeated on days 3, 7, 14, and 28. For adults, the vaccination should always be administered in the deltoid area rather than the gluteal area. HDCV injections into the gluteal result in lower neutralizing antibody titers.[155] In small children, vaccination may be given in the lateral thigh. Other schedules are available for use; physicians not familiar with their use should consult local public health authorities and review the most recent WHO and CDC recommendations.[1,146] The varying immunogenicity of different regimens, and their interaction with the response to immunoglobulin,[156] raises the possibility of treatment failure if the recommendations are not carefully followed. The vaccine must not be given in the same region as the immunoglobulin. Intradermal vaccine administration was previously recommended for preexposure prophylaxis only, but WHO recommends it as an alternative for PET in areas where the cost of IM administration is prohibitive.[1] Patients who have been previously vaccinated receive 1.0 mL IM on days 0 and 3 only, without rabies immune globulin.

A single case of transient false-positive enzyme-linked immunosorbent assay (ELISA) results for human immunodeficiency virus (HIV) after HDCV immunization was reported in 1994.[157] Subsequent screening of samples from people recently immunized against rabies revealed no similar cases,[158,159] but in view of similar phenomena with other vaccines, physicians should be aware of this possibility.

Personnel who care for patients with rabies should practice standard universal and respiratory precautions. In addition, when they perform routine care duties without exposure to potentially contaminated materials, they should receive a preexposure immunization sequence and maintain a serum antirabies antibody titer of 0.5 IU/mL.[160] Exposures to potentially contaminated secretions or tissues should lead to standard PET.

Treatment

Only one case exists of complete recovery from rabies in a patient who had not received rabies prophylaxis either before or after illness onset.[161] The patient was a 15-year-old girl from Wisconsin who had a bat bite 1 month before symptom onset. The patient was admitted with fever, obtundation, ataxia, myoclonus, and dysarthria. The patient was placed into electrographic burst suppression with ketamine and midazolam. Antiviral therapy commenced with ribavirin and amantadine. Neither rabies vaccine nor rabies immune globulin was administered because the patient had an immune response in both the serum and the cerebrospinal fluid. The patient was discharged to home on the 76th day after admission with persistent choreoathetosis and ballismus. Twenty-seven months after exposure, the patient was taking college courses and attending to her own activities of daily living, with only mild neurologic deficits.[162]

Several case reports are found of subsequent treatment of human rabies with the Wisconsin protocol described previously, but all described patients ultimately died of the virus or complications of treatment.[163] No established, specific treatment exists for rabies once symptoms have begun. Despite excellent intensive care, almost all patients die of the disease or its complications within a few weeks of onset. The three patients in the 1970s who survived, two of whom made apparently complete recoveries,[164-166] represent very unusual occurrences. Each of these patients had undergone some form of PET, and this treatment seems likely to have modified the course. Another case with partial recovery was reported in 1994 in a child who received rabies vaccine without immunoglobulin.[121] Trials of many agents have been undertaken in clinical rabies, including interferons, interferon-inducing agents, ribavirin, and cytosine arabinoside, without beneficial effects.[160] A review of issues regarding possible treatment is available.[167]

A link to the Wisconsin protocol is available under the Health Care Professionals tab at http://www.cdc.gov/rabies.

REFERENCES

1. Available at http://www.who.int/immunization/topics/rabies/en/index.html.
2. Baer GM. Rabies: An historical perspective. *Infect Agents Dis.* 1994;3:168-180.
3. Blancou J, Aubert MFA, Artois M. Fox rabies. In: Baer GM, ed. *The Natural History of Rabies.* 2nd ed. Boca Raton, Fla: CRC Press; 1991:257-290.
4. Baer GM. Vampire bat and bovine paralytic rabies. In: Baer GM, ed. *The Natural History of Rabies.* 2nd ed. Boca Raton, Fla: CRC Press; 1991:389-403.
5. Rupprecht CE, Smith JS, Fekadu M, et al. The ascension of wildlife rabies: A cause for public health concern or intervention? *Emerging Infect Dis.* 1995;1:107-114.
6. Negri A. Zur Aetiologie der Tollwuth. Die Diagnose der Tollwuth auf Grund der neuen Befunde. *Z Hyg Infectionskr.* 1903;44:519-540.
7. Goldwasser RA, Kissling RE. Fluorescent antibody staining of street and fixed rabies virus antigens. *Proc Soc Exp Biol Med.* 1958;98:219-223.
8. Foord AJ, Heine HG, Pritchard LI, et al. Molecular diagnosis of lyssaviruses and sequence comparison of Australian bat lyssavirus samples. *Aust Vet J.* 2006;84:225-230.
9. Kuzmin IV, Niezgoda M, Frank R, et al. Possible emergence of west Caucasian bat virus in Africa. *Emerg Infect Dis.* 2008;14:1887-1999.
10. Botvinkin AD, Poleschuk EM, Kuzmin IV, et al. Novel lyssaviruses isolated from bats in Russia. *Emerg Infect Dis.* 2003;9:1623-1625.
11. Reif JS, Webb PA, Monath TP, et al. Epizootic vesicular stomatitis in Colorado, 1982: Infection in occupational risk groups. *Am J Trop Med Hyg.* 1987;36:17-82.
12. Stoeckle MY. Rhabdoviridae. In: Mandell GM, Bennett JE, Dolin R, eds. *Principles and Practice of Infectious Diseases.* New York: Churchill Livingstone; 1994:1526-1527.
13. Wunner WH. The chemical composition and molecular structure of rabies viruses. In: Baer GM, ed. *The Natural History of Rabies.* 2nd ed. Boca Raton, Fla: CRC Press; 1991:31-67.
14. Sokol F, Schlumberger HD, Wiktor TK, et al. Biochemical and biophysical studies on the nucleocapsid and on the RNA of rabies virus. *Virology.* 1969;38:651-665.
15. Dietzschold B, Rupprecht CE, Fu ZF, et al. Rhabdoviruses. In: Fields BN, Knipe DM, Howley PM, et al, eds. *Fields Virology.* 3rd ed. Philadelphia: Lippincott Raven; 1996:1137-1159.
16. Tordo N, Poch O, Ermine A, et al. Walking along the rabies genome: Is the large G-L intergenic region a remnant gene? *Proc Natl Acad Sci U S A.* 1986;83:3914-3918.
17. Bleck TP, Rupprecht CE. Rhabdoviruses. In: Richman DD, Whitley RJ, Hayden FG, eds. *Clinical Virology.* 2nd ed. Washington, DC: ASM Press; 2002:857-873.
18. Yang J, Koprowski H, Dietzschold B, et al. Phosphorylation of rabies virus nucleoprotein regulates viral RNA transcription and replication by modulating leader RNA encapsidation. *J Virol.* 1999;73:1661-1664.
19. Wu X, Gong X, Foley HD, et al. Both viral transcription and replication are reduced when the rabies virus nucleoprotein is not phosphorylated. *J Virol.* 2002;76:4153-4161.
20. Goto H, Minimoto N, Ito H, et al. Expression of the nucleoprotein of rabies virus in *Escherichia coli* and mapping of antigenic sites. *Arch Virol.* 1995;140:1061-1074.
21. Blumberg BM, Giorgi C, Kolakofsky D. N protein of vesicular stomatitis virus selectively encapsidates leader RNA in vitro. *Cell.* 1983;32:559-567.
22. Tordo N, Poch O, Ermine A, et al. Completion of the rabies virus genome sequence determination: Highly conserved domains among the L (polymerase) proteins of unsegmented negative-strand RNA viruses. *Virology.* 1988;165:565-576.
23. Levy JA, Fraenkel-Conrat H, Owens RA. *Virology.* Englewood Cliffs, NJ: Prentice Hall; 1994:77-85.
24. Coll JM. The glycoprotein G of rhabdoviruses. *Arch Virol.* 1995;140:827-851.
25. Mebatsion T, Weiland F, Conzelmann KK. Matrix protein of rabies virus is responsible for the assembly and budding of bullet-shaped particles and interacts with the transmembrane spike glycoprotein G. *J Virol.* 1999;73:242-250.
26. Finke S, Mueller-Waldeck R, Conzelmann KK. Rabies virus matrix protein regulates the balance of virus transcription and replication. *J Gen Virol.* 2003;84:1613-1621.
27. Finke S, Conzelmann KK. Dissociation of rabies virus matrix protein functions in regulation of viral RNA synthesis and virus assembly. *J Virol.* 2003;77:12074-12082.
28. Rupprecht CE, Dietzschold B, Wunner WH, et al. Antigenic relationships of lyssaviruses. In: Baer GM, ed. *The Natural History of Rabies.* 2nd ed. Boca Raton, Fla: CRC Press; 1991:69-100.
29. Seif I, Coulon P, Rollin PE, et al. Rabies virulence: Effect on pathogenicity and sequence characterization of rabies virus mutations affecting antigenic site III of the glycoprotein. *J Virol.* 1985;53:926-934.
30. Morimoto K, Ni Y-J, Kawai A. Syncytium formation is induced in the murine neuroblastoma cell cultures which produce pathogenic G proteins of the rabies virus. *Virology.* 1992;189:203-216.
31. Otvos L, Krivulka GR, Urge L, et al. Comparison of the effects of amino acid substitutions and the β-*N*- vs. α-*O*-glycosylation on the T-cell stimulatory activity and conformation of an epitope on the rabies virus glycoprotein. *Biochim Biophys Acta.* 1995;1267:55-64.
32. Kawai A, Morimoto K. Functional aspects of lyssavirus proteins. In: Rupprecht CE, Dietzschold B, Koprowski H, eds. *Lyssaviruses.* Berlin: Springer-Verlag; 1994:27-42.
33. Thoulouze MI, Lafage M, Schachner M, et al. The neural cell adhesion molecule is a receptor for rabies virus. *J Virol.* 1998;72:7181-7190.
34. Burrage TG, Tignor GH, Smith AL. Rabies virus binding at neuromuscular junctions. *Virus Res.* 1985;2:273-289.
35. Gosztonyi G. Reproduction of lyssaviruses: Ultrastructural composition of lyssaviruses and functional aspects of pathogenesis. In: Rupprecht CE, Dietzschold B, Koprowski H, eds. *Lyssaviruses.* Berlin: Springer-Verlag; 1994:43-68.
36. Murphy FA, Bauer SP, Harrison AK, et al. Comparative pathogenesis of rabies and rabies-like viruses: Infection of the central nervous system and centrifugal spread to peripheral tissues. *Lab Invest.* 1973;29:1-16.
37. Available at http://www.who.int/rabies/rabnet/en.
38. Turner GS. A review of the world epidemiology of rabies. *Trans R Soc Trop Med Hyg.* 1976;70:175-178.
39. *Rabies vaccine WHO position paper.* WHO Weekly Epidemiological Record, December 7, 2007. No. 49/50: 425-436.
40. Meslin F-X, Fishbein DB, Matter HC. Rationale and prospects for rabies elimination in developing countries. In: Rupprecht CE, Dietzschold B, Koprowski H, eds. *Lyssaviruses.* Berlin: Springer-Verlag; 1994:1-26.
41. Blanton JD, Palmer D, Christin KA, et al. Rabies surveillance in the United States during 2007. *JAVMA.* 2008;884-897.
42. Velasco-Villa A, Messenger SL, Orciari LA, et al. Identification of new rabies virus variant in Mexican immigrant. *Emerg Infect Dis.* 2008;14:1906-1908.
43. Blanton JD, Hanlon CA, Ruppreсt CE. Rabies surveillance in the United States during 2006. *JAVMA.* 2007;231:540-556.
44. Centers for Disease Control and Prevention. First human death associated with raccoon rabies: Virginia, 2003. *MMWR Morb Mortal Wkly Rep.* 2003;52:1102-1103.
45. Rupprecht CE, Smith JS. Raccoon rabies: The re-emergence of an epizootic in a densely populated area. *Semin Virol.* 1994;5:155-164.
46. Krebs JW, Strine TW, Smith JS, et al. Rabies surveillance in the United States during 1994. *J Am Vet Med Assoc.* 1995;297:1562-1575.
47. Childs JE, Trimarchi CV, Krebs JW. The epidemiology of bat rabies in New York State, 1988-92. *Epidemiol Infect.* 1994;113:501-511.
48. Centers for Disease Control and Prevention. Human rabies: Connecticut, 1995. *MMWR Morb Mortal Wkly Rep.* 1996;45:207-209.
49. Clark KA, Neill SU, Smith JS, et al. Epizootic canine rabies transmitted by coyotes in south Texas. *J Am Vet Med Assoc.* 1994;204:536-540.
50. East ML, Hofer H, Cox JH, et al. Regular exposure to rabies virus and lack of symptomatic disease in Serengeti spotted hyenas. *Proc Natl Acad Sci U S A.* 2001;98:15026-15031.
51. Echevarria JE, Avellon A, Juste J, et al. Screening of active lyssavirus infection in wild bat populations by viral RNA detection on oropharyngeal swabs. *J Clin Microbiol.* 2001;39:3678-3683.
52. Nadin-Davis SA, Loza-Rubio E. The molecular epidemiology of rabies associated with chiropteran hosts in Mexico. *Virus Res.* 2006;117:215-226.
53. Leslie MJ, Messenger S, Rohde RE, et al. Bat-Associated rabies virus in Skunks. *Emerg Infect Dis.* 2006;12:1274-1277.
54. Centers of Disease Control and Prevention. Human rabies: Alabama, Tennessee, and Texas, 194. *MMWR Morb Mort Wkly Rep.* 1995;44:269-272.
55. Schmida TO. Resurgence of rabies. *Arch Pediatr Adolesc Med.* 1995;149:1043.
56. Murphy FA, Bauer SP, Harrison AK, et al. Comparative pathogenesis of rabies and rabies-like viruses: Virus infection and transit from inoculation site to the central nervous system. *Lab Invest.* 1973;28:361-376.
57. Watson HD, Tignor GH, Smith AL. Entry of rabies virus into the peripheral nerves of mice. *J Gen Virol.* 1981;56:371-382.
58. Lentz TL, Burrage TG, Smith AL, et al. Is the acetylcholine receptor a rabies virus receptor? *Science.* 1982;215:182-184.
59. Lentz TL, Wilson PT, Hawrot E, et al. Amino acid sequence similarity between rabies virus glycoprotein and snake venom curaremimetic neurotoxins. *Science.* 1984;226:847-848.
60. Kelly RM, Strick PL. Rabies as a transneuronal tracer of circuits in the central nervous system. *J Neurosci Methods.* 2000;103:63-71.
61. Raux H, Flamand A, Blondel D. Interaction of the rabies virus P protein with the LC8 dynein light chain. *J Virol.* 2000;74:10212-10216.
62. Bleck TP, Brauner JS. Tetanus. In: Scheld WM, Whitley RJ, Marra CM, eds. *Infections of the Central Nervous System.* 3rd ed. New York: Lippincott Williams & Wilkins; 2004:625-648.
63. Ugolini G. Specificity of rabies virus as a transneuronal tracer of motor networks: Transfer from hypoglossal motoneurons to connected second-order and higher order central nervous system cell groups. *J Comp Neurol.* 1995;356:457-480.
64. Jackson AC. Rabies virus infection: An update. *J Neurovirol.* 2003;9:253-258.
65. Charlton KM. The pathogenesis of rabies and other lyssaviral infections: Recent studies. In: Rupprecht CE, Dietzschold B, Koprowski H, eds. *Lyssaviruses.* Berlin: Springer-Verlag; 1994:95-119.
66. Koschel K, Munzel P. Inhibition of opiate receptor-mediated signal transmission by rabies virus in persistently infected NG-108-15 mouse neuroblastoma: Rat glioma hybrid cells. *Proc Natl Acad Sci U S A.* 1984;81:950-954.
67. Hooper DC, Ohnishi ST, Kean R, et al. Local nitric oxide production in viral and autoimmune diseases of the central nervous system. *Proc Natl Acad Sci U S A.* 1995;92:5312-5316.
68. Morimoto K, Hooper DC, Spitsin S, et al. Pathogenicity of different rabies virus variants inversely correlates with apoptosis and rabies virus glycoprotein expression in infected primary neuron cultures. *J Virol.* 1999;73:510-518.
69. Baloul L, Lafon M. Apoptosis and rabies virus neuroinvasion. *Biochimie.* 2003;85:777-788.
70. Esiri MM, Kennedy PGE. Virus diseases. In: Adams JH, Duchen LW, eds. *Greenfield's Neuropathology.* New York: Oxford University Press; 1992:335-399.
71. Dupont JR, Earle KM. Human rabies encephalitis: A study of forty-nine fatal cases with a review of the literature. *Neurology.* 1965;15:1023-1034.
72. De Brito T, Araujo MD, Tiriba A. Ultrastructure of the Negri body in human rabies. *J Neurol Sci.* 1973;20:363-372.
73. Sung JH, Hayano M, Mastri AR, et al. A case of human rabies and ultrastructure of the Negri body. *J Neuropath Exp Neurol.* 1976;35:541-559.
74. Jackson AC, Ye H, Ridaura-Sanz C, et al. Quantitative study of the infection in brain neurons in human rabies. *J Med Virol.* 2001;65:614-618.
75. Chopra JS, Banerjee AK, Murthy JMK, et al. Paralytic rabies: A clinicopathologic study. *Brain.* 1980;103:789-802.
76. Cohen SL, Gardner S, Lanyi C, et al. A case of rabies in man: Some problems of diagnosis and management. *Br Med J.* 1976;1:1041-1042.
77. de Fatima Araujo M, de Brito T, Machado CG. Myocarditis in human rabies. *Rev Inst Med Trop Sao Paulo.* 1971;13:99-102.
78. Metze K, Feiden W. Rabies virus ribonucleoprotein in the heart. *N Engl J Med.* 1991;324:1814-1815.
79. Wiktor TJ, Doherty PC, Koprowski H. Suppression of cell mediated immunity by street rabies virus. *J Exp Med.* 1977;145:1617-1622.
80. Kasempimolporn S, Hemachudha T, Khawplod P, et al. Human immune response to rabies nucleocapsid and glycoprotein antigens. *Clin Exp Immunol.* 1991;84:195-199.
81. Hemachudha T, Phanuphak P, Sriwanthana B. Immunologic study of human encephalitic and paralytic rabies: A preliminary study of 16 patients. *Am J Med.* 1988;84:673-677.
82. Hemachudha T, Wacharapluesadee S, Lumlertdaecha B, et al. Sequence analysis of rabies virus in humans exhibiting encephalitic or paralytic rabies. *J Infect Dis.* 2003;188:960-966.
83. Haour F, Marquette C, Ban E, et al. Receptors for interleukin-1 in the central nervous system and neuroendocrine systems. *Ann Endocrinol (Paris).* 1995;56:173-179.
84. Ray NB, Ewalt LC, Lodmell DL. Rabies virus replication in primary murine bone marrow macrophages and in human and murine macrophage-like cell lines: Implications for viral persistence. *J Virol.* 1995;69:764-772.
85. Whitley RJ, Middlebrooks M. Rabies. In: Scheld WM, Whitley RJ, Durack DT, eds. *Infections of the Central Nervous System.* New York: Raven Press; 1991:127-144.
86. Constantine DG. *Rabies transmission by air in bat caves.* United States Public Health Service Publication; 1617:1967.

87. Sureau P, Portnoi D, Rollin D, et al. Prévention de la transmission inter-humaine de la rage greffe de cornée. *C R Seances Acad Sci*. 1981;293:689-692.

88. Houff SA, Burton RC, Wilson RW, et al. Human-to-human transmission of rabies virus by corneal transplant. *N Engl J Med*. 1979;300:603-604.

89. Update: Investigation of rabies infections in organ donor and transplant recipients: Alabama, Arkansas, Oklahoma, and Texas, 2004. *MMWR*. 2004;53(Dispatch):1.

90. Johnson N, Brookes SM, Fook AR, et al. Review of human rabies cases in the UK and Germany. *The Veterinary Record*. 2005; 157:715.

91. Srinivasan A, Burton EC, Kuehnert MJ, et al. Transmission of Rabies Virus from an Organ Donor to Four Transplant Recipients. *N Engl J Med*. 2005;352:1103-1111.

92. Fishbein DB, Bernard KW. Rabies virus. In: Mandell GM, Bennett JE, Dolin R, eds. *Principles and Practice of Infectious Diseases*. New York: Churchill Livingstone; 1994:1527-1543.

93. Hemachuda T, Phanthumchinda K, Phanuphak P, et al. Myoedema as a clinical sign in paralytic rabies. *Lancet*. 1987;1:1210.

94. Gode GR, Saksena R, Batra RK, et al. Treatment of 54 clinically diagnosed rabies patients with two survivals. *Indian J Med Res*. 1988;88:564-566.

95. Noah DL, Drenzek CL, Smith JS, et al. Epidemiology of Human Rabies in the United States, 1980-1996. *Annals of Internal Medicine*. 1998;128:922-930.

96. Gowers WR. *A manual of diseases of the nervous system*. Philadelphia: Blakiston; 1888:1237-1254.

97. Warrell DA, Davidson NM, Pope HM, et al. Pathophysiologic studies in human rabies. *Am J Med*. 1976;60:180-190.

98. Cheetham HD, Hart J, Coghill NF, et al. Rabies with myocarditis: Two cases in England. *Lancet*. 1970;1:921-922.

99. Dutta JK. Rabies presenting with priapism (Letter). *J Assoc Physicians India*. 1994;42:430.

100. Human Rabies: California, Georgia, Minnesota 2000. *MMWR*. 2000;29:1111-1115.

101. Willoughby RE, Roy-Burman A, Martin KW, et al. Generalized cranial artery spasm in human rabies. *Develop Biol*. 2008;131:367-375.

102. Willoughby RE, Opladen T, Maier T, et al. Tetrahydrobiopterin deficiency in human rabies. *J Inherit Metab Dis*. 2008 [Epub ahead of print.]

103. Jackson AC, Ye H, Phelan CC, et al. Extraneural organ involvement in human rabies. *Lab Invest*. 1999;79:945-951.

104. Jogai S, Radotra BD, Banerjee AK. Rabies viral antigen in extracranial organs: A post-mortem study. *Neuropathol Appl Neurobiol*. 2002;28:334-338.

105. Bhatt DR, Hattwick MAW, Gerdson R, et al. Human rabies: Diagnosis, complications, and prognosis. *Am J Dis Child*. 1974;127:862-869.

106. Warrell DA. The clinical picture of rabies in man. *Trans R Soc Trop Med Hyg*. 1976;701:188-195.

107. World Health Organization. *Sixth report of the expert committee on rabies: Technical report series 523*. Geneva: World Health Organization; 1973.

108. Baer GM, ed. *The Natural History of Rabies*. 2nd ed. Boca Raton, Fla: CRC Press; 1991.

109. Bleck TP, Rupprecht CE. Rabies. In: Richman DD, Whitley RJ, Hayden FG, eds. *Clinical Virology*. New York: Churchill Livingstone; 1997:879-897.

110. Lewis RL. A 10-year-old boy evacuated from the Mississippi Gulf coast after Hurricane Katrina presents with agitation, hallucinations, and fever. *J Emerg Nurs*. 2007;33:42-44.

111. Human Rabies: Minnesota, 2007. *MMWR*. 2008;57:460-462.

112. Bryceson AD, Greenwood BM, Warrell DA, et al. Demonstration during life of rabies antigen in humans. *J Infect Dis*. 1975;131:71-74.

113. Blenden DC, Creech W, Torres-Anjel MJ. Use of immunofluorescence examination to detect rabies virus in the skin of humans with clinical encephalitis. *J Infect Dis*. 1986;154: 698-701.

114. Crepin P, Audry L, Rotivel Y, et al. Intravital diagnosis of human rabies by PCR using saliva and cerebrospinal fluid. *J Clin Microbiol*. 1998;36:1117-1121.

115. Arai YT, Yamada K, Kameoka Y, et al. Nucleoprotein gene analysis of fixed and street rabies virus variants using RT-PCR. *Arch Virol*. 1997;142:1787-1796.

116. Nadin-Davis SA. Polymerase chain reaction protocols for rabies virus discrimination. *J Virol Methods*. 1998;75:1-8.

117. Whitby JE, Johnstone P, Sillero-Zubiri C. Rabies virus in the decomposed brain of an Ethiopian wolf detected by nested reverse transcription-polymerase chain reaction. *J Wildl Dis*. 1997;33:912-915.

118. Albas A, Ferrari CI, da Silva LH, et al. Influence of canine brain decomposition on laboratory diagnosis of rabies. *Rev Soc Bras Med Trop*. 1999;32:19-22.

119. Zaidman GW, Billingsley A. Corneal impression test for the diagnosis of acute rabies encephalitis. *Ophthalmology*. 1998;105: 249-251.

120. Smith JS, Yager PA, Baer GM. A rapid reproducible test for determining rabies neutralizing antibody. *Bull WHO*. 1973;48:535-541.

121. Alvarez L, Fajardo R, Lopez E, et al. Partial recovery from rabies in a nine-year-old boy. *Ped Infect Dis J*. 1994;13:1154-1155.

122. Laothamatas J, Hemachuda T, Mitrabhakdi E, et al. MR imaging in human rabies. *AJNR Am J Neuroradiol*. 2003;24:1102-1109.

123. Desai RV, Jani V, Singh P, et al. Radiculomyelitic rabies: Can MR imaging help? *AJNR Am J Neuroradiol*. 2002;23:632-634.

124. Whitley RJ. Viral encephalitis. *N Engl J Med*. 1990;323: 242-250.

125. Johnson RT. Slow infections of the central nervous system caused by conventional viruses. In: Björnsson J, Carp RI, Löve A, Wisniewski HM, eds. Slow infections of the central nervous system. *Ann N Y Acad Sci*. 1994;724:6-13.

126. Bundza A, Charlton KM. Comparison of spongiform lesions in experimental scrapie and rabies in skunks. *Acta Neuropathol*. 1988;3:275-280.

127. Bleck TP, Alston SR. Prion diseases. In: Bleck TP, ed. *Central Nervous System and Ocular Infections*. In: Mandell GM, series editor. Atlas of Infectious Diseases. New York: Churchill Livingstone; 1995:11.1-11.16.

128. Warrell MJ, Looareesuwan S, Manatsathit S, et al. Rapid diagnosis of rabies and post-vaccinal encephalitides. *Clin Exp Immunol*. 1988;71:229-234.

129. Murthy JM. MRI in acute disseminated encephalomyelitis following Semple antirabies vaccine. *Neuroradiology*. 1998;40: 420-423.

130. Mani J, Reddy BC, Borgohain R, et al. Magnetic resonance imaging in rabies. *Postgrad Med J*. 2003;79:352-354.

131. Fishbain DA, Barsky S, Goldberg M. Monosymptomatic hypochondriacal psychosis: Belief of contracting rabies. *Int J Psychiatry Med*. 1992;22:3-9.

132. Centers for Disease Control and Prevention. Compendium of animal rabies control, 1999. *J Am Vet Med Assoc*. 1999;214: 198-202.

133. Conti LA, Tucker G, Heston S. Rabies in a dog vaccinated by its owner (Letter). *J Am Vet Med Assoc*. 1994;205:1301.

134. Eng TR, Fishbein DB, Talamante HE, et al. Immunogenicity of rabies vaccines used during an urban epizootic of rabies in Mexico. *Vaccine*. 1994;12:1259-1306.

135. Schneider LG. Rabies virus vaccines. *Dev Biol Stand*. 1995;84:49-54.

136. Rupprecht CE, Hanlon CA, Niezgoda M, et al. Recombinant rabies vaccines: Efficacy assessment in free-ranging animals. *Onderstepoort J Vet Res*. 1993;60:463-468.

137. Brochier B, Boulanger D, Costy F, et al. Toward rabies elimination in Belgium by fox vaccination using a vaccinia-rabies glycoprotein recombinant virus. *Vaccine*. 1994;12:1368-1371.

138. Matter HC, Kharmachi H, Haddad N, et al. Test of three bait types for oral immunization of dogs against rabies in Tunisia. *Am J Trop Med Hyg*. 1995;52:489-495.

139. Petricciani JC. Ongoing tragedy of rabies. *Lancet*. 1993;342: 1067-1068.

140. Extension of the raccoon rabies epizootic: United States, 1992. *MMWR Morb Mortal Wkly Rep*. 1992;41:661-664.

141. Kreindel SM, McGuill M, Meltzer M, et al. The cost of rabies postexposure prophylaxis: One state's experience. *Public Health Rep*. 1998;113:247-251.

142. Dean DJ. Pathogenesis and prophylaxis of rabies in man. *N Y State J Med*. 1963;63:3507-3513.

143. Anderson LJ, Winkler WG. Aqueous quaternary ammonium compounds and rabies treatment. *J Infect Dis*. 1979;139: 494-495.

144. Griego RD, Rosen T, Orengo IF, Wolf JE. Dog, cat, and human bites: A review. *J Am Acad Dermatol*. 1995;33:1019-1029.

145. Mann JM, Burkhart MJ, Rollag OJ. Anti-rabies treatment in New Mexico: Impact of a comprehensive consultations-biologics system. *Am J Public Health*. 1980;70:128-132.

146. Manning SE, Rupprecht CE, Fishbein D, et al. Human Rabies Prevention: United States, 2008; Recommendations of the Advisory Committee on Immunization Practices. *MMWR*. 2008;57;1-26, 28.

147. Chutivongse S, Wilde H, Benjavongkulchai M, et al. Postexposure rabies vaccination during pregnancy: Effect on 202 women and their infants. *Clin Infect Dis*. 1995;20:818-820.

148. Wilde H, Sirikawin S, Sabcharoen A, et al. Failure of postexposure treatment of rabies in children. *Clin Infect Dis*. 1996;22: 228-232.

149. Bakker AB, Python C, Kissling CJ, et al. First administration to humans of a monoclonal antibody cocktail against rabies virus: Safety, tolerability, and neutralizing activity. *Vaccine*. 2008;26: 5922-5927.

150. Arya SC. Transmissible spongiform encephalopathies and sheep-brain derived rabies vaccines (Letter). *Biologicals*. 1994;22:73.

151. Bernard KW, Smith PW, Kader FJ, et al. Neuroparalytic illness and human diploid cell rabies vaccine. *JAMA*. 1982;248: 3136-3138.

152. Hemachuda T, Mitrabhakdi E, Wilde H, et al. Additional reports of failure to respond to treatment after rabies exposure in Thailand. *Clin Infect Dis*. 1999;28:143-144.

153. Brookes SM, Parsons G, Johnson N. Rabies human diploid cell vaccine elicits cross-neutralising and cross-protecting immune responses against European and Australian bat lyssavirus. *Vaccine*. 2005;23:4101-4109.

154. Ewald B, Durrheim D. Australian bat lyssavirus: examination of exposure in NSW. *NSW Public Health Bulletin*. 2008;19:104-107.

155. Fishbein DB, Sayer LA, Reid-Sanden FL, et al. Administration of human diploid cell rabies vaccine in the gluteal area. *N Engl J Med*. 1988;318: 124-125.

156. Lang J, Simanjuntak GH, Soerjosembodo S, et al. Suppressant effect of human or equine rabies immunoglobulins on the immunogenicity of post-exposure rabies vaccination under the 2-1-1 regimen: A field trial in Indonesia. MAS054 Clinical Investigator Group. *Bull World Health Organ*. 1998;76: 491-495.

157. Pearlman E, Ballas S. False-positive human immunodeficiency virus screening test related to rabies vaccination. *Arch Pathol Lab Med*. 1994;118:805-806.

158. Plotkin SA, Loupi E, Blondeau C. False-positive human immunodeficiency virus screening test related to rabies vaccination (Letter). *Arch Pathol Lab Med*. 1995;119:679.

159. Henderson S, Leibnitz G, Turnbull M, et al. False-positive human immunodeficiency virus seroconversion is not common following rabies vaccination. *Clin Diagn Lab Immunol*. 2002;9:942-943.

160. Dutta JK, Dutta TK. Treatment of clinical rabies in man: Drug therapy and other measures. *Clin Pharmacol Therapeut*. 1994; 32:594-597.

161. Willoughby RE, Tieves KS, Hoffman GM, et al. Survival after treatment for rabies with induction of coma. *NEJM*. 2005;352(24):2508-2514.

162. Hu WT, Willoughby RE, Dhonau H, et al. Long-term follow-up after treatment of rabies by induction of coma. *N Engl J Med*. 2007;357;945-946.

163. Human rabies: Indiana and California 2006. *MMWR*. 2007;56: 361-365.

164. Hattwick MA, Weis TT, Stechschulte CJ, et al. Recovery from rabies: A case report. *Ann Intern Med*. 1972;76: 931-942.

165. Porras C, Barboza JJ, Fuenzalida E, et al. Recovery from rabies in man. *Ann Intern Med*. 1976;85:44-48.

166. Rabies in a laboratory worker: New York. *MMWR Morb Mortal Wkly Rep*. 1977:26:183.

167. Jackson AC, Warrell MJ, Rupprecht CE, et al. Management of human rabies. *Clin Infect Dis*. 2003;36:60-63.

164

Marburg and Ebola Virus Hemorrhagic Fevers

C. J. PETERS

Filoviruses are uncommonly encountered, and their natural history is only now being understood. Because of the serious human disease they cause and our lack of predictive information about them, they require our attention.[1] These agents cause a severe, unrelenting viral hemorrhagic fever with high mortality. The identification of Marburg virus in 1967 was the first of only a handful of independent isolations of Marburg virus or the related Ebola virus from humans.[1,2] Most episodes have been characterized by the mysterious emergence of a filovirus with no traces of its origin detectable and the subsequent spread of a single genotype because of the low levels of hygiene in African hospitals. Recent cave-related epidemics have suggested that bats may be the reservoir with multiple introductions of differing genotypes. Primates (humans, monkeys, chimpanzees, gorillas) are the major disease targets. Viral epidemics have originated from Africa and apparently from a source in the Philippines. The name of the viral family comes from their characteristic threadlike (filo, Latin for "filament") morphology, and this has made their recognition in tissues or clinical samples unusually readily achieved with the electron microscope.

Viral Characterization

Filoviruses are elongated structures 80 nm in diameter. The basic length of the replicative form is 790 nm for Marburg virus and 970 nm for Ebola virus, but long, branching convoluted structures are often formed (Fig. 164-1).[3,4] The 50-nm helical nucleocapsid is surrounded by a spike-studded membrane formed as the virus buds from the host cell. Inclusions of nucleocapsid aggregates can be visualized by electron microscopy of thin sections and are often visible as magenta-staining cytoplasmic structures in ordinary pathologic sections.

The virion genetic material is a single strand of negative-sense RNA of 4.2×10^6 daltons that produces monocistronic messages during infection. These properties and the gene organization, virion structure, and viral sequence information place these viruses in a distinct family, Filoviridae, in the order Mononegavirales. The glycoprotein (GP) gene codes for the 125-kDa (Ebola) or 170-kDa (Marburg) transmembrane spike protein that is highly glycosylated and is antigenically most characteristic for each virus.[3,4] Other virion proteins include a polymerase (180 kD), a nucleocapsid protein (96 to 104 kD), a matrix protein (40 kD), and three smaller proteins. Ebola viruses also code for a truncated glycoprotein species that is produced in soluble form.[5]

There are five known species of Ebola that differ significantly from one another,[2,5] and a single Marburg species with one subtype has been recognized (Fig. 164-2). Comparison of 1172 nucleotides from the GP gene shows more than a 40% difference between any pair of the three subtypes from Sudan, Zaire, Ivory Coast, Reston, and Bundibugyo. Marburg viral strains differ from Ebola viruses in their genome organization, the size of their structural proteins, their glycosylation patterns, and their virion length, and they are classified as a separate genus.[4]

No serologic cross-reactivity has been demonstrated between the Marburg and Ebola viruses. The Ebola subtypes share varied degrees of cross-reactivity by the commonly used indirect fluorescent antibody or the enzyme-linked immunosorbent assay (ELISA) test.[4] No hemagglutinin has been demonstrated. An unusual biologic feature of filoviruses has been the difficulty in demonstrating neutralization in cell culture or animals by convalescent sera.

Epidemiology

BASIC ECOLOGY

The natural history of filoviruses remained a mystery until recently.[1] Each filovirus case or epidemic has been investigated for the source of the virus, but without success, whether Ebola (Fig. 164-3) or Marburg (Fig. 164-4). In the case of epidemics, it has usually been possible to trace the epidemic back to a human or nonhuman primate index case, but no further. Suspects have included spiders, soft ticks, bats, and monkeys, but without field evidence to incriminate any of these. Recently, however, there have been two epidemics of Marburg virus with a series of primary infections originating from cave exposure; this, combined with reverse transcriptase-polymerase chain reaction (RT-PCR)–positive reactions from bats, particularly Rousettus aegyptiacus, and suggestions of prolonged infection in experimentally infected bats, places fruit bats as a focus of interest as possible reservoirs.[6,7]

MARBURG VIRUS

In 1967, African green monkeys were brought from Uganda to Europe for use in vaccine production and biomedical research. They were infected with a "new" virus that resulted in deaths among the monkeys and transmission to humans. Seven deaths occurred among the 25 primary and 6 secondary human cases.[8] After 3 other isolated human cases with limited transmission, a major epidemic occurred in Angola with 252 cases and a 90% case-fatality rate. The case-fatality rate was surprisingly high because in the former epidemics, only about one third of cases died. It is not known why this virus appeared to be so virulent but fell well within the phylogenetic group (see Fig. 164-2) of the major clade of Marburg viruses, although the virulence in macaques appears to be higher than other strains.

A second large Marburg virus epidemic occurred over a prolonged period from 1998 to 2000.[9] This outbreak was epidemiologically linked to an underground gold mine and had multiple introductions of Marburg viruses of different phylogenetic lineages. This provided a major opportunity to implicate bats as reservoirs, and indeed RT-PCR products and antibody were found in several bats and represented slightly different genotypes.

EBOLA VIRUS (ZAIRE, SUDAN, AND CÔTE D'IVOIRE SUBTYPES)

Ebola virus was first recognized in 1976, when two unrelated epidemics occurred in northern Zaire and 850 km away in southern Sudan; 88% of the patients in 318 recognized cases died in the former, and 53% of 284 in the latter.[10,11] Disease recurred in the same area of the Sudan in 1979.[12] Ebola hemorrhagic fever was not recognized again for almost two decades. Then, in 1995 and 1996, an additional Ebola subtype (Côte d'Ivoire) was isolated from a human patient,[13] three separate Zaire subtype epidemics were recognized in Gabon,[14] and a major epidemic (315 cases, 81% case-fatality rate) from the Zaire subtype occurred in Kikwit, Zaire.[15] Notably, one Gabon patient made his way from Libreville, where he fell ill, to a modern hospital in South Africa.[16] Despite the fact that his infection was not recognized as Ebola, he transmitted the disease to only a single nurse. The secondary infection was unfortunately fatal, but the entire episode illustrates the low risk in a modern hospital setting. More recently, smoldering outbreaks of

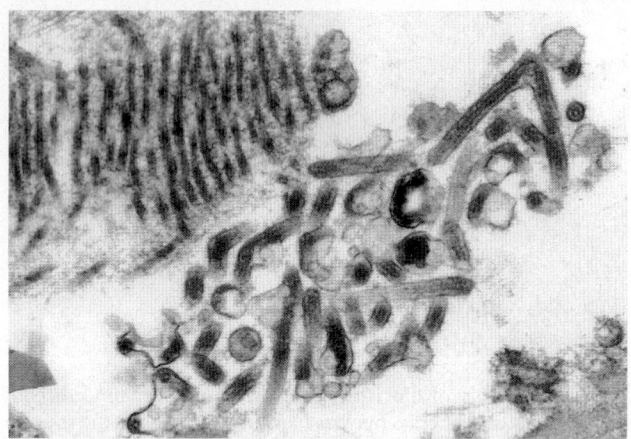

Figure 164-1 Ebola virus, Zaire subtype, human lung—Kikwit, Zaire (now Democratic Republic of the Congo), 1995. Longitudinal and cross sections showing filamentous nucleocapsid, viral envelope, and surface projections. Original magnification, ×17,000. *(Courtesy of Cynthia Goldsmith and Pierre Rollin, Special Pathogens Branch, Centers for Disease Control and Prevention.)*

Sudan and Zaire virus subtypes have occurred in Uganda[3] and Congo,[2] respectively.

EBOLA VIRUS (RESTON SUBTYPE)

In 1989 to 1991, another subtype was discovered in Reston, Virginia, among dying cynomolgus monkeys imported from Manila, Philippines.[17] This virus proved to be highly virulent for macaques, but the four animal caretakers who were infected suffered no overt disease. Fortunately, the quarantine regulations put in place after Marburg virus was first recognized in 1967 prevented the movement of infected animals outside the receiving facility. Other episodes occurred in Italy in 1992 and in the United States in 1996.[18] All these events were traced

to the facility of a single exporter, but the ultimate source of the virus has never been ascertained, although Mindanao was the origin of the monkeys taken for conditioning and resale.

In 2009, an outbreak of Reston Ebola virus was discovered in pigs in the Philippines, and antibody evidence of human infection was also found.[18] The source has not been found, but interestingly, the Reston, Virginia outbreak was associated with simultaneous transmission of the arterivirus simian hemorrhagic fever, and the recent outbreak in the Philippines is with concurrent circulation of porcine respiratory and reproductive syndrome arterivirus. It is not known what role the arterivirus plays in pig disease, but in the Reston, Virginia epidemic it was shown that *Reston ebolavirus* and simian hemorrhagic fever arterivirus are independently pathogenic for cynomolgous macaques.

TRANSMISSION TO HUMANS

In the original Marburg, Germany, importation, close contact with monkey blood or with cell cultures was present in all primary cases. Secondary cases were mainly among hospital staff and were associated with blood exposure.[8] The 1976 Zaire Ebola epidemic in particular was driven by the use of improperly sterilized needles and syringes, resulting in much of the geographic spread of infection. Interhuman spread of Ebola virus in the African epidemics was extensive among medical staff, often resulting in closure of hospitals and clinics. Transmission to household contacts ranged between 3% and 17%, involved up to five generations of infection, and was associated with close contact with sick patients and their body fluids. The epidemics subsided with the use of properly sterilized equipment, closure of hospitals, education of the populace, and institution of mask-gown-glove precautions.[10,15,19,20] In the Reston, Virginia epizootic among imported monkeys, there was transmission between monkeys by droplet and possibly small-particle aerosol; spread to three of the humans caring for the monkeys was thought to be by droplets or small-particle aerosols, and a fourth suffered a scalpel accident during a monkey necropsy.[17]

The exact routes by which filoviruses may be spread are not intimately known. Parenteral inoculation with contaminated needles or syringes has been efficient and carries an enhanced mortality.[19] Skin

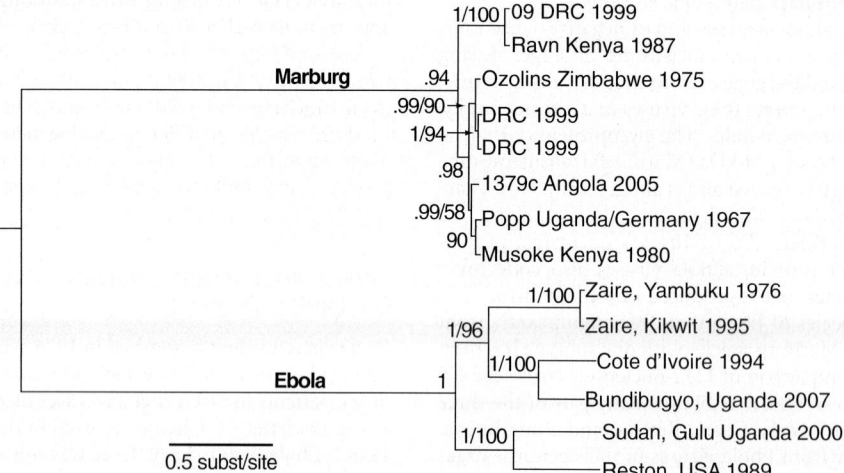

Figure 164-2 Phylogenetic tree of filoviruses. Marburg virus and Ebola virus are two clearly distinct genera. Within the Ebola virus genus, the five distinct species are represented. Note that the Yambuku and Kikwit, Zaire viruses are virtually identical even though separated by two decades and hundreds of kilometers. Virtually every virus sequenced from each of those two epidemics is identical over the part of the genome examined. This is typical of the pattern seen with single introductions followed by human-to-human passage through needle or close contact in an African hospital. In the Marburg virus branch of the tree, a major clade is shown, with a slightly divergent group characterized by the Ravn 1987 Kenya isolate. All the viruses from the major Angola 2005 outbreak are represented by a single virus because the sequences in this human-to-human epidemic were virtually identical. However, in the Democratic Republic of the Congo (DRC) 1999 outbreak resulting from multiple independent infections following cave entry, two viruses with slightly different phylogeny are represented within the major group, and there is even another virus within the Ravn subgroup. These sequences were selected from hundreds performed at the Centers for Disease Control and Prevention and elsewhere. *(Data adapted from references 2, 4, 9, and 19.)*

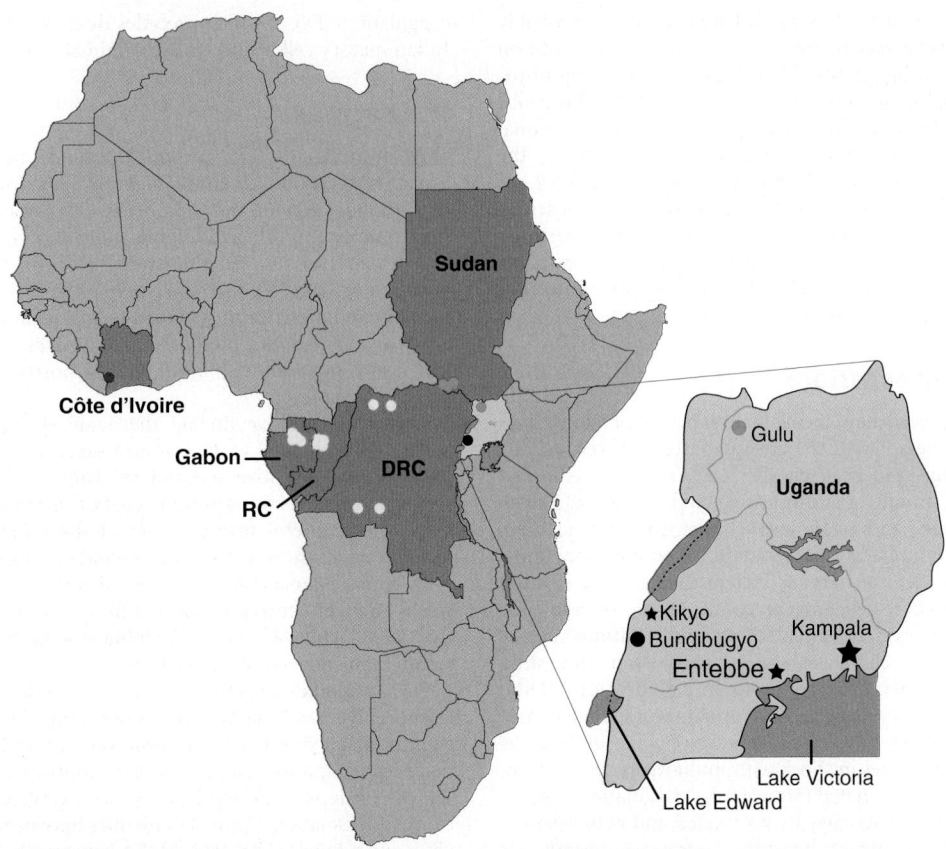

Figure 164-3 **Geography of Ebola virus species.** Dot colors represent the species: yellow, Zaire; green, Sudan; red, Ivory Coast; black, Bundibugyo. These species are spread throughout or adjacent to the Central African primary or secondary forest. Even Ebola virus Ivory Coast was isolated in the Tai forest reserve. The amplified map of Uganda shows a closer view of the zone along the Democratic Republic of the Congo (former Zaire) border with the site of the newest species, Bundibugyo. The Bundibugyo epidemic was also noted in the nearby town of Kikyo. These are tourist destinations and close to the capital, Kampala. Philippine sites of Reston not shown.

Figure 164-4 **Geography of Marburg virus identifications.** Red dots indicate a case or an epidemic. Uige, Angola is remarkable in that it experienced the largest Marburg epidemic (252 cases), with a 90% mortality rate.[9] The Angolan strains differed by only 0% to 0.07% at the nucleotide level (see Fig. 146-2). The Durba outbreak lasted 3 years and was characterized by multiple introductions into men entering a subterranean mine. Nine distinct lineages were detected, and one was in the rather distant (21%) Ravn lineage. Red dots in Gabon indicate detection of virus in bats by polymerase chain reaction. Not shown on this map are recent (2007-2008) human Marburg virus cases acquired in southern Uganda near Lake Edward (see Ebola map, Fig. 164-3, for location).

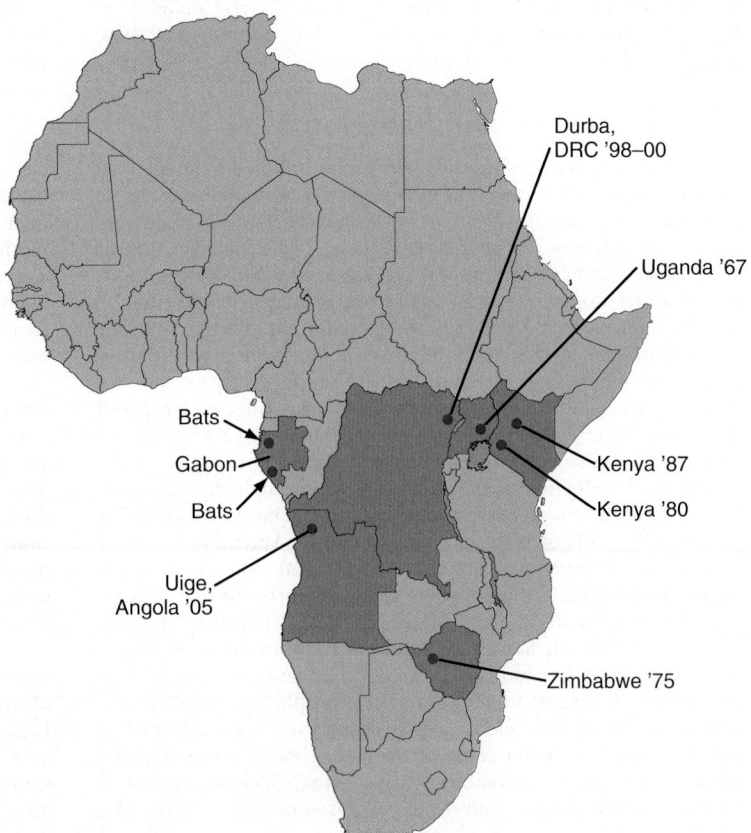

or mucous membrane contact with virus-laden materials has probably been responsible for most recognized human infections. In addition to high titers of virus in blood, the skin of patients, including fibroblasts and other dermal structures, is extensively infected[21]; this probably accounts for the additional risk to those participating in traditional burial preparation of the cadaver[10] and mourners touching the cadaver.[20] Experimental studies of filoviruses establish that they are stable[22] and highly infective[23] in small-particle aerosols, and observations of intermonkey transmission have suggested aerosol transmission. In addition, virions have been visualized in alveoli of humans and aerosol-infected monkeys.[17,24] Nevertheless, airborne infection plays a minor role, if any, in interhuman spread.

Clinical Manifestations

Filovirus hemorrhagic fevers have an incubation period of 5 to 10 days (range, 2 to 19) and begin with the abrupt onset of fever, usually accompanied by myalgia and headache.[5,8,10-13,19,25] The fever is joined by some combination of nausea and vomiting, abdominal pain, diarrhea, chest pain, cough, and pharyngitis. Other common features include photophobia, lymphadenopathy, conjunctival injection, jaundice, and pancreatitis. Central nervous system involvement is often manifested by somnolence, delirium, or coma. As the disease progresses, wasting becomes evident, and bleeding manifestations such as petechiae, hemorrhages, ecchymoses around needle puncture sites, and mucous membrane hemorrhages occur in half or more of the patients. Around day 5, most patients develop a maculopapular rash, prominent on the trunk. In the second week, the patient defervesces and improves markedly or dies in shock with multiorgan dysfunction, often accompanied by disseminated intravascular coagulation, anuria, and liver failure. Convalescence may be protracted and accompanied by arthralgia, orchitis, recurrent hepatitis, transverse myelitis, or uveitis.[8,26]

The mortality rate of Marburg infection is about 25%, Ebola Sudan subtype about 50%, and Ebola Zaire subtype 80% to 90%. Studies during epidemics suggest that subclinical infections with these viruses are uncommon, although a small percentage of the normal population has antibodies reactive in the immunoglobulin G (IgG) ELISA.[20,27,28] The limited number of Ebola Reston subtype infections observed have been subclinical.

Pathogenesis and Pathology

Filovirus disease has findings that are similar in human patients and nonhuman primate models. The viremia persists throughout the acute period, and its disappearance coincides with clinical improvement and usually the appearance of antibodies in blood.[28] The effective immune response is probably not humoral because passive convalescent antibody transfer does not protect against experimental inoculation.[26,29] Possible explanations for the failure to mount an effective immune response in fatal cases include the presence of a putatively immunosuppressive amino acid sequence in the filovirus glycoprotein,[30] the secretion of a soluble glycoprotein by Ebola virus–infected cells,[6] and the extensive lymphoid damage evident in postmortem examination.[24] In addition, Ebola-infected cells have a deficient response to added interferon,[4,31] induction of the antiviral state, and induction of interferon or activation of downstream pathways. One major filovirus protein, VP35, is known to be responsible for the latter.[32]

Important morphologic lesions include focal necrosis in many organs, particularly the liver, where Councilman bodies are present, and the lymphoid organs, where prominent follicular necrosis occurs.[10,11,24] Necrotic lesions are found in conjunction with antigen and viral particles in endothelial, mononuclear, and parenchymal cells of virtually all organs. In addition to the morphologic basis for the multiorgan functional defects, cytokines are extensively activated in sick humans.[33,34] A major cause of the pathogenesis in experimental monkey infections is activation of tissue factor, which occurs first in monocyte-macrophages, and leads to disseminated intravascular

coagulation (DIC), which precedes direct viral endothelial damage.[35] Inflammatory cell infiltrates are minimal.

Diagnosis

Travel to rural sub-Saharan Africa (and now perhaps the Philippines) or exposure to nonhuman primates is a historical clue. The presence of thrombocytopenia and leukopenia with elevated transaminase levels (aspartate aminotransferase levels more elevated than alanine aminotransferase levels) is characteristic of filovirus disease and some other viral hemorrhagic fevers, but a severe progressive course with abdominal pain and diarrhea should lead to suspicion of a filovirus. Elevated amylase and D-dimer levels are common, as is reduced albumin.[34,36] The rash is not seen with other viral hemorrhagic fevers, except occasionally Lassa fever.

Culture is positive during the acute stages, and seroconversion occurs around day 8 to 12. Antigen detection or RT-PCR provides a practical and sensitive method of diagnosis.[27,28] Negative stains of serum and thin sections of buffy coat or fixed tissue (liver, kidney) are helpful, but careful measurement of the putative virions and their internal structure is necessary to exclude artifacts.

In convalescence, virus has been isolated from semen for several weeks and from anterior chamber fluid in a case of late uveitis. Negative semen cultures should be obtained from patients before they resume unprotected sexual activity.

IgM antibodies detected in capture ELISA are useful in early convalescence.[28] IgG serologic testing has not been reliable. False-positive and irreproducible results are common when the indirect fluorescent antibody test is applied. For this reason, confirmation, even of apparent seroconversions, is desirable; only cases verified by viral isolation or from viral-isolation–verified epidemics have been included in the previous discussion. The IgG ELISA appears to have decreased this problem but still requires further verification.[26,27]

Prevention and Treatment

Although some drugs have shown promise in animal studies, no antivirals are available, nor does convalescent plasma hold much promise.[26,29] Interferon has not been effective and may lead to fever and other symptoms that would complicate management. Whole-blood transfusions from recently convalesced patients were used in the 1995 Zaire epidemic, but a lack of concomitant controls precluded evaluation of their efficacy, and retrospective analysis taking into account the day of initial treatment and other variables suggested they were not useful.[35] A DNA vaccine prepared against GP induces protective cellular immunity against Zaire strain challenge in guinea pigs but not in monkeys.[29] A vesicular stomatitis virus–based construct using Ebola Zaire or Marburg GP successfully protected mice and monkeys, including postexposure treatment in some settings.[37] While this type of construct has never been used in humans, no ill effects were seen. A prototype adenovirus vaccine expressing this antigen has successfully protected monkeys and demonstrated a good safety profile in phase I studies in humans.[38,39]

Prevention of epidemics rests on early recognition of initial cases and prompt institution of barrier nursing.[15] Increased clinical awareness should lead to the institution of barrier nursing, which can be done with means appropriate to the African health care setting.[40] Fatal cases can be recognized readily by immunohistochemical staining of postmortem skin samples, obviating the need for cold preservation of samples and providing a safe and inexpensive diagnostic modality in these high-mortality diseases.[21]

Management of the patient should be supportive, with minimal trauma and careful maintenance of hydration, realizing the possibility of myocardial compromise and increased lung vascular permeability. Replacement of coagulation factors and platelets is indicated. Heparin or other treatment of DIC should be undertaken if laboratory evidence shows it to be present, and if adequate hematologic support is available. In the severe Zaire Ebola virus monkey model, activated protein

C improves survival, and this licensed drug should be considered for human therapy.[41] In addition, a recombinant inhibitor of the tissue factor–activated factor VII complex improves survival and should also be considered.[42]

At the community level, properly sterilized injection equipment, protection from body fluids and skin contact during preparation of the dead, and routine barrier nursing precautions are probably adequate in most cases.[15,16] In the United States, where more aggressive therapeutic procedures may be practiced, strict isolation, barrier nursing, staff training to avoid parenteral exposures, and, when practical, respirator protection should be routine.[43,44]

Extensive quarantine precautions are now in place to prevent the movement of infected monkeys into the United States and to prevent contamination of vaccines or cell cultures. Nevertheless, the potential for the emergence of filoviruses as a significant public health problem exists,[1] and concern by U.S. clinicians is warranted when suspicious cases with an epidemiologic link to Africa or nonhuman primates occur.

Note: Useful sources for information of the basic biology of filoviruses are the books that followed the Marburg outbreak[8] and the 1976 Ebola outbreak[45]; a 1999 journal supplement with much of the 1995 Kikwit, Zaire, outbreak and other data[26] (available at http://www.journals.uchicago.edu/JID/journal/contents/v179nS1.html); a 1999 review volume[5]; and a more recent 2007 journal supplement (available at http://www.journals.uchicago.edu/toc/jid/2007/196/s2).[46] These compendia have been referenced freely here to limit the size of the reference list.

REFERENCES

1. Murphy FA, Peters CJ. Ebola virus: Where does it come from and where is it going? In: Krause RM, ed. *Emerging Infections.* New York: Academic Press; 1998;375-410.
2. Towner JS, Sealy TK, Khristova ML, et al. Newly discovered Ebola virus associated with hemorrhagic fever outbreak in Uganda. *PLoS Pathog.* 2008;4:e1000212.
3. Klenk H-D, ed. Marburg and Ebola Viruses. *Curr Top Microbiol Immunol.* 1999;235:1-225.
4. Sanchez A, Khan AS, Zaki SR, et al. Filoviridae: Marburg and Ebola viruses. In: Knipe DM, Howley PM, eds. *Fields' Virology.* 4th ed. Philadelphia: Lippincott, Williams, and Wilkins; 2001; 1279-1304.
5. Sanchez A, Trappier SG, Mahy BWJ, et al. The virion glycoproteins of Ebola viruses are encoded in two reading frames and are expressed through transcriptional editing. *Proc Natl Acad Sci U S A.* 1996;93:3602.
6. Ksiazek TG, Rollin PE, Jahrling PB, et al. Enzyme-linked immunosorbent assays for the detection of antibodies to Ebola viruses. *J Infect Dis.* 1999;179(Suppl 1):S192-S198.
7. Swanepoel R, Leman PA, Burt FJ, et al. Experimental inoculation of plants and animals with Ebola virus. *Emerg Infect Dis.* 1996;2: 321-325.
8. Martini GA, Siegert R, eds. *Marburg Virus Disease.* Berlin: Springer-Verlag; 1971:1-230.
9. Towner JS, Khristova ML, Sealy TK, et al. Marburgvirus genomics and association with a large hemorrhagic fever outbreak in Angola. *J Virol.* 2006;80:6497-6516.
10. World Health Organization. Ebola haemorrhagic fever in Zaire, 1976: Report of an international commission. *Bull World Health Organ.* 1978;56:271-293.
11. World Health Organization. Ebola haemorrhagic fever in Sudan, 1976: Report of a WHO/international study team. *Bull World Health Organ.* 1978;56:247-270.
12. Baron RC, McCormick JB, Zubeir OA. Ebola hemorrhagic fever in southern Sudan: Hospital dissemination and intrafamilial spread. *Bull World Health Organ.* 1983;6:997-1003.
13. Formenty P, Hatz C, Stoll A, et al. Human infection due to Ebola Côte d'Ivoire: Clinical and biological presentation. *J Infect Dis.* 1999;179(Suppl 1):S48-S53.
14. Georges A, Leroy EB, Renaut AA, et al. Recent Ebola outbreaks in Gabon from 1994 to 1997: Epidemiological and health control issues. *J Infect Dis.* 1999;179(Suppl 1):S65-S75.
15. Khan AS, Kweteminga TF, Heymann DH, et al. The reemergence of Ebola hemorrhagic fever (EHF), Zaire, 1995. *J Infect Dis.* 1999;179(Suppl 1):S76-S86.
16. Richards GA, Murphy S, Jobson R, et al. Unexpected Ebola virus in a tertiary setting: Clinical and epidemiologic aspects. *Crit Care Med.* 2000;28:240-244.

17. Peters CJ, Johnson ED, Jahrling PB, et al. Filoviruses. In: Morse S, ed. *Emerging Viruses.* New York: Oxford University Press; 1991:159-175.
18. Rollin PE, Williams J, Bressler D, et al. Ebola (subtype Reston) virus among quarantined non-human primates recently imported from the Philippines to the United States. *J Infect Dis.* 1999;179(Suppl 1):S108-S114.
19. Bausch DG, Nichol ST, Muyembe-Tamfum JJ, et al. Marburg hemorrhagic fever associated with multiple genetic lineages of virus. *N Engl J Med.* 2006;355:909-919.
20. Dowell SF, Mukunu R, Ksiazek TG, et al. Transmission of Ebola hemorrhagic fever: A study of risk factors in family members, Kikwit, Zaire 1995. *J Infect Dis.* 1999;179(Suppl 1):S87-S91.
21. Zaki S, Greer PW, Shieh WJ, et al. A novel immunohistochemical assay for detection of Ebola virus in skin: Implications for diagnosis and surveillance of Ebola hemorrhagic fever. *J Infect Dis.* 1999;179(Suppl 1):S36-S37.
22. Belanov YF, Muntyanov VP, Kryuk VD, et al. Retention of Marburg virus infecting capability on contaminated surfaces and in aerosol particles (in Russian). *Vopr Virusol.* 1996;41:32-34.
23. Bazhutin NB, Belanov EF, Spiridonov VA, et al. The influence of the methods of experimental infection with Marburg virus on the features of the disease process in green monkeys. *Vopr Virusol.* 1992;37:153-156.
24. Zaki SR, Goldsmith CS. Pathologic features of filovirus infections in humans. *Curr Top Microbiol Immunol.* 1999;235:97-116.
25. Bwaka MA, Bonnet M, Calain P, et al. Ebola hemorrhagic fever in Kikwit, Democratic Republic of Congo (former Zaire): Clinical observations. *J Infect Dis.* 1999;179(Suppl 1):S1-S7.
26. Peters CJ, LeDuc JW, ed. Ebola: The virus and the disease. *J Infect Dis.* 1999;179(Suppl 1):S1-S288.
27. Busico KM, Marshall KL, Ksiazek TG, et al. Prevalence of IgG antibodies to Ebola virus in individuals during an Ebola outbreak, Democratic Republic of the Congo, 1995. *J Infect Dis.* 1999; 179(Suppl 1):S102-S107.
28. Ksiazek TG, Rollin PE, Williams AJ, et al. Clinical virology of Ebola hemorrhagic fever (EHF): Virus, virus antigen, and IgG and IgM antibody findings among EHF patients in Kikwit, Democratic Republic of the Congo, 1995. *J Infect Dis.* 1999;179(Suppl 1):S177-S187.
29. Xu L, Sanchez A, Yang Z, et al. Genetic immunization for Ebola virus infection. *Nat Med.* 1998;4:37.
30. Yaddanapudi K, Palacios G, Towner JS, et al. Implication of a retrovirus-like glycoprotein peptide in the immunopathogenesis of Ebola and Marburg viruses. *FASEB J.* 2006;20:2519-2530.
31. Harcourt BH, Sanchez A, Offerman MK. Ebola virus selectively inhibits responses to interferons, but not to IL-1beta in endothelial cells. *J Virol.* 1999;73:3491-3496.

32. Hartman AL, Ling L, Nichol ST, et al. Whole-genome expression profiling reveals that inhibition of host innate immune response pathways by Ebola virus can be reversed by a single amino acid change in the VP35 protein. *J Virol.* 2008;82:5348-5358.
33. Villinger F, Rollin PE, Brar SS, et al. Markedly elevated levels of IFN-gamma/alpha, IL-2, IL-10 and TNF-alpha associated with fatal Ebola virus infection. *J Infect Dis.* 1999;179(Suppl 1): S188-S191.
34. Hutchinson KL, Rollin PE. Cytokine and chemokine expression in humans infected with Sudan Ebola virus. *J Infect Dis.* 2007; 196(Suppl 2):S357-S363.
35. Sadek RF, Kilmarx PH, Khan AS, et al. Outbreak of Ebola hemorrhagic fever, Zaire, 1995: A closer numerical look. *J Infect Dis.* 1999;179(Suppl 1):S24-S27.
36. Rollin PE, Bausch DG, Sanchez A. Blood chemistry measurements and D-dimer levels associated with fatal and nonfatal outcomes in humans infected with Sudan Ebola virus. *J Infect Dis.* 2007;196(Suppl 2):S364-S371.
37. Geisbert TW, Daddario-Dicaprio KM, Geisbert JB, et al. Vesicular stomatitis virus-based vaccines protect nonhuman primates against aerosol challenge with Ebola and Marburg viruses. *Vaccine.* 2008;26:6894-6900.
38. Sullivan NJ, Geisbert TW, Geisbert JB, et al. Accelerated vaccination for Ebola virus haemorrhagic fever in non-human primates. *Nature.* 2003;424:681-684.
39. Dery M, Bausch DG, et al. A DNA vaccine for the prevention of Ebola virus infection. *Curr Opin Mol Ther.* 2008;10:285-293.
40. Lloyd ES, Zaki SR, Rollin PE, et al. Long-term disease surveillance in Bandundu region, Democratic Republic of the Congo: A model for early detection and prevention of Ebola hemorrhagic fever. *J Infect Dis.* 1999;179(Suppl 1):S274-S280.
41. Hensley LE, Stevens EL, Yan SB, et al. Recombinant human activated protein C for the postexposure treatment of Ebola hemorrhagic fever. *J Infect Dis.* 2007;196(Suppl 2):S390-S399.
42. Geisbert TW, Hensley LE, Jahrling PB, et al. Treatment of Ebola virus infection with a recombinant inhibitor of factor VIIa/tissue factor: A study in rhesus monkeys. *Lancet.* 2003;362:1953-1958.
43. Centers for Disease Control and Prevention. Update: Management of patients with suspected viral hemorrhagic fever—United States. *MMWR Morb Mortal Wkly Rep.* 1995;44:475-479.
44. Updated CDC website May 29, 2005. Interim Guidance for managing patients with suspected viral hemorrhagic fevers in U.S. Hospitals. Available at: <http://www.cdc.gov/ncidod/dhqp/bp_ vhf_interimGuidance.html>.
45. Pattyn SR, ed. *Ebola Virus Haemorrhagic Fever.* Amsterdam: Elsevier North-Holland; 1978.
46. Filoviruses: Recent Advances and Future Challenges. *A supplement to The Journal of Infectious Diseases.* 11-15-2007;196(s2):i-S443.

165

Influenza Viruses, Including Avian Influenza and Swine Influenza

JOHN J. TREANOR

Influenza is an acute, usually self-limited, febrile illness caused by infection with influenza type A or B virus that occurs in outbreaks of varying severity almost every winter. The attack rates during such outbreaks may be as high as 10% to 40% over a 5-week to 6-week period. The most common clinical manifestations are fever, malaise, and cough. Two unique features of influenza are the epidemic nature of the disease and the mortality that results in part from its pulmonary complications.

History

Influenza virus has caused recurrent epidemics of febrile respiratory disease every 1 to 3 years for at least the past 400 years. Although the disease is not associated with a characteristic manifestation such as rash, the high attack rate, the explosive nature of the epidemic, and the frequency of cough allow the identification of past epidemics. For example, Hirsch[1] tabulated 299 outbreaks that occurred at an average interval of 2.4 years between 1173 and 1875. The greatest pandemic in recorded history occurred in 1918 to 1919 when, during three waves of influenza, 21 million deaths were recorded worldwide, among them 549,000 in the United States.[2]

The modern understanding of influenza was ushered in by Smith and associates[3] when they isolated influenza A virus in ferrets in 1933. Influenza B virus was isolated by Francis[4] in 1939, and influenza C virus by Taylor[5] in 1950. The discovery by Burnet in 1936 that influenza virus could be grown in embryonated hen eggs allowed extensive study of the properties of the virus and the development of inactivated vaccines.[6] Animal cell culture systems for the growth of influenza viruses were developed in the 1950s.[7] The phenomenon of hemagglutination, which was discovered by Hirst[8] in 1941, led to simple and inexpensive methods for the measurement of virus and specific antibody.

Evidence of the protective efficacy of inactivated vaccines was developed in the 1940s.[9] The use of live vaccines for influenza was first suggested shortly after the virus was discovered,[10] but the first live vaccine was not licensed in the United States until 2003, approximately 70 years later. Finally, four antiviral agents in two classes have been approved for prevention and treatment of influenza. These agents include the M2 inhibitors, amantadine in the mid 1960s, rimantadine in 1993, and the neuraminidase inhibitors zanamivir and oseltamivir in 2000.

The Viruses

CLASSIFICATION

Influenza viruses belong to the family Orthomyxoviridae and are classified into three distinct types, influenza A, influenza B, and influenza C virus, on the basis of major antigenic differences. In addition, significant differences are found in genetic organization, structure, host range, epidemiology, and clinical characteristics between the three influenza virus types (Table 165-1). However, all three viruses share certain features, including the presence of a host-cell derived envelope, envelope glycoproteins of critical importance in virus entry and egress from cells, and a segmented genome of negative sense (i.e., opposite

of message sense) single-stranded RNA. The standard nomenclature for influenza viruses includes the influenza type, place of initial isolation, strain designation, and year of isolation. For example, the influenza A virus isolated by Francis from a patient in Puerto Rico in 1934 is given the strain designation A/Puerto Rico/8/34, sometimes referred to as PR8 virus. Influenza A viruses are further divided into subtypes on the basis of their hemagglutinin (H or HA) and neuraminidase (N or NA) activity (e.g., H1N1 or H3N2).

MORPHOLOGIC CHARACTERISTICS

Influenza viruses are enveloped viruses that may exist in spherical or filamentous forms of 80 to 120 nm (Fig. 165-1), with surface projections that consist of HA and NA spikes. A schematic diagram of an influenza A virus is shown in Figure 165-2.

Eight structural proteins have been identified in influenza A viruses. Each rod-shaped HA spike measures approximately 4 nm in diameter by 14 nm in length. They can be removed from the intact virion with sodium dodecyl sulfate, bromelain, or chymotrypsin. Each spike is a trimer composed of three HA polypeptides, each with a molecular weight of 75,000 to 80,000, which results in a trimer with a molecular weight of approximately 224,640.[11] The HA is synthesized as a monomer (HA_0), which is cleaved by host-cell proteases into HA_1 and HA_2 components that remain linked together. Antigenic sites and sites for binding to cells are located in the globular head of the molecule.

The viral NA is an enzyme that catalyzes the removal of terminal sialic acids (N-acetyl neuraminic acid) from sialic acid–containing glycoproteins. The NA spike is shaped like a mushroom rather than a rod and has a molecular weight of 240,000. The intact NA consists of a tetramer of NA polypeptides, each with a molecular weight of 58,000.[12] As in HA, the antigenic sites and the enzyme active site are located in the mushroom-shaped head.

At least 16 highly divergent, antigenically distinct HAs have been described in influenza A viruses (H1 to H16), as well as at least nine distinct NAs (N1 to N9). A third integral membrane protein, the M2 protein, is also present in small amounts on the viral envelope.[13]

Interior to the envelope is the matrix, or M1, protein. This protein provides structure to the virion and is important for virus assembly. Within the virion are eight physically discrete nucleocapsid segments (Table 165-2). Each nucleocapsid is composed of a single segment of genomic RNA intimately associated with the viral nucleoprotein (NP), with the three polymerase proteins PB1, PB2, and PA bound to one end. Two nonstructural viral proteins, NS1 and NS2 (also referred to as the nuclear export protein [NEP]), are also found within infected cells. Small amounts of NEP are present within virions.

Epidemiology

DISEASE IMPACT

Influenza epidemics are regularly associated with excess morbidity and mortality, usually expressed in the form of excess rates of pneumonia and influenza-associated hospitalizations and deaths during epidemics. For an estimate of the mortality burden of influenza, observed pneumonia-related and influenza-related deaths during periods of

TABLE 165-1	Differences among Influenza A, B, and C Viruses		
	Influenza A	*Influenza B*	*Influenza C*
Genetics	8 gene segments	8 gene segments	7 gene segments
Structure	10 viral proteins	11 viral proteins	9 viral proteins
	M2 unique	NB unique	HEF unique
Host range	Humans, swine, equine, avian, marine mammals*	Humans only	Humans and swine
Epidemiology	Antigenic shift and drift	Antigenic drift only; two main lineages cocirculate	Antigenic drift only; multiple variants
Clinical features	May cause large pandemics with significant mortality in young persons	Severe disease generally confined to older adults or persons at high risk; pandemics not seen	Mild disease without seasonality

*Recently, influenza viruses have also been isolated from dogs and cats.
HEF, hemagglutination, esterase, and fusion activity; NB, membrane protein.

influenza epidemic activity are compared with an expected seasonal baseline derived from a time-series regression model, and the excess mortality attributable to influenza is calculated. A tabulation of levels of these excess pneumonia and influenza deaths attributable to influenza epidemics[14] is shown in Table 165-3, as is the estimated percentage of isolates that were typed as influenza A (H3N2), A (H1N1), or B in each year. Generally, the level of excess mortality is highest in years when influenza A (H3N2) viruses predominate, but influenza B and to a lesser extent H1N1 viruses also can be associated with excess mortality. Because not all influenza-related deaths are manifested as pneumonia, the pneumonia and influenza mortality statistics probably underestimate the true impact of influenza on the population. Table 165-3 also lists the all-cause excess mortality, defined as deaths from any cause, above a similarly derived baseline, that occur during periods of influenza epidemic activity. Although less precise than the pneumonia-related and influenza-related deaths, all-cause mortality is probably a more accurate reflection of the total burden of influenza. Recent studies suggest that even higher levels of mortality might be attributable to influenza, potentially as high as 51,000 deaths annually in the United States.[15]

Mortality is only the most severe manifestation of influenza impact, and similar techniques can be used to estimate excess morbidity from influenza epidemics.[16] Data from the Tecumseh Community Health

TABLE 165-2	Genes and Protein Products of Influenza A Virus		
RNA Segment Number	*Gene Product Description*	*Name of Protein*	*Proposed Functions*
1	PB1 PB1-F2	Basic polymerase 1	RNA transcriptase Proapoptotic
2	PB2	Basic polymerase 2	Cap binding, endonucleolytic cleavage
3	PA	Acidic polymerase	Unknown
4	HA	Hemagglutinin	Viral attachment to cell membranes; membrane fusion
5	NA	Neuraminidase	Cleaves sialic acid from cell surface; released from membranes; prevents aggregation
6	NP	Nucleoprotein	Encapsidates RNA; regulation of transcription/replication
7	M	Matrix	Surrounds viral core; controls nuclear export of RNA
	M2	Matrix 2	Ion channel; necessary for uncoating
8	NS1	Nonstructural	Antagonizes type I interferons, may be involved in regulation of mRNA transport from nucleus
	NEP (NS2)	Nuclear export protein	Transport of newly assembled RNP from nucleus to cytoplasm

Study have been used to estimate that influenza is responsible for 13.8 to 16.0 million excess respiratory illnesses per year in the United States among individuals less than 20 years of age and for 4.1 to 4.5 million excess illnesses in older individuals.[16]

Influenza is usually associated with a U-shaped epidemic curve. Attack rates are generally highest in the young, whereas mortality is generally highest among older adults (Fig. 165-3). Excess morbidity and mortality rates are particularly high in individuals with certain

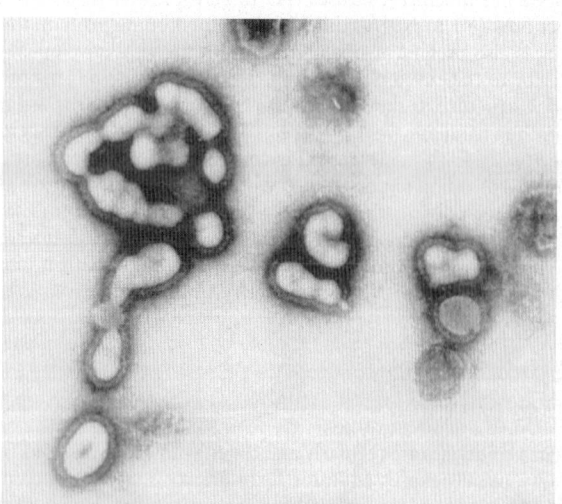

Figure 165-1 Electron micrograph of influenza A/USSR/77 H1N1 (magnification, ×189,000).

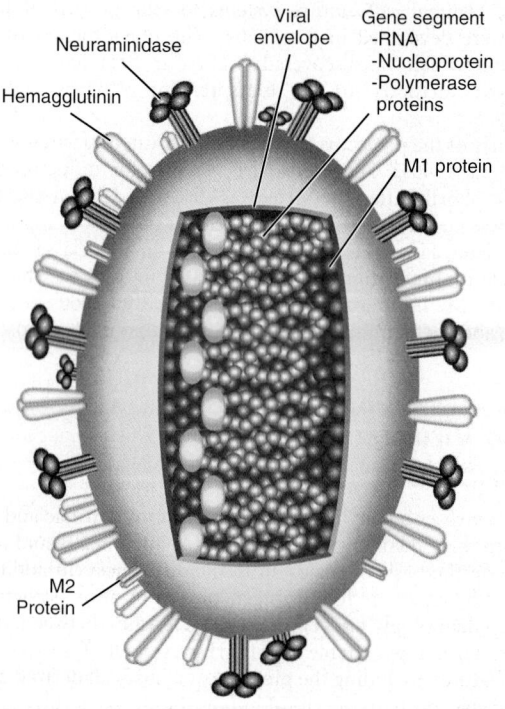

Figure 165-2 Schematic model of influenza A virus.

TABLE 165-3	Estimated Excess Pneumonia-Related and Influenza-Related Deaths and Excess Mortality of All Causes during Influenza Epidemics				
	Percentage of Isolates That Were of Following (Sub) Type			Pneumonia-Related and Influenza-Related Excess Deaths (Range)	All-Cause Excess Deaths (Range)
Year	*H3N2*	*H1N1*	*B*		
1972/1973	90	0	10	7,900 (5,500-10,300)	18,300 (1,200-35,000)
1973/1974	20	0	80	0	0
1974/1975	100	0	0	6,500 (4,100-8,900)	15,100 (0-32,100)
1975/1976	70	0	30	11,800 (9,200-14,400)	24,600 (3,400-45,900)
1976/1977	5	0	95	0	0
1977/1978	60	26	14	8,300 (6,000-10,500)	46,200 (19,800-72,700)
1978/1979	0	98	2	0	0
1979/1980	2	1	97	5,100 (3,500-6,700)	17,300 (600-34,100)
1980/1981	77	23	0	11,700 (9,100-14,200)	47,200 (27,800-66,600)
1981/1982	1	24	75	2,100 (600-3,700)	0
1982/1983	79	10	11	4,700 (2,800-6,700)	9,600 (0-19,200)
1983/1984	5	50	45	3,500 (1,600-5,400)	8,200 (0-17,600)
1984/1985	97	0	3	8,100 (6,600-9,600)	36,200 (17,700-54,700)
1985/1986	24	0	76	6,700 (4,900-8,500)	34,000 (6,800-61,200)
1986/1987	—	—	—	1,800 (1,100-2,500)	16,800 (1,900-31,700)
1987/1988	0	80	20	7,400 (5,600-9,100)	33,400 (12,900-53,800)
1988/1989	45	45	10	5,100 (3,600-6,600)	10,500 (800-20,200)
1989/1990	90	1	9	10,100 (8,500-11,700)	43,600 (27,600-59,600)
1990/1991	4	3	93	4,200 (2,400-6,100)	23,000 (0-46,000)
1991/1992	19	81	0	6,600 (5,600-7,700)	41,700 (19,600-63,700)

Data from Table 153-3 in Treanor JL. Influenza virus. In: Mandell GL, Bennett JE, Dolin R, eds. *Mandell, Douglas, and Bennett's Principles and Practice of Infectious Diseases.* ed. 5. Philadelphia: Saunders; 2000:1826; and Simonsen L, Clarke MJ, Williamson DW, et al. The impact of influenza epidemics on mortality. Introducing a severity index. *Am J Public Health.* 1947;87:1944-1950.

high-risk medical conditions, including adults and children with cardiovascular and pulmonary conditions such as asthma; those who need regular medical care because of chronic metabolic disease, renal dysfunction, hemoglobinopathies, or immunodeficiency; and those with neurologic conditions that compromise handling of respiratory

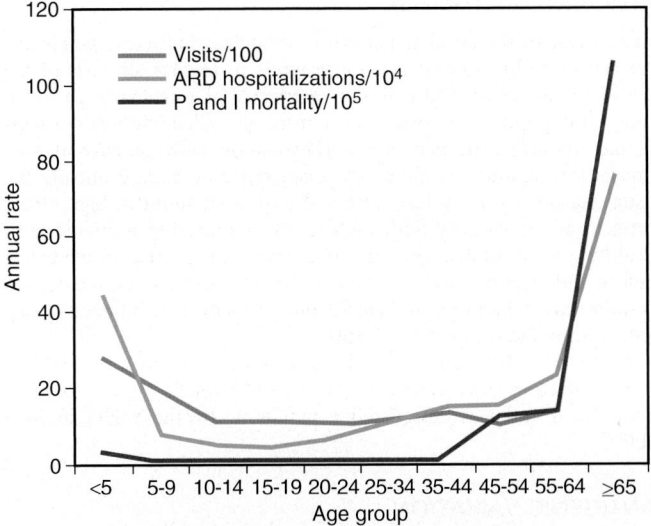

Figure 165-3 Typical epidemic curve in interpandemic era. The graph shows rates of medically attended illness (*green line;* rate per 100), hospitalizations for acute respiratory disease (ARD) (*blue line;* rate per 10,000), and pneumonia-related and influenza-related mortality (*red line;* rate per 100,000) by age for several seasons of influenza in Houston. Attack rates and hospitalizations occur at both extremes of age, but mortality occurs largely in those older than 65 years. (*Data from Glezen WP, Keitel WA, Taber LH, et al. Age distribution of patients with medically attended illnesses caused by sequential variants of influenza A/H1N1: Comparison to age-specific infection rates, 1978-1989. Am J Epidemiol. 1991;133:296-304.*)

secretions.[17] Influenza-related death rates in nursing home residents with comorbid conditions are as high as 2.8% per year.[18]

Influenza also results in more severe disease and significant mortality in individuals with human immunodeficiency virus (HIV) infection[19,20] and in women in the second or third trimester of pregnancy.[21] Influenza is increasingly recognized as an important health problem in young children. Rates of influenza-related hospitalizations are particularly high in healthy children less than 2 years of age, where rates approach those of older children with high-risk conditions.[22,23] In addition, a high rate of secondary complications, particularly otitis media and pneumonia, occur in children with influenza infection.[24] Although rare, influenza-related deaths occur each year in previously healthy children.[17]

Much of the impact of influenza is related to the malaise and consequent disability that it produces, even in young healthy individuals. A typical case of influenza, on average, has been estimated to be associated with 5 to 6 days of restricted activity, 3 to 4 days of bed disability, and about 3 days lost from work or school.[25] The average number of medical visits for cases in which medical attention was sought was from 1.1 to 3.6 per year, depending on severity of the outbreak and age of the patient. In children, outpatient visits are 10 to 250 times more common than hospitalizations.[26] Direct medical costs of illness account for only about 20% of the total expenses of a case of influenza, with a major proportion (30% to 50%) of the economic impact a result of loss of productivity.[27] In one study, influenza in schoolchildren resulted in 37 missed school days by children and 20 days of missed work by parents, per 100 children.[28] Influenza is also associated with decreased job performance in working adults[29] and reduced levels of independent functioning in older adults.[30]

EPIDEMIC INFLUENZA

An *epidemic* is an outbreak of influenza confined to one location, such as a city, town, or country. In a given community, epidemics of influenza A virus infection have a characteristic pattern. A graphic description of a typical and well-characterized epidemic due to influenza A (H3N2) in 1976 is shown in Figure 165-4. The epidemic began abruptly, reached a sharp peak in 2 to 3 weeks, and lasted 5 to 6

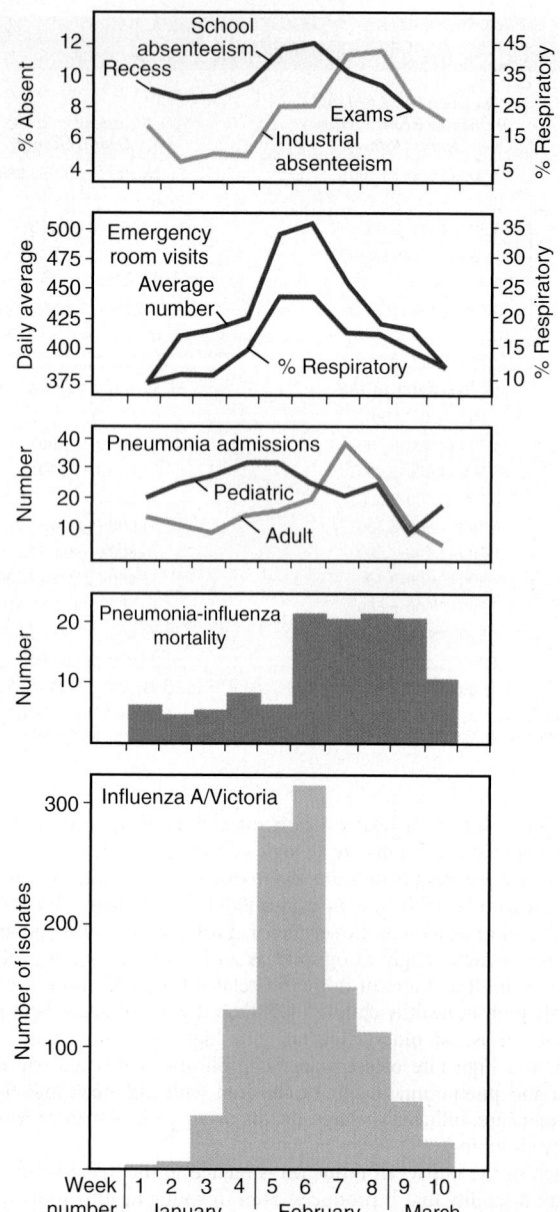

Figure 165-4 **Correlation of nonvirologic indexes of epidemiologic influenza with number of isolates of A/Victoria virus according to week, Houston, 1976.** Industrial absenteeism is determined by percentage with respiratory symptoms. *(From Glezen WP, Couch RB. Interpandemic influenza in the Houston area, 1974-1976. N Engl J Med. 1978;298:587-593, with permission.)*

weeks.[31] The first indicator of influenza activity was reports of increased numbers of children with febrile respiratory illness, followed by the occurrence of influenza-like illnesses among adults. These reports were subsequently followed by increased hospital admissions for patients with pneumonia, exacerbation of chronic obstructive pulmonary disease, croup, and congestive heart failure and finally by increased school and industrial absenteeism. Although an increased number of deaths from pneumonia is a highly specific indicator of influenza, it lags behind the other indications because of the time from the onset of illness to time of death and the delay involved in reporting deaths to public health officials. An increase in Internet searches for topics related to influenza has also been observed to be an early indicator of influenza activity in a community.[32]

During epidemics, attack rates in unvaccinated populations are estimated to be 10% to 20%, but rates as high as 40% to 50% have been

reported.[33] The factors that lead to termination of an outbreak in any given location are unclear, because usually the outbreak ceases before the supply of susceptible individuals is exhausted.

Seasonal influenza viruses are transmitted from person to person through contact with infected respiratory secretions. The relative roles of large-particle and small-particle aerosols (<10 μm mass median diameter) in transmission are uncertain and remain controversial. Transmission is generally considered to be predominantly by large particles (i.e., those that travel relatively short distances through the air).[34,35] Thus, isolation precautions typically include private rooms or cohorting, contact and droplet precautions, and the use of masks.[34] However, in experimental influenza in volunteers, 100-fold lower doses of virus are necessary to infect via an aerosol route than via intranasal drops.[36,37] In addition, several descriptions of outbreaks in closed settings, such as aircraft, can best be explained with small-particle aerosol transmission.[35,38]

In temperate climates in either hemisphere, epidemics occur almost exclusively in the winter months (generally November to April in the Northern Hemisphere, and May to September in the Southern Hemisphere); influenza may be seen year round in the tropics. The reasons for these seasonal changes are not entirely clear but might be the result of more favorable environmental conditions for virus survival.[39] Studies in a model of transmission of influenza in guinea pigs have also supported a role for conditions of cold temperature and low humidity in facilitating transmission.[40] Colder temperatures are also associated with behavioral changes that may increase transmission, such as indoor crowding or school attendance.

Generally, a single strain of influenza virus is the predominant cause of cases during an epidemic. However, this is not always the case, and in some seasons, two different lineages or strains within a single subtype or two different influenza A subtypes (H1N1 and H3N2) or concomitant outbreaks of influenza A and B have occurred. In some years, the end of the influenza epidemic season is characterized by cases from a new strain. These limited outbreaks, which have been referred to as a *herald wave*, sometimes predict the predominant strain in the next influenza season.[41]

PANDEMIC INFLUENZA

In contrast to the familiar pattern of epidemic influenza, *pandemics* are severe outbreaks that rapidly progress to involve all parts of the world and are associated with the emergence of a new virus to which the overall population possesses no immunity. Characteristics of pandemics include extremely rapid transmission with concurrent outbreaks throughout the globe; the occurrence of disease outside the usual seasonality, including during the summer months; high attack rates in all age groups, with high levels of mortality particularly in healthy young adults; and multiple waves of disease immediately before and after the main outbreak. The interval between pandemics is quite variable and unpredictable, but pandemics of influenza likely will continue to occur in the future.

In March 2009, an outbreak of a novel influenza A (H1N1) virus infection was noted in Mexico,[41a] which rapidly became widespread and was designated a pandemic by the WHO in June 2009.[41b]

ANTIGENIC VARIATION

One of the unique and most remarkable features of influenza virus is the frequency with which changes in antigenicity occur, collectively referred to as *antigenic variation*. Alteration of the antigen structure of the virus leads to infection with variants to which little or no resistance is present in the population at risk. The phenomenon of antigenic variation helps explain why influenza continues to be a major epidemic disease of humans. Antigenic variation involves principally the two external glycoproteins of the virus, HA and NA, and is referred to as antigenic drift or antigenic shift, depending on whether the variation is small or great.

ANTIGENIC DRIFT

Antigenic drift refers to relatively minor antigenic changes that occur frequently within the HA or NA of the virus. Drift has been studied most intensively for the HA and is the result of gradual accumulation of amino acid changes in one or more of the five identified major antigenic sites on the HA molecule.[42] Because antibody generated by exposure to previous strains does not neutralize the antigenic variant as effectively, immunologic selection takes place, and the variant supplants previous strains as the predominant virus in the epidemic. Antigenic variants can be produced in cell culture in the presence of limiting amounts of antibody, and these variants have single amino acid sequences in the HA similar to those of drift variants.[43]

Although not studied as intensively, antigenic drift also occurs with amino acid substitutions in the antibody epitopes in the NA.[44] A phenomenon analogous to antigenic drift has also been described for some epitopes recognized by cellular immune effectors.[45] Fitness costs to the virus, and the diversity of human leukocyte antigen (HLA) types in the population, have been speculated to limit the extent of such variability.[46]

Comparison of the HA gene sequences of influenza viruses isolated in successive years reveals differences in the patterns of HA evolution between influenza A, B, and C viruses. Generally, a single lineage, or relatively few lineages, of influenza A virus circulate in humans, and the accumulation of point mutations in the HA is linear, with each strain replacing the previously circulating one. This is particularly true of H3 influenza A viruses.[47] In contrast, multiple lineages of influenza C virus cocirculate, as shown by sequence comparisons of the HEF gene. The evolution of influenza B viruses is somewhere between these two examples, with relatively few lineages of the HA gene (but more than one) cocirculating.[48] Currently, two antigenically distinct lineages of influenza B viruses, referred to as the Yamagata lineage and the Victoria lineage, are cocirculating worldwide.

Although a very tight correlation between genetic changes and antigenic distance generally exists,[49] the antigenic significance of any individual mutation can be more difficult to assess. Usually, significant antigenic changes occur when mutations arise in two or more antigen binding sites within the HA.

ANTIGENIC SHIFT

The major *antigenic shifts* that herald pandemic influenza presumably result from a different mechanism. These viruses are "new" viruses to which the population has no immunity. Very little or no serologic relationship exists between the HA (or NA) antigens of the "old" and "new" viruses; hence, in nomenclature, each receives a different designation. The schema shown in Figure 165-5 ties together the concepts of antigenic shift and antigenic drift in relation to population immu-

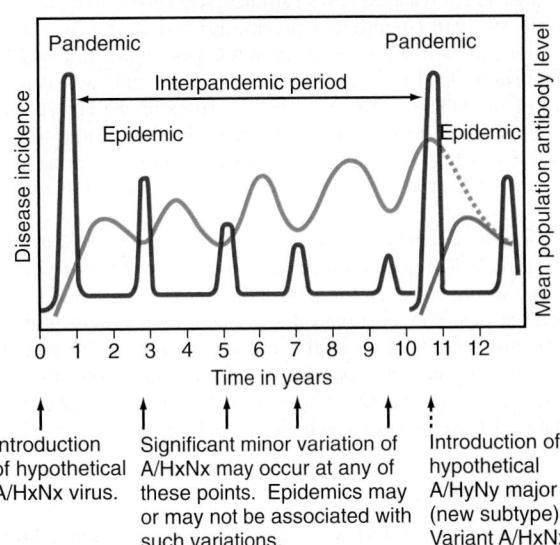

Figure 165-5 **Schema of occurrence of influenza pandemics and epidemics in relation to level of immunity in the population.** A/HxNx and A/HyNy represent influenza viruses with completely different hemagglutinins and neuraminidases. *(Modified from Kilbourne ED. The epidemiology of influenza. In: Kilbourne ED, ed. The Influenza Viruses and Influenza. New York: Academic Press; 1975:483, with permission.)*

nity.[50] When a new virus, here called HxNx, to which antibody is lacking is introduced into a population, pandemic influenza results. After one or more waves of pandemic influenza, the proportion of immune individuals in the population increases. This situation favors the emergence of viruses with antigenic changes in the HA or NA, whose spread through the partially immune population is thus facilitated. This phenomenon is repeated with subsequent epidemics from strains of influenza A/HxNx that exhibit some antigenic drift. After 10 to 30 years of circulation of variants with this given subtype, the level of immunity in the population to all variants within the subtype is very high, and the conditions for the spread of a new virus, HyNy, become favorable, with the emergence of a new pandemic of influenza.

The pattern of replacement of HA and NA subtypes during the most recent century of pandemics is shown in Figure 165-6 and is based

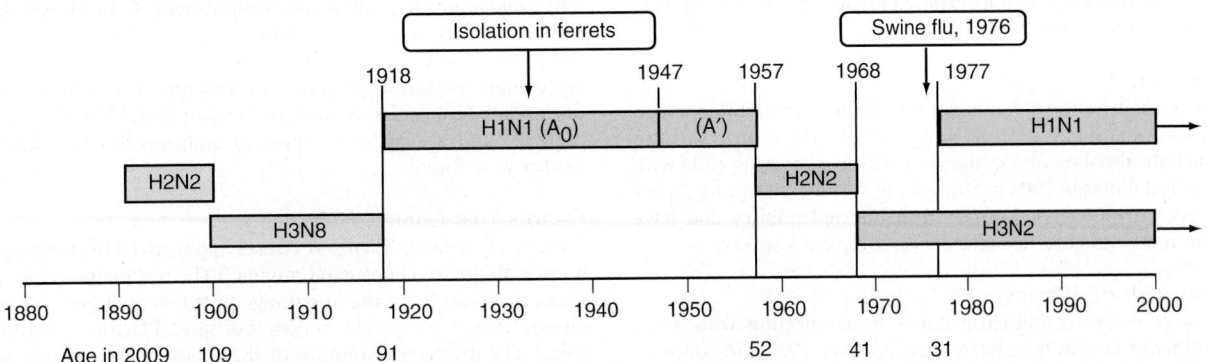

Figure 165-6 **Recent pandemics of influenza.** Duration of circulation of viruses of various subtypes is shown with boxes. Because the nature of influenza epidemics before 1918 is known only by serologic means, those boxes are *shaded tan*. Below the time line are given ages of individuals in 2009 who were alive during the various epidemic periods of earlier influenza subtypes. For example, individuals currently living who are between the ages of 52 and 91 years probably experienced their first influenza A infection with H1N1 virus. Individuals who are 41 years of age or younger have never been infected with H2N2 viruses. A pandemic associated with a novel A (H1N1) virus began in 2009 (see text).

both on virus isolation and serologic studies of individuals who lived through previous pandemics. Such studies suggest that the pandemic of 1889 was associated with viruses of an H3 subtype.[51] Virologic and polymerase chain reaction (PCR) studies have shown that the Spanish pandemic of 1918 (mentioned previously) was caused by an H1N1 virus, which in turn was supplanted in the Asian pandemic of 1957 by H2N2 viruses. In 1968, the Hong Kong pandemic was caused by viruses of the H3N2 subtype. In 1977, viruses of the H1N1 subtype were reintroduced through an unknown mechanism. These viruses are genetically identical to the H1N1 viruses that were circulating in 1950. Since 1977, influenza A viruses of both the H1N1 and H3N2 subtypes have cocirculated.

The degree of genetic difference between subtypes, 30% or greater, precludes their arising by simple point mutation, and the origin of new pandemic strains has been the subject of intense interest and study, for obvious reasons. The most plausible explanation for their origin takes into account three features of this phenomenon: that the virus has a segmented genome, that pandemics occur only with influenza A viruses, and that influenza A viruses, but not other influenza viruses, maintain a large reservoir of genetic diversity primarily in birds.

AVIAN INFLUENZA

Influenza A viruses infect a variety of species, including humans, swine, horses, marine mammals, and in particular, birds. In fact, no less than 16 unique HA subtypes (H1 to H16) and nine NA subtypes (N1 to N9) have been identified in avian influenza viruses. These avian viruses very likely can serve as the source for novel hemagglutinins associated with pandemic influenza in humans. Consequently, intense interest has been seen in sporadic infections of humans with avian influenza viruses that have occurred with increasing frequency during the last 10 years. These infections have involved primarily viruses of the H7, H9, and particularly H5 subtypes.[51a]

Infections with H7 Viruses
The most characteristic finding in human cases has been conjunctivitis. During an outbreak of H7N7 viral pneumonia that involved seals, a marine worker had conjunctivitis develop after being splashed in the eye with secretions from an infected seal.[52] A culture of the conjunctival swab grew the H7N7 virus. Another case of conjunctivitis caused by the H7N7 subtype virus was reported in which a pet duck was implicated as the source of the virus.[53] In 2003, a large outbreak of H7N7 infection involved poultry in the Netherlands.[54] Conjunctivitis was also the most common clinical presentation in this outbreak, but one fatal case of progressive pneumonia was reported in a veterinarian who had visited the poultry farm. In 2004, two farm workers in the Fraser Valley of British Columbia had conjunctivitis develop after an outbreak of H7N3 influenza virus infection among poultry.[55] In addition, serologic evidence of apparently asymptomatic infection has been observed in farm workers in Italy exposed to birds during an outbreak of H7N3 in poultry from 1999 to 2003.[56]

Infections with H9 Viruses
The H9N2 virus infection of humans was described in two children with mild influenza-like illness in Hong Kong in 1999.[57] H9N2 virus was also isolated in cultures of nasopharyngeal aspirate from another child with similar clinical illness in 2003 in Hong Kong.[58] These infections appear to have been acquired via contact with infected poultry and have resulted in mild influenza-like illness with complete recovery.

Infections with H5 Viruses
Human cases of severe influenza illness from infection with avian H5N1 influenza viruses have been reported since 1997 and continue to raise concerns about the potential for a new human pandemic. The highly lethal H5N1 viruses have become well established in migratory waterfowl throughout Asia and have undergone considerable diversification, with the development of at least 10 antigenically distinct clades and multiple subclades, as defined with phylogeny of HA gene sequences. Initial human infections involved viruses subsequently

assigned to clade 3. A second wave of infections was noted in 2004 from viruses of clade 1, and in the most recent years, human infections have primarily been from clade 2 viruses.

Clinical Features of H5N1 in Humans. Descriptions of the signs and symptoms of H5N1 infection are mostly from hospitalized patients.[59] Most patients have nonspecific symptoms of fever, cough, and shortness of breath. In many of the patients, a progression of symptoms leads to respiratory failure that necessitates ventilation and other supportive measures. Atypical symptoms like nausea, vomiting, encephalopathy, and bleeding gums and nose have been reported.[60] Watery diarrhea may be present before the onset of respiratory symptoms. Most patients have abnormal chest radiographic results with diffuse and multifocal or patchy infiltration, but pleural effusions are rare.

Laboratory abnormalities include significant lymphopenia and leucopenia, mild to moderate thrombocytopenia, and elevated transaminase levels. These abnormalities are poor prognostic signs.[61] Most patients have had negative bacteriologic cultures of sputum and blood. Pathologic changes include diffuse alveolar damage in the lungs, reactive hemophagocytosis in the marrow, and lymphoid depletion with atypical lymphocytosis in the spleen and lymphoid tissues.[62] Centrilobular hepatic necrosis and acute tubular necrosis have been reported.

Epidemiologic Features. Patients with symptomatic H5N1 infections have ranged in age from 3 months to 75 years, with a median age of 20 years.[63] Half of all cases have been in people aged less than 20 years, and 90% of cases have been in those less than 40 years of age. The median duration from onset of illness to hospitalization has been 4 days (range, 0 to 18 days). The case fatality rates have been highest for those in the 10 to 19 year age group, lowest for people 50 years or older, and in between for children aged less than 10 years, with an overall rate of 58%.

Most cases have had close contact with ill poultry a week before the onset of illness. Activities like plucking and preparing diseased birds, playing with birds (especially asymptomatically infected ducks), and handling fighting cocks are risk factors for infection.[59] Other apparent modes of acquisition have included eating undercooked poultry or drinking raw duck blood. Transmission of infection to felines from feeding of raw chicken to tigers and leopards has been documented in zoos in Thailand.[64] However, the risk of infection to humans from consumption of appropriately cooked poultry[65] or drinking of adequately treated water from natural reservoirs is likely negligible.

Asymptomatic infections appear to be rare,[66] and significant person-to-person transmission has not been reported. Fifteen family clusters of infection that involved two or more family members have been documented.[67] The largest cluster identified thus far has been in the village of Kubu Sembelang in northern Sumatra in Indonesia in May 2006 where seven confirmed cases occurred in extended family members of a 37-year-old woman who died of an acute respiratory illness and was buried before the establishment of a diagnosis. Sequence comparisons of viruses from human cases and those of concurrent avian cases have established that at least some of the cases in the cluster represented person-to-person transmission. In addition, one well-documented transmission of virus from an ill child in Thailand to her mother[68] and a suggestive report of transmission to a health care worker were found.

Factors That Control Host Range
Fortunately, avian influenza A viruses appear to be relatively restricted in their ability to replicate in humans.[69] The precise molecular mechanisms responsible for the host-range preferences of avian influenza A viruses are not completely known, but several factors probably play a role.[70] The divergent evolution of the genes of these viruses in avian hosts could have resulted in less efficient interactions between undefined viral and mammalian host-cell components. The relative attenuation of avian-human influenza reassortants for humans[71] supports a role for non-HA genes in this restriction. In addition, the HAs of avian and mammalian influenza viruses display a different host-cell receptor specificity, with avian viruses preferring receptors that contain sialic

acid–galactose linkages of the α2→3 variety and mammalian viruses tending toward α2→6 linkages.

Extensive sequence analysis has suggested at least two mechanisms by which avian viruses can circumvent these barriers to interspecies transmission. These studies have shown significant sequence similarity between the HA, NA, and PB1 gene segments of the pandemic H2N2 virus and avian viruses[72] and between the H3 and PB1 gene segments of the pandemic H3N2 virus and avian viruses,[72,73] which suggests that in some circumstances, new pandemic viruses arise by reassortment between avian viruses, which provide novel surface glycoproteins, and human viruses, which provide genes that allow efficient replication in humans. Reassortment is facilitated by the presence of a third species that is susceptible to infection with both avian and human viruses, such as the pig, which contains both types of receptors.[74] However, constraints on what types of reassortants are viable are likely; in particular, it has been suggested that the hemagglutinins of recent human influenza A viruses are not compatible with the matrix genes of current avian viruses,[75] and phenomena of this type may limit the possibilities for generation of pandemic viruses by reassortment.

A second mechanism involves adaptation of avian viruses to the human host by evolution in swine; this is supported by sequence analysis that shows that the 1918 pandemic was most likely the result of direct introduction of an avian or swine influenza A virus into humans.[76]

SWINE INFLUENZA

Swine-origin influenza viruses that represent triple reassortants with human viruses have been circulating among pigs since the late 1990s, with occasional infection of humans, most often after close contact with pigs.[76a,b] In March 2009, a novel influenza A (H1N1) virus was detected, which was a reassortant between previously circulating swine viruses and a Eurasian swine virus.[76c] This novel virus contains neuraminidase and matrix genes from the Eurasian virus and is also referred to as S-OIV (swine origin influenza virus). S-OIV now has the ability to spread efficiently from person to person and has led to a pandemic, which, as of June 15, 2009, has resulted in more than 35,900 laboratory-confirmed cases in 76 countries.[76d] The clinical symptomatology appears to be similar to that of seasonal influenza, perhaps with more frequent vomiting and diarrhea. At this time, disease has been relatively mild. Hospitalization occurred among 2% to 5% of confirmed cases in the United States and Canada,[76e,f,g] and in Mexico, 108 deaths occurred in 6241 laboratory-confirmed cases.[76e] Some 60% of cases have been in individuals 18 years of age or younger, as is typical for seasonal influenza.[76h] Whether earlier infection or immunization with previously circulating A (H1N1) viruses will provide protection against S-OIV is unclear. However, a study of individuals older than 60 years showed that one third had significant microneutralization titers (≥160) against S-OIV.[76h]

Pathogenesis and Host Response

CELLULAR PATHOGENESIS

Influenza virus infection is acquired by a mechanism that involves the transfer of virus-containing respiratory secretions from an infected to a susceptible person. Once virus is deposited on the respiratory tract epithelium, it can attach to and penetrate columnar epithelial cells if not prevented from doing so by specific secretory antibody (immunoglobulin A [IgA]), by nonspecific mucoproteins to which virus may attach, or by the mechanical action of the mucociliary apparatus. After adsorption, virus replication begins and leads to cell death through several mechanisms. A dramatic shutoff of host-cell protein synthesis occurs at several levels. Newly synthesized cellular messenger RNAs (mRNAs) are degraded (probably because cleavage by the virus cap endonuclease renders these transcripts susceptible to hydrolysis by cellular nuclease), whereas translation of already-synthesized cytoplasmic mRNAs is blocked at both initiation and elongation. Finally, expression of the influenza virus PA protein has been shown to induce generalized degradation of coexpressed proteins.[77]

Ultimately, the loss of critical cellular proteins very likely contributes to cell death.

In addition to effects that lead to cell necrosis, infection of cells with influenza A and B viruses causes cell death by apoptosis.[78] Bronchiolar epithelial and alveolar cells harvested from experimentally infected mice also exhibit apoptotic changes, which suggests that this mechanism of cell death may be important in the pathogenesis of influenza in vivo.[79] The specific mechanism by which influenza virus induces apoptosis is unclear, but it may be related to induction of Fas antigen by double-stranded RNA during virus replication.[80] An unusual viral protein of influenza A viruses, encoded by a second open reading frame in the PB1 gene and therefore referred to as PB1-F2, also plays a role in induction of apoptosis by poisoning mitochondria.[81]

Virus release continues for several hours before cell death ensues. Released virus then may initiate infection in adjacent and nearby cells, so within a few replication cycles, a large number of cells in the respiratory tract are releasing virus and dying as a result of the virus replication. The time between the incubation period and the onset of illness and virus shedding varies from 18 to 72 hours depending in part on the inoculum dose.[82]

Influenza virus infection of peripheral blood mononuclear cells, including polymorphonuclear leukocytes (PMNs), lymphocytes, and monocytes, is nonproductive but is associated with measurable defects in cellular function that may be relevant to the pathogenesis of influenza-related infectious complications. These include defects in PMN chemotaxis and phagocytosis[83] and decreased proliferation and costimulation by mononuclear cells.[84] The effects are mediated by virus replication and possibly by a direct toxic effect of certain virus proteins, including hemagglutinin, neuraminidase, and nucleoprotein.[85] The short portion of the sequence of the influenza A virus NP is homologous to a naturally occurring peptide found in normal bronchoalveolar lavage fluid that inhibits PMN chemotaxis and oxidative burst,[86] and exposure of PMNs to influenza virus suppressed endocytosis by these cells.[87]

VIRUS SHEDDING

Quantitation of virus in respiratory tract specimens reveals a characteristic pattern (Fig. 165-7). Virus is first detected just before the onset of illness (within 24 hours), rapidly rises to a peak of 3.0 to 7.0 $\log_{10}$ tissue-culture infective dose (TCID)$_{50}$/mL, remains elevated for 24 to 48 hours, and then rapidly decreases to low titers.[88] Usually, virus is no longer detectable after 5 to 10 days of virus shedding. However, because of the relative lack of immunity in the young, more prolonged shedding of higher titers of virus is seen in children.

The severity of illness correlates temporally with quantities of virus shed in experimental influenza in volunteers, thus suggesting that a major mechanism in the production of illness is cell death from viral replication. Although the clinical manifestations of influenza are dominated by systemic symptoms, viral replication is limited to the respiratory tract. Instead, systemic symptoms are probably the result of the release of potent cytokines, such as type I interferons, tumor necrosis factor, and interleukins (ILs), by infected cells and responding lymphocytes.[88]

HISTOPATHOLOGY

Bronchoscopy of individuals with typical uncomplicated acute influenza has revealed diffuse inflammation of the larynx, trachea, and bronchi, with mucosal injection and edema.[89,90] Biopsy in these cases has revealed a range of histologic findings, from vacuolization of columnar cells with cell loss, to extensive desquamation of the ciliated columnar epithelium down to the basal layer of cells (Fig. 165-8).[90] Individual cells show shrinkage, pyknotic nuclei, and a loss of cilia. Viral antigen can be seen in epithelial cells.[91] Generally, the tissue response becomes more prominent as one moves distally in the airway.[91] Epithelial damage is accompanied by cellular infiltrates primarily composed of lymphocytes and histiocytes. Histologic findings on autopsy in more severe cases show extensive necrotizing tracheo-

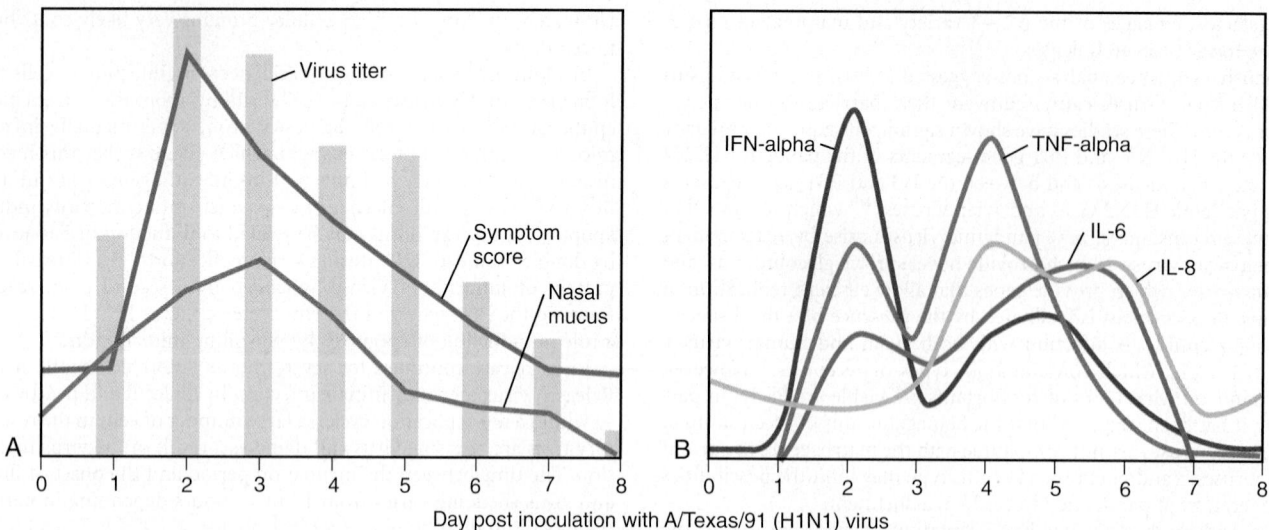

Figure 165-7   Time course of virus shedding, symptoms, and cytokine responses of healthy adults after experimental inoculation with wild-type A/Texas/36/91 (H1N1) virus via nasal drops. A, Mean $\log_{10}$ virus titer ($TCID_{50}$/mL nasal secretions), clinical symptom scores, and nasal mucus weights (in grams). **B,** Nasal cytokine levels measured with ELISA (pg/mL lavage fluid, corrected for collection efficiency). In both graphs, multiple measurements have been combined for illustration, so that y axes are relative values only. Peak values reported in each assay are approximately as follows: virus titer, 3.6 $\log_{10}$ $TCID_{50}$/mL nasal secretions; symptom score, 7.0; nasal mucus weight, 7.0 g; IL-6, 450 pg/mL; IFN-α, 150 pg/mL; tumor necrosis factor (TNF)-α, 270 pg/mL; IL-8, 9000 pg/mL. *(Data from Hayden FG, Fritz R, Lobo MC, et al. Local and systemic cytokine responses during experimental human influenza A virus infection: Relation to symptom formation and host defense. J Clin Invest. 1998;101:643-649.)*

bronchitis, with ulceration and sloughing of the bronchial mucosa,[92] extensive hemorrhage, hyaline membrane formation, and a paucity of PMN infiltration (Fig. 165-9). Patients with secondary bacterial pneumonia have the changes characteristic of bacterial pneumonia in addition to the tracheobronchial findings of influenza (Fig. 165-10). Recovery is associated with rapid regeneration of the epithelial cell layer and with pseudometaplasia.

PATHOPHYSIOLOGY

Abnormalities of pulmonary function are frequently seen in otherwise healthy, nonasthmatic young adults with uncomplicated (nonpneumonic) acute influenza. Demonstrated defects include diminished forced flow rates, increased total pulmonary resistance, and decreased density-dependent forced flow rates consistent with generalized increased resistance in airways less than 2 mm in diameter,[93,94] and increased responses to bronchoprovocation.[93] In addition, abnormalities of carbon monoxide diffusing capacity[95] and increases in the alve-

olar-arterial oxygen gradient[96] have been seen. Of note, pulmonary function defects can persist for weeks after clinical recovery. Influenza in patients with asthma[97] or in patients with chronic obstructive disease[98] may result in acute declines in forced expiratory vital capacity (FVC) or forced expiratory volume in 1 second (FEV_1). Individuals with acute influenza may be more susceptible to bronchoconstriction from air pollutants such as nitrates.[99]

Primary viral pneumonia is an uncommon but frequently severe complication of acute influenza. In this situation, virus infection reaches the lung either via contiguous spread from the upper respiratory tract or via inhalation. The trachea and bronchi contain bloody fluid, and the mucosa is hyperemic.[100] Tracheitis, bronchitis, and bronchiolitis are seen, with loss of normal ciliated epithelial cells. Submucosal hyperemia, focal hemorrhage, edema, and cellular infiltrate are present. The alveolar spaces contain varying numbers of neutrophils and mononuclear cells admixed with fibrin and edema fluid. The alveolar capillaries may be markedly hyperemic with intraalveolar hemorrhage. Acellular hyaline membranes line many of the alveolar

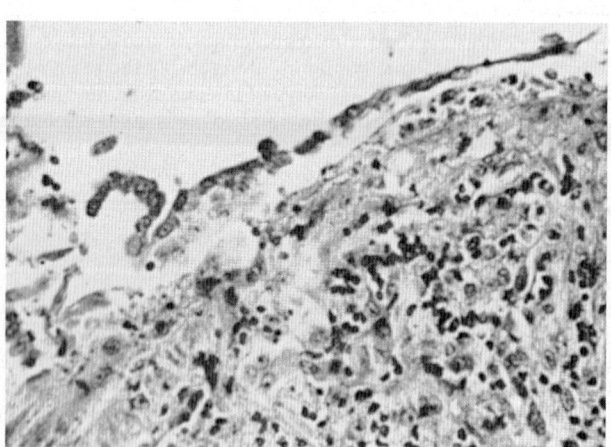

Figure 165-8   Small bronchus in acute influenza A infection shows ulceration and attempted regeneration of epithelium (hematoxylin and eosin [H&E], ×100). *(Courtesy of I. D. Stuard, Reading, PA.)*

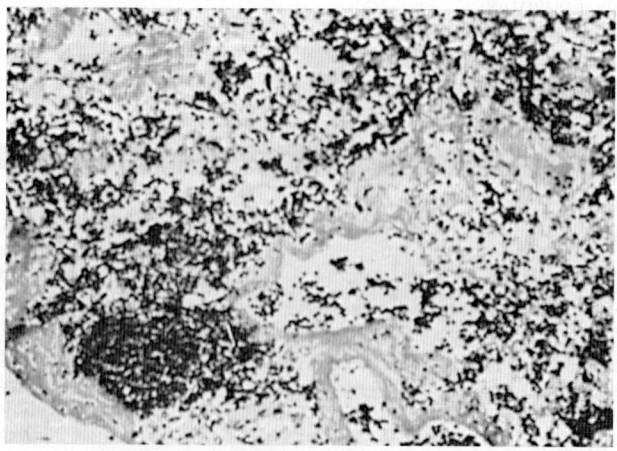

Figure 165-9   Lung parenchyma in primary influenza viral pneumonia shows extensive hemorrhage, acellular hyaline membrane lining alveolar ducts and alveoli, and paucity of inflammatory cells within the alveoli (H&E, ×400). *(Courtesy of I. D. Stuard, Reading, PA.)*

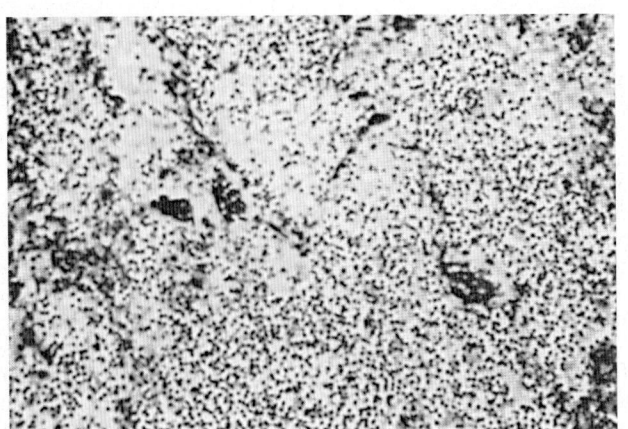

Figure 165-10 **Lung parenchyma in secondary bacterial infection (*S. pneumoniae*) complicating influenza A virus infection.** Note marked intraalveolar polymorphonuclear cell exudate (H&E, ×400). *(Courtesy of I. D. Stuard, Reading, PA.)*

ducts and alveoli.[100] Pathologic findings seen with biopsy of lung in nonfatal cases are similar to those described in fatal cases.[101]

Bacterial superinfection is a well-recognized complication of viral pneumonia and accounts for a large proportion of the morbidity and mortality of viral lower respiratory tract disease, especially in adults. Consequently, the spectrum of disease and pathophysiology of bacterial superinfection has been studied intensively, and a number of factors have been identified in viral respiratory disease that could play a role in increasing the risk of bacterial infection. Uncomplicated influenza is associated with significant abnormalities in ciliary clearance mechanisms.[102] In addition, increased adherence of bacteria to virus-infected epithelial cells has been shown.[103] The disruption of the normal epithelial cell barrier to infection and loss of mucociliary clearance undoubtedly enhance bacterial pathogenesis. In addition, influenza infection may upregulate certain cell surface receptors involved in bacterial adherence.[104] Alterations in PMNs and mononuclear cells may also contribute to enhanced bacterial infection.

VIRAL FACTORS THAT INFLUENCE PATHOGENICITY

Clinical characteristics of illness during the 1918 influenza pandemic differed from those of subsequent pandemics with higher mortality rates in young adults. The viral factors, if any, that might have been responsible for this behavior remain unknown. Extensive analysis of genetic sequences recovered from preserved specimens of material from victims of the pandemic have not revealed obvious differences between the 1918 influenza virus and more conventional influenza viruses, but investigations are continuing. Since that time, little direct evidence has been found for major inherent differences in viral strains with regard to pathogenic potential in humans. Instead, the severity of epidemics is most likely determined largely by the status of immunity in the population. However, in certain situations, individual viral proteins have been shown to have a significant impact on pathogenicity, which is particularly true for the HA and NS1 proteins.

An essential feature of influenza A virus replication is that proteolytic cleavage of the HA is necessary to generate infectious virus; this plays a role in the most clear-cut demonstration of the effect of an individual influenza virus protein in pathogenicity. Infection of fowl with avian influenza viruses can result in a relatively avirulent, asymptomatic infection limited to the respiratory and gastrointestinal mucosa or in a virulent, rapidly progressive, fatal systemic infection with involvement of the brain and other visceral organs. Comparison of the HAs of virulent and avirulent strains of H5 subtype and H7 subtype influenza A viruses has shown that the structure of the HA cleavage site is critical in determination of the virulence phenotype in this model. Proteases capable of cleaving the HA of avirulent viruses,

such as tryptase Clara,[105] are restricted in distribution to cells of the respiratory and gastrointestinal mucosa, thereby limiting replication to these areas. However, addition of several basic amino acids to the cleavage site[106] renders the hemagglutinin capable of cleaving by ubiquitous cellular furin-like proteases[107] and allows these viruses to escape the confines of the mucosa and replicate systemically in chickens.[108]

Lethal human infections with H5 and H7 containing highly cleavable HA have been described. Although some of these viruses also have a high level of lethality in mice, to date, no convincing evidence has been found of replication of these viruses outside the respiratory tract in humans. Thus, the potential role of HA cleavability in pathogenesis in humans is currently unknown. Evaluation of the nucleotide sequence of the HA from the 1918 pandemic virus did not reveal this virus to have the highly cleavable type of HA.[76]

Both influenza A and influenza B viruses use the NS1 protein as a mechanism to circumvent the host type-I interferon response. The NS gene antagonizes the action of type-I interferons through an unknown mechanism, and absence of the NS1 protein renders the virus incapable of growth in interferon-competent systems. The NS gene of the H5 avian viruses appears to be especially potent in this regard, which may provide a partial explanation for its enhanced virulence in mice. Recent reports have suggested that H5 viruses associated with fatal cases in humans have changes in nucleotide sequences in the NS1 gene that result both in increased resistance to the action of interferon and in the ability to induce proinflammatory cytokines.[109] In contrast, when the NS gene of the 1918 pandemic human virus was placed in the background of an avirulent influenza virus and administered to mice, more attenuated disease, rather than enhanced disease, was the result, which suggests the effect is host specific.

Multiple additional animal models have been described in which generation of influenza viruses with altered levels of pathogenicity is possible. A variety of classic genetic and molecular biologic techniques have been used to evaluate the role of specific viral genes or gene products in determination of the virulence of influenza viruses in these models. An exhaustive review of these studies is beyond the scope of this chapter, but results have generally shown that virulence is a multigenic trait with a specific basis that varies with the virus strains and the models used.[110]

IMMUNOLOGY

Epidemiologic and experimental observations in humans have shown that infection with influenza virus results in long-lived resistance to reinfection with the homologous virus. In addition, variable degrees of cross-protection within a subtype have been observed. Some epidemiologic data, particularly evidence that recent prior infection with H1N1 virus seemed to provide some protection to adults against H2N2 in the Cleveland family study,[111] have raised the possibility of heterosubtypic protection in humans, but the mechanism is undefined. Infection induces both systemic and local antibody and cytotoxic T-cell responses, each of which plays a role in recovery from infection and resistance to reinfection.

ANTIBODY RESPONSES

Systemic Antibody Responses
Infection with influenza virus results in the development of antibody to the influenza virus envelope glycoproteins HA and NA and to the structural M and NP proteins. Some individuals may have antibody to the M2 protein develop as well.[112] As measured with enzyme-linked immunosorbent assay (ELISA), serum immunoglobulin M (IgM), IgA, and immunoglobulin G (IgG) antibody to the HA appear simultaneously within 2 weeks of inoculation of virus. The antibody response is more rapid after reinfection. The development of anti-NA antibodies parallels that of hemagglutinin-inhibiting (HAI) antibodies.[113] Peak antibody responses are seen at 4 to 7 weeks after infection and decline slowly thereafter; titers can still be detected years after infection even without reexposure.

Antibody to the HA can be measured with standard HAI tests or a variety of ELISAs, and it neutralizes virus infectivity.[114] Because of the cost and requirement for cell cultures for the neutralizing test, the HAI test is the primary method of detection of antigenic relatedness among hemagglutinins of influenza viruses. Antihemagglutinin antibody protects against both disease and infection with the homologous virus.[115] Although no exact correlation exists, serum HAI titers of 1:40 or greater, or serum neutralizing titers of 1:8 or greater, are associated with protection against infection; HAI titers of 1:20 or 1:10 are associated with lesser degrees of protection.

Antibody to the NA can be measured with NA inhibition or ELISA. In contrast to anti-HA antibody, anti-NA antibody does not neutralize virus infectivity but instead reduces efficient release of virus from infected cells, which results in decreased plaque size with in vitro assays[116] and in reductions in the magnitude of virus shedding in infected animals.[117,118] Observations on the relative protection of those with anti-N2 antibody during the A/Hong Kong/68 (H3N2) pandemic[113,119] and experimental challenge studies in humans[120] have shown that anti-NA antibody can be protective against disease and results in decreased virus shedding and severity of illness but that it is infection permissive.[121]

Antibodies to other influenza viral proteins have also been evaluated for potential protection. Antibody to M2 reduces plaque size in vitro, and passive transfer studies in mice have also suggested that antibody to the M2 protein of influenza A viruses may be partially protective if present in large enough amounts.[122] The mechanism of protection in vivo is related to mediation of antibody-dependent cytotoxicity.[123] Because the extracellular domain of influenza A viral proteins is highly conserved, this has generated interest as a potentially cross-protective vaccine. Antibodies to internal viral proteins such as M or NP are also cross reactive among type A viruses, but they are nonneutralizing. Studies in mice have suggested that such nonneutralizing but cross-reactive antibodies may mediate protection under some circumstances.[124] The mechanism by which antibodies to viral proteins that are not exposed on the surface can mediate protection is unclear.

Mucosal Antibody Responses

Most studies of mucosal responses to influenza in humans have concentrated on measurement of HA responses with ELISA or neutralization tests because nonspecific inhibitors of hemagglutination present in nasal mucus interfere with the standard HAI test. These studies have shown significant mucosal responses to infection with wild-type virus or live-attenuated influenza vaccines. Both IgA and IgG are found in nasal secretions. Nasal HA-specific IgG is predominantly IgG$_1$, and its levels correlate well with serum levels of HA-specific IgG$_1$, which suggests that nasal IgG originates via passive diffusion from the systemic compartment.[125] Nasal HA-specific IgA is predominantly polymeric and IgA$_1$, which suggests local synthesis. Serum HA-specific IgA is also mostly polymeric IgA$_1$. The origin of serum IgA after mucosal infection is unclear but may derive from seeding of peripheral lymphoid tissue by memory cells derived from the mucosa.[115]

Studies in mice and ferrets have emphasized the importance of local IgA antibody in resistance to infection, particularly in protection of the upper respiratory tract. Polymeric IgA was shown to be specifically transported into the nasal secretions of mice and to protect against nasal challenge. Protection could be abrogated with intranasal administration of antiserum against IgA but not IgM or IgG.[126] Local antibody has also been shown to play a role in protection against antigenic variants in mice.[127] Studies in humans have also suggested that the resistance to reinfection induced by virus infection is mediated predominantly by local HA-specific IgA, whereas that induced by parenteral immunization with inactivated virus depends on systemic IgG.[128] Importantly, either mucosal or systemic antibody alone can be protective if present in high enough concentrations, and optimal protection occurs when both serum and nasal antibodies are present.[129,130]

CELLULAR RESPONSES

The induction of cellular response to influenza virus infection has been studied intensively in murine models, and such studies suggest that B cells, CD4$^+$ T cells, and CD8$^+$ T cells all play a role, in addition to antibody, in protection against disease and recovery from infection. A large number of HLA class I (CD8$^+$ T cell) and HLA class II (CD4$^+$ T cell) epitopes have been described, and in situations in which those epitopes are on relatively well-conserved proteins such as NP and M, the cellular responses are cross reactive between subtypes.

Cytotoxic T lymphocyte responses to influenza also develop in humans after influenza virus infections and generally peak on about day 14 after infection. Although not studied extensively, the presence of virus-specific prechallenge, class I–restricted cytotoxic T lymphocytes has been shown to correlate with reductions in the duration and level of virus replication in adults with low levels of serum HA and NA antibodies who were challenged with influenza A virus.[131] The role of cytotoxic T lymphocytes directed against internal viral proteins in protection against severe disease in humans is unclear, as the internal virus proteins were shared between viruses that caused the pandemics of 1957 and 1968 and the viruses in circulation immediately before these pandemics. Memory T-lymphocyte responses may play a role in ameliorating the severity of disease and speeding recovery after infection, as suggested by the finding of more severe influenza in individuals with severe defects in cell-mediated immunity.

Clinical Findings

UNCOMPLICATED INFLUENZA

Typical uncomplicated influenza often begins with an abrupt onset of symptoms after an incubation period of 1 to 2 days. Many patients can pinpoint the hour of onset. Initially, systemic symptoms predominate, including feverishness, chilliness or frank shaking chills, headaches, myalgia, malaise, and anorexia. However, a more gradual onset of signs and symptoms may also occur. In more severe cases, prostration is observed. Usually, myalgia or headache is the most troublesome symptom, and the severity is related to the height of the fever. Myalgia may involve the extremities or the long muscles of the back. In children, calf muscle myalgia may be particularly prominent. Severe pain in the eye muscles can be elicited with lateral gazing, and arthralgia but not frank arthritis is commonly observed. Other ocular symptoms include tearing and burning. The systemic symptoms usually persist for 3 days, the typical duration of fever. Respiratory symptoms, particularly a dry cough, severe pharyngeal pain, and nasal obstruction and discharge are also usually present at the onset of illness but are overshadowed by the systemic symptoms. The predominance of systemic symptoms is a major feature that distinguishes influenza from other viral upper respiratory infections. Hoarseness and a dry or sore throat may also be present, but these symptoms tend to appear as systemic symptoms diminish; thus, they become more prominent as the disease progresses and persist 3 to 4 days after the fever subsides. Cough is the most frequent and troublesome of these symptoms and may be accompanied by substernal discomfort or burning. Older adults may simply present with high fever, lassitude, and confusion without the characteristic respiratory symptoms, which may not occur at all. In addition, a wide range of symptomatology is found in healthy adults, ranging from classic influenza to mild illness or asymptomatic infection.

Fever is the most important physical finding. The temperature usually rises rapidly to a peak of 100°F to 104°F, and occasionally to 106°F, within 12 hours of onset, concurrent with the development of systemic symptoms. Fever is usually continuous but may be intermittent, especially if antipyretics are administered. On the second and third days of illness, the temperature elevation is usually 0.5°F to 1.0°F lower than on the first day, and as the fever subsides, the systemic symptoms diminish. Typically, the duration of fever is 3 days, but it may last 4 to 8 days.

Early in the course of illness, the patient appears toxic, the face is flushed, and the skin is hot and moist. The eyes are watery and reddened. A clear nasal discharge is common, but nasal obstruction is uncommon. The mucous membranes of the nose and throat are hyperemic, but exudate is not observed. Small, tender cervical lymph nodes are often present. Transient scattered rhonchi or localized areas of rales are found in less than 20% of cases. A convalescent period of 1, 2, or more weeks to full recovery then ensues. Cough, lassitude, and malaise are the most frequent symptoms during this period.

At the extremes of age, prominent differences in influenza are found. Influenza attack rates are higher in children than in adults. Maximal temperatures tend to be higher among children, and cervical adenopathy is more frequent among children than among adults. Croup associated with influenza virus infection occurs only among children.[132,133] Among older adults, fever remains a frequent finding, although the height of the febrile response may be lower than among children and young adults. Pulmonary complications are far more frequent in older adults than in any other age group.

COMPLICATIONS OF INFLUENZA

Pulmonary Complications

Two manifestations of pneumonia associated with influenza are well recognized: primary influenza viral pneumonia and secondary bacterial infection. In addition, less distinct and milder pulmonic syndromes often occur during an outbreak of influenza and may represent tracheobronchitis, localized viral pneumonia, or possibly mixed viral and bacterial pneumonia. Comparative features of these clinical syndromes are shown in Table 165-4.

Primary Influenza Viral Pneumonia. The syndrome of *primary influenza viral pneumonia* was first well documented in the 1957 to 1958 outbreak. However, clearly, some deaths of young healthy adults in the 1918 to 1919 outbreak were the result of this syndrome. In outbreaks since 1918, primary influenza viral pneumonia has occurred predominantly among persons with cardiovascular disease, especially rheumatic heart disease with mitral stenosis, and to a lesser extent in others with chronic cardiovascular and pulmonary disorders. The illness begins with a typical onset of influenza, followed by a rapid progression of fever, cough, dyspnea, and cyanosis. Physical examination and chest radiographic results reveal bilateral findings consistent with the adult respiratory disease syndrome but no consolidation. Blood gas studies show marked hypoxia, Gram stain of the sputum fails to reveal significant bacteria, and bacterial culture yields sparse growth of normal flora, whereas viral cultures yield high titers of influenza A virus. Such patients do not respond to antibiotics, and mortality is high. At autopsy, findings consist of tracheitis, bronchitis, diffuse hemorrhagic pneumonia, hyaline membranes lining alveolar ducts and alveoli, and a paucity of inflammatory cells within the alveoli (see Figs. 165-9 and 165-10). At the present time, late in the interpandemic era, severe primary influenza viral pneumonia is rare.

Secondary Bacterial Pneumonia. *Secondary bacterial pneumonia* often produces a syndrome that is clinically indistinguishable from that which occurs in the absence of influenza.[134,135] The patients (most often older adults or those with chronic pulmonary, cardiac, and metabolic or other disease) have a classic influenza illness followed by a period of improvement that lasts usually 4 to 14 days. Recrudescence of fever is associated with symptoms and signs of bacterial pneumonia such as cough, sputum production, and an area of consolidation detected on physical examination and chest radiograph. Gram staining and culture of sputum reveal a predominance of a bacterial pathogen, most often *Streptococcus pneumoniae* or *Haemophilus influenzae,* and notably, an increased frequency of *Staphylococcus aureus,* which is otherwise an uncommon cause of community-acquired pneumonia. Recently, community-acquired, methicillin-resistant *S. aureus* has been seen in children after influenza outbreaks.[136]

During an outbreak of influenza, many patients do not clearly fit into either of the aforementioned categories. The disease is not relentlessly progressive, and yet the fever pattern may not be biphasic. These patients may have primary viral, secondary bacterial, or mixed viral and bacterial infection of the lung. In addition, milder forms of influenza viral pneumonia involving only one lobe or segment have been described that do not invariably lead to death and that are more likely to be confused with pneumonia caused by *Mycoplasma pneumoniae* than to pneumonia produced by bacterial infection.

In children, pneumonia may occur, but it is less common than in adults. Bronchiolitis may also occur as a result of influenza A or B virus infection, but respiratory syncytial virus and parainfluenza virus type 3 are more important causes of bronchiolitis.

Pulmonary Complications in Patients with Immunosuppression. Influenza has been noted to cause severe disease with an increased incidence of pneumonia in children with cancer with immunosuppression compared with age-matched individuals without immunosuppression.[137] Severe disease associated with pneumonia and death has been reported, particularly in hematopoietic stem cell transplant recipients and patients with leukemia.[138,139] Individuals with relatively more immunosuppression early after transplantation appear to be at greater risk. Influenza virus shedding can be quite prolonged in children with immunosuppression,[140] particularly those with HIV and low CD4+ counts.[141] Because of the prolonged, unchecked replication of influenza viruses in these individuals, resistance to antiviral drugs eventually occurs in many treated patients.[142,143]

Other Pulmonary Complications. In addition to pneumonia, other pulmonary complications of influenza have been recognized.

TABLE 165-4	Comparative Features of Pulmonary Complications of Influenza			
	Primary Viral Pneumonia	*Secondary Bacterial Pneumonia*	*Mixed Viral and Bacterial Pneumonia*	*Localized Viral Pneumonia*
Setting	Cardiovascular disease; pregnancy; young adult	Age, >65 y; pulmonary disease	Any associated with A or B	?Normal
Clinical history	Relentless progression from classic 3-day influenza	Improvement, then worsening after 3-day influenza	Features of both primary and secondary pneumonia	Continuation of classic 3-day syndrome
Physical examination	Bilateral findings, no consolidation	Consolidation	Consolidation	Area of rales
Sputum bacteriology	Normal flora	*Pneumococcus, Staphylococcus, H. influenzae*	*Pneumococcus, Staphylococcus, H. influenzae*	Normal flora
Chest radiography	Bilateral findings	Consolidation	Consolidation	Segmental infiltrate
White blood cell count	Leukocytosis with shift to left	Leukocytosis with shift to left	Leukocytosis with shift to left	Usually normal
Isolation of influenza virus	Yes	No	Yes	Yes
Response to antibiotics	No	Yes	Often	No
Mortality	High	Low	Variable	Very low

Croup. Significant numbers of cases of croup occur in influenza A and B outbreaks.[132] Croup associated with influenza A virus appears to be more severe but less frequent than that associated with parainfluenza virus types 1 or 3 or respiratory syncytial virus infections (see Chapters 156 and 158).

Exacerbation of Chronic Pulmonary Disease. Acute exacerbation of chronic bronchitis is a common complication of influenza and may result in a permanent loss of pulmonary function.[144] Exacerbations of asthma and worsening pulmonary function in children with cystic fibrosis may also occur.[145]

Nonpulmonary Complications

Myositis. Myositis and myoglobinuria with tender leg muscles and elevated serum creatine phosphokinase (CPK) levels have been reported, mostly in children but in adults as well.[146] Symptoms may be sufficiently severe to interfere with walking.

Cardiac Complications. Both myocarditis and pericarditis have been rarely associated with influenza A or B virus infection.[147,148] Some investigators have associated influenza with myocardial infarction. However, neither myocarditis nor pericarditis is commonly observed at autopsy among those who died of primary influenza viral pneumonia.[100] In patients with cardiac disease, the acquisition of influenza provides a significant risk of death.[149]

Toxic Shock Syndrome. In recent outbreaks of influenza A or B, a toxic shock–like syndrome has occurred in previously healthy children or adults, presumably because viral infection changed colonization and replication characteristics of the toxin-producing staphylococcus.[150,151]

Central Nervous Complications. Guillain-Barré syndrome has been reported to occur after influenza A infection, as it has after numerous other infections, but no definite etiologic relationship has been established. In addition, cases of transverse myelitis and encephalitis have occurred rarely.[152] An etiologic association of these syndromes with influenza virus infection has only infrequently been proven, and influenza infection accounts at most for only a small proportion of cases of each of these symptoms.

Reye's Syndrome. Reye's syndrome is associated with many viral infections, prominently including influenza and varicella in children. The classic manifestation is a change in mental status that occurs several days after a typical respiratory illness. Manifestations range from lethargy to delirium, obtundation, seizures, and respiratory arrest. Lumbar puncture reveals normal protein values and normal cell counts, confirming the presence of encephalopathy rather than encephalitis or meningoencephalitis. The most frequent laboratory abnormality is elevation of the blood ammonia value, which occurs in almost all patients. Reye's syndrome is almost exclusively seen in children who have been given aspirin to treat febrile illnesses from influenza and other viruses, and use of other antipyretics such as nonsteroidal anti-inflammatory drugs in this situation is important. Children who need continuous aspirin therapy are an important target group for influenza vaccination to reduce the risks of Reye's syndrome.

Diagnosis

VIRUS ISOLATION

Virus can be isolated readily from nasal swab specimens, throat swab specimens, nasal washes, or combined nose and throat swab specimens. The general consensus is that throat swab alone is probably less sensitive for detection than other samples. Virus can also be isolated from sputum samples, if these are produced.[153] Samples should be placed into containers of viral transport medium and transported to the laboratory as soon as possible. Specimens for influenza are inocu-

lated onto rhesus monkey kidney, cynomolgus monkey kidney, or Madin-Darby canine kidney cell cultures, where virus is detected with cytopathic effect or hemadsorption. Less commonly, embryonated eggs can be used for virus isolation. More than 90% of positive cultures can be detected within 3 days of inoculation[154] and the remainder by 5 to 7 days.

RAPID DIAGNOSIS

A variety of techniques have been used for rapid diagnosis. The most widely used tests are based on immunologic detection of viral antigen in respiratory secretions. In each of these tests, a sample of respiratory secretions is treated with a mucolytic agent and then tested, either on a filter paper, in an optical device, or with a dipstick in which reaction with specific antibody results in a color change. Individual tests vary with regard to whether they differentiate influenza A and influenza B, but none of the current tests distinguish between influenza A (H1N1) and influenza A H3N2 viruses. All of these rapid tests are relatively simple to perform and can provide results within 30 minutes; some tests are eligible for Clinical Laboratory Improvement Amendment of 1998 (CLIA) waiver. Additional tests are in development, and updated information is available at http://www.cdc.gov/flu/professionals/labdiagnosis.htm.

The reported sensitivities of each test in comparison with cell culture have ranged between 40% and 80%, and they are somewhat dependent on the nature of the samples tested and the patients from whom they were derived. In general, sensitivities in adults and older adult patients tend to be lower than those reported in young children, who shed much larger quantities of virus in nasal secretions and therefore have much higher concentrations of antigen in their samples. Similarly, sensitivity is likely to be higher early in the course of illness, when viral shedding is maximal. Although all types of respiratory samples can be used in such tests, the sensitivity appears to be better with nasopharyngeal swabs and aspirates than with throat swabs or gargles.[155,156]

A variety of approaches to direct detection of viral nucleic acids in clinical specimens have also been explored for rapid diagnosis, including nucleic acid hybridization and PCR amplification. PCR in particular has the advantage of being potentially more sensitive than cell culture, and it may allow detection of virus in samples in which the virions have lost viability. In addition, multiplex techniques are possible to devise so that a single test can detect a number of different agents.[157] However, because PCR techniques are more labor intensive and technically demanding and require specialized laboratory equipment, they generally have not supplanted antigen detection for rapid diagnosis in clinical laboratories.

Laboratory diagnosis of the recently detected S-OIV should be made by real-time PCR, available through the CDC or state laboratories. Updated recommendations for testing can be found at http://www.cdc.gov/swineflu/.

SEROLOGY

Serologic tests, such as complement fixation and hemagglutination inhibition, can be used to retrospectively establish a diagnosis of influenza infection. Because most individuals have been previously infected with influenza viruses, a single serum is generally not adequate, and paired serum specimens, consisting of an acute and a convalescent sera obtained 10 to 20 days later, should be submitted for testing.

EPIDEMIOLOGIC DIAGNOSIS

A diagnosis can also be made on epidemiologic grounds. That is, when the presence of influenza virus is confirmed in a region or community, healthy adults with acute influenza-like illness most commonly have influenza. In fact, several studies have shown that the accuracy of a clinical diagnosis in healthy adults in the setting of an influenza outbreak is as high as 80% to 90%.[158-160] In an analysis of symptoms in young adults assessed for entry into studies of influenza virus treatment, the best multivariate predictors of laboratory-confirmed influenza virus infection were cough and fever,[159] with an increasing predictive value with increasing levels of fever. However, the predictive value of such a symptom complex may be less in older adults[161] and in children.[162] In nursing homes, the presence of cocirculating pathogens (such as respiratory syncytial virus) that can result in identical symptoms can clearly complicate the ability to make a clinical diagnosis of influenza specifically.[163,164]

ROLE OF RAPID DIAGNOSIS IN CLINICAL DECISION MAKING

The optimal use of rapid diagnostic tests in patient management is yet to be defined. Such tests are most clearly useful in the rapid identification of outbreaks within institutions or in the community, where the testing of multiple specimens can compensate for the relative lack of sensitivity of the test for any single specimen. The utility of rapid testing in other situations depends on a number of factors beyond the specific performance of the test, including the extent of influenza epidemic activity (i.e., the a priori likelihood of infection) and the potential consequences of a positive or negative result.

▦ Treatment

Four antiviral drugs are currently available for the prevention and treatment of influenza. A comparison of the basic pharmacology and antiviral activity of these agents is given in Table 165-5; they are described in detail subsequently (also see Chapter 41). Certain general principles apply regardless of the specific form of therapy chosen. Individuals with an intact immune system who have had previous influenza infections have rapid limitation of replication of these viruses. Therefore, the opportunity to impact viral replication with antiviral agents is limited, and effective use of these agents requires early initiation of therapy. No studies have ever shown a benefit of antiviral therapy begun after 48 hours or more of symptoms, and the greatest effect is typically seen when therapy is started in the first 24 hours. The question of whether delayed therapy may be useful in selected populations, such as individuals with immunosuppression, remains unanswered.

M2 INHIBITORS: AMANTADINE AND RIMANTADINE

Mechanism of Action and Activity
The M2 inhibitors amantadine and rimantadine are related primary symmetrical amines and are active against influenza A virus in a variety of cell culture systems and animal models. In cell culture, inhibitory

levels for influenza A virus range from 0.2 to 0.4 μg/mL for amantadine and from 0.1 to 0.4 μg/mL for rimantadine.

The antiviral activity of these drugs is the result of inhibition of the M2 ion channel activity of susceptible viruses. The function of the M2 ion channel in viral replication is to acidify the interior of the virion, disrupting the interaction between the matrix and nucleoproteins and allowing the ribonucleoproteins to be transported to the nucleus, where replication occurs.[165] Thus, the antiviral effect is primarily manifested in cell culture as inhibition of virus uncoating. Similar ion channels have been described for influenza B and C viruses; however, at clinically achievable levels, these drugs are active against only influenza A.

Pharmacology and Side Effects
Although the mechanism of action and spectrum of activity for amantadine are similar to those for rimantadine, important pharmacokinetic differences are found between the two drugs. Amantadine does not undergo metabolic change and is excreted unchanged in the urine with a half-life of 12 to 18 hours. This leads to rapid accumulation of amantadine in two settings: patients with renal failure and older adults with reduced renal function because of age. In older adults, the dosage of amantadine is recommended to be reduced to no more than 100 mg daily, and perhaps even to 100 mg every other day after the first few days, although extensive evidence of the efficacy for these lower doses is not available. By contrast, rimantadine undergoes extensive metabolism. Less than 15% of the drug is excreted in the urine unchanged, and the remainder is excreted as metabolic product. A dosage reduction to a maximum of 100 mg/day in older adults is also recommended for rimantadine. For equivalent dosages, blood levels of amantadine are higher than for rimantadine, but rimantadine concentrations in the sputum are higher.

The most common side effects of amantadine are minor and reversible central nervous system (CNS) side effects such as insomnia, dizziness, and difficulty with concentration. These side effects may be more troublesome in older adults, in whom confusion is noted in about 18% of recipients. In addition, amantadine use has been associated with seizures in individuals with prior seizure disorder.[166] Minor gastrointestinal symptoms have also been reported. The CNS effects of amantadine are increased when these drugs are coadministered with anticholinergics or antihistamines. In addition, trimethoprim-sulfamethoxazole may inhibit tubular secretion of amantadine and increase the potential for CNS toxicity.[167] No other significant drug interactions with amantadine are known. However, coadministration of amantadine with drugs known to have CNS side effects may exacerbate those effects and thus should be avoided.

TABLE 165-5	Antiviral Agents for Influenza			
	Amantadine	*Rimantadine*	*Zanamivir*	*Oseltamivir*
Protein target	M2	M2	Neuraminidase	Neuraminidase
Activity	A only	A only	A and B	A and B
Side effects	CNS (13%)	GI (6%)	?Bronchospasm	GI (9%)
	GI (3%)	GI (3%)		
Metabolism	None	Multiple (hepatic)	None	Hepatic
Excretion	Renal	Renal + others	Renal	Renal (tubular secretion)
Drug interactions	Antihistamines, anticholinergics	None	None	Probenecid (increased levels of oseltamivir)
Dose adjustments needed	≥65 years old	≥65 years old	None	CrCl <30 mL/min
	CrCl <50 mL/min	CrCl <10 mL/min		Severe liver dysfunction
Contraindications	Acute-angle glaucoma	Severe liver dysfunction	Underlying airway disease	
FDA-Approved Indications				
Therapy	Adults and children ≥1 year of age	Adults only	Adults and children ≥7 years of age	Adults and children ≥1 year of age*
Prophylaxis	Yes	Yes	No	Adults and children ≥13 years of age†

*FDA has authorized treatment of S-OIV with oseltamivir in children ≥3 months of age.
†FDA has authorized prophylaxis for S-OIV with oseltamivir in children ≥1 year of age.
CrCl, creatinine clearance; FDA, U.S. Food and Drug Administration; GI, gastrointestinal.

Rimantadine is associated with a considerably reduced rate of CNS side effects, and in comparative studies of long-term administration, the rate of CNS side effects was not significantly different from the rate with placebo.[168] No known drug interactions significantly affect the levels or metabolism of rimantadine.

Efficacy

Both amantadine and rimantadine are effective in the therapy of experimentally induced and naturally occurring influenza A. Amantadine treatment of H3N2 influenza A during the 1968 pandemic within the first 48 hours of illness was associated with decreases in the duration of fever by about 24 hours[169] and with a greater proportion of "rapid resolvers."[170,171] In addition, treated individuals had more rapid decreases in individual symptoms of cough, sore throat, and nasal obstruction. Treatment with amantadine results in significantly more rapid improvement in small airways dysfunction in healthy adults with uncomplicated H3N2 influenza.[93,172]

Additional trials of amantadine therapy were performed with similar results when H1N1 viruses reappeared in the late 1970s. Early amantadine therapy of influenza A/USSR/77 in otherwise healthy adults was shown to result in a more rapid decrease in fever and in a higher frequency of subjects with improved symptoms at 48 hours compared with placebo.[173] In addition, treated subjects were less likely to shed virus at 48 hours. In a second study conducted in young adults infected with A/Brazil/78, amantadine therapy was associated with a more rapid decrease in symptoms compared with aspirin therapy[174] and with decreased virus shedding.

Studies of rimantadine therapy of acute influenza in otherwise healthy adults with uncomplicated influenza have shown levels of benefit essentially identical to those seen with amantadine. Treatment of adults with H1N1[173] and H3N2[175] influenza A resulted in improved symptoms, decreased fever, and reduced virus shedding compared with placebo. When rimantadine and amantadine were directly compared in a randomized trial,[173] the efficacies of the two drugs were essentially identical.

Neither amantadine nor rimantadine has been subjected to extensive efficacy evaluation in high-risk subjects. One placebo-controlled study carried out among nursing home residents showed more rapid reduction in fever and in symptoms in rimantadine recipients. Furthermore, physicians who were caring for these patients, but who were blinded to study drug status, prescribed significantly fewer antipyretics, antitussives, and antibiotics and obtained fewer chest radiographs for the rimantadine recipients.[176]

Rimantadine has also been evaluated in the treatment of influenza A in children and shown to reduce the level of virus shedding early in infection when compared with acetaminophen. More variable effects on clinical symptom scores have been seen, with one study showing a decrease in scores and fever compared with acetaminophen[177] and the other, in which illness was relatively mild, showing no significant difference.[178]

Drug Resistance

Drug resistance has been a factor in limiting the use of these antiviral agents. Resistant viruses emerge frequently in treated individuals, particularly children, in whom subpopulations of resistant virus can be detected after treatment in virtually all cases.[179] Resistance is the result of single point mutations in the membrane-spanning region of the M2 protein most commonly at amino acid 31, and it confers complete cross resistance between amantadine and rimantadine.[180] Resistant virus can be transmitted to, and can cause disease in, susceptible contacts. Prolonged shedding of resistant viruses may occur in patients with immunocompromise, particularly children, and may continue even after therapy is terminated,[181] consistent with the relative fitness of these resistant viruses. Although previously rare, a rapid increase in the prevalence of de novo resistance to M2 inhibitors was noted in 2005, and essentially all H3N2 viruses are now resistant to these agents as of 2008 to 2009.[182,183] However, most influenza A (H1N1) viruses currently remain sensitive.[184] An exception are the pandemic circulating A (H1N1) viruses (S-OIV), which are resistant to the adamantanes.[184a]

NEURAMINIDASE INHIBITORS: ZANAMIVIR AND OSELTAMIVIR

Mechanism of Action and Activity

The neuraminidase inhibitors act by inhibiting the functioning of the influenza virus neuraminidase. This enzyme cleaves terminal sialic acid from sialic acid–containing glycoproteins that serve as host-cell receptors for attachment of influenza viruses. As virus replication proceeds within the cell, neuraminidase is synthesized and transported to the cell surface, where it removes the sialic acid from these cell surface glycoproteins. Destruction of these receptors by neuraminidase is critical in allowing newly formed viruses to subsequently egress from the cell and spread to other cells. Studies with mutant, neuraminidase-deficient viruses have shown that in the absence of a functional neuraminidase, virus remains attached to the host cell and to other virions.[185] In addition, neuraminidase may be important in facilitation of the penetration of virus through secretions in the respiratory tract, which are rich in sialic acid–containing macromolecules.[186]

Neuraminidase inhibitors are active against influenza viruses at millimolar concentrations or less. Activity against clinical isolates assessed in plaque inhibition tests ranges from concentrations of 0.01 to 16 μmol/mL. Influenza B viruses are approximately 10-fold less sensitive than influenza A viruses, but they are still sensitive well within clinically achievable concentrations. Among the influenza viruses sensitive to neuraminidase inhibitors are avian viruses with all nine known neuraminidase subtypes.

Pharmacology and Side Effects

Although zanamivir and oseltamivir have identical mechanisms of action and similar profiles of antiviral activity, they have different pharmacologic properties. Zanamivir (4-guanidino-Neu5Ac2en) is a polar molecule that is not orally bioavailable. Therefore, effective use of this agent requires local administration. The drug is currently supplied as a dry powder for oral inhalation, with the Diskhaler device (GlaxoSmithKline, Research Triangle Park, NC) also used commonly for a variety of asthma-related medications. Oseltamivir carboxylate is an orally bioavailable ethyl ester prodrug of oseltamivir phosphate, a carbocyclic transition-state–based inhibitor of the influenza virus neuraminidase.[187]

Oseltamivir is rapidly absorbed from the gastrointestinal tract and is converted in the liver by hepatic esterases to the active metabolite, oseltamivir carboxylate. The metabolite is excreted unchanged in the urine via tubular secretion, with a serum half-life of 6 to 10 hours. Administration of the drug with food may improve tolerability without impacting drug levels. Zanamivir is not bioavailable via the oral route and must be administered topically to be effective. The drug is supplied in blister packs in which each blister contains 5 mg of zanamivir and 20 mg of lactose carrier. The standard dose is therefore two inhalations twice a day. Approximately 4 mg of drug is estimated to be actually delivered with each inhalation. Intravenous dosing of zanamivir has also been studied, although this formulation is not currently available for clinical use. In one small study, an intravenous dose of 600 mg twice daily was well tolerated and was effective in prevention of experimental infection of adults with influenza A (H1N1) virus.[188]

Both drugs have been well tolerated in clinical trials. The major adverse effects reported for oseltamivir have been gastrointestinal upset, probably irritation from rapid release of the drug in the stomach. Rates of nausea can be substantially reduced if the drug is taken with food. The most commonly reported adverse effects in individuals treated with zanamivir have been diarrhea, nausea, and nasal signs and symptoms, which have occurred at essentially the same rate as in placebo recipients. In one study in which zanamivir was used in patients with influenza infection with asthma or chronic obstructive pulmonary disease, the frequency of significant changes in FEV$_1$ or peak flow rates was higher in zanamivir than in placebo recipients. For this reason, individuals with these pulmonary conditions should have ready access to a rapidly acting bronchodilator when using zanamivir, in the event that the drug precipitates bronchospasm.

The dose of oseltamivir should be reduced to 75 mg once daily in individuals with renal impairment (i.e., with creatinine clearance of less than 30 mL/min). No data are available regarding the use of the drug in individuals with more significant levels of renal impairment. Likewise, no information is available regarding the use of oseltamivir in individuals with hepatic impairment. Clinically significant drug interactions have not been reported. Because oseltamivir is eliminated via tubular secretion, probenecid increases serum levels of the active metabolite approximately two-fold. However, dosage adjustments are not necessary in individuals taking probenecid. Coadministration of cimetidine, amoxicillin, or acetaminophen has no effect on serum levels of oseltamivir or oseltamivir carboxylate.[189]

Although significant increases in the serum half-life of zanamivir are seen in the presence of renal failure, the small amounts of the drug that are absorbed systemically suggest that dosage adjustments are not necessary. Studies of the pharmacokinetics of the drug in the presence of impaired hepatic function have not been reported.

Efficacy
Zanamivir and oseltamivir, the two available neuraminidase inhibitors, have shown similar results in clinical trials. Both drugs were initially evaluated in the human experimental challenge model. Studies in which oseltamivir was administered 28 hours after experimental infection showed reductions in viral shedding, reduced symptom scores, and decreased frequencies of middle ear abnormalities compared with placebo.[190] Zanamivir given via drops or spray as late as 50 hours after infection also showed reduced viral shedding, symptom scores, nasal mucus weights, and middle ear abnormalities.[191] Similar effects were seen with oseltamivir in adults experimentally infected with influenza B virus.

In studies of naturally occurring, uncomplicated influenza in healthy adults, therapy with oseltamivir initiated within the first 36 hours of symptoms resulted in 30% to 40% reductions in the duration of symptoms and severity of illness and reduced rates of prolonged coughing.[192,193] In addition, early therapy is associated with a significantly earlier return to work or other normal activities. Similarly, in healthy adults, early therapy of uncomplicated influenza A or B with inhaled zanamivir has been shown to result in a reduction of approximately 0.8 to 1.5 days in the duration of influenza symptoms and an earlier return to normal activities.[194,195] Early treatment of healthy adults with zanamivir may also reduce the frequency of complications, with reductions in the use of antibacterials and in hospitalization.[196]

Both oseltamivir and zanamivir have been evaluated as therapy for children. Administration of oseltamivir liquid at a dose of 2 mg/kg per dose twice daily for 5 days was well tolerated and resulted in a 36-hour reduction in the duration of symptoms in children with influenza A.[197] In addition, the use of oseltamivir was associated with a 44% reduction in the frequency of otitis media complicating influenza and with reductions in antibiotic prescriptions in children with influenza infection. Similarly, therapy for children 5 to 12 years old with symptomatic influenza A and B virus infection who were treated within 36 hours with inhaled zanamivir (10 mg twice a day) resulted in relief of symptoms 1.25 days earlier than with placebo recipients and a more rapid return to normal activities.[198]

Neuraminidase inhibitor therapy of influenza in adults with risk factors for influenza complications has not been evaluated extensively. However, both drugs have shown trends toward efficacy in such populations.[195,199] The results of metaanalyses of the pooled data from phase III studies have indicated that early treatment with inhaled zanamivir is associated with a median reduction of illness of 2.5 days in older adult and high-risk subjects and a 3-day earlier return to normal activities.[200] In these pooled analyses, early treatment of high-risk adults and older adults resulted in a 43% reduction in the rates of complications requiring antimicrobials.

Drug Resistance
Analysis of drug-resistant viruses has revealed two basic mechanisms of resistance that illustrate the interactive roles of the viral HA and NA in binding to and release from infected cells. Mutations within the catalytic framework of the NA that abolish binding of the drugs have been described.[201,202] The specific mutations that confer resistance are dependent on the specific NA; that is, common resistance mutations in N1 (e.g., H274Y) are different than the ones seen in the N2 (e.g., R292K or E119V) or influenza B (e.g., D198N). In addition, depending on the location of the mutation, these viruses may be specifically resistant to only one inhibitor.[203] Resistance mutations in the NA may be associated with altered characteristics of the enzyme with significantly reduced activity.[204,205]

A second type of mutation associated with cell cultured resistant viruses involves mutations in the receptor binding region of the hemagglutinin. HA mutations associated with resistance to neuraminidase inhibitors reduce the affinity of the HA for its receptor, allowing cell-to-cell spread of virus in the absence of NA activity.[201,206] Generation is even possible of inhibitor-dependent viruses, in which the affinity for the receptor is apparently so low that NA activity must be inhibited to allow the virus to bind at all. Resistant viruses with HA mutations exhibit cross resistance to these drugs in cell culture but may retain susceptibility in animal models. Many of these viruses also exhibit reduced virulence in animals.

Some resistant viruses appear to have reduced fitness, with reduced levels of replication, attenuation in animals, and reduced ability to be transmitted from animal to animal.[207-210] Therefore, there had been hope that resistance would not be the same limiting issue with NA inhibitors that it has been for the M2 inhibitors. Drug resistant viruses were isolated infrequently from individuals with oseltamivir treatment in clinical trials and were seen in less than 2% of treated adults and 5.6% of children.[197] Subsequently, resistant viruses could be detected in up to 18% of treated children with sensitive PCR techniques to pick up minor subpopulations.[211]

Beginning in 2006, spontaneously resistant H1N1 viruses carrying the H274Y mutation began to be detected in viruses from individuals who did not have a history of exposure to oseltamivir. These viruses remain sensitive to zanamivir. Until March 2009, essentially 100% of H1N1 viruses isolated in the United States have been resistant to oseltamivir, although H3N2 viruses remain sensitive.[184] However, the newly circulating A (H1N1) pandemic viruses (S-OIV) are sensitive to zanamivir and oseltamivir,[184a] although a few resistant isolates to oseltamivir have been noted, and the drugs can be used in prophylaxis or treatment of infection with S-OIV. Updated treatment recommendations for S-OIV infection are available at www.cdc.gov/h1n1flu/recommendations.htm.

For influenza infection with viruses other than S-OIV, the emerging resistance patterns have made treatment recommendations difficult. Influenza B viruses remain sensitive to both zanamivir and oseltamivir; therefore, oseltamivir or zanamivir may be used in influenza B infections. No zanamivir-resistant influenza A viruses have been detected, so that this drug remains an option for treatment of individuals infected with influenza A for whom the drug is licensed. If zanamivir is not licensed for a patient group or is not available, treatment choices must be made based on knowledge of current resistance patterns and locally circulating strains. For influenza A (H1N1) other than S-OIV, rimantadine or amantadine may be used. For influenza A (H3N2), oseltamivir may be used. If the subtype of influenza A virus cannot be ascertained, clinicians could consider treatment with the combination of oseltamivir and rimantadine or amantadine.[212]

TREATMENT OF COMPLICATIONS

Supportive care, including fluid and electrolyte management, is important. For patients with proven or suspected bacterial superinfection, appropriate antibiotics for the specific organism should be administered. Because of the rapidly advancing nature of many cases of pneumonia that occur during an influenza epidemic, therapy to cover the potential pathogens, including *S. pneumoniae* and *H. influenzae*, and possibly *S. aureus*, is indicated if an etiologic diagnosis cannot be made from a Gram stain of the sputum.

No controlled studies have been seen of antiviral therapy for the treatment of influenza viral pneumonia, so use for this condition is based on extrapolation from the benefits in uncomplicated influenza and anecdotal case reports of benefit. In a small controlled study, no difference was found in outcome between hospitalized adults treated with the combination of rimantadine and zanamivir and those treated with rimantadine alone, although both drugs were well tolerated.[213]

Treatment of Avian Influenza A (H5N1)

The efficacy of antiviral therapy for avian influenza A (H5N1) in humans has not been established. Clade 1 and most clade 2 H5N1 viruses from Indonesia and Southeast Asia are fully resistant to the M2 inhibitors, whereas clade 2 viruses from other parts of Eurasia and Africa are usually susceptible.[214] Clade 1 and clade 2 H5N1 viruses are usually sensitive to oseltamivir, although resistant viruses have been detected after therapy with oseltamivir[215] and occasionally before any therapy.[216,217] Based on information from in vitro and experimental animal data, and small observational studies, panels of experts convened by the World Health Organization (WHO) in 2006 and 2007 made the following series of recommendations for therapy of human cases of avian influenza A (H5N1).[216]

Treatment should be begun with oseltamivir, possibly at a higher dose (150 mg twice daily [bid]) and for a longer duration (10 days) than standard therapy. Because the best results appeared to be associated with early therapy, the drug should be started as soon as possible. Inhaled zanamivir is not recommended because of the lack of data in human cases of influenza A (H5N1).[214] Adamantanes are not recommended as first-line therapy, but combinations of oseltamivir and amantadine or rimantadine might be considered if the viral isolate is likely to be susceptible to M2 inhibitors.[217] Supportive care with correction of hypoxemia and treatment of nosocomial complications is essential in the management of patients. Corticosteroids have not been shown to be beneficial and may be harmful.[214,216]

Prevention

VACCINES

Inactivated Influenza Vaccine

The most effective measure available for the control of influenza is the annual administration of influenza vaccines. Chemically inactivated influenza virus vaccines were first licensed in the United States in 1943. The original vaccine, which consisted of formalin-inactivated whole virions grown in embryonated chicken eggs, was shown to have a protective efficacy of 70% in healthy adults.[9] Since then, although several important advances have occurred in the techniques for producing vaccine, the basic vaccine strategy has remained the same. The development of the zonal gradient centrifuge allowed more efficient production and more highly purified vaccines from which reactogenic contaminants had been removed. Treatment of the whole virus with solvents to create split vaccines, or with detergents to create subunit vaccines, has resulted in a vaccine with fewer adverse reactions, particularly fever, than the whole-cell vaccine. The efficiency of vaccine production has also been improved through the development of techniques to create so-called high-yield reassortant strains adapted to grow in high yield from hens' eggs.[218] The current vaccine is generally formulated as a trivalent preparation, containing one example each of influenza A (H1N1) virus, A (H3N2) virus, and influenza B virus thought to be most likely to cause disease in the upcoming season on the basis of epidemiologic and antigenic analysis of currently circulating strains. Since the late 1970s, the vaccine has been standardized to

contain at least 15 μg of each hemagglutinin (HA) antigen as assessed with single radial immunodiffusion (SRID).

Safety. Influenza vaccine is generally well tolerated in adults. Rates of mild local soreness after administration of inactivated influenza vaccine have been documented in the range of 60% to 80% in multiple studies.[219,220] Local side effects are slightly more common in women than in men.[219] Systemic reactions, including malaise, flulike illnesses, and fever, are relatively uncommon. Rates of transient, low-grade fever have varied from 2% to 10% of recipients in these studies; these rates are only marginally increased above the rates in placebo recipients. Although whole-virus and split-product vaccines are similarly reactogenic in adults, whole-virus vaccines are associated with higher rates of febrile adverse events in children[221,222] and are no longer available in the United States.

Severe, life-threatening, immediate hypersensitivity reactions to parenteral inactivated vaccine have been rare. However, hypersensitivity to hen eggs, in which the vaccine virus is grown, is a contraindication to vaccination. Generally, if persons can eat eggs or egg-containing products, vaccination is safe. Although vaccine is usually not administered to patients with a genuine anaphylactic hypersensitivity to egg products, such individuals can be desensitized and safely vaccinated if necessary.[223,224]

During the 1976 National Immunization Program against swine influenza, 45 million persons received influenza vaccine. In the first 4 to 6 weeks after vaccination, the incidence of Guillain-Barré syndrome (GBS) among vaccinees exceeded that among persons who did not receive the vaccine.[225] The estimated risk of GBS during that vaccination program was 1 in 100,000 vaccinations; the mortality rate for those with GBS was 5% (i.e., 1 in 2,000,000 vaccinations), and another 5% to 10% had some residual neurologic abnormality. Very slight increases in the risk of GBS were seen after the 1992 to 1993 and 1993 to 1994 vaccines, representing an excess of approximately one case per million persons vaccinated.[226]

Immune Response. Increases in HAI antibody are seen in about 90% of healthy adult recipients of vaccine. Only a single dose of vaccine is necessary in individuals who were previously vaccinated or who experienced prior infection with a related subtype, but a two-dose schedule is needed in unprimed individuals.[221,227] Primed individuals also generally respond with antibody that recognizes a broader range of antigenic variants than do unprimed individuals.[228] Serum antibodies peak between 2 and 4 months after vaccination but fall quickly, reaching near baseline before the next influenza season.[229] Mucosal anti-influenza antibodies are not generated efficiently by parenteral inactivated influenza vaccine.[230,231] Cellular responses, including HLA class II–restricted CD4 responses, are also noted.[232] Although the induction of HAI antibody is generally accepted as a correlate of vaccine protection, in some populations such as the elderly, induction of cellular responses has been suggested to also correlate with protection.[233]

Groups of adults with potentially decreased responses to inactivated influenza vaccine include older adults, individuals on immunosuppressive therapy, those with renal disease, and transplant recipients. For maximal effectiveness, immunizations should be given before transplantation, should avoid the nadir of white counts, and should include vaccination of close contacts.[234] The responsiveness to influenza vaccination in individuals with HIV is related to the degree of immunosuppression.[235,236] Most patients with chronic lung disease respond reasonably well to vaccination, and steroids at doses commonly used to treat reactive airways disease do not appear to preclude vaccine responses.[237,238]

Efficacy and Effectiveness. Inactivated influenza vaccine has been shown to be effective in the prevention of influenza A in controlled studies conducted in young adults, with levels of protection of 70% to 90% if there is a good antigenic match between the vaccine and the epidemic virus. For example, the efficacy of trivalent inactivated influenza vaccine (TIV) for prevention of culture-proven influenza A illness in adults was 76% (95% confidence interval [CI], 58% to 87%) for H1N1 and 74% (95% CI, 52% to 86%) for H3N2 in a controlled trial that compared live and inactivated vaccines.[239] A subanalysis of efficacy in children in this trial showed efficacy of 91% and 77% in prevention of symptomatic, culture-positive influenza A (H1N1) and A (H3N2) illness, respectively, compared with placebo. Vaccination of adults is also associated with decreased absenteeism from work or school and is significantly cost effective,[27] but these benefits may not be seen in years without a good match between vaccine and circulating viruses.[240] In children, TIV has reduced the rates of otitis media in some,[241,242] but not all,[243] studies.

Relatively few prospective trials of protective efficacy have been conducted in high-risk populations. In one placebo-controlled prospective trial in an older adult population, inactivated vaccine was approximately 58% effective in prevention of laboratory-documented influenza.[244] Vaccine has also been shown to be protective in limited studies in other high-risk groups, including those with HIV infection.[245]

An alternative approach to assessment of vaccine effectiveness in high-risk populations has been the observation of cohorts in which information about vaccine status can be linked to disease outcomes. Studies of this type have confirmed the effectiveness of inactivated influenza vaccines in older adults[246,247] and suggested that use of vaccine is accompanied by a decrease in all-cause mortality[248] and in rates of coronary events or stroke during the influenza season.[249] However, because such studies are not randomized, they are susceptible to biases introduced by undetected differences between vaccinated and unvaccinated populations (e.g., relatively higher degrees of frailty among unvaccinated subjects or relatively greater health maintenance behavior among vaccinated patients) that might partly or completely account for the protective effects seen.[250,251]

Live-Attenuated (Cold-Adapted) Influenza Vaccine

Live-attenuated influenza vaccine, cold-adapted influenza vaccine–trivalent (CAIV-T), is licensed for use in the United States in the age group from 5 to 49 years. The use of live-attenuated viruses as influenza vaccine offers several potential advantages over parenteral inactivated vaccine, including induction of a mucosal immune response and a nasal route of administration that might be more acceptable to patients, particularly in certain age groups.

Development of these vaccines takes advantage of the principle of reassortment to generate rapidly attenuated vaccines for new antigenic variants (Fig. 165-11). In this case, the master vaccine viruses are the cold-adapted influenza A/Ann Arbor/6/60 (H2N2) and B/Ann Arbor/1/66 viruses, developed by Dr. John Maassab at the University of Michigan in the 1960s.[252] The process of cold adaptation is the repetitive passage of a virus at gradually decreasing temperature until a virus is isolated that replicates efficiently at a low temperature at which the replication of the original wild-type virus is significantly restricted.

The use of live, attenuated virus as a vaccine for influenza was suggested very shortly after influenza virus was first recognized as the cause of the human disease,[10] and this approach has been pursued more or less vigorously since that time. The currently licensed live vaccine takes advantage of the segmented nature of the influenza virus genome to generate reassortant viruses in which the gene segments encoding attenuation are derived from the well-characterized master donor A/Ann Arbor/6/60 and B/Ann Arbor/1/66 viruses developed by Dr. John Maassab.[252] These cold-adapted viruses and their reassortants display three characteristic phenotypes: 1, the cold-adapted (ca) phenotype, defined as the ability to replicate efficiently at 25°C, a restrictive temperature for wild-type (wt) influenza viruses; 2, the temperature-sensitive (ts) phenotype, defined as significant (>2 $\log_{10}$) restriction of virus replication at 38°C to 39°C; and 3, the attenuation (att) phenotype, defined as restricted replication in the lower respiratory tract of experimental animals.[253]

Multiple mutations are involved in the attenuation of both donor viruses. In the case of the cold-adapted A/Ann Arbor/6/60 virus, mutations have been shown in all six internal gene segments.[253,254] Studies with single gene reassortants have shown that at least three of these

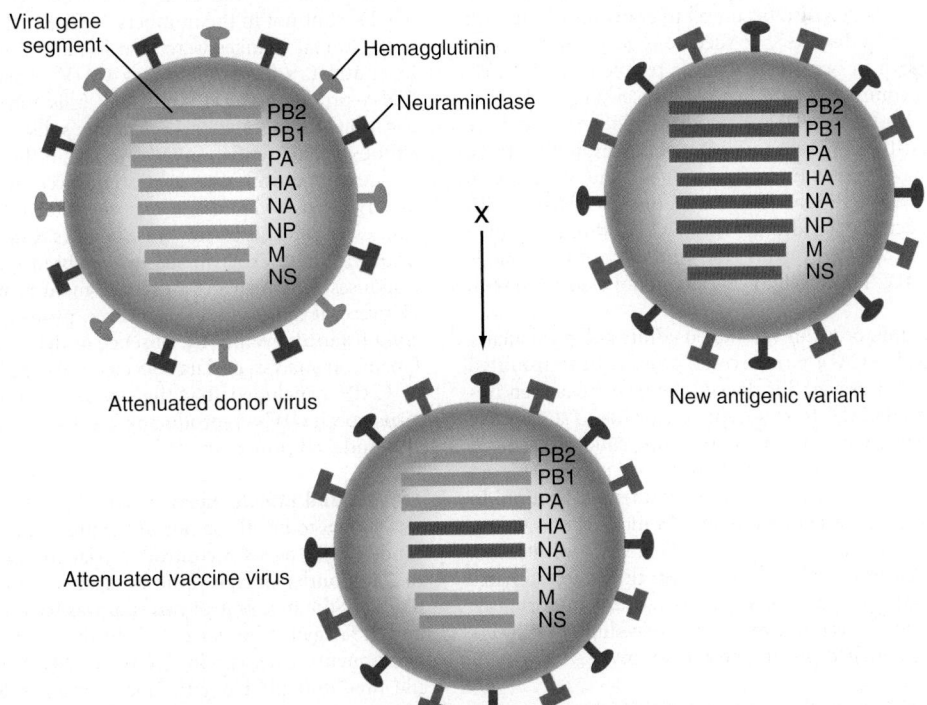

Figure 165-11 Genetic reassortment is used to generate new live-attenuated vaccine viruses. Genetic basis of attenuation of the "master donor virus" is encoded in gene segments other than hemagglutinin (HA) or neuraminidase (NA). With use of either mixed infection in cell culture or reverse genetics techniques, the genes encoding HA and NA of new antigenic variants can be inserted into the background of the master donor virus to rapidly create a new attenuated vaccine virus.

gene segments (PB1, PB2, and PA) participate in the attenuation of the cold-adapted influenza A virus in both animals and healthy seronegative human subjects.[255,256] When individual mutations were placed in the genome with reverse genetics techniques, the ts phenotype of the cold-adapted influenza A/Ann Arbor/6/60 virus was mapped to five sites, three in PB1, one in PB2, and one in NP.[257]

The PA, NP and PB2 gene segments all independently contribute to the cold-adapted phenotype of the cold-adapted B/Ann Arbor/1/66 virus.[258] Unique mutations involved in the ts and ca phenotype include two sites in NP and one in PA. These changes plus two additional changes in M1 are involved in the attenuation phenotype as assessed in the ferret model.[259] These findings are consistent with analysis of laboratory-derived revertant viruses that also implicate the PA gene segment as playing an important role in attenuation.[260,261] Because both donor viruses are attenuated at multiple sites, the vaccines are predicted to be phenotypically stable even after prolonged replication in seronegative children; this has been shown in clinical studies.[262]

Safety. Cold-adapted influenza vaccine–trivalent or closely related formulations of CAIV have been well tolerated in adults, with rates of mild nasal symptoms (runny nose, nasal congestion, or coryza) and sore throat that occur at rates slightly in excess of those in placebo recipients. These vaccines have also been shown to be safe and well tolerated in children, although children less than 8 years of age have had slightly increased but variable rates of low-grade fever, runny nose, and abdominal symptoms in the 7 days after vaccination compared with placebo recipients. However, when considering all the pediatric studies in aggregate, no consistent symptom was significantly more common in CAIV recipients compared with placebo recipients. In older children, 11 to less than 16 years of age, sore throat was observed slightly more frequently in CAIV recipients than in recipients of inactivated influenza.

Safety has also been shown in some high-risk patient groups. No significant vaccine-related adverse events were seen in studies of children with cystic fibrosis or asthma, and vaccinated children with asthma did not have significant changes in FEV$_1$, use of beta-adrenergic rescue medications, or asthma symptom scores compared with placebo recipients.[263] CAIV has also been well tolerated in adults with chronic obstructive airway disease.[264,265] Vaccine is very well tolerated in older adults, although in one study, vaccine recipients had a 13% excess of sore throats compared with those who received placebo.[266]

Young children with advanced HIV infection were reported to have difficulty clearing wild-type influenza virus from the respiratory tract, and several reports have been found of prolonged virus shedding in highly immunosuppressed individuals, including children with acquired immunodeficiency syndrome (AIDS). However, in small studies in adults[267] and children[268] with HIV who did not have manifestations of AIDS, CAIV-T was well tolerated and not associated with prolonged shedding.

Shedding of CAIV does occur in vaccinated adults and particularly in children. Therefore, live CAIV viruses could possibly be transmitted to susceptible contacts. However, this does not appear to happen frequently. Transmission of CAIV from vaccine recipients to susceptible contacts has been rarely detected in studies of young children involved in daycare-like settings where CAIV and placebo recipients played together for up to 8 hours a day for 7 to 10 days after vaccination. In the largest study, 197 children between 8 and 36 months of age in a daycare setting were randomized to receive trivalent CAIV or placebo, and CAIV was detected in one placebo recipient; thus, the estimates of transmissibility in this age group were 0.6% to 2.0%.[269] Importantly, samples of vaccine virus recovered from vaccinated volunteer subjects have all retained the attenuated phenotype and genotype.[270]

Immune Response. Studies of the immunogenicity of cold-adapted reassortant vaccines have been carried out in children, adults, and older adults. The results of these studies are consistent with the hypothesis that the replication of cold-adapted vaccines in the upper respiratory tract, and hence, their immunogenicity, is influenced by the susceptibility of the host at the time of vaccination. The frequency and magnitude of immune responses to vaccination are therefore highest in young children, intermediate in adults, and lowest in older adult subjects who have been repeatedly infected with influenza viruses throughout their lifetime. In addition, the mucosally administered CAIV is generally more effective than parenterally administered inactivated influenza vaccine at inducing nasal HA-specific IgA, whereas inactivated vaccine usually induces higher serum titers of HAI and HA-specific IgG antibody.[271]

Most susceptible children have measurable serum and mucosal HA-specific antibody responses. Mucosal responses have been shown in up to 85% of young children after CAIV-T.[272] In contrast, adults generally have a low rate of serum antibody response after CAIV[273,274] and relatively lower rates of mucosal responses.[275] Even in those subjects prescreened to have low prevaccination vaccine-specific influenza antibody, the rates of serum antibody responses to intranasal CAIV in adults and older adults are low.[274] Immune responses in elderly subjects are relatively rare.[276,277] However, the significance of these findings is unclear, as protection can be seen in some circumstances in the absence of detectable mucosal responses,[129] and the specific levels of mucosal antibody necessary for protection are unknown.

B cell responses to both TIV and CAIV in infants, children, and adults have recently been reported.[278] Influenza-specific IgA and IgG antibody-secreting cells (ASCs) peak on days 7 to 12 after either CAIV or TIV in both adults and older children, consistent with other studies in adults that show peak of ASCs after TIV around days 7 to 8.[279-281] In contrast to children, IgG ASCs were significantly higher in adults after TIV than CAIV. Antibody responses were also significantly lower after CAIV than TIV in both adults and children, and generally, development of ASCs seemed to be a more sensitive indicator of vaccine taken after CAIV than was antibody response. The levels of prevaccination memory B cells were low in all age groups, but numbers of prevaccination memory B cells were higher in adults than children. TIV, but not CAIV, increased the numbers of circulating memory B cells at 1 month.

Influenza-specific interferon-γ (IFN-γ)–producing CD4$^+$ and CD8$^+$ lymphocytes have also been detected after both CAIV and TIV.[282,283] In children 5 to 9 years of age, TIV resulted in increases in the numbers of CD4$^+$ but not in the numbers of CD8$^+$ cells on day 10 after vaccination. No real changes were seen in natural killer (NK) cells after TIV. In contrast, administration of CAIV resulted in increases in both IFN-γ–producing CD4$^+$ and CD8$^+$ cells and in NK cells. In adults, no consistent changes were seen in any subset after either TIV or CAIV, although much variability was found in the responses.

The mechanism of protection induced by cold-adapted vaccine has mostly been evaluated in experimental infection studies, including studies conducted by our investigators. Cold-adapted vaccine is protective in these experiments in the absence of significant serum HAI responses, which suggests that the main protective effect is induction of mucosal antibodies.[130] However, protection can be seen in some circumstances even in the absence of detectable mucosal responses.[129] Finally, an analysis of data collected during a large field trial evaluation of CAIV concluded that the postvaccination numbers of influenza virus-specific IFN-γ–producing T cells were the best correlate of vaccine-induced protection.[284]

Efficacy and Effectiveness. Cold-adapted influenza vaccine–trivalent was shown to be efficacious in the prevention of influenza in a 2-year, randomized, placebo-controlled trial conducted in 1314 children 15 to 74 months of age. Efficacy against culture-confirmed influenza illness in the first year of this trial was 95% against influenza A/H3N2 and 91% against influenza B.[285] In the second year of the trial, the H3 component of the vaccine (A/Wuhan/93) was not a close match with the predominant H3 virus that season, A/Sydney/95. However, the efficacy of CAIV against this variant was 86% (95% CI, 75% to 92%),[286] which suggests that CAIV can induce protective immunity against drift variants.

Efficacy of CAIV-T in adults has been shown in the experimental infection model, in which the combined efficacy of CAIV-T in prevention of laboratory-documented influenza illness was 85%,[274] consistent with observations from previous experimental infection studies conducted with monovalent CAIV. In addition, in a large, 5-year field trial in Nashville, Tenn,[239] the efficacy of bivalent CAIV was 85% (95% CI, 70% to 92%) against A/H1N1 illness and 58% (95% CI, 29% to 75%) against A/H3N2 illness. Use of CAIV-T in adults has also been shown to reduce rates of severe febrile illness of any cause during the influenza season.[287]

No studies of the protective efficacy of CAIV alone have been conducted in older adults because of the possibly reduced immunogenicity of the vaccine in this age group. However, the combination of local live-attenuated influenza vaccine and parenteral inactivated vaccine administered together was shown to result in an approximately 60% decrease in cases of laboratory-confirmed influenza in an older adult nursing home population, compared with inactivated vaccine alone.[288]

Comparisons with Inactivated Vaccine. Although relatively few randomized direct comparisons of the efficacy of live and inactivated vaccines have been performed, the available studies are consistent with the observed effects of age and prior influenza experience on immunogenicity. When these vaccines have been compared in young children 12 months to 59 months of age, CAIV-T has shown consistently superior protection, with an approximately 50% greater protective efficacy than inactivated vaccine.[289,290] In contrast, studies that have directly compared the vaccines in adults have suggested that the vaccines have similar efficacy or that inactivated vaccine is slightly more efficacious than live vaccine,[239,291] although the numbers of subjects involved have been small. A recent observational study in military personnel suggested that TIV was associated with fewer medical encounters related to pneumonia and influenza compared with CAIV.[292]

Vaccines for Pandemic Influenza

Candidate inactivated pandemic influenza vaccines are currently in development, and one such vaccine has been licensed in the United States. Generally, inactivated vaccines have been found to be relatively inefficient at generating functional serum antibody responses, with multiple high doses necessary.[293-295] Although aluminum does not appear to be a useful adjuvant, considerable enthusiasm is found for squalene-based oil-in-water emulsions, which have been reported to generate higher titered and more broadly cross-reactive antibody responses at lower doses.[296] Examples include Novartis' MF59, GSK's AS03, and sanofi's AF03. In addition, some subjects who did not manifest detectable immune responses to the primary vaccination appear to have been primed for responses to subsequent administrations of vaccine many years later,[297] which suggests some utility to priming certain segments of the population.

Live, cold-adapted pandemic vaccine candidates have also been evaluated. Genetically engineered H5N1 viruses with a modified HA cleavage site representing a variety of A/Hong Kong/97 (clade 0) viruses and the A/Hong Kong/213/03 (clade 1) and A/Vietnam/1203/04 (clade 1) viruses have been generated with plasmid rescue.[298,299] These candidate vaccines demonstrate temperature sensitivity and trypsin-dependent plaque formation in vitro and are nonpathogenic in chickens.

In murine models, these viruses are attenuated but are immunogenic. Because ferrets have a relatively high body temperature, cold-adapted, temperature-sensitive viruses tend to be restricted in ferrets. However, administration of very high doses directly to the lung is associated with pulmonary inflammation in ferrets.[300] Importantly, these vaccines are highly protective in mice and also provide excellent protection against antigenic variants within the H5 subtype. Similar cold-adapted H9N2 (G9) vaccine candidates been generated[301,302] and are also attenuated and provide protective efficacy in murine models.

Limited clinical trials of candidate cold-adapted pandemic vaccines have been performed in isolation conditions to prevent transmission of vaccine virus to others. On the basis of the available information, the cold-adapted A/VN/1203/04 vaccine virus appears to exhibit extremely restricted replication in humans.[303] Despite nasal drop

TABLE 165-6	Groups Targeted for Influenza Immunization

Recommendations for Children and Adolescents Aged 6 Months to 18 Years

1. *Children and adolescents at high risk for influenza complications*
   - All children aged 6 months to 4 years
   - Children with chronic pulmonary (including asthma), cardiovascular (except hypertension), renal, hepatic, hematologic, or metabolic disorders (including diabetes mellitus)
   - Children with immunosuppression, including children with HIV and those taking immunosuppressive medications
   - Children with a condition that can compromise respiratory function or handling of respiratory secretions that can increase the risk for aspiration (e.g., cognitive dysfunction, spinal cord injuries, seizure disorders, or other neuromuscular disorders)
   - Children who are undergoing long-term aspirin therapy and who therefore might be at risk of Reye's syndrome
   - Children who are residents of chronic care facilities
   - Individuals who will be pregnant during the influenza season
2. *All children 5 years to 18 years, beginning in 2008-2009 if feasible, but no later than 2009-2010*

Recommendations for Adults

1. *Adults at high risk for influenza-related complications*
   - Persons aged 50 years or greater
   - Women who will be pregnant during the influenza season
   - Persons with chronic pulmonary (including asthma), cardiovascular (except hypertension), renal, hepatic, hematologic, or metabolic disorders (including diabetes mellitus)
   - Persons who have immunosuppression (including immunosuppression from medication or HIV infection)
   - Persons with any condition that can compromise respiratory function or the handling of respiratory secretions or increase the risk of aspiration
   - Residents of nursing homes and other chronic care facilities
2. *Persons who can transmit influenza to others at high risk*
   - Health care personnel
   - Household contacts and caregivers of children aged < 5 years and adults aged ≥ 50 years, with particular emphasis on vaccination of contacts of children aged < 6 months
   - Household contacts and caregivers of persons with medical conditions that put them at high risk for severe complications from influenza
3. *Any person who wishes to avoid influenza*

Adapted from CDC Prevention and Control of Influenza. Recommendations of the Advisory Committee on Immunization Practices (ACIP), 2008. *MMWR* 2008;57:1-60.

administration of 10^7 TCID$_{50}$ to susceptible young adults, virus can be detected with PCR only, and only on the first day after administration, likely representing input virus. Relatively few serum antibody responses have been detected, although mucosal and cellular immune response data have not been reported. Data from preliminary results of candidate cold-adapted H7 and H9 viruses have been promising.[303,304] Although virus replication still appears to be severely compromised, higher frequencies of antibody responses were seen. The most immunogenic vaccine appeared to be the A/chicken/British Columbia/CN-6/2004 (H7N3) vaccine, which is reported to have induced neutralizing antibody responses in 10 of 18 subjects and serum IgA responses in 15 of 21 subjects. IgG and IgA antibody-secreting cells were also detected in peripheral blood after the first dose.[304]

Development of vaccines against S-OIV is currently under way, including both egg-based and cell culture–derived vaccines.

Recommendations for Vaccine Use

The main goals of the strategy for use of influenza vaccine in the United States are to reduce the overall disease impact of seasonal influenza by targeting vaccine to those individuals at highest risk of influenza-related hospitalizations or death and to reduce the exposure of such individuals to influenza by vaccinating their contacts. Table 165-6 lists those groups for whom annual influenza vaccination is currently recommended, including individuals identified at higher risk on the basis of age and the presence of chronic conditions known to increase the risk of influenza complications.

An additional benefit of widespread vaccination of young children could be interruption of transmission of influenza in the community. Relatively little direct evidence supports the use of influenza vaccine for this purpose, but in one study, mass vaccination of school-aged children resulted in reduced rates of influenza in teachers and parents compared with a control community in which children were not vaccinated.[305] Vaccination of children in daycare has been reported to reduce the rates of febrile respiratory illnesses in unvaccinated household contacts.[306] In addition, influenza-related mortality rates among older adults have increased in Japan, coincident with discontinuation of that country's policy of universal vaccination of school children.[307] Such observations suggest that high rates of vaccine coverage in children could be a reasonable approach to reducing the impact of influenza in the whole community.

A critical target group for vaccination is health care workers.[308] At a minimum, universal vaccination of heath care workers will reduce workplace absences and prevent disruptions in care.[309] In addition, supportive evidence shows that vaccination of health care workers reduces the risk of nosocomial influenza in hospitals.[310] In nursing homes, vaccination of staff reduces mortality in residents independently of the vaccination status of the residents themselves.[311,312]

CHEMOPROPHYLAXIS

All four of the available antiviral agents are effective at prevention of influenza prophylaxis, provided drug is administered continuously throughout the period of exposure. Several schemes for such prophylaxis have been evaluated, including seasonal prophylaxis, where the drug is administered throughout the influenza epidemic season, generally 4 to 6 weeks; family prophylaxis, where the drug is administered to family members for a short period of time after recognition of an index case in the family; and outbreak-initiated prophylaxis in institutions, which could be considered to be a variation on the theme of family prophylaxis. In addition, short-term antiviral prophylaxis can be considered for high-risk individuals who are vaccinated during the influenza season.

Seasonal Prophylaxis
Seasonal prophylaxis with amantadine and rimantadine has been shown to provide similar levels of protection against influenza A, ranging from 70% to 90%.[168] Both zanamivir and oseltamivir have also been shown to be protective in seasonal prophylaxis. In healthy adults, inhaled zanamivir was shown to have about 67% efficacy for prevention of confirmed influenza,[313] and in a similar study, the efficacy of oral oseltamivir was 74%.[314] Both drugs were well tolerated with prolonged use.

Relatively less information is available about the use of any of the influenza antivirals for prophylaxis in older adult or high-risk populations. In one study, seasonal prophylaxis was highly effective in prevention of laboratory-documented influenza in older adult residents of retirement communities.[315] Importantly, 80% of the subjects had previously been vaccinated, and prophylaxis resulted in a 91% reduction in influenza in this group. Thus, vaccine and chemoprophylaxis had an additive protective effect in older adults.

Family Prophylaxis
Results of outbreak prophylaxis in the family setting with amantadine or rimantadine have depended on whether both the index case and the contacts are treated. When the index case is not treated with amantadine, protection of family contacts has been seen; however, if the index case is treated with amantadine at the same time that contacts receive prophylaxis, no protection is seen because of the rapid generation and transmission of resistant virus. This problem has not been seen in studies of family prophylaxis with oseltamivir[316] or zanamivir.[317] Generally, the drug is administered to contacts for 5 to 7 days after recognition of the index case. Treated individuals remain susceptible to infection from outside the family after such prophylaxis is discontinued.

Outbreak Prophylaxis
Probably one of the most common uses of antiviral agents for influenza is termination of the transmission of influenza within institutions such as nursing homes during outbreaks. Although this has not been subject to formal, placebo-controlled study, many anecdotal reports support the efficacy of amantadine, zanamivir, and oseltamivir in this setting. When M2 inhibitors are used for outbreak prophylaxis, individuals who receive treatment with amantadine should be isolated from those who receive prophylaxis. Failure to adhere to this practice is associated with the development and transmission of resistant viruses within the institution.[318,319] One preliminary report has suggested that prophylactic administration of zanamivir was successful in terminating an outbreak of influenza in a nursing home in which cases continued to occur despite amantadine prophylaxis.

REFERENCES

1. Hirsch A. Handbook of Geographical and Historical Pathology. 2nd ed. London: New Syndenham Society; 1883.
2. Crosby AW. Epidemic and Peace, 1918. part IV. Westport, CT: Greenwood Press; 1976.
3. Smith W, Andrewes CH, Laidlaw PP. A virus obtained from influenza patients. Lancet. 1933;2:66-68.
4. Francis T Jr. A new type of virus from epidemic influenza. Science. 1940;92:405-408.
5. Taylor RM. A further note on 1233 ("influenza C") virus. Arch Gesamte Virusforsch. 1951;4:485-495.
6. Burnet FM. Influenza virus on the developing egg I. changes associated with the development of an egg-passage strain of virus. Br J Exper Pathol. 1936;17:282-295.
7. Mogabgab WJ, Green IJ, Dierkhising OC. Primary isolation and propagation of influenza virus in cultures of human embryonic renal tissue. Science. 1954;120:320-321.
8. Hirst GK. The agglutination of red cells by allantoic fluid of chick embryos infected with influenza virus. Science. 1941;94:22-23.
9. Francis T Jr, Salk JE, Pearson HE, et al. Protective effect of vaccination against influenza A. Proc Soc Exp Biol Med. 1944;55:104-105.
10. Smorodintseff AA, Tushinsky kMD, Drobyshevskaya AI, et al. Investigation of volunteers infected with the influenza virus. Am J Med Sci. 1937;194:159-170.
11. Wilson IA, Skehel JJ, Wiley DG. Structure of the hemagglutinin membrane glycoprotein of influenza virus at 3A resolution. Nature. 1981;289:366.
12. Colman PM, Varghese JN, Laver WG. Structure of the catalytic and antigenic sites in influenza virus neuraminidase. Nature. 1983;303:41-44.
13. Zebedee SL, Lamb RA. Influenza A virus M2 protein: Monoclonal antibody restriction of virus growth and detection of M2 in virions. J Virol. 1989;62:2762-2772.
14. Simonsen L, Clarke MJ, Williamson DW, et al. The impact of influenza epidemics on mortality: introducing a severity index. Am J Pub Health. 1997;87:1944-1950.
15. Thompson WW, Shay DK, Weintraub E, et al. Mortality associated with influenza and respiratory syncytial virus in the United States. JAMA. 2003;289:179-186.
16. Sullivan KM, Monto AS, Longini IM. Estimates of the US health impact of influenza. Am J Pub Health. 1993;83:1712-1716.
17. Bhat N, Wright JG, Broder KR, et al. Influenza-associated deaths among children in the United States, 2003-2004. N Engl J Med. 2005;353:2559-2567.
18. Ellis SE, Coffey CS, Mitchel EF Jr, et al. Influenza- and respiratory syncytial virus-associated morbidity and mortality in the nursing home population. J Am Geriatr Soc. 2003;51:761-767.
19. Neuzil KM, Reed GW, Mitchel EF Jr, et al. Influenza-associated morbidity and mortality in young and middle-aged women. JAMA. 1999;281:901-907.
20. Lin JC, Nichol KL. Excess mortality due to pneumonia or influenza during influenza seasons among persons with acquired immunodeficiency syndrome. Arch Intern Med. 2001; 161:441-446.
21. Neuzil KM, Reed GW, Mitchel EF, et al. The impact of influenza on acute cardiopulmonary hospitalizations in pregnant women. Am J Epidemiol. 1998;148:1094-1102.
22. Neuzil KM, Mellen BG, Wright PF, et al. The effect of influenza on hospitalizations, outpatient visitis, and courses of antibiotics in children. N Engl J Med. 2000;342:225-231.
23. Izurieta HS, Thompson WW, Kramarz P, et al. Influenza and the rates of hospitalization for respiratory disease among infants and young children. [see comments]. N Engl J Med. 2000; 342:232-239.
24. Silberry GK. Complications of influenza infection in children. Pediatr Ann. 2000;29:683-690.
25. Kavet J. A perspective on the significance of pandemic influenza. Am J Pub Health. 1977;67:1063-1070.
26. Poehling KA, Edwards KM, Weinberg GA, et al. The under-recognized burden of influenza in young children. N Engl J Med. 2006;355:31-40.
27. Nichol KL, Lind A, Margolis KL, et al. The effectiveness of vaccination against influenza in healthy, working adults. N Engl J Med. 1995;333:889-893.
28. Neuzil KM, Hohlbein C, Zhu Y. Illness among schoolchildren during influenza season: effect on school absenteeism, parental absenteeism from work, and secondary illness in families. Arch Pediatr Adolesc Med. 2002;156:986-991.
29. Keech M, Scott AJ, Ryan PJJ. The impact of influenza and influenza-like illness on productivity and healthcare resource utilization in a working population. Occupational Med. 1998; 48:85-90.
30. Barker WH, Borisute H, Cox C. A study of the impact of influenza on the functional status of frail older people. Arch Intern Med. 1998;158:645-650.
31. Glezen WP, Couch RB. Interpandemic influenza in the Houston area, 1974-1976. N Engl J Med. 1978;298:587-593.
32. Ginsberg J, Mohebbi MH, Patel RS, et al. Detecting influenza epidemics using search engine query data. 2008.
33. Monto AS, Kioumehr F. The Tecumseh study of respiratory illness. IX. Occurrence of influenza in the community, 1966-1971. Am J Epidemiol. 1975;102:553-559.
34. Buxton-Bridges C, Kuehnert MJ, Hall CB. Transmission of influenza: implication for control in health care settings. J Infect Dis. 2003;37:1094-1101.
35. Brankston G, Gitterman L, Hirji Z, et al. Transmission of influenza A in human beings. Lancet Infect Dis. 2007;7:257-265.
36. Alford RH, Kasel JA, Gerone PJ, et al. Human influenza resulting from aerosol inhalation. Proc Soc Exper Biol Med. 1966; 122:800-804.

37. Little JW, Douglas RG Jr, Hall WJ, et al. Attenuated influenza produced by experimental intranasal inoculation. *J Med Virol.* 1979;3:177-188.
38. Moser MR, Bender TR, Margolis HS, et al. An outbreak of influenza aboard a commercial airliner. *J Epidemiol.* 1979; 110:1-6.
39. Schaffer FL, Soergel ME, Straube DC. Survival of airborne influenza virus: Effects of propagating host, relative humidity, and composition of spray fluids. *Arch Virol.* 1976;54: 263-273.
40. Lowen AC, Mubareka S, Steel J, et al. Influenza virus transmission is dependent on relative humidity and temperature. *PLoS Pathogens.* 2007;3:e151.
41. Glezen WP, Couch RB, Six HR. The influenza herald wave. *Am J Epidemiol.* 1982;116:589-598.
41a. Outbreak of swine-origin influence A (H1N1) virus infection—Mexico, March-April 2009. *MMWR Morb Mortal Wkly Rep.* 2009;58:467.
41b. World Health Organization. World now at the start of 2009 influenza pandemic. http://www.who.int/mediacentre/news/statements/2009/h1n1_pandemic_phase6_20090611/en/index.html (Accessed June 18, 2009).
42. Wilson IA, Cox NJ. Structural basis of immune recognition of influenza virus hemagglutinin. *Ann Rev Immunol.* 1990;8: 737-771.
43. Webster RG, Laver WG. Determination of the number of non-overlapping antigenic areas on Hong Kong (H3N2) influenza virus hemagglutinin with monoclonal antibodies and the selection of variants with potential epidemiological significance. *Virology.* 1980;104:139-148.
44. Xu X, Cox NJ, Bender CA, et al. Genetic variation in the neuraminidase genes of influenza A (H3N2) viruses. *Virology.* 1996;224:175-183.
45. Rimmelzwaan GF, Boon AC, Voeten JT, et al. Sequence variation in the influenza A virus nucleoprotein associated with escape from cytotoxic T lymphocytes. *Virus Res.* 2004;103: 97-100.
46. Berkhoff EG, de Wit E, Geelhoed-Mieras MM, et al. Fitness costs limit escape from cytotoxic T lymphocytes by influenza A viruses. *Vaccine.* 2006;24:6594-6596.
47. Hay AJ, Gregory V, Douglas AR, et al. The evolution of human influenza viruses. *Phil Trans Royal Soc London B.* 2001;356:1861-1869.
48. Yamashita M, Krystal M, Fitch WM, et al. Influenza B virus evolution: co-circulating lineages and comparison of evolutionary patterns with those of influenza A and C viruses. *Virology.* 1988;163:112-122.
49. Smith DJ, Lapedes AS, de Jong JC, et al. Mapping the antigenic and genetic evolution of influenza virus. *Science.* 2004;305: 371-376.
50. Kilbourne ED. *Influenza.* New York: Plenum Publishing; 1987.
51. Masurel N, Marine WM. Recycling of Asian and Hong Kong influenza A virus hemagglutinins in man. *Am J Epidemiol.* 1973;97:44-49.
51a. Rajagopal S, Treanor J. Pandemic (avian) influenza. *Sem Resp Crit Care Med.* 2007;28:159-170.
52. Webster RG, Geraci J, Petursson G, et al. Conjunctivitis in human beings caused by influenza A virus of seals. *N Engl J Med.* 1981;304:911.
53. Kurtz J, Manvell RJ, Banks J. Avian influenza virus isolated from a woman with conjunctivitis. *Lancet.* 1996;384:901-902.
54. Koopmans M, Wilbrink B, Conyn M, et al. Transmission of H7N7 avian influenza A virus to human beings during a large outbreak in commercial poultry farms in the Netherlands. *Lancet.* 2004;363:587-593.
55. Tweed SA, Skowronski DM, David ST, et al. Human illness from avian influenza H7N3, British Columbia. *Emerg Infect Dis.* 2004;10:2196-2199.
56. Puzelli S, DiÂ Trani L, Fabiani C, et al. Serological analysis of serum samples from humans exposed to avian H7 influenza viruses in Italy between 1999 and 2003, doi:10.1086/444390. *J Infect Dis.* 2005;192:1318-1322.
57. Peiris M, Yuen KY, Leung CW, et al. Human infection with influenza H9N2. *Lancet.* 1999;354:916-917.
58. Butt KM, Smith GJD, Chen H, et al. Human Infection with an Avian H9N2 Influenza A Virus in Hong Kong in 2003. *J Clin Microbiol.* 2005;43:5760-5767.
59. WHO. Avian influenza A (H5N1) infection in humans. *N Engl J Med.* 2005;353:1374-1385.
60. de Jong MD, Cam BV, Qui PT, et al. Fatal avian influenza A (H5N1) in a child presenting with diarrhea followed by coma. *N Engl J Med.* 2005;352:686-691.
61. Chotpitayasunondh T, Ungchusak K, Hanshaoworakul W, et al. Human disease from influenza A(H5N1), Thailand 2004. *Emerg Infect Dis.* 2005;11:201-209.
62. To K, Paul KS, Chan K-F, et al. Pathology of fatal human infection associated with avian influenza A H5N1 virus. *J Med Virol.* 2001;63:242-246.
63. Anonymous. Epidemiology of WHO-confirmed human cases of avian influenza A (H5N1) infection. *Weekly Epidemiologic Record.* 2006;81:249-257.
64. Keawcharoen J, Oraveerakul K, Kuiken T, et al. Avian influenza H5N1 in tigers and leopards. *Emerg Infect Dis.* 2004;10:2189-2191.
65. Mounts AW, Kwong H, Izurieta HS, et al. Case-control study of risk factors for avian influenza A (H5N1) disease, Hong Kong, 1997. *J Infect Dis.* 1999;180:505-508.
66. Katz JM, Lim W, Bridges CB, et al. Antibody response in individuals infected with avian influenza A (H5N1) viruses and detection of anti-H5 antibody among household and social contacts. *J Infect Dis.* 1999;180:1763-1770.
67. Olsen SJ, Ungchusak K, Sovann T, et al. Family clustering of avian influenza A (H5N1). *Emerg Infect Dis.* 2005;11:1799-1801.
68. Ungchusak K, Auewarakul P, Dowell SF, et al. Probable person-to-person transmission of avian influenza A (H5N1). *N Engl J Med.* 2005;352:333-340.
69. Beare AS, Webster RG. Replication of avian influenza viruses in humans. *Arch Virol.* 1991;119:37-42.
70. Naffakh N, Tomoiu A, Rameix-Welti MA, et al. Host restriction of avian influenza viruses at the level of the ribonucleoproteins. *Ann Rev Microbiol.* 2008;62:403-424.
71. Murphy BR, Buckler-White AJ, London WT, et al. Avian-human reassortant influenza A viruses derived by mating avian and human influenza A viruses. *J Infect Dis.* 1984;150:841-850.
72. Kawaoka Y, Krauss S, Webster RG. Avian-to-human transmission of the PB1 gene of influenza A viruses in the 1957 and 1968 pandemics. *J Virol.* 1989;63:4603-4608.
73. Bean WJ, Schell M, Katz J, et al. Evolution of the H3 hemagglutinin from human and nonhuman hosts. *J Virol.* 1992;66: 1129-1138.
74. Ito T, Couceiro JN, Kelm S, et al. Molecular basis for the generation in pigs of influenza A viruses with pandemic potential. *J Virol.* 1998;72:7367-7373.
75. Scholtissek C, Stech J, Krauss S, et al. Cooperation between the hemagglutinin of avian viruses and the matrix protein of human influenza A viruses. *J Virol.* 2002;76:1781-1786.
76. Taubenberger JK, Reid AH, Krafft AE, et al. Initial genetic characterization of the 1918 "Spanish" influenza virus. *Science.* 1997;275:1793-1796.
76a. Vincent AL, Ma W, Lager KM, et al. Swine influenza viruses: a North American perspective. *Adv Virus Res.* 2008;72:127-154.
76b. Shinde V, Bridges CB, Uyeki TM, et al. Triple-reassortant swine influenza A (H1) in humans in the United States, 2005-2009. *N Engl J Med.* 2009;360:2616-2625.
76c. Novel Swine-Origin Influenza A (H1N1) Investigation Team. Emergence of a novel swine-origin influenza A (H1N1) virus in humans. *N Engl J Med.* 360:2605-2615.
76d. World Health Organization. Influenza A (H1N1)—update 49, 15 June 2009. http://www.who.int/csr/don/2009_06_15/en/index.html (Accessed June 16, 2009).
76e. Update: Novel influenza A (H1N1) virus infections—worldwide, May 6, 2009. *MMWR Morb Mortal Wkly Rep.* 2009;58:453.
76f. World Health Organization. Human infection with new influenza A (H1N1) virus: clinical observations from Mexico and other affected countries, May 2009. *Wkly Epidemiol Rec.* 2009; 84:185-189.
76g. Hospitalized patients with novel influenza A (H1N1) virus infection—California, April-May 2009. *MMWR Morb Mortal Wkly Rep.* 2009;58:536.
76h. Serum cross-reactive antibody response to a novel influenza A (H1N1) virus after vaccination with seasonal influenza vaccine. *MMWR Morb Mortal Wkly Rep.* 2009;58:521.
77. Sanz-Esquerro JJ, De La Luna S, Ortin J, et al. Individual expression of the influenza virus PA protein induces degradation of coexpressed proteins. *J Virol.* 1995;69:2420-2426.
78. Hinshaw VS, Olsen CW, Dybdahl-Sissoko N, et al. Apoptosis: a mechanism of cell killing by influenza A and B viruses. *J Virol.* 1994;68:3667-3673.
79. Mori I, Komatsu T, Takeuchi K, et al. In vivo induction of apoptosis by influenza virus. *J Gen Virol.* 1995;76:2869-2873.
80. Takizawa T, Fukuda R, Miyawaki T, et al. Activation of the apoptotic Fas antigen-encoding gene upon influenza virus infection involving spontaneously produced beta-interferon. *Virology.* 1995;209:288-296.
81. Chen W, Calvo PA, Malide D, et al. A novel influenza A virus mitochondrial protein that induces cell death. *Nat Med.* 2001;7:1306-1312.
82. Jordan WS, Badger GF, Dingle JH. A study of illness in a group of Cleveland families. XVI. The epidemiology of inlfuenza 1948-1953. *Am J Hygeine.* 1958;68:169-189.
83. Larson HE, Parry RP, Tyrrell DAJ. Impaired polymorphonuclear leucocyte chemotaxis after influenza virus infection. *Br J Dis Chest.* 1980;74:56-62.
84. Roberts NJ, Steigbigel RT. Effect of in vitro virus infection on response of human monocytes and lymphocytes to mitogen stimulation. *J Immunol.* 1978;121:1052-1058.
85. Cooper JA Jr, Carcelen R, Culbreth R. Effects of influenza A nucleoprotein on polymorphonuclear neutrophil function. *J Infect Dis.* 1996;173:279-284.
86. Cooper JA Jr, Culbreth RR. Characterization of a neutrophil inhibitor peptide harvested from human bronchiolar lavage: homology to influenza A nucleoprotein. *Am J Resp Cell Molec Biol.* 1996;15:207-215.
87. Abramson JS, Wheeler JG, Parce JW, et al. Suppression of endocytosis in neutrophils by influenza A virus in vitro. *J Infect Dis.* 1986;154:456-463.
88. Hayden FG, Fritz R, Lobo MC, et al. Local and systemic cytokine responses during experimental human influenza A virus infection. Relation to symptom formation and host defense. *J Clin Invest.* 1998;101:643-649.
89. Martin CM, Kunin CM, Gottlieb LS, et al. Asian influenza A in Boston, 1957-1958. *Arch Intern Med.* 1959;103:516-531.
90. Walsh JJ, Dietlein LF, Low FN, et al. Bronchotracheal response in human influenza. *Arch Intern Med.* 1961;108:376-388.
91. Guarner J, Shieh WJ, Dawson J, et al. Immunohistochemical and in situ hybridization studies of influenza A virus infection in human lungs. *Am J Clin Pathol.* 2000;114:227-233.
92. Oseasohn R, Adelson L, Kaji M. Clinicopathologic study of thirty-three fatal cases of Asian influenza. *N Engl J Med.* 1959;11:509-518.
93. Little JW, Hall WJ, Douglas RG Jr, et al. Airway hyperreactivity and peripheral airway dysfunction in influenza A infection. *Am Rev Respir Dis.* 1978;118:295-303.
94. Hall WJ, Douglas RG Jr, Hyde RW, et al. Pulmonary mechanics after uncomplicated influenza A infection. *Am Rev Respir Dis.* 1976;113:141-147.
95. Horner GJ, Gray FD Jr. Effect of uncomplicated, presumptive influenza on the diffusing capacity of the lung. *Am Rev Respir Dis.* 1973;108:866-869.
96. Johanson WGJ, Pierce AK, Sanford JP. Pulmonary function in uncomplicated influenza. *Am Rev Respir Dis.* 1969;100: 141-146.
97. Kondo S, Abe K. The effects of influenza virus infection on FEV1 in asthmatic children. *Chest.* 1991;100:1235-1238.
98. Smith CB, Kanner RE, Goldern CA, et al. Effect of viral infections on pulmonary function in patients with chronic obstructive pulmonary diseases. *J Infect Dis.* 1980;141:271-279.
99. Utell MJ, Aquilina AT, Hall WJ, et al. Development of airway reactivity to nitrates in subjects with influenza. *Am Rev Respir Dis.* 1980;121:233-241.
100. Louria DB, Blumenfeld HL, Ellis JT, et al. Studies on influenza in the pandemic of 1957-1958. II. pulmonary complications of influenza. *J Clin Invest.* 1959;38:213-265.
101. Yelandi AV, Colby TV. Pathologic features of lung biopsy specimens from influenza pneumonia cases. *Hum Pathol.* 1994;25: 47-53.
102. Levandowski RA, Gerrity TR, Garrard CS. Modifications of lung clearance mechanisms by acute influenza A infection. *J Lab Clin Med.* 1985;106:428-432.
103. George RC, Broadbent DA, Drasar BS. The effect of influenza virus on the adherence of *Haemophilus influenzae* to human cells in tissue culture. *Br J Exper Pathol.* 1983;64:655-659.
104. McCullers JA, Rehg JE. Lethal synergism between influenza virus and Streptococcus pneumoniae: characterization of a mouse model and the role of platelet-activating factor receptor. *J Infect Dis.* 2002;186:341-350.
105. Kido H, Yokogoshi Y, Sakai K, et al. Isolation and characterization of a novel trypsin-like protease found in rat bronchiolar Clara cells: a possible activator of the viral fusion glycoprotein. *J Biolog Chem.* 1992;267:13573-13579.
106. Kawaoka Y, Webster RG. Sequence requirements for cleavage activation of influenza virus hemagglutinin expressed in mammalian cells. *Proc Natl Acad Sci U S A.* 1988;85:324-328.
107. Stieneke-Grober A, Vey M, Angliker H, et al. Influenza virus hemagglutinin with multibasic cleavage site is activated by furin, a subtilisin-like endoprotease. *EMBO J.* 1992;11:2407-2414.
108. Horimoto T, Kawaoka Y. Reverse genetics provides direct evidence for a correlation of hemagglutinin cleavability and virulence of an avian influenza A virus. *J Virol.* 1994;68:3120-3128.
109. Cheung C, Poon L, Lau A, et al. Induction of proinflammatory cytokines in human macrophages by influenza A (H5N1) viruses: a mechanism for the unusual severity of human disease? *Lancet.* 2002;360:1831-1837.
110. Brown EG. Increased virulence of a mouse-adapted variant of influenza A/FM/1/47 virus is controlled by mutations in genome segments 4, 5, 7, and 8. *J Virol.* 1990;64:4523-4533.
111. Epstein SL. Prior H1N1 influenza infection and susceptibility of Cleveland Family Study participants during the H2N2 pandemic of 1957: and experiment of nature. *J Infect Dis.* 2006;193: 49-53.
112. Black RA, Rota PA, Gorodkova N, et al. Antibody response to the M2 protein of influenza A virus expressed in insect cells. *J Gen Virol.* 1993;74:143-146.
113. Murphy BR, Kasel JA, Chanock RM. Association of serum anti-neuraminidase antibody with resistance to influenza in man. *N Engl J Med.* 1972;286:1329-1332.
114. Virelizier J-L. Host defenses against influenza virus: the role of anti-hemagglutinin antibody. *J Immunol.* 1975;115:434-439.
115. Murphy BR, Clements ML. The systemic and mucosal immune response of humans to influenza A virus. *Curr Top Microbiol Immunol.* 1989;146:107-116.
116. Webster RG, Reay PA, Laver WG. Protection against lethal influenza with neuraminidase. *Virology.* 1988;164:230-237.
117. Schulman JL, Khakpour M, Kilbourne ED. Protective effects of specific immunity to viral neuraminidase on influenza virus infection of mice. *J Virol.* 1968;2:778-786.
118. Schulman JL, Khakpour M, Kilbourne ED. Protective effects of hemagglutinin and neuraminidase antigens on influenza virus: Distinctiveness of hemagglutinin antigens of Hong Kong—68 virus. *J Virol.* 1968;2:778.
119. Monto AS, Kendal AP. Effect of neuraminidase antibody on Hong Kong influenza. *Lancet.* 1973;7804:623-625.
120. Clements ML, Betts RF, Tierney EL, et al. Resistance of adults to challenge with influenza A wild-type virus after receiving live or inactivated virus vaccine. *J Clin Microbiol.* 1986;23:73-76.
121. Johansson BE, Grajower B, Kilbourne ED. Infection-permissive immunization with influenza virus neuraminidase prevents weight loss in infected mice. *Vaccine.* 1993;11:1037-1039.

122. Treanor JJ, Tierney EL, Zebedee SL, et al. Passively transferred monoclonal antibody to the M2 protein inhibits influenza A virus replication in mice. *J Virol.* 1990;64:1375-1377.
123. Jegerlehner A, Schmitz N, Storni T, et al. Influenza A vaccine based on the extracellular domain of M2: Weak protection mediated via antibody-dependent NK cell activity. *J Immunol.* 2004;172:5598-5605.
124. Carragher DM, Kaminski DA, Moquin A, et al. A novel role for non-neutralizing antibodies against nucleoprotein in facilitating resistance to influenza virus. *J Immunol.* 2008;181:4168-4176.
125. Wagner DK, Clements ML, Reimer CB, et al. Analsyis of immunoglobulin G antibody responses after administration of live and inactivated influenza A vaccine indicates that nasal wash immunoglobulin G is a transudate from serum. *J Clin Microbiol.* 1987;25:559-562.
126. Renegar KB, Small PAJ. Passive transfer of local immunity to influenza virus by IgA antibody. *J Immunol.* 1991;146:1972-1978.
127. Liew FY, Russell SM, Appleyard G, et al. Cross-protection in mice infected with influenza A virus by the respiratory route is correlated with local IgA antibody rather than serum antibody or cytotoxic T cell activity. *Eur J Immunol.* 1984;14:409-413.
128. Clements ML, Betts RF, Tierney EL, et al. Serum and nasal wash antibodies associated with resistance to experimental challenge with influenza A wild-type virus. *J Clin Microbiol.* 1986; 24:157-160.
129. Belshe RB, Gruber WC, Mendelman PM, et al. Correlates of immune protection induced by live attenuated, cold-adapted, trivalent, intranasal influenza virus vaccine. *J Infect Dis.* 2000;181:1133-1137.
130. Treanor J, Wright PF. Immune correlates of protection against influenza in the human challenge model. *Dev Biol.* 2003; 115:97-105.
131. McMichael AJ, Gotch FM, Noble GR, et al. Cytotoxic T-cell immunity to influenza. *N Engl J Med.* 1983;309:13-17.
132. Howard JB. Influenza A2 virus as a cause of croup requiring tracheostomy. *J Pediatr.* 1972;81:1148-1150.
133. Glezen WP, Paredes A, Taber LH. Influenza in children. Relationship to other respiratory agents. *JAMA.* 1980;243:1345-1349.
134. Schwarzmann SW, Adler JL, Sullivan RFJ, et al. Bacterial pneumonia during the Hong Kong influenza epidemic of 1968-1969. *Arch Intern Med.* 1971;127:1037-1041.
135. Bisno AL, Griffin JP, VanEpps KA. Pneumonia and Hong Kong influenza: a prospective study of the 1968-1969 epidemic. *Am J Med Sci.* 1971;261:251-274.
136. Centers for Disease Control. Severe methicillin-resistant *Staphylococcus aureus* community-acquired pneumonia associated with influenza—Louisiana and Georgia, December 2006. *MMWR.* 2007;56:325-339.
137. Kempe A, Hall CB, MacDonald NE, et al. Influenza in children with cancer. *J Pediatr.* 1989;115:33-39.
138. Whimbey E, Eling LS, Couch RB, et al. Influenza A virus infection among hospitalized adult bone marrow transplant recipients. *Bone Marrow Transpl.* 1994;13:437-440.
139. Yousuf HM, Englund J, Couch R, et al. Influenza among hospitalized adults with leukemia. *Clin Infect Dis.* 1997;24:1095-1099.
140. Klimov AI, Rocha E, Hayden FG, et al. Prolonged shedding of amantadine-resistant influenzae A viruses by immunodeficient patients: detection by polymerase chain reaction-restriction analysis. *J Infect Dis.* 1995;172:1352-1355.
141. Evans KM, Kline MW. Prolonged influenza A infection responsive to rimantadine therapy in a human immunodeficiency virus-infected child. *Pediatr Infect Dis J.* 1995;14:332-334.
142. Gubareva LV, Matrosovich MN, Brenner MK, et al. Evidence for zanamivir resistance in an immunocompromised child infected with influenza B virus. *J Infect Dis.* 1998;178:1257-1262.
143. Ison MG, Gubareva LV, Atmar RL, et al. Recovery of drug-resistant influenza virus from immunocompromised patients: A case series. *J Infect Dis.* 2006;193:760-764.
144. Monto AS, Ross HW. The Tecumseh study of respiratory illness. X. Relation of acute infections to smoking, lung function, and chronic symptoms. *Am J Epidemiol.* 1978;107:57-64.
145. Ferson MJ, Morton JR, Robertson PW. Impact of influenza on morbidity in children with cystic fibrosis. *J Paedtr Child Health.* 1991;27:308-311.
146. Crum-Cianflone NF. Bacterial, Fungal, Parasitic, and Viral Myositis. *Clin Microbiol Rev.* 2008;21:473-494.
147. Karjalainen J, Nieminen MS, Heikkila J. Influenza A1 myocarditis in conscripts. *Act Med Scand.* 1980;207:27-30.
148. Craver RD, Sorrells K, Gohd R. Myocarditis with influenza B infection. *Pediatr Infect Dis J.* 1997;16:629-630.
149. Barker WH, Mullooly JP. Pneumonia and influenza deaths during epidemics: implications for prevention. *JAMA.* 1982;142:85-89.
150. MacDonald KL, Osterholm MT, Hedberg CW, et al. Toxic shock syndrome: a newly recognized complication of influenza and influenza like illness. *JAMA.* 1987;257:1053-1058.
151. Sperber SJ, Francis JB. Toxic shock during an influenza outbreak. *JAMA.* 1987;257:1086-1089.
152. Edelen JS, Bender TR, Chin TDY. Encephalopathy and pericarditis during an outbreak of influenza. *Am J Epidemiol.* 1974;100:79-83.
153. Kimball AM, Foy HM, Cooney MK, et al. Isolation of respiratory syncytial and influenza viruses from the sputum of patients hospitalized with pneumonia. *J Infect Dis.* 1983;147: 181-184.
154. Newton DW, Mellen CF, Baxter BD, et al. Practical and sensitive screening strategy for detection of influenza virus. *J Clin Microbiol.* 2002;40:4353-4356.
155. Covalciuc KA, Webb KH, Carlson CA. Comparison of four clinical specimen types for detection of influenza A and B viruses by optical immunoassay (FLU OIA test) and cell culture methods. *J Clin Microbiol.* 1999;37:3971-3974.
156. Ryan-Poirier KA, Katz JM, Webster RG, et al. Application of Directigen FLU-A for the detection of influenza A virus in human and non-human specimens. *J Clin Microbiol.* 1992;30:1072-1075.
157. Coiras MT, Perez-Brena P, Garcia ML, et al. Simultaneous detection of influenza A, B, and C viruses, respiratory syncytial virus, and adenoviruses in clinical samples by multiplex reverse transcription nested-PCR assay. *J Med Virol.* 2003;69:132-144.
158. Boivin G, Hardy I, Tellier G, et al. Predicting influenza infections during epidemics with use of a clinical case definition. *Clin Infect Dis.* 2000;31:1166-1169.
159. Monto AS, Gravenstein S, Elliott M, et al. Clinical signs and symptoms predicting influenza infection. *Arch Intern Med.* 2000;160:3243-3247.
160. Zambon M, Hays J, Webster A, et al. Diagnosis of influenza in the community: relationship of clinical diagnosis to confirmed virological, serologic, or molecular detection of influenza. *Arch Intern Med.* 2001;161:2116-2122.
161. Walsh EE, Cox C, Falsey AR. Clinical features of influenza A virus infection in older hospitalized persons. *J Am Geriatr Soc.* 2002;50:1498-1503.
162. Ruest A, Michaud S, Deslandes S, et al. Comparison of the Directigen flu A+B test, the QuickVue influenza test, and clinical case definition to viral culture and reverse transcription-PCR for rapid diagnosis of influenza virus infection. *J Clin Microbiol.* 2003;41:3487-3493.
163. Falsey AR. Noninfluenza respiratory virus infection in long-term care facilities. *Infect Control Hosp Epidemiol.* 1991;12: 602-608.
164. Drinka PJ, Gravenstein S, Krause P, et al. Non-influenza respiratory viruses may overlap and obscure influenza activity. *J Am Geriatr Soc.* 1999;47:1087-1093.
165. Bui M, Whittaker G, Helenius A. Effect of M1 protein and low pH on nuclear transport of influenza virus ribonucleoproteins. *J Virol.* 1996;70:8391-8401.
166. Atkinson WL, Arden NH, Patriarca PA, et al. Amantadine prophylaxis during an institutional outbreak of type A (H1N1) influenza. *Arch Intern Med.* 1986;146:1751-1756.
167. Speeg KV, Leighton JA, Maldonado AL. Case report: toxic delerium in a patient taking amantadine and trimethoprim-sulfamethoxazole. *Am J Med Sci.* 1989;298:410-412.
168. Dolin R, Reichman RC, Madore HP, et al. A controlled trial of amantadine and rimantadine in the prophylaxis of influenza A in humans. *N Engl J Med.* 1982;307:580-584.
169. Galbraith AW, Oxford JS, Schild GC, et al. Therapeutic effect of 1-adamantanamine hydrochloride in naturally occurring influenza A2/Hong Kong infection. *Lancet.* 1971;1:113-115.
170. Togo Y, Hornick RB, Felitti VJ, et al. Evaluation of the therapeutic efficacy of amantadine in patients with naturally occurring A2 influenza. *JAMA.* 1970;211:1149-1156.
171. Hornick RB, Togo Y, Mahler S, et al. Evaluation of amantadine hydrochloride in the treatment of A2 influenzal disease. *Bull WHO.* 1969;41:671-676.
172. Little J, Hall W, Douglas RG Jr, et al. Amantadine effect on peripheral airways abnormalities in influenza. *Ann Intern Med.* 1976;85:177-182.
173. Van Voris LP, Betts RF, Hayden FG, et al. Successful treatment of naturally occurring influenza A/USSR/77 H1N1. *JAMA.* 1981;245:1128-1131.
174. Younkin SW, Betts RF, Roth FK, et al. Reduction in fever and symptoms in young adults with influenza A/Brazil/78 H1N1 infection after treatment with aspirin or amantadine. *Antimicrob Agents Chemother.* 1983;23:577-582.
175. Hayden FG, Monto AS. Oral rimantadine hydrochloride therapy of influenza A virus H3N2 subtype infection in adults. *Antimicrob Agents Chemother.* 1986;29:339-341.
176. Betts RF, Treanor J, Braman P, et al. Antiviral agents to prevent or treat influenza in the elderly. *J Respir Dis.* 1987;8:S56-S59.
177. Hall CB, Dolin R, Gala CL, et al. Children with influenza A infection: treatment with rimantadine. *Pediatrics.* 1987; 80:275-282.
178. Thompson J, Fleet W, Lawrence E, et al. A comparison of acetaminophen and rimantadine in the treatment of influenza A infection in children. *J Med Virol.* 1987;21:249-255.
179. Shiraishi K, Mitamura K, Sakai Y, et al. High frequency of resistant viruses harboring different mutations in amantadine-treated children with influenza. *J Infect Dis.* 2003;188:57-61.
180. Hay AJ, Wolstenholme AJ, Skehel JJ, et al. The molecular basis of the specific anti-influenza action of amantadine. *EMBO J.* 1985;4:3021-3024.
181. Boivin G, Goyette N, Bernatchez H. Prolonged excretion of amantadine-resistant influenza A virus quasi species after cessation of antiviral therapy in an immunocompromised patient. *Clin Infect Dis.* 2002;34:E23-E25.
182. Bright RA, Medina M-j, Xu X, et al. Incidence of adamantane resistance among influenza A (H3N2) viruses isolated worldwide from 1994 to 2005: a cause for concern. *Lancet.* 2005;366:1175-1181.
183. Bright RA, Shay DK, Shu B, et al. Adamantane Resistance Among Influenza A Viruses Isolated Early During the 2005-2006 Influenza Season in the United States. *JAMA.* 2006;295: 891-894.
184. CDC. Update: Influenza Activity: United States, September 28, 2008-January 31, 2009. *MMWR.* 2009;58:115-119.
184a. Centers for Disease Control and Prevention. Update: Drug susceptibility of swine-origin influenza A (H1N1) viruses. *MMWR Morb Mortal Wkly Rep.* 2009;58:433-435.
185. Mitnaul LJ, Castrucci MR, Murti KG, et al. The cytoplasmic tail of influenza A virus neuraminidase (NA) affects NA incorporation into virions, virion morphology, and virulence in mice but is not essential for virus replication. *J Virol.* 1996;70:873-879.
186. Matrosovich MN, Matrosovich TY, Gray T, et al. Neuraminidase is important for the initiation of influenza virus infection in human airway epithelium. *J Virol.* 2004;78:12665-12667.
187. Kim CU, Lew W, Williams MA, et al. Influenza neuraminidase inhibitors possessing a novel hydrophobic interaction in the enzyme active site: Design, synthesis, and structural analysis of carbocyclic sialic acid analogues with potent anti-influenza activity. *J Am Chem Soc.* 1997;119:681-690.
188. Calfee DP, Peng AW, Cass LM, et al. Safety and efficacy of intravenous zanamivir in preventing experimental human influenza a virus infection. *Antimicrob Agents Chemother.* 1999;43: 1616-1620.
189. Hill G, Cihlar T, Oo C, et al. The anti-influenza drug oseltamivir exhibits low potential to induce pharmacokinetic drug interactions via renal secretion-correlation of in vivo and in vitro studies. *Drug Metabolism Disposition.* 2002;30:13-19.
190. Hayden FG, Treanor JJ, Fritz RS, et al. Use of the oral neuraminidase inhibitor oseltamivir in experimental human influenza: Randomized controlled trials for prevention and treatment. *JAMA.* 1999;282:1240-1246.
191. Walker JB, Hussey EK, Treanor JJ, et al. Effects of the neuraminidase inhibitor Zanamivir on otologic manifestations of experimental human influenza. *J Infect Dis.* 1997;176:1417-1422.
192. Treanor JJ, Hayden FG, Vrooman PS, et al. Efficacy and safety of the oral neuraminidase inhibitor oseltamivir in treating acute influenza: a randomized, controlled trial. *JAMA.* 2000;283: 1016-1024.
193. Nicholson KG, Aoki FY, Osterhaus ADME, et al. Efficacy and safety of oseltamivir in treatment of acute influenza: a randomized controlled trial. *Lancet.* 2000;355:1845-1850.
194. Hayden FG, Osterhaus ADME, Treanor JJ, et al. Efficacy and safety of the neuraminidase inhibitor zanamivir in the treatment of influenzavirus infections. *N Engl J Med.* 1997;337:874-880.
195. MIST. Randomised trial of efficacy and safety of inhaled zanamivir in treatment of influenza A and B virus infections. *Lancet.* 1998;352:1877-1881.
196. Kaiser L, Wat C, Mills T, et al. Impact of oseltamivir treatment on influenza-related lower respiratory tract complications and hospitalizations. *Arch Intern Med.* 2003;163:1667-1672.
197. Whitley RJ, Hayden FG, Reisinger KS, et al. Oral oseltamivir treatment of influenza in children. *Pediatr Infect Dis J.* 2001;20:127-133.
198. Hedrick JA, Barzilai A, Behre U, et al. Zanamivir for treatment of symptomatic influenza A and B infection in children five to twelve years of age: a randomized controlled trial. *Pediatr Infect Dis J.* 2000;19:410-417.
199. McClellan K, Perry CM. Oseltamivir: a review of its use in influenza. *Drugs.* 2001;61:263-283.
200. Lalezari J, Campion K, Keene O, et al. Zanamivir for the treatment of influenza A and B infection in high-risk patients: a pooled analysis of randomized controlled trials. *Arch Intern Med.* 2001;161:212-217.
201. Gubareva LV, Bethell R, Hart GJ, et al. Characterization of mutants of influenza A selected with the neuraminidase inhibitor 4-guanidino-Neu5Ac2en. *J Virol.* 1996;70:1818-1827.
202. Gubareva LV, Robinson MJ, Bethell RC, et al. Catalytic and framework mutations in the neuraminidase active site of influenza viruses that are resistant to 4-guanidino-neu5ac2en. *J Virol.* 1997;71:3385-3390.
203. Moscona A. Oseltamivir resistance: disabling our influenza defenses. *N Engl J Med.* 2005;353:2633-2636.
204. McKimm-Breschkin JL, Sahasrabudhe A, Blick TJ, et al. Mutations in a conserved residue in the influenza virus neuraminidase active site decreases sensitivity to neu5acen-derived inhibitors. *J Virol.* 1998;72:2456-2462.
205. Goto H, Bethell RC, Kawaoka Y. Mutations affecting the sensitivity of the influenza virus neuraminidase to 4-guanidino-2,4-dideoxy-2,3-dehydro-*N*-acetylneuraminic acid. *Virology.* 1997; 238:265-272.
206. Blick TJ, Sahasrabudhe A, McDonald M, et al. The interaction of neuraminidase and hemagglutinin mutations in influenza virus in resistance to 4-guanidino-neu5Ac2en. *Virology.* 1998; 246:95-103.
207. Ives JA, Carr JA, Mendel DB, et al. The H274Y mutation in the influenza A/H1N1 neuraminidase active site following oseltamivir phosphate treatment leave virus severely compromised both in vitro and in vivo. *Antiviral Res.* 2002;55:307-317.
208. Carr J, Ives J, Kelly L, et al. Influenza virus carrying neuraminidase with reduced sensitivity to oseltamivir carboxylate has altered properties in vitro and is compromised for infectivity and replicative ability in vivo. *Antiviral Res.* 2002;54:79-88.

209. Herlocher ML, Carr J, Ives J, et al. Influenza virus carrying an R292K mutation in the neuraminidase gene is not transmitted in ferrets. *Antiviral Res.* 2002;54:99-111.
210. Herlocher ML, Truscon R, Elias S, et al. Influenza viruses resistant to the antiviral drug oseltamivir: transmission studies in ferrets. *J Infect Dis.* 2004;190:1627-1630.
211. Kiso M, Mitamura K, Sakai-Tagawa Y, et al. Resistant influenza A viruses in children treated with oseltamivir: descriptive study. *Lancet.* 2004;364:759-765.
212. CDC Health Advisory. CDC Issues Interim Recommendations for the Use of Influenza Antiviral Medications in the Setting of Oseltamivir Resistance among Circulating Influenza A (H1N1) Viruses, 2008-09 Influenza Season. available at <http://www2a.cdc.gov/HAN/ArchiveSys/ViewMsgV.asp?AlertNum=00249>; accessed March 10, 2009.
213. Ison MG, Gnann J, Nagy-Agren S, et al. Safety and efficacy of nebulized zanamivir in hospitalized patients with serious influenza. *Antiviral Ther.* 2003;8:183-190.
214. Writing Committee of the Second World Health Organization Consultation on Clinical Aspects of Human Infection with Avian Influenza A (H5N1) Virus. Update on avian influenza A (H5N1) virus infection in humans. *N Engl J Med.* 2008; 358:261-273.
215. de Jong MD, Thanh TT, Khanh TH, et al. Oseltamivir resistance during treatment of influenza A (H5N1) infection. *N Engl J Med.* 2005;353:2667-2672.
216. World Health Organization. Summary of the second WHO consultation on clinical aspects of human infection with avian influenza A (H5N1) virus. (Accessed December 20, 2007, at http://www.who.int/csr/disease/avian_influenza/meeting19_03_2007/en/index.html)
217. Ilyushina NA, Hoffmann E, Solomon R, et al. Amantadine-oseltamivir combination therapy for H5N1 influenza virus infection in mice. *Antivir Ther.* 2007;12:363-370.
218. Kilbourne ED, Schulman JL, Schild GC, et al. Correlated studies of a recombinant influenza-virus vaccine. I. Derivation and characterization of virus and vaccine. *J Infect Dis.* 1971; 124:449-462.
219. Nichol KL, Margolis KL, Lind A, et al. Side effects associated with influenza vaccination in healthy working adults. A randomized, placebo-controlled trial. *Arch Intern Med.* 1996; 156:1546-1550.
220. Margolis KL, Poland GA, Nichol KL, et al. Frequency of adverse reactions after influenza vaccination. *Am J Med.* 1990; 88:27-30.
221. Wright PF, Thompson J, Vaughn WT, et al. Trials of influenza A/New Jersey/76 virus vaccine in normal children: an overview of age-related antigenicity and reactogenicity. *J Infect Dis.* 1977;136:S731-S741.
222. Gross PA, Ennis FA, Gaerlan PF, et al. A controlled double-blind comparison of reactogenicity, immunogenicity, and protective efficacy of whole-virus and split-product influenza vaccines in children. *J Infect Dis.* 1977;136:623-632.
223. Murphy DR, Strunk RC. Safe administration of influenza vaccine in asthmatic children hypersensitive to egg proteins. *J Pediatr.* 1985;106:931-933.
224. Bierman CW, Shapiro GG, Pierson WE, et al. Safety of influenza vaccination in allergic children. *J Infect Dis.* 1977;136:S652-S655.
225. Schonberger LB, Bregman DJ, Sullivan-Bolyai JZ, et al. Guillan-Barré syndrome following vaccination in the national influenza immunization program, United States, 1976-1977. *Am J Epidemiol.* 1979;110:105-123.
226. Lasky T, Tarracciano GJ, Magder L, et al. The Guillan-Barré syndrome and the 1992-1993 and 1993-1994 influenza vaccines. *N Engl J Med.* 1998;339:1797-1802.
227. Wright PF, Cherry JD, Foy HM, et al. Antigenicity and reactogenicity of influenza A/USSR/77 virus vaccine in children—a multicentered evaluation of dosage and toxicity. *Rev Infect Dis.* 1983;5:758-764.
228. Levandowski RA, Regnery HL, Staton E, et al. Antibody responses to influenza B viruses in immunologically unprimed children. *Pediatrics.* 1991;88:1031-1036.
229. Lerman SJ, Wright PJ, Patil KD. Antibody decline in children following A/New Jersey/76 influenza virus immunization. *J Pediatr.* 1980;96:271-274.
230. Zahradnik JM, Kasel JA, Martin RR, et al. Immune responses in serum and respiratory secretions following vaccination with a live cold-recombinant (CR35) and inactivated A/USSR/77 (H1N1) influenza virus vaccine. *J Med Virol.* 1983;11:277-285.
231. Bokstad KA, Eriksson J-C, Cox RJ, et al. Parenteral vaccination against influenza does not induce a local antigen-specific immune response in the nasal mucosa. *J Infect Dis.* 2002; 185:878-884.
232. Danke NA, Kwok WW. HLA class II–restricted CD4+ T cell responses directed against influenza viral antigens postinfluenza vaccination. *J Immunol.* 2003;171:3163-3169.
233. McElhaney JE, Xie D, Hager WD, et al. T cell responses are better correlates of vaccine protection in the elderly. *J Immunol.* 2006;176:6333-6339.
234. Duchini A, Goss JA, Karpen S, et al. Vaccinations for adult solid-organ transplant recipients: current recommendations and protocols. *Clin Microbiol Rev.* 2003;16:357-364.
235. Nelson KE, Clements ML, Miotti P, et al. The influence of human immunodeficiency virus (HIV) infection on antibody responses to influenza vaccines. *Ann Intern Med.* 1988; 109:383-388.
236. Kroon FP, van Dissel JT, de Jong JC, et al. Antibody response after influenza vaccination in HIV-infected individuals: a consecutive 3-year study. *Vaccine.* 2000;18:3040-3049.
237. Kubiet MA, Gonzalez-Rothi RJ, Cottey R, et al. Serum antibody response to influenza vaccine in pulmonary patients receiving corticosteroids. *Chest.* 1996;110:367-370.
238. Park CL, Frank AL, Sullivan M, et al. Influenza vaccination of children during acute asthma exacerbation and concurrent prednisone therapy. *Pediatrics.* 1996;98:196-200.
239. Edwards KM, Dupont WD, Westrich MK, et al. A randomized controlled trial of cold-adapted and inactivated vaccines for the prevention of influenza A disease. *J Infect Dis.* 1994;169: 68-76.
240. Bridges CB, Thompson WW, Meltzer MI, et al. Effectiveness and cost-benefit of influenza vaccination of healthy working adults: A randomized controlled trial. [see comments]. *JAMA.* 2000;284:1655-1663.
241. Heikkinen T, Ruuskanen O, Waris M, et al. Influenza vaccination in the prevention of acute otitis media in children. *Am J Dis Child.* 1991;145:445-448.
242. Clements DA, Langdon L, Bland C, et al. Influenza A vaccine decreases the incidence of otitis media in 6- to 30- month old children in day care. *Arch Pediatr Adolesc Med.* 1995;149:1113-1117.
243. Hoberman A, Greenberg DP, Paradise JL, et al. Effectiveness of inactivated influenza vaccine in preventing acute otitis media in young children: a randomized controlled trial. *JAMA.* 2003;290:1608-1616.
244. Govaert TM, Thijs CT, Masurel N, et al. The efficacy of influenza vaccination in elderly individuals. A randomized double-blind placebo-controlled trial. *JAMA.* 1994;272:1956-1961.
245. Tasker SA, Treanor JJ, Paxton WB, et al. Efficacy of influenza vaccination in HIV-infected persons: a randomized, double-blind, placebo-controlled trial. *Ann Intern Med.* 1999;131: 430-433.
246. Gross PA, Quinnan GV, Rodstein M, et al. Association of influenza immunization with reduction in mortality in an elderly population: a prospective study. *Arch Intern Med.* 1988;148:562-565.
247. Nichol KL, Nordin J, Nelson DB, et al. Effectiveness of influenza vaccine in the community-dwelling elderly. *N Engl J Med.* 2007;357:1373-1381.
248. Fedson DS, Wajda A, Nicol JP, et al. Clinical effectiveness of influenza vaccination in Manitoba. *JAMA.* 1993;270:1956-1961.
249. Nichol KL, Nordin J, Mullooly J, et al. Influenza vaccination and reduction in hospitalizations for cardiac disease and stroke among the elderly. *N Engl J Med.* 2003;348:1322-1332.
250. Jackson LA, Nelson JC, Benson P, et al. Functional status is a confounder of the association of influenza vaccine and risk of all cause mortality in seniors. *Int J Epidemiol.* 2006;35: 345-352.
251. Jackson LA, Jackson ML, Nelson JC, et al. Evidence of bias in estimates of influenza vaccine effectiveness in seniors. *Int J Epidemiol.* 2006;35:337-344.
252. Maassab HF. Biologic and immunologic characteristics of cold-adapted influenza virus. *J Immunol.* 1969;102:728-732.
253. Murphy BR, Coelingh K. Principles underlying the development and use of live attenuated cold-adapted influenza A and B virus vaccines. *Viral Immunol.* 2002;15:295-323.
254. Herlocher LM, Clavo AC, Maasab HF. Sequence comparisons of the A/AA/6/60 influenza viruses: mutations which may contribute to attenuation. *Virus Res.* 1996;42:11-25.
255. Snyder MH, Betts RF, DeBorde D, et al. Four viral genes independently contribute to attenuation of live influenza A/Ann Arbor/6/60 (H2N2) cold-adapted reassortant virus vaccines. *J Virol.* 1988;62:488-495.
256. Subbarao EK, Perkins M, Treanor JJ, et al. The attenuation phenotype conferred by the M gene of the influenza A/Ann Arbor/6/60 cold-adapted virus (H2N2) on the A/Korea/82 (H3N2) reassortant virus results from a gene constellation effect. *Virus Res.* 1992;25:37-50.
257. Jin H, Lu B, Zhou H, et al. Multiple amino acid residues confer temperature sensitivity to human influenza virus vaccine strains (FluMist) derived from cold-adapted A/Ann Arbor/6/60. *Virology.* 2003;306:18-24.
258. Chen Z, Aspelund A, Kemble G, et al. Genetic mapping of the cold-adapted phenotype of B/Ann Arbor/1/66, the master donor virus for live attenuated influenza vaccines (FluMist(R)). *Virology.* 2006;345:416-423.
259. Hoffman E, Mahmood K, Chen Z, et al. Multiple gene segments control the temperature sensitivity and attenuation phenotypes of ca B/Ann Arbor/1/66. *J Virol.* 2005;79:11014-11021.
260. Donabedian AM, DeBorde DC, Maassab HF. Genetics of cold-adapted B/Ann Arbor/1/66 influenza virus reassortants: The acidic polymerase (PA) protein gene confers temperature sensitivity and attenuated virulence. *Microbiol Pathol.* 1987;3:97-108.
261. Donabedian AM, DeBorde DC, Cook S, et al. A mutation in the PA protein gene of cold-adapted B/Ann Arbor/1/66 influenza virus associated with reversion of temperature sensitivity and attenuated virulence. *Virology.* 1988;163:444-451.
262. Buonagurio DA, O'Neill RE, Shutyak L, et al. Genetic and phenotypic stability of cold-adapted influenza viruses in a trivalent vaccine administered to children in a day care setting. *Virology.* 2006;347:296-306.
263. Redding G, Walker RE, Helssel C, et al. Safety and tolerability of cold-adapted influenza virus vaccine in children and adolescents with asthma. *Pediatr Infect Dis J.* 2002;21: 44-48.
264. Gorse GJ, Belshe RB, Munn NJ. Local and systemic antibody responses in high-risk adults given live attenuated and inactivated influenza A virus vaccines. *J Clin Microbiol.* 1988;26:911-918.
265. Atmar RL, Bloom K, Keitel W, et al. Effect of live attenuated, cold recombinant (CR) influenza virus vaccines on pulmonary function in healthy and asthmatic adults. *Vaccine.* 1990;8:217-224.
266. Jackson LA, Holmes SJ, Mendelman PM, et al. Safety of a trivalent live attenuated intranasal vaccine, FluMist, administered in addition to parenteral trivalent inactivated influenza vaccine to seniors with chronic medical conditions. *Vaccine.* 1999;17:1905-1909.
267. King JC, Treanor J, Fast PE, et al. Comparison of the safety, vaccine virus shedding, and immunogenicity of influenza virus vaccine, trivalent, types A and B, live cold-adapted, administered to human immunodeficiency virus (HIV)-infected and non-HIV-infected adults. *J Infect Dis.* 2000;181: 725-728.
268. King JC Jr, Fast PE, Zangwill KM, et al. Safety, vaccine virus shedding and immunogenicity of trivalent, cold-adapted, live attenuated influenza vaccine administered to human immunodeficiency virus-infected and noninfected children. *Pediatr Infect Dis J.* 2001;20:1124-1131.
269. Vesikari T, Karvonen A, Korhonen T, et al. A randomized, double-blind study of the safety, transmissibility, and phenotypic and genotypic stability of cold-adapted influenza virus vaccine. *Pediatr Infect Dis J.* 2006;25:590-597.
270. Cha TA, Kao K, Zhao J, et al. Genotypic stability of cold-adapted influenza virus vaccine in an efficacy clinical trial. *J Clin Microbiol.* 2000;38:839-845.
271. Beyer WEP, Palache AM, de Jong JC, et al. Cold-adapted live influenza vaccine versus inactivated vaccine: systemic vaccine reactions, local and systemic antibody response, and vaccine efficacy: a meta-analysis. *Vaccine.* 2002;20:1340-1353.
272. Boyce TG, Gruber WC, Coleman-Dockery SD, et al. Mucosal immune response to trivalent live attenuated intranasal influenza vaccine in children. *Vaccine.* 1999;18:82-88.
273. Keitel WA, Couch RB, Quarles JM, et al. Trivalent attenuated cold-adapted influenza virus vaccine: reduced viral shedding and serum antibody responses in susceptible adults. *J Infect Dis.* 1993;167:305-311.
274. Treanor JJ, Kotloff K, Betts RF, et al. Evaluation of trivalent, live, cold-adapted (CAIV-T) and inactivated (TIV) influenza vaccines in prevention of virus infection and illness following challenge of adults with wild-type influenza A (H1N1), A (H3N2), and B viruses. *Vaccine.* 1999;18:899-906.
275. Clements ML, Murphy BR. Development and persistence of local and systemic antibody responses in adults given live attenuated or inactivated influenza A virus vaccine. *J Clin Microbiol.* 1986;23:66-72.
276. Powers DC, Fries LF, Murphy BR, et al. In elderly persons live attenuated influenza A virus vaccines do not offer an advantage over inactivated virus vaccine in inducing serum or secretory antibodies or local immunologic memory. *J Clin Microbiol.* 1991;29:498-505.
277. Powers DC, Murphy BR, Fries L, et al. Reduced infectivity of cold-adapted influenza A H1N1 viruses in the elderly: correlation with serum and local antibodies. *J Am Geriatr Soc.* 1992;40:163-167.
278. Sasaki S, Jaimes MC, Holmes TH, et al. Comparison of the influenza-specific effector and memory B cell responses to immunization of children and adults with live attenuated or inactivated influenza vaccines. *J Virol.* 2007;81:215-228.
279. Brokstad KA, Eriksson J-C, Cox RJ, et al. Parenteral vaccination against influenza does not induce a local antigen-specific immune response in the nasal mucosa. *J Infect Dis.* 2002;185:878-885.
280. Cox RJ, Brokstad KA, Zuckerman MA, et al. An early humoral immune response in peripheral blood following parenteral influenza vaccination. *Vaccine.* 1994;12:993-999.
281. el-Madhun AS, Cox RJ, Soreide A, et al. Systemic and mucosal immune response in young children and adults after parenteral influenza vaccination. *J Infect Dis.* 1998;178:933-939.
282. He X-S, Holmes TH, Zhang C, et al. Cellular Immune Responses in Children and Adults Receiving Inactivated or Live Attenuated Influenza Vaccines. *J Virol.* 2006;80:11756-11766.
283. He X-S, Holmes TH, Mahmood K, et al. Phenotypic changes in influenza-specific CD8+ T cells after immunization of children and adults with influenza vaccines. *J Infect Dis.* 2008;197:803-811.
284. Forrest BD, Pride MW, Dunning AJ, et al. Correlation of cellular immune responses with protection against culture-confirmed influenza virus in young children. *Clin Vaccine Immunol.* 2008;15:1042-1053.
285. Belshe RB, Mendelman PM, Treanor J, et al. The efficacy of live attenuated cold-adapted trivalent, intranasal influenzavirus vaccine in children. *N Engl J Med.* 1998;358:1405-1412.
286. Belshe RB, Gruber WC, Mendelman PM, et al. Efficacy of vaccination with live attenuated, cold-adapted, trivalent, intranasal influenza virus vaccine against a variant (A/Sydney) not contained in the vaccine. *J Pediatr.* 2000;136:168-175.

287. Nichol KL, Mendelman PM, Mallon KP, et al. Effectiveness of live, attenuated intranasal influenza virus vaccine in healthy, working adults: a randomized controlled trial. *JAMA.* 1999;282:137-144.

288. Treanor JJ, Mattison HR, Dumyati G, et al. Protective efficacy of combined live intranasal and inactivated influenza A virus vaccines in the elderly. *Ann Intern Med.* 1992;117:625-633.

289. Ashkenazi S, Vertruyen A, Aristegui J, et al. Superior relative efficacy of live attenuated influenza vaccine compared with inactivated influenza vaccine in young children with recurrent respiratory tract infections. *Pediatr Infect Dis J.* 2006;25:870-879.

290. Belshe RB, Edwards KM, Vesikari T, et al. Live attenuated versus inactivated influenza vaccine in infants and young children. *N Engl J Med.* 2007;356:685-696.

291. Ohmit SE, Victor JC, Rotthoff JR, et al. Prevention of antigenically drifted influenza by inactivated and live attenuated vaccines. *N Engl J Med.* 2006;355:2513-2522.

292. Wang Z, Tobler S, Roayaei J, et al. Live attenuated or inactivated influenza vaccines and medical encounters for respiratory illnesses among US military personnel. *JAMA.* 2009;301:945-953.

293. Treanor JJ, Campbell JD, Zangwill KM, et al. Safety and immunogenicity of an inactivated subvirion influenza A (H5N1) vaccine. *N Engl J Med.* 2006;354:1343-1351.

294. Treanor JJ, Wilkinson BE, Masseoud F, et al. Safety and immunogenicity of a recombinant hemagglutinin vaccine for H5 influenza in humans. *Vaccine.* 2001;19:1732-1737.

295. Bresson J-L, Perronne C, Launay O, et al. Safety and immunogenicity of an inactivated split-virion influenza A/Vietnam/1194/2004 (H5N1) vaccine: phase I randomized trial. *Lancet.* 2006;367:1657-1664.

296. Leroux-Roels I, Borkowski A, Vanwolleghem T, et al. Antigen sparing and cross-reactive immunity with an adjuvanted rH5N1 prototype pandemic influenza vaccine: a randomised controlled trial. *Lancet.* 2007;370:580-589.

297. Goji NA, Nolan C, Hill H, et al. Immune responses of healthy subjects to a single dose of intramuscular inactivated influenza A/Vietnam/1203/04 (H5N1) vaccine after priming with an antigenic variant. *J Infect Dis.* 2008;198:635-641.

298. Li S, Liu C, Klimov A, et al. Recombinant influenza A virus vaccines for the pathogenic human A/Hong Kong/97 (H5N1) viruses. *J Infect Dis.* 1999;179:1132-1138.

299. Suguitan AL Jr, McAuliffe J, Mills KL, et al. Live, attenuated influenza A H5N1 candidate vaccines provide broad cross-protection in mice and ferrets.[see comment]. *PLoS Med Public Library Sci.* 2006;3:1541-1555.

300. Jin H, Manetz S, Leininger J, et al. Toxicological evaluation of live attenuated, cold-adapted H5N1 vaccines in ferrets. *Vaccine.* 2007;25:8664-8672.

301. Chen H, Matsuoka Y, Swayne D, et al. Generation and characterization of a cold-adapted influenza A H9N2 reassortant as a live pandemic influenza virus vaccine candidate. *Vaccine.* 2003;21:4430-4436.

302. Chen H, Subbarao K, Swayne D, et al. Generation and evaluation of a high-growth reassortant H9N2 influenza A virus as a pandemic vaccine candidate. *Vaccine.* 2003;21:1974-1979.

303. Karron R, Callahan K, Luke C, et al. Phase I evaluation of live attenuated H5N1 and H5N1 ca reassortant vaccines in healthy adults. In: Third WHO meeting on evaluation of pandemic influenza prototype vaccines in clinical trials, 15-16 February 2007; 2007; Geneva, Switzerland; 2007.

304. Karron RA. Clinical evaluation of live attenuated pandemic influenza virus vaccines. In: Fourth WHO meeting on evaluation of pandemic influenza prototype vaccines in clinical trials, 14-15 February 2008; 2008; Geneva, Switzerland; 2008.

305. Monto AS, Davenport FM, Napier JA, et al. Modification of an outbreak of influenza in Tecumseh, Michigan by vaccination of schoolchildren. *J Infect Dis.* 1970;122:16-25.

306. Hurwitz ES, Haber M, Chang A, et al. Effectiveness of influenza vaccination of day care children in reducing influenza-related morbidity among household contacts. *JAMA.* 2000;284:1677-1682.

307. Reichert TA, Sugaya N, Fedson DS, et al. The Japanese experience with vaccinating schoolchildren against influenza. *N Engl J Med.* 2001;344:889-896.

308. CDC. Influenza vaccination of health care personnel. *MMWR.* 2006;55:1-12.

309. Wilde JA, McMillan JA, Serwint J, et al. Effectiveness of influenza vaccine in health care professionals: a randomized trial. *JAMA.* 1999;281:908-913.

310. Salgado CD, Gianetta ET, Hayden FG, et al. Preventing nosocomial influenza by improving the vaccine acceptance rate of clinicians. *Infect Control Hosp Epidemiol.* 2004;25:923-928.

311. Potter J, Stott DJ, Roberts MA, et al. Influenza vaccination of health care workers in long-term-care hospitals reduces the mortality of elderly patients. *J Infect Dis.* 1997;175:1-6.

312. Carman WF, Elder AG, Wallace LA, et al. Effects of influenza vaccination of health-care workers on mortality of elderly people in long-term care: a randomised controlled trial [see comments]. *Lancet.* 2000;355:93-97.

313. Monto AS, Robinson DP, Herlocher ML, et al. Zanamivir in the prevention of influenza among healthy adults: a randomized controlled trial. *JAMA.* 1999;282:31-35.

314. Hayden FG, Atmar RL, Schilling M, et al. Use of the selective oral neuraminidase inhibitor oseltamivir to prevent influenza. *N Engl J Med.* 1999;341:1336-1346.

315. Peters Jr PH, Gravenstein S, Norwood P, et al. Long-term use of oseltamivir for the prophylaxis of influenza in a vaccinated frail older population. *J Am Geriatr Soc.* 2001;49:1025-1031.

316. Welliver R, Monto AS, Carewicz O, et al. Effectiveness of oseltamivir in preventing influenza in household contacts: a randomized controlled trial. *JAMA.* 2001;285:748-754.

317. Hayden FG, Gubareva LV, Monto AS, et al. Inhaled zanamivir for the prevention of influenza in families. *N Engl J Med.* 2000;343:1282-1289.

318. Mast EE, Harman MW, Gravenstein S, et al. Emergence and possible transmission of amantadine-resistant viruses during nursing home outbreaks of influenza A(H3N2). *Am J Epidemiol.* 1991;134:988-997.

319. Degelau J, Somani SK, Cooper SL, et al. Amantadine-resistant influenza A in a nursing facility. *Arch Intern Med.* 1992;152:390-392.

166

California Encephalitis, Hantavirus Pulmonary Syndrome, and Bunyavirid Hemorrhagic Fevers

C. J. PETERS

The family Bunyaviridae comprises more than 200 animal viruses classified into four major genera (*Bunyavirus, Phlebovirus, Nairovirus,* and *Hantavirus*) readily distinguished by genetic, morphologic, biochemical, and immunologic characteristics.[1] The circulation of the viruses in nature via arthropod–vertebrate cycles or chronic infection of vertebrates leads to disease distributions that are determined by ecologic circumstances, can be highly focal, and depend on weather and climatic variables. Caused by viruses in the genus *Bunyavirus,* California encephalitis (CE) is the common childhood central nervous system (CNS) disease reported every year, making CE second in importance only to West Nile viral encephalitis among the mosquito-borne viral diseases in the United States. La Crosse (LAC) virus is responsible for most cases of CE, although a number of other antigenically related viruses make up the CE group, including California[2] and Jamestown Canyon[3] viruses. Although not endemic in the Americas, Rift Valley fever (RVF),[4] Crimean-Congo hemorrhagic fever (CCHF),[5] and Hantaan (HTN) viruses[6] cause serious and fatal, acute disease with hemorrhagic manifestations (hemorrhagic fever with renal syndrome [HFRS]) on other continents. Relatives of HTN virus, isolated initially in Korea in 1978, are present in wild rodents throughout Eurasia, where they also cause HFRS, and other relatives in the Americas (e.g., Sin Nombre virus [SNV]) are implicated as causes of severe pulmonary edema and shock.[6,7] Salient features of these agents including genus assignment and associated diseases are summarized in Table 166-1. Emphasis in the following presentation is given primarily to LAC and SNV viruses with comparative properties for HTN, RVF, and CCHF viruses where appropriate. A few emerging agents are mentioned.

Viral Characterization

STRUCTURE, GENETICS, AND ANTIGENIC RELATIONSHIPS

Bunyaviridae are spherical, lipid membrane-enclosed viruses 90 to 110 nm in diameter. They contain three negative-sense RNA segments that code for six or fewer proteins. The molecular weights of the proteins and RNA vary by genus, but the small RNA codes for a viral nucleoprotein and the middle RNA codes for two glycosylated envelope proteins.[8] Nonstructural proteins are usually found, and the large RNA is thought to encode a viral polymerase present in the lipid enveloped viruses. In general, the G1 or G2 protein, or both, are responsible for viral neutralization, fusion of infected cells, and hemagglutination.[8] The nucleocapsid protein is thought to be the most important source of immunologic relationships observed within and across genera of the family. In general, the fluorescent antibody (FA) test is the most cross-reactive with hemagglutination inhibition and particularly the neutralization tests providing greater specificity. The latter is of greatest use in distinguishing individual viruses. Increasingly, enzyme-linked immunosorbent assay (ELISA) tests are used for diagnosis of acute or resolving (immunoglobulin M [IgM]) or retrospective (IgG) infections.

MORPHOGENESIS

Viral morphogenesis usually occurs intracellularly, with virions maturing by budding from the Golgi complex and endoplasmic reticulum into vesicles. Exceptions include RVF virus, which also buds through the outer cell membrane of hepatocytes, and SNV, which matures at the cytoplasmic membrane.[9]

Epidemiology

BASIC ECOLOGY AND DISTRIBUTION

California Encephalitis Viruses

LAC virus is medically the most significant CE virus in the United States, and its principal vector is *Aedes triseriatus,* a forest-dwelling, tree-hole-breeding mosquito of the north-central and northeastern regions of the country. LAC virus is maintained in this mosquito via transovarial transmission supplemented by intraspecific venereal transmission and amplification during summer by mosquitoes feeding on viremic chipmunks, squirrels, foxes, and woodchucks.[10,11]

Female mosquitoes infected by any of these mechanisms are capable of transmitting virus via a bite. The virus survives during the winter in mosquito eggs.[12] LAC virus and human encephalitis were first recognized in the upper Mississippi and Ohio River valleys. Most cases have been reported from Wisconsin, Minnesota, Iowa, Indiana, Ohio, and Illinois.[13,14] However, recognition of the disease in West Virginia and Georgia[13] has led to an understanding that viral transmission occurs throughout the eastern United States, and during 2003-2007, West Virginia had the greatest number of cases (95) in the United States.[15] Studies in Tennessee suggest recent extension into that state.[14] Other vectors are not of major importance except focally. The Asian mosquito *Aedes albopictus* is an efficient vector and is capable of horizontal and vertical transmission in the laboratory.[16] Its strongly anthropophilic biting habits and its documented extension into areas where LAC virus is endemic raise concern, particularly as the virus has been isolated from field collections of *A. albopictus.*[17]

Other CE viruses have distinct ecologic cycles based on an element of transovarial transmission in mosquitoes, and human disease is uncommon and usually, but not always, mild.[2,3]

Rift Valley Fever and Crimean-Congo Hemorrhagic Fever

RVF virus is maintained in sub-Saharan Africa via transovarial transmission in certain floodwater-breeding *Aedes* mosquitoes, notably *Aedes mcintoshi.*[18] Infected eggs can remain dormant but viable in soil for years while awaiting heavy rains for subsequent hatching. Other mosquitoes are important during epizootics and epidemics; large domestic ungulates such as sheep or cattle serve as amplifiers because they experience high viremia during infection.[19] In 1977, the virus was introduced into Egypt, producing widespread epidemic disease in humans and domestic animals; it has reappeared in the 1990s. After

TABLE 166-1	Some Characteristics of Severe Diseases Caused by Bunyaviridae					
Disease	Genus and Viruses	Vector	Transmission to Humans	Disease Pattern and Annual Incidence	Major Clinical Features
California encephalitis	Bunyavirus La Crosse California encephalitis Jamestown Canyon	Aedes triseriatus Transovarial transmission, amplification by chipmunks	Mosquito bite	Summer–fall. Northern United States: 60-130 cases	Meningoencephalitis, seizures, cerebral edema
Rift Valley fever	Phlebovirus Rift Valley fever	Aedes mcintoshi Transovarial transmission Horizontal transmission in other arthropods	Mosquito bite. Aerosol or contact with fresh carcasses, domestic animals	Endemic in rainy season sub-Saharan Africa: hundreds of cases. Occasional epidemics associated with exceptional rainfall	Acute febrile illness with occasional retinitis, hemorrhagic fever, or encephalitis
Crimean-Congo hemorrhagic fever	Nairovirus Crimean-Congo hemorrhagic fever	Hyalomma ticks Amplified by hares, domestic animals	Tick bite, contact with blood of humans or domestic animals	Spring–summer. Former Soviet Union, Middle East, Africa: 50-200 cases	Severe hemorrhagic fever
Hemorrhagic fever with renal syndrome	Hantavirus Hantaan Dobrava Seoul Puumala	Chronic infection of striped field mouse, yellow-necked mouse, rat, or bank vole	Aerosols from rodent excreta	Endemic and epidemic. Season depends on local conditions. Asia, Europe: 100,000 cases	Fever, shock, bleeding, renal failure
Hantavirus pulmonary syndrome	Hantavirus Sin Nombre Others	Chronic infection of deer mouse and other rodents	Aerosols from rodent excreta	Discovered 1993. Dozens of cases annually in North and South America	Fever, shock, pulmonary edema

an extensive epidemic in Kenya in 1997-1998, it was introduced into the Arabian peninsula, where it also caused epidemic disease in animals and humans.[20,21] Heavy rainfall in East Africa resulted in a major recurring epidemic in 2006-2007.[22] It is likely that other receptive areas such as North America would experience the same fate if an introduction should occur.[4]

CCHF virus is transmitted by ticks. The principal vectors belong to the genus Hyalomma. Immature stages feed on hares, hedgehogs, and ground-feeding birds, whereas adults parasitize large wild and domestic animals. This virus is widely distributed in southwestern Russia, the Balkans, the Middle East, central Asia, western China, and Africa.[5]

Hantaviruses

These agents are fundamentally parasites of wild rodents and insectivores.[6] As such, hantaviruses are the exception to the general rule that Bunyaviridae members are arthropod-borne viruses. Although many rodent species worldwide have been shown to be infected, each of the presently recognized viral species has a single major rodent host species. This species becomes chronically infected despite an immune response that eliminates viremia, and its members excrete virus in urine and saliva for weeks or months.[23,24] Mechanisms of intraspecific transmission depend largely on horizontal transmission between sexually mature animals.[6,24] HTN virus, the cause of severe hemorrhagic fever with renal syndrome (HFRS) in Korea, China, and eastern Russia, is carried by the striped field mouse, Apodemus agrarius.[6] A. agrarius is found in or near cultivars of humans; rodent breeding seasons and human agricultural practices result in fall and spring disease peaks.[8,25,26] Dobrava virus associated with Aedes flavicollis is the major cause of severe HFRS in the Balkans, and related viruses cause similarly severe disease in other areas of the former Soviet Union. Another hantavirus, Seoul virus, is found worldwide in Rattus norvegicus. Although the virus is found wherever the reservoir sewer rat occurs, disease has rarely, if ever, been identified in the United States.

Bank voles, Clethrionomys glareolus, are the reservoir-vectors of Puumala virus, the cause of a milder form of HFRS termed nephropathia epidemica in Scandinavia, the western former Soviet Union, and Europe. These small rodents are found in forests and agricultural hedgerows, have highly fluctuating populations, and disperse into rural and suburban gardens and dwellings particularly in the fall and winter of years when their populations reach peaks.[25,26]

Many native North and South American rodents (family Muridae, subfamily Sigmodontinae) host phylogenetically distinct hantaviruses associated with hantavirus pulmonary syndrome (HPS).[27] HPS is a

disease of the Americas and is probably more important in South America than in North America. The most important North American virus is SNV. The reservoir of SNV is the deer mouse, Peromyscus maniculatus, a species that is widespread in the United States and readily enters homes and other structures. On the East Coast, the closely related New York virus causes chronic infection of the white-footed mouse, Peromyscus leucopus. Somewhat more distantly related viruses are Bayou and Black Creek Canal viruses found in the southern United States and Florida, respectively, and associated with a degree of renal failure in their clinical picture. The most important South American virus is Andes virus, which is a common cause of disease in Argentina and Chile and is the only hantavirus that has caused person-to-person transmission.[27]

TRANSMISSION TO HUMANS

California Encephalitis Viruses

LAC virus transmission occurs through the bite of female mosquitoes that have viral infection of their salivary glands. Human infection occurs mainly during the summer and early fall in persons entering forested areas for recreation or those living near forests. Members of A. triseriatus range a considerable distance from forest across open terrain in search of a blood meal and breed effectively in some manufactured containers such as abandoned tires, bringing the mosquito range closer to human habitation.[28]

Rift Valley Fever and Crimean-Congo Hemorrhagic Fever

RVF in Africa has two main modes of transmission. It is recognized as a disease of farmers, veterinarians, and abattoir workers who have close contact with blood shed from sick domestic livestock or fresh carcasses containing a high concentration of virus.[19] Another major route of transmission to humans is from mosquito bites, particularly during epidemics. Infrequent years of heavy precipitation trigger the dormant transovarially infected eggs, and other secondary vectors widely disseminate virus.[4,19] CCHF virus infects humans principally by the bite of adult Hyalomma ticks. Milkers and shepherds are frequent victims. Asymptomatically viremic sheep and cattle have been implicated in transmission to abattoir workers, even outside known endemic areas,[29] and it is also hazardous to crush infected ticks. Highly infectious blood from patients also has caused several alarming nosocomial outbreaks with fatalities in medical personnel, particularly when the correct diagnosis of the index case was not suspected.[30-32]

Hantaviruses

Aerosols of virus-contaminated rodent urine or perhaps feces are thought to represent the principal vehicle for the transmission of hantaviruses; disease has also followed the bite of infected rodents (saliva contains virus).[6,33] Infections from *Apodemus* or *Clethrionomys* are acquired principally by persons visiting or working in forests and on farms. Depending on the circumstances, the incidence may be highest in summer or in fall and early winter. Disease is maximal in "high-rodent" years, when suburban residents may be exposed to disposing of infected rodents.[6,25-27,34]

Infection with Seoul virus from *Rattus norvegicus* may occur on farms or in residential areas. Indeed, cases of HFRS, traced to nontraveling residents of urban Seoul, Korea, were the first clues to the existence of the virus. Rat-borne disease has striking seasonal prevalence (winter–spring) in China and Russia.[34] In addition, infection, human disease, and even death have been linked to infected laboratory rats in Korea, Japan, Belgium, France, and the United Kingdom.[33] Rat colonies are apparently infected by the introduction of infected laboratory rats or by contact with wild rats bearing the virus. The United States has been spared this problem because rat stocks imported for research are cesarean delivered and barrier maintained.

Deer mice are numerous and readily enter human dwellings and outbuildings, particularly when mouse populations are high or in autumn when food and cover are scarce. Abundant rodent populations led to a large number of cases in the southwestern United States in the summer of 1993 and resulted in the first discovery of the virus. Most hantavirus epidemic years have been associated with increased rodent populations.[6,26,27]

Clinical Manifestations

CALIFORNIA ENCEPHALITIS VIRUSES

Infection of humans by CE viruses is most commonly asymptomatic. After an incubation period of 3 to 7 days, however, individuals may experience mild febrile illness, encephalitis, or meningoencephalitis. More than 90% of acute CNS disease caused by LAC virus occurs in children younger than 15 years; males are affected more often than females, and the mortality in acute CNS disease is about 1%.[1,13,35-37] LAC infection has caused encephalitis in an immunocompromised adult with a presentation resembling herpes encephalitis.[36] Clinically and pathologically, CE is difficult to distinguish from other acute viral infections of the CNS. It can range in severity from mild aseptic meningitis to a severe disease mimicking herpes encephalitis. Computed tomography scans are abnormal in a minority of cases, magnetic resonance imaging is sometimes positive, and either can yield focal images;[13] the electroencephalogram is usually abnormal and often focally so, even with periodic lateralizing epileptiform discharges (PLEDs) that lead to a suspicion of herpes encephalitis.[37] PLEDs often localize to the temporal lobe and are associated with more severe disease (convulsions, intubation, prolonged intensive care unit stay) as well as sequelae (epilepsy, cognitive and memory deficits).[38] Fever, headache, nausea, and vomiting are present in most patients. Lethargy, aphasia, incoordination, and focal motor abnormalities, even paralysis, may be present, but the outstanding serious finding is convulsions, which occur in about one half of cases. The spinal fluid generally shows a modest pleocytosis (<100 white blood cells/mm³) that occasionally is largely granulocytic and exhibits a normal or slightly increased protein concentration. Peripheral leukocytosis in excess of 15,000 white blood cells/mm³ is not uncommon. Although most patients make uneventful recoveries, abnormal electroencephalographic findings 1 to 5 years later are present in 75%, emotional lability is persistent in 10%, and epilepsy is a chronic problem in 6% to 10% of all diagnosed cases. Frank neurologic deficit is uncommon but does occur.[35] Thus, the residua of La Crosse encephalitis may be more serious than is generally appreciated. Recently, a possible congenital infection with LAC virus has been reported, without apparent abnor-

malities to the newborn infant. LAC infection during pregnancy has been associated with teratogenic effects in rabbits, gerbils, and sheep.[39-41]

RIFT VALLEY FEVER AND CRIMEAN-CONGO HEMORRHAGIC FEVER

RVF infection in humans causes undifferentiated febrile disease in the great majority of instances. Perhaps 10% of patients experience macular and perimacular retinitis and vasculitis that may cause a permanent loss of vision. In as much as 1% of infections, fulminant disease with hemorrhage, jaundice, and hepatitis may develop at the end of a 3- to 6-day febrile episode with a high mortality.[42] Other infections (<1%) lead to severe, frequently fatal encephalitis directly related to viral invasion of the CNS.

CCHF is a severe hemorrhagic fever with shock, disseminated intravascular coagulation, frequent extensive bleeding, and severe thrombocytopenia.[5,30-32] The virus infects the reticuloendothelial system and frequently involves hepatocytes extensively, leading to icteric hepatitis.[43] Mortality rates range from 20% to 35%. The virus is distributed from western China continuing to the west across the central Asian republics, the Middle East, the Balkans, and all across Africa. There are distinct geographic phylogenetic clusters, with the possibility of reassortment and distant transport occurring, but there is relatively little known about the relation to virulence.[44]

HANTAVIRUSES

Hemorrhagic Fever with Renal Syndrome

The hallmarks of clinical infection by HTN, Dobrara, Seoul, and Puumala viruses as well as other Eurasian hantaviruses are fever, thrombocytopenia, and acute renal insufficiency pathologically typical of acute interstitial nephritis. The incubation period, typically 2 weeks, may vary from 5 to 42 days. In the severe form of HFRS exemplified by HTN virus infection or Dobrava virus in Europe, patients who survive full-blown disease progress through febrile (toxic), hypotensive, oliguric, and polyuric clinical stages and may require weeks or months to recover from general asthenia.[45-47]

In the toxic phase, patients complain of headache, abdominal and lower back pain, dizziness, and, often, blurred vision.[42-45] Conjunctival injection and petechiae occur over the upper trunk and soft palate. An erythematous flush that blanches on pressure is characteristically seen on the torso and face. Leukocyte levels are normal or more likely elevated, often exceeding 20,000/mm³. The differential count shows a left shift, immature myeloid cells, and atypical lymphocytes as well, confirming the decreased thrombocyte count. At the end of the febrile period (4 to 7 days), many patients experience severe clinical shock. Those surviving then must endure varied grades of renal insufficiency that can include anuria, oliguria, mucosal bleeding diathesis, electrolyte and acid-base abnormalities, hypertension, and pneumonitis complicated by pulmonary edema. After 3 to 10 days, polyuria begins with its attendant stresses on the fluid and electrolyte balance. The fatality rate in severe HFRS caused by Hantaan or Dobrava viruses averages about 5%: one third during the shock phases and two thirds (cerebrovascular accidents and pulmonary edema) during the renal phases of illness. Hemodynamic changes result from massive, acute capillary leak syndrome of uncertain cause and equally poorly understood shock-inducing mechanisms. The renal lesions, predominantly in medullary tubules, are possibly related to systemic and intrarenal hemodynamic factors and the influence of immunopathologically released kinins and cytokines.[48]

The milder form of HFRS caused by Puumala virus and often referred to as nephropathia epidemica is rarely hemorrhagic and is fatal in less than 1% of clinical cases. Abdominal pain and hyposphenuria may be manifestations. Up to 90% of Puumala virus infections are asymptomatic. Proteinuria, creatinine level elevation, and leukocytosis, although common, are much less severe than for HTN virus infection.

Seoul virus also causes a mild to moderately severe HFRS in Eurasia with more prominent hepatic involvement than classic HFRS.[45]

Hantavirus Pulmonary Syndrome

HPS begins with a febrile prodrome followed by a severe increase in pulmonary vascular permeability and shock.[48-50] If hypoxia is managed and shock is not fatal, the vascular leak reverses in a few days and recovery is virtually complete, although renal and other sequelae have been suggested.[51] The first symptoms are fever of sudden onset and generalized myalgia. This prodrome resembles the initial phases of HFRS and may also be accompanied by abdominal pain and gastrointestinal disturbances.[49] About 4 to 5 days later (range of 1 to 10 days), the patient presents with respiratory symptoms, which usually consist of modest cough and dyspnea. Examination may be unrevealing, but generally fever, tachycardia, and tachypnea are present, perhaps with mild hypotension. Laboratory abnormalities commonly found at this time or developing within 1 to 2 days thereafter are an elevated hematocrit; leukocytosis, left shift, or both; abnormal (atypical) lymphocytes and immature myeloid cells on smear; mild thrombocytopenia; a prolonged activated partial thromboplastin time; and mildly elevated aspartate aminotransferase or lactate dehydrogenase levels. Mild increases in serum creatinine levels and proteinuria occur in some cases,[27] but the severe renal lesions seen in HFRS are not a regular feature of this syndrome.[48,52] Respiratory involvement can progress from mild desaturation and interstitial pulmonary edema to florid pulmonary edema with respiratory failure in a matter of hours.[50,53] HPS should be suspected when an otherwise healthy adult develops unexplained pulmonary edema or is suspected of adult respiratory distress syndrome without one of the known causes of this syndrome being present; thrombocytopenia or a falling platelet count is a particularly useful finding early in the course.[50] Extracorporeal membrane oxygenation may improve survival but has never been tested in a controlled trial.[54]

The histopathologic findings of interstitial infiltrates of T lymphocytes and alveolar pulmonary edema without marked necrosis or polymorphonuclear leukocyte involvement plus the rapid resolution of the lesion suggest that the major abnormality may be the induction of a functional vascular permeability increase via an immunopathologic mechanism.[52,55]

Diagnosis

The diagnosis of CE is immunologic because virus is not present in blood or secretions during the phase of clinical CNS disease. The diagnosis can be rapidly and specifically achieved with ELISA tests for antiviral IgM antibodies in blood and cerebrospinal fluid, which are usually, but not always, positive at the time of admission.[13,56] A licensed indirect FA test is available for IgG and IgM antibodies to LAC and may be useful in the diagnosis.[14] Virtually all hantavirus patients have both IgM and IgG ELISA antibodies present when admitted to the hospital.[4,6,46] Hantaviruses can be recovered only with difficulty in cell culture or animal hosts,[24] but the agent can be detected in blood or tissues by reverse transcription–polymerase chain reaction or in tissues by immunohistochemical staining.[6,7,52,55]

RVF and CCHF viruses are readily recovered from the blood of acutely ill patients in cell cultures or suckling mice. Antigen-detection ELISA is useful in diagnosis, particularly of severe cases. The polymerase chain reaction provides additional sensitivity with no loss of specificity. Antibodies detectable by a variety of methods generally appear within 5 to 14 days of onset and coincide with clinical improvement. ELISA detection of IgM antibodies is a reliable, definitive method.[5,6,19,29,30] Because of the aerosol hazard to laboratory personnel, acute samples must be handled with care, and attempts to isolate these two agents should be restricted to facilities with maximal containment.

Prevention and Treatment

With the exception of RVF, for which there is an investigational inactivated vaccine and an investigational live-attenuated vaccine,[57] prevention of these diseases is accomplished only by personal means (e.g., avoidance of rodent contact, use of mosquito and tick repellents) and perhaps in the case of La Crosse virus by the elimination of manufactured containers leading to mosquito breeding together with aerial spraying of slow-release insecticides over forested areas of known high *A. triseriatus* reproduction.[58]

Ribavirin, a guanosine analogue, was effective in the treatment of HFRS in a double-blind placebo-controlled study in China using the intravenous dosing regimen established for Lassa fever (see Chapter 167). Intensive monitoring and frequent dialysis even without ribavirin result in very low mortality. Studies in vitro and in laboratory animals suggest that ribavirin also might be effective in the treatment of severe RVF and CCHF, and clinical experience with the drug in CCHF supports its use.[59,60] An open-label trial of ribavirin failed to show any efficacy in HPS patients, perhaps because death typically occurs within 24 to 48 hours of hospitalization.[51] Effective supportive care is important in all of the severe Bunyavirus diseases. Careful management of coma, cerebral edema, and seizures is critical in CE patients; there is danger in too vigorous use of phenobarbital in children with status epilepticus.[13,37,61] LAC virus is sensitive in vitro to ribavirin, and treatment of one unusual case diagnosed with brain biopsy has been reported.[61] Early management of hantavirus patients should avoid excessive administration of fluids in these febrile, hemoconcentrated, hypotensive patients. Vascular leak leads to extravasation into retroperitoneal tissues (HFRS) or lung (HPS); cardiotonic drugs should be used early because of the hemodynamic profile of decreased cardiac output and increased systemic vascular resistance.[48] Patients with severe HFRS may require hemodialysis or peritoneal dialysis during the oliguric phase, and plasma protein or whole blood, or both, may be useful in treating hemorrhage or shock, or both, in this and other hemorrhagic fevers. Heparin is not recommended for the treatment of presumptive or incipient disseminated intravascular coagulation in HFRS. Patients with mild HFRS due to Puumala virus rarely require dialysis.

Other Bunyaviridae of Concern

JAMESTOWN CANYON VIRUS

This California group Bunyavirus is more important than was previously recognized and has been implicated in encephalitis in several adults.[2] Antibodies are not often sought in encephalitis patients and cross-react with other CE antigens in some tests. It is distributed widely across North America and is transmitted by *Culiseta inornata* and several species of *Aedes* mosquitoes, and often-burgeoning populations of white-tailed deer are suspected as the vertebrate amplifier.[62]

OROPOUCHE VIRUS

Another Bunyavirus (Simbu group) has caused epidemics in towns and cities of Brazil, Panama, and Peru but also has a much wider distribution in the forest.[63,64] Infection of humans results in an abrupt onset of fever, chills, headache, myalgia, and often vomiting and arthralgia. Aseptic meningitis has been reported in some cases. The disease is self-limiting, but prolonged asthenia and arthralgia may occur. The natural forest cycle is unknown, but in urban areas the rainy season leads to breeding of biting midges, and epidemics involve thousands of humans.

TOSCANA VIRUS

The classic sand fly fevers (Sicilian and Naples viruses) are acute febrile illnesses with headache and myalgias and were common in the broad

European and Asian range of their vector, *Phlebotomus papatasi*, until DDT campaigns against malaria virtually eliminated this sand fly in much of Europe. Another sand fly, *Phlebotomus perniciosus*, spreads the related but distinct Phlebovirus Toscana, which appears to be an important cause of febrile disease, aseptic meningitis, and mild encephalitis in both adults and children in the Tuscany area, where it may be a more common cause of aseptic meningitis than enteroviruses.[65,66] CNS infections are common in the circum-Mediterranean distribution of the vector in Europe from Cyprus to Portugal and Spain and are often causes of disease in returning travelers.[65,67,68]

NGARI VIRUS

During the 1997-1998 RVF outbreak in Kenya, a virus belonging to the *Bunyavirus* genus was isolated from putative hemorrhagic fever cases and reverse transcription–polymerase chain reaction was positive in 12 sera. The virus was found to have the S and L RNA segments of Bunyamwera virus, but the M segment was derived from another *Bunyavirus*, Ngari virus.[69] Thus, this virus should be considered in other viral hemorrhagic fever epidemics and is a cautionary example of the emergence of novel pathogens through viral reassortment.[70]

REFERENCES

1. Peters CJ, Le Duc JW. Bunyaviridae: Bunyaviruses, phleboviruses, and related viruses. In: Belshe RB, ed. *Textbook of Human Virology*. St. Louis: Mosby-Year Book; 1991:571.
2. Eldridge BF, Glaser C, Pedrin RE, et al. The first reported case of California encephalitis in more than 50 years. *Emerg Infect Dis*. 2001;7:451-452.
3. Huang CW, Campbell L, Grady I, et al. Diagnosis of Jamestown Canyon encephalitis by polymerase chain reaction. *Clin Infect Dis*. 1999;28:1294-1297.
4. Peters CJ. Emergence of Rift Valley fever. In: Saluzzo JF, Dodet B, eds. *Factors in the Emergence of Arbovirus Diseases*. Paris: Elsevier; 1997:253.
5. Swanepoel R. Crimean-Congo haemorrhagic fever. In: Palmer SR, Soulsby EJL, Simpson DIH, eds. *Zoonoses*. Oxford: Oxford University Press; 1998:461-470.
6. Peters CJ, Mills JN, Spiropoulou C, et al. Hantavirus infections. In: Guerrant RL, Walker DH, Weller PF, eds. *Tropical Infectious Diseases – Principles, Pathogens and Practice*. 2nd ed. Philadelphia: Elsevier Churchill Livingstone; 2006:762-780.
7. Nichol ST, Spiropoulou CF, Morzunov S, et al. Genetic identification of a hantavirus associated with an outbreak of acute respiratory illness. *Science*. 1993;262:914-917.
8. Schmaljohn C. Bunyaviridae: the viruses and their replication. In: Knipe D, Howley P, eds. *Fields' Virology*. 5th ed. Philadelphia: Wolters Kluwer Health/Lippincott Williams and Wilkins; 2007:1741-1790.
9. Goldsmith CS, Elliott LH, Peters CJ, et al. Ultrastructural characteristics of Sin Nombre virus, causative agent of hantavirus pulmonary syndrome. *Arch Virol*. 1995;140:2107.
10. Thompson WH: Vector-Virus Relationship. In: Calisher CH, Thompson WH, eds. *California Serogroup Viruses, Proceedings of an International Symposium*. New York: Alan R Liss; 1983:57.
11. Yuill TM. The role of mammals in the maintenance and dissemination of La Crosse virus. In: Calisher CH, Thompson WH, eds. *California Serogroup Viruses, Proceedings of an International Symposium*. New York: Alan R Liss; 1983:77.
12. Watts DM, Thompson WH, Yuill TM, et al. Overwintering of La Crosse virus in *Aedes triseriatus*. *Am J Trop Med Hyg*. 1974;23:694.
13. McJunkin JE, Khan RR, Tsai TF. California-La Crosse encephalitis. *Infect Dis Clin North Am*. 1998;12:83.
14. Jones TF, Erwin PC, Craig AS, et al. Serological survey and active surveillance for La Crosse virus infections among children in Tennessee. *Clin Infect Dis*. 2000;31:1284-1287.
15. Centers for Disease Control and Prevention. Possible congenital infection with La Crosse encephalitis virus—West Virginia, 2006-2007. *MMWR*. 2009;58:4-7.
16. Cully JF, Streit TG, Geard PB. Transmission of La Crosse virus by four strains of *Aedes albopictus* and from the eastern chipmunk (*Tamias striatus*). *J Am Mosquito Control Assoc*. 1992;8:237.
17. Gerhardt RR, Gottfried KL, Apperson CS, et al. First isolation of La Crosse virus from naturally infected *Aedes albopictus*. *Emerg Infect Dis*. 2001;7:807-811.
18. Lithicum KJ, Davies FG, Kairo A, et al. Rift Valley fever virus (family Bunyaviridae, genus *Phlebovirus*). Isolation from Diptera collected during an interepizootic period in Kenya. *J Hyg (Lond)*. 1985;95:197.
19. Swanepoel R, Coetzer JAW. Rift Valley fever. In: Coetzer JAW, Tustin RC, eds. *Infectious Diseases of Livestock*. 2nd ed. Oxford: Oxford University Press; 2004:1037-1070.
20. Woods CW, Karpati AM, Grein T, et al. An outbreak of Rift Valley fever in Northeastern Kenya, 1997-98. *Emerg Infect Dis*. 2002;8:138-144.
21. Fagbo SF. The evolving transmission pattern of Rift Valley fever in the Arabian Peninsula. *Ann N Y Acad Sci*. 2002;969:201-204.
22. Bird BH, Githinji JW, Macharia JM, et al. Multiple virus lineages sharing recent common ancestry were associated with a large Rift Valley fever outbreak among livestock in Kenya during 2006-2007. *J Virol*. 2008;82:11152-11166.
23. Lee HW, Lee PW, Baek LJ, et al. Intraspecific transmission of Hantaan virus, etiotogic agent of Korean hemorrhagic fever, in the rodent *Apodemus agrarius*. *Am J Trop Med Hyg*. 1981;30:1106.
24. Hutchinson KL, Rollin PE, Peters CJ. Pathogenesis of a North American hantavirus, Black Creek Canal virus, in experimentally infected *Sigmodon hispidus*. *Am J Trop Med Hyg*. 1998;59:58.
25. Korpela H, Lahdevirta J. The role of small rodents and patterns of living in the epidemiology of nephropathia epidemica. *Scand J Infect Dis*. 1978;10:303.
26. Niklasson B, Hornfeldt B, Lindkvist A, et al. Temporal dynamics of Puumala virus antibody prevalence in voles and of nephropathia epidemica incidence in humans. *Am J Trop Med Hyg*. 1995;53:134.
27. Peters CJ. Hantavirus pulmonary syndrome in the Americas. In: Scheld WM, Craig WA, Hughes JM, eds. *Emerging Infections II*. Washington, DC: ASM Press; 1998:7-64.
28. Mather TN, DeFoliart GR. Dispersion of gravid *Aedes triseriatus* (Diptera: Culcicidae) from woodlands into open terrain. *J Med Entomol*. 1984;21:384.
29. Rodriguez LL, Maupin GO, Ksiazek TG, et al. Molecular investigation of a multisource outbreak of Crimean-Congo hemorrhagic fever in the United Arab Emirates. *Am J Trop Med Hyg*. 1997;57:512.
30. Burney MI, Ghafoor A, Saleen M, et al. Nosocomial outbreak of viral hemorrhagic fever—Congo virus in Pakistan, January 1976. *Am Trop Med Hyg*. 1980;29:941.
31. Van Eeden PJ, Joubert JR, van de Wal BW, et al. A nosocomial outbreak of Crimean-Congo haemorrhagic fever at Tygerberg hospital. I. Clinical features. *S Afr Med J*. 1985;68:711-717
32. Papa A, Bino S, Llagami A, et al. Crimean-Congo hemorrhagic fever in Albania, 2001. *Eur J Clin Microbiol Infect Dis*. 2002;21:603-606.
33. Kawamata J, Yamanouchi T, Dohmae K, et al. Control of laboratory acquired hemorrhagic fever with renal syndrome (HFRS) in Japan. *Lab Anim Sci*. 1987;37:431.
34. Chen HX, Qiu FX, Dong BJ, et al. Epidemiologic studies in hemorrhagic fever with renal syndrome in China. *J Infect Dis*. 1986;154:394.
35. McJunkin JE, los Reyes EC, Irazuzta JE, et al. La Crosse encephalitis in children. *N Engl J Med*. 2001;344:801-807.
36. Wurtz R, Paleologos N. La Crosse encephalitis presenting like herpes simplex encephalitis in an immunocompromised adult. *Clin Infect Dis*. 2000;31:1113-1114.
37. Deering WM. Neurological aspects and treatment of La Crosse encephalitis. In: Calisher CH, Thompson WH, eds. *California Serogroup Viruses. Proceedings of an International Symposium*. New York: Alan R Liss; 1983:187.
38. de los Reyes EC, McJunkin JE, Glauser TA, et al. Periodic lateralized epileptiform discharges in La Crosse encephalitis, a worrisome subgroup: clinical presentation, electroencephalogram (EEG) patterns, and long-term neurologic outcome. *J Child Neurol*. 2008;23:167-172.
39. Tsai TF. Congenital arboviral infections: something new, something old. *Pediatrics*. 2006;117:936-939.
40. Osorio JE, Schoepp RJ, Yuill TM. Effects of La Crosse infection on pregnant domestic rabbits and Mongolian gerbils. *Am J Trop Med Hyg*. 1996;55:384-390.
41. Edwards JF, Karabatsos N, Collisson EW, et al. Ovine fetal malformations induced by in utero inoculation with main drain, San Angelo, and Lacrosse viruses. *Am J Trop Med Hyg*. 1997;56:171-176.
42. Al Hazmi M, Ayoola EA, Abdurahman M, et al. Epidemic Rift Valley fever in Saudi Arabia: a clinical study of severe illness in humans. *Clin Infect Dis*. 2003;36:245-252.
43. Burt FJ, Swanepoel R, Shieh W-J, et al. Immunohistochemical and in situ localization of Crimean-Congo hemorrhagic fever virus in human tissues and pathogenic implications. *Arch Pathol Lab Med*. 1997;121:839.
44. Deyde VM, Khristova ML, Rollin PE, et al. Crimean-Congo hemorrhagic fever virus genomics and global diversity. *J Virol*. 2006;80:8834-8842.
45. Lee JS, Cho BY, Lee MC, et al. Clinical features of serologically proven Korean hemorrhagic fever patients. *Seoul J Med*. 1980;21:163.
46. Earle DP. Symposium on epidemic hemorrhagic fever. *Am J Med*. 1954;16:617.
47. Bruno P, Harrison HL, Brown J, et al. The protean manifestations of hemorrhagic fever with renal syndrome. A retrospective review of 26 cases from Korea. *Ann Intern Med*. 1990;113:385.
48. Peters CJ, Simpson G, Levy H. Spectrum of hantavirus infection: hemorrhagic fever with renal syndrome and hantavirus pulmonary syndrome. *Annu Rev Med*. 1999;50:531-545.
49. Duchin JS, Koster F, Peters CJ, et al. Hantavirus pulmonary syndrome: clinical description of disease caused by a newly recognized hemorrhagic fever virus in the southwestern United States. *N Engl J Med*. 1994;330:949.
50. Moolenaar RL, Dalton C, Lipman HB, et al. Clinical features that differentiate hantavirus pulmonary syndrome from three other acute respiratory illnesses. *Clin Infect Dis*. 1995;21:643.
51. Pergam SA, Schmidt DW, Nofchissey RA, et al. Potential renal sequelae in survivors of hantavirus cardiopulmonary syndrome. *Am J Trop Med Hyg*. 2009;80:279-285.
52. Peters CJ, Khan AS: Hantavirus pulmonary syndrome: the new American hemorrhagic fever. *Clin Infect Dis*. 2002;34:1224-1231.
53. Ketai LH, Williamson MR, Telepak RJ, et al. Hantavirus pulmonary syndrome: radiographic findings in 16 patients. *Radiology*. 1994;191:665.
54. Dietl CA, Wernly JA, Pett SB, et al. Extracorporeal membrane oxygenation support improves survival of patients with severe Hantavirus cardiopulmonary syndrome. *J Thorac Cardiovasc Surg*. 2008;135:579-584.
55. Zaki SR, Greer PW, Coffield LM, et al. Hantavirus pulmonary syndrome: pathogenesis of an emerging infectious disease. *Am J Pathol*. 1995;146:552.
56. Calisher CH, Pretzman CI, Muth DJ, et al. Serodiagnosis of La Crosse virus infections in humans by detection of immunoglobulin M class antibodies. *J Clin Microbiol*. 1986;12:667.
57. Pittman PR, Liu CT, Cannon TL, et al. Immunogenicity of an inactivated Rift Valley fever vaccine in humans: a 12-year experience. *Vaccine*. 1999;18:181-189.
58. Francy DB. Mosquito control for prevention of California (La Crosse) encephalitis. In: Calisher CH, Thompson WH, eds. *California Serogroup Viruses. Proceedings of an International Symposium*. New York: Alan R Liss; 1983:365.
59. Peters CJ, Reynolds JA, Slone TW, et al. Prophylaxis of Rift Valley fever with antiviral drugs, immune serum, an interferon inducer, and a macrophage activator. *Antiviral Res*. 1986;6:285.
60. Mardani M, Jahromi MK, Naieni KH, et al. The efficacy of oral ribavirin in the treatment of Crimean-Congo hemorrhagic fever in Iran. *Clin Infect Dis*. 2003;36:1613-1618.
61. McJunkin JE, Khan R, de los Reyes EC, et al. Treatment of severe La Crosse encephalitis with intravenous ribavirin following diagnosis by brain biopsy. *Pediatrics*. 1997;99:261.
62. Andreadis TG, Anderson JF, Armstrong PM, et al. Isolations of Jamestown Canyon Virus (Bunyaviridae: Orthobunyavirus) from field-collected mosquitoes (Diptera: Culicidae) in Connecticut, USA: a ten-year analysis, 1997-2006. *Vector Borne Zoonotic Dis*. 2008;8(2):175-188.
63. Watts DM, Phillips I, Callahan JD, et al. Oropouche virus transmission in the Amazon River basin of Peru. *Am J Trop Med Hyg*. 1997;56:148.
64. Bernardes-Terzian AC, de-Moraes-Bronzoni RV, Drumond BP, et al. Sporadic oropouche virus infection, acre, Brazil. *Emerg Infect Dis*. 2009;15(2):348-350.
65. Nicoletti L, Ciufolini MG, Verani P. Sandfly fever viruses in Italy (Review). *Arch Virol*. 1996;(Suppl 11):41.
66. Nicoletti L, Verani P, Caciolli S, et al. Central nervous system involvement during infection by Phlebovirus Toscana of residents in natural foci in central Italy (1977-1988). *Am J Trop Med Hyg*. 1991;45:429.
67. Braito A, Ciufolini MG, Pippi L, et al. Phlebotomus-transmitted toscana virus infections of the central nervous system: a seven-year experience in Tuscany. *Scand J Infect Dis*. 1998;30:505-508.
68. Echevarria JM, de Ory F, Guisasola ME, et al. Acute meningitis due to Toscana virus infection among patients from both the Spanish Mediterranean region and the region of Madrid. *J Clin Virol*. 2003;26:79-84.
69. Gerrard SR, Li L, Barrett AD, Nichol ST. Ngari virus is a Bunyamwera virus reassortant that can be associated with large outbreaks of hemorrhagic fever in Africa. *J Virol*. 2004;78:8922-8926.
70. Bowen MD, Trappier SG, Sanchez AJ, et al. A reassortant bunyavirus isolated from acute hemorrhagic fever cases in Kenya and Somalia. *Virology*. 2001;291:185-190.

167

Lymphocytic Choriomeningitis Virus, Lassa Virus, and the South American Hemorrhagic Fevers

C. J. PETERS

The arenavirus family is characterized by a single-stranded RNA genome, a unique morphology, and the usual use of rodents as virus reservoirs. These viruses include lymphocytic choriomeningitis (LCM) virus, Lassa virus, and American viruses that belong to the Tacaribe complex. The viruses can be divided into two major phylogenetic and antigenic groups corresponding to (1) LCM, Lassa, and close relatives from Old World rodents (family Muridae, subfamily Murinae), and (2) the Tacaribe complex from New World or American rodents (family Muridae, subfamily Sigmodontinae); the correspondence between the phylogeny of the hosts and that of the viruses suggests a long association and coevolution.[1,2] The New World complex can be further divided into three distinct clades designated A, B, and C. Tacaribe virus isolated from bats is the only member of the family that is not known to be a chronic, inapparent infection of rodents. Significant human disease is associated with several of the viruses (Table 167-1). The family prototype, LCM virus, was first isolated in 1933 during serial monkey passage of human material obtained from a fatal infection in the first documented epidemic of St. Louis encephalitis.[3] Junin, Machupo, Lassa, Guanarito, Sabia, and Chapare viruses were first recovered during investigations of human disease in 1958,[4] 1963,[5] 1969,[6] 1989,[7] 1990,[8] and 2003,[9] respectively.

Viral Characterization

Virions are round, oval, or pleomorphic particles averaging about 110 to 130 nm in diameter but ranging from 50 to 300 nm.[10] The viral envelope is formed by budding from the viral glycoprotein-bearing host plasma membrane. The surface of the particle bears 6- to 10-nm spikes, and the interior shows variable numbers of characteristic dense granules, 20 to 25 nm in diameter, which have been shown to be host cell ribosomes (Fig. 167-1). These unique structures resembling grains of sand are responsible for the family name (Latin *arenosos,* or "sandy"). Arenaviruses contain a segmented RNA genome with 31- and 22-S strands. Host ribosomal RNA of 28, 18, and 4 to 6 S is also present but apparently is not biologically functional.

The S, or small, RNA of arenaviruses codes for three virion proteins in a unique manner. The 60- to 70-kDa nucleocapsid protein (N) is read first in a conventional negative sense, and later a glycoprotein precursor polypeptide (GPC) is transcribed from genomic sense messenger RNA. This pattern has been termed *ambisense.* The GPC protein is then glycosylated and cleaved to form the spike glycoproteins G1 and G2, typically 35 to 45 kDa and 40 to 60 kDa, respectively. Arenavirus L, or large, RNA is also ambisense and codes for a viral polymerase of about 200 kDa and a zinc-finger protein.[2] The Z protein is a virion component important in budding[11] and other intracellular functions.

Epitopes mediating neutralization and antibody-complement cell lysis have been localized to the glycoproteins, particularly G1, which is also more genetically and antigenically variable among viral species.[12,13] The most serologically cross-reactive protein is N, which is usually measured in the diagnostic indirect fluorescent antibody (IFA) test. Protective T-cell epitopes are coded by the genes for N and GPC and probably other proteins as well.[13] Old World and clade C New World viruses attach to host cells through α-dystroglycan, possibly with other receptors, and the pathogenic American arenaviruses use the human transferrin receptor as a virus receptor.[14] Arenaviruses then fuse, interiorize, and uncoat within an acidic compartment.[12-16] Replication is usually not accompanied by overt cytopathic effects.

Epidemiology and Epizootiology

Arenaviruses are parasites of rodents. They exhibit high species specificity, and a single rodent species is the reservoir for a given agent. Chronic viral infection without obvious disease occurs with the release of virus into excreta, especially urine, resulting in transmission to humans. Among rodents, both vertical transmission and horizontal intraspecific spread are important to varied degrees.[2] Thus, human arenaviral disease is determined by viral pathogenicity, by the geographic distribution of a particular reservoir rodent, and by rodent-human ecologic factors that permit contact with excreted virus, particularly in aerosolized urine.

LYMPHOCYTIC CHORIOMENINGITIS

Although LCM virus infection may occur worldwide, human infection has been conclusively demonstrated only in Europe and the Americas.[17] Moreover, in regions where the virus is known to exist, infection in the two closely related nonoverlapping reservoir species, *Mus domesticus* and *Mus musculus,* is highly focal. Studies conducted in Baltimore, Boston, and Washington, DC revealed a spotty distribution of virus-positive mice in houses.[18,19] Similarly, in Germany, much higher murine infection rates prevail in the west-central than in the southern or northern portions of the country.[20]

Human cases of LCM are most common in autumn. This pattern is the result of seasonal population densities of rodents and the movement of mice into homes and barns during cold weather. In addition, seasonal variation in infection rates of *Mus* species or differential survival of excreted virus related to the temperature and relative humidity may be involved. It has been shown that aerosolized arenaviruses survive better at lower humidity.[21] Situations associated with wild mouse infection of humans include substandard housing such as mobile homes or inner-city dwellings, the cleaning of rodent-infested barns or outbuildings, and the autumn entry of wild mice into dwellings. Most human LCM infections occur among young adults, although persons of all ages have been affected.

The mode of transmission in most sporadic human infections is not definitely known; however, experimental and epidemiologic observations implicate aerosols, direct contact with rodents, and rodent bites (in that order) as the most likely vehicles.[2,18,22,23] The incubation period of human LCM disease is variable, but it most often ranges from 5 to 10 days. Patients not seeking medical care for the nonspecific febrile illness that begins at this time, but who may later present with acute meningitis, generally are found to have been exposed 2 to 3 weeks before the onset of nervous system signs.

Although most sporadic LCM cases are attributed to contact with infected wild mice, outbreaks of disease have been traced to infected

TABLE 167-1	Arenaviruses and Human Disease					
Virus	**Disease**	**Geography**	**Reservoir**	**Pathogenesis**	**Specific Therapy**	**Prevention**
Lymphocytic choriomeningitis	Aseptic meningitis; other organ involvement	North and South America, Europe, and wherever *Mus* is introduced	*Mus domesticus* and *Mus musculus* (house mice)	Systemic infection; when CNS invasion occurs, immunopathologic CNS disease follows	None	House mouse control and avoidance, particularly by pregnant women; monitor mouse and hamster suppliers
Lassa	Lassa fever	West Africa, particularly Sierra Leone, Guinea, Liberia, and Nigeria	*Mastomys* (multimammate mouse)	Vascular leak, multiorgan dysfunction, shock; bleeding and CNS involvement occur but not as common as in South American diseases	Intravenous ribavirin	Rodent avoidance and control in houses may be of ancillary benefit; strict isolation of hospitalized patients
Junin	Argentine HF	Argentine pampas	*Calomys musculinis*	As Lassa fever, except encephalopathy and thrombocytopenia are common, as is hemorrhage	Convalescent plasma; ribavirin probably efficacious	Effective live-attenuated vaccine
Machupo	Bolivian HF	Bolivia, Beni Department	*Calomys callosus*	As Argentine HF	Ribavirin or convalescent plasma	Elimination of rodents from home; laboratory evidence for cross-protection by Junin vaccine
Chapare	Chapare HF	Bolivia, Cochabamba Department	Unknown	Unknown, resembles Argentine HF or Sabia infection	Unknown, ribavirin suggested	Unknown
Guanarito	Venezuelan HF	Venezuela, Portuguesa State	*Zygodontomys brevicauda*	As Argentine HF	Unknown; ribavirin or convalescent plasma suggested	Unknown; rodent control?
Sabia	Brazilian HF	Brazil	Unknown	Resembles Argentine HF; patient in single naturally occurring case had severe hepatitis	Unknown; ribavirin suggested	Unknown

CNS, central nervous system; HF, hemorrhagic fever.

laboratory mice or Syrian hamsters *(Mesocricetus auratus)*. Several of these were the result of the introduction of LCM virus into hamsters through infected tumor cell lines.[23] An epidemic resulted from chronic infection of nude, athymic mice by stored infected hamster tumors.[24] Other outbreaks in the United States and Europe resulted from exposure in the home to pet hamsters obtained from breeders with infected stock.[25,26]

LASSA FEVER

Lassa fever is a disease of West Africa; however, with the contemporary ease of international travel, it may occur anywhere in the world. This disease is distinguished from other arenaviral diseases by its occasional ability to spread from person to person. Lassa fever was initially recognized in a Nigerian hospital where three nurses developed illness

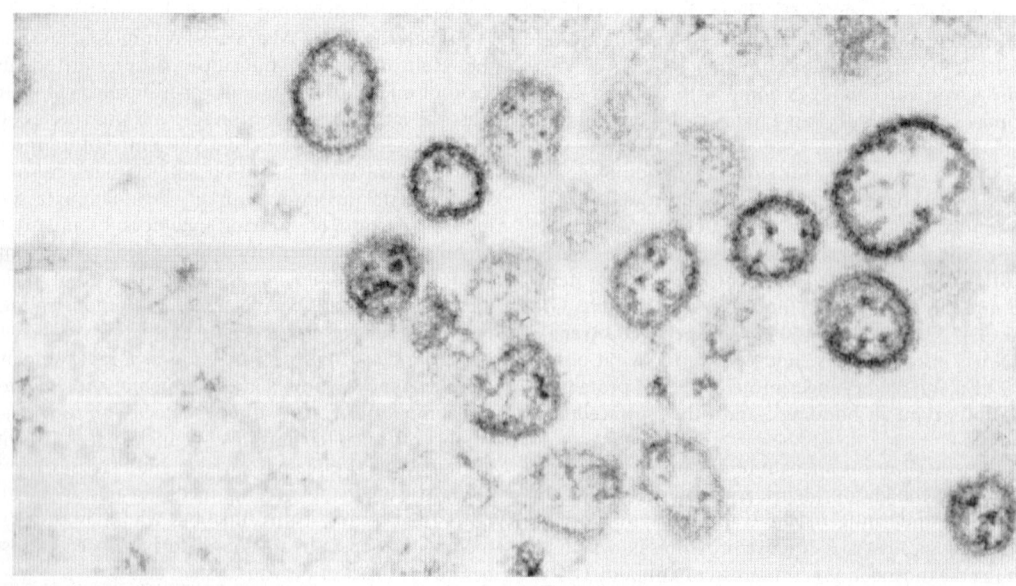

Figure 167-1 **Lassa virus.** Electron micrograph of Lassa virus in the first Vero cell passage envelope; electron-dense interior granules can be seen (original magnification, ×121,000).

successively.[27] Since then, extensive transmission, with occasional nosocomial outbreaks, has been reported from Nigeria, Liberia, Sierra Leone, and Guinea. Serologic studies and occasional cases have shown its presence in every country of West Africa between Nigeria and Senegal. West Africa, however, represents only a small part of the range of *Mastomys* rodents, which serve as viral reservoirs[6], and different species of these are found throughout the continent south of the Sahara Desert. Further work is needed to define the species of the genus *Mastomys* and their viruses, but clearly at least two species are infected in Sierra Leone.[28]

Most of the nosocomial outbreaks of Lassa fever have occurred during the dry season (January to April). Endemic transmission occurs throughout the year, with more cases during dry than during wet periods.[28,29] All ages and both sexes are infected equally; in some villages in Sierra Leone, infection rates may reach 10% to 20% per year. Based on serologic data, there may be 20 mild or inapparent infections for each hospitalized case.[28] In contrast, retrospective studies among white missionaries suggest, but do not yet prove, that moderately severe or even fatal illness usually follows infection.[30] Outbreaks typically include a few health care workers because of their close exposure to patients and infectious body fluids without barrier nursing precautions and because of their residence in the endemic area.

The modes of Lassa virus transmission are not precisely known, but they are almost certainly multiple. Endemic transmission is related to infected rodents by aerosol and direct contact, and most probably to person-to-person spread in homes.[31] Capture of rodents as a supplemental food source is another high risk factor for infection, until the rodents are cooked. *Mastomys* are common rodents in houses and in the nearby bush. In some areas, they are found in virtually all homes with high infection rates,[31] but in others, infection is less intensive, and infected rodents tend to cluster in individual houses,[32,33] not unlike the distribution of LCM virus in urban *Mus*.[19] Given the pervasive nature of *Mastomys,* control campaigns cannot be expected to prevent the disease, although model intensive efforts in a village in Sierra Leone resulted in a temporary fourfold reduction in transmission to humans. During nosocomial outbreaks, parenteral inoculation of body fluids (e.g., surgery or autopsy accidents), contact with infected body fluids, and aerosols generated by patients have all been incriminated.[29] Tertiary and quaternary cases in outbreaks are less numerous than are secondary cases, which suggests that only the unusual patient is very infectious.

The incubation period varies from 3 to 16 days (usually 7 to 12 days) when infection is transmitted from person to person. It is assumed to be similar in rodent-transmitted infection.

OTHER AFRICAN ARENAVIRUSES

Several other African rodent species are infected with distinct arenaviruses, but until recently, none had been associated with human disease. In 2008, a safari-booking agent from Zambia was medically evacuated to South Africa with a viral hemorrhagic fever (HF) and died, as did three secondary cases. A single tertiary case received ribavirin and, apparently, survived.[34] The virus has been identified as a distinctive arenaviral agent and named Lujo virus, but little other information is available. Although the chain of transmission and case-fatality rate are alarming, the initial recognition of these events to those of Lassa fever was similar,[27] so more evidence is needed to understand the potential of this newly recognized virus.

SOUTH AMERICAN HEMORRHAGIC FEVERS

The South American HFs are local public health problems in Argentina, Bolivia, and Venezuela and are caused by Junin, Machupo, and Guanarito viruses. Another lethal arenavirus, Sabia virus, was discovered in 1990 in São Paulo State, Brazil, but its health impact and reservoir are not yet known.[8] A burst of human HF cases in 2003 to 2004 led to the isolation of another new human pathogen, Chapare arenavirus. The issues of host, epidemiology, and clinical picture are sketchy,

but Chapare originates from higher altitudes near Cochabamba, Bolivia, 400 kilometers from the epicenter of Machupo virus activity in the low-lying Beni Department of Bolivia.[9]

In Argentina, the principal reservoir rodent is *Calomys musculinus*.[35] Argentine HF initially occurred mainly in an expanding zone within the rich agricultural pampas of northern Buenos Aires province. Now cases are found within an enlarged zone encompassing two more provinces and putting 5 million people at risk. *Calomys* populations reach their highest density in the cornfields during the austral fall (February to May); the disease thus affects principally men engaged in harvesting corn. Roughly 200 to 2000 cases are reported annually, and the numbers did not change substantially despite the change from manual to mechanized harvesting techniques. Introduction of effective vaccination has had a marked impact on the incidence of the disease, which has fallen below 100 cases annually.[36] Infectious aerosols are thought to be the most common mode of transmission, although food contamination and the direct contact of abraded fingers with blood and tissues of rodents crushed by machinery may also occur.

Bolivian HF is restricted to the tropical savanna of the Beni Department in northeastern Bolivia. The small reservoir rodent *Calomys callosus*[37] freely enters homes and gardens in this region, and most infections are house acquired. The incidence of cases is greatest from April to July (late rainy and early dry season), but the dominant feature of the epidemiologic pattern is that of small outbreaks in different villages and ranches with several years of quiescence thereafter. In town epidemics, all ages and both sexes are equally affected. On remote ranches and in fields, adult male patients predominate. Transmission is thought to occur by aerosols from infected rodents or possibly by contact with food contaminated by infectious rodent urine. Both nosocomial[38] and person-to-person[39] transmission have occurred, although these routes are not usual.

The mechanisms underlying the annual variations in both Bolivian and Argentine HF incidence and the extension of the endemic zone in Argentina are unknown. Rodent population density correlates with horizontal spread among rodents and human infection.[40]

In the Portuguesa state of Venezuela, cases of HF were noted in September 1989. The causative agent, named Guanarito virus for the municipality where most of the cases were found,[7] has the cane mouse (*Zygodontomys brevicauda*)[41] as reservoir. The main affected population was settlers moving into cleared forest areas to practice small-hold agriculture. The carrier rodents are well adapted to open grasslands and readily invaded fields, pastures, and peridomestic habitats.

Sabia virus has caused a single natural human infection that was fatal, as well as two laboratory infections.[8,42]

After parenteral exposures, the incubation period of South American HF may be only 2 to 6 days. The estimated interval after natural exposure to either Junin or Machupo virus (and presumably other South American arenaviruses as well) ranges from 5 to 19 days, with a mode of 7 to 12 days.

OTHER ARENAVIRUSES

Several African viruses related to Lassa and LCM viruses have been discovered (Mopeia, Mobala, Ippy), but no human disease, and in many cases no human infection, has been identified. They are attenuated for nonhuman primates and guinea pigs.[1,2,43] Similarly, there is a growing group of viruses in the Tacaribe complex that have not been associated with human disease in both South America and North America.[44] Some have caused human infections in the laboratory without inducing disease (Pichinde virus), but most are under continuing study, including Whitewater Arroyo virus, possibly associated with fatal human disease in the western United States.

Pathogenesis

RODENTS

Arenavirus infection of rodent hosts is chronic but clinically benign. The age of the host, route of infection, and strain of virus are important variables. In natural murine infections with LCM virus, the newborn or fetal animal becomes chronically viremic but has normal growth and fertility; despite widespread infection of many organs, there is no inflammatory response. Peripheral inoculation of adult mice results in a transient immunizing infection.

Laboratory-manipulated strains of LCM virus exhibit different pathogenicity for inbred strains of laboratory mice, and this infection has been extremely important for studying viral immunopathology and CD8[+] T-cell function. Infection of newborn mice results in chronic viremic infection in which T-cell immunity is suppressed. Depending on the murine genotype, different quantities of antiviral antibodies are produced and complex with viral antigens, leading to the development of chronic glomerulonephritis.[45] The artificial intracerebral inoculation of adult mice produces an acute fatal choriomeningitis with extensive mononuclear cell infiltrate mediated by immune cytotoxic T cells.[46]

The responses of natural reservoir *Calomys* rodents experimentally infected with Junin or Machupo virus somewhat resemble the mouse-LCM virus outcomes.[2,35,37] The differences are that lethal infection is not inducible by any route at any age, that antigen-antibody complexes are not demonstrable, and that some adult rodents develop chronic viremic infection exactly like that observed in very young mice inoculated with LCM. In addition, chronic infection with Machupo virus induces a microcytic hemolytic anemia (Coombs test negative) that results in chronic splenomegaly, a useful field marker for infection.

Mastomys rodents infected with Lassa virus similarly show no acute signs, do not develop inflammatory responses, and exhibit chronic infection or an effective immune response depending on age.[47] Field studies suggest that carrier *Mastomys* have little or no antibody but have sufficiently large quantities of virus to be readily detected in antigen tests.[32]

Arenavirus infection of nonreservoir rodents results in benign, self-limited infection and immunity. Guinea pigs, however, may experience severe acute disease and provide useful models for arenaviral HFs.[43]

NONHUMAN PRIMATES

Monkeys are good but not perfect models for the pathogenesis and experimental therapy of arenavirus infections in humans.[3,21,43,47-49] Macaque monkeys are readily infected by the inhalation of LCM virus, and the resulting disease resembles HF rather than central nervous system disease. Marmosets are also susceptible to fatal disease from LCM virus, including zoo animals fed infected newborn mice.[48]

Lassa virus induces a fatal disease in rhesus monkeys infected by small-particle aerosols, establishing the aerosol infectivity of the virus; the monkeys also have a pathologic appearance similar to that of humans.[21,49] Machupo and Junin viruses are also pathogenic for nonhuman primates, and these models, as well as the less expensive guinea pig models, have provided considerable information on the pathogenesis of human HF.[43,47,49,50]

HUMANS

Few data are available regarding the histopathology of fatal cases of human LCM infection, which is commonly lethal. Two fatal cases associated with early studies of the virus in monkeys displayed hemorrhagic necrosis much more typical of other arenavirus HFs[51]; they are regarded as aberrant human infections with this agent. A single fatal human encephalitis case was particularly well studied, and the patient showed a marked neuronal pattern of viral infection.[52]

Fatal Lassa virus infection in humans shows relatively few lesions. Variable necrosis with little or no inflammatory response has been observed in liver, spleen, and adrenal glands.[53] Focal liver necrosis is always found, but in no instance was the hepatic abnormality sufficient to cause death.[54] The degree of histologic change rarely seems sufficient to explain the clinical severity of the disease on a morphologic basis. Studies in animal models suggest that direct viral infection of endo-

thelial cells, as well as mediators possibly released from infected macrophages, may be extremely important in causing the vascular dysfunction and shock of these viral HFs.[50,55] Immunopathologic events seem less likely to be involved because immunosuppression fails to ameliorate the disease in animal models.[56]

Patients dying of Argentine or Bolivian HF have few prominent findings. There is no vasculitis and virtually no inflammatory response in any organ, but a pattern of small focal hemorrhages is present, primarily in mucosal surfaces. Hepatic necrosis, on the average, is more severe in Lassa than in Junin or Machupo infections, but Councilman-like bodies are readily discernible in all three diseases. Bronchopneumonia, either primary viral or, more commonly, secondary bacterial, is often found as well.

Patients with Argentine HF virus exhibit extremely high concentrations of circulating endogenous interferon-α that reach a maximum at 6 to 12 days of illness. The highest levels were observed in fatal cases.[57] Experimental and clinical studies support the concept that interferons may prove to be detrimental rather than beneficial in arenavirus infections.[58] High levels of circulating proinflammatory cytokines are present as well.[59]

At autopsy, tissues of humans and monkeys infected by Lassa, Junin, or Machupo virus contain large amounts of virus, viral antigen, and, in some instances, virions as in liver in Lassa infection. Spleen, nodes, and bone marrow are major replication sites for Junin and Machupo viruses, whereas Lassa virus is found in many viscera and, notably, in the placentas of pregnant women. Prominent infection of mesothelial surfaces may well be important in the frequent development of serous effusions.[55]

The paucity of histologic lesions in fatal cases and the lack of evidence of immunopathology suggest cytokines as candidates for the mediators of arenavirus HF.[60] The high levels seen in Lassa[61,62] and arenavirus HF,[57,59] as well as the induction of cytokines by in vitro infection of monocytes,[63] lend support to this idea, but the data are not entirely consistent and require further clinical and experimental studies.

Clinical Manifestations

Clinically apparent infections with all the arenaviruses are similar in presenting manifestations. Fever is typically insidious in onset and is accompanied by headache and significant myalgia and malaise. Relative bradycardia is common, as is dysesthesia, particularly hyperesthesia of the skin. Thereafter, the various diseases pursue different courses.

LYMPHOCYTIC CHORIOMENINGITIS VIRUS

LCM virus infections are most commonly febrile illnesses with headache and systemic symptoms and are associated with leukopenia and thrombocytopenia.[2,17,18,22-24,64] After 3 to 5 days of nonspecific illness, occasionally with lymphadenopathy and a maculopapular rash, the fever subsides, but it frequently recurs in 2 to 4 days with several days of even more severe headache. Patients may exhibit frank meningitis during this second febrile period. Cerebrospinal fluid (CSF) pressure usually is elevated, occasionally even with papilledema; the protein concentration ranges from 50 to 300 mg/dL; and several hundred lymphocytes per cubic millimeter are commonly observed. Hypoglycorrachia is found in less than one third of the cases. Encephalomyelitic infection may present as encephalitis, psychosis, paraplegia, or disturbances of cranial, sensory, or autonomic nervous function. Ependymal inflammation has resulted in transient aqueductal stenosis.

Occasionally, patients develop orchitis, myocarditis, arthritis, or alopecia. Orchitis develops 1 to 3 weeks after the onset of the illness; it is usually unilateral and painful and resolves within 2 weeks. Myocarditis is revealed by electrocardiographic changes and labile tachycardia during and after the second febrile period. Arthritis occurs occasionally during convalescence, principally affects the metacarpophalangeal and proximal interphalangeal joints, and is marked by minimal swelling and redness; it generally resolves within a few weeks.

The second febrile episode, as well as some of the complications of convalescence, has long been thought to represent immunopathologic phenomena. Antibodies detectable by immunofluorescence appear at about this time, and the lymphocytes in the CSF presumably are analogues of the T lymphocytes that cause LCM disease in the intracerebrally inoculated adult mouse.[64]

Recently, additional data supporting this idea have gained support from unexpected findings in the renal transplantation field. Thirteen recipients of kidney, lung, or liver transplants from four organ donors developed severe disease with multiorgan involvement and clear evidence of LCMV infection.[65-67] None developed classic LCMV aseptic meningitis. All except one died with severe disease and disseminated infection not unlike that seen in Lassa fever. This pattern has also been described in tumor patients receiving LCMV as a supposed oncolytic therapy.[68] The only survivor had a decrease in immunosuppression and received intravenous ribavirin. Only one of the donors had documented contact with a rodent, and it was a hamster shown to be infected with LCMV and coming from LCMV-infected pet suppliers.[69]

LASSA FEVER

Most Lassa virus infections in Africa are mild or subclinical.[28] Severe multisystem disease occurs only in 5% to 10% of infections. Case-fatality rates in hospitalized patients average 15% to 25%.[70] Clinical manifestations are varied, and differential diagnosis is difficult.[27,30,61,70,71] In a case-control study of patients hospitalized with Lassa fever in Sierra Leone, the frequencies of selected findings were as follows: retrosternal chest pain, 74%; sore throat, 60%; back pain, 62%; cough, 62%; abdominal pain, 50%; vomiting, 49%; diarrhea, 26%; conjunctivitis, 25%; facial edema, 10%; and proteinuria, 43%. Mucosal bleeding at any time was noted in just 17% of patients. These findings were present in many febrile patients not infected with Lassa virus, which rendered a clinical diagnosis in many instances impossible. A combination of fever, pharyngitis, retrosternal pain, and proteinuria correctly predicted 70% of laboratory-confirmed Lassa fever cases and 80%, by exclusion, of the control illnesses.[60] Central nervous system involvement has been described with encephalopathy, encephalitis, meningeal signs, and convalescent cerebellar syndromes.[70,72,73]

Lassa virus infection also causes serious disease and death in children, although manifestations may be even more protean or clinically confusing than among adults.[74] Four cases (three were fatal) of a distinctive syndrome consisting of severe generalized edema, abdominal distention, and bleeding were recorded in children younger than 2 years in Liberia.[75]

Concentrations of virus and serum aspartate transaminase in the blood at admission are highly reliable, objective predictors of the outcome of infection. Patients with at least 10^3 median tissue culture infective doses of virus per milliliter and 150 IU of aspartate transaminase per liter experienced a mortality rate of 78%, whereas 83% of those with lower values survived.[76,77] The clinical manifestations associated with death, however, generally occur during the second week of illness. These consist of hypotension, peripheral vasoconstriction, reduced urinary output, facial and pulmonary edema, and, in some cases, pleural effusions and ascites. These events, often accompanied by minor hemorrhages from mucosal surfaces, strongly suggest a lesion of diffuse capillary leakage. Myocardial depression may contribute to the circulatory defect.

Patients who do not develop a capillary leak syndrome may experience other complications during the second or third week of illness. Chief among these is eighth-nerve deafness, which may be unilateral or bilateral and has been seen in almost one third of hospitalized cases.[78] Some of the patients have mild lesions or will improve, but village surveys confirm a major impact of Lassa infection on hearing loss in the community. About 3% to 5% of male patients suffer pericarditis detected by auscultation that resolves clinically in 7 to 10 days; all such patients survive. Less common complications include uveitis and orchitis. Many hospitalized Lassa fever patients undergo some degree of transient alopecia during convalescence.

SOUTH AMERICAN HEMORRHAGIC FEVERS

Argentine and Bolivian HFs are remarkably similar clinically, and the mortality rate in each is about 15% to 30%.[35,79,80] Reported Venezuelan HF cases have been similar.[7,81] The onset of the illness is insidious, with progressive fever, malaise, and myalgia often centered over the lower back. There may be epigastric pain, retro-orbital pain, dizziness, photophobia, and constipation. Conjunctival infection, flushing of the face and upper portion of the trunk, and orthostatic hypotension also are common. An exanthema consisting of petechiae or small vesicles, or both, on the palate and fauces is present in most patients, as are skin petechiae, particularly in the axilla, and generalized lymphadenopathy. Early diagnosis is facilitated by the frequent findings of dizziness, leukopenia, thrombocytopenia, tremor, and early signs of hemorrhage such as petechial rash.

Fever is unremitting, and some patients become progressively ill with one of a combination of syndromes of vascular or neurologic disease. Vascular disease consists of (1) increasing evidence of a capillary leak syndrome; (2) proteinuria, rising hematocrit, and the onset of gingival, gastrointestinal, nasal, and other membrane hemorrhages; (3) narrowing pulse pressure; and (4) vasoconstriction and clinical shock. There may be signs of pulmonary infiltration due to a vascular leak or to secondary bacterial infection, which is a common complication, or both. Such patients are extremely difficult to manage. Plasma expanders may precipitate refractory pulmonary edema. Neurologic disease is common and is heralded by the development of hyporeflexia followed by gait abnormalities, palmomental reflex, tremors of the tongue and upper extremities, and other cerebellar signs. If these changes are followed by clonic seizures and coma, the prognosis is extremely grave.

Convalescence requires several weeks but occurs without sequelae. Alopecia and nail furrows are common, as is postural hypotension for 1 to 2 weeks.

INTRAUTERINE INFECTION

Arenaviruses readily invade the fetus, whether in their natural reservoir, laboratory animals, or in humans. In Lassa fever, pregnant women often abort and have a high mortality rate,[82] and similar observations have been made in Argentine and Bolivian HFs. LCM virus infection of pregnant women leads to fetal infection, hydrocephalus, microcephaly, chorioretinitis, or all of these.[83-86] Because viral antibody rates indicate that about 5% of adults in large cities of the United States have been infected with LCM virus, congenital infection may be more common than appreciated.[2,87]

Diagnosis

The diagnosis of past infection with arenaviruses is best done through serologic tests with enzyme-linked immunosorbent assay (ELISA) because of the sensitivity of the test. Until more data are obtained confirming ELISA specificity, cell culture plaque-reduction neutralization tests should be used as a supplement because of their known sensitivity and specificity.

The diagnosis of acute illness, by contrast, has features unique to each agent. In the case of LCM, virus is found in the blood early and in the CSF late in disease. The most sensitive test is to inoculate young adult mice in the brain.[17] Fluorescent immunostaining of inoculated cell cultures reveals virus earlier than mouse inoculation in most instances. Immunoglobulin M (IgM) ELISA of serum and CSF is an effective method of diagnosis and is supplanting IFA and other serologic tests.[88]

Virus can be recovered from the blood of acutely ill patients in all arenavirus HFs, but titers are highest in Lassa fever. The viremic interval ranges from 3 to 20 days, with Lassa fever being the most persistent.

Patients with LCM and Lassa fever who exhibit meningeal signs have increased protein, leukocytes, and virus in spinal fluids.[18,72,73,76]

Lassa fever virus is easily isolated from blood during the first 7 to 10 days of illness by inoculating cell cultures.[76,89] Junin virus was recovered from 96% of patients by cocultivation of patients' blood mononuclear cells with Vero cell cultures, whereas cell cultures of suckling mice were only about 50% positive when whole blood was tested.[90] Isolation of some strains of Machupo virus is difficult, but other strains are readily recovered in cell culture.[5,38] Throat swabs are frequently positive in patients with Lassa fever and LCM, and late shedding of Lassa virus is often observed, even up to 67 days.[76,91] Biopsy or autopsy specimens of lymphoid tissues, marrow, and liver usually yield virus, often in concentrations greatly exceeding those found in blood.

Serodiagnosis of Lassa fever by detection of IgM antibodies by IFA or ELISA is rapid and sensitive.[76,89,92] In Sierra Leone, 75% of patients were positive on IFA on admission (mean duration of illness, 8.5 days). In recent studies, either Lassa antigen or IgM antibodies were detectable in the blood of virtually all acutely ill patients, and the degree of antigenemia was correlated with poor prognosis. Antibodies detectable by IFA appear about 2 weeks after the onset of LCM illness.[88]

Reverse transcription of extracted RNA followed by polymerase chain reaction amplification has been used successfully in all the arenavirus infections and is highly sensitive provided broadly reactive primers are chosen and cross-contamination with plasmids is avoided.[1,2,93]

Prevention and Treatment

Prevention of arenavirus infection may be approached by interdicting transmission from rodents to humans, from person to person, and from infected specimens to laboratory workers, or by passive or active immunization. Community rodent control completely halted a major outbreak of Bolivian HF[94]; elimination of infected laboratory hamsters controlled LCM outbreaks.[23,24] A household rodent control study of Lassa infection, however, gave disappointing results.[31]

Person-to-person spread within hospitals has been a problem with Lassa fever. In endemic situations such as in Sierra Leone, partial spatial isolation of patients and the use of "enteric precautions" such as gloves, gowns, and careful disposal of patient wastes and fomites have generally served to prevent nosocomial outbreaks. Segregation of patients on the basis of the risk for death and likely content of virus in blood and body fluids by measuring aspartate transaminase levels should be of value. Rarely, hospital outbreaks appear to have been caused by infectious aerosols.[29,38] Thus, wherever practical, it is advisable to place patients in single rooms with isolated negative-pressure airflow and to provide medical staff with goggles and positive-pressure filtered air respirators or absolute filter respirators.[95] All potentially contaminated refuse or specimens should be double-bagged and the outer bag rinsed with 0.6% sodium hypochlorite before removal from the patient's room. Isolation of patients should continue until multiple blood and urine specimens are virus negative. Condoms should be used for a period in convalescence because of the occasional sexual transmission of arenavirus HF. In the recognized cases of Lassa fever that have been exported from Africa, no secondary transmission has yet been detected in contacts or in medical staff, indicating that a conservative approach to isolation provides a reasonable standard of safe care in most cases.

Laboratory-acquired infection is a major problem because all arenaviruses are infectious as aerosols. Several infections, some fatal, have occurred in laboratory workers. Thus, it is imperative that work with all arenaviruses except LCM be conducted in special laboratories with BSL 4 containment. Clinical pathologic tests, particularly in Lassa fever patients, also present problems. Aerosols must be minimized or contained. Acid treatment inactivates virus for leukocyte counts, and alcohol fixation is useful for blood smears; heating serum at 60° C for 1 hour is feasible for measuring heat-stable substances.[96]

There are no arenavirus vaccines licensed in the United States. A number of immunogens have shown promise in laboratory studies, including adenovirus or vaccinia virus vectored genes. Field trials with a live-attenuated Argentine HF vaccine showed greater than 95% efficacy and virtually no side effects.[97] More than 250,000 doses have been used in the endemic area, and the vaccine is manufactured and licensed in Argentina.[98] Work in laboratory animals suggests the Junin vaccine would be efficacious against Machupo, but not Guanarito or Sabia, viruses.[43]

Convalescent human plasma was proved effective in the treatment of Argentine HF (16% placebo versus 1% treated mortality rates) provided adequate amounts of neutralizing antibodies were given before the ninth day of illness.[99] Cerebellar signs, usually transient and possibly the result of virus multiplication in the central nervous system, occurred in 10% of those receiving this treatment. Immune plasma treatment of Lassa fever has not been as successful, and experiments in animals suggest that this may be related to the fact that neutralizing antibodies after Lassa fever (as well as LCM[88]) appear weeks after recovery and are generally of low titer and avidity.[43]

Ribavirin, a purine nucleoside with broad-spectrum antiviral properties, was found to be highly effective in monkeys lethally infected with Lassa and other arenaviruses.[43] The intravenous administration of this compound to Lassa patients admitted to the hospital in Sierra Leone with aspartate transaminase elevations of at least 150 IU reduced the mortality rate from 55% to 5% when treatment was begun before day 7 of the disease.[77] A positive effect on survival was achieved, however, at all stages of infection. After a 30-mg/kg loading dose, patients were given 15 mg/kg every 6 hours for 4 days and then 7.5 mg/kg 3 times daily for 6 additional days. Reversible anemia, not requiring transfusions, was the only adverse effect associated with treatment. Ribavirin has been used with apparent success in aborting a Sabia laboratory infection,[42] in treating Bolivian HF patients,[39] and in late therapy of Argentine HF patients.[99] Given the similarities to Lassa virus and similar preclinical test efficacy, the drug should be considered for any serious arenavirus infection. Close contacts of patients with arenavirus infections or possible bioterrorist exposures should not be given prophylactic ribavirin but rather should be monitored for the appearance of fever.[100] Ribavirin therapy should be begun expectantly if fever is confirmed. Intravenous ribavirin is not licensed in the United States, and arenavirus treatment is not a U.S. Food and Drug Administration–recognized indication for the oral drug.

Supportive care may be lifesaving in HFs. Fluid balance should be maintained orally as long as possible. Cautious volume replacement therapy with the judicious use of colloid should be started before the appearance of clinical shock, and electrolyte balance should be maintained.

The reader who desires to delve more deeply into arenaviruses should consult one of the following. The biology of arenaviruses, including clinical descriptions, has been reviewed in an excellent volume published in 1993[101] and more recently in two slim but thorough collections of reviews in 2002.[102,103] Two other textbooks also provide additional information regarding the viruses.[2,44]

REFERENCES

1. Bowen MD, Peters CJ, Nichol ST. The phylogeny of New World (Tacaribe complex) arenaviruses. *Virology.* 1996;219:285-290.
2. Enria D, Bowen M, Mills JN, et al. Arenaviruses. In: Guerrant RL, Walker DH, Weller PF, eds. *Tropical Infectious Diseases: Principles, Pathogens, and Practice.* Philadelphia: Elsevier Health Sciences; 2005:Chapter 110.
3. Armstrong C, Lillie RD. Experimental lymphocytic choriomeningitis of monkeys and mice produced by a virus encountered in studies of the 1933 St Louis encephalitis epidemic. *Public Health Rep.* 1934;49:1019-1027.
4. Parodi AS, Greenway DJ, Rugiero HR. Sobre la etiologia del brote epidemico de Junin. *El Dia Medico.* 1958;30:2300-2301.
5. Johnson KM, Wiebenga NH, Mackenzie RB, et al. Virus isolations from human cases of hemorrhagic fever in Bolivia. *Proc Soc Exp Biol Med.* 1965;118:113-118.
6. Buckley SM, Casals J. Lassa fever, a new virus disease of man from West Africa. III. Isolation and characterization of the virus. *Am J Trop Med Hyg.* 1970;19:680-691.
7. Salas R, de Manzione N, Tesh RB, et al. Venezuelan hemorrhagic fever. *Lancet.* 1991;338:1033-1036.
8. Coimbra TLM, Nassar ES, Burattini MN, et al. New arenavirus isolated in Brazil. *Lancet.* 1994;343:391-392.

9. Delgado S, Erickson BR, Agudo R, et al. Chapare virus, a newly discovered arenavirus isolated from a fatal hemorrhagic fever case in Bolivia. *PLoS Pathog.* 2008;4:e1000047. doi:10.1371/journal.ppat.1000047.
10. Murphy FA, Whitfield SG. Morphology and morphogenesis of arenaviruses. *Bull World Health Organ.* 1975;52:409-419.
11. Strecker T, Eichler R, Meulen J, et al. Lassa virus Z protein is a matrix protein sufficient for the release of virus-like particles. *J Virol.* 2003;77:10700-10705.
12. Burns JW, Buchmeier MJ. Glycoproteins of the arenaviruses. In: Salvato MS, ed. *The Arenaviridae.* New York: Plenum; 1993: 17-31.
13. Klavinskas LS, Whitton JL, Oldstone MBA. Molecular anatomy of the cytotoxic T-lymphocyte responses to lymphocytic choriomeningitis virus. In: Salvato MD, ed. *The Arenaviridae.* New York: Plenum; 1993:225-242.
14. Rojek JM, Kunz S. Cell entry by human pathogenic arenaviruses. *Cell Microbiol.* 2008;10:828-835.
15. Cao W, Henry MD, Borrow P, et al. Identification of alpha-dystroglycan as a receptor for lymphocytic choriomeningitis virus and Lassa fever virus. *Science.* 1998;282:2079-2081.
16. Spiropoulou CF, Kunz S, Rollin PE, et al. New World arenavirus clade C, but not clade A and B viruses, utilizes alpha-dystroglycan as its major receptor. *J Virol.* 2002;76:5140-5146.
17. Lehmann-Grube F. *Lymphocytic Choriomeningitis Virus.* New York: Springer; 1971.
18. Farmer TW, Janeway CA. Infection with the virus of lymphocytic choriomeningitis. *Medicine (Baltimore).* 1942;2:11.
19. Childs JC, Glass GE, Korch GW, et al. Lymphocytic choriomeningitis virus infection and house mouse *(Mus musculus)* distribution in urban Baltimore. *Am J Trop Med Hyg.* 1992;47:27-34.
20. Ackermann R, Bloedhorn H, Kupper B, et al. Über die Verbreiting des Virus der lymphocytaren Choriomeningitis unter den Mausen in Westdeutschland. I. Utersuchungen uberwiegend an Hausmauden *(Mus musculus). Zentrabl Bakteriol.* 1964;194:407.
21. Stephenson EH, Larson EW, Dominik JW. Effect of environmental factors on aerosol induced Lassa virus infection. *J Med Virol.* 1984;14:295.
22. Hinman AR, Fraser DW, Douglas RG, et al. Outbreak of lymphocytic choriomeningitis virus infection in medical center personnel. *Am J Epidemiol.* 1975;101:103.
23. Baum SG, Lewis AM, Rowe WP, et al. Epidemic nonmeningitic lymphocytic choriomeningitis virus infection. *N Engl J Med.* 1966;274:934.
24. Dykewitz CA, Dato VM, Fisher-Hoch SF, et al. Lymphocytic choriomeningitis outbreak associated with nude mice in a research institute. *JAMA.* 1992;267:1349-1353.
25. Biggar RJ, Woodall JP, Walter PD, et al. Lymphocytic choriomeningitis outbreak associated with pet hamsters: Fifty-seven cases from New York State. *JAMA.* 1975;232:494.
26. Ackermann R, Stille W, Blumenthal W, et al. Syrische Goldhamster als Ubertrager von lymphozytarer Choriomeningitis. *Dtsch Med Wochenschr.* 1972;97:1725.
27. Frame JD, Baldwin JM Jr, Gocke DJ, et al. Lassa fever, a new virus disease of man from West Africa. I. Clinical description and pathological findings. *Am J Trop Med Hyg.* 1970;19:670.
28. McCormick JB, Webb PA, Krebs JW, et al. A prospective study of the epidemiology and ecology of Lassa fever. *J Infect Dis.* 1987;155:437.
29. Monath TP. Lassa fever: Review of epidemiology and epizootology. *Bull World Health Organ.* 1975;52:577.
30. Frame JD. Surveillance of Lassa fever in missionaries stationed in West Africa. *Bull World Health Organ.* 1975;52:593.
31. Keenlyside RA, McCormick JB, Webb PA, et al. Case-control study of *Mastomys natalensis* and humans in Lassa virus-infected households in Sierra Leone. *Am J Trop Med Hyg.* 1983;32: 829-837.
32. Demby AH, Inapogui A, Kargbo K, et al. Lassa fever in Guinea: II. Distribution and prevalence of Lassa virus infection in small mammals. *Vector Borne Zoonotic Dis.* 2001;1:283-297.
33. Keenlyside RA, McCormick JB, Webb PA, et al. Case-control study of *Mastomys natalensis* and humans in Lassa virus-infected households in Sierra Leone. *Am J Trop Med Hyg.* 1983;32:829-837.
34. Briese T, Paweska JT, McMullan LK, et al. Genetic detection and characterization of Lujo virus, a new hemorrhagic fever-associated arenavirus from southern Africa. *PLoS Pathog.* 2009;5:e1000455.
35. Sabattini MS, Maiztegui JI. Fiebre hemorrhagica argentina. *Medicina (Buenos Aires).* 1970;30(suppl):111.
36. Enria DA, Barrera Oro JG. Junin virus vaccines. *Curr Top Microbiol Immunol.* 2002;263:239-261.
37. Johnson KM, Kuns ML, Mackenzie RB, et al. Isolation of Machupo virus from wild rodent *Calomys callosus. Am J Trop Med Hyg.* 1966;15:103.
38. Peters CJ, Kuehne RW, Mercado R, et al. Hemorrhagic fever in Cochabamba, Bolivia, 1971. *Am J Epidemiol.* 1974;99:425-433.
39. Kilgore PE, Peters CJ, Mills JN, et al. Prospects for the control of Bolivian hemorrhagic fever. *Emerg Infect Dis.* 1995;1:97-100.
40. Mills JN, Ellis BA, McKee KT, et al. A longitudinal study of Junin virus activity in the rodent reservoir of Argentine hemorrhagic fever. *Am J Trop Med Hyg.* 1992;47:749-763.
41. Fulhorst CF, Bowen MD, Salas RA, et al. Isolation and characterization of Pirital virus, a newly discovered South American arenavirus. *Am J Trop Med Hyg.* 1997;56:548-553.
42. Barry M, Russi M, Armstrong L, et al. Treatment of a laboratory-acquired Sabia virus infection. *N Eng J Med.* 1995;333:294-296.
43. Peters CJ, Jahrling PB, Liu CT, et al. Experimental studies of arenaviral hemorrhagic fevers. *Curr Top Microbiol Immunol.* 1987;134:5.
44. Buchmeier MJ, Peters CJ, de la Torre JC. Arenaviridae: the viruses and their replication. In: Knipe DM, Holey PM, eds. Fields virology, 5th ed., vol. 2. Philadelphia: Lippincott Williams & Wilkins; 2007:1792-1827.
45. Oldstone MBA, Dixon FJ. Pathogenesis of chronic disease associated with persistent lymphocytic choriomeningitis infection. II. Relationship of the antilymphocytic choriomeningitis virus immune response to tissue injury in chronic lymphocytic choriomeningitis disease. *J Exp Med.* 1970;131:1.
46. Nathanson N, Monjan AA, Panitch HS, et al. Virus-induced cell-mediated immunopathological disease. In: Notkins AL, ed. *Viral Immunology and Immunopathology.* New York: Academic Press; 1975:357-391.
47. Walker DH, Wulff H, Lange JV, et al. Comparative pathology of Lassa virus infection in monkeys, guinea pigs, and *Mastomys natalensis. Bull World Health Organ.* 1975;52:523.
48. Montali RJ, Scanga CA, Perkikoff D, et al. A common-source outbreak of callitrichid hepatitis in captive tamarins and marmosets. *J Infect Dis.* 1993;167:946-950.
49. McKee KT Jr, Mahlandt BG, Maiztegui JI, et al. Experimental Argentine hemorrhagic fever in rhesus monkeys: Viral strain-dependent clinical response. *J Infect Dis.* 1985;152:218.
50. Peters CJ. Pathogenesis of viral hemorrhagic fevers. In: Nathanson N, Ahmed R, Gonzalez-Scarano F, et al, eds. *Viral Pathogenesis.* Philadelphia: Lippincott-Raven; 1997:779-799.
51. Smadel JE, Green RH, Paltauf RM, et al. Lymphocytic choriomeningitis: Two human fatalities following an unusual febrile illness. *Proc Soc Exp Biol Med.* 1942;49:683.
52. Warkel RL, Rinaldi CF, Bancroft WH, et al. Fatal acute meningoencephalitis due to lymphocytic choriomeningitis virus. *Neurology.* 1973;23:198-202.
53. Walker DH, McCormick JB, Johnson KM, et al. Pathologic and virologic study of fatal Lassa fever in man. *Am J Pathol.* 1982; 107:349.
54. McCormick JB, Walker DB, King IJ, et al. Lassa virus hepatitis: A study of fatal Lassa fever in humans. *Am J Trop Med Hyg.* 1986;35:401.
55. Zaki SR, Peters CJ. Viral hemorrhagic fevers. In: Connor DH, Chandler FW, Schwartz DA, et al, eds. *The Pathology of Infectious Diseases.* Norwalk, CT: Appleton & Lange; 1997:347-364.
56. Kenyon RH, Green DE, Peters CJ. Effect of immunosuppression on experimental Argentine hemorrhagic fever in guinea pigs. *J Virol.* 1985;53:75-80.
57. Levis SC, Saavedra MC, Ceccoli C, et al. Correlation between endogenous interferon and the clinical evolution of patients with Argentine hemorrhagic fever. *J Interferon Res.* 1985;5:383.
58. Vilcek J. Adverse effects of interferon in virus infections, autoimmune diseases and acquired immunodeficiency. *Prog Med Virol.* 1984;30:62.
59. Marta RF, Montero VF, Hack CE, et al. Proinflammatory cytokines and elastase-alpha-1-antitrypsin in Argentine hemorrhagic fever. *Am J Trop Med Hyg.* 1999;60:85-89.
60. Vanzee BE, Douglas RG, Betts RF, et al. Lymphocytic choriomeningitis in university hospital personnel. *Am J Med.* 1975;58:803-807.
61. Schmitz H, Kohler B, Laue T, et al. Monitoring of clinical and laboratory data in two cases of imported Lassa fever. *Microbes Infect.* 2002;4:43-50.
62. Mahanty S, Bausch DG, Thomas RL, et al. Low levels of interleukin-8 and interferon-inducible protein-10 in serum are associated with fatal infections in acute Lassa fever. *J Infect Dis.* 2001;183:1713-1721.
63. Lukashevich IS, Maryankova R, Vladyko AS, et al. Lassa and Mopeia virus replication in human monocytes/macrophages and in endothelial cells: Different effects on IL-8 and TNF-alpha gene expression. *J Med Virol.* 1999;59:552-560.
64. Peters CJ. Arenavirus diseases. In: Porterfield JS, ed. *Kass Handbook of Infectious Diseases. Exotic Viral Infections.* New York: Chapman and Hall Medical; 1995:227-246.
65. Fischer SA, Graham MB, Kuehnert MJ, et al. Transmission of lymphocytic choriomeningitis virus by organ transplantation. *N Engl J Med.* 2006;354:2235-2249.
66. Palacios G, Druce J, Du L, et al. A new arenavirus in a cluster of fatal transplant-associated diseases. *N Engl J Med.* 2008;358: 991-998.
67. Brief report: Lymphocytic choriomeningitis virus transmitted through solid organ transplantation—Massachusetts, 2008. *MMWR Morb Mortal Wkly Rep.* 2008;57:799-801.
68. Peters CJ. Lymphocytic choriomeningitis virus: An old enemy up to new tricks. *N Engl J Med.* 2006;354:2208-2211.
69. Amman BR, Pavlin BI, Albarino CG, et al. Pet rodents and fatal lymphocytic choriomeningitis in transplant patients. *Emerg Infect Dis.* 2007;13:719-725.65.
70. McCormick JB, King IJ, Webb PA, et al. A case-control study of the clinical diagnosis and course of Lassa fever. *J Infect Dis.* 1987;155:445.
71. Bausch DG, Demby AH, Coulibaly M, et al. Lassa fever in Guinea: I. Epidemiology of human disease and clinical observations. *Vector Borne Zoonotic Dis.* 2001;1:269-281.
72. Solbrig MV. Lassa virus and central nervous system diseases. In: Salvato MS, ed. *The Arenaviridae.* New York: Plenum; 1993: 325-330.
73. Gunther S, Weisner B, Roth A, et al. Lassa fever encephalopathy: Lassa virus in cerebrospinal fluid but not in serum. *J Infect Dis.* 2001;184:345-349.
74. Webb PA, McCormick JB, King IJ, et al. Lassa fever in children in Sierra Leone, West Africa. *Trans R Soc Trop Med Hyg.* 1986; 80:577.
75. Monson MH, Cole AK, Frame JD, et al. Pediatric Lassa fever: A review of 33 Liberian cases. *Am J Trop Med Hyg.* 1987;36:408.
76. Johnson KM, McCormick JB, Webb PA, et al. Clinical virology of Lassa fever in hospitalized patients. *J Infect Dis.* 1987;155:456.
77. McCormick JB, King IB, Webb PA, et al. Lassa fever: Effective therapy with ribavirin. *N Engl J Med.* 1986;314:20.
78. Cummins D, McCormick JB, Bennett D, et al. Acute sensorineural deafness in Lassa fever. *JAMA.* 1990;264:2093-2096.
79. Maiztegui JI. Clinical and epidemiological patterns of Argentine haemorrhagic fever. *Bull World Health Organ.* 1975;52:567.
80. Stinebaugh BJ, Schloeder FX, Johnson KM, et al. Bolivian hemorrhagic fever: A report of four cases. *Am J Med.* 1966;40:217.
81. de Manzione N, Salas RA, Paredes H, et al. Venezuelan hemorrhagic fever: clinical and epidemiological studies of 165 cases. *Clin Infect Dis.* 1998;26:308-313.
82. Price ME, Fisher-Hoch SP, Craven RB, et al. A prospective study of maternal and fetal outcome in acute Lassa fever infection during pregnancy. *BMJ.* 1988;297:584-587.
83. Barton LL, Budd SC, Morfitt WS, et al. Congenital lymphocytic choriomeningitis virus infection in twins. *Pediatr Infect Dis J.* 1993;12:942-946.
84. Ackermann R, Korver G, Turss R, et al. Pranatale Infektion mit dem Virus der lymphozytaren Choriomeningitis. *Dtsch Med Wochenschr.* 1974;99:629-632.
85. Wright R, Johnson D, Neumann M, et al. Congenital lymphocytic choriomeningitis virus syndrome: A disease that mimics congenital toxoplasmosis or cytomegalovirus infection. *Pediatrics.* 1997;100:E9.
86. Barton LL, Mets MB, Beauchamp CL. Lymphocytic choriomeningitis virus: Emerging fetal teratogen. *Am J Obstet Gynecol.* 2002;187:1715-1716.
87. Childs JE, Glass GE, Ksiazek TG, et al. Human-rodent contact and infection with lymphocytic choriomeningitis and Seoul viruses in an inner-city population. *Am J Trop Med Hyg.* 1991; 44:117-121.
88. Lehmann-Grube F, Kallay M, Ibscher B, et al. Serologic diagnosis of human infections with lymphocytic choriomeningitis virus: Comparative evaluation of seven methods. *J Med Virol.* 1979;4:125-136.
89. Bausch DG, Rollin PE, Demby AH, et al. Diagnosis and clinical virology of Lassa fever as evaluated by enzyme-linked immunosorbent assay, indirect fluorescent-antibody test, and virus isolation. *J Clin Microbiol.* 2000;38:2670-2677.
90. Ambrosio AM, Enria DA, Maiztegui JI. Junin virus isolation from lymphomononuclear cells of patients with Argentine hemorrhagic fever. *Intervirology.* 1986;25:97.
91. Emond RTD, Bannister B, Lloyd G, et al. A case of Lassa fever: Clinical and virological findings. *BMJ.* 1982;285:1001.
92. Nicklasson BS, Jahrling PB, Peters CJ. Detection of Lassa virus antigens and Lassa virus-specific immunoglobulins G and M by enzyme-linked immunosorbent assay. *J Clin Microbiol.* 1984; 20:239.
93. Park JY, Peters CJ, Rollin PE, et al. Development of an RT-PCR assay for diagnosis of lymphocytic choriomeningitis virus (LCMV) infection and its use in a prospective surveillance study. *J Med Virol.* 1997;51:107-114.
94. Mackenzie RB. Epidemiology of Machupo virus infection. I. Pattern of human infection, San Joaquin, Bolivia, 1962-1965. *Am J Trop Med Hyg.* 1965;14:808.
95. CDC update: Management of patients with suspected viral hemorrhagic fever—United States. *MMWR Morb Mortal Wkly Rep.* 1995;44:475-479.
96. Mitchell SW, McCormick JB. Physicochemical inactivation of Lassa, Ebola, and Marburg viruses and effect on clinical laboratory analyses. *J Clin Microbiol.* 1984;20:486.
97. Maiztegui JI, McKee KT, Barrera Oro JG, et al. Protective efficacy of a live attenuated vaccine against Argentine hemorrhagic fever. *J Infect Dis.* 1998;177;277-283.
98. Enria DA, Barrera Oro JG. Junin virus vaccines. *Curr Top Microbiol Immunol.* 2002;263:239-261.
99. Enria DA, Briggiler AM, Sanchez Z. Treatment of Argentine hemorrhagic fever. *Antiviral Res.* 2008;78:132-139.
100. Borio L, Inglesby T, Peters CJ, et al. Hemorrhagic fever viruses as biological weapons: medical and public health management. *JAMA.* 2002;287:2391-2405.
101. Salvato MS, ed. *The Arenaviridae.* New York: Plenum; 1993.
102. Oldstone MB, ed. Arenaviruses. I. The epidemiology molecular and cell biology of arenaviruses. *Curr Top Microbiol Immunol.* 2002;262:1-197.
103. Oldstone MB, ed. Arenaviruses. II. The molecular pathogenesis of arenavirus infections. *Curr Top Microbiol Immunol.* 2002;263: 1-268.

168

Human T-Cell Lymphotropic Virus Types I and II

EDWARD L. MURPHY | HOPE H. BISWAS

Human T-cell lymphotropic virus type I (HTLV-I), the first recognized human retrovirus, was described in 1979 by Poiesz and co-workers,[1,2] who isolated retroviral particles with type C morphology and budding from fresh cultured lymphocytes of a 28-year-old American man with a diagnosis of cutaneous T-cell lymphoma similar to cases seen in the Caribbean. Soon thereafter, Yoshida and colleagues[3] and Watanabe and colleagues[4] similarly isolated a new retrovirus from cases of adult T-cell leukemia (ATL), which had been recognized as common in southwestern Japan, and the two isolates were subsequently found to be the same virus. The long-standing search for a human homologue to cancer-causing retroviruses of animals, first discovered at the beginning of the 20th century, ended at a time when most researchers had abandoned this quest and focused instead on viral transforming genes that occur as oncogenes in human tumors. HTLV type II (HTLV-II) was identified 2 years later.[5] The techniques used to isolate and characterize these viruses provided the intellectual and technical basis for the discovery of the human immunodeficiency virus (HIV) in 1983,[6,7] which was shown to be the cause of acquired immunodeficiency syndrome in 1984.[8]

Within the taxa of DNA and RNA reverse-transcribing viruses, the HTLV viruses, along with bovine leukemia virus, are classified in the subfamily Retroviridae within the genus *Deltaretrovirus* (formerly termed *Oncovirus*).[9] The oncogenic properties of these viruses and their molecular structure distinguish them from retroviruses HIV type 1 (HIV-1) and HIV type 2 (HIV-2), which are members of the genus *Lentivirus*. Both *oncoviruses* and *lentiviruses* are capable of prolonged asymptomatic infection.[9] In vitro, however, HIV-1 and HIV-2 have cytopathic effects on human T cells, whereas HTLV-I and HTLV-II are capable of transforming T cells, resulting in immortalized cell lines.

HTLV-I has been shown to be associated with ATL, as well as a unique form of progressive neurologic disease known as HTLV-associated myelopathy (HAM), also known as tropical spastic paraparesis. HTLV-II is associated with HAM, but is not known to cause leukemia or lymphoma, although it may have other, more subtle, disease associations.[10]

Structure and Molecular Organization

HTLV-I and HTLV-II are approximately 100 nm in diameter, with a thin electron-dense outer envelope and an electron-dense, roughly spherical core (Fig. 168-1). Its genomic structure is illustrated in Figure 168-2. The total provirus genome consists of roughly 9000 nucleotides with two flanking identical sequences termed *long terminal repeats* (LTRs) at the 5′ and 3′ ends of the genome, which mediate proviral integration and contain *cis*-acting regulatory elements important for viral transcription, viral mRNA processing, and reverse transcription. There is 65% overall nucleotide homology between sequenced HTLV-I and HTLV-II isolates. Homology is lowest within the LTRs (30%) and highest within the 3′ Tax and Rex regulatory genes (75% to 80%).[11-13] Retroviral genes generally code for large overlapping polyproteins that are processed by a virally encoded protease and cellular proteases into functional peptide products. The HTLV viruses share with other replication-competent retroviruses the three main genomic regions of *gag* (group-specific antigen), *pol* (protease/polymerase/integrase), and *env* (envelope) (Table 168-1). However, unlike other vertebrate leukemia viruses, these deltaretroviruses have an additional region called pX that

contains four small open reading frames (ORFs): pX-I, pX-II, pX-III, and pX-IV.[14] The pX ORFs III and IV encode two transcriptional regulatory proteins, the Tax and Rex proteins, which are involved in regulation of virus expression. As shown in Figure 168-2, two overlapping reading frames are involved in the expression of both of these gene products translated from a doubly spliced messenger RNA (mRNA) involving the initiation codon from *env* and the remaining sequences from the pX region. HIV-1 uses a similar strategy for expressing Tat and Rev proteins that share similar regulatory functions. Despite similar function, the Tax and Rex proteins bear little amino acid homology with the corresponding proteins encoded by the transcriptional and posttranscriptional regulators Tat and Rev in HIV-1. The pX ORFs I and II code for other accessory and regulatory genes whose protein products appear to involve cell-cycle regulation.[15] Recently, an anti-sense transcription factor named HTLV-I basic zipper factor (HBZ), transcribed from the minus strand of the 3′ LTR, has been discovered.[16] Its role is still undefined, but it may be involved in the regulation of HTLV-I proviral load or even of lymphocyte proliferation.

The LTR is organized into three regions: (1) U5, R, U3; (2) Rex-responsive elements (RxREs), and (3) 21-base pair (bp) response element. The U3 region contains sequences that control transcription of the provirus. The 21-bp repeats are necessary for *trans*-activating transcriptional activation involving Tax protein. The U3 region also contains sequences responsible for termination and polyadenylation of mRNAs. In addition, the 5′ part of the U3 region encodes the carboxyl terminus of the Tax protein. Comparisons of the LTRs of HTLV-I and HTLV-II reveal that these elements are critical for viral gene expression. The R and U5 regions are unusually long compared with other retroviruses. These regions form the leader sequence encoded at the 5′ end of the mRNAs.

GAG, POL, AND ENV

The Gag proteins function as structural proteins of the nucleocapsid, capsid, and matrix, also named p15, p24, and p19 Gag proteins, respectively. The *pol* gene encodes several enzymes: protease, which cleaves Gag and Gag/Pol polypeptides into proteins of the mature virion; reverse transcriptase, which generates a double-stranded DNA from the RNA genome; and integrase, which integrates viral DNA into the host-cell chromosomes. The polymerase region contains the largest ORF in the HTLV genome, potentially able to encode an 896-amino acid product for HTLV-I and a 982-amino acid product for HTLV-II. The polymerase genes of HTLV-I and HTLV-II share only 56% homology based on their predicted amino acid sequences. The *env* gene encodes the major components of the viral coat: the surface glycoprotein of 46,000 molecular weight (gp46) and the transmembrane glycoprotein of 21,000 molecular weight (gp2l). Although HTLV-I and HTLV-II share the same overall genetic organization, they show some diversity at the nucleotide level, exhibiting a variable degree of amino acid homology between viral capsid and envelope proteins.

Production of the Gag proteins derives from the translation of the full-length mRNA, which yields a large precursor polypeptide that is subsequently cleaved by the virally coded protease. For the Pol proteins, production depends on translation made possible when the stop

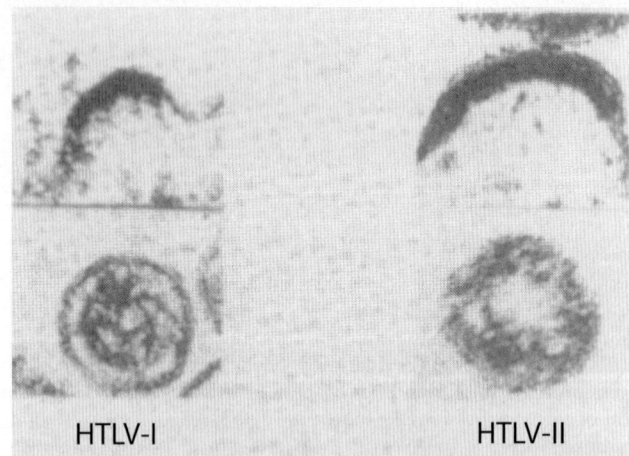

Figure 168-1 Electron micrographs of human T-cell lymphotropic virus type I (HTLV-I) and II. HTLV-I and -II have a diameter of approximately 100 nm. The budding particles are shown for each virus (*top*), and the mature virion (*bottom*). The HTLV-I and -II viruses have a roughly spherical electron-dense core.

TABLE 168-1	**Major Structural and Regulatory Proteins of Human T-Cell Lymphotropic Virus Type I**	

Viral Gene	Gene Product (Protein Size [kDa])	Function
LTR		Regulation of viral gene expression, integration of provirus into host genetic material, and regulation of virion production
3′ LTR	HBZ	HBZ mRNA is found in ATL tumor tissue and is responsible for lymphocyte proliferation
Gag	p15	Nucleocapsid is a small basic protein found in the virion in association with the genome RNA characterized by zinc-finger motifs associated with nucleic acid binding
Gag	p19	Matrix protein forms close linkage to internal surface of viral envelope via myristic acid
Gag	p24	Capsid protein forms the major internal structural feature of the core shell of the virion
Gag	p53	Precursor protein for other gag
Pol	Integrase	Integrates viral DNA into the host-cell chromosomes
Pol	Reverse transcriptase (95 kDa)	Reverse transcriptase generates a double-stranded DNA from the RNA genome
Pro	Protease (p14)	Cleaves Gag and Gag-Pol polypeptides into proteins of the mature virion
Env	p21e	Envelope transmembrane protein
PX	Tax (p40)	Transactivator for enhanced transcription of viral and cellular gene products
PX	Rex (p27/p21)	Regulator of expression of virion proteins for HTLV; stabilizes viral mRNAs and modulates the splicing and transport from the nucleus of viral RNA
PX	ORF I (p12^I)	Activation of STAT5 and interference with major histocompatibility complex class I trafficking; elevation of cytoplasmic calcium, which is antecedent to T-cell activation
PX	ORF II (p30^{II}, p13^{II})	Inhibition of acetyltransferase activity of P/CAF on histones and stabilization of p53. p13″ localizes to the mitochondria; p30″ localizes to the nucleolus

P/CAF, P^{300}/CREB binding protein–associated factor.

codon of the *gag* gene is bypassed, leading to a large polypeptide including *gag*- and *pol*-related proteins, which are subsequently cleaved into functional proteins by the viral protease. Production of the Env surface and transmembrane proteins involves translation of a spliced message (see Fig. 168-2), which results in an envelope precursor cleaved into the subunits. The precursor proteins have characteristic molecular weights that Western blot (WB) analysis can detect immunologically.

TAX

HTLV-I Tax is a 40-kDa protein (p40), and HTLV-II Tax is a 37-kDa protein (p37).[17,18] These proteins localize primarily to the nucleus of infected cells, although small amounts of Tax have been found in the

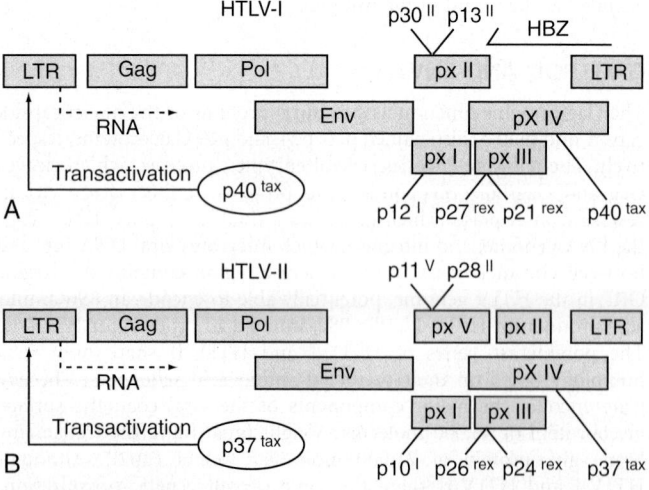

Figure 168-2 Genomic structures of human T-cell lymphotropic virus type I (HTLV-I) (A) and HTLV-II (B). *env*, envelope gene; *gag*, group-specific antigen whose products form the skeleton of the virion (matrix, capsid, nucleocapsid, nucleic acid binding protein); HBZ, antisense transcribed HTLV-I basic zipper gene involved in cell proliferation; LTR, long terminal repeat; *pol/pro*, gene for reverse transcriptase, integrase, and protease; *rex*, viral regulatory gene involved in promoting genomic RNA production; *tax*, transactivator gene.

cytoplasm. The Tax proteins are responsible for enhanced transcription of viral and cellular gene products and are essential for transformation of human T lymphocytes.[19] The Tax viral regulatory protein for HTLV-I, like its counterpart Tat of HIV-1, plays an important role in promoting viral growth and disease pathogenesis. Both promote *trans*-acting, transcriptional activation of the LTR, but the effect of Tax appears to be mediated via expression of cellular growth factors that are abundantly activated by Tax through its *trans*-activation properties. This *trans*-activation of cellular genes by Tax not only facilitates viral replication, but also has emerged as a cofactor in disease pathogenesis. The *tax* gene is responsible for the *trans*-activation of virus transcription via *tax*-responsive elements of a number of regulatory enhancers, such as the 21-bp enhancer, the nuclear factor-κB binding site, and serum-responsive element. Such promoter interactions lead to the activation of a number of cellular genes, such as those encoding interleukin-2 (IL-2) and the IL-2 receptor (IL-2R), which promote cell proliferation. Additionally, *tax* activates the proto-oncogenes c-*fos* and c-*erg*, as well as the gene for granulocyte-macrophage colony-stimulating factor, an array of early response genes, the human lymphotoxin gene, and parathyroid hormone–related protein gene, whereas it *trans*-represses the β-polymerase gene. Overproduction of interferon-γ via this pathway has been implicated in promoting the chronic inflammation that characterizes diseases such as HAM.[20] The mechanism by which Tax interacts with a variety of cell regulatory elements involves nuclear regulatory elements (the nuclear factor-κB pathway); Tax also operates cytoplasmically through the induction of nuclear translocation of active transcriptional factors, but not via pathways typical of other oncoviral proteins that target tumor suppressor genes.[21]

REX PROTEINS

The *rex* gene of HTLV-I and HTLV-II encodes two protein species in each virus. In HTLV-I, a 27-kDa protein (p27) and a 21-kDa protein (p21) seem to result from the use of alternative initiator methionine codons. In HTLV-II, however, a 26-kDa protein appears to be formed by phosphorylation of a serine residue in a 24-kDa protein.[22] Unlike the products of the *tax* gene, *rex* does not directly regulate RNA transcription but instead appears to act chiefly at a posttranscriptional level to regulate viral gene expression. The Rex (regulator of expression of virion proteins for HTLV) stabilizes viral mRNA and is essential for export of full-length *gag/pol* and single-spliced *env* mRNA from the nucleus to the cytoplasm.[23] This function is analogous to that of Rev in HIV-1 and HIV-2.[24-26] Rex localizes to the nucleus and specifically to the nucleoli of infected cells.[27,28] Phosphorylated Rex binds with high affinity to *cis*-acting RNA sequences, called Rex-responsive elements, in the viral mRNA.[29-31] This interaction facilitates the export of mRNA. Rex binding may also inhibit mRNA splicing by preventing early steps in spliceosome assembly.[32] As a consequence of the accumulation of Rex in the cell, there is an accumulation of unspliced and single-spliced mRNA, favoring the production of structural proteins (Gag and Env). This is accompanied by a decrease in the levels of double-spliced mRNA encoding Tax and Rex. Rex accumulation may also inhibit *tax*, thus slowing viral transcription.[33] A fine balance between *tax* and *rex* expression and function may dictate the rate of viral replication within infected cells.

OTHER PROTEINS ENCODED BY THE pX REGION

pX ORF I, produced by a double-splicing mechanism similar to that of the gene products of pX ORF III and IV, codes for a hydrophobic 12-kDa protein, p12[I], and pX ORF II results in the production of two nuclear proteins, p13[II] and p30[II].[15] In addition to activating nuclear factor of activated T cells,[34] p12[I] localizes in the endoplasmic reticulum and *cis*-Golgi apparatus and elevates cytoplasmic calcium that is antecedent to T-cell activation and essential for establishing persistent infection.[35] Other major structural and regulatory proteins of HTLV-I are summarized in Table 168-1. The gene products of pX ORF I and II also appear to affect cell proliferation and modulate host immune responses to HTLV-1 infection.[36] Tax and the ORF I and II gene products may play an integral role in the pathogenesis of HTLV-associated diseases through their effects on cyclins, which regulate cell growth. Recently, an anti-sense transcription factor named HTLV basic zipper factor transcribed from the minus strand of the 3′ LTR was discovered.[16] Analyses of T-cell lines transfected with mutated HTLV-I basic zipper genes showed that HTLV-I basic zipper promotes T-cell proliferation in its RNA form, whereas HTLV-I basic zipper protein suppresses Tax-mediated viral transcription through the 5′ LTR.[37]

Biology

The replication strategy of the HTLVs involves a life cycle typical of all members of the Retroviridae (Fig. 168-3), whereby the RNA genome undergoes reverse transcription into a DNA provirus that integrates into the host genome. Subsequently, new virions are produced via this integrated DNA template under the regulation of viral regulatory genes. The HTLV-I receptor was determined to be the ubiquitous glucose transporter GLUT-1,[38] consistent with the infection by HTLV-I of a wide range of cells in vitro, including endothelial cells and fibroblasts.[39] Additionally, a number of animal species can be infected either

experimentally (mice, rats, rabbits, and New World primate species) or naturally (Old World primates).[40] The natural host range for HTLV is therefore humans and Old World nonhuman primates.

Although HTLV-I can infect a number of different cell types in vitro, its growth and propagation in vivo are supported mainly by CD4+ cells and to a lesser extent CD8+ cells, as determined by real-time quantitative polymerase chain reaction (PCR) performed on flow cytometry-sorted T cells from patients with HAM.[41] In contrast, HTLV-II preferentially infects CD8+ cells over CD4+ cells.[42]

Based on epidemiologic data demonstrating that HTLV-I transmission is strongly cell associated and through in vitro studies in which cocultivation is required for efficient infection of target cells, transmission of HTLV is mediated by live cells and not via cell-free body fluids. For this reason, HTLV-I is not an easily transmitted virus, and universal biohazard precautions are adequate for the inactivation of potentially infectious blood or bodily secretions. Procedures that remove or kill lymphocytes, such as leukoreduction or refrigerated storage of blood products and freeze/thawing of expressed breast milk, have been shown to reduce the risk of HTLV-I transmission.[43-45] Because HTLV-I is highly cell-associated, the means for viral attachment are not well characterized but similar to other retroviruses, fusion of the virion with the cell membrane results in uncoating of the diploid RNA genome of the virus (see Fig. 168-3). Igakura and co-workers[46] found that additional cell surface-adhesion proteins and cell-cell contacts/interface (virologic synapse) are important for facilitating virus transmission. Cytoskeletal reorganization in the infected cells and segregation of virus particles to the interface between the infected and uninfected cells can be observed by immunofluorescence microscopy.[46-48]

Once in the cell, the virally encoded RNA-dependent DNA polymerase (reverse transcriptase) complexed to the genomic RNA of the virus transcribes viral RNA into double-stranded DNA. This double-stranded viral cDNA is transported to the nucleus as a ribonucleoprotein complex that includes the p24 capsid protein, as well as integrase and reverse transcriptase. Once there, the cDNA, through a complex process mediated by the viral integrase, is inserted into the host genome. The genomic integration of HTLV-I establishes a lifelong infection and is integral to both the virus replication cycle and amplification of provirus.

Elements in the viral LTR are essential to integration and replication, as they form the sites for covalent attachment of the provirus to cellular DNA and provide important regulatory components for transcription. Additional key regulatory elements of HTLV are *tax*, which activates transcription of the viral genome, and *rex*, which modulates the processing of the viral RNA expressing unspliced forms of the viral mRNA. When the DNA provirus is expressed (transcribed by a cellular RNA polymerase), viral genomic, mRNA, and subsequently viral proteins are made by the cell. Under the influence of Rex, which stabilizes viral mRNAs and regulates their splicing and transport, new genomic RNA is assembled at the cell membrane and packaged for release. During the budding process, the envelope incorporates some of the cell's lipid bilayer, producing an infectious virion of about 100 nm (see Figs. 168-1 and 168-3).

Laboratory Detection

No gold standard exists for diagnosis of HTLV infection.

VIRUS ISOLATION

Direct detection of virus by culture is intensive, expensive, and time-consuming, often requiring several weeks for results. The ability to culture retroviruses has been improved by co-cultivation of patients' T cells with human peripheral blood-mononuclear cells that have been stimulated in vitro with mitogens (e.g., phytohemagglutinin) and growth factors (e.g., IL-2), as well as by the removal of patients' CD8+ suppressor cells from the coculture. The number of infected cells present in the blood of an infected individual is generally relatively low; mean proviral loads are 3.28 log[10] copies per million peripheral

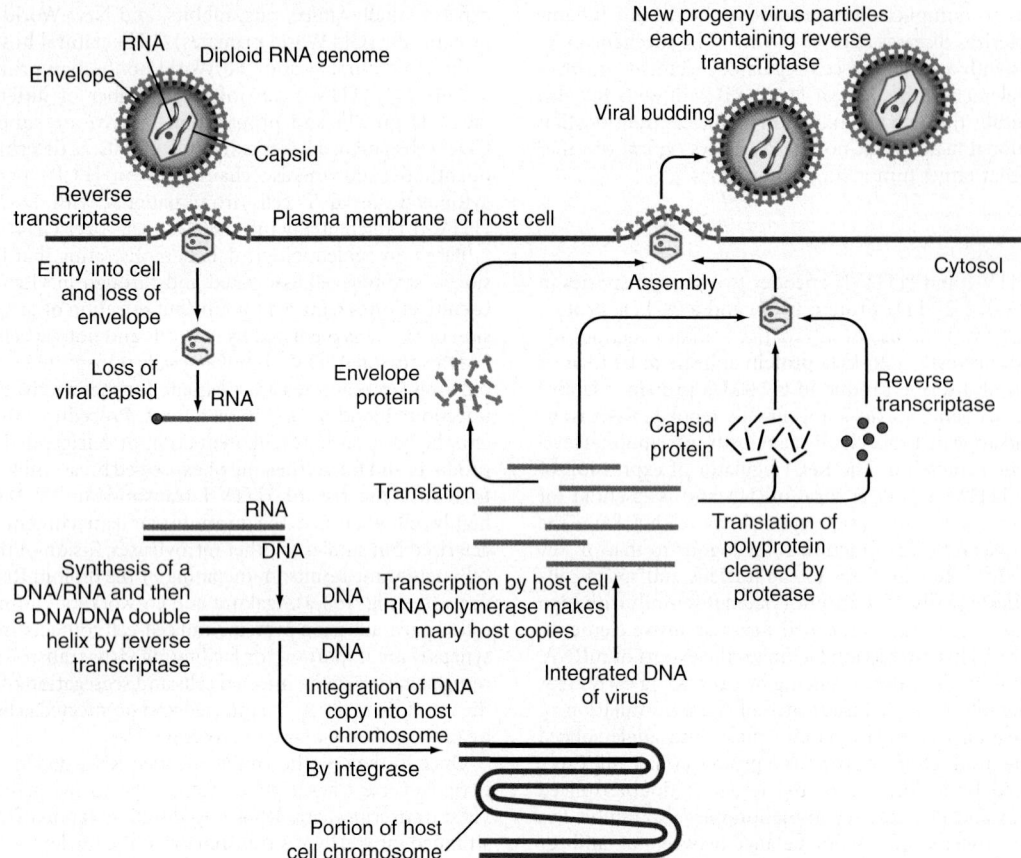

Figure 168-3 Life cycle of human T-cell lymphotropic virus type I (HTLV-I). Virus infection involves initial binding to cell surface of target CD4 cell, uncoating, and release of viral genetic material. Virally encoded reverse transcriptase creates a DNA copy (provirus) that is integrated into the host genome under the influence of viral integrase. Viral replication involves production of both genomic RNA and polyproteins that are cleaved by the viral protease resulting in virion assembly at the cell surface. See text for details. *(Adapted from Alberts B, Bray D, Johnson A, et al., eds. Essential Cell Biology: An Introduction to the Molecular Biology of the Cell. New York: Garland Science Publishing; 2004. Reproduced by permission of Garland Science/Taylor & Francis Books, Inc.)*

blood mononuclear cells (range, 0.5-5.3) for HTLV-I and 2.60 log^{10} copies per million peripheral blood mononuclear cells (range, 0.05-5.95) for HTLV-II.[49] The ability to isolate HTLV is dependent on viral load, immune status, and stage of disease. In infants and children, the small volume of blood available for culture and low virus load make virus isolation especially challenging.

SEROLOGIC ASSAYS AND ANTIGEN DETECTION

The primary test for HTLV-I/II infection is detection of the presence of antibody. A variety of techniques are used to detect antibodies to HTLV-I. Because resolution of HTLV infection has not been described, confirmed HTLV-I antibody positivity can be interpreted as infection with HTLV provirus. Samples are first screened with one of several assays that use whole virus lysates or recombinant HTLV-I and -II antigens. The most widely used assay for the detection of HTLV-I in the United States is the enzyme immunoassay (EIA) technique, using whole disrupted virus and recombinant antigens.[50] These assays have performed with high sensitivity and specificity in the clinical setting, but do not discriminate between HTLV-I and HTLV-II because of cross-reactive antibodies.[51] Nevertheless, because false-positive results are common when using EIAs in low-prevalence populations such as blood donors, repeating the EIA and retesting repeatedly reactive EIAs with a different supplemental test is strongly recommended before informing the patient.

For HTLV-I and -II, a combination of a screening EIA followed by a confirmatory WB is the standard approach, although some investigators and blood banks prefer alternative strategies incorporating a par-

ticle agglutination test for screening or an immunofluorescence assay for confirmation.[52-54] The inclusion of synthetic peptides in EIA and supplemental assays has improved performance.[53-55]

A modified WB has been developed that contains both group-specific conserved motifs from the transmembrane protein and type-specific motifs from the external glycoproteins (recombinant gp46) of HTLV-I (MTA1) and HTLV-II (K55) (Fig. 168-4A). They are coated onto the strips, which allows a simultaneous confirmation and differentiation of both HTLV-I and HTLV-II in 98% of the cases.[56] In a recent line immunoassay, antigens are purified and fixed onto a nylon membrane including two Gag bands (p19 I/II, p24 I/II) and two Env (gp46 I/II, gp21 I/II) as non–type-specific antigens to confirm the presence of antibodies against HTLV I/II (see Fig. 168-4B). The type-specific antigens Gag p19-I and Env gp46-I (specific for HTLV-I) and Env gp46-II (specific for HTLV-II) enable differentiation of HTLV-I and HTLV-II infections.[57] Because of the small anticipated market, neither the modified WB nor the line immunoassay has been licensed for diagnostic use in the United States, posing regulatory problems for U.S. blood banks.

The criterion for WB positivity varies by manufacturer, but should include the presence of reactivity to both a *gag* and an *env* gene product. In the case of *env*, this usually entails a recombinantly produced antigen because of the paucity of HTLV envelope antigens in whole virus preparations. The evolution of WB band patterns in a seroconverting patient is shown in Figure 168-5.

The radioimmunoprecipitation assay, a more difficult procedure based on radiolabeled virus-infected whole cells, is more sensitive for Env antibodies. Confirmatory testing by an immunofluorescence assay

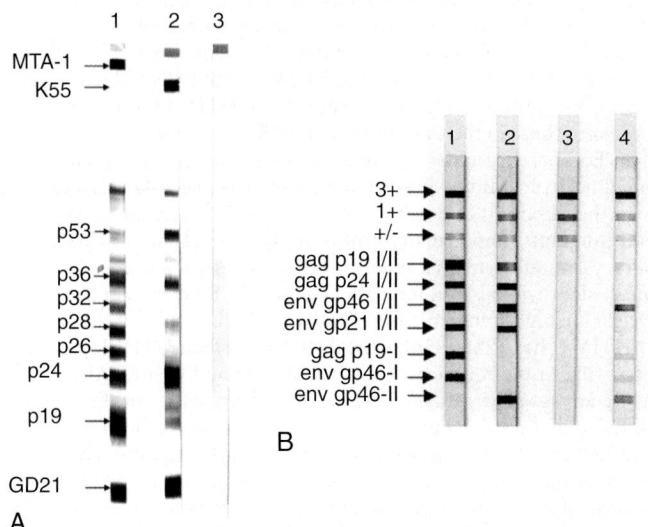

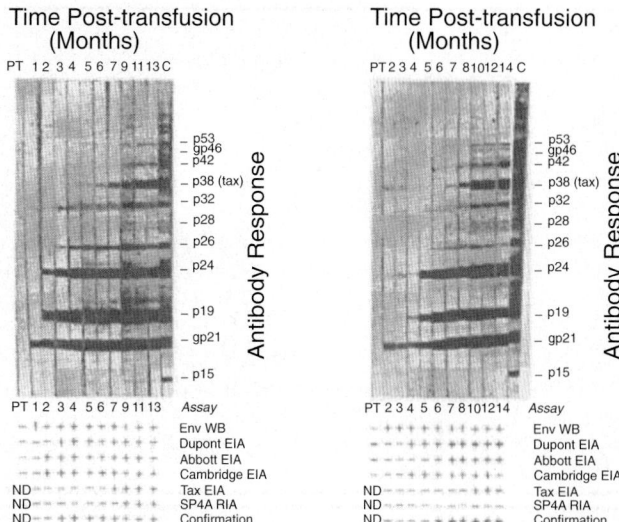

Figure 168-4 **A,** Modified human T-cell lymphotropic virus type I (HTLV-I) and II (HTLV-II) Western blot including recombinant type-specific peptides MTA-1 for HTLV-I and K55 for HTLV-II in addition to other viral antigens. Lane 1 shows an HTLV-I–positive serum, lane 2 shows an HTLV-II–positive serum, and lane 3 shows a negative control serum. *(Adapted with permission from Meertens L et al. J Virol. 76:259-268, 2002.)* **B,** HTLV-I and HTLV-II line immunoassay including type-specific HTLV-I gag p19, HTLV-I env gp46, and HTLV-II env gp46 antigens, in addition to shared gag p19, gag p24, env gp46, and env gp21 antigens. Lane 1 shows an HTLV-I–positive serum, lane 2 shows an HTLV-II–positive serum, lane 3 shows a negative control serum, and lane 4 shows an HTLV-III–positive serum from an African pygmy. *(Adapted with permission from Calattini S et al. Retrovirology. 2005;2:30.)*

Figure 168-5 Sequential serum samples from two transfused patients after exposure to human T-cell lymphotropic virus type I (HTLV-I)–infected blood products. The time course (in months) of seroconversion is revealed by the sequential appearance of bands on a standard HTLV-I Western blot (top) and reactivity (+/–, ND) on a battery of other Western blot, enzyme immunoassay, and radioimmunoassay tests. ND, not done; PT, pretransfusion.

is also possible, although this assay is not suited for high-throughput operations because it is labor-intensive and subjective. Titration to allow quantification of antibody is possible by testing serial dilutions of serum with EIA, particle agglutination or immunofluorescence assays. In tropical countries, particularly Africa, repeatedly reactive EIA reactive samples exhibit a high frequency of indeterminate WB results. Typically, these indeterminate sera show an HTLV Gag indeterminate profile: Gag p19, p26, p28, and p30 without p24 or Env gp21 and gp46, which may be related to endemic *Plasmodium falciparum* infection.[58] To avoid overestimating the rate of HTLV-I/II seroprevalence in these regions, PCR may be useful.[59-61]

NUCLEIC ACID DETECTION

PCR assays have been developed to distinguish virus type and to quantify viral presence. In PCR, proviral DNA is amplified enzymatically and subsequently detected using a system of specific nucleotide primers and probes.[62] The limit of detection is approximately one infected cell per million peripheral blood mononuclear cells.[63] With the addition of a reverse-transcription step before amplification, PCR has been used in the research setting to detect viral mRNA in infected cells, which helps to identify actively replicating virus, although mRNA has not been convincingly demonstrated in ex vivo plasma samples. Although exquisitely sensitive in the best laboratories, PCR remains a research technique; it is under consideration for use as a screening assay as new technologies are evolving. PCR has proved especially valuable in enigmatic situations such as cases of seroindeterminate WBs (i.e., cases from Africa and Melanesia). If used with degenerate primers capable of detecting a variant of HTLV, PCR can rule out the presence of a new exogenous retrovirus.[58] However, PCR has only occasional clinical utility in the diagnosis of HTLV infection in low-risk populations because it is subject to false-positive results. With a low pretest prob-

ability (nonendemic area, no risk factors), individuals with positive EIA and indeterminate WB results have only a 1% to 2% probability of true HTLV infection, so PCR is not recommended.[64] Conversely, PCR is useful in the diagnosis of neonatal HTLV infection because passively transferred maternal antibody makes antibody testing unreliable.[65]

The PCR technique has also been useful to facilitate epidemiologic research studies.[62,66] Theoretically, virus-positive, antibody-negative individuals could be missed by antibody tests and the true prevalence of virus may be underestimated. In fact, several surveys using PCR have not detected large numbers of virus-positive, antibody-negative individuals, although some instances have been reported.[67-70] The recent development of quantitative real-time PCR has allowed the measurement of HTLV proviral DNA in peripheral blood mononuclear cells from infected individuals in the research setting.[49,63,71,72] Unfortunately, proviral load has not yet been characterized as a useful prognostic marker, and these assays are not yet available clinically.[73,74]

Serologic Epidemiology

GEOGRAPHIC DISTRIBUTION

Figure 168-6 shows the different geographic distributions of HTLV-I and HTLV-II. Endemic clusters of HTLV-I infection are present in southern Japan, the islands of the Ryukyu Chain, including Okinawa, and some isolated villages in the north of Japan among aboriginal Ainu populations; most of the seropositives in northern Japan are among immigrants from endemic areas in the south.[75-77] Rates of infection among persons older than 40 years of age exceed 15% in these areas.[76-78] The People's Republic of China, Hong Kong, Korea, Taiwan, and Vietnam are largely free of infection[79,80]; the high rates (>15%) in Melanesia are attributed to a variant HTLV-I strain.[81] Another major endemic focus of HTLV-I infection occurs in the Caribbean, where rates of seropositivity in Jamaica, Trinidad and Tobago, Barbados, Haiti, and the Dominican Republic range between 5% and 14%.[82-84] Foci of seropositivity are present in South and Central America, including Brazil (especially Bahia and the northeast), Colombia, Venezuela, Guyana, Surinam, Panama, and Honduras.[85] In Trinidad and

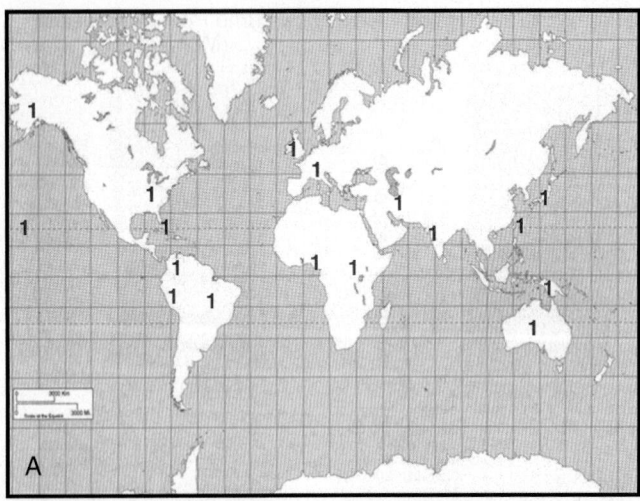

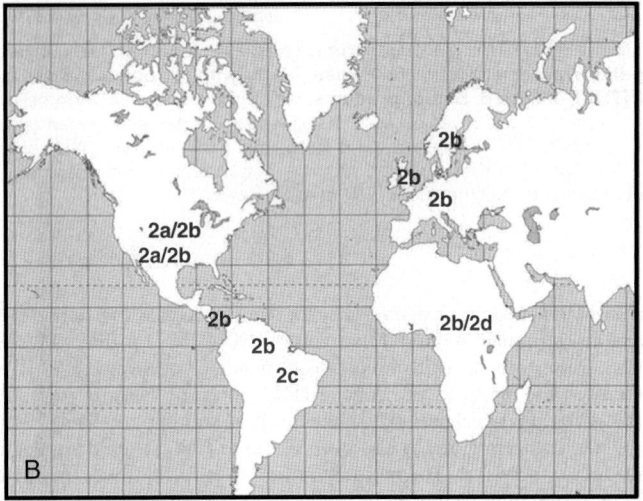

Figure 168-6 A, Geographic distribution of human T-cell lympho-tropic virus type I (HTLV-I) infection. HTLV-I endemic populations are shown in red type, and areas with sporadic cases of HTLV-I often due to immigration from endemic areas are shown in blue type. **B,** Geographic distribution of HTLV-II molecular subtypes 2a, 2b, 2c, and 2d. Areas with endemic human T-cell lymphotropic virus type II (HTLV-II)–infected Native American and African populations are shown in red type, and areas with HTLV-II infection among intravenous drug users and their sexual partners are shown in blue type. *(From Beilke MA, Murphy EL. The human T-lymphotropic leukemia viruses 1 and 2. In: Volberding PA, Palefsky J, eds. Viral and Immunological Malignancies. Hamilton, Ontario: BC Decker; 2006:328 and 330.)*

Tobago, seropositivity (5% to 14%) is restricted almost exclusively to persons of African descent, even though individuals of Indo-Asian ethnic background have shared a common environment for more than a century.[86] In Jamaica, varying rates of seropositivity occur in different regions, with the highest rates (10%) of positivity observed in the lowland, high-rainfall areas.[87] Seropositivity is found more frequently in persons of lower socioeconomic class and those who lack formal education.[82,83,88-90] Men and women attending clinics for sexually trans-mitted infections have the highest rate of seropositivity (>15%).[89]

In the United States, large-scale blood supply screening has docu-mented rates of HTLV-I/II of 0.3 to 0.4 per 1000. Of the donors who test HTLV seropositive, one half to two thirds are HTLV-II infected.[91-93] In a significant proportion of HTLV-I–positive cases, the donor either has links to an endemic area or a history of risk behaviors, such as blood transfusion or multiple sexual partners.[91] Smaller regional surveys and studies of military populations show patterns similar to Trinidad and Tobago; persons of African ancestry have higher rates of seropositivity. Migrant populations from Okinawa to Hawaii, from the Caribbean to

the United States, and from the Caribbean to the United Kingdom are at risk of HTLV positivity, as are those who experience exposure through sexual contact or blood transfusion in viral endemic areas.[88,94-98] Surveys from the Ivory Coast, Ghana, Nigeria, Democratic Republic of Congo, Kenya, and Tanzania document that rates of HTLV-I seropositivity are similar to those in the Caribbean region (5% to 14%).[99,100]

In Europe, occasional infections are detected among migrants from endemic areas. Middle East survey results have been largely negative, with the exception of Iranian Jews from northeastern Iran (Mashhad) and emigrants from that area now residing in Israel and New York.[101,102] Surveys in southern India and Indonesia have identified some HTLV-I–infected individuals, but not endemic foci; the Seychelles in the Indian Ocean are highly endemic for HTLV-I (>15%).[103]

HTLV-II has a more restricted distribution than HTLV-I, primarily occurring in the Americas and parts of West and Central Africa.[104-106] A major reservoir exists in injection drug users in the United States and southern Europe, with rates ranging from 10% to 15% and higher.[107,108] Amerindians residing in North, Central, and South America have varying rates of positivity for HTLV-II (5% to 30%). Pockets of infection are present among the Seminoles in south Florida and the Pueblo and Navajo in New Mexico, but not among various tribes in Alaska.[109-111] In Central America, the Guaymi Indians residing in northeastern Panama near the Costa Rican border have high sero-positive rates (>15%), but this does not hold true for the Guaymi living in southwest Panama. Finally, HTLV-II has been identified in Africa, primarily among pygmy populations living in Central and Western rain forest areas.[105,112]

DEMOGRAPHIC PATTERNS

HTLV-I seroprevalence rates are strongly age- and sex-dependent, with higher rates associated with older age and with female sex (Fig. 168-7).[75,83,113] The increasing prevalence with age may be due to the accumulation of infections over the lifetime of the individuals sur-veyed or an age-cohort effect due to declining HTLV-I seroprevalence over the past decades.[114] The higher prevalence in females may be the result of more efficient male-to-female sexual transmission, as dis-cussed later, or differences in sociodemographic or behavioral factors, such as duration of breast-feeding or frequency of condom use.

For HTLV-II, there is also a characteristic age-dependent increase in seroprevalence in endemic Amerindian populations (Fig. 168-8).[115] In contrast, prevalence among U.S. blood donors shows an HTLV-II age-specific prevalence that peaks at age 40 to 50, consistent with a birth cohort effect due to injection drug use in the 1960s and 1970s, with secondary sexual transmission.[93]

▓ Molecular Epidemiology

HUMAN T-CELL LYMPHOTROPIC VIRUS TYPE I

Phylogenetic analysis has been used to classify HTLV-I into five major molecular and geographic subtypes: (1) a cosmopolitan (C) subtype isolated all over the world (endemic to Caribbean, South America), (2) a Japanese (J) subtype, (3) a West African (WA) subtype, (4) a Central African (CA) subtype, and (5) a Melanesian (M) subtype (Papua New Guinea, Melanesia, and Australian aborigines).[116] Other authors pos-tulate six HTLV-I subtypes, with a broad Cosmopolitan subtype A redefined to include all Japanese isolates, four subtypes (B, D, E, and F) in Africa, and the Melanesian subtype C.[117] HTLV-I isolates from different parts of the world show a high degree of nucleotide sequence conservation, in contrast to HIV-1 and HIV-2, in which considerable genomic variability occurs. Isolates of HTLV-I from Japan, the West Indies, the Americas, and Africa share 97% or greater homology.[118-120] Even the most divergent HTLV-I, isolated in Melanesia, is 92% homol-ogous with a prototypic Japanese isolate.[121] The majority of the nucleo-tide differences are single point mutations that do not correlate with specific disease patterns. Studies of the LTR by restriction fragment length polymorphisms covering the major HTLV-I endemic area have

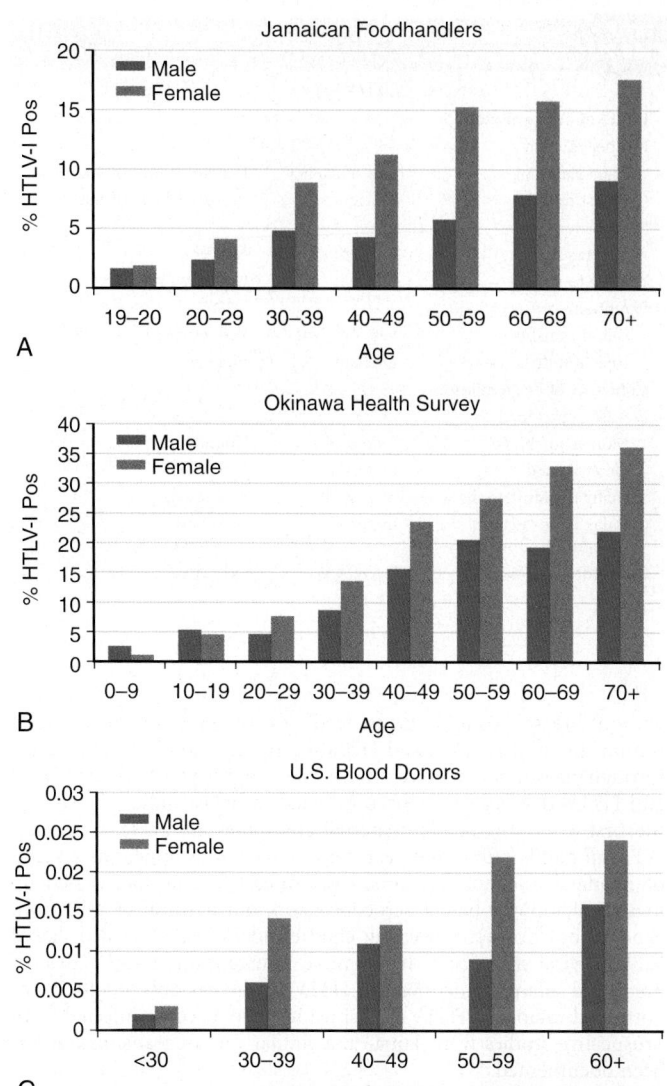

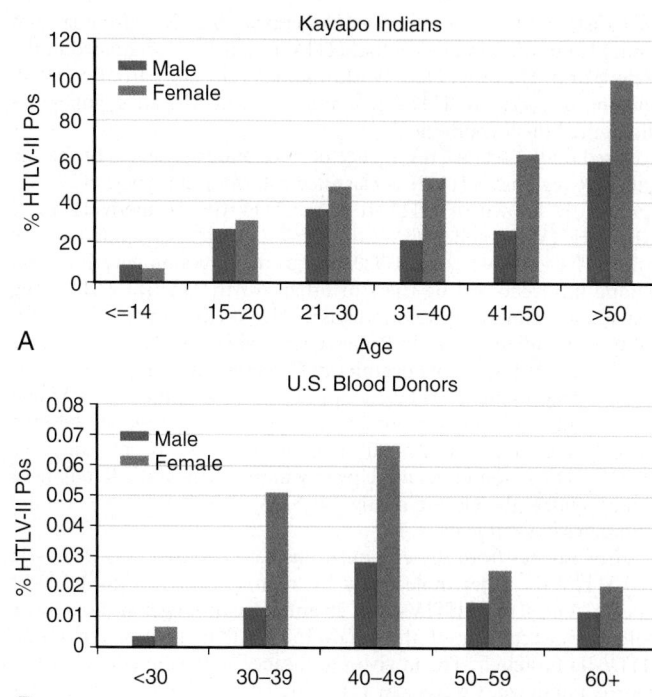

Figure 168-8 **Age- and sex-specific sewer prevalence of human T-cell lymphotropic virus type II (HTLV-II). A,** The highly endemic Kayapo Indians of Brazil, consistent with ongoing mother-to-child and sexual transmission within a closed population (data from Maloney et al.[115]). **B,** U.S. blood donors with very low HTLV-II seroprevalence show a pattern that suggests a birth cohort effect due to intravenous drug use in secondary sexual transmission in the 1960s and 1970s (data from Murphy et al.[93]). *(From Beilke MA, Murphy EL. The human T-lymphotropic leukemia viruses 1 and 2. In: Volberding PA, Palefsky J, eds. Viral and Immunological Malignancies. Hamilton, Ontario: BC Decker; 2006:332.)*

Figure 168-7 **Age- and sex-specific seroprevalence of human T-cell lymphotropic virus type I (HTLV-I) in several population groups showing the characteristic higher female prevalence and increasing prevalence with age. A,** Jamaicans employed in food handling occupations (data from Murphy et al.[83]). **B,** Participants in a community health survey in Okinawa, Japan (data from Kajiyama et al.[75]). **C,** U.S. blood donors with very low HTLV-I seroprevalence (data from Murphy et al.[93]). *(From Beilke MA, Murphy EL. The human T-lymphotropic leukemia viruses 1 and 2. In: Volberding PA, Palefsky J, eds. Viral and Immunological Malignancies. Hamilton, Ontario: BC Decker; 2006:329.)*

demonstrated that variations are more linked to the geographic origin of the infected individuals than the patient's clinical status.[122-124] In addition, simian T-cell lymphotropic virus type I (STLV-I) isolates cluster more closely with human isolates in the same geographic region than with STLV-I isolates from different geographic regions, suggesting multiple instances of trans-species transmission.[125-128] Thus, the genetic variability of HTLV-I appears to reflect a combination of multiple trans-species transmission episodes and migration patterns of ancient populations carrying the virus.

An African origin of most HTLV-I subtypes is supported by the occurrence of many HTLV-I clusters in Africa[60,99,129] and among persons of African descent residing in the Caribbean, but not among other migrant populations residing in the region.[86] The cosmopolitan subtype was likely dispersed throughout the world during the slave trade or early maritime explorations of European countries. The high prevalence of this HTLV subtype in southwestern Japan remains unex-

plained and could be due either to importation by maritime trade with Portugal and Holland starting in the 16th century or to prehistoric dissemination of the cosmopolitan subtype among some ancient ethnic people of Japan.[116,130]

A rare HTLV-I variant, subtype D, was isolated from seropositive individuals in various parts of Melanesia.[131] The original isolate was obtained from an unacculturated hunter-gatherer tribe, the Hagahai, residing in the highlands of Papua, New Guinea. Their only contact with the outside world had occurred within weeks of the original blood sample collection. These viruses differ by as much as 9% to 10% from the prototype Japanese strain and by as much as 4% to 6% from the viruses isolated in Australia and the Solomon Islands.[131-133] HTLV-I subtype D clusters closely with STLV-I isolated from a stump-tailed macaque (*Macacca arctoides*), providing strong evidence of multiple cross-species transmissions.[134] In some cases, these strains have been isolated from persons with ATL[122] and HAM.[135]

HUMAN T-CELL LYMPHOTROPIC VIRUS TYPE II

Compared with HTLV-I, the geographic origin of HTLV-II is less certain. HTLV-II was first documented in and is highly prevalent among intravenous drug users in the United States and Italy.[108,136-140] A natural reservoir was subsequently discovered among various Amerindian populations residing in North, Central, and South America.[109,111,115,141-147] The current bimodal distribution of HTLV-II in the New World probably represents an original transmission from an endemic Amerindian to an intravenous drug user, followed by amplification of prevalence by the efficient transmission within the latter group. The presence of HTLV-II infection in culturally and geographically distinct Indian groups in North America, Central America

(Panama), and South America (Argentina, Brazil, Colombia, and Chile) led to the speculation that HTLV-II may have originated in the New World. However, New World monkeys do not harbor STLV-II, and the discovery of HTLV-II among Central African pygmies has discounted this hypothesis.[105,112]

Based on the relative divergence of nucleotide sequences of the *env* and LTR regions, HTLV-II is classified into four subtypes: HTLV-IIa (previously known as HTLV-II Mo), HTLV-IIb (formerly HTLV-II NRA), HTLV-IIc, and HTLV-IId.[117,144,148-151] Molecular epidemiologic studies have shown that HTLV-IIa is the predominant infection among intravenous drug users in urban North America and among some North American Amerindians.[152] HTLV-IIb is the predominant subtype in Indian groups in Panama, Colombia, and Argentina, but is also found among Bakola pygmies in Cameroon and European intravenous drug users.[105] HTLV-IIc appears to be confined to Brazilian Indian and urban populations and is supported as a separate subtype by LTR region phylogeny, but not *env* gene phylogenic analyses. HTLV-II D was found in an Efe pygmy in the Democratic Republic of Congo and is the closest relative to STLV-II isolated from Bonobo chimpanzees (*Pan paniscus*).[112]

Virus isolates from these populations have revealed that HTLV-IIa and HTLV-IIb differ molecularly by approximately 2% to 4%.[153,154] The tax-2 protein of HTLV-IIb is 25 amino acids longer and is a more potent transactivator of the HTLV-II LTR than the corresponding HTLV-IIa protein.[150] The in vivo significance of this functional difference is unknown. Conversely, HTLV-IIc has LTR and env sequences related to HTLV-IIa and tax sequences similar to those of HTLV-IIb.[144] The identical sequence of the 456 base pair *tax* gene of HTLV-IIb isolates from a Cameroonian pygmy and a Colombian Wayuu Indian support an African origin for HTLV-II.[117] This, taken together with the close similarity of HTLV-IId and STLV-II, supports a scenario whereby HTLV-II evolved into subtypes a, b, and d in Africa and was then transported to the New World, whereas HTLV-IIc represents a more recent variant within subtype a.

HUMAN T-CELL LYMPHOTROPIC VIRUSES TYPES III AND IV

Notwithstanding the initial nomenclature of HTLV-III for the virus subsequently renamed HIV, recently, two new HTLV types have been isolated from a handful of Central Africans living in close contact with nonhuman primates. These viruses were discovered simultaneously by two teams working on samples derived from central African inhabitants. Wolfe and colleagues[155] described two different viral isolates from bush meat hunters, which they termed HTLV-III and HTLV-IV. Callatini and colleagues[156] described an HTLV-III isolate that seems to be identical to the HTLV-III described by Wolfe and colleagues.[155] To date, there is no evidence that these new types are broadly distributed, and they may represent limited instances of simian to human transmission that have not become established in the human population. There has been no evidence that either of these new isolates is widely prevalent in Africa or present at all outside of Africa, and current commercially available tests have not yet been adapted to detect these new HTLV types.

Routes of Transmission

Table 168-2 summarizes the routes, mechanisms, and cofactors associated with HTLV-I and -II transmission. The three major routes of HTLV-I transmission are mother-to-child transmission, sexual transmission, and parenteral transmission. Although the routes of HTLV-II transmission have been less well studied, the available evidence suggests that they are similar to those of HTLV-I.

MOTHER-TO-CHILD TRANSMISSION

In contrast to mother-to-child transmission of HIV-1, wherein as many as 25% of offspring of positive mothers can acquire infection

TABLE 168-2	Transmission of Human T-Cell Lymphotropic Virus Types I and II	
	HTLV Type I	*HTLV Type II*
Route of Transmission		
Mother to child		
Transplacental	Low efficiency	Probable, but not quantified
Breast milk	Efficient	Probable, but not quantified
Sexual		
Heterosexual	Efficient	Efficient
Male to male	Efficient	Unknown
Parenteral		
Blood transfusion	Very efficient	Very efficient
Injection drug use	Efficient	Efficient
Cofactors of Transmission		
Elevated virus load		
Mother to child	Increased	Unknown
Heterosexual	Increased	Increased
Sexually transmitted diseases	Increased	Unknown
Cellular versus plasma transfusion products	Increased	Increased
Cold storage of blood	Decreased	Decreased

without breast-feeding,[157] breast-feeding is the predominant route of mother-to-child HTLV-I and HTLV-II transmission[158-161] and occurs through ingestion of infected milk-borne lymphocytes.[162] Both HTLV-I and HTLV-II viruses have been detected in breast milk.[163-165] During the first 6 months of life, maternal antibodies are present; in serial WBs, all bands often disappear before new bands appear as a result of neonatal infection. In some cases, breast-feeding had ceased up to several months before seroconversion, but a study of cells from exposed but nonseroconverting children identified none with latent HTLV-I viral infection.[67] In Japanese intervention trials,[159] 20% of breast-fed infants seroconvert to HTLV-I, whereas only 1% to 2% of bottle-fed infants of HTLV-I–positive mothers become infected.[159] In prospective studies from Jamaica, a similar rate of transmission has been documented.[163]

The major predictor of maternal-to-child transmission is the proviral load of the mother as measured by antibody titer and viral antigen level on short-term culture.[73,166] The presence of antibody to HTLV Tax[167,168] and/or Env has also been associated with transmission.[163,169,170] Furthermore, the duration and timing of breast-feeding were strongly associated with the efficiency of transmission.[158,160,162,171,172] In a prospective study conducted in Jamaica, among children born of HTLV-I–positive mothers in follow-up for more than 2 years, 32% of children breast-fed for 12 months or longer were HTLV-I seropositive compared with 9% of those breast-fed for less than 12 months.[162] These data strongly suggest that limiting the duration of breast-feeding to less than 6 months may significantly reduce mother-to-child transmission of HTLV-I. Follow-up studies indicated that seroconversion typically occurs in infants at the age of 1 to 3 years, with approximately 2% to 5% of HTLV-I infections resulting from mother-to-child transmission in the first few years of life.[173,174] In many studies, no infants or children became newly infected after 2 years of age.[161] The early life infection may have considerable significance for subsequent risk of disease, particularly adult T-cell leukemia.[175,176]

HTLV-II transmission from mother to child also appears to occur through breast-feeding, but has been less studied.[177] In a small study of infected mothers, 1 of 7 breast-fed children was seropositive for HTLV-II, whereas 1 of 28 non–breast-fed children was seropositive.[178] In another study, no HTLV-II transmissions were found among 19 infected mothers and 20 non–breast-fed children.[179] Among the Gran Chaco Indians of Argentina and the Kayapo Indians of Brazil, high rates of mother-to-child transmission have been observed (30% and 46%, respectively), suggesting the predominant role of breast-feeding in maternal-to-child transmission in these populations.[145,180] Additionally, among the Guaymi Indians of Panama, there is a 1% to 2% prevalence among preadolescent children.[181] This is consistent with early life infection and an excess of seropositive children when the mother is seropositive compared with the virtual absence of seropositive children when the mother is negative.[173,176]

SEXUAL TRANSMISSION

Several markers of sexual activity have been associated with transmission of HTLV-I infection, including the number of lifetime sexual partners[89,182] and ulcerative (syphilis, herpes simplex virus type 2, and chancroid) and nonulcerative (gonorrhea and *Chlamydia*) sexually transmitted diseases.[89,183-185] Virus-positive mononuclear cells have been detected in semen, which suggests that seminal fluid is a likely vehicle for transmission.[186] The presence of HTLV-I DNA has also been found in cervicovaginal secretions from infected commercial sex workers in Peru.[187,188] Although some studies have suggested that male-to-female transmission occurs more efficiently than female-to-male,[189-192] this difference may be less than previously thought.[193] In a 10-year follow-up study of 30 discordant heterosexual couples, the incidence of HTLV-I infection was 0.9 per 100 person-years (95% confidence interval, 0.1-3.3), with one male-to-female and one female-to-male transmission.[193] Male-to-male sexual transmission may also occur and is supported by the higher prevalence of HTLV-I among men who have sex with men (15%) in Trinidad compared with the general population prevalence of 2.4%.[182] HIV-1 shares these routes of infection, but appears to be an order of magnitude more infectious than HTLV-I.[182,183] This may reflect differences in viral load or that HTLV-I is highly cell associated, whereas HIV-1 is both cell-associated and cell-free.

There are also other risk factors associated with sexual transmission of HTLV-I. In a study of married couples, there was a nearly 12-fold higher risk of infection in wives of seropositive husbands older than 60 years of age, possibly because of increased viremia with age or postmenopausal changes in the vaginal epithelium.[189] Higher proviral load and duration of relationship are also associated with increased transmission. In a prospective study of HTLV-infected men and their female sex partners, transmitters had higher proviral loads and had been in their relationships longer than nontransmitters.[191] Another prospective study demonstrated that HTLV-I proviral loads were 2 $\log_{10}$ lower in newly infected partners than in their positive partners who transmitted HTLV, suggesting that a small dose of sexually transmitted HTLV produces a lower proviral load setpoint.[193] In addition, the presence of anti-tax antibody has been shown to be associated with heightened transmission, possibly related to a state of virus proliferation induced by tax and measured indirectly by anti-tax antibody.[194] Host-related factors may also play an important role in determining HTLV-I viral load. A study evaluating the sequence of the gp46 coding region among 13 infected patients and their partners revealed that, although the gp46 sequences were identical in each married couple, the level of HTLV-I proviral DNA in the spouses often differed.[195]

Sexual transmission of HTLV-II has been difficult to study because of the frequent coincidence of injection drug use in the study populations. However, a recent 10-year cohort study of 55 serodiscordant heterosexual couples reported two HTLV-II transmissions, with one male-to-female and one female-to-male transmission (0.5 per 100 person-years), not statistically different from those seen for HTLV-I.[193] In this study, all newly infected sex partners denied any history of intravenous drug use or other parenteral exposure. Previous studies have documented an association between a history of receiving money for sex, total lifetime sex partners,[196,197] and length of sexual relationships with HTLV-II seropositivity.[191,192,197] In one study of female prostitutes, intravenous drug use was the major risk factor for seropositivity.[198] In a serosurvey of Guaymi Indians, it was demonstrated that among women, early age at first intercourse (younger than 13 years), higher number of lifetime sexual partners, and higher number of long-term sexual relationships were significantly associated

with HTLV-II positivity.[199] Among men, intercourse with prostitutes was associated with HTLV-II seropositivity.

PARENTERAL TRANSMISSION

Parenteral transmission, either through transfusion or injection drug use, is another major route of HTLV transmission. Because the HTLV viruses are cell-associated, transmission via transfusion of cellular components (e.g., whole blood, packed cells, platelet concentrates) is highly efficient. Seroconversion rates of 44% to 63% have been reported in recipients of HTLV-I–infected cellular components in endemic areas,[200-204] but seroconversion has not been associated with plasma or cryoprecipitate. Donor units of whole blood or packed cells are less likely to be associated with transmission the longer they are stored in the blood bank, presumably because of the loss of white blood cell viability at refrigerator temperature. In retrospective surveys, the rate of transmission decreased to near zero when blood components were stored for more than 14 days compared with 47% transmission for a storage period of 14 days or less.[43,201]

Transmission of HTLV-II has been well documented in 50% of the recipients of known units of positive blood.[205] Parenteral drug abuse has been associated with transmission of both HTLV-I and -II, but most HTLV-positive drug abusers are HTLV-II infected.[206] Risk factors for seroconversion include sharing of drug abuse paraphernalia and "booting," i.e., aspirating blood into the drug-filled syringe prior to injection. This circumstance may help to explain the exceptionally high rates of seropositivity in older heroin-injecting drug users, suggesting a birth cohort effect linked to an HTLV-II epidemic among U.S. injection drug users in the 1960s and 1970s.[206] Transmission involving casual contact does not seem to occur.

Although rare, HAM and ATL have both been linked to HTLV-I transfusion transmission.[207,208] In recognition of the risk of these diseases, testing of donated blood for HTLV viruses has been routine in the United States since 1988.[50] HTLV seroprevalence is generally low among hemophiliacs unless they were multiply transfused with cellular blood products before the institution of routine screening.[209,210] In developing countries, however, blood transfusions remain a major risk factor for HTLV infection. A case of HTLV-I infection in several transplant recipients sharing the same donor has been documented.[211] Genomic sequencing revealed 100% homology in these cases.

▣ Immunology of Human T-Cell Lymphotropic Virus Infections

HUMORAL IMMUNE RESPONSES

Antibodies to the various antigens of HTLV-I occur at high levels in carriers and among patients with ATL and HAM. During primary infection, the pattern of antibody responses (see Fig. 168-5) demonstrates that the first specific antibodies to emerge after primary HTLV infection are directed against the gp21 transmembrane Env protein and various regions of the Gag polyprotein. Over several weeks to months, anti-gp46 Env antibodies appear, and about 50% of infected individuals develop detectable antibodies to p38/40 Tax protein.[194,212] Antibody titers vary from patient to patient and are significantly higher in patients with HAM and among those at risk of this disease. Antibody titers correlate with the proviral burden, explaining the HAM finding as well as the paradoxical finding of high antibody titers among women who transmit HTLV-I to their infants through prolonged breast-feeding.[163,213] Transplacental maternal antibodies apparently protect the infant from infection in the first months of life, but subsequently the infant becomes infected via maternal virus in the breast milk. Miyoshi and co-workers[214] have shown that passive immunization with high-titer human anti-HTLV globulin is protective against experimental HTLV infection in rabbits. Antibody response is also elicited by immunization with experimental DNA or peptide HTLV-I vaccines.[215] However, there is little evidence that humoral immune response controls HTLV-I proliferation or prevents disease in humans.

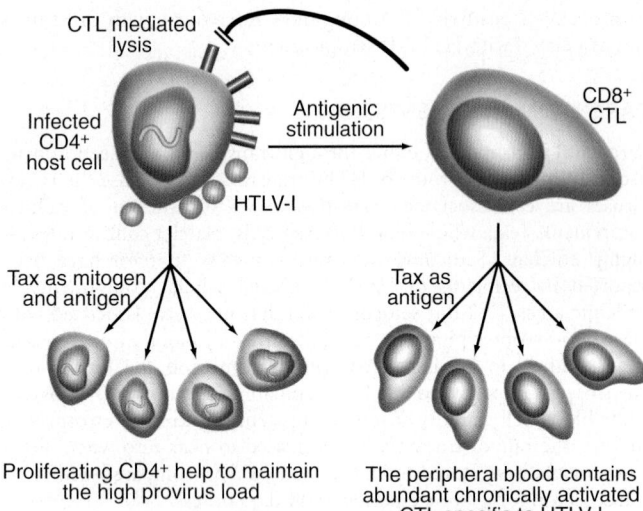

Figure 168-9 A model of CD8⁺ cytotoxic T-lymphocyte–mediated control of human T-cell lymphotropic virus type I (HTLV-I) infection. HTLV-I infects CD4⁺ T lymphocytes with expansion of infection primarily via cell replication. As HTLV-I–specific antigens, particularly tax, are expressed, a robust CD8⁺ cytotoxic T-lymphocyte response is generated. The inability of some persons to control HTLV-I expansion is thought to contribute to disease pathogenesis. See text for details. *(From Bangham CRM. HTLV-1 infections. J Clin Pathol. 1999;53:581-586, with permission.)*

TABLE 168-3	Human T-Cell Lymphotropic Virus-Associated Diseases		
Disease		*HTLV Type I*	*HTLV Type II*
Children			
Infective dermatitis		++++	No
Lymphadenopathy		++	++
Adults			
Adult T-cell leukemia/lymphoma		++++	No
HTLV-associated myelopathy		++++	+++
Infective dermatitis		+++	No
Polymyositis		++	Unknown
Uveitis		+++	Unknown
HTLV-associated arthritis		++	++
Sjögren's syndrome		++	Unknown
Strongyloidiasis		++	Unknown
Pulmonary infiltrative pneumonitis		++	++
Invasive cervical cancer		+	Unknown

++++, very strong evidence; +++, strong evidence; ++, possible association; +, weak association; No, evidence does not support association; Unknown, no data to support association or lack of association.

■ Clinical Manifestations of Human T-Cell Lymphotropic Virus Infections

Clinical disease associated with HTLV-I is rare. ATL develops in 2% to 4% and HAM in 1% to 2% of carriers over their lifetime.[227,228] The risk of the development of disease is related to age and route of infection and the immune competency of the host. Acute seroconversion is associated with no recognized clinical syndrome; the time from infection to seroconversion can vary from 1 to 2 months, as seen with transfusion cases. The time from seroconversion to disease can vary from years to decades, with rare cases of HAM occurring soon after blood transfusion. As summarized in Table 168-3, there is a wide range of clinical conditions linked to HTLV-I, with some caused by virally induced cell transformation and others mediated by immunologic response to the virus.

HUMAN T-CELL LYMPHOTROPIC VIRUS TYPE I–ASSOCIATED MALIGNANCIES

ATL was first recognized in 1977, before the discovery of HTLV-I, as an aggressive leukemia/lymphoma of mature T lymphocytes with varied clinical manifestations: generalized lymphadenopathy, visceral involvement, hypercalcemia, cutaneous skin involvement, lytic bone lesions, and peripheral blood involvement with cells manifesting pleiotropic features ("flower cells") in a large number of cases.[229] The skin lesions seen in ATL are varied and include localized or diffuse papules, nodules (Fig. 168-10A), plaques (see Fig. 168-10B), erythematous patches, and diffuse erythroderma. Biopsy specimens of skin lesions reveal dermal or epidermal infiltration with malignant lymphocytes. So-called Pautrier's microabscesses may also be noted in the dermis, as in mycosis fungoides. Biopsy specimens of bone lytic lesions reveal osteoclast activation and bone resorption (Fig. 168-11), often without infiltration by ATL cells. It has been suggested that Tax transactivation and production of parathyroid hormone-related protein and other cytokines are responsible for the hypercalcemia, osteoclast activation, and lytic bone lesions seen in this disorder.[230,231] The lifetime risk of development of ATL in HTLV-I carriers is estimated at 2% to 4%, and the latent period from infection to development of disease is estimated to be 30 to 50 years.[227,232]

The Lymphoma Study Group in Japan[233] has classified ATL into four clinical types based on clinical features and cell morphology: smoldering (5%), chronic (19%), lymphoma/leukemia (19%), and acute (57%) types. Transformation from the smoldering or chronic phase to the acute form can occur at any point during the course of the

CELLULAR IMMUNITY

Cytotoxic T-lymphocytes targeting viral antigens play an essential role in the regulation of HTLV-I viral burden.[216] Among chronic carriers, infected individuals mount a strong cell-mediated immune response to the virus and as many as 1% of CD8⁺ cytotoxic T-lymphocytes can recognize at least one epitope of HTLV.[217-222] Freshly isolated cells have substantial expression of activation markers, indicating that these cells have recently encountered the Tax antigen.[216,218,219] A proposed model of this viral interaction with the host cell–mediated immune response is shown in Figure 168-9. In this model, the dynamic equilibrium between viral replication and immune destruction is mediated through Tax overexpression, causing CD4⁺ target cell proliferation and a robust cell-mediated response to the antigen in particular, resulting in cytotoxic T-lymphocyte–mediated lysis of these HTLV-I–infected CD4⁺ cells.[218,219,222,223] As a consequence of ongoing Tax proliferation, there is an expansion of HTLV-I–infected CD4⁺ cells and a compensatory expansion of CD8⁺ cytotoxic T-lymphocytes. As the number of infected CD4⁺ cells expands, HTLV-I antigens are expressed on the cell surface and become targets for CD8⁺ T cell–mediated cytotoxic killing. The role of CD8⁺ T cell–mediated killing as the primary means of viral suppression may explain the epidemiologic observation that recipients of HTLV-I–infected blood products who are also receiving exogenous immunosuppressive medications are more susceptible to infection, likely because a diminished cell-mediated immune response is unable to clear the initial virus infection.[204]

The role of CD4⁺-mediated T-helper 1 responses in upregulating the cytotoxic T-lymphocyte response is not well characterized. However, an association between class I HLA haplotypes and protection against HAM suggests that carriers of certain antigen-presenting motifs augment the efficient control of HTLV-I–containing cells. HTLV-I carriers with the HLA-A 02 haplotype have lower HTLV-I proviral loads and are less likely to develop HAM, most likely because they are able to mount a stronger cell-mediated immune response to HTLV-I infection.[222,224-226]

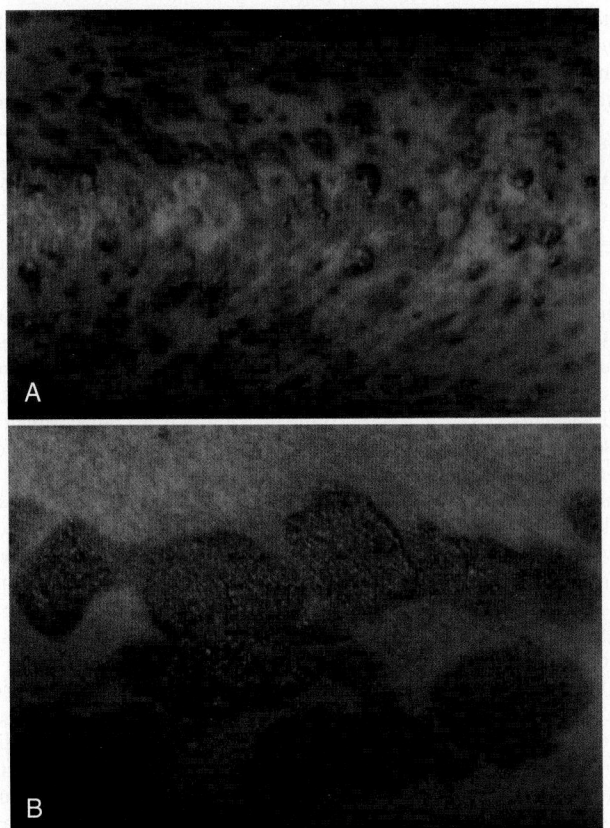

Figure 168-10 Multiple skin papules and nodules (A) and red plaques (B) in patients with adult T-cell leukemia.

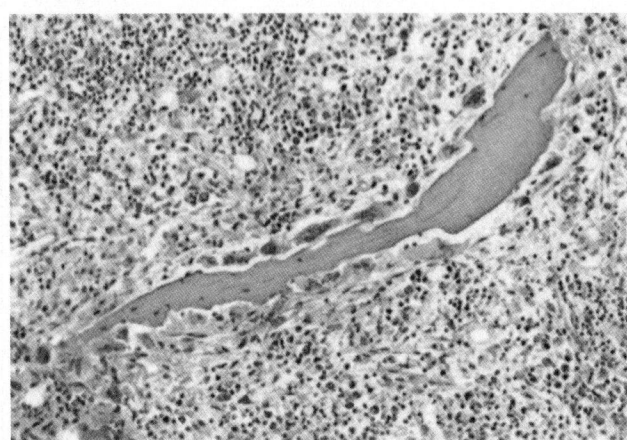

Figure 168-11 A biopsy specimen of lytic bone lesions from a patient with adult T-cell leukemia reveals osteoclast proliferation and bone resorption.

disease progression. Figure 168-12 shows the characteristic morphologic features of the leukemia cells observed in ATL.

Smoldering ATL is characterized by 5% or more abnormal T cells in the peripheral blood with a normal total lymphocyte count, the presence of skin lesions, and, occasionally, pulmonary involvement. There is no hypercalcemia, lymphadenopathy, or other visceral involvement. Serum lactate dehydrogenase levels may be elevated. This phase is often indolent and may last for years. Smoldering ATL may clinically resemble mycosis fungoides/Sézary syndrome with cutaneous involvement presenting as erythema or as infiltrative plaques or tumors, and Pautrier's microabscesses may be observed.

Chronic ATL is characterized by an absolute lymphocytosis (≥4 × 10^9/L) with a T-cell lymphocytosis (>3.5 × 10^9/L) that resembles chronic T-lymphocytic leukemia. Lactate dehydrogenase may be increased as much as twice the normal limit. Cells from chronic ATL patients are relatively uniform in size and nuclear configuration. Patients may have lymphadenopathy, hepatomegaly, splenomegaly, and skin and pulmonary involvement. No hypercalcemia, ascites, pleural effusion, or involvement of the central nervous system, bone, or gastrointestinal tract is present. The median survival time for patients with chronic ATL is 24 months.

Lymphoma/leukemia ATL is characterized by lymphadenopathy in the absence of lymphocytosis. Lymph node involvement with ATL must be histologically proved. The median survival time is approximately 10 months.

Acute ATL is distinguished by increased numbers of leukemic T cells with characteristic pleomorphic morphology, skin lesions, systemic lymphadenopathy, hepatosplenomegaly, and metabolic disorders, especially hypercalcemia. Lytic bone lesions and visceral involvement are common. Acute ATL has a poor prognosis, with a median survival time of 6.2 months.

Most patients with the acute and lymphoma types die within 6 months of diagnosis (Fig. 168-13), particularly if hypercalcemia is a presenting sign.[234] In general, the smoldering type is the least aggressive; the chronic type has a relatively poor prognosis, with death occurring within a few years of diagnosis.[233] The cause of death is usually an explosive growth of tumor cells, hypercalcemia, bacterial sepsis, and other infections observed in patients with immunodeficiency. Sometimes ATL presents as a T-cell non-Hodgkin's lymphoma with no other clinical features of ATL except for monoclonal integration of HTLV-I in the proviral DNA of the tumor cells. These cases are termed lymphoma-type ATL and are indistinguishable from peripheral T-cell lymphomas.

The malignant T cells of ATL are mature (terminal deoxynucleotide transferase negative) CD4+/CD8− and have increased IL-2R α-chain (CD25/TAC antigen) expression.[235-237] All subtypes have a monoclonal integration of HTLV-I proviral DNA into the cellular genome, indicating that the malignant T cells are monoclonal and originated from a single HTLV-I–infected T cell.[238] Southern blot analyses show frequent detection of defective provirus, but fail to demonstrate consistency of HTLV-I integration site in tumors from different patients, suggesting that integration site does not determine leukemogenesis.[239] More

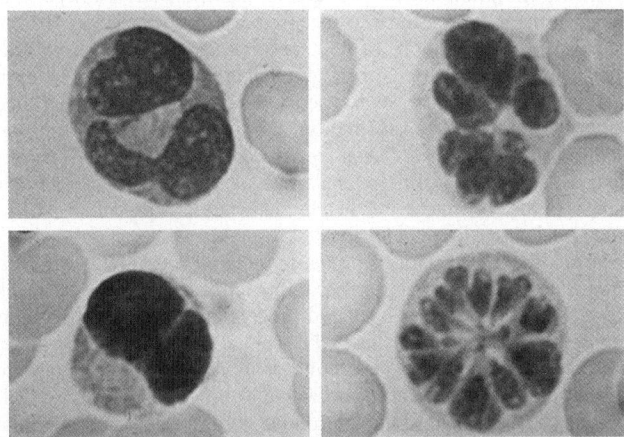

Figure 168-12 Photomicrographs of typical peripheral blood lymphocytes from patients with adult T-cell leukemia. The characteristic cleaved nucleus can result in either a bilobed shape or the archetypical "flower cell" appearance. Low numbers of flower cells can also be seen in occasional human T-cell lymphotropic virus type I seropositive patients without any sign of leukemia or lymphoma.

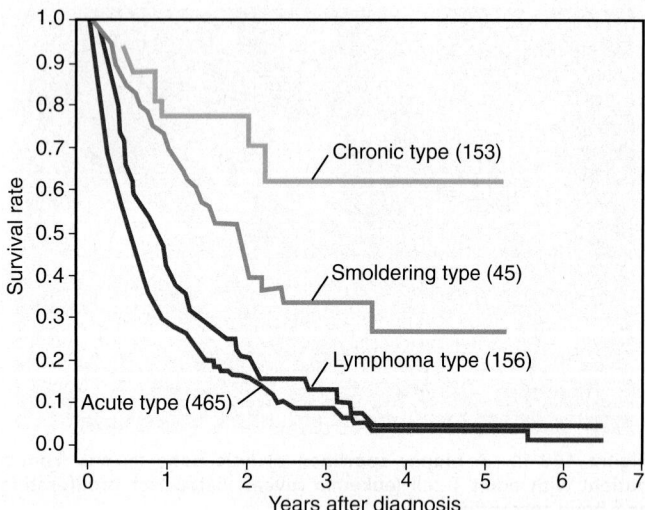

Figure 168-13 **Survival patterns of adult T-cell leukemia (ATL) subtypes after standard chemotherapy.** Acute and lymphoma-type ATL have the poorest prognosis (see text). *(From Tsukasaki K, Ikeda S, Murata K, et al. Characteristics of chemotherapy-induced clinical remission in long survivors with aggressive adult T-cell leukemia/lymphoma. Leuk Res. 1993;17:157-166, with permission.)*

recently, reverse-transcriptase PCR has been used to determine the specific genomic location of integration, since HTLV-I integration sites are more likely to occur in gene-coding than noncoding regions of the genome and near transcriptional start sites in leukemic cells.[240-242] However, no specific proviral integration sites have been linked to the development of ATL.[243] Tanaka and colleagues[244] showed multiple, small HTLV-positive T-cell clonal populations in recently infected persons compared with fewer, larger clonal populations in persons thought to have been infected since birth. Current thinking is that HTLV-I–driven lymphocyte proliferation results in the accumulation of additional somatic DNA mutations at one or more leukemogenic sites, either flanking the HTLV-I proviral integration site or elsewhere.[245,246] Chromosomal additions and deletions are common in ATL and may be related to prognosis; however, there has been little progress in characterizing the function of these additional mutations.[247]

The transcription factor p53 guards against DNA damage, and mutations of the *p53* gene have been reported in more than 50% of human cancers. Mutations of *p53* are not common in ATL, but Tax inhibits the function of *p53* through other mechanisms.[248-250] Ubiquitination of Tax attenuates its transcriptional activity.[251,252] As opposed to in vitro models of transformation, Tax is not expressed in approximately 60% of ATL cases.[253] Analyses of HTLV-I provirus in ATL cases showed three mechanisms to inactivate Tax expression: (1) genetic changes of the *tax* gene,[253,254] (2) DNA methylation of the 5′LTR,[253,255,256] and (3) deletion of the 5′LTR.[257,258]

Pneumocystis jirovecii pneumonia, cryptococcal meningitis, disseminated fungal infections, and other opportunistic infections are often present[259] and contribute to a rapid progression to death for patients with acute and lymphoma-type ATL. The fact that *Strongyloides stercoralis* seems to be a common concurrent infection[260-262] has led to speculation that *Strongyloides* infection may be a cofactor in the development of ATL.[263] The state of immune compromise resulting from HTLV-I infection is not due to the type of immune ablation observed in HIV-1, even though CD4 cells are infected by HTLV-I; rather, the immunodeficiency is associated with rapidly proliferating malignancy and the pattern of opportunistic infections is typical for those reported in patients with other types of aggressive non-Hodgkin's lymphomas. In nonendemic regions, the diagnosis of ATL is suggested by the presence of HTLV-I antibodies in serum from patients with the char-

acteristic features of T-cell malignancy, and is confirmed by the demonstration of monoclonal integration of HTLV-I provirus in tumor tissue or leukemic lymphocytes. Measurement of HTLV-I proviral load is not helpful because levels in ATL are not consistently elevated as they are in HAM, and therefore do not discriminate among ATL, HAM, or a subset of healthy carriers. In some cases of ATL in patients from high-risk areas with typical clinical features, antibody is absent, but a defective integrated virus with retained *tax* function can be detected with PCR.[264]

There is little evidence that HTLV-I is associated with solid tumors or hematologic malignancies other than ATL. Arisawa and colleagues[265] reported a 6-year prospective study of 4297 adults, including 1063 HTLV-I seropositives, living in 4 towns in the Nagasaki Prefecture in southwestern Japan. After excluding ATL, there were 129 neoplasms and HTLV-I was not associated with an increased risk of cancer mortality (relative risk = 1.1; 95% confidence interval, 0.77-1.7). Previous case-control studies that showed associations between HTLV-I infection and cancer may have been confounded by blood transfusion or genetic predisposition.[266,267] Of interest, a recent study found a lower risk of gastric carcinoma in HTLV-I patients: 61.7% of HTLV-I–positive subjects were positive for *Helicobacter pylori* antibodies, compared with 71.6% of the HTLV-I–negative group.[268] There were only 14 cases (2.8%) of gastric cancer in the HTLV-I–positive subjects compared with 35 cases (7%) in the HTLV-I–negative group (adjusted odds ratio = 0.38; 95% confidence interval, 0.21-0.70).

The differential diagnosis of ATL includes other T-cell malignancies, such as non-Hodgkin's lymphoma, mycosis fungoides, and Sézary syndrome. ATL should be suspected in any patient with a T-cell malignancy who is from an endemic population or has risk factors for HTLV-I. The presence of circulating flower cells, hypercalcemia, and skin lesions is highly suggestive. Leukemic cells are characteristically terminal deoxynucleotide-transferase negative CD4$^+$ and CD25$^+$. Laboratory detection and confirmation can be based on testing for anti–HTLV-I antibody or demonstrating via Southern blot or reverse transcriptase–PCR monoclonal integration of HTLV-I proviral DNA in the malignant cells.

HUMAN T-CELL LYMPHOTROPIC VIRUS-ASSOCIATED MYELOPATHY

HAM, or tropical spastic paraparesis, is a chronic progressive demyelinating disease that affects the spinal cord and white matter of the CNS.[269-273] The incidence of HAM in HTLV-I carriers is estimated to be less than 4%.[228] HAM has been linked to blood transfusion, and some cases are acutely progressive.[207,274,275] Familial clusters have also been reported. Although HAM mainly affects adults, particularly females, cases occasionally occur in children under the age of 10. The overrepresentation of females may reflect a higher occurrence of HAM following sexually acquired rather than vertical infection.[276]

The typical time of disease onset is in the fourth decade of life. The onset is often subtle, and the florid clinical picture of HAM is not always seen at first presentation. A single symptom or physical sign may be the only evidence of early HAM. Patients often present with a stiff gait,[277] progressing (usually slowly) to increasing spasticity and lower extremity weakness,[278] back pain, urinary incontinence,[279,280] and impotence in men. Patients may report sensory symptoms such as tingling, "pins and needles," and burning. Vibration sense is frequently impaired.[281] Hyperreflexia of lower limbs, often with clonus and Babinski's sign, is frequently found. Hyperreflexia of the upper limbs is less common, but may occur in severe cases, whereas upper limb weakness is rare. Exaggerated jaw jerk is seen in some patients, and ataxia may develop.

Nuclear magnetic resonance images may be normal or show atrophy of the spinal cord and nonspecific lesions in the brain.[279,282-284] The syndrome is significantly different from classic multiple sclerosis. HAM follows a slow course without the waxing and waning of symptoms, changes in affect, or multiple nuclear magnetic resonance scan abnormalities characteristic of multiple sclerosis. Varying degrees of brain parenchymal degeneration have also been described, with reactive astrocytosis and perivascular mononuclear cell infiltration.[270] These mononuclear cells are predominantly CD8+ lymphocytes,[271,285] suggesting that an immune mechanism may play a role in the development of HAM. The high frequency of cytolytic T cells with specificity directed against major histocompatibility class I–restricted epitopes derived from the Tax protein has also been observed.[286]

It is possible that HTLV-I induces an autoimmune-like process through molecular mimicry (an autoimmune model) or through indirect effects on immune function (a cytotoxic model). In the former model, it is postulated that HTLV-I infection activates autoreactive T cells, which then cause autoimmune destruction within the CNS.[287,288] In the latter model, it is postulated that HTLV-I infects glial cells, which subsequently induces a cytotoxic immune response against these cells, leading to demyelination.[285]

HAM patients characteristically have HTLV-I antibodies or antigens in the blood and cerebrospinal fluid. Cerebrospinal fluid may show mild lymphocytic pleocytosis; lobulated lymphocytes with morphologic similarity to ATL cells (flower cells) (see Fig. 168-12) also may be present in the blood and cerebrospinal fluid.[278] Mild to moderate increases in protein may be observed in the CSF, and oligoclonal bonds with specific reactivity to HTLV-I antigens have been detected.[277,278] Lymphokines such as IL-6, tumor necrosis factor-α, and IL-2 are increased in the CSF. However, attempts to document the presence of HTLV-I in the demyelinated lesion have not demonstrated a direct role of the virus in neurons.

Differential diagnoses of HAM include multiple sclerosis, spinal-cord tumors or extrinsic compression, toxic neuropathies, malnutrition, and HIV or syphilis infection. The diagnosis is suspected in unexplained central nervous system disease with loss of pyramidal tract functions and is confirmed by testing sera for HTLV-I antibodies. In contrast to lymphocytes in ATL, HTLV-I–infected lymphocytes in HAM are oligoclonal or polyclonal rather than monoclonal.[289]

Neurologic abnormalities other than HAM have also been reported with HTLV-I infection, including sensory neuropathy,[290-292] gait abnormalities,[293,294] bladder dysfunction,[290,293-296] erectile dysfunction,[297,298] amyotrophic lateral sclerosis,[299] mild cognitive deficits,[300] and, rarely, motor neuropathies.[290,292,297,301-303] It is unclear whether these abnormalities indicate future progression to HAM or that HAM is simply the "tip of the iceberg" of a broader spectrum of neurologic manifestations associated with HTLV infection.[304]

OTHER DISEASES ASSOCIATED WITH HUMAN T-CELL LYMPHOTROPIC VIRUS TYPE I

Polymyositis of skeletal muscle is rarely associated with HTLV-I seropositivity in viral endemic areas.[303,305] These cases are indistinguishable from polymyositis seen in HTLV-I nonendemic areas. A large joint polyarthropathy has been reported in Japan among elderly patients.[306,307] A distinguishing feature of these cases is the presence of HTLV-I–producing cells in the synovial infiltrate. Recently, a unique form of uveitis has been observed in HTLV-I–positive individuals. These cases account for about 30% to 40% of idiopathic uveitis in HTLV-I endemic areas.[308] The first evidence of an association of HTLV-I infection with uveitis was reported by Ohba and colleagues in Japan, who detected ocular involvement in patients with ATL and HAM and asymptomatic carriers.[309] The ocular manifestations were then classified into three groups: (1) opportunistic infections and tumor infiltration in ATL patients; (2) ocular alterations in HAM patients, including Sjögren's syndrome, retinal pigmentary degeneration, optic atrophy, vitreous opacities, cotton-wool spots, and retinal vasculitis; and (3) HTLV-I uveitis in asymptomatic carriers. Proviral DNA of HTLV-I was identified in 60% of T cells from intraocular fluid of these patients.[309,310] HTLV-I–associated infiltrative pneumonitis has also been reported in some individuals in Japan.[311,312]

The association of HTLV-I with parasitic infestations (e.g., *Strongyloides*) refractory to treatment has also been interpreted to suggest that HTLV-I may have immunosuppressive effects.[261,313,314] A variety of sub-

clinical perturbations in hematologic markers, such as depressed hemoglobin and lymphopenia, have been reported in healthy HTLV-I carriers.[315] In addition, a recent study showed that HTLV-I subjects had higher platelet counts (+16,544 cells/mm³) than seronegative subjects.[316]

The infective dermatitis syndrome was first shown to be HTLV-I associated in Jamaica.[317] It has also been seen in Trinidad and Tobago,[318] Colombia,[319] the Dominican Republic,[320] Brazil,[321] and Africa,[322] but very rarely in Japan, despite the high frequency of HTLV-I carriers.[323] It seems to represent the first childhood HTLV-I syndrome. Patients are born of HTLV-I–positive mothers and experience a failure to thrive syndrome. They are prone to refractory generalized eczema and infection with saprophytic *Staphylococcus* and *Streptococcus* bacteria that are suppressed by long-term antibiotic therapy and recur when the therapy is stopped. This syndrome usually emerges early in life, in the first few years after birth, and may persist into adulthood. Anecdotal cases emerging in adolescence suggest that some infective dermatitis cases may result from infection at an older age. It is postulated that infective dermatitis is an immunodeficiency syndrome induced by HTLV-I. Interestingly, some patients go on to develop ATL and HAM.[323,324] Further study of the pathogenesis of this syndrome should provide valuable insights into the pathogenesis of HTLV-I–associated diseases.

Other possible consequences of HTLV-I infection include persistent lymphadenopathy in offspring of HTLV-I–positive women (including HTLV uninfected children),[163] and waxing and waning lymphadenopathy seen in adult carriers.[294] This lymphadenopathy may be a manifestation of a primary or secondary immune response to HTLV infection. The influence of HTLV-I/HIV-1 on the progression to AIDS is controversial because soluble factors produced by HTLV-I–infected cells can either enhance or inhibit replication of HIV-I. The findings of several epidemiologic and in vitro studies have been mixed,[182,325-332] suggesting that differences in study outcomes may be due to phenotypic differences in HIV-1 clinical disease.[333] It is noteworthy that HTLV-I/HIV-1 coinfected persons have increased CD4 counts, but still develop opportunistic infections.[334]

DISEASES ASSOCIATED WITH HUMAN T-CELL LYMPHOTROPIC VIRUS TYPE II

Although the disease associations with HTLV-II are less clear than those with HTLV-I, there is accumulating evidence showing a link to HAM, as well as to other neurologic abnormalities.[10] Prospective studies of former blood donors who are HTLV-II infected have shown that they are at increased risk of developing HAM,[335] although their incidence is lower than that reported for HTLV-I carriers.[275,336] Among these infected individuals, HTLV-II proviral loads appeared to be lower than HTLV-I proviral loads, which may explain why HTLV-II has been less associated with the development of disease.[275,337] There have been four cases of HTLV-II HAM in the HTLV Outcomes Study,[228] and there are a number of HTLV-II HAM case reports in the literature.[338-344] Sensory neuropathy has been observed with HTLV-II alone[345] and with HIV coinfection.[345-348] In addition, a spinocerebellar syndrome has been documented in HTLV-II–infected patients.[349]

HTLV-II infection has also been diagnosed in certain rare hematologic malignancies, including atypical hairy cell leukemia[5,350] and with some cases of large granular lymphocytic leukemia[351] and mycosis fungoides.[352] Systematic surveys have not identified a clear association of these lymphoid malignancies with HTLV-II, suggesting that these patients may be coincidentally infected. One retrospective study of HTLV-II–positive drug users showed an excess of asthma-related deaths and an increased frequency of skin and soft tissue infections.[353] In a prospective cohort study, HTLV-II has been associated with pulmonary disease, arthritis, and urinary symptoms.[63] HTLV-II subjects also had higher mean lymphocyte counts (+7%) and platelet counts over 14 years of follow-up.[316] Finally, HTLV-II has been associated with increased overall mortality, although a single cause of death did not predominate.[354]

In contrast to the possible association between HTLV-I and accelerated HIV-1/AIDS progression, some studies of HTLV-II/HIV-1 coinfected persons suggest a neutral or protective effect, especially among those with high HTLV-II proviral loads, possibly as a result of chemokine overproduction.[355,356] Further studies are needed to confirm these findings.

Treatment

Although first-generation nucleoside analogues, such as zidovudine and lamivudine, have long been recognized to have activity against HTLV reverse transcription in vitro, there is little clinical evidence of their efficacy in vivo.[357] This, together with the asymptomatic nature of HTLV-I and -II and the low penetrance of HTLV diseases, means that treatment of asymptomatic HTLV carriers is not indicated. Furthermore, the exact role of HTLV-I in disease pathogenesis has not been clearly defined. In ATL, active viral replication does not appear to play a role in established malignant disease and tumor cells harbor oncogenic mutations in cell-regulatory genes that may not be reversible by treating the virus. HAM, with its high viral load and substantial cell-mediated immune response to HTLV-I, would appear to be a better candidate for antiviral treatment. A combination of zidovudine and lamivudine was used in a clinical trial of HAM treatment, but no clinical improvement was seen, and there was no effect on HTLV-I proviral load or immunologic markers.[358] Therapy that targets the immune response itself may afford an equally attractive avenue for the experimental treatment of HAM. Because of the shared routes of exposure, there is a potential opportunity to investigate the impact of antiviral therapy on persons coinfected with HTLV-I or -II and HIV-1. In fact, HTLV-II proviral load actually increased after highly active antiretroviral therapy in patients with HIV-1/HTLV-II coinfection.[359] The increase in HTLV-II proviral load appeared to correlate with the magnitude of CD4+ lymphocyte proliferation after successful control of HIV viral load, suggesting a clonal rebound of HTLV-II–infected lymphocytes.

ASYMPTOMATIC HUMAN T-CELL LYMPHOTROPIC VIRUS TYPES I AND II CARRIERS

Evaluation and treatment of asymptomatic HTLV-I and HTLV-II carriers are the most frequently encountered clinical situations and generally follow HTLV diagnostic screening of asymptomatic blood, tissue, sperm, or oocyte donors. The first step is to confirm HTLV infection, either by review of positive screening EIA and confirmatory tests performed by a reputable testing laboratory or by submission of another specimen. False-positive results are common using EIA alone in low-risk patients; these patients may be relieved of a burdensome diagnosis by the simple performance of a confirmatory assay. Typing of the infection as HTLV-I or HTLV-II is important because of the different disease outcomes associated with the two viral types. This can be done either by type-specific WB or slot blot, differential titration on immunoassay, or PCR. A clinical history regarding risk factors for HTLV infection is important in establishing the pretest probability of infection and can be helpful in typing the infection. Familial or sexual contact with people from HTLV-I endemic areas favors that infection, whereas a history of injection drug use or sex with an injection drug user is more consistent with HTLV-II infection. As mentioned earlier, patients with indeterminate WB results are also unlikely to be infected if they have no risk factors for HTLV infection.

Asymptomatic seropositive patients should be followed by their primary care or infectious disease physician with annual to biannual return visits. Medical history should elicit symptoms of leukemia, lymphoma, or neurologic disease. Physical examination is directed at the skin, lymph nodes, and neurologic system to detect manifestations of HTLV dermatitis, ATL, or HAM. Laboratory evaluation may be limited to a complete blood count. Whereas increases in the absolute lymphocyte and platelet counts have been described in prospective studies of HTLV-I and -II carriers, there is no indication that these

have clinical significance.[316] It is more important to rule out subclinical leukemia by a normal lymphocyte count and absence of flower cell morphology. In general, asymptomatic carriers or those with nonspecific symptoms should be reassured by reminding them of the low penetrance of hematologic and neurologic disease. Attention should be devoted to counseling regarding the prevention of further HTLV transmission by the use of condoms and safe sexual practices and by the avoidance of breast-feeding newborn infants born to HTLV-infected women (at least in developed countries). There is also substantial psychological and social morbidity associated with chronic HTLV infection, and the physician needs to probe for and address these issues.[360]

ADULT T-CELL LEUKEMIA

ATL patients are treated with antitumor chemotherapy, using therapies that are routinely used for non-HTLV-I–positive lymphoproliferative diseases. Patients with chronic and smoldering ATL are not treated or are given prednisone with or without cyclophosphamide; aggressive treatment of these relatively indolent forms of ATL leads to high rates of complicating infections. The acute and lymphoma types of ATL are aggressive high-grade lymphomas with a generally poor prognosis, although prolonged remissions are seen.[233,259,361] In Japan, large trials of vincristine, cyclophosphamide, prednisolone, and doxorubicin with the addition of methotrexate, as well as more complex 9- and 10-drug regimens, have shown some success without prolonging long-term survival.[361,362] Initial response rates, even for the poorest risk categories, are more than 50%, and complete remissions are achieved in 20% of patients, but these responses can be short-lived with relapses occurring in weeks to months.[361] Poor prognostic factors include poor performance status at diagnosis, age over 40 years, extensive disease, hypercalcemia, and high serum lactate dehydrogenase level. Approximately 13% to 15% of patients with such aggressive cases experience long-term survival (>2 years), which in one study was associated with several factors: complete remission, longer time to remission, and total doxorubicin dose. Relapses in these long-term survivors often occurred in the central nervous system and proved refractory to subsequent therapy. Studies using combinations of doxorubicin and etoposide have demonstrated complete remission rates of 40%.

Substantial improvements in therapy have been achieved with newer regimens combining zidovudine and interferon-α.[363] Although its mechanism of action is not well defined, this combination produces a high rate of complete responses and prolongs survival.[364-367] Recently adopted therapy approaches for high-grade lymphomas, such as allogeneic bone marrow transplantation and autologous stem cell transplantation, have resulted in remission and should be strongly considered in younger patients.[368] One case showed reappearance of cells harboring the integration of HTLV-I previously observed in his leukemia cells, but the patient continued in clinical remission, suggesting a possible reversion to the preleukemic carrier state.[369] Experimental approaches that use arsenic trioxide or toxin-linked monoclonal antibodies targeting the IL-2R specific to ATL cells are being tested, with some evidence of at least partial responses.[237,370,371]

HUMAN T-CELL LYMPHOTROPIC VIRUS TYPE I–ASSOCIATED MYELOPATHY AND TROPICAL SPASTIC PARAPARESIS

Advances in the treatment of HAM have been hindered by the difficulty of performing randomized clinical trials because most cases occur in resource-limited countries. Traditionally, immunosuppressive therapy with corticosteroids,[272,372] cyclophosphamide,[373] or both has been used to some benefit, particularly in acutely progressive cases. However, toxicity limits the long-term use of these drugs. More recently, interferon-α and interferon-β1a have shown some clinical benefit, but fall short of definitive treatment.[374-376] Danazol, an androgenic steroid, has been used for symptomatic treatment of bladder and bowel symptoms resulting from spinal cord involvement in HAM, but it does not reverse the underlying neurologic deficit.[377] Experimental studies, such as the use of anti-TAC antibodies directed against CD25 IL-2R α-chain concurrently with zidovudine[378,379] and therapies currently being implemented for multiple sclerosis, may be of value because the mechanism of immune pathogenesis may be shared in the two diseases. Given the emerging picture of disease pathogenesis with the inability to control high viral expression, therapy with antiviral drugs would seem a promising avenue for research, but initial clinical trials of antiretroviral therapy have not been successful.[358]

Prevention

Guidelines for prevention and counseling have been developed for HTLV-I and HTLV-II by a Centers for Disease Control and Prevention working group.[380] Standard prevention approaches address each of the routes of transmission and are similar for both viruses: screen blood donations before transfusion, eliminate breast-feeding by known infected mothers (or, where this is not feasible, limit breast-feeding to the first 6 months of life), and advise the use of condoms.

The value of blood donor screening has been well documented in Japan, where up to 15% of HTLV-I infections have been eliminated. In areas where the infection is not endemic, such as the United States, the cost-effectiveness of screening has been questioned, but because of the risk of HAM in the transfusion setting, all blood bank units in the United States are screened.

In the United States and Europe, it is recommended that pregnant women who are HTLV-I positive should not breast-feed their infants. However, in developing countries where safe alternatives to breast-feeding may not be available, limiting breast-feeding to the first 6 months may afford some protection via maternal antibodies, although the safety of this approach would need to be studied in clinical trials before a recommendation could be made. The use of condoms is recommended for couples who are serodiscordant for HTLV infection. Given the relatively low frequency of sexual transmission for each sexual encounter, couples who desire a pregnancy could plan to have unprotected sex during periods of maximal fertility. Such decisions require careful discussion between physician and patient, and there are no absolute guidelines in this particular area.

Population-based screening for HTLV infection (except for blood donors) is generally not indicated because of the low penetrance of disease and lack of effective therapies. Counseling seropositive patients should involve a clear discussion of the distinction of HTLV from HIV. In addition, HTLV type should be defined by serologic methods, and the distinctions in disease associations of the two virus types should be emphasized. Because the populations at risk of HIV are also at risk of HTLV-I in viral endemic areas (e.g., persons at risk of sexually transmitted diseases, persons with high rates of partner exchange, commercial sex workers), HIV prevention guidelines also benefit those at risk of HTLV-I. Thus, prevention measures that promote condom use, treatment of sexually transmitted infections, and decrease of high-risk exposures also prevent HTLV-I infection.

There is no therapy for HTLV-I infection and thus no chemoprophylaxis. Passive immunoprophylaxis is hypothetically effective, as noted above in animal studies, but has no practical clinical application, given the low risk of transmission, except through sexual contact, breast-feeding, and transfusion exposure, where other prevention methods are more applicable.

Although vaccines against HTLV-I are feasible, due to the low attack rate for disease, there has been little impetus to develop or market an HTLV-I vaccine. Experimentally, vaccines containing whole virus and recombinant HTLV-I envelope antigens have successfully prevented HTLV-I infection in monkey and rabbit models. Protection correlates with the presence of neutralizing antibodies, indicating that humoral immunity can be an effective barrier against infection even when the challenge is cell-associated.[215,381] The HTLV-I envelope is relatively highly conserved, and neutralizing antibody appears to protect against challenge with even major strain variants, consistent with the conclusion that a single serotype protects against all variants. Thus, a synthetic vaccine against one HTLV-I isolate could protect against other HTLV-I isolates. A vaccine that induces cell-mediated immune responses in nonhuman primate studies has also been shown to be effective. Whether a vaccine will ever be implemented in human populations in endemic areas has been questioned.

Summary

The study of HTLV-I and -II is important for public health, clinical, and scientific reasons. In the years since the discovery of this first human leukemia virus, significant progress has been made in understanding the epidemiology and routes of transmission of HTLV. Routes of transmission for HTLV-I and -II are reasonably well defined and include sexual and parenteral routes, which are being addressed by HIV prevention. Knowledge of the clinical outcomes of HTLV infection has expanded since the discoveries of the relationships between HTLV-I and ATL and between HTLV-I and -II and HAM. A growing array of syndromes related to the virologic or immunologic effects of these retroviruses has been recognized, and prospective observational cohorts of persons infected with HTLV-I and -II will yield additional data on their clinical outcomes. The mortality rate resulting directly from ATL or complications of HAM is approximately 5%, and both diseases have substantial morbidity. With millions of people estimated to be infected by HTLV-I worldwide[382] and a lack of effective therapy, prevention efforts are important. Blood transfusions need to be screened, sexual transmission prevented by condom use, and breast-feeding by HTLV-infected mothers limited, although the latter approach may not be feasible in developing countries.

From a scientific viewpoint, the HTLVs offer interesting models for understanding the interplay between chronic retroviral infection and the human immune system, as well as the pathologic mechanisms of related diseases. Understanding the virology, immunology, and pathogenesis of HTLV infection may be relevant to the study of HIV disease, multiple sclerosis, and leukemia/lymphoma. It is also conceivable that additional viruses of this class with long latency, low-level replication, and specific cellular tropism may be discovered in unexplained autoimmune, neurologic, and malignant diseases.

ACKNOWLEDGMENTS

The authors thank William Blattner, MD, and Manhattan Charurat, PhD, who authored the chapter on this topic in the previous edition.

REFERENCES

1. Poiesz BJ, Ruscetti FW, Gazdar AF, et al. Detection and isolation of type C retrovirus particles from fresh and cultured lymphocytes of a patient with cutaneous T-cell lymphoma. *Proc Natl Acad Sci U S A.* 1980;77:7415-7419.
2. Poiesz BJ, Ruscetti FW, Reitz MS, et al. Isolation of a new type C retrovirus (HTLV) in primary uncultured cells of a patient with Sezary T-cell leukaemia. *Nature.* 1981;294:268-271.
3. Yoshida M, Miyoshi I, Hinuma Y. Isolation and characterization of retrovirus from cell lines of human adult T-cell leukemia and its implication in the disease. *Proc Natl Acad Sci U S A.* 1982;79:2031-2035.
4. Watanabe T, Seiki M, Yoshida M. HTLV type I (U.S. isolate) and ATLV (Japanese isolate) are the same species of human retrovirus. *Virology.* 1984;133:238-241.
5. Kalyanaraman VS, Sarngadharan MG, Robert-Guroff M, et al. A new subtype of human T-cell leukemia virus (HTLV-II) associated with a T-cell variant of hairy cell leukemia. *Science.* 1982;218:571-573.
6. Barre-Sinoussi F, Chermann JC, Rey F, et al. Isolation of a T-lymphotropic retrovirus from a patient at risk for acquired immune deficiency syndrome (AIDS). *Science.* 1983;220: 868-871.
7. Gallo RC, Sarin PS, Gelmann EP, et al. Isolation of human T-cell leukemia virus in acquired immune deficiency syndrome (AIDS). *Science.* 1987;220:865-867.
8. Gallo RC, Salahuddin SZ, Popovic M, et al. Frequent detection and isolation of cytopathic retroviruses (HTLV-III) from patients with AIDS and at risk for AIDS. *Science.* 1984;224: 500-503.
9. van Regenmortel M, Fauquet C, Bishop D, et al. *Virus Taxonomy: The Classification and Nomenclature of Viruses. The Seventh Report of the International Committee on Taxonomy of Viruses.* San Diego: Academic Press; 2000.

10. Araujo A, Hall WW. Human T-lymphotropic virus type II and neurological disease. *Ann Neurol.* 2004;56:10-19.
11. Shimotohno K, Takahashi Y, Shimizu N, et al. Complete nucleotide sequence of an infectious clone of human T-cell leukemia virus type II: an open reading frame for the protease gene. *Proc Natl Acad Sci U S A.* 1985;82:3101-3105.
12. Haseltine WA, Sodroski J, Patarca R, et al. Structure of 3′ terminal region of type II human T-lymphotropic virus: evidence for new coding region. *Science.* 1984;225:419-424.
13. Shimotohno K, Wachsman W, Takahashi Y, et al. Nucleotide sequence of the 3′ region of an infectious human T-cell leukemia virus type II genome. *Proc Natl Acad Sci U S A.* 1984; 81:6657-6661.
14. Seiki M, Hattori S, Hirayama Y, et al. Human adult T-cell leukemia virus: complete nucleotide sequence of the provirus genome integrated in leukemia cell DNA. *Proc Natl Acad Sci U S A.* 1983;80:3618-3622.
15. Lairmore MD, Albrecht B, D'Souza C, et al. In vitro and in vivo functional analysis of human T cell lymphotropic virus type 1 pX open reading frames I and II. *AIDS Res Hum Retroviruses.* 2000;16:1757-1764.
16. Gaudray G, Gachon F, Basbous J, et al. The complementary strand of the human T-cell leukemia virus type 1 RNA genome encodes a bZIP transcription factor that down-regulates viral transcription. *J Virol.* 2002;76:12813-12822.
17. Slamon DJ, Shimotohno K, Cline MJ, et al. Identification of the putative transforming protein of the human T-cell leukemia viruses HTLV-I and HTLV-II. *Science.* 1984;226:61-65.
18. Lee TH, Coligan JE, Sodroski JG, et al. Antigens encoded by the 3′-terminal region of human T-cell leukemia virus: evidence for a functional gene. *Science.* 1984;226:57-61.
19. Ross TM, Pettiford SM, Green PL. The *tax* gene of human T-cell leukemia virus type 2 is essential for transformation of human T lymphocytes. *J Virol.* 1996;70:5194-5202.
20. Umehara F, Izumo S, Ronquillo AT, et al. Cytokine expression in the spinal cord lesions in HTLV-I-associated myelopathy. *J Neuropathol Exp Neurol.* 1994;53:72-77.
21. Yoshida M. Multiple viral strategies of HTLV-1 for dysregulation of cell growth control. *Annu Rev Immunol.* 2001; 19:475-496.
22. Green PL, Xie YM, Chen IS. The Rex proteins of human T-cell leukemia virus type II differ by serine phosphorylation. *J Virol.* 1991;65:546-550.
23. Kiyokawa T, Seiki M, Iwashita S, et al. p27x-III and p21x-III, proteins encoded by the pX sequence of human T-cell leukemia virus type I. *Proc Natl Acad Sci U S A.* 1985;82:8359-8363.
24. Ahmed YF, Hanly SM, Malim MH, et al. Structure-function analyses of the HTLV-I Rex and HIV-1 Rev RNA response elements: insights into the mechanism of Rex and Rev action. *Genes Dev.* 1990;4:1014-1022.
25. Hanly SM, Rimsky LT, Malim MH, et al. Comparative analysis of the HTLV-I Rex and HIV-1 Rev trans-regulatory proteins and their RNA response elements. *Genes Dev.* 1989;3:1534-1544.
26. Itoh M, Inoue J, Toyoshima H, et al. HTLV-1 Rex and HIV-1 Rev act through similar mechanisms to relieve suppression of unspliced RNA expression. *Oncogene.* 1989;4:1275-1279.
27. Nosaka T, Siomi H, Adachi Y, et al. Nucleolar targeting signal of human T-cell leukemia virus type I Rex-encoded protein is essential for cytoplasmic accumulation of unspliced viral mRNA. *Proc Natl Acad Sci U S A.* 1989;86:9798-9802.
28. Siomi H, Shida H, Nam SH, et al. Sequence requirements for nucleolar localization of human T cell leukemia virus type I pX protein, which regulates viral RNA processing. *Cell.* 1988;55:197-209.
29. Bogerd HP, Tiley LS, Cullen BR. Specific binding of the human T-cell leukemia virus type I Rex protein to a short RNA sequence located within the Rex-response element. *J Virol.* 1992;66:7572-7575.
30. Grassmann R, Berchtold S, Aepinus C, et al. In vitro binding of human T-cell leukemia virus Rex proteins to the Rex-response element of viral transcripts. *J Virol.* 1991;65:3721-3727.
31. Yip MT, Dynan WS, Green PL, et al. Human T-cell leukemia virus (HTLV) type II Rex protein binds specifically to RNA sequences of the HTLV long terminal repeat but poorly to the human immunodeficiency virus type 1 Rev-responsive element. *J Virol.* 1991;65:2261-2272.
32. Bakker A, Li X, Ruland CT, et al. Human T-cell leukemia virus type 2 Rex inhibits pre-mRNA splicing in vitro at an early stage of spliceosome formation. *J Virol.* 1996;70:5511-5518.
33. Watanabe CT, Rosenblatt JD, Bakker A, et al. Negative regulation of gene expression from the HTLV type II long terminal repeat by Rex: functional and structural dissociation from posttive posttranscriptional regulation. *AIDS Res Hum Retroviruses.* 1996;12:535-546.
34. Albrecht B, D'Souza CD, Ding W, et al. Activation of nuclear factor of activated T cells by human T-lymphotropic virus type 1 accessory protein p12(I). *J Virol.* 2002;76:3493-3501.
35. Ding W, Albrecht B, Kelley RE, et al. Human T-cell lymphotropic virus type 1 p12(I) expression increases cytoplasmic calcium to enhance the activation of nuclear factor of activated T cells. *J Virol.* 2002;76:10374-10382.
36. Franchini G. HTLV and immortalization/transformation: current concepts and clinical relevance. *AIDS Res Hum Retroviruses.* 2001;17:S-5.
37. Satou Y, Yasunaga J, Yoshida M, et al. HTLV-I basic leucine zipper factor gene mRNA supports proliferation of adult T cell leukemia cells. *Proc Natl Acad Sci U S A.* 2006;103:720-725.
38. Manel N, Kim FJ, Kinet S, et al. The ubiquitous glucose transporter GLUT-1 is a receptor for HTLV. *Cell.* 2003;115: 449-459.
39. Richardson JH, Edwards AJ, Cruickshank JK, et al. In vivo cellular tropism of human T-cell leukemia virus type 1. *J Virol.* 1990;64:5682-5687.
40. Kinoshita K, Yamanouchi K, Ikeda S, et al. Oral infection of a common marmoset with human T-cell leukemia virus type-I (HTLV-I) by inoculating fresh human milk of HTLV-I carrier mothers. *Jpn J Cancer Res.* 1985;76:1147-1153.
41. Nagai M, Brennan MB, Sakai JA, et al. CD8(+) T cells are an in vivo reservoir for human T-cell lymphotropic virus type I. *Blood.* 2001;98:1858-1861.
42. Ijichi S, Ramundo MB, Takahashi H, et al. In vivo cellular tropism of human T cell leukemia virus type II (HTLV-II). *J Exp Med.* 1992;176:293-296.
43. Donegan E, Lee H, Operskalski EA, et al. Transfusion transmission of retroviruses: human T-lymphotropic virus types I and II compared with human immunodeficiency virus type 1. *Transfusion.* 1994;34:478-483.
44. Cesaire R, Kerob-Bauchet B, Bourdonne O, et al. Evaluation of HTLV-I removal by filtration of blood cell components in a routine setting. *Transfusion.* 2004;44:42-48.
45. Iwahara Y, Takehara N, Kataoka R, et al. Transmission of HTLV-I to rabbits via semen and breast milk from seropositive healthy persons. *Int J Cancer.* 1990;45:980-983.
46. Igakura T, Stinchcombe JC, Goon PK, et al. Spread of HTLV-I between lymphocytes by virus-induced polarization of the cytoskeleton. *Science.* 2003;299:1713-1716.
47. Bangham CR. The immune control and cell-to-cell spread of human T-lymphotropic virus type 1. *J Gen Virol.* 2003;84: 3177-3189.
48. Piguet V, Sattentau Q. Dangerous liaisons at the virological synapse. *J Clin Invest.* 2004;114:605-610.
49. Murphy EL, Lee TH, Chafets D, et al. Higher human T lymphotropic virus (HTLV) provirus load is associated with HTLV-I versus HTLV-II, with HTLV-II subtype A versus B, and with male sex and a history of blood transfusion. *J Infect Dis.* 2004;190:504-510.
50. Centers for Disease Control and Prevention. Licensure of screening tests for antibody to human T-lymphotropic virus type I. *MMWR Morb Mortal Wkly Rep.* 1988;37:736-747.
51. Madeleine MM, Wiktor SZ, Goedert JJ, et al. HTLV-I and HTLV-II world-wide distribution: reanalysis of 4,832 immunoblot results. *Int J Cancer.* 1993;54:255-260.
52. Roberts BD, Foung SK, Lipka JJ, et al. Evaluation of an immunoblot assay for serological confirmation and differentiation of human T-cell lymphotropic virus types I and II. *J Clin Microbiol.* 1993;31:260-264.
53. Kleinman SH, Kaplan JE, Khabbaz RF, et al. Evaluation of a p21e-spiked Western blot (immunoblot) in confirming human T-cell lymphotropic virus type I or II infection in volunteer blood donors. The Retrovirus Epidemiology Donor Study Group. *J Clin Microbiol.* 1994;32:603-607.
54. Lipka JJ, Santiago P, Chan L, et al. Modified Western blot assay for confirmation and differentiation of human T cell lymphotropic virus types I and II. *J Infect Dis.* 1991;164:400-403.
55. Blomberg J, Robert-Guroff M, Blattner WA, et al. Type- and group-specific continuous antigenic determinants of HTLV: use of synthetic peptides for serotyping of HTLV-I and -II infection. *J Acquir Immune Defic Syndr.* 1992;5:294-302.
56. Horal P, Hall WW, Svennerholm B, et al. Identification of type-specific linear epitopes in the glycoproteins gp46 and gp21 of human T-cell leukemia viruses type I and type II using synthetic peptides. *Proc Natl Acad Sci U S A.* 1991;88:5754-5758.
57. Sabino EC, Zrein M, Taborda CP, et al. Evaluation of the INNO-LIA HTLV I/II assay for confirmation of human T-cell leukemia virus-reactive sera in blood bank donations. *J Clin Microbiol.* 1999;37:1324-1328.
58. Mahieux R, Horal P, Mauclere P, et al. Human T-cell lymphotropic virus type 1 gag indeterminate Western blot patterns in Central Africa: relationship to *Plasmodium falciparum* infection. *J Clin Microbiol.* 2000;38:4049-4057.
59. Gallo D, Diggs JL, Hanson CV. Evaluation of two commercial human T-cell lymphotropic virus Western blot (immunoblot) kits with problem specimens. *J Clin Microbiol.* 1994;32:2046-2049.
60. Garin B, Gosselin S, de The G, et al. HTLV-I/II infection in a high viral endemic area of Zaire, Central Africa: comparative evaluation of serology, PCR, and significance of indeterminate Western blot pattern. *J Med Virol.* 1994;44:104-109.
61. Gessain A, Mathieux R. HTLV-I "indeterminate" Western blot patterns observed in sera from tropical regions: the situation revisited. *J Acquir Immune Defic Syndr Hum Retrovirol.* 1995;9:316-319.
62. Heneine W, Khabbaz RF, Lal RB, et al. Sensitive and specific polymerase chain reaction assays for diagnosis of human T-cell lymphotropic virus type I (HTLV-I) and HTLV-II infections in HTLV-I/II-seropositive individuals. *J Clin Microbiol.* 1992;30:1605-1607.
63. Lee TH, Chafets DM, Busch MP, et al. Quantitation of HTLV-I and II proviral load using real-time quantitative PCR with SYBR Green chemistry. *J Clin Virol.* 2004;31:275-282.
64. Busch MP, Laycock M, Kleinman SH, et al. Accuracy of supplementary serologic testing for human T-lymphotropic virus types I and II in US blood donors: retrovirus Epidemiology Donor Study. *Blood.* 1994;83:1143-1148.
65. Furnia A, Lal R, Maloney E, et al. Estimating the time of HTLV-I infection following mother-to-child transmission in a breast-feeding population in Jamaica. *J Med Virol.* 1999; 59:541-546.
66. Defer C, Coste J, Descamps F, et al. Contribution of polymerase chain reaction and radioimmunoprecipitation assay in the confirmation of human T-lymphotropic virus infection in French blood donors: Retrovirus Study Group of the French Society of Blood Transfusion. *Transfusion.* 1995;35:596-600.
67. Pate EJ, Wiktor SZ, Shaw GM, et al. Lack of viral latency of human T-cell lymphotropic virus type I. *N Engl J Med.* 1991;325:284.
68. Saito S, Ando Y, Furuki K, et al. Detection of HTLV-I genome in seronegative infants born to HTLV-I seropositive mothers by polymerase chain reaction. *Jpn J Cancer Res.* 1989; 80:808-812.
69. Rios M, Khabbaz RF, Kaplan JE, et al. Transmission of human T cell lymphotropic virus (HTLV) type II by transfusion of HTLV-I-screened blood products. *J Infect Dis.* 1994;170: 206-210.
70. Liu H, Shah M, Stramer SL, et al. Sensitivity and specificity of human T-lymphotropic virus (HTLV) types I and II polymerase chain reaction and several serologic assays in screening a population with a high prevalence of HTLV-II. *Transfusion.* 1999;39:1185-1193.
71. Wattel E, Vartanian JP, Pannetier C, et al. Clonal expansion of human T-cell leukemia virus type I-infected cells in asymptomatic and symptomatic carriers without malignancy. *J Virol.* 1995;69:2863-2868.
72. Yamano Y, Nagai M, Brennan M, et al. Correlation of human T-cell lymphotropic virus type 1 (HTLV-1) mRNA with proviral DNA load, virus-specific CD8(+) T cells, and disease severity in HTLV-1-associated myelopathy (HAM/TSP). *Blood.* 2002;99:88-94.
73. Manns A, Miley WJ, Wilks RJ, et al. Quantitative proviral DNA and antibody levels in the natural history of HTLV-I infection. *J Infect Dis.* 1999;180:1487-1493.
74. Kwaan N, Lee TH, Chafets DM, et al. Long-term variations in human T lymphotropic virus (HTLV)-I and HTLV-II proviral loads and association with clinical data. *J Infect Dis.* 2006;194:1557-1564.
75. Kajiyama W, Kashiwagi S, Nomura H, et al. Seroepidemiologic study of antibody to adult T-cell leukemia virus in Okinawa, Japan. *Am J Epidemiol.* 1986;123:41-47.
76. Hinuma Y, Komoda H, Chosa T, et al. Antibodies to adult T-cell leukemia-virus-associated antigen (ATLA) in sera from patients with ATL and controls in Japan: a nation-wide sero-epidemiologic study. *Int J Cancer.* 1982;29:631-635.
77. Tajima K. The 4th nation-wide study of adult T-cell leukemia/lymphoma (ATL) in Japan: estimates of risk of ATL and its geographical and clinical features. *Int J Cancer.* 1990;45: 237-243.
78. Mueller N, Tachibana N, Stuver SO, et al. Epidemiologic perspectives of HTLV-I. Blattner WA, ed. *Human Retrovirology: HTLV.* Philadelphia: Lippincott-Raven; 1990:281-293.
79. Geng L, Zai N, Xiao Y, et al. Search for human T-lymphotropic virus type I carriers among northeastern Chinese. *J Dermatol Sci.* 1998;18:30-34.
80. Au WY, Lo JY. HTLV-1-related lymphoma in Hong Kong Chinese. *Am J Hematol.* 2005;78:80-81.
81. Yanagihara R, Jenkins CL, Alexander SS, et al. Human T lymphotropic virus type I infection in Papua New Guinea: high prevalence among the Hagahai confirmed by Western analysis. *J Infect Dis.* 1990;162:649-654.
82. Blattner WA, Saxinger C, Riedel D, et al. A study of HTLV-I and its associated risk factors in Trinidad and Tobago. *J Acquir Immune Defic Syndr.* 1990;3:1102-1108.
83. Murphy EL, Figueroa JP, Gibs WN, et al. Human T-lymphotropic virus type I (HTLV-I) seroprevalence in Jamaica: I. Demographic determinants. *Am J Epidemiol.* 1991;133: 1114-1124.
84. Riedel DA, Evans AS, Saxinger C, et al. A historical study of human T lymphotropic virus type 1 transmission in Barbados. *Infect Control Hosp Epidemiol.* 1989;159:603-609.
85. Carneiro-Proietti AB, Catalan-Soares B, Proietti FA. Human T cell lymphotropic viruses (HTLV-I/II) in South America: should it be a public health concern? *J Biomed Sci.* 2002;9:587-595.
86. Bartholomew C, Charles W, Saxinger C, et al. Racial and other characteristics of human T cell leukaemia/lymphoma (HTLV-I) and AIDS (HTLV-III) in Trinidad. *Br Med J.* 1985;290: 1243-1246.
87. Maloney EM, Murphy EL, Figueroa JP, et al. Human T-lymphotropic virus type I (HTLV-I) seroprevalence in Jamaica: II. Geographic and ecologic determinants. *Am J Epidemiol.* 1991;133:1125-1134.
88. Blattner WA, Nomura A, Clark JW, et al. Modes of transmission and evidence for viral latency from studies of human T-cell lymphotrophic virus type I in Japanese migrant populations in Hawaii. *Proc Natl Acad Sci U S A.* 1986;83:4895-4898.
89. Murphy EL, Figueroa JP, Gibbs WN, et al. Sexual transmission of human T-lymphotropic virus type I (HTLV-I). *Ann Intern Med.* 1989;111:555-560.
90. Chen YM, Ting ST, Lee CM, et al. Community-based molecular epidemiology of HTLV type I in Taiwan and Kinmen: implication of the origin of the cosmopolitan subtype in northeast Asia. *AIDS Res Hum Retroviruses.* 1999;15:229-237.

91. Williams AE, Fang CT, Slamon DJ, et al. Seroprevalence and epidemiological correlates of HTLV-I infection in U.S. blood donors. *Science*. 1988;240:643-646.
92. Lee HH, Swanson P, Rosenblatt JD, et al. Relative prevalence and risk factors of HTLV-I and HTLV-II infection in U.S. blood donors. *Lancet*. 1991;337:1435-1439.
93. Murphy EL, Watanabe K, Nass CC, et al. Evidence among blood donors for a 30-year-old epidemic of human T lymphotropic virus type II infection in the United States. *J Infect Dis*. 1999;180:1777-1783.
94. Dosik H, Denic S, Patel N, et al. Adult T-cell leukemia/lymphoma in Brooklyn. *JAMA*. 1988;259:2255-2257.
95. Cruickshank JK, Richardson JH, Morgan OS, et al. Screening for prolonged incubation of HTLV-I infection in British and Jamaican relatives of British patients with tropical spastic paraparesis. *Br Med J*. 1990;300:300-304.
96. Catovsky D, Greaves MF, Rose M, et al. Adult T-cell lymphoma-leukaemia in Blacks from the West Indies. *Lancet*. 1982; 1:639-643.
97. Ho G, Nomura A, Nelson K, et al. Declining HTLV-I seroprevalence in Japanese immigrant population in Hawaii. *Am J Epidemiol*. 1991;134:981-987.
98. Blattner WA, Kalyanaraman VS, Robert-Guroff M, et al. The human type-C retrovirus, HTLV, in Blacks from the Caribbean region, and relationship to adult T-cell leukemia/lymphoma. *Int J Cancer*. 1982;30:257-264.
99. Delaporte E, Dupont A, Peeters M, et al. Epidemiology of HTLV-I in Gabon (Western Equatorial Africa). *Int J Cancer*. 1988;42:687-689.
100. Verdier M, Denis F, Sangare A, et al. Prevalence of antibody to human T cell leukemia virus type 1 (HTLV-1) in populations of Ivory Coast, West Africa. *J Infect Dis*. 1989;160:363-370.
101. Farid R, Etermadi M, Baradaran H, et al. Seroepidemiology and virology of HTLV-I in the city of Mashhad, northeastern Iran. *Serodiagn Immunother Infect Dis*. 1993;5:251.
102. Sidi Y, Meytes D, Shohat B, et al. Adult T-cell lymphoma in Israeli patients of Iranian origin. *Cancer*. 1990;65:590-593.
103. Lavanchy D, Bovet P, Hollanda J, et al. High seroprevalence of HTLV-I in the Seychelles. *Lancet*. 1991;337:248-249.
104. Gessain A, de The G. What is the situation of human T cell lymphotropic virus type II (HTLV-II) in Africa? Origin and dissemination of genomic subtypes. *J Acquir Immune Defic Syndr Hum Retrovirol*. 1996;13:S228-S235.
105. Gessain A, Mauclere P, Froment A, et al. Isolation and molecular characterization of a human T-cell lymphotropic virus type II (HTLV-II), subtype B, from a healthy Pygmy living in a remote area of Cameroon: an ancient origin for HTLV-II in Africa. *Proc Natl Acad Sci U S A*. 1995;92:4041-4045.
106. Goubau P, Liu HF, de Lange GG, et al. HTLV-II seroprevalence in Pygmies across Africa since 1970. *AIDS Research and Human Retroviruses*. 1993;9:709-713.
107. Lee HH, Weiss SH, Brown LS, et al. Patterns of HIV-1 and HTLV-I/II in intravenous drug abusers from the middle atlantic and central regions of the USA. *J Infect Dis*. 1990;162:347-352.
108. Biggar RJ, Buskell-Bales Z, Yakshe PN, et al. Antibody to human retroviruses among drug users in three East Coast American cities, 1972-1976. *J Infect Dis*. 1991;163:57-63.
109. Levine PH, Jacobson S, Elliott R, et al. HTLV-II infection in Florida Indians. *AIDS Res Hum Retroviruses*. 1993;9: 123-127.
110. Biggar RJ, Taylor ME, Neel JV, et al. Genetic variants of human T-lymphotrophic virus type II in American Indian groups. *Virology*. 1996;216:165-173.
111. Hjelle B, Scalf R, Swenson S. High frequency of human T-cell leukemia-lymphoma virus type II infection in New Mexico blood donors: determination by sequence-specific oligonucleotide hybridization. *Blood*. 1990;76:450-454.
112. Vandamme AM, Salemi M, Van Brussel M, et al. African origin of human T-lymphotropic virus type 2 (HTLV-2) supported by a potential new HTLV-2d subtype in Congolese Bambuti Efe Pygmies. *J Virol*. 1998;72:4327-4340.
113. Mueller N, Okayama A, Stuver S, et al. Findings from the Miyazaki Cohort Study. *J Acquir Immune Defic Syndr Hum Retrovirol*. 1996;13:S2-S7.
114. Proietti FA, Carneiro-Proietti AB, Catalan-Soares BC, et al. Global epidemiology of HTLV-I infection and associated diseases. *Oncogene*. 2005;24:6058-6068.
115. Maloney EM, Biggar RJ, Neel JV, et al. Endemic human T cell lymphotropic virus type II infection among isolated Brazilian Amerindians. *J Infect Dis*. 1992;166:100-107.
116. Vidal AU, Gessain A, Yoshida M, et al. Phylogenetic classification of human T cell leukaemia/lymphoma virus type I genotypes in five major molecular and geographical subtypes. *J Gen Virol*. 1994;75:3655-3666.
117. Slattery JP, Franchini G, Gessain A. Genomic evolution, patterns of global dissemination, and interspecies transmission of human and simian T-cell leukemia/lymphotropic viruses. *Genome Res*. 1999;9:525-540.
118. Gessain A, Gallo RC, Franchini G. Low degree of human T-cell leukemia/lymphoma virus type I genetic drift in vivo as a means of monitoring viral transmission and movement of ancient human populations. *J Virol*. 1992;66:2288-2295.
119. Komurian F, Pelloquin F, De The G. In vivo genomic variability of human T-cell leukemia virus type I depends more upon geography than upon pathologies. *J Virol*. 1991;65:3770-3778.
120. Malik KT, Even J, Karpas A. Molecular cloning and complete nucleotide sequence of an adult T cell leukaemia virus/human T cell leukaemia virus type I (ATLV/HTLV-I) isolate of Caribbean origin: relationship to other members of the ATLV/HTLV-I subgroup. *J Gen Virol*. 1988;69:1695-1710.
121. Gessian A, Yanagihara R, Franchini G, et al. Highly divergent molecular variants of human T-lymphotropic virus type I from isolated populations in Papua New Guinea and the Solomon Islands. *Proc Natl Acad Sci U S A*. 1991;88:7694-7698.
122. Song KJ, Nerurkar VR, Pereira-Cortez AJ, et al. Sequence and phylogenetic analyses of human T cell lymphotropic virus type 1 from a Brazilian woman with adult T cell leukemia: comparison with virus strains from South America and the Caribbean basin. *Am J Trop Med Hyg*. 1995;52:101-108.
123. Yang YC, Hsu TY, Liu MY, et al. Molecular subtyping of human T-lymphotropic virus type I (HTLV-I) by a nested polymerase chain reaction-restriction fragment length polymorphism analysis of the envelope gene: two distinct lineages of HTLV-I in Taiwan. *J Med Virol*. 1997;51:25-31.
124. Voevodin A, al-Mufti S, Farah S, et al. Molecular characterization of human T-lymphotropic virus, type 1 (HTLV-1) found in Kuwait: close similarity with HTLV-1 isolates originating from Mashhad, Iran. *AIDS Res Hum Retroviruses*. 1995;11: 1255-1259.
125. Koralnik IJ, Boeri E, Saxinger WC, et al. Phylogenetic associations of human and simian T-cell leukemia/lymphotropic virus type I strains: evidence for interspecies transmission. *J Virol*. 1994;68:2693-2707.
126. Liu HF, Goubau P, Van Brussel M, et al. The three human T-lymphotropic virus type I subtypes arose from three geographically distinct simian reservoirs. *J Gen Virol*. 1996;77: 359-368.
127. Vandamme AM, Liu HF, Van Brussel M, et al. The presence of a divergent T-lymphotropic virus in a wild-caught pygmy chimpanzee (Pan paniscus) supports an African origin for the human T-lymphotropic/simian T-lymphotropic group of viruses. *J Gen Virol*. 1996;77:1089-1099.
128. Mahieux R, Chappey C, Georges-Courbot MC, et al. Simian T-cell lymphotropic virus type 1 from Mandrillus sphinx as a simian counterpart of human T-cell lymphotropic virus type 1 subtype D. *J Virol*. 1998;72:10316-10322.
129. Wiktor SZ, Piot P, Mann JM, et al. Human T cell lymphotropic virus type I (HTLV-I) among female prostitutes in Kinshasa, Zaire. *J Infect Dis*. 1990;161:1073-1077.
130. Hinuma Y. Seroepidemiology of adult T-cell leukemia virus (HTLV-I/ATLV): origin of virus carriers in Japan. *AIDS Res*. 1986;2:S17-S22.
131. Sherman MP, Saksena NK, Dube DK, et al. Evolutionary insights on the origin of human T-cell lymphoma/leukemia virus type I (HTLV-I) derived from sequence analysis of a new HTLV-I variant from Papua New Guinea. *J Virol*. 1992;66:2556-2563.
132. May JT, Stent G, Schnagl RD. Antibody to human T-cell lymphotropic virus type I in Australian Aborigines. *Med J Aust*. 1988;149:104.
133. Bastian I, Gardner J, Webb D, et al. Isolation of a human T-lymphotropic virus type I strain from Australian Aboriginals. *J Virol*. 1993;67:842-851.
134. Mahieux R, Pecon-Slattery J, Gessain A. Molecular characterization and phylogenetic analyses of a new, highly divergent simian T-cell lymphotropic virus type 1 (STLV-1marc1) in Macaca arctoides. *J Virol*. 1997;71:6253-6258.
135. Ajdukiewicz A, Yanagihara R, Garruto RM, et al. HTLV-I myeloneuropathy in the Solomon Islands. *N Engl J Med*. 1989;321:615-616.
136. Robert-Guroff M, Weiss SH, Giron JA, et al. Prevalence of antibodies to HTLV-I, -II, and -III in intravenous drug abusers from an AIDS endemic region. *JAMA*. 1986;255:3133-3137.
137. Lee H, Swanson P, Shorty VS, et al. High rate of HTLV-II infection in seropositive IV drug abusers in New Orleans. *Science*. 1989;244:471-475.
138. Cantor KP, Weiss SH, Goedert JJ, et al. HTLV-I/II seroprevalence and HIV/HTLV coinfection among U.S. intravenous drug users. *J Acquir Immune Defic Syndr*. 1991;4:460-467.
139. Khabbaz RF, Hartel D, Lairmore M, et al. Human T-lymphotropic virus type II (HTLV-II) infection in a cohort of New York intravenous drug users: an old infection? *J Infect*. 1991;163:252-256.
140. Calabro ML, Luparello M, Grottola A, et al. Detection of human T lymphotropic virus type II/b in human immunodeficiency virus type 1-coinfected persons in southeastern Italy. *J Infect Dis*. 1993;168:1273-1277.
141. Lairmore MD, Jacobson S, Gracia F, et al. Isolation of human T-cell lymphotropic virus type 2 from Guaymi Indians in Panama. *Proc Natl Acad Sci U S A*. 1990;87:8840-8844.
142. Heneine W, Kaplan JE, Gracia F, et al. HTLV-II endemicity among Guaymi Indians in Panama. *N Engl J Med*. 1991;324:565.
143. Ishak R, Harrington WJ Jr, Azevedo VN, et al. Identification of human T cell lymphotropic virus type IIa infection in the Kayapo, an indigenous population of Brazil. *AIDS Res Hum Retroviruses*. 1995;11:813-821.
144. Eiraku N, Novoa P, da Costa Ferreira M, et al. Identification and characterization of a new and distinct molecular subtype of human T-cell lymphotropic virus type 2. *J Virol*. 1996;70:1481-1492.
145. Ferrer JF, Esteban E, Dube S, et al. Endemic infection with human T cell leukemia/lymphoma virus type IIB in Argentinean and Paraguayan Indians: epidemiology and molecular characterization. *J Infect Dis*. 1996;174:944-953.
146. Ferrer JF, Del Pino N, Esteban E, et al. High rate of infection with the human T-cell leukemia retrovirus type II in four Indian populations of Argentina. *Virology*. 1993;197:576-584.
147. Ijichi S, Zaninovic V, Leon FE, et al. Identification of human T cell leukemia virus type IIb infection in the Wayu, an Aboriginal population of Colombia. *Jpn J Cancer Res*. 1993;84:1215-1218.
148. Lee H, Idler KB, Swanson P, et al. Complete nucleotide sequence of HTLV-II isolate NRA: comparison of envelope sequence variation of HTLV-II isolates from U.S. blood donors and U.S. and Italian IV drug users. *Virology*. 1993;196:57-69.
149. Takahashi H, Zhu SW, Ijichi S, et al. Nucleotide sequence analysis of human T cell leukemia virus, type II (HTLV-II) isolates. *AIDS Res Hum Retroviruses*. 1993;9:721-732.
150. Pardi D, Kaplan JE, Coligan JE, et al. Identification and characterization of an extended Tax protein in human T-cell lymphotropic virus type II subtype b isolates. *J Virol*. 1993;67:7663-7667.
151. Lewis MJ, Novoa P, Ishak R, et al. Isolation, cloning, and complete nucleotide sequence of a phenotypically distinct Brazilian isolate of human T-lymphotropic virus type II (HTLV-II). *Virology*. 2000;271:142-154.
152. Switzer WM, Pieniazek D, Swanson P, et al. Phylogenetic relationship and geographic distribution of multiple human T-cell lymphotropic virus type II subtypes. *J Virol*. 1995;69:621-632.
153. Hall WW, Takahashi H, Liu C, et al. Multiple isolates and characteristics of human T-cell leukemia virus type II. *J Virol*. 1992;66:2456-2463.
154. Kubo T, Zhu SW, Ijichi S, et al. Molecular characterization of human T-cell leukemia virus, type II (HTLV-II). *AIDS Res Hum Retroviruses*. 1994;10:465.
155. Wolfe ND, Heneine W, Carr JK, et al. Emergence of unique primate T-lymphotropic viruses among central African bushmeat hunters. *Proc Natl Acad Sci U S A*. 2005;102:7994-7999.
156. Calattini S, Chevalier SA, Duprez R, et al. Discovery of a new human T-cell lymphotropic virus (HTLV-3) in Central Africa. *Retrovirology*. 2005;2:30.
157. Kourtis AP, Lee FK, Abrams EJ, et al. Mother-to-child transmission of HIV-1: timing and implications for prevention. *Lancet Infect Dis*. 2006;6:726-732.
158. Ando Y, Nakano S, Saito K, et al. Transmission of adult T-cell leukemia retrovirus (HTLV-I) from mother to child: comparison of bottle- with breast-fed babies. *Jpn J Cancer Res*. 1987;78:322-324.
159. Hino S, Katamine S, Kawase K, et al. Intervention of maternal transmission of HTLV-1 in Nagasaki, Japan. *Leukemia*. 1994;8:S68-S70.
160. Kinoshita K, Amagasaki T, Hino S, et al. Milk-borne transmission of HTLV-I from carrier mothers to their children. *Jpn J Cancer Res*. 1987;78:674-680.
161. Ando Y, Matsumoto Y, Nakano S, et al. Long-term follow up study of vertical HTLV-I infection in children breast-fed by seropositive mothers. *J Infect*. 2003;46:177-179.
162. Wiktor SZ, Pate EJ, Rosenberg PS, et al. Mother-to-child transmission of human T-cell lymphotropic virus type I associated with prolonged breast-feeding. *J Hum Virol*. 1997;1:37-44.
163. Wiktor SZ, Pate EJ, Murphy EL, et al. Mother-to-child transmission of human T-cell lymphotropic virus type I (HTLV-I) in Jamaica: association with antibodies to envelope glycoprotein (gp46) epitopes. *J Acquir Immune Defic Syndr*. 1993;6:1162-1167.
164. Kinoshita K, Hino S, Amagaski T, et al. Demonstration of adult T-cell leukemia virus antigen in milk from three sero-positive mothers. *Gann*. 1984;75:103-105.
165. Heneine W, Woods T, Green D, et al. Detection of HTLV-II in breastmilk of HTLV-II infected mothers. *Lancet*. 1992; 340:1157-1158.
166. Ureta-Vidal A, Angelin-Duclos C, Tortevoye P, et al. Mother-to-child transmission of human T-cell-leukemia/lymphoma virus type I: implication of high antiviral antibody titer and high proviral load in carrier mothers. *Int J Cancer*. 1999;82:832-836.
167. Hirata M, Hayashi J, Noguchi A, et al. The effects of breastfeeding and presence of antibody to p40tax protein of human T cell lymphotropic virus type-I on mother to child transmission. *Int J Epidemiol*. 1992;21:989-994.
168. Sawada T, Tohmatsu J, Obara T, et al. High risk of mother-to-child transmission of HTLV-I in p40tax antibody-positive mothers. *Jpn J Cancer Res*. 1989;80:506-508.
169. Hino S, Katamine S, Miyamoto T, et al. Association between maternal antibodies to the external envelope glycoprotein and vertical transmission of human T-lymphotropic virus type I: maternal anti-Env antibodies correlate with protection in non-breast-fed children. *J Clin Invest*. 1995;95:2920-2925.
170. Yoshinaga M, Yashiki S, Oki T, et al. A maternal risk factor for mother-to-child HTLV-I transmission: viral antigen-producing capacities in culture of peripheral blood and breast milk cells. *Jpn J Cancer Res*. 1995;86:649-654.
171. Hino S, Yamaguchi K, Katamine S, et al. Mother-to-child transmission of human T-cell leukemia virus type-I. *Jpn J Cancer Res*. 1985;76:474-480.
172. Tsuji Y, Doi H, Yamabe T, et al. Prevention of mother-to-child transmission of human T-lymphotropic virus type-I. *Pediatrics*. 1990;86:11-17.
173. Nyambi PN, Ville Y, Louwagie J, et al. Mother-to-child transmission of human T-cell lymphotropic virus types I and II

(HTLV-I/II) in Gabon: a prospective follow-up of 4 years. *J Acquir Immune Defic Syndr Hum Retrovirol.* 1996;12:187-192.
174. Kusuhara K, Sonoda S, Takahashi K, et al. Mother-to-child transmission of human T-cell leukemia virus type I (HTLV-I): a fifteen-year follow-up study in Okinawa, Japan. *Int J Cancer.* 1987;40:755-757.
175. Sugiyama H, Doi H, Yamaguchi K, et al. Significance of postnatal mother-to-child transmission of human T-lymphotropic virus type-I on the development of adult T-cell leukemia/lymphoma. *J Med Virol.* 1986;20:253-260.
176. Wilks R, Hanchard B, Morgan O, et al. Patterns of HTLV-I infection among family members of patients with adult T-cell leukemia/lymphoma and HTLV-I associated myelopathy/tropical spastic paraparesis. *Int J Cancer.* 1996;65:272-273.
177. Andersson S, Dias F, Mendez PJ, et al. HTLV-I and -II infections in a nationwide survey of pregnant women in Guinea-Bissau, West Africa. *J Acquir Immune Defic Syndr Hum Retrovirol.* 1997;15:320-322.
178. Van Dyke RB, Heneine W, Perrin ME, et al. Mother-to-child transmission of human T-lymphotropic virus type II. *J Pediatr.* 1995;127:924-928.
179. Kaplan JE, Abrams E, Shaffer N, et al. Low risk of mother-to-child transmission of human T lymphotropic virus type II in non-breast-fed infants. *J Infect Dis.* 1992;166:892-895.
180. Black FL, Biggar RJ, Neel JV, et al. Endemic transmission of HTLV type II among Kayapo Indians of Brazil. *AIDS Res Hum Retroviruses.* 1994;10:1165-1171.
181. Vitek CR, Gracia FI, Giusti R, et al. Evidence for sexual and mother-to-child transmission of human T lymphotropic virus type II among Guaymi Indians, Panama. *J Infect Dis.* 1995;171:1022-1026.
182. Bartholomew C, Saxinger WC, Clark JW, et al. Transmission of HTLV-I and HIV among homosexual men in Trinidad. *JAMA.* 1987;257:2604-2608.
183. Figueroa JP, Ward E, Morris J, et al. Incidence of HIV and HTLV-1 infection among sexually transmitted disease clinic attenders in Jamaica. *J Acquir Immune Defic Syndr Hum Retrovirol.* 1997;15:232-237.
184. Nakashima K, Kashiwagi S, Kajiyama W, et al. Sexual transmission of human T-lymphotropic virus type I among female prostitutes and among patients with sexually transmitted diseases in Fukuoka, Kyushu, Japan. *Am J Epidemiol.* 1995;141:305-311.
185. Figueroa JP, Morris J, Brathwaite A, et al. Risk factors for HTLV-I among heterosexual STD clinic attenders. *J Acquir Immune Defic Syndr Hum Retrovirol.* 1995;9:81-88.
186. Nakano S, Ando Y, Ichijo M, et al. Search for possible routes of vertical and horizontal transmission of adult T-cell leukemia virus. *Gann.* 1984;75:1044-1045.
187. Belec L, Georges-Courbot MC, Georges A, et al. Cervicovaginal synthesis of IgG antibodies to the immunodominant 175-199 domain of the surface glycoprotein gp46 of human T-cell leukemia virus type I. *J Med Virol.* 1996;50:42-49.
188. Zunt JR, Dezzutti CS, Montano SM, et al. Cervical shedding of human T cell lymphotropic virus type I is associated with cervicitis. *J Infect Dis.* 2002;186:1669-1672.
189. Stuver SO, Tachibana N, Okayama A, et al. Heterosexual transmission of human T cell leukemia/lymphoma virus type I among married couples in southwestern Japan: an initial report from the Miyazaki cohort study. *J Infect Dis.* 1993;167:57-65.
190. Larsen O, Andersson S, da Silva Z, et al. Prevalences of HTLV-1 infection and associated risk determinants in an urban population in Guinea-Bissau, West Africa. *J Acquir Immune Defic Syndr.* 2000;25:157-163.
191. Kaplan JE, Khabbaz RF, Murphy EL, et al. Male-to-female transmission of human T-cell lymphotropic virus types I and II: association with viral load. The Retrovirus Epidemiology Donor Study Group. *J Acquir Immune Defic Syndr Hum Retrovirol.* 1996;12:193-201.
192. Vlahov D, Khabbaz RF, Cohn S, et al. Incidence and risk factors for human T-lymphotropic virus type II seroconversion among injecting drug users in Baltimore, Maryland, U.S.A. *J Acquir Immune Defic Syndr Hum Retrovirol.* 1995;9:89-96.
193. Roucoux DF, Wang B, Smith D, et al. A prospective study of sexual transmission of human T lymphotropic virus (HTLV)-I and HTLV-II. *J Infect Dis.* 2005;191:1490-1497.
194. Chen YA, Okayama A, Lee TH, et al. Sexual transmission of human T-cell leukemia virus type I associated with the presence of anti-tax antibody. *Proc Natl Acad Sci U S A.* 1991;88:1182-1186.
195. Iga M, Okayama A, Stuver S, et al. Genetic evidence of transmission of human T cell lymphotropic virus type 1 between spouses. *J Infect Dis.* 2002;185:691-695.
196. Khabbaz RF, Heneine W, Grindon A, et al. Indeterminate HTLV serologic results in U.S. blood donors: are they due to HTLV-I or HTLV-II? *J Acquir Immune Defic Syndr.* 1992;5:400-404.
197. Schreiber GB, Murphy EL, Horton JA, et al. Risk factors for human T-cell lymphotropic virus types I and II (HTLV-I and -II) in blood donors: the Retrovirus Epidemiology Donor Study. NHLBI Retrovirus Epidemiology Donor Study. *J Acquir Immune Defic Syndr Hum Retrovirol.* 1997;14:263-271.
198. Khabbaz RF, Onorato IM, Cannon RO, et al. Seroprevalence of HTLV-1 and HTLV-2 among intravenous drug users and persons in clinics for sexually transmitted diseases. *N Engl J Med.* 1992;326:375-380.
199. Maloney EM, Armien B, Gracia F, et al. Risk factors for human T cell lymphotropic virus type II infection among the Guaymi Indians of Panama. *J Infect Dis.* 1999;180:876-879.
200. Okochi K, Sato H, Hinuma Y. A retrospective study on transmission of adult T cell leukemia virus by blood transfusion: seroconversion in recipients. *Vox Sang.* 1984;46:245-253.
201. Kleinman S, Swanson P, Allain JP, et al. Transfusion transmission of human T-lymphotropic virus types I and II: serologic and polymerase chain reaction results in recipients identified through look-back investigations. *Transfusion.* 1993;33:14-18.
202. Sullivan MT, Williams AE, Fang CT, et al. Transmission of human T-lymphotropic virus types I and II by blood transfusion: a retrospective study of recipients of blood components (1983 through 1988). The American Red Cross HTLV-I/II Collaborative Study Group. *Arch Intern Med.* 1991;151:2043-2048.
203. Kamihira S, Nakasima S, Oyakawa Y, et al. Transmission of human T cell lymphotropic virus type I by blood transfusion before and after mass screening of sera from seropositive donors. *Vox Sang.* 1987;52:43-44.
204. Manns A, Wilks RJ, Murphy EL, et al. A prospective study of transmission by transfusion of HTLV-I and risk factors associated with seroconversion. *Int J Cancer.* 1992;51:886-891.
205. Cohen ND, Munoz A, Reitz BA, et al. Transmission of retroviruses by transfusion of screened blood in patients undergoing cardiac surgery. *N Engl J Med.* 1989;320:1172-1176.
206. Feigal E, Murphy E, Vranizan K, et al. Human T cell lymphotropic virus type I and II in intravenous drug users in San Francisco: risk factors associated with seropositivity. *J Infect Dis.* 1991;164:36-42.
207. Gout O, Baulac M, Gessain A, et al. Rapid development of myelopathy after HTLV-I infection acquired by transfusion during cardiac transplantation. *N Engl J Med.* 1990;322:383-388.
208. Chen YC, Wang CH, Su IJ, et al. Infection of human T-cell leukemia virus type I and development of human T-cell leukemia lymphoma in patients with hematologic neoplasms: a possible linkage to blood transfusion. *Blood.* 1989;74:388-394.
209. Dekaban G, Inwood M, Waters D, et al. Absence of human T-lymphotropic virus types I and II infection in an Ontario hemophilia population. *Transfusion.* 1992;32:513-516.
210. Canavaggio M, Leckie G, Allain JP, et al. The prevalence of antibody to HTLV-I/II in United States plasma donors and in United States and French hemophiliacs. *Transfusion.* 1990;30:780-782.
211. Gonzalez-Perez MP, Munoz-Juarez L, Cardenas FC, et al. Human T-cell leukemia virus type I infection in various recipients of transplants from the same donor. *Transplantation.* 2003;75:1006-1011.
212. Manns A, Murphy EL, Wilks R, et al. Detection of early human T-cell lymphotropic virus type I antibody patterns during seroconversion among transfusion recipients. *Blood.* 1991;77:896-905.
213. Cho I, Sugimoto M, Mita S, et al. In vivo proviral burden and viral RNA expression in T cell subsets of patients with human T lymphotropic virus type-1-associated myelopathy/tropical spastic paraparesis. *Am J Trop Med Hyg.* 1995;53:412-418.
214. Miyoshi I, Takehara N, Sawada T, et al. Immunoglobulin prophylaxis against HTLV-I in a rabbit model. *Leukemia.* 1992;6:24-26.
215. Kazanji M, Heraud JM, Merien F, et al. Chimeric peptide vaccine composed of B- and T-cell epitopes of human T-cell leukemia virus type 1 induces humoral and cellular immune responses and reduces the proviral load in immunized squirrel monkeys (Saimiri sciureus). *J Gen Virol.* 2006;87:1331-1337.
216. Jacobson S, Gupta A, Mattson D, et al. Immunological studies in tropical spastic paraparesis. *Ann Neurol.* 1990;27:149-156.
217. Daenke S, Kermode AG, Hall SE, et al. High activated and memory cytotoxic T-cell responses to HTLV-1 in healthy carriers and patients with tropical spastic paraparesis. *Virology.* 1996;217:139-146.
218. Parker CE, Daenke S, Nightingale S, et al. Activated, HTLV-1-specific cytotoxic T-lymphocytes are found in healthy seropositives as well as in patients with tropical spastic paraparesis. *Virology.* 1992;188:628-636.
219. Hanon E, Hall S, Taylor GP, et al. Abundant Tax protein expression in CD4+ T cells infected with human T-cell lymphotropic virus type I (HTLV-I) is prevented by cytotoxic T lymphocytes. *Blood.* 2000;95:1386-1392.
220. Bieganowska K, Hollsberg P, Buckle GJ, et al. Direct analysis of viral-specific CD8+ T cells with soluble HLA-A2/Tax11-19 tetramer complexes in patients with human T cell lymphotropic virus-associated myelopathy. *J Immunol.* 1999;162:1765-1771.
221. Elovaara I, Koenig S, Brewah AY, et al. High human T cell lymphotropic virus type 1 (HTLV-1)-specific precursor cytotoxic T lymphocyte frequencies in patients with HTLV-1-associated neurological disease. *J Exp Med.* 1993;177:1567-1573.
222. Jacobson S, Shida H, McFarlin DE, et al. Circulating CD8+ cytotoxic T lymphocytes specific for HTLV-I pX in patients with HTLV-I associated neurologic disease. *Nature.* 1990;348:245-248.
223. Jacobson S, Reuben JS, Streilein RD, et al. Induction of CD4+, human T lymphotropic virus type-1-specific cytotoxic T lymphocytes from patients with HAM/TSP: recognition of an immunogenic region of the gp46 envelope glycoprotein of human T lymphotropic virus type-1. *J Immunol.* 1991;146:1155-1162.
224. Bangham C, Kermode A, Hall S, et al. The cytotoxic T-lymphocyte response to HTLV-I: the main determinant of disease? *Virology.* 1996;7:41-48.
225. Kubota R, Kawanishi T, Matsubara H, et al. HTLV-I specific IFN-gamma+ CD8+ lymphocytes correlate with the proviral load in peripheral blood of infected individuals. *J Neuroimmunol.* 2000;102:208-215.
226. Jeffery KJ, Usuku K, Hall SE, et al. HLA alleles determine human T-lymphotropic virus-I (HTLV-I) proviral load and the risk of HTLV-I-associated myelopathy. *Proc Natl Acad Sci U S A.* 1999;96:3848-3853.
227. Murphy EL, Hanchard B, Figueroa JP, et al. Modelling the risk of adult T-cell leukemia/lymphoma in persons infected with human T-lymphotropic virus type I. *Int J Cancer.* 1989;43:250-253.
228. Orland JR, Engstrom J, Fridey J, et al. Prevalence and clinical features of HTLV neurologic disease in the HTLV Outcomes Study. *Neurology.* 2003;61:1588-1594.
229. Uchiyama T, Yodoi J, Sagawa K, et al. Adult T-cell leukemia: clinical and hematologic features of 16 cases. *Blood.* 1977;50:481-492.
230. Richard V, Lairmore MD, Green PL, et al. Humoral hypercalcemia of malignancy: severe combined immunodeficient/beige mouse model of adult T-cell lymphoma independent of human T-cell lymphotropic virus type-1 tax expression. *Am J Pathol.* 2001;158:2219-2228.
231. Mori N, Ejima E, Prager D. Transactivation of parathyroid hormone-related protein gene expression by human T-cell leukemia virus type I tax. *Eur J Haematol.* 1996;56:116-117.
232. Tajima K, Kuroishi T. Estimation of rate of incidence of ATL among ATLV (HTLV-I) carriers in Kyushu, Japan. *Jpn J Clin Oncol.* 1985;15:423-430.
233. Shimoyama M. Diagnostic criteria and classification of clinical subtypes of adult T-cell leukaemia-lymphoma: a report from the Lymphoma Study Group (1984-87). *Br J Haematol.* 1991;79:428-437.
234. Gibbs WN, Lofters WS, Campbell M, et al. Non-Hodgkin lymphoma in Jamaica and its relation to adult T-cell leukemia-lymphoma. *Ann Intern Med.* 1987;106:361-368.
235. Hattori T, Uchiyama T, Toibana T, et al. Surface phenotype of Japanese adult T-cell leukemia cells characterized by monoclonal antibodies. *Blood.* 1981;58:645-647.
236. Waldmann TA, Greene WC, Sarin PS, et al. Functional and phenotypic comparison of human T cell leukemia/lymphoma virus positive adult T cell leukemia with human T cell leukemia/lymphoma virus negative Sezary leukemia, and their distinction using anti-Tac: monoclonal antibody identifying the human receptor for T cell growth factor. *J Clin Invest.* 1984;73:1711-1718.
237. Waldmann TA, White JD, Goldman CK, et al. The interleukin-2 receptor: a target for monoclonal antibody treatment of human T-cell lymphotrophic virus I-induced adult T-cell leukemia. *Blood.* 1993;82:1701-1712.
238. Yoshida M, Seiki M, Yamaguchi K, et al. Monoclonal integration of human T-cell leukemia provirus in all primary tumors of adult T-cell leukemia suggests causative role of human T-cell leukemia virus in the disease. *Proc Natl Acad Sci U S A.* 1984;81:2534-2537.
239. Kamihira S, Sugahara K, Tsuruda K, et al. Proviral status of HTLV-1 integrated into the host genomic DNA of adult T-cell leukemia cells. *Clin Lab Haematol.* 2005;27:235-241.
240. Ozawa T, Itoyama T, Sadamori N, et al. Rapid isolation of viral integration site reveals frequent integration of HTLV-1 into expressed loci. *J Hum Genet.* 2004;49:154-165.
241. Hanai S, Nitta T, Shoda M, et al. Integration of human T-cell leukemia virus type 1 in genes of leukemia cells of patients with adult T-cell leukemia. *Cancer Sci.* 2004;95:306-310.
242. Doi K, Wu X, Taniguchi Y, et al. Preferential selection of human T-cell leukemia virus type I provirus integration sites in leukemic versus carrier states. *Blood.* 2005;106:1048-1053.
243. Derse D, Crise B, Li Y, et al. Human T-cell leukemia virus type 1 integration target sites in the human genome: comparison with those of other retroviruses. *J Virol.* 2007;81:6731-6741.
244. Tanaka G, Okayama A, Watanabe T, et al. The clonal expansion of human T lymphotropic virus type 1-infected T cells: a comparison between seroconverters and long-term carriers. *J Infect Dis.* 2005;191:1140-1147.
245. Ohshima K, Ohgami A, Matsuoka M, et al. Random integration of HTLV-1 provirus: increasing chromosomal instability. *Cancer Lett.* 1998;132:203-212.
246. Mortreux F, Leclercq I, Gabet AS, et al. Somatic mutation in human T-cell leukemia virus type 1 provirus and flanking cellular sequences during clonal expansion in vivo. *J Natl Cancer Inst.* 2001;93:367-377.
247. Tsukasaki K, Krebs J, Nagai K, et al. Comparative genomic hybridization analysis in adult T-cell leukemia/lymphoma: correlation with clinical course. *Blood.* 2001;97:3875-3881.
248. Akagi T, Ono H, Tsuchida N, et al. Aberrant expression and function of p53 in T-cells immortalized by HTLV-I Tax1. *FEBS Lett.* 1997;406:263-266.
249. Mulloy JC, Kislyakova T, Cereseto A, et al. Human T-cell lymphotropic/leukemia virus type 1 Tax abrogates p53-induced cell

cycle arrest and apoptosis through its CREB/ATF functional domain. *J Virol.* 1998;72:8852-8860.
250. Reid RL, Lindholm PF, Mireskandari A, et al. Stabilization of wild-type p53 in human T-lymphocytes transformed by HTLV-I. *Oncogene.* 1993;8:3029-3036.
251. Chiari E, Lamsoul I, Lodewick J, et al. Stable ubiquitination of human T-cell leukemia virus type 1 tax is required for proteasome binding. *J Virol.* 2004;78:11823-11832.
252. Peloponese JM Jr, Iha H, Yedavalli VR, et al. Ubiquitination of human T-cell leukemia virus type 1 tax modulates its activity. *J Virol.* 2004;78:11686-11695.
253. Takeda S, Maeda M, Morikawa S, et al. Genetic and epigenetic inactivation of tax gene in adult T-cell leukemia cells. *Int J Cancer.* 2004;109:559-567.
254. Furukawa Y, Kubota R, Tara M, et al. Existence of escape mutant in HTLV-I tax during the development of adult T-cell leukemia. *Blood.* 2001;97:987-993.
255. Koiwa T, Hamano-Usami A, Ishida T, et al. 5′-long terminal repeat-selective CpG methylation of latent human T-cell leukemia virus type 1 provirus in vitro and in vivo. *J Virol.* 2002;76:9389-9397.
256. Taniguchi Y, Nosaka K, Yasunaga J, et al. Silencing of human T-cell leukemia virus type I gene transcription by epigenetic mechanisms. *Retrovirology.* 2005;2:64.
257. Miyazaki M, Yasunaga J, Taniguchi Y, et al. Preferential selection of human T-cell leukemia virus type 1 provirus lacking the 5′ long terminal repeat during oncogenesis. *J Virol.* 2007;81:5714-5723.
258. Tamiya S, Matsuoka M, Etoh K, et al. Two types of defective human T-lymphotropic virus type I provirus in adult T-cell leukemia. *Blood.* 1996;88:3065-3073.
259. Bunn PA Jr, Schechter GP, Jaffe E, et al. Clinical course of retrovirus-associated adult T-cell lymphoma in the United States. *N Engl J Med.* 1983;309:257-264.
260. Newton RC, Limpuangthip P, Greenberg S, et al. *Strongyloides stercoralis* hyperinfection in a carrier of HTLV-I virus with evidence of selective immunosuppression. *Am J Med.* 1992;92:202-208.
261. Nakada K, Yamaguchi K, Furugen S, et al. Monoclonal integration of HTLV-I proviral DNA in patients with strongyloidiasis. *Int J Cancer.* 1987;40:145-148.
262. Sato Y, Shiroma Y. Concurrent infections with *Strongyloides* and T-cell leukemia virus and their possible effect on immune responses of host. *Clin Immunol Immunopathol.* 1989;52:214-224.
263. Ratner L, Grant C, Zimmerman B, et al. Effect of treatment of *Strongyloides* infection on HTLV-1 expression in a patient with adult T-cell leukemia. *Am J Hematol.* 2007;82:929-931.
264. Miyoshi I, Takemoto S, Taguchi H, et al. Adult T-cell leukemia with cyclic neutropenia in a seronegative patient carrying only the tax gene of HTLV-I. *Am J Hematol.* 2002;71:137-138.
265. Arisawa K, Sobue T, Yoshimi I, et al. Human T-lymphotropic virus type-I infection, survival and cancer risk in southwestern Japan: a prospective cohort study. *Cancer Causes Control.* 2003;14:889-896.
266. Asou N, Kumagai T, Uekihara S, et al. HTLV-I seroprevalence in patients with malignancy. *Cancer.* 1986;58:903-907.
267. Kozuru M, Uike N, Muta K, et al. High occurrence of primary malignant neoplasms in patients with adult T-cell leukemia/lymphoma, their siblings, and their mothers. *Cancer.* 1996;78:1119-1124.
268. Matsumoto S, Yamasaki K, Tsuji K, et al. Human T lymphotropic virus type 1 infection and gastric cancer development in Japan. *J Infect Dis.* 2008;198:10-15.
269. Osame M, Usuku K, Izumo S, et al. HTLV-I associated myelopathy, a new clinical entity [letter]. *Lancet.* 1986;1:1031-1032.
270. Akizuki S, Setoguchi M, Nakazato O, et al. An autopsy case of human T-lymphotropic virus type I-associated myelopathy. *Hum Pathol.* 1988;19:988-990.
271. Bhigjee AI, Wiley CA, Waschsman W, et al. HTLV-I-associated myelopathy: clinicopathologic correlation with localization of provirus to spinal cord. *Neurology.* 1991;41:1990-1992.
272. Ohama E, Horikawa Y, Shimizu T, et al. Demyelination and remyelination in spinal cord lesions of human lymphotropic virus type I-associated myelopathy. *Acta Neuropathol.* 1990;81:78-83.
273. Gessain A, Barin F, Vernant JC, et al. Antibodies to human T-lymphotropic virus type-I in patients with tropical spastic paraparesis. *Lancet.* 1985;2:407-410.
274. Osame M, Janssen R, Kubota H, et al. Nationwide survey of HTLV-I-associated myelopathy in Japan: association with blood transfusion. *Ann Neurol.* 1990;28:50-56.
275. McFarlin DE. Neurological disorders related to HTLV-I and HTLV-II. *J Acquir Immune Defic Syndr.* 1993;6:640-644.
276. Kramer A, Maloney EM, Morgan OS, et al. Risk factors and cofactors for human T-cell lymphotropic virus type I (HTLV-I)-associated myelopathy/tropical spastic paraparesis (HAM/TSP) in Jamaica. *Am J Epidemiol.* 1995;142:1212-1220.
277. Vernant JC, Maurs L, Gessain A, et al. Endemic tropical spastic paraparesis associated with human T-lymphotropic virus type I: a clinical and seroepidemiological study of 25 cases. *Ann Neurol.* 1987;21:123-130.
278. Osame M, Matsumoto M, Usuku K, et al. Chronic progressive myelopathy associated with elevated antibodies to human T-lymphotropic virus type I and adult T-cell leukemialike cells. *Ann Neurol.* 1987;21:117-122.
279. Gessain A, Gout O. Chronic myelopathy associated with human T-lymphotropic virus type I (HTLV-I). *Ann Intern Med.* 1992;117:933-946.
280. Shibasaki H, Endo C, Kuroda Y, et al. Clinical picture of HTLV-I associated myelopathy. *J Neurol Sci.* 1988;87:15-24.
281. Roman GC, Roman LN. Tropical spastic paraparesis: a clinical study of 50 patients from Tumaco (Colombia) and review of the worldwide features of the syndrome. *J Neurol Sci.* 1988;87:121-138.
282. Gout O, Gessain A, Bolgert F, et al. Chronic myelopathies associated with human T-lymphotropic virus type I: a clinical, serologic, and immunovirologic study of ten patients in France. *Arch Neurol.* 1989;46:255-260.
283. Levin MC, Lehky TJ, Flerlage AN, et al. Immunologic analysis of a spinal cord-biopsy specimen from a patient with human T-cell lymphotropic virus type I-associated neurologic disease. *N Engl J Med.* 1997;336:839-845.
284. Tournier-Lasserve E, Gout O, Gessain A, et al. HTLV-I, brain abnormalities on magnetic resonance imaging, and relation with multiple sclerosis. *Lancet.* 1987;2:49-50.
285. Moore GR, Traugott U, Scheinberg LC, et al. Tropical spastic paraparesis: a model of virus-induced, cytotoxic T-cell-mediated demyelination? *Ann Neurol.* 1989;26:523-530.
286. Koenig S, Woods RM, Brewah YA, et al. Characterization of MHC class I restricted cytotoxic T cell responses to tax in HTLV-1 infected patients with neurologic disease. *J Immunol.* 1993;151:3874-3883.
287. Hollsberg P, Hafler DA. Seminars in medicine of the Beth Israel Hospital, Boston: pathogenesis of diseases induced by human lymphotropic virus type I infection. *N Engl J Med.* 1993;328:1173-1182.
288. Levin MC, Lee SM, Kalume F, et al. Autoimmunity due to molecular mimicry as a cause of neurological disease. *Nat Med.* 2002;8:509-513.
289. Cavrois M, Gessain A, Wain-Hobson S, et al. Proliferation of HTLV-1 infected circulating cells in vivo in all asymptomatic carriers and patients with TSP/HAM. *Oncogene.* 1996;12:2419-2423.
290. Leite AC, Mendonca GA, Serpa MJ, et al. Neurological manifestations in HTLV-I-infected blood donors. *J Neurol Sci.* 2003;214:49-56.
291. Shimazaki R, Ueyama H, Mori T, et al. Chronic sensory neuronopathy associated with human T-cell lymphotropic virus type I infection. *J Neurol Sci.* 2002;194:55-58.
292. Leite AC, Silva MT, Alamy AH, et al. Peripheral neuropathy in HTLV-I infected individuals without tropical spastic paraparesis/HTLV-I-associated myelopathy. *J Neurol.* 2004;251:877-881.
293. Morgan DJ, Caskey MF, Abbehusen C, et al. Brain magnetic resonance imaging white matter lesions are frequent in HTLV-I carriers and do not discriminate from HAM/TSP. *AIDS Res Hum Retroviruses.* 2007;23:1499-1504.
294. Murphy EL, Wang B, Sacher RA, et al. Respiratory and urinary tract infections, arthritis, and asthma associated with HTLV-I and HTLV-II infection. *Emerg Infect Dis.* 2004;10:109-116.
295. Rocha PN, Rehem AP, Santana JF, et al. The cause of urinary symptoms among human T lymphotropic virus type I (HLTV-I) infected patients: a cross sectional study. *BMC Infect Dis.* 2007;7:15.
296. Castro NM, Rodrigues Jr W, Freitas DM, et al. Urinary symptoms associated with human T-cell lymphotropic virus type I infection: evidence of urinary manifestations in large group of HTLV-I carriers. *Urology.* 2007;69:813-818.
297. Caskey MF, Morgan DJ, Porto AF, et al. Clinical manifestations associated with HTLV type I infection: a cross-sectional study. *AIDS Res Hum Retroviruses.* 2007;23:365-371.
298. Castro N, Oliveira P, Freitas D, et al. Erectile dysfunction and HTLV-I infection: a silent problem. *Int J Impot Res.* 2005;17:364-369.
299. Silva MT, Leite AC, Alamy AH, et al. ALS syndrome in HTLV-I infection. *Neurology.* 2005;65:1332-1333.
300. Silva MT, Mattos P, Alfano A, et al. Neuropsychological assessment in HTLV-1 infection: a comparative study among TSP/HAM, asymptomatic carriers, and healthy controls. *J Neurol Neurosurg Psychiatry.* 2003;74:1085-1089.
301. Sawa H, Nagashima T, Nagashima K, et al. Clinicopathological and virological analyses of familial human T-lymphotropic virus type I-associated polyneuropathy. *J Neurovirol.* 2005;11:199-207.
302. Arakawa K, Umezaki H, Noda S, et al. Chronic polyradiculoneuropathy associated with human T-cell lymphotropic virus type I infection. *J Neurol Neurosurg Psychiatry.* 1990;53:358-359.
303. Douen AG, Pringle CE, Guberman A. Human T-cell lymphotropic virus type 1 myositis, peripheral neuropathy, and cerebral white matter lesions in the absence of spastic paraparesis. *Arch Neurol.* 1997;54:896-900.
304. Araujo AQ, Silva MT. The HTLV-1 neurological complex. *Lancet Neurol.* 2006;5(12):1068-1076.
305. Morgan OS, Rodgers-Johnson PE, Gibbs WN, et al. Abnormal peripheral lymphocytes in tropical spastic paraparesis. *Lancet.* 1987;2:403-404.
306. Morgan OS, Rodgers-Johnson P, Mora C, et al. HTLV-I and polymyositis in Jamaica. *Lancet.* 1989;2:1184-1187.
307. Nishioka K, Maruyama I, Sato K, et al. Chronic inflammatory arthropathy associated with HTLV-I. *Lancet.* 1989;1:441.
308. Mochizuki M, Tajima K, Watanabe T, et al. Human T lymphotropic virus type 1 uveitis. *Br J Ophthalmol.* 1994;78:149-154.
309. Ohba N, Matsumoto M, Sameshima M, et al. Ocular manifestations in patients infected with human T-lymphotropic virus type I. *Jpn J Ophthalmol.* 1989;33:1-12.
310. Sagawa K, Mochizuki M, Masuoka K, et al. Immunopathological mechanisms of human T cell lymphotropic virus type 1 (HTLV-I) uveitis: detection of HTLV-I-infected T cells in the eye and their constitutive cytokine production. *J Clin Invest.* 1995;95:852-858.
311. Sugimoto M, Nakashima H, Matsumoto M, et al. Pulmonary involvement in patients with HTLV-I-associated myelopathy: increased soluble IL-2 receptors in bronchoalveolar lavage fluid. *Am Rev Respir Dis.* 1989;139:1329-1335.
312. Mita S, Sugimoto M, Nakamura M, et al. Increased human T lymphotropic virus type-1 (HTLV-1) proviral DNA in peripheral blood mononuclear cells and bronchoalveolar lavage cells from Japanese patients with HTLV-1-associated myelopathy. *Am J Trop Med Hyg.* 1993;48:170-177.
313. Robinson RD, Lindo JF, Neva FA, et al. Immunoepidemiologic studies of *Strongyloides stercoralis* and human T lymphotropic virus type I infections in Jamaica. *J Infect Dis.* 1994;169:692-696.
314. Nakada K, Kohakura M, Komoda H, et al. High incidence of HTLV antibody in carriers of *Strongyloides stercoralis*. *Lancet.* 1984;1:633.
315. Ho GY, Nelson K, Nomura AM, et al. Markers of health status in an HTLV-I-positive cohort. *Am J Epidemiol.* 1992;136:1349-1357.
316. Bartman MT, Kaidarova Z, Hirschkorn D, et al. Long-term increases in lymphocytes and platelets in human T-lymphotropic virus type II infection. *Blood.* 2008;112:3995-4002.
317. LaGrenade L, Hanchard B, Fletcher V, et al. Infective dermatitis of Jamaican children: a marker for HTLV-I infection. *Lancet.* 1990;336:1345-1346.
318. Daisley H, Charles W, Suite M. Crusted (Norwegian) scabies as a pre-diagnostic indicator for HTLV-1 infection. *Trans Royal Soc Trop Med Hygiene.* 1993;87:295.
319. Blank A, Herrera M, Lourido MA, et al. Infective dermatitis in Colombia. *Lancet.* 1995;346:710.
320. Mahe A, Chollet-Martin S, Gessain A. HTLV-I-associated infective dermatitis. *Lancet.* 1999;354:1386.
321. Oliveira MS, Fraga AG, Torrado E, et al. Infection with *Mycobacterium ulcerans* induces persistent inflammatory responses in mice. *Infect Immun.* 2005;73:6299-6310.
322. Mahe A, Meertens L, Ly F, et al. Human T-cell leukaemia/lymphoma virus type 1-associated infective dermatitis in Africa: a report of five cases from Senegal. *Br J Dermatol.* 2004;150:958-965.
323. Tsukasaki K, Yamada Y, Ikeda S, et al. Infective dermatitis among patients with ATL in Japan. *Int J Cancer.* 1994;57:293.
324. Hanchard B, LaGrenade L, Carberry C, et al. Childhood infective dermatitis evolving into adult T-cell leukaemia after 17 years. *Lancet.* 1991;338:1593-1594.
325. Beilke MA, Theall KP, O'Brien M, et al. Clinical outcomes and disease progression among patients coinfected with HIV and human T lymphotropic virus types 1 and 2. *Clin Infect Dis.* 2004;39:256-263.
326. Page JB, Lai S, Chitwood DD, et al. HTLV-I/II seropositivity and death from AIDS among HIV-1 seropositive intravenous drug users. *Lancet.* 1990;335:1439-1441.
327. Schechter M, Harrison LH, Halsey NA, et al. Coinfection with human T-cell lymphotropic virus type I and HIV in Brazil. Impact on markers of HIV disease progression. *JAMA.* 1994;271:353-357.
328. Gotuzzo E, Escamilla J, Phillips IA, et al. The impact of human T-lymphotrophic virus type I/II infection on the prognosis of sexually acquired cases of acquired immunodeficiency syndrome. *Arch Intern Med.* 1992;152:1429-1432.
329. Harrison LH, Quinn TC, Schechter M. Human T cell lymphotropic virus type I does not increase human immunodeficiency virus viral load in vivo. *J Infect Dis.* 1997;175:438-440.
330. Beilke MA, Traina-Dorge VL, Sirois M, et al. Relationship between human T lymphotropic virus (HTLV) type 1/2 viral burden and clinical and treatment parameters among patients with HIV type 1 and HTLV-1/2 coinfection. *Clin Infect Dis.* 2007;44:1229-1234.
331. Pagliuca A, Williams H, Salisbury J, et al. Prodromal cutaneous lesions in adult T-cell leukaemia/lymphoma. *Lancet.* 1990;335:733-734.
332. Fantry L, De Jonge E, Auwaerter PG, et al. Immunodeficiency and elevated CD4 T lymphocyte counts in two patients coinfected with human immunodeficiency virus and human lymphotropic virus type I. *Clin Infect Dis.* 1995;21:1466-1468.
333. Casoli C, Pilotti E, Bertazzoni U. Molecular and cellular interactions of HIV-1/HTLV coinfection and impact on AIDS progression. *AIDS Rev.* 2007;9:140-149.
334. Harrison LH, Schechter M. Coinfection with HTLV-I and HIV: increase in HTLV-I-related outcomes but not accelerated HIV disease progression? *AIDS Patient Care STDs.* 1998;12:619-623.
335. Murphy EL, Fridey J, Smith JW, et al. HTLV-associated myelopathy in a cohort of HTLV-I and HTLV-II-infected blood donors: the REDS investigators. *Neurology.* 1997;48:315-320.

336. Hjelle B, Appenzeller O, Mills R, et al. Chronic neurodegenerative disease associated with HTLV-II infection. *Lancet.* 1992;339:645-646.

337. Bhagavati S, Ehrlich G, Kula RW, et al. Detection of human T-cell lymphoma/leukemia virus type I DNA and antigen in spinal fluid and blood of patients with chronic progressive myelopathy. *N Engl J Med.* 1988;318:1141-1147.

338. Black FL, Biggar RJ, Lal RB, et al. Twenty-five years of HTLV type II follow-up with a possible case of tropical spastic paraparesis in the Kayapo, a Brazilian Indian tribe. *AIDS Res Hum Retroviruses.* 1996;12:1623-1627.

339. Lehky TJ, Flerlage N, Katz D, et al. Human T-cell lymphotropic virus type II-associated myelopathy: clinical and immunologic profiles. *Ann Neurol.* 1996;40:714-723.

340. Toro C, Blanco F, Garcia-Gasco P, et al. Human T lymphotropic virus type 1-associated myelopathy/tropical spastic paraparesis in an HIV-positive patient coinfected with human T lymphotropic virus type 2 following initiation of antiretroviral therapy. *Clin Infect Dis.* 2007;45:e118-e120.

341. Harrington Jr WJ, Sheremata W, Hjelle B, et al. Spastic ataxia associated with human T-cell lymphotropic virus type II infection. *Ann Neurol.* 1993;33:411-414.

342. Sheremata WA, Harrington Jr WJ, Bradshaw PA, et al. Association of "(tropical) ataxic neuropathy" with HTLV-II. *Virus Res.* 1993;29:71-77.

343. Jacobson S, Lehky T, Nishimura M, et al. Isolation of HTLV-II from a patient with chronic, progressive neurological disease clinically indistinguishable from HTLV-I-associated myelopathy/tropical spastic paraparesis. *Ann Neurol.* 1993;33:392-396.

344. Biglione MM, Pizarro M, Salomon HE, et al. A possible case of myelopathy/tropical spastic paraparesis in an Argentinian woman with human T lymphocyte virus type II. *Clin Infect Dis.* 2003;37:456-458.

345. Dooneief G, Marlink R, Bell K, et al. Neurologic consequences of HTLV-II infection in injection-drug users. *Neurology.* 1996;46:1556-1560.

346. Zehender G, De Maddalena C, Osio M, et al. High prevalence of human T cell lymphotropic virus type II infection in patients affected by human immunodeficiency virus type 1-associated predominantly sensory polyneuropathy. *J Infect Dis.* 1995;172:1595-1598.

347. Zehender G, Colasante C, Santambrogio S, et al. Increased risk of developing peripheral neuropathy in patients coinfected with HIV-1 and HTLV-2. *J Acquir Immune Defic Syndr.* 2002;31:440-447.

348. Berger JR, Svenningsson A, Raffanti S, et al. Tropical spastic paraparesis-like illness occurring in a patient dually infected with HIV-1 and HTLV-II. *Neurology.* 1991;41:85-87.

349. Castillo LC, Gracia F, Roman GC, et al. Spinocerebellar syndrome in patients infected with human T-lymphotropic virus types I and II (HTLV-I/HTLV-II): report of 3 cases from Panama. *Acta Neurol Scand.* 2000;101:405-412.

350. Rosenblatt JD, Golde DW, Wachsman W, et al. A second isolate of HTLV-II associated with atypical hairy-cell leukemia. *N Engl J Med.* 1986;315:372-377.

351. Loughran Jr TP, Coyle T, Sherman MP, et al. Detection of human T-cell leukemia/lymphoma virus, type II, in a patient with large granular lymphocyte leukemia. *Blood.* 1992;80:1116-1119.

352. Zucker-Franklin D, Hooper WC, Evatt BL. Human lymphotropic retroviruses associated with mycosis fungoides: evidence that human T-cell lymphotropic virus type II (HTLV-II) as well as HTLV-I may play a role in the disease. *Blood.* 1992;80:1537-1545.

353. Modahl LE, Young KC, Varney KF, et al. Are HTLV-II-seropositive injection drug users at increased risk of bacterial pneumonia, abscess, and lymphadenopathy? *J Acquir Immune Defic Syndr Hum Retrovirol.* 1997;16:169-175.

354. Orland JR, Wang B, Wright DJ, et al. Increased mortality associated with HTLV-II infection in blood donors: a prospective cohort study. *Retrovirology.* 2004;1:4.

355. Ciancianaini P, Magnani G, Barchi E, et al. Serological and clinical follow-up of an Italian IVDU cohort of HTLV-II/HIV-1 co-infected patients. Evidence of direct relationship between CD4 count and HTLV-II proviral load. *AIDS Res Hum Retroviruses.* 2001;17:S-70.

356. Turci M, Pilotti E, Ronzi P, et al. Coinfection with HIV-1 and human T-cell lymphotropic virus type II in intravenous drug users is associated with delayed progression to AIDS. *J Acquir Immune Defic Syndr.* 2006;41:100-106.

357. Matsushita S, Mitsuya H, Reitz MS, et al. Pharmacological inhibition of in vitro infectivity of human T lymphotropic virus type I. *J Clin Invest.* 1987;80:394-400.

358. Taylor GP, Goon P, Furukawa Y, et al. Zidovudine plus lamivudine in human T-lymphotropic virus type-I-associated myelopathy: a randomised trial. *Retrovirology.* 2006;3:63.

359. Murphy EL, Grant RM, Kropp J, et al. Increased human T-lymphotropic virus type II proviral load following highly active retroviral therapy in HIV-coinfected patients. *J Acquir Immune Defic Syndr.* 2003;33:655-656.

360. Guiltinan AM, Murphy EL, Horton JA, et al. Psychological distress in blood donors notified of HTLV-I/II infection. Retrovirus Epidemiology Donor Study. *Transfusion.* 1998;38:1056-1062.

361. Tsukasaki K, Ikeda S, Murata K, et al. Characteristics of chemotherapy-induced clinical remission in long survivors with aggressive adult T-cell leukemia/lymphoma. *Leuk Res.* 1993;17:157-166.

362. Taguchi H, Kinoshita KI, Takatsuki K, et al. An intensive chemotherapy of adult T-cell leukemia/lymphoma: CHOP followed by etoposide, vindesine, ranimustine, and mitoxantrone with granulocyte colony-stimulating factor support. *J Acquir Immune Defic Syndr Hum Retrovirol.* 1996;12:182-186.

363. Bazarbachi A, Ghez D, Lepelletier Y, et al. New therapeutic approaches for adult T-cell leukaemia. *Lancet Oncol.* 2004;5:664-672.

364. Matutes E, Taylor GP, Cavenagh J, et al. Interferon alpha and zidovudine therapy in adult T-cell leukaemia lymphoma: response and outcome in 15 patients. *Br J Haematol.* 2001;113:779-784.

365. Ezaki K, Hirano M, Ohno R, et al. A combination trial of human lymphoblastoid interferon and bestrabucil (KM2210) for adult T-cell leukemia-lymphoma. *Cancer.* 1991;68:695-698.

366. Gill PS, Harrington Jr W, Kaplan MH, et al. Treatment of adult T-cell leukemia-lymphoma with a combination of interferon alfa and zidovudine. *N Engl J Med.* 1995;332:1744-1748.

367. Bazarbachi A, Nasr R, El-Sabban ME, et al. Evidence against a direct cytotoxic effect of alpha interferon and zidovudine in HTLV-I associated adult T cell leukemia/lymphoma. *Leukemia.* 2000;14:716-721.

368. Matutes E. Adult T-cell leukaemia/lymphoma. *J Clin Pathol.* 2007;60:1373-1377.

369. Tajima K, Amakawa R, Uehira K, et al. Adult T-cell leukemia successfully treated with allogeneic bone marrow transplantation. *Int J Hematol.* 2000;71:290-293.

370. Waldmann TA, White JD, Carrasquillo JA, et al. Radioimmunotherapy of interleukin-2R alpha-expressing adult T-cell leukemia with Yttrium-90-labeled anti-Tac. *Blood.* 1995;86:4063-4075.

371. Dbaibo GS, Kfoury Y, Darwiche N, et al. Arsenic trioxide induces accumulation of cytotoxic levels of ceramide in acute promyelocytic leukemia and adult T-cell leukemia/lymphoma cells through de novo ceramide synthesis and inhibition of glucosylceramide synthase activity. *Haematologica.* 2007;92:753-762.

372. Matsuo H, Nakamura T, Tsujihata M, et al. Plasmapheresis in treatment of human T-lymphotropic virus type-I associated myelopathy. *Lancet.* 1988;2:1109-1113.

373. Matsuo H, Nakamura T, Shibayama K, et al. Long-term follow-up of immunomodulation in treatment of HTLV-I-associated myelopathy. *Lancet.* 1989;1:790.

374. Izumo S, Goto I, Itoyama Y, et al. Interferon-alpha is effective in HTLV-I-associated myelopathy: a multicenter, randomized, double-blind, controlled trial. *Neurology.* 1996;46:1016-1021.

375. Shibayama K, Nakamura T, Nagasato K, et al. Interferon-alpha treatment in HTLV-I-associated myelopathy studies of clinical and immunological aspects. *J Neurol Sci.* 1991;106:186-192.

376. Oh U, Yamano Y, Mora CA, et al. Interferon-beta1a therapy in human T-lymphotropic virus type I-associated neurologic disease. *Ann Neurol.* 2005;57:526-534.

377. Harrington WJ, Sheremata WA, Snodgrass SR, et al. Tropical spastic paraparesis/HTLV-1-associated myelopathy (TSP/HAM): treatment with an anabolic steroid danazol. *AIDS Res Hum Retroviruses.* 1991;7:1031-1034.

378. Gout O, Gessain A, Iba-Zizen M, et al. The effect of zidovudine on chronic myelopathy associated with HTLV-1. *J Neurol.* 1991;238:108-109.

379. Sheremata WA, Benedict D, Squilacote DC, et al. High-dose zidovudine induction in HTLV-I-associated myelopathy: safety and possible efficacy. *Neurology.* 1993;43:2125-2129.

380. Guidelines for counseling persons infected with human T-lymphotropic virus type I (HTLV-I) and type II (HTLV-II). Centers for Disease Control and Prevention and the U.S.P.H.S. Working Group. *Ann Intern Med.* 1993;118:448-454.

381. Kazanji M, Tartaglia J, Franchini G, et al. Immunogenicity and protective efficacy of recombinant human T-cell leukemia/lymphoma virus type 1 NYVAC and naked DNA vaccine candidates in squirrel monkeys (Saimiri sciureus). *J Virol.* 2001;75:5939-5948.

382. de The G, Bomford R. An HTLV-I vaccine: why, how, for whom? *AIDS Res Hum Retroviruses.* 1993;9:381-386.

169

Human Immunodeficiency Viruses

MARVIN S. REITZ, JR. | **ROBERT C. GALLO**

Infection with human immunodeficiency virus type 1 (HIV-1) and its end stage, acquired immunodeficiency syndrome (AIDS), is the major public health challenge of modern times, with over 25 million persons already dead and 30 to 40 million living with HIV/AIDS, most whom are without access to therapy. AIDS was first recognized in the United States in 1981 with reports of unexplained opportunistic infections, including *Pneumocystis jirovecii* pneumonia and Kaposi's sarcoma (KS), among homosexual men in New York and San Francisco.[1-3] On the basis of the epidemiologic features, association with the loss of CD4+ lymphocytes and immunosuppression, and likely infectious cause, a new human retrovirus was postulated as a causal agent. The field of retrovirology had markedly advanced just a decade earlier with the description of reverse transcriptase (RT) and with the discovery of human T-cell lymphotropic virus types I and II (HTLV-I and HTLV-II), the first two known human retroviruses, in 1979 and 1981 (reported in 1980 and 1982, respectively).[4,5] The discovery of interleukin-2 or T-cell growth factor[6,7] allowed the culture of blood T lymphocytes from early cases of AIDS; by 1984, the detection, isolation, and propagation of HIV-1,[8-12] had led to the development of a diagnostic test, an increasingly detailed understanding of the molecular biology of this virus, and, most important, the introduction of a rational basis for antiviral therapy.[13] After a long era of expanding research, new therapeutic combinations (RT and protease inhibitors), combined with the ability to measure circulating viral RNA and resistance to drugs, have led to a dramatically improved clinical course for persons fortunate enough to have access to therapy. More recently, inhibitors of virus-cell fusion, viral entry into the host cell, and integration of viral DNA into host chromosomal DNA are becoming available. Within a brief period, technologic advances have provided a clearer understanding of viral dynamics and the disease process, focusing attention on viral replication, host immune responses, and T-cell dynamics while confirming and elaborating the causal role of the virus. Equally dramatic has been the elucidation of how HIV enters cells, using both the CD4 molecule and a chemokine receptor as a dual-receptor system, as well as the mapping of the three-dimensional structure of the viral envelope protein. Contemporary retrovirology is largely devoted to the study of HIV-1 and of HIV-associated diseases. The molecular and cellular biology of this virus is now better understood than that of almost any other in history. Research on HIV has shown that rational antiviral therapy is possible, thereby pointing the way toward therapy for other viral diseases. Although this information has yet to be completely translated into greater progress in the areas of prevention, therapy, vaccines, and immune reconstitution for much of the developing world, where most HIV is transmitted, the Presidential Emergency Plan for AIDS Relief (PEPFAR) and other programs have greatly facilitated the institution of effective therapies in many parts of Africa.

Viruses are obligate intracellular parasites, and every aspect of the virus is in some way relevant to virus-host relationships. This chapter outlines the life cycle, molecular and cellular biology, structure, and regulation of HIV-1 and includes some discussion of pathogenesis and outcome of infection. Although the division of the chapter into sections is useful for organization of the information presented, in reality these subjects cannot be separated from one another; from the perspective of both virus and host, the process of infection is a continuous series of connected interactions.

Origin and Classification of Human Retroviruses

Current knowledge places retroviral infection of humans as zoonoses that originated in primate-to-human species-jumping events. For HIV-1 and HIV-2, these events occurred in Central and West Africa, most likely at multiple times, with the more recent attaining major epidemic significance. Simian immunodeficiency virus of chimpanzees (SIV_{cpz}) is the immediate precursor to HIV-1.[14] It now appears likely that similar species-jumping events occurred between certain types of monkeys and chimpanzees.[15]

Retroviruses have been classified by a number of different biologic features into at least seven genera. Oncogenic retroviruses occur in all classes of vertebrates. The first infectious agents that produced cancer in chickens were isolated by Ellerman and Bang (1908)[16] and by Peyton Rous (1911).[17] These workers were considerably ahead of their time, and the biologic systems to culture and study these viruses had not yet been described. Rous eventually won a Nobel Prize for his work in 1966. The pioneering work of Ludwig Gross in the 1950s stimulated renewed interest by demonstrating that oncogenic viruses could produce tumors in mammals,[18] but for the next 3 decades it remained orthodoxy for most scientists that human retroviruses did not exist. We now know that the pathogenic human retroviruses include lentiviruses (HIV-1 and -2) and oncoviruses (HTLV-I and -II). Human endogenous retroviruses, present in the human germ line, are often replication-defective and have not yet been shown to cause any disease.

As a replication strategy, retroviruses use the reverse transcription of viral RNA into linear double-stranded DNA, with subsequent integration into the host genome. The characteristic enzyme used for this process, an RNA-dependent DNA polymerase that reverses the flow of genetic information, is known as reverse transcriptase. The discovery of this enzyme altered the "central dogma" of molecular biology—namely, that genetic information must necessarily flow from DNA to RNA[19,20]—and helped initiate the modern era of molecular biology. This enzyme is error-prone; with the massive turnover of virions in the infected host, these errors accumulate in the viral DNA, accounting for the relatively high mutability of HIV-1. The lifestyle of the retrovirus therefore involves two forms, a DNA provirus and RNA-containing infectious virion.

The discovery of HTLV-I and its etiologic association, first with adult T-cell leukemia, an aggressive T-cell lymphoma,[21-23] and later with a neurologic disease, tropical spastic paraparesis/HTLV-I–associated myelopathy (TSP/HAM),[24] were pivotal events in modern medicine. Although there is relatively little variation among HTLV-I isolates, HTLV-II, the second human retrovirus, is 50% identical to HTLV-I at the genomic level.[4] Similarly, HIV-2, the fourth human retrovirus, was identified as a serologic variant of HIV-1, the third human retrovirus, and was isolated from patients in western Africa.[25,26] Some types of SIV are so closely related to HIV-2 that they may form an overlapping continuum with recent common ancestors. HIV-2 is known to infect several monkey species, including the sooty mangabey, its natural host, and SIV has been known to be transmitted, albeit rarely, to laboratory workers. SIVs and SIV/HIV hybrids (SHIVs) have been used extensively to study animal models of immunodeficiency. Other species, including cats (feline leukemia virus [FeLV] and feline immunodeficiency virus [FIV]) and cattle (bovine leukemia virus [BLV] and bovine immunodeficiency virus [BIV]), harbor retroviruses

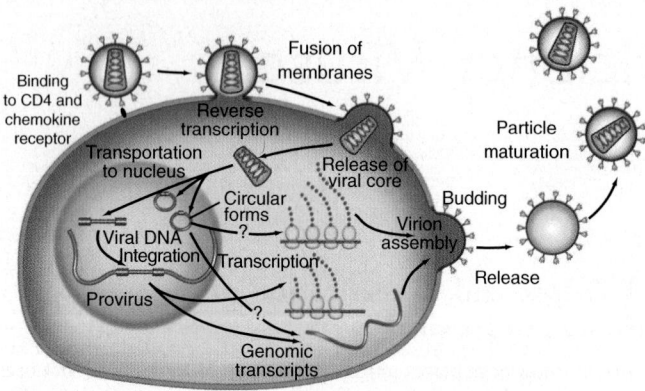

Figure 169-1 **The life cycle of human immunodeficiency virus type 1 (HIV-1).**

analogous to those of humans and some African primates. HIV-related retroviruses, known as lentiretroviruses, also include the ungulate viruses, maedi-visna virus of sheep, caprine arthritis-encephalitis virus, and equine infectious anemia virus.

As RNA viruses, retroviruses have the survival advantage of great genetic diversity. As viruses with a DNA intermediate in their replication cycle, they also have the advantage of latency, as do many DNA viruses, but even more so because the DNA provirus is integrated into the chromosomal DNA of the infected cell. As a CD4⁺ T-cell and macrophage-tropic virus, HIV also has the advantage of reducing the effectiveness of the host immune response.

Retroviruses are typically 100 nm in diameter and contain two single strands of RNA, which permits recombination between the strands (Fig. 169-1). The typical genome is approximately 10 kilobases (kb) or less in size and contains three major structural genes, namely *gag, pol,* and *env.* HIV-1 also contains several additional genes; these "extra" genes were first described in HTLV-I. In both viruses, some of these extra genes are essential to viral replication, whereas others may modulate interactions of the virus with its host. Figure 169-2 outlines the genome composition of HIV-1 and HTLV-I.

Viral Transmission and Life Cycle

BIOLOGY OF TRANSMISSION

The infectious life cycle of HIV can be described both at the molecular, single-cell level and at the level of a host organism infected with a

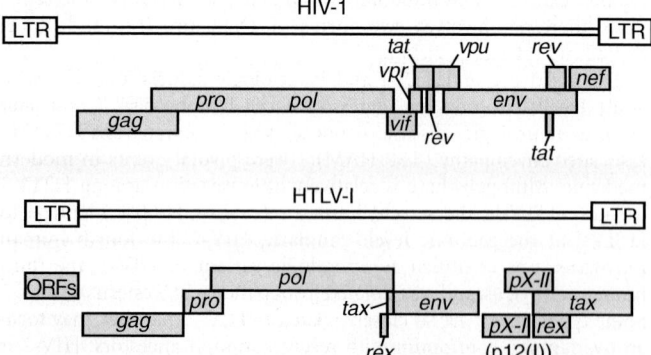

Figure 169-2 **Genomic organization of human retroviruses.** A comparison of the genomes of human T-cell lymphotropic virus type I (HTLV-I) and human immunodeficiency virus (HIV) is shown. Studies of HTLV genes and gene products laid the foundation for an understanding of their functional homologues subsequently found in HIV (e.g., *tat* and *rev*), although there is little sequence homology of these genes between HTLV and HIV.

"swarm" of closely related viral species. Multiple variables, including route of exposure, dose, immunogenetic background, and concomitant infections, influence the probability of transmission. The biologic events during exposure and successful infection of the host are only partially elucidated. The most common modes of infection are sexual transmission at the genital or colonic mucosa, exposure to other infected fluids such as blood or blood products, transmission from mother to infant and, occasionally, accidental occupational exposure. Transmitted viruses typically use the interaction of the viral glycoprotein gp120 with the cellular receptor CD4 and the chemokine receptor CCR5 to gain cell entry, thus selecting for macrophage-tropic *non–syncytia-forming* variants. This finding explains why persons who lack a functional CCR5 receptor are relatively resistant to infection by sexual transmission. Non–macrophage-tropic strains, also called *syncytia-inducing* (SI), are typically found late in infection. These strains use another chemokine receptor, CXCR4, to facilitate entry and are apparently not readily transmitted from person to person. In a model of acute infection in the macaque, the first cellular targets of intravaginal inoculation of the virus are Langerhans cells, tissue dendritic cells in the lamina propria, which then fuse with lymphocytes. However, direct infection of T cells has also been described. Infected cells can be found in draining lymph nodes within 2 days and in plasma by 5 days.[27]

In HIV-1–infected persons, there is a rapid rise in the degree of plasma viremia within days, with high viral titers and widespread dissemination, probably targeting lymphoid organs and the central nervous system (CNS). This acute stage of HIV infection is sometimes manifested as a transient symptomatic illness characterized by a maculopapular rash and flulike symptoms. This phase is followed by a marked reduction in virus to steady-state levels, probably because of vigorous antivirus cellular responses. The immune response probably accounts for the mononucleosis-like acute syndrome seen in approximately half of patients. Initially, perhaps within hours of infection, at least three HIV inhibitory chemokines (notably the chemokines MIP 1α, MIP 1β, and RANTES [regulated on activation, normal T-cell expressed and secreted]) may be produced. As is the case for many infections with viruses that establish chronic infections, this response is at least partially successful in controlling replication. Levels of HIV-1–specific cytotoxic T lymphocytes (CTLs) are inversely correlated with plasma viral RNA levels.[28] High levels of potent CTL virus-specific cells targeted to the viral Env protein and soluble factors produced by these cells early in infection may correlate with the decline of virus, even before a neutralizing antibody can be detected.[29]

A great deal of variability in peak viral RNA plasma levels is seen during the first 120 days after infection. By 3 to 6 months after infection, viral levels reach a temporary steady state, sometimes called a *viral set point.* This level is highly correlated with subsequent disease progression in that lower viral steady-state level is correlated with slower disease progression. Thus, early in the course of infection, virus-host interactions are established that are predictive of subsequent disease.[30]

Intervention to control infection during this initial period has been shown to decrease the risk of subsequent infection in health care workers after needlestick exposure.[31] Treatment of infected mothers and exposed neonates has also shown a dramatic effect in decreasing the incidence of maternal-fetal transmission. The theory underlying the use of antiretroviral prophylaxis following sexual exposure is biologically plausible, but currently lacks direct proof of efficacy in controlled studies.[32]

LIFE CYCLE

The life cycle of HIV-1 can be considered in two distinct phases (see Fig. 169-1). The initial early events include viral attachment, entry into the cytoplasm, reverse transcription, entry into the nucleus, and integration of the double-stranded DNA (the provirus). The second phase occurs over the lifetime of the infected cell as viral and cellular proteins regulate the production of viral proteins and new infectious virions.

Infection is initiated by the binding of the virion gp120 Env surface protein to the CD4 molecule found on some T cells, macrophages, and microglial cells. Both SIV and HIV-2 also use this molecule. CD4 was first identified as a viral receptor in a number of studies showing the susceptibility of CD4-bearing cells to infection and the ability to block infection with anti-CD4 monoclonal antibodies in culture. Transfection of human CD4$^-$ HeLa cells with CD4 DNA rendered them permissive for infection.[33] Successful in vitro experiments blocking this interaction with soluble CD4 used laboratory strains adapted to cell lines and led to therapeutic attempts using immunoglobulin CD4, which were not successful. Subsequent experiments have shown that primary isolates are not sensitive to soluble CD4 and highlighted the necessity of using primary rather than laboratory-adapted isolates in studying virus-host interactions.

Early experiments demonstrated that as with other lentiretroviruses, macrophages could also be infected with HIV, but strains differed in their ability to infect T-cell lines or monocytes.[34] Binding to CD4 is not sufficient for entry of HIV into human or nonhuman cells, and the fact that small changes in the V3 loop of envelope gp120 (see later) could determine tropism of the virus for either macrophage or T-cell lines suggested that a second receptor was present. The first important clue for the basis of this tropism was the unexpected finding that a group of chemokines (RANTES, MIP-1α, and MIP-1β), small extracellular proteins naturally produced by CD8$^+$ T cells, inhibited macrophage-tropic but not T-cell line–adapted strains.[35] This discovery at once explained the nature of a long-sought CD8 viral suppressor factor and suggested a previously unexpected role for chemokine receptors. The independent identification of an orphan chemokine receptor, CXCR4, as the second receptor for T-cell line–tropic strains[36] was followed by a rapid series of reports demonstrating CCR5 to be the principal second receptor for macrophage-tropic strains and CXCR4 for T-cell line–adapted strains.[37-40] Crystallographic evidence indicates that CD4 binds in a recessed pocket on gp120, which includes a deep cavity that binds to phenylalanine-43 of CD4. Previous mutagenesis studies had shown this phenylalanine to be a crucial residue for binding.[41] Other studies have also indicated a role for sugar molecules, glycosaminoglycans, in the binding of gp120, which influences interactions with the chemokine receptor.[42] Binding to CD4 triggers a conformational change in gp120 that allows it to then bind to CCR5 or CXCR4. This second binding event exposes the fusion domain of the gp41 transmembrane protein, allowing fusion of the viral and cellular membranes followed by viral entry into the target cell.

Events that occur immediately after viral entry—collectively, the disassembly process—are not simply the reverse of viral assembly. For example, studies have shown that HIV-1 must incorporate a cellular protein, cyclophilin A, which binds to the viral capsid protein p24. Failure to incorporate this cellular protein results in a profound postentry block during the next viral entry. Coincidentally, cyclophilin (peptidyl-prolyl isomerase) is the binding protein for cyclosporine, an inhibitor of T-cell activation, suggesting that activation-related cellular processes are involved in viral disassembly.[43,44] In addition, Vif and Nef, accessory viral proteins, may also be required.[45]

Reverse transcription begins in the cytoplasm, as DNA synthesis is initiated from the transfer RNA primer bound to the viral genomic RNA just downstream of the 5′ long terminal repeat (LTR). Reverse transcription proceeds in an orderly fashion in a similar manner in all retroviruses. Briefly, the transcription complex begins at the 5′ end, copies the U5 and R regions of the 5′ LTR, and then jumps to the 3′ end of the RNA, where the newly synthesized R region DNA binds to the R region of the 3′ LTR. Reverse transcription continues through the U3 region of the 3′ LTR and then through the remainder of the viral RNA, which gives a complete minus strand of DNA. The RNA is degraded by the viral ribonuclease H, except for two resistant purine-rich tracts in the middle and toward the 3′ end of the viral RNA. These then serve as the primers for formation of the DNA plus strand.[46] Because reverse transcription takes place in the cytoplasm, local concentrations of nucleotides may be a limiting factor, particularly in

nondividing cells. This is the rationale for using the ribonucleoside reductase inhibitor hydroxyurea to limit viral replication.[47,48]

During the formation of double-stranded DNA, the uncoated nucleoprotein complex, termed the *preintegration complex*, is imported into the nucleus.[47,48] This is an energy-requiring process that uses nuclear localization signals present on viral Gag, Vpr, and integrase (IN) proteins. Unlike most retroviruses, which integrate into the host cellular DNA as the nuclear membrane is disrupted during cell division, HIV-1 can be imported into the nucleus and integrate into nondividing cells. This may be especially important in the infection of monocytes and macrophages, which are essentially nondividing cells.

IN-negative mutants of HIV do not integrate and do not produce infectious virus.[49,50] Integration does not appear to be site-directed. However, HIV preferentially integrates into or near active genes, particularly those that are activated following infection by HIV-1.[51] Integration of the provirus appears to be an essential step in every replication cycle. Unintegrated viral DNA may survive, however, particularly in quiescent cells. This may provide a stable intermediate form in cells that are temporarily not permissive for infection; if cell activation occurs when these forms are present, viral infection may then proceed to completion. Integration of viral DNA establishes a linear copy of the viral genome within the genome of the cell, and replication of the virus then occurs along with cell replication. Integration is generally for the life of the cell and, with the cell and its progeny, for the life of the organism.

Synthesis of new viral RNA genomes and proteins is accomplished in a highly regulated manner using host cell proteins. A high level of viral production from several different cellular compartments can be maintained throughout the course of infection. The high number of replication cycles allow the generation of variants and selection by drugs or the immune system. The half-life of virus-producing CD4$^+$ T cells is approximately 0.7 day and the generation time of HIV-1 in vivo is approximately 2 days.[52] HIV-1 pathogenesis is the result of a complex interplay between the virus and the immune system, particularly the mechanisms responsible for T-cell homeostasis and regeneration. Protracted loss of CD4$^+$ T cells results from early viral destruction of selected memory T-cell populations, followed by a combination of profound increases in overall memory T-cell turnover, damage to the thymus and other lymphoid tissues, and physiologic limitations in peripheral CD4$^+$ T-cell renewal.[53] Equally important are indirect hematopoietic and immunoregulatory effects of viral components (see later).

Once integration has occurred, virus production depends on the presence of cellular and viral factors required for activation of viral promoters. External factors, including coinfection with other agents, production of inflammatory cytokines, and cellular activation, may enhance viral replication.[54] The molecular mechanisms regulating virus production include cellular pathways involving factors, such as the nuclear factor-κB (NF-κB) family of inducible transcription factors, that result in a cascade of events leading to viral genome expression.[55]

A unique feature of HIV-1 is that expression of different viral RNA species is temporally regulated. Using cellular enzymes, such as RNA polymerase II, transcription of the provirus is initiated at the viral promoter, at the junction of the U3-R regions in the LTR, as a single complete message. The viral messenger RNA (mRNA) and genomic RNA transcripts, processed by cellular machinery, are spliced, capped, polyadenylated, and transported to the cytoplasm for translation into viral proteins (see Fig. 169-2). Differential splicing of this complete RNA, controlled in part by the viral protein Rev, determines the type of message and protein that is produced. Early after infection, activated cells produce 2-kb mRNAs for viral regulatory proteins that can be detected by Northern blot analysis[56]; using even more sensitive reverse transcription–polymerase chain reaction (PCR) techniques, expression can be detected within 6 hours.[57] These messages include the unique doubly spliced RNA for Tat, Rev, and Nef proteins.[58] Tat protein induces a markedly enhanced activity of the viral promoter, chiefly by facilitating the elongation of nascent short viral transcripts, resulting in greatly increased RNA and protein production. The Rev protein serves to decrease the production of double-spliced messages. With the accumulation of Rev protein, there is a switch to enhanced expression of unspliced and singly spliced mRNAs that encode the late viral proteins, including the virion proteins Gag, Pol, and Env and Vpu, Vpr, and Vif, as well as genomic RNA. The delayed transit from early to late viral genes probably reflects a requirement for threshold levels of Rev needed to bind and form multimers of the protein complexed with the Rev regulatory element (RRE) located in incompletely spliced mRNAs. Packaging of the genomic RNA within a virus particle requires the presence of a specific packaging signal located between the major splice donor at the 5' end of the genome and the initiation codon for the Gag precursor polyprotein. In the absence of this signal, mature particles are formed that are devoid of RNA. The incorporation of genomic RNA requires two zinc-finger domains found in the p7 Gag nucleocapsid protein. Assembly of mature viral particles occurs at the cell membrane with the association of the Gag matrix protein p17 with the cytoplasmic domain of the envelope transmembrane protein gp41, which in turn binds to the viral gp120 on the outer surface. Assembled virions include the viral envelope proteins, cell membrane and associated cellular proteins, a matrix composed mainly of Gag p17, and a capsid composed of the p24 capsid protein and RNA, RT, IN, Gag proteins p6 and p7, and Vpr. The mature viral particle characteristically buds from the cell surface into the surrounding

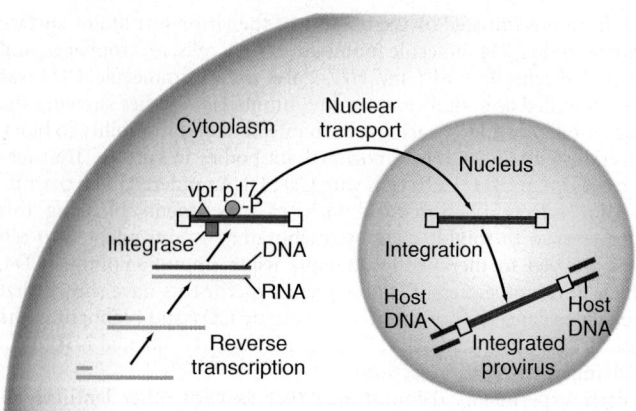

Figure 169-4 **Viral proteins required for nuclear transport and integration.** Following entry, formation of the reverse transcription complex and reverse transcription human immunodeficiency virus infection involves the formation of the preintegration complex, consisting of the newly synthesized viral DNA and several HIV proteins—the matrix protein (p17), integrase, reverse transcriptase, and viral protein R (vpr).

media, completing the life cycle of the virus. Budding of HIV-1 virions occurs at highly specialized membrane microdomains known as lipid rafts.[59] These domains are characterized by a distinct lipid composition that includes high concentrations of cholesterol, sphingolipids, and glycolipids.

The Pathogen

The mature infectious virus particle buds from a cell membrane forming a sphere with an outer lipid bilayer and a nucleocapsid with a dense, cone-shaped core (Fig. 169-3). The core appears to be attached to the viral outer envelope at its narrow end.[60] The outer membrane contains up to 72 spiked knobs, which are assembled as trimers of the outer envelope protein gp120 bound to the transmembrane portion gp41. The viral membrane is cholesterol-rich and includes cellular proteins.[61]

Each mature virion is composed of two molecules of single-stranded RNA surrounded by three *gag* gene cleavage products: the p17 matrix protein; the p24 major capsid protein, which forms the capsid shell; and the p7 nucleoprotein, which binds tightly to the viral RNA. The matrix contains the myristoylated matrix protein p17, which is critical for virion formation and is localized between the capsid protein p24 of the viral core and envelope. The p7 protein binds the two positive-strand copies of complete viral RNA attached at the packaging site, and it also binds to p24. A number of other viral proteins required for the early phases of infection are incorporated with the virion (Fig. 169-4): protease, which is essential for viral assembly; RT and IN, which are needed after entry for viral DNA synthesis and integration; tRNA^{lys} at the 5' end of the RNA, which serves as the primer for initiation of negative-strand DNA synthesis; and Vpr. The latter is a small protein that contains a nuclear localization signal and is associated with the nucleocapsid in large quantities. The virus encodes at least five other regulatory and/or accessory genes of diverse function. Some have been discussed already, and most are present in the infected cell but not in the mature virion. A list of HIV genes and associated proteins is presented in Table 169-1.

GENETIC ORGANIZATION

The HIV-1 proviral DNA integrated into the host cell is 9.7 kb in length and follows the basic genomic structure common to most retroviruses: *gag-pol-env* genes flanked by two complete viral LTRs (see Fig. 169-2). The provirus is symmetrically flanked at either end by the viral LTR and by cellular sequences representing the site of integration. These LTRs

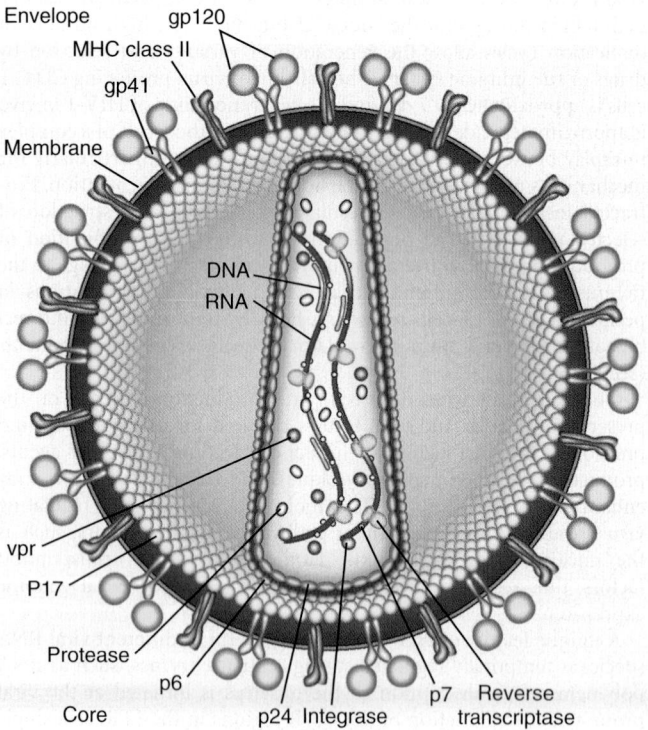

Figure 169-3 **Structure of the human immunodeficiency virus type 1 (HIV-1) virion.** The viral envelope is formed from the host cell membrane, into which the HIV-1 envelope proteins gp41 and gp120 have been inserted and may include several host cell proteins, most significantly the major histocompatibility complex (MHC) class II proteins. The matrix between the envelope and the core is formed predominantly from Gag protein p17. The core contains the viral RNA, closely associated with Gag protein p7, in addition to RT and integrase. It has also been shown that virions contain complementary DNA, as shown, synthesized by the Rt. The major structural proteins of the core are Gag proteins p24 and p6. Also present within the virion are the protease and two cleavage products from the Gag precursor protein (p1 and p2, not shown) of undetermined position within the virion. Vpr is also packaged in the virion and is thought to be localized within the core, as shown.

TABLE 169-1	Genes and Gene Products of Human Immunodeficiency Virus (HIV)-1 and HIV-2		
Gene	*Proteins*	*Size (kDa)*	*Function/Properties*
gag	p17		Matrix protein; interacts with gp41
	p24		Core protein
	p6		Core protein; binds to Vpr
	p7		Nucleocapsid; binds to RNA
	p1		
	p2		
pol	Protease	10	Proteolytic cleavage of Gag and Pol
	Reverse transcriptase	66, 51	Polymerase and RNase H activity (p66 only)
	Integrase	32	Integration into chromosome
env	gp120		Envelope; viral entry into cell
	gp41		Transmembrane protein; cell fusion
vif	Virion infectivity protein	23	Efficient cell-free transmission
vpr	Viral protein R	18	Enhances viral replication in primary cells, virion-associated protein; G_2/M phase arrest; nuclear localization
tat	*Trans*-activator of transcription	14	Major viral *trans*-activator, immune suppression
rev	Regulator of expression of virion protein	19	Enhances expression of unspliced and singly spliced RNAs
vpu*	Viral protein U	15-16	Enhances virion release from cells; downregulates CD4 and MHC class I surface expression
nef	Negative regulatory factor	27	Inhibits or enhances viral replication depending on strain and cell type
			Downregulates CD4; MHC class I
			Antiapoptosis
vpx†	Virion protein x	25	Packaged into the virion

*HIV-1 only.
†HIV-2 only.
MHC, major histocompatibility complex; RNase H, ribonuclease H.

contain transcriptional regulatory sequences, RNA processing signals, packaging sites, and the integration sites. The 5′ end begins with the *gag* gene, which encodes core and matrix proteins, the *pol* gene, which begins in an overlapping frame encoding viral protease, RT, and IN, and then the *env* gene, which encodes the outer and transmembrane envelope proteins. A complex series of open reading frames encode the accessory proteins. *vif* is partly contained within the *pol* coding region and partly downstream, and *vpr* is located downstream from *vif*. The first coding exons for *tat* and *rev* are co-linear and located between *vpr* and *env*, and their second exons, located in the *env* gene, are joined to the first exons by RNA splicing. The *vpu* gene is co-linear with the 5′ region of the *env* gene; *nef* is located downstream from the *env* gene and extends into the downstream LTR sequence.

Transcription of a single unspliced RNA is initiated at the 5′ end by the cellular RNA polymerase II. The unspliced mRNA serves as a template for translation of the Gag and Gag-Pol precursor polypeptides. This message is also spliced to produce single-spliced transcripts for Vif, Vpr, and Vpu proteins and the Env precursor polypeptide, and doubly spliced transcripts for Tat, Rev, and Nef. The precursor polyproteins are then cleaved by cellular or viral enzymes; the Gag and Gag-Pol precursors are cleaved by the viral protease, which is itself transcribed from the unspliced viral message. The Env precursor polypeptide is cleaved by cellular proteases (Fig. 169-5).

Virion Structural Proteins

GAG PROTEINS

The cleavage of the Gag precursor protein by viral protease produces the structural components of the viral core and matrix. To form the virus capsid structure, a large polyprotein is made from the viral mRNA. This 55-kDa Gag precursor protein (sometimes called p55) is cleaved into at least five structural proteins by the viral 34-kb protease encoded at the 5′ end of the *pol* gene. Lack of protease function, either through inhibition by drugs or following transfection of the p55 gene into a cell that lacks protease, results in the formation of noninfectious viral particles.[62]

The p55 protein is seen on Western blot preparations made from whole-cell lysates but not on those made from mature virions. During

or shortly after self-assembly, the viral protease is activated and the precursor is cleaved into three principal proteins and two smaller peptides. These proteins undergo extensive post-translational modification by cellular enzymes. After translation, the initiating methionine residue is removed, p17 is myristoylated, p17 and p24 are

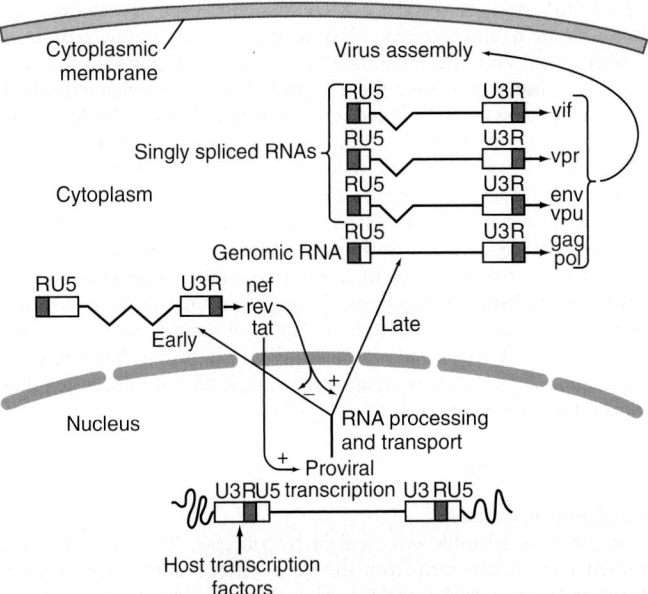

Figure 169-5 The role of RNA splicing in the life cycle of human immunodeficiency virus type 1 (HIV-1). The early mRNA transcripts of HIV-1 are doubly spliced and produce viral regulatory proteins Tat, Rev, and Nef. The function of HIV Rev is to facilitate the expression of the late transcripts of HIV-1. These can be divided into two categories, unspliced and singly spliced. The unspliced HIV-1 mRNA has two functions; it is translated into the structural precursor polyproteins for the *gag* and *pol* gene products and it is incorporated into virions as genomic RNA. The different singly spliced mRNAs of HIV-1 are translated into the envelope proteins gp120 and gp41, as well as Vif, Vpr, and Vpu.

phosphorylated by cellular kinases, and p7 (the nucleocapsid protein, or NC) binds to two zinc ions to form the zinc fingers that bind to RNA. Although the virus depends on cellular systems for many functions, it requires the virally encoded protease for the cleavage of the Gag proteins. Gag proteins are sufficient to form particles when expressed from transfected cells. These self-assembled particles are noninfectious. The p17 matrix protein, MA (molecular weight, 17,000), contains about 130 amino acids and is myristoylated on a glycine at its amino terminus by the host cell enzyme *N*-myristoyl transferase.[63,64] The first 31 amino acids target the myristoylated protein to the cell membrane, and nonmyristoylated proteins cannot form infectious virions. In addition to viral assembly at the cell surface, MA functions as part of the preintegration complex targeting viral DNA to the cell nucleus and enabling HIV-1 to infect and integrate into nondividing cells such as macrophages.[65] p17 has extracellular functions via binding to a receptor on peripheral blood mononuclear cells (PBMCs), including T cells, and increases their production of proinflammatory cytokines and counteracts the inhibitory activity of interleukin-4 (IL-4) on these cells.[66]

The p24 capsid protein, CA, is produced by two cleavages to form a 240–amino acid hydrophobic protein that forms the major subunits of the viral capsid and self-associates to form dimers and higher order structures. This protein binds the cellular cyclophilins, a process that may be important for viral replication.[67] A major homology region of 29 amino acids is shared with many retroviruses.[68,69] p24 Gag is typically the easiest protein to detect using sera from infected patients, and serologic detection in retrovirus-infected animals gave the name *group antigen* (Gag) to these proteins. The carboxyl-terminal sequences encode a 70–amino acid hydrophilic protein, NC, that binds both viral RNA and the capsid p24 protein, intertwining approximately one molecule with four to six nucleotides of RNA.[70] A zinc-finger domain binds RNA, whereas the NC recognizes the packaging site on Gag.[71,72] Two small proteins of unknown function, p2 and p1, are also found in the viral core.

A recently discovered intracellular antiviral mechanism targets the capsid protein and is mediated by the tripartite motif (TRIM) family.[73] The TRIM motif consists of a RING domain at the N-terminus, a B box-2 domain, and a coiled coil domain,[74] and apparently represents a widespread and ancient innate host defense mechanism. TRIM5α appears to be functionally similar to the Fv1 restriction element, which regulates permissivity of murine cells of different genetic backgrounds for infection with different strains of tropic murine leukemia viruses (MuLV), and was identified 40 years ago.[75] The restriction by both human TRIM5α and murine Fv1-B of N-tropic MuLV infection depends on residue 110 of the MuLV capsid protein.[76] HIV-1, however, is only partially sensitive to human TRIM5α (depending on allelic variants),[77] perhaps helping to account for its successful cross-species transmission from chimpanzees, although macaque TRIM5α strongly restricts HIV-1.[73,76] TRIM5α binds to viral capsid hexamers[78] and inhibits replication at a postentry step. The precise mechanism is not clear and may be mediated at more than one level, but may dysregulate viral capsid uncoating.[78,79]

VIRAL ENZYMES

Pol *Gene Products*

The *pol* gene encodes three enzymes, protease, RT, and IN. These proteins are synthesized from the same mRNA as the Gag proteins through a ribosomal translational frameshift. The cleavage of the 160-kDa precursor polyprotein is essential for viability. Because of the inefficiency of the frameshift, which is important in regulating the relative levels of viral proteins, there are about 2000 copies of each Gag protein and 100 copies of each Pol protein per virion.

Protease

Protease is a 10-kDa 99–amino acid protein that is fully active as a dimer. It is autocatalytically cleaved from the precursor protein during the viral assembly process. Site-specific mutagenesis has demonstrated

that noninfectious particles containing uncleaved Gag and Gag-Pol proteins are produced if this enzyme is inactivated. The similarity of viral protease to other aspartyl proteases such as angiotensin-converting enzyme (ACE) has greatly facilitated the design of potent antiviral drugs, including inhibitors of dimerization and molecules that bind to the active catalytic site.[62,80]

Reverse Transcriptase

Viral RT is an RNA-dependent DNA polymerase. This highly versatile enzyme is capable of synthesizing DNA copies from both RNA and DNA templates and degrading viral RNA from RNA-DNA hybrids. RT and its RNase H activity are required for viral replication. The protein is first cleaved from the precursor polyprotein to form a p66 homodimer and, after a second cleavage, forms a p66-p51 heterodimer with identical amino-terminal ends.

The structure of the RT heterodimer revealed the enzymatic mechanism of reverse transcription and the molecular basis of resistance to antiviral drugs.[81] The p66 and p51 assemble in an unusual head-to-tail heterodimer. Four domains of the p66 protein are similar in shape to a clenched right hand and therefore are designated as the fingers, palm, and thumb. These are joined to the RNase H domain. The cleft between them contains the highly conserved catalytic site Tyr-Met-Asp-Asp. Although the p51 subunit is derived from the same protein, it maintains a different conformation.[82,83]

RT plays a major role in the generation of genetic diversity in retroviruses. The fidelity of the enzyme has been determined for a variety of retroviruses by measuring misincorporation rates on defined templates. For HIV-1, this rate ranges from 1:1700 to 1:4000 misincorporations per nucleotide per replication, somewhat higher than for other retroviruses, and considerably greater than for the host cell polymerases. For the 9.7-kb HIV-1 genome, the in vivo error rate is estimated to be one misincorporation per replication cycle.[84] Variants produced by RT generate sequence diversity that may emerge under the selective pressure of immune responses or antiviral drugs and allow the virus to change cell tropism. However, the same lack of fidelity also allows nucleoside analogues to be preferentially incorporated into viral rather than cellular DNA.

Integrase

IN is a 288–amino acid, 32-kDa viral enzyme that mediates the linkage of double-stranded viral DNA into the host cell genome. Integration occurs following the translocation of a large complex derived from the viral core from the cytoplasm into the nucleus.[85] IN is part of this complex and catalyzes the cleavage of viral DNA and ligation to host cell DNA. A large central acidic domain of IN is highly conserved in retroviruses and retrotransposons. Once integrated, the provirus can be considered for most purposes to be a stable genetic element remaining for the life of the cell and, through cellular replication, for the life of the individual. Integrase is required for viral replication, and integrase inhibitors such as raltegravir are one of the most recent class of antiretroviral drugs entering clinical use (see Chapter 128).

ENVELOPE GLYCOPROTEINS AND VIRAL FUSION

The *env* gene of HIV-1 encodes a single-spliced viral RNA transcript that encodes both Vpu and a 160-kDa precursor that is synthesized in the late stages of viral replication. This 850–amino acid polyprotein is cleaved by cellular proteases at amino acids 512 and 513 to form the external surface gp120 and transmembrane gp41 proteins. Proteolytic cleavage is essential for viral infectivity. There is extensive *N*-linked glycosylation on asparagine residues with high-mannose complex oligosaccharide groups. Selective removal of glycosylation sites reduces infectivity. These proteins, especially gp120, are the targets of neutralizing antibodies. The extensive variation among different strains of HIV-1, especially in gp120, and the ability of the virus to evolve during the course of a single infection and to adapt to drugs and immunologic attack rapidly present problems in therapy and vaccine development. Most of the variability among strains of HIV occurs in the envelope sequence in five variable domains of gp120, designated V1 through V5 (comprising amino acids 128 to 152, 182 to 195, 300 to 330, 395 to 415, and 460 to 467, respectively).[86] The third variable region, called the V3 loop (formed by joining two cysteine residues), is a dominant antibody-neutralizing domain of gp120 and plays an important role in determining viral tropism. Four regions that are relatively invariant have been designated C1 through C4 (amino acids 33 to 60, 87 to 126, 231 to 276, and 460 to 467). These regions presumably maintain essential viral structures.

Although some structure-function relationships have been deduced from secondary structure, biochemical, mutagenic, and immunologic analyses, the solution of the crystal structure of the gp120 protein and of part of the gp41 protein has literally put a new face on the virus, with implications for cell fusion mechanisms and immune evasion. The crystal structure of gp120 at 2.5-Å resolution reveals a cavity-laden gp120–CD4 interface and a conserved binding site for the chemokine receptor, with evidence for a conformational change on CD4 binding. gp120 is visualized as two domains joined by a bridge. The V3 loop, together with conserved regions that remain unexposed until CD4 binding occurs, is a principal determinant of chemokine receptor variability. An understanding of the structural basis that enables HIV to evade humoral responses while maintaining function may help in vaccine design.[87,88] One of the most daunting issues in designing vaccines to elicit neutralizing antibodies is the extreme variability of the outer surface of the envelope. Binding to CD4, however, exposes the co-receptor binding site, which is structurally constrained by its functional requirements. Recent efforts to target this region have resulted in the generation of remarkably broadly neutralizing antibodies, suggesting that this approach has promise.[89] The approach may also be important, as recent trials of a vaccine based strictly on eliciting CTL activity failed to show any protection.[90]

Virus-Cell Fusion

The viral envelope ultimately must be understood as a fusion machine that allows viral entry into target cells. Fusion depends on sequential binding of gp120 to CD4 and the chemokine receptors, but the fusogenic domain is located in gp41. The fusion peptide that is inserted into the target cell membrane is formed at the new amino terminus created by proteolytic cleavage of the gp160 precursor protein.[91] However, this hydrophobic tip must be kept in an inactive state until juxtaposed to the target cell membrane. Premature triggering of the fusion peptide would result in an inactive virus. The core structure of gp41 has been crystallized from peptide fragments.[92]

The core structure that mediates the fusion-active state between virus and cell is formed from a trimer of gp41 molecules composed of two α-helical regions within each gp41 that form a six-helix bundle characteristic of "coiled coils." The crystallized complex shows striking structural homology with the low pH-induced fusogenic conformation of the influenza virus hemagglutinin protein (HA), which contains three antiparallel helices packed in a central trimeric coiled coil. The conformational change in HIV-1 is not mediated by endocytic uptake into the low pH compartment as it is for HA, however. The binding of gp120 to the second receptor likely triggers the conformational change that leads to cell fusion and virus uptake. The transition from a loop structure to a coiled coil state is the basis for the spring-loaded model of activation for membrane fusion. The fusion-active state has been identified using synthetic viral peptides to block fusion following triggering [93] (Fig. 169-6). Synthetic peptides that span all or part of these domains can inhibit HIV cell fusion and infection.[94]

VIRAL REGULATORY AND ACCESSORY GENES

In addition to the structural genes, HIV has six accessory genes: *tat* (coding for the *trans*-activator of transcription), *rev* (encoding the regulator of viral expression), *vif* (encoding the virion infectivity factor), *vpr* (encoding the viral protein R), *vpu* (encoding viral protein U), and *nef* (encoding the "negative" regulatory factor, which is a misnomer). These genes enable the virus to usurp host cell processes

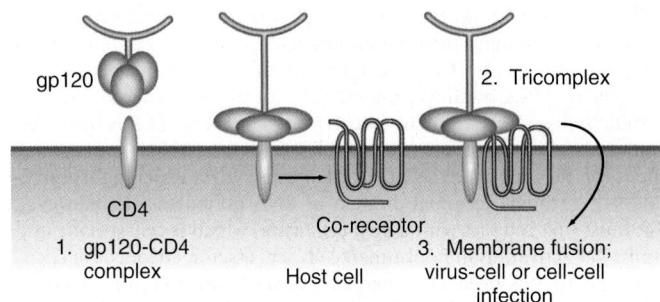

Figure 169-6 **The human immunodeficiency virus type 1 (HIV-1) infection process at the cell surface.** On first infection and after initial binding of gp120 of HIV to the cell surface CD4 molecule, an envelope conformational change occurs that fosters binding to the chemokine co-receptor (e.g., CCR5 or CXCR4). This interaction involves specific portions of gp120 including the V3 region.

and to achieve efficient replication under host-selective pressure, thus contributing to disease progression.[45] Expression of Nef in infected macrophages activates T cells through the CD2 stimulatory pathway, rendering the T cells susceptible to infection.[95] Of these genes, only *tat* and *rev* are necessary for high levels of viral expression in culture. Tat augments viral RNA levels by greatly increasing transcription, primarily by permitting elongation of otherwise blocked short nascent RNA chains. Rev regulates the splicing and transport of RNA. Vif is required for efficient cell-free transmission of virus and acts as an antagonist against APOBEC3G,[96] a deoxycytidine deaminase that acts on newly synthesized viral DNA to induce its degradation and hypermutation and that may represent a general antiretroviral defense mechanism.[97] APOBEC3G may also inhibit reverse transcription. Nef has been found to be crucial to virulence and immune evasion and downregulates surface expression of CD4, presumably to allow efficient expression of gp120 on the cell surface. As noted, expression of Nef in macrophages may be important in rendering neighboring T cells permissive to infection. Vpr also downregulates surface expression of CD4; it is the only accessory protein found abundantly in the mature virion.

As a presumed example of convergent evolution, *tax* and *rex* genes present in HTLV-I (and related viruses) encode two proteins, Tax (*trans*-activator of transcription) and Rex (regulator of viral expression); these genes function analogously to *tat* and *rev*. Similar genes are present in HIV-2, which lacks *vpu* but has *vpx*, which encodes a unique protein Vpx (viral protein X). Accessory genes formed by complex splicing arrangements are not generally found in all retroviruses, suggesting that retroviruses could be classified as simple or complex, depending on the presence or absence of these genes.

Early in infection, a *rev*-independent pathway removes introns from the viral transcript. The multiply spliced messages of *tat* and *rev* are transported and translated and, as proteins, are shuttled back to the nucleus. As Tat acts and Rev accumulates in the nucleus, additional unspliced and single-spliced messages for *gag*, *gag-pol*, and *env* and viral accessory genes *vpu*, *vpr*, and *vif* are transported out of the nucleus.[98]

The Tat protein is translated from a transcript that contains three exons, the first of which is noncoding. The *tat* reading frame overlaps both the *rev* and *env* genes. Tat is a small nuclear (14- to 16-kDa) protein that varies in size, containing 86 to 102 amino acids, depending on the strain of HIV-1. The first 72 amino acids contained in the second exon are required for full activity, whereas all the length variation occurs at the carboxyl-terminal end of the protein.[99] Tat binds to the Tat activation response element (TAR) region found in all HIV-1 mRNAs, in conjunction with cellular factors, to stabilize the nascent mRNA and enhance its rate of elongation up to 1000-fold. However, Tat activation is downregulated after periods of several hours, suggesting that these cellular cofactors may be present in limited amounts and that negative regulatory factors may downmodulate Tat function.

The Tat protein has three functional domains. A highly conserved cysteine-rich domain between amino acids 22 and 37 contains seven cysteine residues and two zinc-finger motifs, as is characteristic of a number of DNA-binding proteins. Loss of any one of six cysteines results in loss of activity. The interaction of Tat with TAR is mediated through a basic domain between nucleic acids 48 and 56. One requirement for Tat activity is the CDC2-like kinase CD9, which phosphorylates the carboxyl-terminal domain of RNA polymerase II. However, Tat must first interact with a host cell factor, which is cell-specific and limits Tat activation in nonhuman cells. This factor, encoded on chromosome 12, has been identified as a novel 87-kDa cyclin C–related protein named cyclin T.[100] Overexpression of this protein, along with CD4 and chemokine receptors, may permit virus infection and expression in nonpermissive cells.

Tat also contains an RGD (arginine-glycine-aspartate) motif at amino acids 78 to 80 that is common to proteins that bind to integrin receptors. This feature is consistent with the finding that Tat may be secreted by cells into the media and induce extracellular effects. Binding of HIV-1 Tat to cells derived from KS lesions, mediated in part through the RGD motif, enhances the growth of these cells. Tat is released from infected cells[101] and extracellular Tat has been shown to induce KS-like lesions in nude mice.[102] Tat contains a stretch of basic amino acids that functions as a protein transduction domain, conferring the ability to be rapidly taken up into uninfected cells from the medium.[101,103] Fusion of this domain with other proteins confers the ability to internalize into cells.[104]

All three functional domains of Tat are highly conserved among HIV-1 isolates. HIV-2/SIV Tat has an additional 30 amino acids in the amino-terminal sequence but lacks the RGD region. Tat should be an inviting target for blocking viral replication, although in some situations cellular factors may allow virus to be expressed without Tat.[105] Extracellular Tat may also be immunosuppressive, as well as promoting increased HIV replication.[106] Both Tat and interferon (IFN)-α inhibit antigen-stimulated T-cell proliferation, and specific anti-Tat and/or anti–IFN-α antibodies prevent generation of HIV-1–induced suppressor cells. It is possible that high-titer anti-Tat and/or anti–IFN-α antibodies, neutralizing extracellular Tat, and/or IFN-α, including those induced by vaccines, antagonize HIV-1–induced immunosuppression.[107]

Tat can affect the expression of heterologous and cellular genes, including the promoters of the human polyomaviruses, human papillomaviruses, and cytokines, such as tumor necrosis factor (TNF)-α and IL-2. The first exon of Tat has been shown to downregulate major histocompatibility complex (MHC) class I expression. The demonstration that another viral protein, Nef, also functions to downregulate this protein suggests that these proteins are important because the immune system is exerting significant selective pressure on the virus. It also illustrates how single viral proteins may have multiple or complex functions that contribute to immunosuppression.

The *rev* gene encodes a serine phosphorylated protein, Rev, that ranges in size from 106 to 123 amino acids but is most commonly 116 amino acids, with a molecular weight of 19 kDa. This protein is translated from a unique doubly spliced mRNA, with the second splice acceptor located downstream from the Tat translation initiation site.[108] Expression of Rev results in the accumulation of viral structural proteins encoded by the Gag, Pol, Env, Vpu, Vpr, and Vif mRNAs. In contrast, multiple-spliced viral messages for Tat, Rev, and Nef are efficiently expressed without Rev protein. In the absence of Rev, most viral mRNA is processed to multiply spliced forms, thereby limiting the production of virions. Rev protein accumulates in the nucleolus and shuttles back and forth to the cytoplasm. Although it binds to unspliced genomic RNA, it does not appear in the mature virion. Rev binds to a unique RNA element located in the Env coding region of HIV-1 RNA. This Rev regulatory element, RRE, is found in all unspliced and singly spliced mRNAs.

Rev contains at least two functional domains, an arginine-rich region at amino acids 35 to 50, which is conserved and required for nucleolar localization and specific RRE binding, and a multimerization

domain. After initial RRE binding, multiple additional Rev molecules bind to each other, and this oligomerization is required for activity.[109]

The *nef* gene product is a 206–amino acid myristoylated protein that inserts into the cell membrane. The Nef protein may have many different properties that depend in part on the experimental methodology used to analyze them. The original observation that T-cell–tropic, Nef-deleted viruses replicated to high levels led to the term *negative factor*. Downregulation of CD4 requires myristoylation and membrane targeting of Nef to the cytoplasmic domain of CD4 and increases CD4 endocytosis. The protection of HIV-1–infected cells by Nef protein against killing by CTL correlates with downregulation of MHC class I.[110] Nef appears to be important in maintaining high virus loads associated with rapid progression to immunodeficiency. As mentioned earlier, Nef leads to activation of T cells when it is expressed in macrophages.

Viruses with Nef deleted appear to be less virulent than wild-type viruses but equally infectious, both in tissue culture and in rhesus macaques. The possible role of Nef as a virulence factor has led to the use of Nef-deleted virus as a potential live vaccine in rhesus macaques. These "attenuated" viruses were able to protect against infection by challenge with other virulent SIV strains. However, the Nef-deleted viruses are not entirely benign and are themselves able to cause disease in both newborn animals and adults.[111,112]

The immune response to Nef may exert considerable selection pressure. When T cells capable of CTL activity against Nef were transferred to HIV-infected patients, a Nef-deleted variant emerged and, although there was apparent successful immunologic intervention, the patient's disease progressed.[113] Nef-deleted viruses detected in several human clusters have been associated with little or no disease, raising the possibility that they represent less virulent viruses.[114] However, long-term follow-up of these cases has demonstrated that definite, albeit slower, disease progression does indeed occur.[115]

Vif is a 193–amino acid viral protein of 23 to 27 kDa with no N-linked glycosylation sites. The infectivity of Vif deletion mutants is decreased up to 1000-fold in some cell lines compared with that of wild-type virus. The deleted virus is capable of cell entry and initiating reverse transcription, but double-stranded DNA is not produced. As noted, Vif likely blocks the activity of deoxycytidine deaminase APOBEC3G.[96]

Vpr is a 96–amino acid protein translated from a single-spliced mRNA and, like Vif, its expression is dependent on Rev function. Vpr is abundantly present in the mature virion associated with capsid protein. Expression of p55 Gag and Vpr in transfected cells is sufficient for incorporation and export of viral proteins. Vpr plays a role in the nuclear localization of the preintegration complex.[116,117] In addition, in transfected human muscle cells, Vpr blocks proliferation and induces differentiation, suggesting a nuclear role for Vpr in regulation of gene expression. Vpr causes arrest of cell cycle progression at the G_2/M interface, presumably through an effect on cyclin CDC2 activity, which correlates with the ability to activate HIV transcription.[118,119] In addition, Vpr causes massive ruptures in cell nuclei.[120] A gene encoding a second homologous protein, VpX, is found in HIV-2 and several SIV strains but not in nonprimate lentiviruses.

Vpu is an amphipathic integral membrane protein.[121] The first 27 amino acids are hydrophobic, whereas the remainder of this small, 81–amino acid 16-kDa protein is hydrophilic. A single-spliced message overlaps with the *env* gene in a different reading frame.[122] The protein forms oligomeric complexes localized to the perinuclear region. Cells infected with Vpu-defective mutants show large accumulations of intracellular vesicles, in contrast with those infected with wild-type virus. Vpu along with Nef is associated with the rapid degradation of CD4, which may in part eliminate CD4–gp160 intracellular complexes that interfere with virus production. The CD4 cytoplasmic tail is required for targeting the degradation of CD4 by Vpu. Vpu has structural similarities to the influenza virus M2 protein, an ion channel protein that modulates the pH of the *trans*-Golgi.[123]

VIRUS REGULATION AND THE LONG TERMINAL REPEAT

The LTR of all retroviruses is located at each end of the provirus as a direct repeat containing U3, R, and U5 region. It functions as an eukaryotic transcription unit (Fig. 169-7). The U3 region contains the viral promoter and enhancer elements. The R region includes the mRNA initiation site (+1) used by all viral messages and ends at a polyadenylation termination site. The function of the U5 region is not well understood. It separates the R region from the tRNA primer binding site used to initiate reverse transcription. HIV-1 uses tRNA^{lys} as a primer. Once the virus has formed a double-stranded DNA copy, it depends on cellular machinery for transcription and translation. However, the control of virus expression results from a complex set of interactions between viral elements and cellular proteins. Small changes in these regions may result in profound differences in virus behavior. *cis*-Acting control elements of the virus (TAR, TATAA, SP1, and enhancer and negative regulatory regions, located within the U3 and R regions) interact with cellular and viral proteins. These interactions, which occur at both the DNA and the RNA levels, are crucial in controlling the level of viral expression in both resting and activated cells.

The TATAA box, located at −27 (relative to the RNA initiation site), binds the critical cellular transcription factor TFIID to initiate transcription. The promoter region, the binding site of the cellular polymerase, lies farther 5′ (between −45 and −77) and contains three binding sites for the cellular SP1 transcription factor.[124]

An enhancer element is still further 5′, mapping to nucleotides −82 to −105, and contains a consensus sequence also found in the immunoglobulin κ, IL-2, and IL-2R enhancer regions. This region binds an inducible cellular transcription factor, NF-κB. Although originally described in B lymphocytes, this factor or family of factors is also expressed in activated T cells and stimulates HIV expression.[55,125]

In addition to NF-κB, other factors can increase HIV-1 promoter activity by interactions in the region. These include cellular cytokines, such as TNF-α and IL-1, and heterologous viral proteins, such as HTLV-I Tax. Such observations indicate molecular mechanisms whereby other viruses could interact with HIV; however, the relevance of such interactions in vivo is unknown.

Farther 5′ are the binding sites for additional cellular factors (AP-1, NFAT-1) that lie within a negative regulatory element (NRE). Removing this region from a functional provirus enhances virus expression, again suggesting that viral production is carefully modulated both negatively and positively.

The R region of the LTR codes for the 5′ untranslated leader sequence shared by all HIV-1 mRNAs and for the TAR, essential for the activity of the potent virally coded HIV-1 *trans*-activating protein, Tat. The TAR is available in the LTR transcript as a unique stem loop structure. Of interest, the structure of the HIV-2 LTR is significantly different from that of the HIV-1 LTR and may contribute to distinctly different biologic activities of these two human retroviruses.

Virus-Host Interactions

VIRAL RECEPTORS, CHEMOKINES, RECEPTORS, AND TROPISM

Chemokines and their receptors constitute a complex signaling system essential for orchestrating angiogenic, inflammatory, and chemotactic responses. Over 40 chemokines are grouped into two principal families, C-C and C-X-C; there are at least 14 known seven-transmembrane spanning G protein–coupled chemokine receptors. These molecules have been exploited by some bacterial and viral pathogens as their receptors to gain entry to or activate cells, and virally encoded antagonists often subvert chemokine function.[126,127]

The revelation that chemokine receptors are essential for HIV cell fusion has brought together several distinct areas of viral research: how CD8$^+$ T cell–derived factors suppress HIV-1 replication, the mechanisms of cell entry and viral tropism, and host genetic determinants of infection. Three CC (or β) cytokines released by CD8$^+$ T cells—RANTES, MIP-1α, and MIP-1β—bind to the CCR5 receptor and potently suppress HIV macrophage-tropic virus.[128,129] The first co-receptor identified, the CXCR4 molecule, known at the time only as an "orphan receptor," was discovered using a complementary DNA (cDNA) screening approach for receptor activity mediating cell-cell fusion.[36] A group of reports rapidly followed, showing that a recently identified receptor, CCR5, that could use the identified suppressor molecules as ligands, was the main co-receptor for primary isolates and macrophage-tropic strains.[37-40] Although the number of receptors that may function as co-receptors continues to expand, CXCR4 appears to be the only other co-receptor of consequence. Dual-tropic strains can use both co-receptors.[130] The role of other receptors, such as CX3CR1, expressed in the brain, or CCR8, expressed in the thymus, is not known, but is probably not major. Some strains of monocyte-tropic virus may use CCR2 or CCR3, at least in vitro. Chemokine co-receptor use may be a determinant of viral virulence and disease progression.[131] Additionally, studies have pointed to the critical role of cholesterol in the cell membrane in HIV-1 co-receptor function; removal of cellular cholesterol rendered primary cells and cell lines highly resistant to HIV-1–mediated syncytium formation and to infection by CXCR4- and CCR5-specific viruses.[132]

A mutant CCR5 gene that encodes a defective protein that is unable to bind virus has been found in exposed but uninfected persons, strongly suggesting that a functional CCR5 protein is required for infection.[133] Homozygosity for this mutant[134] is a strong protective factor, but rare infections by CCR5-independent viruses have been documented in a person with hemophilia and in another person following sexual transmission. Heterozygous adults and children are not protected from infection but may take a longer time to develop disease.[135,136]

PATHOGENESIS, T-CELL DEPLETION, AND VIRAL LOAD

Understanding the rates of HIV-1 production and associated loss of T cells has been dramatically advanced by the ability to measure the changes produced by potent new drug combinations. HIV-1 produc-

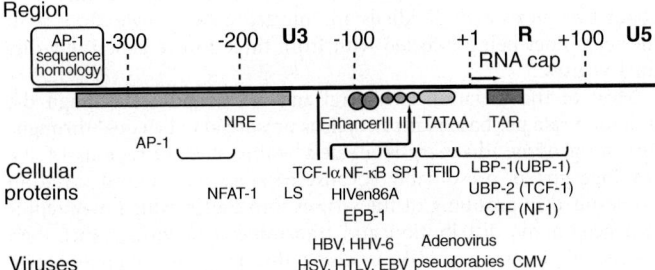

Figure 169-7 The human immunodeficiency virus type 1 (HIV-1) long terminal repeat (LTR). Like other retroviruses, the LTR of HIV-1 is composed of three regions—U3, R, and U5. Integrated proviral DNA is flanked by two complete LTRs, whereas genomic viral RNA transcripts contain partial LTRs at either end, with the 5′ end containing the R and U5 regions, and the 3′ end containing the U3 and R regions. The untranslated 5′ (U3) region contains the major regulatory domains of the LTR, including a negative regulatory element (NRE) and the major binding sites for cellular enhancers of HIV-1 transcription, nuclear factor-κB (NF-κB) and SP1. A number of cellular and viral proteins interact directly or indirectly with the LTRs. The R region of the LTR includes the Tat activation response element (TAR), which (as RNA) binds the HIV-1 transcriptional activator, Tat, and a number of cellular factors that also enhance transcriptional activity. EBV, Epstein-Barr virus; HBV, hepatitis B virus; HHV-6, human herpesvirus 6; HSV, herpes simplex virus; HTLV, human T-cell lymphotropic virus.

tion and T-cell turnover constitute a continuous dynamic process.[137,138] Mathematical modeling of virus production has suggested that a continuous battle is being waged between the virus and host. Production of billions of virions and T-cell turnover estimated at a billion cells/day may help account for the very rapid emergence of viral variants and the fluctuating and progressive nature of T-cell depletion. Virus may be distributed across different cellular compartments, with different rates of turnover and production. Even in the steady state that may occur during periods of clinical latency, hordes of virus freshly infecting T cells lead to a highly activated immune system that is attempting both to control virus replication and to renew itself.[139] The increase in CD4+ T cells with highly active antiretroviral therapy (HAART) is probably due to the result of a combination of initial redistribution of memory T cells and a continuous but slow repopulation with newly produced naive T cells.[140]

Although no similar measure of T-cell turnover in uninfected individuals is available, bromodeoxyuridine labeling of CD4+ and CD8+ T-cell populations in SIV-infected macaques has suggested a generalized state of activation and rapid T-cell turnover compared with uninfected animals.[141]

The mathematical models that have been proposed, however, grossly oversimplify the real dynamics of infection, and are no longer widely accepted as a valid major explanation for HIV pathogenesis and T cell loss. Several other pathologic mechanisms, including indirect viral killing and activation-induced apoptosis, have been suggested to play a role. For example, circulating Tat protein, along with abnormally high levels of IFN-α in those who are HIV-infected, appears to suppress cell-mediated immunity.[106] Uninfected CD8+ T cells turn over as rapidly as CD4+ T cells but are not initially depleted.[142] The eventual loss of noninfected CD8+ T cells may be mediated by gp120 binding to CXCR4.[143] Eventually, viral escape from immune control and emergence of T-cell–tropic viruses using CXCR4 may lead to immunodeficiency,[144] although progression to AIDS often occurs in the absence of detectable variants using CXCR4. All these models incorporate two common assumptions—a demonstrated quantitative association between virus production and T-cell depletion, and a compartmentalization of virus production and cell turnover at different rates.

The significance of virus integration for the natural history of HIV-1 infection has been vividly demonstrated by the effects of combination therapy on virus production from different populations of cells and has helped define what is meant by latent infection. Potent antiretroviral regimens that include a combination of RT and protease inhibitors can produce sustained reductions of plasma viral RNA to below detectable limits.[145] Patients with detectable viral plasma RNA, even if the level is greatly reduced, have viral loads in their lymph nodes similar to those in the nodes of patients who did not receive treatment, reflecting ongoing viral replication and emergence of drug resistance.[146] However, even in those with no detectable plasma RNA, viral DNA could be detected in lymph nodes and PBMCs, and virus could be grown from PBMCs after removal of CD8+ cells and activation. Furthermore, no new mutations associated with drug resistance were detected from these isolates recovered after 2 years of therapy. This strongly suggests that virus persisted in a long-lived and latently infected T-cell population. This pool of latently infected cells is probably established very early during primary HIV-1 infection. Even though plasma viremia could be suppressed, initiation of HAART therapy as early as 10 days after onset of symptoms did not prevent generation of latently infected CD4+ lymphocytes.[147] Although the frequency of these cells is low, on the order of 16/million PBMCs, the fact that virus may survive by hiding out in these cells may represent a significant factor in long-term therapy and shape strategies to eliminate virus.[148] Indeed, therapy may need to be continued for 60 to 70 years to eradicate the reservoir of long-lived latently infected cells.

Similar to the impairment or killing of infected cells, there are several distinct mechanisms whereby bystander cells can be affected that can be demonstrated in vitro. For example, HIV-1–infected PBMCs taken directly from patients or obtained through infection of normal PBMCs with HIV-1 in vitro have shown a marked impairment of proliferative responses, even though only a small fraction of T cells are infected.[149-151] Other possible indirect (bystander) effects include impaired hematopoiesis leading to cytopenias of several blood cell lines, impaired thymopoiesis, anergy and apoptosis of uninfected immune cells, likely through increased levels of cytokines such as TNF-α, IFN-α, and transforming growth factor-beta (TGF-β), and hyperactivation and apoptosis of uninfected immune cells by the effects of extracellular Tat.

VIRAL VARIATION: GENETIC AND PHENOTYPIC VARIATION

On the basis of phylogenetic analysis, HIV strains can be separated into major (M) subgroups A through J and more distant groups N and O. Within the M group are multiple subtypes A, B, C, D, F, G, H, J, and K and numerous circulating recombinant forms, including CRF 01 AE/B and CRF 02 A/G.[152] A subspecies of chimpanzees (Pan troglodytes troglodytes) has been identified as the likely source of HIV-1.[153,154] Transmission appears to have occurred on at least three occasions, with one such transmission in southeastern Cameroon being the origin of the most widespread HIV-1 group, HIV-1(M). It is likely that this has happened on other occasions, that the transmitted viruses failed to survive as infectious human agents, and that the three successful cross-species transmissions are the only ones that have been reported. Data has been recently presented[155] suggesting that following its introduction into humans in Africa, HIV-1 was introduced into Haiti and subsequently into the United States in the 1960s, from where it spread to many other countries, giving rise to clade B HIV-1(M), which is highly prevalent in the United States and Europe, as well as other areas. Clade C is the most prevalent in many parts of Africa and in India.

One of the most striking characteristics of HIV-1 is its remarkable variability, contributing to phenotype diversity and resulting in altered cell tropism, immune escape, and resistance to RT and protease inhibitors. As a consequence of the underlying variation by mutation, high rates of virus turnover and selection of viral variants cause viral evolution in individual hosts with time, as well as among populations of infected individuals. Most affected persons have been thought to be infected with a single strain that evolves into a swarm of related viruses or quasispecies during the course of infection.[156,156] Recently, however, deep sequencing and phylogenetic analyses of viruses from recently infected individuals have suggested that only about two thirds of individuals are infected with a single virus, with the remainder being infected with from three to five genetically distinct viruses.[157]

Most of the variation is neutral and not adaptive. Although the mutation rate per base pair per cycle is presumed to be equal throughout the genome, diversity is greatest within distinct regions of the envelope gp120, presumably because of selection. Neutral variation has resulted in grouping of the viruses into clades, which may represent geographic distribution and transmission of virus rather than functional differences. HIV is going through rapid epidemiologic changes, even as the virus is being studied. Thus, genetic relatedness of viruses can be used to track transmission of the virus as well as the relatedness of different viruses. This information is often presented in the form of a viral phylogenetic tree.[158,159]

Malignancies and Human Immunodeficiency Virus

Although cancer is not common in the young adults most frequently exposed to HIV, KS has been recognized as a defining clinical presentation of AIDS. Previously known as a rare and usually indolent vascular tumor, the incidence of KS in patients with HIV infection may be 10% to 20%, more than 10,000 times that in the general population. Several forms of KS have been described: classic KS, endemic KS, non–HIV-associated KS, transplantation-associated KS, and AIDS-associated KS.

The tumor appears to be a vascular proliferation characterized by the presence of spindle cells, vascular channels, and a mixed cellular infiltrate. The "malignant" cell is most likely a population of activated endothelial cells, which are sometimes clonal and sometimes not. These cells themselves and factors produced from them, such as basic fibroblast growth factor and vascular endothelial cell growth factor, can induce vascular lesions in nude mice. The HIV protein Tat can bind to KS spindle cells and stimulate their growth.[160] Moreover, Tat can cooperate synergistically with a G protein–coupled receptor encoded by human herpesvirus 8 (HHV-8; see later) in inducing KS-like lesions in nude mice.[161] Although the importance of immunodeficiency and viral proliferation in the etiology of KS is well established, the mechanism is not certain, and KS may occur early in the course of HIV infection.

Within the group of HIV-infected individuals, KS occurs predominantly in homosexuals and bisexuals, leading to the hypothesis that a previously undescribed infectious agent might cause KS. In 1994, using DNA subtraction hybridization, DNA representing a novel herpesvirus was obtained from KS lesions, which led to the isolation of HHV-8[162] (see Chapter 141). Also known as KS herpesvirus, it is related to other gamma herpesviruses such as Epstein-Barr virus (EBV). HHV-8 has also been identified in an EBV-transformed B-cell line and from a unique form of B-cell lymphoma known as body cavity lymphoma. This large virus contains many genes that interact with host cells, including several chemokine and cytokine homologues that can induce vascular growth.[163] Seroepidemiologic studies have made a strong association between this virus and KS. HHV-8 was found to be associated with all forms of KS, and seroconversion precedes the appearance of KS in HIV-infected persons. The prevalence of HHV-8 is far greater than the incidence of KS, however, and the relationship of the virus to the disease is not likely to be simple. HHV-8 thus appears to be necessary but not sufficient to cause KS. A review discusses this and other aspects of KS that are not clear at present.[164] The incidence of KS in AIDS continues to decrease and established lesions may respond to HAART only.

B-cell lymphoma is the second most common cancer associated with AIDS, occurring in approximately 3% to 4% of individuals as their first AIDS-defining diagnosis. One type, primary effusion lymphoma, is caused by HHV-8. The most common lymphoma is that of the brain (primary brain lymphoma). However, in contradistinction to KS, lymphoma appears to be a late manifestation of HIV disease, with rates rising directly with length of time infected. Up to 16% of AIDS patients eventually die from this condition.

Also in contradistinction to KS, non-Hodgkin's lymphoma (NHL) appears to occur approximately at equal rates in all HIV-1 risk groups. In 53,042 AIDS patients from 21 European countries, approximately 2.6% of injection drug users, 3.2% of transfusion recipients, 3.4% of homosexual men, 3.9% of hemophiliacs, and 2.6% of those who acquired HIV through heterosexual contact eventually developed AIDS-related lymphoma.[165]

In the United States, data from the Multi-State AIDS Cancer Match Registry have demonstrated a significantly increased risk of lymphoma in patients with a prior AIDS diagnosis, compared with population control subjects who had not been diagnosed with AIDS.[166] The relative risk of all NHL was increased approximately 113-fold. Although the greatest risk is for NHL, there is a 10-fold increase of Hodgkin's disease in the infected group as well.

These tumors are predominantly extranodal and often of high grade, with small cell noncleaved histologic features[167] (see Chapter 125). EBV is found in almost all primary CNS tumors, but high rates of dysregulated B-cell turnover may account for increased cellular turnover, which predisposes to lymphoma. Rates of EBV-associated primary brain lymphoma have fallen off markedly in the era of HAART, but the same cannot be said for systemic lymphoma, which appears to be increasing in frequency as people live longer with HIV.[168]

Several other rare tumors, including leiomyosarcoma, have also been reported.[169] Cervical cancer, almost universally associated with human papillomavirus (HPV) infection, is accepted as an AIDS-defining illness.[170] High rates of HPV-associated anal intraepithelial neoplasia (AIN) have been documented among HIV-infected homosexual men, and routine screening for AIN is being considered, using the same methodology as Pap smears, with samples obtained through anoscopy.[171] However, the incidence of common cancers does not appear to be greatly increased among HIV patients. Most of the cancers seen appear to be associated directly or indirectly with viral proliferation, suggesting that the role of the immune system may be more directly related to viral expression than to immune control of tumor.

Conclusion

Antiretroviral therapy directed at HIV-1 has continued to develop rapidly (see Chapter 128). Significant advances in the ability to treat individual cases, propelled by an understanding of the biology of the virus, have led to the control of viral replication and have altered the course of disease progression. At present, patients have been maintained on combination therapy for several years, with a low rate of relapse because of the development of resistance and low viral burdens. Immune restoration and long-term biologic control or complete eradication of the viral burden with minimal toxicity remain elusive goals, but intense efforts continue to focus on new anti-HIV therapies. As we have learned, retroviral disease has important social aspects that as much as viral biology, determine the extent of viral transmission and the dimensions of the epidemic; this results in a series of epidemics, each with a unique sociobiology. Moreover, despite remarkable progress, the full social and economic effects of the global HIV epidemic are materializing vividly in sub-Saharan Africa, with devastating losses of population life expectancy and productivity. Renewed emphasis on the development of an effective anti-HIV vaccine that might stem an ongoing epidemic or ameliorate the course of disease has been the subject of intensive study in nonhuman primates and in clinical trials. (see Chapter 130). The history of retrovirology has been filled with remarkable, often serendipitous, discoveries based on scientific imagination supported by technologic advances. There is every reason to expect that continued advances will deepen our understanding of fundamental biologic processes and that we will meet the challenges presented by HIV and the inevitability of the emergence of new pathogens.

ACKNOWLEDGMENT

This updated chapter is based on a previous chapter in the sixth edition of Principles and Practice of Infectious Diseases, *co-authored by Dr. Mika Popovic and Dr. Farley Cleghorn of the Institute of Human Virology. We gratefully acknowledge their support.*

REFERENCES

1. Masur H, Michelis MA, Greene JB, et al. An outbreak of community-acquired Pneumocystis carinii pneumonia: Initial manifestation of cellular immune dysfunction. *N Engl J Med.* 1981;305:1431-1438.
2. Gottlieb MS, Schroff R, Schanker HM, et al. Pneumocystis carinii pneumonia and mucosal candidiasis in previously healthy homosexual men: Evidence of a new acquired cellular immunodeficiency. *N Engl J Med.* 1981;305:1425-1431.
3. Durack DT. Opportunistic infections and Kaposi's sarcoma in homosexual men. *N Engl J Med.* 1981;305:1465-1467.
4. Kalyanaraman VS, Sarngadharan MG, Robert-Guroff M, et al. A new subtype of human T-cell leukemia virus (HTLV-II) associated with a T-cell variant of hairy cell leukemia. *Science.* 1982;218:571-573.
5. Poiesz BJ, Ruscetti FW, Gazdar AF, et al. Detection and isolation of type C retrovirus particles from fresh and cultured lymphocytes of a patient with cutaneous T-cell lymphoma. *Proc Natl Acad Sci U S A.* 1980;77:7415-7419.
6. Ruscetti FW, Morgan DA, Gallo RC. Functional and morphologic characterization of human T cells continuously grown in vitro. *J Immunol.* 1977;119:131-138.
7. Morgan DA, Ruscetti FW, Gallo R. Selective in vitro growth of T lymphocytes from normal human bone marrows. *Science.* 1976;193:1007-1008.
8. Barre-Sinoussi F, Chermann JC, Rey F, et al. Isolation of a T-lymphotropic retrovirus from a patient at risk for acquired immune deficiency syndrome (AIDS). *Science.* 1983;220:868-871.
9. Gallo RC, Salahuddin SZ, Popovic M, et al. Frequent detection and isolation of cytopathic retroviruses (HTLV-III) from patients with AIDS and at risk for AIDS. *Science.* 1984;224:500-503.

10. Popovic M, Sarngadharan MG, Read E, et al. Detection, isolation, and continuous production of cytopathic retroviruses (HTLV-III) from patients with AIDS and pre-AIDS. *Science.* 1984;224:497-500.
11. Sarngadharan MG, Popovic M, Bruch L, et al. Antibodies reactive with human T-lymphotropic retroviruses (HTLV-III) in the serum of patients with AIDS. *Science.* 1984;224:506-508.
12. Schupbach J, Popovic M, Gilden RV, et al. Serological analysis of a subgroup of human T-lymphotropic retroviruses (HTLV-III) associated with AIDS. *Science.* 1984;224:503-505.
13. Mitsuya H, Weinhold KJ, Furman PA, et al. 3'-Azido-3'-deoxythymidine (BW A509U): An antiviral agent that inhibits the infectivity and cytopathic effect of human T-lymphotropic virus type III/lymphadenopathy-associated virus in vitro. *Proc Natl Acad Sci U S A.* 1985;82:7096-7100.
14. Santiago ML, Lukasik M, Kamenya S, et al. Foci of endemic simian immunodeficiency virus infection in wild-living eastern chimpanzees (Pan troglodytes schweinfurthii). *J Virol.* 2003;77:7545-7562.
15. Bailes E, Gao F, Bibollet-Ruche F, et al. Hybrid origin of SIV in chimpanzees. *Science.* 2003;300:1713.
16. Ellerman V, Bang O. Experimentelle leukämie bei hühnern. *Zentralbl Bakteriol Parasitenkd Infectionskr Hyg Abt Orig.* 1908;46:595.
17. Rous P. A transmissible avian neoplasm (Sarcoma of the common fowl). *J Exp Med.* 1910;12:696.
18. Gross L. Neck tumors, or leukemia, developing in adult C3H mice following inoculation, in early infancy, with filtered (Berkefeld N), or centrifugated (144,000 X g), Ak-leukemic extracts. *Cancer.* 1953;6:948-958.
19. Baltimore D. RNA-dependent DNA polymerase in virions of RNA tumour viruses. *Nature.* 1970;226:1209-1211.
20. Temin HM, Mizutani S. RNA-dependent DNA polymerase in virions of Rous sarcoma virus. *Nature.* 1970;226:1211-1213.
21. Kalyanaraman VS, Sarngadharan MG, Bunn PA, et al. Antibodies in human sera reactive against an internal structural protein of human T-cell lymphoma virus. *Nature.* 1981;294:271-273.
22. Robert-Guroff M, Nakao Y, Notake K, et al. Natural antibodies to human retrovirus HTLV in a cluster of Japanese patients with adult T cell leukemia. *Science.* 1982;215:975-978.
23. Yoshida M, Miyoshi I, Hinuma Y. Isolation and characterization of retrovirus from cell lines of human adult T-cell leukemia and its implication in the disease. *Proc Natl Acad Sci U S A.* 1982;79:2031-2035.
24. Gessain A, Barin F, Vernant JC, et al. Antibodies to human T-lymphotropic virus type-I in patients with tropical spastic paraparesis. *Lancet.* 1985;2:407-410.
25. Clavel F, Guetard D, Brun-Vezinet F, et al. Isolation of a new human retrovirus from West African patients with AIDS. *Science.* 1986;233:343-346.
26. Kanki PJ, Barin F, M'Boup S, et al. New human T-lymphotropic retrovirus related to simian T-lymphotropic virus type III (STLV-IIIAGM). *Science.* 1986;232:238-243.
27. Kahn JO, Walker BD. Acute human immunodeficiency virus type 1 infection. *N Engl J Med.* 1998;339:33-39.
28. Ogg GS, Jin X, Bonhoeffer S, et al. Quantitation of HIV-1-specific cytotoxic T lymphocytes and plasma load of viral RNA. *Science.* 1998;279:2103-2106.
29. Musey L, Hughes J, Schacker T, et al. Cytotoxic-T-cell responses, viral load, and disease progression in early human immunodeficiency virus type 1 infection. *N Engl J Med.* 1997;337:1267-1274.
30. Schacker TW, Hughes JP, Shea T, et al. Biological and virologic characteristics of primary HIV infection. *Ann Intern Med.* 1998;128:613-620.
31. Cardo DM, Culver DH, Ciesielski CA, et al. A case-control study of HIV seroconversion in health care workers after percutaneous exposure. Centers for Disease Control and Prevention Needlestick Surveillance Group. *N Engl J Med.* 1997;337:1485-1490.
32. Katz MH, Gerberding JL. The care of persons with recent sexual exposure to HIV. *Ann Intern Med.* 1998;128:306-312.
33. Maddon PJ, McDougal JS, Clapham PR, et al. HIV infection does not require endocytosis of its receptor, CD4. *Cell.* 1988;54:865-874.
34. Gartner S, Markovits P, Markovitz DM, et al. The role of mononuclear phagocytes in HTLV-III/LAV infection. *Science.* 1986;233:215-219.
35. Cocchi F, DeVico AL, Garzino-Demo A, et al. Identification of RANTES, MIP-1 alpha, and MIP-1 beta as the major HIV-suppressive factors produced by CD8+ T cells. *Science.* 1995;270:1811-1815.
36. Feng Y, Broder CC, Kennedy PE, et al. HIV-1 entry cofactor: Functional cDNA cloning of a seven-transmembrane, G protein-coupled receptor. *Science.* 1996;272(5263):872-877.
37. Alkhatib G, Combadiere C, Broder CC, et al. CC CKR5: A RANTES, MIP-1alpha, MIP-1beta receptor as a fusion cofactor for macrophage-tropic HIV-1. *Science.* 1996;272:1955-1958.
38. Choe H, Farzan M, Sun Y, et al. The beta-chemokine receptors CCR3 and CCR5 facilitate infection by primary HIV-1 isolates. *Cell.* 1996;85:1135-1148.
39. Deng H, Liu R, Ellmeier W, et al. Identification of a major co-receptor for primary isolates of HIV-1. *Nature.* 1996;381:661-666.
40. Dragic T, Litwin V, Allaway GP, et al. HIV-1 entry into CD4+ cells is mediated by the chemokine receptor CC-CKR-5. *Nature.* 1996;381:667-673.

41. Wyatt R, Sodroski J. The HIV-1 envelope glycoproteins: Fusogens, antigens, and immunogens. *Science.* 1998;280:1884-1888.
42. Reitter JN, Means RE, Desrosiers RC. A role for carbohydrates in immune evasion in AIDS. *Nat Med.* 1998;4:679-684.
43. Sherry B, Zybarth G, Alfano M, et al. Role of cyclophilin A in the uptake of HIV-1 by macrophages and T lymphocytes. *Proc Natl Acad Sci U S A.* 1998;95:1758-1763.
44. Braaten D, Franke EK, Luban J. Cyclophilin A is required for an early step in the life cycle of human immunodeficiency virus type 1 before the initiation of reverse transcription. *J Virol.* 1996;70:3551-3560.
45. Emerman M, Malim MH. HIV-1 regulatory/accessory genes: Keys to unraveling viral and host cell biology. *Science.* 1998;280:1880-1884.
46. Peliska JA, Benkovic SJ. Mechanism of DNA strand transfer reactions catalyzed by HIV-1 reverse transcriptase. *Science.* 1992;258:1112-1118.
47. Lori F, Malykh A, Cara A, et al. Hydroxyurea as an inhibitor of human immunodeficiency virus-type 1 replication. *Science.* 1994;266:801-805.
48. Rutschmann OT, Opravil M, Iten A, et al. A placebo-controlled trial of didanosine plus stavudine, with and without hydroxyurea, for HIV infection. The Swiss HIV Cohort Study. *AIDS.* 1998;12:F71-F77.
49. Cara A, Cereseto A, Lori F, et al. HIV-1 protein expression from synthetic circles of DNA mimicking the extrachromosomal forms of viral DNA. *J Biol Chem.* 1996;271:5393-5397.
50. Wiskerchen M, Muesing MA. Human immunodeficiency virus type 1 integrase: Effects of mutations on viral ability to integrate, direct viral gene expression from unintegrated viral DNA templates, and sustain viral propagation in primary cells. *J Virol.* 1995;69:376-386.
51. Schroder AR, Shinn P, Chen H, et al. HIV-1 integration in the human genome favors active genes and local hotspots. *Cell.* 2002;110:521-529.
52. Markowitz M, Louie M, Hurley A, et al. A novel antiviral intervention results in more accurate assessment of human immunodeficiency virus type 1 replication dynamics and T-cell decay in vivo. *J Virol.* 2003;77:5037-5038.
53. Douek DC, Picker LJ, Koup RA. T cell dynamics in HIV-1 infection. *Annu Rev Immunol.* 2003;21:265-304.
54. Honda Y, Rogers L, Nakata K, et al. Type I interferon induces inhibitory 16-kD CCAAT/ enhancer binding protein (C/EBP) beta, repressing the HIV-1 long terminal repeat in macrophages: pulmonary tuberculosis alters C/EBP expression, enhancing HIV-1 replication. *J Exp Med.* 1998;188:1255-1265.
55. Kawakami K, Scheidereit C, Roeder RG. Identification and purification of a human immunoglobulin-enhancer-binding protein (NF-kappa B) that activates transcription from a human immunodeficiency virus type 1 promoter in vitro. *Proc Natl Acad Sci U S A.* 1988;85:4700-4704.
56. Kim SY, Byrn R, Groopman J, et al. Temporal aspects of DNA and RNA synthesis during human immunodeficiency virus infection: Evidence for differential gene expression. *J Virol.* 1989;63:3708-3713.
57. Klotman ME, Kim S, Buchbinder A, et al. Kinetics of expression of multiply spliced RNA in early human immunodeficiency virus type 1 infection of lymphocytes and monocytes. *Proc Natl Acad Sci U S A.* 1991;88:5011-5015.
58. Robert-Guroff M, Popovic M, Gartner S, et al. Structure and expression of tat-, rev-, and nef-specific transcripts of human immunodeficiency virus type 1 in infected lymphocytes and macrophages. *J Virol.* 1990;64:3391-3398.
59. Liao Z, Cimakasky LM, Hampton R, et al. Lipid rafts and HIV pathogenesis: Host membrane cholesterol is required for infection by HIV type 1. *AIDS Res Hum Retroviruses.* 2001;17:1009-1019.
60. Hoglund S, Ofverstedt LG, Nilsson A, et al. Spatial visualization of the maturing HIV-1 core and its linkage to the envelope. *AIDS Res Hum Retroviruses.* 1992;8:1-7.
61. Arthur LO, Bess JW Jr, Sowder RC, et al. Cellular proteins bound to immunodeficiency viruses: Implications for pathogenesis and vaccines. *Science.* 1992;258:1935-1938.
62. Flexner C. HIV-protease inhibitors. *N Engl J Med* 1998;338:1281-1292.
63. Pal R, Reitz MS Jr, Tschachler E, et al. Myristoylation of gag proteins of HIV-1 plays an important role in virus assembly. *AIDS Res Hum Retroviruses.* 1990;6:721-730.
64. Bryant M, Ratner L. Myristoylation-dependent replication and assembly of human immunodeficiency virus 1. *Proc Natl Acad Sci U S A.* 1990;87:523-527.
65. Bukrinsky MI, Haggerty S, Dempsey MP, et al. A nuclear localization signal within HIV-1 matrix protein that governs infection of non-dividing cells. *Nature.* 1993;365:666-669.
66. De Francesco MA, Baronio M, Fiorentini S, et al. HIV-1 matrix protein p17 increases the production of proinflammatory cytokines and counteracts IL-4 activity by binding to a cellular receptor. *Proc Natl Acad Sci U S A.* 2002;99:9972-9977.
67. Luban J, Bossolt KL, Franke EK, et al. Human immunodeficiency virus type 1 Gag protein binds to cyclophilins A and B. *Cell.* 1993;73:1067-1078.
68. Mammano F, Ohagen A, Hoglund S, et al. Role of the major homology region of human immunodeficiency virus type 1 in virion morphogenesis. *J Virol.* 1994;68:4927-4936.
69. Dorfman T, Bukovsky A, Ohagen A, et al. Functional domains of the capsid protein of human immunodeficiency virus type 1. *J Virol.* 1994;68:8180-8187.

70. Karpel RL, Henderson LE, Oroszlan S. Interactions of retroviral structural proteins with single-stranded nucleic acids. *J Biol Chem.* 1987;262:4961-4967.
71. South TL, Blake PR, Sowder RC III, et al. The nucleocapsid protein isolated from HIV-1 particles binds zinc and forms retroviral-type zinc fingers. *Biochemistry.* 1990;29:7786-7789.
72. Sakaguchi K, Zambrano N, Baldwin ET, et al. Identification of a binding site for the human immunodeficiency virus type 1 nucleocapsid protein. *Proc Natl Acad Sci U S A.* 1993;90:5219-5223.
73. Stremlau M, Owens CM, Perron MJ, et al. The cytoplasmic body component TRIM5alpha restricts HIV-1 infection in Old World monkeys. *Nature.* 2004;427:848-853.
74. Reymond A, Meroni G, Fantozzi A, et al. The tripartite motif family identifies cell compartments. *EMBO J.* 2001;20:2140-2151.
75. Lilly F. Susceptibility to two strains of Friend leukemia virus in mice. *Science.* 1967;155:461-462.
76. Perron MJ, Stremlau M, Song B, et al. TRIM5alpha mediates the postentry block to N-tropic murine leukemia viruses in human cells. *Proc Natl Acad Sci U S A.* 2004;101:11827-11832.
77. Javanbakht H, An P, Gold B, et al. Effects of human TRIM5alpha polymorphisms on antiretroviral function and susceptibility to human immunodeficiency virus infection. *Virology.* 2006;354:15-27.
78. Stremlau M, Perron M, Lee M, et al. Specific recognition and accelerated uncoating of retroviral capsids by the TRIM5alpha restriction factor. *Proc Natl Acad Sci U S A.* 2006;103:5514-5519.
79. Yap MW, Dodding MP, Stoye JP. Trim-cyclophilin A fusion proteins can restrict human immunodeficiency virus type 1 infection at two distinct phases in the viral life cycle. *J Virol.* 2006;80:4061-4067.
80. Roberts NA, Martin JA, Kinchington D, et al. Rational design of peptide-based HIV proteinase inhibitors. *Science.* 1990;248:358-361.
81. Huang H, Chopra R, Verdine GL, et al. Structure of a covalently trapped catalytic complex of HIV-1 reverse transcriptase: implications for drug resistance. *Science.* 1998;282:1669-1675.
82. Arnold E, Jacobo-Molina A, Nanni RG, et al. Structure of HIV-1 reverse transcriptase/DNA complex at 7 A resolution showing active site locations. *Nature.* 1992;357:85-89.
83. Kohlstaedt LA, Wang J, Friedman JM, et al. Crystal structure at 3.5 A resolution of HIV-1 reverse transcriptase complexed with an inhibitor. *Science.* 1992;256:1783-1790.
84. Lukashov VV, Goudsmit J. HIV heterogeneity and disease progression in AIDS: A model of continuous virus adaptation. *AIDS.* 1998;12(Suppl A):S43-S52.
85. Bukrinsky MI, Sharova N, McDonald TL, et al. Association of integrase, matrix, and reverse transcriptase antigens of human immunodeficiency virus type 1 with viral nucleic acids following acute infection. *Proc Natl Acad Sci U S A.* 1993;90:6125-6129.
86. Starcich BR, Hahn BH, Shaw GM, et al. Identification and characterization of conserved and variable regions in the envelope gene of HTLV-III/LAV, the retrovirus of AIDS. *Cell.* 1986;45:637-648.
87. Kwong PD, Wyatt R, Robinson J, et al. Structure of an HIV gp120 envelope glycoprotein in complex with the CD4 receptor and a neutralizing human antibody. *Nature* 1998;393:648-659.
88. Wyatt R, Kwong PD, Desjardins E, et al. The antigenic structure of the HIV gp120 envelope glycoprotein. *Nature.* 1998;393:705-711.
89. DeVico A, Fouts T, Lewis GK, et al. Antibodies to CD4-induced sites in HIV gp120 correlate with the control of SHIV challenge in macaques vaccinated with subunit immunogens. *Proc Natl Acad Sci U S A.* 2007;104:17477-17482.
90. Buchbinder SP, Mehrotra DV, Duerr A, et al. Efficacy assessment of a cell-mediated immunity HIV-1 vaccine (the Step Study): A double-blind, randomised, placebo-controlled, test-of-concept trial. *Lancet.* 2008;372:1881-1893.
91. White JM. Membrane fusion. *Science.* 1992;258:917-924.
92. Chan DC, Fass D, Berger JM, et al. Core structure of gp41 from the HIV envelope glycoprotein. *Cell.* 1997;89:263-273.
93. Furuta RA, Wild CT, Weng Y, et al. Capture of an early fusion-active conformation of HIV-1 gp41. *Nat Struct Biol.* 1998;5:276-279.
94. Wild CT, Shugars DC, Greenwell TK, et al. Peptides corresponding to a predictive alpha-helical domain of human immunodeficiency virus type 1 gp41 are potent inhibitors of virus infection. *Proc Natl Acad Sci U S A.* 1994;91:9770-9774.
95. Swingler S, Brichacek B, Jacque JM, et al. HIV-1 Nef intersects the macrophage CD40L signalling pathway to promote resting-cell infection. *Nature.* 2003;424:213-219.
96. Sheehy AM, Gaddis NC, Choi JD, et al. Isolation of a human gene that inhibits HIV-1 infection and is suppressed by the viral Vif protein. *Nature.* 2002;418:646-650.
97. Harris RS, Bishop KN, Sheehy AM, et al. DNA deamination mediates innate immunity to retroviral infection. *Cell.* 2003;113:803-809.
98. Garrett ED, Tiley LS, Cullen BR. Rev activates expression of the human immunodeficiency virus type 1 vif and vpr gene products. *J Virol.* 1991;65:1653-1657.
99. Fisher AG, Feinberg MB, Josephs SF, et al. The trans-activator gene of HTLV-III is essential for virus replication. *Nature.* 1986;320:367-371.
100. Wei P, Garber ME, Fang SM, et al. A novel CDK9-associated C-type cyclin interacts directly with HIV-1 Tat and mediates its

high-affinity, loop-specific binding to TAR RNA. *Cell.* 1998;92:451-462.

101. Ensoli B, Buonaguro L, Barillari G, et al. Release, uptake, and effects of extracellular human immunodeficiency virus type 1 Tat protein on cell growth and viral transactivation. *J Virol.* 1993;67:277-287.

102. Ensoli B, Gendelman R, Markham P, et al. Synergy between basic fibroblast growth factor and HIV-1 Tat protein in induction of Kaposi's sarcoma. *Nature.* 1994;371:674-680.

103. Frankel AD, Pabo CO. Cellular uptake of the tat protein from human immunodeficiency virus. *Cell.* 1988;55:1189-1193.

104. Fawell S, Seery J, Daikh Y, et al. Tat-mediated delivery of heterologous proteins into cells. *Proc Natl Acad Sci U S A.* 1994;91:664-668.

105. Luznik L, Kraus G, Guatelli J, et al. Tat-independent replication of human immunodeficiency viruses. *J Clin Invest.* 1995;95:328-332.

106. Zagury D, Lachgar A, Chams V, et al. Interferon alpha and Tat involvement in the immunosuppression of uninfected T cells and C-C chemokine decline in AIDS. *Proc Natl Acad Sci U S A.* 1998;95:3851-3856.

107. Gallo RC, Burny A, Zagury D. Targeting Tat and IFN(alpha) as a therapeutic AIDS vaccine. *DNA Cell Biol.* 2002;21:611-618.

108. Sodroski J, Goh WC, Rosen C, et al. A second post-transcriptional trans-activator gene required for HTLV-III replication. *Nature.* 1986;321:412-417.

109. Malim MH, Bohnlein S, Hauber J, et al. Functional dissection of the HIV-1 Rev trans-activator—derivation of a trans-dominant repressor of Rev function. *Cell.* 1989;58:205-214.

110. Collins KL, Chen BK, Kalams SA, et al. HIV-1 Nef protein protects infected primary cells against killing by cytotoxic T lymphocytes. *Nature.* 1998;391:397-401.

111. Hofmann-Lehmann R, Vlasak J, Williams AL, et al. Live attenuated, nef-deleted SIV is pathogenic in most adult macaques after prolonged observation. *AIDS.* 2003;17:157-166.

112. Jekle A, Schramm B, Jayakumar P, et al. Coreceptor phenotype of natural human immunodeficiency virus with nef deleted evolves in vivo, leading to increased virulence. *J Virol.* 2002;76:6966-6973.

113. Koenig S, Conley AJ, Brewah YA, et al. Transfer of HIV-1-specific cytotoxic T lymphocytes to an AIDS patient leads to selection for mutant HIV variants and subsequent disease progression. *Nat Med.* 1995;1:330-336.

114. Deacon NJ, Tsykin A, Solomon A, et al. Genomic structure of an attenuated quasi species of HIV-1 from a blood transfusion donor and recipients. *Science.* 1995;270:988-991.

115. Birch MR, Learmont JC, Dyer WB, et al. An examination of signs of disease progression in survivors of the Sydney Blood Bank Cohort (SBBC). *J Clin Virol.* 2001;22:263-270.

116. Oberste MS, Gonda MA. Conservation of amino-acid sequence motifs in lentivirus Vif proteins. *Virus Genes.* 1992;6:95-102.

117. Heinzinger NK, Bukinsky MI, Haggerty SA, et al. The Vpr protein of human immunodeficiency virus type 1 influences nuclear localization of viral nucleic acids in nondividing host cells. *Proc Natl Acad Sci U S A.* 1994;91:7311-7315.

118. Felzien LK, Woffendin C, Hottiger MO, et al. HIV transcriptional activation by the accessory protein, VPR, is mediated by the p300 co-activator. *Proc Natl Acad Sci U S A.* 1998;95:5281-5286.

119. Poon B, Grovit-Ferbas K, Stewart SA, et al. Cell cycle arrest by Vpr in HIV-1 virions and insensitivity to antiretroviral agents. *Science.* 1998;281:266-269.

120. de Noronha CM, Sherman MP, Lin HW, et al. Dynamic disruptions in nuclear envelope architecture and integrity induced by HIV-1 Vpr. *Science.* 2001;294:1105-1108.

121. Maldarelli F, Chen MY, Willey RL, et al. Human immunodeficiency virus type 1 Vpu protein is an oligomeric type I integral membrane protein. *J Virol.* 1993;67:5056-5061.

122. Schwartz S, Felber BK, Fenyo EM, et al. Env and Vpu proteins of human immunodeficiency virus type 1 are produced from multiple bicistronic mRNAs. *J Virol.* 1990;64:5448-5456.

123. Pinto LH, Holsinger LJ, Lamb RA. Influenza virus M2 protein has ion channel activity. *Cell.* 1992;69:517-528.

124. Jones KA, Peterlin BM. Control of RNA initiation and elongation at the HIV-1 promoter. *Annu Rev Biochem.* 1994;63:717-743.

125. Nabel G, Baltimore D. An inducible transcription factor activates expression of human immunodeficiency virus in T cells. *Nature.* 1987;326:711-713.

126. Pease JE, Murphy PM. Microbial corruption of the chemokine system: An expanding paradigm. *Semin Immunol.* 1998;10:169-178.

127. Premack BA, Schall TJ. Chemokine receptors: Gateways to inflammation and infection. *Nat Med.* 1996;2:1174-1178.

128. Cocchi F, DeVico AL, Yarchoan R, et al. Higher macrophage inflammatory protein (MIP)-1alpha and MIP-1beta levels from CD8+ T cells are associated with asymptomatic HIV-1 infection. *Proc Natl Acad Sci U S A.* 2000;97:13812-13817.

129. Garzino-Demo A, DeVico AL, Cocchi F, et al. Beta-chemokines and protection from HIV type 1 disease. *AIDS Res Hum Retroviruses.* 1998;14(Suppl 2):S177-S184.

130. Doranz BJ, Rucker J, Yi Y, et al. A dual-tropic primary HIV-1 isolate that uses fusin and the beta-chemokine receptors CKR-5, CKR-3, and CKR-2b as fusion cofactors. *Cell.* 1996;85:1149-1158.

131. Connor RI, Sheridan KE, Ceradini D, et al. Change in coreceptor use correlates with disease progression in HIV-1–infected individuals. *J Exp Med.* 1997;185:621-628.

132. Nguyen DH, Hildreth JE. Evidence for budding of human immunodeficiency virus type 1 selectively from glycolipid-enriched membrane lipid rafts. *J Virol.* 2000;74:3264-3272.

133. Liu R, Paxton WA, Choe S, et al. Homozygous defect in HIV-1 coreceptor accounts for resistance of some multiply-exposed individuals to HIV-1 infection. *Cell.* 1996;86:367-377.

134. O'Brien TR, Goedert JJ. Chemokine receptors and genetic variability: Another leap in HIV research. *JAMA.* 1998;279:317-318.

135. Wei X, Ghosh SK, Taylor ME, et al. Viral dynamics in human immunodeficiency virus type 1 infection. *Nature.* 1995;373:117-122.

136. Misrahi M, Teglas JP, N'Go N, et al. CCR5 chemokine receptor variant in HIV-1 mother-to-child transmission and disease progression in children. French Pediatric HIV Infection Study Group. *JAMA.* 1998;279:277-280.

137. Ho DD, Neumann AU, Perelson AS, et al. Rapid turnover of plasma virions and CD4 lymphocytes in HIV-1 infection. *Nature.* 1995;373:123-126.

138. Coffin JM. HIV population dynamics in vivo: Implications for genetic variation, pathogenesis, and therapy. *Science.* 1995;267:483-489.

139. Pakker NG, Notermans DW, de Boer RJ, et al. Biphasic kinetics of peripheral blood T cells after triple combination therapy in HIV-1 infection: A composite of redistribution and proliferation [see comments]. *Nat Med.* 1998;4:208-214.

140. Mohri H, Bonhoeffer S, Monard S, et al. Rapid turnover of T lymphocytes in SIV-infected rhesus macaques. *Science.* 1998;279:1223-1227.

141. de Boer RJ, Mohri H, Ho DD, et al. Turnover rates of B cells, T cells, and NK cells in simian immunodeficiency virus-infected and uninfected rhesus macaques. *J Immunol.* 2003;170:2479-2487.

142. Herbein G, Mahlknecht U, Batliwalla F, et al. Apoptosis of CD8+ T cells is mediated by macrophages through interaction of HIV gp120 with chemokine receptor CXCR4. *Nature* 1998;395:189-194.

143. Zagury D. A naturally unbalanced combat. *Nat Med.* 1997;3:156-157.

144. Gulick RM, Mellors JW, Havlir D, et al. Treatment with indinavir, zidovudine, and lamivudine in adults with human immunodeficiency virus infection and prior antiretroviral therapy. *N Engl J Med.* 1997;337:734-739.

145. Wong JK, Gunthard HF, Havlir DV, et al. Reduction of HIV-1 in blood and lymph nodes following potent antiretroviral therapy and the virologic correlates of treatment failure. *Proc Natl Acad Sci U S A.* 1997;94:12574-12579.

146. Wong JK, Hezareh M, Gunthard HF, et al. Recovery of replication-competent HIV despite prolonged suppression of plasma viremia. *Science.* 1997;278:1291-1295.

147. Chun TW, Engel D, Berrey MM, et al. Early establishment of a pool of latently infected, resting CD4(+) T cells during primary HIV-1 infection. *Proc Natl Acad Sci U S A.* 1998;95:8869-8873.

148. Finzi D, Hermankova M, Pierson T, et al. Identification of a reservoir for HIV-1 in patients on highly active antiretroviral therapy. *Science.* 1997;278:1295-1300.

149. Zagury D, Bernard J, Leonard R, et al. Long-term cultures of HTLV-III–infected T cells: A model of cytopathology of T-cell depletion in AIDS. *Science.* 1986;231:850-853.

150. Gougeon ML, Garcia S, Heeney J, et al. Programmed cell death in AIDS-related HIV and SIV infections. *AIDS Res Hum Retroviruses.* 1993;9:553-563.

151. Oyaizu N, McCloskey TW, Coronesi M, et al. Accelerated apoptosis in peripheral blood mononuclear cells (PBMCs) from human immunodeficiency virus type-1 infected patients and in CD4 cross-linked PBMCs from normal individuals. *Blood.* 1993;82:3392-3400.

152. McCutchan FE. Understanding the genetic diversity of HIV-1. *AIDS.* 2000;14(Suppl 3):S31-S44.

153. Gao F, Bailes E, Robertson DL, et al. Origin of HIV-1 in the chimpanzee Pan troglodytes troglodytes. *Nature.* 1999;397:436-441.

154. Keele BF, Van HF, Li Y, et al. Chimpanzee reservoirs of pandemic and nonpandemic HIV-1. *Science.* 2006;313:523-526.

155. Gilbert MT, Rambaut A, Wlasiuk G, et al. The emergence of HIV/AIDS in the Americas and beyond. *Proc Natl Acad Sci U S A.* 2007;104:18566-18570.

156. Wolinsky SM, Wike CM, Korber BT, et al. Selective transmission of human immunodeficiency virus type-1 variants from mothers to infants. *Science.* 1992;255:1134-1137.

157. Keele BF, Giorgi EE, Salazar-Gonzalez JF, et al. Identification and characterization of transmitted and early founder virus envelopes in primary HIV-1 infection. *Proc Natl Acad Sci U S A.* 2008;105:7552-7557.

158. Yusim K, Peeters M, Pybus OG, et al. Using human immunodeficiency virus type 1 sequences to infer historical features of the acquired immune deficiency syndrome epidemic and human immunodeficiency virus evolution. *Philos Trans R Soc Lond B Biol Sci.* 2001;356:855-866.

159. Foley BT. An overview of the molecular phylogeny of lentiviruses. In: Kuiken C, McCutchan F, Foley B, et al, eds. *HIV Sequence Compendium 2000.* Los Alamos, NM, Theoretical Biology and Biophysics Group, Los Alamos National Laboratory, 2000;35-43.

160. Ensoli B, Barillari G, Salahuddin SZ, et al. Tat protein of HIV-1 stimulates growth of cells derived from Kaposi's sarcoma lesions of AIDS patients. *Nature.* 1990;345:84-86.

161. Guo HG, Pati S, Sadowska M, et al. Tumorigenesis by human herpesvirus 8 vGPCR is accelerated by human immunodeficiency virus type 1 Tat. *J Virol.* 2004;78:9336-9342.

162. Chang Y, Cesarman E, Pessin MS, et al. Identification of herpesvirus-like DNA sequences in AIDS-associated Kaposi's sarcoma. *Science.* 1994;266:1865-1869.

163. Arvanitakis L, Geras-Raaka E, Varma A, et al. Human herpesvirus KSHV encodes a constitutively active G-protein-coupled receptor linked to cell proliferation. *Nature.* 1997;385:347-350.

164. Gallo RC. The enigmas of Kaposi's sarcoma. *Science.* 1998;282(5395):1837-1839.

165. Serraino D, Salamina G, Franceschi S, et al. The epidemiology of AIDS-associated non-Hodgkin's lymphoma in the World Health Organization European Region. *Br J Cancer.* 1992;66:912-916.

166. Cote TR, Biggar RJ, Rosenberg PS, et al. Non-Hodgkin's lymphoma among people with AIDS: Incidence, presentation and public health burden. AIDS/Cancer Study Group. *Int J Cancer.* 1997;73:645-650.

167. Beral V, Peterman T, Berkelman R, et al. AIDS-associated non-Hodgkin lymphoma. *Lancet.* 1991;337:805-809.

168. Flinn IW, Ambinder RF. AIDS primary central nervous system lymphoma. *Curr Opin Oncol.* 1996;8:373-376.

169. McClain KL, Leach CT, Jenson HB, et al. Association of Epstein-Barr virus with leiomyosarcomas in children with AIDS. *N Engl J Med.* 1995;332:12-18.

170. Williams AB, Darragh TM, Vranizan K, et al. Anal and cervical human papillomavirus infection and risk of anal and cervical epithelial abnormalities in human immunodeficiency virus–infected women. *Obstet Gynecol.* 1994;83:205-211.

171. Palefsky JM, Shiboski S, Moss A. Risk factors for anal human papillomavirus infection and anal cytologic abnormalities in HIV-positive and HIV-negative homosexual men. *J Acquir Immune Defic Syndr.* 1994;7:599-606.

170

Introduction to the Enteroviruses and Parechoviruses

JOHN F. MODLIN

Classification

Enteroviruses and parechoviruses are genera in the Picornaviridae, a large family of morphologically identical, single-stranded RNA viruses that share similar genomic and structural organizations. Originally, the human enteroviruses were divided into five subgenera based on differences in host range and pathogenic potential: polioviruses, group A coxsackieviruses (CAV), group B coxsackieviruses (CBV), echoviruses, and "newer" enteroviruses (Table 170-1).[1,2] All enteroviruses discovered since 1970 have been assigned to the enterovirus subgenus. A classification scheme based on RNA homology within the VP1 capsid protein coding region that has been widely adopted divides the non-polio enteroviruses into four classes, designated A through D (Table 170-2).[3] More than 90 unique enterovirus serotypes are distinguished from one another on the basis of neutralization, with each serotype designated according to the traditional taxonomy.[4] Of the original 72 serotypes identified, 64 remain after recognition of redundant serotypes and reclassification of others (see Table 170-1). Isolates of the same serotype characteristically diverge in the VP1 region by less than 25% within corresponding nucleotide sequences and by less than 12% within amino acid sequences.[3]

The parechoviruses are members of a more recently established genus that includes two species: Ljungan virus is a virus of rodents, and human parechoviruses infect humans.[5] Two serotypes formerly considered to be in the echovirus subgenus, echovirus 22 and 23, have been reclassified as members of the parechovirus genus, human parechovirus 1 (HPeV1) and HPeV2,[6] based on certain biophysical and biochemical properties that differ from those of enteroviruses (see later discussion). In addition, 12 new serotypes of HPeV have been described and are discussed in Chapter 172.

ENTEROVIRUSES

Virology

PHYSICAL CHARACTERISTICS

Enterovirus virions are non-enveloped, icosahedral capsids of approximately 30 nm, composed of 60 structural subunits; the subunits are formed from four polypeptides, with an aggregate molecular weight of 80 to 140 kDa, that surround the single-stranded RNA genome.[7] Unlike other picornaviruses (e.g., rhinoviruses), enteroviruses are stable over a wide range of pH (3 to 10), permitting them to retain infectivity during transit through the gastrointestinal tract. Lacking a lipid envelope, enteroviruses are resistant to ether, chloroform, and alcohol. However, they are readily inactivated by ionizing radiation, formaldehyde, or phenol.[7] Molar $MgCl_2$ reduces the thermolability of enteroviruses across a wide range of temperatures; this feature allows live, attenuated oral poliomyelitis (OPV) vaccines to maintain potency when refrigeration is suboptimal or unavailable.

The capsid encloses a linear RNA genome of approximately 7.4 kilobases that is divided into three regions: a 5′ end region of 743 nucleotides, a continuous-coding region of approximately 6625 nucleotides, and a 3′ poly(A) end region of variable length. The 5′ terminus is covalently linked to a small virus-coded protein of approximately 7 kDa (VPg), which is required for the initiation of RNA synthesis. Removal of the poly(A) 3′ terminus renders the RNA noninfectious. The most conserved regions of the genome are the 5′ noncoding region and those regions that code for the VPg protein and the RNA polymerase.[8] The regions coding for the structural proteins are less conserved, and there is considerable variation within the regions that code for epitopes that bind neutralizing antibody.

MOLECULAR BIOLOGY

The RNA genomes of naturally occurring polioviruses, attenuated polioviruses, and many non-polio enteroviruses have been fully sequenced, and the replication of polioviruses in primate cells has been studied in extensive detail.[9] Poliovirus type 1 RNA has been subjected to reverse transcription, and the complementary DNA sequences have been cloned and transfected into cultured cells, resulting in progeny virions.[10,11] The molecular structure and intracellular replicative events appear to be similar for all the human enteroviruses.

Host cell susceptibility to enteroviral infection is defined by the presence of specific membrane receptor proteins that bind enteroviruses generally along taxonomic lines[12,13] (Table 170-3). The three poliovirus serotypes share a common receptor (PVR), a member of the immunoglobulin superfamily that is coded on human chromosome 19.[14-16] Both decay-accelerating factor (DAF, or CD55), a complement regulatory protein, and intercellular adhesion molecule 1 (ICAM-1) play a role in coxsackievirus A21 cell entry.[17] The CBVs also interact with two different cell membrane proteins, the 49-kDa coxsackievirus-adenovirus receptor (CAR) and DAF.[18,19] The presence of CAR permits binding and cell entry by all six CBV serotypes,[19] whereas antibodies to DAF block binding and infection by serotypes 1, 3, and 5.[18,20,21] DAF also appears to be a major echovirus receptor, binding many echovirus serotypes,[22] whereas echovirus serotypes 1 and 8 bind to the α_2-subunit of the very late antigen (VLA) integrin molecule.[23,24]

The processes of penetration, uncoating, and release of the nucleic acid into the cytoplasm occur within minutes at 37° C. RNA synthesis begins within 30 minutes, leading to an exponential increase of minus-strand complementary and plus-strand progeny RNA until 2.5 hours after infection, when there is a switch to a linear accumulation of mainly progeny RNA.[9] The full-length RNA functions as a monocistronic messenger whose translational product, a polyprotein of molecular weight of 250 kDa, is encoded by a single open reading frame involving about 90% of the entire genome. The polyprotein undergoes specific cleavages to form three polypeptides, P1, P2, and P3. Subsequent cleavage of P2 and P3 results in eight nonstructural proteins,

TABLE 170-1 Conventional Classification and Host Range of Human Enteroviruses

Subgenera	No. of Serotypes	Host Range††		
		Primates	Newborn Mice	Cell Culture
Polioviruses*	1-3	++	0	++
Group A coxsackieviruses†,‡	1-24	0	+++	±
Group B coxsackieviruses†,§	1-6	0	+++	++
Echoviruses¶	1-34	0	0	++
Enteroviruses§,**	68-72	Variable	Variable	Variable

*Polioviruses generally replicate only in primates or primate cell cultures, although rare strains such as the type 2 Lansing strain have been adapted to rodents. Although polioviruses multiply in the alimentary tract of some subhuman primates, the hallmark of these viruses is the characteristic histopathologic lesions produced by direct inoculation of the central nervous system.

†The coxsackieviruses were first recovered from the feces of children with poliomyelitis in the town of Coxsackie, New York.[141] Unlike polioviruses, they produce paralysis and death in experimentally infected suckling mice.

‡All group A coxsackieviruses produce generalized myositis of skeletal muscle and flaccid hind limb paralysis in suckling mice,[142] and coxsackievirus A7 is pathogenic for the primate central nervous system. However, most group A coxsackieviruses, except serotypes A9 and A16, grow poorly in cell culture. Coxsackievirus A23 has been reclassified as echovirus 9, leaving 23 coxsackievirus serotypes.

§The group B coxsackieviruses are distinguished by their ability to produce focal myositis and generalized infection of the myocardium, brown fat, pancreas, and central nervous system in suckling mice, resulting in spastic paralysis. The group B coxsackieviruses are commonly isolated in cultured primate cells.

¶The echoviruses (enteric cytopathic human orphan) viruses were originally discovered in fecal specimens of healthy children.[143,144] They cause cytopathic effects in primate cell culture but are generally nonpathogenic for suckling mice (except for echovirus 21) and primates. Echovirus 10 has been reclassified as reovirus 1, and echovirus 28 as rhinovirus 1. Echovirus 34 is a variant of coxsackievirus A24. Echoviruses 22 and 23 have been assigned to the genus *Parechovirus* as parechovirus serotypes 1 and 2, respectively.[83] Therefore, a total of 29 of the original 34 serotypes of echovirus remain.

§The human enteroviral serotypes recognized since 1970 are designated by serial numbers only.[145]

**Hepatitis A virus was briefly classified as enterovirus 72, until genetic sequence data led to its reclassification as a hepadnavirus.[146]

††Replicative capacity.

whose known functions include polymerase activity, proteolytic cleavage of the translational products, and inhibition of host cell protein synthesis.[9]

The 5′ product, P1, undergoes subsequent cleavages to form the viral capsid, which proceeds by aggregation of five copies each of VP1, VP3, and VP0 (a precursor of VP2 and VP4) into subunits and assembly of 12 of these pentamers into the complete dodecahedral capsid shell. Encapsidation of the viral RNA is associated with a final cleavage of the VP0 protein to VP2 and VP4. The latter is an internal protein closely associated with the RNA. The complete virion contains 60 copies of each of the four structural proteins.[9]

Host protein and RNA synthesis are severely compromised by 3 hours after infection. After about 6 to 7 hours, virions are visible by

TABLE 170-2 Classification of Enteroviruses by RNA Homology

Enterovirus Class	Serotypes
A	CAV2-CAV8, CAV10, CAV12, CAV14, CAV16 EV71, EV76, EV89-EV91
B	CAV9 CBV1-CBV6 E1-E7, E9, E11- E21, E24- E27, E29-E33 EV69, EV73-EV75, EV77-EV88, EV100, EV101
C	CAV1, CAV11, CAV13, CAV15, CAV17, CAV18-CAV22, CAV24, PV1-PV3
D	EV68, EV70

CAV, group A coxsackievirus; CBV, group B coxsackievirus; E, echovirus; EV, enterovirus; PV, poliovirus.
Adapted from Centers for Disease Control and Prevention. Enterovirus surveillance—United States, 1970-2005. *MMWR Morb Mortal Wkly Rep.* 2006;55:1.

TABLE 170-3 Enterovirus and Parechovirus Cell Membrane Receptors

Serotype	Receptor Protein
Enteroviruses	
Polioviruses 1-3	Poliovirus receptor (PVR)
Coxsackieviruses A13, A18, A21	Intercellular adhesion molecule 1 (ICAM-1)
Coxsackieviruses B1-B6	Coxsackie-adenovirus receptor (CAR)
Coxsackieviruses B1, B3, B5	Decay accelerating factor (DAF)
Echoviruses 1, 8	Very late antigen 2 ($\alpha_2\beta_1$)
Echoviruses 6, 7, 11, 12, 13, 20, 21, 29, 33	DAF
Enterovirus 70	DAF
Parechoviruses	
Human parechovirus 1 (HPeV1)	$\alpha_V\beta_1$, $\alpha_V\beta_3$ integrins

electron microscopy within the cytoplasm, and they are subsequently released by lysis of the cell, resulting in a yield of 10^4 to 10^5 virions per cell. The number of infectious virions is 10- to 1000-fold lower.[9]

Pathogenesis and Immunity in Enteroviral Infections

PATHOGENESIS

The pathogenesis of poliovirus infection has been extensively investigated in primates experimentally infected with neurovirulent strains and in humans infected with vaccine strains,[25-28] and it is widely assumed that the early pathophysiologic events of non-polio enterovirus infections are similar. Studies of coxsackievirus infection in mice have produced much information about the influence of various host and environmental factors on the ability of the virus to replicate in the heart, brain, and other organs and about the mechanism of vertical transmission of enteroviruses from infected pregnant animals to their offspring.

Enteroviruses infect humans via direct or indirect contact with virus shed from the gastrointestinal tract or upper respiratory tract. Whereas ingested virus implants and replicates in the pharynx and the distal small bowel, volunteer studies have shown that attenuated polioviruses replicate most efficiently in the distal small intestine.[25] The precise site of viral entry has long been the subject of conjecture. Studies have demonstrated that microfold cells (M cells) expressing the PVR serve to transport polioviruses across the intestinal mucosa.[29,30] Enteroviral replication in ileal lymphoid tissue is detectable 1 to 3 days after the ingestion of virus. The quantity of virus recoverable from the tonsils is much less than that in Peyer's patches, where it may reach 10^7 to 10^8 tissue culture infective doses (TCID$_{50}$) per gram. The maximal duration of viral excretion is 3 to 4 weeks from the pharynx and 5 to 6 weeks in the feces.

After multiplication in submucosal lymphatic tissues, enteroviruses pass to regional lymph nodes and give rise to a transient "minor viremia." This leads to infection and viral replication in reticuloendothelial tissue including liver, spleen, and bone marrow. The most common result is a subclinical infection, in which viral replication is contained by host defense mechanisms. In a minority of infected persons, however, further replication of virus occurs in these reticuloendothelial sites, leading to a sustained "major" viremia that coincides with the onset of the "minor illness" of poliomyelitis and probably of the nonspecific febrile illnesses associated with other enterovirus infections. Prodromal viremia has been demonstrated with wild strains of poliovirus[28,31] and echovirus 9[32] but is uncommon with Sabin OPV strains except for type 2.[33]

The major viremia results in dissemination to target organs such as the central nervous system, heart, and skin, where tissue necrosis and inflammation occurs in proportion to the level of viral replication.

Histopathologic lesions usually are not seen in the gastrointestinal tract, even though the small bowel is the site of initial viral replication. The severity of infection in experimental animals can be enhanced by induced exercise, cold exposure, malnutrition, pregnancy, and immune suppression with corticosteroids or radiation.

VIRAL MUTATION DURING NATURAL INFECTION

Enteroviruses undergo a high rate of mutation during replication in the human gastrointestinal tract, and transcription errors occur with a frequency of 1 per 10^4 bases, approximately one error per genome. As a result, single-site mutations are commonly observed in the 5′ noncoding region of attenuated polioviruses within days after feeding to young infants, and such changes are associated with longer excretion and increased neurovirulence.[34,35] Serial isolates of the same enterovirus serotype excreted over many years by patients with B-cell immunodeficiency syndromes exhibit continuous genetic variation, which can be characterized by oligonucleotide fingerprinting[36,37] and RNA sequencing[38] and permits estimation of the duration of infection. In addition, RNA sequencing has led to the discovery of virulent vaccine-derived polioviruses (VDPV) that have caused outbreaks of paralytic disease among underimmunized populations in a number of countries previously free of poliomyelitis.[39-45]

Dual infection with different enteroviral strains may produce recombinant progeny virus if the parent strains are in the same class. Intertypia can be demonstrated in 1 in 10^4 to 1 in 10^5 infectious virions in vitro[46] and also in the feces of infants fed trivalent OPV.[43] Most VDPVs isolated to date are OPVs that have recombined with class C non-polio enteroviruses.[40]

IMMUNITY AND THE IMMUNE RESPONSE

Immunity to enteroviral infections is serotype specific. Antibody-mediated immune mechanisms operate in the alimentary tract to prevent mucosal infection and in the blood to prevent dissemination to target organs. Neutralizing antibodies target epitopes on VP1, the dominantly exposed viral capsid protein. As early as 1 to 3 days after enteroviral challenge, immunoglobulin M (IgM) humoral antibodies are produced; they predominate in serum during the first month and disappear within 2 to 3 months.[27] IgG antibody, which is typically detected by 7 to 10 days after infection, is mostly of the IgG_1 and IgG_3 subtypes.[47] Neutralizing IgG antibodies in serum persist for life after natural infection with enteroviruses.

Small concentrations of humoral type-specific neutralizing antibodies prevented poliovirus viremia and paralysis in experimentally infected primates,[48] and passive immunity to paralytic disease in humans can be achieved by the administration of immune serum globulin before exposure to neurovirulent polioviruses.[49,50] However, passively administered immune globulin does not modify the outcome of established central nervous system poliovirus disease[51]; at this late stage of infection, patients have detectable serum antibody. There is no proven role for immune globulin treatment of other systemic enterovirus infections.

IgA antibody appears in nasal and alimentary secretions 2 to 4 weeks after the administration of live-attenuated OPV and persists for at least 15 years.[27] However, mucosal immunity is relative: on reexposure to infectious virus, high titers of secretory IgA antibodies prevent or substantially reduce poliovirus shedding, whereas lower titers are associated with more extensive oropharyngeal replication of virus and longer viral shedding.[27] The elaboration of virus-specific IgA antibodies by the small intestine depends on local immunocompetent tissues, as was demonstrated in experiments in infants with double-barrel colostomies who were fed live-attenuated poliovirus through the colostomy and generated secretory IgA antibodies only in the distal loop of the colostomy, not in the pharynx or the proximal loop.[52] Antibodies are present in the colostrum and milk of immune women who are nursing and may interfere with the replication of OPV given to breastfed neonates.[51] Maternal antibodies passively acquired trans-placentally or via milk prevent or modify enteroviral infections of early infancy.[53,54]

Humoral antibodies have an important role in the recovery from enteroviral infection, as evidenced by the development of persistent infections in persons with significant B-cell immunodeficiency.[55] However, there is both clinical and laboratory evidence that humoral antibody alone is not sufficient to limit enteroviral replication in target organs. Macrophages predominate in the early stages and play a critical role in viral clearance; in experimental animals, ablation of macrophage function enhances the severity of CBV infections.[56] Inhibition of T-lymphocyte function has little effect on virus replication in vivo,[57] and persons with abnormal cell-mediated immunity are not predisposed to serious or prolonged enterovirus infections unless they have accompanying B-cell dysfunction.

Even though T lymphocytes do not contribute to the inhibition of enteroviral replication, there is evidence that certain immunopathologic events after enterovirus infection are mediated by T-cell activity. In the murine myocarditis model, expression of proinflammatory cytokines and an acute inflammatory infiltration follow peak viral replication,[58-62] and induction of natural killer cell activity and T-lymphocyte immune responses contributes to necrosis of infected cardiac myocytes[57,63,64] (see Chapter 81). An inflammatory response may persist long after viral replication has ceased, and ongoing cardiac damage may be mediated by virus-induced antibodies against cardiac antigens[65] or by cytotoxic T-lymphocyte–mediated myocyte lysis.[61,63,66,67]

Epidemiology of Enteroviral Infections

Enteroviruses are distributed worldwide. Infection rates vary with season, geography, and age and socioeconomic status of the population sampled. Enteroviral infections occur throughout the year, but in temperate climates infections are more prevalent in the summer and autumn months (June to October in the Northern Hemisphere).[68-71] This seasonal periodicity is less pronounced in southern latitudes and disappears altogether in the tropics, where enteroviruses are endemic the year round. In surveys of southern and southwestern cities of the United States, 7% to 15% of children sampled during the year excreted enteroviruses in feces, compared with fewer than 5% of comparable populations in New York, Buffalo, and Minneapolis.[72]

AGE AND SOCIOECONOMIC STATUS

Three fourths of enteroviral infections occur in children younger than 15 years of age.[70] In the United States, attack rates for both infection and illness with non-polio enteroviruses are highest in infants during their first year of life.[73,74] During the annual peak period of enteroviral transmission in Rochester, New York, the incidence of infection was found to be 12.8% during the first month of life.[75] Rates of symptomatic enteroviral infection drop after the second month of life[76] but remain higher for infants and toddlers compared with older children and adults. Enteroviral infections are more prevalent among children of lower socioeconomic status, probably because of crowding, poor hygiene, and opportunities for fecal contamination. Simultaneous infection by more than one serotype is common under these circumstances. In a study of infants in Karachi, Pakistan, 80% had rectal swabs with at least one enterovirus.[77]

The frequency with which different enterovirus serotypes cause infection varies markedly. In the United States, one to three enteroviral serotypes predominate in a given location in each season, although there is variation from one region to another and from year to year. Some prevalent serotypes are continuously isolated from year to year,[69,78,79] whereas others may emerge for the first time or reemerge after years of relative inactivity.[78,80] Wild-type polioviruses now circulate only in a diminishing number of developing countries (see Chapter 171), whereas vaccine strains are commonly isolated in countries that continue to use OPV for poliomyelitis prevention. Global epidemics

TABLE 170-4	Most Common Enterovirus Serotypes Submitted by State and Local Public Health Laboratories to the Centers for Disease Control and Prevention, 1970-2005	
Enterovirus Serotype	**Percentage of Enterovirus Isolates**	
Echovirus 9	11.8	
Echovirus 11	11.4	
Echovirus 30	10.1	
Coxsackievirus B5	8.7	
Echovirus 6	6.1	
Coxsackievirus B2	5.2	
Coxsackievirus A9	4.8	
Echovirus 4	4.6	
Coxsackievirus B4	4.2	
Echovirus 7	4.0	
Total	70.9	

Adapted from Centers for Disease Control and Prevention. Enterovirus surveillance—United States, 1970-2005. *MMWR Morb Mortal Wkly Rep.* 2006;55:1.

of non-polio enteroviruses occasionally occur, such as the worldwide outbreak of echovirus 9 disease in the late 1950s and the explosive pandemics of acute hemorrhagic conjunctivitis due to enterovirus 70 and coxsackievirus A24 that have occurred over the past three decades. Infection with some serotypes, such as coxsackievirus B6 and enteroviruses 68 and 69, is rarely recognized.

The reasons why individual serotypes of enteroviruses appear and disappear and behave as either endemic or epidemic pathogens are not well understood. Some epidemic echovirus strains spread rapidly and exhaust susceptible individuals in the population beyond a "critical mass" necessary for continued transmission; endemic strains that are recovered over a number of years may be less contagious. In addition, periodic reappearances of the same enteroviral serotype may occur because the new enterovirus strain is poorly neutralized by antibodies raised in response to earlier strains.[81-83] Over the 35-year period between 1970 and 2005, 10 serotypes, all group B enteroviruses, represented 71% of all enterovirus isolates submitted from state and local public health laboratories to the National Enterovirus Surveillance System of the Centers for Disease Control and Prevention (Table 170-4).[84]

MOLECULAR EPIDEMIOLOGY

Southern blotting, two-dimensional oligonucleotide gel RNA electrophoresis, and amplification and identification of defined RNA sequences by polymerase chain reaction (PCR) have been used to differentiate between live vaccine and naturally occurring poliovirus strains[85,86] and to trace the routes of spread of polioviruses[87] and other enteroviruses by comparison of RNA relatedness among epidemiologically distinct isolates.[88-91] Genomic RNA sequencing has proved the most adept technique for characterizing the evolutionary relationships among poliovirus isolates of the same serotype. "Genotypes" are distinguished from one another by greater than 15% divergence among the RNA nucleotides in the homologous portions of the genomes that are sequenced.[86] The application of genomic sequencing has detected circulating OPV-derived polioviruses (cVDPV) in Haiti and other locations[39,40] and has traced the pandemic spread of acute hemorrhagic conjunctivitis caused by enterovirus 70 and coxsackievirus A24 in the 1980s.[89,92,93]

TRANSMISSION

Enteroviruses are shed in feces and in respiratory tract secretions. Transmission may occur as a result of direct person-to-person contact or indirectly from exposure to environmental sources contaminated by enteroviruses. The relative importance of each route of transmission depends on viral factors and hygienic conditions. Direct transmission from a respiratory source has been demonstrated in volunteer

studies using coxsackievirus A21 as a challenge virus,[94] and it is likely that other coxsackieviruses which are frequently shed simultaneously from the upper respiratory tract and in the feces are also transmitted in this manner.[95] However, fecal contamination of the household environment is responsible for the very high rates of infection demonstrated with polioviruses and many other enterically shed enteroviruses in poor hygienic conditions. Sampling of sewage in most cities, especially in summer months, usually yields several enteroviral serotypes.[96] Clams in seawater polluted by sewage concentrate enteroviruses 10- to 60-fold, and swimming in contaminated seawater was the apparent cause of a recently reported outbreak of enterovirus infection among tourists returning from Mexico. Enterovirus 70, the agent of acute hemorrhagic conjunctivitis, is spread by fomites, fingers, and ophthalmologic instruments contaminated with virus in tears.[97]

Longitudinal studies have shown substantial clustering of enterovirus infections in families.[95] Once the virus has been introduced into the household, secondary attack rates for infection among seronegative family members are 90% to 100% for wild-type polioviruses and approximately 75% for coxsackieviruses.[95] Secondary attack rates for echoviruses are less than 50%, probably because these viruses tend to be shed only in feces and for shorter periods. Infants in diapers who shed virus in the feces are the most efficient disseminators of infection. Mothers and infant siblings are at greater risk of acquiring infection than are fathers and teenaged siblings.[95] For all enteroviruses, the period of maximal contagiousness corresponds to the period of maximal viral excretion in the feces. When reinfection with the same enterovirus serotype occurs, the duration of excretion of virus is considerably shorter than in the primary infection.[95,98]

INCIDENCE OF INFECTION AND ILLNESS

Approximately 95% of infections caused by wild-type polioviruses and at least 50% to 80% of non-polio enteroviral infections are asymptomatic. When illness occurs, it usually takes the form of an undifferentiated febrile illness lasting only a few days, often accompanied by symptoms of upper respiratory tract infection.[99] These illnesses may be caused by virtually any enteroviral serotype and are clinically indistinguishable from infection by many other viruses. Disease syndromes characteristic of enteroviruses (e.g., aseptic meningitis, pericarditis) are unusual manifestations of infection. A 4-year longitudinal family-based study in New York City detected 291 enteroviral infections, none producing "characteristic" illnesses, and only 6 with exanthems.[95]

The risk of some enterovirus-related clinical syndromes varies with age and sex. Aseptic meningitis is most commonly recognized in very young infants, whereas some other illnesses, such as pleurodynia and myopericarditis, are seen predominantly in adolescents and young adults. Symptomatic enteroviral infections in elderly persons are uncommon. Among young children, boys are at greater risk of illness (but not infection) than are girls.[74] Aseptic meningitis and poliomyelitis occur almost twice as often in boys. After puberty, the reverse is true, perhaps because women have greater exposure than men to children shedding virus.[95,100] Pregnancy may enhance the severity of enteroviral infections. The incidence of paralytic poliomyelitis was two to three times higher in pregnant women than in age-matched nonpregnant women in Boston before the control of poliomyelitis.[101] There are also clinical and epidemiologic data demonstrating that enteroviral illnesses are more frequent[102] and more severe[103] in persons who exercise vigorously before the onset of symptoms. Although these data are anecdotal, they are supported by evidence that exercise enhances the severity of CBV infection in the murine model.[104]

Although the incidence of non-polio enteroviral disease has been measured in selected populations, the overall incidence in the United States is unknown. Serologic surveys encompassing all known enteroviral serotypes are not feasible. Antibody prevalence rates measured for a few serotypes indicate that, after the decline of passively acquired maternal antibodies after the age of 6 months, the fraction of immune persons in the population rises progressively with age, so that 15% to 90% of the adult population have type-specific neutralizing antibodies for each serotype tested, depending on the serotype and the characteristics of the population surveyed.[74,95]

INCUBATION PERIOD AND PERIOD OF COMMUNICABILITY

The incubation period for illness due to enteroviral infections can rarely be determined precisely. Because the source of infection is often an asymptomatic person who transmits virus as readily as one who is ill, the time of exposure is usually unknown. Although the incubation period may range from 2 days to 2 weeks, it is usually 3 to 5 days. Patients with enteroviral illnesses typically excrete virus in throat secretions or feces for several days before the onset of symptoms and continue to excrete virus in feces for several weeks thereafter. Although the period of communicability is therefore potentially long, maximal communicability is believed to occur early in illness, when viral shedding is greatest.

LABORATORY DIAGNOSIS OF ENTEROVIRAL INFECTIONS

The laboratory diagnosis of enteroviral infection is accomplished by virus isolation in cell culture, PCR, or retrospectively by serologic methods. Cell culture is still performed by many academic medical center and public health laboratories and remains the method to which other techniques are compared. However, because cell culture is laborious and relatively slow, it has been gradually supplanted by more rapid and sensitive PCR-based assays.

Viral Isolation

A presumptive diagnosis of enteroviral infection can usually be reported by the laboratory within 2 to 5 days by identification of a characteristic cytopathic effect (CPE) in any of three or four appropriately chosen cell lines.[105] Primary monkey kidney cell lines and human embryonic fibroblast cell lines support the growth of most polioviruses, CBVs, and echoviruses. The inclusion of Buffalo green monkey kidney cells and human rhabdomyosarcoma cells enhances recovery of CBVs and of echoviruses, respectively.[105] Only a few serotypes of the CAVs (e.g., A9, A16) grow readily in routinely used cell lines. Although the use of specialized cell lines such as rhabdomyosarcoma[106] or guinea pig embryo[107] may aid the recovery of some CAVs in cell culture, inoculation of newborn mice remains the method of choice for recovery of this subgroup of enteroviruses.[108]

Isolates demonstrating CPE may be confirmed as enteroviruses with the use of a monoclonal antibody to a broadly reactive VP1 epitope.[109] The serotype of an enterovirus isolated in cell culture is determined by neutralization in cell culture by type-specific antisera or by genomic sequencing. Unless a small number of serotypes is suspected, serotype identification by neutralization requires the use of the Lim-Benyesh-Melnick intersecting antiserum pools,[110] a time-consuming assay that is performed mainly by research and reference laboratories. Because the equine sera that constitute the Lim Benyesh-Melnick pools were harvested against enterovirus strains prevalent more than 30 years ago, their ability to identify contemporary isolates has gradually diminished.[8-10]

The opportunity to recover a virus in cell culture is optimized by sampling of multiple sites. Late in the course of enteroviral illnesses, viral cultures of feces are useful because the lower intestine may be the only site from which the agent is still being excreted. An etiologic diagnosis can be confirmed by the isolation of virus from cerebrospinal fluid, pericardial fluid, tissue, or blood, depending on the clinical syndrome. Isolation of virus from the upper respiratory tract or stool is considered by some to be less definitive, because intercurrent asymptomatic enterovirus infections etiologically unrelated to the observed illness may produce a false-positive result. However, in developed countries, background rates of asymptomatic infection are generally low enough that isolation of an enterovirus from a throat or stool specimen is strong evidence of causation.

Polymerase Chain Reaction and Genomic Sequencing

Reverse transcription–PCR is a rapid, sensitive, and specific method of detecting enterovirus RNA in clinical specimens. Most reported PCR protocols amplify a highly conserved portion of the 5′ nontranslated region of the genome, enabling the detection of most enteroviruses.[111,112] Subgroup-specific primers distinguish the polioviruses from other enteroviruses.[113,114] With cerebrospinal fluid specimens from patients with aseptic meningitis, PCR detects enteroviral RNA in 66% to 86%, compared with viral isolation rates of approximately 30%.[115-117] Experience with specimens other than cerebrospinal fluid is more limited. PCR has detected enteroviral RNA from throat swabs, serum, urine, and stool, although the sensitivity with urine specimens is somewhat lower than with other specimens.[118,119] PCR has detected enteroviral RNA in only a minority of endomyocardial biopsy specimens from patients with acute myopericarditis.[115,116] Further characterization of enteroviruses isolated in cell culture or detected by PCR can be accomplished by sequencing the portions of the capsid-coding regions of the viral RNA, including identification of serotype and assignment of non-polio enterovirus isolates to one of four classes according to the new taxonomy.[3,9,120,121]

Serology

The microneutralization test is the most widely used method for determination of antibodies to enteroviruses. However, microneutralization is serotype specific and therefore has limited usefulness in the routine diagnosis of non-polio enteroviral infections, because the feasibility of testing with multiple live viral antigens is low, and because methods based on neutralization are relatively insensitive, poorly standardized, and labor intensive. Type-specific immunoassays are more versatile and are now offered in commercial laboratories for assay of antibodies against the more common enteroviral serotypes. Serum IgM antibody to the CBVs can often be detected early in the course of illness, but the assay is not serotype specific, and positive test results may occur during infections with enteroviruses of other classes.[117] Epitopes on capsid proteins have been described that are common to many different enteroviral serotypes,[122,123] and monoclonal antibodies are reported to detect VP1 capsid antigens common to many enteroviruses.[109,124] However, identification of a common antigen that is sufficiently immunogenic to form the basis of a broadly reactive serologic assay has not been reported.

Treatment and Prevention of Enteroviral Infections

Most enterovirus infections are self-limited and do not require antiviral therapy. Exceptions include encephalitis, acute myocarditis, and infections in neonates and B-cell–deficient hosts that may be life-threatening. The therapeutic options for these more serious infections are quite limited. Serum immune globulin and intravenous immune globulin have been given to persistently infected B-cell–deficient patients with mixed results[55,125] and have been used in nonrandomized trials in children with myocarditis with uncertain effect.[120]

An effective antiviral drug to treat serious enterovirus infections has not been licensed, even though several agents have shown activity against enteroviruses in animal models and in early clinical trials.[121] The most promising of these are compounds that bind to a pocket in the viral capsid, altering virus attachment and uncoating.[126] The best studied of the capsid-binding drugs is pleconaril, which inhibits replication of most enterovirus serotypes at concentrations of less than 0.1 μg/mL in vitro[127] and which has a favorable pharmacologic profile[128] (see Chapter 41). Placebo-controlled trials of pleconaril in patients with enterovirus meningitis have shown some reductions in the duration and severity of headache and other symptoms and a shorter period of viral shedding when the drug was administered within 24 hours after symptom onset.[129-132] Uncontrolled experience with pleconaril for B-cell–deficient patients with persistent enterovirus infections and patients with potentially fatal infections, including neonates and persons of all ages with acute myocarditis, suggests possible clinical benefit.[133] Pleconaril has also shown mild benefit in the treatment of rhinovirus-induced colds,[134] but it was not approved by the U.S. Food and Drug Administration (FDA) for this indication. The drug induces cytochrome P-450 3A isoenzymes[134] and therefore has raised concern for multiple drug interactions.

The preexposure administration of immune globulin is known to reduce the risk of paralytic poliomyelitis.[50] It is very likely that immune globulin would also prevent non-polio enteroviral disease, but this strategy is rarely applicable to clinical practice. The successful vaccine approach against paralytic poliomyelitis is detailed in Chapter 171. In the setting of a community epidemic or a patient hospitalized with enteroviral illness, simple hygienic measures such as hand washing and careful disposal or autoclaving of potentially infected feces and secretions should be practiced. Gown and mask procedures or isolation of the patient is unwarranted, except in the newborn nursery. Pregnant women, especially those near term, should be advised to avoid contact with people suspected of having an enteroviral illness.

PARECHOVIRUSES

The parechoviruses have many properties in common with other picornaviruses, but they also have biochemical and biophysical differences that have led to their designation as a separate genus of Picornaviridae. The properties of parechoviruses are reviewed in the following paragraphs.

Virology

Parechoviruses have the typical appearance of picornaviruses. They are small (27 to 30 nm), round, and non-enveloped and have icosahedral symmetry.[135] The capsid consists of 12 capsomers. Virions have a buoyant density in CsCl of 1.36 g/cm³. The genome of parechoviruses is contained in a nonsegmented, linear, single-stranded RNA of positive sense. The complete genome is 7500 nucleotides long. The 5′-end of the genome has a genome-linked protein (VPg). The 5′-terminus has a poly(C) tract, and the 3′-terminus has a poly(A) tract.[135] The nucleoside sequence of the genome shows no more than 30% amino acid identity with other picornaviruses.[136]

The genome encodes a single polyprotein, which in most picornaviruses undergoes cleavage into four capsid proteins (VP1 through VP4). However, in contrast to enteroviruses, cleavage into VP4 and VP2 does not occur, and parechoviruses only have three structural proteins: VP0, VP1, and VP3.[137] A number of nonstructural proteins are also generated, including an RNA-dependent RNA polymerase, VPg, and a probable helicase.[137] Receptors for HPeV1 appear to be the $\alpha_v\beta_1$, $\alpha_v\beta_3$ integrins (see Table 170-3).[136,138]

VIRUS TYPES

Because of the relatively laborious and difficult process of determining neutralization of parechoviruses in tissue culture, relatively little information is available on the designation of serotypes among parechoviruses. Rather, molecular techniques, such as PCR, are employed to designate genotypes.[139] Fourteen genotypes have been proposed.[140]

VIRAL DIAGNOSIS

As discussed previously regarding enteroviruses, isolation of virus in tissue culture is still carried out primarily in academic centers, but the availability and advantages of PCR techniques are changing this situation. Serologic responses are infrequently used, but determination of virus-specific IgG or IgM neutralizing responses is occasionally used to establish the occurrence of infection.[137]

Epidemiology

The most extensive study of the epidemiology of parechoviruses has been carried out for HPeV1 (formerly known as echovirus 22), which appears to be widely distributed and mainly infects young children. Infection with HPeV2 (formerly echovirus 23) appears to be much more limited.[137]

The epidemiology and clinical manifestations of parechovirus infections are discussed in Chapter 172.

REFERENCES

1. Melnick JL. Discovery of the enteroviruses and the classification of poliovirus among them. *Biologicals.* 1993;21:305.
2. King AMQ, Brown F, Christian P, et al. Picornaviridae. In: Van Regenmortel MHV, Fauquet CM, Bishop DHL, eds. *Seventh Report of the International Committee on Taxonomy of Viruses.* New York: Academic Press; 2000.
3. Oberste MS, Maher K, Kilpatrick DR, et al. Typing human enteroviruses by partial sequencing of VP1. *J Clin Microbiol.* 1999;37:1288.
4. Oberste MS, Maher K, Michele SM, et al. Enteroviruses 76, 89, 90 and 91 represent a novel group within the species human enterovirus A. *J Gen Virol.* 2005;86:445.
5. Stanway G, Hyypiä T, Minireview: Parechoviruses. *J Virol.* 1999; 73:5249.
6. Al-Sunaidi M, William CH, Hughes PJ, et al. Analysis of a new human parechovirus allows the definition of parechovirus types and the identification of RNA structural domains. *J Virol.* 2007; 81:1013.
7. Melnick JL. Portraits of viruses: The picornaviruses. *Intervirology.* 1983;20:61.
8. Werner G, Rosenwirth B, Bauer E, et al. Molecular cloning and sequence determination of the genomic regions encoding pro- tease and genome-linked protein of three picornaviruses. *J Virol.* 1986;57:1084.
9. Rueckert RR. Picornaviridae and their replication. In: Fields BN, Knipe DM, eds. *Virology.* 2nd ed. New York: Raven Press; 1990:507.
10. Racaniello VR, Baltimore D. Cloned poliovirus complentary DNA is infectious in mammalian cells. *Science.* 1981;214:916.
11. Racaniello VR, Baltimore D. Molecular cloning of poliovirus cDNA and determination of the complete nucleotide sequence of the viral genome. *Proc Nat Acad Sci U S A.* 1981;78:4887.
12. Holland JJ. Receptor affinities as major determinants of enterovirus tissue tropisms in humans. *Virology.* 1961;15:312.
13. Rotbart HA, Kirkegaard K. Picornavirus pathogenesis: Viral access, attachment and entry into susceptible cells. *Sem Virol.* 1992;3:483.
14. Mendelsohn CL, Johnson B, Lionetti KA, et al. Transformation of a human poliovirus receptor gene into mouse cells. *Proc Nat Acad Sci U S A.* 1986;83:7845.
15. Mendelsohn CL, Wimmer E, Racaniello VR. Cellular receptor for poliovirus: Molecular cloning, nucleotide sequence, and expression of a new member of the immunoglobulin super family. *Cell.* 1989;56:855.
16. Miller DA, Miller OJ, Vaithilingam GD, et al. Human chromosome 19 carries a poliovirus receptor gene. *Cell.* 1974;1:167.
17. Shafren DR, Dorahy DJ, Ingham RA, et al. Coxsackievirus A21 binds to decay-accelerating factor, but requires intracellular adhesion molecule 1 for cell entry. *J Virol.* 1997;71:4736.
18. Shafren DR, Bates RC, Agrez MV, et al. Coxsackieviruses B1, B3, and B5 use decay accelerating factor as a receptor for cell attachment. *J Virol.* 1995;69:3873.
19. Bergelson JM, Cunningham JA, Droguett G, et al. Isolation of a common receptor for coxsackie B viruses and adenoviruses 2 and 5. *Science.* 1997;275:1320.
20. Crowell RL, Field AK, Schleif WA, et al. Monoclonal antibody that inhibits infection of HeLa and rhabdomyosarcoma cells by selected enteroviruses through receptor blockade. *J Virol.* 1986;57:438.
21. Hsu K-HL, Lonberg-Holm K, Alstein B, et al. A monoclonal antibody specific for the cellular receptor for the group B coxsackieviruses. *J Virol.* 1988;62:1647.
22. Bergelson JM, Chan M, Solomon K, et al. Decay-accelerating factor (CD55), a glycosylphosphatidylinositol-anchored complement regulatory protein, is a receptor for several echoviruses. *Proc Nat Acad Sci U S A.* 1994;91:6245.

23. Bergelson JM, Shepley MP, Chan BMC, et al. Identification of the integrin VLA-2 as a receptor for echovirus 1. *Science.* 1992;255:1718.
24. Bergelson JM, St. John N, Kawaguchi S, et al. Infection by echoviruses 1 and 8 depends on the a2 subunit of human VLA-2. *J Virol.* 1993;67:6847.
25. Sabin AB. Behavior of chimpanzee-avirulent poliomyelitis viruses in experimentally infected human volunteers. *Am J Med Sci.* 1955;230:1.
26. Sabin AB. Pathogenesis of poliomyelitis: Reappraisal in light of new data. *Science.* 1956;123:1151.
27. Ogra PL, Karzon DT. Formation and function of poliovirus antibody in different tissues. *Prog Med Virol.* 1971;13:157.
28. Horstmann DM, McCollum RW. Poliomyelitis virus in human blood during the "minor" illness and asymptomatic infection. *Proc Soc Exp Biol Med.* 1953;82:434.
29. Iwasaki A, Welker R, Mueller S, et al. Immunofluorescence analysis of poliovirus receptor expression in Peyer's patches of humans, primates, and CD155 transgenic mice: Implications for poliovirus infection. *J Infect Dis.* 2002;186:585.
30. Ouzilou L, Caliot E, Pelletier I, et al. Poliovirus transcytosis through M-like cells. *J Gen Virol.* 2002;83:2177.
31. Davis DC, Melnick JL. Two additional examples of viremia in asymptomatic poliomyelitis infection. *Pediatrics.* 1957;20:975.
32. Yoshioka I, Horstmann DM. Viremia in infection due to echo virus type 9. *N Engl J Med.* 1961;262:224.
33. Horstmann DM, Opton EM, Klemperer R, et al. Viremia in infants vaccinated with oral poliovirus vaccine (Sabin). *Am J Hyg.* 1964;79:47.
34. Minor PD, John A, Ferguson M, Icenogle JP. Antigenic and molecular evolution of the vaccine strain of type 3 poliovirus during the period of excretion by a primary vaccinee. *J Gen Virol.* 1986;67:693.
35. Jameson BA, Bonin J, Wimmer E, et al. Natural variants of the Sabin type 1 vaccine strains of poliovirus and correlation with a poliovirus neutralization site. *Virology.* 1985;143:337.
36. Yoneyama T, Hagiwara A, Hara M, et al. Alteration in oligonucleotide fingerprint patterns of the viral genome in poliovirus type 2 isolated from paralytic patients. *Infect Immun.* 1982;37:46.
37. O'Neil KM, Pallansch MA, Winkelstein JA, et al. Chronic group A coxsackievirus infection in agammaglobulinemia: Demonstration of genomic variation of serotypically identical isolates persistently excreted from the same patient. *J Infect Dis.* 1988; 157:183.
38. Kew OM, Sutter RW, Nottay BK, et al. Prolonged replication of a type 1 vaccine-derived poliovirus in an immunodeficient patient. *J Clin Microbiol.* 1998;36:2893.
39. Centers for Disease Control and Prevention. Update on vaccine-derived polioviruses—Worldwide, January 2006-August 2007. *MMWR Morb Mortal Wkly Rep.* 2007;56:996.
40. Kew O, Morris-Glasgow V, Landaverde M, et al. Outbreak of poliomyelitis in Hispaniola associated with circulating type 1 vaccine-derived poliovirus. *Science.* 2002;296:356.
41. Kew OM, Wright PF, Agol VI, et al. Circulating vaccine-derived polioviruses: Current state of knowledge. *Bull WHO.* 2004;82:16.
42. Estivariz CF, Watkins MA, Handoko D, et al. A large vaccine-derived poliovirus outbreak on Madura Island—Indonesia, 2005. *J Infect Dis.* 2008;197:347.
43. Centers for Disease Control and Prevention. Circulation of a type 2 vaccine-derived poliovirus—Egypt, 1982-1993. *MMWR Morb Mortal Wkly Rep.* 2001;50:41.
44. Centers for Disease Control and Prevention. Public health dispatch: Acute flaccid paralysis associated with circulating vaccine-derived poliovirus—Philippines, 2001. *MMWR Morb Mortal Wkly Rep.* 2001;50:874.
45. Centers for Disease Control and Prevention. Poliomyelitis—Madagascar, 2002. *MMWR Morb Mortal Wkly Rep.* 2002;51:622.
46. Tolskaya EA, Romanova LI, Kolesnikova MS, et al. Intertypic recombination in poliovirus: Genetic and biochemical studies. *Virology.* 1983;124:121.
47. Torfason EG, Reimer CB, Keyserling HL. Subclass restriction of human enterovirus antibodies. *J Clin Microbiol.* 1987;25:1376.
48. Bodian D, Nathanson N. Inhibitory effects of passive antibody on virulent poliovirus excretion and on immune response in chimpanzees. *Bull J Hopkins Hosp.* 1960;107:143.
49. Hammon WM, Coriell LI, Stokes J Jr. Evaluation of Red Cross gamma globulin as a prophylactic agent for poliomyelitis. *J Am Med Assn.* 1952;150:139.
50. Stevens KM. Estimate of molecular equivalent of antibody required for prophylaxis and therapy of poliomyelitis. *J Hyg.* 1959;57:198.
51. Bahlke AM, Perkins JE. Treatment of preparalytic poliomyelitis with gamma globulin. *J Am Med Assn.* 1945;129:1146.
52. Ogra PL, Karzon DT. Distribution of poliovirus antibody in serum, nasopharynx, and alimentary tract following segmental immunization of the lower alimentary tract with poliovaccine. *J Immunol.* 1969;102:1423.
53. Warren RJ, Lepow ML, Bartsch GE, et al. The relationship of maternal antibody, breast feeding, and age to the susceptibility of newborn infants to infection with attenuated poliovirus. *Pediatrics.* 1964;34:4.
54. Modlin JF, Polk BF, Horton P, et al. Perinatal echovirus 11 infection: Risk of transmission during a community outbreak. *N Engl J Med.* 1981;305:368.
55. McKinney RE, Katz SL, Wilfert CM. Chronic enteroviral meningoencephalitis in agammaglobulinemic patients. *Rev Infect Dis.* 1987;9:334.
56. Rager-Zisman B, Allison AC. The role of antibody and host cells in the resistance of mice against infection by coxsackie B-3 virus. *J Gen Virol.* 1973;19:329.
57. Woodruff JF, Woodruff JJ. Involvement of T lymphocytes in the pathogenesis of coxsackievirus B3 heart disease. *J Immunol.* 1974;113:1726.
58. Rabin ER, Hassan SA, Jenson AB, et al. Coxsackie virus B3 myocarditis in mice. *Am J Path.* 1964;44:775.
59. Woodruff JF, Kilbourne ED. The influence of quantitated post-weanling undernutrition on Coxsackievirus B-3 infection of adult mice: I. Viral persistence and increased severity of lesions. *J Infect Dis.* 1970;121:137.
60. Woodruff JF. Viral myocarditis. *Am J Pathol.* 1980;101:427.
61. Kawai C. From myocarditis to cardiomyopathy: Mechanisms of inflammation and cell death—Learning from the past for the future. *Circulation.* 1999;99:1091.
62. Schmidtke M, Gluck B, Merkle I, et al. Cytokine profiles in heart, spleen, and thymus during the acute stage of experimental coxsackievirus B3-induced chronic myocarditis. *J Med Virol.* 2000;61:518.
63. Huber SA, Job LP, Woodruff JF. In vitro culture of coxsackievirus group B, type 3 immune spleen cells on infected endothelial cells and biological activity of the cultured cells in vivo. *Infect Immun.* 1984;43:567.
64. Godeny EK, Gauntt CJ. Murine natural killer cells limit coxsackievirus B3 replication. *J Immunol.* 1987;139:913.
65. Gauntt CJ. Roles of the humoral immune response in coxsackievirus-B-induced disease. In: Tracy S, Chapman NM, Mahy BWJ, eds. *The Coxsackie B Viruses. Current Topics in Microbiology and Immunology 223.* Berlin: Springer; 1997:259.
66. Liao O, Sindhwani R, Rojkind M, et al. Antibody-mediated autoimmune myocarditis depends on genetically determined target organ sensitivity. *J Exp Med.* 1995;181:1123.
67. Schwimmbeck PL, Huber SA, Schultheiss H-P. Roles of T cells in coxsackievirus B-induced disease. In: Tracy S, Chapman NM, Mahy BWJ, eds. *The Coxsackie B Viruses. Current Topics in Microbiology and Immunology 223.* Berlin: Springer; 1997:283.
68. Gelfand HM. The occurrence in nature of the Coxsackie and ECHO viruses. *Prog Med Virol.* 1961;3:193.
69. Moore M. Enteroviral disease in the United States. *J Infect Dis.* 1982;146:103.
70. Berlin LE, Rorabaugh ML, Heldrich F, et al. Aseptic meningitis in infants less than two years of age: Diagnosis and etiology. *J Infect Dis.* 1993;168:888.
71. Grist NR, Bell EJ, Assad F. Enteroviruses in human disease. *Prog Med Virol.* 1978;24:114.
72. Gelfand HM, Holgium AH, Marchetti GE, et al. A continuing surveillance of enterovirus infections in healthy children in six United States cities. I: Viruses isolated during 1960 and 1961. *Am J Hyg.* 1963;78:358.
73. Dagan R, Powell KR, Hall CB, et al. Identification of infants unlikely to have serious bacterial infection although hospitalized for suspected sepsis. *J Pediatr.* 1985;107:855.
74. Froeschle JE, Feorino PM, Gelfand HM. A continuing surveillance of enterovirus infections in healthy children in six United States cities. II: Surveillance enterovirus isolates from cases of acute central nervous system disease. *Am J Epidemiol.* 1966;83:455.
75. Jenista JA, Dalzell LE, Davidson PW, et al. Outcome studies of neonatal enterovirus infection. *Pediatr Res.* 1984;18:230A
76. Rorabaugh ML, Berlin LE, Heldrich F, et al. Aseptic meningitis among infants less than two years of age: Acute illness and neurologic complications. *Pediatrics.* 1993;92:206.
77. Parks WP, Queiroga LT, Melnick JL. Studies of infantile diarrhea in Karachi, Pakistan. II: Multiple virus isolations from rectal swabs. *Am J Epidemiol.* 1967;85:469.
78. Strikas RA, Anderson LJ, Parker RA. Temporal and geographic patterns of isolates of nonpolio enteroviruses in the United States. *J Infect Dis.* 1986;153:346.
79. Centers for Disease Control and Prevention. Enterovirus surveillance—United States, 2000-2001. *MMWR Morb Mortal Wkly Rep.* 2002;51:1047.
80. Centers for Disease Control and Prevention. Enterovirus surveillance—United States, 1990. *MMWR Morb Mortal Wkly Rep.* 1990;39:788.
81. Hovi T, Cantell K, Huovilainen A, et al. Outbreak of paralytic poliomyelitis in Finland: Widespread circulation of antigenically altered poliovirus type 3 in a vaccinated population. *Lancet.* 1986;1:1427.
82. Huovilainen A, Hovi T, Kinnunen L, et al. Evolution of poliovirus during an outbreak: Sequential type 3 poliovirus isolates from several persons show shifts of neutralization determinants. *J Gen Virol.* 1987;68:1373.
83. Auvinen P, Hyypia T. Echoviruses include genetically distinct serotypes. *J Gen Virol.* 1990;71:2133.
84. Centers for Disease Control and Prevention. Entervirus surveillance—United States, 1970-2005. *MMWR Morb Mortal Wkly Rep.* 2006;55:1.
85. Yang CF, De L, Holloway BP, et al. Detection and identification of vaccine related polioviruses by the polymerase chain reaction. *Vir Res.* 1991;20:159.
86. Kew OM. Applications of molecular epidemiology to the surveillance of poliomyelitis. In: *Poliomyelitis Vaccines: Re-evaluating Policy Options.* Washington, DC: National Academy of Sciences; 1988.
87. Hatch MH, Marchetti GE, Nottay BK, et al. Strain characterization studies of poliovirus type 1 isolates from poliomyelitis cases in the United States in 1979. *Develop Biol Stand.* 1981;47:307.
88. Lin K-H, Wang H-L, Sheu M-M, et al. Molecular epidemiology of a variant of coxsackievirus A24 in Taiwan: Two epidemics caused by phylogenetically distinct viruses from 1985 to 1989. *J Clin Microbiol.* 1993;31:1160.
89. Takeda N, Miyamura K, Ogino T, et al. Evolution of enterovirus type 70: Oligonucleotide mapping analysis of RNA genome. *Virology.* 1984;134:375.
90. Miyamura K, Tanimura M, Takeda N, et al. Evolution of enterovirus 70 in nature: All isolates were recently derived from a common ancestor. *Arch Virol.* 1986;89:1.
91. Hamby BB, Pallansch MA, Kew OM. Reemergence of an epidemic coxsackie B5 genotype. *J Infect Dis.* 1987;156:288.
92. Lin K-H, Chern C-L, Chu P-Y, et al. Genetic analysis of recent Taiwanese isolates of a variant of coxsackievirus A24. *J Med Virol.* 2001;64:269.
93. Ishiko H, Shimada Y, Yonaha M, et al. Molecular diagnosis of human enteroviruses by phylogeny-based classification by use of the VP4 sequence. *J Infect Dis.* 2002;185:744.
94. Couch RB, Douglas RG, Lindgren KM, et al. Airborne transmission of respiratory infection with coxsackievirus A type 21. *Am J Epidemiol.* 1970;91:78.
95. Kogon A, Spigland I, Frothingham TE, et al. The Virus Watch Program: A continuing surveillance of viral infections in metropolitan New York families. *Am J Epidemiol.* 1969;89:51.
96. Horstmann DM, Emmons J, Gimpel L, et al. Enterovirus surveillance following a communitywide oral poliovirus vaccination program: A seven year study. *Am J Epidemiol.* 1973;97:173.
97. Hierholzer JC, Hilliard KA, Esposito JJ. Serosurvey for "acute hemorrhagic conjunctivitis" virus (enterovirus 70) antibodies in the southeastern United States, with review of the literature and some epidemiologic implications. *Am J Epidemiol.* 1975;102:533.
98. Modlin JF, Halsey NA, Thoms ML, et al; and Baltimore Area Polio Vaccine Study Group. Humoral and mucosal immunity in infants induced by three sequential IPV-OPV immunization schedules. *J Infect Dis.* 1997;75:S228.
99. Johnson KM, Bloom HH, Forsyth B, et al. The role of enteroviruses in respiratory disease. *Am Rev Respir Dis.* 1963;88:240.
100. Siegel M, Greenberg M, Bodian J. Presence of children in the household as a factor in the incidence of paralytic poliomyelitis in adults. *N Engl J Med.* 1957;257:958.
101. Weinstein L, Aycock WL, Feemster RF. Relation of sex, pregnancy, and menstruation to susceptibility in poliomyelitis. *N Engl J Med.* 1951;245:54.
102. Baron RC, Hatch MH, Kleeman K, et al. Aseptic meningitis among members of a high school football team: An outbreak associated with echovirus 16 infection. *J Am Med Assn.* 1982;248:1724.
103. Josselson J, Pula T, Sadler JH. Acute rhabdomyolysis associated with echovirus 9 infection. *Arch Intern Med.* 1980;140: 1671.
104. Gatmaitan BG, Chason JL, Lerner AM. Augmentation of the virulence of murine coxsackievirus B-3 myocardiopathy by exercise. *J Exp Med.* 1970;131:1121.
105. Dagan R, Menegus MA. A combination of four cell types for rapid detection of enteroviruses in clinical specimens. *J Med Virol.* 1986;19:219.
106. Schmidt NJ, Ho H, Lennette EH. Propagation and isolation of group A coxsackieviruses in RD cells. *J Clin Microbiol.* 1975;2: 183.
107. Landry ML, Madore HP, Fong CKY, et al. Use of guinea pig embryo cell cultures for isolation and propagation of group A coxsackieviruses. *J Clin Microbiol.* 1981;13:588.
108. Lipson SM, Walderman R, Costello P, et al. Sensitivity of rhabdomyosarcoma and guinea pig embryo cell cultures to field isolates of difficult-to-cultivate group A coxsackieviruses. *J Clin Microbiol.* 1988;26:1298.
109. Trabelsi A, Grattard F, Nejmeddine M, et al. Evaluation of an enterovirus group-specific anti-VP1 monoclonal antibody, 5D8/1, in comparison with neutralization and PCR for rapid identification of enteroviruses in cell culture. *J Clin Microbiol.* 1995;33:2454.
110. Melnick JL, Wimberly IL. Lyophilized combination pools of enterovirus equine antisera: New LBM pools prepared from reserves of antisera stored frozen for two decades. *Bull WHO.* 1985;63:543.
111. Rotbart HA, Sawyer MH, Fast S, et al. Diagnosis of enteroviral meningitis by using PCR with a colorimetric microwell detection assay. *J Clin Microbiol.* 1994;32:2590.
112. Halonen P, Rocha E, Hierholzer J, et al. Detection of enteroviruses and rhinoviruses in clinical specimens by PCR and liquid-phase hybridization. *J Clin Microbiol.* 1995;33:648.
113. Abraham R, Chonmaitree T, McCombs J, et al. Rapid detection of poliovirus by reverse transcription and polymerase chain amplification: Application for differentiation between poliovirus and non-poliovirus enteroviruses. *J Clin Microbiol.* 1993;31: 395.
114. Kilpatrick DR, Nottay B, Yang C-F, et al. Group-specific identification of polioviruses by PCR using primers containing mixed-base or deoxyinosine residues at positions of codon degeneracy. *J Clin Microbiol.* 1996;34:2990.
115. Weiss LM, Movahed LA, Billingham ME, et al. Detection of coxsackievirus B3 RNA in myocardial tissues by polymerase chain reaction. *Am J Pathol.* 1991;138:497.
116. Jin O, Sole MJ, Butany JW, et al. Detection of enterovirus RNA in myocardial biopsies from patients with myocarditis and

cardiomyopathy using gene amplification by polymerase chain reaction. *Circulation.* 1990;82:8.

117. Pozzetto B, Gaudin OG, Aouni M, et al. Comparative evaluation of immunoglobulin M neutralizing antibody response in acute-phase sera and virus isolation for the routine diagnosis of enterovirus infection. *J Clin Microbiol.* 1989;27:705.

118. Nielsen LP, Modlin JF, Rotbart HA. Detection of enteroviruses by polymerase chain reaction in urine samples from patients with aseptic meningitis. *Pediatr Infect Dis J.* 1996;15:625.

119. Rotbart HA, Ahmed A, Hickey S, et al. Diagnosis of enterovirus infection by PCR of multiple specimen types. *Pediatr Infect Dis J.* 1997;16:409.

120. Drucker NA, Colan SD, Lewis AB, et al. g-Globulin treatment of acute myocarditis in the pediatric population. *Circulation.* 1994;89:252.

121. Schiff GM, Sherwood JR. Clinical activity of pleconaril in an experimentally induced coxsackievirus A21 respiratory infection. *J Infect Dis.* 2000;181:20.

122. Romero J, Putnak JR, Wimmer E. Use of poliovirus proteins VP3 and 2C as group antigens for the detection of enterovirus infections by indirect immunofluorescence. *Pediatr Res.* 1986; 20:319.

123. Romero JR, Putnak JR, Wimmer E. Enteroviral capsid protein VP3 as a group antigen for the enteroviruses. *Pediatr Res.* 1988;23:380A

124. Yousef GE, Brown IN, Mowbray JF. Derivation and biochemical characterization of an enterovirus group-specific monoclonal antibody. *Intervirology.* 1987;28:163.

125. Mease PJ, Ochs HD, Wedgewood RJ. Successful treatment of echovirus meningoencephalitis and myositis-fasciitis with intravenous immune globulin therapy in a patient with X-linked hypogammaglobulinemia. *N Engl J Med.* 1981;304:1278.

126. Zhang A, Nanni RG, Oren DA, et al. Three-dimensional structure-activity relationships for antiviral agents that interact with picornavirus capsids. *Sem Virol.* 1992;3:453.

127. Pevear DC, Fancher MJ, Felock PJ, et al. Conformational change in floor of the human rhinovirus canyon blocks adsorption to HeLa cell receptors. *J Virol.* 1989;63:2002.

128. Rotbart HA. Treatment of picornavirus infections. *Antivir Res.* 2002;53:83.

129. Sawyer MH, Saez-Llorez X, Aviles CL, et al. Oral pleconaril reduces the duration and severity of enteviral meningitis in children. In: *Pediatric Academic Societies Annual Meeting, San Francisco, CA, May 1-4, 1999.* The Woodlands, TX: Society for Pediatric Research; 1999.

130. Shafran SD, Halota W, Gilbert D, et al. Pleconaril is effective for enterovirus meningitis in adolescents and adults: A randomized placebo-controlled multicenter trial. In: *39th Interscience Conference on Antimicrobial Agents and Chemotherapy, San Francisco, CA.* Toronto: American Society for Microbiology; 1999.

131. Weiner LB, Rotbart HA, Gilbert DL, et al. *Treatment of "enterovirus" meningitis with pleconaril (VP63843), an antipicornavirus agent. In: 37th Interscience Conference on Antimicrobial Agents and Chemotherapy.* Toronto: American Society for Microbiology; 1997.

132. Rotbart HA. Pleconaril therapy of potentially life-threatening enterovirus infections. In: *36th Annual Meeting of the Infectious Disease Society of American.* Denver, CO: Infectious Disease Society of America; 1998.

133. Rotbart HA. Pleconaril therapy of potentially life-threatening enterovirus infections. In: *36th Annual Meeting of the Infectious Disease Society of America.* Denver, CO: Infectious Disease Society of America; 1998.

134. Hayden FG, Herrington DT, Coats TL, et al. Efficacy and safety of oral pleconaril for treatment of picornavirus colds in adults: Results of two double-blind, randomized, placebo-controlled trials. *Clin Infect Dis.* 2003;36:1523.

135. ICTVdB Management. 00.052.0.06. Parechovirus. In: *ICTVdB—The Universal Virus Database,* version 4. Büchen-Osmond, C. (Ed), New York, USA: Columbia University;

Available at <http://www.ncbi.nlm.nih.gov/ICTVdb/ICTVdB/index.htm> 2006 (accessed April 2009).

136. Racaniello VR. Picornaviridae: The Viruses and Their Replication. In: Knipe DM, Howley PM, Griffin DE, et al., eds. *Fields Virology.* 5th ed. Lippincott Williams & Wilkins, Philadelphia, 2007:795.

137. Stanway G, Joki-Korpela P, Hyypiä T. Human parechoviruses: Biology and clinical significance. *Rev Med Virol.* 2000;10:57.

138. Triantafilou K, Triantafilou M, Takada Y, et al. Human parechovirus 1 utilizes integrins alphavbeta3 and alphavbeta1 as receptors. *J Virol.* 2000;74:5856.

139. Nix WA, Maher K, Johansson ES, et al. Detection of all known parechoviruses by real-time PCR. *J Clin Microbiol.* 2008;46:2519.

140. Human parechovirus. Available at <http://www.picornaviridae.com/parechovirus/hpev/hpev.htm> (accessed April 2009).

141. Dalldorf G, Sickles G. An unidentified, filtrable agent isolated from the feces of children with paralysis. *Science.* 1948;108:61.

142. Melnick JL, Shaw EW, Curnen EC. A virus from patients diagnosed as non-paralytic poliomyelitis or aseptic meningitis. *Proc Soc Exp Biol Med.* 1949;71:344.

143. Melnick JL, Agren K. Poliomyelitis and coxsackie viruses isolated from normal infants in Egypt. *Proc Soc Exp Biol Med.* 1952;81:621.

144. Ramos-Alvarez M, Sabin AB. Characteristics of poliomyelitis and other enteric viruses recovered in tissue culture from healthy American children. *Proc Soc Exp Biol Med.* 1954;87:655.

145. Rosen L, Melnick J, Schmidt NJ, et al. Subclassification of enteroviruses and ECHO virus type 34. *Archiv für die gesamte Virusforschung.* 1970;30:89.

146. Cohen JI, Ticehurst JR, Purcell RH, et al. Complete nucleotide sequence of wild-type hepatitis A virus: Comparison with different strains of hepatitis A and other picornaviruses. *J Virol.* 1987;61:50.

171

Poliovirus

JOHN F. MODLIN

Polioviruses are the cause of poliomyelitis, a systemic viral infection that predominantly affects the central nervous system (CNS), causing paralysis. The name of the disease (*polios*, "gray"; *myelos*, "marrow" or "spinal cord"), now commonly shortened to polio, is descriptive of the pathologic lesions that involve neurons in the gray matter, especially in the anterior horns of the spinal cord. Paralytic poliomyelitis has been completely controlled in the United States and other developed countries through routine childhood immunization with either inactivated poliovirus vaccine (IPV), live-attenuated oral poliovirus vaccine (OPV), or both. However, as of 2009, the goal of worldwide poliomyelitis eradication has not yet been achieved.

History

Sporadic poliomyelitis cases were published as early as 1840 and the first descriptions of the natural history and neurologic complications of poliomyelitis were recorded in Sweden by Karl Oskar Medin in 1890.[1] There is little record of epidemic poliomyelitis until the late 19th century, when outbreaks were first recorded in Scandinavia, western Europe, and the United States. Charles Caverly wrote the first description of epidemic poliomyelitis in the United States, an outbreak of 132 cases near Rutland, Vermont, in 1894.[2] Thereafter, sporadic epidemic disease occurred during the first half of the 20th century and, by the 1950s, epidemic polio occurred regularly, with approximately 25 cases/100,000 population reported annually in the United States. Accompanying the increased incidence was a shift in the peak affected age group from infants to school-aged children and young adults. Both the appearance of epidemic disease and the rising age incidence have been attributed to rising standards of hygiene, which delayed the age of infection beyond infancy and loss of maternal antibody, thus creating a pool of susceptible people large enough to permit the spread of epidemic disease.[3]

In 1908, Landsteiner and Popper demonstrated that polio was caused by a "filterable virus" when they transmitted disease to monkeys from human spinal cord homogenates.[4] Scientific progress remained somewhat limited until the landmark discovery in 1949 by Enders, Weller, and Robbins[5] that poliovirus could be propagated in vitro in cultures of human embryonic tissues of non-neural origin. This discovery facilitated experimental investigation of the pathogenesis of the disease in primates and the development of vaccines. Bodian and associates first recognized the three distinct serotypes of poliovirus.[6] By 1952, Bodian and Horstmann had independently discovered that viremia occurred early in infection, which explained the systemic phase of the illness.[7,8]

Salk reported in 1953 that human subjects could be successfully immunized with formalin-inactivated poliovirus, a discovery that rapidly led to an extensive field trial and licensure of IPV in 1955.[9] The introduction of IPV led to a sudden dramatic reduction in the incidence of paralytic poliomyelitis in the United States to 0.4 cases/100,000 in 1962, when OPV replaced IPV for routine use. The last case of endemic wild-type poliomyelitis occurred in 1979, indicating complete cessation of transmission of naturally occurring polioviruses.[10] However, in addition to rare cases of wild-type disease imported from other countries, the United States continued to experience between 6 and 10 cases of OPV vaccine-associated paralytic poliomyelitis (VAPP) each year until 1997, when IPV was reintroduced into the routine childhood immuni-

zation schedule in combination with OPV. Since 2000, only IPV has been used.

Under the leadership of the Pan American Health Organization, the entire Western Hemisphere became free of paralytic polio by 1991. Worldwide, endemic poliomyelitis has been controlled by all countries except four nations and now is limited to a few areas in sub-Saharan Africa and the Indian subcontinent.[11]

Pathophysiology

VIROLOGY

Polioviruses are prototypic members of the genus *Enterovirus* (see Chapter 170). Three poliovirus serotypes exist and infection with each confers type-specific, lifelong immunity to disease but little or no immunity to infection or disease caused by heterologous serotypes.[12] Before the introduction of poliovirus vaccines, most paralytic disease was caused by type 1.[13] Naturally occurring (wild-type) polioviruses, live-attenuated OPV viruses, and virulent polioviruses derived from OPV strains (vaccine-derived polioviruses [cVDPVs]) may circulate in different populations, depending on whether endemic transmission of wild-type polioviruses has been eliminated, on whether OPV is used, and on the vaccine-induced immunity rates in the population.

Humans are the only natural host and reservoir of polioviruses, although experimental infections and disease can be produced in other primates, and polioviruses can be adapted to replicate in subprimate mammals. Naturally occurring strains vary over a 10^7-fold range in neurovirulence.[14] Rhesus and cynomolgus monkeys are readily paralyzed by most naturally occurring strains, although much higher doses or more virulent strains are required to paralyze chimpanzees and humans. In contrast, polioviruses are more infectious for the human gut than for the gut of lower primates.

Attenuated OPV strains are occasionally able to paralyze rhesus and cynomolgus monkeys but only when injected in high doses directly into the CNS. In addition to low neurovirulence, vaccine strains can often be distinguished from naturally occurring strains by their temperature sensitivity and by subtle antigenic differences. The genomes for each of the attenuated Sabin vaccine strains have been fully sequenced, as well as the genomes of each of the naturally occurring parental strains. The RNA sequences of the vaccine strains differ from the sequences of their naturally occurring parents by less than 1%, with the smallest difference occurring between the type 3 vaccine and parent strains. For all three serotypes, analogous nucleotide substitutions in the 5′-noncoding region are associated with diminished ability to replicate in the gastrointestinal tract and with reduced neurovirulence.[15-17] Attenuating mutations also map to capsid proteins for individual serotypes.

In contrast, cVDPVs are OPV viruses that have been permitted to circulate because of low population immunity for long periods of time and, by continuous mutation, acquire biologic properties indistinguishable from those of naturally occurring wild-type polioviruses.[18-20] The cVDPVs isolated so far have RNA sequences that vary by more than 1.0% from the corresponding OPV parent strain, have undergone genomic recombination with other group C enteroviruses, and have acquired virulence markers characteristic of wild-type poliovirus strains, including virulence in transgenic mice bearing the human poliovirus receptor.[19]

PATHOGENESIS

The early events in the pathogenesis of poliomyelitis are similar to other enterovirus infections described in Chapter 170. After implantation at a mucosal site and replication in the gut and adjacent lymphoid tissues, polioviruses disseminate to susceptible reticuloendothelial tissues via a minor viremia. In asymptomatic infections, the virus is contained at this point and elicits the formation of type-specific antibodies. In a few infected persons, replication in the reticuloendothelial system gives rise to a major viremia, which corresponds temporally with the minor illness and causes the symptoms associated with abortive poliomyelitis. At this point, the course of poliomyelitis deviates from other enteroviral diseases in the ability of polioviruses to infect neurons in the gray matter of the brain and spinal cord. Although the preponderance of evidence indicates that viremia precedes paralysis in both experimental primates and humans, the exact routes whereby the central nervous system (CNS) becomes infected remain uncertain.[21,22] A study in transgenic mice expressing the human poliovirus receptor suggests that polioviruses spread from muscle to CNS via peripheral nerve fibers, rather than directly from the bloodstream.[23] Neuropathologic studies and animal experiments have indicated that spread is neural once the virus reaches the CNS.[24,25]

Poliovirus principally affects motor and autonomic neurons. Neuronal destruction is accompanied by inflammatory lesions consisting of polymorphonuclear leukocytes, lymphocytes, and macrophages that are distributed throughout the gray matter of the anterior horns of the spinal cord and the motor nuclei of the pons and medulla.[24,25] The mesencephalon, cerebellar roof nuclei, and precentral gyrus of the cerebral cortex are less severely involved. Clinical symptoms depend on the severity of lesions rather than on their distribution, which is similar in essentially all cases; almost all fatal cases have involvement of both the spinal cord and cranial nerve nuclei and brain stem, even in the absence of bulbar signs. The dorsal root ganglia are commonly involved pathologically, but this does not result in sensory deficits. Polioviruses can be isolated from the spinal cord for only the first few days after the onset of paralysis, but the inflammatory lesions may persist for months.

🔲 Clinical Features

INCUBATION PERIOD

Best estimates of the incubation period of poliomyelitis are 9 to 12 days (range, 5 to 35 days) measured from presumed contact until the onset of the prodromal symptoms, and 11 to 17 days (range, 8 to 36 days) until the onset of paralysis.[26]

CLINICAL MANIFESTATIONS OF INFECTION

The manifestations of infection by polioviruses range from unapparent illness to severe paralysis and death. Usual estimates of the ratio of unapparent to clinically recognized polio infection, which vary by serotype, range from 60 to 1000:1.[3,27] Figure 171-1 depicts the time course for the clinical manifestations of poliovirus infection. At least 95% of infections are asymptomatic or unapparent and can be recognized only by the isolation of poliovirus from feces or oropharynx or by a rise in antibody titer. *Abortive poliomyelitis*, which occurs in 4% to 8% of infections, is characterized by a 2- to 3-day period of fever, which may be accompanied by headache, sore throat, listlessness, anorexia, vomiting, or abdominal pain. Because the neurologic examination is normal, abortive poliomyelitis cannot be distinguished from other viral infections and can be clinically suspected only during an epidemic. *Nonparalytic poliomyelitis* differs from abortive poliomyelitis by the presence of signs of meningeal irritation. The disease is identical to meningitis caused by other enteroviruses. The systemic manifestations of nonparalytic poliomyelitis are generally more severe than in abortive poliomyelitis.

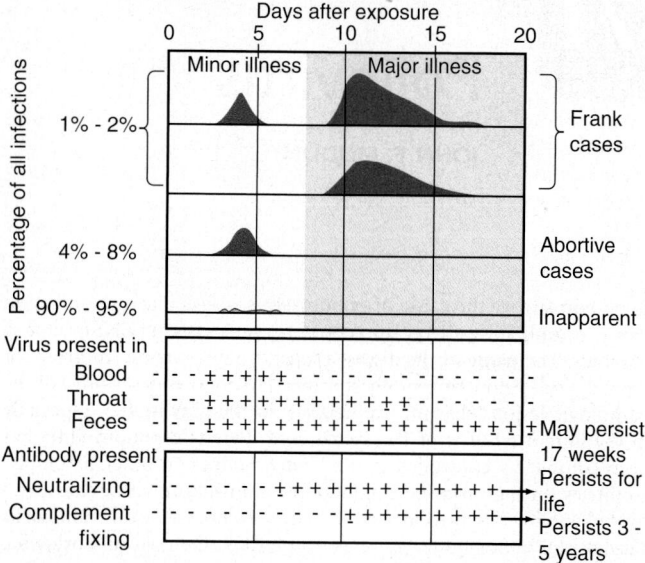

Figure 171-1 **Schema of the clinical and subclinical forms of poliomyelitis.** This graphic representation shows the presence of virus and antibodies in relation to the development and persistence of the infection. *(From Paul JR. History of Poliomyelitis. New Haven, Conn: Yale University Press; 1971.)*

Spinal Paralytic Poliomyelitis

Frank paralysis occurs in roughly 0.1% of all poliovirus infections. A biphasic course with minor and major illnesses is observed in approximately one third of children with paralytic poliomyelitis. The minor illness, coinciding with viremia, corresponds to the symptoms of abortive poliomyelitis and lasts 1 to 3 days. The patient appears to be recovering and remains symptom-free for 2 to 5 days before the abrupt onset of the major illness, which is heralded by symptoms and signs of meningitis, including fever, chills, headache, fever, malaise, vomiting, neck stiffness, and cerebrospinal fluid (CSF) pleocytosis. Adults usually experience a single phase of illness, with a prolonged prodrome of symptoms preceding the gradual onset of paralysis.[28,29] The major illness begins with severe myalgias and occasionally localized cutaneous hyperesthesia, paresthesias, involuntary muscle spasm, or muscular fasciculations. The meningismus and muscle pain are present for 1 to 2 days before frank weakness and paralysis ensue. The severity of the disease varies from weakness of a single portion of one muscle to complete quadriplegia. The paralysis is flaccid; deep tendon reflexes are initially hyperactive and then become absent. The most characteristic feature of the paralysis is its asymmetrical distribution, which affects some muscle groups while sparing others. Proximal muscles of the extremities tend to be more involved than distal muscles, the legs are more commonly involved than the arms, and the large muscle groups of the hand are at greater risk than the small ones. Any combination of limbs may be paralyzed, but the most common pattern is involvement of one leg, followed by one arm, or both legs and both arms. Quadriplegia is almost never observed in infants.[29] Although occasional cases progress from the onset of weakness to complete quadriplegia and bulbar involvement in a few hours, more commonly the paralysis extends over 2 to 3 days. Progression of paralysis stops when the patient becomes afebrile.[28] Paralysis of the bladder is usually associated with paralysis of the legs. It occurs in about 25% of adults but is uncommon in children. Sensory loss in poliomyelitis is very rare[30] and its occurrence should strongly suggest some other diagnosis (e.g., Guillain-Barré syndrome).

Bulbar Paralytic Poliomyelitis

Bulbar poliomyelitis results from paralysis of muscle groups innervated by the cranial nerves, especially those of the soft palate and pharynx, which may present as dysphagia, nasal speech, and some-

most of whom develop paralysis 7 to 21 days after the first feeding of OPV.[86] A similar number of VAPP cases occur among parents, other family members, babysitters, or other household contacts who develop paralysis 20 to 29 days after the administration of OPV to a close contact. For immunocompetent patients, the clinical features and outcome of VAPP differ little from disease caused by naturally occurring polioviruses. More than 80% of recipient and contact cases are associated with the first dose of OPV. OPV virus types 3 and 2 are more common causes of VAPP than type 1.[86]

Approximately 25% of reported VAPP cases occur in children and adults who are immune-deficient.[88] Most of these patients have transient or hereditary B-cell immunodeficiency, severe combined immunodeficiency syndrome, or common variable immunodeficiency. The risk of VAPP in newborn infants with a congenital B-cell immunodeficiency disorder is estimated to be 2000-fold higher than for immunocompetent infants.[29] However, there is little evidence that immunodeficiency states that predominantly affect T-cell function, rather than B-cell function, increase the risk of VAPP. Although one Romanian infant infected with human immunodeficiency virus (HIV) was reported to have developed VAPP,[89] there has been no evidence of neurologic complications among thousands of HIV-infected infants known to have received OPV in the United States and elsewhere.[90,91] Similarly, VAPP is not known to complicate hematologic malignancies, bone marrow transplantation, or solid organ transplantation.

Certain clinical features distinguish VAPP in immunodeficient patients. The interval between the last OPV dose and onset of neurologic disease is unusually long, with a typical range of 1 to 8 months, but it has been documented to be as long as 7 years.[92] The illness is protracted and characterized by chronic meningitis, progressive neurologic dysfunction suggesting involvement of both upper and lower motor neurons, and progression of paralysis over several weeks.[93,94] Immunodeficient patients also have a much higher risk of dying from VAPP than immunocompetent patients. Although fewer than 20% of surviving VAPP patients excrete polioviruses for longer than 6 months,[92] fecal excretion of virus was estimated to occur for as long as 9 years in one immunodeficient patient.[95] Most VAPP cases in immunocompromised children and adults have been associated with type 2 OPV virus.[88]

The mechanism whereby the OPV viruses cause rare cases of paralytic disease is not completely understood. It is well known that OPV virus readily undergoes mutation during the brief period of intestinal replication and that isolates can be recovered that are neurovirulent for primates.[14] Most OPV recipients shed polioviruses that have reverted to the naturally occurring genotype at an analogous codon in the 5′ noncoding region of the genome affecting initiation of transcription, which is strongly associated with attenuation for each of the three OPV serotypes.[96] However, because the attenuated Sabin strains differ from their virulent parent strains at multiple genetic loci, other mutational events probably contribute to reversion to full neurovirulence.[97-101]

USE OF POLIOMYELITIS VACCINES IN THE DEVELOPING WORLD

Trivalent OPV has been used exclusively in underdeveloped nations for routine immunization because of its lower cost and ease of administration, and superior secretory immunity in the gastrointestinal tract. In addition, OPV virus is transmitted by immunized children to nonimmune contacts and is thought to be aided by poor sanitation and crowded living conditions. The WHO Expanded Program on Immunization (EPI) calls for an OPV dose at birth and for three additional OPV doses in the first year of life at 6, 10, and 14 weeks of age.[102,103] Passively acquired maternal antibody present in the infant's circulation and in maternal colostrum blunts the immune response to the birth dose in some infants. However, infants who receive OPV at birth are more likely to have antibody to all three poliovirus types at 4 months of age.[104]

Unfortunately, many infants in tropical countries are left unprotected following receipt of the recommended number of OPV doses. Low seroconversion rates to three OPV doses have been widely documented,[105-109] averaging 73%, 90%, and 70% for types 1, 2, and 3, respectively.[110] This poor response appears to have contributed to poliomyelitis outbreaks in some countries with relatively high immunization rates.[109,111,112] Although the reasons for the lower potency of OPV in tropical areas remains incompletely understood, the effect of concurrent diarrheal illnesses has emerged as an important factor. Studies conducted in Brazil and Bangladesh have shown reduced seroconversion rates to types 2 and 3 OPV in infants with diarrhea at the time of OPV feeding, whereas the response to type 1 was not affected.[113,114] The impact of diarrhea on seroconversion persists despite the administration of three or four OPV doses.

The low effectiveness of trivalent OPV in the presence of intercurrent diarrheal diseases has led to the introduction of other strategies to reduce poliovirus transmission in resource-poor settings. Monovalent types 1 and 3 OPV vaccines have been introduced via supplemental immunization activities into many areas where wild-type polioviruses continue to circulate. A study in Egypt has confirmed the superior immunogenicity of monovalent OPV vaccines for newborn infants[85]; case-control studies in India and Nigeria have demonstrated that monovalent OPV type 1 vaccine is three to four times more effective per dose than trivalent OPV in protecting against paralytic poliomyelitis.[115,116]

Although historically the costs associated with production and delivery, and the requirement for injection, have made the sole use of IPV an undesirable alternative for developing countries, there is now strong interest in using IPV as a supplement to OPV in areas where OPV efficacy is limited by intercurrent diarrheal diseases.[117] In general, IPV is highly immunogenic for infants in developing areas, although seroconversion and antibody titers are diminished with short intervals between doses (e.g., 1 month) and also reduced in the presence of high titers of maternal antibody in young infants.[118-121] IPV has been used as a supplement to OPV immunization in Israel, where type 1 poliovirus continued to cause epidemic disease in the Gaza Strip despite relatively good rates of OPV coverage,[109,122] and in Côte d'Ivoire, where IPV administered at 9 months markedly enhanced seroconversion rates in infants given OPV at 2, 3, and 4 months of age.[123] In a randomized controlled trial in Cuba in which IPV or placebo was administered at 6, 10, and 14 weeks of age, the seroconversion rates were 94%, 83%, and 100% for types 1, 2, and 3 poliovirus, respectively, indicating that three doses of vaccine may mitigate the potential interference of maternal antibody.[120]

Poliomyelitis in Developing Nations and Global Eradication

Even after the introduction of polio vaccines, poliomyelitis was regarded as an epidemic disease of wealthier nations and was ignored in developing countries. However, lameness surveys of schoolchildren in the 1960s and 1970s in more than 20 nations revealed lower limb paralysis prevalence rates of 2 to 11/1000, figures that reflect poliomyelitis incidence rates that equal or exceed those of the peak epidemic years in the United States.[102,124] Most cases of paralytic poliomyelitis in developing countries occur in children between the ages of 6 months and 2 years. Most cases are caused by type 1 poliovirus. In 1974, WHO founded the Expanded Program on Immunization, which provided monetary and technical support for basic immunization against several childhood diseases, including polio, and created a worldwide standard polio immunization policy.[102] There was considerable progress in controlling poliomyelitis, but vaccines still failed to reach many children because of interrupted supplies, disruptions in the cold chain necessary to maintain the potency of OPV, civil strife, and poor political support. In 1983, an international conference held in Bellagio, Italy, soon after smallpox eradication articulated the feasibility of worldwide poliomyelitis eradication.[125] The Pan American Health Organization resolved in 1985 to eradicate poliomyelitis from the Western Hemisphere, a goal that was achieved within 6 years and, in 1988, the World Health Assembly set a goal of global eradication of poliomyelitis by the year 2000.[126,127]

The WHO Global Poliomyelitis Eradication Initiative (GPEI) adopted several successful strategies to control and ultimately eradicate polio from most regions of the world, including encouragement of routine childhood immunization, supplementary immunization activities (SIAs), improvement of laboratory capabilities, intensified surveillance, and rapid response to identified outbreaks.[127,128] SIAs are highly coordinated nationwide or region-wide events in which all children younger than 5 years, regardless of immunization history, receive two doses of OPV given 1 month apart, and have been particularly successful in many areas in rapidly controlling poliomyelitis.[129,130] Seroconversion rates during these mass campaigns are higher than for routine immunization, possibly because of the spread of OPV virus or because they are conducted during the dry season, when diarrheal disease is less prevalent.[131]

These strategies led to a marked global reduction in paralytic poliomyelitis cases from more than 350,000 in 1988 to a low of 784 cases in 2003, including the complete disappearance of all cases caused by wild-type 2 poliovirus.[132] However, just as eradication appeared within reach, a number of unanticipated events have stalled progress, including a temporary but disastrous suspension of all immunization in northern Nigeria in 2003-2004 that led to importation of polio to 27 previously polio-free nations,[11,133] inability to interrupt transmission in some northern Indian states despite high trivalent OPV coverage,[134] civil unrest in some locations, and the emergence of vaccine-derived poliomyelitis viruses in many regions.[135,136] As of early 2009, paralytic polio cases continued to be reported from four nations where polio is considered to be endemic and another 11 countries previously free of polio.[137,138] The greatest challenges to global eradication remain in Nigeria and India, where more than 85% of the world's cases occur.[138]

VACCINE-DERIVED POLIOMYELITIS VIRUSES

During 2000 and 2001, an outbreak of 21 cases of paralytic poliomyelitis on the island of Hispaniola occurred, caused by a virulent strain genetically related to the type 1 Sabin OPV vaccine strain.[19] Since then, other outbreaks of paralytic disease caused by vaccine-derived polioviruses (VDPVs) have been discovered in underimmunized children living in economically deprived regions.[20,139,140] The low immunization rates in these areas have permitted these viruses to circulate for long periods and, by continuous mutation, acquire biologic properties indistinguishable from those of naturally occurring wild polioviruses.[19,136,141,142]

The emergence of VDPV has profoundly influenced plans for the eventual cessation of poliovirus immunization following eradication of poliomyelitis, which will now include a strategy to discontinue OPV use worldwide, introduce IPV into as many countries as feasible, and develop an OPV vaccine stockpile for use anywhere in the world, and a plan for containment of laboratory stocks of naturally occurring and attenuated polioviruses.[135,143,144]

REFERENCES

1. Paul JR. *History of Poliomyelitis*. New Haven: Yale University Press, 1971.
2. Vermont State Department of Public Health. *Infantile Paralysis in Vermont*. Brattleboro, Vt: Vermont Printing, 1924.
3. Nathanson N, Martin JR. The epidemiology of poliomyelitis: Enigmas surrounding its appearance and disappearance. *Am J Epidemiol*. 1979;110:672.
4. Landsteiner K, Popper E. Mikroscopische präparate von einem menschlichen und zwei affenrückemarken. *Wien Klin Wschr*. 1908;21:1830.
5. Enders JF, Weller TH, Robbins FC. Cultivation of the Lansing strain of poliomyelitis virus in cultures of various human embryonic tissue. *Science*. 1949;109:85.
6. Bodian D, Morgan IM, Howe HA. Differentiation of three types of poliomyelitis virus. III. The grouping of fourteen strains into three immunological types. *Am J Hyg*. 1949;49:234.
7. Bodian D. Pathogenesis of poliovirus in normal and passively immunized primates after virus feeding. *Fed Proc*. 1952;11:462.
8. Horstmann DM. Poliomyelitis in the blood of orally infected monkeys and chimpanzees. *Proc Soc Exp Biol Med*. 1952;79:417.
9. Salk JE. Studies in human subjects on active immunization against poliomyelitis. I. A preliminary report of experiments in progress. *JAMA*. 1953;151:1081.
10. Kim-Farley RJ, Bart KJ, Schonberger LB, et al. Poliomyelitis in the USA: Virtual elimination of disease caused by wild virus. *Lancet*. 1984;2:1315.
11. Cochi SL, Kew O. Polio today: Are we on the verge of global eradication? *J Am Med Assn*. 2008;300:839.
12. Bodian D. Second attacks of paralytic poliomyelitis in human beings in relation to immunity, virus types and virulence. *Am J Hyg*. 1951;54:174.
13. Shelokov A, Habel K, McKinstry DW. Relation of poliomyelitis virus types to clinical disease and geographic distribution: A preliminary report. *Ann N Y Acad Sci*. 1955;61:998.
14. Sabin AB. Properties and behavior of orally administered attenuated poliovirus vaccine. *JAMA*. 1957;164:1216.
15. Omata T, Kohara M, Kuge S, et al. Genetic analysis of the attenuation phenotype of poliovirus type 1. *J Virol*. 1986;58:348.
16. Pollard SR, Dunn G, Cammack N, et al. Nucleotide sequence of a neurovirulent variant of the type 2 oral poliovirus vaccine. *J Virol*. 1989;63:4949.
17. Westrop GD, Wareham KA, Evans D, et al. Genetic basis of attenuation of the Sabin type 3 oral poliovirus vaccine. *J Virol*. 1989;63:1338.
18. Centers for Disease Control and Prevention (CDC). Outbreak of poliomyelitis—Dominican Republic and Haiti, 2000. *MMWR Morb Mortal Wkly Rep*. 2000;49:1094.
19. Kew O, Morris-Glasgow V, Landaverde M, et al. Outbreak of poliomyelitis in Hispaniola associated with circulating type 1 vaccine-derived poliovirus. *Science*. 2002;296:356.
20. Centers for Disease Control and Prevention (CDC). Circulation of a type 2 vaccine-derived poliovirus—Egypt, 1982-1993. *MMWR Morb Mortal Wkly Rep*. 2001;50:41.

21. Bodian D. Viremia in experimental poliomyelitis. I. General aspects of infection after intravascular inoculation with strains of high and low invasiveness. *Am J Hyg*. 1954;60:339.
22. Bodian D. Emerging concept of poliomyelitis infection. *Science*. 1955;122:105.
23. Ren R, Costantini F, Gorgacz EJ, et al. Transgenic mice expressing a human poliovirus receptor: A new model for poliomyelitis. *Cell*. 1990;63:353.
24. Bodian D, Howe HA. An experimental study of the role of neurones in the dissemination of poliomyelitis virus in the nervous system. *Brain*. 1940;63:135.
25. Jubelt B, Gallez-Hawkins G, Narayan O, et al. Pathogenesis of human poliovirus infection in mice. II. Age dependency of paralysis. *J Neuropathol Exp Neurol*. 1980;39:138.
26. Horstmann DM, Paul JR. The incubation period in human poliomyelitis and its implications. *JAMA*. 1947;135:11.
27. Melnick JL, Ledinko N. Social serology: Antibody levels in a normal young population during an epidemic of poliomyelitis. *Am J Hyg*. 1951;54:354.
28. Horstmann DM. Clinical aspects of acute poliomyelitis. *Am J Med*. 1949;6:592.
29. Weinstein L, Shelokov A, Seltser R, et al. A comparison of the clinical features of poliomyelitis in adults and children. *N Engl J Med*. 1952;246:297.
30. Plum F. Sensory loss with poliomyelitis. *Neurology*. 1956;6:166.
31. Baker AB. Bulbar poliomyelitis: Its mechanism and treatment. *Am J Med*. 1949;6:614.
32. Ibsen B. The clinical diagnosis and evaluation of respiratory problems in patients with acute poliomyelitis. In: Poliomyelitis Papers and Discussions. *Fourth International Poliomyelitis Conference*. Philadelphia: JB Lippincott, 1958;483-487.
33. Weinstein L. Cardiovascular disturbances in poliomyelitis. *Circulation*. 1957;15:735.
34. Galpine JF, Wilson WCM. Occurrence of myocarditis in paralytic poliomyelitis. *Br Med J*. 1959;2:1379.
35. Neu H. Gastrointestinal complications in poliomyelitis. In: Poliomyelitis Papers and Discussions. *Fourth International Poliomyelitis Conference*. Philadelphia: JB Lippincott, 1958;546.
36. Siegel M, Greenberg M, Bodian J. Presence of children in the household as a factor in the incidence of paralytic poliomyelitis in adults. *N Engl J Med*. 1957;257:958.
37. Weinstein L, Aycock WL, Feemster RF. Relation of sex, pregnancy, and menstruation to susceptibility in poliomyelitis. *N Engl J Med*. 1951;245:54.
38. Anderson GW, Anderson G, Skaar A, Sandler F. Poliomyelitis in pregnancy. *Am J Hyg*. 1952;55:127.
39. Russell WR. Paralytic poliomyelitis: The early symptoms, and the effect of physical activity on the course of disease. *Br Med J*. 1949;1:465.
40. Horstmann DM. Acute poliomyelitis. Relation of physical activity at the time of onset to the course of the disease. *JAMA*. 1950;142:236.

41. Greenberg M, Abramson H, Cooper HM, et al. The relation between recent injections and paralytic poliomyelitis in children. *Am J Public Health*. 1952;42:142.
42. Sutter RW, Patriarca PA, Suleiman AM, et al. Attributable risk of DTP (diphtheria and tetanus toxoids and pertussis vaccine) injection in provoking paralytic poliomyelitis during a large outbreak in Oman. *J Infect Dis*. 1992;165:444.
43. Bodian D. Viremia in experimental poliomyelitis. II. Viremia and the mechanism of the "provoking" effect of injections or trauma. *Am J Hyg*. 1954;60:358
44. Trueta J, Hodes R. Provoking and localizing factors in poliomyelitis. *Lancet*. 1954;1:998.
45. Strebel PM, Nedelcu N-I, Baughman AL, et al. Intramuscular injections within 30 days of immunization with oral poliovirus vaccine—a risk factor for vaccine-associated paralytic poliomyelitis. *N Engl J Med*. 1995;332:500.
46. Eley RC, Flake CG. Acute anterior poliomyelitis following tonsillectomy and adenoidectomy: With special reference to the bulbar form. *J Pediatr*. 1938;13:63.
47. Paffenbarger RS. The effect of prior tonsillectomy on incidence and clinical type of acute poliomyelitis. *Am J Hyg*. 1957;66:131.
48. Sejvar JJ, Leis AA, Stokic DS, et al. Acute flaccid paralysis and West Nile virus infection. *Emerg Infect Dis*. 2003;9:788.
49. Li J, Loeb JA, Shy ME, et al. Asymmetric flaccid paralysis: A neuromuscular presentation of West Nile virus infection. *Ann Neurol*. 2003;53:703.
50. Kew OM. Applications of molecular epidemiology to the surveillance of poliomyelitis. In: Conference Proceedings. *Poliomyelitis Vaccines: Re-Evaluating Policy Options*. Washington, DC: National Academy of Sciences, 1988.
51. Kew OM, Mulders MN, Lipskaya GY, et al. Molecular epidemiology of polioviruses. *Sem Virol*. 1995;6:401.
52. Russell WR, Fischer-Williams M. Recovery of muscular strength after poliomyelitis. *Lancet*. 1954;1:330.
53. Ferris BG Jr, Auld PAM, Cronkhite L, et al. Life threatening poliomyelitis, Boston, 1955. *N Engl J Med*. 1960;262:371.
54. Weinstein L. Diagnosis and treatment of poliomyelitis. *Med Clin North Am*. 1948;32:1377.
55. Bennett RI. Care of the after effects of poliomyelitis. *Am J Med*. 1949;6:620.
56. Dalakas MC, Sever JL, Madden DL, et al. Late postpoliomyelitis muscular atrophy: Clinical, virologic, and immunologic studies. *Rev Infect Dis*. 1984;6:S562.
57. Dalakas MC, Elder G, Hallet M, et al. A long-term follow-up study of patients with post-poliomyelitis neuromuscular symptoms. *N Engl J Med*. 1986;314:959.
58. Ramlow J, Alexander M, LaPorte R, et al. Epidemiology of the post-polio syndrome. *Am J Epidemiol*. 1992;136:769.
59. Johnson RT. Late progression of poliomyelitis paralysis: discussion of pathogenesis. *Rev Infect Dis*. 1984;6:S568.
60. Melnick JL. Advantages and disadvantages of killed and live poliomyelitis vaccines. *Bull WHO*. 1978;56:21.

61. Sabin AB. Oral polio vaccine: History of its development and use and current challenge to eliminate poliomyelitis from the world. *J Infect Dis*. 1985;151:420.
62. Centers for Disease Control and Prevention (CDC). Poliomyelitis prevention in the United States. *MMWR Morb Mortal Wkly Rep*. 2000;49:1.
63. Simoes EA, John TJ. The antibody response of seronegative infants to inactivated poliovirus vaccine of enhanced potency. *Develop Biol Stand*. 1986;14:127.
64. McBean AM, Thoms ML, Albrecht P, et al. The serologic response to oral polio vaccine and enhanced potency inactivated polio vaccines. *Am J Epidemiol*. 1988;128:615.
65. Swartz TA, Roumiantzeff M, Peyron L, et al. Use of a combined DTP-polio vaccine in a reduced schedule. *Develop Biol Stand*. 1986;65:159.
66. Robertson SE, Traverso HP, Drucker JA, et al. Clinical efficacy of a new, enhanced-potency, inactivated poliovirus vaccine. *Lancet*. 1988;1:897.
67. Ogra PL, Karzon DT, Righthand F. Immunoglobulin response in serum and secretions after immunization with live and inactivated poliovaccine and natural infection. *N Engl J Med*. 1968;279:893.
68. Onorato IM, Modlin JF, McBean AM, et al. Mucosal immunity induced by enhanced potency IPV and OPV. *J Infect Dis*. 1991;163:1.
69. Modlin JF, Halsey NA, Thoms ML, et al. Baltimore Area Polio Vaccine Study Group. Humoral and mucosal immunity in infants induced by three sequential IPV-OPV immunization schedules. *J Infect Dis*. 1997;75:S228.
70. Fox JP, Elveback L, Scott W, et al. Herd immunity: Basic concept and relevance to public health immunization practices. *Am J Epidemiol*. 1971;94:179.
71. Stickle G. Observed and expected poliomyelitis in the United States, 1958-1961. *Am J Public Health*. 1964;54:1222.
72. Schaap GJP, Bijkerk H, Coutinho RA, et al. The spread of wild poliovirus in the well-vaccinated Netherlands in connection with the 1978 epidemic. *Prog Med Virol*. 1984;29:124.
73. Expanded programme on immunization. Poliomyelitis surveillance and vaccine efficacy. *Wkly Epidemiol Rec*. 1988;63:249.
74. Robertson HE, Acker MS, Dillenberg HO, et al. Community-wide use of a "balanced" trivalent oral poliovirus vaccine (Sabin). *Can J Public Health*. 1962;53:179.
75. Cohen-Abbo A, Culley BS, Reed GW, et al. Seroresponse to trivalent oral poliovirus vaccine as a function of dosage interval. *Ped Infect Dis J*. 1995;14:100.
76. Hardy GE, Hopkins CC, Linneman CC, et al. Trivalent oral poliovirus vaccine: A comparison of two infant immunization schedules. *Pediatrics*. 1970;45:444.
77. Krugman RD, Hardy GE, Sellers C. Antibody persistence after primary immunization with trivalent oral poliovirus vaccine. *Pediatrics*. 1977;60:80.
78. Bass JW, Halsted SB, Fischer GW, et al. Oral polio vaccine: Effect of booster vaccination one to 14 years after primary series. *JAMA*. 1978;239:2252.
79. Nishio O, Ishihara Y, Sakae K, et al. The trend of acquired immunity with live poliovirus vaccine and the effect of revaccination: follow-up of vaccinees for ten years. *Develop Biol Stand*. 1984;12:1.
80. Ogra PL. Mucosal immune response to poliovirus vaccines in childhood. *Rev Infect Dis*. 1984;6:S361.
81. Ghendon YUZ, Sanakoyeva II. Comparison of the resistance of the intestinal tract to poliomyelitis virus (Sabin's strains) in person after naturally and experimentally acquired immunity. *Acta Virol (Praha)*. 1961;5:265.
82. Kim-Farley RJ, Rutherford G, Lichfield P, et al. Outbreak of paralytic poliomyelitis, Taiwan. *Lancet*. 1984;2:1322.
83. Chen RT, Hausinger S, Dajani AS, et al. Seroprevalence of antibody against poliovirus in inner-city preschool children. *JAMA*. 1996;275:1639.
84. Caceres VM, Sutter RW. Sabin monovalent oral polio vaccines: Review of past experiences and their potential use after polio eradication. *Clin Infect Dis*. 2001;33:531.
85. el-Sayed N, el-Gamal Y, Abbassy AA, et al. Monovalent type 1 oral poliovirus vaccine in newborns. *N Engl J Med*. 2008; 359:1655.
86. Strebel PM, Sutter RW, Cochi SL, et al. Epidemiology of poliomyelitis in the United States one decade after the last reported case of indigenous wild virus-associated disease. *Clin Infect Dis*. 1992;14:568.
87. Prevots DR, Sutter RW, Strebel PM, et al. Completeness of reporting for paralytic poliomyelitis, United States, 1980 through 1991. *Arch Ped Adol Med*. 1994;148:479.
88. Sutter RW, Prevots DR. Vaccine-associated paralytic poliomyelitis among immunodeficient persons. *Infect Med*. 1994;11:426.
89. Ion-Neldescu N, Dobrescu A, Strebel PM, et al. Vaccine-associated paralytic poliomyelitis and HIV infection (letter). *Lancet*. 1994;343:51.
90. von Reyn CF, Clements CJ, Mann JM. Human immunodeficiency virus infection and routine childhood immunisation. *Lancet*. 1987;2:669.
91. Onorato IM, Markowitz LE, Oxtoby MJ. Childhood immunization, vaccine-preventable diseases and infection with human immunodeficiency virus. *Ped Infect Dis J*. 1988;7:588.
92. Khetsuriani N, Prevots DR, Quick L, et al. Persistence of vaccine-derived polioviruses among immunodeficient persons with vaccine-associated paralytic poliomyelitis. *J Infect Dis*. 2003;188: 1845.
93. Davis LE, Bodian D, Price D, et al. Chronic progressive poliomyelitis secondary to vaccination of an immunodeficient child. *N Engl J Med*. 1977;297:241.
94. Wyatt HV. Poliomyelitis in hypogammaglobulinemics. *J Infect Dis*. 1973;128:802.
95. Kew OM, Sutter RW, Nottay BK, et al. Prolonged replication of a type 1 vaccine-derived poliovirus in an immunodeficient patient. *J Clin Microbiol*. 1998;36:2893.
96. Minor P, Dunn G, Begg N, et al. *Poliovirus vaccination schedules and reversion to virulence*. Presented at the 33rd Conference on Antimicrobial Agents and Chemotherapy. New Orleans, October 1993.
97. Stanway G, Hughes PJ, Mountford RC, et al. Comparison of the complete nucleotide sequences of the genomes of the neurovirulent poliovirus P3/Leon/37 and its attenuated Sabin vaccine derivative P3/Leon 12a1b. *Proc Natl Acad Sci U S A*. 1984;81: 1539.
98. Evans DM, Dunn G, Minor PD, et al. Increased neurovirulence associated with a single nucleotide change in a noncoding region of the Sabin type 3 poliovaccine genome. *Nature*. 1985;314:548.
99. Minor PD, John A, Ferguson M, et al. Antigenic and molecular evolution of the vaccine strain of type 3 poliovirus during the period of excretion by a primary vaccinee. *J Gen Virol*. 1986;67:693.
100. Almond JW. The attenuation of poliovirus neurovirulence. *Ann Rev Microbiol*. 1987;41:154.
101. Almond JW, Westrop GD, Evans DM, et al. Studies on the attenuation of the Sabin type 3 oral polio vaccine. *J Virol Methods*. 1987;17:183.
102. Henderson RH. The expanded programme on immunization of the World Health Organization. *Rev Infect Dis*. 1984;6:475.
103. Expanded programme on immunization. Global Advisory Group. *Wkly Epidemiol Rec*. 1985;60:13.
104. Dong D-X, Hu X-M, Liu W-J, et al. Immunization of neonates with trivalent oral poliomyelitis vaccine (Sabin). *Bull WHO*. 1986;64:853.
105. John TJ, Christopher S. Oral polio vaccination of children in the tropics. II. Antibody response in relation to vaccine virus infection. *Am J Epidemiol*. 1975;102:414.
106. John TJ, Jayabal P. Oral polio vaccination of children in the tropics: I. The poor seroconversion rates and the absence of viral interference. *Am J Epidemiol*. 1972;96:263.
107. Domok I, Balayan MS, Fayinka OA, et al. Factors affecting the efficacy of live poliovirus vaccine in warm climates. *Bull WHO*. 1974;51:33.3
108. Hanlon P, Hanlon L, Marsh V, et al. Serological comparisons of approaches to polio vaccination in the Gambia. *Lancet*. 1987;1:800.
109. Lasch EE, Abed Y, Abdulla K, et al. Successful results of a program combining live and inactivated poliovirus vaccines to control poliomyelitis in Gaza. *Rev Infect Dis*. 1984;6:467.
110. Patriarca PA, Wright PF, John TJ. Factors affecting the immunogenicity of oral poliovirus vaccine in developing countries. *Rev Infect Dis*. 1991;13:926.
111. Patriarca PA, Laender F, Palmeira G, et al. Randomised trial of alternative formulations of oral poliovaccine in Brazil. *Lancet*. 1988;1:429.
112. WHO Collaborative Study Group on Oral and Inactivated Poliovirus Vaccines. Combined immunization of infants with oral and inactivated poliovirus vaccines: Results of a randomized trial in the Gambia, Oman, and Thailand. *J Infect Dis*. 1997;175(Suppl 1):S215.
113. Posey DL, Linkins RW, Couto Oliveria MJ, et al. The effect of diarrhea on oral poliovirus vaccine failure in Brazil. *J Infect Dis*. 1997;175:S258.
114. Myaux JA, Unicomb L, Besser RE, et al. Effect of diarrhea on the humoral response to oral polio vaccination. *Ped Infect Dis J*. 1996;15:204.
115. Grassly NC, Wenger J, Durrani S, et al. Protective efficacy of a monovalent oral type 1 poliovirus vaccine: a case-control study. *Lancet*. 2007;369:1356.
116. Jenkins HE, Aylward RB, Gasasira A, et al. Effectiveness of immunization against paralytic poliomyelitis in Nigeria. *N Engl J Med*. 2008;359:1666
117. Introduction of inactivated poliovirus vaccine into oral poliovirus vaccine-using countries. *Wkly Epidemiol Rec*. 2003;78:241.
118. Swartz TA, Ben-Porath E, Ben-Yshai Z, et al. A controlled trial with inactivated poliovaccine. *Dev Biol Stand*. 1981;47:199.
119. Simoes EAF, Padmini B, Steinhoff MC, et al. Antibody response of infants to two doses of inactivated poliovirus vaccine of enhanced potency. *Am J Dis Child*. 1985;139:977.
120. Cuba IPV Study Collaborative Group. Randomized, placebo-controlled trial of inactivated poliovirus vaccine in Cuba. *N Engl J Med*. 2007;356:1536.
121. Asturias EJ, Dueger EL, Omer SB, et al. Randomized trial of inactivated and live polio vaccine schedules in Guatemalan infants. *J Infect Dis*. 2007;196:692.
122. Lasch EE, Abed Y, Marcus O, et al. Combined live and inactivated poliovirus vaccine to control poliomyelitis in a developing country—five years after. *Dev Biol Stand*. 1986;65:137.
123. Morinere BJ, van Loon FPL, Rhodes PH, et al. Immunogenicity of a supplemental dose of oral versus inactivated poliovirus vaccine. *Lancet*. 1993;341:1545.
124. Ofusu-Amaah S. The challenge of poliomyelitis in tropical Africa. *Rev Infect Dis*. 1984;6:318.
125. Rockefeller Foundation. *Protecting the World's Children: Vaccines and Immunization*. Bellagio, Italy: Rockefeller Foundation; 1984.
126. Global eradication of poliomyelitis by the year 2000. *Wkly Epidemiol Rec*. 1988;63:161.
127. Hull HF, Ward NA, Hull BP, et al. Paralytic poliomyelitis: Seasoned strategies, disappearing disease. *Lancet*. 1994;343:1331.
128. Wright PF, Kim-Farley RJ, de Quadros CA, et al. Strategies for the global eradication of poliomyelitis by the year 2000. *N Engl J Med*. 1991;325:1774.
129. John TJ. Poliomyelitis in India: Prospects and problems of control. *Rev Infect Dis*. 1984;6:438.
130. Sabin AB. Strategies for elimination of poliomyelitis in different parts of the world with use of oral poliovirus vaccine. *Rev Infect Dis*. 1984;6:391.
131. Richardson G, Linkins R, Eames M, et al. Immunogenicity of oral poliovirus vaccine administered in mass campaigns versus routine immunization programmes. *Bull WHO*. 1995;73:769.
132. Centers for Disease Control and Prevention (CDC). Apparent global interruption of wild poliovirus type 2 transmission. *MMWR Morb Mortal Wkly Rep*. 2001;50:222.
133. Roberts L. Polio: the final assult? *Science*. 2004;303:1960.
134. Grassly NC, Fraser C, Wenger J, et al. New strategies for the elimination of polio from India. *Science*. 2006;314:1150.
135. Kew OM, Sutter RW, de Gourville EM, et al. Vaccine-derived polioviruses and the endgame strategy for global polio eradication. *Ann Rev Microbiol*. 2005;59:587.
136. Kew OM, Wright PF, Agol VI, et al. Circulating vaccine-derived polioviruses: Current state of knowledge. *Bull WHO*. 2004;82:16.
137. Centers for Disease Control and Prevention (CDC). Progress toward interruption of wild poliovirus transmission—worldwide, January 2007-April 2008. *MMWR Morb Mortal Wkly Rep*. 2008;57:489.
138. Global Polio Eradication Initiative. Wild Poliovirus Weekly Update, 2009. Available at: http://www.polioeradication.org/casecount.asp.
139. Centers for Disease Control and Prevention (CDC). Public health dispatch: Acute flaccid paralysis associated with circulating vaccine-derived poliovirus—Philippines, 2001. *MMWR Morb Mortal Wkly Rep*. 2001;50:874.
140. Centers for Disease Control and Prevention (CDC). Poliomyelitis—Madagascar, 2002. *MMWR Morb Mortal Wkly Rep*. 2002;51:622.
141. Centers for Disease Control and Prevention (CDC). Update on vaccine-derived polioviruses—worldwide, January 2006-August 2007. *MMWR Morb Mortal Wkly Rep*. 2007;56:996.
142. Estivariz CF, Watkins MA, Handoko D, et al. A large vaccine-derived poliovirus outbreak on Madura Island, Indonesia, 2005. *J Infect Dis*. 2008;197:347.
143. Technical Consultative Group to the World Health Organization on the Global Eradication of Poliomyelitis. "Endgame" issues for the global polio eradication initiative. *Clin Infect Dis*. 2002;34:72.
144. World Health Organization. Global Eradication Initiative Strategic Plan, 2004-2008. Available at: http://www.polioeradication.org/content/publications/2004stratplan.pdf.

172

Coxsackieviruses, Echoviruses, Newer Enteroviruses, and Parechoviruses

JOHN F. MODLIN

This chapter covers human disease caused by the group A coxsackieviruses, group B coxsackieviruses, echoviruses, and the newer enteroviruses, which are a subgenera of the genus *Enterovirus*. Diseases caused by *Parechovirus*, a newly designated genus of Picornaviridae (see Chapter 170), are also discussed. These viruses have many physical, epidemiologic, and pathogenetic characteristics in common, as described in Chapter 170. More than 90% of infections caused by the nonpolio enteroviruses are asymptomatic or result only in undifferentiated febrile illness.[1] When disease occurs, the spectrum and severity of clinical manifestations vary with the age, gender, and immune status of the host and with the subgroup, serotype, and even the intratypic enterovirus strain.

Some clinical syndromes (viral meningitis and some exanthems) are caused by many enterovirus serotypes, some are predominately caused by certain enterovirus subgroups (e.g., pleurodynia and myocarditis by the group B coxsackieviruses), and other diseases are mostly associated with individual enterovirus serotypes. Infections caused by the four serotypes representing the subgenus of newer enteroviruses and the newly designated subgenus, *Parechovirus*, are considered at the end of this chapter.

Central Nervous System Infections

ACUTE VIRAL MENINGITIS

Viral infection is the dominant cause of the aseptic meningitis syndrome, and class B enteroviruses (composed mostly of group B coxsackievirus and echovirus serotypes) cause most acute viral meningitis cases in both adults and children.[2,3] Group A coxsackieviruses cause relatively fewer cases.[2] Historically, group B coxsackieviruses 2 through 5 and echoviruses 4, 6, 7, 9, 11, 13, 16, 18, 30, and 33 are the most frequently implicated serotypes. On occasion, a single echovirus serotype may cause widespread outbreaks; for example, echovirus 13 caused outbreaks of aseptic meningitis throughout Europe and the United States in 2000 and 2001,[4] and echovirus 33 caused widespread disease in New Zealand during the winter of 2000.[5] Infection with certain serotypes, particularly the group B coxsackieviruses and echovirus 30, may be more likely to be accompanied by aseptic meningitis than infection with other common enterovirus serotypes.[6]

Clinical Manifestations

Infants younger than 3 months have the highest rates of clinically recognized aseptic meningitis, in part because lumbar punctures are routinely performed for evaluation of fever in this age group.[7] Only a minority of these infants have clinical manifestations suggestive of neurologic disease.[6]

The severity of disease in older children and adults with aseptic meningitis varies widely. The onset may be gradual or abrupt, and the typical patient has a brief prodrome of fever and chills. Headache is usually a prominent complaint. Meningismus, when present, varies from mild to severe. Kernig and Brudzinski signs are present in only about one third of patients. Pharyngitis and other symptoms of upper respiratory tract infections are often present. The illness is sometimes biphasic, as in poliomyelitis; these patients present with a prodromal illness with fever and myalgias, followed by defervescence and absence of symptoms for a few days, and then experience abrupt recurrence of fever with headache and other signs of meningismus. Complications such as febrile seizures, complex seizures, lethargy, coma, and movement disorders occur early in the course of aseptic meningitis in 5% to 10% of patients.[7-9] Adults may experience a more prolonged period of fever and headache than infants and children, and some adult patients may take weeks to return to normal activity.[10,11]

Laboratory Diagnosis

The clinical diagnosis of viral meningitis depends on routine examination of cerebrospinal fluid (CSF). The CSF is clear and under normal or mildly increased pressure. The total CSF cell count is usually 10 to 500/mm³ but may occasionally exceed 1000/mm³. Cell counts less than 10 cells/mm³ may occur in a small minority of cases.[2,12-15] Differential cell counts of the CSF often reveal a high proportion of neutrophils, but the differential typically shifts to a predominance of lymphocytes during the initial 1 to 2 days of illness.[16-18] In general, the CSF glucose concentration is normal, and the CSF protein concentration is normal or slightly elevated. However, the glucose content may be lower than normal in 18% to 33% of cases,[19-21] and values less than 40 mg/dL may occur.[7,20] Uncommonly, it may be difficult to exclude bacterial meningitis on the basis of the CSF profile alone. In some cases, the CSF findings may closely mimic those of tuberculous meningitis.[22]

Polymerase chain reaction (PCR) genomic amplification has replaced cell culture as the primary means of direct detection of enteroviruses in CSF and other specimens. Most PCR protocols amplify a highly conserved portion of the 5′ nontranslated region of the genome, which enables the detection of most enteroviruses. For confirmed or suspected enteroviral meningitis cases, PCR sensitivity ranges from 66% to more than 90%.[23,24-27] The overall sensitivity of virus isolation from the CSF of patients with viral meningitis is typically 30% to 35%,[2,24,28-31] although higher figures have been reported during some echovirus outbreaks.[12,15,32] Concomitant testing of serum, upper respiratory secretions, urine, and stool enhances the likelihood of virus detection by either PCR or cell culture.[2,33,34]

Differential Diagnosis

Bacterial meningitis is the most important disease to be distinguished from enteroviral aseptic meningitis. Although some clinical features of bacterial meningitis that is incompletely treated with antibiotics may overlap those of enteroviral aseptic meningitis when therapy has been instituted before lumbar puncture, several studies have demonstrated that pretreatment of bacterial meningitis alters the CSF minimally. Even when some laboratory indicators are altered by therapy (i.e., change from polymorphonuclear to lymphocytic pleocytosis), others continue to indicate bacterial disease (i.e., low glucose or high protein concentration).[35-37] Arboviruses, lymphocytic choriomeningitis virus, leptospirosis, Lyme borreliosis, and acute human immunodeficiency virus (HIV) infection account for most of the remaining cases of infectious aseptic meningitis. Mumps virus infection was a common cause of aseptic meningitis before the introduction of mumps vaccine in the United States. Aseptic meningitis also occurs with other infectious and noninfectious diseases (see Chapter 84), but the etiology is usually suggested by other clinical features.

Management and Prognosis

Although hospitalization is not necessary for all cases and indeed may not be feasible during summer epidemics of enterovirus infections, it is advisable when disturbances in consciousness, muscle weakness, or a petechial or purpuric rash suggest the possibility of a more serious illness. Pyogenic bacterial meningitis should be excluded by lumbar puncture. When bacterial meningitis cannot be excluded because of prior antibiotic treatment, administration of appropriate antibiotics is advisable after performing Gram stains and bacterial cultures. CSF enterovirus PCR testing may be useful in deciding whether to continue administration of antibiotics if the test can be reported within 1 to 2 days.[38,39]

In most cases, treatment consists only of relief of symptoms. Analgesics are usually given to older children and adults to alleviate headache. Pleconaril, an experimental, orally administered enteroviral capsid-stabilizing drug, modestly reduced the duration of headache and other symptoms in clinical trials but has not been further developed for this purpose.[11] Antiviral therapy may provide significant symptomatic relief to adults and older children, who may experience lassitude and easy fatigability for weeks after the acute illness.[10,11] Treatment studies of infants and young children, who generally experience a shorter duration of symptoms, have been inconclusive.[40]

In one large study of enteroviral aseptic meningitis, subtle disturbances in motor function such as limitation of passive motion, muscle spasm, and poor coordination were observed during convalescence.[8] These abnormalities slowly resolve and are rarely detectable 1 year after infection. In young children, fever and signs of meningeal irritation subside in a few days to 1 week. Infants younger than 3 months may have fewer symptoms of illness and fewer complications than older infants.[7] Although some investigators have suggested that enteroviral meningitis in the first year of life may result in permanent neurologic sequelae,[41,42] studies of larger numbers of children using more rigorous methods indicate that the long-term prognosis for the youngest infants is also excellent.[43,44]

ENCEPHALITIS

Encephalitis is a well-documented, although unusual, manifestation of nonpolio enterovirus central nervous system (CNS) infection. The enteroviruses account for less than 5% of all encephalitis cases and for 11% to 22% of encephalitis cases that are proved to be viral.[28,45-47] Numerous serotypes have been implicated as causes of encephalitis; coxsackievirus types A9, B2, and B5, echovirus types 6 and 9, and enterovirus 71 are the serotypes reported most often, but the evidence linking each of these serotypes to encephalitis is highly variable. In a minority of cases, a specific etiology has been proved by isolating virus from brain tissue or CSF; in others, the cause of encephalitis has been inferred by isolating virus from a non-neurologic site or by serology.

In perinatally acquired enterovirus infection, encephalitis is often only one manifestation of generalized viral disease, but beyond the neonatal period, signs and symptoms are generally limited to the CNS. Children and young adults are most frequently affected. The level and severity of CNS disease varies from relatively mild encephalopathic symptoms in patients with enterovirus meningitis to severe generalized encephalitis with seizures, paresis, and coma. Children with focal encephalitis present with partial motor seizures, hemichorea, and acute cerebellar ataxia,[48-52] features that in some cases have suggested a diagnosis of herpes simplex virus encephalitis.[49,53] Enterovirus 71, and rarely other enterovirus serotypes, are the cause of a severe, often fatal, form of brainstem encephalitis with secondary cardiopulmonary manifestations including noncardiogenic pulmonary edema.[54-56] The CSF findings in enteroviral encephalitis are similar to those in aseptic meningitis. Magnetic resonance imaging of the brain and electroencephalography may demonstrate either generalized or localized abnormal signals reflecting the extent and severity of brain involvement. Most patients with coxsackievirus and echovirus encephalitis beyond the neonatal period recover fully, although permanent neurologic sequelae and rare deaths occur.[28,48,57,58]

PARALYSIS AND OTHER NEUROLOGIC COMPLICATIONS

Sporadic cases of flaccid motor paralysis have been associated with several coxsackievirus and echovirus serotypes and with enterovirus 71, which has been associated with large outbreaks of poliomyelitis-like disease in Russia and eastern Europe and in Thailand and Taiwan. Coxsackievirus A7, which is neuropathogenic in monkeys, and enterovirus 71 have each caused disease with sufficient frequency to be recognized as the etiologic agent in outbreaks of paralysis.[55,59-62] Coxsackievirus A9 was found to be the etiology of 3.1% of poliomyelitis cases in New Delhi, India, over a period of 7 years.[63] In sporadic cases, the serotypes that are most often implicated have been coxsackieviruses A7, A9, and B1 to B5 and echoviruses 6 and 9. Less frequently implicated serotypes are coxsackieviruses A4, A5, and A10 and echoviruses 1 to 4, 7, 11, 14, 16 to 18, and 30.[64-67]

Paralytic disease caused by the nonpolio enteroviruses other than enterovirus 71 is characteristically less severe than poliovirus-associated paralysis. In fact, muscle weakness is more common than flaccid paralysis, and the paresis is not usually permanent. Cranial nerve involvement has occasionally resulted in complete unilateral oculomotor palsy.[68,69] Guillain-Barré syndrome has been reported in a small number of patients in association with coxsackievirus serotypes A2, A5, and A9 and with echovirus serotypes 6 and 22.[29,70,71] In a few cases, the implicated virus has been isolated from CSF or the brainstem.[71] Transverse myelitis was reported in one patient who had a rise in neutralizing antibody to coxsackievirus B4[70] and in another who had echovirus 5 recovered from CSF.[72] Systemic coxsackievirus B2 disease has been reported with many of the clinical features of Reye's syndrome.[73] Furthermore, several children with well-documented Reye's syndrome have had a variety of enteroviruses isolated concurrently from multiple sites, including the brain and CSF[74,75]; however, a clear etiologic or epidemiologic link between enterovirus infection and Reye's syndrome has not been established. Opsoclonus-myoclonus, or the "dancing eyes" syndrome, has been reported in two children with concurrent coxsackievirus B3 infection.[76]

Exanthems

Coxsackieviruses and echoviruses cause a variety of exanthems, which are sometimes associated with enanthems. With the exception of hand-foot-and-mouth (HFM) disease, these rashes are not sufficiently distinctive to permit a reliable etiologic diagnosis on clinical grounds alone. Virus can be isolated from the vesicular lesions of patients with HFM disease, and therefore these lesions appear to be a direct result of viral invasion of the skin after viremia. No attempts at isolation of virus from the skin in cases of maculopapular and petechial exanthems have been reported; consequently, it is not known whether these lesions are also caused by the virus directly or by immunopathologic mechanisms.

Enteroviral exanthems themselves cause little morbidity. They are important as sentinels of the prevalence of coxsackieviruses and echoviruses in the community and because they are often confused with other infective exanthems, some of which have more serious implications. Rashes caused by enteroviruses may be grouped according to the type of exanthem that they mimic: (1) rubelliform or morbilliform, (2) roseoliform, (3) vesicular, and (4) petechial. Some overlap between these types of exanthems may be observed in different patients infected with the same enterovirus or even among different morphologic lesion types in the same patient.

RUBELLIFORM AND MORBILLIFORM EXANTHEMS

Overall, enteroviruses account for about 5% of acute morbilliform exanthems that occur in populations with high measles and rubella vaccine coverage.[77] Maculopapular rashes resembling rubella commonly occur during summer echovirus epidemics. High attack rates have been noted with echovirus 9, the most common serotype associated with rubelliform rash. In one epidemic, 57% of persons younger than 5 years with illness caused by echovirus 9 had rash, 41% of those 5 to 9 years old had rash, but rash affected only 6% of those older than 10 years.[32] The rash, which characteristically appears simultaneously with fever, begins on the face and then spreads to the neck, chest, and extremities. The illness may be distinguished from rubella by the absence of pruritus and posterior cervical lymphadenopathy.[78,79] In occasional patients with an enanthem resembling Koplik spots and a blotchy eruption, the disease may be confused with measles, but the coryza and conjunctivitis characteristic of that disease are absent.[80]

ROSEOLIFORM EXANTHEMS

These enterovirus exanthems are distinctive not in their appearance but in their timing; as in roseola, the rash does not appear until defervescence. The prototype is the "Boston exanthem," the first of the enterovirus exanthems to be recognized and now known to be caused by echovirus 16.[81,82] Multiple cases often occur sequentially in families, with rash developing in as many as one fourth of the children in a household who are mildly ill with low-grade fever and pharyngitis. The fever lasts 24 to 36 hours and then declines simultaneously with the appearance of discrete, nonpruritic, salmon-pink macules and papules about 1 cm in diameter on the face and upper part of the chest. The extremities are less commonly involved. The duration of the rash is 1 to 5 days. Other enterovirus serotypes (coxsackievirus B1 and B5 and echovirus 11 and 25) have also been associated with roseola-like illness.[81,83,84] Exanthem subitum (roseola infantum), a common, nonseasonal exanthem in which the rash typically develops as the fever declines, is caused by human herpesvirus-6 (see Chapter 140).

HERPETIFORM EXANTHEMS

Hand-Foot-and-Mouth Disease

Coxsackievirus A16 is the most common cause of a distinctive vesicular eruption known as HFM disease or vesicular stomatitis with exanthem, although many other enteroviruses are also associated with HFM disease, including coxsackieviruses A4, A5, A6, A7, A9, A10, A24, and B2 to B5, echovirus 18, and enterovirus 71, which has caused large outbreaks in Southeast Asia associated with severe CNS disease and deaths.[56,85-89]

Children younger than 10 years are often affected, and spread to other family members occurs commonly. Most patients complain of sore throat or sore mouth, and affected young children may refuse to eat. Temperatures of 38°C to 39°C last 1 to 2 days and are accompanied in essentially all cases by vesicles in the oral cavity occurring chiefly on the buccal mucosa and tongue. Several lesions may coalesce to form bullae and ulcerate. Peripherally distributed cutaneous lesions occur in roughly 75% of patients.[90] These lesions commonly occur on the extensor surfaces of the hands and feet and sometimes on the buttocks or genitalia. Disseminated lesions have been described in an infant with preexisting atopic eczema and have been given the sobriquet "eczema coxsackium" by analogy with eczema herpeticum and eczema vaccinatum.[91] The lesions are tender and consist of mixed papules and clear vesicles with a surrounding zone of erythema. Skin biopsy demonstrates subepidermal lesions with a mixed lymphocytic and polymorphonuclear inflammatory response and acantholysis of the overlying epidermis.[92] Eosinophilic nuclear inclusions and intracytoplasmic picornavirus particles can be seen microscopically within cells surrounding dermal vessels.[93]

The vesicular lesions of HFM disease superficially resemble those caused by herpes simplex or varicella-zoster virus. Patients with HFM disease invariably have lesions of the oral mucosa. In contrast, oral lesions are less common in patients with chickenpox; moreover, these patients generally appear more ill, and their cutaneous lesions are more extensive and centrally distributed, generally with sparing of the palms and soles. Patients with primary herpetic gingivostomatitis also usually appear more ill and have a higher fever and cervical lymphade-

nopathy; lesions are usually confined to the oral cavity and do not involve the extremities. The enanthem of herpangina also resembles HFM disease, but it occurs in the posterior oropharynx and typically involves the fauces and soft palate.

Other Herpetiform Exanthems

Generalized vesicular eruptions are reported to be caused by coxsackievirus A9[94] and echovirus 11.[95] These eruptions are similar to the lesions of HFM disease, but they occur in crops on the head, trunk, and extremities. Unlike chickenpox, the vesicles do not evolve to form pustules and scabs. Vesicular eruptions caused by echovirus 11 have occurred in immunocompromised adult patients.[95] An acute eruption resembling dermatomal zoster in which echovirus 6 was isolated from the bullous lesions has been reported.[96]

PETECHIAL EXANTHEMS AND OTHER CUTANEOUS MANIFESTATIONS

Petechial and purpuric rashes have been described with echovirus 9[32,97] and coxsackievirus A9[98] infections. When these rashes have a hemorrhagic component, the illness is easily confused with meningococcal disease, especially if aseptic meningitis occurs simultaneously. Occasionally, cutaneous eruptions of coxsackievirus A9 disease have an urticarial nature.[94] One child was reported to have papular acrodermatitis (Gianotti-Crosti syndrome) in association with coxsackievirus A16 infection.[99]

Acute Respiratory Disease

Enteroviruses account for most viruses recovered from children with summertime upper respiratory tract infections, including undifferentiated febrile illnesses ("summer grippe") with sore throat and occasionally cough or coryza.[100,101] Enterovirus upper respiratory tract illnesses are generally clinically indistinguishable from disease caused by other agents such as rhinoviruses and *Mycoplasma pneumoniae*, unless accompanied by aseptic meningitis, exanthem, or other clinical features suggesting enterovirus infection.

Many enterovirus serotypes are associated with upper respiratory tract disease. Among the best characterized enteroviral respiratory viruses are coxsackieviruses A21 and A24, which produce illness resembling the common cold, except for a higher incidence of fever.[102,103] Outbreaks of coxsackievirus A21 illness are reported in military populations. Although epidemics in civilians have not been recognized, sporadic infections presumably account for the observed high antibody prevalence rates in the general population.[102] Unlike most enteroviruses, coxsackievirus A21 is more readily recovered from throat swabs than from feces. In volunteers receiving small-particle aerosols of the virus, illness has included not only coryza and sore throat but also tracheobronchitis and pneumonia.[104] Echoviruses serotypes 4, 8, 9, 11, 20, 22, and 25 are also common causes of respiratory disease.[102] Echovirus 11 produces sore throat, coryza, and cough, and has also been associated with croup. The spectrum of group B coxsackievirus disease includes coryza, laryngotracheobronchitis, bronchiolitis, and pneumonia.[70,105] Pneumonia, which may be interstitial or a patchy bronchopneumonia, has occurred in children[106] and rarely in adults.[107] Severe lower respiratory tract enterovirus infections are uncommon, although some enteroviruses, notably echoviruses 6, 9, 11, and 33 and enterovirus 71, have been isolated after death from infants and young children with severe pneumonia.[5,56,108-110]

HERPANGINA

Herpangina (herpes = vesicular eruption; angina = quinsy, or inflammation of the throat) is a well-characterized vesicular enanthem of the fauces and soft palate that is accompanied by fever, sore throat, and pain on swallowing. Summer outbreaks of herpangina typically affect children 3 to 10 years old and, less commonly, adolescents and young adults. Group A coxsackieviruses (serotypes 1 to 10, 16, and 22) have been the most common viruses recovered from herpangina patients. Other serotypes include group B coxsackieviruses 1 to 5, echoviruses 3, 6, 9, 16, 17, 25, and 30, and enterovirus 71.[89,111]

Clinical Manifestations

Herpangina begins suddenly with fever, vomiting, myalgia, and headache. Sore throat and pain on swallowing are prominent symptoms that precede appearance of the enanthem by several hours to a day. Examination of the throat reveals erythema and mild exudate of the tonsils, and the characteristic enanthem, which begins as punctate macules and evolves over a 24-hour period to 2- to 4-mm erythematous papules that vesiculate and then ulcerate centrally. The moderately painful lesions, which are usually small in number, are located on the soft palate and uvula, and less commonly on the tonsils, the posterior pharyngeal wall, or the buccal mucosa. The fever subsides in 2 to 4 days, but the ulcers may persist for up to a week. Patients with herpangina do not appear very ill and require only symptomatic treatment for sore throat.

A variant of the herpangina termed acute lymphonodular pharyngitis has been described in association with coxsackievirus A10 infection.[112] Lesions occur in the same distribution as herpangina but consist of tiny nodules of packed lymphocytes that eventually recede without undergoing vesiculation or ulceration.

Differential Diagnosis

Herpangina is most often confused with bacterial tonsillitis or other viral causes of pharyngitis, herpetic gingivostomatitis, HFM disease, and aphthous stomatitis. HSV gingivostomatitis occurs in the anterior oral cavity, especially on the inner aspects of the lips, the buccal mucosa, and the tongue. Gingivitis, prominent systemic toxicity, and cervical lymphadenitis are additional features of primary herpes simplex infection that are not seen in herpangina. In HFM disease, lesions also occur on the extremities in most cases. Aphthous stomatitis is characterized by recurrent large ulcerative lesions of the lips, tongue, and buccal mucosa among older children, adolescents, and adults.

▦ Myositis

PLEURODYNIA

Pleurodynia (Bornholm disease) is an acute enteroviral infection of skeletal muscle characterized by fever and sharp, spasmodic pain in the chest or upper part of the abdomen that has been usually observed during infrequent outbreaks. Pleurodynia was first described in 1872 by Daae and by Homann as an outbreak of "acute muscular rheumatism spread by contagion" in Norway. Subsequent reports from Scandinavia included a paper by Ejnar Sylvest, a Danish general practitioner, in 1933, in which he described his experience with the disease on the island of Bornholm in the Baltic Sea. This monograph received worldwide attention after it was translated into English in 1934,[113] and little has been added to Sylvest's descriptions of the disease and its epidemiology, pathogenesis, and complications. The etiologic role of group B coxsackieviruses, the most important cause of epidemic pleurodynia, was established in 1949.[114,115] Other agents rarely implicated in pleurodynia include echoviruses 1, 6, 9, 16, and 19 and group A coxsackieviruses 4, 6, 9, and 10.[66,67,116,117]

Epidemiology

Published reports of major epidemics have come primarily from Europe and North America. These epidemics have been reported at infrequent intervals, often 10 to 20 years, and attack rates have been higher in sparsely populated areas than in cities. Persons with pleurodynia are somewhat older than those with most other diseases caused by coxsackieviruses and echoviruses. Multiple family members may be attacked almost simultaneously or in rapid succession separated by several days.

Pathogenesis

Although pleurodynia probably results from direct viral invasion of thoracic and abdominal muscles after viremia, direct virologic evidence supporting this hypothesis is lacking. Tenderness mimicking spontaneously occurring pain can be elicited by pressure on affected muscles in most cases; in addition, palpable, often visible muscle swelling is a subtle finding in some cases.[113] A pleural friction rub has been rare or absent in most epidemics, although this sign has occasionally been noted in 7% or more of patients.[118,119]

Clinical Manifestations

Pleurodynia has no prodrome and begins with an abrupt onset of spasmodic pain, typically over the lower part of the rib cage or the upper abdominal region. Fever, sore throat, and headache may occur, but cough and coryza are notably absent. Aseptic meningitis and orchitis occur in a small number of patients with pleurodynia, generally less than 10%.[113,120,121] Pericarditis and pneumonia are rare.[118]

The pain, which varies in intensity, is variously described as lancinating, stabbing, constricting, or viselike. Patients asked to localize the pain are likely to indicate a broad area with the palm of the hand rather than a specific point with the finger. The most common location is the vicinity of the costal margin on one or both sides or occasionally the subxiphoid region. About half the patients have pain primarily in muscles of the thorax, especially the intercostals, the trapezius, and occasionally the erector spinae or pectoralis major. In the remainder, pain is primarily in the upper part of the abdomen, especially the hypochondrium (internal and external obliques and transversus abdominis) or the epigastrium (rectus abdominis). Periumbilical pain and pain in the lower abdominal quadrants are also seen, especially in children, in whom abdominal localization of pain is the rule.[103,119] A few patients experience pain in neither the chest nor the abdomen but instead in the neck or limbs[120]; in these cases, the diagnosis can be made only by association with other typical cases in the family. Whatever the localization of the pain, it is usual for an individual patient to experience this pain in only one or two areas of the body.

Although the location and severity vary, it is the spasmodic and paroxysmal character of the pain that is its hallmark. If the pain is mild and the patient ambulatory, the patient stoops forward or leans to the side to splint the chest. With more severe pain, the patient lies still in bed and appears acutely ill and apprehensive. Motion produces pain, and patients resist being turned in bed. Chest pain limits deep inspiration, and respirations are shallow and rapid. Auscultation of the chest reveals no abnormalities. Pain can be elicited by pressure on the involved muscles in most patients. Swelling is seen or felt only occasionally and by careful, sequential observations.

Most patients are ill for 4 to 6 days. Children have milder disease than adults, who are often confined to bed. The first paroxysm is the most severe, and subsequent paroxysms are shorter and accompanied by less fever. Although dull aching of involved muscles usually persists between bouts of sharp pain, the patient may look and feel entirely healthy between paroxysms. About one fourth of patients experience multiple recurrences, often after they have been free of pain for a day or more and have felt well enough to return to work or school.[113,120] In about half of these persons, recurrence of pain is at the same site; in the remainder, a new site is attacked. Late relapses occur in some patients after they have been free of symptoms for a month or longer.[120]

Diagnosis

The severity, location, and other characteristics of the pain are so protean that pleurodynia is readily confused with other illnesses. Pain in the chest may mimic pneumonia, pulmonary infarction, myocardial ischemia, and the pre-eruptive phase of zoster. Abdominal pain in epidemic pleurodynia may resemble that in acute abdomen of a variety of causes. Normal auscultatory examination of the chest, together with the characteristic spasmodic and relapsing character of the pain, is helpful in excluding pneumonia. A negative chest radiographic film is also helpful, although pleural effusions may rarely be present.

Management and Prognosis

Analgesics and the application of heat to affected muscles are useful in relieving pain in most cases; in some, opiate analgesics are required for adequate pain control. Despite the distressing tendency of the disease to relapse, all patients eventually recover completely. Debility out of all proportion to the apparent severity of the illness is occasionally observed for several months during convalescence.[113,121]

OTHER SKELETAL MYOSITIS

Enteroviruses have been implicated as a cause of acute myositis not confined to the torso in some patients,[122-129] although the diagnosis has rarely been proved virologically. Echovirus 11 has been recovered from clinically involved skeletal muscle of a 3-month-old infant with a fatal systemic infection.[122] In other cases, coxsackievirus A9, group B coxsackievirus types 2 and 6, and echovirus 9 have been etiologically linked to myositis on the basis of serology, recovery of virus from the throat or feces, or demonstration of viral antigen in muscle by immunofluorescence. Both generalized polymyositis and focal myositis have been noted, the latter sometimes localized to the thighs. Clinical myositis is manifested by fever, chills, weakness, hypotonia, tenderness, and edema of the involved muscle groups. Myoglobinemia, myoglobinuria, and an elevated creatine phosphokinase level are often found. Most reported patients have recovered rapidly.

A dermatomyositis-like illness occurs in B-cell–deficient immunocompromised patients with persistent enterovirus infections (see later).

Myopericarditis

Because enteroviruses rarely, if ever, infect the pericardium alone without involving the subepicardial myocardium, the term *myopericarditis* best describes the disease caused by these viruses when they affect the heart (see Chapter 81).[130] In the clinical setting, however, signs of either myocarditis or pericarditis often predominate. In older children and adults, the severity of myopericarditis varies from asymptomatic cardiac involvement to severe disease with intractable heart failure and death. Myocarditis that occurs with generalized enterovirus infection in the newborn is discussed separately in the section on neonatal infections.

An epidemic of coxsackievirus B5 myopericarditis occurred in Finland in autumn 1965 when 18 patients were admitted to a single hospital.[131] Epidemic myopericarditis appears to be exceptional, however, and most reported cases beyond the neonatal period have been sporadic, probably because involvement of the heart is a relatively uncommon manifestation of illness even during substantial enterovirus epidemics.

ETIOLOGY AND PATHOGENESIS

Enteroviruses account for at least half of all cases of acute viral myopericarditis.[132-135] However, the strength of the evidence linking a given enterovirus serotype with myopericarditis varies considerably. Proof of causation exists for all group B coxsackievirus serotypes, group A coxsackievirus types 4 and 16, and echovirus types 9 and 22 by demonstration of infectious virus or viral antigen in myocardium or pericardial fluid.[67,136-139] The evidence is less substantive for group A coxsackievirus types 1, 2, 5, 8, and 9 and echovirus types 1 to 4, 6 to 8, 11, 14, 19, 25, and 30.[135-138,140-149] These serotypes have been recovered from noncardiac sources during an episode of acute myopericarditis, some with a significant increase in neutralizing antibody titer to the isolated virus.

Many other viruses and bacteria have been associated with myopericarditis, although adenovirus,[150-152] influenza A virus,[153] parvovirus B19,[154] mumps virus,[155] and vaccinia virus[156] are the principal nonenterovirus agents that have been detected directly in pericardial fluid or myocardial tissue. The weight of clinical evidence suggests that *M. pneumoniae*, respiratory syncytial virus, Epstein-Barr virus, varicellazoster virus, and measles virus also cause myopericarditis.

Group B coxsackieviruses and other enteroviruses reach the heart during the viremia that follows replication in the gastrointestinal or respiratory tract (see Chapter 170). Experimental studies in a murine model demonstrate that virus replication of myocytes results in scattered myocyte necrosis followed by focal infiltration of polymorphonuclear leukocytes, lymphocytes, plasma cells, and macrophages.[157] The chronic inflammatory response that may persist for weeks to months has been a subject of keen interest. German investigators have demonstrated the presence of enterovirus RNA in biopsy samples of cardiac tissue for months after the acute episode.[158] Some investigators consider the late-phase inflammatory response to be due to virus-induced, cytotoxic T-lymphocyte destruction of myocytes.[159] Others have postulated the development of a myocardial neoantigen[160] or cross-reactivity between viral and myocardial cell antigens.[161] Healing is accompanied by a variable degree of interstitial fibrosis and evidence of myocyte loss.

CLINICAL MANIFESTATIONS

Enteroviral myocarditis occurs at all ages but has a special predilection for physically active adolescents and young adults. The incidence in males is at least twice that in females.[132,135] In two thirds of cases, an upper respiratory tract illness precedes the onset of cardiac manifestations by 7 to 14 days.[135] Common initial symptoms include dyspnea, chest pain, fever, and malaise.[131,135,162-164] Pain in the precordial area is usually dull, but it may resemble angina pectoris or be sharp, pleuritic, and exacerbated by recumbency when pericarditis is present. A pericardial friction rub, often transient, has been observed in 35% to 80% of cases. Enlargement of the cardiac silhouette on chest radiograph films, present in about 50%, may be due to either pericardial effusion or cardiac dilatation. A gallop rhythm and other signs of frank congestive heart failure are observed in roughly 20%.[163,164]

Electrocardiographic abnormalities, including ST-segment elevation or nonspecific ST-segment and T-wave abnormalities, are invariably present. More severe myocardial disease leads to the development of Q waves, ventricular tachyarrhythmias, and all degrees of heart block. Echocardiography may confirm the presence of acute ventricular dilation or a diminished cardiac ejection fraction. Serum levels of myocardial enzymes are frequently elevated. Other clinical manifestations of systemic enteroviral disease sometimes occur with myopericarditis and include aseptic meningitis, pleurodynia, hepatitis, and orchitis.

Acute myocardial infarction associated with chest pain, arrhythmias, and congestive heart failure may be difficult to distinguish from myopericarditis. Patients suspected of having acute myocardial infarction sometimes have evidence of concurrent group B coxsackievirus infection,[165-167] and focal myocarditis has been proved in at least one case of acute coxsackievirus B5 infection.[168] Some patients presenting with suspected myocardial infarction who have normal coronary angiographic studies have been shown to have myocarditis by radiolabeled antimyosin antibody cardiac scanning.[169]

DIAGNOSIS

Although coxsackieviruses have been isolated on numerous occasions from pericardial fluid or heart muscle at autopsy[132] or by open biopsy procedures,[170] in practice, these specimens are rarely available. Cardiac tissue infrequently yields a viral isolate when cultured. The likelihood of a positive PCR result may depend on the number of potential viral pathogens included in the assay.[154,171,172] In the absence of identification of virus in cardiac tissue, the diagnosis often rests on circumstantial evidence provided by recovery of the agent from the oropharynx or feces or on serologic evidence of recent infection by a group B coxsackievirus.

MANAGEMENT

Supportive treatment consists of bed rest, pain relief, and medical management of arrhythmias and heart failure.[173] Although one study reported improved cardiac function and a trend toward increased survival for children with acute myocarditis who received intravenous immune globulin (IVIG) compared with historical controls,[174] randomized trials of immunosuppressive therapy, including IVIG, prednisone, and other drugs, have failed to show any consistent treatment effect.[175-177] Compassionate release of the experimental antiviral agent pleconaril has been associated with favorable outcomes in a small number of patients,[178] but controlled studies have not been done, and the drug is no longer available for that purpose.

COURSE AND PROGNOSIS

Persistent electrocardiographic abnormalities (10% to 20%), cardiomegaly (5% to 10%), and chronic congestive heart failure are indications of permanent myocardial injury that occur overall in about one third of adult patients identified with acute myopericarditis; these abnormalities may ultimately lead to a diagnosis of dilated cardiomyopathy.[135,163,164] Chronic constrictive pericarditis has occurred after intervals of 5 weeks to 1 year.[179-181]

The prognosis for children with acute myocarditis is better than for adults. Fewer than 15% of children die during the acute illness from intractable heart failure or uncontrolled arrhythmias, and fewer than 10% develop persistent or recurrent compromise from dilated cardiomyopathy requiring cardiac transplantation.[182] The risk for developing long-term cardiac sequelae may be higher in children with less severe acute myocarditis.[183]

DILATED CARDIOMYOPATHY

Chronic dilated cardiomyopathy, which is second only to ischemic heart disease as a cause of chronic congestive heart failure, is the final result of multiple infectious and noninfectious cardiac insults,[184] including up to one third of cases of acute myopericarditis and, in some instances, unrecognized past enterovirus infection.[135,163,164] Some investigators have detected enterovirus RNA in cardiac tissue months to years after the onset of dilated cardiomyopathy, but others who have employed similar methods have not detected enteroviral RNA.[158,185-193]

■ Coxsackievirus and Echovirus Disease in the Newborn

The human neonate is uniquely susceptible to enterovirus disease. Although many enterovirus serotypes cause the same self-limited clinical syndromes in neonates as in older persons (e.g., aseptic meningitis, exanthems), some serotypes are capable of producing fulminant, frequently fatal disease in the newborn infant. Group B coxsackievirus serotypes 1 to 5 and echovirus 11 are most frequently associated with overwhelming systemic neonatal infections. Rare cases of serious neonatal disease are reported with group A coxsackievirus serotypes 3, 9, and 16.[194-196]

EPIDEMIOLOGY

Although most neonatal enteroviral infections are directly transmitted from the mother, some infections are acquired by a nosocomial route. The first description of group B coxsackievirus disease in newborn infants followed outbreaks occurring in nurseries in South Africa, Zimbabwe, and the Netherlands.[197] Numerous nursery outbreaks of neonatal echovirus infection have been recorded, with the severity of neonatal disease varying according to the viral serotype.[198,199] Introduction of infection into the nursery has been traced to an infected parent or to hospital personnel. Infant-to-infant spread within nurseries probably occurs by the hands of personnel engaged in mouth care, gavage feeding, and other activities requiring close direct contact.[200]

Because most neonatal enterovirus infections are sporadic rather than nosocomial, the incidence and severity of neonatal enteroviral infection generally reflect the occurrence of enteroviral disease in the community. Although many cases occur sporadically during the enterovirus season, clusters of vertically transmitted neonatal infection sometimes occur during community outbreaks with a single enterovirus serotype.[201,202] During the 20-year period between 1983 and 2003, group B coxsackieviruses 1 through 4 and echovirus serotypes 11 and 25 were reported to the Centers for Disease Control and Prevention (CDC) significantly more commonly among neonates than among persons older than 1 month.[203] In 2007 and 2008, a markedly increased number of cases of serious neonatal disease caused by coxsackievirus B1 were reported to the CDC, reflecting both widespread circulation of this virus nationally and a higher attack rate in infants compared with other circulating enteroviruses.[204]

PATHOPHYSIOLOGY

Most newborns with life-threatening enterovirus disease are infected by vertical transmission from the infected mother in the perinatal period.[198,205] About 60% to 70% of women who give birth to infected infants have a febrile illness during the last week of pregnancy.[13,198] Experimental evidence indicates that the fetus is relatively protected by the placenta during maternal infection,[205,206] but the newborn has a high risk for infection,[111,207] perhaps as a result of exposure to either virus-positive cervical secretions[208,209] or viremic maternal blood.[210] Although most vertically transmitted enterovirus infections are probably acquired during delivery, some infants are infected before delivery, as evidenced by the recovery of virus from cord blood[208] and the development of disease within the first 2 days of life.[198,211]

In the infected neonate, enteroviruses spread systemically through the bloodstream. Tropism for and replication within specific organs of the neonatal host depend on both virus and host factors. Experimental evidence suggests that some neonatal tissues are innately more susceptible to infection with some enteroviruses than the corresponding tissues from an adult host.[212] In addition, the neonatal immune system is insufficient to control the replication and spread of virulent enteroviruses. Both premature and term human infants respond adequately to enterovirus infection with humoral neutralizing antibody.[213] However, macrophage function, which does not mature sufficiently until several weeks of age in the human neonate, is necessary to limit initial enteroviral replication.[214,215]

The outcome of neonatal infection is also strongly influenced by the presence or absence of passively acquired maternal antibody specific for the infecting enterovirus serotype.[206,207,216] Thus, the timing of maternal infection in relation to the development of maternal immunoglobulin G (IgG) antibody and delivery of the infant may be the most critical factor in determining the outcome of neonatal enterovirus infection.

CLINICAL MANIFESTATIONS

Symptoms develop in most neonates with generalized enterovirus disease between 3 and 10 days of life.[198,211] A small number have signs of illness in the delivery room or within the first 1 to 2 days of life[198,211]; conversely, the onset of fatal infection has been documented in infants as old as 3 months.[122] Male infants and premature infants are overrepresented among infants with serious illness. Early symptoms are generally mild and nonspecific and include listlessness, anorexia, and transient respiratory distress. Fever may or may not be present. About one third of patients have a biphasic illness with a period of 1 to 7 days of apparent well-being interspersed between the initial symptoms and the appearance of more serious manifestations.

Generalized enterovirus disease in the newborn most often occurs in one of two characteristic clinical syndromes, either myocarditis or fulminant hepatitis. Neonatal myocarditis, which is often accompanied by encephalitis and sometimes by hepatitis, is characteristically a manifestation of group B coxsackievirus infection[67,197] and less commonly echovirus 11 infection.[148,217] Fulminant hepatitis is characterized by hypotension, profuse bleeding, jaundice, and multiple organ failure. Echovirus 11 is responsible for a large proportion of cases, but well-documented cases of severe hepatitis in neonates have resulted from echovirus serotypes 4, 6, 7, 9, 12, 14, 19, 20, 21, 31, and 33.[198,218-222]

Myocarditis

Signs of neonatal myocarditis include rapid onset of heart failure, respiratory distress, tachycardia often exceeding 200 beats/min, cardiomegaly, and electrocardiographic evidence of myocardial injury and arrhythmias. Cyanosis and circulatory collapse develop rapidly in severely affected infants. Fatal cases are often accompanied by disseminated viral infection involving other organs in a pattern resembling that seen in experimentally infected suckling mice; these organs, in order of frequency, are the CNS, liver, pancreas, and adrenal gland. Most affected neonates are lethargic, and seizures, a bulging fontanelle, and CSF pleocytosis indicate the presence of meningoencephalitis. Enlargement of the liver is more often due to congestive heart failure than to viral hepatitis.

The overall mortality rate for neonatal myocarditis is 30% to 50%, and death usually occurs within a week of onset. Myocardial function rapidly improves in surviving infants after defervescence, generally by 1 week, although in a few infants, convalescence is prolonged for several weeks. Pathologic data are limited to information obtained at postmortem examination. Infants dying of myocarditis have enlarged, dilated hearts, extensive myonecrosis, and a variable degree of cardiac inflammation. Lymphocytic infiltration of the brain, meninges, lungs, liver, pancreas, and adrenal glands may also be found.

Hepatitis

The initial symptoms of severe neonatal hepatitis are lethargy, poor feeding, and increasing jaundice. These nonspecific symptoms may initiate an evaluation and therapy for bacterial sepsis. However, within 1 to 2 days, the jaundice progresses, and ecchymoses, bleeding from puncture sites, and signs of metabolic acidosis develop. From this stage, most infected infants rapidly progress downhill with uncontrollable hemorrhage, hepatic failure, acute renal failure, and generalized seizures. Hepatic transaminases rise rapidly to extremely high levels and thrombocytopenia develops. Markedly prolonged prothrombin times and partial thromboplastin times are indicative of profound hepatic failure.

More than half of infants with severe neonatal echovirus hepatitis die within days after the onset of symptoms despite therapy with blood products and intensive supportive care. Some ultimately fatal cases survive for 2 to 3 weeks with supportive care.[201] Postmortem findings include massive hepatic necrosis and extensive hemorrhage into the cerebral ventricles, pericardial sac, renal medullae, and interstitial spaces of many solid organs.[223] Inflammation is commonly limited to the liver and adrenal glands, with sparing of the heart, brain, meninges, and other organs. The long-term prognosis for surviving infants is not well known, although hepatic fibrosis and chronic hepatic insufficiency develop in some early in life.

Pneumonia

Several cases of enterovirus pneumonia occurring in the first few days of life have been reported, all of them fatal and caused by echovirus types 6,[108] 9,[109] and 11,[110] and group A coxsackievirus type 3.

DIAGNOSIS AND DIFFERENTIAL DIAGNOSIS

The diagnosis of neonatal coxsackievirus and echovirus infection is most rapidly made by detection of viral RNA by PCR or isolation of virus in cell culture. Because virus is usually present in the infected neonate in high titer, isolation from oropharyngeal secretions, feces, and urine is relatively rapid; virus may also be recovered

from blood, CSF, ascitic fluid, and multiple tissues obtained at biopsy or autopsy.

Neonatal myocarditis is sometimes mistaken for congenital heart disease because in both conditions murmurs and evidence of congestive heart failure may be present. However, fever and electrocardiographic evidence of acute myocardial injury are absent in patients with congenital heart disease. The early features of myocarditis and severe hepatitis resemble those of bacterial sepsis. Because of liver and CNS involvement in either syndrome, visceral dissemination with perinatally acquired herpes simplex virus in the absence of cutaneous lesions may be suspected.

MANAGEMENT

Management of neonatal enteroviral disease is supportive. Infants in congestive heart failure require judicious fluid management and administration of inotropic agents and diuretics. The profuse bleeding that results from hepatic failure necessitates frequent replacement therapy with packed red blood cells, platelets, and fresh-frozen plasma. Vitamin K should be administered intravenously in pharmacologic doses. Large doses of IVIG, which have been reported to improve outcome in at least one case,[224] may be justified given the extremely poor prognosis, although there is not reliable evidence of efficacy. The experimental antipicornavirus drug pleconaril is under investigation in a phase II trial.[225]

Chronic Meningoencephalitis in Agammaglobulinemic and Other Immunocompromised Patients

The enteroviruses have been responsible for persistent, severe, sometimes fatal infections of the CNS in patients with hereditary or acquired defects in B-lymphocyte function. Most reported patients are children with X-linked agammaglobulinemia, although an increasing number of hematopoietic cell transplant patients and patients treated with anti–B-lymphocyte immunotherapy are now being recorded.[226-228]

ETIOLOGIC AGENTS

Most cases have been caused by echoviruses; single cases caused by group A coxsackievirus serotypes 4, 11, and 15 and by group B coxsackievirus serotypes 2 and 3 are recorded.[226,229]

CLINICAL MANIFESTATIONS

Nervous system manifestations may be totally absent; or mild nuchal rigidity, headache, lethargy, papilledema, seizure disorders, motor weakness, tremors, and ataxia may be present. These neurologic abnormalities may fluctuate in severity, disappear, or steadily progress. The CSF exhibits lymphocytic pleocytosis and a higher protein concentration than is usually seen in cases of acute enterovirus aseptic meningitis. An enterovirus can be repeatedly recovered from the CSF over a period of months to years, usually in high titer. In some cases, virus is isolated only intermittently from the CSF or detected only by PCR. For unknown reasons, it is usually more difficult to isolate virus from the feces than from the CSF. Persistent skeletal muscle involvement causes a dermatomyositis-like syndrome in more than half of these patients, and some also have chronic hepatitis.

Enteroviruses have been recovered from many other sites in these patients, including the brain, lung, liver, spleen, kidney, myocardium, pericardial fluid, skeletal muscle, and bone marrow.[226] Some patients have been infected with more than one enterovirus serotype, either concurrently[230] or sequentially.[226,229] The etiology of the chronic muscle and soft tissue inflammation is not fully understood, but isolation of echovirus from muscle in one case suggests a role for direct virus infection.[231]

In many patients, possibly most, the disease ends fatally. Autopsy findings have included chronic meningitis and encephalitis, with lymphocytic perivascular cuffing, focal loss of neurons, and gliosis of both gray and white matter. However, widespread destruction of motor neurons such as that seen in poliomyelitis has not been observed.

PROPHYLAXIS AND THERAPY

Prophylactic use of IVIG serum globulin reduces the risk for acquiring chronic enterovirus infection by these patients. However, IVIG has been less effective in the treatment of chronic enterovirus meningitis, even when using IVIG lots with relatively high concentrations of specific antibody. Some patients have experienced clinical improvement when IVIG has been injected directly into the ventricles,[226] but relapse of infection may occur even after long-term intraventricular IVIG therapy. The experimental antiviral drug pleconaril has been used in this setting, but the reported experience with it is uncontrolled and limited to a small number of patients.[232]

INFECTIONS IN OTHER IMMUNOCOMPROMISED PATIENTS

Hematopoietic cell allograft recipients have profoundly suppressed immunologic responses during the immediate post-transplantation period, including suppression of the ability to mount a humoral immune response. In some recipients, enterovirus infections have developed in the post-transplantation period that were disseminated, prolonged, and contributed to fatal outcomes.[233-235] One outbreak of coxsackievirus A1 diarrheal illness was observed in a bone marrow transplantation unit in which virus-induced diarrhea was difficult to distinguish from graft-versus-host enteritis.[236] Some patients receiving rituximab (anti-CD20) monoclonal antibody, which profoundly suppresses B-lymphocyte function, have developed paralysis and other complications of CNS infection.[227,228]

Acute Hemorrhagic Conjunctivitis

Acute hemorrhagic conjunctivitis (AHC) is a contagious ocular infection characterized by pain, swelling of the eyelids, and subconjunctival hemorrhage that generally resolves spontaneously within a week. Epidemic or pandemic disease has now occurred in most parts of the world due to enterovirus 70, which has been responsible for tens of millions of cases of AHC. A variant strain of coxsackievirus A24 causes a similar but geographically more restricted disease that has afflicted hundreds of thousands of persons. Some epidemics of conjunctivitis in the Far East have involved both viruses sequentially or concurrently. Although the relative contribution of these two agents has not always been defined, it is clear that enterovirus 70 has accounted for greater total morbidity.

EPIDEMIOLOGY

AHC appeared to emerge as a new disease in 1969 with explosive, pandemic spread from simultaneous foci in Ghana and Indonesia.[237] The initial epidemic caused by enterovirus 70 spread along the coast of West Africa and ultimately involved many countries on the African continent by 1973, as well as England, the former Soviet Union, Holland, France, and Yugoslavia.[238,239] A new strain of coxsackievirus A24 was identified as the etiology of more than 60,000 cases of AHC in Singapore in 1970.[240-242] Subsequently, both viruses circulated in Southeast Asia and the Indian subcontinent, causing large seasonal outbreaks.[243-246] Although the geographic distribution of AHC is wide, large-scale epidemics have occurred predominantly in crowded coastal areas of tropical countries during the hot, rainy season.[247]

Outbreaks in economically developed countries and temperate climates have been much more limited. AHC in the West has been mostly confined to seasonal outbreaks in Central America and the Caribbean. The disease did not appear in the United States until September 1981,

when enterovirus 70 conjunctivitis was first reported in Key West, Florida. Within weeks, about 2500 cases occurred, largely among disadvantaged persons in Miami.[248] With the exception of a few imported cases, AHC activity has not since been noted in the United States.[249] Coxsackievirus A24 AHC cases first appeared in the Western Hemisphere in Trinidad, Jamaica, St. Croix, Panama, and Mexico in 1986.[250] About 31,000 cases occurred in Puerto Rico in 1987.[251]

PATTERNS OF TRANSMISSION

AHC is highly contagious and spreads rapidly. Unlike most other enterovirus infections, AHC is transmitted primarily from fingers or fomites directly to the eye rather than by respiratory secretions or fecal contamination. Both enterovirus 70 and coxsackievirus A24 can be regularly recovered from the conjunctivae early in the illness but only infrequently recovered from respiratory secretions or feces. Both serotypes appear to be naturally occurring, temperature-sensitive viruses whose optimal replication at 33°C to 35°C reflects their adaptation to the temperature of the conjunctiva.[252,253] The observed rapid serial transmission at about 24-hour intervals is consistent with direct spread of virus from hand to eye. During a 1980 enterovirus 70 outbreak in Singapore, the secondary attack rate within affected households was 73%.[254] Contagion is favored by crowding and unsanitary living conditions. AHC occurs substantially more often among the poor than among others living in the same country.[255,256] Reuse of water for bathing and sharing of towels are implicated as factors contributing to the spread of infection. Limited outbreaks of AHC in Europe have been primarily nosocomial, particularly in ophthalmology clinics, where infection appears to have been spread directly by physicians' fingers or by instruments.

Postepidemic antibody prevalence rates of nearly 50% have been observed in Ghana and Indonesia but only 6% in affected populations of Japan. These findings are consistent with less intense spread of AHC in economically developed regions. Antibody prevalence rates are highest in children younger than 10 years, whereas attack rates for clinical disease are greatest in young adults, which indicates that many infections in children must be inapparent or mild.[257,258]

CLINICAL MANIFESTATIONS

The clinical manifestations of AHC begin abruptly and peak within 24 hours. Burning, foreign body sensation, ocular pain, photophobia, eyelid swelling, and watery discharge begin in one eye and rapidly progress to the other eye.[248] Constitutional symptoms such as fever, malaise, and headache are observed in 20% of cases. The most distinctive sign is subconjunctival hemorrhage, which is present in 70% to 90% of patients with AHC caused by enterovirus 70,[258] but it is less frequent in cases caused by coxsackievirus A24.[241,242,244] The hemorrhages may be pinpoint or occupy the entire bulbar conjunctiva and are precipitated by everting the upper lid or by rubbing the eyes. Conjunctival edema is said to be more common in elderly people; hemorrhage is more profuse in young patients.[258] Small follicles appear on the tarsal conjunctiva after 3 to 5 days in 90% of patients. In most cases, corneal erosion or a fine punctate epithelial keratitis can be demonstrated by slit-lamp examination after staining with fluorescein. The ocular discharge is serous or seromucoid and contains abundant neutrophils in the first 24 hours. Preauricular lymph nodes are often enlarged and tender by the second day of illness. Recovery is usually noticeable by the second or third day and is complete in most cases in 10 days, although discoloration from the hemorrhages sometimes persists for many days.

COMPLICATIONS

In severe cases of AHC, keratitis occasionally persists for several weeks but almost never leads to permanent scarring. Uveitis has not been reported. Conjunctivitis may be complicated by secondary bacterial infection.

More than 200 cases of acute motor paralysis have been reported in persons who have recently recovered from AHC in India, Thailand, Taiwan, and Senegal.[245,259-262] This complication is clinically indistinguishable from poliomyelitis except for its temporal association with AHC, which it generally follows by 2 to 5 weeks. Neurologic complications of AHC have been reported only during epidemics caused by enterovirus 70 and not those caused by coxsackievirus A24. Enterovirus 70 has not been recovered from the CSF and has been recovered only once from feces.[259] However, high titers of specific neutralizing antibody to enterovirus 70 have been demonstrated in the CSF of virtually all patients with motor paralysis but not in patients with AHC alone.[262] Neuroparalytic disease has been reproduced clinically and pathologically in monkeys by inoculation of enterovirus 70 into the spinal cord.[237,263]

DIFFERENTIAL DIAGNOSIS

Small outbreaks or sporadic cases may be mistaken for adenovirus infection causing epidemic keratoconjunctivitis (see Chapter 143), which has a longer incubation period (5 to 7 days), peaks several days after onset, and persists for up to 2 or 3 weeks, compared with AHC.

LABORATORY DIAGNOSIS

Enterovirus 70 and coxsackievirus A24 can be recovered from conjunctival swabs or scrapings of patients with AHC during the first 3 days of illness.[240,264] Isolation rates exceeding 90% from conjunctival scrapings have been reported for coxsackievirus A24, but recovery rates for enterovirus 70 have been somewhat lower.[255] Rising antibody titers can be demonstrated in paired sera from patients with conjunctivitis.

TREATMENT AND PREVENTION

Treatment of conjunctivitis is symptomatic. Antimicrobial agents are not indicated. Contagion can be prevented by careful hand washing, use of separate towels, and sterilization of ophthalmologic instruments.

Illnesses in Which the Etiologic Role of Enteroviruses Is Minor or Poorly Defined

GASTROINTESTINAL DISEASES

The liver and the pancreas are both affected in mice infected with group B coxsackieviruses. In humans, acute hepatitis occurring beyond the neonatal period is described in association with group B coxsackievirus and echovirus infections.[265-270] Most cases have been mild and self-limited. Prospective studies indicated that 2% to 20% of patients with acute pancreatitis have concurrent enterovirus infection.[271,272] Group B coxsackievirus types 1 to 5 and echovirus types 6, 11, 22, and 30 are all reported to cause acute pancreatitis.[271-274]

Coxsackieviruses and echoviruses, possibly as a result of their replication in the small bowel, are frequently cited as causes of nonbacterial diarrhea or gastroenteritis. However, conflicting results have been obtained in several studies that compared rates of enteroviral isolation from children with acute diarrheal illness compared with matched healthy control subjects.[67,275-277] Overall, the data favor a variable, generally small excess of enteroviral infections in subjects with diarrhea. Evidence is somewhat stronger that certain echoviruses, particularly types 11, 14, and 18, have occasionally been responsible for epidemic diarrhea in young infants.[67,276,278] Most of these studies were performed before the discovery of toxigenic *Escherichia coli*, rotaviruses, enteric adenoviruses, and caliciviruses, now established as major causes of diarrheal illness. In light of this new knowledge, additional epidemiologic investigations encompassing all these agents are required before the contribution of enteroviruses to diarrheal disease can be accurately assessed. Nonetheless, their role is probably minor. Similarly, the

hemolytic uremic syndrome has been temporally associated with coxsackieviruses A4, B2, and B4 and with echovirus 22 (now parechovirus 1),[279-281] and coxsackievirus B5 has been reported in association with acute renal failure in five patients.[282] Now that a strong link between enterohemorrhagic *E. coli* infection and the hemolytic uremic syndrome exists, the relationship between enterovirus infection and acute renal disease is questionable.

OTHER DISEASES

Orchitis has been observed in adolescent boys during infection with coxsackievirus A9, group B coxsackieviruses 2, 4, and 5, and echovirus 6,[283-287] including coxsackievirus B5 isolation from a testicular biopsy specimen in one case.[283] Splenomegaly and a heterophile-negative mononucleosis-like syndrome have also been reported.[67] Echoviruses have been associated with acute arthritis, including echovirus 11, which was recovered from synovial fluid in one case.[288,289] In separate case reports, echovirus 25[290,291] and an untyped enterovirus resembling a group A coxsackievirus[291] have been recovered from the gastrointestinal tracts of children with acute infectious lymphocytosis; however, further evidence of an etiologic association is lacking.

DIABETES MELLITUS

A gradually accumulating body of epidemiologic, clinical, and experimental evidence suggests an intriguing link between the group B coxsackieviruses and type 1 insulin-dependent diabetes mellitus (IDDM). The reader is referred to several excellent reviews for more detailed analyses.[273,292-296]

The observation that new-onset IDDM cases occur in seasonal patterns[297,298] and sometimes in clusters or small outbreaks[296,299,300] has been cited as evidence for the role of viral disease in the pathophysiology of IDDM. The peak occurrence of new IDDM cases is late in the calendar year, 1 to 2 months later than peak enterovirus activity. However, the occurrence of enterovirus infection and IDDM during the same season could be independent, and at least two studies found no increase in new onset of IDDM after outbreaks of group B coxsackievirus disease.[301,302] Cross-sectional studies in which the prevalence of group B coxsackievirus antibody has been compared in children with IDDM and control subjects are inconclusive. In general, studies that used hospital or neighborhood controls have found a positive association, whereas those using sibling controls have not.[292,294]

Two major theories of the pathophysiology of virus-induced IDDM exist that are not necessarily mutually exclusive. The "direct hit" hypothesis, which posits destruction of pancreatic islets by direct virus infection, derives support from murine studies in which enteroviruses cause specific destruction of β cells in the islets of Langerhans,[273,303] from detection of enterovirus RNA in serum at the onset of IDDM,[304,305] and from postmortem isolation of coxsackievirus serotypes B4[306] and B5[307] from the pancreatic tissue of children dying of ketoacidosis as their initial manifestation of IDDM. Demonstration of group B coxsackievirus IgM antibody in the serum of children with recent-onset IDDM supports the direct-infection hypothesis, although inconsistency regarding this finding has been noted across different studies.[308-312]

A second theory focuses on acute viral infection as a trigger for an autoimmune response to pancreatic islet cells; the autoimmune response is induced by the similarity between viral and islet cell antigens, which may be related to a past viral insult, genetic predisposition, or both.[313] This concept is supported by the induction of chronic islet cell inflammation in genetically susceptible mice by enterovirus infection,[314] by the observation that most children with IDDM have humoral anti–islet cell antibodies at diagnosis, and by one study demonstrating a temporal association between the development of islet cell antibodies and seroconversion to group B coxsackievirus infection.[315] Some investigations suggest that molecular mimicry between a nonstructural coxsackievirus protein and a β-cell enzyme may permit autoimmune destruction of pancreatic islet cell tissue.[316] Although persistent enterovirus infection is also considered a possible mechanism of islet cell damage, no evidence is widely accepted that enteroviruses are capable of persisting in an immunocompetent human host.

Enterovirus 71 Infections

Enterovirus 71 is closely related to coxsackievirus A16, and both viruses cause skeletal myositis in suckling mice and myelitis with paralysis in cynomolgus monkeys.[317,318] Enterovirus 71 was first isolated from young children with encephalitis and aseptic meningitis in California in 1969[319] and has since been found to cause infection globally, including large outbreaks of HFM disease, which have sometimes been associated with aseptic meningitis and serious CNS complications in young children.[54,56,89,320-329] Enterovirus 71 is unique among the non-polio enteroviruses as a cause of epidemic paralysis, in which localized outbreaks have involved small numbers of patients over several years[319,321,330,331] and regional epidemics have involved hundreds to thousands of persons within a single season.[61,62,89,326,332] Infants and young children have developed a brainstem encephalitis associated with high mortality related to rapid cardiovascular collapse and pulmonary edema.[54-56] Other, less common manifestations attributed to enterovirus 71 infection include generalized maculopapular rash,[321] interstitial pneumonia,[56] and myocarditis.[56,62]

Enterovirus 71 has been isolated from vesicle fluid, feces, oropharyngeal secretions, urine, and CSF. Isolation rates are highest from vesicle swabs and lowest from the CSF.[61,62,327] Primary isolation has been most successful in African green monkey kidney cell culture, although a cytopathic effect may take 5 to 8 days to develop and then progress slowly and incompletely.

Treatment of enterovirus 71 infection is symptomatic and supportive. The recent large-scale epidemics occurring in the Far East have generated interest in development of an enterovirus 71 vaccine.[333]

Parechovirus Infections

With the introduction of viral RNA sequencing, it was discovered that the previously designated echovirus serotypes 22 and 23 diverged sufficiently from other enteroviruses to be reassigned to a new picornavirus genus, as parechovirus serotypes 1 and 2, respectively.[334] Parechoviruses differ in capsid protein organization from enteroviruses[335] and utilize a unique cell membrane receptor (see Chapter 170). The 5′ nontranslated end of the genome of parechoviruses differs sufficiently from that of enteroviruses to permit development of specific parechovirus PCRs.[336] Currently, 14 parechovirus serotypes have been proposed.[337-339] The spectrum of diseases attributed to parechoviruses is similar to that of the echoviruses, including respiratory tract infections, exanthems, viral meningitis, encephalitis, myocarditis, and serious neonatal infections.[340,341] The latter have been associated with white matter injury in neonatal encephalitis.[342] As association with mild gastroenteritis has been noted, but the overall significance of parechoviruses as causes of gastrointestinal disease is unknown.[343] A case of fatal pneumonia with human parechovirus 1 in an elderly woman has also been reported.[344] Early studies of the prevalence of parechovirus infections suggest that they are not common,[344,345] but larger scale studies with techniques to identify newly recognized serotypes should provide more definitive information regarding their epidemiology. Studies from the United States suggest that most infections occur during the summer and fall, but the seasonality is not as prominent as for enteroviruses.[346]

REFERENCES

1. Kogon A, Spigland I, Frothingham TE, et al. The Virus Watch Program: A continuing surveillance of viral infections in metropolitan New York families. Am J Epidemiol. 1969;89:51.
2. Berlin LE, Rorabaugh ML, Heldrich F, et al. Aseptic meningitis in infants less than two years of age: diagnosis and etiology. J Infect Dis. 1993;168:888.
3. Kupila L, Vuorinen T, Vainionpaa R, et al. Etiology of aseptic meningitis and encephalitis in an adult population. Neurology. 2006;66:75.
4. Mullins JA, Khetsuriani N, Nix WA, et al. Emergence of echovirus type 13 as a prominent enterovirus. Clin Infect Dis. 2004;38:70.
5. Huang QS, Carr JM, Nix WA, et al. An echovirus type 33 outbreak in New Zealand. Clin Infect Dis. 2003;37:650.
6. Dagan R, Jenista J, Menegus MA. Association of clinical presentation, laboratory findings, and virus serotypes with the presence of meningitis in hospitalized infants with enterovirus infection. J Pediatr. 1988;113:975.
7. Rorabaugh ML, Berlin LE, Heldrich F, et al. Aseptic meningitis among infants less than two years of age: acute illness and neurologic complications. Pediatrics. 1993;92:206.
8. Lepow ML, Coyne N, Thompson LB, et al. A clinical, epidemiologic and laboratory investigation of aseptic meningitis during the four-year period, 1955-1958. II. The clinical disease and its sequelae. N Engl J Med. 1962;266:1188.
9. Bernit E, de Lamballerie X, Zandotti C, et al. Prospective investigation of a large outbreak of meningitis due to echovirus 30 during summer 2000 in Marseilles, France. Medicine. 2004;83:245.
10. Rotbart H, Brennan PJ, Fife KH, et al. Enterovirus meningitis in adults. Clin Infect Dis. 1998;27:896.
11. Desmond RA, Accortt NA, Talley L, et al. Enteroviral meningitis: natural history and outcome of pleconaril therapy. Antimicrobiol Agents Chemother. 2006;50:2409.
12. Haynes RE, Cramblett HG, Kronfol HJ. Echovirus 9 meningoencephalitis in infants and children. JAMA. 1969;208:1657.
13. Lake AM, Lauer BA, Clark JC, et al. Enterovirus infections in neonates. J Pediatr. 1976;89:787.
14. Wenner HA, Abel D, Olson LC, et al. A mixed epidemic associated with echovirus types 6 and 11. Am J Epidemiol. 1981;114:369.
15. Wilfert CM, Lauer BA, Cohen M, et al. An epidemic of echovirus 18 meningitis. J Infect Dis. 1975;131:75.
16. Amir J, Harel L, Frydman M, et al. Shift in cerebrospinal polymorphonuclear cell percentage in the early stage of aseptic meningitis. J Pediatr. 1991;119:938.
17. Feigin RD, Shackelford PG. Value of repeat lumbar puncture in the differential diagnosis of meningitis. N Engl J Med. 1973;289:571.
18. Shah SS, Hodinka RL, Turnquist JL, et al. Cerebrospinal fluid mononuclear cell predominance is not related to symptom duration in children with enteroviral meningitis. J Pediatr. 2006;148:118.
19. Avner E, Satz J, Plotkin SA. Hypoglycorrhachia in young infants with viral meningitis. J Pediatr. 1975;87:883.
20. Singer JI, Mauer PR, Riley JP, et al. Management of central nervous system infections during an epidemic of enteroviral aseptic meningitis. J Pediatr. 1980;96:559.
21. Sumaya CV, Corman LI. Enteroviral meningitis in early infancy: significance in community outbreaks. Pediatr Infect Dis. 1982;3:151.
22. Malcom BS, Eiden JJ, Hendley JO. Echovirus type 9 meningitis simulating tuberculous meningitis. Pediatrics. 1980;65:725.
23. Rotbart HA. Nucleic acid detection systems for enteroviruses. Clin Microbiol Rev. 1991;4:156.
24. Yerly S, Gervaix A, Simonet V, et al. Rapid and sensitive detection of enteroviruses in specimens from patients with aseptic meningitis. J Clin Microbiol. 1996;34:199.
25. Schlesinger Y, Sawyer MH, Storch GA. Enteroviral meningitis in infancy: potential role for polymerase chain reaction in patient management. Pediatrics. 1994;94:157.
26. Rotbart HA, Sawyer MH, Fast S, et al. Diagnosis of enteroviral meningitis by using PCR with a colorimetric microwell detection assay. J Clin Microbiol. 1994;32:2590.
27. Sawyer MH, Holland D, Aintablian N, et al. Diagnosis of enteroviral central nervous system infection by polymerase chain reaction during a large community outbreak. Pediatr Infect Dis J. 1994;13:177.
28. Lennette EH, Magoffin R, Knouf EG. Viral central nervous system disease: An etiologic study conducted at the Los Angeles County General Hospital. JAMA. 1962;179:687.
29. Lepow ML, Carver DH, Wright HT, et al. A clinical, epidemiologic and laboratory investigation of aseptic meningitis during the four-year period, 1955-1958. I. Observations concerning etiology and epidemiology. N Engl J Med. 1962;266:1181.
30. Marier R, Rodriguez W, Chloupek RJ, et al. Coxsackievirus B5 infection and aseptic meningitis in neonates and children. Am J Dis Child. 1975;129:321.
31. Torphy DE, Ray GC, Thompson RS, et al. An epidemic of aseptic meningitis due to echovirus type 30: Epidemiologic features and clinical and laboratory findings. Am J Public Health. 1970;60:1447.
32. Sabin AB, Krumbiegel ER, Wigand R. ECHO type 9 virus disease. Am J Dis Child. 1958;96:197.
33. Rotbart HA, Ahmed A, Hickey S, et al. Diagnosis of enterovirus infection by PCR of multiple specimen types. Pediatr Infect Dis J. 1997;16:409.
34. Kupila L, Vuorinen T, Vainionpaa R, et al. Diagnosis of enteroviral meningitis by use of polymerase chain reaction of cerebrospinal fluid, stool, and serum specimens. Clin Infect Dis. 2005;40:982.
35. Mandal BK. The dilemma of partially treated bacterial meningitis. Scand J Infect Dis. 1976;8:185.
36. Converse GM, Gwaltney JMJ, Strasburg DA, et al. Alteration of cerebrospinal fluid findings by partial treatment of bacterial meningitis. J Pediatr. 1973;83:220.
37. Dalton HP, Allison MJ. Modification of laboratory results by partial treatment of bacterial meningitis. Am J Clin Pathol. 1968;49:410.
38. King RL, Lorch SA, Cohen DM, et al. Routine cerebrospinal fluid enterovirus polymerase chain reaction testing reduces hospitalization and antibiotic use for infants 90 days of age or younger. Pediatrics. 2007;120:489.
39. Robinson CC, Willis M, Meagher A, et al. Impact of rapid polymerase chain reaction results on management of pediatric patients with enteroviral meningitis. Pediatr Infect Dis J. 2002;21:283.
40. Abzug MJ, Cloud G, Bradley J, et al. Double blind placebo-controlled trial of pleconaril in infants with enterovirus meningitis. Pediatr Infect Dis J. 2003;22:335.
41. Farmer K, MacArthur BA, Clay MM. A follow-up study of 15 cases of neonatal meningoencephalitis due to Coxsackie virus B5. J Pediatr. 1975;87:568.
42. Sells CJ, Carpenter RL, Ray CG. Sequelae of central-nervous-system enterovirus infections. N Engl J Med. 1975;293:1.
43. Bergman I, Painter MJ, Wald ER, et al. Outcome in children with enteroviral meningitis during the first year of life. J Pediatr. 1987;110:705.
44. Rorabaugh ML, Berlin LE, Rosenberg L, et al. Absence of Neurodevelopmental Sequelae to Aseptic Meningitis. Baltimore, MD, Society for Pediatric Research, 1992.
45. Fowlkes AL, Honarmand S, Glaser C, et al. Enterovirus-associated encephalitis in the California encephalitis project, 1998-2005. J Infect Dis. 2008;198:1685.
46. Kolski H, Ford-Jones EL, Richardson S, et al. Etiology of acute childhood encephalitis at the Hospital for Sick Children, Toronto, 1994-95. Clin Infect Dis. 1998;26:398.
47. Meyer HM, Johnson RT, Crawford IP, et al. Central nervous system syndromes of viral etiology. A study of 713 cases. Am J Med. 1960;29:334.
48. Chalhub E, Devivo D, Siegel BA, et al. Coxsackie A9 focal encephalitis associated with acute infantile hemiplegia and porencephaly. Neurology. 1977;27:574.
49. Modlin JF, Dagan R, Berlin LE, et al. Focal encephalitis with enterovirus infections. Pediatrics. 1991;88:841.

50. Peters ACB, Vielvoye GJ, Versteeg J, et al. Echo 25 focal encephalitis and subacute hemichorea. *Neurology.* 1979;29:676.
51. Roden VJ, Cantor HE, O'Connor DM, et al. Acute hemiplegia of childhood associated with Coxsackie A9 viral infection. *J Pediatr.* 1975;86:56.
52. Liow K, Spanaki MV, Boyer RS, et al. Bilateral hippocampal encephalitis caused by enteroviral infection. *Pediatr Neurol.* 1999;21:836.
53. Whitley RJ, Cobbs CG, Alford CA, et al. Diseases that mimic herpes simplex encephalitis. *JAMA.* 1989;262:234.
54. Lum LCS, Wong KT, Lam SK, et al. Fatal enterovirus 71 encephalomyelitis. *J Pediatr.* 1998;133:795.
55. Huang C-C, Liu C-C, Chang Y-C, et al. Neurologic complications in children with enterovirus 71 infection. *N Engl J Med.* 1999;341:936.
56. Chan KP, Goh KT, Chong CY, et al. Epidemic hand, foot and mouth disease caused by enterovirus 71, Singapore. *Emerg Infect Dis.* 2003;9:78.
57. Klapper PE, Bailey AS, Longson M, et al. Meningoencephalitis caused by coxsackievirus group B type 2: Diagnosis confirmed by measuring intrathecal antibody. *J Infect.* 1984;8:227.
58. Price RA, Garcia JH, Rightsel WA. Choriomeningitis and myocarditis in an adolescent with isolation of Coxsackie B5 virus. *Am J Clin Pathol.* 1970;53:825.
59. Voroshilova MK, Chumakov MP. Poliomyelitis-like properties of AB-IV-Coxsackie A7 group of viruses. *Prog Med Virol.* 1959;2:106.
60. Grist NR, Bell EJ. Enteroviral etiology of the paralytic poliomyelitis syndrome. *Arch Environ Health.* 1970;21:382.
61. Gilbert GL, Dickson KE, Waters MJ, et al. Outbreak of enterovirus 71 infection in Victoria, Australia, with a high incidence of neurologic involvement. *Pediatr Infect Dis J.* 1988;7:484.
62. Shindarov LM, Chumakov MP, Voroshilova MK, et al. Epidemiological, clinical, and pathophysiological characteristics of epidemic poliomyelitis-like disease caused by enterovirus 71. *J Hygiene Epidemiol Microbiol Immunol.* 1979;23:284.
63. Santhanam S, Choudhury DS. Coxsackie A-9 in the etiology of poliomyelitis-like diseases. *Indian J Pediatr.* 1985;52:405.
64. Assaad F, Cockburn WC. Four year study of WHO virus reports on enteroviruses other than poliovirus. *Bull World Health Organ.* 1972;46:329.
65. Godtfredsen A, Hansen B. A case of mild paralytic disease due to ECHO virus type 11. *Acta Pathol Microbiol Scand.* 1961;53:111.
66. Grist NR, Bell EJ. The epidemiology of enteroviruses. *Scot Med J.* 1975;20:27.
67. Kibrick S. Current status of Coxsackie and ECHO viruses in human disease. *Prog Med Virol.* 1964;6:27.
68. Hertenstein JR, Sarnat HB, O'Connor DM. Acute unilateral oculomotor palsy associated with ECHO 9 viral infection. *J Pediatr.* 1976;89:79.
69. Steigman AJ, Lipton MM. Fatal bulbospinal paralytic poliomyelitis due to ECHO 11 virus. *JAMA.* 1960;174:178.
70. Dery P, Marks MI, Shapera R. Clinical manifestations of coxsackievirus infections in children. *Am J Dis Child.* 1974;128:464.
71. Geer J. Coxsackie virus infections in Southern Africa. *Yale J Biol Med.* 1961;34:289.
72. Barak Y, Schwartz JF. Acute transverse myelitis associated with ECHO type 5 infection (letter). *Am J Dis Child.* 1988;142:128.
73. Kaul A, Cohen ME, Broffman G, et al. Reye-like syndrome associated with Coxsackie B2 virus infection. *J Pediatr.* 1979;94:67.
74. Alvira MM, Mendoza M. Reye's syndrome: A viral myopathy? *N Engl J Med.* 1975;292:1297.
75. Brunberg JA, Bell WE. Reye syndrome. *Arch Neurol.* 1974;30:304.
76. Kuban KC, Ephros MA, Freeman RL, et al. Syndrome of opsoclonus-myoclonus caused by Coxsackie B3 infection. *Ann Neurol.* 1983;13:69.
77. Ramsay M, Reacher M, O'Flynn C, et al. Causes of morbilliform rash in a highly immunised English population. *Arch Dis Child.* 2002;87:202.
78. Bell EJ, Ross CAC, Grist NR. Echo 9 infection in pregnant women with suspected rubella. *J Clin Pathol.* 1975;28:267.
79. Lerner AM, Klein JO, Levin HS, et al. Infections due to Coxsackie virus group A, type 9, in Boston, 1959, with special reference to exanthems and pneumonia. *N Engl J Med.* 1960;263:1265.
80. Annunziato D. Koplik spots and echo 9 virus (letter). *N Y State J Med.* 1987;87:667.
81. Hall CB, Cherry JD, Hatch MH, et al. The return of Boston exanthem: Echovirus 16 infections in 1974. *Am J Dis Child.* 1977;131:323.
82. Neva FA. A second outbreak of Boston exanthem disease in Pittsburgh during 1954. *N Engl J Med.* 1956;254:838.
83. Cherry JD, Lerner AM, Klein JO, et al. Coxsackie B5 infections with exanthems. *Pediatrics.* 1963;31:455.
84. Moritsugu Y, Sawada K, Hinohara M, et al. An outbreak of type 25 echovirus infection with exanthem in an infant home near Tokyo. *Am J Epidemiol.* 1968;87:599.
85. Hughes RO, Roberts C. Hand, foot, mouth disease associated with Coxsackie A9 virus. *Lancet.* 1972;2:751.
86. Lindenbaum JE, Van Dyck PC, Allen RG. Hand, foot and mouth disease associated with coxsackievirus group B. *Scand J Infect Dis.* 1975;7:161.
87. Robinson CR, Doane FW, Rhodes AJ. Report of an outbreak of febrile illness with pharyngeal lesions and exanthem. *Can Med Assn J.* 1958;79:615.
88. Wang S-M, Liu C-C, Tseng H-W, et al. Clinical spectrum of enterovirus 71 infection in children in southern Taiwan, with an emphasis on neurological complications. *Clin Infect Dis.* 1999;29:184.
89. Ho M, Chen E-R, Hsu K-H, et al. An epidemic of enterovirus 71 infection in Taiwan. *N Engl J Med.* 1999;341:929.
90. Adler JL, Mostow SR, Mellin H, et al. Epidemiologic investigation of hand, foot, and mouth disease: Infection caused by coxsackievirus A16 in Baltimore, June through September 1968. *Am J Dis Child.* 1970;120:309.
91. Nahmias AJ, Froeschle JE, Feorino PM, et al. Generalized eruption in a child with eczema due to coxsackievirus A16. *Arch Dermatol.* 1968;97:147.
92. Miller GD. Hand-foot-and-mouth disease. *JAMA.* 1968;203:827.
93. Kimura A, Abe M, Nakao T. Light and electron microscopic study of skin lesions in patients with hand, foot, and mouth disease. *Tohoku J Exp Med.* 1977;122:237.
94. Cherry JD, Lerner AM, Klein JO, et al. Coxsackie A9 infections with exanthems with particular reference to urticaria. *Pediatrics.* 1963;31:819.
95. Deseda-Tous J, Byatt PH, Cherry JD. Vesicular lesions in adults due to echovirus 11 infections. *Arch Dermatol.* 1977;113:1705.
96. Meade RH, Chang TW. Zosterlike eruption due to echovirus 6. *Am J Dis Child.* 1979;133:283.
97. Frothingham TE. ECHO virus type 9 associated with three cases simulating meningococcemia. *N Engl J Med.* 1958;259:484.
98. Cherry JD, Jahn CL. Virologic studies of exanthems. *J Pediatr.* 1966;68:204.
99. James WD, Odom RB, Hatch MH. Gianotti-Crosti-like eruption associated with coxsackievirus A16 infection. *J Am Acad Dermatol.* 1982;6:862.
100. Kepfer P, Hable DA, Smith TF. Viral isolation rates during summer from children with acute upper respiratory tract disease and healthy children. *Am J Clin Pathol.* 1974;61:1.
101. Rotbart HA, McCracken GH, Whitley RJ, et al. The clinical significance of enteroviruses in serious summer febrile illnesses of children. *Pediatr Infect Dis J.* 1999;18:869.
102. Jackson GG, Muidoon RL. Viruses causing common respiratory infections in man. II. Enteroviruses and paramyxoviruses. *J Infect Dis.* 1973;128:387.
103. Johnson KM, Bloom HH, Forsyth B, et al. The role of enteroviruses in respiratory disease. *Am Rev Respir Dis.* 1963; 88:240.
104. Couch RB, Cate TR, Gerone PJ, et al. Production of illness with a small particle aerosol of Coxsackie A21. *J Clin Invest.* 1965; 44:535.
105. Eckert HL, Portnoy B, Salvatore MA, et al. Group B Coxsackie virus infection in infants with acute lower respiratory disease. *Pediatrics.* 1967;39:526.
106. Flewett TH. Histological study of two cases of Coxsackie B virus pneumonia in children. *J Clin Pathol.* 1965;18:743.
107. Jahn CL, Felton OL, Cherry JD. Coxsackie B1 pneumonia in an adult. *JAMA.* 1964;189:236.
108. Boyd MT, Jordan SW, Davis LE. Fatal pneumonitis from congenital echovirus type 6 infection. *Pediatr Infect Dis J.* 1987;6: 1138.
109. Cheeseman SH, Hirsch MS, Keller EW, et al. Fatal neonatal pneumonia caused by echovirus type 9 (letter). *Am J Dis Child.* 1977;131:1169.
110. Toce SS, Keenan WJ. Congenital echovirus 11 pneumonia in association with pulmonary hypertension. *Pediatr Infect Dis J.* 1988;7:360.
111. Cherry JL, Soriano F, Jahn CL. Search for perinatal enterovirus infection. *Am J Dis Child.* 1968;116:245.
112. Steigman AJ, Lipton MM, Braspennickx H. Acute lymphonodular pharyngitis: A newly described condition due to Coxsackie A virus. *J Pediatr.* 1962;61:331.
113. Sylvest E. *Epidemic Myalgia: Bornholm Disease.* London: Oxford University Press; 1934.
114. Curnen EC, Shaw EW, Melnick JL. Disease resembling nonparalytic poliomyelitis associated with virus pathogenic for infant mice. *JAMA.* 1949;141:894.
115. Weller TH, Enders JF, Buckingham M, et al. Etiology of epidemic pleurodynia: Study of two viruses isolated from typical outbreak. *J Immunol.* 1950;65:337.
116. Bell EJ, Grist NR. ECHO viruses, carditis, and acute pleurodynia. *Am Heart J.* 1971;82:133.
117. Madhaven HN, Bedninath S, Chanraseker S. A case of pleurodynia associated with Coxsackie virus type A9. *J Assoc Physicians India.* 1977;25:491.
118. Bain HW, McLean DM, Walker SJ. Epidemic pleurodynia (Bornholm disease) due to Coxsackie B-5 virus: The interrelationship of pleurodynia, benign pericarditis, and aseptic meningitis. *Pediatrics.* 1961;27:889.
119. Disney ME, Howard EM, Wood BSB. Bornholm disease in children. *BMJ.* 1953;1:1351.
120. Warin JF, Davies JBM, Sanders FK, et al. Oxford epidemic of Bornholm disease, 1951. *BMJ.* 1953;i:1345.
121. Gordon RB, Lennette EH, Sandrock RS. The varied clinical manifestations of Coxsackie viral infections. *Arch Intern Med.* 1959;103:63.
122. Halfon N, Spector SA. Fatal echovirus type 11 infections. *Am J Dis Child.* 1981;135:1017.
123. Fukuyama Y, Ando T, Yokota J. Acute fulminant myoglobinuric polymyositis with picornavirus-like crystals. *J Neurol Neurosurg Psychiatry.* 1977;40:775.
124. Gyorkey F, Cabral GA, Gorkey PK, et al. Coxsackievirus aggregates in muscle cells of polymyositis patient. *Intervirology.* 1978;10:69.
125. Schiraldi O, Iandolo E. Polymyositis accompanying Coxsackie virus B2 infection. *Infection.* 1978;6:32.
126. Josselson J, Pula T, Sadler JH. Acute rhabdomyolysis associated with echovirus 9 infection. *Arch Intern Med.* 1980;140:1671.
127. Jehn UW, Fink MW. Myositis, myoglobinemia, and myoglobinuria associated with enterovirus echo 9 infection. *Arch Neurol.* 1980;33:457.
128. Bowles NE, Dubowitz V, Sewry CA, et al. Dermatomyositis, polymyositis, and Coxsackie-B-virus infection. *Lancet.* 1987; i:1004.
129. De Renck J, De Coster W, Inderadjaja N. Acute viral polymyositis with predominant diaphragm involvement. *J Neurol Sci.* 1977;33:453.
130. Smith WG. Adult heart disease due to the Coxsackie virus group B. *Br Heart J.* 1966;28:204.
131. Helin M, Savola J, Lapinleimu K. Cardiac manifestations during a Coxsackie B5 epidemic. *BMJ.* 1968;ii:97.
132. Grist NR. Coxsackie virus infections of the heart. In: Waterson AP, ed. *Recent Advances in Clinical Virology.* Edinburgh: Churchill Livingstone; 1977:141.
133. Grist NR, Bell EJ. A six-year study of coxsackievirus B infections in heart disease. *J Hyg.* 1974;73:165.
134. Ayuthya PSN, Jayavasu JJ, Pongpanich B. Coxsackie group B virus and primary myocardial disease in infants and children. *Am Heart J.* 1974;88:311.
135. Sainani GS, Krompotic E, Slodki SJ. Adult heart disease due to the Coxsackie virus B infection. *Medicine.* 1968;47:133.
136. Russell SJM, Bell EJ. Echoviruses and carditis. *Lancet.* 1970;1:784.
137. Grist NR, Bell EJ. Coxsackieviruses and the heart. *Am Heart J.* 1969;77:295.
138. Lerner AM, Wilson FM. Virus myocardiopathy. *Prog Med Virol.* 1973;15:63.
139. Woodruff JF. Viral myocarditis. *Am J Pathol.* 1980;101:427.
140. Grist NR, Bell EJ. Coxsackie virus and heart diseases. *BMJ.* 1968;3:556.
141. Grist NR, Bell EJ, Assad F. Enteroviruses in human disease. *Prog Med Virol.* 1978;24:114.
142. Meehan WF, Bertrand CA. Ventricular tachycardia associated with echovirus infection. *JAMA.* 1970;212:1701.
143. Schleissner LA, Fiala M, Imagawa DT, et al. Application of systolic time intervals to acute cardiomyopathy with echovirus 2. *Chest.* 1976;69:563.
144. Kanra G, Dogruel N, Tinaztepe K, et al. Myocarditis caused by echovirus 11 virus. *Turk J Pediatr.* 1978;20:24.
145. Lewes D, Rainford DJ, Lane WF. Symptomless myocarditis and myalgia in viral and *Mycoplasma pneumoniae* infections. *Br Heart J.* 1974;36:924.
146. Van Loon GR, Masson AM. Viral pericarditis. *Can Med Assn J.* 1968;99:163.
147. Bell EJ, Grist NR. Echoviruses, carditis, and acute pleurodynia. *Lancet.* 1970;i:326.
148. Berkovich S, Rodriguez-Torres R, Lin J-S. Virologic studies in children with acute myocarditis. *Am J Dis Child.* 1968;115:207.
149. Johnson RT, Portnoy B, Rogers NG, et al. Acute benign pericarditis: virologic study of 34 patients. *Arch Intern Med.* 1961;108: 823.
150. Shimizu C, Rambaud C, Cheron G, et al. Molecular identification of viruses in sudden infant death associated with myocarditis and pericarditis. *Pediatr Infect Dis J.* 1995;14:584.
151. Martin AB, Webber S, Fricker FJ, et al. Acute myocarditis. Rapid diagnosis by PCR in children. *Circulation.* 1994;90:330.
152. Lozinski GM, Davis GG, Krous HF, et al. Adenovirus myocarditis: retrospective diagnosis by gene amplification from formalin-fixed, paraffin-embedded tissues. *Hum Pathol.* 1994; 25:831.
153. Hildebrandt HM, Massab HF, Willis PW. Influenza virus pericarditis. *Am J Dis Child.* 1962;104:579.
154. Mahrholdt H, Wagner A, Deluigi CC, et al. Presentation, patterns of myocardial damage, and clinical course of viral myocarditis. *Circulation.* 2006;114:1581.
155. Centers for Disease Control. Fatal mumps myocarditis in England. *MMWR Morb Mortal Wkly Rep.* 1980;27:425.
156. Caldera R, Sarrut S, Mallet R, et al. Existetil des complications cardiaques de la vaccine? *La Semaine des hôpitaux de Paris.* 1961;37:1281.
157. Woodruff JF, Woodruff JJ. Involvement of T lymphocytes in the pathogenesis of coxsackievirus B3 heart disease. *J Immunol.* 1974;113:1726.
158. Kuhl U, Pauschinger M, Seeberg B, et al. Viral persistence in the myocardium is associated with progressive cardiac dysfunction. *Circulation.* 2005;112:1965.
159. Rose NR, Wolfgram LJ, Herskowitz A, Beisel KW. Postinfectious autoimmunity: Two distinct phases of coxsackievirus B3-induced myocarditis. *Ann N Y Acad Sci.* 1986;475:146.
160. Paque RE, Strauss DC, Nealon TJ, et al. Fractionation and immunologic assessment of KCl-extracted cardiac antigens in coxsackievirus B3 viral-induced myocarditis. *J Immunol.* 1979; 123:358.
161. Gauntt CJ, Arizpe HM, Higdon AL, et al. Anti-coxsackievirus B3 neutralizing antibodies with pathological potential. *Eur Heart J.* 1991;12:124.
162. Sainani GS, Dekate MP, Rao CP. Heart disease caused by coxsackievirus B infection. *Br Heart J.* 1975;37:819.
163. Smith WG. Coxsackie B myopericarditis in adults. *Am Heart J.* 1970;80:34.
164. Koontz CH, Ray CG. The role of Coxsackie group B virus infections in sporadic myopericarditis. *Am Heart J.* 1971;82:750.

165. Woods JD, Nimmo MJ, MacKay-Scollay EM. Acute transmural myocardial infarction associated with active Coxsackie virus B infection. *Am Heart J.* 1975;89:283.
166. Lau RC. Coxsackie B virus-specific IgM responses in coronary care unit patients. *J Med Virol.* 1986;18:193.
167. Griffiths PD, Hannington G, Booth JC. Coxsackie B virus infection and myocardial infarction. *Lancet.* 1980;i:1387.
168. DeSa'Neto A, Bullington JD, Bullington RH, et al. Coxsackie B5 heart disease. Demonstration of inferolateral wall myocardial necrosis. *Am J Med.* 1980;68:295.
169. Narula J, Khaw BA, Dec GW Jr, et al. Brief report: Recognition of acute myocarditis masquerading as acute myocardial infarction. *N Engl J Med.* 1993;328:100.
170. Sutton GC, Harding HB, Truehart RP, et al. Coxsackie B4 myocarditis in an adult: Successful isolation of virus from ventricular myocardium. *Aerospace Med.* 1967;38:66.
171. Jin O, Sole MJ, Butany JW, et al. Detection of enterovirus RNA in myocardial biopsies from patients with myocarditis and cardiomyopathy using gene amplification by polymerase chain reaction. *Circulation.* 1990;82:8.
172. Weiss LM, Movahed LA, Billingham ME, et al. Detection of coxsackievirus B3 RNA in myocardial tissues by polymerase chain reaction. *Am J Pathol.* 1991;138:497.
173. Feldman AM, McNamara D. Myocarditis. *N Engl J Med.* 2000; 343:1388.
174. Drucker NA, Colan SD, Lewis AB, et al. γ-Globulin treatment of acute myocarditis in the pediatric population. *Circulation.* 1994;89:252.
175. Latham RD, Mulrow JP, Virmani R, et al. Recently diagnosed idiopathic dilated cardiomyopathy: incidence of myocarditis and efficacy of prednisone therapy. *Am Heart J.* 1989;117:876.
176. Mason JW, O'Connell JB, Herskowitz A, et al. A clinical trial of immunosuppressive therapy for myocarditis. *N Engl J Med.* 1995;333:269.
177. Garg A, Shaiu J, Guyatt G. The ineffectiveness of immunosuppressive therapy in lymphocytic myocarditis: an overview. *Ann Intern Med.* 1998;129:317.
178. Rotbart HA. Pleconaril therapy of potentially life-threatening enterovirus infections. In: *36th Annual Meeting of the Infectious Disease Society of America.* Denver CO: Infectious Disease Society of America; 1998.
179. Gibbons JE, Goldbloom RB, Dobell ARC. Rapidly developing pericardial constriction in childhood following acute nonspecific pericarditis. *Am J Cardiol.* 1965;15:863.
180. Howard EJ, Maier HC. Constrictive pericarditis following acute Coxsackie viral pericarditis. *Am Heart J.* 1968;75:247.
181. Matthews JD, Cameron SJ, George M. Constrictive pericarditis following Coxsackie virus infection. *Thorax.* 1970;25:624.
182. Lee KJ, McCrindle BW, Bohn DJ, et al. Clinical outcomes of acute myocarditis in childhood. *Heart.* 1999;82:226.
183. McCarthy RE III, Boehmer JP, Hruban RH, et al. Long-term outcome of fulminant myocarditis as compared with acute (nonfulminant) myocarditis. *N Engl J Med.* 2000;342:690.
184. Codd MB, Sugrue DD, Gersh BJ, et al. Epidemiology of idiopathic dilated and hypertrophic cardiomyopathy. A population-based study in Olmsted County, Minnesota, 1975-1984. *Circulation.* 1989;80:564.
185. Weiss LM, Liu XF, Chang KL, et al. Detection of enteroviral RNA in idiopathic dilated cardiomyopathy and other human cardiac tissues. *J Clin Invest.* 1991;90:156.
186. Andreoletti L, Hober D, Decoene C, et al. Detection of enteroviral RNA by polymerase chain reaction in endomyocardial tissue of patients with chronic cardiac diseases. *J Med Virol.* 1996;48:53.
187. Giacca M, Severini GM, Mestroni L, et al. Low frequency of detection by nested polymerase chain reaction of enterovirus ribonucleic acid in endomyocardial tissue of patients with idiopathic dilated cardiomyopathy. *J Am Coll Cardiol.* 1994;24: 1033.
188. de Leeuw N, Melchers WJG, Balk AHMM, et al. No evidence for persistent enterovirus infection in patients with end-stage idiopathic dilated cardiomyopathy. *J Infect Dis.* 1998;178:256.
189. Griffin LD, Kearney D, Ni J, et al. Analysis of formalin-fixed and frozen myocardial autopsy samples for viral genome in childhood myocarditis and dilated cardiomyopathy with endocardial fibroelastosis using polymerase chain reaction (PCR). *Cardiovasc Pathol.* 1995;4:3.
190. Grasso M, Arbustini E, Silini E, et al. Search for coxsackievirus B3 RNA in idiopathic dilated cardiomyopathy using gene amplification by polymerase chain reaction. *Am J Cardiol.* 1992;69:658.
191. Muir P, Nicholson F, Illavia SJ, et al. Serological and molecular evidence of enterovirus infection in patients with end-stage dilated cardiomyopathy. *Heart.* 1996;76:243.
192. Li Y, Bourlet T, Andreoletti L, et al. Enteroviral capsid protein VP1 is present in myocardial tissues from some patients with myocarditis or dilated cardiomyopathy. *Circulation.* 2000;101: 231.
193. Mahon NG, Zal B, Arno G, et al. Absence of viral nucleic acids in early and late dilated cardiomyopathy. *Heart.* 2001;86:687.
194. Baker DA, Phillips CA. Maternal and neonatal infection with coxsackievirus. *Obstet Gynecol.* 1980;55:12.
195. Talsma M, Vegting M, Hess J. Generalized Coxsackie A9 infection in a neonate presenting with pericarditis. *Br Heart J.* 1984;52:683.
196. Wright HT, Landing BH, Lennette EH, et al. Fatal infection in an infant associated with Coxsackie virus group A, type 16. *N Engl J Med.* 1963;268:1041.
197. Gear JHS, Measroch V. Coxsackievirus infection of the newborn. *Prog Med Virol.* 1973;15:42.
198. Modlin JF. Perinatal echovirus infection: Insights from a literature review of 61 cases of serious infection and 16 outbreaks in nurseries. *Rev Infect Dis.* 1986;8:918.
199. Modlin JF, Kinney JS. Perinatal enterovirus infections. In: Aronoff SC, Hughes WT, Kohl S, et al., eds. Advances in Pediatric Infectious Diseases. Vol. 2. Chicago: Year Book Medical Publishers; 1986:57.
200. Kinney JS, McCray E, Kaplan JE, et al. Risk factors associated with echovirus 11 infection in a newborn nursery. *Pediatr Infect Dis J.* 1986;5:192.
201. Modlin JF. Fatal echovirus 11 disease in premature neonates. *Pediatrics.* 1980;66:775.
202. Piraino FF, Sedmak G, Raab K. Echovirus 11 infections of newborns with mortality during the 1979 enterovirus season in Milwaukee, Wis. *Public Health Reports (Washington DC).* 1982;97:346.
203. Khetsuriani N, Lamonte A, Oberste M, et al. Neonatal enterovirus infections reported to the national enterovirus surveillance system in the United States, 1983-2003. *Pediatr Infect Dis J.* 2006;25:889.
204. Centers for Disease Control and Prevention. Increased detections and severe neonatal disease associated with coxsackievirus B1 infection—United States, 2007. *MMWR Morb Mort Wkly Rep.* 2007;57:553.
205. Modlin JF, Kinney JS. Perinatal enterovirus infections. In: Aronoff SC, Hughes WT, Kohl S, et al, eds. Advances in Pediatric Infectious Diseases. Vol. 2. Chicago: Year Book Medical Publishers; 1987.
206. Modlin JF, Bowman M. Perinatal transmission of Coxsackie B3 virus in a murine model. *J Infect Dis.* 1987;156:21.
207. Modlin JF, Polk BF, Horton P, et al. Perinatal echovirus 11 infection: risk of transmission during a community outbreak. *N Engl J Med.* 1981;305:368.
208. Jones MJU, Kolb M, Votava HJ, et al. Intrauterine echovirus type 11 infection. *Mayo Clin Proc.* 1980;55:509.
209. Reyes MP, Ostrea EM, Roskamp J, et al. Disseminated neonatal echovirus 11 disease following antenatal maternal infection with a virus-positive cervix and virus negative gastrointestinal tract. *J Med Virol.* 1983;12:155.
210. Yoshioka I, Horstmann DM. Viremia in infection due to echo virus type 9. *N Engl J Med.* 1961;262:224.
211. Kaplan MH, Klein SW, McPhee J, et al. Group B coxsackievirus infections in infants younger than three months of age: A serious childhood illness. *Rev Infect Dis.* 1983;5:1019.
212. Kunin CM. Virus-tissue union and the pathogenesis of enterovirus infections. *J Immunol.* 1962;88:556.
213. Eichenwald HF, Kotsevalov O. Immunologic responses of premature and full-term infants to infection with certain viruses. *Pediatrics.* 1960;25:829.
214. Rager-Zisman B, Allison AC. The role of antibody and host cells in the resistance of mice against infection by Coxsackie B-3 virus. *J Gen Virol.* 1973;19:329.
215. Woodruff J. Lack of correlation between neutralizing antibody production and suppression of Coxsackie B-3 replication in target organs: evidence for involvement of mononuclear inflammatory cells in host defense. *J Immunol.* 1979;123:31.
216. Berry PJ, Nagington J. Fatal infection with echovirus 11. *Arch Dis Child.* 1982;57:22.
217. Drew JH. Echo 11 virus outbreak in a nursery associated with myocarditis. *Aust J Pediatr.* 1973;9:90.
218. Georgieff MK, Johnson DE, Thompson TR, et al. Fulminant hepatic necrosis in an infant with perinatally acquired echovirus 21 infection. *Pediatr Infect Dis J.* 1987;6:71.
219. Spector SA, Straube RC. Protean manifestations of perinatal enterovirus infection. *West J Med.* 1983;138:847.
220. Speer ME, Yawn DH. Fatal hepatoadrenal necrosis in the neonate associated with echovirus types 11 and 12 presenting as a surgical emergency. *J Pediatr Surg.* 1984;19:591.
221. Wreghitt TG, Gandy GM, King A, et al. Fatal neonatal echo 7 virus infection (letter). *Lancet.* 1984;2:465.
222. Chambon M, Delage C, Bailly J-L, et al. Fatal hepatic necrosis in a neonate with echovirus 20 infection: use of the polymerase chain reaction to detect enterovirus in liver tissue. *Clin Infect Dis.* 1997;24:523.
223. Mostoufizadeh G, Lack EE, Gang DL, et al. Postmortem manifestations of echovirus 11 sepsis in five newborn infants. *Hum Pathol.* 1983;14:819.
224. Johnston JM, Overall JC. Intravenous immunoglobulin in disseminated neonatal echovirus 11 infection. *Pediatr Infect Dis J.* 1989;8:254.
225. Collaborative Antiviral Study Group. *Clinical Trials. Pleconaril enteroviral sepsis syndrome.* Protocol CASG 106 (DMID#99-018). Accessed on: 11/10/08. <http://www.casg.uab.edu/new%20clinical%20trials%20page.htm>.
226. McKinney RE, Katz SL, Wilfert CM. Chronic enteroviral meningoencephalitis in agammaglobulinemic patients. *Rev Infect Dis.* 1987;9:334.
227. Padate BP, Keidan J. Enteroviral meningoencephalitis in a patient with non-Hodgkin's lymphoma treated previously with rituximab. *Clin Lab Haematol.* 2006;28:69.
228. Quartier P, Tournilhac O, Archimbaud C, et al. Enteroviral meningoencephalitis after anti-CD20 (rituximab) treatment. *Clin Infect Dis.* 2003;26:e47.
229. O'Neil KM, Pallansch MA, Winkelstein JA, et al. Chronic group A coxsackievirus infection in agammaglobulinemia: demonstration of genomic variation of serotypically identical isolates persistently excreted from the same patient. *J Infect Dis.* 1988;157:183.
230. Webster ADB. Echovirus disease in hypogammaglobulinaemic patients. *Clin Rheum Dis.* 1984;10:189.
231. Mease PJ, Ochs HD, Wedgewood RJ. Successful treatment of echovirus meningoencephalitis and myositis-fasciitis with intravenous immune globulin therapy in a patient with X-linked hypogammaglobulinemia. *N Engl J Med.* 1981;304:1278.
232. Rotbart HA, Webster ADB. Treatment of potentially life-threatening enterovirus infections with pleconaril. *Clin Infect Dis.* 2001;32:228.
233. Biggs DD, Toorkey BC, Carrigan DR, et al. Disseminated echovirus infection complicating bone marrow transplantation. *Am J Med.* 1990;88:421.
234. Aquino VM, Farah RA, Lee ME, et al. Disseminated Coxsackie A9 infection complicating bone marrow transplantation. *Pediatr Infect Dis J.* 1996;15:1053.
235. Galama JMD, de Leeuw N, Wittebol S, et al. Prolonged enteroviral infection in a patient who developed pericarditis and heart failure after bone marrow transplantation. *Clin Infect Dis.* 1996;22:1004.
236. Townsend TR, Bolyard EA, Yolken RH, et al. Outbreak of Coxsackie A1 gastroenteritis: A complication of bone-marrow transplantation. *Lancet.* 1982;i:820.
237. Kono R. Apollo 11 disease or acute hemorrhagic conjunctivitis: A pandemic of a new enterovirus infection of the eyes. *Am J Epidemiol.* 1975;101:383.
238. Kono R, Sasagawa A, Ishii K, et al. Pandemic of new type of conjunctivitis. *Lancet.* 1972;2:1191.
239. Mirkovic RR, Kono R, Yin-Murphy M, et al. Enterovirus type 70: The etiologic agent of pandemic acute hemorrhagic conjunctivitis. *Bull World Health Organ.* 1973;49:341.
240. Mirkovic RR, Schmidt NJ, Yin-Murphy M, et al. Enterovirus etiology of the 1970 Singapore epidemic of acute conjunctivitis. *Intervirology.* 1974;4:119.
241. Yin-Murphy M, Lim KH, Yo YM. A coxsackievirus type A24 epidemic of acute conjunctivitis. *Southeast Asian J Trop Med Pub Health.* 1976;7:1.
242. Yin-Murphy M, Lim KH. Picornavirus epidemic conjunctivitis in Singapore. *Lancet.* 1972;2:857.
243. Higgins PG, Scott RJ, Davies PM, et al. A comparative study of viruses associated with acute hemorrhagic conjunctivitis. *J Clin Pathol.* 1974;27:292.
244. Christopher S, Theogaraj S, Godbole S, et al. An epidemic of acute hemorrhagic conjunctivitis due to coxsackievirus A24. *J Infect Dis.* 1982;146:16.
245. Kono R, Miyamura K, Tajiri E, et al. Neurologic complications associated with acute hemorrhagic conjunctivitis virus infection and its serologic confirmation. *J Infect Dis.* 1974;129:590.
246. Ray I, Roy IS, Sarkhar JK, et al. Laboratory investigations of an epidemic of conjunctivitis in Calcutta: A preliminary report. *Bull Calcutta Sch Trop Med.* 1972;20:1.
247. Hierholzer JC, Hilliard KA, Esposito JJ. Serosurvey for "acute hemorrhagic conjunctivitis" virus (enterovirus 70) antibodies in the southeastern United States, with review of the literature and some epidemiologic implications. *Am J Epidemiol.* 1975;102:533.
248. Sklar VE, Patriarca PA, Onorato IM, et al. Clinical findings and results of treatment in an outbreak of acute hemorrhagic conjunctivitis in southern Florida. *Am J Ophthalmol.* 1983;95:45.
249. Kuritsky JN, Weaver JH, Bernard KW, et al. An outbreak of acute hemorrhagic conjunctivitis in central Minnesota. *Am J Ophthalmol.* 1983;96:449.
250. Centers for Disease Control. Acute hemorrhagic conjunctivitis caused by coxsackievirus A24—Caribbean. *MMWR Morb Mortal Wkly Rep.* 1987;36:245.
251. Centers for Disease Control. Acute hemorrhagic conjunctivitis caused by coxsackievirus A24 variant—Puerto Rico. *Morb Mortal Wkly Rep.* 1988;37:123.
252. Miyamura K, Tanimura M, Takeda N, et al. Evolution of enterovirus 70 in nature: All isolates were recently derived from a common ancestor. *Arch Virol.* 1986;89:1.
253. Stanton GJ, Langford MP, Baron S. Effect of interferon, elevated temperature, and cell type on replication of acute hemorrhagic conjunctivitis viruses. *Infect Immun.* 1977;18:370.
254. Goh KT, Doraisingham S, Yin-Murphy M. An epidemic of acute conjunctivitis caused by enterovirus-70 in Singapore in 1980. *Southeast Asian J Trop Med Pub Health.* 1981;12:473.
255. Arnow PM, Hierholzer JC, Higbee J, et al. Acute hemorrhagic conjunctivitis: A mixed virus outbreak among Vietnamese refugees on Guam. *Am J Epidemiol.* 1977;105:69.
256. Onorato IM, Morens DM, Schonberger LB, et al. Acute hemorrhagic conjunctivitis caused by enterovirus type 70: an epidemic in American Samoa. *Am J Trop Med Hyg.* 1985;34:984.
257. Kono R, Sasagawa A, Miyamura K, et al. Serologic characterization and seroepidemiologic studies on acute hemorrhagic conjunctivitis (AHC) virus. *Am J Epidemiol.* 1975;101:444.
258. Kono R, Uchida Y. Acute hemorrhagic conjunctivitis. *Ophthalmol Dig.* 1977;39:14.
259. Kono R, Miyamura K, Tajiri E, et al. Virological and serological studies of neurological complications of acute hemorrhagic conjunctivitis in Thailand. *J Infect Dis.* 1977;135:706.
260. Hung TS, Sung SM, Liang HC, et al. Radiculomyelitis following acute hemorrhagic conjunctivitis. *Brain.* 1976;99:771.
261. Katiyar BC, Misra S, Singh RB, et al. Adult polio-like syndrome following Enterovirus 70 conjunctivitis (natural history of the disease). *Acta Neurol Scand.* 1983;67:263.

262. Wadia NH, Katrak SM, Misra VP, et al. Polio-like motor paralysis associated with acute hemorrhagic conjunctivitis in an outbreak in 1981 in Bombay. *J Infect Dis.* 1983;147:660.
263. Kono R, Uchida N, Sasagawa A, et al. Neurovirulence of acute hemorrhagic conjunctivitis virus in monkeys. *Lancet.* 1973;1:61.
264. Yin-Murphy M. Simple tests for the diagnosis of picornavirus epidemic conjunctivitis (acute haemorrhagic conjunctivitis). *Bull World Health Organ.* 1976;54:675.
265. Lansky LL, Krugman S, Huq G. Anicteric Coxsackie B hepatitis. *J Pediatr.* 1979;94:64.
266. Leggiadro RJ, Chwatsky DN, Zucker SW. Echovirus 3 infection associated with anicteric hepatitis. *Am J Dis Child.* 1982; 136:744.
267. O'Shaughnessey WJ, Buechner HA. Hepatitis associated with a Coxsackie B5 virus infection during late pregnancy. *JAMA.* 1962;179:71.
268. Morris JA, Elisberg BL, Pond WL, et al. Hepatitis associated with Coxsackie virus group A, type 4. *N Engl J Med.* 1962;267:1230.
269. Sun NC, Smith VM. Hepatitis associated with myocarditis: Unusual manifestation of infection with Coxsackie virus group B, type 3. *N Engl J Med.* 1966;274:190.
270. Gregor GR, Geller SA, Walker GF, et al. Coxsackie hepatitis in an adult with ultrastructural demonstration of the virus. *Mt Sinai J Med.* 1975;42:575.
271. Arnesjo B, Eden T, Ihse I, et al. Enterovirus infections in acute pancreatitis: a possible etiologic connection. *Scand J Gastroenterol.* 1976;11:645.
272. Imrle CW, Ferguson JC, Sommerville RG. Coxsackie and mumps virus infection in a prospective study of acute pancreatitis. *Gut.* 1977;18:53.
273. Craighead JE. The role of viruses in the pathogenesis of pancreatic disease and diabetes mellitus. *Prog Med Virol.* 1975; 19:162.
274. Ursing B. Acute pancreatitis in Coxsackie B infection. *BMJ.* 1973;iii:524.
275. Ramos-Alvarez M, Olarte J. Diarrheal diseases of children. *Am J Dis Child.* 1964;107:218.
276. Steinhoff MC. Viruses and diarrhea: a review. *Am J Dis Child.* 1978;132:302.
277. Yow DM, Melnick JL, Blattner JR, et al. Enteroviruses in infantile diarrhea. *Am J Hyg.* 1963;77:283.
278. Patel JR, Daniel J, Mathan VI. An epidemic of acute diarrhoea in rural southern India associated with echovirus type 11 infection. *J Hyg.* 1985;95:483.
279. Glasgow LA, Balduzzi P. Isolation of Coxsackie virus group A, type 4, from a patient with hemolytic uremic syndrome. *N Engl J Med.* 1965;273:754.
280. O'Regan S, Robitaille P, Mongeau JG, et al. The hemolytic-uremic syndrome associated with echo 22 infection. *Clin Pediatr.* 1980;19:125.
281. Ray CG, Tucker VL, Harris DJ, et al. Enteroviruses associated with the hemolytic-uremic syndrome. *Pediatrics.* 1970;46:378.
282. Aronson MD, Phillips CA. Coxsackievirus B5 infections in acute oliguric renal failure. *J Infect Dis.* 1975;132:303.
283. Craighead JE, Mahoney EM, Carver DH, et al. Orchitis due to Coxsackie virus group B, type 5. *N Engl J Med.* 1962;267:498.
284. Welliver RC, Cherry JD. Aseptic meningitis and orchitis associated with echovirus 6 infection. *J Pediatr.* 1978;92:239.
285. Ager EA, Felsenstein WC, Alexander ER, et al. An epidemic of illness due to Coxsackie virus group B, type 2. *JAMA.* 1964;187:251.
286. Willems WR, Hornig C, Bauer H, et al. A case of Coxsackie A9 virus infection with orchitis. *J Med Virol.* 1978;3:137.
287. Murphy AM, Simmul R. Coxsackie B4 virus infections in New South Wales during 1962. *Med J Aust.* 1964;2:443.
288. Blotzer JW, Myers AR. Echovirus associated polyarthritis: Report of a case with synovial fluid and synovial histologic characterization. *Arthritis Rheum.* 1978;21:978.
289. Kujala G, Newman JH. Isolation of echovirus type 11 from synovial fluid in acute monocytic arthritis. *Arthritis Rheum.* 1985;28:98.
290. Van der Sar A. Acute infectious lymphocytosis with echovirus type 25. *West Indian Med J.* 1979;28:185.
291. Norwitz MS, Moore GT. Acute infectious lymphocytosis: an etiologic study of an outbreak. *N Engl J Med.* 1968;279:399.
292. Barrett-Connor E. Is insulin-dependent diabetes mellitus caused by coxsackievirus B infection? A review of the epidemiologic evidence. *Rev Infect Dis.* 1985;7:207.
293. Craighead JE, Huber SA, Sriram S. Animal models of picornavirus-induced autoimmune disease: Their possible relevance to human disease. *Lab Invest.* 1990;63:432.
294. Banatvala JE. Insulin-dependent (juvenile-onset, type 1) diabetes mellitus Coxsackie B viruses revisited. *Prog Med Virol.* 1987;34:33.
295. Yoon JW. The role of viruses and environmental factors in the induction of diabetes. *Curr Top Microbiol Immunol.* 1990;164:95.
296. Rewers M, Atkinson M. The possible role of enteroviruses in diabetes mellitus. In: Rotbart HA, ed. *Human Enterovirus Infections.* Washington DC: American Society for Microbiology; 1995:353.
297. Gamble DR, Taylor KW. Seasonal incidence of diabetes mellitus. *BMJ.* 1969;3:631.
298. Gleason RE, Kahn CB, Funk IB, et al. Seasonal incidence of insulin-dependent diabetes in Massachusetts, 1964-1973. *Int J Epidemiol.* 1982;11:39.
299. Rewers M, LaPorte R, Walczak M, et al. Apparent epidemic of insulin-dependent diabetes mellitus in midwestern Poland. *Diabetes.* 1987;36:106.
300. Huff JC, Hierholzer JC, Farris WA. An "outbreak" of juvenile diabetes mellitus: consideration of a viral etiology. *Am J Epidemiol.* 1974;100:277.
301. Hierholzer JC, Farris WA. Follow-up of children infected in a coxsackievirus B3 and B4 outbreak: no evidence of diabetes mellitus. *J Infect Dis.* 1974;129:741.
302. Dippe SE, Bennett PH, Miller M, et al. Lack of causal association between Coxsackie B4 virus infection and diabetes. *Lancet.* 1975;i:1314.
303. Hartig PC, Madge GE, Webb SR. Diversity within a human isolate of Coxsackie B4: relationship to viral-induced diabetes mellitus. *J Med Virol.* 1983;11:23.
304. Andreoletti L, Hober D, Hober-Vandenberghe C, et al. Detection of Coxsackie B virus RNA sequences in whole blood samples from adult patients at the onset of type I diabetes mellitus. *J Med Virol.* 1997;52:121.
305. Clements GB, Galbraith DN, Taylor KW. Coxsackie B virus infection and onset of childhood diabetes. *Lancet.* 1995;346:221.
306. Yoon JW, Austin M, Onodera T, Notkins AL. Virus-induced diabetes mellitus: isolation of a virus from the pancreas of a child with diabetic ketoacidosis. *N Engl J Med.* 1979;300:1173.
307. Gladish R, Hofmann W, Waldherr R. Myocarditis and insulitis in coxsackievirus infection. *Z Kardiol.* 1976;65:835.
308. Helfand RF, Gary HE Jr, Freeman CY, et al., for the Pittsburgh Diabetes Research Group. Serologic evidence of an association between enteroviruses and onset of type 1 diabetes mellitus. *J Infect Dis.* 1995;172:1206.
309. D'Alessio DJ. A case-control study of group B coxsackievirus immunoglobulin M antibody prevalence and HLA-DR antigens in newly diagnosed cases of insulin-dependent diabetes mellitus. *Am J Epidemiol.* 1992;135:1331.
310. Gamble DR, Cumming H. Coxsackie B virus and juvenile-onset diabetes. *Lancet.* 1985;2:455.
311. Tuvemo T, Dahlquist G, Frisk G, et al. The Swedish Childhood Diabetes Study. III. IgM against Coxsackie B viruses in newly diagnosed type 1 (insulin-dependent) diabetic children: no evidence of increased antibody frequency. *Diabetologia.* 1989;32:745.
312. Frisk G, Fohlman J, Kobbah M, et al. High frequency of Virus-B-virus specific IgM in children developing type I diabetes during a period of high diabetes morbidity. *J Med Virol.* 1985;17:219.
313. Oldstone MBA. Molecular mimicry and autoimmune disease. *Cell.* 1987;50:819.
314. See DM, Tilles JG. Pathogenesis of virus-induced diabetes in mice. *J Infect Dis.* 1995;171:1131.
315. Hiltunen M, Hyoty H, Knip M, et al. Islet cell antibody seroconversion in children is temporally associated with enterovirus infections. *J Infect Dis.* 1997;175:554.
316. Solimena M, De Camilli P. Coxsackieviruses and diabetes. *Nat Med.* 1995;1:25.
317. Hagiwara A, Yoneyama T, Takami S, et al. Genetic and phenotypic characteristics of enterovirus 71 isolates from patients with encephalitis and with hand, foot, and mouth disease. *Arch Virol.* 1984;79:273.
318. Hashimoto I, Hagiwara A, Kodama H. Neurovirulence in cynomolgus monkeys of enterovirus 71 isolated from a patient with hand, foot, and mouth disease. *Arch Virol.* 1978;56:257.
319. Schmidt NJ, Lennette EH, Ho HH. An apparently new enterovirus isolated from patients with disease of the central nervous system. *J Infect Dis.* 1974;129:304.
320. Deibel R, Gross L, Collins DN. Isolation of a new enterovirus. *Proc Soc Exp Biol Med.* 1975;148:203.
321. Kennett ML, Birch CJ, Lewis FA, et al. Enterovirus type 71 infection in Melbourne. *Bull World Health Organ.* 1974;51:609.
322. Tagaya I, Takayama R, Hagiwara A. A large-scale epidemic of hand, foot and mouth disease associated with enterovirus 71 infection in Japan in 1978. *Jpn J Med Sci Biol.* 1981;34:191.
323. Bloomberg J, Lycke E, Ahlfors K, et al. New enterovirus type associated with epidemic of aseptic meningitis and/or hand, foot, and mouth disease. *Lancet.* 1974;ii:122.
324. Moses EB, Narian JP, Hatch MH, et al. Isolation of echovirus type 11 and enterovirus type 71 in a day care winter outbreak. *J Arkansas Med Soc.* 1987;83:469.
325. Sohier R. Enterovirus type 71 surveillance: France. World Health Organ *Wkly Epidemiol Rec.* 1979;54:219.
326. Nagy G, Takatsy S, Kukan E, et al. Virological diagnosis of enterovirus type 71 infections: Experiences gained during an epidemic of acute CNS diseases in Hungary in 1978. *Arch Virol.* 1982;71:217.
327. Chumakov MP, Voroshilova MK, Shindarov L, et al. Enterovirus 71 isolated from cases of poliomyelitis-like disease in Bulgaria. *Arch Virol.* 1979;60:329.
328. Alexander JP, Baden L, Pallansch MA, et al. Enterovirus 71 infections and neurologic disease—United States, 1977-1991. *J Infect Dis.* 1994;169:905.
329. Cardosa MJ, Perera D, Brown BA, et al. Molecular epidemiology of human enterovirus 71 strains and recent outbreaks in the Asia-Pacific region: comparative analysis of the VP1 and VP4 genes. *Emerg Infect Dis.* 2003;9:461.
330. Chonmaitree T, Menegus MA, Schervish-Swierkosz EM, et al. Enterovirus 71 infection: Report of an outbreak with two cases of paralysis and a review of the literature. *Pediatrics.* 1981; 67:489.
331. Samuda GM, Chang WK, Yeung CY, et al. Monoplegia caused by enterovirus 71: An outbreak in Hong Kong. *Pediatr Infect Dis J.* 1987;6:206.
332. Miwa C, Ohtani M, Watanabe H, et al. Epidemic of hand, foot and mouth disease in Gifu prefecture in 1978. *Jpn J Med Sci Biol.* 1980;33:167.
333. Modlin JF. Enterovirus déjà vu. *N Engl J Med.* 2007;356:1204.
334. Auvinen P, Hyypia T. Echoviruses include genetically distinct serotypes. *J Gen Virol.* 1990;71:2133.
335. Triantafilou K, Triantafilou M, Takada Y, et al. Human parechovirus 1 utilizes integrins alphavbeta3 and alphavbeta1 as receptors. *J Virol.* 2000;74:5856-5862.
336. Nix WA, Maher K, Johansson ES, et al. Detection of all known parechoviruses by real-time PCR. *J Clin Microbiol.* 2008;46: 2519-2524.
337. *"Human parechovirus."* 15 February 2009 <http://www.picornaviridae.com/parechovirus/hpev/hpev.htm>.
338. Wolthers KC, Benschop KSM, Shinkel J, et al. Human parechoviruses as an important viral cause of sepsislike illness and meningitis in young children. *Clin Infect Dis.* 2008;47:358.
339. de Vries M, Pyrc K, Berkhout R, et al. Human parechovirus type 1, 3, 4, 5, and 6 detection in picornavirus cultures. *J Clin Microbiol.* 2008;46:759.
340. Joki-Korpela P, Hyypia T. Parechoviruses, a novel group of human picornaviruses. *Ann Med.* 2001;33:466.
341. Harvala H, Robertson I, McWilliam Leitch EC, et al. Epidemiology and clinical associations of human parechovirus respiratory infections. *J Clin Microbiol.* 2008;46:3446.
342. Verboon-Maciolek MA, Groenendaal F, Hahn CD, et al. Human parechovirus causes encephalitis with white matter injury in neonates. *Ann Neurol.* 2008;64:266-273.
343. Stanway G, Joki-Korpela P, Hyypiä T. Human parechoviruses: Biology and clinical significance. *Rev Med Virol.* 2000;10: 57-69.
344. Abed Y, Boivin G. Human parechovirus types 1, 2, and 3 infections in Canada. *Emerg Infect Dis.* 2006;12:969-975.
345. van der Sanden S, de Bruin E, Vennema H, et al. Prevalence of human parechovirus in the Netherlands in 2000 to 2007. *J Clin Microbiol.* 2008;46:2884-2889.
346. Khetsuriani N, Lamonte-Fowlkes A, Oberst S., et al. Enterovirus-surveillance–United States, 1970-2005. *MMWR Surveill Summ.* 2006;55:1-20.

173

Hepatitis A Virus

ANNEMARIE WASLEY | STEPHEN M. FEINSTONE | BETH P. BELL*

Hepatitis A is generally an acute, self-limited infection of the liver by an enterically transmitted picornavirus, hepatitis A virus (HAV). Infection may be asymptomatic or result in acute hepatitis. Rarely, fulminant hepatitis can ensue. Although the duration and severity of symptoms vary widely, hepatitis A infections never cause chronic liver disease. The availability of effective vaccines against hepatitis A has markedly affected the epidemiology of hepatitis A in places where the vaccines are widely used, as in the United States (see later).

History

The earliest accounts of contagious jaundice are from ancient China.[1] Although the symptoms that were described are similar to those currently found in people with hepatitis A, it should be remembered that a number of other infections produce similar symptoms. The earliest outbreaks of hepatitis that were almost certainly hepatitis A were documented in Europe in the 17th and 18th centuries, especially during periods of war. From 1855, the disease became known as "catarrhal jaundice" because the pathologists Bamberger and Virchow believed that the disease was caused by blockage of the common bile duct by a plug of inspissated mucus.[2] The first suggestion that the disease was caused by an infectious agent was made by McDonald,[3] who, unable to demonstrate the involvement of enteric bacteria, suggested that the infection might be caused by a virus. Shortly thereafter, Cockayne[4] proposed that the sporadic and the epidemic forms of jaundice were manifestations of the same disease. In 1923, Blumer analyzed a large number of epidemics of hepatitis in the United States and identified its predilection for young adults and children and peak incidence in winter and fall.[5] Hepatitis A had an incubation period of between 15 and 49 days and was transmitted by the fecal-oral route.[6-8] Later studies demonstrated that the virus could be detected in feces or blood during the acute infection, that infection could be transmitted experimentally by both the oral and parenteral routes, and that infection was followed by long-term immunity and could be prevented by previous administration of normal human immunoglobulin (IG).[5,9] In addition, the disease was shown to be associated with a filterable agent resistant to heating at 56°C for 30 minutes and resistant to diethyl ether. In the 1950s and 1960s, Krugman[10] expanded these observations by a series of studies in human volunteers that further defined the incubation period, period of infectivity, and period of viremia, and they developed standardized reagents representing hepatitis A. In 1973, Feinstone and colleagues[11] detected 27-nm virus-like particles in the stools of volunteers infected with hepatitis A and demonstrated that they were aggregated by convalescent but not by preinfection serum, thus indicating that the particles represented the etiologic agent of the disease. The identification of HAV, transmission of the disease to marmosets and chimpanzees, propagation of HAV in cell culture, and molecular cloning of the viral genome ushered in a new era of research that culminated almost two decades later in the development and licensing of effective vaccines.[12-18]

---

*All material in this chapter is in the public domain, with the exception of any borrowed figures or tables.

Classification and Physicochemical and Biologic Properties of Hepatitis A Virus

HAV is a nonenveloped, positive-strand RNA virus member of the Picornaviridae family, which includes the enteroviruses, parechoviruses, and rhinoviruses of humans, as well as the aphthoviruses (foot-and-mouth disease viruses) of hoofed animals and cardioviruses (encephalomyocarditis virus) of mice. Although HAV shares general structure and genomic organization with the other picornaviruses, it has limited nucleotide sequence homology and certain distinguishing characteristics that have resulted in its being classified in its own genus, Hepatovirus.[19-21] Recently, avian encephalomyelitis virus has been tentatively reclassified as a second member of the Hepatovirus genus.[22] Human isolates of HAV are relatively closely related based on partial genomic sequences. However, human HAV strains have been divided into two major genotypes (I and III) and two minor genotypes (II and VII) that differ from each other by 15% to 25% of the nucleotides within a region around the VP1-2A (see later) junction. The other three genotypes, genotypes IV, V, and VI, are all single simian HAV isolates.[23] Phenotypic differences such as disease severity among the genotypes have not been recognized, although mutations in the 2B coding region may be associated with severe and fulminant disease.[24,25] Although antigenic variants exist, among all the genotypes, there is only one recognized serotype of HAV based on cross-neutralization studies.

STRUCTURE

HAV is a 27- to 28-nm spherical, nonenveloped virus[11] (Fig. 173-1) with a surface structure suggesting icosahedral symmetry.[26] High-resolution x-ray crystallography of HAV has not yet been achieved. However, good quality cryoelectron microscopy has confirmed the icosahedral symmetry of the virion with typical picornavirus three- and fivefold axes and 60 repeated pentamers comprising the capsid (Figs. 173-1 and 173-2). The cryoelectron microscopic views of HAV reveal the plateau surrounding the fivefold axis that is typical for picornaviruses, but not the pit or canyon believed to be the receptor binding site of enteroviruses and rhinoviruses (see Fig. 173-2). The prominence at the threefold axis of symmetry is distinct from other picornaviruses and is believed to be the major antigenic site at which neutralizing antibodies are targeted (Holland Cheng, personal communication, 2009).

Purification of virus from clinical samples or tissue culture yields three distinct populations of particles[27]: mature hepatitis A virions that band at 1.32 to 1.34 g/cm³ in cesium chloride and sediment at approximately 160 S (similar to enteroviruses and cardioviruses), a lower density fraction that bands at approximately 1.27 g/cm³ in cesium chloride, and sediments at 70 to 80 S and may represent empty capsids or particles with incomplete genomes and a high-density fraction (1.4 g/cm³) that may represent particles with a more open virion structure that allows increased penetration and binding of cesium chloride to the viral particle. These high-density particles have been shown to contain RNA but tend to be less stable than mature virions.[28,29]

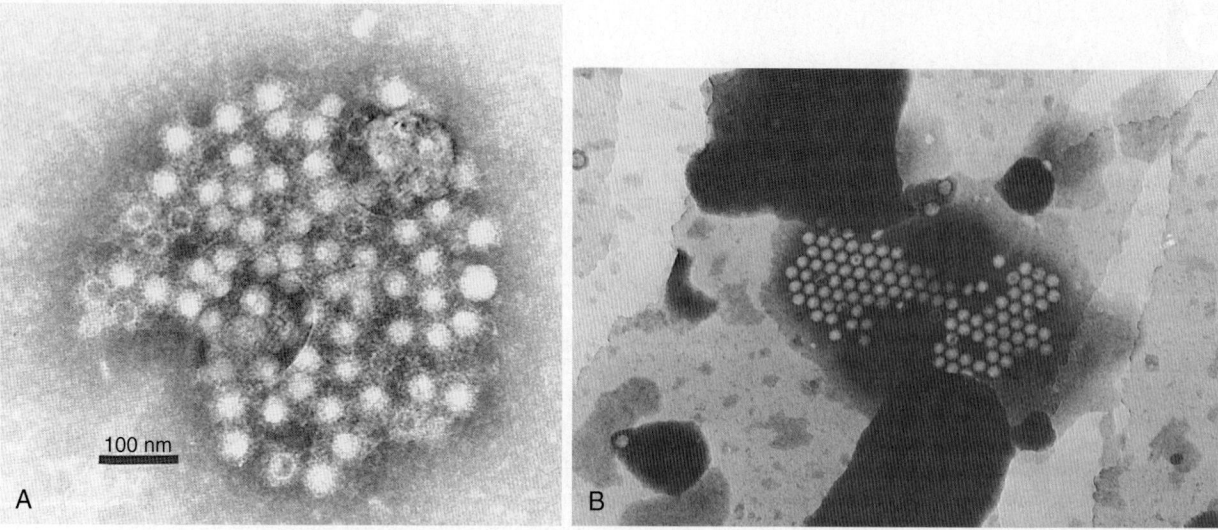

Figure 173-1   Electron micrographs of hepatitis A virus particles (A) aggregated by antibody, 27 to 28 nm in diameter and highly concentrated, purified hepatitis A virus from human feces (B).

RESISTANCE TO PHYSICAL AND CHEMICAL AGENTS

HAV is a relatively stable virus under a variety of environmental conditions. HAV is more resistant to heat than other picornaviruses and may not be completely inactivated (depending on the conditions) by exposure to 60°C for 10 to 12 hours.[30-32] Complete inactivation in food requires heating to higher than 85°C for at least 1 minute.[32] Outbreaks of hepatitis A have been reported after ingestion of steamed shellfish, suggesting that the internal temperature achieved by steaming sometimes may be insufficient to destroy the virus.[33] However, HAV can be reliably inactivated by autoclaving (121°C for 30 minutes).[34] Recent studies have shown that HAV can be inactivated in shellfish by a nonthermal method using high hydrostatic pressure.[35] The virus is resistant to most organic solvents and detergents and to a pH as low as 3.[34,36] HAV can be inactivated by many common disinfecting chemicals including hypochlorite (bleach), and quaternary ammonium formulations containing 23% HCl (found in many toilet bowl cleaners).[34] Currently licensed vaccines are inactivated by 1:4000 formalin at room temperature for at least 15 days to exceed complete inactivation by at least threefold. As a result of several outbreaks of hepatitis A in hemophiliacs who received factor VIII concentrates that had been treated by a solvent detergent method for inactivation of lipid-enveloped viruses, interest has focused on techniques capable of inactivating nonenveloped viruses without compromising the biologic activity of the product.[37] Various manufacturers use different techniques to inactivate or remove HAV as well as human parvovirus B19. These include nanofiltration and other purification techniques, sensitive nucleic acid testing such as polymerase chain reaction (PCR) on minipools of source plasma, pasteurization at of 60°C for 10 hours and dry heat on lyophilized products.

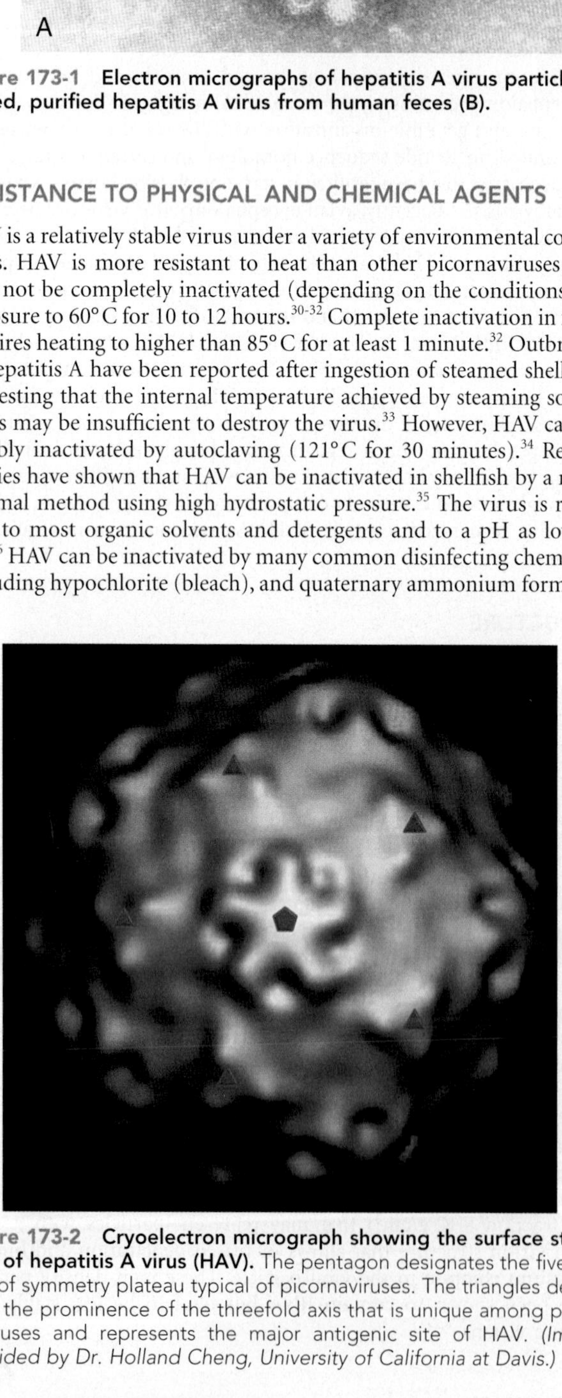

GENOME AND PROTEINS

Although HAV had the characteristics of a picornavirus and indirect tests suggested an RNA genome, molecular cloning and sequence analysis demonstrated that the HAV genome is composed of single-stranded, positive-sense linear RNA of 7478 nucleotides (strain HM175) and a molecular weight of approximately 2.25×10^6, with an overall structure and gene order typical of picornaviruses.[17,19,38]

The 5′ end of the genome does not have a cap structure but instead, as is typical for picornaviruses, has a small, covalently bound protein termed VPg.[39] The genome itself has a long 5′ untranslated region beginning with UU as found in all picornaviruses. This 5′ untranslated region folds to form a highly ordered secondary structure that is important for both replication and translation. These structured regions include an internal ribosome entry site (IRES) that directs the initiation of translation at either of two AUG codons at nucleotide positions 735-737 and 741-743[38] (see Fig. 173-3). The AUG codon initiates a single long open reading frame of 6681 nucleotides that encodes a polyprotein that is 2227 amino acid residues in length. The coding region of picornaviruses has been arbitrarily divided into three parts, termed P1, P2, and P3, and the peptides that are ultimately cleaved from the translation products of these regions are referred to as 1A, 1B, 1C, 2A, 2B, 2C, and so forth, in order of translation from the 5′ to the 3′ end of the genome.[40] The HAV genome ends with a 3′ noncoding region of 63 nucleotides that is followed by a virus encoded poly (A) tail.

The four capsid proteins of mature virus particles are coded by the first 2373 nucleotides (P1) and the nonstructural proteins by the remainder (P2 and P3). The four capsid polypeptides named by analogy with other picornaviruses are referred to in descending order

Figure 173-2   Cryoelectron micrograph showing the surface structure of hepatitis A virus (HAV). The pentagon designates the fivefold axis of symmetry plateau typical of picornaviruses. The triangles designate the prominence of the threefold axis that is unique among picornaviruses and represents the major antigenic site of HAV. (Image provided by Dr. Holland Cheng, University of California at Davis.)

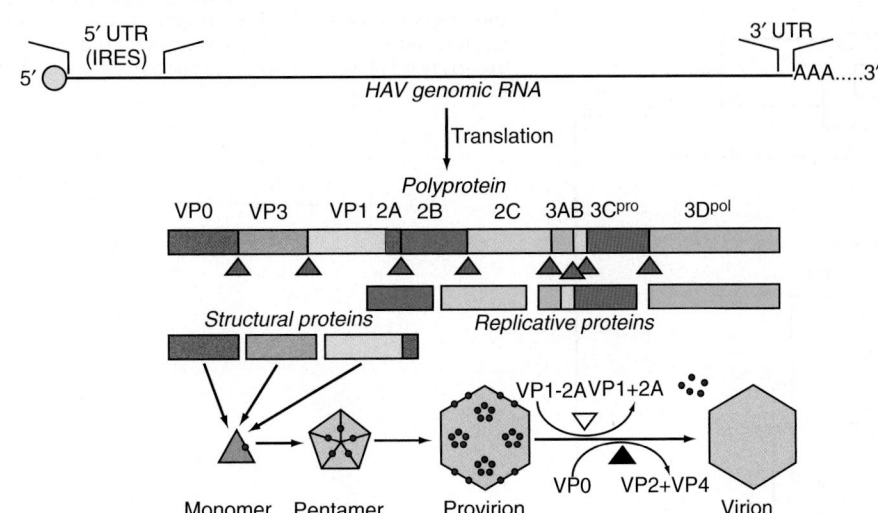

Figure 173-3 **Organization of the RNA genome of hepatitis A virus (HAV), polyprotein cleavage, and viral assembly.** The 7.5-kb positive-strand RNA is covalently attached to VPg (5' end) and has a poly(A) tail. The 5' untranslated region (UTR) of 734 nucleotides functions as an internal ribosome entry site (IRES) to initiate translation (*vertical arrow*) of the precursor polyprotein of 2227 amino acids. Regions of the polyprotein are indicated according to standard nomenclature. The single viral protease, 3C^pro, cleaves itself from the polyprotein, and subsequently cleaves elsewhere in the polyprotein to yield the structural protein precursors VP0, VP3, and VP1-2A (PX) and replicative proteins 2B, 2C, 3A, 3B, and 3D (RNA-dependent RNA polymerase). VP0, VP3, and VP1-2A probably remain associated as a monomer and then form pentamers that are a stable precursor in capsid formation. Assembly of 12 pentamers together with RNA forms the provirion, after which 2A is susceptible to cleavage by host cell protease(s) (*open arrowhead*). The final maturation cleavage of VP0 to VP2 and VP4 (*solid arrowhead*) is dependent on the encapsidated viral RNA.

of size as virion proteins (VP): VP1 = peptide 1D (molecular weight 32,800 Da), VP2 = 1B (24,800 Da), VP3 = 1C (27,300 Da), and VP4 = 1A (2500 Da).[22,41] A VP0 protein (1AB) that is the precursor to VP4 and VP2 can also be detected, especially from cell cultures where immature virions (provirions) may accumulate in large amounts.[42] The VP4 molecule is believed to be liberated during the maturation cleavage of VP0, which converts provirions to virions (see later), but VP4 has never been experimentally determined to be within the virion particle and, at just 23 amino acids, is approximately one third the size of the VP4 proteins of other picornaviruses.

Assembly of HAV particles proceeds through several steps (see Fig. 173-3). Cleavage of the polyprotein by the 3C protease yields three capsid-related proteins, VP0, VP3, and VP1-2A (also known as PX), which constitute a monomer and subsequently assemble into penta-meric subunits. Twelve copies of the pentamer then associate with viral RNA to form provirions or without viral RNA to form empty capsids (procapsids). The involvement of the VP1-2A precursor in assembly is unique to HAV, and it has been shown that the 2A extension is essential for proper processing and assembly of the pentameric subunit.[43-45] After assembly, 2A is removed from VP1 by cellular proteases,[46,47] and in the final maturation step, VP0 is cleaved to yield VP2 and VP4. The VP0 cleavage is dependent on the presence of viral RNA in the particle and procapsids therefore fail to cleave VP0, but HAV procapsids are quite stable and seem to have the same antigenic structure as mature virions.

ANTIGENIC COMPOSITION AND VIRAL DIVERSITY

Although a variety of genotypes of HAV have been identified by analysis of genome sequences (Fig. 173-4), there seems to be only one sero-type.[48-50] This view is supported by the observation that IG prepared in developed countries and monovalent vaccines prepared from strains originating in Australia, Central America, or Europe protect travelers from disease equally well, irrespective of their destination.[51,52]

Neutralization sites for HAV are located primarily on the structural proteins VP1 and VP3, with possibly a minor contribution from VP2.[48] Monoclonal antibodies in competition binding assays and the generation of neutralization escape mutants suggest that the dominant neutralization site is composed of overlapping epitopes on VP1 and VP3 that combine to form a conformational antigenic site at which neutral-

izing antibodies are targeted.[48,50,53] Comparison of nucleic acid sequences in the region around the VP1/2A junction (see Fig. 173-4) from geographically diverse HAV isolates differentiate four genotypes (I, II, III, and VII) plus three additional presumptive simian types (IV, V, and VI).[23,54,55] Most strains recovered from patients in the United States were closely related to each other, whereas viruses recovered in Western Europe belonged to three genotypes, thus suggesting importation from other geographic regions.[23,56] Although individual strains of HAV have differences at the molecular level that may be useful for epidemiologic studies, a high degree of identity in nucleic acid (as high as 90%) and amino acid sequence (as high as 98%) is generally seen between strains.[57,58]

BIOLOGY OF HEPATITIS A VIRUS IN CELL CULTURE

HAV was first propagated in marmoset liver explant cultures and a cloned line of fetal rhesus monkey kidney cells (FRhK-6) with a strain of virus (CR326) that had been adapted by multiple passages in *Sagui-nus mystax* and *Saguinus labiatus* marmosets.[14] Many HAV strains have subsequently been isolated from clinical material, although the procedure may take several weeks. Until recently, only epithelial or fibro-blast cells of primate origin had been shown to support growth of the virus.[15,16,59] However, in a systematic search for cells that would support HAV replication, growth was detected in cells of guinea pig, dolphin, and porcine origin.[60]

The major characteristics of HAV in cell culture are slow growth and low yields relative to other picornaviruses. In addition, the virus remains largely cell associated, does not usually produce a cytopathic effect, and readily leads to persistently infected cell lines.[61] With adaptation, more rapid replication and higher yields can be obtained and cytopathic variants have been selected. These cell culture–adapted viruses are useful for virus titrations, neutralization, inactivation kinetics, and virus replication and have made the production of inactivated vaccines practical.[14,16,62-64]

In one study, direct isolation of a wild-type strain of HAV was achieved through the use of a modified cell line,[65] but it remains to be tested whether these cells will be a universal substrate for rapid viral isolation of wild type HAV. Detection of HAV in either patients' or environmental samples is now done primarily through the use of PCR or other nucleic acid–based technology. The kinetics of viral

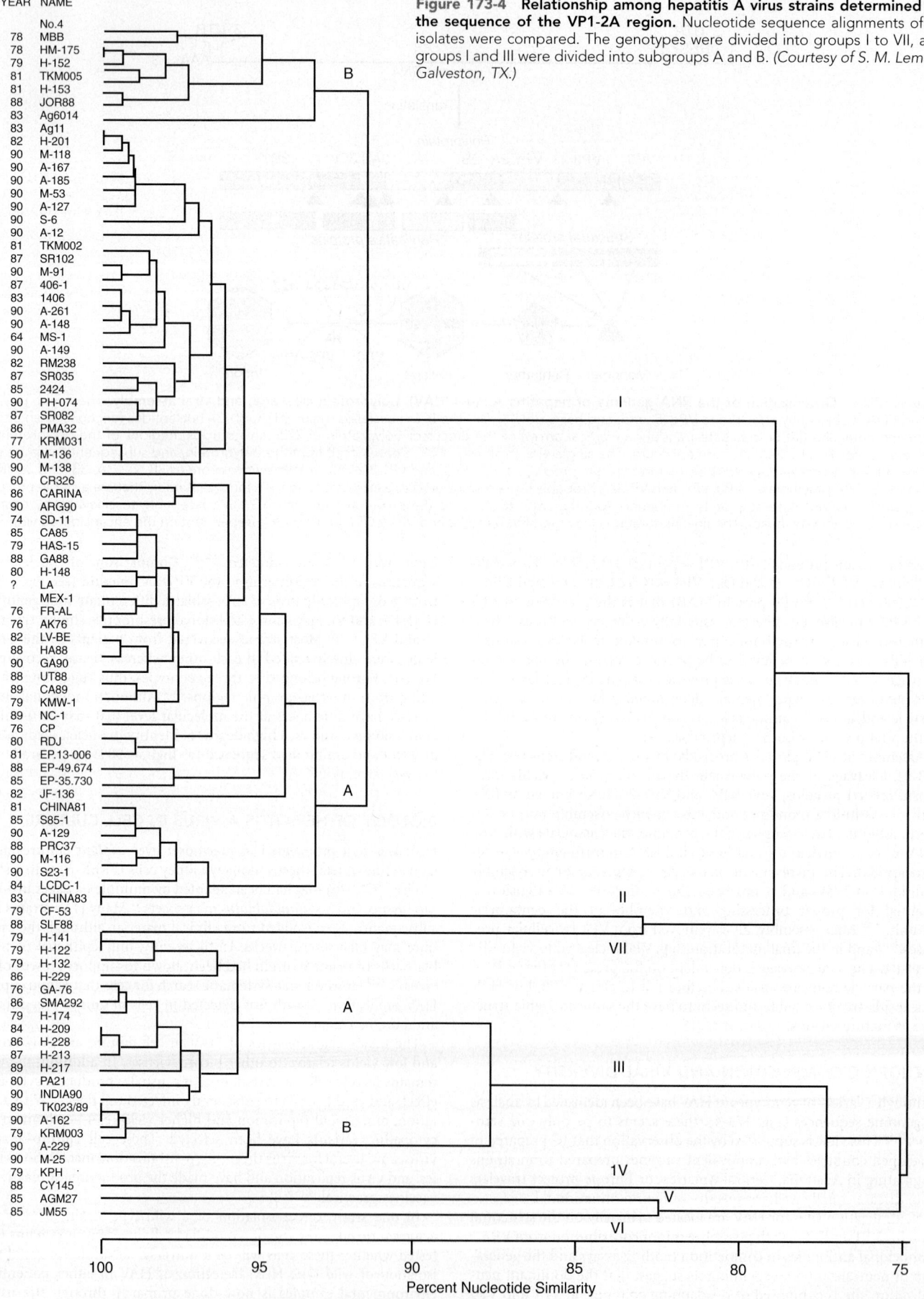

Figure 173-4 Relationship among hepatitis A virus strains determined by the sequence of the VP1-2A region. Nucleotide sequence alignments of 92 isolates were compared. The genotypes were divided into groups I to VII, and groups I and III were divided into subgroups A and B. (Courtesy of S. M. Lemon, Galveston, TX.)

replication and biosynthetic events have been studied in cells infected with cell culture–adapted strains of HAV and reveal a number of differences from most other picornaviruses. After attachment to cells, the uncoating of virus is delayed for more than 8 hours[66,67]; this exceeds the duration of an entire growth cycle for many picornaviruses. The delayed uncoating seems to be related to the protracted maturation cleavage of VP0 to VP2 and VP4 because virions are uncoated more rapidly than provirions.[68] Accumulation of new viral RNA can be detected as early as 12 hours after infection of BS-C-1 cells with a fast-growing, cytopathic variant of strain HM175, but levels of viral replicative intermediates (double-stranded RNAs) remain much lower than in cells infected with other picornaviruses.[66] As outlined previously, translation of the viral polyprotein is directed by the IRES within the 5′ untranslated region, but the IRES of HAV is relatively inefficient, with initiation approximately 1% of that seen for the IRES of encephalomyocarditis virus.[69-71]

The initial proteolytic processing of HAV polyprotein is accomplished by the viral 3C protease, and assembly of viral particles proceeds via monomers and pentamers (see Fig. 173-3).[43] After infection of cell cultures with rapidly replicating and cytopathic variants of HAV, pentamers are first detected at 9 hours post-infection and reach peak levels after approximately 18 hours even though the amount of viral RNA (and presumably viral translation) increases beyond this time.[72] These cells continue to produce virus for 2 to 3 days before cell death, whereas most HAV variants progress to a persistent infection with reduced levels of virus production over many weeks and subsequent cell passages.

Repeated passage in cell culture has been used to apply mutational pressure to HAV to alter the phenotype. For example, HAV variants have been selected that grow more rapidly or are resistant to neutralization by monoclonal antibodies.[64,73,74] Attenuated strains of HAV have been selected by multiple tissue culture passages, and cold adaptation has been achieved by passage at reduced temperature.[26,75] Some of the mutations responsible for these altered phenotypes have been identified by molecular cloning and sequencing of the mutant. Mutations within the 5′ untranslated region and mutations within the 2B and 2C coding regions of HAV RNA have been shown to enhance virus replication in vitro.[74,76,77] However, mutations within the VP1-2A and 2C proteins seem to be most important for attenuation of virulence.[74]

Most viruses initiate infection by first binding to a specific cell surface receptor molecule or, in many cases, may require binding to both receptors and co-receptors to facilitate virus entry and uncoating. Identification of a specific receptor for HAV remained elusive for many years. However, Kaplan and colleagues[78] succeeded in the isolation of one specific receptor molecule, havcr-1, first in cells of simian origin and later in human cells.[79] This molecule is a novel mucin-like class I integral membrane glycoprotein of 451 amino acids, with the N-terminal, cysteine-rich domain responsible for binding to HAV.[79] Because this molecule is expressed on cells from many tissues that are not susceptible to HAV infection, it is likely that specific co-receptors contribute to the organ tropism of HAV. However, a soluble form of havcr-1 has some ability to neutralize particles of HAV directly, which is consistent with roles in both attachment and uncoating of virus.[80]

It remains possible that HAV may use other pathways for cell entry in addition to havcr-1. Recent studies demonstrated that the asialoglycoprotein receptor can also mediate infection of cells with HAV when the virus is first complexed with specific IgA, leading to the interesting hypothesis that IgA may play a role as both carrier and targeting molecule during infection and transmission, particularly in relapsing cases of HAV.[81]

HOST RANGE

Humans are considered to be the only important reservoir of HAV. However, the existence of extra human reservoirs of infection remains possible. In 1961, Hillis[82] described an outbreak of hepatitis A among chimpanzee handlers who apparently contracted the infection from the chimpanzees. Epidemiologic data suggested that the animals had become infected during captivity but before their importation into the United States. Interestingly, although epidemics of hepatitis were recognized in American primate handlers, the disease was rarely seen in Africa, presumably because most handlers were already immune. Widespread screening of nonhuman primates revealed antibodies to HAV in chimpanzees, gorillas, orangutans, gibbons, macaques, owl monkeys, pig tail monkeys, rhesus monkeys, and several species of South American tamarin monkeys.[83,84] It is unclear whether such primates may serve as reservoirs of infection or as transient hosts after exposure to HAV from human sources. However, both the PA21 and AGM-27 strains of HAV seem to be true simian viruses.[55,85] Interestingly, the AGM-27 virus produces attenuated disease in chimpanzees and has been the subject of some study as a potential live attenuated vaccine.[86]

Deinhardt[87] pioneered the use of subhuman primates for hepatitis A studies in both chimpanzees and tamarins (*Saguinas* species). He showed that in chimpanzees, liver function test abnormalities developed upon inoculation with known infectious material of human origin. Since that time, the chimpanzee, several species of tamarins, and the owl monkey have all been shown to be susceptible to HAV infection and to develop hepatitis.[87] These animals have been valuable tools in the study of hepatitis A pathogenesis and for the development of vaccines. Recently, it was shown that guinea pigs express a receptor similar to the human havcr and that both guinea pig cells and guinea pigs can be infected with HAV. However, the animals did not have evidence of hepatitis.[60,88]

◼ Epidemiology

MODES OF TRANSMISSION

HAV replicates in the liver, is excreted in bile, and is found in highest concentrations in stool. Thus, fecal excretion is the primary source of virus. In experimental studies, infectivity of stools was demonstrated for 14 to 21 days before to 8 days after onset of jaundice, but the highest concentrations occur during the 2-week period before jaundice develops or liver enzymes increase, followed by a rapid decrease after the appearance of jaundice[11,89,90] (Fig. 173-5). Data from epidemiologic studies also suggest that peak infectivity occurs during the 2 weeks before the onset of symptoms.[91] Shedding of HAV in stool may continue for longer periods in infected infants and children than adults. HAV RNA has been detected in stool of infected newborns for as long as 6 months after infection.[92] Excretion in older children and adults was demonstrated 1 to 3 months after clinical illness.[52,92] Although chronic shedding of HAV does not occur, the virus has been detected in stool during relapsing illness.[93]

During the period of viremia, which begins during the prodrome and extends through the period of increased liver enzymes (see Fig. 173-5), HAV concentrations in serum are several orders of magnitude lower than in stool.[94-96] However, in experiments conducted in nonhu-

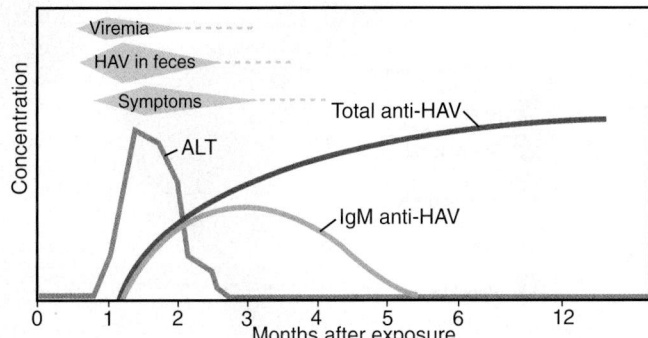

Figure 173-5 Clinical, virologic, and serologic events associated with hepatitis A virus (HAV) infection. ALT, alanine aminotransferase.

man primates, HAV was several orders of magnitude more infectious when administered by the intravenous compared with the oral route, and animals were successfully infected with low concentrations of HAV administered via the intravenous route.[97] Although HAV may occasionally be detected in saliva in experimentally infected animals,[98] transmission by saliva has not been demonstrated.

Enzyme immunoassays and PCR may detect defective as well as infectious viral particles. Thus, the detection of HAV antigen in the stool by enzyme immunoassays or HAV RNA in the serum or stool by PCR does not mean that an infected person is necessarily infectious, and it is likely that the period of infectivity is shorter than the period during which HAV RNA is detectable. For practical purposes, both children and adults with hepatitis A can be assumed to be noninfectious 1 week after jaundice appears.

Person to Person

Person-to-person transmission by the fecal-oral route is the primary means of HAV transmission in the United States and throughout the world.[99,100] Most transmission occurs among close contacts, particularly in households and extended family settings.[101] Young children have the highest rates of infection and are often the source of infection for others because infections in this age group are often asymptomatic and standards of hygiene are generally lower among young children compared with adults.[101-103]

Foodborne and Waterborne

HAV can remain infectious in the environment for long periods of time,[104] allowing for common-source outbreaks and sporadic cases to occur from exposure to fecally contaminated food or water. Many uncooked foods have been recognized as the source of outbreaks. Cooked foods also can transmit HAV if the cooking is inadequate to kill the virus or if the food is contaminated after cooking, as commonly occurs in outbreaks associated with infected food handlers.[105-108] Contaminated shellfish were responsible for a large outbreak in Shanghai, China, in 1988[109,110] and have been implicated as the source of cases in Italy[111-113] but have rarely been associated with outbreaks in the United States in recent years.[114,115] Waterborne outbreaks of hepatitis A are uncommon in developed countries.

Blood-borne

Transfusion-related hepatitis A is rare because HAV does not result in chronic infection, and, in the developed world, blood donors have been screened for many years for elevated aminotransferase levels. However, transmission by transfusion of blood or blood derivatives collected from donors during the viremic phase of their infection has been reported, including outbreaks in Europe and the United States among patients who received factor VIII and IX concentrates prepared using solvent-detergent treatment to inactivate lipid-containing viruses.[37,96,116-118] HAV is resistant to solvent-detergent treatment, and contamination presumably occurred from plasma donors with hepatitis A who donated during the incubation period.

Vertical

Two published case reports describe intrauterine transmission of HAV during the first trimester, resulting in fetal meconium peritonitis.[119,120] After delivery, both infants were found to have a perforated ileum. The risk of transmission from pregnant women who develop hepatitis A in the third trimester of pregnancy to newborns seems to be low.[121] However, newborns who acquire infection in this manner are usually asymptomatic, and an outbreak among hospital staff related to exposure to such an infant has been reported.[122]

WORLDWIDE DISEASE PATTERNS

Hepatitis A occurs worldwide, but major geographic differences exist in endemicity and resulting epidemiologic features (Fig. 173-6). The degree of endemicity is closely related to hygienic and sanitary conditions and other indicators of the level of development. In less developed areas, especially when there is limited access to clean water and inadequate disposal of human feces, HAV infects most people early in life, when infection is rarely clinically apparent (Fig. 173-7). When high standards of hygiene and sanitation apply, the majority of adults remain susceptible. Distinct patterns of HAV infection can be described, each characterized by particular age-specific anti-HAV prevalence and hepatitis A incidence and prevailing environmental (hygienic and sanitary) and socioeconomic conditions[99,123] (see Fig. 173-7).

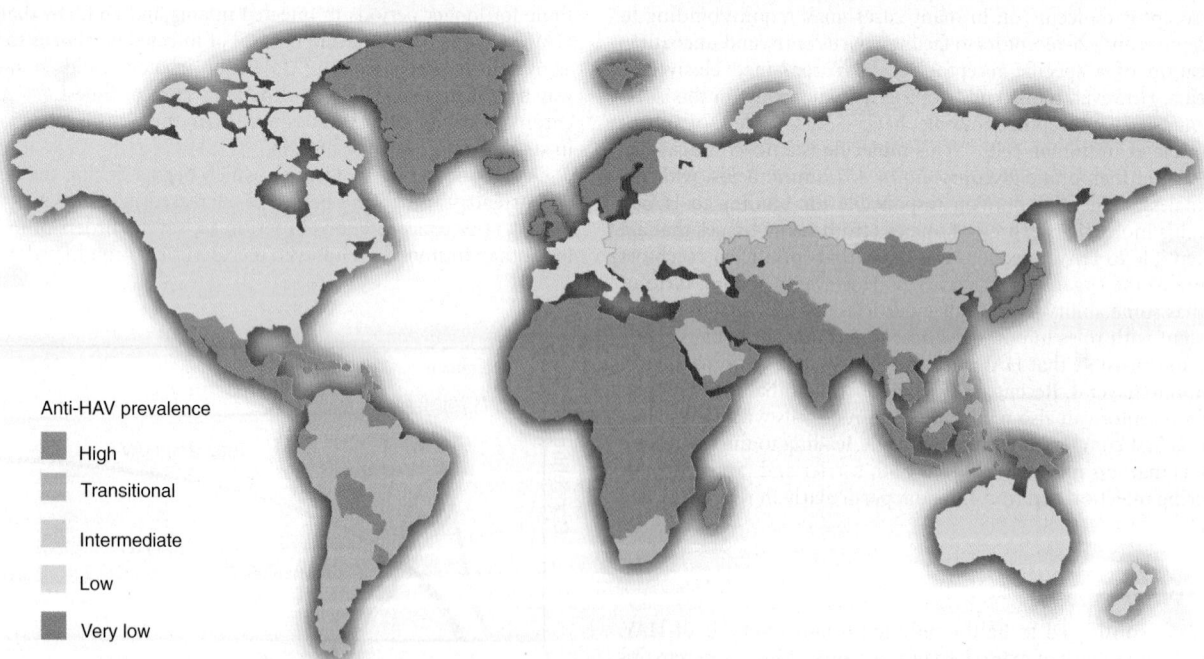

Anti-HAV prevalence

High
Transitional
Intermediate
Low
Very low

Figure 173-6 **World map indicating patterns of endemicity of hepatitis A virus (HAV) infection, generalized from available data.** The patterns of high, transitional, intermediate, low, and very low endemicity are shown.

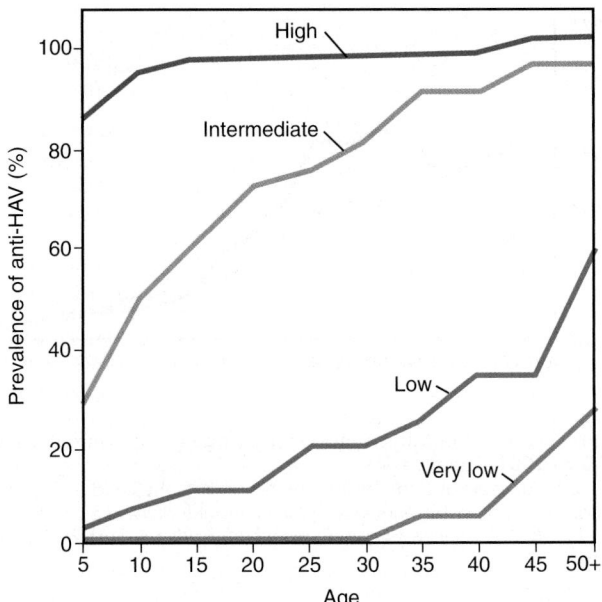

Figure 173-7 **Patterns of hepatitis A virus (HAV) infection worldwide.** Age-specific prevalence of anti-HAV in areas of high, intermediate, low, and very low endemicity is shown.

In areas of high endemicity, represented by the least developed countries (i.e., parts of Africa, Asia, Central and South America), poor hygienic and sanitary conditions allow HAV to spread readily (see Figs. 173-6 and 173-7). Infection is nearly universal in early childhood, when asymptomatic infection predominates, and essentially the entire population is infected before reaching adolescence, as demonstrated by the age-specific prevalence of anti-HAV[124,125] (see Fig. 173-7). Susceptible adults in these areas are at high risk of hepatitis A, but reported disease rates are generally low and outbreaks are rare because most adults are immune. High endemicity patterns can also be seen in some ethnic or geographically defined groups within highly developed countries, such as aboriginal children in the north of Australia.[126]

In areas of moderate endemicity, HAV is not transmitted as readily because of better sanitary and living conditions, and the predominant age at infection is older than in areas of high endemicity[127] (see Figs. 173-6 and 173-7). Paradoxically, the overall incidence and average age of reported cases are often higher than in highly endemic areas because high levels of virus circulate in a population that includes many susceptible older children, adolescents, and young adults who are likely to develop symptoms with HAV infection.[128] Large common-source food- and water-associated outbreaks can occur because of the relatively high rate of virus transmission and large number of susceptible persons, especially among those of higher socioeconomic level. Such an outbreak occurred in Shanghai in 1988, with more than 300,000 cases associated with consumption of clams harvested from water contaminated with human sewage.[109] Nevertheless, person-to-person transmission in communitywide epidemics continues to account for much of the disease in these countries.

Shifts in age-specific prevalence patterns that reflect a transition from high to intermediate endemicity are occurring in many parts of the world (see Fig. 173-6). A feature of this transitional pattern is striking variations in hepatitis A epidemiology among countries and within countries and cities, with some areas displaying a pattern typical of high endemicity and others of intermediate endemicity.[99,129-138] Considerable hepatitis A–related morbidity and associated costs occur with this transition, even in developing countries.[139,140] For example, hepatitis A was the etiology of the fulminant hepatitis of two thirds of children presenting to two hospitals in Argentina during a 15-year

period, and, in one of these hospitals performing liver transplantations, one third of liver transplantations among children were performed for fulminant hepatitis A.[139]

In the United States, Canada, western Europe, and other developed countries, the endemicity of HAV infection is low (see Fig. 173-6). Relatively fewer children are infected, the incidence of disease is generally low, and in countries where hepatitis A vaccine is not used widely, disease often occurs in the context of communitywide and child care center outbreaks.[99,141-144] Population-based seroprevalence surveys show a gradual increase in the prevalence of anti-HAV with increasing age, primarily reflecting declining incidence, changing endemicity, and resultant lower childhood infection rates over time. Some countries (e.g., Scandinavia) currently have very low endemicity, with most cases occurring in defined risk groups such as travelers returning from endemic areas and users of injection drugs.[145]

EPIDEMIOLOGY IN THE UNITED STATES

Hepatitis A epidemiology in the United States can be divided into two time periods, before and after implementation of national recommendations for use of hepatitis A vaccine.

Prevaccine Era
In the prevaccine era, hepatitis A incidence was primarily cyclic, with peaks every 10 to 15 years (Fig. 173-8). Throughout the 1980s and early 1990s in the United States, approximately 25,000 to 35,000 hepatitis A cases were reported annually to the Centers for Disease Control and Prevention,[146] but incidence models indicated that the actual number of infections occurring during that period was likely 10 times greater with an estimated 271,000 infections per year.[103]

The highest hepatitis A rates were among children 5 to 14 years of age, with approximately one third of cases occurring among children younger than 15 years.[147] Furthermore, because young children are more likely to have unrecognized or asymptomatic infection than older individuals, incidence models estimated that more than half of HAV infections occurred among children younger than 10 years old, the majority of which were in children less than 5 years old[103] (Fig. 173-9).

In the prevaccine era, hepatitis A incidence differed among racial and ethnic groups, with rates among Native Americans and Alaska Natives that were more than five times those in other racial/ethnic groups, and rates among Hispanics that were approximately three times higher than those among non-Hispanics (see Fig. 173-11).[148]

Hepatitis A incidence also exhibited striking regional variation with the highest rates and majority of cases consistently occurring in a limited number of states and counties in the western and southwestern United States (see Fig. 173-12). Cases among residents of 11 primarily western states, representing 22% of the U.S. population, on average

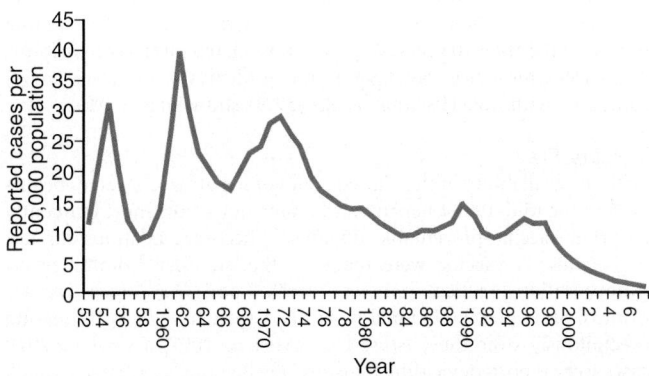

Figure 173-8 **Hepatitis A incidence, United States, 1952 to 2007.** *(From the Centers for Disease Control and Prevention, National Notifiable Diseases Surveillance System, Atlanta, GA.)*

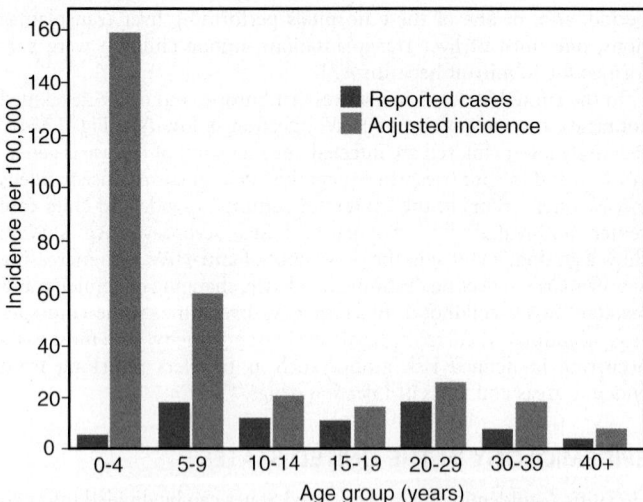

Figure 173-9 Reported and adjusted incidence of hepatitis A in the United States, 1980 to 1999. The purple bars represent the reported age-specific incidence and the brown bars represent the age-specific incidence after adjusting for anicteric infections. *(Modified from Armstrong GL, Bell BP. Hepatitis A virus infections in the United States: model-based estimates and implications for childhood immunization. Pediatrics 2002;109:839-845.)*

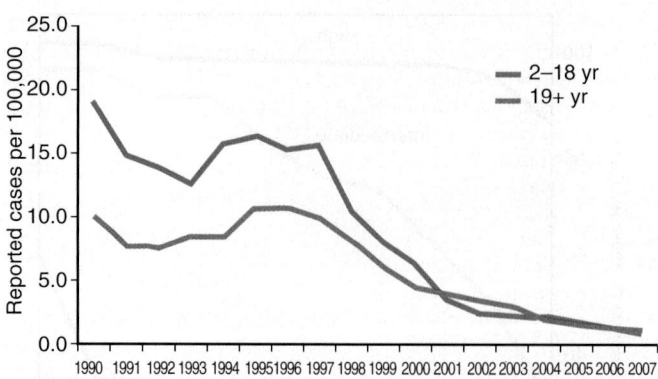

Figure 173-10 Hepatitis A incidence by age group, United States, 1990 to 2007. The blue line represents the incidence among children ages 2 to 18 years and the brown line represents the incidence among persons older than 18 years. *(From the Centers for Disease Control and Prevention, National Notifiable Diseases Surveillance System, Atlanta, GA.)*

VARIATION BY AGE, RACE OR ETHNICITY, AND REGION

Hepatitis A incidence rates among children have decreased more sharply than among adults after the implementation of routine vaccination of children, and since 2002, rates have been similar among adults and children (Fig. 173-10).

Previous disparities in rates across racial/ethnic groups have largely disappeared (Fig. 173-11). By 2000, hepatitis A incidence among

accounted for 50% of reported cases.[149] An additional 18% of cases occurred among residents of six additional states.

In the prevaccine era, most cases of hepatitis A in the United States occurred in the context of communitywide epidemics in which infection was transmitted from person to person in households and extended family settings.[100] In these outbreaks, no single risk group accounted for the majority of cases, and infections among children, many of whom were asymptomatic, played an important role in sustaining transmission. For cases in which a risk factor could be determined, the most frequently reported source of infection was household or sexual contact with another person with hepatitis A, accounting for 12% to 25% of cases. Cyclic outbreaks also occurred in injection and noninjection drug users and among men who have sex with men; as many as 15% of nationally reported cases occurred among persons reporting one or more of these behaviors. Other potential sources of infection such as international travel and foodborne outbreaks accounted for a small proportion of cases. For approximately 50% of reported cases, no source of infection could be identified.

Results of the Third National Health and Nutrition Examination Survey, conducted from 1988 to 1994, indicated that approximately one third of the U.S. population had serologic evidence of previous HAV infection.[150] Anti-HAV prevalence was related directly to age, ranging from 9% among children 6 to 11 years of age to 75% among persons older than 70 years of age and was related inversely to income. Anti-HAV prevalence was highest among Mexican Americans (70%) compared with non-Hispanic blacks (39%) and whites (23%).

Vaccine Era

With the availability in the United States of hepatitis A vaccines beginning in the mid-1990s, hepatitis A became one of the most frequently reported vaccine-preventable diseases.[146] Recommendations for use of hepatitis A vaccine were made by the Advisory Committee on Immunization Practices in 1996,[148] 1999,[149] and 2006[151] (see "Disease Control Strategies"). National hepatitis A rates have been decreasing precipitously over the past several years; in 2007, a total of 2979 cases were reported, yielding a historically low rate of 1.0 per 100,000 (see Fig. 173-8).[152] This remarkable decline in incidence is reflected in other fundamental shifts in hepatitis A epidemiology, as described below.

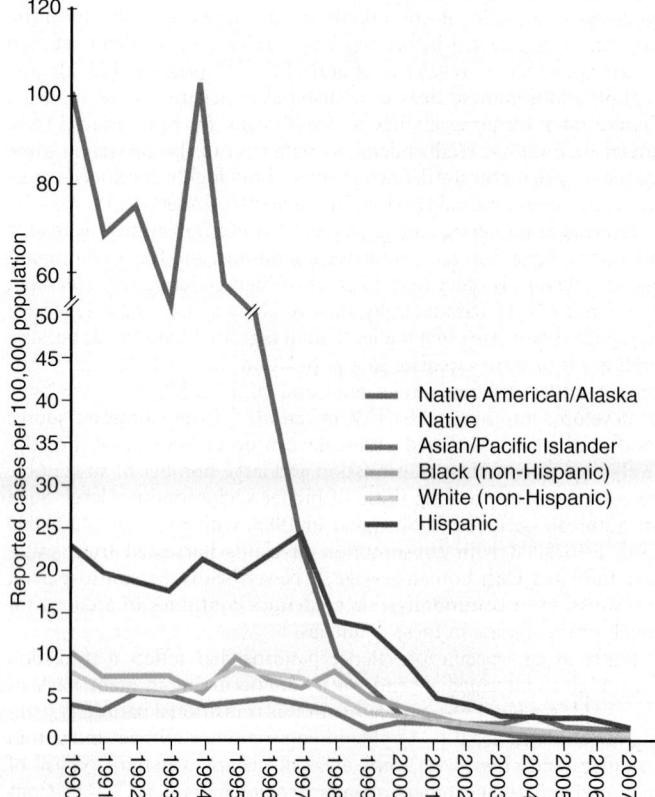

Figure 173-11 Hepatitis A incidence, United States, by race and ethnicity, 1990 to 2007. *(From the Centers for Disease Control and Prevention, National Notifiable Diseases Surveillance System, Atlanta, GA.)*

Native Americans and Alaska Natives had decreased by 97% compared with the beginning of the decade and was lower than the overall U.S. rate (see "Disease Control Strategies").[152,153] The disparity in incidence between Hispanics and non-Hispanics has also decreased, although rates among Hispanics are still twice those among non-Hispanics.

The geographic variations that characterized hepatitis A incidence in the past have also essentially disappeared, presumably due, at least in part, to the implementation of vaccination recommendations.[149,152] Since 2002, the rates in the western states have been similar to those in other regions of the country (Fig. 173-12).

POTENTIAL SOURCES OF INFECTION

Based on data from disease surveillance systems, household or sexual contact with a person who has hepatitis A continues to be a commonly reported potential source of infection (accounting for ~10% to 15% of reported cases), although the proportion of cases with such exposures has been decreasing in recent years[100,152] (Fig. 173-13). Cases occurring among children and employees of child care centers and members of their households, which previously accounted for a substantial proportion of reports, now are uncommon (4%).[100,152] As other sources of transmission have become less common, the proportion of cases accounted for by international travel has increased and is now the most commonly reported risk factor (15%). Suspected foodborne or waterborne outbreaks typically account for a small (5% to 7%) proportion of cases but can vary substantially.[152] Cyclic outbreaks continue to occur among men who have sex with men and users of injection and noninjection drugs.[100,154-157] Historically during outbreak years, these exposures could account for 10% of nationally reported cases and, with the large decreases in incidence among children and their adult contacts, can now account for an even larger proportion of cases. Approximately half of patients with hepatitis A do not have a recognized source of infection[152] but may be contacts with persons, especially children, with asymptomatic infection.

SPECIFIC GROUPS AND SETTINGS

Child Care Centers, Schools, and Institutions
Outbreaks of hepatitis A in child care centers, which historically were a common occurrence, particularly in larger centers and/or in those

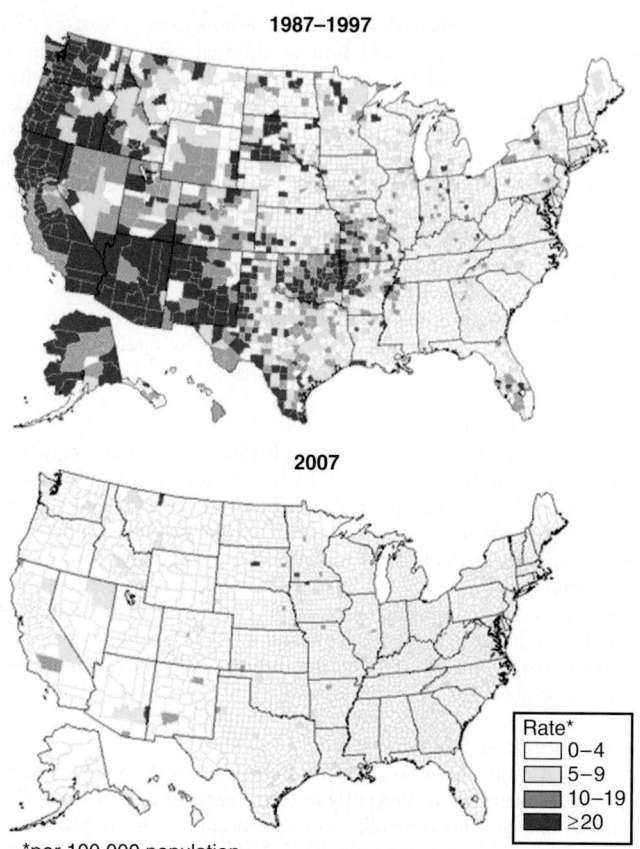

1987–1997

2007

Rate*
☐ 0–4
▨ 5–9
▩ 10–19
■ ≥20

*per 100,000 population

Figure 173-12 Hepatitis A incidence rates by county, United States, 1987 to 1997 and 2007. The top map represents the average incidence from 1987 to 1997; the bottom map represents 2007 incidence. *(From the Centers for Disease Control and Prevention, National Notifiable Diseases Surveillance System, Atlanta, GA.)*

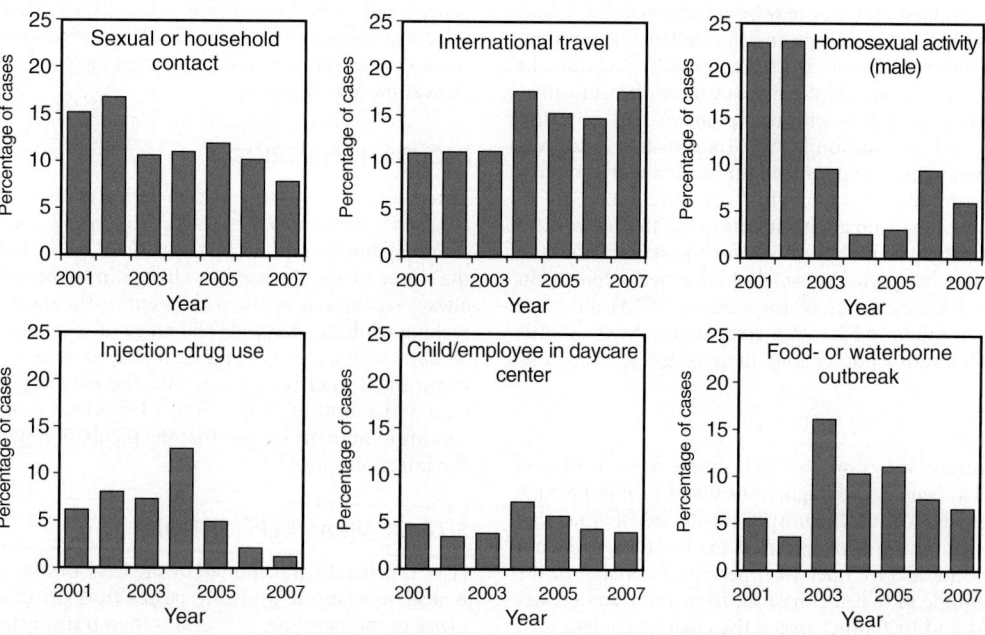

Figure 173-13   Risk factors for hepatitis A among reported cases, United States, 2001 to 2007. *(From the Centers for Disease Control and Prevention, Viral Hepatitis Surveillance Program, Atlanta, GA.)*

that cared for children in diapers,[158-160] are now rare, at least in part because of the routine vaccination of children against hepatitis A. However, the potential for transmission in these settings remains. Outbreaks in child care centers have occasionally been the source of more extensive transmission within a community,[159,161,162] but in most cases, disease in child care centers reflects disease transmission from the community. Similarly, hepatitis A cases among older children in schools usually reflect disease that has been acquired in the community, although multiple cases among children in a school may indicate a common-source outbreak.[163] Historically, HAV infection was endemic in institutions for the developmentally disabled, but with smaller facilities and improved conditions, the incidence and prevalence of infection have decreased and outbreaks are rarely reported in the United States.[164]

Users of Illicit Drugs

During the past two decades, outbreaks have been regularly reported among illicit drug users in North America, Australia, and Europe.[156,157,165-171] In the United States, these outbreaks have frequently involved users of injected and noninjected methamphetamine, who may account for as many as 30% of reported cases in these communities during outbreaks.[100,157,167,172] Cross-sectional serologic surveys have demonstrated that injection drug users have a higher prevalence of anti-HAV than the general U.S. population.[173,174] Transmission among injection drug users probably occurs through both the percutaneous and fecal-oral routes.[167]

Men Who Have Sex with Men

Hepatitis A outbreaks among men who have sex with men have been reported frequently, most recently in urban areas in the United States, Canada, Europe, and Australia, and may occur in the context of an outbreak in the larger community.[100,154,155,175-178] Seroprevalence surveys have not consistently demonstrated an elevated prevalence of anti-HAV compared with a similarly aged general population.[174,179] Some studies conducted during outbreaks and seroprevalence surveys among men who have sex with men have identified specific sex practices associated with illness, whereas others have not demonstrated such associations.[154,174,176]

Transfusions and Other Health Care Settings

Transfusion-related hepatitis A is rare. The risk of infection in patients with hemophilia is not known, but results of one serologic survey of hemophiliac patients suggest that they may be at increased risk,[180] and outbreaks have been reported in Europe and the United States among patients who received factor VIII and IX concentrates.[117,181] Outbreaks have also been reported in neonatal intensive care units after transmission to hospital staff from a neonate with asymptomatic HAV infection acquired from a blood transfusion.[92,182,183] Transmission also was reported in association with an experimental treatment with lymphocytes incubated in serum from a donor with HAV infection.[184]

Nosocomial transmission from adult patients to health care workers is rare because most patients with hepatitis A are hospitalized after the onset of jaundice, when infectivity is low,[89] but it has been reported in association with fecal incontinence of the patient.[185,186] Health care workers have not been found to have an increased prevalence of anti-HAV compared with control populations in serologic surveys conducted in the United States.[187]

International Travel

Hepatitis A is a common infection among travelers from developed countries who travel to regions with high, transitional, or intermediate endemicity[188-190] (see Fig. 173-6). In prospective studies of American and European travelers, the risk of infection for those who did not receive IG was found to be 3 to 5 per 1000 per month of stay, of the same order of magnitude as that for malaria, 10 to 100 times greater than that for typhoid, and 1000 times greater than that for cholera.[191,192] The risk may be higher among travelers staying in areas with poor hygienic conditions,[193] varies according to the region and the length of stay, and seems to be increased even among travelers who reported

observing protective measures and staying in urban areas or luxury hotels (Centers for Disease Control and Prevention, unpublished data, 1996). In the United States and Europe, hepatitis A in persons, especially children, traveling to endemic countries to visit relatives and friends accounts for an increasing proportion of reported cases.[194,195] Compared with persons traveling for work or recreation, these individuals tend to have trips of longer duration, and by staying in family settings rather than hotels, may have greater exposure to HAV circulating in the community.[196] Travelers who acquire hepatitis A during their trip may also transmit to others on their return. Cases of hepatitis A have been reported in nontraveling family members and close contacts of international adoptees upon their arrival from the child's country of origin.[197,198]

Foodborne and Waterborne

Foodborne hepatitis A outbreaks are recognized relatively infrequently in the United States.[107] They are most commonly associated with contamination of food during preparation by a food handler with HAV infection.[105,106,199,200] Implicated foods include those not cooked after handling, such as sandwiches and salads, as well as partially cooked foods.[201-204] Food contaminated before retail distribution, such as lettuce or fruits contaminated at the growing or processing stage, has been increasingly recognized as the source of hepatitis A outbreaks.[163,205-210] Waterborne hepatitis A outbreaks are rare and related to sewage contamination or inadequate treatment of water.[211-213] Outbreaks associated with contaminated shellfish in this country are very rare, but the occurrence of a multistate outbreak linked to oysters from the Gulf of Mexico in 2005 indicates that the potential for these types of transmission remains.[115]

Although the results of some serologic surveys conducted among sewage workers in Europe indicated a possible increased risk of HAV infection, findings have not been consistent.[214-216] In published reports of three serologic surveys conducted among U.S. sewage workers and appropriate comparison populations, no substantial or consistent increase in prevalence of anti-HAV was found among sewage workers.[217-219] No work-related instances of HAV transmission have been reported among sewage workers in the United States.

Pathogenesis

Although HAV shares many virologic characteristics with enteroviruses, it has several differentiating features that influence the pathogenesis and clinical expression of the disease. HAV is resistant to heat, solvents, and acid and grows slowly in living cells, where it has been shown to be relatively noncytolytic and to have little effect on the rate of host protein synthesis.

INCUBATION PERIOD

Determination of the incubation period of disease is imprecise because the early symptoms of hepatitis are often vague and nonspecific. Jaundice may not be noticed by the patient, so the most useful marker of the onset of the disease is a change in urine color, which is almost always recognized by the patient and is the most common reason for seeking medical attention. The range of incubation is between 15 and 50 days, with a mean of approximately 28 days. Although HAV can be transmitted orally or parenterally, the incubation period is independent of the route of inoculation.[220] Experiments in primates and observations in humans suggest that the incubation period is dependent on the infectious dose.[221]

SITE OF VIRAL REPLICATION

HAV is generally transmitted by the fecal-oral route. Because the virus is acid resistant, it probably passes through the stomach, replicates lower in the intestine,[222-224] and is then transported to the liver, which is the major site of replication.[222,225,226] Evidence of replication in the oropharynx has been obtained in chimpanzees.[98] HAV, like many other picornaviruses, is highly organ specific with little evidence of significant replication outside the liver. Virus is shed from infected liver cells into the hepatic sinusoids and canaliculi, passes into the intestine, and is excreted in feces. In humans as well as in nonhuman primates, HAV has been detected in the liver, bile, and feces.[227,228] The first indirect evidence that virus may replicate in the gut was the detection of co-proantibodies in the feces,[229,230] followed by the demonstration of hepatitis A antigen in duodenal lining cells.[222] Nonetheless, the major pathology is restricted to the liver.

PATHOGENESIS

HAV is generally not cytopathic in cell culture, and histopathologic findings in experimental animals and humans do not show widespread hepatocyte necrosis, although the vast majority of hepatocytes at the peak of viral replication appear to be infected by immunohistochemical staining. Therefore, immune mechanisms have been invoked to explain the pathogenesis of the disease.[231] It has been postulated that liver cell damage occurs through a cell-mediated immune response, whereas circulating antibodies are probably more important in limiting the spread of virus to uninfected liver cells and other organs. This hypothesis is consistent with observations in animal models and humans. For example, intravenous inoculation of marmosets with a large dose of HAV resulted in mildly abnormal liver function test results and detectable hepatitis A antigen in hepatocytes within 1 week. Enzyme levels stabilized or even decreased until the third week after inoculation, when a second, higher peak was observed coincident with the appearance of serum antibodies.[232] One explanation is that the early mild hepatitis was due to a direct viral effect, but the second, more severe episode was due to an immune response. The presence of large quantities of virus in hepatocytes before the onset of hepatitis also argues against a major direct cytopathic effect of HAV.[223] It has been suggested that virally elicited T cells target infected liver cells and induce immunopathology. In human studies, Vallbracht and colleagues[231,233] found that lymphocytes from convalescing patients produced cytotoxic effects against autologous epidermal cell lines infected with HAV and that CD8+ T-cell clones demonstrated cytotoxic activity against autologous fibroblasts infected with hepatitis A. These findings are consistent with the hypothesis that CD8+ T lymphocytes mediate liver cell damage. Furthermore, natural killer cells have been demonstrated to be capable of lysing HAV-infected tissue culture cells.[234]

Although liver damage occurs at the time that circulating antibodies become detectable, it has not been proved that the pathology is antibody dependent.[190] Circulating immune complexes containing HAV and specific IgM antibodies have been found during infection. However, IG and complement deposits were not found at the sites of liver cell damage, and resolution of disease occurred even when antibody levels were increasing and hepatitis A antigen could still be detected in the liver.[235-237]

Over the past two decades, there has been a reported dramatic increase in childhood asthma prevalence, which some have hypothesized might be related to improved hygienic conditions leading to fewer childhood infections.[238] At least one study has shown that the prevalence of asthma is lower in children who are seropositive for antibody to HAV.[239] A trait associated with asthma, the T-cell and airway phenotype regulator, which plays a role in controlling the development of airway hyperreactivity, is a member of the T-cell membrane proteins. The human homologue of T-cell membrane protein-1 is the HAV receptor.[79,240] This shared category of membrane proteins is interesting, but appropriate studies to examine any potential association between atopic airway disease and hepatitis A have not been conducted, and no substantial changes in asthma prevalence have been observed in association with the substantial reductions in hepatitis A incidence among U.S. children in recent years.

Clinical Features

Hepatitis A is an acute or a subclinical infection of the liver. Although the clinical expression of infection varies widely, the disease is self-limited, sometimes subclinical, but typically is symptomatic with jaundice. The most important determinant of the likelihood of clinical expression is the age at which infection occurs.[241] The vast majority of infections in children younger than 5 years are silent, and the proportion of symptomatic infections increases with age. The ratio of anicteric to icteric cases has been reported to vary from 12:1 to 1:3.5, depending on the age at which infection occurs.[242] In modeling studies, the estimated average probability of jaundice increased from 7% among children younger than 5 years to 37% among children 5 to 9 years old and to more than 70% among adolescents and adults. In the Greenland epidemic of 1970 to 1974, the frequency of clinically recognizable hepatitis increased from 1% in children younger than 1 year to 24% in 15 year olds.[243,244] Similar low rates of clinical symptoms have been noted in children involved in outbreaks in daycare centers in the United States[245]; however, adults infected in these outbreaks usually became jaundiced.

SYMPTOMS

Patients with hepatitis A often describe a mild illness, the prodrome (see Fig. 173-5), that appears 1 to 7 days before the onset of dark urine, although longer periods have been recorded.[188,241] These symptoms are not usually severe enough to cause the patient to seek medical attention or to stay home from work. In the early stages, flulike symptoms are common; fever (as high as 40°C) may be accompanied by chills, mild headache, malaise, and fatigue. Loss of appetite is a common symptom, with patients reporting that the sight or smell of food, especially fatty foods, is nauseating. Vomiting may occur but is neither severe nor protracted, and weight loss is common. Occasionally, children may experience atypical symptoms such as diarrhea, cough, coryza, and arthralgia.

The first specific sign of disease and the one that causes most patients to seek medical attention is the onset of dark urine. Bilirubinuria is usually followed within a few days by pale or clay-colored feces and yellow discoloration of the sclera, skin, and mucous membranes. The return of color to the stool occurs 2 or 3 weeks after the onset of illness and is an indication of resolution of disease. Itching, a sign of cholestasis, occurs in less than 50% of patients but may be severe enough to require antipruritics or corticosteroids.

On physical examination, the patient's liver may be enlarged and sometimes tender. In adults, the liver can be enlarged up to 14 cm in the vertical axis and has a firm consistency. The spleen is palpable in 5% to 15% of patients. Spider nevi may appear on the trunk and usually disappear during convalescence. Other physical findings occur rarely.

The duration of illness varies, but by the third week, most patients feel better, have lost their hepatomegaly, and have normal or nearly normal levels of serum alanine aminotransferase (ALT) and aspartate aminotransferase. In many patients, the appearance of jaundice is associated with rapid resolution of symptoms. In a study of 59 patients in the United States, approximately two thirds recovered within 2 months, 85% within 3 months, and nearly all by 6 months.[246]

The clinical course and histologic findings do not differ in pregnancy.[247,248] Intrauterine transmission of HAV during the first trimester that resulted in fetal meconium peritonitis has been described in two case reports.[119,120] At delivery, both infants had a perforated ileum. No evidence has suggested that more severe infection or subsequent loss of immunity occurs in the presence of human immunodeficiency virus infection. Although not demonstrated in all published studies, on balance, it seems that HAV infection in persons with chronic liver disease is more severe and more likely to result in fulminant hepatitis A.[249,250,250a]

COMPLICATIONS

Recognized complications of hepatitis A include cholestasis, prolonged and relapsing disease, fulminant hepatitis, triggering of chronic active autoimmune hepatitis, and autoimmune extrahepatic disease.

Cholestatic hepatitis, characterized by fever, pruritus, and prolonged jaundice, has been reported as an occasional complication.

TABLE 173-1	Clinical Manifestations of 8647 Hospitalized Patients, 1988 Shanghai Epidemic					
Symptom	%	*Clinical Findings*	%	*Complications*	%
Jaundice	84	Hepatomegaly	87	Cholestasis	1.6-5.3
Weight loss	82	Splenomegaly	9	Upper gastrointestinal bleeding	0.5-1.2
Malaise	80	Skin rashes	3	Thrombocytopenic purpura	<0.1 (6 cases)
Fever	76	Mild edema	2	Guillain-Barré syndrome	<0.1 (4 cases)
Nausea	69	Petechia	2	Pure red cell aplasia	<0.1 (3 cases)
Vomiting	47	Cardiac arrhythmias	0.8	Autoimmune hemolytic anemia	<0.1 (2 cases)
Abdominal pain	37			Transverse myelitis, optic neuritis	<0.1 (1 case each)
Arthralgia	6				

Data summarized from Yao G. Clinical spectrum and natural history of viral hepatitis A in a 1988 Shanghai epidemic. In: Hollinger FB, Lemon SM, Margolis HS, eds. *Viral Hepatitis and Liver Disease.* Baltimore: Williams & Wilkins; 1991:76-78.

Cholestasis developed in 4 of 59 (7%) patients in a hospital-based study.[246] In a detailed description of six patients, peak serum bilirubin levels of 12 to 29 mg/dL were recorded, and jaundice lasted for 12 to 18 weeks. In each case, peak ALT levels were less than 500 IU/L.[251] Liver biopsy specimens revealed centrilobular cholestasis and portal inflammation. Although the prognosis is universally favorable, a short, rapidly tapered course of corticosteroids has been used to reduce symptoms and hasten resolution.

Relapsing disease has been reported as an occasional complication in both adults and children.[93,246,252] It has been reported that a relapse occurs after a typical initial course in 3% to 20% of cases. Typically, symptoms decrease but may not completely resolve during the recovery phase, and the relapse disease is usually milder than the first. In the study of Tong and colleagues,[246] the mean ALT level was 3500 mIU/mL and the mean bilirubin level was 4.9 mg/dL during the first peak and 1554 mIU/mL and 2.5 mg/dL, respectively, during the second. Viral excretion during the relapse has been detected. Although the pathogenesis of relapses has not been elucidated, it is important to recognize that these cases resolve without sequelae.[252,253] Extrahepatic manifestations of hepatitis A rarely include cardiac involvement, although patients with acute hepatitis may have bradycardia and electrocardiograms may show prolongation of the PR interval and some mild T-wave depression. These changes resolve rapidly during convalescence.[254] HAV infection rarely causes pathology of other organs, but occasional cases of postviral encephalitis, Guillain-Barré syndrome, cholecystitis, acute pancreatitis, acute renal failure secondary to interstitial nephritis, aplastic or hemolytic anemia, agranulocytosis, thrombocytopenic purpura, or pancytopenia have been reported. Several cases of arthritis, vasculitis, and cryoglobulinemia have also been reported.[236,255,256] Some patients may become depressed, and, occasionally, the depression may be severe enough to require treatment, but it is usually mild and self-limited.

The clinical course of hepatitis A is usually benign. Although severe disease is occasionally observed, especially in older patients, long-term sequelae in recovered patients have not been observed. During the 1988 Shanghai epidemic, complications were unusual, mostly involving cholestasis[257] (Table 173-1). Death from hepatitis A is well documented, but unusual. In the Shanghai epidemic that involved primarily adolescents and young adults, 47 deaths were registered among 310,746 cases (0.015%).[257] This is consistent with surveillance data reported to

the Centers for Disease Control and Prevention; in 2006, for example, 5 deaths were identified among approximately 1600 cases, yielding a case-fatality ratio of 0.3% (Table 173-2).[152] In general, the severe clinical manifestations and outcomes (e.g., hospitalizations, fulminant hepatic failure, death) are more common among older adults but also occur among children[152,250a,258,259] (see Table 173-2).

The most serious complication of hepatitis A is fulminant hepatic failure, defined by the appearance of severe acute liver disease with hepatic encephalopathy in a previously healthy person.[260,261] Danger signs include excitability, irritability, insomnia, confusion, and severe vomiting. Laboratory and clinical evidence of deteriorating liver function, especially prolonged prothrombin times, correlates with the histologic picture of almost complete destruction of the hepatic parenchyma, with only a reticulin framework and portal tracts remaining. Occasionally, small groups of surviving hepatocytes can be seen close to the portal tracts, which may represent foci of regeneration. Surprisingly, little indication of a vigorous inflammatory response has been noted. Fulminant hepatitis A is a rare occurrence in the developed world, accounting for 4.5% of cases of fulminant hepatitis in a prospective series of U.S. cases.[261] Spontaneous survival from fulminant hepatitis A occurs more commonly than from fulminant hepatitis of other causes.[261]

Laboratory Diagnosis

Hepatitis A is not clinically distinguishable from other forms of viral hepatitis, although the diagnosis may be suspected in a patient with typical symptoms during an outbreak. Liver function tests (see Fig. 173-5), especially serum levels of ALT and aspartate aminotransferase, are sensitive measures of parenchymal liver damage but are not specific for hepatitis A. In the study by Tong and colleagues,[246] the peak mean ALT level was 1952 mIU/mL and the mean peak aspartate aminotransferase level was 1442 mIU/mL, with the highest ALT level being 9711 mIU/mL, although values greater than 20,000 mIU/mL have been observed. The ALT levels returned to normal by a mean of 7.4 weeks (range, 1 to 29 weeks). Although elevated ALT levels are detected in patients with severe hepatitis, high levels are not necessarily correlated with an adverse outcome. Alkaline phosphatase levels are usually only mildly elevated, and persisting elevated levels suggest hepatitis-associated cholestasis.[251] The highest bilirubin level in the study of Tong and

TABLE 173-2	Hospitalizations and Deaths, by Age (in Years), for Reported Hepatitis A cases, United States, 2006																	
	Age < 5			Age 5-14			Age 15-39			Age 40-59			Age 60+			All		
	n	N	%	n	N	%	n	N	%	n	N	%	n	N	%	n	N	%
Died of hepatitis	0	92	0.0	0	316	0.0	0	567	0.0	1	378	0.3	4	259	1.5	5	1612	0.3
Hospitalized for hepatitis	21	94	22.3	62	319	19.4	188	590	31.9	135	389	34.7	143	273	52.4	549	1665	33.0

Includes all cases with nonmissing relevant data, from among the total of 3579 reported cases of hepatitis A.
From the Centers for Disease Control and Prevention, National Notifiable Diseases Surveillance System, Atlanta, GA.

colleagues was 38 mg/dL and the peak levels of serum bilirubin were positively correlated with age. Elevated levels of total serum IgM, a mild lymphocytosis, and occasional atypical mononuclear cells are commonly found in patients with acute hepatitis A but are not diagnostic of the disease.[246,262]

The diagnosis of acute hepatitis A is most commonly confirmed by detection of specific IgM in a single acute-phase serum sample.[263] The hepatitis A–specific IgM antibody is usually present at the initial evaluation and may be detectable at the time of the first increase in ALT. IgM anti-HAV can be detected in nearly 100% of patients with acute hepatitis A at their first clinical examination and remains positive in most for 3 to 6 months and rarely can be detected for two years or longer. False-positive test results occur particularly among persons who have no other evidence of recent infection, suggesting a low positive predictive value when used to test asymptomatic persons with no known recent HAV exposures.[263a] Assays for total antibody to the virus are of little diagnostic value because IgG persists for many years and may be related to a past infection. Antibodies to naturally acquired HAV are primarily directed against the virion and do not react well with the individual peptides that make up the virion capsid. Low levels of antibodies to nonstructural proteins are found in the serum of convalescing patients and have been used in an attempt to distinguish the antibody response to natural infection from the response to a killed virus preparation.[264,265]

HAV or viral antigen can be detected in the stools of patients 1 to 2 weeks before symptoms develop, but such detection has little place in routine clinical diagnosis because the tests are not widely available and shedding is often complete before the patient seeks medical attention.[266,267] Nucleic acid–based diagnostic techniques, primarily PCR or other nucleic acid amplification assays, have been used in research laboratories when a highly sensitive test for the presence of HAV is required. PCR has been very useful in the study of environmental samples.[268,269] In response to several outbreaks of hepatitis A associated with pooled plasma products, screening by nucleic acid testing of plasma pools intended for manufacture into various plasma components has been instituted by most plasma fractionators for process testing. Although these nucleic acid tests are now commercially available for testing plasma, they are not recommended for use as diagnostics for patients with acute hepatitis. The performance of these assays in the diagnostic setting has not been evaluated. The use of PCR for identifying HAV in stool samples also has not been validated as a diagnostic assay. Many stools have inhibitors of PCR, which could result in false-negative results. Until sufficient studies with nucleic acid testing have been performed, the use of these types of assays for diagnosis cannot be recommended outside the research setting.

Liver biopsy is rarely indicated to establish a diagnosis in acute hepatitis because this procedure is associated with a small, but measurable, risk and the histopathology is not usually diagnostic. In one study done in Japan, where biopsy for acute hepatitis was routine, 86 patients with serologically established acute hepatitis A were evaluated for quantitative and qualitative light microscopic features, together with biopsy samples from 78 patients with acute hepatitis B and from 76 patients with acute hepatitis non-A, non-B. Hepatitis A was characterized by more pronounced portal inflammation than was hepatitis non-A, non-B, but less conspicuous parenchymal changes such as focal necrosis, Kupffer-cell proliferation, acidophil bodies, and ballooning. Nonspecific reactive hepatitis with slightly increased serum transaminase levels was often seen during recovery from hepatitis A and needs to be distinguished from the longer lasting cases of acute hepatitis B and C.[270,271] Hepatitis A antigen and HAV particles can be detected in the cytoplasm of infected cells by immunostaining techniques or thin-section electron microscopy.[227,272]

Immunity

The high prevalence of antibody in older individuals in countries that now have a low incidence of hepatitis A suggests that anti-HAV IgG usually persists for life. Second attacks of hepatitis A have not been documented in the field and have not been induced experimentally. In two sets of experiments involving a total of 19 volunteers, reinoculation with HAV 6 to 9 months after the initial illness failed to induce disease.[5,6]

Passive immunization with IG provides complete protection against hepatitis A, suggesting that serum antibody alone is sufficient to prevent infection. It has been difficult to judge the effect of mucosal immunity because IgA antibodies in saliva or feces either are not detected or are present at very low levels.[273] The antibody response to HAV infection is generally brisk and high titered. Both IgG and IgM can usually be detected at the time of the first expression of clinical illness (see Fig. 173-5). Neutralizing antibody as measured by in vitro tissue culture assays can also be detected early in disease. Because HAV is not usually cytopathic, a radioimmunofocus reduction test was devised that is equivalent to a plaque reduction assay.[274] This highly sensitive test was shown to correlate closely, although it is approximately 100-fold more sensitive than total antibody radioimmunoassay. With this assay, both IgM and IgG have been shown to possess neutralizing activity. It has also been demonstrated that patients convalescing from hepatitis A may have very high titers of in vitro neutralizing antibody. Serum dilutions of 1 : 100,000 to 1 : 500,000 or more are not uncommon.

The role of T lymphocytes in protection from HAV infection has not been fully elucidated. Undoubtedly, T-cell responses do occur, and CD8$^+$ cytotoxic T lymphocytes and possibly natural killer cells are important in pathogenesis.[275-277]

Prevention

The most effective method to control hepatitis A and other enteric infections is through improved standards of hygiene and sanitation, especially the provision of clean water. Good hygienic practices with particular emphasis on hand washing and restriction of activities of workers who are ill are of primary importance in the food preparation industry. Nosocomial infections have been reported but are not common, and transmission usually is from a patient who is not suspected of having hepatitis A.[278,279] Hence, hospitalized patients need only enteric isolation (see Chapter 300). Private rooms, gowns, and masks are not necessary unless the patient is incontinent. Gloves should be worn when handling any material potentially contaminated with feces. Frequent hand washing, whether gloves are worn or not, should be emphasized. Hospital personnel in general do not have a higher prevalence of antibody to HAV than appropriately selected controls do. However, several outbreaks of hepatitis A in hospital nurseries have been reported with transmission to staff.[92,122,279]

Travelers to developing countries should be advised to eat only properly cooked food and be careful of uncooked vegetables and shellfish. Even in the vaccine era, the maxim to prevent traveler's diarrhea, "boil it, cook it, peel it, or forget it," also applies to hepatitis A prevention.

Improvements in sanitary systems, although technologically possible, may not be practical in large parts of the world. In more developed areas, sudden deterioration in living conditions because of war or political or economic instability can rapidly degrade sanitary systems. In the developed world, hepatitis A remains a risk associated with travel. Therefore, considerable effort has been expended in the development of hepatitis A vaccines.

PASSIVE IMMUNIZATION

Before the licensing of hepatitis A vaccines, the mainstay of hepatitis A immunoprophylaxis had been passive immunization with pooled IG, which has been known in the past as gamma globulin or immune serum globulin. IG has proved useful for the prevention of hepatitis A in travelers, Peace Corps volunteers, and military personnel and even for postexposure prophylaxis (PEP) in common-source or family outbreaks. However, IGA has never been successful in altering the epidemiology of hepatitis in a high-risk community because of the transient nature of the protection, coverage rates, and perhaps lack of herd immunity.

IG is manufactured by cold ethanol precipitation from large pools of plasma collected from tens of thousands of donors.[280] At present, the individual plasma units used in these pools are screened for hepatitis B virus, hepatitis C virus, and human immunodeficiency virus by the appropriate serologic and other assays. Minipools of plasma are tested by nucleic acid testing for hepatitis C and human immunodeficiency virus, and the product itself undergoes at least one specific viral inactivation step in its manufacturing process. Because the prevalence of antibody to HAV in the population has been decreasing, concern has been voiced that antibody levels against HAV in IG preparations might drop below effective levels. Although no standard for anti-HAV levels exists in IG preparations in the United States, even though prophylaxis against hepatitis A is the primary use for this product, anti-HAV levels remain adequate at this time to provide protection as indicated.[281] Eventually, the manufacture of IG from selected antibody-positive donors may need to be considered to develop a hyperimmune globulin for hepatitis A prevention analogous to other agent-specific hyperimmune globulins.[282]

The efficacy of IG was first demonstrated in an outbreak at a summer camp in 1944 and has been confirmed many times since.[283,284] Several studies have demonstrated the effectiveness of IG in pre-exposure settings such as among travelers, military personnel,[285] and Peace Corps workers.[286] The rate of HAV infections in Peace Corps volunteers dropped from 1.6 to 2.1 cases per 100 per year before mandatory administering of IG every 4 months, to 0.1 to 0.3 case per 100 per year after the institution of a mandatory program.[286] When administered before exposure or within 2 weeks after exposure, IG is more than 85% effective in preventing hepatitis A.[283,287,288] Whether IG completely prevents infection or leads to asymptomatic infection and the development of persistent anti-HAV (passive-active immunity) is probably related to the amount of time that has elapsed between exposure and IG administration.[283,289]

With the licensure of inactivated hepatitis A vaccines, the use of IG for pre- and postexposure prophylaxis has become more limited, but it remains indicated for some situations. For postexposure prophylaxis, although hepatitis A vaccine is recommended in most circumstances, IG should be used for protecting children younger than 12 months, immunocompromised persons, or persons for whom the vaccine is contraindicated; it is also preferred for persons older than 40 years of age (Table 173-3).[290] Similarly, for pre-exposure prophylaxis such as is needed for travel to endemic areas, IG should be used instead of vaccine for persons who are younger than 12 months of age or who have a contraindication to the vaccine; it is also recommended

that IG be given in addition to vaccine to older or immunocompromised travelers who will depart in 2 weeks or less.[290]

The usual dose of IG is a single intramuscular injection of 0.02 or 0.06 mL/kg. The lower dose is adequate to provide protection for as long as 3 months, and the higher dose is effective for as long as 5 months.[281] Readministration every 5 months is necessary for extended exposures, and hepatitis A vaccine, if not contraindicated, is probably a better choice in such cases. Intramuscular preparations of IG should never be given intravenously, and the intravenous preparations of IG are not intended for hepatitis A prevention and are formulated at a lower globulin concentration.

IG does not interfere with the immune response to oral poliovirus or yellow fever vaccine or, in general, to inactivated vaccines. However, IG can interfere with the immune response to some live attenuated vaccines (e.g., measles, mumps, rubella vaccine; varicella vaccine) (see Chapter 320). Administration of the measles, mumps, rubella vaccine and of varicella-containing vaccines should be delayed for at least 3 months after administration of IG. IG should not be given within 2 weeks after the administration of the measles, mumps, rubella, or varicella-containing vaccines unless the benefits of IG administration are greater than the benefits of vaccination.[291]

Serious adverse events from IG are rare. Because anaphylaxis has been reported after repeated administration to persons with IgA deficiency, these persons should not receive IG.[292] Pregnancy or lactation is not a contraindication to IG administration. For infants and pregnant women, a preparation that does not include thimerosal is preferable.

ACTIVE IMMUNIZATION

Active immunization with hepatitis A vaccines has developed along classic lines similar to the path followed for polio vaccines. Like poliovirus, the initial breakthrough came with the in vitro cultivation of HAV in cell lines suitable for vaccine production.[14] Formalin-inactivated, cell culture–produced, whole-virus vaccines have now been approved in much of the world.

Two HAV inactivated vaccines have been approved for use in the United States and widely throughout the world. Two other inactivated hepatitis A vaccines are available in Europe and other parts of the world.[293,294] Both U.S. licensed vaccines are produced from highly cell culture–adapted virus strains that have also been shown to be highly attenuated in humans, which gives them an extra measure of safety.[295] The entire nucleotide sequences of both the wild-type and the vaccine variant of strain HM175 have been determined.[38] A full-length, infectious complementary DNA clone of the cell culture–adapted virus was made,[38] and the mutations responsible for cell culture adaptation and attenuation have been determined by the molecular construction of chimeric viruses.[76,296] It was found that substitutions and deletions in the 5′ noncoding region and substitutions in the 2B/2C coding regions are highly important for cell culture adaptation and attenuation of virulence. However, mutations throughout the genome contributed to improved in vitro replication.[74]

Both U.S. licensed vaccines, Havrix (GlaxoSmithKline Biologicals) and VAQTA (Merck & Co.), are grown in MRC-5 cells, purified, inactivated by formalin, and formulated with alum as an adjuvant. Both vaccines are licensed in a two-dose series, with the second dose given 6-8 months after the first.

Clinical trials indicate that inactivated hepatitis A vaccines are safe, highly immunogenic, and efficacious.[51,52,293,297] In one study, 1037 healthy seronegative children 2 to 16 years of age in a community experiencing yearly outbreaks of hepatitis A received either a single dose of formalin-inactivated vaccine ($n = 519$) or placebo ($n = 518$). No cases of hepatitis occurred in the vaccinated group, except for a few that appeared within 3 weeks of vaccination. These cases represented patients who were already incubating the infection at the time of vaccination. In the period from 21 days to 103 days, 34 cases of hepatitis A were observed, all in the placebo group, indicating a 100% vaccine protective efficacy during that period of observation[297,298] Vac-

TABLE 173-3	Recommendations for Hepatitis A Postexposure Prophylaxis	
*Group**	*Recommended Prophylaxis†*
Persons 12 mo-40 yr	Single antigen hepatitis A vaccine at age-appropriate dose
Persons > 40 yr	IG 0.02 mL/kg is preferred; vaccine can be used if IG cannot be obtained
Children < 12 mo	IG 0.02 mL/kg‡
Immunocompromised persons, persons who have chronic liver disease, and persons for whom vaccine is contraindicated	IG 0.02 mL/kg‡

*Persons recently exposed to HAV who have not previously received hepatitis A vaccine.

†Postexposure prophylaxis should be given as soon as possible after exposure. The efficacy of immunoglobulin or vaccine if administered more than 2 weeks after exposure has not been established.

‡In the event of ongoing exposure, persons for whom immunoglobulin is recommended should receive immunoglobulin 0.06 mL/kg, repeated every 5 months during exposure.

IG, immunoglobulin.

cination of children at 2 years of age has continued in this community since the time of the original trial. Despite the reintroduction of HAV from unvaccinated individuals joining the community, no new outbreaks have occurred over a 9-year span. In a large field trial of an inactivated vaccine involving more than 40,000 children in Thailand, the vaccine was found to be at least 80% effective compared with placebo and was without serious adverse reactions.[52]

Although the absolute level of antibody required to protect against infection has not been rigorously established, it is accepted based on comparisons with protective antibody levels associated with passive immunization with IG that antibody concentrations of 10 to 20 mIU/mL (depending on the assay used) are protective.[51,299,300] The licensed inactivated hepatitis A vaccines have all been shown to be highly and rapidly immunogenic. They induce seroconversions to protective levels of antibody in as little as 2 weeks after the initial dose.[301,302] The level of antibody after vaccination varies with the dose and schedule of the vaccine. However, after a single dose of vaccine, antibody titers are higher than titers produced by known protective levels of IG but are generally lower than titers measured after natural infection.[303-305] The quality of the antibody response after vaccination has also been studied by comparing antibodies detected by radioimmunoassay, radioimmunoprecipitation, and in vitro neutralization in sera from persons passively immunized with IG and in persons immunized by vaccine. With the antibody normalized between the two groups by radioimmunoassay, the IG recipients had higher neutralization titers but negligible radioimmunoprecipitation titers compared with the group who was vaccinated.[305] However, it has also been shown that IG prepared from the serum of vaccinees could protect a chimpanzee from HAV challenge when the titer of antibody achieved by passive immunization in the chimpanzee was similar to that found in humans receiving IG prophylaxis.[306] It must also be understood that there are no direct correlations between in vitro neutralization assays and seroprotection. Regardless of the results of antibody measurements after vaccination, clinical trials have demonstrated that the vaccine is highly effective within a month after the first dose.

Certain factors may reduce the response to the vaccine. Only approximately 75% of human immunodeficiency virus–positive vaccinees developed protective levels of antibody, and those who responded had lower antibody titers than vaccinees without HIV infection.[307] The final antibody concentrations achieved in patients with chronic liver disease were also lower than in normal subjects, but the seroprotection rates were approximately the same. The common recommended schedule of a single dose followed by a booster dose 6 to 18 months later produces very high levels of antibody, well in excess of that achieved after passive immunization with IG that are known to be effective. After the completed series, it is estimated that protective levels of antibody will persist for at least 20 years.[308] Because the incubation period for hepatitis A average 28-30 days, and the anamnestic responses observed after the second dose are rapid and robust, it has been suggested that vaccinees who have seroconverted will be protected even if their antibody levels have fallen below protective levels.[51] Long-term follow-up studies will have to be performed to confirm this hypothesis.

Live attenuated vaccines based on the CR326 and the HM175 strains have also been tested in primates and to a limited extent in humans, and the H2 strain has been used in extended clinical studies in China.[26,309-312] Both CR326 and HM175 strains have been evaluated as candidate live vaccines and found to be highly attenuated in humans.[310,313] For both strains, an inoculum dose of greater than 10^6 tissue culture infective doses was required to induce an antibody response in volunteers. Even at high doses in the volunteers, it was not possible to prove that the vaccine virus replicated because no vaccine virus was ever isolated from the volunteers and the only evidence for replication was seroconversion, which could have been induced by the antigenic mass contained in the inoculum rather than new antigen produced by replication. It may be difficult to develop a live vaccine that is both adequately immunogenic and attenuated because the properties of replication and pathogenesis may be closely linked.[314-316]

Recommendations for Prevention
POSTEXPOSURE PROPHYLAXIS

For decades, IG has been recommended for postexposure prophylaxis (PEP) to prevent infection after known exposure to HAV. However, with recent data indicating equivalent postexposure efficacy of IG and vaccine in preventing symptomatic hepatitis A among healthy persons 40 years of age or younger[317] and the relative public health advantages of vaccine compared with IG including the induction of active immunity and longer protection, greater ease of administration, and greater acceptability and availability, hepatitis A vaccines are now recommended in most circumstances for postexposure prophylaxis (Table 173-3).[290] When using hepatitis A vaccine alone for PEP, single-antigen vaccine should be used; no data exist regarding the performance of the combination vaccine for prophylaxis after exposure to HAV, and the concentration of HAV antigen in the currently available combination vaccine is half that included in the single-antigen vaccine available from the same manufacturer. IG should still be used for PEP in certain cases. IG (0.02 mL/kg) should be used for children younger than 12 months, immunocompromised persons, persons who have had chronic liver disease diagnosed, and persons for whom vaccine is contraindicated. In addition, IG is preferred for persons older than 40 years of age, although vaccine can be used if IG cannot be obtained. For PEP, the usual dose of IG is a single intramuscular injection of 0.02 mL/kg (see Table 173-3).

PEP with vaccine or IG as described previously is recommended to prevent hepatitis A after exposure in certain settings.[151,290] Household and sexual contacts of patients with hepatitis A should receive appropriate PEP as soon as possible. Casual contacts such as school classmates or co-workers who have not had close physical contact usually do not require PEP. Aggressive use of PEP is indicated to control hepatitis A outbreaks in child care centers when a child or an employee is diagnosed with hepatitis A.[151,160,290] Outbreaks in other settings (e.g., hospitals, facilities for developmentally disabled persons) are rare. When a food handler is identified with hepatitis A, PEP with vaccine or IG should be administered to other food handlers at the food establishment and can be considered for patrons if certain other conditions exist.[105,107,151,290] Once cases are identified that are associated with a food service establishment, it generally is too late to administer PEP to patrons because the 2-week postexposure period during which IG or vaccine is known to be effective will have passed.

PRE-EXPOSURE PROPHYLAXIS

Inactivated hepatitis A vaccine is indicated for pre-exposure protection of susceptible persons 12 months of age or older, persons at increased risk of hepatitis A, and for any person wishing to obtain immunity (Tables 173-4 and 173-5). IG should be used for children younger than 12 months of age or other persons who cannot or choose not to receive hepatitis A vaccine but who require protection against hepatitis A.

Prevaccination serologic testing may be considered to reduce costs by not vaccinating persons with previous immunity, such as older adolescents and adults in certain population groups with a high prevalence of infection (e.g., persons born in areas of high hepatitis A endemicity), but should take into account the cost of testing, vaccine cost, and the likelihood that the person will return for vaccination.[318] Vaccination of immune individuals is not harmful. Postvaccination testing is not indicated because of the high rate of vaccine response. Furthermore, not all commercially available assays can detect the low anti-HAV concentrations generated by immunization.

DISEASE CONTROL STRATEGIES
Routine Vaccination of Children
Soon after hepatitis A vaccines became available in the United States, it was recognized that a strategy of widespread routine vaccination of children had the potential to achieve a sustained reduction in the

TABLE 173-4

TABLE 173-4 Recommendations for Hepatitis A Preexposure Immunoprophylaxis

Age	Exposure Duration	Recommended Prophylaxis
<12 mo	Short term (<3 mo)	IG 0.02 mL/kg
<12 mo	3-5 mo	IG 0.06 mL/kg
<12 mo	>5 mo	IG 0.06 mL/kg repeated every 5 mo
Healthy persons 1-40 yr	Short or long term	Hepatitis A vaccine
Healthy persons >40 yr	Short or long term	Hepatitis A vaccine. Can add IG (0.02 mL/kg) if exposure is expected in ≤2 wk
Immunocompromised persons, and persons with chronic liver disease or other chronic medical conditions	Short or long term	Hepatitis A vaccine. Add IG (0.02 mL/kg) if exposure is expected in ≤2 wk
Persons for whom vaccine is contraindicated or who refuse vaccine	Depending on expected duration of exposure, substitute IG as described above for children <12 mo of age	

IG, immunoglobulin.

overall incidence of hepatitis A by preventing infection among individuals in age groups that accounted for at least one third of cases and eliminating a major source of infection for others. However, hepatitis A vaccines could not be readily incorporated into the routine infant schedule because they were not then licensed for children younger than 2 years of age. To overcome these logistical barriers to widespread use of hepatitis A vaccines among children, a novel vaccination strategy was developed, based on distinct features of hepatitis A epidemiology and experience gathered from demonstration projects and other research involving incremental implementation of routine childhood hepatitis A vaccination.

TABLE 173-5 Recommendations for Routine Preexposure Use of Hepatitis A Virus Vaccine

Group	Comments
Children	Vaccine should be given to all children at age 1 yr (12-23 mo).* Vaccination of children 2-18 yr may also be warranted.†
International travelers‡	Immunoglobulin may be given in addition to or instead of vaccine; children younger than 12 months should receive immunoglobulin (see Table 173-4)
Men who have sex with men	Includes adolescents
Illicit drug users	Includes adolescents
Persons with chronic liver disease	Increased risk of fulminant hepatitis A with HAV infection
Persons receiving clotting factor concentrates	
Persons who work with HAV in research laboratory settings	

*Hepatitis A vaccine is not licensed for children younger than 12 months.
†States and communities with existing vaccination programs for children age 2 to 18 years are encouraged to maintain these programs. Catch-up vaccination for this age group may be warranted elsewhere in the context of ongoing outbreaks among children.
‡Persons traveling to Canada, western Europe, Japan, Australia, or New Zealand are at no greater risk than in the United States.
HAV, hepatitis A vaccine.
From Centers for Disease Control and Prevention. Prevention of hepatitis A through active or passive immunization. Recommendations of the Advisory Committee on Immunization Practices. *MMWR Morb Mortal Wkly Rep.* 2006;55(RR-7):1-23.

Recommendations for use of hepatitis A vaccine were first issued by the Advisory Committee on Immunization Practices of the U.S. Public Health Service, the American Academy of Pediatrics, and other groups in 1996, updated in 1999, and again in 2006 (Table 173-6).[148,149,151,319] The initial recommendations, published in 1996 soon after vaccines became available in the United States, called for routine vaccination of children living in communities with the highest hepatitis A rates (e.g., Native American and Alaska Native communities).[148] Although apparently effective in reducing disease rates in communities covered by the 1996 recommendations, implementation of these recommendations had little impact on overall disease incidence nationwide because only a small proportion of nationally reported cases occurred among persons in such communities. In 1999, the recommendation for routine vaccination of children was extended to include those living in states, counties, and communities with consistently elevated hepatitis A rates,[149] with an average reported incidence of more than 10 cases per 100,000 population in 1987 to 1997. Hepatitis A incidence decreased sharply in the states included in the recommendations for routine vaccination of children, and beginning in 2001, rates were similar across all regions, and the majority of cases were occurring in states that historically had low rates and where hepatitis A vaccination of children had not been widely implemented.[319a] In 2006, after hepatitis A vaccines were licensed for children beginning at age 12 months, to extend the benefits of vaccination to the rest of the country and further reduce transmission of HAV, the recommendations for routine vaccination were expanded to include children 12 to 23 months of age nationwide.[151]

Vaccination of Persons at Increased Risk of Hepatitis A Infection or Severe Consequences

Hepatitis A vaccine is also indicated for persons in the following groups that have an increased risk of HAV infection or of severe consequences if infected (see Table 173-5).[151]

Men Who Have Sex with Men. Adolescent and adult men who have sex with men should be vaccinated, regardless of reported level of sexual activity.[151] Prevaccination serologic testing is not necessary for vaccination of adolescents and young adults, but could be considered for older adults.

Users of Illicit Drugs. Vaccination is recommended for users of injected and noninjected illegal drugs. Prevaccination testing could be considered for adults; the need might depend on the particular characteristics of the population of drug users, including the type and duration of drug use.[173,174,320]

TABLE 173-6 Recommended Doses and Schedules for Inactivated Hepatitis A Vaccines

Age (yr)	Vaccine	Dose	Volume (mL)	No. of Doses	Schedule (mo)*
1-18	Havrix	720 ELU†	0.5	2	0, 6-12
	VAQTA	25 U	0.5	2	0, 6-18
≥19	Havrix	1440 ELU	1.0	2	0, 6-12
	VAQTA	50 U	1.0	2	0, 6-18
≥12	AVAXIM‡	160 antigen units	0.5	2	0, 6-12
1-15	AVAXIM‡	80 antigen units	0.5	2	0, 6-12
≥1	EPAXAL‡	24 IU	0.5	2	0, 6-12

*0 months represents timing of initial dose; subsequent numbers represent months after the initial dose.
†Enzyme-linked immunosorbent assay units.
‡Not licensed in the United States. Licensed ages, doses, and schedules vary among countries.

International Travelers. Susceptible persons who travel to or work in countries where hepatitis A is endemic should be vaccinated or receive IG before departure. Hepatitis A vaccination is preferred, particularly for persons who plan frequent travel or will live in an endemic area. The first dose should be administered as soon as travel is considered. For most healthy persons 1 to 40 years of age, one dose of single-antigen hepatitis A vaccine given any time before departure can provide adequate protection. Older adults, immunocompromised persons, and persons with chronic liver disease or other chronic medical conditions planning to depart to an endemic area in 2 weeks or less should receive the initial dose of the vaccine and also simultaneously can be administered IG (0.02 mL/kg) at a different anatomic injection site (see Table 173-4). Completion of the vaccine series according to the licensed schedule is needed for long-term protection. Prevaccination serologic testing should be considered for older travelers or younger travelers who were born in a country in which hepatitis A is endemic. IG should be given to travelers younger than 1 year of age because hepatitis A vaccine is not licensed for children in this age group to prevent the rare severe cases that occur and to prevent transmission to others after returning from abroad.[151,290] IG should also be used for pre-exposure prophylaxis for travelers who are allergic to vaccine or components.

Regular Recipients of Blood or Plasma-Derived Products. The risk of hepatitis A from a blood transfusion or from plasma derivatives is extremely low, but both have been reported.[37,96] Individuals who receive these products regularly should be immunized against diseases transmitted via blood-borne means with available vaccines. Many recipients of factor VIII, for instance, have been infected by hepatitis C virus or even hepatitis B virus, and they should not undergo another infection of their liver. Currently, these products are treated by a viral inactivation process often based on solvents or heat. Because HAV is resistant to organic solvents and is relatively resistant to heat, cases of hepatitis A associated with factor VIII have caused the manufacturers to begin to develop new methods that would eliminate infectious HAV from their products. Nevertheless, hepatitis A vaccination of persons with clotting factor disorders is recommended.

Persons with Chronic Liver Disease. Although individuals with chronic liver disease are not at increased risk of hepatitis A, acute hepatitis A in such patients can have very serious or fatal consequences.[321] Therefore, it is recommended that all such persons, no matter the cause of their liver disease, be vaccinated against hepatitis A.

Other Groups and Settings. Persons who work with HAV in research settings should be vaccinated.[151]

Hepatitis A Vaccination during Outbreaks

The frequency of large communitywide outbreaks has decreased considerably since implementation of routine childhood immunization, and ongoing vaccination of children should reduce the occurrence of these outbreaks further. Because of logistical difficulties, accelerated vaccination as an additional measure to control outbreaks should be undertaken with caution.[151] Efforts are probably better directed toward sustained routine vaccination of children to maintain high levels of immunity and prevent future epidemics.

The frequency of hepatitis A outbreaks in child care centers has also decreased in recent years and should continue to decrease with ongoing widespread vaccination of children. There is little experience using vaccine to control outbreaks when they do occur.[322] When outbreaks are recognized, aggressive use of PEP for previously unvaccinated persons is effective in limiting transmission.[158] Child care center attendees can be a readily accessible target population for ongoing routine vaccination programs.

The frequency of outbreaks in hospitals, institutions, and schools is not high enough to warrant routine vaccination of persons in these settings, and there are no data with respect to using vaccine

to control outbreaks in these settings. Although persons who work as food handlers are not at increased risk of hepatitis A because of their occupation, they may transmit HAV to others when they contract hepatitis A.[199] To reduce the frequency of evaluations of food handlers with hepatitis A and the need for PEP of patrons, public health officials in some jurisdictions have instituted measures to promote hepatitis A vaccination of food handlers.[323] However, because transmission from infected food handlers accounts for a very small proportion of cases nationwide, vaccination of food handlers is not likely to affect overall disease incidence and has not been found to be cost-effective.[324]

Directions for the Future

At present, hepatitis A vaccination is generally not indicated in developing countries, particularly those with highest endemicity where infection in early childhood is nearly universal and disease is uncommon. Although vaccination strategies could be devised directed at areas within transitional or intermediate endemicity countries where a sizable proportion of adults are likely to be susceptible, such as urban areas with good water and sanitation facilities, the relative cost-effectiveness of hepatitis A vaccination compared with other major public health priorities has not been evaluated. However, the global disease burden associated with hepatitis A will increase in the coming years, particularly in these areas, as a larger proportion of the population remains susceptible to HAV infection into adolescence and adulthood because of continuing improvements in standards of living and sanitary and hygienic conditions.[99] If vaccine was available at a low cost and vaccination was shown to be cost-effective, some countries in which a significant susceptible adolescent and adult population has developed might find it useful to include hepatitis A in their vaccination programs.

In the United States, vaccination of successive cohorts of children should eventually result in a sustained reduction in disease incidence nationwide, providing the opportunity to eliminate HAV transmission. HAV has been considered a target for eradication, but international bodies have not made this recommendation, primarily because of considerations of cost and feasibility.[325] At present, the disease can best be controlled by improving living conditions in the developing world and the wise application of the existing vaccines in other areas.

Therapy and General Management

There is no specific therapy available for hepatitis A, and management is supportive. In the rare event of fulminant hepatitis, identification of patients requiring liver transplantation is difficult because as many as 60% of patients, especially children, with fulminant hepatic failure caused by hepatitis A survive.[261,314] Transplantation is used for the management of carefully selected patients who have a poor prognosis with medical management alone. The survival rate is reported to be 80%, although reinfection has been reported.[315,326]

In most patients with hepatitis A, admission to the hospital is not indicated, provided that patients have access to good care. If hospitalized, fecally incontinent patients, patients with diarrhea, and small children should be given a separate room and toilet. The necessity for bed rest seems to have been overstated because no objective evidence has been provided that bed rest or restriction of physical activity affects the outcome of the disease. Dietary restrictions, including prohibition of even modest amounts of alcohol, also seem to have little effect on outcome. Nevertheless, recommendation of abstention from alcohol has become conventional because alcohol has been linked with relapse of jaundice.[316] Whatever the clinical presentation of any given case of hepatitis A, it is important to recognize that all cases, except the rare event of fulminant hepatitis A, will resolve without any chronic sequelae.

REFERENCES

1. Zuckerman AJ. The history of viral hepatitis from antiquity to the present. In: Deinhardt F, Deinhardt J, eds. *Viral Hepatitis: Laboratory and Clinical Science*. New York: Marcel Dekker; 1983:3-32.
2. Virchow R. Ueber das Vorkommen und den Nachweis des Hepatogenen, Insbesondere des Katarrhalischen Icterus. *Virchows Arch (Pathol Anat)*. 1865;32:117.
3. McDonald S. Acute yellow atrophy of the liver. *Edinb Med J*. 1907;1:83.
4. Cockayne EA. Catarrhal jaundice, sporadic and epidemic, and its relation to acute yellow atrophy of the liver. *Q J Med*. 1912;6:1-29.
5. Havens WP Jr. Immunity in experimentally induced infectious hepatitis. *J Exp Med*. 1946;84:403.
6. Neefe JR, Gellis SS, Stokes J Jr. Homologous serum hepatitis and infectious (epidemic) hepatitis: studies in volunteers bearing on immunological and other characteristics of the etiological agents. *Am J Med*. 1946;1:9.
7. Havens WPJ, Ward R, Drill VA, et al. Experimental production of hepatitis by feeding icterogenic materials. *Proc Soc Exp Biol Med*. 1944;57:206-208
8. MacCallum FO. Transmission of infective hepatitis to human volunteers. *Lancet*. 1944;2:228
9. Gellis SS, Stokes J Jr, Brother GM, et al. The use of immune globulin (gamma globulin) in infectious (epidemic) hepatitis in the Mediterranean theatre of operations. *JAMA*. 1945;128:1062.
10. Krugman S. Viral hepatitis: overview and historical perspectives. *Yale J Biol Med*. 1976;49:199-203.
11. Feinstone SM, Kapikian AZ, Purcell RH. Hepatitis A: detection by immune electron microscopy of a viruslike antigen associated with acute illness. *Science*. 1973;182:1026-1028.
12. Maynard JE, Lorenz D, Bradley DW, et al. Review of infectivity studies in nonhuman primates with virus-like particles associated with MS-1 hepatitis. *Am J Med Sci*. 1975;270:81-85
13. Dienstag JL, Feinstone SM, Purcell RH, et al. Experimental infection of chimpanzees with hepatitis A virus. *J Infect Dis*. 1975;132:532-545.
14. Provost PJ, Hilleman MR. Propagation of human hepatitis A virus in cell culture in vitro. *Proc Soc Exp Biol Med*. 1979;160: 213-221.
15. Frosner GG, Deinhardt F, Scheid R, et al. Propagation of human hepatitis A virus in a hepatoma cell line. *Infection*. 1979;7:303-305.
16. Daemer RJ, Feinstone SM, Gust ID, et al. Propagation of human hepatitis A virus in African green monkey kidney cell culture: primary isolation and serial passage. *Infect Immun*. 1981;32: 388-393.
17. Ticehurst JR, Racaniello VR, Baroudy BM, et al. Molecular cloning and characterization of hepatitis A virus cDNA. *Proc Natl Acad Sci U S A*. 1983;80:5885-5889.
18. Andre FE, D'Hondt E, Delem A, et al. Clinical assessment of the safety and efficacy of an inactivated hepatitis A vaccine: rationale and summary of findings. *Vaccine*. 1992;10(Suppl 1):S160-S168.
19. Cohen JI, Rosenblum B, Ticehurst JR, et al. Complete nucleotide sequence of an attenuated hepatitis A virus: comparison with wild-type virus. *Proc Natl Acad Sci U S A*. 1987;84:2497-2501
20. Martin A, Lemon SM. Hepatitis A virus: from discovery to vaccines. *Hepatology*. 2006;43(2 Suppl 1):S164-S172.
21. Melnick JL. Properties and classification of hepatitis A virus. *Vaccine*. 1992;10(Suppl 1):S24-S26.
22. Tratschin JD, Siegl G, Frosner GG, et al. Characterization and classification of virus particles associated with hepatitis A. III. Structural proteins. *J Virol*. 1981;38:151-156.
23. Robertson BH, Jansen RW, Khanna B, et al. Genetic relatedness of hepatitis A virus strains recovered from different geographical regions. *J Gen Virol*. 1992;73:1365-1377.
24. Fujiwara K, Yokosuka O, Imazeki F, et al. Analysis of the genotype-determining region of hepatitis A viral RNA in relation to disease severities. *Hepatol Res*. 2003;25:124-134.
25. Fujiwara K, Kojima H, Yonemitsu Y, et al. Phylogenetic analysis of hepatitis A virus in sera from patients with hepatitis A of various severities. *Liver Int*. 2008; Nov. 25 [Epub ahead of print].
26. Karron RA, Daemer R, Ticehurst J, et al. Studies of prototype live hepatitis A virus vaccines in primate models. *J Infect Dis*. 1988;157:338-345.
27. Coulepis AG, Locarnini SA, Westaway EG, et al. Biophysical and biochemical characterization of hepatitis A virus. *Intervirology*. 1982;18:107-127.
28. Lemon SM, Jansen RW, Newbold JE. Infectious hepatitis A virus particles produced in cell culture consist of three distinct types with different buoyant densities in CsCl. *J Virol*. 1985;54:78-85.
29. Siegl G, Frosner GG. Characterization and classification of virus particles associated with hepatitis A. II. Type and configuration of nucleic acid. *J Virol*. 1978;26:48-53.
30. Murphy P, Nowak T, Lemon SM, et al. Inactivation of hepatitis A virus by heat treatment in aqueous solution. *J Med Virol*. 1993;41:61-64.
31. Nissen E, Konig P, Feinstone SM, et al. Inactivation of hepatitis A and other enteroviruses during heat treatment (pasteurization). *Biologicals*. 1996;24:339-341
32. Parry JV, Mortimer PP, Murphy P, et al. The heat sensitivity of hepatitis A virus determined by a simple tissue culture method: inactivation of hepatitis A virus by heat treatment in aqueous solution. *J Med Virol*. 1984;14:277-283.
33. Millard J, Appleton H, Parry JV. Studies on heat inactivation of hepatitis A virus with special reference to shellfish. Part 1. Procedures for infection and recovery of virus from laboratory-maintained cockles. *Epidemiol Infect*. 1987;98:397-414.
34. Peterson DA, Hurley TR, Hoff JC, et al. Effect of chlorine treatment on infectivity of hepatitis A virus. *Appl Environ Microbiol*. 1983;45:223-227.
35. Calci KR, Meade GK, Tezloff RC, et al. High-pressure inactivation of hepatitis A virus within oysters. *Appl Environ Microbiol*. 2005;71:339-343.
36. Siegl G, Weitz M, Kronauer G. Stability of hepatitis A virus. *Intervirology*. 1984;22:218-226.
37. Mannucci PM, Gdovin S, Gringeri A, et al. Transmission of hepatitis A to patients with hemophilia by factor VIII concentrates treated with organic solvent and detergent to inactivate viruses. The Italian Collaborative Group. *Ann Intern Med*. 1994;120:1-7.
38. Cohen JI, Ticehurst JR, Purcell RH, et al. Complete nucleotide sequence of wild-type hepatitis A: comparison with different strains of hepatitis A virus and other picornaviruses. *J Virol*. 1987;61:50-59.
39. Weitz M, Baroudy BM, Maloy WL, et al. Detection of a genome-linked protein (VPg) of hepatitis A virus and its comparison with other picornaviral VPgs. *J Virol*. 1986;60:124-130.
40. Rueckert RR, Wimmer E. Systematic nomenclature of picornavirus proteins. *J Virol*. 1984;50:957-959.
41. Updike WS, Tesar M, Ehrenfeld E. Detection of hepatitis A virus proteins in infected BS-C-1 cells. *Virology*. 1991;185:411-418.
42. Bishop NE, Anderson DA. RNA-dependent cleavage of VP0 capsid protein in provirions of hepatitis A virus. *Virology*. 1993;197:616-623.
43. Anderson DA, Ross BC. Morphogenesis of hepatitis A virus: isolation and characterization of subviral particles. *J Virol*. 1990;64:5284-5289.
44. Probst C, Jecht M, Gauss-Muller V. Intrinsic signals for the assembly of hepatitis A virus particles: role of structural proteins VP4 and 2A. *J Biol Chem*. 1999;274:4527-4531.
45. Cohen L, Benichou D, Martin A. Analysis of deletion mutants indicates that the 2A polypeptide of hepatitis A virus participates in virion morphogenesis. *J Virol*. 2002;76:7495-7505.
46. Graff J, Richards OC, Swiderek KM, et al. Hepatitis A virus capsid protein VP1 has a heterogeneous C terminus. *J Virol*. 1999;73:6015-6023.
47. Rachow A, Gauss-Muller V, Probst C. Homogeneous hepatitis A virus particles: proteolytic release of the assembly signal 2A from procapsids by factor Xa. *J Biol Chem*. 2003;278:29744-29751.
48. Stapleton JT, Lemon SM. Neutralization escape mutants define a dominant immunogenic neutralization site on hepatitis A virus. *J Virol*. 1987;61:491-498.
49. Lemon SM, Binn LN. Antigenic relatedness of two strains of hepatitis A virus determined by cross-neutralization. *Infect Immun*. 1983;42:418-420.
50. Ping LH, Lemon SM. Antigenic structure of human hepatitis A virus defined by analysis of escape mutants selected against murine monoclonal antibodies. *J Virol*. 1992;66:2208-2216.
51. Nalin DR, Kuter BJ, Brown L, et al. Worldwide experience with the CR326F-derived inactivated hepatitis A virus vaccine in pediatric and adult populations: an overview. *J Hepatol*. 1993;18(Suppl 2):S51-S55.
52. Innis BL, Snitbhan R, Kunasol P, et al. Protection against hepatitis A by an inactivated vaccine. *JAMA*. 1994;271:1328-1334.
53. Lemon SM, Chao SF, Jansen RW, et al. Genomic heterogeneity among human and nonhuman strains of hepatitis A virus. *J Virol*. 1987;61:735-742.
54. Robertson BH, Khanna B, Nainan OV, et al. Epidemiologic patterns of wild-type hepatitis A virus determined by genetic variation. *J Infect Dis*. 1991;163:286-292.
55. Brown EA, Jansen RW, Lemon SM. Characterization of a simian hepatitis A virus (HAV): antigenic and genetic comparison with human HAV. *J Virol*. 1989;63:4932-4937
56. Jansen RW, Siegl G, Lemon SM. Molecular epidemiology of human hepatitis A virus defined by an antigen-capture polymerase chain reaction method. *Proc Natl Acad Sci U S A*. 1990;87:2867-2871.
57. Nainan OV, Xia G, Vaughan G, et al. Diagnosis of hepatitis a virus infection: a molecular approach. *Clin Microbiol Rev*. 2006;19:63-79.
58. Lemon SM, Jansen RW, Brown EA. Genetic, antigenic and biological differences between strains of hepatitis A virus. *Vaccine*. 1992;10(Suppl 1):S40-S44.
59. Siegl G, Frosner GG, Gauss-Muller V, et al. The physicochemical properties of infectious hepatitis A virions. *J Gen Virol*. 1981;57:331-341.
60. Dotzauer A, Feinstone SM, Kaplan G. Susceptibility of nonprimate cell lines to hepatitis A virus infection. *J Virol*. 1994;68: 6064-6068.
61. Siegl G. Replication of hepatitis A virus and processing of proteins. *Vaccine*. 1992;10(Suppl 1):S32-S35.
62. Cromeans T, Sobsey MD, Fields HA. Development of a plaque assay for a cytopathic, rapidly replicating isolate of hepatitis A virus. *J Med Virol*. 1987;22:45-56.
63. Anderson DA. Cytopathology, plaque assay, and heat inactivation of hepatitis A virus strain HM175. *J Med Virol*. 1987; 22:35-44.
64. Cromeans T, Humphrey C, Sobsey M, et al. Use of immunogold preembedding technique to detect hepatitis A viral antigen in infected cells. *Am J Anat*. 1989;185:314-320.
65. Konduru K, Kaplan GG. Stable growth of wild-type hepatitis A virus in cell culture. *J Virol*. 2006;80:1352-1360.
66. Anderson DA, Ross BC, Locarnini SA. Restricted replication of hepatitis A virus in cell culture: encapsidation of viral RNA depletes the pool of RNA available for replication. *J Virol*. 1988;62:4201-4206.
67. Wheeler CM, Fields HA, Schable CA, et al. Adsorption, purification, and growth characteristics of hepatitis A virus strain HAS-15 propagated in fetal rhesus monkey kidney cells. *J Clin Microbiol*. 1986;23:434-440.
68. Bishop NE, Anderson DA. Uncoating kinetics of hepatitis A virus virions and provirions. *J Virol*. 2000;74:3423-3426.
69. Brown EA, Zajac AJ, Lemon SM. In vitro characterization of an internal ribosomal entry site (IRES) present within the 5′ nontranslated region of hepatitis A virus RNA: comparison with the IRES of encephalomyocarditis virus. *J Virol*. 1994;68:1066-1074.
70. Whetter LE, Day SP, Elroy-Stein O, et al. Low efficiency of the 5′ nontranslated region of hepatitis A virus RNA in directing cap-independent translation in permissive monkey kidney cells. *J Virol*. 1994;68:5253-5263.
71. Borman AM, Bailly JL, Girard M, et al. Picornavirus internal ribosome entry segments: comparison of translation efficiency and the requirements for optimal internal initiation of translation in vitro. *Nucleic Acids Res*. 1995;23:3656-3663.
72. Borovec SV, Anderson DA. Synthesis and assembly of hepatitis A virus-specific proteins in BS-C-1 cells. *J Virol*. 1993;67:3095-3102.
73. Tedeschi V, Purcell RH, Emerson SU. Partial characterization of hepatitis A viruses from three intermediate passage levels of a series resulting in adaptation to growth in cell culture and attenuation of virulence. *J Med Virol*. 1993;39:16-22.
74. Emerson SU, Huang YK, Purcell RH. 2B and 2C mutations are essential but mutations throughout the genome of HAV contribute to adaptation to cell culture. *Virology*. 1993;194:475-480.
75. Provost PJ, Banker FS, Giesa PA, et al. Progress toward a live, attenuated human hepatitis A vaccine. *Proc Soc Exp Biol Med*. 1982;170:8-14.
76. Emerson SU, Huang YK, McRill C, et al. Molecular basis of virulence and growth of hepatitis A virus in cell culture. *Vaccine*. 1992;10(Suppl 1):S36-S39.
77. Funkhouser AW, Purcell RH, D'Hondt E, et al. Attenuated hepatitis A virus: genetic determinants of adaptation to growth in MRC-5 cells. *J Virol*. 1994;68:148-157
78. Kaplan G, Totsuka A, Thompson P, et al. Identification of a surface glycoprotein on African green monkey kidney cells as a receptor for hepatitis A virus. *EMBO J*. 1996;15:4282-4296.
79. Feigelstock D, Thompson P, Mattoo P, et al. The human homolog of HAVcr-1 codes for a hepatitis A virus cellular receptor. *J Virol*. 1998;72:6621-6628.
80. Silberstein E, Dveksler G, Kaplan GG. Neutralization of hepatitis A virus (HAV) by an immunoadhesin containing the cysteine-rich region of HAV cellular receptor-1. *J Virol*. 2001;75:717-725.
81. Dotzauer A, Gebhardt U, Bieback K, et al. Hepatitis A virus-specific immunoglobulin A mediates infection of hepatocytes with hepatitis A virus via the asialoglycoprotein receptor. *J Virol*. 2000;74:10950-10957.
82. Hillis WD. An outbreak of infectious hepatitis among chimpanzee handlers at a United States Air Force Base. *Am J Hyg*. 1961;73:316-328.
83. Maynard JE, Krushak DH, Bradley DW, et al. Infectivity studies of hepatitis A and B in non-human primates. *Dev Biol Stand*. 1975;30:229-235.
84. Hilleman MR, Provost PJ, Villarejos V, et al. Infectious hepatitis (hepatitis A) research in nonhuman primates. *Bull Pan Am Health Organ*. 1977;11:140-152.
85. Emerson SU, McRill C, Rosenblum B, et al. Mutations responsible for adaptation of hepatitis A virus to efficient growth in cell culture. *J Virol*. 1991;65:4882-4886.
86. Emerson SU, Tsarev SA, Govindarajan S, et al. A simian strain of hepatitis A virus, AGM-27, functions as an attenuated vaccine for chimpanzees. *J Infect Dis*. 1996;173:592-597.
87. Deinhardt F. Hepatitis in primates. *Adv Virus Res*. 1976;20: 113-157.
88. Hornei B, Kammerer R, Moubayed P, et al. Experimental hepatitis A virus infection in guinea pigs. *J Med Virol*. 2001;64: 402-409.
89. Skinhoj P, Mathiesen LR, Kryger P. Faecal excretion of hepatitis A virus in patients with symptomatic hepatitis A infection. *Ann Intern Med*. 1987;106:221-226.
90. Tassopoulos NC, Papaevangelou GJ, Ticehurst JR, et al. Fecal excretion of Greek strains of hepatitis A virus in patients with hepatitis A and in experimentally infected chimpanzees. *J Infect Dis*. 1986;154:231-237.

91. Krugman S, Ward R, Giles JP. Infectious hepatitis: detection of virus during the incubation period and in clinically inapparent infection. *N Engl J Med.* 1959;261:729-734.
92. Rosenblum LS, Villarino ME, Nainan OV, et al. Hepatitis A outbreak in a neonatal intensive care unit: risk factors for transmission and evidence of prolonged viral excretion among preterm infants. *J Infect Dis.* 1991;164:476-482.
93. Sjogren MH, Tanno H, Fay O, et al. Hepatitis A virus in stool during clinical relapse. *Ann Intern Med.* 1987;106:221-226.
94. Bower WA, Nainan OV, Han X, et al. Duration of viremia in hepatitis A virus infection. *J Infect Dis.* 2000;182:12-17.
95. Krugman S, Ward R, Giles WP. The natural history of infectious hepatitis. *Am J Med.* 1962;32:717-728.
96. Lemon SM. The natural history of hepatitis A: the potential for transmission by transfusion of blood or blood products. *Vox Sang.* 1994;67(Suppl 4):19-23.
97. Purcell RH, Wong DC, Shapiro M. Relative infectivity of hepatitis A virus by the oral and intravenous routes in 2 species of nonhuman primates. *J Infect Dis.* 2002;185:1668-1771.
98. Cohen JI, Feinstone S, Purcell RH. Hepatitis A virus infection in a chimpanzee: duration of viremia and detection of virus in saliva and throat swabs. *J Infect Dis.* 1989;160:887-890.
99. Bell BP. Global epidemiology of hepatitis A: implications for control strategies. In: Margolis HS, Alter MJ, Liang JT, et al, eds. *Viral Hepatitis and Liver Disease.* London: International Medical Press; 2002:359-365.
100. Bell BP, Shapiro CN, Alter MJ, et al. The diverse patterns of hepatitis A epidemiology in the United States: implications for vaccination strategies. *J Infect Dis.* 1998;178:1579-1584.
101. Staes CJ, Schlenker TL, Risk I, et al. Sources of infection among persons with acute hepatitis A and no identified risk factors during a sustained community-wide outbreak. *Pediatrics.* 2000;106:E54.
102. Smith PF, Grabau JC, Werzberger A, et al. The role of young children in a community-wide outbreak of hepatitis A. *Epidemiol Infect.* 1997;118:243-252.
103. Armstrong GL, Bell BP. Hepatitis A virus infections in the United States: model-based estimates and implications for childhood immunization. *Pediatrics.* 2002;109:839-845.
104. McCaustland KA, Bond WW, Bradley DW, et al. Survival of hepatitis A virus in feces after drying and storage for 1 month. *J Clin Microbiol.* 1982;16:957-958
105. Carl M, Francis DP, Maynard JE. Food-borne hepatitis A: recommendations for control. *J Infect Dis.* 1983;148:1133-1135.
106. Massoudi MS, Bell BP, Paredes V, et al. An outbreak of hepatitis A associated with an infected foodhandler. *Public Health Rep.* 1999;114:157-164.
107. Fiore A. Foodborne hepatitis A. *Clin Infect Dis.* 2004;38:705-715.
108. Centers for Disease Control and Prevention. Foodborne hepatitis A: Alaska, Florida, North Carolina, Washington. *MMWR Morb Mortal Wkly Rep.* 1990;39:228-232.
109. Halliday ML, Kang LY, Zhou TK, et al. An epidemic of hepatitis A attributable to the ingestion of raw clams in Shanghai, China. *J Infect Dis.* 1991;164:852-859.
110. Wang JY, Hu SL, Liu HY, et al. Risk factor analysis of an epidemic of hepatitis A in a factory in Shanghai. *Int J Epidemiol.* 1990;19:435-438.
111. Mele A, Rastelli MG, Gill ON, et al. Recurrent epidemic hepatitis A associated with consumption of raw shellfish probably controlled through public health measures. *Am J Epidemiol.* 1980;130:540-546.
112. Germinario C, Lopalco PL, Chicanna M, et al. From hepatitis B to hepatitis A and B prevention: the Puglia (Italy) experience. *Vaccine.* 2000;18(Suppl):S83-S85.
113. Mele A, Stroffolini T, Palumbe F, et al. Incidence and risk factors for hepatitis A in Italy: public health indications from a 10-year surveillance. *J Hepatol.* 1997;26:743-747.
114. Desenclos JC, Klontz KC, Wilder MH, et al. A multistate outbreak of hepatitis A caused by the consumption of raw oysters. *Am J Public Health.* 1991;81:1268-1272.
115. Bialek SR, George PA, Xia GL, et al. Use of molecular epidemiology to confirm a multistate outbreak of hepatitis A caused by consumption of oysters. *Clin Infect Dis.* 2007;44:838-840.
116. Hollinger FB, Khan NC, Oefinger PE, et al. Posttransfusion hepatitis type A. *JAMA.* 1983;250:2313-2317.
117. Soucie JM, Robertson BH, Bell BP, et al. Hepatitis A virus infections associated with clotting factor concentrate in the United States. *Transfusion.* 1998;38:573-579.
118. Benjamin RJ. Nucleic acid testing: update and applications. *Semin Hematol.* 2001;38:11-16.
119. Leikin E, Lysikiewicz A, Garry D, et al. Intrauterine transmission of hepatitis A virus. *Obstet Gynecol.* 1996;88:690-691.
120. McDuffie RS Jr, Bader T. Fetal meconium peritonitis after maternal hepatitis A. *Am J Obstet Gynecol.* 1999;180:1031-1032.
121. Tong MJ, Thursby M, Rakela J, et al. Studies on the maternal-infant transmission of the viruses which cause acute hepatitis. *Gastroenterology.* 1981;80:999-1004.
122. Watson JC, Fleming DW, Borella AJ, et al. Vertical transmission of hepatitis A resulting in an outbreak in a neonatal intensive care unit. *J Infect Dis.* 1993;167:567-571.
123. Hadler SC. Global impact of hepatitis A virus infection: changing patterns. In: Hollinger FB, Lemon SM, Margolis HS, eds. *Viral Hepatitis and Liver Disease.* Baltimore; Williams & Wilkins; 1991:14-20.
124. Coursaget P, Leboulleux D, Gharbi Y, et al. Etiology of acute sporadic hepatitis in adults in Senegal and Tunisia. *Scand J Infect Dis.* 1995;27:9-11.
125. Tsega E, Mengesha B, Hansson BG, et al. Hepatitis A, B, and delta infection in Ethiopia: a serologic survey with demographic data. *Am J Epidemiol.* 1986;123:344-351.
126. Bowden FJ, Currie BJ, Miller NC, et al. Should aboriginals in the "top end" of the Northern Territory be vaccinated against hepatitis A? *Med J Aust.* 1994;161:372-373.
127. Cianciara J. Hepatitis A shifting epidemiology in Poland and Eastern Europe. *Vaccine.* 2000;18(Suppl 1):S68-S70.
128. Green MS, Block C, Slater PE. Rise in the incidence of viral hepatitis in Israel despite improved socioeconomic conditions. *Rev Infect Dis.* 1989;11:464-469.
129. Lagos R, Potin M, Munoz A, et al. [Serum antibodies against hepatitis A virus among subjects of middle and low socioeconomic levels in urban area of Santiago, Chile]. *Rev Med Chil.* 1999;127:429-436.
130. Gdalevich M, Grotto I, Mandel Y, et al. Hepatitis A antibody prevalence among young adults in Israel: the decline continues. *Epidemiol Infect.* 1998;121:477-479.
131. Innis BL, Snitbhan R, Hoke CH, et al. The declining transmission of hepatitis A in Thailand. *J Infect Dis.* 1991;163:989-995.
132. Kunasol P, Cooksley G, Chan VF, et al. Hepatitis A virus: declining seroprevalence in children and adolescents in Southeast Asia. *Southeast Asian J Trop Med Public Health.* 1998;29:255-262.
133. Pinho JR, Sumita LM, Moreira RC, et al. Duality of patterns in hepatitis A epidemiology: a study involving two socioeconomically distinct populations in Campinas, Sao Paulo State, Brazil. *Rev Inst Med Trop Sao Paulo.* 1998;40:105-106.
134. Poovorawan Y, Vimolkej T, Chongsrisawat V, et al. The declining pattern of seroepidemiology of hepatitis A virus infection among adolescents in Bangkok, Thailand. *Southeast Asian J Trop Med Public Health.* 1997;28:154-157.
135. Das K, Jain A, Gupta S, et al. The changing epidemiological pattern of hepatitis A in an urban population of India: emergence of a trend similar to the European countries. *Eur J Epidemiol.* 2000;16:507-510.
136. Tapia-Conyer R, Santos JI, Cavalcanti AM, et al. Hepatitis A in Latin America: a changing epidemiologic pattern. *Am J Trop Med Hyg.* 1999;61:825-829.
137. Tufenkeji H. Hepatitis A shifting epidemiology in the Middle East and Africa. *Vaccine.* 2000;18(Suppl 1):S65-S67.
138. Wang LY, Cheng YW, Chou SJ, et al. Secular trend and geographical variation in hepatitis A infection and hepatitis B carrier rate among adolescents in Taiwan: an island-wide survey. *J Med Virol.* 1993;39:1-5.
139. Ciocca M. Clinical course and consequences of hepatitis A infection. *Vaccine.* 2000;18(Suppl 1):S71-S74.
140. Shah U, Habib Z, Kleinman RE. Liver failure attributable to hepatitis A virus infection in a developing country. *Pediatrics.* 2000;105:436-438.
141. Gil A, Gonzalez A, Dal Re R, et al. Prevalence of antibodies against varicella zoster, herpes simplex (types 1 and 2), hepatitis B and hepatitis A viruses among Spanish adolescents. *J Infect.* 1998;36:53-56.
142. Shapiro CN, Coleman PJ, McQuillan GM, et al. Epidemiology of hepatitis A seroepidemiology and risk groups in the USA. *Vaccine.* 1992;10(Suppl 1):S59-S62.
143. Prodinger WM, Larcher C, Solder BM, et al. Hepatitis A in western Austria: the epidemiological situation before the introduction of active immunisation. *Infection.* 1994;22:53-55.
144. Termorshuizen F, Dorigo-Zetsma JW, de Melker HE, et al. The prevalence of antibodies to hepatitis A virus and its determinants in the Netherlands: a population-based survey. *Epidemiol Infect.* 2000;124:459-466.
145. Bottiger M, Christenson B, Grillner L. Hepatitis A immunity in the Swedish population: a study of the prevalence of markers in the Swedish population. *Scand J Infect Dis.* 1997;29:99-102.
146. Centers for Disease Control and Prevention. Summary of notifiable diseases, United States, 2000. *MMWR Morb Mortal Wkly Rep.* 2002;49:1-102.
147. Centers for Disease Control and Prevention. *Hepatitis Surveillance Report No. 58.* Atlanta: 2003.
148. Centers for Disease Control and Prevention. Prevention of hepatitis A through active or passive immunization: recommendations of the Advisory Committee on Immunization Practices (ACIP). *MMWR Recomm Rep.* 1996;45:1-30.
149. Centers for Disease Control and Prevention. Prevention of hepatitis A through active or passive immunization: recommendations of the Advisory Committee on Immunization Practices (ACIP). *MMWR Recomm Rep.* 1999;48(RR-12):1-37.
150. Bell BP, Kruszon-Moran D, Shapiro CN, et al. Hepatitis A virus infection in the United States: serologic results from the Third National Health and Nutrition Examination Survey. *Vaccine.* 2005;23:5793-5806.
151. Advisory Committee on Immunization Practices (ACIP), Fiore AE, Wasley A, Bell BP. Prevention of hepatitis A through active or passive immunization: recommendations of the Advisory Committee on Immunization Practices (ACIP). *MMWR Recomm Rep.* 2006;55(RR-7):1-23.
152. Wasley A, Grytdal S, Gallagher K. Surveillance for acute viral hepatitis—United States, 2006. *MMWR Surveill Summ.* 2008;57:1-24.
153. Bialek S, Thoroughman D, Hu D, et al. Hepatitis A incidence and hepatitis A vaccination among American Indians and Alaskan Natives, 1990-2001. *Am J Public Health.* 2004;94:996-1001.
154. Cotter SM, Sansom S, Long T, et al. Outbreak of hepatitis A among men who have sex with men: implications for hepatitis A vaccination strategies. *J Infect Dis.* 2003;187:1235-1240.
155. Friedman MS, Blake PA, Koehler JE, et al. Factors influencing a communitywide campaign to administer hepatitis A vaccine to men who have sex with men. *Am J Public Health.* 2000;90:1942-1946.
156. Harkess J, Gildon B, Istre GR. Outbreaks of hepatitis A among illicit drug users, Oklahoma, 1984-87. *Am J Public Health.* 1989;79:463-466.
157. Hutin YJ, Bell BP, Marshall KL, et al. Identifying target groups for a potential vaccination program during a hepatitis A communitywide outbreak. *Am J Public Health.* 1999;89:918-921.
158. Hadler SC, Webster HM, Erben JJ, et al. Hepatitis A in day-care centers: a community-wide assessment. *N Engl J Med.* 1980;302:1222-1227.
159. Venczel LV, Desai MM, Vertz PD, et al. The role of child care in a community-wide outbreak of hepatitis A. *Pediatrics.* 2001;108:E78.
160. Shapiro CN, Hadler SC. Hepatitis A and hepatitis B virus infections in day-care settings. *Pediatr Ann.* 1991;20:435-441.
161. Desenclos JC, MacLafferty L. Community wide outbreak of hepatitis A linked to children in day care centres and with increased transmission in young adult men in Florida 1988-9. *J Epidemiol Community Health.* 1993;47:269-273.
162. Hadler SC, Erben JJ, Matthews D, et al. Effect of immunoglobulin on hepatitis A in day-care centers. *JAMA.* 1983;249:48-53.
163. Hutin YJ, Pool V, Cramer EH, et al. A multistate, foodborne outbreak of hepatitis A. National Hepatitis A Investigation Team. *N Engl J Med.* 1999;340:595-602.
164. Szmuness W, Purcell RH, Dienstag JL, et al. Antibody to hepatitis A antigen in institutionalized mentally retarded patients. *JAMA.* 1977;237:1702-1705.
165. Shaw DD, Whiteman DC, Merritt AD, et al. Hepatitis A outbreaks among illicit drug users and their contacts in Queensland, 1997. *Med J Aust.* 1999;170:584-587.
166. O'Donovan D, Cooke RP, Joce R, et al. An outbreak of hepatitis A amongst injecting drug users. *Epidemiol Infect.* 2001;127:469-473.
167. Hutin YJ, Sabin KM, Hutwanger LC, et al. Multiple modes of hepatitis A virus transmission among methamphetamine users. *Am J Epidemiol.* 2000;152:186-192.
168. Ngui SL, Granerod J, Jewes LA, et al.; 2002 Hepatitis A Outbreaks Investigation Network. Outbreaks of hepatitis A in England and Wales associated with two co-circulating hepatitis A virus strains. *J Med Virol.* 2008;80:1181-1188.
169. Tjon GM, Götz H, Koek AG, et al. An outbreak of hepatitis A among homeless drug users in Rotterdam, The Netherlands. *J Med Virol.* 2005;77:360-366.
170. Spada E, Genovese D, Tosti ME, et al. An outbreak of hepatitis A virus infection with a high case-fatality rate among injecting drug users. *J Hepatol.* 2005;43:958-964.
171. Roy K, Howie H, Sweeney C, et al. Hepatitis A virus and injecting drug misuse in Aberdeen, Scotland: a case-control study. *J Viral Hepat.* 2004;11:277-382.
172. Vong S, Fiore AE, Haight DO, et al. Vaccination in the county jail as a strategy to reach high risk adults during a community-based hepatitis A outbreak among methamphetamine drug users. *Vaccine.* 2005;23:1021-1028.
173. Ivie K, Spruill C, Bell BP. Prevalence of hepatitis A virus infection among illicit drug users, 1993-1994. *Antiviral Therapy.* 2000;5(Suppl 1):A.7.
174. Villano SA, Nelson KE, Vlahov D, et al. Hepatitis A among homosexual men and injection drug users: more evidence for vaccination. *Clin Infect Dis.* 1997;25:726-728.
175. Stokes ML, Ferson MJ, Young LC. Outbreak of hepatitis A among homosexual men in Sydney. *Am J Public Health.* 1997;87:2039-2041.
176. Henning KJ, Bell E, Braun J, et al. A community-wide outbreak of hepatitis A risk factors for infection among homosexual and bisexual men. *Am J Med.* 1995;99:132-136
177. Centers for Disease Control and Prevention (CDC). Hepatitis A among homosexual men—United States, Canada, and Australia. *MMWR Morb Mortal Wkly Rep.* 1992;41:155, 161-164.
178. Mazick A, Howitz M, Rex S, et al. Hepatitis A outbreak among MSM linked to casual sex and gay saunas in Copenhagen, Denmark. *Euro Surveill.* 2005;10:111-114
179. Katz MH, Hsu L, Wong E, et al. Seroprevalence of and risk factors for hepatitis A infection among young homosexual and bisexual men. *J Infect Dis.* 1997;175:1225-1229.
180. Mah MW, Royce RA, Rathouz PJ, et al. Prevalence of hepatitis A antibodies in hemophiliacs: preliminary results from the Southeastern Delta Hepatitis Study. *Vox Sang.* 1994;67(Suppl 1):21-22.
181. Mannucci PM, Santagostino E, Di Bona E, et al. The outbreak of hepatitis A in Italian patients with hemophilia: facts and fancies. *Vox Sang.* 1994;67(Suppl 1):31-35.
182. Klein BS, Michaels JA, Rytel MW, et al. Nosocomial hepatitis A: a multinursery outbreak in Wisconsin. *JAMA.* 1984;252:2716-2721
183. Noble RC, Kane MA, Reeves SA, et al. Posttransfusion hepatitis A in a neonatal intensive care unit. *JAMA.* 1984;252:2711-2715.

184. Weisfuse IB, Graham DJ, Will M, et al. An outbreak of hepatitis A among cancer patients treated with interleukin-2 and lymphokine-activated killer cells. *J Infect Dis.* 1990;161:647-652.
185. Goodman RA. Nosocomial hepatitis A. *Ann Intern Med.* 1985;103:452-454.
186. Papaevangelou GJ, Roumeliotou-Karayannis AJ, Contoyannis PC. The risk of nosocomial hepatitis A and B virus infections from patients under care without isolation precaution. *J Med Virol.* 1981;7:143-148.
187. Gibas A, Blewett DR, Schoenfeld DA, et al. Prevalence and incidence of viral hepatitis in health workers in the prehepatitis B vaccination era. *Am J Epidemiol.* 1992;136:603-610.
188. Steffen R, Rickenbach M, Wilhelm U, et al. Health problems after travel to developing countries. *J Infect Dis.* 1987;156:84-91.
189. Steffen R. Risk of hepatitis A in travellers. *Vaccine.* 1992;10 (Suppl 1):S69-S72.
190. Mele A, Sagliocca L, Palumbo F, et al. Travel-associated hepatitis A effect of place of residence and country visited. *J Public Health Med.* 1991;13:256-259
191. Steffen R, Kane MA, Shapiro CN, et al. Epidemiology and prevention of hepatitis A in travelers. *JAMA.* 1994;272:885-889.
192. Steffen R. Hepatitis A in travelers: the European experience. *J Infect Dis.* 1995;171(Suppl 1):S24-S28.
193. Lange WR, Frame JD. High incidence of viral hepatitis among American missionaries in Africa. *Am J Trop Med Hyg.* 1990;43:527-533.
194. Weinberg M, Hopkins J, Farrington L, et al. Hepatitis A in Hispanic children who live along the United States-Mexico border: the role of international travel and food-borne exposures. *Pediatrics.* 2004;114:e68-e73.
195. Sonder GJB, Bovee LP, Baayen TD, et al. Effectiveness of a hepatitis A vaccination program for migrant children in Amsterdam, The Netherlands, 1992-2004. *Vaccine.* 2006;24:4962-4968.
196. Gosselin C, De Serres G, Rouleau I, et al. Comparison of trip characteristics of children and adults with travel-acquired hepatitis A infection. *Pediatr Infect Dis J.* 2006;25:1184-1186.
197. Wilson ME, Kimble J. Posttravel hepatitis A: probable acquisition from an asymptomatic adopted child. *Clin Infect Dis.* 2001;33:1083-1085.
198. Fischer G, Teshale EH, Miller C, et al. *Clin Infect Dis.* 2008;47:812-814.
199. Dalton CB, Haddix A, Hoffman RE, et al. The cost of a food-borne outbreak of hepatitis A in Denver, Colo. *Arch Intern Med.* 1996;156:1013-1016.
200. Lowry PW, Levine R, Stroup DF, et al. Hepatitis A outbreak on a floating restaurant in Florida, 1986. *Am J Epidemiol.* 1989;129:155-164.
201. Latham RH, Schable CA. Foodborne hepatitis A at a family reunion: use of IgM-specific hepatitis A serologic testing. *Am J Epidemiol.* 1982;115:640-645.
202. Mishu B, Hadler SC, Boaz VA, et al. Foodborne hepatitis A: evidence that microwaving reduces risk? *J Infect Dis.* 1990;162:655-658.
203. Parkin WE, Marzinsky P, Griffin MR. Foodborne hepatitis A associated with cheeseburgers. *J Med Soc N J.* 1983;80:612-615.
204. Weltman AC, Bennett NM, Ackman DA, et al. An outbreak of hepatitis A associated with a bakery, New York, 1994: the 1968 "West Branch, Michigan" outbreak repeated. *Epidemiol Infect.* 1996;117:333-341.
205. Dentinger CM, Bower WA, Nainan OV, et al. An outbreak of hepatitis A associated with green onions. *J Infect Dis.* 2001;183:1273-1276.
206. Rosenblum LS, Mirkin IR, Allen DT, et al. A multifocal outbreak of hepatitis A traced to commercially distributed lettuce. *Am J Public Health.* 1990;80:1075-1079.
207. Niu MT, Polish LB, Robertson BH, et al. Multistate outbreak of hepatitis A associated with frozen strawberries. *J Infect Dis.* 1992;166:518-524.
208. Reid TM, Robinson HG. Frozen raspberries and hepatitis A. *Epidemiol Infect.* 1987;98:109-112.
209. Wheeler C, Vogt TM, Armstrong GL, et al. An outbreak of hepatitis A associated with green onions. *N Engl J Med.* 2005;353:890-897.
210. Amon JJ, Devasia R, Xia G, et al. Molecular epidemiology of foodborne hepatitis A outbreaks in the United States, 2003. *J Infect Dis.* 2005;192:1323-1330.
211. Bloch AB, Stramer SL, Smith JD, et al. Recovery of hepatitis A virus from a water supply responsible for a common source outbreak of hepatitis A. *Am J Public Health.* 1990;80:428-430.
212. De Serres G, Cromeans TL, Levesque B, et al. Molecular confirmation of hepatitis A virus from well water: epidemiology and public health implications. *J Infect Dis.* 1999;179:37-43.
213. Bergeisen GH, Hinds MW, Skaggs JW. A waterborne outbreak of hepatitis A in Meade County, Kentucky. *Am J Public Health.* 1985;75:170-164.
214. Lerman Y, Chodick G, Aloni H, et al. Occupations at increased risk of hepatitis A: a 2-year nationwide historical prospective cohort. *Am J Epidemiol.* 1999;150:312-320.
215. Glas C, Hotz P, Steffen R. Hepatitis A in workers exposed to sewage: a systematic review. *Occup Environ Med.* 2001;58:762-768.
216. Poole CJ, Shakespeare AT. Should sewage workers and carers for people with learning disabilities be vaccinated against hepatitis A? *Br Med J.* 1993;306:1102.
217. Trout D, Mueller C, Venczel L, et al. Evaluation of occupational transmission of hepatitis A virus among wastewater workers. *J Occup Environ Med.* 2000;42:83-87.
218. Weldon M, Van Engdom MJ, Hendricks KA, et al. Prevalence of antibody to hepatitis A virus in drinking water workers and wastewater workers in Texas from 1996 to 1997. *J Occup Environ Med.* 2000;42:821-826.
219. Venczel L, Brown S, Frumkin H, et al. Prevalence of hepatitis A virus infection among sewage workers in Georgia. *Am J Ind Med.* 2003;43:172-178.
220. Krugman S, Giles JP, Hammond J. Infectious hepatitis: evidence for two distinctive clinical epidemiological and immunological types of infection. *JAMA.* 1967;200:365-373.
221. Purcell RH, Feinstone SM, Ticehurst JR, et al. Hepatitis A virus. In: Vyas GN, Dienstag JL, Hoofnagle JH, eds. *Viral Hepatitis and Liver Disease.* Orlando, FL: Grune & Stratton; 1984:9-22.
222. Karayiannis P, Jowett T, Enticott M, et al. Hepatitis A virus replication in tamarins and host immune response in relation to pathogenesis of liver cell damage. *J Med Virol.* 1986;18:261-276.
223. Karayiannis P, McGarvey MJ, Dry MA, et al. Detection of hepatitis A virus RNA in tissues and feces of experimentally infected tamarins by CDNA-RNA hybridization. In: Zuckerman AJ, ed. *Viral Hepatitis and Liver Disease.* New York: Alan R. Liss; 1988:117-120.
224. Mathiesen LR, Moller AM, Purcell RH, et al. Hepatitis A virus in the liver and intestine of marmosets after oral inoculation. *Infect Immun.* 1980;28:45-48.
225. Mathiesen LR, Feinstone SM, Purcell RH, et al. Detection of hepatitis A antigen by immunofluorescence. *Infect Immun.* 1977;18:524-530.
226. Schulman AN, Dienstag JL, Jackson DR, et al. Hepatitis A antigen particles in the liver, bile and stool of chimpanzees. *J Infect Dis.* 1976;134:80-84.
227. Mathiesen LR, Drucker J, Lorenz D, et al. Localization of hepatitis A antigen in marmoset organs during acute infection with hepatitis A virus. *J Infect Dis.* 1978;138:369-377.
228. Krawczynski KK, Bradley DW, Murphy BL, et al. Pathogenetic aspects of hepatitis A virus infection in enterally inoculated marmosets. *Am J Clin Pathol.* 1981;76:698-706.
229. Locarini SA, Coulepis AG, Westaway EG, et al. Coproantibodies in hepatitis A: detection by enzyme-linked immunosorbent assay and immune electron microscopy. *J Clin Microbiol.* 1980;11:710-716.
230. Yoshizawa H, Itoh Y, Iwakiri S, et al. Diagnosis of type A hepatitis by fecal IgG antibody against hepatitis A antigen. *Gastroenterology.* 1980;78:114-118.
231. Vallbracht A, Gabriel P, Maier K, et al. Cell-mediated cytotoxicity in hepatitis A virus infection. *Hepatology.* 1986;226-230.
232. Feinstone SM, Gust ID. Hepatitis A infection: clinical aspects. In: Seeff LB, Lewis JH, eds. *Current Perspectives in Hepatology.* New York: Plenum; 1989:3-14.
233. Vallbracht A, Fleischer B. Immune pathogenesis of hepatitis A. *Arch Virol.* 1992;4(Suppl):3-4.
234. Kurane I, Binn LN, Bancroft WH, et al. Human lymphocyte responses to hepatitis A virus-infected cells: interferon production and lysis of infected cells. *J Immunol.* 1985;135:2140-2144.
235. Margolis HS, Nainan O. Identification of virus components in circulating immune complexes isolated during hepatitis A virus infection. *Hepatology.* 1990;11:31-37.
236. Inman RD, Hodge M, Johnston MEA, et al. Arthritis, vasculitis, and cryoglobulinemia associated with relapsing hepatitis A virus infection. *Ann Intern Med.* 1986;105:700-703.
237. Thomas HC, de Villiers D, Potter B, et al. Immune complexes in acute and chronic liver disease. *Clin Exp Immunol.* 1978;31:150-157.
238. Umetsu DT, McIntire JJ, Akbari O, et al. Asthma: an epidemic of dysregulated immunity. *Nat Immunol.* 2002;3:715-720.
239. Matricardi PM, Rosmini F, Panetta V, et al. Hay fever and asthma in relation to markers of infection in the United States. *J Allergy Clin Immunol.* 2002;110:381-387.
240. McIntire JJ, Umetsu SE, Akbari O, et al. Identification of Tapr (an airway hyperreactivity regulatory locus) and the linked Tim gene family. *Nat Immunol.* 2001;2:1109-1116
241. Koff RS. Clinical manifestations and diagnosis of hepatitis A virus infection. *Vaccine.* 1992;10(Suppl 1):S15-S17.
242. Mathiesen LR. The hepatitis A virus infection. *Liver.* 1981;1:81-109.
243. Skinhoj P. Natural history of viral hepatitis in Greenland. *Am J Med Sci.* 1975;270:305-307.
244. Skinhoj P, Mikkelsen F, Hollinger FB. Hepatitis A in Greenland: importance of specific antibody testing in epidemiologic surveillance. *Am J Epidemiol.* 1977;105:140-147.
245. Hadler SC, McFarland L. Hepatitis in day care centers: epidemiology and prevention. *Rev Infect Dis.* 1986;8:548-557
246. Tong MJ, el-Farra NS, Grew MI. Clinical manifestations of hepatitis A: recent experience in a community teaching hospital. *J Infect Dis.* 1995;171(Suppl 1):S15-S18.
247. Zhang RL, Zeng JS, Zhang HZ. Survey of 34 pregnant women with hepatitis A and their neonates. *Chin Med J (Engl).* 1990;103:552-555.
248. Mishra L, Seeff LB. Viral hepatitis, A through E, complicating pregnancy. *Gastroenterol Clin North Am.* 1992;21:873-887.
249. Vento S, Garofano T, Renzini C, et al. Fulminant hepatitis associated with hepatitis A virus superinfection in patients with chronic hepatitis C. *N Engl J Med.* 1998;338:286-290.
250. Bianco E, Stroffolini T, Spada E, et al. Case fatality rate of acute viral hepatitis in Italy: 1995-2000: an update. *Dig Liver Dis.* 2003;35:404-408.
250a. VogT TM, Wise ME, Bell BP, Finelli L. Declining hepatitis A mortality in the United States during the era of hepatitis A vaccination. *J Infect Dis.* 2008;197:1282-1288.
251. Gordon SC, Reddy KR, Schiff L, et al. Prolonged intrahepatic cholestasis secondary to acute hepatitis A. *Ann Intern Med.* 1984;101:635-637.
252. Cobden I, James OF. A biphasic illness associated with acute hepatitis A virus infection. *J Hepatol.* 1986;2:19-23.
253. Bornstein JD, Byrd DE, Trotter JF. Relapsing hepatitis A: a case report and review of the literature. *J Clin Gastroenterol.* 1999;28:355-356.
254. Scully LJ, Ryan AE. Urticaria and acute hepatitis A virus infection. *Am J Gastroenterol.* 1993;88:277-278.
255. Kano Y, Kokaji T, Shiohara T. Photo-accentuated eruption and vascular deposits of immunoglobulin A associated with hepatitis A virus infection. *Dermatology.* 2000;200:266-269.
256. Ilan Y, Hillman M, Oren R, et al. Vasculitis and cryoglobulinemia associated with persisting cholestatic hepatitis A virus infection. *Am J Gastroenterol.* 1990;85:586-587.
257. Yao G. Clinical spectrum and natural history of viral hepatitis A in a 1988 Shanghai epidemic. In: Hollinger FB, Lemon SM, Margolis HS, eds. *Viral Hepatitis and Liver Disease.* Baltimore: Williams & Wilkins; 1991:76-78.
258. Willner IR, Uhl MO, Howard SC, et al. Serious hepatitis A: an analysis of patients hospitalized during an urban epidemic in the United States. *Ann Intern Med.* 1998;128:111-114.
259. Hoofnagle JH, Carithers RL Jr, Shapiro C, et al. Fulminant hepatic failure: summary of a workshop. *Hepatology.* 1995;21:240-252.
260. Hann JN, Warnock TH, Shepherd RW, et al. Fulminant hepatitis A in indigenous children in north Queensland. *Med J Aust.* 2000;172;19-21.
261. Schiodt V, Davern TJ, Shakil O, et al. Viral hepatitis-related acute liver failure. *Am J Gastroenterol.* 2003;98:448-453.
262. Norkrans G, Nilsson LA, Frosner G, et al. Serum immunoglobulin levels in hepatitis non-A, non-B: a comparison with hepatitis A and B. *Infection.* 1980;8:98-100.
263. Hoofnagle JH, Di Bisceglie AM. Serologic diagnosis of acute and chronic viral hepatitis. *Semin Liver Dis.* 1991;11:73-83.
263a. Castrodale L, Fiore A, Schmidt T. Detection of immunoglobulin in antibody to hepatitis A virus in Alaska residents without other evidence of hepatitis. *Clin Infect Dis.* 2005;41:e86-e88.
264. Robertson BH, Jia XY, Tian H, et al. Antibody response to nonstructural proteins of hepatitis A virus following infection. *J Med Virol.* 1993;40:76-82.
265. Summers DF, Ehrenfeld E. Host antibody response to viral structural and nonstructural proteins after hepatitis A virus infection. *J Infect Dis.* 1992;165:273-280.
266. Hollinger FB, Bradley DW, Maynard JE, et al. Detection of hepatitis A viral antigen by radioimmunoassay. *J Immunol.* 1975;115:1464-1466.
267. Purcell RH, Wong DC, Moritsugu Y, et al. A microtiter solid-phase radioimmunoassay for hepatitis A antigen and antibody. *J Immunol.* 1976;116:349-356.
268. Tsai YL, Sobsey MD, Sangermano LR, et al. Simple method of concentrating enteroviruses and hepatitis A virus from sewage and ocean water for rapid detection by reverse transcriptase-polymerase chain reaction. *Appl Environ Microbiol.* 1993;59:3488-3491.
269. Le Guyader F, Dubois E, Menard D, et al. Detection of hepatitis A virus, rotavirus, and enterovirus in naturally contaminated shellfish and sediment by reverse transcription-seminested PCR. *Appl Environ Microbiol.* 1994;60:3665-3671.
270. Abe H, Beninger PR, Ikejiri N, et al. Light microscopic findings of liver biopsy specimens from patients with hepatitis type A and comparison with type B. *Gastroenterology.* 1982;82:938-947.
271. Kobayashi K, Hashimoto E, Ludwig J, et al. Liver biopsy features of acute hepatitis C compared with hepatitis A, B, and non-A, non-B, non-C. *Liver.* 1993;13:69-72.
272. Shimizu YK, Mathiesen LR, Lorenz D, et al. Localization of hepatitis A antigen in liver tissue by peroxidase-conjugated antibody method: light and electron microscopic studies. *J Immunol.* 1978;121:1671-1679.
273. Stapleton JT, Lange DK, LeDuc JW, et al. The role of secretory immunity in hepatitis A virus infection. *J Infect Dis.* 1991;163:7-11.
274. Lemon SM, Binn LN, Marchwicki RH. Radioimmunofocus assay for quantitation of hepatitis A virus in cell cultures. *J Clin Microbiol.* 1983;17:834-839.
275. Baba M, Takegawa M, Kaito M, et al. Propagation of hepatitis A virus in a renal cell line JTC-12 P3 of cynomolgus monkey origin. *Acta Virol (Praha).* 1993;37:209-222.
276. Baba M, Fukai K, Hasegawa H, et al. The role of natural killer cells and lymphokine activated killer cells in the pathogenesis of hepatic injury and hepatitis A. *J Clin Lab Immunol.* 1992;38:1-14.
277. Pinto MA, Marchevsky RS, Pelajo-Machado M, et al. Inducible nitric oxide synthase (iNOS) expression in liver and splenic T lymphocyte rise are associated with liver histological damage during experimental hepatitis A virus (HAV) infection in Callithrix jacchus. *Exp Toxicol Pathol.* 2000;52:3-10.

278. Doebbeling BN, Li N, Wenzel RP. An outbreak of hepatitis A among health care workers: risk factors for transmission. *Am J Public Health.* 1993;83:1679-1684.

279. Petrosillo N, Raffaele B, Martini L, et al. A nosocomial and occupational cluster of hepatitis A virus infection in a pediatric ward. *Infect Control Hosp Epidemiol.* 2002;23:343-345.

280. Cohn E, Oncley J, Strong LE. Chemical, clinical, and immunological studies on the products of human plasma fractionation: the characterization of the protein fractions of human plasma. *J Clin Invest.* 1944;23:417-432.

281. Lerman Y, Shohat T, Ashkenazi S, et al. Efficacy of different doses of immune serum globulin in the prevention of hepatitis A: a three-year prospective study. *Clin Infect Dis.* 1993;17:411-414.

282. Smallwood LA, Tabor E, Finlayson JS, et al. Antibodies to hepatitis A virus in immune serum globulin (Letter). *Lancet.* 1980;2:482-483.

283. Stokes J, Neefe JR. The prevention and attenuation of infectious hepatitis by gamma globulin. *JAMA.* 1945;127:144-145.

284. Stapleton JT. Passive immunization against hepatitis A. *Vaccine.* 1992;10(Suppl 1):S45-S47.

285. Weiland O, Niklasson B, Berg R, et al. Clinical and subclinical hepatitis A occurring after immunoglobulin prophylaxis among Swedish UN soldiers in Sinai. *Scand J Gastroenterol.* 1981;16:967-972.

286. Pierce PF, Cappello M, Bernard KW. Subclinical infection with hepatitis A in Peace Corps volunteers following immune globulin prophylaxis. *Am J Trop Med Hyg.* 1990;42:465-469.

287. Kluge I. Gamma globulin in the prevention of viral hepatitis: a study of the effect of medium-size doses. *Acta Med Scand.* 1963;174:469-477.

288. Mosley JW, Reisler DM, Brachott D, et al. Comparison of two lots of immune serum globulin for prophylaxis of infectious hepatitis. *Am J Epidemiol.* 1968;87:539-550.

289. Lemon SM. Type A viral hepatitis: new developments in an old disease. *N Engl J Med.* 1985;313:1059-1067.

290. Advisory Committee on Immunization Practices (ACIP) Centers for Disease Control and Prevention (CDC). Update: Prevention of hepatitis A after exposure to hepatitis A virus and in international travelers. Updated recommendations of the Advisory Committee on Immunization Practices (ACIP). *MMWR Morb Mortal Wkly Rep.* 2007;56:1080-1084.

291. General recommendations on immunization. Recommendations of the Advisory Committee on Immunization Practices (ACIP). *MMWR Recomm Rep.* 2006;55(RR-15):6-8.

292. Ellis EF, Henney CS. Adverse reactions following administration of human gamma globulin. *J Allergy.* 1969;43:45-54.

293. Vidor E, Fritzell B, Plotkin S. Clinical development of a new inactivated hepatitis A vaccine. *Infection.* 1996;24:447-458.

294. Gluck R, Mischler R, Brantschen S, et al. Immunopotentiating reconstituted influenza virus virosome vaccine delivery system for immunization against hepatitis A. *J Clin Invest.* 1992;90:2491-2495.

295. Sjogren MH, Purcell RH, McKee K, et al. Clinical and laboratory observations following oral or intramuscular administration of a live attenuated hepatitis A vaccine candidate. *Vaccine.* 1992;10(Suppl 1):S135-S137.

296. Cohen JI, Rosenblum B, Feinstone SM, et al. Attenuation and cell culture adaptation of hepatitis A virus (HAV): a genetic analysis with HAV cDNA. *J Virol.* 1989;63:5364-5370.

297. Werzberger A, Mensch B, Kuter B, et al. A controlled trial of a formalin-inactivated hepatitis A vaccine in healthy children. *N Engl J Med.* 1992;327:453-457.

298. Werzberger A, Kuter B, Shouval D, et al. Anatomy of a trial: a historical view of the Monroe inactivated hepatitis A protective efficacy trial. *J Hepatol.* 1993;18(Suppl 2):S46-S50.

299. Clemens R, Safary A, Hepburn A, et al. Clinical experience with an inactivated hepatitis A vaccine. *J Infect Dis.* 1995;171(Suppl 1):S44-S49.

300. Dagan R, Amir J, Mijalovsky A, et al. Immunization against hepatitis A in the first year of life: priming despite the presence of maternal antibody. *Pediatr Infect Dis J.* 2000;19:1045-1052.

301. Shouval D, Ashur Y, Adler R, et al. Single and booster dose responses to an inactivated hepatitis A virus vaccine: comparison with immune serum globulin prophylaxis. *Vaccine.* 1993;11(Suppl 1):S9-S14.

302. van Damme P, Mathei C, Thoelen S, et al. Single dose inactivated hepatitis A vaccine: rationale and clinical assessment of the safety and immunogenicity. *J Med Virol.* 1994;44:435-441.

303. Fujiyama S, Iino S, Odoh K, et al. Time course of hepatitis A virus antibody titer after active and passive immunization. *Hepatology.* 1992;15:983-988.

304. Fujiyama S, Odoh K, Kuramoto I, et al. Current seroepidemiological status of hepatitis A with a comparison of antibody titers after infection and vaccination. *J Hepatol.* 1994;21:641-645.

305. Lemon SM, Murphy PC, Provost PJ, et al. Immunoprecipitation and virus neutralization assays demonstrate qualitative differences between protective antibody responses to inactivated hepatitis A vaccine and passive immunization with immune globulin. *J Infect Dis.* 1997;176:9-19.

306. Purcell RH, D'Hondt E, Bradbury R, et al. Inactivated hepatitis A vaccine: active and passive immunoprophylaxis in chimpanzees. *Vaccine.* 1992;10(Suppl 1):S148-S151.

307. Hess G, Clemens R, Bienzle U, et al. Immunogenicity and safety of an inactivated hepatitis A vaccine in anti-HIV positive and negative homosexual men. *J Med Virol.* 1995;46:40-42.

308. Bell BP. Hepatitis A vaccine. *Semin Pediatr Infect Dis.* 2002;13:165-173.

309. Mao JS. Development of live, attenuated hepatitis A vaccine (H2-strain). *Vaccine.* 1990;8:523-524.

310. Sjogren MH, Purcell RH, McKee K, et al. Clinical and laboratory observations following oral or intramuscular administration of a live attenuated hepatitis A vaccine candidate. *Vaccine.* 1992;10(Suppl 1):S135-S137.

311. Midthun K, Ellerbeck E, Gershman K, et al. Safety and immunogenicity of a live attenuated hepatitis A virus vaccine in seronegative volunteers. *J Infect Dis.* 1991;163:735-739.

312. Mao JS, Dong DX, Zhang HY, et al. Primary study of attenuated live hepatitis A vaccine (H2 strain) in humans. *J Infect Dis.* 1989;159:621-624.

313. Cho MW, Ehrenfeld E. Rapid completion of the replication cycle of hepatitis A virus subsequent to reversal of guanidine inhibition. *Virology.* 1991;180:770-780

314. O'Grady J. Management of acute and fulminant hepatitis A. *Vaccine.* 1992;10(Suppl 1):S21-S23.

315. Gane E, Sallie R, Saleh M, et al. Clinical recurrence of hepatitis A following liver transplantation for acute liver failure. *J Med Virol.* 1995;45:35-39.

316. Mijch AM, Gust ID. Clinical, serologic, and epidemiologic aspects of hepatitis A virus infection. *Semin Liver Dis.* 1986;6:42-45.

317. Victor JC, Monto AS, Surdina TY, et al. Hepatitis A vaccine versus immune globulin for postexposure prophylaxis. *N Engl J Med.* 2007;357:1685-1694.

318. Bryan JP, Nelson M. Testing for antibody to hepatitis A to decrease the cost of hepatitis A prophylaxis with immune globulin or hepatitis A vaccines. *Arch Intern Med.* 1994;154:663-668.

319. American Academy of Pediatrics: Hepatitis A. In: Pickering LK, ed. *Red Book: Report of the Committee on Infectious Diseases.* ed. 25. Elk Grove Village, IL: The Academy; 2000:280-289.

319a. Samandari T, Wusley A, Bell BP. Incidence of hepatitis A in the United States in the era of vaccination. *JAMA.* 2005;294:194-201.

320. Ochnio JJ, Patrick D, Ho M, et al. Past infection with hepatitis A virus among Vancouver street youth, injection drug users and men who have sex with men: implications for vaccination programs. *Can Med Assoc J.* 2001;165:293-297.

321. Bell BP. Hepatitis A and hepatitis B vaccination of patients with chronic liver disease. *Acta Gastroenterol Belg.* 2000;63:359-365.

322. Bonanni P, Colombai R, Franchi G, et al. Experience of hepatitis A vaccination during an outbreak in a nursery school of Tuscany, Italy. *Epidemiol Infect.* 1998;121:377-380.

323. Thorburn KM, Bohorques R, Stepak P, et al. Immunization strategies to control a community-wide hepatitis A epidemic. *Epidemiol Infect.* 2001;127:461-467

324. Meltzer JI, Shapiro CN, Mast EE. The economics of vaccinating restaurant workers against hepatitis A. *Vaccine.* 2001;19:2138-2145.

325. Goodman RA, Foster KL, Trowbridge FL, et al. Global disease elimination and eradication as public health strategies. Proceedings of a conference held in Atlanta, Georgia, USA, 23-25 February, 1998. *Bull World Health Organ.* 1998;76:1-162.

326. Fagan E, Yousef G, Brahm J, et al. Persistence of hepatitis A virus in fulminant hepatitis and after liver transplantation. *J Med Virol.* 1990;30:131-136.

174

Rhinovirus

RONALD B. TURNER

The rhinoviruses are among the most common of the pathogens that infect humans. These viruses have been implicated in 30% to 50% of all cases of acute respiratory disease and are the most important cause of the common cold. Historical references to the common cold date from antiquity, but the scientific exploration of rhinovirus infection began in the 20th century. In the early 1900s, colds were induced in volunteers by intranasal inoculation with filtrates of nasal secretions from other volunteers with colds. As a result of these various studies, colds were presumed to be caused by filterable agents (viruses).[1] Subsequent studies of experimental colds in volunteers provided insight into the properties and spread of colds. Many of the nasal secretions used for inducing colds in these volunteers were subsequently shown to contain rhinoviruses.

The initial isolation of rhinovirus is attributed to Pelon and associates[2] and Price[3] and was accomplished by inoculation of nasopharyngeal washings from individuals with colds onto rhesus monkey kidney tissue cultures. These initial isolates, strains 2060 and JH, were shown to be identical and were initially designated echovirus type 28. The name "rhinovirus" was suggested by Andrews, and a description of the group was proposed in 1963. Based on this definition of properties, the original strain was reclassified as rhinovirus type 1A. In retrospect, the isolation of a common cold virus in 1953 was likely the first isolation of rhinovirus, but this isolate was not properly characterized until 1968. In 1960, Tyrrell and Parsons isolated strain HGP by reducing the incubation temperature of cultures to 33° C, lowering the pH of tissue culture media to approximately 7.0, and gently rotating cultures during incubation.[4] The subsequent combination of sensitive strains of human embryonic fibroblast cell cultures and the culture conditions described by the Salisbury group provided a sensitive system for isolation of rhinoviruses.

Once virus isolation techniques had been developed, rapid progress was made in understanding the clinical characteristics and epidemiology of the rhinoviruses.[5,6] The first complete genome sequence was determined for HRV14 in 1984, and the x-ray crystallographic structures of the viral capsids of five serotypes (1A, 2, 3, 14, and 16) were solved soon afterward. Advances in sequencing technology have permitted identification of rhinovirus strains not detectable in cell culture.[7-11] Thus, remarkable progress in rhinovirus research has occurred during a relatively short period of time.

Virology

CLASSIFICATION

The family Picornaviridae consists of nine genera, including four—*Rhinovirus*, *Enterovirus*, *Parechovirus*, and *Hepatovirus*—that cause human infections. The human rhinoviruses have been classified by immunologic serotype, receptor type, antiviral susceptibility, and genotype. Each of these classifications has utility in different situations. Serotyping has been the traditional method of classification. Rhinovirus infectivity is neutralized by specific antisera, and new serotypes are defined by the absence of cross-reactivity with antisera specific for known serotypes. A total of 101 serotypes (1A to A100 and 1B) were identified by 1987, when efforts to identify new serotypes ended. Classification by neutralization testing is limited by the requirement that the virus be cultivated in cell culture—a requirement that is not met by some newly detected rhinovirus strains.

The rhinoviruses may also be classified on the basis of receptor specificity. The "major" receptor group, containing 88 serotypes, uses the intercellular adhesion molecule-1 (ICAM-1; Fig. 174-1C) as receptor for infecting host cells.[12,13] Twelve serotypes, constituting the "minor" receptor group, use the low-density lipoprotein receptor (LDLR) and related proteins as receptors. All members of the minor receptor group are HRVA viruses based on phylogenetic classification, whereas the major receptor group consists of viruses of groups A and B.

Andries and co-workers[14] described two distinct groups of rhinoviruses (A and B) based on variable susceptibility to the capsid-binding agents. These authors also observed that the antiviral group B viruses may be overrepresented among isolates obtained from individuals with colds, suggesting that viruses in this group may be more pathogenic.[14] The antiviral susceptibility group A includes all of the phylogenetic group B strains as well as serotypes 8, 13, 32, 43, 54, and 95 that are classified as phylogenetic group A strains.

The availability of improved sequencing technology and methods has facilitated the genetic characterization of the rhinoviruses. Nucleotide sequences have been determined for the 5′ nontranslated regions and VP4, VP2, and VP1 genes of all serotypes. Complete genome sequences have been determined for 46 serotypes.[15,16] Phylogenetic analysis of these sequences showed that 100 rhinovirus serotypes are divided into two genetic groups or species (A and B),[17] and that HRV87 is actually an enterovirus (EV68). HRV group A (HRVA) consists of 75 serotypes and HRVB of 25 serotypes. Direct sequencing of rhinoviruses in original clinical specimens indicates the existence of previously unrecognized rhinovirus strains and suggests the existence of a new genetic group that has tentatively been designated as group C.[7-11]

MORPHOLOGY AND STRUCTURE

Rhinovirus is composed of an RNA genome packed into a protein shell known as the capsid. In its fully hydrated state, the particle is approximately 30 nm in diameter (Table 174-1). The protein shell is composed of 60 copies of each of four viral proteins, designated VP1 to VP4 (see Fig. 174-1). Protein subunits called protomers, consisting of one copy of each of the four viral proteins, are organized into 12 pentamers. Each of the 12 pentamers contains a prominent depression or "canyon" in VP1 running moatlike around a central plateau (i.e., around the fivefold axis of symmetry). This canyon region contains the binding site for the ICAM-1 receptor, and amino acid residues at the canyon base are more conserved than residues at exposed viral surfaces. Binding of antibody to the virion surface appears to neutralize rhinovirus replication by steric inhibition of this receptor binding. Rhinovirions can also be neutralized by saturation with excess soluble ICAM-1. At the base of the canyon lies a hydrophobic "pocket" (see Fig. 174-1D), which in many rhinoviruses is filled with a still uncharacterized molecule called "pocket factor." This pocket is the binding site for the capsid-binding antivirals.

The rhinoviral genome is a single strand of positive sense RNA of approximately 7200 bases that encodes a single large polyprotein, containing nearly 2200 amino acids. Rhinoviruses have long nontranslated regions (NTRs; 600 to 750 bases) at the 5′ ends with distinctive secondary and tertiary structures, termed internal ribosomal entry sites, that enable ribosomes to initiate translation without the need of the "cap"

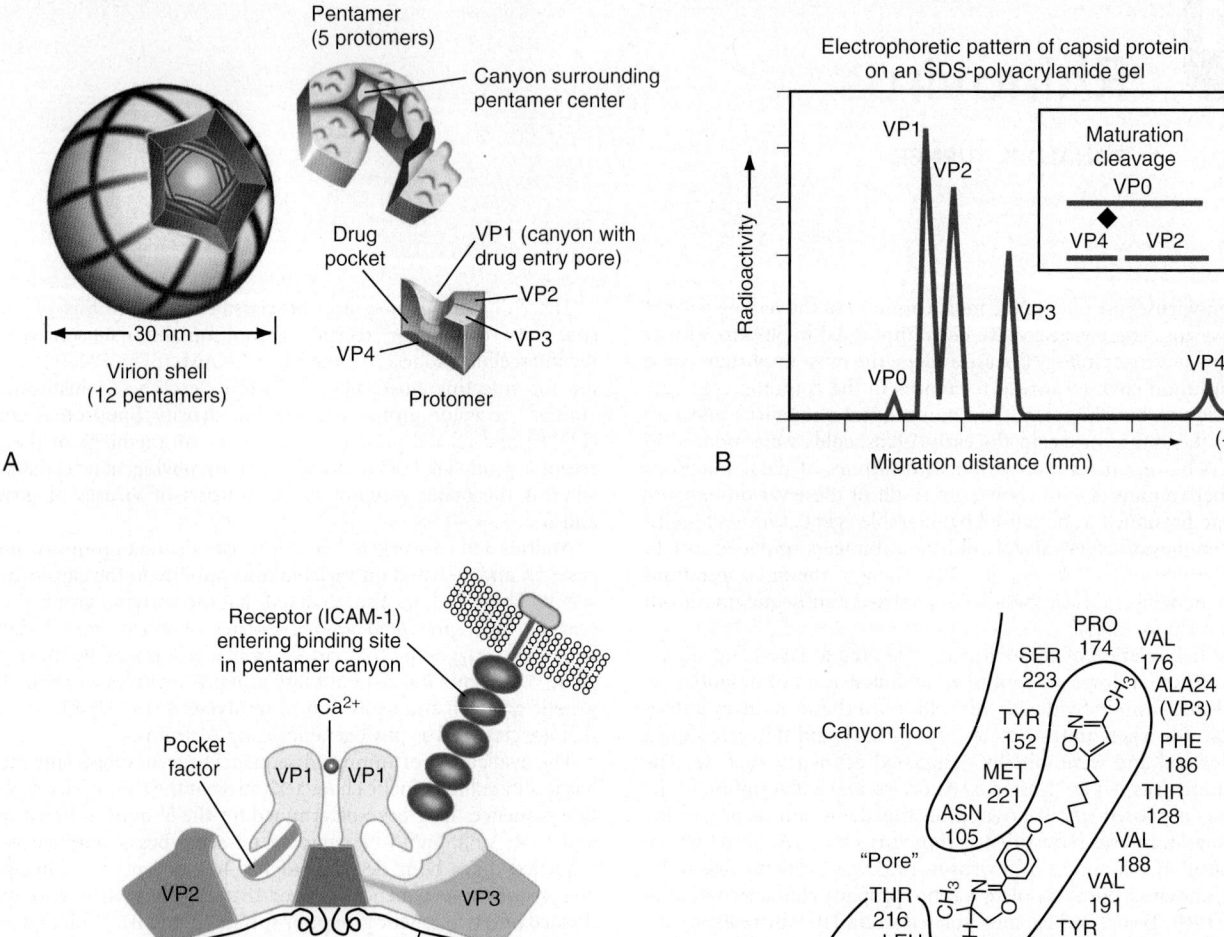

Figure 174-1 **Key features of a human rhinovirus (HRV). A,** The virion shell consists of 12 pentamers, 1 of which has been removed to show the approximate location of the RNA packed tightly into a central cavity. Each pentamer, in turn, consists of five wedge-shaped subunits, called protomers. The canyon *(stippled)* is shown in only 1 of the 12 pentamers. **B,** The virion contains four major proteins (VP1, -2, -3, and -4) plus traces of another, VP0, representing residual precursor following the maturation cleavage *(inset)* required for acquisition of infectivity. **C,** Transverse section through the center of a pentamer depicting entry of its cellular receptor (intercellular adhesion molecule 1 [ICAM-1]) and the location of the drug-binding pocket just beneath the canyon floor. An ion, located at each pentamer center in HRV-1A, -14, and -16, is tentatively identified as calcium, which is necessary for attachment of some rhinoviruses. **D,** Detail showing orientation of a capsid binder (WIN 52084) and identity of amino acid residues lining the canyon floor and drug-binding pocket in a single protomer. In HRV-14, the drug prevents attachment of its receptor, ICAM-1. *(Courtesy of Dr. Roland R. Ruckert.)*

TABLE 174-1	**Characteristics of Rhinovirus**

Size: 30 nm
Shape: nonenveloped capsid with icosahedral symmetry constructed from 60 repeated protomers
Molecular weight: 8.16×10^6 Da
Density: higher in cesium chloride gradient than are other members of the picornavirus group, which suggests a more open capsid structure
Nucleic acid: single-stranded RNA with positive polarity containing approximately 7200 nucleotides
Optimal growth temperature: 33-35°C; growth restricted at 37°C
Replication: virus synthesis and maturation in cell cytoplasm
Antigenicity: type specific

used by most cellular mRNAs. The rhinovirus genome also includes a relatively short 3′-NTR that is required for efficient viral replication.

REPLICATION

Rhinovirus replication is initiated by attachment to the cell via the appropriate receptor. This attachment triggers viral uncoating with delivery of the viral genome to the cytosol of the host cell. The positive strand RNA of the viral genome is translated as a single polyprotein that is then cleaved into the coat proteins and the proteases required for replication of the viral RNA. The positive strand RNA is also transcribed into complementary negative strand replicative intermediates that serve as templates for production of positive strand viral RNA. Early in replication, the new positive strands serve as additional material to amplify the production of the negative strand intermediates, but as positive strands accumulate in the cell, more of these strands are incorporated into virions. Virus is ultimately released by virus-mediated disintegration of the host cell.

HOST RANGE

Rhinoviruses have a high degree of species specificity. Major receptor group viruses do not recognize ICAM-1 from species other than human, with the probable exception of chimpanzees. Although minor group viruses can utilize murine LDLR, only HRV1A and HRV1B can replicate in mouse cells. Chimpanzees can be infected with rhinovirus but do not develop detectable illness.

INACTIVATION BY PHYSICAL AND CHEMICAL AGENTS

The property used to distinguish rhinoviruses from enteroviruses is their acid lability. Inactivation occurs for all rhinoviruses below pH 6, and rapid and complete inactivation occurs at pH 3.[18] In contrast to enteroviruses, most rhinoviruses are thermostable. Rhinoviruses will survive for hours to days on environmental surfaces at 24°C to 37°C; they are stable for years at −70°C.

Rhinoviruses are relatively resistant to lipid solvents such as ethanol, ether, chloroform, and fluorocarbon.[18] Extraction of rhinovirus with diethyl ether has been used for the selective killing of bacterial and fungal contaminants and as a preliminary test to distinguish lipid enveloped viruses from nonenveloped ones. Infectivity is less refractory to extraction with more polar organic solvents such as chloroform, possibly because of the removal of the hydrophobic "pocket factor" or partial solvent denaturation of the protein shell. The rhinoviruses are resistant to nonionic detergents such as Nonidet P40 and sodium deoxycholate, but they are inactivated by sodium dodecyl sulfate. A variety of disinfectants are virucidal for rhinoviruses.[19]

When subjected to any of a variety of treatments including gentle heating, ultraviolet light, high pH, mercurials, phenol, or desiccation, rhinovirions lose their infectivity. Chemicals that alter the nucleic acid include nitrous acid and alkaline reagents such as ammonia. Halogens (chlorine, bromine, and iodine), hydrogen peroxide, and ozone are also commonly used disinfectants.

Epidemiology

GEOGRAPHIC DISTRIBUTION AND PREVALENCE

Rhinoviruses are distributed worldwide. The incidence of rhinovirus infection, based on virus isolation from adults in the United States, is approximately 0.75 infections per person-year.[5,20] The incidence in children is approximately 1.2 infections per year. Studies using polymerase chain reaction (PCR) techniques have reported similar incidence rates, although systematic studies using this technique have not been done.[21-23] A single longitudinal study involving a small number of children reported a rhinovirus infection rate of approximately 6 per year.[24]

Approximately one fourth of rhinovirus infections are asymptomatic. In studies of naturally acquired infection, 12% to 37% of infections detected by virus isolation and 12% to 22% of infections detected by reverse transcriptase (RT)-PCR are asymptomatic. Similarly, 20% to 30% of infections in subjects experimentally infected by intranasal inoculation of rhinovirus are asymptomatic.

SEASONALITY

Rhinovirus infections occur throughout the year, but in temperate climates there are distinct peaks of illness in the fall and spring.[5] The fall peak generally occurs in late August or September in the Northern Hemisphere. By early November, rhinovirus prevalence declines, usually remaining low throughout the late fall, winter, and early spring.[24] A second period of increased rhinovirus activity frequently occurs in April and May. Although the overall incidence of colds is low during the summer months, rhinovirus accounts for up to 50% of the illnesses that occur during this season.[5,24]

The reason for this seasonality is not clear, but it may be a result of both viral biology and human behavior. Rhinovirus survives best in the environment during periods of high humidity.[25] Studies in Charlottesville, Virginia, noted a correlation between the seasons when indoor relative humidity is generally higher than 45% and the increased incidence of rhinovirus infection. Outbreaks of infection also coincide with the times that children are brought together by school attendance.[25,26] The relatively low incidence of infection during the summer months, despite high humidity, may reflect a decrease in transmission during times that school is not in session. In the temperate areas of the Southern Hemisphere, the seasonal incidence of infection mirrors that in the Northern Hemisphere, and in tropical climates rhinovirus activity is detected throughout the year with little relationship to climatic conditions.

TRANSMISSION

Initiation of rhinovirus infection requires that the virus reach the nasal mucosa of a susceptible host. Delivery of virus to the nasal mucosa can potentially occur either by aerosols or by direct contact. Although there is evidence that the rhinovirus genome may be present in small particle aerosols, epidemiologic evidence suggests that small particle aerosols are not an important mechanism of spread. Large particle aerosols, presumably produced by coughs and sneezes and deposited onto the nasal or conjunctival mucosa, have been shown to transmit infection under experimental conditions and may contribute to natural transmission.[27,28] Direct contact, however, appears to be the most efficient mechanism of transmission of rhinovirus. Under experimental conditions, rhinovirus is recovered from the fingers of approximately 65% of infected volunteers after finger-to-nose contact, and the contaminating virus survives for several hours on skin.[29,30] Contact with the contaminated fingers reliably transfers virus to the skin of a recipient individual, and once the fingertips of the recipient are contaminated, infection is readily induced by self-inoculation of the nasal mucosa by rubbing the nose or the eyes. The role of fomites in the transmission of virus is less clear. Virus contaminating the hands is readily transferred to objects in the environment and can be transferred to skin by contact; however, there is substantial loss of infectious virus at each step. An attempt to document transmission of infection from fomites under experimental conditions that would favor transmission was unsuccessful, suggesting that this mechanism may not be efficient for spread of rhinovirus infections.[31]

Studies in the natural setting support the direct contact route of rhinovirus transmission. Virus is recovered from the skin of the hands of approximately 40% of individuals with natural rhinovirus colds and from 6% to 15% of objects in their environment.[29,30] Individuals in the natural setting routinely make finger-to-eye or finger-to-nose contact in a manner that would transfer virus to the nasal mucosa. Despite these suggestive data, assessment of the mechanism of transmission of virus under natural conditions can only be determined by blocking transmission in the natural setting, using an intervention that is specific for a particular route. A single trial found that regular applications of 2% aqueous iodine to the fingers by mothers who had been exposed to a child with a fresh cold in the home reduced colds by 67% compared to placebo. None of 11 mothers using iodine became infected with the same rhinovirus serotype recovered from the index case, compared to 31% of mothers using placebo.[29]

Rhinovirus transmission is most likely when virus concentrations in nasal secretions are highest and symptoms are the most severe. Under experimental conditions, transmission of infection between susceptible individuals living together was most likely when the infected individual had greater than 1000 tissue culture infective dose (TCID$_{50}$) of virus in nasal washings, virus on the hands and anterior nares, and symptoms of at least a moderately severe cold.[32] In most instances, these conditions occurred only on the second and third days after virus inoculation.

Pathogenesis in Humans

Rhinovirus preferentially infects the upper respiratory tract. Rhinovirus grows best in cell culture at approximately 33°C, and this preferential growth at lower temperature has long been cited to suggest that rhinovirus might not infect the lower airways. This concept was also supported by early studies demonstrating that infection was more readily produced when virus was administered by intranasal drops than by aerosol. Recent studies have established that rhinovirus can replicate in the lower respiratory tract, but the frequency of lower tract involvement during natural infection remains unknown.[33] Infection of the upper respiratory tract includes involvement of the paranasal sinuses. Abnormalities of the sinuses are frequently detected by computerized tomography or magnetic resonance imaging during both natural colds and experimentally induced rhinovirus colds, and rhinovirus is detected in the sinus secretions by PCR.[34-36]

Following experimental inoculation into the nasal cavity, rhinovirus is detected initially in the posterior nasopharynx.[37] The infection becomes more generalized in the nose as the cold progresses, but biopsies of the nasal mucosa and nasopharynx demonstrate only small foci of infection interspersed among large areas of uninfected cells.[37,38] Ciliated epithelial cells are the primary cells involved, but nonciliated cells are also infected. The apparent paucity of rhinovirus-infected cells in the epithelium may be a result of desquamation of infected cells into the nasal secretions.[39] Examination of specimens of the nasal epithelium by light or electron microscopy reveals no consistent lesions, and no morphologic changes are seen in monolayers of human nasal epithelium infected with rhinovirus.[40,41]

In contrast to the absence of histopathologic evidence of infection, symptomatic infections are reliably associated with both a local and a systemic cellular inflammatory response. The peripheral white blood cell count increases, as a result of an increase in the concentration of neutrophils, in infected, ill subjects during the first 2 or 3 days after virus challenge.[42] Infected non-ill subjects have no change in the white blood cell count. A similar polymorphonuclear leukocyte response to rhinovirus infection is seen in the nasal mucosa and nasal secretions.[43,44] As with the changes in peripheral neutrophil count, the increase in polymorphonuclear leukocytes is seen in infected symptomatic subjects but not in asymptomatically infected individuals.[44] The correlation between lymphocytic response to rhinovirus infection and symptomatic illness is less clearly characterized. There are conflicting data on the effect of rhinovirus infection on the peripheral lymphocyte count. Modest increases in T-lymphocyte concentrations have been reported in both the nasal mucosa and nasal secretions during rhinovirus infection.[45,46]

The observations summarized previously suggest that nonspecific host inflammatory responses may play a role in symptom expression. Challenge of respiratory epithelial cells in vitro results in elaboration of a number of proinflammatory cytokines. The signaling pathways by which these mediators are stimulated by rhinovirus are unknown, and multiple pathways may be involved. Elaboration of the cytokines is biphasic, and the early phase of elaboration appears to be independent of virus replication, in contrast to late phase elaboration, which appears to be dependent on virus replication and may be mediated by different signaling pathways than the early phase.[47,48] The mediators of these signaling pathways are not known, but virus-induced oxidant stress, toll-like receptor 3, phosphatidylinositol 3-kinase, and mitogen-activated protein kinase pathways have been implicated.[48-51] Rhinovirus also interacts with ceramide-enriched cell membrane platforms that may play a role in stimulating relevant signaling pathways.[52,53] The relevance of these studies to the pathogenesis of rhinovirus infection in vivo remains to be determined.

The interleukins (ILs) IL-1β, IL-6, and IL-8 are present in increased concentrations in the nasal secretions of symptomatic subjects with experimental rhinovirus colds. The concentration of these proteins increases and then decreases, coincident with symptom severity. The concentrations of IL-6 and IL-8 in nasal secretions appear to be directly correlated with the severity of the common cold symptoms.[54,55] Intra-

nasal challenge of normal volunteers with IL-8 produces an influx of neutrophils, a transient increase in nasal resistance to airflow, and a significant increase in nasal symptom scores compared to placebo challenged subjects.[56] Despite these data demonstrating an association between symptoms and inflammatory mediators, the role of these mediators in pathogenesis will not be clear until specific inhibitors are available for use in clinical trials.

The kinins, bradykinin and lysylbradykinin, have been found in the nasal secretions of volunteers with rhinovirus colds, both experimentally induced and naturally acquired.[44,57] The concentration and time course of the production of kinins were roughly correlated with the severity and time course of symptoms in these subjects. Subjects who were infected with rhinovirus but who did not develop symptoms did not have an increase in nasal secretion kinin concentration. Intranasal challenge of uninfected volunteers with bradykinin resulted in symptoms of nasal obstruction, rhinorrhea, and sore throat.[58] However, the role of kinins in the pathogenesis of common cold symptoms is less clear in light of the failure of a bradykinin antagonist to moderate common cold symptoms.[59] Similarly, steroid therapy significantly reduced the concentration of kinins in nasal washes but had no effect on symptoms.[60]

Although antihistamines are commonly used for treatment of rhinovirus colds, there is no evidence that histamine is an important inflammatory mediator in these illnesses.[44] Prostaglandin D₂, another mast cell-derived mediator, also cannot be detected in the nasal secretions of rhinovirus-infected subjects.[44,61] Treatment with a second-generation antihistamine that has antihistaminic activity but reduced anticholinergic activity has no effect on rhinovirus colds.[62] These studies suggest that it is unlikely that histamine or other mast cell mediators make an important contribution to the pathogenesis of rhinovirus colds.

Neurogenic mechanisms also appear to play a role in the expression of illness during rhinovirus infections. The parasympathetic nervous system controls the secretory activity of nasal seromucous glands. These glands, in association with plasma transudation, provide most of the nasal fluid produced during a rhinovirus cold.[61] Drugs with anticholinergic activity, such as atropine methonitrate and ipratropium bromide, given intranasally, and first-generation antihistamines given orally, reduce mean nasal fluid volumes by approximately 30% in volunteers with rhinovirus colds.[63-65] These findings support the role of the parasympathetic nervous system in rhinovirus pathogenesis.

The result of these inflammatory processes is increased vascular permeability with leakage of serum into the nasal mucosa and nasal secretions. Swelling of the nasal mucosa is a major contributor to the nasal obstruction associated with the cold, and serum is a major component of the nasal secretions early in the cold.[61] The contribution of glandular secretions from the nose to the rhinorrhea becomes more important later in the course of the illness.[61]

It has become increasingly clear that rhinovirus is an important cause of wheezing illnesses and exacerbations of asthma.[66,67] The pathogenesis of this lower respiratory tract involvement is not clear. Studies in asthmatics infected with rhinovirus in both the natural setting and experimental challenge models have suggested that an exacerbation is most likely when the acute insult associated with rhinovirus infection is superimposed on allergic airway inflammation, as measured by serum immunoglobulin E (IgE) concentration or airway eosinophilia.[68,69] Whether the viral insult is mediated by inflammatory or neurologic responses generated by nasal infection or whether there is infection of the lower airway in these patients is not known.

Immune Response and Protection from Infection

The inflammatory response with elaboration of inflammatory mediators and polymorphonuclear leukocyte infiltration that is seen in symptomatic rhinovirus infection does not appear to play a role in the control of the infection. Viral shedding is less in asymptomatic individuals, who also have a decreased inflammatory response, and the time to final viral clearance is comparable in symptomatic and asymptomatic individuals. Peak virus shedding occurs at approximately the same time as the peak of symptoms, and virus concentrations in secretions decrease coincidentally with the resolution of symptoms. Low levels of virus shedding continue for 2 or 3 weeks, however, and the termination of viral shedding and protection from subsequent infection is most closely correlated with the appearance of neutralizing antibody.

Both local and serum antibody responses are produced in response to infection.[70] The proportion of rhinovirus-infected individuals who develop a serum neutralizing antibody response varies from 37% to 92% in different studies. Once present, serum neutralizing antibody persists for years, with antibody levels of 16 or higher associated with solid immunity.[70] The dominant serum antibody response is in the IgG$_1$ subclass. Most of the antibody that develops in the nasal secretions is of the IgA class.

The dynamics and the role of neutralizing antibody during acute illness vary depending on the antibody status of the host. During the acute phase of rhinovirus colds, there is considerable transudation of serum proteins into nasal secretions, and transudation of preexisting serum neutralizing antibody may modify the severity of the illness.[71,72] In seronegative people, rhinovirus neutralizing antibody appears in serum and nasal secretions approximately 2 weeks after onset of infection, and titers increase rapidly during the third and fourth weeks, at which time viral shedding in nasal secretions is no longer detectable.[37,70] Viral neutralizing activity, apparently associated with IgA, first appears in nasal secretions 2 or 3 weeks after infection, at approximately the same time that neutralizing activity is detected in serum.

Although it appears that neutralizing antibody is important in complete elimination of rhinovirus shedding from nasal secretions, recovery from illness and the initial reduction in the viral load in nasal secretions occur before specific antibody appears. It also appears that patients with IgA deficiency or with deficiency of serum antibody recover normally from rhinovirus-associated illnesses. The host factors that terminate the inflammatory response and produce the initial reduction in virus replication are not known. Interferon-α may play a role in some individuals but is detected in the nasal secretions during only one third of infections. Preinfection interferon-γ concentrations are inversely correlated with both severity of illness and duration of virus shedding during experimental colds.[73] It is likely that other, as yet undetermined, mechanisms are involved in the resolution of symptoms associated with rhinovirus infections.

The most important host factor that determines susceptibility to infection is the presence or absence of homologous type-specific antibody to the virus. There is no evidence that climatic conditions, chilling, underlying allergic disease, or stress influence the likelihood of infection. A series of studies suggest that host psychological or personality factors may influence the severity of illness. These studies suggest that chronic stress is associated with the development of more severe symptoms.[74] Other studies suggest that personality type may also impact symptom severity. Introverted individuals are reported to have more severe illness.[75] In contrast, a positive emotional style, associated with vigor and a feeling of well-being, is associated with a reduction in symptom severity.[76] The biologic basis of these observed associations is not clear.

Clinical Manifestations

The major clinical syndrome associated with rhinovirus infection is an upper respiratory illness that is traditionally characterized as "the common cold." Rhinovirus colds frequently begin as a sore or "scratchy" throat that is followed closely by development of nasal obstruction and rhinorrhea. During the course of the illness, the signs and symptoms of rhinovirus colds typically include various combinations of sneezing, rhinorrhea, nasal obstruction, facial pressure, sore/scratchy throat, hoarseness, cough, headache, malaise, chilliness, and feverishness (Fig. 174-2).[6] Cough occurs in approximately 30% of

colds and frequently appears after the onset of nasal symptoms and often persists longer. The clinical features of rhinovirus colds are similar in adults and children.

Rhinovirus illness is quite variable in severity and duration; natural rhinovirus colds have shown durations ranging from 1 to 33 days in prospective epidemiologic studies.[6] The median duration of these colds was 7 days, with approximately one fourth lasting 2 weeks. Resolution of the most severe symptoms occurs quite rapidly in most cases, and lingering minor symptoms generally account for the prolonged duration of illness reported by some individuals.

Imaging studies show that sinus involvement is an inherent feature of colds; thus, a rhinovirus cold is more accurately characterized as a viral rhinosinusitis.[34] Rhinovirus has been recovered from sinus aspirates of patients with acute community-acquired sinusitis, and rhinovirus RNA has also been detected in brushings from the sinus cavity.[77] Patients with sinus involvement typically recover from their illness without specific intervention.

Rhinovirus infection also results in abnormalities of the eustachian tube and middle ear. Abnormalities in middle ear pressures are seen in approximately three fourths of patients with rhinovirus colds, sometimes in association with middle ear effusions. Rhinovirus has been recovered alone and in combination with bacteria in middle ear fluids from 24% of patients with otitis media.[78] It is unclear whether viral invasion of the middle ear is required for the development of the eustachian tube and middle ear abnormalities.

There are no specific laboratory findings associated with rhinovirus infections, and routine laboratory tests are not useful in the clinical evaluation of patients with suspected rhinovirus colds. During experimental rhinovirus infection, there is a modest increase in blood neutrophils, and there is a moderate elevation of the erythrocyte sedimentation rate in some volunteers.[42] A predominance of polymorphonuclear leukocytes in the nasal secretions is characteristic of uncomplicated colds and does not aid in the diagnosis of bacterial superinfection.

Complications

ACUTE BACTERIAL SINUSITIS

The incidence of secondary acute bacterial sinusitis is difficult to ascertain, given the changes that occur in the sinuses in uncomplicated rhinovirus colds. Various reports have estimated that 0.5% to 8% of viral colds are complicated by bacterial sinusitis.[79] The factors leading to secondary bacterial invasion of the sinus cavity during colds are incompletely understood. Nose-blowing propels nasal secretions into the sinuses, and occlusion of the ethmoid infundibulum in many patients with colds may trap nasopharyngeal bacteria in the sinus cavity in some patients, thus leading to secondary bacterial infection.

ACUTE BACTERIAL OTITIS MEDIA

Acute bacterial otitis media complicates an estimated 2% of colds in adults and up to 30% of colds in children.[79,80] A high incidence of eustachian tube dysfunction has been reported during the common cold, and bacteria presumably reach the middle ear by a mechanism similar to that described previously for sinusitis.

EXACERBATIONS OF CHRONIC BRONCHITIS

Up to 40% of exacerbations of chronic bronchitis have been associated with rhinovirus infections. The episodes are characterized by fever, increased purulence of the sputum, and worsening of ventilation. One longitudinal study of patients with chronic obstructive pulmonary disease documented viral infections in 23% of hospitalizations; rhinovirus was the most frequently identified agent. The pathogenesis of these abnormalities is unknown but could involve direct viral invasion of the large airways or reflex mechanisms from upper respiratory tract disease.

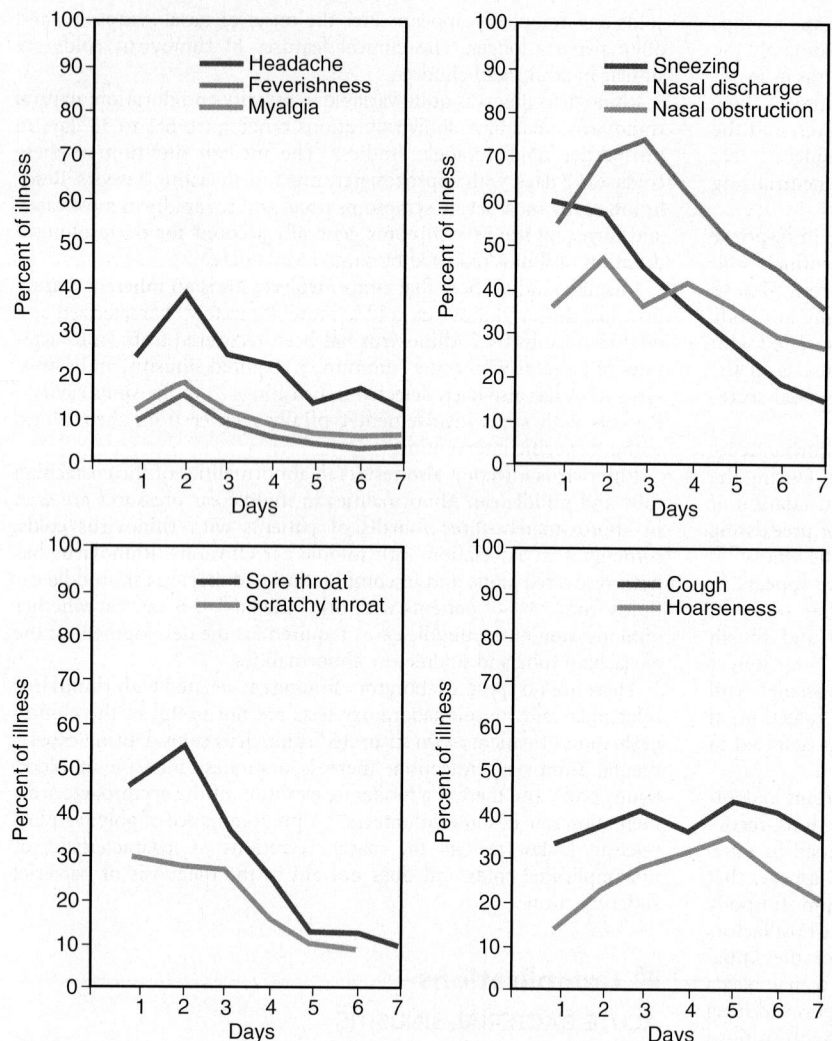

Figure 174-2 **Rhinovirus cold symptoms (139 adults with natural infection).**

ASTHMA

Rhinovirus is the principal virus implicated in precipitating asthma attacks in older children and adults and is associated with 60% to 70% of the asthma exacerbations in school-aged children.[66,67] Both a fall peak of asthma exacerbation and a fall increase in the incidence of rhinovirus infection have been reported in association with the start of the school year.[25,26] Rhinovirus is particularly important in precipitating episodes of asthma in children older than 2 years, in whom the infection is often associated with allergen-specific IgE. The timing of the asthma peak may be due to a convergence of rhinovirus infection spread among schoolchildren and seasonal allergen exposure.[26] The mechanisms by which rhinovirus infection induce wheezing are not well understood.

OTHER LOWER RESPIRATORY SYNDROMES

Rhinoviruses can be isolated from a small fraction of children admitted to hospitals with a diagnosis of bronchiolitis or pneumonia. A higher proportion of rhinovirus infections have been reported in studies that have used RT-PCR techniques for detection of rhinovirus. In one study, rhinovirus was the only pathogen detected in 10% of children younger than 1 year with acute bronchiolitis.[81] Another study of bronchiolitis in children younger than 3 years found rhinovirus in 21% of patients, but it was isolated as the sole pathogen in only 4 of 192

patients (2%).[82] Rhinovirus has also been detected in the upper respiratory tract of patients with pneumonia. One study reported that 24% of children with pneumonia had rhinovirus detected in the upper respiratory tract by RT-PCR,[83] although more than half of these patients had evidence of a concurrent bacterial infection. These data demonstrate an association between rhinovirus and lower respiratory tract disease in immunocompetent children, but the frequency of rhinovirus infection in the general population makes assessment of a causal role for rhinovirus in the lower tract disease difficult.

INFECTIONS IN IMMUNOCOMPROMISED PATIENTS

Rhinovirus has been isolated from the lower respiratory tract of a small number of immunocompromised patients. The significance of these isolates has been questioned, given the prevalence of rhinovirus in the general population, the potential for contamination of the lower airway specimens by upper respiratory secretions, and the fact that most of the rhinovirus isolates were associated with concurrent isolation of more typical lower respiratory pathogens. A recent study, however, has provided definitive evidence for active and persistent infection of the lower respiratory tract in patients following lung transplantation.[84] This observation adds to the growing body of evidence that rhinovirus does infect the lower respiratory tract and is consistent with a conclusion that rhinovirus is a real, although uncommon, cause of lower respiratory disease in this patient population.

Diagnosis

The physical findings in the common cold are limited to the upper respiratory tract. Increased nasal secretion is frequently obvious. A change in the color or consistency of the secretions is common during the course of the illness and is not an indication of bacterial superinfection. Examination of the nasal cavity may reveal swollen, erythematous nasal turbinates; however, this finding is nonspecific and of limited diagnostic usefulness.

Colds are different from episodes of allergic rhinitis, in which persistent sneezing, thin nasal discharge, watery eyes, and sensation of mucosal itch are more common. Also, other symptoms of colds, such as sore throat, cough, malaise, and headache, are less common with allergic or vasomotor rhinitis. When viral culture and nasal smear eosinophilia were used as criteria of diagnosis, adults were able to reliably distinguish colds from allergic rhinitis.

The clinical features of rhinovirus infection do not allow reliable differentiation from respiratory infections caused by other viral pathogens. Knowing the seasonal prevalence of the different respiratory viruses helps in suspecting the specific viral etiology of a cold, but a firm diagnosis depends on identification by laboratory methods, which is usually not practical or necessary for routine patient care.

Distinguishing the rhinosinusitis of a rhinovirus cold from a secondary acute bacterial sinusitis is often difficult. Two clinical presentations of acute bacterial sinusitis can be recognized. First, the classical features of acute bacterial sinusitis include fever and facial pain, swelling, or tenderness. There may also be maxillary toothache if the infection is of dental origin. The features of this presentation, although specific, are often not present and thus lack sensitivity. The second and more common presentation of acute bacterial sinusitis is that of an acute respiratory illness that begins as a cold or "flu" but lasts longer than expected. Most natural rhinovirus colds end after 12 to 14 days, and almost all colds improve by 1 week.[6,80,85] Therefore, in acute respiratory illnesses that have not improved or are worse after 10 days, the diagnosis of secondary bacterial sinusitis should be suspected. Radiographic imaging for diagnosis of bacterial sinusitis is of limited utility,[34] and the imaging abnormalities seen with viral and bacterial sinusitis are often indistinguishable.

Laboratory Diagnosis

VIRUS ISOLATION

Rhinovirus is found primarily in respiratory secretions from the upper airway, with the highest concentration in nasal fluids. Nasopharyngeal swabs or aspirates, or nasal washes, are all appropriate specimens for detection of rhinovirus. Rhinovirus isolation from the blood is rare but has been reported in 3 children with respiratory disease and 2 infants who died of sudden infant death syndrome. One study reported detection of rhinovirus RNA in the plasma of 10 of 88 (11%) normal children with rhinovirus infection.[86] The detection of rhinovirus RNA in plasma was not associated with evidence of systemic illness, and it is not clear that this observation reflects a true systemic infection with the virus.

Isolation of virus in cell culture is most readily accomplished using strains of human diploid embryonic lung (HEL) cells (e.g., WI-38 and MRC-5). Different lots of these cells may vary in their sensitivity to rhinovirus, and cell cultures should be monitored for sensitivity when used for growing rhinovirus. Rhinovirus grows best at temperatures of 33° or 34°C under conditions of motion (e.g., roller drum), and cultures are typically held for 10 to 14 days after inoculation. Blind passage has been shown to improve isolation rates in HeLa cells but not in HEL cells. The typical cytopathic effect of rhinoviruses is readily apparent in sensitive cells (Fig. 174-3). The use of tracheal organ cultures may improve the sensitivity of isolation for some rhinoviruses, but the use of organ culture for routine laboratory detection of rhinoviruses is impractical.

ANTIGEN DETECTION

Detection of rhinovirus can be accomplished by immunofluorescence or immunoperoxidase using serotype-specific antibody.[39] Similarly, enzyme-linked immunosorbent assay methods have been attempted. These techniques, which are serotype specific and thus of no use for detection of virus in the natural setting, have been used only for research purposes. An immunoassay using antibody directed against the 3C protease of rhinovirus, which is highly conserved among different serotypes, was too insensitive for diagnostic use.[87]

NUCLEIC ACID DETECTION

RT-PCR has become the standard diagnostic tool for the detection of rhinoviruses in clinical specimens because it is more sensitive, faster, and easier to perform than traditional virus isolation. The 5′-NTR of the rhinoviral genomic RNA has several short stretches of sequence that are almost completely conserved among all 100 serotypes.[88] The RT-PCR primers based on these conserved sequences have been used for sensitive and specific detection of all rhinoviruses as a group. Recently, a molecular typing assay was developed for rapid identification of individual rhinovirus serotypes or strains in original clinical samples. This assay uses sensitive pan-HRV primers and seminested PCR to amplify a 260-bp variable region in the 5′-NTR of the rhinoviral genome for sequence determination. The serotype or strain is then determined by phylogenetic comparisons of the resulting sequence to homologous reference sequences of 100 known serotypes.[88] In situ hybridization using rhinovirus-specific probes has been used to locate the anatomic sites and cell types that support viral replication in the airways of infected subjects,[38,89] making it useful to study pathogenesis.

SEROLOGIC ASSAYS

Detection of neutralizing antibody is the only available serologic method for diagnosis of rhinovirus infections. Given the large number of serotypes, however, serologic diagnosis is practical only when the serotype of the infecting virus is known or suspected, as in experimental virus challenge studies or in family studies in which a rhinovirus has been recovered from a family member. Rhinovirus neutralizing antibody in human serum and nasal washes is measured by mixing the test material with a small inoculum (3 to 30 TCID$_{50}$) of virus to detect the relatively low concentration of antibody in these specimens.

Prevention and Treatment

Nonspecific and symptomatic treatments for rhinovirus infection are similar for all causes of the common cold. These treatments are reviewed in Chapter 53.

VACCINES

Soon after the discovery of the rhinoviruses, efforts were begun to develop inactivated vaccines against these pathogens. Both monovalent and multivalent inactivated vaccines were evaluated against artificial challenge in volunteers. Some preparations induced antibody titers comparable to those after natural infection, and vaccination with these preparations reduced virus shedding and severity of illness, although neither infection nor illness was prevented. As the large number of different serotypes became apparent, efforts to develop rhinovirus vaccines were abandoned.

INTERFERON-α

Leukocyte interferon was first used to prevent rhinovirus infection in 1973. This initial effort demonstrated efficacy for both infection and illness, but the lack of a ready supply delayed the systematic study of interferon in rhinovirus colds until recombinant interferon became

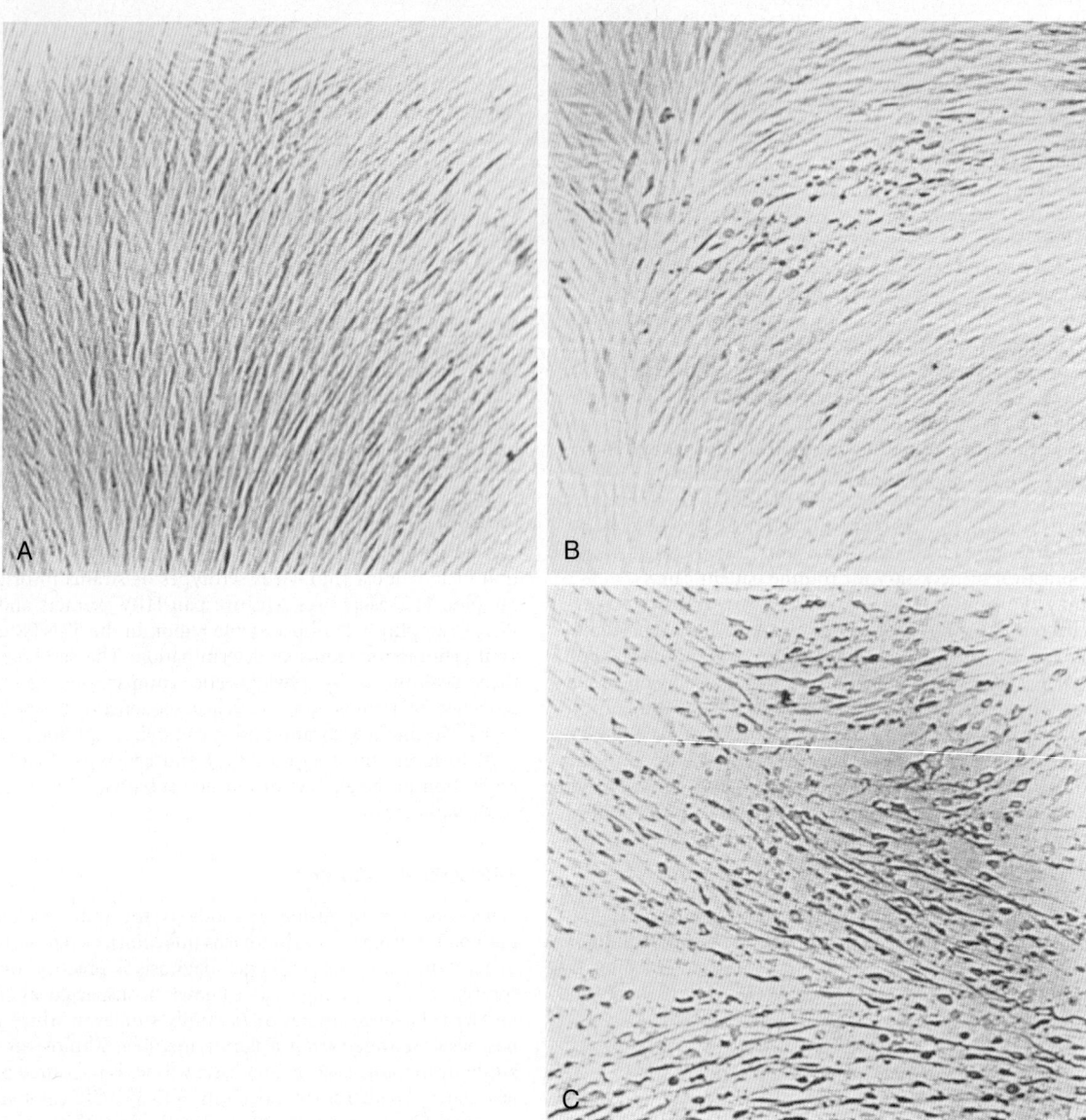

Figure 174-3 Rhinovirus cytopathic effect in human embryonic lung cells (WI-38). A, Uninfected cell cultures (original magnification, ×160). **B,** Cytopathic effect of rhinovirus type 39 at 48 hours. **C,** Cytopathic effect at 72 hours.

available in the early 1980s. A large number of studies were subsequently done in both natural and experimental rhinovirus infections using both prophylactic and treatment designs (reviewed in Arruda[90]). These studies established that interferons were effective for prophylaxis but were ineffective for treatment. The use of interferon for prevention of rhinovirus infection was associated with nasal toxicity. For this reason, and because of the prohibitive cost of the material, the effort to develop interferon as a preventative for rhinovirus infection was abandoned.

BLOCKADE OF ICAM-1 RECEPTOR

The observation that ICAM-1 was the cellular receptor for a large majority of the rhinoviruses suggested that inhibition of attachment might provide an attractive target for prevention of rhinovirus infection.[12,13] Subsequent studies showed that rhinovirus infection could be prevented in vitro by blocking access to the ICAM-1 receptor with monoclonal antibody. Based on these observations, prophylaxis with intranasal monoclonal antibody to ICAM-1 was attempted in experimental colds in volunteers.[91] In the most successful of these studies, the treatment reduced symptoms and viral shedding during the time

the medication was being administered. However, when the medication was discontinued, the amount of virus shedding increased and symptoms became more severe. An alternate approach to receptor blockade was explored in studies using truncated forms of ICAM-1 created by deleting the transmembrane and intracellular domains of the protein. Studies in vitro confirmed that these so-called soluble ICAMs prevented infection by a broad spectrum of rhinovirus serotypes in a variety of different cell lines. A subsequent human clinical trial of sICAM using the experimental rhinovirus challenge model found that when treatment was started either 7 hours before or 12 hours after rhinovirus challenge, there was no effect on the incidence of infection, but symptoms were reduced.[92] There have been no subsequent studies of this approach.

CAPSID-BINDING AGENTS

The capsid-binding agents bind to rhinovirus in a hydrophobic pocket formed by VP1 that lies underneath the canyon region of the virus.[93] The mechanism of the antiviral effect of these compounds is complex. Attachment of rhinovirus to the cellular receptor, subsequent movement of the virus into the host cell, and uncoating of the viral protein coat to release the infectious RNA are all critical events in the initiation of rhinovirus infection that appear to be inhibited in different viral serotypes by these agents. A large number of different molecules that bind in the hydrophobic pocket were found to have antiviral activity; however, pleconaril, a molecule that has favorable pharmacokinetics, is metabolically stable, and has broad and potent antiviral activity, was the most extensively studied of these compounds. Pleconaril was shown to reduce illness in two large studies of natural rhinovirus infection, but the drug was not approved for systemic use because of safety concerns after it was found to induce cytochrome P-450 3A enzymes.[94]

3C PROTEASE INHIBITORS

The rhinovirus genome encodes a single large polyprotein that is cleaved to produce the individual structural and enzymatic proteins of the virus. The 3C protease participates in many of these cleavage reactions. The importance of this protease to rhinovirus replication, and the fact that the active site of the protease appears to be highly conserved in all rhinovirus serotypes, suggested that this enzyme was a potential target for antiviral therapies. A 3C protease inhibitor, ruprintrivir, was subsequently designed and advanced to clinical trials. These clinical trials in experimental human rhinovirus infections revealed a modest effect on infection rates and illness severity.[95] No further studies of this treatment have been published.

VIRUCIDAL TREATMENTS

The observation that direct contact is the predominant mechanism of spread for the rhinovirus suggests that handwashing might be a simple and effective method for prevention of these infections. A 2% aqueous iodine hand treatment appeared useful as prophylaxis against rhinovirus infection, but the cosmetic properties of the iodine solution prevent its practical use as a virucidal finger treatment.[29] Commonly used hand sanitizers containing 62% ethanol are effective for reducing the titer of virus on skin, but studies in the natural setting have not demonstrated efficacy for prevention of colds.[96,97]

The acid lability of the rhinoviruses has been explored as a possible target for prevention or treatment of rhinovirus infections. Initial efforts focused on virucidal tissues that contained citric acid, malic acid, and sodium lauryl sulfate. Studies of these tissues in the natural setting found little impact on the incidence of colds.[98] Recently, organic acids have been incorporated into hand treatments that have been shown in experimental studies to have potent virucidal activity that persists for several hours after application.[99] Whether these agents are effective for prevention of rhinovirus infection in the natural setting has not been determined. The use of a low pH nasal spray for inactivation of rhinovirus in the nasal cavity has been evaluated in a single small study and found to produce a very modest reduction in virus titer and no effect on symptoms.[100]

Thus, despite considerable effort, there are currently no commercially available interventions with proven efficacy for prevention or treatment of rhinovirus infection. Rhinovirus infections are self-limited and usually benign and of short duration. As a result, treatments for these infections must be rapidly effective, inexpensive, and virtually without toxicity or side effects. No treatment to date has met these challenges. The recent observations of more severe consequences of infection in some patient populations may provide an increased urgency for development of effective treatments. A better understanding of the pathogenesis of rhinovirus infection, especially elucidation of the signaling pathways involved in the inflammatory response, may provide new targets for these efforts.

REFERENCES

1. Dochez AR, Shibley GS, Mills KC. Studies on the common cold: IV. Experimental transmission of the common cold to anthropoid apes and human beings by means of a filtrable agent. *J Exp Med.* 1930;52:701-716.
2. Pelon W, Mogabgab WJ, Phillips IA, et al. A cytopathogenic agent isolated from naval recruits with mild respiratory illnesses. *Proc Soc Exp Biol Med.* 1957;94:262-267.
3. Price WH. The isolation of a new virus associated with respiratory clinical disease in humans. *Proc Natl Acad Sci U S A.* 1956;42:892-896.
4. Tyrrell DA, Parsons R. Some virus isolations from common colds: III. Cytopathic effects in tissue cultures. *Lancet.* 1960;1:239-242.
5. Gwaltney Jr JM, Hendley JO, Simon G, et al. Rhinovirus infections in an industrial population: I. The occurrence of illness. *N Engl J Med.* 1966;275:1261-1268.
6. Gwaltney Jr JM, Hendley JO, Simon G, et al. Rhinovirus infections in an industrial population: II. Characteristics of illness and antibody response. *J Am Med Assoc.* 1967;202:494-500.
7. Kistler A, Avila PC, Rouskin S, et al. Pan-viral screening of respiratory tract infections in adults with and without asthma reveals unexpected human coronavirus and human rhinovirus diversity. *J Infect Dis.* 2007;196:817-825.
8. Lamson D, Renwick N, Kapoor V, et al. MassTag polymerase-chain-reaction detection of respiratory pathogens, including a new rhinovirus genotype, that caused influenza-like illness in New York State during 2004-2005. *J Infect Dis.* 2006;194:1398-1402.
9. Lee WM, Kiesner C, Pappas T, et al. A diverse group of previously unrecognized human rhinoviruses are common causes of respiratory illnesses in infants. *PLoS ONE.* 2007;2:e966.
10. McErlean P, Shackelton LA, Lambert SB, et al. Characterisation of a newly identified human rhinovirus, HRV-QPM, discovered in infants with bronchiolitis. *J Clin Virol.* 2007;39:67-75.
11. Renwick N, Schweiger B, Kapoor V, et al. A recently identified rhinovirus genotype is associated with severe respiratory-tract infection in children in Germany. *J Infect Dis.* 2007; 196:1754-1760.
12. Greve JM, Davis G, Meyer AM, et al. The major human rhinovirus receptor is ICAM-1. *Cell.* 1989;56:839-847.
13. Staunton DE, Merluzzi VJ, Rothlein R, et al. A cell adhesion molecule, ICAM-1, is the major surface receptor for rhinoviruses. *Cell.* 1989;56:849-853.
14. Andries K, Dewindt B, Snoeks J, et al. Two groups of rhinoviruses revealed by a panel of antiviral compounds present sequence divergence and differential pathogenicity. *J Virol.* 1990;64:1117-1123.

15. Tapparel C, Junier T, Gerlach D, et al. New complete genome sequences of human rhinoviruses shed light on their phylogeny and genomic features. *BMC Genomics.* 2007;8:224.
16. Kistler AL, Webster DR, Rouskin S, et al. Genome-wide diversity and selective pressure in the human rhinovirus. *Virol J.* 2007;4:40.
17. Savolainen C, Blomqvist S, Mulders MN, et al. Genetic clustering of all 102 human rhinovirus prototype strains: serotype 87 is close to human enterovirus 70. *J Gen Virol.* 2002; 83:333-340.
18. Gwaltney Jr JM, Colonno RJ, Hamparian VV, et al. Rhinoviruses. In: Schmidt NJ, Emmons RW, eds. *Diagnostic Procedures for Viral Rickettsial and Chlamydial Infections.* 6th ed. Washington, DC: American Public Health Association; 1989:579-614.
19. Hendley JO, Mika LA, Gwaltney Jr JM. Evaluation of virucidal compounds for inactivation of rhinovirus on hands. *Antimicrob Agents Chemother.* 1978;14:690-694.
20. Fox J, Cooney M, Hall C, et al. Rhinoviruses in Seattle families, 1975-1979. *Am J Epidemiol.* 1985;122:830-846.
21. Blomqvist S, Roivainen M, Puhakka T, et al. Virological and serological analysis of rhinovirus infections during the first two years of life in a cohort of children. *J Med Virol.* 2002;66:263-268.
22. Kusel MM, de Klerk NH, Holt PG, et al. Role of respiratory viruses in acute upper and lower respiratory tract illness in the first year of life: a birth cohort study. *Pediatr Infect Dis J.* 2006;25:680-686.
23. van Benten I, Koopman L, Niesters B, et al. Predominance of rhinovirus in the nose of symptomatic and asymptomatic infants. *Pediatr Allergy Immunol.* 2003;14:363-370.
24. Winther B, Hayden FG, Hendley JO. Picornavirus infections in children diagnosed by RT-PCR during longitudinal surveillance with weekly sampling: association with symptomatic illness and effect of season. *J Med Virol.* 2006;78:644-650.
25. Gwaltney Jr JM. The Jeremiah Metzger lecture. Climatology and the common cold. *Trans Am Clin Climatol Assoc.* 1984;96:159-175.
26. Johnston NW, Johnston SL, Norman GR, et al. The September epidemic of asthma hospitalization: school children as disease vectors. *J Allergy Clin Immunol.* 2006;117:557-562.
27. Dick EC, Jennings LC, Mink KA, et al. Aerosol transmission of rhinovirus colds. *J Infect Dis.* 1987;156:442-448.
28. Gwaltney Jr JM, Moskalski PB, Hendley JO. Hand-to-hand transmission of rhinovirus colds. *Ann Intern Med.* 1978; 88:463-467.
29. Hendley JO, Gwaltney Jr JM. Mechanisms of transmission of rhinovirus infections. *Epidemiol Rev.* 1988;10:243-258.

30. Reed SE. An investigation of the possible transmission of rhinovirus colds through indirect contact. *J Hygiene.* 1975; 75:249-258.
31. Jennings LC, Dick EC, Mink KA, et al. Near disappearance of rhinovirus along a fomite transmission chain. *J Infect Dis.* 1988;158:888-892.
32. D'Alessio DJ, Peterson JA, Dick CR, et al. Transmission of experimental rhinovirus colds in volunteer married couples. *J Infect Dis.* 1976;133:28-36.
33. Papadopoulos NG, Sanderson G, Hunter J, et al. Rhinoviruses replicate effectively at lower airway temperatures. *J Med Virol.* 1999;58:100-104.
34. Gwaltney Jr JM, Phillips CD, Miller RD, et al. Computed tomographic study of the common cold. *N Engl J Med.* 1994;330: 25-30.
35. Turner RB. Elaboration of interleukin 8 from fibroblast cells and human nasal epithelium in response to rhinovirus challenge [abstract B43]. In: *34th Interscience Conference on Antimicrobial Agents and Chemotherapy.* Orlando, FL: American Society for Microbiology; 1994.
36. Pitkaranta A, Arruda E, Malmberg H, et al. Detection of rhinovirus in sinus brushings of patients with acute community-acquired sinusitis by reverse transcription-PCR. *J Clin Microbiol.* 1997;35:1791-1793.
37. Winther B, Gwaltney Jr JM, Mygind N, et al. Sites of rhinovirus recovery after point inoculation of the upper airway. *JAMA.* 1986;256:1763-1767.
38. Arruda E, Boyle TR, Winther B, et al. Localization of human rhinovirus replication in the upper respiratory tract by in situ hybridization. *J Infect Dis.* 1995;171:1329-1333.
39. Turner RB, Hendley JO, Gwaltney Jr JM. Shedding of infected ciliated epithelial cells in rhinovirus colds. *J Infect Dis.* 1982;145:849-853.
40. Winther B, Brofeldt S, Christensen B, et al. Light and scanning electron microscopy of nasal biopsy material from patients with naturally acquired common colds. *Acta Otolaryngol (Stockh).* 1984;97:309-318.
41. Winther B, Gwaltney Jr JM, Hendley JO. Respiratory virus infection of monolayer cultures of human nasal epithelial cells. *Am Rev Respir Dis.* 1990;141:839-845.
42. Douglas Jr RG, Alford RH, Cate TR, et al. The leukocyte response during viral respiratory illness in man. *Ann Intern Med.* 1966;64:521-530.
43. Winther B, Farr B, Turner RB, et al. Histopathologic examination and enumeration of polymorphonuclear leukocytes in the nasal mucosa during experimental rhinovirus colds. *Acta Otolaryngol (Stockh).* 1984;413(Suppl):19-24.

44. Naclerio RM, Proud D, Lichtenstein LM, et al. Kinins are generated during experimental rhinovirus colds. J Infect Dis. 1988;157:133-142.

45. Winther B. Effects on the nasal mucosa of upper respiratory viruses (common cold). Danish Med Bull. 1994;41:193-204.

46. Levandowski RA, Weaver CW, Jackson GG. Nasal-secretion leukocyte populations determined by flow cytometry during acute rhinovirus infection. J Med Virol. 1988;25:423-432.

47. Newcomb DC, Sajjan US, Nagarkar DR, et al. Human rhinovirus 1B exposure induces phosphatidylinositol 3-kinase-dependent airway inflammation in mice. Am J Respir Crit Care Med. 2008;177:1111-1121.

48. Griego SD, Weston CB, Adams JL, et al. Role of p38 mitogen-activated protein kinase in rhinovirus-induced cytokine production by bronchial epithelial cells. J Immunol. 2000;165:5211-5220.

49. Newcomb DC, Sajjan U, Nanua S, et al. Phosphatidylinositol 3-kinase is required for rhinovirus-induced airway epithelial cell interleukin-8 expression. J Biol Chem. 2005;280:36952-36961.

50. Kaul P, Biagioli MC, Singh I, et al. Rhinovirus-induced oxidative stress and interleukin-8 elaboration involves p47-phox but is independent of attachment to intercellular adhesion molecule-1 and viral replication. J Infect Dis. 2000;181:1885-1890.

51. Sajjan US, Jia Y, Newcomb DC, et al. H. influenzae potentiates airway epithelial cell responses to rhinovirus by increasing ICAM-1 and TLR3 expression. FASEB J. 2006;20:2121-2123.

52. Grassme H, Riehle A, Wilker B, et al. Rhinoviruses infect human epithelial cells via ceramide-enriched membrane platforms. J Biol Chem. 2005;280:26256-26262.

53. Dumitru CA, Dreschers S, Gulbins E. Rhinoviral infections activate p38MAP-kinases via membrane rafts and RhoA. Cell Physiol Biochem. 2006;17:159-166.

54. Turner RB, Weingand KW, Yeh C-H, et al. Association between nasal secretion interleukin-8 concentration and symptom severity in experimental rhinovirus colds. Clin Infect Dis. 1998;26:840-846.

55. Zhu Z, Tang W, Gwaltney Jr JM, et al. Rhinovirus stimulation of interleukin-8 in vivo and in vitro: role of NF-kappaB. Am J Physiol. 1997;273:L814-L824.

56. Douglass JA, Dhami D, Gurr CE, et al. Influence of interleukin-8 challenge in the nasal mucosa in atopic and nonatopic subjects. Am J Respir Crit Care Med. 1994;150:1108-1113.

57. Proud D, Naclerio RM, Gwaltney Jr JM, et al. Kinins are generated in nasal secretions during natural rhinovirus colds. J Infect Dis. 1990;161:120-123.

58. Proud D, Reynolds CJ, LaCapra S, et al. Nasal provocation with bradykinin induces symptoms of rhinitis and a sore throat. Am Rev Respir Dis. 1988;137:613-616.

59. Higgins PG, Barrow GI, Tyrrell DA. A study of the efficacy of the bradykinin antagonist, NPC 567, in rhinovirus infections in human volunteers. Antiviral Res. 1990;14:339-344.

60. Gustafson LM, Proud D, Hendley JO, et al. Oral prednisone therapy in experimental rhinovirus infections. J Allergy Clin Immunol. 1996;97:1009-1014.

61. Igarashi Y, Skoner DP, Doyle WJ, et al. Analysis of nasal secretions during experimental rhinovirus upper respiratory infections. J Allergy Clin Immunol. 1993;92:722-731.

62. Muether PS, Gwaltney Jr JM. Variant effect of first- and second-generation antihistamines as clues to their mechanism of action on the sneeze reflex in the common cold. Clin Infect Dis. 2001;33:1483-1488.

63. Gaffey MJ, Gwaltney Jr JM, Dressler WE, et al. Intranasally administered atropine methonitrate treatment of experimental rhinovirus colds. Am Rev Respir Dis. 1987;135:241-244.

64. Hayden FG, Diamond L, Wood PB, et al. Effectiveness and safety of intranasal ipratropium bromide in common colds: a randomized, double-blind, placebo-controlled trial. Ann Intern Med. 1996;125:89-97.

65. Gwaltney Jr JM, Druce HM. Efficacy of brompheniramine maleate for the treatment of rhinovirus colds. Clin Infect Dis. 1997;25:1188-1194.

66. Johnston SL, Pattemore PK, Sanderson G, et al. Community study of role of viral infections in exacerbations of asthma in 9-11 year old children. BMJ. 1995;310:1225-1229.

67. Rakes GP, Arruda E, Ingram JM, et al. Rhinovirus and respiratory syncytial virus in wheezing children requiring emergency care: IgE and eosinophil analyses. Am J Respir Crit Care Med. 1999;159:785-790.

68. Duff AL, Pomeranz ES, Gelber LE, et al. Risk factors for acute wheezing in infants and children: viruses, passive smoke, and IgE antibodies to inhalant allergens. Pediatrics. 1993;92:535-540.

69. Zambrano JC, Carper HT, Rakes GP, et al. Experimental rhinovirus challenges in adults with mild asthma: response to infection in relation to IgE. J Allergy Clin Immunol. 2003; 111:1008-1016.

70. Cate TR, Rossen RD, Douglas Jr R, et al. The role of nasal secretion and serum antibody in the rhinovirus common cold. Am J Epidemiol. 1966;84:352-363.

71. Alper CM, Doyle WJ, Skoner DP, et al. Prechallenge antibodies moderate disease expression in adults experimentally exposed to rhinovirus strain hanks. Clin Infect Dis. 1998;27:119-128.

72. Alper CM, Doyle WJ, Skoner DP, et al. Prechallenge antibodies: moderators of infection rate, signs, and symptoms in adults experimentally challenged with rhinovirus type 39. Laryngoscope. 1996;106:1298-1305.

73. Gern JE, Vrtis R, Grindle KA, et al. Relationship of upper and lower airway cytokines to outcome of experimental rhinovirus infection. Am J Respir Crit Care Med. 2000;162:2226-2231.

74. Cohen S, Frank E, Doyle WJ, et al. Types of stressors that increase susceptibility to the common cold in healthy adults. Health Psychol. 1998;17:214-223.

75. Cohen S, Doyle WJ, Turner R, et al. Sociability and susceptibility to the common cold. Psychol Sci. 2003;14:389-395.

76. Cohen S, Doyle WJ, Turner RB, et al. Emotional style and susceptibility to the common cold. Psychosom Med. 2003;65:652-657.

77. Pitkaranta A, Starck M, Savolainen S, et al. Rhinovirus RNA in the maxillary sinus epithelium of adult patients with acute sinusitis. Clin Infect Dis. 2001;33:909-911.

78. Pitkaranta A, Virolainen A, Jero J, et al. Detection of rhinovirus, respiratory syncytial virus, and coronavirus infections in acute otitis media by reverse transcriptase polymerase chain reaction. Pediatrics. 1998;102:291-295.

79. Revai K, Dobbs LA, Nair S, et al. Incidence of acute otitis media and sinusitis complicating upper respiratory tract infection: the effect of age. Pediatrics. 2007;119:e1408-e1412.

80. Wald ER, Guerra N, Byers C. Upper respiratory tract infections in young children: duration of and frequency of complications. Pediatrics. 1991;87:129-133.

81. Papadopoulos NG, Moustaki M, Tsolia M, et al. Association of rhinovirus infection with increased disease severity in acute bronchiolitis. Am J Respir Crit Care Med. 2002;165:1285-1289.

82. Jacques J, Bouscambert-Duchamp M, Moret H, et al. Association of respiratory picornaviruses with acute bronchiolitis in French infants. J Clin Virol. 2006;35:463-466.

83. Juven T, Mertsola J, Waris M, et al. Etiology of community-acquired pneumonia in 254 hospitalized children. Pediatr Infect Dis J. 2000;19:293-298.

84. Kaiser L, Aubert JD, Pache JC, et al. Chronic rhinoviral infection in lung transplant recipients. Am J Respir Crit Care Med. 2006;174:1392-1399.

85. Butler CC, Kinnersley P, Hood K, et al. Clinical course of acute infection of the upper respiratory tract in children: cohort study. BMJ. 2003;327:1088-1089.

86. Xatzipsalti M, Kyrana S, Tsolia M, et al. Rhinovirus viremia in children with respiratory infections. Am J Respir Crit Care Med. 2005;172:1037-1040.

87. Ostroff R, Ettinger A, La H, et al. Rapid multiserotype detection of human rhinoviruses on optically coated silicon surfaces. J Clin Virol. 2001;21:105-117.

88. Lee WM, Grindle K, Pappas T, et al. High-throughput, sensitive, and accurate multiplex PCR-microsphere flow cytometry system for large-scale comprehensive detection of respiratory viruses. J Clin Microbiol. 2007;45:2626-2634.

89. Pitkaranta A, Puhakka T, Makela MJ, et al. Detection of rhinovirus RNA in middle turbinate of patients with common colds by in situ hybridization. J Med Virol. 2003;70:319-323.

90. Arruda E, Hayden FG. Clinical studies of antiviral agents for picornavirus infections. In: Jeffries DJ, De Clercq E, eds. Antiviral Chemotherapy. New York: Wiley; 1995.

91. Hayden FG, Gwaltney Jr JM, Colonno RJ. Modification of experimental rhinovirus colds by receptor blockade. Antiviral Res. 1988;9:233-247.

92. Turner RB, Wecker MT, Pohl G, et al. Efficacy of tremacamra, a soluble intercellular adhesion molecule 1, for experimental rhinovirus infection. J Am Med Assoc. 1999;281:1797-1804.

93. Smith TJ, Kremer MJ, Luo M, et al. The site of attachment in human rhinovirus 14 for antiviral agents that inhibit uncoating. Science. 1986;233:1286-1293.

94. Hayden FG, Herrington DT, Coats TL, et al. Efficacy and safety of oral pleconaril for treatment of colds due to picornaviruses in adults: results of 2 double-blind, randomized, placebo-controlled trials. Clin Infect Dis. 2003;36:1523-1532.

95. Hayden FG, Turner RB, Gwaltney JM, et al. Phase II, randomized, double-blind, placebo-controlled studies of ruprintrivir nasal spray 2-percent suspension for prevention and treatment of experimentally induced rhinovirus colds in healthy volunteers. Antimicrob Agents Chemother. 2003;47:3907-3916.

96. Sattar SA, Abebe M, Bueti AJ, et al. Activity of an alcohol-based hand gel against human adeno-, rhino-, and rotaviruses using the fingerpad method. Infect Control Hosp Epidemiol. 2000;21:516-519.

97. Sandora TJ, Taveras EM, Shih MC, et al. A randomized, controlled trial of a multifaceted intervention including alcohol-based hand sanitizer and hand-hygiene education to reduce illness transmission in the home. Pediatrics. 2005;116: 587-594.

98. Farr BM, Hendley JO, Kaiser DL, et al. Two randomized controlled trials of virucidal nasal tissues in the prevention of natural upper respiratory infections. Am J Epidemiol. 1988; 128:1162-1172.

99. Turner RB, Biedermann KA, Morgan JM, et al. Efficacy of organic acids in hand cleansers for prevention of rhinovirus infections. Antimicrob Agents Chemother. 2004;48:2595-2598.

100. Gern JE, Mosser AG, Swenson CA, et al. Inhibition of rhinovirus replication in vitro and in vivo by acid-buffered saline. J Infect Dis. 2007;195:1137-1143.

175

Noroviruses and Other Caliciviruses

RAPHAEL DOLIN | JOHN J. TREANOR

Acute gastrointestinal disease is an exceedingly common and widespread illness throughout the world. According to the National Health Interview Survey, the incidence of acute gastroenteritis in American families is 6% per year, with an estimated 21.2 days lost from work or school per 100 persons annually.[1] About 612,000 hospitalizations and 3000 deaths in adults are estimated to occur annually owing to acute gastroenteritis in the United States.[2] Worldwide, it has been estimated that acute diarrheal disease accounts for nearly 2 million deaths in children younger than 5 years.[3] Although the etiology of much of this disease remains unknown, evidence suggests that many cases result from viral infections.[4-6] Two new virus families, the Caliciviridae and the Astroviridae (see Chapter 176), have emerged as important causes of gastroenteritis in adults and children.[7]

History

The failure to isolate causative agents, bacterial or viral, from apparently infectious outbreaks of diarrhea or vomiting, or both, led to the widely held assumption that undetected viruses were responsible for such disease. In 1945, Reimann and co-workers[8] transmitted disease to volunteers by administering bacteria-free filtrates of throat washings, stool filtrates, or both from naturally occurring cases. Gordon[9] and Jordan[10] and their associates also induced disease in normal volunteers with bacteria-free material. These studies described two transmissible agents of sub-bacterial size, the Marcy and FS agents, that appeared to be antigenically distinct. However, these workers were unable to detect viral agents in vitro with techniques available at that time. Despite extensive virologic investigations in laboratories throughout the world, relatively little progress was made in this area until 1972 when the Norwalk virus, the prototype of this group, was described and partially characterized.[11,12] This virus was initially detected in diarrheal stools obtained from an outbreak of gastroenteritis in Norwalk, Ohio, that involved students in an elementary school and family contacts. Subsequently, additional viruses with similar properties were described, including the Hawaii,[13] Montgomery County (MC),[14] Taunton,[15] and Snow Mountain[16] viruses, also named by the geographical region in which they were first recognized. All these viruses had a similar small round structured morphology on electron microscopy, were of a similar size and density, did not grow in any in vitro propagation system, and were responsible for acute gastroenteritis, commonly in epidemic form with high secondary attack rates.[4] At the same time, viruses with more readily identifiable morphology on electron microscopy, referred to as *human caliciviruses*,[17] were observed in the stools of individuals, primarily children, with gastroenteritis.

A major advance in this field occurred when polymerase chain reaction (PCR) techniques were applied to amplify the genome of the Norwalk virus from virion-containing stool samples.[18,19] These studies identified the Norwalk virus as a member of the Caliciviridae family and allowed determination of the complete nucleotide sequence of this virus.[20] Subsequent molecular studies have clearly identified all these viruses as caliciviruses and established them as major causes of gastrointestinal disease in both adults and children worldwide.

Virology

The name *calicivirus* is derived from the characteristic appearance of the viral particles under the electron microscope, which consists of a scalloped border with cuplike indentations on its surface (Fig. 175-1), from which the Latin name *chalice* or *calyx* is derived.[21,22] Caliciviruses have been detected in a variety of animal species, including marine mammals, swine, felines, and rabbits, as well as humans. Although many animal caliciviruses replicate efficiently in cell culture, no practical in vitro method has been described for the propagation of noroviruses or sapoviruses responsible for gastroenteritis. Recently, transfection of viral RNA from noroviruses in human embryonic kidney cells [23,24] and infection of human intestinal organoid culture[25] with noroviruses have been reported and may provide additional information regarding the molecular events of norovirus replication. However, much of the current information on noroviruses is based on physical properties determined by electron microscopic visualization or physicochemical manipulation, or both, of infectious inocula. Because of the small numbers of virions characteristically found in stool samples, it is sometimes necessary to enhance electron microscopic visualization of the particles through the addition of immune serum, which obscures the typical morphologic features (Fig. 175-2).

Characteristics of the noroviruses include a single-stranded positive-sense RNA genome with a polyadenlylated 3′ tail[20,26] and a single capsid polypeptide of 59- to 62-kDa molecular mass.[27] The virions are 26 to 34 nm in diameter, have cubic symmetry with a buoyant density in cesium chloride (CsCl) of 1.34 to 1.41 g/mL, and are relatively heat and acid stable and ether resistant.[12]

The genomic organization of the Norwalk virus is shown in Figure 175-3.[28] Three long open reading frames (ORFs) are present. The first ORF encodes a protein of about 57-kDa molecular weight, and has the viral RNA polymerase and helicase and protease functions.[7,20] The second ORF encodes the viral capsid protein (VP1) of 58-kDa molecular weight, which determines the antigenic phenotype and interacts with host cell receptors.[29] When expressed in insect cells by a recombinant baculovirus, the capsid protein spontaneously assembles into virus-like particles (VLPs), which are immunogenic and react specifically with convalescent human sera.[29] The three-dimensional structure of these empty capsids has been studied by electron cryomicroscopy, which suggests that the capsid has icosahedral symmetry with T = 3.[30] The x-ray crystallographic structure of these VLPs shows that the capsid contains two domains, a shell (S) domain and a protruding (P) domain that may be involved in binding to susceptible cells.[28,31] Finally, the third ORF encodes a minor structural protein (VP2) of 12 to 29 kDa molecular weight,[20,32] which may add to particle stability.

Genetic analysis of a large number of human and animal caliciviruses has led to the designation of four genera within the Caliciviridae: *Vesivirus*, which cause vesicular diseases in swine, cats, and marine mammals; *Lagovirus*, which cause hemorrhagic diseases in rabbits; and two genera responsible for gastroenteritis in humans, *Norovirus* and *Sapovirus*.[33,34] The prototypic *Norovirus* is the Norwalk virus, and the prototypic *Sapovirus* is the Sapporo virus. A fifth genus, *Nebovirus*, has been proposed for consideration.[33] In addition to sequence differences, the genera differ in minor details of genome organization.

The noroviruses have been further subdivided based on phylogenetic analysis into at least five genogroups designated GI-GV,[35] and gene clusters are recognized within the genogroups.[34,36] Most of the strains implicated in human disease fall into genogroups GI and GII.[34] The GI genogroup includes the Norwalk virus, whereas the Snow Mountain and Hawaii viruses belong to genogroup GII. Individual strains are designated by arabic numeral after the genogroup designation: for example, GI.1 (Norwalk) or GII.1 (Hawaii).

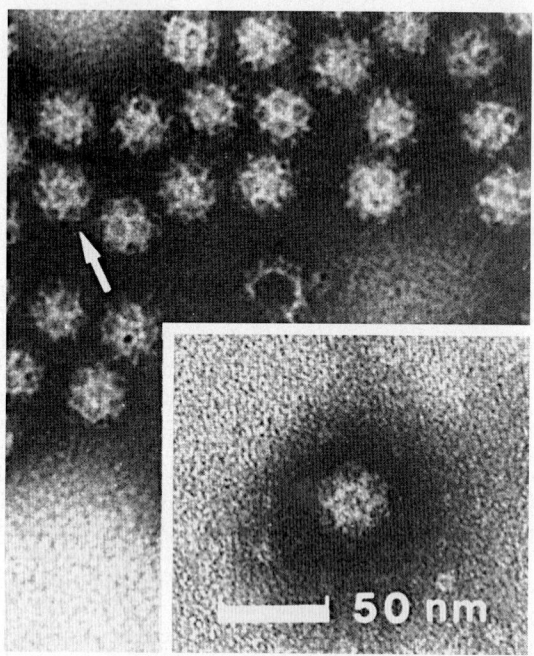

Figure 175-1 **Calicivirus particles** *(arrow)* **in a fecal extract from a child with gastroenteritis.** *Inset is higher magnification of particle indicated by arrow. (From Chiba S, Sakuma Y, Kogasaka R, et al. An outbreak of gastroenteritis associated with calicivirus in an infant home. J Med Virol. 1979;4:249-254. Reprinted by permission of Wiley-Liss, Inc., a subsidiary of John Wiley & Sons, Inc. Copyright © 1979 Wiley-Liss, Inc.)*

Because of the lack of a convenient in vitro propagation system, antigenic characterization of these viruses is less straightforward. Not unexpectedly, predicted amino acid homology within the capsid region is less than that within the polymerase region.[35] Thus, phylogenetic trees based on capsid sequence have a slightly different structure than those based on polymerase structure.[37] Virus-like particles have been generated by expression of the capsid regions of many of the noroviruses, including Norwalk[29] and Desert Sheild[38] viruses (genogroup GI) and MX,[39] Lordsdale,[40] Snow Mountain,[37] Hawaii,[41] and Toronto[42] viruses (genogroup GII), as well as the prototype sapovirus Sapporo.[43] In general, hyperimmune animal sera raised against capsids are very specific. However, tests of postinfection human sera have suggested a significant degree of cross-reactivity among viruses within a genogroup.

The most clear-cut antigenic distinction between these viruses is between the Norwalk and Hawaii viruses because these agents have been compared through cross-challenge experiments in human subjects.[44] In these studies, infection with the Norwalk virus provided

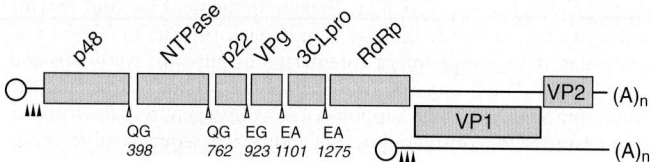

Figure 175-3 Norovirus genome organization (Norwalk strain). Nonstructural proteins in ORF1 are labeled, and protease cleavage sites are indicated by *open arrowheads*. Amino acids numbers below the cleavage sites are the P1 residues of the recognition dipeptides. *Filled arrowheads* mark translation initiation codons. The VPg-linked subgenomic RNA encoding VP1 and VP2 is indicated below the ORFs. VPg is depicted as a *circle* linked to both genomic and subgenomic RNA. *(From Hardy ME. Norovirus protein structure and function. FEMS Microbiol Lett. 2005;253:1-8.)*

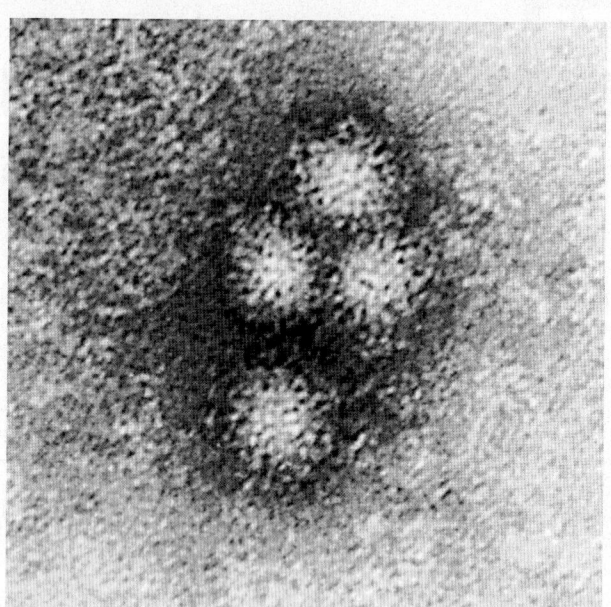

Figure 175-2 **Snow Mountain agent in stool filtrate from a volunteer with experimentally induced disease as visualized by immune electron microscopy.** Particles are 27 nm in diameter and are stained with 2% phosphotungstic acid.

short-term protection against rechallenge with the Norwalk virus but not against the Hawaii virus, and vice versa. Because this type of experiment is the closest analogue to virus neutralization that is available, this is the best evidence that there are at least two distinct norovirus serotypes, roughly corresponding to the GI and GII genogroups described earlier.

The role of antigenic variation in the epidemiology of these viruses remains an area of continued investigation. Generally, antibody to viruses within genogroup II appear to be more common than that to viruses within genogroup I.[45] Typically, a large number of diverse genotypes cocirculate,[46-48] with significant variation from year to year in the predominant genotypes of viruses associated with illness.[49,50] However, occasionally a single predominant strain arises that is responsible for most cases over a widespread distribution.[51] The causes of this phenomenon are unknown.

Epidemiology

With the advent of efficient means for their detection (see later), noroviruses have emerged as major, worldwide causes of gastroenteritis in diverse populations and in both children and adults. Noroviruses are the most common cause of epidemic gastroenteritis and account for more than 90% of outbreaks of viral gastroenteritis and for about 50% of all-cause outbreaks worldwide.[6,34,52-56] Although less well documented, noroviruses are also important causes of sporadic cases of gastroenteritis, and account for 4.4% to 30.7% of children younger than 5 years hospitalized with gastroenteritis throughout the world.[34,57] The Centers for Disease Control and Prevention estimate that noroviruses cause 40% to 50% of foodborne outbreaks of gastroenteritis in the United States and overall account for 23 million cases of gastroenteritis annually in the United States.[58]

In developed countries, serum antibody to the noroviruses is first noted at ages 3 to 4 years, with antibody prevalence gradually rising to greater than 50% by the fifth decade of life.[59-62] Studies using recombinant Norwalk antigen have suggested that significant increases in antibody prevalence occur in infancy, on entry into primary schools, and in young adulthood.[63] Seroepidemiologic studies of the sapoviruses carried out in Japan, Southeast Asia, and the United Kingdom indicate that antibody is acquired in early childhood and can be detected in up to 90% of older children and adults.[64-66] Antibody appears to be acquired more rapidly in developing countries[59] and may be rare or nonexistent in some isolated populations.[59,67] Transmission of noroviruses occurs year-round, but with a higher incidence of disease in the winter months in temperate climates.[68]

The experimental induction of illness in normal volunteers suggests that the major route of person-to-person transmission is fecal-oral. Epidemiologic reports have also implicated vomitus as a vehicle of transmission,[69,70] and virus has been detected in vomitus on electron microscopy[71] and PCR.[72] Airborne transmission has also occasionally been implicated,[73,74] but limited attempts to experimentally transmit virus with nasopharyngeal washings from an ill volunteer were unsuccessful.[12] It has been estimated that fewer than 100 viral particles are required for infection of a susceptible individual.[75]

Incubation periods are generally 24 to 48 hours, although ranges from 18 to 72 hours have been observed. Virus shedding in stools is maximal over the first 24 to 48 hours after illness.[14,16] In volunteer studies, virus has been rarely detected beyond 72 hours after the onset of vomiting or diarrhea[14,16] by immunoelectron microscopy. However, virus can be detected for up to 3 weeks after illness using sensitive enzyme-linked immunosorbent assay techniques[76] or PCR.[77,78] The clinical significance of the prolonged detection of virus in stools is unclear, but epidemiologic data have implicated individuals who are not symptomatic in the transmission of illness.[79]

Noroviruses were first recognized in association with point-source outbreaks of gastroenteritis, and such outbreaks remain the most common situation in which noroviruses have been implicated as etiologic agents. There are several features that are characteristic of such outbreaks that may be useful in empirical diagnosis. These include a short-lived illness of 2 to 3 days' duration with vomiting as a prominent symptom in most affected individuals, an incubation period of 24 to 48 hours, high secondary attack rates, and lack of identifiable pathogens on routine examinations of stool samples.[80] The application of modern diagnostic techniques has shown that the frequency of norovirus infection in such outbreaks is extremely high.[46]

Outbreaks of norovirus gastroenteritis are particularly common in closed settings such as in hospitals, nursing homes, ships, schools, and the military.[81-84] Secondary transmission is a prominent feature of such outbreaks. Although most of these outbreaks will terminate spontaneously after 1 to 2 weeks, some may be quite prolonged. For example, up to 12 recurrent outbreaks of norovirus gastroenteritis have been reported on cruise ships despite stringent attempts to determine the source and disinfect the ship between cruises.[85]

Almost any type of food that has contact with contaminated water or is contaminated by food handlers may serve as a vehicle for outbreaks of norovirus gastroenteritis. The most common foods implicated in norovirus outbreaks are sandwiches and salads, particularly those that require handling, but not subsequent cooking. Contamination of lettuce and salad greens with noroviruses accounts for nearly 25% of all produce-associated outbreaks.[34,86] Outbreaks have also been associated with drinking contaminated water, or even swimming in pools or lakes in which ill individuals have also been swimming,[87,88] indicative of the highly infectious nature of these viruses. Of note, these viruses appear to be relatively resistant to inactivation by chlorine.[70] Because such products as shellfish or contaminated commercial ice[89] can be distributed to multiple sites, these outbreaks can encompass a wide geographic area.[90] Contamination of foodstuffs has been traced to both presymptomatic[91] and postsymptomatic[79] food handlers, complicating infection control recommendations.

Shellfish, such as clams and oysters, are filter feeders and efficiently concentrate microorganisms from contaminated water. When consumed, these foods are frequently implicated in the transmission of enteric viruses in general and of norovirus gastroenteritis in particular.[92] Because noroviruses are relatively resistant to heat inactivation, steaming of shellfish does not entirely eliminate the risk for transmission.[93,94]

Recommendations for evaluation and control of nosocomial outbreaks[75] include identification and elimination of common sources

and the use of handwashing and barrier methods to prevent secondary transmission. Exclusion of ill employees may be important in limiting the spread of nosocomial outbreaks.[95] These methods have generally been found to be more effective in limiting the spread of outbreaks from unit to unit within an institution than in terminating an outbreak in an individual unit once it has begun.[96,97] The Viral Gastroenteritis Section of the Centers for Disease Control and Prevention is available for advice regarding such outbreaks (see http://www.cdc.gov/ncidod/dvrd/revb/gastro/faq.htm).

Although noroviruses were initially recognized primarily in association with outbreaks of acute gastroenteritis mostly involving adults, there has been an increasing recognition of the role of these viruses as causes of sporadic gastroenteritis in children in various parts of the world.[17,21,98-102] Toronto virus has been reported to be the second most common virus detected in the stools of young children with gastroenteritis.[103] The frequency of norovirus gastroenteritis has been estimated at between 10% and 100% of that of rotavirus in children where direct comparisons have been made.[104-106] In one study, 49% of prospectively followed Finnish infants and children seroresponded to norovirus over a 2-year period.[107] Sapoviruses and noroviruses have also been detected in community-wide, daycare,[108] and nosocomial outbreaks of gastroenteritis in children.[109]

Norovirus outbreaks occur throughout the year but tend to peak during cold weather months in temperate climates.[110,111] Frequency, seasonality, and geographic location of outbreaks may vary substantially from year to year, and the factors related to this variation are unclear. The markedly increased number of outbreaks reported in 1995, 2002, 2004, and 2006 were associated with the emergence of novel GII.4 strains.[6,111]

Pathogenesis

Although norovirus infection of nonhuman primates and gnotobiotic piglets has been accomplished,[6] convenient animal models for gastroenteritis induced by the Norwalk viruses are not available, and therefore information about the pathogenesis of this illness is based largely on studies of experimentally induced disease in normal volunteers. Acute infection with Norwalk and Hawaii viruses results in a reversible histopathologic lesion in the jejunum,[13,112-114] with apparent sparing of the stomach[115] and rectum (Fig. 175-4). The villi are blunted, but the mucosa is otherwise intact. Round cells and polymorphonuclear leukocytic infiltration are seen in the lamina propria. On electron microscopy, the epithelial cells are similarly intact, microvilli are shortened, and widened intercellular spaces are noted. These histopathologic changes appear within 24 hours after virus challenge, are present at the

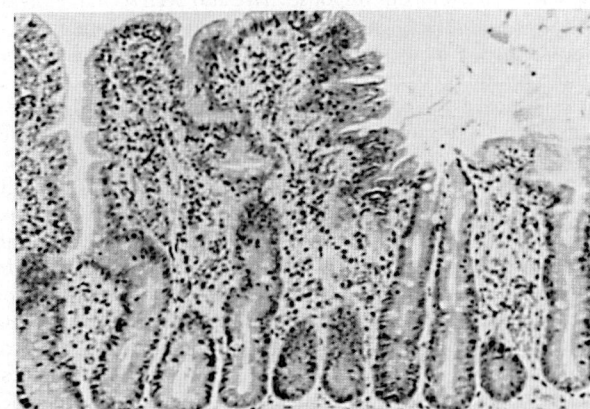

Figure 175-4 Hawaii virus–induced disease. Light micrograph of a jejunal mucosal biopsy specimen from a volunteer with Hawaii virus–induced disease 48 hours after challenge. Blunted villi and inflammatory cell infiltrate in the lamina propria are present (hematoxylin-eosin stain; original magnification, ×140).

height of illness, and persist for a variable period of time after the illness. The histopathologic changes have generally cleared within 2 weeks after the onset of illness, although some jejunal changes have been noted as late as 6 weeks after challenge. Histopathologic changes have been described in both clinical and subclinical cases of infection[113,114] and appear to be indistinguishable between Norwalk virus– and Hawaii virus–induced disease.

Diarrhea induced by the Norwalk virus is associated with a transient malabsorption of D-xylose and fat[116] and with decreased activity of brush-border enzymes, including alkaline phosphatase and trehalase.[112] Absorption and brush-border enzyme levels return to normal values within 2 weeks after challenge. During acute illness, a variable amount of intestinal fluid is produced, but infection with Norwalk and Hawaii agents has not been associated with detectable enterotoxin production. Adenylate cyclase levels in jejunal biopsy specimens appear to be normal during infection.[117] Thus, the precise mechanisms of virus-induced diarrhea, vomiting, or both remain unknown at the present. Calicivirus infections of animals have been associated with atrophy of the small intestinal mucosa along with a mild inflammatory infiltrate in the lamina propria.[118,119]

Susceptibility to infection with certain norovirus strains has been associated with the presence of H blood group carbohydrate antigens, which are also expressed on gastrointestinal epithelial cells.[120-124] These observations, along with in vitro studies demonstrating binding of noroviruses to these carbohydrate antigens, within a pocket of the P2 domain of the viral capsid,[125] have suggested that these carbohydrates may represent or be related to cellular receptors for noroviruses. These findings may explain, at least in part, the observations of a poorly defined long-term resistance to norovirus infection seen in previous challenge studies, in which some individuals consistently remained well despite repeated challenge with virus.[126]

Immune Response

Infection with the Norwalk virus results in the induction of virus-specific serum immunoglobulin G (IgG), IgA, and IgM antibody,[127-130] even in the presence of previous exposure. IgA and IgM responses appear to be relatively short-lived, whereas elevations in Norwalk-specific serum IgG persist for months.[129,130] In addition to recognizing the infecting strain of norovirus, serum antibody responses to infection may recognize other variants within the same genogroup, although generally to lower titer.[131] Such heterologous antibody responses are more common within a genogroup than between genogroups.[128,132] Serum IgM and IgA antibody may be more specific for the infecting strain of virus.[128,133] Using baculovirus-expressed capsid proteins, it has been demonstrated that responses to viruses within genogroup GI may be more specific than responses to infection with viruses within genogroup GII.[134] Heterologous responses have also been seen in individuals infected with the sapoviruses.[65] These broad responses are in contrast to the extremely specific antibody response of animals hyperimmunized with capsid antigen[135] and may in part reflect the extensive prior exposure of most adults to related viruses. The significance of such heterologous responses with respect to protection against reinfection is not clear.

Mucosal immune responses have not been studied extensively, but jejunal IgA synthesis has been shown to be elevated in biopsy specimens obtained 2 weeks after challenge with the Norwalk agent,[136] and fecal IgA responses after Norwalk infection have also been reported.[137] Limited studies of cell-mediated immune responses in these infections indicate that acute illness is associated with a transient lymphopenia that involves thymus-derived, bone marrow–derived, and null cell subpopulations.[138] Antigen-specific cellular responses to the capsid have been demonstrated in peripheral blood after experimental infection and are predominantly of the Th1 type.[139] Such responses are also cross-reactive within a genogroup.

Parameters defining protective immunity to the Norwalk viruses are poorly understood. After infection with Norwalk virus, most individuals manifest resistance to reinfection that persists for at least 4 to 6

months.[126,140] Multiple exposure appears to increase this resistance.[140] This short-term resistance does not appear to extend to other, antigenically distinct viruses.[44] Infection-induced resistance eventually wanes, and after 2 to 3 years, such individuals are susceptible to reinfection with the same virus.[126] As noted earlier, the absence of secretion of HBO blood-group antigens is associated with resistance to infection with the Norwalk strain, and these antigens may represent or be related to cellular receptors for noroviruses.[6]

Studies of the role of serum antibody in mediating this protection have yielded conflicting results. In most studies in adults, infection and illness induced by Norwalk-like agents occur in the presence of a wide range of preexisting serum antibody levels, which thus correlate poorly with protection.[128,140] However, after repeated experimental exposure of adults[140] and in epidemiologic studies of norovirus and sapovirus in children,[141-143] there has been a better correlation between the presence of serum antibody and protection from illness. Protection may also be related to other host defense factors such as a local mucosal antibody. However, direct measurements of intestinal antibody have failed to show a correlation with protection from Norwalk-induced illness,[144] and the presence of prechallenge Norwalk-specific fecal IgA was also not protective against challenge.[77] Studies of related animal viruses have also suggested a role for innate immunity in resistance to norovirus infection.[145]

Clinical Manifestations

Clinical characteristics of illness induced by the noroviruses appear to be similar in both naturally occurring and experimentally induced disease (Fig. 175-5), and there are no apparent differences in clinical findings between genogroups. However, clinically evident sapovirus infections appear to be largely restricted to children younger than 5 years[78] and may be somewhat milder than those seen with norovirus infection.[106] The onset of symptoms can be either gradual or abrupt, and most persons complain first of abdominal cramps or nausea. Generally both vomiting and diarrhea occur, although either can be

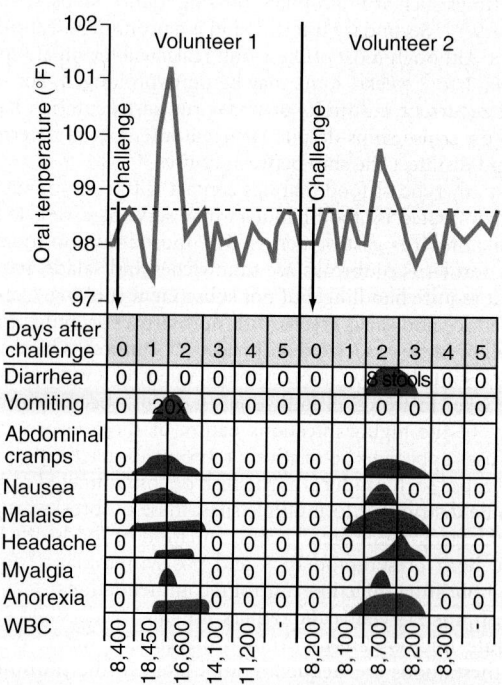

Figure 175-5 **Clinical response of two normal volunteers after the oral administration of the Norwalk agent.** The height of the *shaded curve* is proportional to the severity of the sign or symptom. (From Blacklow NR, Dolin R, Fedson DS, et al. Acute infectious non-bacterial gastroenteritis: Etiology and pathogenesis. Ann Int Med. 1972;76: 993-1008.)

present alone. Myalgias, malaise, and occasional headaches are also seen. Low-grade fever (with temperatures of 101° to 102° F) occurs in about half of cases. Diarrheal stool is generally moderate in amounts, with four to eight nonbloody stools being produced over a period of 24 hours. Disease manifestations generally last 48 to 72 hours and usually remit without sequelae.

More severe disease has been reported in elderly patients, including deaths, which have been observed in nursing home outbreaks.[146,147] Prolonged symptomatic infection and virus shedding of noroviruses have been reported in pediatric oncology patients[148] and in transplant recipients.[7,149]

Diagnosis

A clinical diagnosis of norovirus-related illness can be suspected on the basis of epidemiologic information and on the absence of other documented pathogens. However, the signs and symptoms of illness are not sufficiently characteristic to enable a diagnosis to be made on clinical grounds alone. Routine laboratory tests are also generally not helpful in making a specific diagnosis of norovirus infection. Peripheral white blood cell counts are normal or slightly elevated, with a relative polymorphonuclear leukocytosis and lymphopenia but with otherwise unremarkable white cell morphology. The results of liver function tests, blood urea nitrogen and creatinine determinations, and urinalysis are generally within normal limits. The absence of fecal leukocytes, as determined by microscopic examination of stools stained with methylene blue,[150] is a useful tool with which to exclude infection with enteroinvasive pathogens such as *Shigella* sp.

Specific diagnosis requires laboratory confirmation. Because these agents currently cannot be cultivated in vitro, a variety of methods have been developed to detect virus directly in stool samples.[151] Immune electron microscopy, in which immune sera is used to aggregate and highlight virions in stool suspensions (see Fig. 175-2), was the method used originally to identify these viruses.[16,152] The technique has the advantage of being readily adaptable to the detection of new virus types and can be used both for the detection of virus and for antibody determination but cannot be used conveniently for routine diagnosis.

Enzyme immunoassays (EIA) to detect norovirus antigens in stool have been developed and are commercially available.[34,153,154] These assays are sensitive for detection of homologous virus but lack sensitivity for detection of antigenic variants.[135] The sensitivity of EIAs may also vary according to genogroup.

Highly sensitive and specific reverse transcriptase–polymerase chain reaction (RT-PCR) techniques have been developed for detection of noroviruses and sapoviruses.[155-160] The success of this strategy depends on the ability to remove inhibitors of reverse transcription from the samples, and the choice of primers in relatively conserved regions of the genome to widen the scope of viruses detected.[161,162] Conversely, carefully selected primers within relatively more divergent regions can

be used to genotypically differentiate virus strains.[163] RT-PCR may be particularly useful for detecting contamination of food and environmental samples.[72,164-168]

Immunoassay techniques have also been adapted for the detection of antibody to noroviruses and are useful for the serologic diagnosis of infection. Because virus excretion in stools is limited and collection of stool samples in outbreaks can be problematic, serologic techniques are often used for diagnostic purposes.[169] Serum antibody titer rises can be detected within 10 to 14 days after the onset of illness.[170,171]

Treatment and Prevention

Specific antiviral therapy is not available, and therefore treatment consists entirely of supportive measures. Oral fluid replacement with isotonic liquids is generally adequate to replace fluid losses. Rarely, parenteral intravenous therapy may be required if severe vomiting and diarrhea develop. Symptomatic treatment of headache, myalgias, and nausea with analgesics and antiemetics may provide relief. In one study, the administration of bismuth subsalicylate reduced gastrointestinal symptoms in Norwalk virus–induced disease in normal volunteers, but had no effect on the number or character of stools or on virus shedding.[172] Although antiperistaltic agents are frequently prescribed to control diarrhea, their effect on the disease course and on excretion of virus has not been rigorously evaluated. Development of antivirals against noroviruses has been hampered by the inability to cultivate them in vitro. Recently, the cultivation of a murine norovirus (MVM) in tissue culture has enabled studies of potential antiviral compounds to be undertaken.[173]

There are multiple obstacles to successful development of a vaccine to prevent norovirus gastroenteritis.[174] As described earlier, infection does not appear to induce long-term protective immunity, although short-term protection has been demonstrated. The likely presence of multiple antigenic types is also a challenge, and progress has been further hampered by lack of in vitro propagation systems and a suitable animal model. However, some progress has been made using virus-like particles. Norwalk VLPs have been shown to be immunogenic when administered orally to human volunteers, inducing serum IgG, mucosal IgA, and cellular responses that resemble those seen after infection, although of substantially lower magnitude.[175,176] In addition, Norwalk virus has proved to be an excellent model to evaluate expression of vaccine antigens in plants as a method for oral immunization.[177]

The primary control measures for norovirus outbreaks are prevention of contamination of water and food supplies by proper hygiene procedures, including restriction of the activity of symptomatic food handlers. Because of the resistance of noroviruses to freezing, heating, and standard cleaning solutions, decontamination procedures should use EPA-recommended disinfectants, such as chlorine bleach with a concentration of 1000 to 5000 ppm (1:50 to 1:10 dilution of household bleach).[178]

REFERENCES

1. Adams PF, Hendershot GE, Marano MA. Current estimates from the National Health Interview Survey, 1996. National Center for Health Statistics, Vital Health Stat 10. 1999.
2. Mounts AW, Holman RC, Clarke MJ, et al. Trends in hospitalizations associated with gastroenteritis among adults in the United States, 1979-1995. *Epidemiol Infect*. 1999;123:1-8.
3. Bryce J, Boschi-Pinto C, Shibuya K, et al. WHO estimates of the causes of death in children. *Lancet* 2005;365:1147-1152.
4. Dolin R, Treanor J, Madore HP. Novel agents of viral enteritis in humans. *J Infect Dis*. 1987;155:365-375.
5. Blacklow NR, Greenberg HB. Viral gastroenteritis. *N Engl J Med*. 1991;325:252-264.
6. Dolin R. Noroviruses—challenges to control. *N Engl J Med*. 2007;357:1072-1073.
7. Green K. *Caliciviridae*: The noroviruses. In: Knipe DM, Howley PM, eds. *Fields Virology*. 5th ed. Philadelphia: Lippincott-Raven; 2007:949-979.
8. Reimann HA, Price AH, Hodges JH. The cause of epidemic diarrhea, nausea, and vomiting (viral dysentery?). *Proc Soc Exp Biol Med*. 1945;59:8-9.

9. Gordon I, Ingraham HS, Korns RF. Transmission of epidemic gastroenteritis to human volunteers by oral administration of fecal filtrate. *J Exp Med*. 1947;86:409-422.
10. Jordan WS, Gordon I, Dorrance WR. A study of illness in a group of Cleveland families. VII. Transmission of acute nonbacterial gastroenteritis to volunteers: Evidence for two different etiologic agents. *J Exp Med*. 1953;98:461-475.
11. Kapikian AZ, Gerin JL, Wyatt RG, et al. Density in cesium chloride of the Norwalk agent: Determination by ultracentrifugation and immune electron microscopy. *Proc Soc Exp Biol Med*. 1973;142:874-877.
12. Dolin R, Blacklow NR, DuPont H, et al. Biological properties of Norwalk agent of acute infectious nonbacterial gastroenteritis. *Proc Soc Exp Biol Med*. 1972;140:578-583.
13. Dolin R, Levy AG, Wyatt RG, et al. Viral gastroenteritis induced by the Hawaii agent: Jejunal histopathology and serologic response. *Am J Med*. 1975;59:768-771.
14. Thornhill TS, Wyatt RG, Kalica AR, et al. Detection by immune electron microscopy of 26-27 nm virus-like particles associated with two family outbreaks of gastroenteritis. *J Infect Dis*. 1977;138:20-27.

15. Caul EO, Ashley C, Pether JVS. Norwalk-like particle in epidemic gastroenteritis in the U.K. *Lancet*. 1979;2:1292.
16. Dolin R, Reichman RC, Roessner KD, et al. Detection by immune electron microscopy of the Snow Mountain agent of acute viral gastroenteritis. *J Infect Dis*. 1982;146:184-189.
17. Flewett TH, Davies H. Caliciviruses [Letter]. *Lancet*. 1976;1:311.
18. Jiang X, Graham DY, Wang K, et al. Norwalk virus genome cloning and characterization. *Science*. 1990;250:1580-1583.
19. Matsui S, Kim JP, Greenberg HB, et al. The isolation and characterization of a Norwalk virus-specific cDNA. *J Clin Invest*. 1991;87:1456-1461.
20. Jiang X, Wang M, Wang K, et al. Sequence and genomic organization of Norwalk virus. *Virology*. 1993;195:51-61.
21. Chiba S, Sakuma Y, Kogasaka R, et al. An outbreak of gastroenteritis associated with calicivirus in an infant home. *J Med Virol*. 1979;4:249-254.
22. Chiba S, Sakuma Y, Kagasaka R, et al. Fecal shedding of virus in relation to the days of illness in infantile gastroenteritis due to calicivirus. *J Infect Dis*. 1980;142:247-249.

23. Asanaka M, Atmar RL, Ruvolo V, et al. Replication and packaging of Norwalk virus RNA in cultured mammalian cells. *Proc Natl Acad Sci.* 2005;102:10327-10332.
24. Katayama K, Hansman GS, Oka T, et al. Investigation of norovirus replication in a human cell line. *Arch Virol.* 2006;151:1291-1308.
25. Straub TM, Höner Zu, Bentrup K, Orosz-Coghlan P, et al. In vitro cell culture infectivity assay for human noroviruses. *Emerg Infect Dis.* 2007;13:396-403.
26. Hardy ME, Estes MK. Completion of the Norwalk virus genome sequence. *Virus Genes.* 1996;12:287-290.
27. Greenberg HB, Valdesuso J, Kalica AR. Proteins of Norwalk virus. *J Virol.* 1981;37:994-999.
28. Hardy ME. Norovirus protein structure and function. *FEMS Microbiol Lett.* 2005;253:1-8.
29. Jiang X, Wang M, Graham DY, et al. Expression, self-assembly, and antigenicity of the Norwalk virus capsid protein. *J Virol.* 1992;66:6527-6532.
30. Prasad BV, Rothnagel R, Jiang X, et al. Three-dimensional structure of baculovirus-expressed Norwalk virus capsids. *J Virol.* 1994;68:5117-5125.
31. Prasad BV, Hardy ME, Dokland T, et al. X-ray crystallographic structure of the Norwalk virus capsid. *Science.* 1999;286:287-290.
32. Glass PJ, White LJ, Ball JM, et al. Norwalk virus open reading frame 3 encodes a minor structural protein. *J Virol.* 2000;74:6581-6591.
33. Green KY, Ando T, Balayan MS, et al. Taxonomy of the caliciviruses. *J Infect Dis.* 2000;181(Suppl 2):S322-S330.
34. Patel MM, Hall AJ, Vinjé J, et al. Noroviruses: A comprehensive review. *J Clin Virol.* 2009;44:1-8.
35. Lew JF, Kapikian AZ, Valdesuso J, et al. Molecular characterization of the Hawaii virus and other Norwalk-like viruses: Evidence for genetic polymorphism among human caliciviruses. *J Infect Dis.* 1994;170:535-542.
36. Ando T, Noel JS, Fankhauser RL. Genetic classification of "Norwalk-like viruses. *J Infect Dis.* 2000;181(Suppl 2):S336-S348.
37. Hardy ME, Kramer SF, Treanor JJ, et al. Human calicivirus genogroup II capsid sequence diversity revealed by analysis of the prototype Snow Mountain agent. *Arch Virol.* 1997;142:1469-1479.
38. Lew JF, Kapikian AZ, Jiang X, et al. Molecular characterization and expression of the capsid protein of a Norwalk-like virus recovered from a Desert Shield troop with gastroenteritis. *Virology.* 1994;200:319-325.
39. Jiang X, Matson DO, Ruiz-Palacios GM, et al. Expression, self-assembly, and antigenicity of a Snow Mountain agent-like calicivirus capsid protein. *J Clin Microbiol.* 1995;33:1452-1455.
40. Dingle KE, Lambden PR, Caul EO, et al. Human enteric *Caliciviridae*: the complete genome sequence and expression of virus-like particles from a genetic group II small round structured virus. *J Gen Virol.* 1995;76:2349-2355.
41. Green KY, Kapikian AZ, Valdesuso J, et al. Expression and self-assembly of recombinant capsid protein from the antigenically distinct Hawaii human calicivirus. *J Clin Microbiol.* 1997;35:1909-1914.
42. Leite JP, Ando T, Noel JS, et al. Characterization of Toronto virus capsid protein expressed in baculovirus. *Arch Virol.* 1996;141:865-875.
43. Numata K, Hardy ME, Nakata S, et al. Molecular characterization of morphologically typical human calicivirus Sapporo. *Arch Virol.* 1997;142:1537-1552.
44. Wyatt RG, Dolin R, Blacklow NR, et al. Comparison of three agents of acute infectious nonbacterial gastroenteritis by virus challenge in volunteers. *J Infect Dis.* 1974;129:709-714.
45. Cubitt WD, Green KY, Payment P. Prevalence of antibodies to the Hawaii strain of human calicivirus as measured by a recombinant protein based immunoassay. *J Med Virol.* 1998;54:135-139.
46. Fankhauser RL, Noel JS, Monroe SS, et al. Molecular epidemiology of "Norwalk-like viruses" in outbreaks of gastroenteritis in the United States. *J Infect Dis.* 1998;178:1571-1578.
47. Fankhauser RL, Monroe SS, Noel JS, et al. Epidemiologic and molecular trends of "Norwalk-like viruses" associated with outbreaks of gastroenteritis in the United States. *J Infect Dis.* 2002;186:1-7.
48. Gonin P, Couillard M, d'Halewyn MA. Genetic diversity and molecular epidemiology of Norwalk-like viruses. *J Infect Dis.* 2000;182:691-697.
49. Lewis DC, Hale A, Jiang X, et al. Epidemiology of Mexico virus, a small round-structured virus in Yorkshire, United Kingdom, between January 1992 and March 1995. *J Infect Dis.* 1997;175:951-954.
50. Vinje J, Altena SA, Koopmans MP. The incidence and genetic variability of small round-structured viruses in outbreaks of gastroenteritis in the Netherlands. *J Infect Dis.* 1997;176:1374-1378.
51. Noel JS, Fankhauser RL, Ando T, et al. Identification of a distinct common strain of "Norwalk-like viruses" having a global distribution. *J Infect Dis.* 1999;179:1334-1344.
52. Widdowson MA, Sulka A, Bulens SN, et al. Norovirus and food-borne disease, United States, 1991-2000. *Emerg Infect Dis.* 2005;11(1):95-102.
53. Ike AC, Brockmann SO, Hartelt K, et al. Molecular epidemiology of norovirus in outbreaks of gastroenteritis in southwest Germany from 2001-2004. *J Clin Microbiol.* 2006;44(4):1262-1267.
54. Lopman BA, Reacher MH, van Duijnhoven Y, et al. Viral gastroenteritis outbreaks in Europe, 1995-2000. *Emerg Infect Dis.* 2003;9:90-96.
55. Reuter G, Krisztalovics K, Vennema H, et al. Evidence of the etiological predominance of norovirus in gastroenteritis outbreaks-emerging new variant and recombinant noroviruses in Hungary. *J Med Virol.* 2005;76:598-607.
56. van Duynhoven YT, de Jager CM, Kortbeek LM, et al. A one-year intensified study of outbreaks of gastroenteritis in the Netherlands. *Epidemiol Infect.* 2005;133:9-21.
57. Patel MM, Widdowson MA, Glass RI, et al. Systematic literature review of role of noroviruses in sporadic gastroenteritis. *Emerg Infect Dis.* 2008;14:1224-1231.
58. Centers for Disease Control and Prevention, Viral Gastroenteritis Section. Norovirus: Technical fact sheet. Available at: http://www.cdc.gov/ncidod/dvrd/revb/gastro/norovirus-factsheet.htm.
59. Greenberg HB, Valdesuso J, Kapikian AZ, et al. Prevalence of antibody to the Norwalk virus in various countries. *Infect Immun.* 1979;26:270-273.
60. Dolin R, Roessner KD, Treanor J, et al. Radioimmunoassay for detection of Snow Mountain agent of viral gastroenteritis. *J Med Virol.* 1985;19:11-18.
61. Hinkula J, Ball JM, Lofgren S, et al. Antibody prevalence and immunoglobulin IgG subclass pattern to Norwalk virus in Sweden. *J Med Virol.* 1995;47:52-57.
62. Numata K, Nakata S, Jiang X, et al. Epidemiologic study of Norwalk virus infections in Japan and Southeast Asia by enzyme-linked immunosorbent assays with Norwalk virus capsid protein produced by the baculovirus expression system. *J Clin Microbiol.* 1994;32:121-126.
63. Gray JJ, Jiang X, Morgan-Capner P, et al. Prevalence of antibodies to Norwalk virus in England: Detection by enzyme-linked immunosorbent assay using baculovirus-expressed Norwalk virus capsid antigen. *J Clin Microbiol.* 1993;31:1022-1025.
64. Sakuma Y, Chiba S, Kogasaka R, et al. Prevalence of antibody to human calicivirus in general population of northern Japan. *J Med Virol.* 1981;7:221-225.
65. Cubitt WD, Blacklow NR, Herrmann JE. Antigenic relationships between human caliciviruses and Norwalk virus. *J Infect Dis.* 1987;156:806-814.
66. Nakata S, Chiba S, Terashima H, et al. Prevalence of antibody to human calicivirus in Japan and Southeast Asia determined by radioimmunoassay. *J Clin Microbiol.* 1985;22:519-521.
67. Gabbay YB, Glass RI, Monroe SS, et al. Prevalence of antibodies to Norwalk virus among Amerindians in isolated Amazonian communities. *Am J Epidemiol.* 1994;139:728-733.
68. Mounts AW, Ando T, Koopmans M, et al. Cold weather seasonality of gastroenteritis associated with Norwalk-like viruses. *J Infect Dis.* 2000;181(Suppl 2):S284-S287.
69. Chadwick PR, McCann R. Transmission of a small round structured virus by vomiting during a hospital outbreak of gastroenteritis. *J Hosp Infect.* 1994;26:251-259.
70. Patterson W, Haswell P, Fryers PT, et al. Outbreak of small round structured virus gastroenteritis arose after kitchen assistant vomited. *Commun Dis Rep CDR Rev.* 1997;7:R101-R103.
71. Greenberg HB, Wyatt RG, Kapikian AZ. Norwalk virus in vomitus. *Lancet.* 1979;1:55.
72. Kilgore PE, Belay ED, Hamlin DM, et al. A university outbreak of gastroenteritis due to a small round-structured virus. Application of molecular diagnostics to identify the etiologic agent and patterns of transmission. *J Infect Dis.* 1996;173:787-793.
73. Sawyer LA, Murphy JJ, Kaplan JE, et al. 25- to 30-nm virus particle associated with a hospital outbreak of acute gastroenteritis with evidence for airborne transmission. *Am J Epidemiol.* 1988;127:1261-1271.
74. Caul EO. Small round structured viruses: Airborne transmission and hospital control. *Lancet.* 1994;343:1240-1242.
75. Centers for Disease Control and Prevention. Norwalk-like viruses: public health impact and outbreak management. *MMWR Morb Mortal Wkly Rep.* 2001;50:1-17.
76. Graham DY, Jian X, Tanaka T, et al. Norwalk virus infection of volunteers: New insights based on improved assays. *J Infect Dis.* 1994;170:34-43.
77. Okhuysen PC, Jiang X, Ye L, et al. Viral shedding and fecal IgA response after Norwalk virus infection. *J Infect Dis.* 1995;171:566-569.
78. Rockx B, De Wit M, Vennema H, et al. Natural history of human calicivirus infection: A prospective cohort study. *Clin Infect Dis.* 2002;35:246-253.
79. Patterson T, Hutching P, Palmer S. Outbreak of SRSV gastroenteritis at an international conference traced to food handled by a post-symptomatic caterer. *Epidemiol Infect.* 1993;111:157-162.
80. Kaplan JE, Feldman R, Campbell DS, et al. The frequency of a Norwalk-like pattern of illness in outbreaks of acute gastroenteritis. *Am J Public Health.* 1982;72:1329-1332.
81. Khan AS, Moe CL, Glass RI, et al. Norwalk virus-associated gastroenteritis traced to ice consumption aboard a cruise ship in Hawaii: Comparison and application of molecular method-based assays. *J Clin Microbiol.* 1994;31:318-322.
82. Bourgeois AL, Gardiner CH, Thornton SA, et al. Etiology of acute diarrhea among United States military personnel deployed to South America and West Africa. *Am J Trop Med Hyg.* 1993;48:243-248.
83. Hyams KC, Bourgeois AL, Merrell BR, et al. Diarrheal disease during Operation Desert Shield. *N Engl J Med.* 1991;325:1423-1428.
84. Centers for Disease Control and Prevention. Norovirus outbreak in an elementary school—District of Columbia, February 2007. *MMWR Morb Mortal Wkly Rep.* 2008;56:1340-1343.
85. Ho MS, Glass RI, Monroe SS. Viral gastroenteritis aboard a cruise ship. *Lancet.* 1989;2:961-965.
86. Hedlund KO, Rubilar-Abreu E, Svensson L. Epidemiology of calicivirus infections in Sweden, 1994-1998. *J Infect Dis.* 2000;181(Suppl. 2):S275-S280.
87. Baron RC, Murphy FD, Greenberg HB. Norwalk gastrointestinal illness: An outbreak associated with swimming in a recreational lake with secondary person-to-person transmission. *Am J Epidemiol.* 1982;115:163-172.
88. Koopman JS, Eckert EA, Greenberg HB. Norwalk virus enteric illness acquired by swimming exposure. *Am J Epidemiol.* 1982;115:173-177.
89. Cannon RO, Poliner JR, Hirschhorn RB, et al. A multistate outbreak of Norwalk virus gastroenteritis associated with consumption of commercial ice. *J Infect Dis.* 1991;164:860-863.
90. Hedberg CW, Osterholm MT. Outbreaks of food-borne and waterborne viral gastroenteritis. *Clin Microbiol Rev.* 1993;6:199-210.
91. Lo SV, Connolly AM, Palmer SR, et al. The role of the pre-symptomatic food handler in a common source outbreak of food-borne SRSV gastroenteritis in a group of hospitals. *Epidemiol Infect.* 1994;113:513-521.
92. Stafford R, Strain D, Heymer M, et al. An outbreak of Norwalk virus gastroenteritis following consumption of oysters. *Commun Dis Intell.* 1997;21:317-320.
93. McDonnell S, Kirkland KB, Hlady WG, et al. Failure of cooking to prevent shellfish-associated viral gastroenteritis. *Arch Intern Med.* 1997;157:111-116.
94. Kirkland KB, Meriwether RA, Leiss JK, et al. Steaming oysters does not prevent Norwalk-like gastroenteritis. *Public Health Rep.* 1996;111:527-530.
95. Rodriguez EM, Parrott C, Rolka H, et al. An outbreak of viral gastroenteritis in a nursing home: Importance of excluding ill employees. *Infect Control Hosp Epidemiol.* 1996;17:587-592.
96. Augustin AK, Simor AE, Shorrock C, et al. Outbreaks of gastroenteritis due to Norwalk-like virus in two long-term care facilities for the elderly. *Can J Infect Control.* 1995;10:111-113.
97. Russo PL, Spelman DW, Harrington GA, et al. Hospital outbreak of Norwalk-like virus. *Infect Control Hosp Epidemiol.* 1997;18:576-579.
98. Kjeldsberg E. Small spherical viruses in faeces from gastroenteritis patients. *Acta Pathol Microbiol Immunol Scand.* 1977;85:351-354.
99. Spatt HC, Marks MI, Gomersall M, et al. Nosocomial infantile gastroenteritis associated with mini-rotavirus and calicivirus. *J Pediatr.* 1978;93:922-926.
100. Oishi I, Maeda A, Yamazaki K, et al. Calicivirus detected in outbreaks of acute gastroenteritis in school children. *Biken J.* 1980;23:163-168.
101. Steele AD, Phillips J, Smit TK, et al. Snow mountain-like virus identified in young children with winter vomiting disease in South Africa. *J Diarrh Dis Res.* 1997;15:177-182.
102. Levett PN, Gu M, Luan B, et al. Longitudinal study of molecular epidemiology of small round-structured viruses in a pediatric population. *J Clin Microbiol.* 1996;34:1497-1501.
103. Middleton PJ, Szymanski MT, Petric M. Viruses associated with acute gastroenteritis in young children. *Am J Dis Child.* 1977;131:733.
104. Wolfaardt M, Taylor MB, Booysen HF, et al. Incidence of human calicivirus and rotavirus infection in patients with gastroenteritis in South Africa. *J Med Virol.* 1997;51:290-296.
105. Pang XL, Honma S, Nakata S, et al. Human caliciviruses in acute gastroenteritis of young children in the community. *J Infect Dis.* 2000;181(Suppl 2):S288-S294.
106. Sakai Y, Nakata S, Honma S, et al. Clinical severity of Norwalk virus and Sapporo virus gastroenteritis in children in Hokkaido, Japan. *Pediatr Infect Dis J.* 2001;20:849-853.
107. Lew JF, Valdesuso J, Vesikari T, et al. Detection of Norwalk virus or Norwalk-like virus infections in Finnish infants and young children. *J Infect Dis.* 1994;169:1364-1367.
108. Grohmann G, Glass RI, Gold J, et al. Outbreak of human calicivirus gastroenteritis in a day-care center in Sydney, Australia. *J Clin Microbiol.* 1991;29:544-550.
109. Struve J, Bennet R, Ehrnst AE, et al. Nosocomial calicivirus gastroenteritis in a pediatric hospital. *Pediatr Infect Dis J.* 1994;13:882-885.
110. Mounts AW, Ando T, Koopmans M, et al. Cold weather seasonality of gastroenteritis associated with Norwalk-like viruses. *J Infect Dis.* 2000;181(Suppl 2):S284-S287.
111. Blanton LH, Adams SM, Beard RS, et al. Molecular and epidemiologic trends of caliciviruses associated with outbreaks of acute gastroenteritis in the United States, 2000-2004. *J Infect Dis* 2006;193:413-421.
112. Agus SG, Dolin R, Wyatt RG, et al. Acute infectious nonbacterial gastroenteritis: Intestinal histopathology. *Ann Intern Med.* 1973;79:18-25.

113. Schreiber DS, Blacklow NR, Trier JS. The mucosal lesion of the proximal small intestine in acute infectious nonbacterial gastroenteritis. *N Engl J Med.* 1973;288:1318-1323.

114. Schreiber DS, Blacklow NR, Trier JS. The small intestinal lesion induced by Hawaii agent acute infectious nonbacterial gastroenteritis. *J Infect Dis.* 1974;129:705-708.

115. Widerlite L, Trier J, Blacklow N, et al. Structure of the gastric mucosa in acute infectious nonbacterial gastroenteritis. *Gastroenterology.* 1975;70:321-325.

116. Blacklow NR, Dolin R, Feson DS, et al. Acute infectious nonbacterial gastroenteritis: Etiology and pathogenesis. *Ann Intern Med.* 1972;76:993-1000.

117. Levy AG, Widerlite L, Schwartz CJ, et al. Jejunal adenylate cyclase activity in human subjects during viral gastroenteritis. *Gastroenterology.* 1976;70:321-325.

118. Woode GN, Bridger JC. Isolation of small viruses resembling astroviruses and caliciviruses from acute enteritis of calves. *J Med Microbiol.* 1978;11:441-452.

119. Saif LJ, Bohl EH, Theil KW, et al. Rotavirus-like, calicivirus-like, and 23-nm virus-like particles associated with diarrhea in young pigs. *J Clin Microbiol.* 1980;12:105-111.

120. Marionneau S, Ruvoen N, Le Moullac-Vaidye B, et al. Norwalk virus binds to histo-blood group antigens present on gastroduodenal epithelial cells of secretor individuals. *Gastroenterology.* 2002;122:1967-1977.

121. Hutson AM, Atmar RL, Marcus DM, et al. Norwalk virus-like particle hemagglutination by binding to histo-blood group antigens. *J Virol.* 2003;77:405-415.

122. Huang P, Farkas T, Marionneau S, et al. Noroviruses bind to human ABO, Lewis, and secretor histo-blood group antigens: Identification of 4 distinct strain-specific patterns. *J Infect Dis.* 2003;188:19-31.

123. Tan M, Huang P, Meller J, et al. Mutations within the P2 domain of Norovirus capsid affect binding to human histo-blood group antigens: Evidence for a binding pocket. *J Virol.* 2003;77:12562-12571.

124. Hutson AM, Atmar RL, Graham DY, et al. Norwalk virus infection and disease is associated with ABO histo-blood group type. *J Infect Dis.* 2002;185:1335-1337.

125. Lindesmith L, Moe C, Marionneau S, et al. Human susceptibility and resistance to Norwalk virus infection. *Nat Med.* 2003;9:548-553.

126. Parrino TA, Schreiber DS, Trier JS, et al. Clinical immunity in acute gastroenteritis caused by Norwalk agent. *N Engl J Med.* 1977;291:86-89.

127. Cukor G, Nowak NA, Blacklow NR. Immunoglobulin M responses to the Norwalk virus of gastroenteritis. *Infect Immun.* 1982;37:463-468.

128. Treanor JJ, Jiang X, Madore HP, et al. Subclass-specific serum antibody responses to recombinant Norwalk virus capsid antigen (rNV) in adults infected with Norwalk, Snow Mountain, or Hawaii viruses. *J Clin Microbiol.* 1993;31:1630-1634.

129. Erdman DD, Gary GW, Anderson LJ. Development and evaluation of an IgM capture enzyme immunoassay for diagnosis of recent Norwalk virus infection. *J Virol Methods.* 1989;24:57-66.

130. Erdman DD, Gary GW, Anderson LJ. Serum immunoglobulin A response to Norwalk virus infection. *J Clin Microbiol.* 1989;27:1417-1418.

131. Farkas T, Thornton SA, Wilton N, et al. Homologous versus heterologous immune responses to Norwalk-like viruses among crew members after acute gastroenteritis outbreaks on 2 US Navy vessels. *J Infect Dis.* 2003;187:187-193.

132. Madore HP, Treanor JJ, Buja R, et al. Antigenic relatedness among the Norwalk-like agents by serum antibody rises. *J Med Virol.* 1990;32:96-101.

133. Hale AD, Lewis DC, Jiang X, Brown DW. Homotypic and heterotypic IgG and IgM antibody responses in adults infected with small round structured viruses. *J Med Virol.* 1998;54:305-312.

134. Noel JS, Ando T, Leite JP, et al. Correlation of patient immune responses with genetically characterized small round-structured viruses involved in outbreaks of nonbacterial acute gastroenteritis in the United States, 1990 to 1995. *J Med Virol.* 1997;53:372-383.

135. Jiang X, Wang J, Estes MK. Characterization of SRSVs using RT-PCR and a new antigen ELISA. *Arch Virol.* 1995;140:363-374.

136. Agus S, Falchuk ZM, Sessoms CS, et al. Increased jejunal IgA synthesis in vitro during acute infectious nonbacterial gastroenteritis. *Am J Digest Dis.* 1974;19:127-131.

137. Okhuysen P, Jiang X, Tenjaria G, et al. Detection of Norwalk specific fecal IgA in challenged volunteers utilizing ELISA with baculovirus expressed Norwalk particles as coating antigens. Abstract 1392. In: *32nd Interscience Conference on Antimicrobial Agents and Chemotherapy, 1992.* Anaheim, CA: American Society for Microbiology; 1992:343.

138. Dolin R, Reichman RC, Fauci AS. Lymphocyte populations in acute viral gastroenteritis. *Infect Immunol.* 1976;14:422-428.

139. Lindesmith L, Moe C, LePendu J, et al. Cellular and humoral immunity following Snow Mountain virus challenge. *J Virol.* 2005;79:2900-2909.

140. Johnson PC, Mathewson JJ, DuPont HL, et al. Multiple-challenge study of host susceptibility to Norwalk gastroenteritis in US adults. *J Infect Dis.* 1990;161:18-21.

141. Black RE, Greenberg HB, Kapikian AZ, et al. Acquisition of serum antibody to Norwalk virus and rotavirus and relation to diarrhea in a longitudinal study of young children in rural Bangladesh. *J Infect Dis.* 1982;145:483-489.

142. Ryder RW, Singh N, Reeves WC, et al. Evidence of immunity induced by naturally acquired rotavirus and Norwalk virus infection on two remote Panamanian islands. *J Infect Dis.* 1985;135:20-27.

143. Nakata S, Chiba A, Terashima H, et al. Humoral immunity in infants with gastroenteritis caused by human calicivirus. *J Infect Dis.* 1985;152:274-279.

144. Greenberg HB, Wyatt RG, Kalica AR, et al. New insights in viral gastroenteritis. *Perspect Virol.* 1981;11:163-187.

145. Karst SM, Wobus CE, Lay M, et al. STAT1-dependent innate immunity to a Norwalk-like virus. *Science.* 2003;299:1575-1578.

146. Dedman D, Laurichesse H, Caul EO, et al. Surveillance of small round structured virus (SRSV) infection in England and Wales, 1990-5. *Epidemiol Infect.* 1998;121:139-149.

147. Chadwick PR, Beards G, Brown D, et al. Management of hospital outbreaks of gastro-enteritis due to small round-structured viruses. *J Hosp Infect.* 2000;45:1-10.

148. Simon A, Schildgen O, Maria Eis-Hubinger A, et al. Norovirus outbreak in a pediatric oncology unit. *Scand J Gastroenterol.* 2006;41:693-699.

149. Westhoff TH, Vergoulidou M, Loddenkemper C, et al. Chronic norovirus infection in renal transplant recipients. *Nephrol Dial Transplant.* 2009;24:1051-1053.

150. Harris JC, DuPont HL, Hornick RB. Fecal leukocytes in diarrheal illness. *Ann Intern Med.* 1972;76:697-703.

151. Atmar RL, Estes MK. Diagnosis of noncultivatable gastroenteritis viruses, the human caliciviruses. *Clin Microbiol Rev.* 2001;14:15-37.

152. Kapikian Z, Wyatt RG, Dolin R, et al. Visualization of 27 nm particle associated infectious nonbacterial gastroenteritis. *J Virol.* 1972;10:1075-1081.

153. De Bruin E, Duizer E, Vennema H, et al. Diagnosis of norovirus outbreaks by commercial ELISA or RT-PCR. *J Virol Methods* 2006;137:259-264.

154. Gray JJ, Kohli E, Ruggeri FM, et al. European multicenter evaluation of commercial enzyme immunoassays for detecting norovirus antigen in fecal samples. *Clin Vaccine Immunol.* 2007;14:1349-1355.

155. Jiang X, Wang J, Graham DY, et al. Detection of Norwalk virus in stool by polymerase chain reaction. *J Clin Microbiol.* 1992;30:2529-2534.

156. De Leon R, Matsui SM, Baric RS, et al. Detection of Norwalk virus in stool specimens by reverse transcriptase-polymerase chain reaction and nonradioactive oligoprobes. *J Clin Microbiol.* 1992;30:3151-3157.

157. Willcocks MM, Silcock JG, Carter MJ. Detection of Norwalk virus in the UK by the polymerase chain reaction. *FEMS Microbiol Lett.* 1993;112:7-12.

158. Moe CL, Gentsch J, Ando T, et al. Application of PCR to detect Norwalk virus in fecal specimens from outbreaks of gastroenteritis. *J Clin Microbiol.* 1994;32:642-648.

159. Honma S, Nakata S, Sakai Y, et al. Sensitive detection and differentiation of Sapporo virus, a member of the family Caliciviridae, by standard and booster nested polymerase chain reaction. *J Med Microbiol.* 2001;65:413-417.

160. Vinje J, Vennema H, Maunula L, et al. International collaborative study to compare reverse transcriptase PCR assays for detection and genotyping of noroviruses. *J Clin Microbiol* 2003;41:1423-1433.

161. Jiang X, Huang PW, Zhong WM, et al. Design and evaluation of a primer pair that detects both Norwalk- and Sapporo-like caliciviruses by RT-PCR. *J Virol Methods.* 1999;83:145-154.

162. Kojima S, Kageyama T, Fukushi S, et al. Genogroup-specific PCR primers for detection of Norwalk-like viruses. *J Virol Methods.* 2002;100:107-114.

163. Ando T, Monroe SS, Gentsch JR, et al. Detection and differentiation of antigenically distinct small round-structured viruses (Norwalk-like viruses) by reverse transcription-PCR and southern hybridization. *J Clin Microbiol.* 1995;33:64-71.

164. Atmar RL, Metcalf TG, Neill FH, et al. Detection of enteric viruses in oysters by using the polymerase chain reaction. *Appl Environ Microbiol.* 1993;59:631-635.

165. Gouvea V, Santos N, Timenetsky M, et al. Identification of Norwalk virus in artificially seeded shellfish and selected foods. *J Virol Methods.* 1994;8:177-187.

166. Beller M, Ellis A, Lee SH, et al. Outbreak of viral gastroenteritis due to a contaminated well: International consequences. *JAMA.* 1997;278:563-568.

167. Le Guyader F, Neill FH, Estes MK, et al. Detection and analysis of a small round-structured virus strain in oysters implicated in an outbreak of acute gastroenteritis. *Appl Environ Microbiol.* 1996;62:4268-4272.

168. Shieh Y, Monroe SS, Fankhauser RL, et al. Detection of Norwalk-like virus in shellfish implicated in illness. *J Infect Dis.* 2000;181(Suppl 2):S360-S366.

169. Gary GW, Anderson LJ, Keswick BH, et al. Norwalk virus antigen and antibody response in an adult volunteer study. *J Clin Microbiol.* 1987;25:2001-2003.

170. Brinker JP, Blacklow NR, Estes MK, et al. Detection of Norwalk virus and other genogroup 1 human caliciviruses by a monoclonal antibody, recombinant-antigen-based immunoglobulin M capture enzyme immunoassay. *J Clin Microbiol.* 1998;36:1064-1069.

171. Brinker JP, Blacklow NR, Jiang X, et al. Immunoglobulin M antibody test to detect genogroup II Norwalk-like virus infection. *J Clin Microbiol.* 1999;37:2983-2986.

172. Steinhoff MC, Douglas RG Jr, Greenberg HB, et al. Bismuth subsalysylate therapy of viral gastroenteritis. *Gastroenterology.* 1980;78:1495-1499.

173. Wobus CE, Thackray LB, Virgin HW IV. Murine norovirus: A model system to study norovirus biology and pathogenesis. *J Virol.* 2006;80:5104-5112.

174. Estes MK, Ball JM, Guerrero RA, et al. Norwalk virus vaccines: Challenges and progress. *J Infect Dis.* 2000;181(Suppl 2):S367-S373.

175. Ball JM, Graham DY, Opekun AR, et al. Recombinant Norwalk virus-like particles given orally to volunteers: Phase I study. *Gastroenterology.* 1999;117:40-48.

176. Tacket CO, Sztein MB, Losonsky G, et al. Humoral, mucosal, and cellular immune responses to oral Norwalk virus-like particles in volunteers. *Clin Immunol.* 2003;108:241-247.

177. Tacket CO, Mason HS, Losonsky G, et al. Human immune responses to a novel Norwalk virus vaccine delivered in transgenic potatoes. *J Infect Dis.* 2000;182:302-305.

178. Centers for Disease Control and Prevention. Norovirus activity—United States, 2006-2007. *MMWR Morb Mortal Wkly Rep.* 2007;56:842-846.

176

Astroviruses and Picobirnaviruses

RAPHAEL DOLIN | JOHN J. TREANOR

In addition to caliciviruses, several newly described viruses have been implicated as causes of gastroenteritis in adults and children. The greatest evidence to support this role exists for astroviruses. Other viruses that may be responsible for some cases of gastroenteritis include the toroviruses (see Chapter 155) and the picobirnaviruses (PBVs).

Astroviruses

Astroviruses are members of a newly described virus family, the Astroviridae, which consists of two genera, *Mamastrovirus*, which infects mammals and includes the human astroviruses, and *Avastrovirus*, which includes avian viruses. Astroviruses are now recognized as important causes of gastroenteritis in children and adults. Together with the Caliciviridae (see Chapter 175), these small RNA viruses account for much of the gastroenteritis that had previously been of unknown etiology and was presumed to be caused by undetected viral agents.

VIROLOGY

Astroviruses are small positive-strand RNA viruses that are found in a wide variety of animal species, including humans. The virions are nonenveloped, display icosahedral symmetry, and are about 28 to 30 nm in diameter. Under the electron microscope, the particles in stool samples have a characteristic morphology that consists of round smooth edges with multiple triangular electron-lucent areas and an electron-dense center that results in the appearance of a five- or six-pointed star from which the virus derives its name (Fig. 176-1).[1,2] Analysis of virus grown in cell culture has shown the virus particles to exhibit a layer of 41-nm spikelike projections on the surface.[3] The human astroviruses have a density of 1.35 to 1.37 g/mL in cesium chloride (CsCl) and contain a positive-sense, single-stranded 35 S RNA genome with a 3′ polyadenylated tail.[4] The genomic organization includes three open reading frames (ORFs): ORF1a encodes the protease region; ORF1b encodes the polymerase; and ORF2 encodes a polyprotein that is cleaved into capsid proteins.[5-8] The capsid is translated from a subgenomic polyadenylated RNA in infected cells.[9,10] The number of viral structural proteins appears to vary with the serotype, with between one and three reported for the human viruses,[11,12] possibly reflecting differences in the processing of the capsid precursor.[13]

Astrovirus serotypes can be distinguished by immunofluorescence or plaque neutralization techniques,[14,15] whereas considerable cross-reactivity exists by enzyme immunoassay[16] due to the presence of a group antigen. Eight serotypes of human astroviruses have been recognized,[17-19] denoted HAstV-1 to HAstV-8. The availability of molecular detection techniques (reverse transcriptase–polymerase chain reaction [RT-PCR], see later) has led to the description of genotypes, as well, depending on the region of the genome that is being probed. Genotypes defined by the amino acid sequence of the carboxyl-terminal region of the structural polyprotein correlate well with the eight HAstV serotypes that have been described.[2] These molecular techniques are now being used widely to define the epidemiology of astrovirus infection.[20] An important step in the study of astroviruses has been the propagation of astroviruses in cell culture systems, including primary HEK cells and a variety of monkey cell lines.[16,21,22]

EPIDEMIOLOGY

Astrovirus infection is widely distributed, and all eight HAstV serotypes or genotypes have been detected throughout the world.[18-20] HAstV-1 appears to be the most common based on both serotypic[23-25] and genotypic surveys.[20,26-29]

Astroviruses have been detected in the stools of children with diarrhea brought to medical attention in a variety of settings (Table 176-1). Rates of 2% to 16% have been found in hospital-based studies and 5% to 17% in community-based studies.[30-32] Outbreaks have been described in schools, daycare settings, and pediatric wards.[33-36] Illness has most often been seen in individuals younger than 2 years, although outbreaks in healthy adults[37,38] and in elderly populations[39] have also been described. Astroviruses have also been detected in the stools of immunosuppressed patients with diarrhea, including human immunodeficiency virus (HIV)–infected patients,[40] following hematopoietic cell transplantation,[41] and in children with primary immunodeficiencies[42] or hematologic malignancies.[43] However, the severity of illness in HIV-infected children with astrovirus is no greater than that seen in other children.[44,45]

A winter predilection has been noted in temperate climates in some studies,[12,46] whereas infection occurs throughout the year in tropical climates,[47] similar to the pattern reported for rotaviruses. Transmission is presumably by the fecal-oral route, and astrovirus infection has been induced by oral administration of stool filtrates to normal volunteers.[11] Seroprevalence studies in the United States and elsewhere have shown that more than 90% of children have antibody to HastV-1 by age 9 years,[23] suggesting that infection, largely asymptomatic, is common.

PATHOGENESIS

The pathogenesis of astrovirus-induced illness is not well understood. Astrovirus infections in animals have been associated with small intestinal villus shortening and with mild inflammatory infiltrates in the lamina propria.[48,49] Astrovirus infection may result in decreased intestinal disaccharidase activity and subsequent osmotic diarrhea,[50] similar to the mechanism postulated for rotavirus. As noted previously, stool filtrates that contain astroviruses can infect volunteers after oral administration, but in contrast to noroviruses, astroviruses induce illness very infrequently,[11,51] which suggests that they may be less "pathogenic" in adults than the noroviruses.

CLINICAL ILLNESS

Illness attributed to astroviruses consists primarily of diarrhea, headache, malaise, and nausea, whereas vomiting appears to be less common.[2] In general, the symptoms are similar to those seen in rotavirus infection in children but are milder, and children with astrovirus gastroenteritis are less likely to be dehydrated than those with rotavirus.[52] Low-grade fever is frequently present. The incubation period of illness has been estimated to be 3 to 4 days, and in the absence of coexisting pathogens, disease manifestations usually last 5 days or less, with occasional longer duration. The duration of virus shedding as assessed by PCR may be longer than by enzyme immunoassay (EIA), as long as 35 days.[53]

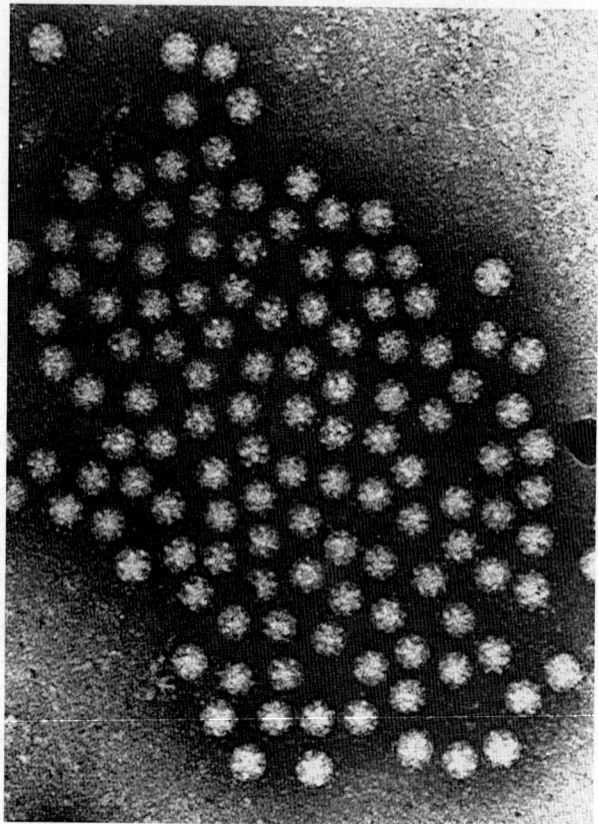

Figure 176-1 **Astrovirus in the intestinal contents of gnotobiotic lambs.** Particles are 30 nm in diameter. *(From Snodgrass DR, Gray W. Detection and transmission of 30 nm virus particles [astroviruses] in the faeces of lambs with diarrhoea. Arch Virol. 1977;55:287-291.)*

	Percentage of Samples in which Astroviruses Were Detected in Subjects		
Geographic Location	*With Illness*	*Without Illness*	*Reference*
Baltimore	2.7	1.4	55
Phoenix	4.0	2.4	24
Providence	6.8	0.0	43
Thailand	8.6	2.0	56
Guatemala	7.3	2.4	35
Korea	1.9	2.2	57
Peru	2.9	2.5	57

TABLE 176-1 **Detection of Astroviruses in Children with Diarrhea**

to detect astroviruses, and they are significantly more sensitive than EIA or IEM.[53,55]

Illness associated with these agents is generally self-limited, and treatment, if required at all, is supportive and directed at maintaining hydration and electrolyte balance. Although the parameters of immunity to astroviruses are not well understood, epidemiologic observations suggest that infection is associated with at least short-term protection against reinfection with the same serotype,[56] raising the possibility of vaccine strategies at some point in the future. Infection is also associated with the development of astrovirus-specific Th1-type CD4 cells in the gut mucosa.[57]

▣ Picobirnaviruses

The PBVs are small icosahedral viruses with a segmented double-stranded RNA genome consisting of two segments. The genomes have been characterized into two types or profiles[58,59]: a large profile (2.3 to 2.6 kbp for the large segment) and a small profile (1.75-1.55 kbp), which are now being used for molecular epidemiologic studies.[60] Their exact taxonomic position is unclear, and they derive their name from the observation that they (usually) have a *bi*segmented double-stranded RNA genome similar to the *Birnaviridae*, but are smaller (pico), with a virion size of 30 to 40 nm.[61] They were first observed in the stools of humans[62] in the course of studies using polyacrylamide gel electrophoresis (PAGE) to detect rotavirus. Picobirnavirus genomes have been found in the stools of a variety of animals and in children and adults with diarrhea, including HIV-infected adults.[40,60,63-65] However, the role of these viruses as causative agents of gastroenteritis is unclear because the prevalence of PBVs in stools of individuals with and without diarrhea is similar.[66]

Toroviruses are newly described viral agents that cause gastroenteritis. They are members of the Coronaviridae family and are discussed in Chapter 155.

DIAGNOSIS, TREATMENT, AND PREVENTION

In contrast to other recently described viral agents of gastroenteritis, astroviruses are often shed in large amounts in stool and can be readily detected by electron microscopy even without immune aggregation. Detection of astroviruses in cell culture has been carried out by immune electron microscopy (IEM) or by immunofluorescence, and an enzyme immunoassay technique[54] that detects the astrovirus group antigen has been used widely in epidemiologic studies. EIA is of comparable sensitivity (91%) and specificity (98%) to IEM.[2] RT-PCR techniques have been developed and are the most widely used techniques

REFERENCES

1. Snodgrass DR, Gray W. Detection and transmission of 30 nm virus particles (astroviruses) in the faeces of lambs with diarrhoea. *Arch Virol.* 1977;55:287-291.
2. Méndez E, Arias CF. Astroviruses. In: Knipe DM, Howley PM, eds. *Fields Virology.* 5th ed. Philadelphia: Lippincott Williams & Wilkins; 2007:981-1000.
3. Risco C, Carrascosa JL, Pedregosa AM, et al. Ultrastructure of human astrovirus serotype 2. *J Gen Virol.* 1995;76:2075-2080.
4. Herring AJ, Gray EW, Snodgrass DR. Purification and characterization of bovine astrovirus. *J Gen Virol.* 1981;53:47-55.
5. Jiang B, Monroe SS, Koonin EV, et al. RNA sequence of astrovirus: Distinctive genomic organization and a putative retrovirus-like ribosomal frameshifting signal that directs the viral replicase synthesis. *Proc Natl Acad Sci. U S A.* 1993;90:10539-10543.
6. Willcocks MM, Brown TDK, Madeley CR, et al. The complete sequence of a human astrovirus. *J Gen Virol.* 1994;75:1785-1788.
7. Caballero S, Guix S, Ribes E, et al. Structural requirements of astrovirus virus-like particles assembled in insect cells. *J Virol.* 2004;78(23):13285-13292.
8. Dalton RM, Pastrana EP, Sanchez-Fanquier A. Vaccinia virus recombinant expressing an 87-kilodalton polyprotein that is suf-

ficient to form astrovirus-like particles. *J Virol.* 2003;77:9094-9098.
9. Monroe SS, Stine SE, Gorelkin L, et al. Temporal synthesis of proteins and RNAs during human astrovirus infection of cultured cells. *J Virol.* 1991;65:641-648.
10. Matsui SM, Kim JP, Greenberg HB, et al. Cloning and characterization of human astrovirus immunoreactive epitopes. *J Virol.* 1993;67:1712-1715.
11. Midthun K, Greenberg HB, Kurtz JB, et al. Characterization and seroepidemiology of a type 5 astrovirus associated with an outbreak of gastroenteritis in Marin County, California. *J Clin Microbiol.* 1993;31:955-962.
12. Monroe SS, Glass RI, Noah N, et al. Electron microscopic reporting of gastrointestinal viruses in the United Kingdom, 1985-1987. *J Med Virol.* 1991;33:193-198.
13. Belliot G, Laveran H, Monroe SS. Capsid protein composition of reference strains and wild isolates of human astroviruses. *Virus Res.* 1997;49:49-57.
14. Kurtz JB, Lee TW. Human astrovirus serotypes [Letter]. *Lancet.* 1984;2:1405.
15. Hudson RW, Herrmann JE, Blacklow NR. Plaque quantitation and virus neutralization assays for human astroviruses. *Arch Virol.* 1989;108:33-38.

16. Herrmann JE, Hudson RW, Perron-Henry DM, et al. Antigen characterization of cell-cultivated astrovirus serotypes and development of astrovirus-specific monoclonal antibodies. *J Infect Dis.* 1988;158:182-185.
17. Lee TW, Kurtz JB. Prevalence of human astrovirus serotypes in the Oxford region 1976-1992, with evidence for two new serotypes. *Epidemiol Infect.* 1994;112:187-193.
18. Noel JS, Lee TW, Kurtz JB, et al. Typing of human astroviruses from clinical isolates by enzyme immunoassay and nucleotide sequencing. *J Clin Microbiol.* 1995;33:797-801.
19. Taylor MB, Walter J, Berke T, et al. Characterisation of a South African human astrovirus as type 8 by antigenic and genetic analyses. *J Med Virol.* 2001;64:256-261.
20. Gabbay YB, Linhares AC, Cavalcante-Pepino EL, et al. Prevalence of human astrovirus genotypes associated with acute gastroenteritis among children in Bélem, Brazil. *J Med Virol.* 2007;79:530-538.
21. Willcocks MM, Carter MJ, Laidler FR, et al. Growth and characterisation of human faecal astrovirus in a continuous cell line. *Arch Virol.* 1990;113:73-81.
22. Yamashita T, Kobayashi S, Sakae K, et al. Isolation of cytopathic small round viruses with BS-C-1 cells from patients with gastroenteritis. *J Infect Dis.* 1991;164:954-957.

23. Mitchell DK, Matson DO, Cubitt WD, et al. Prevalence of antibodies to astrovirus types 1 and 3 in children and adolescents in Norfolk, Virginia. *Pediatr Infect Dis J.* 1999;18:249-254.
24. Kriston S, Willcocks MM, Carter MJ, et al. Seroprevalence of astrovirus types 1 and 6 in London, determined using recombinant virus antigen. *Epidemiol Infect.* 1996;117:159-164.
25. Koopmans MP, Bijen MH, Monroe SS, et al. Age-stratified seroprevalence of neutralizing antibodies to astrovirus types 1 to 7 in humans in the Netherlands. *Clin Diagn Lab Immunol.* 1998;5:33-37.
26. Espul A, Martinez N, Noel JS, et al. Prevalence and characterization of astroviruses in Argentinean children with acute gastroenteritis. *J Med Virol.* 2004;72:75-82.
27. Guix S, Caballero S, Villena C, et al. Molecular epidemiology of astrovirus infection in Barcelona, Spain. *J Clin Microbiol.* 2002;40:133-139.
28. Resque HR, Munford V, Castilho JG, et al. Molecular characterization of astrovirus in stool samples from children in São Paulo, Brazil. *Mem Inst Oswaldo Cruz.* 2007;102:969-974.
29. Nguyen TA, Hoang L, Pham LD, et al. Identification of human astrovirus infections among children with acute gastroenteritis in the Southern part of Vietnam during 2005-2006. *J Med Virol.* 2008;80:298-305.
30. Polombo EA, Bishop RF. Annual incidence, serotype distribution, and genetic diversity of astrovirus isolates from hospitalized children in Melbourne, Australia. *J Clin Microbiol.* 1996;34:1750-1753.
31. Walter JE, Mitchell DK. Role of astroviruses in childhood diarrhea. *Curr Opin Pediatr.* 2000;12:275-279.
32. Méndez-Toss M, Griffin DD, Calva J, et al. Prevalence and genetic diversity of human astroviruses in Mexican children with symptomatic and asymptomatic infections. *J Clin Microbiol.* 2004;42:151-157.
33. Madeley CR, Cosgrove BP. 28 nm particles in faeces in infantile gastroenteritis [Letter]. *Lancet.* 1975;2:451.
34. Esahli H, Breback K, Bennet R, et al. Astroviruses as a cause of nosocomial outbreaks of infant diarrhea. *Pediatr Infect Dis J.* 1991;10:511-515.
35. Svraka S, Duizer E, Vennema H, et al. Etiological role of viruses in outbreaks of acute gastroenteritis in the Netherlands from 1994 through 2005. *J Clin Microbiol.* 2007;45:1389-1394.
36. Lyman WH, Walsh JF, Kotch JB, et al. Prospective study of etiologic agents of acute gastroenteritis outbreaks in child care centers. *J Pediatri.* 2009;154:253-257.
37. Oishi I, Yamazaki K, Kimoto T, et al. A large outbreak of acute gastroenteritis associated with astrovirus among students and teachers in Osaka, Japan. *J Infect Dis.* 1994;170:439-443.
38. Belliot G, Laveran H, Monroe SS. Outbreak of gastroenteritis in military recruits associated with serotype 3 astrovirus infection. *J Med Virol.* 1997;51:101-106.
39. Gray JJ, Wreghitt TG, Cubitt WD, et al. An outbreak of gastroenteritis in a home for the elderly associated with astrovirus type 1 and human calicivirus. *J Med Virol.* 1987;23:377-381.
40. Grohmann GS, Glass RI, Pereira HG, et al. Enteric viruses and diarrhea in HIV-infected patients. Enteric Opportunistic Infections Working Group. *N Engl J Med.* 1993;329:14-20.
41. Cox GJ, Matsui SM, Lo RS, et al. Etiology and outcome of diarrhea after marrow transplantation: A prospective study. *Gastroenterology.* 1994;107:1398-1407.
42. Gallimore CI, Taylor C, Gennery AR, et al. Use of a heminested reverse transcriptase PCR assay for detection of astrovirus in environmental swabs from an outbreak of gastroenteritis in a pediatric primary immunodeficiency unit. *J Clin Microbiol* 2005;43:3890-3894.
43. Coppo P, Scieux C, Ferchal F, et al. Astrovirus enteritis in a chronic lymphocytic leukemia patient treated with fludarabine monophosphate. *Ann Hematol.* 2000;79:43-45.
44. Liste MB, Natera I, Suarez JA, et al. Enteric virus infections and diarrhea in healthy and human immunodeficiency virus-infected children. *J Clin Microbiol.* 2000;38:2873-2877.
45. Giordano MO, Martinez LC, Rinaldi D, et al. Diarrhea and enteric emerging viruses in HIV-infected patients. *AIDS Res Hum Retrovir.* 1999;15:1427-1432.
46. Lew JF, Glass RI, Petric M, et al. Six-year retrospective surveillance of gastroenteritis viruses identified at ten electron microscopy centers in the United States and Canada. *Pediatr Infect Dis J.* 1990;9:709-714.
47. Cruz JR, Bartlett AV, Herrmann JE, et al. Astrovirus-associated diarrhea among Guatemalan ambulatory rural children. *J Clin Microbiol.* 1992;30:1140-1144.
48. Snodgrass DR, Angus KW, Gray EW, et al. Pathogenesis of diarrhoea caused by astrovirus infection in lambs. *Arch Virol.* 1979;60:217-226.
49. Woode GN, Bridger JC. Isolation of small viruses resembling astroviruses and caliciviruses from acute enteritis of calves. *J Med Microbiol.* 1978;11:441-452.
50. Thouvenelle ML, Haynes JS, Sell JL, et al. Astrovirus infection in hatchling turkeys: Alterations in intestinal maltase activity. *Avian Dis.* 1995;39:343-348.
51. Kurtz JB, Lee TW, Craig JW, et al. Astrovirus infection in volunteers. *J Med Virol.* 1979;3:221-230.
52. Dennehy PH, Nelson SM, Spangenberger S, et al. A prospective case-control study of the role of astrovirus in acute diarrhea among hospitalized young children. *J Infect Dis.* 2001;184:10-15.
53. Mitchell DK, Monroe SS, Jiang X, et al. Virologic features of an astrovirus diarrhea outbreak in a day care center revealed by reverse transcriptase-polymerase chain reaction. *J Infect Dis.* 1995;172:1437-1444.
54. Herrmann JE, Nowak NA, Perron-Henry DM, et al. Diagnosis of astrovirus gastroenteritis by antigen detection with monoclonal antibodies. *J Infect Dis* 1990;161:226-229.
55. Major ME, Eglin RP, Easton AJ. 3' Terminal nucleotide sequence of human astrovirus type 1 and routine detection of astrovirus nucleic acid and antigens. *J Virol Methods.* 1992;3:217-225.
56. Naficy AB, Rao MR, Holmes JL, et al. Astrovirus diarrhea in Egyptian children. *J Infect Dis.* 2000;182:685-690.
57. Molberg O, Nilsen EM, Sollid LM, et al. CD4+ T cells with specific reactivity against astrovirus isolated from normal human small intestine [see comments]. *Gastroenterology.* 1998;114:115-122.
58. Wakuda M, Pongsuwanna Y, Taniguchi K. Complete nucleotide sequences of two RNA segments of human picobirnaviruses. *J Virol Methods.* 2005;126:165-169.
59. Taniguchi K, Wakuda M. Picobirnavirus. *Uirusu.* 2005;55:297-302.
60. Bhattacharya R, Sahoo GC, Nayak MK, et al. Molecular epidemiology of human picobirnaviruses among children of a slum community in Kolkata, India. *Infect Genet Evol.* 2006;6:453-458.
61. Chandra R. Picobirnavirus, a novel group of undescribed viruses of mammals and birds: A minireview. *Acta Virol.* 1997;41:59-62.
62. Pereira HG, Fialho AM, Flewett TH, et al. Novel viruses in human faeces. *Lancet.* 1988;2:103-104.
63. Giordano MO, Masachessi G, Martinez LC, et al. Two instances of large genome profile picobirnavirus occurrence in Argentinian infants with diarrhea over a 26-year period (1977-2002). *J Infect.* 2008;56:371-375.
64. Giordano MO, Martinez LC, Rinaldi D, et al. Detection of picobirnavirus in HIV-infected patients with diarrhea in Argentina. *J Acquir Immune Defic Syndr Hum Retrovirol.* 1998;18:380-383.
65. Gonzalez GG, Pujol FH, Liprandi F, et al. Prevalence of enteric viruses in human immunodeficiency virus seropositive patients in Venezuela. *J Med Virol.* 1998;55:288-292.
66. Gallimore CI, Appleton H, Lewis D, et al. Detection and characterisation of bisegmented double-stranded RNA viruses (picobirnaviruses) in human faecal specimens. *J Med Virol.* 1995;45:135-140.

177

Hepatitis E Virus

DAVID A. ANDERSON

Hepatitis E virus (HEV) is the causative agent of hepatitis E[1] and the type member of a distinct virus family. HEV is enterically transmitted and causes an acute and generally self-limiting infection of the liver but with a higher mortality in general than for infections with hepatitis A virus (HAV), which is transmitted via the same route. HEV is unique among the hepatitis viruses because of a high mortality during pregnancy. Clinical hepatitis E is of most importance in developing countries, where it represents the most common form of acute hepatitis that occurs in both sporadic and epidemic forms. Clinical hepatitis E is rare in developed countries, but zoonotic infections are presumed to be responsible for the rare cases that are locally acquired in these countries. Practical and accurate diagnostic assays are available, and an effective vaccine has been developed but is not yet available commercially.

History

Evidence for an enterically transmitted form of viral hepatitis distinct from viral hepatitis A came from serologic studies of waterborne epidemics of hepatitis in India in the late 1970s. Khuroo[2] and Wong and colleagues[3] showed that patients involved in such epidemics of hepatitis in the Kashmir region and in Delhi, India, respectively, lacked serologic evidence of recent HAV infection. In fact, all the patients were found to have immunoglobulin G (IgG)–class but not immunoglobulin M (IgM)–class antibodies to HAV, which indicated that they had been infected with HAV in the past and were presumably immune to reinfection. Therefore, the investigators concluded that another agent must have caused the hepatitis. Three years later, Balayan and co-workers[4] confirmed the existence of a new hepatitis virus with transmission of hepatitis to a volunteer from a patient involved in an outbreak of enterically transmitted non-A, non-B hepatitis in central Asia. The volunteer had preexisting antibody to HAV, developed a severe hepatitis, shed virus-like particles in his feces, and developed antibodies to the virus-like particles during convalescence. Balayan and co-workers[4] also inoculated cynomolgus monkeys with the new virus and again showed virus-like particles and an immune response to the particles in this primate species. The new form of non-A, non-B hepatitis came to be known as epidemic non-A, non-B hepatitis or enterically transmitted non-A, non-B hepatitis, and serologic cross-reactivity between virus particles isolated around the world established that one class of viruses was responsible for most if not all cases.[5] Subsequently, the name of the disease was changed to *hepatitis E* to conform with the accepted nomenclature for the other types of viral hepatitis, and the virus was designated *hepatitis E virus*. The subsequent isolation of molecular clones of parts of the HEV genome by Reyes and colleagues[1] provided the basis for development of the first practical tools for diagnosis of the disease.

Virus

MOLECULAR VIROLOGY

Virions of HEV are nonenveloped, icosahedral particles of around 32-nm diameter, without any obvious distinguishing morphology (Fig. 177-1). HEV has a buoyant density of 1.35 to 1.40 g/cm³ in CsCl[4] and a sedimentation coefficient of 183 S.[5] The virus appears to be relatively stable to environmental and chemical agents.[6] HEV is not present in large amounts in clinical material (bile and feces), and yields from

cell culture are generally very low, which has limited the opportunities for characterization of authentic viral particles. However, cell culture systems now reveal many molecular details of virus replication. Propagation of HEV was first seen in primary macaque hepatocytes,[7] but more robust cell culture systems have been reported in recent years. The first of these uses a subclone of hepatocyte-derived HepG2 cells, and although virus yields remain low, it has allowed some key questions of virus replication to be addressed[8-11] and has provided a system for the study of virus neutralization.[12] Growth and serial passage of a particular isolate of HEV has also been described in hepatocyte-derived PLC/PRF/5 cells[13]; this system has allowed some preliminary characterization of progeny virus particles.[14]

Hepatitis E virus has a single-stranded RNA genome of positive polarity that contains three open reading frames (ORFs), organized as 5'-ORF1-ORF3-ORF2-3' (Fig. 177-2), with ORF3 and ORF2 largely overlapping. The prototype infectious complementary DNA (cDNA) clone of the SAR55 strain is 7204 nucleotide (nt).[15] Full-length HEV sequences deposited in Genbank range in size up to 7251 nt plus the poly A tail. The 5' end of the genome has a 7-methylguanosine cap[16] that is essential for infectivity,[15] and the genome contains short, highly conserved 5' and 3' untranslated regions (UTRs) of 35 and 68 to 75 nt, respectively.

Early studies described the presence of two subgenomic viral RNAs in the liver of infected macaques that were presumed to encode the ORF2 and ORF3 proteins separately.[17] However, the development of functional replicons of HEV RNA has recently allowed the identification of a single subgenomic RNA that functions as a bicistronic messenger RNA (mRNA) for translation of both ORF2 and ORF3 proteins.[11]

Translation of ORF1 yields a polyprotein (PORF1) of approximately 186 kd that contains sequence motifs consistent with methyltransferase, papain-like protease, RNA helicase, and RNA-dependent RNA polymerase (RDRP) activities.[17] The putative HEV protease may require other cofactors because expression of PORF1 alone in HepG2 cells or in an in vitro translation system failed to show any proteolytic processing into mature products.[18]

The PORF3 is a basic protein with an isoelectric point around 12.5 and is the most variable protein between HEV strains. PORF3 appears to be initiated from the third in-frame AUG codon,[19] with a mass of around 11 to 13 kd. PORF3 is associated with the cytoskeleton and is phosphorylated at serine residue 80 by mitogen activated protein kinase.[20] A large number of host cell protein interactions have been reported for PORF3,[21-25] but the specific biologic role of these interactions has not been determined.

The role of PORF3 in viral replication remained unclear for many years, with conflicting results on whether the protein was essential for replication. This conflict was resolved with the discovery of a specific RNA structure that is essential for replication, the cis-reactive element (CRE) in the open reading frame for PORF3.[26] Mutations that abolished PORF3 synthesis without affecting the RNA structure of the CRE allowed replication in cell culture,[10] but translation of PORF3 was essential for infectivity in nonhuman primates.[26] PORF3 may play a role in virus release to allow amplification in the liver,[10] with some recent data that provided evidence for PORF3 associated with HEV virions from cell culture[14] consistent with this putative role. Phosphorylation does not appear to be essential for these functions.[26]

The capsid protein (PORF2) is translated as a 660 amino acid (aa) protein. A large proportion of the nascent protein is modified by

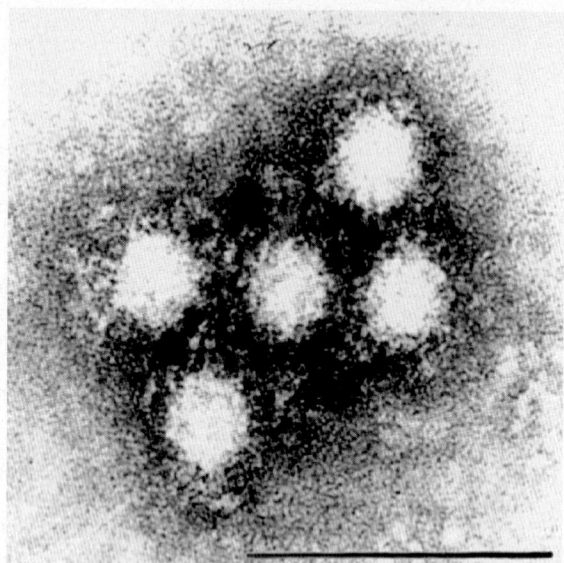

Figure 177-1 Antibody-coated hepatitis E virus particles detected in feces of a patient with hepatitis E in Pakistan (immune electron microscopy). *(Modified from Ticehurst J, Popkin TJ, Bryan JP, et al. Association of hepatitis E virus with an outbreak of hepatitis in Pakistan: Serologic responses and pattern of virus excretion. J Med Virol. 1992;36:84-92.)*

N-glycosylation after heterologous expression in mammalian cells,[27] but this glycosylated form of the protein is highly unstable.[28] When PORF2 is expressed in insect cells, it is cleaved at a predominant site between aa 111 and 112 and at various sites within the C-terminus of the protein. At least some of these truncated forms of PORF2 have the ability to self assemble into virus-like particles (VLPs) or subviral particles (SVPs),[29-32] and cryoelectron microscopy has revealed structural details of such particles.[33,34] Conversely, a protein the size of full-length, nonglycosylated PORF2 has been detected in HEV replicon cell lines.[35] Further studies of native virus particles are necessary to determine whether the native capsid protein is full-length or truncated, and glycosylated or nonglycosylated, but yields from cell culture remain too low for detailed studies.

Expression of truncated PORF2 (aa 112 to 636) in the baculovirus system leads to the formation of HEV VLPs.[29,36,37] These VLPs are smaller than the intact virus particle (27 versus 32 nm), but cryoelectron microscopy[33,34,38] suggests that HEV VLPs are assembled as a T = 1, icosahedral particle that contains 30 dimeric subunits of 50 kd PORF2, with the potential to form an intact virion of the correct size with a T = 3 arrangement of 90 dimeric subunits.[33] PORF2 dimerization appears to be the result of noncovalent interactions in the C-terminal part of the protein.[34,39,40]

CLASSIFICATION

Hepatitis E virus was tentatively assigned to the Caliciviridae family for some years on the basis of its particle structure and overall genome organization. However, detailed analysis of the viral genome showed that it had many features that were inconsistent with classification in any existing virus family,[41] and HEV has now been assigned to the new genus *Hepevirus*, family Hepeviridae.[42] A related virus of chickens (avian HEV)[43,44] is the only other family member known at this time.

GEOGRAPHIC DISTRIBUTION AND GENETIC VARIATION

Although rare cases of sporadic HEV have been reported from many developed countries, the major disease burden of HEV is in developing countries, consistent with its enteric transmission. The Indian subcon-

tinent, Egypt, and parts of China are recognized as highly endemic areas, with HEV the most common cause of acute hepatitis in these countries. HEV has been responsible for major epidemics in refugee settings in Darfur, Sudan, over the past several years.[45-47] Sporadic HEV has been reported in South Africa, Chad, Tunisia, and Morocco[45-47] and is likely to be prevalent throughout the African continent. The prevalence of HEV in South America has been the subject of only isolated studies,[48-50] but studies in Cuba have shown quite high prevalence of clinical HEV infection.[51,52] Epidemic HEV has also been reported in Mexico.[53] In many developing countries, the incidence and prevalence of HEV infection has not been examined, and countries with poor sanitation should be assumed to have a high risk for endemic HEV infection and disease. The distribution of HEV within endemic countries can be highly variable, providing ideal conditions for epidemics in conditions of population displacement when combined with poor sanitary conditions, such as in refugee camps or in army recruits.

Strains of HEV recovered from within one geographic region generally are genetically similar and characteristic of that region and differ from strains indigenous to other regions.[54-60] However, all human strains recovered to date appear to belong to the same serotype.[5] Comparison of HEV sequences provides the basis for classification of strains into genotypes, with around 75% nucleotide identities between genotypes (Fig. 177-3).[61-64] Genotype 1 includes the prototype Burmese HEV[1,17] and related strains (including most Chinese strains), and genotype 2 is represented by the Mexican strain[65] and has also been detected in Africa,[66,67] where it cocirculates with genotype 1.[68] Genotype 3 includes the prototype swine HEV strain discovered in the United States[69] and closely related strains isolated from patients infected in the United States.[58] Genotype 4 includes isolates from a minority of patients in China (T1 strain)[61] and both patients and swine in Taiwan.[70,71] The strong relationship between swine and human HEV isolates in the United States,[58,69] Taiwan,[70,71] Korea,[72] and Japan[73,74] is

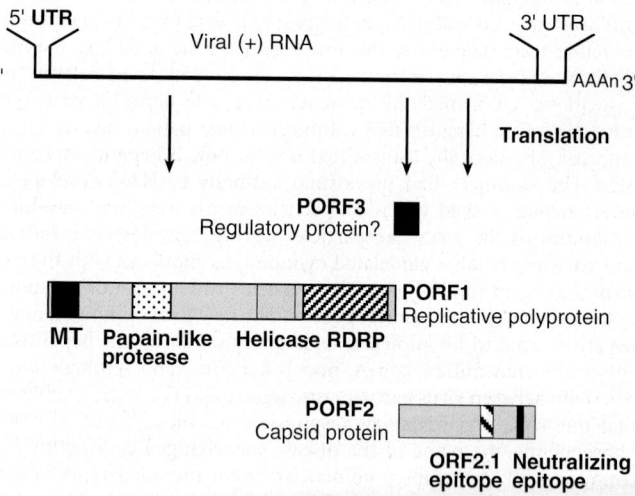

Figure 177-2 Genome organization and major antigenic domains of HEV. Genome of around 7200 nucleotides contains 5′ 7-methylguanosine cap and highly conserved 5′ and 3′ untranslated regions (UTRs) of 35 and 68 to 75 nt, respectively. Three open reading frames (ORFs), organized as 5′-ORF1-ORF3-ORF2-3′, encode viral proteins. PORF1 polyprotein contains replicative proteins. PORF2 is the major capsid protein, and the function of PORF3 is unknown but dispensable for replication in vitro. Both PORF2 and PORF3 are translated from single bicistronic, subgenomic RNA. Linear antigenic domains have been identified with peptide scanning throughout each of the three proteins; within PORF2, a conformational, immunodominant epitope (ORF2.1 epitope) is found between aa 394 to 457, and a conformational, neutralizing epitope is found between aa 578 to 607. *(Modified from Anderson DA, Shrestha IL. Hepatitis E virus. In: Richman DD, Whitley RJ, Hayden FG, eds. Clinical Virology. Washington, DC: ASM Press; 2008:1127-1143.)*

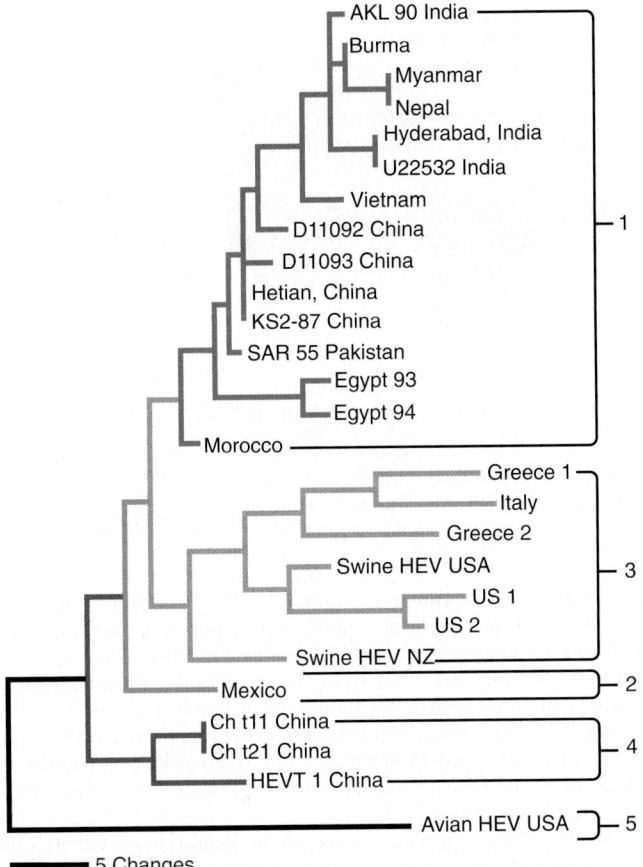

5 Changes

Figure 177-3 Genetic diversity of hepatitis E virus strains. Five major genotypes have been identified. Genotype 1 is found in Asia, the Middle East, and North Africa. Genotype 2 has been found in Mexico and Nigeria. Genotype 3 has been recovered from humans in North and South America, Europe, and Japan and from swine in North America, Europe, Asia, and New Zealand. Genotype 4 has been recovered from humans and swine in Asia. Genotype 5 has been recovered from chickens in North America and Australia. *(Modified from Haqshenas G, Shivaprasad HL, Woolcock PR, et al. Genetic identification and characterization of a novel virus related to human hepatitis E virus from chickens with hepatitis- splenomegaly syndrome in the United States. J Gen Virol. 2001;82:2449-2462.)*

consistent with presumed zoonotic exposure and shows the importance of viral genotypes in helping to understand the epidemiology of HEV infection, especially in nonendemic countries. Avian HEV shares only around 50% nucleotide sequence identity but also shows some antigenic cross-reactivity with human and swine strains.[44] Avian HEV has not yet been formally classified; it is currently considered as genotype 5 in the *Hepevirus* genus (see Fig. 177-3) but might also be considered to represent a separate genus, as in the case of the mammalian and avian hepatitis B viruses.

ANTIGENIC COMPOSITION

The capsid (PORF2) protein is the major, if not only, structural protein of HEV and represents the most relevant antigen for diagnosis and prevention. Mammalian genotypes of HEV exist as a single serotype with cross-genotype serologic protection. Immunization of macaques with recombinant PORF2 proteins of 55 kd (soluble, 112 to 607 aa) or 62 kd (VLP, 112 to 636 aa) expressed with a baculovirus system confers immunity to both homologous and heterologous virus challenge,[37,75-77] which suggests that major protective epitopes are common among HEV genotypes. A major neutralizing epitope has been identified in

the region of amino acids 458 to 607 in PORF2 and shows equivalent reactivity with all genotypes.[78] The enzyme-linked immunosorbent assay (ELISA) based on this antigen should prove useful in clinical vaccine development.

A distinct immunodominant, conformational PORF2 epitope has also been identified in the region of amino acids 394 to 457,[79] although its formation is dependent on expression of the longer HEV fragment from 394 to approximately 660 because of the requirement for dimerization. This ORF2.1 epitope is highly conserved between HEV strains and represents as much as 60% of the total HEV-specific antibody repertoire,[79] properties that have contributed to development of improved commercial diagnostic tests.[80-82]

In contrast to these conserved epitopes, type-specific epitopes in PORF2 and PORF3 were first reported by Yarbough and colleagues[83] in comparisons of the Burmese and Mexican strains of HEV. Antibody responses to these type-specific epitopes also vary between patients infected with the same types, which compromises their performance in diagnostic assays. However, pools of type-specific peptide epitopes (PORF2 and PORF3) are used in a number of commercially available diagnostic assays, and a mosaic protein that encodes multiple peptide epitopes[84,85] has also shown some utility.

Cell culture neutralization assays have been reported but are difficult to perform.[12,86] However, these have provided further evidence for the existence of a single serotype with cross-neutralization of genotype 1 virus seen with sera from animals infected with each of the four genotypes.[12,86]

EPIDEMIOLOGY

Developing Countries

In endemic countries, sporadic HEV infection is often the most common form of viral hepatitis on an annual basis (Fig. 177-4). HEV is responsible for at least 25% of sporadic hepatitis between epidemics in northern India,[87] with other estimates as high as 70% in Kathmandu, Nepal.[88]

Major epidemics also occur with a period of around 7 to 10 years. For example, HEV was responsible for 16 of 17 epidemics of enterically transmitted hepatitis in India.[89] In general, epidemics are associated with the wet season (summer in most endemic countries). Large outbreaks of HEV were seen after flooding that coincided with the conflict and displacement of 1.8 million civilians in the Darfur region of Sudan.[45,46] From July to December 2004, 2621 hepatitis E cases were recorded in the Mornay refugee camp of 78,800 inhabitants (an attack rate of 3.3%), with an overall case-fatality rate of 1.7%.

In many studies, the prevalence of anti-HEV in infants and children has been much lower than expected for a virus transmitted via the fecal-oral route.[90-92] The greatest incremental increase in the prevalence of anti-HEV has generally been found among young adults, the age group at the highest risk of clinical disease (Figs. 177-5 and 177-6).[90-94] In older adults from regions in which the virus is endemic, the prevalence of anti-HEV is relatively constant (10% to 40%), with little or no difference in the prevalence between men and women.[90-92] Although such a pattern of age-specific anti-HEV might suggest a cohort effect representing the disappearance of HEV from endemic regions, as was seen for HAV previously,[95] similar age-specific anti-HEV patterns have been reported for sera collected 10 years apart from the same population in an area that is highly endemic for HEV (see Fig. 177-5).[90-92] Thus, HEV appears to have epidemiologic characteristics that are quite different from those of most viruses, such as HAV, that are transmitted via the fecal-oral route.

In many developing countries with endemic HEV, most of the population has been exposed to HAV during childhood (see Fig. 177-5), when clinical attack rates are low. As such, clinical hepatitis in young and older adults is more likely to be hepatitis E than hepatitis A. However, in countries with endemic HEV and intermediate rates of HAV exposure (such as Cuba), sporadic cases and outbreaks can result from contamination of water supplies with both enterically transmitted viruses, resulting in dual infection.[52]

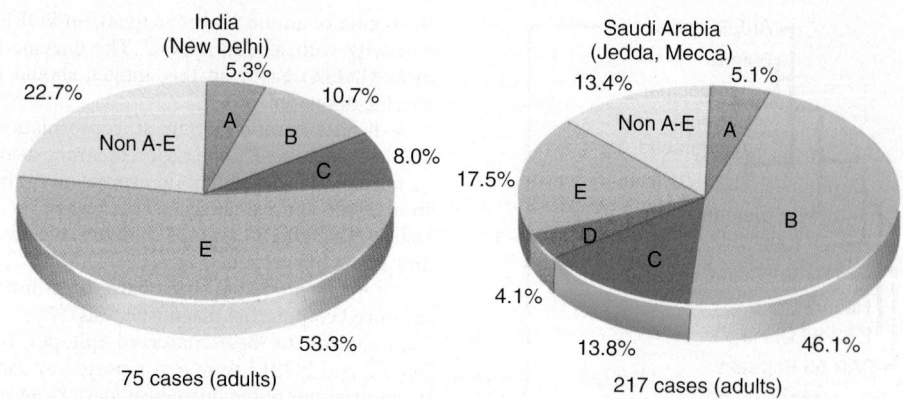

Figure 177-4 **Importance of hepatitis E virus (HEV) in etiology of viral hepatitis in regions where the virus is endemic.** HEV is the most important cause of sporadic hepatitis among adults (and the second most important cause among children) in Asia and the second most important cause among adults (after hepatitis B virus) in the Middle East and North Africa. Hepatitis of unknown etiology is important in both regions. *(Adapted from Das K, Agarwal A, Andrew R, et al. Role of hepatitis E and other hepatotropic virus in aetiology of sporadic acute viral hepatitis: A hospital-based study from urban Delhi. Eur J Epidemiol. 2000;16:937-940; and Ghabrah TM, Strickland GT, Tsarev S, et al. Acute viral hepatitis in Saudi Arabia: Seroepidemiological analysis, risk factors, clinical manifestation, and evidence for a sixth hepatitis agent. Clin Infect Dis. 1995;21:621-627.)*

Developed Countries

In developed countries, sporadic clinical HEV is rare, and epidemics have not been reported. Clinical HEV infection in nonendemic, developed countries is often associated with recent travel to endemic areas, but indigenous cases are also detected. Swine HEV strains have a worldwide distribution, and infection in pigs from both commercial farms and wild populations is almost ubiquitous.[70,72,73,96-99] Swine HEV has been shown to cross species,[100] and the close genetic relationship between swine HEV and strains isolated from some patients in the United States,[58,69] Taiwan,[70,71] Korea,[72] and Japan[73,74] is consistent with a zoonotic source of these indigenous infections, although swine may not be the only reservoir. As such, HEV infection should be considered a possibility in patients with acute hepatitis who do not have a relevant travel history or markers of other hepatitis viruses.

The true rate of subclinical HEV infections in developed countries remains controversial. Serologic assays based on truncated PORF2 protein (aa 112 to 660) expressed with the baculovirus system have yielded seroprevalence rates of more than 20% in blood donors from Baltimore,[101] similar to the rates observed in Saudi Arabia with pre-sumed high rates of endemic infection.[102] These assays may therefore overestimate exposure rates in nonendemic populations. Conversely, with an ELISA based on the ORF2.1 protein (aa 394 to 660) expressed in *Escherichia coli*, rates of less than 2% were found in Australian blood donors compared with more than 35% in highly endemic Nepal.[103] This assay also showed significant differences in exposure rates between urban (low-risk) and indigenous rural (high-risk) populations in Malaysia.[104] The ORF2.1-based assays may therefore provide a better estimate of exposure to HEV.

The avian HEV appears to share some antigenic cross-reactivity with human HEV strains,[43,105] and rats have also been implicated as a potential reservoir of HEV.[106] Exposure to these HEV-like viruses and cross-reactive antibody may contribute to the high seroprevalence estimates in developed countries with some assays. Further studies are needed to resolve the true rate of HEV exposure in these populations.

MODES OF TRANSMISSION

Hepatitis E is transmitted via the fecal-oral route. Consumption of water contaminated with human fecal waste is by far the most common route of transmission for clinical cases in countries where HEV is endemic, although foodborne outbreaks had been reported in China before the advent of specific serologic assays for HEV infection.

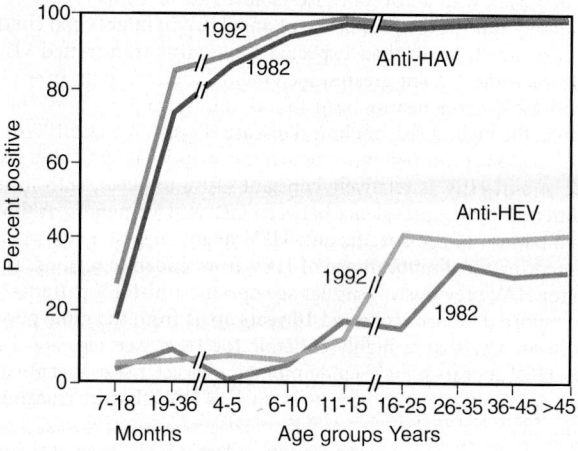

Figure 177-5 **Age-specific prevalences of antibodies to hepatitis A virus and hepatitis E virus in a population in Pune, India.** Antibodies were measured with enzyme-linked immunosorbent assay (ELISA). Infection with hepatitis A virus occurred at an earlier age and in a higher proportion of the population than infection with hepatitis E virus. *(Modified from Arankalle VA, Tsarev SA, Chadha MS, et al. Age-specific prevalence of antibodies to hepatitis A and E viruses in Pune, India, 1982 and 1992. J Infect Dis. 1995;171:447-450.)*

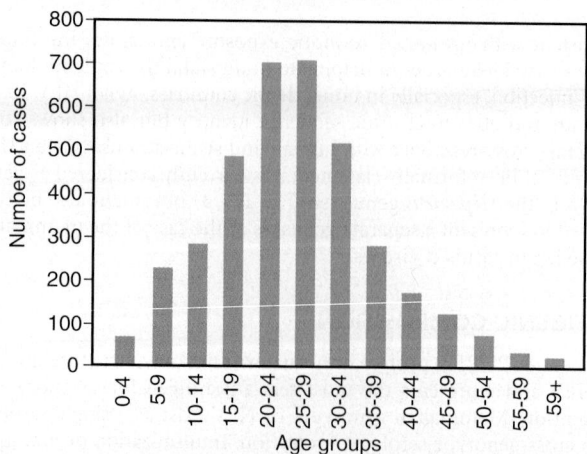

Figure 177-6 **Age-specific clinical attack rate of hepatitis in a large, waterborne epidemic of hepatitis in Delhi, India, 1955 to 1956.** Epidemic was caused by hepatitis E virus. *(Modified from Viswanathan R. Epidemiology. Indian J Med Res. 1957;45:1-29. Copyright © 1957 Indian Council of Medical Research.)*

Most human isolates of HEV in countries where the virus is not considered endemic are found to be more closely related to swine HEV strains (Meng[107] provides a comprehensive review of zoonotic HEV infection). Clearly defined cases of zoonotic HEV infection in Japan have been associated with consumption of HEV-infected pig or deer meat, and swine HEV has been detected in both wild pigs and deer in Japan.[73,99,108-110] However, in most nonendemic countries, the true rate of zoonotic infection remains unclear because of limited testing.

Hepatitis E is not commonly transmitted via person-to-person contact (in contrast to hepatitis A), so household transmission is therefore not a significant risk factor. Nosocomial infections with HEV are probably rare, but transfusion-associated HEV has been reported in Japan[111] and is likely to be more common in countries in which the virus is endemic, with viremia of up to 45 to 112 days detected with polymerase chain reaction (PCR) in naturally infected patients.[112,113]

HOST RANGE: EXPERIMENTAL TRANSMISSION TO ANIMALS

Human strains of HEV can readily infect and cause disease in many nonhuman primates, with cynomolgus macaques (*Macaca fascicularis*) and rhesus macaques (*Macaca mulatta*) widely used for experimental purposes and New World monkeys (owl monkeys, squirrel monkeys, and tamarins) also susceptible. The swine HEV was first detected in pigs in the United States[69] and subsequently shown to be endemic in swine worldwide, and in wild deer in Japan.[73,99,108-110] Swine HEV has been transmitted to macaques, and human HEV (genotype 3) to swine.[100,107] Swine do not appear to have clinical or biochemical disease develop after infection with either swine or human isolates of HEV.[114] Rodents and sheep have been reported to be susceptible to experimental infection,[115,116] but these studies need confirmation.

The course of infection in experimentally infected primates is similar to that in humans.[117] The incubation period to peak liver enzyme levels is generally 3 to 8 weeks but can be quite variable, depending on the dose of virus administered.[31,117-120] Peak viremia and peak shedding of virus in the feces occur during the incubation period and early acute phase of disease. The detection of HEV antigens in the liver parallels the detection of viremia in the serum and feces, and histologic changes in the liver generally parallel biochemical evidence of hepatitis.[121] As in humans, hepatitis E in nonhuman primates is acute and self-limiting. Unlike experimental hepatitis caused by the other human hepatitis viruses, experimental hepatitis E is dose dependent: high doses of virus are associated with histologic and biochemical evidence of hepatitis, whereas lower doses of virus (1000 infectious doses) are more likely to be associated with a normal histologic appearance and normal serum liver enzyme values.[122] Infection with HEV protects nonhuman primates from hepatitis E after reexposure to the virus.[123-125] Evidence for fetal wastage was detected in one study but not in a second study of experimental HEV infection of pregnant rhesus monkeys.[126,127]

HEPATITIS E VIRUS INFECTION IN ANIMALS

Although a number of species including rats, sheep, and domestic cattle have been reported to have serologic evidence of exposure to HEV, unequivocal evidence for HEV infection in animals has relied on the detection of virus with PCR. This detection was first achieved in the landmark studies by Meng and colleagues[69] in which an HEV strain isolated from young domestic swine in the United States was experimentally transmissible to other swine. This virus was genetically distinct from all previously recovered human strains and probably represents the first recognized nonhuman strain of HEV. Interestingly, two isolates of HEV from patients with human hepatitis E in Tennessee and Minnesota were shown to be closely related to swine HEV, and one of these was experimentally transmitted to swine.[58,69,128] Because swine HEV and the two human United States isolates were genetically very similar (including sharing specific nucleotide insertions) and

because they came from the same geographic region, all three of the viruses are possibly of swine origin. Although no direct epidemiologic linkage could be drawn between these first identified cases in the United States and exposure to swine, clearly defined cases of zoonotic HEV infection in Japan have been associated with consumption of HEV-infected pig or deer meat.[73,74,99,108-110]

Conversely, zoonotic infection likely plays only a minor role in circulation of HEV in countries where the virus is endemic in human populations. In India, genotype 1 circulates in humans, whereas genotype 4 circulates in swine in the same region.[129,130] However, differences have been observed in the magnitude of antibody responses among patients with acute hepatitis E during the epidemic versus interepidemic season in Nepal, which could possibly represent exposure to zoonotic strains (genotypes 3 and 4) with somewhat lower antibody reactivity to the human genotype 1 proteins used in the assay.[131]

The transmission of animal viruses to humans via transplantation of animal organs and tissues to humans is a potential threat. The prospects for such transmissions have been greatly increased with improvements in procedures to control immediate and delayed rejection of animal organs by the human immune system. With the control of rejection a possibility, growing interest is seen in the xenotransplantation of animal organs and tissues because of the shortage of suitable clinical materials of human origin. The discovery of swine HEV has added another virus to the list of viruses that must be excluded from swine herds before tissues and organs from those herds can be considered for xenotransplantation (Meng[107] provides a more extensive review of HEV risk in xenotransplantation).

Pathogenesis

INCUBATION PERIOD

The incubation period from exposure to the onset of clinical disease is approximately 28 to 40 days, based on analysis of waterborne epidemics in which the time of exposure was identified.[132] In experimental HEV transmission studies in humans, liver enzyme values peaked 42 to 46 days after ingestion of the virus,[4] and in experimental infections of macaques with intravenous challenge and high doses of virus, disease can be evident as early as 2 weeks after exposure[122,133,134] and viremia is detectable with reverse transcriptase-polymerase chain reaction (RT-PCR) as early as 9 days after exposure.[122,134]

VIRAL REPLICATION

Although some progress has been made in understanding the replication cycle of HEV with use of animal models, cell culture systems, and infectious cDNA clones, most aspects of viral replication in vivo can only be inferred (Fig. 177-7). After ingestion of HEV, the virus may be absorbed directly through the gastrointestinal mucosa into the circulation to reach the liver or after one or more rounds of amplification in enterocytes. However, no evidence has been obtained for replication of HEV at this site, in contrast to HAV for which replication in enterocyte-derived Caco2 cells is well established.[135] HEV is likely to interact with one or more specific receptors/coreceptors leading to penetration and uncoating of the virus, and the input viral RNA then serves as mRNA for PORF1. The PORF1 polyprotein is then cleaved by viral (and perhaps cellular) proteases to yield the mature replicative proteins, but the viral protease activity has not been directly demonstrated. The viral RNA-dependent RNA polymerase (RDRP) then copies the input viral genome to yield negative-strand RNA, which in turn serves as a template for the transcription of further positive-strand RNA molecules, including new genomes and the subgenomic, bicistronic RNA encoding ORF2 and ORF3 proteins. Genomic RNA assembles together with PORF2, although the precise form involved in particle assembly (full-length or truncated, glycosylated or nonglycosylated) is unclear. PORF3 may also associate with the virus particle during assembly,[14] although it is dispensable for replication in vitro. The virus is then released from the hepatocyte via unknown mechanisms.

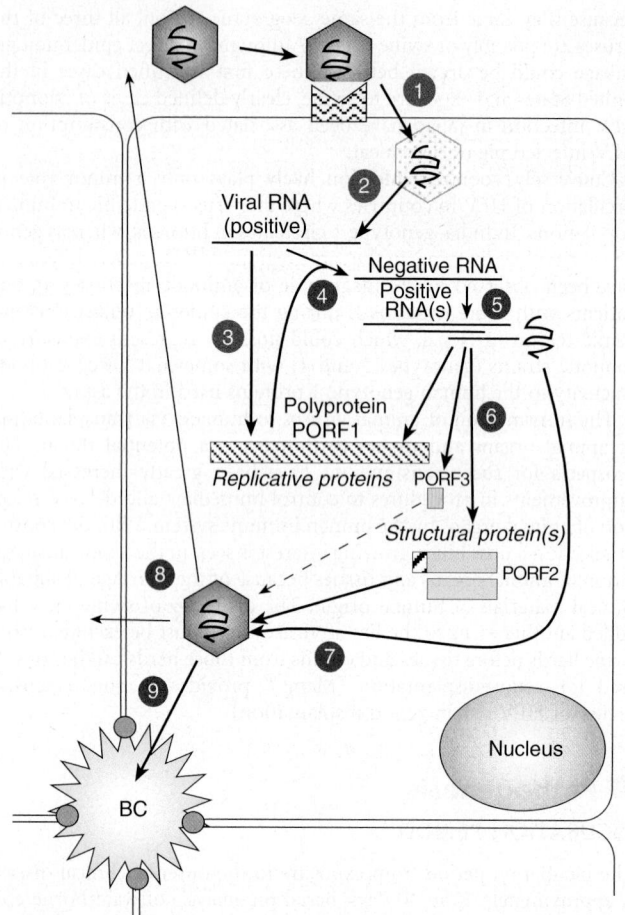

Figure 177-7 Putative replication cycle of hepatitis E virus. After oral ingestion, HEV particles reach the liver where they attach to an unidentified receptor on the basolateral domain of hepatocytes, leading to virus penetration (step 1) and uncoating of the genome (step 2) within the cell. Translation of the input genome (step 3) yields the PORF1 polyprotein, which is cleaved at unknown sites to yield the replicative proteins, which copy the input genome to yield full-length negative strand RNAs (step 4), followed by subgenomic positive strand (messenger) RNAs and full-length positive strand RNAs (new viral genomes; step 5). These subgenomic RNAs are translated to yield further molecules of PORF1, PORF2 (capsid), and PORF3 (regulatory) proteins (step 6). PORF2 and new viral genomes assemble into virions (step 7); whether virions contain full-length or truncated PORF2 products is not known, and the role of membranes and PORF3 in assembly is unclear. Release of progeny virus through basolateral domains of the infected cell (step 8) may result in viremia and infection of distal hepatocytes or infection of neighboring hepatocytes, but transmission to new hosts through the environment is achieved via release of progeny through the apical domain (step 9) to the bile canaliculi (BC) and ultimately the feces. *(Modified from Anderson DA, Shrestha IL. Hepatitis E virus. In: Richman DD, Whitley RJ, Hayden FG, eds. Clinical Virology. Washington, DC: ASM Press; 2008:1127-1143.)*

A small amount of HEV is found in plasma during infection, consistent with release of progeny virus through the basolateral domains of hepatocytes leading to spread through the liver, but most of the virus is likely to be excreted through the biliary system to complete the transmission cycle,[126,134] consistent with release of virus through the apical domain of hepatocytes. Interestingly, however, HAV shows preferential release through the basolateral domain of hepatocytes in vitro, contrary to the similar expectation of its apical release into the biliary system, which suggests an indirect route for excretion of that virus.[136]

Hepatitis E virus replication has not been observed in tissues other than liver, but a low level of replication is likely to occur in enteric epithelium before infection of the liver, as for HAV. Low amounts of HEV can be detected in serum during the late incubation period and for 2 to 6 weeks after the onset of illness. HEV is excreted in feces; virus has not been reported in other excretions.

PATHOLOGY

Histopathologic studies of liver specimens obtained from patients in epidemics have shown that infection with HEV can produce morphologic changes in the liver that comprise both cholestatic and classical acute hepatitis,[137-139] but these features are not unique or diagnostic in hepatitis E. Typical histopathologic changes include lobular disarray with enlargement of portal tracts, Kupffer cell proliferation, focal hepatocyte necrosis and bridging necrosis, ballooning of hepatocytes and acidophilic degeneration of hepatocytes, and mononuclear cell infiltration. Within hepatocytes, dilation occurs of the cisternae of the endoplasmic reticulum with an increase in the number and size of lysosomes within the cytoplasm. Condensation of the matrix within mitochondria together with dilation of the outer mitochondrial membrane has also been reported.

Cholestatic hepatitis E is characterized by bile stasis in canaliculi and gland-like transformation of hepatocytes, degeneration of hepatocytes, and intralobular and portal tract infiltrates of lymphocytes and polymorphonuclear leukocytes. A prominent feature is the presence of cholestasis and glandular transformation of the liver cell plates, with the cholestatic changes persisting until clinical recovery occurs. These histopathologic changes gradually resolve over a period of 3 to 6 months.

Patients with fulminant hepatitis E infection have necrosis of parenchyma with collapse of liver lobules; swelling of hepatocytes, which have a foamy appearance; arrangement of hepatocytes into an acinar pattern; proliferation of small bile ductules; phlebitis of portal and central veins; and portal inflammation with lymphocytic and polymorphonuclear leukocyte infiltration.[138,140,141] HEV replication has also been found also in bile epithelial cells in rhesus monkeys and in many extrahepatic sites in swine,[142,143] but the significance of these extrahepatic sites is unclear.

The average severity of HEV infections is somewhat greater than that of hepatitis A infections, with a mortality rate of around 1%, compared with 0.2% in hepatitis A. However, HEV infection during pregnancy is associated with a high mortality rate from fulminant hepatitis, around 25% in the third trimester.[141,144,145] The mortality rate appears to increase with each succeeding trimester of pregnancy.[146-148]

IMMUNE RESPONSE

The patterns of IgG-class and IgM-class antibody responses during HEV infection are shown in Figure 177-8. These responses are typical of those detected with the 55 to 63 kd ORF2 antigens expressed with a baculovirus system and the ORF2.1 protein expressed in *E. coli*, which can detect specific IgG and IgM responses in most patients. Typically, both IgG and IgM antibodies are detectable at the onset of disease, which allows serologic diagnosis of infection at the time of presentation of the patient; IgM declines to undetectable levels over a period of 2 to 6 months, and an approximately 10-fold decline in IgG levels is seen over this period. Levels then stabilize, but the duration of protective immunity is unknown.

In contrast to the anti-HEV responses shown in Figure 177-8, as few as one in three macaques challenged with a common source inoculum have a detectable IgG response to homologous HEV PORF3 and to many of the linear epitopes in PORF2, and this response is transient.[133] As a result, assays based on these proteins are not suitable for seroepidemiologic studies.

Immunoglobulin A (IgA) responses to HEV (as a correlate of mucosal immunity) have been detected in around 50% of patients[149]; these antibodies rapidly declined to undetectable levels, although IgA may persist somewhat longer than IgM.[150,151] The role of IgA in immunity to HEV infection is unknown, but because passive immunization

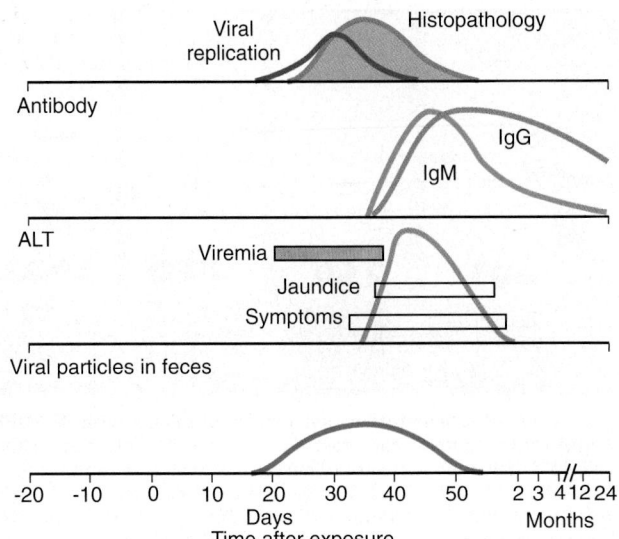

Figure 177-8 Diagram of clinical and serologic events in typical case of acute hepatitis E. Antibody patterns are based on enzyme-linked immunosorbent assay (ELISA) results; viremia and fecal shedding are based on polymerase chain reaction data. After reaching high levels during the acute phase, HEV PORF2-specific IgG declines rapidly over 6 to 12 months and might not persist at protective levels for life, and HEV-specific IgM disappears over 3 to 6 months and is diagnostic for acute HEV infection. *(Modified from Purcell RH, Hoofnagle JH, Ticehurst J, et al. Hepatitis viruses. In: Schmidt NJ, Emmons RW, eds. Diagnostic Procedures for Viral, Rickettsial and Chlamydial Infections. 6th ed. Washington, DC: American Public Health Association; 1989:957-1065.)*

with IgG appears to be sufficient for protection,[75] IgA is likely not essential. Detection of IgA (in addition to IgM) may have some value in diagnosis of HEV, but further studies are needed.[150,151]

Cellular immune responses during HEV infection have not been extensively studied. In patients with HEV, T-cell responses (proliferation) to peptide libraries derived from the PORF2 and PORF3 proteins are observed with peptide pools derived from PORF2 but not PORF3.[152]

Clinical Manifestations

SYMPTOMS

Hepatitis E is clinically indistinguishable from other forms of acute viral hepatitis. The clinical presentation of acute viral hepatitis commonly begins with nonspecific, flu-like prodromal symptoms that last from 1 to 10 days and consist of fatigue, malaise, anorexia, nausea, vomiting, and some alteration in taste and smell. A low-grade fever between 38°C and 39°C is common.

The first distinctive signs of hepatitis are often dark urine and pale clay-colored stools followed by onset of clinical jaundice. With the appearance of clinical jaundice, the prodromal symptoms usually subside; however, some patients may not show visible signs of jaundice despite severe symptoms. Abdominal examination may reveal enlarged and tender liver associated with pain and discomfort in the right upper quadrant. Spleen may be enlarged in 10% to 15% of patients. Occasionally, patients may present with cholestasis, which is more common in pregnant women.

Resolution of HEV is accompanied by normalization of biochemical markers (serum alanine aminotransferase [ALT] levels, bilirubin) over a period of 6 weeks in most patients, whereas histologic changes may persist for up to 6 months without overt disease. Small numbers of patients appear to have a protracted course of disease, with resolution taking many months.

Hepatitis E virus infection during pregnancy is associated with a high mortality rate from fulminant hepatitis that peaks at around 25% in the third trimester.[141,144,145] The basis of the high mortality during pregnancy is not understood; studies in pregnant macaques have not shown any increase in disease severity.[127] Although hormonal factors may contribute to pathogenesis during pregnancy, other factors may also be important, such as the underlying general health status or chronic infection with hepatitis B or C in patients at the time of HEV infection.[153,154] No specific pathogenic factors have yet been identified. Vertical transmission of HEV with severe hepatitis in the infant has been seen.[153,154] HEV has not been associated with congenital abnormalities.

Liver function tests are an important adjunct to diagnosis of acute HEV. The serum aminotransferases ALT and aspartate aminotransferase (AST) show variable increases during the prodromal phase. The ALT level peaks at the onset of symptoms before the serum bilirubin begins to increase. Peak levels of ALT vary from 1000 U/L to 2000 U/L at the onset. ALT levels progressively diminish during the recovery phase. Some patients with anicteric acute HEV infection have only raised ALT levels.

Jaundice is visible in sclera or skin when the serum total bilirubin level exceeds 2.5 mg/dL, usually following the peak levels of ALT. Peak serum total bilirubin levels range from 5 to 25 mg/dL; both conjugated and unconjugated fractions are increased. In cholestatic HEV infection (around 10% of patients), serum bilirubin may remain elevated for prolonged periods.

Prothrombin time may be increased in acute viral hepatitis, especially in fulminant hepatitis, indicating extensive hepatocellular necrosis and a worse prognosis. Similarly, a reduction in the serum albumin level may occur. Reduced blood glucose levels leading to hypoglycemia may be observed in patients with prolonged nausea, vomiting, and inadequate carbohydrate intake. Neutropenia, lymphopenia and atypical lymphocytes may occasionally be observed during the acute phase of viral hepatitis.

COMPLICATIONS

The risk and severity of clinical HEV disease increases with age at exposure, as with hepatitis A. Fever as the presenting sign of hepatitis E may be more common in the young. A major complication of HEV infection is fulminant hepatitis, observed in less than 1% of patients from the general population but in up to 30% during the third trimester of pregnancy, with a death rate as high as 100%.[153,154] Cholestatic hepatitis is seen in around 10% to 25% of patients,[155] with a prolonged period of cholestasis observed in some studies. Evidence shows that HEV infection contributes to fetal death and other complications when the mother has symptomatic hepatitis E,[141,145] but the situation with subclinical infections is unclear.

Laboratory Diagnosis

Acute hepatitis E has no distinguishing clinical characteristics that allow a differential diagnosis from other forms of acute viral hepatitis, and the detection of rare cases of locally acquired HEV in nonendemic countries argues for HEV to be considered in many cases of acute hepatitis, even without a relevant travel history to regions where the virus is endemic. Because of their identical clinical presentation and predominant modes of transmission, hepatitis E may be suspected in the same circumstances as hepatitis A. However, despite declining rates of hepatitis A infection through widespread use of inactivated hepatitis A vaccines, HAV infection remains more common than HEV infection in most developed countries because of much higher rates of HAV transmission through personal contact. Although more sensitive serologic assays are now available for detection of HEV IgM as a marker of acute infection, a low level of false-positive results (around 0.3% to 2%) is still detected in these assays, and the more common agents (HAV, hepatitis B virus, hepatitis C virus) should first be excluded for patients in nonendemic countries who do not have a relevant travel history or other exposure risk. Conversely, in endemic countries, HEV is often the most common cause of acute hepatitis and should be a first-line test. In those developing countries in which improved public health has resulted in a high prevalence of young adults who remain susceptible to HAV infection, waterborne epidemics may be caused by HAV or HEV. Unusually severe hepatitis in pregnant women suggests hepatitis E, but tests for both viruses may be prudent, given their potential for cocirculation in some populations.[52] Early detection of epidemic HEV can also allow improved public health responses, in particular the protection of pregnant women from exposure to contaminated water where possible.

Specific diagnosis of HEV infection remains problematic. A variety of serologic and molecular assays are used in research laboratories,[62] but routine (commercial) diagnostic assays vary widely in sensitivity and specificity. Virus isolation and detection of viral antigen are not appropriate for diagnosis of HEV because of low sensitivity.

SEROLOGIC TESTS

A number of research and commercial immunoassays are available in various countries but have shown major differences in sensitivity and specificity.[156] More recent commercial assays appear to have improved on this performance through the use of better recombinant antigens and assay formats (detailed subsequently), but first-generation and second-generation tests are still commercially available in most parts of the world. The appropriate use and interpretation of serologic assays for HEV infection must take into account the quality of different tests and the widely varying prevalence of clinical HEV infection worldwide.[88]

Diagnosis of Hepatitis E Virus Infection in Areas of Low or Intermediate Prevalence

In areas with a low incidence of clinical HEV infection (such as the United States, Australia, and western Europe) or intermediate prevalence (such as Japan, Korea, and Taiwan), assay specificity has a large impact on the predictive value of HEV serologic tests. Diagnostic assays for the detection of HEV-specific IgG (manufactured by Genelabs Diagnostics/MP Biomedicals Asia Pacific, Singapore, and Abbott Diagnostics, Chicago) have considerable value for the diagnosis of acute hepatitis in travelers returned from endemic areas,[157] among whom the incidence rate may be higher than the background rate of reactivity, around 2% in the healthy population. However, with the recognition that HEV should be considered in the diagnosis of sporadic acute hepatitis *without* a travel history to recognized endemic regions,[58,158] the need for more specific tests becomes evident.

The detection of HEV-specific IgM should therefore become the method of choice for serologic diagnosis of acute HEV infection in areas of low prevalence. Until recently, a single HEV IgM assay was commercially available in most countries (Genelabs Diagnostics/MP Biomedicals Asia Pacific), based on the same recombinant HEV antigens as the widely available IgG tests. This assay had a reported false-positive rate in U.S. blood donors of 26/856 (3%) (Genelabs, 1998 technical bulletin), which made it no more suitable than HEV IgG for diagnosis in nonendemic areas. Published studies have also shown that the recombinant antigens used in this assay may fail to detect antibody in around 40% of patients with acute HEV infection.[36]

Enzyme-linked immunosorbent assays with improved reactivity are in use in research laboratories, based on recombinant antigens derived from baculovirus-based[29,30,36,78,159] or *E. coli*–based expression systems,[84,103] but these have not been widely adopted for commercially available assays. However, the ORF2.1 antigen, representing amino acids 394 to 660 derived from a Chinese strain of HEV expressed in *E. coli*,[103,133,160] has been shown to represent immunodominant and highly conserved epitopes of HEV[79] and forms the basis of the recently developed commercial HEV IgM ELISA 3.0 and the ASSURE rapid point of care (RPOC) tests produced by MP Biomedicals Asia Pacific (formerly Genelabs Diagnostics). In the first published study of these new tests, the IgM ELISA 3.0 showed sensitivity of 99.3% (150/151

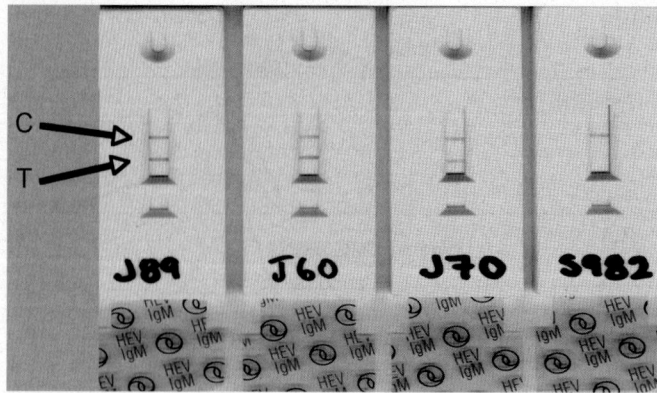

Figure 177-9 **Representative test results obtained with ASSURE HEV IgM rapid point of care test.** Sample with no detectable HEV-specific IgM (S982) shows single line (control, C), and samples with HEV-specific IgM (J89, J60, J70) show both control and test (T) lines (data from the authors' laboratories). *(Modified from Anderson DA, Shrestha IL. Hepatitis E virus. In: Richman DD, Whitley RJ, Hayden FG. Clinical Virology. Washington, DC: ASM Press; 2008:1127-1143.)*

patients with HEV infection) and specificity of 97.6% (203/208 control subjects), and the RPOC test showed slightly reduced sensitivity (96.7%; 146/151) and slightly higher specificity (98.6%; 205/208) on the same samples.[80] In a separate study of the HEV IgM RPOC test, in which the comparator assay was an in-house quantitative IgM ELISA based on baculovirus-expressed HEV antigen,[159] the RPOC assay was also found to have high sensitivity (93%; 186/200) and specificity (99.7%; 320/321).[161] The RPOC test takes around 5 minutes in total and requires minimal training and no specialized equipment; representative assay results with the ASSURE HEV IgM test are shown in Figure 177-9. The sensitivity of both the HEV IgM ELISA 3.0 and the ASSURE HEV IgM tests is clearly adequate for diagnosis of acute HEV infection, but the likely false-positive rate of between 0.3% and 2.4% urges some caution in the interpretation of positive results from patients without a history of travel outside areas of lowest endemicity. Where available, RT-PCR can provide useful confirmation.

Compared with the United States and most of western Europe, larger numbers of HEV cases have been reported from Taiwan,[70,71] Korea,[72] and Japan.[73,74] Serologic diagnosis with HEV IgM tests is likely to have a higher positive predictive value in these populations than in the United States and other countries of lowest endemicity.

Serologic detection of HEV infection in animals also poses a challenge; the quality of species-specific antibody conjugates and variable background reactivity can be problematic. Hu and colleagues[82] have recently described a double-antigen sandwich-based ELISA for total anti-HEV antibodies, in which ET2.1 antigen (equivalent to ORF2.1) and its peroxidase-labeled counterpart are able to detect antibody from patients and from pigs; this assay should prove useful in the search for potential zoonotic reservoirs of HEV or HEV-like viruses.

Diagnosis of Hepatitis E Virus Infection in Areas of High Prevalence

Although the titer of HEV-specific IgG tends to decline markedly in the first year after infection, this relationship is not reliable enough to form the basis of differential diagnosis.[102,103] The detection of HEV-specific IgG is therefore of little use for diagnosis of acute infection in developing countries where HEV is endemic and where large numbers of patients have antibody from past infections. Detection of HEV-specific IgM must therefore be the method of choice in endemic areas.

Because HEV accounts for as much as 70% of the acute sporadic hepatitis in endemic countries, the specificity of assays is less critical than assay sensitivity in these settings. In addition, HEV often is seen in areas where standard equipment, such as ELISA washers and readers, is not available. In this context, the ASSURE HEV IgM rapid point of care test (see Fig. 177-9) appears especially suitable for use in HEV-endemic areas, with sensitivity and specificity substantially equivalent to both the commercial IgM ELISA 3.0 based on the same antigen[80] and a quantitative research ELISA.[161] Although these studies have been performed with pedigreed sera and plasma samples, the ASSURE test is designed for use with fresh whole blood, which further enhances its utility for resource-poor and emergency settings. Further studies are necessary to confirm the expected performance of the test in these settings.

Although the HEV IgM RPOC test can offer equivalent performance to ELISAs, many laboratories have a preference for the more traditional ELISA format for serologic tests. The MP Biomedicals HEV IgM ELISA 3.0 based on ORF2.1 antigen shows greatly improved sensitivity over the former Genelabs Diagnostics/MP Biomedicals HEV IgM ELISA[80] and is progressively replacing that test in most countries, although it is not currently available in the United States. Commercially available ELISA-based HEV IgM kits manufactured by ADALTIS (Italy) and BIOKIT (Spain) are available in many developing countries, but to date, no published evaluations of assay performance for these tests have been seen.

MOLECULAR TESTS

Detection of HEV RNA in serum with reverse transcription-polymerase chain reaction (RT-PCR) provides the gold standard in specificity for diagnosis of acute hepatitis E but is not suitable for routine use, especially in most areas where the virus is endemic or in refugee settings. RT-PCR has been useful in research situations for the detection of divergent HEV strains where the serologic responses may not have been detected with some assays.[61,67,68,71,158] RT-PCR remains an important research-level confirmatory assay for positive HEV IgM tests in nonendemic countries,[62] but its sensitivity is constrained by the limited duration and level of viremia and the stability of HEV RNA in samples. In addition, primers for RT-PCR must be selected carefully because HEV is genetically heterogeneous. Primers located in highly conserved regions of the genome or degenerate primers must be used to ensure detection of all recognized variants of HEV.

Immunity

Antibody is sufficient for protection against clinical hepatitis E, as shown with successful passive immunization of macaques.[75] In addition, the presence of anti-HEV IgG was found to correlate with resistance to clinical hepatitis in cohorts exposed to HEV in waterborne epidemics.[162] However, the duration of antibody-based protection is not known and may not be lifelong in view of the declining levels of total IgG seen in most patients over time (see Fig. 177-8).

Prevention

GENERAL SANITATION

The most significant influence on HEV infection in developing countries is protection of water supplies from contamination with human fecal waste, although zoonotic reservoirs may play a minor role in these settings. Many epidemics in developing countries have occurred from leakage of sewerage pipes into municipal water supply pipes laid in the same or adjacent trenches. A barrier between these two supplies is essential for long-term prevention. Chlorination and filtration systems are generally inadequate if the source water is contaminated. Travelers to endemic regions must take precautions against the consumption of contaminated water. Although infection via food appears to be much less common for hepatitis E than for hepatitis A, travelers must maintain vigilance about the risks of contaminated water, ice, and food. Women should avoid unnecessary travel to endemic areas during pregnancy.

Outbreaks are most often associated with massive contamination of water supplies, commonly from weather conditions that cannot be controlled. This situation is especially problematic in refugee or other emergency settings. The Darfur outbreaks of 2004 were explosive, with the first cases occurring in July and reaching a peak only 6 weeks later.[45,46] Little opportunity is offered for active immunization in control of outbreaks once they have commenced. The recommended procedures for chlorination of water supplies appeared to be inadequate to control HEV in this outbreak, although no bacteria were present in the chlorinated water samples tested.[46] Special efforts should be taken to supply pregnant women with safe water during outbreaks. These studies highlight the need for timely detection of acute HEV in such settings, and the ASSURE HEV IgM rapid test has proven suitable for this purpose (Greg Armstrong, Centers for Disease Control [CDC], personal communication, 2005).

High levels of public sanitation together with the low secondary transmission rate of HEV contribute to the low incidence of clinical HEV infection in developed countries. Interestingly, one study found no association between risk factors for enterically transmitted viruses and the high rate of HEV seroprevalence observed with the baculovirus-based HEV IgG assay in populations from the Untied States,[101] which suggests that exposure to HEV or HEV-like viruses in this setting may represent a different route of transmission, unrelated to poor sanitation.

IMMUNOPROPHYLAXIS

Passive immunization has the potential to protect against disease,[75] but gamma globulin prepared in nonendemic countries is ineffective, and even pools prepared in endemic countries may offer little or no protective efficacy.[53,163] Protective neutralizing monoclonal antibodies[12,164,165] and epitopes[12,164,165] have now been characterized. The development of an ELISA specific for the protective epitopes[78] may allow identification of suitable high-titer plasma pools in the future, and the neutralizing monoclonal antibodies could possibly provide the basis for passive immunoprophylaxis.

Prospects for active immunization are promising. Vaccines based on the PORF2 protein (amino acids 112 to 607 or 660) expressed in insect cells are clearly protective in animal studies.[37,76,77,166,167] The recombinant 56 kDa vaccine represents amino acids 112 to 607, and studies of this vaccine in Army recruits in Nepal showed that the vaccine was highly effective in this population.[168] A group of 1794 healthy HEV-seronegative adults received three doses of either the 56 kDa vaccine or placebo at months 0, 1, and 6 and was followed for a median of 804 days. Hepatitis E developed in 66 of 896 placebo recipients versus three of 898 vaccine recipients, with an efficacy of 95.5%.[168] The vaccine is hoped to eventually be available for use in countries where HEV poses the greatest disease burden. The duration of vaccine protection is an important consideration for use in endemic populations, and the recent development of an ELISA that appears to be specific for the major neutralizing antibody species in HEV, based on the peptide 458 to 607 (minimum neutralization site), is likely to provide an important tool for such studies.[78]

Other approaches to vaccine development for hepatitis E have been attempted.[169,170] After DNA vaccination with the ORF2 gene, two of four macaques were protected against HEV infection.[170] Codelivery of cytokine genes is reported to augment the immune response to ORF2 DNA.[171] However, any further progress on DNA-based vaccine approaches for HEV is likely to be many years in the future.

Therapy

No specific therapy exists for hepatitis E. Patients should be treated symptomatically as for hepatitis A. Because hepatitis E does not progress to chronicity, attempts to treat with antiviral agents are not warranted.

Sections of this chapter are based in part on the chapter in the 6th edition of Principles and Practice of Infectious Diseases, *coauthored by Robert H. Purcell and Suzanne A. Emerson.*

REFERENCES

1. Reyes GR, Purdy MA, Kim JP, et al. Isolation of a cDNA from the virus responsible for enterically transmitted non-A, non-B hepatitis. *Science*. 1990;247:1335-1339.
2. Khuroo MS. Study of an epidemic of non-A, non-B hepatitis. Possibility of another human hepatitis virus distinct from post-transfusion non-A, non-B type. *Am J Med*. 1980;68:818-824.
3. Wong DC, Purcell RH, Sreenivasan MA, et al. Epidemic and endemic hepatitis in India: evidence for a non-A, non-B hepatitis virus aetiology. *Lancet*. 1980;2:876-879.
4. Balayan MS, Andjaparidze AG, Savinskaya SS, et al. Evidence for a virus in non-A, non-B hepatitis transmitted via the fecal-oral route. *Intervirology*. 1983;20:23-31.
5. Bradley D, Andjaparidze A, Cook EH Jr, et al. Aetiological agent of enterically transmitted non-A, non-B hepatitis. *J Gen Virol*. 1988;69:731-738.
6. Jothikumar N, Aparna K, Kamatchiammal S, et al. Detection of hepatitis E virus in raw and treated wastewater with the polymerase chain reaction. *Applied Environ Microbiol*. 1993;59: 2558-2562.
7. Tam AW, White R, Reed E, et al. In vitro propagation and production of hepatitis E virus from in vivo-infected primary macaque hepatocytes. *Virology*. 1996;215:1-9.
8. Emerson SU, Nguyen H, Graff J, et al. In vitro replication of hepatitis E virus (HEV) genomes and of an HEV replicon expressing green fluorescent protein. *J Virol*. 2004;78:4838-4846.
9. Graff J, Nguyen H, Kasorndorkbua C, et al. In vitro and in vivo mutational analysis of the 3'-terminal regions of hepatitis e virus genomes and replicons. *J Virol*. 2005;79:1017-1026.
10. Emerson SU, Nguyen H, Torian U, et al. ORF3 protein of hepatitis E virus is not required for replication, virion assembly, or infection of hepatoma cells in vitro. *J Virol*. 2006;80:10457-10464.
11. Graff J, Torian U, Nguyen H, et al. A bicistronic subgenomic mRNA encodes both the ORF2 and ORF3 proteins of hepatitis E virus. *J Virol*. 2006;80:5919-5926.
12. Emerson SU, Clemente-Casares P, Moiduddin N, et al. Putative neutralization epitopes and broad cross-genotype neutralization of Hepatitis E virus confirmed by a quantitative cell-culture assay. *J Gen Virol*. 2006;87:697-704.
13. Tanaka T, Takahashi M, Kusano E, et al. Development and evaluation of an efficient cell-culture system for Hepatitis E virus. *J Gen Virol*. 2007;88:903-911.
14. Takahashi M, Yamada K, Hoshino Y, et al. Monoclonal antibodies raised against the ORF3 protein of hepatitis E virus (HEV) can capture HEV particles in culture supernatant and serum but not those in feces. *Arch Virol*. 2008;153:1703-1713.
15. Emerson SU, Zhang M, Meng XJ, et al. Recombinant hepatitis E virus genomes infectious for primates: importance of capping and discovery of a cis-reactive element. *Proc Natl Acad Sci U S A*. 2001;98:15270-15275.
16. Kabrane-Lazizi Y, Meng XJ, Purcell RH, et al. Evidence that the genomic RNA of hepatitis E virus is capped. *J Virol*. 1999; 73:8848-8850.
17. Tam AW, Smith MM, Guerra ME, et al. Hepatitis E virus (HEV): molecular cloning and sequencing of the full-length viral genome. *Virology*. 1991;185:120-131.
18. Ansari IH, Nanda SK, Durgapal H, et al. Cloning, sequencing, and expression of the hepatitis E virus (HEV) nonstructural open reading frame 1 (ORF1). *J Med Virol*. 2000;60:275-283.
19. Huang YW, Opriessnig T, Halbur PG, et al. Initiation at the third in-frame AUG codon of open reading frame 3 of the hepatitis E virus is essential for viral infectivity in vivo. *J Virol*. 2007;81:3018-3026.
20. Zafrullah M, Ozdener MH, Panda SK, et al. The ORF3 protein of hepatitis E virus is a phosphoprotein that associates with the cytoskeleton. *J Virol*. 1997;71:9045-9053.
21. Kar-Roy A, Korkaya H, Oberoi R, et al. The hepatitis E virus open reading frame 3 protein activates ERK through binding and inhibition of the MAPK phosphatase. *J Biol Chem*. 2004;279: 28345-28357.
22. Korkaya H, Jameel S, Gupta D, et al. The ORF3 protein of hepatitis E virus binds to Src homology 3 domains and activates MAPK. *J Biol Chem*. 2001;276:42389-42400.
23. Moin SM, Panteva M, Jameel S. The hepatitis E virus Orf3 protein protects cells from mitochondrial depolarization and death. *J Biol Chem*. 2007;282:21124-21133.
24. Chandra V, Kar-Roy A, Kumari S, et al. The hepatitis E virus ORF3 protein modulates epidermal growth factor receptor trafficking, STAT3 translocation, and the acute-phase response. *J Virol*. 2008;82:7100-7110.
25. Ratra R, Kar-Roy A, Lal SK. The ORF3 protein of hepatitis E virus interacts with the b beta chain of fibrinogen resulting in decreased fibrinogen secretion from HuH-7 cells. *J Gen Virol* 2009;90:1359-1370.
26. Graff J, Nguyen H, Yu C, et al. The open reading frame 3 gene of hepatitis E virus contains a cis-reactive element and encodes a protein required for infection of macaques. *J Virol*. 2005; 79:6680-6689.
27. Jameel S, Zafrullah M, Ozdener MH, et al. Expression in animal cells and characterization of the hepatitis E virus structural proteins. *J Virol*. 1996;70:207-216.
28. Torresi J, Li F, Locarnini SA, et al. Only the non-glycosylated fraction of hepatitis E virus capsid (open reading frame 2) protein is stable in mammalian cells. *J Gen Virol*. 1999;80:1185-1188.
29. Li TC, Yamakawa Y, Suzuki K, et al. Expression and self-assembly of empty virus-like particles of hepatitis E virus. *J Virol*. 1997; 71:7207-7213.
30. Robinson RA, Burgess WH, Emerson SU, et al. Structural characterization of recombinant hepatitis E virus ORF2 proteins in baculovirus-infected insect cells. *Protein Expr Purif*. 1998; 12:75-84.
31. Tsarev SA, Tsareva TS, Emerson SU, et al. ELISA for antibody to hepatitis E virus (HEV) based on complete open-reading frame-2 protein expressed in insect cells: identification of HEV infection in primates. *J Infect Dis*. 1993;168:369-378.
32. Zhang Y, McAtee P, Yarbough PO, et al. Expression, characterization, and immunoreactivities of a soluble hepatitis E virus putative capsid protein species expressed in insect cells. *Clin Diagn Lab Immunol*. 1997;4:423-428.
33. Xing L, Kato K, Li T, et al. Recombinant hepatitis E capsid protein self-assembles into a dual-domain T = 1 particle presenting native virus epitopes. *Virology*. 1999;265:35-45.
34. Anderson DA, Cheng RH. Hepatitis E: structure and molecular virology. In: Thomas HC, Lemon S, Zuckerman AJ, eds. *Viral Hepatitis*. 3rd ed. Malden: Blackwell Publishing; 2005.
35. Thakral D, Nayak B, Rehman S, et al. Replication of a recombinant hepatitis E virus genome tagged with reporter genes and generation of a short-term cell line producing viral RNA and proteins. *J Gen Virol*. 2005;86:1189-1200.
36. Yarbough PO, Garza E, Tam AW, et al. Assay development of diagnostic tests for IgM and IgG antibody to hepatitis E virus. In: Buisson Y, Coursaget P, Kane M, eds. *Enterically-Transmitted Hepatitis Viruses*. Joue-les-Tours: La Simarre; 1996:294-296.
37. Yarbough PO, Krawczynski K, Tam AW, et al. Prevention of hepatitis E using r62K ORF 2 subunit vaccine: full protection against heterologous HEV challenge in cynomolgus macaques. In: Rizzetto M, Purcell RH, Gerin JL, Verme G, eds. *Viral Hepatitis and Liver Disease*. Turin: Edizioni Minervi Medica; 1997:650-655.
38. Li TC, Takeda N, Miyamura T, et al. Essential elements of the capsid protein for self-assembly into empty virus-like particles of hepatitis E virus. *J Virol*. 2005;79:12999-13006.
39. Anderson DA, Riddell MA, Chandler JD, et al. Molecular biology of hepatitis E virus. In: Margolis H, ed. *Viral Hepatitis and Liver Disease*. London: International Medical Press; 2002: 82-89.
40. Tyagi S, Jameel S, Lal SK. The full-length and N-terminal deletion of ORF2 protein of hepatitis E virus can dimerize. *Biochem Biophys Res Commun*. 2001;286:214-221.
41. Koonin EV, Gorbalenya AE, Purdy MA, et al. Computer-assisted assignment of functional domains in the nonstructural polyprotein of hepatitis E virus: delineation of an additional group of positive-strand RNA plant and animal viruses. *Proc Natl Acad Sci U S A*. 1992;89:8259-8263.
42. Emerson SU, Anderson D, Arankalle A, et al. Hepevirus. In: Fauquet CM, Mayo MA, Maniloff J, et al, eds. *Virus Taxonomy: Eighth Report of the ICTV*. London: Elsevier/Academic Press; 2005:851-855.
43. Haqshenas G, Huang FF, Fenaux M, et al. The putative capsid protein of the newly identified avian hepatitis E virus shares antigenic epitopes with that of swine and human hepatitis E viruses and chicken big liver and spleen disease virus. *J Gen Virol*. 2002;83:2201-2209.
44. Huang FF, Sun ZF, Emerson SU, et al. Determination and analysis of the complete genomic sequence of avian hepatitis E virus (avian HEV) and attempts to infect rhesus monkeys with avian HEV. *J Gen Virol*. 2004;85:1609-1618.
45. Boccia D, Guthmann JP, Klovstad H, et al. High mortality associated with an outbreak of hepatitis E among displaced persons in Darfur, Sudan. *Clin Infect Dis*. 2006;42:1679-1684.
46. Guthmann JP, Klovstad H, Boccia D, et al. A large outbreak of hepatitis E among a displaced population in Darfur, Sudan, 2004: the role of water treatment methods. *Clin Infect Dis*. 2006;42:1685-1691.
47. Tucker TJ, Kirsch RE, Louw SJ, et al. Hepatitis E in South Africa: evidence for sporadic spread and increased seroprevalence in rural areas. *J Med Virol*. 1996;50:117-119.
48. Munne MS, Vladimirsky S, Otegui L, et al. Identification of the first strain of swine hepatitis E virus in South America and prevalence of anti-HEV antibodies in swine in Argentina. *J Med Virol*. 2006;78:1579-1583.
49. Pujol FH, Favorov MO, Marcano T, et al. Prevalence of antibodies against hepatitis E virus among urban and rural populations in Venezuela. *J Med Virol*. 1994;42:234-236.
50. Schlauder GG, Frider B, Sookoian S, et al. Identification of 2 novel isolates of hepatitis E virus in Argentina. *J Infect Dis*. 2000;182:294-297.
51. Quintana A, Sanchez L, Larralde O, et al. Prevalence of antibodies to hepatitis E virus in residents of a district in Havana, Cuba. *J Med Virol*. 2005;76:69-70.
52. Rodriguez Lay Lde L, Quintana A, Villalba MC, et al. Dual infection with hepatitis A and E viruses in outbreaks and in sporadic clinical cases: Cuba 1998-2003. *J Med Virol*. 2008;80: 798-802.
53. Velazquez O, Stetler HC, Avila C, et al. Epidemic transmission of enterically transmitted non-A, non-B hepatitis in Mexico, 1986-1987. *JAMA*. 1990;263:3281-3285.
54. Chatterjee R, Tsarev S, Pillot J, et al. African strains of hepatitis E virus that are distinct from Asian strains. *J Med Virol*. 1997;53:139-144.
55. Gouvea V, Snellings N, Cohen SJ, et al. Hepatitis E virus in Nepal: similarities with the Burmese and Indian variants. *Virus Res*. 1997;52:87-96.
56. Huang R, Nakazono N, Ishii K, et al. Existing variations on the gene structure of hepatitis E virus strains from some regions of China. *J Med Virol*. 1995;47:303-308.
57. Meng J, Pillot J, Dai X, et al. Neutralization of different geographic strains of the hepatitis E virus with anti-hepatitis E virus-positive serum samples obtained from different sources. *Virology*. 1998;249:316-324.
58. Schlauder GG, Dawson GJ, Erker JC, et al. The sequence and phylogenetic analysis of a novel hepatitis E virus isolated from a patient with acute hepatitis reported in the United States. *J Gen Virol*. 1998;79:447-456.
59. van Cuyck-Gandre H, Zhang HY, Tsarev SA, et al. Characterization of hepatitis E virus (HEV) from Algeria and Chad by partial genome sequence. *J Med Virol*. 1997;53:340-347.
60. Yin S, Purcell RH, Emerson SU. A new Chinese isolate of hepatitis E virus: comparison with strains recovered from different geographical regions. *Virus Genes*. 1994;9:23-32.
61. Wang Y, Ling R, Erker JC, et al. A divergent genotype of hepatitis E virus in Chinese patients with acute hepatitis. *J Gen Virol*. 1999;80:169-177.
62. Mushahwar IK. Hepatitis E virus: molecular virology, clinical features, diagnosis, transmission, epidemiology, and prevention. *J Med Virol*. 2008;80:646-658.
63. Schlauder GG, Mushahwar IK. Genetic heterogeneity of hepatitis E virus. *J Med Virol*. 2001;65:282-292.
64. Zanetti AR, Schlauder GG, Romano L, et al. Identification of a novel variant of hepatitis E virus in Italy. *J Med Virol*. 1999;57:356-360.
65. Huang CC, Nguyen D, Fernandez J, et al. Molecular cloning and sequencing of the Mexico isolate of hepatitis E virus (HEV). *Virology*. 1992;191:550-558.
66. Buisson Y, Grandadam M, Nicand E, et al. Identification of a novel hepatitis E virus in Nigeria. *J Gen Virol*. 2000;81: 903-909.
67. Maila HT, Bowyer SM, Swanepoel R. Identification of a new strain of hepatitis E virus from an outbreak in Namibia in 1995. *J Gen Virol*. 2004;85:89-95.
68. van Cuyck H, Juge F, Roques P. Phylogenetic analysis of the first complete hepatitis E virus (HEV) genome from Africa. *FEMS Immunol Med Microbiol*. 2003;39:133-139.
69. Meng X-J, Purcell RH, Halbur PG, et al. A novel virus in swine is closely related to the human hepatitis E virus. *Proc Natl Acad Sci U S A*. 1997;94:9860-9865.
70. Hsieh SY, Meng XJ, Wu YH, et al. Identity of a novel swine hepatitis E virus in Taiwan forming a monophyletic group with Taiwan isolates of human hepatitis E virus. *J Clin Microbiol*. 1999;37:3828-3834.
71. Hsieh SY, Yang PY, Ho YP, et al. Identification of a novel strain of hepatitis E virus responsible for sporadic acute hepatitis in Taiwan. *J Med Virol*. 1998;55:300-304.
72. Ahn JM, Kang SG, Lee DY, et al. Identification of novel human hepatitis E virus (HEV) isolates and determination of the seroprevalence of HEV in Korea. *J Clin Microbiol*. 2005;43:3042-3048.
73. Sonoda H, Abe M, Sugimoto T, et al. Prevalence of hepatitis E virus (HEV) Infection in wild boars and deer and genetic identification of a genotype 3 HEV from a boar in Japan. *J Clin Microbiol*. 2004;42:5371-5374.
74. Matsuda H, Okada K, Takahashi K, et al. Severe hepatitis E virus infection after ingestion of uncooked liver from a wild boar. *J Infect Dis*. 2003;188:944.
75. Tsarev SA, Tsareva TS, Emerson SU, et al. Successful passive and active immunization of cynomolgus monkeys against hepatitis E. *Proc Natl Acad Sci U S A*. 1994;91:10198-10202.
76. Tsarev SA, Tsareva TS, Emerson SU, et al. Recombinant vaccine against hepatitis E: dose response and protection against heterologous challenge. *Vaccine*. 1997;15:1834-1838.
77. Purcell RH, Nguyen H, Shapiro M, et al. Pre-clinical immunogenicity and efficacy trial of a recombinant hepatitis E vaccine. *Vaccine*. 2003;21:2607-2615.
78. Zhou YH, Purcell RH, Emerson SU. An ELISA for putative neutralizing antibodies to hepatitis E virus detects antibodies to genotypes 1, 2, 3, and 4. *Vaccine*. 2004;22:2578-2585.
79. Riddell MA, Li F, Anderson DA. Identification of immunodominant and conformational epitopes in the capsid protein of hepatitis E virus by using monoclonal antibodies. *J Virol*. 2000;74:8011-8017.
80. Chen HY, Lu Y, Howard T, et al. Comparison of a new immunochromatographic test to enzyme-linked immunosorbent assay for rapid detection of immunoglobulin m antibodies to hepatitis e virus in human sera. *Clin Diagn Lab Immunol*. 2005;12:593-598.
81. Myint KS, Endy TP, Gibbons RV, et al. Evaluation of diagnostic assays for hepatitis E virus in outbreak settings. *J Clin Microbiol*. 2006;44:1581-1583.

82. Hu WP, Lu Y, Precioso NA, et al. Double-antigen enzyme-linked immunosorbent assay for detection of hepatitis E virus-specific antibodies in human or swine sera. *Clin Vaccine Immunol.* 2008;15:1151-1157.
83. Yarbough PO, Tam AW, Fry KE, et al. Hepatitis E virus: identification of type-common epitopes. *J Virol.* 1991;65:5790-5797.
84. Favorov MO, Khudyakov YE, Mast EE, et al. IgM and IgG antibodies to hepatitis E virus (HEV) detected by an enzyme immunoassay based on an HEV-specific artificial recombinant mosaic protein. *J Med Virol.* 1996;50:50-58.
85. Khudyakov YE, Favorov MO, Khudyakova NS, et al. Artificial mosaic protein containing antigenic epitopes of hepatitis E virus. *J Virol.* 1994;68:7067-7074.
86. Meng J, Dubreuil P, Pillot J. A new PCR-based seroneutralization assay in cell culture for diagnosis of hepatitis E. *J Clin Microbiol.* 1997;35:1373-1377.
87. Kar P, Budhiraja S, Narang A, Chakravarthy A. Etiology of sporadic acute and fulminant non-A, non-B viral hepatitis in north India. *Indian J Gastroenterol.* 1997;16:43-45.
88. Anderson DA. Waterborne hepatitis. In: Specter SC, Hodinka RL, Young SA, eds. *Clinical Virology Manual.* Washington: ASM Press; 2000:295-305.
89. Arankalle VA, Chadha MS, Tsarev SA, et al. Seroepidemiology of water-borne hepatitis in India and evidence for a third enterically-transmitted hepatitis agent. *Proc Natl Acad Sci U S A.* 1994;91:3428-3432.
90. Arankalle VA, Tsarev SA, Chadha MS, et al. Age-specific prevalence of antibodies to hepatitis A and E viruses in Pune, India, 1982 and 1992. *J Infect Dis.* 1995;171:447-450.
91. Lee SD, Wang YJ, Lu RH, et al. Seroprevalence of antibody to hepatitis E virus among Chinese subjects in Taiwan. *Hepatology (Baltimore, Md).* 1994;19:866-870.
92. Lok AS, Kwan WK, Moeckli R, et al. Seroepidemiological survey of hepatitis E in Hong Kong by recombinant-based enzyme immunoassays. *Lancet.* 1992;340:1205-1208.
93. Clayson ET, Shrestha MP, Vaughn DW, et al. Rates of hepatitis E virus infection and disease among adolescents and adults in Kathmandu, Nepal. *J Infect Dis.* 1997;176:763-766.
94. Clayson ET, Vaughn DW, Innis BL, et al. Association of hepatitis E virus with an outbreak of hepatitis at a military training camp in Nepal. *J Med Virol.* 1998;54:178-182.
95. Purcell RH, Ticehurst JR. Enterically transmitted non-A, non-B hepatitis: Epidemiology and clinical characteristics. In: Zuckerman AJ, ed. *Viral Hepatitis and Liver Disease.* New York: Alan R Liss; 1988:131-137.
96. Clayson ET, Innis BL, Myint KS, et al. Detection of hepatitis E virus infections among domestic swine in the Kathmandu Valley of Nepal. *Am J Tropical Med Hygiene.* 1995;53:228-232.
97. Meng XJ, Dea S, Engle RE, et al. Prevalence of antibodies to the hepatitis E virus in pigs from countries where hepatitis E is common or is rare in the human population. *J Med Virol.* 1999;59:297-302.
98. Wu JC, Chen CM, Chiang TY, et al. Clinical and epidemiological implications of swine hepatitis E virus infection. *J Med Virol.* 2000;60:166-171.
99. Michitaka K, Takahashi K, Furukawa S, et al. Prevalence of hepatitis E virus among wild boar in the Ehime area of western Japan. *Hepatol Res.* 2007;37:214-220.
100. Meng XJ, Halbur PG, Shapiro MS, et al. Genetic and experimental evidence for cross-species infection by swine hepatitis E virus. *J Virol.* 1998;72:9714-9721.
101. Thomas DL, Yarbough PO, Vlahov D, et al. Seroreactivity to hepatitis E virus in areas where the disease is not endemic. *J Clin Microbiol.* 1997;35:1244-1247.
102. Ghabrah TM, Tsarev S, Yarbough PO, et al. Comparison of tests for antibody to hepatitis E virus. *J Med Virol.* 1998;55:134-137.
103. Anderson DA, Li F, Riddell MA, et al. ELISA for IgG-class antibody to hepatitis E virus based on a highly conserved, conformational epitope expressed in *Eschericia coli. J Virol Methods.* 1999;81:131-142.
104. Seow H-F, Mahomed NMB, Mak J-W, et al. Seroprevalence of antibodies to hepatitis E virus in the normal blood donor population and two aboriginal communities in Malaysia. *J Med Virol* 1999 (in press).
105. Guo H, Zhou EM, Sun ZF, et al. Identification of B-cell epitopes in the capsid protein of avian hepatitis E virus (avian HEV) that are common to human and swine HEVs or unique to avian HEV. *J Gen Virol.* 2006;87:217-223.
106. Kabrane-Lazizi Y, Fine JB, Elm J, et al. Evidence for widespread infection of wild rats with hepatitis E virus in the United States. *Am J Tropical Med Hygiene.* 1999;61:331-335.
107. Meng XJ. Swine hepatitis E virus: cross-species infection and risk in xenotransplantation. *Curr Top Microbiol Immunol.* 2003;278:185-216.
108. Masuda J, Yano K, Tamada Y, et al. Acute hepatitis E of a man who consumed wild boar meat prior to the onset of illness in Nagasaki, Japan. *Hepatol Res.* 2005;31:178-183.
109. Takahashi K, Kitajima N, Abe N, et al. Complete or near-complete nucleotide sequences of hepatitis E virus genome recovered from a wild boar, a deer, and four patients who ate the deer. *Virology.* 2004;330:501-505.
110. Tei S, Kitajima N, Takahashi K, et al. Zoonotic transmission of hepatitis E virus from deer to human beings. *Lancet.* 2003;362:371-373.
111. Matsubayashi K, Nagaoka Y, Sakata H, et al. Transfusion-transmitted hepatitis E caused by apparently indigenous hepatitis E virus strain in Hokkaido, Japan. *Transfusion.* 2004;44:934-940.
112. Clayson ET, Myint KS, Snitbhan R, et al. Viremia, fecal shedding, and IgM and IgG responses in patients with hepatitis E. *J Infect Dis.* 1995;172:927-933.
113. Nanda SK, Ansari IH, Acharya SK, et al. Protracted viremia during acute sporadic hepatitis E virus infection. *Gastroenterology.* 1995;108:225-230.
114. Halbur PG, Kasorndorkbua C, Gilbert C, et al. Comparative pathogenesis of infection of pigs with hepatitis e viruses recovered from a pig and a human. *J Clin Microbiol.* 2001;39:918-923.
115. Maneerat Y, Clayson ET, Myint KS, et al. Experimental infection of the laboratory rat with the hepatitis E virus. *J Med Virol.* 1996;48:121-128.
116. Usmanov RK, Balaian MS, Dvoinikova OV, et al. [An experimental infection in lambs by the hepatitis E virus]. *Voprosy virusologii.* 1994;39:165-168.
117. Purcell RH, Emerson SU. Animal models of hepatitis A and E. *ILAR J/Natl Res Council, Institute of Laboratory Animal Resources.* 2001;42:161-177.
118. Bradley DW, Krawczynski K, Cook EHJ, et al. Enterically transmitted non-A, non-B hepatitis: serial passage of disease in cynomolgus macaques and tamarins and recovery of disease-associated 27- to 34-nm viruslike particles. *Proc Natl Acad Sci U S A.* 1987;84:6277-6281.
119. Ticehurst J, Rhodes LL Jr, Krawczynski K, et al. Infection of owl monkeys (Aotus trivirgatus) and cynomolgus monkeys (Macaca fascicularis) with hepatitis E virus from Mexico. *J Infect Dis.* 1992;165:835-845.
120. Uchida T, Win KM, Suzuki K, et al. Serial transmission of a putative causative virus of enterically transmitted non-A, non-B hepatitis to Macaca fascicularis and Macaca mulatta. *Japan J Exp Med.* 1990;60:13-21.
121. Tsarev SA, Emerson SU, Tsareva TS, et al. Variation in course of hepatitis E in experimentally infected cynomolgus monkeys. *J Infect Dis.* 1993;167:1302-1306.
122. Tsarev SA, Tsareva TS, Emerson SU, et al. Infectivity titration of a prototype strain of hepatitis E virus in cynomolgus monkeys. *J Med Virol.* 1994;43:135-142.
123. Arankalle VA, Chadha MS, Chobe LP, et al. Cross-challenge studies in rhesus monkeys employing different Indian isolates of hepatitis E virus. *J Med Virol.* 1995;46:358-363.
124. Arankalle VA, Favorov MO, Chadha MS, et al. Rhesus monkeys infected with hepatitis E virus (HEV) from the former USSR are immune to subsequent challenge with an Indian strain of HEV. *Acta Virologica.* 1993;37:515-518.
125. Bradley DW, Krawczynski K, Cook EHJ, et al. Enterically transmitted non-A, non-B hepatitis; Etiology of disease and laboratory studies in nonhuman primates. In: Zuckerman AJ, ed. *Viral Hepatitis and Liver Disease.* New York: Alan R Liss; 1988:138-147.
126. Arankalle VA, Chadha MS, Banerjee K, et al. Hepatitis E virus infection in pregnant rhesus monkeys. *Indian J Med Res.* 1993;97:4-8.
127. Tsarev SA, Tsareva TS, Emerson SU, et al. Experimental hepatitis E in pregnant rhesus monkeys: failure to transmit hepatitis E virus (HEV) to offspring and evidence of naturally acquired antibodies to HEV. *J Infect Dis.* 1995;172:31-37.
128. Kwo PY, Schlauder GG, Carpenter HA, et al. Acute hepatitis E by a new isolate acquired in the United States. *Mayo Clin Proc.* 1997;72:1133-1136.
129. Arankalle VA, Chobe LP, Joshi MV, et al. Human and swine hepatitis E viruses from Western India belong to different genotypes. *J Hepatol.* 2002;36:417-425.
130. Shukla P, Chauhan UK, Naik S, et al. Hepatitis E virus infection among animals in northern India: an unlikely source of human disease. *J Viral Hepatitis.* 2007;14:310-317.
131. Anderson DA, Shrestha IL. Hepatitis E virus. In: Richman DD, Whitley RJ, Hayden FG, eds. *Clinical Virology.* 4th ed. Washington, DC: ASM Press; 2008:1127-1143.
132. Viswanathan R. Epidemiology. *Indian J Med Res.* 1957;45:1-29.
133. Li F, Zhuang H, Kolivas S, et al. Persistent and transient antibody responses to hepatitis E virus detected by Western immunoblot using open reading frame 2 and 3 and glutathione S-transferase fusion proteins. *J Clin Microbiol.* 1994;32:2060-2066.
134. Tsarev SA, Emerson SU, Reyes GR, et al. Characterization of a prototype strain of hepatitis E virus. *Proc Natl Acad Sci U S A.* 1992;89:559-563.
135. Blank CA, Anderson DA, Beard M, et al. Infection of polarized cultures of human intestinal epithelial cells with hepatitis A virus: vectorial release of progeny virions through apical cellular membranes. *J Virol.* 2000;74:6476-6484.
136. Snooks MJ, Bhat P, Mackenzie J, et al. Vectorial entry and release of hepatitis A virus in polarized human hepatocytes. *J Virol.* 2008;82:8733-8742.
137. Bradley DW. Hepatitis E: epidemiology, aetiology and molecular biology. *Rev Med Virol.* 1992;2:19-28.
138. Krawczynski K. Hepatitis E. *Hepatology (Baltimore, Md).* 1993;17:932-941.
139. Zhuang H. Hepatitis E and strategies for its control. *MonogrVirol.* 1992;19:126-139.
140. Asher LV, Innis BL, Shrestha MP, et al. Virus-like particles in the liver of a patient with fulminant hepatitis and antibody to hepatitis E virus. *J Med Virol.* 1990;31:229-233.
141. Hamid SS, Jafri SM, Khan H, et al. Fulminant hepatic failure in pregnant women: acute fatty liver or acute viral hepatitis? *J Hepatol.* 1996;25:20-27.
142. Kawai HF, Koji T, Iida F, et al. Shift of hepatitis E virus RNA from hepatocytes to biliary epithelial cells during acute infection of rhesus monkey. *J Viral Hepatitis.* 1999;6:287-297.
143. Williams TP, Kasorndorkbua C, Halbur PG, et al. Evidence of extrahepatic sites of replication of the hepatitis E virus in a swine model. *J Clin Microbiol.* 2001;39:3040-3046.
144. Hussaini SH, Skidmore SJ, Richardson P, et al. Severe hepatitis E infection during pregnancy. *J Viral Hepatitis.* 1997;4:51-54.
145. Tsega E, Krawczynski K, Hansson BG, et al. Hepatitis E virus infection in pregnancy in Ethiopia. *Ethiop Med J.* 1993;31:173-181.
146. Jaiswal SP, Jain AK, Naik G, et al. Viral hepatitis during pregnancy. *Int J Gynaecol Obstet Official Organ Int Federation Gynaecol Obstet.* 2001;72:103-108.
147. Khuroo MS, Kamili S. Aetiology, clinical course and outcome of sporadic acute viral hepatitis in pregnancy. *J Viral Hepatitis.* 2003;10:61-69.
148. Tsega E, Hansson BG, Krawczynski K, et al. Acute sporadic viral hepatitis in Ethiopia: causes, risk factors, and effects on pregnancy. *Clin Infect Dis.* 1992;14:961-965.
149. Chau KH, Dawson GJ, Bile KM, et al. Detection of IgA class antibody to hepatitis E virus in serum samples from patients with hepatitis E virus infection. *J Med Virol.* 1993;40:334-338.
150. Tian DY, Chen Y, Xia NS. Significance of serum IgA in patients with acute hepatitis E virus infection. *World J Gastroenterol.* 2006;12:3919-3923.
151. Zhang S, Tian D, Zhang Z, et al. Clinical significance of anti-HEV IgA in diagnosis of acute Genotype 4 hepatitis E virus infection negative for anti-HEV IgM. *Digest Dis Sci.* 2009; in press.
152. Aggarwal R, Shukla R, Jameel S, et al. T-cell epitope mapping of ORF2 and ORF3 proteins of human hepatitis E virus. *J Viral Hepatitis.* 2007;14:283-292.
153. Khuroo MS, Kamili S, Jameel S. Vertical transmission of hepatitis E virus. *Lancet.* 1995;345:1025-1026.
154. Singh S, Mohanty A, Joshi YK, et al. Mother-to-child transmission of hepatitis E virus infection. *Indian J Pediatr.* 2003;70:37-39.
155. Khuroo MS, Rustgi VK, Dawson GJ, et al. Spectrum of hepatitis E virus infection in India. *J Med Virol.* 1994;43:281-286.
156. Mast EE, Alter MJ, Holland PV, et al. Evaluation of assays for antibody to hepatitis E virus by a serum panel. Hepatitis E Virus Antibody Serum Panel Evaluation Group. *Hepatology (Baltimore, MD).* 1998;27:857-861.
157. Dawson GJ, Mushahwar IK, Chau KH, et al. Detection of long-lasting antibody to hepatitis E virus in a US traveller to Pakistan. *Lancet.* 1992;340:426-427.
158. Schlauder GG, Desai SM, Zanetti AR, et al. Novel hepatitis E virus (HEV) isolates from Europe: evidence for additional genotypes of HEV. *J Med Virol.* 1999;57:243-251.
159. Seriwatana J, Shrestha MP, Scott RM, et al. Clinical and epidemiological relevance of quantitating hepatitis E virus-specific immunoglobulin M. *Clin Diagn Lab Immunol.* 2002;9:1072-1078.
160. Li F, Torresi J, Locarnini SA, et al. Amino-terminal epitopes are exposed when full-length open reading frame 2 of hepatitis E virus is expressed in *Escherichia coli*, but carboxy-terminal epitopes are masked. *J Med Virol.* 1997;52:289-300.
161. Myint KS, Guan M, Chen HY, et al. Evaluation of a new rapid immunochromatographic assay for serodiagnosis of acute hepatitis E infection. Am *J Tropical Med Hygiene.* 2005;73:942-946.
162. Bryan JP, Iqbal M, Tsarev S, et al. Epidemic of hepatitis E in a military unit in Abbotrabad, Pakistan. Am *J Tropical Med Hygiene.* 2002;67:662-668.
163. Khuroo MS, Dar MY. Hepatitis E: evidence for person-to-person transmission and inability of low dose immune serum globulin from an Indian source to prevent it [see comments]. *Indian J Gastroenterol.* 1992;11:113-116.
164. Schofield DJ, Glamann J, Emerson SU, et al. Identification by phage display and characterization of two neutralizing chimpanzee monoclonal antibodies to the hepatitis E virus capsid protein. *J Virol.* 2000;74:5548-5555.
165. Schofield DJ, Purcell RH, Nguyen HT, et al. Monoclonal antibodies that neutralize HEV recognize an antigenic site at the carboxyterminus of an ORF2 protein vaccine. *Vaccine.* 2003;22:257-267.
166. McAtee CP, Zhang Y, Yarbough PO, et al. Purification and characterization of a recombinant hepatitis E protein vaccine candidate by liquid chromatography-mass spectrometry. *J Chromatogr B Biomed Appl.* 1996;685:91-104.
167. Zhang M, Emerson SU, Nguyen H, et al. Recombinant vaccine against hepatitis E: duration of protective immunity in rhesus macaques. *Vaccine.* 2002;20:3285-3291.
168. Shrestha MP, Scott RM, Joshi DM, et al. Safety and efficacy of a recombinant hepatitis E vaccine. *N Engl J Med.* 2007;356:895-903.
169. Fuerst TR, Yarbough PO, Zhang Y, et al. Prevention of hepatitis E using a novel ORF-2 subunit vaccine. In: Buisson Y, Coursaget P, Kane M, eds. *Enterically-Transmitted Hepatitis Viruses.* Joue-Les-Tours, France: La Simarre; 1996:384-392.
170. Kamili S, Spelbring J, Carson D, et al. Protective efficacy of hepatitis E virus DNA vaccine administered by gene gun in the cynomolgus macaque model of infection. *J Infect Dis.* 2004;189:258-264.
171. Tuteja R, Li TC, Takeda N, et al. Augmentation of immune responses to hepatitis E virus ORF2 DNA vaccination by codelivery of cytokine genes. *Viral Immunol.* 2000;13:169-178.

178

Prions and Prion Diseases of the Central Nervous System (Transmissible Neurodegenerative Diseases)

PATRICK J. BOSQUE | KENNETH L. TYLER

Prions are the transmissible agents of a class of neurodegenerative diseases that afflict humans and other mammals. Prions are composed mainly, perhaps only, of abnormally folded and aggregated forms of a normally expressed protein called the *prion protein* (PrP). The human forms of prion disease are most commonly referred to as Creutzfeldt-Jakob disease, although some specific clinical forms carry other names, notably Gerstmann-Straussler-Scheinker syndrome (GSS) and fatal familial insomnia (FFI). The most important prion diseases of animals are scrapie in sheep, bovine spongiform encephalopathy (BSE) in cattle, and chronic wasting disease (CWD) of deer and related species.

Scrapie is the prototypic prion disease. It was first recognized as a distinct clinical entity in 18th-century western Europe.[1] Studies on scrapie in the late 19th through mid-20th century, particularly those of Cuillé and Chelle, established that the disease was transmissible by a filterable agent after unusually long incubation periods that sometimes extended to many years following inoculation outside the central nervous system (CNS).[2,3] Later studies uncovered the extraordinary resistance of the scrapie agent to ionizing radiation and other physical and chemical treatments that ordinarily inactivate viruses. This led Alper and colleagues to suggest in 1966 that the agent might replicate despite lacking nucleic acid.[4]

Gajdusek and co-workers' studies of kuru,[5,6] a neurodegenerative condition endemic in certain cannibalistic tribes in the highlands of New Guinea, led to the recognition of human prion disease.[7] They were aided in this discovery by the insights of the veterinary neuropathologist Hadlow, who remarked on the histopathologic similarity of kuru to scrapie, triggering the search for the potential transmissibility of kuru.[8,9] The similarities between kuru and scrapie that first drew Hadlow's attention included the "soap bubble"-like vacuolation of the neuropil, profound neurodegeneration, an intense reactive astrogliosis, and the absence of an associated inflammatory response. Modern neuropathologists would add only the immunohistochemical detection of abnormal forms of PrP to this list of key pathologic features of prion diseases.

Prusiner and colleagues founded the molecular era of prion biology by purifying the infectious agent.[10-12] Long incubation times and great expense hampered early studies of scrapie in sheep. Even after the scrapie agent was adapted to rodents, an end point titration might take more than 6 months. The incubation time interval assay,[13,14] which is based on the observation that as the infective dose of prions in a test inoculum increases, the time to the appearance of symptoms decreases, markedly accelerated scrapie research. Using this assay with hamster-adapted scrapie, Prusiner discovered that a previously unidentified protein was the chief component of a highly infectious fraction purified from brains. This led him in 1982 to propose the name *prion* for the agent responsible for scrapie and related neurodegenerative diseases.[15] The protein that comprised the dominant component of the infection fraction was thus named the "prion protein." The term *prion* initially was chosen to emphasize the hypothesis that the causative agents in these diseases were *pro*teinaceous *in*fectious particles that could be distinguished from viruses and viroids by their apparent lack of nucleic acid.

Since the word "prion" was coined, understanding of the biochemistry of these agents has evolved. Nowadays, the term refers to an alternatively folded and probably aggregated form of a protein normally produced by the organism. The aggregated form of the protein is capable of self-propagating by incorporating the normally nonaggregated normal host protein form into the pathologic aggregates.[16] Prions formed of PrP remain the only known mammalian prions, but a number of fungal proteins engage in prion-like behavior. The exact mechanism leading to the conversion of the normal prion protein to its pathologic isoform, the high-resolution structure of the prion form of proteins, and the mechanism by which the mammalian prion leads to neuronal cell death are subjects of active investigation and continued controversy.

Molecular Biology of Prion Diseases

PRION PROTEIN

PrP is a constitutively expressed cell surface glycoprotein. It is transcribed off a chromosomal gene (20p13 in humans).[17,18] The gene consists of a 10-kb intron, followed by a long open reading frame contained within a single exon encoding a 253–amino-acid polypeptide.[17,19] PrP mRNA transcription begins by embryonic day 14 in the mouse brain, and PrP levels increase during postnatal development.[20] In the adult, PrP^C is constitutively expressed at high levels in the brain, and mRNA levels are comparable in neurons, oligodendrocytes, and astrocytes.[21] The protein is also expressed at high levels in certain cells of the reticuloendothelial system, a distribution that is important in the pathogenesis of epidemic prion disease. Other tissues known to produce PrP include peripheral nerve, skeletal and heart muscle, and salivary gland tissues. The expression of the PrP mRNA does not differ between healthy and scrapie-infected animals.[17,19]

During PrP biosynthesis, the carboxyl-terminal 23 amino acids of PrP are removed and a phosphatidylinositol glycolipid (GPI) moiety is added (Fig. 178-1).[22] An amino-terminal signal sequence of 22 amino acids is also removed, presumably by the signal peptidase complex within the endoplasmic reticulum.[23] There are two asparagine-linked oligosaccharides, which subsequently are sialylated within the Golgi apparatus.[24] Forms of PrP with no, one, or two asparagines glycosylated are produced, so that PrP usually resolves into three distinct bands on Western immunoblots. A single disulfide bond links the two cysteine residues in the mature protein. In populations of European ancestry, a common polymorphism at codon 129 codes for methionine in approximately 60% of alleles and valine in the remainder. Another distinctive feature is the presence of a degenerate sequence of 8 amino acids repeated five times at the amino terminus of the protein. PrP^C is attached to the extracellular plasma membrane by the GPI anchor. A small fraction of PrP polypeptides may span the cell membrane, and these forms may play a role in neurodegenerative processes.[25,26]

The normal function of the prion protein remains obscure. Among the candidate functions for PrP^C are cell adhesion, laminin binding,

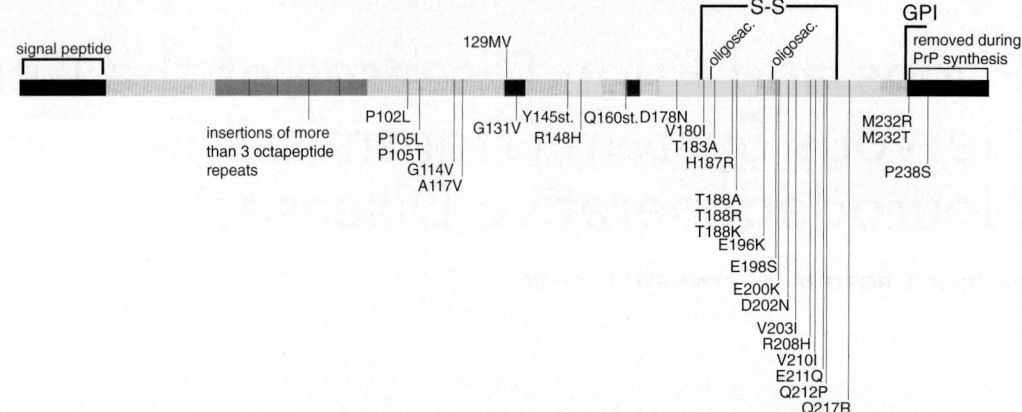

Figure 178-1 Schematic depiction of structural elements of PrP and mutations associated with genetic human prion disease. The PrP polypeptide is depicted as a horizontal bar running from the amino terminus on the left to the carboxyl terminus on the right. Amino and carboxyl termini removed in postranslational processing are shown in black, and the locations of the five octapeptide repeats are shown in dark gray. The elements of regular secondary structure in recombinant PrP^C are the α-helix (*yellow*) and two short β-strands (*red*). The sites of covalent modifications are shown above the bar, as is the location of the common codon 129MV polymorphism. PrP mutations associated with human prion disease are shown below the bar. Not shown are rare, apparently nonpathogenic polymorphisms.

neurite genesis, and synaptic function.[27-30] Several lines of evidence suggest a role in copper metabolism and a role in regulating cuproenzymes, such as superoxide dismutase activity.[31-33] Still, mice in which production of PrP is abolished by disruption of the PRNP gene show no gross abnormalities. They may have subtle signs of brain dysfunction, such as altered sleep patterns.[34] On the other hand, the PrP sequence is highly conserved evolutionarily, so it presumably confers a survival benefit. The pattern of expression, which is constitutive and widespread, with highest levels in the CNS and in certain cells of the reticuloendothelial system, conveys no obvious clue as to the protein's function.

PrP and two other structurally similar genes make up the prion protein family. "Doppel" is a 179–amino-acid protein encoded by a gene (*PRND*) located approximately 16 kb downstream of the gene encoding PrP (*PRNP*).[35-37] Doppel's structure and amino acid sequence are strongly similar to the carboxyl terminus of PrP. It is found in the testis and plays a role in the function of the male reproductive system. It is not normally expressed in the CNS, and ectopic expression there results in cerebellar degeneration due to apoptotic death of granule cells.[35,38] "Shadoo" is coded on a gene (*SPRN*) found on chromosome 10 in humans.[37] In contrast to doppel, shadoo shares sequence and structural motifs with the amino terminus of PrP. It is expressed in the CNS, and like the other members of the prion protein family, its precise function is unknown. Neither shadoo nor doppel have been associated with any naturally occurring neurodegenerative disease.

INFECTIOUS PRIONS

Prion diseases are marked by the appearance of a pathologic isoform of the normal prion protein designated PrP^{Sc} (Table 178-1). Neither inactivation studies with ionizing radiation nor attempts at direct isolation have found evidence for a specific nucleic acid or any specific macromolecule other than PrP in the infectious agent.[39] The proposition that a protein could act as an infectious agent was initially branded as heretical because it appeared to violate the central dogma of molecular biology—that sequence information proceeds from nucleic acid to protein, and never the reverse. The central dogma was spared, however, by the discovery that a chromosomal gene codes for PrP.[17,18] No differences have been detected in the organization or coding sequence of the PrP gene in healthy and experimentally infected animals.[40]

In Prusiner's original procedure, scrapie infectivity co-purified with a protease-resistant protein of 27 to 30 kD in molecular weight, designated PrP 27-30. This is the protease-resistant core generated by hydrolysis of the amino-terminus of the scrapie-associated isoform of

PrP, designated PrP^{Sc}.[17,41] Resistance of PrP^{Sc} to digestion with the serine endopeptidase proteinase K featured in the discovery of the protein because the original empirical fractionation procedure included a proteinase K digestion step. The normal form of the prion protein, found in uninfected animals and designated PrP^C, is rapidly hydrolyzed in the presence of proteases. Generation of protease-resistant carboxyl-terminal fragments of characteristic size continues to be the most widely used assay for the pathogenic form of the prion protein. The exact size of the protease-resistant fragment varies in different forms of prion disease. In sporadic and iatrogenic human prion diseases, the protease-resistant fragment typically extends either from residue 82 to the carboxyl terminus to yield a 21-kD (type 1) fragment or from residue 97 to yield a 19-kD (type 2) fragment.[42] The differences between these two forms relate to the "strain" properties of prions. In

TABLE 178-1	Properties of the Normal and Scrapie-Associated PrP Isoforms	
Property	*PrP^C (Normal Isoform)*	*PrP^{Sc} (Scrapie Isoform)*
Encoded on *PRNP* gene on chromosome 20	Yes	Yes
Present in normal brain	Yes	No
Present in scrapie-infected brain	Yes	Yes
Covalent modifications	GPI anchor, Asn-linked oligosaccharides, single intramolecular disulfide bond	Probably identical to PrP^C
Soluble in mild detergent	Yes	No
Effect of protease	Hydrolyzed to small peptides	Protease-resistant carboxyl-terminal portion of variable length
Secondary structure	~40% α-helical, little β-sheet	30% β-sheet, 20% α-helix
Tertiary structure	Three α-helical regions, unstructured amino terminus	Not determined
Quaternary structure	Monomeric or few-subunit oligomer	Aggregated

GPI, phosphatidylinositol glycolipid.
After Riesner D. Biochemistry and structure of PrP(C) and PrP(Sc). *Br Med Bull.* 2003;66:21-33.

hereditary prion disease with the GSS phenotype, type 1 and type 2 fragments are often not prominent, and smaller fragments of 7 to 14 kD, formed by both amino- and carboxyl-terminal cleavage, are found.[43] Some protease-resistant fragments of PrP may form in situ in prion-infected animals, presumably through the action of endogenous cellular proteases.[44] The degree of resistance of the carboxyl-terminal portion of PrP^{Sc} to proteolysis also varies among strains. Finally, a substantial portion of PrP^{Sc} within prion-infected animals is protease sensitive. The relative amounts of protease-resistant and -sensitive PrP may also be a marker of prion strains.[45]

PrP^C is readily soluble in mild non-ionic detergents, whereas PrP^{Sc} is not. This strongly suggests that PrP^{Sc} exists mainly in a highly aggregated state, whereas PrP^C is monomeric or oligomeric. Treatment of brain homogenates from infected, but not uninfected, animals with certain detergents yields fibrillary structures referred to as "scrapie-associated fibrils" that are composed of PrP^{Sc}.[46,47] Conformation-specific antibodies have been developed that selectively bind PrP^C but only bind PrP^{Sc} after the protein has been treated with denaturing agents.[45] Other antibodies specifically bind PrP^{Sc}, and binding is lost when the protein is denatured.[48] Taken together, these data indicate that although PrP^C and PrP^{Sc} are identical in their "primary" structure (i.e., amino-acid sequence and covalent attachments), they differ in higher order architecture, and at least a substantial portion of PrP^{Sc} is bound up in large insoluble aggregates. The precise nature of conformational differences between PrP^C and PrP^{Sc} is a major focus of ongoing research.

High-resolution structures for PrP^C have been obtained by nuclear magnetic resonance (NMR) spectroscopy and x-ray crystallography. These show PrP^C to be a globular protein composed of three α-helical segments and two short β-strands that form a small anti-parallel β-sheet. A curious feature of the protein is the absence of any regular structure of the purified protein in the amino terminus (amino acids 23 to 121) (see Fig. 178-1).[49-51] Presumably, this region assumes some more regular structure in vivo through association with other macromolecules or small molecule ligands. The structure of PrP^{Sc} has proven more difficult to determine, in part because available methods for high-resolution determination of protein structure require that the protein be soluble. Circular dichroism and infrared spectroscopy indicate that PrP^{Sc} contains approximately 40% β-sheet, in contrast to PrP^C, which contains only a very short β-sheet.[52] These tertiary structural characteristics of PrP^{Sc} suggest that it aggregates via intermolecular β-sheet formation between PrP molecules.

Because the conformation of PrP^{Sc} appears to be central to the process of prion propagation, efforts to decipher this structure using advanced techniques are under way. PrP in the detergent-extracted and protease-treated infectious fraction of hamster brains can form two-dimensional crystalline arrays. These have been examined by electron microscopy,[53,54] and 12-Å resolution images reveal a trimeric structure, hypothesized to be formed of monomers containing left-handed β-helices—triangular loops of the polypeptide chain stabilized by intramolecular β-sheets. In this model, the subunits of the trimer would associate along the two faces of the β-helix. This model contrasts with evidence from structural studies of yeast prions, which appear to assemble as in-register (i.e., each amino acid is aligned with the same amino acid on the neighboring chain) parallel (i.e., amino-termini aligned) β-sheets.[55] Likewise, amyloid formed of recombinant prion protein by a process that produced minimally infectious prions predominantly assumes an in-register parallel sheet conformation.[56]

Fragments of the prion protein have been induced to aggregate into fibrils in vitro, and the fiber structure has been analyzed by solid-state NMR, atomic force microscopy, x-ray diffraction of microcrystal, and other techniques. In general, these studies have used only short fragments of PrP, and only one of the studied fragments, comprising residues 89 to 143, is known to be infectious in vivo. Several groups report that the PrP fragments assemble into parallel, in-register β-sheets. The amino-acid side chains in these structures form a "steric zipper"—an interface where residues in adjacent chains tightly interdigitate like teeth on a zipper.[57,58] This type of structure is seen in short polypeptide fragment aggregates from several amyloidogenic proteins,[57] including Sup25, the substrate of a yeast prion. In contrast, solid-state NMR studies of the large 80 to 143 fragment of PrP suggest that the β-strands are neither parallel nor in register.[59] These findings are also not compatible with the "left-hand β-helix" predicted from two-dimensional crystals of PrP studied by electron microscopy.

The term *amyloid* is defined histopathologically as an accumulation of protein that binds the dye Congo red and alters its staining properties so that it exhibits an apple-green color under certain angles of polarized light. This occurs because amyloid is formed of fibrils composed of protein monomers, bound together in β-sheets, oriented perpendicularly to the long axis of the fibril. Molecules of Congo red intercalating into amyloid fibrils are aligned in such a way as to display the birefringence described above. A more general biophysical definition of amyloid is any fibril formed of proteins bound in β-sheets oriented perpendicular to the long axis of the fibril. Amyloids of the classical and biophysical definition seem to play a central pathogenic role in many neurodegenerative diseases, including, in addition to prion disease, Alzheimer's, Parkinson's, and Huntington's disease. The kinetics of amyloid fiber formation in vitro suggests a mechanism for prion propagation. Typically, a pure solution of monomers of an amyloidogenic peptide will exhibit a lag phase, often days in duration, before the rapid conversion of monomers into amyloid fibrils. If a small "seed" fibril is introduced into a solution of monomeric peptides, the lag phase is eliminated, and the monomers rapidly polymerize. This "seeded polymerization" is a popular mechanistic model for prion propagation, although other models exist.[60,61] Amyloid of the histopathologically defined type (amyloid plaques) is seen in some forms of human and animal prion disease, and amyloid fibrils may be present in all forms of prion disease. Uncertainty persists over whether fibrils or a preamyloid protofibrillary state may be the actual infectious moiety of prion diseases.[61-63]

Some molecule other than PrP might form a minor but important part of the infectious prion.[64,65] Immunopurified PrP^C from hamster brains was induced to form infectious prions through an in vitro process of sonication and incubation known as *protein misfolding cyclic amplification* (PMCA), but this process required the presence of single-stranded nucleic acids: polyadenosine RNA or polythymidine DNA. The highly purified samples were contaminated with small amounts of lipid as well. Remarkably, this process was able to spontaneously generate infectious prions: A mixture of highly purified brain-derived hamster PrP^C and polyadenosine RNA subject to intermittent sonication and incubation at 37°C produced PrP that, like brain-derived PrP^{Sc}, was protease resistant, was insoluble, and transmitted scrapie to hamsters. This indicates that the infectious prion might be composed of as little as PrP and nonspecific linear polyanions such as RNA. It is worth noting that the ratio of prion infectivity to protease-resistant PrP in these studies was lower than with PrP^{Sc} derived from scrapie-infected animals. One possible explanation for this discrepancy is that more highly infectious prion particles produced in vivo may have a more complex composition. An entirely synthetic PrP polypeptide, folded into an amyloid conformation in vitro, triggered prion disease in transgenic mice overexpressing the PrP gene.[66] This experiment strongly supports the "prion hypothesis," and many have taken this as its final proof. However, these "synthetic prions" did not transmit illness to wild-type mice, and in the transgenic mice incubation times were long, indicating that the synthetic prions were inefficient.

One early line of evidence implicating PrP in the pathogenesis of prion disease was the discovery that mutations in the *PRNP* coding region are responsible for genetic cases of human prion disease.[67] Several lines of transgenic mice expressing mutant human transgenes or their mouse homologues have been made. Some develop neurodegenerative disease, but it is not clear to what extent the disease in these transgenic mice mimics human prion disease.[68] Transgenic mice have proven quite useful in exploring the "species barrier" to prion transmission. Typically, prion disease transmits inefficiently across different mammalian species. Studies in transgenic mice demonstrated that this barrier to transmission could be abrogated by the introduction of a gene directing expression of PrP of the prion donor species into the host mouse.[68,69] Mice expressing the human PrP sequence have largely replaced subhuman primates as laboratory models of human prion strains.[70] Intracerebral inoculation of transgenic mice expressing bovine, ovine, human, or cervid prion proteins is used to assay for the presence of prions from the appropriate species.[68] As discussed later, the species barrier depends not only on host and donor PrP sequence differences but also on the particular prion strain involved.

Other proteins, although not part of the infectious particle, may play a role in the conversion of PrP^C to PrP^{Sc}. In the yeast prion state [PSI+], which is mediated by aggregates of the protein Sup35, the protein chaperone HSP104, as well as chaperones of the HSP70 and HSP40 families, can catalyze or inhibit the formation of prions.[71,72] A perhaps similar effect occurs in mice that overexpress HSP70 and manifest prolonged mouse-adapted scrapie incubation times relative to wild-type mice.[73] The propagation of human prions in mice expressing human PrP is inhibited by the coexpression of mouse PrP. This has been taken as evidence that a factor, termed "protein X," facilitates the conversion of PrP^C to PrP^{Sc} in mice and that this factor binds mouse PrP^C with greater avidity than human PrP^C.[74,75] Despite these lines of indirect evidence, no protein other than PrP has been proven to participate in mammalian prion propagation.

The mechanism by which propagation of PrP^{Sc} leads to neurodegeneration remains unknown. Although the phenotypic expression of yeast prions is in several instances due to the loss of the protein's normal function, this does not appear to be the case with mammalian prions. Rather, the conversion of PrP^C to PrP^{Sc} causes a toxic "gain of function."[76] The nature of this toxic function remains poorly understood. Toxicity requires expression of PrP,[76] and this PrP must be GPI anchored because transgenic mice expressing only a secreted form of PrP lacking a GPI anchor do not undergo neurodegeneration. These mice do produce infectious prions when inoculated with prions, with the conversion of the anchorless extracellular PrP^C to PrP^{Sc}.[77] As with other neurodegenerative diseases associated with protein aggregates, dysfunction of the ubiquitin-proteosome system has been invoked as a cause of neurodegeneration in prion disease.[78]

Only a small proportion of all cases of human prion disease are infectiously transmitted, but this is the major cause of prion disease in animals. The reticuloendothelial system plays a major role in the initial propagation of prions outside the CNS and in carrying infection to the CNS. After oral challenge with scrapie, prion titers rise first in gut-associated lymphoid tissue. Mice deficient in the number of functional Peyer's patches show increased resistance to oral scrapie challenge.[79] Similarly, a number of studies document that follicular dendritic cells are necessary for mice inoculated intraperitoneally with scrapie to propagate prions in the brain and develop scrapie.[80] Prion infection is carried to the brain from lymphoid tissue by axoplasmic transport in neurons of the sympathetic nervous system.[81-85] Sympathectomized mice have reduced susceptibility to prion disease, and mice with hyperinnervation of lymphoid tissue show enhanced susceptibility.[86] In some models of scrapie infection, the vagus nerve is also important to spread infection to the CNS. The "drowsy" strain of hamster scrapie spreads to the brain without infecting lymphoreticular tissue after inoculation in the tongue, apparently by spreading through the motor neurons of the hypoglossal nerve and the gustatory sensory neurons of the nucleus of the solitary tract.[87]

Because follicular dendritic cells and perhaps other components of the lymphoreticular system can efficiently propagate prions to high levels, inflammatory states can lead to the accumulation of PrP^{Sc} in tissues in which prions are not normally found.[88] For example, coincident nephritis and prion infection leads to the shedding of infectious prions in urine,[89] and highly sensitive assays are reported to detect prions in urine late in scrapie infections.[90]

One of the most enigmatic features of prion diseases is the existence of what are termed prion "strains."[91] These are isolates distinguishable by clinical, pathologic, and biochemical features even in genetically identical hosts (Table 178-2). Because the prion consists only of host-derived PrP and perhaps other host-derived components, the means

	Strain	
Property	*Hyper*	*Drowsy*
Incubation time[308]	65 days	165 days
Clinical signs[308]	Hyperexcitability and ataxia	Lethargy
Size of protease-resistant fragment (nonglycosylated band)[309]	21 kD	20 kD
Sensitivity of resistant carboxyl-terminal fragment to prolonged exposure to protease[309]	Present after 24 hr of digestion	Hydrolyzed after 12 hr
Resistance to denaturation (concentration of guanidine HCl that denatures 50% of PrP^{Sc})[310]	1.5 M	1.1 M
Distribution of PrP^{Sc} in the brain of clinically affected hamsters[311]	Most in medial geniculate nucleus and deep cerebellar nuclei	Most in regions of hippocampus, cerebellar granular layer, and occipital cortex
Distribution of PrP^{Sc} outside the CNS[93]	In spleen and other lymphoreticular organs	Not found in lymphoreticular system
Species barrier[308]	Nonpathogenic in mink	Pathogenic in mink

TABLE 178-2 Comparison of Two Hamster Prion Strains*

*Perhaps the two most well-studied prion strains are "hyper" and "drowsy," which are adapted to hamsters from transmissible mink encephalopathy, a prion disease of mink. The two strains are typically propagated in Syrian golden hamsters. Some characteristic properties are compared in the table. The number of potential strains that can exist on a single genetic background is not known, but evidence indicates that it is more than two.[310]

CNS, central nervous system.

by which the properties of individual strains are maintained is puzzling. Upon intracerebral inoculation, a particular strain of prions will reliably cause all inoculated animals to fall ill within a remarkably narrow range of incubation times—typically varying by only a few percent between individual animals. In contrast, mice inoculated with different strains may display markedly different incubation times.[92] For example, in certain inbred lines of mice, inoculation of scrapie 139A strain results in incubation times of approximately 200 days, whereas the same line of mice inoculated with scrapie strain 87A have an incubation time of nearly 600 days. The clinical features of disease can also differ between scrapie strains: The well-studied "hyper" and "drowsy" strains (derived from mink transmissible spongiform encephalopathy but propagated in hamsters) are so named because of the behavior of the hamsters at the time of onset of illness. The fact that PrP^{Sc} accumulation and neurodegeneration are greatest in differing regions of the brain for different strains presumably underlies the difference in clinical signs. The differences in regional and cell type distribution between strains can be profound: Like many prion strains, hyper accumulates in the spleen of infected animals. In contrast, drowsy does not propagate or accumulate in lymphoid tissue at all.[93] Strains can differ in many features (see Table 178-2). Of particular interest from the perspective of public health, the propensity of prions in one mammalian species to infect another species (the "species barrier") varies depending on the strain involved.[91] The role of strain differences with regard to disease transmission is discussed further with respect to BSE and variant Creutzfeldt-Jakob Disease (vCJD) later.

The biochemical basis of prion strain variety is understood poorly, but it appears to reflect conformational differences between the PrP^{Sc} associated with the various strains (Fig. 178-2). The size of the protease-resistant carboxyl-terminal fragment can differ slightly between strains. Other studies show that strains differ in their susceptibility to denaturation with chaotropic salts. The relative resistance of the carboxyl-terminal fragment to complete hydrolysis also varies among strains. Taken together, these observations indicate that subtle confor-

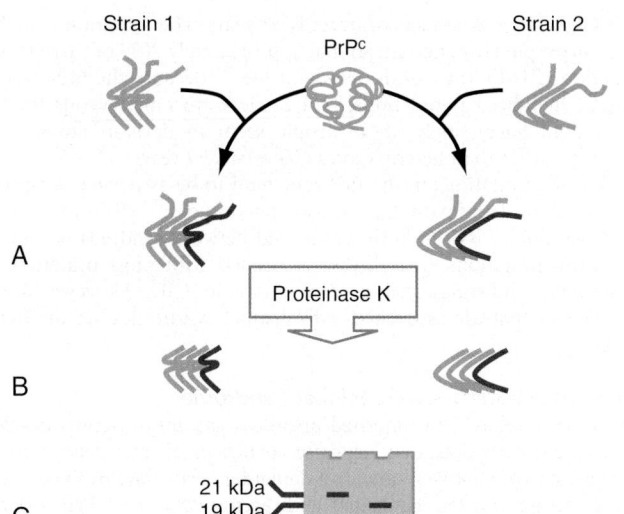

Figure 178-2 Schematic representation of prion strain propagation and strain analysis. A, Strains differ in the conformation of the pathogenic aggregate. PrP^C can be recruited into the PrP^{Sc} aggregate of different strains and thus adopt the conformation of that strain. The number of strains that potentially exist is unknown. **B,** In one technique of strain analysis, protease treatment is used to hydrolyze the amino-terminal end of PrP^{Sc}. The length of the hydrolyzed segment varies slightly between strains. **C,** When the protease-treated fragments are disaggregated and separated on a polyacrylamide gel, the protease-resistant fragment of strain 1 is revealed to be slightly larger than that of strain 2. The figure depicts only the nonglycosylated form of the protein. Generally, non-, mono-, and diglycosylated forms occur.

mational differences between PrP^{Sc} associated with the various strains somehow dictate the clinical and pathologic differences.

YEAST PRIONS

Wickner first proposed that certain epigenetic traits of yeast could be manifestations of a process anologous to that which occurs in mammalian prion diseases.[94] To date, at least three yeast prions ([PSI+], [URE3], and [PIN+]) and one prion of the filamentous fungus *Podospora anserina* ([Het-s]) have been identified. These traits are transmitted through cytoplasmic exchange but are not linked to the mitochondrial genome.[95-97] Each trait is linked to a particular protein, encoded by the nuclear genome, that is found to be in an aggregated state when the prion trait is expressed.[98] Unlike the mammalian PrP prion, the phenotype of at least some yeast prions is equivalent to an inactivating mutation in the cognate protein. The [Het-s] prion is particularly interesting in that it appears to convey a useful property, mating incompatibility, upon its host. Yeast prions are intensively studied as models of mammalian prions and the processes of protein folding and aggregation in general. Yeast prions do not play any role in the initiation or transmission of mammalian prion diseases.

▓ Human Prion Diseases

Traditionally, human prion diseases have been classified by a combination of epidemiology, clinical features, histopathology, and family history. This has led to a proliferation of named syndromes that fundamentally share a similar pathophysiology. A more useful and consistent classification considers the various manifestations of human prion disease in terms of origin: sporadic, genetic, or infectiously transmitted. Generally, the term *Creutzfeldt-Jakob disease* refers to human prion disease and includes sporadic, genetic, and infectiously acquired forms that have not been given another name. The substantial diversity of prion disease not accounted for by the previous classification may represent the manifestation of different strains of prions.

However, typing of human prion strains is an emerging technology, and the basis of prion strain differences is only incompletely understood. It is not clear whether the diverse manifestations of human prion disease can be attributed to differences in the properties of the initiating prion strains or result from other as yet unidentified factors. Human genetic diversity and the variety of circumstances in which human prion disease develops or is acquired are greater than in laboratory models of prion disease, and these factors likely contribute to variance in clinical and pathologic presentation.

SPORADIC CREUTZFELDT-JAKOB DISEASE

In the early 1920s, the German neurologists Creutzfeldt and Jakob separately described a puzzling series of cases of neurodegenerative disease.[99,100] The neuropathologist Spielmeyer was the first to use the eponym *Creutzfeldt-Jakob disease*, a designation now solidified by historical usage, although modern review of the available pathologic material from Creutzfeldt and Jakob's original cases suggests that many were examples of other diseases, and only a few of the original cases likely would be diagnosed as CJD today. CJD is a rare disease, with an annual prevalence and incidence of approximately 1 case per 1 million people worldwide. In several countries, the reported rate of CJD has increased since the mid-1990s. This most likely is the result of improved surveillance in response to the outbreak of BSE and vCJD.[101-105] In the United States, studies have found a substantially lower rate of CJD among African Americans and other nonwhites than among whites.[106,107] Whether this reflects reduced ascertainment in these groups or a truly reduced incidence is not certain. Sporadic CJD (sCJD) comprises approximately 85% to 94% of human prion disease,[108,109] and in most populations, virtually all the remainder are genetic cases.

sCJD serves as the prototype of all human prion diseases. sCJD shows no gender predilection. Mean age at onset is 57 to 66 years, although patients as young as 17 years and older than 80 years with classic CJD have been reported.[109] Several studies found a peak incidence, approaching 6 per 1 million, in the eighth decade and then a distinct decline in incidence in those older than 80 years.[108,109] This is unusual for neurodegenerative diseases, the incidences of which tend to steadily increase with age.

The most distinctive clinical feature of sCJD is the pace of its progression, typically described as "rapid" or "subacute." In the context of neurodegenerative conditions, these terms refer to perceptible declines in cognitive and motor function that are obvious over a period of a few weeks. In contrast, in more common neurodegenerative conditions such as Alzheimer's or Parkinson's disease, decline is typically only apparent over periods ranging from months to years. Some observers have noted that the pace of decline in CJD accelerates until the later stages of akinetic mutism, when neurologic dysfunction is so severe that it is difficult to appreciate further decline. A second distinctive feature of CJD is the prominent involvement of multiple brain systems, in which motor signs such as ataxia, bradykinesia, or spasticity are combined with memory and other cognitive deficits. There is a great deal of variability in the clinical manifestations of CJD, and this has led to attempts to describe a variety of clinical subtypes, including those with predominance of visual,[110] cerebellar,[111] thalamic,[112] and striatal[113,114] features. The existence of these syndromes indicates that CJD may affect particular brain regions disproportionately. In some cases, as with sporadic fatal insomnia (discussed later), the specific regional predominance of pathology may reflect the strain of prion involved.

In many patients with sCJD, there is a prodromal phase of psychiatric disturbance before the onset of neurologic signs. Of 126 mostly sporadic cases of CJD, 26% of patients had psychiatric signs in the prodromal or presenting phase.[115] Most common were sleep disturbance, depression, and anxiety. In approximately one third of patients, predominant initial visual or cerebellar symptoms may overshadow dementia. Mental deterioration typically is rapidly progressive, and the average duration of illness from onset of symptoms to death is 7 to 9 months. Unusual cases of longer duration have been described.[116] In addition to profound and rapidly progressive mental deterioration, another very common feature is myoclonus. However, myoclonus in demented patients is not pathognomonic of CJD. It can occasionally occur in Alzheimer's disease and is common in Lewy body dementia. Extrapyramidal symptoms and signs, including hypokinesia and rigidity, and cerebellar signs and symptoms, including nystagmus, tremor, and ataxia, ultimately develop in approximately two thirds of patients. Approximately 40% to 80% of patients have signs of corticospinal tract dysfunction, including hyperreflexia, spasticity, and extensor plantar responses. Prominent visual disturbances, which can include visual field cuts, cortical blindness, and visual agnosia, occur in 50% of CJD patients.

Certain neurologic disturbances occur only rarely as prominent features in CJD, and their presence should prompt clinicians to consider other diagnostic possibilities. Although seizures occur in 10% to 20% of cases, they are rarely a dominant feature and typically are amenable to therapy. Cranial nerve involvement is never prominent, although isolated cases have been reported with involvement of the pupils; extraocular movements; and trigeminal, auditory, and vestibular systems.[117]

Some patients have vague sensory complaints, including pruritus and aching limbs. It is uncertain if these sensations are of peripheral or central origin.[118] Signs of a motor or sensory peripheral neuropathy are occasionally found in sCJD, although these signs are almost always overshadowed by the dramatic signs of CNS dysfunction. One study found clinical evidence of peripheral neuropathy in approximately 20% of cases examined and electrophysiologic abnormalities in 14 of 16 surveyed cases of sCJD.[119] Occasionally, signs of sensory or motor neuropathy may dominate the early disease course. Rarely, fasciculations and muscle wasting—signs of motor nerve or motor neuron damage—will be so prominent as to suggest amyotrophic lateral sclerosis.[120,121] Some cases of CJD also have been reported in which the clinical features indicated prominent autonomic nervous system involvement. These features included hypohidrosis, bowel dysfunction, abnormal pupillary responses to autonomic drugs, abnormal diurnal blood pressure variation, and electrocardiogram abnormalities.[117] Such findings are a cardinal feature in FFI.

GENETIC CREUTZFELDT-JAKOB DISEASES

Approximately 10% of cases of human prion disease are caused by some nonconservative (i.e., amino-acid sequence-changing) mutation in PRNP, although the precise proportion varies among countries.[108] PRNP mutations are found in all cases from families with a history of inherited prion disease, as well as approximately 5% of apparently sporadic cases. Familial prion diseases are transmitted in an autosomal-dominant pattern, but the penetrance differs between mutations. No mutation or polymorphism in any other gene has been identified as a risk factor for human prion disease.

At least 30 distinct mutations in the PRNP gene are known to be associated with the inherited prion diseases (see Fig. 178-1).[122,123] These include least 28 missense mutations, two premature stop mutations at codons 160 and 145, and several expansions in the number of a series of five repeats of a degenerate sequence of eight amino acids at the amino terminus of the protein. Not all patients with genetic forms of prion disease present with a family history of dementia.[124] In a large European survey of prion disease, a family history of a CJD-like dementia was elicited in only half of genetic cases.[125] The frequency of various PRNP mutations varies markedly in different regions of the world. The most common mutation worldwide is a lysine-for-glutamic acid substitution in codon 200 (E200K).[123] This mutation has been found in geographic clusters of familial CJD in Slovakia and Chile and among Sephardic Jews in Greece, Libya, Tunisia, and Israel. Before the mutation was discovered to be prevalent in Libyan Jews, the high rate of CJD in this group was misattributed to the consumption of sheep brains or eyeballs.[126] This form of familial CJD usually manifests with signs and symptoms indistinguishable from the common presentation

of sCJD. The median age of onset is 58 years. The mutation is highly but incompletely penetrant so that approximately 80% of carriers will develop CJD by the eighth decade of life.[127] Because the mutation is found in inbred populations, rare carriers are homozygous for the mutation. Surprisingly, these people seem to develop illness only slightly earlier than heterozygotes (50 versus 59 years).[128]

Specific mutations in the PrP gene tend to be associated with particular clinical and pathologic disease phenotypes.[125] However, significant variability is seen both within and between kindreds harboring identical mutations. The disease associated with most mutations is essentially indistinguishable from sporadic CJD. However, some mutations that are associated with distinct syndromes are discussed next.

Gerstmann-Sträussler-Scheinker Syndrome

In some families with inherited prion disease, most victims develop prominent early ataxia and signs of corticospinal tract degeneration. Progression is relatively slow, and dementia occurs late in the disease. This picture is often associated with accumulations of PrP in large amyloid plaques, composed of PrP, in the CNS.[129,130] This clinico-pathologic picture is known as the GSS. The syndrome is linked to several different mutations in PRNP. The most common is a missense mutation that substitutes a lysine for a proline at codon 102 (P102L). Other associated mutations are P105L, A117V, Q187H, F198S, D202N, Q212P, Q217R, Y145STOP, and an insertion of eight or nine octapeptide repeats.[131] The duration of illness ranges from 3 months to 13 years, with a mean of 5 or 6 years.[131-133] Sporadic cases of human prion disease with GSS-like plaque formation occur in the absence of PRNP mutations. Likewise, a subset of patients with dura mater graft-associated CJD in Japan present with a GSS-like clinicopathologic picture.[134]

Neuropathologic findings of GSS are typical of other prion diseases except that patients have widespread amyloid plaques. Within the cerebellum, where the concentration is typically the most dense, plaques are found in the molecular layer, are often multicentric, and are associated with a microglial reaction. The multicentric morphology of GSS plaques distinguishes them from plaques seen in kuru, which are typically unicentric.[135] The degree of spongiform change is variable, ranging from substantial and severe to completely absent. Atypical kindreds have been reported in whom prion amyloid plaques are prominent throughout the telencephalon and are not limited to the cerebellum and in whom neurofibrillary tangles are prominent.[136] Cases of this type may have been mischaracterized previously as familial Alzheimer's disease. The availability of immunostaining now allows the amyloid plaques associated with prion diseases to be distinguished clearly from the senile plaques characteristic of Alzheimer's disease.

Fatal Familial Insomnia

FFI first was reported as a human disease in 1986,[137] although there is clinical and pathologic overlap between FFI and cases described earlier as "thalamic dementia."[138] In the early 1990s, the immunohistochemical detection of abnormal PrP and the subsequent recognition of a D178N mutation in PRNP marked FFI as a prion disease with unusual features.[139] The D178N mutation can occur in two different PRNP allele forms, with either a methionine or a valine coded for on the polymorphic codon 129. The D178N/129M allele associates with FFI, whereas a syndrome more closely resembling typical sCJD occurs in patients carrying the D178N/129V allele. Although the first reports of FFI were all in Italian families, currently a total of approximately 27 families with FFI have been reported from the United Kingdom, Europe, the United States, Finland, Australia, China, and Japan.[140]

In the typical form of FFI, patients develop insomnia as a prominent and early complaint, associated with signs of autonomic hyperactivity (increased sweating, tearing, salivation, mild nocturnal hyperthermia, tachycardia, and hypertension). Motor disturbances develop later and can include ataxia, myoclonus, spasticity, hyperreflexia, and dysarthria.[139-141] Marked memory impairment is not prominent early in the disease, although a delirium-like hallucinosis may occur. The mean age of onset in FFI is 50 to 56 years, somewhat younger than in sCJD.[125,142-144] Cases in patients as young as 19 years and as old as 83 years of age have been reported.[125] Series of patients with the FFI genotype have found substantial clinical heterogeneity. Ataxia and psychiatric signs such as depression, apathy, or anxiety are common initial complaints, and insomnia is not always noted by the patient, family, or clinicians.[142,143] Polysomnography is a sensitive test for FFI, being abnormal in almost all cases, but investigations have shown this is true for sCJD as well.[145] In both forms of prion diseases, there are marked reductions or absence of both rapid eye movement (REM) and normal non-REM sleep.

Neuropathologic changes, including neuronal loss and reactive gliosis, are found consistently in the anterior ventral and mediodorsal nuclei of the thalamus, the inferior olives, and, less strikingly, the cerebellar and cerebral cortex.[139,141,146] Immunostaining of brain material for PrP^{Sc} is positive, although the concentration of protein is 5 to 10 times less than that seen in sCJD.

A rare sporadic form of human prion disease presents with clinical and histopathologic features identical to those of FFI (sporadic fatal insomnia [sFI]).[147] By definition, no *PRNP* mutation is present in sFI cases, but the protease-resistant PrP^{Sc} fragment associated with sFI is identical to that seen in FFI. Both FFI and sFI can be transmitted to transgenic mice expressing wild-type human PrP. The clinical and histopathologic properties of the disease in these mice, as well as the biochemical properties of the PrP^{Sc} produced, are identical, and they are distinct from those of sCJD.[148] Thus, the prions associated with sFI and FFI are a distinct strain, different from that which causes typical sCJD.

Long-Duration Disease

Certain PRNP mutations frequently cause disease with exceptionally slow progression. These include large expansions in the octapeptide repeat region and the missense mutations T183A and H187R.[149-151] Some mutations may be associated with lifelong psychiatric disturbances that precede the onset of progressive dementia by decades.[150]

Polymorphisms in PRNP

Polymorphisms at codon 129 of the PrP gene play a role in CJD expression and susceptibility. In European populations, approximately 60% to 70% of alleles have methionine at this position, and the rest have valine. The alleles are in Hardy-Weinberg equilibrium, so genotypes in the general population are approximately 42% 129MM, 46% MV, and 12% VV.[152] In contrast, 95% of patients who develop sCJD exhibit homozygosity (either MM or VV) at this locus.[153,154] Codon 129 allele distributions vary across ethnic groups, but the tendency for overrepresentation of homogzygotes in CJD cases holds.[155]

PrP polymorphisms might influence the risk of neurodegenerative conditions other than CJD. Some, but not all, investigations have found an overrepresentation of the PRNP 129M allele in Alzheimer's disease, particularly in early onset disease.[156-158] Other investigators found that the heterozygous 129MV genotype was overrepresented in patients with primary progressive aphasia.[157] Currently, such associations are not convincing.

INFECTIOUSLY TRANSMITTED HUMAN PRION DISEASE

In most countries, less than 1% of human prion disease is infectiously acquired. Yet study of an epidemic of infectious prion disease in New Guinea led to the recognition of prions as a cause of neurodegenerative illness in humans, and transmission of prion disease from animals or humans to humans continues to be an issue of great concern.

KURU

Kuru was the first of the human prion diseases to be studied in detail.[5-7,159-162] It was endemic within the Fore linguistic tribal group of the Eastern Highlands of Papua New Guinea. Epidemiologic studies suggest that the disease likely was transmitted through the practice of ritual endocannibalism at funeral feasts.[163] No one born since the cessation of this practice has developed kuru.[163] The mean incubation period was 10 to 13 years, with 90% of cases occurring within 21 to 27 years of exposure. Incubation period was likely related to exposure dose and was shorter in women than in men and shorter in older women than in younger women, reflecting the likelihood of participation in cannibalistic practices.[164] Rare cases of kuru continue to occur, likely as a result of exposure before ritual cannibalism ceased in 1960. Thus, in some cases the incubation period for kuru can exceed 50 years.[163]

Kuru remains important conceptually, even as it disappears as a clinical entity, as the largest outbreak of human-to-human transmission of a prion disease and as an example of human prion disease transmitted via the oral route. In its clinical and pathologic manifestations, it is distinct from most human prion disease. Kuru typically begins insidiously with a prodrome of headaches and aching limbs that may last for several months.[165] This prodrome is followed by the development of an inexorably progressive neurologic disease resulting in death within 3 to 24 months of onset, usually from intercurrent pneumonia and malnutrition. Typical disease duration is 12 months.[165] The cardinal clinical features include cerebellar ataxia, action tremor, and involuntary movements (choreoathetosis, myoclonic jerks, and coarse fasciculations). Cranial nerve abnormalities, motor weakness, and sensory loss are absent or occur only in the late stages of the disease. Dementia is usually not noted until late in the illness, 8 or more months after the onset of ataxia.

Neuropathologic examination of kuru brains shows neuronal loss, astrogliosis, and the accumulation of PrP^{Sc}, all findings typical of prion disease.[160,166-168] The pathologic hallmark of kuru is the presence of PrP-reactive plaques, predominantly in cerebellar tissue. These plaques are usually unicentric, located in the granular layer of the cerebellum, and often associated with microglial cells. Molecular analyses of *PRNP* and of the characteristics of the PrP^{Sc} derived from brain material from kuru patients are limited. Kuru cases show a higher than expected incidence of MM homozygosity at polymorphic codon 129 of the *PRNP* gene, as is seen in sCJD. In contrast, older women who potentially were exposed to infected brain material during the era of cannibalism and survived without developing kuru show a higher than expected frequency of heterozygosity at codon 129. Thus, this heterozygosity may have played a protective role against the transmission of prion diseases in the Fore and other ancient populations practicing cannibalism. It has been suggested, not without controversy, that the wide geographic prevalence of codon 129 heterozygosity is indirect evidence that cannibalism may have been more widespread among ancient human populations than previously believed, although environmental exposure to prion diseases from other sources (e.g., tainted animal meat) also would have provided a survival benefit for maintaining codon 129 heterozygosity.[169]

Variant Creutzfeldt-Jakob Disease

Beginning in 1995, cases of a new variant of CJD were reported from the United Kingdom.[170-172] As of February 2009, a total of 165 cases have been reported to the UK Creutzfeldt-Jakob Disease Surveillance Unit (see http://www.cjd.ed.ac.uk/ for latest case totals). This includes three symptomatic "secondary" cases transmitted through blood transfusions.[173-175] An additional 44 cases have occurred outside the United Kingdom, with 23 of these in France and the remainder in the Republic of Ireland, Italy, the Netherlands, Portugal, Spain, Japan, Saudi Arabia, the United States, and Canada.[176] The four North American cases appear to be due to exposure of the victims to infected beef products in the United Kingdom or Saudi Arabia.[177] Retrospective review of available autopsy material suggests that vCJD did emerge as a new disease entity in 1995; no current evidence suggests that cases occurred earlier.[178,179] It is likely that millions of people were exposed to BSE-infected food.[180] However, fears of a large epidemic of vCJD have proven unfounded. The largest number of annual cases, 28, was reported in 2000. There were five cases in Great Britain in 2007, and modeling of the epidemic there predicts fewer than five new cases annually for the next several years.[181] In recent years, more cases have occurred outside the United Kingdom than inside.

The epidemiologic, clinical, and pathologic features of the vCJD cases set them apart from typical sCJD.[182,183] Patients with vCJD have been considerably younger than patients with sCJD, with a mean age at onset of 26 years (range, 12 to 74 years) compared with 65 years for sCJD. Ninety percent of vCJD patients are younger than 40 years at the onset of their disease. The reason for this striking age dependence is not clear, but it appears to be due to greater susceptibility in the young rather than greater exposure to BSE-contaminated foodstuffs.[184] The duration of illness in vCJD is longer (average of 14 months) than in sCJD (average of 4.5 months). This longer duration may be a reflection of the younger age of the patients because younger patients with sporadic CJD have a similar duration of illness.[185,186]

Patients with vCJD frequently present with sensory disturbances and psychiatric manifestations. Such symptoms are not unusual in young-onset sCJD, but in vCJD they are more prominent, perhaps because dementia and more obvious neurologic signs supervene later than in sCJD.[185] Among the sensory symptoms are vague pain, cold sensation, or paresthesias involving the face and limbs or in a hemisensory distribution. Most studied patients have had normal electromyography or mild abnormalities that do not point to a peripheral origin for the sensory disturbance.[118] It is speculated that they may be of thalamic origin.[187] Psychiatric manifestations frequently include dysphoria, withdrawal, anxiety, irritability, insomnia, and loss of interest in usual activities.[188,189] These symptoms often prompt an initial diagnosis of psychiatric illness. Neurologic signs and symptoms are uncommon within 4 months of onset. As disease progresses, the most frequent neurologic signs include dysarthria and gait disturbance. In the later stages of disease (>6 months after onset), prominent neurologic signs include hyperreflexia, myoclonus, incoordination, or other cerebellar signs.[188]

Blood transfusion has transmitted vCJD on at least four occasions. These transmissions occurred among a group of 66 individuals who were identified as having received blood components from donors who later developed vCJD. Only 33 of the transfusion recipients survived more than 5 years after transfusion, with the rest dying of conditions other than CJD or dementia.[174,190-192] In the four cases of vCJD infection in the remaining 33 patients, the donors had developed signs of vCJD from 16 months to 3.5 years after donation, whereas the recipients developed signs of vCJD 6 to 8 years after transfusion. One donor was linked to two vCJD cases in recipients who had received his blood products. All cases received non-leukodepleted red blood cells. The rate of vCJD in transfusion recipients from donors who later developed vCJD, 4/66 or 6%, is more than 20,000-fold higher than the rate of vCJD in the British population, conclusively implicating the transfusion as the cause of disease. In one transmitted case, the patient died without signs of vCJD but was found to have PrP^Sc in his spleen and a cervical lymph node. Remarkably, in an autopsied symptomatic case, PrP^Sc was found in the tonsils, suggesting that the tonsillar accumulation of PrP^Sc that is found in most vCJD cases is not due to the alimentary route of exposure but, rather, is a tropism inherent in the vCJD prion strain.[173]

The neuropathologic features of vCJD are strikingly different than those of sCJD.[171] The most characteristic differences between the neuropathology of vCJD and sCJD seem to be the prominent involvement of the cerebellum in almost all cases of vCJD compared with only a subset of cases with sCJD (Brownell-Oppenheimer variant and GSS cases). vCJD cases also show typical spongiform change, neuronal loss, and astrogliosis in cortex, basal ganglia, and thalamus, but these do not distinguish vCJD from sCJD. vCJD cases have prominent amyloid plaques distributed throughout the cerebrum and cerebellum and, to a lesser extent, the basal ganglia and thalamus. These plaques have a dense eosinophilic center and pale periphery and are surrounded by vacuoles in the neuropil arranged about the plaque like petals on a flower (hence the name "florid plaques"). The plaques stain strongly

positive for PrP^Sc. This flower-like morphology is common in plaques from vCJD but infrequently seen in other plaque-forming types of human prion disease such as GSS, kuru, and some sporadic cases of CJD.[193] Patients with vCJD also have a consistent pattern of electrophoretic mobility of PrP^Sc protein (type 4 isoform) that is distinct from the mobility patterns encountered in sCJD and is similar to the pattern seen in BSE PrP^Sc.[194-196]

It is interesting to compare the pathology of vCJD to that of kuru, the only other human prion disease known to be caused by oral exposure to the infectious agent. In both diseases, plaques are prominent, whereas in sCJD plaques are rare, although the plaque morphology differs in the two conditions.[166] It has been suggested that brain plaque formation may be caused by peripheral exposure to prions. Indeed, plaques seem more common in growth hormone-associated cases,[197] but unlike kuru or vCJD, they are not always present.[198,199] Unlike vCJD, which has only occurred in persons homozygous for methionine at PRNP codon 129, kuru is found in all three (MM, MV, and VV) codon 129 genotypes. Molecular typing of PrP^Sc from three kuru cases found both Collinge type 2MM and type 3MV (corresponding to Parchi types 1MM and 2MV)—both forms encountered in cases of sCJD—but no type 4 forms associated with vCJD.[200] (Molecular types are discussed later; see also Fig. 178-2). Kuru causes pathology similar to typical sCJD when transmitted to mice.[200] A single careful autopsy of a kuru victim surprisingly found no evidence of PrP^Sc in lymphoreticular tissue.[167] This is unlike vCJD and further indicates that lymphoreticular involvement with vCJD prions is not due to the route of inoculation.

A compelling body of evidence indicates that vCJD is the result of bovine-to-human transmission of BSE.[195,201-204] From an epidemiologic standpoint, cases of vCJD followed a massive epidemic of BSE in the United Kingdom with a lag period that is consistent with the known incubation period of prions. During the BSE epidemic, the first cases of which were recognized retrospectively as early as April 1985, it was estimated that several hundred thousand BSE-infected cattle might have entered the human food chain.[205-207] The number of BSE-infected cattle peaked during 1992 and 1993 and subsequently declined steadily. This decline has been attributed to bans on using ruminant protein for ruminant feeds (July 1988) and on using bovine brain, spinal cord, and other specified offal as feed for nonruminant animals and poultry (September 1990). Another ban prohibited use of certain bovine tissues for human consumption (November 1989). It has been suggested that the BSE epidemic was triggered by changes in the rendering process, particularly the abandonment of the use of organic solvents.[208]

Additional evidence for a BSE-vCJD link comes from the close neuropathologic similarities ("signature") between the two diseases. Transgenic mice expressing bovine PrP develop indistinguishable neurologic illness and neuropathologic changes after a similar incubation period when injected with brain material from either cattle with BSE or humans with vCJD, and this differs from the pattern and incubation time seen after inoculation with scrapie.[204] In addition, the PrP^Sc protein isoforms isolated from the brains of the BSE-inoculated or vCJD-inoculated mice show an identical fragment size and glycosylation pattern, which differs from that seen after scrapie inoculation.[203] Furthermore, macaques inoculated with BSE prions develop florid plaques histologically indistinguishable from those seen in vCJD, whereas those inoculated with sporadic CJD prions do not develop plaques.[202] Finally, the susceptibility of mice expressing murine PrP, or transgenic mice expressing PrP of humans, to vCJD more closely resembles the susceptibility of these same mice to BSE than to other forms of human prion disease.[209] In fact, mice of the nontransgenic RIII strain, inoculated with brain homogenate from sCJD victims, show no reduction in survival compared to saline-inoculated controls (although late in life they do begin to accumulate PrP^Sc), whereas vCJD-inoculated mice uniformly fall ill approximately 350 days after inoculation, as do BSE-inoculated mice.[204] Thus, the human-derived vCJD prion can readily cross the species barrier into mice, whereas human sCJD prions do so poorly. This and similar observations dem-

TABLE 178-3	Case Definitions for Sporadic and Variant CJD

Sporadic CJD

Possible
  Progressive dementia and
  EEG atypical or not known and
  Duration <2 years and
  At least two of the following clinical features:
    Myoclonus
    Visual or cerebellar disturbance
    Pyramidal/extrapyramidal dysfunction
    Akinetic mutism
Probable (in the absence of an alternative diagnosis from routine
  investigation)
  Progressive dementia and
  At least two of the following four clinical features:
    Myoclonus
    A typical EEG, whatever the clinical duration of the disease, and/or
    A positive 14-3-3 assay for CSF, and
    A clinical duration to death <2 years
Definite CJD
  Neuropathologic confirmation and/or
  Confirmation of protease-resistant prion protein (immunocytochemistry or
    Western blot) and/or
  The presence of scrapie-associated fibrils

Variant CJD

I   A Progressive neuropsychiatric disorder
    B Duration of illness >6 months
    C Routine investigations do not suggest an alternative diagnosis
    D No history of potential iatrogenic exposure
    E No evidence of a familial form of TSE
II A Early psychiatric symptoms
    B Persistent painful sensory symptoms
    C Ataxia
    D Myoclonus or chorea or dystonia
    E Dementia
III A EEG does not show the typical appearance of sporadic CJD (or no EEG
       performed)
    B MRI brain scan shows bilateral symmetrical pulvinar high signal
IV A Positive tonsil biopsy
Definite: I A *and* neuropathologic confirmation of variant CJD
Probable: I *and* 4/5 of II *and* III A *and* III B *OR* I *and* IV A
Possible: I and 4/5 of II and III A

CSF, cerebrospinal fluid; EEG, electroencephalography; TSE, transmissible spongiform encephalopathy.

Source: World Health Organization. *WHO Manual for Surveillance of Human Transmissible Spongiform Encephalopathies Including Variant Creutzfeldt-Jakob Disease.* Geneva: World Health Organization; 2003.

onstrate that species barriers depend not only on sequence differences in PrP between species but also on the particular prion strain in question.

No vCJD patients tested to date have had mutations in the *PRNP* gene, but all have shown homozygosity for methionine at polymorphic codon 129 (129M).[172,194] One young patient in Great Britain with the 129VV genotype developed CJD with clinical and pathologic features not typical of sporadic or variant CJD. Protease-resistant PrP^Sc from this patient showed a size and glycoform pattern identical to that found in vCJD.[210] Whether this was a sporadic case or, like vCJD, caused by exposure to BSE prions is undetermined.

Diagnosis of vCJD should be considered when patients with a history of residence in a BSE endemic area, such as the United Kingdom, develop a progressive neurodegenerative disease. Table 178-3 lists the World Health Organization criteria for vCJD. These criteria identified vCJD cases with 77% sensitivity and 100% specificity.[183]

Iatrogenic CJD

Examples of iatrogenic person-to-person spread are exceedingly rare, but such spread has followed transplantation of dural grafts,[211-214] corneal transplantation,[211] liver transplantation, use of dura mater material in radiographic embolization procedures,[215,216] use of contaminated neurosurgical instruments or stereotactic depth electrodes,[211] and, in cases of vCJD, blood transfusions. Although the numbers are evolving constantly as new cases are identified, a review

in 2006 identified 198 cases of iatrogenic CJD (iCJD) associated with human pituitary hormone administration, 196 cases associated with cadaver lyophilized dural transplants, 6 cases associated with contaminated neurosurgical instruments or intracortically implanted electroencephalography (EEG) depth electrodes, and 2 cases associated with cadaver corneal transplantation.[212] The important issue of sterilizing neurosurgical instruments after operations on patients with possible CJD is discussed in Chapter 301.

In the case of dura mater grafts, most, but not all, implicated grafts have been Lyodura, the product of a single German commercial producer, Braun. More cases (132 as of February 2008) have been reported from Japan than from all other countries worldwide.[212,213] Cases have occurred in at least 17 additional countries, however, including at least 7 cases from Canada and the United States.[213,217,218] The incubation period in these cases has ranged from 16 months to 25 years (median, approximately 12 years).[213] In Japan, two distinct clinicopathologic forms of dura graft-associated CJD are reported. Approximately 75% of cases present very similarly to typical sCJD, with rapid progression, myoclonus, periodic sharp waves on the EEG, and a diffuse cortical distribution of PrP^Sc.[219] One fourth of cases present with a picture reminiscent of GSS with slower progression, absent myoclonus, absent or late appearance of sharp waves on the EEG, and deposition of PrP in amyloid plaques, some with a "florid" pattern like that seen in vCJD cases.[134] Neither the common MV129 polymorphism nor an EK219 polymorphism, which is more common in the Japanese population, correlate with the clinicopathologic forms.

At least 114 cases of iCJD have been reported in young patients who received cadaver-derived human growth hormone for the treatment of endocrine disorders, including panhypopituitarism,[211,212,220] with at least 4 additional cases in women receiving cadaver pituitary gonadotropin for infertility,[211,212] practices that have been discontinued. Patients with human growth hormone–associated CJD typically received injections of growth hormone prepared from pools of 15,000 pituitary glands, several times weekly for several years. The risk of developing CJD differs among countries and cannot be absolutely determined because new cases continue to occur, even though several decades have passed since the use of human pituitary-derived growth hormone ceased. In a cohort of 6107 people who received human pituitary-derived growth hormone between 1963 and 1985 in the United States, 26 had developed CJD by 2002.[221] In this group, the median incubation period was 21.5 years. France has an exceptionally high rate of CJD among growth hormone recipients, in part because patients continued to receive the pituitary-derived product for several years after other countries halted the practice.[222] One recently reported patient received human growth hormone in low dose on one occasion for diagnostic purposes and developed iCJD 38 years later, suggesting that even longer incubation periods are possible in cases with low inoculum exposure.[198]

CJD has been reported in 10 recipients of corneal transplants from 1974 to 2006 worldwide. However, in only two of those cases was the donor known to have had CJD. When the large number of corneal transplants performed annually is taken into account, it has been estimated that sporadic CJD might coincidentally occur in a corneal graft recipient every 1.5 years in the United States alone.[223] Thus, most of the 10 reported cases are likely coincidental.

Five cases of iCJD have followed surgery with contaminated neurosurgical instruments, four from the United Kingdom[224] and one from France.[225] The incubation period after surgery ranged from 12 to 28 months (median, 17 months). In two cases from Switzerland,[226] intracortically implanted stereotactic depth electrodes for EEG monitoring were implicated. The incubation period was 16 and 20 months in the two affected patients. Documented cases of neurosurgical transmission are remarkably rare, despite the large number of neurosurgical procedures performed. The results of epidemiologic studies have been mixed, but several show an increased risk of CJD in those who have undergone any of a variety of surgical procedures.[227-230] Many of these studies may have been contaminated with recall and other biases, but a case-control study based on national hospital discharge registries in

Sweden and Denmark also found an approximately twofold risk of CJD in those who had undergone major surgery, again of various sorts. Consistent with known CJD incubation periods, the risk in this and other studies was highest in those who had undergone surgery 10 or more years earlier.[227-229] A twofold increased relative risk for a rare disease such as CJD translates into only a small increase in absolute risk, and the increased risk observed after surgery, even if real, does not necessarily implicate an infectious etiology.

Several hospitals in the United States, Canada, and the United Kingdom have reported incidents in which neurosurgical instruments were inadvertently reused in other patients after having been used initially for diagnostic brain biopsies in patients who subsequently were found to have CJD. Despite these medical mishaps, no patient so exposed is known to have developed iCJD, although the time since surgery in most of these instances is insufficient to exclude absolutely the possibility that this may occur in the future. The Joint Commission on Accreditation of Healthcare Organizations has issued a Sentinel Event Alert concerning this risk.[231] Hospitals should be aware of this potential and should establish guidelines for the handling, quarantine, and tracking of neurosurgical instruments in patients undergoing brain biopsy for dementia or other unknown neurodegenerative illnesses. In such cases, disposable instruments can be used if practicable, reducing the need for quarantine and tracking.

As discussed previously, four cases of human-to-human transmission of vCJD through blood transfusion have occurred. In contrast, many epidemiologic studies have failed to find a convincing link between blood transfusions and any other form of human prion disease,[232] and a history of preceding transfusion does not seem to increase the risk for CJD in epidemiologic studies.[227,228,230,232-234] The reasons for this remarkable divergence are unknown. Animal transmission studies suggest that whole blood, serum, or buffy coat derived from patients with vCJD, cattle with BSE, deer with CWD, or animals experimentally inoculated with prions can transmit prion disease to at least some IV inoculated animals.[232]

Isolated cases of CJD have occurred in at least 24 physicians and other health care workers,[235] including 2 neurosurgeons, 1 pathologist, 9 nurses, and 2 histology technicians. Despite the natural concern these reports produce among some health care professionals, the incidence of CJD in this group does not seem to exceed what would be expected by chance alone. There have been no documented reports of clear-cut transmission of disease from patients to hospital or mortuary staff. Similarly, although isolated cases of conjugal CJD have been reported, there does not seem to be any increased risk to spouses or other family members from exposure to CJD. As noted previously, the presence of familial cases of CJD seems invariably to result from genetic factors rather than from person-to-person spread of illness.

Prion Disease in Ruminants
Overwhelming evidence implicates the transmission of BSE from cattle to humans as the cause of vCJD. Prion disease is also endemic or epidemic in other ruminant species consumed by humans, including caprinae (sheep and goats) and cervidae (deer, elk, and related species). The risk that prions in these species pose to humans appears low but is under active study. Intensive surveillance for prion disease in cattle and sheep has uncovered what appear to be forms of prion disease other than classic BSE and scrapie.

Two unusual forms of bovine prion disease, known as BASE (or sometimes BSE-L) and BSE-H, were first described in 2004 and have been found in a total of 36 cattle to date.[236-238] These forms are histopathologically distinct from classic BSE, and the protease-resistant fragments migrate differently from classic BSE on Western immunoblots. Early data from transmission studies in various lines of transgenic and nontransgenic mice also support the notion that these forms are strains of prions different from that which causes classic BSE.[239] Whether BASE and BSE-H represent spontaneous (i.e., sporadic) prion disease in cattle, strain divergence of classic BSE, or another phenomenon is not known. In this regard, a single case of genetic BSE has been found in cattle.[240] PrP^{Sc} from this animal had a BSE-H pattern

of migration on Western immunoblotting. Sequencing of the *PRNP* found an E211K mutation. This mutation is homologous to the E200K mutation, which is the most common cause of genetic CJD in humans. A concern with these recently discovered strains of BSE prions is that they may be more pathogenic for humans than the classic BSE strain.[236,241]

Scrapie has long been endemic in sheep, and evidence indicates that the disease is either not transmitted to humans or transmits at a very low rate.[242] As with BSE, intensive surveillance in recent years has revealed previously unrecognized strains of scrapie in domesticated sheep. Nor98 is the most distinctive of these strains, with an unusual 12-kD protease-resistant core and a characteristic neuropathologic profile in sheep and in transgenic mice expressing ovine PrP.[243,244] Unlike classic scrapie, it is not clear if Nor98 is horizontally transmitted within flocks. Published studies of potential transmissibility to primates are lacking.

Chronic wasting disease (CWD) is epidemic in certain populations of deer and elk in North America. The greatest number of infected animals is found in regions of northern Colorado and southern Wyoming, but the disease has been discovered in free-ranging deer in many states and provinces, including Utah, Wisconsin, New York, Alberta, and Saskatchewan.[245] CWD is remarkable for the high rate of horizontal transmission among deer. In northern Colorado, as many as 5% of all mule deer are infected, and in captive populations infection rates have exceeded 30%.[246] Human hunters and others have certainly consumed infected animals, but fortunately it appears that CWD is not readily transmissible to humans. In Colorado, there has been no outbreak of unusual forms of CJD, and the rate of CJD seems to be no higher in the northern part of the state, where most infected deer are hunted and consumed, than in the southern part of the state.[247] Transgenic mice expressing human PrP do not develop prion disease when inoculated with CWD prions,[248,249] and in vitro conversion studies also suggest a species barrier between the common CWD strain in deer and humans.[250] Nonetheless, the dynamics of interspecies transmission of prion diseases are poorly understood, so humans should avoid consuming CWD-contaminated cervids.

Laboratory Diagnosis of Prion Disease

Currently, the certain diagnosis of human prion disease requires finding PrP^{Sc} in the CNS by biopsy or autopsy. However, some less invasive laboratory tests can provide supportive evidence. All such tests have less than perfect specificity. CJD is rare, so ancillary tests, if applied indiscriminately, will have poor positive predictive value, even if the specificity and sensitivity of these tests are high. A number of rare but treatable conditions mimic the clinical features of CJD, but CJD itself is untreatable and universally fatal. Therefore, the most important goal of the diagnostic process is to search for these other treatable causes of subacute dementia.

Routine laboratory and diagnostic tests may be useful in excluding other diagnostic possibilities. Prion disease is not itself an inflammatory condition. Elevated white blood cell count, sedimentation rate, or C-reactive protein or other signs of inflammation or autoimmunity should prompt the clinician to consider other diagnoses. In patients with CJD, the cerebrospinal fluid (CSF) is acellular and has a normal glucose concentration and a normal or mildly elevated protein content. The presence of a significant pleocytosis or hypoglycorrhachia should prompt a search for other diagnostic possibilities.

The presence of elevated levels of certain proteins in CSF may serve as useful diagnostic tests for CJD. The first evidence for this possibility came when abnormalities were noted in the CSF protein profile of patients with CJD after two-dimensional isoelectric focusing.[251,252] One of the abnormal CSF proteins is the 14-3-3 protein. Specific Western immunoblot and enzyme-linked immunosorbent assays for CSF 14-3-3 protein have been developed.[253,254] Testing for CSF 14-3-3 protein is available through commercial laboratories,[255] but interpretation of 14-3-3 results is not standardized, so more reliable results may be available through the large central prion disease laboratories of the United States (National Prion Disease Pathology Surveillance Center at http://www.cjdsurveillance.com), the United Kingdom, and the European Union. Early studies reported elevated 14-3-3 protein in 95% to 97% of patients with definite sCJD and in 93% of patients with probable sCJD. In subsequent practice, the sensitivity of the study has proven somewhat lower. In most studies, the test has a sensitivity of approximately 80% to 90% and a specificity of 90% or higher. However, CJD is a rare disease. In a group of 3756 patients referred to the French CJD Surveillance System, 365 were ultimately found to have CJD.[256] In this group, the positive predictive value of the 14-3-3 assay was only 53%. In contrast, negative predictive values were greater than 98%. Several conditions that may mimic CJD also may elevate the CSF 14-3-3 level. These include frontotemporal dementia, Alzheimer's disease, vascular dementia, dementia with Lewy bodies, metabolic encephalopathy, intracerebral metastatic cancer and carcinomatous meningitis, paraneoplastic encephalitis, hypoxic encephalopathy, herpes simplex encephalitis, Hashimoto's encephalopathy, and Morvan's syndrome.[257,258] In general, the specificity and sensitivity of the test are increased in patients with typical clinical syndromes. An elevated CSF 14-3-3 protein is useful to support the diagnosis in such cases, and a negative 14-3-3 test in a patient thought to have CJD should prompt reconsideration of the diagnosis. The specificity of the test is reduced in patients with presentations unusual for CJD, so the test should not be used to confirm the diagnosis in atypical cases.

Levels of a variety of proteins, including neuron-specific enolase and tau protein,[259-261] may also be elevated in the CSF of patients with CJD, although the sensitivity and specificity of these tests in clinical situations are not fully defined. Similar to assays of 14-3-3 protein, these tests have the disadvantage that elevated values can be found in a variety of neurologic diseases, some of which can present with a CJD-like subacute dementia. Whether combinations of these proteins may provide a "fingerprint" to distinguish CJD from other conditions is an area of active research.[262-264]

Infectious prions accumulate not just in the brain but also often in other tissues and fluids, such as CSF, blood, lymphatic tissue, and muscle.[265-267] PrP^{Sc} levels in these components are often too low for detection with the immunohistochemical techniques and Western blots that are typically used to find PrP^{Sc} in brain tissue. Highly sensitive methods to detect PrP^{Sc} are now available or in development. It is possible that such assays might be applied to CSF, blood, lymphatic tissue, muscle, or other tissue or fluids to diagnose at least in some cases of human prion disease, but such tests are not routinely available. Several assays rely on recently developed methods to amplify PrP^{Sc} in vitro. Foremost among these is protein misfolding cyclic amplification (PMCA).[268] Under certain conditions, it is possible to increase minute amounts of PrP^{Sc}, as low as the equivalent of a single infectious unit, to detectable levels with this technique.[269] In experimental animals, PMCA has successfully detected PrP^{Sc} in the blood and spinal fluid of scrapie-infected hamsters.[270,271]

Brain MRI is the most useful imaging technique in the diagnosis of CJD (Fig. 178-3).[272,273] Diffusion-weighted imaging (DWI) is probably the most sensitive MRI sequence for detecting characteristic abnormalities associated with sporadic CJD. Fluid-attenuated inversion recovery (FLAIR) may be superior to DWI for variant CJD. In sporadic CJD, the most common abnormality seen on standard MRI sequences is increased T_2, DWI, or FLAIR signal in the striatum. Ribbon-like increased signal intensity in cerebral cortex is also common.[272] Increased signal intensity in the basal ganglia has been reported to have 67% sensitivity and 93% specificity for diagnosis of sCJD. In a study of 193 consecutive cases of suspect CJD, sensitivity of MRI changes ranged from 50% to 70%, depending on the evaluator, whereas specificity was approximately 80%.[274] The neuropathologic substrate for DWI abnormalities has not been characterized fully, although these abnormalities correlate with areas of severe neuropathologic change, including spongiform degeneration.[272] MRI is particularly useful in the diagnosis of vCJD.[275] In a prospective study of 368 MRI scans of patients with clinical histories suspicious for CJD, the presence of the "pulvinar sign" identified 74 of 82 patients eventually proven by neuropathologic

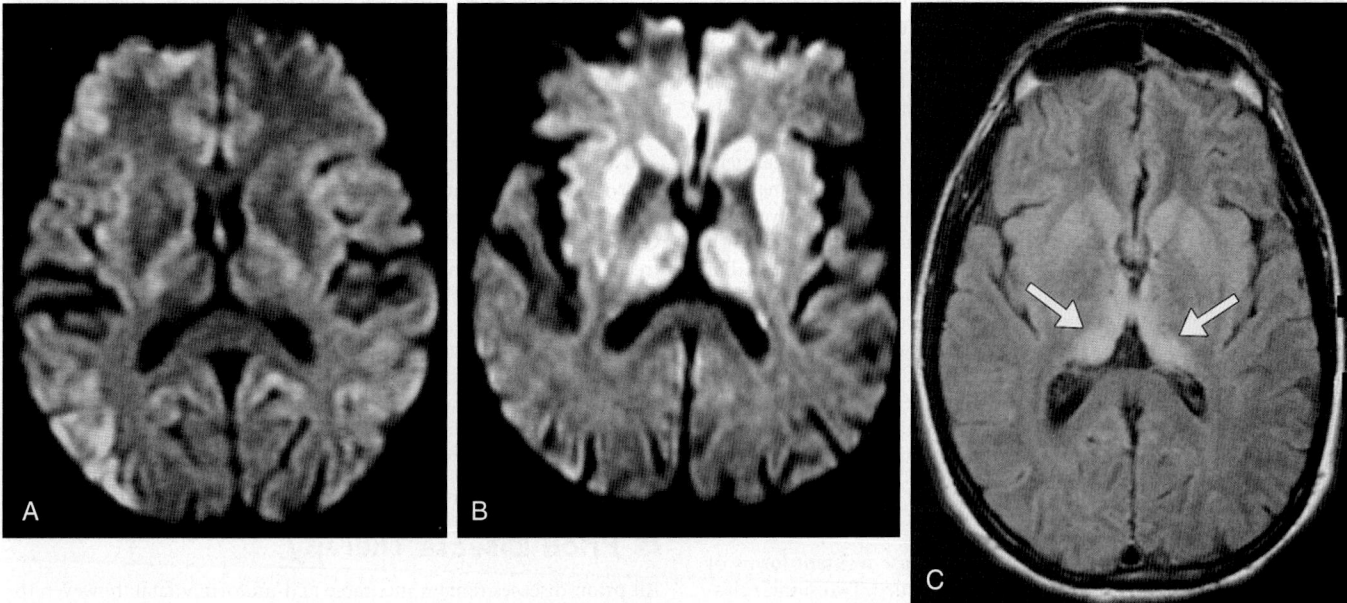

Figure 178-3   MRI appearance of CJD. The images depict DWI sequences from MRIs of three patients with CJD. **A,** Restricted diffusion in a cortical ribbon pattern in a patient with sporadic CJD. **B,** Restricted diffusion in the deep cerebral gray matter in a different case of sporadic CJD. **C,** Restricted diffusion in the posterior thalamus (the pulvinar), indicated by arrows, in a patient with vCJD. ADC mapping confirms that hyperintense areas on DWI represent restricted diffusion (not shown). Similar, but generally less obvious, abnormalities can be seen on FLAIR and T_2-weighted images. (*A and B, from Kallenberg K, Schulz-Schaeffer WJ, Jastrow U, et al. Creutzfeldt-Jakob disease: comparative analysis of MR imaging sequences. AJNR Am J Neuroradiol. 2006;27:1459-62;* **C,** *from Tschampa HJ, Zerr I, Urbach H. Radiological assessment of Creutzfeldt-Jakob disease. Eur Radiol. 2007;17:1200-11.*)

studies to have vCJD. The FLAIR sequence was most sensitive, with the sign recognized in 30 of 30 vCJD patients in whom the FLAIR images were obtained. The pulvinar sign consists of increased signal in the posterior thalamus, usually seen on image sequences sensitive to T_2 effects, including T_2, proton density, FLAIR, and DWI. Rarely, T_1 hyperintensity is recognized in the pulvinar as well. When strictly defined as greater hyperintensity in the posterior thalamus relative to other deep brain nuclei, the pulvinar sign is specific for vCJD. Increased pulvinar and other deep gray matter hyperintensity occurs in some cases of sporadic CJD; however, in these cases, the signal in other nuclei, especially the anterior putamen, is greater than in the pulvinar.

Computed tomography is usually not helpful in the diagnosis of CJD, except that it may exclude some other conditions. Studies evaluating neuroimaging techniques such as positron emission tomography[276] and single-photon emission computed tomography[277] are too few to determine the sensitivity or specificity of these tests.

Patients with CJD often have characteristic abnormalities on EEG,[278-281] and this test may be helpful as a diagnostic tool. The classic EEG pattern, which ultimately appears in 67% to 95% of patients, consists of a slow background interrupted by generalized, bilaterally synchronous biphasic or triphasic periodic sharp wave complexes (PSWCs). These occur at intervals of 0.5 to 2.5 seconds and have a duration of 100 to 600 msec. PSWCs may be absent early in disease, may disappear in the terminal stages, and often are more dramatic during periods of alertness, but they may disappear during sleep or under the influence of certain drugs. It has been suggested that the presence of PSWCs, identified according to strict criteria in blinded EEG readings, has a sensitivity of approximately 65% and a specificity of 74% to 86% for the diagnosis of CJD.[280,281] Obtaining serial EEGs in patients suspected of having CJD may be useful if PSWCs are absent on an initial EEG study.[279] Certain forms of human prion disease, including GSS, fatal insomnia, and vCJD, do not usually display periodic EEG abnormalities.

Examination of brain material remains the gold standard for diagnosis of prion diseases. The classic neuropathologic features of neuronal loss, reactive gliosis, and vacuolation of the neuropil (spongiform change), with an absence of inflammatory changes, typically are present in such cases and are consistent with the diagnosis. However, the modern diagnosis of prion disease rests on the immunohistochemical demonstration of abnormal forms of PrP. A variety of techniques have been developed to immunostain for PrP^{Sc} in paraffin-embedded brain material. The general strategy in these techniques is to hydrolyze PrP^{C} while enhancing the antigenicity of PrP^{Sc} by partially denaturing the aggregates. A widely used protocol includes autoclaving tissue sections in water (hydrolytic autoclaving), followed by treatment with formic acid and then a chaotropic salt (guanidine thiocyanate).[282] With these techniques, a variety of PrP staining patterns have been identified in CJD brain tissue.[283] This tissue may show positive PrP staining limited to plaques or a more diffuse staining pattern that co-localizes with synaptic markers (e.g., synaptophysin) throughout the gray matter or a combination of both patterns.[284,285] In the United States, the National Prion Disease Pathology Surveillance Center at Case Western Reserve University in Cleveland, Ohio, assists clinicians and pathologists in analyzing fixed brain material for characteristic histopathology and the presence of PrP^{Sc} and performs PrP^{Sc} immunohistochemistry and prion isoform analysis on frozen brain tissue from patients with suspected prion diseases. Instructions for shipping material are available at the center's website (http://www.cjdsurveillance.com).

If frozen tissue is available, analysis of protease-resistant forms of PrP by Western immunoblot is generally performed. Two similar classification schemes correlate the clinical features of sporadic human prion disease with the biochemical properties of the PrP^{Sc} that accumulates in these cases. In these schemes, patients are classified by (1) the size of the protease-resistant fragment of PrP^{Sc} isolated from the brain and (2) the genotype at the polymorphic codon 129 of PrP (MM, MV, or VV). These "molecular" types are then correlated to the patients' clinical syndromes. In the scheme of Parchi and collabora-

tors, the protease-resistant fragment is of either 21 kD (type 1) or 19 kD (type 2) in size. Thus, there are six possible molecular types of human prion disease under this scheme (MM1, MM2, MV1, etc.). In the scheme originally proposed by Collinge and collaborators, three PrP^{Sc} size variants are recognized (with type 1 and type 2 being close in size to Parchi's type 1).[195] The subtle differences between the schemes may be an artifact.[286] At any rate, the molecular types do correlate to clinical syndromes, with distinct differences in age of onset, duration, and dominant clinical symptoms between the types.[194,287] For example, under the Parchi scheme, patients with the MM1 molecular type have a mean age of onset of 66 years and a duration of 4 months, whereas those with the rare VV1 type have a mean onset of 40 years and a duration of 15 months. These molecular types likely reflect in part the same sorts of biochemical differences in the PrP^{Sc} seen between well-characterized animal prion strains with an additional, incompletely understood influence from the PrP genotype. Different relative amounts of the three PrP^{Sc} glycoforms also associate with clinical properties and probably reflect prion strain differences.[147,195]

Unlike most sporadic CJD cases, in vCJD lymphoid tissue of the tonsils, spleen, and appendix contains immunohistochemically detectable PrP^{Sc}.[288,289] It has been suggested that analysis of PrP from extraneural lymphoreticular tissue might provide a less invasive method than brain biopsy for definitive diagnosis of vCJD. Highly sensitive immunoblotting assays are now available that enable detection of small quantities of PrP^{Sc} from patients with vCJD.[290] In an autopsy study, 19 of 20 (95%) appendices removed at autopsy from patients with vCJD tested positive for PrP,[291] although a subsequent report found only 1 positive case among 4 tested (25%).[292] If future studies confirm the sensitivity and specificity of tonsil and lymphoreticular tissue biopsy for diagnosis of vCJD, this may become an important diagnostic tool.

In a symptomatic patient with a family history of prion disease, finding a *PRNP* gene mutation can be taken as definitive evidence of CJD. A family history of unusual dementia is absent in as many as 46% of patients with a genetic prion disease.[125] Such cases can be due to new mutations, incomplete family history, incomplete penetrance, or misidentified paternity. Thus, it may be worth obtaining the sequence of the *PRNP* coding region in patients with undiagnosed subacute or otherwise unusual dementias. Genetic techniques are highly specific but insensitive when used for diagnosis of isolated cases of prion disease because approximately 90% of prion disease patients will have no PRNP mutation.

The World Health Organization has published criteria for the clinical diagnosis of CJD (see Table 178-3).

Despite the high specificity of available diagnostic clinical criteria and associated ancillary testing, some patients ultimately prove to have alternate diagnoses, including rapidly progressive forms of Alzheimer's disease, frontotemporal dementia, and dementia with Lewy bodies.[109,293] Of more concern are patients with treatable or at least potentially treatable disorders that can mimic sCJD. These include encephalopathies due to toxic levels of therapeutic agents such as lithium[294,295] or bismuth[296,297]; autoimmune encephalitides including Hashimoto's encephalitis and Morvan's fibrillary chorea (rare conditions diagnosed by finding elevated levels against, respectively, thyroid antigens[298-300] and voltage-gated potassium channels[301,302]); nonconvulsive status epilepticus[303]; cerebral vasculitis[109]; paraneoplastic encephalitis[109]; intravascular lymphoma[304]; hyperparathyroidism[109]; and normal pressure hydrocephalus.[109]

Prion Disease Therapy

All prion diseases remain incurable and uniformly fatal; however, the availability of excellent animal models of prion disease has encouraged investigation of a large number of different therapeutic strategies. These strategies include immunotherapies such as antibodies and immunization against PrP, various small molecule inhibitors of PrP^{Sc} propagation identified by in vitro screening methods, polyanionic and polycationic compounds, and iRNA and other inhibitors of PrP translation (reviewed by Trevitt and Collinge[305]). Several of these treatments are able to abolish scrapie infection in cultured cells. A number can delay the onset of clinical illness in rodents when administered prior to inoculation and in some cases after inoculation but before the emergence of clinical signs. However, no treatment significantly alters the course of disease after the appearance of obvious clinical signs—the situation that would be most useful for treatment of sporadic human prion disease. Four compounds have been tried in series of humans symptomatic with prion disease.[306] Pentosan polysulfate by intraventricular infusion may have slowed disease progression in some patients, but the studies are uncontrolled. Likewise, studies of orally administered quinacrine treatment generally suggest no substantial benefit. Amantadine may have transiently improved symptoms in some patients, but it probably provides no clinically important benefit. Only one randomized trial has been reported. In this study, in which 28 CJD patients were randomized to flupirtine or placebo, the drug may have slowed cognitive decline.[307]

REFERENCES

1. Brown P, Bradley R. 1755 and all that: a historical primer of transmissible spongiform encephalopathy. *BMJ.* 1998;317:1688-1692.
2. Cuillé J, Chelle P-L. La maladie dite "tremblante" du mouton; est-elle inoculable? *Compte Rend Acad Sci.* 1936;203:1552.
3. Cuillé J, Chelle PL. Experimental transmission of trembling to the goat. *CR Seances Acad Sci.* 1939;208:1058-1060.
4. Alper T, Haig DA, Clarke MC. The exceptionally small size of the scrapie agent. *Biochem Biophys Res Commun.* 1966;22:278-284.
5. Gajdusek DC, Zigas V. Clinical, pathological and epidemiological study of an acute progressive degenerative disease of the central nervous system among natives of the eastern highlands of New Guinea. *Am J Med.* 1959;26:442-469.
6. Gajdusek DC, Zigas V. Degenerative disease of the central nervous system in New Guinea? The endemic occurrence of "kuru" in the native population. *N Engl J Med.* 1957;257:974-978.
7. Gajdusek DC, Gibbs Jr CJ, Alpers M. Experimental transmission of a kuru-like syndrome to chimpanzees. *Nature.* 1966;209:794-796.
8. Hadlow WJ. Scrapie and kuru. *Lancet.* 1959;2:289-290.
9. Hadlow WJ. Neuropathology and the scrapie-kuru connection. *Brain Pathol.* 1995;5:27-31.
10. Prusiner SB, Hadlow WJ, Eklund CM, et al. Sedimentation properties of the scrapie agent. *Proc Natl Acad Sci U S A.* 1977;74:4656-4660.
11. Prusiner SB. An approach to the isolation of biological particles using sedimentation analysis. *J Biol Chem.* 1978;253:916-921.
12. Prusiner SB, Groth DF, Cochran SP, et al. Gel electrophoresis and glass permeation chromatography of the hamster scrapie agent after enzymatic digestion and detergent extraction. *Biochemistry.* 1980;19:4892-4898.
13. Prusiner SB, Groth DF, Cochran SP, et al. Molecular properties, partial purification, and assay by incubation period measurements of the hamster scrapie agent. *Biochemistry.* 1980;21:4883-4891.
14. Prusiner SB, Cochran SP, Groth DF, et al. Measurement of the scrapie agent using an incubation time interval assay. *Ann Neurol.* 1982;11:353-358.
15. Prusiner SB. Novel proteinaceous infectious particles cause scrapie. *Science.* 1982;216:136-144.
16. Chien P, Weissman JS, DePace AH. Emerging principles of conformation-based prion inheritance. *Annu Rev Biochem.* 2004;73:617-656.
17. Oesch B, Westaway D, Wälchli M, et al. A cellular gene encodes scrapie PrP 27-30 protein. *Cell.* 1985;40:735-746.
18. Prusiner SB. Molecular biology of prion diseases. *Science.* 1991;252:1515-1522.
19. Chesebro B, Race R, Wehrly K, et al. Identification of scrapie prion protein-specific mRNA in scrapie-infected and uninfected brain. *Nature.* 1985;315:331-333.
20. Manson J, West JD, Thomson V, et al. The prion protein gene: a role in mouse embryogenesis? *Development.* 1992;115:117-122.
21. Moser M, Colello RJ, Pott U, et al. Developmental expression of the prion protein gene in glial cells. *Neuron.* 1995;14:509-517.
22. Stahl N, Borchelt DR, Hsiao K, et al. Scrapie prion protein contains a phosphatidylinositol glycolipid. *Cell.* 1987;51:229-240.
23. Taraboulos A, Raeber AJ, Borchelt DR, et al. Synthesis and trafficking of prion proteins in cultured cells. *Mol Biol Cell.* 1992;3:851-863.
24. Bolton DC, Meyer RK, Prusiner SB. Scrapie PrP 27-30 is a sialoglycoprotein. *J Virol.* 1985;53:596-606.
25. Hegde RS, Mastrianni JA, Scott MR, et al. A transmembrane form of the prion protein in neurodegenerative disease. *Science.* 1998;279:827-834.
26. Hegde RS, Tremblay P, Groth D, et al. Transmissible and genetic prion diseases share a common pathway of neurodegeneration. *Nature.* 1999;402:822-826.
27. Schmitt-Ulms G, Legname G, Baldwin MA, et al. Binding of neural cell adhesion molecules (N-CAMs) to the cellular prion protein. *J Mol Biol.* 2001;314:1209-1225.
28. Rieger R, Edenhofer F, Lasmézas CI, et al. The human 37-kDa laminin receptor precursor interacts with the prion protein in eukaryotic cells. *Nat Med.* 1997;3:1383-1388.
29. Lledo P-M, Tremblay P, DeArmond SJ, et al. Mice deficient for prion protein exhibit normal neuronal excitability and synaptic transmission in the hippocampus. *Proc Natl Acad Sci U S A.* 1996;93:2403-2407.
30. Graner E, Mercadante AF, Zanata SM, et al. Cellular prion protein binds laminin and mediates neuritogenesis. *Mol Brain Res.* 2000;76:85-92.
31. Brown DR, Qin K, Herms JW, et al. The cellular prion protein binds copper in vivo. *Nature.* 1997;390:684-687.
32. Whittal RM, Ball HL, Cohen FE, et al. Copper binding to octarepeat peptides of the prion protein monitored by mass spectrometry. *Protein Sci.* 2000;9:332-343.
33. Brown DR, Besinger A. Prion protein expression and superoxide dismutase activity. *Biochem J.* 1998;334:423-429.
34. Tobler I, Gaus SE, Deboer T, et al. Altered circadian activity rhythms and sleep in mice devoid of prion protein. *Nature.* 1996;380:639-642.
35. Moore RC, Lee IY, Silverman GL, et al. Ataxia in prion protein (PrP) deficient mice is associated with upregulation of the novel PrP-like protein doppel. *J Mol Biol.* 1999;292:797-817.
36. Silverman GL, Qin K, Moore RC, et al. Doppel is an *N*-glycosylated, glycosylphosphatidylinositol-anchored protein. *J Biol Chem.* 2000;275:26834-26841.
37. Watts JC, Westaway D. The prion protein family: diversity, rivalry, and dysfunction. *Biochem Biophys Acta.* 2007;1772:654-672.
38. Moore RC, Mastrangelo P, Bouzamondo E, et al. Doppel-induced cerebellar degeneration in transgenic mice. *Proc Natl Acad Sci U S A.* 2001;98:15288-15293.
39. Safar JG, Kellings K, Serban A, et al. Search for a prion-specific nucleic acid. *J Virol.* 2005;79:10796-10806.
40. Basler K, Oesch B, Scott M, et al. Scrapie and cellular PrP isoforms are encoded by the same chromosomal gene. *Cell.* 1986;46:417-428.
41. Meyer RK, McKinley MP, Bowman KA, et al. Separation and properties of cellular and scrapie prion proteins. *Proc Natl Acad Sci U S A.* 1986;83:2310-2314.
42. Parchi P, Castellani R, Capellari S, et al. Molecular basis of phenotypic variability in sporadic Creutzfeldt-Jakob disease. *Ann Neurol.* 1996;39:767-778.
43. Parchi P, Chen SG, Brown P, et al. Different patterns of truncated prion protein fragments correlate with distinct phenotypes in P102L Gerstmann-Straussler-Scheinker disease. *Proc Natl Acad Sci U S A.* 1998;95:8322-8327.
44. Yadavalli R, Guttmann RP, Seward T, et al. Calpain-dependent endoproteolytic cleavage of PrPSc modulates scrapie prion propagation. *J Biol Chem.* 2004;279:21948-21956.
45. Safar J, Wille H, Itri V, et al. Eight prion strains have PrP^{Sc} molecules with different conformations. *Nat Med.* 1998;4:1157-1165.
46. Merz PA, Somerville RA, Wisniewski HM, et al. Abnormal fibrils from scrapie-infected brain. *Acta Neuropathol (Berlin).* 1981;54:63-74.
47. Merz PA, Kascsak RJ, Rubenstein R, et al. Antisera to scrapie-associated fibril protein and prion protein decorate scrapie-associated fibrils. *J Virol.* 1987;61:42-49.
48. Korth C, Stierli B, Streit P, et al. Prion (PrP^{Sc})-specific epitope defined by a monoclonal antibody. *Nature.* 1997;389:74-77.
49. Hornemann S, Korth C, Oesch B, et al. Recombinant full-length murine prion protein, *m*PrP(23-231): purification and spectroscopic characterization. *FEBS Lett.* 1997;413:277-281.
50. Riek R, Hornemann S, Wider G, et al. NMR characterization of the full-length recombinant murine prion protein, *m*PrP(23-231). *FEBS Lett.* 1997;413:282-288.
51. Donne DG, Viles JH, Groth D, et al. Structure of the recombinant full-length hamster prion protein PrP(29-231): the N terminus is highly flexible. *Proc Natl Acad Sci U S A.* 1997;94:13452-13457.
52. Pan K-M, Baldwin M, Nguyen J, et al. Conversion of α-helices into β-sheets features in the formation of the scrapie prion proteins. *Proc Natl Acad Sci U S A.* 1993;90:10962-10966.
53. Govaerts C, Wille H, Prusiner SB, et al. Evidence for assembly of prions with left-handed beta-helices into trimers. *Proc Natl Acad Sci U S A.* 2004;101:8342-8347.
54. Wille H, Michelitsch MD, Guenebaut V, et al. Structural studies of the scrapie prion protein by electron crystallography. *Proc Natl Acad Sci U S A.* 2002;99:3563-3568.
55. Wickner RB, Dyda F, Tycko R. Amyloid of Rnq1p, the basis of the [PIN+] prion, has a parallel in-register beta-sheet structure. *Proc Natl Acad Sci U S A.* 2008;105:2403-2408.
56. Cobb NJ, Sonnichsen FD, McHaourab H, et al. Molecular architecture of human prion protein amyloid: a parallel, in-register beta-structure. *Proc Natl Acad Sci U S A.* 2007;104:18946-18951.
57. Sawaya MR, Sambashivan S, Nelson R, et al. Atomic structures of amyloid cross-beta spines reveal varied steric zippers. *Nature.* 2007;447:453-457.
58. Lee SW, Mou Y, Lin SY, et al. Steric zipper of the amyloid fibrils formed by residues 109-122 of the Syrian hamster prion protein. *J Mol Biol.* 2008;378:1142-1154.
59. Lim KH, Nguyen TN, Damo SM, et al. Solid-state NMR structural studies of the fibril form of a mutant mouse prion peptide PrP89-143(P101L). *Solid State Nucl Magn Reson.* 2006;29:183-190.
60. Harper JD, Lansbury Jr PT. Models of amyloid seeding in Alzheimer's disease and scrapie: mechanistic truths and physiological consequences of the time-dependent solubility of amyloid proteins. *Annu Rev Biochem.* 1997;66:385-407.
61. Stohr J, Weinmann N, Wille H, et al. Mechanisms of prion protein assembly into amyloid. *Proc Natl Acad Sci U S A.* 2008;105:2409-2414.
62. Nazor KE, Kuhn F, Seward T, et al. Immunodetection of disease-associated mutant PrP, which accelerates disease in GSS transgenic mice. *EMBO J.* 2005;24:2472-2480.
63. Silveira JR, Raymond GJ, Hughson AG, et al. The most infectious prion protein particles. *Nature.* 2005;437:257-261.
64. Deleault NR, Harris BT, Rees JR, et al. Formation of native prions from minimal components in vitro. *Proc Natl Acad Sci U S A.* 2007;104:9741-9746.
65. Geoghegan JC, Valdes PA, Orem NR, et al. Selective incorporation of polyanionic molecules into hamster prions. *J Biol Chem.* 2007;282:36341-36353.
66. Legname G, Baskakov IV, Nguyen HO, et al. Synthetic mammalian prions. *Science.* 2004;305:673-676.
67. Hsiao K, Baker HF, Crow TJ, et al. Linkage of a prion protein missense variant to Gerstmann-Sträussler syndrome. *Nature.* 1989;338:342-345.
68. Telling GC. Transgenic mouse models of prion diseases. *Methods Mol Biol.* 2008;459:249-263.
69. Scott M, Foster D, Mirenda C, et al. Transgenic mice expressing hamster prion protein produce species-specific scrapie infectivity and amyloid plaques. *Cell.* 1989;59:847-857.
70. Telling GC, Scott M, Hsiao KK, et al. Transmission of Creutzfeldt-Jakob disease from humans to transgenic mice expressing chimeric human-mouse prion protein. *Proc Natl Acad Sci U S A.* 1994;91:9936-9940.
71. Sadlish H, Rampelt H, Shorter J, et al. Hsp110 chaperones regulate prion formation and propagation in *S. cerevisiae* by two discrete activities. *PLoS ONE.* 2008;3:e1763.
72. Shorter J, Lindquist S. Hsp104, Hsp70 and Hsp40 interplay regulates formation, growth and elimination of Sup35 prions. *EMBO J.* 2008;27:2712-2724.
73. Tamguney G, Giles K, Glidden DV, et al. Genes contributing to prion pathogenesis. *J Gen Virol.* 2008;89:1777-1788.
74. Kaneko K, Zulianello L, Scott M, et al. Evidence for protein X binding to a discontinuous epitope on the cellular prion protein during scrapie prion propagation. *Proc Natl Acad Sci U S A.* 1997;94:10069-10074.
75. Telling GC, Scott M, Mastrianni J, et al. Prion propagation in mice expressing human and chimeric PrP transgenes implicates the interaction of cellular PrP with another protein. *Cell.* 1995;83:79-90.
76. Aguzzi A, Sigurdson C, Heikenwaelder M. Molecular mechanisms of prion pathogenesis. *Annu Rev Pathol.* 2008;3:11-40.
77. Chesebro B, Trifilo M, Race R, et al. Anchorless prion protein results in infectious amyloid disease without clinical scrapie. *Science.* 2005;308:1435-1439.
78. Kristiansen M, Messenger MJ, Klohn PC, et al. Disease-related prion protein forms aggresomes in neuronal cells leading to caspase activation and apoptosis. *J Biol Chem.* 2005;280:38851-38861.
79. Prinz M, Huber G, Macpherson AJ, et al. Oral prion infection requires normal numbers of Peyer's patches but not of enteric lymphocytes. *Am J Pathol.* 2003;162:1103-1111.
80. Klein MA, Frigg R, Flechsig E, et al. A crucial role for B cells in neuroinvasive scrapie. *Nature.* 1997;390:687-690.
81. Chiocchetti R, Mazzuoli G, Albanese V, et al. Anatomical evidence for ileal Peyer's patches innervation by enteric nervous

system: a potential route for prion neuroinvasion? *Cell Tissue Res.* 2008;332:185-194.
82. Hoffmann C, Ziegler U, Buschmann A, et al. Prions spread via the autonomic nervous system from the gut to the central nervous system in cattle incubating bovine spongiform encephalopathy. *J Gen Virol.* 2007;88:1048-1055.
83. Kimberlin RH, Walker CA. Pathogenesis of scrapie in mice after intragastric infection. *Virus Res.* 1989;12:213-220.
84. McBride PA, Beekes M. Pathological PrP is abundant in sympathetic and sensory ganglia of hamsters fed with scrapie. *Neurosci Lett.* 1999;265:135-138.
85. Prinz M, Heikenwalder M, Junt T, et al. Positioning of follicular dendritic cells within the spleen controls prion neuroinvasion. *Nature.* 2003;425:957-962.
86. Glatzel M, Heppner FL, Albers KM, et al. Sympathetic innervation of lymphoreticular organs is rate limiting for prion neuroinvasion. *Neuron.* 2001;31:25-34.
87. Bartz JC, Dejoia C, Tucker T, et al. Extraneural prion neuroinvasion without lymphoreticular system infection. *J Virol.* 2005;79:11858-11863.
88. Heikenwalder M, Zeller N, Seeger H, et al. Chronic lymphocytic inflammation specifies the organ tropism of prions. *Science.* 2005;307:1107-1110.
89. Seeger H, Heikenwalder M, Zeller N, et al. Coincident scrapie infection and nephritis lead to urinary prion excretion. *Science.* 2005;310:324-326.
90. Gonzalez-Romero D, Barria MA, Leon P, et al. Detection of infectious prions in urine. *FEBS Lett.* 2008;582:3161-3166.
91. Collinge J, Clarke AR. A general model of prion strains and their pathogenicity. *Science.* 2007;318:930-936.
92. Bruce ME. TSE strain variation. *Br Med Bull.* 2003;66:99-108.
93. Bartz JC, Aiken JM, Bessen RA. Delay in onset of prion disease for the HY strain of transmissible mink encephalopathy as a result of prior peripheral inoculation with the replication-deficient DY strain. *J Gen Virol.* 2004;85:265-273.
94. Wickner RB. [URE3] as an altered URE2 protein: evidence for a prion analog in *Saccharomyces cerevisiae*. *Science.* 1994;264:566-569.
95. Aigle M, Lacroute F. Genetical aspects of [URE3], a non-Mendelian, cytoplasmically inherited mutation in yeast. *Mol Gen Genet.* 1975;136:327-335.
96. Coustou V, Deleu C, Saupe S, et al. The protein product of the *het-s* heterokaryon incompatibility gene of the fungus *Podospora anserina* behaves as a prion analog. *Proc Natl Acad Sci U S A.* 1997;94:9773-9778.
97. Cox BS. PSI, a cytoplasmic suppressor of super-suppressor in yeast. *Heredity.* 1965;20:505-521.
98. Wickner RB, Chernoff YO. Prions of fungi: [URE3], [PSI], and [Het-s] discovered as heritable traits. In: Prusiner SB, ed. *Prion Biology and Diseases.* Cold Spring Harbor, NY: Cold Spring Harbor Laboratory Press; 1999:229-272.
99. Creutzfeldt HG. Über eine eigenartige herdförmige Erkrankung des Zentralnervensystems. Z. Gesamte Neurol. *Psychiatrie.* 1920;57:1-18.—[Translated by Richardson EP Jr. In: Rottenberg DA, Hochberg FH, eds. Neurological Classics in Modern Translation. New York: Hafner; 1977:97-112.]
100. Jakob A. Über eine der multiplen Sklerose klinisch nahestehende Erkrankung des Zentralnervensystems (spastische Pseudosklerose) mit bemerkenswertem anatomischem Befunde. Mitteilung eines vierten Falles. *Med Klin.* 1921;17:372-376.—[Translated by Richardson EP, Jr. In: Rottenberg DA, Hochberg FH, eds. *Neurological Classics in Modern Translation.* New York: Hefner; 1977:113-125.]
101. Stoeck K, Hess K, Amsler L, et al. Heightened incidence of sporadic Creutzfeldt-Jakob disease is associated with a shift in clinicopathological profiles. *J Neurol.* 2008;255:1464-1472.
102. Klug GM, Boyd A, Lewis V, et al. Surveillance of Creutzfeldt-Jakob disease in Australia: 2008. *Commun Dis Intell.* 2008;32:232-236.
103. Papacostas S, Malikides A, Petsa M, et al. Ten-year mortality from Creutzfeldt-Jakob disease in Cyprus. *East Mediterr Health J.* 2008;14:715-719.
104. Gelpi E, Heinzl H, Hoftberger R, et al. Creutzfeldt-Jakob disease in Austria: an autopsy-controlled study. *Neuroepidemiology.* 2008;30:215-221.
105. Van Everbroeck B, Michotte A, Sciot R, et al. Increased incidence of sporadic Creutzfeldt-Jakob disease in the age groups between 70 and 90 years in Belgium. *Eur J Epidemiol.* 2006;21:443-447.
106. Maddox RA, Holman RC, Belay ED, et al. Creutzfeldt-Jakob disease among American Indians and Alaska Natives in the United States. *Neurology.* 2006;66:439-441.
107. Gibbons RV, Holman RC, Belay ED, et al. Creutzfeldt-Jakob disease in the United States: 1979-1998. *JAMA.* 2000;284:2322-2323.
108. Ladogana A, Puopolo M, Croes EA, et al. Mortality from Creutzfeldt-Jakob disease and related disorders in Europe, Australia, and Canada. *Neurology.* 2005;64:1586-1591.
109. Heinemann U, Krasnianski A, Meissner B, et al. Creutzfeldt-Jakob disease in Germany: a prospective 12-year surveillance. *Brain.* 2007;130:1350-1359.
110. Heidenhain A. Klinische und anatomische Untersuchungen über eine eigenartige Erkrankung des Zentralnervensystems im Praesenium. *Z Neurol Psychiatry.* 1929;118:49-114.
111. Brownell B, Oppenheimer DR. An ataxic form of subacute presenile polioencephalopathy (Creutzfeldt-Jakob disease). *J Neurol Neurosurg Psychiatry.* 1965;28:350-361.
112. Stern K. Severe dementia associated with bilateral symmetrical degeneration of the thalamus. *Brain.* 1939;62:157-171.
113. Garcin R, Brion S, Khochneviss AA. Le syndrome de Creutzfeldt-Jakob et les syndromes corticostries du presenium (a l'occasion de 5 observations anatomo-cliniques). *Rev Neurol (Paris).* 1963;109:419-441.
114. Kirschbaum W. *Jakob-Creutzfeldt Disease.* New York: Elsevier; 1968.
115. Wall CA, Rummans TA, Aksamit AJ, et al. Psychiatric manifestations of Creutzfeldt-Jakob disease: a 25-year analysis. *J Neuropsychiatry Clin Neurosci.* 2005;17:489-495.
116. Brown P, Rodgers-Johnson P, Cathala F, et al. Creutzfeldt-Jakob disease of long duration: clinicopathological characteristics, transmissibility, and differential diagnosis. *Ann Neurol.* 1984;16:295-304.
117. Guiroy DC, Shankar SK, Gibbs CJ, et al. Neuronal degeneration and neurofilament accumulation in the trigeminal ganglia in Creutzfeldt-Jakob disease. *Ann Neurol.* 1989;25:102-106.
118. Macleod MA, Stewart GE, Zeidler M, et al. Sensory features of variant Creutzfeldt-Jakob disease. *J Neurol.* 2002;249:706-711.
119. Niewiadomska M, Kulczycki J, Wochnik-Dyjas D, et al. Impairment of the peripheral nervous system in Creutzfeldt-Jakob disease. *Arch Neurol.* 2002;59:1430-1436.
120. Kovacs T, Aranyi Z, Szirmai I, et al. Creutzfeldt-Jakob disease with amyotrophy and demyelinating polyneuropathy. *Arch Neurol.* 2002;59:1811-1814.
121. Worrall BB, Rowland LP, Chin SS, et al. Amyotrophy in prion diseases. *Arch Neurol.* 2000;57:33-38.
122. Kovacs GG, Trabattoni G, Hainfellner JA, et al. Mutations of the prion protein gene phenotypic spectrum. *J Neurol.* 2002;249:1567-1582.
123. Mead S. Prion disease genetics. *Eur J Hum Genet.* 2006;14:273-281.
124. Goldman JS, Miller BL, Safar J, et al. When sporadic disease is not sporadic: the potential for genetic etiology. *Arch Neurol.* 2004;61:213-216.
125. Kovacs GG, Puopolo M, Ladogana A, et al. Genetic prion disease: the EUROCJD experience. *Hum Genet.* 2005;118:166-174.
126. Herzberg L, Herzberg BN, Gibbs Jr CJ, et al. Creutzfeldt-Jakob disease: hypothesis for high incidence in Libyan Jews in Israel. *Science.* 1974;186:848.
127. Spudich S, Mastrianni JA, Wrensch M, et al. Complete penetrance of Creutzfeldt-Jakob disease in Libyan Jews carrying the E200K mutation in the prion protein gene. *Mol Med.* 1995;1:607-613.
128. Simon ES, Kahana E, Chapman J, et al. Creutzfeldt-Jakob disease profile in patients homozygous for the PRNP E200K mutation. *Ann Neurol.* 2000;47:257-260.
129. Tagliavini F, Prelli F, Ghiso J, et al. Amyloid protein of Gerstmann-Sträussler-Scheinker disease (Indiana kindred) is an 11 kd fragment of prion protein with an N-terminal glycine at codon 58. *EMBO J.* 1991;10:513-519.
130. Giaccone G, Verga L, Bugiani O, et al. Prion protein preamyloid and amyloid deposits in Gerstmann-Sträussler-Scheinker disease, Indiana kindred. *Proc Natl Acad Sci U S A.* 1992;89:9349-9353.
131. Collins S, McLean CA, Masters CL. Gerstmann-Straussler-Scheinker syndrome, fatal familial insomnia, and kuru: a review of these less common human transmissible spongiform encephalopathies. *J Clin Neurosci.* 2001;8:387-397.
132. Colucci M, Moleres FJ, Xie ZL, et al. Gerstmann-Straussler-Scheinker: a new phenotype with "curly" PrP deposits. *J Neuropathol Exp Neurol.* 2006;65:642-651.
133. Cervenakova L, Buetefisch C, Lee HS, et al. Novel PRNP sequence variant associated with familial encephalopathy. *Am J Med Genet.* 1999;88:653-656.
134. Noguchi-Shinohara M, Hamaguchi T, Kitamoto T, et al. Clinical features and diagnosis of dura mater graft associated Creutzfeldt Jakob disease. *Neurology.* 2007;69:360-367.
135. Liberski PP, Bratosiewicz J, Walis A, et al. A special report I. Prion protein (PrP)—amyloid plaques in the transmissible spongiform encephalopathies, or prion diseases revisited. *Folia Neuropathol.* 2001;39:217-235.
136. Amano N, Yagishita S, Yokoi S, et al. Gerstmann-Straussler syndrome—a variant type: amyloid plaques and Alzheimer's neurofibrillary tangles in cerebral cortex. *Acta Neuropathol.* 1992;84:15-23.
137. Lugaresi E, Medori R, Montagna P, et al. Fatal familial insomnia and dysautonomia with selective degeneration of thalamic nuclei. *N Engl J Med.* 1986;315:997-1003.
138. Petersen RB, Tabaton M, Berg L, et al. Analysis of the prion protein gene in thalamic dementia. *Neurology.* 1992;42:1859-1863.
139. Medori R, Tritschler H-J, LeBlanc A, et al. Fatal familial insomnia, a prion disease with a mutation at codon 178 of the prion protein gene. *N Engl J Med.* 1992;326:444-449.
140. Montagna P, Gambetti P, Cortelli P, et al. Familial and sporadic fatal insomnia. *Lancet Neurol.* 2003;2:167-176.
141. Manetto V, Medori R, Cortelli P, et al. Fatal familial insomnia: clinical and pathological study of five new cases. *Neurology.* 1992;42:312-319.
142. McLean CA, Storey E, Gardner RJM, et al. The D178N (cis-129M) "fatal familial insomnia" mutation associated with diverse clinicopathologic phenotypes in an Australian kindred. *Neurology.* 1997;49:552-558.
143. Zarranz JJ, Digon A, Atares B, et al. Phenotypic variability in familial prion diseases due to the D178N mutation. *J Neurol Neurosurg Psychiatry.* 2005;76:1491-1496.
144. Krasnianski A, Bartl M, Sanchez Juan PJ, et al. Fatal familial insomnia: clinical features and early identification. *Ann Neurol.* 2008;63:658-661.
145. Landolt HP, Glatzel M, Blattler T, et al. Sleep-wake disturbances in sporadic Creutzfeldt-Jakob disease. *Neurology.* 2006;66:1418-1424.
146. Gambetti P, Medori R, Manetto V, et al. Fatal familial insomnia: a prion disease with distinctive histopathological and genotype features. In: Guilleminault C, Lugaresi E, Montagna P, et al, eds. *Fatal Familial Insomnia: Inherited Prion Diseases, Sleep, and the Thalamus.* New York: Raven Press; 1994:27-32.
147. Parchi P, Capellari S, Chin S, et al. A subtype of sporadic prion disease mimicking fatal familial insomnia. *Neurology.* 1999;52:1757-1763.
148. Mastrianni JA, Nixon R, Layzer R, et al. Prion protein conformation in a patient with sporadic fatal insomnia. *N Engl J Med.* 1999;340:1630-1638.
149. Butefisch CM, Gambetti P, Cervenakova L, et al. Inherited prion encephalopathy associated with the novel PRNP H187R mutation: a clinical study. *Neurology.* 2000;55:517-522.
150. Hall DA, Leehey MA, Filley CM, et al. PRNP H187R mutation associated with neuropsychiatric disorders in childhood and dementia. *Neurology.* 2005;64:1304-1306.
151. Nitrini R, Rosemberg S, Passos-Bueno MR, et al. Familial spongiform encephalopathy associated with a novel prion protein gene mutation. *Ann Neurol.* 1997;42:138-146.
152. Dyrbye H, Broholm H, Dziegiel MH, et al. The M129V polymorphism of codon 129 in the prion gene (PRNP) in the Danish population. *Eur J Epidemiol.* 2008;23:23-27.
153. Palmer MS, Dryden AJ, Hughes JT, et al. Homozygous prion protein genotype predisposes to sporadic Creutzfeldt-Jakob disease. *Nature.* 1991;352:340-342.
154. Windl O, Dempster M, Estibeiro JP, et al. Genetic basis of Creutzfeldt-Jakob disease in the United Kingdom: a systematic analysis of predisposing mutations and allelic variation in the PRNP gene. *Hum Genet.* 1996;98:259-264.
155. Jeong BH, Lee KH, Kim NH, et al. Association of sporadic Creutzfeldt-Jakob disease with homozygous genotypes at PRNP codons 129 and 219 in the Korean population. *Neurogenetics.* 2005;6:229-232.
156. Riemenschneider M, Klopp N, Xiang W, et al. Prion protein codon 129 polymorphism and risk of Alzheimer disease. *Neurology.* 2004;63:364-366.
157. Li X, Rowland LP, Mitsumoto H, et al. Prion protein codon 129 genotype prevalence is altered in primary progressive aphasia. *Ann Neurol.* 2005;58:858-864.
158. Jeong BH, Lee KH, Jeong YE, et al. Polymorphisms at codons 129 and 219 of the prion protein gene (PRNP) are not associated with sporadic Alzheimer's disease in the Korean population. *Eur J Neurol.* 2007;14:621-626.
159. Zigas V, Gajdusek DC. Kuru: clinical study of a new syndrome resembling paralysis agitans in natives of the Eastern Highlands of Australian New Guinea. *Med J Aust.* 1957;2:745-754.
160. Klatzo I, Gajdusek DC, Zigas V. Pathology of kuru. *Lab Invest.* 1959;8:799-847.
161. Gajdusek DC. Kuru. *Trans R Soc Trop Med Hyg.* 1963;57:151-169.
162. Beck E, Daniel PM, Alpers M, et al. Experimental "kuru" in chimpanzees: a pathological report. *Lancet.* 1966;2:1056-1059.
163. Collinge J, Whitfield J, McKintosh E, et al. Kuru in the 21st century—an acquired human prion disease with very long incubation periods. *Lancet.* 2006;367:2068-2074.
164. Huillard d'Aignaux JN, Cousens SN, Maccario J, et al. The incubation period of kuru. *Epidemiology.* 2002;13:402-408.
165. Collinge J, Whitfield J, McKintosh E, et al. A clinical study of kuru patients with long incubation periods at the end of the epidemic in Papua New Guinea. *Philos Trans R Soc London B Biol Sci.* 2008;363:3725-3739.
166. McLean CA. Review: the neuropathology of kuru and variant Creutzfeldt-Jakob disease. *Philos Trans R Soc London B Biol Sci.* 2008;363:3685-3687.
167. Brandner S, Whitfield J, Boone K, et al. Central and peripheral pathology of kuru: pathological analysis of a recent case and comparison with other forms of human prion disease. *Philos Trans R Soc London B Biol Sci.* 2008;363:3755-3763.
168. Boone K. An account of the last autopsy carried out on a kuru patient. *Philos Trans R Soc London B Biol Sci.* 2008;363:3630.
169. Mead S, Stumpf MP, Whitfield J, et al. Balancing selection at the prion protein gene consistent with prehistoric kurulike epidemics. *Science.* 2003;300:640-643.
170. Britton TC, Al-Sarraj S, Shaw C, et al. Sporadic Creutzfeldt-Jakob disease in a 16-year-old in the UK [letter]. *Lancet.* 1995;346:1155.
171. Will RG, Ironside JW, Zeidler M, et al. A new variant of Creutzfeldt-Jakob disease in the UK. *Lancet.* 1996;347:921-925.
172. Zeidler M, Stewart GE, Barraclough CR, et al. New variant Creutzfeldt-Jakob disease: neurological features and diagnostic tests. *Lancet.* 1997;350:903-907.
173. Wroe SJ, Pal S, Siddique D, et al. Clinical presentation and premortem diagnosis of variant Creutzfeldt-Jakob disease associated with blood transfusion: a case report. *Lancet.* 2006;368:2061-2067.
174. Hewitt PE, Llewelyn CA, Mackenzie J, et al. Creutzfeldt-Jakob disease and blood transfusion: results of the UK Transfusion

Medicine Epidemiological Review study. *Vox Sang.* 2006; 91:221-230.
175. Health Protection Agency. 4th case of variant CJD infection associated with blood transfusion. Available at <http://www.hpa.org.uk/webw/HPAweb&HPAwebStandard/HPAweb_C/1195733711457?p=1171991026241>; January 18, 2007.
176. National Creutzfeldt-Jakob Disease Surveillance Unit. Variant Creutzfeldt-Jakob disease. Available at <http://www.cjd.ed.ac.uk>; September, 2008.
177. Editorial team. Third case of vCJD reported in the United States. *Euro Surveill.* 2006;11:E061207.2.
178. Hillier CE, Salmon RL, Neal JW, et al. Possible underascertainment of variant Creutzfeldt-Jakob disease: a systematic study. *J Neurol Neurosurg Psychiatry.* 2002;72:304-309.
179. Will RG, Knight RS, Ward HJ, et al. vCJD: the epidemic that never was. New variant Creutzfeldt-Jakob disease: the critique that never was. *BMJ.* 2002;325:102.
180. Scientific Steering Committee. Opinion of the scientific steering committee on the human exposure risk (HER) via food with respect to BSE. European Commission; December 10, 1999.
181. Ghani AC, Donnelly CA, Ferguson NM, et al. Updated projections of future vCJD deaths in the UK. *BMC Infect Dis.* 2003;3:4.
182. Will RG, Ironside JW, Zeidler M, et al. A new variant of Creutzfeldt-Jakob disease in the UK. *Lancet.* 1996;347:921-925.
183. Will RG, Zeidler M, Stewart GE, et al. Diagnosis of new variant Creutzfeldt-Jakob disease. *Ann Neurol.* 2000;47:575-582.
184. Boelle PY, Cesbron JY, Valleron AJ. Epidemiological evidence of higher susceptibility to vCJD in the young. *BMC Infect Dis.* 2004;4:26.
185. Boesenberg C, Schulz-Schaeffer WJ, Meissner B, et al. Clinical course in young patients with sporadic Creutzfeldt-Jakob disease. *Ann Neurol.* 2005;58:533-543.
186. Pocchiari M, Puopolo M, Croes EA, et al. Predictors of survival in sporadic Creutzfeldt-Jakob disease and other human transmissible spongiform encephalopathies. *Brain.* 2004;127: 2348-2359.
187. Chazot G, Broussolle E, Lapras CI, et al. New variant of Creutzfeldt-Jakob disease in a 26-year-old French man. *Lancet.* 1996;347:1181.
188. Spencer MD, Knight RS, Will RG. First hundred cases of variant Creutzfeldt-Jakob disease: retrospective case note review of early psychiatric and neurological features. *BMJ.* 2002;324: 1479-1482.
189. Zeidler M, Johnstone EC, Bamber RW, et al. New variant Creutzfeldt-Jakob disease: psychiatric features. *Lancet.* 1997;350:908-910.
190. Hewitt PE, Llewelyn CA, Mackenzie J, et al. Three reported cases of variant Creutzfeldt-Jakob disease transmission following transfusion of labile blood components. *Vox Sang.* 2006;91:348.
191. Llewelyn CA, Hewitt PE, Knight RS, et al. Possible transmission of variant Creutzfeldt-Jakob disease by blood transfusion. *Lancet.* 2004;363:417-421.
192. Editors. Fourth case of transfusion-associated vCJD infection in the United Kingdom. *Euro Surveill.* 2007;12:E070118.14.
193. Sikorska B, Liberski PP, Sobow T, et al. Ultrastructural study of florid plaques in variant Creutzfeldt-Jakob disease: a comparison with amyloid plaques in kuru, sporadic Creutzfeldt-Jakob disease and Gerstmann-Straussler-Scheinker disease. *Neuropathol Appl Neurobiol.* 2009;35:46-59.
194. Hill AF, Joiner S, Wadsworth JD, et al. Molecular classification of sporadic Creutzfeldt-Jakob disease. *Brain.* 2003;126: 1333-1346.
195. Collinge J, Sidle KCL, Meads J, et al. Molecular analysis of prion strain variation and the aetiology of "new variant" CJD. *Nature.* 1996;383:685-690.
196. Parchi P, Capellari S, Chen SG, et al. Typing prion isoforms [letter]. *Nature.* 1997;386:232-233.
197. Billette de Villemeur T, Gelot A, Deslys JP, et al. Iatrogenic Creutzfeldt-Jakob disease in three growth hormone recipients: a neuropathological study. *Neuropathol Appl Neurobiol.* 1994;20:111-117.
198. Croes EA, Roks G, Jansen GH, et al. Creutzfeldt-Jakob disease 38 years after diagnostic use of human growth hormone. *J Neurol Neurosurg Psychiatry.* 2002;72:792-793.
199. Lewis AM, Yu M, DeArmond SJ, et al. Human growth hormone-related iatrogenic Creutzfeldt-Jakob disease with abnormal imaging. *Arch Neurol.* 2006;63:288-290.
200. Wadsworth JD, Joiner S, Linehan JM, et al. Kuru prions and sporadic Creutzfeldt-Jakob disease prions have equivalent transmission properties in transgenic and wild-type mice. *Proc Natl Acad Sci U S A.* 2008;105:3885-3890.
201. Hill AF, Desbruslais M, Joiner S, et al. The same prion strain causes vCJD and BSE. *Nature.* 1997;389:448-450.
202. Lasmézas CI, Deslys J-P, Demaimay R, et al. BSE transmission to macaques. *Nature.* 1996;381:743-744.
203. Scott MR, Will R, Ironside J, et al. Compelling transgenetic evidence for transmission of bovine spongiform encephalopathy prions to humans. *Proc Natl Acad Sci U S A.* 1999;96: 15137-15142.
204. Bruce ME, Will RG, Ironside JW, et al. Transmissions to mice indicate that "new variant" CJD is caused by the BSE agent. *Nature.* 1997;389:498-501.
205. Collee JG, Bradley R. BSE: a decade on—Part 1. *Lancet.* 1997;349:636-641.
206. Collee JG, Bradley R. BSE: a decade on—Part 2. *Lancet.* 1997;349:715-721.
207. Anderson RM, Donnelly CA, Ferguson NM, et al. Transmission dynamics and epidemiology of BSE in British cattle. *Nature.* 1996;382:779-788.
208. Nathanson N, Wilesmith J, Griot C. Bovine spongiform encephalopathy (BSE): cause and consequences of a common source epidemic. *Am J Epidemiol.* 1997;145:959-969.
209. Lasmezas CI, Fournier JG, Nouvel V, et al. Adaptation of the bovine spongiform encephalopathy agent to primates and comparison with Creutzfeldt-Jakob disease: implications for human health. *Proc Natl Acad Sci U S A.* 2001;98:4142-4147.
210. Mead S, Joiner S, Desbruslais M, et al. Creutzfeldt-Jakob disease, prion protein gene codon 129VV, and a novel PrPSc type in a young British woman. *Arch Neurol.* 2007;64:1780-1784.
211. Brown P, Preece M, Brandel JP, et al. Iatrogenic Creutzfeldt-Jakob disease at the millennium. *Neurology.* 2000;55: 1075-1081.
212. Brown P, Brandel JP, Preece M, et al. Iatrogenic Creutzfeldt-Jakob disease: the waning of an era. *Neurology.* 2006;67: 389-393.
213. Centers for Disease Control and Prevention. Update: Creutzfeldt-Jakob disease associated with cadaveric dura mater grafts—Japan, 1978-2008. *MMWR Morb Mortal Wkly Rep.* 2008;57:1152-1154.
214. Heath CA, Barker RA, Esmonde TF, et al. Dura mater-associated Creutzfeldt-Jakob disease: experience from surveillance in the UK. *J Neurol Neurosurg Psychiatry.* 2006;77:880-882.
215. Antoine JC, Michel D, Bertholon P, et al. Creutzfeldt-Jakob disease after extracranial dura mater embolization for a nasopharyngeal angiofibroma. *Neurology.* 1997;48:1451-1453.
216. Defebvre L, Destee A, Caron J, et al. Creutzfeldt-Jakob disease after an embolization of intercostal arteries with cadaveric dura mater suggesting a systemic transmission of the prion agent. *Neurology.* 1997;48:1470-1471.
217. Lane KL, Brown P, Howell DN, et al. Creutzfeldt-Jakob disease in a pregnant woman with an implanted dura mater graft. *Neurosurgery.* 1994;34:737-740.
218. Blossom DB, Maddox RA, Beavers SF, et al. A case of Creutzfeldt-Jakob disease associated with a dura mater graft in the United States. *Infect Control Hosp Epidemiol.* 2007;28: 1396-1397.
219. Iwasaki Y, Mimuro M, Yoshida M, et al. Clinicopathologic characteristics of five autopsied cases of dura mater-associated Creutzfeldt-Jakob disease. *Neuropathology.* 2008;28:51-61.
220. Billette de Villemeur T, Deslys J-P, Pradel A, et al. Creutzfeldt-Jakob disease from contaminated growth hormone extracts in France. *Neurology.* 1996;47:690-695.
221. Mills JL, Schonberger LB, Wysowski DK, et al. Long-term mortality in the United States cohort of pituitary-derived growth hormone recipients. *J Pediatr.* 2004;144:430-436.
222. Spurgeon B. French doctors are tried for treating children with infected growth hormone. *BMJ.* 2008;336:348-349.
223. Maddox RA, Belay ED, Curns AT, et al. Creutzfeldt-Jakob disease in recipients of corneal transplants. *Cornea.* 2008;27:851-854.
224. Will RG, Matthews WB. Evidence for case-to-case transmission of Creutzfeldt-Jakob disease. *J Neurol Neurosurg Psychiatry.* 1982;45:235-238.
225. el Hachimi KH, Chaunu MP, Cervenakova L, et al. Putative neurosurgical transmission of Creutzfeldt-Jakob disease with analysis of donor and recipient: agent strains. *C R Acad Sci III.* 1997;320:319-328.
226. Bernoulli C, Siegfried J, Baumgartner G, et al. Danger of accidental person-to-person transmission of Creutzfeldt-Jakob disease by surgery. *Lancet.* 1977;1:478-479.
227. Ward HJ, Everington D, Croes EA, et al. Sporadic Creutzfeldt-Jakob disease and surgery: a case-control study using community controls. *Neurology.* 2002;59:543-548.
228. Ward HJ, Everington D, Cousens SN, et al. Risk factors for sporadic Creutzfeldt-Jakob disease. *Ann Neurol.* 2008;63: 347-354.
229. Mahillo-Fernandez I, de Pedro-Cuesta J, Bleda MJ, et al. Surgery and risk of sporadic Creutzfeldt-Jakob disease in Denmark and Sweden: registry-based case-control studies. *Neuroepidemiology.* 2008;31:229-240.
230. Collins S, Law MG, Fletcher A, et al. Surgical treatment and risk of sporadic Creutzfeldt-Jakob disease: a case-control study. *Lancet.* 1999;353:693-697.
231. Joint Commission. Sentinel event alert: Exposure to Creutzfeldt-Jakob disease. *Joint Commission Perspect.* 2001;21:10-11.
232. Zou S, Fang CT, Schonberger LB. Transfusion transmission of human prion diseases. *Transfus Med Rev.* 2008;22: 58-69.
233. van Duijn CM, Delasnerie-Laupretre N, Masullo C, et al. Case-control study of risk factors of Creutzfeldt-Jakob disease in Europe during 1993-95. European Union (EU) Collaborative Study Group of Creutzfeldt-Jakob disease (CJD). *Lancet.* 1998;351:1081-1085.
234. Wientjens DP, Davanipour Z, Hofman A, et al. Risk factors for Creutzfeldt-Jakob disease: a reanalysis of case-control studies. *Neurology.* 1996;46:1287-1291.
235. Berger JR, David NJ. Creutzfeldt-Jakob disease in a physician: a review of the disorder in health care workers. *Neurology.* 1993;43:205-206.
236. Kong Q, Zheng M, Casalone C, et al. Evaluation of the human transmission risk of an atypical bovine spongiform encephalopathy prion strain. *J Virol.* 2008;82:3697-3701.
237. Biacabe AG, Laplanche JL, Ryder S, et al. Distinct molecular phenotypes in bovine prion diseases. *EMBO Rep.* 2004;5:110-115.
238. Casalone C, Zanusso G, Acutis P, et al. Identification of a second bovine amyloidotic spongiform encephalopathy: molecular similarities with sporadic Creutzfeldt-Jakob disease. *Proc Natl Acad Sci U S A.* 2004;101:3065-3070.
239. Beringue V, Bencsik A, Le Dur A, et al. Isolation from cattle of a prion strain distinct from that causing bovine spongiform encephalopathy. *PLoS Pathog.* 2006;2:e112.
240. Richt JA, Hall SM. BSE case associated with prion protein gene mutation. *PLoS Pathog.* 2008;4:e1000156.
241. Comoy EE, Casalone C, Lescoutra-Etchegaray N, et al. Atypical BSE (BASE) transmitted from asymptomatic aging cattle to a primate. *PLoS ONE.* 2008;3:e3017.
242. Bosque PJ. Bovine spongiform encephalopathy, chronic wasting disease, scrapie, and the threat to humans from prion disease epizootics. *Curr Neurol Neurosci Rep.* 2002;2:488-495.
243. Benestad SL, Arsac JN, Goldmann W, et al. Atypical/Nor98 scrapie: properties of the agent, genetics, and epidemiology. *Vet Res.* 2008;39:19.
244. Le Dur A, Beringue V, Andreoletti O, et al. A newly identified type of scrapie agent can naturally infect sheep with resistant PrP genotypes. *Proc Natl Acad Sci U S A.* 2005;102:16031-16036.
245. Sigurdson CJ. A prion disease of cervids: chronic wasting disease. *Vet Res.* 2008;39:41.
246. Williams ES. Chronic wasting disease. *Vet Pathol.* 2005;42:530-549.
247. Mawhinney S, Pape WJ, Forster JE, et al. Human prion disease and relative risk associated with chronic wasting disease. *Emerg Infect Dis.* 2006;12:1527-1535.
248. Kong Q, Huang S, Zou W, et al. Chronic wasting disease of elk: transmissibility to humans examined by transgenic mouse models. *J Neurosci.* 2005;25:7944-7949.
249. Tamguney G, Giles K, Bouzamondo-Bernstein E, et al. Transmission of elk and deer prions to transgenic mice. *J Virol.* 2006;80:9104-9114.
250. Raymond GJ, Bossers A, Raymond LD, et al. Evidence of a molecular barrier limiting susceptibility of humans, cattle and sheep to chronic wasting disease. *EMBO J.* 2000;19:4425-4430.
251. Harrington MG, Merril CR, Asher DM, et al. Abnormal proteins in the cerebrospinal fluid of patients with Creutzfeldt-Jakob disease. *N Engl J Med.* 1986;315:279-283.
252. Blisard KS, Davis LE, Harrington MG, et al. Pre-mortem diagnosis of Creutzfeldt-Jakob disease by detection of abnormal cerebrospinal fluid proteins. *J Neurol Sci.* 1990;99:75-81.
253. Hsich G, Kenney K, Gibbs CJ, et al. The 14-3-3 brain protein in cerebrospinal fluid as a marker for transmissible spongiform encephalopathies. *N Engl J Med.* 1996;335:924-930.
254. Zerr I, Bodemer M, Gefeller O, et al. Detection of 14-3-3 protein in the cerebrospinal fluid supports the diagnosis of Creutzfeldt-Jakob disease. *Ann Neurol.* 1998;43:32-40.
255. Geschwind MD, Martindale J, Miller D, et al. Challenging the clinical utility of the 14-3-3 protein for the diagnosis of sporadic Creutzfeldt-Jakob disease. *Arch Neurol.* 2003;60:813-816.
256. Peoc'h K, Delasnerie-Laupretre N, Beaudry P, et al. Diagnostic value of CSF 14-3-3 detection in sporadic CJD diagnosis according to the age of the patient. *Eur J Neurol.* 2006;13:427-428.
257. Chapman T, McKeel Jr DW, Morris JC. Misleading results with the 14-3-3 assay for the diagnosis of Creutzfeldt-Jakob disease. *Neurology.* 2000;55:1396-1397.
258. Geschwind MD, Shu H, Haman A, et al. Rapidly progressive dementia. *Ann Neurol.* 2008;64:97-108.
259. Skinningsrud A, Stenset V, Gundersen AS, et al. Cerebrospinal fluid markers in Creutzfeldt-Jakob disease. *Cerebrospinal Fluid Res.* 2008;5:14.
260. Otto M, Stein H, Szudra A, et al. S-100 protein concentration in the cerebrospinal fluid of patients with Creutzfeldt-Jakob disease. *J Neurol.* 1997;244:566-570.
261. Otto M, Wiltfang J, Cepek L, et al. Tau protein and 14-3-3 protein in the differential diagnosis of Creutzfeldt-Jakob disease. *Neurology.* 2002;58:192-197.
262. Bahl JM, Heegaard NH, Falkenhorst G, et al. The diagnostic efficiency of biomarkers in sporadic Creutzfeldt-Jakob disease compared to Alzheimer's disease. *Neurobiol Aging.* 2008.
263. Brechlin P, Jahn O, Steinacker P, et al. Cerebrospinal fluid-optimized two-dimensional difference gel electrophoresis (2-D DIGE) facilitates the differential diagnosis of Creutzfeldt-Jakob disease. *Proteomics.* 2008;8:4357-4366.
264. Goodall CA, Head MW, Everington D, et al. Raised CSF phospho-tau concentrations in variant Creutzfeldt-Jakob disease: diagnostic and pathological implications. *J Neurol Neurosurg Psychiatry.* 2006;77:89-91.
265. Bosque PJ, Telling GC, Cayetano J, et al. Evidence for prion replication in skeletal muscle. *Ann Neurol.* 1997;42:986.
266. Eklund CM, Kennedy RC, Hadlow WJ. Pathogenesis of scrapie virus infection in the mouse. *J Infect Dis.* 1967;117:15-22.
267. Brown P, Gibbs Jr CJ, Rodgers-Johnson P, et al. Human spongiform encephalopathy: the National Institutes of Health series of 300 cases of experimentally transmitted disease. *Ann Neurol.* 1994;35:513-529.
268. Saborio GP, Permanne B, Soto C. Sensitive detection of pathological prion protein by cyclic amplification of protein misfolding. *Nature.* 2001;411:810-813.
269. Saa P, Castilla J, Soto C. Ultra-efficient replication of infectious prions by automated protein misfolding cyclic amplification. *J Biol Chem.* 2006;281:35245-35252.

270. Atarashi R, Moore RA, Sim VL, et al. Ultrasensitive detection of scrapie prion protein using seeded conversion of recombinant prion protein. *Nat Methods.* 2007;4:645-650.

271. Saa P, Castilla J, Soto C. Presymptomatic detection of prions in blood. *Science.* 2006;313:92-94.

272. Macfarlane RG, Wroe SJ, Collinge J, et al. Neuroimaging findings in human prion disease. *J Neurol Neurosurg Psychiatry.* 2007;78:664-670.

273. Collie DA, Sellar RJ, Zeidler M, et al. MRI of Creutzfeldt-Jakob disease: imaging features and recommended MRI protocol. *Clin Radiol.* 2001;56:726-739.

274. Tschampa HJ, Kallenberg K, Urbach H, et al. MRI in the diagnosis of sporadic Creutzfeldt-Jakob disease: a study on interobserver agreement. *Brain.* 2005;128:2026-2033.

275. Collie DA, Summers DM, Sellar RJ, et al. Diagnosing variant Creutzfeldt-Jakob disease with the pulvinar sign: MR imaging findings in 86 neuropathologically confirmed cases. *AJNR Am J Neuroradiol.* 2003;24:1560-1569.

276. Henkel K, Zerr I, Hertel A, et al. Positron emission tomography with [(18)F]FDG in the diagnosis of Creutzfeldt-Jakob disease (CJD). *J Neurol.* 2002;249:699-705.

277. Watanabe N, Seto H, Shimizu M, et al. Brain SPECT of Creutzfeldt-Jakob disease. *Clin Nucl Med.* 1996;21:236-241.

278. Levy SR, Chiappa KH, Burke CJ, et al. Early evolution and incidence of electroencephalographic abnormalities in Creutzfeldt-Jakob disease. *J Clin Neurophysiol.* 1986;3:1-21.

279. Aguglia U, Farnarier G, Tinuper P, et al. Subacute spongiform encephalopathy with periodic paroxysmal activities: clinical evolution and serial EEG findings in 20 cases. *Clin Electroencephalogr.* 1987;18:147-158.

280. Steinhoff BJ, Racker S, Herrendorf G, et al. Accuracy and reliability of periodic sharp wave complexes in Creutzfeldt-Jakob disease. *Arch Neurol.* 1996;53:162-166.

281. Zerr I, Pocchiari M, Collins S, et al. Analysis of EEG and CSF 14-3-3 proteins as aids to the diagnosis of Creutzfeldt-Jakob disease. *Neurology.* 2000;55:811-815.

282. Bell JE, Gentleman SM, Ironside JW, et al. Prion protein immunocytochemistry—UK five centre consensus report. *Neuropathol Appl Neurobiol.* 1997;23:26-35.

283. Budka H, Aguzzi A, Brown P, et al. Neuropathological diagnostic criteria for Creutzfeldt-Jakob disease (CJD) and other human spongiform encephalopathies (prion diseases). *Brain Pathol.* 1995;5:459-466.

284. Hauw JJ, Sazdovitch V, Laplanche JL, et al. Neuropathologic variants of sporadic Creutzfeldt-Jakob disease and codon 129 of PrP gene. *Neurology.* 2000;54:1641-1646.

285. Kitamoto T, Shin RW, Doh-ura K, et al. Abnormal isoform of prion proteins accumulates in the synaptic structures of the central nervous system in patients with Creutzfeldt-Jakob disease. *Am J Pathol.* 1992;140:1285-1294.

286. Cali I, Castellani R, Yuan J, et al. Classification of sporadic Creutzfeldt-Jakob disease revisited. *Brain.* 2006;129:2266-2277.

287. Parchi P, Giese A, Capellari S, et al. Classification of sporadic Creutzfeldt-Jakob disease based on molecular and phenotypic analysis of 300 subjects. *Ann Neurol.* 1999;46:224-233.

288. Hill AF, Zeidler M, Ironside J, et al. Diagnosis of new variant Creutzfeldt-Jakob disease by tonsil biopsy. *Lancet.* 1997;349:99-100.

289. Hill AF, Butterworth RJ, Joiner S, et al. Investigation of variant Creutzfeldt-Jakob disease and other human prion diseases with tonsil biopsy samples. *Lancet.* 1999;353:183-189.

290. Wadsworth JD, Joiner S, Hill AF, et al. Tissue distribution of protease resistant prion protein in variant Creutzfeldt-Jakob disease using a highly sensitive immunoblotting assay. *Lancet.* 2001;358:171-180.

291. Hilton DA, Ghani AC, Conyers L, et al. Accumulation of prion protein in tonsil and appendix: review of tissue samples. *BMJ.* 2002;325:633-634.

292. Joiner S, Linehan J, Brandner S, et al. Irregular presence of abnormal prion protein in appendix in variant Creutzfeldt-Jakob disease. *J Neurol Neurosurg Psychiatry.* 2002;73:597-598.

293. Tschampa HJ, Neumann M, Zerr I, et al. Patients with Alzheimer's disease and dementia with Lewy bodies mistaken for Creutzfeldt-Jakob disease. *J Neurol Neurosurg Psychiatry.* 2001;71:33-39.

294. Finelli PF. Drug-induced Creutzfeldt-Jakob like syndrome. *J Psychiatry Neurosci.* 1992;17:103-105.

295. Primavera A, Brusa G, Poeta MG. A Creutzfeldt-Jakob like syndrome due to lithium toxicity. *J Neurol Neurosurg Psychiatry.* 1989;52:423.

296. Supino-Viterbo V, Sicard C, Risvegliato M, et al. Toxic encephalopathy due to ingestion of bismuth salts: clinical and EEG studies of 45 patients. *J Neurol Neurosurg Psychiatry.* 1977;40:748-752.

297. Von Bose MJ, Zaudig M. Encephalopathy resembling Creutzfeldt-Jakob disease following oral, prescribed doses of bismuth nitrate. *Br J Psychiatry.* 1991;158:278-280.

298. Brain L, Jellinek EH, Ball K. Hashimoto's disease and encephalopathy. *Lancet.* 1966;2:512-514.

299. Shaw PJ, Walls TJ, Newman PK, et al. Hashimoto's encephalopathy: a steroid-responsive disorder associated with high antithyroid antibody titers—report of 5 cases. *Neurology.* 1991;41:228-233.

300. Seipelt M, Zerr I, Nau R, et al. Hashimoto's encephalitis as a differential diagnosis of Creutzfeldt-Jakob disease. *J Neurol Neurosurg Psychiatry.* 1999;66:172-176.

301. Tan KM, Lennon VA, Klein CJ, et al. Clinical spectrum of voltage-gated potassium channel autoimmunity. *Neurology.* 2008;70:1883-1890.

302. Geschwind MD, Tan KM, Lennon VA, et al. Voltage-gated potassium channel autoimmunity mimicking Creutzfeldt-Jakob disease. *Arch Neurol.* 2008;65:1341-1346.

303. Floel A, Reilmann R, Frese A, et al. Anticonvulsants for Creutzfeldt-Jakob disease? *Lancet.* 2003;361:224.

304. Albrecht R, Krebs B, Reusche E, et al. Signs of rapidly progressive dementia in a case of intravascular lymphomatosis. *Eur Arch Psychiatry Clin Neurosci.* 2005;255:232-235.

305. Trevitt CR, Collinge J. A systematic review of prion therapeutics in experimental models. *Brain.* 2006;129:2241-2265.

306. Stewart LA, Rydzewska LH, Keogh GF, et al. Systematic review of therapeutic interventions in human prion disease. *Neurology.* 2008;70:1272-1281.

307. Otto M, Cepek L, Ratzka P, et al. Efficacy of flupirtine on cognitive function in patients with CJD: A double-blind study. *Neurology.* 2004;62:714-718.

308. Bessen RA, Marsh RF. Identification of two biologically distinct strains of transmissible mink encephalopathy in hamsters. *J Gen Virol.* 1992;73:329-334.

309. Bessen RA, Marsh RF. Biochemical and physical properties of the prion protein from two strains of the transmissible mink encephalopathy agent. *J Virol.* 1992;66:2096-2101.

310. Peretz D, Scott M, Groth D, et al. Strain-specified relative conformational stability of the scrapie prion protein. *Protein Sci.* 2001;10:854-863.

311. Bessen RA, Marsh RF. Distinct PrP properties suggest the molecular basis of strain variation in transmissible mink encephalopathy. *J Virol.* 1994;68:7859-7868.

Introduction to *Chlamydia* and *Chlamydophila*

WALTER E. STAMM | BYRON E. BATTEIGER

Chlamydia and *Chlamydophila* are nomotile, obligate intracellular prokaryotic organisms with a unique biphasic life cycle.[1] Although there is disagreement in the field about the most appropriate taxonomic classification of these organisms, in the current schema they are classified in the order Chlamydiales, which contains only one family, the Chlamydiaceae, and two genera, *Chlamydia* and *Chlamydophila*. Within this family are four currently recognized species: *Chlamydophila pecorum*,[2] *Chlamydophila psittaci*, *Chlamydia trachomatis*, and *Chlamydophila pneumoniae*. All except *C. pecorum* have been associated with human disease (Table 179-1). Although the chlamydiae were originally classified taxonomically on the basis of their phenotypic properties, Everett and colleagues have proposed, based on sequence analysis of 16Sr ribonucleic acid (RNA), that there is sufficient divergence between the *C. trachomatis* group organisms and the *C. psittaci*, *C. pecorum*, and *C. pneumoniae* group organisms to divide these groups at the genus level into *Chlamydia* and *Chlamydophila*, respectively. Both the new and older classifications are currently in use in the literature. From a clinician's perspective, the most important conclusions from this debate are that (1) all Chlamydiales belong to a distinct bacterial division that is widely separated from other bacterial divisions and has a direct phylogenetic root that diverges very early in the evolution of eubacteria, and (2) the known *Chlamydia* and three *Chlamydophila* species—namely, *C. trachomatis*, *C. pneumoniae*, *C. pecorum*, and *C. psittaci*—form coherent and distinct groups based on phenotypic characteristics and rRNA sequence comparisons. Based on ribosomal RNA sequencing, the current species *C. psittaci* contains four distinct genetic groups of strains that may eventually be proposed as separate species.[3,4] Deoxyribonucleic acid (DNA) sequence homology confirms these insights.[5,6] The multiple strains of *C. psittaci* exhibit from less than 10% to 60% homology with each other and from less than 5% to approximately 20% homology with *C. trachomatis* strains. The human strains of *C. trachomatis* are almost 100% homologous with each other and approximately 30% homologous with the mouse biovar. The latter does not cause human disease, and it has also been suggested that the mouse biovar be classified as a separate species.[4,5] *C. pneumoniae* shows 10% or less homology with either of the other two species and so far appears to consist of only a single strain, TWAR.[7,8]

C. trachomatis has been the most extensively studied species because of its association with ocular trachoma and its importance as a sexually transmitted pathogen. Three biovars have been identified: the trachoma biovar associated with oculogenital disease, the lymphogranuloma venereum biovar associated with proctitis and systemic infections, and the mouse pneumonitis biovar, which appears to contain only a single strain. *C. pneumoniae* may be even more prevalent a human pathogen than *C. trachomatis*. This species was only recognized in 1992,[9] and the full extent and spectrum of disease attributable to it remain to be defined. Current evidence suggests, however, that *C. pneumoniae* is an extremely common pathogen on a global basis, most likely infecting nearly everyone and often causing recurrent infections throughout life. Most of these infections initially involve the upper or lower respiratory tract, but recent evidence also suggests that the organism may infect macrophages within the respiratory tract that later transport chlamydiae via the bloodstream to other distant sites. This likely includes the vascular endothelium, where endothelial cells, smooth muscle cells, and macrophages may be infected. The pathogenic role of *C. pneumoniae* in atherosclerotic cardiovascular disease has been extensively studied but remains unestablished.[10] There are multiple strains of *C. psittaci* that primarily infect birds and other nonhuman mammalian hosts. Transmission to humans occasionally occurs, usually after exposure to avian strains.[11]

Chlamydiae are prokaryotes that all share a common biology and life cycle. The organisms grow only within a specialized vacuole in eukaryotic cells called an inclusion (Fig. 179-1). They have extremely small genomes (e.g., 894 protein coding genes for *C. trachomatis*) and are auxotrophic for many amino acids and nucleotides, depending on the host cell for these molecules. They exhibit morphologic and structural similarities to gram-negative bacteria, including a trilaminar outer membrane that contains lipopolysaccharide and several membrane proteins that are structurally and functionally analogous to those found in *Escherichia coli*. Chlamydiae appear to lack classic peptidoglycan,[1,12] a macromolecule that provides most prokaryotes with structural rigidity and osmotic stability, despite the fact that the chlamydial genome contains all the genes necessary for peptidoglycan synthesis.[13]

All chlamydiae have a unique life cycle that uses an extracellular infectious form, the elementary body (EB), and an intracellular replicative form, the reticulate body (RB). The extracellular form, the EB, exhibits extensive disulfide cross-linking between cysteine residues both within and between outer membrane proteins.[14,15] The result is an almost sporelike structure that is metabolically inert. The life cycle is initiated when an EB attaches to a susceptible epithelial cell. A number of candidate chlamydial adhesins have been proposed, and putative membrane protein candidates have been identified in the chlamydial genome, but the precise identity of adhesins and associated epithelial cell receptors remains uncertain. The EB enters the epithelial cell by receptor-mediated endocytosis via clathrin-coated pits,[16,17] but evidence also exists for other mechanisms, including pinocytosis via noncoated pits and the use of heparin-like bridging molecules. It is likely that chlamydiae exploit several adhesin ligand entry mechanisms. EBs appear to facilitate their own entry after attachment by secreting a preformed protein (Tarp, CT456), which is phosphorylated by the host and signals cytoskeletal rearrangements leading to endocytosis.[18] A unique feature of all chlamydiae is their ability to inhibit lysosomal fusion by undefined mechanisms, allowing the infecting EB to reside in a protected membrane-bound vesicle called an inclusion. The EB, which is approximately 350 nm in diameter, then undergoes reorganization into the much larger replicative form, the RB, which is about 800 to 1000 nm in diameter.[19] The initial events triggering this reorganization have not been defined precisely, but early events include synthesis of new chlamydial proteins, reduction of disulfide bonds so that membrane proteins are no longer cross-linked,[15] and activation of an adenosine triphosphatase.[20]

During growth and replication, chlamydiae obtain high-energy phosphate compounds from the host cell.[21] They also require some amino acids from the host cell but are able to synthesize others. RBs are osmotically unstable and incapable of infecting another cell. They divide by binary fission to produce an enlarging inclusion (Fig. 179-2) that eventually fills the infected cells. The intracellular regulatory signals that control EB to RB and RB to EB conversion are not known.[22] Condensation of RBs into EBs leads to extensive shedding of mem-

TABLE 179-1	Comparative Aspects of Chlamydial Species Causing Human Infections						
Species	*Serovars*	*Natural Host*	*Transmission*	*Tropism*	*Acute Infection*	*Long-Term Complications*	*Prevention/Control*
C. trachomatis	A-C	Human	Hand-eye, fomites, flies	Conjunctiva	Conjunctivitis	Blindness	SAFE strategy
C. trachomatis	D-K	Human	Sexual, perinatal	Anogenital mucosa: urethra, cervix, rectum	Nongonococcal urethritis, mucopurulent cervicitis, acute proctitis	PID, TFI, EP, SARA, CA	Screen, treat; behavioral modifications, condoms
C. trachomatis	L1, L2, L3	Human	Sexual	Genital mucosa, lymphocyte, monocyte	Genital ulcers, lymphadenopathy	LGV, rectal scarring, lymphatic fistulae	None
C. pneumoniae	One	Human	Direct-indirect respiratory droplets	Respiratory epithelium	Upper respiratory infection, community-acquired pneumonia	Atherosclerotic cardiovascular disease? asthma?	None
C. psittaci	Many	Birds, mammals	Aerosol, respiratory	Systemic	Community-acquired pneumonia	Hepatitis	Identify and eliminate animal reservoir

CA, cancer; EP, ectopic pregnancy; PID, pelvic inflammatory disease; SARA, sexually acquired reactive arthritis; SAFE, surgery, antibiotics, facial cleanliness, and environmental improvement; TFI, tubal factor infertility.

brane blebs containing lipopolysaccharide[23] and compaction of the chromatin into an electron-dense nucleoid. The latter is mediated by a histone-like protein and is associated with a decrease in transcription.[24] Depending on the species, the cell membrane proteins are cross-linked during condensation or later during cell lysis and release. Release of the organisms from infected cells apparently can be accomplished by cell lysis,[25] extrusion of intact inclusions,[26] or a process resembling exocytosis.[27] The release of the infectious elementary bodies permits infection of new cells and the potential for transmission to a new host.

Numerous advances in our understanding of the chlamydiae and their cell biology are emerging now that more than a dozen chlamydial genomes have been sequenced. For example, a new family of polymorphic outer membrane proteins (POMPs) has been identified. In addition, chlamydiae express proteins that localize in the cytoplasmic surface of the inclusion membrane; its prototype is IncA.[28] Such exported proteins may be involved in the trafficking of inclusions into the exocytic pathway,[29,30] the trafficking of host cell lipids into chlamydial membranes by intercepting exocytic vesicles[31] and directing cytoplasmic lipid droplets into the inclusion,[32] and the inhibition of apoptosis.[33] Such proteins are hypothesized to enter the host cell from the inclusion by a type III secretion mechanism,[34] similar to systems used by *Yersinia* and other gram-negative species to inject effector proteins into eukaryotic cells. *C. trachomatis* has been shown to possess type III secretion genes,[13,34] including potential effectors such as phosphatases and kinases used by other bacteria to influence eukaryotic cell signaling. On electron microscopy, chlamydia possess surface projec-

tions[35] that are outwardly similar to structures in *Salmonella* known to be composed of type III secretion components. It is speculated that the surface projections of chlamydiae may constitute the chlamydial type III secretion apparatus.[36]

Chlamydiae primarily infect columnar epithelial cells, but studies have indicated that a wide range of cells can be productively infected, including endothelial cells, smooth muscle cells, lymphocytes, and monocytes and macrophages. In macrophages, some strains of *C. psittaci* exhibit productive growth.[37] Conversely, macrophages restrict the growth of both the lymphogranuloma venereum and trachoma biovars of *C. trachomatis,* although they are more permissive for lymphogranuloma venereum.[38] Human polymorphonuclear leukocytes ingest and destroy *C. trachomatis* and *C. psittaci* fairly efficiently. However, a small proportion of organisms remain viable and potentially able to perpetuate infection.[39] Infection of host epithelial cells causes secretion of a variety of cytokines, including interleukin-6 (IL-6) and tumor necrosis factor (TNF).

The chlamydial genome has a molecular mass of only 660×10^3 kDa, which is smaller than that of any other prokaryote except *Mycoplasma* spp.[13] The complete genome sequence of *C. trachomatis* serovar D, 1.043 million base pairs, was the first chlamydial genome to be completed.[13] Based on the sequence, certain metabolic pathways are missing from this small genome, including amino acid and purine-pyrimidine biosynthesis, anaerobic fermentation, and transformation competence proteins.[40] However, complete glycolytic and glycogen degrading pathways are present, and a full synthetic capacity for fatty acids, phospholipids, lipopolysaccharide, and peptidoglycan is repre-

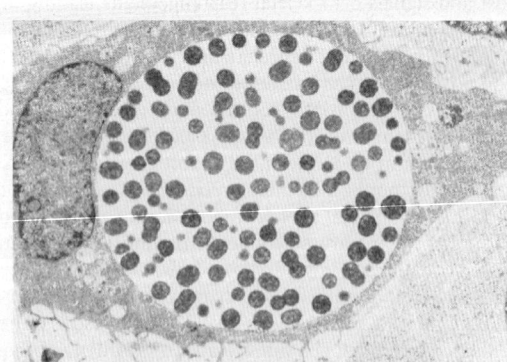

Figure 179-1 **Electron photomicrograph of *Chlamydia trachomatis* growing in tissue culture.** The larger reticulate bodies (RBs) have more diffuse chromatin. One of the RBs appears to be dividing, and the trilaminar outer membrane is evident in some areas. The smaller dense bodies are elementary bodies. *(Courtesy of Robert Suchland, Seattle.)*

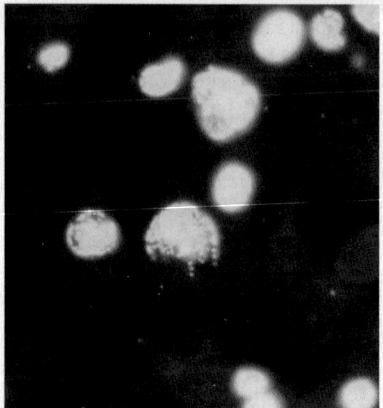

Figure 179-2 *Chlamydia trachomatis* **inclusions in a McCoy cell monolayer.** (Stained with a genus-reactive mouse monoclonal antibody followed by fluorescein conjugated rabbit antimouse immunoglobulin.) *(Courtesy of Robert Suchland, Seattle.)*

sented.[13] The subsequent completion of additional chlamydial genomes has demonstrated that there are striking similarities among the chlamydiae both in terms of gene content and order. This may indicate that there is little opportunity for horizontal genetic exchange between chlamydiae and other microorganisms, which might be expected given the intracellular location of its replicative cycle. However, gene exchange could occur via plasmids or bacteriophage, which some chlamydiae have. In addition, recent studies using antibiotic resistance markers have demonstrated horizontal exchange between two chlamydial strains coinfecting the same monolayer and epithelial cells.[41,42]

C. pneumoniae does not appear to contain any extrachromosomal genetic material,[7] whereas some strains of *C. psittaci*[43] and most strains of *C. trachomatis* contain a plasmid of approximately 7.5 kb. Slight sequence variations exist between plasmids from different strains within *C. trachomatis* and more extensive variations among the plasmids from *C. psittaci*.[44] Although the extensive conservation implies a critical function and, based on sequence homology with *E. coli* genes, it has been suggested that it may play a role in DNA replication,[45] the function of the plasmid remains unknown.

Phenotypically, the three chlamydial species that cause human disease differ antigenically, metabolically, and in host cell preference, antibiotic susceptibility, and inclusion morphology. Shared antigenic determinants are present in the lipopolysaccharide and some of the membrane proteins.[1,7] In addition, several outer membrane proteins contain species and subspecies determinants. Strain-specific determinants reside primarily in the major outer membrane protein. All strains of *C. trachomatis* are sensitive to sulfonamides, whereas *C. pneumoniae* and most strains of *C. psittaci* are not. The morphology of the elementary and reticulate bodies of *C. psittaci* and *C. trachomatis* are very similar to each other. Also, the RBs of all four species appear morphologically identical. However, the elementary bodies of *C. pneumoniae* are often pear-shaped, with a relatively large periplasmic space that contains electron-dense structures that are not seen in the other two species and whose function is unknown. *C. psittaci* forms multiple small inclusions in a single infected cell, with each infective EB forming its own inclusion. In cells infected with multiple *C. trachomatis* EBs, the organism-containing vesicles usually fuse so that each infected cell ultimately contains only one or two inclusions.[23] However, nonfusogenic variants of *C. trachomatis* have been described whose inclusions appear to lack IncA.[46] The inclusions of *C. pneumoniae* resemble those of *C. psittaci* but are less variable in shape. Only *C. trachomatis* accumulates glycogen in its inclusions, a property that allows their staining with iodine.

Despite the relative uniformity of their life cycle, genomes, and physiology, chlamydiae exhibit a wide range of host and tissue tropism, modes of transmission, and disease causation. *C. trachomatis* and *C. pneumoniae* appear to be exclusively human pathogens, except for the mouse pneumonitis biovar of *C. trachomatis*, which does not infect humans. Lymphogranuloma venereum strains of *C. trachomatis*, as well as those associated with oculogenital disease, are generally spread by sexual contact, during birth, or by autoinoculation of the eye with infected genital secretions. The strains associated with ocular trachoma are spread by fingers, fomites, and on the feet of flies. Transfer of respiratory secretions by droplets or hands is probably the primary mode of transmission of *C. pneumoniae*.[9] Strains of *C. psittaci* associated with human disease are shed in feces, urine, and secretions of infected birds, aerosolized, and transmitted by the respiratory route.

Most chlamydial species produce an initial acute infection often limited to the mucosal epithelium and generally producing minimal or no symptoms. Many such infections may spontaneously resolve but others appear to persist in an asymptomatic state. Initial infections by LGV strains of *C. trachomatis* or by *C. psittaci* are generally more invasive, producing severe or systemic infections, or both, in the initial phase.

The natural history of chlamydial infections is poorly defined in most cases. However, a growing body of data suggests that chronic asymptomatic or persistent infections are frequent. This appears to be the case for *C. psittaci* in animals[5] and for both *C. trachomatis*[46-48] and *C. pneumoniae*[49] in humans. Reinfection with *C. trachomatis* or *C. pneumoniae* also appears to be frequent, suggesting that infection-induced immunity is incompletely protective, short-lived, or both. Chronic persistent infection or exogenous reinfection is thought to play an important role in inducing the immunopathologic responses that are important in the pathogenesis of the major complications associated with chlamydial infections—namely, blinding trachoma or upper genital tract fibrosis and inflammation causing pelvic inflammatory disease (PID), infertility, and ectopic pregnancy. Moreover, considerable evidence now suggests that chronic endovascular *C. pneumoniae* infections may play a role in atherosclerosis and coronary artery disease.[9,50]

ACKNOWLEDGMENT

The authors acknowledge and appreciate the major contributions of Robert B. Jones, MD, PhD, to earlier editions of this chapter.

REFERENCES

1. Moulder JW. Looking at chlamydiae without looking at their hosts. *Am Soc Microbiol News.* 1984;50:353-362.
2. Fukushi H, Hirai K. 1989. Proposal of *Chlamydia pecorum* sp. nov. for *Chlamydia* strains derived from ruminants. *Int J Syst Bacteriol.* 1992;42:306-308.
3. Everett KDE, Bush RM, Andersen AA. Emended description of the order Chlamydiales, proposed of Parachlamydiaceae fam. nov and Simkaniaceae fam. nov, each containing one monotypic genus, revised taxonomy of the family Chlamydiaceae, including a new genus and five new species and standards for the identification of organisms. *Int J Syst Bacteriol.* 1999;49:415-440.
4. Pudjiatmoko, Fukushi H, Ochiai Y, et al. Phylogenetic analysis of the genus *Chlamydia* based on 16S rRNA gene sequences. *Int J Syst Bacteriol.* 1997;47:425-431.
5. Moulder JW. Interaction of chlamydiae and host cells in vitro. *Microbiol Rev.* 1991;55:143-190.
6. Herring AJ. The molecular biology of chlamydia—a brief overview. *J Infect.* 1992;25(Suppl 1):1-10.
7. Kalman S, Mitchell W, Marathe R, et al. Comparative genomes of *Chlamydia pneumoniae* and *Chlamydia trachomatis. Nat Genet.* 1999;21:385-389.
8. Pettersson B, Andersson A, Leitner T, et al. Evolutionary relationships among members of the genus *Chlamydia* based on 16S ribosomal DNA analysis. *J Bacteriol.* 1997;179:4195-4205.
9. Kuo CC, Jackson LA, Campbell LA, et al. *Chlamydia pneumoniae. Clin Microbiol Rev.* 1995;8:451-461.
10. Campbell LA, Kuo CC. Chlamydia pneumoniae–an infectious risk factor for atherosclerosis. *Nature Reviews.* 2004;2:23-32.
11. Yung AP, Grayson ML. Psittacosis—a review of 135 cases. *Med J Aust.* 1988;148:228-233.

12. Fox A, Robers JC, Gilbart J, et al. Muramic acid is not detectable in *Chlamydia psittaci* or *Chlamydia trachomatis* by gas chromatography–mass spectrometry. *Infect Immun.* 1990;58:835-837.
13. Stephens RS, Kalman S, Lammel C, et al. Genome sequence of an obligate intracellular pathogen of humans: *Chlamydia trachomatis. Science.* 1998;282:754-759.
14. Newhall WJV, Jones RB. Disulfide-linked oligomers of the major outer membrane protein of chlamydiae. *J Bacteriol.* 1983;154:998-1001.
15. Hatch TP, Miceli M, Sublett JE. Synthesis of disulfide-bonded outer membrane proteins during the developmental cycle of *Chlamydia psittaci* and *Chlamydia trachomatis. J Bacteriol.* 1986;165:379-385.
16. Rockey DD. Chlamydial interactions with host cells. In: Schachter J, Christiansen G, Clarke IN, et al, eds. *Chlamydial Infections: Proceedings of the Tenth International Symposium on Human Chlamydial Infection.* San Francisco: International Chlamydial Symposium; 2002:35-45.
17. Wyrick PB, Choong J, Davis CH, et al. Entry of genital *Chlamydia trachomatis* into polarized human epithelial cells. *Infect Immun.* 1989;57:2378-2389.
18. Clifton DR, Fields KA, Grieshabe SS, et al. A chlamydial type III translocated protein is tyrosine-phosphorylated at the site of entry and is associated with the recruitment of actin. *Proc Natl Acad Sci U S A.* 2004;101:10166-10171.
19. Schachter J, Caldwell HD. Chlamydiae. *Ann Rev Microbiol.* 1980;34:285-309.
20. Peeling R, Peeling J, Brunham R. High-resolution ³¹P nuclear magnetic resonance study of *Chlamydia trachomatis*: Induction

of ATPase activity in elementary bodies. *Infect Immun.* 1989;57:3338-3344.
21. Hatch TP, Al-Hossainy E, Silverman JA. Adenine nucleotide and lysine transport in *Chlamydia psittaci. J Bacteriol.* 1982;150:662-670.
22. Kaul R, Wenman WM. Cyclic AMP inhibits developmental regulation of *Chlamydia trachomatis. J Bacteriol.* 1986;168:722-777.
23. Stirling P, Richmond SJ. Production of outer membrane blebs during chlamydial replication. *FEMS Microbiol Lett.* 1980;9:103-105.
24. Barry CE, Hayes SF, Hackstadt T. Nucleoid condensation in *Escherichia coli* that express a chlamydial histone homolog. *Science.* 1992;256:377-379.
25. Todd WJ, Storz J. Ultrastructural cytochemical evidence for the activation of lysosomes in the cytocidal effect of *Chlamydia psittaci. Infect Immun.* 1975;12:638-646.
26. De la Maza LM, Peterson EM. Scanning electron microscopy of McCoy cells infected with *Chlamydia trachomatis. Exp Mol Pathol.* 1982;36:217-226.
27. Todd WJ, Caldwell HD. The interaction of *Chlamydia trachomatis* with host cells: Ultrastructural studies of the mechanism of release of a biovar II strain from HeLa 229 cells. *J Infect Dis.* 1985;151:1037-1044.
28. Rockey DD, Grosenbach D, Hruby DE, et al. *Chlamydia psittaci* IncA is phosphorylated by the host cell and is exposed on the cytoplasmic face of the developing inclusion. *Mol Microbiol.* 1997;24:217-228.
29. Hackstadt T, Scidmore MA, Rockey DD. Lipid metabolism in *Chlamydia trachomatis*–infected cells: Directed trafficking of

Golgi-derived sphingolipids to the chlamydial inclusion. *Proc Natl Acad Sci U S A*. 1995;92:4877-4881.

30. Heinzen RA, Scidmore MA, Rockey DD, et al. Differential interaction with endocytic and exocytic pathways distinguish parasitophorous vacuoles of *Coxiella burnetii* and *Chlamydia trachomatis*. *Infect Immun*. 1996;64:796-809.

31. Wylie JL, Hatch GM, McClarty G. Host cell phospholipids are trafficked to and then modified by *Chlamydia trachomatis*. *J Bacteriol*. 1997;179:7233-7242.

32. Cocchoriaro JL, Kumar Y, Fischer ER, et al. Cytoplasmic lipid droplets are translocated into the lumen of the Chlamydia trachomatis parasitophorous vacuole. *Proc Natl Acad Sci U S A*. 2008;105:9379-9384.

33. Read TD, Fraser CM, Hsia R-C, et al. Comparative analysis of Chlamydia bacteriophages reveals variation localized to a putative receptor binding domain. *Microb Comp Genomics*. 2000;5:223-231.

34. Hsia R-C, Pannekoek Y, Ingerowski E, et al. Type III secretion genes identify a putative virulence locus of *Chlamydia*. *Mol Microbiol*. 1997;25:351-359.

35. Matsumoto A. Structural characteristics of chlamydial bodies. In: Barron AL, ed. *Microbiology of Chlamydia*. Boca Raton, Fla: CRC Press; 1998:21-46.

36. Bavoil PB, Hsia R-C. Type III secretion in *Chlamydia*: A case of deja vu? *Mol Microbiol*. 1998;28:860-862.

37. Wyrick PB, Brownridge EA. Growth of *Chlamydia psittaci* in macrophages. *Infect Immun*. 1978;19:1054-1060.

38. Kuo C-C. Cultures of *Chlamydia trachomatis* in mouse peritoneal macrophages: Factors affecting organism growth. *Infect Immun*. 1978;20:439-445.

39. Register KB, Morgan PA, Wyrick PB. Interaction between *Chlamydia* spp. and human polymorphonuclear leukocytes in vitro. *Infect Immun*. 1986;52:664-670.

40. Rockey DD, Lenart J, Stephens RS, Genome sequencing and our understanding of chlamydiae. *Infect Immun*. 2000;68:5473-5479.

41. DeMars R, Weinfurter J, Guex E, et al. Lateral gene transfer in vitro in the intracellular pathogen *Chlamydia trachomatis*. *J Bacteriol*. 2007;189:991-1003.

42. Suchland RJ, et al. Horizonatal transfer of rifampin, ofloxacin and tetracycline resistance among Chlamydia spp. (In review.)

43. McClenaghan M, Honeycombe JR, Bevan BJ, et al. Distribution of plasmid sequences in avian and mammalian strains of *Chlamydia psittaci*. *J Gen Microbiol*. 1988;134:559-565.

44. Comanducci M, Ricci S, Cevenini R, et al. Diversity of the *Chlamydia trachomatis* common plasmid in biovars with different pathogenicity. *Plasmid*. 1990;23:149-154.

45. Hatt C, Ward ME, Clarke IN. Analysis of the entire nucleotide sequence of the cryptic plasmid of *Chlamydia trachomatis* serovar L1. Evidence for involvement in DNA replication. *Nucleic Acids Res*. 1988;16:4053-4067.

46. Suchland RJ, Rockey DD, Bannantine JP, et al. Isolates of *Chlamydia trachomatis* that occupy nonfusogenic inclusions lack IncA, a protein localized to the inclusion membrane. *Infect Immun*. 2000;68:360-367.

47. Campbell LA, Patton DL, Moore DE, et al. Detection of *Chlamydia trachomatis* deoxyribonucleic acid in women with tubal infertility. *Fertil Steril*. 1993;59:45-50.

48. Dean D, Suchland RJ, Stamm WE. Evidence for long-term persistence of *Chlamydia trachomatis* by omp1 genotyping. *J Infect Dis*. 2000;182:909-916.

49. Hammerschlag MR, Chirgwin K, Roblin PM, et al. Persistent infection with *Chlamydia pneumoniae* following acute respiratory illness. *Clin Infect Dis*. 1992;14:178-182.

50. Kalayoglu MV, Libby P, Byrne GI. *Chlamydiae pneumoniae* as an emerging risk factor in cardiovascular disease. *JAMA*. 2002;288:2724-2731.

180

Chlamydia trachomatis (Trachoma, Perinatal Infections, Lymphogranuloma Venereum, and Other Genital Infections)

WALTER E. STAMM | **BYRON E. BATTEIGER**

Chlamydia trachomatis infections, which are among the most common of bacterial infections, impose a tremendous burden on humans globally.[1-4] It has been estimated that worldwide at least 500 million people are affected by ocular trachoma and approximately 7 million to 9 million are blind as a result.[5] Ocular trachoma is considered the most common cause of preventable blindness worldwide. Although the disease has disappeared from many parts of the developed world coincident with improved sanitation, access to water, and reduced crowding, it remains common in many developing areas of the world. Genital tract infections with *C. trachomatis* are even more prevalent and have as major complications pelvic inflammatory disease (PID), ectopic pregnancy, infertility, and infant pneumonia. Because of a lack of universal testing and reporting, reliable incidence and prevalence data are not available (Fig. 180-1). However, the Centers for Disease Control and Prevention (CDC) estimated that there are approximately 4 million new *C. trachomatis* infections per year in the United States.[6] The World Health Organization (WHO) estimated that 90 million cases occur annually on a global basis. On the basis of selective screening of target populations of sexually active young women, the proportion infected ranges from 8% to 40%, with a median of about 15%.[7] Approximately 10% of sexually active asymptomatic men are infected.[8] Prevalence studies demonstrate that the disease is most prevalent in adolescents and is found worldwide.

Life Cycle

As discussed in the preceding chapter, chlamydiae have a unique biphasic life cycle.[9] The elementary body, which is the transmissible form of the organism capable of extracellular survival, attaches to a susceptible epithelial cell to initiate the cycle (Fig. 180-2). Neither the eukaryotic receptors nor the chlamydial surface structures responsible for attachment and entry have been fully defined, although possible candidates have been identified.[10-13] The two primary candidates are the major outer membrane protein (MOMP) and the chlamydial 60-kD cysteine-rich protein OmcB[12]; other candidates include members of the polymorphic membrane protein family of autotransporters (pmps).[13] It may well be that different chlamydial species and serovars utilize different and perhaps multiple means for initial attachment and entry.[14] It appears that in some instances, cells may be infected with more than one strain simultaneously.[15] Stephens and co-workers have demonstrated that the chlamydial outer membrane protein OmcB and MOMP bind heparin.[16] Consequently, because heparin reduces chlamydial infectivity in cell culture, a potential role has been hypothesized for host cell heparan sulfate glycosaminoglycans that may serve as a molecular bridge between chlamydiae and host cells.[16] However, Stephens and colleagues have more recently used a cell line specifically lacking heparan sulfate glycosaminoglycans to demonstrate that host cell surface heparan sulfate does not serve an essential function in chlamydial infectivity.[16]

C. trachomatis can enter cells by phagocytosis, pinocytosis, or receptor-mediated endocytosis.[10] The last is the pathway by which eukaryotic cells internalize and transport macromolecules to specific sites within the cell. Convincing data that receptor-mediated endocytosis is also the pathway primarily used by the trachoma biovar of *C. trachomatis* come from microscopic observations using polarized human genital epithelial cells.[17] In this model, infecting chlamydial elementary bodies are found predominantly in clathrin-coated pits and vesicles that are associated with receptor-mediated endocytosis.[18] The clathrin-coated pit invaginates and becomes an endocytic vesicle containing the chlamydial elementary body.[17] Other experimental approaches using either RNA-interference or dominant-negative mutants of clathrin-mediated endocytosis suggest that clathrin-coated vesicles may not be required for chlamydial entry.[19] However, a comparative study in non-phagocytic host cells using RNA-interference methods to knock down expression of proteins essential for various modes of entry suggests that clathrin and its accessory factors are required for chlamydial entry, whereas caveola-mediated endocytosis (lipid rafts), phagocytosis, and macropinocytosis are not.[20]

Despite the uncertainties surrounding mechanisms of entry and host cell receptors and chlamydial ligands, considerable progress has been made regarding other initial aspects of infection. The time from attachment to internalization of elementary bodies is about 1.5 minutes[19]; during this time, a pedestal-like structure is formed resulting from actin recruitment to the site of entry. The elementary body contains a preformed protein TARP (translocated actin-recruiting phosphoprotein), which is delivered to the host cell via a type 3 secretion mechanism.[21] TARP is rapidly phosphorylated and is involved in signaling actin recruitment[21] via Rac GTPase activation.[22] TARP activates Rac by binding guanine nucleotide exchange factors, which requires TARP phosphorylation.[23] In addition, TARP is capable of serving as an actin nucleator.[24]

The elementary body has stores of adenosine triphosphate (ATP) and an adenosine triphosphatase (ATPase)[25] that is activated in the presence of reducing agents.[26] ATPase activation and reduction of the disulfide bonds that cross link membrane proteins are early events in reorganization of elementary bodies into reticulate bodies.[26,27] The MOMP is a porin that is extensively cross linked by disulfide bonds both internally and with two other cysteine-rich membrane proteins in elementary bodies but not in reticulate bodies.[28,29] Reduction of these bonds may be a key factor in initiation of reorganization. *C. trachomatis* binding and infectivity are markedly reduced in CHO6 cells lacking a functional protein disulfide isomerase at the cell surface.[30]

The reticulate body is the intracellular and replicative form of the organism. As it divides, it fills the endosome, now a cytoplasmic inclusion, with its progeny and with glycogen. When an epithelial cell is infected with more than one elementary body of *C. trachomatis*, the endosomes usually fuse so that each cell eventually contains only one inclusion (see Fig 180-2). The yield of new infectious units per host cell ranges from less than 100 to more than 1000,[31] representing the equivalent of 8 to 12 doublings of a single organism. Synthesis of specific proteins is temporally regulated throughout the life cycle.[32] Proteins thought to be associated with conversion of elementary to reticulate bodies are synthesized early,[33] followed by the MOMP and then late in the cycle by the other cysteine-rich proteins[29] and DNA-binding proteins.[34] Regulation of the cycle appears at least in part to

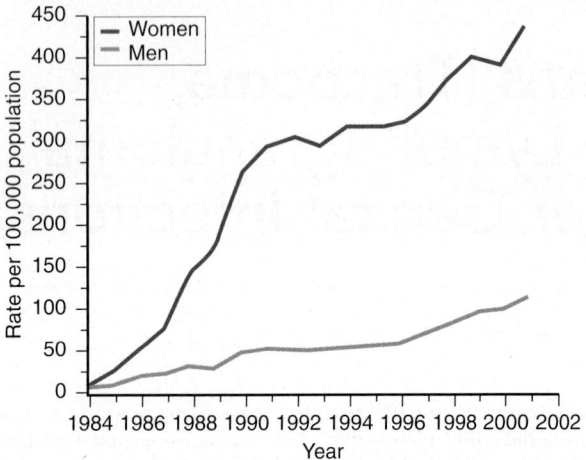

Figure 180-1 Reported incidence of *Chlamydia trachomatis* in the United States. *(Data from Centers for Disease Control and Prevention. Sexually Transmitted Disease Surveillance 2001 Supplement, Chlamydia Prevalence Monitoring Project. Atlanta, Ga: Centers for Disease Control and Prevention; 2002.)*

be at a transcriptional level. Growth cycle-specific messenger RNA (mRNA) has been identified,[35] and multiple promoters for several different genes have been described.[36] Binding of subunits of RNA polymerase to the different promoters may serve as a key regulatory mechanism.[36] Two of the DNA-binding proteins of *C. trachomatis* have extensive sequence homology with eukaryotic histone H₁ (Hc1 and Hc2). They are expressed concomitantly with nucleoid condensation and cessation of transcription as the reticulate body forms an elementary body. They may provide global regulation of gene expression rather than conventional transcriptional regulation.[37] Regulators of Hc1 expression and Hc1 and Hc2 DNA binding have been described. A small regulatory RNA (encoded by *IhtA*) found in reticulate bodies negatively regulates Hc1 synthesis[38] during vegetative growth, whereas a metabolite of the methylerythritol phosphate pathway (key synthetic

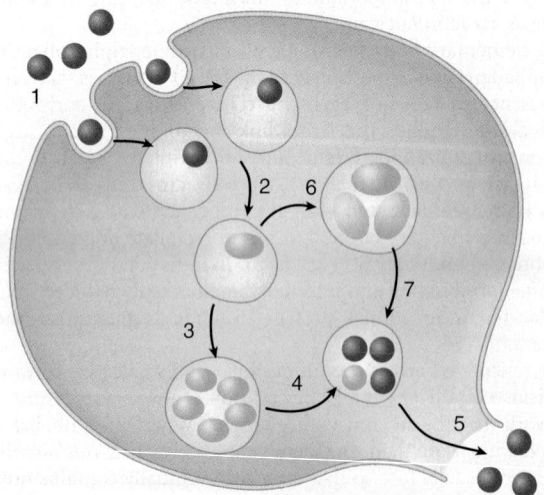

Figure 180-2 Life cycle of *Chlamydia trachomatis* in cell culture. (1) Electron-dense elementary bodies (EBs) attach to and are taken up by epithelial cells. (2) Inclusions fuse and EBs differentiate into reticulate bodies (RBs). (3) RBs divide by binary fission. (4) RBs re-form into EBs. (5) EBs released, often with cell death, to infect other cells. (6) Alternate course under stressful conditions (i.e., IFN-γ exposure) leading to large, metabolically inactive persistent forms. (7) With removal of stress, return to replication and infectious state.

enzyme encoded by *IspE*) dissociates Hc1 and Hc2 from chlamydial chromatin at elementary body germination.[39,40]

Studies have demonstrated the complex and intimate array of interactions between chlamydia and the infected host cell throughout the life cycle.[11] These activities include endocytosis, tyrosine phosphorylation events, cytoskeletal rearrangement, and alterations in host cell macromolecular biosynthesis.[41] Chlamydiae have been found to possess a type III secretion system (T3SS) comparable to that found in other gram-negative bacteria. The system serves as a means of transporting chlamydial proteins both across the host plasma membrane on elementary body attachment from an extracellular location (as with TARP) and across the inclusion membrane from an intracellular location, whether into the host cytoplasm or for insertion into the inclusion membrane. Once transported, these T3SS effectors likely regulate host cell transcription, perhaps facilitating key events such as regulation of vesicular transport or inhibition of fusion of the chlamydial inclusion with host cell lysosomes. Using a shigella expression system, Subtil and colleagues demonstrated that chlamydial Inc proteins can be secreted by the type III secretion apparatus.[42] Substances that induce T3SS in other gram-negative bacteria are capable of activating cell-free elementary bodies to secrete TARP.[43] The importance of T3SS is further established in cell culture systems in which inhibitors of T3SS reversibly disrupt chlamydial development.[44] Protein components of the needle apparatus (injectisome) have been identified.[45] Whereas in most bacteria T3SS genes are clustered in chromosomal pathogenicity islands or virulence-associated plasmids, chlamydial T3SS genes are chromosomal but scattered. Hefty and Stephens[46] described 10 operons preceded by sigma 70-like promoters, and more than 20 proteins of bacterial origin have been localized to the host cell cytosol.[47] The regulation of developmental stage-specific expression of T3SS is undefined.

In cell culture, the entire life cycle takes between 48 and 72 hours, with some strains or serovars growing faster than others. In particular, strains of the lymphogranuloma venereum (LGV) biovar usually complete their life cycle more rapidly than those of the trachoma biovar. Hybiske and Stephens[48] carefully described two mechanisms by which chlamydiae exit the host cell at the end of the growth cycle. The first is lysis, which is an ordered series of membrane ruptures, starting with the inclusion membrane and then the nuclear membrane and, finally, the plasma membrane. The lysis pathway is mediated by proteases, most likely calcium-activated cysteine proteases. It is not known whether the proteases are of chlamydial or cellular origin. The second mechanism is extrusion, where the inclusion protrudes through the plasma membrane and is constricted into separate compartments. Over several hours, the exterior compartment becomes tethered and then separates from the cell.[48] The extrusions are bounded by both the inclusion and plasma membranes, and the inclusion may be partially or completely extruded from the cell. Extrusion requires a variety of host cell factors, including actin polymerization.[48] Interestingly, serovars D and L2 used both pathways at an approximately equal frequency, whereas *Chlamydia caviae* (guinea pig inclusion conjunctivitis agent) less commonly used extrusion.

Largely on the basis of work done in cell culture systems, a modification of the chlamydial life cycle has been proposed incorporating a persistent state.[49] In cell culture systems, a state of persistence can be induced by exposure of chlamydia-infected cells to interferon-γ (IFN-γ), to penicillin, or to tryptophan depletion. Under these conditions, viable chlamydiae undergo a growth cycle arrest characterized by lack of replication, conversion of reticulate to elementary bodies, or viability. During persistence, enlarged atypical reticulate bodies are seen; synthesis of MOMP and the 60-kD cysteine-rich proteins is reduced, but synthesis of the chlamydial 60-kD heat shock protein continues. Removal of the IFN-γ or other inciting factor results in reestablishment of the normal life cycle and chlamydial viability.[49] Although chlamydial persistence seemingly fits with current understanding of the epidemiology and biology of chlamydial infections, further study of whether and how often persistence actually occurs in vivo is needed.

Antigenic and Chemical Composition

Isolates of *C. trachomatis* from the LGV and trachoma biovars were originally classified into 15 serovars (see Chapter 179) on the basis of antigenic cross-reactivity in the microimmunofluorescence test of Wang and Grayston.[50] Three serovars—L_1, L_2, and L_3—are associated either with clinical LGV or with proctocolitis in homosexual men and are rarely recovered in other circumstances. These strains rarely produce asymptomatic infection. The remaining 12 serovars are associated with oculogenital disease: strains A, B, Ba, and C with ocular trachoma and strains D through K with genital tract disease and with inclusion conjunctivitis. Occasionally, serovars B and Ba have been isolated from the genital tract, but A and C have not. Cross-reactivity patterns originally revealed two subgroups within the oculogenital group: B complex (B, Ba, D, E, L_1, and L_2) and C complex (C, J, H, I, A, K, and L_3). Serovars F and G bridge the two complexes, although they are more closely related to the B complex.[49] These relationships were subsequently confirmed and further defined by monoclonal antibodies that identified genus-, species-, subspecies-, and serovar (strain)-specific antigens and by defining the molecular sequence of the MOMP genes for prototype strains.[51] In addition, they led to recognition of three new serovars (Da, Ia, and L_{2a}).[52]

The molecular basis for chlamydial tissue tropism is partly understood for the trachoma and the genital serovars of *C. trachomatis*.[53] Thus, all of the trachoma serovar strains tested to date (both wild-type and reference strains) lack a functional tryptophan synthase gene because of either mutational inactivation (serovars A and C) or loss of the entire operon (serovar C). In contrast, all genital isolates retain functional enzymes that can synthesize tryptophan from indole.[53] Genomic analysis of the trachoma serovar A and the genital isolate D has established that the genomes share 99.6% identity.[54] The primary differences are related to the tryptophan synthase operon and to the *C. trachomatis* cytotoxin locus.[55] The other differences among strains relate to variable numbers of repeat sequences within TARP and a higher concentration of single nucleotide polymorphisms (SNPs) within the polymorphic membrane protein family of autotransporters.[54] Rare strains of *C. trachomatis* lack the cryptic 7.5-kb plasmid, and an L2 strain lacking the plasmid is less virulent in a mouse model of genital infection[56] by virtue of transcriptional downregulation of chromosomal genes. A parallel finding has been reported with a plasmidless *Chlamydia muridarum* strain, which although capable of producing lower genital tract infection, fails to cause upper tract disease in the mouse oviduct.[57] Finally, variations in observed disease severity and organism shedding of human trachoma strains in ocular infections in nonhuman primates appear to be related to SNPs or insertion/deletion events in 22 genes, some of which encode hypothetical proteins of unknown function.[58]

The epitopes reactive with species-, subspecies-, and serovar-specific antibodies are located in four variable sequence regions of the MOMP.[59] The serovar-specific epitopes are found mostly in variable sequence regions 1 and 2, whereas the more broadly shared epitopes cluster in variable region 4.[59] However, some serovars contain more than one serovar-specific epitope, and serovar-specific epitopes are found in variable region 4 as well.[60] Classification of strains on the basis of nucleotide sequencing of the MOMP gene (*ompA*) has revealed variation within serovars[61,62] that may reflect immunologic pressure[63] and that has been useful in defining the molecular epidemiology of trachoma[64] and genital infection.[65] However, these variations in *ompA* in general do not correlate with disease groups (trachoma, genital, and LGV) or symptoms.[62,66] Genus-reactive epitopes have been demonstrated in the MOMP,[67] the 60-kD cysteine-rich protein,[67] and in a 60-kD heat shock protein (HSP60).[68] However, the immunodominant genus-reactive epitope is in lipopolysaccharide. Chlamydial lipopolysaccharide is closely related to the lipopolysaccharide of other gram-negative bacteria, particularly the deep rough (Re) mutants of *Salmonella minnesota* and *Salmonella typhimurium*. However, it contains a 3-deoxy-D-manno-octulosonic acid trisaccharide in a 2,4 and 2,8 linkage, with the latter being unique to the genus *Chlamydia*.[69]

The chlamydial genome of serovar D was the initial complete genome sequenced, as was an LGV isolate, and the data are available on the Internet.[70,71] At least a dozen other genomes have now also been completed. Previously, a number of individual genes had been cloned and sequenced, including the genes for the MOMP,[72] the 60-kD cysteine-rich outer membrane protein,[73] the 60-kD heat shock protein,[68] enzymes involved in lipopolysaccharide synthesis,[69] and the S7 and S12 ribosomal proteins.[74] Information derived from comparative genomic analysis includes confirmation of the antigenic relationships predicted by serologic and monoclonal antibody studies[75] and a molecular basis for some of the antigenic variation observed within serovars.[76,77] In addition, sequence analysis of 16S ribosomal RNA genes has confirmed the eubacterial nature of chlamydiae and established their singularity (see Chapter 179).[78] By this measure, their closest relatives are the *Planctomyces*, an obscure group of bacteria that also lack peptidoglycan. A new antigenic family, the polymorphic membrane protein family of autotransporters, has also been described as a result of genomic analysis (see Chapter 179), and pmpD has been shown to be a species-specific neutralizing epitope.[79] Further studies[80,81] confirm the outer membrane location and autotransporter characteristics of pmpD. Sequence analysis of another of these genes, *C. trachomatis* pmpH, indicates that it has evolved in parallel with the three disease groups (trachoma, genital, and LGV), suggesting that the protein may play a role in pathogenesis.[80]

Pathogenesis

The mechanisms by which *C. trachomatis* induces inflammation and tissue destruction are poorly understood. The LGV biovar of *C. trachomatis* gains entrance through breaks in the skin or infects epithelial cells of the mucous membranes of the genital tract or rectum. It is then carried by lymphatic drainage to the regional lymph nodes, where it multiplies inside mononuclear phagocytes.[82] Bacteremic spread may also occur, and the central nervous system may be infected. The characteristic histopathology is that of granuloma formation with development of small abscesses that may become necrotic or coalesce into suppurative foci.[83]

The target cells of the trachoma biovar of *C. trachomatis* are the squamocolumnar epithelial cells of the endocervix and upper genital tract in women and the conjunctiva, urethra, and rectum in men and women. In men, the epididymis and perhaps the prostate can be infected, whereas in infants the columnar epithelial cells of the respiratory tract are also commonly infected.[82] Regardless of the site, the initial response to infection appears to be primarily a polymorphonuclear leukocyte response.[84-86] Epithelial cells infected in vitro produce interleukin-8 (IL-8) and other proinflammatory cytokines, stimulating the initial neutrophilic response.[87] Lipopolysaccharide may be the predominant chlamydial antigen capable of inducing proinflammatory cytokines.[88]

Studies have shed light on the mechanisms by which infected epithelial cells produce cytokines that direct the initial innate and acquired responses to chlamydial infection. In immortalized human cells, IL-8 induction depends on host cell signaling,[89] in part via extracellular signal-regulated kinase.[90] Independently, IL-8 is also induced via the pattern response receptor NOD1.[91] In a mouse cell culture model employing oviduct epithelial cell lines, *C. muridarum* infection induces a wide variety of cytokines, including IL-1α, IL-6, tumor necrosis factor-α, and cytokines that augment gamma interferon production, including IFN-α/β and IL-12-p70.[92] Toll-like receptor (TLR) 2 is the principal pattern response receptor responsible for induction of acute phase cytokines in this model.[93] IFN-β, a type I interferon, is produced by infected oviduct epithelial cells, even though chlamydiae are not known to possess a classic pathogen-associated molecular pattern to engage TLR3.[94] In the mouse *C. muridarum* model of genital infection, Darville and colleagues have shown using TLR2 knockout mice that TLR2 is an important mediator of the innate response by playing a role in production of both acute phase mediators and chronic inflammatory pathology.[95] The same group studied mice deficient in receptors for type I interferons (α and β) and found that these animals had reduced duration and shedding of organisms during infection, less oviduct pathology, and enhanced CD4 recruitment to cervical tissue compared to wild-type mice, suggesting that induction of type I interferons exacerbates infection by inhibiting the specific CD4 response to chlamydiae.[96]

The initial neutrophilic infiltration is followed by tissue infiltration with lymphocytes, macrophages, plasma cells, and eosinophils.[82] In ocular and genital infections, plasma cells are generally present in large numbers,[97,98] whereas in infant pneumonia, eosinophils and neutrophils predominate.[85] In ocular and genital disease with the trachoma biovar, lymphoid follicles (aggregates of lymphocytes and macrophages in the submucosa) form as the acute inflammation begins to subside. There is thinning or loss of epithelium overlying the follicles, and they may become necrotic as the disease progresses.[82] They are clinically apparent in the conjunctiva as raised avascular lesions. Epithelial proliferation leads to formation of papillae and papillary hypertrophy. As the infection then begins to resolve, fibrosis and scarring occur.

Initial infection of the eye in humans[82] and of the eye[98] and genital tract in monkeys[99] resolves with little or no residual tissue damage. However, in both settings recurrent infection produces an accelerated and more intense inflammatory response with scarring and tissue damage. The potentially important role of reinfection in chlamydial disease was first recognized during human trachoma vaccine trials in which volunteers were immunized and then subsequently challenged with live organisms.[100,101] In these and other studies in humans and monkeys, limited serovar-specific protection against infection could be induced. However, when infection did occur after immunization, it was more severe than in unvaccinated people, and the increased severity was not serovar specific.[1,101]

Multiple episodes of reinfection or persistent infection appear to be required for the development of ocular trachoma, and much of the inflammation and tissue damage appears to be due to the host immune response to the organism.[101] Thus, marked inflammation can be induced in the eyes of previously infected monkeys by application of an extract of *C. trachomatis* containing the chlamydial 60-kD heat shock protein (cHSP60).[102] Furthermore, the presence of serum antibodies reactive with HSP60 is associated with ectopic pregnancy and infertility in women as well as with persistent upper genital tract infection and with perihepatitis.[103-105] There is considerable sequence homology between cHSP60 and analogous proteins from other species including humans,[106,107] and human sera reactive with cHSP60 also react with an analogous human protein.[106,108] Consequently, it has been suggested that the pathogenesis of chlamydial disease may be in part autoimmune, with cHSP60 being the sensitizing antigen.[107-109] In mice, the antibody response to HSP60 is restricted at the major histocompatibility locus[110]; that is, the genetic background of the mouse regulates the response. If the same is true in humans, it might explain some of the variability observed in both the antibody response and morbidity in infected individuals.[110] More recent data have confirmed the relationship between antibody response to cHSP60 and risk of PID[111] and scarring trachoma.[112]

Chlamydiae are able to induce cytokine production, one consequence of which is the production of IFN-γ.[113] IFN-γ inhibits chlamydial replication[114] and in animal models shortens the duration of infection.[115] In cell culture systems, it induces a dose-related persistent infection in which synthesis of cHSP60 continues out of proportion to structural membrane components.[49] However, subsequent removal of the IFN-γ allows the infectious organisms to be rescued and viable once again. Long-lasting infections are now known to occur relatively frequently in the absence of treatment in women[116,117] and perhaps in men as well.[118] The in vivo bacterial and inclusion morphology of these long-lasting infections in people is unknown. However, it is possible that cyclic changes in inhibitory cytokines, chlamydial replication, antigen production, and hypersensitivity response could explain the chronic inflammation and scarring often associated with chlamydial infections.[119]

■ Immunity

Natural infection with *C. trachomatis* appears to confer little protection against reinfection, and the limited protection that is conferred is short lived. Multiple or persistent infections are an essential factor in the pathogenesis of ocular trachoma.[120] Moreover, rates of recurrent infection are also quite high in young, sexually active individuals with genital tract infections: 29% during a 3½-year period in men and women attending a sexually transmitted disease clinic[121] and 38.4% in adolescent women who were observed prospectively for up to 2 years.[122] However, other data suggest that genital tract infections confer at least partial immunity against reinfection. In women with endocervical infection, the presence of secretory immunoglobulin A (IgA) correlated inversely with the numbers of organisms shed.[123] Men experiencing their first episode of nongonococcal urethritis (NGU) are more likely to have *C. trachomatis* recovered from their urethra than are men with a prior history of NGU.[124] Also, individuals at risk for a chlamydial infection who have either a prior history of any sexually transmitted disease or a documented chlamydial infection within the preceding 6 months are at lower risk for a chlamydial infection than those without such a history.[125] In a study of female sex workers in Nairobi, protective immunity against incident infection was observed and correlated with cHSP60-specific IFN-γ production in peripheral blood mononuclear cells.[126] In the trachoma vaccine trials mentioned previously, partial serovar-specific immunity could be elicited, but protection lasted for only 1 or 2 years.[101,120]

In mouse models, CD4 lymphocytes of the Th1 type that traffic to the genital mucosa are crucial for restriction of intracellular growth and resolution of infection.[127] Antibodies directed at epitopes on the MOMP are neutralizing and may play a role in reducing acquisition of infection.[128] Antibodies may also influence the severity of upper genital tract pathology in the mouse.[129] Antibodies against MOMP or lipopolysaccharide protect against reinfection but not primary infections in the mouse, indicating that the protective effect is dependent on CD4-mediated adaptive immunity acquired at the initial infection.[130] IgA antibodies are not absolutely required for protective immunity in this model.[131] Both antibody and cell-mediated mechanisms are important in protective immunity in the guinea pig model.[132] It is possible that antigen presentation in natural mucosal infection may be relatively ineffective in producing strong protective immunity because dendritic cells pulsed in vitro with inactivated chlamydiae are capable of conferring protective immunity in the mouse model.[133] The current consensus is that CD4+ T cells and B cells are most critical in mediating recall immunity to *C. trachomatis* infection and CD8+ T cells are less important. The latter may exert antichlamydial activity by production of IFN-γ rather than by cytotoxic activity.

Increasing evidence suggests that *C. trachomatis* is capable of downregulating the host immune responses to promote long-lasting infection. One example is the chlamydial protein CPAF (chlamydial protease-like activity factor), originally described by Zhong and coworkers.[134] CPAF appears to be secreted into the host cell cytoplasm and proteolytically degrades host transcription factors USF1 and RFX5, which are needed by the host to transcribe HLA class I and class II molecules, respectively. CPAF has also been shown to degrade CD1d, which is an MHC-like molecule expressed on epithelial cells that can signal innate immune responses by natural killer and natural killer T cells.[135] CPAF also displays other activities that may contribute to virulence in addition to immune-modulatory effects. For example, CPAF degrades the host adherens junction molecule nectin-1 in genital epithelial cells[136] and degrades pro-apoptotic BH3-only proteins.[137] Antibodies from infected people can neutralize the proteolytic activity of CPAF[138]; mice immunized with recombinant CPAF with IL-12[139] or CpG[140] are protected against genital challenge, making CPAF an attractive vaccine candidate.

Because of the combination of protective and deleterious effects seen with whole organism infection or vaccination, current vaccine development efforts have been directed at defining relevant epitopes that could be used as components in some form of synthetic or genetically engineered vaccine.[141] Studies of DNA vaccines utilizing the *ompA* gene of *C. muridarum* showed reduced organism burden and mortality in a mouse pneumonia model,[142] but similar studies have not demonstrated an influence on the course of experimental genital infection in mice.[143] Vaccines composed of native conformations of trimeric MOMP of *C. muridarum* compounded with human vaccine adjuvants have been shown to induce partial protection in genital tract challenge in mice.[144]

Laboratory Diagnosis

Among *C. trachomatis* infections, only classic trachoma can be diagnosed on clinical grounds alone and then only in the proper epidemiologic setting. Although other chlamydial infections are often associated with specific clinical syndromes, syndromic diagnosis is imprecise and laboratory confirmation is required for definitive diagnosis. Laboratory procedures of value include cytologic examination for intracytoplasmic inclusions, isolation of *C. trachomatis* in cell culture, demonstration of chlamydial antigen by enzyme-linked immunosorbent assay or by immunofluorescent staining, and demonstration of nucleic acid by direct hybridization or by amplification techniques.[145]

CYTOLOGIC DIAGNOSIS

In infant inclusion conjunctivitis and in ocular trachoma, typical intracytoplasmic inclusions can often be identified in Giemsa-stained cell scrapings from the conjunctiva. However, the technique is relatively insensitive in mild disease, with inclusion-bearing cells found in 10% to 30% of scrapings collected from patients with active trachoma.[146] Stained scrapings are positive in infants with neonatal conjunctivitis and in adults with inclusion conjunctivitis in as many as 90% and 50%, respectively. Cytology has also been used to evaluate endocervical scrapings, including those obtained for Papanicolaou smears. However, interpretation is difficult, and sensitivity and specificity have been low.[147] Cytologic diagnosis has largely been replaced by the much more sensitive and specific nucleic acid amplification tests.

ISOLATION IN CELL CULTURE

C. trachomatis grows well in a variety of cell lines that can be maintained in culture. Most commonly used are McCoy or HeLa cells, which are grown either on glass cover slips in 12-mm-diameter vials or on the bottom of polystyrene microtiter plate wells.[148] Incubation in cell culture ranges from 40 to 72 hours, depending on the cell type and biovar. Intracytoplasmic inclusions can be detected after staining with Giemsa, Macchiavello, or Gimenez stains or by immunofluorescence. Inclusions can also be detected in McCoy cells by staining with iodine, which stains glycogen.[146] However, immunofluorescent staining with monoclonal antibodies is clearly the most sensitive and specific means of detecting inclusions and has largely replaced other methods (see Chapter 179).[149] The quantity of infectious chlamydiae in a specimen is usually expressed as inclusion-forming units. Proper handling of clinical specimens before cell culture inoculation is critical for optimal recovery of organisms but limits the utility of this method.[150] For example, specimens must be maintained at 4°C and inoculated into tissue culture within 24 hours from the time they are obtained.[151] Alternatively, they can be frozen and stored at −70°C before inoculation, but this results in loss of some organisms and in false-negative results in some specimens containing low numbers of inclusion-forming units.[152] Sensitivity of the culture method is enhanced by blind passage of monolayers after incubation or by inoculation of multiple monolayers with a single specimen.[150] Although its specificity approaches 100%, even under optimal conditions the sensitivity of culture is estimated at between 70% and 80% in experienced laboratories and may be as low as 40% to 50% in some settings.[153] These estimates have been derived from studies comparing the results of culture with those of the more sensitive nucleic acid amplification

tests.[145] Because of its high specificity, cell culture has been recommended when testing is used to establish the presence or absence of infection in situations with legal implications (e.g., rape or sexual assault).[6] However, the 2006 Sexually Transmitted Diseases Treatment Guidelines also support use of Food and Drug Administration (FDA)-approved nucleic acid amplification tests (NAATs) for this purpose, which offer the advantage of increased sensitivity of detection of *C. trachomatis*.[154]

The numbers of viable organisms shed by infected individuals and the isolation rates in cell culture parallel each other. Both are affected by the clinical situation.[155] For example, the highest isolation rates and highest numbers of recoverable inclusion-forming units are found in ocular infections such as active trachoma and neonatal or adult inclusion conjunctivitis. Rates are lower in mild or chronic ocular disease. In genital infections, many more organisms are usually recovered from the endocervix than from the male urethra, and even fewer are recovered from the female urethra.[156] More organisms generally accompany infections associated with symptoms or signs, and higher inclusion counts are also generally seen in younger patients.[157] When women at risk for infection have cultures of both the endocervix and the urethra, as opposed to the endocervix alone, the increase in identification of infected women is approximately 20%[156]; that is, 20% of infected women have positive urethral and negative endocervical cultures. In LGV, the organism can be recovered by culture from bubo pus in approximately 30% of cases and less frequently from sites such as the cervix or the urethra.[158] In appropriate clinical settings, *C. trachomatis* has been recovered from the nasopharynx and rectum,[159] bronchoalveolar lavage fluid and lung biopsy tissue,[160] endometrium, fallopian tubes,[161] epididymis,[162] peritoneal cavity,[163] and donor semen.[164]

ANTIGEN DETECTION AND NUCLEIC ACID HYBRIDIZATION

Given the limited availability and variable sensitivity of *C. trachomatis* cultures as well as the technical impediments associated with their use, considerable effort has been directed at developing better diagnostic tests for chlamydia.[165] Several tests that do not require culture for detection of chlamydiae are commercially available. These tests are based on (1) antigen detection by direct fluorescent antibody (DFA) staining, (2) antigen detection by enzyme-linked immunosorbent assay, or (3) detection of chlamydial ribosomal RNA by hybridization with a DNA probe. Published evaluations have been based primarily on MicroTrak DFA (Syva Co., Palo Alto, Calif.) and Chlamydiazyme (Abbott Laboratories, North Chicago, Ill.), although a number of similar tests have been approved by the FDA.[6] Most studies evaluating these tests have reported sensitivities greater than 70% and specificities of 97% to 99% in populations of men and women with a prevalence of infection of 5% or more.[6] Although these performance characteristics offer acceptable positive and negative predictive values for most diagnostic purposes,[6] they have largely been replaced with NAATs. In general, nonculture tests are more sensitive in patients who are symptomatic and shedding large numbers of organisms than in patients who are asymptomatic and may be shedding fewer organisms.[155,165] All of these tests require invasive collection procedures (i.e., a cervical swab in women or a urethral swab in men) and cannot utilize urine or self-collected vaginal swabs because of low sensitivity with these approaches when used with these tests.

In low-prevalence populations (i.e., <5% infected), a significant proportion of positive test results are false positives. For example, if 1000 patients have a prevalence of 3%, 30 are infected. A test with a sensitivity of 80% and a specificity of 99% detects 24 of the infected people but falsely identifies 10 (1% of 1000) uninfected people as infected. Consequently, the interpretation of a positive test result must be handled with care in counseling patients, and verification may be desirable in this situation. Verification of a positive test result can be accomplished by (1) culture, (2) a second nonculture test that identifies a different chlamydial antigen or nucleic acid sequence than the first test, or (3) a blocking antibody or competitive probe.[6] However, as noted previously, only culture or FDA-approved NAATs should be used if there are potential legal consequences associated with misdiagnosis of a chlamydial infection.[6,154]

Each of these tests and formats has its own advantages and disadvantages. DFA allows assessment of the quality of the specimen (by observation of the presence of epithelial cells) in addition to the presence or absence of organisms but requires a highly skilled microscopist for proper interpretation.[165] Tests using antibodies directed against the MOMP are species specific, whereas those using antilipopolysaccharide antibodies can cross react with other bacteria, including other species of chlamydiae.[6] Performance of the enzyme immunoassay tests requires personnel with fewer skills, but these tests generally take longer to perform. To differentiate false-positive from true-positive reactions, some manufacturers provide reagents for the test to be repeated on the same specimen with blocking antibody present.[166] The DNA hybridization techniques are relatively easy to perform and interpret. Although considerably fewer comparative data have been published on the DNA hybridization techniques than on the other formats, their sensitivity and specificity generally appear similar to those of the enzyme immunoassay tests.[167,168]

NUCLEIC ACID AMPLIFICATION TESTS

NAATs based on the detection of chlamydial DNA or RNA using amplification procedures such as polymerase chain reaction (PCR), ligase chain reaction, chlamydial ribosomal RNA using transcription-mediated amplification, or other methods are now available. A review of studies establishes that these tests are considerably more sensitive than culture and are nearly as specific.[145,169-172] Because of their excellent sensitivity, these tests have provided a major breakthrough in chlamydial diagnosis as they are the first tests that exceed culture in their sensitivity. In general, these tests are 15% to 20% more sensitive than high-quality culture systems, but they may be up to 40% to 50% more sensitive than some culture or enzyme immunoassay tests (Table 180-1). Moreover, the NAATs can be used to detect *C. trachomatis* in urine or in self-collected vaginal swab specimens,[173] with a sensitivity comparable to that obtained with urogenital swab specimens. Thus, these tests make noninvasive testing for chlamydial infections possible for the first time.[172,174] Studies of military recruits,[175] adolescents,[176] high school students,[177] job training participants,[178] and juvenile detainees demonstrate the utility of these tests in diagnosing infection without pelvic examination or collection of swab specimens and outside traditional screening sites. Such testing makes both population-based research projects and community-based prevention programs utilizing widespread screening programs feasible. However, the NAATs are expensive and may not be affordable by health departments for comprehensive screening. In addition, they may be technically demanding for some routine laboratory settings, leading to erroneous false-positive or false-negative results. What remains to be determined is the most cost-effective way to employ NAATs in screening situations to ensure the greatest impact on the adverse consequences of undiagnosed chlamydial infections. Considerations include selective screening, pooling of specimens, and combined use of less expensive enzyme immunoassays followed by NAAT confirmation. Approaches to development of appropriate quality control procedures must also be delineated. The choice of the most appropriate NAAT or approach to screening will likely vary with the clinical setting, the facilities available, and the relative cost.

In 2006, a new variant strain of *C. trachomatis* was discovered in Sweden, where an unexpected plateau in chlamydial prevalence prompted a reevaluation of NAATs then in use.[179] This strain has a 377-base pair deletion in the cryptic plasmid, encompassing the very sequences amplified by the two NAATs (Roche Amplicor PCR and Abbott m200 real-time PCR) then employed for routine screening in Sweden. Although infections caused by these strains give negative assays using these NAATs, assays using different target sequences such as 16S or 23S rRNA reliably detect them.[180,181] In one study in Stockholm, the variant strains constituted 23% of diagnosed chlamydia cases.[182] However, preliminary studies indicate that these strains are largely localized to Sweden.[183] Regardless, this is a fascinating demonstration of the ability of the organism to gain a competitive advantage, in this case by escaping diagnostic detection.

SEROLOGY

Chlamydial serologic tests are of limited value in the diagnosis of most common oculogenital chlamydial infections. A complement fixation test is commercially available that measures antibodies against group-reactive antigens (i.e., lipopolysaccharide) in people infected with *C. trachomatis*, *Chlamydia pneumoniae*, or *Chlamydia psittaci*. Virtually 100% of individuals with LGV or psittacosis have complement-fixing antibody titers greater than 1:16 after infection.[184] Patients with LGV often present 3 or 4 weeks after the onset of their illness, at which time their antibody titer is stable. Consequently, in an appropriate clinical setting a complement fixation titer of 1:64 or greater is strongly supportive of a diagnosis of LGV, although confirmation requires a fourfold or greater titer rise between acute and convalescent specimens.[184] The complement fixation test may also become positive, however, in patients with recently acquired *C. pneumoniae* infections or some patients with oculogenital infections and thus it lacks specificity. Titers are low or nonexistent in this test among most patients with chlamydial urethritis, cervicitis, or conjunctivitis; thus, it has little diagnostic utility in these settings.

The other serologic test that is available primarily in research laboratories is the microimmunofluorescence test. In its most common format, elementary bodies from each of the 15 serovars are employed as antigens, and antibodies against cell wall components of the organisms are detected.[50] When done in an experienced laboratory, this test is more sensitive than the complement fixation test, and because the target MOMP antigens are species specific, it can differentiate infections caused by *C. trachomatis*, *C. pneumoniae*, and *C. psittaci*. The test, when used on acute and convalescent sera, demonstrates a fourfold rise in antibody in the majority of adult patients with eye or genital infection. Titers are especially high in women with PID or perihepatitis, in whom its diagnostic sensitivity may be highest. Likewise, anti-*Chlamydia* IgM is present in approximately 30% of infants with neonatal inclusion and in nearly all infants with chlamydial pneumonia.[184] Consequently, an IgM titer of 1:32 or greater in the microimmunofluorescence test can be diagnostic of infant chlamydial pneumonia in an appropriate clinical setting.

Anti-*Chlamydia* IgM is uncommon in adults with genital tract infection. The prevalence of anti-*Chlamydia* IgG is high in sexually active adults (30% to 60%), even in those who do not have an active infection, and it is probably due to past infection. There may be an association between chlamydia-specific serum IgA and active disease.

TABLE 180-1	Comparative Performances of Selected Diagnostic Tests in the Detection of *Chlamydia trachomatis*		
Test	Sensitivity Relative to Expanded Gold Standard (%)*	Specificity (%)	Detectability Level (Elementary Bodies)
Enzyme immunoassay	40-60	99.5[†]	1,000-10,000
Nonamplified genetic probe	40-65	99.0	1,000-10,000
Direct fluorescent antibody	50-80	99.8	50-1,000
Cell culture	50-90	99.9	10-100
Nucleic acid amplification tests	Cervix 81-100 F urine 80-96 M urine 90-96	99.7	1-10

*Defined using a combination of different test methodologies, including culture, direct fluorescent antibody, and polymerase chain reaction (PCR) or ligase chain reaction (LCR) directed against a target sequence distinct from that used in the routine PCR or LCR assays.
[†]Specificity using confirmatory assays.
F, female; M, male.

However, the sensitivity, specificity, and predictive values of this test are not high enough to make it clinically useful in the diagnosis of active disease.[185] Thus, chlamydial serologies are not recommended for diagnosis of active disease except in suspected cases of LGV, psittacosis, and infants with pneumonia.

Clinical Manifestations

C. trachomatis infections can be divided into four clinical categories: (1) classic ocular trachoma, (2) LGV, (3) other oculogenital diseases in adults, and (4) perinatal infections.

OCULAR TRACHOMA

Ocular trachoma has been recognized since antiquity. Therapy for trachoma and its complications was described in China in the 27th century BC and in Egypt in the 19th century BC.[1] In areas in which trachoma is endemic, the first infection usually occurs early in life (generally before age 2 years), and active disease persists for several years. Although initial infections may resolve spontaneously, they are frequently complicated by reinfection or by superimposed bacterial conjunctivitis. In its initial stages, trachoma manifests as a chronic follicular conjunctivitis with papillary hypertrophy and inflammatory infiltration. As the disease progresses, scarring of the conjunctiva occurs, and there is involvement of the cornea. In addition, as the inner surface of the lids becomes scarred, the eyelashes turn in and abrade the cornea, resulting in ulceration, scarring, and visual loss. Children with mild disease are left with some conjunctival scarring and pannus formation (fibrovascular infiltrate), whereas others develop badly scarred conjunctivae and corneas. The latter may not occur until well into adult life.[186] The WHO's simplified grading scheme for trachoma is presented in Table 180-2.

Treatment

In endemic areas, the primary reservoir is children with ocular infection.[187] Transmission occurs by hand-to-eye contact between children and their caregivers or by contact with the feet of flies who feed on the exudate from children with active conjunctivitis.[188,189] Hygienic factors that seem to be particularly important in control of disease include facial cleanliness, access to water, and reduction of household fly density. Topical antibiotic therapy is of only marginal benefit,[186] perhaps because extraocular sites such as the nasopharynx and rectum are infected in children with trachoma.[188] Systemic antibiotic therapy is effective in individuals and possibly in communities in which the incidence of disease is relatively low.[186] However, compliance with erythromycin is poor, and doxycycline is contraindicated in young children. Trials of mass treatment with azithromycin at the village level indicate that both infection and clinical disease are markedly decreased at 6 and 12 months after such treatment.[190-193] Programs involving lid

TABLE 180-2	World Health Organization Simplified Grading Scheme for Trachoma

Trachomatous inflammation—follicular (TF): There are five or more follicles in the upper tarsal conjunctiva (follicles must be at least 0.05 mm in diameter).

Trachomatous inflammation—intense (TI): Pronounced inflammatory thickening of the tarsal conjunctiva, which obscures half of the normal deep tarsal vessels.

Trachomatous conjunctival scarring (TS): The presence of easily visible scars in the tarsal conjunctiva.

Trachomatous trichiasis (TT): At least one eyelash rubs on the eyeball. Evidence of recent removal of inturned lashes was also graded as trichiasis.

Corneal opacity (CO): Easily visible corneal opacity present over the pupil, which was so dense that at least part of the pupil margin was blurred when seen through the opacity.

Adapted from Thylefors B, Dawson CR, Jones BR, et al. A simple system of the assessment of trachoma and its complications. *Bull World Health Organ.* 1987;65:477-483.

surgery teams for the prevention of blindness related to lid deformities that cause continuing corneal damage are also of value.[186] Because of the importance of hygienic factors, there is a strong historic link between improvement in socioeconomic conditions and disappearance of endemic trachoma.

The WHO has initiated a program to eliminate blinding trachoma by 2020.[189] The objective is not necessarily to eliminate the trachoma serovars of chlamydiae (A, B, Ba, and C) but to eliminate or at least markedly reduce clinically active disease. The key elements of the S-A-F-E strategy are surgery for deformed eyelids, periodic mass treatment of villages with the antibiotic azithromycin, face washing and hygiene, and environmental improvements to control flies by such techniques as building latrines outside villages. In a study performed in Nepal, an annual treatment of all children 1 to 10 years old with azithromycin was associated with a marked reduction in both clinically evident trachoma and evidence of chlamydial infection by PCR.[191] In some areas, trachoma appears to be disappearing coincident with economic gains and without the introduction of specific control programs.

LYMPHOGRANULOMA VENEREUM

LGV is a sexually transmitted disease caused by the LGV serovars of *C. trachomatis*. It is endemic in Africa, India, Southeast Asia, South America, and the Caribbean and occurs as a sporadic disease elsewhere. There are three distinct stages in classic LGV. The first stage is formation of a primary lesion, usually on the genital mucosa or adjacent skin. *C. trachomatis* cannot infect squamous epithelial cells, and when the primary lesion occurs on the external genitalia or in the vagina, the organism probably gains entry through minute lacerations or abrasions.[158] The primary lesion is usually a small papule or herpetiform ulcer that produces few or no symptoms and is generally not noticed. It appears between 3 and 30 days after acquisition of infection[83] and heals rapidly without leaving a scar. Initial infection can also be intraurethral, producing a symptomatic urethritis; cervical, producing cervicitis; or rectal, causing proctitis.

The secondary stage occurs days to weeks after the primary lesion and is characterized by lymphadenopathy and systemic symptoms. The lymph nodes involved are those that drain the area of the primary lesion and thus depend on its location. In men, the primary lesion is usually on the penis or in the urethra, and thus the inguinal lymph nodes are the main ones affected. Lymphadenopathy is unilateral in two thirds of patients.[83] Similarly, when the site of primary infection is vulvar, inguinal and femoral nodes are affected. When the primary infection is rectal, the affected nodes are the deep iliac nodes, and when it is upper vaginal or cervical, the obturator and iliac nodes are infected.[157]

Inguinal lymphadenopathy, however, is the most characteristic manifestation of the secondary stage and the one most frequently recognized. Initially, the lymph nodes are discrete and tender with overlying erythema, but because of extensive periadenitis the inflammatory process spreads from the lymph nodes into the surrounding tissue, forming an inflammatory mass. Abscesses within the mass coalesce, forming a bubo that may rupture spontaneously with development of loculated abscesses, fistulas, or sinus tracts.[194]

Systemic manifestations are often associated with this phase, including fever, headache, and myalgias. Meningitis may occur, and in some cases the organism has been recovered from blood or cerebrospinal fluid.[157] Rupture of the fluctuant inflammatory mass (bubo) relieves pain and fever,[158] although sinus tracts may continue to drain thick, yellowish pus for several weeks or months before fully resolving.[194] Excised inguinal nodes often have a characteristic inflammatory response, with central stellate coalescing abscesses that contain neutrophils and necrotic debris surrounded by a zone of palisaded epithelioid cells, macrophages, and occasional multinucleated giant cells. Surrounding this, there is an outer layer of lymphocytes and plasma cells. With time, the nodal architecture is effaced and replaced by progressive fibrosis. This histopathologic presentation is suggestive of the diagnosis of LGV or cat-scratch disease but is not unique to these entities.

Healing leaves some scarring in the inguinal region but does not result in significant sequelae in most cases. Relapse occurs in approximately 20% of untreated cases.[158] Only approximately one third of buboes become fluctuant and rupture. The others harden and form inguinal masses, which gradually involute over time.[194] Femoral nodes are also frequently affected, and the division between the femoral and inguinal nodes by the inguinal ligament produces the "groove" sign described as characteristic of LGV.[158] Inguinal or femoral lymphadenopathy may be misdiagnosed as inguinal hernia, whereas deep iliac node involvement may raise a question of appendicitis. Only 20% to 30% of women present with inguinal lymphadenopathy as their primary manifestation. Other common presentations in women and in homosexual or bisexual men are symptoms consistent with proctitis, proctocolitis, or complaints of lower abdominal and back pain related to involvement of deep pelvic and lumbar lymph nodes.[194]

In the third stage, complications include *esthiomene* (Greek, "eating away"), which refers to hypertrophic chronic granulomatous enlargement with ulceration of the external genitalia (either the vulva or scrotum and penis).[194] Lymphatic obstruction may also lead to elephantiasis of the male or female genitalia.

The differential diagnosis of inguinal lymphadenopathy in the age group likely to be infected includes herpes simplex virus, syphilis, chancroid, and, occasionally, lymphoma.[195] Mild leukocytosis, with an increase in monocytes and eosinophils, frequently accompanies early bubonic and anogenital rectal LGV.[158] Significant polymorphonuclear leukocytosis suggests bacterial adenitis or superinfection with pyogenic bacteria. The diagnosis can be made on the basis of a positive chlamydial serology, isolation of LGV from infected tissue, or histopathology. A skin test (the Frei test) has been used in the past but is no longer available.[158,196] C. trachomatis can be recovered from bubo aspirates, genital tissue, or rectal tissue in only approximately 30% of cases.[158] The utility of newer diagnostic techniques such as NAATs has not been extensively studied, but limited experience indicates high sensitivity. Histopathologic changes in LGV are not specific but, when combined with serologic results in an appropriate clinical setting, are usually sufficient to make a presumptive diagnosis.

LGV manifesting as inguinal lymphadenopathy can be distinguished from genital herpes by the presence of the multiple painful ulcers at the site of the primary herpes infection, in contrast to the painless primary lesion of LGV, and by matting of the lymph nodes in LGV. Also, lymphadenopathy is frequently bilateral in herpes but not in LGV. A diagnosis of syphilis is suggested by a primary lesion with indurated margins (chancre) and bilateral and nontender inguinal lymphadenopathy. Large ulcers that are multiple and extremely tender in association with lymphadenopathy suggest chancroid. The pseudobuboes that occur in granuloma inguinale are nodules in the skin and subcutaneous tissue, with lymph node involvement being the result of secondary infection.[83] However, the clinical presentation of sexually transmitted agents causing inguinal lymphadenopathy clearly overlaps, and appropriate laboratory tests are usually required to distinguish among them. When an ulcer is present, a darkfield examination should be performed for *Treponema pallidum* and serologic tests for syphilis obtained.[83,156,195]

Treatment of Lymphogranuloma Venereum

Although sulfonamides have in vitro activity against *C. trachomatis* and some clinical efficacy, they do not produce bacteriologic cures reliably.[196] Tetracycline, doxycycline, minocycline, chloramphenicol, erythromycin, and rifampin have been used with good effect in the treatment of primary and secondary stages of LGV.[158,197,198] Few comparative studies of therapy have been done, but current recommendations by the CDC are for 21 days of doxycycline, 100 mg twice daily, with erythromycin or sulfisoxazole listed as alternative regimens.[199] In addition, fluctuant buboes should be aspirated to prevent rupture and sinus tract formation.[158] Antibiotic therapy results in rapid abatement of constitutional symptoms but has only a limited effect on bubo resolution.[158] Effects on late complications such as strictures are variable.[83,158]

OCULOGENITAL DISEASE IN ADULTS

C. trachomatis serovars D through K, and occasionally B and Ba, produce a wide variety of oculogenital infections (Fig. 180-3).

Inclusion Conjunctivitis

In the adult, chlamydial eye infection manifests as an acute follicular conjunctivitis, often with a foreign body sensation in the eye. Symptoms are usually unilateral. The clinical picture in the first 2 weeks is dominated by hyperemia and a mucoid discharge that becomes purulent.[200] This is followed by lymphoid follicle formation (frequently with corneal lesions and epithelial keratitis[201,202]), as well as invasion of the cornea by blood vessels (pannus), and is indistinguishable from early ocular trachoma. Preauricular lymphadenopathy and otitis media may be present.[201] Untreated or improperly treated, the condition may persist for many months but usually resolves without complications.[203]

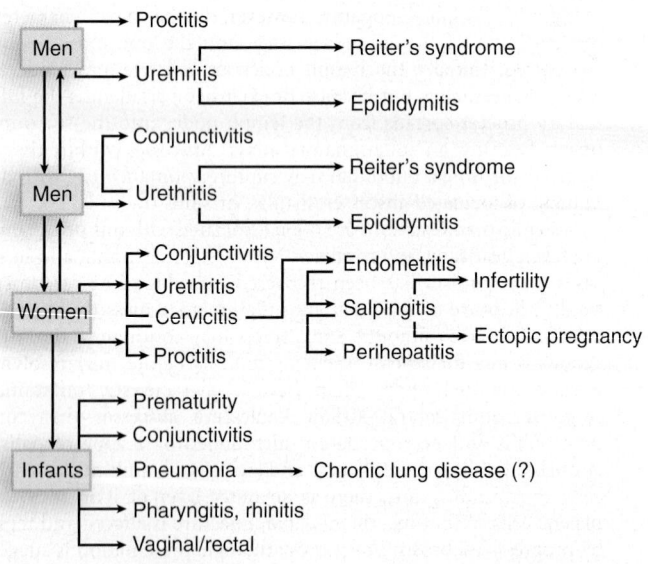

Figure 180-3 **Clinical manifestations of *Chlamydia trachomatis* and patterns of transmission.**

Scarring similar to that seen in mild trachoma may occur in occasional cases.

Slightly more than half of adults with inclusion conjunctivitis have documented concurrent genital tract infections with *C. trachomatis*.[203,204] In such individuals, the presumed mode of transmission is autoinoculation with infected genital secretions or, in some cases, direct inoculation from an infected partner. More difficult to explain is the acquisition of infection by individuals who do not have concurrent genital tract infections. Spread between individuals from eye to eye by transfer of infected secretions without sexual contact may also occur and account for some cases.[204] Many such cases may be due to asymptomatic or unrecognized genital infection. Although as many as 9% of patients with keratoconjunctivitis who are 16 to 20 years of age have chlamydial ocular infection, eye involvement is still seen in less than 1% of individuals with proven genital tract infection.[203,204]

The differential diagnosis is primarily conjunctivitis caused by adenovirus or other viruses.[202] A definitive diagnosis can be made only by demonstration of the organism by culture, NAATs, or another test. The condition responds promptly to the administration of appropriate systemic antibiotics such as azithromycin or doxycycline with decrease in discharge, hyperemia, and symptoms from keratitis within 48 hours.[200] Evaluation and treatment of the patient and partners for genital tract infection should also be undertaken.

Urogenital Infections

The risk of aquisition of *C. trachomatis* with a single episode of sexual intercourse with an infected partner is not known. However, it appears to be substantially less than that for *Neisseria gonorrhoeae*.[205] On the basis of extrapolation of data from partner notification programs and from couples with discordant cell culture-proven infection, the transmission probability has been estimated as 0.39 from men to women and as 0.32 from women to men.[206] Based on results of a more sensitive diagnostic test, PCR, transmission probability has been estimated as approximately 0.68 in both directions.[207] However, these estimates are based on the average frequency of intercourse among pairs rather than a single encounter. Partners of asymptomatic individuals identified through a screening program are less likely to be infected than partners of symptomatic individuals,[208] and in one study, recent exposure to a new partner was much more strongly associated with gonococcal than with chlamydial infection.[209] Furthermore, in adolescents, chlamydial infection is strongly associated with frequency of intercourse, both in those reporting only one lifetime partner and in those reporting more than one lifetime partner.[210] Thus, in contrast to gonococcal infections, genital infections with *C. trachomatis* have more characteristics of a prevalent than an incident disease. Most individuals infected with *N. gonorrhoeae* develop symptoms and seek care quickly, whereas many men and most women infected with *C. trachomatis* are either asymptomatic or minimally symptomatic and are diagnosed as a result of screening or because a contact is symptomatic.[209]

C. trachomatis is recovered more often from women who acquire gonorrhea than from similarly exposed women who do not acquire gonorrhea.[211] In individuals with gonorrhea, the recurrence rate of *C. trachomatis* infection with the same serovar is significantly greater than can be explained by variables related to likely exposure.[212] Furthermore, individuals infected with both *C. trachomatis* and *N. gonorrhoeae* shed larger numbers of *C. trachomatis* than those infected with *C. trachomatis* alone.[155] These data suggest that acquisition of a gonococcal infection either reactivates a persistent chlamydial infection or increases the susceptibility of the host to acquisition of chlamydiae.

Urethritis

There is little information on the natural history of untreated urethral infection. Several small studies suggest that in men untreated chlamydial infection at the urethra may persist for as many as 6 months.[118,213,214] Only one of eight infected men who were observed without treatment for a minimum of 21 days developed symptomatic urethritis.[215] Although asymptomatic infections are common in men, *C. trachomatis* is also the cause of between 30% and 50% of cases of

symptomatic NGU and an even higher proportion of cases of postgonococcal urethritis.[216] Other causes of NGU include *Ureaplasma urealyticum* (not *Ureaplasma parvum*), *Trichomonas vaginalis*, *Mycoplasma genitalium*, and herpes simplex virus.[217,218] *C. trachomatis* can also be recovered from approximately 20% of men with gonococcal urethritis.[219] When men who are dually infected are treated only with single-dose therapy for their gonorrhea, most develop postgonococcal urethritis, which manifests as a persistence or recurrence of their urethritis. In the United States, the incidence of NGU exceeds that of gonococcal urethritis by ratios greater than 2 to 1 in most sexually transmitted diseases clinics, with even higher ratios in many private practice settings.[7] Risk factors for chlamydial urethritis in men include age younger than 20 years, black race, and heterosexual orientation.[220]

The incubation period for symptomatic chlamydial urethritis is usually between 7 and 14 days, in contrast to that for gonococcal urethritis, which is approximately 4 days. Patients present with dysuria and urethral discharge, which is usually white, gray, or sometimes clear, in contrast to the more purulent discharge observed with gonococcal urethritis.[220] The discharge may be so slight as to be demonstrable only after penile stripping or only in the morning. Some patients may deny the presence of discharge but may note stained underwear in the morning resulting from scant discharge overnight. However, there is sufficient overlap between the signs and symptoms of gonococcal urethritis and NGU that a reliable distinction between them cannot be made on clinical grounds alone. An average of 4 or more polymorphonuclear leukocytes per oil immersion field (1000×) in a Gram stain of an endourethral swab specimen establishes a diagnosis of urethritis.[221] The absence of organisms with the typical morphology of *N. gonorrhoeae* and the subsequent failure to culture *N. gonorrhoeae* establish a diagnosis of NGU. In adolescent males, more than 10 leukocytes per high-power field in the initial 15 to 20 mL of a first-catch urine specimen is also strongly suggestive of urethritis,[222] as is a positive urine leukocyte esterase test result.[223] The primary complications of chlamydial urethritis in men are (1) epididymitis; (2) sexually reactive arthritis, including Reiter's syndrome; and (3) transmission to women.

Epididymitis and Prostatitis

C. trachomatis and *N. gonorrhoeae* are the most frequent causes of epididymitis in men younger than 35 years, whereas Enterobacteriaceae (primarily *Escherichia coli*) are the usual pathogens in men older than 35 years.[224] In younger men, urethritis is usually also present but may be asymptomatic and demonstrable only on examination. However, its absence does not exclude chlamydial infection or gonorrhea as the etiologic agent. Most men with *E. coli* as the etiologic agent, in addition to being older, have other risk factors for urinary tract infection, including recent catheterization, urologic surgery, or rectal insertive intercourse. Chlamydial epididymitis is often associated with oligospermia during the acute phase,[224] but there are no data indicating that future fertility is impaired. In addition, epididymitis is usually unilateral, and attempts to correlate chlamydial infections with male factor infertility have been unsuccessful.[225] A presumptive diagnosis of NGU can be confirmed as chlamydial in etiology utilizing a first void urine specimen tested by a NAAT (Table 180-3).

Typically, epididymitis arises with a unilateral swollen epididymis or testicle or both, dysuria, fever, and, in some cases, shaking chills. Many patients can be managed in the outpatient setting, but others require hospitalization for parenteral antibiotics, scrotal elevation, analgesia, and observation. The diagnosis of testicular torsion should always be considered in young men with acute onset of severe unilateral scrotal pain and should be ruled out with radionuclide studies.

The role of chlamydia in prostatic infection remains controversial. From available data, it does not appear to play a role in acute prostatitis; these cases are mainly attributable to *E. coli*, other gram-negative rods, or enterococci. Its role in chronic nonbacterial prostatitis remains more controversial. Although some investigators have recovered *C. trachomatis* from prostatic expressate or biopsies of such patients,

TABLE 180-3	Clinical Characteristics of Common *Chlamydia trachomatis* Infections				
	Infection	Symptoms and Signs	Presumptive Diagnosis	Definitive Diagnosis	Treatment
Men	Nongonococcal urethritis	Urethral discharge, dysuria	Urethral leukocytosis; no gonococci seen	Urine or urethral NAAT	Azithromycin, 1 g PO (single dose) *or* Doxycycline, 100 mg PO bid, for 7 days
	Epididymitis	Unilateral epididymal tenderness, swelling; pain; fever, presence of NGU	Urine or urethral NAAT	Urethral leukocytosis; pyuria on urinalysis	Outpatient: levofloxacin, 500 mg bid for 10 days *or* Ceftriaxone, 1 g IM, plus doxycycline, 100 mg PO bid, for 10 days
	Proctitis	Rectal pain, discharge, bleeding; history of receptive anal intercourse	≥1 PMN/OIF on rectal Gram stain; no gonococci seen	Urine or urethral NAAT; rectal culture or NAAT	Doxycycline, 100 mg PO bid, for 7 days
	Conjunctivitis	Ocular pain, redness, discharge; simultaneous genital infection	Gram stain of conjunctival swab negative for bacterial pathogens; PMNs on smear	Rectal culture or NAAT; NAAT of conjunctivae	Azithromycin, 1 g PO (single dose) *or* Doxycycline, 100 mg PO bid, for 7 days
Women	Cervicitis	Mucopurulent cervical discharge; ectopy, easily induced bleeding	≥20 PMN/OIF on cervical Gram stain	Urine or cervical NAAT	Azithromycin, 1 g PO (single dose) *or* Doxycycline, 100 mg PO bid, for 7 days
	Urethritis	Dysuria, frequency; no hematuria	Pyuria on UA; negative urine Gram stain and culture	Urine, cervical, or urethral NAAT	Azithromycin, 1 g PO (single dose) *or* Doxycycline, 100 mg PO bid, for 7 days
	Salpingitis	Lower abdominal pain, adnexal pain, cervical motion tenderness	Evidence of mucopurulent cervicitis	Urine or cervical NAAT	Outpatient: Ofloxacin, 400 mg PO bid, plus metronidazole, 500 mg PO bid, for 14 days *or* Ceftriaxone, 250 g IM plus doxycycline, 100 mg PO bid, for 14 days
Adult	Conjunctivitis	Ocular pain, redness, discharge; simultaneous genital infection	Gram stain of conjunctival swab negative for bacterial pathogens; PMNs on smear	DFA or NAAT on conjunctival swab	Azithromycin, 1 g PO (single dose) *or* Doxycycline, 100 mg PO bid, for 7 days
Newborn	Conjunctivitis	Ocular pain, redness, discharge; simultaneous genital infection	Gram stain of conjunctival swab negative for bacterial pathogens; PMNs on smear	DFA or NAAT on conjunctival swab; vagina, rectum, pharynx also often positive	Erythromycin base 50 mg/kg/day, orally divided into four doses daily for 14 days, evaluate and treat parents as well
	Pneumonia	Staccato cough, tachypnea, hyperinflation	Diffuse interstitial infiltrate, eosinophilia	Nasopharyngeal NAATs or culture; MIF serology (IgM)	Erythromycin base 50 mg/kg/day, orally divided into four doses daily for 14 days, evaluate and treat parents as well

DFA, direct fluorescent antibody; IgM, immunoglobulin M; MIF, microimmunofluorescence; NAAT, nucleic acid amplification test; NGU, nongonococcal urethritis; OIF, oil immersion field; PMN, polymorphonuclear neutrophil; UA, urinalysis.

convincing evidence that chlamydia plays an etiologic role in chronic nonbacterial prostatitis has yet to be developed and antibiotic therapy is not recommended.[226]

Proctitis and Proctocolitis

Although asymptomatic rectal carriage of the non-LGV serovars of *C. trachomatis* occurs in both infants[159] and adults,[227] *C. trachomatis* is also a common cause of symptomatic proctitis and proctocolitis in homosexual men.[228] Proctitis can result from direct inoculation of the rectum in either men or women through anal intercourse or secondary spread of secretions from the cervix. In LGV, lymphatic spread from the posterior vaginal wall or cervix through lymphatics may occur.[158,229] Severity and extent of disease are related to the infecting serovars. In infection with serovars D through K, the primary manifestations are anal pruritus and a mucous rectal discharge that may become mucopurulent. The infection remains superficial, is limited to the rectum,

and closely resembles gonococcal proctitis. In many patients, infection is asymptomatic. Leukocytes are usually present on rectal Gram stain even in asymptomatic patients with *C. trachomatis* infection.[228,230] With the LGV strains, rectal pain, tenesmus, rectal bleeding, and fever are present. Epidemiologic studies have called attention to an apparent increase in the number of cases of LGV strain proctitis in men who have sex with men, mostly in the setting of concomitant human immunodeficiency virus (HIV) infection.[231] The disease extends into the colon. The rectal and colonic mucosa become ulcerated, and a granulomatous inflammatory process is present in the bowel wall, with both noncaseating granulomas and crypt abscesses. As the disease related to LGV strains progresses, muscle layers are replaced by fibrous tissue, which contracts to form rectal strictures. Sinus tract formation can lead to rectovaginal fistulas in women.[194,229] The inflammatory process as seen on sigmoidoscopy may be localized to one segment or may occur at several different levels concurrently. Involvement of the distal rectal mucosa can lead to perirectal abscesses and anal fissures. Outgrowths of lymphatic tissue resembling hemorrhoids occur as a result of lymphatic obstruction. The clinical and histologic similarity between LGV strain infection and other inflammatory bowel diseases, such as Crohn's disease, can lead to misdiagnosis and inappropriate therapy.[228]

Sexually Reactive Arthritis

Reactive arthritis by definition is an immune-mediated inflammatory response in the joints to a primary infection at a distant mucosal site.[232] Although enteric infections such as salmonella, shigella, campylobacter, or yersinia can provoke reactive arthritis, chlamydial infections appear to be a very common triggering event as well. Approximately 1% of men presenting with NGU develop an acute aseptic arthritis syndrome referred to as sexually reactive arthritis. One third of these have the full complex of Reiter's syndrome, namely, arthritis, conjunctivitis, urethritis, and skin lesions.[233] In men with untreated Reiter's syndrome who have urethritis, *C. trachomatis* can be recovered from the urethra in as many as 69% at the onset of the acute arthritis.[234] Reiter's syndrome patients have elevated synovial and serum antibody levels to *C. trachomatis*,[234] and it has been reported that patients who develop Reiter's syndrome after chlamydial urethritis have antibodies in sera and synovial fluid directed against cHSP60.[235] Approximately 80% of Reiter's syndrome patients also have the histocompatibility marker HLA-B27.[233] Furthermore, in addition to Reiter's syndrome, there appears to be an association between chlamydial infection, HLA-B27, and undifferentiated oligoarthritis.[236]

Synovial lymphocytes from Reiter's syndrome patients show higher proliferative responses in vitro to chlamydial antigens than do peripheral blood lymphocytes from the same patients or synovial fluid lymphocytes from control patients.[232] These and other data suggest that *C. trachomatis* may be present in the joints of afflicted patients but in a form that either cannot be cultured or is very difficult to culture. Early reports suggested that *C. trachomatis* could be recovered by culture from the synovial membranes of at least some patients with Reiter's syndrome,[237,238] but recent studies have not confirmed this even with improvements in isolation technique.[232] However, organisms with morphology consistent with *Chlamydia* have been identified in the synovium of Reiter's syndrome patients by electron microscopy, immunocytochemical staining,[232,234] and molecular hybridization and amplification techniques,[232] suggesting that *Chlamydia* may persist in some form in the synovial membranes of patients with Reiter's syndrome. Similar studies have been done with enteric organisms associated with reactive arthritis. Chlamydial DNA was found in synovial biopsies together with mRNA detected by reverse transcriptase–PCR, suggesting that the detectable forms and DNA represent viable, persistent organisms.[239] These persistent chlamydiae exhibit aberrant gene expression, with no *OMP1* mRNA detected but with detectable cHSP60 mRNA.[239] A double-blind study comparing lymecycline (tetracycline-L-methylene lysine) and placebo in patients with reactive arthritis suggested that 3 months of treatment was efficacious in arthritis associated with chlamydial infection but not in reactive arthritis associated with other causes.[240] Furthermore, when patients with Reiter's syndrome were treated for genitourinary infections with antichlamydial antibiotics, the incidence of arthritic relapses was significantly reduced compared with that observed in patients left untreated or treated with penicillin.[241] These data have led some to suggest that patients with Reiter's syndrome should receive prompt antichlamydial therapy for arthritic recurrences and any genitourinary complaints suggestive of a chlamydial infection.[242]

Genital Infection in Women

Although most infected women are asymptomatic, it is women who suffer the most serious consequences of genital chlamydial infections. Risk factors for infection vary in different population groups, but in most circumstances being a sexual partner of a man with either gonococcal urethritis or NGU confers a risk of infection in excess of 30%.[7,219] In the United States, higher prevalence rates in sexually active individuals have been associated with younger age, African American ethnicity, unmarried status, new or multiple sexual partners, and oral contraceptive use.[6,7,243] Higher rates are also seen in the southeastern part of the country. Young age is the single factor most strongly associated with increased risk of chlamydial infection among sexually active females. In addition, young age is associated with an increased risk of repeated infection[244] and with an associated increased risk of PID, ectopic pregnancy, and infertility.[245] Oral contraceptives may truly increase susceptibility or ease detection because of an increase in cervical ectopy in exposed susceptible cells. Alternatively, oral contraceptive use may be a surrogate marker for increased sexual activity.[243] In some studies,[246] but not others,[209] a recent change of sexual partners and increased numbers of partners have also been associated with increased prevalence.

The natural history of endocervical infection with *C. trachomatis* in women is not fully known. In most animal models, including primates, an immune response is mounted after infection or reinfection, and the organism can no longer be cultured.[247] It is likely that this occurs in a substantial proportion of infected women as well, or the women may inadvertently receive effective antichlamydial therapy for some other indication. However, other data suggest that chlamydiae can persist in an asymptomatic state for prolonged periods of time in the female genital tract. In 14 infected college women who were observed for a minimum of 15 months without specific treatment, 7 remained infected.[248] Likewise, 68 of 85 (80%) infected adolescent women who remained asymptomatic were still infected when reevaluated 2 months or more after their initial evaluation.[249] Two epidemiologic studies indicate that untreated genital infection persists for 1 year in 45% to 50% in women.[116,117] Other examples of persistent infection in humans include a case of LGV from which the organism was recovered after 20 years,[250] persistence of organisms in the synovium of patients with Reiter's syndrome,[232,239] detection of chlamydial DNA in fallopian tube biopsy specimens from infertile women,[251] infants persistently infected for up to 28 months,[252] young women persistently infected with genetically identical strains for up to 5 years,[253] and recovery of *C. trachomatis* from the fallopian tubes and endometrium of infertile women in circumstances in which recent acquisition of infection was unlikely.[161]

Cervicitis and Urethritis

Mucopurulent cervicitis caused by *C. trachomatis* has been called the female counterpart of male NGU. Approximately 70% of women with endocervical infection have no symptoms or have only mild symptoms such as vaginal discharge, bleeding, mild abdominal pain, or dysuria.[7] Dysuria may reflect concurrent urethral infection. A vaginal discharge in such women is attributable to endocervical rather than vaginal infection because *C. trachomatis* cannot infect the squamous epithelium of the adult vagina. However, it can cause vaginitis before puberty when the vagina is lined with transitional cell epithelium. On examination, the cervix may appear normal or may exhibit edema, erythema, and hypertrophy with a mucopurulent discharge from the os.[84] Studies employing colposcopy emphasize the follicular nature of the cervicitis as well as erythema, ectopy, and easily induced mucosal bleeding.[254]

The acute urethral syndrome is defined as dysuria and frequency with fewer than 10^5 organisms per milliliter of urine.[255] In one study of 59 women with this syndrome, 42 also had pyuria and 11 of the 42 were infected with *C. trachomatis*, as were 3 of 66 women without symptoms and 1 of 35 women with cystitis related to *E. coli*. Most of the remainder of the women with pyuria and the urethral syndrome had low urine concentrations of *E. coli* or *Staphylococcus saprophyticus* demonstrated by culture of urine obtained by suprapubic aspiration.[255] Women with this clinical syndrome respond to appropriate antibiotics such as doxycycline. *C. trachomatis* has also been isolated from the Bartholin glands in women with bartholinitis. Although case-control studies have found an association between cervical dysplasia or neoplasia and *C. trachomatis* infection,[256,257] considerable evidence now supports the role of specific oncogenic types of human papillomavirus in the etiology of cervical cancer. Furthermore, in prospective studies of women with human papillomavirus infections, concurrent chlamydial infection had little apparent effect on the course of their cervical lesions.[258] It is still possible that *C. trachomatis* may play an important role as a cofactor in the development of cervical neoplasia. Studies indicating that specific strains of *C. trachomatis* may be associated with cervical cancer support such a role.[259] In addition, coinfection with *C. trachomatis* was found to be associated with more prolonged shedding of human papillomavirus in a longitudinal study of adolescents.[260]

Of potentially far greater concern is the possible association between chlamydial cervicitis and acquisition of HIV infection by women.[261] In a case-control study of female prostitutes in Zaire, the adjusted odds ratio for HIV seroconversion with *C. trachomatis* infection was 3.6, with a 95% confidence interval of 1.4 to 9.1. Other data also support the idea that infections with *C. trachomatis* and other sexually transmitted agents increase shedding of HIV in genital secretions,[262] although not all studies have demonstrated this.[262] However, the finding that infection with agents that produce genital mucosal inflammation would increase the risk of acquisition of HIV is not surprising and has substantial public health implications for control of the spread of HIV among heterosexuals.[262]

Endometritis and Salpingitis

The proportion of women with endocervical *C. trachomatis* infections who develop acute salpingitis has been estimated to be 8% but probably varies by population group.[7] Eighteen of 109 (16.5%) infected asymptomatic adolescent women observed for 2 months or more became symptomatic, but only 2 (1.8%) developed clinical PID.[249] However, when women infected with both *C. trachomatis* and *N. gonorrhoeae* were treated for gonorrhea with penicillin only, 6 of 20 (30%) developed acute salpingitis during a 7-day follow-up interim.[263] The broader term *pelvic inflammatory disease* is preferable to *salpingitis* because the clinical entity usually encompasses clinically suspected endometritis, salpingitis, peritonitis, or a combination of these, and the presence of salpingitis has not been confirmed pathologically or by direct visual inspection of the fallopian tubes in most patients (e.g., laparoscopically).[264] The proportion of women presenting with acute PID from whom chlamydiae can be isolated from the urogenital tract ranges between 5% and 51%, depending on the population studied and the techniques used, but is most often approximately 20%.[7] Histologic evidence of plasma cell endometritis is present in most cases of laparoscopically verified salpingitis, suggesting early spread of the infection from the cervix to the endometrium in most patients.[265] Endometritis is also present in 40% of women with mucopurulent cervicitis and presumably progresses to salpingitis if untreated.[97]

The spectrum of PID associated with *C. trachomatis* infection ranges from acute, severe disease resembling gonococcal salpingitis, with associated perihepatitis and ascites, to completely or largely asymptomatic or "silent" salpingitis.[266] Subclinical, undiagnosed salpingitis appears to be far more common than acute disease. When women with chlamydial salpingitis are compared with women with gonococcal or with nongonococcal nonchlamydial salpingitis, those in the chlamydial group are more likely to experience a chronic, subacute course with a longer duration of abdominal pain before seeking medical care. Yet, they have as much or more tubal inflammation at laparoscopy.[267] In a prospective study of women randomly assigned to normal care or to chlamydial screening, routine screening of asymptomatic women for chlamydial infection followed by treatment of those identified as infected reduced the incidence of PID in a health maintenance organization setting.[268]

Infertility and Ectopic Pregnancy

The long-term consequences of both acute PID and silent, subclinical disease are tubal infertility, ectopic pregnancy, and chronic pelvic pain syndrome.[266] In developed countries, infertility affects approximately one in six couples, with tubal occlusion being a factor in 10% to 30%.[264] The mechanisms responsible for the tubal occlusion are not understood. In the case of *Chlamydia*, presumably they involve a combination of chronic inflammation and scarring induced by either recurrent or persistent infection. In a nonhuman primate model,

repeated endocervical infections followed by a direct tubal inoculation of *C. trachomatis* produced peritubular adhesions as well as plasma cell endometritis.[269] Furthermore, women with nongonococcal salpingitis are more likely to have an adverse reproductive outcome than women with gonococcal salpingitis.[270]

In a prospective study of women who underwent laparoscopy for suspected PID,[271] those with verified salpingitis were observed for a mean of 94 months. Sixteen percent of the patients and 2.7% of the control subjects failed to conceive. Ten percent of patients and none of the control subjects had confirmed tubal factor infertility. Tubal factor infertility increased with increasing severity of infection as judged at the time of the index laparoscopy from 0.6% after a case of mild PID to 21.4% after a case of severe PID. It also increased with the number of episodes of PID, from 8% after one episode to 19% after two and 40% after three. The ectopic pregnancy rate was 9.1% among patients versus 1.4% among control subjects.[271]

Most women with infertility related to tubular disease do not have a prior history of a sexually transmitted disease or of PID. However, a strong association between tubal infertility and serologic evidence of prior chlamydial infection has been a consistent observation in multiple studies.[7] Furthermore, *Chlamydia* has been recovered from fallopian tube biopsies in women undergoing microtuboplasty for surgical correction of damaged tubes,[161,163] and chlamydial DNA and antigens have been demonstrated by in situ hybridization in the fallopian tubes of infertile women from whom *Chlamydia* could not be recovered by culture.[272]

Case-control studies have also shown a strong association between ectopic pregnancy and serologic evidence of past chlamydial infection,[7] and in one study 22% of women experiencing ectopic pregnancy had histologic evidence of plasma cell salpingitis as well as antichlamydial antibodies.[273] Moreover, 81% of women experiencing ectopic pregnancy who had high titers of antichlamydial antibodies had specific antibody to cHSP60,[105] suggesting that hypersensitivity induced by this protein may play a role in tubal damage. In addition, the presence of cHSP60 antibodies predicted a two- or threefold increased risk of PID.[111] However, further studies are needed to define the role of persistent, as opposed to prior, infection in ectopic pregnancy.

Pregnancy Complications

Women experiencing recurrent spontaneous abortions were found to have high titers of antichlamydial IgG but negative endocervical cultures for *C. trachomatis*,[274] raising the possibility that prior or persistent *C. trachomatis* infection of the endometrium may be associated with some spontaneous abortions. Existing data on the effect of *C. trachomatis* infections on pregnancy outcome are conflicting. Several studies found no association between adverse outcome and *C. trachomatis* infection, although a subset of women with IgM antibody against *C. trachomatis* (indicating recent infection) had infants with lower birth weight than those of women lacking specific IgM.[275,276] Other investigators found an association between chlamydial infection and prematurity and premature rupture of the membranes.[277,278]

In one large treatment study, a comparison of pregnancy outcomes was carried out in 1110 women who were infected with *C. trachomatis* but not treated, 1323 infected women who were treated with erythromycin, and 9111 uninfected, untreated women.[279] There was a significant association between treatment and a decrease in premature rupture of the membranes with an odds ratio of 0.56 (range, 0.37 to 0.85). In addition, there was a trend toward increased perinatal survival with an odds ratio of 2.21 (range, 0.89 to 5.49; $P < .08$).

Pregnancy outcomes have also been compared in 244 treated women who were cured of a *C. trachomatis* infection and 79 treated women who had a persistent or recurrent infection.[280] Successful treatment was found to decrease the frequency of premature rupture of the membranes and small-for-gestational-age infants.

These studies suggest that identification and treatment of *C. trachomatis* infection in pregnancy are likely to improve pregnancy outcome as well as prevent infant infection. However, more definitive data are needed. A major difficulty in such studies is the potential interaction of many infections that may influence pregnancy outcomes, including mycoplasmas, urinary tract infections, and vaginal colonization with gram-negative rods, herpesviruses such as cytomegalovirus, trichomonas, and bacterial vaginosis. Studies need to evaluate and analyze all of these factors comprehensively, which make such studies both large and complex.[281]

Other Infections
Pneumonia caused by *C. trachomatis* is primarily a disease of infants, although there have been isolated reports of *C. trachomatis* pneumonia in immunocompromised patients.[282] In addition, pulmonary infection may occur in laboratory workers exposed to relatively high concentrations of LGV serovars. Previously reported serologic associations with community-acquired pneumonia[283] probably reflected cross-reacting antibody with then-unrecognized *C. pneumoniae*. *C. trachomatis* has also been associated in case reports or in case-control studies serologically with meningoencephalitis,[284] myocarditis,[285] and endocarditis.[286]

Treatment of Genital and Ocular Infections in Adults
The antibiotics that have excellent activity against *Chlamydia* in cell culture include the tetracyclines, macrolides and related compounds, rifampin, and some of the fluoroquinolones.[287] Although chlamydiae lack peptidoglycan, ampicillin and penicillin, both of which penetrate eukaryotic cells to a limited degree, have some activity, whereas cephalosporins and aminocyclitols do not. Considerable clinical data are available on the treatment of uncomplicated urogenital tract infections in both men and women. These data have been utilized to develop guidelines for the prevention and management of *C. trachomatis* infections.[288] For many years, standard therapy for uncomplicated genital tract infection has been doxycycline, 100 mg orally, twice daily for 7 days, with erythromycin as the first alternative. However, azithromycin given as a single 1-g dose has been found to be as effective as a 7-day course of doxycycline[289] and is the recommended regimen in the most recent guidelines for the treatment of sexually transmitted diseases from the CDC. This is the only antimicrobial agent effective against *C. trachomatis* infection as single-dose therapy, which eliminates lack of compliance as a source of treatment failure. However, studies indicate that there may be early recurrences of chlamydial infection in as many as 5% to 13% of adolescents treated with azithromycin.[290,291] Reinfection probably accounts for some of these early recurrences, but persistent infection despite treatment may have occurred in some cases.[291] To date, antimicrobial resistance among wild-type chlamydiae has not been demonstrated to be a clinically important problem.[292] Resistance can be induced in the laboratory to fluoroquinolones, ritfampicin, and other drugs, however. Azithromycin has also been shown to be effective in the treatment of the NGU syndrome, whether related to *C. trachomatis,* genital mycoplasmas, or neither.[293] Ofloxacin at a dose of 300 mg twice daily for 7 days has been approved by the FDA for uncomplicated *C. trachomatis* infections; levofloxacin at 500 mg once daily for 7 days is included in the 2006 CDC treatment guidelines.[154] However, it should not be used in adolescents younger than 18 years or in pregnant women.[6] Azithromycin is considerably more expensive than doxycycline, and relative costs are a consideration in choice of therapy. Given the excellent efficacy achieved with doxycycline in compliant patients, it may be preferable in such groups. Cost-effectiveness studies have suggested that despite its higher purchase price, azithromycin is cost-effective in the long term because of complications averted with improved compliance.

Guidelines from the CDC now recommend azithromycin, 1 g orally, as the preferred drug for treatment of chlamydia in pregnancy.[288] Alternatively, amoxicillin, 500 mg orally three times a day for 7 to 10 days can be used. Amoxicillin appears to be more effective overall than erythromycin as an alternative agent because of a lower frequency of side effects and better compliance.[294,295] Clindamycin is only partially effective in eradicating *C. trachomatis* in men with NGU,[296] but it appears to be as efficacious as erythromycin in both pregnant[297] and nonpregnant women.[298] Doxycycline and levofloxacin are contraindicated in pregnancy.

Clinical conditions in which the likelihood of a chlamydial infection is high enough to warrant presumptive treatment for *C. trachomatis* in both the patient and sexual partners are NGU (heterosexual men), PID, epididymitis in men younger than 35 years, and gonococcal infection in either men or women.[6] Presumptive treatment of mucopurulent cervicitis alone is more controversial, and current guidelines suggest diagnostic testing with treatment based on test results as a reasonable approach.[199]

Proctitis in homosexual men and the acute urethral syndrome in women may be managed either by presumptive therapy or by therapy based on test results. Empirical therapy of both proctitis and epididymitis should include treatment for gonorrhea—for example, ceftriaxone, 250 mg intramuscularly, in a single dose, followed by 7 to 10 days of doxycycline, 100 mg orally twice daily.[199] When chlamydial infection is proved or strongly suspected, partners with whom the person has had recent sexual contact should be treated.[6]

The management of PID, even when gonorrhea is present, should always include therapy directed against *C. trachomatis* as well as *N. gonorrhoeae* and anaerobic bacteria. Some experts recommend that initial therapy should be parenteral, followed by oral administration after initial improvement.[199] Recommended regimens include cefoxitin or cefotetan along with doxycycline, with the latter continued for a total of 14 days, or, alternatively, clindamycin and an aminoglycoside, again followed by doxycycline to complete a total of 14 days of therapy. An alternative to doxycycline is to continue clindamycin orally at a dose of 450 mg four times a day to complete 14 days of therapy.[199] Outpatient regimens include initial, single-dose, intramuscular therapy with a second- or third-generation cephalosporin plus 14 days of doxycycline. Alternatively, ofloxacin, 400 mg orally twice daily, or levofloxacin, 500 mg orally once daily, plus oral metronidazole may be given.[199]

Few comparative data exist on the treatment of adult inclusion conjunctivitis, but tetracycline and its congeners (e.g., doxycycline) are effective when given for a 2- or 3-week period of time.[299] Erythromycin is an effective alternative.

PERINATAL INFECTIONS

Neonatal Inclusion Conjunctivitis
Before the introduction of perinatal ocular prophylaxis for gonorrhea, it was assumed that all neonatal conjunctivitis was gonococcal in origin. However, even after prophylaxis for gonorrhea was introduced, neonatal conjunctivitis continued to occur, and conjunctival scrapings from neonates with conjunctivitis were shown to contain cells with cytoplasmic inclusions identical to those seen in patients with ocular trachoma. Subsequently, inclusions were demonstrated in cells from the cervix of the mother and the urethra of the father of an infected infant and in urethral scrapings from men with NGU. Infant infection is usually acquired during passage through an infected birth canal. Exceptions include occasional infants who seem to have acquired an infection perinatally despite birth by cesarean section[300] and infants who acquire the organism postnatally from an infected caregiver by hand-to-eye contact. Between 22% and 44% of infants born to infected women develop neonatal conjunctivitis, although approximately 60% have serologic evidence of infection.[301] The usual incubation period is 5 to 12 days from birth, although the onset may be as late as 6 weeks of age.[302] Typically, a watery ocular discharge appears, which becomes progressively more purulent. The eyelids swell and the conjunctivae become erythematous and thickened. At birth, the conjunctiva lacks a lymphoid layer, and so follicles do not develop initially but may become apparent after 3 to 6 weeks.

The progression of the disease is very similar to that described for adults, with spontaneous resolution occurring in most untreated infants after 3 to 12 months.[303] However, mild or subclinical infection may persist for several years,[252] and late sequelae such as scars and corneal lesions occur in a small proportion of cases.[304] A mucopurulent rhinitis, and in female infants vulvovaginitis, is often associated with the conjunctivitis. The primary differential diagnosis in a newborn is gonococcal ophthalmia, which is uncommon in children who receive ocular prophylaxis at birth but does still occur.[305] Ocular prophylaxis does not seem to be effective against *C. trachomatis* infection even when erythromycin or tetracycline is applied topically.[305]

Infant Pneumonia

Between 11% and 20% of infants born to infected mothers develop pneumonia caused by *C. trachomatis*.[306] Infected infants usually become symptomatic before 8 weeks of age with nasal obstruction or discharge or both, tachypnea, and cough.[307] Presentation for care is usually between 4 and 11 weeks, and, characteristically, the infants have been symptomatic for 3 or more weeks before presentation. Most are only moderately ill and are afebrile.[308] A history of conjunctivitis is present in approximately half of infants and middle ear abnormalities in more than half.[307] Paroxysms of staccato coughing that interfere with sleeping and eating are sometimes present. Auscultation may reveal scattered crackles, but breath sounds are usually good and wheezing is usually absent. Chest radiographs show bilateral interstitial infiltrates with hyperinflation (Fig. 180-4).[307] Peripheral eosinophilia, arterial hypoxemia, and elevated serum immunoglobulins are characteristic.[307-309] *C. trachomatis* can usually be recovered from nasopharyngeal swab specimens, and antichlamydial IgM titers are elevated.[306]

Untreated, the course is protracted, often lasting weeks to months.[308] Especially in very young infants, the initial respiratory manifestations of *C. trachomatis* infection may be more severe and include prolonged spells of apnea or respiratory failure.[310,311] Although published reports emphasize more serious disease, it is likely that most patients with *C. trachomatis* infant pneumonia are treated as outpatients, often without laboratory confirmation of diagnosis. However, follow-up for as long as 8 years of children who had chlamydial pneumonia in the first 6 months of life has demonstrated a higher than normal frequency of obstructive airway disease (by pulmonary function testing) and of physician-diagnosed asthma.[312,313] Thus, long-term respiratory sequelae may be significant.

Perinatally acquired *C. trachomatis* infection may persist in the nasopharynx, urogenital tract, or rectum for more than 2 years.[252] Consequently, differentiating infection acquired at birth from infection related to sexual abuse may be particularly difficult in younger children. In older children, oropharyngeal infection with *C. trachomatis* needs to be differentiated from that with *C. pneumoniae*. For this reason and because of problems with sensitivity and specificity of nonculture tests (nonamplified probes, enzyme immunoassay, and direct fluorescent antibody test), cell culture testing using *C. trachomatis*-specific fluorescent antibody to detect inclusions should be used for diagnosis of infections in the genitalia, rectum, or pharynx in children.[199] The most recent CDC guidelines in 2006 also support the use of culture because data supporting the use of NAATs in this setting are insufficient. However, when culture is unavailable, FDA-approved NAATs may be an alternative when confirmation with a second FDA-approved NAAT targeting a different sequence than the initial test is available.[154]

Prevention and Treatment of Infant Infections

Topical treatment of inclusion conjunctivitis is not recommended primarily because of difficulty in application and failure to eliminate concurrent nasopharyngeal carriage.[314] The latter can result in recurrent conjunctivitis, pneumonia, or both.[314] Recommended therapy is oral erythromycin in doses of 50 mg/kg of body weight per day in four divided doses for 10 to 14 days. The efficacy of therapy is approximately 80%, and a second course may be required.[315] The course of therapy for *C. trachomatis* pneumonia is the same as that for conjunctivitis, and the efficacy is also approximately 80%. Mothers of infants with *C. trachomatis* should be evaluated and treated appropriately, as should their sexual partners.

Prenatal screening for chlamydia and treatment of infected women is approximately 90% effective in preventing their infants from acquiring infection.[315] However, in populations at high risk for reinfection,

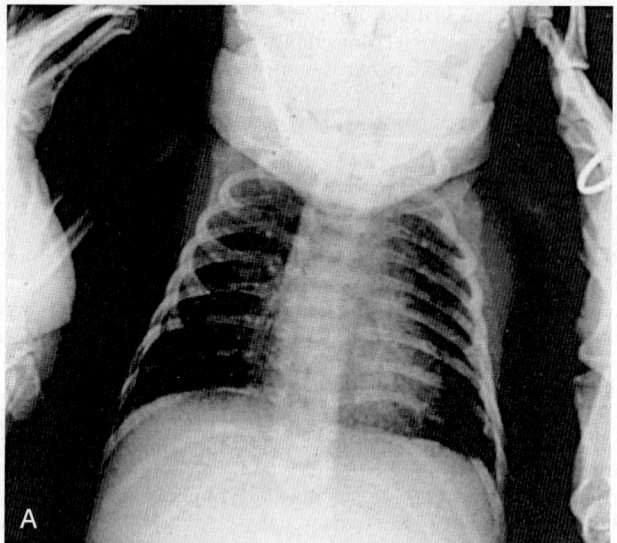

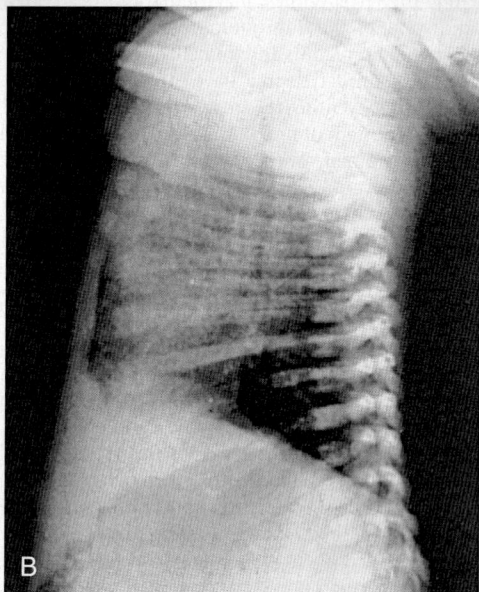

Figure 180-4 **A** and **B**, Chest radiographs of a 2-month-old infant with *Chlamydia trachomatis* pneumonia demonstrate typical patchy interstitial infiltrates and flattened diaphragms. *(Courtesy of Dr. John Gaebler, Indianapolis, Ind.)*

particularly adolescents, reacquisition of infection after the first trimester is frequent,[316] and repeated prenatal screening may be warranted in this population.

Prevention Strategies

Primary prevention strategies involve (1) inducing behavioral changes that reduce the risk of acquisition of chlamydial infections as well as other sexually transmitted diseases and (2) identification and treatment of people with genital infection before they can transmit the infection. Behaviors that reduce risk of infection include delaying age of first intercourse, decreasing numbers of partners, and use of condoms. The use of vaginal microbicides such as vaginal sponges containing the spermicide nonoxynol-9 was previously thought to be of value.[6,317-319] Nonoxynol-9 has in vitro activity against *C. trachomatis*[320] and in two controlled trials was shown to reduce male-to-female transmission.[317,318] However, a controlled trial showed that nonoxynol-9 did not reduce the rate of male-to-female new chlamydial infection.[321] Furthermore, a meta-analysis of multiple trials of nonoxynol-9 concluded that it was ineffective in preventing cervical gon-

TABLE 180-4	Screening for Chlamydial Infection, U.S. Preventive Services Task Force, 2007

Screen all sexually active women ≤25 years old.

Screen other high-risk women.*

Screen pregnant women ≤25 years old.

Screen older high-risk pregnant women.*

Insufficient evidence to recommend male screening at present.

*High-risk women as defined in various populations can include women ≤ 25 years old, unmarried, African American, prior sexually transmitted disease, new or multiple sexual partners, cervical ectopy, and inconsistent use of barrier contraceptives.

orrhea, chlamydial infection, or HIV infection.[322] In addition, nonoxynol-9 exhibits in vitro toxicity to cervical cells,[320,323] increases the likelihood of vaginal yeast infection,[318] and may increase the risk of HIV transmission.[154,322,323] Other microbicides are under development that may be more effective and less toxic than nonoxynol-9, but none are yet available.

Most developed countries have initiated programs to reduce transmission of *C. trachomatis* by screening high-risk populations for asymptomatic infections and by aggressive partner notification and treatment programs. Indications for screening women have been published and are summarized in Table 180-4 and most recently by the U.S. Preventive Services Task Force.[324]

Because of the high frequency of repeated chlamydial infections within the first several months after treatment of an initial infection,[291,325] more frequent (e.g., every 6 months) screening of asymptomatic sexually active adolescents may be important in some populations.[326] The advantages of employing noninvasive screening (i.e., urine testing or use of self-collected vaginal swabs) of sexually active young men and women have been proved using NAATs, particularly in nontraditional settings such as high schools, military intake centers, juvenile detention centers, and other nonclinic sites in the community.[175-177,327] Also promising is the potential use of the leukocyte esterase test to identify asymptomatic adolescent men with pyuria for further evaluation with more expensive amplification tests.[223,328] The benefits of screening women have been assessed primarily in ecologic studies in which a declining prevalence of infection and of PID has been observed in the screened population during the first several years of implementation of screening. However, subsequent analyses have demonstrated an unexpected increase in chlamydial prevalence in these same populations as screening continued. Despite the increase in prevalence, rates of complications appear to be continuing to decline.[329] The explanation for these unexpected findings is not clear but may be due to early identification and treatment of infections before immunity can fully develop, leaving the individual more susceptible to reinfection. Further studies addressing this issue are ongoing. In the most clear-cut example of the advantages of screening to date, a randomized trial of screening using selective screening criteria in a health maintenance organization demonstrated a 60% reduction in PID among screened women during 12 months of follow-up.[268]

Notification and treatment of sexual partners are also effective in reducing infection and can be shown to be cost-effective despite the resources required.[330,331] Innovative approaches to improve the effectiveness of sex partner management are under study, including partner delivered therapy, which is provision of empirical single-dose antibiotic therapy through the index case, often with solicitation of mailed-in urine or swabs for NAAT testing. Randomized trials have demonstrated the effectiveness of this approach.[332]

ACKNOWLEDGMENT

The authors recognize and thank Robert B. Jones for this excellent contributions to earlier editions of this chapter.

REFERENCES

1. Schachter J, Dawson CR. *Human Chlamydial Infections.* Littleton, Mass: PSG Publishing; 1978:63-96.
2. Institute of Medicine Committee on Prevention and Control of Sexually Transmitted Diseases. In: Eng T, Butler E, eds. *The Hidden Epidemic: Confronting Sexually Transmitted Diseases.* Washington, DC: National Academy Press; 1997: 1-411.
3. Centers for Disease Control and Prevention. *Sexually Transmitted Disease Surveillance 2004.* Atlanta, Ga: U.S. Department of Health and Human Services; 2005.
4. Centers for Disease Control and Prevention. *Tracking the Hidden Epidemics: Trends in STDs in the United States 2000.* Atlanta, Ga: Centers for Disease Control and Prevention; 2001:1-31.
5. Thylefors B. Development of trachoma control programs and the involvement of national resources. *Rev Infect Dis.* 1985;7:774-776.
6. Centers for Disease Control and Prevention. *Sexually Transmitted Disease Surveillance 2001 Supplement, Chlamydia Prevalence Monitoring Project.* Atlanta, Ga: Centers for Disease Control and Prevention; 2002.
7. Cates W Jr, Wasserheit JN. Genital chlamydial infections: epidemiology and reproductive sequelae. *Am J Obstet Gynecol.* 1991;164:1771-1781.
8. Podgore JK, Holmes KK, Alexander ER. Asymptomatic urethral infections due to *Chlamydia trachomatis* in male U.S. military personnel. *J Infect Dis.* 1982;146:828.
9. Abdelrahman YM, Belland RJ. The chlamydial developmental cycle. *FEMS Microbiol Rev.* 2005;29:949-959.
10. Rockey DD. Chlamydial interactions with host cells. In: Schachter J, Christiansen G, Clarke IN, et al, eds. *Chlamydial Infections: Proceedings of the 10th International Symposium on Human Chlamydial Infection.* San Francisco: International Chlamydia Symposium; 2002:35-44.
11. Duensing TD, Wing JS, van Putten JP. Sulfated polysaccharide-directed recruitment of mammalian host proteins: a novel strategy for microbial pathogenesis. *Infect Immun.* 1999;67: 4463-4468.
12. Stephens RS. The cellular paradigm of chlamydial pathogenesis. *Trends Microbiol.* 2003;11:44-51.
13. Wehrl W, Brinkmann V, Jungblut PR, et al. From the inside out—processing of the chlamydial autotransporter pmpD and its role in bacterial adhesion and activation of human host cells. *Mol Microbiol.* 2004;51:319-334.
14. Dautry-Varsat A, Subtil A, Hackstadt T. Recent insights into the mechanisms of *Chlamydia* entry. *Cell Microbiol.* 2005;7: 1714-1722.

15. Suchland RJ, Jeffrey BM, Xia M, et al: Identification of concomitant infection with *Chlamydia trachomatis* Inc-A negative mutant and wild type strains. *Infect Immun.* 2008;76: 5438-5446.
16. Stephens RS, Koshiyama K, Lewis E, et al. Heparin-binding outer membrane of chlamydiae. *Mol Microbiol.* 2001;40: 691-699.
17. Wyrick PB, Choong J, Davis CH, et al. Entry of genital *Chlamydia trachomatis* into polarized human epithelial cells. *Infect Immun.* 1989;57:2378-2389.
18. Hodinka RL, Davis CH, Choong J, et al. Ultrastructural study of endocytosis of *Chlamydia trachomatis* by McCoy cells. *Infect Immun.* 1988;56:1456-1463.
19. Stephens RS, Poteralski JM, Olinger L. Interaction of *Chlamydia trachomatis* with mammalian cells is independent of host cell surface heparin sulfate glycosaminoglycans. *Infect Immun.* 2006;74:1795-1799.
20. Hybiske K, Stephens RS. Mechanisms of *Chlamydia trachomatis* entry into nonphagocytic cells. *Infect Immun.* 2007;75: 3925-3934.
21. Clifton DR, Fields KA, Grieshaber SS, et al. A chlamydial type III translocated protein is tyrosine-phosphorylated at the site of entry and associated with recruitment of actin. *Proc Natl Acad Sci U S A.* 2004;10166-10171.
22. Carabeo RA, Grieschaber SS, Hasenkrug A, et al. Requirement for the Rac GTPase in *Chlamydia trachomatis* invasion of nonphagocytic cells. *Traffic.* 2004;5:418-425.
23. Lane BJ, Mutchler C, Al Khodor S, et al. Chlamydial entry involves TARP binding of guanine nucleotide exchange factors. *PLoS Pathog.* 2008;4:e1000014.
24. Jewett TJ, Fischer ER, Mead DJ, et al. Chlamydial TARP is a bacterial nucleator of actin. *Proc Natl Acad Sci U S A.* 2006;103:15599-155604.
25. Tipples G, McClarty G. The obligate intracellular bacterium *Chlamydia trachomatis* is auxotrophic for three of the four ribonucleoside triphosphates. *Mol Microbiol.* 1993;8:1105-1114.
26. Peeling R, Peeling J, Brunham R. High-resolution ³¹P nuclear magnetic resonance study of *Chlamydia trachomatis*: induction of ATPase activity in elementary bodies. *Infect Immun.* 1989;57:3338-3344.
27. Hatch TP, Miceli M, Sublett JE. Synthesis of disulfide-bonded outer membrane proteins during the developmental cycle of *Chlamydia psittaci* and *Chlamydia trachomatis. J Bacteriol.* 1986;165:379-385.
28. Bavoil P, Ohlin A, Schachter J. Role of disulfide bonding in outer membrane structure and permeability in *Chlamydia trachomatis. Infect Immun.* 1984;44:479-485.

29. Newhall WJ. 5th Biosynthesis and disulfide cross-linking of outer membrane components during the growth cycle of *Chlamydia trachomatis. Infect Immun.* 1987;55:162-168.
30. Conant CG, Stephens RS. *Chlamydia* attachment to mammalian cells requires protein disulfide isomerase. *Cell Microbiol.* 2007;9:222-232.
31. Moulder JW. Interaction of chlamydiae and host cells in vitro. *Microbiol Rev.* 1991;55:143-190.
32. Belland RJ, Zhong G, Crane DD, et al. Genomic transcriptional profiling of the developmental cycle of *Chlamydia trachomatis. Proc Natl Acad Sci U S A.* 2003; 100:8040-8042.
33. Gerard HC, Krausse-Opatz B, Wang Z, et al. Expression of *C. trachomatis* genes encoding products required for DNA synthesis and cell division during active vs. persistent infection. *Mol Microbiol.* 2001;41:731-741.
34. Nicholson TL, Olinger L, Chong K, et al. Global stage-specific gene regulation during the developmental cycle of *Chlamydia trachomatis. J Bacteriol.* 2003;185:3179-3189.
35. Crenshaw RW, Fahr MJ, Wichlan DG, et al. Developmental cycle-specific host-free RNA synthesis in *Chlamydia* spp. *Infect Immun.* 1990;58:3194-3201.
36. Rockey DD, Stephens RS. Genome sequencing and our understanding of *Chlamydia. Infect Immun.* 2000;68:5473-5479.
37. Barry CE, Hayes SF, Hackstadt T. Nucleoid condensation in *Escherichia coli* that express a chlamydial histone homolog. *Science.* 1992;256:377-379.
38. Grieschaber NA, Grieshaber SS, Fischer ER, et al. A small RNA inhibits translation of the histone-like protein Hc1 in *Chlamydia trachomatis. Mol Microbiol.* 2006;59:541-550.
39. Grieshaber NA, Sager JB, Dooley CA, et al. Regulation of the *Chlamydia trachomatis* histone H1-like protein Hc2 is IspE dependent and IhtA independent. *J Bacteriol.* 2006;188:5289-5292.
40. Grieschaber NA, Fischer ER, Mead DJ, et al. Chlamydial histone-DNA interactions are disrupted by a metabolite in the methylerythritol phosphate pathway of isoprenoid biosynthesis. *Proc Natl Acad Sci U S A.* 2004;101:7451-7456.
41. Bavoil PM, Hsia R, Ojicius DM. Closing in on *Chlamydia* and its intracellular bag of tricks. *Microbiology.* 2000;146: 2723-2731.
42. Subtil A, Blocker A, Dantry-Varsat A. Type III secretion system in *Chlamydia* species: Identified members and candidates. *Microbes Infect.* 2000;2:367-369.
43. Jamison WP, Hackstadt T. Induction of type III secretion by cell-free *Chlamydia trachomatis* elementary bodies. *Microb Pathog.* 2008;45:435-440.

44. Wolf K, Betts HJ, Chellas-Gery B, et al. Treatment of *Chlamydia trachomatis* with a small molecule inhibitor of the Yersinia type III secretion system disrupts progression of the chlamydial developmental cycle. *Mol Microbiol.* 2006;61:1543-1555.
45. Betts HJ, Twiggs LE, Sal MS, et al. Bioinformatic and biochemical evidence for the identification of the type III secretion system needle protein of *Chlamydia trachomatis*. *J Bacteriol.* 2008;190:1680-1690.
46. Hefty PS, Stephens RS. Chlamydial type III secretion system is encoded on ten operons preceded by signma 70-like promoter elements. *J Bacteriol.* 2007;189:198-206.
47. Kleba B, Stephens RS. Chlamydial effector proteins localized to the host cell cytoplasmic compartment. *Infect Immun.* 2008;76:4842-4850.
48. Hybiske K, Stephens RS. Mechanisms of host cell exit by the intracellular bacterium *Chlamydia*. *Proc Natl Acad Sci U S A.* 2007;104:11430-11435.
49. Beatty WL, Byrne GL, Morrison RP. Morphologic and antigenic characterization of IFN-γ mediated persistent *C. trachomatis* infection in vitro. *Proc Natl Acad Sci U S A.* 1993;90:3998-4002.
50. Wang SP, Grayston JT. Microimmunofluorescence antibody responses in *Chlamydia trachomatis* infection, a review. In: Mardh PA, Holmes KK, Oriel JD, et al, eds. *Chlamydial Infections.* Amsterdam: Elsevier Biomedical Press; 1982:301-316.
51. Wang SP, Kuo CC, Barnes RC, et al. Immunotyping of *Chlamydia trachomatis* with monoclonal antibodies. *J Infect Dis.* 1985;152:791-800.
52. Wang SP, Grayston JT. Three new serovars of *Chlamydia trachomatis*: Da, Ia, and L2a. *J Infect Dis.* 1991;163:403-405.
53. Fehlner-Gardiner C, Roshick C, Carlson JH, et al. Molecular basis defining human *C. trachomatis* tissue tropism: a possible role for tryptophan synthase. *J Biol Chem.* 2002;13:468-476.
54. Carlson JH, Porcella SF, McClarty G, et al. Comparative genomic analysis of *Chlamydia trachomatis* oculotropic and genitotropic strains. *Infect Immun.* 2005;73:6407-6418.
55. Carlson JH, Hughes S, Hogan D, et al. Polymorphisms in the *Chlamydia trachomatis* cytotoxin locus associated with ocular and genital isolates. *Infect Immun.* 2004;72:7063-7072.
56. Carlson JH, Whitmire WM, Crane DD, et al. The *Chlamydia trachomatis* plasmid is a transcriptional regulator of chromosomal genes and a virulence factor. *Infect Immun.* 2008;76:2273-2283.
57. O'Connell CM, Ingalls RR, Andrews Jr CW, et al. Plasmid-deficient *Chlamydia muridarum* fail to induce immune pathology and protect against oviduct disease. *J Immunol.* 2007;179:4027-4034.
58. Kari L, Whitmire WM, Carlson JH, et al. Pathogenic diversity among *Chlamydia trachomatis* ocular strains in nonhuman primates is affected by subtle genomic variations. *J Infect Dis.* 2008;197:449-456.
59. Stephens RS, Wagar EA, Schoolnik GK. High-resolution mapping of serovar-specific and common antigenic determinants of the major outer membrane protein of *Chlamydia trachomatis*. *J Exp Med.* 1988;167:817-831.
60. Batteiger BE. The major outer membrane protein of a single *Chlamydia trachomatis* serovar can possess more than one serovar-specific epitope. *Infect Immun.* 1996;64:542-547.
61. Dean D, Millman K. Molecular and mutation trends analyses of omp1 alleles for serovar E of *Chlamydia trachomatis*. *J Clin Invest.* 1997;99:475-483.
62. Stothard DR, Boguslawski G, Jones RB. Phylogenetic analysis of the *Chlamydia trachomatis* major outer membrane protein and examination of potential pathogenic determinants. *Infect Immun.* 1998;66:3618-3625.
63. Brunham RC, Plummer FA, Stephens RS. Bacterial antigenic variation, host immune response, and pathogen-host coevolution. *Infect Immun.* 1993;61:2273-2276.
64. Hayes LJ, Pecharatana S, Bailey RL, et al. Extent and kinetics of genetic change in the omp1 gene of *Chlamydia trachomatis* in two villages with endemic trachoma. *J Infect Dis.* 1995;172:268-272.
65. Brunham RC, Kimani J, Bwayo J, et al. The epidemiology of *Chlamydia trachomatis* within a sexually transmitted diseases core group. *J Infect Dis.* 1996;173:950-956.
66. Millman K, Black CM, Stamm WE, et al. Population-based genetic epidemiologic analysis of *Chlamydia trachomatis* serotypes and lack of association between ompA polymorphisms and clinical phenotypes. *Microbes Infect.* 2006;8:604-611.
67. Mondesire RR, Maclean IW, Shewen PE, et al. Identification of genus-specific epitopes on the outer membrane complexes of *Chlamydia trachomatis* and *Chlamydia psittaci* immunotypes 1 and 2. *Infect Immun.* 1989;57:2914-2918.
68. Yuan Y, Lyng K, Zhang YX, et al. Monoclonal antibodies define genus-specific, species-specific and cross-reactive epitopes of the chlamydial 60-kilodalton heat shock protein (hsp60): specific immunodetection and purification of chlamydial hsp60. *Infect Immun.* 1992;60:2288-2296.
69. Belunis CJ, Mdluli KE, Raetz CRH, et al. A novel 3-deoxy-D-manno-octulosonic acid transferase from *Chlamydia trachomatis* required for expression of the genus-specific epitope. *J Biol Chem.* 1992;267:18702-18707.
70. Stephens RS, Kalman S, Fenner C, et al. *Chlamydia Genome Project.* Available at http://www.ncbi.nlm.nih.gov/pubmed/10192388?dopt=Abstract.
71. Thompson NR, holden MT, Cardner C, et al. *Chlamydia trachomatis*: genome sequence analysis of LGV isolates. *Genome Res.* 2008;18:161-171.
72. Stephens RS, Mullenbach G, Sanchez Pescador R, et al. Sequence analysis of the major outer membrane protein gene from *Chlamydia trachomatis* serovar L2. *J Bacteriol.* 1986;168:1277-1282.
73. Allen JE, Stephens RS. Identification by sequence analysis of two-site posttranslational processing of the cysteine-rich outer membrane protein 2 of *Chlamydia trachomatis* serovar L2. *J Bacteriol.* 1989;171:285-291.
74. Wagar EA, Pang M. The gene for the S7 ribosomal protein of *Chlamydia trachomatis*: characterization within the chlamydial str operon. *Mol Microbiol.* 1992;6:327-335.
75. Yuan Y, Zhang YX, Watkins NG, et al. Nucleotide and deduced amino sequences for the four variable domains of the major outer membrane proteins of the 15 *Chlamydia trachomatis* serovars. *Infect Immun.* 1989;57:1040-1049.
76. Dean D, Patton M, Stephens RS. Direct sequence evaluation of the major outer membrane protein gene variant regions of *Chlamydia trachomatis* subtypes D′, I′, and L2′. *Infect Immun.* 1991;59:1579-1582.
77. Lampe MF, Schland RJ, Stamm WE. Nucleotide sequence of the variable domains within the major outer membrane protein gene from serovariants of *Chlamydia trachomatis*. *Infect Immun.* 1993;61:213-219.
78. Weisburg WG, Hatch TP, Woese CR. Eubacterial origin of chlamydiae. *J Bacteriol.* 1986;167:570-574.
79. Crane DD, Carlson ER, Fischer ER, et al. *Chlamydia trachomatis* polymorphic membrane protein D is a species-common pan-neutralizing antigen. *Proc Natl Acad Sci U S A.* 2006;103;1894-1899.
80. Kiselev AO, Stamm WE, Yates JR, et al. Expression, processing, and localization of pmpD of *Chlamydia trachomatis* serovar L2 during the chlamydial developmental cycle. *PLoS ONE.* 2007;2:e568.
81. Swanson KA, Taylor LD, Frank SD, et al. *Chlamydia trachomatis* polymorphic membrane protein D is an oligomeric autotransporter with higher-ordered structure. *Infect Immun.* 2009;77:508516.
82. Kuo CC. Host response. In: Barron AL, ed. *Microbiology of Chlamydia*. Boca Raton, Fla: CRC Press; 1988:193-208.
83. Schachter J, Dawson CR. *Human Chlamydial Infections.* Littleton, Mass: PSG Publishing; 1978:45-62.
84. Brunham RC, Paavonen J, Stevens CE, et al. Mucopurulent cervicitis: the ignored counterpart in women of urethritis in men. *N Engl J Med.* 1984;311:1-6.
85. Griffin M, Pushpanathan C, Andrews W. *Chlamydia trachomatis* pneumonitis: a case study and literature review. *Pediatr Pathol.* 1990;10:843-852.
86. Braley AE. Inclusion blennorrhea. *Am J Ophthalmol.* 1938;21:1203-1207.
87. Rasmussen SJ, Eckmann L, Quayle AJ, et al. Secretion of proinflammatory cytokines by epithelial cells in response to *Chlamydia* infection suggests a central role for epithelial cells in chlamydial pathogenesis. *J Clin Invest.* 1997;99:77-87.
88. Ingalls RR, Rice PA, Qureshi N, et al. The inflammatory cytokine response to *Chlamydia trachomatis* infection is endotoxin mediated. *Infect Immun.* 1995;63:3125-3130.
89. Buchholz KR, Stephens RS. Activation of the host cell proinflammatory interleukin-8 response by *Chlamydia trachomatis*. *Cell Microbiol.* 2006;8:1768-1779.
90. Buchholz KR, Stephens RS. The extracellular signal-regulated kinase/mitogen-activated protein kinase pathway induces the inflammatory factor interleukin-8 following *Chlamydia trachomatis* infection. *Infect Immunn.* 2007;75:5924-5929.
91. Buchholz KR, Stephens RS. The cytosolic pattern recognition receptor NOD1 induces inflammatory interleukin-8 during *Chlamydia trachomatis* infection. *Infect Immun.* 2008;76:3150-3155.
92. Johnson RM. Murine oviduct epithelial cell cytokine responses to *Chlamydia muridarum* infection include interleukin-12-p70 secretion. *Infect Immun.* 2004;72:3951-3960.
93. Derbigny WA, Kerr MS, Johnson RM. Pattern recognition molecules activated by *Chlamydia muridarum* infection of cloned murine oviduct epithelial cell lines. *J Immunol.* 2005;175:6065-6075.
94. Derbigny WA, Hong SC, Kerr MS, et al. *Chlamydia muridarum* infection elicits a beta interferon response in murine oviduct epithelial cells dependent on interon regulatory fact 3 and TRIF. *Infect Immun.* 2007;75:1280-1290.
95. Darville T, O'Neill JM, Andrews Jr CW, et al. Toll-like receptor-2, but not Toll-like receptor-4, is essential for development of oviduct pathology in chlamydial genital tract infection. *J Immunol.* 2003;171:6187-6197.
96. Nagarajan UM, Prantner D, Sides JD, et al. Type I interferon signaling exacerbates *Chlamydia muridarum* genital infection in a murine model. *Infect Immun.* 2008;76:4642-4648.
97. Paavonen J, Kiviat N, Brunham RC, et al. Prevalence and manifestations of endometritis among women with cervicitis. *Am J Obstet Gynecol.* 1985;152:280-286.
98. Patton DL, Taylor HR. The histopathology of experimental trachoma: ultrastructural changes in the conjunctival epithelium. *J Infect Dis.* 1986;153:870-878.
99. Patton DL, Kuo CC, Wang SP, et al. Distal tubal obstruction induced by repeated *Chlamydia trachomatis* salpingeal infections in pigtailed macaques. *J Infect Dis.* 1987;155:1292-1299.
100. Grayston JT, Wang SP, Lin HM, et al. Trachoma vaccine studies in volunteer students of the National Defense Medical Center. II. Response to challenge eye inoculation of egg grown trachoma virus. *Chin Med J (Republic of China).* 1961;8:312-318.
101. Grayston JT, Wang S. New knowledge of chlamydiae and the diseases they cause. *J Infect Dis.* 1975;132:87-105.
102. Taylor HR, Maclean IW, Brunham RC, et al. Chlamydial heat shock proteins and trachoma. *Infect Immun.* 1990;58:3061-3063.
103. Brunham RC, Peeling R, Maclean I, et al. *Chlamydia trachomatis*-associated ectopic pregnancy: serologic and histologic correlates. *J Infect Dis.* 1992;165:1076-1081.
104. Eckert LO, Hawes SE, Wölner-Hanssen P, et al. Prevalence and correlates of antibody to chlamydial heat shock protein in women attending sexually transmitted disease clinics and women with confirmed pelvic inflammatory disease. *J Infect Dis.* 1997;175:1453-1458.
105. Money DM, Hawes SE, Eschenbach DA, et al. Antibodies to the chlamydial 60 kd heat-shock protein are associated with laparoscopically confirmed perihepatitis. *Am J Obstet Gynecol.* 1997;176:870-877.
106. Cerrone MC, Ma JJ, Stephens RS. Cloning and sequence of the gene for heat shock protein 60 from *Chlamydia trachomatis* and immunological reactivity of the protein. *Infect Immun.* 1991;59:79-90.
107. Morrison RP, Belland RJ, Lyng K, et al. Chlamydial disease pathogenesis: 57 kD chlamydial hypersensitivity antigen is a stress response protein. *Exp Med.* 1989;170:1271-1283.
108. Yi Y, Zhong G, Brunham RC. Continuous B cell epitopes in *Chlamydia trachomatis* heat shock protein 60. *Infect Immun.* 1993;61:1117-1120.
109. Domeika M, Domeika K, Paavonen J, et al. Humoral immune response to conserved epitopes of *Chlamydia trachomatis* and human 60-kDa heat-shock protein in women with pelvic inflammatory disease. *J Infect Dis.* 1998;177:714-719.
110. Zhong G, Brunham RC. Antibody responses to chlamydial heat shock proteins hsp60 and hsp70 are H2 linked. *Infect Immun.* 1992;60:3143-3149.
111. Peeling RW, Kimani J, Plummer F, et al. Antibody to chlamydial hsp60 predicts an increased risk for chlamydial pelvic inflammatory disease. *J Infect Dis.* 1997;175:1153-1158.
112. Peeling RW, Bailey RL, Conway DJ, et al. Antibody response to the 60-kDa chlamydial heat-shock protein is associated with scarring trachoma. *J Infect Dis.* 1998;177:256-259.
113. Zhong G, Peterson EM, Czarniecki CW, et al. Role of endogenous gamma interferon in host defense against *Chlamydia trachomatis* infections. *Infect Immun.* 1989;57:152-157.
114. Rothermel CD, Byrne GI, Havell EA. Effect of interferon on the growth of *Chlamydia trachomatis* in mouse fibroblasts (L cells). *Infect Immun.* 1983;39:362-370.
115. Rank RG, Ramsey KH, Pack EA, et al. Effect of gamma interferon on resolution of murine chlamydial genital infection. *Infect Immun.* 1992;60:4427-4429.
116. Morre S, van den Brule AJC, Rozendaal L, et al. The natural course of asymptomatic *Chlamydia trachomatis* infections: 45% clearance and no development of clinical PID after one-year follow-up. *Int J STD AIDS.* 2002;13(suppl 2):12-18.
117. Molano M, Meijer CJLM, Weiderpass E, et al. The natural course of *Chlamydia trachomatis* infection in asymptomatic Colombian women: a 5-year follow-up study. *J Infect Dis.* 2005;191:907-916.
118. van den Brule AJC, Munk C, Winter JF, et al. Prevalence and persistence of asymptomatic *Chlamydia trachomatis* infections in urine specimens from Danish male military recruits. *Int J STD AIDS.* 2002;13(suppl 2):19-22.
119. Morrison RP. New insights into a persistent problem—chlamydial infections. *J Clin Invest.* 2003;111:1647-1649.
120. Grayston JT, Wang SP, Yeh LJ, et al. Importance of reinfection in the pathogenesis of trachoma. *Rev Infect Dis.* 1985;7:717-725.
121. Katz BP, Caine VA, Batteiger BE, et al. A randomized trial to compare 7- and 21-day tetracycline regimens in the prevention of recurrence of infection with *Chlamydia trachomatis*. *Sex Transm Dis.* 1991;18:36-40.
122. Blythe MJ, Katz BP, Batteiger BE, et al. Recurrent genitourinary chlamydial infections in sexually active female adolescents. *J Pediatr.* 1992;121:487-493.
123. Brunham RC, Kuo CC, Cles L, et al. Correlation of host immune response with quantitative recovery of *Chlamydia trachomatis* from the human endocervix. *Infect Immun.* 1983;39:1491-1494.
124. Alani MD, Darougar S, Burns DC, et al. Isolation of *Chlamydia trachomatis* from the male urethra. *Br J Vener Dis.* 1977;53:88-92.
125. Katz BP, Batteiger BE, Jones RB. Effect of prior sexually transmitted disease on the isolation of *Chlamydia trachomatis*. *Sex Transm Dis.* 1987;14:160-164.
126. Cohen CR, Koochesfahani KM, Meier AS, et al. Immunoepidemiologic profile of *Chlamydia trachomatis* infection: Importance of heat-shock protein 60 and interferon gamma. *Infect Immun.* 2005;192:591-599.
127. Igietseme JU, Ramsey KH, Magee DM, et al. Resolution of murine chlamydial genital infection by the adoptive transfer of a biovar-specific, Th1 clone. *Reg Immunol.* 1994;5:317-324.
128. Su H, Feilzer K, Caldwell HD, et al. *Chlamydia trachomatis* genital tract infection of antibody-deficient gene knockout mice. *Infect Immun.* 1997;65:1993-1999.
129. Cotter TW, Meng Q, Shen ZL, et al. Protective efficacy of major outer membrane protein specific immunoglobulin A (IgA) and IgG murine monoclonal antibodies in a murine model of *Chla-*

mydia trachomatis genital tract infection. *Infect Immun.* 1995;63:4704-4714.
130. Morrison SG, Morrison RP. A predominant role for antibody in acquired immunity to chlamydial genital tract reinfection. *J Immunol.* 2005;175:7536-7542.
131. Morrison SG, Morrison RP. The protective effect of antibody in immunity to murine chlamydial genital tract reinfection is independent of immunoglobulin A. *Infect Immun.* 2005;73: 6183-6186.
132. Igietseme JU, Black CM, Caldwell HD. *Chlamydia* vaccines—Strategies and status. *Biodrugs.* 2002;16:19-35.
133. Su H, Messer R, Whitmire W, et al. Vaccination against chlamydial genital tract infection after immunization with dendritic cells pulsed ex vivo with nonviable *Chlamydiae. J Exp Med.* 1998;188:809-818.
134. Zhong G, Fan P, Ji H, et al. Identification of a chlamydial protease-like activity factor responsible for the degradation of host transcription factors. *J Exp Med.* 2001;193:935-942.
135. Kawana K, Quayle AJ, Ficarra M, et al. CD1d degradation in *Chlamydia trachomatis*-infected epithelial cells is the result of both cellular and chlamydial proteasomal activity. *J Biol Chem.* 2007;282:7368-7375.
136. Sun J, Schoborg RV. The host adherens junction molecule nectin-1 is degraded by chlamydial protease-like activity factor (CPAF) in *Chlamydia trachomatis*-infected genital epithelial cells. *Microbes Infect.* 2009;11:12–19.
137. Pirbhai M, Dong F, Zhong Y, et al. The secreted protease factor CPAF is responsbile for degrading pro-apoptotic BH3-only proteins in *Chlamydia trachomatis*-infected cells. *J Biol Chem.* 2006;281:31495-31501.
138. Sharma J, Dong F, Pirbhai M, et al. Inhibition of proteolytic activity of a chlamydial proteasome/protease-like activity factor by antibodies from humans infected with *Chlamydia trachomatis. Infect Immun.* 2005;73:4414-4419.
139. Murthy AK, Chambers JP, Meier PA, et al. Intranasal vaccination with a secreted chlamydial protein enhances resolution of genital *Chlamydia muridarum* infections, protects against oviduct pathology, and is highly dependent upon endogenous gamma interferon production. *Infect Immum.* 2007;75: 666-676.
140. Cong Y, Jupelli M, Guentzel MN, et al. Intranasal immunization with chlamydial protease-like activity factor and CpG deoxynucleotides enhances protective immunity against genital *Chlamydia muridarum* infection. *Vaccine.* 2007;25:3773-3780.
141. de la Maza L, Peterson EM. Vaccines for *Chlamydia trachomatis* infections. *Curr Opin Investig Drugs.* 2002;3:980-986.
142. Zhang D, Yang X, Berry J, et al. DNA vaccination with the major outer membrane protein gene induces acquired immunity to *Chlamydia trachomatis* (mouse pneumonitis) infection. *J Infect Dis.* 1997;176:1035-1040.
143. Pal S, Barnhart KM, Abai AM, et al. Immunization of mice with expression plasmids containing DNA sequences corresponding to the *C. trachomatis* MOPN MOMP failed to protect against a genital challenge. In: Stephens RS, Byrne GI, Christiansen G, et al, eds. *Chlamydial Infections: Proceedings of the Ninth International Symposium on Human Chlamydial Infection.* San Francisco: International Chlamydial Symposium; 1998:438-441.
144. Pal S, Peterson EM, Rappuoli R, et al. Immunization with the *Chlamydia trachomatis* major outer membrane protein, using adjuvants developed for human vaccines, can induce partial protection in a mouse model against a genital challenge. *Vaccine.* 2006;24:766-775.
145. Black CM. Current methods of laboratory diagnosis of *Chlamydia trachomatis* infections. *Clin Microbiol Rev.* 1997;10: 160-184.
146. Schachter J, Dawson CR. *Human Chlamydial Infections.* Littleton, Mass: PSG Publishing; 1978:181-219.
147. Dorman SA, Danos LM, Wilson DJ, et al. Detection of chlamydial cervicitis by Papanicolaou-stained smears and culture. *Am J Clin Pathol.* 1983;79:421-425.
148. Yoder BL, Stamm WE, Koester CM, et al. Microtest procedure for isolation of *Chlamydia trachomatis. J Clin Microbiol.* 1981;13:1036-1039.
149. Stamm WE, Tam M, Koester M, et al. Detection of *Chlamydia trachomatis* inclusions in McCoy cell cultures with fluorescein-conjugated monoclonal antibodies. *J Clin Microbiol.* 1983;17: 666-668.
150. Jones RB, Van Der Pol B, Katz BP. Effect of differences in specimen processing and passage technique on recovery of *Chlamydia trachomatis. J Clin Microbiol.* 1989;27:894-898.
151. Mahony JB, Chernesky MA. Effect of swab type and storage temperature on the isolation of *Chlamydia trachomatis* from clinical specimens. *J Clin Microbiol.* 1985;22:865-867.
152. Lin JL, Jones WE, Yan L, et al. Underdiagnosis of *Chlamydia trachomatis* infection: diagnostic limitations in patients with low-level infection. *Sex Transm Dis.* 1992;19:259-265.
153. Stamm WE. *Chlamydia trachomatis*: The persistent pathogen: Thomas Parran Award Lecture. *Sex Transm Dis.* 2001;28: 684-689.
154. Centers for Disease Control and Prevention. *Sexually Transmitted Diseases Treatment Guidelines, 2006.* Atlanta, Ga: Centers for Disease Control and Prevention; 2006.
155. Barnes RC, Katz BP, Rolfs RT, et al. Quantitative culture of endocervical *Chlamydia trachomatis. J Clin Microbiol.* 1990; 28:774-780.
156. Jones RB, Katz BP, Van Der Pol PB, et al. Effect of blind passage and multiple sampling on recovery of *Chlamydia trachomatis* from urogenital specimens. *J Clin Microbiol.* 1986;24:1029-1033.
157. Geisler WM, Suchland RJ, Whittington WLH, et al. Quantitative culture of *Chlamydia trachomatis*: relationship of inclusion-forming units produced in culture to clinical manifestations and acute inflammation in urogenital disease. *J Infect Dis.* 2001;184:1350-1354.
158. Perine PL, Osoba AO. Lymphogranuloma venereum. In: Holmes KK, Mardh PA, Sparling PF, et al, eds. *Sexually Transmitted Diseases.* 2nd ed. New York: McGraw-Hill; 1990: 195-204.
159. Schachter J, Grossman M, Holt J, et al. Infection with *Chlamydia trachomatis*: involvement of multiple anatomic sites in neonates. *J Infect Dis.* 1979;139:232-234.
160. Moncada JV, Schachter J, Wofsy C. Prevalence of *Chlamydia trachomatis* lung infection in patients with acquired immune deficiency syndrome. *J Clin Microbiol.* 1986;23:986.
161. Shepard MK, Jones RB. Recovery of *Chlamydia trachomatis* from endometrial and fallopian tube biopsies in women with infertility of tubal origin. *Fertil Steril.* 1989;52:232-238.
162. Berger RE, Alexander ER, Monda GD, et al. *Chlamydia trachomatis* as a cause of acute "idiopathic" epididymitis. *N Engl J Med.* 1978;298:301-304.
163. Henry-Suchet J, Catalan F, Loffredo V, et al. *Chlamydia trachomatis* associated with chronic inflammation in abdominal specimens from women selected for tuboplasty. *Fertil Steril.* 1981;36:599-605.
164. Sherman JK, Jordan GW. Cryosurvival of *Chlamydia trachomatis* during cryopreservation of human spermatozoa. *Fertil Steril.* 1985;43:664-666.
165. Stamm WE. Diagnosis of *Chlamydia trachomatis* genitourinary infections. *Ann Intern Med.* 1988;108:710-717.
166. Moncada J, Schachter J, Bolan G, et al. Confirmatory assay increases specificity of the Chlamydiazyme test for *Chlamydia trachomatis* infection of the cervix. *J Clin Microbiol.* 1990;28:1770-1773.
167. Clarke LM, Sierra MF, Daidone BJ, et al. Comparison of the Syva MicroTrak enzyme immunoassay and Gen-Probe PACE 2 with cell culture for diagnosis of cervical *Chlamydia trachomatis* infection in a high-prevalence female population. *J Clin Microbiol.* 1993;31:968-971.
168. Chapin-Robertson K. Use of molecular diagnostics in sexually transmitted diseases: critical assessment. *Diagn Microbiol Infect Dis.* 1993;16:173-184.
169. Ossewaarde JM, Rieffe M, Rozenberg-Arska M, et al. Development and clinical evaluation of polymerase chain reaction test for detection of *Chlamydia trachomatis. J Clin Microbiol.* 1992;30:2122-2128.
170. Viscidi RP, Bobo L, Hook EW, et al. Transmission of *Chlamydia trachomatis* among sex partners assessed by polymerase chain reaction. *J Infect Dis.* 1993;168:488-492.
171. Dille BJ, Butzen CC, Birkenmeyer LG. Amplification of *Chlamydia trachomatis* by ligase chain reaction. *J Clin Microbiol.* 1993;31:729-731.
172. Mahony JB, Luinstra KE, Waner J, et al. Interlaboratory agreement study of a double set of PCR plasmid primers for detection of *Chlamydia trachomatis* in a variety of genitourinary specimens. *J Clin Microbiol.* 1994;32:87-91.
173. Hook EW III, Smith K, Mullen C, et al. Diagnosis of genitourinary *Chlamydia trachomatis* infections by using the ligase chain reaction on patient-obtained vaginal swabs. *J Clin Microbiol.* 1997;35:2133-2135.
174. Bauwens JE, Clark AM, Loeffelholz MJ, et al. Diagnosis of *Chlamydia trachomatis* urethritis in men by polymerase chain reaction assay of first-catch urine. *J Clin Microbiol.* 1993; 31:3013-3016.
175. Gaydos CA, Howell MR, Pare B, et al. *Chlamydia trachomatis* infections in female military recruits. *N Engl J Med.* 1998; 339:739-744.
176. Rietmeijer CA, Yamaguchi KJ, Ortiz CG, et al. Feasibility and yield of screening urine for *Chlamydia trachomatis* by polymerase chain reaction among high-risk male youth in field-based and other nonclinic settings. *Sex Transm Dis.* 1997;24:429-435.
177. Cohen DA, Nsuami M, Etame RB, et al. A school-based *Chlamydia* control program using DNA amplification technology. *Pediatrics.* 1998;101:E1.
178. Lifson AR, Halcon LL, Hannan P, et al. Screening for sexually transmitted infections among economically disadvantaged youth in a national job training program. *J Adolesc Health.* 2001;28:190-196.
179. Ripa T, Nilsson PA. A *Chlamydia trachomatis* strain with a 277-bp deletion in the cryptic plasmid causing false-negative nucleic acid amplification test. *Sex Transm Dis.* 2007;34: 255-256.
180. Moller JK, Pedersen LN, Persson K. Comparison of Gen-probe transcription-mediated amplification, Abbott PCR, and Roche PCR assays for detection of wild-type and mutant plasmid strainst of *Chlamydia trachomatis* in Sweden. *J Clin Microbiol.* 2008;46:3892-3895.
181. Hadad R, Fredlund H, Unemo M. Evaluation of the new COBAS TaqMan CT test v2.0 and the impact on the proportion of the new variant of *Chlamydia trachomatis* (nvCT) by introduction of diagnostics detection nvCT (LightMix 480HT PCR) in Orebro county, Sweden. *Sex Transm Dis.* 2008 Dec 5. [Epub ahead of print.]
182. Marions L, Rotzen-Ostlund M, Grillner L, et al. High occurrence of a new variant of *Chlamydia trachomatis* escaping diagnostic tests among STI clinic patients in Stockholm, Sweden. *Sex Transm Dis.* 2008; 35:61-64.
183. Schachter J. The *Chlamydia trachomatis* plasmid deletion mutant: what does it mean to us? *Sex Transm Dis.* 2007;34:257.
184. Schachter J. Chlamydiae. In: Rose NR, Friedman H, eds. *Manual of Clinical Immunology.* 2nd ed. Washington, DC: American Society for Microbiology; 1980:700-706.
185. Mattila A, Miettinen A, Heinonen PK, et al. Detection of serum antibodies to *Chlamydia trachomatis* in patients with chlamydial and nonchlamydial pelvic inflammatory disease by the IPAzyme *Chlamydia* and enzyme immunoassay. *J Clin Microbiol.* 1993;31:998-1000.
186. Dawson CR, Schachter J. Strategies for treatment and control of blinding trachoma: cost effectiveness of topical or systemic antibiotics. *Rev Infect Dis.* 1985;7:768-773.
187. Baral K, Osaki S, Shresta B, et al. Reliability of clinical diagnosis in identifying infectious trachoma in a low prevalence area of Nepal. *Bull World Health Organ.* 1999;11:461-466.
188. Taylor HR, Siler JA, Mkocha HA, et al. The natural history of endemic trachoma: A longitudinal study. *Am J Trop Med Hyg.* 1992;46:552-559.
189. Bailey R, Lietman T. The SAFE strategy for the elimination of trachoma by 2020—will it work? *Bull World Health Organ.* 2001;79:233-236.
190. Kuper H, Solomon AW, Buchan J, et al. A critical review of the SAFE strategy for preventing blinding trachoma. *Lancet Infect Dis.* 2003;3:372-379.
191. Gaynor BD, Miao Y, Cevallos V, et al. Eliminating trachoma in areas with limited disease. *Emerg Infect Dis.* 2003;9:596-598.
192. Baily RL, Arullendraw P, Whittle HC, et al. Randomized controlled trial of single-dose azithromycin in treatment of trachoma. *Lancet.* 1993;342:453-456.
193. Schachter J, West SK, Mabey D, et al. Azithromycin in control of trachoma. *Lancet.* 1999;354:630-635.
194. D'Aunoy R, von Haam E. General reviews: venereal lymphogranuloma. *Arch Pathol.* 1939;27:1032-1082.
195. Perine PL, Stamm WE. Lymphogranuloma venereum. In: Holmes KK, Sparing PF, et al, eds. *Sexually Transmitted Diseases.* 3rd ed. New York: McGraw-Hill; 1999:423-432.
196. Coutts WE. Lymphogranuloma venereum: a general review. *Bull World Health Organ.* 1950;2:545-562.
197. Greenblatt RB. Antibiotics in treatment of lymphogranuloma venereum and granuloma inguinale. *Ann NY Acad Sci.* 1952; 55:1082-1089.
198. Greaves AB, Hilleman MR, Taggart SR, et al. Chemotherapy in bubonic lymphogranuloma venereum: a clinical and serological evaluation. *Bull World Health Organ.* 1957;16:277-289.
199. Centers for Disease Control and Prevention. Sexually transmitted diseases treatment guidelines 2002. *MMWR Recomm Rep.* 2002;51:1-80.
200. Schachter J, Dawson CR. *Human Chlamydial Infections.* Littleton, Mass: PSG Publishing; 1978:97-109.
201. Dawson CR, Schachter J. TRIC agent infections of the eye and genital tract. *Am J Ophthalmol.* 1967;63(suppl):1288-1298.
202. Stenson S. Adult inclusion conjunctivitis: clinical characteristics and corneal changes. *Arch Ophthalmol.* 1981;99:605-608.
203. Rönnerstam R, Persson K, Hansson H, et al. Prevalence of chlamydial eye infection in patients attending an eye clinic, a VD clinic, and in healthy persons. *Br J Ophthalmol.* 1985;69: 385-388.
204. Stenberg K, Mardh PA. Genital infection with *Chlamydia trachomatis* in patients with chlamydial conjunctivitis: Unexplained results. *Sex Transm Dis.* 1991;18:1-4.
205. Lycke E, Löwhagen GB, Hallhagen G, et al. The risk of transmission of genital *Chlamydia trachomatis* infection is less than that of genital *Neisseria gonorrhoeae* infection. *Sex Transm Dis.* 1980;7:6-10.
206. Katz BP, Caine VA, Jones RB. Estimation of transmission probabilities for chlamydial infection. In: Bowie WR, Caldwell HD, Jones RP, et al, eds. *Chlamydial Infections.* Cambridge, UK: Cambridge University Press; 1990:567-570.
207. Quinn TC, Gaydos C, Shepherd M, et al. Epidemiologic and microbiologic correlates of *Chlamydia trachomatis* infection in sexual partnerships. *JAMA.* 1996;276:1737-1742.
208. Ramstedt K, Forssman L, Giesecke J, et al. Epidemiologic characteristics of two different populations of women with *Chlamydia trachomatis* infection and their male partners. *Sex Transm Dis.* 1991;18:205-210.
209. Hook EW 3rd, Reichart CA, Upchurch DM, et al. Comparative behavioral epidemiology of gonococcal and chlamydial infections among patients attending a Baltimore, Maryland, sexually transmitted disease clinic. *Am J Epidemiol.* 1992;136:662-672.
210. Blythe MJ, Katz BP, Orr DP, et al. Historical and clinical factors associated with *Chlamydia trachomatis* genitourinary infection in female adolescents. *J Pediatr.* 1988;112:1000-1004.
211. Oriel JD, Ridgway GL. Studies of the epidemiology of chlamydial infection of the human genital tract. In: Mardh PA, Holmes KK, Piot P, et al, eds. *Chlamydial Infections.* Amsterdam: Elsevier Biomedical Press; 1982:425-428.
212. Batteiger BE, Fraiz J, Newhall WJ, et al. Association of recurrent chlamydial infection with gonorrhea. *J Infect Dis.* 1989;159: 661-669.
213. Geisler WM, Wang C, Morrison SG, et al. The natural history of untreated *Chlamydia trachomatis* infection in the interval

between screening and returning for treatment. *Sex Transm Dis.* 2008;35:119-123.
214. Joyner JL, Douglas Jr JM, Foster M, et al. Persistence of *Chlamydia trachomatis* infection detected by polymerase chain reaction in untreated patients. *Sex Transm Dis.* 2002;29:196-200.
215. Stamm WE, Cole B. Asymptomatic *Chlamydia trachomatis* urethritis in men. *Sex Transm Dis.* 1986;13:163-165.
216. Bowie WR, Alexander ER, Holmes KK. Etiologies of postgonococcal urethritis in homosexual and heterosexual men: roles of *Chlamydia trachomatis* and *Ureaplasma urealyticum*. *Sex Transm Dis.* 1978;5:151-154.
217. Krieger JN, Verdon M, Siegel N, et al. Risk assessment and laboratory diagnosis of trichomoniasis in men. *J Infect Dis.* 1992;166:1362-1366.
218. Martin DH. Nongonococcal urethritis: new views through the prism of modern molecular biology. *Curr Infect Dis Rep.* 2008;10:128-132.
219. Nettleman MD, Jones RB, Roberts SD, et al. Cost effectiveness of culturing for *Chlamydia trachomatis*. A study in a clinic for sexually transmitted diseases. *Ann Intern Med.* 1986; 105:189-196.
220. Stamm WE, Koutsky LA, Benedetti JK, et al. *Chlamydia trachomatis* urethral infections in men: prevalence, risk factors, and clinical manifestations. *Ann Intern Med.* 1984;100:47-51.
221. Bowie WR. Approach to men with urethritis and urologic complications of sexually transmitted diseases. *Med Clin North Am.* 1990;74:1543-1557.
222. Adger H, Sweet RL, Shafer MA, et al. Screening for *Chlamydia trachomatis* and *Neisseria gonorrhoeae* in adolescent males: value of first-catch urine examination. *Lancet.* 1984;2:944-945.
223. Shafer MA, Schachter J, Moscicki AB, et al. Urinary leukocyte esterase screening test for asymptomatic chlamydial and gonococcal infections in males. *JAMA.* 1989;262:2562-2566.
224. Berger RE, Alexander ER, Harnisch JP, et al. Etiology, manifestations and therapy of acute epididymitis: prospective study of 50 cases. *J Urol.* 1979;121:750-754.
225. Ruijs GJ, Kauer FM, Jager S, et al. Is serology of any use when searching for correlations between *Chlamydia trachomatis* infection and male infertility? *Fertil Steril.* 1990;53:131-136.
226. Shortliffe LMD, Sellers RG, Schachter J. The characterization of the nonbacterial prostatitis: search for an etiology. *J Urol.* 1992;148:1461-1466.
227. Jones RB, Rabinovitch RA, Katz BP, et al. Recovery of *Chlamydia trachomatis* from the pharynx and rectum of heterosexual patients at risk for genital infection. *Ann Intern Med.* 1985;6: 757-762.
228. Quinn TC, Goodell SE, Mkrtichian E, et al. *Chlamydia trachomatis* proctitis. *N Engl J Med.* 1981;305:195-200.
229. Annamunthodo H. Rectal lymphogranuloma venereum in Jamaica. *Ann R Coll Surg Engl.* 1961;28:141-159.
230. Stamm WE. *Chlamydia trachomatis* infections of the adult. In: Holmes KK, Mardh PA, Sparling PF, et al, eds. *Sexually Transmitted Diseases.* 3rd ed. New York: McGraw-Hill; 1999:407-422.
231. Spaargaren J, Fennema HAS, Morre SA. New lymphogranuloma venereum *Chlamydia trachomatis* variant Amsterdam. *Emerging Infect Dis.* 2005;11:1090-1094.
232. Rahman MU, Hudson AP, Schumacher Jr HR. *Chlamydia* and Reiter's syndrome (reactive arthritis). *Rheum Dis Clin North Am.* 1992;18:67-79.
233. Keat A, Thomas BJ, Taylor-Robinson D. Chlamydial infection in the aetiology of arthritis. *Br Med Bull.* 1983;39:168-174.
234. Keat A. Extragenital *Chlamydia trachomatis* infection as sexually-acquired reactive arthritis. *J Infect.* 1992;25(suppl 1): 47-49.
235. Inman RD, Morrison RP. Immunoblot analysis of reactivity to chlamydial 57-kD heat shock protein in Reiter's syndrome [abstract]. *Arthritis Rheum.* 1990;33:S26.
236. Sieper J, Braun J, Brandt J, et al. Pathogenetic role of *Chlamydia, Yersinia* and *Borrelia* in undifferentiated oligoarthritis. *J Rheumatol.* 1992;19:1236-1242.
237. Schachter J. Isolation of Bedsoniae from human arthritis and abortion tissues. *Am J Ophthalmol.* 1967;63(suppl):1082-1086.
238. Vilppula AH, Yli-Kerttula UI, Ahlroos AK, et al. Chlamydial isolation and serology in Reiter's syndrome. *Scand J Rheumatol.* 1981;10:181-185.
239. Gerard HC, Branigan PJ, Schumacher Jr HR, et al. Synovial *Chlamydia trachomatis* in patients with reactive arthritis/Reiter's syndrome are viable but show aberrant gene expression. *J Rheumatol.* 1998;25:734-742.
240. Lauhio A, Leirisalo-Repo M, Lähdevirta J, et al. Double-blind, placebo-controlled study of three-month treatment with lymecycline in reactive arthritis, with special reference to *Chlamydia* arthritis. *Arthritis Rheum.* 1991;34:6-14.
241. Bardin T, Enel C, Cornelis F, et al. Antibiotic treatment of venereal disease and Reiter's syndrome in a Greenland population. *Arthritis Rheum.* 1992;35:190-194.
242. Bardin T, Schumacher HR. Should we treat postvenereal Reiter's syndrome by antibiotics [editorial]? *J Rheumatol.* 1991;18: 1780-1782.
243. Washington AE, Gove S, Schachter J, et al. Oral contraceptives, *Chlamydia trachomatis* infection, and pelvic inflammatory disease. *JAMA.* 1985;253:2246-2250.
244. Hillis SD, Nakashima A, Marchbanks PA, et al. Risk factors for recurrent *Chlamydia trachomatis* infections in women. *Am J Obstet Gynecol.* 1994;170:801-806.
245. Hillis SD, Owens LM, Marchbanks PA, et al. Recurrent chlamydial infections increase the risks of hospitalization for ectopic pregnancy and pelvic inflammatory disease. *Am J Obstet Gynecol.* 1997;176:103-107.
246. Handsfield HH, Jasman LL, Roberts PL, et al. Criteria for selective screening for *Chlamydia trachomatis* infection in women attending family planning clinics. *JAMA.* 1986;255:1730-1734.
247. Wolner-Hanssen P, Patton DL, Holmes KK. Protective immunity in pigtailed macaques after cervical infection with *Chlamydia trachomatis*. *Sex Transm Dis.* 1991;18:21-25.
248. McCormack WM, Alpert S, McComb DE, et al. Fifteen-month follow-up study of women infected with *Chlamydia trachomatis*. *N Engl J Med.* 1979;300:123-125.
249. Rahm VA, Gnarpe H, Odlind V. *Chlamydia trachomatis* among sexually active teenage girls: lack of correlation between chlamydial infection, history of the patient and clinical signs of infection. *Br J Obstet Gynaecol.* 1988;95:916-919.
250. Dan M, Rotmensch HH, Eylan E, et al. A case of lymphogranuloma venereum of 20 years' duration. *Br J Vener Dis.* 1980; 56:344-346.
251. Campbell LA, Patton DL, Moore DE, et al. Detection of *Chlamydia trachomatis* deoxyribonucleic acid in women with tubal infertility. *Fertil Steril.* 1993;59:45-50.
252. Bell TA, Stamm WE, Wang SP, et al. Chronic *Chlamydia trachomatis* infections in infants. *JAMA.* 1992;267:400-402.
253. Dean D, Suchland RJ, Stamm WE. Evidence for long-term persistence of *C. trachomatis* by Omp-1 genotyping. *J Infect Dis.* 2000;182:909-916.
254. Dunlop EMC, Garner A, Darougar S, et al. Colposcopy, biopsy, and cytology results in women with chlamydial cervicitis. *Genitourin Med.* 1989;65:22-31.
255. Stamm WE, Wagner KF, Amsel R, et al. Causes of the acute urethral syndrome in women. *N Engl J Med.* 1980;303: 409-415.
256. Hare MJ, Taylor-Robinson D, Cooper P. Evidence for an association between *Chlamydia trachomatis* and cervical intraepithelial neoplasia. *Br J Obstet Gynaecol.* 1982;89:489-492.
257. Schachter J, Hill EC, King EB, et al. *Chlamydia trachomatis* and cervical neoplasia. *JAMA.* 1982;248:2134-2138.
258. Yliskoski M, Tervahauta A, Saarikoski S, et al. Clinical course of cervical human papillomavirus lesions in relation to coexistent cervical infections. *Sex Transm Dis.* 1992;19:137-139.
259. Anttila T, Saikku P, Koskela P, et al. Serotypes of *C. trachomatis* and risk for development of cervical squamous cell carcinoma. *JAMA.* 2001;285:47-51.
260. Shew ML, Fortenberry JD, Tu W, et al. Association of condom use, sexual behaviors, and sexually transmitted infections with the duration of genital human papillomavirus infection among adolescent women. *Arch Pediatr Adolesc Med.* 2006;160: 151-156.
261. Laga M, Manoka A, Kivuvu M, et al. Nonulcerative sexually transmitted diseases as risk factors for HIV-1 transmission in women: results from a cohort study. *AIDS.* 1993;7:95-102.
262. Centers for Disease Control and Prevention. HIV prevention through early detection and treatment of other sexually transmitted diseases—United States. *MMWR Morb Mortal Wkly Rep.* 1998;47:2-4.
263. Stamm WE, Guinan ME, Johnson C, et al. Effect of treatment regimens for *Neisseria gonorrhoeae* on simultaneous infection with *Chlamydia trachomatis*. *N Engl J Med.* 1984;310:545-549.
264. Cates W Jr, Rolfs RT Jr, Aral SO. Sexually transmitted diseases, pelvic inflammatory disease, and infertility: an epidemiologic update. *Epidemiol Rev.* 1990;12:199-220.
265. Paavonen J, Aine R, Teisala K, et al. Comparison of endometrial biopsy and peritoneal fluid cytologic testing and laparoscopy in the diagnosis of acute pelvic inflammatory disease. *Am J Obstet Gynecol.* 1985;151:645-650.
266. Paavonen J. Genital *Chlamydia trachomatis* infections in the female. *J Infect.* 1992;25(suppl 1):39-45.
267. Svenssen L, Westrom L, Ripa KT, et al. Differences in some clinical and laboratory parameters in acute salpingitis related to culture and serologic findings. *Am J Obstet Gynecol.* 1980; 138:1017-1021.
268. Scholes D, Stergachis A, Heidrich FC, et al. Prevention of pelvic inflammatory disease by screening for cervical chlamydial infection. *N Engl J Med.* 1996;334:1362-1366.
269. Patton DL, Wölner-Hanssen P, Cosgrove SJ, et al. The effects of *Chlamydia trachomatis* on the female reproductive tract of the *Macaca nemestrina* after a single tubal challenge following repeated cervical inoculations. *Obstet Gynecol.* 1990;76: 643-650.
270. Brunham RC, Binns B, Guijon F, et al. Etiology and outcome of acute pelvic inflammatory disease. *J Infect Dis.* 1988; 158:510-517.
271. Weström L, Joesoef R, Reynolds G, et al. Pelvic inflammatory disease and fertility: a cohort study of 1,844 women with laparoscopically verified disease and 657 control women with normal laparoscopic results. *Sex Transm Dis.* 1992;19:185-192.
272. Campbell LA, Patton DL, Moore DE, et al. Detection of *Chlamydia trachomatis* deoxyribonucleic acid in women with tubal infertility. *Fertil Steril.* 1993;59:45-50.
273. Brunham RC, Binns F, McDowell J, et al. *Chlamydia trachomatis* infection in women with ectopic pregnancy. *Obstet Gynecol.* 1986;67:722-726.
274. Witkin SS, Ledger WJ. Antibodies to *Chlamydia trachomatis* in sera of women with recurrent spontaneous abortions. *Am J Obstet Gynecol.* 1992;167:135-139.
275. McGregor JA, French JI. *Chlamydia trachomatis* infection during pregnancy. *Am J Obstet Gynecol.* 1991;164:1782-1789.
276. Berman SM, Harrison HR, Boyce WT, et al. Low birth weight, prematurity, and postpartum endometritis: Association with prenatal cervical *Mycoplasma hominis* and *Chlamydia trachomatis* infections. *JAMA.* 1987;257:1189-1194.
277. Gravett MG, Nelson HP, DeRouen T, et al. Independent associations of bacterial vaginosis and *Chlamydia trachomatis* infection with adverse pregnancy outcome. *JAMA.* 1986;256:1899-1903.
278. Martius J, Krohn MA, Hillier SL, et al. Relationships of vaginal *Lactobacillus* species, cervical *Chlamydia trachomatis*, and bacterial vaginosis to preterm birth. *Obstet Gynecol.* 1988;71:89-95.
279. Ryan Jr GM, Abdella TN, McNeeley SG, et al. *Chlamydia trachomatis* infection in pregnancy and effect of treatment on outcome. *Am J Obstet Gynecol.* 1990;162:34-39.
280. Cohen I, Vielle JC, Calkins BM. Improved pregnancy outcome following successful treatment of chlamydial infection. *JAMA.* 1990;263:3160-3163.
281. Hillier SL, Nugent RP, Eschenbach DA, et al. Association between bacterial vaginosis and preterm delivery of a low birth-weight infant. The Vaginal Infections and Prematurity Study Group. *N Engl J Med.* 1995;333:1737-1742.
282. Meyers JD, Hackman RC, Stamm WE. *Chlamydia trachomatis* infection as a cause of pneumonia after human marrow transplantation. *Transplantation.* 1983;36:130-134.
283. Komaroff AL, Aronson MD, Schachter J. *Chlamydia trachomatis* infection in adults with community-acquired pneumonia. *JAMA.* 1981;245:1319-1322.
284. Myhre EB, Mardh PA. *Chlamydia trachomatis* infection in a patient with meningoencephalitis. *N Engl J Med.* 1981; 304:910-911.
285. Grayston JT, Mordhorst CH, Wang SP. Childhood myocarditis associated with *Chlamydia trachomatis* infection. *JAMA.* 1981;246:2823-2837.
286. van der Bel-Kahn JM, Watanakunakorn C, Menefee MG, et al. *Chlamydia trachomatis* endocarditis. *Am Heart J.* 1978;95: 627-636.
287. Suchland RJ, Geisler WM, Stamm WE. Methodologies and cell lines used for antimicrobial susceptibility testing of *Chlamydia* spp. *Antimicrob Agents Chemother.* 2003;47:636-642.
288. Centers for Disease Control and Prevention. *MMWR Morb Mortal Wkly Rep.* 2006;1-94.
289. Martin DH, Mroczkowski TF, Dalu ZA, et al. A controlled trial of a single dose of azithromycin for the treatment of chlamydial urethritis and cervicitis. *N Engl J Med.* 1992;327:921-925.
290. Hillis SD, Coles B, Litchfield B, et al. Doxycycline and azithromycin for prevention of chlamydial persistence or recurrence one month after treatment in women: a use-effectiveness study in public health settings. *Sex Transm Dis.* 1998;25:5-11.
291. Fortenberry JD, Brizendine EJ, Katz BP, et al. Subsequent STDs among adolescent women with *C. trachomatis, N. gonorrhoeae* or *T. vaginalis*. *Sex Transm Dis.* 1999;26:26-32.
292. Stamm WE, Geisler WM, Suchland RJ. Assessment of antimicrobial resistance in *C. trachomatis* strains associated with treatment failure or same strain recurrence. In: Schachter J, Christiansen G, Clarke IN, et al, eds. *Chlamydial Infections, Proceedings of the Tenth International Symposium on Human Chlamydial Infections.* San Francisco: International Chlamydial Symposium; 2002.
293. Stamm WE, Hicks CB, Martin DH, et al. Azithromycin for empirical treatment of the nongonococcal urethritis syndrome in men: a randomized double-blind study. *JAMA.* 1995;274: 545-549.
294. Magat AH, Alger LS, Nagey DA, et al. Double-blind randomized study comparing amoxicillin and erythromycin for the treatment of *Chlamydia trachomatis* in pregnancy. *Obstet Gynecol.* 1993;81:745-749.
295. Crombleholme WR, Schachter J, Grossman M, et al. Amoxicillin therapy for *Chlamydia trachomatis* in pregnancy. *Obstet Gynecol.* 1990;75:752-756.
296. Bowie WR, Yu JS, Jones HD. Partial efficacy of clindamycin against *Chlamydia trachomatis* in men with nongonococcal urethritis. *Sex Transm Dis.* 1986;13:76-80.
297. Alger LS, Lovchik JC. Comparative efficacy of clindamycin versus erythromycin in eradication of antenatal *Chlamydia trachomatis*. *Am J Obstet Gynecol.* 1991;165:375-381.
298. Campbell WF, Dodson MG. Clindamycin therapy for *Chlamydia trachomatis* in women. *Am J Obstet Gynecol.* 1990; 162:343-347.
299. Viswalingam ND, Daroughar S, Yearsley P. Oral doxycycline in the treatment of adult chlamydial ophthalmia. *Br J Ophthalmol.* 1986;70:301-304.
300. Shariat H, Young M, Abedin M. An interesting case presentation: a possible new route for perinatal acquisition of *Chlamydia*. *J Perinatol.* 1992;12:300-302.
301. Hammerschlag MR. Chlamydial infections in infants and children. In: Holmes KK, Mardh PA, Sparling PF, et al, eds. *Sexually Transmitted Diseases.* 3rd ed. New York: McGraw-Hill; 1999;1155-1164.
302. Chandler JW, Alexander ER, Pheiffer TA, et al. *Ophthalmia neonatorum* associated with maternal chlamydial infections. *Trans Am Acad Ophthalmol Otolaryngol.* 1977;83:302-308.
303. Schachter J, Dawson CR. *Human Chlamydial Infections.* Littleton, Mass: PSG Publishing; 1978:111-120.
304. Persson K, Rönnerstam R, Svanberg L, et al. Neonatal chlamydial eye infection: an epidemiological and clinical study. *Br J Ophthalmol.* 1983;67:700-704.

305. Hammerschlag MR, Cummings C, Roblin PM, et al. Efficacy of neonatal ocular prophylaxis for the prevention of chlamydial and gonococcal conjunctivitis. *N Engl J Med.* 1989;320: 769-772.

306. Schachter J, Grossman M, Sweet RL, et al. Prospective study of perinatal transmission of *Chlamydia trachomatis. JAMA.* 1986;255:3374-3377.

307. Tipple MA, Beem MO, Saxon EM. Clinical characteristics of the afebrile pneumonia associated with *Chlamydia trachomatis* infection in infants less than six months of age. *Pediatrics.* 1979;63:192-197.

308. Beem MO, Saxon EM. Respiratory tract colonization and a distinctive pneumonia syndrome in infants infected with *Chlamydia trachomatis. N Engl J Med.* 1977;296:306-310.

309. Harrison HR, English MG, Lee CK, et al. *Chlamydia trachomatis* infant pneumonitis: comparison with matched controls and other infant pneumonitis. *N Engl J Med.* 1978;288:702-708.

310. Wheeler WB, Kurachek SC, Lobas JG, et al. Acute hypoxemic respiratory failure caused by *Chlamydia trachomatis* and diagnosed by flexible bronchoscopy. *Am Rev Respir Dis.* 1990;142: 471-473.

311. Broadbent R, O'Leary L. Chlamydial infections in young infants—A cause for concern. *N Z Med J.* 1988;101:44-45.

312. Brasfield DM, Stagno S, Whitley RJ, et al. Infant pneumonitis associated with cytomegalovirus, *Chlamydia, Pneumocystis,* and *Ureaplasma:* follow-up. *Pediatrics.* 1987;79:76-83.

313. Weiss SG, Newcomb RW, Beem MO. Pulmonary assessment of children after chlamydial pneumonia of infancy. *J Pediatr.* 1986;108:659-664.

314. Heggie AD, Jaffe AC, Stuart LA, et al. Topical sulfacetamide vs oral erythromycin for neonatal chlamydial conjunctivitis. *Am J Dis Child.* 1985;139:564-566.

315. Pereira LH, Embil JA, Haase DA, et al. Cytomegalovirus infection among women attending a sexually transmitted disease clinic: association with clinical symptoms and other sexually transmitted diseases. *Am J Epidemiol.* 1990;131: 683-692.

316. Oh MK, Cloud GA, Baker SL, et al. Chlamydial infection and sexual behavior in young pregnant teenagers. *Sex Transm Dis.* 1993;20:45-50.

317. Louv WC, Austin H, Alexander WJ, et al. A clinical trial of nonoxynol 9 for preventing gonococcal and chlamydial infections. *J Infect Dis.* 1988;158:518-523.

318. Rosenberg MJ, Rojanapithayakorn W, Feldblum PJ, et al. Effect of contraceptive sponge on chlamydial infection, gonorrhea, and candidiasis: a comparative clinical trial. *JAMA.* 1987; 257:2308-2312.

319. Addiss DG, Vaughn ML, Ludka D, et al. Decreased prevalence of *Chlamydia trachomatis* infection associated with a selective screening program in family planning clinics in Wisconsin. *Sex Transm Dis.* 1993;20:28-35.

320. Patton DL, Wang SK, Kuo CC. In vitro activity of nonoxynol 9 on HeLa 229 cells and primary monkey cervical epithelial cells infected with *Chlamydia trachomatis. Antimicrob Agents Chemother.* 1992;36:1478-1482.

321. Roddy RE, Zekeng L, Ryan KA, et al. A controlled trial of nonoxynol 9 film to reduce male-to-female transmission of sexually transmitted diseases. *N Engl J Med.* 1998;339:504-510.

322. Wilkinson D, Tholandi M, Ramjee G, et al. Nonoxynol-9 spermicide for prevention of vaginally acquired HIV and other sexually transmitted infections: systematic review and meta-analysis of randomised controlled trials including more than 5000 women. *Lancet Infect Dis.* 2002;2:613-617.

323. Hillier SL, Moench T, Shattock R, et al. In vitro and in vivo: The sotyr of nonoxynol 9. *J Acquir Immune Defic Syndr.* 2005;39: 1-8.

324. U.S. Preventive Services Task Force. Screening for chlamydial infection: U.S. Preventive Services Task Force recommendation statement. *Ann Intern Med.* 2007;147;128-134.

325. Burstein GR, Gaydos CA, Diener-West M, et al. Incident *Chlamydia trachomatis* infection among inner-city adolescents. *JAMA.* 1998;280:521-526.

326. Orr DP, Fortenberry JD. Screening adolescents for sexually transmitted infections. *JAMA.* 1998;280:654-655.

327. Screening tests to detect *C. trachomatis* and *N. gonorrheal* infections—2002. *MMWR Recomm Rep.* 2002;51:1-38.

328. Bowden FJ. Reappraising the value of urine leukocyte esterase testing in the age of nucleic acid amplification. *Sex Transm Dis.* 1998;25:322-326.

329. Brunham RC, Pourbohloul B, Mak S, et al. The unexpected impact of a *Chlamydia trachomatis* infection control program on susceptiblity to reinfection. *J Infect Dis.* 2005;195:1836-1844.

330. Katz BP, Danos CS, Quinn TS, et al. Efficiency and cost effectiveness of field follow-up for patients with *Chlamydia trachomatis* infection in a sexually transmitted diseases clinic. *Sex Transm Dis.* 1988;15:11-16.

331. Ripa T. Epidemiologic control of genital *Chlamydia trachomatis* infections. *Scand J Infect Dis.* 1990;69(suppl):157-167.

332. Golden MR, Whittington WLH, Handsfield HH, et al. Effect of expedited treatment of sex partners on recurrent or persistent gonorrhea or chlamydial infection. *N Engl J Med.* 2005;352: 676-685.

181

Chlamydophila (Chlamydia) psittaci (Psittacosis)

DAVID SCHLOSSBERG

Psittacosis is a systemic infection that frequently causes pneumonia. Its relationship to bird exposure has been known for more than 100 years. In 1879, Ritter studied an outbreak in Switzerland and called it pneumotyphus.[1] Morange applied the term *psittacosis* (from the Greek word for parrot) in 1892 after studying cases associated with sick parrots. In 1930, the organism was identified in several laboratories, by Bedson in the United Kingdom, Kromwede in the United States, and Levinthal in Germany.[2]

The name psittacosis has persisted, even though the term *ornithosis* more accurately depicts the potential for all birds to spread this infection. In fact, even mammals, including humans, are rare sources of psittacosis.

The causative agent of psittacosis is *Chlamydophila psittaci*. Under a proposed classification, *C. psittaci* would now be grouped with *C. pneumoniae, C. pecorum, C. abortus, C. caviae,* and *C. felis* in the genus *Chlamydophila* of the family Chlamydiaceae.[3]

Epidemiology

C. psittaci is common in birds and domestic animals. Infection is therefore a hazard to pet owners, pet shop employees, poultry farmers (turkey-associated psittacosis has the highest attack rate in psittacosis epidemics), workers in abattoirs and processing plants (psittacosis is the most common abattoir-associated pneumonia), and veterinarians. However, anyone in contact with an infected bird or animal is at risk. Human cases occur both sporadically and as outbreaks.[4]

Most patients with psittacosis have had some contact with a bird, usually as a pet. In fact, the importation of exotic birds (sometimes illegal) has been correlated with an increase in human psittacosis in the United States, Sweden, England, and Wales. Often, the bird was recently acquired or was ill. Bird contact may achieve surprising levels of intimacy. Patients have acquired psittacosis by kissing their parrot or by performing mouth-to-mouth resuscitation on a dying bird. Other patients have had more trivial or transient exposure, such as visits to public bird parks, transporting pigeons by car, passing through a room in which infected birds were sitting, sharing a stage with a parrot, or guarding crates of pigeons at a railroad depot. Still, some patients (25%) have had no avian exposure.[5]

Birds transmit the infection to their nestlings, which in turn shed the organism during periods of both illness and good health. In bird populations studied, there is a baseline prevalence of 5% to 8% of *C. psittaci* carriage. This may increase to 100% when birds are subjected to the stress of shipping, crowding, and breeding.[2,5]

It is likely that all birds are susceptible. More than 130 avian species have been documented as hosts of *C. psittaci*.[2] These include members of the parrot family (macaws, cockatoos, parakeets, budgerigars), finches (canaries, bullfinches, goldfinches, sparrows), poultry (hens, ducks, geese, turkeys), pigeons, pheasants, egrets, seagulls, and puffins.

Infection may appear in birds years after exposure. Infected birds may be asymptomatic or obviously sick. In the latter case, birds may exhibit shivering, depression, anorexia, emaciation, dyspnea, and diarrhea, frequently with closed eyes and ruffled feathers. Spontaneous relapse and remittance of the illness may occur, although it is during periods of illness that infected birds excrete the largest numbers of organisms. Discharge from their beaks and eyes and feces and urine are all infective; their feathers and the dust around their cage become contaminated.

The infection is generally spread by the respiratory route, by direct contact or aerosolization of infective discharges or dust. Rarely, the bird may spread the infection by a bite. If untreated, 10% of infected birds become chronic asymptomatic carriers.[5]

Strains from turkeys and psittacine birds are the most virulent for humans. Although most human exposure comes from avian strains of *C. psittaci*, disease has occurred in ranchers after exposure to infected tissues from parturient cows, goats, and sheep. Endocarditis has been attributed to avian and nonavian strains, and cats have spread feline pneumonitis to humans and other mammals. The growing practice of pet-associated therapy in nursing homes has produced a new epidemiologic risk for psittacosis.[6]

Human-to-human[7] and nosocomial[8] transmissions are rare and it is therefore thought unnecessary to isolate patients in the hospital or to give antibiotic prophylaxis to contacts. However, cases acquired from humans tend to be more severe than avian-acquired disease. Environmental sanitation is important because the organism is resistant to drying and can remain viable for months at room temperature.[2,5]

Clinical Findings and Differential Diagnostic Considerations

The disease begins after an incubation period of 5 to 15 days. Onset may be insidious or abrupt, and the clinical manifestations tend to be nonspecific. Several syndromes may result. The infection may be subclinical, or it may resemble a nonspecific viral illness with fever and malaise or a mononucleosis-like syndrome with fever, pharyngitis, hepatosplenomegaly, and adenopathy. A typhoidal form manifests as fever, bradycardia, malaise, and splenomegaly. Finally, the presentation most suggestive of the cause is that of atypical pneumonia, with nonproductive cough, fever, headache, and chest film abnormalities more dramatic than would be suggested by the physical findings. The illness ranges in severity from an inapparent or mild disease to a fatal systemic illness with prominent respiratory symptoms.

Because many patients have an illness with nonspecific findings, the list of initial diagnoses for which patients have been referred to hospitals is extensive. This list reflects the various organ systems that may be involved in *C. psittaci* infection and includes the diagnoses of meningitis, tonsillitis, pneumonia, pulmonary embolism, myocardial infarction, gastroenteritis, hepatitis, peritonitis, pancreatic carcinoma, urinary tract infection, endocarditis, vasculitis, septicemia, malaria, brucellosis, fever of unknown origin, and polymyositis.[6,9]

The list of considerations in the differential diagnosis is extensive, and the diagnostic possibilities depend on the presentation. A typhoidal picture suggests the mononucleosis syndrome, typhoid fever, brucellosis, tularemia, influenza, or subacute bacterial endocarditis. Respiratory signs and symptoms plus headache and myalgias should orient the clinician to causes of atypical pneumonia, such as viral pneumonia, Q fever, legionellosis, and infection with mycoplasma and *C. pneumoniae*. Helpful clues to a diagnosis of psittacosis, when present, are relative bradycardia, rash, hemoptysis, epistaxis, and splenomegaly.

The most common symptom is fever, occurring in 50% to 100% of patients. Cough has been reported in 50% to 100%, but often it appears late in the illness and is not present initially. Headache, myalgias, and chills are reported in 30% to 70% of patients. The nonspecificity of these signs and symptoms may be puzzling until cough supervenes. Even then, the long list of other signs and symptoms that occur in less than half the patients may be particularly confusing: diaphoresis, photophobia, tinnitus, ataxia, deafness, anorexia, nausea and vomiting, abdominal pain, diarrhea, constipation, sore throat, dyspnea, hemoptysis, epistaxis, arthralgia, and rash. Chest soreness is reported, but true pleuritic pain is rare.[4,5,9,10]

The signs most frequently reported are fever, pharyngeal erythema, rales or other abnormalities on chest auscultation, and hepatomegaly. These occur in more than half of cases. Fewer than 50% of patients show the signs of somnolence, confusion, tachycardia, relative bradycardia, pleural rub, splenomegaly (this occurs toward the end of the first week and is helpful diagnostically), adenopathy, palatal petechiae, herpes labialis, Horder's spots (see later), and muscle tenderness.[4,5,9]

Specific end-organ involvement reflects the systemic nature of psittacosis. The organ most commonly involved in humans is the lung. This is manifested clinically by cough, dyspnea, and a variety of nonspecific auscultatory findings on physical examination. Occasionally, the pneumonitis may progress to acute respiratory distress syndrome (ARDS). Cardiac manifestations include pericarditis (rarely with effusion and tamponade), myocarditis, idiopathic dilated cardiomyopathy,[11] and "culture-negative" endocarditis. *C. psittaci* endocarditis is associated with preexisting heart disease and may cause valvular destruction. Arterial embolism to major vessels occurs rarely. The source of these emboli and the mechanism are unknown; some are attributed to endocarditis or mural thrombi.[12]

Hepatitis may develop, sometimes with jaundice. Anemia may result from hemolysis (both Coombs' test positivity and cold agglutinins are reported) and from a reactive hemophagocytosis, in which case pancytopenia may be present. Disseminated intravascular coagulation (DIC) also complicates psittacosis.[13,14] Reactive arthritis occurs 1 to 4 weeks after the initial illness. Although most of the described cases are polyarticular, monoarticular arthritis has also been described.

Neurologic abnormalities include cranial nerve palsy (including sensorineural hearing loss), cerebellar involvement, transverse myelitis, confusion, meningitis, encephalitis, transient focal neurologic signs, and seizures. Results of cerebrospinal fluid examination on lumbar puncture are usually normal; a small number of white cells (predominantly lymphocytes) may be seen, and the protein level on occasion is greatly elevated.[15-19]

Dermatologic phenomena include Horder's spots, which are a pink, blanching, maculopapular eruption resembling the rose spots of typhoid fever. Also described are erythema multiforme, erythema marginatum, erythema nodosum, and urticaria, as well as acrocyanosis, subungual splinter hemorrhages, and superficial venous thromboses. Acute glomerulonephritis, acute tubulointerstitial nephritis, and acute tubular necrosis have been reported. Psittacosis has severe consequences in pregnancy and often causes DIC, hepatic dysfunction, and placentitis, with fetal compromise.[20,21] Additional clinical complications of psittacosis include phlebitis, pancreatitis, and thyroiditis. Bacteremia has been demonstrated in a patient with a sarcoid-like illness.

Recent observations have suggested that *C. psittaci* is associated with ocular adnexal lymphomas involving orbital soft tissue, lacrimal glands, and conjunctiva. *C. psittaci* has been detected in lymphoma biopsies by polymerase chain reaction (PCR) assay, and tumors in some patients have regressed after treatment with doxycycline. However, the prevalence of *C. psittaci* in these lymphomas varies, particularly geographically,[22-24] and some tumors with no evidence of *C. psittaci* have also responded to doxycycline therapy, suggesting either that *C. psittaci* detection methods are inadequate or that other doxycycline-responsive organisms may cause this malignancy.[25,26]

There is no documented protection after infection, and second infections have been seen in spite of elevated levels of complement-fixing antibodies.[2] Treated birds can also be reinfected.

Laboratory Findings

The total white blood cell count is usually normal or slightly elevated. Two thirds of patients have a leftward shift. Eosinophilia has been seen in convalescence. Results on liver function testing are mildly abnormal in 50% of cases and may suggest cholestasis. Culture of the organism is possible from blood in the first 4 days of illness and from sputum in the first 2 weeks. However, although the organism can be isolated in cell culture and by animal inoculation, these methods are dangerous, and serologic diagnosis is preferred (see later).

Appearance on the chest film is abnormal in approximately 75% of patients (range, 50% to 90%) and is usually more abnormal than auscultation would predict. The most frequent finding is consolidation in a single lower lobe, seen in 90% of the abnormal chest films. However, a variety of patterns have been reported, including a homogeneous ground-glass appearance, a patchy reticular pattern radiating from the hila, segmental or lobar consolidation with or without atelectasis, a miliary pattern, and unilateral or bilateral hilar enlargement. These chest film findings may take as long as 20 weeks to resolve, with resolution occurring by 6 weeks on average. Pleural effusions are seen in up to 50% of cases but are usually small and asymptomatic.[4] As noted, hilar enlargement may be present but never as the sole manifestation of disease.

Pathologic Findings

Birds show involvement predominantly in the liver, spleen, and pericardium, but in humans the lung is most frequently and characteristically involved. The trachea and bronchi become inflamed, with widespread mucous plugging. The inflammation spreads from respiratory bronchioles to the alveoli in a lobular pattern. Alveolar and then interstitial exudate accumulates; this is composed of mononuclear cells with a few polymorphonuclear leukocytes, red blood cells, epithelial cells, and fibrin. There is hyperplasia, proliferation, and desquamation of alveolar lining cells, which contain basophilic intracytoplasmic inclusions. Hilar lymph nodes swell, and the lungs become rubbery and solid. The classic sequence of congestion, edema, and red and then gray hepatization is seen.

The brain is congested and edematous, with diffuse arachnoiditis. Meningeal exudate contains macrophages with intracytoplasmic inclusions. The heart shows monocytic infiltration, edema, fatty degeneration, and subendocardial hemorrhage. The pathologic findings in acute glomerulonephritis include hyaline glomerular occlusion, with subepithelial electron-dense deposits on electron microscopy. The liver may show nonspecific hepatitis or granulomas. Infected placental tissue shows intervillositis with trophoblastic cytoplasmic inclusions.[20] In emboli, polymorphonuclear leukocytes, platelets, and fibrin are seen, but not organisms or chlamydial antigen.[14]

Diagnosis

Culture from sputum, pleural fluid, and clotted blood is possible but dangerous, and direct identification in tissue specimens is not standardized, so diagnosis depends on serology. The Centers for Disease Control and Prevention (CDC)[5] consider a confirmed case one with a compatible clinical illness plus laboratory confirmation by one of the following: a titer of 1:16 with microimmunofluorescence (MIF) IgM, culture from respiratory secretions, or a fourfold or greater rise in complement-fixing (CF) or MIF antibody to a titer of 1:32 in specimens drawn 2 weeks apart. A probable case is one associated with a compatible illness linked epidemiologically to a confirmed human case or a titer of at least 1:32 in a single specimen by CF or MIF. There are false-positive and false-negative reactions. Also, the complement fixation test is only genus-specific and does not distinguish *C. psittaci* from *C. trachomatis* or *C. pneumoniae*, both of which are common pathogens. MIF testing has greater sensitivity and specificity and is therefore preferable to the CF, but cross-reactions still occur. Thus, serologic testing remains imperfect. In addition, antibiotic therapy can delay or diminish the antibody response. PCR assay can detect *C. psittaci* in avian and human tissues[27-29] and has been used for real-time diagnosis in both birds and humans.[27,30] However, PCR is not routinely available and may yield false-negative results. Thus, none of the diagnostic methods is both reliable and rapid, and therapy for psittacosis should be initiated on the basis of clinical suspicion.

Treatment

The treatment of choice is tetracycline hydrochloride, 500 mg PO four times daily, or doxycycline, 100 mg PO twice daily, for 10 to 21 days. Some observers recommend the longer course to prevent relapse, but this is controversial. Erythromycin therapy is the alternative treatment but may be less efficacious in severe cases and may not protect the fetus when treating pregnant patients.

Anecdotal reports have suggested possible efficacy of azithromycin and chloramphenicol, and some of the newer quinolones demonstrate activity in vitro and in animal models. For example, an in vitro study of 10 strains of *C. psittaci* demonstrated a moxifloxacin minimal inhibitory concentration (MIC) range of 0.06 to 0.125 mg/L; the minimal bactericidal concentration (MBC) range was identical. MIC_{50} was 0.06 mg/L and MIC_{90} was 0.125 mg/L.[31] In a mouse model of psitta-cosis, sitafloxacin, sparfloxacin, and tosufloxacin showed promising therapeutic potency, with in vitro MIC ranges of 0.031 to 0.063 mg/L for sitafloxacin and sparfloxacin and 0.125 to 0.125 mg/L for tosufloxa-cin. MBC ranges were identical to those of the corresponding MIC. The authors also studied ofloxacin (MIC range, 0.5 to 1.0 mg/L; MBC, 0.5 to 2.0 mg/L) and ciprofloxacin (MIC range, 1.0 to 2.0 mg/L; MBC, 1.0 to 4.0 mg/L).[32] The usefulness of these latter agents awaits further clinical evaluation.

Most patients respond within 24 hours subjectively. Without treatment, the fatality rate is approximately 20%; with treatment, it drops to 1%. The best therapy for endocarditis is valve replacement and prolonged antimicrobial therapy.[5,12]

Prevention

Infected birds should be treated with tetracycline, chlortetracycline, or doxycycline for at least 45 consecutive days. The U.S. Department of Agriculture (USDA) requires that imported birds be quarantined for 30 days to prevent introduction of Newcastle disease. During this period, birds are treated with chlortetracycline. The USDA recommends that importers continue treatment for an additional 15 days, but this is not always done, and, if treated for fewer than 45 days, some infected birds will continue to shed the organism.[5]

REFERENCES

1. Harris RL, Williams TW. Contribution to the question of pneumotyphus: A discussion of the original article by J. Ritter in 1880. *Rev Infect Dis.* 1985;7:119-122.
2. Macfarlane JT, Macrae AD. Psittacosis. *Med Bull.* 1983;39:163-167.
3. Everett KD, Bush RM, Andersen AA. Emended description of the order Chlamydiales, proposal of Parachlamydiaceae fam. nov. and Simkaniaceae fam. nov., each containing one monotypic genus, revised taxonomy of the family Chlamydiaceae, including a new genus and five new species and standards for the identification of organisms. *Int J Syst Bacteriol.* 1999;49:415-440.
4. Schlossberg D, Delgado J, Moore MM, et al. An epidemic of avian and human psittacosis. *Arch Intern Med.* 1993;153:2594-2596.
5. Centers for Disease Control and Prevention. Compendium of measures to control Chlamydia psittaci infection among humans (psittacosis) and pet birds (avian chlamydiosis). *MMWR Recomm Rep.* 2000 Jul 14;49(RR-8):3-18.
6. Guay DR. Pet-assisted therapy in the nursing home setting: Potential for zoonosis. *Am J Infect Control.* 2001;29:178-186.
7. Ito I, Ishida T, Mishima M, et al. Familial cases of psittacosis: Possible person-to-person transmission. *Intern Med.* 2002;41:580-583.
8. Hughes C, Maharg P, Rosario P, et al. Possible nosocomial transmission of psittacosis. *Infect Control Hosp Epidemiol.* 1997;18:165-168.
9. Yung AP, Grayson ML. Psittacosis: A review of 135 cases. *Med J Aust.* 1988;148:228-233.
10. Schaffner W, Drutz DJ, Duncan GW, et al. The clinical spectrum of endemic psittacosis. *Arch Intern Med.* 1967;119:433-443.
11. Schinkel AFL, Bax JJ, van der Wall EE, et al. Echocardiographic follow-up of Chlamydia psittaci myocarditis. *Chest.* 2000;117:1203-1205.
12. Patel RT, Jekinson LR, Wheeler MH, et al. Arterial embolism associated with psittacosis. *J R Soc Med.* 1991;84:374-375.
13. Timmerman R, Bieger R. Haemolytic anemia due to cold agglutinins caused by psittacosis. *Neth J Med.* 1989;34:306-309.
14. Wong KF, Chan JKC, Chan CH, et al. Psittacosis-associated hemophagocytic syndrome. *Am J Med.* 1991;91:204-205.
15. Zumla A, Lipscomb G, Lewis D. Sixth cranial nerve palsy complicating psittacosis. *J Neurol Neurosurg Psychiatry.* 1988;51:1462.
16. Newton P, Lalvani A, Conlon CP. Psittacosis associated with bilateral 4th cranial nerve palsies. *J Infect.* 1996;32:63-65.
17. Crook T, Bannister B. Acute transverse myelitis associated with Chlamydia psittaci infection. *J Infect.* 1996;32:151-152.
18. Brewis C, McFerran J. Farmer's ear: Sudden sensorineural hearing loss due to Chlamydia psittaci infection. *J Laryngol Otol.* 1997;111:855-857.
19. Shee CD. Cerebellar disturbance in psittacosis. *Postgrad Med J.* 1988;64:382-383.
20. Hyde SR, Benirschke K. Gestational psittacosis: Case report and literature review. *Mod Pathol.* 1997;10:602-607.
21. Jorgensen DM. Gestational psittacosis in a Montana sheep rancher. *Emerg Infect Dis.* 1997;3:191-194.
22. Husain A, Roberts D, Pro B, et al. Meta-analyses of the association between Chlamydia psittaci and ocular adnexal lymphoma and the response of ocular adnexal lymphoma to antibiotics. *Cancer.* 2007;110:809-815.
23. Chanudet E, Zhou Y, Bacon CM, et al. Chlamydia psittaci is variably associated with ocular adnexal MALT lymphoma in different geographical regions. *J Pathol.* 2006;209:344-351.
24. Vargas RL, Fallone E, Felgar RE, et al. Is there an association between ocular adnexal lymphoma and infection with Chlamydia psittaci? The University of Rochester experience. *Leuk Res.* 2006;30:547-551.
25. Zucca E, Bertoni F. Chlamydia or not Chlamydia, that is the question: which is the microorganism associated with MALT lymphomas of the ocular adnexa? *J Natl Cancer Inst.* 2006;98:1348-1349.
26. Ferreri AJ, Ponzoni M, Guidoboni M, et al. Bacteria-eradicating therapy with doxycycline in ocular adnexal MALT lymphoma: a multicenter prospective trial. *Natl Cancer Inst.* 2006;98:1375-1382.
27. Branley JM, Roy B, Dwyer DE, et al. Real-time PCR detection and quantitation of Chlamydophila psittaci in human and avian specimens from a veterinary clinic cluster. *Eur J Clin Microbiol Infect Dis.* 2008;27:269-273.
28. Laroucau K, Trichereau A, Vorimore F, et al. A pmp genes-based PCR as a valuable tool for the diagnosis of avian chlamydiosis. *Vet Microbiol.* 2007;121:150-157.
29. Sareyyupoglu B, Cantekin Z, Bas B. Chlamydophila psittaci DNA detection in the faeces of cage birds. *Zoonoses Public Health.* 2007;54:237-242.
30. Heddema ER, van Hannen EJ, Duim B, et al. An outbreak of psittacosis due to Chlamydophila psittaci genotype A in a veterinary teaching hospital. *J Med Microbiol.* 2006;55(Pt 11):1571-1575.
31. Donati M, Rodriguez FM, Olmo A, et al. Comparative in vitro activity of moxifloxacin, minocycline and azithromycin against Chlamydia spp. *J Antimicrob Chemother.* 1999;43:825-827.
32. Miyashita N, Niki Y, Matsushima T. In vitro and in vivo activities of sitafloxacin against Chlamydia spp. *Antimicrob Agents Chemother.* 2001;45:3270-3272.

182

Chlamydophila (Chlamydia) pneumoniae

MARGARET R. HAMMERSCHLAG | STEPHAN A. KOHLHOFF | PETRA M. APFALTER

Chlamydiae are obligate intracellular bacterial pathogens whose entry into mucosal epithelial cells is necessary for intracellular survival and subsequent growth. Chlamydiae cause a variety of diseases in animal species at virtually all phylogenic levels, from amphibians and reptiles to birds and mammals. The order originally contained one genus, Chlamydia, with four recognized species: Chlamydia trachomatis, Chlamydia psittaci, Chlamydia pneumoniae, and Chlamydia pecorum. C. trachomatis and C. pneumoniae are the most important as human pathogens. Taxonomic analysis with the 16S and 23S ribosomal RNA (rRNA) genes have found that the order Chlamydiales contains at least four distinct groups at the family level and that within the family Chlamydiaceae are two distinct lineages.[1] This analysis has suggested splitting the genus Chlamydia into two genera, Chlamydia and Chlamydophila. Two new species, Chlamydia muridarum (formerly MoPn, the agent of mouse pneumonitis) and Chlamydia suis (gastrointestinal infection in swine), would join C. trachomatis. Chlamydophila contains C. pecorum (infection in cattle, sheep and koalas), C. pneumoniae, and C. psittaci (infection primarily in avian species; causes psittacosis in humans) and three new species split off from C. psittaci: Chlamydia abortus (ovine and bovine abortion), Chlamydia caviae (formerly C. psittaci guinea pig conjunctivitis strain), and Chlamydia felis (keratoconjunctivitis in cats). Continuing controversy surrounds this reclassification, but for the purposes of this chapter, we continue to refer to Chlamydophila as Chlamydia.

History

The first isolates of C. pneumoniae were serendipitously obtained during trachoma studies in the 1960s. After the recovery of a similar isolate from the respiratory tract of a college student with pneumonia in Seattle, Grayston and colleagues[2] applied the designation TWAR after their first two isolates, TW-183 and AR-39. On the basis of inclusion morphology and staining characteristics in cell culture, C. pneumoniae was initially considered to be a novel strain of C. psittaci; however, subsequent analyses showed that this organism is distinct from both C. psittaci and C. trachomatis.[3] Ultrastructural studies showed that the elementary bodies (EB) of C. pneumoniae had a pear-shaped appearance caused by a loose periplasmic membrane, whereas the elementary bodies of C. trachomatis and C. psittaci are round.[4] The presence of pear-shaped EBs does not appear to be a consistent species-defining characteristic because other C. pneumoniae isolates have been found to have round EBs. Only one serotype of C. pneumoniae has been identified so far. Genetic studies have found a high degree of genetic relatedness (greater than 98%) among human C. pneumoniae isolates tested.[5]

Microbiology

Chlamydiae have a Gram-negative envelope without detectable peptidoglycan; however, recent genomic analysis has revealed that both C. trachomatis and C. pneumoniae encode for proteins that form a nearly complete pathway for synthesis of peptidoglycan, including penicillin-binding proteins.[6] Chlamydiae also share a group-specific lipopolysaccharide antigen and use host adenosine triphosphate (ATP) for the synthesis of chlamydial protein.[6] Although chlamydiae are auxotrophic for three of four nucleoside triphosphates, they do encode functional glucose-catabolizing enzymes, which can be used for generation

of ATP.[6] As with peptidoglycan synthesis, for some reason, these genes are turned off, which may be related to their adaptation to the intracellular environment. All chlamydiae also encode an abundant protein called the major outer membrane protein (MOMP or OmpA) that is surface exposed in C. trachomatis and C. psittaci but apparently not in C. pneumoniae.[6] The MOMP is the major determinant of the serologic classification of C. trachomatis and C. psittaci isolates. Chlamydiae are susceptible to antibiotics that interfere with DNA and protein synthesis, including tetracyclines, macrolides, and quinolones.

Chlamydiae have a unique developmental cycle with morphologically distinct infectious and reproductive forms: elementary body (EB) and reticulate body (RB; Fig. 182-1). After infection, the infectious EBs, which are 200 to 400 nm in diameter, attach to the host cell by a process of electrostatic binding and are taken into the cell by endocytosis that does not depend on the microtubule system. EBs are spore-like; they are metabolically inactive but stable in the extracellular environment. Within the host cell, the EB remains within a membrane-lined phagosome with inhibition of phagosomal-lysosomal fusion. The inclusion membrane is devoid of host cell markers, but lipid markers traffic to the inclusion, which suggests a functional interaction with the Golgi apparatus. Chlamydiae appear to circumvent the host endocytic pathway, inhabiting a nonacidic vacuole, which is dissociated from late endosomes and lysosomes. EBs then differentiate into RBs that undergo binary fission. After approximately 36 hours, the reticulate bodies differentiate back into elementary bodies. Despite the accumulation of 500 to 1000 infectious EBs in the inclusion, host cell function is minimally disrupted. At about 48 hours, release may occur via cytolysis or a process of exocytosis or extrusion of the whole inclusion, leaving the host cell intact. This strategy is very successful and enables the organism to cause essentially silent chronic infection.

A number of in vitro studies have challenged this biphasic paradigm. Chlamydiae may enter a persistent state in vitro after treatment with certain cytokines such as gamma-interferon (IFN-γ); treatment with antibiotics, specifically penicillin; restriction of certain nutrients, including iron, glucose, and amino acids; infection in monocytes; and heat shock.[7] While in the persistent state, metabolic activity is reduced and the organism is often refractory to antibiotic treatment. These different systems produce similar growth characteristics, including loss of infectivity and development of small inclusions that contain fewer EBs and RBs and ultrastructural findings, specifically morphologically abnormal RBs, which suggests that they are somehow altered during their otherwise normal development. These abnormal RBs are often called aberrant bodies (ABs). Restriction of certain nutrients has also been shown to induce persistence in chlamydiae. Ultrastructural analysis of IFN-γ–treated C. pneumoniae also reveals atypical inclusions that contain large reticulate-like aberrant bodies with no evidence of redifferentiation into EBs.

Another model of persistent C. pneumoniae infection is long-term continuous infection. In contrast to the previously described models, continuous cultures become spontaneously persistent when both chlamydiae and host cells multiply freely in the absence of stress. C. pneumoniae infection was maintained in HEp-2 and A549 cells for more than 4 years without centrifugation, addition of cycloheximide, or IFN-γ.[8] Infection levels in these infected cells were high (70% to 80%). Ultrastructural studies revealed three types of inclusions in these cells. Approximately 90% were typical large inclusions that ranged approxi-

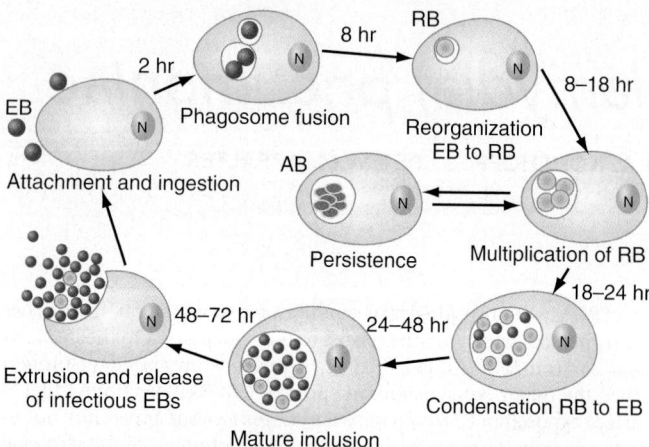

Figure 182-1 Life cycle of Chlamydiae in epithelial cells. EB, elementary body; N, nucleus; RB, reticulate body. *(Modified from Hammerschlag MR, Kohlhoff SA, Darville T:* Chlamydia pneumoniae *and* Chlamydia trachomatis. *In Fratamico PM, Smith JL, Brogden KA, editors:* Post-Infectious Sequelae and Long-Term Consequences of Infectious Diseases, *Washington, DC, 2008, American Society for Microbiology.)*

mately from 5 to 12 μm in diameter. The second type (altered inclusions) contained both normal EBs and RBs, but in considerably lower numbers than typical inclusions, and pleomorphic aberrant bodies, which were up to four to five times the size of normal RBs (2.5 μm in diameter); their cytoplasm was homogeneous.

The third type of inclusion was small aberrant inclusions, on average 4 μm in diameter, that contained about 60 aberrant bodies (ABs) that were similar in size to normal RBs but appeared electron dense and no longer retained smooth spherical shape. These dense ABs retained the characteristic chlamydial outer membrane structure, with very little periplasmic space, and the membranes more tightly bound to the chlamydial body, similar to normal RBs. No EBs were observed in these inclusions. These findings show that the developmental cycle of *C. pneumoniae* can combine the typical development forms with the persistent phase in tissue culture.

Another possible mechanism of chlamydial persistence could be through direct effect on the host cell, possibly through an effect on apoptosis, which is an important regulator of cell growth and tissue development. Apoptosis is a genetically programmed, tightly controlled process, unlike necrosis, which involves nonspecific inflammation and tissue damage and intracellular enzymes, condensation of nucleus, and cytoplasm and fragmentation. Many microbial pathogens, including chlamydia, have been found to modulate cellular apoptosis to survive and multiply. *Chlamydia* spp. have been shown to both induce and inhibit host cell apoptosis, depending on the stage of the chlamydial developmental cycle.[9] Chlamydiae protect infected cells against apoptosis as a result of external stimuli during early stages of infection and induce apoptosis of the host cell during later stages. Thus, chlamydiae may protect infected cells against cytotoxic mechanisms of the immune system, and the apoptosis observed at the end of the infection cycle may contribute to the inflammatory response, as apoptotic cells secrete proinflammatory cytokines, and facilitate the release of the organism from the infected cells. Studies with IFN-γ–treated cultures have reported that cells infected with *C. trachomatis* and *C. pneumoniae* resist apoptosis as the result of external ligands, via inhibition of caspace activation. Data from studies with the long-term continuously infected cell model showed marked differences in the effect of *C. pneumoniae* on apoptosis in acute and chronically infected A-549 cells.[9] Acute *C. pneumoniae* infection *induced* apoptotic changes in A-549 cells within the first 24 and 48 hours after infection. Induction of apoptosis in acute infection may facilitate release of *C. pneumoniae* from the host cell. Chronic *C. pneumoniae* infection *inhibited* apoptotic changes within the first 24 hours and up to 7 days. These results

suggest that inhibition of apoptosis may help to protect the organism when it is in the persistent state.

Laboratory Testing for *C. pneumoniae*

Although numerous methods can be used to detect *C. pneumoniae* in clinical samples, in practice, detection is very difficult, primarily because of the lack of standardized well-validated methods. Determination of whether *C. pneumoniae* infection is acute primary infection or reinfection, a chronic persistent stage, or past infection is also very difficult. Cell culture, immunohistochemistry (IHC), and nucleic acid amplification techniques detect living bacteria, antigen, or nucleic acid, respectively. These techniques are primarily used in research settings or require at least experienced specialized laboratories. Thus, in clinical settings and everyday routine diagnosis of *C. pneumoniae*, infection is still based on results of serologic testing to identify anti–*C. pneumoniae* immunoglobulin G, A, and M antibodies. This approach is problematic for a number of reasons subsequently outlined in detail.

CELL CULTURE

C. pneumoniae, as an obligate intracellular parasite, can be isolated by means of cell culture, but the organism is fastidious and slow growing. *C. pneumoniae* has been isolated from the respiratory tract (nasopharyngeal and throat cultures, bronchoalveolar lavage fluids) and tissue biopsies, including lung and adenoids. The organism can also be isolated from sputum, but sputum can be toxic to cell culture and often is contaminated by overgrowing fungi or bacteria. If nasopharyngeal or pharyngeal swab specimens are collected, use of aluminum or plastic-shafted Dacron tip swabs is mandatory because calcium alginate or cotton tips and those with wooden shafts may inhibit the growth of the organism in tissue culture and may be toxic to cells. Specimens for culture must be stored in a suitable transport medium optimized for chlamydia. A suitable medium is sucrose-phosphate-glutamic (SPG) buffer with antibiotics and fetal calf serum, but ready-to-use media are also commercially available.

Specimens that can be processed within 24 hours should be kept refrigerated at 4°C and shipped on wet ice. Samples that cannot be processed within 24 hours should be held at 4°C before freezing at −70°C because more rapid freezing decreases the titer of viable organisms. Specimens need to be centrifuged onto the cell monolayers to facilitate absorption.

Before centrifugation and inoculation, specimens also need to be treated with sterile glass beads or sonification to disrupt cells that potentially contain chlamydiae. Usually cell cultures (various cell types are possible; most studies were performed with HEp-2 cells) are incubated at 37°C with 5% CO_2 for at least 72 hours per passage. Culture confirmation is assessed with immunofluorescence staining, which requires a high level of experience to avoid false misinterpretation of unspecific staining from overlaying material from clinical specimens as chlamydial inclusions or elementary bodies (Fig. 182-2). Depending on specimen and cell culture type, more than one subculture may be necessary for isolation; thus, culture is not a straightforward attempt to diagnose the microorganism in a timely fashion. In addition to preanalytic shortcomings and special growth requirements of this fastidious pathogen, another possible reason for the low isolation rate may be the loss of infectivity of *C. pneumoniae* under in vitro conditions.

ANTIGEN DETECTION

C. pneumoniae has also been detected in tissue sections or cells with monoclonal antibodies labeled with a peroxidase (immunohistochemistry) or fluorescent (immunofluorescent) marker. Antigen detection testing, in general, allows preservation of tissue morphology. On the other hand, interpretation of the staining pattern to distinguish the organism from background or nonspecific staining is subjective and influenced by a number of technical issues.[5] In complex biologic

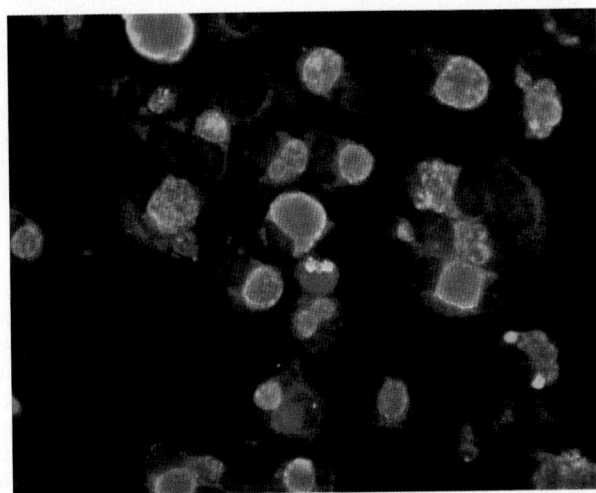

Figure 182-2 Direct immunofluorescence staining of cell culture 72 hours after infection. The *apple-green C. pneumoniae* inclusion bodies are seen in *red* counterstained HEp-2 cells. Magnification, ×600. *(Courtesy of P. Apfalter.)*

samples, IHC gives rise to cross reactions between antitarget antibodies and nontarget proteins that produce nonspecific signals (e.g., immunoreactivity for *C. pneumoniae* was frequently present in atheroma and nonatheroma sections of vessel walls). The sites with positive results with *C. pneumoniae* IHC assays precisely matched the sites with autofluorescent ceroid deposits.[10] The interpretation of IHC staining must be performed with uttermost caution.

NUCLEIC ACID AMPLIFICATION TECHNIQUES

In 2000, a group of experts suggested a few conventional polymerase chain reaction (PCR) assays to create highly accurate results for detection of *C. pneumoniae* DNA.[5] Nearly a decade later, however, these tests turned out to be highly prone to false-positive results.[11,12] As of November 2008, not a single nucleic acid amplification technique (NAAT) for the detection of *C. pneumoniae* was listed in the in vitro diagnostic (IVD) database of the Food and Drug Administration (http://www.accessdata.fda.gov/ scripts/cdrh/cfdocs/cfivd/index.cfm). First CE-marked (approval to offer in vitro diagnostic tests in the European Common Market) PCR-based tests for *C. pneumoniae* are commercially available, but clinical validation in defined clinical settings (e.g., community-acquired pneumonia) is scarce. For this reason, numerous in-house PCR-based tests still are performed, but these assays range from those that are well validated to those that are not validated at all. Although NAATs offer the promise of exquisite sensitivity, theoretically allowing for detection of a single organism in a clinical sample, both false-negative and -positive results can and do occur because of a large number of technical issues that were summarized recently.[13]

Currently, real-time PCR technology for the detection of *C. pneumoniae* should be used. Only a few centers have published data on how protocols were evaluated in terms of specificity, sensitivity, and reproducibility of test results, also enrolling various patient specimens,[14,15] which seems to be most important because the analytic sensitivity of an assay for detection of *C. pneumoniae* does not necessarily predict the ability to detect its target in clinical specimens.[16] Real-time PCR offers significant advantages over conventional PCR in its rapidity, the ease with which it can be automated, the potential decreased risk of carryover contamination, and the potential provision of a quantitative result. The clinical value of the latter remains to be clarified. To date, at least 12 real-time PCR-based protocols for the detection of *C. pneumoniae* have been published (http://www.chlamydiae.com/restricted/docs/Methods/tech_quantitative_pcr.asp.). Specimens for PCR testing include nasopharyngeal swabs, secretions from the respiratory tract

inclusive sputum and bronchoalveolar lavage fluid (BAL), tissue, and peripheral blood mononuclear cells. Swabs should be sent in tubes without transport medium. Sputum, BAL, and tissue should also be collected in a sterile device without transport medium. If necessary, sputum can be diluted by homogenizing it with TRIS-EDTA buffer. Tissue has to be homogenized before DNA extraction. If DNA extraction for PCR is performed within 24 hours, storage at 4°C is sufficient; otherwise, specimens should be kept at least at –20°C.

SEROLOGIC TESTING

Several types of serologic assays are currently commercially available for the detection of antibodies to *C. pneumoniae*. However, none are currently approved by the US Food and Drug Administration (FDA) for this indication. The test used most frequently and recommended by the Centers for Disease Control and Prevention (CDC) remains the micro-immunofluorescence (MIF) assay.[5] Tests based on an enzyme-linked immunosorbent assay (ELISA) format are in particular easy to perform and do not need sophisticated laboratory equipment, which makes them the preferentially offered diagnostic chlamydial tool for laboratories. *C. pneumoniae*, however, is an intracellular pathogen, and the poor correlation between direct detection (e.g., with culture or NAAT) and serologic results is not surprising. Besides specificity issues, which classes and titers of antibodies might represent acute first or reinfection, chronic, persistent, or past *C. pneumoniae* infection is not clear at all.[5] This is true for complement fixation tests (measurement of antibodies to chlamydial lipopolysaccharide; therefore, not specific for *C. pneumoniae*), ELISA-based tests (purified *C. pneumoniae* elementary bodies or recombinant antigens detected; specificity unclear), and also the gold standard MIF (formalinized *C. pneumoniae* elementary bodies fixed onto glass slides). A serologic test can only be as specific as the antigen used. Cross reactivity between *C. pneumoniae* and other *Chlamydia* species has been shown with the MIF test. Factors like strain type, purity, and concentration of antigen used and the assay procedure itself might contribute to the fact that the MIF is less specific for *C. pneumoniae* than thought 20 years ago. Data also show significant problems with subjective interpretation and intralaboratory and interlaboratory reproducibility.[17] The problems in context with *C. pneumoniae* serology have been discussed in detail in two recently published review articles.[18,19] For an example of the complexity of this issue, consider: Two multicenter pneumonia treatment studies showed that although 7% to 13% of the patients in the study had positive culture results and 7% to 18% met the serologic criteria with the MIF for acute infection, they were not the same patients. Only 1% to 3% of the patients with positive culture results met the serologic criteria, and approximately 70% with positive culture results for *C. pneumoniae* were seronegative.[20] Another problem with serologic diagnosis of *C. pneumoniae* infection is that the MIF method used to detect serum antibodies is not standardized; recent studies have shown substantial interlaboratory variation in the performance of these tests.[17] In summary, serology seems not only to be insufficient for diagnosis of *C. pneumoniae* respiratory tract infection but also to be an inadequate methodology to study associations between *C. pneumoniae* and other diseases.

Chlamydiae are a unique group of obligate intracellular bacteria that compose important pathogens of vertebrates and symbionts of free-living amoebae. In this context, it is important to know that new environmental *Chlamydia* species are steadily described.[21,22] Ample evidence exists for a huge diversity and wide distribution of *Chlamydiae* in nature—and men are exposed to that diversity of species. As an example, the recovery of a novel environmental *Chlamydia* strain from activated sludge with cocultivation with *Acanthamoeba* sp. was reported; it was shown to also invade mammalian cells. These new environmental *Chlamydiae* (i.e., *Simkania*, *Waddlia*, and *Parachlamydia*) may significantly interfere with diagnostic testing for traditional *Chlamydiaceae* (i.e., *Chlamydophila* and *Chlamydia*).

In summary, *C. pneumoniae* serology is most problematic in terms of specificity and reproducibility and what titer, even if prospectively defined, may mean what in a given clinical picture or disease.

Epidemiology

C. pneumoniae appears to be a common human respiratory pathogen; however, the organism has also been isolated from nonhuman species, including a horse, koalas, bandicoots, and amphibians. The role these infections may play in human disease is unknown.[23] The mode of transmission remains uncertain but probably occurs through infected respiratory secretions. Acquisition of infection via droplet aerosol was described during a laboratory accident.[24] *C. pneumoniae* can remain viable on Formica countertops for 30 hours and can survive small-particle aerosolization.[25] Spread within families and enclosed populations, such as military recruits and nursing homes, has been described.[26]

Several serologic surveys have documented rising chlamydial antibody prevalence rates, beginning in school-aged children and reaching 30% to 45% by adolescence.[2] Seroprevalence rate of antibody, as determined with the MIF method, can exceed 80% in some adult populations.[27,28] The proportion of community-acquired pneumonia in children and adults associated with *C. pneumoniae* infection has ranged from 0 to more than 44%, varying with geographic location, the age group examined, and the diagnostic methods used (Table 182-1).[29] Early studies that relied on serology suggested that infection in children younger than 5 years of age was rare; however, subsequent studies with culture or PCR have found the prevalence rate of infection in children beyond early infancy to be similar to that found in adults.[29] Approximately 50% or more children with culture-documented *C. pneumoniae* respiratory infection (pneumonia and asthma) show seronegativity with the MIF.[20,29] Prolonged respiratory infection, documented with culture, that lasts from several weeks to several years after acute infection has been reported.[30]

Coinfections with other organisms, specifically *Streptococcus pneumoniae* and *Mycoplasma pneumoniae*, may occur frequently.[31] Clinically, these patients cannot be differentiated from those infected with a single organism. In these cases, *C. pneumoniae* may not be the primary cause of the pneumonia but might disrupt the normal clearance mechanisms and enable other pathogens to invade. Asymptomatic respiratory infection may occur in 2% to 5% of adults and children.[27,32] What role asymptomatic carriage plays in the epidemiology of *C. pneumoniae* is not known. Acute respiratory infection with *C. pneumoniae* does not appear to vary by season, but no systematic surveillance for *C. pneumoniae* infection exists in the United States.

Clinical Manifestations

Most respiratory infections from *C. pneumoniae* are probably mild or asymptomatic. Initial reports emphasized mild atypical pneumonia clinically resembling that associated with *M. pneumoniae*.[2] Subsequent studies have found that pneumonia associated with *C. pneumoniae* has been clinically indistinguishable from other pneumonias.[27,31] *C. pneumoniae* has been associated with severe illness and even death, although the role of preexisting chronic conditions as contributing factors in many of these patients is difficult to assess. *C. pneumoniae* can be a serious pathogen even in the absence of underlying disease. *C. pneumoniae* was isolated from the respiratory tract and the pleural fluid of a previously healthy adolescent boy with severe pneumonia complicated by respiratory failure and pleural effusions.[33]

The role of host factors remains to be determined. Although *C. pneumoniae* has been detected in bronchoalveolar lavage fluid from 10% of a group of patients with AIDS and pneumonia, its clinical role in these patients is uncertain because most were coinfected with other well-recognized pathogens such as *Pneumocystis carinii* and *Mycobacterium tuberculosis*.[34] Gaydos and colleagues[35] identified *C. pneumoniae* infection with PCR in 11% of a group of immunocompromised adults with HIV infection, malignant neoplasms, and other immune disorders, including systemic lupus erythematosus, sarcoidosis, and common variable immunodeficiency. *C. pneumoniae* appeared to be responsible for six of 31 episodes (19%) of acute chest syndrome in children with sickle cell disease.[36] *C. pneumoniae* infection in these patients appeared to be associated with more severe hypoxia than was infection with *M. pneumoniae*.

The relationship of *C. pneumoniae* and upper respiratory infections, including pharyngitis, sinusitis, and otitis media, is less clear.

Treatment

Data on treatment of *C. pneumoniae* respiratory infection are limited. *C. pneumoniae* is susceptible to antibiotics that affect DNA and protein synthesis, including macrolides; azalide, specifically azithromycin; tetracyclines; and quinolones (Table 182-2). However, in vitro activity may not always predict in vivo efficacy. Most published pneumonia treatment studies have used serology alone for diagnosis of *C. pneumoniae* infection, which is at best a clinical endpoint. Results of several multicenter treatment studies that used culture showed 70% to 86% efficacy of treatment with erythromycin, clarithromycin, azithromycin, levofloxacin, and moxifloxacin in eradicating *C. pneumoniae* from the nasopharynx of children and adults with community-acquired pneumonia.[37] Most patients had clinical improvement despite persistence of the organism. Persistence did not appear to be the result of the development of antibiotic resistance because the minimum inhibitory concentrations (MICs) of the isolates obtained after treatment did not change. Antibiotic resistance is unusual in chlamydiae. Investigators were unable to select for macrolide resistance after passage of *C.*

TABLE 182-1	Summary of Selected Studies of Respiratory Infection from *C. pneumoniae* in Adults and Children Published Since 2001			
Location	*Age (No. Tested)*	*Diagnostic Methods*	*No. Positive*	*Comments*
United Kingdom	>16 y (316)	Serology,* gene amplification	55 (17%)	All positive with serology
Netherlands	1-88 y (159)	EIA, PstI-based PCR	5 (3.1%)	All positive with serology alone
Netherlands	≥18 y (107)	Conventional test or PCR†	0	Test not described
Taiwan	17-99 y (168)	MIF	12 (7.1%)	
Sweden†	Adults Patients: (125) Controls: (113)	MIF, multiplex PCR	Patients: 3 (1.3%) Controls: 0	Multiplex PCRs may have lower sensitivity
Japan	17-99 y (232)	MIF, PCR, culture	15 (6.5%)	Proportion of results positive with each test not stated
Germany	≥18 y (546)	MIF, PCR	5 (0.9%)	All 5 positive with 2 different PCR assays, negative with MIF
Italy	2-14 y (613)	MIF, nested MOMP based PCR	87 (14.1%)	52 positive with serology, of which 13 confirmed with PCR and 35 with PCR alone
Thailand	1 m-15 y (333)	MIF	149 (44.7%)	14 of 149 positive with single titers
United States	6 wk-18 y (154)	MIF, EIA	14 (9%)	Proportion positive with MIF and EIA not stated

EIA, enzyme immunoassay; MIF, microimmunofluorescence; MOMP, major outer membrane protein; PCR, polymerase chain reaction.
*PCR or serology method not described.
†Study enrolled both patients and age-matched controls.
Modified from Kumar S, Hammerschlag MR. Acute respiratory infection due to *Chlamydia pneumoniae*: Current status of diagnostic methods. *Clin Infect Dis.* 2007;44:568-576.

| TABLE 182-2 | Comparative In Vitro Activities of Currently Available Antimicrobials against *C. pneumoniae* |

TABLE 182-2	Comparative In Vitro Activities of Currently Available Antimicrobials against *C. pneumoniae*

Antimicrobial Agent	MIC Range (μg/mL)
Doxycycline	0.015-0.5
Tigecylcine	0.125-0.25
Erythromycin	0.015-0.25
Roxithromycin	0.0625-2
Azithromycin	0.05-0.25
Clarithromycin	0.004-0.03
Telithromycin	0.015-0.25
Ciprofloxacin	1-4
Levofloxacin	0.25-1
Moxifloxacin	0.125-1
Gatifloxacin	0.125-0.25
Rifampin	0.0075-0.03
Trimethoprim	≥128
Sulfamethoxazole	≥500

Modified from Kumar S, Kutlin S, Roblin P, et al. Isolation and antimicrobial susceptibilities of chlamydial isolates from western barred bandicoots. *J Clin Microbiol.* 2007;45:392-394.

pneumoniae in subinhibitory concentrations of azithromycin.[38] In contrast, resistance to quinolones has been selected in vitro after passage of *C. pneumoniae* in subinhibitory concentrations of moxifloxacin.[39] These isolates were found to have a point mutation in the GyrA gene.[39] Studies with long-term continuously infected cells suggest that *C. pneumoniae* may be refractory to antibiotics when in the persistent state.[40]

On the basis of these few data, the following regimens can be used for respiratory infection from *C. pneumoniae*: in adults, doxycycline, 100 mg orally twice daily for 14 to 21 days; tetracycline, 250 mg orally four times daily for 14 to 21 days; azithromycin, 1.5 g orally over 5 days; clarithromycin, 500 mg orally twice a day for 10 days; levofloxa-cin, 500 mg, intravenously or orally once a day for 7 to 14 days; or moxifloxacin, 400 mg orally once a day for 10 days. For children, erythromycin suspension, 50 mg/kg per day for 10 to 14 days; clarithromycin suspension, 15 mg/kg per day for 10 days; or azithromycin suspension, 10 mg/kg once a day followed by 5 mg/kg once daily for 4 days. Some patients may need retreatment.

C. PNEUMONIAE AND CHRONIC DISEASE IN HUMANS

One of the distinguishing characteristics of chlamydiae is the ability to cause persistent, often subclinical infections. From a clinical standpoint, chlamydia may be the persistent infection par excellence, capable of persisting in the host for months to years, often without causing obvious illness. From a microbiologic standpoint, persistence also refers to long-term intracellular infection that can be detected with antigen, microscopy, or nucleic acid-based amplification methods. Chronic persistent infection with *C. pneumoniae* has been implicated in the pathogenesis of several chronic diseases, initially not thought to be infectious, including asthma, arthritis, and atherosclerosis. However, studies of the association of *C. pneumoniae* and these disorders have been hampered with difficulty in diagnosis of chronic persistent infection with the organism, which, in turn, makes determination of the efficacy of interventions, especially with antibiotics, difficult.

C. PNEUMONIAE AND ASTHMA

Infection with *C. pneumoniae* has been linked to asthma by a large number of epidemiologic and clinical studies. The controversy about definition of infection and diagnostic tests contributes to the difficulty in interpretation and comparison of studies. The field is further complicated by differences in study populations in regard to asthma phenotype and the presence of acute symptoms. Table 182-3 summarizes selected studies that have examined the association of *C. pneumoniae* infection and asthma. The wide range of positivity illustrates the some-

TABLE 182-3	Summary of Clinical Studies of the Role of *C. pneumoniae* in Asthma

Population (Year)	No. with Asthma/ Control	Culture+ Asthma/ Control (%)	PCR+ Asthma/ Control (%)	Serology– MIF Asthma/Control	Comments
United States, adults (1991)	365	–	–	Positive correlation between IgG titers (MIF) and wheezing	
Italy, adults (1994)	74/–	–	–	IgG seroconversion (10%/–)	Asthmatics with acute exacerbation
United States, children (1994)	118/41	11/4.9	–	No significant difference in IgG titers between groups; 58% of culture+ asthmatics without IgG/IgM response	Asthmatics with acute exacerbation
Japan, adults (1998)	168/108	1.2/0	5.4/0.9	Higher prevalence rate of IgG and IgA in asthmatics (85%/68% and 48%/17%); mean IgG titers: 39/18	Asthmatics with acute exacerbation
Great Britain, adults (1998)	123/1518	–	–	No difference in prevalence rate of IgG titers (≥512 and ≥64-256) between groups (5.7%/5.7% and 15%/13%, respectively)	IgG ≥ 64-256 more common in subgroup of severe asthmatics (34.8%)
New Zealand, children, adults (2000)	96/102	–	–	No positive correlation between diagnosis of asthma and IgG titer at 11 y and 21 y of age	Asthma-enriched birth cohort; self-reported asthma
Italy, children (2000)	71/80	–	8/2.5	Serologic response consistent with acute infection: 13%/0%	Asthmatics with acute exacerbation
United States, adults (2001)	55/11	0/0	12.7*/0	Serologic response consistent with acute infection in 42% of PCR+ asthmatics	Stable asthmatics
Great Britain, adults (2004)	74/74	–	22†/9†	–	Cases: stable atopic asthmatics; Controls: nonatopic spouses
Finland, adults (2005)	83/162	–	–	No difference in titers or conversion rates	Population-based cohort
Finland, adults (2006)	103/30	–	21‡/37	–	Stable asthmatics

*Respiratory specimens obtained from lower airway (bronchoalveolar lavage, biopsy, or airway brushing).
†Positivity rate during 3-month (October to December) longitudinal study (at least one positive sample obtained on repeat sampling).
‡Positivity rate in mild asthmatics: 20.8%; moderate asthmatics: 22%.
Ig, immunoglobulin; MIF, microimmunofluorescence; PCR, polymerase chain reaction.
Modified from Hammerschlag MR, Kohlhoff SA, Darville T. *Chlamydia pneumoniae* and *Chlamydia trachomatis.* In Fratamico PM, Smith JL, Brogden KA, editors. *Post-Infectious Sequelae and Long-Term Consequences of Infectious Diseases.* Washington, DC: American Society for Microbiology; 2008.

times contradictory findings regarding an association between *C. pneumoniae* and asthma, some of which may be explained by differences in populations and diagnostic methods.

In 1991, Hahn and colleagues[41] reported an association between serologic evidence of acute *C. pneumoniae* infection and adult-onset asthma and asthmatic bronchitis in the United States. Studies that have shown an association or lack of association between the presence of antibodies (immunoglobulins G, M, and A [IgG, IgM, and IgA, respectively]) and higher antibody titers (IgG) against *C. pneumoniae* with asthma have been reported since then in a variety of populations.[42] Studies that used direct detection methods (culture or PCR) were more consistent in establishing a role of *C. pneumoniae* in exacerbations of asthma (see Table 182-2). Evidence for infection with *C. pneumoniae* of up 22% with PCR, alone or in combination with *M. pneumoniae*, in patients with stable asthma symptoms may suggest chronic infection.[42] The clinical implications of *C. pneumoniae* infection in patients with asthma who have no acute symptoms are not clear; the obvious concern is that the persistent presence of the pathogen may lead to ongoing inflammation and thus contribute to severity and progression of asthma.[43] Currently, minimal data exist to examine the immunologic basis for the association between *C. pneumoniae* and asthma pathology. Persistent infection with *C. pneumoniae*, which has been shown in patients with asthma, might be the result of an insufficient Th1 response in these patients, which is critical for clearance of the intracellular bacterium.[32,44] In analogy to the correlation of abnormal host immune response to *C. trachomatis* infection and tissue sequelae, a similar relationship may conceivably exist between respiratory infection with *C. pneumoniae* and asthma pathology.[45] Abnormal cellular immune responses to respiratory infections with *C. pneumoniae* in patients with asthma may in part be related to genetic variation in immune mediator genes.[46] Differences in *C. pneumoniae* IgG antibody responses were seen in children with asthma depending on variant mannose-binding lectin alleles.[47] In addition, human T lymphocyte clones raised against *C. pneumoniae* elementary body antigens showed IFN-γ production in the context of the human leukocyte antigen (HLA) DR4 molecule, and interleukin (IL)–4 production was linked to antigen recognition in the context of the HLA DR15 molecule.[48] An association between wheezing and anti–*C. pneumoniae* immunoglobulin E (IgE) in children infected with *C. pneumoniae* was shown, which suggests a Th2 response to the bacterium in patients with asthma.[49] The role of stress and host genetics in delayed or suboptimal Th1 response to chlamydial infection and development of complications in certain individuals, and the role of specific *C. pneumoniae* antigens eliciting harmful immune responses in patients with asthma, is unclear.

Treatment

If infection with *C. pneumoniae* contributes to inflammation in patients with allergic asthma, diagnosis and treatment of these infections is important. Interactions may also exist between *C. pneumoniae* infection and asthma drugs. Treatment of asthma exacerbations frequently includes systemic steroids, which have been shown to enhance the in vitro infectivity of *C. pneumoniae*[50]; this was reflected in significant increases of inclusions but did not affect the in vitro activities of azithromycin, erythromycin, and doxycycline against *C. pneumoniae*.[50]

Several studies have addressed the question of whether antibiotic treatment of *C. pneumoniae* infection in patients with asthma leads to improvement in disease activity. Study design has been complicated by the fact that macrolides, quinolones, and tetracyclines all have immunomodulatory activity independent of their antimicrobial activity.[51,52] Any positive treatment outcomes may therefore be the result of antichlamydial or immunomodulatory effects, or a combination of the two. Several uncontrolled studies showed beneficial effects of antibiotics on patients with asthma with proven or presumed *C. pneumoniae* infection.[32,53] Subsequent placebo-controlled trials attempted to confirm the benefits suggested by these preliminary studies. A placebo-controlled 6-week trial of roxithromycin in patients with asthma who were seropositive for *C. pneumoniae* showed significantly higher

morning peak expiratory flow in the treatment group at the end of treatment, but not at subsequent time points.[54] In the absence of clear evidence that patients with asthma in this study had persistent *C. pneumoniae* infection, one could conclude that the treatment effect was the result of the anti-inflammatory action of roxithromycin, which disappeared after stopping the drug. A double-blind, randomized, placebo-controlled study of telithromycin in patients with acute exacerbations of asthma found reduction of asthma symptoms among those treated with the active drug; however, the study could not adequately assess the effect of infection because only one of 278 enrolled patients was positive for *C. pneumoniae* with PCR of upper airway samples.[55] A randomized controlled trial of minocycline in patients with allergic asthma showed improved asthma symptoms and reduced total serum IgE, a beneficial effect, that did not appear to be the result of a respiratory infection with *C. pneumoniae*; seropositivity for *C. pneumoniae* was not significantly different between patients and controls, and no patient had positive nasopharyngeal cultures for *C. pneumoniae*.[56]

Comparison of studies of antibiotic treatment of patients with asthma is complicated by the use of different criteria of *C. pneumoniae* infection status (culture, PCR, serology, or combination of these tests), use of nonstandard methods, and the unclear definition of chronic infection. Most studies have been underpowered to show effects of infections status. In conclusion, although diagnosis and treatment of *C. pneumoniae* infections in patients with asthma with signs and symptoms of an airway infection are recommended, the benefits of using antibiotics with activity against atypical bacteria in patients with asthma without acute infection remain controversial.

C. PNEUMONIAE AND OTHER CHRONIC DISEASES

Persistent *C. pneumoniae* infection has also been implicated in the pathogenesis of several chronic diseases, initially not thought to be infectious, including atherosclerosis, multiple sclerosis (MS), temporal arteritis, stroke, Alzheimer's disease, lung cancer, and macular degeneration.[42] Studies in mice have shown that *C. pneumoniae* disseminates to the spleen and other organs after respiratory infection via macrophages.[57] However, this effect has not been conclusively shown to occur in humans. In addition, studies of the association of *C. pneumoniae* and these disorders have been hampered by difficulty in diagnosis of chronic persistent infection with the organism; no validated serologic or other surrogate markers exist for chronic *C. pneumoniae* infection.[5] The high prevalence of chlamydial infections and transient immunity after infection makes differentiation of persistent infection from reinfection or even past infection difficult. This, in turn, makes determination of the efficacy of any therapeutic intervention difficult.

C. pneumoniae and Atherosclerosis

Conventional risk factors including cigarette smoking, hypertension, and high serum lipid levels do not fully explain the incidence, prevalence, and distribution of coronary artery disease (CVD). Inflammation of the vessel wall plays an essential role in the initiation and progression of atherosclerosis, erosion, fissure, and eventual rupture of the atheromatous plaques.[58] Various markers of systemic inflammation, including C-reactive protein, have been found to predict future cardiovascular events, including nonfatal and fatal myocardial infarction and stroke. Although inflammation is present, the exact cause is still not known. Infectious agents including cytomegalovirus, human herpes viruses, enteroviruses, *Helicobacter pylori*, bacteria involved with periodontal disease, and *C. pneumoniae* have also been investigated as possible causes for this inflammation. The first report that suggested a possible association between *C. pneumoniae* infection and CVD came from a case-control study from Finland published in 1988 that showed that patients with proven CVD were significantly more likely to have antibodies to *C. pneumoniae* than controls selected at random.[59] This report was quickly followed by additional seroepidemiologic studies and studies that identified *C. pneumoniae* in atheroma with various methods, including culture, immunohistochemical staining (IHS), and PCR.[18,19] Animal studies have shown that *C. pneumoniae* can either induce or enhance the development of atherosclerosis in mice.[60] In vitro studies have shown that *C. pneumoniae* can infect and replicate within monocytes, macrophages and vascular endothelial and smooth muscle cells and that all are important components of atherosclerotic plaque.[58,61] In vitro infection also results in oxidation of cellular low-density lipoprotein (LDL), the production of proinflammatory cytokines involved in atherogenesis, including tumor necrosis factor-alpha (TNF-α), IL-6, IL-1β, and interferon-α (INF-α); and the transendothelial migration of neutrophils and monocytes.[58,61] *C. pneumoniae* can induce human macrophage foam cell formation in vitro, a key event in early atheroma development.[62] However, this may not be specific because the key component appears to be the chlamydia lipopolysaccharide, which is conserved in all chlamydial species, including *C. trachomatis.*

However, no single serologic, PCR, or IHS assay has been used consistently across all studies, and these assays are not standardized. In 2002, Boman and Hammerschlag[18] reviewed 14 seroepidemiologic studies published from 1992 to 2000 and found a great deal of heterogeneity among these studies in terms of the serologic tests used and the criteria for seropositivity. In some studies, an IgG or IgA titer of 1:64 or more was used as an indicator of chronic infection; in others, the same criteria were used as indicators of *past* infection. Nine of these studies used the MIF assay; all were in-house tests. The antigen used was only specified in four of the MIF assays. The remaining studies used a variety of other methods, including genus-specific enzyme immunoassays and whole-cell immunofluorescence. As stated previously, MIF assays are not standardized and are subject to significant operator variation.[17] Background seropositivity rates in the general population often exceed 70%, which can also make demonstration of an association between the presence of *C. pneumoniae* antibodies and CVD difficult. Earlier case-controlled studies that showed an association were generally small and based on single serum samples, which do not take into account that antibody titers fluctuate over time. A meta-analysis of 12 studies only found combined odds ratios (ORs) of 1.15 and 1.13 for IgG and IgA antibodies, respectively.[63]

Boman and Hammerschlag[18] analyzed 43 studies published from 1992 through 2000 that examined 2679 samples of atheromatous tissue for presence of *C. pneumoniae* with culture, electron microscopy, PCR, and IHS. The overall rates of detection of *C. pneumoniae* ranged from 0 to 100%, with 49.7% being positive by at least one method. However, when specimens were analyzed with more than one method, the prevalence rate of specimens positive by at least two methods (usually IHS and PCR) was only 15.14%. As with the serologic studies, major variation was found in the methods, including the antibodies and techniques for IHS and PCR. IHS has also been found to have problems with interpretation and reproducibility. Studies from Hoymans and colleagues[10] reported that ceroid, an insoluble lipid present in plaque, could cause nonspecific reactions with IHS.

The extent of interlaboratory variation with performance of PCR was shown by Apfalter and colleagues,[11] who sent a panel of 15 homogenized clinical atheroma specimens (carotid and coronary) and controls to nine laboratories in Europe and the United States for detection with PCR. The positivity rate in the clinical specimens ranged from 0 to 60%, and three laboratories identified *C. pneumoniae* in negative controls. The concordance between the assays was only 25% for one specimen. Subsequently, Apfalter and colleagues[12] showed that contamination was practically impossible to avoid with nested PCR assays. Ieven and Hoymans[19] published an analysis of studies reported since 2000, many of which used real-time PCR and were found to be predominantly negative. Real-time PCR is much less subject to contamination from amplicon carryover. Ieven and Hoymans[19] also noted that in studies where serology was done in addition to PCR, no correlation was found between presence of *C. pneumoniae* in the atheroma tissue and presence of anti–*C. pneumoniae* antibodies in individual patients.

With extrapolation from the observation that *C. pneumoniae* can disseminate systemically in mice after intranasal inoculation,[57] the presence of *C. pneumoniae* in peripheral blood mononuclear cells (PBMCs) has been suggested to act as a surrogate marker for infection with *C. pneumoniae* in individuals with cardiovascular and other diseases.[18,19] More than 20 studies that examined the presence of *C. pneumoniae* DNA in PBMCs have been published, and as seen with studies of vascular tissue, the reported prevalence rate of *C. pneumoniae* DNA in PBMCs has also varied significantly, from 0 to 59% of patients with CVD and 0 to 46% of healthy blood donors.[64] Kohlhepp and others[65] examined PBMCs from more than 300 blood donors either younger than 20 years of age or older than 60 years. The samples were divided and sent to two different laboratories where they were tested for *C. pneumoniae* DNA with real-time, touchdown, and nested PCR assays. Only two samples from the younger than 20-year-old group were positive in one of the laboratories but negative in the second. None of the samples for the more than 60-year-old group was positive in either laboratory. This study showed that two different laboratories, with different extraction methods and real-time PCR targets, did not detect *C. pneumoniae* DNA in both cohorts of patients, but evidence of interlaboratory discrepancy was found with two specimens.

Results of the initial seroepidemiologic and organism detection studies led to several preliminary studies that investigated the efficacy of antibiotic treatment directed at *C. pneumoniae* for the prevention of secondary cardiac events. The results of these preliminary studies suggested an effect but were underpowered and raised questions about the antibiotic regimens used and methods of identification of patients with *C. pneumoniae* infection. The major assumption of many of the seroepidemiologic studies of the association of *C. pneumoniae* and atherosclerosis and other chronic conditions is that the presence of anti–*C. pneumoniae* antibody implies the presence of the organism somewhere in the body. However, earlier studies of patients with respiratory infection often found a poor correlation between serology and isolation of the organism from the respiratory tract.[37]

Gupta and others[66] randomized 60 men with prior myocardial infarction who were seropositive with MIF (IgG ≥ 8) to receive either azithromycin 500 mg/d for 3 or 6 days or placebo. They found that the patients who received azithromycin showed a decrease in MIF IgG titers and had a lower risk of a secondary adverse cardiac event than the patients who received placebo. The antibiotic regimen used by Gupta and colleagues[66] was never studied for treatment of *C. pneumoniae* infections. A meta-analysis of 11 randomized trials, which enrolled a total of 19,217 patients, was published in 2005.[67] Seven of these trials used azithromycin; length of treatment ranged from 500 mg/d for 3 to 6 days to 500 to 600 mg/wk for 6 weeks to 1 year. Three studies used roxithromycin for 30 days to 6 weeks; one used clarithromycin, 500 mg/d for 85 days; and one used gatifloxacin 400 mg/d per month for 2 years. The duration of follow-up ranged from 3 months to 2 years. The results of two of six of the earlier small studies (≤150 patients in each arm) favored antibiotic, but all of the remaining five large studies favored placebo for all endpoints including total mortality, subsequent myocardial events including infarction, and unstable angina. Also, no relationship was found between outcome and *C. pneumoniae* serologic status. A similar analysis with similar results was published by Baker and Couch in 2007.[68]

A number of possible reasons have been proposed for the failure to show a positive effect of antibiotic treatment, including populations studied, trial design, and duration of treatment. Given lack of a reliable marker for endovascular *C. pneumoniae* infection and the largely negative results in recent organism detection studies, additional studies are unlikely to show any benefit of long-term antibiotic treatment in reducing mortality or cardiovascular events in patients with CVD.

C. pneumoniae *and Multiple Sclerosis*

During the past 60 years, 20 different bacteria and viruses have been proposed to be associated with MS. The results were often inconsistent. The possible association of *C. pneumoniae* and MS was first described in a case study from researchers at Vanderbilt University Medical Center (VUMC); this study was then followed by a series of patients from VUMC in which the researchers claimed that they identified organism with culture and PCR.[69] The hypothesis of how *C. pneumoniae* might cause MS was not clear. The results of subsequent studies from a number of other groups were conflicting, some finding *C. pneumoniae* DNA in approximately 30% to more than 80% of cerebrospinal fluid (CSF) from patients with MS and in approximately 20% of CSF from patients with other neurologic diseases and others finding none in CSF and brain tissue with culture and PCR.[70,71]

In an effort to deal with the issue of laboratory-to-laboratory differences in methods used to detect *C. pneumoniae* in studies of MS, prospectively collected CSF samples from patients with MS and other neurologic diseases were sent to laboratories at VUMC, Johns Hopkins University (JHU), and the University of Umea (UU) in Sweden and subsequently also to the Centers for Disease Control and Prevention (CDC).[72] Thirty specimens from patients with MS and 22 controls were tested; none was positive with PCR at JHU, UU, and the CDC, but 73% of the CSF from patients with MS and 23% of the controls were positive with PCR at VUMC. Reasons for these discrepant results were discussed and included poor sensitivities of the assays used by JHU, UU, and the CDC or specificity problems with the assays used by VUMC. The primer sets used by VUMC in the multicenter study were analyzed at the CDC and were found to have high sequence similarity to human DNA, as determined with a BLAST (basic local alignment search tool), suggesting that they were not specific for *C. pneumoniae*.

REFERENCES

1. Everett KDE, Bush RM, Anderson AA. Emended description of the order *Chlamydiales*, proposal of *Parachlamydiaceae* fam. nov. and *Simkaniaceae* fam. nov., each containing one monotypic genus, revised taxonomy of the family *Chlamydiaceae*, including a new genus and five new species, and standards for identification of organisms. *Int J Syst Bacteriol.* 1999;49:425-440.
2. Grayston JT, Campbell LA, Kuo C-C, et al. A new respiratory tract pathogen: *Chlamydia pneumoniae* strain TWAR. *J Infect Dis.* 1990;61:618-625.
3. Kalman S, Mitchell W, Marathe R, et al. Comparative genomes of *Chlamydia pneumoniae* and *C. trachomatis*. *Nature Gen.* 1999;21:385-389.
4. Chi EY, Kuo C-C, Grayston JT. Unique ultrastructure in the elementary body of *Chlamydia* sp. strain TWAR. *J Bacteriol.* 1987;169:3757-3763.
5. Dowell SF, Peeling RW, Boman J, et al. Standardizing *Chlamydia pneumoniae* assays: Recommendations from the Centers for Disease Control and Prevention (USA) and the Laboratory Centre for Disease Control (Canada). *Clin Infect Dis.* 2001;33:492-503.
6. Rockey DD, Lenart J, Stephens RS. Genome sequencing and our understanding of chlamydiae. *Infect Immun.* 2000;68:5473-5479.
7. Beatty WL, Morrison RP, Byrne GL. Persistent chlamydiae: from cell culture to a paradigm form chlamydial pathogenesis. *Microbiol Rev.* 1994;58:689-694.
8. Kutlin A, Flegg C, Stenzel D, et al. Ultrastructural study of *Chlamydia pneumoniae* in a continuous infection model. *J Clin Microbiol.* 2001;39:3721-3723.
9. Kohlhoff SA, Kutlin A, Riska P, et al. In vitro models of acute and long- term continuous infection of human respiratory epithelial cells with *Chlamydophila pneumoniae* have opposing effects on host cell apoptosis. *Microb Pathogen.* 2008;44:34-42.
10. Hoymans VY, Bosmans JM, Ursi D, et al. Immunohistostaining assays for detection of *Chlamydia pneumoniae* in atherosclerotic arteries indicate cross-reactions with nonchlamydial plaque constituents. *J Clin Microbiol.* 2004;42:3219-3224.
11. Apfalter P, Blasi F, Boman J, et al. Multicenter comparison trial of DNA extraction methods and PCR assays for detection of *Chlamydia pneumoniae* in endarterectomy specimens. *J Clin Microbiol.* 2001;39:519-524.
12. Apfalter P, Assadian O, Blasi F, et al. Reliability of nested PCR for the detection of *Chlamydia pneumoniae* DNA in atheromas: results from a multicenter study applying standardized protocols. *J Clin Microbiol.* 2002;40:4428-4434.
13. Apfalter P, Reischl U, Hammerschlag MR. In-house nucleic acid amplification assays in research: How much quality control is needed before one can rely upon the results? *J Clin Microbiol.* 2005;43:5385-5841.
14. Kuoppa Y, Boman J, Scott L, et al. Quantitative detection of respiratory *Chlamydia pneumoniae* infection by Real-Time PCR. *J Clin Microbiol.* 2002;40:2273-2274.
15. Tondella ML, Talkington DF, Holloway BP, et al. Development and evaluation of Real-Time PCR-based fluorescence assays for detection of *Chlamydia pneumoniae*. *J Clin Microbiol.* 2002;40:575-583.
16. Apfalter P, Barousch W, Nehr M, et al. Comparison of a new quantitative ompA-Real-Time PCR TaqMan Assay for detection of *Chlamydia pneumoniae* in respiratory specimens with four conventional PCR assays. *J Clin Microbiol.* 2003;41:592-600.
17. Littman AJ, Jackson LA, White E, et al. Interlaboratory reliability of microimmunofluorescence test for measurement of *Chlamydia pneumoniae*-specific immunoglobulin A and G antibody titers. *J Clin Microbiol.* 2004;11:615-617.
18. Boman J, Hammerschlag MR. *Chlamydia pneumoniae* and atherosclerosis: a critical assessment of diagnostic methods and the relevance to treatment studies. *Clin Microbiol Rev.* 2002;15:1-20.
19. Ieven MM, Hoymans VY. Involvement of *Chlamydia pneumoniae* in atherosclerosis: more evidence for lack of evidence. *J Clin Microbiol.* 2005;43:19-24.
20. Hammerschlag MR. *Chlamydia pneumoniae* and the lung. *Eur Resp J.* 2000;16:1001-1007.

21. Collingro A, Toenshoff E, Taylor MW, et al. Recovery of an environmental *Chlamydia* strain from activated sludge by co-cultivation with *Acanthamoeba* sp. *Microbiology.* 2005;151:301-309.
22. Griffiths E, Petrich AK, Gupta RS. Conserved indels in essential proteins that are distinctive characteristics of *Chlamydiales* and provide novel means for their identification. *Microbiology.* 2005;151:2647-2657.
23. Kumar S, Kutlin S, Roblin P, et al. Isolation and antimicrobial susceptibilities of chlamydial isolates from western barred bandicoots. *J Clin Microbiol.* 2007;45:392-394.
24. Hyman CL, Augenbraun MH, Roblin PM, et al. Asymptomatic respiratory tract infection with *Chlamydia pneumoniae* (Strain TWAR). *J Clin Microbiol.* 1991;29:2082-2083.
25. Falsey AR, Walsh EE. Transmission of *Chlamydia pneumoniae*. *J Infect Dis.* 1993;168:493-496.
26. Kleemola M, Saikku P, Visakorpi R, et al. Epidemics of pneumonia caused by TWAR, a new *Chlamydia* organism, in military trainees in Finland. *J Infect Dis.* 1988;157:230-236.
27. Hyman CL, Roblin PM, Gaydos CA, et al. Prevalence of asymptomatic nasopharyngeal carriage of *Chlamydia pneumoniae* in subjectively healthy adults: Assessment by polymerase chain reaction-enzyme immunoassay and culture. *Clin Infect Dis.* 1995;20:1174-1178.
28. Kern DG; Neill MA, Schachter J. A seroepidemiologic study of *Chlamydia pneumoniae* in Rhode Island. *Chest.* 1993;104:208-213.
29. Kumar S, Hammerschlag MR. Acute respiratory infection due to *Chlamydia pneumoniae*: Current status of diagnostic methods. *Clin Infect Dis.* 2007;44:568-576.
30. Hammerschlag MR, Chirgwin K, Roblin PM, et al: Persistent infection with *Chlamydia pneumoniae* following acute respiratory illness. *Clin Infect Dis.* 1992;14:178-182.
31. Kauppinen MT, Herva E, Kujula P, et al. The etiology of community-acquired pneumonia among hospitalized patients during a *Chlamydia pneumoniae* epidemic in Finland. *J Infect Dis.* 1995;172:1330-1335.
32. Emre U, Roblin PM, Gelling M, et al. The association of *Chlamydia pneumoniae* infection and reactive airway disease in children. *Arch Pediatr Adolesc Med.* 1994;148:727-732.
33. Augenbraun MH, Roblin PM, Mandel LJ, et al: *Chlamydia pneumoniae* pneumonia, with pleural effusion: Diagnosis by culture. *Am J Med.* 1991;43:437-438.
34. Augenbraun MH, Roblin PM, Chirgwin K, et al. Isolation of *Chlamydia pneumoniae* from the lungs of patients infected with the human immunodeficiency virus. *J Clin Microbiol.* 1991;29:401-402.
35. Gaydos CA, Fowler CL, Gill VJ, et al. Detection of *Chlamydia pneumoniae* by polymerase chain reaction-enzyme immunoassay in an immunocompromised population. *Clin Infect Dis.* 1993;17:718-723.
36. Miller ST, Hammerschlag MR, Chirgwin K, et al. The role of *Chlamydia, pneumoniae* in acute chest syndrome of sickle cell disease. *J Pediatr.* 1991;118:30-33.
37. Hammerschlag MR. Advances in the management of *Chlamydia pneumoniae* infections. *Expert Rev Anti-Infect Ther.* 2003;1:493-504.
38. Riska PF, Kutlin A, Ajiboye P, et al. Genetic and culture-based approaches for detecting macrolide resistance in *Chlamydia pneumoniae*. *Antimicrob Agents Chemother.* 2004;48:3586-3690.
39. Rupp J, Gebert A, Solbach W, et al. Serine-to-asparagine substitution in the GyrA gene leads to quinolone resistance in moxifloxacin-exposed *Chlamydia pneumoniae*. *Antimicrob Agents Chemother.* 2005;49:406-407.
40. Kutlin A, Roblin PM, Hammerschlag MR. Effect of prolonged treatment with azithromycin, clarithromycin and levofloxacin on *Chlamydia pneumoniae* in a continuous infection model. *Antimicrob Agents Chemother.* 2002;46:409-412.
41. Hahn DL, Dodge RW, Golubjatnikov R. Association of *Chlamydia pneumoniae* (strain TWAR) infection with wheezing, asthmatic bronchitis, and adult-onset asthma. *JAMA.* 1991;266:225-230.

42. Hammerschlag MR, Kohlhoff SA, Darville T. *Chlamydia pneumoniae* and *Chlamydia trachomatis*. In: Fratamico PM, Smith JL, Brogden KA, eds. *Post-Infectious Sequelae and Long-Term Consequences of Infectious Diseases.* Washington, DC: American Society for Microbiology; in press, 2008.
43. Von Hertzen LC. Role of persistent infection in the control and severity of asthma: focus on *Chlamydia pneumoniae*. *Eur Respir J.* 2002;19:546-556.
44. Biscione GL, Corne J, Chauhan AJ, et al. Increased frequency of detection of *Chlamydophila pneumoniae* in asthma. *Eur Resp J.* 2004;24:745-749.
45. Holland MJ, Bailey RL, Conway DJ, et al. T-helper type 1 (Th1)/Th2 profiles of peripheral blood mononuclear cells (PBMC); responses to antigens of *Chlamydia trachomatis* in subjects with severe trachomatous scarring. *Clin Exp Immunol.* 1996;105:429-435.
46. Hoffjan S, Ostrovnaja I, Nicolae D, et al. Genetic variation in immunoregulatory pathways and atopic phenotypes in infancy. *J Allergy Clin Immunol.* 2004;113:511-518.
47. Nagy A, Kozma GT, Keszei M, et al. The development of asthma in children with *Chlamydia pneumoniae* is dependent on the modifying effect of mannose-binding lectin. *J Allergy Clin Immunol.* 2003;112:729-734.
48. Halme S, Saikku P, Surcel HM. Characterization of *Chlamydia pneumoniae* antigens using human T cell clones. *Scand J Immunol.* 1997;45:378-384.
49. Emre U, Sokolovskaya N, Roblin PM, et al. Detection of anti-*Chlamydia pneumoniae* IgE in children with reactive airway disease. *J Infect Dis.* 1995;172:265-267.
50. Tsumura N, Emre U, Roblin P, et al. The effect of hydrocortisone succinate on the growth of *Chlamydia pneumoniae* in vitro. *J Clin Microbiol.* 1996;34:2379-2381.
51. Schultz MJ. Macrolide activities beyond their antimicrobial effects: macrolides in diffuse panbronchiolitis and cystic fibrosis. *J Antimicrob Chemother.* 2004;54:21-28.
52. Williams AC, Galley HF, Watt AM, et al. Differential effects of three antibiotics on T helper cell cytokine expression. *J Antimicrob Chemother.* 2005;56:502-506.
53. Kraft M, Cassell GH, Pak J, et al. *Mycoplasma pneumoniae* and *Chlamydia pneumoniae* in asthma: effect of clarithromycin. *Chest.* 2002;121:1782-1788.
54. Black PN, Blasi F, Jenkins CR, et al. Trial of roxithromycin in subjects with asthma and serological evidence of infection with *Chlamydia pneumoniae*. *Am J Respir Crit Care Med.* 2001;164:536-541.
55. Johnston SL, Blasi F, Black PN, et al. The effect of telithromycin in acute exacerbations of asthma. *N Engl J Med.* 2006;354:1589-1600.
56. Daoud A, Gloria CJ, Taningco G, et al. Minocycline treatment results in reduced oral steroid requirements in adult asthma. *Allergy Asthma Proc.* 2008;29:286-294.
57. Moazed TC, Kuo CC, Grayston JT, et al. Evidence of systemic dissemination of *Chlamydia pneumoniae* via macrophages in the mouse. *J Infect Dis.* 1998;177:1322-1325.
58. Kalayoglu MV, Libby P, Byrne GI. *Chlamydia pneumoniae* as an emerging risk factor in cardiovascular disease. *JAMA.* 2002;288:2724-2731.
59. Saikku P, Leinonen M, Mattila K, et al. Serological evidence of an association of a novel *Chlamydia*, TWAR, with chronic coronary heart disease and acute myocardial infarction. *Lancet.* 1988;2:983-986.
60. de Kruif MD, van Gorp EC, Keller TT, et al. *Chlamydia pneumoniae* infections in mouse models: relevance for atherosclerosis research. *Cardiovasc Res.* 2005; 65:317-327.
61. Byrne GI, Skarlotos SI, Grunfeld C, et al. Collaborative multidisciplinary workshop report: Interface of lipid metabolism, atherosclerosis and *Chlamydia* infection. *J Infect Dis.* 2000;181:S490-S491.
62. Kalayoglu MV, Byrne GI. A *Chlamydia pneumoniae* component that induces macrophage foam cell formation is chlamydial lipopolysaccharide. *Infect Immun.* 1998;66:5067-5072.

63. Danesh J, Whincup P, Walker M, et al. *Chlamydia pneumoniae* IgG titres and coronary heart disease: prospective study and meta-analysis. *BMJ.* 2000;321:208-213.
64. Smieja M, Mahoney J, Petrich A, et al. Association of circulating *Chlamydia pneumoniae* DNA with cardiovascular disease: a systematic review. *BMC Infect Dis.* 2002;2:21, <http://www.biomedcentral.com/1471-2334/2/21> [last accessed June 1, 2009].
65. Kohlhepp SJ, Hardick J, Gaydos CA. *Chlamydia pneumoniae* in peripheral blood mononuclear cells from individuals younger than 20 years and older than 60 years. *J Clin Microbiol.* 2005;43:3030.
66. Gupta S, Leatham EW, Carrington D, et al. Elevated *Chlamydia pneumoniae* antibodies, cardiovascular events, and azithromycin in male survivors of myocardial infarction. *Circulation.* 1997;96:404-407.
67. Andraws R, Berger JS, Brown DL. Effects of antibiotic therapy on outcomes of patients with coronary artery disease. A meta-analysis of randomized controlled trials. *JAMA.* 2005;293:2641-2647.
68. Baker WL, Couch KA. Azithromycin for secondary prevention of coronary artery disease: A meta-analysis. *Am J Health-Syst Pharm.* 2007;64:830-836.
69. Sriram S, Mitchell W, Stratton C. Multiple sclerosis associated with *Chlamydia pneumoniae* infection of the CNS. *Neurology.* 1998;50:571-572.
70. Swanborg RH, Whittum-Hudson JA, Hudson AP. Infectious agents and multiple sclerosis-are *Chlamydia pneumoniae* and human herpes virus 6 involved? *J Neuroimmunol.* 2003;135:1-8.
71. Hammerschlag MR, Gaydos GA. *Chlamydia pneumoniae* and multiple sclerosis: fact or fiction. *Lancet Neurol.* 2006;5:892-893.
72. Kaufman M, Gaydos CA, Sriram S, et al. Is *Chlamydia pneumoniae* found in spinal fluid samples from multiple sclerosis patients? Conflicting results. *Multiple Sclerosis.* 2002;8:289-294.

183

Introduction to *Mycoplasma* and *Ureaplasma*

STEPHEN G. BAUM

Mycoplasma organisms are ubiquitous as pathogens and colonizing agents in the plant, animal, and insect kingdoms.[1] They represent the smallest known free-living forms, but because they have fastidious growth requirements, they are often difficult to culture on a cell-free medium. On the other hand, the presence of several species of *Mycoplasma* as commensals in animals and on human oral and genital mucosa has in the past produced frequent contamination of cell cultures.[2] Such contamination has in turn led to the false implication of mycoplasmas as causative agents in many human diseases, both trivial and life-threatening. Knowledge of the true range of diseases that these organisms cause is, however, expanding rapidly with the advent of immunohistochemical and nucleic acid probe techniques used to detect mycoplasmas directly in tissue specimens. To date, more than 120 species of *Mycoplasma* and seven species of *Ureaplasma* have been identified.[3]

Description of the Organism

Mycoplasma organisms are prokaryotes that lack a cell wall. They are bounded by a cell membrane containing sterols, substances not found in other bacteria or viruses. Because of their small size (150 to 250 nm) and deformable membrane, they are able to pass through filters with pore sizes that retain other bacteria. Therefore, when first discovered, they were thought to be viruses.[4] However, their ability to grow in cell-free medium and the fact that they contain both RNA and DNA clearly set them apart from this class of microorganisms. DNA homology studies have failed to demonstrate a significant relationship between mycoplasmas and known bacteria, although mycoplasmas probably devolved from gram-positive bacteria through reductive evolution[1] (Table 183-1).

The small size of these organisms suggests that they require many exogenous nutrients for growth, including vitamins, amino acids, nucleic acid precursors and, in particular, lipids. The latter are provided by the addition of serum or cholesterol to growth medium. Energy is supplied by carbohydrate metabolism. Some nonfermenting mycoplasmas derive energy from amino acid (arginine) metabolism. As the name implies, *Ureaplasma* organisms can split urea, but it is unclear whether urea splitting is their sole source of energy.[5]

Most mycoplasmas grown on agar form colonies with a dense central zone and a less dense peripheral zone. The resultant colony has been likened to the shape of a fried egg (Fig. 183-1A). An important exception is *Mycoplasma pneumoniae*, the most significant human pathogen of the genus. This mycoplasma forms no peripheral halo, and colonies have been likened to a mulberry (see Fig. 183-1B).

Other characteristics of *Mycoplasma* growth in vitro include adsorption of erythrocytes from a number of animal species and hemolysis of erythrocytes in blood agar through the elaboration of hydrogen peroxide.

Taxonomy and Distribution

Mycoplasmas have now been assigned taxonomically to their own class, Mollicutes, which has five families: Mycoplasmataceae, which encompasses organisms infecting and colonizing humans and animals,

including *Ureaplasma*; Spironoplasmataceae, the plant mycoplasmas; and Acholeplasmataceae, most of which are isolated primarily from birds. A fourth family, Anaeroplasmataceae, consists of strict anaerobes that have been isolated from bovine and ovine rumen; they are not known to infect humans. A fifth family, Entomoplasmataceae, infects insects and plants. It is likely that all complex living organisms are or can be colonized by mycoplasmas. Species specificity is less restrictive than was once believed.[6]

The family Mycoplasmataceae is composed of two genera responsible for human infection, *Mycoplasma* and *Ureaplasma;* the genus *Mycoplasma* has more than 13 species that infect humans, as shown in Figure 183-2.[1,6] Ureaplasmas were previously referred to as T-strain mycoplasmas because of the tiny colonies that they formed on agar.[7] One serovar of *Ureaplasma*, *U. parvum*, has now been designated as a new species.[8] Based on studies of 16SrRNA homology, increasing numbers of unculturable organisms are being classified as mycoplasmas.[9]

Pathogenesis

Mycoplasmas appear to cause infection primarily as extracellular parasites. They attach to the surface of ciliated and nonciliated epithelial cells. Some mycoplasmas, such as *M. pneumoniae, M. penetrans,* and *M. genitalium,* have special attachment organelles containing adhesin molecules, but many that effectively penetrate cells, such as *M. fermentans* and *M. hominis*, do not.[10] The lipid-associated membrane proteins present on the mycoplasmal surface are recognized by Toll-like receptors on cells, and the interraction between these entities may provoke an inflammatory response to the organism.[3,11] Subsequent events are unclear but may include direct cytotoxicity of such elaborated substances as hydrogen peroxide,[12] or they may involve cytolysis via an inflammatory response mediated through chemotaxis of mononuclear cells, upregulation or downregulation of inflammatory cytokines, or antigen-antibody reactions.[13,14]

Mycoplasma organisms are very common contaminants of tissue cultures.[2,15] In these cases, they are most often intracellular parasites. This fact may contribute to the difficulty in eradicating mycoplasmas from contaminated cultures. Their presence has been shown to markedly alter cellular and viral molecular events, a fact that has prompted some to question many of the molecular biologic results derived from tissue culture experiments.[2] A more complete discussion of mycoplasma molecular biology and pathogenesis in provided in a comprehensive review by Razin and associates.[1]

UNCOMMON *MYCOPLASMA* ASSOCIATED WITH HUMAN DISEASE

Mycoplasma incognitus (a variant of *M. fermentans*), *Mycoplasma penetrans,* and *Mycoplasma pirum* have been associated with severe disease in healthy people and those with acquired immunodeficiency syndrome (AIDS).[16-18] *M. fermentans* was first isolated by Lo and colleagues from the blood, organs, and Kaposi's sarcoma lesions of

TABLE 183-1	Defining Characteristics of Mycoplasmas and Ureaplasmas
General	
Prokaryotic	
Small size: 150-250 nm	
No cell wall	
Trilayered cell membrane	
Most are aerobic	
Fastidious growth requirements	
Form fried egg colonies on agar	
Differentiation from bacteria and L-forms	
Sterols in membrane	
No DNA homology with known bacteria	
Low guanine + cytosine content	
Low-molecular-weight genome (580 to ~2200 kb)	
No reversion to walled forms	
Differentiation from viruses	
Contain both DNA and RNA	
Free-living—cell-free growth on defined media in vitro	
Extracellular parasitism in vivo	

patients with AIDS and has since been reported to cause fulminant multisystem infection in presumably healthy patients.[19] The organism was first believed to be a virus,[16,17] then was identified as the mycoplasma *M. penetrans*,[1,18] and ultimately was shown by immunohistochemistry, DNA homology, electron microscopy, and in situ hybridization to be a mycoplasma closely related to *M. fermentans*.[19]

The organism has been identified at the advancing margins of lesions in the liver, brain, spleen, lymph nodes, and thymus of infected patients.[20] *M. penetrans* has been isolated from the urogenital tract and *M. pirum* from the blood of patients with human immunodeficiency virus (HIV) infection.[17] In addition, *Mycoplasma amphoriforme* has

been isolated from respiratory tracts of antibody-deficient patients with chronic bronchitis and bronchiectasis.[3]

Cultivation of these organisms directly from patient material on cell-free medium has proved to be difficult, and prior animal and tissue culture passage is required. This difficulty in direct culturing has fueled controversy over whether these organisms are pathogens or contaminants in these patients.

Mycoplasma found in humans are usually susceptible in vitro to tetracycline, chloramphenicol, clindamycin, and the quinolones. Sensitivity to the macrolides appears to be very limited.[21]

ANIMAL *MYCOPLASMA* ORGANISMS AS HUMAN PATHOGENS

Case reports have recently appeared of human infections caused by mycoplasmas previously thought to infect only animals. Fatal septicemia involving *M. arginini* (a commensal in cattle, sheep, and goats) occurred in an immunocompromised slaughterhouse worker[22] and *M. phocicerebrale* causes "seal finger" in seal hunters.[6]

GENITAL *MYCOPLASMA* ORGANISMS CAUSING NONGENITAL INFECTION

A number of reports have indicated that the genital mycoplasmas (*Mycoplasma hominis*, *Mycoplasma genitalium*, and *Ureaplasma urealyticum* and *U. parvum*) can cause serious infections involving the respiratory tract, heart, bloodstream, central nervous system, sternotomy wounds, and prosthetic valves and joints of infants and adults.[23-34] The urogenital Mycoplasmataceae are discussed in detail in Chapter 185.

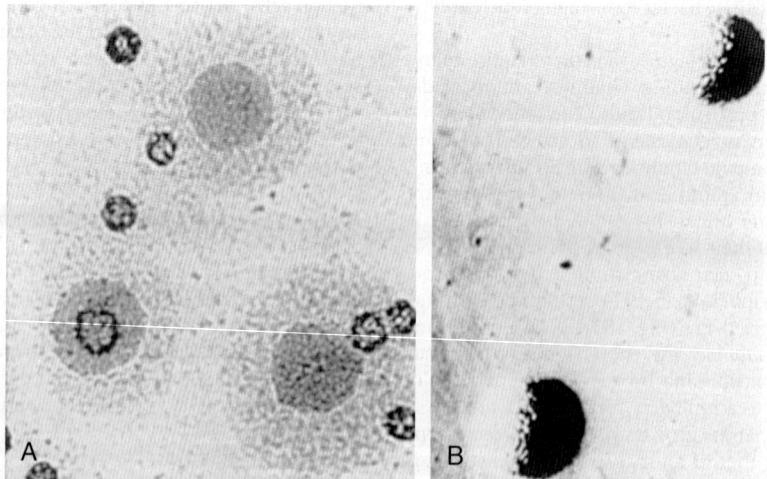

Figure 183-1 Photomicrograph of colonies of mycoplasma growing on agar medium. **A,** *Mycoplasma salivarium* colonies growing with fried egg appearance. **B,** *Mycoplasma pneumoniae* colonies with mulberry colony formation.

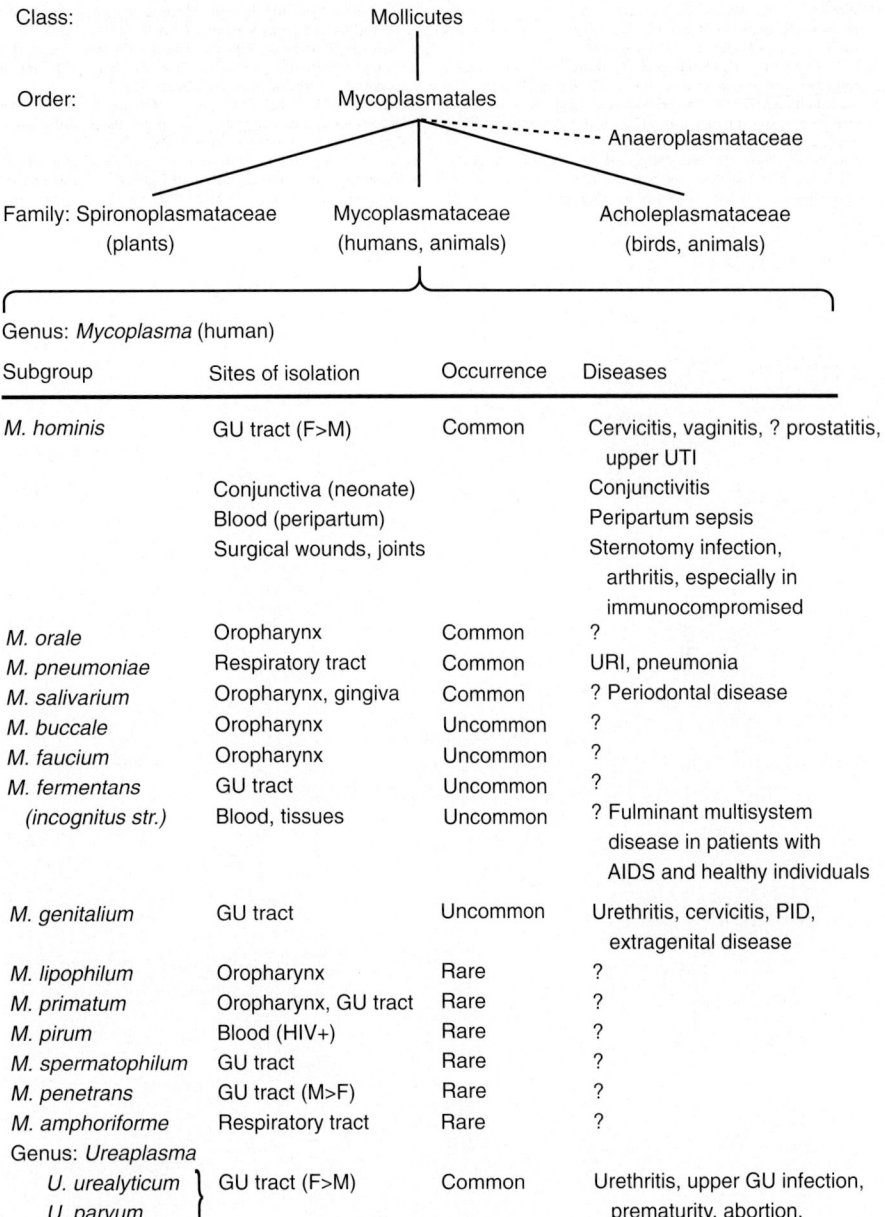

Figure 183-2 Taxonomy and distribution of the class Mollicutes. AIDS, acquired immunodeficiency syndrome; F, female; GU, genitourinary; HIV, human immunodeficiency virus; M, male; PID, pelvic inflammatory disease; UTI, urinary tract infection. *(Adapted from Somerson NL, Cole BC. The mycoplasma flora of human and nonhuman primates. In: Tully JG, Whitcomb RF, eds. The Mycoplasmas, vol 2. New York: Academic Press; 1979;191-216.)*

REFERENCES

1. Razin S, Yogev D, Naot Y. Molecular biology and pathogenicity of mycoplasmas. *Microbiol Mol Biol Rev.* 1998;62:1094-1156.
2. Barile MF, Hopps HE, Grabowski MW, et al. The identification and sources of mycoplasmas isolated from contaminated cell cultures. *Ann N Y Acad Sci.* 1973;25:251-264.
3. Waites KB, Taylor-Robinson E. *Mycoplasma* and *Ureaplasma*. In: Murray PR, Baron EJ, Jorgensen JH, et al, eds. *Manual of Clinical Microbiology*, 9th ed. Washington, DC: ASM Press; 2007:1004-1020.
4. Eaton MD, Meiklejohn G, van Herick W, et al. Studies on the etiology of primary atypical pneumonia. II. Properties of the virus isolated and propagated in chick embryos. *J Exp Med.* 1945;82:317.
5. Waites KB, Rikihisa Y, Taylor-Robinson D. *Mycoplasma and Ureaplasma*. In: Murray PR, Baron EJ, Jorgensen JH, et al, eds. *Manual of Clinical Microbiology*, 8th ed. Washington, DC: ASM Press; 2003:972-990.
6. Pitcher DG, Nichols RAJ. Mycoplasma host specificity: fact or fiction? *Vet J.* 2005;170:300-306.
7. Razin S, Freundt EA. The mycoplasmas. In: Krieg NR, Holt JG, eds. *Bergey's Manual of Systematic Microbiology*, vol 1. Baltimore: Williams & Wilkins; 1984:740-793.
8. Taylor-Robinson D. The role of Mycoplasmas in pregnancy outcome. *Best Pract Res Clin Obstet Gynaecol.* 2007;21:425-438.
9. Neimark HC, Kocan KM. The cell wall-less rickettsia *Eperythrozoon wenyoni* is a mycoplasma. *FEMS Microbiol Lett.* 1997;156:287-291.
10. Krause DC, Balish MF. Cellular engineering in a minimal microbe: Structure and assembly of the terminal organelle of *Mycoplasma pneumoniae*. *Molec Microbiol.* 2004;51:917-924.
11. You XM, Zeng YM, Wu YM. Interactions between mycoplasma lipid-associated membrane proteins and the host cells. *J Zhejiang Univ Sci B.* 2006;7:342-350.
12. Clyde WA Jr. *Mycoplasma pneumoniae* infections of man. In: Tully JG, Whitcomb RF, eds. *The Mycoplasmas*, vol 2. New York: Academic Press; 1979:275-306.
13. Chmura K, Lutz RD, Chiba H, et al. *Mycoplasma pneumoniae* antigens stimulate interleukin-8. *Chest.* 2003;123(Suppl):425S.
14. Tanaka H, Narita M, Teramoto S, et al. Role of interleukin-18 and T-helper type 1 cytokines in the development of *Mycoplasma pneumoniae* pneumonia in adults. *Chest.* 2002;121:1493-1497.
15. Taylor-Robinson D, Davies HA, Sarathchandra P, et al. Intracellular location of mycoplasmas in cultured cells demonstrated by immunochemistry and electron microscopy. *Int J Exp Pathol.* 1991;72:705-714.
16. Mycoplasma incognitus: A workshop. *Am J Trop Med Hyg.* 1990;42:399-402.
17. Lo SC, Dawson MS, Newton PB III, et al. Association of the virus-like infectious agent originally reported in patients with AIDS with acute fatal disease in previously healthy non-AIDS patients. *Am J Trop Med Hyg.* 1989;41:364-376.
18. Wang RY-H, Shih JW-K, Grandinetti T, et al. High frequency of antibodies to *Mycoplasma penetrans* in HIV-infected patients. *Lancet.* 1992;340:1312-1316.
19. Hawkins RE, Rickman LS, Vermund SH, et al. Detection of amplified *Mycoplasma fermentans* DNA in blood. *J Infect Dis.* 1992;165:581-585.
20. Lo SC, Dawson M, Wong DM. Identification of *Mycoplasma incognitus* infection in patients with AIDS: An immunohistochemical, in-situ hybridization and ultrastructural study. *Am J Trop Med Hyg.* 1989;41:601-616.
21. Waites KB, Crabb DM, Duffy LB. In vitro activities of ABT-773 and other antimicrobials against human mycoplasmas. *Antimicrob Agents Chemother.* 2003;47:39-42.
22. Yechouron A, Lefebvre J, Robson HG. Fatal septicemia due to *Mycoplasma arginini*: A new human zoonosis. *Clin Infect Dis.* 1992;15:434-438.
23. Cassell GH, Waites KB, Krause DT. Perinatal mycoplasmal infections. *Clin Perinatol.* 1991;18:241-262.

24. Alonso-Vega C, Wauters N, Vermeylen D, et al. A fatal case of *Mycoplasma hominis* meningoencephalitis in a full-term newborn. *J Clin Microbiol*. 1997;35:286-287.

25. Cohen JI, Sloss LJ, Kundsin R, et al. Prosthetic valve endocarditis caused by *Mycoplasma hominis*. *Am J Med*. 1989;86:819-821.

26. Mohiuddin AA, Coren J, Harbeck RJ, et al. *Ureaplasma urealyticum* chronic osteomyelitis in a patient with hypogammaglobulinemia. *J Allergy Clin Immunol*. 1991;87:104-107.

27. Parides GC, Bloom JW, Ampel NM, et al. *Mycoplasma* and *Ureaplasma* in bronchoalveolar lavage fluids from immunocompromised hosts. *Diagn Microbiol Infect Dis*. 1988;9:55-57.

28. Smeller H, Wellborne F, Barile MF, et al. Prosthetic joint infection with *Mycoplasma hominis*. *J Infect Dis*. 1986;153:174-175.

29. Baseman JB, Dallo SF, Tully JG, et al. Isolation and characterization of *Mycoplasma genitalium* strains from the human respiratory tract. *J Clin Microbiol*. 1988;26:2266-2269.

30. Pinna GS, Skevaki CL, Kafetzis DA. The significance of *Ureaplasma urealyticum* as a pathogenic agent in the paediatric population. *Curr Opin Infect Dis*. 2006;19:283-289.

31. Jensen JS. *Mycoplasma genitalium*: The aetiologic agent of urethritis and other sexually transmitted diseases. *J European Acad of Derm and Venereology*. 2004;18:1-11.

32. Sielaff TD, Everett JE, Shumway SJ, et al. *Mycoplasma hominis* infections occurring in cardiovascular surgical patients. *Ann Thorac Surg*. 1996;61:99-103.

33. Luttrell LM, Kanj SS, Corey GR, et al. *Mycoplasma hominis* septic arthritis: Two case reports and review. *Clin Infect Dis*. 1994;19:1067-1070.

34. Waites KB, Katz B, Schelonka RL. Mycoplasmas and Ureaplasmas as neonatal pathogens. *Clin Microbiol Rev*. 2005;18:757-789.

184

Mycoplasma pneumoniae and Atypical Pneumonia

STEPHEN G. BAUM

The concept of atypical pneumonia arose at the onset of the antibiotic era. In the early 1940s, sulfonamides and then penicillins were introduced into clinical practice. At that time, it was recognized that some cases of pneumonia did not respond to these antibiotics and that these were the pneumonias that could not be attributed by Gram stain or culture to a known bacterial cause. The condition was designated primary atypical pneumonia (PAP). The prefix *primary* indicated that no causative agent could be determined.

In the intervening years, with the advent of virology and better techniques for identifying fastidious bacterial and protozoan agents, it has become clear that the atypical pneumonia syndrome can be caused by influenza virus, adenovirus, respiratory syncytial virus, cytomegalovirus, *Chlamydophila* sp., *Legionella* sp., *Pneumocystis jirovecii*, *Mycoplasma pneumoniae*, the newly described coronavirus variant causing severe acute respiratory syndrome (SARS),[1] and probably numerous other agents. Because we now can identify many of the agents, the prefix *primary* should be discarded. In addition, some of these agents do respond to antimicrobial drugs.

Despite the identification of multiple causes, "atypical pneumonias" share two unifying features. The first is a nonlobar, patchy, or interstitial pattern on chest radiography, and the other is the failure to identify a causative organism on Gram stain or culture of sputum as routinely performed. Because the organisms involved are difficult to identify at the time the patient presents to the physician, it is unlikely that the designation *atypical pneumonia* will disappear from the infectious diseases or pulmonary medicine lexicon any time soon. The term *community-acquired pneumonia* (CAP) is not synonymous because it may include common bacterial pneumonias such as pneumococcal pneumonia.

History

From the time of the description of the atypical pneumonia syndrome in the mid-1940s until the early 1960s, the cause of this syndrome was in question. Bacteria other than the pneumococci, viruses such as influenza, and other as yet unidentified agents were all implicated at one time or another. However, one organism, *M. pneumoniae*, is probably responsible for a large percentage of PAP cases.

In 1945, Eaton and colleagues described an agent that passed through virus filters and caused focal areas of pneumonia when inoculated in several species of rodents.[2] The agent, initially thought to be a virus, could be serially passaged in chick embryos but could not be grown in culture. The relation of this agent to the PAP syndrome was suggested by the fact that human serum from some patients recovering from PAP neutralized the agent.[3] Serum from about 50% to 70% of these patients also was found by Finland and colleagues to agglutinate red blood cells when a mixture of the two was exposed to the cold (4°C).[4] When serum from patients with PAP caused by a known etiologic agent (e.g., influenza virus) was used, cold agglutinins were not demonstrable, and there was no neutralization of Eaton agent.[5] This provided a link between Eaton agent and a proportion of PAP cases of unknown cause. However, serum from this same group of patients also had antibodies to *Streptococcus* sp. This and other nonspecific antibody formation in these patients served to confuse matters for a time and to detract from the evidence that Eaton agent was a major cause of PAP.

By 1946, the disease could be transmitted to human volunteers by ultrafiltrates from patients,[5] but the firm link to Eaton agent came in 1961 with the evidence that convalescent serum from volunteers inoculated with PAP ultrafiltrate neutralized Eaton's chick embryo "virus."[6] Subsequently, further definition of the organism came from Clyde,[7] who grew the agent in tissue culture; Goodburn and Marmion,[8] who described its morphology; and Chanock and co-workers,[9] who, in 1962, were the first to grow the organism on cell-free artificial medium. The ultimate proof of the role of Eaton agent in PAP was the demonstration that the organism isolated in cell-free culture produced the syndrome in volunteers.[10]

Because Eaton agent passed through virologic filters and could be grown only in chick embryos, it was believed throughout most of two decades after its discovery that the agent was a virus. In the early 1960s, it was established that the organism had many characteristics in common with those that caused pneumonia in cattle, hence the transiently used term *pleuropneumonia-like organism*.[11] These organisms were soon shown to be mycoplasmas[12] of the class Mollicutes, described in Chapter 183.

Description of the Organism

M. pneumoniae exhibits most of the biologic and metabolic characteristics described for the Mycoplasmataceae described in Chapter 183. It is capable of growth on cell-free defined medium, setting it apart from all but one (*Legionella* sp.) of the common causative organisms of the atypical pneumonia syndrome. *M. pneumoniae*, unlike most of the other human mycoplasmas, grows well aerobically and ferments glucose as its primary energy source, producing acid.[9,13]

This organism is also unusual among human mycoplasmas in being able to reduce the dye tetrazolium from a blue to a yellow color, adsorb guinea pig and chick erythrocytes to growing colonies, and lyse red blood cells incorporated into the growth agar by means of the elaboration of hydrogen peroxide. Detection of each of these unique characteristics has been used to establish presumptive identification of this organism in culture.

M. pneumoniae is a short rod (about 10 × 200 nm) and has at one end an organelle that is responsible for attachment of the organism to cell membranes.[14] The major adhesion proteins of this organelle (P1, P30, P116, and HMW1-3) have been identified and confer on *M. pneumoniae* its affinity for respiratory epithelium. Actions of these adhesion proteins are primarily responsible for the organism's pathogenesis.[15] *M. pneumoniae* is prokaryotic and has a very small genome (about 800,000 base pairs).[15] The organism is bounded by a trilamellar membrane containing sterols. It divides by binary fission, with a doubling time of more than 6 hours.[16] This long doubling time makes culturing of *M. pneumoniae* a slow process (5 to 20 days), compared with bacteria.[13] Colonies of *M. pneumoniae* differ in morphology from those of other mycoplasmas. They have no outer halo and grow in a dense mulberry shape (see Fig. 183-1 in Chapter 183). Because they lack a cell wall, mycoplasmas including *M. pneumoniae* are not affected by β-lactam antibiotics and are not visible on Gram staining.

Epidemiology

Most cases of mycoplasma respiratory infection occur singly or as family outbreaks with a high rate of secondary infection. In closed populations such as military recruit camps and boarding schools, mycoplasma can cause miniepidemics and may represent from 25% to 75% of pneumonias in such settings.[17] Serologically based epidemiologic studies throughout the world have documented the high incidence of mycoplasma respiratory infection. In the United States, it is estimated that each year at least one case of mycoplasma pneumonia occurs for each 1000 persons, or more than 2 million cases annually. The incidence of mycoplasma nonpneumonic respiratory infection may be 10 to 20 times this high.[18,19] The highest attack rates are in individuals 5 to 20 years old, but *M. pneumoniae* infection can occur at any age and may cause particularly severe disease in neonates.[20]

A few studies have reported a peak incidence in the fall in temperate climates.[21-23] This is not surprising given the peak age-related incidence and the fact that late summer and fall represent the time of return to schools. Most surveys, however, show little or no seasonal preponderance in sporadic cases. Distribution of the disease is worldwide.[24,25]

There appears to be an age-related incidence of upper versus lower respiratory tract infection caused by *M. pneumoniae*. Children younger than 3 years of age develop primarily upper respiratory tract infection,[26] whereas those 5 to 20 years old tend to develop bronchitis and pneumonia. In older infected adults, pneumonia is relatively common.[27]

Transmission

M. pneumoniae infection is spread from one patient to another by respiratory droplets produced by coughing. Relatively close association with the index case appears to be required. The disease is usually introduced into families by a young child, and in some studies, most of the adults who were infected were the parents of young children.[20,28,29]

As opposed to most viral respiratory infections, which are clinically manifest 1 to 3 days after infection, mycoplasma has an incubation period of 2 to 3 weeks.[29] Therefore, a careful history showing several weeks between cases within a family may give an important clue to mycoplasmal etiology. In experimental situations, the incubation period seemed to be shorter (7 to 10 days), but this may have resulted from the use of large inocula to induce disease.[10]

Organisms can be cultured from the sputum of infected individuals for weeks to months after clinically effective treatment,[30] and the extent of the effect of treatment of an index case on subsequent transmission to family members is unclear but may be beneficial.[17]

Clinical Disease

In view of the high incidence of mycoplasma pneumonia when studied epidemiologically in large populations and the rarity of individual sporadic diagnoses, it would appear that specific, confirmed diagnosis of this entity is not often accomplished in routine clinical practice. There are probably four reasons for this. The first is that mycoplasma pneumonia is usually self-limited and rarely fatal. This fact dampens the zeal to establish the cause of infection. Second, mycoplasmas are relatively fastidious and slow growing; therefore, culture results, if obtained at all, often return after the patient is well. Third, *M. pneumoniae* responds to the empirical antimicrobial therapy suggested for CAP, and finally, there is deficient knowledge of the epidemiology and clinical manifestations of infection, so that the diagnosis is often not considered.

RESPIRATORY INFECTION

Epidemiologic studies indicate that most *M. pneumoniae* infections lead to clinically apparent disease rather than to subclinical infection, and most involve only the upper respiratory tract.[20] After a 2- to

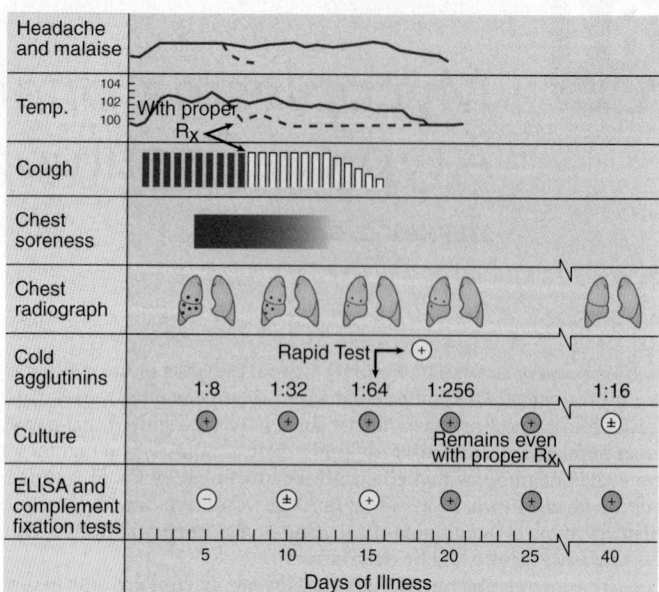

Figure 184-1 **Major clinical and laboratory manifestations of mycoplasmal pneumonia.** ELISA, enzyme-linked immunosorbent assay. *(Adapted from Baum SG. Mycoplasmal infections. In: Wyngaarden JB, Smith LH Jr, eds.* Cecil Textbook of Medicine, *17th ed. Philadelphia; WB Saunders; 1985:1506.)*

3-week incubation period, the disease has an insidious onset manifested by fever, malaise, headache, and cough. The latter is the clinical hallmark of *M. pneumoniae* infection (Fig. 184-1). The frequency and severity of cough increase over the next 1 to 2 days and may become debilitating. The gradual onset of symptoms is in contradistinction to the often acute presentation of respiratory infection caused by influenza, adenovirus, and other respiratory viruses.

In 5% to 10% of patients, depending somewhat on age, the infection progresses to tracheobronchitis or pneumonia. In these cases, the original manifestations persist, and the cough becomes more severe. It is usually relatively nonproductive but may yield white or occasionally blood-flecked sputum. Gram staining of this sputum reveals evidence of inflammatory cells but no predominant bacterial species. With continued cough, the patient may develop parasternal chest soreness due to muscle strain, but true pleuritic pain is unusual. Fever is usually at the level of 101° to 102° F and may be associated with chilly sensations. As opposed to pneumonia caused by *Streptococcus pneumoniae*, that caused by *M. pneumoniae* rarely involves true shaking chills. In comparison with influenza, which can also manifest as an atypical pneumonia syndrome, myalgias and gastrointestinal complaints of nausea and vomiting are unusual. Diarrhea, sometimes a concomitant of adenoviral pneumonia (see Chapter 143), is uncommon in mycoplasmal infection.

On physical examination, the general appearance is that of a patient who is not terribly ill. In fact, this disease is the paradigm of the term *walking pneumonia*. The pharynx may be injected and erythematous, usually without the marked cervical adenopathy seen in group A streptococcal pharyngitis. *M. pneumoniae* is not a common cause of isolated pharyngitis in the pediatric or adult population.[29] Much has been made of the finding of bullous myringitis in this disease. This abnormality was associated with experimentally induced *M. pneumoniae* infection in about 20% of volunteers.[31] However, true bullous myringitis in naturally occurring mycoplasma disease is rare. In a study of a pediatric population, otitis was rarely associated with isolation of mycoplasma and, on the contrary, was often associated with bacterial and viral upper respiratory tract pathogens.[32,33] The important synthesis of these data is that the absence of myringitis, bullous or otherwise, should not dissuade one from a diagnosis of mycoplasma pneumonia.

Examination of the chest in patients with mycoplasma pneumonia is often unrevealing, even in those patients with severe, productive cough. There may be no auscultative or percussive findings, or only minimal rales may be present. Disparity between physical findings and radiographic evidence of pneumonia in this condition may be the greatest of any of the atypical pneumonia syndromes. Although wheezing can occur in this disease, in one study of asthmatic patients, the presence of wheezing had a negative correlation with the isolation of *M. pneumoniae,* compared with viral respiratory pathogens.[34] *M. pneumoniae* also does not seem to be a common pathogen in patients with preexisting chronic obstructive lung disease.[28] Bacterial superinfection following *M. pneumoniae* respiratory infection is rare.

Pleural effusion (usually small) occurs in 5% to 20% of patients with *M. pneumoniae* infection.[35] This low incidence of pleural inflammation is consistent with the rarity of pleuritic pain. If effusion is present, thoracentesis reveals serous fluid that is exudative with minimal inflammatory reaction. The cell differential count in the fluid is variable,[36] and bloody effusions are rare. It is unusual to isolate *M. pneumoniae* from effusions when they do occur, but several reports of such isolation exist.[36]

Although pneumonia is usually mild and self-limited, fulminant, severe, and lethal cases have been reported in normal children, and young adults and may be underdiagnosed.[37,38]

The role of *M. pneumoniae* in asthma remains controversial, but there is increasing evidence, based primarily on molecular probe nucleic acid detection, that infection with this organism may initiate or exacerbate asthma.[39]

EXTRAPULMONARY INVOLVEMENT

Abnormalities in almost every organ system have been described as examples of the extrapulmonary manifestations of *M. pneumoniae* infection.[40] The frequency of these extrapulmonary manifestations varies greatly from one report to another and is much less common when viewed as part of a prospective epidemiologic study rather than as the sum of isolated case reports. The lesson from this appears to be that the high prevalence of mycoplasma infection in most populations predisposes to the reporting of many concurrent *but perhaps unrelated* events as if they were part of the mycoplasmal disease. Therefore, single case reports, particularly those confirmed only by serologic response, have not been included in this chapter. Several clinical syndromes have been reported with sufficient frequency to provide some support for a causal relationship.

DERMATOLOGIC INVOLVEMENT

A wide variety of transient dermatologic conditions have been reported in conjunction with mycoplasma pneumonia. These include macular, morbilliform, and papulovesicular eruptions as well as erythema nodosum and urticaria.[41] Again, the variety and high incidence of these rashes in the absence of mycoplasma infection makes it difficult to define the causal relationships, if any, among these occurrences. Further, the role that concurrent antibiotic therapy plays in the development of the exanthems seen during *M. pneumoniae* infection is unknown.

One skin condition that occurs often enough in concert with *M. pneumoniae* infection to provide some basis for relatedness is erythema multiforme major, or Stevens-Johnson syndrome (Fig. 184-2A). This has been reported in up to 7% of patients with mycoplasma pneumonia.[42-44] Erythema multiforme major consists of erythematous vesicles, plaques, and bullae involving the skin, with particular localization at mucocutaneous junctions. The conjunctivae may also be involved,[45] as may organs of the gastrointestinal and genitourinary tracts and the joints.[42]

These manifestations have been associated in isolated cases with many other infections, including some that can manifest as the atypical pneumonia syndrome, including legionnaires' pneumonia,[46] adenovirus conjunctivitis,[47] and influenza B infection.[48] However, among pos-

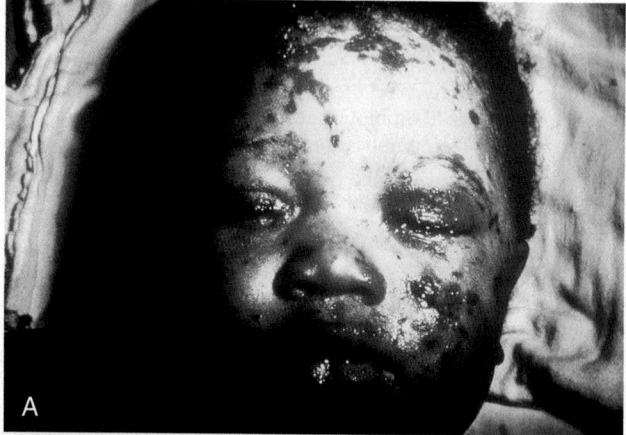
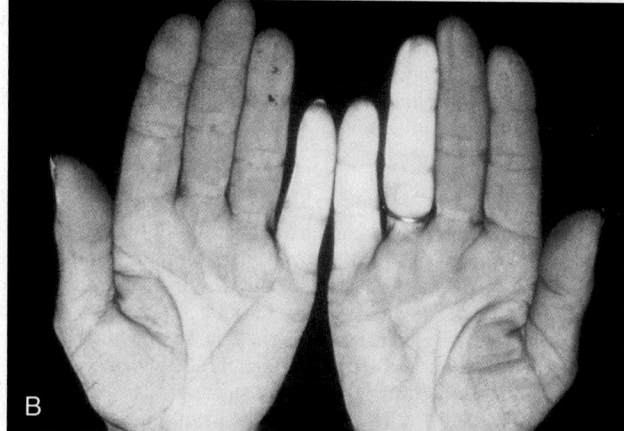
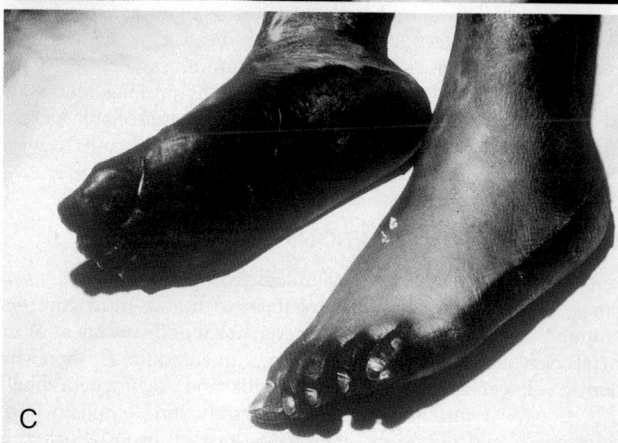

Figure 184-2 Skin conditions associated with *Mycoplasma pneumoniae* infection. A, Stevens-Johnson syndrome in a child with *M. pneumoniae* infection. **B,** Raynaud phenomenon in a young woman with *M. pneumoniae* infection and high titers of cold agglutinins. **C,** Necrosis of distal extremities in a patient with sickle cell disease who contracted *M. pneumoniae* infection accompanied by very high cold agglutinin titers.

sible associations of Stevens-Johnson syndrome with infectious diseases, the association with *M. pneumoniae* infection is by far the most common.[49] This complication tends to occur in the younger patients with mycoplasma pneumonia and has a definite male predominance (2:1 to 4:1) in this disease.

The pathogenesis of this syndrome in any of the diseases in which it occurs is unclear. It has long been supposed that immunity plays a major role,[43,50,51] but several reports have noted culture of *M. pneumoniae* from the lesions.[52,53] The relationship to the level of cold agglutinins in this disease is variable. It has been suggested that development of Stevens-Johnson syndrome may be the result of augmented sensitivity to antibiotics in the presence of *M. pneumoniae* infection,[54] but some patients develop erythema multiforme major in the absence of prior or concurrent antibiotic therapy. Corticosteroid therapy has been suggested for this complication, but data in support of the usefulness of this therapy are lacking.[55] Most patients clear the lesions in 1 to 2 weeks without scarring unless impetiginization supervenes.

RAYNAUD PHENOMENON

Although transient reversible vasospasm of the digits on exposure to the cold is not technically a dermatologic syndrome, it is manifested in the skin (see Fig. 184-2B). This phenomenon occurs in many people, usually women, without any association with infection. It has been reported in patients with acute mycoplasma pneumonia whether or not these patients manifested this syndrome before infection.[41,56] Although the pathophysiology of this phenomenon in *M. pneumoniae* infection is unclear, it may be related to in vivo action of cold agglutinins (see "Immunology," later).[57,58] Other vascular complications reported in *M. pneumoniae* infection include internal carotid artery occlusion and cerebral infarction.[59]

CARDIAC COMPLICATIONS

Cardiac abnormalities are among the most commonly reported extrapulmonary manifestations of *M. pneumoniae* infection. Most studies have involved hospitalized patients, so the true incidence of cardiac changes may be overestimated or underestimated.[60-62] The signs and symptoms suggesting involvement of the heart are arrhythmia, congestive failure, chest pain, and electrocardiographic abnormalities, particularly conduction defects. One report suggests that a loud third heart sound may be the only clue to cardiac involvement.[63] Although cardiac abnormalities have been reported in as many as 10% of cases of *M. pneumoniae* infection, other reports indicate a much lower prevalence. Cardiac complications are more common as the age of the patients studied increases. These complications prolong illness and have led to death[64] but generally do not appear to appreciably increase mortality. The mechanism of heart damage is unknown, but *M. pneumoniae* has been isolated from the pericardial fluid of one patient.[65]

NEUROLOGIC COMPLICATIONS

There are increasing reports of neurologic complications of *M. pneumoniae* infection, and some believe them to be the most common extrapulmonary manifestations. However, proof of involvement of the central nervous system in mycoplasma pneumonia is somewhat tenuous.[17] Encephalitis, aseptic meningitis and meningoencephalitis,[66,67] transverse myelitis,[68] brain stem dysfunction,[67] Guillain-Barré syndrome,[69,70] and peripheral neuropathy have all been reported. In aggregate, these central nervous system manifestations occur no more frequently than 1 per 1000 cases and are most often noted in hospitalized patients.[71] The cerebrospinal fluid findings in these cases are variable, but cellular response is usually minimal, with slightly elevated protein and normal to slightly depressed glucose. Most often, diagnosis of mycoplasma-related central nervous system involvement is made on exclusion of other causes, presence of antecedent or intercurrent respiratory illness, and a rise in antibody titer to *M. pneumoniae* in the serum.[67] Occasionally, mycoplasma-specific antibodies have been demonstrated in the cerebrospinal fluid, but these titers have paralleled serum antibody titers.

Neurologic complications are usually reversible when associated with mycoplasma infection, but the mortality of patients with central nervous system involvement is higher than that of others. Although *M. pneumoniae* has been isolated from a few of these patients,[72] polymerase chain reaction (PCR) failed to detect *M. pneumoniae* DNA in the cerebrospinal fluid of 11 patients deemed to have *M. pneumoniae*–related central nervous system disease on serologic grounds.[73] There-

fore, immune mechanisms of neural damage have been suggested.[70,74] Some mycoplasmas elaborate a neurotoxin, but this has not been described for *M. pneumoniae*.[67,75]

MUSCULOSKELETAL, RENAL, AND HEMATOPOIETIC COMPLICATIONS

Polyarthralgias are common in mycoplasma pneumonia, but arthritis is rare.[76] Immune mechanisms have been postulated for this complication, but there have been a few reports of isolation of *M. pneumoniae* from joint fluid.[77] When present, arthritis may be monoarticular or migratory. Several of the cases of frank arthritis have been reported in patients with hypogammaglobulinemia.[40] Nonhuman mycoplasmas probably cause arthropathy in several animal species and *Mycoplasma hominis* has been associated with human arthritis (see Chapter 183). Rhabdomyolysis also has been reported.[78]

Renal complications associated with immune complex deposition and high-titer cold agglutinins have been reported (see "Immunology," later).[79] There are several case reports of *M. pneumoniae*–associated aplastic anemia.[80]

CONDITIONS LEADING TO INCREASED SUSCEPTIBILITY

Several reports have emphasized the unusually high severity of *M. pneumoniae* infection in patients with sickle cell disease[81] or sickle-related hemoglobinopathies.[82,83] These patients may develop large pleural effusions and marked respiratory distress. Functional asplenia and its attendant opsonization deficiencies may contribute to overwhelming infection with *M. pneumoniae*, as they do to *S. pneumoniae* infection. It is interesting in this regard that some patients with sickle cell disease and *M. pneumoniae* infection who develop extremely high cold agglutinin titers may experience digital necrosis, as they do with *S. pneumoniae*. One such patient is shown in Figure 184-2C, and a hypothesis on pathogenesis is given in the discussion on cold agglutinins later under "Immunology."

Patients with immune deficiency syndromes have been the subjects of case reports of *M. pneumoniae* infection.[84] Because mycoplasma infections are so common in normal children, the contribution of the immune deficiency is unclear. *M. pneumoniae* does not seem to be a common opportunistic agent in the acquired immunodeficiency syndrome (AIDS),[84] but another mycoplasma, *Mycoplasma fermentans* (*incognitus* strain), has been identified in these patients.[85]

Unusually severe *M. pneumoniae* infection has also been reported in children with Down syndrome.[86] All these patients survived infection.

Immunology

Mycoplasmas are active in stimulating several components of the immune system. They can act as polyclonal T-cell and B-cell activators[87,88] and can cause capping of lymphocytes.[89] Macrophages can also be stimulated by some mycoplasmas in vitro.[90] *M. pneumoniae* is capable of inducing many proinflammatory and anti-inflammatory cytokines and chemokines in vitro and in vivo, including granulocyte-macrophage colony-stimulating factor,[91] interferon,[92] tumor necrosis factor-α, and transforming growth factor-β.[13,88,92,93] The elaboration of particular cytokines is tissue specific in vitro, and their interaction and proinflammatory or anti-inflammatory interaction in vivo is not well understood.[92]

In the course of *M. pneumoniae* infection, several classes of antibody are produced. Some of these fulfill the desired role of antibody production in infection—neutralization of the agent[94]—and others appear to be autoantibodies. The latter include agglutinins to lung, brain, cardiolipins, and smooth muscle.[73,92] The best studied of these autoagglutinins are the cold isohemagglutinins.

In 1943, Finland and colleagues described the presence of cold agglutinins in 50% to 70% of patients with Eaton agent pneumonia.[4,95,96] These agglutinins were capable of clumping erythrocytes at 4°C. Agglutination was reversible by warming the serum–erythrocyte mixture to 37°C and, unlike hemagglutination by myxoviruses and paramyxoviruses, was repeatable with the same sample, indicating that receptor-destroying enzyme (neuraminidase) played no role in the dissociation at 37°C.

Cold agglutinins in *M. pneumoniae* infection have been shown to be oligoclonal IgM antibodies directed against an altered I antigen on the surface of erythrocytes of *M. pneumoniae*–infected patients.[97] The I antigen is one of the blood group antigens, but unlike the A and B isoantigens, it appears to be common to almost all mature erythrocytes. Fetal erythrocytes have i antigen instead. Like other IgM antibodies, the mycoplasma-induced cold agglutinins develop early in the disease (7 to 10 days) and therefore are often present by the time the patient seeks medical attention. The titer of these agglutinins peaks at 2 to 3 weeks and persists for 2 to 3 months.

There are several theories on the factors triggering formation of cold agglutinins in mycoplasma pneumonia. One is that the organism alters the I antigen so as to make it antigenic to the patient. Hydrogen peroxide elaborated by *M. pneumoniae* could be responsible for this alteration. One study indicates that the I antigen in a sialated state may serve as a receptor for *M. pneumoniae* and that the cold agglutinins are directed at the modified receptor.[98] Other studies indicate that the cold agglutinins are directed at mycoplasma substructures themselves and merely cross-react with the I antigen on red cells.[99] The role in pathogenesis that these antibodies play is unclear. Given their apparent target, they could either contribute to cytolysis and exacerbate infection or interfere with cell-to-cell spread by blocking or disrupting the cell receptor for the mycoplasma.

There is a report of chronic renal failure associated with *M. pneumoniae*–induced cold agglutinins. Fluctuating severity of the renal failure correlated with variations in cold agglutinin titer; respiratory infection associated with complement-fixing antibodies to *M. pneumoniae* preceded the renal failure. There were no immunohistologic analyses done in this case, and the role of cold agglutinins in this patient's renal disease remains speculative.[79,80] High titers of cold agglutinins also have been associated with hemolysis, presumably as a result of the activation of complement-mediated erythrocyte destruction.[4] The direct Coombs test is positive in many of these patients.[100,101] Although clinically significant hemolysis is uncommon, subclinical levels of red cell destruction are common.

A fascinating syndrome seen in some patients with mycoplasma pneumonia that could be related to cold agglutinins is Raynaud phenomenon, described previously. A unifying hypothesis would relate capillary obstruction in extremities exposed to the cold to erythrocyte autoagglutination in the microcirculation of these patients with high-titer cold agglutinins. In support of this hypothesis is the severe vascular damage that occurs in patients with sickle cell disease who contract mycoplasma pneumonia accompanied by high titers of cold agglutinins. The extremities of one such patient, who had a cold agglutinin titer greater than 1:20,000, are shown in Figure 184-2C. The hypothetical pathogenesis of vasculopathy in this condition would then extend from reversible in vivo cold agglutination in microvasculature exposed to the cold (Raynaud), to irreversible vascular damage in patients who have underlying microvascular compromise that is exacerbated and leads to digital necrosis (sickle cell disease).

M. pneumoniae infection leads to the production of complement-fixing antibodies as well. These arise early in the disease (2 to 3 weeks) and persist for 2 to 3 months. Assay of *M. pneumoniae*–specific complement-fixing antibodies has been the standard for retrospective serologic confirmation of infection with this organism.

Clearly, antibody production of both IgG and IgA classes plays a part in protection against the disease.[94] However, second cases of *M. pneumoniae* infection are not rare in apparently immunocompetent individuals.[102] Polymorphonuclear leukocytes and pulmonary macrophages also play a role in containing infection, but they appear to have relative difficulty in clearing the organism, in comparison with the cellular killing of most bacteria.[103]

Pathology and Pathophysiology

Because of two fortunate aspects of mycoplasma pneumonia—its low severity and low mortality—there is relatively little information on pathologic findings in this disease, and knowledge rests on relatively few specimens. As stated previously, sickle cell disease, sickle-related hemoglobinopathies, and hypogammaglobulinemia predispose to increased severity and to mortality. Some of the available pathologic data therefore may be influenced by the pathophysiology of these underlying conditions.

When deaths have occurred, they have been in cases of diffuse pneumonia, adult respiratory distress syndrome, thromboembolism, and disseminated intravascular coagulopathy.[39,88,104-106]

A clinicopathologic presentation described a previously healthy man who succumbed to *M. pneumoniae* infection; autopsy revealed diffuse alveolar pneumonia with hyaline membrane formation and multiple pulmonary infarctions. Other evidence of diffuse intravascular coagulopathy included thrombosis and infarction of kidneys, liver, spleen, and brain.[107] Other pathologic findings have included myocarditis[108] and diffuse interstitial fibrosis.[109]

In nonfatal cases in which lung biopsy was performed, the inflammatory process involved primarily the trachea, bronchioles, and peribronchial tissues.[41,110] The lumen of the respiratory tree was filled with purulent exudate rich in polymorphonuclear leukocytes. The lining of the bronchial and bronchiolar walls showed metaplastic cells, and the walls themselves were infiltrated with monocytic elements, especially plasma cells. There was widening of the peribronchial septa and hyperplasia of type II pneumocytes.

Tracheal organ culture has demonstrated that, on inoculation of *M. pneumoniae*, first ciliary action is stopped, and then loss of cilia and complete desquamation of ciliated epithelial cells into the lumen occur.[111] This sloughing of cells is doubtless responsible for the cough that defines the clinical presentation. Histologic findings in human lung biopsy mirror the findings of ciliated cell damage seen in the animal experiments.[110]

Several characteristics of *M. pneumoniae* probably play a direct role in the respiratory pathogenicity of this organism. The first is the relatively great affinity of *M. pneumoniae* for respiratory epithelial cells. Attachment appears to be between a terminal organelle at one end of the filamentous organism[13,14] and a sialated glycoprotein (I-FI) on the surface of both respiratory epithelium and erythrocytes,[112-114] which acts as a receptor. The mycoplasmal terminal adhesion proteins (P1, P30, P65, P116, and high molecular weight [HMW] auxiliary proteins 1 to 3) have been purified and are the primary pathogenic elements of *M. pneumoniae*. Adherence-deficient mutants are avirulent.[15] *M. pneumoniae* attaches to ciliated epithelial cells at the base of cilia and appears to produce most of its physiologic and cytolytic changes while remaining extracellular. Hydrogen peroxide, which only *M. pneumoniae* of all the human mycoplasmas produces, may be responsible for some in vivo cell damage, as it is for the hemolysis seen when the organisms are grown on blood agar plates. Proinflammatory cytokine upregulation, as described earlier, plays a role in inflammation-related cell destruction.[13,16,88,92,93]

Diagnosis

Culture of the organism from respiratory secretions or body fluids should be the gold standard for diagnosis. However, mycoplasmas are fastidious in their growth requirements, and culture of *M. pneumoniae* is an elaborate and time-consuming procedure requiring specialized media (see Chapter 183). Because of this and the relative infrequency of requests for culture, most hospital microbiology laboratories are not set up to culture mycoplasmas. If culture is successfully performed, *M. pneumoniae* grown on agar produces a "mulberry" colony as opposed to a "fried-egg" appearance, as shown in Figure 183-1 in Chapter 183. Further identification can be established by other growth characteristics and by specific direct immunofluorescence.[115] Culture requires 1 to 2 weeks for definitive results. Although there are methods using pH

TABLE 184-1	Identifying Properties of *Mycoplasma pneumoniae*

Slow growth on cell-free media
Both aerobic and anaerobic growth
"Mulberry" rather than "fried-egg" colonies
Ferments glucose as major nutritional source, producin g acid
Hemadsorption to colonies
Hemolysis by hydrogen peroxide
Affinity for respiratory epithelium
Infection leads to cold agglutinin formation
Resistance to cell wall inhibitors
Inhibited by macrolides, tetracyclines, and quinolones

and dye indicators that provide presumptive results more rapidly, even these require at least 4 to 5 days. Table 184-1 lists identifying properties of *M. pneumoniae*.

Because culture is rarely carried out, there has been considerable interest in developing rapid diagnostic tests with high sensitivity and specificity for *M. pneumoniae*. These assays fall into three categories: detection of *M. pneumoniae*–specific immunoglobulins in serum and detection of *M. pneumoniae*–specific antigens or mycoplasmal nucleotide sequences directly in clinical specimens.

Diagnostically, the most useful *M. pneumoniae*–specific immunoglobulin to detect is IgM because it is most likely to indicate recent infection. Enzyme-linked immunoassays have been developed to detect IgM and IgG directed against *M. pneumoniae*.[116] Both immunoglobulins have been chosen as targets of the assay because adults with *M. pneumoniae* infection (presumably reinfection) may elaborate only an IgG response. When used in patients with positive assays for complement-fixing antibodies, the enzyme immunoassay had a specificity of more than 99% and a sensitivity of 98%. Specificity was retained, but sensitivity dropped to only 46% when IgG alone was the target. Variations on this theme detect IgM antibodies directed at specific *M. pneumoniae* antigens.[117] The tests are simple to perform and have high sensitivity and specificity but are limited in that they do not become positive until 1 to 2 weeks into the infection. One study compared three assays designed to detect antimycoplasma IgM: a particle agglutination test, a mu-capture enzyme-linked immunosorbent assay, and indirect immunofluorescence.[118] All three assays were about equally sensitive when compared with a standard complement fixation assay, but the particle agglutination assay appeared to give more false-positive results. In that all these tests are designed to detect IgM antibody, they may all be negative early (<7 to 10 days) into infection. Therefore, they do not provide the desired confirmation early enough to guide initial therapy in many cases.

Detection of *M. pneumoniae* antigens directly in sputum specimens has been accomplished with the use of an antigen-capture, indirect enzyme immunoassay.[119] The specificity of the assay was high, the reagents reacting only with *M. pneumoniae* and *M. genitalium*. Sensitivity was also relatively high (91%) when the assay was used on sputum and nasopharyngeal aspirates from patients who were shown either by culture or serology to have *M. pneumoniae* infection.[120]

The high sensitivity and specificity of the real-time PCR, performed on sputum, nasopharyngeal aspirate, or throat swab material, suggest that this test could serve as a specific and rapid diagnostic method.[121-124] Detection of *M. pneumoniae*–specific nucleotide sequences directly in clinical material has been accomplished with the use of tests developed locally or by large reference laboratories.[125] The tests, which can be completed in a few hours, detect either *M. pneumoniae* DNA (PCR) or ribosomal RNA (reverse transcriptase nucleic acid amplification). When compared with PCR as the gold standard of proven infection, few of the available antibody assays had acceptable sensitivity and specificity.[116] On the other hand, although the nucleic acid probe assays show excellent specificity, they failed to detect infection in some antibody-positive patients,[117] and sensitivity varied considerably depending on the source of the specimen tested. It was highest when sputum

was used, but lower when nasophayngeal aspirate or throat swab material was used.[126] This latter point is important when evaluating comparative studies, many of which use different specimen sources for their assays.

The cold agglutinin assay, once the mainstay of confirmative tests in suspected *M. pneumoniae* infection is neither very sensitive (50% to 70%) nor specific. The cold agglutination phenomenon is not unique to patients with mycoplasma pneumonia, and many patients with mycoplasma pneumonia never develop demonstrable cold agglutinins. A titer of 1:32 or greater is highly suggestive of infection with *M. pneumoniae*. Other diseases that can give rise to cold agglutinins are mononucleosis caused by Epstein-Barr virus (anti-i),[127] cytomegalovirus (anti-I),[128] some other viral diseases, and lymphoma.

A rapid bedside version of this test can be performed easily by any health care provider. In this test, 1 mL of the patient's blood is drawn into a tube containing anticoagulant. The type of tube used to collect specimens for prothrombin determination is preferred. Before cooling, examination shows a smooth coating of the tube by red cells. The blood is cooled to 4°C by placing it on liquid ice or in a standard refrigerator. After 3 to 4 minutes, the tube is examined for the presence of macroscopic agglutination. The tube is then rewarmed to 37°C in an incubator, or by exposure to body heat, and reexamined. The agglutination should dissociate at 37°C. This temperature-associated agglutination and dissociation can be repeated many times on the same sample. A positive result in the "bedside" test correlates with a laboratory titer of 1:64 or greater and is therefore less sensitive than the laboratory test. It can be accomplished in minutes, however, and if positive, it is highly suggestive of mycoplasma-related cold agglutination. The presence of cold agglutinins can also artifactually give rise to macrocytic indices as measured by the Coulter counter method. This is secondary to in vitro clumping of erythrocytes. In this case, the red cell distribution width would be high, indicating heterogeneity in measured red cell size.

Finally, although the PCR should become the gold standard for diagnosis because of its high sensitivity and specificity and the rapidity with which results can be produced, the test is not available or rarely ordered, even in microbiology laboratories serving major children's hospitals (personal communication). There is no commercially available kit for this test, and specimens generally are sent out to large diagnostic laboratories. Even when a home-grown test is available on site, low frequency of requests forces only periodic testing of bundled specimens. Both of these situations undermine the inherent timeliness of PCR diagnostic results.

In summary, the most promising molecular modalities for the diagnosis of acute infection are the nucleic acid amplification techniques (PCR) coupled with serology. They provide the best opportunity for specific diagnosis of current or recent *M. pneumoniae* infection.[119,120,129] However, at present, it would appear that most *M. pneumoniae* infections are treated empirically and either escape clinical diagnosis or, if considered clinically, never receive laboratory confirmation.

Treatment

Despite the number and variety of tests for the diagnosis of *M. pneumoniae* infection, most cases are encountered in the ambulatory setting, and institution of antimicrobial therapy remains empirical as part of CAP therapy, or based on clinical recognition of the explicit syndrome.

Antimicrobial therapy is not necessary for mycoplasmal upper respiratory tract infection, and the mycoplasmal etiology of this syndrome probably most often goes undiagnosed. Pneumonia due to mycoplasma is self-limited and not life-threatening in most cases. However, treatment with effective antimicrobials can markedly shorten the illness and, by reducing cough and the number of organisms per unit volume of sputum, can perhaps reduce the spread of infections in contacts.[17]

As would be predicted by the lack of a cell wall the entire class of mycoplasmas including, *M. pneumoniae* is unaffected by treatment with β-lactam antibiotics such as the penicillins and cephalosporins and by glycopeptides. Aminoglycosides are effective in vitro but have not been evaluated for efficacy in vivo.

The mainstays of treatment for *M. pneumoniae* respiratory tract infection are macrolides and tetracyclines. Use of either of these antimicrobials shortens the duration of illness. The radiographic findings may take a week or longer to resolve, even with appropriate therapy (see Fig. 184-1). In addition, studies have shown that organisms may continue to be identified from the sputum for several weeks after a complete course of clinically effective treatment.[30] This may be a result of the fact that, although *M. pneumoniae* causes respiratory disease as an extracellular parasite, it has the capacity to reside intracellularly as well. Intracellular residence may make it difficult to eradicate the organism in vivo, as it does in cell cultures. The effect of therapy on extrapulmonary manifestations is less certain.

Although the tetracyclines are active against *M. pneumoniae*, their use is precluded in young children because of adverse effects of the drug on developing teeth and bones. Furthermore, erythromycin is poorly tolerated by many people because of its gastrointestinal side effects. Erythromycin also raises theophylline levels, a consideration in the few asthmatic patients who may be still taking this drug.

Because of the adverse effects of erythromycin and tetracycline, there is considerable interest in the antimycoplasmal efficacy of other agents. Doxycycline is somewhat better tolerated than tetracycline and can be administered in two daily doses rather than three. In vitro, doxycycline is as effective as tetracycline against *M. pneumoniae* but, again, is contraindicated in children.[130]

Several other classes of antimicrobials have been found to have significant in vitro and in vivo activity against *M. pneumoniae* and other *Mycoplasma* species. These include the fluoroquinolones[88,131] and members of the macrolide-lincomycin-streptogramin-ketolide (MLSK) class of antimicrobials.[132,133] There are no good data on the optimal duration of therapy needed to minimize carriage and relapse with these agents.

The macrolides are more active in vitro than the tetracyclines. Fluoroquinolones are more active than the tetracyclines but are at least 100 times less active than the macrolides. Nevertheless, the fluoroquinolones have adequate activity for treatment of these infections. The streptogramins are also less active than the macrolides but more active than the tetracyclines.[132] There is a significant cost differential in the use of these drugs. The newer macrolides and quinolones are 50 to 60 times more expensive than the tetracyclines and 6 to 10 times more costly than erythromycin. Quinolones are relatively contraindicated in children because of their adverse effects on weight-bearing joints in young animals.[131] *M. pneumoniae* is generally susceptible to the MLSK class of antibiotics. However, starting in 2000, Japanese investigators recognized the emergence of macrolide-resistant *M. pneumoniae*.[134] The prevalence of these resistant organisms rose steadily over the next

few years and represented more than 30% of isolates in children in Japan by the year 2006. Adult isolates remained macrolide sensitive and, although the duration of illness in children was increased by about 2 days, there have been no treatment failures, and the clinical significance of this resistance has thus far not been appreciable. The basis of this resistance appears to be a mutation in 23S rRNA. Macrolide resistance has been identified in Europe, associated with sequence variation in the P1 adhesin gene, but remains rare.[135] Nonetheless, in cases of severe proven *M. pneumoniae* extrapulmonary infection, it might be wise to switch to a nonmacrolide antimicrobial agent such as a quinolone.

Recommended standard therapy for mycoplasmal pneumonia in teenagers and adults would include doxycycline, 100 mg every 12 hours, or an extended-spectrum macrolide such as azithromycin, 500 mg on day 1, and then 250 mg every 24 hours. The usual duration of therapy is 7 to 14 days. Young children should be given erythromycin, 10 mg/kg every 6 hours, or an extended spectrum macrolide (azithromycin), 10 to 12 mg/kg on day 1, followed by 5 mg/kg daily for 10 to 14 days. Infection of extrapulmonary sites may require prolonged treatment at higher doses.

Prevention

Because of outbreaks of *M. pneumoniae* respiratory infection among military recruits, there was for a time great enthusiasm and activity to produce a vaccine to protect against this organism. The vaccines did induce specific antibody responses, but protection against infection was limited to no more than 50% of vaccine recipients.[136,137] Live vaccines using attenuated wild-type and temperature-sensitive mutant mycoplasma have proved no more effective.[138,139]

In one study, volunteers who received vaccine but did not mount an antibody response developed more severe disease when rechallenged with wild-type mycoplasma than did nonvaccinated personnel.[140] Although *M. pneumoniae* continues to be perhaps the leading cause of the atypical pneumonia syndrome in closed populations, the enthusiasm for vaccine development for this disease appears to have waned. Vaccine development technology involving DNA expression-library immunization has proved successful in animal studies with nonhuman mycoplasmas.[141] These methods may breathe new life into *M. pneumoniae* vaccine development.

Secondary family cases definitely feed community outbreaks.[17] Examination of the effects of prophylactic antibiotic use in family members exposed to mycoplasma has shown a decrease in clinical disease in these patients, but seroconversion was not prevented.[142] A study showed that azithromycin prophylaxis, given as a 500-mg loading dose and 250 mg/day on days 2 through 5, significantly reduced the secondary attack rate of *M. pneumoniae* infection in a long-term care facility.[143]

REFERENCES

1. Drosten C, Gunther S, Preiser W, et al. Identification of a novel coronavirus in patients with severe acute respiratory syndrome. *N Engl J Med.* 2003;348:1967-1976.
2. Eaton MD, Meikeljohn G, van Herick W, et al. Studies on the etiology of primary atypical pneumonia: II. Properties of the virus isolated and propagated in chick embryos. *J Exp Med.* 1945;82:317.
3. Eaton MD, van Herick W, Meikeljohn G. Studies on the etiology of primary atypical pneumonia: III. Specific neutralization of the virus by human serum. *J Exp Med.* 1945;82:329.
4. Finland M, Peterson OL, Allen HE, et al. Cold agglutinins: I. Occurrence of cold isohaemagglutinins in various conditions. *J Clin Invest.* 1945;24:451.
5. Marmion BP. Eaton agent—Science and scientific acceptance: A historical commentary. *Rev Infect Dis.* 1990;12:338.
6. Chanock RM, Mufson MA, Bloom HH, et al. Eaton agent pneumonia. *JAMA.* 1961;175:213.
7. Clyde WA Jr. Demonstration of Eaton's agent in tissue culture. *Proc Soc Exp Biol Med.* 1961;107:715.
8. Goodburn GM, Marmion BP. Study of properties of Eaton's primary atypical pneumonia organism. *J Gen Microbiol.* 1962;29:271.
9. Chanock RM, Hayflick L, Barile MF. Growth on artificial medium of an agent associated with atypical pneumonia and its

identification as a PPLO. *Proc Natl Acad Sci U S A.* 1962; 48:41.
10. Chanock RM, Rifkind D, Dravetz HM, et al. Respiratory disease in volunteers infected with Eaton agent: A preliminary report. *Proc Natl Acad Sci U S A.* 1961;47:887.
11. Marmion BP, Goodburn GM. Effect of an organic gold salt on Eaton's primary atypical pneumonia organism and other observations. *Nature.* 1961;189:247.
12. Conference on Newer Respiratory Disease Viruses, *US Public Health Service.* Bethesda, Md: National Institutes of Health; 1962:198.
13. Razin S, Yogev D, Naot Y. Molecular biology and pathogenicity of mycoplasmas. *Microbiol Mol Biol Rev.* 1998;62:1094-1156.
14. Krause DC, Balish MF. Cellular engineering in a minimal microbe: Structure and assembly of the terminal organelle of *Mycoplasma pneumoniae.* *Molec Microbiol.* 2004;51:917-924.
15. Chaudhry R, Varshney A, Malhotra P. Adhesion proteins of *Mycoplasma pneumoniae.* *Front Biosci.* 2007;12:609-699.
16. Rottem S. Interaction of mycoplasmas with host cells. *Physiol Rev.* 2003;83:417-432.
17. Walter ND, Grant GB, Bandy U, et al. Community outbreak of *Mycoplasma pneumoniae* infection: School-based cluster of neurologic disease associated with household transmission of respiratory illness. *J Infect Dis.* 2008;198:1365-1374.

18. Foy HM, Kenny GE, Cooney MK, et al. Long term epidemiology of infections with *Mycoplasma pneumoniae.* *J Infect Dis.* 1979;139:681.
19. Chanock RM. Mycoplasma infections of man. *N Engl J Med.* 1965;273:1199.
20. Waites KB. New Concepts of *Mycoplasma pneumoniae* infections in children. *Pediatr Pulmonol.* 2003;36:267-278.
21. Foy HM, Kenny GE, McMahan R, et al. *Mycoplasma pneumoniae* pneumonia in an urban area. *JAMA.* 1970;214:1966.
22. Foy HM, Alexander ER. *Mycoplasma pneumoniae* infections in childhood. *Adv Pediatr.* 1969;16:301.
23. Denny FW, Clyde WA, Glenzen WP. *Mycoplasma pneumoniae* disease: clinical spectrum, pathophysiology, epidemiology and control. *J Infect Dis.* 1971;123:74.
24. Noah ND. *Mycoplasma pneumoniae* infections in the United Kingdom—1967-73. *Br Med J.* 1974;2:544.
25. Toma S. Isolation of *Mycoplasma pneumoniae* from respiratory tract specimens in Ontario. *Can Med Assoc J.* 1987;137:48.
26. Fernald GW, Collier AM, Clyde WA. Respiratory infections due to *Mycoplasma pneumoniae* in infants and children. *Pediatrics.* 1975;55:327.
27. McIntosh JC, Gutierrez HH. *Mycoplasma* infections. In: Smith TF, ed. *Immunology and Allergy Clinics of North America: Respiratory Infections.* Philadelphia: WB Saunders; 1993:43.

28. Alexander ER, Foy HM, Kenny GE, et al. Pneumonia due to *Mycoplasma pneumoniae*. *N Engl J Med*. 1966;275:131.
29. Foy HM, Grayston JT, Kenny GE, et al. Epidemiology of *Mycoplasma pneumoniae* infection in families. *JAMA*. 1966;197:859.
30. Smith CB, Friedewald WT, Chanock RM. Shedding of *Mycoplasma pneumoniae* after tetracycline and erythromycin therapy. *N Engl J Med*. 1967;276:1172.
31. Ritkind D, Chanock R, Kravetz H, et al. Ear involvement (myringitis) and primary atypical pneumonia following inoculation of volunteers with Eaton agent. *Am Rev Respir Dis*. 1962;85:479.
32. Klein JO, Teele DW. Isolation of viruses and mycoplasmas from middle ear effusions: A review. *Ann Otol Rhinol Laryngol*. 1976;85:140.
33. Sobeslavsky O, Syrucek L, Bruckaya M, et al. The etiologic role of *Mycoplasma pneumoniae* in otitis media in children. *Pediatrics*. 1965;35:652.
34. Nagayama Y, Sakurai N, Yamamota K, et al. Isolation of *Mycoplasma pneumoniae* from children with lower-respiratory-tract infections. *J Infect Dis*. 1988;157:911.
35. Mansel JK, Rosenow EC III, Smith TF, et al. *Mycoplasma pneumoniae* pneumonia. *Chest*. 1989;95:639.
36. Loo VG, Richardson S, Quinn P. Isolation of *Mycoplasma pneumoniae* from pleural fluid. *Diagn Microbiol Infect Dis*. 1991;14:443.
37. Wang R-S, Wang S-Y, Hsieh K-S, et al. Necrotizing pneumonitis caused by *Mycoplasma pneumoniae* in pediatric patients. *Pediatr Infect Dis J*. 2004;23:564-567.
38. Chan ED, Welsh CH. Fulminant *Mycoplasma pneumoniae* pneumonia. *West J Med*. 1995;162:133-142.
39. Nisar N, Guleria R, Kumar S, et al. *Mycoplasma pneumoniae* and its role in asthma. *Postgrad Med J*. 2007;83:100-104.
40. Sanchez-Vargas FM, Gomez-Duarte OG. *Mycoplasma pneumoniae*—an emerging extra-pulmonary pathogen. *Clin Microbiol Infect Dis*. 2008;14:105-115.
41. Murray HW, Masur H, Senterfit LB, et al. The protean manifestations of *Mycoplasma pneumoniae* in adults. *Am J Med*. 1975;58:229.
42. Levy M, Shear NH. *Mycoplasma pneumoniae* infections and Stevens-Johnson syndrome. *Clin Pediatr (Phila)*. 1991;30:42.
43. Schalock PC, Dinulos JGH. *Mycoplasma pneumoniae*–induced Stevens-Johnson syndrome without skin lesions: Fact or fiction? *J Am Acad Dermatol*. 2005;52:312-315.
44. Lyell A, Dick HM, Gordon AM, et al. Mycoplasmas and erythema multiforme. *Lancet*. 1967;2:1116.
45. Arstikaitis MJ. Ocular aftermath of Stevens-Johnson syndrome. *Arch Ophthalmol*. 1973;90:376.
46. Anderson R, Bergan T, Halvorsen K, et al. Legionnaires' disease combined with erythema multiforme in a 3 year old boy. *Acta Pediatr Scand*. 1981;70:427.
47. Kierman JP, Schanzlin DJ, Leveille AS. Stevens-Johnson syndrome associated with adenovirus conjunctivitis. *Am J Ophthalmol*. 1981;92:543.
48. Baine WB, Luby JB, Martin SM. Severe illness with influenza B. *Am J Med*. 1980;68:181.
49. Tay Y-K, Huff JC, Weston WL. *Mycoplasma pneumoniae* infection is associated with Stevens-Johnson syndrome, not erythema multiforme (von Hebra). *J Am Acad Dermatol*. 1996;35:757-760.
50. Kazmierowski JA, Wuepper KD. Erythema multiforme: Clinical spectrum and immunopathogenesis. *Springer Semin Immunopathol*. 1981;4:45.
51. Goldsmith DP. The erythema syndromes: Erythema multiforme and the Stevens-Johnson syndrome. *Pract Pediatr*. 1980;3:1.
52. Stutman HR. Stevens-Johnson syndrome and *Mycoplasma pneumoniae*: Evidence for cutaneous infection. *J Pediatr*. 1987;111:845.
53. Meseguer MA, de Rafael L, Vidal ML. Stevens-Johnson syndrome with isolation of *Mycoplasma pneumoniae* from skin lesions. *Eur J Clin Microbiol*. 1986;5:167.
54. McCormack JG. *Mycoplasma pneumoniae* and the erythema multiforme–Stevens-Johnson syndrome. *J Infect*. 1981;3:32.
55. Easterly NB. Corticosteroids for erythema multiforme? *Pediatr Dermatol*. 1989;6:229.
56. Feizi T, Maclean H, Sommerville RG, et al. Studies on an epidemic of respiratory disease caused by *Mycoplasma pneumoniae*. *Br Med J*. 1967;1:457.
57. Schubothe H. The cold hemagglutinin disease. *Semin Hematol*. 1966;3:27.
58. Furioli J, Bourdon C, Le Loc'h H. *Mycoplasma pneumoniae* infection: Manifestation in a 3 year old child by Raynaud's phenomenon. *Arch Fr Pediatr*. 1985;42:313.
59. Visudhiphan P, Chiemchanya S, Sirinavin S. Internal carotid artery occlusion associated with *Mycoplasma pneumoniae* infection. *Pediatr Neurol*. 1992;8:237.
60. Sands MJ, Satz JE, Soloff LA. Pericarditis and perimyocarditis associated with active *Mycoplasma pneumoniae* infection. *Ann Intern Med*. 1977;86:544.
61. Ponka A. Carditis associated with *Mycoplasma pneumoniae* infection. *Acta Med Scand*. 1979;11:1.
62. Fenollar F, Gauduchon V, Casalta J-P, et al. Mycoplasma endocarditis: Two case reports and a review. *Clin Infect Dis*. 2004;38:e21-e24.
63. Karjalainen J. A loud third heart sound and asymptomatic myocarditis during *Mycoplasma pneumoniae* infection. *Eur Heart J*. 1990;11:960.
64. Sands MJ Jr, Rosenthal R. Progressive heart failure and death associated with *Mycoplasma pneumoniae*. *Chest*. 1982;81:763.
65. Meseguer MA, Perez-Molina J, Fernández-Bustamante J, et al. *Mycoplasma pneumoniae* pericarditis and cardiac tamponade in a ten-year-old girl. *Pediatr Infect Dis J*. 1996;15:829-831.
66. Daxboeck F, Blacky A, Seidl R, et al. Diagnosis, treatment, and prognosis of *Mycoplasma pneumoniae* childhood encephalitis: systematic review of 58 cases. *J Child Neurol*. 2004;19:865-871.
67. Tsiodras S, Kelesidis I, Kelesidis T, et al. Central nervous system manifestations of *Mycoplasma pneumoniae* infections. *J Infection*. 2005;51:343-354.
68. Mills RW, Schoolfield L. Acute transverse myelitis associated with *Mycoplasma pneumoniae* infection: A case report and review of the literature. *Pediatr Infect Dis J*. 1992;11:228.
69. Tsiodras S, Kelesidis T, Kelesidis I, et al. *Mycoplasma pneumoniae*-associated myelitis: a comprehensive review. *Eur J Neurol*. 2006;13:112-124.
70. Daxboeck F. *Mycoplasma pneumoniae* central nervous system infections. *Current Opinion in Neurol*. 2006;19:374-378.
71. Guleria R, Nisar N, Chawla TC, et al. *Mycoplasma pneumoniae* and central nervous system complications: a review. *J Lab Clin Med*. 2005;146:55-63.
72. Abramovitz P, Schvartzman P, Harel D, et al. Direct invasion of the central nervous system by *Mycoplasma pneumoniae:* A report of two cases. *J Infect Dis*. 1987;155:482.
73. Fink CG, Sillis M, Read SJ, et al. Neurologic disease associated with *Mycoplasma pneumoniae* infection: PCR evidence against a direct invasive mechanism. *Clin Mol Pathol*. 1995;48:51-54.
74. Kusunoki S, Shiina M, Kanazawa I. Anti-Gal-C antibodies in GBS subsequent to mycoplasma infection: Evidence for molecular mimicry. *Neurology*. 2001:57:736-738.
75. Thomas L, Alen F, Bitensky MW, et al. The neurotoxin of *Mycoplasma neurolyticum*. *J Exp Med*. 1966;124:1967.
76. Ponka A. Arthritis associated with *Mycoplasma pneumoniae* infection. *Scand J Rheumatol*. 1979;8:27.
77. Davis CP, Cochran S, Lisse J, et al. Isolation of *Mycoplasma pneumoniae* from synovial fluid samples in a patient with pneumonia and polyarthritis. *Arch Intern Med*. 1988;148:969.
78. Minami K, Maeda H, Yanagawa T, et al. Rhabdomyolysis associated with *Mycoplasma pneumoniae* infection. *Pediatr Infect Dis J*. 2003;22:291-293.
79. Vitullo BV, O'Regan S, de Chadarevian JP, et al. *Mycoplasma pneumoniae* associated with acute glomerulonephritis. *Nephron*. 1978;21:284.
80. Stephan JL, Galambrun C, Pozzetto B, et al. Aplastic anemia after *Mycoplasma pneumoniae* infection: A report of two cases. *J Pediatr Hematol Oncol*. 1999;21:299-302.
81. Shulman ST, Barlett J, Clyde WA, et al. The unusual severity of mycoplasmal pneumonia in children with sickle-cell disease. *N Engl J Med*. 1972;287:164.
82. Solanki DL, Berdoff RL. Severe mycoplasma pneumonia with pleural effusions in a patient with sickle cell-hemoglobin C (SC) disease. *Am J Med*. 1979;66:707.
83. Chusid MJ, Lachman BS, Lazerson J. Severe mycoplasma pneumonia and vesicular eruption in SC hemoglobinopathy. *J Pediatr*. 1978;93:449.
84. Foy HM. Infections caused by *Mycoplasma pneumoniae* and possible carrier state in different populations of patients. *Clin Infect Dis*. 1993;17(Suppl 1):S37-S46.
85. Lo SC, Dawson M, Wong DM. Identification of *Mycoplasma incognitus* infection in patients with AIDS: An immunohistochemical, in-situ hybridization and ultrastructural study. *Am J Trop Med Hyg*. 1989;41:601.
86. Orlieck SL, Walker MS, Kuhls TL. Severe mycoplasma pneumonia in young children with Down syndrome. *Clin Pediatr (Phila)*. 1992;31:409.
87. Biberfeld G, Gronowicz E. *Mycoplasma pneumoniae* is a polyclonal B-cell activator. *Nature*. 1976;261:238.
88. Waites KB, Talkington DF. *Mycoplasma pneumoniae* and its role as a human pathogen. *Clin Microbiol Rev*. 2004;17:697-728.
89. Stanbridge EJ, Weiss RL. Mycoplasma capping on lymphocytes. *Nature*. 1978;276:583.
90. Dietz JN, Cole BC. Direct activation of the J774.1 murine macrophage cell line by *Mycoplasma arthritidis*. *Infect Immun*. 1981;37:811.
91. Mahkoul N, Merchav S, Tatarsky I, et al. Mycoplasma-induced in vitro production of interleukin-2 and colony-stimulating activity. *Isr J Med Sci*. 1987;23:480.
92. Yang J, Hooper W, Phillips D, et al. Cytokines in *Mycoplasma pneumoniae* infections. *Cytokine Growth Factor Rev*. 2004;15:157-168.
93. Tanaka H, Mitsuo N, Shin T, et al. Role of interleukin-18 and T-helper type 1 cytokines in the development of *Mycoplasma pneumoniae* pneumonia in adults. *Chest*. 2002;121:1493-1497.
94. Brunner H, Greenberg HB, James WD, et al. Antibody to *Mycoplasma pneumoniae* in nasal secretions and sputa of experimentally infected human volunteers. *Infect Immun*. 1973;8:612.
95. Peterson OL, Ham TH, Finland M. Cold agglutinins (autohaemagglutinins) in primary atypical pneumonias. *Science*. 1943;97:167.
96. Turner JC. Development of cold agglutinins in atypical pneumonia. *Nature*. 1943;151:419.
97. Feizi T, Taylor-Robinson D. Cold agglutinin anti-I and *Mycoplasma pneumoniae*. *Immunology*. 1967;13:405.
98. Konig AL, Kreft H, Hengge U. Coexisting anti-I and anti-FI/Gd cold agglutinins in infections by *Mycoplasma pneumoniae*. *Vox Sang*. 1988;55:176.
99. Costea N, Yakulis VJ, Heller P. Inhibition of cold agglutinins (anti-I) by *M. pneumoniae* antigens. *Proc Soc Exp Biol Med*. 1972;139:476.
100. Feizi T. Cold agglutinins, the direct Coombs' test and serum immunoglobulins in *Mycoplasma pneumoniae* infection. *Ann N Y Acad Sci*. 1967;143:801.
101. Jacobson LB, Longstreth GF, Edington TS. Clinical and immunologic features of transient cold agglutinin hemolytic anemia. *Am J Med*. 1973;54:514.
102. Foy HM, Kenny GE, Sefi R, et al. Second attacks of pneumonia due to *Mycoplasma pneumoniae*. *J Infect Dis*. 1977;135:673.
103. Erb P, Bredt W. Interaction of *Mycoplasma pneumoniae* with alveolar macrophages: Viability of adherent and ingested mycoplasmas. *Infect Immun*. 1979;25:11.
104. Koletsky RJ, Weinstein AJ. Fulminant mycoplasma pneumonia infection: Report of a fatal case and a review of the literature. *Am Rev Respir Dis*. 1980;122:491.
105. Nilsson IM, Rausing A, Dennenberg T, et al. Intravascular coagulation and acute renal failure in a child with mycoplasma infection. *Acta Med Scand*. 1971;189:359.
106. Meyers BR, Hirshman SZ. Fatal infections associated with *Mycoplasma pneumoniae:* Discussion of three cases with necropsy findings. *Mt Sinai J Med*. 1972;39:258.
107. Scully RE, ed. Case records of the Massachusetts General Hospital: Mycoplasma pneumonia with diffuse alveolar damage and disseminated intravascular coagulation. *N Engl J Med*. 1992;326:324.
108. Pickens S, Catterall JR. Disseminated intravascular coagulation and myocarditis associated with *Mycoplasma pneumoniae* infection. *Br Med J*. 1978;23:1526.
109. Kaufman JM, Cuvelier CA, Van der Staeten M. Mycoplasma pneumonia with fulminant evolution into diffuse interstitial fibrosis. *Thorax*. 1980;35:140.
110. Rollin S, Colby T, Clayton F. Open lung biopsy in mycoplasma pneumonia. *Arch Pathol Lab Med*. 1986;110:34.
111. Hu PC, Collier AM, Baseman JB. Interaction of virulent *Mycoplasma pneumoniae* with hamster tracheal organ cultures. *Infect Immun*. 1976;14:217.
112. Brunner H, Feldner J, Bredt W. Effect of monoclonal antibodies to the attachment tip on experimental *Mycoplasma pneumoniae* infection of hamsters. *Isr J Med Sci*. 1984;20:878.
113. Baseman JB, Banai M, Kahane I. Sialic acid residues mediate *Mycoplasma pneumoniae* attachment to human and sheep erythrocytes. *Infect Immun*. 1982;38:389.
114. Hengge VR, Kirschfink M, Konig AL, et al. Characterization of I/F1 glycoprotein as a receptor for *Mycoplasma pneumoniae*. *Infect Immun*. 1992;60:79.
115. Del Giudice RA, Robillard NF, Carski TR. Immunofluorescence identification of mycoplasma on agar by use of incident illumination. *J Bacteriol*. 1967;93:1205.
116. Beersma MFC, Dirven K, van Dam AP, et al. Evaluation of 12 commercial tests and the complement fixation test for *Mycoplasma pneumoniae*-specific immunoglobulin G (IgG) and IgM antibodies, with PCR used as the "Gold Standard." *J Clin Microbiol*. 2005;43:2277-2285.
117. Kim NH, Lee JA, Eun BW, et al. Comparison of polymerase chain reaction and the indirect particle agglutination antibody test for the diagnosis of *Mycoplasma pneumoniae* pneumonia in children during two outbreaks. *Pediatric Infect Dis J*. 2007;26:897-903.
118. Barker CE, Sillis M, Wreghitt TG. Evaluation of Serodia, Myco II particle agglutination test for detecting *Mycoplasma pneumoniae* antibody: Comparison with mu-capture ELISA and indirect fluorescence. *J Clin Pathol*. 1990;43:163.
119. Daxboeck F, Krause R, Wenisch C. Laboratory diagnosis of *Mycoplasma pneumoniae* infection. *Clin Microbiol Infect Dis*. 2003;9:263-273.
120. Loens K, Beck T, Ursi D, et al. Evaluation of different nucleic acid amplification techniques for the detection of *M. pneumoniae, C. pneumoniae* and *Legionella* spp. in respiratory specimens from patients with community acquired pneumonia. *J Microbiol Methods*. 2008;73:257-262.
121. Van Kuppeveld FJ, Johansson KE, Galoma JM, et al. 16S mRNA based polymerase chain reaction compared with culture and serologic methods for diagnosis of *Mycoplasma pneumoniae* infection. *Eur J Clin Microbiol Infect Dis*. 1994;13:401-405.
122. Ramirez JA, Ahkee S, Tolentino A, et al. Diagnosis of *Legionella pneumophila, Mycoplasma pneumoniae* or *Chlamydia pneumoniae* lower respiratory infection using the polymerase chain reaction on a single throat swab specimen. *Diagn Microbiol Infect Dis*. 1996;24:7-14.
123. Shelhamer JH, Gill VJ, Quinn TC, et al. The laboratory evaluation of opportunistic pulmonary infections. *Ann Intern Med*. 1996;124:585-599.
124. Schluger NW, Rom WN. The polymerase chain reaction in the diagnosis and evaluation of pulmonary infections. *Am J Respir Crit Care Med*. 1995;152:11-16.
125. Dular R, Kajioka R, Kusatiya S. Comparison of Gen-Probe commercial kit and culture technique for the diagnosis of *Mycoplasma pneumoniae* infection. *J Clin Microbiol*. 1988;26:1068.
126. Räty R, Rönkkö E, Kleemola M. Sample type is crucial to the diagnosis of mycoplasma pneumoniae pneumonia by PCR. *J Med Microbiol*. 2005;54:287-291.
127. Rosenfield RE, Schmidt PJ, Calvo RC, et al. Anti-i, a frequent cold agglutinin in infectious mononucleosis. *Vox Sang*. 1965;10:631.

128. Lind K, Spencer ES, Anderson HK. Cold agglutinin production and cytomegalovirus infection. *Scand J Infect Dis.* 1974;6:109.

129. Baum SG. Mycoplasma infection: Immunologic and molecular biologic diagnostic techniques. In: Rose NR, de Macario EC, Folds JD, et al, eds. *Manual of Clinical Laboratory Immunology: Infections Caused by Bacteria, Mycoplasmas, Chlamydiae and Rickettsiae.* Washington, DC: American Society for Microbiology; 1997:547-557.

130. Rylander M, Hallander HO. In vitro comparison of the activity of doxycycline, tetracycline, erythromycin and a new macrolide, CP 62993, against *Mycoplasma pneumoniae, Mycoplasma hominis* and *Ureaplasma urealyticum. Scand J Infect Dis.* 1988;53(Suppl):12.

131. Pereyre S, Renaudin H, Bébéar C, et al. In vitro activities of the newer quinolones garenoxacin, gatifloxacin, and gemifloxacin against human mycoplasmas. *Antimicrob Agents Chemother.* 2004;48:3165-3168.

132. Bébéar C, Pereyre S. Mechanisms of drug resistance in *Mycoplasma pneumoniae. Curr Drug Targets Infect Disord.* 2005;5: 263-271.

133. Waites KB, Crabb DM, Duff LB. In vitro activities of ABT-773 and other antimicrobials against human mycoplasmas. *Antimicrob Agents Chemother.* 2003;47:39-42.

134. Morozumi M, Iwata S, Hasegawa K, et al. Increased macrolide resistance of *Mycoplasma pneumoniae* in pediatric patients with community-acquired pneumonia. *Antimicrob Agents Chemother.* 2008;52:348-350.

135. Pereyre S, Charron A, Renaudin H, et al. First report of macrolide-resistant strains and description of a novel nucleotide sequence variation in the P1 adhesin gene in *Mycoplasma pneumoniae.* Clinical strains isolated in France over 12 years. *J Clin Microbiol.* 2007;45:3534-3539.

136. Wenzel RP, Craven RB, Davies JA, et al. Field trial on an inactivated *Mycoplasma pneumoniae* vaccine: I. Vaccine efficacy. *J Infect Dis.* 1976;134:571.

137. Smith CB, Friedewald WT, Chanock RM. Inactivated *Mycoplasma pneumoniae* vaccine. *JAMA.* 1967;199:353.

138. Couch RB, Cate TR, Chanock RM. Infection with artificially propagated Eaton agent (*Mycoplasma pneumoniae*). *JAMA.* 1964;187:442.

139. Greenberg H, Helms CM, Brunner H, et al. Asymptomatic infection of adult volunteers with a temperature sensitive mutant of *Mycoplasma pneumoniae. Proc Natl Acad Sci U S A.* 1974;71:4015.

140. Smith CB, Chanock RM, Friedewald WTK, et al. *Mycoplasma pneumoniae* infections in volunteers. *Ann N Y Acad Sci.* 1967;143:471.

141. Barry M, Lai WC, Johnston SA. Protection against mycoplasma infection using expression-library immunization. *Nature.* 1995;377:632-635.

142. Jensen KE, Senterfit LB, Scully WE, et al. *Mycoplasma pneumoniae* infections in children: An epidemiological appraisal in families treated with oxytetracycline. *Am J Epidemiol.* 1967;86:419.

143. Klausner JD, Passaro D, Rosenberg J. Enhanced control of an outbreak of *Mycoplasma pneumoniae* pneumonia with azithromycin prophylaxis. *J Infect Dis.* 1998;177:161-166.

185

Genital Mycoplasmas: *Mycoplasma genitalium, Mycoplasma hominis*, and *Ureaplasma* Species

GEORGE E. KENNY

The microbial flora of the human genital tract is complex, including organisms that are difficult to cultivate and detect and most likely organisms that have yet to be discovered.[1] Mycoplasmas and ureaplasmas fit into the difficult-to-grow category. To date, eight species of mycoplasmas and ureaplasmas have been identified in the genital tract (Table 185-1). Although six species are classified in the genus *Mycoplasma*, they are far more heterogeneous than their classification implies. *Mycoplasma genitalium* has the smallest genome of any mycoplasma (580 kb) and is closely related to *Mycoplasma pneumoniae* despite its much larger genome (816 kb).[2] Metabolically, they are also diverse. *Mycoplasma hominis, Mycoplasma primatum*, and *Mycoplasma spermatophilum* metabolize arginine to ornithine with the production of ammonia but do not utilize glucose. *M. genitalium* utilizes glucose with the production of acid but does not utilize arginine. *Mycoplasma fermentans* and *Mycoplasma penetrans* utilize both arginine and glucose. *Ureaplasma urealyticum* (biovar 2) and *Ureaplasma parvum* (biovar 1) are the most unusual because they both require and hydrolyze urea with the production of energy, CO_2, and NH_3.[2] No other microorganism has such a requirement. They are also unusual in that they grow only in medium that is pH 6.5 or lower. The features that mycoplasmas and ureaplasmas have in common are small size (0.2 or 0.3 μm), small genome (580 to 1170 kb),[2] no cell wall, and a requirement for a highly enriched medium containing animal serum. The generation times in broth culture are 1 or 2 hours for ureaplasmas and most mycoplasmas, but *M. genitalium* grows very slowly, with initial estimates of its doubling time of 12 hours or more for the established strain G-37.[3]

Prevalence of Genital Mycoplasmas in Healthy People

M. hominis and ureaplasmas have been most studied because of their relative ease of cultivation. Ureaplasmas are highly prevalent in the genital tracts of healthy sexually active women, with infection rates of 60% to 70%.[4] *U. parvum* strains account for 70% of ureaplasmas detected.[5] The prevalence of ureaplasmas in the male urethra is lower at 10% to 20%.[6] Infants can be infected with ureaplasmas at birth. The organisms persist for a while and disappear by age 2 years.[7] Ureaplasmas become prevalent with the onset of sexual activity in both males and females. Taken as a whole, the high prevalence of ureaplasmas and *M. hominis* in healthy people indicates that they are not prime pathogens. It is not known how long an individual ureaplasmal serovar or biovar persists in carriers or if there are changes in types over time. *M. penetrans* has been found in people with human immunodeficiency virus infection.[8] *M. spermatophilum* has been reported in several people.

Mycoplasmas and Nongonococcal Urethritis in Men

The diagnosis of nongonococcal urethritis (NGU) arose when it was recognized that urethritis persisted in some cases after treatment with penicillin and elimination of gonococci. Mycoplasmas and ureaplasmas have no cell walls and thus are not susceptible to antimicrobial agents, such as penicillin, that target the cell wall of bacteria. Ureaplasmas were discovered in the late 1950s and were suspected of having a role in NGU because of their prevalence, resistance to penicillin, susceptibility to tetracyclines, and the fact that they were sexually transmitted. However, another group of bacteria, the chlamydiae, were subsequently found to have a major role in NGU, accounting for as much as 30% of disease.[6,9] There was some evidence that ureaplasmas were involved in cases of urethritis in young men experiencing their first sexual encounters.[10] Now that it is possible to identify ureaplasmal biovars by the polymerase chain reaction (PCR), it appears that *U. urealyticum*, but not *U. parvum*, may have a role in NGU biovar 2.[11] With the advent of simple and effective PCR assays, it appears clear that *M. genitalium* may account for as much as 15% to 20% of NGU.[3,6,12,13] Chlamydiae and *M. genitalium* are independent agents of NGU.[6,14] Detection of *M. genitalium* is not associated with the presence of other mycoplasmas and ureaplasmas. *M. hominis* is found as often in the control populations as in NGU cases. It is not possible to determine whether *U. urealyticum* or *U. parvum* is associated with disease from the literature because nearly all historical isolates were identified as *U. urealyticum* before it was divided into two species. If chlamydiae are associated with 30% of NGU and *M. genitalium* with 20%, then these two organisms are the major cause of NGU.

Mycoplasmal Infections in Women

The high prevalence of ureaplasmas in the vagina of healthy sexually active women (~66%)[4,6,15] indicates that they are commensals and normal flora. *M. hominis* is less prevalent at approximately 10% in healthy women. Concentrations of *M. hominis* are high in bacterial vaginosis.[16] Studies of the association of *M. genitalium* with genital diseases in women are just beginning, and only a few case-control studies have been carried out. *M. genitalium* was detected in 7% of 719 women with mucopurulent cervicitis.[17] The relative risk was 3.3-fold, indicating that *M. genitalium* may have a role in cervicitis. Similar results were obtained for endometritis, in which 16% of cases were positive for *M. genitalium*, with 2% positive in the control subjects.[16] In a study of pelvic inflammatory disease, 13% of 45 cases had *M. genitalium* compared with none in 37 control subjects.[18] Twenty-seven percent were positive for *Chlamydia trachomatis*. There is serologic evidence that as many as 40% of women with pelvic inflammatory disease showed antibody increases to *M. genitalium*.[14] Overall, *M. genitalium* is associated with a proportion of the same diseases that *C. trachomatis* is associated with. On premature rupture of membranes, there is invasion of the uterus not only by ureaplasmas but also by the numerous bacterial species normally found in the vagina.[16]

CULTIVATION AND DETECTION

Mycoplasma medium for isolation contains peptones, yeast extract, and 20% serum. Horse serum is most frequently used, although some formulations call for fetal calf serum. *M. hominis* grows readily on both agar plates and broth cultures. *M. genitalium* grows slowly, with the

TABLE 185-1	The Human Genital Ureaplasmas and Mycoplasmas				
Species	Prevalence in Genital Tract of Healthy People	Substrate Utilization	Atmosphere for Isolation	pH for Growth	Growth from Specimens
Ureaplasma urealyticum	++	Urea	Indifferent	6.0-6.5	Rapid (2-4 days)
Ureaplasma parvum	++++	Urea	Indifferent	6.0-6.5	Rapid (2-4 days)
Mycoplasma hominis	+++	Arginine	Indifferent	6.5-8.0	Rapid (2-5 days)
Mycoplasma genitalium	Unknown	Glucose	Aerobic	7.0-7.5	Tissue culture required
Mycoplasma fermentans	+?	Glucose and arginine	Anaerobic	7.0-8.0	Slow (5-10 days)
Mycoplasma penetrans	Rare	Glucose and arginine	?	7.0-8.0?	?
Mycoplasma spermatophilum	Rare	Arginine	?	7.0-8.0?	?
Mycoplasma primatum	Rare	Arginine	?	7.0-8.0?	?

Adapted from Razin S, Yogev D, Naot Y. Molecular biology and pathogenicity of mycoplasmas. *Microbiol Mol Biol Rev*. 1998;62:1094.

prototype strain G37 producing colonies in 6 days or more (Fig. 185-1). However, strains from specimens cannot be directly cultured on agar but require tissue culture enrichment (see Table 185-1). *M. hominis* forms microscopically visible colonies in 2 to 5 days. It occasionally is recognized as minute colonies on conventional blood agar. In broth cultures, *M. hominis* forms only a faint haze. Growth in broth is usually detected visually by identifying the alkaline products of arginine hydrolysis with a pH indicator. Minute ureaplasmal colonies appear in 2 to 5 days on a special medium of pH 6.5 or lower. In broth culture, the alkaline reaction from hydrolysis of urea is used to monitor growth. *M. fermentans* is isolated best on mycoplasma agar or broth under anaerobic or microaerophilic conditions. Initial isolation may take 10 days or more. *M. spermatophilum* and *M. penetrans* have seldom been isolated in clinical studies. Overall, diagnosis of mycoplasmal and ureaplasmal infections by culture is slow and difficult compared with isolation of *Neisseria gonorrhoeae*. As a consequence, PCR methods have been developed[19-22] and are the assays of choice. Determining the quantity of organisms present has proved useful for assessing the disease-causing ability of mycoplasmas and ureaplasmas.[10,23] Real-time PCR addresses this problem.

DETECTION OF MYCOPLASMA GENITALIUM

The initial isolation of *M. genitalium* on SP-4 medium was reported in 1981.[24] No subsequent isolates were recovered from the genital tract until 1996, when Jensen and colleagues[25] reported isolation of the organism on agar using tissue culture as an enrichment culture for eventual growth on Friis medium, a process that took as much as 1 year. As a consequence, detection is carried out by PCR. Urine appears to be as good a sample in men as urethral swabs and is much easier to collect. In women, vaginal or cervical swabs are used. The most commonly used primers are directed at the 110-kD attachment protein.[6,19,21] Because PCR contamination is a major problem, strains may be genotyped, which permits identification of specific strains and excludes the possibility of contamination with stock strains.[26] Culture is important for obtaining organisms for susceptibility testing and is a topic of continuing research. A tissue culture method has been devised for susceptibility testing.[27]

Infections Outside the Genital Tract

M. hominis and ureaplasmas appear to be opportunists when they infect beyond the lower genital tract. Both are associated with mild self-limiting postpartum fevers.[28] *M. hominis* has been recovered from a variety of extragenital diseases,[23,29,30] including infection of the kidneys, joints, surgical wounds, and other sites, particularly in immunocompromised individuals.[30] *M. fermentans* is a rare isolate from the genital tract. It has been associated with rheumatoid arthritis, but proof that it is an independent cause is lacking. It was thought to be a cofactor in the development of the acquired immunodeficiency syndrome (AIDS). However, the organism can be detected as often in the bloodstream of healthy people as in those with AIDS.[20] The significance of the frequent detection of *M. fermentans* DNA in the bloodstream from apparently healthy people is not understood and may be a promising avenue for further study.

SERODIAGNOSIS

The procedures used by mycoplasmologists to determine antibody levels include indirect immunofluorescence, Western blotting, enzyme-linked immunosorbent assay (ELISA), and metabolic inhibition testing. The metabolic inhibition test relies on the ability of patients' serum to prevent growth of mycoplasmas as evidenced by the failure to produce a metabolic product. A major problem for diagnosis of *M. genitalium* infections is its strong cross-reactivity with *M. pneumoniae*. A cloned *M. genitalium*–specific protein[31] may have utility for specific measurement of antibodies, which could be carried out by ELISA.

INTERPRETATION OF LABORATORY RESULTS

M. hominis detected in the vagina or male urethra can best be interpreted as normal flora. Determination of the significance of detection of ureaplasmas requires the ability to distinguish the two species. Detection of *M. genitalium* from these sites implies potential disease that should be treated with the same concern as chlamydial infections. Detection of ureaplasmas or mycoplasmas in the bloodstream, joints, wound lesions, and other extragenital sites is significant. Mycoplasmas and ureaplasmas should be searched for in putatively infected sites where conventional bacteria cannot be found. Overall, detection of mycoplasmas by conventional culture is slow; it takes 2 or more days to detect any colonies and several more days to identify species. More widespread use of PCR will facilitate timely diagnosis of mycoplasmal infections.

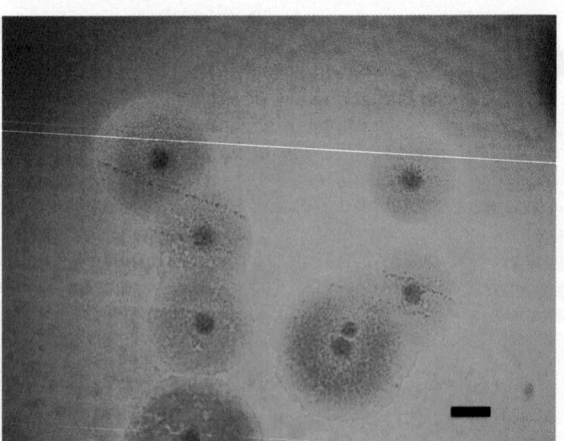

Figure 185-1 Light micrograph of *Mycoplasma genitalium* strain G37 on H agar[41] after 14 days of incubation. Scale bar = 100 μm.

SUSCEPTIBILITY TO ANTIMICROBIAL AGENTS

Mycoplasmas in general are susceptible to tetracyclines and quinolones.[32-36] Because they have no cell wall, they are not susceptible to penicillins or cephalosporins. The susceptibilities of *M. genitalium* parallel those of *M. pneumoniae* in that both are highly susceptible to macrolides.[35,36] *M. hominis* is intrinsically resistant to erythromycin and other macrolides[31] but moderately susceptible to josamycin and lincomycin.

Ureaplasmas show limited susceptibility to erythromycin and other macrolides[32] but are resistant to lincomycin. Because macrolide susceptibility is less as pH decreases,[32] macrolides are less effective in the acid environment of the genital tract. In vitro, azithromycin and clarithromycin are significantly more active than erythromycin.[32]

Some clinical strains of both ureaplasmas and *M. hominis* show high-level tetracycline resistance because of the transposon TetM.[37,38] Treatment with azithromycin but not tetracycline has resulted in clearance of *M. genitalium* from people with NGU.[39] Treatment of extragenital *M. hominis* infections is difficult. Tetracycline resistance is becoming more common, and tetracycline is bacteriostatic so that infections tend to recur even with susceptible strains. The mutation rate for quinolone resistance is high in *M. hominis*, and resistant strains have already been recognized.[32] Approved quinolones with the highest in vitro activity relative to achievable blood levels should be used to minimize chances for mutation because mutation to high-level resistance is a multistep process.[40]

REFERENCES

1. Krieger JN, Riley DE, Roberts MC, et al. Prokaryotic DNA sequences in patients with chronic idiopathic prostatitis. *J Clin Microbiol.* 1996;34:3120.
2. Razin S, Yogev D, Naot Y. Molecular biology and pathogenicity of mycoplasmas. *Microbiol Mol Biol Rev.* 1998;62:1094.
3. Hamasuna R, Osada Y, Jensen JS. Isolation of *Mycoplasma genitalium* from first-void urine specimens by co-culture with Vero cells. *J Clin Microbiol.* 2007;45:847.
4. Tsunoe H, Tanaka M, Nakayama H, et al. High prevalence of *Chlamydia trachomatis*, *Neisseria gonorrhoeae* and *Mycoplasma genitalium* in female commercial sex workers in Japan. *Int J STD AIDS.* 2000;12:790.
5. Abele-Horn M, Wolf C, Dressel P, et al. Association of *Ureaplasma urealyticum* biovars with clinical outcome for neonates, obstetric patients and gynecological patients with pelvic inflammatory disease. *J Clin Microbiol.* 1997;35:1199.
6. Totten PA, Schwartz MA, Sjostrom KE, et al. Association of *Mycoplasma genitalium* with nongonococcal urethritis in heterosexual men. *J Infect Dis.* 2001;183:269.
7. Foy HM, Kenny GE, Levinsohn EM, et al. Acquisition of mycoplasmata and T-strains during infancy. *J Infect Dis.* 1970;121:579.
8. Hussain AI, Robson WLM, Kelley R, et al. *Mycoplasma penetrans* and other mycoplasmas in urine of human immunodeficiency virus-positive children. *J Clin Microbiol.* 1999;37:1518.
9. Johannisson G, Enstrom Y, Lowhagen GB, et al. Occurrence and treatment of *Mycoplasma genitalium* in patients visiting STD clinics in Sweden. *Int J STD AIDS.* 2000;11:324.
10. Bowie WR, Wang SP, Alexander ER. Etiology of non-gonococcal urethritis: evidence for *Chlamydia trachomatis* and *Ureaplasma urealyticum. J Clin Invest.* 1977;59:735.
11. Povlsen K, Bjørnelius E, Lidbrink P, et al. Relationship of *Ureaplasma urealyticum* biovar 2 to nongonococcal urethritis. *Eur J Clin Microbiol Infect Dis.* 2002;21:97.
12. Jensen JS, Orsum R, Dohn B, et al. *Mycoplasma genitalium*: a cause of male urethritis? *Genitourin Med.* 1993;69:265.
13. Martin DH. Non-gonococcal urethritis: new views through the prism of modern molecular microbiology. *Curr Infect Dis Rep.* 2008;10:128.
14. Taylor-Robinson D, Gilroy CB, Hay PE. Occurrence of *Mycoplasma genitalium* in different populations and its clinical significance. *Clin Infect Dis.* 1993;17(suppl 1):S66.
15. Taylor-Robinson D. *Ureaplasma urealyticum, Mycoplasma hominis,* and *Mycoplasma genitalium.* In: Mandell GL, Bennet JE, Dolin R, eds. *Principles and Practice of Infectious Diseases.* 5th ed. Philadelphia: Churchill Livingstone; 2000:2027.
16. Germain M, Krohn MA, Hillier SL, et al. Genital flora in pregnancy and its association with intrauterine growth retardation. *J Clin Microbiol.* 1994;32:2162.
17. Manhart LE, Critchlow CW, Holmes KK, et al. Mucopurulent cervicitis and *Mycoplasma genitalium. J Infect Dis.* 2003;187:650.
18. Simms I, Eastick K, Mallinson H, et al. Associations between *Mycoplasma genitalium, Chlamydia trachomatis,* and pelvic inflammatory disease. *Sex Transm Infect.* 2003;79:154.
19. Jensen JS, Uldum SA, Sondergard-Andersen J, et al. Polymerase chain reaction for detection of *Mycoplasma genitalium* in clinical samples. *J Clin Microbiol.* 1991;29:46.
20. Kovacic R, Launay V, Tuppin P, et al. Search for the presence of six *Mycoplasma* species in peripheral blood mononuclear cells of subjects seropositive and seronegative for human immunodeficiency virus. *J Clin Microbiol.* 1996;34:1808.
21. Palmer HM, Gilroy CB, Claydon EJ, et al. Detection of *Mycoplasma genitalium* in the genitourinary tract of women by the polymerase chain reaction. *Int J STD AIDS.* 1991;4:261.
22. Yoshida T, Macda S-I, Deguchi T, et al. Rapid detection of *Mycoplasma genitalium, Mycoplasma hominis, Ureaplasma parvum,* and *Ureaplasma urealyticum* organisms in genitourinary samples by PCR-microtiter plate hybridization assay. *J Clin Microbiol.* 2003;41:1850.
23. Heggie AD, Bar-Shain D, Boxerbaum B, et al. Identification and quantification of ureaplasmas colonizing the respiratory tract and assessment of their role in the development of chronic lung disease in preterm infants. *Pediatr Infect Dis J.* 2001;20:854.
24. Tully J, Taylor-Robinson D, Cole RM, et al. A newly discovered mycoplasma in the human genital tract. *Lancet.* 1981;1:1288.
25. Jensen JS, Hansen HT, Lind K. Isolation of *Mycoplasma genitalium* strains from the male urethra. *J Clin Microbiol.* 1996;34:286.
26. Hjorth SV, Bjornelius E, Lidbrink P, et al. Sequence-based typing of *Mycoplasma genitalium* reveals sexual transmission. *J Clin Microbiol.* 2006;44:2078.
27. Hamasuna R, Osada Y, Jensen SK. Antibiotic susceptibility testing of *Mycoplasma genitalium* by TaqMan 5′ nuclease real-time PCR. *Antimicrob Agents Chemother.* 2005;49:4993.
28. Eschenbach DA. *Ureaplasma urealyticum* as a cause of postpartum fever. *Pediatr Infect Dis J.* 1986;5(6 Suppl):S258.
29. Madoff S, Hooper DC. Nongenitourinary infections caused by *Mycoplasma hominis* in adults. *Rev Infect Dis.* 1988;3:602.
30. Meyer RD, Clough W. Extragenital *Mycoplasma hominis* infections in adults: emphasis on immunosuppression. *Clin Infect Dis.* 1993;17(suppl 1):S243.
31. Clausen HF, Fedder J, Drasbek M, et al. Serological investigation of *Mycoplasma genitalium* in infertile women. *Hum Reprod.* 2001;16:866.
32. Kenny GE, Cartwright FD. Susceptibilities of *Mycoplasma hominis, M. pneumoniae* and *Ureaplasma urealyticum* to GAR 936, dalfopristin, dirithromycin, evernimicin, gatifloxacin, linezolid, moxifloxacin, quinupristin-dalfopristin and telithromycin compared to their susceptibilities to reference macrolides, tetracyclines and quinolones. *Antimicrob Agents Chemother.* 2001;45:3604.
33. Cakan H, Polat E, Kocazeybek B, et al. Assessment of antibiotic susceptibility of *Ureaplasma urealyticum* from prostitutes and outpatient clinic patients using the E-test and agar dilution method. *Chemotherapy.* 2003;49:39.
34. Bebear CM, Renaudin H, Charron A, et al. In vitro activity of trovafloxacin compared to those of five antimicrobials against mycoplasmas including *Mycoplasma hominis* and *Ureaplasma urealyticum* fluoroquinolone-resistant isolates that have been genetically characterized. *Antimicrob Agents Chemother.* 2000;44:2557.
35. Hannan PC. Comparative susceptibilities of various AIDS-associated and human mycoplasmas and strains of *Mycoplasma pneumoniae* to 10 classes of antibiotics in vitro. *J Med Microbiol.* 1998;47:1115.
36. Taylor-Robinson D, Bebear C. Antibiotic susceptibilities of mycoplasmas and treatment of mycoplasmal infections. *J Antimicrob Chemother.* 1997;40:622.
37. Roberts MC, Kenny GE. Dissemination of the tetM tetracycline resistance determinant to *Ureaplasma urealyticum. Antimicrob Agents Chemother.* 1986;29:350.
38. Roberts MC, Koutsky LA, Holmes KK, et al. Tetracycline-resistant *Mycoplasma hominis* strains contain streptococcal tetM sequences. *Antimicrob Agents Chemother.* 1985;28:141.
39. Falk L, Fredlund H, Jensen JS. Tetracycline treatment does not eradicate *Mycoplasma genitalium. Sex Transm Infect.* 2003;79: 318.
40. Kenny GE, Young PA, Cartwright FD, et al. Sparfloxacin selects gyrase mutations in first-step *Mycoplasma hominis* mutants whereas ofloxacin selects topoisomerase IV mutations. *Antimicrob Agents Chemother.* 1999;43:2493.
41. Kenny GE, Kaiser GG, Cooney MK, et al. Diagnosis of *Mycoplasma pneumoniae* pneumonia: sensitivities and specificities of serology with lipid antigen and isolation of the organism on soy peptone medium for identification of infections. *J Clin Microbiol.* 1999;37:1518.

186

Introduction to Rickettsioses, Ehrlichioses, and Anaplasmosis

DIDIER RAOULT

Bacteriology

The definition of the Rickettsiaceae family has been based mainly on nonspecific phenotypic characters. Originally, small gram-negative bacteria, associated (or not) with arthropods and necessitating (or not) eukaryotic cells from growth, were considered Rickettsiaceae. During the past 20 years, gene sequencing and genetic phylogeny have deeply challenged this classification. The controversy has centered around how much difference between strains should constitute a sub-species.[1-5] Among the agreed-upon changes, *Orientia* was created from an independent branch of its phylum. The Ehrlichia group has been reclassified[6] into four genera, with *Ehrlichia* and *Anaplasma* being associated with ticks, *Neorickettsia* with helminths, and *Wolbachia* with both arthropods and helminths. This chapter is limited to the Rickettsiales (*Rickettsia*, *Ehrlichia*, and *Anaplasma* genera). All are intracellular alpha proteobacteria associated with eukaryotic hosts (arthropods or helminths). Based on antigenic and genetic data, pathogenic Rickettsiae are traditionally divided into three groups—the spotted fever group, the typhus group, and the scrub typhus group (Table 186-1). The spotted fever group accounts for most tick-borne rickettsioses. The typhus group comprises two human pathogens transmitted by insects. Epidemic typhus is caused by *Rickettsia prowazekii* and is transmitted by the body louse. Murine typhus is caused by *Rickettsia typhi* and is transmitted by rat and cat fleas. The scrub typhus group is composed of *Orientia tsutsugamushi* only and is transmitted by "chiggers."

History and Emerging Diseases

New genetic tools, as well as the use of cell culture assays, have allowed the description of many new rickettsioses and ehrlichioses during the past 20 years (Table 186-2).[7] Three ehrlichioses and 12 rickettsioses have been described since 1980. Three major conditions determined the description and separation of these species. Some were discovered after clinical description in countries where spotted fever had been unknown (Japan and *Rickettsia japonica*, Flinder's Island and *Rickettsia honei*, and Russia and Astrakhan fever). Some were recognized by bacterial identification based on culture and polymerase chain reaction (PCR) in places where the new pathogen was confounded with another known rickettsial pathogen (*Rickettsia africae* with *Rickettsia conorii*, *Rickettsia heilongjiianghensis* with *Rickettsia sibirica*, *R. sibirica mongolitimonae* and *Rickettsia aeschlimannii* with *R. conorii*, *Rickettsia felis* with *R. typhi*, and *Anaplasma phagocytophilum* and *Ehrlichia ewingii* with *Ehrlichia chaffeensis*). Some were identified through association by physicians and microbiologists when an atypical unknown disease (*E. chaffeensis*, *Rickettsia slovaca*, *Rickettsia raoultii*, and *Rickettsia helvetica*) was being explored.[7]

In addition to the description of new species, some old diseases, such as epidemic typhus or scrub typhus, reemerged apparently because of lack of social control or ecologic changes. These diseases, which were the more deadly rickettsioses for the human species, remain a threat. Recent studies in Asia found that rickettsioses such as murine typhus and scrub typhus were among the most common causes of fever.[8]

Wolbachia, an essential symbiont of human filarial worms, has been shown to play a major role in the pathology and clinical manifestations of filariasis. It introduces a completely new concept in infectious diseases.[9] It appears that inflammatory reactions of patients during the disease and during the treatment of filariasis are caused by the release of lipopolysaccharide-like molecules from the symbiotic *Wolbachia*.

Many rickettsiae were found in their vectors long before a particular disease could be associated with them. The denomination *nonpathogenic rickettsia* that is used for bacteria found only in ticks is misleading.[7] Among famous pathogens first classified as nonpathogenic rickettsiae are *Legionella pneumophila*; *Coxiella burnetii*, the agent of Q fever; *Rickettsia parkeri*[10]; and *R. africae*. Several rickettsiae have been found in ticks throughout the world, the pathogenic potential of which remains unknown.

Pathophysiology

Rickettsia, *Ehrlichia*, and *Anaplasma* are host-associated pathogens. These pathogens depend on their environment for the supply of many nutriments. *Rickettsia* species escape rapidly from the phagosome to multiply within the cytoplasm. Spotted fever rickettsiae, which are motile in the cytoplasm through actin polymerization,[11] invade neighboring cells. *R. prowazekii* is devoid of such motility and is released only by destruction of the host cell. I suspect that phospholipase D may play a key role in cellular invasion.[12]

The target cell of *Rickettsia* is the vascular endothelial cell, except for *Rickettsia akari* and *O. tsutsugamushi*, which multiply in monocytic cells. *E. chaffeensis* multiplies in monocytic cells; *A. phagocytophilum* and *E. ewingii* multiply in polymorphonuclear cells. Some animal ehrlichiae multiply in blood platelets.

Genetics

The complete gene sequences of *R. prowazekii*,[13] *R. conorii*,[14] *R. typhi*, *R. akari*, *R. sibirica sibirica*, *R. felis*, *Rickettsia bellii*, *Rickettsia massiliae*, and *R. africae* have been published. Genomes of *E. chaffeensis*, *Ehrlichia ruminantium*, *A. phagocytophilum*, *Anaplasma marginale*, *Wolbachia pipientis*, and *Neorickettsia senetsu* have also been released. Analysis shows that *R. prowazekii* is genetically a subset of *R. conorii*.

Epidemiology

The geographic and temporal distribution of rickettsioses and ehrlichioses is mainly determined by their vectors (see Table 186-1). Louse-transmitted diseases occur worldwide, and the human louse is distributed worldwide. Lice parasitize poor people, preferentially in cold places and during wars. Common fleas such as cat and dog fleas (*Ctenocephalides felis* and *Ctenocephalides canis*) and rat fleas (*Xenopsylla cheopis* and *Pulex irritans*) are also worldwide, as are their transmitted diseases—murine typhus (*R. typhi*) and flea-borne spotted fever (caused by *R. felis*). Tick species are highly dependent on their environment; very few are found worldwide, with the exception of

TABLE 186-1	Rickettsiosis, Ehrlichiosis, and Anaplasmosis of Humans and Their Vectors				
	Tick-borne	Flea-borne	Louse-borne	Mite-borne	Helminth-borne
Rickettsiae					
Spotted fever group	R. rickettsii	R. felis		R. akari	
	R. conorii				
	R. japonica				
	R. sibirica				
	R. australis				
	R. slovaca				
	R. africae				
	R. honei				
	R. aeschlimanii				
	R. helvetica				
	R. parkeri				
	R. heilongjianghensis				
	R. raoultii				
Typhus group		R. typhi	R. prowazekii		
Scrub typhus group (Orientia)				O. tsutsugamushi	
Anaplasma	A. phagocytophilum				
Ehrlichia	E. chaffeensis				
	E. ewingii				
	E. canis*				

*A single asymptomatic patient was reported as infected.

Rhipicephalus sanguineus—the dog tick, vector of *R. conorii* in the Old World and *R. rickettsii* in the United States and of *R. massiliae* and *Ehrlichia canis* worldwide. Tick-transmitted diseases are usually restricted to areas of the world where they can be transmitted by the local fauna. Among rickettsioses and ehrlichioses transmitted by ticks, only *A. phagocytophilum* is currently found worldwide.

Tick behavior may determine the targeted human population and the seasonality. It may also influence the clinical presentation. For example, *Amblyomma* ticks are aggressive hunting ticks. They frequently attack in groups. This behavior explains grouped cases and several inoculation eschars per patient. *Dermacentor* species wait for their host in an ambush strategy, falling onto a hairy host from a height of 1 m.[15] Therefore, they bite frequently in the hair, and children are a primary target. As a consequence, *Dermacentor*-transmitted rickettsioses, such as Rocky Mountain spotted fever (RMSF), and infections by *R. slovaca* more frequently involve children than do other rickettsial diseases.[16] Wide variations in the annual incidence of tick-transmitted diseases, such as RMSF and Mediterranean spotted fever, have been observed. A worldwide increase was noticed during the 1970s, followed by a decrease in the 1980s and a dramatic increase since 1990, which is not understood.[17] It was hypothesized that this was caused by increased exposure, better use of diagnostic tests, or a shift from effective to ineffective empirically prescribed antibiotics.

Clinical Findings

Fever, rash, and headache were considered for years the diagnostic clue for rickettsial diseases. Indeed, this remains a major triad, but spotless RMSF has been reported, and many of the newly described rickettsial diseases have no rash.[18] Major findings in rickettsioses and ehrlichioses include fever in a patient with exposure to a potential vector that may be associated with rash, inoculation eschar, or localized lymphadenopathy (Table 186-3). Biologically, neutropenia, thrombocytopenia, and moderate increases in transaminases are common. This may prompt a diagnostic test and eventually treatment with doxycycline.

The severity of these diseases varies with the causative agent and the host. Some *Rickettsia* species, such as *R. rickettsii* and *R. prowazekii*, and *O. tsutsugamushi* are often more severe. Some variations in the same disease are seen between regions for scrub typhus and RMSF.

Currently, the RMSF fatality rate reported by the Centers for Disease Control and Prevention is very low, possibly suggesting misdiagnosis.[5] Host factors also play a role in severity. Old age, alcoholism, and deficit in glucose-6-phosphate dehydrogenase have been associated with more severe disease.[19] In such patients, a multiple-organ dysfunction syndrome can be observed that usually leads to a fatal outcome. Gangrene of the extremities can also be observed in severe cases.

Diagnosis

Culture remains extremely difficult for these organisms, and diagnosis mainly relies on serology and PCR. The reference technique for serology is immunofluorescence. Many cross-reactions are observed, and precise species determination of the infecting agent may be difficult. Testing of several antigens on the same slide to compare reactivity may help in discriminating among cross-reacting agents. Western blot may be more specific in early sera. Cross-absorption may help to resolve these problems, but it is technically demanding and expensive.[7]

PCR has been effectively used for the diagnosis of ehrlichiosis and anaplasmosis with the use of blood samples. Observation of morula in monocytes or neutrophils in blood smear has also been helpful in the diagnosis of those infections. With rickettsiosis, biopsies of skin lesions are preferable because biopsies can also be used for immunohistochemistry.[20,21] PCR may also be of value for the serum testing of patients with rickettsial disease.[22]

Treatment

The most useful drug in children and in adults is doxycycline. It can be prescribed in short courses (1 day for typhus, scrub typhus, and Mediterranean spotted fever). Dental problems should not be a problem for children if fewer than three courses of several days of doxycycline are prescribed during childhood. Chloramphenicol should not be prescribed as first-line therapy because it is not active for ehrlichioses[23] and it is less active than doxycycline for RMSF.[24] However, it remains widely used in Asia, where rickettsioses and typhoid are common. Quinolones, which have been disappointingly inactive in cases of typhus and scrub typhus despite good in vitro efficacy (see Chapters 190 and 191), are not effective for ehrlichiosis.

TABLE 186-2	Historical Data on Diseases Caused by *Rickettsia* Species (First and Senior Authors)	
Year	*Discovery*	*Authors*
1760	Description of exanthematic typhus	Boissier de Sauvage
1879	First report of scrub typhus	Nagayo
1899	Description of RMSF	Maxcy
1906	Isolation of *R. rickettsii*	Ricketts
1909	Role of body lice in typhus	Nicolle (Nobel prize)
1909	Description of MSF	Conor et al
1910	Serology test based on *Proteus*	Wilson
1911	Isolation of *R. prowazekii*	Nicolle
1914	Tick role in MSF	Wilson
1916	Weil-Felix test	Weil and Felix
1921	Identification of *R. typhi*	Mooser
1925	Description of the tâche noire in MSF	Pieri
1930	First isolation of *Orientia tsutsugamushi* (*R. orientalis*)	Nagayo
1930	Role of chiggers in scrub typhus	Kawarimura
1930	Role of fleas in murine typhus	Dyer
1932	Isolation of *R. conorii*	Brumpt
1935	Description of Siberian tick typhus	Shmatikov et al
1938	Isolation of *R. sibirica*	Krontovuka et al
1940	*R. phagocytophila*	Gordon
1946	Description of rickettsialpox	Huebner
1946	Isolation of *R. akari*	Huebner
1946	Isolation of *R. australis*	Plotz and Smadel
1946	Queensland tick typhus	Plotz and Smadel
1956	*Ehrlichia sennetsu*	Kobayashi
1968	Isolation of *R. slovaca*	Brezina et al
1974	Culture of *R. conorii*	Goldwasser
1979	Isolation of *R. helvetica*	Burgdorfer and Peter
1981	*Ehrlichia chaffeensis*	Anderson
1984	Japanese spotted fever	Mahara
1985	Culture of *R. heilongjianghensis*	Udida and Walker
1987	First case of human erhlichiosis in United States	Maeda and McDade
1989	Culture of *R. japonica*	Lov
1990	First human cases of granulocytic erhlichioses	Bakken
1990	Isolation of *R. africae*	Kelly
1991	Flinder's Island spotted fever	Stewart
1992	Molecular identification of *Ehrlichia ewingii*	Anderson
1992	First case of infection by *R. africae*	Kelly and Raoult
1992	Culture and identification of *R. conorii*	Tarasevitch and Raoult
1992	Culture of *R. honei*	Baird et al
1993	Culture and identification of *R. sibirica mongolitimonae*	Yu and Raoult
1994	First case of flea-borne spotted fever	Schriefer and Azad
1996	Infection by *R. sibirica mongolitimonae*	Raoult et al
1997	First infection by *R. slovaca*	Raoult et al
1997	Culture of *R. aeschlimanii*	Beati and Raoult
1999	Astrakhan fever	Tarasevitch and Raoult
1999	First human cases of infection with *E. ewingii*	Buller
2000	Role of *Wolbachia* in filariasis	Taylor
2000	First case of acute infection by *R. helvetica*	Fournier and Raoult
2000	Culture of *R. felis*	Raoult et al
2002	First case of infection by *R. aeschlimanii*	Raoult et al
2004	First case of infection by *R. parkeri*	Paddock et al
2006	Description of infection by *R. heilongjianghensis* (Far Eastern spotted fever)	Mediannikov et al*
2008	Formal description of *R. raoultii*	Mediannikov et al†

*Mediannikov O, Sidelnikov Y, Ivanov L, et al. Far Eastern tick-borne rickettsiosis: identification of two new cases and tick vector. *Ann N Y Acad Sci.* 2006;1078:80-88.
†Mediannikov O, Matsumoto K, Samoylenko I, et al. *Rickettsia raoultii* sp. nov., a spotted fever group rickettsia associated with *Dermacentor* ticks in Europe and Russia. *Int J Syst Evol Microbiol.* 2008;58:1635-1639.
MSF, Mediterranean spotted fever; RMSF, Rocky Mountain spotted fever.

TABLE 186-3	Clinical Findings and Target Cells for Rickettsiosis, Ehrlichiosis, and Anaplasmosis				
Disease	Rash	Rash Specificity	Eschar	Enlarged Lymph Nodes	Target Cells
Rocky Mountain spotted fever (*R. rickettsii*)	90%	45% purpuric	No	No	Endothelial cells
Mediterranean spotted fever (*R. conorii*)	97%	10% purpuric	72%	Rare	Endothelial cells
Siberian tick typhus (*R. sibirica sibirica*)	100%	Macular	77%	Yes	Endothelial cells
Queensland tick typhus (*R. australis*)	100%	Vesicular	65%	Yes	Endothelial cells
Israeli spotted fever (*R. conorii israelensis*)	100%	Macular	Rare	No	Endothelial cells
Flinder's Island spotted fever (*R. honei*)	85%	8% purpuric	28%	Yes	Endothelial cells
Astrakhan fever (*R. conorii caspiensis*)	100%	Macular	23%	No	Endothelial cells
African tickbite fever (*R. africae*)	30%	Vesicular	100% multiple	Yes	Endothelial cells
Japanese spotted fever (*R. japonica*)	100%	Macular	90%	No	Endothelial cells
Lymphangitis-associated rickettsiosis (*R. sibirica mongolitimonae*)	Yes	Macular	Yes (could be multiple)	No	Endothelial cells
Tick-borne lymphadenopathy (TIBOLA) (*R. slovaca, R. raoultii*)	No	Macular	Yes	Yes	Endothelial cells
Rickettsia helvetica	No	—	No	No	Endothelial cells
Far Eastern spotted fever (*R. heilongjianghensis*)	Yes	Macular	Yes	Yes	Endothelial cells
R. aeschlimanii	Yes	—	Yes	No	Endothelial cells
Flea-borne spotted fever (*R. felis*)	Yes	Macular	Yes	?	?
Rickettsialpox (*R. akari*)	100%	Vesicular	100%	Yes	Macrophages/monocytes
Epidemic typhus (*R. prowazekii*)	50%	Macular	No	No	Endothelial cells
Murine typhus (*R. typhus*)	50%	Macular	No	No	Endothelial cells
Scrub typhus (*O. tsutsugamushi*)	30%	Macular	50% (could be multiple)	Yes	Macrophages/monocytes
Ehrlichiosis (*E. chaffeensis*)	36%	Macular	No	25%	Macrophages/monocytes
Anaplasmosis (*A. phagocytophylum*)	<10%	Macular	No	No	Polymorphonuclear cells
Infection by *Ehrlichia ewingii*	—	—	—	—	Polymorphonuclear cells

REFERENCES

1. Roux V, Raoult D. Phylogenetic analysis and taxonomic relationships among the genus *Rickettsia*. In: Raoult D, Brouqui P, eds. *Rickettsiae and Rickettsial Diseases at the Turn of the Third Millennium*. Marseille: Elsevier; 1999:52-66.
2. Walker DH, Bouyer DH. *Rickettsia* and *Orientia*. In Murray PR, Baron JE, Jorgensen JH, et al, eds. *Manual of Clinical Microbiology*. Washington, DC: ASM Press; 2007:1036-1045.
3. Zhu Y, Fournier PE, Eremeeva M, et al. Proposal to create subspecies of *Rickettsia conorii* based on multi-locus sequence typing and an emended description of *Rickettsia conorii*. BMC Microbiol. 2005;5:11.
4. Fournier PE, Zhu Y, Yu X, et al. Proposal to create subspecies of *Rickettsia sibirica* and an emended description of *Rickettsia sibirica*. Ann N Y Acad Sci. 2006;1078:597-606.
5. Raoult D, Parola P. Rocky Mountain spotted fever in the USA: a benign disease or a common diagnostic error? Lancet Infect Dis. 2008;8:587-589.
6. Dumler JS, Barbet AF, Bekker CPJ, et al. Reorganisation of genera in the families Rickettsiaceae and Anaplasmataceae in the order Rickettsiales: Unification of some species of *Ehrlichia* with *Anaplasma*, *Cowdria* with *Ehrlichia* and *Ehrlichia* with *Neorickettsia*; descriptions of six new species combinations and designation of *Ehrlichia equi* and "HGE agent" as subjective synonyms of *Ehrlichia phagocytophila*. Int J Syst Evol Microbiol. 2001; 51:2145-2165.
7. Raoult D, Roux V. Rickettsioses as paradigms of new or emerging infectious diseases. Clin Microbiol Rev. 1997;10:694-719.

8. Phongmany S, Rolain JM, Phetsouvanh R, et al. Rickettsial infections and fever, Vientiane, Laos. Emerg Infect Dis. 2006;12: 256-262.
9. Cross HF, Haarbrink M, Egerton G, et al. Severe reactions to filarial chemotherapy and release of *Wolbachia* endosymbionts into blood. Lancet. 2001;358:1873-1875.
10. Paddock CD, Sumner JW, Comer JA, et al. *Rickettsia parkeri*: a newly recognized cause of spotted fever rickettsiosis in the United States. Clin Infect Dis. 2004;38:805-811.
11. Teysseire N, Chiche-Portiche C, Raoult D. Intracellular movements of *Rickettsia conorii* and *R. typhi* based on actin polymerization. Res Microbiol. 1992;143:821-829.
12. Renesto P, Dehoux P, Gouin E, et al. Identification and characterization of a phospholipase D-superfamily gene in rickettsiae. J Infect Dis. 2003;188:1276-1283.
13. Andersson SG, Zomorodipour A, Andersson JO, et al. The genome sequence of *Rickettsia prowazekii* and the origin of mitochondria. Nature. 1998;396:133-140.
14. Ogata H, Audic S, Renesto-Audiffren P, et al. Mechanisms of evolution in *Rickettsia conorii* and *R. prowazekii*. Science. 2001;293:2093-2098.
15. Parola P, Raoult D. Ticks and tickborne bacterial diseases in humans: an emerging infectious threat. Clin Infect Dis. 2001;32:897-928.
16. Raoult D, Lakos A, Fenollar F, et al. Spotless rickettsiosis caused by *Rickettsia slovaca* and associated with *Dermacentor* ticks. Clin Infect Dis. 2002;34:1331-1336.

17. Walker DH, Raoult D. *Rickettsia rickettsii* and other spotted fever group rickettsiae (Rocky Mountain spotted fever and other spotted fevers). In: Mandell GL, Bennett JE, Dolin R, eds. *Principles and Practice of Infectious Diseases*. 4th ed. New York: Churchill Livingstone; 1995:1721-1727.
18. Sexton DJ, Kaye KS. Rocky Mountain spotted fever. Med Clin North Am. 2002;86:351-360, VII, VIII.
19. Walker DH. The role of host factors in the severity of spotted fever and typhus rickettsioses. Ann N Y Acad Sci. 1990;590: 10-19.
20. La Scola B, Raoult D. Diagnosis of Mediterranean spotted fever by cultivation of *Rickettsia conorii* from blood and skin samples using the centrifugation-shell vial technique and by detection of *R. conorii* in circulating endothelial cells: a 6 year follow-up. J Clin Microbiol. 1996;34:2722-2727.
21. Walker DH, Feng H-M, Ladner S, et al. Immunohistochemical diagnosis of typhus rickettsioses using an anti-lipopolysaccharide monoclonal antibody. Mod Pathol. 1997;10:1038-1042.
22. Raoult D, Fournier PE, Fenollar F, et al. *Rickettsia africae*, a tick-borne pathogen in travelers to sub-Saharan Africa. N Engl J Med. 2001;344:1504-1510.
23. Maurin M, Bryskier A, Raoult D. Antibiotic susceptibilities of *Parachlamydia acanthamoeba* in amoebae. Antimicrob Agents Chemother. 2002;46:3065-3067.
24. Paddock CD, Holman RC, Krebs JW, et al. Assessing the magnitude of fatal Rocky Mountain spotted fever in the United States: comparison of two national data sources. Am J Trop Med Hyg. 2002;67:349-354.

187

Rickettsia rickettsii and Other Spotted Fever Group Rickettsiae (Rocky Mountain Spotted Fever and Other Spotted Fevers)

DAVID H. WALKER

The spotted fevers comprise a large group of tick-, mite-, and flea-borne zoonotic infections that are caused by closely related rickettsiae. These include Rocky Mountain spotted fever, boutonneuse fever, African tick bite fever, North Asian tick typhus, lymphangitis associated rickettsiosis, Queensland tick typhus, Flinders Island spotted fever, Japanese spotted fever, tick-borne lymphadenopathy, Far Eastern spotted fever, flea-borne spotted fever, and rickettsialpox. Rickettsiae are emerging or reemerging pathogens in many parts of the world.[1-28] Associated diseases have a broad spectrum of severity; the most virulent, Rocky Mountain spotted fever, historically in Montana exhibited a case fatality rate of 66%.[29] Even young and previously healthy people may die of Rocky Mountain spotted fever. In recent years, the wide distribution and potential severity of the other spotted fevers have been recognized, especially in Europe, Africa, Australia, Asia, and Japan. Early diagnosis remains deceptively difficult.

Rocky Mountain Spotted Fever

THE PATHOGEN

Rocky Mountain spotted fever (RMSF) was first described in Idaho in the late 19th century.[30] Ricketts established the infectious nature of the illness and demonstrated the role of ticks as the vector in western Montana in 1906.[30,31] Wolbach in 1919 clearly identified the causative rickettsiae in endothelial cells.[32,33] The causative agent was designated *Rickettsia rickettsii*. Geographic origin, clinicoepidemiologic observations, and serotyping were the historical basis for species designation of subsequent rickettsial isolates. Phylogenetic analyses have more accurately revealed the evolutionary relationships among the rapidly increasing number of clinical and environmental isolates. It is likely that virulence was a relatively late mechanism of evolutionary survival for *Rickettsia*, which arose as vertically transmitted symbiotes of insects, arachnids, leeches, and amebas.[34] Contemporary phylogenomics based on whole genome sequences have defined the ancestral, typhus, transitional, and spotted fever groups.[35] *Rickettsia australis, R. felis,* and *R. akari* are members of the transitional group. Criteria for species designation of *Rickettsia* based on historically named species, an approach considered inappropriate by some respected taxonomists,[36] have been proposed to be determined by the divergence of 16S rRNA, citrate synthase, outer membrane proteins A and B, and Sca 4 of the most closely related, previously named species.[37] These criteria have resulted in proposals for species designation of rickettsial strains that are much more closely related than other bacterial species. For example, a proposed criterion of 0.2% divergence of the 16S rRNA gene would create many more species names than the usual 1% to 1.3% divergence of other bacterial taxa.[38,39] An attractive approach, concatenated phylogeny based on multilocus sequence typing using eight loci of *Rickettsia* genes, has revealed that species designation of *R. sibirica, R. africae,* and *R. parkeri,* should be subject to further discussion.[40] The spotted fever group (SFG) rickettsial strains that have been strongly or weakly associated with human infections (*R. rickettsii, R. conorii, R. africae, R. sibirica,* including the mongolitimonae strain, *R. honei, R. japonica, R. slovaca, R. parkeri, R. massiliae, R. monacensis, R. aeschlimannii, R. heilongjiangensis, R. amblyommii,* and *R. helvetica*) definitely merit identification that is useful for clinical and epidemiologic purposes. It is controversial whether they and a rapidly growing number of candidates merit separate designations as different at the species level.

Virulence Factors

SFG rickettsiae are obligately intracellular bacteria that reside in the cytosol and less often in the nuclei of host cells. These rickettsiae are small, measuring approximately 0.3 by 1.0 μm. They have one of the smallest bacterial genomes, ranging between 1.1 and 1.6 Mb. The cell wall, which has the ultrastructural appearance of a gram-negative bacterium, contains peptidoglycan and lipopolysaccharide (LPS). Rickettsiae are difficult to stain with ordinary bacterial stains but are conveniently stained by the Gimenez method or with acridine orange. They have not been cultivated in cell-free medium. Growth requires living host cells, such as the yolk sac of embryonated eggs, experimental animals, or cell culture (e.g., Vero, HEL, and L-929 cells). Rickettsiae have undergone remarkable genome reduction with exploitation of their cytosolic environment by being highly adapted for intracellular survival with effective transport systems for adenosine triphosphate (ATP), amino acids, and phosphorylated sugars, as well as their own independent metabolic enzymes. Rickettsiae exhibit a large family of surface proteins, autotransporters, that are a major source of antigenic differences.[41] Among these OmpA (190 kDa) and OmpB (135 kDa) contain conformational epitopes that are targets of humoral immunity and are the antigenic basis for serotyping; other antigens are also shared among the SFG.[42] The LPS of SFG rickettsiae contains highly immunogenic antigens that are strongly cross-reactive among all members of the group. However, antibodies to LPS do not provide protection against infection.[43]

Epidemiology

The role of a tick bite in the transmission of RMSF was demonstrated by McCalla and Brereton and reported in 1908[30]; a tick obtained from a patient suffering from RMSF transmitted the disease to two volunteers. The seasonal distribution of RMSF parallels tick activity. The tick is both the vector and the main reservoir.[44] *Dermacentor variabilis*, the American dog tick, is the prevalent vector in the eastern two thirds of the United States and the Far West; *Dermacentor andersoni*, the Rocky Mountain wood tick, in the western states; *Rhipicephalus sanguineus*, in Mexico and Arizona[45]; and *Amblyomma cajennense* and *A. aureolatum* in South America. Causes for the variation in infection rates among populations of ticks are not clear, although in *Dermacentor*, only a small portion of ticks (generally 4%) carry any rickettsiae, and fewer than 1 in 1000 ticks carry virulent *R. rickettsii*. One limiting factor is the deleterious effect that *R. rickettsii* has on ticks; another is the inhibition of establishment of transovarial transmission of *R. rickettsii* by the presence of another *Rickettsia* species in the tick.[46,47] Humidity, climatic variations, human activities altering the vegetation and fauna, and the use of insecticides have been suspected to play a role in the fluctuation of tick populations and the prevalence of human rickettsiosis.

R. rickettsii is transmitted trans-stadially (stage to stage) and transovarially in ticks, thus maintaining the agent in nature. Horizontal transmission through vertebrate hosts would also appear to occur to a small degree and to be a necessary factor for the maintenance of *R. rickettsii* in nature.[44] In most mammals, rickettsemia is of very short duration and low titer, allowing for infection of only a small proportion of feeding ticks. Of the three tick stages—larva, nymph, and adult—only adult *Dermacentor* ticks feed on humans. The prevalence of pathogenic rickettsiae in various populations of ticks is variable. Many rickettsiae of unknown pathogenicity have been isolated and characterized in the United States, including *R. bellii*, *R. montanensis*, *R. rhipicephali*, and *R. peacockii*.[47,48]

The tick transmits the disease to humans during a prolonged period of feeding that may last for 1 to 2 weeks. The bite is painless and frequently goes unnoticed. After the attached tick has fed for 6 to 10 hours, rickettsiae begin to be injected from the salivary glands. An even longer period may be required for reactivation of rickettsial virulence in unfed ticks. Humans can also be infected by exposure to infective tick hemolymph during the removal of ticks from persons or domestic animals, especially when the tick is crushed between the fingers.

Laboratory-acquired infection[49] transmitted by infectious aerosols or parenteral inoculation of *R. rickettsii* may be prevented by careful technique and the use of biohazard containment hoods, masks, and gloves. *R. rickettsii* is covered by the Select Agents Act, which restricts its possession, investigation, transfer, and shipment, because of its potential use as an aerosol-transmitted agent of bioterrorism.[50]

From the 1870s until 1931, RMSF was recognized as existing only in the western United States. At present, the prevalence of the disease is higher in the South Atlantic states and in the South Central regions than in the Rocky Mountain states (Fig. 187-1).[51-53] Local prevalence in highly endemic areas such as North Carolina has been as great as 14.59/100,000.[53] Moreover, although the incidence of infection may be decreasing in one area, it is increasing simultaneously in another region. The report of a focus in the South Bronx emphasizes that the ecologic conditions that permit the establishment of RMSF are widely distributed.[54] Most cases are diagnosed during late spring and summer. However, especially in the southern states, a few cases occur during the winter.

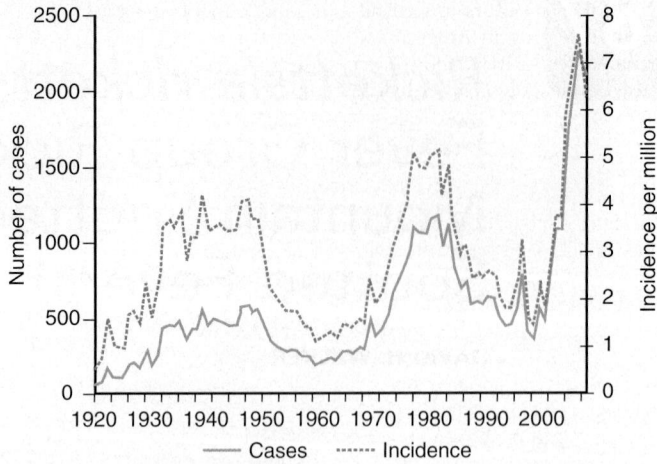

Figure 187-2 **Reported Rocky Mountain spotted fever cases in the United States (1920 to 2007).**

In the southern states, incidence is highest in children, adults 60 to 69 years old, and patients who are known to be exposed more often to ticks than are matched controls.[55] In the western states, because of transmission by the wood tick *D. andersoni*, a higher proportion of men contract the disease because of occupational exposure. The case-fatality rates are significantly higher for progressively older age groups.[29]

Consistent with unexplained 30- to 40-year cycles of waxing and waning incidence of RMSF, the number of cases reported to the Centers for Disease Control and Prevention (CDC) has skyrocketed (2288 cases in 2006; Fig. 187-2). Problematic issues are the low proportion of laboratory-confirmed cases (15%, with only 5% with specific evidence for *R. rickettsii*), a significant population of healthy persons with serum antibodies reactive with *R. rickettsii*, which shares antigens with other SFG rickettsiae, discovery that *R. parkeri* transmitted by *Amblyomma maculatum* causes human infections, evidence that highly prevalent *R. amblyommii* carried by *Amblyomma americanum* ticks causes mild or subclinical infections, and a reported RMSF case-fatality rate of 0.5% compared with 23% in the preantibiotic era and 5% in recent years.[14,56-62] It is likely that many of these patients had human monocytotropic ehrlichiosis and were misdiagnosed based on the presence of antibodies stimulated at a previous time by *R. amblyommii*. Some of them likely were infected with *R. parkeri*.[2]

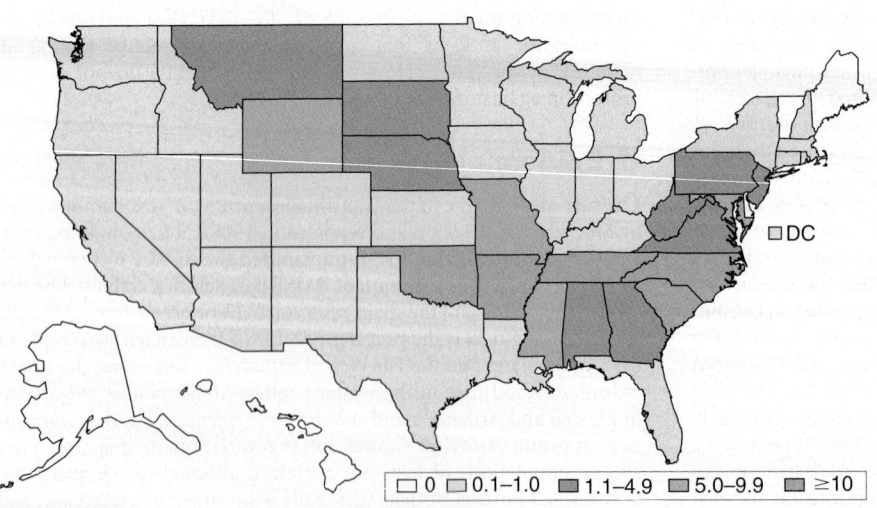

Figure 187-1 **Average reported annual U.S. incidence of Rocky Mountain spotted fever (1997 to 2002).**

| 0 | 0.1–1.0 | 1.1–4.9 | 5.0–9.9 | ≥10 |

Per 1,000,000 persons per year.

RMSF also occurs in Central and South America, where it is currently emerging in Argentina and re-emerging in Brazil, Colombia, Panama, Costa Rica, and Mexico, largely unrecognized and misdiagnosed as dengue or other febrile exanthems.[10,11,15,16] *R. rickettsii* infections appear to be more severe in these regions.

PATHOGENESIS

Rickettsiae introduced into the skin apparently spread via lymphatics and small blood vessels to the systemic and pulmonary circulation where, by means of OmpA and OmpB, they attach to and induce phagocytosis by their target cells—the vascular endothelium—to establish numerous disseminated foci of infection.[63-69] Comparison of the genomes of two highly passaged isolates of *R. rickettsii*, one virulent and the other attenuated, has revealed numerous deletions and amino acid substitutions in both isolates but only four genes that were expressed less in the attenuated strain.[70] The most notable mutations were disruption of *ompA*, leading to absence of its expression and four amino acid substitutions in OmpB, which does not undergo normal post-translational processing. After entry, the rickettsiae escape rapidly from the phagosome into the cytosol in association with expression of membranolytic phospholipase D and hemolysin C,[71] and less frequently invade the nucleus. Rickettsiae proliferate intracellularly by binary fission. The movement of spotted fever rickettsiae within the cytoplasm, into projections invaginating into the nucleus, and into cell projections from which they are released extracellularly or spread into the adjacent cell, is caused by propulsion by the host cell's actin filaments.[72] SFG rickettsial protein Rick A is associated with activation of Arp2/3 and polymerization of actin at one pole of the rickettsiae.[73-76]

The consequence of cell-to-cell spread in the body is a focal network of hundreds of contiguous infected endothelial cells corresponding to the lesions (e.g., maculopapular rash). The presence of greater quantities of rickettsiae in damaged cells supports the concept of direct cell injury.[73] No convincing data support endotoxin or exotoxin as a pathogenic mechanism. Rickettsial injury to the host cell is caused, at least in part, by free radical–induced damage to host cell membranes and rickettsial phospholipase and protease activities.[77-82] The major pathophysiologic effect of endothelial cell injury is increased vascular permeability, which in turn results in edema, hypovolemia, hypotension, and hypoalbuminemia.[83] Endothelial cells produce prostaglandins that may contribute to vasodilatation and increased vascular permeability.[84] Hyponatremia is the result of secretion of antidiuretic hormone as an appropriate response to hypovolemia.[85] High quantities of rickettsiae infecting the pulmonary microcirculation are associated with increased vascular permeability and cause noncardiogenic pulmonary edema.[86,87] Vascular injury and the subsequent host lymphohistiocytic response correspond to the distribution of rickettsiae and include interstitial pneumonia, interstitial myocarditis, encephalitis, and similar vascular lesions in the rash, gastrointestinal tract, pancreas, liver, skeletal muscles, and kidneys. However, even severe vascular injury rarely leads to clinically significant hemorrhage. Platelets are consumed locally in numerous foci of infection; consequently, thrombocytopenia is observed in 32% to 52% of patients.[88,89] A procoagulant state ensues, including endothelial injury, release of procoagulant components, activation of the coagulation cascade with thrombin generation, platelet activation, increased antifibrinolytic factors, consumption of natural anticoagulants, activation of the kallikrein-kinin system, and secretion of coagulation-promoting cytokines.[90-97] These observations are supported by numerous studies of endothelial cells in culture, such as the demonstration that tissue factor is secreted by *Rickettsia*-infected endothelial cells,[98,99] but true disseminated intravascular coagulation occurs only rarely, and occlusive vascular thrombosis is not the basic pathophysiologic event.[93,100]

The host immune and inflammatory responses are critical for clearance of infection, but cytokines may contribute also to increased vascular permeability and T regulatory cells may contribute to suppression of immunity in overwhelming fatal illness.[101-103]

T lymphocytes (particularly CD8 cells) are important effectors of immune clearance of rickettsiae, and interferon-γ and tumor necrosis factor-α activate infected endothelial cells to kill intracellular rickettsiae.[63,104-107] Dendritic cells stimulated via Toll-like receptor 4 activate natural killer (NK) cells in the early innate immune response, which secrete interferon-γ that dampens the rickettsial burden[101,108,109]; cytotoxic T lymphocytes are crucial to the clearance of rickettsial infection.[110] OmpA and OmpB cell wall proteins are important immunogens.[111-114]

CLINICAL MANIFESTATIONS

The incubation period of RMSF ranges from 2 to 14 days, with a median of 7 days. Variation in incubation time may be related in part to inoculum size. The disease usually begins with fever, myalgia, and headache, most likely the effects of proinflammatory cytokines (Table 187-1). The temperature is higher than 102°F (38.9°C) in 63% of patients during the first 3 days and in 90% later.[88] The variable incidences of reported headache and myalgia in different series are likely related to the proportion of young children who may not articulate the concept of pain. Other signs and symptoms are frequently prominent early in the course before the onset of rash, at

TABLE 187-1	Features of Rocky Mountain Spotted Fever, Boutonneuse Fever, and African Tick Bite Fever		
Feature	**RMSF (%)**	**BF (%)**	**ATBF (%)**
Fever	99-100	100	81-88
Headache	79-91	56	83
Rash	88-90	97	26-46
Vesicular rash			16-45
Tache noire	<1	72	32-95
Multiple eschars	0	0	21-54
Myalgia	72-83	36	63-87
Nausea, vomiting	56-60		
Abdominal pain	35-52		
Petechial rash	45-49	10	
Conjunctivitis	30	9	
Lymphadenopathy	27		43-49
Stupor	21-26	10	
Diarrhea	19-20		
Edema	18-20		
Ataxia	5-18		
Meningismus	18	11	
Splenomegaly	14-16	6	
Hepatomegaly	12-15	13	
Jaundice	8-9	2	
Pneumonitis	12-17		
Cough	33	10	
Dyspnea		21	
Coma	9-10		
Seizures	8		
Shock, hypotension	7-17		
Decreased hearing	7		
Arrhythmia	7-16		
Myocarditis	5-26	11	
Death	4-8	2.5	
Increased AST level	36-62	39	
Thrombocytopenia	32-52	35	
Anemia	5-24		
Hyponatremia	19-56	25	
Azotemia	12-14	6	

AST, aspartate transaminase; ATBF, African tick bite fever; BF, boutonneuse fever; RMSF, Rocky Mountain spotted fever.

which time gastrointestinal involvement with nausea, vomiting, abdominal pain, diarrhea, and abdominal tenderness occurs in substantial numbers of patients; this may suggest gastroenteritis or an acute surgical abdomen.

The rash, the major diagnostic sign, appears in a small fraction of patients on the first day of the disease and in only 49% during the first 3 days, usually appearing 3 to 5 days after the onset of fever and occurring in 88% to 90% of patients overall. Rocky Mountain "spotless" fever occurs more often in older patients and in black patients.[88] A delay in diagnosis is occasionally associated with the absence or late onset of rash. The rash typically begins around the wrists and ankles but may start on the trunk or be diffuse at the onset. Involvement of the palms and soles is considered characteristic, but it occurs in only 36% to 82% of patients who have a rash; it often appears late in the course (Figs. 187-3 and 187-4). Skin necrosis or gangrene develops in only 4% of cases as a result of rickettsial damage to the microcirculation.[89] Gangrene involves the digits or limbs and occasionally requires amputation. Careful examination seldom reveals an eschar at the site of the tick bite in RMSF.[115] Headache is usually quite severe. Focal neurologic deficits, transient deafness, meningismus, and photophobia may suggest meningitis or meningoencephalitis. The cerebrospinal fluid (CSF) contains increased leukocytes in one third of patients, with either lymphocytic or polymorphonuclear predominance[89]; CSF protein concentration is increased in one third of patients. However, glucose concentration is low in the CSF of only 8% of patients.

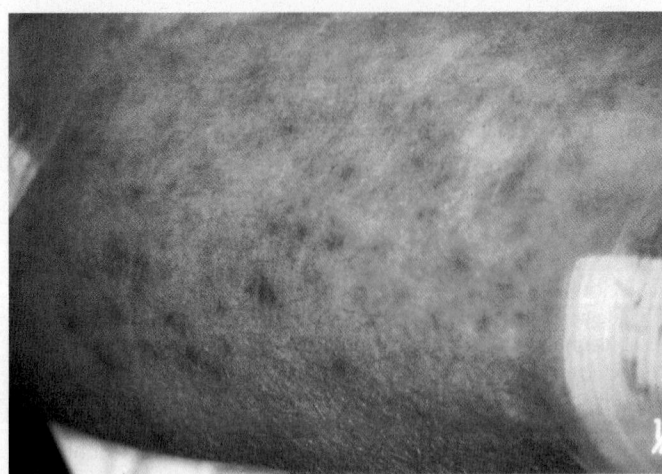

Figure 187-4 **Late acute stage of Rocky Mountain spotted fever.** The lower portion of the arm shows a florid petechial rash.

The electroencephalogram (EEG) may show diffuse cortical dysfunction. Generally, neurologic involvement portends a bad prognosis. Among 37 patients followed for 1 to 8 years after acute RMSF, including those in the preantibiotic era, 21 had residual neurologic abnormalities.[116] These sequelae were headache and other subjective findings, but 12 involved electroencephalographic abnormalities. In a recent series of cases of children with RMSF, 15% of survivors had neurologic deficits at discharge, including global encephalopathy, ataxia, and blindness.[117] Sequelae occur less often in patients with early antibiotic treatment. On funduscopic examination, retinal vein engorgement, arterial occlusion, flame hemorrhage, and papilledema without increased CSF pressure have been noted. These changes may reflect retinal vasculitis with increased permeability and focal thrombosis. Renal failure is an important problem in severe RMSF.[118] Prerenal azotemia related to hypovolemia responds to IV hydration; however, acute tubular necrosis may require hemodialysis. Pulmonary involvement is suggested by cough and radiologic changes such as alveolar infiltrates, interstitial pneumonia, and pleural effusion.[119] Pulmonary edema with impairment of pulmonary function or adult respiratory distress syndrome may require oxygen therapy and ventilatory assistance. Echocardiographic studies reveal minimal myocardial dysfunction,[120] and normal pulmonary capillary wedge pressure measurements document the noncardiogenic nature of the pulmonary edema.

In classic RMSF, death occurs 7 to 15 days after the onset of symptoms when appropriate therapy is not given in a timely manner. In fulminant RMSF, death occurs within the first 5 days. Several features account for the extreme difficulty associated with the diagnosis of fulminant RMSF—the course is rapid, the rash develops shortly before death if at all, antibodies to *R. rickettsii* do not have time to develop, and the pathologic lesions even appear different, containing more thrombi and lacking the characteristic lymphohistiocytic component.[121] Fulminant RMSF is more often observed in black males with glucose-6-phosphate dehydrogenase (G6PD) deficiency, apparently because of an unidentified secondary effect of the usually moderate degree of hemolysis. After hemolysis has depleted the older red blood cells (RBCs) with low G6PD content, evaluation of hemolysis by plasma haptoglobin may be more revealing than assay of G6PD activity in the remaining RBCs. Hemolysis may be the pathogenic factor rather than the reduced G6PD enzyme activity itself. Other risk factors for a lethal outcome in classic RMSF include older age and possibly alcoholism.

Characteristic laboratory data may support the clinical diagnosis of classic RMSF but are relatively nonspecific.[88,89] The white blood cell count is generally normal, but increased quantities of immature myeloid cells occur frequently. Anemia is observed in 5% to 30% of cases. Thrombocytopenia occurs in more severe cases, but also in some

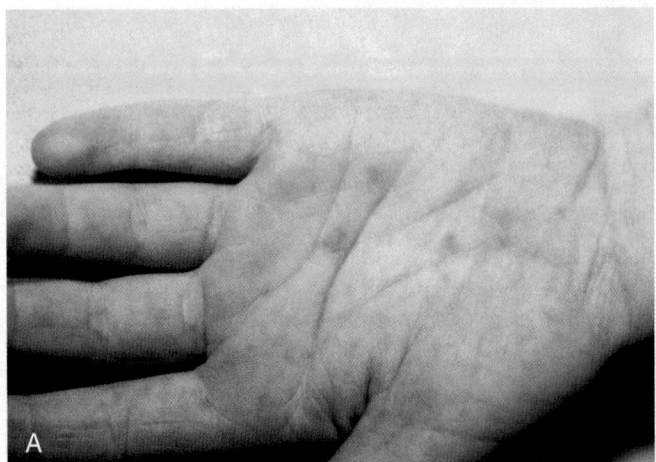

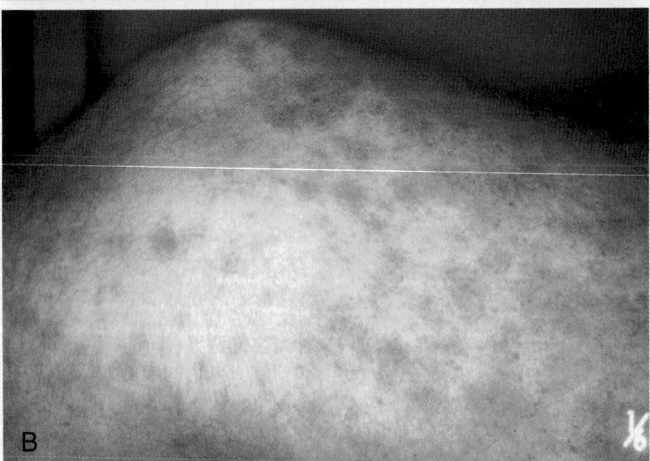

Figure 187-3 **Rocky Mountain spotted fever rash. A,** The wrist and palm manifest the rash of Rocky Mountain spotted fever with central petechiae in some of the maculopapules. **B,** Early petechial rash on arm.

patients with mild disease. Coagulopathy with prolonged coagulation times and decreased concentrations of fibrinogen and other clotting factors occurs infrequently because the hemostatic system usually functions effectively to prevent severe bleeding from vascular lesions, and generally does not contribute importantly to the pathologic state.[93] Disseminated intravascular coagulation is rarely documented. Hyponatremia is observed in half of patients with RMSF. Increased concentrations of serum lactate dehydrogenase, creatine kinase, and other enzymes are related to diffuse tissue injury, such as multifocal rhabdomyonecrosis.

The prognosis in RMSF is largely related to the timeliness of initiation of appropriate therapy. The intervals between onset of disease and appearance of the rash, clinical diagnosis, and effective antibiotic treatment are significantly longer in dying patients than in surviving patients.[29,88] Fatal cases more frequently have hepatomegaly, jaundice, stupor, and renal insufficiency and report a history of tick exposure less often.[122] Patients who survive RMSF have solid immunity to *R. rickettsii*. Long-term sequelae are mainly neurologic or result from amputation of gangrenous limbs.[123,124]

DIAGNOSIS

The diagnosis of RMSF before the onset of rash is clinical and epidemiologic. The differential diagnosis at the first consultation includes typhoid fever, measles, rubella, respiratory tract infection, gastroenteritis, acute surgical abdomen, enteroviral infection, meningococcemia, disseminated gonococcal infection, secondary syphilis, leptospirosis, immune complex vasculitis, immune thrombocytopenic purpura, thrombotic thrombocytopenic purpura, infectious mononucleosis, drug reaction, ehrlichiosis, anaplasmosis, and other rickettsial diseases. Laboratory diagnosis of RMSF may be achieved by isolation of *R. rickettsii* from the blood. Few laboratories undertake isolation of *R. rickettsii* in guinea pigs, embryonated hen's eggs, or cell culture because of the biohazard; however, a centrifugation-enhanced cell culture system—the shell vial assay—has been successfully applied to rickettsial isolation.[125] Some hospitals and public health laboratories can demonstrate *R. rickettsii* in cutaneous biopsy specimens by immunohistochemistry, a timely diagnostic method used during the acute phase for patients with a rash.[126-128] Serology, the usual method for confirmation of the diagnosis, is retrospective; serum antibodies usually become detectable during convalescence. Serology does not allow discrimination of the particular causative SFG *Rickettsia* species unless Western immunoblotting and cross-absorption with appropriately selected antigens are performed.[129] The Weil-Felix test using *Proteus* OX-19 and OX-2 agglutination is not to be relied on. This method lacks sensitivity and specificity. Antibodies to rickettsial antigens are detected by indirect immunofluorescence and enzyme immunoassay. The diagnostic titer is 1:64 for indirect immunofluorescence assay, which is the most sensitive and specific test. Indirect immunofluorescence and dot enzyme immunoassay have commercially available reagents. Polymerase chain reaction (PCR) amplification of *R. rickettsii* DNA has not proved to be a sensitive diagnostic method for blood samples, except late in the course, particularly for fatal cases.[130,131] However, improved methods, including real-time PCR, offer potentially increased sensitivity, and PCR has been successfully applied to other SFG rickettsioses, such as skin biopsies during Mediterranean spotted fever (MSF).[129,132] Primers used amplify genes of the 17-kDa protein, citrate synthase, OmpA, and OmpB and allow the identification of rickettsiae. Early clinical diagnosis remains essential for this life-threatening disease.

TREATMENT

Doxycycline is the treatment of choice. Since the introduction of chloramphenicol and the tetracyclines, including doxycycline, the lethality of the disease has decreased dramatically but remains significant at 3%.[52] In vitro and in ovo, *R. rickettsii* is susceptible not only to chloramphenicol and tetracycline but also to rifampin, some quinolone

compounds, including ciprofloxacin, and the macrolide clarithromycin. Clinical experience with these agents has been insufficient to enable recommendation of their use for RMSF.[133,134] Dogs infected with *R. rickettsii* have been effectively treated with enrofloxacin. The organism is resistant to β-lactam antibiotics, aminoglycosides, and trimethoprim-sulfamethoxazole. Erythromycin has a minimal inhibitory concentration (MIC) of 3 to 8 μg/mL and is not effective.

RMSF responds to treatment with oral tetracycline (25 to 50 mg/kg/day) or chloramphenicol (50 to 75 mg/kg/day) given in four divided doses. Tetracyclines such as doxycycline are superior to chloramphenicol, which is associated with a higher case-fatality rate.[135] Doxycycline, 100 mg every 12 hours, is the drug of choice, except for pregnant patients or those with hypersensitivity to the drug. The selected antibiotic is usually administered for 7 days and is continued for 2 days after the patient has become afebrile. Single-day treatment with 200 mg doxycycline has proved to be safe and efficient in adults and children with MSF but has not been tested and is not recommended for RMSF. Treatment should be given intravenously to patients with nausea and vomiting and to those who are seriously ill. Chloramphenicol is preferred during pregnancy because of the effects of tetracycline on fetal bones and teeth, although this drug is not considered to be effective in ehrlichiosis, an infection that closely resembles RMSF. Tetracyclines have been avoided in young children because of concerns for staining the teeth, but it is recommended that doxycycline be used for suspected RMSF in children of all ages because of the life-threatening nature of RMSF and the unlikelihood that a single course of doxycycline would stain the teeth.[136] Avoidance of therapeutic delay is critical for a favorable prognosis.[29,137] Severely ill patients require intensive supportive care. Fluid maintenance is critical for maintenance of organ perfusion. Because of increased vascular permeability and risk of extravasation of fluid into pulmonary alveoli, a Swan-Ganz catheter may be needed to monitor hemodynamics in some patients. Glucocorticoids are sometimes given to severely ill patients, but no documentation of efficacy has occurred and they are not recommended, although in experimentally infected dogs treated simultaneously with doxycycline, no detrimental effects of prednisolone treatment were noted.[138]

PREVENTION

Although no vaccine is available currently, immunodominant surface proteins have been identified, and the major surface protein antigens (OmpA and OmpB) of *R. rickettsii* and *R. conorii* are candidate vaccine antigens. Immunization of guinea pigs with OmpA provided protective immunity against a virulent challenge, and protective fragments of OmpB have been identified.[111-114] The presence of antibodies to OmpA or OmpB are associated with protection.[43] A vaccine may be developed that would protect against all SFG rickettsiae, or even typhus group and SFG rickettsiae, but currently no vaccine is available for any of the SFG rickettsiae.[139,140]

Currently, the best means of prevention remains the avoidance of contact with ticks through the use of repellents and protective clothing. In the hot weather usually associated with the tick season, these techniques are often impractical. Regular checks of the body, including scalp, pubic, and axillary hair, allow removal of the tick before rickettsial transmission. To remove an attached tick, one should use forceps to detach the intact tick without leaving mouth parts in the skin. The tick bite wound should be cleansed.

▣ Other Spotted Fever Group Rickettsioses

Other SFG rickettsioses have been given a variety of names, including geographic names, that often do not indicate their full distribution (e.g., Flinders Island spotted fever, which also occurs in mainland Australia and southeastern Asia),[12,141] and clinically descriptive names (e.g., tick-borne lymphadenopathy).[3] Aside from the latter highly distinctive disease, the other SFG rickettsioses form a spectrum of similar clinical illnesses with indistinguishable symptoms at onset and subsequent courses with overlapping clinical manifestations, such as varying in severity from occasionally life-threatening to nonfatal, in incidence of the rash from almost all to only half, in characteristics of the rash (usually maculopapular; in some illnesses, occasionally vesicular-pustular, frequently petechial to never petechial), in incidence of eschars, in incidence of regional lymphadenopathy that may be painful (from frequently to never), and in incidence of lymphangitis (from almost half to never). The severity of illness is associated with both the particular *Rickettsia* species or strain and host factors. Among the 15 other SFG *Rickettsia* species reported with evidence to have caused infection of humans (*R. conorii, R. sibirica, R. japonica, R. australis, R. honei, R. africae, R. parkeri, R. slovaca, R. aeschlimannii, R. massiliae, R. parkeri, R. heilongjiangensis, R. helvetica, R. felis,* and *R. akari*), the first 13 are transmitted by tick bite. SFG cross-reactive protein and LPS antigens are detected serologically, and cross-protection is shared among SFG rickettsiae.[139,142] *R. conorii,* a typical SFG rickettsia with high genetic homology with *R. rickettsii,* appears to have greater intraspecies antigenic and genetic diversity than *R. rickettsii* and consists of four strains.[143,144] *R. sibirica* has two distinct strains.[145] The proposal to designate the strains as subspecies is controversial because several already named species are so closely related that some taxonomists would combine them into one. This situation could create the rationale to convert some former species names into subspecies.

R. felis is maintained transovarially in fleas, largely cat fleas, and is presumably transmitted by them.[6] The last, *R. akari,* is discussed in Chapter 188. In addition, numerous distinct SFG rickettsiae (e.g., *R. amblyommii, R. montanensis, R. peacockii,* and *R. rhipicephali*) have been identified only in ticks.[1] Some of these may prove to be pathogenic for humans, even if they cause only a short, nonexanthematous, febrile illness or asymptomatic seroconversion.[61]

The most severe SFG rickettsiosis other than RMSF is boutonneuse fever, caused by *R. conorii.* Infection has been designated by many geographic names—Marseilles fever, Mediterranean spotted fever, Kenya tick typhus, Israeli tick typhus, Astrakhan spotted fever, and Indian tick typhus. Historically, boutonneuse fever was first described by Conor and Bruch in 1909 in Tunisia, although the *tache noire* (black spot)—that is, the eschar at the site of the bite—was not described until 1923 by Pieri in Marseilles. *R. conorii* has been identified in India, Pakistan, Israel, Russia, Georgia, Ukraine, Ethiopia, Kenya, South Africa, Morocco, and southern Europe. The epidemiology of boutonneuse fever and ecology of *R. conorii* are closely related to *Rhipicephalus sanguineus* ticks. *R. conorii* is maintained transovarially in ticks and is transmitted to humans by tick bite. The frequent absence of a history of tick bite is likely because of transmission by immature larvae and nymphs, which are often not noticed. Cases occur mainly in the warm months, with peak incidences in July, August, and September in many Mediterranean locations. Imported cases occur in travelers returning to the United States and northern Europe from southern Europe. The pathogenic basis for tissue injury in the spotted fevers is well elucidated in the tache noire or eschar at the site of the infective tick bite. Dermal and epidermal necrosis and perivascular edema are the consequences of endothelial injury by *R. conorii.*[146] Necropsies of fatal cases of boutonneuse fever reveal disseminated vascular infection and injury by *R. conorii,* including meningoencephalitis and vascular lesions in kidneys, lungs, gastrointestinal tract, liver, pancreas, heart, spleen, and skin.[147,148] Hepatic biopsy specimens reveal focal hepatocellular necrosis and granuloma-like lesions.[149] In a large series of well-documented cases, patients infected with the *R. conorii* Israeli spotted fever (ISF) strain were more severely ill than those infected with the Malish strain.[132] Although eschars were present in many patients with both strains, tick bite inoculation lesions occurred more often with Malish strain. Severity and fatality were manifested by more frequent petechial rash, gastrointestinal symptoms, obtundation, dehydration, tachypnea, hepatomegaly, leukocytosis, coagulopathy, acute renal failure, hyperbilirubinemia, and elevated serum transaminase and creatine kinase levels.[132] Host factors that are risks for severity include diabetes mellitus, cardiac insufficiency, alcoholism, old age, and G6PD deficiency.[132,150,151] The disease is milder in children. In France, Israel, and

Spain, the death rate among hospitalized patients ranges from 1.4% to 5.6%, similar to that of RMSF.[71] In contrast, SFG rickettsiosis in northeastern Spain documented by cross-reactive serology is a milder illness, suggesting that another strain might be the actual agent.[152] Other rickettsiae that share antigens and cause similar disease in Europe include *R. massiliae, R. monacensis, R. sibirica* mongolitimonae strain, and *R. akari.*[18,20,23,153] Boutonneuse fever is associated with a procoagulant state,[91–94,154] and 9.6% of cases are complicated by deep venous thrombosis late in the course.[155] Plasma levels of tumor necrosis factor rise during infection.[97] After a mean incubation period of 7 days, fever, myalgias, and headache characterize the onset (see Table 187-1). Careful clinical examination may reveal a tache noire, which facilitates the clinical diagnosis.

Rickettsia sibirica was discovered in the 1930s in eastern Russia and subsequently in China, Mongolia, and Pakistan. A genomic variant considered a strain or a subspecies, named mongolitimonae, has been found in Europe, Asia, and Africa. *R. sibirica* causes North Asian or Siberian tick typhus closely resembling RMSF. Nearly half of patients infected with *R. sibirica* mongolitimonae strain manifest a very unusual ropelike lymphangitis between an inoculation eschar and the draining lymph node.[20] This clinical feature led to the term *lymphangitis-associated rickettsiosis. Rickettsia australis* is limited to eastern Australia, and *Rickettsia honei,* the causative agent of Flinders Island spotted fever, also causes human infections on mainland Australia and Thailand.[12,24,141]

Although Japanese spotted fever has been described as a typically moderate SFG rickettsial illness (fever 100%, rash 100%, and eschar 90%), more severe illness, including meningoencephalitis, respiratory failure, shock, and even death associated with elevated proinflammatory cytokines does occur.[156–159] *R. heilongjiangensis,* the agent of Far Eastern spotted fever, is present in eastern Russia, Thailand, and China.[25] It causes typical non–life-threatening SFG rickettsiosis, with some patients exhibiting ropelike lymphangitis.

Rickettsia africae is prevalent throughout sub-Saharan Africa, where the vector ticks—*Amblyomma hebraeum* and *Amblyomma variegatum*—are present.[24] The identification of *R. africae* infections in the West Indies apparently conforms to the distribution of *A. variegatum.*[26] African tick bite fever is the only tick-transmitted rickettsiosis in which several inoculation eschars are observed in a high proportion of cases.[26] *R. africae,* the most frequently imported rickettsiosis, is often observed in patients who have hunted or traveled in the bush in southern Africa.[26,160] The attack rate in an exposed group can be rather high. Patients with African tick bite fever typically have headache, fever, and myalgia, as well as acute-stage elevations of serum tumor necrosis factor-α, interleukin-6 (IL-6), IL-8, IL-13, interferon gamma, RANTES (*r*egulated upon *a*ctivation *n*ormal *T* cell *e*xpressed and *s*ecreted), and MIP1α (macrophage inflammatory protein 1-α).[161] Rash may be vesicular, maculopapular, sparse, or even absent in more than half of patients. Distinctive features include frequent regional lymphadenitis that drains the region of the eschars. The infection is common among native Africans, in whom it is frequently suspected to be malaria or typhoid fever.[21]

R. parkeri infection has been documented recently in the United States,[162] transmitted by the Gulf Coast tick (*Amblyomma maculatum*) and appears to be associated with human infections in Uruguay, Brazil, and Argentina.[2,13,14,59] It causes a spotted fever very similar to African tick bite fever, caused by the agent to which *R. parkeri* is closely related. It is likely one of the causes of cases reported as RMSF based on serology, though *R. parkeri* infection may be less severe than RMSF. As another possible difference from RMSF, all 12 patients in a recent report had an eschar.[162]

Human infections with *R. slovaca* in Europe are called TIBOLA (*ti*ck-*bo*rne *l*ymph*a*denopathy), a SFG rickettsiosis with different clinical manifestations.[3,19,27] *R. slovaca* is transmitted to humans most often by the bite of adult *Dermacentor marginatus* ticks during winter and early spring. The illness is characterized by an eschar, typically on the scalp, and enlarged, often tender, draining cervical lymph nodes. Fewer than half of patients manifest a fever, and rash occurs rarely. The eschar site may have prolonged alopecia. There is a persistent asthenia in a small fraction of patients, despite response to antirickettsial treatment. The possibility of chronic illness associated with a SFG rickettsial infection has also been suggested in patients in Australia.[163] The fact that SFG rickettsiae can cause an eschar in an otherwise healthy person[164]—the mildest manifestation of illness, short of asymptomatic seroconversion—has been demonstrated for *R. aeschlimanii*.[4] Another case of *R. aeschlimannii* infection presenting as typical SFG rickettsiosis has also been reported.[17] *R. massiliae* infects *Rhipicephalus sanguineus* ticks worldwide and has been isolated from a patient in Sicily.[23] A patient with acute febrile illness in Sweden was reported with molecular and serologic evidence of *R. helvetica* infection.[28]

R. felis, the agent of flea-borne spotted fever, was the first *Rickettsia* shown to contain a plasmid.[165-167] *R. felis* infections have been documented by PCR assay in the United States, Mexico, Brazil, and Germany and by serology in France, Brazil, and Mexico.[5-8] The cat flea host, *Ctenocephalides felis*, is cosmopolitan, suggesting a worldwide distribution. *R. felis* has been identified in North and South America, Europe, and Asia.[168] Six *R. felis* infections documented by PCR have manifested fever in all cases, maculopapular rash (four cases), headache (three cases), neurologic involvement (photophobia, stupor, and meningismus in one case each), myalgia (two cases), abdominal pain (two cases), vomiting (two cases), eschar with lymphadenopathy (one case), and cough with radiologic infiltrates (one case).

The diagnosis of SFG rickettsiosis may be established by immunohistologic demonstration of organisms in skin biopsy; PCR assay has been used with blood or skin biopsy for *R. conorii*, *R. africae*, *R. slovaca*, *R. felis*, and *R. japonica*.[5,6,129,132,146,147,169] Pitfalls associated with ascribing an illness to a causative agent by PCR are emphasized in the dubious association of *R. helvetica* with sarcoidosis and chronic myopericarditis.[170,171] A novel approach that can be used to diagnose boutonneuse fever before the onset of rash is immunofluorescent detection of *R. conorii* in circulating endothelial cells captured by immunomagnetic beads coated with a monoclonal antibody to the human endothelial cell surface.[126,130,172] Timely diagnosis can also be established by isolating SFG rickettsiae in a shell vial cell culture system.[125] During the convalescent phase, production of antibodies to SFG rickettsiae can be demonstrated by the use of microimmunofluorescence, latex agglutination, enzyme immunoassay, Western blot, or complement fixation. Antibodies to *R. africae* appear late in convalescence in African tick bite fever.[173]

Successful treatment is achieved with doxycycline (200 mg/day), tetracycline (50 mg/kg/day), chloramphenicol (2 g/day for 7 to 10 days), or ciprofloxacin (1.5 g/day for 5 to 7 days).[174-176] Single-dose treatment with 200 mg doxycycline has been proposed, as has treatment with josamycin, a macrolide compound, for children and pregnant women, or with clarithromycin or azithromycin for children with mild disease.[177]

REFERENCES

1. Galvao MA, Dumler JS, Mafra CL, et al. Fatal spotted fever rickettsiosis, Minas Gerais, Brazil. *Emerg Infect Dis.* 2003;9:1402-1405.
2. Paddock CD, Sumner JW, Comer JA, et al. *Rickettsia parkeri*: A newly recognized cause of spotted fever rickettsiosis in the United States. *Clin Infect Dis.* 2004;38:805-811.
3. Raoult D, Lakos A, Fenollar F, et al. Spotless rickettsiosis caused by *Rickettsia slovaca* and associated with *Dermacentor* ticks. *Clin Infect Dis.* 2002;34:1331-1336.
4. Pretorius A-M, Birtles RJ. *Rickettsia aeschlimanii*: A new spotted fever group rickettsia, South Africa. *Emerg Infect Dis.* 2002;8:874.
5. Zavala-Velazquez JE, Ruiz-Sosa JA, Sanchez-Elias RA, et al. *Rickettsia felis* rickettsiosis in Yucatán. *Lancet.* 2000;356:1079-1080.
6. Pérez-Osorio CE, Zavala-Velázquez, Aria León JJ, et al. *Rickettsia felis* as emergent global threat for humans. *Emerg Infect Dis.* 2008;14:1019-1023.
7. Raoult D, La Scola B, Enea M, et al. A flea-associated rickettsia pathogenic for humans. *Emerg Infect Dis.* 2001;7:73-81.
8. Richter J, Fournier P-E, Petridou J, et al. *Rickettsia felis* infection acquired in Europe and documented by polymerase chain reaction. *Emerg Infect Dis.* 2002;8:207-208.
9. Parola P, Paddock CD, Raoult D. Tick-borne rickettsioses around the world: Emerging diseases challenging old concepts. *Clin Microbiol Rev.* 2005;18:719-756.
10. Estripeaut D, Aramburu MG, Saez-Llorens X, et al. Rocky Mountain spotted fever, Panama. *Emerg Infect Dis.* 2007;13:1763-1765.
11. Hidalgo M, Orejuela L, Fuya P, et al. Rocky Mountain spotted fever, Colombia. *Emerg Infect Dis.* 2007;13:1058-1060.
12. Jiang J, Sangkasuwan V, Lerdthusnee K, et al. Human Infection with *Rickettsia honei*, Thailand. *Emerg Infect Dis.* 2005;11:1473-1475.
13. Seijo A, Picollo M, Nicholson W, et al. [Fiebre manchada por rickettsias en el Delta del Parana una enfermedad emergente.] *Medicina (Buenos Aires).* 2007;67:723-726.
14. Conti-Diaz IA. [Rickettsiosis por *Rickettsii conorii* (fiebre botonosa de Mediterraneo o fiebre de Marsella). Estado actual en Uruguay.] *Rev Med Uruguay.* 2001;119-124.
15. Paddock CD, Fernandez S, Echenique GA, et al. Rocky Mountain spotted fever in Argentina. *Am J Trop Med Hyg.* 2008;78:687-692.
16. Zavala-Castro JE, Dzul-Rosado KR, Arias Leon JJ, et al. An increase in human cases of spotted fever rickettsiosis in Yucatan, Mexico, involving children. *Am J Trop Med Hyg.* 2008; 79:907-910
17. Raoult D, Fournier P-E, Abboud P, et al. First documented human *Rickettsia aeschlimannii* infection. *Emerg Infect Dis.* 2002;8:748-749.
18. Jado I, Oteo JA, Aldamiz M, et al. *Rickettsia monacensis* and human disease, Spain. *Emerging Infectious Diseases.* 2007;13:1405-1407.
19. Oteo JA, Ibarra V, Blanco JR, et al. Dermacentor-borne necrosis erythema and lymphadenopathy: Clinical and epidemiological features of a new tick-borne disease. *Clin Microbiol Infect.* 2004;10:327-331.
20. Fournier P-E, Gouriet F, Brouqui P, et al. Lymphangitis-associated rickettsiosis, a new rickettsiosis caused by *Rickettsia sibirica* mongolotimonae: Seven new cases and review of the literature. *Clin Infect Dis.* 2005;40:1435-1444.
21. Ndip LM, Fokam EB, Bouyer DH, et al. Detection of *Rickettsia africae* in patients and ticks along the coastal region of Cameroon. *Am J Trop Med Hyg.* 2004;71:363-366.
22. Ndip LM, Bouyer DH, Travassos da Rosa APA, et al. Acute spotted fever rickettsiosis among febrile patients, Cameroon. *Emerg Infect Dis.* 2004;10:432-437.
23. Vitale G, Mansuelo S, Rolain JM, et al. *Rickettsia massiliae* human isolation. *Emerg Infect Dis.* 2006;12:174-175.
24. Stewart RS. Flinders Island spotted fever: A newly recognized endemic focus of tick typhus in Bass Strait. *Med J Aust.* 1991;154:94-99.
25. Mediannikov OY, Sidelnikov Y, Ivanov L, et al. Acute tick-borne rickettsiosis caused by *Rickettsia heilongjiangensis* in Russian Far East. *Emerg Infect Dis.* 2004;10:810-817.
26. Raoult D, Fournier P-E, Fenollar F, et al. *Rickettsia africae*, a tick-borne pathogen in travelers to sub-Saharan Africa. *N Engl J Med.* 2001;344:1501-1510.
27. Casola C, Enea M, Lucht F, et al. First isolation of *Rickettsia slovaca* from a patient, France. *Emerg Infect Dis.* 2003;9:135.
28. Nilsson K. Septicemia with *Rickettsia helvetica* in a patient with acute febrile illness, rash and myasthenia. *J Infect.* 2009;58:79-82.
29. Childs JE, Paddock CD. Passive surveillance as an instrument to identify risk factors for fatal Rocky Mountain spotted fever: is there more to learn? *Am J Trop Med Hyg.* 2002;66:842-847.
30. Ricketts HT. A micro-organism which apparently has a specific relationship to Rocky Mountain spotted fever. *JAMA.* 1909;52:379-380.
31. Walker DH. Ricketts creates rickettsiology. *J Infect Dis.* 2004;189:938-955.
32. Harden VA. *Rocky Mountain Spotted Fever: History of a Twentieth Century Disease.* Baltimore: Johns Hopkins University Press; 1990.
33. Wolbach SB. Studies on Rocky Mountain spotted fever. *J Med Res.* 1919;41:2-197.
34. Perlman SJ, Hunter MS, Zchori-Fein E. The emerging diversity of *Rickettsia*. *Proc R Soc B.* 2006;273:2097-2106.
35. Gillespie JJ, Williams K, Shukla M, et al. *Rickettsia* phylogenomics: Unwinding the intricacies of obligate intracellular life. *PLoS One.* 2008;3:e2018.
36. Gevers D, Cohan FM, Lawrence JG, et al. Re-evaluating prokaryotic species. *Nat Rev Microbiol.* 2005;3:733-739.
37. Fournier P-E, Dumler JS, Greub G, et al. Gene sequence-based criteria for identification of new *Rickettsia* isolates and description of *Rickettsia heilongjiangensis* sp.nov. *J Clin Microbiol.* 2003;41:5456-5465.
38. Achtman M, Wagner M. Microbial diversity and the genetic nature of microbial species. *Nature Rev Microbiol.* 2008;6:431-440.
39. Medini D, Serruto D, Parkhill J, et al. Microbiology in the post-genomic era. *Nat Rev Microbiol.* 2008;6:419-430.
40. Vitorino L, Chelo IM, Bacellar F, et al. Rickettsial phylogeny: A multigenic approach. *Microbiology.* 2007;153:160-168.
41. Blanc G, Ogata H, Robert C, et al. Lateral gene transfer between obligate intracellular bacteria: Evidence from the *Rickettsia massiliae* genome. *Genome Res.* 2007;17:1657-1664.
42. Xu WB, Raoult D. Taxonomic relationships among spotted fever group rickettsiae as revealed by antigenic analysis with monoclonal antibodies. *J Clin Microbiol.* 1998;36:887-896.
43. Feng H-M, Olano JP, Whitworth T, et al. Fc-dependent polyclonal antibodies and antibodies to outer membrane proteins A and B, but not to lipopolysaccharide, protect SCID mice against fatal *Rickettsia conorii* infection. *Infect Immun.* 2004;72:2222-2228.
44. McDade JE, Newhouse VF. Natural history of *Rickettsia rickettsii*. *Annu Rev Microbiol.* 1986;40:287-309.
45. Demma LJ, Traeger MS, Nicholson WL, et al. Rocky Mountain spotted fever from an unexpected tick vector in Arizona. *N Engl J Med.* 2005;353:587-593.
46. Niebylski ML, Peacock MG, Schwan TG. Lethal effect of *Rickettsia rickettsii* on its tick vector (*Dermacentor andersoni*). *Appl Environ Microbiol.* 1999;65:773-777.
47. Niebylski ML, Schrumpf ME, Burgdorfer W, et al. *Rickettsia peacockii* sp. nov., a new species infecting wood ticks, *Dermacentor andersoni*, in western Montana. *Int J Syst Bacteriol.* 1997;47:446-452.
48. Philip RN, Casper EA, Anacker RL, et al. *Rickettsia bellii* sp. nov.: A tick-borne rickettsia, widely distributed in the United States, that is distinct from the spotted fever and typhus biogroups. *Int J Syst Bacteriol.* 1983;33:94-106.
49. Johnson JE, Kadull PJ. Rocky Mountain spotted fever acquired in a laboratory. *N Engl J Med.* 1967;227:842-846.
50. Walker DH. Rocky Mountain spotted fever and other rickettsioses. In: Engleberg NC, DiRita V, Dermody TS, eds. *Schaechter's Mechanisms of Microbial Disease.* Baltimore: Lippincott William & Wilkins; 2007:292-299.
51. Walker DH, Fishbein DB. Epidemiology of rickettsial diseases. *Eur J Epidemiol.* 1991;7:237-245.
52. Treadwell TA, Holman RC, Clarke MJ, et al. Rocky Mountain spotted fever in the United States, 1993-1996. *Am J Trop Med Hyg.* 2000;63:21-26.
53. Wilfert CM, McCormack JN, Kleeman K, et al. Epidemiology of Rocky Mountain spotted fever as determined by active surveillance. *J Infect Dis.* 1984;150:469-479.
54. Salgo MP, Telzak EE, Currie B, et al. A focus of Rocky Mountain spotted fever within New York City. *N Engl J Med.* 1988;318:1345-1348.
55. Chapman AS, Murphy SM, Demma LJ, et al. Rocky Mountain spotted fever in the United States, 1997-2002. *Vector Borne Zoonotic Dis.* 2006;6:170-178.
56. Walker DH, Paddock CD, Dumler JS. Emerging and re-emerging tick-transmitted rickettsial and ehrlichial infetions. *Med Clin North Am.* 2008;92:1345-1361.
57. Apperson CS, Engber B, Nicholson WL, et al. Tick-borne diseases in North Carolina: Is "*Rickettsia amblyommii*" a possible cause of rickettsiosis reported as Rocky Mountain spotted fever? *Vector-Borne Zoonotic Dis.* 2008;8:597-606.
58. Marshall GS, Stout GG, Jacobs RF, et al. Antibodies reactive to *Rickettsia rickettsii* among children living in the southeast and south central regions of the United States. *Arch Pediatr Adolesc Med.* 2003;157:443-448.
59. Labruna MB, Pinter A, Szabo MPJ. [*Rickettsia parkeri* infectando um carrapato *Amblyomma triste* em pauliceia, estrado de São Paulo.] *Rev Bras Parasitol.* 2004;13:359.

60. Kardatzke JT, Neidhardt K, Dzuban DP, et al. Cluster of tick-borne infections at Fort Chaffee, Arkansas: Rickettsiae and *Borrelia burgdorferi* in ixodid ticks. *J Med Entomol.* 1992;29:669-672.
61. McCall CL, Curns AT, Rotz LD, et al. Fort Chaffee revisited: The epidemiology of tick-borne rickettsial and ehrlichial diseases at a natural focus. *Vector Borne Zoonotic Dis.* 2001;1:119-127.
62. Yevich SJ, Sanchez JL, DeFraites RF, et al. Seroepidemiology of infections due to spotted fever group rickettsiae and *Ehrlichia* species in military personnel exposed to areas of the United States where such infections are endemic. *J Infect Dis.* 1995;171:1266-1273.
63. Walker DH, Ismail N. Emerging and re-emerging rickettsioses: Endothelial cell infection and early disease events. *Nat Rev Microbiol.* 2008;6:375-386.
64. Uchiyama T, Kawano H, Kusuhara Y. The major outer membrane protein rOmpB of spotted fever group rickettsiae functions in the rickettsial adherence to and invasion of Vero cells. *Microb Infect.* 2006;8:801-809.
65. Li H, Walker DH. rOmpA is a critical protein for the adhesion of *Rickettsia rickettsii* to host cells. *Microb Pathog.* 1998;24:289-298.
66. Martinez JJ, Seveau S, Veiga E, et al. Ku70, a component of DNA-dependent protein kinase, is a mammalian receptor for *Rickettsia conorii. Cell.* 2005;123:1013-1023.
67. Rydkina E, Turpin LC, Sahni SK. Activation of p38 mitogen-activated protein kinase module facilitates *in vitro* host cell invasion by *Rickettsia rickettsii. J Med Microbiol.* 2008;57(Pt 9):1172-1175.
68. Silverman DJ, Santucci LA, Meyers N, et al. Penetration of host cells by *Rickettsia rickettsii* appears to be mediated by a phospholipase of rickettsial origin. *Infect Immun.* 1992;60: 2733-2740.
69. Martinez JJ, Cossart P. Early signaling events involved in the entry of *Rickettsia conorii* into mammalian cells. *J Cell Sci.* 2004;117:5097-5106.
70. Ellison DW, Clark TR, Sturdevant DE, et al. Genomic comparison of virulent *Rickettsia rickettsii* Shela Smith and avirulent *Rickettsia rickettsii* Iowa. *Infect Immun.* 2008;76: 542-550.
71. Whitworth T, Popov VL, Yu XJ, et al. Expression of the *Rickettsia prowazekii* pld or tlyC gene in *Salmonella* enterica serovar typhimurium mediates phagosomal escape. *Infect Immun.* 2005;73:6668-6673.
72. Teysseire N, Chiche-Portiche C, Raoult D. Intracellular movements of *Rickettsia conorii* and *R. typhi* based on actin polymerization. *Res Microbiol.* 1992;143:821-829.
73. Gouin E, Egile C, Dehoux P, et al. The RickA protein of *Rickettsia conorii* activates the arp2/3 complex. *Nature.* 2004;427:457-461.
74. Ogata H, Audic S, Barbe V, et al. Selfish DNA in protein-coding genes of *Rickettsia. Science.* 2000;290(5490):347-350.
75. Jeng RL, Goley ED, D'alessio JA, et al. A *Rickettsia* wasp-like protein activates the arp2/3 complex and mediates actin-based motility. *Cell Microbiol.* 2004;6:761-769.
76. Simser JA, Rahman MS, Dreher-Lesnick SM, et al. A novel and naturally occurring transposon, ISRpe1 in the *Rickettsia peacockii* genome disrupting the rickA gene involved in actin-based motility. *Mol Microbiol.* 2005;58:71-79.
77. Santucci LA, Gutierrez PL, Silverman DJ. *Rickettsia rickettsii* induces superoxide radical and superoxide dismutase in human endothelial cells. *Infect Immun.* 1992;60:5113-5118.
78. Eremeeva ME, Dasch GA, Silverman DJ. Quantitative analyses of variations in the injury of endothelial cells elicited by 11 isolates of *Rickettsia rickettsii. Clin Diagn Lab Immunol.* 2001;8:788-795.
79. Eremeeva ME, Silverman DJ. Effects of the antioxidant α-lipoic acid on human umbilical vein endothelial cells infected with *Rickettsia rickettsii. Infect Immun.* 1998;66:2290-2299.
80. Walker DH, Firth WT, Ballard JG, et al. Role of phospholipase-associated penetration mechanism in cell injury by *Rickettsia rickettsii. Infect Immun.* 1983;40:840-842.
81. Walker DH, Tidwell RR, Rector TM, et al. Effect of synthetic protease inhibitors of the amidine type on cell injury by *Rickettsia rickettsii. Antimicrob Agents Chemother.* 1984;25: 582-585.
82. Rydkina E, Sahni SK, Santucci LA, et al. Selective modulation of antioxidant enzyme activities in host tissues during *Rickettsia conorii* infection. *Microbiol Pathogen.* 2004;36:293-301.
83. Harrell GT, Aikawa JK. Pathogenesis of circulatory failure in Rocky Mountain spotted fever. Alteration in the blood volume and the thiocyanate space at various stages of the disease. *Arch Intern Med.* 1949;83:331-347.
84. Rydkina E, Sahni A, Baggs RB, et al. Infection of human endothelial cells with spotted fever group Rickettsiae stimulates cyclooxygenase 2 expression and release of vasoactive prostaglandins. *Infect Immun.* 2006;74:5067-5074.
85. Kaplowitz LG, Robertson GL. Hyponatremia in Rocky Mountain spotted fever: Role of antidiuretic hormone. *Ann Intern Med.* 1983;98:334-335.
86. Walker DH, Crawford CG, Cain BG. Rickettsial infection of the pulmonary microcirculation: The basis for interstitial pneumonitis in Rocky Mountain spotted fever. *Hum Pathol.* 1980; 11:263-272.
87. Lankford HV, Glauser FL. Cardiopulmonary dynamics in a severe case of Rocky Mountain spotted fever. *Arch Intern Med.* 1980;140:1357-1360.
88. Helmick CG, Bernard KW, D'Angelo LJ. Rocky Mountain spotted fever: Clinical, laboratory, and epidemiological features of 262 cases. *J Infect Dis.* 1984;150:480-486.
89. Kaplowitz LG, Fischer JJ, Sparling PF. Rocky Mountain spotted fever: A clinical dilemma. In: Remington JB, Swartz HN, eds. Current Clinical Topics in Infectious Diseases. vol 2. New York: McGraw-Hill; 1981:89-108.
90. Rao AK, Schapira M, Clements ML, et al. A prospective study of platelets and plasma proteolytic systems during the early stages of Rocky Mountain spotted fever. *N Engl J Med.* 1988;318:1021-1028.
91. Davi G, Giammarresi C, Vigneri S, et al. Demonstration of *Rickettsia conorii*-induced coagulative and platelet activation in vivo in patients with Mediterranean spotted fever. *Thromb Haemost.* 1995;74:631-634.
92. George F, Brouqui P, Boffa M-C, et al. Demonstration of *Rickettsia conorii*–induced endothelial injury in vivo by measuring circulating endothelial cells, thrombomodulin, and von Willebrand factor in patients with Mediterranean spotted fever. *Blood.* 1993;82:2109-2116.
93. Elghetany TM, Walker DH. Hemostatic changes in Rocky Mountain spotted fever and Mediterranean spotted fever. *Am J Clin Pathol.* 1999;112:159-168.
94. Vicente V, Espana F, Tabernero D, et al. Evidence of activation of the protein C pathway during acute vascular damage induced by Mediterranean spotted fever. *Blood.* 1991;78: 416-422.
95. Vicente V, Estelles A, Moraleda JM, et al. Fibrinolytic changes during acute vascular damage induced by Mediterranean spotted fever. *Fibrinolysis.* 1993;7:324-329.
96. Yamada T, Harber P, Pettit GW, et al. Activation of the kallikrein-kinin system in Rocky Mountain spotted fever. *Ann Intern Med.* 1978;88:764-768.
97. Oristrell J, Amengual MJ, Font-Creus B, et al. Plasma levels of tumor necrosis factor-α in patients with Mediterranean spotted fever: Clinical and analytical correlations. *Clin Infect Dis.* 1994;19:1141-1143.
98. Teysseire N, Arnoux D, George F, et al. Von Willebrand factor release and thrombomodulin and tissue factor expression in *Rickettsia conorii*-infected endothelial cells. *Infect Immun.* 1992;60:4388-4393.
99. Sporn LA, Haidaris PJ, Shi R, et al. *Rickettsia rickettsii* infection of cultured human endothelial cells induces tissue factor expression. *Blood.* 1994;83:1527-1534.
100. Schmaier AH, Srikanth S, Elghetany MT, et al. Hemostatic/fibrinolytic protein changes in C3H/HeN mice infected with *Rickettsia conorii. Thromb Haemost.* 2001;86:871-879.
101 Jordan JM, Woods ME, Olano JP, et al. Absence of TLR4 signaling in C3H/HeJ mice predisposes to overwhelming rickettsial infection and decreased protective Th1 responses. *Infec Immun.* 2008;76:3717-3724.
102. Woods ME, Olano JP. Host defenses to *Rickettsia rickettsii* infection contribute to increased microvascular permeability in human cerebral endothelial cells. *J Clin Immunol.* 2008;28: 174-185.
103. Fang R, Ismail N, Soong L, et al. Differential interaction of dendritic cells with *Rickettsia conorii*: impact on host susceptibility to murine spotted fever rickettsiosis: *Infect Immun.* 2007; 756:3112-3123.
104. Feng H-M, Walker DH. Mechanisms of intracellular killing of *Rickettsia conorii* in infected human endothelial cells, hepatocytes, and macrophages. *Infect Immun.* 2000;68:6729-6736.
105. Feng H-M, Popov VL, Yuoh G, et al. Role of T-lymphocyte subsets in immunity to spotted fever group rickettsiae. *J Immunol.* 1997;158:5314-5320.
106. Feng H-M, Popov VL, Walker DH. Depletion of interferon gamma and tumor necrosis factor alpha in mice with *Rickettsia conorii*-infected endothelium: Impairment of rickettsicidal nitric oxide production resulting in fatal, overwhelming rickettsial disease. *Infect Immun.* 1994;62:1952-1960.
107. De Sousa R, Ismail N, Nobrega SD, et al. Intralesional expression of mRNA of interferon-γ, tumor necrosis factor-α, interleukin-10, nitric oxide synthase, indoleamine-2,3-dioxygenase, and rantes is a major immune effector in Mediterranean spotted fever rickettsiosis. *J Infect Dis.* 2007;196:770-781.
108. Jordan JM, Woods ME, Soong L, et al. Rickettsiae stimulate dendritic cells through TLR4, leading to enhanced NK cell activation in vivo. *J Infect Dis.* 2009;199:236-242.
109. Billings AN, Feng H-M, Olano JP, et al. Rickettsial infection in murine models activates an early anti-rickettsial effect mediated by NK cells and associated with production of gamma interferon. *Am J Trop Med Hyg.* 2001;65:52-56.
110. Walker DH, Olano JP, Feng H-M. Critical role of cytotoxic T lymphocytes in immune clearance of rickettsial infection. *Infect Immun.* 2001;69:1841-1846.
111. Sumner JW, Sims KG, Jones DC, et al. Protection of guinea-pigs from experimental Rocky Mountain spotted fever by immunization with baculovirus-expressed *Rickettsia rickettsii* rOmpA protein. *Vaccine.* 1995;13:29-35.
112. Vishwanath S, McDonald GA, Watkins NG. A recombinant *Rickettsia conorii* vaccine protects guinea pigs from experimental boutonneuse fever and Rocky Mountain spotted fever. *Infect Immun.* 1990;58:646-653.
113. Crocquet-Valdes PA, Diaz-Montero CM, Feng H-M, et al. Immunization with a portion of rickettsial outer membrane protein A stimulates protective immunity against spotted fever rickettsiosis. *Vaccine.* 2002;20:979-988.
114. Díaz-Montero CM, Feng H-M, Crocquet-Valdes PA, et al. Identification of protective components of two major outer membrane proteins of spotted fever group rickettsiae. *Am J Trop Med Hyg.* 2001;65:371-378.
115. Walker DH, Gay RM, Valdes-Dapena M. The occurrence of eschars in Rocky Mountain spotted fever. *J Am Acad Dermatol.* 1981;4:571-576.
116. Rosenblum MJ, Masland RL, Harrell GT. Residual effects of rickettsial disease on the central nervous system. *Arch Intern Med.* 1952;90:444-445.
117. Buckingham SC, Marshall GS, Schutze GE, et al. Clinical and laboratory features, hospital course, and outcome of Rocky mountain spotted fever in children. *J Pediatr.* 2007;150: 180-184.
118. Walker DH, Mattern WD. Acute renal failure in Rocky Mountain spotted fever. *Arch Intern Med.* 1979;139:443-448.
119. Donohue JF. Lower respiratory tract involvement in Rocky Mountain spotted fever. *Arch Intern Med.* 1980;140:223-227.
120. Feltes TF, Wilcox WD, Feldman WE, et al. M-mode echocardiographic abnormalities in Rocky Mountain spotted fever. *South Med J.* 1984;787:1130-1132.
121. Walker DH, Hawkins HL, Hudson P. Fulminant Rocky Mountain spotted fever. Its pathologic characteristics associated with glucose-6-phosphate dehydrogenase deficiency. *Arch Pathol Lab Med.* 1983;107:121-125.
122. Dalton MJ, Clarke MJ, Holman RC, et al. National surveillance for Rocky Mountain spotted fever, 1981-1992: Epidemiologic summary and evaluation of risk factors for fatal outcome. *Am J Trop Med Hyg.* 1995;52:405-413.
123. Archibald LK, Sexton DJ. Long-term sequelae of Rocky Mountain spotted fever. *Clin Infect Dis.* 1995;20:1122-1125.
124. Kirkland KB, Marcom PK, Sexton DJ, et al. Rocky Mountain spotted fever complicated by gangrene: Report of six cases and review. *Clin Infect Dis.* 1993;16:629-634.
125. LaScola B, Raoult D. Diagnosis of Mediterranean spotted fever by cultivation of *Rickettsia conorii* from blood and skin samples using the centrifugation-shell vial technique and by detection of *R. conorii* in circulating endothelial cells: A 6-year follow-up. *J Clin Microbiol.* 1996;34:2722-2727.
126. Walker DH, Burday MS, Folds JD. Laboratory diagnosis of Rocky Mountain spotted fever. *South Med J.* 1980;73: 1443-1447.
127. Kaplowitz LG, Lange JV, Fischer JJ, et al. Correlation of rickettsial titers, circulating endotoxin, and clinical features in Rocky Mountain spotted fever. *Arch Intern Med.* 1983;143:1149-1151.
128. Dumler JS, Gage WR, Pettis GL, et al. Rapid immunoperoxidase demonstration of *Rickettsia rickettsii* in fixed cutaneous specimens from patients with Rocky Mountain spotted fever. *Am J Clin Pathol.* 1990;93:410-414.
129. LaScola B, Raoult D. Laboratory diagnosis of rickettsioses: Current approaches to diagnosis of old and new rickettsial diseases. *J Clin Microbiol.* 1997;35:2715-2727.
130. Tzianabos T, Anderson BE, McDade JE. Detection of *Rickettsia rickettsii* DNA in clinical specimens using polymerase chain reaction technology. *J Clin Microbiol.* 1989;27:2866-2868.
131. Sexton DJ, Kanj SS, Wilson K, et al. The use of a polymerase chain reaction as a diagnostic test for Rocky Mountain spotted fever. *Am J Trop Med Hyg.* 1994;50:59-63.
132. de Sousa R, Franca A, Nobrega DS. Host and microbial risk factors and pathophysiology of fatal *Rickettsia conorii* infection in Portuguese patients. *J Infect Dis.* 2008;198:576-585.
133. Walker DH, Sexton D. Rickettsia rickettsii. In: Yu VL, Merigan TC, Barriere SL, eds. *Antimicrobial Therapy and Vaccines.* 2nd ed. Baltimore: Williams & Wilkins; 2002:899-906.
134. Rolain JM, Maurin M, Vestris G, et al. In vitro susceptibilities of 27 rickettsiae to 13 antimicrobials. *Antimicrob Agents Chemother.* 1998;42:1537-1541.
135. Holman RC, Paddock CD, Curns AT, et al. Analysis of risk factors for fatal Rocky Mountain spotted fever: Evidence for superiority of tetracyclines for therapy. *J Infect Dis.* 2002;184:1437-1444.
136. American Academy of Pediatrics, Committee on the Control of Infectious Diseases. Rocky Mountain spotted fever. In: Pickering LK, ed. *2000 Red Book: Report of the Committee on Infectious Diseases.* 25th ed. Elk Grove Village, Ill: American Academy of Pediatrics; 2000:491-493.
137. Kirkland KB, Wilkinson WE, Sexton DJ. Therapeutic delay and mortality in cases of Rocky Mountain spotted fever. *Clin Infect Dis.* 1995;20:1118-1121.
138. Breitschwerdt EB, Davidson MG, Hegarty BC, et al. Prednisolone at anti-inflammatory or immunosuppressive dosages in conjunction with doxycycline does not potentiate the severity of *Rickettsia rickettsii* infection in dogs. *Antimicrob Agents Chemother.* 1997;41:141-147.
139. Feng H-M, Walker DH. Cross-protection between distantly related spotted fever group rickettsiae. *Vaccine.* 2003;21: 3901-3905.
140. Valbuena G, Jordan JM, Walker DH. T cells mediate cross-protective immunity between spotted group rickettsiae and spotted fever group rickettsiae. *J Infect Dis.* 2004;190: 1221-1227.
141. Dyer JR, Einsiedel L, Ferguson PE, et al. A new focus of *Rickettsia honei* spotted fever in South Australia. *MJA.* 2005;182:231-234.
142. Vishwanath S. Antigenic relationships among the rickettsiae of the spotted fever and typhus groups. *FEMS Microbiol Lett.* 1991;81:341-344.

143. Walker DH, Feng H, Saada JI, et al. Comparative antigenic analysis of spotted fever group rickettsiae from Israel and other closely related organisms. *Am J Trop Med Hyg.* 1995;52:569-576.

144. Zhu Y, Fournier PE, Eremeeva M, et al. Proposal to create subspecies of *Rickettsia conorii* based on multi-locus sequence typing and an emended description of *Rickettsia conorii*. *BMC Microbiol.* 2005;5:11.

145. Fournier PE, Zhu Y, Yu X, et al. proposal to create subspecies of *Rickettsia sibirica* and an emended description of *Rickettsia sibirica*. *Ann N Y Acad Sci.* 2006;1078:597-606.

146. Walker DH, Occhino C, Tringali GR, et al. Pathogenesis of rickettsial eschars. The tache noire of boutonneuse fever. *Hum Pathol.* 1988;19:1449-1454.

147. Walker DH, Gear JM. Correlation of the distribution of *Rickettsia conorii*, microscopic lesions, and clinical features in South African tick bite fever. *Am J Trop Med Hyg.* 1985;34:361-371.

148. Walker DH, Herrero-Herrero JI, Ruiz-Beltran R, et al. The pathology of fatal Mediterranean spotted fever. *Am J Clin Pathol.* 1987;87:669-672.

149. Walker DH, Staiti A, Mansueto S, et al. Frequent occurrence of hepatic lesions in boutonneuse fever. *Acta Trop.* 1986;43:175-181.

150. de Sousa R, Nobrega SD, Bacellar F, et al. Mediterranean spotted fever in Portugal: Risk factors for fatal outcome in 105 hospitalized patients. *Ann N Y Acad Sci.* 2003;990:285-294.

151. Raoult D, Zuchelli P, Weiller PJ, et al. Incidence, clinical observations and risk factors in the severe form of Mediterranean spotted fever among patients admitted to the hospital in Marseilles 1983-1984. *J Infect.* 1986;12:111-116.

152. Anton E, Font B, Munoz T, et al. Clinical and laboratory characteristics of 144 patients with Mediterranean spotted fever. *Eur J Clin Microbiol Infect Dis.* 2003;22:126-128.

153. Radulovic S, Feng H-M, Morovic M, et al. Isolation of *Rickettsia akari* from a patient in a region where Mediterranean spotted fever is endemic. *Clin Infect Dise.* 1996;22:216-220.

154. Vicente V, Alberca I, Ruiz R, et al. Coagulation abnormalities in patients with Mediterranean spotted fever. *J Infect Dis.* 1986;153:128-131.

155. Raoult D, Weiller PJ, Chagnon A, et al. Mediterranean spotted fever: Clinical, laboratory and epidemiological features of 199 cases. *Am J Trop Med Hyg.* 1986;35:845-850.

156. Iwasaki H, Mahara F, Takada N, et al. Fulminant Japanese spotted fever associated with hypercytokinemia. *J Clin Microbiol.* 2001;39:2341-2343.

157. Araka M, Takatsuka K, Kawamura J, et al. Japanese spotted fever involving the central nervous system. Two case reports and a literature review. *J Clin Microbiol.* 2002;40:3874-3876.

158. Kodama K, Senba T, Yamauchi H, et al. Fulminant Japanese spotted fever definitively diagnosed by the polymerase chain reaction method. *J Infect Chemother.* 2002;8:266-268.

159. Kodama K, Senba T, Yamauchi H, et al. Clinical studies of Japanese spotted fever and its aggravating factors. *J Infect Chemother.* 2003;9:83-87.

160. McQuiston JH, Paddock CD, Singleton J Jr, et al. Imported spotted fever rickettsioses in United States travelers returning from Africa: A summary of cases confirmed by laboratory testing at the Centers for Disease Control and Prevention, 1999-2002. *Am J Trop Med.* 2004;70:98-101.

161. Jensenius M, Ueland T, Fournier PE, et al. Systemic inflammatory responses in African tick-bite fever. *J Infect Dis.* 2003;187:1332-1336.

162. Paddock CD, Finley RW, Wright CS, et al. *Rickettsia parkeri* rickettsiosis and its clinical distinction from Rocky Mountain Spotted Fever. *Clin Infect Dis.* 2008;47:1188-1196.

163. Unsworth N, Graves S, Nguyen C, et al. Markers of exposure to spotted fever rickettsiae in patients with chronic illness, including fatigue, in two Australian populations. *Q J M.* 2008;101:269-274.

164. Mansueto S, Tringali G, Leo RD, et al. Demonstration of spotted fever group rickettsiae in the *tache noire* of a healthy person in Sicily. *Am J Trop Med Hyg.* 1984;33:479-482.

165. Bouyer DH, Stenos J, Crocquet-Valdes P, et al. *Rickettsia felis*: Molecular characterization of a new member of the spotted fever group. *Int J Syst Evol Bacteriol.* 2001;51:339-347.

166. La Scola B, Meconi S, Fenollar F, et al. Emended description of *Rickettsia felis* (Bouyer et al, 2001), a temperature-dependent cultured bacterium. *Int J Syst Evol Bacteriol.* 2002;52:2035-2041.

167. Ogata H, Renesto P, Audic S, et al. The genome sequence of *Rickettsia felis* identifies the first putative conjugative plasmid in an obligate intracellular parasite. *PLoS Biol.* 2005;3:e248.

168. Perez-Osorio CE, Zavala-Velazuez JE, Arias Leon J, et al. Rickettsia felis as emergent global threat to humans. *Emerg Infect Dis.* 2008;14:1019-1023.

169. Furuya Y, Katayama T, Yoshida Y, et al. Specific amplification of *Rickettsia japonica* DNA from clinical specimens by PCR. *J Clin Microbiol.* 1995;33:487-489.

170. Nilsson K, Lindquist O, Pahlson C. Association of *Rickettsia helvetica* with chronic perimyocarditis in sudden cardiac death. *Lancet.* 1999;354:1169-1173.

171. Nilsson K, Pahlson C, Lukinius A, et al. Presence of *Rickettsia helvetica* in granulomatous tissue from patients with sarcoidosis. *J Infect Dis.* 2002;185:1128-1130.

172. Drancourt M, George F, Brouqui P, et al. Diagnosis of Mediterranean spotted fever by indirect immunofluorescence of *Rickettsia conorii* in circulating endothelial cells isolated with monoclonal antibody-coated immunomagnetic beads. *J Infect Dis.* 1992;166:660-663.

173. Fournier P-E, Jensenius M, Laferl H, et al. Kinetics of antibody responses in *Rickettsia africae* and *Rickettsia conorii* infections. *Clin Diag Lab Immunol.* 2002;9:324-328.

174. Raoult D, Maurin M. *Rickettsia* species. In: Yu VL, Merigan TC, Barriere SL, eds. *Antimicrobial Therapy and Vaccines.* 2nd ed. Baltimore: Williams & Wilkins; 2002:568-574.

175. Raoult D, Gallais H, De Micco C, et al. Ciprofloxacin therapy for Mediterranean spotted fever. *Antimicrob Agents Chemother.* 1986;30:606-607.

176. Ruiz-Beltran R, Herrero-Herrero JI. Evaluation of ciprofloxacin and doxycycline in the treatment of Mediterranean spotted fever. *Eur J Clin Microbiol Infect Dis.* 1992;11:427-431.

177. Cascio A, Colomba C, Di Rosa D, et al. Efficacy and safety of clarithromycin as a treatment for Mediterranean spotted fever in children: A randomized controlled trial. *Clin Infect Dis.* 2001;33:409-411.

188

Rickettsia akari (Rickettsialpox)

DIDIER RAOULT

Rickettsialpox is a worldwide mite-borne rickettsiosis with a vesicular eruption. It is caused by *Rickettsia akari*, associated with mice, and transmitted by its ectoparasite, the mite *Liponyssoides sanguineus*.

Etiology

R. akari is classified among spotted fever group rickettsiae based on antigenic and genetic data. Its genome has recently been sequenced and it harbors a plasmid, as does *R. felis*.[1]

It differs from these in that it is transmitted by the bite of *Liponyssoides sanguineus*, the mouse mite. The epidemiology of rickettsialpox is therefore linked to house mice. Another vector (perhaps the tick or flea) is suspected in that the seroprevalence of *R. akari* is high in New York City dogs.[2] The target cell of *R. akari* is the macrophage and not the endothelial cell, as with other rickettsiae.[3]

Epidemiology

Rickettsialpox was initially described in New York City and has been since reported in eastern Europe, Korea, and South Africa.[4] The recent bioterrorist attack with anthrax directed the attention of physicians to skin eschars and rash and allowed the identification of 34 cases of rickettsialpox in New York City[4] from February 2001 to August 2002. The patients were suspected of suffering cutaneous anthrax or smallpox. The usual yearly incidence in New York City is five cases. A surprisingly high seroprevalence of *R. akari* has been reported in IV drug users from Baltimore[5] and in patients using a free clinic in Los Angeles County.[6] Because this disease is not actively sought, its overall prevalence is completely unknown.

Clinical Manifestations

The typical triad of the disease, which includes fever, rash, and eschar,[7] was found in 92% of patients investigated in New York City (Table 188-1). Indeed, the disease is recognized by only a few physicians; in the New York City cases, half of patients were identified by a single physician, and 75% by three. The incubation period is approximately

7 days. Eschar is the clinical hallmark of the disease.[8] It starts as a primary papule; a vesicle then appears in the center and, when it dries, it leaves a brown or dark eschar (Fig. 188-1). Palpable regional lymph nodes draining this eschar are common and are usually tender.[8] The rash usually appears on the third or fourth day. It is papular at the beginning and becomes vesicular in many patients. The vesicles dry, and each leaves a black crust. Patients typically have 20 to 40 skin lesions. Palm and soles are not involved. The disease is benign, and patients usually recover. A transient leukopenia can be documented, as can thrombocytopenia and elevated aminotransferases.[10] A case was described of a human immunodeficiency virus (HIV)–positive patient who recovered.[11]

Diagnosis

Serology is the easiest tool that can be used for diagnosis. Cross-reactions have been noted between *R. akari* and *Rickettsia rickettsii*. Homologous antigens are more sensitive and are preferable. Immunoglobulin (Ig)M and IgG are detected 7 to 15 days after onset. Immunohistochemistry is of value with skin biopsies and was considered the most efficient tool in the New York City series. A nested polymerase chain reaction (PCR) assay that used DNA sequences that coded for a 17-kDa antigen was used on fresh tissues.[4] Isolation from skin biopsy could be performed on Vero cells in specialized laboratories. Consideration of *R. akari* in the differential diagnosis is critical in that its eschar can be misdiagnosed as inoculation anthrax. Moreover, it is one of the few infections that causes vesicular rashes, along with smallpox, varicella, herpes zoster, herpes simplex, and some other rickettsioses (e.g., Queensland tick typhus and African tick bite fever).

Treatment

Treatment[12] for rickettsialpox is doxycycline (200 mg/day for 7 days). The alternative treatment is chloramphenicol. Although clinical efficacy is unknown, *R. akari* is susceptible to many antibiotics, including azithromycin.

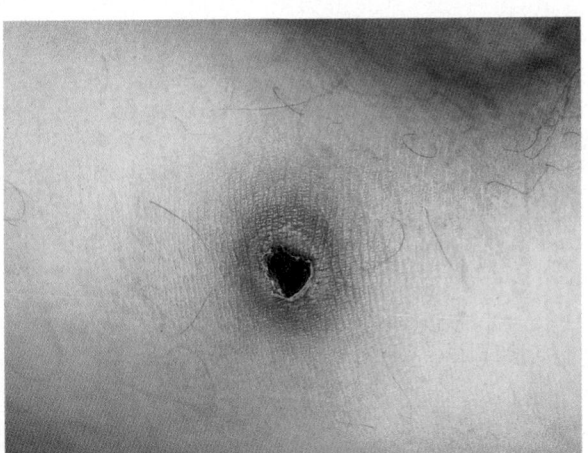

Figure 188-1 **Patient with rickettsialpox in 2002.** *(Courtesy of C. Paddock.)*

TABLE 188-1	Clinical and Epidemiologic Findings in Rickettsialpox		
Series	*Paddock et al*[4]	*Greenberg et al*[9]	*Kass et al*[7]
Number of cases	34	144	13
Year of study	2003	1947	1994
Fever	97%	100%	100%
Mice at residence or work	67%	—	—
Eschars	90%	99.8%	100%
Any rash	100%	100%	100%
Vesicular rash	—	—	92%
Fever plus eschars plus rash	92%	—	100%
Hospitalization	32%	—	—
Headache	NA	90%	100%

REFERENCES

1. Fournier PE, Belghazi L, Robert C, et al. Variations of plasmid content in *Rickettsia felis*. *PLoS ONE.* 2008;3: e2289.
2. Comer JA, Vargas MC, Poshni I, et al. Serologic evidence of *Rickettsia akari* infection among dogs in a metropolitan city. *J Am Vet Med Assoc.* 2001;218:1780-1782.
3. Walker DH, Hudnall SD, Szaniawski WK, et al. Monoclonal antibody-based immunohistochemical diagnosis of rickettsialpox: The macrophage is the principal target. *Mod Pathol.* 1999;12:529-533.
4. Paddock CD, Zaki SR, Koss T, et al. Rickettsialpox in New York City: A persistent urban zoonosis. *Ann N Y Acad Sci.* 2003;990:36-44.
5. Comer JA, Tzianabos T, Flynn C, et al. Serologic evidence of rickettsialpox (*Rickettsia akari*) infection among intravenous drug users in inner-city Baltimore, Maryland. *Am J Trop Med Hyg.* 1999;60:894-898.
6. Bennett SG, Comer JA, Smith HM, et al. Serologic evidence of a *Rickettsia akari*-like infection among wild-caught rodents in Orange County and humans in Los Angeles County, California. *J Vector Ecol.* 2007;32:198-201.
7. Kass EM, Szaniawski WK, Levy H, et al. Rickettsialpox in a New York City hospital, 1980 to 1989. *N Engl J Med.* 1994; 15:1612-1617.
8. Brettman LR, Lewin S, Holzman RS, et al. Rickettsialpox: Report of an outbreak and a contemporary review. *Medicine (Baltimore).* 1981;60:363-372.
9. Greenberg M, Pellitteri O, Klein IF, et al. Rickettsialpox—a newly recognized rickettsial disease. II. Clinical observations. *JAMA.* 1947;133:901-906.
10. Madison G, Kim-Schluger L, Braverman S, et al. Hepatitis in association with rickettsialpox. *Vector Borne Zoonotic Dis.* 2008;8:111-115.
11. Sanders S, Di Costanzo D, Leach J, et al. Rickettsialpox in a patient with HIV infection. *J Am Acad Dermatol.* 2003; 48:286-289.
12. Raoult D, Maurin M. *Rickettsia akari* (Rickettsialpox). In: Yu VL, Weber R, Raoult D, eds. *Antimicrobial Therapy and Vaccine.* 2nd ed. New York: Apple Trees Production; 2002:889-892.

189

Coxiella burnetii (Q Fever)

THOMAS J. MARRIE | DIDIER RAOULT

Q fever is an acute (on occasion chronic) febrile illness that occurs worldwide. The most common animal reservoirs for this zoonosis are cattle, sheep, and goats. These domestic ungulates, when infected, shed the desiccation-resistant organisms in urine, feces, milk, and especially in birth products. The placenta of infected sheep contains up to 10^9 organisms/g of tissue. Humans are infected by inhalation of contaminated aerosols and after an incubation period of 20 days (range, 14 to 39 days) become ill with severe headache, fever, chills, fatigue, and myalgia. There is a dose-response effect on the incubation period with incubation periods as short as 2 days occurring on occasion. Other signs and symptoms depend on the organs involved. In contrast to other rickettsial infections, rash rarely occurs in acute Q fever. However some patients do have a nonspecific erythematous reaction whereas others have urticaria that persists for weeks. The rash in chronic Q fever (endocarditis) is that of palpable purpura related to an immune complex vasculitis. Other differences between Q fever and the usual rickettsial infections are the aerosol route of infection and the lack of cross-reacting antibodies to the *Proteus* X strain (the Weil-Felix reaction).

The Pathogen

Coxiella burnetii, the causative agent of Q fever, is a highly pleomorphic coccobacillus with a gram-negative cell wall (Fig. 189-1). It measures 0.3 to 0.7 μm long[1] but, unlike true rickettsiae, enters the cell by a passive mechanism. Within host cells, it survives within the phagolysosome; the low pH of this environment is necessary for the metabolic functioning of *C. burnetii*. Large and small variants exist, and a spore stage has been described.[2] This spore stage explains the ability of *C. burnetii* to withstand harsh environmental conditions.[3] It survives for 7 to 10 months on wool at 15° to 20°C, for more than 1 month on fresh meat in cold storage, and for more than 40 months in skim milk at room temperature.[4] Although it is destroyed by 2% formaldehyde, the organism has been isolated from infected tissues stored in formaldehyde for up to 4 to 5 months. It has also been isolated from fixed "paraffinized" tissues. Either 1% Lysol or 5% hydrogen peroxide kills *C. burnetii*.

C. burnetii undergoes phase variation.[4] In nature and in laboratory animals it exists in the phase I state, in which organisms react with late (45 days) convalescent guinea pig sera and only slightly with early (21 days) sera.[4] Repeated passage of phase I virulent organisms in embryonated chicken eggs leads to gradual conversion to phase II avirulent forms by chromosomal deletions.[5] There is no morphologic difference between the two phases, although they differ in the sugar composition of their lipopolysaccharides,[6] in their buoyant density in cesium chloride, and in their affinity for hematoxylin and basic fuchsin dyes. *C. burnetii* lipopolysaccharide is nontoxic to chicken embryos at doses higher than 80 mg/embryo, in contrast to *Salmonella typhimurium* smooth- and rough-type lipopolysaccharide, which is toxic in nanogram amounts.[7]

Plasmids have been found in both phase I and phase II cells.[8] Some strains are without plasmid. No specific role in pathogenesis has been associated with the presence of a plasmid.[9]

The genome of *C. burnetii* consists of 1,995,275 base pairs.[10] It contains many genes with potential roles in adhesion, invasion, intracellular trafficking, and host cell modulation.[10] A difference from other intracellular bacteria is the observation that the genome of *C. burnetii* contains 32 insertion sequences dispersed in the chromosome.[10]

Epidemiology

Humans become infected by inhalation of small-particle aerosols containing *C. burnetii*. The resulting illness has been termed *Q fever*. In August 1935, Derrick, a medical officer of health in Queensland, Australia, investigated a febrile illness that affected 20 of 800 employees of a Brisbane meat works.[11] He coined the term *Q* (or query) *fever* for this illness, for which he had no diagnosis but suspected was a new disease. Burnet and Freeman showed that the microorganism isolated from the blood and urine of Derrick's patients was a rickettsia.[12] At about the same time, Davis and Cox isolated a microorganism from ticks (*Dermacentor andersoni*) collected near Nine Mile Creek, Montana.[13] Later, Dyer[14,15] showed that *Rickettsia burnetii* (Burnet and Freeman's organism) was the same as *Rickettsia diaporica* (Cox's organism); it is now known as *Coxiella burnetii*.

C. burnetii has been identified in arthropods, fish, birds, rodents, marsupials, and livestock.[1] Worldwide, the most common animal reservoirs are cattle, sheep, and goats.[16] A variety of other animals may be infected by *C. burnetii* including horses, dogs, swine, camels, water buffalo, pigeons, ducks, geese, turkeys, several species of wild birds, squirrels, deer mice, harvest mice, cats, and rabbits. The epidemiology of *C. burnetii* varies from country to country. For example, collared doves have been suspected of carrying *C. burnetii* from western Europe to Ireland. In Nova Scotia, exposure to infected parturient cats has resulted in several outbreaks of Q fever.[17,18]

Q fever has been reported from at least 51 countries on five continents.[5] It is usually an occupational disease affecting those with direct contact with infected animals, such as farmers, veterinarians, and abattoir workers.[5] However, indirect contact with infected animals has resulted in outbreaks of Q fever, as in Switzerland, where more than 350 persons who lived along a road over which sheep traveled from mountain pastures developed Q fever.[19] Exposure to contaminated straw, manure, or dust from farm vehicles resulted in Q fever in British residents who lived along a road traveled by these vehicles.[20] Exposure may be even more indirect, as in the case of laundry workers who developed Q fever after handling contaminated laundry.[21] Ingestion of contaminated raw milk,[22] exposure to infected parturient cats,[17] and the skinning of infected wild rabbits are also ways in which Q fever may be acquired. *C. burnetii* has also been isolated from human milk[23] and human placentas.[24] *C. burnetii* is known to undergo reactivation during pregnancy in animals other than humans. It is likely that this happens in humans as well, and Q fever complicating human pregnancy is probably underdiagnosed.[25] Laboratory exposure to *C. burnetii*[26] and transport of infected sheep through hospitals to research laboratories have resulted in large outbreaks of Q fever.[27,28]

Rarely, Q fever has been transmitted by blood transfusion.[29] Transmission has occurred during an autopsy[30] but has rarely occurred during clinical care of infected patients. An obstetrician developed Q fever following delivery of a woman infected with *C. burnetii* during pregnancy.[31] There were two reports of transmission of Q fever to attendants during autopsies,[32,33] and one report of apparent human-to-human transmission of Q fever among members of a household.[34]

Q fever was not a notifiable disease in the United States until 1999 when, because of concerns about its potential as a biologic warfare agent, it was added to the list of notifiable diseases.[35] Between 1948 and 1977, a total of 1168 cases were reported to the Centers for Disease Control and Prevention[35,36] (mean, 58.4 cases/year).

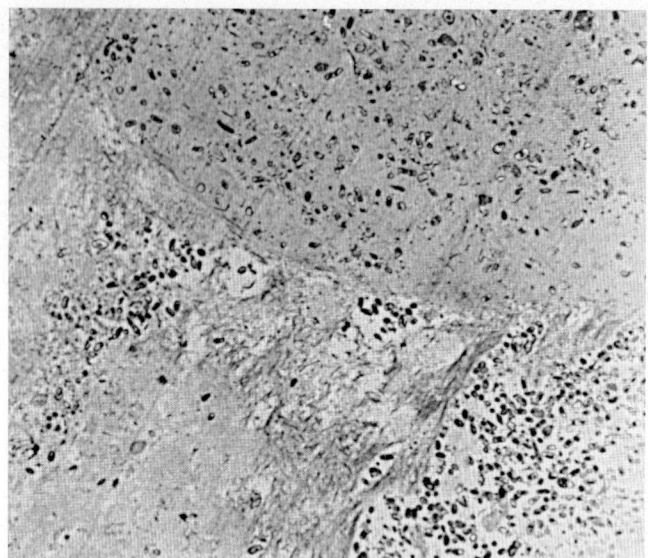

Figure 189-1 Transmission electron micrograph of a vegetation from a patient with Q fever endocarditis. Many *Coxiella burnetii* cells are evident. The electron-dense material within each cell is DNA. (Original magnification, ×46,665.)

McQuiston and Childs[36] have reported that from 1978 to 1999, there were 436 cases of Q fever in the United States, an average of 26 cases/year (range, 6 to 41 cases/year). From 2000 to 2004, there were 255 cases from 37 states, an average of 51 cases/year (range, 18 to 73 cases/year). These investigators noted a seasonal effect, with 39% of cases reported from April through June. Of these, 77% were male, the mean age was 50.5 years, median 51 years, and 92% were white, 6% black, and 2% Asian. The racial distribution of the Q fever cases was proportionally similar to that of the U.S. population. The age distribution of the Q fever cases differed from that of the U.S. population, with the Q fever cases increasing with increasing age and peaking in the 50- to 59-year-old age group. Karakousis and colleagues[37] have reported a case of chronic Q fever and reviewed all the published cases of chronic Q fever from the United States. They could only find seven such cases, likely a gross underestimate, from 1976 to 2004.

McQuiston and Childs[36] noted that sheep and goats in the United States have a higher seroprevalence for *C. burnetii* than cattle. They also noted an extensive U.S. wildlife reservoir for this organism. Various studies have shown varying degrees of seropositivity for coyotes, grey foxes, skunks, raccoons, rabbits, deer, mice, bears, birds and opossums.

There are major lessons from recent events regarding Q fever in Germany. A superspreading infected ewe at a farmers market resulted in hundreds of cases of Q fever.[38] It is also apparent that the urbanization of sheep farming is a major factor in the spread of Q fever in Germany; in one outbreak, those who lived within 50 m of a sheep meadow had an attack rate of 11.8%.[39] Also, an outbreak of Q fever in the Netherlands that is now 2 years in duration and involving over 1000 people will undoubtedly provide additional insights into the epidemiology of Q fever.

Pathogenesis

The most likely sequence of events in the cycle of transmission of *C. burnetii* to humans is that the organism is maintained in ticks or other arthropods. These ectoparasites infect domestic and other animals, including a variety of small mammals, by bite or through contamination of the skin by infected feces. Infected domestic ungulates are usually asymptomatic, although abortion or stillbirth may result. The heavily infected placenta contaminates the environment at the time of parturition. Air samples are positive for up to 2 weeks after parturition,

and viable organisms are present in the soil for periods of up to 150 days.[40-42] Humans are infected by the inhalation of contaminated aerosols. The microorganisms proliferate in the lung or lungs, and bloodstream invasion follows. This invasion results in the onset of systemic symptoms and a variety of clinical manifestations, depending on the dose of the microorganism inhaled and probably on the characteristics of the infecting strain.[43] Depending on the host, primary infection may be symptomatic (acute Q fever) or not. Children and women are less likely to be symptomatic, which may partly be dependent on steroid hormones.[44] Pregnant women are even more commonly asymptomatic following primary infection.[45] The evolution to chronic Q fever does not appear to be related to specific strains[46] but mainly to host factors, and can follow symptomatic or asymptomatic primary infection. When patients have valvular heart disease, the turbulent blood flow could result in an increased rate of apoptopic lymphocytes that could cause an increase of interleukin-10 (IL-10).[47] In the healthy host, multiplication of *C. burnetii* is controlled by macrophages, and granulomas are formed. In some people, the macrophages cannot kill *C. burnetii*, seemingly because of the secretion of IL-10.[48] Patients with chronic Q fever have increased levels of IL-10 secreted by stimulated blood monocytes. Patients with cancer, valve lesions, or arterial aneurysms, or who are pregnant, are at increased risk for chronic Q fever if infected with *C. burnetii*.[9] Polymorphisms in Toll-like receptors 2 and 4 are not associated with disease manifestations in acute Q fever.[49]

Clinical Manifestations

Humans are the only animals known to develop illness regularly as a result of *C. burnetii* infection.[50] In one large series of 207 patients, the mortality rate was 2.4%.[51] There are several clinical syndromes:

1. Self-limited febrile illness (2 to 14 days)
2. Pneumonia
3. Endocarditis
4. Hepatitis
5. Osteomyelitis
6. Q fever in the immunocompromised host
7. Q fever in infancy
8. Neurologic manifestations—encephalitis, aseptic meningitis, toxic confusional states, dementia, extrapyramidal disease
9. Q fever in pregnancy
10. Post–Q fever fatigue syndrome

SELF-LIMITED FEBRILE ILLNESS

Self-limited febrile illness is probably the most common form of Q fever. In many areas, 11% to 12% of individuals have antibodies to *C. burnetii*; most do not recall pneumonia or other severe illness.[52] It is likely that the age at which infection occurs and the dose of the agent determine whether or not Q fever is a mild self-limited febrile illness.[53,54] There is also a suggestion that some infections may be totally asymptomatic.[55] The proportion of all Q fever infections that represent asymptomatic seroconversion is unknown. In the south of Spain, 21% (108 of 505) of adults who had fever longer than 1 week and less than 3 weeks' duration had Q fever.[56] There was no radiographic evidence of pneumonia among these individuals.

PNEUMONIA

There are three presentations of this form of Q fever—atypical pneumonia, rapidly progressive pneumonia, and pneumonia as an incidental finding in a patient with a febrile illness. The last presentation is probably the most common form of Q fever pneumonia.

Atypical pneumonia is a clinical term used to describe pneumonia characterized by a dry nonproductive cough, with blood and sputum cultures negative for conventional bacterial pathogens.[57] Cough is a symptom in only 28% of patients with radiographically confirmed Q fever pneumonia. This illness may be of gradual or sudden onset.[58] Fever occurs in all patients. A severe headache is present in about 75%

of patients and is a useful clue to the diagnosis. Other symptoms and the frequency with which they occur are fatigue, 98%; chills, 88%; sweats, 84%; myalgia, 68%; nausea, 49%; vomiting, 25%; pleuritic chest pain, 28%; and diarrhea, 21%. On occasion, diarrhea may be a presenting feature of Q fever.[59]

Physical examination of the chest is often unremarkable. The most common physical finding is inspiratory crackles.[58] Patients with rapidly progressive pneumonia usually have the physical signs of pulmonary consolidation. About 5% of patients have splenomegaly. Fever and severe headache suggest central nervous system infection, and lumbar puncture is often performed. The spinal fluid is usually normal; however, *C. burnetii* has been isolated from the spinal fluid under such circumstances.[60] It is noteworthy that many patients indicate that the headache associated with Q fever is the most severe headache that they have ever had. The rapidly progressive form of Q fever pneumonia mimics legionnaires' disease and the pneumonic form of tularemia; all the causes of rapidly progressive pneumonia enter the differential diagnosis.

The radiographic picture of Q fever pneumonia is variable (Fig. 189-2). Nonsegmental and segmental pleural-based opacities are common.[61-63] Multiple rounded opacities are very suggestive of Q fever that follows exposure to infected parturient cats (see Fig. 189-2).[61] Pleural effusion is found in 35% of cases and is usually small, but on occasion may be large.[62] Atelectasis, an increase in reticular markings, and hilar adenopathy may occur. In one series, the resolution time ranged from 10 to 70 days, with a mean of 30 days.[62]

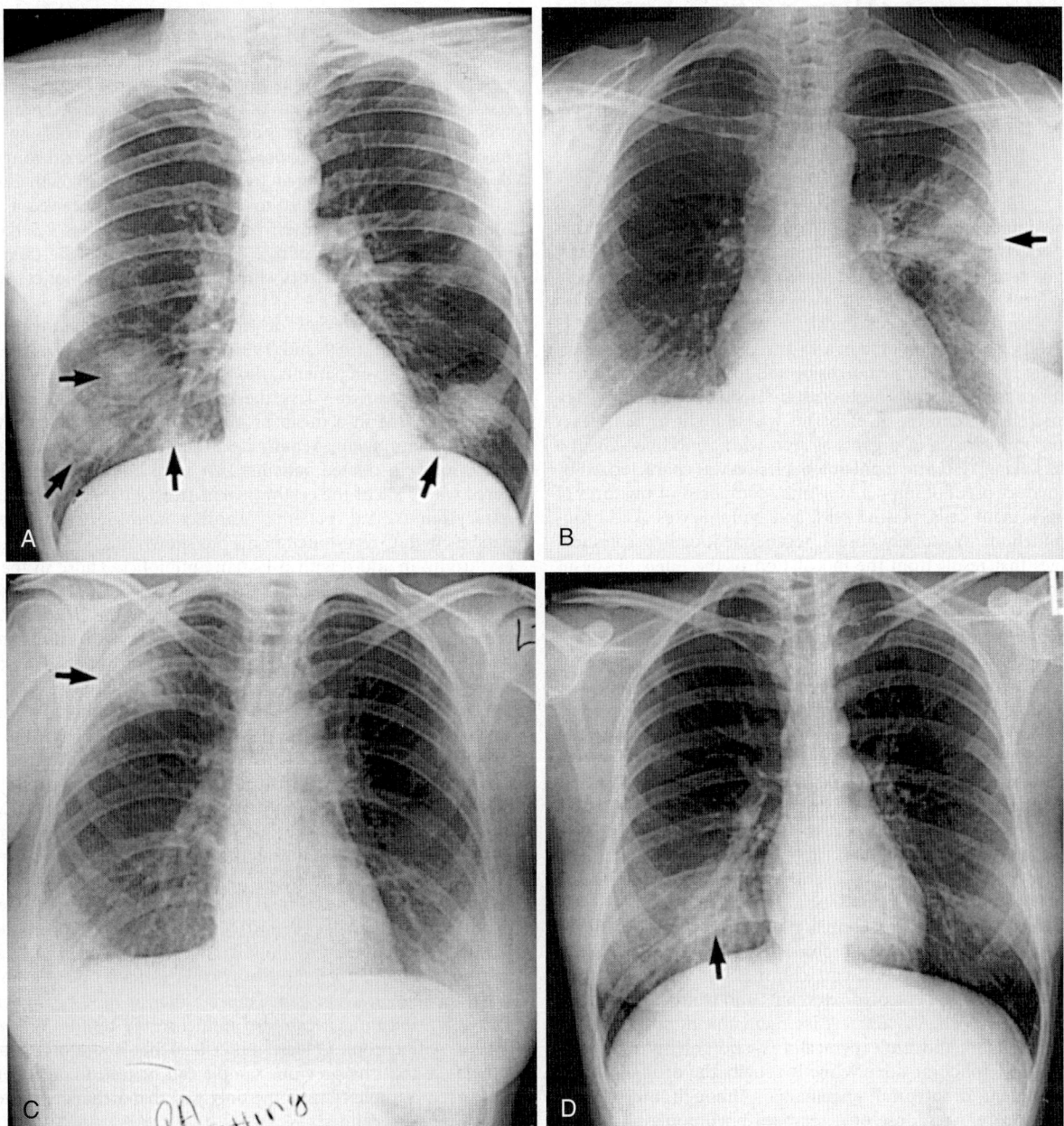

Figure 189-2 **Radiographic manifestations of Q fever pneumonia.** All four patients are members of one family who developed Q fever after exposure to the infected products of feline conception. Their cat gave birth to kittens in their house. **A,** Multiple rounded opacities (*arrows*). **B,** Left upper lobe opacity (*arrow*). **C,** Pleural-based opacity involving the right upper lobe (*arrow*). **D,** Right lower lobe opacity (*arrow*). In an endemic area **A** is characteristic of cat-related Q fever pneumonia, and **C** is suggestive of this diagnosis. However, **B** and **D** are not at all distinctive and could be caused by any pulmonary pathogen.

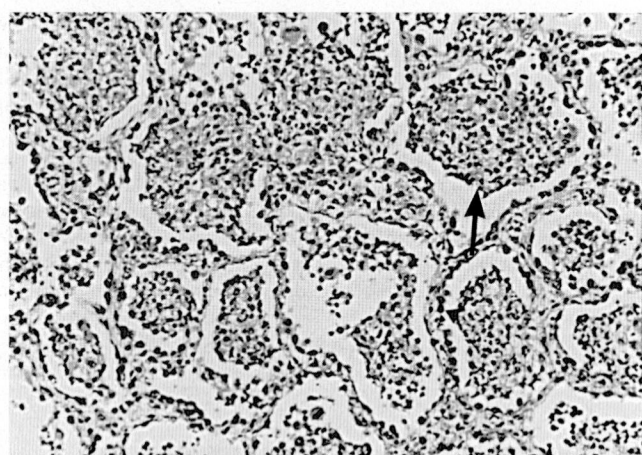

Figure 189-3 **Photomicrograph of an open lung biopsy specimen from a patient with Q fever pneumonia.** The alveolar spaces are filled with an inflammatory exudate consisting of lymphocytes and macrophages (*arrow*). Note the hyperplasia of the alveolar lining cells (*arrowhead*). (Hematoxylin and eosin stain, ×500.)

C. burnetii pneumonia is rarely fatal, and in such instances there is usually a coexisting condition that contributes to the mortality.[63] Information regarding the histology of this form of pneumonia in humans is limited. Pierce and co-workers found small coccobacilli in alveolar macrophages on transbronchial biopsy in a patient with Q fever.[64] A fatal case of pneumonia in a 43-year-old man was characterized by severe intra-alveolar hemorrhagic and focal necrotizing pneumonia, with associated necrotizing bronchitis. Histiocytes, lymphocytes, and plasma cells were in the alveoli. This was thought to be Q fever pneumonia on the basis of organisms seen with a modified Giemsa stain.[65] A resolving, *C. burnetii* pneumonia lesion was characterized by an inflammatory pseudotumor, a lung mass composed of mixtures of macrophages, giant cells, plasma cells, and lymphocytes. The bronchiolar epithelium was focally absent, regenerated, or hyperplastic.[66] The changes that result from the inoculation of the lungs of rhesus monkeys resemble those reported from humans. The resulting consolidation is peribronchial or peribronchiolar.[67] The interstitial infiltrate had more lymphocytes than monocytes (Fig. 189-3).

The white blood cell count is usually normal, but one third of patients have an increased count. Thrombocytopenia and thrombocytosis may occur. The thrombocytosis can be extreme, with platelet counts of 1 million/mm³ or higher. We have treated such patients with aspirin as prophylaxis against thrombotic events. A slight elevation (two to three times normal) of the hepatic transaminase level occurs in almost all patients. The serum bilirubin level is usually normal; however, jaundice may occur. Rarely, the syndrome of inappropriate secretion of antidiuretic hormone occurs.[68]

The treatment of choice for *C. burnetii* pneumonia is tetracycline.[69] Chloramphenicol has been used to treat Q fever.[64] Yeaman and associates performed antibiotic susceptibility testing of *C. burnetii* by using persistently infected L929 fibroblast cells.[70] The most effective agents were quinolones (difloxacin, ciprofloxacin, oxolinic acid) and rifampin. Chloramphenicol, doxycycline, and trimethoprim were somewhat effective, whereas tetracycline, gentamicin, streptomycin, erythromycin, sulfamethoxazole, penicillin G, and polymyxin B were ineffective. A macrolide or doxycycline is usually the drug of choice for the treatment of atypical pneumonia. Although others have reported an apparent response of *C. burnetii* pneumonia to macrolides,[71-74] we have observed that all of our cases of rapidly progressive pneumonia caused by *C. burnetii* have failed to respond to erythromycin therapy, despite dosages of up to 4 g/day. The addition of rifampin, 300 mg twice daily PO, resulted in cure. When tested in vitro, no antibiotic compound was bactericidal against *C. burnetii*.[75] When

several strains were tested, some variation in antibiotic susceptibilities was observed.[76] Doxycycline is usually effective but some strains may be resistant; co-trimoxazole (trimethoprim-sulfamethoxazole), chloramphenicol, and rifampin are consistently efficacious. New macrolide compounds such as the ketolide telithromycin are effective.[77] Erythromycin and quinolones have inconsistent in vitro activities.

There is very little evidence from clinical trials for making recommendations about the optimal therapy of Q fever pneumonia. Sobradillo and colleagues,[78] Basque Country, Spain, carried out a prospective, randomized, double-blind study of doxycycline and erythromycin in the treatment of pneumonia presumed to be caused by Q fever. Forty-eight patients were proven by serologic studies to have Q fever; 23 received 100 mg doxycycline twice daily, and 25 received erythromycin (500 mg, four times daily) for 10 days. Fever resolution was faster in the doxycycline-treated group (3 ± 1.6 days vs. 4.3 ± 2 days for erythromycin-treated patients; $P = .05$). The erythromycin-treated group had more gastrointestinal adverse effects (11 vs. 2 for the doxycycline-treated patients; $P < .01$). By day 40, the chest radiograph was normal in 47 of 48 patients. The authors concluded that doxycycline is more effective than erythromycin, but they recognized the self-limiting and benign nature of most cases of pneumonia caused by Q fever.

Kuzman and associates[74] have studied 64 patients with Q fever pneumonia. Of their patients, 22 were treated with azithromycin (total dosage, 1.5 g administered over 3 to 5 days), 15 with doxycycline (100 mg twice daily for 10 to 14 days), and 15 received a variety of other antibiotics. The mean duration of fever was 2.5 days in the azithromycin-treated group, 2 days in the doxycycline-treated group, and 3.5 days in the patients who received other antibiotics. All patients were cured.

A retrospective review of 130 patients with Q fever pneumonia treated between 1989 and 1995 was carried out by Kofteridis and coworkers.[73] Eleven patients who were treated with tetracycline became afebrile in a mean of 3 days; the 42 patients treated with erythromycin became afebrile in a mean of 4.26 days and the 28 patients treated with β-lactam agents required 6.8 days to become afebrile. Of the clarithromycin-treated patients, 15% were still febrile at 5 days compared with 35% of the erythromycin-treated patients and none of the tetracycline-treated patients. Another retrospective review of 19 patients with Q fever pneumonia has shown that 11 were treated with erythromycin and 8 with β-lactam antibiotics. Those in the erythromycin-treated group became afebrile by day 3, whereas only 2 of the β-lactam-treated group were afebrile by this time ($P < .005$).[79]

From these studies and from the in vitro data, it can be concluded that β-lactams are ineffective. For those who cannot tolerate doxycycline, a macrolide may be as effective as a quinolone.

The diagnosis of Q fever (*C. burnetii*) pneumonia is confirmed serologically because most laboratories do not have the facilities required to isolate *C. burnetii*.[80] The development of primers derived from the *C. burnetii* superoxide dismutase gene has allowed the amplification of *C. burnetii* DNA in clinical specimens using the polymerase chain reaction (PCR) assay.[81] The microagglutination,[82] complement fixation,[83] and microimmunofluorescence tests,[84] as well as the enzyme-linked immunosorbent assay,[85] have all been used in the serologic diagnosis of this illness. The indirect immunofluorescence test is best for the diagnosis of acute and chronic Q fever. Cut-off titers for a positive test may vary by population. For example, in screening for infection with *C. burnetii* in Nova Scotia, Canada one of us used a titer of 1:8 or higher, whereas in France a titer of 1:32 or higher is used. The source of antigen can also influence the results. When treating patients with chronic Q fever, it is critical that laboratories store serum samples so that the previous sample can be tested concurrently with the current sample. This is the only way that a change in titer can be definitively determined.

A fourfold rise in titer between acute and convalescent samples is diagnostic of Q fever. Cross-reactions have been reported between antibodies to *Bartonella* and *Legionella micdadei* and antibodies to *C. burnetii*.[86] Some have advocated using the indirect immunofluorescence test to detect antibodies to immunoglobulin M (IgM) so that a

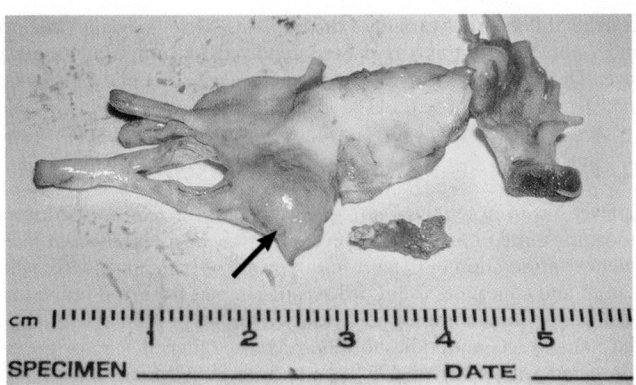

Figure 189-4   Mitral valve of a patient with Q fever endocarditis. The nodule (*arrow*) was full of *Coxiella burnetii* organisms within foamy macrophages. (*From Raoult D, Raza A, Marrie TJ. Q fever endocarditis and other forms of chronic Q fever. In: Marrie TJ, ed. Q Fever—The Disease. Boca Raton, Fla: CRC Press; 1990:179-199, with permission.*)

single serum specimen may be used for the diagnosis of acute Q fever.[86] A titer of 1:50 or higher has a high positive predictive value.[88] However, IgM antibodies may persist for up to 678 days[89] and, in one study,[90] 3% of 162 patients still had a significant IgM antibody level 1 year after the infection. *C. burnetii* is highly infectious, and tissues from patients with Q fever should be processed under biosafety level 3 conditions.

Whether there should be appropriate follow-up after acute Q fever is an issue that is still evolving. The observation of chronic Q fever following cases of acute Q fever, especially in patients with unrecognized or mild valvular heart lesions, has led some to recommend serologic monitoring every 4 months for 2 years.[91] Others have proposed that all patients with acute Q fever should have transthoracic echocardiography to detect valve lesions.[92] The risk of endocarditis in patients with acute Q fever and valvular heart disease is high, 39% in one study.[93] We recommend that these patients be treated with hydroxychloroquine and doxycycline for 1 year and followed closely.

ENDOCARDITIS

It is now recognized that chronic Q fever has a variety of manifestations—endocarditis, infection of a vascular prosthesis, infection of aneurysms, osteomyelitis, hepatitis, interstitial pulmonary fibrosis, prolonged fever, and purpuric eruptions.[94] Endocarditis is the prime manifestation of "chronic" Q fever.[95-114] Usually, abnormal native or prosthetic cardiac valves are affected[113]; however, any part of the vascular tree may become infected,[112] including clot in a left ventricular aneurysm. Such patients have a defective cell-mediated immune response to *C. burnetii*.

The incidence of Q fever endocarditis is increasing, but this may reflect increased recognition of this entity. Turck and colleagues reported 16 cases of chronic Q fever diagnosed between 1968 and 1973; their world literature review yielded 55 cases.[95] Siegman-Igra and associates reported on 408 cases of Q fever from 17 countries in their 1997 review.[114] From 1975 to 1980, 79 cases of Q fever endocarditis were reported to the Public Health Laboratory Service Communicable Disease Surveillance Center in England[108]; from 1975 to 1981, *C. burnetii* accounted for 3% of all cases of endocarditis reported in England and Wales.[107] In France, 229 cases of Q fever endocarditis were diagnosed.[51] The clinical presentation is that of culture-negative endocarditis; however, fever is frequently absent. Q fever endocarditis is rare in children.[111]

Marked clubbing of the fingers and hypergammaglobulinemia are frequently present. Splenomegaly and hepatomegaly are found in slightly more than 50% of patients. A purpuric rash related to leukocytoclastic vasculitis occurs in about 20%. The erythrocyte sedimenta-

tion rate is usually increased; anemia and microscopic hematuria are also found. Arterial emboli complicate the course in one third of patients.

The vegetations in chronic Q fever differ in gross and microscopic appearance from those seen in pyogenic bacterial endocarditis. Figures 189-4 and 189-5 show the gross appearance of the vegetations in Q fever endocarditis. Microscopically, there is a subacute and chronic inflammatory infiltrate. Many large foamy macrophages are present. Characteristic microorganisms are readily seen with electron microscopy (see Fig. 189-1).

The confirmation of the diagnosis in most cases is serologic. A complement fixation titer of 1:200 or higher to phase I antigen is said to be diagnostic of chronic Q fever, although not all patients in the series of Turck and co-workers had this titer.[95] In acute Q fever, complement fixation antibody titers to phase I antigen do not reach this level.

Studies have reported high titers of IgA antibodies to phase I antigen in chronic Q fever (endocarditis and granulomatous hepatitis),[89,115] whereas another study found that patients with acute Q fever also produced IgA antibodies to phase I antigen, albeit in low titer.[89] Fournier and colleagues used a phase I IgG antibody titer of 1:800 or greater by microimmunofluorescence as diagnostic of Q fever endocarditis.[116] They and others have proposed that this be added as a major criterion to the Duke Endocarditis Service criteria for the diagnosis of infective endocarditis.[117,119]

Antibody titers fall slowly with treatment. Western immunoblot testting of serum samples from patients with chronic Q fever shows that there are IgG antibodies to 12 to 15 antigens of phase I *C. burnetii*, whereas serum from patients with acute Q fever reacts with 7 to 10 *C. burnetii* antigens.[119] Antibodies to antigens with a molecular mass of 50, 80, and 160 kD were present only in serum from patients with chronic Q fever.

There is no agreement on the type and duration of antimicrobial therapy for Q fever endocarditis.[89,90] Some authorities recommend that treatment be continued indefinitely.[89] A consensus is emerging that combination antibiotic therapy is necessary to treat chronic Q fever.[120] We have used doxycycline in combination with ciprofloxacin or rifampin for 2 years to treat this infection. Others have successfully used doxycycline with pefloxacin or ofloxacin. Maurin and colleagues have found that the bactericidal effect of doxycycline is enhanced when the phagolysosome is alkalinized with chloroquine or amantadine.[75] Doxycycline and hydroxychloroquine have been successfully used to treat patients with Q fever endocarditis.[121] Hydroxychloroquine is given at a dosage of 200 mg/day, and the dose is adjusted to maintain

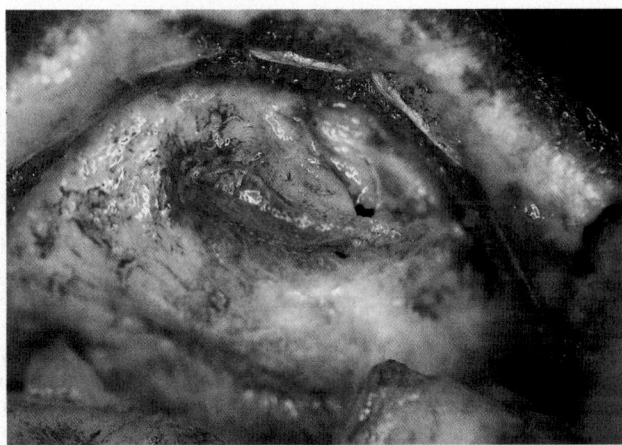

Figure 189-5   Q fever endocarditis on bioprosthetic valve leaflet. The ridge in the center of the photograph is the area infiltrated with *Coxiella burnetii*. (*From Raoult D, Raza A, Marrie TJ. Q fever endocarditis and other forms of chronic Q fever. In: Marrie TJ, ed. Q Fever—The Disease. Boca Raton, Fla: CRC Press; 1990:179-199, with permission.*)

a serum concentration between 0.8 and 1.2 μg/mL. It has been found that doxycycline levels vary among patients and that a serum level of 5 μg/mL should be reached to obtain high success rates.[122] In one patient who failed treatment and died, the minimal inhibitory concentration (MIC) of his *C. burnetii* to doxycycline was 8 μg/mL.[123]

Antibody titers should be determined every 6 months during therapy and every 3 months for the first 2 years after the cessation of therapy. Successful therapy is accompanied by a falling erythrocyte sedimentation rate, correction of anemia, and resolution of hyperglobulinemia. Valve replacement is frequently necessary but should be dictated by the patient's hemodynamic status. Patients are considered cured when the IgG phase I antibody titer is less than 1:800 and IgM and IgA antibody titers are less than 1:50 by microimmunofluorescence. The release of IL-10 and transforming growth factor-β (TGF-β) from unstimulated peripheral blood mononuclear cells is markedly increased in Q fever endocarditis.[124] IL-10 and TGF-β impair the function of macrophages and monocytes. IL-10 counteracts the shift to a protective helper T-cell 1 pattern and also favors the survival of intracellular bacteria.

HEPATITIS

Hepatitis is the most common manifestation of *C. burnetii* infection in France.[51,125,126] In the United States, 61.9% of all cases of Q fever are manifested as hepatitis. Also, hepatitis is more frequent in sheep- and goat-breeding areas. In Nova Scotia, there have been no cases diagnosed as Q fever hepatitis.

There are three presentations of Q fever hepatitis[75,127-132]:

1. An infectious hepatitis–like picture
2. Fever of unknown origin, with characteristic granulomas on liver biopsy
3. As an incidental finding in a patient with acute Q fever pneumonia

In patients with fever of unknown origin related to Q fever, the typical doughnut granuloma is seen on liver biopsy.[128,129] This is a granuloma with a dense fibrin ring surrounded by a central lipid vacuole. These granulomas are highly suggestive of Q fever but may be seen in Hodgkin's disease and infectious mononucleosis. *C. burnetii* has been isolated from the liver of patients with Q fever hepatitis, but the organism has not been visualized within the hepatic parenchyma.[95] Antibiotic treatment for 2 weeks is probably sufficient. The rare cases of Q fever hepatitis with a serologic profile suggestive of chronic Q fever should be treated for longer than 2 weeks. There are no data on which to base a recommendation for the exact duration of therapy. These patients should be observed with serial antibody titers.

NEUROLOGIC MANIFESTATIONS

Severe headache is the most common manifestation and probably represents central nervous system infection, although there is little evidence of serious brain involvement in Q fever.[133-136] Aseptic meningitis, encephalitis, or both complicate 0.2% to 1.3% of cases of Q fever.[134] A review of 16 cases of Q fever meningoencephalitis has revealed that 8 patients had an elevated cerebrospinal fluid white blood cell level, ranging from 18 to 1392 cells/mm³.[137] In all but one case, mononuclear cells predominated. The protein level was usually increased, and the glucose level was normal.[137] The electroencephalogram was abnormal in 5 of 6 patients in whom this investigation was carried out.

In a study from Plymouth, England, Reilly and co-workers have reported an astoundingly high 22% incidence of neurologic complications in 103 patients, of whom 46 had acute Q fever, 5 had chronic Q fever, and 52 had past infections.[138] Of the 45 patients with acute Q fever, 6 had residual neurologic impairment—weakness, recurrent meningismus, blurred vision, residual paresthesias, and sensory loss involving the left leg. The meningoencephalitis of Q fever may be accompanied by seizures and coma.[139] Behavioral disturbance, cerebellar symptoms and signs, cranial nerve palsies, extrapyramidal disease,

and the Miller-Fisher variant of the Guillain-Barré syndrome (areflexia and ophthalmoparesis) have been reported to complicate acute Q fever. Demyelinating polyradiculoneuritis developed in a 71-year-old man 10 weeks after the onset of *C. burnetii* pneumonia.[140]

Q FEVER IN THE IMMUNOCOMPROMISED HOST

Q fever has been reported infrequently as an infection in the immunocompromised host[141-145]; however, this may be a reflection of infrequent consideration of Q fever in this group of patients. Indeed, when Raoult and colleagues examined serum samples from 500 individuals positive for human immunodeficiency virus, they found that 10.4% of the 500 had IgG antibodies to *C. burnetii* in a titer of 1:25 or greater, compared with 4.1% of 925 apparently healthy blood donors (*P* < .001).[145] They also found that from 1987 to 1989, 5 of 68 patients (7.3%) hospitalized with Q fever were positive for human immunodeficiency virus (HIV). They estimated that in those positive for HIV, the number of cases of Q fever was 13 times higher and these patients were symptomatic more frequently than the general population.

In a review of all cases of chronic Q fever in France from 1982 to 1990, the investigators noted that 20% of 84 patients were immunocompromised.[94] These were patients with cancer, chronic myeloid leukemia, acquired immunodeficiency syndrome, renal transplantation, corticosteroid therapy, renal dialysis, postpartum state, and chronic alcoholism.

C. burnetii infection resulted in a fatal interstitial pneumonia in an 11-year-old boy with chronic granulomatous disease.[146]

OTHER MANIFESTATIONS OF Q FEVER

Osteomyelitis is an uncommon manifestation of *C. burnetii* infection.[147] Q fever may also occur in infancy, when it has caused pneumonia, febrile seizures, pyrexia of unknown origin, malaise, and meningeal irritation.[148] Hematologic manifestations include bone marrow necrosis,[149] histiocytic hemophagocytosis,[150] and hemolytic anemia[151] and, on occasion, this disease may have simulated lymphoma.[152] Other hematologic manifestations include transient hypoplastic anemia,[153] reactive thrombocytosis, rarely thrombocytopenia, and splenic rupture.[154] Optic neuritis[155] and erythema nodosum[156] have also rarely been reported in association with *C. burnetii* infection. In the past, it was thought Kawasaki disease might be a variant of Q fever.[157,158] Support for this concept has not materialized.

Q Fever In Pregnancy

Q fever during pregnancy may result in abortion when the infection occurs during the first trimester.[159] Q fever during pregnancy should be treated with trimethoprim-sulfamethoxazole for the duration of the pregnancy. In one retrospective study this approach reduced obstetric complications from 81% to 44%. There were no intrauterine fetal deaths in the trimethoprim-sulfamethoxazole–treated group.[160] Those patients with a chronic Q fever serologic profile should be treated with doxycycline and hydroxychloroquine for 1 year following delivery. Unresolved is whether or not to screen pregnant women for *C. burnetii* infection if an outbreak of Q fever is occurring in a particular region. Support for such an approach is given by the finding that seropositive women have lower birth weight babies than those who are seronegative.[161]

Post–Q Fever Fatigue Syndrome

The designation Q fever fatigue syndrome (QFFS) is used to describe the protracted state of fatigue that can develop in up to 20% of patients who develop acute infection with *C. burnetii*.[162] This syndrome consists of a constellation of symptoms, including fatigue, headaches, sweats, arthralgia, myalgias, blurred vision, muscle fasciculations, and enlarged and painful lymph nodes.[162] In a case-control study 5 years after a large outbreak of Q fever in individuals in a community in the West Midlands, England, Ayres and co-workers[163] found that participants who were diagnosed with acute Q fever during the initial outbreak had more complaints of fatigue, sweats, blurring of vision, and dyspnea than their age, gender, and geographically matched controls and that 42.3% of the infected individuals fulfilled the Centers for Disease Control and Prevention (CDC) criteria for chronic fatigue state. Although not conclusive, there is evidence to suggest that "cytokine dysregulation and immunomodulation from persistence of *C. burnetii*" in the host may be responsible for QFFS.[164,165] In a study conducted in Newfoundland, in which 49 patients with goat-related Q fever were followed and the Short Form 36 Health Survey (SF-36) was used to assess quality of life, 38% (19 of 49) who had acute Q fever during the outbreak had persistent symptoms 3 months later and had significantly lower scores on all components of the SF-36 than those who did not have persistent symptoms.[166] Two years after the initial outbreak, 10 of 33 participants (30%) who had serologic evidence of *C. burnetii* infection continued to report persistent symptoms, compared with 4% (1 of 24) of those who did not have Q fever. Helbig and associates[167] compared variability in phenotype distribution among a range of cytokine and accessory immune response genes in 23 patients with post–Q fever fatigue syndrome and in 42 Red Cross blood donors from Adelaide, Australia. They found that there were significantly more variants in the natural resistance–associated macrophage protein gene among the patients compared with controls. In addition, there were significant differences in the IL-10 promoter and in intron 1 of the interferon-γ gene. HLA DR-11 was present in 19.6% of cases and 4.3% of controls (*P* = .0014). This all indicates that there may be a genetic basis for the post–Q fever fatigue syndrome.

Hickie and co-workers[168] enrolled 253 patients with Epstein-Barr virus (EBV) infection (*n* = 68), Q fever (*n* = 43), Ross River virus (RRV) infection (*n* = 60), and an unconfirmed group (*n* = 82) in a prospective longitudinal study to determine the frequency of chronic fatigue following each of these acute infections and the factors that predict the fatigue state. The incidence for postfatigue syndrome at 6 weeks and 3, 6, and 12 months was 35%, 27%, 12% and 9%, respectively, with no difference in incidence among the initial infecting agents. For the 29 cases with fatigue, the initial infection was as follows: EBV, 5 (7.3%); Q fever, 3 (6.9%); RRV, 13 (21.6%); and unconfirmed infection, 8 (9.7%). They concluded that aspects of the host response, rather than the infecting agent, is the likely determinant of the postinfective fatigue syndrome. In the same population of patients, it was found that ongoing production of cytokines does not play a role in the fatigue state.[169]

PREVENTION

Vaccination of those at risk for infection (e.g., abattoir workers, veterinarians) should be carried out as soon as a safe vaccine is available.[170,171] An investigational inactivated vaccine, made from infected egg yolk sacs, has been used to protect laboratory workers handling live *C. burnetii*. Vaccine may be requested from the Investigational New Drugs from the Commanding Officer, U.S. Army Medical Research Institute for Infectious Diseases, Fort Detrick, Frederick, MD 21701-5011.

Using only seronegative sheep in research facilities prevents outbreaks in these institutions. Because of the lack of person-to-person spread, there is no need to isolate patients hospitalized with Q fever.[172] Simple measures, such as the consumption of only pasteurized milk, serve to eliminate cases of Q fever transmitted in this manner. In Cyprus, the incidence of *C. burnetii* infection among sheep and goats was reduced by a program in which aborted material was destroyed, affected dams isolated, and the premises disinfected.[173] Control of ectoparasites on cattle, sheep, and goats is also important in the control of Q fever. In addition, it seems prudent not to accept blood donors from a region undergoing an outbreak of Q fever, both during the outbreak and for up to 4 weeks following cessation of the outbreak.

A recent study has shown that veterinarians in the United States do not engage in practices that could prevent zoonotic transmission of disease.[174] Instituting such programs in veterinary school would seem to be an appropriate intervention.

REFERENCES

1. Baca OG, Paretsky D. Q fever and *Coxiella burnetii*: A model for host-parasite interaction. *Microbiol Rev.* 1983;47:127-149.
2. McCaul TF, Williams JC. Development cycle of *Coxiella burnetii*: Structure and morphogenesis of vegetative and sporogenic differentiations. *J Bacteriol.* 1981;147:1063-1076.
3. Sawyer LA, Fishbein DB, McDade JE. Q fever: Current concepts. *Rev Infect Dis.* 1987;9:935-946.
4. Q fever. In: Christie AB. *Infectious Diseases, Epidemiology and Clinical Practice.* Edinburgh: Churchill Livingstone; 1974:876-891.
5. Hoover TA, Culp DW, Vodkin MH, et al. Chromosomal DNA deletions explain phenotypic characteristics of two antigenic variants, phase II and RSA 514 (crazy), of the *Coxiella burnetii* nine-mile strain. *Infect Immun.* 2002;70:6726-6733.
6. Schramek S, Mayer H. Different sugar compositions of lipopolysaccharides isolated from phase I and pure phase II cells of *Coxiella burnetii. Infect Immun.* 1982;38:53-57.
7. Hackstadt T, Peacock MG, Hitchcock PJ, et al. Lipopolysaccharide variation in *Coxiella burnetii*: Intrastrain heterogeneity in structure and antigenicity. *Infect Immun.* 1985;48:359-365.
8. Samuel JE, Frazier ME, Mallavia LP. Correlation of plasmid type and disease caused by *Coxiella burnetii. Infect Immun.* 1985;49:775-777.
9. Maurin M, Raoult D. Q fever. *Clin Microbiol Rev.* 1999;12:518-553.
10. Seshadri R, Paulsen IT, Eisen JA, et al. Complete genome sequence of the Q-fever pathogen *Coxiella burnetii. Proc Natl Acad Sci U S A.* 2003;100:5455-5460.
11. Derrick EH. "Q" fever, new fever entity: Clinical features, diagnosis and laboratory investigation. *Med J Aust.* 1937;2:281-299.
12. Burnet FM, Freeman M. Experimental studies on the virus of "Q" fever. *Med J Aust.* 1937;2:299-305.
13. Davis G, Cox HR. A filter-passing infectious agent isolated from ticks: Isolation from *Dermacentor andersoni*, reactions in animals, and filtration experiments. *Public Health Rep.* 1939;53:2259-2267.
14. Dyer RE. A filter-passing infectious agent isolated from ticks. IV. Human infection. *Public Health Rep.* 1939;53:2277-2283.
15. Dyer RE. Similarity of Australian Q fever and a disease caused by an infectious agent isolated from ticks in Montana. *Public Health Rep.* 1939;54:1229-1237.
16. Babudieri B. Q fever: A zoonosis. *Adv Vet Sci.* 1959;5:81-181.

17. Langley JM, Marrie TJ, Covert A, et al. Poker players' pneumonia. An urban outbreak following exposure to a parturient cat. *N Engl J Med.* 1988;319:354-356.
18. Marrie TJ, Durant H, Williams JC, et al. Exposure to parturient cats is a risk factor for acquisition of Q fever in Maritime Canada. *J Infect Dis.* 1988;158:101-108.
19. Centers for Disease Control (CDC). Q fever outbreak—Switzerland. *MMWR Morb Mortal Wkly Rep.* 1984;33:355-361.
20. Salmon MM, Howells B, Glencross EJF, et al. Q fever in an urban area. *Lancet.* 1982;1:1002-1004.
21. Oliphant JW, Gordon DA, Meis A, et al. Q fever in laundry workers presumably transmitted from contaminated clothing. *Am J Hyg.* 1949;49:76-82.
22. Bell JA, Beck MD, Huebner RJ. Epidemiologic studies of Q fever in southern California. *JAMA.* 1950;142:868-872.
23. Kumar A, Yadav MP, Kakkar S. Human milk as a source of Q fever infection in breast-fed babies. *Indian J Med Res.* 1981;73:510-512.
24. Syrucek L, Sobeslavsky O, Gutvirth I. Isolation of *Coxiella burnetii* from human placentas. *J Hyg Epidemiol Microbiol Immunol.* 1958;2:29-35.
25. Raoult D, Fenollar F, Stein A. Q fever during pregnancy: Diagnosis, treatment and follow-up. *Arch Intern Med.* 2002;162:701-704.
26. Johnson JE II, Kadull PJ. Laboratory-acquired Q fever. A report of fifty cases. *Am J Med.* 1966;41:391-403.
27. Hall CJ, Richmond SJ, Caul EO, et al. Laboratory outbreak of Q fever acquired from sheep. *Lancet.* 1982;1:1004-1006.
28. Meiklejohn G, Reimer LG, Graves PS, et al. Cryptic epidemic of Q fever in a medical school. *J Infect Dis.* 1981;144:107-114.
29. Q fever transmitted by blood transfusion—United States [editorial]. *Can Dis Wkly Rep.* 1977;3:210.
30. Harman JB. Q fever in Great Britain: Clinical account of eight cases. *Lancet.* 1949;2:1028-1030.
31. Raoult D, Stein A. Q fever during pregnancy. A risk factor for women, fetuses and obstetricians. *N Engl J Med.* 1994;330:371.
32. Gerth H-J, Leidig U, Reimenschneider TH. [Q-fever epidemic in an institute of human pathology.] *Dtsch Med Wochenschr.* 1982;107:1391-1395.
33. Deutch DL, Peterson ET. Q fever: Transmission from one human being to others. *JAMA.* 1950;143:348-350.
34. Mann JS, Douglas JG, Inglis JN, et al. Q fever: Person to person transmission within a family. *Thorax.* 1986;41:974-975.

35. McQuiston JH, Holman RC, Mccall CL, et al. National surveillance and the epidemiology of q fever in the united states, 1978-2004. *Am J Trop Med hyg.* 2006;75:36-40.
36. McQuiston JH, Childs JE. Q fever in humans and animals in the united states. *Vector Borne Zoonotic Dis.* 2002;2:179-191.
37. Karakousis PC, Trucksis M, Dumler JS. Chronic Q fever in the United States. *J Clin Microbiol.* 2006;44:2238-2287.
38. Porten K, Rissland J, Tigges A, et al. Super-spreading ewe infects hundreds with Q fever at a farmer's market in Germany. *BMC Infect Dis.* 2006;6:147.
39. Gelsdorf A, Kroh C, Grimm S, et al. Large Q fever outbreak due to sheep farming near residential areas, Germany, 2005. *Epidemiol Infect.* 2008;136:1084-1087.
40. Welsh HH, Lennette EH, Abinanti FR, et al. Air-borne transmission of Q fever: The role of parturition in the generation of infective aerosols. *Ann N Y Acad Sci.* 1958;70:528-540.
41. Lennette EH, Welsh HH. Q fever in California. X. Recovery of *Coxiella burnetii* from the air of premises harbouring infected goats. *Am J Hyg.* 1951;54:44-49.
42. Welsh HH, Lennette EH, Abinanti FR, et al. Q fever studies XXI. The recovery of *Coxiella burnetii* from the soil and surface water of premises harbouring infected sheep. *Am J Hyg.* 1959;70:14-20.
43. Baca OG. Pathogenesis of rickettsial infections. Emphasis on Q fever. *Eur J Epidemiol.* 1991;7:222-228.
44. Raoult D, Marrie T, Mege J. natural history and pathophysiology of Q fever. *Lancet Infect Dis.* 2005;5:219-226.
45. Tissot-Dupont H, Vaillant V, Rey S, et al. Role of sex, age, previous valve lesion, and pregnancy in the clinical expression and outcome of Q fever after a large outbreak. *Clin Infect Dis.* 2007;44:232-237.
46. Glazunova O, Roux V, Freylikman O, et al. *Coxiella burnetii* genotyping. *Emerg Infect Dis.* 2005;11:1211-1217.
47. Benoit M, Ghigo E, Capo C, et al. The uptake of apoptotic cells drives *Coxiella burnetii* replication and macrophage polarization: A model for Q fever endocarditis. *PloS Pathog.* 2008;4:e1000066.
48. Honstettre A, Imbert G, Ghigo E, et al. Dysregulation of cytokines in acute Q fever: Role of interleukin-10 and tumor necrosis factor in chronic evolution of Q fever. *J Infect Dis.* 2003;187:956-962.
49. Everett B, Cameron B, Li H, et al. Polymorphisms in toll-like receptors -2 and -4 are not associated with disease manifestations in acute Q fever. *Genes Immun.* 2007;8:699-702.

50. Stoker MGP, Marmion BP. The spread of Q fever from animals to man. The natural history of a rickettsial disease. *Bull World Health Organ.* 1955;13:781-806.
51. Raoult D. Rickettsial diseases. *Medicine (Baltimore).* 1996;24:71-75.
52. Clark WH, Romker MS, Holmes MA, et al. Q fever in California. VIII. An epidemic of Q fever in a small rural community in northern California. *Am J Hyg.* 1951;54:25-34.
53. Gonder JC, Kishimoto RA, Kastello MR, et al. Cynomolgus monkey model for experimental Q fever infection. *J Infect Dis.* 1979;139:191-196.
54. Tigertt WD, Benenson AS, Goscheneur WS. Airborne Q fever. *Bacteriol Rev.* 1961;25:285-293.
55. Luoto L, Casey ML, Pickens EG. Q fever studies in Montana. Detection of asymptomatic infection among residents of infected dairy premises. *Am J Epidemiol.* 1965;81:356-369.
56. Viciana P, Pachon J, Cuello JA, et al. Fever of indeterminate duration in the community. A seven-year study in the south of Spain. Presented at the 32nd Interscience Conference on Antimicrobial Agents and Chemotherapy. American Society for Microbiology. Washington DC, October 11-14, 1992.
57. Cunha BA, Quintiliani R. The atypical pneumonias. A diagnostic and therapeutic approach. *Postgrad Med.* 1979;66:95-102.
58. Feinstein M, Yesner R, Marks JL. Epidemic of Q fever among troops returning from Italy in the spring of 1945. 1. Clinical aspects of the epidemic at Fort Patrick Henry, Virginia. *Am J Hyg.* 1946;44:72-87.
59. Lim KCL, Kang JYU. Q fever presenting with gastroenteritis. *Med J Aust.* 1980;1:327.
60. Robins FC. Q fever in the Mediterranean area: Report of its occurrence in Allied troops. *Am J Hyg.* 1946;12:51-71.
61. Gordon JD, MacKeen AD, Marrie TJ, et al. The radiographic features of epidemic and sporadic Q fever pneumonia. *J Can Assoc Radiol.* 1984;35:293-296.
62. Millar JK. The chest film findings in 'Q' fever—a series of 35 cases. *Clin Radiol.* 1978;329:371-375.
63. Perin TL. Histopathologic observations in a fatal case of Q fever. *Arch Pathol.* 1949;47:361-365.
64. Pierce TH, Yucht SC, Gorin AB, et al. Q fever pneumonitis: Diagnosis by transbronchoscopic lung biopsy. *West J Med.* 1979;130:453-455.
65. Urso FP. The pathologic findings in rickettsial pneumonia. *Am J Clin Pathol.* 1975;64:335-342.
66. Janigan DT, Marrie TJ. An inflammatory pseudotumor of the lung in Q fever pneumonia. *N Engl J Med.* 1983;30:86-88.
67. Lille RD, Perrin TL, Armstrong C. An institutional outbreak of pneumonitis. III. Histopathology in man and rhesus monkeys in the pneumonitis due to the virus of "Q fever." *Public Health Rep.* 1941;56:1419-1425.
68. Biggs BA, Douglas JG, Grant IWB, et al. Prolonged Q fever associated with inappropriate secretion of anti-diuretic hormone. *J Infect.* 1984;8:61-63.
69. Turck WPG. Q fever. In: Braude AL, Davis CE, Fierer J, eds. *Medical Microbiology and Infectious Diseases.* Philadelphia: WB Saunders; 1981:932-937.
70. Yeaman MR, Mitscher LA, Baca OG. In vitro susceptibility of *Coxiella burnetii* to antibiotics, including several quinolones. *Antimicrob Agents Chemother.* 1987;31:1079-1084.
71. D'Angelo LJ, Hetherington R. Q fever treated with erythromycin. *BMJ.* 1979;2:305-306.
72. Ellis ME, Dunbar EM. In vivo response of acute Q fever to erythromycin. *Thorax.* 1982;37:867-868.
73. Kofteridis D, Gikas A, Spiradakis G, et al. Clinical response of Q fever infection to macrolides. Presented at the Fourth International Conference on Macrolides, Azalides, Streptogramins and Ketolides, Barcelona, Spain, January 12-23, 1998.
74. Kuzman I, Schonwald S, Culig J, et al. The efficacy of azithromycin in the treatment of Q fever: A retrospective study. Presented at the Fourth International Conference on Macrolides, Azalides, Streptogramins and Ketolides, Barcelona, Spain, January 21-23, 1998.
75. Maurin M, Benoliel A, Bongrand P, et al. Phagolysosomal alkalinization and the bactericidal effect of antibiotics: The *Coxiella burnetii* paradigm. *J Infect Dis.* 1992;166:1097-1102.
76. Raoult D, Bres P, Drancourt M, et al. In vitro susceptibilities of *Coxiella burnetii, Rickettsia rickettsii,* and *Rickettsia conorii* to the fluoroquinolone Sparfloxacin. *Antimicrob Agents Chemother.* 1991;35:88-91.
77. Rolain JM, Maurin M, Bryskier A, et al. In vitro activities of telithromycin (HMR 3647) against Rickettsia rickettsii, Rickettsia conorii, Rickettsia africae, Rickettsia typhi, Rickettsia prowazekii, Coxiella burnetii, Bartonella henselae, Bartonella quintana, Bartonella bacilliformis, and Ehrlichia chaffeensis. *Antimicrob Agents Chemother.* 2000;44:1391-1393.
78. Sobradillo V, Zalacain R, Capebastegui A, et al. Antibiotic treatment in pneumonia due to Q fever. *Thorax.* 1992;47:276-278.
79. Carcopino X, Raoult D, Bretelle F, et al. Managing Q fever during pregnancy: The benefits of long-term cotrimoxazole therapy. *Clin Infect Dis.* 2007;45:548-555.
80. Huebner RJ, Jellison WL, Beck MD. Q fever, a review of current knowledge. *Ann Intern Med.* 1949;30:495-509.
81. Stein A, Raoult D. Detection of *Coxiella burnetii* by DNA amplification using polymerase chain reaction. *J Clin Microbiol.* 1992;30:2462-2466.
82. Fiset P, Ormsbee RA, Silberman R, et al. A microagglutination technique for detection and measurement of rickettsial antibodies. *Acta Virol.* 1969;13:60-66.
83. Murphy AM, Field PR. The persistence of complement-fixing antibodies to Q fever *(Coxiella burnetii)* after infection. *Med J Aust.* 1970;1:1148-1150.
84. Field PR, Hunt JG, Murphy AM. Detection and persistence of specific IgM antibody to *Coxiella burnetii* by enzyme-linked immunosorbent assay: A comparison with immunofluorescence and complement fixation tests. *J Infect Dis.* 1983;148:477-487.
85. Peter O, Dupuis G, Burgdorfer W, et al. Evaluation of the complement fixation and indirect immunofluorescence test in the early diagnosis of primary Q fever. *Eur J Clin Microbiol.* 1985;4:394-396.
86. Maurin M, Raoult D. Q fever. *Clin Microbiol Rev.* 1999; 12:518-553.
87. Hunt JG, Field PR, Murphy AM. Immunoglobulin responses to *Coxiella burnetii* (Q fever): Single-serum diagnosis of acute infection using an immunofluorescence technique. *Infect Immun.* 1983;39:977-981.
88. Tissot-Dupont H, Thirion X, Raoult D. Q fever serology: Cutoff determination for microimmunofluorescence. *Clin Diagn Lab Immunol.* 1994;1:189-196.
89. Worswick D, Marmion BP. Antibody response in acute and chronic Q fever and in subjects vaccinated against Q fever. *J Med Microbiol.* 1985;119:281-296.
90. Dupuis G, Peter O, Peacock M, et al. Immunoglobulin responses in acute Q fever. *J Clin Microbiol.* 1985;22:484-487.
91. Healy B, Llewelyn M, Westmoreland P, et al. The value of follow-up after acute Q fever. *J Infect.* 2006;52:e109-e112.
92. Fenollar F, Thuny F, Xeridat B, et al. Endocarditis after acute Q fever in patients with previously undiagnosed valvulopathy. *Clin Infect Dis.* 2006;42:818-821.
93. Fenollar F, Fournier P-E, Carrieri MP, et al. Risk factors and prevention of Q fever endocarditis. *Clin Infect Dis.* 2001;33:312-316.
94. Brouqui P, Dupont HT, Drancourt M, et al. Chronic Q fever: Ninety-two cases from France, including 27 cases without endocarditis. *Arch Intern Med.* 1993;153:642-649.
95. Turck WPG, Howitt G, Turnberg LA, et al. Chronic Q fever. *Q J Med.* 1976;45:193-217.
96. Wilson HG, Neilson GH, Galea EG, et al. Q fever endocarditis in Queensland. *Circulation.* 1976;53:680-684.
97. Grist NR. Q fever endocarditis. *Am Heart J.* 1968;75:845-846.
98. Robson AO, Shimin CDGL. Chronic Q fever. 1. Clinical aspects of a patient with endocarditis. *BMJ.* 1959;2:980-953.
99. Varma MPS, Adgey AAJ, Connolly JH. Chronic Q fever endocarditis. *Br Heart J.* 1980;43:695-699.
100. Tobin MH, Cahill N, Gearty G, et al. Q fever endocarditis. *Am J Med.* 1982;72:396-400.
101. Kimbrough RC III, Ormsbee RA, Peacock M, et al. Q fever endocarditis in the United States. *Ann Intern Med.* 1979;91:400-402.
102. Ross PJ, Jacobson J, Muir JR. Q fever endocarditis of porcine xenograft valves. *Am Heart J.* 1983;105:151-153.
103. Wiley RF, Matthews MB, Peutherere JF, et al. Chronic cryptic Q fever infection of the heart. *Lancet.* 1979;2:270-272.
104. Subramanya NI, Wright JS, Khan MAR. Failure of rifampicin and co-trimoxazole in Q fever endocarditis. *Br Med J (Clin Res Ed).* 1982;203:343-344.
105. Marmion BP. Subacute rickettsial endocarditis: An unusual complication of Q fever. *J Hyg Epidemiol Microbiol Immunol.* 1952;6:79-84.
106. Applefield MM, Bellingsley LN, Tucker JH, et al. Q fever endocarditis: A case occurring in the United States. *Am Heart J.* 1977;93:669-670.
107. Palmer SR, Young SEJ. Q fever endocarditis in England and Wales, 1975-81. *Lancet.* 1982;2:1148-1149.
108. Chronic Q fever [editorial]. *J Infect.* 1984;8:1-4.
109. Haldane EV, Marrie TJ, Faulkner RS, et al. Endocarditis due to Q fever in Nova Scotia: Experience with five patients in 1981-1982. *J Infect Dis.* 1983;148:978-985.
110. Raoult D, Etienne J, Massip P, et al. Q fever endocarditis in the south of France. *J Infect Dis.* 1987;155:570-573.
111. Laufer D, Lew PD, Oberhansli I, et al. Chronic Q fever endocarditis with massive splenomegaly in childhood. *J Pediatr.* 1986;108:535-539.
112. Raoult D, Piquet PH, Gallais H, et al. *Coxiella burnetii* infection of a vascular prosthesis. *N Engl J Med.* 1986;315:1358-1359.
113. Tellez A, Sainz C, Echevarria C, et al. Q fever in Spain: Acute and chronic cases, 1981-1985. *Rev Infect Dis.* 1988;10:198-202.
114. Siegman-Igra Y, Kraufman O, Keysary A, et al. Q fever endocarditis in Israel and a worldwide review. *Scand J Infect Dis.* 1997;29:41-49.
115. Peacock MG, Philip RN, Williams JC, et al. Serological valuation of Q fever in humans: Enhanced phase I titers of immunoglobulins G and A are diagnostic for Q fever endocarditis. *Infect Immun.* 1983;41:1089-1098.
116. Fournier PE, Casalta JP, Habib G, et al. Verification of the diagnostic criteria proposed by the Duke Endocarditis Service to permit improved diagnosis of Q fever endocarditis. *Am J Med.* 1996;100:629-633.
117. Durack DT, Lukes AS, Bright DK. New criteria for diagnosis of infective endocarditis: Utilization of specific echocardiographic findings. *Am J Med.* 1994;96:200-209.
118. Li JS, Sexton DJ, Mick N, et al. Proposed modifications to the Duke criteria for the diagnosis of infective endocarditis. *Clin Infect Dis.* 2000;30:633-638.
119. Blondeau JM, Williams JC, Marrie TJ. The immune response to phase I and phase II *Coxiella burnetii* antigens as measured by Western immunoblotting. *Ann N Y Acad Sci.* 1990;590: 187-202.
120. Levy PY, Drancourt M, Etienne J, et al. Comparison of different antibiotic regimens for therapy of 32 cases of Q fever endocarditis. *Antimicrob Agents Chemother.* 1991;35:533-537.
121. Raoult D, Marrie T. Q fever. *Clin Infect Dis.* 1995;20:489-496.
122. Rolain JM, Mallet MN, Raoult D. Correlation between serum doxycycline concentrations and serologic evolution in patients with *Coxiella burnetii* endocarditis. *J Infect Dis.* 2003;188:1322-1325.
123. Rolain JM, Boulos A, Mallet MN, et al. Correlation between ratio of serum doxycycline concentration to MIC and rapid decline of antibody levels during treatment of Q fever endocarditis. *Antimicrob Agents Chemother.* 2005;49:2673-2676.
124. Capo C, Zaffran Y, Zugun F, et al. Production of interleukin-10 and transforming growth factor β by peripheral blood mononuclear cells in Q fever endocarditis. *Infect Immun.* 1996;64:4143-4147.
125. Hofmann CER, Heaton JW Jr. Q fever hepatitis. Clinical manifestations and pathological findings. *Gastroenterology.* 1982;83:474-479.
126. Dupont HL, Hornick EV, Levin HA, et al. Q fever hepatitis. *Ann Intern Med.* 1971;74:198-206.
127. Qizilbash AH. The pathology of Q fever as seen on liver biopsy. *Arch Pathol Lab Med.* 1983;107:364-367.
128. Travis LB, Travis WD, Li C-Y, et al. Q fever. A clinicopathologic study of five cases. *Arch Pathol Lab Med.* 1986;110:1017-1020.
129. Weir WRC, Bannister B, Chambers S, et al. Chronic Q fever associated with granulomatous hepatitis. *J Infect.* 1980;8: 56-60.
130. Pellegrin M, Delsol G, Auvergnat JC, et al. Granulomatous hepatitis in Q fever. *Hum Pathol.* 1980;11:51-57.
131. Voigt JJ, Delsol G, Fabre J. Liver and bone marrow granulomas in Q fever. *Gastroenterology.* 1983;84:887-888.
132. Alkan WJ, Ewenchik Z, Eschar J. Q fever and infectious hepatitis. *Am J Med.* 1965;38:54-61.
133. Harrell GT. Rickettsial involvement of the central nervous system. *Med Clin North Am.* 1953;37:395-422.
134. Bernit E, Pouget J, Janbon F, et al. Neurological involvement in acute Q fever. A report of 29 cases and review of the literature. *Arch Intern Med.* 2002;162:693-700.
135. Gomez-Aranda F, Diaz JKP, Acebol MR, et al. Computed tomographic brain scan findings in Q fever encephalitis. *Neuroradiology.* 1984;26:329-332.
136. Marrie TJ. Pneumonia and meningo-encephalitis due to *Coxiella burnetii. J Infect.* 1985;11:59-61.
137. Marrie TJ, Raoult D. Rickettsial infections of the central nervous system. *Semin Neurol.* 1992;12:213-224.
138. Reilly S, Northwood JL, Caul EO. Q fever in Plymouth, 1972-88. A review with particular reference to neurological manifestations. *Epidemiol Infect.* 1990;105:391-408.
139. Drancourt M, Raoult D, Xeridat B, et al. Q fever meningoencephalitis in five patients. *Eur J Epidemiol.* 1991;7:134-138.
140. Bonetti B, Monaco S, Ferrari S, et al. Demyelinating polyradiculoneuritis following *Coxiella burnetii* infection (Q fever). *Ital J Neurol Sci.* 1991;12:415-417.
141. Heard SR, Ronalds CJ, Heath RB. *Coxiella burnetii* infection in immunocompromised patients. *J Infect.* 1985;11:15-18.
142. Kanfer E, Farraj N, Price C, et al. Q fever following bone-marrow transplantation. *Bone Marrow Transplant.* 1988;3: 165-168.
143. Loudon MM, Thompson EN. Severe combined immunodeficiency syndrome, tissue transplant, leukemia and Q fever. *Arch Dis Child.* 1988;63:207-209.
144. Raoult D, Brouqui P, Gastraut JA, et al. Acute and chronic Q fever in patients with cancer. *Clin Infect Dis.* 1992;14:127-130.
145. Raoult D, Levy P-Y, Dupont HT, et al. Q fever and HIV infection. *AIDS.* 1993;7:81-86.
146. Meis JFGM, Weemaes CRM, Horrevorts AM, et al. Rapidly fatal Q-fever pneumonia in a patient with chronic granulomatous disease. *Infection.* 1992;20:287-289.
147. Ellis ME, Smith CC, Moffatt MAJ. Chronic or fatal Q-fever infection: A review of 16 patients seen in north-east Scotland (1967-1980). *Q J Med.* 1983;205:54-66.
148. Richardus JH, Dumas AM, Huisman J, et al. Q fever in infancy: A review of 18 cases. *Pediatr Infect Dis.* 1985;4:369-373.
149. Brada M, Bellingham AJ. Bone marrow necrosis and Q fever. *BMJ.* 1980;210:1108-1109.
150. Estrov Z, Bruck R, Shtalrid M, et al. Histiocytic hemophagocytosis in Q fever. *Arch Pathol Lab Med.* 1984;108:7.
151. Cardellach F, Font J, Agusti AGN, et al. Q fever and hemolytic anemia. *J Infect Dis.* 1983;148:769.
152. Ramos HS, Hodges RE, Meroney WH. Q fever: Report of a case simulating lymphoma. *Ann Intern Med.* 1957;47:1030-1035.
153. Hitchins R, Cobcroft RG, Hocker G. Transient severe hypoplastic anemia in Q fever. *Pathology.* 1986;18:254-255.
154. Baumbach A, Brehm B, Sauer W, et al. Spontaneous splenic rupture complicating acute Q fever. *Am J Gastroenterol.* 1992;87:1651-1653.
155. Schuil J, Richardus JH, Baarsma GS, et al. Q fever as a possible cause of bilateral optic neuritis. *Br J Ophthalmol.* 1985; 69:580-583.
156. Conger I, Mallolas J, Mensa J, et al. Erythema nodosum and Q fever. *Arch Dermatol.* 1987;123:867.
157. Swaby ED, Fisher-Hoch S, Lambert HP, et al. Is Kawasaki disease a variant of Q fever? *Lancet.* 1980;2:146.

158. Weir WRC, Bouchet VA, Mitford E, et al. Kawasaki disease in European adult associated with serological response to *Coxiella burnetii*. *Lancet*. 1985;2:504.

159. Raoult D, Fenollar F, Stein, A. Q fever during pregnancy: Diagnosis, treatment and follow-up. *Arch Intern Med*. 2002;162:701-704.

160. Carcopino X, Raoult D, Bretelle F, et al. Managing q fever during pregnancy: The benefitis of long-term cotrimoxazole therapy. *Clin Infect Dis*. 2007;45:548-555.

161. Langley JM, Marrie TJ, Leblanc JC, et al. *Coxiella burnetii* seropositivity in parturient women is associated with adverse pregnancy outcomes. *Am J Obstet Gynecol*. 2003;189:228-232.

162. Marmion BP, Shannon M, Meddocks I, et al. Protracted debility and fatigue after acute Q fever. *Lancet*. 1996;347:977-978.

163. Ayres JG, Flint N, Smith EG, et al. Post infection fatigue syndrome following Q fever. *Q J Med*. 1998;91:105-123.

164. Penttila IA, Harris RJ, Storm P, et al. Cytokine dysregulation The post-Q fever fatigue syndrome. *Q J Med*. 1998;91:549-560.

165. Harris RJ, Storm PA, Lloyd A, et al. Long-term persistence of Coxiella burnetii in the host after primary Q fever. *Epidemiol Infect*. 2000;124:543-549.

166. Hatchette TF, Hayes M, Merry H, et al. The effect of Coxiella burnetii on quality of life following an outbreak of Q fever. *Epidemiol Infect*. 2003;130:491-495.

167. Helbig KJ, Heatley SL, Harris RJ, et al. Variation in immune response genes and chronic Q fever: Concepts: Preliminary test with post-Q fever fatigue syndrome. *Genes Immun*. 2003;4:82-85.

168. Hickie I, Davenport T, Wakefield D, et al. Dubbo Infection Outcomes Study Group. Post-infective and chronic fatigue syndromes precipitated by viral and non-viral pathogens: prospective cohort study. *BMJ*. 2006;333:575.

169. Vollmer-Conn U, Cameron B, Hadzi-Pavlovic D, et al. Post-infective fatigue syndrome is not associated with altered cytokine production. *Clin Infect Dis*. 2007;45:732-735.

170. Ascher MS, Berman MA, Ruppaner R. Initial clinical and immunologic evaluation of a new phase I Q fever vaccine and skin test in humans. *J Infect Dis*. 1983;148:214-224.

171. Marmion BP, Ormsbee RAD, Kyrkou M, et al. Vaccine prophylaxis of abattoir-associated Q fever. *Lancet*. 1984;2:1411-1414.

172. Grant CG, Ascher MS, Bernard KW, et al. Q fever and experimental sheep. *Infect Control*. 1985;6:122-123.

173. Polydorou K. Q fever control in Cyprus—recent progress. *Br Vet J*. 1985;141:427-430.

174. Wright JG, Jung S, Holman RC, et al. Infection control practices and zoonotic disease among veterinarians in the United States. *J Am Vet Assoc*. 2008;232:1863-1872.

190

Rickettsia prowazekii (Epidemic or Louse-Borne Typhus)

DAVID H. WALKER | DIDIER RAOULT

*R*ickettsia prowazekii is the only rickettsia that can cause devastating, naturally occurring epidemics capable of killing a substantial proportion of human populations infested with body lice. Epidemics are associated with conditions that prevent bathing and washing of clothes in hot water, such as war and poverty, natural disasters such as earthquakes and floods, displacement of populations, jails, and lack of hygiene. A continued problem in impoverished, louse-infested populations, epidemic typhus threatens to re-emerge as it did during the Civil War in Burundi; an estimated 100,000 persons suffered from typhus in 1997.[1]

Based on his observations of an Italian epidemic in 1528, epidemic typhus was described vividly by Hieronymus Fracastorius as a previously unknown, life-threatening disease—a petechial rash appeared 4 to 7 days after the onset of fever and was accompanied by stupor and delirium. The word *typhus* is derived from the Greek *typhos*, meaning smoky or hazy, which describes the state of confusion accompanied by stupor. Luis de Toro described the same course and signs of an illness that occurred in soldiers on the Iberian Peninsula in 1557, also noting winter seasonality and association with contact with clothing of the ill. The term *exanthematic typhus* was proposed by Boissier de Sauvages in 1760 and differentiated from typhoid.[2] During an epidemic of typhoid fever in Philadelphia in 1836, Gerhard distinguished these diseases by the presence of intestinal lesions in typhoid patients. In 1909, Charles Nicolle experimentally established the fact that typhus was a transmissible infection with the human body louse as its vector. Investigations from 1910 to 1922 by Ricketts, von Prowazek, da Rocha-Lima, and Wolbach used microscopy, xenodiagnosis in lice, and histochemistry to establish that the agent was a bacterium that proliferated in human endothelial cells and louse gut epithelium but could not be cultured axenically.[3]

In 1896 and 1910, Nathan Brill described a series of patients in New York with a mild febrile illness that was shown by Hans Zinsser in 1934 to be a rickettsial infection.[4,5] Zinsser hypothesized correctly that the illness is a recrudescence of long-latent *R. prowazekii*. The distinction of *Rickettsia typhi* as a separate agent that causes an endemic, clinically similar disease transmitted to humans by fleas from a zoonotic cycle involving rats was established by the work of Neill (1917),[6] Mooser (1928),[7] Maxcy (1929),[8] and Dyer (1931).[9] The feared specter of epidemic louse-borne typhus receded with the following: (1) the success of a killed rickettsia vaccine in preventing the deaths of allied soldiers during World War II; (2) the effectiveness of insecticides in curtailing epidemics by louse control; and (3) the effective treatment of illness with tetracyclines and chloramphenicol. Currently, epidemics of typhus are increasingly recognized, lice resistant to various insecticides have been detected, antibiotic-resistant rickettsiae have been developed, and aerosol-transmitted, weaponized *R. prowazekii* has emerged as a biothreat. *R. prowazekii* has been found in *Amblyomma* and *Hyalomma* ticks in Ethiopia and in *Amblyomma imitator* ticks in Mexico.[10,11] Moreover, in 1975, *R. prowazekii* was identified in a highly prevalent zoonotic cycle in flying squirrels in the eastern United States.[12]

Cause

The causative agent of louse-borne typhus, *R. prowazekii*, is an obligately intracellular, small (1 × 0.3 μm) coccobacillus. Its 1.1-Mb genome has undergone considerable reduction and contains a subset of the genes of *R. conorii*. Many biosynthetic functions are provided by its milieu in the resource-rich host cell cytosol to which the organism has adapted by evolutionary selection for transport mechanisms for adenosine triphosphate (ATP), amino acids, and phosphorylated sugars.[13] Its gram-negative cell wall contains an abundant 135-kDa, immunodominant, tetragonally arranged, S-layer surface protein, lipopolysaccharide, and peptidoglycan.[14] It possesses an extracellular dormant form that remains infectious in louse feces for months. Interestingly, no virulence factor specific to this rickettsia has been identified despite its high pathogenicity.

Epidemiology

Typhus has affected the outcomes of wars from the 1500s until the end of the 19th century. During the Russian campaign of 1812, typhus was responsible for the deaths of many of the 700,000 troops of Napoleon.[15] During World War I, the Bolshevik revolution, and its aftermath, an estimated 30 million cases of typhus occurred in the Soviet Union alone, with 3 million deaths.[16] During World War II, epidemics of typhus occurred in eastern Europe, North Africa, concentration camps, and southern Italy, where DDT was used against lice to abort an epidemic in Naples in 1944.

R. prowazekii is transmitted between patients by the human body louse (*Pediculus humanus corporis*), which is strictly adapted to humans, lives in the clothes, and takes a blood meal five times daily.[17] Lice become infected while feeding on the blood of rickettsemic patients. *R. prowazekii* enters the louse gut epithelial cells and replicates by binary fission until the massively infected cells burst[18] and are released into the louse feces 5 to 7 days after ingestion. Lice are not adapted to an elevated body temperature and leave febrile patients for a new host. Rickettsia-laden louse feces are deposited on the skin and clothes and are introduced into the new host by scratching into the louse-bitten skin or by rubbing into mucous membranes such as the conjunctiva; they are also transmitted through inhalation.

Persons who recover from typhus fever remain latently infected and are susceptible to reactivation of the infection and rickettsemia, which can infect body lice and ignite an epidemic under circumstances of crowding, extreme poverty, cold climate, and poor hygiene. This can lead to a high prevalence of louse infestation (Fig. 190-1). The louse population can expand rapidly (11% daily).[18,19] Lice are currently prevalent in poor countries, spreading in the former USSR, and found on homeless persons in developed countries. In France, 35% of members of the homeless population have lice. Risk factors for reactivation of latent infection in humans have not been determined, but waning immunity, poor nutrition, alcoholism, and stress have been hypothesized as potentially important.

Typhus is endemic in the Peruvian Andes, Burundi, and Rwanda, Cases have been diagnosed in Russia, in patients from Algeria and Senegal, and in a homeless person in France.[1,20-22] Given the geographic distribution of latent typhus infection from known historic epidemics, the neglect with which this disease has been handled, and the unavailability of laboratory diagnostic methods, the current epidemiology of louse-borne typhus, particularly in marginal populations of mountainous areas in Asia, South and Central America, and Africa, is unknown.

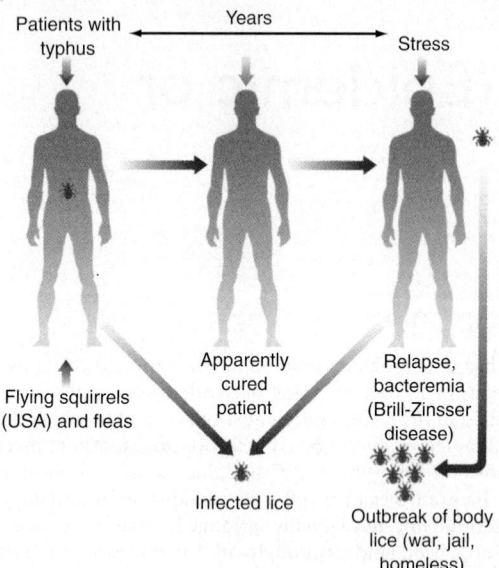

Figure 190-1 **Transmission of typhus.**

An extrahuman reservoir of *R. prowazekii* exists in a large portion of Southern flying squirrels (*Glaucomys volans*), which are distributed from Florida to Maine and westward to Minnesota and east Texas.[12] In stark contrast with the louse-human cycle, in which 15% of humans die and 100% of lice suffer rickettsial destruction of the intestine with extravasation of the red blood meal into the hemocele and death, *R. prowazekii* causes subclinical rickettsemia in flying squirrels and no ill effects on the squirrel's own species of lice and fleas.[23] Infections are apparently transmitted to humans by flying squirrel fleas or mucous membrane or inhalation exposure to the feces of the flea or louse. These illnesses occur mainly during winter, when flying squirrels enter buildings.[24] The role of ticks in transmitting *R. prowazekii* is currently unknown.

Pathogenesis

After inoculation into the skin, *R. prowazekii* spreads throughout the body via the bloodstream. Rickettsiae enter mainly through endothelial cells and, to a lesser extent, through macrophages by induced phagocytosis; they escape from the phagosome into the cytosol, where they proliferate until the cell bursts.[25] Phospholipase D has been found to play a significant role in pathogenesis, with evidence for mediating rickettsial phagosomal escape in concert with rickettsial hemolysin C.[26,27] *R. prowazekii* lacks actin-based mobility that mediates the cell-to-cell spread of spotted fever group rickettsiae. Rickettsial phospholipase A$_2$ activity has been hypothesized to play a role in lysis of infected cells. A gene for patatin-like protein has been identified in *Rickettsia*, with sequence similarity to phospholipase A but without experimental evidence for physiologic activity or pathologic effect.[28,29] The principal pathophysiologic effects of rickettsial infection include increased vascular permeability and petechial hemorrhage. Thrombosis occurs in only a tiny minority of foci of vascular infection and injury, and ischemic necrosis is a rare consequence.[3] The most important vital target organs are the brain and the lung. The petechial maculopapular rash is a manifestation of cutaneous vascular infection by *R. prowazekii*. Classic pathologic lesions are comprised of swollen, infected endothelial cells in the microcirculation, with adjacent perivascular infiltration by lymphocytes and macrophages, which represents the effector host cellular immune response.[3,30] The primary animal model for epidemic typhus is guinea pigs infected intraperitoneally with *R. prowazekii*. Lesions typical of typhus encephalitis are produced.[31] Balb/C mice have been reported to become infected by a narrow dose range of *R. prowazekii*, develop illness associated with growth of *R. prowazekii*, and

mount an effective immune response.[32] Nonhuman primate models have been described that reproduce the pathologic lesions of human typhus.[33,34]

Clinical Manifestations

Experiments in human volunteers during the preantibiotic era demonstrated that after an incubation period of 8 to 16 days (mean, 11.1 days) and a prodrome of 2 days, rash developed in 79% of subjects an average of 4 days after onset of illness, and the fever lasted for 12 days. In an epidemic in Poland after World War I, a prodrome of 1 day or longer occurred in 88%, followed by fever (100%), headache (89%), chills (74%), myalgias (54%), rash (an entry criterion of the study), conjunctival injection (87%), and rales (74%).[3] Erythematous 2- to 6-mm macules appeared most often on the trunk on day 5 and later on the extremities. Without the availability of antibiotics, the course was characterized by marked delirium (48%), severe cough (38%), hemorrhagic rash (34%), gangrene (4%), coma (6%), death (13%) a median of 12.5 days after onset, or defervescence a median of 14 days after onset. Studies from Ethiopia and Burundi have demonstrated a lower incidence of rash in darkly pigmented skin, marked myalgia, variable incidence of stupor, cough, and conjunctivitis (Table 190-1), and a lower case-fatality rate caused by effective antimicrobial treatment in many patients.[1,35] The illness in Burundi was locally called *sutama*, denoting the crouching position that the patient assumed to mitigate the severe muscle pain.

Onset is usually abrupt, with rigors, malaise, and severe headache. The tongue is dry and the patient is constipated. The rash progresses through macules that disappear on pressure to maculopapules with petechiae. The face, palms, and soles are usually spared. In darkly pigmented patients, cutaneous lesions are more easily visible in the axilla. Chest radiographs frequently reveal interstitial pneumonia. Cases have not occurred in settings in which clinical laboratory abnormalities have been studied extensively, except for the Ethiopian series, which demonstrated values characteristic of disseminated rickettsial vascular injury and increased vascular permeability (Table 190-2).[35]

Flying squirrel–associated typhus cases have generally been less severe, with no fatalities recorded. Patients have developed fever (100%), headache (81%), maculopapular rash (66%), confusion (44%), and myalgia (42%).[24,36-38]

In 1910, Brill's clinical description of recrudescent typhus was that of an illness resembling nonfatal typhus, with onset characterized by chills, intense headache, fever, myalgia, nausea, and sometimes vomiting. Patients are prostrate with apathy, dulled sensorium, and persis-

TABLE 190-1	Clinical Manifestations of Epidemic Typhus	
	Place	
Manifestation	*Burundi**	*Ethiopia†*
Number of cases	102	60
Fever > 39° C	100%	100%
Headaches	100%	100%
Any rash	25%	38%
Purpuric rash	11%	33%
Stupor	81%	35%
Coma	4%	—
Cough	70%	38%
Nausea, vomiting	57%	43%
Conjunctivitis	15%	53%
Diarrhea	13%	—
Splenomegaly	8%	13%
Photophobia	—	33%
Myalgias	100%	70%

*Fournier PE, Ndihokubwayo JB, Guidran J, et al. Human pathogens in body and head lice. *Emerg Infect Dis.* 2002;8:1515-1518.

†Perine PL, Chandler BP, Krause DK, et al. A clinico-epidemiological study of epidemic typhus in Africa. *Clin Infect Dis.* 1992;14:1149-1158.

TABLE 190-2	Clinical Laboratory Findings in Patients with Epidemic Typhus	
Finding	**Incidence (%)**	
White blood cell count	Low, 3; elevated, 14	
Thrombocytopenia	43	
Increased serum AST	63	
Increased serum ALT	35	
Increased serum LDH	82	
Increased serum CPK	31	
Increased BUN	31	
Decreased serum protein	38	

ALT, alanine transaminase; AST, aspartate transaminase; BUN, blood urea nitrogen; CPK, creatine phosphokinase; LDH, lactate dehydrogenase.

Adapted from Perine PL, Chandler BP, Krause DK, et al. A clinico-epidemiological study of epidemic typhus in Africa. *Clin Infect Dis.* 1992;14:1149-1158.

tent headache as an overriding symptom. Between the fifth and seventh days of illness, a maculopapular rash appears on the back and abdomen and spreads rapidly. Congested conjunctivae and constipation are prominent features in many cases. The untreated illness lasts about 2 weeks. Brill stated, "In the case of an epidemic of typhus fever, in my opinion, it would be simply impossible to say that these cases which I have described were not mild typhus fever."[4] Twenty-four years later, Hans Zinsser isolated rickettsiae from the blood of similar patients—louse-free immigrants from typhus-endemic regions of Europe. Thus, the eponymic designation, Brill-Zinsser disease, began to be used to refer to recrudescent typhus.[5]

Diagnosis

In the midst of a recognized epidemic, the patient with a late-stage florid rash or even one with fever, severe headache, and myalgia without a rash would likely be diagnosed with louse-borne typhus. The diagnosis of louse-borne typhus early in an outbreak when only a few cases have been reported is more challenging. The most important differential diagnoses are typhoid fever and malaria in tropical countries.[20] The prominent cough and crackles often suggest a diagnosis of pneumonia. Neurologic signs and cerebrospinal fluid (CSF) pleocytosis may lead to consideration of viral or bacterial meningoencephalitis. Nausea, vomiting, and abdominal tenderness raise the diagnostic possibilities of viral or bacterial enterocolitis or acute surgical abdomen. Jaundice and elevated hepatic enzyme levels suggest viral hepatitis. The hemorrhagic rash may lead to diagnostic consideration of arenaviral and filoviral hemorrhagic fevers.[39] Other differential diagnoses include leptospirosis, arboviral and enteroviral infections, meningococcemia, trench fever, relapsing fever, and other rickettsioses.

Other circumstances under which *R. prowazekii* infection should be considered involve immigrants from regions where epidemic typhus has been prevalent, persons who have been exposed to flying squirrels, and homeless persons.[21,24,36] It is unlikely that cases of aerosol-transmitted typhus in a bioterrorist attack would be diagnosed clinically before the onset of rash, if even then.[40]

The laboratory diagnosis of louse-borne typhus generally relies on the detection of antibodies with a fourfold rise in titer in convales-cence. Usually, a diagnostic titer is detected during the second week of illness. The standard serologic method is indirect immunofluorescence assay, and an immunoglobulin (Ig) G titer of 1:128 or an IgM titer of 1:32 confirms the diagnosis. Enzyme immunoassays that yield reliable results have also been developed. Although the *Proteus vulgaris* OX-19 agglutination (Weil-Felix reaction) has been demonstrated to be poorly sensitive and nonspecific, it may be useful when it is the only method available in a developing country. Antibodies stimulated by *R. prowazekii* react with shared antigens of *R. typhi*, allowing for diagnostic detection of cross-reactive antibodies. A fourfold higher titer against *R. prowazekii* than *R. typhi* distinguishes epidemic typhus from murine typhus in fewer than half of cases.[41] The predominance of IgG antibodies and the absence of IgM and Weil-Felix antibodies in recrudescent typhus is controversial.[42]

Although serodiagnosis is retrospective, methods that can establish a diagnosis during the acute stage of infection—namely, the polymerase chain reaction (PCR) assay and immunohistochemical detection of *R. prowazekii* in blood or tissue, respectively—are seldom available in regions where typhus epidemics occur.[43,44] Feasibility has been demonstrated for serodiagnosis on blood spotted onto filter paper and for rickettsial isolation or PCR detection in lice removed from the patient, either of which can be sent to a referral laboratory by mail.[45,46] Rickettsiae may also be isolated most effectively from blood, buffy coat, plasma, or tissue in shell vial cell culture.[47]

Treatment

The treatment of choice for all patients who are not allergic to tetracyclines and who are not pregnant is doxycycline 100 mg twice daily for 7 to 10 days.[48] Under chaotic epidemic conditions and in other situations in which doxycycline availability is limited, a single dose of 200 mg of doxycycline is effective, although a small portion of patients may relapse.[49] Chloramphenicol (60 to 75 mg/kg/day in four divided doses) and tetracycline (25 to 50 mg/kg/day in four divided doses) are also effective. Other antibiotics, including β-lactams, aminoglycosides, and sulfonamides, are ineffective. Although fluoroquinolones, rifampin, and some of the newer macrolides show inhibition of growth of *R. prowazekii* in cell culture, none has been proved to be efficacious clinically.

Prevention

Control of body lice is the mainstay in the prevention of epidemic typhus. When an outbreak of lice appears, the first step is to change all garments and wash them in hot water. Introducing regular washing of clothes will stop outbreaks. Only when this is impossible is delousing using insecticides useful, such as Lindane in powder form. Application of 30 to 50 g of 1% permethrin dusting powder per adult both inside and outside of clothing and on bedding may be repeated every 6 weeks to kill lice.

No vaccine is currently available for the prevention of typhus. However, the identification of the attenuating point mutation of a previously successful live vaccine (E strain) that was prone to reversion offers the opportunity to develop a permanently attenuated protective vaccine against *R. prowazekii*.[50,51]

REFERENCES

1. Raoult D, Ndihokubwayo JB, Tissot-Dupont H, et al. Outbreak of epidemic typhus associated with trench fever in Burundi. *Lancet.* 1998;352:353-358.
2. Bechah Y, Capo C, Mege JL, et al. Epidemic typhus. *Lancet Infect Dis.* 2008;8:417-426.
3. Wolbach SB, Todd JL, Palfrey FW. *The Etiology and Pathology of Typhus.* Cambridge, Mass: Harvard University Press; 1922.
4. Brill NE. An acute infectious disease of unknown origin. *Am J Med Sci.* 1910;139:484.
5. Zinsser H. Varieties of typhus virus and the epidemiology of the American form of European typhus fever (Brill's disease). *Am J Hyg.* 1934;20:513.
6. Neill MH. Experimental typhus fever in guinea pigs. *Public Health Rep.* 1917;21:1105-1108.

7. Mooser H. Experiments relating to the pathology and the etiology of Mexican typhus (Tabardillo). *J Infect Dis.* 1928;43:241-260.
8. Maxcy KF. Typhus fever in the United States. *Public Health Rep.* 1929;44:1735-1743.
9. Dyer RE. Typhus fever. A virus of the typhus type derived from fleas collected from wild rats. *Public Health Rep.* 1931;46:334-338.
10. Reiss-Gutfreund RJ. The isolation of *Rickettsia prowazekii* and *mooseri* from unusual sources. *Am J Trop Med Hyg.* 1966;15:943-949.
11. Medina-Sanchez A, Bouyer DH, Alcantara-Rodriguez V, et al. Detection of a typhus group *Rickettsia* in *Amblyomma* ticks in the state of Nuevo Leon, Mexico. *Ann NY Acad Sci.* 2005;1063:327-332.

12. Bozeman FM, Masiello SA, Williams MS, et al. Epidemic typhus rickettsiae isolated from flying squirrels. *Nature.* 1975;255:545-547.
13. Andersson SG, Zomorodipour A, Andersson JO, et al. The genome sequence of *Rickettsia prowazekii* and the origin of mitochondria. *Nature.* 1998;396:133-140.
14. Moron CG, Bouyer DH, Yu X-J, et al. Phylogenetic analysis of the *rompB* genes of *Rickettsia felis* and *Rickettsia prowazekii* European-human and North American flying-squirrel strains. *Am J Trop Med Hyg.* 2000;62:598-603.
15. Raoult D, Dutour O, Houhamdi L, et al. Evidence for louse-transmitted diseases in soldiers of Napoleon's Grand Army in Vilnius. *J Infect Dis.* 2006;193:112-120.
16. Patterson KD. Typhus and its control in Russia, 1870-1940. *Med Host.* 1993;37:361.

17. Raoult D, Roux V. The body louse as a vector of reemerging human diseases. *Clin Infect Dis.* 1999;29:888-911.
18. Houhamdi L, Fournier PE, Fang R, et al. An experimental model of human body louse infection with *Rickettsia prowazekii. J Infect Dis.* 2000;186:1639-1646.
19. Fournier PE, Ndihokubwayo JB, Guidran J, et al. Human pathogens in body and head lice. *Emerg Infect Dis.* 2002;8:1515-1518.
20. Niang M, Brouqui P, Raoult D. Epidemic typhus imported from Algeria. *Emerg Infect Dis.* 1999;5:716-718.
21. Brouqui P, Raoult D. Arthropod-borne diseases in homeless. *Ann NY Acad Sci.* 2006;1078:223-235.
22. Tarasevich I, Rydkina E, Raoult D. Outbreak of epidemic typhus in Russia. *Lancet.* 1998;352:1151.
23. Sonenshine DE, Bozeman FM, Williams MS, et al. Epizootiology of epidemic typhus *(Rickettsia prowazekii)* in flying squirrels. *Am J Trop Med Hyg.* 1978;27:339-349.
24. Reynolds MG, Krebs JW, Comer JA, et al. Flying squirrel–associated typhus, United States. *Emerg Infect Dis.* 2003;9:1341-1343.
25. Walker TS. Rickettsial interactions with human endothelial cells in vitro: Adherence and entry. *Infect Immun.* 1984;44:205-210.
26. Renesto P, Dehoux P, Gouin E, et al. Identification and characterization of a phospholipase D-superfamily gene in Rickettsiae. *J Infect Dis.* 2003;188:1276-1283.
27. Whitworth TJ, Popov VL, Yu X-J, et al. Expression of the *Rickettsia prowazekii pld* or *tlyC* gene in *Salmonella enterica* serovar typhimurium mediates phagosomal escape. *Infect Immun.* 2005;73:6668-6673.
28. Walker DH, Feng H-M, Popov VL. Rickettsial phospholipase A₂ as a pathogenic mechanism in a model of cell injury by typhus and spotted fever group rickettsiae. *Am J Trop Med Hyg.* 2001;65:936-946.
29. Blanc G, Renesto P, Raoult D. Phylogenic analysis of rickettsial patatin-like protein with conserved phospholipase A2 active site. *Ann NY Acad Sci.* 2005;1063:83-86.
30. Turco J, Winkler HH. Role of nitric oxide synthase pathway in inhibition of growth of interferon-sensitive and interferon-resistant *Rickettsia prowazekii* stains in L929 cells treated with tumor necrosis factor alpha and gamma interferon. *Infect Immun.* 1993;61:4317.
31. Lillie RD, Dyer RE. Brain reaction in guinea pigs infected with endemic typus, epidemic (European) typhus, and Rocky Mountain spotted fever, eastern and western types. *Pub Health Rep.* 1936;51:1293-1307.
32. Bechah Y, Capo C, Grau GE, et al. A murine model of infection with *Rickettsia prowazekii*: implications for pathogenesis of epidemic typhus. *Microbes Infect.* 2007;9:898-906.
33. Gonder JC, Kenyon RH, Pedersen CE. Epidemic typhus infection in cynomolgus monkeys *(Macaca fascicularis).* *Infect Immun.* 1980;30:219-223.
34. Barker LF, Palmer AE, Kirschstein RL, et al. Experimental infection with *Rickettsia prowazekii* in rhesus and vervet monkeys. *J Infect Dis.* 1967;117:285-291.
35. Perine PL, Chandler BP, Krause DK, et al. A clinico-epidemiological study of epidemic typhus in Africa. *Clin Infect Dis.* 1992;14:1149-1158.
36. Centers for Disease Control (CDC). Epidemic typhus associated with flying squirrels—United States. *MMWR Morb Mortal Wkly Rep.* 1982;31:555-556, 561.
37. Duma RJ, Sonenshine DE, Bozeman M, et al. Epidemic typhus in the United States associated with flying squirrels. *JAMA.* 1981;245:2318-2323.
38. McDade JE, Shepard CC, Redus MA, et al. Evidence of *Rickettsia prowazekii* infections in the United States. *Am J Trop Med Hyg.* 1980;29:277-284.
39. Zanetti G, Francioli P, Tagan D, et al. Imported epidemic typhus. *Lancet.* 1998;352:1709.
40. Azad AF. Pathogenic rickettsiae as bioterrorism agents. *Clin Infect Dis.* 2007;45(Suppl 1):S52-S55.
41. LaScola B, Rydkina L, Ndihokubwayo JB, et al. Serological differentiation of murine typhus and epidemic typhus using cross-absorption and Western blotting. *Clin Diagn Lab Immunol.* 2000;7:612-616.
42. Eremeeva ME, Balayeva NM, Raoult D. Serological response of patients suffering from primary and recrudescent typhus: Comparison of complement fixation reaction, Weil-Felix Test, microimmunofluorescence, and immunoblotting. *Clin Diagn Lab Immunol.* 1995;1:318-324.
43. Carl M, Tibbs CW, Dobson ME, et al. Diagnosis of acute typhus infection using the polymerase chain reaction. *J Infect Dis.* 1990;161:791-793.
44. Walker DH, Feng H-M, Ladner S, et al. Immunohistochemical diagnosis of typhus rickettsioses using an anti-lipopolysaccharide monoclonal antibody. *Mod Pathol.* 1997;10:1038-1042.
45. Fenollar F, Raoult D. Diagnosis of rickettsial diseases using samples dried on blotting paper. *Clin Diagn Lab Immunol.* 1999;6:483-488.
46. Roux V, Raoult D. Body lice as tools for diagnosis and surveillance of reemerging diseases. *J Clin Microbiol.* 1999;37:596-599.
47. Birg ML, La Scola B, Roux V, et al. Isolation of *Rickettsia prowazekii* from blood by shell vial cell culture. *J Clin Microbiol.* 1999;37:3722-3724
48. Maurin M, Raoult D. *Rickettsia prowazekii.* In: Mann J, Crabbe MJC, eds. *Bacteria and Antibacterial Agents.* Baltimore: Williams & Wilkins. 2001:558-561.
49. Perine PL, Krause DW, Awoke A, et al. Single-dose doxycycline treatment of louse-borne relapsing fever and epidemic typhus. *Lancet.* 1974;2:742-744.
50. Zhang J-Z, Hao J-F, Walker DH, et al. A mutation inactivating the methyltransferase gene in avirulent Madrid E strain of *Rickettsia prowazekii* reverted to wild type in the virulent revertant strain Evir. *Vaccine.* 2006;24:2317-2323.
51. Fox JP, Jordan ME, Gelfand HM. Immunization of man against epidemic typhus by infection with avirulent *Rickettsia prowazekii* strain E. *J Immunol.* 1957;79:348-354.

191

Rickettsia typhi (Murine Typhus)

J. STEPHEN DUMLER | DAVID H. WALKER

In 1922, Hone first described human infections "closely resembling typhus fever."[1] Since 1926, when Maxcy successfully differentiated among typhus fevers and identified murine typhus as a distinct clinical and epidemiologic entity, and 1931, when Dyer isolated a new typhus group *Rickettsia* from rats and fleas, murine typhus has been recognized as a worldwide zoonotic problem.[2] Often underrecognized and believed to be clinically mild, murine typhus may occur in epidemics or with high prevalence in certain geographic regions.[3-9] Illness may be severe, with death occurring in a small proportion of individuals. The association with both rat and cat fleas is now well established; with fluctuations in human seroprevalence, the changing ecology of this zoonosis complicates both clinical recognition and laboratory diagnosis.[10,11]

Cause

Rickettsia typhi, the causative agent of murine typhus, is an obligate intracellular bacterium that infects endothelial cells in mammalian hosts and midgut epithelial cells in the flea host.[10] A new rickettsial agent, *Rickettsia felis*, has been recognized as sharing some antigenic and genetic components with *R. typhi* but is best phylogenomically characterized as a transitional group bacterium between typhus and spotted fever group rickettsiae.[12,13] As typical for the genus *Rickettsia*, *R. typhi* contains rickettsial outer membrane protein B (OmpB) and Sca4, but its lack of rickettsial outer membrane protein A (OmpA), a characteristic of spotted fever group rickettsiae, resembles the typhus group.[14] In addition to *ompB*, the genome encodes for three other autotransporters, Sca1, Sca2, and Sca3. OmpB is known to mediate adhesion and entry events for other *Rickettsia* spp. and features of Sca2 suggest that it may also function as an adhesin.[14,15] In addition, the *R. typhi* genome encodes at least four potentially membranolytic proteins—*tlyA*, *tlyC*, *pldA*, and *pat-1*—that could facilitate cell invasion or endosomal escape.[13,16] These organisms are well adapted for intracellular life, because they lack enzymes for carbohydrate metabolism, lipid biosynthesis, nucleotide synthesis, and amino acid metabolism, and a complete TCA cycle, but possess several adenosine triphosphate–adenosine diphosphate (ATP-ADP) translocase genes that likely mediate host energy parasitism.[13] In fact, the genome encodes both secA and type IV secretion system components, further suggesting the elaboration of effector proteins delivered into the host cell that influence cell function and fate with *R. typhi* infection.[13,17] Unlike the situation for spotted fever group rickettsiae, *R. typhi* lacks *rickA*, which encodes a protein promoting intracellular motility via actin polymerization.[14]

Epidemiology

Murine typhus is found worldwide and is especially prevalent in tropical and subtropical seaboard regions, where the most important rat reservoirs (*Rattus* spp.) and flea vectors (*Xenopsylla cheopis*) are found.[2,10,18] An important vector in some areas (south Texas and southern California) is the cat flea (*Ctenocephalides felis*), and opossums have been implicated as a potential reservoir in these areas.[8,10,18-20] Thus, residents and visitors to these urban and suburban regions are at risk when flea-bearing animals bring infected fleas into close proximity to humans.

Murine typhus persists at a low but increasing level in the United States, where most cases are seen in south Texas and southern California.[21] Outbreaks are well documented around the world, however, especially in regions with inadequate vector and reservoir control.[2,22-25] Among displaced Khmers at the Thai-Cambodian border with unexplained fever, 70% were cases of murine typhus, with an attack rate of 172/100,000 adult patients,[9] and 11% to 26% of febrile patients in Nepal were retrospectively diagnosed with murine typhus.[26,27] Most patients are adults, although persons of all ages may become ill.[28] Cases are recognized year-round, with a peak prevalence from April through June in Texas[8] and during the warm months of summer and early fall elsewhere.[2,24,29] It is worth remembering that murine typhus can occur in travelers returning from endemic regions throughout the world.[30]

The disease is transmitted after the inoculation of infected flea feces into a flea bite wound. Because predominantly gut epithelial cells are infected in the flea vector, a reservoir of infected fleas is maintained mostly by horizontal transmission from flea to vertebrate host to uninfected flea.[31] Once infected, the flea maintains the rickettsial infection for the duration of its life. *R. typhi* may also infect the flea reproductive organs and foregut tissues, which explains the low levels of transovarial (vertical) transmission.[32] The longevity of fleas is unaffected by gut epithelial cell or disseminated *R. typhi* infection.[10]

Pathology and Pathogenesis

Few accurate descriptions of the histopathology of murine typhus are available, despite the fact that the case-fatality rate ranges between 1% and 4%.[8] Pathologic findings indicate a systemic endothelial infection similar to epidemic typhus and Rocky Mountain spotted fever.[33,34] Lymphohistiocytic vasculitis may affect any organ and, in fatal cases, interstitial pneumonitis, interstitial nephritis, interstitial myocarditis, meningoencephalitis, and portal triaditis may be present. Rickettsiae may be demonstrated in many organs and are especially numerous in foci of vasculitis.[33] This underlying vasculitic lesion and the rickettsia-induced vascular injury account for most of the clinicopathologic abnormalities. As vascular injury accumulates, a substantial loss of intravascular volume, albumin, and electrolytes occurs, and leukocytes and platelets are consumed at foci of infection. With multifocal heavy infection and attendant inflammation, vascular and parenchymal injury may yield localized symptoms, signs, or laboratory findings related to the sites of infection and injury. The induction of hypovolemia insufficiently corrected by normal homeostatic mechanisms further exacerbates tissue perfusion compromise and may lead to renal insufficiency. Mild to moderate hepatic injury is a frequent finding in murine typhus and probably results from multifocal infection of hepatic sinusoidal and portal endothelium, with bystander hepatocyte damage.[8,35] With extensive rickettsial vascular injury and hypoperfusion secondary to volume loss, the result may be renal failure, respiratory failure, central nervous system abnormalities, or multiorgan failure.[8,33]

Immunity to *R. typhi* is mediated mainly by early interactions with and maturation of dendritic cells, and control is provided by natural killer (NK) cells. This is followed by adaptive responses via CD4 and CD8 T lymphocytes, their cytokine products interferon-γ and tumor necrosis factor-α (TNF-α), and antibody, which likely plays an adjunctive role.[36-41]

Clinical Manifestations

SIGNS AND SYMPTOMS

Only a small proportion of patients (median, 4%) with murine typhus recall a flea bite or exposure, and an incubation period of approximately 1 to 2 weeks may transpire before an abrupt onset of illness occurs. The presentation is often nonspecific, and fever (93% to 100%), headache (10% to 91%), myalgia (8% to 10%), and nausea or vomiting (14% to 59%) are the most frequently reported early findings.[8,24,42-46] Rash is noted in up to 18% of patients at presentation, but over the course of the illness, as few as 3% and as many as 80% will develop this sign.[47] As the illness progresses, most patients continue with fever and can have gastrointestinal (nausea, 48%; vomiting, 40%; and anorexia, 35%) or respiratory involvement (cough in 14% to 44%). Some studies record the presence of hepatomegaly and splenomegaly in up to 24% and 10% of patients, respectively.[48,49] Severe neurologic complications occur in up to 17% of patients, usually manifested as confusion, stupor, seizures, or localized findings such as ataxia.[50,51]

The absence of rash or lack of petechiae should not dissuade one from a diagnosis of murine typhus. In fact, when rash is identified, it is described as macular or maculopapular in 75% to 80% of cases, and petechiae are noted in less than 13%.[8,28,47,49] The rash is most often distributed on the trunk (88% of cases), but involvement of the extremities (>45%) is not infrequent. The initial rash distribution is equally frequent on the extremities and on the trunk, and is present on the palms and soles in less than 3% of patients.[24]

The clinical course of murine typhus is usually uncomplicated, and childhood murine typhus is often mild, with one series reporting only nighttime fever with normal daytime activities.[24,43,49] However, occasional patients develop central nervous system abnormalities,[52-56] renal insufficiency,[44] or respiratory failure requiring intubation.[57] Patients are ill enough that 10% require admission to an intensive care facility, and up to 4% of hospitalized adult patients die from the infection.[8]

Once the diagnosis has been considered and appropriate therapy begun, most patients defervesce rapidly (median 3 days). Findings associated with severe illness include leukocytosis, elevated blood urea nitrogen or creatinine level, and a high blood urea nitrogen–to–creatinine ratio. Advanced age and a prolonged interval before the administration of specific antirickettsial therapy are also significantly correlated with severity.[8] One report has suggested a link between hemolytic disorders such as glucose-6-phosphate dehydrogenase deficiency, hemoglobinopathy, and thalassemia and more severe hepatic involvement, including jaundice.[35] A trend toward more severe infection is also noted in patients treated with trimethoprim-sulfamethoxazole.

LABORATORY FEATURES

Early mild leukopenia (which coincides with thrombocytopenia) is seen in 25% to 50% of patients during the first 7 days of illness. Subsequently, leukocytosis develops in less than one third. Prothrombin times are occasionally prolonged, but true disseminated intravascular coagulation with hypofibrinogenemia is infrequently documented. The most frequent laboratory abnormality in murine typhus, a mild to moderate elevation in serum aspartate aminotransferase levels, is present in most patients (67% to 92%), and related indices of hepatic and cellular injury (alanine aminotransferase, alkaline phosphatase, lactate dehydrogenase levels) are often elevated in parallel.[8,24,28,35,47,49] Rickettsia-induced vascular damage frequently leads to hypoproteinemia (45%) and hypoalbuminemia (89%) and is probably responsible in large part for multiple serum electrolyte abnormalities, especially hyponatremia (60%) and hypocalcemia (79%). Even in the presence of symptomatic central nervous system abnormalities, cerebrospinal fluid examination can be normal or reveal pleocytosis and increased protein concentration, resembling the findings in viral or leptospiral meningoencephalitis.[52,53,55]

Diagnosis

Early diagnosis of murine typhus is still based mostly on clinical suspicion. Because timely specific antirickettsial therapy is indicated to avoid severe or potentially fatal infections, treatment should not be withheld while laboratory confirmation is awaited.[8,28] The predominant method of laboratory confirmation is serologic. Because antibodies are infrequently detected during acute illness, serologic diagnosis is retrospective.[49] Obsolete Weil-Felix agglutination reactions have proved insensitive, are intrinsically nonspecific and, as such, should not be used to establish a definitive diagnosis.[58] Instead, sensitive serologic tests that use specific *R. typhi* antigens such as indirect fluorescent antibody are preferable. With the use of a sensitive and specific test such as indirect fluorescent antibody assay, diagnostic titers are present in approximately 50% of murine typhus patients within 1 week and in almost all patients within 15 days after the onset of illness.[8,49] Because typhus group rickettsiae share antigens, routine serologic evaluation does not distinguish between epidemic and murine typhus.[59] In occasional sera, reactions against both typhus and spotted fever groups are observed, creating further serodiagnostic difficulties. Although it affords a definitive diagnosis, culture is rarely attempted because of a reputation of biohazard and difficulty reducing the use of this potentially valuable adjunct to diagnosis.

Methods for laboratory confirmation of rickettsiosis include the immunohistologic demonstration of *R. typhi* in tissues[33,60] and polymerase chain reaction amplification of rickettsial nucleic acids in peripheral blood.[29,61,62] However, none of these methods has been adequately evaluated for the diagnosis of murine typhus and are generally unavailable in clinical laboratories; thus, sensitivities, specificities, and predictive values are unknown.

Most patients are initially investigated for fever of undetermined origin and, less often, patients are investigated for upper or lower respiratory tract infection, urinary tract infection, cerebrovascular accident, gastroenteritis, or neoplasm, among other diagnoses.[8,63] Despite the occasional presence of findings that suggest alternative diagnoses because of isolated organ system involvement, an early clue toward the successful diagnosis of murine typhus is recognition of the systemic manifestations associated with fever. Other rickettsioses may cause considerable difficulty in the differential diagnosis; in the western hemisphere, Rocky Mountain spotted fever is the most frequent, whereas in Europe, Africa, and Asia, other spotted fever rickettsioses or scrub typhus should be considered. Murine typhus and spotted fever rickettsiosis may be distinguished on the basis of the history, clinical presentation, and four-fold differences in titer using specific serologic tests.[64] Many patients with murine typhus are exposed to animals or flea vectors in urban or suburban regions[3,11,29,65] and a small proportion (1% to 40%) report a flea bite or exposure, whereas patients with Rocky Mountain spotted fever often acquire illness after rural exposure or documented tick bites and more often develop rash and petechiae. Eschar is absent in both murine typhus and Rocky Mountain spotted fever, but is more often present in other spotted fever group rickettsioses and scrub typhus. The distribution of rash is of little help in individual cases.[8,28,29,44] The likelihood of monocytic ehrlichiosis or human granulocytic anaplasmosis is diminished if leukopenia and thrombocytopenia are minimal or absent, although serum hepatic transaminase levels may be elevated in murine typhus and ehrlichiosis. Murine typhus, spotted fever rickettsiosis, and ehrlichiosis or anaplasmosis occur during warm seasons, when the arthropod vectors are most active. In contrast, the louse vector of epidemic typhus is most active and likely to spread *R. prowazekii* in cool seasons when layers of clothing are worn, persons are crowded indoors, and personal hygiene diminishes. Differentiation of the sporadic cases of sylvatic typhus caused by *R. prowazekii* from murine typhus may be difficult, but the former illness is suggested when exposure to potential reservoirs (e.g., flying squirrels) is elicited.

There are many differential diagnoses of murine typhus because of its usually nonspecific presentation. Aside from the rickettsioses and ehrlichioses, alternative diagnoses that may need to be considered include meningococcemia, measles, typhoid fever, bacterial and viral meningitis, secondary syphilis, leptospirosis, toxic shock syndrome, and Kawasaki syndrome.

Treatment and Prevention

The preferred drug for treatment of *R. typhi* infection is a tetracycline, such as doxycycline. In vitro, doxycycline, rifampin, chloramphenicol, and the fluoroquinolones—ciprofloxacin, levofloxacin, and pefloxacin—as well as azithromycin, inhibit rickettsial growth, and have ratios of maximal serum concentration (C_{max}) to minimal inhibitory concentration (MIC) (C_{max}/MIC) achievable in human therapy.[66-68] No prospective clinical trials have been conducted regarding treatment of murine typhus; thus, all current recommendations are based on retrospectively analyzed series and cases. The current recommendation is for administration of twice-daily doxycycline, 100 mg orally, or intravenously, in severely ill patients. The use of doxycycline and tetracycline is supported by at least 19 case series that have described treatment in 582 patients.[8,24,28,29,42-49,53,69-75] Although chloramphenicol, 50 to 75 mg/kg/day in four divided doses, has been long advocated as the best alternative treatment for murine typhus, the evidence for its use is derived from 13 case series comprising treatment in only 96 patients.[8,24,28,29,42,43,45,48,53,69,70,73,76] Oral chloramphenicol is not currently available in the United States. Clinical trials of fluoroquinolones for treatment of spotted fever rickettsioses have shown their effectiveness as alternatives to tetracyclines and, for murine typhus, reports of successful treatment [55,77-81] with ciprofloxacin outnumber reports of poor responses,[82] although these data only involved treatment of 37 patients. Corticosteroids are occasionally used for severe central nervous system disease, but no controlled study to evaluate their efficacy has been performed. Infected pregnant patients must be evaluated individually, and doxycycline is preferred (late trimester); alternately, chloramphenicol (early trimester) can be used. Erythromycin has been used twice during pregnancy with murine typhus and resulted in good outcomes.[83,84] Antimicrobial therapy should be continued until 2 to 3 days after defervescence. After initiation of therapy, patients become afebrile at a median interval of 3 days. Single-dose doxycycline therapy was effective in almost 80% of patients in one study[48] but is not routinely advocated because relapse may occur.

Prevention is directed primarily toward the control of flea vectors and potential flea hosts.[10] Because the potential for epidemic spread is associated with foci of infected flea infestations, all suspected cases of murine typhus should be promptly reported to local public health authorities. Although it is usually considered a mild illness, murine typhus may be fatal or severe if misdiagnosed or inadequately treated. Unfortunately, no vaccine of proven effectiveness exists for murine typhus. Recovery from natural infection confers solid, long-lasting immunity to reinfection.

REFERENCES

1. Hone FS. A series of cases closely resembling typhus fever. *Med J Aust.* 1922;1:1-13.
2. Azad AF. Epidemiology of murine typhus. *Annu Rev Entomol.* 1990;35:553-569.
3. Marshall GS. *Rickettsia typhi* seroprevalence among children in the southeast United States. Tick-borne infections in children study (ticks) group. *Pediatr Infect Dis J.* 2000;19:1103-1104.
4. Tay ST, Ho TM, Rohani MY, et al. Antibodies to *Orientia tsutsugamushi, Rickettsia typhi* and spotted fever group rickettsiae among febrile patients in rural areas of Malaysia. *Trans R Soc Trop Med Hyg.* 2000;94:280-284.
5. Lledo L, Gegundez MI, Saz JV, et al. Prevalence of antibodies to *Rickettsia typhi* in an area of the center of Spain. *Eur J Epidemiol.* 2001;17:927-928.
6. Daniel SA, Manika K, Arvanmdou M, et al. Prevalence of *Rickettsia conorii* and *Rickettsia typhi* infections in the population of northern Greece. *Am J Trop Med Hyg.* 2002;66:76-79.
7. Boostrom A, Beier MS, Macaluso JA, et al. Geographic association of *Rickettsia felis*-infected opossums with human murine typhus, Texas. *Emerg Infect Dis.* 2002;8:549-554.
8. Dumler JS, Taylor JP, Walker DH. Clinical and laboratory features of murine typhus in south Texas, 1980 through 1987. *JAMA.* 1991;266:1365-1370.
9. Duffy PE, Le Guillouzic H, Gass RF, et al. Murine typhus identified as a major cause of febrile illness in a camp for displaced Khmers in Thailand. *Am J Trop Med Hyg.* 1990;43:520-526.
10. Azad AF, Radulovic S, Higgins JA, et al. Flea-borne rickettsioses: Ecologic considerations. *Emerg Infect Dis.* 1997;3:319-327.
11. Comer JA, Paddock CD, Childs JE. Urban zoonoses caused by *Bartonella, Coxiella, Ehrlichia*, and *Rickettsia* species. *Vector Borne Zoonotic Dis.* 2001;1:91-118.
12. Bouyer DH, Stenos J, Crocquet-Valdes P, et al. *Rickettsia felis*: Molecular characterization of a new member of the spotted fever group. *Int J Syst Evol Microbiol.* 2001;51(Pt 2):339-347.
13. McLeod MP, Qin X, Karpathy SE, et al. Complete genome sequence of *Rickettsia typhi* and comparison with sequences of other rickettsiae. *J Bacteriol.* 2004;186:5842-5855.
14. Walker DH, Yu XJ. Progress in rickettsial genome analysis from pioneering of *Rickettsia prowazekii* to the recent *Rickettsia typhi*. *Ann N Y Acad Sci.* 2005;1063:13-25.
15. Uchiyama T, Kawano H, Kusuhara Y. The major outer membrane protein rOmpB of spotted fever group Rickettsiae functions in the rickettsial adherence to and invasion of vero cells. *Microbes Infect.* 2006;8:801-809.
16. Radulovic S, Troyer JM, Beier MS, et al. Identification and molecular analysis of the gene encoding *Rickettsia typhi* hemolysin. *Infect Immun.* 1999;67:6104-6108.
17. Rahman MS, Simser JA, Macaluso KR, et al. Functional analysis of *seca* homologues from Rickettsiae. *Microbiology.* 2005;151(Pt 2):589-596.
18. Traub R, Wisseman CL. The ecology of murine typhus—a critical review. *Trop Dis Bull.* 1978;75:237-317.
19. Irons JV, Bohls SW, Thurman DCJ, et al. Probable role of the cat flea, *Ctenocephalides felis*, in transmission of murine typhus. *Am J Trop Med Hyg.* 1944;s1-24:359-362.
20. Civen R, Ngo V. Murine typhus: An unrecognized suburban vectorborne disease. *Clin Infect Dis.* 2008;46:913-918.
21. Texas State Department of Health Services. Murine typhus in Texas, 2008. *EpiLink.* Available at http://www.dshs.state.tx.us/idcu/epilink/volume_65/issue_3/Docs/650305.pdf.
22. Phongmany S, Rolain JM, Phetsouvanh R, et al. Rickettsial infections and fever, Vientiane, Laos. *Emerg Infect Dis.* 2006;12:256-262.
23. Dupont HT, Brouqui P, Faugere B, et al. Prevalence of antibodies to *Coxiella burnetti, Rickettsia conorii*, and *Rickettsia typhi* in seven African countries. *Clin Infect Dis.* 1995;21:1126-1133.
24. Bernabeu-Wittel M, Pachon J, Alarcon A, et al. Murine typhus as a common cause of fever of intermediate duration: A 17-year study in the south of Spain. *Arch Intern Med.* 1999;159:872-876.
25. Hidalgo M, Salguero E, de la Ossa A, et al. Murine typhus in Caldas, Colombia. *Am J Trop Med Hyg.* 2008;78:321-322.
26. Murdoch DR, Woods CW, Zimmerman MD, et al. The etiology of febrile illness in adults presenting to Patan Hospital in Kathmandu, Nepal. *Am J Trop Med Hyg.* 2004;70:670-675.
27. Blacksell SD, Sharma NP, Phumratanaprapin W, et al. Serological and blood culture investigations of Nepalese fever patients. *Trans R Soc Trop Med Hyg.* 2007;101:686-690.
28. Whiteford SF, Taylor JP, Dumler JS. Clinical, laboratory, and epidemiologic features of murine typhus in 97 Texas children. *Arch Pediatr Adolesc Med.* 2001;155:396-400.
29. Gikas A, Doukakis S, Pediaditis J, et al. Murine typhus in Greece: Epidemiological, clinical, and therapeutic data from 83 cases. *Trans R Soc Trop Med Hyg.* 2002;96:250-253.
30. Hassan IS, Ong EL. Fever in the returned traveller. Remember murine typhus! *J Infect Dis.* 1995;31:173-174.
31. Azad AF, Traub R. Experimental transmission of murine typhus by *Xenopsylla cheopis* flea bites. *Med Vet Entomol.* 1989;3:429-433.
32. Farhang-Azad A, Traub R, Baqar S. Transovarial transmission of murine typhus rickettsiae in *Xenopsylla cheopis* fleas. *Science.* 1985;227:543-545.
33. Walker DH, Parks FM, Betz TG, et al. Histopathology and immunohistologic demonstration of the distribution of *Rickettsia typhi* in fatal murine typhus. *Am J Clin Pathol.* 1989;91:720-724.
34. Binford CH, Ecker HD. Endemic (murine) typhus. Report of autopsy findings in three cases. *Am J Clin Pathol.* 1947;17:797-806.
35. Silpapojakul K, Mitarnun W, Ovartlarnporn B, et al. Liver involvement in murine typhus. *QJM.* 1996;89:623-629.
36. Walker DH, Popov VL, Feng HM. Establishment of a novel endothelial target mouse model of a typhus group rickettsiosis: Evidence for critical roles for gamma interferon and CD8 T lymphocytes. *Lab Invest.* 2000;80:1361-1372.
37. Rollwagen FM, Dasch GA, Jerrells TR. Mechanisms of immunity to rickettsial infection: Characterization of a cytotoxic effector cell. *J Immunol.* 1986;136:1418-1421.
38. Crist AE, Jr., Wisseman CL Jr, Murphy JR. Characteristics of lymphoid cells that adoptively transfer immunity to *Rickettsia mooseri* infection in mice. *Infect Immun.* 1984;44:55-60.
39. Murphy JR, Wisseman CL Jr, Fiset P. Mechanisms of immunity in typhus infection: Analysis of immunity to *Rickettsia mooseri* infection of guinea pigs. *Infect Immun.* 1980;27:730-738.
40. Walker DH, Ismail N. Emerging and re-emerging rickettsioses: Endothelial cell infection and early disease events. *Nat Rev Microbiol.* 2008;6:375-386.
41. Feng HM, Whitworth T, Popov V, et al. Effect of antibody on the rickettsia-host cell interaction. *Infect Immun.* 2004;72:3524-3530.
42. Older JJ. The epidemiology of murine typhus in Texas, 1969. *JAMA.* 1970;214:2011-2017.
43. Silpapojakul K, Chupuppakarn S, Yuthasompob S, et al. Scrub and murine typhus in children with obscure fever in the tropics. *Pediatr Infect Dis J.* 1991;10:200-203.
44. Hernandez Cabrera M, Angel-Moreno A, Santana E, et al. Murine typhus with renal involvement in Canary Islands, Spain. *Emerg Infect Dis.* 2004;10:740-743.
45. Koliou M, Psaroulaki A, Georgiou C, et al. Murine typhus in Cyprus: 21 paediatric cases. *Eur J Clin Microbiol Infect Dis.* 2007;26:491-493.
46. Wilde H, Pornsilapatip J, Sokly T, et al. Murine and scrub typhus at Thai-Kampuchean border displaced persons' camps. *Trop Geogr Med.* 1991;43:363-369.
47. Fergie JE, Purcell K, Wanat D. Murine typhus in South Texas children. *Pediatr Infect Dis J.* 2000;19:535-538.
48. Silpapojakul K, Chayakul P, Krisanapan S, et al. Murine typhus in Thailand: Clinical features, diagnosis and treatment. *Q J Med.* 1993;86:43-47.
49. Tselentis Y, Babalis TL, Chrysanthis D, et al. Clinicoepidemiological study of murine typhus on the Greek island of Evia. *Eur J Epidemiol.* 1992;8:268-272.
50. Stuart BM, Pullen RL. Endemic (murine) typhus fever: Clinical observations of 180 cases. *Ann Intern Med.* 1945;23:520-536.
51. Samra Y, Shaked Y, Maier MK. Delayed neurologic display in murine typhus. Report of two cases. *Arch Intern Med.* 1989;149:949-951.
52. Vander T, Medvedovsky M, Valdman S, et al. Facial paralysis and meningitis caused by *Rickettsia typhi* infection. *Scand J Infect Dis.* 2003;35:886-887.
53. Silpapojakul K, Ukkachoke C, Krisanapan S, et al. Rickettsial meningitis and encephalitis. *Arch Intern Med.* 1991;151:1753-1757.
54. Tsiachris D, Deutsch M, Vassilopoulos D, et al. Sensorineural hearing loss complicating severe rickettsial diseases: Report of two cases. *J Infect Dis.* 2008;56:74-76.
55. Vallejo-Maroto I, Garcia-Morillo S, Wittel MB, et al. Aseptic meningitis as a delayed neurologic complication of murine typhus. *Clin Microbiol Infect.* 2002;8:826-827.
56. Hudson HL, Thach AB, Lopez PF. Retinal manifestations of acute murine typhus. *Int Ophthalmol.* 1997;21:121-126.
57. Bernabeu-Wittel M, Villanueva-Marcos JL, de Alarcon-Gonzalez A, et al. Septic shock and multiorganic failure in murine typhus. *Eur J Clin Microbiol Infect Dis.* 1998;17:131-132.
58. Hechemy KE, Stevens RW, Sasowski S, et al. Discrepancies in Weil-Felix and microimmunofluorescence test results for Rocky Mountain spotted fever. *J Clin Microbiol.* 1979;9:292-293.
59. La Scola B, Rydkina L, Ndihokubwayo JB, et al. Serological differentiation of murine typhus and epidemic typhus using cross-adsorption and Western blotting. *Clin Diagn Lab Immunol.* 2000;7:612-616.
60. Walker DH, Feng HM, Ladner S, et al. Immunohistochemical diagnosis of typhus rickettsioses using an anti-lipopolysaccharide monoclonal antibody. *Mod Pathol.* 1997;10:1038-1042.

61. Carl M, Tibbs CW, Dobson ME, et al. Diagnosis of acute typhus infection using the polymerase chain reaction. *J Infect Dis.* 1990;161:791-793.

62. Paris DH, Blacksell SD, Stenos J, et al. Real-time multiplex PCR assay for detection and differentiation of rickettsiae and orientiae. *Trans R Soc Trop Med Hyg.* 2008;102:186-193.

63. Miller ES, Beeson PB. Murine typhus fever. *Medicine.* 1946;25:1-15.

64. Keysary A, Strenger C. Use of enzyme-linked immunosorbent assay techniques with cross-reacting human sera in diagnosis of murine typhus and spotted fever. *J Clin Microbiol.* 1997;35:1034-1035.

65. Sorvillo FJ, Gondo B, Emmons R, et al. A suburban focus of endemic typhus in Los Angeles County: Association with sero-positive domestic cats and opossums. *Am J Trop Med Hyg.* 1993;48:269-273.

66. Keren G, Itzhaki A, Oron C, et al. Evaluation of the anti-rickettsial activity of fluoroquinolones. *Drugs.* 1995;49(Suppl 2):208-210.

67. Keysary A, Itzhaki A, Rubinstein E, et al. The in-vitro anti-rickettsial activity of macrolides. *J Antimicrob Chemother.* 1996;38:727-731.

68. Rolain JM, Maurin M, Vestris G, et al. In vitro susceptibilities of 27 rickettsiae to 13 antimicrobials. *Antimicrob Agents Chemother.* 1998;42:1537-1541.

69. Giroud P, Le Gac P, Rouby M, et al. [Contribution to the study of rickettsial diseases in Oubangui-Chari following brush fire; 4 new cases in Bangui; clinical cases, serological behavior, isolation of strains; spectacular results of antibiotics.] *Bull Soc Pathol Exot Filiales.* 1951;44:871-879.

70. Taylor JP, Betz TG, Rawlings JA. Epidemiology of murine typhus in Texas. 1980 through 1984. *JAMA.* 1986;255:2173-2176.

71. Bitsori M, Galanakis E, Gikas A, et al. *Rickettsia typhi* infection in childhood. *Acta Paediatr.* 2002;91:59-61.

72. Centers for Disease Control. Murine typhus—Hawaii, 2002. *MMWR Morb Mortal Wkly Rep.* 2003;52:1224-1226.

73. Gikas A, Doukakis S, Pediaditis J, et al. Comparison of the effectiveness of five different antibiotic regimens on infection with *Rickettsia typhi*: Therapeutic data from 87 cases. *Am J Trop Med Hyg.* 2004;70:576-579.

74. Letaief AO, Kaabia N, Chakroun M, et al. Clinical and laboratory features of murine typhus in central Tunisia: A report of seven cases. *Int J Infect Dis.* 2005;9:331-334.

75. Gray E, Atatoa-Carr P, Bell A, et al. Murine typhus: A newly recognised problem in the Waikato region of New Zealand. *N Z Med J.* 2007;120:U2661.

76. Smadel JE, Leon AP, Ley HL, et al. Chloromycetin in the treatment of patients with typhus fever. *Proc Soc Exp Biol Med.*1948;68:12-19.

77. Gomez J, Molina Boix M, Banos V, et al. [Murine typhus. Efficacy of treatment with ciprofloxacin.] *Enferm Infecc Microbiol Clin.* 1992;10:377.

78. Eaton M, Cohen MT, Shlim DR, et al. Ciprofloxacin treatment of typhus. *JAMA.* 1989;262:772-773.

79. Strand O, Stromberg A. Ciprofloxacin treatment of murine typhus. *Scand J Infect Dis.* 1990;22:503-504.

80. Van Der Kleij FG, Gansevoort RT, Kreeftenberg HG, et al. Imported rickettsioses: Think of murine typhus. *J Intern Med.* 1998;243:177-179.

81. Raoult D, Drancourt M. Antimicrobial therapy of rickettsial diseases. *Antimicrob Agents Chemother.* 1991;35:2457-2462.

82. Laferl H, Fournier PE, Seiberl G, et al. Murine typhus poorly responsive to ciprofloxacin: A case report. *J Travel Med.* 2002;9:103-104.

83. Koliou M, Christoforou C, Soteriades ES. Murine typhus in pregnancy: A case report from Cyprus. *Scand J Infect Dis.* 2007;39:625-628.

84. Graves SR, Banks J, Dwyer B, et al. A case of murine typhus in Queensland. *Med J Aust.* 1992;156:650-651.

192

Orientia tsutsugamushi (Scrub Typhus)

DIDIER RAOULT

Scrub typhus is a rickettsiosis caused by *Orientia tsutsugamushi* and transmitted by a chigger bite. It is a rural disease prevalent in much of the world. Its distribution is documented in a triangle limited by northern Japan, eastern Australia, and eastern Russia that includes the Indian subcontinent, western Russia, China, and the Far East. It has been known in the Far East for more than 1500 years. One billion people live in the endemic area. As many as 1 million may be infected yearly (Fig. 192-1).

Etiology

O. tsutsugamushi is a rickettsial organism formerly named *Rickettsia tsutsugamushi* (until 1995).[1] This bacterium exhibits a wide heterogenicity that may lead to the defining of several species in this genus. Major serotypes have been identified and must be included in serologic tests to detect scrub typhus, including serotypes Gilliam, Karp, Kato, Boryon, and Kawazaki. *O. tsutsugamushi* is transmitted by the bite of thrombiculid mite larvae (chiggers). It is transmitted transovarially in mites and generates a deviation of the gender ratio in infected females that favors females. Seasonality of the disease is determined by the appearance of larvae. In temperate zones, scrub typhus season is observed mainly in the autumn but also in the spring.

Epidemiology

The disease has been known since ancient times. The first description was documented in 313 AD in China. Scrub typhus is a common disease in endemic areas. A type of mite called chiggers is prevalent in rural areas, and local residents as well as tourists are exposed to their bite. In the past, military personnel, during wars in the Far East, were frequently infected, and it may have been one of the first infections that they experienced. During the Vietnam War, it was the second or third most common cause of fever in American soldiers.[2,3] Its current prevalence is not known, but in Thailand and Laos, along with leptospirosis and murine typhus, it is one of the two most frequent infections reported in hospitalized patients. It is also common in India but is apparently grossly underreported.

Clinical Manifestations

The major signs and symptoms of scrub typhus include fever, mental changes, headache, inoculation eschar, and lymphadenopathy (Table 192-1).[4-5a] Ten or more days after exposure, the onset of the disease is abrupt, with fever, headache, and myalgia. Ability to differentiate the eschar from the mite bite, as with tick-borne disease, highly depends on the investigator. In a survey in Japan, where it was considered prevalent in 50% of cases, a trained physician found it in 100% of cases.[6]

The patient can have several eschars. The rash is macular, pale, and transient and is easily missed. Lymph nodes may be tender and are sometimes limited to the site proximal to the mite bite. Hepatomegaly and splenomegaly can be observed. Mental changes are usual and range from slight intellectual blunting to coma or delirium.[4] Compared to murine typhus, scrub typhus more commonly presents with eschar and lymphadenopathy.[7]

In severe cases, evolution to a multiple-organ dysfunction syndrome with hemorrhage can be observed. After apparent recovery, relapses frequently occur and may also follow short treatment courses. Relapse is usually less severe than the first attack. Surprisingly, scrub typhus has been reported to lead to a diminution of viral load in human immunodeficiency virus (HIV)–1 infected patients and to help restore the immune status of infected patients.[8] A wide variation in prevalence of cutaneous symptoms has been noted, as well as in severity and fatality rate. This varies with published series, year of publication, and country and population studied. The fatality rate during scrub typhus before the advent of chemotherapy was widely variable,[6] from 3% in Taiwan to 60% on the northern coast of Japan. It is still a life-threat-

Figure 192-1 Geographic distribution of scrub typhus. Darker colors indicate areas with a higher incidence.

TABLE 192-1	Scrub Typhus: Prevalence of Signs and Symptoms	
	Phongmany[5a]	*Tattersall*[4]
Year	2006	1945
Number of cases	31	500
Location	Laos	India, Burma
Population	Local residents	Soldiers and local residents
Signs and Symptoms		
Fever	100%	
Mental changes		100%
Headache	95%	100%
Cough	38%	68%
Myalgia	95%	
Nausea	62%	
Adenopathy	59%	92%
Eschar	52%	11%
Splenomegaly	59%	47%
Rash	27%	64%
Case-fatality rate	1.5%	6%

ening disease despite efficient treatment. During pregnancy, scrub typhus frequently leads to spontaneous abortion.[9]

Biologically, lymphocyte count is decreased and the T4 : T8 ratio is diminished. Liver enzyme levels are increased in 60% of cases. Thrombocytopenia may be sufficient to cause bleeding.

Diagnosis

Serology is the preferred diagnostic tool. Immunofluorescence and immunoperoxidase are the most reliable. However there is a wide variety of results in different laboratories.[10] Several strains must be included in the serology because there are wide differences in the antigens and genotypes between strains in different regions, a variability that has also hampered development.[10a] The Weil-Felix test detects cross-reacting antibodies to *Proteus mirabilis* OX-K. The Weil-Felix test is still used because of its low cost. Isolation of *O. tsutsugamushi* can be done in cell culture or in inoculated mice. The organism is visualized in the spleens of infected mice by Giemsa (or Diff-Quick) staining, not by Gimenez stain, as is used for *Rickettsia*. Polymerase chain reaction amplification of blood, skin, or lymph node samples is useful. Usually, the primers are selected from the gene that codes for the 56-kDa protein gene.[11,12]

Treatment

Doxycycline and, overseas, chloramphenicol remain the preferred treatment approaches.[13] Doxycycline is usually given as 100 mg PO twice daily for 7 days but can also be given in a single dose or for short periods (3 to 7 days), although relapse can occur . Doxycycline is recommended for use in children as well. Chloramphenicol is given as 50 to 75 mg/kg per day in four divided doses. Parola and associates[13] have reported that some patients responded poorly to doxycycline and chloramphenicol. Alternative drugs, including rifampin (600 to 900 mg/day) and azithromycin (500 mg the first day and 250 mg/day later),[14] can also be prescribed for pregnant women. Ciprofloxacin, in experience with parturient women in India, is ineffective and should not be used.[9]

Prevention is limited to the use of insect repellents, such as DEET, during travel in rural areas of endemic countries. No vaccine is available.

REFERENCES

1. Tamura A, Ohashi N, Urakami H, et al. Classification of *Rickettsia tsutsugamushi* in a new genus, *Orientia* gen nov, as *Orientia tsutsugamushi* comb. nov. *Int J Syst Bacteriol.* 1995;45:589-591.
2. Deller JJ, Russell PK. An analysis of fevers of unknown origin in American soldiers in Vietnam. *Ann Intern Med.* 1967;66:1129-1143.
3. Berman SJ, Irving GS, Kundin WD, et al. Epidemiology of the acute fevers of unknown origin in South Vietnam: Effect of laboratory support upon clinical diagnosis. *Am J Trop Med Hyg.* 1973;22:796-801.
4. Tattersall RN. *Tsutsugamushi* fever on the India-Burma border. *Lancet.* 1945;2:392-394.
5. Berman SJ, Kundin WD. Scrub typhus in South Vietnam. A study of 87 cases. *Ann Intern Med.* 1973;79:26-30.
5a. Phongmany S, Rolain JM, Phetsouvanh R, et al. Rickettsial infections and fever, Vientiane, Laos. *Emerg Infect Dis.* 2006;12:256-262.
6. Kawamura AJ, Tanaka H, Tamura A. *Tsutsugamushi Disease.* Tokyo: University of Tokyo Press; 1995.
7. Phongmany S, Rolain JM, Phetsouvanh R, et al. Rickettsial infections and fever, Vientiane, Laos. *Emerg Infect Dis.* 2006;12:256-262.
8. Watt G, Kantipong P, de Souza M, et al. HIV-1 suppression during acute scrub-typhus infection. *Lancet.* 2000;356:475-479.
9. Mathai E, Rolain JM, Verghese L, et al. Case reports: Scrub typhus during pregnancy in India. *Trans R Soc Trop Med Hyg.* 2003;97:570-572.
10. Blacksell SD, Bryant NJ, Paris DH, et al. Scrub typhus serologic testing with the indirect immunofluorescence method as a diagnostic gold standard: a lack of consensus leads to a lot of confusion. *Clin Infect Dis.* 2007;44:391-401.
10a. Kelly DJ, Furest PA, Ching W-M, Richards AL. Scrub typhus: the geographic distribution of phenotypic and genotypic variants of *Orientia tsutsugamushi. Clin Infect Dis.* 2009;38:S203-S230.
11. Furuya Y, Yoshida Y, Katayama T, et al. Specific amplification of *Rickettsia tsutsugamushi* DNA from clinical specimens by polymerase chain reaction. *J Clin Microbiol.* 1991;29:2628-2630.
12. Fournier PE, Siritantikorn S, Rolain JM, et al. Detection of new genotypes of Orientia tsutsugamushi infecting humans in Thailand. *Clin Microbiol Infect.* 2008;14:168-173.
13. Parola P, Watt G, Brouqui P. *Orientia tsutsugamushi* (scrub typhus). In: Yu VL, Weber R, Raoult D, eds. *Antimicrobial Therapy and Vaccine.* 2nd ed. New York: Apple Trees Productions; 2002:883-887.
14. Phimda K, Hoontrakul S, Suttinont C, et al. Doxycycline versus azithromycin for treatment of leptospirosis and scrub typhus. *Antimicrob Agents Chemother.* 2007;51:3259-3263.

193

Ehrlichia chaffeensis (Human Monocytotropic Ehrlichiosis), Anaplasma phagocytophilum (Human Granulocytotropic Anaplasmosis), and Other Anaplasmataceae

J. STEPHEN DUMLER | DAVID H. WALKER

Until 1987, infections by members of the family Anaplasmataceae, including the genera *Ehrlichia, Anaplasma,* and *Neorickettsia,* were known mainly as veterinary diseases (Table 193-1). Canine ehrlichiosis was first described in 1935 by Donatien and Lestoquard in Algeria. This disease is produced by *Ehrlichia canis,* which is transmitted to dogs by *Rhipicephalus sanguineus* ticks. The disease was characterized by fever associated with the presence of clusters of small Giemsa-stained organisms in circulating monocytes. *Ehrlichia* spp. generally have a tick vector and tropism for either macrophages or granulocytes where they grow within cytoplasmic membrane-bound vacuoles. Consequently, *Ehrlichia* was recognized as distinct from other genera of obligate intracellular bacteria of medical importance (*Rickettsia, Coxiella,* and *Chlamydia*). In 1937, the genus *Ehrlichia* was suggested in honor of the German bacteriologist Paul Ehrlich.[1] Subsequent phylogenetic studies have shown that two other economically important veterinary pathogens, *Anaplasma marginale* (described in 1910) and *Ehrlichia* (formerly *Cowdria*) *ruminantium* (described in 1925), are also ehrlichiae.[2] The first human disease demonstrated to have an ehrlichial cause was sennetsu neorickettsiosis, an infectious mononucleosis–like illness recognized to have occurred only in western Japan, Malaysia, and Laos. Although human infections caused by all members of the reorganized family Anaplasmataceae have been generically referred to as "ehrlichiosis" and the causative agents are referred to as "ehrlichiae," it is increasingly apparent that the clinical manifestations and causative agents are distinct.

The first diagnosed case of human ehrlichiosis in the United States occurred in a 51-year-old man who became ill in April 1986, 12 to 14 days after tick bites in rural Arkansas.[3] Although initially thought to be caused by the canine pathogen *Ehrlichia canis,* the main causative agent of human monocytotropic ehrlichiosis (HME), *Ehrlichia chaffeensis,* was finally described in 1990.[4] In 1994, *Anaplasma phagocytophilum* was identified as the causative agent of a distinctly different infection, now called human granulocytotropic anaplasmosis (HGA).[5,6]

Etiology

Members of the family Anaplasmataceae are defined predominantly by their genetic similarities and differences but also by phenotypic characteristics and host affinities (see Table 193-1). These are small (0.5-µm) gram-negative bacteria. Their clustered inclusion-like appearance of a microcolony in the host cell vacuole is called a morula, from the Latin word for mulberry (Fig. 193-1).

The taxonomic relationships of *Ehrlichia, Anaplasma, Neorickettsia, Wolbachia, Orientia, Rickettsia, Coxiella,* and *Chlamydia* have been clarified by molecular and metabolic studies. The evolutionary relationships determined by *rrs* (16S ribosomal RNA gene) and *groESL* comparisons indicate that *Ehrlichia, Anaplasma, Neorickettsia, Wolba-*chia, *Orientia,* and *Rickettsia* evolved from a common ancestor[2,4]; in contrast, *Coxiella* and *Chlamydia* are phylogenetically unrelated to ehrlichiae. Ehrlichiae and chlamydiae superficially resemble one another in that both reside within cytoplasmic vacuoles. Unlike chlamydiae, however, ehrlichiae are able to synthesize adenosine triphosphate by metabolism of glutamine, a metabolic characteristic shared with members of the genus *Rickettsia.* The family Anaplasmataceae contains four genera that are actually very different from one another. *E. chaffeensis* shares many antigens and genetic sequences with the canine pathogens, *E. canis* and *Ehrlichia ewingii, Ehrlichia muris* found in Japanese wild mice, voles, and ticks, and the ruminant pathogen, *E. ruminantium.*[4,7-9] A second genus includes a granulocytotropic bacterium that can infect humans, *A. phagocytophilum,* that is related genetically to *Anaplasma platys, A. bovis,* and *A. marginale.*[2,6] The third contains *Neorickettsia sennetsu,* which is closely related to *Neorickettsia risticii, Neorickettsia helminthoeca,* and an unnamed organism found in Japanese fish flukes. The fourth genus, *Wolbachia,* contains bacterial endosymbionts of invertebrates, including insects and helminths, some of which may contribute to disease in human filariasis.

Ehrlichia and *Anaplasma* have two ultrastructural forms, a larger reticulate cell and a smaller, dense core cell, and the cell wall differs from that of *Rickettsia* spp., with thinner outer and inner leaflets reflecting the absence of lipopolysaccharide and lipooligosaccharide.[10] Genes coding for the enzymes required for the biosynthesis of peptidoglycan and lipopolysaccharide are not present in the *E. chaffeensis* or *A. phagocytophilum* genome.[11] The genomes of these obligately intracellular bacteria are small, ranging from 1.2 to 1.6 Mb to as low as 900 kb for *Neorickettsia.* Bacteria in the Anaplasmataceae family possess multiple genes that are members of the pfam01617.8, Surface_Ag_2 gene family, encoding major surface porin proteins responsible for antigenic variation and host cell adhesion in genera as diverse as *Neisseria, Brucella,* and *Pseudomonas. E. chaffeensis, E. canis, E. ewingii,* and *A. phagocytophilum* have gene families that encode more than 19 paralogous, surface-exposed pfam01617.8 proteins of 22 to 30 kDa (p28/Omp-1 family) for *Ehrlichia* and approximately 105 paralogous genes encoding 41 to 49 kDa (major surface protein-2 [Msp2]) for *A. phagocytophilum.*[12-14] In accordance with the pfam01617.8 predictions, roles for *A. phagocytophilum* Msp2 in binding to surfaces of neutrophils and in antigenic variation have been shown,[15,16] and Msp2/p44 and p28/Omp-1 could function as porins in both *A. phagocytophilum* and *E. chaffeensis.*[17,18] Antigenic diversity within a single strain is based on the presence of hypervariable regions in the *Ehrlichia p28/omp1* family, where each gene is transcribed independently yet is dominated by the expression of a single protein in mammalian infection.[19,20] Reinfections with different *E. chaffeensis* and *A. phagocytophilum* strains have been reported, underscoring the role of antigenic diversity in immune protection.[21,22] Similarly, Msp2/p44

Causative Agent	Mammalian Host	Major Target Cell	Vector, Transmission
Ehrlichia chaffeensis	Humans, deer, dogs, coyotes, marsh deer	Macrophages	Ticks (Amblyomma americanum, Dermacentor variabilis, and Ixodes pacificus)
Ehrlichia ewingii	Dogs, humans, deer	Granulocytes	Ticks (A. americanum, D. variabilis)
Ehrlichia muris	Humans, Apodemus mice, vole	Unknown	Ticks (Ixodes persulcatus, Haemaphysalis flava)
Ehrlichia canis	Dogs, humans	Macrophages	Ticks (Rhipicephalus sanguineus)
Ehrlichia ruminantium	Cattle, sheep, wild ruminants	Endothelial cells	Ticks (Amblyomma variegatum)
Anaplasma phagocytophilum	Humans, white-footed mice, wood rats, bank voles, wood mice, yellow-necked mice, horses, dogs, cats, sheep, cattle, white-tailed deer, roe deer, red deer, fallow deer	Granulocytes	Ticks (Ixodes scapularis, Ixodes pacificus, Ixodes ricinus, Ixodes persulcatus)
Anaplasma platys	Dogs	Platelets, macrophages	Unknown
Anaplasma marginale	Cattle, wild ruminants	Erythrocytes	Ticks (e.g., Boophilus, Rhipicephalus)
Neorickettsia sennetsu	Humans	Macrophages	Possibly ingestion of raw fish
Neorickettsia risticii	Horses	Macrophages, enterocytes, mast cells	Unknown
Neorickettsia helminthoeca	Dogs	Macrophages	Ingestion of fluke-infested salmon

TABLE 193-1 Ehrlichiae Causing Medical and Veterinary Diseases

Epidemiology of Human Monocytic Ehrlichiosis

Human ehrlichioses are tick-borne zoonoses.[30,31] Most patients give a history of tick exposure during the month before the onset of illness. The seasonality of HME, with peak incidence in May to August, reflects the tick-transmitted epidemiology.[32] Exposures are predominantly rural and suburban and involve recreational, peridomestic, occupational, and military activities. More than 66% of patients are male. Documented cases of HME have been reported in 47 states, particularly in the south-central and southeastern United States. This region conforms to the distribution of the Lone Star tick, *Amblyomma americanum*; along with white-tailed deer, this maintains the ehrlichiae in nature by acquiring *E. chaffeensis* during feeding as a larva or nymph on persistently infected deer and subsequently transmitting ehrlichiae to nonimmune deer. The pathogen is transmitted transstadially from larvae to nymphs and from nymphs to adults, but not transovarially.[33] On the other hand, *E. chaffeensis* is also found in *Dermacentor variabilis* and *Ixodes pacificus*, potential additional vectors.[34-36] Organisms closely related to *E. chaffeensis* and evidence of human ehrlichial infections have also been reported in South America, Africa, and Eastern Asia.[37-42]

In a prospective study of hospitalized patients in the state of Georgia, 11% with fever of undetermined cause were demonstrated by seroconversion to have HME.[43] An active, prospective, 3-year study in Cape Girardeau, Missouri, revealed 29 cases in a family practice of 7,000 patients, an average annual incidence of 138 cases per 100,000 population.[44] Similarly, selected communities in the Midwest have prevalences as high as 330 cases/100,000 population under permissive ecologic circumstances.[45]

Since 1987, 3687 cases of HME have been reported to the Centers for Disease Control and Prevention (CDC). Currently, most infections are not diagnosed. HME requires hospitalization in 42% of cases and is life-threatening in 17%; thus, it is suspected that asymptomatic seroconversion reflects exposure to another *Ehrlichia* or *Anaplasma* species or another antigenic stimulus. *E. canis* that induces cross-reactive serologic responses has been isolated from patients in South America, and *E. ewingii* is known to cause milder infections that result in serologic cross-reactions with *E. chaffeensis*.[46,47] A single case of

of *A. phagocytophilum* is characterized by conserved domains that flank a hypervariable region, but expression requires gene conversion into a single genomic site. This condition may be further complicated by segmental conversion that generates even greater antigenic complexity.[23-25] Infection in vivo yields a large number of transcriptional and antigenic variants that presumably contribute to persistence in reservoir hosts.[26] In addition, *E. chaffeensis* and *E. canis* have several antigenic surface–exposed proteins such as p120, which contains two to five tandem repeat regions, is differentially expressed on infective dense core cells, and plays a role in adhesion to the target cell.[27,28] Both species express functional type IV secretion systems, and at least one *A. phagocytophilum* substrate, AnkA, has been identified that is translocated into the infected host cell. There it plays a crucial role in bacterial entry by interacting with Abl-interactor 1 (abl-i), which influences epidermal growth factor receptor (EGFR) signal transduction and cytoskeletal changes.[29] AnkA eventually migrates to complex with host nuclear heterochromatin, where it likely influences host gene transcription. Both bacteria also express two-component histidine kinase regulatory systems that influence trafficking of the parasitophorous vacuole after bacterial entry.[18]

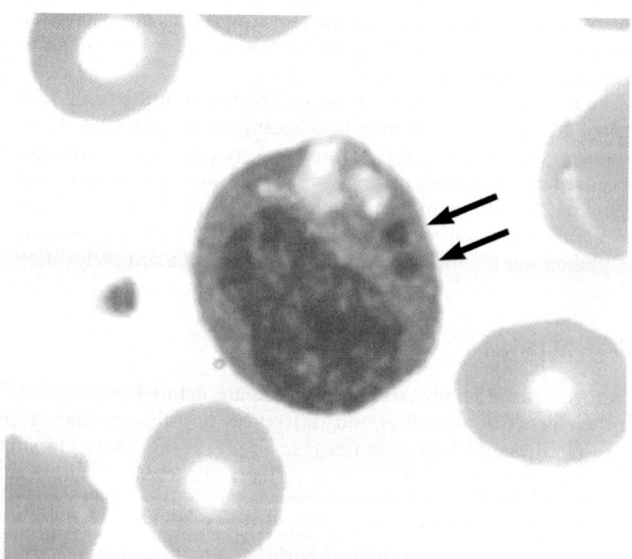

Figure 193-1 Human monocytotropic ehrlichiosis. Peripheral blood smear (buffy coat preparation) showing intracellular inclusions (*arrows*) in mononuclear cells of a patient with human monocytotropic ehrlichiosis (Wright stain, ×400).

infection by an *Ehrlichia ruminantium*–like bacterium, called the Panola Mountain *Ehrlichia*, has been identified in a 31-year-old man from Georgia.[48] Although there is a potential for transfusion-transmitted HME,[49] no specific transfusion-related infections by *E. chaffeensis, E. canis,* or *E. ewingii* have been described.

EPIDEMIOLOGY AND EPIZOOTIOLOGY OF HUMAN GRANULOCYTIC ANAPLASMOSIS

HGA has a seasonal occurrence, peaking in June but persisting through December in the eastern United States, in accordance with the activity of nymphal and adult stages of *Ixodes scapularis* ticks.[50] Although risk for HGA is associated with outdoor activity, a substantial proportion of cases occurs in suburban areas of northeastern and upper Midwestern cities.[51] HGA occurs in specific geographic locations—92% of cases are reported from southern New England, New York, New Jersey, Wisconsin, and Minnesota.[52] The distribution is almost identical to that of Lyme disease because of the shared *Ixodes* spp. tick vectors. HGA has been documented broadly throughout Europe, particularly in Slovenia, Sweden, and Norway, as well as in Asia.[38] Serologic studies have suggested a global distribution in the northern hemisphere for HGA, *A. phagocytophilum,* and its tick vectors.[53,54]

The incidence of HGA is not known; however, active case collection has yielded an incidence of 14 to 16 cases/100,000 population in the upper Midwest between 1990 and 1995, with rates as high as 24 to 58 cases/100,000 population in some northwest Wisconsin counties from 1994 to 1995 and in Connecticut from 1997 to 1999.[50,55] Cross-sectional seroprevalence studies have shown that up to 15% of the population in northwestern Wisconsin, 1% of Connecticut residents and U.S. military personnel, 17% of Slovenians, and 12% of the population of Sweden's Koster Islands have antibodies reactive with *A. phagocytophilum* in the absence of antecedent evidence for HGA.[56-59] Similar high seroprevalence exists in the state of New York but has been attributed to nonspecificity in the analytic method.[60] The demonstration of mildly affected patients who recover spontaneously, even in the absence of specific therapy, suggests that HGA may frequently be subclinical or asymptomatic.[61]

Between 4% and 36% of patients with serologic evidence of *A. phagocytophilum* infection also have serologic evidence of *Borrelia burgdorferi* or *Babesia microti* infection; both agents are also transmitted by *Ixodes* spp. tick bites.[56,60] Concurrent human granulocytic ehrlichiosis and Lyme disease, documented by isolation of both agents, has been reported,[62] although a prospective study has shown only a 2% incidence of coinfection in patients with erythema migrans and Lyme disease.[63] Coinfection with tick-borne encephalitis has been demonstrated in Europe.[64] Whether concurrent infection by these agents results in increased severity, prolonged duration of illness, or more frequent and severe sequelae has yet to be determined.[65]

A. phagocytophilum is transmitted to humans by the bites of nymphal and adult *I. scapularis* ticks in the eastern United States, *I. pacificus* in California, *Ixodes ricinus* in Europe, and presumably *Ixodes persulcatus* in Asia. Although transstadial transmission of the infectious agent occurs, *A. phagocytophilum* is not maintained transovarially, and thus natural maintenance requires horizontal (tick-mammal-tick) transmission.[31] A major proven reservoir host is the white-footed mouse, *Peromyscus leucopus*; however, other small mammals, such as sciurids (squirrels) in the western U.S., and ruminants have been found naturally infected or have serologic evidence of infection, including voles, wood rats, white-tailed deer, red deer, and roe deer.[66-68] Current serologic evidence suggests that larval ticks acquire *A. phagocytophilum* after feeding on small mammals infected earlier in the season by nymphal ticks. White-footed mice develop immunity to *A. phagocytophilum* after a period of bacteremia that may last from several days to weeks; prior immunity reduces small mammal reservoir competence and transmission.[69] Small mammals are not adversely affected by the infection, and some may become persistently infected. The contribution of persistently infected ruminants and cervids as reservoir hosts for *A. phagocytophilum* requires further investigation.

Pathogenesis and Pathology

HUMAN MONOCYTOTROPIC EHRLICHIOSIS

After entering the skin by tick bite inoculation and being spread presumably through lymphatic and blood vessels, ehrlichiae invade target cells of the hematopoietic and lymphoreticular systems. Morulae of *E. chaffeensis* are observed mainly in macrophages and monocytes, less frequently in lymphocytes, and rarely in polymorphonuclear leukocytes.[70-72] Ehrlichial morulae have been identified in peripheral blood, bone marrow, hepatic sinusoids, lymph nodes, splenic cords, splenic sinusoids, splenic periarteriolar lymphoid sheaths, cerebrospinal fluid (CSF) macrophages, and macrophages in perivascular lymphohistiocytic infiltrates in organs such as the kidney, appendix, and heart.

The best studied tissue in HME is bone marrow, largely owing to the frequency of leukopenia, thrombocytopenia, and anemia. Frequent findings include granulomas, myeloid hyperplasia, and megakaryocytosis.[70] Erythrophagocytosis and plasmacytosis occur in smaller proportions of patients with HME. Focal hepatocellular necrosis, hepatic granulomas including ring granulomas, cholestasis, splenic and lymph node necrosis, diffuse mononuclear phagocyte hyperplasia in the spleen, liver, lymph node, and bone marrow, perivascular lymphohistiocytic infiltrates of various organs including kidney, heart, liver, meninges and brain, and interstitial mononuclear cell pneumonitis have also been observed.[71,72] It is worthy of emphasis that endothelial injury and thrombosis have not been described. The observation of erythrophagocytosis, myeloid hyperplasia, and megakaryocytosis in the bone marrow of patients with HME suggests peripheral consumption of blood elements and a compensatory response.

Although *E. chaffeensis* causes a direct cytopathic effect when grown in cell culture,[73] it appears that the host responses account for most of the clinical manifestations. The toxic shock manifestations of HME are likely to be the systemic effects of proinflammatory cytokines, including interleukin-10 (IL-10) and tumor necrosis factor-α (TNF-α).[74] The latter cytokine is produced by hyperactivated CD8 T lymphocytes in murine models and possibly humans and, together with perforin expressed by these cells, results in significant reductions in interferon-γ (IFN-γ) expression and apoptotic tissue injury.[75,76] IFN-γ stimulates macrophage killing of *E. chaffeensis* through the sequestration of iron, and opsonization with immune serum enhances the destruction of ehrlichiae by macrophages.[77,78] Ehrlichial infection is controlled by a combination of NKT, CD4, and CD8 T lymphocytes, antibodies, IFN-γ, IL-10, and TNF-α. *E. chaffeensis* circumvents host defenses by inhibiting the fusion of infected phagosomes with lysosomes and inhibiting the signal transduction pathway of IFN-γ–mediated anti-ehrlichial activity.[79] There is evidence that *E. chaffeensis* also evades immunity by downregulation of other host defense genes of the infected macrophage and manipulation of host cell as a niche favorable to its survival and growth.[80,81]

HUMAN GRANULOCYTOTROPIC ANAPLASMOSIS

A. phagocytophilum is observed predominantly in neutrophils in peripheral blood and tissues from infected individuals.[50,72] Dramatic histopathologic findings involve the presence of opportunistic pathogens, especially severe fungal and viral infections that account for most fatalities. Pathologic findings in humans and animal models include normocellular or hypercellular bone marrow, erythrophagocytosis in mononuclear phagocytic organs, hepatic apoptosis and periportal lymphohistiocytic infiltrates, focal splenic necrosis, and mild interstitial pneumonitis and pulmonary hemorrhage.[82] Vasculitis, endothelial injury, granulomas, and meningeal inflammation have not been described.

A. phagocytophilum disseminate to bone marrow and spleen after a tick bite. In the bone marrow, progenitors of myeloid and monocytic lineages are infected.[83] Endothelial cells can be infected in vitro, and possibly in vivo[84]; a definitive role for endothelial infection in vivo has yet to be shown. With neutrophil infection, the ehrlichiae attach to the cell surface platelet selectin ligand-1 (PSGL-1), and perhaps other ligands, enter an endosome that avoids lysosomal fusion, and replicate.[85,86] In vitro, *A. phagocytophilum* survive by deactivation of the neutrophil antimicrobial response through inhibition of granulocyte *RAC2* and *CYBB* (*gp91^phox*) transcription, downregulation of phagocyte oxidase activity, delay of apoptosis, ineffective binding to and transmigration of activated endothelium, and inhibition of phagocytic activity.[87-90] However, infection also paradoxically stimulates an inflammatory response with neutrophil activation, with chemokine secretion and degranulation.[91] Increased proinflammatory activity allows the recruitment of new neutrophil host cells and localized tissue injury that may further exacerbate inflammatory stimulation when neutrophils cannot generate effective antimicrobial responses. These findings are consistent with the dissociation of bacterial burden and histopathologic evidence of tissue injury in the mouse model, suggesting a role for host immunity in disease.[92] *A. phagocytophilum* infection is initially controlled by IFN-γ, which results in macrophage activation and marked increases in inflammatory tissue injury in mouse models, paralleling evidence of macrophage activation as a mechanism of increased severity in humans.[93]

Clinical Manifestations

HUMAN MONOCYTOTROPIC EHRLICHIOSIS

Signs and Symptoms
The clinical picture of HME in immunocompetent patients is of a mild to severe multisystemic illness, with a median duration of 23 days (Table 193-2).[43,44,94-98] Approximately 12% to 30% of infections have been reported in immunocompromised patients in whom *E. chaffeensis* acts as an opportunistic pathogen and can cause a fatal overwhelming infection.[32,99-103] The median incubation period is 7 days. Symptoms at onset of illness include fever, chills, headache, myalgia, and malaise. Later in the course, patients often develop nausea, anorexia, vomiting, and weight loss. Physical signs are not striking. Fewer than half of patients have a rash, which is maculopapular and may be petechial. Rash is observed much more frequently in children. Adult patients with severe illness are more likely to have a cough, diarrhea, confusion,

and lymphadenopathy, whereas pediatric patients may develop edema of the hands or feet. Severe complications occur in 17% of patients and include adult respiratory distress syndrome (18% require mechanical ventilation), acute renal insufficiency, central nervous system (CNS) abnormalities, including meningoencephalitis, coagulopathy, gastrointestinal hemorrhage, and even death.[72,104,105] CSF pleocytosis usually shows a predominance of lymphocytes and increased protein concentration and can demonstrate the presence of infected cells.[104] Nearly half of patients with chest roentgenographic evaluation have infiltrates. Failure to recognize the frequency of pulmonary and CNS involvement is associated with delayed treatment and greater likelihood of ICU admission and severe complications.[101]

Important laboratory features are thrombocytopenia, mild to moderate leukopenia, and elevations of serum hepatic transaminase levels (see Table 193-2).[95-106] The nadir of leukopenia is usually between 1300 and 4000 cells/μL. Neutropenia, lymphopenia, or both combined account for the leukopenia. Thrombocytopenia occurs concurrently with leukopenia and is usually between 50,000 and 140,000 platelets/μL, although it is occasionally profound (less than 20,000 platelets/μL).

Course
The clinical course of illness ranges from mild illness to a fatal outcome. The higher incidence in older patients suggests that host factors are important in disease severity. A virulent form of HME occurs in human immunodeficiency virus–infected individuals that is often associated with an overwhelming infection, a toxic shock– or sepsis-like syndrome, and fatality.[107] Immune compromise related to corticosteroid therapy or immunosuppression with organ transplantation is also associated with increased severity, although prompt treatment abrogates this increased risk.[21,100,103]

The median duration of hospitalization is about 1 week. Convalescence is often prolonged. Persistent infection has been documented in only one patient with HME.[96] Fatalities occur in approximately 3%.[72] Many patients treated with doxycycline or tetracycline recover rapidly. On the other hand, most patients receiving no effective antiehrlichial treatment also have uncomplicated complete recovery.

Diagnosis
A diagnosis based on epidemiologic and clinical factors offers the opportunity to administer prompt empirical antiehrlichial treatment. However, the physician's index of suspicion must be high or an early diagnosis is not made. Patients presenting with fever, leukopenia, thrombocytopenia, elevated serum transaminase levels, and a history of recent tick bite in endemic regions from May through July should be considered as possibly having HME. No absolute clinical criteria distinguish HME from Rocky Mountain spotted fever, although patients with ehrlichiosis are less likely to have a rash and more likely to have leukopenia (median white blood cell count, 3500/μL). Morulae are observed in less than 7% of patients with HME, most often in immunocompromised patients with overwhelming ehrlichiosis.[102]

The gold standard for causative diagnosis of infectious disease, cultivation of the agent, has been achieved in one large series of cases of HME.[108] Currently, it is only a research tool using specialized methods and unique cell lines and incubating for more than 1 month.

Because of the presence of *E. chaffeensis* in peripheral blood or CSF mononuclear cells during active infection and before the presence of diagnostic levels of serum antibodies, methods to detect bacterial DNA, such as polymerase chain reaction (PCR) assay, are highly sensitive and useful diagnostic tools. There are a large number of potential gene targets that have been used, with sensitivity ranging from 60% to 75%.[108,109] A wider availability of PCR assays and technologic advances such as real-time PCR methods hold great promise for even better sensitivity to support clinical diagnosis, management, and therapy definitively during active infection.[110,111]

At present, the major diagnostic criterion for human ehrlichiosis is serologic, as determined by indirect immunofluorescence assay (IFA) with *E. chaffeensis*–infected cells. To be considered positive, the patient's sera must show a fourfold or higher rise or fall in antibody

TABLE 193-2	Clinical and Laboratory Abnormalities in Human Monocytic Ehrlichiosis (HME) and Human Granulocytic Anaplasmosis (HGA)	
Sign, Symptom, or Laboratory Finding	*HME Patients with Abnormal Findings (%)*	*HGA Patients with Abnormal Findings (%)*
Fever	97	94-100
Headache	81	61-85
Chills or rigors	67	39-98
Myalgia	68	78-98
Malaise	84	98
Nausea	48	39
Anorexia	66	37
Vomiting	37	34
Diarrhea	25	22
Abdominal pain	22	—
Rash	36	2-11
Cough	26	29
Dyspnea	23	—
Lymphadenopathy	25	—
Confusion	20	17
Leukopenia	60	50-59
Thrombocytopenia	68	59-92
Elevated AST	86	69-91
Elevated ALT	80	61
Elevated urea nitrogen	38	—
Elevated creatinine	29	70

ALT, alanine aminotransferase; AST, aspartate aminotransferase.

titer during the course of the disease, with a minimal peak titer of 64.[112] IFA shows a peak geometric mean titer of 1280 at 6 weeks after onset.[113] Only 22% to 44% of the sera tested in the first week of illness have a titer of 80 or higher. Among sera from patients tested in the second week, 68% are diagnostic. Sera tested 4 or more weeks after the onset of illness should demonstrate seroconversion.

DIFFERENTIAL DIAGNOSIS

Early in the course of the disease, when the patient presents with fever, headache, myalgia, and malaise, the differential diagnoses may include various viral syndromes, Rocky Mountain spotted fever, upper respiratory illness, sepsis, and urinary tract infection. If nausea, vomiting, and anorexia are prominent symptoms, gastroenteritis is often suspected. With prominent cough, pneumonia is often considered. CNS signs and symptoms with CSF pleocytosis suggest viral or bacterial meningoencephalitis. On obtaining a history of recent tick bite, the physician may consider a tick-borne febrile illness, such as Rocky Mountain spotted fever, relapsing fever, tularemia, Lyme borreliosis, Colorado tick fever, or babesiosis. Other diagnostic considerations include meningococcemia, toxic shock syndrome, leptospirosis, hepatitis, enteroviral infection, influenza, murine typhus, Q fever, typhoid fever, bacterial sepsis, endocarditis, Kawasaki disease, collagen-vascular diseases, and leukemia. A comparison of the ehrlichioses and Rocky Mountain spotted fever is presented in Table 193-3.

Doxycycline is the drug of choice, even in pregnant patients and children, and is administered to adults at a dose of 100 mg twice daily until the patient has become afebrile and clinically improved. Courses of treatment of 7 to 10 days have yielded a favorable outcome in many patients. *E. chaffeensis* has been demonstrated to be susceptible to rifampin and resistant to fluoroquinolones in cell culture; at present, there are no clinical studies to support the use of rifampin for HME.

EHRLICHIOSIS CAUSED BY *EHRLICHIA EWINGII* AND *EHRLICHIA MURIS*

E. ewingii ehrlichiosis has been diagnosed in Missouri, Tennessee, and Oklahoma, and *E. ewingii* has been identified in *A. americanum* or other ticks in North Carolina, Florida, Georgia, New York, and New Jersey, as well as in deer in Missouri, Arkansas, Kentucky, North Carolina, and South Carolina.[114,115] *E. ewingii* has also been detected in Korea and Cameroon.[40,116] Most infections have been reported in immunocompromised patients. Clinical manifestations are similar to those of HME, with the impression that overall the illness is not as severe, with fewer complications, and no deaths have been reported.[102,103] Diagnosis requires PCR with species-specific primers or probes or with DNA sequencing of amplicons of broad-range PCR. Sera of patients with *E. ewingii* ehrlichiosis react with *E. chaffeensis* IFA antigens, and expression of recombinant *E. ewingii* 28-kDa proteins distinct from those of *E. chaffeensis* may allow creation of a specific serodiagnostic test.

E. muris has been detected in *I. persulcatus* ticks in the Perm region of Russia, where 86 patients with an acute febrile illness had antibody titers of 80 to 1200 against the antigenically related *E. chaffeensis*.[117] In Japan, where *E. muris* is found in *Apodemus* mice and *Haemaphysalis flava* ticks, antibodies were present in 1% of humans in a large serosurvey.[118] No human illness has been reported.

HUMAN GRANULOCYTOTROPIC ANAPLASMOSIS

Human granulocytotropic anaplasmosis was formerly known as human granulocytic ehrlichiosis.

Signs, Symptoms, and Course

Although not a reportable illness in some states, more than 3957 cases have been reported by the CDC in the United States since 1999.[52] Approximately 65 cases have been documented in Europe, where disease manifestations seem less severe.[53] Male patients comprise 57% of infections, and the median age is 51 years, but ranges from younger than 1 to 97 years.[32] After an incubation period of approximately 1 to 2 weeks, HGA arises as a mild to severe illness with fever, headache, malaise, and myalgias in most patients.[50,51,54,119] Nausea, vomiting, diarrhea, cough, arthralgias, stiff neck, and confusion are present in less than half of patients, less than 10% have rash, and most of these reflect erythema migrans with concurrent Lyme disease. Most doxycycline-treated patients are well within 7 days and, if untreated, the median duration of illness is 9 days (range, 1 to 60 days).[120] Severe manifestations include respiratory insufficiency, a septic shock–like illness, rhabdomyolysis, hemorrhage, and opportunistic infections.[32] Meningoencephalitis and CSF pleocytosis are exceedingly rare in documented cases of HGA; however, neurologic sequelae may include facial diplegia, brachial plexopathy, and demyelinating polyneuropathy.[121-123] At least six patients have died after HGA, including three after severe opportunistic fungal or viral infections.[32,72,82]

Laboratory features observed in a substantial portion of cases include thrombocytopenia, leukopenia, mild anemia, and increases in serum hepatic aminotransferase activities within the first 7 days of illness.[50,51] Neutropenia with a left shift and relative lymphocytosis may occur. Leukocyte, erythrocyte, and platelet counts return to normal by 14 days, but the left shift may persist for longer.[124] Doxycycline therapy reverses the decline in leukocyte and platelet counts and blunts the degree of left shift, usually within 5 to 7 days; anemia responds more slowly.

Diagnosis

Unlike the rarity of morulae in circulating mononuclear cells in HME, between 20% and 80% of patients with HGA are reported to have ehrlichial morulae identified in peripheral blood neutrophils (Fig. 193-2).[50,51] Culture of *A. phagocytophilum* is promising but usually requires 1 week or longer and is not routinely available, whereas PCR amplification of *A. phagocytophilum* nucleic acids from blood is between 54% and 86% sensitive and highly specific, and can be performed in a timely manner.[125,126] Serologic diagnosis is most often achieved retrospectively by detection of antibodies reactive with *A. phagocytophilum* in infected tissue culture cells.[127,128] By current criteria, a titer of at least 64 is considered significant, but a fourfold rise

TABLE 193-3	Comparison of Ehrlichiosis and Anaplasmosis in the United States with Rocky Mountain Spotted Fever (RMSF)

Similarities

History of tick attachment

Incubation period of about 1 wk between tick bite and onset of symptoms

Peak incidence in late spring and summer

Acute onset with headache, fever, myalgia, and malaise; cough, dyspnea, and vomiting present less commonly

Severe cases may have coagulopathy, azotemia, and encephalopathy

WBC count usually not elevated, platelet count often low, AST (SGOT) level may be increased

Diagnosis by acute and convalescent serology

Treatment—a tetracycline (chloramphenicol may not be effective for ehrlichioses)

Differences

RMSF—rash is present in 90% of patients and is petechial in about half the cases

Ehrlichiosis and anaplasmosis—rash is present in less than half of adult patients with HME and rarely in HGA, is maculopapular, rarely petechial

Leukopenia and absolute lymphopenia and neutropenia common in hospitalized patients with HME and neutropenia in those with HGA, but uncommon in RMSF

Inclusions (morulae) seen rarely in monocytes and macrophages of patients with HME, occasionally in neutrophils of patients with HGA, but not with RMSF

Histopathologic vasculitis, hallmark of RMSF, not observed in ehrlichioses or anaplasmosis

AST, aspartate aminotransferase; HGA, human granulocytic anaplasmosis; HME, human monocytotropic ehrlichiosis; SGOT, serum glutamate oxaloacetate transaminase; WBC, white blood cell.

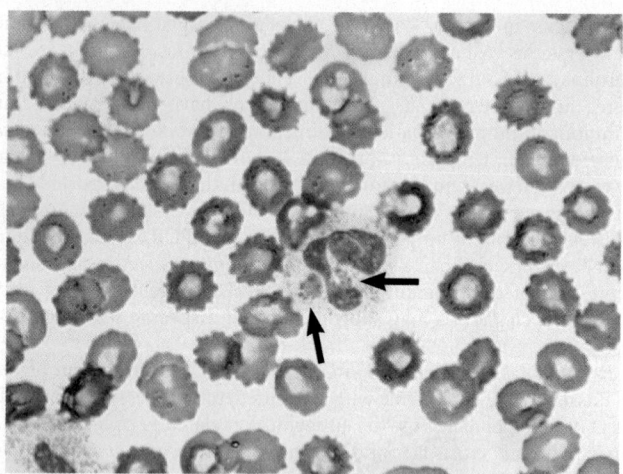

Figure 193-2 Human granulocytic anaplasmosis. Peripheral blood smear showing intracellular inclusion within a neutrophil of a patient with human granulocytic anaplasmosis (*arrows*; Wright stain, ×1000).

provides more definitive evidence for infection because of the fact that 15% to 16% of the population in the upper Midwest and New York State have preexisting serologic reactions.[60] Immunoglobulin M testing may be useful because reactions are demonstrated only during the first 45 to 60 days, but this test lacks sensitivity. A role for Western immunoblot confirmation or use of recombinant antigens for serodiagnosis is not currently defined.

Treatment and Prevention

Doxycycline, 100 mg twice daily, or tetracycline, 500 mg four times a day, has been used successfully. Based on *A. phagocytophilum* cell culture, doxycycline and the rifamycins are bactericidal and chloramphenicol is not effective.[129] The clinical effectiveness of rifampin has not yet been evaluated, but it has been used in children and during pregnancy.[130,131] Although fluoroquinolones have in vitro minimal inhibitory concentration (MIC) values that predict in vivo effectiveness, relapse after use of levofloxacin unrelated to mutations in bacterial *gyrA* has been documented in HGA.[132,133]

Prevention of Ehrlichiosis and Anaplasmosis

At present, prevention of human ehrlichioses and anaplasmosis must rely on avoidance of tick exposure, regular careful search of the body for ticks after exposure, and prompt removal of ticks from the body. Although *A. phagocytophilum* may be transmitted within 4 hours of a tick bite, no analysis of prophylactic antibiotic therapy has been conducted.[134]

Sennetsu Neorickettsiosis

Physicians outside the Far East are unlikely to see a patient with sennetsu neorickettsiosis, which has been documented in Japan, Malaysia, and recently in Laos and is associated with consumption of raw fish and not with arthropod vectors. *N. sennetsu* was isolated in 1953 from the blood, bone marrow, and lymph node of a 25-year-old man who had fever, severe headaches, myalgia, anorexia, lymphadenopathy, and an increased quantity of atypical lymphocytes in his peripheral blood.[135] Organisms isolated in mice were inoculated into human volunteers, who developed a syndrome resembling infectious mononucleosis. Neorickettsiae were recovered from their blood samples.

The average incubation period of 14 days is followed by sudden onset of chills and a fever that lasts for 2 weeks unless treated effectively. Patients also complain of headache and myalgia. Postauricular and posterior cervical lymphadenopathy appears 5 to 7 days after onset. Hepatosplenomegaly occurs in one third to one half of patients. Aseptic meningitis is observed only occasionally and rash very rarely. Early in the illness leukopenia occurs; in the late febrile and convalescent phases, absolute lymphocytosis is observed with 10% or greater atypical lymphocytes. Mild to moderate elevations occur in serum transaminase levels. Laboratory diagnosis can be made by PCR on buffy coat blood or by demonstration of specific serum antibody by IFA. Treatment with one of the tetracycline antimicrobials, including doxycycline or minocycline, results in defervescence after 1 to 2 days.

REFERENCES

1. Silverstein AM. On the naming of rickettsiae after Paul Ehrlich. *Bull Hist Med.* 1998;72:731-733.
2. Dumler JS, Barbet AF, Bekker CP, et al. Reorganization of genera in the families *Rickettsiaceae* and *Anaplasmataceae* in the order *Rickettsiales*: Unification of some species of *Ehrlichia* with *Anaplasma*, *Cowdria* with *Ehrlichia* and *Ehrlichia* with *Neorickettsia*, descriptions of six new species combinations and designation of *Ehrlichia equi* and 'hge agent' as subjective synonyms of *Ehrlichia phagocytophila*. *Int J Syst Evol Microbiol.* 2001;51:2145-2165.
3. Maeda K, Markowitz N, Hawley RC, et al. Human infection with *Ehrlichia canis*, a leukocytic rickettsia. *N Engl J Med.* 1987;316:853-856.
4. Anderson BE, Dawson JE, Jones DC, et al. *Ehrlichia chaffeensis*, a new species associated with human ehrlichiosis. *J Clin Microbiol.* 1991;29:2838-2842.
5. Bakken JS, Dumler JS, Chen SM, et al. Human granulocytic ehrlichiosis in the upper Midwest United States. A new species emerging? *JAMA.* 1994;272:212-218.
6. Chen SM, Dumler JS, Bakken JS, et al. Identification of a granulocytotropic *Ehrlichia* species as the etiologic agent of human disease. *J Clin Microbiol.* 1994;32:589-595.
7. Anderson BE, Greene CE, Jones DC, et al. *Ehrlichia ewingii* sp. nov., the etiologic agent of canine granulocytic ehrlichiosis. *Int J Syst Bacteriol.* 1992;42:299-302.
8. Chen SM, Dumler JS, Feng HM, et al. Identification of the antigenic constituents of *Ehrlichia chaffeensis*. *Am J Trop Med Hyg.* 1994;50:52-58.
9. Wen B, Rikihisa Y, Mott J, et al. *Ehrlichia muris* sp. nov., identified on the basis of 16S rRNA base sequences and serological, morphological, and biological characteristics. *Int J Syst Bacteriol.* 1995;45:250-254.
10. Popov VL, Han VC, Chen SM, et al. Ultrastructural differentiation of the genogroups in the genus *Ehrlichia*. *J Med Microbiol.* 1998;47:235-251.

11. Dunning Hotopp JC, Lin M, Madupu R, et al. Comparative genomics of emerging human ehrlichiosis agents. *PLoS genet.* 2006;2:e21.
12. Ohashi N, Zhi N, Zhang Y, et al. Immunodominant major outer membrane proteins of *Ehrlichia chaffeensis* are encoded by a polymorphic multigene family. *Infect Immun.* 1998;66:132-139.
13. Yu X, McBride JW, Zhang X, et al. Characterization of the complete transcriptionally active *Ehrlichia chaffeensis* 28-kDa outer membrane protein multigene family. *Gene.* 2000;248:59-68.
14. Asanovich KM, Bakken JS, Madigan JE, et al. Antigenic diversity of granulocytic *Ehrlichia* isolates from humans in Wisconsin and New York and a horse in California. *J Infect Dis.* 1997;176:1029-1034.
15. Ijdo JW, Wu C, Telford SR 3rd, et al. Differential expression of the p44 gene family in the agent of human granulocytic ehrlichiosis. *Infect Immun.* 2002;70:5295-5298.
16. Park J, Choi KS, Dumler JS. Major surface protein 2 of *Anaplasma phagocytophilum* facilitates adherence to granulocytes. *Infect Immun.* 2003;71:4018-4025.
17. Huang H, Wang X, Kikuchi T, et al. Porin activity of *Anaplasma phagocytophilum* outer membrane fraction and purified p44. *J Bacteriol.* 2007;189:1998-2006.
18. Kumagai Y, Huang H, Rikihisa Y. Expression and porin activity of p28 and OMP-1F during intracellular *Ehrlichia chaffeensis* development. *J Bacteriol.* 2008;190:3597-3605.
19. Zhang JZ, Guo H, Winslow GM, et al. Expression of members of the 28-kilodalton major outer membrane protein family of *Ehrlichia chaffeensis* during persistent infection. *Infect Immun.* 2004;72:4336-4343.
20. Singu V, Peddireddi L, Sirigireddy KR, et al. Unique macrophage and tick cell-specific protein expression from the p28/p30-outer membrane protein multigene locus In *Ehrlichia chaffeensis* and *Ehrlichia canis*. *Cell Microbiol.* 2006;8:1475-1487.

21. Liddell AM, Sumner JW, Paddock CM, et al. Reinfection with *Ehrlichia chaffeensis* in a liver transplant recipient. *Clin Infect Dis.* 2002;34:1644-1647.
22. Horowitz HW, Aguero-Rosenfeld M, Dumler JS, et al. Reinfection with the agent of human granulocytic ehrlichiosis. *Ann Intern Med.* 1998;129:461-463.
23. Zhi N, Ohashi N, Rikihisa Y. Multiple p44 genes encoding major outer membrane proteins are expressed in the human granulocytic ehrlichiosis agent. *J Biol Chem.* 1999;274:17828-17836.
24. Caspersen K, Park JH, Patil S, et al. Genetic variability and stability of *Anaplasma phagocytophila* msp2 (p44). *Infect Immun.* 2002;70:1230-1234.
25. Barbet AF, Lundgren AM, Alleman AR, et al. Structure of the expression site reveals global diversity in msp2 (p44) variants in *Anaplasma phagocytophilum*. *Infect Immun.* 2006;74:6429-6437.
26. Scorpio DG, Leutenegger C, Berger J, et al. Sequential analysis of *Anaplasma phagocytophilum* msp2 transcription in murine and equine models of human granulocytic anaplasmosis. *Clin Vaccine Immunol.* 2008;15:418-424.
27. Mcbride JW, Yu XJ, Walker DH. Glycosylation of homologous immunodominant proteins of *Ehrlichia chaffeensis* and *Ehrlichia canis*. *Infect Immun.* 2000;68:13-18.
28. Popov VL, Yu X, Walker DH. The 120-kDa outer membrane protein of *Ehrlichia chaffeensis*: Preferential expression on dense-core cells and gene expression in *Escherichia coli* associated with attachment and entry. *Microb Pathog.* 2000;28:71-80.
29. Lin M, Den Dulk-Ras A, Hooykaas PJ, et al. *Anaplasma phagocytophilum* anka secreted by type iv secretion system is tyrosine phosphorylated by abl-1 to facilitate infection. *Cell Microbiol.* 2007;9:2644-2657.
30. Ewing SA, Dawson JE, Kocan AA, et al. Experimental transmission of *Ehrlichia chaffeensis* (Rickettsiales: Ehrlichieae) among white-tailed deer by *amblyomma americanum* (Acari: Ixodidae). *J Med Entomol.* 1995;32:368-374.

31. Telford SR 3rd, Dawson JE, Katavolos P, et al. Perpetuation of the agent of human granulocytic ehrlichiosis in a deer tick-rodent cycle. *Proc Natl Acad Sci U S A.* 1996;93:6209-6214.

32. Demma LJ, Holman RC, McQuiston JH, et al. Epidemiology of human ehrlichiosis and anaplasmosis in the United States, 2001-2002. *Am J Trop Med Hyg.* 2005;73:400-409.

33. Long SW, Zhang X, Zhang J, et al. Evaluation of transovarial transmission and transmissibility of *Ehrlichia chaffeensis* (Rickettsiales: Anaplasmataceae) in *Amblyomma americanum* (Acari: Ixodidae). *J Med Entomol.* 2003;40:1000-1004.

34. Holden K, Boothby JT, Anand S, et al. Detection of *Borrelia burgdorferi*, *Ehrlichia chaffeensis*, and *Anaplasma phagocytophilum* in ticks (Acari: Ixodidae) from a coastal region of California. *J Med Entomol.* 2003;40:534-539.

35. Kramer VL, Randolph MP, Hui LT, et al. Detection of the agents of human ehrlichioses in ixodid ticks from California. *Am J Trop Med Hyg.* 1999;60:62-65.

36. Steiert JG, Gilfoy F. Infection rates of *Amblyomma americanum* and *Dermacentor variabilis* by *Ehrlichia chaffeensis* and *Ehrlichia ewingii* in southwest Missouri. *Vector Borne Zoonotic Dis.* 2002;2:53-60.

37. Calic SB, Galvao MA, Bacellar F, et al. Human ehrlichioses in Brazil: First suspect cases. *Braz J Infect Dis.* 2004;8:259-262.

38. Heo EJ, Park JH, Koo JR, et al. Serologic and molecular detection of *Ehrlichia chaffeensis* and *Anaplasma phagocytophila* (human granulocytic ehrlichiosis agent) in Korean patients. *J Clin Microbiol.* 2002;40:3082-3085.

39. Brouqui P, Le Cam C, Kelly PJ, et al. Serologic evidence for human ehrlichiosis in Africa. *Eur J Epidemiol.* 1994;10:695-698.

40. Ndip LM, Ndip RN, Ndive VE, et al. *Ehrlichia* species in *Rhipicephalus sanguineus* ticks in Cameroon. *Vector Borne Zoonotic Dis.* 2007;7:221-227.

41. Ndip LM, Ndip RN, Esemu SN, et al. Ehrlichial infection in Cameroonian canines by *Ehrlichia canis* and *Ehrlichia ewingii*. *Vet Microbiol.* 2005;111:59-66.

42. Machado RZ, Duarte JM, Dagnone AS, et al. Detection of *Ehrlichia chaffeensis* in Brazilian marsh deer (*Blastocerus dichotomus*). *Vet Parasitol.* 2006;139:262-266.

43. Fishbein DB, Kemp A, Dawson JE, et al. Human ehrlichiosis: Prospective active surveillance in febrile hospitalized patients. *J Infect Dis.* 1989;160:803-809.

44. Olano JP, Walker DH. Human ehrlichioses. *Med Clin North Am.* 2002;86:375-392.

45. Standaert SM, Dawson JE, Schaffner W, et al. Ehrlichiosis in a golf-oriented retirement community. *N Engl J Med.* 1995;333:420-425.

46. Buller RS, Arens M, Hmiel SP, et al. *Ehrlichia ewingii*, a newly recognized agent of human ehrlichiosis. *N Engl J Med.* 1999;341:148-155.

47. Perez M, Bodor M, Zhang C, et al. Human infection with *Ehrlichia canis* accompanied by clinical signs in Venezuela. *Ann N Y Acad Sci.* 2006;1078:110-117.

48. Reeves WK, Loftis AD, Nicholson WL, et al. The first report of human illness associated with the Panola Mountain *Ehrlichia* species: A case report. *J Med Case Reports.* 2008;2:139.

49. McKechnie DB, Slater KS, Childs JE, et al. Survival of *Ehrlichia chaffeensis* in refrigerated, ADSOL-treated RBCs. *Transfusion.* 2000;40:1041-1047.

50. Bakken JS, Krueth J, Wilson-Nordskog C, et al. Clinical and laboratory characteristics of human granulocytic ehrlichiosis. *JAMA.* 1996;275:199-205.

51. Aguero-Rosenfeld ME, Horowitz HW, Wormser GP, et al. Human granulocytic ehrlichiosis: A case series from a medical center in New York State. *Ann Intern Med.* 1996;125:904-908.

52. Centers for Disease Control (CDC). Summary of notifiable diseases—United States, 2006. *MMWR Morbid Mortal Wkly Rep.* 2008;55:1-94.

53. Strle F. Human granulocytic ehrlichiosis in Europe. *Int J Med Microbiol.* 2004;293(Suppl 37):27-35.

54. Blanco JR, Oteo JA. Human granulocytic ehrlichiosis in Europe. *Clin Microbiol Infect.* 2002;8:763-772.

55. IJdo JW, Meek JI, Cartter ML, et al. The emergence of another tickborne infection in the 12-town area around Lyme, Connecticut: Human granulocytic ehrlichiosis. *J Infect Dis.* 2000;181:1388-1393.

56. Magnarelli LA, Dumler JS, Anderson JF, et al. Coexistence of antibodies to tick-borne pathogens of babesiosis, ehrlichiosis, and Lyme borreliosis in human sera. *J Clin Microbiol.* 1995;33:3054-3057.

57. Dumler JS, Dotevall L, Gustafson R, et al. A population-based seroepidemiologic study of human granulocytic ehrlichiosis and Lyme borreliosis on the west coast of Sweden. *J Infect Dis.* 1997;175:720-722.

58. Bakken JS, Goellner P, Van Etten M, et al. Seroprevalence of human granulocytic ehrlichiosis among permanent residents of northwestern Wisconsin. *Clin Infect Dis.* 1998;27:1491-1496.

59. Graf PC, Chretien JP, Ung L, et al. Prevalence of seropositivity to spotted fever group rickettsiae and *Anaplasma phagocytophilum* in a large, demographically diverse U.S. sample. *Clin Infect Dis.* 2008;46:70-77.

60. Aguero-Rosenfeld ME, Donnarumma L, Zentmaier L, et al. Seroprevalence of antibodies that react with *Anaplasma phagocytophila*, the agent of human granulocytic ehrlichiosis, in different populations in Westchester County, New York. *J Clin Microbiol.* 2002;40:2612-2615.

61. Petrovec M, Lotric Furlan S, Zupanc TA, et al. Human disease in Europe caused by a granulocytic *Ehrlichia* species. *J Clin Microbiol.* 1997;35:1556-1559.

62. Nadelman RB, Horowitz HW, Hsieh TC, et al. Simultaneous human granulocytic ehrlichiosis and Lyme borreliosis. *N Engl J Med.* 1997;337:27-30.

63. Steere AC, McHugh G, Suarez C, et al. Prospective study of coinfection in patients with erythema migrans. *Clin Infect Dis.* 2003;36:1078-1081.

64. Lotric-Furlan S, Petrovec M, Avsic-Zupanc T, et al. Concomitant tickborne encephalitis and human granulocytic ehrlichiosis. *Emerg Infect Dis.* 2005;11:485-488.

65. Krause PJ, McKay K, Thompson CA, et al. Disease-specific diagnosis of coinfecting tickborne zoonoses: babesiosis, human granulocytic ehrlichiosis, and Lyme disease. *Clin Infect Dis.* 2002;34:1184-1191.

66. Nicholson WL, Muir S, Sumner JW, et al. Serologic evidence of infection with *Ehrlichia* spp. in wild rodents (Muridae: Sigmodontinae) in the United States. *J Clin Microbiol.* 1998; 36:695-700.

67. Liz JS, Sumner JW, Pfister K, et al. PCR detection and serological evidence of granulocytic ehrlichial infection in roe deer (*Capreolus capreolus*) and chamois (*Rupicapra rupicapra*). *J Clin Microbiol.* 2002;40:892-897.

68. Magnarelli LA, Ijdo JW, Stafford KC 3rd, et al. Infections of granulocytic ehrlichiae and *Borrelia burgdorferi* in white-tailed deer in Connecticut. *J Wildl Dis.* 1999;35:266-274.

69. Levin ML, Fish D. Immunity reduces reservoir host competence of *Peromyscus leucopus* for *Ehrlichia phagocytophila*. *Infect Immun.* 2000;68:1514-1518.

70. Dumler JS, Dawson JE, Walker DH. Human ehrlichiosis: Hematopathology and immunohistologic detection of *Ehrlichia chaffeensis*. *Hum Pathol.* 1993;24:391-396.

71. Dumler JS, Brouqui P, Aronson J, et al. Identification of *Ehrlichia* in human tissue. *N Engl J Med.* 1991;325:1109-1110.

72. Walker DH, Dumler JS. Human monocytic and granulocytic ehrlichioses. Discovery and diagnosis of emerging tick-borne infections and the critical role of the pathologist. *Arch Pathol Lab Med.* 1997;121:785-791.

73. Lee EH, Rikihisa Y. Anti-*Ehrlichia chaffeensis* antibody complexed with *E. chaffeensis* induces potent proinflammatory cytokine mRNA expression in human monocytes through sustained reduction of IkappaB-alpha and activation of NF-kappaB. *Infect Immun.* 1997;65:2890-2897.

74. Ismail N, Stevenson HL, Walker DH. Role of tumor necrosis factor alpha (TNF-alpha) and interleukin-10 in the pathogenesis of severe murine monocytotropic ehrlichiosis: Increased resistance of TNF receptor p55- and p75-deficient mice to fatal ehrlichial infection. *Infect Immun.* 2006;74:1846-1856.

75. Ismail N, Crossley EC, Stevenson HL, et al. Relative importance of T-cell subsets in monocytotropic ehrlichiosis: A novel effector mechanism involved in *Ehrlichia*-induced immunopathology in murine ehrlichiosis. *Infect Immun.* 2007;75:4608-4620.

76. Dierberg KL, Dumler JS. Lymph node hemophagocytosis in rickettsial diseases: A pathogenetic role for CD8 T lymphocytes in human monocytic ehrlichiosis (HME)? *BMC Infect Dis.* 2006;6:121.

77. Barnewall RE, Rikihisa Y. Abrogation of gamma interferon-induced inhibition of *Ehrlichia chaffeensis* infection in human monocytes with iron-transferrin. *Infect Immun.* 1994;62:4804-4810.

78. Winslow GM, Yager E, Shilo K, et al. Antibody-mediated elimination of the obligate intracellular bacterial pathogen *Ehrlichia chaffeensis* during active infection. *Infect Immun.* 2000;68:2187-2195.

79. Lee EH, Rikihisa Y. Protein kinase A–mediated inhibition of gamma interferon-induced tyrosine phosphorylation of Janus kinases and latent cytoplasmic transcription factors in human monocytes by *Ehrlichia chaffeensis*. *Infect Immun.* 1998;66:2514-2520.

80. Zhang JZ, McBride JW, Yu XJ. L-selectin and E-selectin expressed on monocytes mediating *Ehrlichia chaffeensis* attachment onto host cells. *FEMS Microbiol Lett.* 2003;227:303-309.

81. Lin M, Rikihisa Y. *Ehrlichia chaffeensis* downregulates surface Toll-like receptors 2/4, CD14 and transcription factors PU.1 and inhibits lipopolysaccharide activation of NF-kappa B, ERK 1/2 and p38 MAPK in host monocytes. *Cell Microbiol.* 2004;6:175-186.

82. Lepidi H, Bunnell JE, Martin ME, et al. Comparative pathology, and immunohistology associated with clinical illness after *Ehrlichia phagocytophila*-group infections. *Am J Trop Med Hyg.* 2000;62:29-37.

83. Klein MB, Miller JS, Nelson CM, et al. Primary bone marrow progenitors of both granulocytic and monocytic lineages are susceptible to infection with the agent of human granulocytic ehrlichiosis. *J Infect Dis.* 1997;176:1405-1409.

84. Herron MJ, Ericson ME, Kurtti TJ, et al. The interactions of *Anaplasma phagocytophilum*, endothelial cells, and human neutrophils. *Ann N Y Acad Sci.* 2005;1063:374-382.

85. Webster P, IJdo JW, Chicoine LM, et al. The agent of human granulocytic ehrlichiosis resides in an endosomal compartment. *J Clin Invest.* 1998;101:1932-1941.

86. Herron MJ, Nelson CM, Larson J, et al. Intracellular parasitism by the human granulocytic ehrlichiosis bacterium through the P-selectin ligand, PSGL-1. *Science.* 2000;288:1653-1656.

87. Carlyon JA, Chan WT, Galan J, et al. Repression of rac2 mRNA expression by *Anaplasma phagocytophila* is essential to the inhibition of superoxide production and bacterial proliferation. *J Immunol.* 2002;169:7009-7018.

88. Banerjee R, Anguita J, Roos D, et al. Cutting edge: Infection by the agent of human granulocytic ehrlichiosis prevents the respiratory burst by down-regulating gp91phox. *J Immunol.* 2000;164:3946-3949.

89. Yoshiie K, Kim HY, Mott J, et al. Intracellular infection by the human granulocytic ehrlichiosis agent inhibits human neutrophil apoptosis. *Infect Immun.* 2000;68:1125-1133.

90. Choi KS, Garyu J, Park J, et al. Diminished adhesion of *Anaplasma phagocytophilum*-infected neutrophils to endothelial cells is associated with reduced expression of leukocyte surface selectin. *Infect Immun.* 2003;71:4586-4594.

91. Choi KS, Park JT, Dumler JS. *Anaplasma phagocytophilum* delay of neutrophil apoptosis through the p38 mitogen-activated protein kinase signal pathway. *Infect Immun.* 2005;73:8209-8218.

92. Martin ME, Caspersen K, Dumler JS. Immunopathology and ehrlichial propagation are regulated by interferon-gamma and interleukin-10 in a murine model of human granulocytic ehrlichiosis. *Am J Pathol.* 2001;158:1881-1888.

93. Dumler JS, Barat NC, Barat CE, et al. Human granulocytic anaplasmosis and macrophage activation. *Clin Infect Dis.* 2007;45:199-204.

94. Harkess JR, Ewing SA, Crutcher JM, et al. Human ehrlichiosis in Oklahoma. *J Infect Dis.* 1989;159:576-579.

95. Eng TR, Harkess JR, Fishbein DB, et al. Epidemiologic, clinical, and laboratory findings of human ehrlichiosis in the United States, 1988. *JAMA.* 1990;264:2251-2258.

96. Dumler JS, Sutker WL, Walker DH. Persistent infection with *Ehrlichia chaffeensis*. *Clin Infect Dis.* 1993;17:903-905.

97. Harkess JR, Stucky D, Ewing SA. Neurologic abnormalities in a patient with human ehrlichiosis. *South Med J.* 1990;83:1341-1343.

98. Schutze GE, Buckingham SC, Marshall GS, et al. Human monocytic ehrlichiosis in children. *Pediatr Infect Dis J.* 2007;26:475-479.

99. Fichtenbaum CJ, Peterson LR, Weil GJ. Ehrlichiosis presenting as a life-threatening illness with features of the toxic shock syndrome. *Am J Med.* 1993;95:351-357.

100. Marty AM, Dumler JS, Imes G, et al. Ehrlichiosis mimicking thrombotic thrombocytopenic purpura. Case report and pathological correlation. *Hum Pathol.* 1995;26:920-925.

101. Hamburg BJ, Storch GA, Micek ST, et al. The importance of early treatment with doxycycline in human ehrlichiosis. *Medicine (Baltimore).* 2008;87:53-60.

102. Paddock CD, Folk SM, Shore GM, et al. Infections with *Ehrlichia chaffeensis* and *Ehrlichia ewingii* in persons coinfected with human immunodeficiency virus. *Clin Infect Dis.* 2001;33:1586-1594.

103. Thomas LD, Hongo I, Bloch KC, et al. Human ehrlichiosis in transplant recipients. *Am J Transplant.* 2007;7:1641-1647.

104. Dunn BE, Monson TP, Dumler JS, et al. Identification of *Ehrlichia chaffeensis* morulae in cerebrospinal fluid mononuclear cells. *J Clin Microbiol.* 1992;30:2207-2210.

105. Moskovitz M, Fadden R, Min T. Human ehrlichiosis: A rickettsial disease associated with severe cholestasis and multisystemic disease. *J Clin Gastroenterol.* 1991;13:86-90.

106. Fishbein DB, Dawson JE, Robinson LE. Human ehrlichiosis in the United States, 1985 to 1990. *Ann Intern Med.* 1994;120:736-743.

107. Paddock CD, Sumner JW, Shore GM, et al. Isolation and characterization of *Ehrlichia chaffeensis* strains from patients with fatal ehrlichiosis. *J Clin Microbiol.* 1997;35:2496-2502.

108. Standaert SM, Yu T, Scott MA, et al. Primary isolation of *Ehrlichia chaffeensis* from patients with febrile illnesses: Clinical and molecular characteristics. *J Infect Dis.* 2000;181:1082-1088.

109. Olano JP, Masters E, Hogrefe W, et al. Human monocytotropic ehrlichiosis, Missouri. *Emerg Infect Dis.* 2003;9:1579-1586.

110. Doyle CK, Labruna MB, Breitschwerdt EB, et al. Detection of medically important *Ehrlichia* by quantitative multicolor TaqMan real-time polymerase chain reaction of the dsb gene. *J Mol Diagn.* 2005;7:504-510.

111. Sirigireddy KR, Ganta RR. Multiplex detection of *Ehrlichia* and *Anaplasma* species pathogens in peripheral blood by real-time reverse transcriptase-polymerase chain reaction. *J Mol Diagn.* 2005;7:308-316.

112. Childs JE, Sumner JW, Nicholson WL, et al. Outcome of diagnostic tests using samples from patients with culture-proven human monocytic ehrlichiosis: Implications for surveillance. *J Clin Microbiol.* 1999;37:2997-3000.

113. Dawson JE, Fishbein DB, Eng TR, et al. Diagnosis of human ehrlichiosis with the indirect fluorescent antibody test: Kinetics and specificity. *J Infect Dis.* 1990;162:91-95.

114. Arens MQ, Liddell AM, Buening G, et al. Detection of *Ehrlichia* spp. in the blood of wild white-tailed deer in Missouri by PCR assay and serologic analysis. *J Clin Microbiol.* 2003;41:1263-1265.

115. Yabsley MJ, Varela AS, Tate CM, et al. *Ehrlichia ewingii* infection in white-tailed deer (*Odocoileus virginianus*). *Emerg Infect Dis.* 2002;8:668-671.

116. Kim CM, Yi YH, Yu DH, et al. Tick-borne rickettsial pathogens in ticks and small mammals in Korea. *Appl Environ Microbiol.* 2006;72:5766-5776.

117. Ravyn MD, Korenberg EI, Oeding JA, et al. Monocytic *Ehrlichia* in *Ixodes persulcatus* ticks from Perm, Russia. *Lancet.* 1999;353:722-723.

118. Kawahara M, Ito T, Suto C, et al. Comparison of *Ehrlichia muris* strains isolated from wild mice and ticks and serologic survey of humans and animals with *E. muris* as antigen. *J Clin Microbiol.* 1999;37:1123-1129.

119. Bakken JS, Dumler JS. Human granulocytic ehrlichiosis. *Clin Infect Dis.* 2000;31:554-560.

120. Lotric-Furlan S, Petrovec M, Avsic-Zupanc T, et al. Comparison of patients fulfilling criteria for confirmed and probable human granulocytic ehrlichiosis. *Scand J Infect Dis.* 2004;36:817-822.

121. Horowitz HW, Marks SJ, Weintraub M, et al. Brachial plexopathy associated with human granulocytic ehrlichiosis. *Neurology.* 1996;46:1026-1029.

122. Bakken JS, Erlemeyer SA, Kanoff RJ, et al. Demyelinating polyneuropathy associated with human granulocytic ehrlichiosis. *Clin Infect Dis.* 1998;27:1323-1324.

123. Lee FS, Chu FK, Tackley M, et al. Human granulocytic ehrlichiosis presenting as facial diplegia in a 42-year-old woman. *Clin Infect Dis.* 2000;31:1288-1291.

124. Bakken JS, Aguero-Rosenfeld ME, Tilden RL, et al. Serial measurements of hematologic counts during the active phase of human granulocytic ehrlichiosis. *Clin Infect Dis.* 2001;32:862-870.

125. Edelman DC, Dumler JS. Evaluation of an improved PCR diagnostic assay for human granulocytic ehrlichiosis. *Mol Diagn.* 1996;1:41-49.

126. Horowitz HW, Aguero-Rosenfeld ME, McKenna DF, et al. Clinical and laboratory spectrum of culture-proven human granulocytic ehrlichiosis: Comparison with culture-negative cases. *Clin Infect Dis.* 1998;27:1314-1317.

127. Walls JJ, Aguero-Rosenfeld M, Bakken JS, et al. Inter- and intralaboratory comparison of *Ehrlichia equi* and human granulocytic ehrlichiosis (HGE) agent strains for serodiagnosis of HGE by the immunofluorescent-antibody test. *J Clin Microbiol.* 1999;37:2968-2673.

128. Bakken JS, Haller I, Riddell D, et al. The serological response of patients infected with the agent of human granulocytic ehrlichiosis. *Clin Infect Dis.* 2002;34:22-27.

129. Maurin M, Bakken JS, Dumler JS. Antibiotic susceptibilities of *Anaplasma* (*Ehrlichia*) *phagocytophilum* strains from various geographic areas in the United States. *Antimicrob Agents Chemother.* 2003;47:413-415.

130. Buitrago MI, Ijdo JW, Rinaudo P, et al. Human granulocytic ehrlichiosis during pregnancy treated successfully with rifampin. *Clin Infect Dis.* 1998;27:213-215.

131. Krause PJ, Corrow CL, Bakken JS. Successful treatment of human granulocytic ehrlichiosis in children using rifampin. *Pediatrics.* 2003;112:e252-e253.

132. Maurin M, Abergel C, Raoult D. DNA gyrase-mediated natural resistance to fluoroquinolones in *Ehrlichia* spp. *Antimicrob Agents Chemother.* 2001;45:2098-2105.

133. Wormser GP, Filozov A, Telford SR 3rd, et al. Dissociation between inhibition and killing by levofloxacin in human granulocytic anaplasmosis. *Vector Borne Zoonotic Dis.* 2006;6:388-394.

134. des Vignes F, Piesman J, Heffernan R, et al. Effect of tick removal on transmission of *Borrelia burgdorferi* and *Ehrlichia phagocytophila* by *Ixodes scapularis* nymphs. *J Infect Dis.* 2001;183:773-778.

135. Misao T, Kobayashi Y. Studies on infectious mononucleosis (glandular fever). I. Isolation of etiologic agent from blood, bone marrow, and lymph node of a patient with infectious mononucleosis by using mice. *Kyushu J Med Sci.* 1955;6:145-152.

194

Introduction to Bacteria and Bacterial Diseases

MARTIN J. BLASER

Bacteria, the oldest forms of life on earth, are remarkably diverse and exist in astounding numbers. Diseases caused by bacteria include some of the most common infections in the world, as well as some of the most important human scourges, past, present, and probably future. At the same time, each of us is colonized by more bacterial cells than we have human cells in our bodies. Generally, this is a peaceful and even productive (symbiotic) relationship, but occasionally even these well-tolerated residents of the human biosphere cause disease.[1,2]

We are surrounded by and always exposed to bacteria, including those that evolved to live well with us (e.g., *Bacteroides* species), as well as those whose evolution has promoted the tendency to cause disease (e.g., *Mycobacterium tuberculosis*) and death (e.g., *Bacillus anthracis*). In consequence, and not surprisingly, many of the presently recognized infectious diseases are caused by bacteria. It also may be safely predicted that many important illnesses not yet recognized or widespread ("emerging" infectious diseases), will be found to be caused by bacteria,[3] as will some chronic inflammatory diseases of unknown cause (see later). Therefore, knowledge of pathogenic bacteria, the diseases to which they lead, and current preventive and therapeutic strategies are critical for all health care providers, especially specialists in infectious diseases. An emerging concept is that our residential bacteria, part of human physiology and protective against introduced pathogens, are changing,[4] with important health consequences.[5-7]

Classification of Bacteria

Bacteria have been classified according to phenotype, including size, shape, staining properties, and biochemical properties, since the beginning of microbiology. In recent years, classification has been dominated by genotype, especially relying on conserved molecules such as 16S ribosomal RNA.[8] Although there is a considerable degree of overlap between phenotype and genotype, as would be expected, dichotomies occur. In the future, taxonomy, understanding of pathogenesis, and diagnostics will be increasingly based on genotype. Thus, physicians and other students of infectious diseases must broaden their knowledge of molecular biology and taxonomy. As bacteriology advances in its differentiation of genera and species, as subspecies diversity is increasingly appreciated,[9] as variation within individual hosts is better understood, and as the evolution of pathogens is better outlined,[10,11] a grounding in evolutionary biology and ecology also will become more critical. The current National Institutes of Health (NIH) Roadmap Project focusing on the human microbiome will provide a new scientific basis for understanding strain and species variation among the indigenous organisms in human hosts to the biomedical community.[12] Over time, this information will be translated into clinical advances in prevention, diagnosis, and treatment of infectious diseases. I have stated that we will find bacterial roles in diseases that were not previously suspected to have a microbial cause.[3]

Variation in Bacterial Infections

Because all organs of the body are subject to bacterial infection, a recitation of these sites would be exhaustive and thus not useful. However, at the least, bacterial infections may be considered as varying in cause, mechanisms, and time frame. Infections may be caused by gram-positive or gram-negative bacilli or cocci; these were the first recog-

nized bacterial agents of disease. However, this simple taxonomy does not fully account for other causative bacterial agents, including *Mycobacterium* species, treponemes, mycoplasma, rickettsia, chlamydia, and actinomyces, all of which are Eubacteria. Each of these types of organisms has particular stereotypic features that characterize its interactions with hosts, but exceptions and variations abound. In recent years, Archaea, a widespread and ancient group of prokaryotes, most closely resembling bacteria, has been isolated from human specimens[13,14]; whether or not they play roles in human diseases is not yet known.

The mechanisms whereby bacteria cause disease are quite varied (Table 194-1). There is no universal mechanism or principle—the causative organism need not even be present in the human body. For example, food poisoning is commonly caused by the ingestion of preformed toxin produced by *Clostridium botulinum* or *Staphylococcus aureus* when they are growing in food, not in the host. The scope of bacterial infections includes interactions across time frames that vary from minutes to decades, or longer (Table 194-2). The descendants of the organisms that we each acquire from our mother[15] as a newborn can be the cause of our death in old age (e.g., caused by a perforated diverticulum) to carry the argument to the farthest extreme. Each bacterial infection is unique, which increases the difficulty in grasping the underlying concepts; this complexity also makes the practice of infectious diseases so intellectually satisfying.

Polymorphism and Bacterial Infection

From the earliest days of microbiology, when it was recognized that some organisms of the same species were encapsulated and many were not, it has been clear that pathogenic bacteria are polymorphic. With the development of antisera came the recognition that apparently identical organisms showed variation; this information became the basis for typing schemes based on capsular, somatic O-antigen, or flagellar antigenic differences. Such polymorphisms have enabled better classification of virulent (and avirulent) meningococci, pneumococci, and *Escherichia coli*, for example, and have led to diagnostics, therapeutic antisera, and vaccines. However, in recent years especially, has come the understanding that once bacteria begin to multiply in a host, their own populations become polymorphic.[16] Antigenic variation is one subtheme of that phenomenon and has been known since the studies of *Borrelia recurrentis*, the cause of relapsing fever. Increasingly, with the tools provided by the sequencing of whole bacterial genomes, we are learning just how polymorphic are bacteria, often considered as clonal organisms, and how dynamic their changes in relation to individual hosts.[17] Even the most highly clonal bacteria, such as *M. tuberculosis*, have extensive variations at particular loci, often those involving interaction with hosts.[18]

In parallel, we have been learning more about human genetic polymorphisms and their relationship to bacterial diseases. Medical science is rapidly advancing from phenotypes (e.g., blood groups) to genotypes (e.g., alleles of the interleukin-1β [IL-1β] promoter). The genetic composition of each individual helps determine its response to bacterial infections and thus the outcome. Increasingly, these host characteristics will become the focus of the information that clinicians will need when considering prevention, differential diagnosis, and therapy of bacterial infections.[19]

TABLE 194-1	Disease Mechanisms Involved in Bacterial Infections
Mechanism	**Examples**
Pyogenic infection	Pneumococcal pneumonia, staphylococcal abscess
Granulomatous infection	Pulmonary tuberculosis, brucellosis, syphilis
Intoxication (augmentation of host physiology)	Cholera (*Vibrio cholerae*)
Intoxication (tissue destruction)	Gas gangrene (*Clostridium perfringens*), diphtheria (*Corynebacterium diphtheriae*)
Immunologic mediation	Guillain-Barré syndrome following *Campylobacter jejuni* infection; Reiter syndrome following shigellosis; acute rheumatic fever following pharyngitis by *Streptococcus pyogenes*
Neoplasia	Adenocarcinoma of the stomach as a consequence of *Helicobacter pylori* persistence; adenocarcinoma of the esophagus as a consequence of physiologic changes induced by absence of *Helicobacter pylori*

Bacteria As "New" Causes for "Old" Diseases

The finding that an indigenous bacterium, *Helicobacter pylori*, plays pathogenetic roles in two important illnesses, peptic ulcer disease and gastric cancer,[20] has advanced a new paradigm—that many of the diseases that we consider diseases of unknown cause may in fact be infectious diseases.[3] This idea, which gained prominence with the knowledge about the relationship of streptococcal pharyngitis to rheumatic fever, has been growing since the 1930s, and other examples have been recognized. For example, after an episode of enteritis caused by *Campylobacter jejuni*, the Guillain-Barré syndrome may develop.[21] Similarly, more than 20 years ago, it was recognized that acute infection with enterohemorrhagic *E. coli* may lead to the hemolytic uremic syndrome.[22] Thus, acute, transient, and self-limited infections of the respiratory or gastrointestinal tracts may trigger cardiac, neurologic, or systemic diseases, with consequences lasting months or permanently. Importantly, the disease locus (e.g., kidney, peripheral nervous system, heart) may be distant from the original infection at a mucosal surface. How many other examples of parallel phenomena may be present? The uncovering of clinical and epidemiologic associations has led to research that has identified pathogenetic mechanisms, which provide new paradigms for autoimmunity.[23] Could a more persistent bacterial pathogen trigger multiple sclerosis, or Graves' disease?

Diseases such as sarcoidosis, ulcerative colitis, Crohn's disease, Wegener's granulomatosis, and thyroiditis are chronic inflammatory diseases for which a bacterial role in causation is not improbable. Despite a long and inconclusive history, studies again point to *Mycobacteria* being present in sarcoidosis.[24]

Bacterial Evolution

The study of infectious diseases is a dynamic field, at least in part because of the evolving nature of the pathogens we consider. An obvious and absolutely critical aspect of bacterial evolution is the acquisition of resistance to antimicrobial agents. As the prescribing of antimicrobial therapies flourishes—whether they address important, controversial, or even trivial indications—antimicrobial resistance by pathogens and indigenous organisms continues to grow.[25-27] Understanding resistance patterns is pivotal to understanding proper therapeutic approaches.[25] Also importantly, understanding the biology, epidemiology, and mechanisms for resistance will lead to methods that will be needed to prevent and curtail resistance in the populations of microbes that infect and colonize humans, which may provide reservoirs for resistance.[27,28] Physicians, especially those who are specialists in infectious diseases, must be at the forefront of efforts to reduce the development of resistance.

Interestingly, considerations of resistance are useful for understanding other important aspects in the evolution of infectious diseases; we live in a world of natural selection. Resistance is among the easiest phenotypes to detect and understand, but bacteria continue to be selected on the basis of differences in the soaps used (also a function of resistance), sizes of families and other social groups, presence of daycare centers and jet planes, and changing dietary habits (functions of transmission).[29] As the connectivity of human populations increases, there may be greater selection for virulence.[11] We may already be witnessing progressively increasing virulence of *M. tuberculosis*,[30] in addition to its progressively increasing antibiotic resistance.[31] The spontaneous and widespread emergence of hypervirulent *Clostridium difficile* strains of different genotypes but similar phenotypes (hypertoxigenic because of deletions involving regulatory elements) indicates the power of microbes to adapt to strong selective forces.[32,33] Study of bacterial infections provides a rich school, not only for the health care provider but also for the student of human evolutionary biology.[34,35] The lessons learned will also be critical in clinical medicine and epidemiology.

Bacteria As Therapeutics

Since Metchnikoff and earlier, physicians have sought ways to harness bacteria to fight disease. At present, the highly lethal exotoxin of *C. botulinum* is being used as a therapeutic agent for medical and cosmetic purposes. The bacille Calmette-Guérin (BCG) vaccine, an attenuated form of *Mycobacterium bovis*, is used as adjuvant therapy for bladder cancer. Although at first glance such harnessing of bacteria for useful purposes seems extraordinary, it actually makes great sense. The bacteria that live with us, or that attack us, often know us well; their evolution has selected for organisms that exploit chinks in our

TABLE 194-2	Variation in Time Courses for Representative Bacterial Infections			
Time Frame	**Disease**	**Representative Causative Organism**	**Clinical Manifestations**	**Mechanisms**
Minutes	Food poisoning	*Clostridium perfringens*	Vomiting, diarrhea	Preformed enterotoxin
Hours	Necrotizing fasciitis	*Streptococcus pyogenes*	Devitalization of muscle, sepsis	Bacterial spread across tissue planes
Days	Anthrax	*Bacillus anthracis*	Cough, chest pain, fever, dyspnea	Resistance to macrophage killing
Weeks	Lung abscess	Oral anaerobes	Cough, fever, chest pain	Necrotizing pyogenic process
Months	Subacute bacterial endocarditis	α-Hemolytic streptococci	Fever, anemia, stroke, heart failure, uremia	Infection of immunologically privileged site
Years	Whipple's disease	*Tropheryma whipplei*	Fever, diarrhea, weight loss	Resistance to macrophage killing
Decades (persistence)	Osteomyelitis	*Staphylococcus aureus*	Fever, wound discharge, pain	Pyogenic infection of devitalized tissue (± foreign body)
Decades (latency)	Pulmonary tuberculosis	*Mycobacterium tuberculosis*	Cough, fever, weight loss	Reactivation of latent focus into active granulomatous process
Decades (oncogenesis)	Gastric cancer	*Helicobacter pylori*	Cachexia, abdominal pain	Persistent inflammation leading to progressive metaplastic and dysplastic conditions

armor.[11,36] They are skilled cell biologists, immunologists, and physiologists, and are great competitors with one another. Bacteria have potential usefulness as probiotics to treat disease.[37,38] Probiotics, nutrients that provide a substrate for particular bacteria or biochemical processes, extend the concept by another step.[39] Understanding the clinical manifestations and pathogenesis of bacterial infections will

lead to new approaches to medicine—new therapeutics[38] and new preventives.[7] Predictably, each of the new treatments will lead to new complications. A thorough grounding in knowledge about bacterial infections will enable physicians and researchers to develop these new therapeutic modalities, and to predict and treat the expected complications.

REFERENCES

1. Relman DA. The human body as microbial observatory. *Nat Genet.* 2002;30:131-133.
2. Kroes I, Lepp PW, Relman DA. Bacterial diversity within the human subgingival crevice. *Proc Natl Acad Sci U S A.* 1999;96:14547-14552.
3. Blaser MJ. Bacteria and diseases of unknown cause. *Ann Intern Med.* 1994;121:144-145.
4. Blaser MJ. Who are we? Indigenous microbes and the ecology of human diseases. *EMBO Reports.* 2006;7:956-960.
5. Chen Y, Blaser MJ. *Helicobacter pylori* colonization is inversely associated with childhood asthma. *J Infect Dis.* 2008;198:553-560.
6. Blaser MJ. Understanding microbe-induced cancers. *Cancer Prev Res (Phila Pa).* 2008;1:15-20.
7. Blaser MJ. Disappearing microbiota: *Helicobacter pylori* protection against esophageal adenocarcinoma. *Cancer Prev Res (Phila Pa).* 2008;1:308-311.
8. Woese C. Microbiology in transition. *Proc Natl Acad Sci U S A.* 1994;91:1601-1603.
9. Caldwell HD, Wood H, Crane D, et al. Polymorphisms in *Chlamydia trachomatis* tryptophan synthase genes differentiate between genital and ocular isolates. *J Clin Invest.* 2003;111:1757-1769.
10. Walder MK, Mekalanos JJ. Lysogenic conversion by a filamentous phage encoding cholera toxin. *Science.* 1996;272:1910-1914.
11. Blaser MJ, Kirschner D. The equilibria that permit bacterial persistence in human hosts. *Nature.* 2007;449:843-849.
12. Turnbaugh PJ, Ley RE, Hamady M, et al. The human microbiome project. *Nature.* 2007;449:804-810.
13. Eckburg PB, Lepp PW, Relman DA. Archaea and their potential role in human disease. *Infect Immun.* 2003;71:591-596.
14. Gill SR, Pop M, Deboy RT, et al. Metagenomic analysis of the human distal gut microbiome. *Science.* 2006;312:1355-1359.
15. Palmer C, Bik EM, Digiulio DB, et al. Development of the human infant intestinal microbiota. *PLoS Biol.* 2007;5:e177.
16. Blaser MJ, Musser JM. Bacterial polymorphisms and disease in humans. *J Clin Invest.* 2001;107:391-392.
17. Kang J, Blaser MJ. Bacterial populations as perfect gases: genomic integrity and diversification tensions in Helicobacter pylori. *Nat Rev Microbiol.* 2006;4:826-836.
18. Caws M, Thwaites G, Dunstan S, et al. The influence of host and bacterial genotype on the development of disseminated disease with Mycobacterium tuberculosis. *PLoS Pathog.* 2008;4:e1000034.
19. Rossouw M, Nel HJ, Cooke GS, et al. Association between tuberculosis and a polymorphic NFkappaB binding site in the interferon γ gene. *Lancet.* 2003;361:1871-1872.
20. Blaser MJ. The changing relationships of *Helicobacter pylori* and humans: Implications for health and disease. *J Infect Dis.* 1999;179:1523-1530.
21. Rees JH, Soudain SE, Gregson NA, et al. *Campylobacter jejuni* infection and Guillain-Barré syndrome. *N Engl J Med.* 1995;333:1374-1379.
22. Karmali MA, Petric MA, Lim C, et al. The association between idiopathic hemolytic uremic syndrome and infection by verotoxin-producing *Escherichia coli. J Infect Dis.* 1985;151:775-782.
23. Ang CW, Noordzij PG, de Klerk MA, et al. Ganglioside mimicry of *Campylobacter jejuni* lipopolysaccharides determines antiganglioside specificity in rabbits. *Infect Immun.* 2002;70:5081-5085.
24. Drake WP, Pei Z, Pride DT, et al. Molecular analysis of sarcoidosis and control tissues for DNA from *Mycobacterium* species. *Emerg Infect Dis.* 2002;8:1334-1341.
25. Lonks JR, Garau J, Gomez L, et al. Failure of macrolide antibiotic treatment in patients with bacteremia due to erythromycin-resistant *Streptococcus pneumoniae. Clin Infect Dis.* 2002;35:556-564.
26. Fenton KA, Ison C, Johnson AP, et al. Ciprofloxacin resistance in *Neisseria gonorrhoeae* in England and Wales in 2002. *Lancet.* 2003;361:1867-1868.
27. Sjolund M, Andersson DI, Blaser MJ, et al. Long-term persistence of resistant *Enterococcus* species after antibiotic treatment to eliminate *Helicobacter pylori. Ann Intern Med.* 2003;139:483-487.
28. Sjölund M, Tano E, Blaser MJ, et al. Persistence of resistant *Staphylococcus epidermidis* after single course of clarithromycin. *Emerg Infect Dis.* 2005;11:1389-1393.
29. Wilson ME. Infectious diseases: An ecological perspective. *BMJ.* 1995;331:1681-1684.
30. Gagneux S, DeRiemer K, Van T, et al. Variable host-pathogen compatibility in Mycobacterium tuberculosis. *PNAS.* 2006;103:2869-2873.
31. Gagneux S, Burgos MV, DeRiemer K, et al. Impact of bacterial genetics on the transmission of isoniazid-resistant Mycobacterium tuberculosis. *PLoS Pathog.* 2006;2:e61.
32. McDonald LC, Killgore GE, Thompson A, et al. An epidemic, toxin gene-variant strain of Clostridium difficile. *N Engl J Med.* 2005;353:2433-2441.
33. Loo VG, Poirier L, Miller MA, et al. A predominantly clonal multi-institutional outbreak of Clostridium difficile-associated diarrhea with high morbidity and mortality. *N Engl J Med.* 2005;353:2442-2449.
34. Ghose C, Perez-Perez GI, Dominguez-Bello MG, et al. East Asian genotypes of *Helicobacter pylori*: Strains in Amerindians provide evidence for its ancient human carriage. *Proc Natl Acad Sci U S A.* 2002;99:15107-15111.
35. Linz B, Balloux F, Moodley Y, et al. An African origin for the intimate association between humans and Helicobacter pylori. *Nature.* 2007;445:915-918.
36. Collin M, Olsen A. Extracellular enzymes with immunomodulating activities: Variations on a theme in *Streptococcus pyogenes. Infect Immun.* 2003;71:2983-2992.
37. Kalliomaki M, Salminen S, Poussa T, et al. Probiotics and prevention of atopic disease: 4-year follow-up of a randomised placebo-controlled trial. *Lancet.* 2003;361:1869-1870.
38. Tannock G, ed. *Probiotics and Prebiotics: Where Are We Going?* Wymondham, UK: Caister Academic Press; 2002:1-336.
39. Dominguez-Bello MG, Blaser MJ. Do you have a probiotic in your future? *Microbes Infect.* 2008;10:1072-1076.

195

Staphylococcus aureus (Including Staphylococcal Toxic Shock)

YOK-AI QUE | PHILIPPE MOREILLON

Staphylococcus aureus is a highly successful opportunistic pathogen. It is a frequent colonizer of the skin and mucosa of humans and animals (it is present in the anterior nares of up to 30% of the healthy human population) and can produce a wide variety of diseases. These diseases encompass relatively benign skin infections, such as folliculitis and furunculosis, and life-threatening conditions, including erysipelas, deep-seated abscesses, osteomyelitis, pneumonia, sepsis, and endocarditis.[1] In addition to infections in which the organism is physically present at the infected site, *S. aureus* is also capable of producing "distant" diseases, which are mediated by the secretion of toxins.[2] The toxins can be produced *directly* by bacteria that colonize the skin or mucosa or *indirectly* by microorganisms that colonize food or beverages. The former is exemplified by staphylococcal scalded skin syndrome (SSSS),[3] which is the result of mucosal or wound colonization by *S. aureus* producing exfoliative toxin A or B (ETA or ETB), and by staphylococcal toxic shock syndrome (TSS),[4] which is the result of the production of toxic shock syndrome toxin 1 (TSST-1) or exotoxins B or C. The latter is exemplified by *S. aureus* food intoxication, in which the toxin is ingested with the contaminated dish and disease follows shortly thereafter in the form of vomiting and diarrhea. Food intoxication is the result of staphylococcal toxins called *enterotoxins*.[2,5] These toxins are heat stable. Cooking may kill the contaminants but does not denature the toxins. Hence, subsequent culture of the dish may fail to grow the culprit bacterium.

The heterogeneity of these diseases and the unique ability of *S. aureus* to develop antibiotic resistance reflect the extraordinary capacity of this organism to adapt and survive in a great variety of environments. During the last decades, molecular and genetic dissection of *S. aureus* has revealed a great number of surface adhesins, which mediate adherence to and colonization of target tissues, and secreted enzymes and toxins that are responsible for invasion and distant disease (Table 195-1).[1,6-8] The development of genomics and the availability of the complete nucleotide sequence of more than 10 *S. aureus* genomes have helped complete this portrait (e.g., see http://www.ncbi.nlm.nih.gov/genomes/lproks.cgi). Approximately 50% of the *S. aureus* genome shares homology with notoriously nonpathogenic *Bacillus subtilis*, which indicates that the two organisms are quite close and have evolved from a common ancestor.[9,10] Homology searches on the chromosome revealed numerous new surface-attached and secreted factors that might represent additional pathogenic factors. Most interestingly, *S. aureus* harbors a large number of mobile genetic elements (MGEs) from exogenous origin, including insertion sequences, transposons, bacteriophages, pathogenicity islands, and genomic islands, which contain specific determinants responsible for disease and antibiotic resistance.[6,7,10-12] The presence of these exogenous elements attests the high capacity of *S. aureus* to undergo horizontal gene transfer and exchange genetic elements with other organisms, including staphylococcal and nonstaphylococcal genera. Because gene exchange is a key player of evolution, this peculiar genetic plasticity is a likely explanation for the success of *S. aureus,* both as a colonizer and a disease-producing microbe. In the case of superantigens (see subsequent discussion), one of the trading partners is suspected to be *Streptococcus pyogenes.*[4]

The Microorganism

Members of the *Staphylococcus* genus are gram-positive cocci (0.5 to 1.5 µm in diameter) that occur singly and in pairs, tetrads, short chains, and irregular grapelike clusters. Ogston[13] introduced the name *staphylococcus* (from Greek *staphylé*, a bunch of grapes) to describe micrococci responsible for inflammation and suppuration. Staphylococci are nonmotile, non–spore forming, and usually catalase positive, and they are often unencapsulated or have a limited capsule (Fig. 195-1). Most species are facultative anaerobes.[9]

Staphylococci were formerly classified in a common genus with micrococci. However, the organisms are quite different in several aspects, including major differences in guanidine-cytosine (G+C) content (staphylococci have a low G+C content of 30% to 39%, whereas micrococci have a high G+C content of 63% to 73%), in cell wall structure (staphylococci have peptidoglycan-bound teichoic acids, whereas micrococci have no teichoic acids), and in cytochrome and menaquinone composition of respiratory chain.[9] Staphylococci are closer to *Bacillus* spp. and streptococci and belong to the broad *Bacillus-Lactobacillus-Streptococcus* cluster.

The genus *Staphylococcus* contains 36 species, 16 of which are found in humans (Table 195-2). Only a few are pathogenic in the absence of predisposing immunosuppression or implanted foreign material. The most virulent ones include *S. aureus* and *Staphylococcus lugdunensis* in humans, and *S. aureus* and *Staphylococcus intermedius* in animals. Although *Staphylococcus epidermidis, Staphylococcus haemolyticus,* and *Staphylococcus saprophyticus* are commonly responsible for device-related and urinary tract infections, they produce substantially less devastating disease syndromes than *S. aureus.* Pathogenic staphylococci harbor some unique features when compared with their less disease-producing congeners. These include coagulase and clumping factor (or fibrinogen-binding protein), which have laboratory diagnostic value because they help rapidly discriminate between coagulase-positive (i.e., *S. aureus)* and coagulase-negative staphylococci (CoNS; see Table 195-2). Moreover, comparative genomics indicates that *S. aureus* carries between more than 20 and more than 30 adhesin genes and toxin genes, respectively, as compared with 10 or less adhesin genes and no toxin genes for the CoNS mentioned previously.[7,14-16] Thus, *S. aureus* is a distinct pathogen within the *Staphylococcus* genus.

HABITAT

Staphylococci are ubiquitous colonizers of the skin and mucosa of virtually all animals, including mammals and birds.[9] Some species have preferential niches as indicated by their names (see Table 195-2). *S. epidermidis* and *Staphylococcus capitis* are constant colonizers of the skin and scalp, respectively.

S. aureus is widely spread among primates but is not restricted to them. It is a major cause of disease (mastitis) in bovine and ovine herds. In humans, *S. aureus* has a niche preference for the anterior nares, especially in adults,[17,18] and is shed onto healthy skin, including axilla and perineum, where it can be recovered as well. It can exist as a resident or a transient member of the normal flora. Nasal carrier rate

| TABLE 195-1 | *Staphylococcus aureus* Extracellular Factors Involved in Pathogenesis, and Response to Global Regulatory Elements during Bacterial Growth | | | | | | | |

Gene	Location	Product	Activity/Function	Timing*	Action of Regulatory Genes†			
					agr	saeRS	rot	sarA
Surface proteins								
spa	Chromosome	Protein A	Antiimmune, anti-PMN	exp		‡	+	
cna	Chromosome	Collagen BP	Collagen binding	pxp	0			
fnbA	Chromosome	Fibronectin BPA	Fibronectin binding	exp				+
fnbB	Chromosome	Fibronectin BPB	Fibronectin binding	exp				+
clfA	Chromosome	Clumping factor A	Fibrinogen binding	exp	0			
clfB	Chromosome	Clumping factor B / Lactoferrin BP	Fibrinogen binding / Lactoferrin binding	exp	0		+	0
Capsular polysaccharides								
cap5	Chromosome	Polysaccharide capsule type 5	Antiphagocytosis?	pxp	+			+
cap8	Chromosome	Polysaccharide capsule type 8	Antiphagocytosis?	pxp	+			
Cytotoxins								
hla	Chromosome	α-hemolysin	Hemolysin, cytotoxin	pxp	+	+	−	‡
hlb	Chromosome	β-hemolysin	Hemolysin, cytotoxin	pxp	+	+	−	‡
hld	Chromosome	δ-hemolysin	Hemolysin, cytotoxin	xp	+	0		
hlg	Chromosome	γ-hemolysin	Hemolysin, cytotoxin	pxp	+		−	+
lukS/F	PVL phage	PVL*	Leucolysin	pxp	+		−	
Superantigens								
sea	Bacteriophage	Enterotoxin A	Food poisoning, TSS	xp	0			
seb	SaPI3§	Enterotoxin B	Food poisoning, TSS	pxp	+			‡
sec	SaPI4§	Enterotoxin C	Food poisoning, TSS	pxp	+			
sed	Plasmid	Enterotoxin D	Food poisoning, TSS	pxp	+			
eta	ETA phage	Exfoliatin A	Scalded skin syndrome	pxp	+			
etb	Plasmid	Exfoliatin B	Scalded skin syndrome	pxp	+			
tst	SaPI1,2,bov1§	Toxic shock toxin-1	Toxic shock syndrome	pxp	+			‡
Enzymes								
SplA-F	Chromosome	Serine protease-like	Putative protease		+		−	
ssp	Chromosome	V8 protease	Spreading factor	pxp	+	0		−
aur		Metalloprotease (aureolysin)	Processing enzyme?	pxp	+			−
sspB		Cysteine protease	Processing enzyme?		+		−	
scp		Staphopain (protease II)	Spreading, nutrition	pxp	+			−
geh	Chromosome	Glycerol ester hydrolase	Spreading, nutrition	pxp	+	0		‡
lip		Lipase (butyryl esterase)	Spreading, nutrition	pxp	+	0		‡
fme	Chromosome	FAME	Fatty acid esterification	pxp	+			‡
plc		PI-phospholipase C		pxp	+			
nuc	Chromosome	Nuclease	Nutrition	pxp	+	+		
hys	Chromosome	Hyaluronidase	Spreading factor	xp	‡			
coa	Chromosome	Coagulase	Clotting, clot digestion	exp		+	+	+
sak	Bacteriophage	Staphylokinase	Plasminogen activator	pxp	+	0		

*Timing: *xp*, throughout exponential phase; *exp*, early exponential phase only; *pxp*, postexponential phase; *0*, no effect of gene on. Expression: +, upregulated; −, downregulated.
†*agr*, accessory gene regulator; *saeRS*, *S. aureus* exoproteins; *rot*, repressor of toxins; *sarA*, *Staphylococcus* accessory regulator; FAME, fatty acid modifying enzyme; PMN, polymorphonuclear neutrophil.
‡Controversial.
§*SaPI*, *S. aureus* pathogenic island.
BP, binding protein.
Adapted from Cheung AL, Projan SJ, Gresham H. The genomic aspect of virulence, sepsis, and resistance to killing mechanisms in Staphylococcus aureus. *Curr Infect Dis Rep.* 2002;4:400-410; and Novick RP. Autoinduction and signal transduction in the regulation of staphylococcal virulence. *Mol Microbiol.* 2003;48:1429-1449.

varies from 10% to 40% in both the community and the hospital environment. Chronic nasal carriage may put certain populations at an increased risk of infection, such as patients with recurring furunculosis and patients who are subject to medical procedures including hemodialysis, peritoneal dialysis, and surgery (see also Carriage of *S. aureus* section of Clinical Aspects and Epidemiology).[19,20]

Nasal carriage of *S. aureus* has also become a way of persistence and spread of multiresistant staphylococci, especially methicillin-resistant *S. aureus* (MRSA).[17,18] Because MRSA can resist practically all available antibiotics, it has risen to the level of public health threat, in the hospital for three decades and in the community since the beginning of this century.[21,22]

CULTURE AND IDENTIFICATION

Live organisms obtained via cultures are critical for phenotypic diagnosis and revealing emerging antibiotic resistances from as yet unknown mechanisms. On the other hand, molecular diagnosis helps speed up the results, which take a few hours instead of 1 to 3 days with bacterial subculturing. Molecular methods also help detect the presence of noncultivable microbes, mostly when patients have taken antibiotics before sample collection.

Techniques for culture and identification of staphylococci have been described.[9] Specimens should be inoculated both on blood agar and into rich liquid media such as Mueller-Hinton broth. With *S.*

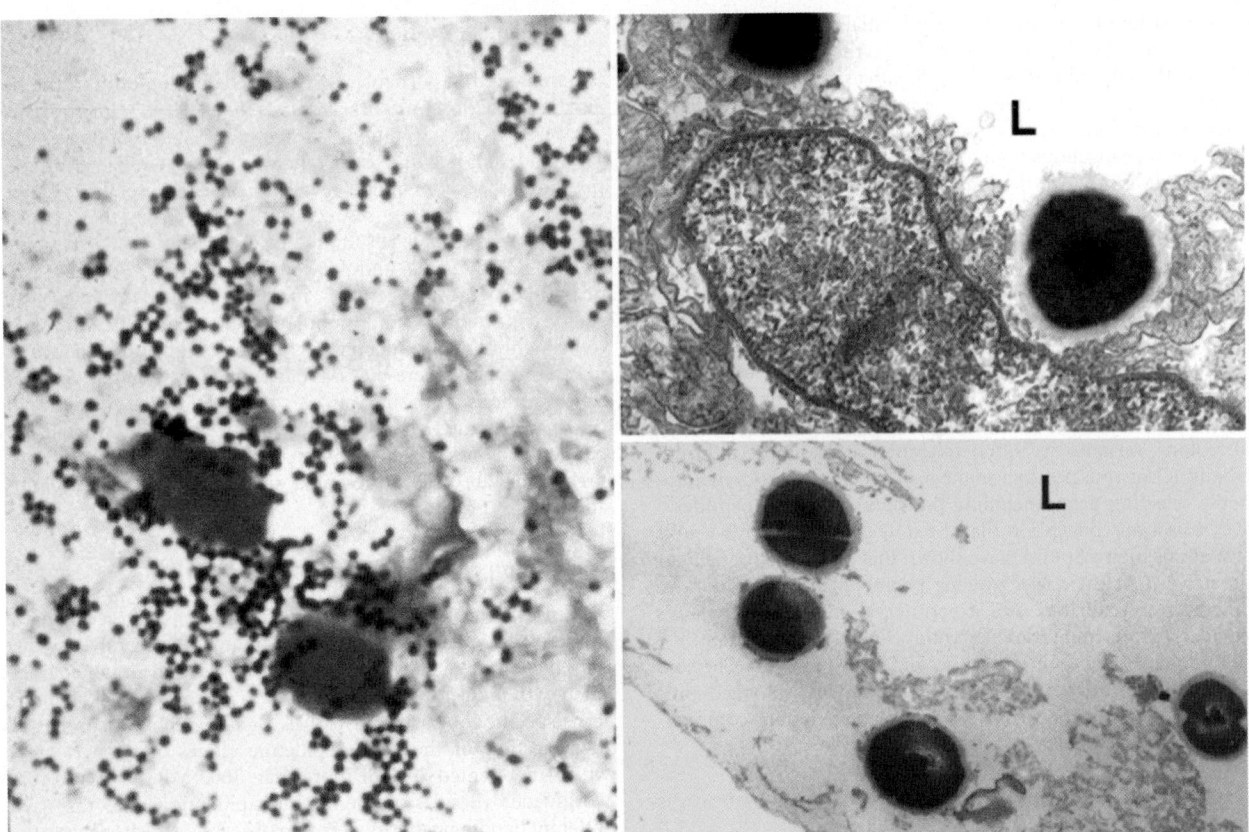

Figure 195-1 **Gram staining and transmission electron microscopy of clinical samples of *S. aureus*.** *Left,* Gram-stained sputum specimen from 20-year-old patient with fulminant hemorrhagic *S. aureus* pneumonia (see also Fig. 195-7). Grapelike clusters of bacteria and eukaryotic cells are visible. *Right,* Electron microscopy images from rat with experimental aortic endocarditis caused by *S. aureus*. *Upper* part depicts *S. aureus* in process of invading valve endothelial cell. *Lower* part depicts endothelial cell that has been lysed by invading bacteria, probably as a result of *S. aureus* hemolysin secretion. *L,* lumen side of endothelium.

TABLE 195-2	Some Staphylococcal Species from Mammals and Relationship between Production of Coagulase and Clumping Factor (Fibrinogen-Binding Protein A) and Potential Virulence			
Host	*Species*	*Coagulase**	*Clumping factor**	*Virulence**
Human and other primates	S. aureus	++	++	+++
	S. epidermidis	−	−	+
	S. capitis	−	−	±
	S. caprae	−	−	±
	S. saccharolyticus	±	−	−
	S. warneri	−	−	−
	S. pasteuri	−	−	−
	S. haemolyticus	−	−	+
	S. hominis	−	−	±
	S. lugnunensis	−	±	+
	S. auricularis	−	−	±
	S. saprophyticus	−	−	+
	S. cohnii	−	−	−
	S. xilosus	−	−	−
	S. simulans	−	−	−
	S. schleiferi	±	+	+
Carnivores	S. intermedius	+	−	++
	S. felis	−	−	++

*Semiquantitative estimate of production of coagulase and clumping factor and relation to virulence.

Adapted from Kloos WE, Schleifer KH, Goetz F. The genus staphylococcus. In Balows A, Trüper HG, Dworkin M, et al, editors. *The Prokaryotes.* 2nd ed. New York: Springer-Verlag; 1992:1369-1420; and Kloos WE, Bannerman TL. *Staphylococcus* and *Micrococcus.* In Murray PR, Baron EJ, Pfaller MA, et al, editors. *Manual of Clinical Microbiology.* 6th ed. Washington, DC: ASM Press; 1995:282-298.

aureus, abundant growth occurs normally within 18 to 24 hours. However, morphology variants (see subsequent discussion) may require prolonged growth periods, and plates should be kept 2 to 3 days to detect them. Colonies should be gram-stained, subcultured, and tested for genus, species, and antibiotic susceptibility when appropriate. Phenotypic tests for species identification include coagulase tests and agglutination tests, which detect the presence of surface determinants, including clumping factor, protein A, and polysaccharides.[23] Molecular specification with polymerase chain reaction (PCR) amplification of the 16S or 23S ribosomal RNA (rRNA) may be necessary in case of unclear phenotypes. Antibiotic-resistance tests vary from agar-diffusion methods (e.g., Kirby-Bauer and E-tests) to automated measurement of metabolic activity or growth rates. Macro broth or agar dilution methods are precise but are not routinely performed in the laboratory.[24]

MORPHOLOGY VARIANTS

Prolonged incubation is particularly important in detection of morphology variants such as *small colony variants* (SCV). SCVs grow into tiny colonies that are difficult to distinguish and may be mistakenly disregarded as contaminants.[25] They are usually recovered from protracted difficult-to-treat infections such as chronic osteomyelitis and infected osteosynthetic prostheses and were recently described in patients with cystic fibrosis.[26]

The most classical type of SCVs is selected during aminoglycoside therapy and results from mutations in the respiratory chain. Such mutants have a lower transmembrane potential, which impedes the intake of the drug.[27] SCVs were recovered from the sputa of up to 20% of patients with cystic fibrosis carrying *S. aureus* and were associated with prior treatment with trimethoprim-sulfamethoxazole.[26] These SCVs carry a mutation in their thymidylate synthase gene *(thyA)* and are dependent on exogenous thymidine to grow.[28]

Many bacteria synthesize thymidine on their own, which requires tetrahydrofolate for thymidine synthase to convert uridine-mono-phosphate into thymidine-monophosphate. Trimethoprim inhibits the synthesis of essential tetrahydrofolate, thus making thymidine synthase useless. Hence, by mutating their *thyA* gene, thymidine-dependent SCVs force themselves to import exogenous thymidine to survive, which makes the bacteria resistant to trimethoprim but forces them to activate thymidine import. Thymidine is available in DNA-rich lung secretions of patients with cystic fibrosis, but thymidine import is rate limiting and thus responsible for slow growth.

Small colony variants are often tolerant (i.e., resistant to drug-induced killing) or resistant to a number of other antibiotics in addition to the selecting drug, including β-lactams and glycopeptides.[26] Moreover, it is a misconception that the slow growth of SCVs results in lower pathogenicity. Studies have shown that SCVs were equally or more infective than their fast growing parent in infections such as experimental osteoarthritis[29] and experimental endocarditis.[30] SCVs are particularly prone to invade eukaryotic cells and persist in them.[25,31] This trait might explain their occurrence in latent infections. They are particularly difficult to eradicate and may necessitate prolonged antibiotic therapy and specific drug combinations, including combinations with rifampin.

▣ Molecular Diagnosis

Molecular diagnosis plays an increasing role in rapid detection of microbial pathogens and identification of drug-resistance determinants. Results can be obtained within a few hours. Identification techniques based on molecular probing were recently reviewed.[32] One of these techniques relies on fluorescent detection of 16S rRNA with a peptide nucleic acid probe *(peptide nucleic acid fluorescence in situ hybridization* [PNA-FISH]). It identified *S. aureus* in positive blood cultures in less than 3 hours with a more than 95% sensitivity and specificity.[33] The method allowed rapid discrimination between *S. aureus* and potential contaminant CoNS, thus improving therapeutic decision making.[34]

In addition to PNA-FISH, *multiplex real-time PCR* is being developed to quantify organisms directly in clinical samples. Genes representative of both species and resistance mechanisms are amplified simultaneously. For MRSA, the resistance gene sought is *mecA*, which encodes low-affinity penicillin-binding protein 2A (PBP2A). However, *mecA* is also present in methicillin-resistant CoNS and thus detects simultaneously both MRSA and commensal methicillin-resistant CoNS. Two studies showed that simultaneous amplification of additional regions that were specific for *S. aureus* could circumvent the problem and was successfully applied to screen MRSA directly from nasal samples.[35,36] In one of these studies, the rightward PCR primer targeted *mecA*, which is shared by both MRSA and methicillin-resistant CoNS, and a leftward primer targeted *orfX*, which is situated further downward and is specific for *S. aureus*.[35] In the other, the amplicons included the *mecA* gene and two versions of the *femA* gene specific for *S. aureus* and *S. epidermidis*, respectively.[36]

A wealth of molecular techniques is being developed and proposed for routine use. In addition to identification of species and resistance genes, quantitative multiplex PCR methods and DNA arrays are being developed for profiling the whole setup of virulence genes. Further high-throughput techniques, including RNomics and proteomics, might provide a comprehensive picture of the "good" and the "bad" staphylococci and help decide which of them must be considered for therapeutic intervention.

MOLECULAR TYPING

S. aureus, and in particular MRSA, are common both in the hospital and in the community. In a survey of 3,309,413 microbial isolates recovered from sterile body sites in 300 U.S. laboratories (between 1998 and 2005), *S. aureus* was the most prevalent bacterium in inpatients and the second most prevalent isolate in outpatients (18.7% and 14.7% of the isolates, respectively).[37] Moreover, the frequency of MRSA was as high as 59% in intensive care unit (ICU) patients, 55% in non-ICU patients, and 48% in outpatients.[22,37] Because MRSA is of particular medical concern, major efforts were devoted to understand its evolution and population structure.[38,39] MRSA appears to be highly clonal, and a few highly successful clones, named according to the place where they were described, can be recovered at multiple locations both nationwide and worldwide (i.e., the Iberian, Brazilian, Hungarian, New York/Japan, Pediatric, and EMRSA-16 pandemic clones).[38] The main typing methods underlying this comprehension are briefly presented subsequently. Phage typing is not addressed.

PULSE FIELD GEL ELECTROPHORESIS

The most widely used method is a restriction-fragment length technique based on large chromosomal fragments generated by digestion with the low-frequency cutting enzyme *Sma*1. The fragments are separated with *pulse field gel electrophoresis* (PFGE) and yield banding patterns specific for particular clones. Banding comparison has allowed identification of the major epidemic clones alluded to previously, which represented 70% of more than 3000 MRSA isolates recovered worldwide.[38] Besides, numerous nonepidemic clones that generated different banding patterns were also observed, which suggests that they were less successful in colonization and spread.

Although extremely useful for following given clones, PFGE does not provide accurate information on the genealogy of the organism. Indeed, the length of chromosomal fragments, and thus the clone-specific banding, may be modified with acquisition or loss of mobile DNA (MGEs) such as transposons, prophages, or pathogenicity islands. The new banding pattern may identify a different clone, which is in fact the same bacterium that has gained or lost MGEs. If the new organism has acquired properties important for successful spread, it may indeed behave as a new clone with its proper behavior. Nevertheless, the phylogenic relation between the new clone and the parent persists.

MULTILOCUS SEQUENCE TYPING

In contrast to PFGE, *multilocus sequence typing* (MLST) is a sequence-based method that allows the unambiguous assignment of the ancestral phylogeny of the staphylococcal population.[39] The technique consists of sequencing a total of seven housekeeping genes (i.e., *arcC, aroF, glpF, gmk, pta, tpi,* and *yqiY*) and submitting the sequences to a central database (www.mls.net) that compares them with the sequences of other isolates. The differentiation is based on allelic diversity based on approximately 500-bp internal gene fragments. Thousands of sequences have been submitted, generating numerous sequence types (STs). Organisms that share all seven alleles are defined as *clones,* those that share five of seven identical alleles are defined as *clonal complexes* (CC), and those that share less than seven alleles are defined as *unrelated.*

Because housekeeping genes are independent of antibiotic-resistance genes, MLST traces resistant staphylococci to their antibiotic susceptible ancestors. Of the seven pandemic clones mentioned previously, six could be traced back to three ancestral methicillin-susceptible *S. aureus* (MSSA; i.e., CC5, CC8, and CC30; Fig. 195-2).[40] Hence, MLST suggests that a few ancestral clones of MSSA already took the lead and successfully colonized humans and animals before antibiotic resistance. Then, acquisition of MGEs carrying drug-resistance or virulence genes helped further adaptation to new conditions (e.g.,

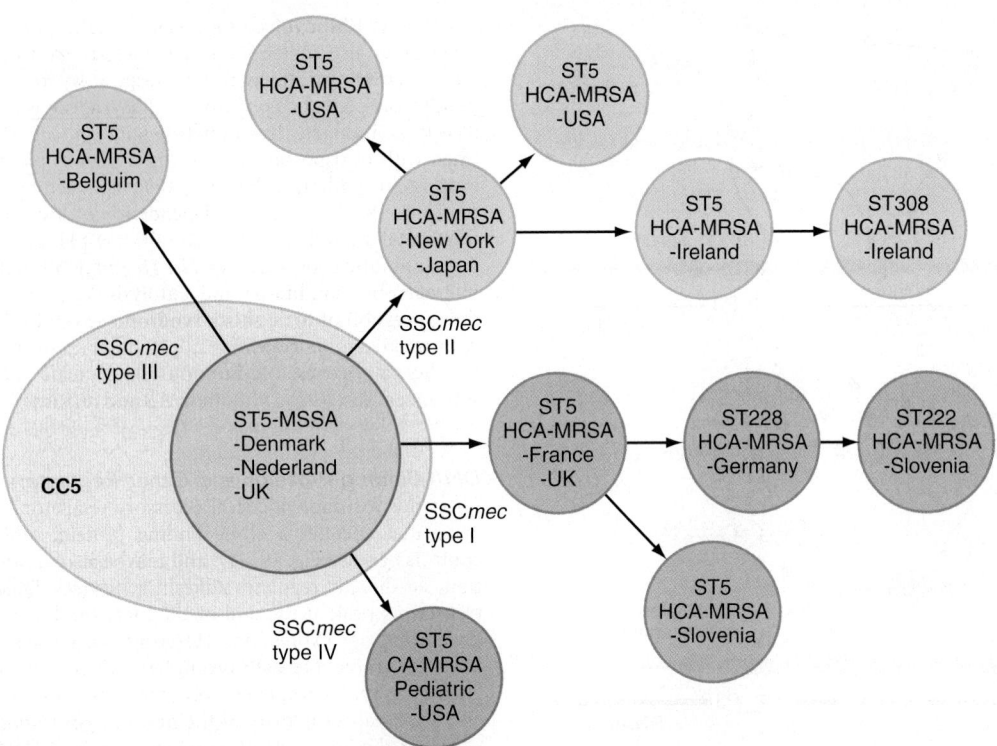

Figure 195-2   Evolution of methicillin-susceptible *Staphylococcus aureus* (MSSA) into methicillin-resistant *S. aureus* (MRSA) as exemplified by sequence type 5 (ST5). ST5 belongs to clonal cluster 5 (CC5), which gathers *S. aureus* isolates sharing homologies in five of the seven genes (*arcC, aroF, glpF, gmk, pta, tpi* and *yqiY*) compared with method of multilocus sequence typing (MLST). Parental ST5 is a MSSA that has been isolated in several countries including Denmark, the Netherlands, and the United Kingdom. It acquired various types of SCC*mec* at several independent occasions, probably from CoNS donor strains. After SCC*mec* acquisition, new MRSA clones followed their own geographic and genetic evolution, spreading either as HCA-MRSA (SCC*mec* I, II or III) or CA-MRSA clones (SCC*mec* IV) and sometimes evolving into new ST types (e.g., ST222, ST228 and ST308). Three clonal clusters (CC5, CC8, and CC30) generated six of the seven major pandemic MRSA clones described over the last three decades. (*Adapted from Robinson DA, Enright MC. Evolutionary models of the emergence of methicillin-resistant* Staphylococcus aureus. Antimicrob Agents Chemother. *2003;47:3926-3934.*)

antibiotic use in hospitals), generating a new PFGE makeup on similar ancestral parents.

SPA TYPING AND DOUBLE-LOCUS *SPA-CLFB* TYPING

These sequence-based methods, *spa typing* and *double-locus spa-clfb typing,* rely on PCR amplification of strain-specific regions within hypervariable segments of the *spa* (protein A) or *clfB* (clumping factor B) genes.[41] The variable regions are made of 24 nucleotide repeats in *spa* and serine-aspartate (SD) repeats in *clfB*, the length of which may vary from duplication or accidental loss of DNA material. Although less discriminative, these simpler methods generate unambiguous data sets that can be compared in multicenter studies.

Typing has become an important part of the comprehension of the *S. aureus* epidemiology. As yet, however, no specific types could be attributed to disease-producing versus mere colonizing strains.[11,42]

■ Pathogenesis I: Regulation and Virulence Determinants

S. aureus is extremely well equipped in surface factors and secreted proteins that mediate host colonization and disease.[1] The principal determinants of this armamentarium are listed in Table 195-1. In addition to these features, *S. aureus* is equipped with regulatory systems that sense environmental conditions and respond by fine tuning the expression of given metabolic and virulence determinants (for review see Cheung and colleagues,[8] Novick,[43] and Pragman and Schlievert[44]).

Some aspects of this subtle adaptation machinery are described subsequently.

REGULATION

At least three families of regulatory elements intertwine to adjust gene expression to specific environmental conditions: first, two-component regulatory systems (TCRS), of which *agr* is a paradigm; second, DNA-binding proteins, largely represented by the Sar family of proteins; and third, small regulatory RNAs.

agr and Other Two-Component Regulatory Systems

The paradigm of TCRS virulence gene regulation is *agr*, which stands for *accessory gene regulator* and is schematized in Figure 195-3.[45] *agr* functions as a quorum sensing control that reacts to bacterial density, allowing the preferential expression of surface adhesins during the exponential phase of growth (low cell density) and switching to the expression of exoproteins during the postexponential and stationary growth phases (high cell density).[43,45] The switch is composed of two divergent operons (see Fig. 195-3). On the left hand, promoter P2 drives the transcription of a series of components that comprises: 1, a transmembrane protein (AgrB); 2, an auto-inducing peptide precursor (AgrD), which is processed and exported by membrane-spanning AgrB; 3, a transmembrane sensor (AgrC), which is the cognate receptor of the AgrD-derived auto-inducing peptide; and 4, a transcription regulator (AgrA) that can be activated by AgrC. At low cell density (exponential growth phase), the P2 promoter is off and the operon is transcribed at a low level. As cell growth proceeds, the concentrations

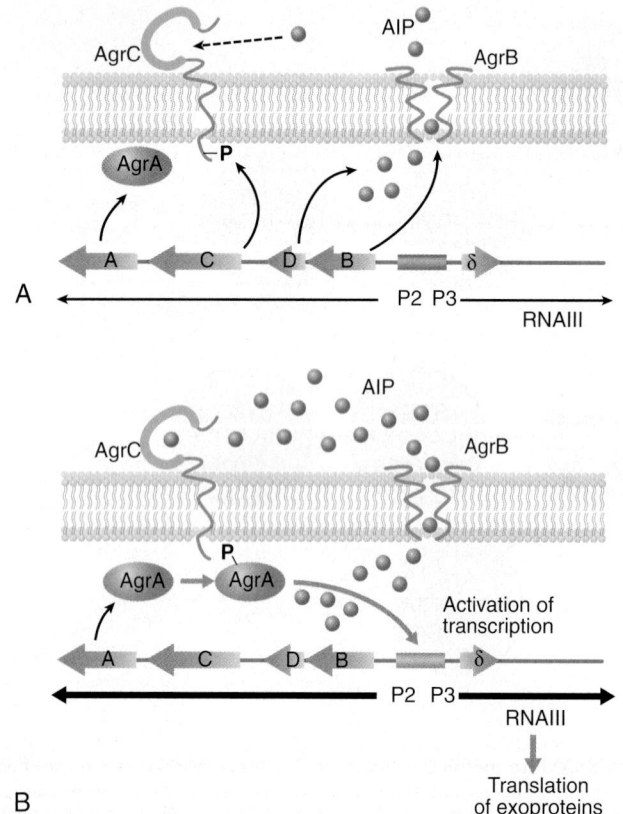

Figure 195-3 **Schematic representation of S. aureus global regulatory system agr (accessory gene regulator). A,** System at rest. It consists of two divergent operons, transcribed from promoters P2 and P3. Promoter P2 encodes putative membrane protein AgrB, precursor of autoinducing peptide (AIP) AgrD, which is processed by AgrB; transmembrane receptor AgrC; and response regulator AgrA. Promoter P3 encodes δ-hemolysin and RNAIII. At low bacterial density, P2 and P3 are off and only a small amount of AIP is secreted because of promoter leakiness **(A)**. As bacterial growth proceeds and bacterial density increases **(B)**, chance of AIP encountering its cognate receptor AgrC increases. On contact, AgrC undergoes conformational change and phosphorylates (or dephosphorylates) response regulator AgrA. Activated AgrA activates transcription from both P2 and P3, resulting in positive feedback. δ-Hemolysin is membrane-active protein toxic for eukaryotic cells. RNAIII is intracellular regulator that acts in trans and regulates expression of many virulence genes, including numerous toxins (see Table 195-1). Although agr is pivotal in quorum-sensing regulation of gene expression, it is not the only regulator of pathogenic determinants in S. aureus. sar, saeRS, rot, and other systems may affect the expression of agr itself or affect virulence genes directly (e.g., sar), or both (see Table 195-1).

of both bacteria and extracellular auto-inducing peptide increase in the milieu, thereby augmenting the chance of auto-inducing peptide to make contact with its cognate AgrC receptor. On contact, AgrC activates the response regulator AgrA, a process that may involve AgrA dephosphorylation.[43]

Activated AgrA is a DNA-binding protein that turns on the transcription from both promoter P2, generating a positive feedback on the system, and promoter P3, which drives the transcription of δ-hemolysin and of a peculiar effector called RNAIII. RNAIII has a reciprocal effect and activates the expression of most secreted proteins while downregulating the expression of surface-bound factors (see Table 195-1). RNAIII has a complex three-dimensional structure and a long half-life (up to 15 minutes). It is believed to regulate gene expression in several ways, including at the translational level by blocking the messenger RNA (mRNA) ribosome-binding site of the target genes.

Other TCRSs involved in global regulation of virulence genes, and most often also metabolic genes, include sae (for S. aureus exoproteins),[46] srrAB (for staphylococcal respiratory response),[47] and arlS (for autolysis-related locus sensor).[48] They affect gene expression either directly or indirectly by interfering with agr (Fig. 195-4). sae was identified with transposon mutation in a pleiotropic mutant defective in exoprotein synthesis other than that regulated by agr (e.g., coagulase; see Table 195-1). sae acts independently of agr and responds to environmental stimuli such as high salt, low pH, glucose, and subinhibitory antibiotic concentrations. srrAB and arlS interfere with growth in microaerobic conditions and autolysis, respectively. srrAB represses the expression of toxic shock syndrome toxin-1 (TSST-1) and protein A in microaerobic conditions,[47] an observation that may be relevant for the pathogenesis of tampon-related toxic shock syndrome (see subsequent discussion).[4] Both srrAB and arlS interact reciprocally with agr.[44,49]

DNA-Binding Proteins and Other Regulators

sar stands for staphylococcal accessory regulator.[50] It is an important locus that encodes a DNA-binding protein, sarA, which positively controls agr (see Fig. 195-4)[8] and maybe also sae and arlS.[43,49] In addition, sar directly regulates adhesin genes (see Table 195-1). The sarA transcripts peak at the end of the logarithmic phase of growth, thus promoting agr expression. Moreover, sarA itself is encoded downstream of three alternate promoters, which can themselves be regulated by as yet incompletely solved factors. This highlights the subtlety and potential complexity of the network governing gene regulation.

sarA is the prototype of a growing family of DNA-binding proteins that may drive a number of transcriptional activities, including the expression of housekeeping genes and phage-related genes. sarA homologues include sarR, sarS, sarT, sarV, sarU, sarY, and rot.[44,49] rot stands for repressor of toxins and counters toxin expression by repressing agr.[51] Inactivation of rot in agr-negative mutants partially restored the agr phenotype, probably by alleviating a repressing effect on the downstream P3 cascade of the agr. This downstream cascade might be the target of several additional regulators that also affect the agr phenotype (see Figure 195-4).

Sigma factors (σ) are another major mechanism of response to environmental stimuli. In bacteria, σ factors combine with and acti-

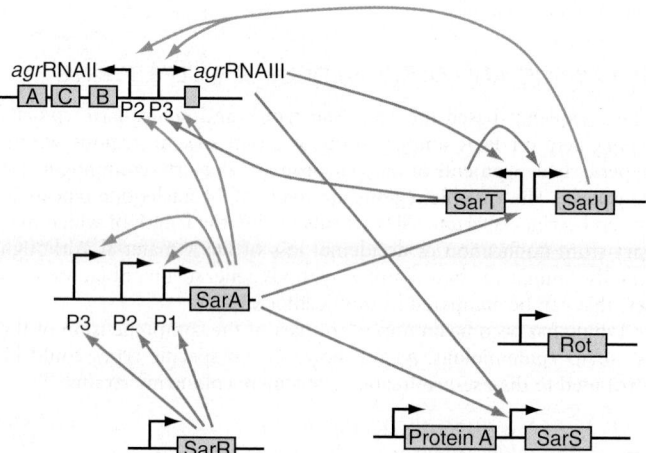

Figure 195-4 **Regulatory network of agr and Sar family of DNA-binding proteins.** Intertwining of activation (green arrows) and repression (red arrows) underlines complexity of system. Gene expression is further modulated by additional factors including alternative σ^B, arlS, sae and srrAB, which can act on agr promoters or directly on specific genes. Gene promoters are denominated P1, P2, and P3 and represented by black lines. (Adapted from Pragman AA, Schlievert PM. Virulence regulation in Staphylococcus aureus: the need for in vivo analysis of virulence factor regulation. FEMS Immunol Med Microbiol. 2004;42:147-154.)

vate RNA polymerase to transcribe specific sets of genes. *S. aureus* contains one σ^A and two alternative σ^B and σ^C. Alternative σ^B is important for the microbial response to a variety of stresses, including temperature, energy depletion, and chemical stimuli.[52] It acts mostly via the global regulatory network but also has some direct effect by activating the expression of coagulase and fibronectin-binding proteins at the early growth phase and downregulating certain secreted proteins in the stationary phase. Increasing the production of surface adhesins suggests that stimulation of σ^B could increase virulence, as suggested in mutants that overexpress σ^B that were tested in experimental endocarditis.[53] But the pathogenic role of σ^B was not shown in other models.

Other Potential Regulatory Factors and Small RNAs
Other factors that influence *agr* may be the RAP and TRAP proteins, which stand for *RNAIII-activating proteins* and *target of RAP*, respectively.[54] The RAP-TRAP complex is proposed to be a TCRS that activates *agr*. It consists of: 1, an autoinducer (RAP), which is an homologue of ribosomal protein L2; 2, an unknown transmembrane sensor (possibly *svrA*)[55]; and 3, an intracellular protein called TRAP. However, recent experiments indicate that the phenotypes of RAP/TRAP and *svrA* mutants might be from simultaneous mutations in the *arg* locus, rather than their regulatory effect on it.[56,57]

Small RNAs (sRNA) are increasingly recognized as major players in regulation of gene expression. They act mainly at the translational level via antisense hybridization with mRNA, where they can either alter mRNA stability, hide ribosome-binding sites (RBS) from ribosome recognition, or conversely reveal RBS that are hidden in secondary mRNA structures by unfolding these very structures. Alternatively, sRNA can also bind regulatory DNA-binding proteins, thus sequestering them from their original gene regulatory function. At least 12 regulatory sRNA have been identified in *S. aureus*,[58] but many more are likely to come. The most prominent of them are RNAIII, which orchestrates the *agr* response, and RNAI, which regulates the replication of multiresistance plasmid pSK41. The role of other sRNA is being actively studied.

This intricate network underlines the subtlety of the bacterial response to environmental stresses. Moreover, it also suggests that dissecting out the role of each of these pathways in disease is an almost impossible task. The regulatory network must be considered as a metabolic hub that integrates both external and internal information and responds in the most appropriate way. Some of these circuitries are likely to complement each other. Interruption of one of them may cause compensation by others, thus introducing biases in the observed phenotype. In this complex system, *agr* appears to be a central switch toward which many other regulators converge (see Fig. 195-4).

Role in Pathogenesis
The intuitive *agr*-based model suggests that scattered growing bacteria produce primarily adhesins, promoting tissue colonization, whereas installed organisms that form dense populations switch to the production of hydrolytic enzymes and toxins for the purpose of feeding and escaping host defenses.[8,43] Accordingly, inactivation of the function of *agr* alone decreased pathogenicity in experimental models of tissue destruction, (e.g., subcutaneous abscesses), where exoprotein production is likely to be important.[59] On the other hand, *agr* inactivation did not influence much the course of experimental endocarditis, where bacterial surface adhesins are critical for valve colonization.[60] Indeed, although *agr*-negative mutants are hampered in exoprotein production, they are still fully equipped with surface-bound colonizing determinants (see Table 195-1). In contrast, inactivation of *sar* decreased infectivity in experimental endocarditis[60] because in addition to its effect on *agr* expression (see Table 195-1; see Fig. 195-3), *sar* also acts directly on expression of surface-bound fibronectin-binding protein A, which promotes experimental endocarditis.[61,62]

In addition, in vivo gene expression revealed a further level of complexity.[44] For instance, although *sar* transcripts were detected in infected vegetations during experimental endocarditis, they were expressed from both P1 and P2 promoters, rather than only from P1

promoter as observed in vitro.[63] Likewise, in vivo expression of several genes appeared dissociated from their control regulator as described in vitro. Although *agr* positively regulates TSST-1 in vitro (see Table 195-1), the toxin was still expressed by an *agr*-negative mutant in a rabbit model of toxic shock syndrome in vivo.[64] This may result from alternative regulation by other regulators that act either downstream of the *agr* locus or directly on the *tss* gene promoter. Eventually, *agr*-negative mutants can be recovered from clinical samples. Such *agr*-negative clinical isolates, and *agr*-negative laboratory mutants, have an increased ability to form biofilms, which are found in chronic infections such as osteomyelitis and device infections.[65] Expression of *agr* might be detrimental to this form of subacute infection.

Hence, the pathogenic implication of regulatory circuitries cannot be drawn merely from in vitro observations. In vivo experimentation reveals the plurality of *S. aureus* infection forms, which may be variously altered by novel antivirulence therapies. For instance, inhibition of the *agr* loop by acting on the auto-inducing peptide impedes acute tissue destruction[59] but might promote biofilm formation and chronic infection.

Ecologic and Epidemiologic Implication of agr
Genetic and functional experiments revealed the existence of at least four *agr* groups in *S. aureus*, which were characterized by specific variations in all three AgrB, AgrD, and AgrC proteins (i.e., the processors-transporter, the auto-inducing peptide precursor, and the receptor, respectively).[66] Although the auto-inducing peptide of a given type stimulated signaling by members of the same group, it either cross inhibited (e.g., group I and group IV) or cross activated (e.g., group I and group II) members of other groups, which suggests that certain antagonistic *agr* groups could be mutually exclusive with attempts to simultaneously colonize the same niche. However, studies regarding this hypothesis gave conflicting results. In particular, patients with cystic fibrosis colonized with *S. aureus* can successfully harbor organisms from two antagonistic *agr* groups.

Although *agr* and other global regulators control the timely expression of pathogenic genes, they are not bona fide pathogenic factor themselves. The *agr* locus has homologues in numerous nonpathogenic staphylococci. A phylogenic study of nonpathogenic CoNS indicated that variations in *agr* genes followed parallel variations in species-specific rRNA genes[67] Thus, *agr* types are not selected by the capacity of one organism to exclude another but rather represent a clonal marker of distinct staphylococcal strains that evolve in distinct environments.

This clonal relation was confirmed when comparing *agr* groups with other epidemiologic markers. Most of the *S. aureus* that produces the TSST-1 toxin or the Panton-Valentine toxin (see subsequent discussion) belongs to *agr* group III; vancomycin-intermediate strains tend to belong to *agr* group II; and the exfoliative toxin A (ETA)–producing strains belong to group IV. Thus, global regulators were originally meant to control the expression of useful metabolic genes. How exogenous virulent genes, which were acquired later, succeeded in taking advantage of such systems remains a fascination question of evolutionary genetics.

CELL SURFACE DETERMINANTS INVOLVED IN PATHOGENESIS

Figure 195-5 depicts the surface constituents believed to be involved in the bacterial-host relationship. Their structure and function in relation to *S. aureus* pathogenesis is discussed subsequently.

Biofilm
Biofilm is an extracellular polysaccharidic and proteinaceous network that gathers bacterial communities within a mechanically cohesive scaffold. It is common in the bacterial world. Biofilm-trapped bacteria are dormant and thus phenotypically tolerant to antibiotic-induced killing. They are a major therapeutic problem.[68] Biofilm-producing staphylococci were mainly described in CoNS but are also formed by

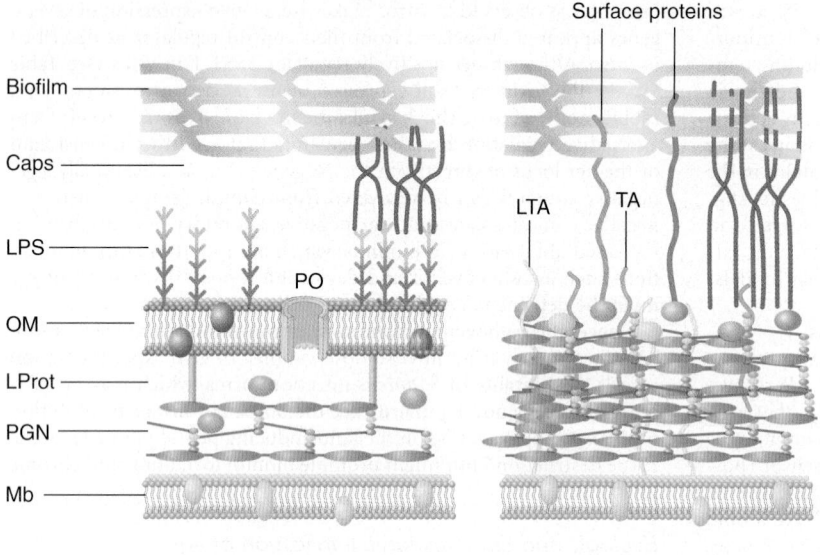

Figure 195-5 Schematic representation of gram-negative *(left)* and gram-positive *(right)* bacterial envelopes. Gram-negative bacteria have very thin peptidoglycan (PGN) and outer membrane (OM), made of lipopolysaccharide (LPS), which is not present in gram-positive bacteria. Gram-positive bacteria have very thick peptidoglycan and teichoic acids (TA) and lipoteichoic acids (LTA) that are not present in gram-negative bacteria. *Caps,* capsule; *Lprot,* lipoprotein; *Mb,* plasma membrane; *PO,* porin.

S. aureus, especially in the settings of colonization and persistence on catheters and biomaterials. Biofilm-producing staphylococci were associated with persistence and virulence in various experimental models, including *Caenorhabditis elegans* and mice with foreign body infection.[69]

Biofilm-formation evolves in two steps, starting with nonspecific adherence of individual cells to the materials, followed by growth and biofilm formation. In CoNS, it is associated with the production of polysaccharide intercellular adhesion (PIA), which consists of β-1,6-glucosamine chains that are *N*-substituted with succinate residues.[70] PIA is synthesized by an operon called *ica* composed of a regulator (*icaR*) and biosynthetic (*icaADBC*) genes.[71]

An *ica* homologue with the ability to produce biofilm was also described in *S. aureus.* Its role in colonizing amorphous surfaces might be identical to that shown in CoNS. However, its role in disease initiation is debated.[72] Biofilm production may possibly be a relatively ancestral mode of colonization, especially used by poorly pathogenic bacteria. The presence of more effective adherence factors in *S. aureus* could mask the contribution of biofilm to colonization. Ideally, the effect of *S. aureus* biofilm should be tested in mutants deficient in other surface colonization factors (e.g., microbial surface component reacting with adherence matrix molecules, see subsequent discussion).

Capsule
More then 90% of clinical isolates of *S. aureus* elaborate a polysaccharidic *capsule,* among which 11 serotypes have been reported.[9] Capsule type 1 and type 2 *S. aureus* produce large quantities of polysaccharides and appear mucoid on culture plates. However, they are rarely found in human clinical samples. In contrast, capsule type 5 and type 8 *S. aureus* are responsible for up to 75% of clinical infections. Type 5 and type 8 capsules are made of various sugars, including mannose and fucose. They are both antiphagocytic and can increase virulence in several animal models. Antibodies against these capsular types are protective in animal models of sepsis, and naturally occurring antibodies are detected in normal human serum. A conjugate vaccine directed against type 5 and type 8 capsules showed transient efficacy in patients for hemodialysis.[73] Thus, the capsule is an antiphagocytic constituent that might be a promising target for vaccination. Nevertheless, no definitive human studies are available on this issue.

Surface Adhesins
S. aureus carry several *surface adhesins* (see Table 195-1; Table 195-3) that confer adherence to a variety of host matrix proteins. These microbial surface component reacting with adherence matrix mole-

cules are reassembled under the acronym MSCRAMM.[74] Most are covalently bound to the cell wall peptidoglycan. Wall anchoring obeys a conserved mechanism in gram-positive bacteria.[75] It involves a membrane-bound enzyme called *sortase* that recognizes a conserved amino acid motif (LPXTG) at the C-terminal end of wall-attached proteins. Sortase covalently binds the threonine residue of LPXTG to a free acceptor in the peptidoglycan side chain, usually a glycine in *S. aureus* (Fig. 195-6). Eleven of these surface proteins were characterized because of their in vitro adherence properties, and 10 additional proteins with screening of the staphylococcal genome for LPXTG-containing sequences (see Table 195-3).[76] Putative MSCRAMMs and their proven in vitro or in vivo implication are listed in Table 195-3.

All these MSCRAMMs obey a relatively similar type of architecture. A *N*-terminal signal sequence is followed by variable functional domains that carry the binding activity and are themselves followed by a series of repeated sequences, a LPXTG wall-anchoring domain, and a membrane-spanning domain, which is cleaved off during wall anchoring by an enzyme called sortase (see Figure 195-6). Relevant MSCRAMMs for pathogenesis include clumping factor B (ClfB) for colonization of nasal epithelia,[77] clumping factor A (ClfA) and fibronectin-binding proteins A and B (FnBPA and FnBPB) for experimental endocarditis[61,78] and ventricular assist device-related infections,[79] collagen-binding protein *(cna)* for osteomyelitis,[80] protein A for immune escape and promotion of experimental osteoarthritis,[81] major histocompatibility complex class II analog protein (MAP) (or extracellular adherence protein [EAP]) as immunomodulator subverting the T-cell response in mice,[82] and the *sasG* and *sasH* products for their relation with epithelial colonization and invasive clinical isolates (see Table 195-3).[76,83]

In this kind of in vivo investigation, the results highly depend on the experimental model used. As for regulatory elements, a perversity comes from the fact that *S. aureus* harbors many MSCRAMMs at the surface. Thus, inactivation of only one might pass undetected because its function might be complemented by others. Such a situation may wrongly underestimate the importance of a given factor in disease. To circumvent this limitation, the suspected gene can be transferred and expressed in a surrogate bacterium devoid of the redundant *S. aureus* background. The recombinant organism is then tested for increased adherence or infectivity in vitro and in vivo. Such experiments were useful to assess the specific pathogenic role of ClfA and FnBPA in experimental endocarditis and ventricular assist device infections.[61,78,79]

Most MSCRAMMs summarized in Table 195-3 are present in all *S. aureus* isolates, with some variation regarding collagen-binding protein

TABLE 195-3	*Staphylococcus aureus* MSCRAMMs Belonging to Sortase-Mediated Cell-Wall Associated Proteins[76,337,338]					
Gene	*Protein*	*AA*	*Sortase*	*Motif*	*Ligand Specificity*	*Potential Implication in Disease*
Spa	Protein A	508	SrtA	LPETG	Antibody Fc fragment (IgG, IgM) von Willebrand's factor, TNFR1, platelets	Experimental sepsis Experimental osteoarthritis
clfA	Clumping factor A	933	SrtA	LPDTG	Fibrinogen Platelets	Experimental endocarditis
clfB	Clumping factor B	913	SrtA	LPETG	Fibrinogen, Cytokeratin 10, Platelets	Colonization of nasal mucosa
Cna	Collagen-binding protein	1183	SrtA	LPKTG	Collagen	Experimental osteomyelitis, Septic arthritis
fnA	Fibronectin-binding protein A	1018	SrtA	LPETG	Fibronectin, Fibrinogen, Elastin Platelets	Experimental endocarditis Cell invasion Experimental mastitis
fnB	Fibronectin-binding protein B	914	SrtA	LPETG	Fibronectin, Fibrinogen, Elastin Platelets	Experimental mastitis
sdrC	Serine-aspartate repeat protein	947	SrtA	LPETG	Undetermined	—
sdrD	Serine aspartate repeat protein	1315	SrtA	LPETG	Undetermined	—
sdrE	Serine aspartate repeat protein	1166	SrtA	LPETG	Platelets	—
pls	Plasmin-sensitive protein	1637	SrtA	LPDTG	Cellular lipids, ganglioside M3; Nasal epithelial cells	Colonization of nasal mucosa
sraP (sasA)	Serin-rich adhesin for platelets	2261	SrtA	LPDTG	Platelets	Experimental endocarditis
IsdA (sasE)	Iron-regulated surface determinant A	354	SrtA	LPKTG	Fibrinogen, Fibronectin Hemoglobin/Transferrin	Nasal colonization
IsdB (sasJ)	Iron-regulated surface determinant B	645	SrtA	LPQTG	Hemoglobin/Hemin	—
isdC	Iron-regulated surface determinant C	227	SrtB	NPQTN	Hemin	—
isdH (harA) (sasI)	Iron-regulated surface determinant H	895	SrtA	LPKTG	Haptoglobin Haptoglobin/Hemoglobin complex	Nasal colonization
sasB	S. aureus surface protein B	937	SrtA	LPDTG	Undetermined	—
sasC	S. aureus surface protein C	2186	SrtA	LPNTG	Undetermined	—
sasD	S. aureus surface protein D	241	SrtA	LPAAG	Undetermined	—
sasF	S. aureus surface protein F	637	SrtA	LPKAG	Undetermined	—
sasG	S. aureus surface protein G	1117	SrtA	LPKTG	Nasal epithelial cells	Associated to invasive disease
sasH	S. aureus surface protein H	308	SrtA	LPKTG	Undetermined	Associated to invasive disease
sasK	S. aureus surface protein K	211	SrtA	LPKTG	Undetermined	—

AA, protein length in amino acids; Srt, sortase; IgM, immunoglobulin M; MSCRAMMs, microbial surface components recognizing adhesive matrix molecules; *TNFR1*, TNF-receptor 1.

(cna). Although implicated in pathogenesis, they are encoded on the chromosome,[6,7,12] which suggests that they have arisen and become stabilized in the genome earlier than MGEs during the *S. aureus* evolution. In comparison, genomes of CoNS contain notoriously fewer MSCRAMM genes (approximately 10 in *S. epidermidis*, six in *S. haemolyticus*, and one in *S. saprophyticus*).[7,14-16]

Teichoic Acids and Lipoteichoic Acids
Teichoic acids represent up to 50% of the dry weight of purified staphylococcal walls. They are constituted of polyribitol-phosphate polymers cross linked to *N*-acetylmuramic acid residues of the peptidoglycan (Fig. 195-7) and decorated with D-alanine and *N*-acetylglucosamine residues.[84] Teichoic acids play an important physiologic role in cell wall metabolism and are likely to be a site of attachment of cell wall active enzymes and other proteins. Teichoic acids have been involved in adherence to nasal epithelia,[85] but their role in invasive infection and host inflammatory response is unclear.[86]

Lipoteichoic acids (LTAs) are the plasma membrane-bound counterparts of teichoic acids. They have a similar general structure except that they contain polyglycerol-phosphates and are linked to a diacyl-

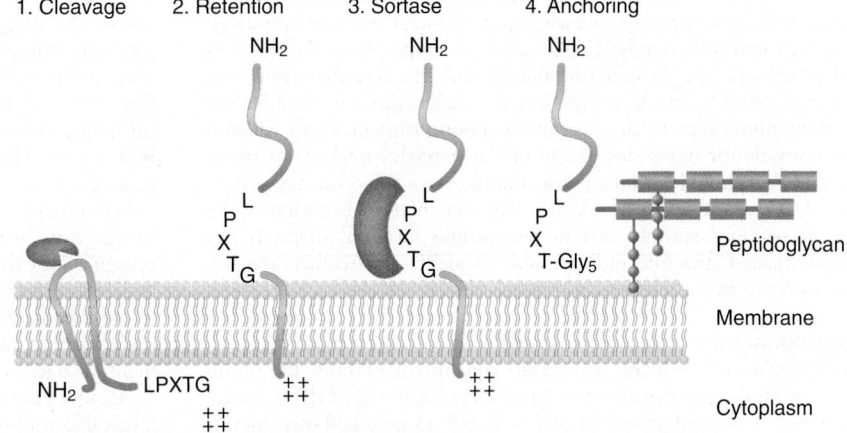

Figure 195-6 Anchoring of gram-positive surface proteins to peptidoglycan through sortase-mediated processing of LPXTG consensus motif. During membrane translocation, *N*-terminal leader sequence is clipped off. Protein is then transiently retained on cell surface through membrane-anchor domain, rich in positively charged amino acids at its intracellular carboxyl-terminal portion. LPXTG consensus region is then processed by sortase that clips between threonine and glycine (*T-G*) and transfers covalent bond to glycine acceptor in peptidoglycan meshwork. (*Adapted from Fischetti VA, Pancholi V, Schneewind O. Conservation of a hexapeptide sequence in the anchor region of surface proteins from gram-positive cocci. Mol Microbiol. 1990;4:1603-1605; Mazmanian SK, Ton-That H, Schneewind O. Sortase-catalysed anchoring of surface proteins to the cell wall of Staphylococcus aureus. Mol Microbiol. 2001;40:1049-1057.*)

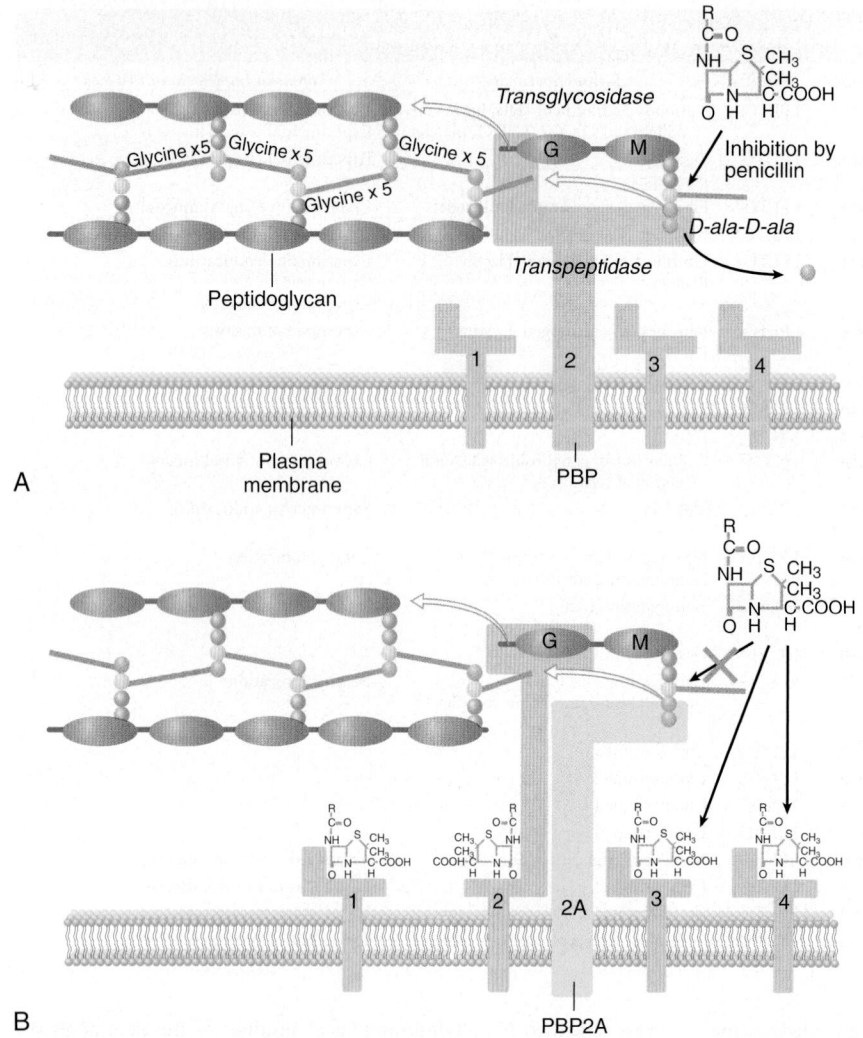

Figure 195-7 **Peptidoglycan assembly in wild-type *S. aureus* (A) and in MRSA (B). A,** Cell wall precursors consist of disaccharide pentapeptides *N*-acetylglucosamine-*N*-acetylmuramic acid-L-ala-D-glu-L-lys-D-ala-D-ala. After membrane translocation, precursors are handled by membrane penicillin-binding proteins (PBPs). High–molecular-weight PBPs are bifunctional enzymes that perform both transglycosidase step, linking incoming *N*-acetylglucosamine (G) to muramic acid (M) in nascent wall, and transpeptidase step, linking penultimate D-ala to glycine acceptor in nascent wall. In *S. aureus*, lysine in position 3 of stem peptide is almost always decorated with pentaglycine side chain (*orange bars*). Penicillin is mechanism-based inhibitor of transpeptidase domain of PBPs. **B,** MRSA carry additional PBP called PBP2A, which has very low affinity for most available β-lactam drugs. Therefore, when β-lactams are present, they block normal PBPs but not PBP2A. PBP2A has only a transpeptidase domain and must "hijack" transglycosidase domain of normal PBP2 to be active. (*From de Lencastre H, Wu SW, Pinho MG, et al. Antibiotic resistance as a stress response: Complete sequencing of a larger number of chromosomal loci in Staphylococcus aureus strain COL that iimpact on the expression of resistance to methicillin. Microb Drug Resist. 1999;5:163-175.*)

glycerol moiety that serves as a plasma membrane anchor. LTAs have been implicated in inflammation by triggering the release of cytokines by macrophages and other players of the innate immune system. In particular, the stereochemistry of the D-alanine decorations and the presence of the diacylglycerol lipid anchor were shown to be determinants for host recognition and subsequent inflammation.[84]

However, although LTAs may facilitate bacterial recognition by host innate immunity, they also protect the microbes from killing by cationic antimicrobial peptides (CAPs) that are produced by professional phagocytes. Native LTA is polyanionic and attracts CAPs. To circumvent the problem, LTAs become decorated with D-alanyl residues by the *dltABC* gene products, which render the structure more positively charged and thus repulse CAPs.[87] Mutants impaired in *dltABC* were also less adherent to endothelial cells and less able than wild type staphylococci to produce experimental endocarditis in rabbits. The same authors showed that membrane-bound protein MprF, which is responsible for lysine decoration of the staphylococcal major membrane phospholipid (which is also anionic), was also critical to protect the cells from attack by host CAPs. Thus, the microbial envelope is not an amorphous scaffold that merely ensures bacterial shape. It is a sophisticated structure indispensable to mediate adherence, sensing, and growth in complex environments.

Peptidoglycan

Peptidoglycan is a highly conserved constituent of both the gram-positive and gram-negative envelopes. It is constituted of glycan chains made of *N*-acetylglucosamine and *N*-acetylmuramic acid disaccharide

subunits, in which the *N*-acetylmuramate moiety is linked to highly conserved pentapeptide or tetrapeptide stems (L-alanine–D-isoglutamine–L-lysine–D-alanine–[D-alanine]; see Fig. 195-7). The position 3 L-lysine is typical of staphylococci and streptococci but can be substituted for diaminopimelic acid in other gram-positive microbes (e.g., in *Bacillus* spp.) and in gram-negative bacteria. Peptidoglycan is a thick structure in gram-positive bacteria (≥10 layers), whereas it is thin (1 or 2 layers) in gram-negative bacteria.[9]

The chains of disaccharide-peptide are cross linked via peptide bridges between the penultimate D-alanine and the diamino acid L-lysine located in position 3 of a neighboring stem peptide. In *S. aureus*, the interpeptide bridge typically contains a polyglycine linking piece that comprises one to five glycine residues. The addition of glycines to the wall precursors is driven by the *femABC* and *fmhB* genes (Fig. 195-8).[88] These determinants are implicated in the plasticity of the wall and are indirectly implicated in staphylococcal resistance to both methicillin and vancomycin (see subsequent Antibiotic Resistance section).

Peptidoglycan is the major scaffold for anchoring most MSCRAMMs. In this sense, it plays a role in pathogenesis. On the other hand, it is recognized by the innate immune system and triggers cytokine release and inflammation, as LTA.[86] Thus, it is probably important for the microorganisms to hide these structures from host recognition, an objective that can be achieved by producing antiphagocytic components such as a capsule, or protein A.

Because peptidoglycan is a critical cell structure, its assembly is the target of antibiotics such as β-lactams and glycopeptides (e.g., vanco-

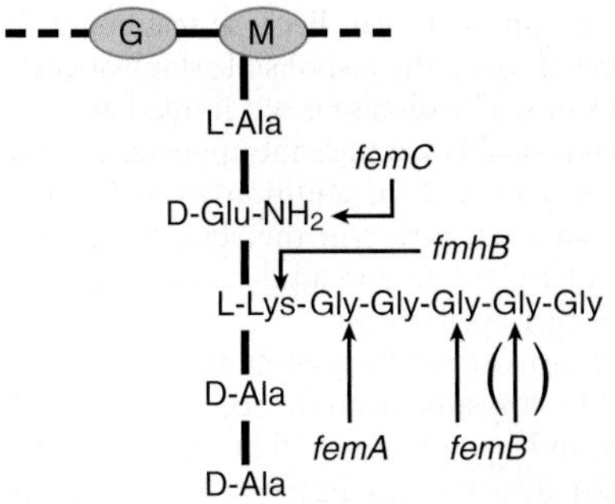

G — M

L-Ala
femC
D-Glu-NH₂
fmhB
L-Lys-Gly-Gly-Gly-Gly-Gly
D-Ala
femA *femB*
D-Ala

Figure 195-8 **In order to be functional, penicillin-binding protein 2A (PBP2A) requires that the cell provide fully decorated precursors, containing both pentaglycine side chain and amidated glutamine.** Inactivation of *femB*, *femA*, and *fhmB* genes blocks addition of pentaglycines and thus decreases expression of methicillin-resistance even though PBP2A is present in bacterial membrane. Inactivation of *femC* has a similar effect. (Adapted from Berger-Bächi B. Expression of resistance to methicillin. Trends Microbiol. 1994;2:389-393.)

mycin). Modification of peptidoglycan synthesis is a response of resistant staphylococci to cell wall–active antibiotics (see subsequent Antibiotic Resistance section).

SECRETED ENZYMES AND HEMOLYSINS

S. aureus produces a number of exoenzymes, membrane-active proteins (hemolysins and leukocidins), and toxins that are involved in disease mechanisms (see Table 195-1).[2-4] *Exoenzymes* encompass proteases and lipases, which are destructive regarding host tissues and useful for getting nutrient to the invading bacterium. Their pathogenic role has not been much studied in animal models, but their contribution to disease is apparent.

Hemolysins

S. aureus has a minimum of four *hemolysins* referred to as α-hemolysin, β-hemolysin, γ-hemolysin, and δ-hemolysin.[9] They can lyse erythrocytes and other eukaryotic cells. α-hemolysin and δ-hemolysin are secreted in nontoxic soluble forms and multimerize on eukaryotic membranes to form lytic pores.[2] α-Hemolysin was shown to be important in experimental endocarditis.[89]

β-Hemolysin is distinctive because it is a sphingomyelinase that damages membranes by enzymatic alteration of their lipid content. γ-Hemolysin is also peculiar. It is composed of two types of proteins called S and F, for slow and fast elution at chromatography. It can lyse white blood cells in addition to other cells and is sometimes referred to as *leukocidin*. It is encoded by two distinct operons, one that encodes a unique *HlgA* (S protein) and another that encodes for one S protein (*HglC*) and one F protein (*HglB*). S and F proteins must assemble to form membrane-perforating complexes. Therefore, this class of hemolysins is also referred to as *synergohymenotrop* toxins. Active γ-hemolysin exists in two bioactive forms: *HlgA-HglB* and *HlgA-HglC*. α-hemolysin, β-hemolysin, δ-hemolysin, and γ-hemolysin are present in most *S. aureus* isolates. They are all encoded on the chromosome and are subject to *agr* regulation (see Table 195-1).

Panton-Valentine Toxin

A few homologues of γ-hemolysin have been described. One was reported in 1932 by Panton and Valentine.[90] The toxin is encoded by two genes, *lukS* and *lukF*, which can assemble either between themselves or with the components of γ-hemolysin, thus producing chimera complexes. Like the other hemolysins, *Panton-Valentine toxin* (PVL) is apparently regulated by *agr* (see Table 195-1). Unlike the other hemolysins, PVL is encoded by a mobile phage (φSLT) that can transfer PVL to other strains. Also unlike the other hemolysins, the prevalence rate of PVL is usually low (≤2%) in MSSA and health

care–associated MRSA (HCA-MRSA),[91] whereas it is present in almost 100% of isolates of community-acquired MRSA (CA-MRSA).[22,92]

Panton-Valentine toxin–producing *S. aureus* is associated with skin and soft tissue infection (SSTI) and severe hemorrhagic pneumonia in children and young adults.[93] In contrast, it is rarely responsible for other infections such as osteomyelitis, septicemia, and endocarditis. The reason for clustering in young patients is unclear. The clustering could be linked to an age-related permissive milieu or permissive immunologic window. Nevertheless, the connection is important; a young adult with recurrent boils and pneumonia should receive particular attention because the mortality rate of hemorrhagic lung disease is high (Fig. 195-9). Moreover, the high representation in CA-MRSA is worrisome.[21,22,40,92]

EXFOLIATIVE TOXINS AND STAPHYLOCOCCAL SCALDED SKIN SYNDROME

Staphylococcal scalded skin syndrome (SSSS) is a superficial skin disorder that varies from local blistering to impressive generalized scalding (Fig. 195-10). It was originally described by the German physician Baron Gotfried Ritter von Rittershain who published a series of 297 cases in young children in 1878.[94] Hence, the syndrome is sometimes referred to as *Ritter's disease*. SSSS clusters in newborns and infants less than 1 year old and rarely in adults. It is typically the result of mucosal or skin colonization (e.g., umbilical cord) with a toxigenic *S. aureus* that produces either exfoliative toxin A (ETA) or B (ETB), encoded by the *eta* and *etb* genes, respectively. The toxin genes are located either on a phage (*eta*)[12] or on a plasmid (*etb*). Two additional isoforms of SSSS toxins (exfoliative toxins C [ETC] and D [ETD]) were isolated through pathologic observations in animals and with genome screen.[95]

Staphylococcal scalded skin syndrome often evolves as small epidemics that result from clonally related strains, usually in nurseries. Nasal carriage of the organism may be found among the medical staff, and all caretakers should be screened for this possibility. A recent study indicates that the proportion of *S. aureus* carrying *eta* or *etb* in overall staphylococcal nasal carriers or clinical isolates is low (0 to 2% of

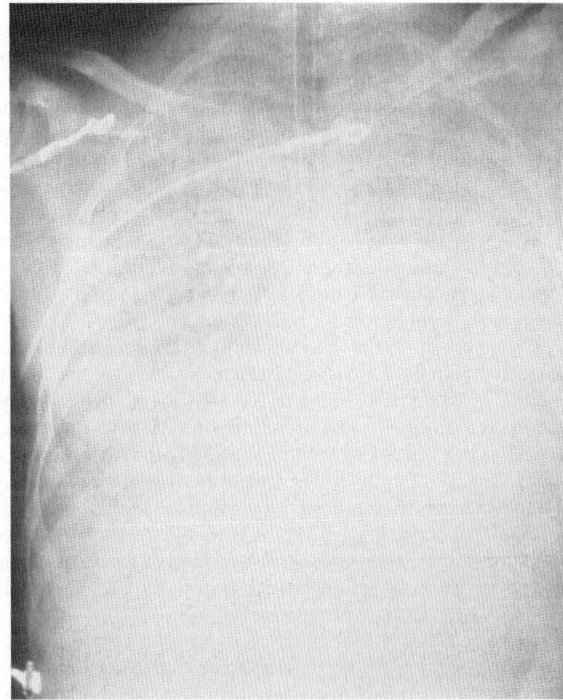

Figure 195-9 **Fulminant hemorrhagic pneumonia in 20-year-old patient infected with Panton-Valentine toxin–producing *S. aureus*.**

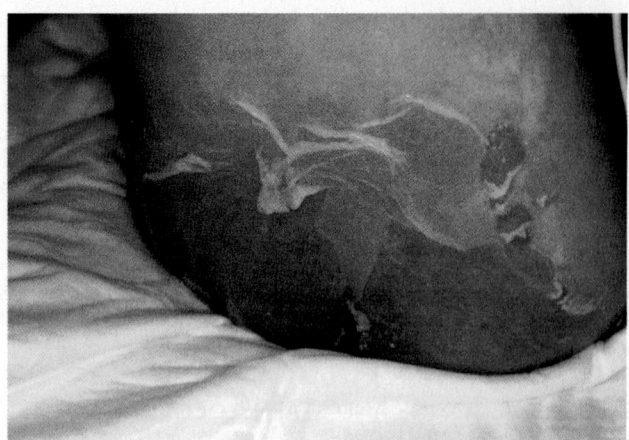

Figure 195-10 Staphylococcal scalded skin syndrome. Blisters are expression of toxin-related (exfoliative toxin A or B) distant disease and usually do not contain microorganisms.

isolates),[96] which may explain the rarity of the disease and its clustering in favorable milieus.

The toxins act by a direct effect on the stratum granulosum of the epidermis. Mucosa are never involved. This consideration is important for differential diagnosis with more severe Lyell's syndrome, which usually involves the mucosa.[3] *Lyell's syndrome,* or toxic epidermal necrolysis, results from cleavage below the dermoepidermal junction. It is associated with a reaction to more than 100 drugs and sometimes vaccination and has a high fatality rate.

Molecular Pathogenesis of Staphylococcal Scalded Skin Syndrome

The molecular pathogenesis of SSSS is complex. The toxin is released by staphylococci locally, passes though the body, and localizes at the level of the strata granulosum. The toxin is a glutamate-specific serine protease whose molecular target is desmoglein-1 (Dsg1). Dsg1 is a transmembrane desmosomal glycoprotein that is important to maintenance of interkeratinocyte adhesion.[97] The human skin harbors four Dsg isoforms (Dsg1 to Dsg4) that are localized in various layers of the epidermis, but only Dsg1 is present at the level of the strata granulosum and only Dsg1 is hydrolyzed by SSSS toxins.

An incompletely solved question is why children are primarily affected by the disease. One hypothesis was that the toxin is targeted to Dsg1 because of the local occurrence of a specific cell membrane ganglioside (GM4), which is only present in the skin of young children or in adults with peculiar skin diseases. This could explain the clustering of SSSS in these particular populations. GM4-like gangliosides are present in the skin of suckling mice and can inhibit the effect of the toxin when coincubated before injection to susceptible animals.[3] The toxin has a serine protease activity, but only after it has reached the skin, which suggests that a locally induced conformational change is needed for activity. Extensive research has lead to the following model.[95,97] The secreted toxin is targeted to the skin of susceptible patients via recognition of Dsg1 (and maybe GM4). Once on site, the toxin specifically cleaves Dsg1 with a specificity that leaves other proteins unaffected. Protein hydrolysis might be triggered by direct protein-protein recognition followed by conformational change and activation of the enzymatic activity. Eventually, whether Dsg1 hydrolysis is responsible for the whole disease process or whether secondary keratinocyte reactions are implicated in skin pealing is as yet unclear.

Clinical Aspects

The two forms of SSSS are a generalized form and a localized form. In the *generalized* form, the toxin spreads throughout the body and localizes at the level of the skin, where it produces generalized scalding (see Fig. 195-10). The skin easily detaches by mere rubbing (Nikolsky's

sign). The blister liquid is clear. Because scalding is the expression of a distantly secreted toxin, the responsible staphylococci are usually not found in the lesions. The disease is self limited and wanes off within 4 to 5 days, which probably parallels the appearance of specific antitoxin immunoglobulins. Indeed, in addition to age-related expression of GM4 or other specific factors in the skin, the presence of antitoxin antibodies in older children and adults also explains the restriction of SSSS to the younger age groups.

The *localized* form of SSSS is sometimes referred to as *bullous impetigo* (Fig. 195-11). It results from the local spread of the toxin around a colonized wound in individuals that already bear some immunity against the toxin, as is the case in newborns (often around the umbilicus), in infants still benefiting from passive maternal immunity, or in older individuals who are already immunized. The presence of antibodies hinders distant dissemination of the toxin but not local spread around the colonized area. Unlike the generalized form, scalding is localized and the blister liquid often contains bacteria and sometimes white blood cells.

Patients may have general symptoms that include fever and lethargy, especially in the generalized form. Treatment includes general measures such as antiseptic wound dressing and fluid support, specific antibiotic therapy to eradicate the causative agent, and screening and decontamination of caretakers, especially in nurseries. If appropriately handled, the prognosis of SSSS in children is usually good with a mortality rate less than 5%. In contrast, the mortality rate can be very high in adults (>50%) and is usually associated with an underlying condition.

As mentioned, the differential diagnosis with Lyell's syndrome (toxic epidermal necrolysis) is critical because the etiology, treatment, and prognosis of the diseases are different. In doubtful cases, skin biopsy is useful to provide the definitive answer.

SUPERANTIGENS

Toxic shock syndrome toxin-1 (TSST-1) and staphylococcal enterotoxins (SEs) are the paradigm of a large family of pyrogenic exotoxins called *superantigens* (SAgs).[2,4,98] SAgs are proteins that do not activate the immune system via normal contact between antigen-presenting cells and T-lymphocytes. Normally, antigens are taken up by antigen-presenting cells, hydrolyzed, and presented as restricted peptides to cognate T-lymphocytes. The peptides are expressed within a grove on the major histocompatibility complex (MCH)-class II receptor on the surface of the antigen-presenting cell. Cognate T-cells recognize the peptide-MHC-class II complex by specific contacts with the five variable domains of the α and β chain of the T-cell receptor (Vβ, Dβ, Jβ, Vα, Jα).

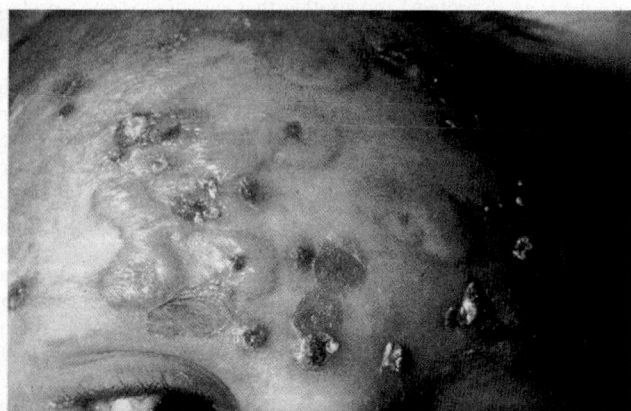

Figure 195-11 Localized staphylococcal scalded skin syndrome, also called bullous impetigo. Disease is caused by local production of exfoliative toxins, and bacteria may be found in blister liquid.

Superantigens can bypass this highly specific interaction. They attach to an external portion of the Vβ domain from large quantities of lymphocytes and directly wedge them to the MHC class II receptors of antigen-presenting cells. This nonspecific contact activates up to 20% of the total pool of T-cells, instead of approximately 1/10,000 during normal antigen presentation. The consequence is a massive burst in cytokine release, which drives an overwhelming inflammatory response that results in endotoxin-like shock, including endothelial leakage, hemodynamic shock, multiorgan failure, and possibly death.

S. aureus can produce a large number of SAgs. Aside from TSST-1, it can produce at least 15 different enterotoxins (SEs A, B, C$_n$, D, E, G, H, I, J, K, L, M, N, O), to which genomic analyses have added an equivalent number of SAg homologues called staphylococcal exotoxins, denominated SET1 to SET15.[99]

Although quite some variation exists in the primary structure of many SAgs, they all share a common architecture as shown with crystallography. They consist of A and B globular domains, which are made of β-sheet barrels and α-helices and rejoined by a discrete linking piece. In TSST-1, the region binding to the Vβ chain of the T-cells receptor has been mapped at the A-B hinge region.

A genealogy of SAgs was built on the base of their sequence homologies. The SAgs studied segregated into five groups.[4] Group I was represented only by TSST-1. Group III contained only staphylococcal SAgs (SEs H, I, K, L, and P), and group IV only streptococcal SAgs (SPs E C, G, and SME Z). On the other hand, groups II and V contained both staphylococcal and streptococcal SAgs. Group II contained staphylococcal SEs B, C, and G and streptococcal SSA and SPE A, and group V contained staphylococcal SEs I, K, L, and P and streptococcal SPs E and H. This underlines the likelihood of horizontal gene transfer between these two genera, a fact that is becoming increasingly apparent with genome comparisons.[2,100]

TOXIC SHOCK SYNDROME

Toxic shock syndrome (TSS) has been sporadically reported as staphylococcal scarlet fever since 1927.[101] Interest in TSS dramatically increased in the early 1980s, when a number of staphylococcal TSS cases occurred in young women who used high-absorbency tampons during menses.[102] The disease was shown to be associated with a toxin called TSST-1 that was secreted locally by toxigenic strains. TSST-1 can cross the mucosal membrane, which is apparently not the case for all SAgs, and then disseminate throughout the body. An experimental study suggests that TSST-1 could activate directly epithelial cells and the innate immune system to promote its translocation.[103] The are two clinical forms of TSS are: menstrual TSS and nonmenstrual TSS.

Menstrual Toxic Shock Syndrome

Menstrual toxic shock syndrome starts within 2 days of the beginning or the end of menses and is primarily associated with the use of high-absorbency tampons. Clinical signs include high fever, capillary-leak syndrome with hypotension and hypoalbuminemia, generalized nonpitting edema, and a morbilliform rash, followed by desquamation after a few days. The toxin is produced locally, and blood culture results are typically negative. The organisms responsible were represented by a single clone in most reported cases.

The disease proceeds by SAg-induced hyperactivation of the immune system (see previous discussion). TSST-1 production is regulated by *agr* (see Table 195-1). However, its expression requires specific conditions that include: 1, an elevated protein level; 2, a relatively neutral pH (6.5 to 8); 3, an elevated partial pressure of CO_2; and 4, an elevated partial pressure of O_2.[47] All four conditions are met when menstruation is combined with the use of high-absorbency tampons. The high protein concentration and neutral pH are provided by blood proteins and their buffering capacity. The high partial pressure in CO_2 is ensured by the higher than atmospheric CO_2 content of blood. Eventually, the high concentration in O_2 is introduced into the vaginal anaerobic flora by the high-absorbency tampon. Thus, the O_2 brought in by the tampon might be the trigger that modifies an otherwise

equilibrated ecosystem and stimulates the production of TSST-1 by colonizing staphylococci.

Toxic shock syndrome toxin-1–producing *S. aureus* is found in up to 20% of isolates from both carrier and clinical specimens.[96] The fact that TSST-1 expression has special requirements may partially explain the comparatively low prevalence rate of the disease (approximately 0.5 to 10 per 100,000 patients per years between normal incidence and tampon-related peaks).[4]

Nonmenstrual Toxic Shock Syndrome

Nonmenstrual TSS has attracted less attention than menstrual TSS. Yet, it can occur in any patient. In addition to TSST-1, non-menstrual TSS can be the result of enterotoxin SEB and SEC, which are *agr*-regulated (see Table 195-1). Responsible organisms may colonize virtually any site of the body, including surgical wounds (surgical TSS), lung (influenza-associated TSS), mucosa or skin (recalcitrant desquamative syndrome in patients with AIDS), contraceptive diaphragms, and dialysis catheters in patients undergoing chronic peritoneal dialysis. The development of general symptoms with high fever and cutaneous rash should suggest the possibility of nonmenstrual TSS in such patients.

A special feature of wound colonization is that the affected tissues often do not appear inflammatory. This is believed to result from the toxin itself, which is able to prevent the influx of professional macrophages.

Predisposing Factors

In addition to the use of high-absorbency tampons or colonization by a toxigenic strain, most patients who are TSS susceptible also lack specific antibodies that block the responsible SAg. In one study, antibody titers considered protective against TSST-1 (≥1:100) were detected in 30% of 2-year-old children and in more than 90% of women and men 25 years of age. However, low or negative titers of anti–TSST-1 antibodies (<5) were found in acute phase sera from 90.5% of patients with menstrual TSS, and less than 50% had positive titers of anti–TSST-1 antibody developed during convalescence.[4,104] Hence, some patients remain susceptible to recurrent TSS.

An interesting feature of SAgs is that they primarily trigger a CD$_4^+$ T-cell response, which privileges a T-helper Th1 cytokine release response without a significant Th2 response. A consequence of the dominant Th1 response is a decreased antibody expression, which could explain the relative lack of antibody response of patients with TSS. An additional explanation for the anergy could be SAg-induced apoptosis of responsive T-cells, which could account for the prolonged anergy toward the deleterious toxin.

Diagnosis

The diagnosis of TSS is based on a constellation of clinical and laboratory signs as proposed by the Centers for Disease Control.[105] Table 195-4 also proposes additional laboratory features, such as isolation of a toxin-producing organism to broaden the diagnostic tools.[4] The criteria of streptococcal TSS, from toxigenic *S. pyogenes* isolates, are presented for comparison. Although both syndromes are the results of similar kinds of SAgs, they differ in two important aspects. First, in contrast to staphylococcal TSS, streptococcal TSS is almost always associated with the presence of streptococci in deep-seated infections, such as erysipelas or necrotizing fasciitis, which has been referred to as flesh-eating disease. Second, although the mortality rate of adequately treated staphylococcal TSS is approximately 5%, the mortality rate of streptococcal TSS is close to 50%, and treatment necessitates urgent and generous surgical débridement of infected tissues, and sometimes amputation.

Treatment and Prevention

Treatment of staphylococcal TSS consists of elimination of the causative agent with antibiotic treatment and appropriate drainage of affected tissues if necessary. Otherwise, supportive care that includes intravenous fluid and vasopressors might be necessary. The immunologic gap that allows the toxin to be active in susceptible patients

Diagnostic Criteria for Staphylococcal and Streptococcal Toxic Shock Syndrome

Staphylococcal Toxic Shock Syndrome*	Streptococcal Toxic Shock Syndrome
Fever	Isolation of group A streptococci from:
Hypotension	
Diffuse macular rash with subsequent desquamation	Sterile site for definite case
	Nonsterile site for probable case
Three of following organ systems involved:	Hypotension
Liver	Two of the following symptoms:
Blood	Renal dysfunction
Renal	Liver involvement
Mucous membranes	Erythematous macular rash
Gastrointestinal	Coagulopathy
Muscular	Soft tissue necrosis
Central nervous system	Adult respiratory distress syndrome
Negative serologies for measles, leptospirosis, and Rocky Mountain spotted fever and negative blood or cerebral spinal fluid cultures for organisms other than S. aureus	

*Proposed revision of diagnostic criteria for staphylococcal toxic shock syndrome (TSS) includes: 1, isolation of *S. aureus* from mucosal or normally sterile site; 2, production of TSS-associated superantigen by isolate; 3, lack of antibody to implicated toxin at time of acute illness; and 4, development of antibody to toxin during convalescence.

Adapted from McCormick JK, Yarwood JM, Schlievert PM. Toxic shock syndrome and bacterial superantigens: An update. *Annu Rev Microbiol.* 2001;55:77-104.

suggests that passive immunotherapy such as intravenous immunoglobulin (IVIG) could be effective. A study done with patients with streptococcal TSS suggests that IVIG combined with antibiotic and supportive therapy may have reduced the fatality rate.[106] Because the mortality rate of staphylococcal TSS is relatively low, immunotherapy is usually not warranted and is held for life-threatening cases of streptococcal TSS.

Prevention is aimed at avoiding the use of hyperabsorbent tampons and preventing staphylococcal colonization of wound and mucosa. In the case of nasal carriage, this is achieved with topical application of antibacterials such as mupirocin. In the case of extranasal colonization, additional complete body washing with antiseptics such as chlorhexidine is recommended for at least 1 week (see Table 195-8). Control cultures should be taken thereafter.

Because up to 20% of natural *S. aureus* colonizers carry the TSST-1 gene,[96] the risk of recolonization with another strain is high. Immunization with a TSST-1 vaccine could circumvent this problem.[107] However, vaccines might be incompletely effective in patients who are intrinsically anergic to the toxin.

ENTEROTOXINS AND FOOD POISONING

S. aureus harbors up to 15 enterotoxins, which are defined as SAgs able to produce gastrointestinal symptoms that include vomiting and diarrhea in primate models.[2,5] Although many of these toxins have potential SAg activity, not all of them have a clear role in human disease. As mentioned, SEB and SEC are associated with nonmenstrual TSS. Likewise, SEA, SEB, and SEC are the most frequent enterotoxins associated with food poisoning.

Food-borne disease is a major public health problem that may account for 6 to 8 million cases per year in the United States. *S. aureus* food poisoning follows ingestion of toxins that have been released into contaminated food stocks or beverages. The toxins are heat stable and thus are not denatured by cooking. The disease typically starts 2 to 6 hours after ingestion with general malaise, nausea, vomiting, abdominal pain, and diarrhea. No fever occurs, but the symptoms may be distressing enough to justify hospital consultation in approximately 10% of patients. The symptoms spontaneously resolve within 6 to 12 hours, and the prognosis is excellent, except in the case of severe dehydration in young children and elderly patients.

Although the mode of action of SAgs at the level of T-lymphocytes is known, their mechanism at the surface of the intestinal mucosa is unclear. TSST-1 and SEB, which may produce TSS, can traverse the mucosa via transcytosis.[103,108] On the other hand, SEA, which is one of the first causes of food intoxication, apparently cannot. Thus, symptoms must be related to some kind of local toxicity.

OTHER IMPLICATIONS OF SUPERANTIGENS

Although SAgs can result in dramatic subversion of the host immune system, they are not ultimate bacterial weapons because they affect only restricted subgroup of anergic patients. Many of these genes are physically contiguous, which suggests that they may have arisen by duplication, maybe for the purpose of diversity.[12,99,100] The versatility of SAgs is further supported by the discovery that one of them (i.e., SHE) develops its SAg activity by binding to the Vα rather than the Vβ domains of the T-cell receptor, thus expanding different sets of T-cell lineages than classical SAgs.[109]

The clinical relevance of this multiplicity of toxins is not entirely understood. Toxin genes are dispensable elements that are not needed for growth in rich media and in the absence of competition. Some SAgs (e.g., TSST-1 and SEs A, B, and C) obviously provide a way for the bacterium to escape host immunity. Carrying multiple toxin variants may be an advantage for survival in specific niches. For instance, SAgs have been involved in the etiology of psoriasis and atopic dermatitis,[110] where toxin-induced skin modification could promote bacterial survival. On the other hand, the survival advantage of provoking allergic diseases including rhinitis and asthma[111] and Kawasaki syndrome[112] is less intuitive. All together, the multiplicity of SAgs could enable *S. aureus* to interfere with the immune response of various animal species, thus broadening its host spectrum.

Pathogenesis II: Pathogenicity (Genomic) Islands and Mobile Genetic Elements

At the time of writing, 12 complete *S. aureus* genomes are available in public databases (e.g., http://www.ncbi.nlm.nih.gov/genomes/lproks.cgi). *S. aureus* genomes are circular and contain approximately 2.8 million bp that represent approximately 2700 coding sequences, plus structural and regulatory RNAs. They are divided in a core genome, which contains mostly housekeeping genes, is quite conserved along various staphylococcal species, and accounts for about 80% of the whole DNA; and an accessory genome that carries mobile DNA (MGEs), contains most *S. aureus* pathogenic and drug-resistance features, and may vary between different species and strains.[12,14-16,100,113] Approximately 50% of predicted proteins encoded by the *S. aureus* chromosome are highly homologous to those of *B. subtilis*,[10] which suggests that these apparently distant organisms have inherited most of their genes from a common ancestor and diverged later on. Divergent genes comprise sporulation genes, which are only present in *B. subtilis*, and pathogenic genes, which are only present in *S. aureus*.

Genome evolution is driven by random point mutations that lead to single nucleotide polymorphism (SNP), larger variations in core genes (e.g., deletions or duplication of repeat regions) that may differ between lineages (core variable genes [CV]), and MGEs that include insertion sequences, transposons, viruses, and pathogenicity island and genomic islands (Table 195-5).[6,7,10-12,14-16,99] Insertion sequences may move throughout the chromosome and turn off or turn on target genes by disruption/restitution of open reading frames or transcription-activation by intrinsic promoters. Transposons often carry resistance determinants against antibiotics or heavy metals. Viruses mostly carry single pathogenic determinants such as exfoliative toxin A[10] and Panton-Valentine leukocidin[12,114] and can transmit these determinants by infecting other strains.

Pathogenicity and genomic islands are continuous structures that vary in size from approximately 15 kb to 70 kb and can harbor many

TABLE 195-5	Summary of Major MGE in Sequenced *Staphylococcus aureus* Strains										
Strain	MRSA252	N315	Mu50	COL	8325	MW2	MSSA476	FPR3757	JH1/JH9	Newman	RF122
Clonal cluster	30	5	5	8	8	1	1	8	5	8	151
Bacteriophage											
ΦSa1			NI								*lukFM*
ΦSa2	NI				NI (Φ12)	PV-*luk*		PV-*luk*	NI		
ΦSa3	*chip scin sak sea*	*chip scin sak sep*	*chip sak sea*		*chip scin sak*	*scin sak sea seg sek*	*scin sak sea seg sek*	*chip scin sak*	*chip scin sak*	*chip scin sak sea*	
ΦSa4							NI		NI		
ΦSa5					NI (Φ11)					NI	
ΦSa6			NI (L54a)						NI	NI	NI
ΦSA7										NI	
ΦSa8											NI
SAPIs											
SAPI1						*seb ear seq sek*		*ear seq sek*			
SAPI2		*sel sec tst*	*sel sec tst*								*mdr*
SAPI3			*fhuD*			*ear sel sec*					
SAPI4	NI						NI				
SAPIbov											*tst sel*
Plasmids											
I	*ble kn**	*ble kn**	*ble kn**	*tet*				*tetK; NI*			
II	*cadAC arsBC**	*cadDX arsBC*				*blaZ cadD*	*blaZ cadD*		*blaZ arsR cadD aac/aph*		
III			*aac/aph qacA*					*erm ileS*			
Transposons											
Tn552	*blaZ*										
Tn554	*erm spc*	*erm spc*	*erm spc*								
Tn5801			*tetM*								
Tn976-like	NI			NI							
SCC											
mec I				*mecA*							
mec II	*mecA*	*mecA*	*mecA*							*mecA*	
mec III											
mec IV						*mecA*		*mecA arc opp*			
non-*mec*							*far1*				

Phage and SaPI families based on homology of integrase genes and insertion site. NI, Element present but no identified virulence or resistance gene. FPR3757 SCC*mec* is fused to ACME element; SaPIS belongs to SaPI1 family based on integrase and insertion site. RF122 has two phage fragments.

*Integrated plasmid.

aac/aph, aminoglycoside resistance; *arc*, arginine catabolism; *arsBC*, arsenic resistance genes; *blaZ*, penicillin resistance; *bsa*, bacteriocin biosynthesis genes; *cadACDX*, cadmium resistance genes; *chip*, chemotaxis inhibitory protein; *ear*, putative β-lactamase type protein; *erm*, erythromycin resistance; *far1*, fusidic acid resistance; *fhuD*, siderophore transporter; *ileS*, mupiricin resistance; *lukFM*, leukocidin; *mdr*, multidrug resistance; *opp*, oligopeptide uptake; *mecA*, penicillin-binding protein 2a conferring resistance to methicillin; *qacA*, quarternary ammonium compound (antiseptic) resistance; *PV-luk*, Panton-Valentine leukocidin; *sak*, staphylokinase; *SaPI*, S. aureus pathogenicity island; *SCC*, staphylococcal cassette chromosome; *scin*, staphylococcal chemotaxis inhibitory protein; *sea* to *sep*, enterotoxin A to enterotoxin P; *spc*, spectinomycin resistance; *tst*, toxic shock syndrome toxin-1 ; *tet* and *tetM*, tetracycline resistance.

Adapted from Lindsay J. *S. aureus* evolution: lineages and mobile genetic elements (MGEs). In Lindsay J, editor. *Staphylococcus aureus Molecular Genetics.* Norfolk, UK: Casiter Academic Press; 2008. p. 45-69.

virulence or resistance genes. They mostly contain heterologous DNA that indicates exogenous acquisition. A common feature of these elements is that they are bracketed by direct or inverted repeats and carry recombinase genes. The repeats serve as attachment site *(att)* for integration into homologous regions of the bacterial chromosome. The recombinase, which is often an integrase, catalyzes integration into the chromosome.[115]

MOBILIZATION OF PATHOGENICITY ISLANDS

A seminal study showed that *S. aureus pathogenicity island* 1 (SaPI1) could be mobilized from the bacterial chromosome by φ80α and φ11 and transferred into naive recipients thereafter (see Table 195-5).[115] During productive phage infection, SaPI1 is first excised from the chromosome, as a result of the phage Xis function, then amplified in the cytoplasm (up to 120 copies in case of φ80α), encapsidated, and

ready for infection of naive recipients. After entering a new *Staphylococcus*, SaPI1 undergoes Campell-like site-specific integration into the chromosome with both its *att* site and its own integrase. Such phage mobilization was observed with other pathogenicity islands (e.g., SaPI2) and is likely to be a general mechanism of gene transfer for these large elements (see Table 195-5). Excision and transfer of such elements are triggered by stresses such as exposure to ultraviolet (UV) light and antibiotics[115,116] and thus could be promoted by antibiotic treatment in the clinical setting.

PATHOGENICITY AND GENOMIC ISLANDS: TYPES AND NOMENCLATURE

S. aureus pathogenicity islands are relatively short (≤15 kb) structures that contain various types of virulence genes (see Table 195-5). Seven SaPIs have described and are reunified in four groups based on the homology of their integrase genes.[11] SaPI1 and SaPI2 harbor the gene for TSST-1 and are responsible for most cases of TSS (one SaPI2-containing clone in particular). SaPI3 and SaPI4 contain numerous enterotoxin genes. SaPIbov encodes for a bovine version of TSST, and SaPIbap encodes for a bovine adherence protein that might play a role in bovine mastitis.

In addition, complete genome analyses revealed the existence of two larger islands that were present in all sequences strains and were always inserted at the same chromosomal location. These more stable elements were designated *genomic islands* and referred to as vSaα and vSa.[10,12,99,117] Although present in all the available sequences, these islands may vary in their gene content. They harbor a variety of staphylococcal exotoxins *(set)* and other virulence genes and thus have been variously referred to as exotoxin gene cluster *(egc)* or virulence gene nursery.[5] The frequency and mechanism of mobilization of staphylococcal genomic island is as yet unclear.

THE RESISTANCE ISLAND STAPHYLOCCOCAL CHROMOSOME CASSETTE *mec*

Methicillin-resistant S. aureus contains one resistance island called *staphylococcal chromosome cassette* (SCC) *mec*, where *mec* is the genetic element that confers resistance to methicillin.[118] SCC*mec* is an exogenous piece of DNA that may vary between 15 and 60 kb. Its boundaries are demarcated by direct and inverted repeats, which allow integration at a homologous site into the chromosome. The SCC*mec* critical genes are the recombinases *ccrA* and *ccrB*, which can mediate mobilization of the whole element, and the *mecA* gene, which mediates β-lactam resistance. The rest of SCC*mec* contains various additional determinants and is referred to as J for junkyard.[119]

mecA encodes for a particular penicillin-binding protein (PBP) called PBP2A, which has a low affinity for methicillin and most other β-lactam drugs.[120] PBP2A is responsible for the intrinsic resistance of MRSA to almost all β-lactams (see subsequent section Mechanism of Methicillin Resistance). The *mecA* gene is preceded or not by the *mecRI* and *mecI* regulator determinants, which are homologues of the *blaRI* and *blaI* regulators of penicillinase *(bla)* genes. *mecRI* (and *blaRI*) encodes for a membrane receptor, and *mecI* (and *blaI*) encodes for a gene repressor. In the presence of penicillin, the extracellular portion of the membrane *mecRI (blaRI)* receptor triggers an autocatalytic cleavage of its intracytoplasmic portion. The liberated intracytoplasmic peptide acts as a metalloprotease, which further cleaves the *mecI (blaI)* repressor, thus derepressing gene expression.[121] The *mecA* gene is bracketed by one or two copies of IS431, which are believed to serve as a gene collector and might promote the local insertion of additional determinants, such as antibiotic resistance genes.[119]

At least six types of SCC*mec* were discriminated on the basis of the structure of their *ccrA-B* and *mecA* complexes.[119,122-125] These six types are likely to mirror major original MRSA clones. Types I, II, and III were shown to belong to health care–associated clones (HCA-MRSA). They harbor multiple resistance determinants, they have relatively large sizes (35 to 60 kb), and they are therefore difficult to mobilize. Types IV, V, and VI were associated with community-associated clones (CA-MRSA).[123,124] They are much smaller (about 15 kb) than their hospital congeners and do not carry multiple antibiotic-resistance genes. On the other hand, they appear to be associated with other elements in the same bacterium, including prophage-related Panton-Valentine toxin and multiple staphylococcal exotoxins *(set)* genes.[12] One particularly successful clone of CA-MRSA (clone USA300 of ST8 lineage) has also acquired a so-called arginine catabolic mobile element (ACME) inserted downstream of the SCC*mec* cassette.[126] ACME was acquired from *S. epidermidis* and confers survival advantages in acidic and maybe other environments. It improved survival and fitness of USA300 in a rabbit model of bacteremia.[127] Together these elements may render the organism particularly fit and virulent.

Health care–associated MRSA is often clonal, carries large SCC*mec* cassettes that contain multiple antibiotic-resistance genes, and is difficult to mobilize. In contrast, CA-MRSA seems to be less clonal (with the notorious exception of clone USA300) and carries small SCC*mec* cassettes, which are more prone to mobilization.[119] It is now clear that CA-MRSA has not arisen from HCA-MRSA that permeated the community but has emerged independently by acquiring its SCC*mec* most likely from CoNS donors. Whether its spread is from the widespread use of β-lactams or because its SCC*mec* and global genetic context provide other advantages to the bacterium is as yet undetermined.

Antibiotic Resistance

S. aureus has developed resistance to virtually all antibiotic classes available for clinical use. These encompass cell wall inhibitors such as β-lactams and glycopeptides; ribosomal inhibitors that include macrolide-lincosamide-streptogramin B (MLS$_B$), aminoglycosides, tetracyclines, fusidic acid, and the new oxazolidinones; the RNA polymerase inhibitor rifampin; the DNA gyrase blocking quinolones; the antimetabolite trimethoprim-sulfamethoxazole; and the newer lipopeptides and lipoglycopeptides.[128,129] The main resistance mechanisms are summarized in Table 195-6. Some are discussed subsequently.

β-LACTAMS

β-lactams inhibit bacterial growth by interfering with cell wall assembly. They bind to the active site of a series of membrane-bound enzymes responsible for inserting the peptidoglycan precursors into the nascent wall (see Fig. 195-7).[130] Certain enzymes are bifunctional and carry both a transglycosidase and a transpeptidase activity. Transpeptidation takes place at the D-ala- D-ala terminal of the precursor. It hydrolyses the covalent bond between the penultimate and the terminal D-ala and then transfers it to a free NH$_2$ terminal (the ε−NH$_2$ of lysine) of neighboring stem peptides. The terminal D-ala is released, and a new stem peptide crosslink is created (see Fig. 195-7A).

Penicillin and other β-lactams are steric analogs of the cell wall D-ala- D-ala terminal of the precursors. They compete with it for binding to the active site of the membrane-bound transpeptidase and act as mechanism-based inhibitors, hence the term *penicillin-binding protein* (PBP) coined for these enzymes.

Resistance to Penicillin

The most common resistance mechanism of *S. aureus* to β-lactams is penicillinase, which is encoded by the *bla* gene usually carried on a plasmid. The gene is inducible and preceded by the *blaRI* and *blaI* regulatory determinants (see previous section The Resistance Island Staphyloccocal Chromosome Cassette *mec*). Penicillinase is a secreted enzyme that hydrolyses penicillin and other penicillinase-susceptible compounds into inactive penicilloic acid. Penicillinase-producing *S. aureus* emerged rapidly after penicillin was introduced as a therapeutic agent in the mid 1940s. It is now prevalent both in the hospital and in the community where it represents close to 80% of the isolates.[128,131]

The minimal inhibitory concentration (MIC) of penicillin G for fully susceptible *S. aureus* is approximately 0.01 mg/L. In contrast, the MIC of penicillinase-stable drugs such as nafcillin or cephalosporins is 10-fold greater. Thus, penicillin G remains one of the best choices against penicillin-susceptible staphylococci.

Methicillin-Resistant S. aureus

The first penicillinase-stable β-lactams such as cephalosporins and semisynthetic methicillin and nafcillin became available in the late 1950s. Ironically, the first MRSA was described at about the same time.[132] The prevalence of MRSA progressively increased thereafter. One survey of the National Nosocomial Infections Surveillance (NNIS) reported that the hospital prevalence rate of MRSA increased from 2.1% in 1975 to 35% in 1991.[133] It is now as high up to 60% in certain centers in the United States,[37] but great geographic variations exist worldwide. In one survey from the SENTRY antimicrobial surveillance program (1997 to 1999), the MRSA prevalence rate varied as follows: Western Pacific region, 46%; United States, 34.2%; Latin America,

TABLE 195-6	*Staphylococcus aureus* Resistance Mechanisms to Major Classes of Antibiotics

	Resistance Mechanisms			Resistance Gene		
Antimicrobials	Target Modification	Drug Inactivation	Decreased Accumulation	Nature	Origin	Location[†]
β-Lactams						
Penicillinase-S	Yes	Yes	No	PBP2A* Penicillinase	Acquired Acquired	Plasmid SCC*mec* (chromosome)
Penicillinase-R	Yes	No	No	PBP2A*	Acquired	SCC*mec* (chromosome)
Glycopeptides						
Intermediate-R	Yes	No	No	Mutations in wall-building genes	Intrinsic	Chromosome
Fully-R	Yes	No	No	*vanA* and *vanH*	Acquired	SCC*mec* (chromosome)
Lipoglycopeptides Daptomycin	Yes	No	No	Mutations in genes involve in wall-building and membrane charges (*mprF*)	Intrinsic	Chromosome
MLS_B						
Macrolides	Yes	No	Yes	*erm* *msrA*	Acquired Acquired	Plasmid or chromosome Plasmid
Lincosamide[‡]	Yes	Yes	No	*erm* *linA'*	Acquired Acquired	Plasmid or chromosome Plasmid or chromosome
Streptogramin B[‡]	Yes	Yes	Yes	*erm* *vgb* (rare) *msrA* (rare)	Acquired Acquired Acquired	Plasmid or chromosome Plasmid or chromosome Plasmid or chromosome
Streptogramin A	No	Yes	Yes	*vat, vatA* (rare)	Acquired	Plasmid or chromosome
Quinupristin-dalfopristin	Yes	Yes	Yes	*vga, vgaB* (rare) Combinations of above (rare)	Acquired	Plasmid or chromosome
Linezolid	Yes	No	No	Mutation in 23S rRNA gene *cfr*	Intrinsic Acquired	Chromosome Plasmid
Tetracyclines	Yes	No	Yes	*tet*(M), *tet*(O) *tet*(K) and *tet*(L)	Acquired Acquired	Plasmid or chromosome Plasmid or chromosome
Gentamicin	No	Yes	Yes	*aac*(6')-*aph*(2″) Respiratory chain mutants	Acquired	Plasmid or chromosome Chromosome
Chloramphenicol	No	Yes	No	*cat*	Acquired	Plasmid or chromosome
Fusidic acid	Yes	No	Yes	*fusA* mutation pUB101	Intrinsic Acquired	Chromosome Plasmid
Rifampin	Yes	No	No	*rpoB* mutation	Intrinsic	Chromosome
Fluoroquinolones	Yes	No	Yes	*grlA* and *gyrA* *norA*	Intrinsic Intrinsic	Chromosome Chromosome
Trimethoprim	Yes	No	No	*dfrA* mutation *dfrA*	Intrinsic Acquired	Chromosome Plasmid or chromosome (acts by mutation or overproduction)
Sulfamethoxazole	Yes	No	No	*dpsA*	Intrinsic Acquired	Chromosome Plasmid (probable) (acts by mutation or overproduction)

*PBP2A, penicillin-binding protein 2A.

[†]SCC*mec*, staphylococcal chromosomal cassette *mec* (see text for details).

[‡]*erm* gene must be induced or constitutively expressed to confer resistance to lincosamides and streptogramines B. Only macrolides are good inducers. Lincosamides and streptogramins do not induce resistance but are inactive against constitutively MLS_B-resistant strains.

vanA and *vanH*, vancomycin resistance A and H genes (see text for details); *mprF*, lysylphophatidylglycerol synthase; *erm*, erythromycin-resistance methylase, mainly *ermA* (chromosome, transposons Tn554) and *ermC* (plasmid); *linA* , lincosamide nucleotidyl transferase; *vgb*, virginiamycin hydrolysis; *msrA*, macrolide-streptogramin resistance, ABC-transporter; *vat* and *vatA*, acetyl transferase genes; *vga* and *vgaB*, streptogramin A efflux gene, ABC-transporter; *cfr (chloramphenicol-florfenicol resistance)*, 23S rRNA methyltransferase; *tet(M) and tet(O)*, responsible for ribosomal-modification and protection; *tet(K) and tet(L)*, responsible for active efflux of tetracyclines; *aac*(6')-*aph*(2″), bifunctional aminoglycoside acetyl-transferase and phosphor-transferase determinant, present on transposons Tn4001; *cat*, chloramphenicol acetyl-transferase; *fusA*, gene encoding elongation factor G (EF-G); pUB101, plasmid encoding penicillin-resistance (penicillinase), cadmium-resistance, and a protein (Far1) conferring impermeability to fusidic acid; *rpoB*, gene encoding for β subunit of RNA polymerase; *grlA* and *gyrA*, genes encoding for the DNA topoisomerase and gyrase, respectively; *norA*, gene encoding for staphylococcal efflux pump; *dfrA*, dihydrofolate reductase gene; *dpsA*, dihydropteroate synthase.

34.9%; Europe, 26.3%; and Canada, 5.7%. Methicillin resistance varied greatly among countries within a region. In Western Pacific countries, percentages of MRSA ranged from 23.6% in Australia to more than 70% in Japan and Hong Kong. In European centers, these percentages varied from less than 2% in the Netherlands to 54.4% in Portugal.[134]

Health Care–Acquired versus Community-Acquired Methicillin-Resistant *S. aureus*. Although originally confined to the hospital environment, MRSA has emerged as a community-acquired infection over the last decade.[21,22,135] *Community-acquired MRSA* is different from *health care-acquired MRSA*, from both epidemiologic and molecular points of view. Case-definition studies showed that HCA-MRSA and CA-MRSA represented different organisms that produced different clinical syndromes.[136,137] HCA-MRSA was associated with risk factors that included recent hospitalization or surgery, living in a nursing home, or carrying an indwelling catheter or device. It pro-

duced mostly hospital-related pneumonia and bacteremia. CA-MRSA was not associated with any risk factors and produced primarily skin and soft tissue infections, and sometimes rapidly fatal necrotizing pneumonia. Recently, it was also described as responsible for necrotizing fasciitis and bone and joint infections.[127,138] In addition, HCA-MRSA was multiresistant and highly clonal, whereas CA-MRSA was pauciresistant and seemingly more polyclonal,[92,119] except for an extremely successful USA300 clone that has become highly prevalent in the United States.[22]

As mentioned, CA-MRSA is also associated with SCC*mec* type VI (and type V and VI in a few cases) and almost always carries the PVL toxin.[22,92] PVL is epidemiologically associated with SSTI and necrotizing pneumonia, but its specific role in disease remains controversial. Experimental studies in models of pneumonia and skin abscesses suggest that it could have a differential activity in various tissues. It is apparently involved in lung injuries[127,139] but might be dispensable for soft tissues infection.[140] Although debate still exists,[141] these issues must be solved because the perspective of blocking the toxin with specific antibodies depends on them.

Thus, HCA-MRSA and CA-MRSA are not alike. Practically, MRSA in patients at risk is likely to be of the multiresistant hospital type, whereas MRSA in patients without risks is likely to more susceptible but more invasive.

Mechanism of Methicillin Resistance. The main mechanism of methicillin-resistance is not mediated by penicillinase but the newly acquired penicillin-binding protein 2A (PBP2A), encoded by *mecA*.[120] The few staphylococci that express borderline methicillin resistance from the overexpression of penicillinase are not clinically relevant. Because of its low β-lactam affinity, PBP2A can take over the cell wall assembly when normal staphylococcal PBPs are blocked by these compounds (see Fig. 195-7B).[142] However, although this confers high intrinsic resistance to virtually all β-lactams, PBP2A has a special requirement for peculiar cell wall precursors. These must contain a pentaglycine decorating side chain attached to the position 3 L-lysine of their stem peptide and other specificities such as an amidated D-glutamine in position 2 of the peptide (see Fig. 195-8).

Provision of this adequate substrate to PBP2A requires the functionality of numerous accessory genes implicated in the normal wall building machinery,[88,143] including 14 or more accessory determinants,[143] some of which (*femABC* and *fmhB*) are responsible for adding the glycine residues critical for the PBP2A function.[88] Any alteration in these elements decreases the expression of methicillin resistance in spite of the fact that PBP2A is present.

Another fragility of PBP2A is that it carries only a transpeptidase domain and misses a transglycosidase activity (see Fig. 195-7B). Thus, for successful assembly of the peptidoglycan, PBP2A needs to hijack the transglycosidase domain of normal staphylococcal PBP, namely PBP2.[144] This is a salient example of heterologous protein cooperation in antibiotic resistance but also represents the Achilles' heel of the system. Because most β-lactams can readily block the normal staphylococcal PBPs, further drug development needs only to target additional PBP2A to be effective. Both experimental work and recent crystallographic evidence indicate that such an approach is feasible.[145] Indeed, successful treatment of experimental endocarditis from MRSA was achieved with an array of older and newer β-lactams with good PBP2A affinity.[146,147] This approach is a driving force for the development of new anti-MRSA compounds,[148] which recently generated some novel molecules of the cephalosporin and carbapenem classes.[149]

GLYCOPEPTIDES

As a general rule, current *glycopeptides* (e.g., vancomycin) are less efficacious than β-lactams against MSSA. Thus, they should not be used as first-line treatment against β-lactam–susceptible organisms.[150] However, vancomycin is still a gold standard against severe MRSA infections, until proof is found of newer anti-MRSA drugs, such as daptomycin and anti-MRSA β-lactams, which are discussed subsequently.

Two types of resistance to glycopeptides were reported in clinical isolates of *S. aureus*. According to the May 2008 U.S. Food and Drug Administration (FDA) policy, the vancomycin breakpoints for *S. aureus* are as follow: 1, intermediate resistance (MIC of vancomycin, 4 to 8 mg/L); and 2, high-level resistance (MIC of vancomycin, ≥16 mg/L). Both phenotypes result from different mechanisms and may be of different clinical and epidemiologic relevance.

Intermediate Resistance to Glycopeptides
Intermediate-resistant *S. aureus* isolates were originally described in Japan and in the United States[151,152] but are ubiquitous. The first isolate,[153] called Mu50, was recovered from a 4-month-old child with MRSA sternal wound infection after cardiac surgery. The infection did not respond to vancomycin treatment. The organism had a minimal inhibitory concentration (MIC) of vancomycin of 8 mg/L, as detected with standard broth dilution methods. At that time, the Clinical and Laboratory Standards Institute (CLSI, formerly National Committee

on Clinical Laboratory Standards [NCCLS]) defined staphylococci for which the MIC of vancomycin was 4 mg/L or less as *susceptible*, for which the MIC was 8 to 16 mg/L as *intermediate*, and for which the MIC was 32 mg/L or more as *resistant*.[24] Therefore, the Mu50 isolate was defined as a vancomycin (or *glycopeptide) intermediate S. aureus* (GISA).

The same author reported a second *S. aureus*, called Mu3, responsible for vancomycin treatment failure in an adult patient with pneumonia.[154] Although the vancomycin MIC for this isolate was 4 mg/L, formally considered as susceptible, Mu3 contained GISA subpopulations (≤10⁻⁶ colony-forming unit [CFU]) that grew in the presence of 5 to 9 mg/L of vancomycin and were not detected with standard drug-susceptibility testing. The term *heteroresistant GISA* (hGISA) was coined to define the Mu3 phenotype. Since then, a number of cases of GISA and hGISA were described worldwide and were associated with vancomycin treatment failures both in animal experiments and in human cases.[155] More recently, failures of vancomycin treatment were associated with MIC of more than 1.5 mg/L, which supports the argument for a more stringent definition of GISA.[156] The revised CLSI breakpoints now classify isolates with an MIC of 4 mg/L vancomycin as GISA.[157]

Intermediate glycopeptide resistance arises from chromosomal mutations that affect the structure of the wall peptidoglycan. In susceptible strains, glycopeptides inhibit cell wall assembly by binding to the D-ala-D-ala terminal of cell wall precursors and block both transpeptidation and transglycosylation. GISA harbors a thickened cell wall that contains an increased number of free uncrosslinked D-ala-D-ala terminals. This increased amount of free D-ala-D-ala is thought to act as a lure and trap glycopeptide molecules before they reach their target.[158] Recent genomic analyses indicate that mutations in a two-component sensing system (*graSR*) are involved.[159,160]

Although GISA may cause glycopeptide treatment failure, its low level of resistance and sometimes heterogeneous phenotype make it hard to detect in the laboratory.[24] However, a recent dual-antibiotic Etest strip assay that contained vancomycin and teicoplanin performed remarkably well. It detected GISA and hGISA with a high sensitivity (95%) and specificity (94%), which was almost identical to much more cumbersome population analysis, which is not performed in routine laboratory testing.[161]

Full Resistance to Glycopeptides
Full vancomycin resistance (MIC ≥ 32 mg/L for species other than *S. aureus*) has been known for more than a decade in *Enterococcus* spp.[162] In these organisms, glycopeptide resistance results from the acquisition of either Tn*1546* or Tn*1547*, two transposons that encode for a series of genes that modify the D-ala-D-ala terminal of the bacterial peptidoglycan precursor, the very target of glycopeptide compounds, to D-ala-D-lactate. The modified D-ala-D-lactate–containing precursor has a low affinity for glycopeptides and thus confers resistance. Tn*1546*, which encodes the so-called VanA resistance phenotype, could be transferred to *S. aureus* experimentally.[163] Thus, the recent emergence of fully vancomycin-resistant *S. aureus* (VRSA) that expresses the VanA phenotype among human clinical isolates is not astonishing. Only seven cases were described in the United States until 2006,[164] but these organisms must be taken seriously. First, all patients had evidence of previous MRSA and enterococcal infection, but not all had received vancomycin. Thus, transfer of the transposon may occur by more generalized triggering effects, maybe involving unrelated antibiotics. Second, the VRSA phenotype may be missed with routine automated antibiotic susceptibility testing[165] and could be more prevalent than observed. Third, two new cases were recently described in hospitals in Iran.[166] So, VRSA warrants constant attention in the diagnostic laboratory.

DAPTOMYCIN

Daptomycin is a relatively new lipopeptide that was recently approved in the United States and elsewhere for *S. aureus*–complicated SSTI, bacteremia, and right-sided infective endocarditis (IE).[129] It is proposed as a replacement for vancomycin against MRSA. Daptomycin is an amphophilic molecule that requires calcium to solubilize as octamer-micelles in liquid phases.[167] Because of its large size, it cannot traverse the outer membrane of gram-negative bacteria, which are naturally resistant to the drug. In gram-positive organisms, it diffuses through the peptidoglycan toward the plasma membrane, where the calcium ions disperse and leave the lipid moiety of daptomycin to interact with the plasma membrane and destabilize its electric potential.[168] Daptomycin is highly bactericidal, but its activity is dose dependent and the dosage of the drug must be large enough to ensure supra-MIC tissue levels. At least 6 mg/kg/d intravenously (and maybe more) should be used for severe infections.[129] Compassionate studies suggest that daptomycin might also be considered against left-sided IE,[169] but definitive studies are missing. On the other hand, daptomycin should not be used against airway-acquired pneumonia because it is inactivated by alveolar surfactant.[170]

Mutants with decreased daptomycin susceptibility (MIC > 4 mg/L) were recovered both in the laboratory and in clinical samples.[129,171] Moreover, a correlation between vancomycin resistance and reduced daptomycin susceptibility was described, for which caution should be used with daptomycin against GISA.[172, 173] Decreased susceptibility might involve more than one mechanism, including alteration of the membrane-modifying enzyme lysylphosphatidylglycerol synthase (*mprF*),[174] and overexpression of the *vraSR* operon and a thickened cell wall, which are also altered in GISA (see previous discussion).[175]

PROTEIN SYNTHESIS INHIBITORS

The *macrolide-lincosamide-streptogramin B* (MLS$_B$) antibiotics and the oxazolidinone linezolid are discussed in this section. The new glycylcycline tigecycline is addressed in the subsequent section Alternative Treatments. MLS$_B$ antibiotics comprise separate classes of molecules (i.e., macrolides, ketolides, lincosamides, and streptogramins B) that all bind to the bacterial ribosome and block protein synthesis. Resistance proceeds by any of the three classic mechanisms: modification of the bacterial drug target, modification-inactivation of the drug itself, and decreasing intracellular accumulation of the drug.

Ribosome Modification

Ribosome modification and drug efflux are the most frequent resistance mechanisms in *S. aureus*.[176] *Ribosome modification* is mediated by the *erm* gene (for erythromycin methylase), which encodes a methylase that adds one or two methyl groups to the 23 S rRNA. This inflicts a steric alteration that greatly decreases the affinity of the drug for its target. The *erm* determinants belong to a family of methylase genes preferentially located on mobile elements such as transposons (e.g., Tn*554* and *ermA*) or plasmids (e.g., pE194 and *ermC*). An additional sophistication in *S. aureus* is that the expression of *erm* is inducible.[176] The *erm* product is synthesized only in the presence of inducing drugs. Thus, the bacterium does not spend worthless metabolic energy in the absence of antibiotic pressure. Among MLS$_B$ drugs, only macrolides are good *erm* inducers. However, once induced, the gene product confers cross resistance to the other members of the group, including the newer ketolides, lincosamides, and streptogramins B (but not streptogramins A). Moreover, mutations that result in constitutive *erm* expression, and hence, global MLS$_B$ resistance, occur at high frequency (10^{-7} to 10^{-8}). Therefore, lincosamides (e.g., clindamycin) should be used with great caution against *erm*-inducible isolates (i.e., resistant to erythromycin, but susceptible to lincosamides and streptogramins B) because the drug might select for constitutive MLS$_B$ mutants, which are resistant to the whole group of compounds.[177]

In the laboratory, the MLS$_B$ resistance phenotype is detected with the disk diffusion D-test in which erythromycin and clindamycin disks are placed at a distance on a plate inoculated with bacteria and the diffusion of erythromycin toward the clindamycin disk induces clindamycin resistance. As a result, the zone of inhibition around the clindamycin disk takes a D-shape.[177] In contrast, constitutive MLS$_B$ resistance yields no inhibition zone at all around the clindamycin.

Drug Efflux

Active macrolide *efflux* has been reported in both streptococci and staphylococci.[178,179] In *S. pyogenes* and *Streptococcus pneumoniae*, efflux is mediated by the *mefA* and *mefE* genes, respectively, which are members of the major facilitator transporter and export only macrolides (M-resistance phenotype). *S. aureus* and coagulase-negative staphylococci may contain *msrA*, which belongs to the complex ABC-transporter (adenosine triphosphate [ATP]–binding cassette) set of genes[178] and confers resistance to both macrolides and streptogramins B (MS-resistance phenotype). In contrast to major facilitators, ABC transporters use ATP hydrolysis as a source of energy for active efflux. The *msrA* complex is located on a plasmid and is frequently observed in MLS$_B$-resistant coagulase-negative staphylococci. It can be transferred into *S. aureus*,[178] but its clinical relevance for MLS$_B$ resistance is unclear. Of note, lincosamides (e.g., clindamycin) are not subject to efflux by these pumps.

Constitutive MLS$_B$ resistance associated or not to drug efflux is extremely frequent (>90%) in HCA-MRSA. Therefore, MLS$_B$ drugs should never be considered against such organisms. The only exception is the quinupristin/dalfopristin combination (streptogramin B and A; see subsequent section Alternative Treatments). In contrast, only 5% of CA-MRSA is reported as clindamycin-resistant, and mostly are the inducible phenotype.[22] Thus, clindamycin remains a therapeutic option against CA-MRSA.

Linezolid

The oxazolidinone *linezolid* prevents initiation of proteins synthesis by binding to the 23S rRNA of the 50S ribosomal subunit, near its interface with the 30S subunit. It is only active against gram-positive bacteria and is essentially bacteriostatic. It is approved in the United States for complicated SSTI and nosocomial pneumonia from susceptible organisms, including MRSA. One study showed that linezolid might be superior to vancomycin in this indication.[180] A systematic review on infective endocarditis from multiresistant bacteria, including 18 MRSA and vancomycin-intermediate *Staphylococcus aureus* (VISA), reported a success rate of about 60%, which suggests that compassionate use of linezolid might be an option in such complicated situations.[181] Success was also reported in compassionate use against MRSA osteomyelitis.[182]

One asset of linezolid is it can be administered orally and thus is useful for outpatient therapy. Another is that it inhibits the secretion of TSST-1 and other toxins, such as clindamycin, and should be considered against toxin-associated infections including CA-MRSA hemorrhagic pneumonia.[183] On the other hand, linezolid is not suitable for long term (>28 days) therapy because prolonged treatment may be associated with thrombocytopenia, sometimes peripheral or optic neuropathy, and lactic acidosis.[184]

Linezolid resistance has been reported episodically in clinical settings. It is primarily the result of mutations is the 23S rRNA gene.[185] Because staphylococci harbor six to seven copies of rRNA genes, mutations in only one of them does not yield high-level resistance at once. MIC increments are progressive, and MICs of such mutants are usually 4 to 8 mg/L compared with a baseline of 2 mg/L. However, plasmid-mediated high-level resistance was recently detected in one clinical isolate of *S. aureus* and one of *S. epidermidis* (MIC, 8 and >257 mg/L, respectively).[186] The resistance gene *(cfr)* encodes a 23S rRNA methylase that confers cross resistance to other drugs that bind at the same site, including chloramphenicol, lincosamides (i.e., clindamycin), and streptogramin A. Although as yet anecdotal, plasmid-mediated resistance to linezolid is potentially transmissible to other organisms and might become a clinical problem.

QUINOLONES

Quinolones are an important class in the antiinfective armamentarium. They originated in the 1960s as a byproduct from the synthesis of antimalarial quinines. Fluorinated derivatives such as ciprofloxacin, norfloxacin, and ofloxacin appeared in the 1980s. They had low MICs (in the order of 0.01 mg/L) for most gram-negative pathogens. However, the MIC for gram-positive bacteria was relatively high (MIC, 0.25 to 2 mg/L for *Staphylococcus* spp. and *Streptococcus* spp.)[187] and close to therapeutic concentrations in the serum of humans (2 mg/L for peak concentration of ciprofloxacin). Use of these borderline active drugs against problematic gram-positive pathogens such as MRSA facilitated the selection for resistant derivatives. The prevalence rate of quinolone resistance in HCA-MRSA has been around 90% for a long time[128] and is close to 40% in CA-MRSA,[22] which makes older and newer quinolones mostly inappropriate against MRSA.

Mechanisms of Resistance

Known quinolone-resistance mechanisms result from chromosomal mutations (see Table 195-6). Plasmid-mediated resistance has been described in gram-negative pathogens and is associated with the *qnr* gene, which protects the quinolone targets.[188] A *qnr*-like gene has been described in *Enterococcus faecalis* and could confer resistance to *S. aureus*.[189] However, such a mechanism is not yet described in clinical isolates.

Quinolone resistance proceeds by two types of mechanisms, including overexpression of the efflux pump NorA[190] and structural mutations in the quinolone targets topoisomerase IV *(grlA* and *grlB)* and gyrase *(gyrA* and *gyrB)* genes.[191] Resistance is acquired stepwise. A first *grlA* mutation, which occurs at frequencies of 10^{-7} to 10^{-8}, produces a moderate increase in MIC (e.g., from 0.5 to 2 mg/L of ciprofloxacin) that is still considered susceptible (<4 mg/mL). However, this first mutation paves the way to a second mutation in the *gyrA* gene, which combined with the *grlA* mutation results in high-level resistance. Because the initial *grlA* mutation jeopardizes the efficacy of quinolones, it is critical to avoid selecting it at first. Therefore, prevention of first-level quinolone resistance by ensuring appropriate drug levels in the tissues is important.

Older quinolones readily select for such alterations, yielding highly resistant organisms after only a few serial exposures to the drug.[192] Newer quinolones with improved anti gram-positive activity (levofloxacin, moxifloxacin, gatifloxacin, garenoxacin) are less selective. However, they still carry the risk of selection, particularly in bacteria that already acquired a first-degree *(grlA* mutant) of ciprofloxacin resistance (MIC, 2 to 8 mg/L).

A series of pharmacokinetics/pharmacodynamics criteria was established to predict both quinolone efficacy and risk of resistance. Efficacy was predicted by peak drug-level/MIC ratios of 8 or more and ratios of area under the curve/MIC of 100 or more.[193] With regard to resistance prevention, in vitro and in vivo experiments suggest that drug dosage might be adjusted on so-called mutation prevention concentration (MPC), which is two to four times higher than the MIC, rather than on MIC.[194] However, the clinical relevance of MPCs has not yet been assessed.

ALTERNATIVE TREATMENTS

Treatment of infections from multiresistant HCA-MRSA may be problematic. The activity of all available drugs must be tested against the isolate to establish whether some could still be used. Evaluation of the severity of the disease is also important because not all drugs are equally appropriate in serious conditions. Superficial and non–life-threatening infections probably respond to a variety of drugs, including trimethoprim-sulfamethoxazole, to which HCA-MRSA and CA-MRSA are often susceptible, combined or not with other substances such as rifampin. On the other hand, a notorious lack of good alternatives is available in the case of deep-seated or life-threatening infection. Vancomycin is one of the first choices in such situations. However, poor response to vancomycin may occur in a substantial proportion of patients[195] because of the relatively poor bactericidal activity of the drug and resistance development. Combining vancomycin with an aminoglycoside increases in vitro bactericidal activity. However, the clinical benefit of this combination is not shown, and both kidney and ototoxicity are a matter of concern.[196] Likewise, com-

bining vancomycin with rifampin gave rather inconclusive results.[197] Other strategies are based on relatively new compounds and require expert supervision.

Quinupristin-Dalfopristin and Tigecycline

Two of the alternative compounds available for clinical use are the protein ribosome inhibitors *quinupristin-dalfopristin* and *tigecycline*. Both compounds have proved efficacious against problematic *S. aureus* infections, but no large double-blinded studies showing their superiority over standard therapy are available.

Quinupristin-dalfopristin is a combination of streptogramin B and streptogramin A.[198] It is active against both MLS_B-susceptible and MLS_B-resistant staphylococci. It is highly bactericidal against MLS_B-susceptible isolates but tends to be less bactericidal in the case of constitutive MLS_B resistance, which is practically always the case in HCA-MRSA (see Table 195-6). Relatively large quantities of the compound (7.5 mg/kg every 8 hours) should be given to ensure efficacy against such organisms. Experimental data indicate that combining quinupristin-dalfopristin with a β-lactam increases its activity against MRSA, even though the β-lactam is inactive on its own.[199] This strategy is awaiting further clinical demonstration. One limitation of quinupristin-dalfopristin is its venotoxicity, which requires the drug to be administered through a central catheter.

Tigecycline is a modified minocycline, from the tetracycline family of molecules. It is almost universally active against gram-negative and gram-positive pathogens, with the notorious exception of *Pseudomonas aeruginosa* and a few other gram-negative organisms that can extrude the drug via efflux pumps.[200] Tigecycline overcomes current *S. aureus* tetracycline-resistance mechanisms, including ribosome protection and active efflux, and thus is effective against all tetracycline-resistant isolates. It is approved in the United States and Europe for the treatment of complicated SSTI. However, it is strictly bacteriostatic, and no trials on *S. aureus*–specific severe infections are available yet. The drug must be administered intravenously.

Beta-Lactams with Improved Penicillin-Binding Protein 2A Affinity

Improving the affinity of β-lactams for MRSA-specific PBP2A has been the purpose of intensive research.[149] Recent work on the structure of PBP2A and potential blocking β-lactams indicates that the active site of the enzyme is closed in resting state and thus difficult to reach with the drug. However, when the enzyme is exposed to cell wall precursors or β-lactams with appropriate pharmacophores, allosteric interactions at other portions of PBP2A trigger opening of the active site, providing access to the precursors or to the blocking drug.[201] The success of this interaction probably depends on the hydrophobic pentaglycine side chain of the precursor (see Fig. 195-8) and thus on the presence of hydrophobic pharmacophores on the β-lactam molecule.[149] This poses solubility problems, which were solved by delivering the compound as a prodrug, as in ceftobiprole medocaril.

Ceftobiprole is the first of these new compounds that is becoming clinically available. It is effective against both MSSA and all major clones of MRSA (MIC, ≤4 mg/L) and was equivalent to vancomycin in two noninferiority complicated SSTI studies of 170 MRSA isolates.[202] Moreover, ceftobiprole and other β-lactams were shown to be synergistic with vancomycin against GISA and VRSA,[203,204] which could add values to such new compounds. Thus, ceftobiprole and other β-lactams with improved PBP2A affinity may represent promising anti-MRSA compounds.

Lipoglycopeptides

Lipoglycopeptides are semisynthetic derivatives of glycopeptides that carry modifications of specific functional groups. The most advanced are *dalbavancin* and *oritavancin*.[205,206] Like vancomycin, they bind to the D-Ala-D-Ala terminal of peptidoglycan precursors, thus inhibiting both transpeptidation and transglycosylation. In addition, the presence of lipophilic pharmacophores allows the molecules to interact with the plasma membrane, which leads to dispersion of membrane potential and rapid bacterial killing. Their lipophilic nature also prolongs their plasma half-life. For instance, dalbavancin can be given only once a week.

Both compounds are active against antibiotic-susceptible and antibiotic-resistant (including vancomycin) gram-positive pathogens and showed efficacy in various animal infection models. In a double-blind complicated SSTI trial, dalbavancin given once weekly for 2 weeks (1 g at week 1 and 0.5 g at week 2, intravenously) was highly effective (success rate, >90%) and comparable with linezolid given twice a day (600 mg every 12 h orally or intravenously) for the same length of time.[207] These drugs are awaiting further clinical evaluation.

PREVENTION AND PROSPECTIVES

Prospective antistaphylococcal strategies encompass prevention of colonization and decolonization of chronic carriers with local antiseptics and the developing new antipathogenesis strategies and new vaccines. Besides new antimicrobial molecules, one reemerging line of interest is *phage therapy*. Phages have been used against bacteria since early 1920 but were abandoned in Western countries at the introduction of penicillin G. Nevertheless, phages were continuously developed in Poland and in the countries of the former Soviet Union, especially Georgia and Russia and particularly at the Elavia Institute in Tbilisi, Georgia.[208] Currently, research is aimed at purifying the lytic enzymes of the phages, rather then using then as a whole.

Antipathogenesis strategies include molecules aimed at blocking *agr*-type regulatory loops and surface adhesins blockage (see Pathogenesis I: Regulation and Virulence Determinants section). Moreover, active work is ongoing on inhibition of the enzyme sortase (see Pathogenesis I: Regulation and Virulence Determinants section), in the aim of blocking the physical expression of staphylococcal surface proteins, including adhesin and essential proteins involved in iron uptake.[209]

Vaccination is an important area of research, both in human and in veterinary medicine. Vaccines pursue one of three aims: blocking the effect of toxins, blocking the function surface adhesins or other relevant proteins, or stimulating phagocytosis. Experimental vaccines have been raised by a variety of means, including DNA vaccines, and against constituents as diverse as the capsule or specific surface determinants, including PBP2A and adhesins. Most of these vaccines conferred some protection in experimental models, and one trial with a conjugated capsular vaccine gave promising results in patients for hemodialysis.[73] However, as yet, no approved antistaphylococcal vaccine is available for clinical use.[210]

▓ Clinical Aspects and Epidemiology

S. aureus is one of the most common bacterial pathogens in hospital-acquired and community-acquired infections.[37] Incidence rates of *S. aureus* infections range between 28.4 and 35.4/ per 100,000 inhabitants per year.[20,211] Its prevalence rate increased from 0.74% of all inpatients admitted to U.S. hospitals in 1998 to 1% in 2003 (annual increasing rate from 7% to 11%), corresponding to a total of nearly 300,000 patients with *S. aureus* infections in U.S. hospitals in 2003.[212] *S. aureus* infection is associated with substantial morbidity and mortality. Infected inpatients had, on average, a three times longer hospital stay (14.3 versus 4.5 days), three times greater charges (US $48,824 versus $14,141), and a five times greater risk of in-hospital death (11.2% versus 2.3%). After controlling for confounders, the annual impact in the United States was estimated to be 2.7 million additional days in hospitals, $9.5 billion excess costs, and at least 12,000 inpatient deaths.[213] Studies on *S. aureus* invasive infections consistently report high mortality rates, from 19% to 34%.[20,214-216] Combined with the increasing problem of multiple antibiotic resistance, these numbers underline the high social and economic burden of this particular pathogen.

CLINICAL SPECTRUM

S. aureus is responsible for an array of infections where it is either present on the infection site or acts at a distance by secreting of toxins (see Pathogenesis I: Regulation and Virulence Determinants section). The SENTRY antimicrobial surveillance program, which collects data from the United States, Canada, Latin America, Europe, and the Western Pacific, reported the following distributions of *S. aureus* infections: 1, 39.2% of SSTI; 2, 23.2% of lower respiratory tract infections; 3, 22% of bloodstream infections, including infective endocarditis; and 4, 15.6% of other infections, including infections of the urinary tract, brain, and abdominal cavity.[134]

S. aureus is a leading cause of nosocomial infections,[217] particularly in the case of surgical site infections (19.5% to 30%),[217,218] catheter-related bacteremia, and ventilator-associated pneumonia (20.5% t o 28%).[217-219] In the community, it is also one of the first causes of native valve (31.6% of cases) and prosthetic valve endocarditis (23% of cases)[220,221] and osteomyelitis (in 50% to 70% of cases)[222,223] and the second cause of community-onset bacteremia after *Escherichia coli* (15% to 23.5%).[37,224]

RISK FACTORS FOR *S. AUREUS* INFECTION

Population-based studies have consistently identified male gender and very young and elderly individuals as at increased risk for *S. aureus* infections. Moreover, two studies showed that the most important risk factor is necessity for dialysis, either peritoneal (relative risk [RR], 150 to 204) or hemodialysis (RR, 257 to 291). Other conditions that increase the risk of invasive *S. aureus* infections include diabetes (RR, 7), cancer (RR, 7.1 to 12.9), rheumatoid arthritis (RR, 2.2 to 9.2), HIV infection (RR, 23.7), intravenous drug use (RR, 10.1), or alcohol abuse (RR, 8.2; (Table 195-7).[20,211]

Rare but classical predisposing factors encompass chemotactic defects and defect in phagocytosis. Inheritable chemotactic defects include Job's syndrome, the Chédiak-Higashi syndrome, the Wiskott-Aldrich syndrome, and Down syndrome. *Job's syndrome* is a condition that involves recurrent eczema with repeated skin infections and cold abscesses. *Chédiak-Higashi syndrome* is defined clinically by albinism and recurrent *S. aureus* infections and cytologically by giant granules in phagocytic and other cells. Acquired chemotactic defects are also relatively rare and include rheumatoid arthritis and decompensated acidotic diabetes mellitus. Opsonic defects, whether inherited or acquired, are predisposing factors for all kinds of pyogenic infections and are not specific for *S. aureus*. They are exemplified by selective or combined hypogammaglobulinemias and various kinds of complement defects.

However, one of the most important factors that independently adds to all these predisposing conditions is chronic *S. aureus* nasal carriage (see sebsequent discussion). Whether they are in the hospital or in the community, patients mostly become infected with their own carriage strain). Thus, it has been proposed to screen patients at high risk for *S. aureus* nasal or cutaneous carriage and decontaminate positive cases with mupirocin ointments or other means (Table 195-8).[225] Implementation of this policy for selected patients admitted to the hospital remains a matter of debate.

THE BURDEN OF ANTIBIOTIC RESISTANCE

Methicillin-resistant *S. aureus* is at present one of the most commonly identified antibiotic-resistant pathogens in many parts of the world, including Europe, the Americas, North Africa, the Middle East, and East Asia.[134,226] Recent studies in the United States show a continuing increase of MRSA infections in hospitals,[226,227] as high as 3.1% per year in ICUs.[228] During the period from 2006 to 2007, the proportion of hospital-onset *S. aureus* infections that were methicillin resistant reached 56.2% in U.S. hospitals,[217] a proportion that is even higher (64.4%) in U.S. ICUs.[228]

TABLE 195-7	Risk of Invasive *Staphylococcus aureus* Infection, Associated with Selected Underlying Conditions, in Adults 20 Years Old or Older			
Underlying Condition	*No. of Patients with ISA Infection (n = 226)*	*Annual Incidence, per 100,000*	*Relative Risk (95% Confidence Interval)*	*P Value*
Hemodialysis	24	7692	257.2 (161.0-393.6)	<.001
Peritoneal dialysis	3	4918	150.0 (30.5-44l.1)	<.001
HIV infection	4	778	23.7 (6.4-61.4)	<.001
Solid organ transplantation	3	683	20.7 (4.2-61.3)	<.001
Heart disease	114	362	20.6 (15.8-27.0)	<.001
Cancer	47	348	12.9 (9.1-17.8)	<.001
Illicit intravenous drug use	13	321	10.1 (5.3-17.7)	<.001
Alcohol abuse	31	241	8.2 (5.4-12.0)	<.001
Diabetes mellitus	48	192	7.0 (5.0-9.7)	<.001
Stroke	16	200	6.4 (3.6-10.6)	<.001
Chronic obstructive pulmonary disease	26	120	3.9 (2.5-5.9)	<.001
Systemic lupus erythematosus	2	80	2.4 (0.3-8.7)	.3
Rheumatoid arthritis	5	74	2.2 (0.7-5.3)	.1

HIV, human immunodeficiency virus; ISA, invasive *S. aureus*.

Adapted from Laupland KB, Church DL, Mucenski M, et al. Population-based study of the epidemiology of and the risk factors for invasive Staphylococcus aureus infections. *J Infect Dis.* 2003;187:1452-1459.

In the health care setting, HCA-MRSA infections are associated with greater lengths of stay, higher mortality, and increased costs.[216] Whether MRSA is more virulent than MSSA is still a matter of debate. The molecular typing of thousand strains of carriage and disease-associated *S. aureus* strains revealed that MRSA did not represent specific lineages and that all types of *S. aureus* can become invasive given the appropriate circumstances.[42] On the other hand, most MRSA infections are mainly of nosocomial origin and manifest themselves as complications of health care procedures or underlying disorders. In this specific context, patient differences could account for the variation in mortality because a greater number of older patients with severe underlying disease contract infections from MRSA.[220] In addition, ineffective or delay in effective antibiotic therapy could also play a large role in suboptimal response to therapy.[150,229]

CA-MRSA has now become the most frequent cause of skin and soft tissue infections acquired in the community.[230] Groups with high-intensity physical contact are particularly affected. This includes competitive athletes, children in daycare centers, military recruits, injections drug users, jailed inmates, and men who have sex with men.[231] CA-MRSA also can cause severe sometimes fatal invasive disease, such as necrotizing pneumoniae,[93] bacteremia,[232] or necrotizing fasciitis.[138] Moreover, CA-MRSA has started to spread from the community into hospitals, where outbreaks of health care–associated hospital-onset infections with typical CA-MRSA have occurred.[232,233] Even if compared with HCA-MRSA, CA-MRSA retained susceptibility to many non–β-lactam antibiotics; the rapid increase of such infections will rapidly become a serious public health challenge.

CARRIAGE OF *S. AUREUS*

Three patterns of carriage can be distinguished: 1, persistent carriers; 2, intermittent carriers; and 3, noncarriers. Approximately 20% (range, 12% to 30%) of healthy people are persistent *S. aureus* nasal carriers, 30% (range, 16% to 70%) are intermittent carriers, and 50% (range, 16% to 69%) are noncarriers.[234] Persistent carriers usually carry the same strain for extended periods of time, whereas intermittent carriers tend to host different strains over time.[18] Those distinctions are important because persistent carriers have higher *S. aureus* loads and are at higher risk of acquiring *S. aureus* infection.[235]

The primary reservoirs of *S. aureus* are the anterior nares, but the organism can be isolated from multiple sites. Some patient subgroups are at increased risk of carriage. Activities such as those that lead to skin lesions are often correlated with higher *S. aureus* nasal carriage rates. They include patients with insulin-dependent diabetes, patients undergoing hemodialysis or peritoneal dialysis, intravenous drug users, patients with recurrent *S. aureus* skin infections, patients with HIV, and healthy patients receiving repeated injections for allergies.[234]

Staphylococcal cell surface-associated molecules are important in colonization efficacy (see Surface Adhesins). ClfB specifically binds to human cytokeratin type 10,[236] and SasG to an unknown ligand[83] of desquamated nasal epithelial cells. Cell wall teichoic acid is also essential for *S. aureus* nasal carriage by mediating interactions with nasal epithelial cells.[237]

Most infants become colonized shortly after birth, usually with the same strain as their mother.[238] Carriage then decreases with age (40% to 60% at 2 months, and 21% to 28% at 6 months), reflecting both the development of an immune response to *S. aureus*[238,239] and the consequence of bacterial competition and interference between microorganisms in the nasopharynx. This is particularly true for *S. aureus* and *S. pneumoniae* because being a *S. pneumoniae* carrier is inversely associated with *S. aureus* carriage and vice versa.[240]

TABLE 195-8	Example of Decontaminating Scheme for Patients Colonized or Infected with Methicillin-Resistant *Staphylococcus aureus* (MRSA)

Protective Measures

Put patient in contact isolation (one or several contaminated patients in single room with restricted access).
Use protective gown and gloves.
Use protective mask and glasses if risk of projection of contaminated liquids.
Clean hands with alcoholic solution at glove removal and between cares.
Leave any disposable in room and discard for sterilization in special containers.

Decontamination Measures

Apply nasal mupirocin (2%) every 8 h for 5 to 7 days.
Apply chlorhexidine-based oral spray 3 to 4 times a day for 5 to 7 days.
Take daily shower or clean body thoroughly with chlorhexidine-based soap for 5 to 7 days.
In the case of dental prostheses, clean and soak daily chlorhexidine-based solution for 5 to 7 days.

Control Cultures and Decision

Take control swabs of any contaminated sites 48 h and 96 h after the end of treatment.
Keep isolation measures until laboratory results.
If no MRSA is present in control cultures, consider decontaminated. Relief isolation and swab weekly for follow-up cultures.
If MRSA is present in control cultures, pursue isolation measures and repeat whole decontamination scheme.

Adapted from Current Recommendations at the University Hospital of Lausanne (CHUV), Switzerland.

Many people change their pattern of carriage between the age of 10 and 20 years. Children and adolescent under 20 years of age seem to have higher persistent carriage rates than adults. Ten percent of children from 0 to 9 years and 24% of children from 10 to 19 years were found to be persistent carriers. Cross-sectional surveys of healthy adult populations used to report carriage rates up to 35% to 50%.[17] Since 2000, the reported prevalence rate of *S. aureus* nasal colonization has decreased to 25% to 35%.[241,242] Explanations for this decline might include improved personal hygiene, changes in socioeconomic class, and smaller families.[18]

Traditionally, control of *S. aureus* has been focused on preventing cross infection between patients.[243] However, at least three sets of observations indicate that nasal carriage of *S. aureus* is an important risk factor for sepsis: 1, carriers have higher rates of infections than noncarriers[235]; 2, a large proportion of nosocomial *S. aureus* infections originate from patients' own flora[19,235]; and 3, eradication of carriage reduces nosocomial infections.[225,234]

Carriage of Methicillin-Resistant S. aureus

Methicillin-resistant *S. aureus* colonization overall has increased from 0.8% in 2001 to 2002 to 1% in 2003 to 2004.[242] MRSA colonization is particularly important in the hospital environment because colonized and infected patients represent the most important reservoir of MRSA in health care facilities.[137] Factors associated with MRSA carriage include prior antibiotic exposure, prolonged hospitalization, surgery, admission to an intensive care unit (ICU), living a nursing home, and close proximity to a patient colonized or infected with MRSA.[244,245]

Despite the increasing CA-MRSA infections, the prevalence rate of MRSA among persons without typical risk factors remains relatively low (≤0.24%), and most MRSA colonization and infection still develops among those who have health care–associated risk factors or contact with other persons who have such risks.[137] When patients known to be colonized with nosocomial MRSA are discharged from the hospital or nursing home into the community, spread to family members or close contacts can occur.[244]

No single measure to control the spread of MRSA within the hospital has proven effective on its own. In contrast, guidelines recommend a combination of effective measures to disrupt the cycle of transmission.[246] An MRSA-control program must thus include a comprehensive set of interventions that include administrative support, such as avoiding overcrowding and understaffing of health care facilities[247]; judicious use of antimicrobials; routine and enhanced surveillance to quickly identify carriers[248]; standard and contact precautions to stop transmission; environmental measures; education (e.g., hand hygiene[243]); and decolonization to eliminate reservoirs.[249,250] Such programs have reported success in controlling or reducing transmission of MRSA nationally, regionally, and institutionally.[251] In this context, infection control measures should always involve the laboratory. Determining the clonality of MRSA recovered from several patients is important to differentiate sporadic cases of MRSA from more problematic epidemic situations. Common typing techniques are described in Molecular Typing.

Decolonization of Individual Carriers

Eradication of MRSA carriage is one important part of the control of MRSA dissemination. Most decontamination regimens recommend a 1-week daily total body washing with a chlorhexidine-based soap, plus nasal mupirocin application (see Table 195-8). Use of systemic antibiotic (e.g., trimethoprim-sulfamethoxazole + rifampin) must be restrained to particular situations. Control cultures should be made thereafter. Routine antibiotic testing must be performed to detect emergence of resistance to the decolonizing agent.

About 5% of health care workers become colonized with MRSA; clinical disease develops in approximately 5% of these workers. Eradicating MRSA carriage from health care workers might thus be performed as well.[252] However, health care workers most frequently act as vectors of transmission, not as main source of MRSA.

Regarding nasal carriers, three regimens have been envisioned: 1, systemic antibiotics; 2, local antibiotics or disinfectants; and 3, bacterial interference. Results with systemic antibiotics, such as rifampin or trimethoprim-sulfamethoxazole, were disappointing because of the emergence of resistance and significant failure rates.

Local disinfection appears more successful. Application of a mupirocin (2%) into the anterior nares is highly efficacious in eliminating *S. aureus* in both healthy carriers and carriers in at-risk groups.[253,254] *Mupirocin* is a topical antibiotic with broad-spectrum activity against gram-positive bacteria, including *S. aureus* and MRSA. It is well tolerated when applied twice daily for up to 5 days. Low-level resistance (MIC, 8 to 256 mg/L) and high-level resistance (MIC, >512 mg/L) exist but are uncommon and usually follow prolonged administration.[255] Currently, intranasal application of mupirocin is the standard for *S. aureus* decolonization of carrier patients (see Table 195-8). Insufficient evidence exists to support the use of topical or systemic antimicrobial therapy for eradicating extranasal MRSA carriage, except in well-defined outbreak settings.[256] Monitoring susceptibility is essential to detect appearance of resistance to the decolonizing agent.

Bacterial interference is an old concept in which a nonpathogenic staphylococcus is used to outcompete a pathogenic species on the patient. However, several complications occurred and the project was abandoned. The concept may become resurgent in the light of recent research on the global regulator *agr* (see Pathogenesis I: Regulation and Virulence Determinants section). No applicable strategy has emerged from this research yet. Possible alternatives include the cell wall lytic enzyme lysostaphin,[257] bacteriophage-derived cell wall autolysins, and an extract from the Australian native plant *Melaleuca alternifolia*.[258]

Clinical Syndromes

Infection begins with the colonization of target tissues by the microbes. Further spread results from more specific invasion processes, during which bacteria interact directly or indirectly (e.g., via toxins) with the host. Once they have broken through the natural skin barrier, bacteria can disseminate to more profound normally sterile sites. Thus, any localized infection has the potential to become the seeding site of a more severe infection, either by contiguous extension or by distant spread via the blood circulation. Toxin-mediated diseases, including TSST-1 and PVL, are addressed in the previous Pathogenesis I: Regulation and Virulence Determinants and Antibiotic Resistance sections. Pyogenic infections are described subsequently.

SKIN AND SOFT TISSUES INFECTIONS

Classification

S. aureus skin and soft tissue infections include primary pyoderma (such as folliculitis, furuncles, carbuncles, and impetigo) and soft tissue infections (i.e., cellulitis, erysipelas, and pyomyositis). They are commonly classified according to the anatomic structure involved (Fig 195-12): (1) infection of the epidermis: impetigo; (2) infection of the superficial dermis: folliculitis; (3) infection of deep dermis: furuncles, carbuncles, and hydradenitis suppurative; and (4) infection of subcutaneous cellular tissues: erysipelas, cellulitis, fasciitis, and pyomyositis.

The diagnosis of an SSTI is most frequently made clinically. The basic anatomic lesion induced by *S. aureus* is a pyogenic exudate or an abscess. The more severe infections tend to be associated with deeper tissue invasion. Superficial infections can often be treated with local care, surgical drainage, and rarely, systemic antibiotics. On the other hand, deeper infections such as erysipelas, lymphangitis, lymphadenitis, cellulitis, and necrotizing fasciitis are severe diseases that may be life threatening. They require hospitalization, systemic antibiotic therapy, and prompt surgical drainage and débridement.

Impetigo. *Impetigo* is a superficial infection of the skin that involves only the epidermis. It affects mostly children, usually on exposed areas

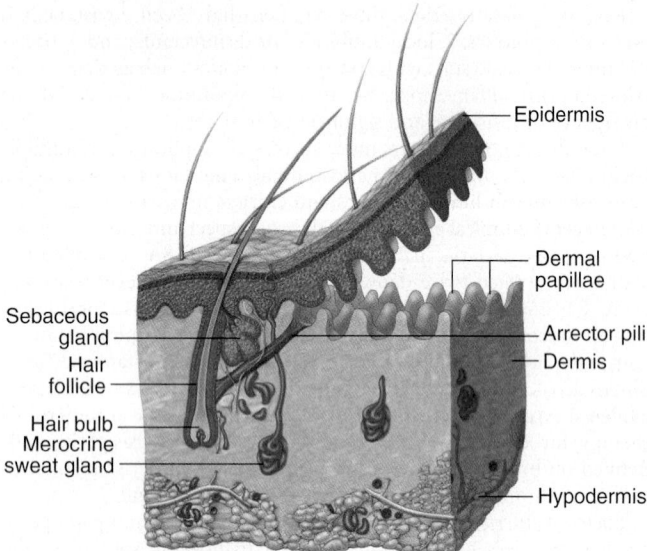

Figure 195-12 **Skin anatomy delineating various levels at which** *Staphylococcus aureus* **infection can occur (see text for details).**

of the body (e.g., the face and the legs). Although *S. pyogenes* was usually considered as the causative agent, most cases of impetigo are now caused by *S. aureus*. *S. pyogenes* is found in only 20% of cases, often in association with *S. aureus*.

The disease usually starts as a red macula that evolves into vesicles that contain cloudy fluid based on the area of erythema (Fig. 195-13). The bullae are the result of epidermolytic toxins of the serine protease family. The vesicles rapidly rupture and leave a yellowish, thick, wet crust with a diameter exceeding 1 cm that is surrounded by erythema. Most affected children present with multiple lesions of various age. General symptoms are absent, but a local inflammatory lymph node reaction is a rule. At the beginning, the differential diagnosis includes other vesicular eruptions, such as herpes simplex and varicella. However, the evolution is typical and rapidly differentiates the diseases. Although of mild severity, the disease is extremely contagious and the affected child should be kept apart from other children until an effective treatment has been applied. A basic treatment that combines disinfection with a chlorhexidine-based or povidone-iodine–based soap and additional bacitracin zinc ointment in patients with limited lesions, or fusidic acid cream (not available in the United States) in cases of more extensive lesions, is generally sufficient. Oral antibiotic are rarely needed. Mupirocin should be reserved for the treatment of *S. aureus* nasal carriage.

Folliculitis. *Folliculitis* is defined as a pyoderma that involves the hair follicle and its immediate surroundings (see Fig. 195-12). It manifests

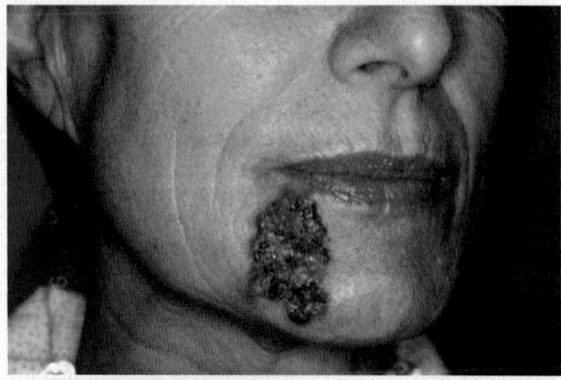

Figure 195-13 **Infective skin lesions in staphylococcal impetigo.**

as a series of raised painful reddish lesions with indurated bases, each of them centered on a hair follicle. Extensive folliculitis of the bearded area of the face is called *sycosis barbae*. General symptoms are usually absent, and local antiseptic measures are the treatment of choice.

Furuncles and Carbuncles. *Furuncles* (boils) represent extension of the infectious process involving the hair follicle and are located, by definition, on the hairy areas of the body, with a predilection for the face, neck, axilla, and buttocks. The disease starts as a painful red nodule and rapidly evolves into a hot, painful, raised, and indurated lesion with a diameter of 1 to 2 cm. Its evolution is characterized by the appearance of a yellowish area in its center. On rupture (either spontaneous or surgical), it liberates a small amount of yellowish creamy discharge of purulent and necrotic material. Secondary foci from autoinoculation are frequent. General symptoms are normally absent. Local treatment is usually sufficient. In case of recurrent episodes, testing for nasal carriage and appropriate eradication may be necessary, although its effectiveness in reducing the risk of recurrence is not clearly shown.

Community-acquired MRSA is a particular issue in furuncles.[259] They are often centered by a necrotic spot, are multiple, and occur in outbreaks. Lesion can progress to abscesses and cellulitis.[260] In young patients with boils and systemic signs of infection, one must remember the risk of severe hemorrhagic pneumonia (see Fig. 195-9)[93] or necrotizing fasciitis[138] (see previous section Pathogenesis I: Regulation and Virulence Determinants for more details).

Another remarkable situation is when furuncles are located around the nares or upper lip. Such lesions may lead to life-threatening septic thrombophlebitis of the intracerebral veins. Therefore, furuncles in this location should be treated with high-dose parenteral antibiotics.

Carbuncles are deep-seated infections that involve several hair follicles and result from the coalescence and spreading of the infectious process into the depths of subcutaneous tissue. They are usually localized at the base of the neck. The disease leads to the development of a central necrotic crater, which heals with the development of a hard hypertrophic violaceous scar. Fever and malaise are generally present. Carbuncles may be the source of bacteremia and require parenteral antibiotic therapy.

Hydradenitis Suppurativa. *Hydradenitis suppurativa* is a pyogenic infection of the apocrine sweat glands that manifests as crops of furuncles that develop in the axillary, perineal, and genital areas. After spontaneous drainage, hypertrophic scarring may occur. As in furunculosis, treatment is primarily limited to local care and topical disinfectants. Administration of oral antimicrobial is only indicated in the case of systemic symptoms.

Mastitis. *Mastitis* occurs in approximately 10% of mothers in the United States who are breastfeeding. The infection develops most commonly during the second or the third week of the puerperium. The diagnosis of mastitis is usually clinical, with patients presenting with focal tenderness in one breast accompanied by fever and malaise. Treatment includes analgesics, changing breast-feeding technique, and reversing milk stasis, often with the assistance of a lactation consultant. Continued breast feeding should be encouraged in the presence of mastitis and generally does not pose a risk to the infant. When antibiotics are needed (i.e., in the presence of acute pain, systemic symptoms, or fever), those effective against *S. aureus* are preferred. Breast abscess is the most common complication of mastitis. It can be prevented with early treatment of mastitis and continued breast feeding. Once an abscess occurs, surgical drainage or needle aspiration is needed.

Surgical Site Infection. Recent Centers for Disease Control (CDC) data indicate that 2.6% of patient operations were associated with *surgical site infection* (SSI), an incidence rate that might be underestimated because of inadequate postdischarge surveillance.[261] *S. aureus* and coagulase-negative staphylococci are the most prevalent pathogens that cause SSI for most types of surgery (in 30% and 14% of the cases, respectively). Gram-negative rods and enterococci are, however, the most prevalent pathogens that cause SSI after abdominal surgery.[217] Most infections are caused by *S. aureus* strains that are carried by the patient on admission to the hospital.[19,235] Hence, nasal carriage of *S. aureus* is a risk factor for subsequent infection in patients undergoing surgery.[18] Although not shown, decontamination of nasal carriers might decrease the risk of SSI.[262]

Surgical site infections are characterized by progressive edema, erythema, and pain around the surgical incision 2 or more days after surgery. General symptoms are frequently associated. Careful inspection of the wound, ulcer, or lesion is essential. If deeper structures are not involved, release of the stitches, repeated cleansing, and antibiotic coverage for 7 to 10 days is usually curative. If the infection involves deeper structures (e.g., bone) or foreign material (e.g., prosthetic devices), prolonged parenteral antibiotic therapy (4 to 6 weeks) may be necessary, and removal of the foreign material is warranted. The evolution of wound infection is highly dependent on the patient's comorbidities. Healing may be delayed particularly in vascular insufficiency and diabetes.

Erysipelas, Cellulitis, and Fasciitis. Superficial or deep extension of infection may result in erysipelas, cellulitis, and fasciitis. Erysipelas and fasciitis are commonly the result of *S. pyogenes*, but this etiology is not exclusive. Fasciitis can arise from hematogenous seeding. An important common feature of all three entities is severe pain. In the case of erysipelas, soreness is associated with typical skin lesions. In the case of cellulitis or fasciitis, on the other hand, severe pain symptoms are disproportional with regard to the visible anatomic lesions (Fig. 195-14). Hence, high fever, severe local pain, and relatively meager clinical findings at visible examination are highly suggestive of one of these entities. The consideration is important because emergency surgical drainage is indicated in the case of fasciitis, and prompt intervention may be delayed because of the confounding picture.

Erysipelas is a superficial cellulitis with prominent lymphatic involvement, with an indurate, "peau d'orange" appearance with a raised border that is demarcated from normal skin. It often complicates edematous extremities and skin ulcers such as in varicose limbs. As in impetigo, it may be the result of mixed *S. pyogenes* and *S. aureus* infection. Clinical signs of sepsis with high fever are present. In most cases, an etiologic diagnosis is not established. Local sampling with puncture may be attempted, and blood cultures must be drawn. Prompt empiric treatment should be started with parenteral antibiotics covering at least both staphylococci and streptococci.

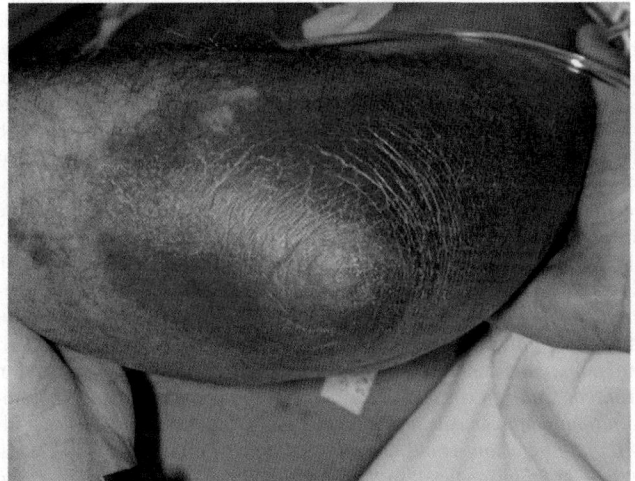

Figure 195-14 *S. aureus* **cellulitis of the elbow in cancer patient with low neutrophil counts.** Pain was disproportional to visual appearance of the lesion. Patient was bacteremic.

In patients with underlying conditions, such as diabetic foot, mixed pictures of erysipelas and cellulitis may occur and may be the result of gram-negative bacteria as well, including *P. aeruginosa*. Therefore, the spectrum of empiric treatment should be broadened to cover these agents until the microbiologic results are available. If gram-negative bacteria or MRSA are suspected, the addition of aminoglycoside or vancomycin to a broad spectrum β-lactam may be warranted.

Cellulitis involves deeper anatomic structures and does not produce the typical geographic skin lesion of erysipelas (see Fig. 195-14). Therefore, it is more confusing and may be mistaken with nonspecific lesions such as trauma. The association of pain and fever are important signs. Cellulitis may be from multiple other organisms, including gram-negative bacteria, especially in patients with immunocompromise. Therefore, microbiologic sampling (including blood cultures) should be promptly followed by broad-spectrum antibiotic therapy with both anti–gram-positive and anti–gram-negative coverage. Radiologic examination is unnecessary in most cases of cellulitis. Computed tomographic (CT) scan is useful when subjacent osteomyelitis is suspected, whereas magnetic resonance imaging (MRI) helps to differentiate cellulitis from necrotizing fasciitis.

Necrotizing fasciitis is the most severe condition that paradoxically presents the least superficial signs at visual observation of the skin and soft tissues. The pain may be so intense that it requires opiate administration for relief. The condition is often the result of *S. pyogenes*, but *S. aureus* may be involved, especially in the presence of CA-MRSA.[138] Gram-negative bacteria, including *P. aeruginosa*, may be responsible, especially in patients with immunocompromise, and must be considered in the choice of initial empiric treatment.

Whatever its cause, fasciitis is an absolute emergency that necessitates immediate and generous surgical débridement and drainage. The evolution is a matter of minutes rather than hours and may rapidly result in amputation or death. Prompt clinical diagnosis and multidisciplinary evaluation is warranted. Imaging may help delineate the lesions, but urgent surgical exploration and fasciotomy should not be delayed. High-dose and broad-spectrum antibiotic therapy is necessary and can be readjusted after isolating the bacterial pathogen. In the case of *S. pyogenes* and severe refractory shock, intravenous immunoglobulins have been proposed[106] (see also Pathogenesis I: Regulation and Virulence Determinants section).

Management of Skin and Soft Tissue Infection

Localized lesions can be handled with disinfectant or topical antibiotics such as fusidic acid. However, increasing rates of resistance to topical agents have been reported. Mupirocin should be reserved for the treatment of *S. aureus* nasal carriage. Extensive lesions should be treated with systemic antibiotic. A decision to hospitalize a patient is made on clinical judgment (large abscesses, signs of systemic infection) and the at-risk characteristics of the patients (age < 6 months, diabetes, or immunodeficiency). Surgical drainage is a major part of treatment, and most benign SSTIs are cured with drainage alone.

Empiric therapy of health care–associated SSTI should cover multiresistant HCA-MRSA and thus include vancomycin or maybe linezolid. Empiric therapy of community-acquired SSTI is complicated by the occurrence of CA-MRSA. β-Lactams should be used with caution and according to the local epidemiology. Unlike HCA-MRSA, CA-MRSA is often susceptible to clindamycin and trimethoprim-sulfamethoxazole, sometimes to tetracyclines, and mostly to linezolid. However, if coinfection with *S. pyogenes* is found and antibiotics are required, first-line treatment should consider linezolid, vancomycin, or maybe tigecycline. If toxin secretion is an issue, linezolid might be preferred.[183]

BLOODSTREAM INFECTION

Bloodstream infection (BSI) is defined as one or several positive blood cultures associated with general symptoms such as fever or hypotension.[263] Its incidence rate has increased from 7.4 episodes per 1000 admissions in the 1950s[264] to 31.2 episodes per 1000 admissions (or

270 episodes per 100,000 inhabitants per year) in 2006.[265] Gram-positive pathogens have overcome the prominent cause of BSI, representing 54.8% of all episodes in one study.[265] This is particularly true for *S. aureus*, with a rate between 20 and 30 episodes per 100,000 inhabitants per year in various parts of the world.[265-268] The increase is especially important in male patients. Mortality related to *S. aureus* BSI is high, ranging from 20% to 30% of the cases,[267,268] and varied as a function of underlying conditions.[214] Despite the increased prevalence of SSTI from CA-MRSA in outpatients in the United States, a paralleled increase of CA-MRSA bacteremia or endocarditis has not yet been reported.[269,270] Recent studies suggest that PVL-positive strains rather infect skin and soft tissues (see previous section).

Bloodstream infection is usually divided in two categories: nosocomial BSI, where positive blood cultures occur 2 days or more after hospital entry; and community-acquired BSI, which occurs in the community or before 2 days of hospitalization. However, the increasing number of individuals treated in outpatient programs makes these two categories progressively overlapping. Hence, community-acquired BSI may be more appropriately referred to as *community-onset BSI*, which is further subdivided in *health care–associated BSI* (HCA-BSI) and *community-associated BSI* (CA-BSI). The subdivision is similar to that made between HCA-MRSA and CA-MRSA.

Community-Onset Bacteremia

Community-onset HCA-BSI is comparable with nosocomial BSI in terms of risk factors of multiresistant organisms. These include intravenous devices, a history of surgical treatment, and dialysis. In contrast, community-onset CA-BSI, which occurs in patients without underlying conditions, is mostly from antibiotic-susceptible organisms and always associated with a detectable infected focus, including SSTI, deep-seated abscesses, or osteoarticular infections, or with infective endocarditis.[268] Of note, patients of dialysis are at a particularly high risk of staphylococcal endocarditis and represent a quasi-new at-risk group for this disease.[221]

Nosocomial and Health Care–Associated Bloodstream Infection

S. aureus is the leading cause of nosocomial and HCA-BSI, together with CoNS.[215,217] These are mostly associated with the presence of intravascular catheters or devices, procedures in contaminated sites, SSI, and sometimes *S. aureus* pneumoniae. Complications involve peripheral metastatic foci, which can reveal themselves later in time. Nosocomial *S. aureus* bacteremia enters in the differential diagnosis of any hospital-related febrile or septic episodes. The risk for patients with catheter-induced *S. aureus* bacteremia to develop infective endocarditis is about 10%.[271,272] Thus, catheter-related *S. aureus* bacteremia must be taken very seriously and consideration given to excluding infective endocarditis with transesophageal echocardiography.[273]

Management of S. aureus Bloodstream Infection

With *S. aureus*, even a single positive blood culture should prompt initiation of antibiotic therapy, sampling of blood for follow-up cultures, and determination of the source and extent of infection.[274] Approximately one third of patients with *S. aureus* BSI have metastatic complications develop, especially in case of prosthetic material. The strongest indicator of clinical complication is a positive result of follow-up blood culture after 48 to 96 hours of treatment.[275]

Removal of the original focus is a golden rule, especially in the case of infected intravascular material or prosthetic devices. Failure to do so is strongly associated with recurrence. In the case of nonremovable implanted catheter, the use of antibiotic locks between infusions may be attempted, but success is variable.[276] In case of removable infection source (e.g., a catheter), a 10-day to 14-day postcatheter removal antibiotic treatment may be appropriate: 1, after the removal of all prosthetic material and endovascular catheter; 2, after the exclusion of endocarditis; 3, as long as the follow-up blood cultures drawn 2 to 4 days after initial positive cultures are negative for *S. aureus*; 4, if the fever has vanished within 72 hours after the initiation of antistaphylo-

coccal therapy; and 5, when the absence of metastatic foci has been confirmed.[274]

Bloodstream infection associated with skin and soft tissue infection usually responds to a 14-day course of antibiotic treatment. Deeper infections, such as arthritis and osteomyelitis and endocarditis, must be treated with antibiotics for 4 to 6 weeks, with or without surgery depending on individual circumstances (see Chapters 77, 78, 102, and 103 for more detailed recommendations). Empiric antibiotic treatment must take into account the probability of methicillin resistance; this prevalence rate can be more than 50%, especially among ICU patients.

INFECTIVE ENDOCARDITIS

Infective endocarditis is one the most severe complications of *S. aureus* bacteremia. The disease is uniformly lethal if not treated with antibiotics with or without surgery. *S. aureus* endocarditis typically follows an acute course with multiple peripheral septic emboli, valve destruction, myocarditis, and mixed cardiogenic and septic shock. Appropriate care involves a multidisciplinary evaluation, including infectious disease and microbiology experts, cardiologists, intensive care specialists, cardiac surgeons, and sometimes neurologists.

Epidemiology

In spite of improved health care, the overall incidence rate of IE remained between 2 and 6 per 100,000 populations per year over the last 30 years.[221] However, risk factors are changing. Chronic rheumatic heart disea34se, which was a prime risk factor in the preantibiotic era, is being replaced by new at-risk groups, including intravenous drug users (IVDUs), elderly people with valve sclerosis, patients with intravascular prostheses,[277] patients with nosocomial-acquired IE, and patients for hemodialysis.[278] As a result, the mean age of patients with IE has increased from 30 years in the 1950s to older than 60 years since the 1990s, and oral streptococci, which are still a leading cause in developing countries, have been supplanted by *S. aureus* and CoNS, especially in industrialized countries.[279] This finding also correlates with the fact that the portal of entry has become more often cutaneous than dental.

Pathogenesis

The Role of Bacterial Adhesins. The pathogenesis of *S. aureus* endocarditis implicates a close relation between certain *S. aureus* surface adhesins (MSCRAMMs) and host proteins present on the surface of damaged or inflamed valves. Physically damaged endothelia are covered by a meshwork of fibrin, platelets, and numerous host matrix proteins.[280]

S. aureus is extremely well equipped with both surface-bound and secreted factors that mediate tissue colonization and invasion. With a system developed in *Lactococcus lactis*,[281] Que and colleagues[61,282] showed that *S. aureus* ClfA was necessary and sufficient for early valve colonization and infection in rats with experimental IE but not sufficient for invasive and persistent disease. The same authors showed that fibronectin-binding protein A (FnBPA) promoted both early valve colonization and persistent infection. FnBPA is a peculiar MSCRAMM that carries at least three binding specificities, to fibronectin, to fibrinogen, and to elastin.[283,284] Constructing truncated and chimera proteins indicated that although fibrinogen binding was necessary and sufficient for early valve colonization, as observed with ClfA, fibronectin binding was necessary for further invasion and persistence. This invasive phenotype was associated with the capacity of fibronectin binding to trigger active internalization of staphylococci into eukaryotic cells, both in vitro and in vivo.[285] Thus, valve infection proceeds through consecutive binding to fibrinogen, for early colonization, and fibronectin, for invasion and persistence.[61] Such interadhesin cooperation could also occur between other MSCRAMMs, adding even more flexibility to the already wealthy set of *S. aureus* surface determinants.[61,62]

In the case of physically intact but inflamed endothelia, *S. aureus* fibronectin-binding proteins might be of primary importance. During inflammation, endothelial cells express integrins of the β₁ family, which can bind plasma fibronectin at the luminal pole of the cell. The resulting fibronectin coat functions as a ligand surface for circulating *S. aureus* that expresses fibronectin-binding proteins. The contact between the adhesin and its ligand triggers the active internalization of *S. aureus* by endothelial cells and by other cells.[286] Once internalized, *S. aureus* may either persist locally, protected from host defenses and antimicrobial therapy, or multiply and secrete hemolysins (see Table 195-1), which lyse the host cell and allow bacteria to spread both locally and to distant organs. This second scenario probably explains many cases of infective endocarditis on anatomically normal valves.

The Role of Platelets. Bacterial-induced platelet aggregation is commonly considered as a pathogenic factor. However, bacteria-induced platelet activation is a double-edged sword. On the one hand, platelets contribute to the formation of the vegetation. On the other hand, platelets also contribute to antiinfective host defenses by releasing antimicrobial peptides and inflammatory mediators.[287] These cationic peptides (CAPs) are contained in the α-granules of thrombocytes and are released in the surrounding on platelet activation. They kill numerous gram-positive organisms by perturbing their membrane potential.

Experimental evidence indicates that platelet-resistant mutants of staphylococci or streptococci have an increased ability to produce endocarditis in animals. In addition, clinical studies indicate that isolates of *S. aureus* recovered from patients with endocarditis are more often resistant to platelet-induced killing than *S. aureus* isolated from other infected sites.[288] Resistance to CAPs in *S. aureus* is caused by a combination of several factors, including enhanced membrane fluidity,[289] reduced membrane potential,[290] a plasmid-encoded efflux pump (*qacA*)[291] via a mode of action independent of efflux,[292] and a high proportion of positively charged groups in the membrane-attached LTA and phosphatidyl-glycerol.[87]

S. aureus bind to and activates platelets via several surface proteins, including fibrinogen-binding clumping factors (ClfA and ClfB), fibronectin-binding proteins (FnBPA), serine aspartate repeat protein SdrE,[293] and a newly described serine-rich protein called SraP (an homologue of the *S. gordonii* Has protein).[294] Adhesion of *S. aureus* to activated platelets may also involve protein A and von Willebrand's factor, or SdrE and complement activation.[295]

Rapid platelet activation mediated by ClfA and FnBPAs requires two mechanisms of bacterial binding to resting platelets: a fibrinogen or fibronectin bridge to the low-activity platelet integrin GPIIb/IIIa, and a concomitant immunoglobulin bridge to the platelet FcγRIIa receptor. *S. aureus* can also activate platelet with a slower mechanism that is independent of fibrinogen and GPIIb/IIIa. This was shown in a non–fibrinogen-binding ClfA mutant of *S. aureus* and with *L. lactis* that expressed staphylococcal SdrE. In both cases, immunoglobulin G (IgG) specific for the surface protein was required to engage FcγRIIa and also to activate complement by the classical pathway.[296]

This raises the question as to whether antiaggregant therapy might be useful as adjuvant therapy in the treatment of IE. Antiaggregant therapy with acetosalicylic acid decreases the severity of experimental endocarditis from *S. aureus*.[297] Although platelet antiaggregants have a potential efficacy, extrapolating these experimental results to the human situation must be tempered by the risk of hemorrhage. This was clearly shown in a randomized, double-blind, placebo-controlled trial in which a daily dose of aspirin (325 mg/d) in addition to the conventional antibiotic therapy did not reduce the risk of embolic events in patients with IE and was even associated with an increased risk of bleeding.[298] Similarly, anticoagulants increase the risk of secondary bleeding at the site of septic emboli, including hemorrhagic stroke, and are not recommended.[299]

Host Defenses and Prevention

The role of host defenses is marginal in infective endocarditis. Once staphylococci have colonized the valves, their intrinsic procoagulant activities (e.g., fibrinogen polymerization by coagulase and platelet activation by fibrinogen-binding protein) trigger further deposition of platelets and fibrin on top of the microorganisms, thus providing a protective niche inside the vegetation. Moreover, *S. aureus* can be internalized into endothelial cells via bridging with fibronectin (see previous discussion). Both cases result in a failure of professional phagocyte to eradicate the organisms.

Killing by T-cell-mediated effectors is not operative in endocarditis. Therefore, the only alternative is antibody-mediated protection, which could act before colonization by blocking *S. aureus* surface adhesins or by increasing the speed of blood clearance via opsonization. Active research is dedicated to such an approach, but little promising results are available yet. The limitation of preventive vaccines in endocarditis might be the short (1-minute to 2-minute) delay between blood invasion and valve colonization, which leaves a small window for antibodies to be active.

Other preventive measures are scarce. Because *S. aureus* is a ubiquitous skin colonizer, prevention starts with hygiene and disinfection. Decontamination of carriers and proper antisepsis at the site of injection and catheter placement is mandatory. Antibiotic prophylaxis may be useful but is limited to the cases of medicosurgical procedures in the area of well-defined infective foci (see Chapters 77, 78, and 80 for details). Thus, detection of patients with risk factors and respect for proper hygiene and antisepsis measures remain the cornerstones of *S. aureus* endocarditis prevention.

Clinical Features

S. aureus IE often presents as an acute septic syndrome with fever, tachycardia, and often hypotension. Dyspnea may be present from congestive heart and from septic pulmonary emboli in the case of right-sided endocarditis (Fig. 195-15). General signs such as arthralgia/myalgia, back pain, and pleuritic pain are present in 10% to 50% of cases. Specific signs include a new cardiac murmur, usually of valve regurgitation, in about 90% of cases; septic emboli in the form of petechiae and Janeway lesions; and central nervous manifestations in up to one third of the patients (Fig. 195-16).

Cardiac failure is a major indication for emergency valve replacement. A defect in atrioventricular conduction may represent a mycotic aneurysm of the sinus of Valsalva, usually the noncoronary cusp. Transoesophageal echocardiography is useful in detecting this complication. Large vegetations (≥1 cm) are relatively frequent in *S. aureus* endocarditis and have been associated with an increased risk of embolization. However, the risk of embolization rapidly decreases within the first days of efficacious therapy.

Vascular Complications. Septic emboli from broken off vegetations can occlude the coronary or peripheral arteries (Fig. 195-17). Small skin lesions from immune-related vasculitis are a delayed sign of relatively chronic infection and are not a usual feature of acute *S. aureus* endocarditis. Mycotic aneurysms are found in up to 15% of patients with bacterial endocarditis, and probably more frequently in *S. aureus* endocarditis. They may arise either from direct invasion of the arterial wall by the infecting organisms, from septic embolization of the vasa vasorum, or from the deposition of immune complexes that trigger local inflammation and weakening of the arterial wall.

Neurologic Complications. Neurologic manifestations, mainly septic emboli and mycotic aneurysms, may occur in up to 40% of cases. However, because patients who have no neurologic symptoms do not undergo specific investigations, the true incidence of neurologic events during endocarditis may be underestimated. Lesions include cerebral infractions, arteritis, abscesses, mycotic aneurysms, intracerebral or subarachnoid hemorrhage, encephalomalacia, cerebritis, and meningitis. Control of the infection is essential because embolization sharply decreases thereafter. Recurrent embolization after the onset of efficacious therapy may be an indication for urgent valve replacement. This decision is difficult because anticoagulation therapy during extracorporeal circulation and after valve replacement puts the patients at

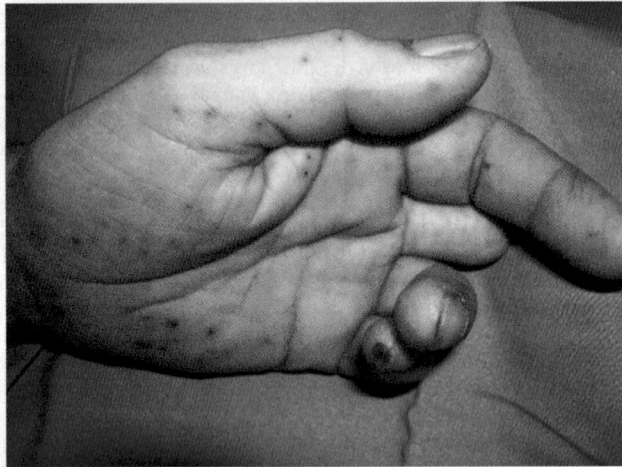

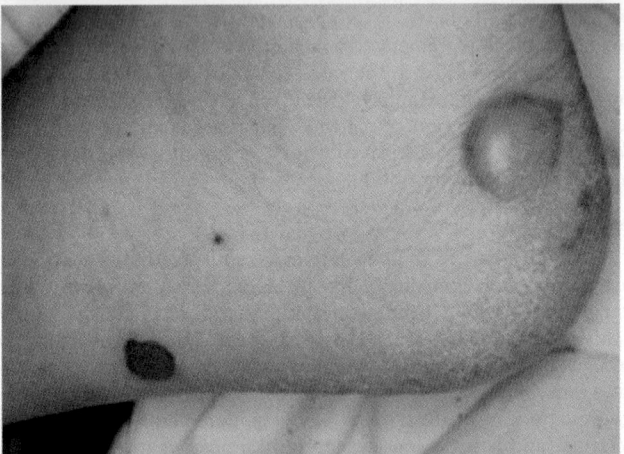

Figure 195-15 Embolic skin lesions (Janeway spots) in framework of acute mitral valve endocarditis caused by *Staphylococcus aureus.*

increased risk of secondary intracerebral hemorrhage. Therefore, the tendency is often to postpone emergency surgery and wait for the patient's condition to stabilize. On the other hand, ongoing studies suggest that earlier intervention, within the first 72 hours of stroke, may be beneficial in selected patients.

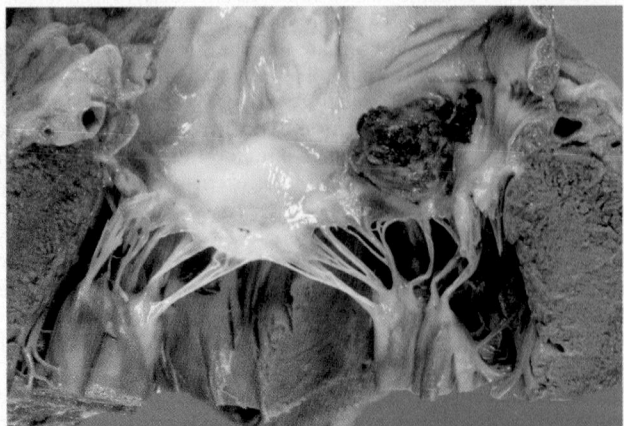

Figure 195-16 *Staphyococcus aureus* **endocarditis of the mitral valve.** Picture shows large ulcerovegetative lesion on anterior leaflet. *(Courtesy of Drs. A. Lobrinus and I. Letovanec, Pathology Institute, Lausanne University.)*

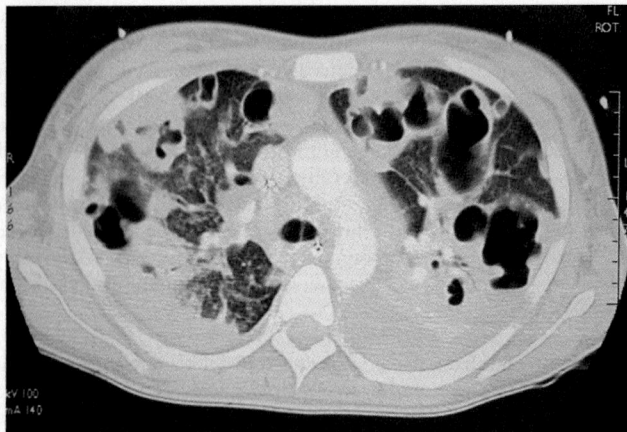

Figure 195-17 Chest computed tomographic scan of 30-year-old intravenous drug addict with tricuspid valve *S. aureus* endocarditis and bilateral lung abscesses and empyema.

Diagnosis

Criteria for the diagnosis of infective endocarditis changed with the use of echocardiography and are discussed in detail in Chapter 77. In *S. aureus* endocarditis, the first two blood cultures are positive in more than 90% of cases. The volume of blood cultures is critical because persistent bacteremia in infective endocarditis is often of low level, representing 1 to 100 bacteria/mL of blood. For each culture, 8 to 12 mL of blood should be drawn with careful antiseptic precaution.

Management of S. aureus Endocarditis

Treatment options are listed in Table 195-9.[273]

Management of Right-Sided Endocarditis in Injection Drug Users. While standard treatment of left-sided *S. aureus* endocarditis requires 4 to 6 weeks of antibiotic therapy (see Table 195-9), the duration of treatment for right-sided endocarditis can be considerably shortened in injection drug users[300] because right-sided endocarditis has a somewhat different physiopathology and is easier to cure or can heal spontaneously in experimental models. Moreover, the prognosis is less severe than left-sided valve infection. Regimens proven appropriate for 2-week treatment of right-sided endocarditis were nafcillin or cloxacillin combined with an effective aminoglycoside to which the organism is susceptible (gentamicin, tobramycin, or amikacin given every 8 hours).[300] If an aminoglycoside is contraindicated, ciprofloxacin may be substituted if the organism is susceptible. Another proposed regimen that may allow intravenous-oral switch therapy is ciprofloxacin plus rifampin.[301] Today, new anti–gram-positive quinolones, combined with rifampin, might be even more effective. Some authors do not start rifampin until 3 days of effective therapy have been given, hoping to reduce the chance of secondary rifampin resistance. Recently, a new lipoglycopeptide daptomycin was accepted as well for right-sided IE therapy (see Chapter 31).[129]

On the other hand, glycopeptides (vancomycin or teicoplanin) combined with aminoglycosides resulted in an unacceptable proportion of failures. Thus, glycopeptides should not be used for short course treatment.

Contraindications to short course therapy in injection drug users include the following: (1) slow clinical or microbiologic response (>96 hours) to the initial antibiotic treatment; (2) complicated right-sided endocarditis with heart failure, valve vegetations, greater than 2 cm, acute respiratory failure, empyema, or septic metastatic foci outside of the lung; (3) therapy with glycopeptides or first-generation cephalosporins; (4) right-sided endocarditis caused by MRSA or polymicrobial infection; and (5) severe immunosuppression (<200 CD4 cells/L) or AIDS.[300]

TABLE 195-9	Suggested Treatment for Native Valve and Prosthetic Valve Endocarditis Caused by Staphylococci			
Antibiotic	*Frequency, Dosage, and Route*	*Duration*	*Comments*	
Native Valves				
Methicillin-Susceptible Staphylococci				
Flucloxacillin (non-USA) or oxacillin, or nafcillin	2 g IV q4h	4-6 wk	Benefit of gentamicin addition is not shown	
with gentamicin (optional)	1 mg/kg IV or IM q8h	3-5 d		
Cefazolin (or other first-generation cephalosporins) with gentamicin	2 g IV q8h	4-6 wk	Alternative for patients allergic to penicillins (not in case of immediate-type penicillin hypersensitivity)	
(optional)	1 mg/kg IV or IM q8h	3-5 d		
Vancomycin	15 mg/kg IV q12h	4-6 wk	Recommended for patients with life-threatening β-lactam allergy	
Methicillin-Resistant Staphylococci				
Vancomycin	15 mg/kg IV q12h	4-6 wk		
Prosthetic Valves				
*Methicillin-Susceptible Staphylococci**				
Flucloxacillin (non-USA) or oxacillin, or nafcillin	2 g IV q4h	≥6 wk	Rifampin increases hepatic metabolism of numerous drugs, including warfarin	
with rifampin and gentamicin	300 mg PO or IV q8h	≥6 wk		
	1 mg/kg IV or IM q8h	2 wk		
	15 mg/kg IV q12h	≥6 wk	Recommended for patients with β-lactam allergy	
Vancomycin plus rifampin and gentamicin	300 mg PO or IV q8h	≥6 wk		
	1 mg/kg IV or IM q8h	2 wk		
Methicillin-Resistant Staphylococci				
Vancomycin	15 mg/kg IV q12h	≥6 wk		
plus rifampin	300 mg PO or IV q8h	≥6 wk		
and gentamicin	1 mg/kg IV or IM q8h	2 wk		

*Rifampin plays special role in prosthetic device infection because it helps kill bacteria attached to foreign material. Rifampin should never be used alone because it selects for resistance at a high frequency (about 10⁻⁶).

IM, intramuscular; IV, intravenous; PO, by mouth; q, every.

Adapted with modifications from Moreillon P, Que YA. Infective endocarditis. *Lancet*. 2004;363:135-149; and Wilson WR, Karchmer AW, Dajani AS, et al. Antibiotic treatment of adults with infective endocarditis due to streptococci, enterococci, staphylococci, and HACEK microorganisms. *JAMA*. 1995;274:1706-1713.

MENINGITIS

S. aureus meningitis is an uncommon disease that accounts for only 1% to 9% of cases of bacterial meningitis.[302,303] Two different modes of pathogenesis have been described: 1, postoperative meningitis, associated with neurosurgical procedures, shunt devices, or head trauma; and 2, spontaneous hematogenous meningitis, from staphylococcal infection outside the central nervous system.

Postoperative and spontaneous *S. aureus* meningitis are two different clinical syndromes. *Postoperative meningitis* usually appears as hospital-acquired infection in young people, and most cases are associated with cerebrospinal fluid shunt devices.[304] On the other hand, *spontaneous meningitis* is a community-acquired infection associated with a variety of clinical sources (primary bacteremia, IE, osteomyelitis) that mainly affects older patients with severe underlying conditions.[303] The mortality rate associated with *S. aureus* meningitis is high, around 50%; the mortality rate of spontaneous meningitis is usually higher than that of postoperative meningitis.[303-305]

PERICARDITIS

Purulent *pericarditis* may result from contiguous contamination during surgery, local extension of a paravalvular infection, or embolization of septic material in the coronary arteries. An autopsy study has shown that up to 22% of pericarditis was caused by *S. aureus*.[306] Installation of sudden chest pain with septic conditions and maybe tamponade or global cardiac dysfunction during staphylococcal infection should suggest the possibility of this potentially lethal complication. Echocardiography to determine the status of both the pericardial space and the valves is useful before pericardiocentesis and possible emergency surgery for drainage or valve repair and replacement.

PULMONARY INFECTIONS

Epidemiology

S. aureus is responsible for less than 10% of microbiologically confirmed cases of community-acquired *pneumonia* (CAP)[307] but for 20% to 30% of hospital-acquired pneumonia (HAP).[219,308] *S. aureus* community-acquired pneumonia occurs primarily in elderly patients (>75

years) admitted from nursing homes but also in patients with predisposing factors, such as diabetes and alcoholism, and typically during *influenza* epidemics.[309] Lethality is high, especially when it is associated with acute respiratory distress syndrome or septic shock.

In the hospital, *S. aureus* is becoming the most frequent pathogen responsible for nosocomial pneumonia. It increased from 13% of the cases between 1981 and 1986 to 25% between 2006 and 2007,[217,310] with a proportion of MRSA more than 55%.

Clinical Spectrum

The clinical manifestations of *S. aureus* pneumonia are frequently indistinguishable from those of pneumonia caused by other pathogens, although the pneumonia caused by *S. aureus* is typically a necrotizing infection with rapid progression to tissue destruction and cavitation (see Figure 195-15). The infection may result either from airborne contamination or aspiration or from hematogenous seeding during bacteremia or right-sided endocarditis. In both cases, the pulmonary infection can lead to local complications, such as abscesses and pleural empyema.

Pneumonia in young previously healthy adults with a preceding influenza-like illness characterized by severe respiratory symptoms, hemoptysis, high fever, leukopenia, very high C-reactive protein level (>400 mg/L), hypotension, and a chest radiograph that shows multilobar cavitating alveolar infiltrates should lead one to suspect CA-MRSA infection.[311] The fatality rate of CA-MRSA necrotizing pneumonia can be as high as 60%.[312] Airway bleeding, erythroderma, and leukopenia are strong predictors of mortality.[312] Figure 195-9 illustrates the case of such an acute hemorrhagic pneumonia from PVL toxin-secreting *S. aureus* associated with *Influenza A* infection in a 20-year-old patient (see previous section Pathogenesis II: Pathogenicity (Genomic) Islands and Mobile Genetic Elements).

S. aureus remains one of the most common causes of pleural empyema and still accounts for about one third of the cases.[313] Acute empyema usually arises by direct extension from *S. aureus* pneumonia or lung abscess. It is also often seen as a complication of thoracic surgery. Radiologic findings on CT scan or ultrasound scan confirm the clinical suspicion. Demonstration of a pleural air-fluid level in the absence of a previous thoracocentesis suggests a bronchopleural fistula, another feared complication of *S. aureus* infection. Figure 195-15 demonstrates the case of multiple lung abscesses and pleural effusion in a young patient with right-sided endocarditis.

Treatment

Rapid institution of appropriate antibiotic therapy is essential. Delay is associated with poor outcome.[229] Because the rapid determination of the etiology of severe pneumonia is possible only in a limited number of cases, initial broad-spectrum antibiotic therapy that treats MRSA and other pathogens should be instituted early. However, deescalation therapy should occur whenever possible; in particular, a switch to a more rapidly bactericidal β-lactam agent should be done whenever possible according to susceptibility testing.

For years, vancomycin was the only treatment for MRSA pneumonia, but the cure rate was disappointing. This led to the recommendation of higher vancomycin through serum concentrations (15 to 20 µg/mL). In this context, linezolid, a new oxazolidinone with bacteriostatic activity, appears to be a promising alternative. Clinical outcomes of *S. aureus* HAP and VAP treated with linezolid therapy were found to be significantly better than those treated with vancomycin.[180] For patients with pneumonia caused by MRSA strains with vancomycin MICs of 1.0 mg/mL of more, who require concomitant nephrotoxic therapy or who have preexisting renal failure, linezolid at 600 mg every 12 hours is advised.[314]

The duration of treatment of *S. aureus* pneumonia is determined by the general picture of the disease. The less complicated cases of CAP without overt tissue destruction and without associated deep-seated infections respond to appropriate antibiotic therapy in 10 to 15 days. With the exception of MRSA pneumonia, 7 to 8 days of treatment is sufficient for most patients with HAP or VAP without bacteremia.[315] In the case of surgical drainage of empyema, the treatment duration is adjusted to cultures and persistence of the pleural effusion. In the case of right-sided endocarditis, therapy is prolonged to 4 weeks according to standard recommendations for endocarditis treatment (see previous discussion).

OSTEOMYELITIS

Epidemiology

Osteomyelitis has been known since antiquity. Its epidemiology, however, is constantly changing together with the emergence of resistant bacterial strains (e.g., CA-MRSA), the disappearance of causative organisms after the introduction of community immunization programs (i.e., *Haemophilus influenzae*), and the improved ability to isolate specific organisms (i.e., *Kingella kingae*). *S. aureus* continues to be the leading organism, isolated in 50% to 70% of cases (Table 195-10).[222,223]

Both the mortality and incidence of osteomyelitis have markedly decreased since the introduction of antibacterial therapy. In one pediatric case review, the mortality rate decreased from more than 30% before the introduction of sulfa derivatives (years 1936 to 1940) to approximately 13% afterward (from 1941 to 1945).[316] The mortality

rate from osteomyelitis continued to decline with modern antibiotics and is now close to zero. The incidence is declining as well. In children (<13 years) in the area of the Greater Glasgow Board Health Center (United Kingdom), the incidence rate of osteomyelitis declined by about three times over the last 30 years and by two times during the 1990s. It was 2.9 per 100,000 populations per year in 1997,[223] which is comparable with the lowest estimates for infective endocarditis.[221] This decrease was almost exclusively related to a decline in acute hematogenous forms, which reflects a better handling of banal *S. aureus* skin and soft tissue infections, which are often the source of transient bacteremia.

However, the incidence of osteomyelitis varies with the presence of underlying risk factors. In one large study (454 patients), men were affected twice as much as women, and 90% of cases were the result of contiguous infections. Patients with diabetes had a 4.9-times greater risk of bone infection than the normal population, followed by a two-times greater risk in patients with vascular diseases.[222] Other risk groups include individuals with an increased risk of bacteremia, such as patients for hemodialysis.

For the last several years, medical centers around the world began to report an increasing incidence and severity of musculoskeletal infections in children.[223,317-319] Concurrent to this phenomenon was the rise in the incidence of MRSA as the causative organism in most complicated cases.[317,318,320] Deep venous thrombosis also became recognized as a complication increasingly associated with osteomyelitis in children,[317] especially that associated with CA-MRSA.

Pathogenesis

The two ways by which bacteria can infect the bones are: 1, hematogenous seeding; and 2, contiguous contamination. Both have epidemiologic and pathogenic correlates. Bone infection requires certain predisposing circumstances. In children with hematogenous osteomyelitis, the disease is usually located at the distal end of the long bone metaphysis, including the humerus, femur, and tibia. The nature of the blood flow close to the growing plate may be responsible. Terminal arterioles followed by stagnant blood in the venous sinusoids may facilitate the settlement of blood-borne staphylococci. A similar model may apply for vertebral osteomyelitis (Fig. 195-18A), where blood flow at the vertebral interface is somewhat similar. In addition, micro (or macro) bone trauma may facilitate infection as well, by affecting the local blood supply or exposing host matrix proteins to which staphylococci can adhere.

On the bacterial side, *S. aureus* is equipped with several surface adhesins or MSCRAMMs (see previous Pathogenesis I: Regulation and Virulence Determinants section), including collagen-binding protein and sialoprotein-binding protein, which were shown to promote experimental osteoarticular infection (see Table 195-1). After local settlement, secreted proteases and hemolysins promote tissue destruction and invasion, as indicated by a decreased virulence of *sar* and *agr* mutants that are affected in toxin secretion (see previous Pathogenesis I: Regulation and Virulence Determinants section).[321] The combined effect of both *S. aureus* factors and immune cell-mediated production of oxygen radicals and cytokines results in local necrosis and abscess formation. If adequate antibacterial therapy is given, the nascent abscess can heal totally. Alternatively, bone necrosis can extend and circumscribe devitalized bone fragments, or sequestra, floating in the abscess cavity (see Fig. 195-18B). The formation of necrosis and sequestra exemplifies the evolution of acute osteomyelitis to the chronic form (see subsequent discussion) and requires the combination of antibiotics and surgical débridement and sequestrectomy for successful treatment.

Clinical Features

Osteomyelitis is conventionally divided into acute and chronic disease. *Acute osteomyelitis* is defined as a first episode that responds to medical treatment within 6 weeks.[322] It is usually hematogenous and predominant in children and elderly patients. Symptoms are those of an acute septic syndrome with chills, high fever, malaise, and local pain and

TABLE 195-10	Frequency of Osteomyelitis Caused by Various Microorganisms[222,223]		
	Frequency of Osteomyelitis (%)		
Microorganisms			
Staphylococcus aureus	54.2	65	50
Coagulase-negative staphylococci	13.9	5	13
Non-group D streptococci	13.7	30	23
Pseudomonas aeruginosa	4.4	ND	ND
Other	13.8	0	14
Total	100	100	100
Demography			
No. of patients/episodes	454	20	62
Median age (y; average)	6-92 (51)	0.1-12 (5.4)	0.1-13 (4)
References	(222)	(223)	(341)

ND, not determined.

swelling. Blood cultures are positive in about 50% of cases, and blood plus tissue cultures in 65% of cases.

Chronic osteomyelitis infection is considered in all other situations, including the relapse of a previously treated or untreated disease and infection arising by contiguity. The process can evolve over months or even years and is characterized by low-grade inflammation, the presence of necrosis, sequestra, pus, fistula, and recurrences.

Aside from open-wound fractures, contiguous osteomyelitis involves diabetes-related and unrelated vascular diseases and prosthesis-related osteomyelitis. Diabetes-related osteomyelitis and vascular-related osteomyelitis principally involve the feet. They complicate chronic ulcers, which may be paradoxically painless because of associated neuritis. The ulcerative lesion should be explored gently, but in depth, with a surgical probe. If the probe encounters the bone surface, osteomyelitis is present.[323] Other investigations involve radiology and surgical biopsy. Cultures of deep tissues and bone biopsy are mandatory for microbiologic diagnosis. Cultures of surface swabs and fistula fluids mostly yield skin contaminants but not the responsible pathogen.

Prosthetic Joint Infections

With the use of perioperative antimicrobial prophylaxis and laminar airflow operating rooms, *prosthetic joint infections* are fairly rare. The infection rate after primary joint replacement is usually less than 1% in hip and shoulder prostheses, less than 2% in knee prostheses, and less than 9% in elbow prostheses.[324] Infection rates after surgical revision are usually considerably higher.

Implant-associated infections are typically caused by microorganisms that grow in structures known as *biofilms*. *S. aureus* is the second cause of infection after coagulase-negative staphylococci.[324] Infections within the 12 first weeks after implantation are considered as early, or acute; infections that occur from 12 weeks to 24 months after implantation are considered as delayed, or low-grade, infections; and those that occur after 24 months are considered as late, or chronic.[324]

S. aureus is mostly responsible for early infection. As for prosthetic heart valves, the organisms usually originate from the skin and are likely to be introduced at the time of operation. Although early symptoms may be acute, patients with low-grade or chronic infection may have few general symptoms and the clinical signs may crystallize around local pain and loosening of the prosthesis. Prosthetic joints remain susceptible to hematogenous seeding during their entire lifetime. The overall risk for prosthetic joint infection after bacteremia from all pathogens was only 0.3%.[325] However, in the case of *S. aureus* bacteremia, this risk was as high as 34% for prosthetic joints and 7% for nonarticular prosthetic devices.[325]

Blood culture results are often negative. Cultures of the fluid from the artificial joint are critical but can have negative results as well. Molecular diagnosis with PCR should be considered (see previous Culture and Identification section). If the prosthesis is surgically removed, multiple microbiologic samples should be taken at various sites of the prosthesis and bone cavity because bacteria may remain clustered in circumscribed areas.

The suggested treatment duration is 3 months for hip prostheses and 6 months for knee prostheses. Intravenous therapy should be administrated for the first 2 to 4 weeks. The addition of rifampin to conventional antistaphylococcal regimen appeared clearly useful in patients with prosthetic joint infections. Rifampin has an excellent activity on slow-growing and adherent staphylococci. In general, retention of the implant should not be attempted. Débridement with retention is an option only for patients with early postoperative or acute hematogenous infection; if duration of clinical signs and symptoms is less than 3 weeks, the implant is stable and effective therapy against biofilm microorganisms is available. The prerequisites for one-stage exchange are satisfactory condition of soft tissue, the absence of severe coexisting illnesses, and the absence of difficult-to-treat bacteria. In all other cases, a two-stage exchange is preferred, with a 2-week to 4-week interval between both procedures (see Chapter 103).[326]

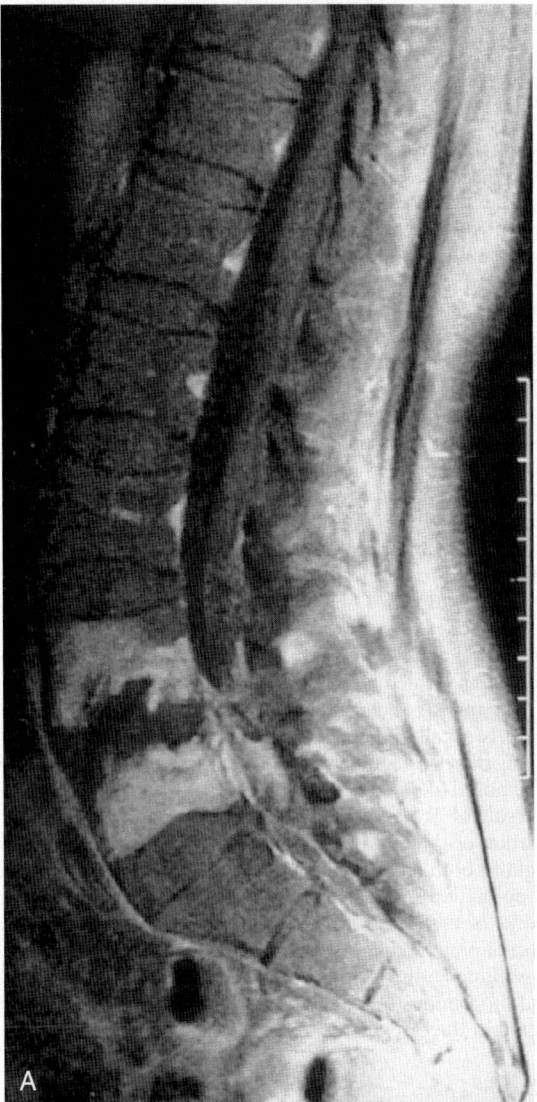

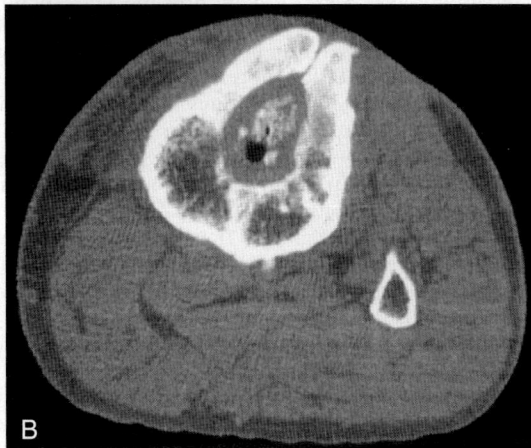

Figure 195-18 Osteomyelitis imaging. A, Nuclear magnetic resonance imaging of L4-L5 lumbar osteomyelitis after injection of gadolinium contrast medium (T1 view). **B,** Chronic osteomyelitis of left tibia. A vast necrotic cavern containing sequestrum surrounded by air can be seen. A fistula with drainage to the skin is present.

Diagnosis

Diagnosis of osteomyelitis integrates clinical signs, radiology, and microbiology. However, clinical signs may be scarce in chronic infection. Current radiology techniques include standard radiograph, [99m]technetium (Tc)-methylene-diphosphonate bone scan, CT scan, and nuclear magnetic resonance imaging (MRI), with MRI being the most useful. Less useful amd infrequently used techniques include [111In]Tc-labeled or ^{99m}Tc-labeled granulocytes, ^{99m}Tc-labeled antigranulocyte antibodies, ^{99m}Tc-labeled polyclonal immunoglobulins, ^{99m}Tc-labeled ciprofloxacin, and gallium-67-citrate scan.[327]

Conventional radiographic results may be negative within the first 10 days of acute osteomyelitis because necrosis, decalcification, and peripheral sclerosis are not yet apparent. In one study, results were positive in only 50% of acute osteomyelitis cases. However, it is still useful to follow the healing process. ^{99m}Tc-bone scan and MRI are very sensitive, and results were positive in more than 80% in the same study. ^{99m}Tc-bone scan is also sensitive in chronic osteomyelitis. However, because it detects bone remodeling, interpretation of results may be difficult when underlying osteosynthetic prostheses or degenerative bone lesions are present.

Microbiologic cultures are indispensable to guide therapy. Whenever possible, both blood cultures and tissue cultures should be performed. Importantly, chronic infection may be associated with persistent forms of *S. aureus,* such as small colony variants, especially if aminoglycosides have been used in conjunction with osteosynthetic material (see previous Culture and Identification section).[328] The diagnostic laboratory should be made aware of this possibility so appropriate measures may be taken.

Treatment

Rapid institution of antibiotic therapy is mandatory to prevent bone necrosis and the passage of acute osteomyelitis to more problematic chronic disease. The duration of drug treatment in most studies is 4 and 6 weeks but may vary up to 10 weeks or more in complicated situations. Empiric treatment of osteomyelitis should include adequate coverage of MRSA in areas where CA-MRSA is endemic. Adequate representative cultures should be obtained to ensure the early identification of MRSA.

The classical regimens are as follows: (1) for penicillin-susceptible *S. aureus*: intravenous penicillin G, 4 millions units every 6 hours; (2) for penicillin-resistant *S. aureus*: intravenous nafcillin, cloxacillin, or, outside the United States, flucloxacillin, 2 g every 6 hours; and (3) for MRSA: intravenous vancomycin, 1 g every 12 hours. Clindamycin might be a good alternative to vancomycin in the presence of susceptible CA-MRSA.

The question of a proven "best" antibiotic treatment for osteomyelitis was addressed in a metaanalysis of 22 trials encompassing 927 episodes.[329] The results indicated that almost any of the drugs or drug combinations tested (including β-lactams, glycopeptides, clindamycin, and quinolones) were equivalent. However, the analysis also disclosed that the comparative trials were generally of poor quality (see Chapter 103).

In children with hematogenous *S. aureus* osteomyelitis, a relatively short course (4 to 7 days) of intravenous treatment is often followed by oral therapy with amoxicillin or penicillin-stable β-lactams for 4 to 6 weeks, with outpatient therapy allowed.[330] Oral treatment is currently not recommended in adults, although newer quinolones may be appropriate because of their high bioavailability. However, outpatient therapy is also increasingly used. This may be achieved with ceftriaxone (2 g once a day), which was shown to be effective against *S. aureus* osteomyelitis in two studies.[222,331] In one of these studies, ceftriaxone and penicillin-stable β-lactams performed significantly better than vancomycin.[332]

Finally, osteomyelitis from multiresistant MRSA remains difficult to treat. Insufficient clinical trials exist to suggest whether quinupristin-dalfopristin, linezolid, daptomycin, or other newer molecules are more effective than standard alternatives (mostly vancomycin).

SEPTIC ARTHRITIS, SEPTIC BURSITIS, AND PYOMYOSITIS

Septic Arthritis

S. aureus remains the most frequent cause of *septic arthritis* in children and in nongonococcal arthritis of adults.[333] Rheumatoid arthritis and diabetes are risk factors. The disease may follow both hematogenous seeding and local trauma and may be of iatrogenic nature in the case of joint puncture or arthroscopy. Symptoms associated are acute pain and joint swelling. Joint destruction occurs within a few days from both bacterial and host inflammatory factors and probably also ischemic lesions from the increased intraarticular hydrostatic pressure. Therefore, patients with underlying arthritis with acute pain in a single joint should undergo aspiration immediately and the fluid examined for cell count, chemistry, and culture.

The prognosis of hematogenous arthritis in children is good. In adults, the prognosis is mostly associated with that of the underlying disease (i.e., rheumatoid arthritis or endocarditis or other deep-seated condition responsible for the initial bacteremia). Medical treatment is identical to that of osteomyelitis. Open joint drainage is usually unnecessary, except for hip infections in children, where it may help prevent necrosis of the femoral head.[334]

Septic Bursitis

Septic bursitis is an acute infection that involves the periarticular bursa. It is most often located in pressure areas such as the olecranon and the patella. It manifests as an acute juxtaarticular inflammation. The overlying skin is usually inflamed. Unlike arthritis and osteomyelitis, the underlying bone and joint are usually painless at pressure or mobilization. The portal of entry is likely to be local. More than 80% of bursitis is the result of *S. aureus*.[335] Diagnosis is made with puncture and examination of the bursa fluid. Importantly, septic bursitis may be at the origin of both local and distant septic complication. Thus, careful clinical evaluation is mandatory. The prognosis is good but requires 2 to 3 weeks of appropriate antibiotic therapy. Repeated aspiration of the bursa is preferable to incision and drainage for patient with persistent swelling and pain. Complicated cases may require hospitalization and intravenous treatment. Surgical excision of the bursa may be considered in the case of recurrences.

Pyomyositis

Primary *pyomyositis*, also called tropical myositis, infective myositis, pyogenic myositis, and myositis purulenta tropica, is a rare subacute infection of skeletal muscles. It does not follow contiguous contamination and is most probably of hematogenous origin. The rarity of the disease is attributed to the resistance of muscles to infection. A history of muscle trauma is often reported.

Pyomyositis is frequently seen in Africa and South Pacific, but it is rare in the Northern Hemisphere. Hence, it could be related to particular local conditions or bacterial properties. In a review of 676 cases, the disease occurred in all age groups. However, it was about twice as frequent in children and adults below the age of 30 years than in older adults, and males were predominantly affected.[336] Any muscle may be involved, but the quadriceps and iliopsoas muscles were most often implicated, in 26% and 14%, respectively. *S. aureus* was the etiologic agent in about 80% of cases.

Clinical symptoms evolve in three stages. They first start with the insidious onset of dull cramping and low-grade fever, general malaise, and muscle aches. Because only the aponeurosis is innervated, overt muscle pain may be delayed for 1 or 2 weeks, before frank abscess formation. Second, the formation of muscle abscess becomes symptomatic, with pain, muscle swelling, tenderness, and sepsis. Most patients are seen at this stage. If left untreated, the disease evolves to the third stage, with muscle destruction, local extension with osteomyelitis, or osteoarthritis, septicemia, and distant dissemination. Diagnosis involves radiographic imaging (CT scan and MRI) and bacteriologic diagnosis with blood cultures and muscle puncture. Treatment is essentially based on antibiotic therapy. Treatment duration is a matter of debate. Parenteral treatment is often recommended for 7 to 14 days, followed by oral treatment for up to 6 weeks. The prognosis before stage 3 is usually excellent.

This work was supported by the grant 3200B0-113854 from the Swiss National Science Foundation and by the grant PASMP3-123226 / 1 from both the Swiss Foundation for Grants in Biology and Medicine and the Swiss Medical Association.

REFERENCES

1. Gordon RJ, Lowy FD. Pathogenesis of methicillin-resistant *Staphylococcus aureus* infection. *Clin Infect Dis.* 2008;46:S350-S359.
2. Dinges MM, Orwin PM, Schlievert PM. Exotoxins of *Staphylococcus aureus*. *Clin Microbiol Rev.* 2000;13:16-34.
3. Ladhani S, Joannou CL, Lochrie DP, et al. Clinical, microbial, and biochemical aspects of the exfoliative toxins causing staphylococcal scalded-skin syndrome. *Clin Microbiol Rev.* 1999;12:224-242.
4. McCormick JK, Yarwood JM, Schlievert PM. Toxic shock syndrome and bacterial superantigens: an update. *Annu Rev Microbiol.* 2001;55:77-104.
5. Jarraud S, Peyrat MA, Lim A, et al. egc, a highly prevalent operon of enterotoxin gene, forms a putative nursery of superantigens in *Staphylococcus aureus*. *J Immunol.* 2001;166:669-677.
6. Novick RP. Mobile genetic elements and bacterial toxinoses: the superantigen-encoding pathogenicity islands of *Staphylococcus aureus*. *Plasmid.* 2003;49:93-105.
7. Feng Y, Chen CJ, Su LH, et al. Evolution and pathogenesis of *Staphylococcus aureus*: lessons learned from genotyping and comparative genomics. *FEMS Microbiol Rev.* 2008;32:23-37.
8. Cheung AL, Projan SJ, Gresham H. The genomic aspect of virulence, sepsis, and resistance to killing mechanisms in *Staphylococcus aureus*. *Curr Infect Dis Rep.* 2002;4:400-410.
9. Gotz F, Bannerman T, Schleifer K-H. The genera *Staphylococcus* and *Macrococcus*. In: Balows A, Truper AG, Dworkin M, et al, eds. *The Prokaryotes*. ed 3. New York: Springer Science+Business Media; 2006:1-75.
10. Kuroda M, Ohta T, Uchiyama I, et al. Whole genome sequencing of meticillin-resistant *Staphylococcus aureus*. *Lancet.* 2001;357:1225-1240.
11. Lindsay JA, Holden MT. Understanding the rise of the superbug: investigation of the evolution and genomic variation of *Staphylococcus aureus*. *Funct Integr Genomics.* 2006;6:186-201.
12. Baba T, Takeuchi F, Kuroda M, et al. Genome and virulence determinants of high virulence community-acquired MRSA. *Lancet.* 2002;359:1819-1827.
13. Ogston A. *Micrococcus* poisoning. *J Anat Physiol (London)*. 1883;17:24-58.
14. Kuroda M, Yamashita A, Hirakawa H, et al. Whole genome sequence of *Staphylococcus saprophyticus* reveals the pathogenesis of uncomplicated urinary tract infection. *Proc Natl Acad Sci U S A.* 2005;102:13272-13277.
15. Takeuchi F, Watanabe S, Baba T, et al. Whole-genome sequencing of *Staphylococcus haemolyticus* uncovers the extreme plasticity of its genome and the evolution of human-colonizing staphylococcal species. *J Bacteriol.* 2005;187:7292-7308.
16. Gill SR, Fouts DE, Archer GL, et al. Insights on evolution of virulence and resistance from the complete genome analysis of an early methicillin-resistant *Staphylococcus aureus* strain and a biofilm-producing methicillin-resistant *Staphylococcus epidermidis* strain. *J Bacteriol.* 2005;187:2426-2438.
17. Kluytmans J, van Belkum A, Verbrugh H. Nasal carriage of *Staphylococcus aureus*: epidemiology, underlying mechanisms, and associated risks. *Clin Microbiol Rev.* 1997;10:505-520.
18. The role of nasal carriage in *Staphylococcus aureus* infections. (2005).
19. von Eiff C, Becker K, Machka K, et al. Nasal carriage as a source of *Staphylococcus aureus* bacteremia. Study Group. *N Engl J Med.* 2001;344:11-16.
20. Laupland KB, Church DL, Mucenski M, et al. Population-based study of the epidemiology of and the risk factors for invasive *Staphylococcus aureus* infections. *J Infect Dis.* 2003;187:1452-1459.
21. Dufour P, Gillet Y, Bes M, et al. Community-acquired methicillin-resistant *Staphylococcus aureus* infections in France: emergence of a single clone that produces Panton-Valentine leukocidin. *Clin Infect Dis.* 2002;35:819-824.
22. Moran GJ, Krishnadasan A, Gorwitz RJ, et al. Methicillin-resistant *S. aureus* infections among patients in the emergency department. *N Engl J Med.* 2006;355:666-674.
23. Compernolle V, Verschraegen G, Claeys G. Combined use of Pastorex Staph-Plus and either of two new chromogenic agars, MRSA ID and CHROMagar MRSA, for detection of methicillin-resistant *Staphylococcus aureus*. *J Clin Microbiol.* 2007;45:154-158.
24. Walsh TR, Bolmstrom A, Qwarnstrom A, et al. Evaluation of current methods for detection of staphylococci with reduced susceptibility to glycopeptides. *J Clin Microbiol.* 2001;39:2439-2444.
25. Proctor RA, Balwit JM, Vesga O. Variant subpopulations of *Staphylococcus aureus* as cause of persistent and recurrent infections. *Infect Agents Dis.* 1994;3:302-312.
26. Besier S, Smaczny C, von Mallinckrodt C, et al. Prevalence and clinical significance of *Staphylococcus aureus* small-colony variants in cystic fibrosis lung disease. *J Clin Microbiol.* 2007;45:168-172.
27. Baumert N, von Eiff C, Schaaff F, et al. Physiology and antibiotic susceptibility of *Staphylococcus aureus* small colony variants. *Microb Drug Resist.* 2002;8:253-260.
28. Chatterjee I, Kriegeskorte A, Fischer A, et al. In vivo mutations of thymidylate synthase (encoded by thyA) are responsible for thymidine dependency in clinical small-colony variants of *Staphylococcus aureus*. *J Bacteriol.* 2008;190:834-842.
29. Jonsson IM, von Eiff C, Proctor RA, et al. Virulence of a hemB mutant displaying the phenotype of a *Staphylococcus aureus* small colony variant in a murine model of septic arthritis. *Microb Pathog.* 2003;34:73-79.
30. Bates DM, Eiff Cv C, McNamara PJ, et al. *Staphylococcus aureus* menD and hemB mutants are as infective as the parent strains, but the menadione biosynthetic mutant persists within the kidney. *J Infect Dis.* 2003;187:1654-1661.
31. Vaudaux P, Francois P, Bisognano C, et al. Increased expression of clumping factor and fibronectin-binding proteins by hemB mutants of *Staphylococcus aureus* expressing small colony variant phenotypes. *Infect Immun.* 2002;70:5428-5437.
32. Tenover FC. Rapid detection and identification of bacterial pathogens using novel molecular technologies: infection control and beyond. *Clin Infect Dis.* 2007;44:418-423.
33. Oliveira K, Brecher SM, Durbin A, et al. Direct identification of *Staphylococcus aureus* from positive blood culture bottles. *J Clin Microbiol.* 2003;41:889-891.
34. Forrest GN, Mehta S, Weekes E, et al. Impact of rapid in situ hybridization testing on coagulase-negative staphylococci positive blood cultures. *J Antimicrob Chemother.* 2006;58:154-158.
35. Huletsky A, Lebel P, Picard FJ, et al. Identification of methicillin-resistant *Staphylococcus aureus* carriage in less than 1 hour during a hospital surveillance program. *Clin Infect Dis.* 2005;40:976-981.
36. Harbarth S, Masuet-Aumatell C, Schrenzel J, et al. Evaluation of rapid screening and pre-emptive contact isolation for detecting and controlling methicillin-resistant *Staphylococcus aureus* in critical care: an interventional cohort study. *Crit Care.* 2006;10:R25.
37. Styers D, Sheehan DJ, Hogan P, Sahm DF. Laboratory-based surveillance of current antimicrobial resistance patterns and trends among *Staphylococcus aureus:* 2005 status in the United States. *Ann Clin Microbiol Antimicrob.* 2006;5:2.
38. Oliveira DC, Tomasz A, de Lencastre H. Secrets of success of a human pathogen: molecular evolution of pandemic clones of meticillin-resistant *Staphylococcus aureus*. *Lancet Infect Dis.* 2002;2:180-189.
39. Enright MC, Robinson DA, Randle G, et al. The evolutionary history of methicillin-resistant *Staphylococcus aureus* (MRSA). *Proc Natl Acad Sci U S A.* 2002;99:7687-7692.
40. Robinson DA, Enright MC. Evolutionary models of the emergence of methicillin-resistant *Staphylococcus aureus*. *Antimicrob Agents Chemother.* 2003;47:3926-3934.
41. Kuhn G, Francioli P, Blanc DS. Double-locus sequence typing using clfB and spa, a fast and simple method for epidemiological typing of methicillin-resistant *Staphylococcus aureus*. *J Clin Microbiol.* 2007;45:54-62.
42. Natural population dynamics and expansion of pathogenic clones of *Staphylococcus aureus*. (2004).
43. Novick RP. Autoinduction and signal transduction in the regulation of staphylococcal virulence. *Mol Microbiol.* 2003;48:1429-1449.
44. Pragman AA, Schlievert PM. Virulence regulation in *Staphylococcus aureus*: the need for in vivo analysis of virulence factor regulation. *FEMS Immunol Med Microbiol.* 2004;42:147-154.
45. Novick RP, Ross HF, Projan SJ, et al. Synthesis of staphylococcal virulence factors is controlled by a regulatory RNA molecule. *EMBO J.* 1993;12:3967-3975.
46. Giraudo AT, Cheung AL, Nagel R. The sae locus of *Staphylococcus aureus* controls exoprotein synthesis at the transcriptional level. *Arch Microbiol.* 1997;168:53-58.
47. Yarwood JM, McCormick JK, Schlievert PM. Identification of a novel two-component regulatory system that acts in global regulation of virulence factors of *Staphylococcus aureus*. *J Bacteriol.* 2001;183:1113-1123.
48. Fournier B, Hooper DC. A new two-component regulatory system involved in adhesion, autolysis, and extracellular proteolytic activity of *Staphylococcus aureus*. *J Bacteriol.* 2000;182:3955-3964.
49. Cheung AL, Bayer AS, Zhang G, et al. Regulation of virulence determinants in vitro and in vivo in *Staphylococcus aureus*. *FEMS Immunol Med Microbiol.* 2004;40:1-9.
50. Cheung AL, Koomey JM, Butler CA, et al. Regulation of exoprotein expression in *Staphylococcus aureus* by a locus (*sar*) distinct from *agr*. *Proc Natl Acad Sci U S A.* 1992;89:6462-6466.
51. Said-Salim B, Dunman PM, McAleese FM, et al. Global regulation of *Staphylococcus aureus* genes by Rot. *J Bacteriol.* 2003;185:610-619.
52. Chan PF, Foster SJ. The role of environmental factors in the regulation of virulence-determinant expression in *Staphylococcus aureus* 8325-4. *Microbiology.* 1998;144:2469-2479.
53. Entenza JM, Moreillon P, Senn MM, et al. Role of sigmaB in the expression of *Staphylococcus aureus* cell wall adhesins ClfA and FnbA and contribution to infectivity in a rat model of experimental endocarditis. *Infect Immun.* 2005;73:990-998.
54. Balaban N, Goldkorn T, Nhan RT, et al. Autoinducer of virulence as a target for vaccine and therapy against *Staphylococcus aureus*. *Science.* 1998;280:438-440.
55. Garvis S, Mei JM, Ruiz-Albert J, Holden DW. *Staphylococcus aureus* svrA: a gene required for virulence and expression of the *agr* locus. *Microbiology.* 2002;148:3235-3243.
56. Chen J, Novick RP. svrA, a multi-drug exporter, does not control *agr*. *Microbiology.* 2007;153:1604-1608.
57. Adhikari RP, Arvidson S, Novick RP. A nonsense mutation in agrA accounts for the defect in *agr* expression and the avirulence of *Staphylococcus aureus* 8325-4 traP::kan. *Infect Immun.* 2007;75:4534-4540.
58. Pichon C, Felden B. Small RNA genes expressed from *Staphylococcus aureus* genomic and pathogenicity islands with specific expression among pathogenic strains. *Proc Natl Acad Sci U S A.* 2005;102:14249-14254.
59. Mayville P, Ji G, Beavis R, et al. Structure-activity analysis of synthetic autoinducing thiolactone peptides from *Staphylococcus aureus* responsible for virulence. *Proc Natl Acad Sci U S A.* 1999;96:1218-1223.
60. Cheung AL, Eberhardt KJ, Chung E, et al. Diminished virulence of a *sar-/agr-* mutant of *Staphylococcus aureus* in the rabbit model of endocarditis. *J Clin Invest.* 1994;94:1815-1822.
61. Que YA, Haefliger JA, Piroth L, et al. Fibrinogen and fibronectin binding cooperate for valve infection and invasion in *Staphylococcus aureus* experimental endocarditis. *J Exp Med.* 2005;201:1627-1635.
62. The fibrinogen- and fibronectin-binding domains of *Staphylococcus aureus* fibronectin-binding protein A synergistically promote endothelial invasion and experimental endocarditis. (2008).
63. Cheung AL, Nast CC, Bayer AS. Selective activation of *sar* promoters with the use of green fluorescent protein transcriptional fusions as the detection system in the rabbit endocarditis model. *Infect Immun.* 1998;66:5988-5993.
64. Yarwood JM, McCormick JK, Paustian ML, et al. Repression of the *Staphylococcus aureus* accessory gene regulator in serum and in vivo. *J Bacteriol.* 2002;184:1095-1101.
65. Boles BR, Horswill AR. Agr-mediated dispersal of *Staphylococcus aureus* biofilms. *PLoS Pathog.* 2008;4:e1000052.
66. Ji G, Beavis R, Novick RP. Bacterial interference caused by autoinducing peptide variants. *Science.* 1997;276:2027-2030.
67. Dufour P, Jarraud S, Vandenesch F, et al. High genetic variability of the *agr* locus in *Staphylococcus* species. *J Bacteriol.* 2002;184:1180-1186.
68. Patel R. Biofilms and antimicrobial resistance. *Clin Orthop Relat Res.* 2005:41-47.
69. Begun J, Gaiani JM, Rohde H, et al. Staphylococcal biofilm exopolysaccharide protects against *Caenorhabditis elegans* immune defenses. *PLoS Pathog.* 2007;3:e57.
70. Gerke C, Kraft A, Sussmuth R, et al. Characterization of the N-acetylglucosaminyltransferase activity involved in the biosynthesis of the *Staphylococcus epidermidis* polysaccharide intercellular adhesin. *J Biol Chem.* 1998;273:18586-18593.
71. Heilmann C, Schweitzer O, Gerke C, et al. Molecular basis of intercellular adhesion in the biofilm-forming *Staphylococcus epidermidis*. *Mol Microbiol.* 1996;20:1083-1091.
72. Francois P, Tu Quoc PH, Bisognano C, et al. Lack of biofilm contribution to bacterial colonisation in an experimental model of foreign body infection by *Staphylococcus aureus* and *Staphylococcus epidermidis*. *FEMS Immunol Med Microbiol.* 2003;35:135-140.
73. Shinefield H, Black S, Fattom A, et al. Use of a *Staphylococcus aureus* conjugate vaccine in patients receiving hemodialysis. *N Engl J Med.* 2002;346:491-496.
74. Patti JM, Allen BL, McGavin MJ, et al. MSCRAMM-mediated adherence of microorganisms to host tissues. *Annu Rev Microbiol.* 1994;48:585-617.
75. Fischetti VA, Pancholi V, Schneewind O. Conservation of a hexapeptide sequence in the anchor region of surface proteins from gram-positive cocci. *Mol Microbiol.* 1990;4:1603-1605.

76. Roche FM, Massey R, Peacock SJ, et al. Characterization of novel LPXTG-containing proteins of *Staphylococcus aureus* identified from genome sequences. *Microbiology*. 2003;149:643-654.
77. Wertheim HF, Walsh E, Choudhurry R, et al. Key role for clumping factor B in *Staphylococcus aureus* nasal colonization of humans. *PLoS Med*. 2008;5:e17.
78. Piroth L, Que YA, Widmer E, et al. The fibrinogen- and fibronectin-binding domains of *Staphylococcus aureus* fibronectin-binding protein A synergistically promote endothelial invasion and experimental endocarditis. *Infect Immun*. 2008;76:3824-3831.
79. Arrecubieta C, Asai T, Bayern M, et al. The role of *Staphylococcus aureus* adhesins in the pathogenesis of ventricular assist device-related infections. *J Infect Dis*. 2006;193:1109-1119.
80. Patti JM, Allen BL, McGavin MJ, et al. MSCRAMM-mediated adherence of microorganisms to host tissues. *Annu Rev Microbiol*. 1994;48:585-617.
81. Palmqvist N, Foster T, Tarkowski A, et al. Protein A is a virulence factor in *Staphylococcus aureus* arthritis and septic death. *Microb Pathog*. 2002;33:239-249.
82. Lee LY, Miyamoto YJ, McIntyre BW, et al. The *Staphylococcus aureus* Map protein is an immunomodulator that interferes with T cell-mediated responses. *J Clin Invest*. 2002;110:1461-1471.
83. Roche FM, Meehan M, Foster TJ. The *Staphylococcus aureus* surface protein SasG and its homologues promote bacterial adherence to human desquamated nasal epithelial cells. *Microbiology*. 2003;149:2759-2767.
84. Deininger S, Stadelmaier A, Von Aulock S, et al. Definition of structural prerequisites for lipoteichoic Acid-inducible cytokine induction by synthetic derivatives. *J Immunol*. 2003;170:4134-4138.
85. Weidenmaier C, Kokai-Kun JF, Kristian SA, et al. Role of teichoic acids in *Staphylococcus aureus* nasal colonization, a major risk factor in nosocomial infections. *Nat Med*. 2004;10:243-245.
86. Majcherczyk PA, Rubli E, Heumann D, et al. Teichoic acids are not required for *Streptococcus pneumoniae* and *Staphylococcus aureus* cell walls to trigger the release of tumor necrosis factor by peripheral blood monocytes. *Infect Immun*. 2003;71:3707-3713.
87. Weidenmaier C, Peschel A, Kempf VA, et al. DltABCD- and MprF-mediated cell envelope modifications of *Staphylococcus aureus* confer resistance to platelet microbicidal proteins and contribute to virulence in a rabbit endocarditis model. *Infect Immun*. 2005;73:8033-8038.
88. Berger-Bächi B. Expression of resistance to methicillin. *Trends Microbiol*. 1994;2:389.
89. Bayer AS, Ramos MD, Menzies BE, et al. Hyperproduction of alpha-toxin by *Staphylococcus aureus* results in paradoxically reduced virulence in experimental endocarditis: a host defense role for platelet microbicidal proteins. *Infect Immun*. 1997;65:4652-4660.
90. Panton P, Valentine F. Staphylococcal toxins. *Lancet*. 1932;222:506-508.
91. von Eiff C, Friedrich AW, Peters G, et al. Prevalence of genes encoding for members of the staphylococcal leukotoxin family among clinical isolates of *Staphylococcus aureus*. *Diagn Microbiol Infect Dis*. 2004;49:157-162.
92. Vandenesch F, Naimi T, Enright MC, et al. Community-acquired methicillin-resistant *Staphylococcus aureus* carrying Panton-Valentine leukocidin genes: worldwide emergence. *Emerg Infect Dis*. 2003;9:978-984.
93. Lina G, Piemont Y, Godail-Gamot F, et al. Involvement of Panton-Valentine leukocidin-producing *Staphylococcus aureus* in primary skin infections and pneumonia. *Clin Infect Dis*. 1999;29:1128-1132.
94. Von Rittershain GR. Die exfloliative Dermatitis jungere Senglinge. *Z Kinderheilkd*. 1878;2(3-23).
95. Ladhani S. Understanding the mechanism of action of the exfoliative toxins of *Staphylococcus aureus*. *FEMS Immunol Med Microbiol*. 2003;39:181-189.
96. Becker K, Friedrich AW, Lubritz G, et al. Prevalence of genes encoding pyrogenic toxin superantigens and exfoliative toxins among strains of *Staphylococcus aureus* isolated from blood and nasal specimens. *J Clin Microbiol*. 2003;41:1434-1439.
97. Nishifuji K, Sugai M, Amagai M. Staphylococcal exfoliative toxins: "molecular scissors" of bacteria that attack the cutaneous defense barrier in mammals. *J Dermatol Sci*. 2008;49:21-31.
98. Fraser JD, Proft T. The bacterial superantigen and superantigen-like proteins. *Immunol Rev*. 2008;225:226-243.
99. Fitzgerald JR, Reid SD, Ruotsalainen E, et al. Genome diversification in *Staphylococcus aureus*: Molecular evolution of a highly variable chromosomal region encoding the Staphylococcal exotoxin-like family of proteins. *Infect Immun*. 2003;71:2827-2838.
100. Hiramatsu K, Cui L, Kuroda M, et al. The emergence and evolution of methicillin-resistant *Staphylococcus aureus*. *Trends Microbiol*. 2001;9:486-493.
101. Stevens F. The occurrence of *Staphylococcus aureus* infection with a scarlatiniform rash. *JAMA*. 1927;88:1957-1958.
102. Shands KN, Schmid GP, Dan BB, et al. Toxic-shock syndrome in menstruating women: association with tampon use and *Staphylococcus aureus* and clinical features in 52 cases. *N Engl J Med*. 1980;303:1436-1442.
103. Peterson ML, Ault K, Kremer MJ, et al. The innate immune system is activated by stimulation of vaginal epithelial cells with *Staphylococcus aureus* and toxic shock syndrome toxin 1. *Infect Immun*. 2005;73:2164-2174.
104. Stolz SJ, Davis JP, Vergeront JM, et al. Development of serum antibody to toxic shock toxin among individuals with toxic shock syndrome in Wisconsin. *J Infect Dis*. 1985;151:883-889.
105. Reingold AL, Hargrett NT, Shands KN, et al. Toxic shock syndrome surveillance in the United States, 1980 to 1981. *Ann Intern Med*. 1982;96:875-880.
106. Darenberg J, Ihendyane N, Sjolin J, et al. Intravenous immunoglobulin G therapy in streptococcal toxic shock syndrome: a European randomized, double-blind, placebo-controlled trial. *Clin Infect Dis*. 2003;37:333-340.
107. Narita K, Hu DL, Tsuji T, et al. Intranasal immunization of mutant toxic shock syndrome toxin 1 elicits systemic and mucosal immune response against *Staphylococcus aureus* infection. *FEMS Immunol Med Microbiol*. 2008;52:389-396.
108. Hamad AR, Marrack P, Kappler JW. Transcytosis of staphylococcal superantigen toxins. *J Exp Med*. 1997;185:1447-1454.
109. Petersson K, Pettersson H, Skartved NJ, et al. Staphylococcal enterotoxin H induces V alpha-specific expansion of T cells. *J Immunol*. 2003;170:4148-4154.
110. Yarwood JM, Leung DY, Schlievert PM. Evidence for the involvement of bacterial superantigens in psoriasis, atopic dermatitis, and Kawasaki syndrome. *FEMS Microbiol Lett*. 2000;192:1-7.
111. Semic-Jusufagic A, Bachert C, Gevaert P, et al. *Staphylococcus aureus* sensitization and allergic disease in early childhood: population-based birth cohort study. *J Allergy Clin Immunol*. 2007;119:930-936.
112. Matsubara K, Fukaya T. The role of superantigens of group A Streptococcus and *Staphylococcus aureus* in Kawasaki disease. *Curr Opin Infect Dis*. 2007;20:298-303.
113. Holden MT, Feil EJ, Lindsay JA, et al. Complete genomes of two clinical *Staphylococcus aureus* strains: evidence for the rapid evolution of virulence and drug resistance. *Proc Natl Acad Sci U S A*. 2004;101:9786-9791.
114. Kaneko J, Kimura T, Narita S, et al. Complete nucleotide sequence and molecular characterization of the temperate staphylococcal bacteriophage phiPVL carrying Panton-Valentine leukocidin genes. *Gene*. 1998;215:57-67.
115. Lindsay JA, Ruzin A, Ross HF, et al. The gene for toxic shock toxin is carried by a family of mobile pathogenicity islands in *Staphylococcus aureus*. *Mol Microbiol*. 1998;29:527-543.
116. Ubeda C, Maiques E, Knecht E, et al. Antibiotic-induced SOS response promotes horizontal dissemination of pathogenicity island-encoded virulence factors in staphylococci. *Mol Microbiol*. 2005;56:836-844.
117. Novick RP, Subedi A. The SaPIs: mobile pathogenicity islands of *Staphylococcus*. *Chem Immunol Allergy*. 2007;93:42-57.
118. Katayama Y, Ito T, Hiramatsu K. A new class of genetic element, staphylococcus cassette chromosome mec, encodes methicillin resistance in *Staphylococcus aureus*. *Antimicrob Agents Chemother*. 2000;44:1549-1555.
119. Ito T, Okuma K, Ma XX, et al. Insights on antibiotic resistance of *Staphylococcus aureus* from its whole genome: genomic island SCC. *Drug Resist Updat*. 2003;6:41-52.
120. Chambers HF, Hartman BJ, Tomasz A. Increased amounts of a novel penicillin binding protein in a strain of methicillin-resistant *Staphylococcus aureus*. *J Clin Invest*. 1985;76:325-331.
121. Zhang HZ, Hackbarth CJ, Chansky KM, et al. A proteolytic transmembrane signaling pathway and resistance to beta-lactams in staphylococci. *Nature*. 2001;291:1962-1965.
122. Ito T, Katayama Y, Asada K, et al. Structural comparison of three types of staphylococcal cassette chromosome mec integrated in the chromosome in methicillin-resistant *Staphylococcus aureus*. *Antimicrob Agents Chemother*. 2001;45:1323-1336.
123. Ma XX, Ito T, Tiensasitorn C, et al. Novel type of staphylococcal cassette chromosome mec identified in community-acquired methicillin-resistant *Staphylococcus aureus* strains. *Antimicrob Agents Chemother*. 2002;46:1147-1152.
124. Ito T, Ma XX, Takeuchi F, et al. Novel type V staphylococcal cassette chromosome mec driven by a novel cassette chromosome recombinase, ccrC. *Antimicrob Agents Chemother*. 2004;48:2637-2651.
125. Oliveira DC, Milheirico C, de Lencastre H. Redefining a structural variant of staphylococcal cassette chromosome mec, SCCmec type VI. *Antimicrob Agents Chemother*. 2006;50:3457-3459.
126. Diep BA, Gill SR, Chang RF, et al. Complete genome sequence of USA300, an epidemic clone of community-acquired meticillin-resistant *Staphylococcus aureus*. *Lancet*. 2006;367:731-739.
127. Diep BA, Stone GG, Basuino L, et al. The arginine catabolic mobile element and staphylococcal chromosomal cassette mec linkage: convergence of virulence and resistance in the USA300 clone of methicillin-resistant *Staphylococcus aureus*. *J Infect Dis*. 2008;197:1523-1530.
128. Nimmo GR, Bell JM, Mitchell D, et al. Antimicrobial resistance in *Staphylococcus aureus* in Australian teaching hospitals, 1989-1999. *Microb Drug Resist*. 2003;9:155-160.
129. Fowler VG Jr, Boucher HW, Corey GR, et al. Daptomycin versus standard therapy for bacteremia and endocarditis caused by *Staphylococcus aureus*. *N Engl J Med*. 2006;355:653-665.
130. Goffin C, Ghuysen JM. Multimodular penicillin-binding proteins: an enigmatic family of orthologs and paralogs. *Microbiol Mol Biol Rev*. 1998;62:1079-1093.
131. Gillespie MT, May JW, Skurray RA. Antibiotic resistance in *Staphylococcus aureus* isolated at an Australian hospital between 1946 and 1981. *J Med Microbiol*. 1985;19:137-147.
132. Jevons MP. "Celbenin"-resistant staphylococci. *Br Med J*. 1961;1:124-125.
133. Panlilio AL, Culver DH, Gaynes RP, et al. Methicillin-resistant *Staphylococcus aureus* in U.S. hospitals, 1975-1991. *Infect Control Hosp Epidemiol*. 1992;13:582-586.
134. Diekema DJ, Pfaller MA, Schmitz FJ, et al. Survey of infections due to *Staphylococcus* species: frequency of occurrence and antimicrobial susceptibility of isolates collected in the United States, Canada, Latin America, Europe, and the Western Pacific region for the SENTRY Antimicrobial Surveillance Program, 1997-1999. *Clin Infect Dis*. 2001;32:S114-S132.
135. Centers for Disease Control and Prevention. Public health dispatch: outbreaks of community-associated methicillin-resistant *Staphylococcus aureus* skin infections: Los Angeles County, California, 2002-2003. *JAMA*. 2003;289:1377.
136. Dietrich DW, Auld DB, Mermel LA. Community-acquired methicillin-resistant *Staphylococcus aureus* in southern New England children. *Pediatrics*. 2004;113:e347-e352.
137. Salgado CD, Farr BM, Calfee DP. Community-acquired methicillin-resistant *Staphylococcus aureus*: a meta-analysis of prevalence and risk factors. *Clin Infect Dis*. 2003;36:131-139.
138. Miller LG, Perdreau-Remington F, Rieg G, et al. Necrotizing fasciitis caused by community-associated methicillin-resistant *Staphylococcus aureus* in Los Angeles. *N Engl J Med*. 2005;352:1445-1453.
139. Labandeira-Rey M, Couzon F, Boisset S, et al. *Staphylococcus aureus* Panton-Valentine leukocidin causes necrotizing pneumonia. *Science*. 2007;315:1130-1133.
140. Voyich JM, Otto M, Mathema B, et al. Is Panton-Valentine leukocidin the major virulence determinant in community-associated methicillin-resistant *Staphylococcus aureus* disease? *J Infect Dis*. 2006;194:1761-1770.
141. Diep BA, Otto M. The role of virulence determinants in community-associated MRSA pathogenesis. *Trends Microbiol*. 2008;16:361-369.
142. de Jonge BL, Sidow T, Chang YS, et al. Altered muropeptide composition in *Staphylococcus aureus* strains with an inactivated femA locus. *J Bacteriol*. 1993;175:2779-2782.
143. de Lencastre H, Tomasz A. Reassessment of the number of auxiliary genes essential for expression of high-level methicillin resistance in *Staphylococcus aureus*. *Antimicrob Agents Chemother*. 1994;38:2590-2598.
144. Pinho MG, de Lencastre H, Tomasz A. An acquired and a native penicillin-binding protein cooperate in building the cell wall of drug-resistant staphylococci. *Proc Natl Acad Sci U S A*. 2001;98:10886-10891.
145. Lim D, Strynadka NC. Structural basis for the beta lactam resistance of PBP2a from methicillin-resistant *Staphylococcus aureus*. *Nat Struct Biol*. 2002;9:870-876.
146. Francioli M, Bille J, Glauser MP, et al. Beta-lactam resistance mechanisms of methicillin-resistant *Staphylococcus aureus*. *J Infect Dis*. 1991;163:514-523.
147. Que YA, Entenza JM, Francioli P, et al. The impact of penicillinase on cefamandole treatment and prophylaxis of experimental endocarditis due to methicillin-resistant *Staphylococcus aureus*. *J Infect Dis*. 1998;177:146-154.
148. Tomasz A. "Intelligence coup" for drug designers: crystal structure of *Staphylococcus aureus* beta-lactam resistance protein PBP2A. *Lancet*. 2003;361:795-796.
149. Guignard B, Entenza JM, Moreillon P. Beta-lactams against methicillin-resistant *Staphylococcus aureus*. *Curr Opin Pharmacol*. 2005;5:479-489.
150. Chang FY, Peacock JE Jr, Musher DM, et al. *Staphylococcus aureus* bacteremia: recurrence and the impact of antibiotic treatment in a prospective multicenter study. *Medicine (Baltimore)*. 2003;82:333-339.
151. Hiramatsu K, Aritaka N, Hanaki H, et al. Dissemination in Japanese hospitals of strains of *Staphylococcus aureus* heterogeneously resistant to vancomycin [see comments]. Comment in: Lancet 1997;351:601-602, Comment in: Lancet 1997;351:602, Comment in: Lancet 1997;350:1644-1645, Comment in: Lancet 1998;351:1212. *Lancet*. 1997;350:1670-1673.
152. Sieradzki K, Roberts RB, Haber SW, et al. The development of vancomycin resistance in a patient with methicillin-resistant *Staphylococcus aureus* infection. *N Engl J Med*. 1999;340:517-523.
153. Hiramatsu K, Hanaki H, Ino T, et al. Methicillin-resistant *Staphylococcus aureus* clinical strain with reduced vancomycin susceptibility. *J Antimicrob Chemother*. 1997;40:135-136.
154. Hiramatsu K, Aritaka N, Hanaki H, et al. Dissemination in Japanese hospitals of strains of *Staphylococcus aureus* heterogeneously resistant to vancomycin. *Lancet*. 1997;350:1670-1673.
155. Charles PG, Ward PB, Johnson PD, et al. Clinical features associated with bacteremia due to heterogeneous vancomycin-intermediate *Staphylococcus aureus*. *Clin Infect Dis*. 2004;38:448-451.
156. Soriano A, Marco F, Martinez JA, et al. Influence of vancomycin minimum inhibitory concentration on the treatment of methicillin-resistant *Staphylococcus aureus* bacteremia. *Clin Infect Dis*. 2008;46:193-200.
157. Institute CaLS. Methods for dilution antimicrobial susceptibility tests for bacteria that grow aerobically. In: CLSI, ed. *Approved standards CLSA document M7-A7*. ed 7. Wayne, PA: Clinical Laboratory Standards Institute; 2006.
158. Pereira PM, Filipe SR, Tomasz A, et al. Fluorescence ratio imaging microscopy shows decreased access of vancomycin to cell wall synthetic sites in vancomycin-resistant *Staphylococcus aureus*. *Antimicrob Agents Chemother*. 2007;51:3627-3633.

159. Neoh HM, Cui L, Yuzawa H, et al. Mutated response regulator graR is responsible for phenotypic conversion of *Staphylococcus aureus* from heterogeneous vancomycin-intermediate resistance to vancomycin-intermediate resistance. *Antimicrob Agents Chemother.* 2008;52:45-53.
160. Howden BP, Stinear TP, Allen DL, et al. Genomic analysis reveals a point mutation in the two-component sensor gene graS that leads to intermediate vancomycin resistance in clinical *Staphylococcus aureus. Antimicrob Agents Chemother.* 2008;52: 3755-3762.
161. Yusof A, Engelhardt A, Karlsson A, et al. Evaluation of a new Etest vancomycin-teicoplanin strip for detection of glycopeptide-intermediate *Staphylococcus aureus* (GISA), in particular, heterogeneous GISA. *J Clin Microbiol.* 2008;46:3042-3047.
162. Arthur M, Courvalin P. Genetics and mechanisms of glycopeptide resistance in enterococci. *Antimicrob Agents Chemother.* 1993;37:1563-1571.
163. Noble WC, Virani Z, Cree RG. Co-transfer of vancomycin and other resistance genes from *Enterococcus faecalis* NCTC 12201 to *Staphylococcus aureus. FEMS Microbiol Lett.* 1992;72: 195-198.
164. Sievert DM, Rudrik JT, Patel JB, et al. Vancomycin-resistant *Staphylococcus aureus* in the United States, 2002-2006. *Clin Infect Dis.* 2008;46:668-674.
165. Centers for Disease Control. Vancomycin-resistant *Staphylococcus aureus*: New York, 2004. *MMWR Morb Mortal Wkly Rep.* 2004;53:322-323.
166. Aligholi M, Emaneini M, Jabalameli F, et al. Emergence of high-level vancomycin-resistant *Staphylococcus aureus* in the Imam Khomeini Hospital in Tehran. *Med Princ Pract.* 2008;17:432-434.
167. Scott WR, Baek SB, Jung D, et al. NMR structural studies of the antibiotic lipopeptide daptomycin in DHPC micelles. *Biochim Biophys Acta.* 2007;1768:3116-3126.
168. Baltz RH, Miao V, Wrigley SK. Natural products to drugs: daptomycin and related lipopeptide antibiotics. *Nat Prod Rep.* 2005;22:717-741.
169. Levine DP, Lamp KC. Daptomycin in the treatment of patients with infective endocarditis: experience from a registry. *Am J Med.* 2007;120:S28-S33.
170. Silverman JA, Mortin LI, Vanpraagh AD, et al. Inhibition of daptomycin by pulmonary surfactant: in vitro modeling and clinical impact. *J Infect Dis.* 2005;191:2149-2152.
171. Rose WE, Leonard SN, Sakoulas G, et al. Daptomycin activity against *Staphylococcus aureus* following vancomycin exposure in an in vitro pharmacodynamic model with simulated endocardial vegetations. *Antimicrob Agents Chemother.* 2008;52: 831-836.
172. Patel JB, Jevitt LA, Hageman J, et al. An association between reduced susceptibility to daptomycin and reduced susceptibility to vancomycin in *Staphylococcus aureus. Clin Infect Dis.* 2006;42:1652-1653.
173. Cui L, Tominaga E, Neoh HM, Hiramatsu K. Correlation between reduced daptomycin susceptibility and vancomycin resistance in vancomycin-intermediate *Staphylococcus aureus. Antimicrob Agents Chemother.* 2006;50:1079-1082.
174. Friedman L, Alder JD, Silverman JA. Genetic changes that correlate with reduced susceptibility to daptomycin in *Staphylococcus aureus. Antimicrob Agents Chemother.* 2006;50:2137-2145.
175. Camargo IL, Neoh HM, Cui L, et al. Serial daptomycin selection generates daptomycin-nonsusceptible *Staphylococcus aureus* strains with a heterogeneous vancomycin-intermediate phenotype. *Antimicrob Agents Chemother.* 2008;52:4289-4299.
176. Weisblum B. Erythromycin resistance by ribosome modification. *Antimicrob Agents Chemother.* 1995;39:577-585.
177. Levin TP, Suh B, Axelrod P, et al. Potential clindamycin resistance in clindamycin-susceptible, erythromycin-resistant *Staphylococcus aureus*: report of a clinical failure. *Antimicrob Agents Chemother.* 2005;49:1222-1224.
178. Ross JI, Eady EA, Cove JH, et al. Identification of a chromosomally encoded ABC-transport system with which the staphylococcal erythromycin exporter MsrA may interact. *Gene.* 1995;153: 93-98.
179. Clancy J, Petitpas J, Dib-Hajj F, et al. Molecular cloning and functional analysis of a novel macrolide-resistance determinant, mefA, from *Streptococcus pyogenes. Mol Microbiol.* 1996;22: 867-879.
180. Linezolid vs Vancomycin: Analysis of two double-blind studies of patients with methicillin-resistant *Staphylococcus aureus* Nosocomial Pneumonia. (2003).
181. Falagas ME, Manta KG, Ntziora F, et al. Linezolid for the treatment of patients with endocarditis: a systematic review of the published evidence. *J Antimicrob Chemother.* 2006;58:273-280.
182. Chen CJ, Chiu CH, Lin TY, et al. Experience with linezolid therapy in children with osteoarticular infections. *Pediatr Infect Dis J.* 2007;26:985-988.
183. Stevens DL, Ma Y, Salmi DB, et al. Impact of antibiotics on expression of virulence-associated exotoxin genes in methicillin-sensitive and methicillin-resistant *Staphylococcus aureus. J Infect Dis.* 2007;195:202-211.
184. Beekmann SE, Gilbert DN, Polgreen PM. Toxicity of extended courses of linezolid: results of an Infectious Diseases Society of America Emerging Infections Network survey. *Diagn Microbiol Infect Dis.* 2008;62:407-410.
185. Meka VG, Gold HS. Antimicrobial resistance to linezolid. *Clin Infect Dis.* 2004;39:1010-1015.
186. Mendes RE, Deshpande LM, Castanheira M, et al. First report of cfr-mediated resistance to linezolid in human staphylococcal clinical isolates recovered in the United States. *Antimicrob Agents Chemother.* 2008;52:2244-2246.
187. Dholakia N, Rolston KV, Ho DH, et al. Susceptibilities of bacterial isolates from patients with cancer to levofloxacin and other quinolones. *AntimicrobialAgents & Chemotherapy.* 1994;38: 848-852.
188. Jacoby GA. Mechanisms of resistance to quinolones. *Clin Infect Dis.* 2005;41:S120-S126.
189. Arsene S, Leclercq R. Role of a qnr-like gene in the intrinsic resistance of *Enterococcus faecalis* to fluoroquinolones. *Antimicrob Agents Chemother.* 2007;51:3254-3258.
190. Yoshida H, Bogaki M, Nakamura S, et al. Nucleotide sequence and characterization of the *Staphylococcus aureus* norA gene, which confers resistance to quinolones. *J Bacteriol.* 1990; 172:6942-6949.
191. Fournier B, Hooper DC. Mutations in topoisomerase IV and DNA gyrase of *Staphylococcus aureus*: novel pleiotropic effects on quinolone and coumarin activity. *Antimicrobial Agents Chemother.* 1998;42:121-128.
192. Entenza JM, Vouillamoz J, Glauser MP, et al. Levofloxacin versus ciprofloxacin, flucloxacillin, or vancomycin for treatment of experimental endocarditis due to methicillin-susceptible or -resistant *Staphylococcus aureus. Antimicrob Agents Chemother.* 1997;41:1662-1667.
193. Craig WA. Does the dose matter? *Clin Infect Dis.* 2001;33: S233-S237.
194. Cui J, Liu Y, Wang R, et al. The mutant selection window in rabbits infected with *Staphylococcus aureus. J Infect Dis.* 2006; 194:1601-1608.
195. Moise PA, Schentag JJ. Vancomycin treatment failures in *Staphylococcus aureus* lower respiratory tract infections. *Int J Antimicrob Agents.* 2000;16:S31-S34.
196. Falagas ME, Matthaiou DK, Bliziotis IA. The role of aminoglycosides in combination with a beta-lactam for the treatment of bacterial endocarditis: a meta-analysis of comparative trials. *J Antimicrob Chemother.* 2006;57:639-647.
197. Levine DP, Fromm BS, Reddy BR. Slow response to vancomycin or vancomycin plus rifampin in methicillin-resistant *Staphylococcus aureus* endocarditis. *Ann Intern Med.* 1991;115:674-680.
198. Cocito C, Di Giambattista M, Nyssen E, et al. Inhibition of protein synthesis by streptogramins and related antibiotics. [Review]. *J AntimicrobialChemother.* 1997;39:13.
199. Vouillamoz J, Entenza JM, Feger C, et al. Quinupristin-dalfopristin combined with beta-lactams for treatment of experimental endocarditis due to *Staphylococcus aureus* constitutively resistant to macrolide-lincosamide-streptogramin B antibiotics. *Antimicrob Agents Chemother.* 2000;44:1789-1795.
200. Chopra I. Glycylcyclines: third-generation tetracycline antibiotics. *Curr Opin Pharmacol.* 2001;1:464-469.
201. Fuda C, Hesek D, Lee M, et al. Mechanistic basis for the action of new cephalosporin antibiotics effective against methicillin- and vancomycin-resistant *Staphylococcus aureus. J Biol Chem.* 2006;281:10035-10041.
202. Deresinski SC. The efficacy and safety of ceftobiprole in the treatment of complicated skin and skin structure infections: evidence from 2 clinical trials. *Diagn Microbiol Infect Dis.* 2008;61:103-109.
203. Climo MW, Patron RL, Archer GL. Combinations of vancomycin and beta-lactams are synergistic against staphylococci with reduced susceptibilities to vancomycin. *Antimicrob Agents Chemother.* 1999;43:1747-1753.
204. Perichon B, Courvalin P. Synergism between beta-lactams and glycopeptides against VanA-type methicillin-resistant *Staphylococcus aureus* and heterologous expression of the vanA operon. *Antimicrob Agents Chemother.* 2006;50:3622-3630.
205. Billeter M, Zervos MJ, Chen AY, et al. Dalbavancin: a novel once-weekly lipoglycopeptide antibiotic. *Clin Infect Dis.* 2008; 46:577-583.
206. Allen NE, Nicas TI. Mechanism of action of oritavancin and related glycopeptide antibiotics. *FEMS Microbiol Rev.* 2003;26: 511-532.
207. Jauregui LE, Babazadeh S, Seltzer E, et al. Randomized, double-blind comparison of once-weekly dalbavancin versus twice-daily linezolid therapy for the treatment of complicated skin and skin structure infections. *Clin Infect Dis.* 2005;41: 1407-1415.
208. Mann NH. The potential of phages to prevent MRSA infections. *Res Microbiol.* 2008;159:400-405.
209. Maresso AW, Schneewind O. Sortase as a target of anti-infective therapy. *Pharmacol Rev.* 2008;60:128-141.
210. Projan SJ, Nesin M, Dunman PM. Staphylococcal vaccines and immunotherapy: to dream the impossible dream? *Curr Opin Pharmacol.* 2006;6:473-479.
211. Jacobsson G, Dashti S, Wahlberg T, et al. The epidemiology of and risk factors for invasive *Staphylococcus aureus* infections in western Sweden. *Scand J Infect Dis.* 2007;39:6-13.
212. National trends in *Staphylococcus aureus* infection rates: impact on economic burden and mortality over a 6-year period (1998-2003). (2007).
213. The burden of *Staphylococcus aureus* infections on hospitals in the United States: an analysis of the 2000 and 2001 Nationwide Inpatient Sample Database. (2005).
214. Mylotte JM, Tayara A. *Staphylococcus aureus* bacteremia: predictors of 30-day mortality in a large cohort. *Clin Infect Dis.* 2000;31:1170-1174.
215. Nosocomial bloodstream infections in US hospitals: analysis of 24,179 cases from a prospective nationwide surveillance study. (2004).
216. The impact of methicillin resistance in *Staphylococcus aureus* bacteremia on patient outcomes: mortality, length of stay, and hospital charges. (2005).
217. NHSN annual update: antimicrobial-resistant pathogens associated with healthcare-associated infections: annual summary of data reported to the National Healthcare Safety Network at the Centers for Disease Control and Prevention, 2006-2007. (2008).
218. Antimicrobial-resistant pathogens in intensive care units in Canada: results of the Canadian National Intensive Care Unit (CAN-ICU) study, 2005-2006. (2008).
219. Hoban DJ, Biedenbach DJ, Mutnick AH, et al. Pathogen of occurrence and susceptibility patterns associated with pneumonia in hospitalized patients in North America: results of the SENTRY Antimicrobial Surveillance Study (2000). *Diagn Microbiol Infect Dis.* 2003;45:279-285.
220. *Staphylococcus aureus* endocarditis: a consequence of medical progress. (2005).
221. Infective endocarditis. (2004).
222. Tice AD, Hoaglund PA, Shoultz DA. Risk factors and treatment outcomes in osteomyelitis. *J Antimicrob Chemother.* 2003;51: 1261-1268.
223. Blyth MJ, Kincaid R, Craigen MA, et al. The changing epidemiology of acute and subacute haematogenous osteomyelitis in children. *J Bone Joint Surg Br.* 2001;83:99-102.
224. Laupland KB, Gregson DB, Flemons WW, et al. Burden of community-onset bloodstream infection: a population-based assessment. *Epidemiol Infect.* 2007;135:1037-1042.
225. Mupirocin ointment for preventing *Staphylococcus aureus* infections in nasal carriers. (2008).
226. Emergence and resurgence of meticillin-resistant *Staphylococcus aureus* as a public-health threat. (2006).
227. Antimicrobial resistance trends and outbreak frequency in United States hospitals. (2004).
228. Changes in the epidemiology of methicillin-resistant *Staphylococcus aureus* in intensive care units in US hospitals, 1992-2003. (2006).
229. Shorr AF, Micek ST, Kollef MH. Inappropriate therapy for methicillin-resistant *Staphylococcus aureus*: resource utilization and cost implications. *Crit Care Med.* 2008;36:2335-2340.
230. Methicillin-resistant *S. aureus* infections among patients in the emergency department. (2006).
231. Epidemiology of methicillin-resistant *Staphylococcus aureus.* (2008).
232. Seybold U, Kourbatova EV, Johnson JG, et al. Emergence of community-associated methicillin-resistant *Staphylococcus aureus* USA300 genotype as a major cause of health care-associated blood stream infections. *Clin Infect Dis.* 2006;42:647-656.
233. Davis SL, Rybak MJ, Amjad M, et al. Characteristics of patients with healthcare-associated infection due to SCCmec type IV methicillin-resistant *Staphylococcus aureus. Infect Control Hosp Epidemiol.* 2006;27:1025-1031.
234. Kluytmans J, van Belkum A, Verbrugh H. Nasal carriage of *Staphylococcus aureus*: epidemiology, underlying mechanisms, and associated risks. *Clin Microbiol Rev.* 1997;10:505-520.
235. Risk and outcome of nosocomial *Staphylococcus aureus* bacteraemia in nasal carriers versus non-carriers. (2004).
236. Walsh EJ, O'Brien LM, Liang X, et al. Clumping factor B, a fibrinogen-binding MSCRAMM (microbial surface components recognizing adhesive matrix molecules) adhesin of Staphylococcus aureus, also binds to the tail region of type I cytokeratin 10. *J Biol Chem.* 2004;279:50691-50699.
237. Role of teichoic acids in *Staphylococcus aureus* nasal colonization, a major risk factor in nosocomial infections. (2004).
238. Determinants of acquisition and carriage of *Staphylococcus aureus* in infancy. (2003).
239. Dynamics and Determinants of *Staphylococcus aureus* Carriage in Infancy. The Generation R Study. (2008).
240. Colonisation by *Streptococcus pneumoniae* and *Staphylococcus aureus* in healthy children. (2004).
241. Prevalence of *Staphylococcus aureus* nasal colonization in the United States, 2001-2002. (2006).
242. Changes in the prevalence of nasal colonization with *Staphylococcus aureus* in the United States, 2001-2004. (2008).
243. Pittet D, Hugonnet S, Harbarth S, et al. Effectiveness of a hospital-wide programme to improve compliance with hand hygiene. Infection Control Programme. *Lancet.* 2000;356: 1307-1312.
244. Spread of methicillin-resistant *Staphylococcus aureus* (MRSA) among household contacts of individuals with nosocomially acquired MRSA. (2003).
245. Lucet JC, Chevret S, Durand-Zaleski I, et al. Prevalence and risk factors for carriage of methicillin-resistant *Staphylococcus aureus* at admission to the intensive care unit: results of a multicenter study. *Arch Intern Med.* 2003;163:181-188.
246. Control of endemic methicillin-resistant *Staphylococcus aureus*—recent advances and future challenges. (2006).
247. Overcrowding and understaffing in modern health-care systems: key determinants in meticillin-resistant *Staphylococcus aureus* transmission. (2008).
248. Wernitz MH, Swidsinski S, Weist K, et al. Effectiveness of a hospital-wide selective screening programme for methicillin-resistant *Staphylococcus aureus* (MRSA) carriers at hospital admission to prevent hospital-acquired MRSA infections. *Clin Microbiol Infect.* 2005;11(6):457-465.
249. 2007 Guideline for Isolation Precautions: Preventing Transmission of Infectious Agents in Health Care Settings. (2007).

250. Guidelines for the control and prevention of meticillin-resistant *Staphylococcus aureus* (MRSA) in healthcare facilities. (2006).
251. Management of multidrug-resistant organisms in health care settings, 2006. (2007).
252. Health-care workers: source, vector, or victim of MRSA? (2008).
253. Fernandez C, Gaspar C, Torrellas A, et al. A double-blind, randomized, placebo-controlled clinical trial to evaluate the safety and efficacy of mupirocin calcium ointment for eliminating nasal carriage of *Staphylococcus aureus* among hospital personnel. *J Antimicrob Chemother.* 1995;35:399-408.
254. Laupland KB, Conly JM. Treatment of *Staphylococcus aureus* colonization and prophylaxis for infection with topical intranasal mupirocin: an evidence-based review. *Clin Infect Dis.* 2003;37:933-938.
255. Walker ES, Vasquez JE, Dula R, et al. Mupirocin-resistant, methicillin-resistant *Staphylococcus aureus*: does mupirocin remain effective? *Infect Control Hosp Epidemiol.* 2003;24: 342-346.
256. Loeb M, Main C, Walker-Dilks C, Eady A. Antimicrobial drugs for treating methicillin-resistant *Staphylococcus aureus* colonization. Cochrane Database Syst Rev. 2003: CD003340.
257. Kokai-Kun JF, Walsh SM, Chanturiya T, Mond JJ. Lysostaphin cream eradicates *Staphylococcus aureus* nasal colonization in a cotton rat model. *Antimicrob Agents Chemother.* 2003;47: 1589-1597.
258. Halcón L, Mikus K. *Staphylococcus aureus* and wounds: a review of tea tree oil as a promising antimicrobial. *Am J Infect Control.* 2004;32:402-408.
259. Frazee BW, Lynn J, Charlebois ED, et al. High prevalence of methicillin-resistant *Staphylococcus aureus* in emergency department skin and soft tissue infections. *Ann Emerg Med.* 2005;45:311-320.
260. Zetola N, Francis JS, Nuermberger EL, et al. Community-acquired methicillin-resistant *Staphylococcus aureus*: an emerging threat. *Lancet Infect Dis.* 2005;5:275-286.
261. Wilson MA. Skin and soft-tissue infections: impact of resistant gram-positive bacteria. *Am J Surg.* 2003;186:35S-41S; discussion 2S-3S, 61S-64S.
262. van Rijen MM, Bonten M, Wenzel RP, Kluytmans JA. Intranasal mupirocin for reduction of *Staphylococcus aureus* infections in surgical patients with nasal carriage: a systematic review. *J Antimicrob Chemother.* 2008;61:254-261.
263. Eggimann P, Sax H, Pittet D. Catheter-related infections. *Microbes Infect.* 2004;6:1033-1042.
264. McGowan JE Jr, Barnes MW, Finland M. Bacteremia at Boston City Hospital: Occurrence and mortality during 12 selected years (1935-1972), with special reference to hospital-acquired cases. *J Infect Dis.* 1975;132:316-335.
265. Rodríguez-Créixems M, Alcalá L, Muñoz P, et al. Bloodstream infections: evolution and trends in the microbiology workload, incidence, and etiology, 1985-2006. *Medicine (Baltimore).* 2008;87:234-249.
266. Uslan DZ, Crane SJ, Steckelberg JM, et al. Age- and sex-associated trends in bloodstream infection: a population-based study in Olmsted County, Minnesota. *Arch Intern Med.* 2007;167:834-839.
267. Benfield T, Espersen F, Frimodt-Møller N, et al. Increasing incidence but decreasing in-hospital mortality of adult *Staphylococcus aureus* bacteraemia between 1981 and 2000. *Clin Microbiol Infect.* 2007;13:257-263.
268. Laupland KB, Ross T, Gregson DB. *Staphylococcus aureus* bloodstream infections: risk factors, outcomes, and the influence of methicillin resistance in Calgary, Canada, 2000-2006. *J Infect Dis.* 2008;198:336-343.
269. Tsigrelis C, Armstrong MD, Vlahakis NE, et al. Infective endocarditis due to community-associated methicillin-resistant *Staphylococcus aureus* in injection drug users may be associated with Panton-Valentine leukocidin-negative strains. *Scand J Infect Dis.* 2007;39:299-302.
270. Ellington MJ, Hope R, Ganner M, et al. Is Panton-Valentine leucocidin associated with the pathogenesis of *Staphylococcus aureus* bacteraemia in the UK? *J Antimicrob Chemother.* 2007;60:402-405.
271. Gouello JP, Asfar P, Brenet O, et al. Nosocomial endocarditis in the intensive care unit: an analysis of 22 cases. *Crit Care Med.* 2000;28:377-382.
272. Chang FY, MacDonald BB, Peacock JE Jr, et al. A prospective multicenter study of *Staphylococcus aureus* bacteremia: incidence of endocarditis, risk factors for mortality, and clinical impact of methicillin resistance. *Medicine (Baltimore).* 2003;82:322-332.
273. Baddour LM, Wilson WR, Bayer AS, et al. Infective endocarditis: diagnosis, antimicrobial therapy, and management of complications: a statement for healthcare professionals form the Committee on Rheumatic Fever, Endocarditis, and Kawasaki Disease, Council on Cardiovascular Disease in the Young, and the Councils on Clinical Cardiology, Stroke, and Cardiovascular Surgery and Anesthesia, American Heart Association: endorsed by the Infectious Diseases Society of America. *Circulation.* 2005;111:e394-e434.
274. Cosgrove SE, Fowler VG Jr. Management of methicillin-resistant *Staphylococcus aureus* bacteremia. *Clin Infect Dis.* 2008;46:S386-S393.
275. Fowler VG Jr, Olsen MK, Corey GR, et al. Clinical identifiers of complicated *Staphylococcus aureus* bacteremia. *Arch Intern Med.* 2003;163:2066-2072.
276. Berrington A, Gould FK. Use of antibiotic locks to treat colonized central venous catheters. *J Antimicrob Chemother.* 2001;48:597-603.
277. Wang A, Athan E, Pappas PA, et al. Contemporary clinical profile and outcome of prosthetic valve endocarditis. *JAMA.* 2007;297:1354-1361.
278. Kamalakannan D, Pai RM, Johnson LB, et al. Epidemiology and clinical outcomes of infective endocarditis in hemodialysis patients. *Ann Thorac Surg.* 2007;83:2081-2086.
279. Fowler VG Jr, Miro JM, Hoen B, et al. *Staphylococcus aureus* endocarditis: a consequence of medical progress. *JAMA.* 2005;293:3012-3021.
280. Moreillon P, Que YA, Bayer AS. Pathogenesis of streptococcal and staphylococcal endocarditis. *Infect Dis Clin North Am.* 2002;16:297-318.
281. Que Y, Haefliger J, Francioli P, et al. Expression of *Staphylococcus aureus* clumping-factor A in *Lactococcus lactis cremoris* using a new shuttle vector. *Infect Immun.* 2000;68:3516-3522.
282. Que YA, François P, Haefliger JA, et al. Reassessing the role of *Staphylococcus aureus* clumping-factor and fibronectin-binding protein by expression in *Lactococcus lactis. Infect Immun.* 2001;69:6296-6302.
283. Wann ER, Gurusiddappa S, Hook M. The fibronectin-binding MSCRAMM FnbpA of *Staphylococcus aureus* is a bifunctional protein that also binds to fibrinogen. *J Biol Chem.* 2000;275: 13863-13871.
284. Roche FM, Downer R, Keane F, et al. The N-terminal A domain of fibronectin-binding proteins A and B promotes adhesion of *Staphylococcus aureus* to elastin. *J Biol Chem.* 2004;279: 38433-38440.
285. Sinha B, François P, Nuesse O, et al. Fibronectin-binding protein acts as *Staphylococcus aureus* invasin via fibronectin bridging to integrin α_5–β_1. *Cellular Microbiology.* 1999;1: 101-117.
286. Sinha B, Francois P, Que YA, et al. Heterologously expressed *Staphylococcus aureus* fibronectin-binding proteins are sufficient for invasion of host cells. *Infect Immun.* 2000;68:6871-6878.
287. Yeaman MR. The role of platelets in antimicrobial host defense. *Clin Infect Dis.* 1997;25:951-968; quiz 69-70.
288. Fowler VG Jr, McIntyre LM, et al. In vitro resistance to thrombin-induced platelet microbicidal protein in isolates of *Staphylococcus aureus* from endocarditis patients correlates with an intravascular device source. *J Infect Dis.* 2000;182:1251-1254.
289. Bayer AS, Prasad R, Chandra J, et al. In vitro resistance of *Staphylococcus aureus* to thrombin-induced platelet microbicidal protein is associated with alterations in cytoplasmic membrane fluidity. *Infect Immun.* 2000;68:3548-3553.
290. Bayer AS, McNamara P, Yeaman MR, et al. Transposon disruption of the complex I NADH oxidoreductase gene (snoD) in *Staphylococcus aureus* is associated with reduced susceptibility to the microbicidal activity of thrombin-induced platelet microbicidal protein 1. *J Bacteriol.* 2006;188:211-222.
291. Kupferwasser LI, Skurray RA, Brown MH, et al. Plasmid-mediated resistance to thrombin-induced platelet microbicidal protein in staphylococci: role of the qacA locus. *Antimicrob Agents Chemother.* 1999;43:2395-2399.
292. Bayer AS, Kupferwasser LI, Brown MH, et al. Low-level resistance of *Staphylococcus aureus* to thrombin-induced platelet microbicidal protein 1 in vitro associated with qacA gene carriage is independent of multidrug efflux pump activity. *Antimicrob Agents Chemother.* 2006;50:2448-2454.
293. O'Brien L, Kerrigan SW, Kaw G, et al. Multiple mechanisms for the activation of human platelet aggregation by *Staphylococcus aureus*: roles for the clumping factors ClfA and ClfB, the serine-aspartate repeat protein SdrE and protein A. *Mol Microbiol.* 2002;44:1033-1044.
294. Siboo IR, Chambers HF, Sullam PM. Role of SraP, a serine-rich surface protein of *Staphylococcus aureus*, in binding to human platelets. *Infect Immun.* 2005;73:2273-2280.
295. Fitzgerald JR, Foster TJ, Cox D. The interaction of bacterial pathogens with platelets. *Nat Rev Microbiol.* 2006;4:445-457.
296. Fitzgerald JR, Foster TJ, Cox D. The interaction of bacterial pathogens with platelets. *Nat Rev Microbiol.* 2006;4:445-457.
297. Kupferwasser LI, Yeaman MR, Shapiro SM, et al. Acetylsalicylic acid reduces vegetation bacterial density, hematogenous bacterial dissemination, and frequency of embolic events in experimental *Staphylococcus aureus* endocarditis through antiplatelet and antibacterial effects. *Circulation.* 1999;99:2791-2797.
298. Chan KL, Dumesnil JG, Cujec B, et al. A randomized trial of aspirin on the risk of embolic events in patients with infective endocarditis. *J Am Coll Cardiol.* 2003;42:775-780.
299. Tornos P, Almirante B, Mirabet S, et al. Infective endocarditis due to *Staphylococcus aureus*: deleterious effect of anticoagulant therapy. *Arch Intern Med.* 1999;159:473-475.
300. Miro JM, Moreno A, Mestres CA. Infective endocarditis in intravenous drug abusers. *Curr Infect Dis Rep.* 2003;5: 307-316.
301. Heldman AW, Hartert TV, Ray SC, et al. Oral antibiotic treatment of right-sided staphylococcal endocarditis in injection drug users: prospective randomized comparison with parenteral therapy. *Am J Med.* 1996;101:68-76.
302. Hussein AS, Shafran SD. Acute bacterial meningitis in adults. A 12-year review. *Medicine (Baltimore).* 2000;79:360-368.
303. Jensen AG, Espersen F, Skinhoj P, et al. Staphylococcus aureus meningitis. A review of 104 nationwide, consecutive cases. *Arch Intern Med.* 1993;153:1902-1908.
304. Pintado V, Meseguer MA, Fortun J, et al. Clinical study of 44 cases of *Staphylococcus aureus* meningitis. *Eur J Clin Microbiol Infect Dis.* 2002;21:864-868.
305. Pedersen M, Benfield TL, Skinhoej P, et al. Haematogenous *Staphylococcus aureus* meningitis. A 10-year nationwide study of 96 consecutive cases. *BMC Infect Dis.* 2006;6:49.
306. Klacsmann PG, Bulkley BH, Hutchins GM. The changed spectrum of purulent pericarditis: an 86 year autopsy experience in 200 patients. *Am J Med.* 1977;63:666-673.
307. File TM. Community-acquired pneumonia. *Lancet.* 2003;362: 1991-2001.
308. Weber DJ, Rutala WA, Sickbert-Bennett EE, et al. Microbiology of ventilator-associated pneumonia compared with that of hospital-acquired pneumonia. *Infect Control Hosp Epidemiol.* 2007;28:825-831.
309. Sethi S. Bacterial pneumonia. Managing a deadly complication of influenza in older adults with comorbid disease. *Geriatrics.* 2002;57:56-61.
310. Lynch JP III. Hospital-acquired pneumonia: risk factors, microbiology, and treatment. *Chest.* 2001;119:373S-384S.
311. Morgan MS. Diagnosis and treatment of Panton-Valentine leukocidin (PVL)-associated staphylococcal pneumonia. *Int J Antimicrob Agents.* 2007;30:289-296.
312. Gillet Y, Vanhems P, Lina G, et al. Factors predicting mortality in necrotizing community-acquired pneumonia caused by *Staphylococcus aureus* containing Panton-Valentine leukocidin. *Clin Infect Dis.* 2007;45:315-321.
313. Bryant RE, Salmon CJ. Pleural empyema. *Clin Infect Dis.* 1996;22:747-762; quiz 63-64.
314. Rubinstein E, Kollef MH, Nathwani D. Pneumonia caused by methicillin-resistant *Staphylococcus aureus. Clin Infect Dis.* 2008;46:S378-S385.
315. Chastre J, Wolff M, Fagon JY, et al. Comparison of 8 vs 15 days of antibiotic therapy for ventilator-associated pneumonia in adults: a randomized trial. *JAMA.* 2003;290:2588-2598.
316. White M, Dennison WM. Acute heamatogeneous osteitis in childhood: a review of 212 cases. *J Bone Joint Surg (Br).* 1952;34-B:608-623.
317. Martinez-Aguilar G, Avalos-Mishaan A, Hulten K, et al. Community-acquired, methicillin-resistant and methicillin-susceptible *Staphylococcus aureus* musculoskeletal infections in children. *Pediatr Infect Dis J.* 2004;23:701-706.
318. Goergens ED, McEvoy A, Watson M, et al. Acute osteomyelitis and septic arthritis in children. *J Paediatr Child Health.* 2005;41:59-62.
319. Gafur OA, Copley LA, Hollmig ST, et al. The impact of the current epidemiology of pediatric musculoskeletal infection on evaluation and treatment guidelines. *J Pediatr Orthop.* 2008;28:777-785.
320. Arnold SR, Elias D, Buckingham SC, et al. Changing patterns of acute hematogenous osteomyelitis and septic arthritis: emergence of community-associated methicillin-resistant *Staphylococcus aureus. J Pediatr Orthop.* 2006;26:703-708.
321. Blevins JS, Elasri MO, Allmendinger SD, et al. Role of sarA in the pathogenesis of *Staphylococcus aureus* musculoskeletal infection. *Infect Immun.* 2003;71:516-523.
322. Cunha BA. Osteomyelitis in elderly patients. *Clin Infect Dis.* 2002;35:287-293.
323. Grayson ML, Gibbons GW, Balogh K, et al. Probing to bone in infected pedal ulcers. A clinical sign of underlying osteomyelitis in diabetic patients. *JAMA.* 1995;273:721-723.
324. Trampuz A, Zimmerli W. Prosthetic joint infections: update in diagnosis and treatment. *Swiss Med Wkly.* 2005;135:243-251.
325. Ainscow DA, Denham RA. The risk of haematogenous infection in total joint replacements. *J Bone Joint Surg Br.* 1984;66: 580-582.
326. Zimmerli W, Trampuz A, Ochsner PE. Prosthetic-joint infections. *N Engl J Med.* 2004;351:1645-1654.
327. Malamitsi J, Giamarellou H, Kanellakopoulou K, et al. Infecton: a 99mTc-ciprofloxacin radiopharmaceutical for the detection of bone infection. *Clin Microbiol Infect.* 2003;9:101-109.
328. von Eiff C, Bettin D, Proctor RA, et al. Recovery of small colony variants of *Staphylococcus aureus* following gentamicin bead placement for osteomyelitis. *Clin Infect Dis.* 1997;25:1250-1251.
329. Stengel D, Bauwens K, Sehouli J, et al. Systematic review and meta-analysis of antibiotic therapy for bone and joint infections. *Lancet Infect Dis.* 2001;1:175-188.
330. Vinod MB, Matussek J, Curtis N, et al. Duration of antibiotics in children with osteomyelitis and septic arthritis. *J Paediatr Child Health.* 2002;38:363-367.
331. Guglielmo BJ, Luber AD, Paletta D Jr, et al. Ceftriaxone therapy for staphylococcal osteomyelitis: a review. *Clin Infect Dis.* 2000;30:205-207.
332. Annane D, Aegerter P, Jars-Guincestre MC, et al. Current epidemiology of septic shock: the CUB-Rea Network. *Am J Respir Crit Care Med.* 2003;168:165-172.
333. Shirtliff ME, Mader JT. Acute septic arthritis. *Clin Microbiol Rev.* 2002;15:527-544.
334. Broy SB, Schmid FR. A comparison of medical drainage (needle aspiration) and surgical drainage (arthrotomy or arthroscopy) in the initial treatment of infected joints. *Clin Rheum Dis.* 1986;12:501-522.
335. Zimmermann B III, Mikolich DJ, Ho G Jr. Septic bursitis. *Semin Arthritis Rheum.* 1995;24:391-410.
336. Bickels J, Ben-Sira L, Kessler A, et al. Primary pyomyositis. *J Bone Joint Surg Am.* 2002;84-A:2277-2286.
337. Clarke S, Foster S. Surface adhesins of *Staphylococcus aureus. Adv Microb Physiol.* 2006;51:187-224.
338. Dedent A, Marraffini L, Schneewind O. Staphylococcal sortases and surface proteins. In: Fischetti V, Novick RP, Ferretti J, et al, eds. *Gram-positive pathogens.* ed 2. Washington, DC: ASM Press; 2006:486-495.

196

Staphylococcus epidermidis and Other Coagulase-Negative Staphylococci

MARK E. RUPP | PAUL D. FEY

Coagulase-negative staphylococci, with over 40 recognized species and subspecies, are the most abundant microbes inhabiting normal human skin and mucous membranes. They infrequently cause primary invasive disease and are most commonly encountered by clinicians as contaminants of microbiological cultures. However, because of relatively recent changes in the practice of medicine and changes in underlying host populations, coagulase-negative staphylococci, most notably *Staphylococcus epidermidis*, have arisen to become formidable pathogens.[1] At the present time, *S. epidermidis* is the most common cause of primary bacteremia and is frequently encountered in infections of indwelling medical devices.[2,3] *S. epidermidis* owes its pathogenic success to two major features—its natural niche on human skin, thus resulting in ready access to any device inserted or implanted across the skin, and its ability to adhere to biomaterials and form a biofilm.[2-5] Infections caused by *S. epidermidis* are often indolent and may be clinically difficult to diagnose. Differentiation of culture contamination from true infection can be challenging. Treatment is made more difficult by increasing rates of antibiotic resistance in coagulase-negative staphylococci and by the effect of biofilms on host defense and antimicrobial susceptibility. Unfortunately, infected prosthetic devices must often be removed to exact cure. Because the use of indwelling medical devices will most likely continue to increase, it is anticipated that the clinical significance of coagulase-negative staphylococci will similarly increase.

Microbiology and Ecology

The staphylococci are members of the family Micrococcaceae that also includes *Micrococcus*, *Stomatococcus*, and *Planococcus*. These bacteria are catalase-positive, gram-positive cocci that divide in irregular clusters producing a "grapelike cluster" appearance when viewed under the microscope. The *Staphylococcus* are comprised of 46 described species and subspecies (Table 196-1).[6] In the clinical microbiology laboratory, staphylococci are typically categorized as those that have the ability to coagulate rabbit plasma (i.e., coagulase-positive staphylococci or *S. aureus*) and those that do not (i.e., coagulase-negative staphylococci). The most common coagulase-negative staphylococci associated with human disease include *S. epidermidis*, *S. saprophyticus*, *S. lugdunensis*, and *S. haemolyticus*. However, numerous other species have less commonly been associated with disease (see Table 196-1). An alternative to the coagulase test commonly used in clinical microbiology laboratories includes rapid agglutination kits (containing antibody bound to beads) that target specific *S. aureus* antigens. The ability to identify coagulase-negative staphylococci to the species level correctly is difficult because of the number of tests needed to yield accurate results.[7] However, most systems used in clinical laboratories today can accurately identify those species most commonly isolated from human disease, including *S. aureus*, *S. epidermidis*, *S. haemolyticus*, and *S. saprophyticus*. A simplified scheme has been recently introduced to rapidly identify *S. lugdunensis* from other coagulase-negative staphylococci that includes a positive pyrrolidonyl aminopeptidase (PYR) and ornithine decarboxylase test.[8] In addition, molecular methods have been developed that identify *Staphylococcus* to the species level through the phylogenetic analyses of several conserved DNA sequences.[9]

Coagulase-negative staphylococci are normal commensal skin and mucous membrane microbes and are indigenous to a variety of mammalian hosts. Depending on the anatomic site, healthy human skin or mucous membranes support from 10^1 to 10^6 colony-forming units (CFU)/cm^2 of coagulase-negative staphylococci . Aptly named, *S. epidermidis* is the most prevalent species found on human skin, with the average person consistently carrying 10 to 24 different strains.[7] Because of varying characteristics of human skin, including varying moisture content, nutrient substances, pH range, and temperature, *S. epidermidis* must adapt to a variety of environmental conditions. Certain species of coagulase-negative staphylococci are well adapted to exist in specialized niches such as *S. capitis* (human scalp), *S. auricularis* (human ear canal), and *S. saprophyticus* (human alimentary and genitourinary tracts).

Antibiotic Resistance

Coagulase-negative staphylococci isolated from nosocomial environments are almost always resistant to multiple antimicrobial agents. In a large surveillance study from North America, 87.5% of isolates were resistant to oxacillin, 93.5% were resistant to penicillin, 65.6% were resistant to ciprofloxacin, 73% resistant to erythromycin, 52% resistant to clindamycin, and 48% resistant to trimethoprim-sulfamethoxazole.[10] Similar results were obtained from the United Kingdom.[11] Although *vanA*-positive coagulase-negative staphylococci have not been isolated to date, elevated minimal inhibitory concentrations (MICs) to glycopeptide antibiotics, especially within *S. haemolyticus*, have been reported.[12-15]

Phenotypic expression of methicillin (oxacillin)-resistance in coagulase-negative staphylococci is much more heterotypic than that observed in *S. aureus*, meaning that the percentage of the population that expresses high-level oxacillin resistance is smaller. To address this expression difference, the MIC break point to detect oxacillin resistance is lower for coagulase-negative staphylococci (except *S. lugdunensis*) than *S. aureus* (≥0.5 μg/mL vs. >4 μg/mL, respectively).[16] Regardless of the degree of heterotypy observed, all isolates containing *mecA* (the gene conferring oxacillin resistance) are clinically resistant to all β-lactam antibiotics.[17] Alternative methods to detect oxacillin resistance include a cefoxitin disk test, which is used as a surrogate to detect *mecA*-mediated oxacillin-resistance,[16] polymerase chain reaction (PCR) assay for *mecA* detection,[18] and commercial assays to detect PBP2A production (gene product of *mecA*).[19] However, in some coagulase-negative staphylococci, PBP2A is detected only after oxacillin induction.

Fortunately, several newer antibiotics that have been successfully introduced to the market have good antibacterial activity against staphylococci, including daptomycin,[20] linezolid,[21] and tigecycline.[22,23] In addition, several agents in various stages of development awaiting final regulatory approval also have potency against coagulase-negative staphylococci; these include dalbavancin,[24] televancin,[25] oritavancin,[26] iclaprim,[27] ceftibiprole,[28] and ceftaroline.[29] A particular onerous aspect of treatment of most coagulase-negative staphylococcal infections is their ability to form biofilms on biomaterials (e.g., catheters, prostheses; see later). Tolerance to antibiotics and persister cells is a common theme with staphylococci and other bacteria growing within a biofilm;

TABLE 196-1	Taxonomy of Coagulase-Negative Staphylococci	
Human		*Animal*
Species Frequently Associated with Disease		*Staphylococcus arlettae*
Staphylococcus epidermidis		*Staphylococcus caseolyticus*
Staphylococcus haemolyticus		*Staphylococcus chromogenes*
Staphylococcus lugdunensis		*Staphylococcus condimenti*
Staphylococcus saprophyticus		*Staphylococcus delphini*
		Staphylococcus equorum
Species Rarely Associated with Human Disease		*Staphylococcus felis*
		Staphylococcus fleurettii
Staphylococcus auricularis		*Staphylococcus gallinarum*
Staphylococcus capitis		*Staphylococcus hyicus*
Staphylococcus caprae		*Staphylococcus intermedius*
Staphylococcus carnosus		*Staphylococcus kloosii*
Staphylococcus cohnii		*Staphylococcus lentus*
Staphylococcus hominis		*Staphylococcus lutrae*
Staphylococcus pasteuri		*Staphylococcus muscae*
Staphylococcus pettenkoferi		*Staphylococcus nepalensis*
Staphylococcus pulvereri		*Staphylococcus piscifermentans*
Staphylococcus saccharolyticus		*Staphylococcus pseudintermedius*
Staphylococcus simulans		*Staphylococcus sciuri*
Staphylococcus schleiferi		*Staphylococcus simiae*
Staphylococcus warneri		*Staphylococcus succinus*
Staphylococcus xylosus		*Staphylococcus vitulinus*

these facts need to be taken into consideration during treatment.[30] Studies testing the effectiveness of antibiotics against staphylococci growing in a biofilm have demonstrated that they are significantly less effective than when treating planktonic cells.[31] However, antibiotic combinations containing rifampin seem promising in treating staphylococcal biofilm infections (examples include rifampin-vancomycin-gentamicin and rifampin-ciprofloxacin-fusidic acid).

Molecular Epidemiology

Pulsed-field gel electrophoresis (PFGE) is the gold standard methodology for addressing the short-term molecular epidemiology of *S. epidermidis* and other coagulase-negative staphylococci. There is extreme diversity in pulsed-field patterns when studying *S. epidermidis* epidemiology.[32,33] Therefore, the finding of indistinguishable PFGE patterns within the context of an outbreak assessment is highly relevant. Longer term relationships and trends are better addressed by multilocus sequence typing (MLST) analysis, which suggests that the population structure of *S. epidermidis* is epidemic in structure and that nine clonal lineages are disseminated worldwide.[34] One major clone, CC2, represented 74% of isolates worldwide in one study; similar results were found in other MLST studies.[34-37] However, rapid evolution (and thus PFGE patterns) occurs through frequent transfer of mobile genetic elements and recombination, possibly through insertion sequence elements. Other molecular typing methodologies, including sequence analysis of repeat regions of *sdrG/aap* genes and MLVA (multiple-locus variable-number tandem repeat analysis), have been developed, which yield similar discriminatory power as MLST or PFGE.[38,39]

Pathogenesis

In contrast to *S. aureus*, which produces an array of toxins and adherence factors, there are few defined virulence factors in *S. epidermidis* (Table 196-2) and other coagulase-negative staphylococci. However, significant advances have been made in the past 10 years that have helped define the pathogenesis of infections caused by *S. epidermidis*. The ability of *S. epidermidis* to adhere and form biofilm on the surface of biomaterials is thought to be the most significant virulence factor associated with this bacterium.[40-42] However, other factors, such as the secretion of poly-gamma-DL-glutamic acid (PGA)[43] and phenol-soluble modulins (PSMs),[44] appear to complement and increase virulence.

VIRULENCE FACTORS

Biofilm

Biofilm formation is thought to occur in three stages—adherence, maturation, and dispersal (Fig. 196-1). It is well established that bacteria growing within a biofilm are unique compared with those growing exponentially in the planktonic phase. Microarray studies have demonstrated that both *S. epidermidis* and *S. aureus* growing in a biofilm state have unique transcriptional responses compared with cells growing exponentially.[45-47] For example, these experiments have shown that staphylococci growing in a biofilm shift their physiology toward anaerobic or microaerobic metabolism and downregulate protein, cell wall, and DNA synthesis. Although these experiments have been extremely helpful in defining the "average" transcriptional response of biofilm growth (as all cells growing in a biofilm were examined), it is also well established that cells growing within a biofilm have spatial and temporal responses to their immediate environment (e.g., nutrient and oxygen availability and interactions with metabolic waste).[48] For example, *S. epidermidis* growing within a biofilm consists of at least four metabolic states: aerobic growth, anaerobic growth, dormant cells and dead cells.[49] It is hypothesized that these unique physiologic states found within a biofilm allow for tolerance to antibiotics and development of persister and/or dormant cells.[30]

Adherence. Biomaterials placed within a human host are rapidly coated with serum matrix proteins, including fibrinogen and fibronectin. Genome and functional analyses have suggested that *S. epidermidis* possesses at least the ability to bind fibrinogen, fibronectin, collagen,

TABLE 196-2	Defined and Proposed Virulence Factors of *Staphylococcus epidermidis*
Defined and Putative Virulence Factors	*Proposed Mechanism*
Biofilm	**Immune System Avoidance, Antimicrobial Tolerance**
Polysaccharide intercellular adhesin (PIA)	Polysaccharide component of biofilm
Accumulation associated protein (Aap)	Accumulation of biofilm
Bap homologue protein (Bhp)	Accumulation of biofilm
Extracellular DNA	Structure of biofilm
Adhesin Molecules	**Adherence to Host Proteins or Plastic**
Autolysin, adhesin (Aae)	Binds fibrinogen, vitronectin, fibronectin
Autolysin (AtlE)	Binds vitronectin
Bap homologue protein (Bhp)	Binds polystyrene
Elastin binding protein (Ebp)	Binds elastin
Extracellular matrix binding protein (EmbP)	Binds fibronectin
Fibrinogen-binding protein (Fbe)	Binds fibrinogen
Glycerol ester hydrolase (GehD)	Binds collagen
Staphylococcal conserved antigen (ScaA)	Binds fibrinogen, vitronectin, fibronectin
Staphylococcal conserved antigen (ScaB)	Binds undefined ligand
Serine aspartate repeat protein F (SdrF)	Binds collagen
Serine aspartate repeat protein G (SdrG)	Binds fibrinogen
Staphylococcal surface protein 1 (Ssp-1)	Binds polystyrene
Staphylococcal surface protein 2 (Ssp-2)	Binds polystyrene
Teichoic acid	Binds fibronectin
Other Putative Virulence Factors	**Mechanisms**
Peptidoglycan, lipoteichoic acid	Stimulates cytokine production
Phenol-soluble modulins	Immune system modulation, biofilm dispersion
Poly-D-glutamic acid	Immune system avoidance, resistance to antimicrobial peptides
Delta toxin	Immune system avoidance
Exoenzymes	
Fatty acid–modifying enzyme (FAME)	Inactivates fatty acids on skin, skin colonization
Lipases	Skin and wound colonization
Proteases	Destruction of host tissue
Elastase	Immune modulation, skin colonization
Lantibiotics	
Epidermin, epilancin, epicidin, Pep5, K7	Bacterial interference and skin colonization

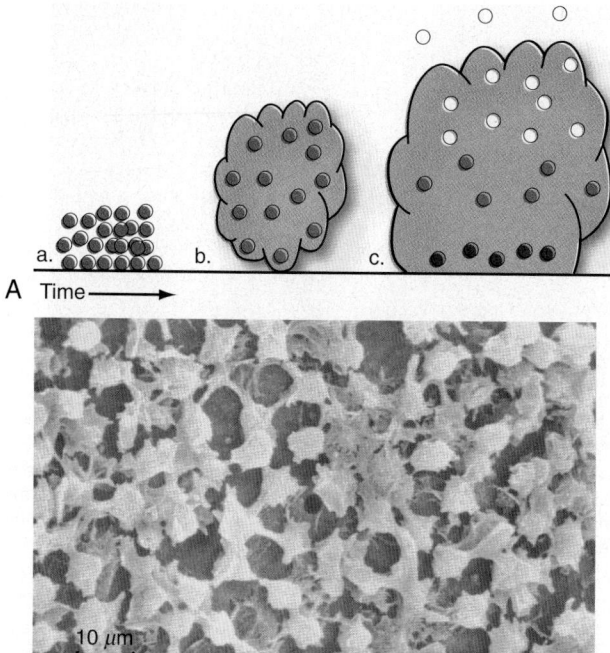

A, Time ⟶

B

10 µm

Figure 196-1 **Biofilm formation in *Staphylococcus epidermidis*.**
A, Model of biofilm formation in *S. epidermidis*. Staphylococci initially adhere to biomaterial by binding to serum matrix proteins coated on the biomaterial and through direct biomaterial interactions (a). Once bound, *S. epidermidis* produces extracellular polymeric substances (PIA, eDNA) and other proteinaceous factors (Aap, Bap), which facilitate intercellular adherence (b). A mature biofilm has multiple metabolic states, including cells growing under aerobic conditions (white cells), microaerobic or anaerobic conditions (bright red cells), and dormant cells (dark red cells) (c). Through the action of phenol soluble modulins, cells disperse from the biofilm, which facilitates colonization at other sites. **B,** Scanning electron micrograph of *S. epidermidis* biofilm adhering to a tissue cage in a guinea pig model (×1360).

vitronectin, and elastin.[50-55] Furthermore, there is evidence that *S. epidermidis* autolysins have the ability to bind directly to plastic and contain matrix protein binding sites.[56,57] Lipase (GehD), in addition to its enzymatic function, has also been shown to bind collagen.[54] Lastly, mutants that do not have the ability to bind fibrinogen or produce autolysin are less virulent in pertinent in vivo models, suggesting that initial adherence to serum matrix proteins is critical.[58,59]

Maturation. Following adherence to the biomaterial, intercellular adherence of the bacteria is primarily mediated by polymeric molecules. It has recently been shown that eDNA (extracellular DNA) is a major component of both *S. aureus* and *S. epidermidis* biofilms and mutants defective in DNA release produce deficient biofilms.[60,61] *S. epidermidis* biofilm contains an abundance of polysaccharide intercellular adhesin (PIA), whereas it is a minor component of a *S. aureus* biofilm.[62] PIA (or poly-*N*-acetylglucosamine [PNAG]) is a β-1,6-linked *N*-acetylglucosamine[63] synthesized by the *ica* operon gene products.[42] The *ica* operon is composed of four genes, *icaA*, *icaD*, *icaB*, and *icaC*. A divergently transcribed repressor, *icaR*, is found just upstream of *ica*.[64] PIA appears to be important in *S. epidermidis* surface colonization, biofilm formation, and immune system evasion.[65,66] Regulation of *icaADBC* transcription has been an intense area of study and involves SarA, SarZ, σB, IcaR, and the TCA cycle, among others.[67-73] In *S. aureus*, PIA (also known as PNAG) is essential for virulence in murine systemic disease models and is a vaccine candidate for both

S. aureus and *S. epidermidis*.[74-77] It should be noted that some clinically relevant strains of *S. epidermidis* do not contain the *icaADBC* operon and other alternative, proteinaceous biofilm strategies exist (e.g., AAP, Bap).[36,78-80] Furthermore, allelic replacement of *icaADBC* confers increased fitness during colonization of human skin as compared with the isogenic wild-type isolate.[81] Therefore, although production of PIA is highly advantageous to the organism during the infection process, PIA production may be deleterious to the organism during colonization of human skin.

Dispersal. As shown in Figure 196-1, the last stage of biofilm development is dispersal and subsequent spread to other potential sites. The production of PSMs by *S. epidermidis* has been shown in flow cell biofilm experiments to mediate the detachment of the upper layers of the biofilm.[46] PSMs, which are regulated by the quorum-sensing global regulator *agr*, act as surfactants, leading to loss of cellular clusters. In addition, *S. epidermidis* PSMs are proinflammatory and have been shown to recruit, activate, and lyse human neutrophils during infection with *S. aureus*.[44,82-84]

Other Virulence Factors

Poly-Gamma-DL-Glutamic Acid (PGA). A somewhat surprising finding is that in contrast to *S. aureus*, multiple species of coagulase-negative staphylococci, including *S. epidermidis*, produce PGA.[43] PGA is a cell surface–associated, antiphagocytic polymer first described as a virulence factor in *Bacillus anthracis*.[85] PGA appears to have a bifunctional role in *S. epidermidis* and functions to inhibit innate host defense as well as facilitate colonization of human skin.

Lantibiotics. *S. epidermidis* produces several lantibiotics (e.g., epidermin, Pep5, epilancin, epicidin), which are bacteriocins. These thioether amino acid–containing antimicrobial peptides are active against a variety of bacteria and may play a role in bacterial interference and successful colonization and persistence on human skin.[5,86]

Other Coagulase-Negative Species

Because of the lack of well-developed genetic systems within other coagulase-negative staphylococci, investigations of virulence mechanisms in other staphylococcal species is limited. However, significant progress has been made with the uropathogen *S. saprophyticus* and *S. lugdunensis*. *S. saprophyticus* shows strong adherence to uroepithelial cells, erythrocytes, and produces urease, facilitating the growth of this pathogen in urine.[87-91] In addition, genome sequencing reveals that *S. saprophyticus* ATCC15305 is particularly adapted to growth in urine because of expansion of systems involved in osmotolerance and inorganic ion transport.[88] *S. lugdunensis* does not produce toxins and adherence factors similar to *S. aureus* despite its apparently increased virulence.[8] However, several studies have found that *S. lugdunensis* does bind human host matrix proteins, including collagen, IgG, fibrinogen, laminin, vitronectin, fibronectin, thrombospondin, von Willebrand factor, and plasminogen.[51,92-94] In addition, although it contains the *icaADBC* locus, *S. lugdunensis* appears to produce protein-dependent biofilms that are not PIA-dependent.

■ Epidemiology and Clinical Syndromes

Previously disregarded as nonvirulent contaminants, coagulase-negative staphylococci have more recently been increasingly recognized as true pathogens. Coagulase-negative staphylococci cause a wide variety of clinical infections, many related to foreign bodies and prosthetic medical devices.

BACTEREMIA

Coagulase-negative staphylococci account for approximately 30% of health care–associated bloodstream infections. Most of these infections are caused by involvement of intravascular catheters or other prosthetic medical devices. Immunosuppressed patients, particularly those with severe neutropenia, are at increased risk of coagulase-negative staphylococci bloodstream infection. In addition to intravascular catheters, mucosal breakdown caused by cytotoxic chemotherapy may precipitate infection in these patients.

Because coagulase-negative staphylococci, particularly *S. epidermidis*, occupy such a prominent position in the commensal flora of human skin and mucous membranes, they are frequently encountered as culture contaminants. Approximately 1% to 6% of blood cultures are contaminated and coagulase-negative staphylococci are responsible in 70% to 80% of cases.[95,96] Typically, rates of true bacteremia range from 10% to 25% when coagulase-negative staphylococci are isolated from blood cultures.[97]

Determining the clinical significance of coagulase-negative staphylococci isolated from blood cultures is difficult and a variety of clinical and laboratory parameters should be examined when making this determination. This is not a trivial issue, because contaminants treated as true pathogens result in unnecessary antibiotic treatment, emergence of antibiotic resistance, excessive use of laboratory resources, antibiotic-associated side effects and toxicity, and greater expense. Many clinicians use fever or other signs of infection (e.g., leukocytosis or leukopenia, hypotension) to assist with the interpretation of blood cultures that yield coagulase-negative staphylococci and a number of studies have offered support.[95,96,98] However, most blood cultures are obtained because of a clinical suspicion of bacteremia, and other investigators have not found clinical signs and symptoms helpful in differentiating contamination from infection.[99] Another parameter often used is the number or proportion of cultures that yield coagulase-negative staphylococci. Most studies relate that the likelihood of true bacteremia increases when multiple cultures are obtained and yield coagulase-negative staphylococci,[100] but this has not been universally observed.[101] The problem is compounded in neonates from whom it is common practice to obtain only one blood culture when entertaining the possible diagnosis of bacteremia. Similarly, a shorter time to growth or a greater burden of bacteria in quantitative blood cultures has been used to differentiate true bacteremia from contamination, with mixed success.[102] In general, a time to positivity of less than 24 hours is considered consistent with true bacteremia.

In differentiating intravascular catheter-associated coagulase-negative staphylococci bloodstream infection from bacteremia from other sources, the differential time for a blood culture to become positive between peripheral blood and catheter blood can now be readily determined with most automated blood culture methods. When the catheter blood is positive 2 or more hours sooner than the peripheral blood, this can be taken as indicator that the catheter is the source of bacteremia.[103] Other laboratory parameters that may have some usefulness for differentiating contaminants from pathogens in certain settings include C-reactive protein[104] and serum procalcitonin levels,[105] molecular typing,[106,107] antibiogram,[108] and biofilm production.[109]

Methods that have been used to prevent blood culture contamination include use of effective skin antiseptics, phlebotomy teams, culture bottle preparation, blood culture kits, and double-needle bottle inoculation.[95,96,110,111]

In general, blood cultures should be obtained using careful aseptic technique in persons in whom a clinical suspicion for bacteremia exists. Paired cultures should be drawn and, if a central venous catheter (CVC) source is being considered, one of the blood samples should be obtained from the catheter. The site (catheter or periphery) and time of obtainment should be recorded. Patients with clinical signs of sepsis, with multiple positive cultures that reveal growth in less than 24 hours, are more likely to have true bacteremia.

Intravascular Catheter Infections

This subject is discussed more fully in Chapter 302. Approximately 180 million peripheral intravascular catheters and 7 million central venous catheters are used in the United States annually and, as a result, approximately 250,000 persons experience catheter-associated bloodstream infection (Fig. 196-2). Coagulase-negative staphylococci are the most common cause of these infections. A detailed discussion of the

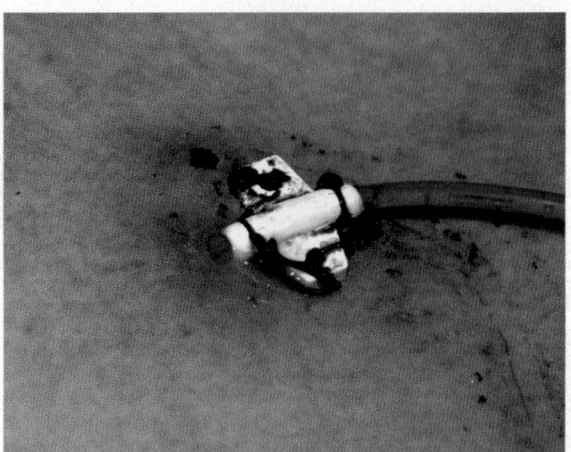

Figure 196-2   Infected central venous catheter. Although many infected central venous catheters appear innocuous, this *S. epidermidis*–infected implanted catheter site exhibits erythema, tenderness, and purulent drainage at the skin exit site.

pathogenesis of central venous catheter-associated bloodstream infection is beyond the scope of this chapter. Briefly, for peripheral intravascular catheters and nontunneled CVCs, infection most commonly results from coagulase-negative staphylococci entering via the cutaneous surface of the catheter to the bloodstream. For tunneled CVCs, hub colonization and passage of organisms along the lumen appears to be an important route of infection. The ability of coagulase-negative staphylococci to adhere to the catheter and elaborate biofilm are crucial traits that allow them to cause infection of vascular catheters.[112]

The diagnosis of coagulase-negative staphylococci CVC bloodstream infection can be difficult because most infected CVCs have no obvious local evidence of inflammation or infection[112] and, as already discussed, coagulase-negative staphylococci are most often clinically encountered as blood culture contaminants. In the past, diagnosis of CVC-associated bloodstream infection was considered to require removal of the catheter and semiquantitative or quantitative culture of the catheter tip.[113,114] Many clinicians take advantage of automated, continuously monitored blood culture systems and use a 2-hour cutoff differential time to positivity assessment on blood cultures drawn from the periphery and CVC.[103] The limitations of this technique are discussed in detail in Chapter 302.

In general, short-term, nontunneled CVCs infected with coagulase-negative staphylococci should be removed. In patients with coagulase-negative staphylococci–infected tunneled CVCs who do not exhibit signs of severe sepsis, it is permissible to attempt catheter salvage. If the central venous catheter is retained, it is advisable to use systemic antimicrobials through all the lumens of the catheter for 10 to 14 days.[115] If fever or bacteremia persists for more than 3 days after initiating therapy, the CVC usually should be removed. Most health care–associated coagulase-negative staphylococci are methicillin-resistant, and vancomycin is most frequently used to treat these infections. If once-daily daptomycin is used, each dose should be distributed among all the lumens of a multiport catheter. If the catheter is retained, the clinician should be alert for relapse because this occurs in a substantial minority of patients.[116] Tunnel track or port pocket infections require catheter removal, whereas exit site infections can usually be successfully treated with the CVC in place.

Endocarditis

Prosthetic valve endocarditis (PVE), although uncommon, is caused by coagulase-negative staphylococci in 15% to 40% of cases.[117-119] The infection is usually health care–related (resulting from inoculation at the time of surgery) and manifests within 12 months of valve placement. These isolates are likely to be methicillin-resistant. The cases of PVE that present after this time period are less commonly caused by the coagulase-negative staphylococci, usually associated with trauma to mucosal surfaces or incidental infection and, if caused by coagulase-negative staphylococci, are more apt to be methicillin-susceptible.[120] Patients may present in an acute or more indolent fashion. An acute presentation is characterized by fever and physical evidence of valve dysfunction, whereas peripheral stigmata of endocarditis are more commonly observed in patients exhibiting a more indolent course. The diagnosis is usually confirmed by documenting repeatedly positive blood cultures and vegetations on transesophageal echocardiography. Heart failure occurs in 54% of cases and more than 80% have complications, including prosthetic valve dysfunction and intracardiac abscesses. Typically, antibiotic therapy consists of vancomycin and rifampin for at least 6 weeks combined with gentamicin for the first 2 weeks (see Chapter 78).[121] Isolates susceptible to penicillinase-stable penicillins should be treated with oxacillin or nafcillin instead of vancomycin. There is increasing concern regarding vancomycin "MIC creep" and clinicians are sometimes turning to daptomycin or other vancomycin alternatives. Valve replacement surgery is usually necessary. Despite aggressive therapy, the mortality caused by coagulase-negative staphylococci PVE remains high, at approximately 25%.

Unlike PVE, native valve endocarditis caused by coagulase-negative staphylococci is relatively rare, occurring in only 5% to 8% of endocarditis cases.[117,122] This infection is the result of hematogenous seeding of previously damaged heart valves and endocardium. Many of these cases are health care–associated, most often caused by the use of intravascular catheters and cardiac devices, and the causative isolates are usually methicillin-resistant. Prolonged symptoms and physical signs (fever, vascular, or immunologic findings) prior to diagnosis are relatively common[122] and patients often have a very complicated clinical course because of embolic events, rhythm conduction abnormalities, and congestive heart failure.[123] More than half of these cases require valve replacement and, despite aggressive combined medical-surgical treatment, mortality continues to be approximately 25%.

Cardiac Devices

Cardiac electrophysiologic device infection (pacemakers, defibrillators) occurs in 1% to 2% of device placement procedures (see Chapter 79); coagulase-negative staphylococci (predominantly *S. epidermidis*) account for approximately 50% to 60% of these infections.[124-127] Infection can be limited to the pocket or can spread via intravascular leads to involve endocardial tissue. One fourth of pacemaker infections present acutely within 1 month of insertion, but delays of up to 1 to 2 years are commonly observed. Factors implicated in increased risk of infection include diabetes, concomitant corticosteroid therapy, urgent electrode repositioning, and skin diseases. Clinically, most patients present with inflammation at the pocket site, whereas systemic symptoms are less frequently observed. Diagnosis is generally made by culture of the generator pocket, culture of the device itself, or multiple positive sequential blood cultures with the same strain of coagulase-negative staphylococci. However, only one third of patients with implantable cardiac device infection were bacteremic in one study.[126] Transesophageal echocardiography is recommended for all patients and is much more sensitive than transthoracic echocardiography.[125,128] Successful treatment generally requires complete removal of the device. Relapse rates and mortality are substantially increased if complete removal of the device is not accomplished.[125-128] Antibiotic therapy typically consists of vancomycin or daptomycin, with or without rifampin, continued for 14 days after device removal for patients with infection limited to the pocket and for 6 weeks for patients with bacteremia, lead involvement, or endocarditis. Device reimplantation, if necessary, should be at a new site when the patient is no longer bacteremic.

Vascular Grafts

Although infection is a relatively rare complication of arterial reconstruction (lower than 1%), coagulase-negative staphylococci are one of the most common causes (20% to 30%) of this feared entity.[129-131] The coagulase-negative staphylococci, usually *S. epidermidis*, causing these infections are thought to be inoculated at the time of surgery from the patient's skin. Major risk factors include a groin incision, diabetes, emergency aortic aneurysm repair, steroid therapy, and remote infections. Most cases of vascular graft infection caused by coagulase-negative staphylococci present in an indolent fashion, months to years after surgery and manifest as a false aneurysm, fistula or sinus tract formation, or hemorrhage at the anastomotic site. Diagnosis is usually entertained based on local physical findings and supported by radiographic modalities, such as computed tomography (CT), magnetic resonance imaging (MRI), or ultrasound. Blood cultures are often negative because infection may not extend to the graft lumen. Confirmation of the causative role of coagulase-negative staphylococci is maximized by sonication of the explanted graft at the time of surgery to recover biofilm-associated organisms.[132] Optimum treatment requires a combined medical and surgical approach. Intensive and prolonged antibiotic therapy is important, but surgery is required for cure. Surgical strategy can be summarized as graft excision with extra-anatomic bypass or graft excision with in situ reconstruction using a prosthetic conduit, allograft, or autogenous tissue. These techniques have been summarized elsewhere, but are all associated with mortality of approximately 10% to 25%. As expected, in situ reconstruction is associated with less risk of amputation, but an increased risk (15% to 20%) of recurrent infection. There is some support for the use of antibiotic-treated or silver-coated grafts in the treatment of vascular graft infection or, similar to their application in orthopedic surgery, the placement of antibiotic-impregnated beads into the infected tissue bed.[133] A systematic review and meta-analysis of perioperative strategies to prevent infection in patients undergoing peripheral arterial reconstruction has confirmed the beneficial role of prophylactic antibiotics but did not find benefit associated with rifampin-bonded Dacron grafts, suction groin wound drainage, or perioperative bathing with antiseptic agents.[130]

Orthopedic Prosthetic Device Infections

Coagulase-negative staphylococci, usually *S. epidermidis*, are responsible for 30% to 43% of cases, and are the most common cause of infection of prosthetic orthopedic devices (see Chapter 104).[134,135] These organisms are generally inoculated at the time of the arthroplasty and, because of their relatively avirulent nature, may be quite indolent in their clinical presentation. Risk factors consistently observed include previous joint surgery, perioperative wound complications, and rheumatoid arthritis.[136] Risk factors observed in some studies but not others include history of malignancy, diabetes, corticosteroid use, obesity, age, nutritional status, infection at remote site at time of surgery, psoriasis, hemophilia, sickle cell anemia, dialysis, acquired immunodeficiency syndrome (AIDS), and solid organ transplantation. Infections can be classified as early (within 3 months of surgery and are often caused by *S. aureus*); delayed (3 months to 2 years postoperatively; most frequently caused by coagulase-negative staphylococci); and late (longer than 2 years after surgery; usually caused by hematogenous inoculation of organisms from some other source). Delayed infections caused by coagulase-negative staphylococci are usually indolent and manifest as pain at the affected joint, without fever or other systemic manifestations. The diagnosis is supported by the presence of an elevated erythrocyte sedimentation rate or C-reactive protein level. Radiographic imaging studies may be helpful but are often limited by poor sensitivity and specificity or imaging artifact caused by metallic components of the implant. Aspiration and synovial fluid analysis or tissue biopsy may also be helpful, but can be limited by the localized nature of inflammation or infection and potential contamination. The recovery of organisms can be optimized by sonication of the prosthesis at the time of removal.[134] Coagulase-negative staphylococci may also be a prominent cause of culture-negative prosthetic joint infection manifest as aseptic loosening of the joint.[137] It is thought that prior antibiotic therapy and the presence of a metabolically quiescent population of coagulase-negative staphylococci encased in biofilm may explain this condition. Eradication of infection is best achieved by a two-stage exchange procedure combined with 6 weeks of antibiotic treatment. Vancomycin is most frequently used, often in combination with rifampin. There are limited data regarding treatment with vancomycin alternatives such as linezolid[138] or daptomycin,[139] and clinical trials are ongoing (see http://clinicaltrials.gov/archive/NCT00428844/2009_02_11). Prevention strategies include the use of laminar flow operating suites, antimicrobial prophylaxis, and antibiotic-impregnated bone cement.[140-142]

Cerebrospinal Fluid Shunt Infections

Infection is one of the most significant complications associated with cerebrospinal fluid shunt implantation, ranging in incidence between 1.5% and 38%, but more recently occurring in approximately 5% of patients (see Chapter 85). Coagulase-negative staphylococci, most predominantly *S. epidermidis*, are the most common cause and are responsible for approximately half of cases. Risk factors predisposing for infection include age younger than 6 months, shunt revision surgery, scalp dermatitis, duration of procedure, proficiency of the surgeon, and intraoperative use of a neuroendoscope. Patients who receive a short-term ventriculostomy (external ventricular drain) are at substantial risk (approximately 10%) of developing ventriculitis or meningitis and coagulase-negative staphylococci are the predominant pathogens,[143] although some reports have indicated a shift toward gram-negative pathogens.[144] The duration of catheterization appears to be the major risk factor for infection that is not substantially modified by catheter exchange or prophylactic antibiotics. Signs and symptoms of shunt infection typically develop within 2 months of shunt insertion and should be suspected in patients with local signs of inflammation, nausea, or vomiting, signs of increased intracranial pressure, or shunt malfunction. The diagnosis is confirmed by isolation of coagulase-negative staphylococci from cerebrospinal fluid obtained from the shunt. A modest pleocytosis is usually evident, accompanied by an elevated protein level. Positive blood cultures are observed in patients with infected ventriculoatrial shunts.

Most infections are caused by methicillin-resistant strains of coagulase-negative staphylococci, and combination therapy with vancomycin, gentamicin, and rifampin is a traditional regimen. Vancomycin and gentamicin are often delivered intraventricularly. Rifampin achieves excellent cerebrospinal fluid concentration with systemic administration. Experience with newer anti-staphylococcal agents, such as linezolid or daptomycin, is limited. Successful treatment usually requires shunt removal.[145] In patients with coagulase-negative staphylococcal infections and normal cerebrospinal fluid findings, reshunting can be performed on the third day after shunt removal. If cerebrospinal fluid abnormalities are present, 7 days of therapy are generally recommended before reshunting as long as repeat cerebrospinal fluid cultures are sterile and the cerebrospinal fluid protein level is lower than 200 mg/dL.

In a systematic review and meta-analysis of 17 trials involving 2134 patients, the administration of perioperative (24 hours) prophylactic antibiotics in cerebrospinal fluid shunt surgery significantly decreased the risk of infection.[146] Additional reduction in infection was observed through application of strict operative aseptic technique,[147] but use of antibiotic-impregnated shunt catheters has been associated with inconsistent results.[148,149]

Surgical Site Infections

Surgical site infections caused by the coagulase-negative staphylococci occur frequently and are second only to *S. aureus* as a causative agent.[150] Coagulase-negative staphylococci are more often causative of superficial incisional infections rather than deep incisional infections and rarely cause organ or space infections. A notable exception is mediastinitis after median sternotomy for cardiac surgery (see Chapter 82). In addition, coagulase-negative staphylococci are more likely to cause infections involving clean procedures rather than those classified as contaminated (e.g., bowel, genitourinary). Superficial incisional infec-

tions generally manifest within 5 to 10 days postprocedure and usually result from inoculation of organisms from the patient's endogenous flora or, less frequently, from the operating personnel or environment. Risk factors include duration of the surgical procedure, host factors (e.g., extremities of age, obesity, nutritional status), and experience of the surgeon and surgical staff. Signs and symptoms of a surgical site infection include pain, tenderness, swelling, warmth, erythema, drainage at the incisional site, leukocytosis, and fever. The causative pathogen is confirmed by recovery of coagulase-negative staphylococci from wound cultures. Culture results require careful interpretation because coagulase-negative staphylococci are commonly regarded as contaminants or colonizers. Generally, coagulase-negative staphylococci are interpreted to be the causative agent of the infection if they are the predominant or only isolate from purulent drainage and/or are repeatedly cultured from the same source. Treatment depends on the severity of the infection and ranges from topical wound care alone to surgical débridement and parenteral antibiotics. Preventive measures should be emphasized, and detailed guidelines are available (see Chapter 317 and Mangram et al[150]).

Peritoneal Dialysis Catheter-Associated Infections

Coagulase-negative staphylococci, accounting for 25% to 50% of cases, are the most frequent cause of peritonitis in patients undergoing peritoneal dialysis.[151] *S. epidermidis* is responsible for 50% to 80% of infections caused by coagulase-negative staphylococci, with a wide variety of other coagulase-negative staphylococcal species less frequently observed; clonal spread of coagulase-negative staphylococci has been documented at some centers.[152,153] Coagulase-negative staphylococci gain access to the peritoneum from the patient's skin via the intraluminal route or from the exit site via the periluminal route.

Clinically, compared with infection by *S. aureus*, coagulase-negative staphylococci peritonitis is relatively benign and infrequently leads to catheter removal. Signs and symptoms of infection include abdominal pain and tenderness, fever, nausea, and vomiting. Diagnosis is confirmed by documenting more than 100 white blood cells/mL in dialysate fluid and recovery of coagulase-negative staphylococci in cultures of the fluid. When culturing the dialysate, it is necessary to culture large volumes of fluid (more than 100 mL) or to use a filter technique or broth enrichment to detect small numbers of organisms. However, care must be taken because it may be difficult to differentiate contaminants from causative pathogens.[151] Although historically most of these infections were caused by methicillin-susceptible strains, the antimicrobial susceptibility pattern has recently shifted and most causative strains are now methicillin-resistant.[154] Treatment with vancomycin via the dialysate fluid is a relatively convenient dosing method and is often successful. Recalcitrant peritonitis is an indication for catheter removal.

Prevention of infection depends on proper catheter placement, exit site care, infusion with Y sets and twin bag systems, and careful training of patients regarding aseptic practices.[155] Perioperative antibiotic prophylaxis significantly reduces the risk of early peritonitis but not exit site or tunnel infections.[156]

Endophthalmitis

Coagulase-negative staphylococci are readily recovered from conjunctival cultures of preophthalmologic surgery patients,[157] and thus it is not surprising that they are the most frequent cause of postoperative endophthalmitis, responsible for 60% to 70% of cases (see Chapter 112).[158,159] Symptoms typically develop within 1 week of surgery and usually consist of pain, redness, and decreased visual acuity. Fever is generally absent and leukocyte count is normal. The physical examination reveals conjunctival injection and a hypopyon. Optimal treatment consists of vitrectomy and intravitreal administration of antibiotics.[160] Vancomycin is usually administered at an intravitreal dose of 1 mg and bactericidal concentrations usually persist for 2 to 3 days.[161] Intraocular lens removal is generally not required. Although prognosis largely depends on presenting visual acuity, residual visual impairment is frequently observed.

Urinary Tract Infection

Urinary tract infections caused by the coagulase-negative staphylococci fall into two major groups. The first is caused by *S. saprophyticus,* which is covered more fully in a separate section of this chapter (also see Chapter 69). The second group is uncommon and occurs almost exclusively in hospitalized patients with underlying urinary tract complications. Most of these patients have a urinary catheter in place and have recently undergone urinary tract surgery, kidney transplantation, experienced kidney stone disease, or have a neurogenic bladder or obstructive uropathy. Coagulase-negative staphylococci cause approximately 3% of nosocomial urinary tract infections, with *S. epidermidis* responsible for 90% of these isolates.[162] Additional risk factors include advanced age and extended length of hospital stay. Approximately 1% of urinary tract infections in outpatients are caused by coagulase-negative staphylococci.[163] Infection with coagulase-negative staphylococci is associated with a lesser degree of pyuria than infection with gram-negative bacilli (mean urine leukocyte count, of 39 vs. 121 white blood cells/mL) and most of these patients are asymptomatic.[164] Coagulase-negative staphylococci causing nosocomial urinary tract infections are usually methicillin-resistant and treatment, if required, should be based on the susceptibility profile of the organism.

Infections of Genitourinary Prostheses

S. epidermidis is responsible for 35% to 60% of infections of synthetic urinary sphincters and penile prostheses in which an overall infection rate of 2% to 4% is observed.[165] Coagulase-negative staphylococcal infections of penile prostheses are often indolent and may take up to a year from the date of implantation to manifest clinically. Those with infected prostheses exhibit local pain, swelling, induration, and erythema of the penis. Occasionally, fistula formation is observed and malfunction or impairment of the device is frequent. Rarely do systemic signs of infection occur. Diagnosis is made clinically and by culture of any drainage or of the device itself. Surgical removal of the device is required, accompanied by 10 to 14 days of systemic antibiotics for uncomplicated infection.[166] In addition to fastidious surgical technique and antibiotic prophylaxis, the use of antibiotic-coated prostheses appears promising as a means to prevent infection.[167]

Infections of Breast Implants

Infection associated with breast implant surgery occurs in approximately 1% to 2% of patients and is often caused by coagulase-negative staphylococci.[168,169] *S. epidermidis* inhabits the glandular tissue ducts of the breast and from there may gain access to the space surrounding the implant.[170] Infection may present acutely or may be very indolent. Signs and symptoms are predominantly localized and include erythema, tenderness, pain, swelling, induration, and drainage. Acute infections are often associated with systemic findings such as fever and leukocytosis. Diagnosis is confirmed by culture of the drainage or fluid surrounding the implant or of the implant itself. Treatment consists of antibiotic therapy and a two-stage replacement procedure.[166] Capsular contracture remains the most common complication following breast augmentation. Although controversial, chronic low-grade or subclinical infection with coagulase-negative staphylococci may be a cause for capsular contracture.

Miscellaneous Prosthetic Device and Implant Infections

Almost any biomaterial or device that is inserted or implanted across the skin or mucous membranes can become colonized or infected by coagulase-negative staphylococci. Miscellaneous devices that have been associated with infections caused by coagulase-negative staphylococci include ventricular assist devices, coronary stents, hemodialysis shunts and catheters, implantable neurologic stimulators, cochlear implants, fracture fixation devices and other orthopedic implants, ureteral or urethral stents, and surgical mesh. It can be anticipated that infection caused by coagulase-negative staphylococci will parallel the increasing use of such devices.

■ Patient Populations at Increased Risk of Infection by Coagulase-Negative Staphylococci

TRANSPLANT PATIENTS AND NEUTROPENIC HOSTS

Solid organ or hematopoietic stem cell transplant patients are susceptible to coagulase-negative staphylococcal infections caused by immunosuppression, intravascular catheterization, and mucosal or skin breakdown.[171] These infections most often manifest as a *S. epidermidis* bloodstream infection and are due to an infected intravenous catheter. Mucositis and the breakdown of gastrointestinal mucosal integrity, related to cytotoxic chemotherapy or radiation therapy, may be an alternate source for coagulase-negative staphylococcal bacteremia.[172] Interleukin-2 therapy has been associated with an increased risk of *S. epidermidis* bacteremia.[173] Cardiac transplant patients are at increased risk of sternal wound infections and mediastinitis caused by coagulase-negative staphylococci (see Chapter 82).

NEONATES

Approximately 20% of very low birth weight preterm infants (less than 1500 g) experience late-onset neonatal sepsis (more than 3 days after birth).[174,175] Half of these infections are caused by coagulase-negative staphylococci and are associated with a mortality rate of 9%. *S. epidermidis* accounts for 60% to 93% of the infections caused by coagulase-negative staphylococci, with lesser contributions by *S. haemolyticus, S. hominis, S. warneri, S. saprophyticus, S. cohnii,* and *S. capitis.*

Neonates become colonized with coagulase-negative staphylococci on their skin and in their nares, umbilicus, and pharynx within days of their admission to the neonatal intensive care unit (NICU) and, in most cases, these organisms do not originate from the mother but are acquired from the hospital environment and health care workers. In one study using multiple molecular epidemiologic typing methods, 62% of NICU nurses harbored methicillin-resistant strains of coagulase-negative staphylococci that were identical to bacteremic strains.[176] In addition, endemic strains of coagulase-negative staphylococci can persist in the NICU for many years.[177] Risk factors for developing coagulase-negative staphylococcal bacteremia include low birth weight, the presence and duration of use of CVCs and umbilical catheters, mechanical ventilation and total parenteral nutrition, especially with IV lipid emulsions.[174,178,179] The rate of catheter-associated bloodstream infection in level II and III NICUs ranges from 2.4/1000 to 5.9/1000 central venous line days, depending on birth weight.[180] Similarly, the rate of bloodstream infection caused by umbilical catheters ranges from 0.9/1000 umbilical catheter days for infants weighing more than 2500 g to 6.9/1000 umbilical catheter days for infants less than 750 g.

Coagulase-negative staphylococcal bacteremia is often indolent and signs of infection may include abdominal distention, apnea, bradycardia, inability to maintain body temperature, feeding difficulties, lethargy, neutropenia, thrombocytopenia, hyperglycemia, and metabolic acidosis.[174,178] Although most bloodstream infections occur in infants with indwelling catheters, some cases are also found when there are no IV catheters present. These may be the result of skin lesions or respiratory or gastrointestinal colonization by these organisms. Differentiating true bacteremia from contamination is made even more difficult in neonates for several reasons, including the difficulty in obtaining blood from low-birth-weight infants, the small volume of blood generally obtained (0.1 to 1 mL), and the common practice of obtaining a single sample of blood for culture to preserve blood volume.[181] It is usually necessary to correlate other laboratory findings along with the clinical presentation and the blood culture results to arrive at the correct diagnosis. In addition to bacteremia, coagulase-negative staphylococci can also cause skin infections, pneumonia, urinary tract infections, and meningitis in the newborn. Erythema toxicum neonatorum, a benign self-limited eruption, may be caused by an innate immune response to coagulase-negative staphylococci that have colonized the hair follicles. Similarly, there are data associating delta toxin–producing *S. epidermidis* to neonatal necrotizing enterocolitis.[182] However, causation remains conjectural.[183] Coagulase-negative staphylococcal infections in the neonate infrequently result in mortality but are often associated with morbidity requiring many additional days of care in the hospital while receiving antimicrobial therapy.

Prevention of coagulase-negative staphylococcal infection in neonates has largely concentrated on prevention of intravascular catheter–associated infection. Catheters should be inserted with meticulous attention to aseptic practices. Staff should adhere to appropriate protocol in caring for the catheter site and in accessing the catheter, including thorough disinfection of the catheter connector valve or hub.[184] Other preventive measures have included use of prophylactic antibiotics or antimicrobial flush solutions. A meta-analysis of five randomized controlled trials that evaluated the safety and efficacy of prophylactic vancomycin in preventing late-onset sepsis in neonates has confirmed a beneficial effect.[185] However, mortality and length of stay were not significantly different between the two groups. There were insufficient data to evaluate the risk of development of vancomycin-resistant organisms. Similarly, a trial of a vancomycin–heparin catheter lock solution proved beneficial in preventing bloodstream infections.[186]

Non–*S. epidermidis* Species of Coagulase-Negative Staphylococci

In addition to *S. epidermidis*, there are several other species of coagulase-negative staphylococci that should be specifically discussed because of their pathogenic potential and other unique features.

STAPHYLOCOCCUS HAEMOLYTICUS

S. haemolyticus is typically the second or third most common species of coagulase-negative staphylococci to be incriminated as a cause of infection. These infections are usually nosocomial bloodstream infections related to intravascular catheters, but descriptions of skin and soft tissue infection, urinary tract infection, meningitis, endocarditis, and a variety of device-associated infections have been described.[187-190] *S. haemolyticus* has been implicated in outbreaks, most often in neonatal intensive care units. *S. haemolyticus* contains several putative virulence genes, including lipases, proteases, and lyases. The most noteworthy feature of *S. haemolyticus* is that it is often resistant to multiple antibiotics, including glycopeptides.[191,192] The glycopeptide-resistant strains possess highly cross-linked peptidoglycans with serine instead of glycine in their cross bridges.

STAPHYLOCOCCUS LUGDUNENSIS

S. lugdunensis, first described in 1988, is a constituent of the normal human skin flora and an infrequent, but not rare, human pathogen.

S. lugdunensis behaves clinically in a manner similar to *S. aureus* and has been described to cause fulminant native valve endocarditis, prosthetic valve endocarditis, skin and soft tissue infection, bacteremia, ocular infection, urinary tract infection, central nervous system infection, bone and joint infection, and peritonitis.[8,193,194] It is thought that *S. lugdunensis* is more virulent than other coagulase-negative staphylococci because of the production of several virulence factors, including a delta toxin–like hemolytic peptide, a variety of adhesins promoting adherence to collagen, fibronectin, fibrinogen, laminin, and vitronectin, a variety of enzymes including DNase and lipase, lysozyme resistance, and biofilm formation.[8] Its prominent role in native valve endocarditis may be the result of the production of a von Willebrand factor–binding protein that allows it to bind to endothelial lesions.[51] In addition, it possesses an accessory gene regulator system (*agr* locus) similar to *S. aureus*.

Identification of this species by the clinical laboratory can be difficult. *S. lugdunensis* can be easily confused with *S. aureus* if identification is only based on the latex agglutination test, because the production of clumping factor by *S. lugdunensis* will yield a positive test result.[8] Fortuitously, the organism is generally susceptible to most antistaphylococcal antibiotics because β-lactamase production is found in only about 25% of strains and methicillin resistance is uncommon. Infections with *S. lugdunensis* are treated similarly to those with *S. aureus*. Although similar putative virulence determinants have been described in *S schleiferi*, this species is only rarely associated with disease in humans.[5] However, it appears to be a significant cause of skin disease and otitis in companion animals.[195]

STAPHYLOCOCCUS SAPROPHYTICUS

S. saprophyticus colonizes the rectum or urogenital tracts of approximately 5% to 10% of women[196] and is second only to *E. coli* as the causative agent of uncomplicated urinary tract infections in young, sexually active women.[197,198] These urinary tract infections have a seasonal predilection (late summer and fall), often follow sexual intercourse or menstruation, and may occur concomitantly with vaginal candidiasis.[199] 90% of patients with *S. saprophyticus* urinary tract infections are symptomatic, with dysuria, frequency, or urgency, and 80% have pyuria or hematuria. *S. saprophyticus* possesses a unique adhesion protein, UafA, which allows it to adhere to human uroepithelial cells and mediates hemagglutination.[88] In addition, this bacterium encodes several transport proteins, enabling it to adjust rapidly to osmotic and pH changes, and it produces abundant urease, allowing it to proliferate in urine.[90] *S. saprophyticus* can be differentiated from other coagulase-negative staphylococci because of its resistance to novobiocin. However, it remains susceptible to other antimicrobial agents and *S. saprophyticus* urinary tract infections are usually successfully treated with urinary tract antimicrobials, with only rarely reported sequelae. Rare cases of native valve endocarditis, endophthalmitis, and septicemia have been cited in the literature.

REFERENCES

1. Rupp ME, Archer GL. Coagulase-negative staphylococci: Pathogens associated with medical progress. *Clin Infect Dis.* 1994;19:231-243.
2. Rogers KL, Fey PD, Rupp ME. Epidemiology of infections due to coagulase-negative staphylococci. In: Crossley KB, Jefferson KK, Archer G, Fowler VG Jr, eds. *The Staphylococci in Human Disease.* 2nd ed. Blackwell Publishing; 2009:310-332.
3. Mack D, Horstkotte MA, Rhode H, et al. Coagulase-negative staphylococci. In: Pace JL, Rupp ME, Finch RG, eds. *Biofilms, Infection, and Antimicrobial Therapy.* Boca Raton, Fla: Taylor & Francis; 2006:109-153.
4. O'Gara JP, Humphreys H. *Staphylococcus epidermidis* biofilms: importance and implications. *J Med Microbiol.* 2001;50:582-587.
5. von Eiff C, Peters G, Heilmann C. Pathogenesis of infections due to coagulase-negative staphylococci. *Lancet Infect Dis.* 2002;2:677-685.
6. Bannerman TL, Peacock SJ. Staphylococcus, micrococcus, and other catalase-positive cocci. In: Murray PR, Baron EJ, Jorgensen JH, et al, eds. *Manual of Clinical Microbiology.* Washington, DC: American Society for Microbiology; 2007:390-411.
7. Kloos WE, Musselwhite MS. Distribution and persistence of *Staphylococcus* and *Micrococcus* species and other aerobic bacteria on human skin. *Appl Microbiol.* 1975;30:381-385.
8. Frank KL, Del Pozo JL, Patel R. From clinical microbiology to infection pathogenesis: How daring to be different works for *Staphylococcus lugdunensis*. *Clin Microbiol Rev.* 2008;21:111-133.
9. Ghebremedhin B, Layer F, Konig W, et al. Genetic classification and distinguishing of *Staphylococcus* species based on different partial gap, 16S rRNA, hsp60, rpoB, sodA, and tuf gene sequences. *J Clin Microbiol.* 2008;46:1019-1025.
10. Streit JM, Jones RN, Sader HS, et al. Assessment of pathogen occurrences and resistance profiles among infected patients in the intensive care unit: report from the SENTRY Antimicrobial Surveillance Program (North America, 2001). *Int J Antimicrob Agents.* 2004;24:111-118.
11. Hope R, Livermore DM, Brick G, et al. Non-susceptibility trends among staphylococci from bacteraemias in the UK and Ireland, 2001-06. *J Antimicrob Chemother.* 2008;62(Suppl 2):ii65-ii74.
12. Sieradzki K, Villari P, Tomasz A. Decreased susceptibilities to teicoplanin and vancomycin among coagulase-negative methi-

cillin-resistant clinical isolates of staphylococci. *Antimicrob Agents Chemother.* 1998;42:100-107.
13. Sieradzki K, Roberts RB, Serur D, et al. Heterogeneously vancomycin-resistant *Staphylococcus epidermidis* strain causing recurrent peritonitis in a dialysis patient during vancomycin therapy. *J Clin Microbiol.* 1999;37:39-44.
14. Nunes AP, Teixeira LM, Iorio NL, et al. Heterogeneous resistance to vancomycin in *Staphylococcus epidermidis*, *Staphylococcus haemolyticus* and *Staphylococcus warneri* clinical strains: Characterisation of glycopeptide susceptibility profiles and cell wall thickening. *Int J Antimicrob Agents.* 2006;27:307-315.
15. Froggatt JW, Johnston JL, Galetto DW, et al. Antimicrobial resistance in nosocomial isolates of *Staphylococcus haemolyticus*. *Antimicrob Agents Chemother.* 1989;33:460-466.
16. Clinical and Laboratory Standards Institute. *Performance Standards for Antimicrobial Susceptibility Testing: Eighteenth Information Supplement.* CLSI Document M100-S18. Wayne, Pa: Clinical and Laboratory Standards Institute; 2008.
17. Vazquez GJ, Archer GL. Antibiotic therapy of experimental *Staphylococcus epidermidis* endocarditis. *Antimicrob Agents Chemother.* 1980;17:280-285.

18. Prere MF, Baron O, Cohen Bacrie S, et al. Genotype MRSA, a new genetic test for the rapid identification of staphylococci and detection of mecA gene. *Pathol Biol (Paris).* 2006;54:502-505.

19. Knausz M, Ghidan A, Grossato A, et al. Rapid detection of methicillin resistance in teicoplanin-resistant coagulase-negative staphylococci by a penicillin-binding protein 2′ latex agglutination method. *J Microbiol Methods.* 2005;60:413-416.

20. Petersen PJ, Bradford PA, Weiss WJ, et al. In vitro and in vivo activities of tigecycline (GAR-936), daptomycin, and comparative antimicrobial agents against glycopeptide-intermediate *Staphylococcus aureus* and other resistant gram-positive pathogens. *Antimicrob Agents Chemother.* 2002;46:2595-2601.

21. Noskin GA, Siddiqui F, Stosor V, et al. In vitro activities of linezolid against important gram-positive bacterial pathogens including vancomycin-resistant enterococci. *Antimicrob Agents Chemother.* 1999;43:2059-2062.

22. Sader HS, Jones RN, Dowzicky MJ, et al. Antimicrobial activity of tigecycline tested against nosocomial bacterial pathogens from patients hospitalized in the intensive care unit. *Diagn Microbiol Infect Dis.* 2005;52:203-208.

23. Gales AC, Jones RN, Andrade SS, et al. In vitro activity of tigecycline, a new glycylcycline, tested against 1,326 clinical bacterial strains isolated from Latin America. *Braz J Infect Dis.* 2005;9:348-356.

24. Lin G, Credito K, Ednie LM, et al. Antistaphylococcal activity of dalbavancin, an experimental glycopeptide. *Antimicrob Agents Chemother.* 2005;49:770-772.

25. King A, Phillips I, Kaniga K. Comparative in vitro activity of telavancin (TD-6424), a rapidly bactericidal, concentration-dependent anti-infective with multiple mechanisms of action against gram-positive bacteria. *J Antimicrob Chemother.* 2004;53:797-803.

26. Micek ST. Alternatives to vancomycin for the treatment of methicillin-resistant *Staphylococcus aureus* infections. *Clin Infect Dis.* 2007;45(Suppl 3):S184-S190.

27. Kohlhoff SA, Sharma R. Iclaprim. *Expert Opin Investig Drugs.* 2007;16:1441-1448.

28. Bogdanovich T, Ednie LM, Shapiro S, et al. Antistaphylococcal activity of ceftobiprole, a new broad-spectrum cephalosporin. *Antimicrob Agents Chemother.* 2005;49:4210-4219.

29. Parish D, Scheinfeld N. Ceftaroline fosamil, a cephalosporin derivative for the potential treatment of MRSA infection. *Curr Opin Investig Drugs.* 2008;9:201-209.

30. Lewis K. Persister cells, dormancy and infectious disease. *Nat Rev Microbiol.* 2007;5:48-56.

31. Saginur R, Stdenis M, Ferris W, et al. Multiple combination bactericidal testing of staphylococcal biofilms from implant-associated infections. *Antimicrob Agents Chemother.* 2006;50:55-61.

32. Miragaia M, Carrico JA, Thomas JC, et al. Comparison of molecular typing methods for characterization of *Staphylococcus epidermidis*: proposal for clone definition. *J Clin Microbiol.* 2008;46:118-129.

33. Jamaluddin TZ, Kuwahara-Arai K, Hisata K, et al. Extreme genetic diversity of methicillin-resistant *Staphylococcus epidermidis* strains disseminated among healthy Japanese children. *J Clin Microbiol.* 2008;46:3778-3783.

34. Miragaia M, Thomas JC, Couto I, et al. Inferring a population structure for *Staphylococcus epidermidis* from multilocus sequence typing data. *J Bacteriol.* 2007;189:2540-2552.

35. Wisplinghoff H, Rosato AE, Enright MC, et al. Related clones containing SCCmec type IV predominate among clinically significant *Staphylococcus epidermidis* isolates. *Antimicrob Agents Chemother.* 2003;47:3574-3579.

36. Kozitskaya S, Olson ME, Fey PD, et al. Clonal analysis of *Staphylococcus epidermidis* isolates carrying or lacking biofilm-mediating genes by multilocus sequence typing. *J Clin Microbiol.* 2005;43:4751-4757.

37. Wang XM, Noble L, Kreiswirth BN, et al. Evaluation of a multilocus sequence typing system for *Staphylococcus epidermidis*. *J Med Microbiol.* 2003;52:989-998.

38. Johansson A, Koskiniemi S, Gottfridsson P, et al. Multiple-locus variable-number tandem repeat analysis for typing of *Staphylococcus epidermidis*. *J Clin Microbiol.* 2006;44:260-265.

39. Francois P, Hochmann A, Huyghe A, et al. Rapid and high-throughput genotyping of *Staphylococcus epidermidis* isolates by automated multilocus variable-number of tandem repeats: a tool for real-time epidemiology. *J Microbiol Methods.* 2008;72:296-305.

40. Rupp ME, Ulphani JS, Fey PD, et al. Characterization of *Staphylococcus epidermidis* polysaccharide intercellular adhesin/hemagglutinin in the pathogenesis of intravascular catheter-associated infection in a rat model. *Infect Immun.* 1999;67:2656-2659.

41. Rupp ME, Ulphani JS, Fey PD, et al. Characterization of the importance of polysaccharide intercellular adhesin/hemagglutinin of *Staphylococcus epidermidis* in the pathogenesis of biomaterial-based infection in a mouse foreign body infection model. *Infect Immun.* 1999;67:2627-2632.

42. Heilmann C, Schweitzer O, Gerke C, et al. Molecular basis of intercellular adhesion in the biofilm-forming *Staphylococcus epidermidis*. *Mol Microbiol.* 1996;20:1083-1091.

43. Kocianova S, Vuong C, Yao Y, et al. Key role of poly-gamma-DL-glutamic acid in immune evasion and virulence of *Staphylococcus epidermidis*. *J Clin Invest.* 2005;115:688-694.

44. Vuong C, Durr M, Carmody AB, et al. Regulated expression of pathogen-associated molecular pattern molecules in *Staphylococcus epidermidis*: Quorum-sensing determines pro-inflamma-

tory capacity and production of phenol-soluble modulins. *Cell Microbiol.* 2004;6:753-759.

45. Resch A, Rosenstein R, Nerz C, et al. Differential gene expression profiling of *Staphylococcus aureus* cultivated under biofilm and planktonic conditions. *Appl Environ Microbiol.* 2005;71:2663-2676.

46. Yao Y, Sturdevant DE, Otto M. Genomewide analysis of gene expression in *Staphylococcus epidermidis* biofilms: Insights into the pathophysiology of S. epidermidis biofilms and the role of phenol-soluble modulins in formation of biofilms. *J Infect Dis.* 2005;191:289-298.

47. Beenken KE, Dunman PM, McAleese F, et al. Global gene expression in *Staphylococcus aureus* biofilms. *J Bacteriol.* 2004;186:4665-4684.

48. Stewart PS, Franklin MJ. Physiological heterogeneity in biofilms. *Nat Rev Microbiol.* 2008;6:199-210.

49. Rani SA, Pitts B, Beyenal H, et al. Spatial patterns of DNA replication, protein synthesis, and oxygen concentration within bacterial biofilms reveal diverse physiological states. *J Bacteriol.* 2007;189:4223-4233.

50. Zhang YQ, Ren SX, Li HL, et al. Genome-based analysis of virulence genes in a non-biofilm-forming *Staphylococcus epidermidis* strain (ATCC 12228). *Mol Microbiol.* 2003;49:1577-1593.

51. Nilsson M, Bjerketorp J, Guss B, et al. A fibrinogen-binding protein of *Staphylococcus lugdunensis*. *FEMS Microbiol Lett.* 2004;241:87-93.

52. Hartford O, O'Brien L, Schofield K, et al. The Fbe (SdrG) protein of *Staphylococcus epidermidis* HB promotes bacterial adherence to fibrinogen. *Microbiology.* 2001;147:2545-2552.

53. Gill SR, Fouts DE, Archer GL, et al. Insights on evolution of virulence and resistance from the complete genome analysis of an early methicillin-resistant *Staphylococcus aureus* strain and a biofilm-producing methicillin-resistant *Staphylococcus epidermidis* strain. *J Bacteriol.* 2005;187:2426-2438.

54. Bowden MG, Visai L, Longshaw CM, et al. Is the GehD lipase from *Staphylococcus epidermidis* a collagen binding adhesin? *J Biol Chem.* 2002;277:43017-43023.

55. Bowden MG, Heuck AP, Ponnuraj K, et al. Evidence for the "dock, lock, and latch" ligand binding mechanism of the staphylococcal microbial surface component recognizing adhesive matrix molecules (MSCRAMM) SdrG. *J Biol Chem.* 2008;283:638-647.

56. Heilmann C, Thumm G, Chhatwal GS, et al. Identification and characterization of a novel autolysin (Aae) with adhesive properties from *Staphylococcus epidermidis*. *Microbiology.* 2003;149:2769-2778.

57. Heilmann C, Hussain M, Peters G, et al. Evidence for autolysin-mediated primary attachment of *Staphylococcus epidermidis* to a polystyrene surface. *Mol Microbiol.* 1997;24:1013-1024.

58. Rupp ME, Fey PD, Heilmann C, et al. Characterization of the importance of *Staphylococcus epidermidis* autolysin and polysaccharide intercellular adhesin in the pathogenesis of intravascular catheter-associated infection in a rat model. *J Infect Dis.* 2001;183:1038-1042.

59. Guo B, Zhao X, Shi Y, et al. Pathogenic implication of a fibrinogen-binding protein of *Staphylococcus epidermidis* in a rat model of intravascular-catheter-associated infection. *Infect Immun.* 2007;75:2991-2995.

60. Qin Z, Ou Y, Yang L, et al. Role of autolysin-mediated DNA release in biofilm formation of *Staphylococcus epidermidis*. *Microbiology.* 2007;153:2083-2092.

61. Rice KC, Mann EE, Endres JL, et al. The cidA murein hydrolase regulator contributes to DNA release and biofilm development in *Staphylococcus aureus*. *Proc Natl Acad Sci U S A.* 2007;104:8113-8118.

62. Izano EA, Amarante MA, Kher WB, et al. Differential roles of poly-N-acetylglucosamine surface polysaccharide and extracellular DNA in *Staphylococcus aureus* and *Staphylococcus epidermidis* biofilms. *Appl Environ Microbiol.* 2008;74:470-476.

63. Mack D, Fischer W, Krokotsch A, et al. The intercellular adhesin involved in biofilm accumulation of *Staphylococcus epidermidis* is a linear beta-1,6-linked glucosaminoglycan: purification and structural analysis. *J Bacteriol.* 1996;178:175-183.

64. Conlon KM, Humphreys H, O'Gara JP. Regulation of icaR gene expression in *Staphylococcus epidermidis*. *FEMS Microbiol Lett.* 2002;216:171-177.

65. Vuong C, Kocianova S, Voyich JM, et al. A crucial role for exopolysaccharide modification in bacterial biofilm formation, immune evasion, and virulence. *J Biol Chem.* 2004;279:54881-54886.

66. Gotz F. Staphylococcus and biofilms. *Mol Microbiol.* 2002;43:1367-1378.

67. Xu L, Li H, Vuong C, et al. Role of the luxS quorum-sensing system in biofilm formation and virulence of *Staphylococcus epidermidis*. *Infect Immun.* 2006;74:488-496.

68. Wang L, Li M, Dong D, et al. SarZ is a key regulator of biofilm formation and virulence in *Staphylococcus epidermidis*. *J Infect Dis.* 2008;197:1254-1262.

69. Vuong C, Kidder JB, Jacobson ER, et al. *Staphylococcus epidermidis* polysaccharide intercellular adhesin production significantly increases during tricarboxylic acid cycle stress. *J Bacteriol.* 2005;187:2967-2973.

70. Tormo MA, Marti M, Valle J, et al. SarA is an essential positive regulator of *Staphylococcus epidermidis* biofilm development. *J Bacteriol.* 2005;187:2348-2356.

71. Jefferson KK, Cramton SE, Gotz F, et al. Identification of a 5-nucleotide sequence that controls expression of the ica locus

in *Staphylococcus aureus* and characterization of the DNA-binding properties of IcaR. *Mol Microbiol.* 2003;48:889-899.

72. Handke LD, Slater SR, Conlon KM, et al. SigmaB and SarA independently regulate polysaccharide intercellular adhesin production in *Staphylococcus epidermidis*. *Can J Microbiol.* 2007;53:82-91.

73. Conlon KM, Humphreys H, O'Gara JP. icaR encodes a transcriptional repressor involved in environmental regulation of ica operon expression and biofilm formation in *Staphylococcus epidermidis*. *J Bacteriol.* 2002;184:4400-4408.

74. McKenney D, Pouliot KL, Wang Y, et al. Broadly protective vaccine for *Staphylococcus aureus* based on an in vivo-expressed antigen. *Science.* 1999;284:1523-1527.

75. Kropec A, Maira-Litran T, Jefferson KK, et al. Poly-N-acetylglucosamine production in *Staphylococcus aureus* is essential for virulence in murine models of systemic infection. *Infect Immun.* 2005;73:6868-6876.

76. Kelly-Quintos C, Cavacini LA, Posner MR, et al. Characterization of the opsonic and protective activity against *Staphylococcus aureus* of fully human monoclonal antibodies specific for the bacterial surface polysaccharide poly-N-acetylglucosamine. *Infect Immun.* 2006;74:2742-2750.

77. Cerca N, Maira-Litran T, Jefferson KK, et al. Protection against *Escherichia coli* infection by antibody to the *Staphylococcus aureus* poly-N-acetylglucosamine surface polysaccharide. *Proc Natl Acad Sci U S A.* 2007;104:7528-7533.

78. Rohde H, Burandt EC, Siemssen N, et al. Polysaccharide intercellular adhesin or protein factors in biofilm accumulation of *Staphylococcus epidermidis* and *Staphylococcus aureus* isolated from prosthetic hip and knee joint infections. *Biomaterials.* 2007;28:1711-1720.

79. Rohde H, Kalitzky M, Kroger N, et al. Detection of virulence-associated genes not useful for discriminating between invasive and commensal *Staphylococcus epidermidis* strains from a bone marrow transplant unit. *J Clin Microbiol.* 2004;42:5614-5619.

80. Cucarella C, Solano C, Valle J, et al. Bap, a Staphylococcus aureus surface protein involved in biofilm formation. *J Bacteriol.* 2001;183:2888-2896.

81. Rogers KL, Rupp ME, Fey PD. The presence of icaADBC is detrimental to the colonization of human skin by *Staphylococcus epidermidis*. *Appl Environ Microbiol.* 2008;74:6155-6157.

82. Wang R, Braughton KR, Kretschmer D, et al. Identification of novel cytolytic peptides as key virulence determinants for community-associated MRSA. *Nat Med.* 2007;13:1510-1514.

83. Otto M, O'Mahoney DS, Guina T, et al. Activity of *Staphylococcus epidermidis* phenol-soluble modulin peptides expressed in *Staphylococcus carnosus*. *J Infect Dis.* 2004;190:748-755.

84. Mehlin C, Headley CM, Klebanoff SJ. An inflammatory polypeptide complex from *Staphylococcus epidermidis*: Isolation and characterization. *J Exp Med.* 1999;189:907-918.

85. Little SF, Ivins BE. Molecular pathogenesis of *Bacillus anthracis* infection. *Microbes Infect.* 1999;1:131-139.

86. Kupke T, Gotz F. Expression, purification, and characterization of EpiC, an enzyme involved in the biosynthesis of the lantibiotic epidermin, and sequence analysis of *Staphylococcus epidermidis* epiC mutants. *J Bacteriol.* 1996;178:1335-1340.

87. Szabados F, Kleine B, Anders A, et al. *Staphylococcus saprophyticus* ATCC 15305 is internalized into human urinary bladder carcinoma cell line 5637. *FEMS Microbiol Lett.* 2008;285:163-169.

88. Kuroda M, Yamashita A, Hirakawa H, et al. Whole genome sequence of *Staphylococcus saprophyticus* reveals the pathogenesis of uncomplicated urinary tract infection. *Proc Natl Acad Sci U S A.* 2005;102:13272-13277.

89. Hell W, Meyer HG, Gatermann SG. Cloning of aas, a gene encoding a *Staphylococcus saprophyticus* surface protein with adhesive and autolytic properties. *Mol Microbiol.* 1998;29:871-881.

90. Gatermann S, John J, Marre R. *Staphylococcus saprophyticus* urease: Characterization and contribution to uropathogenicity in unobstructed urinary tract infection of rats. *Infect Immun.* 1989;57:110-116.

91. Gatermann S, Marre R. Cloning and expression of *Staphylococcus saprophyticus* urease gene sequences in *Staphylococcus carnosus* and contribution of the enzyme to virulence. *Infect Immun.* 1989;57:2998-3002.

92. Nilsson M, Bjerketorp J, Wiebensjo A, et al. A von Willebrand factor-binding protein from *Staphylococcus lugdunensis*. *FEMS Microbiol Lett.* 2004;234:155-161.

93. Mitchell J, Tristan A, Foster TJ. Characterization of the fibrinogen-binding surface protein Fbl of Staphylococcus lugdunensis. *Microbiology.* 2004;150:3831-3841.

94. Minhas T, Ludlam HA, Wilks M, et al. Detection by PCR and analysis of the distribution of a fibronectin-binding protein gene (fbn) among staphylococcal isolates. *J Med Microbiol.* 1995;42:96-101.

95. Weinstein MP, Towns ML, Quartey SM, et al. The clinical significance of positive blood cultures in the 1990s: A prospective comprehensive evaluation of the microbiology, epidemiology, and outcome of bacteremia and fungemia in adults. *Clin Infect Dis.* 1997;24:584-602.

96. Hall KK, Lyman JA. Updated review of blood culture contamination. *Clin Microbiol Rev.* 2006;19:788-802.

97. Souvenir D, Anderson DE Jr, Palpant S, et al. Blood cultures positive for coagulase-negative staphylococci: antisepsis, pseudobacteremia, and therapy of patients. *J Clin Microbiol.* 1998;36:1923-1926.

98. Beekmann SE, Diekema DJ, Doern GV. Determining the clinical significance of coagulase-negative staphylococci isolated from blood cultures. *Infect Control Hosp Epidemiol.* 2005;26: 559-566.

99. Shafazand S, Weinacker AB. Blood cultures in the critical care unit: Improving utilization and yield. *Chest.* 2002;122: 1727-1736.

100. Tokars JI. Predictive value of blood cultures positive for coagulase-negative staphylococci: implications for patient care and health care quality assurance. *Clin Infect Dis.* 2004;39: 333-341.

101. Mirrett S, Weinstein MP, Reimer LG, et al. Relevance of the number of positive bottles in determining clinical significance of coagulase-negative staphylococci in blood cultures. *J Clin Microbiol.* 2001;39:3279-3281.

102. Haimi-Cohen Y, Shafinoori S, Tucci V, et al. Use of incubation time to detection in BACTEC 9240 to distinguish coagulase-negative staphylococcal contamination from infection in pediatric blood cultures. *Pediatr Infect Dis J.* 2003;22:968-974.

103. Raad I, Hanna HA, Alakech B, et al. Differential time to positivity: A useful method for diagnosing catheter-related bloodstream infections. *Ann Intern Med.* 2004;140:18-25.

104. Santolaya ME, Cofre J, Beresi V. C-reactive protein: A valuable aid for the management of febrile children with cancer and neutropenia. *Clin Infect Dis.* 1994;18:589-595.

105. Schuetz P, Mueller B, Trampuz A. Serum procalcitonin for discrimination of blood contamination from bloodstream infection due to coagulase-negative staphylococci. *Infection.* 2007;35:352-355.

106. Seo SK, Venkataraman L, DeGirolami PC, et al. Molecular typing of coagulase-negative staphylococci from blood cultures does not correlate with clinical criteria for true bacteremia. *Am J Med.* 2000;109:697-704.

107. Sharma M, Riederer K, Johnson LB, et al. Molecular analysis of coagulase-negative Staphylococcus isolates from blood cultures: Prevalence of genotypic variation and polyclonal bacteremia. *Clin Infect Dis.* 2001;33:1317-1323.

108. Khatib R, Riederer KM, Clark JA, et al. Coagulase-negative staphylococci in multiple blood cultures: strain relatedness and determinants of same-strain bacteremia. *J Clin Microbiol.* 1995;33:816-820.

109. de Silva GD, Kantzanou M, Justice A, et al. The ica operon and biofilm production in coagulase-negative Staphylococci associated with carriage and disease in a neonatal intensive care unit. *J Clin Microbiol.* 2002;40:382-388.

110. Spitalnic SJ, Woolard RH, Mermel LA. The significance of changing needles when inoculating blood cultures: a meta-analysis. *Clin Infect Dis.* 1995;21:1103-1106.

111. Schifman RB, Strand CL, Meier FA, et al. Blood culture contamination: A College of American Pathologists Q-Probes study involving 640 institutions and 497134 specimens from adult patients. *Arch Pathol Lab Med.* 1998;122:216-221.

112. Rupp ME. Infections associated with intravascular catheters. In: Baddour L, Gorbach SL, eds. *Therapy of Infectious Diseases.* Philadelphia: WB Saunders; 2003:141-151.

113. Sherertz RJ, Heard SO, Raad II. Diagnosis of triple-lumen catheter infection: Comparison of roll plate, sonication, and flushing methodologies. *J Clin Microbiol.* 1997;35:641-646.

114. Maki DG, Weise CE, Sarafin HW. A semiquantitative culture method for identifying intravenous catheter–related infection. *N Engl J Med.* 1977;296:1305-1309.

115. Mermel LA, Farr BM, Sherertz RJ, et al. Guidelines for the management of intravascular catheter-related infections. *Clin Infect Dis.* 2001;32:1249-1272.

116. Raad I, Davis S, Khan A, et al. Impact of central venous catheter removal on the recurrence of catheter-related coagulase-negative staphylococcal bacteremia. *Infect Control Hosp Epidemiol.* 1992;13:215-221.

117. Demitrovicova A, Hricak V, Karvay M, et al. Endocarditis due to coagulase-negative staphylococci: Data from a 22-years national survey. *Scand J Infect Dis.* 2007;39:655-656.

118. Lalani T, Kanafani ZA, Chu VH, et al. Prosthetic valve endocarditis due to coagulase-negative staphylococci: Findings from the International Collaboration on Endocarditis Merged Database. *Eur J Clin Microbiol Infect Dis.* 2006;25:365-368.

119. Wang A, Athan E, Pappas PA, et al. Contemporary clinical profile and outcome of prosthetic valve endocarditis. *Jama.* 2007;297:1354-1361.

120. Karchmer AW, Archer GL, Dismukes WE. Staphylococcus epidermidis causing prosthetic valve endocarditis: microbiologic and clinical observations as guides to therapy. *Ann Intern Med.* 1983;98:447-455.

121. Baddour LM, Wilson WR, Bayer AS, et al. Infective endocarditis: Diagnosis, antimicrobial therapy, and management of complications: A statement for health care professionals from the Committee on Rheumatic Fever, Endocarditis, and Kawasaki Disease, Council on Cardiovascular Disease in the Young, and the Councils on Clinical Cardiology, Stroke, and Cardiovascular Surgery and Anesthesia, American Heart Association: endorsed by the Infectious Diseases Society of America. *Circulation.* 2005;111:e394-e434.

122. Chu VH, Woods CW, Miro JM, et al. Emergence of coagulase-negative staphylococci as a cause of native valve endocarditis. *Clin Infect Dis.* 2008;46:232-242.

123. Caputo GM, Archer GL, Calderwood SB, et al. Native valve endocarditis due to coagulase-negative staphylococci. Clinical and microbiologic features. *Am J Med.* 1987;83:619-625.

124. Chambers ST. Diagnosis and management of staphylococcal infections of pacemakers and cardiac defibrillators. *Intern Med J.* 2005;35(Suppl 2):S63-S71.

125. del Rio A, Anguera I, Miro JM, et al. Surgical treatment of pacemaker and defibrillator lead endocarditis: The impact of electrode lead extraction on outcome. *Chest.* 2003;124: 1451-1459.

126. Chua JD, Wilkoff BL, Lee I, et al. Diagnosis and management of infections involving implantable electrophysiologic cardiac devices. *Ann Intern Med.* 2000;133:604-608.

127. Gandelman G, Frishman WH, Wiese C, et al. Intravascular device infections: Epidemiology, diagnosis, and management. *Cardiol Rev.* 2007;15:13-23.

128. Baddour LM, Bettmann MA, Bolger AF, et al. Nonvalvular cardiovascular device-related infections. *Circulation.* 2003;108: 2015-2031.

129. Perera GB, Fujitani RM, Kubaska SM. Aortic graft infection: Update on management and treatment options. *Vasc Endovascular Surg.* 2006;40:1-10.

130. Stewart AH, Eyers PS, Earnshaw JJ. Prevention of infection in peripheral arterial reconstruction: a systematic review and meta-analysis. *J Vasc Surg.* 2007;46:148-155.

131. Chambers ST. Diagnosis and management of staphylococcal infections of vascular grafts and stents. *Intern Med J.* 2005;35(Suppl 2):S72-S78.

132. Bergamini TM, Bandyk DF, Govostis D, et al. Identification of Staphylococcus epidermidis vascular graft infections: A comparison of culture techniques. *J Vasc Surg.* 1989;9:665-670.

133. Batt M, Magne JL, Alric P, et al. In situ revascularization with silver-coated polyester grafts to treat aortic infection: Early and midterm results. *J Vasc Surg.* 2003;38:983-989.

134. Trampuz A, Piper KE, Jacobson MJ, et al. Sonication of removed hip and knee prostheses for diagnosis of infection. *N Engl J Med.* 2007;357:654-663.

135. Zimmerli W, Trampuz A, Ochsner PE. Prosthetic-joint infections. *N Engl J Med.* 2004;351:1645-1654.

136. Steckelberg JM, Osmon DR. Prosthetic joint infections. In: Waldvogel FA, Bisno AL, eds. *Infections Associated with Indwelling Medical Devices.* 3rd ed. Washington DC: ASM Press; 2000:173-210.

137. Berbari EF, Marculescu C, Sia I, et al. Culture-negative prosthetic joint infection. *Clin Infect Dis.* 2007;45:1113-1119.

138. Bassetti M, Vitale F, Melica G, et al. Linezolid in the treatment of Gram-positive prosthetic joint infections. *J Antimicrob Chemother.* 2005;55:387-390.

139. Antony SJ. Combination therapy with daptomycin, vancomycin, and rifampin for recurrent, severe bone and prosthetic joint infections involving methicillin-resistant *Staphylococcus aureus.* *Scand J Infect Dis.* 2006;38:293-295.

140. Laurent F, Bignon A, Goldnadel J, et al. A new concept of gentamicin loaded HAP/TCP bone substitute for prophylactic action: In vitro release validation. *J Mater Sci Mater Med.* 2008;19:947-951.

141. Norden CW. Prevention of bone and joint infections. *Am J Med.* 1985;78:229-232.

142. Lidgren L. Joint prosthetic infections: A success story. *Acta Orthop Scand.* 2001;72:553-556.

143. Lozier AP, Sciacca RR, Romagnoli MF, et al. Ventriculostomy-related infections: a critical review of the literature. *Neurosurgery.* 2002;51:170-181.

144. Arabi Y, Memish ZA, Balkhy HH, et al. Ventriculostomy-associated infections: Incidence and risk factors. *Am J Infect Control.* 2005;33:137-143.

145. Tunkel AR, Hartman BJ, Kaplan SL, et al. Practice guidelines for the management of bacterial meningitis. *Clin Infect Dis.* 2004;39:1267-1284.

146. Ratilal B, Costa J, Sampaio C. Antibiotic prophylaxis for preventing meningitis in patients with basilar skull fractures. *Cochrane Database Syst Rev.* 2006(1):CD004884.

147. Pirotte BJ, Lubansu A, Bruneau M, et al. Sterile surgical technique for shunt placement reduces the shunt infection rate in children: Preliminary analysis of a prospective protocol in 115 consecutive procedures. *Childs Nerv Syst.* 2007;23:1251-1261.

148. Sciubba DM, Stuart RM, McGirt MJ, et al. Effect of antibiotic-impregnated shunt catheters in decreasing the incidence of shunt infection in the treatment of hydrocephalus. *J Neurosurg.* 2005;103:131-136.

149. Ritz R, Roser F, Morgalla M, et al. Do antibiotic-impregnated shunts in hydrocephalus therapy reduce the risk of infection? An observational study in 258 patients. *BMC Infect Dis.* 2007;7:38.

150. Mangram AJ, Horan TC, Pearson ML, et al. Guideline for prevention of surgical site infection, 1999. Hospital Infection Control Practices Advisory Committee. *Infect Control Hosp Epidemiol.* 1999;20:250-278.

151. Vas S, Oreopoulos DG. Infections in patients undergoing peritoneal dialysis. *Infect Dis Clin North Am.* 2001;15: 743-774.

152. Monsen T, Olofsson C, Ronnmark M, et al. Clonal spread of staphylococci among patients with peritonitis associated with continuous ambulatory peritoneal dialysis. *Kidney Int.* 2000;57:613-618.

153. de Lourdes Ribeiro de Souza da Cunha M, Montelli AC, Fioravante AM, et al. Predictive factors of outcome following staphylococcal peritonitis in continuous ambulatory peritoneal dialysis. *Clinical Nephrology.* 2005;64:378-382.

154. Zelenitsky S, Barns L, Findlay I, et al. Analysis of microbiological trends in peritoneal dialysis-related peritonitis from 1991 to 1998. *Am J Kidney Dis.* 2000;36:1009-1013.

155. Bender FH, Bernardini J, Piraino B. Prevention of infectious complications in peritoneal dialysis: Best demonstrated practices. *Kidney Int Suppl.* 2006:S44-S54.

156. Bonifati C, Pansini F, Torres DD, et al. Antimicrobial agents and catheter-related interventions to prevent peritonitis in peritoneal dialysis: Using evidence in the context of clinical practice. *Int J Artif Organs.* 2006;29:41-49.

157. de Kaspar HM, Kreidl KO, Singh K, et al. Comparison of preoperative conjunctival bacterial flora in patients undergoing glaucoma or cataract surgery. *J Glaucoma.* 2004;13:507-509.

158. Mollan SP, Gao A, Lockwood A, et al. Postcataract endophthalmitis: Incidence and microbial isolates in a United Kingdom region from 1996 through 2004. *J Cataract Refract Surg.* 2007;33:265-268.

159. Recchia FM, Busbee BG, Pearlman RB, et al. Changing trends in the microbiologic aspects of postcataract endophthalmitis. *Arch Ophthalmol.* 2005;123:341-346.

160. Hanscom TA. Postoperative endophthalmitis. *Clin Infect Dis.* 2004;38:542-546.

161. Haider SA, Hassett P, Bron AJ. Intraocular vancomycin levels after intravitreal injection in post cataract extraction endophthalmitis. *Retina.* 2001;21:210-213.

162. National Nosocomial Infections Surveillance (NNIS) System report, data summary from October 1986-April 1998, issued June 1998. *Am J Infect Control.* 1998;26:522-533.

163. Zhanel GG, Hisanaga TL, Laing NM, et al. Antibiotic resistance in outpatient urinary isolates: Final results from the North American Urinary Tract Infection Collaborative Alliance (NAUTICA). *Int J Antimicrob Agents.* 2005;26:380-388.

164. Tambyah PA, Maki DG. The relationship between pyuria and infection in patients with indwelling urinary catheters: A prospective study of 761 patients. *Arch Intern Med.* 2000;160:673-677.

165. Carson CC. Diagnosis, treatment and prevention of penile prosthesis infection. *Int J Impot Res.* 2003;15(Suppl 5):S139-S146.

166. Darouiche RO. Treatment of infections associated with surgical implants. *N Engl J Med.* 2004;350:1422-1429.

167. Abouassaly R, Angermeier KW, Montague DK. Risk of infection with an antibiotic-coated penile prosthesis at device replacement for mechanical failure. *J Urol.* 2006;176:2471-2473.

168. Brown SL, Hefflin B, Woo EK, et al. Infections related to breast implants reported to the Food and Drug Administration, 1977-1997. *J Long Term Eff Med Implants.* 2001;11:1-12.

169. Kjoller K, Holmich LR, Jacobsen PH, et al. Epidemiological investigation of local complications after cosmetic breast implant surgery in Denmark. *Ann Plast Surg.* 2002;48:229-237.

170. Pittet B, Montandon D, Pittet D. Infection in breast implants. *Lancet Infect Dis.* 2005;5:94-106.

171. Rupp ME. Hematopoietic stem cell transplantation. In: Carrico R, ed. *APIC Text of Infection Control and Epidemiology.* 2nd ed, vol 2. Washington DC: Association for Professionals in Infection Control and Epidemiology; 2005:43C1-13.

172. Costa SF, Barone AA, Miceli MH, et al. Colonization and molecular epidemiology of coagulase-negative Staphylococcal bacteremia in cancer patients: A pilot study. *Am J Infect Control.* 2006;34:36-40.

173. Richards JM, Gilewski TA, Vogelzang NJ. Association of interleukin-2 therapy with staphylococcal bacteremia. *Cancer.* 1991;67:1570-1575.

174. Kaufman D, Fairchild KD. Clinical microbiology of bacterial and fungal sepsis in very-low-birth-weight infants. *Clin Microbiol Rev.* 2004;17:638-680, table of contents.

175. Stoll BJ, Hansen N, Fanaroff AA, et al. Late-onset sepsis in very low birth weight neonates: The experience of the NICHD Neonatal Research Network. *Pediatrics.* 2002;110:285-291.

176. Patrick CH, John JF, Levkoff AH, et al. Relatedness of strains of methicillin-resistant coagulase-negative Staphylococcus colonizing hospital personnel and producing bacteremias in a neonatal intensive care unit. *Pediatr Infect Dis J.* 1992;11: 935-940.

177. Huebner J, Pier GB, Maslow JN, et al. Endemic nosocomial transmission of *Staphylococcus epidermidis* bacteremia isolates in a neonatal intensive care unit over 10 years. *J Infect Dis.* 1994;169:526-531.

178. Strunk T, Richmond P, Simmer K, et al. Neonatal immune responses to coagulase-negative staphylococci. *Curr Opin Infect Dis.* 2007;20:370-375.

179. Freeman J, Goldmann DA, Smith NE, et al. Association of intravenous lipid emulsion and coagulase-negative staphylococcal bacteremia in neonatal intensive care units. *N Engl J Med.* 1990;323:301-308.

180. Edwards JR, Peterson KD, Andrus ML, et al. National Healthcare Safety Network (NHSN) Report, data summary for 2006, issued June 2007. *Am J Infect Control.* 2007;35:290-301.

181. Venkatesh MP, Placencia F, Weisman LE. Coagulase-negative staphylococcal infections in the neonate and child: An update. *Semin Pediatr Infect Dis.* 2006;17:120-127.

182. Scheifele DW, Bjornson GL, Dyer RA, et al. Delta-like toxin produced by coagulase-negative staphylococci is associated with neonatal necrotizing enterocolitis. *Infect Immun.* 1987;55:2268-2273.

183. Gupta S, Morris JG Jr, Panigrahi P, et al. Endemic necrotizing enterocolitis: Lack of association with a specific infectious agent. *Pediatr Infect Dis J.* 1994;13:728-734.

184. O'Grady NP, Alexander M, Dellinger EP, et al. Guidelines for the prevention of intravascular catheter-related infections. Centers for Disease Control and Prevention. *MMWR Recomm Rep.* 2002;51(RR-10):1-29.

185. Craft AP, Finer NN, Barrington KJ. Vancomycin for prophylaxis against sepsis in preterm neonates. Cochrane Database Syst Rev. 2000(2):CD001971.

186. Garland JS, Alex CP, Henrickson KJ, et al. A vancomycin-heparin lock solution for prevention of nosocomial bloodstream infection in critically ill neonates with peripherally inserted central venous catheters: A prospective, randomized trial. *Pediatrics.* 2005;116:e198-e205.

187. Raimundo O, Heussler H, Bruhn JB, et al. Molecular epidemiology of coagulase-negative staphylococcal bacteraemia in a newborn intensive care unit. *J Hosp Infect.* 2002;51:33-42.

188. Carretto E, Barbarini D, Couto I, et al. Identification of coagulase-negative staphylococci other than *Staphylococcus epidermidis* by automated ribotyping. *Clin Microbiol Infect.* 2005;11: 177-184.

189. Shittu A, Lin J, Morrison D, et al. Isolation and molecular characterization of multiresistant *Staphylococcus sciuri* and *Staphylococcus haemolyticus* associated with skin and soft-tissue infections. *J Med Microbiol.* 2004;53:51-55.

190. Huang CR, Lu CH, Wu JJ, et al. Coagulase-negative staphylococcal meningitis in adults: Clinical characteristics and therapeutic outcomes. *Infection.* 2005;33:56-60.

191. Biavasco F, Vignaroli C, Varaldo PE. Glycopeptide resistance in coagulase-negative staphylococci. *Eur J Clin Microbiol Infect Dis.* 2000;19:403-417.

192. Takeuchi F, Watanabe S, Baba T, et al. Whole-genome sequencing of *Staphylococcus haemolyticus* uncovers the extreme plasticity of its genome and the evolution of human-colonizing staphylococcal species. *J Bacteriol.* 2005;187:7292-7308.

193. Herchline TE, Ayers LW. Occurrence of *Staphylococcus lugdunensis* in consecutive clinical cultures and relationship of isolation to infection. *J Clin Microbiol.* 1991;29:419-421.

194. Patel R, Piper KE, Rouse MS, et al. Frequency of isolation of *Staphylococcus lugdunensis* among staphylococcal isolates causing endocarditis: A 20-year experience. *J Clin Microbiol.* 2000;38:4262-4423.

195. May ER, Hnilica KA, Frank LA, et al. Isolation of *Staphylococcus schleiferi* from healthy dogs and dogs with otitis, pyoderma, or both. *J Am Vet Med Assoc.* 2005;227:928-931.

196. Rupp ME, Soper DE, Archer GL. Colonization of the female genital tract with *Staphylococcus saprophyticus.* *J Clin Microbiol.* 1992;30:2975-2979.

197. Raz R, Colodner R, Kunin CM. Who are you—Staphylococcus saprophyticus? *Clin Infect Dis.* 2005;40:896-898.

198. Latham RH, Running K, Stamm WE. Urinary tract infections in young adult women caused by *Staphylococcus saprophyticus.* *JAMA.* 1983;250:3063-3066.

199. Mardh PA, Hovelius B. Staphylococcus saprophyticus infections. *Lancet.* 1977;2:875.

197

Classification of Streptococci

KATHRYN L. RUOFF | ALAN L. BISNO

Members of the genus *Streptococcus* are catalase-negative, gram-positive bacteria that form oval or coccoid cells arranged in pairs and chains. Streptococci are nutritionally fastidious and require complex media, preferably supplemented with blood, for optimal growth. They are homofermentative lactic acid bacteria, producing lactic acid without gas as the major end product of glucose metabolism. Although streptococci are referred to as facultative anaerobes, growing both aerobically and anaerobically, streptococci do not use oxygen metabolically. In addition, some strains are capnophilic, whereas others grow better under anaerobic conditions. This large and heterogeneous group of parasites of humans and animals harbors relatively avirulent normal flora organisms as well as some of the most impressive human pathogens.[1]

Early attempts to classify streptococci of clinical importance centered around their action on blood-containing agars[2] and antigens contained in their cell walls.[3] Some streptococci (β-hemolytic) can lyse blood cells and cause complete clearing of blood in the vicinity of their growth (Fig. 197-1). Other strains cause no change in blood agar (γ- or nonhemolytic), whereas the remainder of the streptococci (α-hemolytic) reduce hemoglobin and cause a greenish discoloration of the agar (Fig. 197-2). Lancefield,[3] concentrating initially on virulent, β-hemolytic streptococci, found that they could be subdivided based on cell wall antigens. It was thought that β-hemolytic organisms with the same Lancefield antigen were closely related, but this correlation was not always valid for non–β-hemolytic strains. Other phenotypic traits of

streptococci were also examined and catalogued throughout the 20th century, giving rise to various classification schemes. In 1937, Sherman[4] classified the streptococci into the pyogenic, viridans, enterococcal, and lactic divisions, based on phenotypic traits. Subsequent molecular studies generally upheld these basic divisions,[5] but revealed multiple genera among organisms traditionally thought to be streptococci.

By the mid-1980s, the enterococcal streptococci (Lancefield group D, bile esculin-positive and salt-tolerant) had taken up residence in their own newly created *Enterococcus* genus and the "dairy" or "lactic" streptococci (Lancefield group N, occasionally documented in human infection) were moved to the new *Lactococcus* genus. Ensuing studies of streptococci isolated from human and animal infections gave rise to updated classification schemes based on 16S ribosomal RNA sequences and other molecular information. These investigations also aided accurate differentiation of genera of streptococcal-like, catalase-negative, gram-positive cocci (e.g., *Leuconostoc, Pediococcus,* and numerous others) that had previously been unrecognized in clinical specimens. Many, but not all, β-hemolytic streptococci were found to be members of the pyogenic group, whereas the viridans streptococci were divided into five species groups. Although the viridans strains, normal flora of the oral cavity and gastrointestinal tract, were traditionally characterized as α-hemolytic, it was realized that some members of this group also displayed β-hemolysis. Organisms considered to be nutritionally variant streptococci (also referred to as pyridoxal-dependent or satelliting streptococci) were reclassified in two new genera, *Abiotrophia* and *Granulicatella*.[6-8] It became apparent that the hemolytic reactions, Lancefield antigens, and other phenotypic characteristics relied on in the past were not always accurate predictors of genetic relatedness among strains. These characteristics are, however, still useful to clinical laboratorians for the presumptive identification of many commonly encountered streptococci. Table 197-1 summarizes currently described streptococcal species and species groups that are frequently isolated from humans. Streptococci normally associated with animals that are infrequently isolated from human infection are presented in Table 197-2.

Figure 197-1 Group A streptococci growing in pure culture on a sheep blood–agar plate. Individual colonies are surrounded by zones of complete β-hemolysis. Subsurface hemolysis (agar stab) is caused in part by the action of streptolysin O, which is oxygen-labile. The zone of inhibition around a low-potency bacitracin disk is a presumptive test for group A organisms.

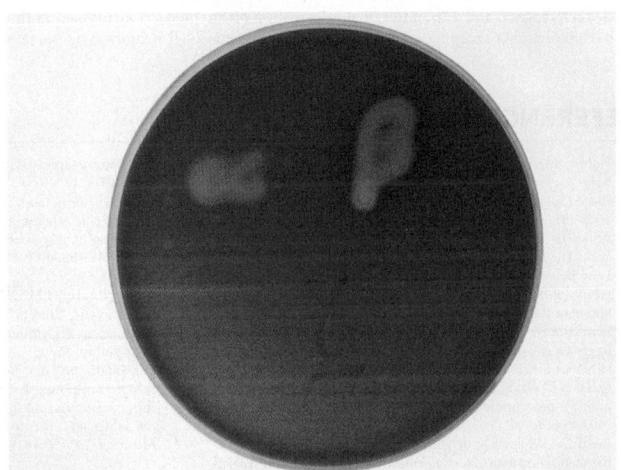

Figure 197-2 Sheep blood–agar plate with α-, β-, and γ-hemolytic streptococci.

TABLE 197-1	Classification of Streptococci Commonly Isolated from Humans*		
Species	**Lancefield Antigen(s)**	**Hemolytic Reaction(s)**	**Comments**
S. pyogenes	A	β	Pyogenic; can be differentiated from β-hemolytic anginosus group strains with the group A antigen by the formation of relatively large colonies and other phenotypic traits; agent of pharyngitis and respiratory, skin, and other infections; can cause nonsuppurative sequelae (acute rheumatic fever, acute glomerulonephritis)
S. agalactiae	B	β, γ	Pyogenic; hemolytic reaction is weak; agent of chorioamnionitis, puerperal sepsis, neonatal sepsis and meningitis, and infections in nonpregnant adults
S. dysgalactiae subsp. equisimilis	C, G[†]	β	Pyogenic; formerly named S. equisimilis; can be differentiated from β-hemolytic S. anginosus group strains with the C or G antigen by the formation of relatively large colonies and other phenotypic traits; agent of respiratory and deep tissue infections, cellulitis, and septicemia
S. pneumoniae	No detectable antigen	α	Closely related to members of the viridans S. mitis species group; agent of respiratory infections, otitis media, and meningitis
S. anginosus species group	A, C, F, G, or no detectable antigen	α, β, γ	Viridans streptococcal group composed of three species, S. anginosus, S. constellatus, and S. intermedius; two subspecies of S. constellatus, S. constellatus subsp. constellatus and S. constellatus subsp. pharyngis, have been described[9]; formerly known as S. milleri; β-hemolytic strains form small colonies compared with those of pyogenic β-hemolytic group A, C, and G streptococci and also differ in other phenotypic traits; agents of purulent infections
S. bovis species group	D	α, γ	Viridans streptococcal group formerly known as group D nonenterococcal streptococci; species commonly isolated from humans have been reclassified as S. gallolyticus subsp. gallolyticus (formerly S. bovis biotype I), S. gallolyticus subsp. pasteurianus (formerly S. bovis biotype II/2), S. infantarius subsp. Infantarius, and S. lutetiensis (formerly S. bovis biotype II/1)[10-12]; some strains produce extracellular polysaccharides[‡]; agents of endocarditis; isolated from blood in patients with colonic cancer
S. mutans species group	Not useful for differentiation	α, γ, occasionally β	Viridans streptococcal group; S. mutans and S. sobrinus species commonly isolated from humans; produce extracellular polysaccharides[‡]; agents of dental caries and endocarditis
S. salivarius species group	Not useful for differentiation	α, γ	Viridans streptococcal group; S. salivarius and S. vestibularis species commonly isolated from humans; strains in the S. salivarius group may react with Lancefield's group K antiserum and may produce extracellular polysaccharides[‡]; infrequent opportunists in compromised hosts
S. mitis species group	Not useful for differentiation	α	Viridans streptococcal group; species commonly isolated from humans include S. mitis, S. oralis, S. sanguinis, and S. gordonii; strains in S. mitis group may react with Lancefield's group H antiserum and may produce extracellular polysaccharides[‡]; agents of endocarditis and systemic infection in neutropenic patients

*See references 6 and 7 for additional information on streptococci mentioned in this table.
[†]Isolates with the group A antigen have also been described.
[‡]Extracellular polysaccharides (dextran, levan) are thought to aid colonization and may play a role in virulence.

TABLE 197-2	Streptococci Primarily Isolated from Animals that May Occasionally Cause Human Infection*		
Species	**Lancefield Antigen(s)**	**Hemolytic Reaction**	**Comments**
S. dysgalactiae subsp. dysgalactiae	C, L	α, β, γ	Pathogen of domesticated animals; participation in human infections not well documented
S. equi subsp. equi	C	β	Agent of equine strangles; participation in human infections not well documented
S. equi subsp. zooepidemicus	C	β	Agent of bovine mastitis and infection in other domesticated animals; implicated in outbreaks of nephritis in humans
S. porcinus	E, P, U, V	β	Swine are usual hosts; isolated from human female genital tract; may cross-react with commercially available group B streptococcal grouping reagents
S. canis	G	β	Dogs and other animals are usual hosts; documented as infrequent human pathogen
S. suis	R, S, T	α, β[†]	Swine are usual hosts; isolated infrequently from cases of human meningitis
S. iniae	No detectable antigen	β	Fish are usual hosts; isolated infrequently from cutaneous and systemic infection in humans

*See references 6 and 7 for additional information on streptococci mentioned in this table.
[†]α-Hemolytic on sheep blood agar, but some strains may be β-hemolytic on horse blood agar.

REFERENCES

1. Hardie JM. *Streptococcus Rosenbach* 184,22AL. In: Sneath PHA, Mair NS, Sharpe ME, Holt JG, eds. *Bergey's Manual of Systematic Bacteriology*. Baltimore, Md: Williams & Wilkins; 1986: 1042-1071.
2. Brown JH. *The Use of Blood Agar for the Study of Streptococci*. New York: The Rockefeller Institute for Medical Research; 1919.
3. Lancefield RC. A serological differentiation of human and other groups of hemolytic streptococci. *J Exp Med*. 1933;57:571-595.
4. Sherman JM. The Streptococci. *Bacteriol Rev*. 1937;1:3-97.
5. Bentley RW, Leigh JA, Collins MD. Intrageneric structure of *Streptococcus* based on comparative analysis of small-subunit rRNA sequences. *Int J Syst Bacteriol*. 1991;41:487-494.
6. Facklam R. What happened to the streptococci: Overview of taxonomic and nomenclature changes. *Clin Microbiol Rev*. 2002;15:613-630.
7. Ruoff KL, Whiley RA, Beighton D. *Streptococcus*. In: Murray PR, Baron EJ, Jorgensen JH, et al, eds. *Manual of Clinical Microbiol-*

ogy. Washington, DC: American Society for Microbiology; 2003:405-421.
8. Ruoff KL. *Aerococcus, Abiotrophia*, and other infrequently isolated aerobic catalase-negative, Gram positive cocci. In: Murray PR, Baron EJ, Jorgensen JH, et al, eds. *Manual of Clinical Microbiology*. Washington, DC: American Society for Microbiology; 2007:443-454.
9. Whiley RA, Hall LMC, Hardie JM, et al. A study of small-colony, β-haemolytic, Lancefield group C streptococci within the anginosus group: description of *Streptococcus constellatus* subsp. *pharyngis* subsp. nov., associated with the human throat and pharyngitis. *Int J Syst Bacteriol*. 1999;49:1443-1449.
10. Schlegel L, Grimont F, Collins MD, et al. *Streptococcus infantarius* subsp. *infantarius* subsp. nov. and *Streptococcus infantarius* subsp. *coli* subsp. nov., isolated from humans and food. *Int J Syst Evol Microbiol*. 2000;50:1425-1434.

11. Schlegel L, Grimont F, Ageron E, et al. Reappraisal of the taxonomy of the *Streptococcus bovis/Streptococcus equinus* complex and related species: description of *Streptococcus gallolyticus* subsp. *gallolyticus* subsp. nov., *S. gallolyticus* subsp. *macedonicus* subsp. nov. and *S. gallolyticus* subsp. *pasteurianus* subsp. nov. *Int J Syst Evol Microbiol*. 2003;53:631-645.
12. Poyart C, Quesne G, Trieu-Cuot T. Taxonomic dissection of the *Streptococcus bovis* group by analysis of manganese-dependent superoxide dismutase gene (*sodA*) sequences: reclassification of "*Streptococcus infantarius* subsp. *coli*" as *Streptococcus lutetiensis* sp. nov. and of *Streptococcus bovis* biotype II.2 as *Streptococcus pasteurianus* sp. nov. *Int J Syst Evol Microbiol*. 2002;52:1247-1255.

198

Streptococcus pyogenes

ALAN L. BISNO | DENNIS L. STEVENS

Streptococcus pyogenes (group A *Streptococcus*) is one of the most important bacterial pathogens of humans. This ubiquitous organism is the most frequent bacterial cause of acute pharyngitis, and it also gives rise to a variety of cutaneous and systemic infections. Its unique place in medical microbiology stems from its propensity to initiate two nonsuppurative sequelae, acute rheumatic fever (ARF) and poststreptococcal acute glomerulonephritis (AGN). The former malady has been responsible for suffering, disability, and mortality in all parts of the world.

History

Streptococci were demonstrated in cases of erysipelas and wound infections by Billroth in 1874 and in the blood of a patient with puerperal sepsis by Pasteur in 1879. Fehleisen, in 1883, isolated chain-forming organisms in pure culture from erysipelas lesions and then demonstrated that these organisms could induce typical erysipelas in humans. Rosenbach applied the designation *Streptococcus pyogenes* to these organisms in 1884.

Initial progress toward a rational classification of streptococci dates from the description by Schötmuller in 1903 of the blood agar technique for differentiating hemolytic from nonhemolytic streptococci. In 1919, Brown[1] made a systematic study of patterns of hemolysis and introduced the terms α-, β-, and γ-hemolysis (see Chapter 197).

Lancefield's classification of β-hemolytic streptococci into distinct serogroups in 1933[2] was a major turning point in our understanding of the epidemiology of streptococcal infections. Most strains pathogenic for humans were found to belong to serogroup A (*S. pyogenes*). Systems of serotyping group A streptococci were developed on the basis of M protein precipitin reactions (Lancefield) or T protein agglutination reactions (Griffith). In addition, Lancefield established the critical role of M protein in streptococcal virulence and the type-specific nature of protective immunity to group A streptococcal infection. Studies by Dochez and collaborators and by George and Gladys Dick in the 1920s established the relationship of scarlet fever to hemolytic streptococcal infection. A few years later, Todd's description of the method for titration of anti–streptolysin O (ASO) in serum added still another important tool to the armamentarium available for study of the immunology and epidemiology of streptococcal disease. Such tools were used by a number of investigators, including Coburn, Collis, Rammelkamp, Stollerman, and Wannamaker, to establish the relationship of group A streptococcal infection to ARF and AGN. Much of our knowledge of the detailed epidemiology of streptococcal infections and of ARF derives from the pioneering studies performed at Warren Air Force Base, Wyoming, during 1949 to 1951 by Rammelkamp, Wannamaker, and Denny.[3-5]

Description of the Pathogen

Group A streptococci (GAS) grow as spherical or ovoid cells 0.6 to 1.0 μm in diameter and occur as pairs or as short to moderate-sized chains in clinical specimens. When growing in broth media enriched with serum or blood, long chains are frequently formed, and many strains produce capsules of hyaluronic acid. The organisms are gram-positive, nonmotile, non–spore-forming, catalase-negative, and facultatively anaerobic. Group A streptococci are nutritionally fastidious and are usually cultivated in complex media, often supplemented with blood or serum.

When cultured on blood agar plates, *S. pyogenes* appears as white to gray colonies 1 to 2 mm in diameter surrounded by zones of complete (β) hemolysis. (Strains that fail to produce such hemolysis occur but are rare.) Strains that produce copious amounts of the hyaluronate capsular material appear mucoid, at times resembling a water drop on the plate. Less mucoid strains assume a crinkled, so-called matte appearance. Small opaque colonies of organisms that lack capsules and detectable M protein are termed *glossy*.

The complete genome sequences from several distinct *S. pyogenes* serotypes have been reported, and this genome information is beginning to provide insight into the subtle genetic differences among streptococcal types that arm them to produce specific syndromes. A large number of somatic constituents and extracellular products of group A streptococci have been identified. The most important of these are indicated in the following sections.

SOMATIC CONSTITUENTS

The organism is enveloped in a hyaluronic acid capsule that serves as an accessory virulence factor in retarding phagocytosis by polymorphonuclear leukocytes and macrophages of the host.[6,7] Streptococcal strains vary greatly in their degree of encapsulation, and those with the most exuberant capsule production have a mucoid appearance when cultivated on blood agar plates. In certain heavily encapsulated GAS strains, the capsule may take precedence over M protein in mediating resistance to phagocytosis.[7] GAS capsular hyaluronate is chemically similar to that found in human connective tissue. For this reason, it is a poor immunogen, and antibodies to GAS hyaluronic acid have not been demonstrated in humans.

The cell wall is a complex structure containing many different antigenic substances. The group-specific carbohydrate of group A strains is a dimer of rhamnose and *N*-acetylglucosamine in a ratio of approximately 2 : 1. The mucopeptide (peptidoglycan) layer provides rigidity to the cell wall; it is composed of polymers of repeating subunits of *N*-acetylglucosamine and *N*-acetylmuramic acid connected by amino acid side chains.

M protein is the major somatic virulence factor of group A streptococci. Strains rich in this protein are resistant to phagocytosis by polymorphonuclear leukocytes, multiply rapidly in fresh human blood, and are capable of initiating disease. Strains that do not express M protein are avirulent.[8] GAS may be divided into serotypes on the basis of antigenic differences in M protein molecules, and more recently into genotypes on the basis of nucleotide differences in the *emm* gene encoding the molecule. More than 120 such serotypes and/or genotypes are currently recognized.[9] Acquired human immunity to streptococcal infection is based on the development of opsonic antibodies directed against the antiphagocytic moiety of M protein. Such immunity is type-specific and quite durable, lasting for many years and perhaps indefinitely.

M protein is a filamentous macromolecule that exists as a stable dimer with an α-helical coiled coil structure.[10] The molecule, which is anchored to the cell membrane, traverses and penetrates the cell wall. The more proximal portion of the molecule contains epitopes widely conserved among group A streptococci, whereas the more distal

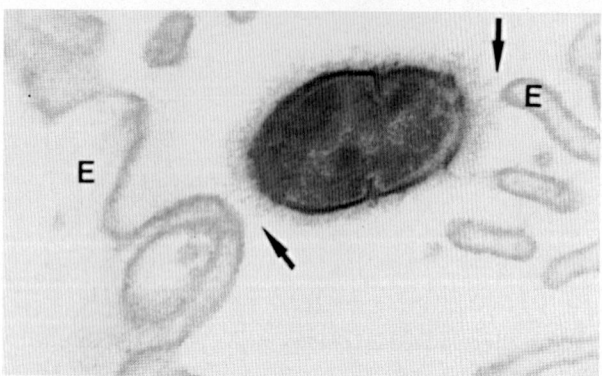

Figure 198-1 **Electron micrograph of group A streptococci.** Surface fibrils contain type-specific, antiphagocytic epitopes of M protein. Lipoteichoic acid and fibronectin binding proteins facilitate adherence of streptococci to the membrane (arrows) of a human oral epithelial cell (E; ×67,500). *(From Beachey EH, Ofek I. Epithelial cell binding of group A streptococci by lipoteichoic acid on fimbriae denuded of M protein. J Exp Med. 1976;143:759-771, with permission.)*

portion contains type-specific epitopes.[11] This configuration localizes the type-specific moiety on the tips of fibrils protruding from the cell surface (Fig. 198-1). In the nonimmune host, M protein exerts its antiphagocytic effect by inhibiting activation of the alternate complement pathway on the cell surface.[12,13] Such inhibition appears to be mediated by the binding to the M protein molecule of host proteins, among which are complement control proteins (factor H, a factor H–like protein, and human C4b-binding protein)[14-16] and fibrinogen.[17-19] The antiphagocytic effect is nullified in the presence of adequate concentrations of type-specific antibody. There is evidence that immunity caused by opsonic anti–M-type antibody may be strain- and not type-specific.[20,21] M proteins analogous to those of GAS are present in many strains of groups C[22] and G[23] streptococci.

Additional surface proteins related to M protein have now been identified. Although their structure is overall similar to that of M protein, they differ in the types of repeats and in their ability to interact with different human proteins. Genes encoding these proteins (e.g., *enn*, *mrp*, *fcrA*, *arp*, *protH*) have been designated as members of the *emm* gene superfamily. A number of the M-like proteins bind IgG or IgA at the non–antigen-binding site and appear to be cooperative with M protein in antiphagocytic effect.[24,25] Indeed, a notable function of the M protein family is its ability to bind to a wide range of host proteins, including, among others, albumin, fibrinogen, and plasminogen. Still other antiopsonic surface proteins continue to be described.[26] For example, Mac, a secreted group A streptococcal protein with homology to a human β_2-integrin, binds to CD16 on the surface of human polymorphonuclear leukocyte (PML) and inhibits phagocytosis and bacterial killing.[27] An additional surface protein, streptococcal hemeassociated protein (Shp) has been found in M1 strains of GAS, which likely has a role in transport of iron intracellularly. Antibody against Shp has been found in convalescent sera and has opsonic capability.[28] These observations underscore the extreme virtuosity with which the bacterium develops multiple mechanisms to evade phagocytic killing.

A protein antigen very closely associated with the M protein molecule of group A streptococci is the so-called serum opacity factor (OF). This factor is an α-lipoproteinase that is detected by its ability to opacify horse serum and that also has fibronectin-binding properties.[29] Strains of a minority of the currently identified M types elaborate this antigen.[30] OF itself is antigenic and type-specific—that is, its ability to opacify serum can be specifically inhibited by antiserum raised against homologous but not heterologous M types. Type-specific and non–type-specific immune responses to streptococcal M protein are generally weaker after pharyngeal infection with OF-positive than with OF-negative types.[31] The former importance of this substance as an

ancillary typing system for strains that could not be M serotyped has been obviated by the advent of *emm* genotyping. Interestingly, antibody against OF has opsonic activity and has been shown to synergize with anti–M protein antibody in protecting mice against challenge with OF-positive strains.[32]

A number of somatic streptococcal constituents play critical roles in the first step of colonization, namely, adherence to the surface of human epithelial cells. At least 17 adhesin candidates have been described,[33] but the most extensively studied have been lipoteichoic acid (LTA), M protein, and fibronectin binding proteins. It is believed that through hydrophobic interactions, LTA serves as a "first-step" adhesin, bringing the organisms into close contact with host cells and then allowing other adhesins to promote high-affinity binding.[34] Although M protein does not appear to promote adhesion to human buccal or tonsillar epithelial cells,[35,36] it does mediate adherence to skin keratinocytes via the attachment of the C repeat region to keratinocyte membrane cofactor CD46.[37,38] Group A streptococcal surface proteins that bind fibronectin have been studied extensively and are important in adherence to both throat and skin. These include protein F1 (PrtF1),[39] also known as SfbI (streptococcal fibronectin-binding protein I),[40] and related proteins known as SbfII,[41] FBP54,[42] protein F2,[43] and PFBB.[44]

Moreover, the expression of these adhesins has been reported to be environmentally regulated.[45] Expression of protein F1 is enhanced in an O_2-rich environment, whereas that of M protein is greater at higher partial pressures of CO_2.[46] Thus, teleologically, it might be postulated that the organism displays protein F1 on its surface when it seeks to adhere to the cutaneous surface but expresses M protein in the deeper tissues, where it is more likely to encounter phagocytic cells.

EXTRACELLULAR PRODUCTS

During the course of growth in vitro or in vivo, GAS elaborate numerous extracellular products, only a limited number of which have been well characterized. Two distinct hemolysins have been elaborated. Streptolysin O derives its name from its oxygen lability. It is reversibly inhibited by oxygen and irreversibly inhibited by cholesterol. In addition to its effect on erythrocytes, it is toxic to a variety of cells and cell fractions, including polymorphonuclear leukocytes, platelets, tissue culture cells, lysosomes, and isolated mammalian and amphibian hearts. Streptolysin O is produced by almost all strains of *S. pyogenes* (as well as many group C and G organisms) and is antigenic. Measurement of ASO antibodies in human sera has proved exceedingly useful as an indicator of recent streptococcal infection.

Streptolysin S is a hemolysin produced by streptococci growing in the presence of serum (hence the "S") or in the presence of a variety of other substances such as serum albumin, α-lipoprotein, ribonucleic acid, or detergents such as Tween. Streptolysin S is nonantigenic, or at least no antibody to it has been detected that neutralizes its hemolytic activity. Streptolysin S shares with streptolysin O the capacity to damage the membranes of polymorphonuclear leukocytes, platelets, and subcellular organelles. Unlike streptolysin O, it is not inactivated by oxygen, but it is quite thermolabile. Most strains of *S. pyogenes* produce both hemolysins. Hemolysis on the surface of blood agar plates is primarily caused by streptolysin S, whereas streptolysin O exerts its hemolytic effect best in subsurface colonies, in pour plates, or in anaerobic cultures. An occasional strain may produce only one of the two hemolysins. Rarely, strains are encountered that lack both hemolysins.

Several extracellular products may theoretically serve to facilitate the liquefaction of pus and the spreading of streptococci through tissue planes characteristic of streptococcal cellulitis and necrotizing fasciitis. These include the following: (1) four antigenically distinct enzymes that participate in the degradation of deoxyribonucleic acid (DNases A, B, C, and D); (2) hyaluronidase, which enzymatically degrades hyaluronic acid found in the ground substance of connective tissue; (3) streptokinase, which promotes the dissolution of clots by catalyzing the conversion of plasminogen to plasmin; (4) streptococcal pyrogenic exotoxin B (SpeB), which is a potent protease; and (5) C5a peptidase, which specifically cleaves the human chemotaxin C5a at the PML binding site.[47,48] SpeB also cleaves IgG bound to GAS, thus interfering with ingestion and killing by phagocytes.[49]

The streptococcal pyrogenic exotoxins (Spe) are a family of bacterial superantigens believed to be associated with streptococcal toxic shock syndrome (strep TSS), necrotizing fasciitis, and other severe infections. This family includes the bacteriophage-encoded SpeA[50] and SpeC, historically known as the scarlatinal toxins because of their association with scarlet fever, as well as the cysteine protease SpeB; a number of additional pyrogenic exotoxins (e.g., mitogenic factor [MF, SpeF], and streptococcal superantigen [SSA]) have more recently been identified.[51]

Superantigens are potent immunostimulators able to bind simultaneously to the major histocompatibility complex (MHC) class II molecules and the T-cell receptor.[52] This binding results in activation of a large number of T cells expressing specific V-β subsets of the T-cell repertoire. Superantigen activation of T cells leads to increased secretion of proinflammatory cytokines. This issue is discussed in more detail in the section on pathogenesis of streptococcal toxic shock syndrome (see later).

Emerging concepts regarding the molecular biology of streptococcal virulence, colonization, and tissue invasion have been reviewed.[51,53] Control of the expression of the heretofore-mentioned virulence factors over time and under diverse environmental circumstances depends on a complex system of genetic modulation. Of the known transcriptional regulators in *S. pyogenes*, the two most intensively studied are Mga[54] (multiple gene regulator) or Mry, the regulator of M protein expression, and a two-component regulatory system known as CsrRS[55] (capsule synthesis regulator) or, alternatively, CovRS[56] (control of virulence genes), which represses the synthesis of the capsule and several exotoxins.[57]

Streptococcal Pharyngitis

EPIDEMIOLOGY

Streptococcal sore throat is among the most common bacterial infections of childhood. Group A streptococci are responsible for the great majority of such infections, but strains of other serogroups, especially groups C and G,[58] are occasionally involved. The disease occurs primarily among children 5 to 15 years of age, with the peak incidence occurring during the first few years of school. All age groups are susceptible, however, and severe epidemics are common in military training facilities. There is no gender predilection. The disease is ordinarily spread by direct person-to-person contact, most likely via droplets of saliva or nasal secretions. Crowding such as occurs in schools or barracks favors interpersonal spread of the organism (Fig. 198-2) and may also enhance its virulence by processes of natural selection analogous to those that occur during mouse passage in the laboratory. The effect of crowding in facilitating transmission may account in part for the increased incidence of streptococcal pharyngitis in northern latitudes during the colder months of the year. Explosive foodborne or waterborne outbreaks are also well documented. Contamination of dust, clothing, blankets, or other fomites does not appear to play a significant role in contagion.

Group A streptococci frequently colonize the throats of asymptomatic persons. Pharyngeal carriage rates among normal schoolchildren vary with geographic location and season of the year. Carriage rates as high as 15% to 20% have been noted in several studies. The carriage rate among adults is considerably lower.

Studies of experimentally induced human infections and of transmission in military barracks have shed considerable light on the variables involved in interpersonal spread. During the acute phase of tonsillopharyngeal infection, M-typeable group A streptococci are frequently present in large numbers in both the nose and throat. In untreated infections, organisms may persist for many weeks, although the signs and symptoms of illness abate within a few days. During

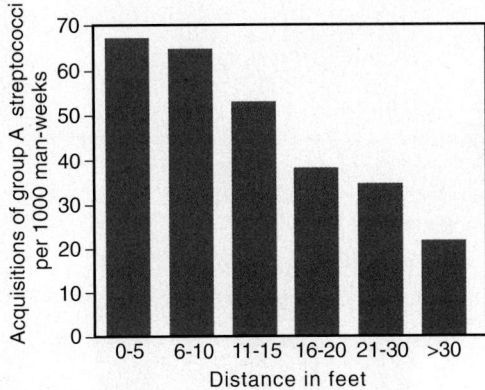

Figure 198-2 **Transmission of group A streptococci in a military barracks according to bed distance from the nearest carrier.** *(From Wannamaker LW. The epidemiology of streptococcal infection. In: McCarty M, ed. Streptococcal Infections. New York: Columbia University Press; 1953:157-175, with permission.)*

convalescence, the organisms decrease in numbers and tend to disappear from the anterior nares sooner than from the throat. In addition, the M protein content and virulence of persisting organisms gradually decline. The result of these qualitative and quantitative changes is that convalescent carriers are much less likely to transmit the organism to close contacts than acutely infected persons.

In patients who do not receive effective antibiotic therapy for acute streptococcal pharyngitis, type-specific antibodies are frequently detectable in the serum between 4 and 8 weeks after the infection. These opsonic antibodies protect against subsequent infection with organisms of the same M type, but the person remains susceptible to infection by heterologous types. Prompt and effective antibiotic therapy may ablate the type-specific immune response.

CLINICAL MANIFESTATIONS

The usual incubation period of streptococcal pharyngitis is 2 to 4 days. The onset of illness is heralded by the rather abrupt onset of sore throat accompanied by malaise, feverishness, and headache. Nausea, vomiting, and abdominal pain are common in children. Prominent physical findings include redness, edema, and lymphoid hyperplasia of the posterior portion of the pharynx, enlarged, hyperemic tonsils, patchy discrete tonsillopharyngeal exudates (Fig. 198-3), enlarged, tender lymph nodes at the angles of the mandibles, and a temperature of 101°F or higher. In the absence of these symptoms and signs, simple coryza, hoarseness, cough, or conjunctivitis does not suggest the presence of streptococcal infection. Laboratory findings include a positive throat culture for β-hemolytic streptococci and a total white blood cell count usually exceeding 12,000/mm^3, with increased numbers of polymorphonuclear leukocytes. The test for C-reactive protein is usually positive.[59]

Not all patients with streptococcal pharyngitis have the full-blown syndrome just described. Endemically occurring infections in open populations manifest a wide spectrum of clinical severity. For example, only approximately 50% of such patients with sore throats and positive throat cultures have tonsillar or pharyngeal exudates. Patients who have undergone tonsillectomy tend to experience a milder clinical syndrome. In infants, the response to streptococcal infection is much less sharply focalized to the lymphoid tissue of the faucial and posterior pharyngeal area. Rhinorrhea, suppurative complications, low-grade fever, and a more protracted course tend to characterize infections at this age. Exudative pharyngitis in children younger than 3 years is rarely streptococcal in cause.

In the absence of suppurative complications, the disease is self-limited. Fever abates within 3 to 5 days. Almost all acute signs and symptoms subside within 1 week, although several additional weeks

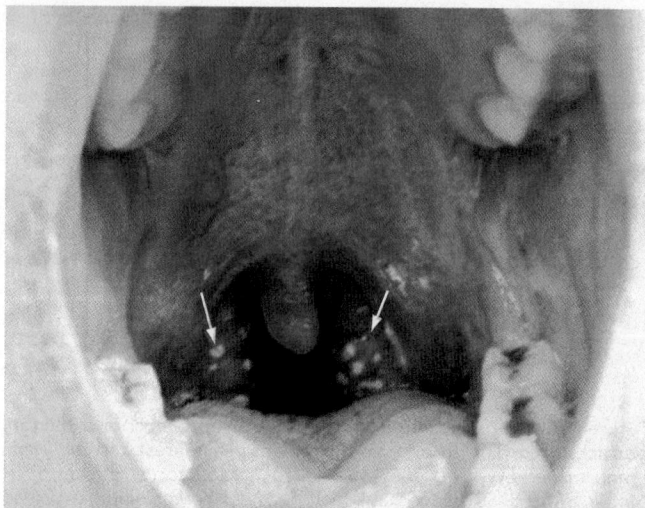

Figure 198-3 Streptococcal tonsillopharyngitis. Exudates (*arrows*) are present on the enlarged erythematous tonsils. *(From Nimishikavi S, Stead I. Images in clinical medicine. Streptococcal pharyngitis. N Engl J Med. 2005;352(11):e10, with permission. Copyright @2005, Massachusetts Medical Society. All rights reserved.)*

may be required for tonsils and lymph nodes to return to their usual size. Penicillin shortens the period of fever, toxicity, and infectivity.[60-62] Given the rather brief time course of untreated disease, however, such shortening of the clinical syndrome may not be striking unless therapy is initiated within the first 24 hours of illness.

SCARLET FEVER

Scarlet fever results from infection with a streptococcal strain that elaborates streptococcal pyrogenic exotoxins (erythrogenic toxins). Although this disease is usually associated with pharyngeal infections, it may follow streptococcal infections at other sites, such as wound infections or puerperal sepsis. The clinical syndrome is similar in most respects to that associated with nontoxigenic strains, save for the scarlatinal rash. The latter must be differentiated from those of viral exanthems, drug eruptions, staphylococcal toxic shock syndrome, and Kawasaki disease.

The rash usually appears on the second day of clinical illness as a diffuse red blush, with many points of deeper red that blanch on pressure. It is often first noted over the upper part of the chest and then spreads to the remainder of the trunk, neck, and extremities. The palms, soles, and usually the face are spared. Skin folds in the neck, axillae, groin, elbows, and knees appear as lines of deeper red (Pastia's lines). There are scattered petechiae, and the Rumpel-Leeds test of capillary fragility is positive. Occlusion of sweat glands imparts a sandpaper texture to the skin, a particularly helpful finding in dark-skinned patients.

The face appears flushed, except for marked circumoral pallor. In addition to findings of exudative pharyngitis and tonsillitis, patients display an enanthem characterized by small, red, hemorrhagic spots on the hard and soft palates. The tongue is initially covered with a yellowish white coat through which may be seen the red papillae (white strawberry tongue). Later, the coating disappears, and the tongue is beefy red in appearance (red strawberry tongue). The skin rash fades over the course of 1 week and is followed by extensive desquamation lasting for several weeks. A modest eosinophilia may be present early in the course of the illness.

Severe forms of scarlet fever, either associated with local and hematogenous spread of the organism (septic scarlet fever) or with profound toxemia (toxic scarlet fever), are characterized by high fever and marked systemic toxicity. The course may be complicated by arthritis, jaundice, and, very rarely, hydrops of the gallbladder. Such severe forms of the disease are infrequent in the antibiotic era.

Suppurative Complications

Inflammation in the faucial area induced by acute streptococcal infection may affect structures that are directly contiguous to the pharynx or that drain that site. Such relatively rare complications include peritonsillar cellulitis, peritonsillar abscess, retropharyngeal abscess, suppurative cervical lymphadenitis, mastoiditis, acute sinusitis, and otitis media.[63] Peritonsillar or retropharyngeal abscesses, however, frequently contain a variety of other oral flora, including anaerobes, with or without group A streptococci.[64] Group A streptococci are responsible for only a small minority of cases of otitis media or sinusitis.

Extension up the cribriform plate of the ethmoid or via the mastoid bone may cause meningitis, brain abscess, or thrombosis of the intracranial venous sinuses. Streptococcal pneumonia, another potential suppurative complication, is discussed later. Finally, bacteremic spread of the streptococci may result in a variety of metastatic foci of infection, such as suppurative arthritis, endocarditis, meningitis, brain abscess, osteomyelitis, or liver abscess. Such complications of streptococcal pharyngitis are extremely rare since the advent of effective chemotherapy.

Nonsuppurative Complications

The nonsuppurative complications of streptococcal pharyngitis, acute rheumatic fever and acute post–streptococcal glomerulonephritis, are discussed in Chapter 199. The role of streptococci vis-à-vis other infectious and noninfectious agents in initiating certain other acute inflammatory disorders such as erythema nodosum and anaphylactoid purpura remains unresolved.

DIAGNOSIS

Pharyngitis and tonsillitis may be caused by infectious agents other than *S. pyogenes*.[58,65] Among these are streptococci of groups C[66,67] and G.[68-70] *Corynebacterium diphtheriae*, the other major bacterial pathogen associated with exudative pharyngitis, is now extremely rare in the United States[71] and, when it occurs in the classic form, is differentiated by the appearance of the diphtheritic membrane, respiratory embarrassment, severe systemic toxicity, and myocardial and neurologic manifestations. Other bacterial agents such as *Neisseria gonorrhoeae* and perhaps *Neisseria meningitidis* occasionally cause pharyngitis, as does *Mycoplasma pneumoniae*.

Pharyngitis due to *Arcanobacterium* (formerly *Corynebacterium*) *hemolyticum*, although rare, may closely mimic that caused by *S. pyogenes*.[72,73] *Arcanobacterium hemolyticum* affects primarily teenagers and young adults, and the patients may exhibit both an exudative pharyngitis and a scarlatiniform rash. The organism is more readily identified on rabbit or human blood agar than on sheep blood agar. Another rare cause of acute pharyngitis is *Yersinia enterocolitica*.[74] Patients infected with this organism may appear quite ill and may or may not have associated enteric symptoms. When *Y. enterocolitica* pharyngitis is associated with disseminated yersiniosis, the mortality rate may be appreciable. Diagnosis depends on clinical clues because the organism is unlikely to be detected on routine throat cultures and antistreptococcal therapy is unavailing (see Chapter 229). The oropharyngeal form of tularemia is characterized by severe sore throat, exudative and ulcerative tonsillopharyngitis, and cervical adenopathy (see Chapter 227).

Acute pharyngitis is more frequently caused by viruses than by bacteria. Infectious mononucleosis and adenovirus infections frequently give rise to exudative pharyngitis and thus may closely mimic streptococcal sore throat. Herpes simplex viruses 1 and 2,[75-77] influenza,[78] and parainfluenza viruses may also simulate streptococcal pharyngitis, as may initially the acute retroviral syndrome in human immunodeficiency virus infection. Pharyngitis associated with the acute retroviral syndrome is, however, not exudative.[79] Even when careful microbiologic techniques are used to detect bacteria, mycoplasma, and viruses, no causative agent can be detected in a substantial proportion of all cases of acute sore throat.[80] A more complete discussion of the differential diagnosis of acute pharyngitis may be found in Chapter 54.

Approximately one fourth to one third of all children complaining of sore throat have a positive throat culture for group A streptococci. Of these, about half can be demonstrated to have immunologically significant infection, as judged by a significant rise in serum titer of one or more antistreptococcal antibodies. Many of the remainder are likely to be asymptomatic carriers, because the average carriage rate among school-aged children in temperate climates during the winter months may approximate 15%. Such asymptomatic carriers are at no risk of developing suppurative and nonsuppurative complications and do not require antibiotic therapy. Although acutely infected individuals tend to have more strongly positive throat cultures, this distinction cannot be made with confidence in patients whose signs and symptoms are compatible with those of streptococcal pharyngitis.

Numerous studies have tested the precision with which physicians may differentiate between streptococcal and nonstreptococcal sore throat by clinical criteria alone. In the presence of a classic scarlatinal rash or during a documented epidemic of streptococcal infections, such differentiation is usually easy. On the other hand, in the case of endemically occurring infections, the problem is much more complex. Certain clinical findings, particularly tonsillopharyngeal exudate and tender, enlarged lymph nodes at the angles of the jaws, have a statistically significant correlation with the presence of positive throat cultures for group A streptococci.[81] Such findings are not diagnostic, however. Although only approximately 50% of patients with immunologically proven streptococcal sore throat have tonsillar exudate, a substantial proportion of cases of exudative pharyngitis are nonstreptococcal in cause.

It is possible to identify individual patients in which "strep throat" can be effectively excluded on a combination of epidemiologic (see earlier) and clinical grounds. For example, symptoms of the common cold are not caused by *S. pyogenes*. Similarly, the presence of hoarseness and conjunctivitis and the absence of fever or pharyngeal erythema make streptococcal pharyngitis very unlikely. A number of investigators have developed clinical algorithms in children and adults to assist in determining the likelihood that a particular patient has group A streptococcal pharyngitis.[81-87] These algorithms are useful and accurate in identifying patients whose risk of streptococcal infection is so low as to obviate the need for further microbiologic testing. Otherwise, such testing should be performed.

One published practice guideline[88,89] has suggested that in adults with features strongly suggestive of streptococcal pharyngitis, empirical antimicrobial therapy without microbiologic confirmation is an acceptable alternative. That guideline uses an algorithm, developed by Centor and co-workers[87] using four clinical criteria—presence of tonsillar exudates, presence of swollen tender anterior cervical nodes (i.e., cervical lymphadenitis), lack of cough, and history of fever—that have been reported to be independently associated with the likelihood of a positive throat culture for group A streptococci.[90] A subsequent cost-effectiveness analysis[91] and two prospective clinical studies[92,93] have concluded that such empirical therapy is neither the most effective nor least expensive strategy for diagnosis of strep throat in adults. Furthermore, empirical therapy in adults leads to considerable overuse of antibiotics.[94] This is of particular concern in view of the fact that 73% of the 6.7 million adults visiting primary care providers annually in the United Sates with the complaint of sore throat receive a prescription for antibiotics.[95]

Thus, for adults and children, expert panels of the Infectious Diseases Society of America,[96] American Heart Association,[97] and American Academy of Pediatrics[98] recommend that the presence of group A streptococci in the pharynx should be documented by a throat culture or rapid antigen detection test (RADT).[96-98]

Throat Culture

Throat culture remains the gold standard for diagnosing streptococcal pharyngitis. Failure to isolate β-hemolytic streptococci in a carefully obtained and accurately interpreted throat culture rules out the diagnosis of streptococcal sore throat for practical purposes. In cases in which doubt exists as to the validity of a negative culture, it may be preferable to repeat the culture rather than to treat empirically with antimicrobial agents.

Although a negative culture eliminates the necessity for therapy, a positive culture does not differentiate between acute infection and asymptomatic carriage. Serum antibody titers do not rise until convalescence and thus are of no help in short-term management. Although the degree of positivity of the throat culture may assist in making this differentiation, it is best to assume that all positive cultures in patients with acute pharyngitis are significant and to treat accordingly while recognizing that, even with the use of the throat culture, some degree of overtreatment is inevitable.

Detailed instructions for obtaining and processing a throat culture have been published by the American Heart Association.[99] Sheep blood agar is preferred because clear-cut patterns of hemolysis are obtained using this medium. In regard to isolation of group A streptococci, there is controversy in the literature as to the relative merits of plain sheep blood agar plates versus plates to which trimethoprim-sulfamethoxazole has been added to suppress competing normal pharyngeal flora. Similar controversy exists about the optimal atmosphere for incubation—aerobic, aerobic in the presence of 5% to 10% carbon dioxide, or anaerobic. Detailed analyses of these issues have been published.[100,101] If blood agar plates are not immediately available, the swab may be placed in a dry sterile tube for transportation to the laboratory. After overnight incubation at 35°C to 37°C, culture plates from patients with streptococcal pharyngitis show colonies surrounded by clear zones of hemolysis as well as β-hemolysis around the agar stab. Plates that are negative on first reading should be reexamined after an additional 24 hours of incubation. Serologic grouping of β-hemolytic streptococcal isolates may now be readily performed by using commercially available kits. Fluorescent antibody techniques provide excellent results and specifically identify group A organisms. No quantitative information is gained about the degree of positivity of the culture. A less expensive screening procedure, the bacitracin sensitivity test, is best performed once the organism has been isolated in pure culture. This susceptibility procedure is based on the observation that more than 95% of all group A streptococcal strains are inhibited by low-potency (0.04 unit) bacitracin disks, whereas 80% to 90% of non–group A strains are resistant.

Because no group A streptococci resistant to penicillin or cephalosporins have yet been detected, antibiotic testing is unnecessary if these drugs are to be used. The same holds true in general for macrolides because group A streptococci resistant to this drug are rare in the United States at this time[102] (see later, "Treatment," for caveats).

Rapid Antigen Detection Tests

These tests allow detection of the presence of the group A carbohydrate antigen directly from throat swabs. Unlike the throat culture, which requires overnight or longer to yield a definitive result, RADTs can be completed in a matter of minutes. By facilitating early diagnosis and therapy, an RADT may possibly shorten the duration of illness, decrease secondary spread of the organism, and allow earlier return of patients and parents to school and work. Earlier tests based on latex agglutination methodology have been largely replaced by enzyme immunoassays that are easier to interpret and more sensitive. More recently, tests using optical immunoassay (OIA) and chemiluminescent DNA probes have become available.

Most currently commercially available RADTs are highly specific (95% or higher), so a positive result obviates the need for a throat culture. Unfortunately, the sensitivity of these tests is lower than that of the conventional throat culture, and therefore they may be negative in patients in whom conventional culture proves to be positive. Some investigators[103,104] have found newer tests such as OIA to have a sensitivity equivalent to that of culture, but others have reached opposite conclusions.[105-107] At present, the American Academy of Pediatrics recommends that a negative RADT be confirmed with a throat culture. In view of conflicting data about sensitivity of commercially available RADTs, as well as the paucity of studies directly comparing the various tests with each other, physicians who elect to use any RADT in children and adolescents without culture back-up of negative results should do so only after confirming in their own practice that the rapid test is comparable in sensitivity to the throat culture.[98]

In considering appropriate laboratory diagnostic testing for adults, certain epidemiologic distinctions from pediatric disease deserve consideration. The group A streptococcus causes 15% to 30% of cases of acute pharyngitis in pediatric patients but only approximately 10% of such illnesses in adults.[86,108,109] However, the risk of streptococcal pharyngitis may be higher in parents of school-aged children and adults whose occupation brings them into close association with children. Moreover, the risk of a first attack of acute rheumatic fever is extremely low in adults in the United States and most other developed countries, even if they experience an undiagnosed and untreated episode of streptococcal pharyngitis. These facts make performance of RADT without culture back-up of negative results an acceptable alternative to throat culture.[96,97] The generally high specificity of RADTs should minimize overprescribing of antimicrobials for adults. This later point is of particular importance in view of national data indicating that antibiotics are prescribed for approximately 75% of adults consulting community primary care physicians for the complaint of sore throat and that the prescription of more expensive, broader-spectrum antibiotics is frequent.[95] Physicians who wish to ensure they are achieving maximal sensitivity in diagnosis may continue to use the conventional throat culture or to back up a negative RADT with a culture. However, in one recent adult study,[93] OIA without culture back-up was performed in adults exhibiting two or more Centor criteria.[87] When compared with throat culture, this strategy led to nearly optimal treatment (94%) and antibiotic prescription (37%), with minimal antibiotic overuse (3%) and underuse (3%).

TREATMENT

Antimicrobial therapy is indicated for individuals with symptomatic pharyngitis after the presence of the organism in the throat is confirmed by culture or RADT. The goals of antimicrobial therapy are (1) prevention of acute rheumatic fever, (2) prevention of suppurative complications, (3) improvement in clinical symptoms and signs, and (4) rapid decrease in infectivity so as to reduce transmission of group A β-hemolytic streptococci to family members, classmates, and other close contacts and to allow the rapid resumption of usual activities. There is no firm evidence that post–streptococcal acute glomerulonephritis is preventable by treatment of the antecedent streptococcal infection.[110]

Treatment of group A streptococcal sore throat as long as 9 days after onset is still effective for the prevention of rheumatic fever.[111] Thus, if the patient is seen early in the course of his illness, the delay in initiation of therapy occasioned by obtaining a positive throat culture is not ordinarily a matter of concern in this regard. As noted, patients with signs and symptoms of acute pharyngitis and a positive rapid test (properly performed and interpreted) for group A carbohydrate antigen should receive appropriate antimicrobial therapy.

In the minority of patients who are severely ill or toxic at presentation and in whom there is clinical and epidemiologic evidence resulting in a high index of suspicion, oral antimicrobial therapy can be initiated while awaiting the results of the throat culture (either as a primary diagnostic tool or in confirmation of a negative RADT). If oral therapy is prescribed, a positive throat culture serves as a guide to the necessity of completion of a full antimicrobial course or, alternatively, of recalling the patient for an injection of penicillin G benzathine. Early initiation of antimicrobial therapy results in faster resolution of the signs and symptoms,[60-62] but group A streptococcal pharyngitis is usually a self-limited disease; fever and constitutional symptoms are markedly diminished within 3 or 4 days of onset, even without antimicrobial therapy.[112] Thus, antimicrobial therapy initiated within the first 48 hours of onset hastens symptomatic improvement by only 1 to 2 days.

The drug of choice in the treatment of streptococcal infection is penicillin, because of its efficacy in the prevention of rheumatic fever, safety, narrow spectrum, and low cost[96-98] (Table 198-1). Prevention of acute rheumatic fever is believed to require eradication of the infecting streptococcus from the pharynx, an effect that depends on prolonged rather than high-dose penicillin therapy. This objective may be accomplished by the administration of a single injection of 1.2 million units of penicillin G benzathine. For children weighing 60 pounds or less, the dose is reduced to 600,000 units. Most physicians in the United States, however, elect to administer oral therapy. In this case, penicillin V, in one of the regimens listed in Table 198-1, must be continued for a full 10 days. Amoxicillin is often prescribed in preference to penicillin V in children requiring liquid medication because of poor palatability of oral suspensions of penicillin V. Once-daily amoxicillin therapy is effective for the treatment of group A streptococcal pharyngitis[113-115] in children. An oral time-release formulation of amoxicillin has recently been approved by the FDA for once-daily treatment of GAS pharyngitis in adolescents and adults. Because of its convenience, low cost, and relatively narrow spectrum, once-daily amoxicillin is an acceptable

TABLE 198-1	Primary Prevention of Rheumatic Fever (Treatment of Streptococcal Tonsillopharyngitis)*		
Agent	**Dose**	**Mode**	**Duration (days)**
Penicillins			
Penicillin V (phenoxymethyl penicillin)	Children: 250 mg two to three times daily for ≤27 kg (60 lb); children > 27 kg (60 lb), adolescents, and adults: 500 mg two to three times daily	Oral	10
or			
Amoxicillin	50 mg/kg once daily (maximum, 1 g)	Oral	10
or			
Benzathine penicillin G	600,000 U for patients ≤27 kg (60 lb); 1,200,000 U for patients > 27 kg (60 lb)	Intramuscular	Once
For Individuals Allergic to Penicillin			
Narrow-spectrum cephalosporin† (cephalexin, cefadroxil)	Variable	Oral	10
or			
Clindamycin	20 mg/kg/day divided in three doses (maximum, 1.8 g/day)	Oral	10
or			
Azithromycin	12 mg/kg once daily (maximum, 500 mg)	Oral	5
or			
Clarithromycin	15 mg/kg/day divided bid (maximum 250 mg bid)	Oral	10

*The following are not acceptable: sulfonamides, trimethoprim, tetracyclines, and fluoroquinolones.
†To be avoided in those with immediate (type I) hypersensitivity to a penicillin.
From Gerber M, Baltimore R, Eaton C, et al. Prevention of Rheumatic Fever and Diagnosis of Acute Streptococcal Pharyngitis. A scientific statement from the American Heart Association Rheumatic Fever, Endocarditis, and Kawasaki Disease Committee, Council on Cardiovascular Disease in the Young, and Quality of Care and Outcomes Research Interdisciplinary Working Group. *Circulation.* 2009;119:1541-1551. Reprinted with permission, © 2009, American Heart Association, Inc.

alternative regimen for the treatment of group A β-hemolytic streptococcal pharyngitis.[97]

A variable percentage of patients continue to harbor group A streptococci of the originating serotype in their pharynx after completion of a course of oral penicillin.[116] Such bacteriologic treatment failures are sometimes associated with symptomatic relapse. Because penicillin is ineffective in eradicating asymptomatic streptococcal pharyngeal carriage, apparent treatment failures may actually represent persistence of such carriage in patients with superimposed viral pharyngitis.[117]

Oral cephalosporins are highly effective in the treatment of streptococcal pharyngitis, and meta-analyses have suggested that streptococcal eradication rates and clinical cure rates attained with these agents are slightly higher in children and adults than those achieved with penicillin.[116,118,119] These analyses have, however, been strongly challenged on methodologic grounds.[120,121] It does appear that cephalosporins are more effective than penicillin in eradicating asymptomatic group A streptococcal carriage. Penicillin remains the recommended drug of choice.[96-98] In penicillin-allergic patients, macrolide (erythromycin or clarithromycin) or azalide (azithromycin) antimicrobials, clindamycin, or first-generation cephalosporins are the agents of choice.[96] The latter should be avoided in those with immediate (type I) penicillin hypersensitivity (see Table 198-1). Cephalosporins should not be administered to patients with a history of immediate (anaphylactic-type) hypersensitivity to penicillin. The physician should bear in mind the possibility of an increased risk of allergic reactions to cephalosporins when treating penicillin-allergic patients.

Erythromycin is less expensive than clarithromycin or azithromycin but may be associated with more gastrointestinal side effects. Although there have been reports of relatively high levels of resistance to macrolide antimicrobials from several countries,[122-124] as well as isolated reports of increased rates of macrolide resistance in certain localized areas of the United States,[125,126] such resistance does not appear to be widespread in this country at present. Three multistate surveillance studies conducted during 2002 and 2003 detected overall macrolide resistance rates of 3.8%,[127] 5.2%,[128] and 6.8%.[129] However, given the increasing use of azalides for upper and lower respiratory tract infections, the situation may change. Physicians should therefore be cognizant of local patterns of antimicrobial resistance. In areas in which macrolide resistance is known to be prevalent, antimicrobial susceptibility testing should be performed if these agents are used to treat group A streptococcal infections. Furthermore, continued surveillance of national trends in macrolide susceptibility is warranted.

There has been considerable recent interest in abbreviated courses of antimicrobial therapy. It has been reported that second- and third-generation cephalosporins such as cefuroxime,[130,131] cefixime,[132] ceftibuten,[133] cefdinir,[134] cefpodoxime,[135] and cefditoren[136] are effective in eradication of group A streptococci from the pharynx when administered for 5 days, although not all of these are approved for a 5-day course of therapy for acute streptococcal pharyngitis by the U.S. Food and Drug Administration (FDA) at the time of this writing. Although such shortened courses might theoretically enhance patient compliance, the potential ecologic effects of using these broad-spectrum agents to treat such a common bacterial infection are of great concern. This is particularly true should these agents be used as first-line therapy for strep throat. Moreover, even when administered for short courses, they are considerably more expensive than penicillin.

Similar favorable results of short-course therapy have also been reported for the newer macrolides or azalides, clarithromycin,[137] and azithromycin.[138-141] Because of its long intracellular half-life and slow release from tissue sites, a 5-day course of azithromycin is approved by the American Heart Association[97] for use in penicillin-allergic patients. As noted, promiscuous use of macrolides has been associated with development of resistance by group A streptococci.[122,123]

Because tetracycline-resistant group A streptococci are prevalent in many areas, this drug is not recommended. Sulfonamides, which are effective for the secondary prophylaxis of rheumatic fever (see Chapter 199), are ineffective for the eradication of pharyngeal organisms or the prevention of rheumatic fever when used as therapy for acute pharyngeal infections.

Patients with more severe suppurative infections such as those involving the mastoid or ethmoid may require higher doses of penicillin or other β-lactam antibiotics administered parenterally. When streptococcal upper respiratory infection is complicated by the development of abscesses associated with suppurative cervical adenitis or in the peritonsillar or retropharyngeal soft tissues, aspiration or incision and drainage are usually required.

Because prevention of rheumatic fever appears to require eradication of the streptococcus from the pharynx, treatment failures are of concern. In addition to true treatment failure (i.e., reisolation of the original infecting streptococcal serotype shortly after completion of a full course of antibiotic therapy), causes of post-treatment culture positivity include failure of compliance with oral medication schedules and reinfection with the same or different streptococcal types in the home or school environment. Apparent failure may also occur when the patient is in reality a streptococcal carrier suffering from an acute viral pharyngitis. In everyday practice, it is often impossible to differentiate among these alternatives.

Nevertheless, routine reculture of the throat after a course of antistreptococcal therapy in an asymptomatic patient is not advised[96] because the cost-benefit ratio of such cultures continues to decline in parallel with the incidence of acute rheumatic fever in developed countries. Such cultures should be undertaken in high-risk circumstances (e.g., if the patient or a family member has a history of rheumatic fever) or when symptoms compatible with streptococcal infection persist or recur. When an increased incidence of acute rheumatic fever is detected in a community, as happened in a number of U.S. cities during the 1980s, the approach to streptococcal infection must be particularly rigorous, and serious consideration should be given to routine performance of post-treatment cultures. If reculture is undertaken, only a single retreatment course is warranted for patients who still harbor group A streptococci. Retreatment with an oral cephalosporin might be considered in view of the slightly increased eradication rates observed with these agents.

The presence of persistently but weakly positive throat cultures after repeated courses of antibiotic therapy in an otherwise asymptomatic patient is not a cause for alarm. Such persons are streptococcal carriers[117] who are neither at risk of developing rheumatic fever nor likely to spread their infection to others. Their most frequent problem is anxiety produced by multiple medical consultations associated with the streptococcal colonization. In the event in which, for medical or psychological reasons, eradication of chronic streptococcal carriage becomes highly desirable, clindamycin,[142] amoxicillin-clavulanate,[143] or azithromycin may be efficacious.[96,144]

Streptococcal acquisition rates of 25% or higher have been recorded in family contacts. Certainly, family contacts with symptoms of upper respiratory infection should be cultured and treated appropriately if positive. Asymptomatic family contacts should also be cultured in high-risk circumstances, such as a family member who has had rheumatic fever or known cases of rheumatic fever or poststreptococcal glomerulonephritis occurring in the general area. In situations of lesser risk, routine culture of asymptomatic family contacts is not recommended.[96,97] The advisability of culture and/or prophylaxis of household contacts of patients with invasive group A streptococcal infection is discussed later.[144]

There is no firm evidence to suggest that tonsillectomy reduces the incidence of rheumatic fever, either in healthy persons or in persons who have had rheumatic fever and faithfully maintained continuous antibiotic prophylaxis. In certain patients with recurrent bouts of tonsillopharyngitis, however, tonsillectomy may decrease the frequency of incapacitating acute infections.[145,146] Tonsillectomy should be considered only for the most severely affected patients.[147]

Streptococcal Pyoderma

Pyoderma, *impetigo*, and *impetigo contagiosa* are terms used synonymously to describe discrete purulent lesions that are primary infections of the skin and that are extremely prevalent in many parts of the world. In the great majority of cases, pyoderma is caused by β-hemolytic streptococci and/or *Staphylococcus aureus*.

EPIDEMIOLOGY

Pyoderma occurs most frequently in economically disadvantaged children dwelling in tropical or subtropical climates. It is also prevalent in northern climates during the summer months.[148] The peak incidence of impetigo is in children aged 2 to 5 years. This disorder also occurs among older children and adults whose recreational activities or occupation results in cutaneous cuts or abrasions.[149,150,150a] There is no gender predilection, and all races appear to be susceptible. The prevalence of streptococcal pyoderma is markedly influenced by several factors, the most important of which appear to be climate and level of hygiene.

Meticulous prospective studies of streptococcal impetigo have demonstrated that the responsible microorganisms initially colonize the unbroken skin,[148] an observation that probably explains the influence of personal hygiene on disease incidence. Development of skin colonization with a given streptococcal strain precedes the development of impetiginous lesions by an average interval of 10 days. The mechanism of production of skin lesions is unproved, but it is most likely caused by intradermal inoculation of surface organisms by abrasions, minor trauma, or insect bites. Frequently, there is a transfer of the streptococcal strains from the skin and/or pyoderma lesions to the upper respiratory tract. The interval between colonization of the skin and colonization of nose and/or throat averages 2 to 3 weeks.

BACTERIOLOGY AND IMMUNOLOGY

Streptococci isolated from pyodermal lesions are primarily group A, but occasionally representatives of other serogroups such as C and G are responsible. Group A streptococci that cause impetigo differ in several respects from those usually associated with tonsillitis and pharyngitis. Skin strains belong to different M serotypes or genotypes from the classic throat strains; because most have been identified more recently, they tend to comprise the higher numbered M types. Throat and skin strains can also be differentiated by genetic markers.[151] A relatively small number of serotypes seem capable of regularly initiating both pharyngitis and pyoderma.[152]

Assays of streptococcal antibodies are of no value in the diagnosis and management of impetigo, but they provide helpful supporting evidence of recent streptococcal infection in patients suspected of having post–streptococcal glomerulonephritis. The ASO response is weak in patients with streptococcal impetigo,[153,154] presumably because the activity of streptolysin O response is inhibited by skin lipids (cholesterol),[155] whereas anti–DNase B levels are elevated.[153,154]

CLINICAL MANIFESTATIONS

The lesion of streptococcal pyoderma begins as a papule that rapidly evolves into a vesicle surrounded by an area of erythema. The vesicular lesions are evanescent and rarely recognized clinically; they give rise to pustules that gradually enlarge and then break down over a period of 4 to 6 days to form characteristic thick crusts (Fig. 198-4). The lesions heal slowly and leave depigmented areas. A deeply ulcerated form of impetigo is known as *ecthyma*.

Streptococcal impetigo occurs on exposed areas of the body, most frequently on the lower extremities or face. The lesions remain well localized but are frequently multiple. Although regional lymphadenitis may occur, systemic symptoms are not ordinarily present.

In the past, the lesions described above could be rather confidently diagnosed as streptococcal. This was the predominant form of impe-

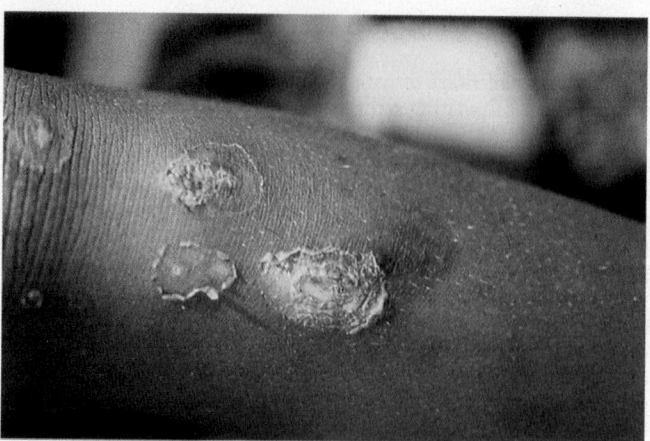

Figure 198-4 **Multiple pyoderma lesions on the lower extremities of a child in rural Mississippi.** *(Courtesy of Dr. K. Nelson, Baltimore.)*

tigo and could be distinguished from bullous impetigo caused by phage group II *S. aureus*. Although bullous impetigo remains almost exclusively staphylococcal in cause, the bacteriology of nonbullous impetigo has changed.[156] *S. aureus*, either alone or in combination with *S. pyogenes*, is now the predominant causative agent.[157-159] Almost all such staphylococci are penicillinase producers. Therefore, treatment with penicillin, which in the past had been highly effective against nonbullous impetigo, even when both streptococci and staphylococci were isolated from the lesions, now frequently fails.[158]

TREATMENT AND PREVENTION

Because of the current frequency of isolation of *S. aureus* from nonbullous impetigo lesions and concomitant reports of penicillin failures,[158,160,161] penicillinase-resistant penicillins or first-generation cephalosporins are preferred.[158] Erythromycin has long been a mainstay of pyoderma therapy, but its use may be lessened in areas in which erythromycin-resistant strains of *S. aureus* or, more recently, *S. pyogenes* are prevalent. Topical therapy with mupirocin is equivalent to oral systemic antimicrobials[162,163] and may be used when lesions are limited in number. It is expensive, however, and some strains of staphylococci may be resistant.[164] Retapamulin, a novel pleuromutilin antibacterial, has recently been approved by the FDA for treatment of bullous and nonbullous impetigo caused by GAS and methicillin-susceptible strains of *S. aureus* in children 9 months of age or older.[165-167] In vitro data have suggested that it may be more effective than mupirocin against methicillin-resistant *Staphylococcus aureus* (MRSA).

Adherence to good regimens of personal hygiene is the most effective measure currently available for prevention of impetigo.

COMPLICATIONS

Suppurative complications are uncommon. For as yet unexplained reasons, rheumatic fever has never been shown to occur after streptococcal pyoderma. On the other hand, cutaneous infections with nephritogenic strains of group A streptococci are the major antecedent of poststreptococcal glomerulonephritis in many areas of the world. There are as yet no conclusive data to indicate that treatment of an individual case of pyoderma prevents the subsequent occurrence of nephritis in these patients. Such therapy is nevertheless important as an epidemiologic measure in eradicating nephritogenic strains from the environment.

Invasive Streptococcal Infections of Skin and Soft Tissues

In the mid-1980s, outbreaks of acute rheumatic fever began to occur throughout the United States, concomitant with the reappearance of certain streptococcal strains exhibiting characteristics known to be associated with rheumatogenicity (see Chapter 199). Shortly thereafter, invasive streptococcal infections, of a frequency and severity not seen in the preceding decades, began to be reported both in the United States and abroad.[168-171] Although strains of a number of group A streptococcal M types have been isolated from invasive infections, there has been a definite and consistent tendency for M types 1 and 3 to be associated with life-threatening infections.[169-173] A high proportion of these cases has occurred in adults, and the portal of entry is frequently the skin or soft tissues. In some cases, the infections give rise to shock and multiorgan failure, features that simulate in certain respects the staphylococcal toxic shock syndrome.[174] This entity has thus been termed *strep TSS*. Clinical features of serious streptococcal skin and soft tissue infections and TSS are described later.

ERYSIPELAS

Erysipelas is a superficial cutaneous process, usually restricted to the dermis but with prominent lymphatic involvement. It is distinguished clinically from other forms of cutaneous infection by three features: the lesions are raised above the level of the surrounding skin, there is a clear line of demarcation between involved and uninvolved tissue, and the lesions are a brilliant salmon-red color. This disorder is more common in infants, young children, and older adults. It is almost always caused by β-hemolytic streptococci. In most cases the infecting agent is the group A streptococci, but similar lesions can be caused by streptococci of group C or G. Rarely, group B streptococci or *S. aureus* may be the culprits. In older reports, erysipelas was described as characteristically involving the butterfly area of the face (Fig. 198-5), but at present the lower extremities are more frequently involved (see Fig. 198-6). In patients with facial erysipelas, there is frequently a history of preceding streptococcal sore throat, although the exact mode of

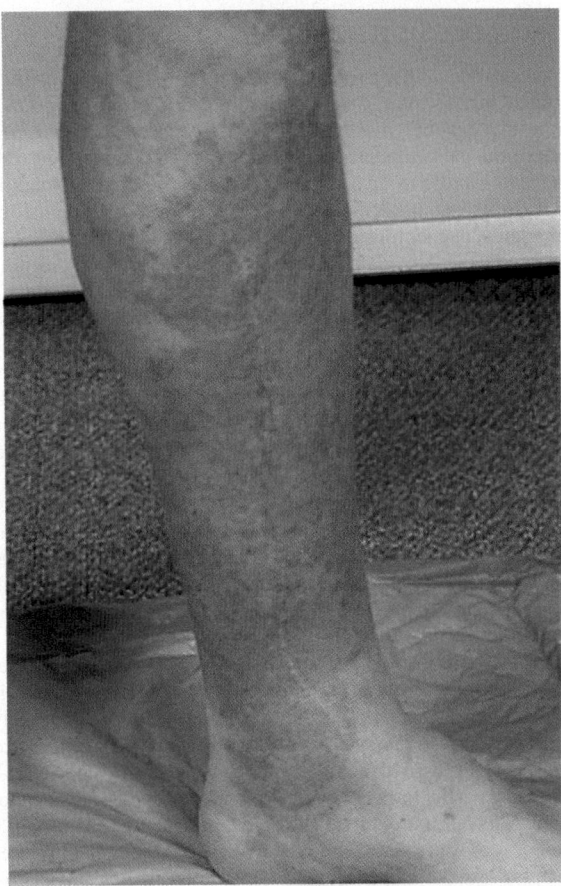

Figure 198-6 **Erysipelas in saphenous venectomy limb.** This patient had undergone coronary artery bypass grafting.

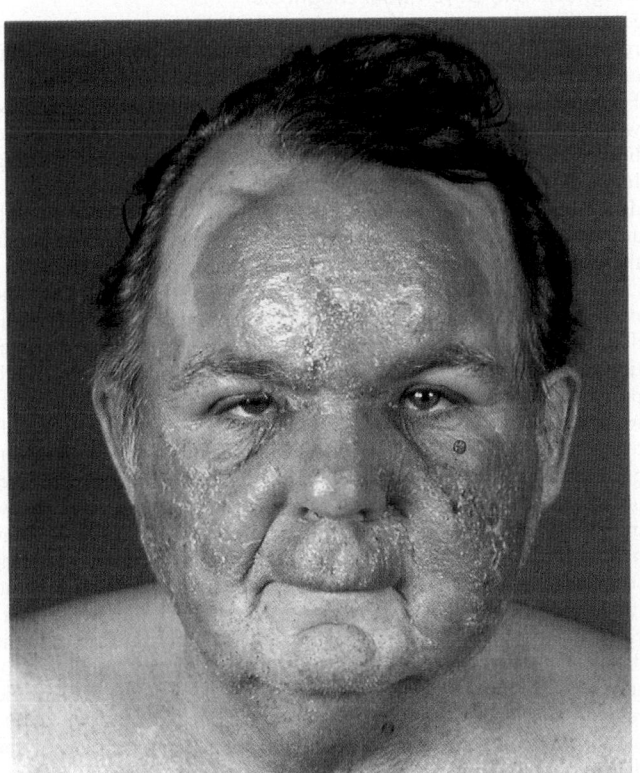

Figure 198-5 **Facial erysipelas.** The lesion is well demarcated from surrounding skin and illustrates the typical butterfly distribution. *(From Bisno AL. Cutaneous infections: Microbiologic and epidemiologic considerations. Am J Med. 1984;76:172-179, with permission.)*

spread to the skin is unknown. When erysipelas involves the extremities, breaks in the cutaneous barrier serve as portals of entry; these include surgical incisions, trauma or abrasions, dermatologic diseases such as psoriasis, or local fungal infections.

The cutaneous lesion begins as a localized area of erythema and swelling and then spreads rapidly with advancing red margins, which are raised and well demarcated from adjacent normal tissue. There is marked edema, often with bleb formation, and in facial erysipelas the eyes are frequently swollen shut. The lesion may demonstrate central resolution while continuing to extend on the periphery. The cutaneous inflammation is accompanied by chills, fever, and toxicity.

The differential diagnosis is limited. Early on, the lesions of facial herpes zoster, contact dermatitis, or giant urticaria may be confused with erysipelas. Lesions resembling erysipelas may occur in patients with familial Mediterranean fever. Cutaneous lesions similar in appearance to those of erysipelas may occur on the hands of patients who sustain cuts or abrasions while handling fish or meats. This entity, known as erysipeloid of Rosenbach and caused by *Erysipelothrix rhusiopathiae*, is usually unaccompanied by fever or systemic symptoms.

With early diagnosis and treatment, the prognosis is excellent. Rarely, however, the process may spread to deeper levels of the skin and soft tissues. Penicillin, either parenterally or orally, depending on clinical severity, is the treatment of choice. If staphylococcal infection is suspected, a penicillinase-resistant semisynthetic penicillin or cephalosporin should be selected. In a randomized, prospective multicenter trial,[175] roxithromycin, a macrolide antimicrobial, was equivalent to penicillin. Increased levels of macrolide resistance among group A streptococci, however, have been detected in certain areas of the United States.[125,126]

STREPTOCOCCAL CELLULITIS

Streptococcal cellulitis, an acute spreading inflammation of the skin and subcutaneous tissues, results from infection of burns, wounds, or surgical incisions but may also follow mild trauma. Clinical findings include local pain, tenderness, swelling, and erythema. The process may extend rapidly to involve large areas of skin. Systemic manifestations include fever, chills, and malaise, and there may be associated lymphangitis, bacteremia, or both. In contrast to erysipelas, the lesion is not raised, the demarcation between involved and uninvolved skin is indistinct and lesions are more pink than salmon red in color. Often, however, the clinical differentiation between these entities is not clear-cut.

Two predisposing causes of streptococcal cellulitis deserve special mention. One is the parenteral injection of illicit drugs.[176-178] These cases are often associated with bacteremia and deep tissue infections such as septic thrombophlebitis, suppurative arthritis, osteomyelitis, and occasionally infective endocarditis. Second, patients who have impaired lymphatic drainage from upper or lower extremities are prone to recurrent episodes of streptococcal cellulitis. Examples include individuals with filariasis and women who have undergone radical mastectomy with axillary node dissection.[179] It is speculated that repetitive infection further damages local lymphatics and worsens lymphatic stasis.[180]

Recurrent episodes of severe cellulitis have also been reported in certain patients who have undergone coronary artery bypass grafting.[181] The lesion invariably occurs in the extremity from which the saphenous vein was removed, and at times it may exhibit features of erysipelas (Fig. 198-6). Patients with tinea pedis of the venectomy limb appear to be particularly at risk.[182-184] As with other forms of cellulitis, pathogenic bacteria are difficult to recover during these episodes. The appearance of the lesions and the response to penicillin therapy suggest, however, a streptococcal cause. The few β-hemolytic streptococci that have been recovered and characterized often belong to serogroups other than A.[185]

Disruption of the cutaneous barrier (leg ulcers, wounds, dermatophytosis) is a risk factor for the development of cutaneous streptococcal infection.[186] There is suggestive evidence that local dermatophyte infection (i.e., athlete's foot) may serve as a reservoir for β-hemolytic streptococci that initiate episodes of erysipelas or cellulitis of the lower extremities.[182,187] Thus, care should be taken to eradicate such fungal infections in patients who experience recurrent bouts of erysipelas or cellulitis. Another potential reservoir is anal streptococcal colonization.[188] Other risk factors include venous insufficiency, edema, and obesity.[186] Not surprisingly, an increased risk of recurrent cellulitis has also been reported in homeless persons.[189]

Cellulitis may be caused by infection with a variety of bacterial pathogens (see Chapter 90), but most cases are caused by *S. pyogenes* (or, occasionally, streptococci of groups B, C, or G) or by *S. aureus*. In the absence of positive blood cultures, which are present in only 5% of cases of cellulitis, a specific microbiologic diagnosis is often not possible. Aspirate or biopsy samples from sites of active cellulitis are helpful when positive on smear or culture, but unfortunately such specimens are usually negative in adult patients.[190-192]

It is often impossible to differentiate streptococcal from staphylococcal cellulitis on initial presentation confidently. In this case a semisynthetic penicillinase-resistant penicillin should be used. In penicillin-allergic patients, a first-generation cephalosporin may be used if the hypersensitivity is not of the immediate type. Clindamycin or vancomycin may be used in patients who manifest anaphylactic hypersensitivity to β-lactam antibiotics, and the latter should be administered if there is reason to suspect infection with MRSA strains. Patients with milder cases of streptococcal cellulitis may be switched to oral medications after an initial favorable response to parenteral therapy.

The role of continuous antimicrobial prophylaxis[193-195] in patients prone to frequent recurrences remains unsettled. At present, such prophylaxis seems justified only for patients with very frequent or severe episodes, and the optimal regimen has not been established.

NECROTIZING FASCIITIS (STREPTOCOCCAL GANGRENE)

Necrotizing fasciitis is an infection of the deeper subcutaneous tissues and fascia, characterized by extensive and rapidly spreading necrosis and by gangrene of the skin and underlying structures. As detailed in Chapter 90, this entity may arise in several distinct epidemiologic settings, may be caused by multiple aerobic and anaerobic microorganisms, and may vary in clinical manifestations. The present discussion is limited to necrotizing fasciitis caused by the group A streptococcus[196] and described by Meleney[197] in 1924 as hemolytic streptococcal gangrene. Characteristically, streptococcal gangrene begins at a site of trivial or even inapparent trauma or in an operative incision. The initial lesion may appear only as an area of mild erythema but over the next 24 to 72 hours undergoes a rapid evolution. The inflammation becomes more pronounced and extensive, the skin becomes dusky and then purplish, and bullae containing yellow or hemorrhagic fluid appear. Bacteremia is frequently present, and metastatic abscesses may occur. By the fourth to fifth day, frank gangrenous changes are evident in the affected skin,[198] followed by extensive sloughing. The process may march inexorably over large bodily areas unless measures are taken to contain it. The patient with streptococcal gangrene appears perilously ill, with high fever and extreme prostration. Mortality rates are high, even with appropriate treatment.[198] Fournier's gangrene, a form of necrotizing fasciitis involving the male genital area, may rarely be caused by group A streptococci.

The course of necrotizing fasciitis today appears to be much more fulminant than that described by Meleney. Specifically, ecchymoses and bullae may appear within 2 to 3 days and associated myonecrosis is more common. In addition, the mortality rate in 1924 was 20%, whereas mortality rates of 20% to 70% have been reported in the current era. This difference is even more remarkable because antibiotics, IV fluids, ventilators, and dialysis were not available in 1924.

Diagnosis and Differential Diagnosis

Successful management of necrotizing fasciitis is dependent on early recognition, yet early in their course, patients may present with fever and toxicity when the cutaneous lesion may appear relatively benign.[199] Fever and severe pain are the first manifestations of disease. In those with a defined portal of entry such as a surgical incision, burn, insect bite, or varicella lesion, there is redness of the skin, pain, and swelling. In the 50% of patients who develop necrotizing fasciitis without a defined portal of entry, the infection begins deep to the skin, frequently at the site of a hematoma, muscle strain, or traumatic joint injury. In these, crescendo pain is the most reliable clinical clue.

Routine radiographs, computed tomography (CT) scanning, and magnetic resonance imaging (MRI) may show localized swelling of the deep structures but characteristically do not show frank abscess formation or gas in the tissue and *thus are not definitive procedures*. This is particularly problematic in those patients without a portal of entry who have deep infection at the site of recent trauma such as muscle tear, hematoma, or prior surgery, in which the clinician cannot distinguish the cause of the deep swelling. Unfortunately, imaging studies often serve to delay rather than facilitate a diagnosis. Fever and increasingly severe pain are the best and earliest signs of infection. Some patients do not present with fever,[199] and others may have taken nonsteroidal anti-inflammatory (NSAIDs) drugs that mask fever and reduce pain. Unexplained tachycardia, marked left shift, and an elevated creatine phosphokinase level are also important clues to the diagnosis of necrotizing fasciitis, and their presence should prompt surgical inspection of the deep tissues. Gram stains of aspirated fluid reveal chains of gram-positive cocci that contain few, if any, white blood cells. Similarly, a biopsy with frozen section may aid in the diagnosis of necrotizing fasciitis.[200,201]

MYOSITIS AND MYONECROSIS

Most cases of purulent muscle infection occur in the tropics, and *S. aureus* is the predominant causative agent. Myositis caused by group

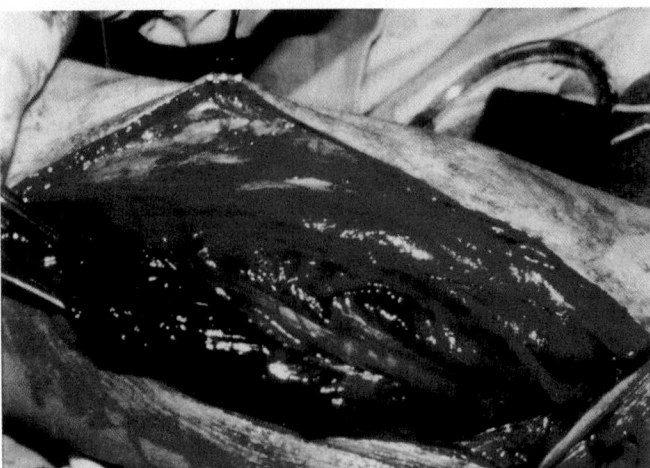

Figure 198-7 Surgical exploration of patient with streptococcal toxic shock syndrome. This patient had necrotizing fasciitis and myositis that occurred spontaneously, with no prior injury to the site. *(From Stevens D. Streptococcal toxic shock syndrome. Infect Med. 1992;9:33-39, with permission.)*

TABLE 198-2	Case Definition for the Streptococcal Toxic Shock Syndrome*

I. Isolation of group A streptococci (*Streptococcus pyogenes*)
  A. From a normally sterile site (e.g., blood, cerebrospinal, pleural, or peritoneal fluid, tissue biopsy, surgical wound)
  B. From a nonsterile site (e.g., throat, sputum, vagina, superficial skin lesion)

II. Clinical signs of severity
  A. Hypotension: systolic blood pressure ≤ 90 mm Hg in adults or below fifth percentile for age in children
    and
  B. Two or more of the following signs:
    1. Renal impairment: creatinine ≥ 177 µmol/L (≥2 mg/dL) for adults or ≥2× the upper limit of normal for age. In patients with preexisting renal disease, a twofold or greater elevation over the baseline level
    2. Coagulopathy: platelets ≤ 100 × 10^9/L (≤ 100,000/mm^3) or disseminated intravascular coagulation defined by prolonged clotting times, low fibrinogen level, and the presence of fibrin degradation products
    3. Liver involvement: serum aspartate aminotransferase (AST), alanine aminotransferase (ALT), or total bilirubin levels ≥2× the upper limit of normal for age. In patients with preexisting liver disease, a twofold or greater elevation over the baseline level.
    4. Adult respiratory distress syndrome defined by acute onset of diffuse pulmonary infiltrates and hypoxemia in the absence of cardiac failure, or evidence of diffuse capillary leak manifested by acute onset of generalized edema, or pleural or peritoneal effusions with hypoalbuminemia
    5. A generalized erythematous macular rash that may desquamate
    6. Soft tissue necrosis, including necrotizing fasciitis or myositis, or gangrene

*An illness fulfilling criteria IA and II (A and B) can be defined as a definite case. An illness fulfilling criteria IB and II (A and B) can be defined as a probable case if no other cause for the illness is identified.

From The Working Group on Severe Streptococcal Infections. Defining the group A streptococcal toxic shock syndrome: Rationale and consensus definition. *JAMA* 1993;269:390-391, with permission.

A streptococci has been rare but occurs in many patients with necrotizing fasciitis and strep TSS. Most of these cases occur after blunt nonpenetrating trauma or occur spontaneously. Most likely, bacteria are translocated to the deep tissue hematogenously from the throat. Systemic toxicity is common and mortality as high as 80% has been reported.[202] Destruction of tissue is poorly understood, but infection and inflammation within the confined muscle compartment space may result in pressures exceeding arterial pressure, necessitating emergent fasciotomy and débridement (Fig. 198-7). There is much overlap in the clinical features of necrotizing fasciitis and myonecrosis,[198,202] and the differentiation must be made by surgical inspection or biopsy.

STREPTOCOCCAL TOXIC SHOCK SYNDROME

Strep TSS is defined as described in Table 198-2 but, simply put, it is any streptococcal infection associated with the sudden onset of shock and organ failure. Such cases were first described in the mid to late 1980s, and reports of strep TSS have subsequently emanated from North America, Europe, Australia, and Asia.[169,174,175,203-211] Most cases have occurred sporadically. The highest incidence of invasive streptococcal disease occurred in a small Minnesota community, where 26 cases/100,000 population were recorded.[210] In addition, outbreaks of invasive group A streptococcal infections have occurred in closed environments such as nursing homes[212-216] and hospitals.[217] Secondary cases of strep TSS are unusual, but transmission to family members[217,218] or health care workers[217,219] has been well documented by demonstrating identical pulsed-field gel electrophoresis patterns from cross-infecting strains. Although many of the studies cited earlier described strep TSS in adults, several reports have documented that this disorder also occurs in children.[204,209,210,220,221] Thus, persons of all ages can be afflicted and, although some have underlying medical conditions such as diabetes and alcoholism,[204,206,222-226] many have no predisposing medical condition and are not immunocompromised. This contrasts sharply with reviews of group A streptococcal bacteremia from several decades ago[222-224] that found the disease to occur primarily among the very young, the very old, or patients with predisposing conditions such as cancer, renal failure, leukemia, severe burns, or iatrogenic immunosuppression.

The portals of entry for streptococci are the vagina, pharynx, mucosa, and skin in 50% of cases.[173] Surgical procedures such as suction lipectomy, hysterectomy, vaginal delivery, bunionectomy, reduction mammoplasty, hernia repair, bone pinning, and vasectomy have provided portals in other cases (Table 198-3). Rarely, infection occurs secondary to streptococcal pharyngitis.[227-229] Virus infections such as varicella and influenza have provided portals of entry in other cases.[173,209,227]

Additional factors that increase the risk of invasive group A streptococcal infection, including bacteremia, strep TSS, and necrotizing fasciitis, are listed in Table 198-3. Three studies have demonstrated that a high or increasing prevalence of M-1 or M-3 strains among throat isolates may signal an increased incidence of strep TSS in a community.[209,225,230] NSAIDs taken for problems such as muscle strain, trauma, or postpartum pain may mask the early signs and symptoms of streptococcal infection or possibly predispose to more severe infection, such as necrotizing fasciitis or strep TSS.[173,231,232]

Pathogenesis

Entry of group A streptococci into the deeper tissues and bloodstream may occur as a result of breach of a barrier, or the organism itself may penetrate intact mucous membranes such as the pharyngeal mucosa.

TABLE 198-3	Factors That Increase the Likelihood of Developing Streptococcal Toxic Shock Syndrome

Age (neonates and older adults)

Diabetes

Alcoholism

Surgical procedures

Trauma
  Penetrating (insect bites, lacerations, slivers, abrasions, burns)
  Nonpenetrating (hematoma, bruise, muscle strain, hemarthrosis)

Varicella
  Contact with a case
  High prevalence of invasive strains in the community

Nonsteroidal anti-inflammatory drugs*

*Based on limited evidence.

Although bacteremia is a very uncommon phenomenon in streptococcal pharyngitis, transient bacteremia must occur in those 50% of patients who develop invasive infections without a portal of entry. In either case, group A streptococci avoid phagocytosis largely because of the antiphagocytic properties of M protein.[8] Adherence of group A streptococci to pharyngeal mucosal cells is a prerequisite to colonization or infection and has been related to surface structures, such as lipoteichoic acid and fibronectin-binding proteins. Penetration or translocation of group A streptococci through respiratory epithelial cells has been demonstrated for M-1 types of group A streptococci. Some have suggested that those M-1 strains possessing an invasin (inv+) gene penetrate more efficiently.[233] If penetration of mucosal barriers occurs commonly, it does not result in clinically detectable bacteremia in the vast majority of patients, because the incidence of invasive infection is very low—that is, 3.5 cases/100,000 population.[234] Thus, clearance of group A streptococci must be highly efficient in the vast majority of humans either because of preexisting type-specific immunity or nonspecific clearance mechanisms in the reticuloendothelial system. Recent studies have suggested that following colonization of mucosa or skin, SpeB may play a role in attenuation of the local host response because of its proteolytic activity. Later in the growth cycle, some GAS production of SpeB is curtailed through alteration of the CovR (control of virulence regulator), allowing these particular strains to bind plasminogen, evade the immune system, and switch to an invasive phenotype.[235]

The enigma is how and why GAS cause deep infection of traumatized muscle and fascia in the absence of penetrating injury. Recent studies have demonstrated that injured muscle cells express vimentin on their surface during the healing and repair process and that GAS bind vimentin.[236] In addition, intravenously injected GAS home to the site of muscle injury and this process is augmented in the presence of NSAIDs.[237]

Mechanisms of Shock and Organ Failure: Cytokine Induction

Within the deeper tissues and bloodstream, the induction of cytokine synthesis plays a critically important role in the production of shock and organ failure. Pyrogenic exotoxins (scarlatina toxins, erythrotoxins) have the ability to cause fever, enhance susceptibility to endotoxin, suppress IgM antibody synthesis, and act as superantigens. These toxins, like the staphylococcal enterotoxins (A, B, C) and TSST-1, can stimulate T-cell responses through their ability to bind to both the MHC class II complex of antigen-presenting cells and the V-β region of the T-cell receptor.[238] The net effect is the induction of monocyte cytokines (tumor necrosis factor-α [TNF-α], interleukin [IL]-1β, and IL-6) as well as the lymphokines (TNF-β, IL-2, and interferon-γ).[239-245] There is evidence that M protein fragments may also act as superantigens.[243] Pyrogenic exotoxins C and MF, as well as SSA and several new Spe, are also capable of inducing massive quantities of proinflammatory cytokines, as well as lymphokines,[244] that contribute to shock and organ failure. Some clinical studies have suggested that variation in human leukocyte antigen (HLA) haplotype may predispose worse outcomes in some patients with strep TSS.[245]

Other streptococcal virulence factors are also capable of inducing proinflammatory cytokines such as TNF-α and IL-1β. Specifically, SpeB, a potent cysteine protease, causes release of IL-1β from preformed intracellular pools.[246] Streptolysin O also stimulates mononuclear cells to produce TNF-α and IL-1β and, in the presence of SpeA, has synergistic effects on IL-1β production.[247] Heat-killed group A streptococci, as well as peptidoglycan and lipoteichoic acid, are also potent inducers of TNF-α and IL-1β.[248,249] Noncytokine mechanisms of shock may also play a role. A cysteine protease produced by group A streptococci was shown to release bradykinin from a high-molecular-weight kininogen.[250] Bradykinin is a potent vasodilator of systemic and pulmonary vasculature and could be responsible, at least in part, for the early hypotension observed in strep TSS.[250]

Thus, there are likely many streptococcal and host factors that contribute to the shock and organ failure characteristic of strep TSS. That

TNF plays a central role is supported by two observations. First, high levels of TNF are observed in a baboon model of group A streptococcal bacteremia at a point in time when profound hypotension is manifest.[251] Second, in that model, a neutralizing monoclonal antibody against TNF restored normal blood pressure and reduced mortality by 50%.[251] Diffuse capillary leak contributes to volume depletion and hypotension and is likely related to cytokine release but may also be related to circulating M protein–fibrinogen complexes.[252]

Clinical Manifestations

The first phase of strep TSS begins with an influenza-like prodrome characterized by fever, chills, myalgias, nausea, vomiting, and diarrhea that precedes hypotension by 24 to 48 hours.[173] Confusion and/or combativeness is present in 55% of patients. Where there is a defined or superficial portal of entry such as a laceration, suspicion of streptococcal infection or frank evidence of infection may be present at this phase of infection. In contrast, in patients without a portal of entry (50% of cases) and who subsequently develop necrotizing fasciitis, postpartum infection, peritonitis, or joint space infection, pain that progressively increases in severity is the most common initial symptom that prompts patients to seek medical care and, interestingly, precedes clinical evidence of localized infection by 12 to 24 hours.[173] In both children[209] and adults.[173] the soft tissues are the most common primary site of infection. In the remaining cases, pneumonia, meningitis, endophthalmitis, meningitis, peritonitis, myocarditis, joint infection, and intrauterine infection have been described.[173,209]

Phase 2 of strep TSS is characterized by tachycardia, tachypnea, persistent fever and, in patients who subsequently have necrotizing fasciitis or myonecrosis, increasingly severe pain at the site of infection. In others, fever and severe pain are the best early clinical clues.[253] In children, toxicity during varicella or persistence of fever longer than 4 days should also prompt careful evaluation. Many patients are seen in emergency departments at this stage and frequently sent home on one or two occasions with mistaken diagnoses, such as deep vein thrombophlebitis, muscle strain, viral gastroenteritis, dehydration, and sprained ankle.[199] High fever and excruciating pain, particularly in individuals with no risk factors for deep vein thrombosis, should arouse suspicion of a deep-seated infection. The laboratory tests described later are helpful, and CT and MRI may be useful to define the level of tissue injury but are not specific (see earlier discussion of necrotizing fasciitis).

Phase 3 of strep TSS is characterized by the symptoms and signs mentioned but with the sudden onset of shock and organ failure. Many patients are in florid shock at the time of admission, but in almost 50% hypotension is apparent during the first 4 to 8 hours after admission. Clinical evidence of necrotizing fasciitis is frequently a late finding, often occurring after hypotension is present. The appearance of purple bullae and dusky-appearing skin is a bad prognostic sign and should prompt emergent surgical exploration (see earlier discussion of necrotizing fasciitis). It should be noted that currently, the progression of necrotizing fasciitis from red skin to purple bullae may take place within a 24-hour period, whereas that described by Meleney in 1924 took 7 to 10 days. In addition, the rapidity with which shock and multiorgan failure can progress is impressive, and many patients die within 24 to 48 hours of hospitalization.[173]

Laboratory tests should be performed in patients with aggressive soft tissue infections or patients with severe pain and fever who appear toxic. The serum creatinine measurement is particularly useful because renal impairment (creatinine level more than twice normal) is apparent even during phase 2, before hypotension is apparent. In addition, creatine phosphokinase levels in serum are markedly elevated in those with necrotizing fasciitis and myonecrosis. The white blood count is usually normal or elevated at admission but with a profound left shift that includes myelocytes and metamyelocytes. Finally, serum albumin and calcium levels are usually low on admission and drop precipitously as a diffuse capillary leak syndrome develops. Thrombocytopenia does not develop until later in the course but is the earliest sign of disseminated coagulopathy.[173] Profound metabolic acidosis develops early in phase 3, and serum bicarbonate, lactate, and blood gas pH determinations are crucial tests to follow therapeutic progress. Because the acute respiratory distress syndrome (ARDS) develops in 55% of patients with strep TSS, pulse oximetry and, later, blood gas levels are necessary to evaluate the need for intubation and ventilation.

MANAGEMENT

Source Control
Prompt and aggressive surgical exploration and débridement of suspected deep-seated streptococcal infection are mandatory. It is as important to establish the cause of the infection as it is to determine the extent of necrosis. CT and MRI are helpful to locate the primary site of infection, but because the group A streptococci do not form gas or frank abscess, radiologist interpretations are frequently not definitive. Such findings in a patient with extreme pain and fever or who is toxic should prompt surgical consultation. Once necrosis is established, extensive débridement is necessary, because shock and organ failure continue to progress if devitalized tissue remains.

Fluid Resuscitation
If several liters of crystalloid intravenous fluid challenge do not rapidly improve blood pressure (mean arterial pressure more than 60 mm Hg) or tissue perfusion, then invasive monitoring is indicated. The goal should be to maintain a pulmonary artery occlusion pressure of 12 to 16 mm Hg.[254] If this goal is reached but hypotension persists, the serum albumin concentration and hematocrit should be checked, because profoundly low albumin levels are common and because hemolysins produced by GAS can cause dramatic drops in circulating red cell mass. Thus, transfusion with packed red blood cells, with or without albumin, may be useful to improve blood pressure and preserve tissue perfusion.

Because of intractable hypotension and diffuse capillary leak, massive amounts of IV fluids (10 to 20 L/day) in an adult may be required. Albumin replacement may be necessary because many patients' serum albumin levels drop to lower than 2.0 g/dL.

Antimicrobial Treatment
Prompt antimicrobial therapy is mandatory, and empirical broad-spectrum coverage for septic shock should be instituted initially. Once the streptococcal cause is confirmed, high-dose penicillin and clindamycin should be given. This recommendation is based on the following information: (1) all strains of group A streptococci remain sensitive to penicillin; (2) resistance to erythromycin is currently found in less than 5% of group A streptococci in the United States, but the rate is higher in certain locales, and there have been rare reports of resistance to clindamycin; (3) clindamycin and erythromycin are more active in experimental models of necrotizing fasciitis and myonecrosis; (4) penicillin-binding proteins are not expressed during stationary-phase growth of group A streptococci, and thus penicillin is ineffective in severe deep infections in which large numbers of bacteria are present; (5) clindamycin suppresses exotoxin and M protein production by group A streptococci; (6) clindamycin has a much longer half-life; (7) combinations of penicillin and clindamycin have indifferent interaction against group A streptococci in vitro at clinically relevant concentrations of antibiotics (no antagonistic effects were found)[255]; and (8) clindamycin and azithromycin suppress cytokine production by human mononuclear cells.[256,257]

Management in the Intensive Care Unit
In patients with persistent hypotension, monitoring of cardiac outputs, pulmonary artery occlusion pressure, and mean arterial pressure is important. Intubation and ventilator support are usually required because of the high incidence of ARDS (55%) in patients with strep TSS. Pressors such as dopamine are used frequently, although no controlled trials have been performed in strep TSS. In patients with intractable hypotension, high doses of dopamine, epinephrine, or phenylephrine have been used, but caution should be exercised in

those with evidence of disseminated intravascular coagulation (DIC) and in particular in those with cold, cyanotic digits. Symmetrical gangrene involving all 20 digits and toes, the tip of the nose, and the breast areola have been described. In addition, amputation of one, two, three, and even four extremities has been observed (our unpublished data). In these cases, both excessive pressors and DIC likely contribute to symmetrical gangrene.

Dialysis and Hemoperfusion
Either of these methodologies may be necessary because more than 50% of patients develop acute renal failure. Both dialysis and hemoperfusion may also nonspecifically reduce the concentrations of circulating toxins. It is interesting that a study from Sweden that used hemofiltration achieved the lowest mortality rate in patients with strep TSS ever recorded.[226] Finally, a polystyrene superantigen absorbing device (SAAD) was developed in Japan and shown to be highly efficacious in absorbing pyrogenic exotoxin A or toxic shock syndrome toxin 1 (TSST-1) from plasma and, when used extracorporeally in animals infused with TSST-1 and lipopolysaccharide (LPS), mortality improved from 100% to 50%.[258]

Intravenous Immune Globulin
The rationale for the use of intravenous immune globulin (IVIG) in the treatment of strep TSS is based on the data implicating extracellular exotoxins as mediators of shock and organ failure. George and Gladys Dick in 1924 demonstrated that convalescent sera from patients with scarlet fever neutralized scarlatina toxins and that when passively administered, attenuated the course of severe scarlet fever.[259] Just as penicillin was becoming available, antiscarlatina toxin horse serum became commercially available in the United States, but because of the availability of penicillin and the decline in the severity of scarlet fever, it was never used. Several reports have described the successful use of IVIG in patients with strep TSS.[260-262] The largest treatment group (15 patients) showed a significant reduction in mortality compared with matched historical controls.[263] The mortality rate of 70% in the control group was among the highest ever reported, whereas the rate was 30% in the IVIG group. This rate is similar to that of some series that did not use IVIG.[173] A double-blind clinical trial was undertaken in northern Europe comparing IVIG with albumin in patients with strep TSS. All patients received clindamycin. The mortality rate in the IVIG group was 16%, whereas that in the albumin group was 32%.[264] Unfortunately, the study was stopped because of low enrollment and only seven or eight patients with proved GAS infections were in each group. Thus, the differences were not significant. A retrospective study in patients with strep TSS has also shown no benefit of IVIG on mortality.[265] It is hoped that further double-blind studies with sufficient numbers of cases will resolve the continuing dilemma regarding the potential efficacy of IVIG.[266] It is clear that if IVIG were to be used, it should be given early and probably more than one dose should be given, because batches of IVIG have variable neutralizing activity against streptococcal exotoxins.[244,267]

There have been no comparative trials describing the efficacy of hyperbaric oxygen treatment in strep TSS, although some state that such treatment reduces mortality and the need for further débridements.[268] Certainly, use of this modality should not delay or be used in preference to surgical débridement when the latter is indicated.

Bacteremia

Group A streptococcal bacteremia has been relatively uncommon in the antibiotic era.[269] Before the mid-1980s, bacteremia occurred predominantly at the extremes of life and was usually community acquired. Occasional cases were seen in young and middle-aged adults associated with surgical wound infections and endometritis.

During the past decade, however, there has been an increase in the number of reported cases of group A streptococcal bacteremia, reflecting the changing epidemiology and clinical patterns of invasive streptococcal infection as noted earlier. Many of the patients were previously healthy adults between the ages of 20 and 50 years. There has been an apparent increase in cases associated with parenteral injection of illicit drugs,[173,178,224] as well as nosocomial outbreaks in nursing homes.[212-216]

Bacteremia in children may emanate from an upper respiratory infection, but it is more commonly associated with cutaneous foci, including burns and varicella.[219] Older patients with streptococcal bacteremia present with a variety of chronic illnesses; their relation to the bacteremia is often unclear. Diabetes mellitus and peripheral vascular disease do appear, however, to be predisposing factors in older adults and, as in children, the portal of entry is usually the skin. Malignancy and immunosuppression are risk factors in both age groups.[198,270] Although group A streptococcal bacteremia may at times be transient and relatively benign,[271] it is more often fulminant. The onset is abrupt, with chills, high fever, and prostration. Rarely, patients may present with acute abdominal pain.[271,272] Mortality in five modern series[222,271-274] has ranged from 27% to 38%.

Other Streptococcal Infections

Lymphangitis may accompany cellulitis or may occur after clinically minor or inapparent skin infection. Lymphangitis is readily recognized by the presence of red, tender, linear streaks directed toward enlarged, tender, regional lymph nodes. It is accompanied by systemic symptoms such as chills, fever, malaise, and headache. Puerperal sepsis follows abortion or delivery when streptococci colonizing the patient herself or transmitted from medical personnel invade the endometrium and surrounding structures, lymphatics, and bloodstream. The resulting endometritis and septicemia may be complicated by pelvic cellulitis, septic pelvic thrombophlebitis, peritonitis, or pelvic abscess. This disease was associated with high mortality in the preantibiotic era. Although endocarditis caused by *S. pyogenes* was relatively common in the preantibiotic era, it is now rarely seen.[275,276] Meningitis caused by *S. pyogenes* usually follows upper respiratory infection, including sinusitis or otitis,[277] or neurosurgical conditions.[278] It is indistinguishable clinically from other forms of acute pyogenic meningeal infection.[279]

Pneumonia caused by *S. pyogenes* is frequently associated with preceding viral infections such as influenza, measles, or varicella or with chronic pulmonary disease. Numerous epidemics have been described in military recruit populations.[280,281] An increased number of cases has been reported over the past few years in association with the resurgence of invasive streptococcal infections. In one third or fewer of the cases, there was a history of preceding streptococcal upper respiratory infection. The onset is typically abrupt and the disease is characterized by chills, fever, dyspnea, cough productive of blood-streaked sputum, pleuritic chest pain and, in more severe cases, cyanosis. The pulmonary picture is that of bronchopneumonia, with consolidation being uncommon. Empyema develops in 30% to 40% of cases, tends to appear early in the disease, and typically consists of copious amounts of thin serosanguineous fluid. Bacteremia occurs in 10% to 15% of cases. Complications include mediastinitis, pericarditis, pneumothorax, and bronchiectasis, and the clinical course of the disease is often prolonged. Mortality has generally been low with penicillin therapy and adequate drainage of empyema, perhaps reflecting its occurrence in healthy military recruits. However, in a recent Canadian report of 222 cases of community-acquired pneumonia among adults (median age, 56 years), the case-fatality ratio was 38%.[282] Interestingly, a recent review of deaths in the 1918 pandemic of influenza has demonstrated that the major cause of death was secondary bacterial pneumonia.[283] Whereas *S. pneumoniae* was the most common, group A streptococcus was second and *S. aureus* third. Among patients with empyema complicating pneumonia, group A streptococcus was first. Investigators have demonstrated in a mouse model that a nonlethal influenza infection greatly enhanced the severity and mortality of secondary respiratory infection after challenge with group A streptococcus.[284]

Group A streptococcal perianal cellulitis and vulvovaginitis are symptomatic but benign disorders primarily affecting children.[285,286] Asymptomatic carriage of group A streptococci in the vagina, anus, scalp or, rarely, upper respiratory tract of adults has, however, been the source of outbreaks of nosocomial streptococcal infection.[287]

PROPHYLAXIS AND RISK OF SECONDARY CASES OF STREPTOCOCCAL TOXIC SHOCK SYNDROME

Strep TSS is most commonly community-acquired and sporadic in nature, yet clusters of invasive cases have been described in nursing homes,[212-216] families,[217,218] and hospital workers.[219,288] In San Francisco, 23 hospital workers became colonized or infected with GAS as a result of contact from a single case of strep TSS.[288] This example, as well as many historical studies in schools, military posts, and nursing homes, have taught us that group A streptococci are highly contagious. Luckily, mere contact or colonization is usually not sufficient to cause a secondary case of invasive GAS infection. Epidemiologic studies by the Centers for Disease Control and Prevention found one secondary case of invasive infection among more than 1500 contacts.[144] This would extrapolate to 66/100,000 population/year for secondary cases.[289] As noted, the current incidence of primary cases of invasive GAS infections in the United States is 3.5/100,000 population/year. Thus, the risk to contacts is roughly 20 times greater than that for the general population, but is still very low. Given the relative infrequency of these infections and the lack of a clearly effective chemoprophylactic regimen, routine screening for and prophylaxis against streptococcal infection are not recommended for household contacts of index patients. In deciding who should receive prophylaxis, the clinician needs to factor in the duration of contact, intimacy of contact, and underlying host factors of individual contacts. Specifically, contacts with open wounds, recent surgery, recent childbirth, concurrent viral infections such as varicella or influenza, or immunodeficiency diseases should receive prophylaxis. In a multicenter study of adults aged 18 to 45 years, human immunodeficiency virus infection and injecting drug use were independently associated with an increased risk of invasive group A streptococcal disease. In those aged 45 years of age or older, diabetes, cardiac disease, cancer, and corticosteroid use were significant risk factors.[290] Moreover, persons aged 65 years or older are at increased risk of mortality should they contract invasive disease. Thus, it may be prudent to initiate prophylaxis in households with older adults or those with the above-mentioned risk factors.

Lacking firm data on which to base antimicrobial prophylaxis, it seems reasonable to choose those agents that have achieved highest rates of pharyngeal eradication in asymptomatic individuals; among these are clindamycin and azithromycin. Specific regimens have been published elsewhere.[144]

REFERENCES

1. Brown JH. *The Use of Blood Agar for the Study of Streptococci.* New York: The Rockefeller Institute for Medical Research; 1919.
2. Lancefield RC. A serological differentiation of human and other groups of hemolytic streptococci. *J Exp Med.* 1933;57:571-595.
3. Rammelkamp CH. Epidemiology of streptococcal infections. *Harvey Lect.* 1955;51:113-142.
4. Wannamaker LW. The epidemiology of streptococcal infection. In: McCarty M, ed. *Streptococcal Infections.* New York: Columbia University Press; 1953:157-175.
5. Rammelkamp CH, Denny FW, Wannamaker LW. Studies on the epidemiology of rheumatic fever in the armed services. In:

Thomas L, ed. *Rheumatic Fever.* Minneapolis: University of Minnesota Press; 1952:72-89.
6. Moses AE, Wessels MR, Zalcman K, et al. Relative contributions of hyaluronic acid capsule and M protein to virulence in a mucoid strain of the group A *Streptococcus. Infect Immun.* 1997;65:64-71.
7. Dale JB, Washburn RG, Marques MB, et al. Hyaluronate capsule and surface M protein in resistance to opsonization of group A streptococci. *Infect Immun.* 1996;64:1495-1501.
8. Lancefield RC. Current knowledge of type-specific M antigens of group A streptococci. *J Immunol.* 1962;89:307-313.

9. Facklam RF, Martin DR, Lovgren M, et al. Extension of the Lancefield classification for group A streptococci by addition of 22 new M protein gene sequence types from clinical isolates: emm103 to emm124. *Clin Infect Dis.* 2002;34:28-38.
10. Phillips GN Jr, Flicker PF, Cohen C, et al. Streptococcal M protein: Alpha-helical coiled-coil structure and arrangement on the cell surface. *Proc Natl Acad Sci U S A.* 1981;78:4689-4693.
11. Jones KF, Manjula BN, Johnston KH, et al. Location of variable and conserved epitopes among the multiple serotypes of streptococcal M protein. *J Exp Med.* 1985;161:623-628.

12. Bisno AL. Alternate complement pathway activation by group A streptococci: Role of M protein. *Infect Immun*. 1979;26: 1172-1176.
13. Peterson PK, Schmeling D, Cleary PP, et al. Inhibition of alternative complement pathway opsonization by group A streptococcal M protein. *J Infect Dis*. 1979;139:575-585.
14. Horstmann RD, Sievertsen HJ, Knobloch J, et al. Antiphagocytic activity of streptococcal M protein: Selective binding of complement control protein factor H. *Proc Natl Acad Sci U S A*. 1988;85:1657-1661.
15. Kihlberg BM, Collin M, Olsen A, et al. Protein H, an antiphagocytic surface protein in Streptococcus pyogenes. *Infect Immun*. 1999;67:1708-1714.
16. Morfeldt E, Berggard K, Persson J, et al. Isolated hypervariable regions derived from streptococcal M proteins specifically bind human C4b-binding protein: Implications for antigenic variation. *J Immunol*. 2001;167:3870-3877.
17. Whitnack E, Dale JB, Beachey EH. Common protective antigens of group A streptococcal M proteins masked by fibrinogen. *J Exp Med*. 1984;159:1201-1212.
18. Whitnack E, Beachey EH. Biochemical and biological properties of the binding of human fibrinogen to M protein in group A streptococci. *J Bacteriol*. 1985;164:350-358.
19. Whitnack E, Beachey EH. Inhibition of complement-mediated opsonization and phagocytosis of *Streptococcus pyogenes* by D fragments of fibrinogen and fibrin bound to cell surface M protein. *J Exp Med*. 1985;162:1983-1997.
20. de Malmanche SA, Martin DR. Protective immunity to the group A streptococcus may be only strain specific. *Med Microbiol Immunol*. 1994;183:299-306.
21. Villasenor SA, McShan WM, Salmi D, et al. Variable susceptibility to opsonophagocytosis of group A streptococcus M-1 strains by human immune sera. *J Infect Dis*. 1999;180:1921-1928.
22. Bisno AL, Collins CM, Turner JC. M proteins of group C streptococci isolated from patients with acute pharyngitis. *J Clin Microbiol*. 1996;34:2511-2515.
23. Campo RE, Schultz DR, Bisno AL. M proteins of group G streptococci: Mechanisms of resistance to phagocytosis. *J Infect Dis*. 1995;171:601-606.
24. Podbielski A, Schnitzler N, Beyhs P, et al. M-related protein (Mrp) contributes to group A streptococcal resistance to phagocytosis by human granulocytes. *Mol Microbiol*. 1996;19: 429-441.
25. Ji Y, Schnitzler N, DeMaster E, et al. Impact of M49, Mrp, Enn, and C5a peptidase proteins on colonization of the mouse oral mucosa by Streptococcus pyogenes. *Infect Immun*. 1998;66: 5399-5405.
26. Dale JB, Chiang EY, Liu S, et al. New protective antigen of group A streptococci. *J Clin Invest*. 1999;103:1261-1268.
27. Lei B, DeLeo FR, Hoe NP, et al. Evasion of human innate and acquired immunity by a bacterial homolog of CD11b that inhibits opsonophagocytosis. *Nat Med*. 2001;7:1298-1305.
28. Lei B, Smoot LM, Menning HM, et al. Identification and characterization of a novel heme-associated cell surface protein made by Streptococcus pyogenes. *Infect Immun*. 2002;70: 4494-4500.
29. Rakonjac JV, Robbins JC, Fischetti VA. DNA sequence of the serum opacity factor of group A streptococci: Identification of a fibronectin-binding repeat domain. *Infect Immun*. 1995; 63:622-631.
30. Johnson DR, Kaplan EL. A review of the correlation of T-agglutination patterns and M protein typing and opacity factor production in the identification of group A streptococci. *J Med Microbiol*. 1993;38:311-315.
31. Widdowson JP, Maxted WR, Notley CM, et al. The antibody responses in man to infection with different serotypes of group A streptococci. *J Med Microbiol*. 1974;7:483-496.
32. Courtney HS, Hasty DL, Dale JB. Serum opacity factor (SOF) of Streptococcus pyogenes evolkes antibodies that opsonize homologous and heterologous SOF-positive serotypes of group A streptococci. *Infect Immun*. 2003;71;5097-5103.
33. Courtney HS, Hasty DL, Dale JB. Molecular mechanisms of adhesion, colonization, and invasion of group A streptococci. *Ann Med*. 2002;34:77-87.
34. Hasty DL, Ofek I, Courtney HS, et al. Multiple adhesins of streptococci. *Infect Immun*. 1992;60:2147-2152.
35. Ofek I, Beachey EH, Jefferson W, et al. Cell membrane–binding properties of group A streptococcal lipoteichoic acid. *J Exp Med*. 1975;187:1161-1167.
36. Caparon MG, Stephens DS, Olsen A, et al. Role of M protein in adherence of group A streptococci. *Infect Immun*. 1991;59: 1811-1817.
37. Okada N, Pentland AP, Falk P, et al. M protein and protein F act as important determinants of cell-specific tropism of *Streptococcus pyogenes* in skin tissue. *J Clin Invest*. 1994;94:965-977.
38. Okada N, Liszewski MK, Atkinson JP, et al. Membrane cofactor protein (CD46) is a keratinocyte receptor for the M protein of the group A streptococcus. *Proc Natl Acad Sci U S A*. 1995;92: 2489-2493.
39. Hanski E, Caparon M. Protein F, a fibronectin-binding protein, is an adhesin of the group A streptococcus *Streptococcus pyogenes*. *Proc Natl Acad Sci U S A*. 1992;89:6172-6176.
40. Talay SR, Valentin-Weigand P, Jerlstrom PG, et al. Fibronectin-binding protein of *Streptococcus pyogenes*: Sequence of the binding domain involved in adherence of streptococci to epithelial cells. *Infect Immun*. 1992;60:3837-3844.
41. Kreikemeyer B, Talay SR, Chhatwal GS. Characterization of a novel fibronectin-binding surface protein in group A streptococci. *Mol Microbiol*. 1995;17:137-145.
42. Courtney HS, Dale JB, Hasty DL. Differential effects of the streptococcal fibronectin-binding protein, FBP54, on adhesion of group A streptococci to human buccal cells and HEp-2 tissue culture cells. *Infect Immun*. 1996;64:2415-2419.
43. Jaffe J, Natanson-Yaron S, Caparon MG, et al. Protein F2, a novel fibronectin-binding protein from Streptococcus pyogenes, possesses two binding domains. *Mol Microbiol*. 1996;21:373-384.
44. Rocha CL, Fischetti VA. Identification and characterization of a novel fibronectin-binding protein on the surface of group A streptococci. *Infect Immun*. 1999;67:2720-2728.
45. Gibson C, Fogg G, Okada N, et al. Regulation of host cell recognition in *Streptococcus pyogenes*. *Dev Biol Stand*. 1995;85: 137-144.
46. Caparon MG, Geist RT, Perez-Casal J, et al. Environmental regulation of virulence in group A streptococci: Transcription of the gene encoding M protein is stimulated by carbon dioxide. *J Bacteriol*. 1992;174:5693-5701.
47. Yinduo J, McLandsborough L, Kondagunta A, et al. C5a peptidase alters clearance and trafficking of group A streptococci by infected mice. *Infect Immun*. 1996;64:503-510.
48. Wexler DE, Chenoweth DE, Cleary PP. Mechanism of action of the group A streptococcal C5a inactivator. *Proc Natl Acad Sci U S A*. 1985;82:8144-8148.
49. Eriksson A, Norgren M. Cleavage of antigen-bound immunoglobulin G by SpeB contributes to streptococcal persistence in opsonizing blood. *Infect Immun*. 2003;71:211-217.
50. Baker M, Gutman DM, Papageorgiou AC, et al. Structural features of a zinc binding site in the superantigen strepococcal pyrogenic exotoxin A (SpeA1): Implications for MHC class II recognition. *Protein Sci*. 2001;10:1268-1273.
51. Bisno AL, Brito MO, Collins CM. Molecular basis of group A streptococcal virulence. *Lancet Infect Dis*. 2003;3:191-200.
52. Marrack P, Kappler J. The staphylococcal enterotoxins and their relatives. *Science*. 1990;248:705-711.
53. Cunningham MW. Pathogenesis of group A streptococcal infections. *Clin Microbiol Rev*. 2000;13:470-511.
54. Perez-Casal J, Caparon MG, Scott JR. Mry, a *trans*-acting positive regulator of the M protein gene of *Streptococcus pyogenes* with similarity to the receptor proteins of two-component regulatory systems. *J Bacteriol*. 1991;173:2617-2624.
55. Levin JC, Wessels MR. Identification of csrR/csrS, a genetic locus that regulates hyaluronic acid capsule synthesis in group A Streptococcus. *Mol Microbiol*. 1998;30:209-219.
56. Federle MJ, McIver KS, Scott JR. A response regulator that represses transcription of several virulence operons in the group A streptococcus. *J Bacteriol*. 1999;181:3649-3657.
57. Heath A, DiRita VJ, Barg NL, et al. A two-component regulatory system, CsrR-CsrS, represses expression of three Streptococcus pyogenes virulence factors, hyaluronic acid capsule, streptolysin S, and pyrogenic exotoxin B. *Infect Immun*. 1999;67:5298-5305.
58. Bisno AL. Acute pharyngitis: Etiology and diagnosis. *Pediatrics*. 1996;97(Pt 2):949-954.
59. Kaplan EL, Wannamaker LW. C-reactive protein in streptococcal pharyngitis. *Pediatrics*. 1977;60:28-32.
60. Randolph MF, Gerber MA, DeMeo KK, et al. Effect of antibiotic therapy on the clinical course of streptococcal pharyngitis. *J Pediatr*. 1985;106:870-875.
61. Krober MS, Bass JW, Michels GN. Streptococcal pharyngitis: Placebo-controlled double-blind evaluation of clinical response to penicillin therapy. *JAMA*. 1985;253:1271-1274.
62. Nelson JD. The effect of penicillin therapy on the symptoms and signs of streptococcal pharyngitis. *Pediatr Infect Dis J*. 1984;3:10-13.
63. Shulman ST. Complications of streptococcal pharyngitis. *Pediatr Infect Dis J*. 1994;13:S70-S74.
64. Shoemaker M, Lampe RM, Weir MR. Peritonsillitis: Abscess or cellulitis? *Pediatr Infect Dis J*. 1986;5:435-439.
65. Alcaide ML, Bisno AL. Pharyngitis and epiglottitis. *Infect Dis Clin North Am*. 2007;21:449-469.
66. Turner JC, Fox A, Fox K, et al. Role of group C beta-hemolytic streptococci in pharyngitis: Epidemiologic study of clinical features associated with isolation of group C streptococci. *J Clin Microbiol*. 1993;31:808-811.
67. Meier FA, Centor RM, Graham L Jr, et al. Clinical and microbiological evidence for endemic pharyngitis among adults due to group C streptococci. *Arch Intern Med*. 1990;150:825-829.
68. Hill HR, Caldwell GG, Wilson E, et al. Epidemic of pharyngitis due to streptococci of Lancefield group G. *Lancet*. 1969;2: 371-374.
69. McCue JD. Group G streptococcal pharyngitis: Analysis of an outbreak at a college. *JAMA*. 1982;248:1333-1336.
70. Cimolai N, Elford RW, Bryan L, et al. Do the beta-hemolytic non-group A streptococci cause pharyngitis? *Rev Infect Dis*. 1988;10:587-601.
71. Bisgard KM, Hardy IR, Popovic T. Respiratory diphtheria in the United States, 1980-1995. *Am J Public Health*. 1998;88:787-791.
72. Miller RA, Brancato F, Holmes KK. *Corynebacterium hemolyticum* as a cause of pharyngitis and scarlatiniform rash in young adults. *Ann Intern Med*. 1986;105:867-872.
73. Karpathios T, Drakonaki S, Zervoudaki A, et al. *Arcanobacterium haemolyticum* in children with presumed streptococcal pharyngotonsillitis or scarlet fever. *J Pediatr*. 1992;121:735-737.
74. Tacket CO, Davis BR, Carter GP, et al. *Yersinia enterocolitica* pharyngitis. *Ann Intern Med*. 1983;99:40-42.
75. Glezen WP, Fernald GW, Lohr JA. Acute respiratory disease of university students with special reference to the etiologic role of *Herpesvirus hominis*. *Am J Epidemiol*. 1975;101:111-121.
76. McMillan JA, Weiner LB, Higgins AM, et al. Pharyngitis associated with herpes simplex virus in college students. *Pediatr Infect Dis J*. 1993;12:280-284.
77. Young EJ, Vainrub B, Musher DM, et al. Acute pharyngotonsillitis caused by herpesvirus type 2. *JAMA*. 1978;239:1885-1886.
78. McMillan JA, Sandstrom C, Weiner LB, et al. Viral and bacterial organisms associated with acute pharyngitis in a school-aged population. *J Pediatr*. 1986;109:747-752.
79. Vanhelms P, Allard R, Cooper DA, et al. Acute human immunodeficiency virus type 1 disease as a mononucleosis-like illness: Is the diagnosis too restrictive? *Clin Infect Dis*. 1997;24: 965-970.
80. Glezen WP, Clyde WAJ, Senior RJ, et al. Group A streptococci, mycoplasmas, and viruses associated with acute pharyngitis. *JAMA*. 1967;202:455-460.
81. Kaplan EL, Top FH Jr, Dudding BA, et al. Diagnosis of streptococcal pharyngitis: Differentiation of active infection from the carrier state in the symptomatic child. *J Infect Dis*. 1971;123:490-501.
82. Breese BB. A simple score card for the tentative diagnosis of streptococcal pharyngitis. *Am J Dis Child*. 1977;131:514-517.
83. Wald ER, Green MD, Schwartz B, et al. A streptococcal score card revisited. *Pediatr Emerg Care*. 1998;14:109-111.
84. Walsh BT, Bookheim WW, Johnson RC, et al. Recognition of streptococcal pharyngitis in adults. *Arch Intern Med*. 1975;135:1493-1497.
85. McIsaac WJ, White D, Tannenbaum D, et al. A clinical score to reduce unnecessary antibiotic use in patients with sore throat. *Can Med Assoc J*. 1998;158:75-83.
86. Komaroff AL, Pass TM, Aronson MD, et al. The prediction of streptococcal pharyngitis in adults. *J Gen Intern Med*. 1986;1:1-7.
87. Centor RM, Witherspoon JM, Dalton HP, et al. The diagnosis of strep throat in adults in the emergency room. *Med Decis Making*. 1981;1:239-246.
88. Cooper JR, Hoffman JR, Bartlett JG, et al. Principles of appropriate antibiotic use for acute pharyngitis in adults: Background. *Ann Intern Med*. 2001;134:509-517.
89. Snow V, Mottur-Pilson C, Cooper RJ, et al. Principles of appropriate antibiotic use of acute pharyngitis in adults. *Ann Intern Med*. 2001;134:506-508.
90. Ebell MH, Smith MA, Barry HC, et al. The rational clinical examination. Does this patient have strep throat? *JAMA*. 2000;284:2912-2918.
91. Neuner JM, Hamel MB, Phillips RS, et al. Diagnosis and management of adults with pharyngitis. A cost-effectiveness analysis. *Ann Intern Med*. 2003;139:113-122.
92. McIsaac WJ, Kellner JD, Aufricht P, et al. Empirical validation of guidelines for the management of pharyngitis in children and adults. *JAMA*. 2004;291:1587-1595.
93. Humair JP, Revaz SA, Bovier P, et al. Management of acute pharyngitis in adults: reliability of rapid streptococcal tests and clinical findings. *Arch Intern Med*. 2006;166:640-644.
94. Bisno AL. Diagnosing strep throat in the adult patient: Do clinical criteria really suffice? *Ann Intern Med*. 2003;139:150-151.
95. Linder JA, Stafford RS. Antibiotic treatment of adults with sore throat by community primary care physicians: A national survey, 1989-1999. *JAMA*. 2001;286:1181-1186.
96. Bisno AL, Gerber MA, Gwaltney JM Jr, et al. Practice guidelines for the diagnosis and management of group A streptococcal pharyngitis. Infectious Diseases Society of America. *Clin Infect Dis*. 2002;35:113-125.
97. Gerber M, Baltimore R, Eaton C, et al. Prevention of rheumatic fever and diagnosis and treatment of acute streptococcal pharyngitis. A scientific statement from the American Heart Association Rheumatic Fever, Endocarditis, and Kawasaki Disease Committee of the Council on Cardiovascular Disease in the Young, the Interdisciplinary Council on Functional Genomics and Translational Biology, and the Interdisciplinary Council on Quality of Care and Outcomes Research. *Circulation*. 2009;119:1541-1550.
98. Committee on Infectious Diseases. Group A streptococcal infections. In: Pickering LK, ed. *Red Book: 2006 Report of the Committee on Infectious Diseases*. Elk Grove Village, Ill, American Academy of Pediatrics; 2006:610-620.
99. Rheumatic Fever Committee, American Heart Association. *Throat Cultures for Rational Treatment of Sore Throat*. New York: American Heart Association; 1972.
100. Kellogg JA, Manzella JP. Detection of group A streptococci in the laboratory or physician's office. *JAMA*. 1986;255:2638-2642.
101. Kellogg JA. Suitability of throat culture procedures for detection of group A streptococci and as reference standards for evaluation of streptococcal antigen detection kits. *J Clin Microbiol*. 1990;28:165-169.
102. Freeman AF, Shulman ST. Macrolide resistance in group A Streptococcus. *Pediatr Infect Dis J*. 2002;21:1158-1160.
103. Gerber MA, Tanz RR, Kabat W, et al. Optical immunoassay test for group A beta-hemolytic streptococcal pharyngitis. An office-based, multicenter investigation. *JAMA*. 1997;277:899-903.
104. Fries SM. Diagnosis of group A streptococcal pharyngitis in a private clinic: Comparative evaluation of an optical immunoassay method and culture. *J Pediatr*. 1995;126:933-936.

105. Schlager TA, Hayden GA, Woods WA, et al. Optical immunoassay for rapid detection of group A beta-hemolytic streptococci. *Arch Pediatr Adolesc Med.* 1996;150:245-248.
106. Baker DM, Cooper RM, Rhodes C, et al. Superiority of conventional culture technique over rapid detection of group A *Streptococcus* by optical immunoassay. *Diagn Microbiol Infect Dis.* 1995;21:61-64.
107. Gieseker KE, Mackenzie T, Roe MH, et al. Comparison of two rapid Streptococcus pyogenes diagnostic tests with a rigorous culture standard. *Pediatr Infect Dis J.* 2002;21:922-927.
108. Poses RM, Cebul RD, Collins M, et al. The accuracy of experienced physicians' probability estimates for patients with sore throats: implications for decision making. *JAMA.* 1985; 254:925-929.
109. Bisno AL. Acute pharyngitis. *N Engl J Med.* 2001;344:205-211.
110. Weinstein L, Le Frock J. Does antimicrobial therapy of streptococcal pharyngitis or pyoderma alter the risk of glomerulonephritis? *J Infect Dis.* 1971;124:229-231.
111. Catanzaro FJ, Stetson CA, Morris AJ, et al. The role of streptococcus in the pathogenesis of rheumatic fever. *Am J Med.* 1954;17:749-756.
112. Brink WR, Rammelkamp CH Jr, Denny FW, et al. Effect of penicillin and aureomycin on the natural course of streptococcal tonsillitis and pharyngitis. *Am J Med.* 1951;10:300-308.
113. Shvartzman P, Tabenkin H, Rosentzwaig A, et al. Treatment of streptococcal pharyngitis with amoxycillin once a day. *BMJ.* 1993;306:1170-1172.
114. Feder HMJ, Gerber MA, Randolph MF, et al. Once-daily therapy for streptococcal pharyngitis with amoxicillin. *Pediatrics.* 1999;103:47-51.
115. Lennon DR, Farrell E, Martin DR, et al. Once-daily amoxicillin versus twice daily penicillin V in group A beta-haemolytic streptococcal pharyngitis. *Arch Dis Child.* 2008;93:474-478.
116. Pichichero ME, Margolis PA. A comparison of cephalosporins and penicillins in the treatment of group A beta-hemolytic streptococcal pharyngitis: A meta-analysis supporting the concept of microbial copathogenicity. *Pediatr Infect Dis J.* 1991;10:275-281.
117. Kaplan EL, Gastanaduy AS, Huwe BB. The role of the carrier in treatment failures after antibiotic therapy for group A streptococci in the upper respiratory tract. *J Lab Clin Med.* 1981; 98:326-335.
118. Pichichero ME. Cephalosporins are superior to penicillin for treatment of streptococcal tonsillopharyngitis: Is the difference worth it? *Pediatr Infect Dis J.* 1993;12:268-274.
119. Casey JR, Pichichero M. Meta-analysis of cephalosporin versus penicillin treatment of group A streptococcal tonsillopharyngitis in adults. *Clin Infect Dis.* 2004;38:1526-1534.
120. Shulman ST, Gerber MA, Tanz RR, et al. Streptococcal pharyngitis: the case for pencillin therapy. *Pediatr InfectDis J.* 1994;13:1-7.
121. Bisno AL. Are cephalosporins superior to penicillin for treatment of acute streptococcal pharyngitis? *Clin Infect Dis.* 2004;38:1535-1537.
122. Cresti S, Lattanzi M, Zanchi A, et al. Resistance determinants and clonal diversity in group A streptococci collected during a period of increasing macrolide resistance. *Antimicrob Agents Chemother.* 2002;46:1816-1822.
123. Seppala H, Klaukka T, Vuopio-Varkila J, et al. The effect of changes in the consumption of macrolide antibiotics on erythromycin resistance in group A streptococci in Finland. *N Engl J Med.* 1997;337:441-446.
124. Cornaglia G, Ligozzi M, Mazzariol A, et al. Resistance of *Streptococcus pyogenes* to erythromycin and related antibiotics in Italy. *Clin Infect Dis.* 1998;27(suppl 1):S87-S92.
125. Martin JM, Green M, Barbadora KA, et al. Erythromycin-resistant group A streptococci in schoolchildren in Pittsburgh. *N Engl J Med.* 2002;346:1200-1206.
126. York MK, Gibbs L, Perdreau-Remington F, et al. Characterization of antimicrobial resistance in Streptococcus pyogenes isolates from the San Francisco Bay area of northern California. *J Clin Microbiol.* 1999;37:1727-1731.
127. Tanz RR, Shulman ST, Shortridge VD, et al. Community-based surveillance in the united states of macrolide-resistant pediatric pharyngeal group A streptococci during 3 respiratory disease seasons. *Clin Infect Dis.* 2004;39:1794-1801.
128. Green MD, Beall B, Marcon MJ, et al. Multicentre surveillance of the prevalence and molecular epidemiology of macrolide resistance among pharyngeal isolates of group A streptococci in the USA. *J Antimicrob Chemother.* 2006;57:1240-1243.
129. Richter SS, Heilmann KP, Beekmann SE, et al. Macrolide-resistant Streptococcus pyogenes in the United States, 2002-2003. *Clin Infect Dis.* 2005;41:599-608.
130. Mehra S, van Moerkerke M, Welck J, et al. Short course therapy with cefuroxime axetil for group A streptococcal tonsillopharyngitis in children. *Pediatr Infect Dis J.* 1998;17:452-457.
131. Adam D, Scholz H, Helmerking M. Comparison of short-course (5-day) cefuroxime axetil with a standard 10-day oral penicillin V regimen in the treatment of tonsillopharyngitis. *J Antimicrob Chemother.* 2000;45(Suppl):23-30.
132. Adam D, Hostalek U, Troster K. 5-Day therapy of bacterial pharyngitis and tonsillitis with cefixime: Comparison with 10-day treatment with penicillin V. *Klinische Padiatrie.* 1996;208: 310-313.
133. Boccazzi A, Tonelli P, DeAngelis M, et al. Short-course therapy with ceftibutin versus azithromycin in pediatric streptococcal pharyngitis. *Pediatr Infect Dis J.* 2000;19:963-967.
134. Tack KJ, Henry DC, Gooch WM, et al. Five-day cefdinir treatment for streptococcal pharyngitis. Cefdinir Pharyngitis Study Group. *Antimicrob Agents Chemother.* 1998;42: 1073-1075.
135. Pichichero ME, Gooch WM, Rodriguez W, et al. Effective short-course treatment of acute group A beta-hemolytic streptococcal tonsillopharyngitis: Ten days of penicillin vs 5 days or 10 days of cefpodoxime therapy in children. *Arch Pediatr Adolesc Med.* 1994;148:1053-1060.
136. Ozaki T, Nishimura N, Suzuki M, et al. Five-day oral cefditoren pivoxil versus 10-day oral amoxicillin for pediatric group A streptococcal pharyngotonsillitis. *J Infect Chemother.* 2008; 14:213-218.
137. McCarty J, Hedrick JA, Gooch WM. Clarithromycin suspension vs penicillin V suspension in children with streptococcal pharygitis. *Adv Ther.* 2000;17:14-26.
138. Still JG. Management of pediatric patients with group A beta-hemolytic *Streptococcus* pharyngitis: Treatment options. *Pediatr Infect Dis J.* 1995;14:S57-S61.
139. Hamill J. Multicentre evaluation of azithromycin and penicillin V in the treatment of acute streptococcal pharyngitis and tonsillitis in children. *J Antimicrob Chemother.* 1993;31(suppl E): 89-94.
140. Weippl G. Multicentre comparison of azithromycin versus erythromycin in the treatment of paediatric pharyngitis or tonsillitis caused by group A streptococci. *J Antimicrob Chemother.* 1993;31(suppl E):95-101.
141. Hooton TM. A comparison of azithromycin and penicillin V for the treatment of streptococcal pharyngitis. *Am J Med.* 1991; 91(suppl 3A):3A-23A.
142. Tanz RR, Poncher JR, Corydon KE, et al. Clindamycin treatment of chronic pharyngeal carriage of group A streptococci. *J Pediatr.* 1991;119:123-128.
143. Kaplan EL, Johnson DR. Eradication of group A streptococci from the upper respiratory tract by amoxicillin with clavulanate after oral penicillin V treatment failure. *J Pediatr.* 1988;113: 400-403.
144. Prevention of Invasive Group A Streptococcal Infections Workshop Participants. Prevention of invasive group A streptococcal disease among household contacts of case patients and among postpartum and postsurgical patients: Recommendations from the Centers for Disease Control and Prevention. *Clin Infect Dis.* 2002;35:950-959.
145. Paradise JL, Bluestone CD, Bachman RZ, et al. Efficacy of tonsillectomy for recurrent throat infection in severely affected children: Results of parallel randomized and nonrandomized clinical trials. *N Engl J Med.* 1984;310:674-683.
146. Alho OP, Koivunen P, Penna T, et al. Tonsillectomy versus watchful waiting in recurrent streptococcal pharyngitis in adults: randomised controlled trial. *BMJ.* 2007;334:939.
147. Paradise JL, Bluestone CD, Colborn DK, et al. Tonsillectomy and adenotonsillectomy for recurrent throat infection in moderately affected children. *Pediatrics.* 2002;110(Pt 1):7-15.
148. Ferrieri P, Dajani AS, Wannamaker LW, et al. Natural history of impetigo. I. Site sequence of acquisition and familial patterns of spread of cutaneous streptococci. *J Clin Invest.* 1972;51: 2851-2862.
149. Adams BB. Dermatologic disorders of the athlete. *Sports Med.* 2002;32:309-321.
150. Fehrs LJ, Flanagan K, Kline S, et al. Group A beta-hemolytic streptococcal skin infections in a US meat-packing plant. *JAMA.* 1987;258:3131-3134.
150a. Wasserzug O, Valinsky L, Kement E, et al. A cluster of ecthyma outbreaks caused by a single clone of invasive and highly infective *Streptococcus pyogenes*. *Clin Infect Dis.* 2009;49:1213-1219.
151. Fiorentino TR, Beall B, Mshar P, et al. A genetic-based evaluation of the principal tissue reservoir for group A streptococci isolated from normally sterile sites. *J Infect Dis.* 1997; 176:177-182.
152. Anthony BF, Kaplan EL, Wannamaker LW, et al. The dynamics of streptococcal infections in a defined population of children: Serotypes associated with skin and respiratory infections. *Am J Epidemiol.* 1976;104:652-666.
153. Kaplan EL, Anthony BF, Chapman SS, et al. The influence of the site of infection on the immune response to group A streptococci. *J Clin Invest.* 1970;49:1405-1414.
154. Bisno AL, Nelson KE, Waytz P, et al. Factors influencing serum antibody responses in streptococcal pyoderma. *J Lab Clin Med.* 1973;81:410-420.
155. Kaplan EL, Wannamaker LW. Suppression of the antistreptolysin O response by cholesterol and by lipid extracts of rabbit skin. *J Exp Med.* 1976;144:754-767.
156. Barnett BO, Frieden IJ. Streptococcal skin diseases in children. *Semin Dermatol.* 1992;11:3-10.
157. Gonzalez A, Schachner LA, Cleary T, et al. Pyoderma in children. *Adv Dermatol.* 1989;4:127-142.
158. Demidovich CW, Wittler RR, Ruff ME, et al. Impetigo. Current etiology and comparison of penicillin, erythromycin, and cephalexin therapies. *Am J Dis Child.* 1990;144:1313-1315.
159. Rasmussen JE. The changing nature of impetigo. *Patient Care.* 1992;15:233-239.
160. Dagan R, Bar-David Y. Comparison of amoxicillin and clavulanic acid (augmentin) for the treatment of nonbullous impetigo. *Am J Dis Child.* 1989;143:916-918.
161. Barton LL, Friedman AD. Impetigo: A reassessment of etiology and therapy. *Pediatr Dermatol.* 1987;4:185-188.
162. Barton LL, Friedman AD, Sharkey AM, et al. Impetigo contagiosa III. Comparative efficacy of oral erythromycin and topical mupirocin. *Pediatr Dermatol.* 1989;6:134-138.
163. Britton JW, Fajardo JE, Krafte-Jacobs B. Comparison of mupirocin and erythromycin in the treatment of impetigo. *J Pediatr.* 1990;117:827-829.
164. Yun HJ, Lee SW, Yoon GM, et al. Prevalence and mechanisms of low- and high-level mupirocin resistance in staphylococci isolated from a Korean hospital. *J Antimicrob Chemother.* 2003;51:619-623.
165. Retapamulin (Altabax)—a new topical antibiotic. *Med Lett Drugs Ther.* 2008;50:13-15.
166. Yang LP, Keam SJ. Retapamulin: A review of its use in the management of impetigo and other uncomplicated superficial skin infections. *Drugs.* 2008;68:855-873.
167. Koning S, van der Wouden JC, Chosidow O, et al. Efficacy and safety of retapamulin ointment as treatment of impetigo: Randomized double-blind multicentre placebo-controlled trial. *Br J Dermatol.* 2008;158:1077-1082.
168. Hoge CW, Schwartz B, Talkington DF, et al. The changing epidemiology of invasive group A streptococcal infections and the emergence of streptococcal toxic shock-like syndrome. A retrospective population-baseD study. *JAMA.* 1993;269: 384-389.
169. Martin PR, Hoiby EA. Streptococcal serogroup A epidemic in Norway. 1987-1988. *Scand J Infect Dis.* 1990;22:421-429.
170. Stromberg A, Romanus V, Burman LG. Outbreak of group A streptococcal bacteremia in Sweden: An epidemiologic and clinical study. *J Infect Dis.* 1991;164:595-598.
171. Demers B, Simor AE, Vellend H, et al. Severe invasive group A streptococcal infections in Ontario, Canada: 1987-1991. *Clin Infect Dis.* 1993;16:792-800.
172. Johnson DR, Stevens DL, Kaplan EL. Epidemiologic analysis of group A streptococcal serotypes associated with severe systemic infections, rheumatic fever, or uncomplicated pharyngitis. *J Infect Dis.* 1992;166:374-382.
173. Stevens DL, Tanner MH, Winship J, et al. Severe group A streptococcal infections associated with a toxic shock-like syndrome and scarlet fever toxin A. *N Engl J Med.* 1989;321:1-7.
174. Bartter T, Dascal A, Carroll K, Curley FJ. "Toxic strep syndrome": A manifestation of group A streptococcal infection. *Arch Intern Med.* 1988;148:1421-1424.
175. Eriksson BK, Andersson J, Holm SE, et al. Epidemiological and clinical aspects of invasive group A streptococcal infections and the streptococcal toxic shock syndrome. *Clin Infect Dis.* 1998;27:1428-1436.
176. Lentnek AL, Giger O, O'Rourke E. Group A beta-hemolytic streptococcal bacteremia and intravenous substance abuse: A growing clinical problem? *Arch Intern Med.* 1990;150:89-93.
177. Barg NL, Kish MA, Kauffman CA, et al. Group A streptococcal bacteremia in intravenous drug abusers. *Am J Med.* 1985;78 :569-574.
178. Craven DE, Rixinger AI, Bisno AL, et al. Bacteremia caused by group G streptococci in parenteral drug abusers: Epidemiological and clinical aspects. *J Infect Dis.* 1986;153:988-992.
179. Simon MS, Cody RL. Cellulitis after axillary lymph node dissection for carcinoma of the breast. *Am J Med.* 1992;93:543-548.
180. de Godoy JM, de Godoy MF, Valente A, et al. Lymphoscintigraphic evaluation in patients after erysipelas. *Lymphology.* 2000;33:177-180.
181. Baddour LM, Bisno AL. Recurrent cellulitis after saphenous venectomy for coronary bypass surgery. *Ann Intern Med.* 1982;97:493-496.
182. Semel JD, Goldin H. Association of athlete's foot with cellulitis of the lower extremities: Diagnostic value of bacterial cultures of ipsilateral interdigital space samples. *Clin Infect Dis.* 1996;23:1162-1164.
183. Greenberg J, DeSanctis RW, Mills RM Jr. Vein-donor-leg cellulitis after coronary artery bypass surgery. *Ann Intern Med.* 1982;97:565-566.
184. Baddour LM, Bisno AL. Recurrent cellulitis after coronary bypass surgery: Association with superficial fungal infection in saphenous venectomy limbs. *JAMA.* 1984;251:1049-1052.
185. Baddour LM, Bisno AL. Non–group A beta-hemolytic streptococcal cellulitis: Association with venous and lymphatic compromise. *Am J Med.* 1985;79:155-159.
186. Dupuy A, Benchikhi H, Roujeau JC, et al. Risk factors for erysipelas of the leg (cellulitis): Case-control study. *BMJ.* 1999;318:1591-1594.
187. Roldan YB, Mata-Essayag S, Hartung C. Erysipelas and tinea pedis. *Mycoses.* 2000;43:181-183.
188. Eriksson BK. Anal colonization of group G beta-hemolytic streptococci in relapsing erysipelas of the lower extremity. *Clin Infect Dis.* 1999;29:1319-1320.
189. Lewis SD, Peter GS, Gomez-Marin O, et al. Risk factors for recurrent lower extremity cellulitis in a U.S. veterans medical center population. *Am J Med Sci.* 2006;332:304-307.
190. Hook EWI, Hooton TM, Horton CA, et al. Microbiologic evaluation of cutaneous cellulitis in adults. *Arch Intern Med.* 1986;146:295-297.
191. Howe PM, Fajardo JE, Orcutt MA. Etiologic diagnosis of cellulitis: Comparison of aspirates obtained from the leading edge and the point of maximal inflammation. *Pediatr Infect Dis J.* 1987;6:685.
192. Newell PM, Norden CW. Value of needle aspiration in bacteriologic diagnosis of cellulitis in adults. *J Clin Microbiol.* 1988; 26:401-404.

193. Wang JH, Liu YC, Cheng DL, et al. Role of benzathine penicillin G in prophylaxis for recurrent streptococcal cellulitis of the lower legs. *Clin Infect Dis*. 1997;25:685-689.
194. Sjoblom AC, Eriksson B, Jorup-Ronstrom C, et al. Antibiotic prophylaxis in recurrent erysipelas. *Infection*. 1993;21:390-393.
195. Kremer M, Zuckerman R, Avraham Z, et al. Long-term antimicrobial therapy in the prevention of recurrent soft-tissue infections. *J Infect*. 1991;22:37-40.
196. Bisno AL, Stevens DL. Streptococcal infections of skin and soft tissues. *N Engl J Med*. 1996;334:240-244.
197. Meleney FL. Hemolytic streptococcus gangrene. *Arch Surg*. 1924;9:317-364.
198. Stevens DL. Invasive group A streptococcus infections. *Clin Infect Dis*. 1991;14:2-13.
199. Bisno AL, Cockerill FR III, Bermudez CT. The initial outpatient-physician encounter in group A streptococcal necrotizing fasciitis. *Clin Infect Dis*. 2000;31:607-608.
200. Stamenkovic I, Lew PD. Early recognition of potentially fatal necrotizing fasciitis: The use of frozen-section biopsy. *N Engl J Med*. 1984;310:1689-1693.
201. Majeski J, Majeski E. Necrotizing fasciitis: Improved survival with early recognition by tissue biopsy and aggressive surgical treatment. *South Med J*. 1997;90:1065-1068.
202. Adams EM, Gudmundsson S, Yocum DE, et al. Streptococcal myositis. *Arch Intern Med*. 1985;145:1020-1023.
203. Holm SE. Invasive group A streptococcal infections [editorial, comment]. *N Engl J Med*. 1996;335:590-591.
204. Wheeler MC, Roe MH, Kaplan EL, et al. Outbreak of group A streptococcus septicemia in children: Clinical, epidemiologic, and microbiological correlates. *JAMA*. 1991;266:533-537.
205. Gaworzewska ET, Hallas G. Group A streptococcal infections and a toxic shock–like syndrome. *N Engl J Med*. 1989;321: 1546.
206. Schwartz B, Facklam RR, Breiman RF. Changing epidemiology of group A streptococcal infection in the USA. *Lancet*. 1990;336:1167-1171.
207. Hribalova V. Streptococcus pyogenes and the toxic shock syndrome. *Ann Intern Med*. 1988;108:772.
208. Greenberg RN, Willoughby BG, Kennedy DJ, et al. Hypocalcemia and "toxic" syndrome associated with streptococcal fasciitis. *South Med J*. 1983;76:916-918.
209. Kiska DL, Thiede B, Caracciolo J, et al. Invasive group A streptococcal infections in North Carolina: Epidemiology, clinical features, and genetic and serotype analysis of causative organisms. *J Infect Dis*. 1997;176:992-1000.
210. Cockerill FR, MacDonald KL, Thompson RL. An outbreak of invasive group A streptococcal disease associated with high carriage rates of the invasive clone among school-aged children. *JAMA*. 1997;277:38-43.
211. Davies HD, McGreer A, Schwartz B, et al. Invasive group A streptococcal infections in Ontario, Canada. *N Engl J Med*. 1996;335:547-554.
212. Thigpen MC, Richards CL Jr, Lynfield R, et al. Invasive group A streptococcal infection in older adults in long-term care facilities and the community, United States, 1998-2003. *Emerg Infect Dis*. 2007;13:1852-1859.
213. Hohenboken JJ, Anderson F, Kaplan EL. Invasive group A streptococcal (GAS) serotype M-1 outbreak in a long-term care facility (LTCF) with mortality. Presented at the 34th Interscience Conference on Antimicrobial Agents and Chemotherapy, Orlando, Fla, October 1994.
214. Jordan HT, Richards CL, Burton DC, et al. Group A streptococcal disease in Long-term care facilities: Descriptive epidemiology and potential control measures. *Clin Infect Dis*. 2007;45:742-752.
215. Harkness GA, Bentley DW, Mottley M, et al. *Streptococcus pyogenes* outbreak in a long-term care facility. *Am J Infect Control*. 1992;20:142-148.
216. Ruben FL, Norden CW, Heisler B, et al. An outbreak of *Streptococcus pyogenes* infections in a nursing home. *Ann Intern Med*. 1984;101:494-496.
217. DiPersio JR, File TM Jr, Stevens DL, et al. Spread of serious disease-producing M3 clones of group A streptococcus among family members and health care workers. *Clin Infect Dis*. 1996;22:490-495.
218. Gamba MA, Martinelli M, Schaad HJ. Familial transmission of a serious disease-producing group A streptococcus clone: Case reports and review. *Clin Infect Dis*. 1997;24:1118-1121.
219. Valenzuela TD, Hooton TM, Kaplan EL, et al. Transmission of "toxic strep" syndrome from an infected child to a firefighter during CPR. *Ann Emerg Med*. 1991;20:90-92.
220. Givner LB, Abramson JS, Wasilauskas B. Apparent increase in the incidence of invasive group A beta-hemolytic streptococcal disease in children. *J Pediatr*. 1991;118:341-346.
221. Brogan TV, Nizet V, Waldhausen JHT, et al. Group A streptococcal necrotizing fasciitis complicating primary varicella: A series of fourteen patients. *Pediatr Infect Dis J*. 1995;14:588-594.
222. Francis J, Warren RE. *Streptococcus pyogenes* bacteraemia in Cambridge—a review of 67 episodes. *Q J Med*. 1988;68: 603-613.
223. Barnham M. Invasive streptococcal infections in the era before the acquired immune deficiency syndrome: A 10 years' compilation of patients with streptococcal bacteraemia in North Yorkshire. *J Infect*. 1989;18:231-248.
224. Braunstein H. Characteristics of group A streptococcal bacteremia in patients at the San Bernardino County Medical Center. *Rev Infect Dis*. 1991;13:8-11.
225. Holm SE, Norrby A, Bergholm AM, et al. Aspects of pathogenesis of serious group A streptococcal infections in Sweden, 1988-1989. *J Infect Dis*. 1992;166:31-37.
226. Stegmayr B, Bjorck S, Holm S, et al. Septic shock induced by group A streptococcal infection: Clinical and therapeutic aspects. *Scand J Infect Dis*. 1992;24:589-597.
227. Herold AH. Group A beta-hemolytic streptococcal toxic shock from a mild pharyngitis. *J Fam Pract*. 1990;31:549-551.
228. Bradley JS, Schlievert PM, Peterson BM. Toxic shock-like syndrome, a complication of strep throat. *Pediatr Infect Dis J*. 1991;10:790.
229. Chapnick EK, Gradon JD, Lutwick LI, et al. Streptococcal toxic shock syndrome due to noninvasive pharyngitis. *Clin Infect Dis*. 1992;14:1074-1077.
230. Sellers BJ, Woods ML, Morris SE, et al. Necrotizing group A streptococcal infections associated with streptococcal toxic shock syndrome. *Am J Med*. 1996;172:523-528.
231. Stevens DL. Could nonsteroidal antiinflammatory drugs (NSAIDs) enhance the progression of bacterial infections to toxic shock syndrome? *Clin Infect Dis*. 1995;21:977-980.
232. Barnham M. Nonsteroidal anti-inflammatory drugs: Concurrent or causative drugs in serious infection? *Clin Infect Dis*. 1997;25:1272-1273.
233. LaPenta D, Rubens C, Chi E, et al. Group A streptococci efficiently invade human respiratory epithelial cells. *Proc Natl Acad Sci U S A*. 1994;91:12115-12119.
234. O'Brien KL, Beall B, Barrett NL, et al. Epidemiology of invasive group A streptococcus disease in the United States, 1995-1999. *Clin Infect Dis*. 2002;35:268-276.
235. Walker MJ, Hollands A, Sanderson-Smith ML, et al. DNase Sda1 provides selection pressure for a switch to invasive group A streptococcal infection. *Nat Med*. 13:981-985, 2007.
236. Bryant AE, Bayer CR, Huntington JD, et al. Group A streptococcal myonecrosis: Increased vimentin expression after skeletal-muscle injury mediates the binding of Streptococcus pyogenes. *J Infect Dis*. 2006;193:1685-1692.
237. Hamilton SM, Bayer CR, Stevens DL, et al. Muscle injury, vimentin expression, and nonsteroidal anti-inflammatory drugs predispose to cryptic group a streptococcal necrotizing infection. *J Infect Dis*. 2008;198:1692-1698.
238. Mollick JA, Rich RR. Characterization of a superantigen from a pathogenic strain of *Streptococcus pyogenes*. *Clin Res*. 1991; 39:213A.
239. Hackett SP, Stevens DL. Superantigens associated with staphylococcal and streptococcal toxic shock syndrome are potent inducers of tumor necrosis factor-beta synthesis. *J Infect Dis*. 1993;168:232-235.
240. Fast DJ, Schlievert PM, Nelson RD. Toxic shock syndrome-associated staphylococcal and streptococcal pyrogenic toxins are potent inducers of tumor necrosis factor production. *Infect Immun*. 1989;57:291-294.
241. Norrby-Teglund A, Newton D, Kotb M, et al. Superantigenic properties of the group A streptococcal exotoxin SpeF (MF). *Infect Immun*. 1994;62:5227-5233.
242. Norrby-Teglund A, Norgren M, Holm SE, et al. Similar cytokine induction profiles of a novel streptococcal exotoxin, MF, and pyrogenic exotoxins A and B. *Infect Immun*. 1994;62: 3731-3738.
243. Kotb M, Ohnishi H, Majumdar G, et al. Temporal relationship of cytokine release by peripheral blood mononuclear cells stimulated by the streptococcal superantigen pep M5. *Infect Immun*. 1993;61:1194-1201.
244. Norrby-Teglund A, Basma H, Andersson J, et al. Varying titres of neutralizing antibodies to streptococcal superantigens in different preparations of normal polyspecific immunoglobulin G (IVIG): Implications for therapeutic efficacy. *Clin Infect Dis*. 1998;26:631-638.
245. Kotb M, Norrby-Teglund A, McGeer A, et al. An immunogenetic and molecular basis for differences in outcomes of invasive group A streptococcal infections. *Nat Med* 2002;8:1398-1404.
246. Kapur V, Majesky MW, Li LL, et al. Cleavage of interleukin-1beta (IL-1beta) precursor to produce active IL-1beta by a conserved extracellular cysteine protease from *Streptococcus pyogenes*. *Proc Natl Acad Sci U S A*. 1993;90:7676-7680.
247. Hackett SP, Stevens DL. Synthesis of tumor necrosis factor and interleukin-1 by monocytes stimulated with pyrogenic exotoxin A and streptolysin O. *J Infect Dis*. 1992;165:885.
248. Hackett S, Ferretti J, Stevens D. Cytokine induction by viable group A streptococci: Suppression by streptolysin O. Presented at the 94th Annual Meeting of the American Society for Microbiology, Las Vegas, Nev, May 1994.
249. Muller-Alouf H, Alouf JE, Gerlach D, et al. Comparative study of cytokine release by human peripheral blood mononuclear cells stimulated with *Streptococcus pyogenes* superantigenic erythrogenic toxins, heat-killed streptococci, and lipopolysaccharide. *Infect Immun*. 1994;62:4915-4921.
250. Herwald H, Collin M, Muller-Esterl W, et al. Streptococcal cysteine proteinase releases kinins: A novel virulence mechanism. *J Exp Med*. 1996;184:665-673.
251. Stevens DL, Bryant AE, Hackett SP, et al. Group A streptococcal bacteremia: The role of tumor necrosis factor in shock and organ failure. *J Infect Dis*. 1996;173:619-626.
252. Herwald H, Cramer H, Morgelin M, et al. M protein, a classical bacterial virulence determinant, forms complexes with fibrinogen that induces vascular leakage. *Cell*. 2004;116:367-379.
253. Stevens DL. Streptococcal toxic-shock syndrome: Spectrum of disease, pathogenesis, and new concepts in treatment. *Emerg Infect Dis*. 1995;1:69-78.
254. Cruz K, Hollenberg S. Update on septic shock: The latest approaches to treatment. *J Crit Illness*. 2003;18:162-168.
255. Stevens DL, Madaras-Kelly KJ, Richards DM. In vitro antimicrobial effects of various combinations of penicillin and clindamycin against four strains of *Streptococcus pyogenes*. *Antimicrob Agents Chemother*. 1998;42:1266-1268.
256. Stevens DL, Bryant AE, Hackett SP. Antibiotic effects on bacterial viability, toxin production and host response. *Clin Infect Dis*. 1995;20(suppl 2):S154-S157.
257. Stevens DL, Hackett SP, Bryant AE. Suppression of mononuclear cell synthesis of tumor necrosis factor by azithromycin. Presented at the Annual Meeting of the Infectious Disease Society of America, San Francisco, September 1997.
258. Miwa K, Fukuyama M, Ida N, et al. Preparation of a superantigen-adsorbing device and its superantigen removal efficacies in vitro and in vivo. *Int J Infect Dis*. 2003;7:21-26.
259. Dick GF, Dick GH. Therapeutic results with concentrated scarlet fever antitoxin. *JAMA*. 1925;84:803.
260. Lamothe F, D'Amico P, Ghosn P, et al. Clinical usefulness of intravenous human immunoglobulins in invasive group A streptococcal infections: Case report and review. *Clin Infect Dis*. 1995;21:1469-1470.
261. Barry W, Hudgins L, Donta ST, et al. Intravenous immunoglobulin therapy for toxic shock syndrome. *JAMA*. 1992;267: 3315-3316.
262. Stevens DL. Rationale for the use of intravenous gamma globulin in the treatment of streptococcal toxic shock syndrome [editorial response]. *Clin Infect Dis*. 1998;26:639-641.
263. Kaul R, McGeer A, Norrby-Teglund A, et al. Intravenous immunoglobulin therapy for streptococcal toxic shock syndrome—a comparative observational study. *Clin Infect Dis*. 1999; 28:800-807.
264. Darenberg J, Ihendyane N, Sjolin J, et al. Intravenous immunoglobulin G therapy in streptococcal toxic shock syndrome: A European randomized, double-blind, placebo-controlled trial. *Clin Infect Dis*. 2003;37:333-340.
265. Beaulieu A, McGeer A, Muller MP, et al. Intravenous immunoglobulin for group A streptococcal toxic shock syndrome: A reassessment of efficacy. Presented at the 48th Annual Interscience Conference on Antibicrobial Agents and Chemotherapy and The Infectious Disease Society of America 46th Annual Meeting. Washington, DC, October 23-28, 2008.
266. Stevens DL. Dilemmas in the treatment of invasive Streptococcus pyogenes infections. *Clin Infect Dis*. 2003;37:341-343.
267. Norrby-Teglund A, Kaul R, Low DE, et al. Evidence for the presence of streptococcal-superantigen-neutralizing antibodies in normal polyspecific immunoglobulin G. *Infect Immun*. 1996;64:5395-5398.
268. Riseman JA, Zamboni WA, Curtis A, et al. Hyperbaric oxygen therapy for necrotizing fasciitis reduces mortality and the need for debridements. *Surgery*. 1990;108:847-850.
269. Weinstein MP, Reller B, Murphy JR, et al. The clinical significance of positive blood cultures: A comparative analysis of 500 episodes of bacteremia and fungemia in adults. I. Laboratory and epidemiologic observations. *Rev Infect Dis*. 1983;5: 35-53.
270. Duma RJ, Weinberg AN, Medrek TF, et al. Streptococcal infections: A bacteriological and clinical study of streptococcal bacteremia. *Medicine*. 1969;48:87-127.
271. Dan M, Maximova S, Siegman-Igra Y, et al. Varied presentations of sporadic group A streptococcal bacteremia: Clinical experience and attempt at classification. *Rev Infect Dis*. 1990; 12:537-542.
272. Ispahani P, Donald FE, Aveline AJ. Streptococcus pyogenes bacteraemia: An old enemy subdued, but not defeated. *J Infect*. 1988;16:37-46.
273. Bucher A, Martin PR, Hoiby EA, et al. Spectrum of disease in bacteraemic patients during a *Streptococcus pyogenes* serotype M-1 epidemic in Norway in 1988. *Eur J Clin Microbiol Infect Dis*. 1992;11:416-426.
274. Burkert T, Watanakunakorn C. Group A streptococcal bacteremia in a community teaching hospital—1980-1989. *Clin Infect Dis*. 1992;14:29-37.
275. Ramirez CA, Naraqi S, McCulley DJ. Group A beta-hemolytic streptococcus endocarditis. *Am Heart J*. 1984;108:1383-1386.
276. Baddour LM. Infective endocarditis caused by beta-hemolytic streptococci. The Infectious Diseases Society of America's Emerging Infections Network.
277. van de Beek D, de Gans J, Spanjaard L, et al. Group A streptococcal meningitis in adults: Clin Infect Dis. 1998;26:66-71.Report of 41 cases and a review of the literature. *Clin Infect Dis*. 2002;34:e32-e36.
278. Sommer R, Rohner P, Garbino J, et al. Group A beta-hemolytic streptococcus meningitis: Clinical and microbiological features of nine cases. *Clin Infect Dis*. 1999;29:929-931.
279. Murphy DJ Jr. Group A streptococcal meningitis. *Pediatrics*. 1983;71:1-5.
280. Basiliere JL, Bistrong HW, Spence WF. Streptococcal pneumonia: Recent outbreaks in military recruit populations. *Am J Med*. 1968;44:580-589.
281. Crum NF, Russell KL, Kaplan EL, et al. Pneumonia outbreak associated with group A streptococcus species at a military training facility. *Clin Infect Dis*. 2005;40:511-518.

282. Muller MP, Low DE, Green KA, et al. Clinical and epidemiologic features of group A streptococcal pneumonia in Ontario, Canada. *Arch Intern Med.* 2003;163:467-472.

283. Morens DM, Taubenberger JK, Fauci AS. Predominant role of bacterial pneumonia as a cause of death in pandemic influenza: Implications for pandemic influenza preparedness. *J Infect Dis.* 2008;198:962-970.

284. Okamoto S, Kawabata S, Nakagawa I, et al. Influenza A virus-infected hosts boost an invasive type of Streptococcus pyogenes Infection in mice. *J Virol.* 2003;77:4104-4112.

285. Petersen JP, Kaltoft MS, Misfeldt JC, et al. Community outbreak of perianal group A streptococcal infection in Denmark. *Pediatr Infect Dis J.* 2003;22:105-109.

286. Mogielnicki NP, Schwartzman JD, Elliott JA. Perineal group A streptococcal disease in a pediatric practice. *Pediatrics.* 2000;106(Pt 1):276-281.

287. Mastro TD, Farley TA, Elliott JA, et al. An outbreak of surgical wound infections due to group A *Streptococcus* carried on the scalp. *N Engl J Med.* 1990;323:968-972.

288. Kakis A, Gibbs L, Eguia J, et al. An outbreak of group A streptococcal infection among health care workers. *Clin Infect Dis.* 2002;35:1353-1359.

289. Robinson KA, Rothrock G, Phan Q, et al. Risk for severe group A streptococcal disease among patients' household contacts. *Emerg Infect Dis.* 2003;9:443-447.

290. Factor SH, Levine OS, Schwartz B, et al. Invasive group A streptococcal disease: Risk factors for adults. *Emerg Infect Dis.* 2003;9:970-977.

199

Nonsuppurative Poststreptococcal Sequelae: Rheumatic Fever and Glomerulonephritis

ALAN L. BISNO

▓ Rheumatic Fever

Acute rheumatic fever (ARF) is a disease characterized by nonsuppurative inflammatory lesions involving primarily the heart, joints, subcutaneous tissues, and central nervous system. In its classic form, ARF is acute, febrile, and largely self-limited. However, damage to heart valves may occur, and such damage may be chronic and progressive and lead to severe cardiac failure, total disability and death many years after the acute attack. The manifestations of ARF are extremely variable; the disorder remains for the most part a clinical syndrome for which no specific diagnostic test exists. All cases of ARF follow group A streptococcal upper respiratory tract infection, although the exact mechanisms mediating development of the disease remain speculative. Persons who have suffered an attack of ARF are predisposed to recurrent episodes after subsequent group A streptococcal infections.

HISTORY

Guillaume de Baillou (1538-1616), also known as Ballonius, first clearly distinguished acute arthritis from gout. Thomas Sydenham (1624-1689) described chorea but failed to associate this entity with other manifestations of ARF. Raymond Vieussens (1641-1715) published pathologic descriptions of mitral stenosis and aortic insufficiency. It remained, however, for William Charles Wells in 1812 to emphasize the association of rheumatism and carditis and to provide the first clear description of subcutaneous nodules. Jean-Baptiste Bouillard in 1836 and Walter B. Cheadle in 1889 published extensive studies of rheumatic arthritis and carditis that have come to be regarded as classic works in this field, and form the basis for modern clinical concepts of ARF. In 1904, Ludwig Aschoff described the specific rheumatic lesion in the myocardium.

In 1880, J. K. Fowler pointed out the association between sore throat and rheumatic fever and, shortly after the dawn of the 20th century, Bela Schick identified ARF as one of the "nachkrankheiten" of scarlet fever. The introduction of Rebecca Lancefield's grouping system for β-hemolytic streptococci allowed clarification of the epidemiology of the disease by a number of investigators in the United States and the United Kingdom, including Coburn, Collis, Rammelkamp, Wannamaker, Massell, and Stollerman. Finally, the widespread introduction of antibiotic agents after World War II resulted in the development of strategies for primary and secondary prevention of rheumatic fever.[1]

ETIOLOGY AND PATHOGENESIS

ARF is a delayed nonsuppurative sequela of upper respiratory infection caused by group A streptococci, a conclusion firmly supported by several lines of evidence. There is a close temporal relationship between epidemics of streptococcal sore throat and scarlet fever and epidemics of ARF. Most patients with ARF relate a history of preceding pharyngitis; even in the absence of such clear-cut evidence, elevated serum levels of antistreptococcal antibodies almost always document recent streptococcal infection. Prospective studies of primary and recurrent ARF have shown that this disease occurs only after an immunologically significant streptococcal infection. Finally, continuous antimicrobial prophylaxis, when successful in preventing intercurrent streptococcal infections, also effectively prevents ARF recurrences in rheumatic persons.

An intriguing and as yet unexplained aspect of the host-parasite relationship is the fact that, insofar as is known, cutaneous streptococcal infections do not initiate ARF. This may indicate a requirement for the pharyngeal site, with its rich endowment of lymphoid tissue, for initiation of the disease process, or it may result from a lack of rheumatogenicity among the so-called pyoderma strains of group A streptococci.

A substantial body of evidence indicates that group A streptococci do vary in their rheumatogenic potential. Studies of outbreaks of streptococcal pharyngitis have revealed that strains of certain M serotypes or genotypes are strongly and repeatedly associated with ARF[2] (Table 199-1), whereas strains of other equally prevalent types fail to initiate the disease or even to reactivate it in exquisitely susceptible hosts.[3] Investigations of endemic ARF cases in Trinidad[4] and Chile[5] have indicated that streptococci causing ARF belong to different serotypes than those causing acute glomerulonephritis (AGN) occurring simultaneously in the same population. Strains of group A streptococci isolated from ARF patients may, however, differ widely in different geographic locales.[6] Although the association of pyoderma strains of group A streptococci (see Chapter 198) with ARF has been postulated,[6,7] such strains have never been definitively associated with ARF[8,9] even when, as frequently occurs, they colonize the throat.

Variations in the rheumatogenicity of prevalent group A streptococci likely account for the striking temporal and geographic fluctuations in the incidence of ARF. For example, strains of mucoid group A streptococci that were genetically identical, or almost so, were prevalent in Salt Lake City, Utah during two peak periods of rheumatic fever incidence occurring 12 years apart.[10,11]

Rheumatogenic streptococcal strains exhibit distinct biologic characteristics. Their M protein molecules share a particular surface-exposed antigenic domain[12] against which ARF patients mount a strong IgG response.[13] These strains fail to elaborate α_1-lipoproteinase (so-called streptococcal opacity factor), and they are frequently heavily encapsulated.[14,15] The latter feature is manifested by the formation of mucoid colonies in blood agar plates. Whether such strains express a unique rheumatogenic antigen, however, remains unknown.

It is probable that not all strains of rheumatogenic serotypes are equally dangerous. The propensity of a given strain to cause ARF may well depend on its degree of virulence, a reflection of quantitative factors such as expression of M protein, hyaluronate, or other less well-defined biologic properties. Virulence is likely to be enhanced in epidemiologic settings that favor rapid person-to-person transmission.

Although the group A streptococcus is known to be the causative agent of rheumatic fever, the exact mechanism whereby this microorganism induces the disease remains unexplained. Several theories have

TABLE 199-1	M Serotypes of Group A Streptococci Associated with Nonsuppurative Sequelae in the Western Hemisphere*		
ARF	**Pharyngitis-Associated AGN**		**Pyoderma-Associated AGN**
1	1		2
3	4		49[†]
5	12		55[†]
6	25		57
14			59
18			60
19			61
24			

*This list represents the major serotypes known to be associated with ARF and AGN in the Western Hemisphere, but it is not all-inclusive. M types of streptococcal strains isolated from various geographic areas vary widely.[6,189]

[†]M types 49 and 55 have also been reported on occasion to cause pharyngitis-associated AGN.

AGN, Acute glomerulonephritis; ARF, acute rheumatic fever.

been advanced. These include the following: (1) toxic effects of streptococcal products, particularly streptolysins S or O, which are known to be capable of inducing tissue injury; (2) serum sickness–like reaction mediated by antigen-antibody complexes, perhaps localized to sites of tissue injury; and (3) autoimmune phenomena induced by similarity or identity of certain streptococcal antigens to a wide variety of human tissue antigens.[16]

Although none of these theories has been unequivocally proved or refuted, most attention has been focused on the concept of autoimmunity or, more precisely, molecular mimicry.[17] Interest in this mechanism has been spurred by the identification of antibodies in the sera of patients with ARF or rheumatic heart disease that react with the human heart in a variety of test systems. These so-called heart-reactive antibodies (HRAs) are also present, albeit in much lower titer, in sera of patients with uncomplicated streptococcal pharyngitis. The presence of bound immunoglobulin and complement in the myocardia of children dying of rheumatic carditis suggests that circulating HRAs may have pathogenetic significance.

Improved methods of purifying M protein have been developed, and molecular biology techniques have been used in studies on the relationship between specific peptides of the M protein molecule and human tissues. Epitopes of streptococcal M proteins have been identified that share antigenic determinants with cardiac myosin,[18,19] sarcolemmal membrane proteins,[20] synovium, and articular cartilage.[21]

Goldstein and colleagues[22] have described a cross-reaction between group A polysaccharide and a structural glycoprotein isolated from human and bovine heart valves. Such a cross-reaction might explain the observation that serum levels of antibodies to group A carbohydrate appear to remain elevated for many years in patients with rheumatic valvulitis, but not in rheumatic patients without valvulitis,[23] and decline remarkably if valve resection is performed.

Chronic remittent nodular lesions have been observed in dermal connective tissue after injection into experimental animals of a streptococcal mucopeptide-polysaccharide cell wall complex.[24] Antibodies raised in rabbits against streptococcal hyaluronate cross react with human hyaluronate.[25] Many children with Sydenham's chorea have circulating antibodies that react both with neurons of the caudate and subthalamic nuclei and with group A streptococcal cell membranes.[26] Taken together, these cross-reactive and toxic phenomena could explain most of the individual manifestations of ARF. On the other hand, it should be emphasized that no direct proof exists that these systems play any role in the pathogenesis of rheumatic fever.

Much of the work reviewed in the preceding paragraphs, particularly that related to HRAs and group A carbohydrate, has focused on humoral immune responses to streptococci. Indeed, serum antibody responses to streptolysin O, non–type-specific M antigens, and almost every other streptococcal antigen are, on average, more vigorous in patients with ARF than in those with uncomplicated streptococcal infections. However, it is likely that delayed hypersensitivity responses to streptococcal antigens also play a critical role in the etiology of ARF.[27,28] Preparations of streptolysin S contain a nonspecific mitogen that is closely related but separable from the hemolytic activity. In rheumatic persons, lymphocyte reactivity to streptococcal cell walls and membranes is heightened, but the reactivity to membranes is more striking and persists for several years after an acute attack.[29] During active rheumatic carditis, both the number of helper (CD4) lymphocytes and the ratio of CD4 to CD8 cells are increased in heart valves as well as in peripheral blood.[30,31] Production of interleukin-1[32] and interleukin-2[32,33] has been reported to be enhanced. The recognition that both M protein[34] and streptococcal pyrogenic exotoxins[35] function as superantigens suggests a potential mechanism mediating the unrestrained immunologic assault postulated to cause ARF.

A complete elucidation of the pathogenesis of ARF obviously requires an understanding not only of the peculiarities of the causative agent but also of the nature of the susceptible host. The fact that even in severe epidemics of exudative pharyngitis, rheumatic fever affects only a small proportion of infected persons, coupled with the known familial aggregation of ARF cases, has long suggested the possibility of a genetic predisposition to rheumatic attacks. Studies of the distribution of class 1 HLA antigens in rheumatic individuals compared with controls have been inconclusive. A statistically significant association has been reported between certain of the class II HLA antigens (HLA-DR2 in blacks[36] and HLA-DR4 in whites[36,37]) and rheumatic fever. An intriguing potential link between the genetic constitution of the human host and susceptibility to ARF is the identification of certain alloantigens that are expressed in a higher proportion of circulating B lymphocytes of rheumatic subjects and their family members than of patients with AGN or normal controls.[38,39]

PATHOLOGIC FINDINGS

Rheumatic fever is characterized pathologically by the presence of exudative and proliferative inflammatory lesions of connective tissue, most notably the heart, joints, blood vessels, and subcutaneous tissue.[40] In the early stages of the disease, there is fragmentation of collagen fibers, cellular infiltration that is predominantly lymphocytic, and fibrinoid deposition. This is followed shortly by the appearance of the myocardial Aschoff nodule. The Aschoff nodule is a perivascular focus of inflammation that consists of an area of central necrosis surrounded by a rosette of large mononuclear and giant multinuclear cells. The nuclei of these cells may contain a clear area just within the nuclear membrane (owl-eyed nucleus) or present a serrated (caterpillar) appearance, depending on their orientation in microscopic cross section. Such cells are known as Anichkov myocytes, although immunohistochemical studies have demonstrated that they are of macrophage-histiocyte origin.[41,42] Cardiac findings may include pericarditis, myocarditis, or endocarditis. Endocarditis involves the left side of the heart in most instances. A thickened and roughened area is frequently seen in the left atrium above the base of the posterior leaflet of the mitral valve (MacCallum's patch). Valvular lesions begin as edema and cellular infiltration of the leaflets and chordae, with small verrucae along the line of closure. As healing progresses, the valves may become thickened and deformed, the chordae shortened, and the valve commissures fused, thereby resulting in valvular stenosis or insufficiency.

The joint lesions are characterized by fibrinous exudate over the synovial membrane and serous effusion without joint destruction. Histologic findings include cellular infiltration and fibrinoid degeneration. Subcutaneous nodules resemble Aschoff bodies in many features. They consist of a central zone of fibrinoid necrosis surrounded by histiocytes and fibroblasts; perivascular accumulations of lymphocytes and polymorphonuclear leukocytes are also apparent. Although scattered areas of arteritis and petechial hemorrhages have been found in the brain, their relationship to Sydenham's chorea remains uncertain.

EPIDEMIOLOGY

Acute rheumatic fever is most frequent in children aged 5 to 15 years old. Only approximately 5% of cases occur in children younger than 5 years.[43] Indeed, its relative rarity in infants and preschool-aged children has led some observers to question whether repeated "primary" infections might be a precondition for the development of this disease. Both initial and recurrent episodes also occur in adults.[44-46] There is no clear-cut gender predilection, although a female preponderance exists in certain clinical manifestations, notably mitral stenosis and Sydenham's chorea when the latter occurs after puberty. In temperate climates, rheumatic fever tends to occur less frequently during the summer.

The attack rate of rheumatic fever after untreated streptococcal exudative tonsillitis in military recruit camps has been carefully studied and has been shown consistently to be approximately 3%.[47] The ARF attack rate is considerably lower after endemically occurring infections in open populations of school-aged children. Siegel and colleagues[48] studied 519 untreated children with pharyngitis associated with throat cultures positive for group A streptococci. The attack rate of ARF was found to be 0.4%. Among those patients with an immunologically significant infection, as judged by a rise in the serum titer of antistreptolysin O (ASO), the attack rate was 0.9%. In that study, ARF was observed to occur only in the group of 81 patients with exudative pharyngitis, throat cultures positive for group A streptococci, ASO titer increases, and prolonged convalescent streptococcal carriage. In this group, the ARF attack rate, 2.5%, approximated that seen in military recruit camps. These and other data suggest that ARF is more likely to occur after more severe forms of streptococcal throat infection, as judged by clinical, bacteriologic, and immunologic criteria. Nevertheless, one third or more of ARF cases occur after asymptomatic streptococcal infection.

It may be difficult for physicians trained in North America to comprehend the magnitude of the problem of ARF in developing countries. The disease is rampant in the Middle East, the Indian subcontinent, and selected areas of Africa and South America.[49,50] The World Health Association has estimated that approximately a half-million individuals worldwide acquire rheumatic fever annually, of whom 300,000 will go on to develop rheumatic heart disease (RHD). Over 15 million persons have been estimated to be living with this disease, and 233,000 die each year from RHD or its complications.[51] Extraordinarily high rates of ARF and rheumatic heart disease are seen in Aboriginal populations such as those in New Zealand and Australia. Between 1989 and 1993, the annual incidence of ARF in Aboriginal children aged 5 to 14 years in Australia's Northern Territory was 254/100,000, and the point prevalence of rheumatic heart disease among the Aboriginal population was 9.6/1000.[52]

The overall incidence of ARF in the United States cannot be ascertained precisely because of inherent difficulties in diagnosing the disease and because most states no longer maintain operational rheumatic fever registries. There is general agreement, however, that the incidence of ARF and rheumatic heart disease declined markedly over the course of the 20th century in the United States and Western Europe. The rate of decline appears to have been particularly steep during the 1960s and 1970s. A survey in Memphis, Tennessee,[53] indicated that during 1977 through 1981, the incidence of ARF in white suburban schoolchildren was only 0.5/100,000 annually. Similar rates have been reported from many geographic areas of the United States.[54] Traditionally, ARF in the United States was largely a disease of lower socioeconomic groups. The incidence has been much higher in blacks than whites,[53,55] a fact that appears to relate to basic environmental conditions rather than to any genetic predisposition of blacks for the development of rheumatic fever. The major predisposing environmental condition that has been identified is crowding. The degree of crowding markedly influences the acquisition rate of group A streptococci (see Chapter 198) and hence the risk of development of ARF.[54]

In the mid-1980s, a resurgence of ARF occurred in many communities in the United States.[56] Beginning in early 1985, an epidemic of the disease occurred in Salt Lake City, Utah, and the surrounding intermountain area.[54,57] By the year 2000, more than 500 cases had been diagnosed at the Primary Children's Medical Center in Salt Lake City. Smaller clusters of ARF, ranging from 15 to 40 cases, were reported during approximately the same time period from the following regions: Columbus and Akron, Ohio; Pittsburgh, Pennsylvania; Nashville and Memphis, Tennessee; Kansas City, Missouri; Morgantown and Charleston, West Virginia; Dallas, Texas; and New York City, New York. Moreover, for the first time in many years, outbreaks occurred in army and navy training camps.[58,59]

Quite surprisingly, a number of the 1980s civilian outbreaks[54,60] involved children of middle-class families residing in suburban or rural settings. The group A streptococcal strains most strongly associated epidemiologically with these ARF outbreaks belong to the well-recognized rheumatogenic serotypes (e.g., types 1, 3, 5, 6, and 18); particularly prominent in this regard were highly mucoid strains of M18.[15,61]

Persons who have suffered an initial attack of rheumatic fever have a marked predilection to develop recurrences after subsequent episodes of streptococcal pharyngeal infection. The risk of recurrence after streptococcal infection is highest within the first few years after the initial attack and then declines. It is unclear whether the reason for this decline is the length of time since the preceding attack or the older age of the patient. Nevertheless, rheumatic patients remain at an increased risk of recurrence well into adult life. Two other factors positively correlated with a risk of rheumatic recurrences after streptococcal infection are the magnitude of the ASO response and the presence of preexisting heart disease. In the classic studies conducted at Irvington House, New York,[62] for example, 56% of streptococcal infections occurring in persons with RHD and accompanied by four-tube or higher ASO titer rises induced ARF recurrences.

CLINICAL MANIFESTATIONS

Rheumatic fever manifests itself as a variety of signs and symptoms that may occur singly or in combination. The most important of these, in terms of diagnosis, have been termed the *major manifestations* and include carditis, polyarthritis, chorea, subcutaneous nodules, and erythema marginatum. Certain additional findings that are frequently present in ARF but are nonspecific in nature constitute the so-called *minor manifestations*—fever, arthralgia, heart block, and acute-phase reactants in the blood (C-reactive protein, elevation of the leukocyte count, and erythrocyte sedimentation rate).

The latent period between the onset of preceding streptococcal sore throat and the onset of ARF averages 19 days.[63] The range has been difficult to establish precisely but appears to be between 1 and 5 weeks. The average latent period is the same for recurrent attacks as for initial episodes.

The mode of onset is variable. If acute polyarthritis is the initial complaint, the disease may have a rather abrupt onset and may be marked by fever and toxicity. On the other hand, when isolated mild carditis is the initial manifestation, the onset of ARF may be insidious or even subclinical.

Most attacks begin with polyarthritis, although occasionally this may be preceded by abdominal pain. Carditis, if it appears, usually does so early in the course of the disease. Overall, arthritis occurs in approximately 75% of first attacks of ARF, clinically evident carditis in 40% to 50%, chorea in 15%, and subcutaneous nodules and erythema marginatum in fewer than 10%.[64,65] These incidences vary with age; carditis occurs most frequently when ARF strikes younger children, whereas the proportion of cases with arthritis increases with the age of the patient.

Carditis is the only manifestation of ARF that has the potential to cause long-term disability or death. Heart involvement in ARF is frequently a pancarditis involving the endocardium, myocardium, and pericardium. Nevertheless, in the absence of high fever or symptoms of acute pericarditis or congestive heart failure, it may be asymptomatic. Carditis almost always manifests itself within the first 3 weeks of an attack of ARF if it appears at all. The clinical signs of carditis include the development of organic heart murmur(s) not previously present, cardiac enlargement, congestive heart failure, pericardial friction rubs, or signs of effusion.

Intractable heart failure may cause death in the acute phase of the disease, but fortunately, this occurrence is rare. Echocardiographic studies have shown that patients with rheumatic fever and congestive heart failure have preserved left ventricular systolic function and severe mitral and/or aortic regurgitation.[66-69] Serum levels of cardiac troponin I are not elevated in ARF patients with congestive failure.[66,70] Thus, the cause of heart failure appears to be acute valvular dilatation and not myocarditis.[71]

Chronic inflammatory changes involving the myocardium and endocardium may lead to the delayed development of chronic rheumatic heart disease (Fig. 199-1). Endocarditis involves the mitral valve more frequently than the aortic valve. There are three characteristic murmurs of acute rheumatic carditis: a high-pitched blowing holosystolic apical murmur of mitral regurgitation, a low-pitched apical middiastolic flow murmur (Carey Coombs murmur), and a high-pitched decrescendo diastolic murmur of aortic regurgitation heard at the secondary and primary aortic areas. Murmurs of mitral and aortic stenosis are associated with chronic but not with acute rheumatic valvular disease. The tricuspid valve is involved much less frequently and pulmonic valve very rarely. Delayed atrioventricular conduction, as manifested by first-degree or even greater degrees of heart block,[72]

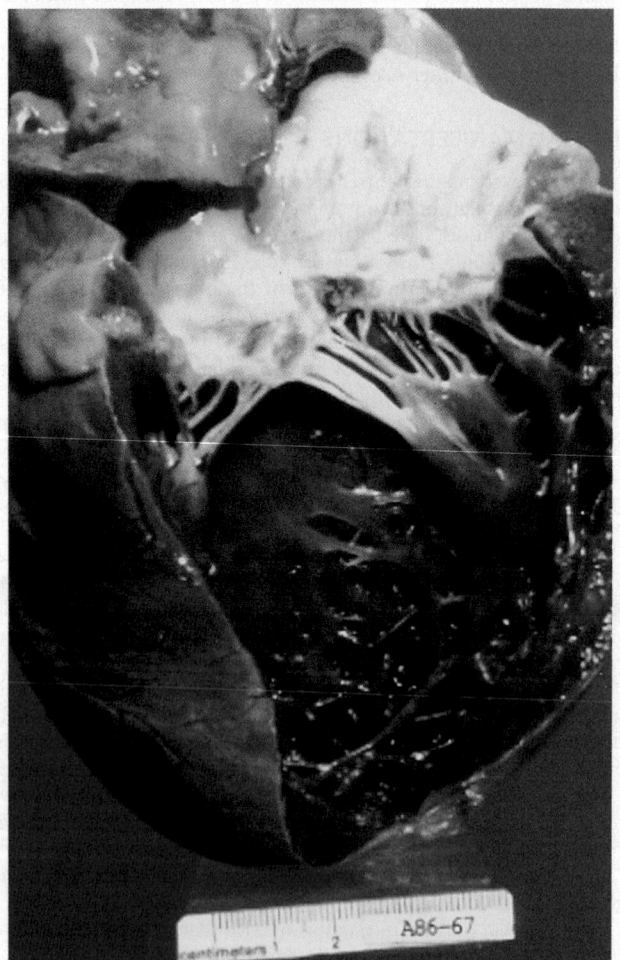

Figure 199-1   Chronic rheumatic valvular heart disease. The mitral valve leaflets and chordae are thickened, fibrotic, and distorted; intercommissural adhesions are present. *(Courtesy of Dr. L. Alvarez, VA Medical Center, Miami.)*

is a toxic phenomenon associated with ARF but is not in itself diagnostic of rheumatic carditis.

Joint involvement in ARF ranges from arthralgia without objective findings to frank arthritis characterized by heat, swelling, redness, and exquisite tenderness. There is an inverse relationship between the severity of joint involvement and risk of development of carditis.[73] The most frequently involved joints are the knees, ankles, elbows, and wrists. The small joints of the hands are less frequently affected, and the spine is only rarely involved. When the course of the illness is not suppressed by anti-inflammatory drugs, multiple joints are usually involved; approximately 50% of patients develop arthritis in more than six joints. Arthritis in ARF is classically migratory in nature—that is, the inflammation travels from joint to joint. Once a joint becomes involved, inflammation begins to subside within a few days to a week and disappears within 2 to 3 weeks. The evolution of arthritis in individual joints tends to overlap, so multiple joints may be inflamed at the same time. The typical migratory polyarthritis pattern may not be present, however, if effective anti-inflammatory therapy is administered early in the course of the disease. Moreover, the classic migratory pattern is not invariable. In some cases, the pattern may initially be additive, persisting in several joints simultaneously or, even rarely, monoarthritic.[74]

In most cases, the entire bout of polyarthritis subsides within 4 weeks, leaving no residual articular damage. One possible exception to this has been claimed by several authors, who report the very rare occurrence of the so-called Jaccoud form of periarticular fibrosis after rheumatic arthritis.

The existence of a reactive poststreptococcal arthritis distinct from ARF has been postulated to occur in certain patients whose arthritis is atypical in time of onset or duration,[46] is nonmigratory, is unaccompanied by other major manifestations of rheumatic fever, and fails to respond promptly to salicylate therapy.[75-77] The ultimate prognosis of such cases is unknown, but in some cases rheumatic heart disease has ensued.[78-80] Although the issue remains controversial,[81] it seems prudent to consider all cases of poststreptococcal polyarthritis that fulfill the diagnostic criteria of Jones as representing ARF,[76] providing that other common causes of polyarthritis have been excluded.[82-84]

Subcutaneous nodules usually are associated with severe carditis and tend to occur several weeks after its onset. They are firm and painless and vary in size from a few millimeters to 2.0 cm. Such nodules are usually found over bony surfaces or prominences and over tendons. Common sites are adjacent to elbows, knees, wrists, or ankles and over Achilles tendons, the occiput, or spinous processes of the vertebrae. Their number varies from one to a few dozen. They usually persist for 1 or 2 weeks. Somewhat similar but more persistent lesions are seen in rheumatoid arthritis.

Erythema marginatum is a nonpruritic, nonpainful erythematous eruption usually seen on the trunk or proximal aspects of the extremities. The individual lesions are evanescent, moving over the skin in serpiginous patterns that change before the observer's eyes and are often likened to smoke rings, with a tendency to advance at the margins while clearing in the center (Fig. 199-2). The lesions are usually macular with raised margins and appear to be more a vasomotor phenomenon than a manifestation of cutaneous pathologic changes. Individual lesions may come and go in minutes to hours, but the process may go on intermittently for weeks to months.

Sydenham's chorea (St. Vitus dance) is a neurologic disorder characterized by emotional lability, muscular weakness, and rapid, uncoordinated, involuntary purposeless movements. The choreiform movements disappear during sleep and may be partially suppressed by sedation. The nonrhythmic movements are most notable in the face, hands, and feet. Sensation remains intact. Detailed descriptions of the nature of the choreiform movements can be found elsewhere.[1,85] Individual attacks in hospitalized patients usually last 2 to 4 months.

Chorea may occur in relatively close association with other rheumatic manifestations or in isolated form (pure chorea). In cases of pure chorea, laboratory evidence of acute inflammation (C-reactive protein, elevated erythrocyte sedimentation rate) or recent streptococcal infec-

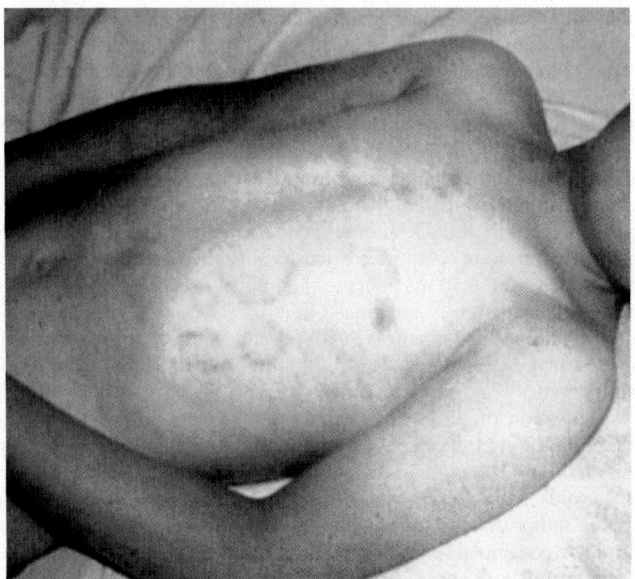

Figure 199-2 **Annular plaques (complete rings) of varying sizes with macular centers and erythematous, raised margins.** Note the serpiginous borders formed by coalescence of several partial rings. *(Courtesy Dr. M. Tyrell, Saskatoon, Canada; From Bisno AL. Noncardiac manifestations of rheumatic fever. In: Narula J, Vrmani R, Reddy KS, Tandon R, eds. Rheumatic Fever. Washington, DC: Armed Forces Institute of Pathology; 1999;245-256.)*

tion (elevated levels of antistreptococcal antibodies) may be lacking. This observation, which led investigators in the past to question the relationship of ARF to pure chorea, is now known to result from the fact that Sydenham's chorea often occurs with a longer latent period than the other manifestations of ARF. Relapses of pure chorea may occur in some patients despite faithful adherence to prophylaxis with intramuscular benzathine penicillin.[86,87] Some patients with pure chorea are found on follow-up to have RHD manifested primarily by mitral stenosis.[88]

Interest has focused on the possibility that certain other neurologic conditions, including tics, obsessive-compulsive disorder, and Tourette's syndrome, may be poststreptococcal sequelae.[89,90] This entity has been termed *poststreptococcal autoimmune neuropsychiatric disorders associated with streptococci* (PANDAS). A prospective blinded cohort study of patients meeting suggested diagnostic criteria for PANDAS found that, following group A streptococcal infection, exacerbations of childhood tics and obsessive-compulsive disorders were more frequent in cases than controls. However, streptococcal infection was not the only or even the most common antecedent of such exacerbations.[91] Studies of this putative entity are continuing.

Several clinical manifestations of ARF occur with some frequency but are not in themselves specific enough to be considered major manifestations. These include fever, which accompanies almost all ARF attacks at their onset, arthralgia, abdominal pain, and epistaxis. The pulmonary parenchyma in ARF may be involved by a variety of pathologic processes, including pulmonary edema, atelectasis, pulmonary embolism, or thromboses. Some observers think that in addition, a specific rheumatic pneumonia may occur in rare cases.[92]

The average duration of an attack, in the absence of anti-inflammatory therapy, is approximately 3 months. Fewer than 5% of the cases persist for longer than 6 months, justifying the designation of "chronic" rheumatic fever. Stollerman[1] listed the criteria for continuing clinical activity as follows: joint symptoms, new organic murmurs, changing heart size, congestive heart failure in the absence of long-standing valvular disease, subcutaneous nodules, sleeping pulse rate higher than 100 beats/min, erythema marginatum, chorea, positive test for C-reactive protein, and a rectal temperature of 100.4°F or higher for 3 or more consecutive days.

DIAGNOSIS

Because ARF can have such diverse manifestations (acute polyarthritis, congestive heart failure, chorea, or combinations of these) and because there is no specific diagnostic test for the disease, the differential diagnostic possibilities in an individual case may be extensive. Among the diseases that most frequently need to be differentiated are rheumatoid arthritis, juvenile rheumatoid arthritis, systemic lupus erythematosus, serum sickness, sickle cell crisis or cardiopathy, rubella arthritis, septic arthritis (especially gonococcal arthritis in adolescent patients), Lyme disease,[93] infective endocarditis, viral myocarditis, and early stages of Henoch-Schönlein purpura. Less frequent differential diagnostic considerations include gout, sarcoidosis, Hodgkin's disease, and leukemia. Choreiform movements have been described in patients with systemic lupus erythematosus,[94] neoplasms involving the basal ganglia,[95] legionnaires' disease,[96] hypoparathyroidism,[97] antiphospholipid syndrome,[98] Wilson's disease, and Huntington's disease. Chorea is also seen occasionally in women taking oral contraceptives,[99] and during pregnancy (chorea gravidarum).[100]

Arriving at the correct diagnosis is particularly important in ARF, not only in terms of prescribing appropriate therapy for the acute attack and formulating an accurate prognosis but also because of the necessity for prescribing continuous antistreptococcal prophylaxis. To minimize over- and underdiagnosis, the criteria originally formulated by Jones,[101] and updated and modified by a committee of the American Heart Association in 1992,[83] have been generally accepted as the basis for reaching a diagnosis of ARF (Table 199-2). The updated criteria are to be applied most stringently to the diagnosis of an initial ARF attack. Although most patients with recurrences fulfill the criteria, the diagnosis of recurrent ARF may be less apparent. In a patient with established rheumatic heart disease, for example, it may be difficult to diagnose recurrent carditis confidently unless a previously normal valve is affected. The updated criteria therefore allow a presumptive diagnosis of recurrent ARF to be made if clinical findings are suggestive and there is supporting evidence of recent streptococcal infection.

Certain patients with acute rheumatic fever have echocardiographic evidence of valvular regurgitation in the absence of an audible murmur. Although valvular regurgitation can also be detected in normal individuals by two-dimensional echo Doppler and color flow Doppler techniques, criteria for discriminating physiologic from pathologic regurgitation have been proposed by experienced investigators.[54,102-104] In a recent study from India, 333 patients suspected of having ARF

TABLE 199-2	Guidelines for the Diagnosis of Initial Attack of Rheumatic Fever (Jones Criteria, Updated 1992)*

Major Manifestations
Carditis
Polyarthritis
Chorea
Erythema marginatum
Subcutaneous nodules

Minor Manifestations
Clinical findings
  Arthralgia
  Fever
Laboratory findings
  Elevated acute phase reactants
    Erythrocyte sedimentation rate
    C-reactive protein
  Prolonged PR interval

Supporting Evidence of Antecedent Group A Streptococcal Infection
Positive throat culture or rapid streptococcal antigen test
Elevated or rising streptococcal antibody titer

*If supported by evidence of preceding group A streptococcal infection, the presence of two major manifestations or of one major and two minor manifestations indicates a high probability of acute rheumatic fever.

From Dajani AS, Ayoub E, Bierman FZ, et al. Guidelines for the diagnosis of rheumatic fever: Jones criteria, updated 1992. *Circulation.* 1993; 87:302-307.

were investigated using stringent echocardiographic criteria, and 15% were judged to have evidence of subclinical carditis.[105] At present, so-called echocarditis is not considered diagnostic of rheumatic carditis by the American Heart Association for the purpose of fulfilling the Jones criteria,[106] and its long-term prognostic significance remains uncertain. The issue, however, remains controversial,[71,107] and in some areas of the world with a high incidence of ARF, positive echocardiographic evidence is considered to establish the diagnosis of carditis.[108,109]

The Jones criteria are not infallible, particularly when the diagnosis rests on the presence of acute polyarthritis as the sole major criterion with supporting evidence of fever plus an elevated erythrocyte sedimentation rate or a positive test result for C-reactive protein. For this reason, it is important to recognize that evidence of recent streptococcal infection must be obtained to satisfy the revised Jones criteria. Such evidence might include a recent microbiologically documented episode of streptococcal pharyngitis, a positive throat culture or rapid streptococcal antigen test for group A streptococci (although here the differentiation of infection from colonization presents a problem), or the demonstration of an elevated serum titer of antistreptococcal antibodies. In most cases, physicians rely on the latter criterion.

If a serum sample is obtained within 2 months of onset, approximately 80% of patients with ARF will have an ASO titer higher than 200 Todd units/mL. If a second streptococcal antibody test is performed on the same serum specimen, the proportion of patients with ARF with at least one elevated titer will rise to 90%.[110] Although an elevated antistreptococcal antibody titer is certainly not diagnostic of ARF, failure to demonstrate evidence of recent immunologically significant streptococcal infection using ASO and anti-DNase B tests makes the diagnosis of ARF doubtful. An exception to this statement must be made for the patient with pure chorea whose antibody titers may have declined to the normal range because of the long latent period between the antecedent streptococcal infection and the onset of this manifestation. Similarly, the onset of isolated carditis may be difficult to date; if recognition of isolated carditis is delayed, immunologic evidence of recent streptococcal infection may have disappeared.

TREATMENT AND PROGNOSIS

The objectives of therapy in ARF are to relieve inflammation, decrease fever and toxicity, and control cardiac failure. The mainstays of treatment are salicylates and corticosteroids. Neither of these agents prevents or modifies the development of chronic rheumatic heart disease.[111] A suggested treatment schedule is outlined in Table 199-3. Analgesics without anti-inflammatory properties are recommended for patients with mild disease. This allows complete expression of the clinical manifestations to aid in diagnosis and also avoids post-therapeutic rebounds. Most patients require salicylates. If the high doses of

Clinical Severity	Treatment
Arthralgia or mild arthritis; no carditis	Analgesics only, such as codeine or propoxyphene
Moderate or severe arthritis; no carditis, or carditis *with or without* cardiomegaly, but without failure	Aspirin, 90-100 mg/kg/day for 2 wks increased if necessary; 60-70 mg/kg/day for the subsequent 6 wk
Carditis with failure, with or without joint manifestations	Prednisone, 40-60 mg/day, increased, if necessary; methylprednisone sodium succinate IV in fulminating cases; after 2-3 wk, slow withdrawal to be completed in 3 more wk; aspirin to be continued for 1 month after discontinuation of prednisone

TABLE 199-3 Suggested Schedule of Anti-inflammatory Therapy in Rheumatic Fever

From Stollerman GH. *Rheumatic Fever and Streptococcal Infection.* New York: Grune & Stratton, 1975.

salicylates required cannot be tolerated because of gastric irritation or if symptoms of salicylism develop, a reduction in the aspirin dosage or a change to corticosteroids is necessary. The more potent anti-inflammatory action of corticosteroids should be brought to bear whenever salicylates fail to control the inflammatory process or whenever carditis with congestive heart failure is present. The reader is referred elsewhere for a more detailed description of the therapeutic regimen.[1] Although nonsteroidal anti-inflammatory drugs (NSAIDs) would appear to be a reasonable alternative for patients who do not tolerate salicylates but do not require corticosteroids, there is a paucity of data on the use of these agents in acute rheumatic fever. Two small studies, one using naproxen[112] and one tolmetin,[113] reported NSAIDs to be equivalent to aspirin in efficacy with fewer side effects. Further experience with these agents is required before specific recommendations can be made.

Reactivation of clinical or laboratory manifestations of rheumatic inflammation may occur after cessation of anti-inflammatory therapy. This "rebound" phenomenon is more frequent after therapy with corticosteroids than with aspirin. For this reason, therapy should be tapered rather than discontinued abruptly, and aspirin administration should be continued for 1 month after treatment with adrenal steroids is discontinued.

Heart failure should be treated by conventional measures. The potential risk of digitalis-induced arrhythmias in the patient with active myocarditis must be kept in mind. As noted, in the absence of preexisting valvular disease, congestive heart failure in ARF patients is usually attributable primarily to valvular dilatation and not to myocardial failure. Patients with chorea require a quiet, nonstimulatory environment and sedation. Agents such as phenobarbital or diazepam may be used. In patients with severe and debilitating hyperkinesis, haloperidol has been given. A recent review has suggested valproic acid as first-line treatment and risperidone for nonresponders.[114] There is also recent evidence to suggest that corticosteroids may be beneficial in decreasing both the intensity and duration of the manifestations.[115] The potential role of plasmapheresis and IV immunoglobulin for the rare cases of intractable chorea is under investigation.[116]

The only long-term sequela of ARF is RHD. The prognosis in rheumatic patients has been greatly improved by our ability to prevent recurrent attacks, with their concomitant threat of additional valvular damage. The ultimate prognosis of an individual attack is related to the severity of cardiac involvement during the acute phase. This was best studied in the United Kingdom–United States report.[117] In that study, only 6% of patients with no carditis or with only questionable carditis during their attack of ARF were found to have heart murmurs when reexamined 10 years later. Heart disease was present at follow-up in 30% of the patients initially found to have only apical systolic murmurs, in 40% of those with basal diastolic murmurs during the acute phase, and in 68% of those who initially suffered from congestive heart failure, pericarditis, or both. Patients with pure chorea appear to have a relatively high incidence of late development of rheumatic heart disease, even if carditis is not recognized at the time of the initial attack. These finding may, however, have to be reevaluated in the echocardiographic era.

Our concepts of the prevalence of rheumatic heart disease in developing countries may require revision in view of the results of echocardiographic screening of some 5800 randomly selected schoolchildren in Columbia and Mozambique.[118] The authors reported the prevalence of rheumatic heart disease to be approximately 10-fold greater than that recognized by conventional clinical screening. If confirmed by other investigators, prospective follow-up of these children will be required to determine the functional implications of these imaging studies.

PREVENTION

Prevention of ARF in persons without a prior history of this disease depends on accurate diagnosis and appropriate treatment of the antecedent streptococcal infection. This approach (so-called primary pre-

TABLE 199-4	Secondary Prevention of Rheumatic Fever (Prevention of Recurrent Attacks)	
Agent	**Dose**	**Mode**
Benzathine penicillin G	600,000 U for children ≤27 kg (60 lb), 1.2 million U for those >27 kg (60 lb) every 4 wks*	Intramuscular
Penicillin V	250 mg twice daily	Oral
Sulfadiazine	0.5 g once daily for patients ≤27 kg (60 lb) 1.0 g once daily for patients >27 kg (60 lb)	Oral
For individuals allergic to penicillin and sulfadiazine:		
Macrolide or azalide	Variable	Oral

*In high-risk situations, administration every 3 weeks is justified and recommended.
From Gerber MA, Baltimore RS, Eaton CB, et al. Prevention of rheumatic fever and diagnosis and treatment of acute streptococcal pharyngitis. *Circulation*. 2009;191:1541-1551. Copyright 2009, American Heart Association, Inc. Reprinted with permission.

vention) is outlined in Chapter 198. It is effective,[119] but suffers from the limitation that one third or more of ARF cases follow streptococcal infections that are entirely subclinical or too mild to bring them to medical attention.

Rheumatic patients are at extremely high risk of developing recurrent ARF after immunologically significant streptococcal upper respiratory infections. These persons require continuous prophylaxis to prevent intercurrent streptococcal infections. The recommended regimen[120] for most patients in the United States and other countries in which ARF incidence is low consists of a single injection of penicillin G benzathine administered every 4 weeks (Table 199-4). In the most comprehensive study reported to date,[121] children following this regimen experienced a rheumatic fever recurrence rate of only 0.4/100 patient-years of observation. In areas of the world in which ARF and RHD remain very highly prevalent, ARF recurrence rates have been found to be even lower when injections of penicillin G benzathine are administered every 3 weeks rather than every 4 weeks.[122] A similar regimen may be appropriate for high-risk individuals, such as those with rheumatic heart disease. The possible benefits of the 3-week regimen must be balanced against the potential decrease in patient compliance and increase in associated costs.

Oral sulfadiazine or penicillin V are also acceptable prophylactic agents but are less effective than penicillin G benzathine (see Table 199-4). The lesser efficacy of oral regimens is at least in part the result of the extreme difficulty of enforcing compliance. Patients allergic to penicillin and sulfadiazine may be given erythromycin. Patients requiring protection for many years are often begun on a regimen of penicillin G benzathine, which is changed to oral prophylaxis later when the risk of recurrence is deemed to be lower.

The optimal duration of continuous antimicrobial prophylaxis remains controversial. The risk of ARF recurrence is neither continuous nor uniform. It declines with the age of the patient and the number of years since the most recent attack. It is positively correlated with the number of previous attacks and with the presence and severity of preexisting rheumatic heart disease. Thus, the risk of recurrence becomes low in older adults without heart disease who are not in intimate contact with school-aged children. In view of these facts, the physician must make the decision as to when and if to discontinue prophylaxis after discussion with the patient and after careful assessment of the patient's risk of acquiring a streptococcal infection, the anticipated recurrence rate per infection, and the likely consequences of such recurrence. Even when all these factors are favorable, prophylaxis should not be discontinued until the patient has reached his or her early 20s and at least 5 years have elapsed since the most recent rheumatic attack.[123] Recommendations of the American Heart Association are given in Table 199-5.

Investigative efforts are currently being directed toward the development of a safe, effective M-protein vaccine for the prevention of streptococcal infection and ARF. Such a vaccine would have to provide

protection against the major serotypes associated with ARF and deeply invasive infections.[124,125]

Glomerulonephritis

Poststreptococcal AGN is an acute inflammatory disorder of the renal glomerulus characterized pathologically by diffuse proliferative glomerular lesions and clinically by edema, hypertension, hematuria, and proteinuria. The disease is a delayed nonsuppurative sequela of pharyngeal or cutaneous infection with certain nephritogenic group A streptococcal strains belonging to a limited number of serotypes.

HISTORY

Richard Bright (1789-1858) clearly differentiated cardiac from renal dropsy. He also noted the association between acute diseases, particularly scarlet fever, and AGN.[126] Subsequently, many investigators confirmed the relationship between β-hemolytic streptococcal infections and AGN. Schick,[127] in 1907, commented on the similarity of the latent period in serum sickness to that in AGN, thus suggesting the possibility of an immunologic basis for the latter disease. Rammelkamp and Weaver[128] explained the puzzling variations in attack rate of AGN after group A streptococcal infection by proposing that only certain serotypes of *Streptococcus pyogenes* were nephritogenic. Detailed prospective studies of the epidemiology, bacteriology, immunology, and natural history of pyoderma-associated nephritis by Wannamaker[129] in Minnesota, Potter and colleagues[130] in south Trinidad, and Dillon and co-workers[131] in Alabama have added greatly to our understanding of this disease.

ETIOLOGY AND PATHOGENESIS

Poststreptococcal AGN follows infection with a limited number of group A streptococcal serotypes (see Table 199-1). Type 12 is the most frequent M serotype causing AGN after pharyngitis or tonsillitis, whereas M-49 is the type most frequently related to pyoderma-associated nephritis. Not all streptococcal strains belonging to these serotypes are nephritogenic, however. As yet, there are no reliable biologic markers to differentiate nephritogenic from non-nephritogenic streptococci. Poststreptococcal AGN is almost always caused by strains of serogroup A. Well-documented outbreaks caused by group C organisms (*Streptococcus equi* subsp. *zooepidemicus*) have been reported, however.[132-134]

The precise mechanism whereby streptococcal infection gives rise to AGN has not been delineated. The weight of evidence favors the view that the renal injury is immunologically mediated. Such evidence includes the latent period between infection and the development of AGN, the associated hypocomplementemia, and the fact that immunoglobulins, complement components, and antigens that react with streptococcal antisera are present in the renal glomerulus early in the course of the disease.[135-138] It is possible that antibodies elicited

TABLE 199-5	Duration of Secondary Rheumatic Fever Prophylaxis
Category	**Duration After Last Attack**
Rheumatic fever with carditis and residual heart disease (persistent valvular disease*)	10 yr or until age 40, whichever is longer; sometimes lifelong prophylaxis (see text)
Rheumatic fever with carditis but no residual heart disease (no valvular disease*)	10 yr or until age 21, whichever is longer
Rheumatic fever without carditis	5 yr or until age 21, whichever is longer

*Clinical or echocardiographic evidence.
From Gerber MA, Baltimore RS, Eaton CB, et al. Prevention of rheumatic fever and diagnosis and treatment of acute streptococcal pharyngitis. *Circulation*. 2009;191:1541-1551. Copyright 2009, American Heart Association, Inc. Reprinted with permission.

by nephritogenic streptococci react with renal tissues in such a way as to produce glomerular injury. Indeed, antigenic similarities between constituents of the streptococcus and the human kidney have been described.[139-141] On the other hand, the electron microscopic finding of nodular subepithelial "humps" in renal biopsy specimens from patients with AGN suggests that the renal injury may be caused by deposition of preformed complexes consisting of streptococcal antigen and host antibody within the glomerulus. Such subepithelial nodular deposits are a characteristic feature of experimentally induced disease caused by circulating immune complexes. Several groups[142-144] have detected circulating immune complexes in AGN. The possible role of cellular immune mechanisms has not yet been adequately explored.

The identity of the streptococcal constituent(s) involved in the pathogenesis of AGN remains unknown. M protein is an obvious candidate because of the close association of nephrotogenicity and the M serotype. Monoclonal antibodies raised against human glomeruli have been found to cross react with streptococcal M protein.[141] Moreover, in an animal model of nephritis induced by nephritogenic type 12 streptococci, eluted bound glomerular antibodies were found to be directed against type 12 M protein but not against other streptococcal and renal antigens.[145] Others, however, have described cross-reactions between fragments of streptococcal cell membrane and human glomerular basement membrane[139]; proliferative glomerular lesions in rhesus monkeys have been produced by immunization with streptococcal membrane fragments or by IV injection of antibodies to these fragments.[146]

Two antigens isolated from nephritogenic streptococci are currently under investigation in regard to their role in the pathogenesis of AGN—streptococcal pyrogenic exotoxin B and its zymogen precursor[147-150] and a nephritis-associated plasmin-receptor (NAPlr).[151] The latter demonstrates both plasmin(ogen)-binding activity and glyceraldehyde phosphate dehydrogenase (GAPDH) activity. Both these substances have affinity for the glomeruli and induce long-lasting antibody responses. Another nephritis strain–associated protein, initially identified as an extracellular product of nephritogenic streptococci, has been characterized as a streptokinase. Streptokinase production has been postulated to play a role in the pathogenesis of AGN[152] and has been found to be essential for development of the disease in a mouse model.[153] However, there is no unique reactivity to group A streptokinase in sera of AGN patients, nor has streptokinase deposition been demonstrated in biopsy specimens obtained early in the disease.[154]

PATHOLOGIC CHARACTERISTICS

In the acute phase of illness, light microscopic examination of renal biopsy specimens demonstrates a marked increase in glomerular intracapillary cellularity caused by endothelial and mesangial cell proliferation. These changes involve almost all the glomeruli, which appear enlarged and bloodless, tending to fill the Bowman space.[155] In addition to this diffuse proliferative endocapillary process, a variable degree of polymorphonuclear leukocytic exudation is observed. Proliferation of parietal and visceral epithelial cells only occurs to a modest degree and is rarely extensive enough to give rise to well-developed crescent formation. Thin sectioning and special strains may reveal discrete deposits on the epithelial side of the basement membrane that correspond to the humps visible on electron microscopy. Focal degeneration, interstitial edema, and cellular infiltration also occur in the renal tubular cells, but these tubular changes are far less prominent than is the glomerulitis. Arterioles are normal or almost normal in most cases of AGN.

Immunofluorescence technique demonstrates considerable variability in the pattern of deposition of immunoglobulin and complement components. C3 is almost always present in the glomeruli, and deposits of IgG are also frequently demonstrable. These substances are present in the form of discrete deposits similar in size and location to the subepithelial humps visualized under the electron microscope,[136,137]

although deposits of C3 may also occur in an interrupted linear pattern along the basement membrane or in the mesangium.[137] Deposits of IgM, C1q, C4, and fibrin are found less commonly. The rather weak and inconsistent deposition of early complement components suggests that activation of the alternate complement pathway may play a role in the immunopathology of AGN.

EPIDEMIOLOGY

It has been estimated that over 470,000 cases of AGN occur annually worldwide, with approximately 5000 deaths.[156] The great majority of these occur in less developed countries. The epidemiologic characteristics of AGN largely reflect those of the antecedent group A streptococcal infection—that is, pharyngitis or pyoderma (Table 199-6). Thus, the classic streptococcal sore throat occurs primarily among school-age children during the cooler months of the year. Pyoderma is largely a disease of children aged 2 to 6 years and, in temperate climates, occurs during the summer and early fall. Studies have suggested that, given a skin infection with a nephritogenic strain, the attack rate of AGN is higher in children 6 years of age or younger than in older children.[157] AGN can also follow cutaneous infections other than pyoderma.[158,159] The latent period of AGN is variable but averaged 10 days after pharyngeal infection in the studies of Stetson and colleagues[160]; prospective studies at Red Lake Indian Reservation in Minnesota have indicated the usual latent period of pyoderma-associated AGN to be 3 weeks or longer.[157]

Although the attack rate of AGN after throat or skin infection with a nephritogenic strain is substantial (i.e., 10% to 15%),[157,161] the disease differs dramatically from acute rheumatic fever in that recurrences are rare. This is attributable at least in part to the relatively limited number of streptococcal strains that are nephritogenic and presumably also to the acquisition of type-specific protective immunity to the serotype that elicited the initial attack. When second attacks of AGN do occur, they are clinically and histologically indistinguishable from the initial attack.[162] A more commonly recognized phenomenon than recurrent AGN attacks is the propensity for streptococcal infections to precipitate exacerbations of chronic glomerulonephritis.[163] Such exacerbations often occur after a relatively brief latent period of 1 to 4 days. The coexistence of ARF and AGN in the same patient after pharyngeal infection is rare, but a few such cases have been reported.[164,165]

The introduction of a highly nephritogenic strain into a family unit may result in multiple cases. When systematic screening of sibling contacts for hypertension, urinary abnormalities, and serum complement levels has been performed, the incidence of proven and suspected cases of AGN in sibling contacts has been extremely variable,[166-169] with estimates ranging as high as 20%.[170]

TABLE 199-6	Epidemiologic Characteristics of Pharyngitis-Associated and Pyodermia-Associated Acute Glomerulonephritis	
Feature	*Pharyngitis-Associated AGN*	*Pyoderma-Associated AGN*
Age	Early school age	Preschool age
Gender	Male-to-female ratio ≅ 2:1	Equally distributed
Season	Winter and spring	Late summer and early fall
Geographic distribution	North and south	Predominantly south
Familial occurrence	Common	Common
Latent period	10 days	3 wk
Attack rate*	10%-15%	10%-15%
Serologic types	Limited types	Also limited, but different types
Recurrences	Rare	Rare

*After infection with known nephritogenic strain.
AGN, Acute glomerulonephritis.
From Wannamaker LW. Differences between streptococcal infections of the throat and of the skin. *N Engl J Med.* 1970;282:23-31.

CLINICAL AND LABORATORY FEATURES

The typical clinical features of AGN, as seen in children entering the hospital with this disease, include edema, hypertension, and smoke- or rust-colored urine. Patients also exhibit pallor and may complain of lethargy, malaise, weakness, anorexia, headache, and dull back pain. Fever is not a prominent finding.

Facial and periorbital edema are usually present, especially on arising in the morning, but edema also involves dependent areas such as the feet and legs, scrotum, and sacrum. In severe cases, ascites or pleural effusions may occur. Another manifestation of fluid overload is circulatory congestion, which may give rise to dyspnea, orthopnea, rales at the lung bases, distended neck veins, and even frank pulmonary edema. Manifestations of circulatory overload tend to be particularly prominent in the occasional cases of AGN occurring in older adults and, in these patients, may obscure the correct diagnosis if urinary findings are not properly interpreted.

Hypertension occurs in most patients but is usually of modest degree. Hypertensive retinopathy or heart failure do not ordinarily complicate the clinical picture. On the other hand, a small proportion of AGN patients, perhaps 5% to 10%, develop severe hypertension complicated by signs and symptoms of encephalopathy. These range from headache and vomiting to confusion, somnolence, and convulsions.

Although these clinical features are typical of hospitalized patients, many cases of AGN are so mild as to escape detection unless those at risk are tested prospectively for urinary sediment abnormalities and serum complement levels. Two studies that included renal biopsy data have concluded that in epidemic situations, as many as 50% of cases of AGN may be subclinical.[167,170] Whatever the exact proportion might be, and chances are that this varies considerably in differing epidemiologic settings, it seems clear that subclinical episodes of AGN are by no means rare.

Laboratory findings include a mild normocytic normochromic anemia, elevated erythrocyte sedimentation rate, slight hypoproteinemia, and elevations of the blood urea nitrogen and serum creatinine concentrations. Hypercholesterolemia and hyperlipemia may also be present. Serum levels of total hemolytic complement and C3 complement are markedly reduced in the great majority of patients with clinically apparent AGN. Urine volume may be significantly diminished, and the urine itself is smoky, rusty, or brownish, with a high specific gravity and positive test findings for protein and hemoglobin. Total urinary protein excretion is usually less than 3 g/day.[171] Microscopic examination of the urine reveals erythrocytes, leukocytes, and hyaline, granular, and red blood cell casts.

The urinary abnormalities in AGN must be distinguished from the mild hematuria and proteinuria that may be seen during the acute phase of acute streptococcal infection and other febrile illnesses. The relationship, if any, of these early urinary findings to the development of AGN is at present unknown.[172] Finally, diagnostic confusion is almost inevitable in the rare cases in which pronounced clinical manifestations of AGN occur in patients with minimal or no urinary sediment abnormalities.[173]

DIAGNOSIS

The diagnosis of AGN is based on the clinical history, physical findings, and confirmatory evidence of antecedent streptococcal infection. The latter may include a recent history of scarlet fever, isolation of group A streptococci from throat or skin lesions, or demonstration of elevated serum titers of streptococcal antibodies. Even in the absence of bacteriologic isolation of streptococci, the presence of skin lesions morphologically compatible with streptococcal impetigo is highly suggestive.

It is almost always possible to demonstrate an elevated level of streptococcal antibodies in AGN although, in cases with relatively short latent periods, serial bleedings may be necessary. It must be recalled that in pyoderma-associated nephritis ASO responses are weak and it is frequently necessary to perform serum titrations of anti-DNase B. Although anti–Streptozyme titers rise in pyoderma nephritis, technical problems limit the reliability of the test. Finally, if renal biopsy is performed, the demonstration of diffuse proliferative glomerulonephritis with subepithelial electron-dense deposits is a very helpful confirmatory finding.

Poststreptococcal acute glomerulonephritis must be differentiated from other infectious processes involving the kidney. It is, for example, often extremely difficult to differentiate an acute exacerbation of chronic glomerulonephritis, such as may be precipitated by streptococci or by other intercurrent infections, from a true attack of AGN. A short latent period of 1 to 4 days suggests that the episode is an exacerbation of preexisting renal disease. Patients with subacute bacterial endocarditis tend to develop high serum levels of circulating immune complexes and may develop diffuse proliferative or focal glomerulonephritis, both of which may be confused clinically with poststreptococcal nephritis. Other bacterial and protozoan illnesses such as pneumococcal pneumonia, typhoid fever, leptospirosis, syphilis, toxoplasmosis, and *Plasmodium falciparum* malaria have been reported on occasion to be associated with nephritis. Viral infections such as hepatitis B and C, infectious mononucleosis, measles, mumps, and togaviral and enteroviral disease have similarly been implicated as causes of viruria, transient renal dysfunction, or actual glomerulonephritis.[174] In addition to the development of focal and segmental glomerulosclerosis, patients infected with the human immunodeficiency virus may rarely develop an immune complex glomerulonephritis.[175] Other entities that may at times mimic AGN are Henoch-Schönlein disease, systemic lupus erythematosus, polyarteritis nodosa, acute tubular necrosis, focal glomerulonephritis with hematuria, hereditary nephritis, rapidly progressive glomerulonephritis, idiopathic nephrotic syndrome, and malignant hypertension.

TREATMENT

Because no form of treatment is known to alter the long-term prognosis of AGN, therapy is directed toward management of the acute problems. Attention is directed to what is ordinarily the most immediate problem—namely, circulatory overload. In most cases, this is handled adequately by salt and fluid restriction alone, but at times diuretics are required. Digitalis is not indicated because the risk of toxicity is substantial and usually myocardial function is intact.[176] Specific antihypertensive therapy is usually unnecessary, but in cases of severe hypertension and hypertensive encephalopathy, potent parenteral agents are required. Patients developing acute pulmonary edema or severe and prolonged oliguria require measures conventionally used in these conditions.

All nonallergic patients should receive penicillin, preferably penicillin G benzathine (see Chapter 198 for dosage schedule), to eradicate the nephritogenic streptococcal strain. Penicillin-allergic patients should receive one of the alternative regimens listed in Chapter 198. In addition to urinalysis and serum C3 complement determination, family contacts should have cultures of throat and skin lesions. Persons with positive cultures for group A streptococci should be treated appropriately. Such treatment is for epidemiologic purposes only and will not modify the course of preexistent AGN nor, in all probability, abort the disease in persons who are within the latent period (see later).

With skillful use of the supportive measures outlined in the preceding, mortality during the acute phase of AGN is now rare. Perhaps 1% or fewer of patients develop severe and irreversible renal failure. In the remainder, signs and symptoms often begin to abate within a few days after admission. Serum complement levels return to normal within a month, but microscopic hematuria and cylindruria frequently persist for months, despite the patient's general feeling of well-being.

PREVENTION

Although penicillin treatment of the antecedent streptococcal infection is highly efficacious in preventing acute rheumatic fever, the same does not appear to be the case in AGN. Stetson and colleagues,[160] in a controlled study of an epidemic of pharyngitis-associated (type 12) AGN in a military population, found a small but not statistically significant[177] preventive effect of penicillin. Uncontrolled observations during an epidemic of nephritis in Israel[178] (both throat and skin infections caused by M type 55) documented the occurrence of AGN in a number of subjects who had received prior antibiotic therapy according to different dosage regimens. Moreover, there was no difference in the clinical severity of AGN between subjects who had and those who had not received antibiotic therapy. Data available at present are not adequate to determine whether penicillin might have a small effect on the primary prevention of AGN, but such an effect, at any rate, is not striking.[179]

As noted, penicillin is nevertheless effective in epidemiologic attempts to eradicate nephritogenic strains by treatment of AGN patients and their colonized family contacts. In appropriate high-risk settings during epidemics of AGN, universal penicillin prophylaxis of selected populations might be considered in a manner somewhat analogous to that used in U.S. military recruit camps for rheumatic fever control. Such universal prophylaxis is rarely indicated and should be used only after careful consideration of the specific epidemiologic parameters involved.

Because recurrent episodes of AGN are so rare, continuous antistreptococcal prophylaxis, such as that used in the secondary prevention of rheumatic fever, is unnecessary.

PROGNOSIS

One of the most important issues relating to poststreptococcal glomerulonephritis is the frequency with which patients afflicted with the disease eventually develop chronic glomerulonephritis. In a certain group of AGN patients constituting only a small percentage of its victims, the acute attack is never resolved and the disease enters a subacute phase, leading to an almost complete loss of renal function within 6 months to 2 years. It is the ultimate fate of the remainder of the patients in whom the illness appears to have resolved clinically that remains controversial. Most observers now agree that the long-term prognosis in children is excellent. A 10-year follow-up of 61 patients involved in an epidemic at Red Lake, Minnesota,[180] revealed no cases

of chronic glomerulonephritis. Moreover, in a 12- to 17-year follow-up of 534 Trinidadians convalescent from AGN,[181] only 3.5% of the subjects had persistent urine abnormalities, 3.7% were hypertensive, and none had serum creatinine values higher than 1.25 mg/dL. These figures are not in excess of what would be expected in surveys of normal populations. Almost all the Trinidadian patients had been children at the time of their attack of AGN. There was no difference in outcome of sporadic AGN cases as opposed to those associated with epidemics. A report from Australia, however, noted increased prevalences of albuminuria and hematuria in Aboriginal children several years convalescent from two epidemics of AGN. There were no significant differences between patients and controls in blood pressure, serum creatinine level, or calculated glomerular filtration rate.[182]

These data stand in sharp contrast to Baldwin's findings, who followed 168 subjects for periods up to 18 years and concluded that "irreversible renal damage has ensued in 50% of these patients, as evidenced by the presence of proteinuria and/or hypertension,"[183] although clinical uremia occurred in only 6 patients. Renal biopsy specimens from the subjects in this series showed that proliferative changes had decreased, whereas glomerulosclerosis of marked degree was present in more than half of the specimens. Their study population contained a high proportion of adults, who are generally agreed to have a worse prognosis than children.[184] Moreover, the results presented have been challenged because of the difficulty of sorting out exacerbations of chronic nephritis from true de novo attacks of AGN in studies of sporadically occurring disease[185] and because of the paucity of published data documenting the poststreptococcal cause of the cases studied.[186] More recently, however, a follow-up of Brazilian adults who contracted AGN from consumption of cheese contaminated with *Streptococcus zooepidemicus* revealed a high rate of hypertension and renal abnormalities, with some patients having reached end-stage renal disease.[134,187]

Based on the bulk of currently available data, it seems likely that more than 90% of children with AGN make an uneventful recovery, and that this disease in the pediatric age group is not an important precursor of chronic glomerulonephritis or hypertension. The prognosis appears more guarded in adult patients,[134,188] but the proportion who might be left with residual renal function impairment is at present unknown.

REFERENCES

1. Stollerman GH. *Rheumatic Fever and Streptococcal Infection.* New York: Grune & Stratton, 1975.
2. Bisno AL. The concept of rheumatogenic and non-rheumatogenic group A streptococci. In: Read SE, Zabriskie JB, eds. *Streptococcal Diseases and the Immune Response.* New York: Academic Press; 1980:789-803.
3. Kuttner AG, Krumwiede E. Observations on the effect of streptococcal upper respiratory infections on rheumatic children: A three-year study. *J Clin Invest.* 1941;20:273-287.
4. Potter EV, Svartman M, Mohammed I, et al. Tropical acute rheumatic fever and associated streptococcal infections compared with concurrent acute glomerulonephritis. *J Pediatr.* 1978;92:325-333.
5. Berrios X, Quesney F, Morales A, et al. Acute rheumatic fever and poststreptococcal glomerulonephritis in an open population: Comparative studies of epidemiology and bacteriology. *J Lab Clin Med.* 1986; 108:535-542.
6. Martin DR, Voss LM, Walker SJ, et al. Acute rheumatic fever in Auckland, New Zealand: Spectrum of associated group A streptococci different from expected. *Pediatr Infect Dis J.* 1994;13:264-269.
7. McDonald M, Currie BJ, Carapetis JR. Acute rheumatic fever: A chink in the chain that links the heart to the throat? *Lancet Infect Dis.* 2004;4:240-245.
8. Bisno AL, Pearce IA, Wall HP, et al. Contrasting epidemiology of acute rheumatic fever and acute glomerulonephritis: Nature of the antecedent streptococcal infection. *N Engl J Med.* 1970;283:561-565.
9. Bisno AL, Pearce IA, Stollerman GH. Streptococcal infections that fail to cause recurrences of rheumatic fever. *J Infect Dis.* 1977;136:278-285.
10. Smoot JC, Barbian KD, Van Gompel JJ, et al. Genome sequence and comparative microarray analysis of serotype M18 group A Streptococcus strains associated with acute rheumatic fever outbreaks. *Proc Natl Acad Sci U S A.* 2002;99:4668-4673.
11. Smoot JC, Korgenski EK, Daly JA, et al. Molecular analysis of group A Streptococcus type emm18 isolates temporally associ-

ated with acute rheumatic fever outbreaks in Salt Lake City, Utah. *J Clin Microbiol.* 2002;40:1805-1810.
12. Bessen DE, Fischetti VA. Differentiation between two biologically distinct classes of group A streptococci by limited substitutions of amino acids within the shared region of M protein-like molecules. *J Exp Med.* 1990;172:1757-1764.
13. Bessen DE, Veasy LG, Hill HR, et al. Serologic evidence for a class I group A streptococcal infection among rheumatic fever patients. *J Infect Dis.* 1995;172:1608-1611.
14. Stollerman GH, Dale JB. The importance of the group a streptococcus capsule in the pathogenesis of human infections: a historical perspective. *Clin Infect Dis.* 2008; 46:1038-1045.
15. Veasy LG, Tani LY, Daly JA, et al. Temporal association of the appearance of mucoid strains of Streptococcus pyogenes with a continuing high incidence of rheumatic fever in Utah. *Pediatrics.* 2004; 113(Pt 1):e168-e172.
16. Stollerman GH. Rheumatogenic streptococci and autoimmunity. *Clin Immunol Immunopathol.* 1991;61:131-142.
17. Froude J, Gibofsky A, Buskirk DR, et al. Cross-reactivity between streptococcus and human tissue: A model of molecular mimicry and autoimmunity. *Curr Top Microbiol Immunol.* 1989;145:5-26.
18. Cunningham MW. T cell mimicry in inflammatory heart disease. *Mol Immunol.* 2004;40:1121-1127.
19. Dale JB, Beachey EH. Epitopes of streptococcal M proteins shared with cardiac myosin. *J Exp Med.* 1985;162:583-591.
20. Dale JB, Beachey EH. Protective antigenic determinant of streptococcal M protein shared with sarcolemmal membrane protein of human heart. *J Exp Med.* 1982;156:1165-1176.
21. Baird RW, Bronze MS, Kraus W, et al. Epitopes of group A streptococcal M protein shared with antigens of articular cartilage and synovium. *J Immunol.* 1991;146: 3132-3137.
22. Goldstein I, Rebeyrotte P, Parlebas J, et al. Isolation from heart valves of glycopeptides which share immunological properties with *Streptococcus haemolyticus* group A polysaccharides. *Nature.* 1968;219:866-868.

23. Dudding BA, Ayoub EM. Persistence of streptococcal group A antibody in patients with rheumatic valvular disease. *J Exp Med.* 1968;128:1081-1098.
24. Schwab JH, Cromartie WJ. Immunological studies on a C polysaccharide complex of group A streptococci having a direct toxic effect on connective tissue. *J Exp Med.* 1960;111:295-307.
25. Fillit HM, McCarty M, Blake M. Induction of antibodies to hyaluronic acid by immunization of rabbits with encapsulated streptococci. *J Exp Med.* 1986;164:762-776.
26. Husby G, van de Rijn I, Zabriskie JB, et al. Antibodies reacting with cytoplasm of subthalamic and caudate nuclei neurons in chorea and rheumatic fever. *J Exp Med.* 1976;144:1094-1110.
27. Zabriskie JB. T-cells and T-cell clones in rheumatic fever valvulitis: Getting to the heart of the matter? *Circulation.* 1995;92:281-282.
28. Carreno-Manjarrez R, Visvanathan K, Zabriskie JB. Immunogenic and genetic factors in rheumatic fever. *Curr Infect Dis Rep.* 2000;2:302-307.
29. Read SE, Fischetti VA, Utermohlen V, et al. Cellular reactivity studies to streptococcal antigens. Migration inhibition studies in patients with streptococcal infections and rheumatic fever. *J Clin Invest.* 1974;54:439-450.
30. Morris K, Mohan C, Wahi PL, et al. Increase in activated T cells and reduction in suppressor/cytotoxic T cells in acute rheumatic fever and active heart disease: A longitudinal study. *J Infect Dis.* 1993;167:979-983.
31. Kemeny E, Grieve T, Marcus R, et al. Identification of mononuclear cells and T cell subsets in rheumatic valvulitis. *Clin Immunol Immunopathol.* 1989;52:225-237.
32. Morris K, Mohan C, Wahi PL, et al. Enhancement of IL-1, IL-2 production and IL-2 receptor generation in patients with acute rheumatic fever and active rheumatic heart disease; a prospective study. *Clin Exp Immunol.* 1993;91:429-436.
33. Zedan MM, el-Shennawy FA, Abou-Bakr HM, et al. Interleukin-2 in relation to T cell subpopulations in rheumatic heart disease. *Arch Dis Child.* 1992;67:1373-1375.

34. Tomai M, Kotb M, Majumdar G, et al. Superantigenicity of streptococcal M protein. *J Exp Med*. 1990;172:359-362.
35. Schlievert PM. Role of staphylococcal and streptococcal pyrogenic-toxin superantigens in human disease. *Mediguide Infect Dis*. 1993;13:1-7.
36. Ayoub EM, Barrett DJ, Maclaren NK, et al. Association of class II human histocompatibility leukocyte antigens with rheumatic fever. *J Clin Invest*. 1986;77: 2019-2026.
37. Anastasiou-Nana MI, Anderson JL, Carlquist JF, et al. HLA-DR typing and lymphocyte subset evaluation in rheumatic heart disease: A search for immune response factors. *Am Heart J*. 1986;112:992-997.
38. Khanna AK, Buskirk DR, Williams RC Jr, et al. Presence of a non-HLA B cell antigen in rheumatic fever patients and their families as defined by a monoclonal antibody. *J Clin Invest*. 1989;83:1710-1716.
39. Gibofsky A, Khanna A, Suh E, et al. The genetics of rheumatic fever: Relationship to streptococcal infection and autoimmune disease. *J Rheumatol (Suppl)*. 1991;30:1-5.
40. Virmani R, Farb A, Burke AP, et al. Pathology of acute rheumatic carditis. In: Narula J, Virmani R, Reddy KS, Tandon R, eds. *Rheumatic Fever*. Washington, DC: Armed Forces Institute of Pathology; 1999:217-234.
41. Chopra P, Wanniang J, Kumar AS. Immunochemical and histochemical profile of Aschoff bodies in rheumatic carditis in excised left atrial appendages: An immunoperoxidase study in fresh and paraffin-embedded tissue. *Int J Cardiol*. 1992;34:199-207.
42. Husby GH, Arora R, Williams RC, et al. Immunofluorescent studies of florid rheumatic Aschoff lesions. *Arthritis Rheum*. 1986;29:207-211.
43. Tani LY, Veasy LG, Minich LL, et al. Rheumatic fever in children younger than 5 years: Is the presentation different? *Pediatrics*. 2003;112:1065-1068.
44. Ben-Dov I, Berry E. Acute rheumatic fever in adults over the age of 45 years: An analysis of 23 patients together with a review of the literature. *Semin Arthritis Rheum*. 1980;10:100-110.
45. Feuer J, Spiera H. Acute rheumatic fever in adults: A resurgence in the Hasidic Jewish community. *J Rheumatol*. 1997;24: 337-340.
46. Deighton C. Beta haemolytic streptococci and reactive arthritis in adults. *Ann Rheum Dis*. 1993;52:475-482.
47. Rammelkamp CH, Denny FW, Wannamaker LW. Studies on the epidemiology of rheumatic fever in the armed services. In: Thomas L, ed. *Rheumatic Fever*. Minneapolis: University of Minnesota Press; 1952:72-89.
48. Siegel AC, Johnson EE, Stollerman GH. Controlled studies of streptococcal pharyngitis in a pediatric population. I. Factors related to the attack rate of rheumatic fever. *N Engl J Med*. 1961;265:559-566.
49. WHO Cardiovascular Diseases Unit and Principal Investigators. WHO programme for the prevention of rheumatic fever/rheumatic heart disease in 16 developing countries: Report from Phase I (1986-90). *Bull World Health Organ*. 1992;70:213-218.
50. Eisenberg MJ. Rheumatic heart disease in the developing world: Prevalence, prevention, and control. *Eur Heart J*. 1993;14:122-128.
51. Carapetis JR, McDonald M, Wilson NJ. Acute rheumatic fever. *Lancet*. 2005; 366:155-168.
52. Carapetis JR, Wolff DR, Currie BJ. Acute rheumatic fever and rheumatic heart disease in the top end of Australia's Northern Territory. *Med J Aust*. 1996;164:146-149.
53. Land MA, Bisno AL. Acute rheumatic fever: A vanishing disease in suburbia. *JAMA*. 1983;249:895-898.
54. Veasy LG, Wiedmeier SE, Orsmond GS, et al. Resurgence of acute rheumatic fever in the intermountain area of the United States. *N Engl J Med*. 1987;316:421-427.
55. Ferguson GW, Shultz JM, Bisno AL. Epidemiology of acute rheumatic fever in a multi-ethnic, multi-racial U.S. urban community: The Miami-Dade experience. *J Infect Dis*. 1991;164:720-725.
56. Bisno AL. The resurgence of acute rheumatic fever in the United States. *Annu Rev Med*. 1990;41:319-329.
57. Veasy LG, Tani LY, Hill HR. Persistence of acute rheumatic fever in the intermountain area of the United States. *J Pediatr*. 1994;124:9-16.
58. Wallace MR, Garst PD, Papadimos TJ, et al. The return of acute rheumatic fever in young adults. *JAMA*. 1989;262:2557-2561.
59. Centers for Disease Control (CDC). Acute rheumatic fever among Army trainees—Fort Leonard Wood, Missouri, 1987-1988. *Morbid Mortal Wkly Rep MMWR*. 1988;37:519-522.
60. Zangwill KM, Wald ER, Londino AV Jr. Acute rheumatic fever in western Pennsylvania: A persistent problem into the 1990s. *J Pediatr*. 1991;118:561-563.
61. Bisno AL. Group A streptococcal infections and acute rheumatic fever. *N Engl J Med*. 1991;325:783-793.
62. Taranta A, Wood HF, Feinstein AR, et al. Rheumatic fever in children and adolescents. A long-term epidemiologic study of subsequent prophylaxis, streptococcal infections, and clinical sequelae. IV. Relation of the rheumatic fever recurrence rate per streptococcal infection to the titers of streptococcal antibodies. *Ann Intern Med*. 1964;60(Suppl 5):47-57.
63. Rammelkamp CH Jr, Stolzer BL. The latent period before the onset of acute rheumatic fever. *Yale J Biol Med*. 1961;34:386-398.
64. Sanyal SK, Thapar MK, Ahmed SH, et al. The initial attack of acute rheumatic fever during childhood in North India; a prospective study of the clinical profile. *Circulation*. 1974; 49:7-12.
65. Ravisha MS, Tullu MS, Kamat JR. Rheumatic fever and rheumatic heart disease: clinical profile of 550 cases in India. *Arch Med Res*. 2003; 34:382-387.
66. Kamblock J, Payot L, Iung B, et al. Does rheumatic myocarditis really exists? Systematic study with echocardiography and cardiac troponin I blood levels. *Eur Heart J*. 2003;24: 855-862.
67. Gentles TL, Colan SD, Wilson NJ, et al. Left ventricular mechanics during and after acute rheumatic fever: Contractile dysfunction is closely related to valve regurgitation. *J Am Coll Cardiol*. 2001;37:201-207.
68. Vasan RS, Shrivastava S, Vijayakumar M, et al. Echocardiographic evaluation of patients with acute rheumatic fever and rheumatic carditis. *Circulation*. 1996;94:73-82.
69. Essop MR, Wisenbaugh T, Sareli P. Evidence against a myocardiac factor as the cause of left ventricular dilation inactive rheumatic carditis. *J Am Coll Cardiol*. 1993;22:826-829.
70. Williams RV, Minich LL, Shaddy RE, et al. Evidence for lack of myocardial injury in children with acute rheumatic carditis. *Cardiol Young*. 2002;12:519-523.
71. Minich LL, Tani LY, Veasy LG. Role of echocardiography in the diagnosis and follow-up evaluation of rheumatic fever. In: Narula N, Virmani R, Reddy KS, Tandon R, eds. *Rheumatic Fever*. Washington, DC: Armed Forces Institute of Pathology; 1999:307-318.
72. Reddy DV, Chun LT, Yamamoto LG. Acute rheumatic fever with advanced degree AV block. *Clin Pediatr*. 1989;28: 326-328.
73. Feinstein AR, Spagnuolo M. The clinical patterns of acute rheumatic fever: A reappraisal. *Medicine*. 1962;41:279-305.
74. Carapetis JR, Currie BJ. Rheumatic fever in a high incidence population: The importance of monoarthritis and low grade fever. *Arch Dis Child*. 2001;85:223-227.
75. Arnold MH, Tyndall A. Poststreptococcal reactive arthritis. *Ann Rheum Dis*. 1989;48:686-688.
76. Tutar E, Atalay S, Yilmaz E, et al. Poststreptococcal reactive arthritis in children: Is it really a different entity from rheumatic fever? *Rheumatol Int*. 2002;22:80-83.
77. Barash J, Mashiach E, Navon-Elkan P, et al. Differentation of post-streptococcal reactive arthritis from acute rheumatic fever. *J Pediatr*. 2008; 153:696-699.
78. de Cunto CL, Giannini EH, Fink CW, et al. Prognosis of children with poststreptococcal reactive arthritis. *Pediatr Infect Dis J*. 1988;7:683-686.
79. Shulman ST, Ayoub EM. Poststreptococcal reactive arthritis. *Curr Opin Rheumatol*. 2002;14:562-565.
80. Lehman TJ, Edelheit BS. Clinical trials for post-streptococcal reactive arthritis. *Curr Rheumatol Rep*. 2001;3:363-364.
81. Iglesias-Gamarra A, Mendez EA, Cuellar ML, et al. Poststreptococcal reactive arthritis in adults: Long-term follow-up. *Am J Med Sci*. 2001;321:173-177.
82. Herold BC, Shulman ST. Poststreptococcal arthritis. *Pediatr Infect Dis J*. 1988;4:681-682.
83. Dajani AS, Ayoub E, Bierman FZ, et al. Guidelines for the diagnosis of rheumatic fever: Jones criteria, updated 1992. *Circulation*. 1993;87:302-307.
84. Ayoub EM, Majeed HA. Poststreptococcal reactive arthritis. *Curr Opin Rheumatol*. 2000;12:306-310.
85. Taranta A. Rheumatic fever: Clinical aspects. In: Hollander JL, McCarty DJ Jr, eds. *Arthritis and Allied Conditions*. Philadelphia: Lea & Febiger; 1972:764-820.
86. Berrios X, Quesney F, Morales A, et al. Are all recurrences of "pure" Sydenham's chorea true recurrences of acute rheumatic fever? *J Pediatr*. 1985;107:867-872.
87. Terreri MT, Roja SC, Len CA, et al. Sydenham's chorea—clinical and evolutive characteristics. *Sao Paulo Med J*. 2002;120:16-19.
88. Bland EF. Chorea as a manifestation of rheumatic fever: A long-term perspective. *Trans Am Clin Climatol Assoc*. 1961;73:209-213.
89. Murphy ML, Pichichero ME. Prospective identification and treatment of children with pediatric autoimmune neuropsychiatric disorder associated with group A streptococcal infection (PANDAS). *Arch Pediatr Adolesc Med*. 2002;156:356-361.
90. Leonard HL, Swedo SE. Paediatric autoimmune neuropsychiatric disorders associated with streptococcal infection (PANDAS). *Int J Neuropsychopharmacol*. 2001;4:191-198.
91. Kurlan R, Johnson D, Kaplan EL. Streptococcal infection and exacerbations of childhood tics and obsessive-compulsive symptoms: A prospective blinded cohort study. *Pediatrics*. 2008;121:1188-1197.
92. Burgert SJ, Classen DC, Burke JP, et al. Rheumatic pneumonia: Reappearance of a previously recognized complication of acute rheumatic fever. *Clin Infect Dis*. 1995;21:1020-1022.
93. Dlesk A, Balian AA, Sullivan BJ, et al. Diagnostic dilemma for the 1990s: Lyme disease versus rheumatic fever. *Wis Med J*. 1991;90:632-634.
94. Herd JK, Medhi M, Uzendoski DM, et al. Chorea associated with systemic lupus erythematosus: Report of two cases and review of the literature. *Pediatrics*. 1978;61:308-315.
95. Thompson HG, Jr, Carpenter MB. Hemichorea due to metastatic lesion in the subthalamic nucleus. *Arch Neurol*. 1960;2:83-87.
96. Bamford JM, Hakin RN. Chorea after legionnaire's disease. *Br Med J (Clin Res Ed)*. 1982;284:1232-1233.
97. McKinney AS. Idiopathic hypoparathyroidism presenting as chorea. *Neurology*. 1962;12:485-491.
98. Figueroa F, Berrios X, Gutierrez M, et al. Anticardiolipin antibodies in acute rheumatic fever. *J Rheumatol*. 1992;19:1175-1180.
99. Riddoch D, Jefferson M, Bickerstaff ER. Chorea and the oral contraceptives. *Br Med J*. 1971;4:217-218.
100. Jonas S, Spagnuolo M, Kloth HH. Chorea gravidarum and streptococcal infection. *Obstet Gynecol*. 1972;39:77-79.
101. Jones TD. The diagnosis of rheumatic fever. *JAMA*. 1944;126:481-484.
102. Veasy LG, Dajani AS, Allen HD, et al. Echocardiography for diagnosis and management of rheumatic fever. *JAMA*. 1993;269:2084.
103. Minich LL, Tani LY, Pagotto LT, et al. Doppler echocardiography distinguishes between physiologic and pathologic "silent" mitral regurgitation in patients with rheumatic fever. *Clin Cardiol*. 1997;20:924-926.
104. Figueroa FE, Fernandez MS, Valdes P, et al. Prospective comparison of clinical and echocardiographic diagnosis of rheumatic carditis: Long term follow up of patients with subclinical disease. *Heart*. 2001;85:407-410.
105. Vijayalakshmi IB, Vishnuprabhu RO, Chitra N, et al. The efficacy of echocardiographic criterions for the diagnosis of carditis in acute rheumatic fever. *Cardiol Young*. 2008;18:586-592.
106. Ferrieri P. Proceedings of the Jones Criteria workshop. *Circulation*. 2002;10:2521-2523.
107. Lanna CC, Tonelli E, Barros MV, et al. Subclinical rheumatic valvitis: a long-term follow-up. *Cardiol Young*. 2003; 13:431-438.
108. Atatoa-Carr P, Lennon D, Wilson N. Rheumatic fever diagnosis, management, and secondary prevention: a New Zealand guideline. *N Z Med J*. 2008;121:59-69.
109. Carapetis JR, Brown A, Wilson NJ, et al. An Australian guideline for rheumatic fever and rheumatic heart disease: an abridged outline. *Med J Aust*. 2007;186:581-586.
110. Stollerman GH, Lewis AJ, Schultz I, et al. Relationship of immune response to group A streptococci to the course of acute, chronic and recurrent rheumatic fever. *Am J Med*. 1956;20:163-169.
111. Cilliers AM, Manyemba J, Saloojee H. Anti-inflammatory treatment for carditis in acute rheumatic fever. Cochrane Database Syst Rev. 2003;(2):CD003176.
112. Uziel Y, Hashkes PJ, Kassem E, et al. The use of naproxen in the treatment of children with rheumatic fever. *J Pediatr*. 2000;137:269-271.
113. Karademir S, Oguz D, Senocak F, et al. Tolmetin and salicylate therapy in acute rheumatic fever: Comparison of clinical efficacy and side-effects. *Pediatr Int*. 2003;45:676-679.
114. Cardoso F. Sydenham's chorea. *Curr Treat Options Neurol*. 2008;10:230-235.
115. Paz JA, Silva CA, Marques-Dias MJ. Randomized double-blind study with prednisone in Sydenham's chorea. *Pediatr Neurol*. 2006;34:264-269.
116. Garvey MA, Snider LA, Leitman SF, et al. Treatment of Sydenham's chorea with intravenous immunoglobulin, plasma exchange, or prednisone. *J Child Neurol*. 2005;20:424-429.
117. United Kingdom and United States Joint Report on Rheumatic Heart Disease. The treatment of acute rheumatic fever in children. A cooperative clinical trial of ACTH, cortisone and aspirin. *Circulation*. 1955;11:343-377.
118. Marijon E, Ou P, Celermajer DS, et al. Prevalence of rheumatic heart disease detected by echocardiographic screening. *N Engl J Med*. 2007;357:470-476.
119. Gordis L. Effectiveness of comprehensive care programs in preventing rheumatic fever. *N Engl J Med*. 1973;289:331-335.
120. Gerber MA, Baltimore RS, Eaton CB, et al. A scientific statement from the American Heart Association Rheumatic Fever, Endocarditis, and Kawasaki Disease Committee of the Council on Cardiovascular Disease in the Young, the Interdisciplinary Council on Functional Genomics and Translational Biology, and the Interdisciplinary Council on Quality of Care and Outcomes Research. *Circulation*. 2009;119:1541-1551.
121. Wood HF, Feinstein AR, Taranta A, et al. Rheumatic fever in children and adolescents. A long-term epidemiologic study of subsequent prophylaxis, streptococcal infections, and clinical sequelae. III. Comparative effectiveness of three prophylaxis regimens in preventing streptococcal infections and rheumatic recurrences. *Ann Intern Med*. 1964;60(Suppl 5):31-46.
122. Lue HC, Wu MH, Wang JK, et al. Three- versus four-week administration of benzathine penicillin G: Effects of incidence of streptococcal infections and recurrences of rheumatic fever. *Pediatrics*. 1996;97(Suppl):984-988.
123. Berrios X, del Campo E, Guzman B, et al. Discontinuing rheumatic fever prophylaxis in selected adolescents and young adults: A prospective study. *Ann Intern Med*. 1993;118:401-406.
124. Bisno AL, Rubin FA, Cleary PP, et al. Prospects for a group A streptococcal vaccine: Rationale, feasibility, and obstacles—report of a National Institute of Allergy and Infectious Diseases workshop. *Clin Infect Dis*. 2005;41:1150-1156.
125. McNeil SA, Halperin SA, Langley JM, et al. Safety and immunogenicity of 26-valent group A streptococcus vaccine in healthy adult volunteers. *Clin Infect Dis*. 2005;41:1114-1122.
126. Bright R. Cases and observations, illustrative of renal disease accompanied with the secretion of albuminous urine. *Guys Hosp Rep*. 1936;1:338-400.
127. Schick B. Die nachkrankheiten des Schariach. *Jb Kinderheilk*. 1907;65:132-173.

128. Rammelkamp CH, Jr, Weaver RS. Acute glomerulonephritis: The significance of the variations in the incidence of the disease. *J Clin Invest.* 1953;32:345-358.

129. Wannamaker LW. Differences between streptococcal infections of the throat and of the skin. *N Engl J Med.* 1970;282:23-31.

130. Potter EV, Ortiz JS, Sharrett R, et al. Changing types of nephritogenic streptococci in Trinidad. *J Clin Invest.* 1971;50:1197-1205.

131. Dillon HC, Derrick CW, Dillon MS. M-antigens common to pyoderma and acute glomerulonephritis. *J Infect Dis.* 1974;130:257-267.

132. Duca E, Teodorovici G, Radu C, et al. A new nephritogenic streptococcus. *J Hyg.* 1969;67:691-698.

133. Barnham M, Thornton TJ, Lange K. Nephritis caused by *Streptococcus zooepidemicus* (Lancefield group C). *Lancet.* 1983;1:945-948.

134. Sesso R, Pinto SW. Five-year follow-up of patients with epidemic glomerulonephritis due to Streptococcus zooepidemicus. *Nephrol Dial Transplant.* 2005;20:1808-1812.

135. Seegal BC, Andres GA, Hsu KC, et al. Studies on the pathogenesis of acute and progressive glomerulonephritis in man by immunofluorescein and immunoferritin technique. *Fed Proc.* 1965;24:100-108.

136. Michael AF, Drummond KN, Good RA, et al. Acute poststreptococcal glomerulonephritis: Immune deposit disease. *J Clin Invest.* 1966;45:237-248.

137. Michael AF, Hoyer JR, Westberg NG, et al. Experimental models for the pathogenesis of acute poststreptococcal glomerulonephritis. In: Wannamaker LW, Masten JM, eds. *Streptococci and Streptococcal Disease.* New York: Academic Press; 1972:481-500.

138. Zabriskie JB. The role of streptococci in human glomerulonephritis. *J Exp Med.* 1971;134(Suppl):180S-192S.

139. Lange CF. Chemistry of cross-reactive fragments of streptococcal cell membrane and human glomerular basement membrane. *Transplant Proc.* 1969;1:959-963.

140. Bisno AL, Wood JW, Lawson J, et al. Antigens in urine of patients with glomerulonephritis and in normal human serum which cross-react with group A streptococci: Identification and partial characterization. *J Lab Clin Med.* 1978;91:500-513.

141. Goroncy-Bermes P, Dale JB, Beachey EH, et al. Monoclonal antibody to human renal glomeruli cross-reacts with streptococcal M protein. *Infect Immun.* 1987;55:2416-2419.

142. Ooi YM, Vallota EH, West CD. Serum immune complexes in membranoproliferative and other glomerulonephritides. *Kidney Int.* 1977;11:275-283.

143. Tung KSK, Woodroffe AJ, Ahlin TD, et al. Application of the solid phase C1q and raji cell radioimmune assays for the detection of circulating immune complexes in glomerulonephritis. *J Clin Invest.* 1978;62:61-72.

144. van de Rijn J, Fillit H, Brandeis WE, et al. Serial studies on circulating immune complexes in post-streptococcal sequelae. *Clin Exp Immunol.* 1978;34:318-325.

145. Lindberg LH, Vosti KL. Elution of glomerular bound antibodies in experimental streptococcal glomerulonephritis. *Science.* 1969;166:1032-1033.

146. Markowitz AS, Horn D, Aseron C, et al. Streptococcal related glomerulonephritis. 3. Glomerulonephritis in rhesus monkeys immunologically induced both actively and passively with a soluble fraction from nephritogenic streptococcal protoplasmic membranes. *J Immunol.* 1971;107:504-511.

147. Cu GA, Mezzano S, Bannan JD, et al. Immunohistochemical and serological evidence for the role of streptococcal proteinase

in acute post-streptococcal glomerulonephritis. *Kidney Int.* 1998;54:819-826.

148. Parra G, Rodriguez-Iturbe B, Batsford S, et al. Antibody to streptococcal zymogen in the serum of patients with acute glomerulonephritis: A multicentric study. *Kidney Int.* 1998;54:509-517.

149. Batsford SR, Mezzano S, Mihatsch M, et al. Is the nephritogenic antigen in post-streptococcal glomerulonephritis pyrogenic exotoxin B (SPE B) or GAPDH? *Kidney Int.* 2005;68:1120-1129.

150. Ahn SY, Ingulli E. Acute poststreptococcal glomerulonephritis: An update. *Curr Opin Pediatr.* 2008;20:157-162.

151. Rodriguez-Iturbe B. Postinfectious glomerulonephritis. *Am J Kidney Dis.* 2000;35:xlvi-xlviii.

152. Johnson KH, Zabriskie JB. Purification and partial characterization of the nephritis strain–associated protein from *Streptococcus pyogenes*, group A. *J Exp Med.* 1986;163:697-712.

153. Nordstrand A, Norgren M, Ferretti JJ, et al. Streptokinase as a mediator of acute post-streptococcal glomerulonephritis in an experimental mouse model. *Infect Immun.* 1998;66:315-321.

154. Mezzano S, Burgos E, Mahabir R, et al. Failure to detect unique reactivity to streptococcal streptokinase in either the sera or renal biopsy specimens of patients with acute poststreptococcal glomerulonephritis. *Clin Nephrol.* 1992;38:305-310.

155. Lewy JE, Salinas-Madrigal L, Herdson PB, et al. Clinicopathologic correlations in acute poststreptococcal glomerulonephritis. A correlation between renal functions, morphologic damage and clinical course of 46 children with acute poststreptococcal glomerulonephritis. *Medicine.* 1971;50:453-501.

156. Carapetis JR, Steer AC, Mulholland EK, et al. The global burden of group A streptococcal diseases. *Lancet Infect Dis.* 2005;5:685-694.

157. Anthony BF, Kaplan EL, Wannamaker LW, et al. Attack rates of acute nephritis after type 49 streptococcal infection of the skin and of the respiratory tract. *J Clin Invest.* 1969;48:1697-1704.

158. Tasic V, Polenakovic M. Acute poststreptococcal glomerulonephritis following circumcision. *Pediatr Nephrol.* 2000;15:274-275.

159. Nair S, Schoeneman MJ. Acute glomerulonephritis with group A streptococcal vulvovaginitis. *Clin Pediatr (Philadelphia).* 2000;39:721-722.

160. Stetson CA, Rammelkamp CH, Jr, Krause RM, et al. Epidemic acute nephritis: Studies on etiology, natural history and prevention. *Medicine.* 1955;34:431-450.

161. Lange K, Ahmed U, Kleinberger H, et al. A hitherto unknown streptococcal antigen and its probable relation to acute poststreptococcal glomerulonephritis. *Clin Nephrol.* 1976;5:207-215.

162. Roy S, Wall HP, Etteldorf JN. Second attacks of acute glomerulonephritis. *J Pediatr.* 1969;75:758-767.

163. Seegal D, Lyttle JD, Loeb EN, et al. On the exacerbation in chronic glomerulonephritis. *J Clin Invest.* 1940;19:569-589.

164. Bisno AL. The coexistence of acute rheumatic fever and acute glomerulonephritis. *Arthritis Rheum.* 1989;32:230-232.

165. Matsell DG, Baldree LA, DiSessa TG, et al. Acute poststreptococcal glomerulonephritis and acute rheumatic fever: Occurrence in the same patient. *Child Nephrol Urol.* 1990;10:112-114.

166. Poon-King T, Mohammed I, Cox R, et al. Recurrent epidemic nephritis in South Trinidad. *N Engl J Med.* 1967;277:728-733.

167. Kaplan EL, Anthony BF, Chapman SS, et al. Epidemic acute glomerulonephritis associated with type 49 streptococcal pyoderma. *Am J Med.* 1970;48:9-27.

168. Derrick CW, Reeves MS, Dillon HC Jr. Complement in overt and asymptomatic nephritis after skin infection. *J Clin Invest.* 1970;49:1178-1187.

169. Sharrett AR, Poon-King T, Potter EV, et al. Subclinical nephritis in South Trinidad. *Am J Epidemiol.* 1971;94:231-245.

170. Dodge WF, Spargo BH, Travis LB. Occurrence of acute glomerulonephritis in sibling contacts of children with sporadic acute glomerulonephritis. *Pediatrics.* 1967;40:1029-1030.

171. Schwartz WB, Kassirer JP. Clinical aspects of acute poststreptococcal glomerulonephritis. In: Strauss MB, Welt LG, eds. *Disease of the Kidney.* Boston: Little, Brown; 1971:419-462.

172. Freedman P, Meister HP, Lee HJ, et al. The renal response to streptococcal infection. *Medicine.* 1970;49:433-463.

173. Berman LB, Vogelsang P. Poststreptococcal glomerulonephritis without proteinuria. *N Engl J Med.* 1963;268:1275-1277.

174. Smith RD, Aquino J. Viruses and the kidney. *Med Clin North Am.* 1971;55:89-106.

175. Humphreys MH. Renal complications of HIV infection. In: Sande MA, Volbercling PA, eds. *The Medical Management of AIDS.* Philadelphia: WB Saunders, 1997.

176. Balat A, Baysal K, Kocak H. Myocardial functions of children with acute poststreptococcal glomerulonephritis. *Clin Nephrol.* 1993;39:151-155.

177. Kassirer JP, Schwartz WB. Acute glomerulonephritis. *N Engl J Med.* 1961;265:686-692.

178. Lasch EE, Frankel V, Vardy PA, et al. Epidemic glomerulonephritis in Israel. *J Infect Dis.* 1971;124:141-147.

179. Weinstein L, Le Frock J. Does antimicrobial therapy of streptococcal pharyngitis or pyoderma alter the risk of glomerulonephritis? *J Infect Dis.* 1971;124:229-231.

180. Perlman LV, Herdman RC, Kleinman H. Poststreptococcal glomerulonephritis: A ten-year follow-up of an epidemic. *JAMA.* 1965;194:63-70.

181. Potter EV, Lipschultz SA, Abidh S, et al. Twelve- to seventeen-year follow-up of patients with poststreptococcal acute glomerulonephritis in Trinidad. *N Engl J Med.* 1982;307:725-729.

182. White AV, Hoy WE, McCredie DA. Childhood post-streptococcal glomerulonephritis as a risk factor for chronic renal disease in later life. *Med J Aust.* 2001;174:492-496.

183. Baldwin DS. Poststreptococcal glomerulonephritis. A progressive disease? *Am J Med.* 1977;62:1-11.

184. Jennings RB, Earle DP. Post-streptococcal glomerulonephritis: Histopathologic and clinical studies of the acute, subsiding acute and early chronic latent phases. *J Clin Invest.* 1961;40:1525-1595.

185. Kurtzman NA. Does acute poststreptococcal glomerulonephritis lead to chronic renal disease? *N Engl J Med.* 1978;298:795-796.

186. Kaplan EL, Vernier RL. Progressive nephritis after strep infection questioned. *Am J Med.* 1978;64:910-911.

187. Pinto SW, Sesso R, Vasconcelos E, et al. Follow-up of patients with epidemic poststreptococcal glomerulonephritis. *Am J Kidney Dis.* 2001;38:249-255.

188. Richmond DE, Doak PB. The prognosis of acute post infectious glomerulonephritis in adults: A long-term prospective study. *Aust N Z J Med.* 1990;20:215-219.

189. Kaplan EL, Johnson DR, Nanthapisud P, et al. A comparison of group A streptococcal serotypes isolated from the upper respiratory tract in the USA and Thailand: Implications. *Bull World Health Organ.* 1992;70:433-437.

200

Streptococcus pneumoniae

DANIEL M. MUSHER*

Long recognized as a major cause of pneumonia, meningitis, sinusitis, and otitis media, *Streptococcus pneumoniae* is an important bacterial pathogen in humans; it is a less frequent cause of endocarditis, septic arthritis, and peritonitis and an uncommon cause of a variety of other infectious diseases.

History

A brief review of the history of *S. pneumoniae*, also known as pneumococcus, documents the important role of this organism in the history of microbiology.[1-3] In 1881, the organism was identified concurrently in the Old and New Worlds; Pasteur, in France named it *Microbe septicemique du salive*, and Sternberg, in the United States, called it *Micrococcus pasteuri*. By the late 1880s, the term *pneumococcus* was generally used because this bacterium had come to be recognized as the most common cause of lobar pneumonia. The name *Diplococcus pneumoniae* was assigned in 1926 because of its appearance in Gram-stained sputum, and in 1974 the organism was renamed once again, this time as *Streptococcus pneumoniae*, because of its morphology during growth in liquid medium.

S. pneumoniae was the first organism to be shown to behave as what is now regarded as a prototypic extracellular bacterial pathogen. In the absence of antibody, this bacterium resists phagocytosis and replicates extracellularly in mammalian tissues. In the early 1890s, Felix and Georg Klemperer showed that immunization with killed pneumococci protected animals against subsequent pneumococcal challenge and, furthermore, that protection could be transferred by infusing serum ("humoral" substance) from immunized mice into naive recipients. Subsequently, serum from persons who had recovered from pneumococcal pneumonia was found to confer the same degree of protection. The basis for this immunity was shown by Neufeld and Rimpau to be the presence of factor(s) in serum that facilitated ingestion by white blood cells (WBCs), a process that these investigators called opsonization, derived from the Greek word for preparing food. These observations provided the basis for what we now call humoral immunity. Serotypes were also recognized after observing that injection of killed organisms into a rabbit stimulated the production of serum antibody that agglutinated and caused capsular swelling of the immunizing strain, as well as some, but not all other pneumococcal isolates. Early in the 20th century, three serotypes were distinguished, called serotypes 1, 2, and 3; all other pneumococci were called group 4.

In the first decade of the 20th century, Maynard, Lister, Wright, and others applied the concepts of humoral immunity to the problem of epidemic lobar pneumonia that each year affected as many as 1 in 10 African miners.[1,4] Inoculation of killed pneumococci caused a substantial reduction in the incidence of pneumonia. In the 1920s, Heidelberger and Avery[5] demonstrated that the protective antibody was reactive with surface capsular polysaccharides. Felton[6] prepared the first purified pneumococcal capsular polysaccharides for immunization of human subjects, and a preparation of type 1 polysaccharide was used to abort an epidemic of pneumonia at a state hospital in Massachusetts in the winter of 1937-1938.[7] Taken together, these studies showed that a specific bacterial polysaccharide antigen could be used to stimulate humoral antibodies that conferred protection against epidemic human infection. Further confirmation was provided

during World War II, when MacLeod and colleagues[8] found that vaccinating military recruits with capsular material from four serotypes of *S. pneumoniae* greatly reduced the incidence of pneumonia caused by serotypes in the vaccine, but not by other pneumococcal serotypes.

S. pneumoniae also played a central role in the discovery of DNA. Experiments done by Griffith[9] in the 1920s had shown that intraperitoneal injection of live unencapsulated (mutant) pneumococci, together with heat-killed encapsulated pneumococci, into mice led to the emergence of viable, encapsulated bacteria; he called this process transformation. This observation remained unexplained until the 1940s, when Avery and associates[10] provided conclusive evidence that these mutants had recovered the capacity to produce capsule by taking up DNA from killed virulent organisms—in other words, that DNA is responsible for the observed transformation and is, in fact, the genetic material that encodes for phenotype.

Microbiology

S. pneumoniae is a gram-positive coccus that replicates in chains in liquid medium. The organism is catalase-negative but generates H_2O_2 via a flavoenzyme system, and therefore grows better in the presence of a source of catalase such as red blood cells. Pneumococci produce pneumolysin (formerly called α-hemolysin), which breaks down hemoglobin into a green pigment; as a result, pneumococcal colonies are surrounded by a green zone during growth on blood agar plates. This property is still termed α-hemolysis, although properly speaking it should not be, because lysis of red blood cells is not responsible. This point becomes readily apparent when one observes the greenish yellow color that appears around colonies of *S. pneumoniae* during growth on chocolate agar, a medium in which red blood cells were already lysed during preparation. Growth of pneumococci is inhibited by ethyl hydrocupreine (Optochin), and the organisms are lysed by bile salts. Thus, pneumococci are identified in the microbiology laboratory by four reactions: (1) α-hemolysis of blood agar; (2) catalase negativity; (3) susceptibility to Optochin; and (4) solubility in bile salts. Some pneumococci are Optochin-resistant,[11] and a newly recognized species, *Streptococcus pseudopneumoniae*, which is associated with exacerbation of chronic obstructive pulmonary disease (COPD) or pneumonia, is Optochin-susceptible during growth in room air at 37°C but Optochin-resistant when grown in the presence of increased CO_2.[12] These factors have led to greater reliance on the use of bile solubility for definitive identification. A highly reliable probe that detects rRNA sequences unique to *S. pneumoniae* is also commercially available.

Anatomy and Physiology

Peptidoglycan and teichoic acid are the principal constituents of the pneumococcal cell wall[13] (Fig. 200-1). Peptidoglycan consists of long chains of alternating *N*-acetyl-D-glucosamine and *N*-acetylmuramic acid, from which extend chains of four to six amino acids called stem peptides. Stem peptides are cross-linked by pentaglycine bridges, which provides substantial strength to the cell wall. Teichoic acid, a carbohydrate polymer that contains phosphorylcholine, is covalently linked to the peptidoglycan on the outermost surface of the bacterial wall and protrudes into the capsule. This teichoic acid, together with tightly adherent fragments of peptidoglycan, makes up C-polysaccharide, a substance that is present in all pneumococci and is otherwise detected only in a few species of viridans streptococci. C-polysaccharide reacts with proteins that appear in the blood stream

---

*All material in this chapter is in the public domain, with the exception of any borrowed figures or tables.

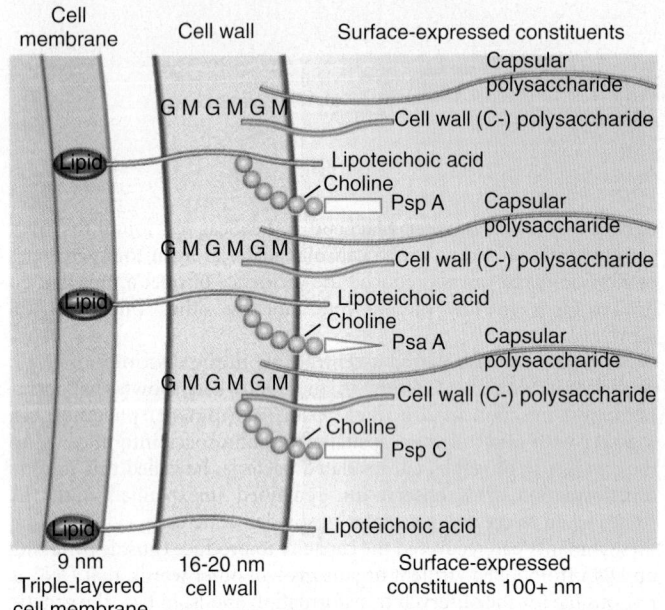

Figure 200-1 **Representation of the cell membrane, cell wall, and capsule of *Streptococcus pneumoniae*.** Within the cell wall, M = *N*-acetylmuramic acid and G = *N*-acetyl-D-glucosamine. The stem peptides and the cross-linked pentaglycine bridges that extend from the long M-G-M-G chains are not shown. Cell wall (C−) polysaccharide consists of teichoic acid with peptidoglycan and phosphorylcholine (not shown). F antigen is the lipid–teichoic acid moiety in the cell membrane that extends into the cell wall.

in inflammatory conditions (called acute-phase reactants or C-reactive proteins). Many proteins are expressed on the pneumococcal cell surface. Of particular importance in pathogenesis of disease are those that bind to choline, including pneumococcal surface proteins A and C, pneumococcal surface adhesin (choline-binding protein) A, choline-binding protein C, and proteins involved in competence, all of which will be discussed later in this chapter because of their potential role in pathogenicity. The characteristic three-layered cell membrane consists of lipid and teichoic acid and is called F antigen because of cross-reactivity with Forssman antigens.

Almost every clinical isolate of *S. pneumoniae* contains an external capsule; unencapsulated isolates have mainly been implicated in outbreaks of conjunctivitis.[14] Capsules[15] (see Fig. 200-1) are made up of repeating oligosaccharides that are synthesized within the cytoplasm, polymerized, and transported to the bacterial surface by cell membrane transferases. These polysaccharides are covalently bound to peptidoglycan and C-polysaccharide, which explains the difficulty of separating capsular from cell wall polysaccharide. Genetic control of this complex set of events has been elucidated for some serotypes; for example, a cassette of 15 genes that functions as a single transcriptional unit is responsible for encapsulation in serogroup 19.[16] Ninety-one serotypes of *S. pneumoniae* have been identified on the basis of antigenic differences in their capsular polysaccharides. Among the genes that encode capsule production, some are specific for individual polysaccharides, whereas others are conserved among almost all pneumococci and even some other streptococci.[17] Immunization of rabbits with a pneumococcus of a specific capsular type stimulates the appearance of antibodies that cause agglutination and microscopic demonstrability of the capsule; in the latter reaction, called the Quellung reaction, antibody renders the capsule refractile and therefore more readily visible, which visibility is often, but erroneously, referred to as capsular swelling. Because serum antibody is the basis for identifying these types of pneumococcus, they are called serotypes. In the American numbering system, serotypes are numbered from 1 to 91 in the order in which they were identified. The more widely accepted Danish

numbering system distinguishes 46 serogroups, with the groups containing antigenically related serotypes. For example, Danish serogroup 19 includes serotypes 19F, 19A, 19B, and 19C (the letter F indicates the first member of the group to be identified, followed by A, B, and C), which in the American system would be serotypes 19, 57, 58, and 59, respectively. Serotypes that most frequently cause human disease were the earliest to be identified and assigned numbers, which explains why the lower numbered serotypes are more likely to be implicated in human infection. Serotyping was clinically relevant in the 1930s, when antisera were administered for therapy, and is of great interest from epidemiologic and public health standpoints today, especially as new vaccines are being developed, but has little relevance for the clinician in an individual case of pneumococcal infection.

An important property of *S. pneumoniae* is its capacity, as part of its quorum-sensing mechanism, to express a competence-sensing protein and internalize DNA from other pneumococci or from other bacterial species.[18] This transfer of genetic information to pneumococci is called transformation, and it enables pneumococci to acquire new traits—for example, the ability to make a different capsular polysaccharide. Transformation of capsular types occurs under experimental conditions but, more importantly, also occurs during colonization or infection of humans.[19-21]

Epidemiology

As with many other microorganisms, *S. pneumoniae* finds its ecologic niche in colonizing the nasopharynx. On a single occasion, appropriate culturing yields pneumococci in 5% to 10% of healthy adults and 20% to 40% of healthy children. With repeated attempts at culture, the percentage increases in all age groups, rising to 40 to 60% or greater[22] in toddlers and young children in daycare. For reasons that remain unclear, the rate of colonization is seasonal, with an increase in the midwinter period, although pneumococci can be recovered from healthy children and adults throughout the year. A careful prospective study in infants in the United States[23] has shown that the first pneumococcus to colonize an infant is generally acquired at around 6 months of age and can be detected for a mean of about 4 months. In contrast, infants from select populations, such as native Americans, aboriginal Australians, or disadvantaged members of developed societies,[24] are more likely to be colonized, and with high numbers of pneumococci, even within the first few weeks of life. In adults, an individual serotype persists for shorter periods, usually 2 to 4 weeks,[25] but sometimes much longer.[1]

Population-based studies carried out in different parts of the world have shown that the overall rate of invasive pneumococcal disease, defined as the isolation of *S. pneumoniae* from a normally sterile site such as blood, pleural fluid, or cerebrospinal fluid (CSF), is about 15/100,000 persons/year.[26] This figure reflects extensive data obtained before the widespread use of conjugate pneumococcal vaccine in infants and toddlers; the incidence has been reduced substantially in countries in which this vaccine is used. Furthermore, this number reflects the averaging of rates of disease in different age groups and populations. Invasive pneumococcal disease is relatively common in newborns and infants up to 2 years of age and much less in teenage children and young adults, again increasing in adults older than 65 years[27,28] (Fig. 200-2); for example, in South Carolina before conjugate pneumococcal vaccine was used,[28] the incidence was 160, 5, and 70/100,000 persons, respectively, among infants, young adults, and those 70 years of age or older. Interestingly, although the overall incidence of pneumococcal infection in the population is vastly reduced when compared with the preantibiotic era, this relationship to age has not changed. In certain populations, including African Americans,[29] Native Americans[30] (especially Alaskans[31]), and Australian Aboriginals,[32] the incidence may be up to 10-fold greater, although it is unclear to what extent genetic or environmental factors are responsible (Table 200-1).[33] Most cases of pneumococcal bacteremia in adults are caused by pneumonia, and probably three to four cases of nonbacteremic pneumonia occur for every case of bacteremic pneumonia, thus

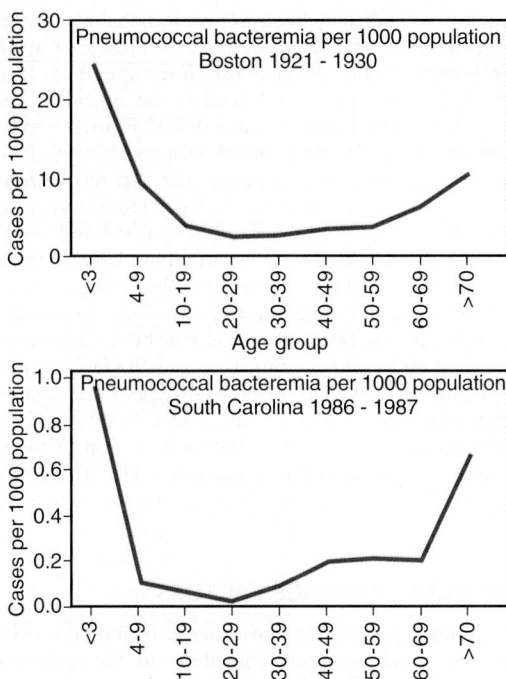

TABLE 200-1 Invasive Pneumococcal Disease in U.S. Racial Groups*

| | Age (yr) | |
Group	18-64	≧65
White	10	57
Black	44	82
Navajo	56	190

*Data are presented as rates/100,000 persons/year for 1989-1998 (before licensing of conjugate pneumococcal vaccination). These results reflect the impact of genetic and environmental factors.[33]

Adapted from Watt JP, O'Brien KL, Benin AL, et al. Invasive pneumococcal disease among Navajo adults, 1989-1998. *Clin Infect Dis.* 2004;38:496-501.

Figure 200-2 Relationship between pneumococcal bacteremia and age is shown for two studies, widely separated in time. A, Data published in the preantibiotic era. **B,** Includes data from South Carolina obtained in 1986 and 1987.[30] Interestingly, the shape of the curve is remarkably similar to that in **A,** although the vertical axis in the lower curve shows a vastly reduced incidence when compared with that in the upper one. More recent studies continue to confirm these earlier findings. (**A** adapted from Heffron R. Pneumonia: With Special Reference to Pneumococcus Lobar Pneumonia. © 1939 by the Commonwealth Fund. © 1979 by the President and Fellows of Harvard College. Reprinted by permission of Harvard University Press.)

The occurrence of pneumococcal otitis media[34,35] or bacteremia[36,37] is related to season, perhaps because of the association with viral respiratory illnesses. A November through April clustering with a clear peak in February was apparent for otitis media in the study of Gray and Dillon.[23] In Houston, Texas, invasive disease in children occurred mainly during September through May, thus coinciding with the school year and sparing the summer months, but with no clear midwinter peak (Fig. 200-3). In contrast, invasive disease in adults clearly reaches a peak in the middle of winter, inversely related to ambient temperature and directly associated with the peak of viral respiratory disease.[36,37]

Pneumococci are transmitted from one individual to another as a result of close contact,[38] but infection is generally not regarded as contagious because so many factors intervene between acquisition of the organism (colonization) and development of disease. Daycare centers are very likely to be places for spread of these organisms in toddlers.[39-41] In adults, close crowded living conditions such as in military camps,[42] prisons,[43] shelters for the homeless,[44] and nursing homes,[45] are associated with epidemics, but contact in schools or in the workplace is generally not.[38] The common feature for outbreaks is that in addition to crowding and close contact, the population has some additional feature(s) that contribute(s) to susceptibility to infection such as fatigue, malnutrition, or intercurrent viral infection.

Pathogenetic Mechanisms

To cause disease, pneumococci, like other extracellular bacterial pathogens, must adhere to mammalian cells; replicate in situ; be carried to, replicate in, and fail to be cleared from anatomic areas that are normally free of them, escape phagocytosis; and damage tissue by

leading to estimates of 25 cases of pneumococcal pneumonia/100,000 young adults and 280/100,000 older adults each year. Because of lack of confirmation, the true incidence may be several times greater. By contrast, in the preantibiotic era, about 700 cases of pneumonia occurred in 100,000 young adults each year.[1]

Figure 200-3 Invasive pneumococcal disease. Each bar shows the number of cases of invasive pneumococcal disease at four tertiary care hospitals (adult and pediatric) in Houston during a 2-week period. A fall, winter, and early spring predominance is noted. The line graph[36] is the number of specimens from patients thought to have a viral syndrome, obtained by a consortium of physicians in cooperation with the Influenza Research Center of the Baylor College of Medicine, Houston.

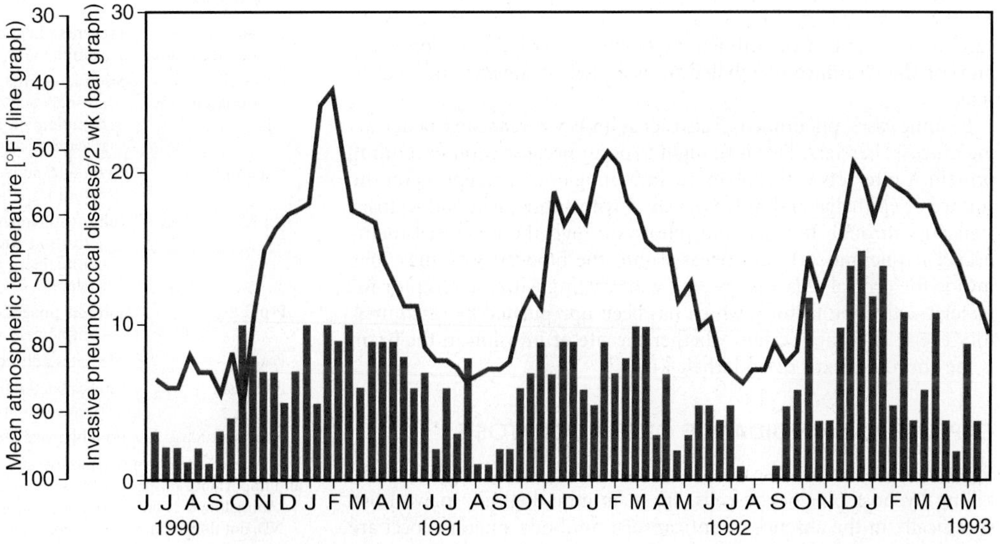

causing inflammation and/or producing substances that directly damage cells. Many of these reactions are governed at a molecular level by bacterial and host properties.[46-48] Unlike certain other organisms such as *Streptococcus pyogenes,* which produce a variety of tissue-damaging substances, *S. pneumoniae* produces few toxins, of which pneumolysin is the principal one. Rather, this organism causes disease because of its capacity to an intense inflammatory response. In most organs—for example, the lungs, middle ear, and central nervous system—this inflammatory response is the disease.

ADHERENCE, COLONIZATION, INVASION

The prevalence of pneumococcal colonization attests to the adaptational success of this organism in adhering to mammalian cells and replicating in the nasopharynx. *S. pneumoniae* attaches to human pharyngeal cells through a variety of mechanisms involving the specific interaction of bacterial surface adhesins (e.g., pneumococcal surface antigen A, choline-binding proteins) and epithelial cell receptors such as platelet-activating factor.[49] Rhinovirus infection, for example, is followed by increased adherence of pneumococci to cultured human tracheal cells, and this reaction is inhibited by blocking platelet activating factor.[50] Pneumococci also become invasive as a result of the interaction with platelet-activating factor on the surface of epithelial cells.[51] Epithelial cell glycoconjugates containing the disaccharide GlcNAcb1-4Gal[52] or asialo-GM glycolipid[53] are other possible binding sites. Phase variation of pneumococci may also play a role. On culture in vitro, a mixed population of transparent and opaque colonies can be identified. Organisms from transparent colonies have greatly increased quantities of phosphorylcholine and choline binding protein A, which contribute to their capacity to adhere to mammalian cells.[54] When an opaque colony is inoculated intranasally into an experimental animal, only those organisms that make transparent colonies persist. In contrast, intraperitoneal inoculation of opaque colonies may be lethal, whereas transparent colonies are less likely to be lethal; increased capsule production by opaque forms may in part be responsible. The recently demonstrated adhesin PsrP does not affect nasopharyngeal colonization but is necessary for pneumococci to adhere to and persist in the lungs of mice after tracheal challenge; antibody to this protein protects mice against challenge with *S. pneumoniae* serotype 4.[55]

Once nasopharyngeal colonization has taken place, infection may result if the organisms are carried into cavities from which they are not readily cleared. Under normal circumstances, when bacteria find their way into eustachian tubes, sinuses, or bronchi, clearance mechanisms, chiefly ciliary action, lead to their rapid removal. If allergy or coexisting viral infection, for example, has caused edema that obstructs the opening of the eustachian tube into the pharynx or the ostium of a paranasal sinus, clinically recognizable infection may result. Similarly, damage to ciliated bronchial cells or increased production of mucus, whether chronic (e.g., from cigarette smoking or occupational exposure) or acute (e.g., from influenza or some other viral infection), may prevent the clearance of inhaled or aspirated organisms and lead to infection.

In some cases, pneumococci also act as invasive organisms, penetrating mucosal barriers. This is thought to occur because choline-binding protein A interacts with polymeric immunoglobulin receptors on the surface of epithelial and mucosal cells,[56] with subsequent endocytosis, transport through the cell, and release through the inner cell membrane. If pneumococci are released into the bloodstream, they may invade the central nervous system by interacting with the receptor for platelet-activating factor,[57] which has been upregulated by inflammatory events. It is not certain whether the site of invasion in the brain is the choroid plexus or endothelial cells.[58]

CAPSULE AND AVOIDANCE OF PHAGOCYTOSIS

S. pneumoniae causes disease because it is able to avoid ingestion and killing by host phagocytic cells. In an immunologically naive host, specifically in the absence of anticapsular antibody, pneumococci are poorly ingested and killed by the host's professional phagocytes, polymorphonuclear leukocytes (PMNs), and macrophages. Capsule plays a central role in preventing phagocytosis. Interruption of capsule production in *S. pneumoniae* type 3 renders the organism essentially avirulent, with the lethal dose in mice shifted from 2–3 to $>3 \times 10^7$ colony-forming units.[59] Possible contributing mechanisms include (1) the absence of receptors on phagocytic cells that recognize capsular polysaccharides, (2) the presence of electrochemical forces that repel phagocytic cells, (3) the masking of antibody to cell wall constituents and C3b that may have fixed to the cell wall but beneath the capsule, and (4) the inactivation of complement.[60] A close relationship has been observed between the absolute amount of capsule produced and the virulence of pneumococcal strains, as well as between the amount of anticapsular antibody infused into mice and the level of protection against challenge with each of several serotypes of *S. pneumoniae.*[61] PspA prevents deposition and activation of C3b by interfering with complement factor B[62,63] and PspC blocks activation of the complement cascade by binding complement factor H.[64] These effects are attenuated or blocked by antibody to these surface-expressed proteins.

NONCAPSULAR VIRULENCE FACTORS

As noted, noncapsular protein constituents, including pneumolysin, surface proteins, and autolysin, contribute to the pathogenesis of pneumococcal disease. Genetically engineered mutants that lack the ability to produce one or more of these substances have generally been shown to have diminished virulence, and immunization with the purified substance has stimulated the production of antibodies that confer protection in experimental animals (Table 200-2). It needs to be emphasized, however, that despite the current interest in these and other protein constituents of *S. pneumoniae,*[65,66] at the time of this writing (April, 2009), only indirect evidence of a protective effect of antibody to any of these substances has been found in humans.

All serotypes of *S. pneumoniae* produce pneumolysin, a thiol-activated toxin that inserts into the lipid bilayer of cell membranes via its interaction with cholesterol. Pneumolysin is cytotoxic for phagocytic and respiratory epithelial cells and causes inflammation by

TABLE 200-2	Role of Pneumococcal Constituents as Virulence Factors*		
		Strength of Evidence as Virulence Factor	
Pneumococcal Constituent	**Mechanism**	*Antibody Prevents Disease[†]*	*Mutants Lack Virulence*
Capsular polysaccharide	Prevents phagocytosis; activates complement	4+	4+
Cell wall polysaccharide	Stimulates inflammation by strongly activating complement and stimulating release of cytokines	0	ND
Pneumolysin	Cytotoxic; activates complement, cytokines	2-3+	2-3+
PspA	Inhibits phagocytosis by blocking activation and deposition of complement on bacterial surface	2+	2+
PspC	Inhibits phagocytosis by binding complement factor H	1-2+	1-2+
PsaA	Mediates adherence	1-2+	1-2+
Autolysin	Causes bacterial disintegration; releases components	1+	2+
Neuraminidase	Possibly mediates adherence	0-1+	0-1+

*The grading system is subjective and indicates (on a scale of 1+ to 4+) the stringency and importance of the demonstrated effect. For discussion and references, see the text.
[†]Animal models only, except capsular polysaccharides.
ND, not done; Psa, pneumococcal surface adhesin; Psp, pneumococcal surface protein.

activating complement and inducing the production of tumor necrosis factor-α and interleukin-1 (IL-1).[67,68] Injection of pneumolysin into rat lung causes all the histologic findings of pneumonia,[69] and immunization of mice with this substance before pneumococcal infection[70] or challenge with genetically engineered pneumococci that do not produce it[71] is associated with a significant reduction in virulence. Different regions of the pneumolysin molecule are responsible for cytotoxic and complement activity properties, and studies using strains with defined point mutations have shown that the cytotoxic activity is dominant in causing disease after intraperitoneal but not necessarily after intranasal challenge of mice.[72] When human macrophages are infected in vitro, altered expression can be demonstrated in a large number of genes; in the great majority, observed alterations specifically reflect the response to pneumolysin.[73] Human antibody to pneumolysin increases after pneumococcal pneumonia; the presence of this antibody is associated with a decreased likelihood of bacteremic infection, and it protects mice against pneumococcal challenge.[74]

Proteins on the pneumococcal surface that bind to choline residues may mediate attachment to and penetration of mammalian cells, especially if these cells have been upregulated by prior cytokine exposure.[57] Pneumococcal surface protein A is present on the surface of almost all pneumococci and exerts an antiphagocytic force, perhaps by blocking deposition of complement.[75] Despite some antigenic variability, antibody raised against pneumococcal surface protein A protects experimental animals to a greater or lesser extent against challenge with the same or different strain,[76] and genetically engineered mutants that lack it have reduced virulence for mice.[77] Human antibody to this protein protects mice against pneumococcal infection[78] and may protect humans against pneumococcal colonization.[79] This substance is a major constituent of a vaccine that is currently in development (see later). Pneumococcal surface adhesin A, a surface-expressed permease, is universally present in *S. pneumoniae*. This protein shows very little antigenic variability. Antibody to it reduces pneumococcal colonization of the nasopharynx in mice,[80] perhaps by blocking attachment[81]; this antibody may also be associated with a reduced risk of otitis media.[82] It may be involved in colonization of the nasopharynx, but it appears to contribute to virulence in other, as yet undetermined ways. Autolysin[71] disrupts the bacterial wall at the site of attachment of stem proteins. In nature, this enzyme contributes to cell wall remodeling. In infection, it probably contributes to disease by releasing peptidoglycan components that more vigorously activate complement, as well as substances (e.g., pneumolysin) to which the tissues of the infected host might otherwise not be exposed. As with other putative virulence factors, strains that lack autolysin are less virulent in experimental animals, and antibody to autolysin is modestly protective.[83] Pneumococci produce neuraminidase, which may contribute to bacterial adherence and colonization by cleaving sialic acid on mucous membrane surfaces and exposing GlcNAc-Gal, to which *S. pneumoniae* adheres more readily. Immunization of mice with neuraminidase has also provided modest protection against parenteral pneumococcal challenge, perhaps suggesting a role in virulence other than inhibition of colonization. All pneumococci also produce hyaluronidase, but a role in pathogenesis has not been clearly demonstrated.

Innate Immunity to Pneumococcus

Natural immune mechanisms are those that require no prior exposure to an infecting organism to exert their protective effect. This section discusses activation of complement, the pattern recognition receptors on human cells, and B-1 cells. Nonimmunologic mechanisms that protect against pneumococcal infection, such as glottal reflex and ciliary activity of bronchial epithelial cells, are discussed later, under host mechanisms of defense.

ACTIVATION OF COMPLEMENT

The cell wall of *S. pneumoniae*, including both teichoic acid and peptidoglycan constituents, activates complement by the alternative pathway.[84,85] Injection of either of these substances into the subarachnoid space causes an inflammatory reaction that has the characteristics of bacterial meningitis, although the kinetics vary with the substance injected.[85] C-reactive protein may also play an active part.[86] Polysaccharide capsule in addition appears to activate the alternative pathway in vitro,[87,88] albeit to a somewhat lesser extent. The classic pathway is activated by almost universally present antibody to cell wall polysaccharides, even in the absence of anticapsular antibody.[88] To the extent that complement is fixed on bacterial surfaces and is accessible to phagocytic cells, such activation may be protective. Polymorphisms in the complement receptor on phagocytic cells are associated with a greater likelihood of having bacteremic pneumococcal infection.[89] Complement activation is associated with the release of C5a so that, whether or not complement is fixed on the bacterial surface, C5a, a potent attractant for PMNs, is released to the surrounding medium. Thus, an intense inflammatory response fueled by vigorous activation of both the alternative and classic complement pathways accompanies pneumococcal infection of an immunologically naive host.

OTHER INNATE MECHANISMS

Pathogen recognition receptors on the surface of mammalian cells play a major role in innate immunity.[48] Peptidoglycan and lipoteichoic acid interact with CD14, stimulating Toll-like receptor 2,[90,91] and pneumolysin interacts with Toll-like receptor 4 to induce nuclear factor kappa B (NF-κB).[92] The result could be regarded as a two-edged sword. These stimuli facilitate uptake of pneumococci in the absence of antibody to any of its constituents.[93] At the same time, they stimulate a vigorous inflammatory response by upregulating production of inflammatory cytokines IL-1, IL-6, and TNF-α, thereby contributing to pneumococcal disease that is largely a result of inflammation and is often severe in direct proportion to the intensity of the inflammatory response. A C-type lectin, SIGN-R1, expressed by macrophages, specifically interacts with some capsular polysaccharides, facilitating ingestion of pneumococci.[94] Serum proteins that react with cell wall polysaccharide (C-reactive protein) might play a modest role in protection by activating complement and exerting an opsonizing effect.[86] A recently recognized line of B-1a cells make IgM antibody to polysaccharides without regard to prior exposure to bacteria[95]; this natural antibody, present in germ-free mice, provides some protection against pneumococcal challenge.[48,96] Finally, a host deficiency of serum mannose-binding lectin may reduce innate immune responses and contribute to lethal infection in humans.[97]

Immunologically Specific Mechanisms of Immunity

ANTIBODY TO PNEUMOCOCCAL CAPSULE

Ample evidence has shown that in humans, anticapsular antibody is protective against pneumococcal infection, with little or no evidence to date to support a role for antibody to other bacterial constituents: (1) antibody to capsule appears in the bloodstream 5 to 8 days after the onset of infection, which is when that fever spontaneously resolves in the absence of treatment[1]; (2) in the preantibiotic era, administration of serum that contained type-specific antibody was moderately effective in treating pneumococcal pneumonia[98]; and (3) various assays all seem to show greatly increased uptake and killing of pneumococci in vitro in the presence of anticapsular antibody.[27,99,100] In contrast, except for indirect data suggesting an association between antibody to pneumolysin[74] or pneumococcal surface adhesin a,[82] there are few data in humans to support a protective role for antibody to other substances. Epidemiologic evidence supports the notion that immune mechanisms other than antibody to capsule are responsible for protection in the population.[101] It is important to note, however, that in the preantibiotic era, some proportion of patients recovered from pneumococcal pneumonia without producing measurable amounts of anticapsular antibody. Furthermore, some adults lack the capacity to make antibody to most pneumococcal capsules,[102] yet live long and healthy lives free of pneumococcal disease.

Although IgG antibody to capsular polysaccharides, as measured by enzyme-linked immunosorbent assay (ELISA), generally predicts protection of experimental animals and opsonophagocytosis activity in vitro, such is not uniformly the case. Older adults[103,104] or those admitted for pneumococcal pneumonia[105] may have relatively high levels of anticapsular antibody, but the antibody may not opsonize pneumococci for phagocytosis or protect mice against experimental challenge. The precise reason for the lack of protection is not known; perhaps the IgG antibody is relatively less avid for capsular material. Significant differences in kappa and lambda gene usage have been shown in older versus younger subjects.[104] Thus, when present, anticapsular antibody is regarded as a generally good, but not ideal, surrogate marker of immunity. The converse—namely, that the absence of such antibody indicates a relative degree of susceptibility—is probably true, even though many other factors (e.g., innate immunity, antibody to other pneumococcal constituents, general level of health, host receptors for pneumococcal constituents) enter into protection against pneumococcal disease.

PREVALENCE OF ANTICAPSULAR ANTIBODY

In the late 1980s, before the introduction of a pediatric pneumococcal vaccine, a sensitive and specific ELISA technique[106,107] showed that the great majority of 19-year-old military recruits lack antibody to most pneumococcal serotypes[108]; the average subject had type-specific anticapsular IgG to only 15% of commonly infecting serotypes. Around this same time (which also preceded wide-scale pneumococcal vaccination of adults) the average working adult or older man was likely to have antibody to no more than one third of common pneumococcal serotypes. To the extent that immunity is greatly enhanced by the presence of anticapsular antibody, these data suggest that unvaccinated healthy adults of all ages tend to be susceptible to most serotypes of *S. pneumoniae* that commonly cause infection.

EMERGENCE OF ANTIBODY DURING COLONIZATION OR SUBCLINICAL INFECTION

Pneumococcal colonization stimulates production of anticapsular antibody. Studies of families carried out in the preantibiotic era[109] and of infants and toddlers in the 1970s[23] suggested that the acquisition of antibody also follows colonization. Serotype-specific antibody developed within 30 days in about two thirds of military personnel who became colonized during an outbreak of pneumococcal pneumonia.[108] After pneumococcal infection, antibody to the infecting serotype, as measured in older studies by agglutination in vitro or mouse protection, appears in the serum of adults in about two thirds of cases with some variability, depending on the serotype.[110] In children, the rate of appearance of antibody may be lower,[111-113] but these studies need to be repeated with ELISA. The reason(s) for the failure of detectable levels of antibody to develop after infection remain unclear. One explanation is a genetically mediated incapacity to recognize as foreign the relevant capsular polysaccharide and, therefore, to make antibody to it.[102] Failure to switch to IgG synthesis or to make certain IgG subclasses may also be implicated.[114]

COLONIZATION AND IMMUNITY

The best explanation for the low incidence of pneumococcal disease despite the relatively high rate of colonization and the low prevalence of detectable antipneumococcal antibody in the adult population is that antibody to the capsular polysaccharide of a colonizing organism is likely to appear before infection. However, in those who aspirate pharyngeal contents or who have diminished mechanisms of lower airway clearance, exposure to a high inoculum of organisms is more likely to occur before antibody is produced. Of course, those individuals who have a diminished capacity to form antibody remain susceptible as long

as they are colonized, which explains the high rate of pneumococcal pneumonia in patients with multiple myeloma, acquired immunodeficiency syndrome (AIDS), and other such conditions.

THE SPLEEN IN DEFENSE OF PNEUMOCOCCAL INFECTION

The principal organ that clears unopsonized pneumococci from the bloodstream is the spleen.[115,116] Experiments in human subjects have shown that highly opsonized particles are removed from the circulation by the liver but, with decreasing opsonization, the spleen increasingly assumes the role of clearance.[117] Presumably, the slow passage of blood through the spleen and prolonged contact time with reticuloendothelial cells in the cords of Billroth and the splenic sinuses allow for the relatively less efficient removal of nonopsonized particles through natural immune mechanisms (see earlier).[118] Overwhelming pneumococcal infection occurs in children and adults from whom the spleen has been removed or does not function normally. The heralding event in an outbreak of pneumococcal pneumonia in a metropolitan[43] prison was the rapid septic death of two prisoners, both of whom had previously undergone splenectomy. Pneumococcal disease progressed so rapidly in these cases that pneumonia was not initially detectable clinically or even with certainty by chest radiographs, although it was seen at autopsy. The 100-fold increase in the incidence of pneumococcal bacteremia or meningitis in children with sickle cell disease is probably caused by splenic dysfunction, although other factors such as complement abnormalities may also contribute.[115,119]

Factors That Predispose to Pneumococcal Infection

S. pneumoniae is a prototypic extracellular bacterial pathogen; host defenses against infection rely heavily on the interaction between humoral factors such as antibody and complement and phagocytic cells, specifically PMNs. A representative listing of conditions that affect the immunologic capacity of the host and predispose to pneumococcal infection is shown in Table 200-3. Specific conditions associated with pneumococcal pneumonia are shown in Table 200-4.

Defective antibody formation, whether congenital or acquired, has the greatest impact on susceptibility to pneumococcal infection. Bruton's original description of congenital agammaglobulinemia stressed the prominence of *S. pneumoniae* as an infecting agent. Pneumococcus is also a major cause of serious infection in acquired agammaglobulinemia (common variable immunodeficiency)[120] and perhaps in IgG subclass deficiency[121] as well; subtle defects may also be responsible.[114] Homozygous expression of the R131 allele of the FCγII receptor on PMNs, a receptor that binds the Fc of IgG$_2$ only poorly, or absence of the mannose-binding protein may be associated with susceptibility to pneumococcal bacteremia.[122]

The incidence of invasive pneumococcal disease (isolation of *S. pneumoniae* from a normally sterile site) in adults is about 9/100,000 in healthy subjects—51 in diabetes, 63 in chronic lung disease, 94 in chronic heart disease, and 100 in alcohol abuse. The incidence rises further to 300 in patients with solid cancer, 423 in HIV/AIDS, and 503 in hematologic malignancies.[123] Pneumococcus continues to be the most common bacterial pathogen to infect persons who have multiple myeloma, lymphoma, or chronic lymphocytic leukemia, before chemotherapy and hospitalization tip the balance toward gram-negative infections.[124] In these conditions, as well as in HIV infection, there are probably immunologic defects at several points in the host defense, but defective antibody production predominates in the predisposition to pneumococcal infection. Just to place these numbers in perspective, if three to four nonbacteremic cases of pneumonia occur for each invasive (bacteremic) case, almost 1 in 25 HIV-infected persons may be expected to have pneumococcal pneumonia in a given year. Some authorities have recommended that bacteremic pneumonia or unusual pneumococcal infections in young adults[125,126] should trigger a search for HIV infection.

TABLE 200-3	Conditions That Predispose to Pneumococcal Infection

Defective antibody formation
  Primary
    Congenital agammaglobulinemia
    Common variable (acquired) hypogammaglobulinemia
    Selective IgG subclass deficiency
  Secondary
    Multiple myeloma
    Chronic lymphocytic leukemia
    Lymphoma
    HIV infection
Defective complement (primary or secondary)
  Decreased or absent C1, C2, C3, C4
Insufficient numbers of PMNs
  Primary
    Cyclic neutropenia
  Secondary
    Drug-induced neutropenia
    Aplastic anemia
Poorly functioning PMNs
  Alcoholism
  Cirrhosis of the liver
  Diabetes mellitus
  Glucocorticosteroid treatment
  Renal insufficiency
    Poorly avid receptors for FCγII (R131 allele)
Defective clearance of pneumococcal bacteremia
  Primary
    Congenital asplenia, hyposplenia
  Secondary
    Splenectomy
    Sickle cell disease (autosplenectomy)
Multifactorial and/or uncertain
  Infancy and aging
  Glucocorticosteroid treatment
  Malnutrition
  Cirrhosis of the liver
  Renal insufficiency
  Diabetes mellitus
  Alcoholism
  Chronic disease, hospitalization
  Fatigue
  Stress
  Cold exposure
Excess likelihood of exposure
  Daycare centers
  Military training camps
  Prisons
  Shelters for the homeless
Prior respiratory infection
  Influenza
  Other
Inflammatory condition
  Cigarette smoking
  Asthma
  COPD

COPD, chronic obstructive pulmonary disease; HIV, human immunodeficiency virus; PMNs, polymorphonuclear leukocytes.

Of the many possible defects in complement, only those factors required to generate C3b are associated with pneumococcal infection. Because pneumococci are not killed by serum, the host response is unaffected by defects in C6, C7, C8, or C9, which result in decreased membrane attack complexes. In contrast, deficiencies in C1, C2, and C4, whether congenital or acquired, are expected to be associated with increased susceptibility to pneumococcal infection, although cases documenting the association are reported only rarely.[127]

Neutropenia of whatever cause is associated with *S. pneumoniae* infection although, somewhat surprisingly, leukocyte adhesion deficiency syndrome (Mac-1 deficiency) is generally not.[128] One study[129] has shown that at the time of initial hospitalization for acute leukemia, patients are more likely to have infection caused by more ordinary gram-positive pathogenic bacteria, probably analogous to the pretreatment situation in multiple myeloma.[124] Defective bacterial killing by PMNs as seen in chronic granulomatous disease does not predispose to infection with *S. pneumoniae*; the absence of catalase renders this organism susceptible to the interaction between its endogenous H_2O_2 and myeloperoxidase and the halide present in PMNs.

The susceptibility of older adults to pneumococcal pneumonia is multifactorial, reflecting senescence of the immune system because of diminished production of immunoglobulins (or production of poorly functional ones), impaired response to cytokines, and general debilitation caused by weakening of the gag reflex, malnutrition, and the presence of other diseases. The effect of alcoholism is also multifactorial and involves lifestyle (e.g., cold exposure, malnutrition), suppression of the gag reflex, and possibly deleterious effects on PMN function, although in most cases these alterations have been difficult to attribute to the effect of alcohol alone.[130,131] Heffron[1] has cited studies from the preantibiotic era showing a 30% to 50% incidence of alcohol abuse in patients with pneumococcal pneumonia. More recent studies have continued to find about one third of such patients to have alcoholic-related disease.[27,132,133] A disproportionately high number of patients with pneumococcal infection have diabetes mellitus,[27,132-135] a condition in which PMN chemotaxis is reduced[136] and phagocytic function is defective.[137] Anemia (hemoglobin lower than 10 g/dL) was detected in one third of a series of patients with pneumococcal pneumonia.[133]

Many chronic diseases are associated with pneumococcal pneumonia by virtue of an association with pneumonia of whatever cause, which suggests that the predisposition is a general one rather than being specific for *S. pneumoniae*. Pneumococcal pneumonia follows hospitalization for all causes[138] and has even been observed as a nosocomial infection.[139] Other factors such as cold exposure, stress, and fatigue[21] may predispose to pneumococcal pneumonia by unknown mechanisms.

As noted, prior respiratory viral infection, especially that caused by influenza virus, plays a prominent role in predisposing to pneumococcal infection.[36,37,140,141] Upregulation of surface receptors during viral infection may enhance pneumococcal adherence[142] and invasion. Bacteria are certainly less well cleared from the airways because of viral-induced damage. Pneumococcal disease is greatly increased in people with altered pulmonary clearance, such as those who have chronic bronchitis, asthma, or COPD. Only fairly recently has a study supported clinical observations to associate cigarette smoking with susceptibility to pneumonia.[143] It is an interesting sign of the times that Heffron's classic treatise[1] on pneumococcus, published in 1939, had a section on inhalation of "noxious substances," yet did not mention cigarette smoking. In the United States, invasive pneumococcal disease is more common in certain ethnic groups (e.g., African Americans and Navajo Indians[30]); this prevalence is thought to reflect genetic and environmental factors.[33]

Clinical Syndromes

S. pneumoniae causes infection of the middle ear, sinuses, trachea, bronchi, and lungs by direct spread of organisms from the nasopharyngeal site of colonization and causes infection of the central nervous system, heart valves, bones, joints by hematogenous spread; the peritoneal cavity may be infected by either route (Fig. 200-4). Infection of pleura or peritoneal cavity and of the central nervous system may occur by direct extension or by hematogenous spread. In any individual case, the route of infection cannot usually be determined. Bacteremia that occurs without an apparent source or focus of infection is called primary bacteremia. In a population-based study of adults in Israel,[144] pneumonia was present in 71% of cases of pneumococcal bacteremia, meningitis was present in 8%, and otitis media or sinusitis in 4%; bacteremia was regarded as primary in 18%. Primary bacteremia has always been more common in children than adults; when therapy has been withheld, a focus of infection has often become apparent.

OTITIS MEDIA

Almost every study of acute otitis media in which material from the middle ear has been cultured has shown *S. pneumoniae* to be the most common isolate or second only to nontypeable *Haemophilus influen-*

TABLE 200-4	Factors Predisposing Adults to Invasive Pneumococcal Disease*					
Predisposing Factor	All Invasive Pneumococcal Infection (Sweden)[28]	All Community-Acquired Pneumonia (Pittsburgh)[113]	Pneumococcal Bacteremic Meningitis (Israel)[115]	Bacteremic Pneumococcal Pneumonia (Ohio)[116]	Nonbacteremic Pneumococcal Pneumonia (Houston)[114]	Bacteremic Pneumococcal Pneumonia (Houston)[114]
Alcoholism	32	33	NL	11	35	58
Cigarette smoking	40	55	NL	56	67	69
Chronic lung disease	17	31	19	28	58	42
Congestive heart failure	NL	13	35	16	17	27
Diabetes mellitus	6	13	15	18	12	11
Malignancy	12	29	NL	26	17	25
Kidney disease	1	7	13	4	4	2
Liver disease	2	5	6	NL	21	23
Immunosuppression	NL	36	36	NL	24	32
Recent hospitalization	NL	NL	NL	NL	37	35
No underlying disease	21	31	22	10	0	0

*With the exception of "no underlying disease," the finding of low numbers in some studies and much higher ones in others suggests the possibility of incomplete availability of data in the former. In the Swedish study,[27] 20% of patients with meningitis had prior head injury.
NL, not listed.

zae; Moraxella (Branhamella) catarrhalis is usually a distant third.[145] In these studies, which were usually carried out in children aged 6 months to 4 years and were completed before widespread use of pneumococcal conjugate vaccine, S. pneumoniae was implicated in about 40% to 50% of cases in which a causative agent was isolated or in 30% to 40% of all cases. Pneumococcus is the most prevalent pathogen in otitis media in adults as well.[146] Prior infection by a respiratory virus is thought to play a major contributory role by causing congestion of the opening to the eustachian tube. Prospective longitudinal studies[23,34,147] have shown that when pneumococcal otitis media follows fairly closely after colonization by a new serotype, although most cases of colonization occur without disease. The traditional predominant role of serotypes

6, 14, 19F, and 23F as colonizing and infecting organisms in unvaccinated children may be related to more avid adherence to mammalian cells; important changes that have resulted from widespread use of the conjugate pneumococcal vaccine are discussed later.

SINUSITIS

Acute purulent sinusitis is caused by the same organisms as acute otitis media; thus, S. pneumoniae dominates or is second to H. influenzae.[148] The pathogenesis of infection is also similar, with a prominent predisposing role for congestion of the mucosal membranes caused by viral infection, atmospheric pollutants, or allergens. Accumulation of fluid

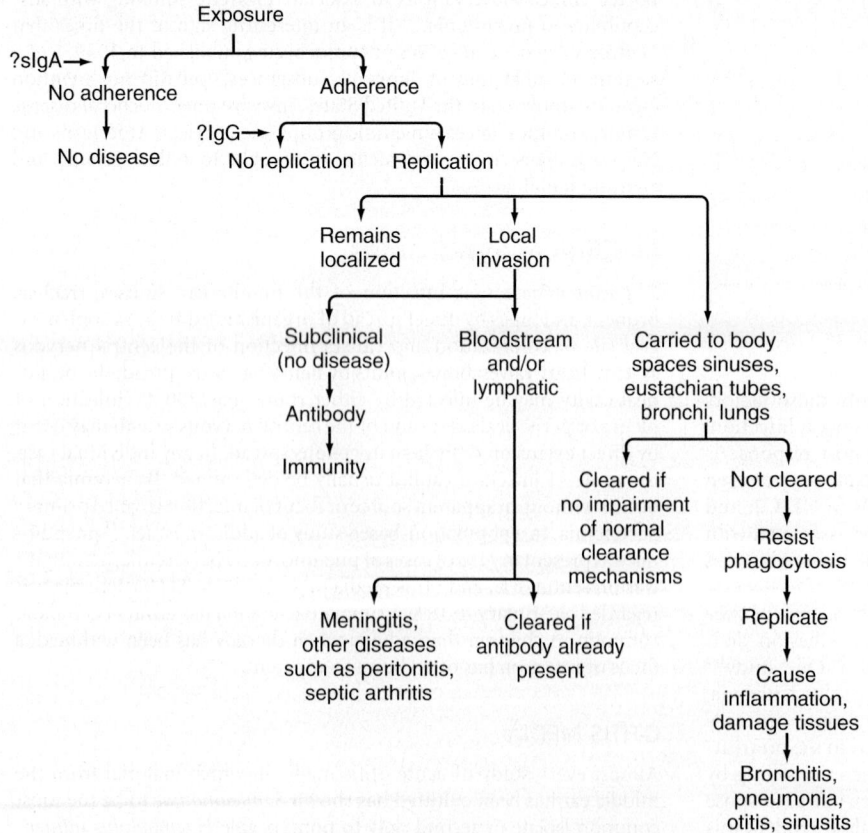

Figure 200-4 Relationship of exposure to development of pneumococcal disease. This is a schematic representation of events that take place between the initial response to pneumococci and eventual development of disease.

in the paranasal sinus cavities, even during simple colds,[149] provides a medium for bacterial proliferation and subsequent acute sinus infection.

MENINGITIS

Except during an epidemic of meningococcal infection, *S. pneumoniae* is the most common cause of bacterial meningitis in adults.[150] In countries that have implemented effective vaccination programs for *H. influenzae* type b, pneumococcus has become the most common sporadic cause of meningitis in children older than 6 months as well.

Meningitis may result from direct extension from the sinuses or middle ear or from bacteremia.[58,151] Favoring the former possibility are the association between acute otitis media or sinusitis and infection of the central nervous system, and the well-documented role of *S. pneumoniae* as the most common cause of recurrent bacterial meningitis associated with head trauma, CSF leak, or a break in the integrity of the dura.[152] Favoring the latter is the high association of pneumococcal pneumonia or bacteremia without a known focus with subsequent meningitis. In addition, an autopsy study of the temporal bones of children who died of bacterial meningitis[153] showed no evidence for extension from the middle ear, which supports the possibility that even when it follows otitis media, meningitis may develop as a result of bacteremia. Although hematogenous spread to the choroid plexus was originally thought to be the pathogenesis in most cases of pneumococcal meningitis, it is now believed that infection upregulates platelet-activating factor on vascular endothelial surfaces in the meninges, and that pneumococci adhere and are internalized by this mechanism.[52] Extension through lymphatics may also contribute.[154] Communication through the cochlear aqueduct between the inner ear and the subarachnoid space may explain deafness, a common complication in patients with hematogenous bacterial meningitis.[154,155]

Once pneumococci appear in the meninges or subarachnoid space, the capabilities to escape phagocytosis and produce inflammation are central to the disease process. As noted, intracisternal injection of cell wall constituents in rabbits, principally peptidoglycan and, to a lesser extent, teichoic acid, causes the CSF abnormalities of bacterial meningitis, presumably through various mediators, including C5a, tumor necrosis factor, IL-1, IL-6, and other active inflammatory peptides.[59,157] Although interaction with Toll-like receptors 2 and 4 may provide some protection, this interaction clearly stimulates further inflammation.[157]

No distinctive clinical or laboratory features of pneumococcal meningitis enable the physician to suspect *S. pneumoniae* over any other causative agent. Using current laboratory techniques for centrifugation of specimens, examination of a Gram-stained specimen of CSF provides the correct diagnosis in almost all cases,[158] unless 3 to 6 hours have passed since the administration of an effective antibiotic, in which case the number of bacteria may be greatly decreased. Immunologic detection of pneumococcal capsular material ("bacterial antigen") generally does not add information beyond what is determined by Gram stain,[159] although nuclear probes are likely to be developed in the near future to help in this situation.

ACUTE EXACERBATION OF CHRONIC BRONCHITIS

Careful microbiologic observation[160,161] has confirmed the clinical impression that *S. pneumoniae* is second to *H. influenzae* as a common cause of exacerbation in patients who have chronic bronchitis. The converse also applies, namely, that a clinically recognizable exacerbation of the chronic disease is highly associated with acquisition of a new pneumococcal strain.[162]

PNEUMONIA

Pathogenesis

If potentially protective mechanisms fail to prevent both the access of pneumococci to the alveoli and their subsequent replication, pneumo-

nia results. Bacteria proliferate in alveolar spaces and spread via the alveolar septa; in these sites, they activate complement, generate cytokine production, and upregulate receptors on vascular endothelial surfaces. Exudative fluid and WBCs accumulate in the septa and alveoli and extend to uninvolved areas through the pores of Kohn. This filling of alveoli with microorganisms and inflammatory exudate defines the presence of pneumonia; a clinical diagnosis is made when fluid accumulation is great enough to allow it to be seen radiographically as a nonlucent region of "infiltration" or "consolidation."

Predisposing Factors

In a prospective study of pneumococcal pneumonia,[133] almost all patients had two or more predisposing conditions such as cigarette smoking, chronic obstructive pulmonary disease, alcohol abuse, neurologic disease (e.g., cerebrovascular accident [CVA], seizures, and dementia), malignancy, liver disease (e.g., hepatitis and/or cirrhosis), recent IV drug use, congestive heart failure, diabetes mellitus, or HIV infection. One third of patients had been discharged from a hospital within the preceding 6 months. The wintertime increase in adult pneumococcal pneumonia and the striking association with viral infections in children and adults has long been noted.[36,42,163,164]

Symptoms and Physical Findings

Cough, fatigue, fever, chills, sweats, and shortness of breath are the most frequent symptoms of pneumonia; these are all more prominent in younger than in older patients.[165,166] Patients with pneumococcal pneumonia usually appear ill and have a grayish, anxious appearance that differs from that of persons with viral or mycoplasmal pneumonia. The temperature may be elevated to 102° to 103° F, the pulse to 90 to 110 beats/min, and the respiratory rate to more than 20/min. Older patients may have only a slight temperature elevation or be afebrile but are more likely to have an increased respiratory rate.[165] The absence of fever in proven pneumococcal pneumonia is associated with increased morbidity and mortality, as is (especially) hypothermia.

Physical examination may reveal diminished respiratory excursion (splinting) on the affected side because of pain. Dullness to percussion is present in about half of cases. Crackling sounds are heard on careful auscultation in almost all cases, but in patients who have chronic lung disease, it is often difficult to be certain that such sounds signify the presence of pneumonia. Increased fremitus is often overlooked, but is very useful in detecting pneumonia. Bronchial or tubular breath sounds may be heard if consolidation is present. Flatness to percussion at the lung base and an inability to detect the expected degree of diaphragmatic motion based on the patient's respiratory excursion suggest the presence of pleural fluid. Unless all the vital signs are normal, which substantially reduces the likelihood of pneumonia, no set of physical findings can reliably replace the chest x-ray in diagnosing the presence or absence of pneumonia.[167] The finding of a heart murmur raises concern about endocarditis, a rare but serious complication. Confusion, obtundation, or especially neck stiffness suggest the presence of meningitis.

Radiographic Findings

In most cases of pneumococcal pneumonia, chest radiography reveals an area of infiltration involving one or more segments within a single lobe.[133] Air space consolidation is detected radiographically in most cases, and is more frequent in bacteremic cases; an air bronchogram, which reflects especially dense air space consolidation, highly correlates with bacteremia.[133,168] Rarely, *S. pneumoniae* infection causes a lung abscess.[169] As emphasized earlier, pneumococci do not produce highly toxic tissue-damaging substances. Thus, abscesses do not generally occur, even at a microscopic level and, if an abscess is seen, concurrent anaerobic infection or an anatomic abnormality such as bronchial obstruction, cancer, or pulmonary infarction should be suspected. Although pleural effusion may be found in 40% of patients with pneumococcal pneumonia by careful search, only 10% have sufficient amounts of fluid to aspirate, and in only a minority of these, perhaps 2% of the total, is empyema present.[170]

General Laboratory Findings

Twenty-five percent of patients with pneumococcal pneumonia have a hemoglobin level of 10 mg/dL or lower.[133] Although most have leukocytosis (WBC count > 12,000/mm³), a substantial proportion may have a normal WBC count, at least at the time of admission. A WBC count lower than 6000/mm³ occurs in 5% to 10% of persons hospitalized for pneumococcal pneumonia and indicates a very poor prognosis.[171] Bone marrow suppression is responsible, resulting from overwhelming infection, sometimes with further contribution by ethanol.[172] The low serum albumin level that often is present may result from malnutrition—and therefore indicate a predisposing condition—or reflect catabolism and fluid shifts that are manifestations of sepsis.[133] The serum bilirubin level may be increased to 3 to 4 mg/dL; the pathogenesis of this abnormality is multifactorial, with hypoxia, hepatic inflammation, and breakdown of red blood cells in the lung all thought to contribute. Levels of lactate dehydrogenase may be elevated. The likelihood that underlying disease is present must always be considered when evaluating abnormal laboratory findings. Laboratory abnormalities in empyema are reviewed in Chapter 65.

Diagnostic Microbiology

The causative role of the pneumococcus in a patient who has pneumonia is strongly suggested by microscopic demonstration of large numbers of PMNs, very few epithelial cells, and numerous, slightly elongated gram-positive cocci in pairs and chains in Gram-stained sputum (Fig. 200-5). If accepted terminology is strictly followed, a presumptive diagnosis of pneumococcal pneumonia is then made if *S. pneumoniae* is identified by sputum culture and the diagnosis is proved if *S. pneumoniae* is identified by blood culture. The argument that the diagnosis is never certain unless the blood culture is also positive is overly restrictive because, even in the preantibiotic era, only about 25% of patients with pneumococcal pneumonia had detectable bacteremia.[1] Ways of interpreting results of blood and sputum culture are shown in Table 200-5.

Attempts to make a diagnosis based on an inadequate sputum specimen[173-175] are largely responsible for studies claiming that microscopic examination and culture of sputum are not reliable. To be reliable, the sputum sample should contain material that on microscopic examination reveals areas with hundreds of WBCs and few epithelial cells at low-power magnification (100×) and at least 10 to 20 WBCs with no epithelial cells under 1000× magnification. At this higher magnification, pneumococci are generally present in large numbers (more than 25/field; see Fig. 200-5), although occasionally as few as 1 to 2 may be seen per field. If sufficient numbers of inflammatory cells are not present, relevant material has not been obtained; if many epithelial cells are detected, the finding of bacteria cannot be trusted to reflect what is present in the bronchi or lungs. A good-quality sputum specimen is far more likely to be obtained by a physician, who best understands its central role in establishing an etiologic diagnosis and

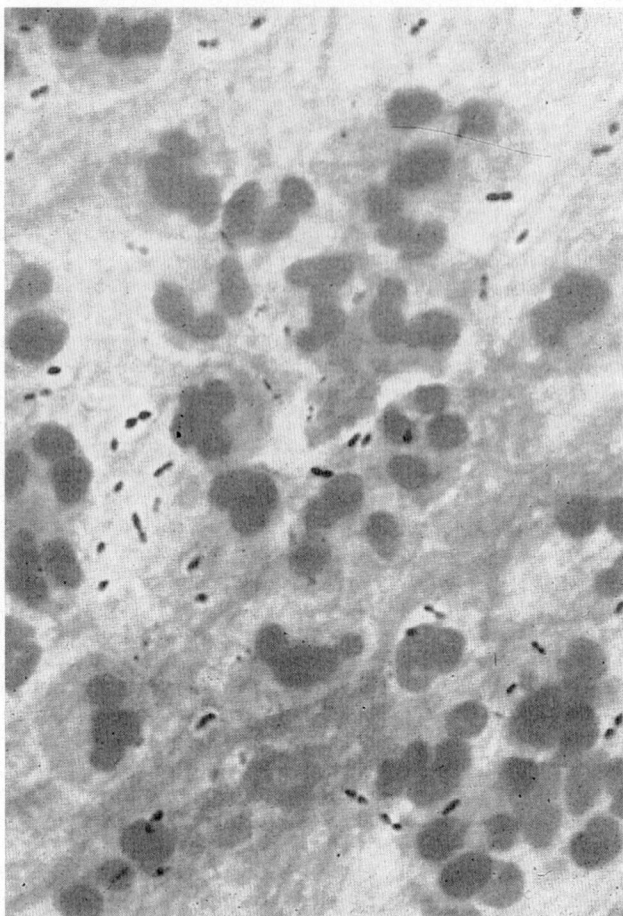

Figure 200-5 **Gram-stained sputum from patient with pneumococcal pneumonia (×1000).** Shown are many polymorphonuclear neutrophils and no epithelial cells, with large numbers of slightly elongated, gram-positive cocci in pairs and chains indicative of *Streptococcus pneumoniae*. A clear area surrounding bacteria indicates the capsule.

determining therapy, than by ancillary personnel, who may not. In our studies,[176] we have found that if patients who cannot provide any specimen or an adequate specimen are excluded, Gram stain and culture identify pneumococci in more than two thirds of cases. With further exclusion of patients who have received antibiotics for 24 hours or longer, Gram stain and culture each are more than 85% likely to reveal

TABLE 200-5	Microscopic Examination and Culture of Sputum for Pneumococci		
Gram Stain	Sputum Culture	Blood Culture	Comment
+	+	+	Generally regarded as conclusive diagnosis of invasive pneumococcal disease (pneumonia), but does not exclude contribution by a contributing cause (e.g., influenza virus infection or lung cancer)
+	+	−	Good evidence for nonbacteremic pneumococcal pneumonia if a clinical syndrome suggesting pneumonia is present, microscopic examination of Gram-stained sputum is characteristic (see Fig. 200-5), and culture shows strongly predominant growth of pneumococci with no other likely pathogenic bacteria
+ or −	−	+	With symptoms and signs of pneumonia and an infiltrate on the chest radiograph, these findings are generally taken to indicate invasive pneumococcal pneumonia, even if organisms are not found in sputum.
+	−	−	In the presence of the appropriate clinical syndrome, still remains suggestive of pneumococcal pneumonia because organisms can be missed on culture as a result of sampling error and overgrowth of streptococci from saliva.
−	+	−	Less suggestive of pneumococcal disease. Pneumococci can be isolated by culture of sputum from persons who are colonized. However, especially in patients already treated with antibiotics, the positive culture may be the only supporting evidence for diagnosis of nonbacteremic pneumococcal pneumonia.
−	−	−	Does not support a diagnosis of pneumococcal pneumonia

pneumococci in expectorated sputum of patients with pneumococcal pneumonia.

When a patient who has pneumonia cannot initially provide an expectorated specimen, the potential problems of empirical therapy should be balanced against the time and trouble that it may take to obtain one (e.g., by nasotracheal suction or hydration, or by having the patient breathe humidified air or hypertonic saline mist). Undue delay (e.g., beyond 6 to 8 hours) should be avoided because it has been shown in large series of cases to be associated with a worse outcome; nevertheless, I believe that many individual patients receive deficient care because the causative organism has not been identified. The recommendation that an antibiotic must be given within 4 hours of a patient's arrival at an emergency room has been recently withdrawn.[177]

Other diagnostic techniques focus on the detection of antigen or antibody. In general, if the sputum is not of sufficiently good quality that the Gram stain is positive, other tests such as coagglutination, antigen detection, or polymerase chain reaction that look for pneumococci in the sputum are not helpful because they are confounded by the potential problem of detecting carriage rather than infection. Pneumococcal cell wall polysaccharide is detected in urine in about 80% of patients with bacteremic pneumococcal pneumonia and a slightly lower percentage of those with pneumococcal bacteremia without pneumonia, or pneumococcal pneumonia without bacteremia. Less than 10% of adults without pneumococcal pneumonia also may have a positive test.[178,179] A strongly positive test in the clinical setting of pneumonia is now regarded as diagnostic of pneumococcal pneumonia in adults.[177] In children, the test is positive with pharyngeal colonization and is not useful diagnostically.[180]

Complications

Empyema, the most common complication of pneumococcal pneumonia in the preantibiotic era, occurred in about 5% of cases and remains the most common today, with an incidence of approximately 2%.[170] As noted, pleural fluid appears in a substantial proportion of cases of pneumonia but is usually reactive. When bacteria reach the pleural space, either hematogenously or as a result of extension of the pneumonia to the visceral pleura with spread via lymphatics, empyema results. Persistence of fever, even if low grade, and leukocytosis after 4 to 5 days of appropriate antibiotic treatment of pneumococcal pneumonia is suggestive of empyema; this diagnosis is even more likely if the radiograph shows persistence of pleural fluid. The presence of frank pus in the pleural space, a positive Gram stain, or fluid with a pH of 7.1 or lower are all indications for aggressive and complete drainage with repeated needle aspiration or prompt insertion of a chest tube. If no response is seen, immediate removal of infected material by pleuroscopy or open thoracotomy is indicated.[181] One study of medical empyema caused by all organisms found that mortality exceeded 30% in two hospitals in which the therapeutic approach was not aggressive but was less than 10% in a third hospital where it was.[182]

We have recently noted an important set of noninfectious complications of pneumococcal pneumonia.[183] In a series of 170 veterans hospitalized for this disease, 33 (19.4%) had at least one major cardiac complication, including 12 (7%) with acute myocardial infarction (MI; of these, 2 also had arrhythmia and 5 had new-onset or worsening congestive heart failure [CHF]), 8 (5%) with new-onset atrial fibrillation or ventricular tachycardia that was transient in every case, and 13 (8%) with newly diagnosed or worsening CHF, without MI or new arrhythmias. Mechanisms for these cardiac events include the following: (1) increased local inflammatory response in vulnerable plaques in coronary arteries with rupture and infarction[184]; (2) decreased oxygen supply because of ventilation-perfusion mismatch; and (3) increased demand on the heart related to the response to fever in the presence of shunting in the lungs.

OTHER INFECTIOUS SYNDROMES

S. pneumoniae can be implicated in a wide variety of infectious states. Isolated or epidemic conjunctivitis may occur, caused (somewhat surprisingly) by unencapsulated pneumococci, essentially the only condition in which unencapsulated pneumococci play a role.[185,186] A case of pneumococcal endocarditis[187] is seen once or twice per decade at a large tertiary care hospital in the United States; 14 cases were identified in Denmark (population, 5 million) in a 10-year period.[188] Alcoholic dependence is common, most infections involve previously normal heart valves, and the disease tends to be rapidly progressive and severe.[187-189] Purulent pericarditis[190] caused by pneumococcus has also become exceedingly rare, whether it occurs as a separate entity or together with endocarditis. Pneumococcal peritonitis occurs by hematogenous or local inoculation of the peritoneal cavity.[191] In patients who have preexisting ascites, pneumococci reach the peritoneum and replicate in the peritoneal fluid, generally in the absence of a documented source of infection elsewhere. Local inoculation occurs in women when pneumococci are carried to the peritoneal cavity via the female reproductive tract, with or without clinically recognizable infection (e.g., salpingitis), or as a result of bowel perforation. Pneumococcal infections of the female reproductive organs[192-194] may occur, with or without peritonitis. Septic arthritis occurs spontaneously in a natural or prosthetic joint or as a complication of rheumatoid arthritis.[195-197] Multiple joints are involved in less than 25% of cases,[198] and the functional outcome is often bad. Osteomyelitis in adults tends to involve the vertebral bones.[199] Epidural and brain abscesses are rarely described.[200] Soft tissue infections[201,202] occur, especially in persons who have connective tissue diseases or HIV infection. Bacteremic pneumococcal cellulitis generally occurs in patients who have severe underlying diseases, and a respiratory focus is often apparent.[203] Finally, the appearance of unusual pneumococcal infections in a young adult might suggest that tests for HIV infection be undertaken.[125]

Antibiotic Susceptibility

Until the mid-1970s, pneumococci were inhibited or killed by readily achievable levels of almost all relevant antibiotics. This remarkable susceptibility allowed for a somewhat cavalier approach to diagnosing and treating otitis, sinusitis, and pneumonia, an approach that has unfortunately not changed, despite the fact that in the past 2 decades, pneumococci have become more resistant to penicillin and other antibiotics. The subject of pneumococcal resistance to penicillin is complicated because the definitions have changed and the susceptibility patterns have evolved.[204] Until the time that pneumococcal resistance was first recognized (importantly, this was in cases of meningitis), no one had ever bothered to apply a definition of susceptibility. Based on the historical knowledge that all isolates had previously been susceptible to ≤0.06 µg/mL, isolates with a minimal inhibitory concentration (MIC) of 0.06 µg/mL (levels readily achievable in CSF with maximum doses of penicillin) were called penicillin-susceptible. Isolates with an MIC ≥ 0.12 to 1.0 µg/mL (levels between 0.5 and 1.0 µg/mL are achieved in some patients) were said to have reduced susceptibility or intermediate resistance, whereas those with an MIC > 1.0 µg/mL were defined as resistant. However, with generally administered doses of IV penicillin, levels achieved in interstitial fluid and in the lungs are far in excess of those achieved in CSF and well above 1 to 2 µg/mL for most of the treatment period. In 2008, the definitions of susceptibility to penicillin changed to reflect the site of infection and the route of therapy.[205]

For infections other than those of the CNS, which are treated with parenteral penicillin, susceptibility, intermediate resistance, and resistance to penicillin are now defined as an MIC ≤ 2, 4, and ≥8 µg/mL, respectively, for infections other than those of the CNS. If oral penicillin is to be used, the old definitions apply, reflecting the substantially lower tissue levels achievable with that therapy. Most importantly, in cases of meningitis, organisms with an MIC ≤ 0.06 µg/mL are susceptible; those with an MIC ≥ 0.12 µg/mL are regarded as resistant. Similar approaches and definitions have been developed to define susceptibility to amoxicillin, ceftriaxone, and other β-lactam antibiotics. For example, MICs for susceptibility, intermediate resistance, and resistance to amoxicillin are defined simply as ≤2, 4, and ≥8 µg/mL, respectively, reflecting the concept that no physician would use oral therapy to treat a CNS infection. For ceftriaxone, there are separate definitions for CNS and non-CNS infections. It is essential to understand these changes in definitions before reading the medical literature on this subject published from 1985 through 2007. Current rates of resistance to these and other antimicrobials are presented in the following section ("Prevalence of Resistance") and summarized in Table 200-6.

Penicillin inhibits the replication of *S. pneumoniae* by binding enzymes needed to synthesize peptidoglycan, including higher molecular weight transpeptidases and a lower molecular weight carboxypeptidase. The binding is covalent, and a serine ester–linked, enzymatically nonactive penicilloyl complex is formed. The reaction with penicillin is used to recognize these enzymes by two general methods: incubating with radiolabeled penicillin, followed by electrophoresis and autoradiography, or incubating with nonlabeled penicillin, followed by electrophoresis and immunoblotting with radiolabeled antipenicilloyl antibody. Six such enzymes have been identified—1A, 1B, 2A, 2B, 2X, and 3. In fully susceptible isolates of *S. pneumoniae*, these six enzymes, which are also called penicillin-binding proteins (PBPs), are identifiable after incubation with low concentrations of penicillin. Resistant isolates have PBPs with decreased affinity for penicillin in a very approximate proportion to the degree of resistance. Changes in the genes that encode these enzymes, with relatively minor alterations in the amino acids at essential loci,[206] may result in the decreased affinity. Alterations in PBP 2B are more likely to account for low-level resistance, whereas mutations in PBP 2X have been associated with high-level resistance.[207]

Pneumococci have become resistant by acquiring genetic material from other bacteria with which they coexist in close proximity. In fact, the altered sequence in the gene for PBP 2B in many penicillin-resistant isolates appears to have originated in *Streptococcus mitis*.[208] The unique capacity of *S. pneumoniae* to acquire genetic material by transformation is a major determinant of this process. Extensive diversity among isolates[209] or within the transpeptide-encoding region of the pneumococcal genome[207,210] indicates that many discrete mutational events have occurred, some of which reflect acquisition and others, rearrangement of DNA. Alterations in several PBPs may eventually appear within an individual isolate, and a mosaic array of PBPs results. Nevertheless, the major source of resistance worldwide has been the geographic spread of a few clones that seem to have special capability to spread and colonize.[211] One well-documented example was the importation into, and rapid spread throughout Iceland of a strain that was prevalent in Spain during the 1992 Olympics.[212] In the United States, the dominant factor in the emergence of antibiotic-resistant pneumococci has been human-to-human spread of relatively

few clonal groups that harbor resistance determinants to multiple classes of antibiotics.[213] These same clones seem to have spread worldwide and may be found, for example, in Korea or Thailand, as well as in Europe.[214] Geographic spread is greatly facilitated by antibiotic pressure, which explains why many of the widespread colonizing clones exhibit antibiotic resistance. A prominent site for this selection is daycare centers. Point prevalence studies in the United States have shown that at any given time, a remarkably high proportion of children in daycare are receiving antibiotics. These conditions (1) suppress susceptible flora, thereby creating a niche for resistant organisms; (2) spare antibiotic-resistant pneumococci; (3) increase the prevalence of antibiotic-resistant viridans streptococci, thus setting the stage for further transformation of pneumococci to antibiotic resistance; and (4) provide close contact among small children, which allows for the spread of organisms. Other situations characterized by close contact and excessive antibiotic use, such as nursing homes, may also serve as breeding grounds for these organisms.

Resistance to penicillin is only the tip of the iceberg. Resistance results from acquisition of a cassette of genetic elements that encode resistance to other antibiotics as well. Many penicillin-resistant strains have alterations in PBPs, especially PBP 2X and 1A,[210] that also render them resistant to third-generation cephalosporins, such as cefotaxime or ceftriaxone. Even low-level increases in MICs for penicillin that still define strains as sensitive are associated with resistance to other widely used antibiotics, including the macrolides, trimethoprim-sulfamethoxazole, tetracyclines, and, to a lesser extent, the quinolones (see Table 200-6).

An understanding of macrolide resistance is important clinically. Macrolides insert into a pocket of the 23S subunit of the 50S ribosome, specifically by attaching at domain V of the peptidyl transferase loop, thereby blocking protein assembly. In doing so, these drugs are bactericidal for *Streptococcus pneumoniae*. (The mechanism for killing of pneumococci is complex; macrolides are generally regarded as bacteriostatic drugs against gram-positive pathogens such as *Staphylococcus aureus*, but are bactericidal against pneumococcus.) Acquisition of genetic material, designated *erm*(B) or *mef*(A), often together with genes that encode penicillin resistance, may lead to resistance:

1. *erm*(B) encodes methylation of a base in domain V of the 23S rRNA (A2058). This methylation essentially blocks the ribosomal pocket; because the macrolide no longer fits into the pocket, increasing its concentration has little effect, and high-level resistance results (≥ 64 µg/mL).
2. *mef*(A) encodes an efflux pump that excludes macrolides. High antibiotic concentrations might be expected to overcome the pump, forcing enough antibiotic into the bacterium to exert an antibacterial effect. This resistance is at a lower level (usually ≤ 16 µg/mL) and, at a sufficient dosage, a macrolide might be expected to be effective.

The debate about whether such resistance is clinically meaningful[215] is based on the fact that most macrolide-resistant isolates in the United States have *mef*(A), and that present doses of macrolides may be effective despite the in vitro finding that an isolate is resistant. Other mutations are responsible for resistance in a small percentage of isolates, causing other base substitutions in domain V or altering protein sequences within or adjacent to the macrolide binding site, especially involving ribosomal proteins L4 and L22.[216]

Prevalence of Resistance

Because the medical literature from 1985 to 2006 used definitions that have now been changed, levels of pneumococcal resistance to β-lactam antibiotics appeared to be much higher than they actually were. Extrapolating from earlier studies, in the United States at present, in treating non-CNS infections caused by *S. pneumoniae*, about 65% of isolates appear to be susceptible to penicillin given orally, 17% are of intermediate resistance, and 17% are resistant (see Table 200-6).[217-220] About 93% of all pneumococci are susceptible to penicillin given parenterally or amoxicillin given orally, 5% are intermediate, and 2% are

TABLE 200-6	Definitions of Susceptibility of Pneumococci to Representative β-Lactam Antibiotics*		
Antibiotic	*Susceptible*	*Intermediate*	*Resistant*
Penicillin (oral)	≥0.06	0.12-1	≥2
Penicillin (parenteral)			
Non-CNS infection	≤2	4	≥8
CNS infection	≤0.06		≥0.12
Amoxicillin†			
Non-CNS	≤2	4	≥8
Ceftriaxone or cefotaxime			
Non-CNS infection	≤1	2	≥4
CNS infection	≤0.5	1	≥2

*Distinguishing between isolates from patients in whom the CNS is or is not involved, according to definitions of the National Committee for Clinical and Laboratory Standards.

†In the case of amoxicillin, no definition is made for CNS infection under the assumption that physicians would not use an oral antibiotic to treat patients for meningitis; parenteral amoxicillin is not available in the United States.

CNS, central nervous system.

resistant.[220] In cases of meningitis, 65% or organisms are susceptible to penicillin and 35% are resistant (no intermediate resistance is defined). For ceftriaxone, in non-CNS infections, 97% of organisms are susceptible, 2% are intermediate, and 1% resistant; in CNS infections, these percentages are 90%, 7%, and 3%, respectively.[221]

Isolates from invasive infection are generally more likely to be antibiotic-susceptible than those from otitis media or nasopharyngeal colonization. Variations occur from city to city and within segments of the population or even within institutions in a single city, so the actual likelihood that a patient will be infected with a resistant strain varies greatly. Rates of resistance are higher in most European countries, with the notable exception of the Netherlands and Germany, where accepted standards of practice strictly limit antibiotic usage,[222] especially among very young children, and are even higher in Korea, Hong Kong, and Thailand, where antibiotic usage is uncontrolled.[223]

Pneumococci with low MICs for penicillin remain susceptible to most other antibiotics. In contrast, as resistance to penicillin increases, organisms are progressively more likely to exhibit resistance to other commonly used antibiotics[219] (Table 200-7). At present, in the United States, about 25% of all pneumococci are resistant to macrolides, 10% to clindamycin, 30% to trimethoprim-sulfamethoxazole, 18% to doxycycline, and 2% to the newer quinolones,[224] again varying with the site of isolation and the geographic region. One third of macrolide-resistant strains have *erm*(B) and are also resistant to clindamycin. In Europe, a higher proportion of pneumococci show some level of macrolide resistance, and *erm*(B) is responsible in most isolates. Rates of resistance are lower in Canada than in the United States and higher in the Far East than in Europe. In general, more than 98% of isolates remain susceptible to fluoroquinolones, probably because these drugs are not used to treat children. In Canada, an increase in resistance has paralleled increased quinolone use[225] and, in high-usage locales, such as chest clinics[226] or nursing homes,[227] the rate of resistance may exceed 5%. Resistance to vancomycin, the oxazolidinones (linezolid), the ketolides (e.g., telithromycin and cethromycin), or the glycylcyclines (e.g., tigecycline) has not yet been documented.

TABLE 200-7	Likelihood (%) of In Vivo Susceptibility of Pneumococcus to Antibiotic Indicated*	
Antibiotic		*Likelihood*
Penicillin (parenteral), ampicillin, piperacillin		93[†]
Amoxicillin		93[†]
Cefuroxime, cefpodoxime, cefdinir		85[†]
Cefotaxime, ceftriaxone, cefepime		97[†]
Imipenem, meropenem, ertapenem		95
Azithromycin, clarithromycin		85[‡]
Clindamycin		93
Telithromycin		100
Trimethoprim-sulfamethoxazole		65
Doxycycline		82
Vancomycin		100
Quinolones[§]		98

*When causing a non-CNS infection such as pneumonia (see text). This is my estimate of the likelihood (%) of a bacteriologic response during treatment with customary doses, based on numerous approximations discussed in the text, as well as by Musher and colleagues.[204] This is not the same as in vitro susceptibility, which is defined by a committee of the National Committee for Clinical and Laboratory Standards (NCCLS), nor is it the same as the likelihood of producing a curve in vivo, which depends in part on bacterial susceptibility but also on other factors, such as the status of the host and the severity of the infection.

[†]With high doses of these drugs, almost all pneumococci are expected to be susceptible.

[‡]This number reflects a balance between the 25% rate of resistance in vitro and clinical experience, which has documented some failures but shows a generally high rate of response. At the time of this writing (November 2008), the precise relationship between in vitro resistance and in vivo failure is still uncertain.

[§]Quinolones = levofloxacin, moxifloxacin.

Treatment

The basic principles of treating pneumococcal infection are similar to those for treating other infections: (1) administer an antibiotic that provides a level sufficient to inhibit or kill the infecting organism; (2) continue treatment at least until the host is able to complete the curing and healing processes; (3) drain infections of closed spaces if necessary; (4) know what response to expect; and (5) be prepared to reevaluate if this response is not observed. These basic principles having been stated, the reader will discover that their application is by no means simple. A few selected factors include the following: (1) for most diseases caused by pneumococcus, when therapy is begun, the causative agent is unknown and, in many cases, no microbiologic studies will be done to reveal it; (2) even if *S. pneumoniae* is believed to be causative, antibiotic susceptibility is not known when treatment is begun; (3) for many common infections, the appropriate duration of therapy has not been established by scientific study; (4) in otitis media and sinusitis, the most common infections caused by *S. pneumoniae*, drainage is not usually done; and (5) many physicians do not clearly understand what response to expect after treatment has begun.

OTITIS MEDIA

In 1998, the Otitis Media Working Group of the Centers for Disease Control and Prevention[145] recommended amoxicillin, 30 mg/kg, three times daily, to treat children with otitis media. The group reasoned that (1) *S. pneumoniae* is the most common identifiable cause of this infection and the one associated with the greatest morbidity; (2) penicillin-susceptible and intermediately resistant pneumococci are likely to respond better to this treatment than to any other; and (3) no other oral therapy is likely to be more effective for resistant pneumococci. The American Academy of Pediatrics has subsequently recommended watchful waiting for children older than 2 years unless severe pain or high fever are present,[228] and these recommendations seem appropriate for adults, as well. Amoxicillin–clavulanic acid, a fluoroquinolone, or ceftriaxone can be used if amoxicillin alone fails. In the absence of a perforated tympanic membrane or some other complication, therapy need not be given for more than 5 days.[229]

SINUSITIS

Because the pathogenesis and causative organisms of acute sinusitis are essentially identical to those of otitis media, the same therapeutic considerations apply. Guidelines have been carefully crafted, and treatment has been related to antibiotic susceptibility patterns, as outlined earlier.[230] Once again, the physician is left with the essential problem of empirical therapy, not knowing whether *S. pneumoniae* is present or, if it is present, whether it is susceptible or resistant to the selected therapy. Amoxicillin is regarded as first-line therapy, with a likely beneficial effect in 80% to 90% of cases; amoxicillin–clavulanic acid, with a slightly higher likelihood of success because of efficacy against β-lactamase–producing *H. influenzae,* is the backup in cases of failure.[230] Unlike children, for whom quinolones have not been approved, adults can be treated with this class of drugs. Ceftriaxone is the fall-back choice, and a failure after this antibiotic has been tried is likely to require referral to an otolaryngologist.

PNEUMONIA

Outpatient Therapy

This section will generally be confined to the selection of therapy for pneumonia caused by *S. pneumoniae* because the broader question of treatment of pneumonia is covered in Chapter 64. Some redundancy is, however, necessary. In outpatients, an attempt is generally not made to establish an etiologic diagnosis; when such attempts are made, *S. pneumoniae* is the predominant agent, accounting for more than half of cases in which a bacterium is cultured and more than one third in which a diagnosis is made (or suspected) by bacteriologic or serologic means. The response generally appears to be excellent, irrespective of the therapy chosen; specifically, penicillins with or without β-lactamase inhibitors, macrolides, doxycycline, or a newer fluoroquinolone all seem to be equally effective,[177] although attention has been called to clinical failures when macrolides are used to treat outpatient pneumonia caused by macrolide-resistant pneumococci.[231] When patients are stratified by risk groups,[232] the mortality reported (without regard to cause) is negligible in most patients who do not require hospitalization.

To treat outpatients for pneumonia, the Infectious Disease Society of America[233] recommends, in no particular order, the use of a macrolide, doxycycline, amoxicillin (with or without clavulanic acid), or a quinolone. There is no certainty of cure in infectious disease practice, and, in my opinion, the cautious physician would do well to try to make the correct diagnosis by microbiologic means. When this cannot be done, patients should be advised of this fact; the physician should keep in close touch with them for the first few days rather than feel content in having "covered" them with empirical antibiotic therapy.

Inpatient Therapy

The importance of the decision to hospitalize or even to admit directly to intensive care cannot be overemphasized. Published guidelines[177] should generally be used, although not followed slavishly. Stratification in accord with recommendations by the Pneumonia Outcomes Research Team[232] should be used to help decide whether hospitalization is needed although, if the physician is in doubt, he or she should hospitalize the patient, at least for the initiation of therapy. The remainder of this section deals with selection of an antibiotic to treat pneumococcal pneumonia.

Pneumococcal pneumonia caused by organisms that are susceptible or intermediately resistant to penicillin responds to treatment with penicillin, 1 million units IV every 4 hours, ampicillin, 1 g every 6 hours, or ceftriaxone, 1 g every 24 hours.[234] The principal concern is whether pneumonia caused by those relatively uncommon pneumococci that are resistant by present definitions responds to such therapy, and also whether the use of higher doses of β-lactam antibiotics or the addition of vancomycin or a fluoroquinolone in such instances seems appropriate.

Patients who are treated for pneumococcal pneumonia with an effective antibiotic generally have substantially reduced fever and feel much better within 48 hours. Based on all the foregoing considerations, if a patient has responded to treatment with a β-lactam antibiotic, this therapy should be continued, even if the antibiotic susceptibility test shows that the causative organism is resistant. If, however, a clear response is not observed and the organism is resistant, therapy should be changed in accordance with susceptibility testing results. A large prospective study[235] has appeared to show that mortality from severe pneumococcal pneumonia is lower in patients who receive two antibiotics (usually a β-lactam and a macrolide) than in those who receive only one (usually a β-lactam). The mortality in the monotherapy arm was excessively high by any standard, even by comparison with data from the early antibiotic era. The authors of that study proposed a role for the anti-inflammatory effect of the macrolide, which was most often the second antibiotic. A more recent prospective study[236] that compared a fluoroquinolone with or without the addition of ceftriaxone has shown no difference. I continue to treat pneumococcal pneumonia with a β-lactam antibiotic.

The optimal duration of therapy for pneumococcal pneumonia is uncertain. Pneumococci are not readily detected in sputum microscopically by culture more than 24 hours after the administration of an effective antibiotic.[175] A small-scale study in the 1950s showed that a single dose of procaine penicillin, which maintains an effective antimicrobial level for as long as 24 hours, could otherwise healthy young adults of pneumococcal pneumonia. Experience obtained early in the antibiotic era showed that 5 to 7 days of therapy sufficed. Nevertheless, the tendency of the medical profession has been to prolong therapy and, in the absence of data to prove additional benefit, most physicians now treat pneumonia for 10 to 14 days. The inclination to prolong therapy entails the risk of emergence of antibiotic-resistant organisms and the onset of complications such as *Clostridium difficile* infection. Three to 5 days of close observation with parenteral therapy for pneumococcal pneumonia and a final few days of oral treatment, in all totaling 7 to 8 days and not exceeding 3 days after a febrile patient has defervesced (temperature lower than 99° F), may be the best approach. Failure of the patient to defervesce within 3 to 5 days should stimulate a review of the organism's antibiotic susceptibility, as well as a search for a loculated infection such as empyema.

MENINGITIS

Pneumococcal meningitis has been treated with 12 to 24 million units of penicillin every 24 hours or 1 to 2 g ceftriaxone every 12 hours. Either regimen is effective against antibiotic-susceptible *S. pneumoniae*; pharmacokinetic considerations and achievable CSF levels favor the use of ceftriaxone. During treatment of resistant strains, β-lactam antibiotics are likely not to achieve therapeutic levels in CSF. This explains why, until susceptibility results are reported, vancomycin is recommended along with the β-lactam antibiotic—the β-lactam because it crosses the blood-brain barrier more reliably and most isolates are susceptible, and the vancomycin because of its potential efficacy against β-lactam-resistant strains. In patients who have major penicillin and cephalosporin allergies, vancomycin can be used; in such cases, addition of a carbapenem should be considered.

Some anecdotal reports have claimed a better outcome when rifampin is added to a β-lactam antibiotic in the treatment of pneumococcal meningitis. In experimental animals, the addition of rifampin to ceftriaxone[237] or vancomycin[238] has not been beneficial, except in the presence of concomitant glucocorticosteroid administration, which may diminish CNS penetration of the antibiotics. Our systematic study in vitro has shown indifference or antagonism when rifampin is added to β-lactam drugs.[239] Although some authorities[156] recommend that rifampin be added when steroids are given together with a third-generation cephalosporin, I believe that the available data do not justify this practice. A study in adults[240] has found, as had been previously shown in children, that addition of dexamethasone, 10 mg four times daily, leads to a distinctly better outcome in pneumococcal meningitis. I use this approach in my practice, although two more recent studies have not confirmed these results. Because of the possibility that steroids may diminish the penetration of antibiotics into the CNS,[241-243] patients receiving these agents should be observed particularly closely; repeat spinal taps may be needed to document abatement of CSF abnormalities, especially if there is any suggestion of a delayed clinical response. Steroid administration should not be continued beyond the recommended 4 days.

MISCELLANEOUS

The use of activated protein C (drotrecogin) has been recommended in patients with severe sepsis. Subgroup analysis suggests that patients with pneumococcal pneumonia and severe sepsis are among those most likely to benefit, with a more than 25% improvement in short- and long-term survival.[244] Pneumococcal endocarditis is associated with rapid destruction of heart valves, and all patients with this disease should be evaluated from the start by a cardiologist and/or a cardiovascular surgeon. Initial therapy should include vancomycin and ceftriaxone until the results of minimal bactericidal concentration testing are known. An aminoglycoside may inhibit the bactericidal activity of β-lactam antibiotics[245] and should not be added unless synergy in vitro is documented to occur.

Prevention

The subject of vaccination to protect against pneumococcal infection has been reviewed extensively.[26,246] Two types of pneumococcal vaccine are now available in the United States. Pneumococcal capsular polysaccharide vaccine, marketed as Pneumovax, contains 25 μg of capsular polysaccharides from each of 23 common infecting serotypes of *S. pneumoniae*. Protein conjugate pneumococcal vaccine, marketed as Prevnar, contains capsular material from seven pneumococcal serotypes that are most commonly implicated in disease of children. This vaccine is released only for pediatric use. In development in the United States, and already in use elsewhere in the world, are vaccines that contain a greater number of conjugated polysaccharides.

ANTIBODY LEVELS POSTVACCINATION

After vaccination with pneumococcal polysaccharide vaccine, a healthy young adult responds with antibody to an average of about three quarters of the antigens.[102] IgG and IgM become detectable within 5 to 7 days after vaccination; in persons with prior exposure, increases in antibody appear according to the same kinetics seen with initial exposure.[108] Although the concept is prevalent that IgM antibody appears first and then production switches to IgG, both classes of antibody appear at the same time in the bloodstream, as well as in lymphocyte cultures in vitro.[108,247] IgG levels then rise to a peak in 4 to 12 weeks, after which they subside over 1 to 2 years but maintain levels significantly higher than those that preceded vaccination for 5 to 10 years. Protection is thought to persist as long as antibody is detectable, but it is not known what level of antibody can be used to determine a threshold for immunity.

Genetic factors govern the ability to make antibody to capsular polysaccharides, and the inheritance is autosomal and dominant.[102] After vaccination, some individuals have high levels of IgG to all capsular polysaccharides, whereas others may fail to respond to most polysaccharides and the IgG levels to the polysaccharide antigens to which they do respond may be very low. Repeated vaccination does not elicit antibody in nonresponders, although IgG to some of the antigens may appear in some subjects after administration of a protein-conjugated vaccine.[248]

The problem with pneumococcal vaccination is that those who need it the most are least likely to make good responses. Older persons may have lower antibody levels after vaccination than younger persons,[103,249] especially those who have chronic lung or heart disease.[99,107] Those who have immunosuppressive conditions that place them at highest risk of pneumococcal infection, such as multiple myeloma, Hodgkin's disease, splenectomy, lymphoma, nephrotic syndrome, renal failure, cirrhosis, sickle cell disease, bone marrow transplantation, and HIV infection, have greatly diminished ability to make IgG to polysaccharide antigens. Persons with acquired AIDS may lose responsiveness to some antigens while retaining relatively normal responses to others.[250,251] A further problem is that many studies have looked only at initial responses. We have recently shown that persons who have recovered from pneumococcal pneumonia respond initially to vaccination, but no longer have detectable antibody at 6 months.[252]

Unlike proteins, polysaccharides do not stimulate long-lived lymphocyte lines that exhibit anamnestic responses—that is, respond to rechallenge with earlier and more vigorous antibody responses. In fact, vaccination induces a suppressive effect that persists for 3 to 4 years, so that revaccination during that time stimulates antibody levels that approach, but do not reach, the original peak.[252]

POSTVACCINATION PROTECTION

Field trials in the first 2 decades of the 20th century showed that vaccination of South African miners with whole killed organisms was protective.[27] Vaccine efficacy with relatively purified preparations of capsular polysaccharide was also demonstrated in civilians and in members of the armed forces in the 1930s and 1940s[253,254]; the reduction in pneumococcal disease was thought to be about 60% in these studies. In subgroups in the population who are thought to be at greatest risk of pneumococcal infection, such as older adults with underlying diseases, some trials have shown similar efficacy,[255,256] but others have failed to find a protective effect.[257-259] For example, in a blinded prospective study carried out under the auspices of the Veterans

Administration,[259] 2354 subjects who were at least 55 years old and had one or more underlying diseases for which vaccine is routinely recommended (principally COPD, alcoholism, chronic renal insufficiency, and congestive heart failure) were randomized to receive 14-valent pneumococcal vaccine or placebo. During almost 3 years of follow-up, no difference in the frequency of pneumococcal pneumonia or bronchitis was noted in the two groups. More recently,[260] a placebo-controlled study of pneumococcal vaccine in those who were discharged from the hospital (a particularly high-risk group) showed a fivefold decrease in pneumococcal bacteremia but no difference in what was called pneumococcal pneumonia based on not well-established serologic techniques.

Other methods of investigation have been used to show the efficacy of pneumococcal vaccine. Use of an indirect cohort method has shown that when organisms causing invasive pneumococcal disease are serotyped, previously vaccinated persons have a significantly lower incidence of infection by vaccine versus nonvaccine serotypes than controls.[261] A retrospective cohort study has shown approximately a 56% reduction in proven pneumococcal bacteremia, but no impact on the overall rate of pneumonia in an older population.[262] Several case-control studies have also shown efficacy.[263-265] In all these studies, the efficacy of vaccine was about 60% to 70%, the same efficacy that had been recorded in prospective field trials. In one large case-control study, the protective effect of pneumococcal vaccine was shown to be greatest in younger adults and to decline slowly with time, persisting for at least 5 years in young adults but not in older adults (Table 200-8).[264]

ANTIBODY EFFICIENCY

Recent laboratory investigations have helped explain why vaccine efficacy might be reduced in those who are in greatest need of it. First, although postvaccination IgG levels are similar in very healthy older and younger adults, antibody levels in the older population at large may be lower because of reduced responses in chronically ill persons. Second, the ability of IgG to opsonize pneumococci for phagocytosis and to protect experimental animals against pneumococcal challenge is diminished in ill and older persons.[103,266] Finally, about one third of adults who are hospitalized with pneumococcal pneumonia have antibody to their infecting serotype at the time of admission, but this antibody is nonopsonic in vitro and does not protect mice against experimental challenge with that organism.[105] Thus, antibody levels may be lower and/or antibody may have lesser ability to protect those who are in greatest need of vaccine.

VACCINE RECOMMENDATIONS

With data demonstrating the safety, low cost, and efficacy of pneumococcal vaccine, failure to use it more widely can be regarded as a missed opportunity in public health policy.[267] The Advisory Committee on Immunization Practices of the Centers for Disease Control and

TABLE 200-8	Case-Control Study: Protection by Pneumococcal Vaccine*			
		Years Since Vaccination		
Age (yr)	Pairs of Subjects	<3	3-5	>5
<55	125	93	89	85
55-64	149	88	82	75
65-74	213	80	71	58
75-84	188	67	53	32
≥85	133	46	33	0

*Results of a case-control study[240] that estimated the efficacy of pneumococcal vaccination by matching infected patients with uninfected controls (pairs of subjects) and examining the incidence of prior vaccination in each group. Data are shown as a percentage indicating efficacy as estimated percent protection.

Prevention has broadened its recommendations to include immunization of all children aged 2 to 23 months with the seven-serotype conjugate vaccine (Prevnar; also see Chapter 320).[268,269] The 23-valent vaccine (Pneumovax) is recommended for all persons older than 2 years who are at substantially increased risk of developing pneumococcal infection and/or a serious complication of such an infection.[270] General categories included within these recommendations are those persons who (1) are older than 65 years; (2) have anatomic or functional asplenia, CSF leak, diabetes mellitus, alcoholism, cirrhosis, chronic renal insufficiency, chronic pulmonary disease (including asthma), or advanced cardiovascular disease; (3) have an immunocompromised condition associated with increased risk of pneumococcal disease, such as multiple myeloma, lymphoma, Hodgkin's disease, HIV infection, organ transplantation, or chronic use of glucocorticosteroids; (4) are genetically at increased risk, such as Native Americans and Alaskans; and (5) who live in special environments in which outbreaks may occur, such as nursing homes.

Recommendations regarding revaccination seem to be somewhat inconsistent because the committee advocates a single revaccination for those older than 65 years. Because antibody levels decline and there is no anamnestic response, it seems more reasonable simply to recommend revaccination at 5- to 7-year intervals, especially in adults older than 65, who will have a minimal local reaction.[271] Persons who are at highest risk of recurring pneumococcal infection are those who have undergone splenectomy or have a CSF leak; in my opinion, these persons should be vaccinated every 5 years.

PROTEIN CONJUGATE VACCINES

The protein conjugate vaccines[246] were developed because children younger than 2 years do not respond well to polysaccharide antigens. However, when pneumococcal capsular polysaccharides have been covalently conjugated to carrier proteins, the resulting antigens are recognized as T-cell–dependent; they stimulate good antibody responses in children younger than 2 years and induce immunologic memory. A series of three or four injections of a vaccine that contained seven commonly infecting pneumococcal serotypes each conjugated to a genetically engineered diphtheria toxoid stimulated good antibody levels in infants; invasive disease (bacteremic infection or meningitis) was almost eliminated by the full set of immunizations.[272] The impact on less clearly proven entities is much less striking, indicating a problem with diagnosis of disease, not with the vaccine. Thus, proven pneumococcal otitis media is reduced by 65%, whereas all-cause otitis is only reduced by 8%[273]; bacteremic pneumococcal pneumonia is reduced by more than 90%, whereas all-cause pneumonia is only reduced by 21%.[274] Conjugate pneumococcal vaccine has a major impact on reducing the rate of carriage of vaccine strains.[272]

In adults, protein conjugate pneumococcal vaccine can induce a response in persons who, on a genetic basis, do not make antibody to polysaccharide antigens[249] and may possibly stimulate higher mean levels of IgG in those who respond normally or are immunocompro-

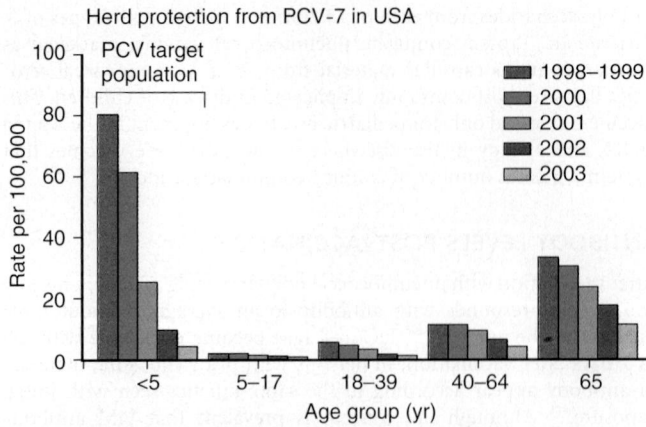

Figure 200-6 **Incidence of pneumococcal disease in all age groups.** An active vaccination program in infants and toddlers using sevenvalent conjugate pneumococcal vaccine (PCV-7) beginning in 2000 greatly reduced the incidence of invasive pneumococcal disease in children each year through 2003.[278] There has also been a striking decline in the incidence of disease among older subjects. Some of the effects in children younger than 5 years and almost all the effects in older adults are attributable to the herd effect (see text).

mised.[276] We have shown that in patients who have recovered from pneumococcal pneumonia, conjugate vaccine stimulates higher levels of antibody that persist better than those following polysaccharide vaccine.[249] Nevertheless, because of the limited number of strains covered and concerns related to suppressed responses after repeated vaccinations, conjugate vaccine is not recommended for adults.

Widespread use of the conjugate vaccine has enormously reduced the incidence of pneumococcal disease in all age groups (Fig. 200-6).[277] In children, this effect is a direct result of vaccination; in nonvaccinated children and adults it represents what is called the "herd effect," in which the protection of the entire population results from reduced nasopharyngeal carriage of infective strains in the vaccinated population.[278] Reduction of carriage of vaccine strains in infants is important in producing the herd effect,[275,279] in which even highly susceptible groups of adults such as those with HIV infection have been protected against invasive disease.[280] An unwanted side effect of widespread vaccination, however, has been the emergence of replacement strains as commonly infecting organisms. These are serotypes that are not included in the vaccine and that were not previously common, such as *S. pneumoniae* types 15, 19A, and 33F.[281] In fact, type 19A has become the most common cause of invasive pneumococcal disease in children, a finding that is particularly worrisome because a disproportionate number of isolates are resistant to penicillin. Interestingly, the prevalent type 19A strain reflects capsule switching because it has the genotype of *S. pneumoniae* type 4.[282]

REFERENCES

1. Heffron R. *Pneumonia with Special Reference to Pneumococcus Lobar Pneumonia.* New York: Commonwealth Fund; 1939 [reprinted by Harvard University Press, 1979].
2. White B, Robinson ES, Barnes LA. *The Biology of the Pneumococcus: The Bacteriological, Biochemical and Immunological Characters and Activities of Diplococcus pneumoniae.* New York: Commonwealth Fund; 1938 [reprinted by Harvard University Press, 1979].
3. Gray BM, Musher DM. The history of pneumococcal disease. In: Siber G, Klugman KP, Makela P, eds. *Pneumococcal Vaccines: The Impact of Conjugate Vaccine.* Washington DC: ASM Press; 2008:3-17.
4. Musher DM, Watson DA, Dominguez EA. Pneumococcal vaccination: Work to date and future prospects. *Am J Med Sci.* 1990;300:45-52.
5. Heidelberger M, Avery OT. The soluble specific substance of pneumococcus. *J Exp Med.* 1923;38:73.
6. Felton LD. Studies on the immunizing substances in pneumococci. *J Immunol.* 1934;27:379-393.
7. Smillie WG, Wornock GH, White HJ. A study of a type I pneumococcus epidemic at the State Hospital at Worcester, Mass. *Am J Publ Health.* 1938;28:293-302.
8. MacLeod CM, Hodges RG, Heidelberger M, et al. Prevention of pneumococcal pneumonia by immunization with specific capsular polysaccharides. *J Exp Med.* 1945;82:445-465.
9. Griffith F. The significance of pneumococcal types. *J Hyg (Lond).* 1928;27:113-159.
10. Avery OT, MacLeod C, McCarty M. Studies on the chemical nature of the substance inducing transformation of pneumococcal types. *J Exp Med.* 1944;79:137-157.
11. Munoz R, Fenoll A, Vicioso D, et al. Optochin-resistant variants of Streptococcus pneumoniae. *Diagn Microbiol Infect Dis.* 1990;13:63-66.
12. Keith ER, Podmore RG, Anderson TP, et al. Characteristics of Streptococcus pseudopneumoniae isolated from purulent sputum samples. *J Clin Microbiol.* 2006;44:923-927.
13. Sorensen UB. Pneumococcal polysaccharide antigens: Capsules and C-polysaccharide. An immunochemical study. *Dan Med Bull.* 1995;42:47-53.
14. Ertugrul N, Rodriguez-Barradas MC, Musher DM, et al. BOX-polymerase chain reaction-based DNA analysis of nonserotypeable Streptococcus pneumoniae implicated in outbreaks of conjunctivitis. *J Infect Dis.* 1997;176:1401-1405.
15. van Dam JE, Fleer A, Snippe H. Immunogenicity and immunochemistry of Streptococcus pneumoniae capsular polysaccharides. *Antonie Van Leeuwenhoek.* 1990;58:1-47.
16. Morona JK, Morona R, Paton JC. Molecular and genetic characterization of the capsule biosynthesis locus of Streptococcus pneumoniae type 19B. *J Bacteriol.* 1997;179:4953-4958.
17. Yother J, Bentley S, Hennessey J Jr. Genetics, biosynthesis and chemistry of pneumococcal capsular polysaccharides. In: Siber G, Klugman KP, Makela P, eds. *Pneumococcal Vaccines: The Impact Of Conjugate Vaccine.* Washington DC: ASM Press; 2008:33-46.

18. Peterson S, Cline RT, Tettelin H, et al. Gene expression analysis of the Streptococcus pneumoniae competence regulons by use of DNA microarrays. *J Bacteriol.* 2000;182:6192-6202.
19. Coffey TJ, Enright MC, Daniels M, et al. Recombinational exchanges at the capsular polysaccharide biosynthetic locus lead to frequent serotype changes among natural isolates of Streptococcus pneumoniae. *Mol Microbiol.* 1998;27:73-83.
20. Coffey TJ, Daniels M, Enright MC, et al. Serotype 14 variants of the Spanish penicillin-resistant serotype 9V clone of Streptococcus pneumoniae arose by large recombinational replacements of the cpsA-pbp1a region. *Microbiology.* 1999;145(Pt 8):2023-2031.
21. Jefferies JM, Smith A, Clarke SC, et al. Genetic analysis of diverse disease-causing pneumococci indicates high levels of diversity within serotypes and capsule switching. *J Clin Microbiol.* 2004;42:5681-5688.
22. Dudley S, Ashe K, Winther B, et al. Bacterial pathogens of otitis media and sinusitis: Detection in the nasopharynx with selective agar media. *J Lab Clin Med.* 2001;138:338-342.
23. Gray BM, Dillon HC Jr. Epidemiological studies of Streptococcus pneumoniae in infants: antibody to types 3, 6, 14, and 23 in the first two years of life. *J Infect Dis.* 1988;158:948-955.
24. Huang SS, Finkelstein JA, Rifas-Shiman SL, et al. Community-level predictors of pneumococcal carriage and resistance in young children. *Am J Epidemiol.* 2004;159:645-654.
25. Ekdahl K, Ahlinder I, Hansson HB, et al. Duration of nasopharyngeal carriage of penicillin-resistant Streptococcus pneumoniae: Experiences from the South Swedish Pneumococcal Intervention Project. *Clin Infect Dis.* 1997;25:1113-1117.
26. Fedson DS, Musher DM. Pneumococcal vaccine. In: Plotkin SA, Orenstein WB, eds. *Vaccines.* 4th ed. Philadelphia: WB Saunders; 2003:529-588.
27. Burman LA, Norrby R, Trollfors B. Invasive pneumococcal infections: Incidence, predisposing factors, and prognosis. *Rev Infect Dis.* 1985;7:133-142.
28. Breiman RF, Spika JS, Navarro VJ, et al. Pneumococcal bacteremia in Charleston County, South Carolina. A decade later. *Arch Intern Med.* 1990;150:1401-1405.
29. Harrison LH, Dwyer DM, Billmann L, et al. Invasive pneumococcal infection in Baltimore, Md: Implications for immunization policy. *Arch Intern Med.* 2000;160:89-94.
30. Watt JP, O'Brien KL, Benin AL, et al. Invasive pneumococcal disease among Navajo adults, 1989-1998. *Clin Infect Dis.* 2004;38:496-501.
31. Davidson M, Parkinson AJ, Bulkow LR, et al. The epidemiology of invasive pneumococcal disease in Alaska, 1986-1990—ethnic differences and opportunities for prevention. *J Infect Dis.* 1994;170:368-376.
32. Torzillo PJ, Hanna JN, Morey F, et al. Invasive pneumococcal disease in central Australia. *Med J Aust.* 1995;162:182-186.
33. Watt JP, O'Brien KL, Benin AL, et al. Risk factors for invasive pneumococcal disease among Navajo adults. *Am J Epidemiol.* 2007;166:1080-1087.
34. Gray BM, Converse GM 3rd, Dillon HC Jr. Epidemiologic studies of *Streptococcus pneumoniae* in infants: Acquisition, carriage, and infection during the first 24 months of life. *J Infect Dis.* 1980;142:923-933.
35. Frenck Jr RW, Glezen WP. Respiratory tract infections in children in day care. *Semin Pediatr Infect Dis.* 1990;1:234-244.
36. Kim PE, Musher DM, Glezen WP, et al. Association of invasive pneumococcal disease with season, atmospheric conditions, air pollution, and the isolation of respiratory viruses. *Clin Infect Dis.* 1996;22:100-106.
37. Dowell SF, Whitney CG, Wright C, et al. Seasonal patterns of invasive pneumococcal disease. *Emerg Infect Dis.* 2003;9:573-579.
38. Musher DM. How contagious are common respiratory infections? *N Engl J Med.* 2003;348:1256-1266.
39. Henderson FW, Gilligan PH, Wait K, et al. Nasopharyngeal carriage of antibiotic-resistant pneumococci by children in group day care. *J Infect Dis.* 1988;157:256-263.
40. Rauch AM, O'Ryan M, Van R, et al. Invasive diease due to multiply resitant *Streptococcus pneumoniae* in a Houston, Texas day care center. *Am J Dis Child.* 1990;144:923-927.
41. Doyle MG, Morrow AL, Van R, et al. Intermediate resistance of *Streptococcus pneumoniae* to penicillin in children in day-care centers. *Pediatr Infect Dis J.* 1992;11:831-835.
42. Hodges R, MacLeod C. Epidemic pneumococcal pneumonia: I. Description of the epidemic. *Amer J Hygiene.* 1946;44:183-192.
43. Hoge CW, Reichler MR, Dominguez EA, et al. An epidemic of pneumococcal disease in an overcrowded, inadequately ventilated jail. *N Engl J Med.* 1994;331:643-648.
44. Mercat A, Nguyen J, Dautzenberg B. An outbreak of pneumococcal pneumonia in two men's shelters. *Chest.* 1991;99:147-151.
45. Gleich S, Morad Y, Echague R, et al. Streptococcus pneumoniae serotype 4 outbreak in a home for the aged: Report and review of recent outbreaks. *Infect Control Hosp Epidemiol.* 2000;21:711-717.
46. Mitchell TJ. Streptococcus pneumoniae: infection, inflammation and disease. *Adv Exp Med Biol.* 2006;582:111-124.
47. Kadioglu A, Weiser JN, Paton JC, et al. The role of Streptococcus pneumoniae virulence factors in host respiratory colonization and disease. *Nat Rev Microbiol.* 2008;6:288-301.
48. Paterson GK, Mitchell TJ. Innate immunity and the pneumococcus. *Microbiology.* 2006;152(Pt 2):285-293.
49. Cundell DR, Pearce BJ, Sandros J, et al. Peptide permeases from Streptococcus pneumoniae affect adherence to eucaryotic cells. *Infect Immun.* 1995;63:493-498.
50. Ishizuka S, Yamaya M, Suzuki T, et al. Effects of rhinovirus infection on the adherence of Streptococcus pneumoniae to cultured human airway epithelial cells. *J Infect Dis.* 2003;188:1928-1939.
51. Fillon S, Soulis K, Rajasekaran S, et al. Platelet-activating factor receptor and innate immunity: uptake of gram-positive bacterial cell wall into host cells and cell-specific pathophysiology. *J Immunol.* 2006;177:6182-6191.
52. Krivan H, Roberts D, Ginsberg V. Many pulmonary pathogenic bacteria bind specifically to the carbohydrate sequence GalNAc B1-4-Gal found in some glycolipids. *Proc Natl Acad Sci U S A.* 1988;85:6157-6161.
53. Sundberg-Kovamees M, Holme T, Sjogren A. Interaction of the C-polysaccharide of *Streptococcus pneumoniae* with the receptor asialo-GM. *Microb Pathog.* 1996;21:223-234.
54. Weiser JN, Markiewicz Z, Tuomanen EI, et al. Relationship between phase variation in colony morphology, intrastrain variation in cell wall physiology, and nasopharyngeal colonization by Streptococcus pneumoniae. *Infect Immun.* 1996;64:2240-2245.
55. Rose L, Shivshankar P, Hinojosa E, et al. Antibodies against PsrP, a novel Streptococcus pneumoniae adhesin, block adhesion and protect mice against pneumococcal challenge. *J Infect Dis.* 2008;198:375-383.
56. Brock SC, McGraw PA, Wright PF, et al. The human polymeric immunoglobulin receptor facilitates invasion of epithelial cells by Streptococcus pneumoniae in a strain-specific and cell type-specific manner. *Infect Immun.* 2002;70:5091-5095.
57. Cundell DR, Gerard NP, Gerard C, et al. Streptococcus pneumoniae anchor to activated human cells by the receptor for platelet-activating factor. *Nature.* 1995;377:435-438.
58. Koedel U, Scheld WM, Pfister HW. Pathogenesis and pathophysiology of pneumococcal meningitis. *Lancet Infect Dis.* 2002;2:721-736.
59. Watson DA, Musher DM. Interruption of capsule production in Streptococcus pneumonia serotype 3 by insertion of transposon Tn916. *Infect Immun.* 1990;58:3135-3138.
60. Angel CS, Ruzek M, Hostetter MK. Degradation of C3 by Streptococcus pneumoniae. *J Infect Dis.* 1994;170:600-608.
61. Musher DM, Johnson Jr B, Watson DA. Quantitative relationship between anticapsular antibody measured by enzyme-linked immunosorbent assay or radioimmunoassay and protection of mice against challenge with Streptococcus pneumoniae serotype 4. *Infect Immun.* 1990;58:3871-3876.
62. Ren B, Szalai AJ, Thomas O, et al. Both family 1 and family 2 PspA proteins can inhibit complement deposition and confer virulence to a capsular serotype 3 strain of Streptococcus pneumoniae. *Infect Immun.* 2003;71:75-85.
63. Ren B, McCrory MA, Pass C, et al. The virulence function of Streptococcus pneumoniae surface protein A involves inhibition of complement activation and impairment of complement receptor-mediated protection. *J Immunol.* 2004;173:7506-7512.
64. Quin LR, Carmicle S, Dave S, et al. In vivo binding of complement regulator factor H by Streptococcus pneumoniae. *J Infect Dis.* 2005;192:1996-2003.
65. Boulnois GJ. Pneumococcal proteins and the pathogenesis of disease caused by Streptococcus pneumoniae. *J Gen Microbiol.* 1992;138(Pt 2):249-259.
66. Paton JC, Berry AM, Lock RA. Molecular analysis of putative pneumococcal virulence proteins. *Microb Drug Resist.* 1997;3:1-10.
67. Rubins JB, Charboneau D, Paton JC, et al. Dual function of pneumolysin in the early pathogenesis of murine pneumococcal pneumonia. *J Clin Invest.* 1995;95:142-150.
68. Rubins JB, Janoff EN. Pneumolysin: A multifunctional pneumococcal virulence factor. *J Lab Clin Med.* 1998;131:21-27.
69. Feldman C, Munro NC, Jeffery PK, et al. Pneumolysin induces the salient histologic features of pneumococcal infection in the rat lung in vivo. *Am J Respir Cell Mol Biol.* 1991;5:416-423.
70. Alexander JE, Lock RA, Peeters CC, et al. Immunization of mice with pneumolysin toxoid confers a significant degree of protection against at least nine serotypes of Streptococcus pneumoniae. *Infect Immun.* 1994;62:5683-5688.
71. Berry AM, Paton JC, Hansman D. Effect of insertional inactivation of the genes encoding pneumolysin and autolysin on the virulence of Streptococcus pneumoniae type 3. *Microb Pathog.* 1992;12:87-93.
72. Berry AM, Alexander JE, Mitchell TJ, et al. Effect of defined point mutations in the pneumolysin gene on the virulence of Streptococcus pneumoniae. *Infect Immun.* 1995;63:1969-1974.
73. Rogers PD, Thornton J, Barker KS, et al. Pneumolysin-dependent and -independent gene expression identified by cDNA microarray analysis of THP-1 human mononuclear cells stimulated by Streptococcus pneumoniae. *Infect Immun.* 2003;71:2087-2094.
74. Musher DM, Phan HM, Baughn RE. Protection against bacteremic pneumococcal infection by antibody to pneumolysin. *J Infect Dis.* 2001;183:827-830.
75. Roche H, Hakansson A, Hollingshead SK, et al. Regions of PspA/EF3296 best able to elicit protection against Streptococcus pneumoniae in a murine infection model. *Infect Immun.* 2003;71:1033-1041.
76. McDaniel LS, Sheffield JS, Delucchi P, et al. PspA, a surface protein of Streptococcus pneumoniae, is capable of eliciting protection against pneumococci of more than one capsular type. *Infect Immun.* 1991;59:222-228.
77. McDaniel LS, Yother J, Vijayakumar M, et al. Use of insertional inactivation to facilitate studies of biological properties of pneumococcal surface protein A (PspA). *J Exp Med.* 1987;165:381-394.
78. Briles DE, Hollingshead SK, King J, et al. Immunization of humans with recombinant pneumococcal surface protein A (rPspA) elicits antibodies that passively protect mice from fatal infection with Streptococcus pneumoniae bearing heterologous PspA. *J Infect Dis.* 2000;182:1694-1701.
79. McCool TL, Cate TR, Tuomanen EI, et al. Serum immunoglobulin G response to candidate vaccine antigens during experimental human pneumococcal colonization. *Infect Immun.* 2003;71:5724-5732.
80. Johnson SE, Dykes JK, Jue DL, et al. Inhibition of pneumococcal carriage in mice by subcutaneous immunization with peptides from the common surface protein pneumococcal surface adhesin a. *J Infect Dis.* 2002;185:489-496.
81. Romero-Steiner S, Pilishvili T, Sampson JS, et al. Inhibition of pneumococcal adherence to human nasopharyngeal epithelial cells by anti-PsaA antibodies. *Clin Diagn Lab Immunol.* 2003;10:246-251.
82. Rapola S, Kilpi T, Lahdenkari M, et al. Do antibodies to pneumococcal surface adhesin a prevent pneumococcal involvement in acute otitis media? *J Infect Dis.* 2001;184:577-581.
83. Lock RA, Hansman D, Paton JC. Comparative efficacy of autolysin and pneumolysin as immunogens protecting mice against infection by Streptococcus pneumoniae. *Microb Pathog.* 1992;12:137-143.
84. Winkelstein JA, Tomasz A. Activation of the alternative complement pathway by pneumococcal cell wall teichoic acid. *J Immunol.* 1978;120:174-178.
85. Tuomanen EI, Liu H, Hengstler B, et al. The induction of meningeal inflammation by components of the pneumococcal cell wall. *J Infect Dis.* 1985;151:859-868.
86. Wolbink GJ, Bossink AW, Groeneveld AB, et al. Complement activation in patients with sepsis is in part mediated by C-reactive protein. *J Infect Dis.* 1998;177:81-87.
87. Winkelstein JA, Bocchini Jr JA, Schiffman G. The role of the capsular polysaccharide in the activation of the alternative pathway by the pneumococcus. *J Immunol.* 1976;116:367-370.
88. Rodriguez-Barradas MC, Das TS, Watson DA, et al. Relative contribution of cell wall and capsular polysaccharides in activating alternative and classical complement pathways by *Streptococcus pneumoniae. Gen Microbiol.* 1993:427-435.
89. Yee AM, Phan HM, Zuniga R, et al. Association between Fcgamma RIIa-R131 allotype and bacteremic pneumococcal pneumonia. *Clin Infect Dis.* 2000;30:25-28.
90. Schroder NW, Morath S, Alexander C, et al. Lipoteichoic acid (LTA) of Streptococcus pneumoniae and Staphylococcus aureus activates immune cells via Toll-like receptor (TLR)-2, lipopolysaccharide-binding protein (LBP), and CD14, whereas TLR-4 and MD-2 are not involved. *J Biol Chem.* 2003;278:15587-15594.
91. Dessing MC, Schouten M, Draing C, et al. Role played by Toll-like receptors 2 and 4 in lipoteichoic acid-induced lung inflammation and coagulation. *J Infect Dis.* 2008;197:245-252.
92. Malley R, Henneke P, Morse SC, et al. Recognition of pneumolysin by Toll-like receptor 4 confers resistance to pneumococcal infection. *Proc Natl Acad Sci U S A.* 2003;100:1966-1971.
93. Texereau J, Chiche JD, Taylor W, et al. The importance of Toll-like receptor 2 polymorphisms in severe infections. *Clin Infect Dis.* 2005;41(Suppl 7):S408-S415.
94. Lanoue A, Clatworthy MR, Smith P, et al. SIGN-R1 contributes to protection against lethal pneumococcal infection in mice. *J Exp Med.* 2004;200:1383-1393.
95. Baumgarth N, Tung JW, Herzenberg LA. Inherent specificities in natural antibodies: a key to immune defense against pathogen invasion. *Springer Semin Immunopathol.* 2005;26:347-362.
96. Alugupalli KR, Gerstein RM. Divide and conquer: division of labor by B-1 B cells. *Immunity.* 2005;23:1-2.
97. Eisen DP, Dean MM, Boermeester MA, et al. Low serum mannose-binding lectin level increases the risk of death due to pneumococcal infection. *Clin Infect Dis.* 2008;47:510-516.
98. Podolsky SH. *Pneumonia Before Antibiotics: Therapeutic Evolution and Evaluation in Twentieth-century America.* Baltimore, Md: Johns Hopkins Press; 2006.
99. Musher DM, Chapman AJ, Goree A, et al. Natural and vaccine-related immunity to Streptococcus pneumoniae. *J Infect Dis.* 1986;154:245-256.
100. Romero-Steiner S, Libutti D, Pais LB, et al. Standardization of an opsonophagocytic assay for the measurement of functional antibody activity against Streptococcus pneumoniae using differentiated HL-60 cells. *Clin Diagn Lab Immunol.* 1997;4:415-422.
101. Lipsitch M, Whitney CG, Zell E, et al. Are anticapsular antibodies the primary mechanism of protection against invasive pneumococcal disease? *PLoS Med.* 2005;2:e15.
102. Musher DM, Groover JE, Watson DA, et al. Genetic regulation of the capacity to make immunoglobulin G to pneumococcal capsular polysaccharides. *J Investig Med.* 1997;45:57-68.
103. Romero-Steiner S, Musher DM, Cetron MS, et al. Reduction in functional antibody activity against *Streptococcus pneumoniae* in vaccinated elderly individuals highly correlates with decreased IgG antibody avidity. *Clin Infect Dis.* 1999;29:281-288.

104. Smithson SL, Kolibab K, Shriner AK, et al. Immune response to pneumococcal polysaccharides 4 and 14 in elderly and young adults: Analysis of the variable light chain repertoire. *Infect Immun.* 2005;73:7477-7484.
105. Musher DM, Phan HM, Watson DA, et al. Antibody to capsular polysaccharide of Streptococcus pneumoniae at the time of hospital admission for Pneumococcal pneumonia. *J Infect Dis.* 2000;182:158-167.
106. Siber GR, Priehs C, Madore DV. Standardization of antibody assays for measuring the response to pneumococcal infection and immunization. *Pediatr Infect Dis J.* 1989;8(Suppl):S84-S91.
107. Musher DM, Luchi MJ, Watson DA, et al. Pneumococcal polysaccharide vaccine in young adults and older bronchitics: Determination of IgG responses by ELISA and the effect of adsorption of serum with non-type-specific cell wall polysaccharide. *J Infect Dis.* 1990;161:728-735.
108. Musher DM, Groover JE, Rowland JM, et al. Antibody to capsular polysaccharides of Streptococcus pneumoniae: Prevalence, persistence, and response to revaccination. *Clin Infect Dis.* 1993;17:66-73.
109. Finland M, Tilghman RC. Bacteriological and immunological studies in families with pneumococci infections: The development of type-specific antibodies in healthy contact carriers. *J Clin Invest.* 1936;15:500-508.
110. Finland M, Winkler AW. Antibody response to infections with type II and with the related type VIII pneumococcus. *J Clin Invest.* 1934;13:97-107.
111. Finland M, Shuman HI. The type-specific agglutinin response of infants and children with pneumococcal pneumonias. *J Immunol.* 1942;45:215-223.
112. Sloyer JLJ, Howie VM, Ploussard JH, et al. Immune response to acute otitis media in children. I. Serotypes isolated and serum and middle ear fluid antibody in pneumococcal otitis media. *Infect Immun.* 1974;9:1028-1032.
113. Prober CG, Frayha H, Klein MJ. Immunologic responses of children to serious infections with *Streptococcus pneumoniae. J Infect Dis.* 1983;148:427-435.
114. Sanders LAM, Rijkers GT, Kuis W, et al. Defective antipneumococcal polysaccharide antibody response in children with recurrent respiratory tract infections. *J Allergy Clin Immunol.* 1993;91:110-119.
115. Wara DW. Host defense against Streptococcus pneumoniae: The role of the spleen. *Rev Infect Dis.* 1981;3:299-309.
116. Styrt B. Infection associated with asplenia: Risks, mechanisms, and prevention. *Am J Med.* 1990;88:33N-42N.
117. Jandl JH, Jones AR, Castle WB. The destruction of red cells by antibodies in man. I. Observations on the sequestration and lysis of red cells altered by immune mechanisms. *J Clin Invest.* 1957;36:1428-1459.
118. Frank MM, Hosea SW, Brown EJ, et al. Opsonic requirements for intravascular clearance after splenectomy. *N Engl J Med.* 1981;304:245-250.
119. Wong WY, Overturf GD, Powars DR. Infection caused by *Streptococcus pneumoniae* in children with sickle cell disease: Epidemiology, immunologic mechanisms, prophylaxis, and vaccination. *Clin Infect Dis.* 1992;14:1124-1136.
120. Cunningham-Rundles C. Clinical and immunologic analyses of 103 patients with common variable immunodeficiency. *J Clin Immunol.* 1989;9:22-33.
121. Umetsu DT, Ambrosino DM, Quinti I, et al. Recurrent sinopulmonary infection and impaired antibody response to bacterial capsular polysaccharide antigen in children with selective IgG subclass deficiency. *N Engl J Med.* 1985;313:1247-1251.
122. Yee AMF, Phan HM, Zuniga R, et al. The FcyRIIa-R131 allotype increases risk for bacteremic pneumococcal infections. *Clin Infect Dis.* 2000;30:25-28.
123. Kyaw MH, Rose Jr CE, Fry AM, et al. The influence of chronic illnesses on the incidence of invasive pneumococcal disease in adults. *J Infect Dis.* 2005;192:377-386.
124. Savage DG, Lindenbaum J, Garrett TJ. Biphasic pattern of bacterial infection in multiple myeloma. *Ann Intern Med.* 1982;96:47-50.
125. Rodriguez Barradas MC, Musher DM, Hamill RJ, et al. Unusual manifestations of pneumococcal infection in human immunodeficiency virus-infected individuals: The past revisited. *Clin Infect Dis.* 1992;14:192-199.
126. Schuchat A, Broome CV, Hightower A, et al. Use of surveillance for invasive pneumococcal disease to estimate the size of the immunosuppressed HIV-infected population. *JAMA.* 1991;265:3275-3279.
127. Figueroa JE, Densen P. Infectious diseases associated with complement deficiencies. *Clin Microbiol Rev.* 1991;4:359-395.
128. Anderson DC, Schmalstieg FC, Finegold MJ, et al. The severe and moderate phenotypes of heritable Mac-1, LFA-1 deficiency: Their quantitative definition and relation to leukocyte dysfunction and clinical features. *J Infect Dis.* 1985;152:668-689.
129. Beam TRJ, Allen JC. Patterns of infection in untreated acute leukemia: Impact of initial hospitalization. *South Med J.* 1979;72:282-286.
130. Gluckman SJ, Dvorak VC, MacGregor RR. Host defenses during prolonged alcohol consumption in a controlled environment. *Arch Intern Med.* 1977;137:1539-1543.
131. Young CL, MacGregor RR. Alcohol and host defenses: Infectious consequences. *Infect Med.* 1989;6:163-175.
132. Fang GD, Fine M, Orloff J, et al. New and emerging etiologies for community-acquired pneumonia with implications for therapy. A prospective multicenter study of 359 cases. *Medicine (Baltimore).* 1990;69:307-316.
133. Musher DM, Alexandraki I, Graviss EA, et al. Bacteremic and nonbacteremic pneumococcal pneumonia. A prospective study. *Medicine (Baltimore).* 2000;79:210-221.
134. Rahav G, Toledano Y, Engelhard D, et al. Invasive pneumococcal infections: A comparison between adults and children. *Medicine (Baltimore).* 1997;76:295-303.
135. Watanakunakorn C, Bailey TA. Adult bacteremic pneumococcal pneumonia in a community teaching hospital, 1992-1996. A detailed analysis of 108 cases. *Arch Intern Med.* 1997;157:1965-1971.
136. Mowat AG, Baum J. Chemotaxis of polymorphonuclear leukocytes from patients with diabetes mellitus. *N Engl J Med.* 1971;284:621-627.
137. Repine JE, Clawson CC, Goetz FC. Bactericidal function of neutrophils from patients with acute bacterial infections and from diabetics. *J Infect Dis.* 1980;142:869-875.
138. Lipsky BA, Boyko EJ, Inui TS, et al. Risk factors for acquiring pneumococcal infections. *Arch Intern Med.* 1986;146:2179-2185.
139. Chang JL, Mylotte JM. Pneumococcal bacteremia: Updated from an adult hospital with a high rate of nosocomial cases. *J Am Geriatr Soc.* 1987;35:747-754.
140. Hodges R, MacLeod C. Epidemic pneumococcal pneumonia. II. The influence of population characteristics and the environment. *Amer J Hygiene.* 1946;44:193-206.
141. Jones EE, Alford PL, Reingold AL, et al. Predisposition to invasive pneumococcal illness following parainfluenza type 3 virus infection in chimpanzees. *J Am Vet Med Assoc.* 1998;185:1351-1353.
142. Fainstein V, Musher DM, Cate TR. Bacterial adherence to pharyngeal cells during viral infection. *J Infect Dis.* 1980;141:172-176.
143. Nuorti JP, Butler JC, Farley MM, et al. Cigarette smoking and invasive pneumococcal disease. Active Bacterial Core Surveillance Team. *N Engl J Med.* 2000;342:681-689.
144. Raz R, Elhanan G, Shimoni Z, et al. Pneumococcal bacteremia in hospitalized Israeli adults: Epidemiology and resistance to penicillin. *Clin Infect Dis.* 1997;24:1164-1168.
145. Dowell SF, Butler JC, Giebink GS, et al. Acute otitis media: Management and surveillance in an era of pneumococcal resistance—a report from the Drug-resistant Streptococcus pneumoniae Therapeutic Working Group. *Pediatr Infect Dis J.* 1999;18:1-9.
146. Schwartz LE, Brown RB. Purulent otitis media in adults. *Arch Intern Med.* 1992;152:2301-2304.
147. Faden H, Duffy L, Wasielewski R, et al. Relationship between nasopharyngeal colonization and the development of otitis media in children. *J Infect Dis.* 1997;175:1440-1445.
148. Gwaltney JMJ, Scheld WM, Sande MA, et al. The microbial etiology and antimicrobial therapy of adults with acute community-acquired sinusitis: A fifteen-year experience at the University of Virginia and review of other selected studies. *J Allergy Clin Immunol.* 1992;90:457-462.
149. Gwaltney JMJ, Phillips CD, Miller RD, et al. Computed tomographic study of the common cold. *N Engl J Med.* 1994;330:25-30.
150. Quagliarello VJ, Scheld WM. Treatment of bacterial meningtis. *N Engl J Med.* 1997;336:708-716.
151. Brandt CT, Holm D, Liptrot M, et al. Impact of bacteremia on the pathogenesis of experimental pneumococcal meningitis. *J Infect Dis.* 2008;197:235-244.
152. Hand WL, Sanford JP. Posttraumatic bacterial meningtis. *Ann Intern Med.* 1970;72:869-874.
153. Eavey RD, Gao Y, Schuknecht HF, et al. Otologic features of bacterial meningtis of childhood. *J Pediatr.* 1985;136:2025-2029.
154. Klein M, Koedel U, Kastenbauer S, et al. Nitrogen and oxygen molecules in meningitis-associated labyrinthitis and hearing impairment. *Infection.* 2008;36:2-14.
155. Bhatt SM, Lauretano A, Cabellos C, et al. Progression of hearing loss in experimental pneumococcal meningtis: Correlation with cerebrospinal fluid cytochemistry. *J Infect Dis.* 1993;167:675-683.
156. Quagliarello V, Scheld WM. Bacterial meningitis: Pathogenesis, pathophysiology, and progress. *N Engl J Med.* 1992;327:864-872.
157. Klein M, Obermaier B, Angele B, et al. Innate immunity to pneumococcal infection of the central nervous system depends on toll-like receptor (TLR) 2 and TLR4. *J Infect Dis.* 2008;198:1028-1036.
158. Dunbar SA, Eason RA, Musher DM, et al. Microscopic examination and broth culture of cerebrospinal fluid in diagnosis of meningitis. *J Clin Microbiol.* 1998;36:1617-1620.
159. Perkins MD, Mirrett S, Reller LB. Rapid bacterial antigen detection is not clinically useful. *J Clin Microbiol.* 1995;33:1486-1491.
160. Chodosh S. Acute bacterial exacerbations in bronchitis and asthma. *Am J Med.* 1987;82:154-163.
161. Chodosh S, McCarty J, Farkas S, et al. Randomized, double-blind study of ciprofloxacin and cefuroxime axetil for treatment of acute bacterial exacerbations of chronic bronchitis. The Bronchitis Study Group. *Clin Infect Dis.* 1998;27:722-7229.
162. Sethi S, Evans N, Grant BJ, et al. New strains of bacteria and exacerbations of chronic obstructive pulmonary disease. *N Engl J Med.* 2002;347:465-471.
163. Ampofo K, Bender J, Sheng X, et al. Seasonal invasive pneumococcal disease in children: Role of preceding respiratory viral infection. *Pediatrics.* 2008;122:229-237.
164. Morens DM, Taubenberger JK, Fauci AS. Predominant role of bacterial pneumonia as a cause of death in pandemic influenza: Implications for pandemic influenza preparedness. *J Infect Dis.* 2008;198:962-970.
165. Murphy TF, Fine BC. Bacteremic pneumococcal pneumonia in the elderly. *Am J Med Sci.* 1984;288:114-118.
166. Metlay JP, Schulz R, Li Y-H, et al. Influence of age on symptoms at presentation in patients with community-acquired pneumonia. *Arch Intern Med.* 1997;157:1453-1459.
167. Metlay JP, Kapoor WN, Fine MJ. Does this patient have community-acquired pneumonia? Diagnosing pneumonia by history and physical examination. *JAMA.* 1997;278:1440-1445.
168. Ort S, Ryan RL, Barden G, et al. Pneumococcal pneumonia in hospitalized patients. *JAMA.* 1983;249:214-2148.
169. Yangco BG, Deresinski SC. Necrotizing or cavitating pneumonia due to *Streptococcus pneumoniae:* Report of four cases and review of the literature. *Medicine (Baltimore).* 1980;59:449-457.
170. Light RW, Girard WM, Jenkinson SG, et al. Parapneumonic effusions. *Am J Med.* 1980;69:507-512.
171. Hook EWI, Horton CA, Schaberg DR. Failure of intensive care unit support to influence mortality from pneumococcal bacteremia. *JAMA.* 1983;249:1055-1057.
172. Perlino CA, Rimland D. Alcoholism, leukopenia, and pneumococcal sepsis. *Am Rev Respir Dis.* 1985;132:757-760.
173. Barrett-Connor E. The nonvalue of sputum culture in the diagnosis of pneumococcal pneumonia. *Am Rev Respir Dis.* 1971;103:845-848.
174. Perlino CA. Laboratory diagnosis of pneumonia due to *Streptococcus pneumoniae. J Infect Dis.* 1984;150:139-144.
175. Musher DM, Montoya R, Wanahita A. Reliability of microscopic examination of gram-stained sputum and sputum culture in patients with bacteremic pneumococcal pneumonia. Clin Infect Dis. 2004;39:165-169.
176. Musher DM, Montoya R, Wanahita A. Diagnostic value of microscopic examination of gram-stained sputum and sputum cultures in patients with bacteremic pneumococcal pneumonia. *Clin Infect Dis.* 2004;39:165-169.
177. Mandell LA, Wunderink RG, Anzueto A, et al. Infectious Diseases Society of America/American Thoracic Society consensus guidelines on the management of community-acquired pneumonia in adults. *Clin Infect Dis.* 2007;44(Suppl 2):S27-S72.
178. Smith MD, Derrington P, Evans R, et al. Rapid diagnosis of bacteremic pneumococcal infections in adults by using the Binax NOW Streptococcus pneumoniae urinary antigen test: A prospective, controlled clinical evaluation. *J Clin Microbiol.* 2003;41:2810-2813.
179. Roson B, Fernandez-Sabe N, Carratala J, et al. Contribution of a urinary antigen assay (Binax NOW) to the early diagnosis of pneumococcal pneumonia. *Clin Infect Dis.* 2004;38:222-226.
180. Dowell SF, Garman RL, Liu G, et al. Evaluation of Binax NOW, an assay for the detection of pneumococcal antigen in urine samples, performed among pediatric patients. *Clin Infect Dis.* 2001;32:824-825.
181. Anstadt MP, Guill CK, Gordon HS, et al. Surgical vs. nonsurgical treatment of empyema: An outcomes analysis. *Am J Med Sci.* 2003;326:9-14.
182. Franco M, Musher DM. Thoracic empyema: The impact of management on outcome [abstract]. *Am Rev Respir Dis.* 1982;124:82.
183. Musher DM, Rueda AM, Kaka AS, et al. The association between pneumococcal pneumonia and acute cardiac events. *Clin Infect Dis.* 2007;45:158-165.
184. Madjid M, Vela D, Khalili-Tabrizi H, et al. Systemic infections cause exaggerated local inflammation in atherosclerotic coronary arteries: Clues to the triggering effect of acute infections on acute coronary syndromes. *Tex Heart Inst J.* 2007;34:11-18.
185. Barker JH, Musher DM, Silberman R, et al. Genetic relatedness among nontypeable pneumococci implicated in sporadic cases of conjunctivitis. *J Clin Microbiol.* 1999;37:4039-4041.
186. Martin M, Turco JH, Zegans ME, et al. An outbreak of conjunctivitis due to atypical Streptococcus pneumoniae. *N Engl J Med.* 2003;348:1112-1121.
187. Powderly WG, Stanley Jr SL, Medoff G. Pneumococcal endocarditis: Report of a series and review of the literature. *Rev Infect Dis.* 1986;8:786-791.
188. Lindberg J, Prag J, Schonheyder HC. Pneumococcal endocarditis is not just a disease of the past: An analysis of 16 cases diagnosed in Denmark 1986-1997. *Scand J Infect Dis.* 1998;30:469-472.
189. Lefort A, Mainardi JL, Selton-Suty C, et al. Streptococcus pneumoniae endocarditis in adults. A multicenter study in France in the era of penicillin resistance (1991-1998). The Pneumococcal Endocarditis Study Group. *Medicine (Baltimore).* 2000;79:327-337.
190. Case Records of the Massachusetts General Hospital. Weekly clinicopathological exercises. Case 49-1990. A 47-year-old Cape Verdean man with pericardial disease. *N Engl J Med.* 1990;323:1614-1624.
191. Dugi 3rd DD, Musher DM, Clarridge 3rd JE, et al. Intraabdominal infection due to Streptococcus pneumoniae. *Medicine (Baltimore).* 2001;80:236-244.

192. Westh H, Skibsted L, Korner B. *Streptococcus pneumoniae* infections of the female genital tract and in the newborn child. *Rev Infect Dis.* 1990;12:416-422.
193. Robinson ENJ. Pneumococcal endometritis and neonatal sepsis. *Rev Infect Dis.* 1990;12:799-801.
194. Rahav G, Ben-David L, Persitz E. Postmenopausal pneumococcal tubo-ovarian abscess. *Rev Infect Dis.* 1991;13:896-897.
195. Ross JJ, Saltzman CL, Carling P, et al. Pneumococcal septic arthritis: Review of 190 cases. *Clin Infect Dis.* 2003;36:319-327.
196. Ryczak M, Sands M, Brown RB, et al. Pneumococcal arthritis in a prosthetic knee. A case report and review of the literature. *Clin Orthop.* 1987;224:224-227.
197. Morley PK, Hull RG, Hall MA. Pneumococcal septic arthritis in rheumatoid arthritis. *Ann Rheum Dis.* 1987;46:482-484.
198. Raad J, Peacock Jr JE. Septic arthritis in the adult caused by Streptococcus pneumoniae: A report of 4 cases and review of the literature. *Semin Arthritis Rheum.* 2004;34:559-569.
199. Turner DP, Weston VC, Ispahani P. Streptococcus pneumoniae spinal infection in Nottingham, United Kingdom: Not a rare event. *Clin Infect Dis.* 1999;28:873-881.
200. Grigoriadis E, Gold WL. Pyogenic brain abscess caused by *Streptococcus pneumoniae:* Case report and review. *Clin Infect Dis.* 1997;25:1108-1112.
201. Peters NS, Eykyn SJ, Rudd AG. Pneumococcal cellulitis: A rare manifestation of pneumococcaemia in adults. *J Infect.* 1989;19:57-59.
202. DiNubile MJ, Albornoz MA, Stumacher RJ, et al. Pneumococcal soft-tissue infections: Possible association with connective tissue diseases. *J Infect Dis.* 1991;163:897-900.
203. Capdevila O, Grau I, Vadillo M, et al. Bacteremic pneumococcal cellulitis compared with bacteremic cellulitis caused by Staphylococcus aureus and Streptococcus pyogenes. *Eur J Clin Microbiol Infect Dis.* 2003;22:337-341.
204. Musher DM, Bartlett JG, Doern GV. A fresh look at the definition of susceptibility of Streptococcus pneumoniae to beta-lactam antibiotics. *Arch Intern Med.* 2001;161:2538-2544.
205. Effects of new penicillin susceptibility breakpoints for *Streptococcus pneumoniae*—United States, 2006-2007. *MMWR Morb Mortal Wkly Rep.* 2008;57:1353-1357.
206. Smith AM, Klugman KP. Alterations in penicillin-binding protein 2B from penicillin-resistant wild-type strains of *Streptococcus pneumoniae. Antimicrob Agents Chemother.* 1995;39:859-867.
207. Smith AM, Klugman KP, Coffey TJ, et al. Genetic diversity of penicillin-binding protein 2B and 2X genes from Streptococcus pneumoniae in South Africa. *Antimicrob Agents Chemother.* 1993;37:1938-1944.
208. Dowson CG, Coffey TJ, Kell C, et al. Evolution of penicillin resistance in Streptococcus pneumoniae; The role of Streptococcus mitis in the formation of a low affinity PBP2B in S. pneumoniae. *Mol Microbiol.* 1993;9:635-643.
209. Versalovic J, Kapur V, Mason Jr EO, et al. Penicillin-resistant Streptococcus pneumoniae strains recovered in Houston: Identification and molecular characterization of multiple clones. *J Infect Dis.* 1993;167:850-856.
210. McDougal LK, Rasheed JK, Biddle JW, et al. Identification of multiple clones of extended-spectrum cephalosporin-resistant Streptococcus pneumoniae isolates in the United States. *Antimicrob Agents Chemother.* 1995;39:2282-2288.
211. Tomasz A. Antibiotic resistance in Streptococcus pneumoniae. *Clin Infect Dis.* 1997;24(Suppl 1):S85-S88.
212. Soares S, Kristinsson KG, Musser JM, et al. Evidence for the introduction of a multiresistant clone of serotype 6B *Streptococcus pneumoniae* from Spain to Iceland in the late l980s. *J Infect Dis.* 1993;168:158-163.
213. Richter SS, Heilmann KP, Coffman SL, et al. The molecular epidemiology of penicillin-resistant Streptococcus pneumoniae in the United States, 1994-2000. *Clin Infect Dis.* 2002;34:330-339.
214. Overweg K, Bogaert D, Sluijter M, et al. Molecular characteristics of penicillin-binding protein genes of penicillin-nonsusceptible Streptococcus pneumoniae isolated in the Netherlands. *Microb Drug Resist.* 2001;7:323-334.
215. Musher DM. Antibiotic resistance of Streptococcus pneumoniae: Macrolides, lincosamides and ketolides. *UpToDate.* 2009.
216. Musher DM, Dowell ME, Shortridge VD, et al. Emergence of macrolide resistance during treatment of pneumococcal pneumonia. *N Engl J Med.* 2002;346:630-631.
217. Whitney CG, Farley MM, Hadler J, et al. Increasing prevalence of multidrug-resistant Streptococcus pneumoniae in the United States. *N Engl J Med.* 2000;343:1917-1924.
218. Thornsberry C, Sahm DF, Kelly LJ, et al. Regional trends in antimicrobial resistance among clinical isolates of Streptococcus pneumoniae, Haemophilus influenzae, and Moraxella catarrhalis in the United States: Results from the TRUST Surveillance Program, 1999-2000. *Clin Infect Dis.* 2002;34(Suppl 1):S4-S16.
219. Karlowsky JA, Thornsberry C, Jones ME, et al. Factors associated with relative rates of antimicrobial resistance among Streptococcus pneumoniae in the United States: Results from the TRUST Surveillance Program (1998-2002). *Clin Infect Dis.* 2003;36:963-970.
220. Sahm DF, Brown NP, Draghi DC, et al. Tracking resistance among bacterial respiratory tract pathogens: Summary of findings of the TRUST Surveillance Initiative, 2001-2005. *Postgrad Med.* 2008;120(Suppl 1):8-15.

221. Hsu HE, Shutt KA, Moore MR, et al. Effect of pneumococcal conjugate vaccine on pneumococcal meningitis. *N Engl J Med.* 2009;360:244-256.
222. Harbarth S, Albrich W, Brun-Buisson C. Outpatient antibiotic use and prevalence of antibiotic-resistant pneumococci in France and Germany: A sociocultural perspective. *Emerg Infect Dis.* 2002;8:1460-1467.
223. Overweg K, Bogaert D, Sluijter M, et al. Genetic relatedness within serotypes of penicillin-susceptible Streptococcus pneumoniae isolates. *J Clin Microbiol.* 2000;38:4548-4553.
224. Doern GV, Richter SS, Miller A, et al. Antimicrobial resistance among Streptococcus pneumoniae in the United States: Have we begun to turn the corner on resistance to certain antimicrobial classes? *Clin Infect Dis.* 2005;41:139-148.
225. Chen DK, McGeer A, de Azavedo JC, et al. Decreased susceptibility of Streptococcus pneumoniae to fluoroquinolones in Canada. Canadian Bacterial Surveillance Network. *N Engl J Med.* 1999;341:233-239.
226. Weiss K, Restieri C, Gauthier R, et al. A nosocomial outbreak of fluoroquinolone-resistant Streptococcus pneumoniae. *Clin Infect Dis.* 2001;33:517-522.
227. Kupronis BA, Richards C, Whitney CG. Invasive pneumococcal disease in older adults residing in long-term care facilities and in the community. *J Am Geriatr Soc.* 2003;51:1520-1525.
228. McCormick DP, Chonmaitree T, Pittman C, et al. Nonsevere acute otitis media: A clinical trial comparing outcomes of watchful waiting versus immediate antibiotic treatment. *Pediatrics.* 2005;115:1455-1465.
229. Hendrickse WA, Kusmiesz H, Shelton S, et al. Five vs. ten days of therapy for acute otitis media. *Pediatr Infect Dis J.* 1988;7:14-23.
230. Anon JB, Jacobs MR, Poole MD, et al. Antimicrobial treatment guidelines for acute bacterial rhinosinusitis. *Otolaryngol Head Neck Surg.* 2004;130(Suppl 1):1-45.
231. Lonks JR, Garau J, Gomez L, et al. Failure of macrolide antibiotic treatment in patients with bacteremia due to erythromycin-resistant Streptococcus pneumoniae. *Clin Infect Dis.* 2002;35:556-564.
232. Fine MJ, Auble TE, Yealy DM, et al. A prediction rule to identify low-risk patients with community-acquired pneumonia. *N Engl J Med.* 1997;336:243-250.
233. Bartlett JG, Dowell SF, Mandell LA, et al. Practice guidelines for the management of community-acquired pneumonia in adults. Infectious Diseases Society of America. *Clin Infect Dis.* 2000;31:347-382.
234. Yu VL, Baddour LM. Infection by drug-resistant Streptococcus pneumoniae is not linked to increased mortality. *Clin Infect Dis.* 2004;39:1086-1087.
235. Baddour LM, Yu VL, Klugman KP, et al. Combination antibiotic therapy lowers mortality among severely ill patients with pneumococcal bacteremia. *Am J Respir Crit Care Med.* 2004;170:440-444.
236. Torres A, Garau J, Arvis P, et al. Moxifloxacin monotherapy is effective in hospitalized patients with community-acquired pneumonia: The MOTIV study—a randomized clinical trial. *Clin Infect Dis.* 2008;46:1499-1509.
237. Friedland IR, Paris M, Shelton S, et al. Time-kill studies of antibiotic combinations against penicillin-resistant and -susceptible Streptococcus pneumoniae. *J Antimicrob Chemother.* 1994;34:231-237.
238. Paris MM, Hickey SM, Uscher MI, et al. Effect of dexamethasone on therapy of experimental penicillin- and cephalosporin-resistant pneumococcal meningitis. *Antimicrob Agents Chemother.* 1994;38:1320-1324.
239. Giron KP, Gross ME, Musher DM, et al. In vitro antimicrobial effect against Streptococcus pneumoniae of adding rifampin to penicillin, ceftriaxone, or 1-ofloxacin. *Antimicrob Agents Chemother.* 1995;39:2798-2800.
240. de Gans J, van de Beek D. Dexamethasone in adults with bacterial meningitis. *N Engl J Med.* 2002;347:1549-1556.
241. Scheld WM. Drug delivery to the central nervous system: General principles and relevance to therapy for infections of the central nervous system. *Rev Infect Dis.* 1989;11(Suppl 7):S1669-S1690.
242. Cabellos C, Martinez-Lacasa J, Martos A, et al. Influence of dexamethasone on efficacy of ceftriaxone and vancomycin therapy in experimental pneumococcal meningitis. *Antimicrob Agents Chemother.* 1995;39:2158-2160.
243. Ahmed A, Jafri H, Lutsar I, et al. Pharmacodynamics of vancomycin for the treatment of experimental penicillin- and cephalosporin-resistant pneumococcal meningitis. *Antimicrob Agents Chemother.* 1999;43:876-881.
244. Laterre PF, Garber G, Levy H, et al. Severe community-acquired pneumonia as a cause of severe sepsis: Data from the PROWESS study. *Crit Care Med.* 2005;33:952-961.
245. Gross ME, Giron KP, Septimus JD, et al. Antimicrobial activities of beta-lactam antibiotics and gentamicin against penicillin-susceptible and penicillin-resistant pneumococci. *Antimicrob Agents Chemother.* 1995;39:1166-1168.
246. Eskola J, Black S, Shinefield H. Pneumococcal conjugate vaccines. In: Plotkin SA, Orenstein WA, eds. *Vaccines.* 4th ed. Philadelphia: WB Saunders; 2004:589-624.
247. Kehrl JH, Fauci AS. Activation of human B lymphocytes after immunization with pneumococcal polysaccharides. *J Clin Invest.* 1983;71:1032-1040.
248. Musher DM, Groover JE, Watson DA, et al. IgG responses to protein-conjugated pneumococcal capsular polysaccharides in

persons who are genetically incapable of responding to unconjugated polysaccharides. *Clin Infect Dis.* 1998;27:1487-1490.
249. Musher DM, Groover JE, Graviss EA, et al. The lack of association between aging and postvaccination levels of IgG antibody to capsular polysaccharides of Streptococcus pneumoniae. *Clin Infect Dis.* 1996;22:165-167.
250. Rodriguez-Barradas MC, Musher DM, Lahart C, et al. Antibody to capsular polysaccharides of *Streptococcus pneumoniae* after vaccination of human immunodeficiency virus-infected subjects with 23-valent pneumococcal vaccine. *J Infect Dis.* 1992;165:553-556.
251. Janoff EN, Breiman RF, Daley CL, et al. Pneumococcal disease during HIV infection. Epidemiologic, clinical, and immunologic perspectives. *Ann Intern Med.* 1992;117:314-324.
252. Musher DM, Rueda AM, Nahm MH, et al. Initial and subsequent response to pneumococcal polysaccharide and protein-conjugate vaccines administered sequentially to adults who have recovered from pneumococcal pneumonia. *J Infect Dis.* 2008;198:1019-1027.
253. Austrian R, Douglas RM, Schiffman G, et al. Prevention of pneumococcal pneumonia by vaccination. *Trans Assoc Am Physicians.* 1976;89:184-194.
254. Austrian R. Some observations on the pneumococcus and on the current status of pneumococcal disease and its prevention. *Rev Infect Dis.* 1981;3(Suppl):S1-S17.
255. Gaillat J, Zmirou D, Mallaret MR, et al. [Clinical trial of an antipneumococcal vaccine in elderly subjects living in institutions.] *Rev Epidemiol Sante Publique.* 1985;33:437-444.
256. Koivula I, Sten M, Leinonen M, et al. Clinical efficacy of pneumococcal vaccine in the elderly: A randomized, single-blind population-based trial. *Am J Med.* 1997;103:281-290.
257. Bentley DW. Pneumococcal vaccine in the institutionalized elderly: Review of past and recent studies. *Rev Infect Dis.* 1981;3(Suppl):S61-S70.
258. Bentley DW, Ha K, Mamot K, et al. Pneumococcal vaccine in the institutionalized elderly: Design of a nonrandomized trial and preliminary results. *Rev Infect Dis.* 1981;3(Suppl):S71-S81.
259. Simberkoff MS, Cross AP, Al-Ibrahim M, et al. Efficacy of pneumococcal vaccine in high-risk patients. Results of a Veterans Administration Cooperative Study. *N Engl J Med.* 1986;315:1318-1327.
260. Ortqvist A, Hedlund J, Burman LA, et al. Randomised trial of 23-valent pneumococcal capsular polysaccharide vaccine in prevention of pneumonia in middle-aged and elderly people. Swedish Pneumococcal Vaccination Study Group. *Lancet.* 1998;351:399-403.
261. Bolan G, Broome CV, Facklam RR, et al. Pneumococcal vaccine efficacy in selected populations in the United States. *Ann Intern Med.* 1986;104:1-6.
262. Jackson LA, Neuzil KM, Yu O, et al. Effectiveness of pneumococcal polysaccharide vaccine in older adults. *N Engl J Med.* 2003;348:1747-1755.
263. Sims RV, Steinmann WC, McConville JH, et al. The clinical effectiveness of pneumococcal vaccine in the elderly. *Ann Intern Med.* 1988;108:653-657.
264. Shapiro ED, Berg AT, Austrian R, et al. The protective efficacy of polyvalent pneumococcal polysaccharide vaccine. *N Engl J Med.* 1991;325:1453-1460.
265. Farr BM, Johnston BL, Cobb DK, et al. Preventing pneumococcal bacteremia in patients at risk. Results of a matched case-control study. *Arch Intern Med.* 1995;155:2336-2340.
266. Rubins JB, Puri AK, Loch J, et al. Magnitude, duration, quality, and function of pneumococcal vaccine responses in elderly adults. *J Infect Dis.* 1998;178:431-440.
267. Fedson DS. Influenza and pneumococcal vaccination in Canada and the United States, 1980-1993: What can the two countries learn from each other? *Clin Infect Dis.* 1995;201371-201376.
268. Centers for Disease Control and Prevention (CDC). Preventing pneumococcal disease among infants and young children: Recommendations of the Advisory Committee on Immunization Practices. *MMWR Morb Mortal Wkly Rep.* 2000;49RR(09):1-38.
269. Centers for Disease Control and Prevention. Pneumococcal conjugate vaccine shortage resolved. *MMWR Morb Mortal Wkly Rep.* 2004;53:851-852.
270. Centers for Disease Control and Prevention. Prevention of pneumococcal disease: Recommendations of the Advisory Committee on Immunization Proctices (ACIP). *MMWR Morb Mortal Wkly Rep.* 1997;46:1-18.
271. Jackson LA, Nelson JC, Whitney CG, et al. Assessment of the safety of a third dose of pneumococcal polysaccharide vaccine in the Vaccine Safety Datalink population. *Vaccine.* 2006;24:151-156.
272. Black S, Shinefield H, Fireman B, et al. Efficacy, safety and immunogenicity of heptavalent pneumococcal conjugate vaccine in children. Northern California Kaiser Permanente Vaccine Study Center Group. *Pediatr Infect Dis J.* 2000;19:187-195.
273. Fireman B, Black SB, Shinefield HR, et al. Impact of the pneumococcal conjugate vaccine on otitis media. *Pediatr Infect Dis J.* 2003;22:10-16.
274. Black SB, Shinefield HR, Ling S, et al. Effectiveness of heptavalent pneumococcal conjugate vaccine in children younger than five years of age for prevention of pneumonia. *Pediatr Infect Dis J.* 2002;21:810-815.

275. O'Brien KL, Millar EV, Zell ER, et al. Effect of pneumococcal conjugate vaccine on nasopharyngeal colonization among immunized and unimmunized children in a community-randomized trial. *J Infect Dis.* 2007;196:1211-1220.

276. Feikin DR, Elie CM, Goetz MB, et al. Randomized trial of the quantitative and functional antibody responses to a 7-valent pneumococcal conjugate vaccine and/or 23-valent polysaccharide vaccine among HIV-infected adults. *Vaccine.* 2001;20: 545-553.

277. Direct and indirect effects of routine vaccination of children with 7-valent conjugate vaccine on incidence of invasive pneumococcal disease—United States 1998-2003. *CDC.* 2005; 54:893-897.

278. Musher DM. Pneumococcal vaccine–direct and indirect ("herd") effects. *N Engl J Med.* 2006;354:1522-1524.

279. Hammitt LL, Bruden DL, Butler JC, et al. Indirect effect of conjugate vaccine on adult carriage of Streptococcus pneumoniae: An explanation of trends in invasive pneumococcal disease. *J Infect Dis.* 2006;193:1487-1494.

280. Flannery B, Heffernan RT, Harrison LH, et al. Changes in invasive Pneumococcal disease among HIV-infected adults living in the era of childhood pneumococcal immunization. *Ann Intern Med.* 2006;144:1-9.

281. Hicks LA, Harrison LH, Flannery B, et al. Incidence of pneumococcal disease due to non-pneumococcal conjugate vaccine (PCV7) serotypes in the United States during the era of widespread PCV7 vaccination, 1998-2004. *J Infect Dis.* 2007; 196:1346-1354.

282. Brueggemann AB, Pai R, Crook DW, et al. Vaccine escape recombinants emerge after pneumococcal vaccination in the United States. *PLoS Pathog.* 2007;3:e168.

201

Enterococcus Species, Streptococcus bovis Group, and Leuconostoc Species

CESAR A. ARIAS | BARBARA E. MURRAY

Historical Remarks

The first time that the term *entérocoque* was used appears to have been in an article in the French literature in 1899.[1] The manuscript was referring to a "diplococcus" found as commensal of the gastrointestinal tract that had the potential to become pathogenic for humans. The first clinical and pathologic description of an enterococcal infection was published the same year (1899)[2] concerning a patient admitted "in Dr. Osler's Service" with a clinical picture of endocarditis who succumbed to the infection. The authors isolated gram-positive cocci in "pairs and short chains" from the patient's blood and several other organs (postmortem). The virulence properties of the organism were confirmed after inoculating it into several animal models and reproducing the pathologic findings observed in the patient. This organism was initially designated "*Micrococcus zymogenes*" because of its fermentative properties. In 1906, Andrews and Horder[3] described in detail a study of streptococci pathogenic for humans and used for the first time the name "*Streptococcus faecalis*" to denote the most common species of streptococci present in the intestine of humans and other vertebrates. In fact, they refer to previous environmental experiments performed by themselves and Houston[3] in London, which indicated that the most common microorganisms collected from London's air were "intestinal streptococci," which probably originated from horse dung, "which forms so large of a part of the organic contamination of London's air." In December, 1937, James Sherman, addressing the Society of American Bacteriologists, indicated that the "the enterococcus" was an unspecific term used for streptococci isolated from the gut, which was "a screen behind which the investigator could hide his ignorance of the organisms with which he worked."[4] That year, he proposed to group the enterococci as *S. faecalis*, *S. faecalis* var. *hemolyticus*, *S. faecalis* var. *zymogenes*, *S. faecalis* var. *liquefaciens*, and *S. durans*, all of which displayed the common phenotypic characteristics that included growth in the presence of 6.5% NaCl and pH 9.6 and growth temperature.[4] In the 1940s and 1950s, studies showed that an organism initially identified in 1919 as *S. faecium*[5] had in fact distinct characteristics that differentiated it from *S. faecalis*,[6,7] and in 1970, a formal proposal that the enterococcal streptococci be considered a new genus was put forward, based on their distinct phenotypic characteristics.[8] However, it was not until 1984 that *Enterococcus* was widely confirmed as a separate genus from *Streptococcus* after DNA hybridization experiments were performed and, subsequently, genetic tools were applied to differentiate the different species of enterococci.[9]

Microbiology and Taxonomy

Organisms belonging to the genus *Enterococcus* are gram-positive, facultatively anaerobic, usually appear oval in shape, and can be seen as single cells, pairs, short chains, or even very long chains (Fig. 201-1). They are capable of growing in medium containing 6.5% NaCl and in temperatures between 10° and 45°C and are able to hydrolyze esculin in the presence of 40% bile salts, produce a leucine aminopeptidase and a pyrrolidonylarylamidase (PYR) (except for *E. cecorum*, *E. columbae*, *E. pallens*, and *E. saccarolyticus*). Enterococci are usually α- or γ-hemolytic on trypticase soy and 5% sheep blood agar (Table 201-1); some are β-hemolytic on horse, rabbit, or human blood; most react with the Lancefield group D antisera and some with group Q antisera;

and some of them are motile (e.g., *E. casseliflavus* and *E. gallinarum*). Table 201-2 shows species of enterococci isolated from human infections; most clinical infections are produced by two species (*E. faecalis* and *E. faecium*), and clinical laboratories usually will not identify enterococci at the species level. However, in certain clinical scenarios or in epidemiology studies, it may be important to differentiate between these two species because they appear to differ in their virulence and antibiotic resistance profile (see later).

Conventional methods to identify enterococci at the species level include manual biochemical differentiation based on several tests (e.g., acid formation and hydrolysis of arginine); nonetheless, because of the laboriousness of this approach, laboratories usually rely on automated methods or rapid biochemical methods (such as the API system), which appear to be accurate for *E. faecalis* but not for other enterococcal species. Because of this limitation, several molecular techniques have been developed, although they are not used routinely by clinical laboratories; amongst the most popular, amplification of *ddl* genes,[10] amplification and probe of the *ace* gene,[11] and sequencing of the 16S recombinant RNA gene appear to reliably differentiate the relevant enterococcal species.

Colonization, Virulence, and Genomics

Enterococci are organisms that have developed well-adapted mechanisms to survive in the gastrointestinal tract of humans. The human colonic flora comprises about 10^{14} commensal bacteria per gram of contents encompassing more than 100 culturable bacterial species with a predominance of anaerobes.[12] Enterococci are clearly outnumbered by the amount of anaerobic commensals, and in a normal host, they appear to establish a symbiotic relationship with the immune system and the other bacteria. However, one of the main effects that antibiotics have in the human gut is to alter the dynamics of colonization in favor of enterococci, which are naturally tolerant to a number of antimicrobial compounds (see later). Antibiotics that are excreted in the bile or have substantial antianaerobic activity without inhibiting enterococci (e.g., various cephalosporins) have been shown to increase colonization of the gastrointestinal tract by enterococci (e.g., vancomycin-resistant enterococci, VRE).[13-15] Moreover, it has been shown that the administration of broad-spectrum antibiotics also favors the emergence of vancomycin-resistant enterococci by downregulating the intestinal expression of the intestinal antimicrobial peptide RegIIIγ (a bactericidal lectin produced by intestinal epithelial and Paneth cells), which has activity against gram-positive intestinal organisms. This effect appears to be due to broad-spectrum antibiotics eradicating the competing gram-negative organisms (mainly anaerobic) in the gut that are responsible for the activation of the signals necessary for the production of the RegIIIγ peptide through the lipopolysaccharide present in their outer membranes.[16] Other factors that may also play a role in favoring outgrowth of enterococci in the gut include the increased stomach pH, usually secondary to the administration of proton pump inhibitors, a strategy commonly used in critically ill patients to reduce the incidence of aspiration pneumonitis.

Once enterococci are established, they can gain access to the lymphatics and bloodstream through mechanisms that are not fully elucidated. Considerable research has been performed in the investigation

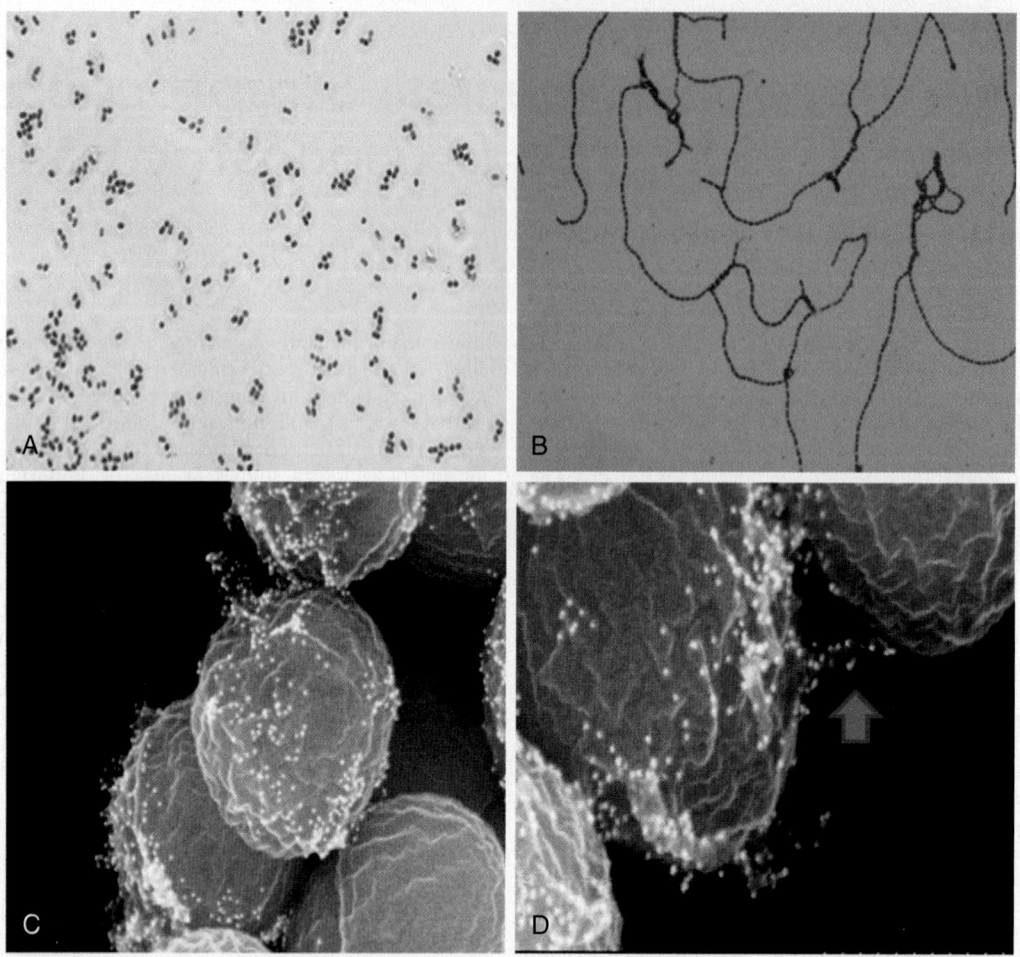

Figure 201-1 **Gram stains and scanning electron microscopy (SEM) of** *Enterococcus faecalis* **isolates. A,** Gram stain of *E. faecalis* V583 stained after growth in brain-heart infusion broth for 5 hours, exhibiting pairs, single cells, and short chains (original magnification ×100). **B,** *E. faecalis* TX0623, an isolate that produces β-lactamase showing very long chains (original magnification ×50) after growth using the same conditions indicated in A. **C and D,** Immunogold labeling and SEM of *E. faecalis* pili stained with anti-Ebp antibodies (one of the pilus proteins) (original magnification ×90,000 and ×150,000, respectively). Pili are seen as projections from the cell surface (*arrow* in D).

of pathogenic determinants that increase the ability of enterococci to cause disease by enhancing their survival or colonizing capacity in the human hosts. The study of enterococcal virulence has been possible since the development of animal models for the study of specific pathogenic determinants. It has been known since 1899[2] that enterococci are able to produce disease in mice, rats, and rabbits. Therefore, models such as mouse peritonitis and urinary tract infection, rat and rabbit endocarditis, and rabbit endophthalmitis, among others, have been useful in the study of enterococcal pathogenesis. Additionally,

nonvertebrate models such as the worm *Caenorhabditis elegans*, the moth *Galleria mellonella*, and in vitro cell culture systems have also yielded valuable information in the characterization of pathogenic determinants.

Several possible pathogenic determinants have been studied in enterococci, including cytolysin, gelatinase, serine protease, and Gls24 proteins, which have been characterized in *E. faecalis*.[17-19] A plasmid gene encoding a protein with a hyaluronidase domain has been postulated as an important virulence factor in *E. faecium*.[20] The cytolysin-

					Phenotypic Characteristics					
Genus	*VAN*	*Gas*	*BE*	*PYR*	*LAP*	*NaCl*	*10°C*	*45°C*	*HEM*	*Lancefield Grouping*
Enterococcus spp.	S/R	– –	+ +	+ +	+ +	+ +	+ +	+ +	α/γ	D
Leuconostoc spp.	R	+ +	+	– –	– –	+	–	–	α/γ	None
Streptococcus bovis group[a]	S[b]	– –	+ +	– –	+ +	– –	–	+ +	α/γ	D (+)

TABLE 201-1 **Phenotypic Differentiation between Enterococci,** *Leuconostoc,* **and** *Streptococcus bovis* **Group**

VAN, vancomycin susceptibility; Gas, production of gas in MRS broth; BE, hydrolysis of esculin in the presence of bile; PYR, production of pyrrolidonylarylamidase; LAP, production of leucine aminopeptidase; NaCl, growth in medium containing 6.5% NaCl; 10°C and 45°C, growth at 10°C and 45°C, respectively; HEM, hemolysis in sheep blood agar; S, susceptible; R, resistant; ++, positive in ≥85% of isolates; +, positive in 50% to 84% of isolates; –, positive in 16% to 49% of isolates; — —, positive in ≤15% of isolates.
[a]Includes *S. gallolyticus* subsp. *gallolyticus*, *S. gallolyticus* subsp. *pasteurianus*, and *S. infantarius* subsp. *coli*.
[b]Vancomycin-resistant isolates carrying the *vanB* gene cluster have been described.
Adapted from Facklam RR, Carvalho M, Teixeira L. History, taxonomy, biochemical characteristics and antibiotic susceptibilities testing of enterococci. In: Gilmore MS, ed. *The Enterococci: Pathogenesis, Molecular Biology and Antibiotic Resistance*. Washington, DC: ASM Press; 2002:1-54.

TABLE 201-2	Enterococcal Species Isolated from Human Infections

E. faecalis
E. faecium
E. gallinarum
E. durans
E. avium
E. raffinosus
E. pallens
E. gilvus
E. cecorum
E. malodoratus
E. italicus
E. sanguinicola
E. mundtii
E. casseliflavus/flavescens
E. dispar
E. hirae
E. pseudoavium
E. bovis

hemolysin is a bacterial toxin often encoded by pheromone-responsive plasmids capable of lysing eukaryotic (and prokaryotic) cells and shown to contribute to *E. faecalis* virulence.[17] The gelatinase and serine proteases are bacterial enzymes that may contribute to virulence in *E. faecalis* by several mechanisms that include, among others: (1) the facilitation of microbial invasion by altering immunoglobulins or complement molecules[21,22]; (2) processing of virulence factors to regulate autolysis and release of high-molecular-weight extracellular DNA, a critical component for the development of *E. faecalis* biofilms[23]; and (3) degradation of host connective tissues exposing ligands for bacterial attachment and possibly providing nutrients for the cell. The expression of gelatinase and serine protease genes is regulated by the *fsr* system, a two-component quorum-sensing regulatory system that is a global regulator of the expression of a number of genes in *E. faecalis* and is similar to the *agr* system of *Staphylococcus aureus*.[24,25] Gls24 is a general stress protein that has been shown to be important in virulence of *E. faecalis* in both mouse peritonitis[19] and rat endocarditis[26] models. Although its function has not been elucidated, Gls24 is associated with the resistance of *E. faecalis* to bile salts. In *E. faecium*, a hyaluronidase-like gene has been found in a virulence plasmid that has been highly associated with clinical strains versus commensal colonizer isolates.[20] The gene is present within a cluster encoding proteins predicted to be involved in sugar metabolism.

Cell surface components are important factors in bacterial virulence because they are usually the first molecules to interact with the host tissue or immune system. Aggregation substance (AS) of *E. faecalis* is encoded by pheromone-responsive plasmids that are involved in a particular type of conjugative plasmid transfer as well as virulence (i.e., endocarditis). AS proteins increase the adherence and internalization of enterococci into several eukaryotic cells (phagocytes, renal, intestinal, and epithelial cells) and enhance the adherence to serum and extracellular matrix proteins such as fibrin, fibronectin, thrombospondin, vitronectin, and collagen type I.[27] The *E. faecalis* surface protein (Esp) (and its homologue in *E. faecium*) is a protein that appears to function as an adhesin involved in the formation of biofilms in a glucose-dependent manner.[28] Ace, an adhesin to collagen of *E. faecalis*, belongs to the family designated MSCRAMMs, for *m*icrobial *s*urface *c*omponents *r*ecognizing *a*dhesive *m*atrix *m*olecules, and was the first of this class identified in *E. faecalis*. The Ace protein binds to collagen through what has been called the *collagen hug model*, in which the protein embraces the collagen molecule after initial docking.[29] A similar protein has also been identified in *E. faecium* (Acm) and shown to be important in the pathogenesis of endocarditis and implicated in the recent emergence of *E. faecium* as an important nosocomial pathogen.[30] Another surface protein found to be important in enterococcal pathogenesis is ElrA (for enterococcal leucin-rich repeat-containing protein). This polypeptide is a member of the WxL family of surface proteins. Deletion of the gene encoding this protein produced attenuation of *E. faecalis* virulence in a mouse peritonitis model, decreasing the ability of the organism to infect macrophages and decreasing sub-

sequent interleukin-6 response in vivo.[31] The characterization of pili on the surface of gram-positive pathogens has been a major step in the understanding of bacterial virulence. In *E. faecalis*, the presence of pili was demonstrated (see Fig. 201-1), and the characterization of genes encoding the pili subunits led to establishing that these structures play a major role in biofilm formation and are important in the pathogenesis of experimental endocarditis and urinary tract infection (UTI).[32,33] Genes encoding the pili subunits have also been identified in *E. faecium*,[34] indicating that the pili are ubiquitous structures of enterococci.

Polysaccharides on bacterial surfaces may be important pathogenic determinants and may affect leukocyte-mediated killing of bacteria. Certain *E. faecium* strains are resistant to polymorphonuclear cell killing, a characteristic that might be due to a carbohydrate-containing moiety.[35] Additionally, antibody to a capsular polysaccharide component purified from an *E. faecalis* strain enhanced phagocytosis and killing of both *E. faecalis* and *E. faecium* strains; it was also suggested that the capsular material would have vaccine potential because a reduction in bacterial numbers recovered from different organs of immunized mice was obtained compared with nonimmunized controls.[36,37] Using rabbit antisera for the typing of *E. faecalis*, four capsular serotypes (1, 2, 4, and 7) were found to be present in most clinical isolates,[38] and at least two types of gene clusters for the production of polysaccharide have been characterized (designated the epa[39] and cps[40] loci).

Sequencing of enterococcal genomes has been another useful tool to facilitate the understanding of the complicated pathway from which enterococci evolved from a commensal to a pathogen. Sequencing of the genome of the first vancomycin-resistant *E. faecalis* strain isolated in the United States (designated V583) indicated that more than one fourth of the genome is mobile DNA (more than any other bacterial genome). A pathogenicity island, which is a large genetic element carrying a set of putative virulence-associated genes,[41] a transposon carrying the *vanB* gene cluster, three plasmids with antibiotic resistance determinants, and insertion sequences were found among the most prominent and potentially mobile elements of V583.[42] The pathogenicity island encodes factors that may enable enterococci to gain advantage in the gut such as the cytolysin, which has antibacterial properties, several surface adhesins, several carbohydrate utilization pathways, and enzymes that may permit colonization of certain areas of the intestine. It has been postulated that this pathogenicity island was acquired by an ancestral *E. faecalis* clonal strain that evolved to acquire antibiotic resistance determinants, thus becoming equipped to cause problematic infections in humans. Similarly, sequencing of the entire genome of another *E. faecalis* strain (*E. faecalis* OG1RF) revealed that a considerable amount of variation in gene content is present in this species. As opposed to V583, *E. faecalis* OG1RF lacks plasmids and the pathogenicity island but is still able to cause infection in animal models. This strain lacks the mobile elements typical of V583 but harbors additional genes predicted to encode proteins involved in adherence, defense against bacteriophages, metabolism of myoinositol, and novel surface proteins.[43]

Epidemiology of Enterococcal Infections

The two most common species responsible for most enterococcal infections are *E. faecalis* and *E. faecium*. The only other species of enterococci known to be responsible for outbreaks and nosocomial spread, albeit uncommon, is *E. gallinarum*.[44] Enterococci are among the leading causes of nosocomial infections in the United States (second or third), and it is estimated that in 2004, 521,285 hospital discharges were associated with enterococcal infections.[45,46] The study of the dynamics of acquisition and infection with VRE has yielded information crucial for better understanding the epidemiology of enterococcal infections. VRE now accounts for about 30% of enterococcal infections, with most VRE isolates being *E. faecium* (>90%).[47] The first step in the infectious process appears to involve colonization by hospital-associated strains of the gastrointestinal tract, which may persist for months or years, although direct inoculation onto intravenous or urinary catheters, intravenous stopcock sets used in the anesthesia work area, or thermometers has been documented. It has also been shown that the hospital environment can be heavily colonized with VRE, including bed rails, linen, doorknobs, bedpans, urinals, blood pressure cuffs, stethoscopes, and monitoring equipment amongst others.[48] Risk factors associated with increased VRE colonization include the presence of immunosuppression or serious comorbid condition (e.g., diabetes, renal failure, high APACHE score), increased hospital stay, residence in a long-term care facility, proximity to another colonized or infected patient (including sharing a room) or hospitalization in a room previously occupied by a patient colonized with VRE, invasive procedures, and administration of broad-spectrum antibiotics (e.g., cephalosporins) or vancomycin.[49,50] The hands of health care workers appear to be the most common source of transmission of VRE, and the Society for Health Epidemiology of America has published specific guidelines to curtail this transmission.[51] The organisms are capable of surviving on the hands, gloves, and gowns of health care workers for prolonged periods of time, and independent risk factors for glove and gown contamination include contact with a colonized patient's catheter or drain, trunk, or lower extremity.[52]

After a patient becomes colonized with VRE, the risk for developing a subsequent bloodstream infection with the same VRE colonizing strain appears to increase,[53] although some studies have not found the same association. Rates of bloodstream infections in patients colonized with VRE have ranged from 0% to 34% and appear to be higher among cancer patients and solid and bone marrow transplant recipients. The risk factors associated with developing a VRE bloodstream infection in an already VRE colonized patient include cancer or diabetes (relative risk [RR], 3.91), gastrointestinal procedure (RR, 4.56), acute renal failure (RR, 3.1), exposure to vancomycin (RR, 1.95), and infection of an additional site other than blood (OR, 3.9).[54] Among patients with leukemia, concurrent *Clostridium difficile* infection was associated with increased risk for developing a VRE bloodstream infection.[55] Additionally, two meta-analyses have evaluated the mortality of patients with bacteremia with VRE compared with those with vancomycin-susceptible enterococci (VSE).[56,57] Both studies concluded that patients with bacteremia with VRE were about 2.5 times more likely to die than those with VSE bacteremia, indicating that the development of vancomycin resistance is a poor prognostic sign in critically ill patients.

Clinical Presentations of Enterococcal Disease

BACTEREMIA AND ENDOCARDITIS

Bacteremia and endocarditis are common presentations of enterococcal disease. Bacteremia without endocarditis is by far the more frequent of the two presentations, and enterococci are currently one of the leading causes of nosocomial bacteremias.[58] Frequent sources of the bacteremia are usually the genitourinary and gastrointestinal tracts in cases originating outside the hospital (endocarditis should always be ruled out). Intravascular or urinary catheters are the most common source in nosocomial bacteremias, and intra-abdominal, pelvic, biliary tract, wounds (including in burned patients), and bone have also been documented as sources of the bacteremia. Enterococcal bacteremia often occurs in debilitated patients who have received antibiotics and have serious underlying conditions, and polymicrobial bacteremia can be seen in up to about 50% of cases.[59] Recent data suggest that *E. faecium* bloodstream infection may have a worse prognosis than *E. faecalis*, likely because these organisms are much more resistant to antibiotics and are increasingly difficult to treat.[60] Enterococcal bacteremia and meningitis (see later) have also been associated with the *Strongyloides* hyperinfection syndrome.[61]

The percentage of patients who have endocarditis as the cause of detectable enterococcal bacteremia varies according to the study and population studied, ranging from about 1% to 32%. Enterococci are

the second or third cause of endocarditis, depending on the series and patients examined, accounting for 5% to 20% of cases of endocarditis. In a recent prospective observational cohort study that included 193 patients with endocarditis, *E. faecalis* was the second most common organism isolated after *S. aureus*.[62] The organisms can affect both native and prosthetic valves and can cause both community- and nosocomial-associated endocarditis, with *E. faecalis* being recovered much more frequently than *E. faecium* or other enterococcal species. The disease usually occurs in the setting of damaged heart valves, and the mitral and aortic are the valves usually involved, although endocarditis of apparently intact valves has also been reported.[63,64] Most patients tend to be male and elderly with comorbidities, although enterococcal endocarditis in women of childbearing age has been well documented. The infection usually originates from the genitourinary or gastrointestinal tract and procedures associated with the development of enterococcal endocarditis include cystoscopy, cesarean section, prostatectomy, transrectal prostatic biopsy, transjugular intrahepatic portosystemic shunt (TIPS), extracorporeal shock wave lithotripsy, colonoscopy, fiberoptic sigmoidoscopy, and liver biopsy.[7,64] Malignant and inflammatory lesions of the gut and biliary tract may also be the source of endocarditis. Most patients with enterococcal endocarditis display a subacute course, and the most common clinical manifestations include fevers, presence of a murmur, and constitutional symptoms such as weight loss, generalized aches, and malaise. Peripheral signs of endocarditis such as petechiae, Osler nodes, and Roth spots have been found less frequently (about 15%) than in endocarditis caused by other organisms.[64] Atypical manifestations include polyarthritis, spondylodiscitis, dementia, metastatic abscesses to the spleen, and empyema. The most common complication of enterococcal endocarditis is heart failure, which occurs in about half of the patients, with a significant percentage requiring valve replacement. Embolization occurs in 27% to 43% of patients,[64,65] and the brain appears to be the most common end organ. Mortality ranges from 11% to 35%, usually due to heart failure or embolization.

URINARY TRACT INFECTIONS

Enterococcal UTIs in young, healthy women without history of urinary tract instrumentation or anatomic abnormalities is infrequent (<5% of all UTIs) and was first reported in 1906.[3,7] Conversely, enterococcal UTIs are well documented in the hospital and usually associated with indwelling catheters, instrumentation, and abnormalities of the genitourinary tract. Recent data from the National Healthcare Safety Network from 463 hospitals across the United States indicate that enterococci are the third most common organism isolated from catheter-associated UTIs, with *E. faecium*, *E. faecalis*, and other enterococcal species accounting for 40%, 25%, and 35% of the total enterococcal organisms isolated, respectively.[46] It is sometimes difficult to differentiate between infection and colonization in the hospital setting; therefore, the isolation of more than 10^5 colony-forming units (CFUs) of *Enterococcus* spp. from urine may represent colonization, and removal of the catheter may suffice to eradicate the presence of the organism. Recurrent UTIs and previous antibiotic treatment have also been associated with enterococcal UTIs. The infection appears to be more common in older men, and associated prostatitis and epididymitis have been documented. Enterococci can also cause complicated UTIs with the development of pyelonephritis and perinephric abscesses that can lead to bacteremic episodes.[7]

MENINGITIS

Enterococci are uncommon causes of meningitis accounting for about 0.3% to 4% of meningitis cases according to different series.[66,67] Two presentations are usually described: spontaneous and postoperative meningitis. *E. faecalis* is the most common species isolated, followed by *E. faecium*, *E. gallinarum*, *E. avium*, and *E. casseliflavus*. Spontaneous meningitis is a community-associated infection that often presents in patients with severe comorbidities such as diabetes, chronic renal failure, pulmonary or cardiovascular disease, immunosuppression (including steroid use and HIV), malignancies, transplantation, and splenectomy. In some cases, meningitis can present in apparently healthy individuals with no clear focus of infection.[67,68] In children, spontaneous meningitis has been reported associated with central nervous system (CNS) pathology (neural tube defects and hydrocephalus), prematurity, recent surgery, or congenital heart disease. Meningitis in the setting of disseminated strongyloidosis has also been well characterized. Postoperative meningitis is a hospital-associated infection, and the presence of shunt devices appears to be the most important predisposing factor. In rare instances, enterococcal meningitis has been associated as a complication of lumbar or ventricular tap, placement of CNS electrodes, and epidural anesthesia.[67]

The clinical characteristics of meningitis are similar in both presentations (spontaneous and postoperative). Patients have an acute course with fever, altered mental status, and signs of meningeal irritation (coma, petechial rash, shock, and focal deficits are uncommon). Cerebrospinal fluid (CSF) findings include pleocytosis, increased protein levels, and low glucose. In a series of 140 patients with enterococcal meningitis, the median CSF leukocyte count was 533 mm^3, and only 35% had a leukocyte count of less than 200 mm^3, with a positive Gram stain seen in up to 40% of cases.[67] Accompanying bacteremia can be found in more than half of cases of spontaneous meningitis. Complications of enterococcal meningitis include hydrocephalus, stroke, and brain abscesses. The overall mortality rate approaches 20%, and poor prognostic factors include seizures, altered consciousness, advanced age, respiratory failure, septic shock, and the presence of hypoglycorrhachia or decreased white count in the CSF[66]; residual sequelae can be seen in about 17% of patients.

INTRA-ABDOMINAL AND PELVIC INFECTIONS

Enterococci are commensals of the gastrointestinal and genitourinary tracts and are commonly isolated from abdominal and pelvic infections, usually with other Gram-negative and anaerobic organisms; the role of enterococci in these infections has been the subject of controversy.[69] An analysis of six clinical trials with the objective of examining the use of antibiotics without enterococcal activity in the treatment of intra-abdominal infections did not find any case of treatment failure despite evidence of the presence of enterococci in 20% to 30% of initial cultures.[70] Similarly, several studies have shown that community-associated, complicated intra-abdominal infections with mixed flora that include enterococci can be treated with surgery and antibiotics that do not exhibit in vitro activity against enterococci. Moreover, data from animal experiments indicate that enterococci alone do not cause intra-abdominal sepsis when injected intraperitoneally unless other substances or organisms that promote abscess formation are added.[71] Nonetheless, several well-conducted studies have demonstrated that enterococci are able to cause treatment failures and adverse outcomes, including a randomized, prospective, double-blind trial involving 330 patients, which concluded that the isolation of enterococcal isolates from intra-abdominal collections was a predictor of treatment failure.[72] Several other series have confirmed these observations, concluding that the presence of enterococci increases the rates of postoperative infectious complications and also the mortality of these patients. Although the bulk of evidence indicates that the use of antienterococcal antibiotics may not be necessary in most initial treatments of acute intra-abdominal infections, the apparent increased frequency of isolation of nosocomial multidrug-resistant enterococci indicates that antienterococcal therapy should be considered for immunocompromised and severely ill patients with nosocomial peritonitis and abdominal sepsis or persistent collections who have received broad-spectrum antibiotics that do not have activity against enterococci (e.g., cephalosporins) and patients with peritonitis and damaged or prosthetic heart valves (to prevent endocarditis).[69] Enterococci are also capable of producing spontaneous peritonitis and empyema in cirrhotic and chronic renal failure patients and have also been reported as etiologic agents in peritonitis associated with chronic ambulatory peritoneal dialysis.[7]

NEONATAL INFECTIONS

Enterococci are part of the normal adult vaginal flora and can be acquired by neonates during delivery. The organisms have been implicated in about 6% of late-onset sepsis, 5% of pneumonias, 9% of surgical site infections, 10% of bacteremias, and 17% of UTIs in neonatal units.[73] In the case of late-onset sepsis, enterococcal infections are usually hospital associated and may be polymicrobial. Affected patients usually have a prolonged hospital stay, low birth weight, prior antibiotic therapy, and several invasive procedures. The clinical presentation of sepsis is usually associated with localized sites of infection or necrotizing enterocolitis. Endocarditis is rare in the neonatal period but can be seen in infants with prolonged enterococcal bacteremia.[73]

Several outbreaks of neonatal sepsis have been documented in the literature. In 1982, an outbreak of *E. faecium* was documented in Virginia[74]; the infants had severe underlying conditions with the presence of endovascular devices and nasogastric tubes and were premature. Similarly, a 6-month outbreak of *E. faecalis* neonatal sepsis was documented in Colorado in 1987; most of the infants were also premature with low birth weight and intravascular devices and had undergone bowel surgery.[75] Outbreaks of vancomycin-resistant enterococci causing sepsis in neonates have also been well characterized in different parts of the world.

SKIN, SOFT TISSUE, AND OTHER INFECTIONS

Enterococci have been associated with skin and soft tissue (including wounds) infections. When found in clinical samples from soft tissues, they are usually accompanied by other microorganisms; therefore, their pathogenic potential in these infections is debatable. Decubitus and diabetic foot ulcers are the usual lesions associated with the presence of enterococci, and in some cases, the organisms have been isolated from bone, causing osteomyelitis.[76] Enterococci are rare causes of soft tissue abscesses; however, liver, lung, and even brain abscesses have been reported.[77] The authors have seen a breast abscess caused by *E. faecium* in a patient hospitalized in the critical care unit. Enterococcal pneumonia and spontaneous empyema are also uncommon but have been occasionally described.

Therapy and Antimicrobial Resistance

The main hurdle the clinician faces in the treatment of enterococcal infections is that these organisms are intrinsically resistant to a number of compounds and also have an ability to recruit antibiotic resistance genes. These therapeutic problems have long been recognized, and in the past, about 60% of failures in the treatment of enterococcal endocarditis occurred when penicillin was used as monotherapy in these infections,[7] as opposed to endocarditis caused by streptococci. Bactericidal therapy is needed for optimal cure rates in endocarditis and other endovascular infections, which is usually not achieved with available single agents; therefore, combination therapy is usually given (Figs. 201-2 and 201-3) (Table 201-3). The emergence of resistance to various antimicrobial agents poses enormous clinical problems because the bactericidal goal may not be achieved.

β-LACTAM AND AMINOGLYCOSIDES

β-lactam antibiotics inhibit the penicillin-binding proteins (PBPs) of susceptible bacteria, interfering with the cell wall synthesis, and this class of antibiotics should be the first choice for the treatment of susceptible enterococcal isolates (see Table 201-3). Relative resistance to β-lactams with minimal inhibitory concentration (MIC) of penicillin 10 to 100 times or more those of streptococci is a well-described characteristic of enterococci. Many strains are also tolerant to β-lactams, that is, are not killed with concentrations of antibiotics 16 times higher than the MIC.[78] The most potent activity is observed with the aminopenicillins (e.g., ampicillin) and ureidopenicillins, followed by penicillin G and carbapenems. Although the MIC breakpoint defined by the

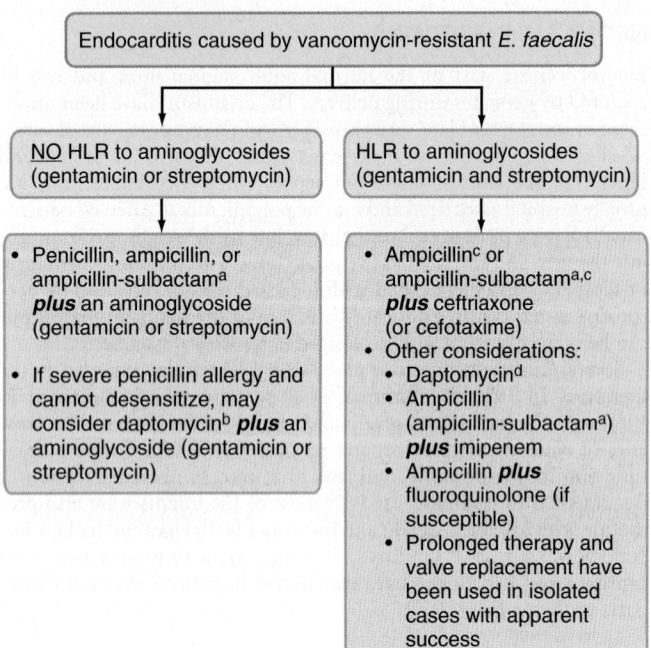

Figure 201-2 **Possible therapeutic alternatives for the treatment of endocarditis caused by vancomycin-resistant *E. faecalis*.** HLR, high-level resistance. [a]In rare cases of β-lactamase–producing isolates, the American Heart Association (AHA) recommends ampicillin-sulbactam 12 g/day. [b]High-dose daptomycin (8-10 mg/kg) may be preferable to 6 mg/kg. [c]Continuous infusion of ampicillin or ampicillin-sulbactam as monotherapy is preferred by some. [d]Because of concern of lack of efficacy of 4 or 6 mg/kg, high-dose daptomycin with the addition of another active agent (e.g., ampicillin, fluoroquinolone) might be considered. None of these indications is approved by the U.S. Food and Drug Administration, nor have prospective, randomized trials been conducted. Recommendations are based on literature review and personal opinion. A duration of therapy of 4 to 6 weeks for both native and prosthetic valves should be considered, and extending the treatment to 8 weeks or longer is recommended in case a β-lactam agent cannot be used because of resistance (rare) or allergy. (Adapted from Arias CA, Murray BE. Emergence and management of drug-resistant enterococcal infections. Exp Rev Anti Infect Ther. 2008;6:637-655.)

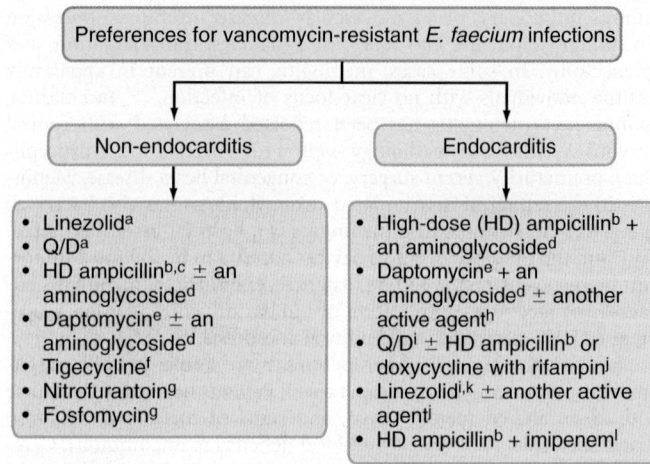

Figure 201-3 **Possible therapeutic alternatives for the treatment of infections caused by vancomycin-resistant *E. faecium*.** Q/D, quinupristin-dalfopristin. [a]U.S. Food and Drug Administration (FDA) approved for non-endocarditis vancomycin-resistant *E. faecium* infections. Linezolid and Q/D have been successfully used in meningitis caused by resistant isolates of *E. faecium*. [b]If MIC is ≤64 μg/mL, high-dose ampicillin up to 30 g/day could be considered. [c]Because of high urine concentrations obtained with high-dose ampicillin therapy, ampicillin is likely to be effective in lower urinary tract infections even when caused by organisms with MICs ≥128 μg/mL (plus catheter removal). [d]If the organism lacks high-level resistance (HLR) to gentamicin and streptomycin. [e]High-dose daptomycin (8 to 10 mg/kg) may be preferable to 6 mg/kg. [f]Not approved for any *E. faecium* infection but active in vitro; concerns exist in the treatment of bacteremia due to low serum levels. [g]Urinary tract infections only. [h]High-dose ampicillin (MIC ≤64 μg/mL) and rifampin have been used; daptomycin plus tigecycline in one case report. [i]Q/D or linezolid are listed in the American Heart Association (AHA) recommendations for the treatment of vancomycin and ampicillin-resistant *E. faecium*. [j]If susceptible to each agent. [k]Concerns over reports of lack of efficacy or development of resistance with monotherapy. [l]If imipenem MIC ≤32 μg/mL. The recommendations for compounds that are not FDA approved are based on literature review and personal opinion. No prospective, randomized trials have been conducted. (Adapted from Arias CA, Murray BE. Emergence and management of drug-resistant enterococcal infections. Exp Rev Anti Infect Ther. 2008;6:637-655.)

Clinical and Laboratory Standards Institute (CLSI) for ampicillin susceptibility is less than 16 mg/L, high doses of ampicillin can achieve plasma concentrations of more than 150 mg/L, which has led to the suggestion that isolates with ampicillin MIC of 64 mg/L or less may be successfully treated with doses of 18 to 30 g/day of ampicillin or ampicillin-sulbactam,[79] usually combined with an aminoglycoside (see later), although there are few safety data for use of this high-dose β-lactam regimen.

Resistance to penicillins and carbapenems is usually found in clinical isolates of *E. faecium* and rarely in *E. faecalis*. The mechanisms of resistance in *E. faecium* involve mutations or overexpression of the *pbp5* gene, which decrease the affinity of its product for ampicillin.[80] A laboratory strain of *E. faecium* with a PBP-independent mechanism of β-lactam resistance involving a novel transpeptidation pathway of peptidoglycan has also been reported,[81] although no clinical isolates have so far been found to exhibit this mechanism. β-Lactam resistance in *E. faecalis* can be mediated by the production of a β-lactamase enzyme[82]; although rare, occasional outbreak strains harboring this enzyme have been reported, mainly in the United States and Argentina. It is important to note that the presence of this enzyme is not detected by routine susceptibility testing; therefore, testing specifically for β-lactamase in endocarditis or serious enterococcal infections should always be considered.[83]

A bactericidal regimen should be used for the treatment of enterococcal endocarditis (see Figs. 201-2 and 201-3) and is also recom-

mended for any other endovascular infection. However, as mentioned previously, β-lactams are not readily bactericidal for enterococci; hence, a synergistic and bactericidal effect is usually achieved with the addition of an aminoglycoside. In vitro synergism in enterococci is defined as a 2 $\log_{10}$ or higher increase in killing at 24 hours by the combination compared with the β-lactam (or glycopeptides, see later) alone when the concentration of the aminoglycoside does not have any effect on the growth curve of the microorganism and a 99.9% decrease from the starting inoculum resulting from the antibiotic combination is achieved. The aminoglycosides gentamicin and streptomycin are the only two compounds recommended for achieving this synergistic effect in clinical practice. The use of other aminoglycosides for this purpose is discouraged (see later).

High-level resistance (HLR) to aminoglycosides is defined by growth at concentrations of 2000 mg/L and 500 mg/L of streptomycin and gentamicin, respectively, on brain-heart infusion agar (BHI) or 1000 mg/L of streptomycin when using BHI broth. The presence of HLR to both gentamicin and streptomycin abolishes the synergistic effect of these compounds in clinical practice. The emergence of HLR to both aminoglycosides was reported in 1983[84] and has increased since then in both *E. faecalis* and *E. faecium*. HLR to gentamicin is mostly due to the presence of a bifunctional aminoglycoside modifying enzyme, AAC(6′)-Ie-APH(2″)-Ia, which confers high-level resistance to gentamicin (as well as HLR or resistance to synergism with tobra-

TABLE 201-3 Treatment of Nonendovascular Infections Due to β-Lactam and Glycopeptide-Susceptible Enterococcal Species

Disease	Suggested Regimen	Dosage and Duration
Bacteremia[a]	Ampicillin[b] *or* Penicillin G *or* Vancomycin	9-12 g daily in divided doses q 4-6 h for 14 days[c] 18-30 million units daily divided q 4-6 h for 14 days 30 mg/kg daily divided q 6-12 h for 14 days
Meningitis[d]	Ampicillin[e] *or* Penicillin G[e] *plus* Gentamicin *or* Streptomycin	12-20+ g daily in divided doses q 4 h for 14 days 18-30 million units daily in divided doses q 4 h for 14 days 5.1-7 mg/kg single daily dose for 14 days 15 mg/kg single daily dose for 14 days
Urinary tract infections	Nitrofurantoin, fosfomycin, amoxicillin[f]	100 mg PO q 6 h for 5 days 3 g PO (single dose) 875 mg PO q 12 h for 5 days

[a]Adding an aminoglycoside for synergistic therapy (gentamicin, 1 mg/kg q 8 h, or streptomycin, 7.5 mg/kg q 12 h) with a cell wall agent should be considered in seriously ill patients or with high risk for developing endocarditis.

[b]In rare β-lactamase-producing isolates, ampicillin-sulbactam (12 g daily in divided doses) should be considered.

[c]In catheter-associated bacteremias, a shorter duration of therapy (5-7 days) may be sufficient after removal of the catheter.

[d]In refractory cases, linezolid has been reported successful; intrathecal vancomycin or gentamicin may be considered in cases of postoperative meningitis or with failure to respond to systemic antibiotics.

[e]For patients with penicillin allergy, vancomycin IV, 500-750 mg q 6 h, is recommended.

[f]For β-lactamase producers, amoxicillin-clavulanate can be used.

mycin, netilmicin, sisomicin, kanamycin, and amikacin, but not streptomycin). HLR to streptomycin can be due to mutations in the 30S ribosomal subunit[85] and to the presence of a streptomycin adenylyltransferase.[84] The evaluation of the presence of HLR is therefore critical for the treatment of all enterococcal isolates causing endovascular or severe infections. As a caveat, rare isolates of both *E. faecalis* and *E. faecium* (and *E. gallinarum*) whose MIC of gentamicin is lower than 500 mg/L (i.e., reported as not HLR to gentamicin) may be resistant to the synergistic effect of the combination with a cell wall agent owing to the presence of the APH(2″)-Ic enzyme or other yet unidentified mechanisms. Hence, this situation must be considered in patients who do not respond appropriately to combination therapy with gentamicin, that is, in isolates reported as not having HLR to this aminoglycoside.

Other compounds of the aminoglycoside class are not recommended for the treatment of enterococcal infections (except possibly arbekacin [in Japan] and tobramycin in *E. faecalis* with no HLR to gentamicin; see later) because (1) as stated earlier, the common mechanism of resistance to gentamicin in clinical isolates is mediated by the AAC(6′)-Ie-APH (2″)-Ia enzyme, which confers resistance to synergism with all aminoglycosides commonly available in the United States, except streptomycin; (2) *E. faecium* possess an aminoglycoside 6′-acetyltransferase (6′-AAC) enzyme (as a species characteristic), which results in a higher MIC of tobramycin, as well as kanamycin, netilmicin, and sisomicin, resulting in loss of the synergistic effect with cell wall agents; and (3) the *aph(3′)-IIIa* gene (encoding a kanamycin-neomycin phosphotransferase) is commonly found in enterococci and confers HLR resistance or resistance to synergism with amikacin and kanamycin. In Japan, the aminoglycoside arbekacin is approved for clinical use, and this compound appears to be more stable to the action of the AAC(6′)-Ie-APH (2″)-Ia enzyme. It has also been shown that arbekacin exhibited synergism in vitro when combined with ampicillin against 40% of enterococci possessing the bifunctional enzyme.[86]

Therefore, this compound may be useful for certain isolates with HLR to aminoglycosides.

Typically, the cephalosporins have weak activity against all species of enterococci with exceptions: ceftriaxone or cefotaxime in combination with ampicillin for the treatment of endocarditis produced by isolates of *E. faecalis* exhibiting HLR to all aminoglycosides (see Fig. 201-2).[87] In an open-label and nonrandomized trial in Spain, patients with *E. faecalis* endocarditis were treated successfully (clinical cure rate at 3 months was 67.4%) with the combination of ceftriaxone (2 g every 12 hours) and ampicillin (2 g every 4 hours), given for 6 weeks if the isolates exhibited HLR to aminoglycosides or toxicity precluded their use.[87] The rationale of this approach is based on the observation that low concentrations of an aminopenicillin may be capable of partially saturating low-molecular-weight PBP-4 and PBP-5, but not PBP-2 and PBP-3, which then could actively participate in the synthesis of the bacterial cell wall. The addition of cefotaxime (or ceftriaxone) could produce total saturation of PBP-2 and PBP-3, producing the bactericidal synergistic effect[88] in *E. faecalis* (this effect is not observed in clinical isolates of *E. faecium*). Ceftobiprole and ceftaroline are examples of a new generation of cephalosporins with increased affinity for PBPs of many resistant species (mainly PBP-2a of methicillin-resistant *S. aureus* [MRSA]), which have relatively good activity against clinical isolates of *E. faecalis* (but not ampicillin-resistant *E. faecium*).[89] Ceftobiprole has potent activity against β-lactamase–producing and vancomycin-resistant strains of *E. faecalis*, has exhibited synergism with aminoglycosides against selected isolates of *E. faecalis*, and has activity comparable to that of ampicillin in an in vivo mouse peritonitis model.[89]

GLYCOPEPTIDES AND LIPOGLYCOPEPTIDES

The two glycopeptides currently used in clinical practice to treat enterococcal infections are vancomycin and teicoplanin. The mechanism of action of these compounds includes the inhibition of the last steps of peptidoglycan synthesis, which involves transglycosylation and transpeptidation of the pentapeptide units. Glycopeptides have been mainly used in the past in the treatment of β-lactam–resistant *E. faecium*. However, the increased prevalence of vancomycin resistance has reduced the clinical use of these compounds against enterococci. Oritavancin (formerly, LY333328) is a semisynthetic glycopeptide antibiotic derived from chloroeremomycin, which is in the late stages of clinical development. Oritavancin has potent dose-dependent bactericidal activity against enterococci, including VRE with MIC ranging between 1 and 2 mg/L.[90,91] This antibiotic shares a similar mechanism of action with glycopeptides; additionally, it appears to produce depolarization of the cell membrane, which increases its bactericidal activity.[92] Initial clinical trials testing oritavancin in human infections indicate that the antibiotic is safe and fulfilled the noninferiority criteria against the comparators, and pharmacologic studies indicate that the antibiotic is well tolerated in healthy human volunteers. Telavancin appears to have limited activity against glycopeptide-resistant enterococci with MIC$_{90}$ for vancomycin-resistant *E. faecalis* and *E. faecium* ranging between 4 and 16 mg/L and 2 and 16 mg/L, respectively (although the MICs are several-fold lower than those of vancomycin). Phase III studies[93] indicate that this compound may be useful in the treatment of skin and soft tissue infections in which VSE play a role.

DAPTOMYCIN

This lipopeptide antibiotic was approved by the U.S. Food and Drug Administration (FDA) in September 2003 for the treatment of complicated skin and soft tissue infections, including vancomycin-susceptible *E. faecalis*, and it was granted an additional indication in 2006 for *S. aureus* (including MRSA) bacteremia and right-sided endocarditis. Daptomycin is not FDA approved for the treatment of *E. faecium* (regardless of susceptibility) or for VRE infections. The molecular events involved in its antibacterial action have not yet been completely elucidated, and it is thought that daptomycin inserts into the bacterial cell membrane in a calcium-dependent manner and then subsequently produces an alteration of the membrane potential, which eventually leads to bacterial cell death by an unknown mechanism. In vitro, daptomycin exhibits rapid concentration-dependent bactericidal killing of enterococci, and in vivo, the AUC (free drug)/MIC ratio appears to be the best parameter that correlates with clinical success.[94] The activity of daptomycin in vivo appears to be affected by its high binding affinity to albumin (90% to 94%), and the unbound fraction might be crucial in the treatment of endovascular enterococcal infections when bactericidal therapy is a requirement, which has led to the suggestion that a higher dose (8 to 10 mg/kg day) may be of benefit (see Figs. 201-2 and 201-3). Combination therapies that include daptomycin have been used in recalcitrant enterococcal infections. For example, failure of daptomycin monotherapy in the treatment of *E. faecium* endocarditis was overcome by the use of a combination of high-dose daptomycin (8 mg/kg/day), high-dose ampicillin, and gentamicin.[95] Similarly, the combination of daptomycin, gentamicin, and rifampin successfully treated a case of prosthetic valve endocarditis caused by a vancomycin-resistant isolate of *E. faecium* that failed linezolid,[96] and in vivo experiments have demonstrated that the renal toxicity of gentamicin appears to be attenuated by the concomitant use of daptomycin. An additional anecdotal successful combination used in the treatment of endocarditis caused by a multidrug-resistant (including HLR to aminoglycosides) *E. faecium* included the combination of daptomycin (6 mg/kg every 48 hours) and tigecycline.[97] Resistance to daptomycin in enterococci has been well documented (daptomycin MICs range from 6 to >32 mg/L), although remains relatively rare. Daptomycin resistance emerging during prolonged therapy (average exposure to daptomycin of 18 days) has been documented in *E. faecalis*, *E. faecium*, and *E. durans* isolates, although it has also been documented in isolates without previous exposure to the antibiotic.[98] All patients had a certain degree of immunosuppression and were treated for bacteremia or endocarditis. Little is known about the mechanisms of resistance in these enterococcal strains.

LINEZOLID

The efficacy of linezolid against enterococci (including VRE) has been evaluated in several clinical trials and in a recent meta-analysis.[99] In the case of endocarditis, controversial reports can be found in the literature regarding the outcomes of these patients because the antibiotic has been used when other recommended options have failed or when resistance or allergies to approved agents have been documented. In an intention-to-treat analysis of 22 patients with VRE endocarditis treated with linezolid in a compassionate use basis, cure was achieved in only 10 (45%) of the patients. Conversely, linezolid was used as a single agent in the treatment of five patients with endocarditis caused by *E. faecalis* (three were vancomycin-resistant) and four with *E. faecium* (all vancomycin-resistant). The overall cure or improvement rate was 78% (7 out of 9 patients), with the development of thrombocytopenia in 33% of patients. Of note, the American Heart Association (AHA) recommends linezolid as one of two drugs that can be used as first-line therapy for endocarditis caused by *E. faecium* resistant to β-lactams, glycopeptides, and aminoglycosides[100] (evidence is "expert opinion"). We suggest that linezolid should be used with caution in the treatment of VRE enterococcal endocarditis and only when combinations of β-lactams and aminoglycosides, high-dose daptomycin, or daptomycin plus aminoglycosides cannot be used, because of resistance, toxicity, or therapeutic failure. In patients allergic to β-lactams, desensitization should be considered in severe infections due to *E. faecalis* (see Fig. 201-2). Linezolid has also been successfully used in the treatment of enterococcal meningitis caused by different species, but no clinical trials have been conducted because of the paucity of cases.

Linezolid resistance appears to be increasing, and horizontal spread of specific linezolid-resistant outbreak strains has been reported,[101] including in patients without previous exposure to the antibiotic. Risk factors for the acquisition of nosocomial linezolid-resistant strains included peripheral vascular disease, receipt of a solid organ transplant, total parenteral nutrition, and the administration of piperacillin-tazobactam, cefepime, or both. The common mechanism of resistance involves mutations in the central loop of domain V of the 23S rRNA. The mutation G2576T (*Escherichia coli* 23S rRNA gene numbering) is commonly found in resistant strains and other mutations (G2505A, G2512T, G2513T, C2610G) have also been found in enterococci, mainly in vitro. The rRNA mutations appear to interfere with the oxazolidinone interaction with its target at the core of the ribosomal peptidyl-transferase center. *E. faecalis* and *E. faecium* contain 4 and 6 copies of the rRNA operons, respectively, and the increase in MIC to linezolid has been associated with the number of mutated rRNA genes[102] in which homologous recombination may play a crucial role. Studies in the gastrointestinal tract of gnotobiotic mice also indicate that the dose and duration of linezolid exposure directly influence the number of mutated rRNA genes. Nonmutational resistance to linezolid has been characterized in clinical isolates of staphylococci from animal and human clinical sources. Resistance is mediated by the presence of a gene designated *cfr* (for chloramphenicol-florfenicol resistance), which was originally described on a plasmid in an animal isolate of *Staphylococcus sciuri* and encodes an enzyme capable of methylating position A2503 of the 23S rRNA of bacterial ribosomes. It has been postulated that the *cfr* gene may have been transferred from enterococci to a clinical human isolate of MRSA.[103,104]

TIGECYCLINE

Tigecycline is FDA approved for the treatment of complicated skin and soft tissue infections and abdominal infections caused by susceptible organisms, including vancomycin-susceptible *E. faecalis*. Animal models of peritonitis and endocarditis have documented the efficacy of tigecycline against enterococci regardless of the presence of vancomycin or tetracycline resistance. It is thought that its prolonged half-life, postantibiotic effect, and homogeneous diffusion into the cardiac vegetation could enhance the in vivo activity of this compound against enterococci in valvular vegetations. However, no clinical data are available to support the use of tigecycline monotherapy in enterococcal endocarditis or any other endovascular infections, and concerns over the use of tigecycline for the treatment of bloodstream infections have been raised because only low serum concentrations are achieved at the recommended dose. Furthermore, emergence of resistance to tigecycline during therapy has been documented in an enterococcal isolate (*E. faecalis*) from the urine of a patient who was receiving treatment for a respiratory infection caused by *Stenotrophomonas maltophilia*,[105] but the mechanism of resistance remains to be elucidated. Nonetheless, in phase III trials of complicated skin and soft tissue and intra-abdominal infections, tigecycline was not inferior to the comparators (vancomycin-aztreonam and imipenem-cilastatin, respectively) against vancomycin-susceptible *E. faecalis*, supporting the potential clinical usefulness of tigecycline against enterococci.[106]

QUINUPRISTIN-DALFOPRISTIN (Q/D)

Q/D is a parenteral, semisynthetic antibiotic combination of streptogramin type A (dalfopristin) and type B (quinupristin), which was the first FDA-approved antibiotic for the treatment of VRE infections. It is important to note that Q/D is not active against *E. faecalis* because of the presence of an ATP-binding cassette (ABC) protein homologue designated Lsa,[107] which is likely to act as an efflux pump for this compound. Nonetheless, certain clinical and laboratory strains of *E. faecalis* appear to be susceptible to Q/D due to mutations in *lsa* or possible modifications of the promoter region. Q/D has been evaluated in patients with severe vancomycin-resistant *E. faecium* infections in two prospective noncomparative, emergency-use studies, with overall success rates (clinical and bacteriological) of about 65%.[108] Q/D side effects such as phlebitis, myalgia-arthralgia, and metabolic abnormalities appear to be the most relevant problems with this compound, which may lead to treatment interruptions. Successful treatment of enterococcal endocarditis caused by a vancomycin-resistant *E. faecium* with several combination therapies in which one of the components was Q/D has been documented and includes Q/D plus doxycycline and rifampin[109] and Q/D plus high-dose ampicillin (24 g/day). As mentioned earlier, Q/D or linezolid is recommended by the AHA for the treatment of enterococcal endocarditis in isolates resistant to β-lactams, aminoglycosides, and glycopeptides[100] (see Figs. 201-2 and 3), and Q/D has also been used successfully in the treatment of enterococcal meningitis.

Nonsusceptibility to Q/D in enterococci is due to several mechanisms and includes (1) the macrolide-lincosamide-streptogramin B (MLS$_B$) type of resistance mediated by the *erm* genes (encoding a 23S rRNA methyltransferase), which appears to decrease the bactericidal activity of Q/D in vitro and in vivo; (2) the presence of the *vat*(D) and *vat*(E) genes, which encode acetyltransferases that inactivate streptogramin A (these genes are usually carried on plasmids and also confer resistance to the related streptogramin, virginiamycin, which is an antibiotic previously used as a growth promoter in the veterinary industry); and (3) efflux pumps, encoding ABC transporter proteins (such as Lsa).

OTHER ANTI-ENTEROCOCCAL ANTIMICROBIALS

Quinolones (mainly ciprofloxacin and moxifloxacin) have been reported as part of combination therapy for the treatment of enterococcal infections (see Fig. 201-2). However, the increased rates of resistance observed, the selection of resistant mutants during therapy, and the lack of effect in certain animal models make the quinolones less appealing for enterococcal infections, particularly as monotherapy. A potential role of quinolones may be as long-term suppressive therapy against fluoroquinolone-susceptible enterococci in endovascular infections in combination with amoxicillin. Tetracyclines (doxycycline and minocycline) also have been sporadically used in enterococcal infections either as monotherapy or in combination with other compounds when isolates are susceptible to these antibiotics.

Although resistance to chloramphenicol in enterococci mediated by the chloramphenicol-acetyl transferase enzyme has been long documented, the prevalence amongst VRE isolates appears to be low, and hence chloramphenicol has been used in the treatment of resistant enterococcal infections. In a case series of 51 patients with VRE bloodstream infections treated with chloramphenicol, 61.1% demonstrated a clinical response, and 79.1% exhibited microbiologic eradication, with no serious side effects that could be definitely attributed to chloramphenicol.[110] Similarly, successful treatment of prosthetic valve endocarditis and meningitis with chloramphenicol plus minocycline and chloramphenicol monotherapy, respectively, has been reported.[111,112] However, blood levels of this antibiotic at doses generally used (50-100 mg/kg/day) may not be appropriate, and treatment failures have occurred; hence, chloramphenicol should only be considered as an alternative in certain clinical settings (when available), and close monitoring for hematologic toxicity is strongly recommended.

Antibiotics that concentrate into the urine, such as β-lactams (very high concentrations of ampicillin may be obtained in urine), could be useful for the treatment of enterococcal urinary tract infections, even in cases of isolates with increased ampicillin MIC. Nitrofurantoin also achieves good levels in urine, and a randomized, open-label trial comparing nitrofurantoin for 5 days with trimethoprim-sulfamethoxazole for 3 days in the treatment of UTIs (including those caused by enterococci), indicated that nitrofurantoin was equivalent to the comparator drug.[113] Successful treatment of UTIs caused by vancomycin and ampicillin-resistant *E. faecium* with nitrofurantoin in an outbreak setting (100 mg every 6 hr) has also been documented.[114] Similarly, fosfomycin tromethamine has activity against enterococci and has an FDA indication for the treatment of UTI caused by *E. faecalis*. In vitro activity against *E. faecium* isolates from UTIs (MIC$_{90}$, 128 mg/L) indicates that it would seem a reasonable option to consider in treatment of

UTIs caused by *E. faecium*, which are susceptible using the *E. faecalis* criteria,[83] although clinical trials are lacking.

Intrathecal antibiotics have been used in the treatment of enterococcal meningitis, mostly combined with systemic therapy. The antibiotics used include vancomycin, teicoplanin, gentamicin, and Q/D. However, no clear clinical data favor the use of intrathecal antibiotics over systemic compounds alone in the management of enterococcal meningitis, and this approach may be considered in cases with multidrug-resistant organisms in which systemic therapy fails and removal of intrathecal catheters or shunts cannot be achieved (see Table 201-3).

Streptococcus bovis Group

Streptococci belonging to the *S. bovis* group are organisms that have been considered opportunistic pathogens in humans. Recent taxonomic reclassification has occurred with the *S. bovis* group, which traditionally had been divided into three different biotypes based on the fermentation of mannitol and the presence of β-glucuronidase activity. The former *S. bovis* biotype I (the most commonly associated with endocarditis and bacteremia) has been designated *S. gallolyticus* subsp. *gallolyticus*; the biotype II/2, *S. gallolyticus* subsp. *pasteurianus*, and the biotype II/1, *S. infantarius* subsp. *coli*.[115] An additional species, *S. gallolyticus* subsp. *macedomius*, has been proposed to include *S. macedomius* and *S. waius* within the biotype II/2 organisms.[115] This change in nomenclature has generated some degree of confusion among clinicians because the important association between *S. bovis* bacteremia-endocarditis and colonic malignancy has been missed because of the lack of recognition of the new species names. The differentiation between these species can be difficult at times, and sequencing of the 16S ribosomal DNA may be the only tool available for accurate identification to the species level. As with other grampositive organisms, the *S. bovis* group of organisms (particularly *S. gallolyticus*, formerly *S. bovis* biotype I) has been found to adhere in vitro to individual proteins of the extracellular matrix (ECM), such as collagen, fibronectin, and fibrin, which is a mechanism thought to be important in the pathogenesis of endocarditis, although a degree of strain variability regarding the ECM binding was observed.[116]

The *S. bovis* group is estimated to cause between 11% and 17% of all cases of endocarditis and about 24% of streptococcal endocarditis. Bacteremia and endocarditis caused by the *S. bovis* group have been highly associated with the presence of colonic malignancy (particularly *S. gallolyticus* subsp. *gallolyticus*) and hepatobiliary disease, although the reason for this association remains obscure. In a study analyzing the clinical characteristics of cases of the *S. bovis* group endocarditis (excluding drug addicts) over 13 years, it was found that these organisms caused about 17% of all cases of endocarditis, with the aortic valve being the most frequent heart valve affected. Simultaneous involvement of two cardiac valves, moderate to severe regurgitation, and embolic events were also commonly found. Of note, colonic neoplasms were documented in 77% of patients.[117]

The AHA recommends the use of a β-lactam (ceftriaxone or penicillin G) plus an aminoglycoside (gentamicin) for 2 weeks or the β-lactam alone (in patients older than 65 years with concomitant impairment of renal function or eighth cranial nerve function) for 4 weeks for the treatment of native valve endocarditis owing to the *S. bovis* group when MICs to penicillin are 0.12 mg/L or less. For isolates with MICs of more than 0.12 but 0.5 mg/L or less, the combination of the β-lactam (4 weeks) and aminoglycoside (2 weeks) should always be considered. Similar recommendations are given for the treatment of prosthetic valve endocarditis, although the duration of the β-lactam therapy should be extended to 6 weeks.[100] For isolates with an MIC of more than 0.5 mg/L, 4 to 6 weeks of therapy with ampicillin or penicillin G plus gentamicin is recommended. Vancomycin should be used in patients unable to tolerate the β-lactams, and a minimum of 4 or 6 weeks of therapy is recommended for native or prosthetic valves, respectively. It is important to note that the *vanB* gene cluster conferring high-level vancomycin resistance has been identified in members of the *S. bovis* group, which indicates that acquisition of these genes from an enterococcal donor was likely. Shorter regimens should be considered for bacteremia without endocarditis, and patients should undergo evaluation of the gastrointestinal tract to rule out malignancies.

Leuconostoc Species

Members of the *Leuconostoc* genus are catalase-negative, gram-positive cocci usually arranged in pairs or chains and often found in plants, dairy products, and foods that were previously considered of low pathogenic potential for humans but have recently emerged as sporadic pathogens. Because *Leuconostoc* spp. are phenotypically similar to *Streptococcus*, *Enterococcus*, *Pediococcus*, and *Lactococcus* spp., they may sometimes be misidentified; their distinguishing characteristics include vancomycin resistance, negative reaction for PYR and leucine aminopeptidase (see Table 201-1), and lack of gas production from glucose. *L. mesenteroides*, *L. pseudomesenteroides*, *L. paramesenteroides*, *L. citreum*, and *L. lactis* are the most common species isolated from human infections. Recently, a taxonomic study using 16S rRNA sequences indicated that members of the *Leuconostoc* genus could be grouped in three subclusters: the *L. mesenteroides* subcluster (which contains most of the human pathogenic species), the *L. fructosum* subcluster (which was proposed to be renamed as *Fructobacillus*), and the *L. fallax* subcluster.[118]

Leuconostoc spp. appear to be normal colonizers of the gastrointestinal tract, which could be the initial portal of entry in human infections. The first report of *Leuconostoc* spp. human infection was in 1985 in two immunocompromised patients with bloodstream infections.[119] Since then, *Leuconostoc* spp. have been implicated in a variety of infections, including bacteremia (including catheter-related), endocarditis, pulmonary infections, meningitis, brain and liver abscesses, and osteomyelitis, among others, affecting both immunocompetent and immunocompromised patients (majority), including children and newborns. It has been postulated that previous antibiotic therapy (e.g., vancomycin), presence of intravascular devices, and underlying gastrointestinal disease may be risk factors for *Leuconostoc* infections. Nosocomial outbreaks of *Leuconostoc* spp. have also been described, suggesting that they have the potential to disseminate in the hospital environment.

Antimicrobial susceptibility testing is crucial for the treatment of *Leuconostoc* infections because these bacteria are resistant to glycopeptides owing to the production of peptidoglycan precursors ending in D-Ala-D-Lac. The organisms are usually susceptible to penicillin G and ampicillin (although MICs tend to be higher than streptococci), which are generally more active than the cephalosporins and should be considered as the treatment of choice. The carbapenems (i.e., imipenem) have good activity, but a carbapenem-resistant isolate from a patient with postoperative meningitis has been documented. Resistance to trimethoprim, sulfonamide, and fosfomycin appears to be common among the members of the genus. Erythromycin, clindamycin, tetracycline, minocycline, and chloramphenicol appear to remain active against most of the clinical isolates. Linezolid MICs are higher for *Leuconostoc* compared with streptococci (MIC_{90}, 4 mg/L), whereas daptomycin is highly active in vitro and has been used successfully in the treatment of catheter-related bacteremia due to *Leuconostoc* in two patients who underwent bone marrow transplantation.[120]

REFERENCES

1. Thiercelin, E. Sur un diplocoque saphrophyte de l'intestin susceptible de devenir pathogene. *C R Soc Biol.* 1899;5:269-271.
2. MacCallum WG, Hastings TW. A case of acute endocarditis caused by *Micrococcus zymogenes* (nov. spec.), with a description of the microorganism. *J Exp Med.* 1899;4:521-534.
3. Andrews F, Horder T. A study of streptococci pathogenic for man. *Lancet.* 1906;2:708-713.
4. Sherman JM. The streptococci. *Bacteriol Rev.* 1937;1:3-97.
5. Orla-Jensen S. The lactic acid bacteria. *Mem Acad Royal Sci Danemark Sect Sci Ser.* 1919;5:81-197.
6. Barnes EM. Tetrazolium reduction as a means of differentiating *Streptococcus faecalis* from *Streptococcus faecium*. *J Gen Microbiol.* 1956;14:57-68.
7. Murray BE. The life and times of the *Enterococcus*. *Clin Microbiol Rev.* 1990;3:46-65.
8. Kalina A. The taxonomy and nomenclature of enterococci. *Int J Syst Bacteriol.* 1970;20:185-189
9. Schleifer KH, Kilpper-Balz R. Transfer of *Streptococcus faecalis* and *Streptococcus faecium* to the genus *Enterococcus* nom. rev. as *Enterococcus faecalis* comb. nov and *Enterococcus faecium* comb. nov. *Int J Syst Bacteriol.* 1984;34:31-34.
10. Dutka-Malen S, Evers S, Courvalin P. Detection of glycopeptide resistance genotypes and identification to the species level of clinically relevant enterococci by PCR. *J Clin Microbiol.* 1995;33:24-27.
11. Duh RW, Singh KV, Malathum K, et al. In vitro activity of 19 antimicrobial agents against enterococci from healthy subjects and hospitalized patients and use of an ace gene probe from *Enterococcus faecalis* for species identification. *Microb Drug Resist.* 2001;7:39-46.
12. Ley RE, Peterson DA, Gordon JI. Ecological and evolutionary forces shaping microbial diversity in the human intestine. *Cell.* 2006;124:837-848.
13. Donskey CJ, Chowdhry TK, Hecker MT, et al. Effect of antibiotic therapy on the density of vancomycin-resistant enterococci in the stool of colonized patients. *N Engl J Med.* 2000;343:1925-1932.
14. Sullivan A, Edlund C, Nord CE. Effect of antimicrobial agents on the ecological balance of human microflora. *Lancet Infect Dis.* 2001;1:101-114.
15. Stiefel U, Pultz NJ, Helfand MS, et al. Increased susceptibility to vancomycin-resistant *Enterococcus* intestinal colonization persists after completion of anti-anaerobic antibiotic treatment in mice. *Infect Control Hosp Epidemiol.* 2004;25:373-379.
16. Brandl K, Plitas G, Mihu CN, et al. Vancomycin-resistant enterococci exploit antibiotic-induced innate immune deficits. *Nature.* 2008;455:804-807.
17. Gilmore MS, Segarra RA, Booth MC, et al. Genetic structure of the *Enterococcus faecalis* plasmid pAD1-encoded cytolytic toxin system and its relationship to lantibiotic determinants. *J Bacteriol.* 1994;176:7335-7344.
18. Singh KV, Qin X, Weinstock GM, et al. Generation and testing of mutants of *Enterococcus faecalis* in a mouse peritonitis model. *J Infect Dis.* 1998;178:1416-1420.
19. Teng F, Nannini EC, Murray BE. Importance of *gls24* in virulence and stress response of *Enterococcus faecalis* and use of the Gls24 protein as a possible immunotherapy target. *J Infect Dis.* 2005;191:472-480.
20. Rice LB, Carias L, Rudin S, et al. A potential virulence gene, hyl_{Efm}, predominates in *Enterococcus faecium* of clinical origin. *J Infect Dis.* 2003;187:508-512.
21. Gilmore MS, Coburn PS, Nallapareddy SR, et al. Enterococcal Virulence. In: Gilmore MS, ed. *The enterococci: pathogenesis, molecular biology and antibiotic resistance*, 1st ed. Washington, DC: ASM Press; 2002:301-354.
22. Park SY, Kim KM, Lee JH, et al. Extracellular gelatinase of *Enterococcus faecalis* destroys a defense system in insect hemolymph and human serum. *Infect Immun.* 2007;75:1861-1869.
23. Thomas VC, Thurlow LR, Boyle D, et al. Regulation of autolysis-dependent extracellular DNA release by *Enterococcus faecalis* extracellular proteases influences biofilm development. *J Bacteriol.* 2008;190:5690-5698.
24. Qin X, Singh KV, Weinstock GM, et al. Characterization of *fsr*, a regulator controlling expression of gelatinase and serine protease in *Enterococcus faecalis* OG1RF. *J Bacteriol.* 2001;183:3372-3382.
25. Bourgogne A, Hilsenbeck SG, Dunny GM, et al. Comparison of OG1RF and an isogenic *fsrB* deletion mutant by transcriptional analysis: the Fsr system of *Enterococcus faecalis* is more than the activator of gelatinase and serine protease. *J Bacteriol.* 2006;188:2875-2884.
26. Nannini EC, Teng F, Singh KV, et al. Decreased virulence of a *gls24* mutant of *Enterococcus faecalis* OG1RF in an experimental endocarditis model. *Infect Immun.* 2005;73:7772-7774.
27. Rozdzinski E, Marre R, Susa M, et al. Aggregation substance-mediated adherence of *Enterococcus faecalis* to immobilized extracellular matrix proteins. *Microb Pathog.* 2001;30:211-220.
28. Tendolkar PM, Baghdayan AS, Shankar N. The N-terminal domain of enterococcal surface protein, Esp, is sufficient for Esp-mediated biofilm enhancement in *Enterococcus faecalis*. *J Bacteriol.* 2005;187:6213-6222.
29. Liu Q, Ponnuraj K, Xu Y, et al. The *Enterococcus faecalis* MSCRAMM Ace binds its ligand by the Collagen Hug model. *J Biol Chem.* 2007;282:19629-19637.
30. Nallapareddy SR, Singh KV, Okhuysen PC, et al. A functional collagen adhesin gene, acm, in clinical isolates of *Enterococcus faecium* correlates with the recent success of this emerging nosocomial pathogen. *Infect Immun.* 2008;76:4110-4119.
31. Brinster S, Posteraro B, Bierne H, et al. Enterococcal leucine-rich repeat-containing protein involved in virulence and host inflammatory response. *Infect Immun.* 2007;75:4463-4471.
32. Nallapareddy SR, Singh KV, Sillanpaa J, et al. Endocarditis and biofilm-associated pili of *Enterococcus faecalis*. *J Clin Invest.* 2006;116:2799-2807.
33. Singh KV, Nallapareddy SR, Murray BE. Importance of the *ebp* (endocarditis- and biofilm-associated pilus) locus in the pathogenesis of *Enterococcus faecalis* ascending urinary tract infection. *J Infect Dis.* 2007;195:1671-1677.
34. Hendrickx AP, Bonten MJ, van Luit-Asbroek M, et al. Expression of two distinct types of pili by a hospital-acquired *Enterococcus faecium* isolate. *Microbiology.* 2008;154:3212-3223.
35. Arduino RC, Jacques-Palaz K, Murray BE, et al. Resistance of *Enterococcus faecium* to neutrophil-mediated phagocytosis. *Infect Immun.* 1994;62:5587-5594.
36. Huebner J, Quaas A, Krueger WA, et al. Prophylactic and therapeutic efficacy of antibodies to a capsular polysaccharide shared among vancomycin-sensitive and -resistant enterococci. *Infect Immun.* 2000;68:4631-4636.
37. Huebner J, Wang Y, Krueger WA, et al. Isolation and chemical characterization of a capsular polysaccharide antigen shared by clinical isolates of *Enterococcus faecalis* and vancomycin-resistant *Enterococcus faecium*. *Infect Immun.* 1999;67:1213-1219.
38. Maekawa S, Yoshioka M, Kumamoto Y. Proposal of a new scheme for the serological typing of *Enterococcus faecalis* strains. *Microbiol Immunol.* 1992;36:671-681.
39. Teng F, Jacques-Palaz KD, Weinstock GM, et al. Evidence that the enterococcal polysaccharide antigen gene (*epa*) cluster is widespread in *Enterococcus faecalis* and influences resistance to phagocytic killing of *E. faecalis*. *Infect Immun.* 2002;70:2010-2015.
40. Hancock LE, Gilmore MS. The capsular polysaccharide of *Enterococcus faecalis* and its relationship to other polysaccharides in the cell wall. *Proc Natl Acad Sci U S A.* 2002;99:1574-1579.
41. Shankar N, Baghdayan AS, Gilmore MS. Modulation of virulence within a pathogenicity island in vancomycin-resistant *Enterococcus faecalis*. *Nature.* 2002;417:746-750.
42. Paulsen IT, Banerjei L, Myers GS, et al. Role of mobile DNA in the evolution of vancomycin-resistant *Enterococcus faecalis*. *Science.* 2003;299:2071-2074.
43. Bourgogne A, Garsin DA, Qin X, et al. Large scale variation in *Enterococcus faecalis* illustrated by the genome analysis of strain OG1RF. *Genome Biol.* 2008;9:R110.
44. Contreras GA, Diazgranados CA, Cortes L, et al. Nosocomial outbreak of *Enteroccocus gallinarum*: untaming of rare species of enterococci. *J Hosp Infect.* 2008;70:346-352.
45. Reik R, Tenover FC, Klein E, et al. The burden of vancomycin-resistant enterococcal infections in US hospitals, 2003 to 2004. *Diagn Microbiol Infect Dis.* 2008;62:81-85.
46. Hidron AI, Edwards JR, Patel J, et al. NHSN annual update: antimicrobial-resistant pathogens associated with healthcare-associated infections: annual summary of data reported to the

National Healthcare Safety Network at the Centers for Disease Control and Prevention, 2006-2007. *Infect Control Hosp Epidemiol.* 2008;29:996-1011.

47. Deshpande LM, Fritsche TR, Moet GJ, et al. Antimicrobial resistance and molecular epidemiology of vancomycin-resistant enterococci from North America and Europe: a report from the SENTRY antimicrobial surveillance program. *Diagn Microbiol Infect Dis.* 2007;58:163-170.
48. Goodman ER, Platt R, Bass R, et al. Impact of an environmental cleaning intervention on the presence of methicillin-resistant *Staphylococcus aureus* and vancomycin-resistant enterococci on surfaces in intensive care unit rooms. *Infect Control Hosp Epidemiol.* 2008;29:593-599.
49. Vergis EN, Hayden MK, Chow JW, et al. Determinants of vancomycin resistance and mortality rates in enterococcal bacteremia: a prospective multicenter study. *Ann Intern Med.* 2001;135:484-492.
50. Furtado GH, Mendes RE, Pignatari AC, et al. Risk factors for vancomycin-resistant *Enterococcus faecalis* bacteremia in hospitalized patients: an analysis of two case-control studies. *Am J Infect Control.* 2006;34:447-451.
51. LeDell K, Muto CA, Jarvis WR, et al. SHEA guideline for preventing nosocomial transmission of multidrug-resistant strains of *Staphylococcus aureus* and *Enterococcus*. *Infect Control Hosp Epidemiol.* 2003;24:639-641.
52. Snyder GM, Thom KA, Furuno JP, et al. Detection of methicillin-resistant *Staphylococcus aureus* and vancomycin-resistant enterococci on the gowns and gloves of healthcare workers. *Infect Control Hosp Epidemiol.* 2008;29:583-589.
53. Weinstock DM, Conlon M, Iovino C, et al. Colonization, bloodstream infection, and mortality caused by vancomycin-resistant enterococcus early after allogeneic hematopoietic stem cell transplant. *Biol Blood Marrow Transplant.* 2007;13:615-621.
54. Olivier CN, Blake RK, Steed LL, et al. Risk of vancomycin-resistant *Enterococcus* (VRE) bloodstream infection among patients colonized with VRE. *Infect Control Hosp Epidemiol.* 2008;29:404-409.
55. Roghmann MC, McCarter RJ Jr, Brewrink J, et al. *Clostridium difficile* infection is a risk factor for bacteremia due to vancomycin-resistant enterococci (VRE) in VRE-colonized patients with acute leukemia. *Clin Infect Dis.* 1997;25:1056-1059.
56. Salgado CD, Farr BM. Outcomes associated with vancomycin-resistant enterococci: a meta-analysis. *Infect Control Hosp Epidemiol.* 2003;24:690-698.
57. DiazGranados CA, Zimmer SM, Klein M, et al. Comparison of mortality associated with vancomycin-resistant and vancomycin-susceptible enterococcal bloodstream infections: a meta-analysis. *Clin Infect Dis.* 2005;41:327-333.
58. National. National Nosocomial Infections Surveillance (NNIS) System Report, data summary from January 1992 through June 2004, issued October 2004. *Am J Infect Control.* 2004;32:470-485.
59. Garrison RN, Fry DE, Berberich S, et al. Enterococcal bacteremia: clinical implications and determinants of death. *Ann Surg.* 1982;196:43-47.
60. Ghanem G, Hachem R, Jiang Y, et al. Outcomes for and risk factors associated with vancomycin-resistant *Enterococcus faecalis* and vancomycin-resistant *Enterococcus faecium* bacteremia in cancer patients. *Infect Control Hosp Epidemiol.* 2007;28:1054-1059.
61. Zeana C, Kubin CJ, Della-Latta P, et al. Vancomycin-resistant *Enterococcus faecium* meningitis successfully managed with linezolid: case report and review of the literature. *Clin Infect Dis.* 2001;33:477-482.
62. Hill EE, Herijgers P, Claus P, et al. Infective endocarditis: changing epidemiology and predictors of 6-month mortality: a prospective cohort study. *Eur Heart J.* 2007;28:196-203.
63. Rice LB, Calderwood SB, Eliopoulos GM, et al. Enterococcal endocarditis: a comparison of prosthetic and native valve disease. *Rev Infect Dis.* 1991;13:1-7.
64. Fernandez Guerrero ML, Goyenechea A, Verdejo C, et al. Enterococcal endocarditis on native and prosthetic valves: a review of clinical and prognostic factors with emphasis on hospital-acquired infections as a major determinant of outcome. *Medicine (Baltimore).* 2007;86:363-377.
65. Anderson DJ, Olaison L, McDonald JR, et al. Enterococcal prosthetic valve infective endocarditis: report of 45 episodes from the International Collaboration on Endocarditis-merged database. *Eur J Clin Microbiol Infect Dis.* 2005;24:665-670.
66. Durand ML, Calderwood SB, Weber DJ, et al. Acute bacterial meningitis in adults. A review of 493 episodes. *N Engl J Med.* 1993;328:21-28.
67. Pintado V, Cabellos C, Moreno S, et al. Enterococcal meningitis: a clinical study of 39 cases and review of the literature. *Medicine (Baltimore).* 2003;82:346-364.
68. Nagai K, Yuge K, Ono E, et al. *Enterococcus faecium* meningitis in a child. *Pediatr Infect Dis J.* 1994;13:1016-1017.
69. Harbarth S, Uckay I. Are there patients with peritonitis who require empiric therapy for enterococcus? *Eur J Clin Microbiol Infect Dis.* 2004;23:73-77.
70. Gorbach SL. Intraabdominal infections. *Clin Infect Dis.* 1993;17:961-965.
71. Onderdonk AB, Bartlett JG, Louie T, et al. Microbial synergy in experimental intra-abdominal abscess. *Infect Immun.* 1976;13:22-26.
72. Burnett RJ, Haverstock DC, Dellinger EP, et al. Definition of the role of *Enterococcus* in intraabdominal infection: analysis of a prospective randomized trial. *Surgery.* 1995;118:716-721; discussion 21-23.
73. Graham PL 3rd. Staphylococcal and enterococcal infections in the neonatal intensive care unit. *Semin Perinatol.* 2002;26:322-331.
74. Coudron PE, Mayhall CG, Facklam RR, et al. *Streptococcus faecium* outbreak in a neonatal intensive care unit. *J Clin Microbiol.* 1984;20:1044-1048.
75. Luginbuhl LM, Rotbart HA, Facklam RR, et al. Neonatal enterococcal sepsis: case-control study and description of an outbreak. *Pediatr Infect Dis J.* 1987;6:1022-1026.
76. Till M, Wixson RL, Pertel PE. Linezolid treatment for osteomyelitis due to vancomycin-resistant *Enterococcus faecium*. *Clin Infect Dis.* 2002;34:1412-1414.
77. Pehlivan Y, Toy MA, Karaoglan I, et al. *Enterococcus avium* cerebral abscess. *Intern Med.* 2007;46:1280.
78. Krogstad DJ, Pargwette AR. Defective killing of enterococci: a common property of antimicrobial agents acting on the cell wall. *Antimicrob Agents Chemother.* 1980;17:965-968.
79. Murray BE. Vancomycin-resistant enterococcal infections. *N Engl J Med.* 2000;342:710-721.
80. al-Obeid S, Gutmann L, Williamson R. Modification of penicillin-binding proteins of penicillin-resistant mutants of different species of enterococci. *J Antimicrob Chemother.* 1990;26:613-618.
81. Mainardi JL, Legrand R, Arthur M, et al. Novel mechanism of beta-lactam resistance due to bypass of DD-transpeptidation in *Enterococcus faecium*. *J Biol Chem.* 2000;275:16490-16496.
82. Murray BE, Mederski-Samoraj B, Foster SK, et al. In vitro studies of plasmid-mediated penicillinase from *Streptococcus faecalis* suggest a staphylococcal origin. *J Clin Invest.* 1986;77:289-293.
83. Clinical and Laboratory Standards Institute. *Performance standards for antimicrobial susceptibility testing, 18th informational supplement. M100-S18.* In: Wayne, PA, ed. Clinical and Laboratory Standards Institute; 2008.
84. Mederski-Samoraj BD, Murray BE. High-level resistance to gentamicin in clinical isolates of enterococci. *J Infect Dis.* 1983;147:751-757.
85. Zimmermann RA, Moellering RC Jr, Weinberg AN. Mechanism of resistance to antibiotic synergism in enterococci. *J Bacteriol.* 1971;105:873-879.
86. Kak V, Donabedian SM, Zervos MJ, et al. Efficacy of ampicillin plus arbekacin in experimental rabbit endocarditis caused by an *Enterococcus faecalis* strain with high-level gentamicin resistance. *Antimicrob Agents Chemother.* 2000;44:2545-2546.
87. Gavalda J, Len O, Miro JM, et al. Brief communication: treatment of *Enterococcus faecalis* endocarditis with ampicillin plus ceftriaxone. *Ann Intern Med.* 2007;146:574-579.
88. Mainardi JL, Gutmann L, Acar JF, et al. Synergistic effect of amoxicillin and cefotaxime against *Enterococcus faecalis*. *Antimicrob Agents Chemother.* 1995;39:1984-1987.
89. Arias CA, Singh KV, Panesso D, et al. Evaluation of ceftobiprole medocaril against *Enterococcus faecalis* in a mouse peritonitis model. *J Antimicrob Chemother.* 2007;60:594-598.
90. Nicas TI, Mullen DL, Flokowitsch JE, et al. Semisynthetic glycopeptide antibiotics derived from LY264826 active against vancomycin-resistant enterococci. *Antimicrob Agents Chemother.* 1996;40:2194-2199.
91. Baltch AL, Smith RP, Ritz WJ, et al. Comparison of inhibitory and bactericidal activities and postantibiotic effects of LY333328 and ampicillin used singly and in combination against vancomycin-resistant *Enterococcus faecium*. *Antimicrob Agents Chemother.* 1998;42:2564-2568.
92. Allen NE, Nicas TI. Mechanism of action of oritavancin and related glycopeptide antibiotics. *FEMS Microbiol Rev.* 2003;26:511-532.
93. Stryjewski ME, Graham DR, Wilson SE, et al. Telavancin versus vancomycin for the treatment of complicated skin and skin-structure infections caused by gram-positive organisms. *Clin Infect Dis.* 2008;46:1683-1693.
94. Dandekar PK, Tessier PR, Williams P, et al. Pharmacodynamic profile of daptomycin against *Enterococcus* species and methicillin-resistant *Staphylococcus aureus* in a murine thigh infection model. *J Antimicrob Chemother.* 2003;52:405-411.
95. Arias CA, Torres HA, Singh KV, et al. Failure of daptomycin monotherapy for endocarditis caused by an *Enterococcus faecium* strain with vancomycin-resistant and vancomycin-susceptible subpopulations and evidence of in vivo loss of the *vanA* gene cluster. *Clin Infect Dis.* 2007;45:1343-1346.
96. Stevens MP, Edmond MB. Endocarditis due to vancomycin-resistant enterococci: case report and review of the literature. *Clin Infect Dis.* 2005;41:1134-1142.
97. Jenkins I. Linezolid- and vancomycin-resistant *Enterococcus faecium* endocarditis: successful treatment with tigecycline and daptomycin. *J Hosp Med.* 2007;2:343-344.
98. Lesho EP, Wortmann GW, Craft D, et al. De novo daptomycin nonsusceptibility in a clinical isolate. *J Clin Microbiol.* 2006;44:673.
99. Falagas ME, Siempos II, Vardakas KZ. Linezolid versus glycopeptide or beta-lactam for treatment of Gram-positive bacterial infections: meta-analysis of randomised controlled trials. *Lancet Infect Dis.* 2008;8:53-66.
100. Baddour LM, Wilson WR, Bayer AS, et al. Infective endocarditis: diagnosis, antimicrobial therapy, and management of complications: a statement for healthcare professionals from the Committee on Rheumatic Fever, Endocarditis, and Kawasaki Disease, Council on Cardiovascular Disease in the Young, and the Councils on Clinical Cardiology, Stroke, and Cardiovascular Surgery and Anesthesia, American Heart Association: endorsed by the Infectious Diseases Society of America. *Circulation.* 2005;111:e394-e434.
101. Herrero IA, Issa NC, Patel R. Nosocomial spread of linezolid-resistant, vancomycin-resistant *Enterococcus faecium*. *N Engl J Med.* 2002;346:867-869.
102. Marshall SH, Donskey CJ, Hutton-Thomas R, et al. Gene dosage and linezolid resistance in *Enterococcus faecium* and *Enterococcus faecalis*. *Antimicrob Agents Chemother.* 2002;46:3334-3336.
103. Toh SM, Xiong L, Arias CA, et al. Acquisition of a natural resistance gene renders a clinical strain of methicillin-resistant *Staphylococcus aureus* resistant to the synthetic antibiotic linezolid. *Mol Microbiol.* 2007;64:1506-1514.
104. Arias CA, Vallejo M, Reyes J, et al. Clinical and microbiological aspects of linezolid resistance mediated by the *cfr* gene encoding a 23S rRNA methyltransferase. *J Clin Microbiol.* 2008;46:892-896.
105. Werner G, Gfrorer S, Fleige C, et al. Tigecycline-resistant *Enterococcus faecalis* strain isolated from a German intensive care unit patient. *J Antimicrob Chemother.* 2008;61:1182-1183.
106. Ellis-Grosse EJ, Babinchak T, Dartois N, et al. The efficacy and safety of tigecycline in the treatment of skin and skin-structure infections: results of 2 double-blind phase 3 comparison studies with vancomycin-aztreonam. *Clin Infect Dis.* 2005;(Suppl 5):S341-S353.
107. Singh KV, Weinstock GM, Murray BE. An *Enterococcus faecalis* ABC homologue (Lsa) is required for the resistance of this species to clindamycin and quinupristin-dalfopristin. *Antimicrob Agents Chemother.* 2002;46:1845-1850.
108. Moellering RC, Linden PK, Reinhardt J, et al. The efficacy and safety of quinupristin/dalfopristin for the treatment of infections caused by vancomycin-resistant *Enterococcus faecium*. Synercid Emergency-Use Study Group. *J Antimicrob Chemother.* 1999;44:251-561.
109. Matsumura S, Simor AE. Treatment of endocarditis due to vancomycin-resistant *Enterococcus faecium* with quinupristin/dalfopristin, doxycycline, and rifampin: a synergistic drug combination. *Clin Infect Dis.* 1998;27:1554-1556.
110. Lautenbach E, Schuster MG, Bilker WB, et al. The role of chloramphenicol in the treatment of bloodstream infection due to vancomycin-resistant *Enterococcus*. *Clin Infect Dis.* 1998;27:1259-1265.
111. Safdar A, Bryan CS, Stinson S, et al. Prosthetic valve endocarditis due to vancomycin-resistant *Enterococcus faecium*: treatment with chloramphenicol plus minocycline. *Clin Infect Dis.* 2002;34:E61-E63.
112. Perez Mato S, Robinson S, Begue RE. Vancomycin-resistant *Enterococcus faecium* meningitis successfully treated with chloramphenicol. *Pediatr Infect Dis J.* 1999;18:483-484.
113. Gupta K, Hooton TM, Roberts PL, et al. Short-course nitrofurantoin for the treatment of acute uncomplicated cystitis in women. *Arch Intern Med.* 2007;167:2207-2212.
114. Panesso D, Ospina S, Robledo J, et al. First characterization of a cluster of VanA-type glycopeptide-resistant *Enterococcus faecium*, Colombia. *Emerg Infect Dis.* 2002;8:961-965.
115. Schlegel L, Grimont F, Ageron E, et al. Reappraisal of the taxonomy of the *Streptococcus bovis/Streptococcus equinus* complex and related species: description of *Streptococcus gallolyticus* subsp. *gallolyticus* subsp. nov., *S. gallolyticus* subsp. *macedonicus* subsp. nov. and *S. gallolyticus* subsp. *pasteurianus* subsp. nov. *Int J Syst Evol Microbiol.* 2003;53:631-645.
116. Sillanpaa J, Nallapareddy, SR, Singh, KV, et al. Adherence characteristics of endocarditis-derived *Streptococcus gallolyticus* subs. *gallolyticus* (*S. bovis* biotype I) isolates to host extracellular matrix proteins. FEMS Microbiol Lett 2009 (in press).
117. Gonzalez-Juanatey C, Gonzalez-Gay MA, Llorca J, et al. Infective endocarditis due to *Streptococcus bovis* in a series of non-addict patients: clinical and morphological characteristics of 20 cases and review of the literature. *Can J Cardiol.* 2003;19:1139-1145.
118. Endo A, Okada S. Reclassification of the genus *Leuconostoc* and proposals of *Fructobacillus fructosus* gen. nov., comb. nov., *Fructobacillus durionis* comb. nov., *Fructobacillus ficulneus* comb. nov. and *Fructobacillus pseudoficulneus* comb. nov. *Int J Syst Evol Microbiol.* 2008;58:2195-2205.
119. Buu-Hoi A, Branger C, Acar JF. Vancomycin-resistant streptococci or *Leuconostoc* spp. *Antimicrob Agents Chemother.* 1985;28:458-460.
120. Huang YT, Liao CH, Teng LJ, et al. Daptomycin susceptibility of unusual gram-positive bacteria: comparison of results obtained by the Etest and the broth microdilution method. *Antimicrob Agents Chemother.* 2007;51:1570-1572.

202

Streptococcus agalactiae (Group B Streptococcus)

MORVEN S. EDWARDS | CAROL J. BAKER

Historical Perspective

Group B streptococci (*Streptococcus agalactiae*) were reported as human pathogens in 1938 by Fry, who described three cases of fatal puerperal sepsis.[1] Before Fry,[1] Lancefield and Hare[2] had identified the organisms in vaginal cultures from asymptomatic postpartum women. Group B streptococcal infections in humans were reported infrequently until the early 1960s, when several authors noted that disease was occurring more commonly than had been appreciated previously.[3-5] By the 1970s, group B streptococcus had become the predominant pathogen causing septicemia and meningitis in neonates and infants younger than 3 months. Initially a concern for pediatricians, group B streptococci also cause substantial pregnancy-related morbidity. Implementation of recommendations for the use of maternal intrapartum chemoprophylaxis in the mid-1990s resulted in a dramatic decrease in early-onset neonatal disease incidence and in a substantial decline in invasive disease during pregnancy.[6]

Invasive group B streptococcal infection in nonpregnant adults is now recognized as a major health concern. In the past two decades, twofold to fourfold increases in the incidence of group B streptococcal disease have been reported in nonpregnant adults, most of whom have underlying medical conditions or are 65 years of age or older.[7,8] Active, population-based surveillance indicates that two thirds of patients with invasive group B streptococcal disease now are nonpregnant adults.[6,9] The highest case-fatality rate as a consequence of group B streptococcal infection is among nonpregnant adults older than 65 years of age. Nursing home residents have a markedly higher incidence of invasive group B streptococcal disease than do community-dwelling residents.[10] These shifts in incidence and outcome suggest that older adults could benefit from immunization with group B streptococcal glycoconjugate vaccines as these become commercially available. Publication in 2002 of the complete genome sequence of serotypes III and V group B streptococci, and more recently serotypes Ia, Ib, II, IV, VI and VIII, opened new avenues for the identification of novel vaccine targets as well as for further elucidating the molecular basis for virulence of the organism.[11,12]

Description

CLASSIFICATION AND MORPHOLOGIC CHARACTERISTICS

S. agalactiae is the species designation for streptococci belonging to Lancefield group B. The serologic differentiation of hemolytic streptococci by groups was described in 1933.[13] It is based on the capillary precipitin reaction between the group-specific carbohydrate cell wall antigen and hyperimmune rabbit antisera. Group B streptococci are facultative, gram-positive diplococci that grow on a variety of bacteriologic media. Isolated colonies on sheep blood agar are 3 to 4 mm in diameter and grayish white. The flat, somewhat mucoid colonies are surrounded by a narrow zone of β-hemolysis that, for some strains, is detectable only on lifting a colony from the agar. One to 2% of strains are nonhemolytic. To enhance the accurate detection of low numbers of group B streptococci from sites such as the genital or gastrointestinal tract, a number of selective broth media have been employed. These usually contain Todd-Hewitt broth with or without sheep red blood cells and antimicrobial agents such as nalidixic acid and gentamicin or colistin.[14]

IDENTIFICATION

Definitive identification of group B streptococci is based on detection of the group B–specific cell wall antigen common to all strains. A number of serologic methods using hyperimmune group B–specific antisera have been developed for the detection of the group B antigen. Latex agglutination is the most widely employed. When the manufacturer's instructions are followed, these products for serogrouping β-hemolytic streptococci are comparable to the Lancefield capillary precipitin method.

Biochemical methods that permit the presumptive identification of group B streptococci include resistance to bacitracin or trimethoprim-sulfamethoxazole, positive sodium hippurate hydrolysis, and the production of an orange pigment during anaerobic growth on certain media. β-Hemolytic streptococci that hydrolyze sodium hippurate belong to either group B or group D; these can be distinguished on the basis of hydrolysis of bile esculin agar. Among group D strains, 99% hydrolyze bile esculin, whereas 99% to 100% of group B strains do not. Production of CAMP factor, which is a thermostable extracellular protein that results in synergistic hemolysis on sheep blood agar with the β-lysin of *Staphylococcus aureus,* is observed in 98% to virtually 100% of group B streptococci. The combination of the CAMP test with bacitracin sensitivity testing and the bile esculin reaction is adequate for presumptive differentiation of group B from other serogroups of β-hemolytic streptococci.

CLASSIFICATION AND TYPING

Group B streptococci are differentiated serologically by capsular polysaccharide type and by cell surface expressed proteins. Lancefield defined two cell wall carbohydrate antigens, the group B–specific or C substance common to all strains and the S substance that allowed classification into types I, II, and III.[15] Later, Lancefield reported distinct differences in type I strains, and these were designated Ia, Ib, and Ic.[16] These strains possess capsular polysaccharide Ia or Ib, and some Ia and all Ib strains also have a surface-protein designated C protein that has α and β components. The nomenclature was revised in 1984 to designate the capsular polysaccharides as type antigens with surface proteins as additional markers.[17] Additional capsular polysaccharide types, IV through VIII and provisional type IX, each with unique polysaccharides alone or with protein antigens, have been defined,[18-22] and additional candidates are being evaluated.

The β C protein binds to human immunoglobulin A (IgA) and is found mainly in type Ib strains. The α C protein is the prototype for a family of proteins (α-like proteins) that includes Rib and Alp1-4 and is found in most group B streptococci. R proteins (R1-4) are found on some strains but genetically are less well defined. Each of the common polysaccharide types has a characteristic protein expression pattern, but there is no genetic linkage, and exceptions occur. For example, Alp1 is found frequently in type Ia strains, Rib is most often associated with type II and III strains, and Alp3 with type V strains.[23]

Antibodies directed against polysaccharide antigens were shown by Lancefield to provide passive protection in mice challenged with homologous—but not heterologous—antigen-containing strains.[24] The α and β C proteins and Rib also can elicit protective antibodies in animals,[25-27] but their role in human infections is not known. Antibodies directed at the group B antigen are not protective.

The classic method for typing group B streptococci is by analysis of capillary precipitin or immunodiffusion in agarose reactions between acid extracts of the organism and hyperimmune rabbit antisera. Molecular approaches to typing of group B streptococci include multilocus sequencing typing and pulsed gel electrophoresis.[28] Sequencing primers also have been designed to allow identification of capsular polysaccharide gene clusters.[29] Polymerase chain reaction–based methods offer the potential for widespread availability of an alternative to conventional typing and also a powerful tool to document the epidemiologic relatedness of group B streptococcal strains. Such methods can determine whether recurrent infections are caused by separate or identical strains and can identify virulent clone families that may be disproportionate causes of invasive disease.[30]

Epidemiology and Transmission

ASYMPTOMATIC COLONIZATION

Group B streptococci have been isolated from genital or lower gastrointestinal tract cultures of pregnant and nonpregnant women at rates ranging from 10% to 40%. These variations in the reported prevalence of asymptomatic colonization relate to sites sampled, methods used for detection of the organism, and demographic differences in populations (Table 202-1). When multiple appropriate sites, such as the lower

vagina or the periurethral area *and* the rectum are sampled and when the selective broth media is used, the colonization rates usually exceed 20%. Group B streptococci can be associated with asymptomatic bacteriuria during pregnancy and bacteriuria is a marker for heavy genital colonization.

Colonization with group B streptococci occurs more frequently among black women than in other racial or ethnic groups.[31,32] Diabetes is also independently associated with higher rates of group B streptococcal colonization during pregnancy.[33] Sexual intercourse is an important risk factor for vaginal acquisition of group B streptococci.[34,35] Multiple partners and frequent or recent sexual intercourse are associated with increased risk for vaginal acquisition over time, possibly because sexual activity alters the vaginal microenvironment to make it more permissive for colonization. Sexual activity and particularly male-to-female oral sex increase the risk for cocolonization with identical group B streptococcal strains in heterosexual college couples.[36] Low genital colonization rates are reported for sexually inexperienced persons.[37] Pregnancy, however, does not influence colonization prevalence.

The principal reservoir for group B streptococci is the lower gastrointestinal tract. Rectal to vaginal isolation ratios exceeding 1 and the rectum as the site most accurately predicting chronicity of carriage support the premise that genital colonization may reflect acquisition from the rectal site.[38] Further, group B streptococci have been isolated from the proximal part of the small intestine of adults. The prevalence of oropharyngeal colonization in adults is about 5% but can approach 20% in men who have sex with men. The colonization rate in healthy older adults is about 20%.[39]

TRANSMISSION TO NEONATES

Colonization of newborns results from vertical transmission from the mother, either in utero by the ascending route or at the time of delivery. Vaginally colonized pregnant women are at an increased risk for premature labor.[40] The rate of vertical transmission among neonates born to women colonized with group B streptococci at the time of delivery is about 50%.[41] A high maternal genital inoculum at delivery significantly increases the likelihood of vertical transmission.[42] Infants born to heavily colonized women also are more likely to develop early-onset (younger than age 7 days) disease. Nosocomial colonization of the neonate can occasionally occur, likely through the hands of caregivers or visitors. The rate of community acquisition of group B streptococci in young infants has not been adequately investigated.

Factors that increase the incidence of invasive early-onset infection among neonates born to colonized mothers include group B streptococcal bacteriuria, delivery at less than 37 weeks of gestation, intrapartum fever or intra-amniotic infection, and rupture of membranes for 18 hours or longer before delivery.[43] Maternal age younger than 20 years and a history of previous miscarriage also are associated with higher attack rates for early-onset neonatal disease.[44] A concordance of serotypes between infant and maternal genital isolates establishes the vertical transmission route for early-onset disease, but in infants with late-onset disease (age 7 to 89 days), one half to two thirds of cases also have isolates concordant with the mother, suggesting that vertical or household acquisition precedes invasive infection.

INCIDENCE AND SEROTYPE DISTRIBUTION OF ISOLATES

The incidence of early-onset group B streptococcal infection in neonates, formerly 1 to 3 per 1000 live births, declined 65% with implementation of maternal antibiotic prophylaxis guidelines and an additional 27% after the 2002 revised early-onset disease prevention guidelines to a rate of 0.34 per 1000 live births in 2003 to 2005.[6,45] The burden of early-onset disease remains disproportionately high in black infants for reasons that are not yet understood. In contrast, use of intrapartum antibiotic prophylaxis has had no impact on late-onset disease incidence, which still occurs in 0.3 to 0.4 per 1000 live births.

TABLE 202-1	Factors Influencing Detection of Group B Streptococcal Colonization		
	Effect on Isolation Rate		
	Increased	*Decreased*	*None*
Method Employed			
Culture medium	Broth media	Agar media	—
	Antibiotic-containing media	Nonselective broth media	—
Sites in women	Lower vagina and rectum	Cervical os	—
Sites in infants and adults	Multiple sites	Single site	—
Interval	Two or more cultures in interval of 6-8 wk	Single sampling time	—
Genital Carriage in Women			
Pregnancy	—	—	+
Time during pregnancy	—	—	+
Day of menstrual cycle	First half	—	—
Age	≤20 yr	—	—
Sexual activity	Active	Virgin	—
Frequency of sexual intercourse or total number of partners	+	—	—
Vaginal discharge	—	—	+
Birth control method	Intrauterine device	—	Oral contraceptives
Parity	Primigravida	More than 3 pregnancies	—
Ethnic origin	Black	Asian	—
Marital status	—	—	+
Socioeconomic group	Lower income	—	—

+, documented to have effect indicated on isolation rate.

Pregnancy-associated group B streptococcal disease is responsible for about 15% to 25% of peripartum febrile morbidity with or without bacteremia.[46] Intrapartum vaginal colonization with group B streptococci is an independent risk factor for chorioamnionitis. Women with heavy colonization are at significantly greater risk for intra-amniotic infection than those with light vaginal colonization.[47] The incidence of invasive disease in pregnancy also has declined significantly in association with the use of intrapartum antibiotic prophylaxis, from 0.29 per 1000 live births in 1993 to 0.11 to 0.14 per 1000 live births in surveillance from 1999 to 2005.[6,45] Among women with invasive group B streptococcal disease for whom pregnancy outcome was known, 61% had a spontaneous abortion or a stillborn infant, 30% had infants without apparent illness, 5% had live-born infants who developed clinical infections, and 4% had induced abortions.

The incidence of invasive group B streptococcal disease among nonpregnant adults has been rising for the past two decades.[9] Nonpregnant adults now account for nearly two thirds of all invasive group B streptococcal disease.[6,48] Most have at least one underlying medical condition, such as diabetes mellitus, chronic liver or renal disease, human immunodeficiency virus (HIV) infection, malignancy, or stroke.[9] The overall incidence increased from 6.0 per 100,000 population in 1999 to 7.9 per 100,000 in 2005.[45] In a recent population-based surveillance report, adults 65 years of age and older represented one third of cases of invasive group B streptococcal disease. Nursing home residents had a markedly higher incidence (72 per 100,000 population) than community residents 65 years of age and older.[10] The biologic basis for the high risk among nursing home residents is not known but is likely to be related to their having a higher proportion of underlying medical conditions that predispose them to invasive infection.

In the 1970s and 1980s, type III strains of group B streptococci accounted for one third of early-onset infections, for nearly 90% of late-onset infections, and for most cases of meningitis regardless of the age at the onset of infection. In the 1990s, the serotype distribution of invasive isolates from infants and adults shifted somewhat. Among neonates with early-onset disease, type Ia predominates and accounts for 30% to 40% of isolates, followed by types III (25% to 30%) and V (15% to 20%).[45,49-51] Late-onset infant disease and meningitis is still caused predominantly by serotype III strains.[45,52] The emergence of serotype V has been echoed in the distribution of isolates that asymptomatically colonize and cause invasive disease in pregnant women. Taken together, serotypes Ia, III, and V represent more than two thirds of colonizing isolates in pregnancy.[53] Serotypes Ia (34%), III (25%), and V (23%) also account for more than 80% of strains from 53 pregnant women with invasive group B streptococcal infection.[51] Among nonpregnant adults, a population-based surveillance found that type V strains predominate, accounting for 31% of almost 5000 cases of invasive disease, followed by types Ia (24%), II (12%), and III (12%).[45] In a recent seroepidemiologic assessment, serotype V accounted for almost half of the strains colonizing healthy older adults.[39] Types IV, VI through VIII, and nontypable isolates are uncommonly associated with invasive infection, but in Japan, serotypes VI and VIII are frequently isolated from pregnant women.[54]

Pathogenetic Mechanisms

To cause disease, group B streptococci, like other extracellular bacterial pathogens, must colonize mucosal surfaces and then breach these surfaces to enter normally sterile sites such as the bloodstream. The presence in group B streptococci of two surface-exposed protective antigens that are components of high-molecular-weight, covalently linked, pilus-like structures has recently been described, and these structures are now known to contribute both to adherence and invasion of host cells.[55,56]

ADHERENCE

Group B streptococci adhere to a number of human cells, including vaginal and intestinal epithelium, placental membranes, respiratory tract epithelium, and the blood-brain barrier endothelium. The requirement for maternal genital tract colonization with group B streptococci at delivery as a prelude to invasive early-onset infection in neonates is well established.[41,57] There is an increased risk for invasive neonatal infection rather than mucosal colonization when exposure is prolonged or intensified by a high maternal genital inoculum or intra-amniotic infection.[42,57] Heavy maternal colonization with group B streptococci increases the risk for delivering a preterm, low-birth-weight infant.[58] However, these factors do not fully explain the low colonization-to-invasion ratio observed among newborns born to colonized mothers.

The nature of the bacterial structures of group B streptococci involved in adhering to human cells is partially elucidated. A role for the α protein is proposed in the interaction between the bacterium and the host cell.[59] The α protein is a prototype for a family of long, tandem repeat-containing surface proteins that are common to serotypes of group B streptococci (Ia, Ib, II, and V) causing most invasive disease. The pilus operon codes for three proteins that contain the conserved amino acid motif, LPXTG, associated with cell wall–anchored proteins together with two genes coding for sortase enzymes.[56] Genes encoding the surface-associated pili have a role in adhering to cell surfaces such as brain endothelium.[60] The widely conserved, surface-exposed fibrinogen receptor FbsA also promotes adherence of group B streptococci to human epithelial cells.[61] Capsular polysaccharide, in contrast, attenuates group B streptococcal adherence to human cells.[62]

INVASION

Group B streptococci can cross the epithelial barrier by a paracellular route, and translocation of epithelial barriers is proposed as the predominant route for dissemination of the of the organism in the human host.[63,64] In support of this mechanism, pili have been shown to locate in the intercellular space ahead of translocating bacteria. That pilus backbone also contributes to paracellular translocation of group B streptococci is supported by experiments in which deletion of the pilus backbone protein reduces the capacity of the organism to transcytose through differentiated human epithelial cells.[65]

Group B streptococci can invade respiratory epithelial and endothelial cells as well as brain microvascular endothelial cells in vitro.[62,66] The invasive capacity of an unencapsulated mutant appears enhanced compared with that of an encapsulated parent strain.[62] However, invasion is independent of capsular polysaccharide expression and can be regulated by growth rate.[67] Growth rate–dependent invasion occurred when group B streptococci were grown in continuous culture under glucose-defined, thiamine-defined, and undefined nutrient limitations. Baron and colleagues[68] have proposed that the α C protein mediates translocation across epithelial barriers by facilitating intracellular invasiveness through binding to glycosaminoglycan on the surface of the host cell. Proper anchoring of lipotechoic acid on the group B streptococcal surface facilitates invasion,[69] and the group B streptococcal pore-forming β-hemolysin/cytolysin also promotes invasion of lung epithelial cells.[70] β-Hemolysin/cytolysin expression also correlates with lung epithelial cell injury and promotes injury of lung microvascular endothelial cells, increasing cell permeability in vitro. This increased permeability contributes to alveolar edema and hemorrhage that may be a feature of group B streptococcal pneumonia.[71] Inhibition studies suggest that the α protein and, in particular, its *N*-terminal region are involved in bacterial entry into epithelial cells.[59] Group B streptococcal fibrinogen-binding protein FbsB also participates in the overall process of host cell entry.

BACTERIAL VIRULENCE FACTORS

Group B streptococci produce a capsule that inhibits complement deposition and phagocytosis. Strains that effectively evade host phagocytes can damage tissues by inducing the release of substances that cause inflammation or by production of substances that directly damage cells. A high quantity of cell-associated sialic acid and its elaboration in supernatant fluid are associated with virulence of type III strains.[72] Transposon mutant strains of type III group B streptococcus have been constructed that are unencapsulated or that express a capsular polysaccharide differing from the wild type in expressing a capsule lacking sialic acid.[73,74] These changes in capsular expression are associated with a loss of virulence in a neonatal rat model of lethal infection, supporting the critical nature of capsular antigen as a virulence factor. The unique capsular structures of group B streptococci also might enhance the invasiveness of one serotype over another. Type III strains, for example, invade brain microvascular endothelial cells more efficiently than strains from other common serotypes (although the capsule itself does not facilitate invasion).[75] The capsular polysaccharides of types Ia, Ib, II, III, IV, and V all contain glucose, galactose, glucosamine, and sialic acid, but their structural arrangements are distinct. Sialic acid, which constitutes the exclusive terminal residue of types Ia, Ib, and III—but not type II or V—group B streptococcal capsular polysaccharide, inhibits activation of the alternative pathway of complement.[76] Types VI and VIII lack glucosamine, and type VIII contains rhamnose.[20,21,77] A novel insertion sequence in the hyaluronidase gene has been identified predominantly in group B streptococcal strains causing endocarditis.[78] The mechanism by which this genetic alteration and the lack of hyaluronidase increases disease potential is speculative.

The capsular polysaccharide is the best defined virulence factor of group B streptococcus.[79] Other virulence factors, such as the pore-forming β-hemolysin/cytolysin, enhance virulence by promoting invasion and cell injury[71] and by inducing cytolysis and apoptosis of phagocytes in concert with shielding by carotenoid of group B streptococci from oxidative damage.[80] Hyperhemolytic variants derived by transposon mutagenesis enhanced lethality and promoted joint injury compared with a nonhemolytic group B streptococcal variant in a murine model of infection.[81] Group B streptococcal β-hemolysin/cytolysin also directly impairs cardiomyocyte viability and function.[82] The organism expresses additional factors that allow it to resist host defenses. A recent report indicated that the surface-localized β protein binds human complement factor H and that the complexed factor H retains its ability to downregulate complement activation.[83] In addition, *cspA*, a novel gene encoding a surface-localized, serine protease–like protein, has been identified.[84] It promotes group B streptococcal survival by evasion of opsonophagocytosis and is required for group B streptococcal cleavage of fibrinogen.

HOST FACTORS

Baker and Kasper reported in 1976 that neonates and young infants at risk for invasive type III group B streptococcal infection were those with low concentrations of passively acquired maternal antibodies to the type III capsular polysaccharide.[79] Premature infants, especially those born before 32 weeks' gestation, are less likely than term infants to acquire protective levels of maternally derived type-specific antibodies. Women colonized with type III group B streptococci and delivering healthy neonates have significantly higher concentrations of type III–specific IgG than women whose infants develop early-onset type III disease.[85] A low concentration of maternal antibodies to capsular polysaccharides Ia, Ib, and II, and probably V, at delivery also is a determinant of neonatal susceptibility to infection caused by these group B streptococcal types.[86-88] Antibody to the group B–specific polysaccharide, however, is not protective against human or animal infection.[89]

The classic complement pathway and heat-stable opsonins are required for maximal opsonic activity of group B streptococcal strains of the major serotypes.[90-92] The alternative complement pathway participates in opsonophagocytosis of type III strains when specific antibody is present in a sufficient concentration. A role for L-ficolin/mannose-binding, lectin-associated serine protease complexes in calcium-dependent, antibody-independent opsonophagocytosis of type III also has been shown.[93] The opsonophagocytic requirements for type

II strains are complex, modulated in part by C proteins, and classic pathway integrity appears essential for effective opsonophagocytosis.[91,94] Opsonization and phagocytosis of type Ia strains can proceed by the classic complement pathway in an antibody-independent fashion.[95] Neutrophil complement and Fc receptors are important in opsonic recognition of group B streptococci. Blockade of complement receptor 3 on neutrophils from adults or neonates inhibits killing of types Ia, III, and V strains of group B streptococci.[92,96] Blockade of neutrophil Fc receptor III inhibits phagocytosis of type III group B streptococci to an even greater extent.[97] In complement-inactivated serum, Fc receptor II also has a substantial role in mediating ingestion of serotype III strains.[98]

INFLAMMATORY MEDIATORS

Group B streptococci induce tumor necrosis factor-α (TNF-α), interleukin-1β, interleukin-6, and interleukin-8.[99-101] In experimental models, elevated levels of TNF-α correlate with the severity of disease and with mortality. Purified group-specific polysaccharide and peptidoglycan, rather than type-specific capsular polysaccharide, induce the proinflammatory cytokine response. Type III group B streptococci interacting with cord blood monocytes induce TNF-α gene expression by host cell transduction pathways that lead to activation of the transcription factors nuclear factor (NF)-κB and activator protein-1 through a pathway that involves phosphorylation of the p38 mitogen-activated protein kinase pathway.[102] Engagement of mammalian Toll-like receptors (TLR-2 and TLR-6), as well as CD14 expression, is essential for cells to respond to the presence of group B streptococci.[103] However, this recognition is due to a novel secreted or shed bacterial product. Whole group B streptococci activate macrophages independently of TLR-2 and TLR-6.

Clinical Manifestations
NEONATAL INFECTIONS
Early-Onset Infection

As the incidence of neonatal group B streptococcal infections rose during the 1970s, a bimodal distribution of cases by age at the onset of symptoms became apparent. Two distinctive clinical syndromes related to age were described by Franciosi and co-workers[104] (acute and delayed) and by Baker and colleagues[105] (early and late onset). Early-onset infection, defined as the development of systemic infection during the first 6 days of life, has a mean age of 12 hours at its onset. Maternal obstetric complications are frequent (50% to 60%), and infants born at less than 37 weeks of gestation have significantly higher attack rates than infants born at term. The three major clinical expressions of infection are bacteremia or septicemia without a focus, pneumonia, and meningitis, and they occur at frequencies of about 80% to 85%, 10%, and 5% to 10%, respectively.[45]

Clinical abnormalities are present at or within a few hours after birth in most infants. The presenting signs of early-onset group B streptococcal infection—lethargy, poor feeding, abnormal temperature, grunting respirations, pallor, and hypotension—are indistinguishable from those in neonates with bacterial infections of other causes. Regardless of the focus of infection, signs of respiratory distress such as apnea, grunting, tachypnea, and cyanosis are observed in most. Pulmonary infiltrates or a radiograph consistent with respiratory distress syndrome or transient tachypnea of the newborn may suggest the diagnosis. Infants with meningitis have a clinical presentation that initially cannot be distinguished from those without meningeal invasion.

Increased awareness of the disease and improvements in supportive therapy have resulted in decreased mortality among infants with early-onset group B streptococcal infection, and present rates range from 5% to 10%. Mortality rates are inversely proportional to birth weight. In the era of maternal screening, virtually all the cases of early-onset disease occur in infants whose mothers had intra-amniotic infection, thereby not allowing prophylaxis, or who either did not receive prophylaxis during preterm labor or were negative for group B streptococcal colonization at screening.[106]

Late-Onset Infection

The late-onset syndrome has an onset between 7 days and 89 days of age, with a median of 36 days.[107] Half of all infants with late-onset disease are now born preterm. Other maternal obstetric complications are uncommon, and the case-fatality ratio is 3% to 5%.[44,45] Bacteremia without a focus and meningitis are common clinical manifestations of late-onset infection, occurring in 65% and 25% to 30% of affected infants, respectively, but a variety of focal infections, including osteomyelitis, septic arthritis, and cellulitis, usually with accompanying bacteremia, also occur. The nonspecific initial signs of late-onset disease, such as lethargy, poor feeding, and irritability, generally occur in association with fever. These infants can present with fulminant infection characterized by rapid progression to a moribund state with septic shock and seizures and sheets of organisms on Gram stains of cerebrospinal fluid (CSF). An increased risk for death or permanent neurologic sequelae occurs in patients with this fulminant presentation.[108] Additional clinical findings that have been associated with a fatal outcome or permanent neurologic sequelae include neutropenia at admission, prolonged seizures, and high concentrations of type III polysaccharide antigen in admission CSF specimens. Among survivors of group B streptococcal meningitis, whether early or late onset, 25% to 50% have permanent neurologic sequelae.[108,109]

Infection beyond Early Infancy

Infants older than 3 months now constitute 10% to 15% of late-onset disease cases.[110] Many of these infections occur among very low birth weight infants who may still be hospitalized for complications of prematurity. The term *late, late onset* is often used in this setting. Healthy older infants occasionally present with occult bacteremia. Congenital heart disease and immune deficiency, including HIV infection, should be considered when group B streptococcal disease is diagnosed beyond early infancy.[111,112]

INFECTIONS IN ADULTS

Invasive group B streptococcal infection causes substantial morbidity and mortality among adults. In a contemporary, prospective, population-based assessment of invasive group B streptococcal disease, men and nonpregnant women accounted for 66% of the total number of cases.[6] Adults with bacteremia unrelated to pregnancy are usually older, but ages range from 18 to 99 years.[113-117] The mean age in one report was 62 years, and 57% were men.[9] The incidence increases with age, is higher in blacks than in other races or ethnicities, and is quadrupled in older adults in nursing homes compared with community-dwelling older adults.[9,10,117]

One or more medical conditions predisposing to infection can be identified in most adults with invasive disease (Table 202-2). In a 2005 multistate, population-based survey, underlying medical conditions included diabetes mellitus (41%), heart disease (36%), and malignancy (17%). Smoking, obesity, neurologic disorders, renal disease, immunosuppressive conditions, liver disease, and lung disease also were common factors associated with disease.[45] Among patients with soft tissue infections, one third report diabetes mellitus as a comorbid condition.[118] Neurologic abnormalities associated with invasive infections include dementia, cerebrovascular disease resulting in alterations of mental status, and paraplegia or quadriplegia. Young adults (20 to 40 years of age) with diabetes, cancer, or HIV infection are at significantly increased risk (28- to 30-fold) for invasive group B streptococcal disease.[9] In a case-control study, diabetes, cirrhosis, stroke, breast cancer, decubitus ulcer, and neurogenic bladder significantly increased the risk for community-acquired group B streptococcal infection. Nosocomial infection was independently associated with the placement of a central venous line, diabetes, congestive heart failure, and a seizure disorder.[119]

TABLE 202-2	Underlying Conditions in Invasive Group B Streptococcal Infections*	
Condition		*n* (%)
Diabetes mellitus		82 (30)
Liver disease or history of alcohol abuse		66 (24)
Neurologic impairment		58 (21)
Malignancy		52 (19)
Renal failure		37 (14)
Cardiovascular disease or heart failure		37 (14)
Pulmonary disease		21 (8)
Urologic disease		11 (4)
Peripheral vascular disease		9 (3)
Human immunodeficiency virus infection		7 (3)
Intravenous catheter-related infection		5 (2)
Gastrointestinal disease		5 (2)
Steroid administration		5 (2)
Hypertension		4 (1)
Functional or surgical splenectomy		3 (1)
Other		7 (3)
None		5 (2)

N = 271 adults. Streptococcal infections listed were not related to pregnancy. Some patients had more than one underlying condition.

From Farley MM. Group B streptococcal disease in nonpregnant adults. *Clin Infect Dis.* 2001;33:556-561; Opal SM, Cross A, Palmo M, et al. Group B streptococcal sepsis in adults and infants: Contrasts and comparisons. *Arch Intern Med.* 1988;148:641-645; Gallagher PG, Watanakunakorn C. Group B streptococcal bacteremia in a community teaching hospital. *Am J Med.* 1985;78:795-800; Verghese A, Mireault K, Arbeit RD. Group B streptococcal bacteremia in men. *Rev Infect Dis.* 1986;8:912-917; Lerner PI, Gopalakrishna KV, Wolinsky E, et al. Group B streptococcus (*S. agalactiae*) bacteremia in adults: Analysis of 32 cases and review of the literature. *Medicine* (Baltimore). 1977;56:457-473; Schwartz B, Schuchat A, Oxtoby MJ, et al. Invasive group B streptococcal disease in adults: A population-based study in metropolitian Atlanta. *JAMA.* 1991;266:1112-1114.

Age 65 years or older is a risk factor for invasive group B streptococcal infection.[120] The incidence doubles when 50- to 64-year-olds are compared with those 65 years of age and older.[118] Among a group of community-dwelling older adults, the age-specific incidence increased steadily and was about threefold higher in those older than 85 years than in the 65- to 74-year-old group.

Mortality is increased in older patients, in those with polymicrobial infection, and in those with diabetes mellitus, liver disease, or malignancy. Case-fatality rates ranging from 8% to 70% previously have been reported,[113-115,121,122] but contemporary case-fatality rates range from 5% to 25% in nonpregnant adults.[6-8,10,118] Adults are more likely than infants to die as a result of group B streptococcal infection.[6] Shock at diagnosis, alcoholism, and cancer are associated independently with an increased risk for dying.[7,123] Nursing home residents are significantly more likely to have a fatal outcome than are community-dwelling older adults.[10] Of 29 adults with bacteremia described by Opal and associates,[113] only 34% acquired infection in the community. Others have described nosocomial acquisition, but case clustering has not been observed.[113-115,121] The latter suggests that endogenous respiratory, genitourinary, or gastrointestinal colonization rather than the acquisition of group B streptococci in the hospital is the source of these bacteremias. About one fourth of patients with group B streptococci isolated from the bloodstream have polymicrobial bacteremia. *S. aureus* is a frequently observed second isolate. The age distribution, mortality rate, and proportion of nosocomial cases does not differ among patients with bacteremia caused only by group B streptococcus and those with polymicrobial bacteremia.[119]

Postpartum bacteremias increased during the 1970s concomitant with neonatal infection, and group B streptococci accounted for up to 10% to 20% of blood culture isolates from women admitted to obstetric services. An uncomplicated outcome after appropriate antimicrobial therapy is the rule for pregnancy-associated infections, although complications such as meningitis or endocarditis have occurred.[46,121]

Most adult group B streptococcal infections are manifested as one of several clinical expressions of infection.

Primary Bacteremia

When no evident site of infection can be established, patients in whom group B streptococcus has been isolated from the bloodstream are classified as having primary bacteremia. In several reports, primary bacteremia is the most frequent diagnosis, accounting for 20% to 50% of cases, but this manifestation carries a high fatality rate.[7,113,116,122] Among survivors, recurrence of infection can be associated with a foci of infection such as endocarditis or osteomyelitis,[124] or another defined ongoing focus.

Infections of the Female Genital Tract

A substantial number of adult infections due to group B streptococcus are associated with pregnancy. The female genital tract is the source of these infections. Group B streptococci alone or as a component of polymicrobial infection is among the most commonly isolated facultative aerobes from women with early postpartum endometritis. Half of cases of bacteremic pregnancy-associated disease currently are associated with infection of the upper genital tract, placenta, or amniotic sac, resulting in fetal death. Other manifestations include bacteremia without a focus in one third of women, endometritis without fetal death, chorioamnionitis without fetal death, pneumonia, and puerperal sepsis.[45] Overall, group B streptococci account for an estimated 15% of cases of peripartum endometritis, 15% of puerperal bacteremias, and up to 15% of wound infections after cesarean section.[125]

Focal signs and symptoms of infection usually develop within 48 hours after delivery. An association between abdominal delivery and endometritis has been noted.[126] Among patients who deliver abdominally, women colonized with group B streptococci have a significantly increased frequency of premature rupture of membranes, postpartum fever, and endometritis when compared with noncolonized women. The clinical findings of endometritis are nonspecific and include fever with or without chills, malaise, moderate uterine tenderness, and normal lochia. Initial lack of symptoms referable to the genital area can be followed by chorioamnionitis.[127] Life-threatening sequelae of endometritis such as pelvic abscess, septic shock, or septic thrombophlebitis are rare.[128] Another manifestation of morbidity from group B streptococcal infection in pregnant women is urinary tract infection. Bacteriuria can be asymptomatic or, less often, can manifest as cystitis or, rarely, pyelonephritis.

The role of group B streptococcus as an etiologic agent causing vaginitis has not been established. It is regarded as a commensal organism in the vagina and does not elicit a vaginal inflammatory response. There are, however, anecdotal reports suggesting the pathogenic potential of group B streptococcus in vaginitis and of resolution of the symptoms of vaginitis in association with a short course of antibiotic administration.[129,130]

Pneumonia

Patients with group B streptococcal pneumonia have in common the apparent inability to limit the spread of the organism from colonizing mucous membrane sites to the bloodstream. The most common underlying medical conditions among patients with group B streptococcal pneumonia include diabetes mellitus and neurologic disease. The seven patients described by Verghese and associates were older (median age, 78 years), debilitated, and bedridden.[131] All patients were febrile, had leukocytosis, and were hypoxic in room air. Chest radiographs showed bilateral or lobar infiltrates. Infection was frequently polymicrobic, although group B streptococcus was the predominant organism. Pleural empyema also has been described in association with the pneumonia.[132] Fatality rates in patients with pneumonia range from 30% to 85%.

Endocarditis

A shift in the clinical expression of group B streptococcal endocarditis was first documented by Lerner and colleagues.[116] In contrast to the predominance of acute endocarditis in pregnant women during the preantibiotic era, cases reported since 1945 have had no gender predilection, have been both acute and subacute in onset, and have occurred in older patients (mean age, about 50 years).[116,133] The mitral valve is most frequently affected (48%); infections involving the aortic (29%), mitral and aortic (10%), and tricuspid valves (5%) have been described. Tricuspid valve involvement typically occurs in injection drug users.[112] An increasing rate of prosthetic valve endocarditis and endocarditis in association with injection drug use has been noted in a contemporary report.[134] Underlying heart disease exists in more than half of the cases reported since 1962, rheumatic heart disease being the most common diagnosis.[133] Valvular disease, atherosclerotic heart disease, and mitral valve prolapse also may be predisposing conditions.[131,135] Large friable vegetations are a frequent feature of group B streptococcal endocarditis. These can resemble atrial myxomas, and embolization may occur early in the clinical course. Rapid valve destruction may occur, necessitating early valve replacement in some patients.[136,137] The mortality rate is about 35% to 50%.

Arthritis

Group B streptococcal arthritis is monoarticular in two thirds of patients and involves more than one joint in the remainder. Polyarticular disease with a central pattern can occur.[116] In a review of 75 adults with group B streptococcal arthritis, the mean age was 58 years, and 45% were men.[138] The most commonly affected joints, in descending order of frequency, were the knee, shoulder, hip, and sternoclavicular and sacroiliac joints. One or more underlying medical conditions were present in three fourths of patients, most commonly diabetes mellitus, malignancy, or chronic liver disease. One third had a nonjoint focus of group B streptococcal infection, such as vertebral osteomyelitis or urinary tract infection. The most common presenting features were fever and joint pain, but about 14% of patients were afebrile. The erythrocyte sedimentation rate, when performed, was more than 30 mm/hr in 95% of patients, and group B streptococci were isolated from blood cultures in two thirds. With appropriate antimicrobial therapy, repeated joint aspirations or surgical débridement, and (usually) removal of a prosthesis, if present, complete recovery was achieved in one half of patients.[139] In the remainder, disease was associated with substantial functional sequelae. The mortality rate is about 10%.

Osteomyelitis

Osteomyelitis occurs as a consequence of adjacent arthritis, peripheral vascular disease, orthopedic surgery, or an adjacent focus of infection such as frontal sinusitis.[140] In a review of 39 cases of group B streptococcal osteomyelitis, half were diagnosed as acute and half as chronic episodes.[141] The mean age was 56 years, one third of patients were older than 65 years, and two thirds were men. The most commonly affected bones were the vertebrae, followed in order of frequency by the foot, bones around the hip, tibia, and toes. Underlying medical conditions were almost invariably present, most commonly diabetes mellitus, previous bone surgery, prosthetic bone or joint, or peripheral vascular disease. Foot bone involvement occurred predominantly in diabetic patients. Bones around the hip were involved in association with prior surgical procedures or trauma to the hip joint.

No specific clinical signs were associated with group B streptococcal osteomyelitis. A majority of patients were afebrile and had a normal erythrocyte sedimentation rate at the time of presentation. Cultures of bone or blood yielded group B streptococci in about 90% and about 40% of patients, respectively.[141] One fourth of infections were polymicrobial, with *S. aureus* the most commonly associated microorganism. Most patients required a combined medical and surgical approach. The mean duration of antibiotic therapy was 10 weeks. Fatal infections were uncommon and were a consequence of associated foci of infection such as endocarditis, but amputation can be required for resolution of infection for diabetics with vascular insufficiency.

Skin and Soft Tissue Infections

Skin and soft tissues are the most common sites of focal group B streptococcal infections in adults, accounting for more than one third of infections in some reports.[9,117,142] Cellulitis, foot ulcers, abscess, and infection of decubitus ulcers are common manifestations. Cellulitis has occurred in association with foreign bodies, such as breast or penile implants. Less common manifestations of skin and soft tissue infections are pyomyositis, blistering dactylitis, and necrotizing fasciitis, on occasion associated with toxic shock–like syndrome.[143-145] There are no features of these latter infections unique to group B streptococci except that predisposing conditions such as diabetes mellitus generally exist. In one report of 37 patients, the mean age (44 years) of the two thirds who had serious underlying conditions was significantly greater than that of otherwise normal hosts (21 years), who often acquired infection in association with minor trauma.[142] Abscess formation was observed in 46% of these infections. Group B streptococcus was the only organism isolated from 71% of patients with an abscess. Appropriate drainage and parenteral antimicrobial therapy effected complete recovery in 89% of these patients.

Meningitis

Meningitis due to group B streptococci has been reported in at least 64 adults, most of whom have had the previously mentioned underlying predisposing comorbid conditions.[5,116,121,146-151] The mean age of nonparturient adults is 52 years; almost one half are men. Several have had proven or possible disruption of the anatomic barrier protecting the brain in consequence of surgery for tumors or chronic sinusitis. The overall case-fatality rate is 34%. Advanced age and overwhelming illness with presenting features such as coma or septic shock are associated with a poor outcome.[150] Deafness, reported in 7% of the survivors, is the most common neurologic sequela.

Uncommon Manifestations of Infection

Group B streptococci, alone or as a component of mixed infection, have been isolated from a number of patients with keratitis or endophthalmitis. These infections were in eyes with severely damaged surfaces; the outcome was poor, with light perception being lost in one half of the affected eyes.[152,153]

Group B streptococci are a cause of urinary tract infections in nonobstetric populations, accounting for about 2% of positive urine cultures in one prospective evaluation.[154] Such infections are most often community acquired, occurring in middle-aged women. Almost all the patients have a predisposing condition, most commonly alterations of urinary flow or stones. Clinical manifestations are referable to the upper or lower urinary tracts in equal numbers. Despite appropriate treatment, the clinical outcome is poor in about one fifth of the patients. Treatment failure or relapse is most likely the result of persistent vaginal or enteric colonization. Group B streptococci also may be a cause of nongonococcal urethritis in men.[155]

Unusual infections caused by group B streptococcus include breast abscess in a nonlactating woman,[156] epiglottic abscess,[157] ventriculoperitoneal shunt infection,[158] myotic aneurysm of the femoral artery,[159] liver abscess,[113,122] peritonitis,[7,116,121] and infection of a pacemaker wire after sigmoidoscopy.[160] Group B streptococcus has also been reported to cause a toxic shock–like syndrome,[161] bacteremia after traumatic splenectomy,[162] bacteremia after cardiac catheterization,[163] and fever of unknown origin.[164]

Recurrent Invasive Group B Streptococcal Infection

About 4% of nonpregnant adults surviving an episode of group B streptococcal bacteremia and followed for at least 1 year have a second episode.[124] The mean interval between episodes of bacteremia is 24 weeks, but the interval is shorter when the recurrent episode is caused by the same strain (mean, 14 weeks) than when it is caused by another strain (mean, 43 weeks between episodes). Several patients in whom primary bacteremia was the diagnosis of the first episode presented with focal infection, such as endocarditis or osteomyelitis, during the second episode. Little is known regarding host factors that predispose adults to developing group B streptococcal infection. Limited data suggest that at least some adults already have relatively high concentrations of antibodies to the infecting capsular polysaccharide when illness occurs.[165] Although anticapsular antibody may be protective in many cases, the susceptibility of some adult patients to group B streptococcal infection may be the result of defects in other aspects of the host defense.

Diagnosis

Isolation of group B streptococcus from blood, CSF, another usually sterile site, or a site of focal suppuration is the only means by which the diagnosis of invasive infection can be documented. Recovery of the organism from mucous membrane sites is of no diagnostic significance.

Intrapartum detection of colonization with group B streptococcus in women presenting for delivery would allow the accurate identification of at-risk patients who might benefit from early chemoprophylaxis or empirical treatment. Gram stains of vaginal or cervical swabs from pregnant women and rapid immunoassays are not sufficiently accurate for routine use in the intrapartum detection of women vaginally colonized with group B streptococci.[166] For women with heavy colonization, the optical immuonassay method is highly sensitive and specific.

Bergeron and colleagues[167] described a fluorogenic real-time polymerase chain reaction (PCR) technique for rapid detection of group B streptococci in pregnant women at delivery that had a sensitivity of 97% and a specificity of 100% when compared with cultures of vaginal and rectal swabs inoculated in selective broth medium. Results were available in 45 minutes, as compared with 100 minutes for conventional PCR and 36 hours or longer for the conventional culture technique. Field testing of such commercially manufactured assays as the Xpert GBS Assay (Cepheid, Sunnyvale, California) that uses automated real-time PCR technology and IDI-StrepB (Infectio Diagnostic, Quebec, Canada) that uses a PCR assay to amplify group B streptococcus–specific DNA and a fluorogenic probe to detect the amplified group B streptococcal target have been performed.[168,169] These assays are sufficiently robust, when compared with conventional culture methods, to be performed for intrapartum patients in point-of-care settings but have not replaced the culture-based method currently in use for antenatal identification of women who are colonized with group B streptococci as candidates for intrapartum antibiotic prophylaxis to prevent early-onset neonatal infection.

Treatment

The antimicrobial regimens recommended for treatment of group B streptococcal infections in infants and adults are summarized in Table 202-3. Group B streptococci remain susceptible to penicillins and cephalosporins in vitro,[170] although several strains with somewhat reduced susceptibility to penicillin have been identified recently in Japan,[171] and penicillin G is the drug of choice after the diagnosis is established.[170] The organism also is susceptible to ampicillin, cephalosporins, vancomycin, and teicoplanin.[170] Meropenem and imipenem have good in vitro activity.[171] Rates of fluoroquinolone resistance are about 5% and are associated with mutations in the gyrase and topoisomerase IV genes.[172] Increasing resistance to erythromycin and clindamycin now precludes their use as empirical treatment for invasive infection or for intrapartum prophylaxis unless susceptibility is established. Resistance rates for colonizing isolates are as high as 42% for erythromycin and 41% for clindamycin.[173] Among isolates from patients with invasive disease, resistance rates for erythromycin range from 7% to 32%, and for clindamycin, from 3% to 20%.[173-175] Most macrolide-resistant strains present an MLS_B phenotype, mainly constitutive, due to *erm* genes.[176] A chromosomally integrated, composite transposon has been defined for *ermB*-type macrolide resistance.[177] Tetracycline resistance has increased to nearly 90%.[178] Group B streptococci are uniformly resistant to nalidixic acid, trimethoprim-sulfamethoxazole, metronidazole, and aminoglycosides.

The initial use of ampicillin and an aminoglycoside for suspected neonatal bacteremia or meningitis due to group B streptococcus is based on their in vitro synergy for these organisms and on the need

TABLE 202-3	Treatment of Group B Streptococcal Infections				
	Antibiotic (IV Dosage)				
Diagnosis	*Neonate and Infant*	*Adult*	*Alternative for Penicillin-Allergic Adults*	*Duration*	
Bacteremia, soft tissue infections	Ampicillin (150 mg/kg/day) plus an aminoglycoside initially, then penicillin G (200,000 U/kg/day)	Penicillin G (10-12 million U/day)	Vancomycin or clindamycin if susceptible strain	10 days	
Meningitis	Ampicillin (300-400 mg/kg/day) plus gentamicin initially, then penicillin G (400,000-500,000 U/kg/day)	Penicillin G (20-30 million U/day)	Vancomycin	14-21 days	
Osteomyelitis	Penicillin G (200,000 U/kg/day)	Penicillin G (10-20 million U/day)	Vancomycin	3-4 wk	
Endocarditis (see Chapter 77)	Penicillin G (400,000 U/kg/day)	Penicillin G (20-30 million U/day) with gentamicin for 2 wk	Vancomycin with gentamicin	4-6 wk	

for broad-spectrum antimicrobial coverage until the diagnosis is established with certainty. Once the diagnosis is established and a clinical response is documented, treatment can be completed with penicillin G alone. Therapy of 10 days' duration is recommended for the treatment of bacteremia, pneumonia, and pyelonephritis, whereas a 14-day minimal duration is recommended for the treatment of soft tissue infections or meningitis, and a 4-week minimum for the treatment of osteomyelitis, endocarditis, or ventriculitis is recommended. In infants, oral therapy is never appropriate. In adults with endocarditis, cardiac surgery early in the course may be necessary because of rapid left-sided valvular destruction.[135] Relapses of infection have occurred in association with both an inadequate dosage and an inadequate duration of therapy. High-dose penicillin therapy does not reliably eliminate mucous membrane infection with group B streptococci, a source that may explain some recurrences.

Prevention

Antibiotic prophylaxis and immunization are the approaches in use or under investigation for prevention of group B streptococcal infections.

INTRAPARTUM ANTIBIOTIC PROPHYLAXIS

Most infants with early-onset sepsis are ill at or within a few hours of birth, rendering prophylaxis for the newborn impractical in most circumstances. The proof that maternal intrapartum antibiotic prophylaxis can prevent neonatal group B streptococcal infection dates to the 1985s when Boyer and Gotoff[179] showed that ampicillin given during labor to antenatally identified colonized parturients significantly reduced the risk for early-onset infant disease. The American College of Obstetricians and Gynecologists (ACOG) and the American Academy of Pediatrics (AAP) each published documents in the early 1990s emphasizing the need to reduce morbidity from group B streptococcal infection, but their approaches to selection of women at risk differed, and neither approach was implemented fully.[180,181] Consensus was reached in 1996 to select women to receive intrapartum prophylaxis based either on antenatal culture screening or by risk factor–based approaches.[182] The impact of maternal antibiotic prophylaxis on the incidence of early-onset group B streptococcal disease was first assessed by active, population-based surveillance in selected counties of eight states and reported in 2000.[6] The incidence of early-onset neonatal disease from 1993 to 1998 decreased by 65%, from 1.7 to 0.6 per 1000 live births, and the incidence of invasive disease in pregnant women declined by 21%. A multistate retrospective cohort comparison found that the culture-based approach was 50% more effective than a risk-based approach in preventing early-onset group B streptococcal infection.[183] The current guidelines for prevention of perinatal group B streptococcal infection were issued in 2002 by the Centers for Disease Control and Prevention, and endorsed by the ACOG and the AAP.[184]

These specify that lower vaginal and rectal swab screening cultures be performed at 35 to 37 weeks of gestation for all pregnant women with the exception of patients with documented group B streptococcal bacteriuria during the current pregnancy or with a previous infant with invasive group B streptococcal disease. The indications for intrapartum prophylaxis are shown in Table 202-4. When the culture status is not known, prophylaxis is indicated when there is preterm labor, when amniotic membranes have been ruptured for 18 hours or longer, and when there is fever during labor.[185] Prophylaxis is not indicated for planned cesarean delivery performed in the absence of labor or membrane rupture, regardless of the maternal group B streptococcal colonization status, or for women colonized in a prior pregnancy.

Penicillin G is the preferred agent for intrapartum prophylaxis because of its narrow spectrum of antimicrobial activity. The recommendation is to administer 5 million units of penicillin G initially and then 2.5 million units every 4 hours until delivery. Ampicillin is an alternative agent, but its use is discouraged because of its broader antimicrobial spectrum and because of its potential impact on incidence of ampicillin-resistant *Escherichia coli* or other forms of non–group B streptococcal sepsis.[186] Because of the increasing resistance

TABLE 202-4	Indications* for Intrapartum Antibiotic Prophylaxis to Prevent Perinatal Group B Streptococcal (GBS) Disease
Intrapartum Prophylaxis Indicated	*Intrapartum Prophylaxis Not Indicated*
Previous infant with invasive GBS disease	Previous pregnancy with a positive GBS screening culture (unless a culture was also positive during the current pregnancy)
GBS bacteriuria during the current pregnancy	
Positive GBS screening culture during current pregnancy	Planned cesarean delivery performed in the absence of labor or membrane rupture (regardless of maternal GBS culture status)
GBS status unknown (culture not done, incomplete, or results unknown) and any of the following: Delivery at <37 weeks' gestation† Amniotic membrane rupture ≥18 hr Intrapartum temperature ≥100.4° F (≥38.0° C)‡	Negative vaginal and rectal GBS screening culture in late gestation during the current pregnancy, regardless of intrapartum risk factors

*Indications are based on a universal prenatal screening strategy that involves obtaining combined vaginal and rectal GBS cultures from *all* pregnant women at 35 to 37 weeks' gestation. (Screening is not necessary if a woman has already been shown to have GBS bacteriuria during the current pregnancy, or if a previous infant had invasive GBS disease. In these cases, prophylaxis is always indicated.)

†If onset of labor or rupture of amniotic membranes occurs at <37 weeks' gestation and there is a significant risk for preterm delivery (as assessed by the clinician), a suggested algorithm for GBS prophylaxis management is provided.[184,185]

‡If amnionitis is suspected, broad-spectrum antibiotic therapy that includes an agent known to be active against GBS should replace GBS prophylaxis.

rates of group B streptococci to erythromycin and clindamycin, cefazolin (2 g initially, then 1 g every 8 hours) is recommended for use in women allergic to penicillin but at low risk for anaphylaxis. Vancomycin (1 g every 12 hours until delivery) is the suggested alternative for penicillin-allergic women at high risk for anaphylaxis, but its ability to penetrate into amniotic fluid or to prevent early-onset disease is not known.[187]

The AAP guidelines provide a detailed algorithm for management of infants born to mothers who have received intrapartum antibiotic prophylaxis.[188] These advocate a full diagnostic evaluation and empirical treatment for infants if intrapartum antibiotics were administered for suspected chorioamnionitis and for infants with signs of neonatal sepsis. The guidelines base a decision to perform a limited sepsis evaluation on a duration of intrapartum prophylaxis with penicillin, ampicillin, or cefazolin of less than 4 hours. A healthy-appearing infant at term gestation whose mother received 4 or more hours of intrapartum prophylaxis can be discharged home after 24 hours of observation if other discharge criteria have been met and a person able to comply fully with instructions for home observation is available.

GROUP B STREPTOCOCCAL VACCINES

Because the risk for invasive group B streptococcal disease in pregnant women and neonates is associated with low concentrations of maternal antibodies to the type-specific capsular polysaccharides of these organisms at delivery,[79,189] immunization to prevent these infections is desirable. Uncoupled group B streptococcal capsular polysaccharides were initially developed and evaluated for safety and immunogenicity in adult volunteers.[190-192] Although the immune responses to these vaccines were robust in adults with preexisting type-specific antibodies, they were inadequate in nonimmune adults.[192] Vaccine-induced capsular type-specific antibodies were predominantly IgG$_1$ and IgG$_2$, crossed the placenta efficiently, and were protective in animal models of lethal infection.[193,194] However, because of the variable immunogenicity of uncoupled type Ia, II, and III polysaccharide vaccines in nonimmune adults, polysaccharide-protein conjugate vaccines were subsequently developed.[195-197] The first, composed of type III polysaccharide covalently linked to tetanus toxoid, was immunogenic in rabbits and mice, and the antibodies elicited were functional in vitro and protective in vivo.[195] In healthy young women, type III group B streptococcal polysaccharide–tetanus toxoid conjugate vaccine was safe and significantly more immunogenic than uncoupled capsular polysaccharide.[198] Additional conjugate vaccines have been developed for capsular types Ia, Ib, II, and V polysaccharides.[199-201] Each of these monovalent conjugate vaccines is safe and significantly more immunogenic than uncoupled capsular polysaccharide when administered as a single dose in healthy nonpregnant adults.[202-204] A type V polysaccharide–tetanus toxoid conjugate vaccine also was safe and immunogenic in healthy adults 65 years of age and older.[205] A type III polysaccharide–tetanus toxoid conjugate vaccine has been administered to healthy women in the third trimester (mean gestation, 31 weeks) of pregnancy.[206] The concentration of capsular polysaccharide–specific IgG was sufficient to provide antibodies transplacentally that were functional in vitro through the first 2 months of life for infants born to these women. The concept that two monovalent conjugate vaccines combined can elicit immune responses comparable to those of the monovalent vaccines alone has been proved by the administration to healthy adults of a bivalent type II and III group B streptococcal conjugate vaccines.[207]

Administration of a multivalent group B streptococcal polysaccharide–tetanus toxoid conjugate vaccine to women during the last third of pregnancy theoretically could provide capsular type-specific antibodies in sufficient concentrations to passively protect neonates from early- and from late-onset disease. Such a multivalent conjugate vaccine tested in a murine model provided protection of pups against lethal infection with multiple group B streptococcal types.[208] This approach to prevention, in contrast to maternal intrapartum chemoprophylaxis, offers a method that is simple, cost-effective, and durable and would not promote antimicrobial resistance. The demonstration that type V group B streptococcal tetanus toxoid conjugate vaccine was well tolerated and immunogenic in healthy older adults also offers promise that immunization could confer protection from invasive infection in at-risk nonpregnant adults, but further studies are needed.[205] The concept that group B streptococcal conjugate vaccines are safe, immunogenic, and elicit functionally active antibodies in vitro has been amply demonstrated.

Meanwhile, the discovery that surface-associated pili are widely distributed among group B streptococci and that these vaccines based on combinations of recombinant pilus components protect mice against lethal challenge with a wide variety of group B streptococcal strains paves the way for design of pilus-based, multivalent vaccines against group B streptococci.[209] Furthermore, pilus islands 1, 2a, and 2b, alone or in combination, were uniformly identified on more than 200 isolates from infants and adults with invasive group B streptococcal disease, and most were highly surface expressed.[210] Other group B streptococcal surface proteins, including Rib and components of C protein, also offer potential as carriers in conjugate vaccines.[211,212] The impact of an immunization program on the group B streptococcal disease burden cannot be realized until development by the pharmaceutical industry is realized.

REFERENCES

1. Fry RM. Fatal infections by haemolytic streptococcus group B. *Lancet*. 1938;1:199-201.
2. Lancefield RC, Hare R. The serological differentiation of pathogenic and nonpathogenic strains of hemolytic streptococci from parturient women. *J Exp Med*. 1935;61:335-349.
3. Hood M, Janney A, Dameron G. Beta hemolytic streptococcus group B associated with problems of perinatal period. *Am J Obstet Gynecol*. 1961;82:809-818.
4. Eickhoff TC, Klein JO, Daly AL, et al. Neonatal sepsis and other infections due to group B beta-hemolytic streptococci. *N Engl J Med*. 1964;271:1221-1228.
5. Butter MNW, DeMoor CE. *Streptococcus agalactiae* as a cause of meningitis in the newborn, and of bacteremia in adults. *Antonie van Leeuwenhoek*. 1967;33:439-450.
6. Schrag SJ, Zywicki S, Farley MM, et al. Group B streptococcal disease in the era of intrapartum antibiotic prophylaxis. *N Engl J Med*. 2000;342:15-20.
7. Muñoz P, Llancaqueo A, Rodriguez-Creixems M, et al. Group B streptococcus bacteremia in nonpregnant adults. *Arch Intern Med*. 1997;157:213-216.
8. Farley MM. Group B streptococcal disease in nonpregnant adults. *Clin Infect Dis*. 2001;33:556-561.
9. Farley MM, Harvey RC, Stull T, et al. A population-based assessment of invasive disease due to group B streptococcus in nonpregnant adults. *N Engl J Med*. 1993;328:1807-1811.
10. Henning KJ, Hall EL, Dwyer DM, et al. Invasive group B streptococcal disease in Maryland nursing home residents. *J Infect Dis*. 2001;183:1138-1142.
11. Glaser P, Rusniok C, Buchrieser C, et al. Genome sequence of *Streptococcus agalactiae*, a pathogen causing invasive neonatal disease. *Mol Microbiol*. 2002;45:1499-1513.
12. Tettelin H, Masignani V, Cieslewicz MJ, et al. Complete genome sequence and comparative genomic analysis of an emerging human pathogen, serotype V *Streptococcus agalactiae*. *Proc Natl Acad Sci U S A*. 2002;99:12391-12396.
13. Lancefield RC. A serological differentiation of human and other groups of hemolytic streptococci. *J Exp Med*. 1933;57:571-595.
14. Baker CJ, Clark DJ, Barrett FF. Selective broth medium for isolation of group B streptococci. *Appl Microbiol*. 1973;26:884-885.
15. Lancefield RC. A serological differentiation of specific types of bovine hemolytic streptococci (group B). *J Exp Med*. 1934;59:441-458.
16. Wilkinson HW, Eagon RG. Type-specific antigens of group B type Ic streptococci. *Infect Immun*. 1971;4:596-604.
17. Henrichsen J, Ferrieri P, Jelinkova J, et al. Nomenclature of antigens of group B streptococci. *Int J Syst Bacteriol*. 1984;34:500.
18. Jelinkova J, Motlova J. Worldwide distribution of two new serotypes of group B streptococci: Type IV and provisional type V. *J Clin Microbiol*. 1985;21:361-362.
19. Wessels MR, DiFabio JL, Benedi V-J, et al. Structural determination and immunochemical characterization of the type V group B streptococcus capsular polysaccharide. *J Biol Chem*. 1991;266:6714-6719.
20. Von Hunolstein C, D'Ascenzi S, Wagner B, et al. Immunochemistry of capsular type polysaccharide and virulence properties of type VI *Streptococcus agalactiae* (group B streptococci). *Infect Immun*. 1993;61:1272-1280.
21. Kogan G, Uhrin D, Brisson J-R, et al. Structure and immunochemical characterization of the type VIII group B streptococcus capsular polysaccharide. *J Biol Chem*. 1996;271:8786-8796.
22. Slotved H-C, Kong F, Lambertsen L, et al. Serotype IX, a proposed new *Streptococcus agalactiae* serotype. *J Clin Microbiol*. 2007;45:2929-2936.
23. Ferrieri P, Flores AE. Surface protein expression in group B streptococcal invasive isolates. *Adv Exp Med Biol*. 1997;418:635-637.
24. Lancefield RC, McCarty M, Everly WN. Multiple mouse-protective antibodies directed against group B streptococci. Special reference to antibodies effective against protein antigens. *J Exp Med*. 1975;142:165-179.
25. Stålhammar-Carlemalm M, Stenberg L, Lindahl G. Protein Rib: A novel group B streptococcal cell surface protein that confers protective immunity and is expressed by most strains causing invasive infections. *J Exp Med*. 1993;177:1593-1603.
26. Michel JL, Madoff LC, Kling DE, et al. Cloned alpha and beta C-protein antigens of group B streptococci elicit protective immunity. *Infect Immun*. 1991;59:2023-2028.
27. Madoff LC, Michel JL, Gong EW, et al. Protection of neonatal mice from group B streptococcal infection by maternal immunization with beta C protein. *Infect Immun*. 1992;60:4989.
28. Ramaswamy SV, Ferrieri P, Flores AE, et al. Molecular characterization of nontypeable group B streptococcus. *J Clin Microbiol*. 2006;44:2398-2403.

29. Kong F, Gowan S, Martin D, et al. Serotype identification of group B streptococci by PCR and sequencing. *J Clin Microbiol.* 2002;40:216-226.
30. Quentin R, Huet H, Wang F-S, et al. Characterization of *Streptococcus agalactiae* strains by multilocus enzyme genotype and serotype: Identification of multiple virulent clone families that cause invasive neonatal disease. *J Clin Microbiol.* 1995;33:2576-2581.
31. Newton ER, Butler MC, Shain RN. Sexual behavior and vaginal colonization by group B streptococcus among minority women. *Obstet Gynecol.* 1996;88:577-582.
32. Campbell JR, Hillier SL, Krohn MA, et al. Group B streptococcal colonization and serotype-specific immunity in pregnant women at delivery. *Obstet Gynecol.* 2000;96:498-503.
33. Ramos E, Gaudier FL, Hearing LR, et al. Group B streptococcus colonization in pregnant diabetic women. *Obstet Gynecol.* 1997;89:257-260.
34. Meyn LA, Moore DM, Hillier SL, et al. Association of sexual activity with colonization and vaginal acquisition of group B streptococcus in nonpregnant women. *Am J Epidemiol.* 2002;155:949-957.
35. Bliss SJ, Manning SD, Tallman P, et al. Group B streptococcus colonization in male and nonpregnant female university students: A cross-sectional prevalence study. *Clin Infect Dis.* 2002;34:184-190.
36. Manning SD, Tallman P, Baker CJ, et al. Determinants of co-colonization with group B streptococcus among heterosexual college couples. *Epidemiology.* 2002;13:533-539.
37. Manning SD, Neighbors K, Tallman PA, et al. Prevalence of group B *Streptococcus* colonization and potential for transmission by casual contact in healthy young men and women. *Clin Infect Dis.* 2004;39:380-388.
38. Dillon HC, Gray E, Pass MA, et al. Anorectal and vaginal carriage of group B streptococci during pregnancy. *J Infect Dis.* 1982;145:794-799.
39. Edwards MS, Rench MA, Palazzi DL, et al. Group B streptococcal colonization and serotype-specific immunity in healthy elderly persons. *Clin Infect Dis.* 2005;40:352-357.
40. Allen U, Nimrod C, MacDonald N, et al. Relationship between antenatal group B streptococcal vaginal colonization and premature labour. *Paediatr Child Health.* 1999;4:465-469.
41. Baker CJ, Barrett FF. Transmission of group B streptococci among parturient women and their neonates. *J Pediatr.* 1973;83:919-925.
42. Ancona RJ, Ferrieri P, Williams PP. Maternal factors that enhance the acquisition of group B streptococci by newborn infants. *J Med Microbiol.* 1980;13:273-280.
43. Schuchat A, Deaver-Robinson K, Plikaytis BD, et al. Multistate case-control study of maternal risk factors for neonatal group B streptococcal disease. *Pediatr Infect Dis J.* 1994;13:623-629.
44. Schuchat A, Oxtoby M, Cochi S, et al. Population-based risk factors for neonatal group B streptococcal disease: Results of a cohort study in metropolitan Atlanta. *J Infect Dis.* 1990;162:672-677.
45. Phares CR, Lynfield R, Farley MM, et al. Epidemiology of invasive group B streptococcal disease in the United States, 1999-2005. *JAMA.* 2008;299:2056-2065.
46. Yancey MK, Duff P, Clark P, et al. Peripartum infection associated with vaginal group B streptococcal colonization. *Obstet Gynecol.* 1994;84:816-819.
47. Krohn MA, Hillier SL, Baker CJ. Maternal peripartum complications associated with vaginal group B streptococci colonization. *J Infect Dis.* 1999;179:1410-1415.
48. Centers for Disease Control and Prevention. Active bacterial core surveillance (ABCs) report emerging infections program network group B streptococcus. 2007. http://www.cdc.gov/ncidod/dbmd/abcs/survreports/gbs07.pdf. Accessed May 24, 2009.
49. Lin F-YC, Clemens JD, Azimi PH, et al. Capsular polysaccharide types of group B streptococcal isolates from neonates with early-onset systemic infection. *J Infect Dis.* 1998;177:790-792.
50. Harrison LH, Elliott JA, Dwyer DM, et al. Serotype distribution of invasive group B streptococcal isolates in Maryland: Implications for vaccine formulation. *J Infect Dis.* 1998;177:998-1002.
51. Zaleznik DF, Rench MA, Hillier S, et al. Invasive disease due to group B streptococcus in pregnant women and neonates from diverse population groups. *Clin Infect Dis.* 1999;30:276-281.
52. Davies HD, Raj S, Adair C, et al. Population-based active surveillance for neonatal group B streptococcal infections in Alberta, Canada: Implications for vaccine formulation. *Pediatr Infect Dis J.* 2001;20:879-884.
53. Davies HD, Adair C, McGeer A, et al. Antibodies to capsular polysaccharides of group B streptococcus in pregnant Canadian women: Relationship to colonization status and infection in the neonate. *J Infect Dis.* 2001;184:285-291.
54. Lachenauer C, Kasper DL, Shimada J, et al. Serotypes VI and VIII predominate among group B streptococci isolated from pregnant Japanese women. *J Infect Dis.* 1999;174:1030-1033.
55. Lauer P, Rinaudo CD, Soriani M, et al. Genome analysis reveals pili in group B *Streptococcus*. *Science.* 2005;309:105.
56. Rosini R, Rinaudo CD, Soriani M, et al. Identification of novel genomic islands coding for antigenic pilus-like structures in *Streptococcus agalactiae*. *Mol Microbiol.* 2006;61:126-141.
57. Pass MA, Gray BM, Khare S, et al. Prospective studies of group B streptococcal infections in infants. *J Pediatr.* 1979; 95:437-443.
58. Regan JA, Klebanoff MA, Nugent RP, et al. Colonization with group B streptococci in pregnancy and adverse outcome. *Am J Obstet Gynecol.* 1996;174:1354-1360.
59. Bolduc GR, Baron MJ, Gravekamp C, et al. The alpha C protein mediates internalization of group B Streptococcus within human cervical epithelial cells. *Cell Microbiol.* 2002;4:751-758.
60. Maisey HC, Hensler M, Nizet V, et al. Group B streptococcal pilus proteins contribute to adherence to and invasion of brain microvascular endothelial cells. *J Bacteriol.* 2007; 189:1464-1467.
61. Schubert A, Zakikhany K, Pietrocola G, et al. The fibrinogen receptor FbsA promotes adherence of *Streptococcus agalactiae* to human cells. *Infect Immun.* 2004;72:6197-6205.
62. Tamura GS, Rubens CE. Host-bacterial interactions in the pathogenesis of group B streptococcal infections. *Curr Opin Infect Dis.* 1994;7:317-322.
63. Soriani M, Santi I, Taddei A, et al. Group B *Streptococcus* crosses human epithelial cells by a paracellular route. *J Infect Dis.* 2006;193:241-250.
64. Pezzicoli A, Santi I, Lauer P, et al. Pilus backbone contributes to group B *Streptococcus* paracellular translocation through epithelial cells. *J Infect Dis.* 2008;198:890-898.
65. Gutekunst H, Eikmanns BJ, Reinscheid DJ. The novel fibrogen-binding protein FbsB promotes *Streptococcus agalactiae* invasion into epithelial cells. *Infect Immun.* 2004;72:3495-3504.
66. Nizet V, Kim KS, Stins M, et al. Invasion of brain microvascular endothelial cells by group B streptococci. *Infect Immun.* 1997;65:5074-5081.
67. Malin G, Paoletti LC. Use of a dynamic in vitro attachment and invasion system (DIVAS) to determine influence of growth rate on invasion of respiratory epithelial cells by group B streptococcus. *Proc Natl Acad Sci U S A.* 2001;98:13335-13340.
68. Baron MJ, Filman DJ, Prophete GA, et al. Identification of a glycosaminoglycan binding region of the alpha C protein that mediates entry of group B streptococci into host cells. *J Biol Chem.* 2007;282:10526-10536.
69. Doran KS, Engelson EJ, Khosravi A, et al. Blood-brain barrier invasion by group B *Streptococcus* depends upon proper cell-surface anchoring of lipoteichoic acid. *J Clin Invest.* 2005;115:2499-2507.
70. Doran KS, Chang JCW, Benoit VM, et al. Group B streptococcal β-hemolysin/cytolysin promotes invasion of human lung epithelial cells and the release of interleukin-8. *J Infect Dis.* 2002;185:196-203.
71. Gibson RL, Nizet V, Rubens CE. Group B streptococcal beta-hemolysin promotes injury of lung microvascular endothelial cells. *Pediatr Res.* 1999;45:626-634.
72. Takahashi S, Adderson EE, Nagano Y, et al. Identification of a highly encapsulated, genetically related group of invasive type III group B streptococci. *J Infect Dis.* 1998;177:1116-1119.
73. Rubens CE, Wessels MR, Heggen LM, et al. Transposon mutagenesis of group B streptococcal type III capsular polysaccharide: Correlation of capsule expression with virulence. *Proc Natl Acad Sci U S A.* 1987;84:7208-7212.
74. Wessels MR, Rubens CE, Benedi V-J, et al. Definition of a bacterial virulence factor: Sialylation of the group B streptococcal capsule. *Proc Natl Acad Sci U S A.* 1989;86:8983-8987.
75. Nizet V, Kim KS, Stins M, et al. Invasion of brain microvascular endothelial cells by group B streptococci. *Infect Immun.* 1997;65:5074-5081.
76. Kasper DL, Baker CJ, Edwards MS, et al. The type III group B streptococcal capsular polysaccharide: Structure, immunospecificity, immunogenicity, and relationship to virulence. In: Weinstein L, Fields BN, eds. *Seminars in Infectious Disease, vol. 4. Bacterial Vaccines.* New York: Thieme-Stratton; 1982: 275-278.
77. Kogan G, Brisson JR, Kasper DL, et al. Structural elucidation of the novel type VII group B streptococcus capsular polysaccharide by high resolution NMR spectroscopy. *Carbohydr Res.* 1995;277:1-9.
78. Granlund M, Oberg L, Sellin M, et al. Identification of a novel insertion element, IS*1548*, in group B streptococci, predominantly in strains causing endocarditis. *J Infect Dis.* 1998;177:967-976.
79. Baker CJ, Kasper DL. Correlation of maternal antibody deficiency with susceptibility to neonatal group B streptococcal infection. *N Engl J Med.* 1976;294:753-756.
80. Liu GY, Doran KS, Lawrence T, et al. Sword and shield: linked group B streptococcal beta-hemolysin/cytolysin and carotenoid pigment function to subvert host phagocyte defense. *Proc Natl Acad Sci U S A.* 2004;101:14491-14496.
81. Puliti M, Nizet V, von Hunolstein C, et al. Severity of group B streptococcal arthritis is correlated with beta-hemolysin expression. *J Infect Dis.* 2000;182:824-832.
82. Hensler ME, Miyamoto S, Nizet V. Group B streptococcal β-hemolysin/cytolysin directly impairs cardiomyocyte viability and function. *PLoS ONE.* 2008;3:e2446-e2452.
83. Areschoug T, Stalhammar-Carlemalm M, Karlsson I, et al. Streptococcal beta protein has separate binding sites for human factor H and IgA-Fc. *J Biol Chem.* 2002;277:12642-12648.
84. Harris TO, Shelver DW, Bohnsack JF, et al. A novel streptococcal surface protease promotes virulence, resistance to opsonophagocytosis, and cleavage of human fibrinogen. *J Clin Invest.* 2003;111:61-70.
85. Baker CJ, Kasper DL, Tager IB, et al. Quantitative determination of antibody to capsular polysaccharide in infection with type III strains of group B streptococcus. *J Clin Invest.* 1977;59: 810-818.
86. Lin F-YC, Philips JB II, Azimi PH, et al. Level of maternal antibody required to protect neonates against early-onset disease caused by group B streptococcus type Ia: A multicenter, seroepidemiology study. *J Infect Dis.* 2001;184:1022-1028.
87. Gotoff SP, Papierniak CK, Klegerman ME, et al. Quantitation of IgG antibody to the type-specific polysaccharide of group B streptococcus type Ib in pregnant women and infected infants. *J Pediatr.* 1984;105:628-630.
88. Gray BM, Pritchard DG, Dillon HC Jr. Seroepidemiological studies of group B streptococcus type II. *J Infect Dis.* 1985;151:1073-1080.
89. Anthony BF, Concepcion NF, Concepcion KF. Human antibody to the group-specific polysaccharide of group B streptococcus. *J Infect Dis.* 1985;151:221-226.
90. Shigeoka AO, Hall RT, Hemming VG, et al. Role of antibody and complement in opsonization of group B streptococci. *Infect Immun.* 1978;21:34-40.
91. Baker CJ, Webb BJ, Kasper DL, et al. The role of complement and antibody in opsonophagocytosis of type II group B streptococci. *J Infect Dis.* 1986;154:47-54.
92. Hall MA, Hickman ME, Baker CJ, et al. Complement and antibody in neutrophil-mediated killing of type V group B streptococcus. *J Infect Dis.* 1994;170:88-93.
93. Aoyagi Y, Adderson EE, Min JG, et al. Role of L-ficolin/mannose-binding lectin-associated serine protease complexes in the opsonophagocytosis of type III group B streptococci. *J Immunol.* 2005;174:418-425.
94. Payne NR, Kim Y, Ferrieri P. Effect of differences in antibody and complement requirements on phagocytic uptake and intracellular killing of "c" protein-positive and -negative strains of type II group B streptococci. *Infect Immun.* 1987;55: 1243-1251.
95. Baker CJ, Edwards MS, Webb BJ, et al. Antibody-independent classical pathway-mediated opsonophagocytosis of type Ia, group B streptococcus. *J Clin Invest.* 1982;63:394-404.
96. Smith CL, Baker CJ, Anderson DC, et al. Role of complement receptors in opsonophagocytosis of group B streptococci by adult and neonatal neutrophils. *J Infect Dis.* 1990;162:489-495.
97. Yang KD, Bathras JM, Shigeoka AO, et al. Mechanisms of bacterial opsonization by immune globulin intravenous: Correlation of complement consumption with opsonic activity and protective efficacy. *J Infect Dis.* 1989;159:701-707.
98. Noya FJD, Baker CJ, Edwards MS. Neutrophil Fc receptor participation in phagocytosis of type III group B streptococci. *Infect Immun.* 1993;61:1415-1420.
99. Vallejo JG, Baker CJ, Edwards MS. Roles of the bacterial cell wall and capsule in induction of tumor necrosis factor alpha by type III group B streptococci. *Infect Immun.* 1996;64:5042-5046.
100. Teti G, Mancuso G, Tomasello F, et al. Production of tumor necrosis factor-α and interleukin-6 in mice infected with group B streptococci. *Circ Shock.* 1992;38:138-144.
101. Rowen JL, Smith CW, Edwards MS. Group B streptococci elicit leukotriene B_4 and interleukin-8 from human monocytes: Neonates exhibit a diminished response. *J Infect Dis.* 1995;172:420-426.
102. Vallejo JG, Knuefermann P, Mann DL, et al. Group B streptococcus induces TNF-α gene expression and activation of the transcription factors NFκB and activator protein-1 in human cord blood monocytes. *J Immunol.* 2000;165:419-425.
103. Henneke P, Takeuchi O, van Strijp JA, et al. Novel engagement of CD14 and multiple toll-like receptors by group B streptococci. *J Immunol.* 2001;167:7069-7076.
104. Franciosi RA, Knostman JD, Zimmerman RA. Group B streptococcal neonatal and infant infections. *J Pediatr.* 1973;82:707-718.
105. Baker CJ, Barrett FF, Gordon RC, et al. Suppurative meningitis due to streptococci of Lancefield group B: A study of 33 infants. *J Pediatr.* 1973;82:724-729.
106. Puopolo KM, Madoff LC, Eichenwald EC. Early-onset group B streptococcal disease in the era of maternal screening. *Pediatrics.* 2005;115:1240-1246.
107. Jordan HT, Farley MM, Craig A, et al. Revisiting the need for vaccine prevention of late-onset neonatal group B streptococcal disease. A multistate, population-based analysis. *Pediatr Infect Dis J.* 2008;27:1057-1064.
108. Edwards MS, Rench MA, Haffar AA, et al. Long-term sequelae of group B streptococcal meningitis in infants. *J Pediatr.* 1985;106:717-722.
109. Wald ER, Bergman I, Taylor HG, et al. Long-term outcome of group B streptococcal meningitis. *Pediatrics.* 1986;77:217-221.
110. Garcia Peña BM, Harper MB, Fleisher GR. Occult bacteremia with group B streptococci in an outpatient setting. *Pediatrics.* 1998;102:67-72.
111. Hussain SM, Luedtke GS, Baker CJ, et al. Invasive group B streptococcal disease in children beyond early infancy. *Pediatr Infect Dis J.* 1995;14:278-281.
112. Alsoub H, Najma F, Robida A. Group B streptococcal endocarditis in children beyond the neonatal period. *Pediatr Infect Dis J.* 1997;16:418-420.
113. Opal SM, Cross A, Palmo M, et al. Group B streptococcal sepsis in adults and infants: Contrasts and comparisons. *Arch Intern Med.* 1988;148:641-645.
114. Gallagher PG, Watanakunakorn C. Group B streptococcal bacteremia in a community teaching hospital. *Am J Med.* 1985;78:795-800.

115. Verghese A, Mireault K, Arbeit RD. Group B streptococcal bacteremia in men. *Rev Infect Dis.* 1986;8:912-917.
116. Lerner PI, Gopalakrishna KV, Wolinsky E, et al. Group B streptococcus *(S. agalactiae)* bacteremia in adults: Analysis of 32 cases and review of the literature. *Medicine (Baltimore).* 1977;56:457-473.
117. Schwartz B, Schuchat A, Oxtoby MJ, et al. Invasive group B streptococcal disease in adults: A population-based study in metropolitan Atlanta. *JAMA.* 1991;266:1112-1114.
118. Tyrrell GJ, Senzilet LD, Spika JS, et al. Invasive disease due to group B streptococcal infection in adults: Results from a Canadian, population-based, active laboratory surveillance study—1996. *J Infect Dis.* 2000;182:168-173.
119. Jackson LA, Hilsdon R, Farley MM, et al. Risk factors for group B streptococcal disease in adults. *Ann Intern Med.* 1995;123:415-420.
120. Edwards MS, Baker CJ. Group B streptococcal infections in elderly adults. *Clin Infect Dis.* 2005;41:839-847.
121. Bayer AS, Chow AW, Anthony BF, et al. Serious infections in adults due to group B streptococci. *Am J Med.* 1976;61:498-503.
122. Colford JM Jr, Mohle-Boetani J, Vosti KL. Group B streptococcal bacteremia in adults: Five years' experience and a review of the literature. *Medicine.* 1995;74:176-190.
123. Blancas D, Santin M, Olmo M, et al. Group B streptococcal disease in nonpregnant adults: Incidence, clinical characteristics, and outcome. *Eur J Clin Microbiol Infect Dis.* 2004;23:168-173.
124. Harrison LH, Ali A, Dwyer DM, et al. Relapsing invasive group B streptococcal infection in adults. *Ann Intern Med.* 1995;123:421-427.
125. Gibbs RS, Roberts DJ. Case records of the Massachusetts General Hospital. Case 27-2007: A 30-year-old pregnant woman with intrauterine fetal death. *N Engl J Med.* 2007;357:918-925.
126. Minkoff HL, Sierra MF, Pringle GF, et al. Vaginal colonization with group B beta-hemolytic streptococcus as a risk factor for post-cesarean section febrile morbidity. *Am J Obstet Gynecol.* 1982;142:992-995.
127. Gibbs RS, Blanco JD. Streptococcal infections in pregnancy: A study of 48 bacteremias. *Am J Obstet Gynecol.* 1981;140:405-411.
128. Duff P. Pathophysiology and management of postcesarean endomyometritis. *Obstet Gynecol.* 1986;67:269-276.
129. Maniatis AN, Palermos J, Kantzanou M, et al. *Streptococcus agalactiae*: A vaginal pathogen? *J Med Microbiol.* 1996;44:199-202.
130. Boyle D, Smith JR. Group B streptococcal vulvovaginitis. *J R Soc Med.* 1997;90:298-299.
131. Verghese A, Berk SL, Boelen LJ, et al. Group B streptococcal pneumonia in the elderly. *Arch Intern Med.* 1982;142:1642-1645.
132. George AL Jr, Savage AM. Fatal group B streptococcal empyema in an adult. *South Med J.* 1987;80:1436-1438.
133. Gallagher PG, Watanakunakorn C. Group B streptococcal endocarditis: Report of seven cases and review of the literature, 1962-1985. *Rev Infect Dis.* 1986;8:175-188.
134. Sambola A, Miro JM, Tornos MP, et al. *Streptococcus agalactiae* infective endocarditis: Analysis of 30 cases and review of the literature, 1962-1998. *Clin Infect Dis.* 2002;34:1576-1584.
135. Watanakunakorn C, Habte-Gabr E. Group B streptococcal endocarditis of tricuspid valve. *Chest.* 1991;100:569-571.
136. Pringle SD, McCartney AC, Marshall DAS, et al. Infective endocarditis caused by *Streptococcus agalactiae*. *Int J Cardiol.* 1989;24:179-183.
137. Scully BE, Spriggs D, Neu HC. *Streptococcus agalactiae* (group B) endocarditis: a description of twelve cases and review of the literature. *Infection.* 1987;15:169-176.
138. Nolla JM, Gómez-Vaquero C, Corbella X, et al. Group B streptococcus *(Streptococcus agalactiae)* pyogenic arthritis in nonpregnant adults. *Medicine.* 2003;82:119-128.
139. Small CB, Slater LN, Lowy FD, et al. Group B streptococcal arthritis in adults. *Am J Med.* 1984;76:367-375.
140. Pischel KD, Weisman MH, Cone RO. Unique features of group B streptococcal arthritis in adults. *Arch Intern Med.* 1985;145:97-102.
141. García-Lechuz JM, Bachiller P, Vasallo FJ, et al. Group B streptococcal osteomyelitis in adults. *Medicine.* 1999;78:191-199.
142. McCarty JM, Haber J. Group B streptococcal soft tissue infections beyond the neonatal period. *West J Med.* 1987;147:558-560.
143. Riefler J III, Molavi A, Schwartz D, et al. Necrotizing fasciitis in adults due to group B streptococcus. *Arch Intern Med.* 1988;148:727-729.
144. Sutton GP, Smirz LR, Clark DH, et al. Group B streptococcal necrotizing fasciitis arising from an episiotomy. *Obstet Gynecol.* 1985;66:733-736.
145. Tang WM, Ho PL, Yau WP, et al. Report of 2 fatal cases of adult necrotizing fasciitis and toxic shock syndrome caused by *Streptococcus agalactiae*. *Clin Infect Dis.* 2000;31:e15-e17.
146. Harburg TD, Leonard HA, Kimbrough RC III, et al. Group B streptococcal meningitis appearing as acute deafness in an adult. *Arch Neurol.* 1984;41:214-216.
147. Sepkowitz KA, Kasemsri T, Brown AE, et al. Meningitis due to β-hemolytic non-A, non-D streptococci among adults at a cancer hospital: Report of four cases and review. *Clin Infect Dis.* 1992;14:92-97.
148. Vartian CV, Septimus EJ. Meningitis caused by group B streptococcus in association with cerebrospinal rhinorrhea. *Clin Infect Dis.* 1992;14:1261-1262.
149. Dunne DW, Quagliarello V. Group B streptococcal meningitis in adults. *Medicine.* 1993;72:1-10.
150. Domingo P, Barquet N, Alvarez M, et al. Group B streptococcal meningitis in adults: Report of twelve cases and review. *Clin Infect Dis.* 1997;25:1180-1187.
151. Guerin JM, Leibinger F, Mofredj A, et al. Streptococcus B meningitis in post-partum. *J Infect.* 1997;34:151-153.
152. Farber BP, Weinbaum DL, Dummer JS. Metastatic bacterial endophthalmitis. *Arch Intern Med.* 1985;145:62-64.
153. Ormerod LD, Paton BG. Severe group B streptococcal eye infections in adults. *J Infect.* 1989;18:29-34.
154. Muñoz P, Coque T, Rodriguez-Creixems M, et al. Group B streptococcus: A cause of urinary tract infection in nonpregnant adults. *Clin Infect Dis.* 1992;14:492-496.
155. Lefevre J-C, Lepargneur J-P, Bauriand R, et al. Clinical and microbiologic features of urethritis in men in Toulouse, France. *Sex Transm Dis.* 1991;18:76-79.
156. Weiss RL, Matsen JM. Group B streptococcal breast abscess. *Arch Pathol Lab Med.* 1987;111:74-75.
157. Ridgeway NA, Perlman PE, Verghese A. Epiglottic abscess due to group B streptococcus. *Ann Otol Rhinol Laryngol.* 1984;93:277-278.
158. Kane JM, Jackson K, Conway JH. Maternal postpartum group B beta-hemolytic streptococcus ventriculoperitoneal shunt infection. *Arch Gynecol Obstet.* 2004;269:139-141.
159. Burnet NG, Wilkinson RC, Evans DS. Mycotic aneurysm caused by group B streptococcus: A cautionary tale of management problems and a rare organism. *Br J Clin Pract.* 1990;44:372-374.
160. Baddour LM, Cox JW Jr. Group B streptococcal infection of a pacemaker wire following sigmoidoscopy. *Clin Infect Dis.* 1992;15:1069.
161. Begley JS, Barnes RC. Group B streptococcus toxic shock-like syndrome in a healthy woman: a case report. *J Reprod Med.* 2007;52:323-325.
162. Raz R, Raichman N, Flatau E. Group B streptococcal bacteremia in a normal splenectomized adult. *Isr J Med Sci.* 1987;23:920-921.
163. Stampfer MJ, Ullman RF, Sacks-Berg A, et al. Group B streptococcal bacteremia after cardiac catheterization. *Crit Care Med.* 1987;15:625-626.
164. O'Mahony D, Hyland CM. Group B streptococcal infection as a pyrexia of unknown origin. *Isr J Med Sci.* 1989;158:233.
165. Wessels MR, Kasper DL, Johnson KD, et al. Antibody responses in invasive group B streptococcal infection in adults. *J Infect Dis.* 1998;178:569-572.
166. Baker CJ. Inadequacy of rapid immunoassays for intrapartum detection of group B streptococcal carriers. *Obstet Gynecol.* 1996;88:51-55.
167. Bergeron MG, Ke D, Ménard C, et al. Rapid detection of group B streptococci in pregnant women at delivery. *N Engl J Med.* 2000;343:175-179.
168. Edwards RK, Novak-Weekley SM, Koty PP, et al. Rapid group B streptococci screening using a real-time polymerase chain reaction assay. *Obstet Gynecol.* 2008;111:1335-1341.
169. Davies HD, Miller MA, Faro S, et al. Multicenter study of a rapid molecular-based assay for the diagnosis of group B *Streptococcus* colonization in pregnant women. *Clin Infect Dis.* 2004;39:1129-1135.
170. Fernandez M, Hickman ME, Baker CJ. Antimicrobial susceptibilities of group B streptococci isolated between 1992 and 1996 from patients with bacteremia or meningitis. *Antimicrob Agents Chemother.* 1998;42:1517-1519.
171. Kimura K, Suzuki S, Wachino J, et al. First molecular characterization of group B streptococci with reduced penicillin susceptibility. *Antimicrob Agents Chemother.* 2008;52:2890-2897.
172. Wehbeh W, Rojas-Diaz R, Li X, et al. Fluoroquinolone-resistant *Streptococcus agalactiae*: Epidemiology and mechanism of resistance. *Antimicrob Agents Chemother.* 2005;49:2495-2497.
173. Borchardt SM, DeBusscher JH, Tallman PA, et al. Frequency of antimicrobial resistance among invasive and colonizing group B streptococcal isolates. *BMC Infect Dis.* 2006;6:57-64.
174. Murdoch DR, Reller LB. Antimicrobial susceptibilities of group B streptococci isolated from patients with invasive disease: 10-year perspective. *Antimicrob Agents Chemother.* 2001;45:3623-3624.
175. Lin F-YC, Azimi PH, Weisman LE, et al. Antibiotic susceptibility profiles for group B streptococci isolated from neonates, 1995-1998. *Clin Infect Dis.* 2000;31:76-79.
176. Aracil B, Miñambres M, Oteo J, et al. Susceptibility of strains of *Streptococcus agalactiae* to macrolides and lincosamides, phenotype patterns and resistance genes. *Clin Microbiol Infect.* 2002;8:745-748.
177. Puopolo KM, Klinzing DC, Lin MP, et al. A composite transposon associated with erythromycin and clindamycin resistance in group B *Streptococcus*. *J Med Microbiol.* 2007;56:947-955.
178. Berkowitz K, Regan JA, Greenberg E. Antibiotic resistance patterns of group B streptococci in pregnant women. *J Clin Microbiol.* 1990;28:5-7.
179. Boyer KM, Gotoff SP. Prevention of early-onset neonatal group B streptococcal disease with selective intrapartum chemoprophylaxis. *N Engl J Med.* 1986;314:1665-1669.
180. American College of Obstetricians and Gynecologists. Group B streptococcal infections in pregnancy. *ACOG Tech Bull.* 1992;170:1-5.
181. Committee on Infectious Diseases and Committee on Fetus and Newborn. Guidelines for prevention of group B streptococcal (GBS) infection by chemoprophylaxis. *Pediatrics.* 1992;90:775-778.
182. Centers for Disease Control. Prevention of perinatal group B streptococcal disease: A public health perspective. *MMWR Morb Mortal Wkly Rep.* 1996;45:1-24.
183. Schrag SJ, Zell ER, Lynfield R, et al. A population-based comparison of strategies to prevent early-onset group B streptococcal disease in neonates. *N Engl J Med.* 2002;347:233-239.
184. Centers for Disease Control and Prevention. Prevention of perinatal group B streptococcal disease. *MMWR Recomm Rep.* 2002;51(RR-11):1-22.
185. American College of Obstetricians and Gynecologists. Committee on Practice Bulletins—Obstetrics. ACOG Practice Bulletin No. 80: Premature rupture of membranes. Clinical management guidelines for obstetrician-gynccologists. *Obstet Gynecol.* 2007;109:1007-1019.
186. Schrag SS, Stoll BJ. Early-onset neonatal sepsis in the era of widespread intrapartum chemoprophylaxis. *Pediatr Infect Dis J.* 2006;25:939-940.
187. Matteson KA, Lievense SP, Catanzaro B, et al. Intrapartum group B streptococci prophylaxis in patients reporting a penicillin allergy. *Obstet Gynecol.* 2008;111:356-364.
188. American Academy of Pediatrics. Group B streptococcal infections. In: Pickering LK, Baker CJ, Long SS, et al., eds. *Red Book 2006: Report of the Committee on Infectious Diseases.* 27th ed. Elk Grove Village, IL: American Academy of Pediatrics; 2006:620-627.
189. Lin FY, Weisman LE, Azimi PH, et al. Level of maternal IgG anti-group B streptococcus type III antibody correlated with protection of neonates against early-onset disease caused by this pathogen. *J Infect Dis.* 2004;190:928-934.
190. Baker CJ, Edwards MS, Kasper DL. Immunogenicity of polysaccharides from type III, group B streptococcus. *J Clin Invest.* 1978;61:1107-1110.
191. Eisenstein TK, DeCuenick BJ, Resavy D, et al. Quantitative determination in human sera of vaccine-induced antibody to type-specific polysaccharides of group B streptococci using an enzyme-linked immunosorbent assay. *J Infect Dis.* 1983;147:847-856.
192. Baker CJ, Kasper DL. Group B streptococcal vaccines. *Rev Infect Dis.* 1985;4:458-467.
193. Baker CJ, Rench MA, Edwards MS, et al. Immunization of pregnant women with a polysaccharide vaccine. *N Engl J Med.* 1988;319:1180-1185.
194. Givner LB, Baker CJ. Pooled human IgG hyperimmune for type III group B streptococci: Evaluation against multiple strains in vitro and in experimental disease. *J Infect Dis.* 1991;163:1141-1145.
195. Wessels MR, Paoletti LC, Kasper DL, et al. Immunogenicity in animals of a polysaccharide-protein conjugate vaccine against type III group B streptococcus. *J Clin Invest.* 1990;86:1428-1433.
196. Paoletti LC, Kasper DL, Michon F, et al. An oligosaccharide-tetanus toxoid conjugate vaccine against type III group B streptococcus. *J Biol Chem.* 1990;265:18278-18283.
197. Madoff LC, Paoletti LC, Tai JY, et al. Maternal immunization of mice with group B streptococcal type III polysaccharide-beta C protein conjugate elicits protective antibody to multiple serotypes. *J Clin Invest.* 1994;94:286-292.
198. Kasper DL, Paoletti LC, Wessels MR, et al. Immune response to type III group B streptococcal polysaccharide–tetanus toxoid conjugate vaccine. *J Clin Invest.* 1996;98:2308-2314.
199. Wessels MR, Paoletti LC, Rodewald AK, et al. Stimulation of protective antibodies against type Ia and Ib group B streptococci by a type Ia polysaccharide–tetanus toxoid conjugate vaccine. *Infect Immun.* 1993;61:4760-4766.
200. Paoletti LC, Wessels MR, Michon F, et al. Group B streptococcus type II polysaccharide–tetanus toxoid conjugate vaccine. *Infect Immun.* 1992;60:4009-4014.
201. Wessels MR, Paoletti LC, Pinel J, et al. Immunogenicity and protective activity in animals of a type V group B streptococcal polysaccharide–tetanus toxoid conjugate vaccine. *J Infect Dis.* 1995;171:879-884.
202. Baker CJ, Paoletti LC, Wessels MR, et al. Safety and immunogenicity of capsular polysaccharide–tetanus toxoid conjugate vaccines for group B streptococcal types Ia and Ib. *J Infect Dis.* 1999;179:142-150.
203. Baker CJ, Paoletti LC, Rench MA, et al. Use of capsular polysaccharide-tetanus toxoid conjugate vaccine for type II group B streptococcus in healthy women. *J Infect Dis.* 2000;182:1129-1138.
204. Baker CJ, Rench MA, Ward ME, et al. Immune response of healthy women to two different type V group B streptococcal capsular polysaccharide-protein conjugate vaccines. *J Infect Dis.* 2004;189:1103.
205. Palazzi DL, Rench MA, Paoletti LC, et al. Group B streptococcal (GBS) type V capsular polysaccharide (CPS)-tetanus toxoid (V-TT) conjugate vaccine (CV) in healthy adults 65 to 85 years of age. *J Infect Dis.* 2004;190:558-564.
206. Baker CJ, Rench MA, McInnes P. Immunization of pregnant women with group B streptococcal type III capsular polysaccha-

ride-tetanus toxoid conjugate vaccine. *Vaccine.* 2003;21:3468-3472.

207. Baker CJ, Rench MA, Fernandez M, et al. Safety and immunogenicity of a bivalent group B streptococcal conjugate vaccine for serotypes II and III. *J Infect Dis.* 2003;188:66-73.

208. Paoletti LC, Wessels MR, Rodewald AK, et al. Neonatal mouse protection against infection with multiple group B streptococcal (GBS) serotypes by maternal immunization with a tetravalent GBS polysaccharide-tetanus toxoid conjugate vaccine. *Infect Immun.* 1994;62:3236-3243.

209. Buccato S, Maione D, Rinaudo CD, et al. Use of *Lactococcus lactis* expressing pili from group B *Streptococcus* as a broad-coverage vaccine against streptococcal disease. *J Infect Dis.* 2006;194:331-340.

210. Margarit I, Rinaudo CD, Galeotti CL, et al. Preventing bacterial infections with pilus-based vaccines: the group B Streptococcus paradigm. *J Infect Dis.* 2009;199:108-115.

211. Yang H-H, Madoff LC, Guttormsen H-K, et al. Recombinant group B *Streptococcus* beta C protein and a variant with the deletion of its immunoglobulin A-binding site are protective mouse maternal vaccines and effective carriers in conjugate vaccines. *Infect Immun.* 2007;75:3455-3461.

212. Larsson C, Lindroth M, Nordin P, et al. Association between low concentrations of antibodies to protein α and Rib and invasive neonatal group B streptococcal infection. *Arch Dis Child Fetal Neonatal Ed.* 2006;91:F403-F408.

203

Viridans Streptococci, Groups C and G Streptococci, and *Gemella* Species

SCOTT W. SINNER | ALLAN R. TUNKEL

Viridans streptococci and the β-hemolytic streptococci constitute a diverse group of organisms with varying environmental niches and pathogenicity. Although these organisms usually reside as commensals in the respiratory and intestinal tracts of animals and humans, they may also invade sterile body sites, resulting in life-threatening diseases. This chapter reviews infections caused by the viridans streptococci, nutritionally variant (deficient) streptococci (NVS, genera *Abiotrophia* and *Granulicatella*), and β-hemolytic streptococci (other than groups A, B, and D) that are associated with human disease. Although the *Streptococcus milleri* group (*S. anginosus, S. intermedius,* and *S. constellatus*) are viridans streptococci, they are discussed in detail elsewhere (see Chapter 204). *Streptococcus iniae, Stomatococcus,* and *Pediococcus* are also discussed in this chapter.

Viridans Group Streptococci

MICROBIOLOGY

Viridans streptococci possess the general characteristics common to all streptococci (see Chapter 197).[1] They are facultatively anaerobic, gram-positive cocci that do not produce catalase or coagulase; on blood agar, their colonies are rarely β-hemolytic. The term *viridans* derives from the Latin word *viridis*, meaning "green." Many species in this group cause partial destruction of erythrocytes, with resultant green discoloration on blood agar (α-hemolysis), whereas others have no effect on blood (γ-hemolysis). Although some isolates react with Lancefield grouping antisera, the species do not conform to specific serogroups, and many isolates are entirely nongroupable. Viridans streptococci can be distinguished from *Streptococcus pneumoniae*, another species producing α-hemolysis on blood agar, by resistance to optochin and lack of bile solubility. They are distinguished from enterococci by their inability to grow in broth containing 6.5% sodium chloride. *Streptococcus bovis*, one of the nonenterococcal group D streptococci, was previously considered a member of the viridans group but has a different habitat and clinical significance (see Chapter 201).

Viridans streptococci are fastidious with respect to their nutritional growth requirements; enriched agars and broths are recommended for optimal recovery from primary cultures. Most strains grow well in conventional blood culture media. On solid agar, viridans streptococci are usually facultatively anaerobic, but some strains are capnophilic and/or microaerophilic. The colonies vary in size and appearance, depending on the composition of the medium and the incubation atmosphere.[1] In broth cultures, streptococci appear as spherical or ovoid cells that form chains or pairs. The organisms are nonmotile and non–spore-forming and ferment carbohydrates with production of acid but not gas.

SPECIES IDENTIFICATION

In the past, terminology applied to the viridans group of streptococci was confusing and inconsistent. When organisms were recovered in clinical laboratories, species designation often sidestepped identification of the isolate in favor of a generic descriptive term such as *nonhemolytic* or *α-hemolytic*. In addition, terms such as *Streptococcus mutans* and *Streptococcus sanguis* were used loosely to refer to groups

of organisms without denoting clear relationships. In the 1970s, two schemes for identification of viridans streptococci were proposed. Colman and Williams suggested classification of the group into five species: *S. milleri, S. mitior, S. mutans, S. salivarius,* and *S. sanguis,* which they termed the *human oral viridans streptococci*.[2] The scheme of Facklam recognized 10 physiologic species: *S. acidominimus, S. mitis, S. morbillorum, S. mutans, S. salivarius, S. sanguis* I and II, *S. uberis,* and two subdivisions of the *S. milleri* group, *S. anginosus-constellatus* and *S. MG-intermedius*.[3] The various species, as defined by these two schemes, were not identical. More recently, molecular approaches, especially application of 16S rRNA gene sequencing,[4] have been applied to define the taxonomy of viridans streptococci based on genetic relatedness. Analyses have resulted in emended descriptions of well-recognized species (e.g., *S. mitis, S. sanguis*), the discovery and description of several new species, and the division of the serotypes of the *S. mutans* group into distinct species. Expanded batteries of phenotypic tests, combined with differences observed between genotypes, have permitted laboratories to identify accurately species for correlation with clinical syndromes. When reviewing older literature pertaining to the viridans group of streptococci, the extensive changes in taxonomy and nomenclature should be taken into consideration.

At present, most clinically significant species of viridans group streptococci can be assigned to one of the following groups (Table 203-1): the *anginosus* group, the *mitis* group, the *mutans* group, the *salivarius* group, and the *sanguinis* group.[4] Some of these species are newly described; others have undergone name changes to comply with rules of nomenclature since publication of prior reviews.[5] All have either been recovered from human clinical specimens or have a potential for causing human disease based on transmission from nonhuman sources. The discovery of new species of viridans streptococci (e.g., *S. sinensis, S. massiliensis*) in recent years has blurred the boundaries of these groups somewhat, because results of various rRNA or DNA sequencing tests have suggested close relationships of these new species to current viridans streptococci that may belong to separate groups.[6,7] Viridans streptococcal species can be distinguished phenotypically by their physiologic and biochemical characteristics, in particular their type of hemolysis on blood agar, result of the Voges-Proskauer reaction, pattern of acid formation from carbohydrates, ability to hydrolyze esculin and arginine, and production of dextran, levan, alkaline phosphatase, hydrogen peroxide, or acetoin (Table 203-2).[1-5,8,9] A simplified scheme, consisting of 14 biochemical tests, has also been proposed.[10] Although rapid automated systems for species identification of streptococci are commercially available, their performance is variable. For some, the databases have not been updated or expanded to include newer species; others require supplemental procedures to ensure that they perform accurately. Conventional biochemical tests remain the most reliable method for identification of these organisms in clinical laboratories,[11] although gene sequence analysis[12] or mass spectroscopy[13] may provide more accurate means for species identification in the future.

S. morbillorum was once considered to be a viridans streptococcus because it failed to produce β-hemolysis on blood agar, lacked distinguishing serogroup antigens, and did not have the biochemical characteristics of enterococci or pneumococci. In Facklam's review of this species, half of the 46 isolates described were associated with serious infections.[3] The organism has been reclassified as the second species

TABLE 203-1	Classification of Viridans Streptococci Other Than S. milleri Group, S. bovis, and S. pneumoniae

Mitis Group	*Salivarius* Group
S. cristatus	S. alactolyticus
S. infantis	S. hyointestinalis
S. mitis	S. infantarius
S. oralis	S. salivarius
S. peroris	S. thermophilus
S. orisratti	S. vestibularis
Mutans Group	**Sanguinis Group**
S. cricetus	S. gordonii
S. downei	S. parasanguinis
S. ferus	S. sanguinis
S. hyovaginalis	
S. macaccae	
S. mutans	
S. ratti	
S. sobrinus	

in the genus *Gemella* (*G. morbillorum*). In the past decade, this genus has grown to six species (*G. bergerie, G. haemolysans, G. morbillorum, G. sanguinis, G. palaticanis,* and *G. cuniculi*). Only the first four listed species have been associated with human infection[14]; the general principles of infection and therapy for these organisms are the same as for the viridans streptococci.

Although NVS were also once thought to be viridans streptococci, they have been shown to form a genetically unrelated group (genera *Abiotrophia* and *Granulicatella;* see later).[15,16]

EPIDEMIOLOGY

Viridans streptococci are an important part of the normal microbial flora of humans and animals. They are indigenous to the upper respiratory tract, the female genital tract, and all regions of the gastrointestinal tract, but are most prevalent in the oral cavity.[1] On average, streptococci represent 28% to 45% of the total culturable flora from assorted regions in the oral cavity, although not in uniform distribution. Gibbons and van Houte have demonstrated that this nonuniform distribution of viridans streptococcal species is determined by their selective adherence to the various oral tissues.[17] Using the emended descriptions of viridans species, the ecology of strains in the oral cavity and oropharynx can now be described as follows: the buccal mucosa is associated with *S. sanguis* and *S. mitis;* the dorsum of the tongue with *S. mitis* and *S. salivarius;* initial dental plaque with *S. sanguis, S. mitis,* and *S. oralis;* mature supragingival plaque with *S. gordonii;* and subgingival plaque with *S. anginosus.*[18]

In healthy persons, adherence of viridans streptococci may provide "colonization resistance" within the oral cavity to prevent establish-

ment of more pathogenic bacteria. Fibronectin, a complex glycoprotein found on the surface of oral epithelial cells, selectively promotes attachment of a number of gram-positive cocci. If fibronectin is lost or diminished, as occurs in chronically ill or hospitalized patients, adherence of organisms such as *Pseudomonas aeruginosa* to oral epithelial cells is increased. Because oropharyngeal colonization with enteric gram-negative bacilli often precedes invasion (e.g., development of gram-negative bacillary pneumonia), selective adherence of viridans streptococci in the oral cavity can be viewed as a protective mechanism for the host.

PATHOGENICITY

Viridans streptococci are considered to be bacteria of low virulence, and do not possess the traditional virulence factors that characterize more pathogenic bacteria. They are not known to produce endotoxin or secrete exotoxins, and they are fully susceptible to lysis by serum and lysosomal enzymes. Although some species make proteolytic enzymes, these enzymes are not clearly related to the pathogenesis of infection. Some strains have been shown to invade and kill human endothelial cells in vitro.[19] This cytotoxicity is mediated by peroxidogenesis and acidogenesis but not by production of protein exotoxins.

The pathogenicity of viridans group streptococci is best exemplified by their ability to produce endocarditis. Extracellular dextran produced by these bacteria plays an important role in adherence and propagation of the organisms on cardiac valves. Clinical observations have noted that after bacteremia caused by dextran-producing streptococci, there is a higher incidence of infective endocarditis than when bacteremia is caused by non–dextran-producing streptococci. Investigators have also shown that the amount of dextran produced by a streptococcal strain correlates with its ability to adhere to cardiac valves in vitro and to induce infective endocarditis in experimental animal models. Pretreatment with dextranase abolishes the differences in pathogenicity of various strains. In addition, production of dextran by the pathogen also mediates the response to antimicrobial therapy. Endocarditis caused by dextran-producing strains is more resistant to penicillin treatment and yields larger vegetations than infection caused by dextran-negative strains. Treatment of experimental endocarditis with penicillin and dextranase results in higher rates of valve sterilization than treatment with penicillin alone. Another bacterial factor that might be related to the pathogenesis of endocarditis is FimA. This surface-associated protein of *S. parasanguinis* has been associated with initial colonization of damaged heart tissue in an endocarditis model. Immunization with recombinant FimA has resulted in antibody-mediated inhibition of bacterial adherence and protection from endocarditis in an animal model.[20]

TABLE 203-2	Biochemical Characteristics for Differentiation of Selected Viridans Streptococci

Organism	Pattern of Hemolysis	Voges-Proskauer	Hydrolysis of Esculin	Hydrolysis of Arginine	Hydrolysis of H₂O₂	Acid Production from Mannitol	Acid Production from Sorbitol	Acid Production from Lactose	Acid Production from Trehalose	Acid Production from Inulin	Acid Production from Raffinose	Production of Alkaline Phosphatase	Production of Dextran	Production of Levan
Streptococcus mutans	α, β, γ	+	+	−	−	+	+	+	+	+	+	−	+	−
S. mitis	α	−	−	−	+	−	−	+	v	−	v	v	−	−
S. oralis	α	−	−	−	+	−	−	+	v	−	v	+	v	−
S. sanguinis	α	−	v	+	+	−	v	+	+	+	v	−	+	−
S. gordonii	α	−	+	+	+	−	−	+	+	+	v	+	+	−
S. cristatus	α	−	−	v	+	−	−	v	+	−	−	−	v	na
S. salivarius	α	+	+	−	−	−	−	v	v	v	+	v	−	+
S. vestibularis	α	v	v	−	+	−	−	v	v	−	−	v	−	−
S. parasanguinis	α	−	v	+	+	−	−	+	v	−	+	+	−	−
Gemella morbillorum	α, γ	na	−	−	na	−	−	−	−	−	−	na	−	na

+, 85% or more of strains positive; −, 85% or more of strains negative; na, not available; v, variable.

Fibronectin, which is secreted by endothelial cells, platelets, and fibroblasts in response to vascular injury, is one possible molecule that mediates adherence of streptococci to cardiac valves. It constitutes about 4% of the mass of a blood clot and has been found on the surfaces of traumatized rabbit valves. Microorganisms more likely to cause endocarditis bind significantly better to fibronectin in vitro than non–endocarditis-producing strains. Lipoteichoic acid appears to be the fibronectin adhesin on streptococci. Exposure of various streptococci to subinhibitory concentrations of antibiotics results in loss of surface lipoteichoic acid and a subsequent decrease in ability to produce endocarditis.[21] Once adherent to the surface of the valve, viridans streptococci induce propagation of the infected vegetation by stimulating production of tissue factor from the underlying valvular tissue and by directly triggering further platelet aggregation. The ability of viridans streptococci to induce release of interleukin-1β (IL-1β) from monocytes has also been shown to be a potential facilitator of deposition of bacteria in fibrin clots by increasing expression of adhesion molecules in endothelial cells.[22]

In addition to causing infective endocarditis, certain species of viridans streptococci, notably *S. mutans,* have a strong association with the development of dental caries. The organism is acquired early in life through horizontal and vertical transmission from mother to infant.[23] Laboratory experiments have shown that caries develop in germ-free animals after infection with *S. mutans.* However, colonization of dental surfaces and production of caries occurs only in the presence of dietary sucrose. The organism uses sucrose to synthesize a number of extracellular polysaccharides, including glucans, that serve to bind it to dental enamel and to other bacteria. The high cariogenic potential of *S. mutans* is thought to be related to its ability to adhere in large masses on teeth, to produce high concentrations of acid from the fermentation of dietary sugars, and then to tolerate this acidic environment. *S. sobrinus,* another cariogenic organism, has been shown to produce an enolase that suppresses a primary immune response against T-cell–dependent antigens and to stimulate production of IL-10, an anti-inflammatory cytokine. These observations suggest that this organism itself can act in ways to interfere with the specific host immune response to its infection.[24]

Occasionally, viridans streptococci produce bacteremia and septic shock in neutropenic patients. The pathogenesis of viridans streptococcal shock appears to be not unlike that of gram-negative septic shock. In vitro studies have shown that clinical isolates of viridans streptococci from shock patients were able to induce tumor necrosis factor-α (TNF-α) in murine macrophages. Production of TNF-α was dose-dependent and followed kinetics similar to that of *Escherichia coli* isolates. In a study of patients with neutropenia and overwhelming infection, serum levels of TNF-α and IL-6 were found to be increased, regardless of whether shock was caused by viridans streptococci or gram-negative bacilli.[25]

CLINICAL MANIFESTATIONS AND THERAPY

Endocarditis

In the preantibiotic era, viridans streptococci accounted for approximately 75% of cases of infective endocarditis. At the present time, their relative frequency in association with infective endocarditis has declined to as low as 20%.[26] This change in epidemiology reflects an increase in the number of patients acquiring staphylococcal endocarditis in association with injection drug use or prosthetic valves, rather than a decrease in the overall incidence of streptococcal endocarditis. Many different viridans streptococcal species have been reported to cause endocarditis, and the clinical manifestations and outcomes associated with the various species causing endocarditis appear to be similar.

Viridans streptococci have been more frequently the cause of endocarditis in patients known to have heart disease (55%) than in those not previously known to have heart disease (29%).[27] In the past, rheumatic and congenital heart disease were the major predisposing factors, accounting for 37% to 76% and 6% to 24% of endocarditis cases,

respectively. With the declining incidence of rheumatic fever, mitral valve prolapse (29%) and degenerative valvular lesions (21%) have assumed a more prominent role.[28] Most cases of viridans streptococcal endocarditis are thought to arise from organisms within the oral cavity, but cases of endocarditis related to such diverse processes as colon cancer[29] and navel piercing[30] have also been described. Among cases of infective endocarditis in injection drug users, viridans streptococci account for a small proportion (6%). In patients with prosthetic valves, the incidence of streptococcal infective endocarditis increases with greater periods of time since valve surgery. In early disease (less than 60 days since valve replacement), only 7% of infections are caused by streptococci; the frequency increases to 30% in patients in whom infection develops 1 year or more after surgery.[31]

Viridans streptococcal endocarditis typically has an insidious onset followed by a subacute but progressive course. In most patients, symptoms develop within 2 weeks of presumed onset; however, it is often 5 weeks or more from the time of initial symptoms until the diagnosis is established. Fever, the single most common finding in endocarditis, is present in almost all patients except those who have preexisting renal failure, congestive heart failure, or concomitant antibiotic use. Constitutional symptoms such as fatigue, anorexia, weight loss, and malaise often accompany the fever. Cardiac murmurs are detected in more than 90% of patients with streptococcal endocarditis, and splenomegaly is noted in up to half of cases. Manifestations of circulating immune complexes such as Osler's nodes, petechiae, and splinter hemorrhages may also occur (28% of cases).[32]

The critical element for diagnosis of infective endocarditis is demonstration of continuous bacteremia. With viridans streptococci, the bacteremia is often low grade (1 to 30 colony-forming units (CFU)/mL of blood). In the absence of recent antimicrobial therapy, 96% of one set of blood cultures and 98% of two sets of blood cultures yield the pathogen. For those patients in whom a microbiologic cause cannot be made by blood cultures (usually because of recent use of antibiotics), nucleic acid amplification tests, such as polymerase chain reaction (PCR) assay and sequencing of 16S ribosomal RNA (rRNA) from tissue samples, may have a role.[33,34] Echocardiography is used as a confirmatory test in patients with blood cultures positive for viridans streptococci; 39% to 72% of patients with endocarditis have vegetations identified on a two-dimensional echocardiogram.[35] Echocardiography can also be used to identify valvular dysfunction, hemodynamic complications, and myocardial abscesses, findings that may indicate the need for surgical intervention. Whether echocardiography provides prognostic information about the risk of systemic emboli is a controversial issue.[36]

Recommended regimens for treatment of streptococcal endocarditis are based largely on clinical observations and studies of antibiotic efficacy in experimental animal models of endocarditis.[37] In an experimental rabbit model, prolonged penicillin therapy adequately sterilized vegetations, but addition of streptomycin or gentamicin led to more rapid eradication of the pathogen.[38,39] Penicillin G remains the mainstay of therapy for viridans streptococcal endocarditis. As with other types of infective endocarditis, the antibiotic is administered in high doses for extended periods, usually 4 weeks. For sensitive organisms, the duration of penicillin therapy can be shortened if given in combination with an aminoglycoside, but this strategy does add the potential for nephrotoxicity and ototoxicity. Although most clinical experience with two-drug regimens has been with streptomycin plus penicillin, gentamicin is now considered interchangeable with streptomycin in the combination, and has become the preferred agent in clinical practice because of the ability to measure serum gentamicin concentrations readily and the convenience of intravenous administration.

Antibiotic regimens that are currently recommended by the American Heart Association are summarized in Table 203-3.[40] For endocarditis caused by streptococcal strains that are highly susceptible to penicillin (minimal inhibitory concentration [MIC] ≤ 0.12 μg/mL), four β-lactam–based regimens are endorsed. All can be expected to achieve very high bacteriologic cure rates. In a review of endocarditis

TABLE 203-3	Antimicrobial Therapy for Adult Native Valve Infective Endocarditis Caused by Viridans and Nutritionally Variant Streptococci		
Organism (Penicillin MIC)	**Antibiotic Regimen Options**	**Dosage and Route[†*]**	**Duration (wk)**
Penicillin-susceptible viridans streptococci and *S. bovis* (≤0.12 μg/mL)	1. Aqueous crystalline penicillin G sodium (PCN)	12-18 million U IV daily, continuously or in four or six equally divided doses	4
	2. Ceftriaxone sodium	2 g IV, IM daily in one dose	4
	3. PCN	As above	2
	plus		
	gentamicin sulfate	3 mg/kg IV/IM daily in one dose	2
	4. Ceftriaxone	As above	2
	plus		
	gentamicin	As above	2
	5. Vancomycin hydrochloride (if unable to tolerate PCN or ceftriaxone)	30 mg/kg IV daily, divided in two equal doses, not to exceed 2 g daily unless serum concentrations are inappropriately low	4
Relatively resistant viridans streptococci and *S. bovis* (>0.12 but ≤0.5 μg/mL)	1. PCN	As above, except 24 million units of penicillin G daily	4
	plus		
	gentamicin	As above	2
	2. Ceftriaxone	As above	4
	plus		
	gentamicin	As above	2
	3. Vancomycin	As above	4
Resistant viridans streptococci and *S. bovis* (>0.5 μg/mL), *Abiotrophia defectiva*, *Granulicatella* spp. and *Gemella* spp.	1. PCN	As above, except 18-30 million units penicillin G daily	4-6[†]
	plus		
	gentamicin	3 mg/kg daily in three equally divided doses	4-6
	2. Ampicillin sodium	12 g IV daily in six equally divided doses	4-6
	plus		
	gentamicin	3 mg/kg daily in three equally divided doses	4-6
	3. Vancomycin	As above	6

*Doses should be adjusted according to renal function and, for gentamicin and vancomycin, by serum concentrations.
[†]4-wk therapy recommended for patients with symptoms of illness ≤3 mo; 6-week therapy recommended for patients with symptoms >3 mo.
MIC, minimal inhibitory concentration; IM, intramuscularly; IV, intravenously.
Adapted from Baddour LM, Wilson WR, Bayer AS, et al. Infective endocarditis: Diagnosis, antimicrobial therapy, and management of complications: A statement for healthcare professionals from the Committee on Rheumatic Fever, Endocarditis, and Kawasaki Disease, Council on Cardiovascular Disease in the Young, and the Councils on Clinical Cardiology, Stroke, and Cardiovascular Surgery and Anesthesia, American Heart Association: Endorsed by the Infectious Diseases Society of America. *Circulation.* 2005;111:e394-e433.

treatment outcomes, Wilson and Geraci found a relapse rate of 0.6% (1 in 154) for patients receiving 4 weeks of penicillin alone, and 2.0% (6 in 295) for those treated with a 2-week course of penicillin plus streptomycin.[41] Ceftriaxone shows similar efficacy,[42] with no cases of microbiologic failure or relapse reported in one noncomparative trial (although 10 of the 55 patients ultimately required valve replacement for congestive heart failure or recurrent embolization).[43] Another study compared the efficacy of a daily 2-g dose of ceftriaxone for 4 weeks with that of a regimen of 2 weeks of ceftriaxone followed by 2 weeks of oral amoxicillin (1 g four times daily), and reported relapse in only 1 of 30 patients.[44] However, a regimen that includes oral therapy cannot yet be endorsed for routine use.

Because relapse is uncommon, selection of a specific antimicrobial regimen should be individualized for each patient. The 2-week regimen is most appropriate for uncomplicated cases of endocarditis occurring in patients at low risk for aminoglycoside toxicity. It is not indicated for patients with extracardiac foci of infection or intracardiac abscess. Courses of treatment longer than 4 weeks may be preferred for patients with protracted illness (symptoms lasting longer than 3 months), aortic insufficiency, moderate to severe congestive heart failure, or who have had a documented relapse.[45] In patients whose infection involves prosthetic valves or other prosthetic material, a 6-week regimen of penicillin or ceftriaxone is recommended, together with gentamicin for at least the first 2 weeks.[40]

Although endocarditis caused by penicillin-resistant viridans streptococci is uncommon,[46] patients infected with such strains may be at higher risk of relapse after antimicrobial therapy. For relatively resistant strains (penicillin MIC 0.12 to ≤ 0.5 μg/mL), gentamicin should be given for the first 2 weeks of a 4-week course of β-lactam therapy

(see Table 203-3). For resistant strains (those requiring >0.5 μg/mL of penicillin for inhibition), treatment is the same as for enterococci, and consists of penicillin plus gentamicin for a full 4 to 6 weeks. This regimen also applies to endocarditis caused by *Abiotrophia*, *Granulicatella*, and *Gemella* species. For any regimens containing an aminoglycoside, serum aminoglycoside concentrations should be monitored during therapy to avoid toxicity.

For patients who have immediate-type hypersensitivity to penicillin, vancomycin is an appropriate alternate regimen. Addition of an aminoglycoside is not required, regardless of whether or not the isolate is resistant to penicillin. Cephalosporins are not indicated in cases in which the pathogen is highly resistant to penicillin (MIC > 0.5 μg/mL).

Bacteremia

Viridans streptococci account for 2.6% of positive blood cultures reported from clinical laboratories. Of these, only 21% are thought to be clinically significant.[47] The remainder have been attributed to contamination, despite the fact that viridans streptococci are not typically part of the normal skin flora. In many cases, failure to ascribe clinical significance to these organisms in blood cultures occurs because of their low virulence and the transient nature of the positive cultures. In contrast, prolonged bacteremia (without endocarditis) has emerged as a genuine problem in patients undergoing cancer chemotherapy, usually occurring in association with aggressive cytoreductive therapy for acute leukemia or allogeneic bone marrow transplantation, especially after high-dose cytosine arabinoside treatment.[48] In some centers, viridans streptococci are now a leading cause of bacteremia in febrile neutropenic patients. At the M.D. Anderson Cancer Center in Houston, the incidence of streptococcal bacteremia increased from 1 case/10,000 admissions in 1972 to 47 cases/10,000 in 1989.[49] In another study, viridans streptococci were recovered from the blood in 35 (17.5%) of 200 consecutive recipients of autologous stem cell transplants, at a median of 6 days after the procedure.[50] Primary viridans streptococcal bacteremia has also been suggested to occur with increased frequency in patients with end-stage liver disease.[51]

In one cancer study in which patients with other gram-positive bacteremias served as controls, the risk of streptococcal infection was reported to increase with profound neutropenia, prophylactic administration of trimethoprim-sulfamethoxazole or a fluoroquinolone, and use of antacids or histamine type 2 (H2) receptor antagonists.[49] Another risk factor strongly implicated is the presence of mucositis.[48] In one noncomparative study of 32 patients, 78% had oral inflammation or ulceration at the time of their infection.[52] Similarly, Bostrom and Weisdorf reported an association of viridans streptococcal bacteremia with increased radiation dose to the oral cavity,[53] and Ringden and colleagues described an association with herpes simplex infection.[54] In the latter study, use of prophylactic acyclovir decreased the frequency of bacteremia after allogeneic bone marrow transplantation. The presence of an indwelling venous catheter poses an additional risk factor for streptococcal bacteremia in neutropenic patients.

In the setting of malignancy, bacteremia with viridans streptococci is more common in children than in adults, typically developing within 15 days of chemotherapy or bone marrow transplantation at the time of profound neutropenia. In a series of 123 patients, 73% presented with fever alone, whereas 27% also had evidence of organ dysfunction.[55] A fulminant shock syndrome characterized by hypotension, rash, palmar desquamation, and adult respiratory distress syndrome has been described in approximately 25% of patients.[49,56] *S. mitis* was the cause in most such cases.[57] Very few cases of viridans streptococcal bacteremia in immunocompromised patients have led to clinically apparent endocarditis.

Despite early initiation of broad-spectrum antibiotics, the mortality rate for viridans streptococcal bacteremia in immunocompromised patients is approximately 6% to 12%.[49,52,55] Fatal cases have been characterized by early, fulminant cardiovascular collapse or secondary central nervous system involvement. In most, the isolates were susceptible in vitro to the selected empiric antimicrobial regimen, usually a β-lactam plus an aminoglycoside. Lack of treatment efficacy is associated with the poor clinical status of patients at the time of antibiotic initiation. Because penicillin susceptibility cannot be assumed, some authorities recommend use of vancomycin for empiric treatment of neutropenic patients in whom streptococcal septicemia is suspected.[57]

Use of antimicrobial agents to prevent streptococcal bacteremia is controversial. At one cancer institute, the incidence of streptococcal bacteremia decreased from 11.5% in 1989 to 2.5% in 1995 after penicillin was introduced for prophylaxis in neutropenic patients.[58] Similarly, in a sequential cohort study of 289 bone marrow transplant recipients, both vancomycin and β-lactam prophylaxis were shown to decrease the incidence of gram-positive bacteremia compared with controls; however, no differences in mortality could be demonstrated.[59] In contrast, Bilgrami and co-workers have found that prophylactic use of ampicillin fails to decrease the incidence of viridans streptococcal sepsis in bone marrow transplant recipients.[50] Regardless of efficacy, a consequence of prophylactic use of β-lactam antibiotics in many of these studies was emergence of resistance. The proportion of penicillin-resistant viridans streptococcal bacteremias increased from 0% in 1989, before any prophylaxis was given to marrow transplant recipients, to 16% in 1991, when quinolones were used for prophylaxis, to 44% when penicillin was added to the quinolones.[58] Fatality rates among neutropenic patients with bacteremia caused by penicillin-resistant viridans streptococci have been shown to be higher than for penicillin-susceptible strains.[48,58,60] Concerns over hypersensitivity reactions and selection of resistant strains should preclude routine use of antibiotic prophylaxis for these infections, except in centers with high infection rates.

Meningitis

Despite the frequency with which viridans streptococci cause bacteremia, they are an uncommon cause of meningitis, accounting for only 0.3% to 5% of culture-proven cases.[61,62] Although species designation was often not provided in the early literature, more recent reports have suggested that *S. salivarius* is most commonly associated with meningitis.[63,64] Infections with *S. mitis* and *S. sanguinis* have also been described.[65,66] Infections occur in patients of all ages, including neonates. Clinical manifestations are typical of acute pyogenic meningitis with signs of meningeal irritation, neurologic deficits, seizures, and altered sensorium.

The source of infection for most cases of viridans streptococcal meningitis is endogenous flora. In instances of neonatal meningitis, the infection was presumed to be acquired perinatally from the mother.[65,66] Portals of entry have been various and not always identifiable. In the largest review of viridans streptococcal meningitis (55 cases), ear, nose, or throat pathology was found in 31% of patients, endocarditis in 13%, primary extracranial infection in 13%, and head trauma or neurosurgery in 8%. No portal for entry was identified in 35% of patients.[61] Other predisposing factors include gastrointestinal pathology, gastrointestinal manipulation such as endoscopy, trauma, ganglionic thermocoagulation, and severe immunocompromise after chemotherapy.[62-64,55] In a review of meningitis occurring after dural puncture, streptococcal species were responsible for over 50% of the 179 cases.[67] Spinal anesthesia, myelography, epidural anesthesia, and diagnostic lumbar puncture were the most common predisposing events, respectively. Iatrogenic meningitis caused by viridans streptococci has been reported in association with failure to adhere to infection control measures while performing lumbar puncture, especially regarding the use of face masks.[68]

When α-hemolytic streptococci other than pneumococci are recovered from cerebrospinal fluid (CSF), they are more likely to be contaminants than true pathogens. In 43 patients from whom various species of α-hemolytic streptococci were isolated on culture of CSF, only eight isolates (19%) were determined to be clinically relevant.[69] The significance of isolation of α-hemolytic streptococci from CSF depends on the clinical setting and the CSF laboratory parameters. CSF protein concentrations and white blood cell differential counts are clearly abnormal in patients with true infection, but CSF glucose levels may be normal. A positive Gram stain is highly significant but occurs in fewer than 50% of patients with viridans streptococcal meningitis. Differentiation of these streptococci from *S. pneumoniae* on the basis of a spinal fluid Gram stain is seldom possible.

The finding of positive blood cultures in association with viridans streptococcal meningitis might suggest underlying endocarditis, but meningitis as a complication of endocarditis is uncommon. Among 41 patients with infective endocarditis who also had symptoms suggestive of meningitis or encephalitis, the organism was recovered on CSF culture in only four cases.[70] Bacteremic meningitis in the absence of cardiac involvement has been described primarily in severely immunocompromised patients.[55]

In the preantibiotic era, viridans streptococcal meningitis was almost uniformly fatal; only nine surviving patients were reported before 1937.[61] After the introduction of antibiotic therapy, mortality rates declined significantly, with most fatalities occurring in patients who were immunocompromised. Penicillin G, 24 million units/day, is the antibiotic of choice for treatment of viridans streptococcal meningitis in patients with normal renal function. Most clinical isolates have MICs of 0.1 μg/mL or less, and thus are extremely sensitive. Meningitis caused by multiple-antibiotic–resistant viridans streptococci has also been described. MICs to penicillin for these strains are 4 μg/mL or higher, similar to those seen with antibiotic-resistant *S. pneumoniae*. Although clinical data are lacking, vancomycin plus a third-generation cephalosporin is the preferred treatment of meningitis caused by such strains, pending full susceptibility test results. Because of the unpredictable susceptibility patterns of viridans streptococci, in vitro susceptibility testing of all CSF isolates is mandatory.

Pneumonia

Although viridans streptococci are often isolated from respiratory tract specimens, they are rarely ascribed clinical significance. Recovery of these organisms from expectorated sputum is usually attributable to their presence as normal oral flora. However, they may also be cultured from lower respiratory tract specimens obtained by transtracheal aspiration or protected bronchial brush. Here, viridans streptococci occur, in association with other oral organisms (e.g., anaerobes), as part of the aspiration pneumonia syndrome. In one study of community-acquired aspiration pneumonia, cultures of transtracheal aspirates yielded streptococci in 9 of 24 patients.[71] In another review, the organism was recovered from 51% of 189 transtracheal aspirations performed on patients with suspected bacterial pneumonia.[72] The relative importance of viridans streptococci in the pathogenesis of these polymicrobial infections is unknown.

Isolation of viridans streptococci as sole pathogens from lower respiratory tract infections has been reported. Pratter and Irwin have described two patients in whom the diagnosis was ascertained by culture of transtracheal aspirate and pleural fluid.[73] Sarkar and associates have reported three cases of acute community-acquired viridans streptococcal pneumonia in which the diagnosis was confirmed by the presence of positive blood cultures.[74] In a series of patients described by Marrie, all seven adult patients with bacteremic viridans streptococcal community-acquired pneumonia were older (49 to 80 years) and had multiple underlying conditions, such as alcoholism, lung carcinoma, and diabetes mellitus.[75] Empyema, with or without an obvious underlying pneumonic process, is still commonly caused by viridans streptococci; alcoholism is not uncommonly a predisposing factor in these patients.[76]

The prognosis for patients with primary viridans streptococcal pneumonia is good. Fatalities are rare in the absence of immunocompromise. Penicillin G has been used successfully as therapy in most cases reported in the literature.

Miscellaneous Infections

Viridans streptococci are associated with a variety of other infections. A pathogenic role in these cases has been confirmed by recovery of the organism in pure culture and often by concurrent presence of bacteremia. Excluding localized purulent collections associated with the *S. anginosus* (*milleri*) group (see Chapter 204), viridans strains have been identified in patients with pericarditis, peritonitis, acute bacterial sialadenitis, orofacial odontogenic infections, endophthalmitis (see Chapter 112), spondylodiscitis, and various upper respiratory tract infections (e.g., otitis media and sinusitis).

ANTIMICROBIAL RESISTANCE AND PRINCIPLES OF THERAPY

Viridans streptococci are inherently susceptible to most antimicrobial agents, including β-lactam antibiotics, macrolides, tetracyclines, and aminoglycosides. Recently, however, resistance has emerged as a significant problem, especially with β-lactams. Among 352 unselected blood culture isolates obtained from across the United States during 1993 and 1994, only 44% were fully susceptible to penicillin (using the National Committee for Clinical Laboratory Standards interpretive criterion of MIC ≤ 0.125 µg/mL).[77] Resistance occurs more frequently in nosocomial bloodstream isolates and in those obtained from immunocompromised patients. In a national surveillance program, 61% of 98 nosocomial bloodstream isolates were susceptible to penicillin,[78] whereas rates as low as 43% were reported in neutropenic cancer patients, apparently because of selection of resistance by use of antimicrobial prophylaxis with cancer chemotherapy. The susceptibility of isolates from patients with endocarditis had not changed appreciably in several decades, although that trend may be changing. In a 2004 review from one U.S. hospital, only 17% of viridans streptococcal endocarditis isolates from a 25-year period showed nonsusceptibility to penicillin.[79] One recent retrospective case series from Taiwan, however, found a 45% rate of penicillin nonsusceptibility among

streptococcal endocarditis isolates; most were from the viridans group.[80]

Some strains of viridans group streptococci exhibit a high level of resistance to penicillin, defined as a penicillin MIC ≥ 4 µg/mL. Note that this breakpoint for resistance, as defined by the National Committee for Clinical Laboratory Standards, differs from the MIC criterion (more than 0.5 µg/mL) used in the American Heart Association guidelines for determining treatment of streptococcal endocarditis (see Table 203-3).[40] Surveys of viridans streptococci from the United States have reported high-level penicillin resistance in 5% to 13% of bloodstream isolates.[77,81] Rates reported from other areas of the world approach 50%, depending on the types of patients and specimens studied. The two reviews of endocarditis isolates mentioned earlier documented only 1 of 50[79] and 3 of 48[80] viridans streptococci with high-level penicillin resistance. Like penicillin-resistant pneumococci, resistant viridans strains are non–β-lactamase-producing and possess altered penicillin-binding proteins. In vitro studies suggest the presence of genes homologous to the pneumococcal PBP 1a and 2b genes. Transfer of resistance determinants between these gram-positive bacteria has been accomplished in vitro and may be an important means of disseminating resistance in nature.

Whether species identity for viridans streptococci can be used to predict antimicrobial susceptibility and thus guide therapeutic selections is controversial.[4] Continuous changes in the taxonomy and nomenclature of these organisms, combined with the incomplete species identification provided in many reports, limit the usefulness of the historical literature. Nevertheless, there do appear to be trends in species-related differences in penicillin susceptibility among viridans group streptococci. *S. mitis* is the least sensitive, with only 40% of isolates inhibited by 0.125 µg/mL or less of penicillin.[82] *S. oralis* is the next most likely to be resistant, especially those isolates recovered from blood cultures of neutropenic cancer patients.[51] *S. sanguinis*, a frequent cause of endocarditis, appears to be the least resistant to β-lactam antibiotics.

Some strains of viridans streptococci exhibit a phenomenon termed *tolerance,* in which the concentration of penicillin required for bactericidal activity is at least 32-fold higher than that required simply to inhibit the organism's growth. In experimental animal models of endocarditis, tolerant strains are eradicated more slowly from vegetations than nontolerant strains, although this effect may be relevant only when low doses of penicillin are used.[83] There are conflicting reports on the incidence of tolerance in viridans streptococci.[84] Tolerance is probably observed in most *S. sanguinis* and *S. gordonii* strains, but it occurs in a minority of *S. mitis* strains and rarely, if at all, in *S. salivarius.* No clinical significance has been attached to tolerance in the treatment of infective endocarditis. Relapse after a 4-week course of high-dose parenteral penicillin is rare and has not been associated with tolerance in the pathogen.[41] Addition of an aminoglycoside may enhance bactericidal activity in vitro, but is not mandatory for organisms with a low penicillin MIC (≤0.12 µg/mL or lower).[40]

Other β-lactam antibiotics have in vitro activity similar to penicillin against viridans streptococci. Generally, community-acquired endocarditis isolates tend to be highly susceptible. In one study, ceftriaxone inhibited 98% of 49 strains at a concentration of 0.1 µg/mL or lower.[42] Among surveys of isolates collected from hospitalized or neutropenic cancer patients, ceftriaxone has been less active, with approximately 15% to 23% of isolates found to be resistant.[78,81] Most such isolates also have high-level resistance to penicillin (MIC > 4 µg/mL) as well as resistance to other antimicrobial agents.

Viridans streptococci are resistant to aminoglycosides when traditional breakpoint concentrations for these agents are applied. However, in vitro studies and experimental models of endocarditis have demonstrated synergistic bactericidal activity for combinations of penicillin and aminoglycosides.[38,39] In strains with a streptomycin MIC of 1000 µg/mL or higher, synergy is lost for streptomycin but not necessarily for gentamicin. The breakpoint for predicting synergy with gentamicin is not clear. Strains with a gentamicin MIC of 16 µg/mL have shown synergy, whereas two strains with MICs of 64 and 128 µg/mL have not.

Antibiotics with consistently excellent in vitro activity against viridans streptococci include chloramphenicol, vancomycin, linezolid, daptomycin, and tigecycline,[85] with resistance very rarely reported to any of these drugs. The fluoroquinolones also demonstrate generally good in vitro activity; among those currently available in the United States, moxifloxacin tends to have the lowest MIC.[77] However, neutropenic cancer patients who receive prophylaxis with a fluoroquinolone antibiotic can develop breakthrough bacteremia with isolates expressing high-level resistance.[86] Therefore, the role of these agents in therapy is uncertain. Tetracycline, clindamycin, and erythromycin have variable activity, often with 25% to 50% of isolates reported as being resistant. Most strains of viridans streptococci are resistant to trimethoprim-sulfamethoxazole.

Nutritionally Variant (Deficient) Streptococci (*Abiotrophia* and *Granulicatella*)

NVS were first described in 1961 as fastidious gram-positive bacteria that grew as satellite colonies around other bacteria. Originally isolated from patients with endocarditis and otitis media, these organisms were deemed to be mutant subspecies of *S. mitis* ("*S. mitior*") because of their sugar fermentation, cell wall composition, and possession of a heat-acid–extractable chromophore, such as that of *S. mitis*. However, despite evidence for similarity between NVS and *S. mitis*, important phenotypic differences were also evident, such as their enzymatic capabilities and patterns of penicillin-binding proteins. Over the past 2 decades, based on DNA-DNA hybridization studies and 16S ribosomal RNA (rRNA) sequence analysis, the names of these organisms have been revised several times. First included in the genus *Streptococcus*, and later assigned to a new genus *Abiotrophia*, they have most recently been placed into two genera, comprising four species that have been identified from human specimens: *Abiotrophia defectiva*, *Granulicatella adiacens*, *Granulicatella elegans*, and *Granulicatella para-adiacens*.[16]

All NVS species require pyridoxal or cysteine for growth and produce leucine aminopeptidase and arylamidase. Species can be differentiated by their patterns of carbohydrate fermentation, production of α- and β-galactosidases and β-glucuronidase, and hydrolysis of hippurate or arginine. They tend to form satellite colonies around *Staphylococcus aureus* and other microbes, including some Enterobacteriaceae and other streptococci. Colonies of NVS are small, measuring 0.2 to 0.5 mm in diameter, and are either nonhemolytic or α-hemolytic on blood agar. On Gram staining, cells may be pleomorphic and may exhibit variable staining characteristics. There appears to be sufficient pyridoxal in human blood to support the growth of NVS in most blood culture media, with the notable exception of unsupplemented tryptic soy broth. For subculture, however, solid media must be supplemented with 0.001% pyridoxal or 0.01% L-cysteine to sustain growth. Alternatively, the subculture plate can be cross-streaked with *S. aureus* to provide these factors and permit growth as satellite colonies. Some studies have suggested that blood cultures suspected of harboring NVS should be subcultured within 48 hours, because viability of the organism may decline with continued incubation.

Given these inherent difficulties with NVS in the clinical microbiology laboratory, novel techniques for their isolation and identification have been developed. In one case, a *G. adiacens* isolate from a patient with septic arthritis was only able to be identified after synovial fluid was inoculated directly into blood culture bottles.[87] Additionally, specific rRNA PCR assays have been developed to aid in the identification of NVS,[88] and have led to the microbiologic diagnosis in cases of culture-negative endocarditis and bacteremia.[89,90]

In vitro antimicrobial susceptibility testing of NVS is beyond the scope of many routine clinical laboratories. Moreover, the results of in vitro susceptibility tests do not correlate well with clinical outcome

in patients treated for endocarditis, the most common serious infection that these organisms cause. Some general comments can be made, however. NVS are less susceptible in vitro to penicillin than other streptococci. Approximately 33% to 67% of strains are relatively resistant (MICs, 0.25 to 2.0 µg/mL), and some isolates are highly resistant to the antibiotic (MIC ≥ 4 µg/mL).[91] Depending on the method used, many strains of NVS also exhibit tolerance to penicillin, although the clinical significance of this is not clear. High-level aminoglycoside resistance (MIC > 500 µg/mL), as seen in enterococci and viridans streptococci, has not been reported in NVS. Synergy between penicillin or vancomycin and an aminoglycoside is observed both in vitro and in experimental animal models of endocarditis for tolerant and non-tolerant strains of NVS. All strains of NVS are susceptible to vancomycin in vitro, and susceptibility rates to fluoroquinolones have remained high. Decreasing susceptibility to other agents, including the third-generation cephalosporins azithromycin and clindamycin, has been reported.[92]

NVS are found as normal flora of the upper respiratory, urogenital, and gastrointestinal tracts of humans. They cause approximately 5% of cases of bacterial endocarditis. Historically, NVS accounted for most cases of culture-negative endocarditis, but with current laboratory media and techniques, recovery of strains is no longer as significant a problem. Among NVS, *A. defectiva* seems especially suited to cause endovascular infection because of its ability to adhere to fibronectin in the extracellular matrix. By contrast, *Granulicatella* species do not adhere well to extracellular matrix, and instead tend to cause primary bacteremias in immunocompromised patients.[93,94] Endocarditis caused by NVS carries greater morbidity and mortality than endocarditis caused by other streptococci. A comparison between 49 patients with NVS endocarditis and 130 patients with infection caused by other oral species revealed a higher mortality rate (14% vs. 5%), more frequent complications of embolization (33% vs. 11%) and congestive heart failure (33% vs. 18%), and an increased rate of surgical intervention (33% vs. 18%).[45] Because of the difficulties in performing susceptibility tests and correlating the results with clinical outcome, it is recommended that all patients with NVS endocarditis be treated with long-term combination therapy (e.g., penicillin plus gentamicin for 4 to 6 weeks; see Table 203-3).[40] Even with this regimen, however, the rates of bacteriologic failure and relapse are high (41% and 17% of cases, respectively, in one review).[95] Even in cases of endocarditis with strains highly susceptible to penicillin, relapses may be seen.

Apart from endocarditis, and bacteremias in immunocompromised patients, the precise role of NVS as pathogens in other disease processes is unknown. Because the organisms grow poorly on solid media, they can easily be overlooked if broth cultures are not performed or not subcultured to appropriately supplemented media. Isolation of NVS as likely pathogens has been reported in a diverse list of infections that can be caused by other streptococci, including otitis media, a variety of ocular infections, pancreatic abscess, prosthetic joint infections,[96] breast implant infections,[97] central nervous system infections,[98] and osteomyelitis.

β-Hemolytic Streptococci (Groups C and G)
MICROBIOLOGY

Confusing and conflicting results from taxonomic studies make it impossible to recommend a practical identification scheme that would correlate with genetic descriptions of the non–group A, B, and D β-hemolytic streptococci. For convenience, these streptococci can initially be divided into groups based on colony size. Small or minute colony types (<0.5 mm in diameter) have been placed into the *S. milleri* group (see Chapter 204). β-Hemolytic streptococci of large colony size (0.5 mm in diameter or larger) can almost always be grouped with Lancefield antisera using latex agglutination or coagglutination directed against the cell wall carbohydrate of groups A, B, C, or G. Although serologic typing according to cell wall components has classically been used to separate streptococci into species, DNA homology studies have shown that this method is not always valid. Nevertheless, this classification remains useful as an aid to identification of clinical isolates. In many diagnostic microbiology laboratories, bacitracin disk susceptibility is also used as a screening test to separate group A streptococci from other *pyogenes*-like organisms. Some studies using the standard 0.04-unit bacitracin disk have demonstrated that less than 10% of groups C and G β-hemolytic streptococci are susceptible. However, other investigators have found greater variation in the bacitracin susceptibility of these streptococcal strains (see later discussion of specific microorganisms).

Large colony-forming β-hemolytic strains not containing group antigens are rarely causative agents of human disease. Those possessing group antigens other than A, B, C, and G have been isolated primarily from animals and environmental sources and may be carried as the normal flora of the pharynx, vagina, or skin of wild or domestic animals. Rare infections in humans have been reported to be caused by other serogroups, including E, F, L, M, N, and O[99,100]; these types are not discussed here. The following sections review in detail the microbiologic and clinical characteristics of groups C and G β-hemolytic streptococci.

Group C Streptococci

Most group C streptococci produce β-hemolysis on sheep blood agar, although all types of hemolysis have been noted. All group C streptococci are common pathogens in domestic animals, birds, rabbits, and guinea pigs. Although bacitracin resistance has historically been seen in most group C streptococcal isolates, this is not a universal characteristic. Therefore, group C streptococci may be misidentified as group A streptococci if sensitivity to bacitracin is used for presumptive identification of group A strains. This indicates the importance of performing Lancefield serologic testing on all bacitracin-sensitive and -resistant β-hemolytic streptococci. Identification by antibiotic screening can be improved with the use of a trimethoprim-sulfamethoxazole disk, to which group C organisms are sensitive and group A organisms resistant.

Traditionally, there were four large-colony species (and a number of potential subspecies) within Lancefield group C—*Streptococcus dysgalactiae*, *S. equi*, *S. equisimilis*, and *S. zooepidemicus*. By current taxonomy, all large-colony organisms previously classified within group C or G (with the exception of *S. canis*) are included within *S. dysgalactiae* subsp. *equisimilis*.[5] In this chapter, however, references to older nomenclature schemes are often made to allow for easier correlation with much of the published literature on these organisms.

Streptococcus dysgalactiae subsp. *equisimilis* ferments trehalose but not sorbitol, and it produces streptokinase and streptolysin O but not streptolysin S. The streptokinase used for human thrombolytic therapy is derived from *S. equisimilis*. Because *S. dysgalactiae* subsp. *equisimilis* produces streptolysin O, infections caused by this organism may result in elevated antistreptolysin O (ASO) antibody titers, which are classically used to screen patients for antecedent group A β-hemolytic streptococcal infection. *S. dysgalactiae* subsp. *equisimilis* has been isolated from the throat, nose, and genital tract of asymptomatic carriers and from the umbilicus of up to two thirds of asymptomatic newborns. Domestic animals (e.g., horses, cattle, pigs, chickens) may also be infected.

Streptococcus equi subsp. *zooepidemicus* causes significant, often epidemic, infections in domestic animals (horses, cattle, sheep, and pigs). Most cases of human infection can be traced to an animal source.[101] It ferments sorbitol but not trehalose, produces a novel hemolysin but not streptolysin O or S, does not produce streptokinase, and is not considered part of the normal human flora. Human infection is uncommon; some cases have been associated with consumption of homemade cheese and unpasteurized cow's milk.[102] In one study from England, *S. equi* subsp. *zooepidemicus* represented 1.4% of 214 isolates recovered from a variety of clinical specimens,[103] although it has been suggested that this organism causes a higher proportion of aggressive

infections than would be expected from its rare occurrence at superficial sites.

Group G Streptococci

β-Hemolytic streptococcal strains carrying the group G antigen were first described by Lancefield and Hare in 1935.[104] The great majority of group G strains demonstrate β-hemolysis when incubated in 5% to 10% carbon dioxide at 35° C for 18 to 48 hours on trypticase soy agar with 5% sheep's blood. Similar to the situation with group C streptococci, bacitracin resistance alone cannot reliably be used to distinguish these organisms from group A streptococci, because a variable percentage of group G streptococci may be sensitive to bacitracin. Group G β-hemolytic streptococci produce a streptolysin that is antigenically similar to the streptolysin O produced by group A β-hemolytic streptococci. Therefore, patients with group G streptococcal pharyngitis may have a significant increase in serum ASO antibody titers. *S. canis* is one species of group G streptococcus that remains separate in taxonomy from the other group C and G streptococci contained in *S. dysgalactiae* subsp. *equisimilis*.[5]

EPIDEMIOLOGY

Group C Streptococci

Group C β-hemolytic streptococci have been identified as part of the normal human flora of the nasopharynx, skin, and genital tract; the organism has also been cultured from umbilical specimens in newborns without signs of infection, and in routine puerperal vaginal cultures. In addition, many animal species are colonized with group C streptococci; some infections in humans have been traced to animal sources. Underlying conditions have been noted in most patients with group C streptococcal infection. In one review of 88 cases of group C streptococcal bacteremia, 73% of the patients had a significant underlying condition (cardiovascular disease in 20%, malignancy in 20%); prior exposure to animals was documented in 24% of cases.[101]

Group G Streptococci

Most types of group G streptococci may be found to colonize the nasopharynx, skin, and genital tract; intestinal colonization has also been reported. Several investigators have noted that up to 65% of patients with group G streptococcal infections have an underlying malignancy.[105] However, a study of 57 cases of group G streptococcal infection in 11 hospitals in northeastern Ohio found that only 21% of patients had an underlying malignancy[106]; 21% were alcohol abusers and 14% had diabetes mellitus. A similar cancer rate was found in another study of 24 patients with group G streptococcal bacteremia, in which the rate of underlying neoplastic disease was 25%.[107]

S. canis has been recognized with increasing frequency as a cause of skin and soft tissue infection in dog owners.[108] One review of 54 cases of human infection found syndromes such as soft tissue infection, primary bacteremia, urinary tract infection, osteomyelitis, and pneumonia.[109] Antibiotic susceptibilities are similar to other group G streptococci (see later discussion of therapy).

CLINICAL MANIFESTATIONS

Numerous reports of groups C and G streptococcal suppurative infections of various organ systems have been published.[101,106,110-112] Infection can be endogenous (i.e., from organisms residing on skin or mucous membranes) or exogenous (i.e., from animal sources). Endogenous infection often occurs in hosts predisposed by age (neonate or older adult), alcoholism, injection drug abuse, diabetes mellitus, immunosuppressive therapy with corticosteroids or cytotoxic drugs, or underlying malignancy. Infections are often severe, resembling those caused by groups A and B β-hemolytic streptococci.

Pharyngitis

Non–group A β-hemolytic streptococci have been associated with outbreaks of pharyngitis, although their precise role in the causation of endemic or sporadic pharyngitis has not been defined.[113,114] In one report of children and adolescents with sporadic pharyngitis, 17% of β-hemolytic isolates were non–group A; of these, fewer than half were groups C and G.

Several studies comparing group C β-hemolytic streptococcal isolation rates among pharyngitis patients versus controls have reported contradictory results.[113] In five studies, group C streptococci were isolated more frequently from patients than from controls, although the results were statistically significant in only one study.[115] In this study, which used optimal laboratory techniques, the isolation rate of group C streptococci was higher in 1425 adult patients than in 284 controls (6% versus 1.4%; *P* = .002). In a carefully done study of 232 college students with pharyngitis,[116] a strong epidemiologic association between group C streptococci and endemic pharyngitis was demonstrated; group C streptococci were isolated significantly more often from patients than from 198 age-matched controls (26% vs. 11%; *P* < .0001). Culture-positive patients also had fever, exudative tonsillitis, and anterior cervical adenopathy more often than culture-negative patients, and quantitative colony counts were generally higher in patients compared with controls. The 11% isolation rate in controls suggests that group C streptococci may represent normal oropharyngeal flora.

The symptoms and signs of pharyngitis caused by group C streptococci are very similar to those caused by group A β-hemolytic streptococci and include fever, mild to moderate sore throat, pharyngeal exudate, and cervical adenopathy. Because of these similarities, patients with an epidemiologic and clinical picture consistent with streptococcal pharyngitis, but with a negative rapid test for *S. pyogenes*, should undergo throat culture.[117] Group C streptococci also have the potential to cause a severe pharyngitis, followed by bacteremia and metastatic infection. Rapid detection of group C streptococci from throat swabs has been attempted. Compared with culture, the rapid test had poor sensitivity (34.4%) but very high specificity (99.4%) in the detection of group C β-hemolytic streptococci[118]; the sensitivity of the test improved with increasing colony counts isolated from throat cultures.

Asymptomatic pharyngeal carriage of group G β-hemolytic streptococci occurs in up to 23% of humans. Symptoms and signs in patients with group G streptococcal pharyngitis range from a mild upper respiratory tract infection with coryza to an exudative pharyngitis with fever and lymphadenopathy. As with group C streptococci, the illness is indistinguishable from pharyngitis caused by group A β-hemolytic streptococci. Initial reports that suggested a causative role of group G streptococci in pharyngitis consisted of anecdotes, small case clusters, and investigations of predominantly food-borne outbreaks (related to consumption of eggs and chicken salad).[113,119] Few of these studies were adequately controlled, and the isolation rate of group G streptococci was too low to demonstrate a statistically significant difference between symptomatic and asymptomatic groups. In an outbreak of pharyngitis in children, throat cultures for group G β-hemolytic streptococci were positive in 56 of 222 patients (25%); DNA fingerprinting revealed identical strains in 75% of cases.[120] Patients with group G streptococcal pharyngitis were comparable to those with group A streptococcal pharyngitis with respect to clinical findings, ASO antibody titer response, and clinical response to antimicrobial therapy. In this study, antimicrobial therapy appeared to have a dramatic impact on the clinical course of group G streptococcal pharyngitis, although other investigators have found no evidence that antimicrobial therapy modifies the duration or severity of symptoms.

Complications of Pharyngitis. Poststreptococcal glomerulonephritis has been associated with group C streptococcal pharyngitis.[121] In these reports, infection was acquired by consumption of unpasteurized milk from cattle with mastitis; the causative agent was *S. zooepidemicus*. The pathogenesis of poststreptococcal glomerulonephritis from group C streptococcal infection is unclear, although certain group C streptococcal strains recovered from throat cultures were found to possess human antibody receptors that were thought to be virulence factors

for these organisms.[122] In addition, endostreptosin, a cytoplasmic polypeptide antigen that plays a role in poststreptococcal glomerulonephritis associated with group A streptococcal infection, was demonstrated in the cytoplasm of infecting group C isolates, and elevated concentrations of antiendostreptosin antibodies were detected in the patients' sera.

Type 12 M-protein antigen, identical to the nephritogenic antigen of the group A streptococcus, has been isolated from the group G streptococcus. However, association of group G β-hemolytic streptococci with acute glomerulonephritis is anecdotal; a causal relation has not yet been established.[123] Group C and G streptococcal pharyngitis has also been associated with sterile reactive arthritis.[124] Group C streptococci, and possibly group G streptococci, can produce a class C1 M protein that may be responsible for the development of streptococcal-associated sequel diseases.[125] Acute rheumatic fever has not been described in association with group C or G streptococcal pharyngitis.

Skin and Soft Tissue Infection
Colonization of human skin with groups C and G streptococci is common, and these organisms have been responsible for various cutaneous and subcutaneous infections, including cellulitis, wound infections, pyoderma, erysipelas, impetigo, and cutaneous ulcers.[110] Breaches in skin integrity may provide a portal of entry leading to bacteremia. As with group A streptococci, group C streptococci have been isolated in patients with cellulitis after vein harvest for coronary artery bypass grafts and in conditions associated with abnormal venous or lymphatic drainage. Accompanying lymphangitis may also be seen.

One recent case-control study has actually found that group G streptococcus is isolated at a higher incidence than group A streptococcus (22% vs. 7%) among patients hospitalized for cellulitis. Pharyngeal carriage was discovered in a small percentage of these patients and their household members, but not in any control subjects.[126] Group G streptococcal bacteremia may occur as a complication of skin and soft tissue infections. In one review of 37 patients with group G streptococcal bacteremia,[106] 73% of patients became bacteremic from a cutaneous source, including 58% of patients with an underlying malignancy. Other reviews of group G streptococcal bacteremia have shown significantly lower percentages of skin and soft tissue infections as the source of the bacteremia.[111]

Arthritis
β-Hemolytic streptococci account for 11% to 28% of cases of nongonococcal septic arthritis, with most cases in children and adults caused by group A streptococci. Group C streptococcal arthritis is quite uncommon, and most frequently occurs in joints with preexisting rheumatologic abnormalities.[127,128] In an extensive literature review of 18 cases of group C streptococcal septic arthritis,[129] underlying conditions, both rheumatic and nonrheumatic, were recognized in 72% of patients. The skin was the presumed portal of entry in five patients, although in most cases the source of infection was not identified. Almost any joint can be involved, and frequently the arthritis is polyarticular (30% of cases in one review). Infective endocarditis was diagnosed in two patients. Antimicrobial therapy (primarily penicillin G) and surgical drainage were used in most cases. Three of the patients died, all of whom were bacteremic.

Group G streptococci are the second most common of the β-hemolytic streptococci to cause septic arthritis.[130,131] In one review of 57 cases,[132] clinical features were known in 46 patients, including 13 with infected prosthetic joints. Of those with group G streptococcal septic arthritis of native joints, 48% had polyarticular involvement. An extra-articular focus of infection was present in more than half of patients; the major foci were cellulitis and endocarditis. Only 4 patients had no underlying conditions or joint abnormalities. Antimicrobial therapy varied, but most often included a β-lactam; length of therapy ranged from 14 to 90 days, with the organism cleared rapidly from the joint in most cases. However, in some patients, the clinical course was protracted, and bacteriologic relapse after medical therapy was common. Surgical drainage was required in 13 patients, including 5 with prosthetic joints. Patients with infected prosthetic joints have been noted to do well even without joint removal. There may be a slow response to antimicrobial therapy despite in vitro susceptibility. Coexistent osteomyelitis may be present, and recurrent sterile joint effusions may also occur.

Osteomyelitis

Isolated reports have described cases of group C streptococcal osteomyelitis.[133,134] A review of the literature described 11 patients with group G streptococcal osteomyelitis,[132] 3 of whom also had septic arthritis. Of 7 patients with group G streptococcal osteomyelitis in this review, 6 had underlying conditions (malignancy, alcoholic cirrhosis, osteoarthritis, internal fixation for fractures, or prostheses); 3 patients were treated with antibiotics and another 3 patients required antimicrobial therapy plus surgery. Two cases of group G streptococcal vertebral osteomyelitis have also been reported,[135] as has a case of postoperative sternal osteomyelitis,[136] and a surprising case of a subacute femoral osteomyelitis that mimicked a bone tumor was reported.[137]

Respiratory Tract Infections

The group C streptococcus is an uncommon cause of pneumonia, but it is associated with significant morbidity and mortality, similar to infection caused by the group A streptococcus.[110,138] Development of pneumonia is often preceded by a viral upper respiratory tract infection. In one review of nine cases,[139] the pneumonia was typically lobar and often heralded by fever, chills, dyspnea, and pleuritic chest pain. Bacteremia was documented in 75% of cases. All patients had pleural effusions. Complications included metastatic infection, empyema, and cavitation. All patients received therapy with intravenous penicillin, sometimes in combination with other antimicrobial agents.

Pneumonia caused by the group G streptococcus is rare. Similar to other group G streptococcal infections, underlying malignancy has been reported with varying frequency.[105,106,111]

Group C streptococcal sinusitis has also been reported. Common to all cases in one review[140] was age younger than 18 years, the presence of suppurative central nervous system complications (perhaps secondary to inadequate medical or surgical therapy), and a delay in initiation of adequate therapy. Of the five patients in this review, three were bacteremic and two died.

Endocarditis

Infective endocarditis caused by groups C and G streptococci is uncommon, accounting for fewer than 1% of total cases and 8.4% of cases caused by β-hemolytic streptococci.[106,110,111,141] In a review of 4705 cases of infective endocarditis,[142] 166 (3.5%) were caused by β-hemolytic streptococci, 8 were group C, and 14 were group G. The likelihood of infective endocarditis appears to be more common with groups C and G streptococcal bacteremia than with groups A and B, even though the latter more often cause bacteremia.

In a review of 88 cases of group C streptococcal bacteremia,[101] patients with endocarditis (24 cases) usually presented subacutely (mean duration of symptoms, 17.4 days). Major emboli were observed in 10 cases; one third of patients died. Response to single-agent β-lactam therapy was poor, leading the authors to favor the use of bactericidal combinations (e.g., penicillin plus gentamicin), although no comparative data were available to make firm recommendations. Four patients required surgical valve replacement for congestive heart failure. In contrast, in another review of group C streptococcal infections in which 20 cases of infective endocarditis were identified,[110] the presentation was typically acute, with a propensity for involvement of normal valves, a high mortality rate (approaching 40% to 50%), and a frequent need for valve replacement. More than half of patients developed cardiac complications, including destruction of the valve leaflets, myocardial abscesses, conduction abnormalities, and severe congestive heart failure. Major systemic emboli occurred in about half of patients. In 12 patients for whom there was information on antimicrobial therapy, there were no bacteriologic failures among those

treated with penicillin, with or without an aminoglycoside. However, patients who received combination therapy required valve replacement less frequently than those treated with penicillin alone. Combination therapy may be more rapidly bactericidal, but the relation of antimicrobial therapy to surgery cannot be adequately assessed given the small number of patients reviewed.

Group G streptococcal endocarditis tends to occur in older patients with multiple underlying disorders.[111,143] Both native and prosthetic valves may be affected, and left-sided disease is more common. The onset is generally abrupt, with rapid valve destruction and perivalvular infection; metastatic foci are not uncommon. In a review of 40 cases of group G streptococcal endocarditis,[144] the mean age of patients was 56 years. Underlying conditions included malignancy, diabetes mellitus, alcohol abuse, and injection drug use. The presentation was acute in 26 of 40 patients. A cutaneous portal of entry was found in almost 50% of cases. Cases were split equally between patients with underlying valvular heart disease and those with previously normal valves. Among the 29 patients in whom complications were reported, 25 had cardiac or embolic complications. The mortality rate was 36%, but it has ranged from 43% to 67% in other studies.[141,143] There was a trend toward improved survival in patients treated with the antimicrobial combination of a β-lactam plus an aminoglycoside for at least 28 days.

Meningitis

Cases of groups C and G streptococcal meningitis have been reported and are often associated with infective endocarditis.[110,145,146] Infection may occur in healthy patients, particularly those with animal contact; cases have been reported in association with ingestion of unpasteurized goat's milk,[147] from head trauma as a result of a kick by a horse,[148] and simply from frequent contact with horses.[149] The clinical presentation is typically acute, and the response to antimicrobial therapy slow. In one review of the literature of 18 previous cases (9 in adults) of group C streptococcal meningitis,[150] the case-fatality rate was 55%. In assessing the approximately 30 cases of group C streptococcal meningitis that have been reviewed overall,[150,151] complications have included bacteremia, pneumonia, sinusitis, subdural empyema, bacterial endocarditis, brain abscess, and otitis media. The mortality rate was high (43%), and most significant at the extremes of age (neonates and older adults).

Puerperal Infection

In their original paper, Lancefield and Hare recovered group G streptococci from 5 of 855 antepartum vaginal swabs and from the blood of a patient with puerperal sepsis who was also infected with *S. aureus*.[104] About 5% of asymptomatic women harbor group G β-hemolytic streptococci in their genital tracts. Both group C and group G streptococci have been associated with epidemic and nonepidemic puerperal sepsis and endometritis.[111,152] When endometritis occurs without bacteremia, it may be relatively mild and associated with few systemic symptoms.

Neonatal Sepsis

Neonatal sepsis caused by group G streptococci occurs in premature or low-birth-weight infants and in the setting of premature rupture of membranes.[153] Infection most likely complicates colonization of the birth canal, with spread to the child after vaginal delivery. The onset of disease is typically within the first week of life. Infection in the child is also associated with a high incidence of maternal obstetric complications. In a review of neonatal sepsis from one institution over a 5-year period, group G streptococci accounted for 7 of 305 cases.[154] Symptoms and signs included hypothermia, irritability, seizures, apnea, bradycardia, and cardiac arrest. Complications such as progressive respiratory distress, shock, and disseminated intravascular coagulation are invariably fatal.

Bacteremia

Group C streptococci are rarely isolated from blood cultures, accounting for fewer than 1% of all bacteremias.[112,155,156] However, in patients with group C streptococcal infections, bacteremia is frequently detected. In one review of 31 cases of group C streptococcal infections,[110] bacteremia was observed in 23 (74%). The bacteremia was polymicrobial in eight patients, with facultative gram-negative bacteria predominating as the second microorganism. In a review of 88 cases of group C streptococcal bacteremia,[101] 27% of patients had infective endocarditis, 10% had meningitis, 9% had cutaneous infections, and 23% had primary bacteremia; 88% of cases were community-acquired. Many of the patients had underlying illnesses, including cardiovascular disease (20%), malignancy (20%), and immunosuppression (15%). Acute illness with fever, chills, and prostration was most common, except in patients with infective endocarditis, who tended to present subacutely in this review,[110] contrasting with an earlier study. Mortality rates were high (25%), especially in older patients and those with endocarditis, meningitis, or disseminated infection. Similar findings were noted in a review of 45 cases, specifically of *S. equi* subsp. *zooepidemicus* septicemia, in which 27% of patients had underlying cardiovascular disease; the overall mortality rate was 22%.[157]

Group G streptococci account for 8% to 11% of all β-hemolytic streptococcal bacteremias[158]; an underlying malignancy has been reported in 21% to 65% of patients.[106,107,111] Polymicrobial bacteremia is not uncommon, with *S. aureus* being the most frequently isolated copathogen. Patients usually have another primary site of infection, such as pneumonia, septic arthritis, ophthalmitis, or meningitis. In a review of 24 cases of group G streptococcal bacteremia over a 29-month period,[107] underlying conditions included alcohol abuse (8 patients), malignancy (6 patients), diabetes mellitus (5 patients), neurologic disease (4 patients), cardiovascular disease (4 patients), and end-stage renal disease (2 patients). The rate of underlying malignancy was 25%, compared with rates as high as 65% in other series.[106] The skin was the portal of entry in 79% of cases. Infective endocarditis was uncommon in this series, documented in only one patient. In another review of 56 cases of group G streptococcal bacteremia from 11 hospitals in northeastern Ohio,[111] polymicrobial infection, including bacteremia, was an important feature. The most common copathogen was *S. aureus*, probably secondary to the presence of skin and soft tissue infection, the background of surgical procedures and invasive diagnostic maneuvers, and the effects of chemotherapy and underlying malignant disease. Mortality (39% in those with only bacteremia) was usually related to the severity of the underlying disease. In a review from the Mayo Clinic,[106] group G streptococci accounted for 0.3% of all bacteremias and 10.8% of those caused by β-hemolytic streptococci; bacteremia was community-acquired in 70% of cases. This series was characterized by a high frequency of underlying malignancy in infected patients and, typically, a cutaneous portal of entry. Cutaneous origin of the bacteremias was related to chronic venous insufficiency, prior lymph node removal, or disruption by surgery, radiation, or tumor. A 12-year retrospective study of 84 patients with group G streptococcal bacteremia found a median age of 62 years, and confirmed previous findings of frequent underlying disease (35% with malignancy and 35% with diabetes mellitus) and a cutaneous portal of entry (61% from cellulitis).[159] A new finding in this review was that of recurrent group G streptococcal bacteremia (16 episodes in 6 patients), seen primarily in patients with chronic regional lymphatic abnormalities and possibly related to specific M protein types on the bacterium's surface.

Miscellaneous Infections

Several other infections have been reported to be caused by groups C and G β-hemolytic streptococci. These include acute group C streptococcal pericarditis,[160] group G streptococcal pericarditis as the initial presentation of colon cancer,[161] group C streptococcal pyomyositis,[162] and group G streptococcal spinal epidural abscess.[163] A toxic shock–like syndrome associated with both group C and group G streptococci has also been reported.[164,165] Although these organisms are not known to secrete any exotoxin, indirect evidence of superantigen toxin production via stimulation of peripheral blood mononuclear cells was described in a case of group C streptococcal soft tissue infection presenting as a toxic shock–like syndrome. Other documented infections caused by group C streptococci include brain abscess and epiglottitis caused by *S. equi* subsp. *equisimilis*, intra-abdominal infections, subdural empyema, infected arteriovenous fistula, peritonitis in dialysis patients, and an aortitis likely acquired from contact with a patient's horse.[110,166-169] Group G streptococci have also been reported to cause endophthalmitis (after a dental procedure),[170] and were found in one case of a polymicrobial brain abscess in a patient infected with the human immunodeficiency virus.[171]

TREATMENT

Group C Streptococci

The antimicrobial agent of choice for group C β-hemolytic streptococci is penicillin G.[172] Other agents with good in vitro activity include amoxicillin, the ureidopenicillins, penicillins, cefazolin, cefotaxime, vancomycin, and linezolid. Oxacillin and nafcillin are not effective therapy.[173] However, aside from vancomycin, the clinical experience with antimicrobial agents other than penicillin is not extensive. In one study, 95% of erythromycin-resistant isolates revealed the presence of the *mefA* or *mefE* drug efflux gene.[174] A recent review of 20 isolates of group C streptococcus has shown that 30% had resistance to tetracycline, 25% had resistance to erythromycin, and 10% had resistance to ciprofloxacin. Two isolates had intermediate susceptibility to clindamycin.[173] A case of pharyngitis caused by penicillin-resistant *S. equi* subsp. *equisimilis* has been reported, although the mechanism of resistance was not clear.[175] Tolerance has been reported in group C streptococci with minimal bactericidal concentrations ranging from 32- to 512-fold higher than the MIC.[176,177] The frequency of tolerance is unclear; it was reported in 2 of 25 cases in one series[172] and in 16 of 17 cases in another.[176]

A marked synergy for in vitro killing of group C streptococci by penicillin plus gentamicin, independent of penicillin tolerance, has been demonstrated. The addition of gentamicin or rifampin to a β-lactam antibiotic or vancomycin has resulted in bactericidal activity against group C streptococci.[176,177] Although the clinical relevance of these findings is uncertain, retrospective reviews of group C streptococcal endocarditis noted a trend to better outcome in those treated with the combination of penicillin plus gentamicin, compared with penicillin alone,[110] leading the authors to recommend combination therapy for patients with severe infections (e.g., endocarditis, meningitis, septic arthritis, or bacteremia in neutropenic hosts) caused by group C streptococci. Tolerance to cephalothin and vancomycin has also been reported for group C streptococci.

Group G Streptococci

Group G streptococci are susceptible in vitro to various antimicrobial agents, including penicillin G, the ureidopenicillins, most cephalosporins, vancomycin, and linezolid[172,173]; the most active drugs are penicillin, ampicillin, and cefotaxime. Oxacillin and nafcillin are not effective therapeutic agents. Clindamycin, erythromycin, and tetracycline have relatively poor bactericidal activity against group G streptococci,[178] with a recent review of 60 isolates demonstrating 8%, 28%, and 27% resistance to these agents, respectively.[173] Combinations of gentamicin with a penicillin, cefotaxime, or vancomycin are synergistic against 80% to 90% of isolates.[179]

Penicillin tolerance is not a major feature of group G streptococci, and it has been demonstrated only in the presence of a high inoculum and stationary growth phase of the organism. When strains were tested at high inocula (10^8 CFU/mL) of stationary-phase cells, there was a marked reduction in killing by penicillin G. This impaired bactericidal effect was not seen at high inocula of logarithmic-phase organisms or at low inocula of stationary-phase organisms. The paradigm of this high inoculum–stationary phase situation is infective endocarditis, which may partially explain the relatively poor clinical outcome seen in group G streptococcal endocarditis caused by sensitive organisms. The end result of this phenomenon was also seen clinically in a case of antibiotic-sensitive group G streptococcal cellulitis that failed to improve with high-dose penicillin, but that improved dramatically with the addition of clindamycin.[180] Vancomycin tolerance has also been reported in group G streptococci, although tolerance to this agent may also depend on the growth phase and laboratory media used.[178] The clinical significance of tolerance is unclear, and its presence does not necessarily predict clinical inefficacy. The combinations of gentamicin with a β-lactam and of gentamicin or rifampin with vancomycin are bactericidal against tolerant strains.[171] Of concern, however, are reports of the emergence of high-level gentamicin resistance in group G streptococci,[181] which may affect the bactericidal therapy required for treatment of serious infections caused by this organism. Surveillance for high-level aminoglycoside resistance must be carefully monitored.

Streptococcus iniae

Streptococcus iniae, a pathogen recognized fairly recently in humans, is a β-hemolytic streptococcus that does not react with any Lancefield grouping sera. The organism was first reported in 1976 as a cause of subcutaneous abscesses in freshwater dolphins.[182]

In the clinical laboratory, *S. iniae* may elude identification. Few commercial laboratory systems include this species in their database, but approximately 70% of isolates from a fish kill in 1999 were correctly identified by the Biolog Microlog system.[183] In addition, the organism's β-hemolysis may be inapparent under certain growth conditions. As a result, isolates are often misidentified as viridans group streptococci and discounted as contaminants. In 6 of the 11 patients reported by Weinstein and co-workers, *S. iniae* isolates were initially misidentified as *S. uberis,* a viridans group streptococcus not typically pathogenic in humans.[184]

To date, most invasive infections caused by *S. iniae* have been confirmed by the presence of bacteremia. Almost all patients have had cellulitis of the hand as the presumed primary site of infection. Handling of live or killed fish, especially tilapia, has been the usual suspected exposure source. Patients have responded readily to therapy with a β-lactam antibiotic.

Stomatococcus and Pediococcus

Stomatococcus mucilaginosus (reclassified as *Rothia mucilaginosa*[185]) is a gram-positive aerobic coccus that was traditionally found as a cause of oral, cutaneous, and central nervous system infections in impaired hosts. Infections in immunocompetent hosts, including meningitis, necrotizing fasciitis, and prosthetic joint infection, have more recently been reported.[186-188] Most strains are susceptible to third-generation cephalosporins, vancomycin, carbapenems, and levofloxacin.

Pediococcus spp. are gram-positive aerobic cocci that have caused nosocomial infections and are often resistant to vancomycin.[189]

REFERENCES

1. Ruoff KL, Whiley RA, Beighton D. *Streptococcus.* In: Murray PR, Baron EJ, Jorgensen JH, et al., eds. *Manual of Clinical Microbiology.* 8th ed. Washington DC: American Society for Microbiology; 2003:405-421.
2. Colman G, Williams REO. Taxonomy of some human viridans streptococci. In: Wannamaker LW, Matsen JM, eds. *Streptococci and Streptococcal Diseases: Recognition, Understanding, and Management.* New York: Academic Press; 1972:281-299.
3. Facklam RR. Physiological differentiation of viridans streptococci. *J Clin Microbiol.* 1977;5:184-201.
4. Facklam R. What happened to the streptococci: Overview of taxonomic and nomenclature changes. *Clin Microbiol Rev.* 2002;15:613-630.
5. Bruckner DA, Colonna P, Bearson BL. Nomenclature for aerobic and facultative bacteria. *Clin Infect Dis.* 1999;29:713-723.
6. Faibis F, Mihaila L, Perna S, et al. *Streptococcus sinensis*: An emerging agent of infective endocarditis. *J Med Microbiol.* 2008;57:528-531.
7. Glazunova OO, Raoult D, Roux V. *Streptococcus massiliensis* sp. nov., isolated from a patient blood culture. *Int J Syst Evol Microbiol.* 2006;56:1127-1131.
8. Kilian M, Mikkelson L, Henrichsen J. Taxonomic study of viridans streptococci: Description of *Streptococcus gordonii* sp. nov. and amended descriptions of *Streptococcus sanguis* (White and Niven 1946), *Streptococcus oralis* (Bridge and Sneath 1982), and *Streptococcus mitis* (Andrews and Horder 1906). *Int J Syst Bacteriol.* 1989;39:471-484.
9. Schleifer KH, Kilpper-Balz R. Molecular and chemotaxonomic approaches to the classification of streptococci, enterococci, and lactococci: A review. *Syst Appl Microbiol.* 1987;10:1-19.
10. Beighton D, Hardie JM, Whiley RA. A scheme for the identification of viridans streptococci. *J Med Microbiol.* 1991;35:367-372.
11. Hinnebusch CJ, Nikolai DM, Bruckner DA. Comparison of API Rapid Strep, Baxter Microscan Rapid Pos ID Panel, BBL Minitek Differential Identification System, IDS RapID STR System, and Vitek GPI to conventional biochemical tests for identification of viridans streptococci. *Am J Clin Pathol.* 1991;96:459-463.
12. Westling K, Julander I, Ljungman P, et al. Identification of species of viridans streptococci in clinical blood culture isolates by sequence analysis of the RNase P RNA gene, *rnpB*. *J Infection.* 2008;56:204-210.
13. Friedrichs C, Rodloff AC, Chhatwal GS, et al. Rapid identification of viridans streptococci by mass spectrometric discrimination. *J Clin Microbiol.* 2007;45:2392-2397.
14. Collins MD, Hutson RA, Falsen E, et al. Description of *Gemella sanguinis* sp. nov., isolated from human clinical specimens. *J Clin Microbiol.* 1998;36:3090-3093.
15. Kawamura Y, Hou XG, Sultana F, et al. Transfer of *Streptococcus adjacens* and *Streptococcus defectivus* to *Abiotrophia* gen. nov. as *Abiotrophia adiacens* comb. nov. and *Abiotrophia defectiva* comb. nov., respectively. *Int J Syst Bacteriol.* 1995;45:798-803.
16. Collins MD, Lawson PA. The genus *Abiotrophia* (Kawamura et al.) is not monophyletic: Proposal of *Granulicatella* gen. nov., *Granulicatella adiacens* comb. nov., *Granulicatella elegans* comb. nov. *and Granulicatella balaenopterae* com. nov. *Int J Syst Evol Microbiol.* 2000;50:365-369.
17. Gibbons RJ, van Houte J. Selective bacterial adherence to oral epithelial surfaces and its role as an ecological determinant. *Infect Immun.* 1971;3:567-573.
18. Frandsen EVG, Pedrazzoli V, Kilian M. Ecology of viridans streptococci in the oral cavity and pharynx. *Oral Microbiol Immunol.* 1991;6:129-133.
19. Stinson MW, Alder S, Kumar S. Invasion and killing of human endothelial cells by viridans group streptococci. *Infect Immun.* 2003;71:2365-2372.
20. Viscount HB, Munro CL, Burnette-Curley D, et al. Immunization with FimA protects against *Streptococcus parasanguis* endocarditis in rats. *Infect Immun.* 1997;65:994-1002.
21. Lowy FD, Chang DS, Neuhaus EG, et al. Effect of penicillin on the adherence of *Streptococcus sanguis* in vitro and in the rabbit model of endocarditis. *J Clin Invest.* 1983;71:668-675.
22. Hahn CL, Best AM, Tew JG. Rapid tissue factor induction by oral streptococci and monocyte-IL-1beta. *J Dent Res.* 2007;86:255-259.
23. Berkowitz RJ. Acquisition and transmission of mutans streptococci. *J Calif Dent Assoc.* 2003;31:135-138.
24. Veiga-Malta I, Duarte M, Dinis M, et al. Enolase from *Streptococcus sobrinus* is an immunosuppressive protein. *Cell Microbiol.* 2004;6:79-88.
25. Engel A, Kern P, Kern WV. Levels of cytokines and cytokine inhibitors in the neutropenic patients with α-hemolytic streptococcus shock syndrome. *J Infect Dis.* 1996;23:785-789.
26. Hoen B, Alla F, Selton-Suty C, et al. Changing profile of infective endocarditis: Results of a 1-year survey in France. *JAMA.* 2002;288:75-81.
27. Van der Meer JTM, Thompson J, Valkenburg HA, et al. Epidemiology of bacterial endocarditis in the Netherlands: Patient characteristics. *Arch Intern Med.* 1992;152:1863-1868.
28. McKinsey DS, Ratts TE, Bisno AL. Underlying cardiac lesions in adults with infective endocarditis: The changing spectrum. *Am J Med.* 1987;82:681-688.
29. Lin CY, Chao PC, Hong GJ, et al. Infective endocarditis from *Streptococcus viridans* associated with colon carcinoma: A case report. *J Card Surg.* 2008;23:263-265.
30. Barkan D, Abu Fanne R, Elazari-Scheiman A, et al. Navel piercing as a cause for *Streptococcus viridans* endocarditis: Case report, review of the literature and implications for antibiotic prophylaxis. *Cardiol.* 2007;108:159-160.
31. Douglas JL, Cobbs CG. Prosthetic valve endocarditis. In: Kaye D, ed. *Infective Endocarditis.* 2nd ed. New York: Raven Press; 1992:375-396.
32. Bush LM, Johnson CC. Clinical syndrome and diagnosis of endocarditis. In: Donald Kaye, ed. *Infective Endocarditis.* 2nd ed. Philadelphia: Raven Press; 1992:99-115.
33. Shin GY, Manuel RJ, Ghori S, et al. Molecular technique identifies the pathogen responsible for culture negative infective endocarditis. *Heart.* 2005;91:e47.
34. Madershahian N, Strauch JT, Breuer M, et al. Polymerase chain reaction amplification as a diagnostic tool in culture-negative multiple-valve endocarditis. *Ann Thor Surg.* 2005;79:e21-e22.
35. Sokil AB. Cardiac imaging in infective endocarditis. In: Kaye D, ed. *Infective Endocarditis.* 2nd ed. New York: Raven Press; 1992:125-150.
36. Steckelberg JM, Murphy JG, Ballard D, et al. Emboli in infective endocarditis: The prognostic value of echocardiography. *Ann Intern Med.* 1991;114:635-640.
37. Tunkel AR, Scheld WM. Experimental models of endocarditis. In: Kaye D, ed. *Infective Endocarditis.* 2nd ed. New York: Raven Press; 1992:37-56.
38. Sande MA, Irvin RG. Penicillin-aminoglycoside synergy in experimental streptococcal viridans endocarditis. *J Infect Dis.* 1974;129:572-576.
39. Carrizosa J, Kaye D. Antibiotic concentration in serum, bactericidal activity, and results of therapy of streptococcal endocarditis in rabbits. *Antimicrob Agents Chemother.* 1977;12:479-483.
40. Baddour LM, Wilson WR, Bayer AS, et al. Infective endocarditis: Diagnosis, antimicrobial therapy, and management of complications: A statement for healthcare professionals from the Committee on Rheumatic Fever, Endocarditis, and Kawasaki Disease, Council on Cardiovascular Disease in the Young, and the Councils on Clinical Cardiology, Stroke, and Cardiovascular Surgery and Anesthesia, American Heart Association: Endorsed by the Infectious Diseases Society of America. *Circulation.* 2005;111:e394-e433.
41. Wilson WR, Geraci JE. Treatment of streptococcal endocarditis. *Am J Med.* 1985;78(Suppl 6B):128-137.
42. Francioli PB. Ceftriaxone and outpatient treatment of infective endocarditis. *Infect Dis Clin North Am.* 1993;7:97-115.
43. Francioli P, Etienne J, Hoigne R, et al. Treatment of streptococcal endocarditis with a single daily dose of ceftriaxone sodium for 4 weeks: Efficacy and outpatient treatment feasibility. *JAMA.* 1992;267:264-279.
44. Stamboulian D, Bonvehi P, Arevalo C, et al. Antibiotic management of outpatients with infectious endocarditis due to penicillin-susceptible streptococci. *Rev Infect Dis.* 1991;13(Suppl 2):S160-S168.
45. Roberts RB. Streptococcal endocarditis: The viridans and β-hemolytic streptococci. In: Kaye D, ed. *Infective Endocarditis.* 2nd ed. New York: Raven Press; 1992:191-208.
46. Levy CS, Kogulan P, Gill VJ, et al. Endocarditis caused by penicillin-resistant viridans streptococci: 2 cases and controversies in therapy. *Clin Infect Dis.* 2001;33:577-579.
47. Swenson FJ, Rubin SJ. Clinical significance of viridans streptococci isolated from blood cultures. *J Clin Microbiol.* 1982;15:725-727.
48. Engelhard D, Elishoov H, Or R, et al. Cytosine arabinoside as a major risk factor for *Streptococcus viridans* septicemia following bone marrow transplantation: A 5-year prospective study. *Bone Marrow Transplant.* 1995;16:565-570.
49. Elting LS, Bodey GP, Keefe BH. Septicemia and shock syndrome due to viridans streptococci: A case-control study of predisposing factors. *Clin Infect Dis.* 1992;14:1201-1207.
50. Bilgrami S, Feingold JM, Dorsky D, et al. *Streptococcus viridans* bacteremia following autologous peripheral blood stem cell transplantation. *Bone Marrow Transplant.* 1998;21:591-595.
51. Bert F, Valla D, Moreau R, et al. Viridans group streptococci causing spontaneous bacterial peritonitis and bacteremia in patients with end-stage liver disease. *Liver Transplant.* 2008;14:710-711.

52. Burden AD, Oppenheim BA, Crowther D, et al. Viridans streptococcal bacteremia in patients with haematological and solid malignancies. *Eur J Cancer*. 1991;27:409-411.
53. Bostrom B, Weisdorf D. Mucositis and α-streptococcal sepsis in bone marrow transplant recipients. *Lancet*. 1984;1:1120-1121.
54. Ringden O, Heimdahl A, Lonnqvist B, et al. Decreased incidence of viridans streptococcal septicaemia in allogeneic bone marrow transplant recipients after the introduction of acyclovir. *Lancet*. 1984;1:744.
55. Villablanca JG, Steiner M, Kersey J, et al. The clinical spectrum of infections with viridans streptococci in bone marrow transplant patients. *Bone Marrow Transplant*. 1990;6:387-393.
56. Martino R, Manteiga R, Sanchez I, et al. Viridans streptococcal shock syndrome during bone marrow transplantation. *Acta Haematol*. 1995;94:69-73.
57. Tunkel AR, Sepkowitz KA. Infections caused by viridans streptococci in patients with neutropenia. *Clin Infect Dis*. 2002;34:1524-1529.
58. Koren P, Krcmery V Jr. Viridans streptococcal bacteremia due to penicillin-resistant and penicillin-sensitive streptococci: Analysis of risk factors and outcome in 60 patients from a single cancer centre before and after penicillin is used for prophylaxis. *Scand J Infect Dis*. 1997;29:245-249.
59. Arns da Cunha C, Weisdorf D, Shu XO, et al. Early gram-positive bacteremia in BMT recipients: Impact of three different approaches to antimicrobial prophylaxis. *Bone Marrow Transplant*. 1998;21:173-180.
60. Mrazova M, Docze A, Buckova E, et al. Prospective national survey of viridans streptococcal bactaeremia risk factors, antibacterial susceptibility and outcome of 120 episodes. *Scand J Infect Dis*. 2005;37:637-641.
61. Hoyne AL, Herzon H. *Streptococcus viridans* meningitis: A review of the literature and report of nine recoveries. *Ann Intern Med*. 1950;33:879-902.
62. Enting RH, deGans J, Blankevoort JP, et al. Meningitis due to viridans streptococci in adults. *J Neurol*. 1997;244:435-438.
63. Leiger JF. *Streptococcus salivarius* meningitis and colonic carcinoma. *South Med J*. 1991;84:1058-1059.
64. Legrand M, Denis J, Drouhin F, et al. Bacterial meningitis following upper gastrointestinal endoscopy in patients with cirrhosis—bear it in mind. *Endoscopy*. 2007;39:E96.
65. Heath RE, Rogers JA, Cheldelin LV, et al. *Streptococcus sanguis* sepsis and meningitis: A complication of vacuum extraction. *Am J Obstet Gynecol*. 1980;138:343-344.
66. Bignardi GE, Isaacs D. Neonatal meningitis due to *Streptococcus mitis*. *Rev Infect Dis*. 1989;11:86-88.
67. Baer ET. Post-dural puncture bacterial meningitis. *Anesthesiology*. 2006;105:381-393.
68. Schneeberger PM, Janssen M. Voss A. α-Hemolytic streptococci: A major pathogen of iatrogenic meningitis following lumbar puncture. *Infection*. 1996;24:29-33.
69. Nachamkin I, Dalton HP. The clinical significance of streptococcal species isolated from cerebrospinal fluid. *Am J Clin Pathol*. 1983;79:195-199.
70. Neal JB, Jackson HW, Appelbaum E. Neurological complications of subacute bacterial endocarditis. *N Y State J Med*. 1936;36:1819.
71. Lorber B, Swenson RM. Bacteriology of aspiration pneumonia. *Ann Intern Med*. 1974;81:329-331.
72. Rose H. Viridans streptococcal pneumonia [letter]. *JAMA*. 1981;245:32.
73. Pratter MR, Irwin RS. Viridans streptococcal pulmonary parenchymal infections. *JAMA*. 1980;243:2515-2517.
74. Sarkar TK, Murarka RS, Gilardi GL. Primary *Streptococcus viridans* pneumonia. *Chest*. 1989;96:831-834.
75. Marrie TJ. Bacteremic community-acquired pneumonia due to viridans group streptococci. *Clin Invest Med*. 1993;16:38-44.
76. Liang SJ, Chen W, Lin YC, et al. Community-acquired thoracic empyema in young adults. *South Med J*. 2007;100:1075-1080.
77. Rodriguez-Avial I, Rodriguez-Avial C, Culebras E, et al. Fluoroquinolone resistance among invasive viridans group streptococci and *Streptococcus bovis* isolated in Spain. *Int J Antimicrob Agents*. 2007;29:478-480.
78. Pfaller MA, Jones RN, Marshall SA, et al. Nosocomial streptococcal bloodstream infections in the SCOPE program: Species occurrence and antimicrobial susceptibility. *Diagn Microbiol Infect Dis*. 1997;29:259-263.
79. Prabhu RM, Piper KE, Baddour LM, et al. Antimicrobial susceptibility patterns among viridans group streptococcal isolates from infective endocarditis patients from 1971 to 1986 and 1994 to 2002. *Antimicrob Agents Chemother*. 2004;48:4463-4465.
80. Hsu RB, Lin FY. Effect of penicillin resistance on presentation and outcome of nonenterococcal streptococcal endocarditis. *Cardiology*. 2006;105:234-239.
81. Pfaller MA, Marshall SA, Jones RN. In vitro activity of cefepime and ceftazidime against 197 nosocomial blood stream isolates of streptococci: A multicenter study. *Diagn Microbiol Infect Dis*. 1997;29:273-276.
82. Tuohy M, Washington JA. Antimicrobial susceptibility of viridans group streptococci. *Diagn Microbiol Infect Dis*. 1997;29:277-280.
83. Lowy FD, Neuhaus EG, Chang DS, et al. Penicillin therapy of experimental endocarditis induced by tolerant *Streptococcus sanguis* and non-tolerant *Streptococcus mitis*. *Antimicrob Agents Chemother*. 1983;28:607-611.
84. Handwerger S, Tomasz A. Antibiotic tolerance among clinical isolates of bacteria. *Rev Infect Dis*. 1985;7:368-386.
85. Moet GJ, Dowzicky MJ, Jones RN. Tigecycline (GAR-936) activity against *Streptococcus gallolyticus (bovis)* and viridans group streptococci. *Diagn Microbiol Infect Dis*. 2007;57:333-336.
86. McWhinney PHM, Patel S, Whiley RA, et al. Activities of potential therapeutic and prophylactic antibiotics against blood culture isolates of viridans group streptococci from neutropenic cancer patients receiving ciprofloxacin. *Antimicrob Agents Chemother*. 1993;37:2493-2495.
87. Hepburn MJ, Fraser SL, Rennie TA, et al. Septic arthritis caused by *Granulicatella adiacens*: Diagnosis by inoculation of synovial fluid into blood culture bottles. *Rheum International*. 2003;23:255-257.
88. Roggenkamp A, Leitritz L, Baus K, et al. PCR for detection and identification of *Abiotrophia* spp. *J Clin Microbiol*. 1998;36:2844-2846.
89. Casalta JP, Habib G, La Scola B, et al. Molecular diagnosis of *Granulicatella elegans* on the cardiac valve of a patient with culture-negative endocarditis. *J Clin Microbiol*. 2002;40:1845-1847.
90. Woo PC, Fung AM, Lau SK, et al. *Granulicatella adiacens* and *Abiotrophia defectiva* bacteraemia characterized by 16S rRNA gene sequencing. *J Med Microbiol*. 2003;52:137-140.
91. Zheng X, Freeman AF, Villafranca J, et al. Antimicrobial susceptibilities of invasive pediatric *Abiotrophia* and *Granulicatella* isolates. *J Clin Microbiol*. 2004;42:4323-4326.
92. Liao CH, Teng LJ, Hsueh PR, et al. Nutritionally variant streptococcal infections at a University Hospital in Taiwan: Disease emergence and high prevalence of beta-lactam and macrolide resistance. *Clin Infect Dis*. 2004;38:452-455.
93. Senn L, Entenza JM, Prod'hom G. Adherence of *Abiotrophia defectiva* and *Granulicatella* species to fibronectin: Is there a link with endovascular infection? *FEMS Immunol Med Microbiol*. 2006;48:215-217.
94. Senn L, Entenza JM, Greub G, et al. Bloodstream and endovascular infections due to *Abiotrophia defectiva* and *Granulicatella* species. *BMC Infect Dis*. 2006;6:9.
95. Stein DS, Nelson KE. Endocarditis due to nutritionally deficient streptococci: Therapeutic dilemma. *Rev Infect Dis*. 1987;9:908-916.
96. Ince A, Tiemer B, Gille J, et al. Total knee arthroplasty infection due to *Abiotrophia defectiva*. *J Med Microbiol*. 2002;51:899-902.
97. del Pozo JL, Garcia-Quetglas E, Hernaez S, et al. *Granulicatella adaciens* breast implant–associated infection. *Diagn Microbiol Infect Dis*. 2008;61:58-60.
98. Cerceo E, Christie JD, Nachamkin I, et al. Central nervous system infections due to *Abiotrophia* and *Granulicatella* species: An emerging challenge? *Diagn Microbiol Infect Dis*. 2004;48:161-165.
99. Foley GE. Further observations on the occurrence of streptococci of groups other than A in human infection. *N Engl J Med*. 1947;237:809-811.
100. Broome CV, Moellering RC Jr, Watson BK. Clinical significance of Lancefield groups L-T streptococci from blood and cerebrospinal fluid. *J Infect Dis*. 1976;133:382-392.
101. Bradley SF, Gordon JJ, Baumgartner DD, et al. Group C streptococcal bacteremia: Analysis of 88 cases. *Rev Infect Dis*. 1991;13:270-280.
102. Centers for Disease Control and Prevention (CDC). Group C streptococcal infection associated with eating homemade cheese—New Mexico. *MMWR Morb Mortal Wkly Rep*. 1983;32:510-516.
103. Barnham M, Kerby J, Chandler RS, et al. Group C streptococci in human infection: A study of 308 isolates with clinical correlations. *Epidemiol Infect*. 1989;102:379-390.
104. Lancefield RC, Hare R. The serological differentiation of pathogenic and non-pathogenic strains of hemolytic streptococci from parturient women. *J Exp Med*. 1935;61:335-349.
105. Armstrong D, Blevins A, Louria DB, et al. Groups B, C, and G streptococcal infections in a cancer hospital. *Ann NY Acad Sci*. 1970;174:511-522.
106. Auckenthaler R, Hermans PE, Washington JA II. Group G streptococcal bacteremia: Clinical study and review of the literature. *Rev Infect Dis*. 1983;5:196-204.
107. Wasky KL, Kollisch N, Densen P. Group G streptococcal bacteremia: The clinical experience at Boston University Medical Center and a critical review of the literature. *Arch Intern Med*. 1985;145:58-61.
108. Lam MM, Clarridge JE III, Young EJ, et al. The other group G streptococcus: Increased detection of *Streptococcus canis* ulcer infections in dog owners. *J Clin Microbiol*. 2007;45:2327-2329.
109. Galperine T, Cazorla C, Blanchard E, et al. *Streptococcus canis* infections in humans: Retrospective study of 54 patients. *J Infect*. 2007;55:23-26.
110. Salata RA, Lerner PI, Shlaes DM, et al. Infections due to Lancefield group C streptococci. *Medicine (Baltimore)*. 1989;68:225-239.
111. Vartian C, Lerner PI, Shlaes DM, et al. Infections due to Lancefield group G streptococci. *Medicine (Baltimore)*. 1985;64:75-88.
112. Mohr DN, Feist DJ, Washington JA II, et al. Infections due to group C streptococci in man. *Am J Med*. 1979;66:450-456.
113. Cimolai N, Elford RW, Bryan L, et al. Do the β-hemolytic non-group A streptococci cause pharyngitis? *Rev Infect Dis*. 1988;10:587-601.
114. Zaoutis T, Attia M, Gross R, et al. The role of group C and group G streptococci in acute pharyngitis in children. *Clin Microbiol Infect*. 2004;10:37-40.
115. Meier FA, Centor RM, Graham L, et al. Clinical and microbiological evidence for endemic pharyngitis among adults due to group C streptococci. *Arch Intern Med*. 1990;150:825-829.
116. Turner JC, Hayden GF, Kiselica D, et al. Association of group C β-hemolytic streptococci with endemic pharyngitis among college students. *JAMA*. 1990;264:2644-2647.
117. Shah M, Centor RM, Jennings M. Severe acute pharyngitis caused by group C streptococcus. *J Gen Intern Med*. 2007;22:272-274.
118. Hayden GF, Turner JC, Kiselica D, et al. Latex agglutination testing directly from throat swabs for rapid detection of β-hemolytic streptococci from Lancefield serogroup C. *J Clin Microbiol*. 1992;30:716-718.
119. McCue JD. Group G streptococcal pharyngitis: Analysis of an outbreak at a college. *JAMA*. 1982;248:1333-1336.
120. Gerber MA, Randolph MF, Martin NJ, et al. Community-wide outbreak of group G streptococcal pharyngitis. *Pediatrics*. 1991;87:598-603.
121. Barnham M, Thorton TJ, Lange K. Nephritis caused by *Streptococcus zooepidemicus* (Lancefield group C). *Lancet*. 1983;1:945-948.
122. Lebrun L, Guibert M, Wallet P, et al. Human Fc(g) receptors for differentiation in throat cultures of group C "*Streptococcus equisimilis*" and group C "*Streptococcus milleri*." *J Clin Microbiol*. 1988;24:705-707.
123. Reid HF, Bassett DC, Poon-King T, et al. Group G streptococci in healthy school-children and in patients with glomerulonephritis in Trinidad. *J Hyg*. 1985;94:61-68.
124. Jansen TL, Janssen M, de Jong AJ. Reactive arthritis associated with group C and group G beta-hemolytic streptococci. *J Rheumatol*. 1998;25:1126-1130.
125. Geyer A, Roth A, Vettermann S, et al. M protein of a *Streptococcus dysgalactiae* human wound isolate shows multiple binding to different plasma proteins and shares epitopes with keratin and human cartilage. *FEMS Immunol Med Microbiol*. 1999;26:11-24.
126. Siljander T, Karppelin M, Vahakuopus S, et al. Acute bacterial, nonnecrotizing cellulitis in Finland: Microbiological findings. *Clin Infect Dis*. 2008;46:855-861.
127. Ike RW. Septic arthritis due to group C streptococcus: Report and review of the literature. *J Rheumatol*. 1990;17:1230-1236.
128. Ortel TL, Kallianos J, Gallis HA. Group C streptococcal arthritis: Case report and review. *Rev Infect Dis*. 1990;12:829-837.
129. Collazos J, Echevarria MJ, Ayarza R, et al. *Streptococcus zooepidemicus* septic arthritis: Case report and review of group C streptococcal arthritis. *Clin Infect Dis*. 1992;15:744-746.
130. Nakata MM, Silvers JH, George WL. Group G streptococcal arthritis. *Arch Intern Med*. 1983;143:1328-1330.
131. Bronze MS, Whitby S, Schaberg DR. Group G streptococcal arthritis: A case report and review of the literature. *Am J Med Sci*. 1997;313:239-243.
132. Burkert T, Watanakunakorn C. Group G streptococcus septic arthritis and osteomyelitis: Report and literature review. *J Rheumatol*. 1991;18:904-907.
133. Asciutto R, Drennan J, Fitzgerald V, et al. Group C streptococcal arthritis and osteomyelitis in an adolescent with a hereditary sensory neuropathy. *Pediatr Infect Dis*. 1985;4:553-554.
134. Barson WJ. Group C streptococcal osteomyelitis. *J Pediatr Orthop*. 1986;6:346-348.
135. Tobias JH, Lee PYC, Bruckner FE. Group G β-haemolytic streptococcal vertebral osteomyelitis. *J Infect*. 1992;25:115-116.
136. Sarria JC, Perez-Verdia A, Kimbrough RC 3rd, et al. Deep sternal wound infection caused by group G streptococcus after open heart surgery. *Am J Med Sci*. 2004;327:253-254.
137. Tong SH, Tang WM, Wong JW. Group G streptococcus—a rare cause of osteomyelitis simulating bone tumour: A case report. *J Orthopaed Surg*. 2003;11:221-223.
138. Stamm AM, Cobbs CG. Group C streptococcal pneumonia: Report of a fatal case and review of the literature. *Rev Infect Dis*. 1980;2:889-898.
139. Dolinski SY, Jones PG, Zabransky RJ, et al. Group C streptococcal pleurisy and pneumonia: A fulminant case and review of the literature. *Infection*. 1990;18:239-241.
140. Gallagher PG, Hyer CM III, Crone K, et al. Group C streptococcal sinusitis. *Am J Otolaryngol*. 1990;11:352-354.
141. Bouza E, Meyer RD, Busch DF. Group G streptococcal endocarditis. *Am J Clin Pathol*. 1978;70:108-111.
142. Blair DC, Martin DB. β-Hemolytic streptococcal endocarditis: Predominance of non–group A organisms. *Am J Med Sci*. 1978;276:269-277.
143. Venezio FR, Gullberg RM, Westenfelder GO, et al. Group G streptococcal endocarditis and bacteremia. *Am J Med*. 1986;81:29-34.
144. Smyth EG, Pallett AP, Davidson RN. Group G streptococcal endocarditis: Two case reports, a review of the literature and recommendations for treatment. *J Infect*. 1988;16:169-176.
145. Low DE, Young MR, Harding GKM. Group C streptococcal meningitis in an adult: Probable acquisition from a horse. *Arch Intern Med*. 1980;140:977-978.
146. Daly MP. Group G streptococcal infection in an elderly patient. *South Med J*. 1992;85:43-44.
147. Edwards AT, Roulson M, Ironside MJ. A milk-borne outbreak of serious infection due to *Streptococcus zooepidemicus* (Lancefield group C). *Epidemiol Infect*. 1988;101:43-51.

148. Downar J, Willey BM, Sutherland JW, et al. Streptococcal meningitis resulting from contact with an infected horse. *J Clin Microbiol.* 2001;39:2358-2359.

149. Ural O, Tuncer I, Dikici N, et al. *Streptococcus zooepidemicus* meningitis and bacteraemia. *Scand J Infect Dis.* 2003;35: 206-207.

150. Mollison LC, Donaldson E. Group C streptococcal meningitis. *Med J Aust.* 1990;152:319-320.

151. Shah S, Matthews RP, Cohen C. Group C streptococcal meningitis: Case report and review of the literature. *Pediatr Infect Dis J.* 2001;20:445-448.

152. Ramsay AM, Gillespie M. Puerperal infection associated with haemolytic streptococci other than Lancefield's group A. *J Obstet Gynecol Br Empire.* 1941;48:569-585.

153. Appelbaum PC, Friedman Z, Fairbrother PF, et al. Neonatal sepsis due to group G streptococci. *Acta Paediatr Scand.* 1980;69:559-562.

154. Dyson AE, Read SE. Group G streptococcal colonization and sepsis in neonates. *J Pediatr.* 1981;99:944-947.

155. Berenguer J, Sampedro I, Cercenado E, et al. Group C β-hemolytic streptococcal bacteremia. *Diagn Microbiol Infect Dis.* 1992;15:151-155.

156. Carmeli Y, Ruoff KL. Report of cases of and taxonomic considerations for large-colony-forming Lancefield group C streptococcal bacteremia. *J Clin Microbiol.* 1995;33:2114-2117.

157. Yuen KY, Seto WH, Choi CH, et al. *Streptococcus zooepidemicus* (Lancefield group C) septicaemia in Hong Kong. *J Infect.* 1990; 21:241-250.

158. Rolston KVI. Group G streptococcal infections. *Arch Intern Med.* 1986;146:857-858.

159. Chen-Poradosu R, Jaffe J, Lavi D, et al. Group G streptococcal bacteremia in Jerusalem. *Emerg Infect Dis.* 2004;10:1455-1460.

160. McClure RS, Burgess JJ, Bayes AJ, et al. Primary purulent pericarditis due to group C streptococcus. *Can J Cardiol.* 2004; 20:1479-1480.

161. Kim NH, Park JP, Jeon SH, et al. Purulent pericarditis caused by group G streptococcus as an initial presentation of colon cancer. *J Korean Med Sci.* 2002;17:571-573.

162. Woo PC, Teng JL, Lau SK, et al. Analysis of a viridans group strain reveals a case of bacteremia due to Lancefield group G alpha-hemolytic *Streptococcus dysgalactiae* subsp *equisimilis* in a patient with pyomyositis and reactive arthritis. *J Clin Microbiol.* 2003;41:613-618.

163. Saeed MU, Gottmukkula R, Kennedy DJ. Group G streptococcus spinal epidural abscess: case report and review of the literature. *Scand J Infect Dis.* 2007;39:1073-1075.

164. Wagner JG, Schlievert PM, Assimacopoulos AP, et al. Acute group G streptococcal myositis associated with streptococcal toxic shock syndrome: A case report and review. *Clin Infect Dis.* 1996;23:1159-1161.

165. Korman TM, Boers A, Gooding TM, et al. Fatal case of toxic shock-like syndrome due to group C streptococcus associated with superantigen exotoxin. *J Clin Microbiol.* 2004;42: 2866-2869.

166. Dinn JJ. Brain abscess due to *Streptococcus equisimilis* in a maltworker. *J Ir Med Assoc.* 1971;64:50-51.

167. Lee TW, Sandoe JA. Epiglottitis caused by group C streptococcus. *Acta Paediatr.* 2001;90;1085.

168. Layton J, McCulley D. Subdural empyema and group C streptococcus. *South Med J.* 1985;78:64-66.

169. Gonzales AJ, Hughes JD, Leon LR Jr. Probable zoonotic aortitis due to group C streptococcal infection. *J Vasc Surg.* 2007;46: 1039-1043.

170. Ziakis NG, Tzetzi D, Boboridis K, et al. Endogenous group G streptococcus endophthalmitis following a dental procedure. *Eur J Ophthalmol.* 2004;14:59-60.

171. Maniglia RJ, Roth T, Blumber EA. Polymicrobial brain abscess in a patient with human immunodeficiency virus. *Clin Infect Dis.* 1997;24:449-451.

172. Rolston KVI, LeFrock JL, Schell RF. Activity of nine antimicrobial agents against Lancefield group C and group G streptococci. *Antimicrob Agents Chemother.* 1982;22:930-932.

173. Lloyd CA, Jacob SE, Menon T. Antibiotic resistant beta-hemolytic streptococci. *Indian J Pediatr.* 2007;74:1077-1080.

174. Kataja J, Seppala H, Skurnik M, et al. Different erythromycin resistance mechanisms in group C and group G streptococci. *Antimicrob Agents Chemother.* 1998;42:1493-1494.

175. Hutchinson NA, Eltringham IL. Therapeutic failure in group C streptococcal pharyngitis [letter]. *Lancet.* 1995;346:1367.

176. Portnoy D, Prentis J, Richards GK. Penicillin tolerance of human isolates of group C streptococci. *Antimicrob Agents Chemother.* 1981;20:235-238.

177. Rolston KVI, Chandraseker PH, LeFrock JL. Antimicrobial tolerance in group C and group G streptococci. *J Antimicrob Chemother.* 1984;13:389-392.

178. Lam K, Bayer AS. Serious infections due to group G streptococci. *Am J Med.* 1983;75:561-570.

179. Lam K, Bayer AS. In vitro bactericidal synergy of gentamicin combined with penicillin G, vancomycin, or cefotaxime against group G streptococci. *Antimicrob Agents Chemother.* 1984;26: 260-262.

180. Pillai A, Thomas S, Williams C. Clindamycin in the treatment of group G beta-haemolytic streptococcal infections. *J Infect.* 2005;51:e207-e211.

181. Faibis F, Fiacre A, Demachy MC. Emergence of high-level gentamicin resistance in group G streptococci. *Eur J Clin Microbiol Infect Dis.* 2001;20:901-902.

182. Pier GB, Madin SH. *Streptococcus iniae* sp. nov., a beta-hemolytic streptococcus isolated from an Amazon freshwater dolphin, *Imia geoffrensis. Int J Syst Bacteriol.* 1976;26:545-553.

183. Roach JC, Levett PN, Lavoie MC. Identification of *Streptococcus iniae* by commercial bacterial identification systems. *J Microbiol Methods.* 2006;67:20-26.

184. Weinstein MR, Litt M, Kert DA, et al. Invasive infections due to a fish pathogen, *Streptococcus iniae. N Engl J Med.* 1997;337: 589-594.

185. Collins MD, Hutson RA, Baverud V, et al. Characterization of a *Rothia*-like organism from a mouse: Description of *Rothia nasimurium* sp. nov. and reclassification of *Stomatococcus mucilaginosus* as *Rothia mucilaginosa* comb. nov. *Int J Syst Evol Microbiol.* 2000;50:1247-1251.

186. Rizvi M, Fatima N, Shukla I, et al. *Stomatococcus mucilaginosus* meningitis in a healthy 2-month-old child. *J Med Microbiol.* 2008;57:382-383.

187. Lowry TR, Brennan JA. *Stomatococcus mucilaginosis* infection leading to early cervical necrotizing fasciitis. *Otolaryngol Head Neck Surg.* 2005;132:658-660.

188. Michels F, Colaert J, Gheysen F, et al. Late prosthetic joint infection due to *Rothia mucilaginosa. Acta Orthopaedica Belgica.* 2007;73:263-267.

189. Barton LL, Rider ED, Coen RW. Bacteremic infection with *Pediococcus*: Vancomycin-resistant opportunist. *Pediatrics.* 2001;107:775-776.

204

Streptococcus anginosus Group

CATHY A. PETTI | CHARLES W. STRATTON IV

Streptococcus intermedius, Streptococcus constellatus, and *Streptococcus anginosus* are three distinct species[1] that constitute the *Streptococcus anginosus* group.[2] This group is also commonly referred to as the *Streptococcus milleri* group.[3] Genetic and phenotypic studies[3-6] have clearly demonstrated that the *S. anginosus* group consists of these three distinct streptococcal species, with *S. constellatus* having two subspecies, *S. constellatus* subsp. *constellatus* and *S. constellatus* subsp. *pharyngis.* These species and subspecies appear to be associated with a number of different body habitats as well as sites and types of clinical infections.[7-9]

Clinically, this group causes invasive pyogenic infections, which usually differentiates them from the other viridans streptococci.[3,8,9] Microbiologically, members of this group are recognized by their microaerophilic or anaerobic growth requirements, their formation of minute colonies, and the frequent presence of a characteristic caramel-like odor.[2] This chapter defines the three species currently making up the *S. anginosus* group and discusses their role in clinical infections.

Bacteriologic Characteristics

Members of the *S. anginosus* group share the phenotypic characteristics of the members of the genus *Streptococcus,* whose classification in general is based on patterns of hemolysis, Lancefield serologic antigenic reactions, growth properties, and biochemical reactions (Fig. 204-1). Like other streptococci, these organisms may be β-hemolytic, α-hemolytic, or γ-hemolytic on sheep blood agar. Members of the *S. anginosus* group often exhibit Lancefield antigens A, C, F, or G, but can be differentiated from Lancefield-grouped streptococci by the small size of their colonies. Strains containing the group F antigen may cross-react with the other grouping sera: Lancefield groupings therefore are of little value in identifying these organisms.[2,9]

Gram staining of *S. intermedius* strains reveals gram-positive spherical or ovoid cells that form short chains or pairs. *S. anginosus* group can be differentiated from other streptococci by a combination of three rapid tests—a positive Voges-Proskauer test for acetoin production, hydrolysis of arginine, and failure to ferment sorbitol.[2,3,9] In addition, the presence of the caramel-like odor, often attributed to the production of a diacetyl metabolite, can be helpful. These characteristics are summarized in Table 204-1.

Taxonomy

The diversity of hemolytic and Lancefield groupings have made identification of these pathogens difficult in many laboratories.[2] Whiley and colleagues[3] have noted that almost all *S. intermedius* strains (93%) are not β-hemolytic, whereas 38% of *S. constellatus* and 12% of *S. anginosus* are β-hemolytic. Of those strains of *S. constellatus* and *S. anginosus* that reacted with Lancefield serologic group F antibody, almost all the former but almost none of the latter were β-hemolytic. Laboratories can readily differentiate the three members of the *S. anginosus* group using phenotypic characteristics that correlate well with molecular taxonomic techniques.[2-9] A number of commercial systems are available for the identification of viridans streptococci, and studies have shown similar performance to manual biochemical testing.[10-12]

Nucleic acid amplification assays have been developed for the identification of clinically relevant viridans group streptococci to the species and group level. Targets for these assays have included the 16S rRNA gene, the 16S-23S rRNA intergenic spacer region, *tuf* gene, *rpoB* gene, or *groEL* gene. Most assays require both amplification and sequencing of the targeted region, making the method impractical for routine use in the clinical laboratory. Additionally, viridans streptococci are naturally competent—that is, they freely exchange genetic material within and between species. This phenomenon makes the taxonomic classification of viridans streptococci by DNA target sequencing and their identification to species level much more challenging. Additionally, non–sequence-based methods for identification, such as matrix-assisted laser desorption ionization–time of light mass spectrometry (MALDI-TOF-MS), have been reported, with promising results.[13]

Normal Habitat

Members of the *S. anginosus* group have been considered harmless commensals of the oropharyngeal, urogenital, and gastrointestinal microbiota.[2] *S. intermedius* is more commonly found in dental plaque whereas *S. anginosus* is more frequently found in the gastrointestinal tract.[7] Spread from the gastrointestinal tract to the vagina with subsequent vaginal colonization is common.[14]

Pathogenicity

The association of the *S. anginosus* group with the tendency to form abscesses has long been recognized.[2] However, the reasons for this pathogenic characteristic are not yet completely understood. Part of the explanation appears to be that mixed infections involving members of the *S. anginosus* group and other microbes (e.g., *Eikenella corrodens* and anaerobes) allow more rapid replication of the streptococci.[15,16] A murine model of pneumonia has been used to demonstrate synergy between members of the *S. anginosus* group and oral anaerobes.[17] This study found that mortality was higher, abscesses or empyema were more frequently noted on histopathologic examination, and viable bacteria were more numerous in the lungs of mice with mixed infections caused by members of the *S. intermedius* group and oral anaerobes than in the lungs of mice with monomicrobial infection. In vitro studies by these investigators have confirmed that anaerobes enhance the growth of *S. anginosus* group organisms. In 45 cases of acute pneumonia and/or pulmonary abscess and 25 cases of thoracic empyema in humans, the predominant species recovered were anaerobic bacteria and members of the *S. anginosus* group,[17] confirming the clinical importance of this phenomenon in pulmonary infections.

Anginosus group streptococci also possess virulence factors that are likely to be involved in their ability to cause serious invasive infections. For example, members of the *S. anginosus* group may express a number of different adhesins on their cell surfaces that facilitate adherence to substrates found in their natural environment.[18-21] All members of the *S. anginosus* group are able to bind fibronectin via a cell surface protein,[19] and some strains are able to bind to platelets, fibrin, fibrin clots, and fibrinogen.[20] This property is thought to be a factor in the ability of these pathogens to cause endocarditis. Fibrinogen binding may, in turn, aid in platelet aggregation, which would also facilitate the development of endocarditis.[21,22] In an experimental rat endocarditis model in which all three species of the *S. anginosus* group were studied, *S. anginosus* strains produced infective vegetations and bacteremia in almost all catheterized rats, *S. constellatus* strains did so less frequently, and *S. intermedius* strains did so only occasionally.[23] Moreover, the vegetations infected with *S. anginosus* strains harbored significantly higher numbers of microorganisms than those infected by other strains.

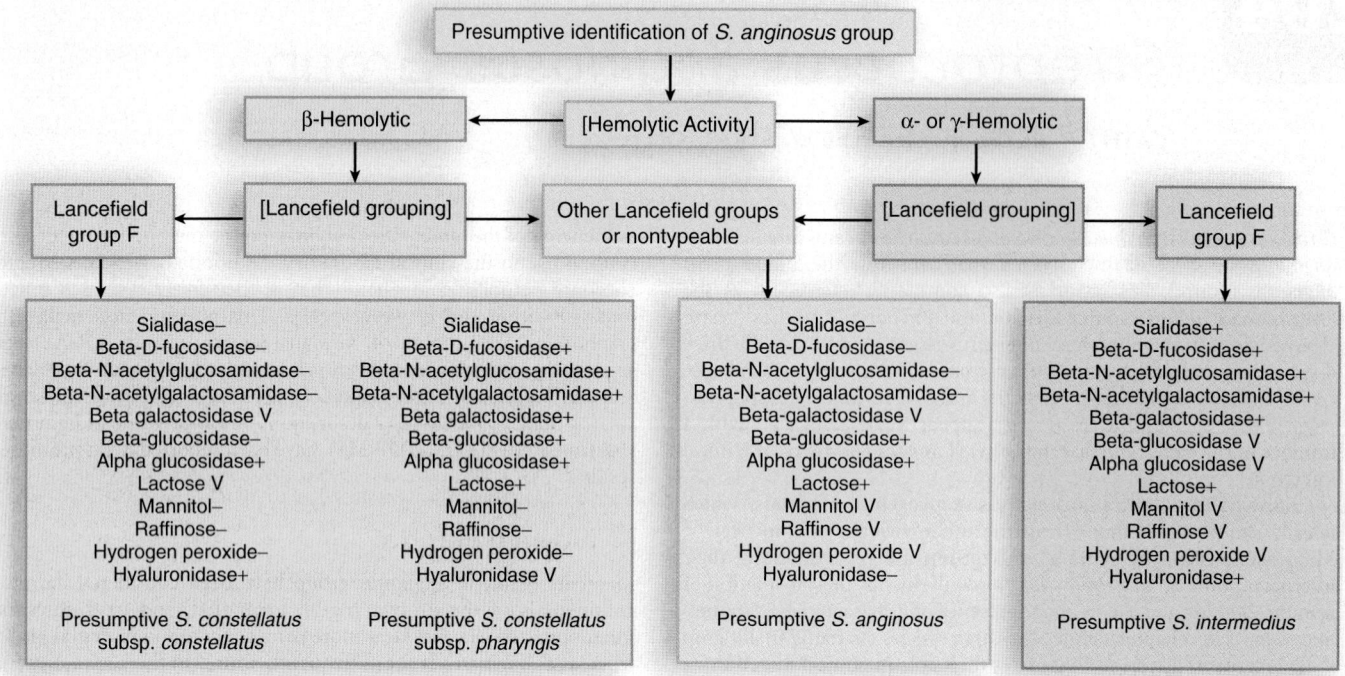

Figure 204-1 **Phenotypic differentiation of the members of the *Streptococcus anginosus* group.** V, Variable; +, at least 90% of strains have a positive reaction; –, at least 90% of strains have a negative reaction. *(Adapted from Whiley RA, Fraser HY, Hardie JM, et al. Phenotypic differentiation of Streptococcus constellatus, Streptococcus intermedius, and Streptococcus anginosus [the Streptococcus milleri group]: Association with different body sites and clinical infections. J Clin Microbiol. 1990;28:1497–1501 and Whiley RA, Hall LMC, Hardie JM, Beighton D. A study of small colony, beta-haemolytic, Lancefield group C streptococci within the anginosus group: Description of Streptococcus constellatus subsp. pharyngis subsp. nov., associated with the human throat and pharyngitis. Int J Syst Bacteriol. 1999;49:1443–1449.)*

Another potential virulence factor is the frequent presence in members of the *S. anginosus* group of a polysaccharide capsule[9] that hinders phagocytosis. The ability to escape phagocytosis would allow these pathogens to replicate after arriving at and adhering to a site of tissue damage. A murine model used to investigate the pathogenicity

TABLE 204-1	Presumptive Identification of Members of the *Streptococcus anginosus* Group

Growth of Minute Streptococcal Colonies Under Microaerophilic-Anaerobic Conditions:

Acid from
• Insulin –
• Sorbitol –
• Salicin +
Hydrolysis of
• Hippurate –
• Esculin +
• Deoxyribonuclease –
• Arginine dihydrolysis +
• Voges-Proskauer test*+
• Caramel-like odor V
↓
Presumptive *S. anginosus* group

+, ≥90% of strains have a positive reaction; –, ≥90% of strains have a negative reaction; V, variable; *, rare exceptions.

Adapted from Spellerberg B, Brandt C. *Streptococcus.* In: Murray PR, Baron EJ, Jorgenson JH, et al, eds. *Manual of Clinical Microbiology.* 9th ed. Washington DC: American Society for Microbiology Press; 2007:412-429; Whiley RA, Fraser HY, Hardie JM, et al. Phenotypic differentiation of *Streptococcus constellatus, Streptococcus intermedius,* and *Streptococcus anginosus* (the *Streptococcus milleri* group): Association with different body sites and clinical infections. *J Clin Microbiol.* 1990;28:1497-1501; and Hinnebusch CJ, Nikolai DM, Bruckner DA. Comparison of API Rapid Strep, Baxter Microscan Rapid Pos ID panel, BBL Minitek Differential Identification System, IDS RapID STR System and Vitek GPI to conventional biochemical tests for identification of viridans streptococci. *Am J Clin Pathol.* 1991;96:459-463.

of *S. constellatus* in pulmonary infections has demonstrated that virulent strains are less likely to be phagocytized and killed than avirulent strains, presumably because of capsular variation.[24]

The production of pyrogenic exotoxins by *Streptococcus* species is well known.[25] A unique cytolytic toxin specific for human cells, intermedilysin, has been described from a strain of *S. intermedius* isolated from a liver abscess.[26] In particular, intermedilysin has been noted to have a potent hemolytic effect on human erythrocytes, suggesting that this or similar exotoxins may be responsible for β-hemolysis on blood agar plates. Moreover, intermedilysin is essential for the invasion of human hepatic cells and is thus an important factor in the pathogenesis of liver abscesses.[27] The intermedilysin gene has been found only in *S. intermedius.*[28] Production of intermedilysin in *S. intermedius* isolates from deep-seated abscesses is higher than that in strains from normal habitats, suggesting that this cytolysin is a virulence factor.[28]

Members of the *S. anginosus* group produce a wide variety of hydrolytic enzymes, including hyaluronidase, deoxyribonuclease, and chondroitin sulfatase.[29] These enzymes may facilitate the spread of these pathogens through tissues, play a role in microbial nutrition, and assist in liquefaction of pus. One of the most prevalent hydrolytic enzymes is hyaluronidase,[30] which has been found in pus[31] and shown to be a growth factor.[32] Another hydrolytic enzyme, chondroitin sulfatase, is produced by *S. intermedius.*[33] In addition, a novel glycosaminoglycan depolymerase isolated from *S. intermedius* acts on both chondroitin sulfate and hyaluronic acid.[34] Yet another enzyme that may play a role in pathogenesis is sialidase (neuraminidase), which is produced by *S. intermedius.*[35] Sialidase production by other bacteria is considered to be an important feature of their pathogenicity. Sialic acid is known to be a nutrient source for these microorganisms; members of the *S. anginosus* group are able to use sialic acid efficiently as a sole carbon source. Sialidase therefore may be a growth factor and may play an important role in the ability of these microorganisms to proliferate in humans.

A number of other possible virulence factors related to the host immune response have been identified. One such factor is an immunosuppressive and B-cell mitogenic protein (P90) that is produced by *S. intermedius*.[36] Mice treated with this protein were 50 times more susceptible to infection by *S. intermedius*. This virulence effect is thought to be mediated by stimulation of suppressor lymphocytes.

Another potentially important virulence factor for members of the *S. anginosus* group in relation to the host immune response may be superantigens. Superantigens are bacterial proteins that bind to major histocompatibility complex class II and T-cell receptor to stimulate large numbers of T cells.[37] Groups C and G *Streptococcus dysgalactiae* subspecies *equisimilis* have been found to possess the superantigen genes *speM*, *ssa*, and *smeZ*,[38] which are thought to be the result of the transfer of these genes from group A streptococci (GAS). In addition, the authors demonstrated the *smeZ* allele in *S. canis*, demonstrating the wide dissemination of the GAS *smeZ* gene in another streptococcal species. It is very possible that these superantigen genes have also been transferred from GAS to members of the anginosus group.

The interaction of the *S. anginosus* group and human polymorphonuclear cells also has been examined because of their striking propensity to cause abscesses. One study has demonstrated that a virulent strain of *S. constellatus* is less likely to be killed by human polymorphonuclear cells than the avirulent strains.[39] A second study has shown that members of the *S. anginosus* group stimulate less chemotaxis than *Staphylococcus aureus*, which may provide an advantage for proliferating bacteria.[40] In the latter study, members of the *S. anginosus* group survived ingestion by polymorphonuclear cells better than strains of *S. aureus*.[40] These characteristics help explain the ability of members of the *S. anginosus* group to cause abscesses.

Clinical Manifestations

HEAD AND NECK INFECTIONS

Members of the *S. anginosus* group were initially recovered from dental abscesses and continue to be recovered from endodontic and periapical dental abscesses.[41] A transient bacteremia may occur with dental abscesses (or with dental procedures) and has been associated with metastatic abscesses.[42] Finally, members of the *S. anginosus* group have been isolated from dental caries and periodontal disease; their role, if any, in these processes is unclear. The periodontal location does allow transient bacteremias to occur during dental procedures, which could predispose to metastatic infections.

The presence of members of the *S. anginosus* group in the oral cavity clearly predisposes to oral and maxillofacial infections[43] as well as head and neck infections.[44] In several series, this group represented the most common microorganisms isolated in sinus-induced intracranial sepsis, and were recovered from intracranial and orbital empyemas in up to 50% of cases.[42,45-47] Because of the potential for metastatic spread, sinusitis caused by *S. anginosus* group isolates requires aggressive management.[47]

BACTEREMIA AND ENDOCARDITIS

Bacteremia caused by *S. anginosus* group isolates has been well documented.[48-50] Most of these bacteremic episodes were associated with an identifiable focus of infection—usually a deep-seated abscess in a visceral organ, implicating the gastrointestinal tract as the source. Such bacteremia, therefore, should alert the clinician to initiate an appropriate investigation for the detection of a possible suppurative focus of infection. Finally, viridans streptococci, including members of the anginosus group, have been recognized as an increasingly important cause of bacteremia in neutropenic cancer patients undergoing chemotherapy.[51]

Bacteremia by *S. anginosus* group isolates may be caused by, or may cause, bacterial endocarditis.[52,53] It is estimated that members of this group represent between 3% and 15% of streptococcal isolates from patients with endocarditis.[3] The propensity for suppuration of these pathogens has resulted in the complication of myocardial abscess or metastatic abscess,[48,49] although these complications do not occur in all patients. Endocarditis most often results from an abnormal heart valve, although the exact attachment mechanism is unknown. *S. anginosus* group strains have been shown to adhere to buccal epithelial cells and also to bind to fibronectin, which may contribute to their pathogenicity in endocarditis.[18-22]

CENTRAL NERVOUS SYSTEM INFECTIONS

S. anginosus group organisms have a strikingly prominent association with brain abscesses and have been isolated in approximately 50% to 80% of these infections.[48,54] These organisms may be isolated in pure or mixed culture. In addition, these organisms have been found in culture-negative intracerebral abscesses by gene sequencing from direct specimens.[55] Factors associated with brain abscesses caused by these isolates include congenital heart defects, sinusitis, otitis media, liver disease, and direct trauma. Of the three members, *S. intermedius* appears to be the one most commonly isolated from brain abscesses. Although *S. intermedius* can be found in the mouth, it has been suggested that most brain abscesses caused by this pathogen originate from the intestine.[48] On rare occasions, *S. anginosus* group organisms cause meningitis; this often is preceded by trauma or purulent infection at another site.[56] Transient or persistent bacteremia often results in epidural abscesses of the spine. Rapid surgical drainage is a critical prognostic factor for effective management of these spinal cord abscesses.

ABDOMINAL INFECTIONS

Given that members of the *S. anginosus* group are considered commensal organisms of the intestinal tract, it is not surprising to find these pathogens causing infections within the abdominal cavity. Such infections include liver abscesses, peritonitis, pelvic abscesses, subphrenic abscesses, appendicitis, abdominal wound infections, and cholangitis.[57-59] The use of antimicrobial drugs with minimal or no activity against the *S. anginosus* group for prophylaxis or therapy involving the abdominal cavity has been associated with the development of infections by these organisms clinically and experimentally.[60] Specifically, metronidazole alone or in combination with gentamicin appears to allow these bacteria to become pathogens. Infections caused by members of the *S. anginosus* group can be seen after abdominal surgery, particularly if prophylactic antibiotics do not cover these pathogens. The proclivity for liver abscess and bacteremia,[57] as well as cholangitis,[58] must be appreciated. Finally, *S. anginosus*[7] and *S. constellatus*[8] are the species in the *S. anginosus* group that are most frequently recovered from infections in the abdominal cavity.

THORACIC INFECTIONS

The presence of *S. anginosus* group organisms in the oropharynx can lead to aspiration pneumonia followed by pulmonary complications such as lung abscess, pleural empyema, or both.[17,24,58,61,62] Such complications are particularly likely to occur with mixed pulmonary infections.[15] Predisposing factors to *S. anginosus* group pulmonary infections include male gender, previous pneumonia, alcoholism, cancer, and possibly cystic fibrosis.[63] Significant morbidity and mortality (death rates of 15% to 30%) has been associated with these pulmonary infections. Management of pulmonary infections caused by the *S. anginosus* group must be aggressive and often requires operative intervention.[64,65] Mediastinitis has also been reported.[66] *S. constellatus* and *S. anginosus* are the species of the group most frequently identified from respiratory tract infections.[7,8]

MISCELLANEOUS INFECTIONS

A number of other infections caused by members of the *S. anginosus* group have been reported. These include osteomyelitis,[67] septic arthritis,[68] and subcutaneous abscess or cellulitis.[58] Drug addicts appear to be at risk for subcutaneous abscesses caused by members of the anginosus group.[69] Finally, peritonsillar abscesses involving anaerobic microorganisms mixed with *S. anginosus* group members have been described.[44]

Antimicrobial Therapy

Most members of the *S. anginosus* group have minimal inhibitory concentrations (MICs) to penicillin G lower than 0.125 μg/mL, with occasional strains with MICs higher than 1.0 μg/mL.[70-74] As noted, streptococci are naturally competent, and the potential for penicillin and cephalosporin resistance clearly exists because of the horizontal transfer of genes among streptococci.[75] In one study, 29% of viridans streptococci overall, including members of the *S. anginosus* group, were tolerant to intermediate concentrations of penicillin G (MIC = 0.25 to 2 μg/mL) and 9% of all strains had a MIC to penicillin G > 4 μg/mL.[74] Other studies continue to report high MICs to penicillin in fewer than 2% of *S. anginosus* group isolates.[71,72] Moreover, resistance to erythromycin and clindamycin has been described.[73,76] When penicillin resistance is seen, it is more common among *S. anginosus* and *S. intermedius* isolates. Although most strains of the *S. anginosus* group are relatively resistant to aminoglycosides, synergy with a β-lactam agent usually can be demonstrated. Therefore, the addition of an aminoglycoside to a β-lactam agent for treatment of endocarditis caused by members of the *S. anginosus* group is a reasonable practice, particularly for strains with intermediate MICs.

Clinically, infections caused by these streptococci have responded well to penicillin G and cephalosporins. Vancomycin and clindamycin have been useful for patients with β-lactam allergies. The recent increase in MICs to penicillin G suggests that initiation of penicillin G combined with gentamicin may be prudent. Alternatively, higher doses of penicillin or vancomycin could be used. Of the cephalosporins that are clinically available, cefepime, cefotaxime, and ceftriaxone have been noted to be superior in potency and spectrum for empirical coverage of patients at risk for streptococcal bacteremias.[71] Macrolides do not appear to be potent enough for such empirical therapy.[76] Finally, it is important to remember that surgical drainage of abscesses is usually indicated as adjunctive therapy.

REFERENCES

1. Whiley RA, Beighton D. Emended description and recognition of *Streptococcus constellatus, Streptococcus intermedius,* and *Streptococcus anginosus* as distinct species. *Int J Syst Bacteriol.* 1991;41:1-5.
2. Spellerberg B, Brandt C. *Streptococcus.* In: Murray PR, Baron EJ, Jorgenson JH, et al, eds. *Manual of Clinical Microbiology.* 9th ed. Washington DC: American Society for Microbiology Press; 2007:412-429.
3. Whiley RA, Fraser HY, Hardie JM, et al. Phenotypic differentiation of *Streptococcus constellatus, Streptococcus intermedius,* and *Streptococcus anginosus* (the *Streptococcus milleri* group): Association with different body sites and clinical infections. *J Clin Microbiol.* 1990;28:1497-1501.
4. Whiley RA, Hall LMC, Hardie JM, et al. A study of small colony beta-hemolytic, Lancefield group C streptococci within the anginosus group: Description of *Streptococcus constellatus* subsp. *pharyngis* subsp. nov associated with the human throat and pharyngitis. *Int J Syst Bacteriol.* 1999;49:1443-1449.
5. Clarridge JE III, Osting C, Jalali M, et al. Genotypic and phenotypic characterization of "*Streptococcus milleri*" group isolates from a Veterans Administration Hospital population. *J Clin Microbiol.* 1999;37:3681-3687.
6. Jacobs JA, Schot CS, Schouls LM. The *Streptococcus anginosus* group comprises five 16S rRNA ribogroups with different phenotypic characteristics and clinical relevance. *Int J Syst Evol Microbiol.* 2000;50:1073-1079.
7. Whiley RA, Beighton D, Winstanley TG, et al. *Streptococcus intermedius, Streptococcus constellatus,* and *Streptococcus anginosus* (the *Streptococcus milleri* group): Association with different body sites and clinical infections. *J Clin Microbiol.* 1992;30:243-244.
8. Clarridge JE III, Attori S, Musher DM, et al. *Streptococcus intermedius, Streptococcus constellatus,* and *Streptococcus anginosus* ("*Streptococcus milleri* group") are of different clinical importance and are not equally associated with abscess. *Clin Infect Dis.* 2001;32:1511-1515.
9. Brogan O, Malone J, Fox C, et al. Lancefield grouping and smell of caramel for presumptive identification and assessment of pathogenicity in the *Streptococcus milleri* group. *J Clin Pathol.* 1997;50:332-335.
10. Hinnebusch CJ, Nikolai DM, Bruckner DA. Comparison of API Rapid Strep, Baxter Microscan Rapid Pos ID panel, BBL Minitek Differential Identification System, IDS RapID STR System and Vitek GPI to conventional biochemical tests for identification of viridans streptococci. *Am J Clin Pathol.* 1991;96:459-463.
11. Flynn CE, Ruoff KL. Identification of "*Streptococcus milleri*" group isolates to the species level with a commercially available rapid test system. *J Clin Microbiol.* 1995;33:2704-2706.
12. Brigante G, Luzzaro F, Bettaccini A, et al. Use of the Phoenix Automated System for identification of *Streptococcus* and *Enterococcus* spp. *J Clin Microiol.* 2006;44:3263-3267.
13. Friedrichs C, Rodloff AC, Chhatwal GS, et al. Rapid identification of viridans streptococci by mass spectrometric discrimination. *J Clin Microbiol.* 2007;45:2392-2397.
14. Ahmet Z, Warren M, Houang ET. Species identification of members of the *Streptococcus milleri* group isolated from the vagina by ID 32 Strep system and differential characteristics. *J Clin Microbiol.* 1995;33:1592-1595.
15. Shinzato T, Saito A. A mechanism of pathogenicity of "*Streptococcus milleri* group" in pulmonary infection: Synergy with an anaerobe. *J Med Microbiol.* 1994;40:118-123.
16. Young KA, Allaker RP, Hardie JM, et al. Interactions between *Eikenella corrodens* and "*Streptococcus milleri*-group" organisms: Possible mechanisms of pathogenicity in mixed infections. *Antonie Van Leeuwenhoek.* 1996;69:371-373.
17. Shinzato T, Saito A. The *Streptococcus milleri* group as a cause of pulmonary infections. *Clin Infect Dis.* 1995;21(Suppl 3): S238-S243.
18. Jenkinson HF, Lamont RJ. Streptococcal adhesion and colonization. *Crit Rev Oral Biol Med.* 1997;8:175-200.
19. Wilcox MD, Knox KW. Surface-associated properties of *Streptococcus milleri* group strains and their potential relation to pathogenesis. *J Med Microbiol.* 1990;31:259-270.
20. Wilcox MD, Oakey HJ, Harty DW, et al. Lancefield group C *Streptococcus milleri* group strains aggregate human platelets. *Microb Pathog.* 1994;16:451-457.
21. Wilcox MD. Potential pathogenic properties of members of the "*Streptococcus milleri*" group in relation to the production of endocarditis and abscesses. *J Med Microbiol.* 1995;43:405-410.
22. Kitada K, Inoue M, Kitano M. Infective endocarditis-inducing abilities of "*Streptococcus milleri*" group. *Adv Exp Med Biol.* 1997;418:161-163.
23. Kitada K, Inoue M, Kitano M. Experimental endocarditis induction and platelet aggregation by *Streptococcus anginosus, Streptococcus constellatus* and *Streptococcus intermedius. FEMS Immunol Med Microbiol.* 1997;19:25-32.
24. Toyoda K, Kusano M, Saito A. Pathogenicity of the *Streptococcus milleri* group in pulmonary infections. *Kansenshogaku Zasshi.* 1995;69:308-315.
25. Bohach GA, Stauffacher CV, Ohlendorf DH, et al. The staphylococcal and streptococcal pyrogenic toxin family. *Adv Exp Med Biol.* 1996;391:131-154.
26. Nagamune H, Ohnishi C, Katsuura A, et al. Intermedilysin: A cytolytic toxin specific for human cells of a *Streptococcus intermedius* isolated from human liver abscess. *Adv Exp Med Biol.* 1997;418:773-775.
27. Sukeno A, Nagamune H, Whiley RA, et al. Intermedilysin is essential for the invasion of hepatoma hepG2 cells by *Streptococcus intermedius. Microbiol Immunol.* 2005;49:681-694.
28. Magamune H, Whiley RA, Goto T, et al. Distribution of intermedilysin gene among the anginosus group streptococci and correlation between intermedilysin production and deep-seated infection with *Streptococcus intermedius. J Clin Microbiol.* 2000;38:220-226.
29. Jacobs JA, Stobberingh EE. Hydrolytic enzymes of *Streptococcus anginosus, Streptococcus constellatus* and *Streptococcus intermedius* in relation to infection. *Eur J Clin Microbiol Infect Dis.* 1995;14:818-820.
30. Shain H, Homer KA, Aduse-Opoku J, et al. A conserved region of a hyaluronidase gene from *Streptococcus intermedius. Adv Exp Med Biol.* 1997;418:769-772.
31. Takao A, Nagashima H, Usui H, et al. Hyaluronidase activity in human pus for which *Streptococcus intermedius* was isolated. *Mirobiol Immunol.* 1997;41:795-798.
32. Homer K, Shain H, Beighton D. The role of hyaluronidase in growth of *Streptococcus intermedius* on hyaluronate. *Adv Exp Med Biol.* 1997;418:681-683.
33. Shain H, Homer KA, Beighton D. Degradation and utilisation of chondroitin sulphate by *Streptococcus intermedius. J Med Microbiol.* 1996;44:372-380.
34. Shain H, Homer KA, Beighton D. Purification and properties of a novel glycosaminoglycan depolymerase for *Streptococcus intermedius. J Med Microbiol.* 1996;44:381-389.
35. Byers HL, Homer KA, Beighton D. Sialic acid utilisation by viridans streptococci. *Adv Exp Med Biol.* 1997;418:713-716.
36. Lima M, Bandeira A, Portnoi D, et al. Protective effect of a T-cell-dependent immunosuppressive, B-cell-mitogenic protein (F3′EP-Si, or P90) produced by *Streptococcus intermedius. Infect Immun.* 1992;60:3571-3578.
37. Fraser J, Proft T. The bacterial superantigen and superantigen-like proteins. *Immunol Rev.* 2008;225:226-243.
38. Igwe EI, Shewmaker PL, Facklam RR, et al. Identification of superantigen genes *speM, ssa,* and *smeZ* in invasive strains of beta-hemolytic group C and G streptococci recovered from humans. *FEMS Microbiol Lett.* 2003;229:259-264.
39. Toyoda K, Kusano N, Saito A. Pathogenicity of the *Steptococcus milleri* group in pulmonary infections—effect on phagocytic killing by human polymorphonuclear neutrophils. *Kansenshogaku Zasshi.* 1995;69:308-315.
40. Wanahita A, Goldsmith EA, Musher DM, et al. Interaction between human polymorphonuclear leukocytes and *Streptococcus milleris* group bacteria. *J Infect Dis.* 2002;185:85-90.
41. Sassone LM, Fidel R, Faveri M, et al. Microbiological evaluation of primary endodontic infections in teeth with and without sinus tract. *Int Endod J.* 2008;41:508-515.
42. Udaondo P, Garcia-Delpech S, Diaz-Llopis M, et al. Bilateral intraorbital abscesses and cavernous sinus thromboses secondary to *Streptococci milleri* with a favorable outcome. *Ophthal Plast Reconstr Surg.* 2008;24:408-410.
43. Bancescu G, Lofthus B, Hofstad T, et al. Isolation and characterization of "*Streptococcus milleri*" group strains from oral and maxillofacial infections. *Adv Exp Med Biol.* 1997;418:165-167.
44. Han JK, Kerschner JE. *Streptococcus milleri:* An organism for head and neck infections and abscess. *Arch Otolaryngol Head Neck Surg.* 2001;127:650-654.
45. Watkins LM, Pasternack MS, Banks M, et al. Bilateral cavernous sinus thromboses and intraorbital abscesses secondary to *Streptococcus milleri. Ophthalmology.* 2003;110:569-574.
46. Greenlee JE. Subdural empyema. *Curr Treat Options Neurol.* 2003;5:13-22.
47. Jones RL, Vioares NS, Chavda SV, et al. Intracranial complications of sinusitis: The need for aggressive management. *J Laryngol Otol.* 1995;109:1061-1062.
48. Casariego E, Rodriguez A, Corredoira JC, et al. Prospective study of *Streptococcus milleri* bacteremia. *Eur J Clin Microbiol Infect Dis.* 1996;15:194-200.
49. Salavert M, Gomez L, Rodgriguez-Carballeira M, et al. Seven-year review of bacteremia caused by *Streptococcus milleri* and other viridans streptococci. *Eur J Clin Microbiol Infect Dis.* 1996;15:365-371.
50. Bert F, Bariou-Lancelin M, Lambert-Zechovsky N. Clinical significance of bacteremia involving the "*Streptococcus milleri*" group: 51 cases and review. *Clin Infect Dis.* 1998;27:385-387.
51. Awada A, van der Auwera P, Meunier F, et al. Streptococcal and enterococcal bacteremia in patients with cancer. *Clin Infect Dis.* 1992;15:33-48.
52. Lefort A, Lortholary O, Casassus P, et al. Comparison between adult endocarditis due to beta-hemolytic streptococci (serogroups A, B, C, and G) and *Streptococcus milleri:* A multicenter study in France. *Arch Intern Med.* 2002;162:2450-2456.
53. Woo PC, Tse H, Chan KM, et al. "*Streptococcus milleri*" endocarditis caused by *Streptococcus anginosus. Diagn Microbiol Infect Dis.* 2004;48:81-88.
54. Mathisen GE, Johnson JP. Brain abscess. *Clin Infect Dis.* 1997;25:763-781.
55. Petti CA, Simmon KE, Bender J, et al. Culture-negative intracerebral abscesses in children and adolescents from *Streptococcus*

anginosus group infection: A case series. *Clin Infect Dis.* 2008;46:1578-1580.

56. Cabellos C, Viladrich PF, Corredoira J, et al. Streptococcal meningitis in adult patients: Current epidemiology and clinical spectrum. *Clin Infect Dis.* 1999;28:1104-1108.

57. Corredoira J, Casariego E, Moreno C, et al. Prospective study of *Streptococcus milleri* hepatic abscess. *Eur J Clin Microbiol Infect Dis.* 1998;17:556-560.

58. Molina J-M, Leport C, Bure A, et al. Clinical and bacterial features of infections caused by *Streptococcus milleri. Scand J Infect Dis.* 1991;23:659-666.

59. Hardwick RH, Taylor A, Thompson MH, et al. Association between *Steptococcus milleri* and abscess formation after appendicitis. *Ann R Coll Surg Engl.* 2000;82:24-26.

60. Onderdonk AB, Cisneros R. Comparison of clindamycin and metronidazole for the treatment of experimental intra-abdominal sepsis produced by *Bacteroides fragilis* and *Streptococcus intermedius. Curr Ther Res Clin Exp.* 1985;38:893-898.

61. Wong CA, Donald F, Macfarlane JT. *Streptococcus milleri* pulmonary disease: A review and clinical description of 25 patients. *Thorax.* 1995;50:1093-1096.

62. Steizmueller I, Biebl M, Berger N, et al. Relevance of group Milleri streptococci in thoracic surgery: a clinical update. *Am Surg.* 2007;73:492-497.

63. Parkins MD, Sibley CD, Surette MG, et al. The *Streptococcus milleri* group—an unrecognized cause of disease in cystic fibrosis: A case series and literature review. *Pediatr Pulmonol.* 2008;43:490-497.

64. Marinella MA, Harrington GD, Standiford TJ. Empyema necessitans due to *Streptococcus milleri. Clin Infect Dis.* 1996;23:203-204.

65. Ripley RT, Cothren CC, Moore EE, et al. *Streptococcus milleri* infections of the pleural space: operative management predominates. *Am J Surg.* 2006;817-821.

66. Shishido H, Watanabe K, Matsumoto K, et al. Primary purulent mediastinitis due to *Streptococcus milleri. Respiration.* 1997;64:313-315.

67. Calza L, Manfredi R, Briganti E, et al. Iliac osteomyelitis and gluteal muscle abscess caused by *Streptococcus intermedius. J Med Microbiol.* 2001;50:480-482.

68. Ortel TL, Kallianos J, Gallis HA. Group C streptococcal arthritis: Case report and review. *Rev Infect Dis.* 1990;12:829-837.

69. Stocker E, Cortes E, Pema K, et al. *Streptococcus milleri* as a cause of anticubital abscess and bacteremia in intravenous drug abusers. *South Med J.* 1994;87:95-96.

70. Limia A, Jimenez ML, Alarcon T, et al. Five-year analysis of antimicrobial susceptibility of the *Streptococcus milleri* group. *Eur J Clin Microbiol Infect Dis.* 1999;18:440-444.

71. Aracil B, Gomez-Garces JL, Alos JL. A study of susceptibility of 100 clinical isolates belonging to the *Streptococcus milleri* group to 16 cephalosporins. *J Antimicrob Chemother.* 1999;43:399-402.

72. Tracy M, Wanahita A, Shuhatovich Y, et al. Antibiotic susceptibilities of genetically characterized *Streptococcus milleri* group strains. *Antimicrob Agents Chemother.* 2001;45:1511-1514.

73. Yamamoto N, Kubota T, Tohyama M, et al. Trends in antimicrobial susceptibility of the *Streptococcus milleri* group. *J Infect Chemother.* 2002;8:134-137.

74. Bantar C, Canigia LF, Relloso S, et al. Species belonging to the "*Streptococcus milleri*" group: Antimicrobial susceptibility and comparative prevalence in significant clinical specimens. *J Clin Microbiol.* 1996;34:2020-2022.

75. Dowson CG, Barcus V, King S, et al. Horizontal gene transfer and the evolution of resistance and virulence determinants in *Streptococcus. Soc Appl Bacteriol Symp Ser.* 1997;26:42-51.

76. Jacobs JA, van Baar GJ, London NH, et al. Prevalence of macrolide resistance genes in clinical isolates of the *Streptococcus anginosus* ("*S. milleri*") group. *Antimicrob Agents Chemother.* 2001;45:2375-2377.

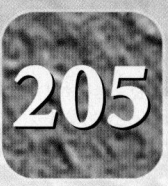

205

Corynebacterium diphtheriae

ROB ROY MacGREGOR

The name *diphtheria* was coined by Bretonneau, from the Greek root for "leather," describing the tough pharyngeal membrane that is the hallmark of the disease. The definition of diphtheria as a unique syndrome, the explanation of its pathogenesis, and its subsequent control parallel the development of the fields of pathology, bacteriology, and immunology. During the first half of the 20th century, it was a major worldwide health problem, then yielded to scientifically grounded vigorous public health control measures. However, the epidemic that occurred in the 1990s in the former Soviet Union and adjacent areas as a result of relaxed immunization practices and social disorganization was a reminder of the need for sustained vigilance.

History

Although clinical descriptions of sore throat, membrane production, and death by suffocation appear in Hippocratic writings, epidemics of "throat distemper" are not described until the 16th century.[1] A major epidemic occurred in New England in the early 1700s, killing an estimated 2.5% of the total population, and up to one third of all children. Thereafter, similar epidemics were reported at about 25-year intervals throughout the 18th and 19th centuries. Diphtheria was not clearly differentiated from other upper respiratory illnesses, viewed collectively as "croup" or "distemper," until an epidemic in southern France in 1821 when the clinician-pathologist Pierre Bretonneau first described its unique clinical characteristics. However, arguments about the differentiation among diphtheria, croup, and other throat distempers continued through most of the 1800s.[2]

The first major advance occurred in 1883 when Klebs described chaining cocci and bacilli in microscopic sections of diphtheritic membranes. The following year, working in Koch's laboratory in Berlin, Friedrich Loeffler first isolated the diphtheria bacillus in pure culture, aided by a culture medium of his own design that is still used today. He then demonstrated that the organism could reproduce the disease in guinea pigs, thus fulfilling his mentor's postulates for proof that it was the etiologic agent for diphtheria.[3] Using his special culture medium, he demonstrated that healthy individuals could carry the organism asymptomatically in their throats, thus establishing the carrier state as an important phenomenon in the maintenance and spread of the disease. He also noted that the organisms remained in the membrane without invading the tissues of the throat or more distant sites, and theorized that the neurologic and cardiologic manifestations of the disease were caused by a toxic substance elaborated by the organism. In 1888, Roux and Yersin, working at the Pasteur Institute, proved Loeffler correct by demonstrating that bacteria-free filtrates of cultures of diphtheria bacilli were able to kill guinea pigs. Two years later, von Behring, also working in Koch's laboratory, demonstrated that antiserum against the toxin was capable of protecting infected animals from death following infection. Then in 1894, after showing that horses were the most efficient animals at producing antitoxin, Roux reported that administration of antiserum reduced mortality from diphtheria among foundlings in Paris from 51% to 24%.

In 1913, Schick reported that an individual's local reaction to injection of toxin into the skin could be used to predict susceptibility to infection (a negative reaction indicated presence of protective antitoxin antibodies). At the same time, Theobald Smith and von Behring successfully immunized children with a toxin-antitoxin mixture, and in 1923, Ramon, at the Pasteur Institute, found that exposure of toxin to formalin and heat rendered it nontoxic to recipients while retaining

the ability to induce an antibody response. The following year, clinical trials showed that injection of this "toxoid" induced a high level of protection among recipients. Problems of antigenic standardization, determining optimal dosage, frequency of administration, needs for boosting, and so forth delayed the widespread use of immunization with toxoid, but between 1930 and 1945, most Western countries established intensive programs of childhood immunization. The result was a dramatic decrease in the incidence of diphtheria, from about 200,000 cases in the United States in 1921 to 0 to 2 cases yearly since 2000. During the 1950s, Freeman, Groman, Barksdale, Pappenheimer, and others demonstrated that toxin production by *Corynebacterium diphtheriae* depended on the presence of a lysogenic ß-phage, and during the following decade, the mechanism by which toxin inhibited protein synthesis was elucidated.[4-6] By the 1980s, diphtheria had become a rare occurrence in most countries that had effective immunization programs, but in 1990, a large epidemic of diphtheria began in the former Soviet Union and extended to eastern Europe and parts of Asia. The reestablishment of vigorous immunization policies and other public health measures after the peak of the epidemic in 1994 again controlled this ancient scourge.[7]

The Pathogen

C. diphtheriae is a nonsporulating, unencapsulated, nonmotile, pleomorphic, gram-positive bacillus. Its name is derived from the Greek *korynee,* or "club," referring to its clubbed ends, and *diphthera,* meaning "leather hide," for the characteristic leathery pharyngeal membrane that it provokes. When inoculated on the nutritionally inadequate medium devised by Loeffler, it initially outgrows other throat flora, so plates should be inspected for growth after 12 to 18 hours. The characteristic metachromatic granules (best seen with methylene blue staining) and "Chinese character" palisading morphology that differentiate it from other corynebacteria are displayed more prominently on smears taken from colonies grown on this medium than with direct smears from clinical specimens. The current selective potassium tellurite media, such as modified Tinsdale, inhibit many of the normal throat flora and identify any *C. diphtheriae* present as brown colonies with brown halos containing reduced tellurite. Tinsdale medium has a short shelf life, and most laboratories do not stock this medium. *C. diphtheriae* will grow on routine blood agar but will not be identified unless the clinician is alerted to the possible diagnosis.

The species is subdivided into four biovars—*gravis, intermedius, mitis,* and *belfanti*—based on differing colonial morphology on tellurite agar, fermentation reactions, and hemolytic potential. Modern molecular techniques have proved to be more sensitive in recent outbreaks for tracking different strains: ribotyping (the use of restriction endonucleases to detect polymorphisms of recombinant RNA genes), pulsed-field gel electrophoresis (PFGE) analysis of genomic DNA, and multilocus enzyme electrophoresis of organism sonicates have shown that an epidemic clone of *C. diphtheriae* emerged in Russia in 1990 and became increasingly common as the epidemic progressed.[8,9] An International *C. diphtheriae* Ribotype Database has been established at the Pasteur Institute in Paris by Professor Patrick Grimont and contains more than 85 distinct *Bst*EII ribotypes of toxigenic and nontoxigenic *C. diphtheriae* submitted from throughout the world.[10]

Exotoxin production by *C. diphtheriae* depends on the presence of a lysogenic β-phage, which carries the gene encoding for toxin (*tox*⁺).[4,6]

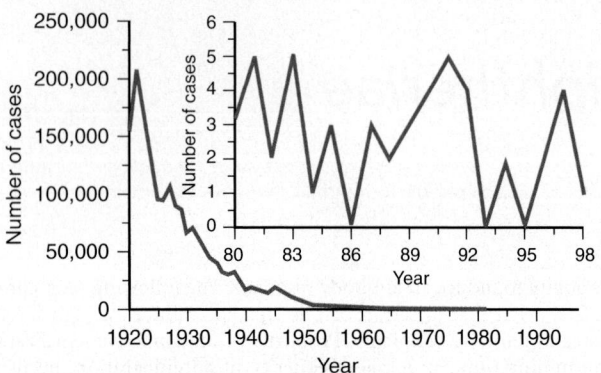

Figure 205-1 **Annual incidence of diphtheria in the United States, 1920-1998.** *(From Golaz A, Hardy IR, Strebel P, et al. Epidemic diphtheria in the Newly Independent States of the former Soviet Union: Implications for diphtheria control in the United States. J Infect Dis. 2000;181[Suppl 1]:S237-S243.)*

In its lysogenic phase, the phage's circular DNA integrates into the host bacteria's genetic material as a prophage, with the result that the host cell now can express the gene necessary for synthesis of the polypeptide toxin. When induced by stimuli such as ultraviolet light, the phage enters a lytic cycle, destroying the host cell and releasing new ß-phage. Strains of *C. diphtheriae* lacking lysogenic phage do not produce toxin, but they can be converted to toxigenicity in the laboratory by infection with the lysogenic *tox*[+] phage ("lysogenization"). Evidence has been found that such conversion also occurs in nature.[11] Even though the frequency of carriage of *tox*[+] lysogenic *C. diphtheriae* currently is very low in the West, there is an ongoing risk that resident nontoxigenic strains could become lysogenized by introduction of a β-phage–bearing strain from another part of the world. (As noted later, strains of *Corynebacterium ulcerans* and *Corynebacterium pseudotuberculosis* can also carry the phage and produce a diphtheria-like illness.) In addition to the *tox*[+] gene, significant toxin production requires that bacterial growth be slowed by exhaustion of iron in the environment. Historically, toxigenicity of individual *C. diphtheriae* strains was demonstrated in vivo by lethality in guinea pigs, but this has been replaced by more rapid in vitro tests (see "Diagnosis").

Epidemiology

Humans are the only known reservoir for *C. diphtheriae*. The primary modes of spread are by airborne respiratory droplets and direct contact with either respiratory secretions or exudate from infected skin lesions. Fomites can play a role in transmission, and epidemics have been caused by contaminated milk. Most respiratory tract disease occurs in the colder months in temperate climates, associated with crowded indoor living conditions and hot, dry air. Asymptomatic respiratory carriage is important in perpetuating both endemic and epidemic diphtheria, and immunization reduces an individual's likelihood of being a carrier. Current reservoirs for disease are obscure. In endemic conditions, 3% to 5% of healthy individuals may harbor the organism in their throat,[12] but in the West, where the disease has become very uncommon, isolation of the organism from healthy individuals has become extremely rare. Skin infection, once thought to be primarily a problem in tropical environments, has caused several recent epidemics in Europe and North America among alcoholics and other disadvantaged groups.[13,14] Thus, skin carriage of *C. diphtheriae* can act as a silent reservoir for the organism, and it has been found that person-to-person spread from infected skin sites is more efficient than from the respiratory tract.[15,16]

The incidence and pattern of diphtheria in the Western world has changed dramatically in the past 50 to 75 years. From 1921 to 1924, it was the leading cause of death among Canadian children aged 2 to 14 years. Since then, the incidence has decreased steadily (Fig. 205-1) to

the point at which diphtheria is a rare event. For example, 147,991 cases were reported in the United States in 1920 (151 cases/100,000 population), and 0 to 2 since 1998 (<0.001/100,000).[17,18] From the 1960s to 1990, similar decreases occurred in Europe[18-20] and, less dramatically, worldwide, although the disease remained endemic in many parts of the Third World (e.g., Brazil, Haiti, Nigeria, Eastern Mediterranean region, the Indian subcontinent, Indonesia, and the Philippines).[18,21] Moreover, pockets of skin and pharyngeal colonization and disease continue to be identified among Native American groups, destitute inner-city dwellers, substance abusers, and homosexual men, giving rise to concern that outbreaks could occur, particularly among adults in the West, where the proportion of adults with protective antibody levels is as low as 50%.[22]

Beginning in 1990, epidemic diphtheria began in Russia (Fig. 205-2) and swiftly spread to all countries of the Newly Independent States (NIS).[7,23] In 1995, 50,425 cases were reported in the Russian Federation, for a yearly rate of 17.3/100,000.[23] The World Health Organization (WHO) and United Nations Children's Fund (UNICEF) formulated a strategic plan to control the epidemic, including (1) mass immunization with at least one dose of toxoid to the whole population, (2) early detection and proper management of cases, and (3) early identification and proper management of close contacts. In response, new cases in the Russian Federation fell from 7196 in 1997, to 1377 in 2001 and to less than 600 in 2005.[18,24] The 2006 WHO summary of vaccine-preventable diseases[18] reported a total of 8229 cases of diphtheria worldwide, roughly stable since 2000. Seventy-eight percent of cases were from the Southeast Asia region, with 89% of those from India. Moreover, more than 30 endemic cases were also reported each from Afghanistan, Haiti and the Dominican Republic, Indonesia, Papua New Guinea, the Philippines, Vietnam, and Nigeria.

A defining characteristic of the Russian epidemic was that half or more of cases occurred among those 15 years of age or older, suggesting that the young remained relatively well protected by the high rates of infant immunization operative in the 1980s, but that older people were vulnerable because either they had not been vaccinated as children or their protective antibody levels had faded in the absence of subsequent boosting by vaccine or colonization.[7,22,25,26]

When it was common in the West, diphtheria primarily affected children younger than 15 years, but recent outbreaks have also involved unimmunized or poorly immunized adults, particularly the urban and rural poor. Minority racial groups have had attack rates 5 to 20 times higher than whites. For example, in 1996, a focus of toxigenic diphtheria was discovered among Native Americans in South Dakota, which by molecular subtyping methods was found to have been endemic in the area since the 1970s. Enhanced surveillance of patients

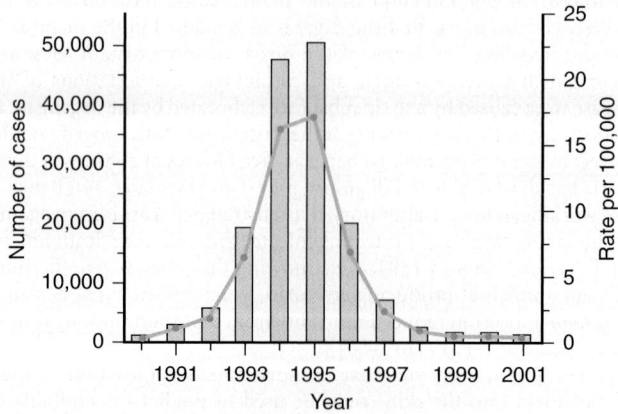

Figure 205-2 **Annual incidence of diphtheria in the Russian Federation and Baltic States, 1990-2001.** Number of reported cases of diphtheria and rate per 100,000 population. *Bars* represent the total yearly number of cases, and *connected dots* represent the yearly rate per 100,000 population.

in this community with upper respiratory symptoms showed that almost 4% of them were carrying toxigenic *C. diphtheriae.*[27,28]

Since 1995, there has been growing awareness of two phenomena: disease caused by nontoxigenic strains of *C. diphtheriae* and that caused by toxin-producing *C. ulcerans.* Nontoxigenic *C. diphtheriae* has produced typical respiratory tract diphtheria, milder pharyngitis and asymptomatic pharyngeal carriage, bacteremia, endocarditis, and bone and joint infections.[13,29-38] Toxigenic *C. ulcerans* can also cause classic respiratory diphtheria and skin lesions.[39,40]

Although immunized individuals can still develop clinical diphtheria, prior immunization reduces the frequency and severity of disease: between 1959 and 1970 in the United States, two thirds of reported cases had received no immunization, 13% more had had one to two doses of toxoid, and only 19% reported receiving three or more doses and could be considered fully immunized.[41] Among cases reported since 1980, *no cases* were fully immunized.[17] Disease was considered severe in 25% of unimmunized patients compared with 6.3% of those fully immunized. Nineteen percent of unimmunized patients died, compared with 1.3% of those fully immunized; even partial immunization reduced morbidity and mortality rates by more than 50%. The benefit of prior immunization has also been demonstrated in the recent Russian epidemic.[42,43]

The full explanation for the dramatic decrease in diphtheria's incidence in immunized populations is not evident. Immunization with toxoid is generally thought to attenuate only the local and systemic effects of toxin without preventing local colonization with the organism. If so, carriage would be expected to remain high in the population, and diphtheria should be an ongoing occurrence among the sizable proportion believed to be inadequately immunized. However, disease has become rare, and surveys show an extremely low incidence of carrier state. Nonetheless, results from the Third National Health and Nutrition Examination Survey (1988 to 1994) showed what are considered subprotective levels of serum antitoxin in 40% of the overall population.[44] The percentage with protective antibody decreased with increasing age, and only 30% of men aged 60 to 69 years were thought to have protective levels. In 1985, the U.S. preschool immunization rate was only 64.9% for diphtheria-pertussis-tetanus (DPT)[45]; fortunately, the 2003 National Immunization Survey showed that 96% of children 19 to 35 months of age had received at least three doses of DPT vaccine.[46] Several factors may contribute to the current low incidence of disease. First, although unproved, historical evidence suggests that diphtheria has occurred in cycles that include gaps of 100 years or more.[1] Second, organisms isolated from immunized individuals are less likely to be toxigenic than are those from unimmunized carriers (64% vs. 94%).[44] If toxin production confers no advantage to the organism in an immunized host, its metabolic cost would put toxigenic organisms at a selective disadvantage, and so loss of this attribute might be predicted.[5] Third, some experts believe that the local elaboration of toxin, in the absence of antibody, enhances an organism's ability to colonize. Immunization with toxoid could counteract this selective advantage of toxigenic strains. Fourth, some virulence factors other than toxin production may exist. For example, in a recent outbreak in Sweden, investigators used genetic probes to demonstrate that all clinical cases were caused by a single strain, although several different toxigenic strains were present in the population.[47] Finally, protection may correlate with lower serum concentrations of antitoxin antibody, or other immune mechanisms may be protective that are not measured. To explain the absence of diphtheria in the West and the occurrence of the recent epidemic in the NIS, the following model has been proposed[22,23,25,43]: absence of an effective immunization program allows for high carriage rates of toxigenic strains which leads to high rates of infant disease, and survivors in such populations are continually immunized by adult colonization with toxigenic strains, which explains low adult disease rates. Pediatric immunization programs reduce carriage rates of toxigenic strains because toxin production does not provide an advantage to the organism, and even nontoxigenic strain carriage falls. As a result, adults lose the opportunity for natural antibody boosting from asymptomatic carriage, so protective antibody levels wane in the adult population immunized only in childhood. Fortunately, good pediatric immunization programs appear to be sufficient to keep toxigenic strains from circulating and causing adult disease. Ultimately, if pediatric programs lapse, the population then contains *both* vulnerable children and adults, a situation that promotes epidemics. Thus, the public health strategy must be to maintain pediatric programs with more than 90% immunization rates and to strongly promote periodic adult boosters.

Pathogenesis

C. diphtheriae is not a very invasive organism, ordinarily remaining in the superficial layers of the respiratory mucosa and skin lesions, where it can induce a mild inflammatory reaction in the local tissue. The major virulence of *C. diphtheriae* results from the action of its potent exotoxin, which inhibits protein synthesis in mammalian cells but not in bacteria. The 62,000-dalton polypeptide toxin is composed of two segments: B, which binds to specific receptors on susceptible cells, and A, the active segment. After proteolytic cleavage of the bound molecule, segment A enters the cell, where it catalyzes inactivation of the transfer RNA (tRNA) translocase, "elongation factor 2," present in eukaryotic cells but not in bacteria. Loss of this enzyme prevents the interaction of messenger RNA and tRNA, stopping further addition of amino acids to developing polypeptide chains.[48] The toxin affects all cells in the body, but the most prominent effects are on the heart (myocarditis), nerves (demyelination), and kidneys (tubular necrosis). Diphtheria toxin is extremely potent: a single molecule can stop protein synthesis in a cell within several hours, and 0.1 µg/kg will kill susceptible animals.

Within the first few days of respiratory tract infection, toxin elaborated locally induces a dense necrotic coagulum composed of fibrin, leukocytes, erythrocytes, dead respiratory epithelial cells, and organisms (Fig. 205-3). Removal of this adherent gray-brown "pseudomembrane" reveals a bleeding edematous submucosa. The membrane can be local (tonsillar, pharyngeal, nasal) or extend widely, forming a cast of the pharynx and tracheobronchial tree. The underlying soft tissue edema and cervical adenitis can be intense, and, particularly in the proportionally smaller airways of children, can cause respiratory embarrassment and a bull-neck appearance. In both adults and children, a common cause of death is suffocation after aspiration of the membrane.

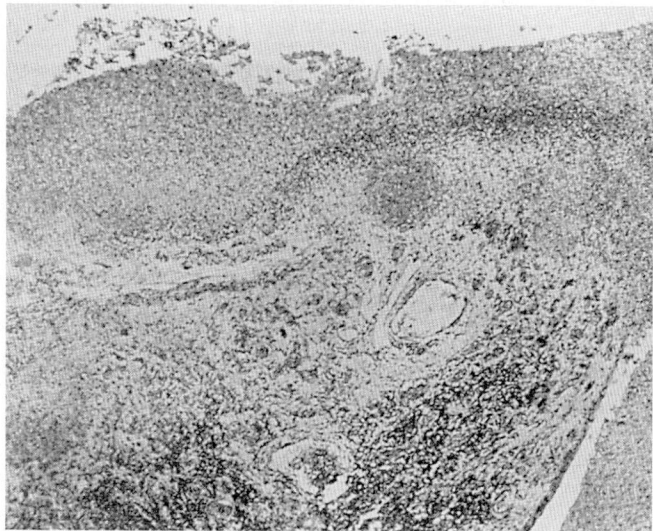

Figure 205-3 **Diphtheria involving a pharyngeal tonsil.** The membrane-tissue junction is clearly marked by intense cellular infiltration. (*From Moore RA. A Textbook of Pathology. Philadelphia: WB Saunders; 1944.*)

Clinical Manifestations

Symptoms of infection with *C. diphtheriae* occur locally in the respiratory tract and skin secondary to noninvasive infection of these two organs and at distant sites secondary to absorption and dissemination of diphtheria toxin. Occasionally, *C. diphtheriae* disseminates from the skin or respiratory tract and causes systemic infections, including bacteremia, endocarditis, and arthritis.

RESPIRATORY TRACT DIPHTHERIA

Asymptomatic upper respiratory tract carriage of the organism occurs commonly in areas where diphtheria is endemic and is an important reservoir for maintenance and spread of the organism in a population. However, in the industrial Western world, throat colonization has become exceedingly rare, except in individuals associated with pockets of infection, such as the inner-city poor and rural poverty areas.

Following an incubation period averaging 2 to 4 days, local signs and symptoms of inflammation can develop at various sites within the respiratory tract.

Anterior Nasal

Infection limited to the anterior nares presents with a serosanguineous or seropurulent nasal discharge often associated with a subtle whitish mucosal membrane, particularly on the septum. The discharge can excite an erosive reaction on the external nares and upper lip, but symptoms generally are mild, and signs indicating toxin effects are rare.

Faucial

Including the posterior structures of the mouth and the proximal pharynx, this area is the most common site for clinical diphtheria. Onset is usually subacute over several days, with low-grade fever (rarely >102.5° F), malaise, sore throat, mild pharyngeal injection, and development of a membrane typically on one or both tonsils, with extension variously to involve the tonsillar pillars, uvula, soft palate, oropharynx, and nasopharynx (Fig. 205-4). The membrane initially appears white and glossy but evolves into a dirty gray color, with patches of green or black necrosis. The extent of the membrane correlates with the severity of symptoms: localized tonsillar disease is often mild, but involvement of the posterior pharynx, soft palate, and periglottal areas is associated with profound malaise, weakness, prostration, cervical adenopathy, and swelling. The latter can distort the normal contour of the submental and cervical area, creating a bull-neck appearance and causing respiratory stridor.

Laryngeal and Tracheobronchial

Pharyngeal infection may spread downward into the larynx, or occasionally the disease may begin there. Symptoms then include hoarseness, dyspnea, respiratory stridor, and a brassy cough. Edema and membrane involving the trachea and bronchi can embarrass respiration further, and a child so afflicted will appear anxious and cyanotic, use accessory muscles of respiration, and demonstrate inspiratory retractions of intercostal, supraclavicular, and substernal tissues. If this state is not relieved promptly by intubation and mechanical removal of membrane, patients become exhausted and die.

Systemic complications are due to diphtheria toxin, which, although toxic to all tissues, has its most striking effects on the heart and nervous system.

Cardiac Toxicity. Subtle evidence of myocarditis can be detected in as many as two thirds of patients, but 10% to 25% develop clinical cardiac dysfunction, with the risk to an individual patient correlating directly with the extent and severity of local disease.[49,50] Cardiac toxicity can be acute, with congestive failure and circulatory collapse, or more insidious, after 1 to 2 weeks of illness with progressive dyspnea, weakness, diminished heart sounds, cardiac dilation, and gallop rhythm. Changes in electrocardiograph (ECG) pattern, particularly ST-T wave changes and first-degree heart block, can progress to more severe forms of block, atrioventricular (AV) dissociation, and other arrhythmias, which carry an ominous prognosis. Because patients without clinical evidence of myocarditis may have significant electrical changes, it is important to monitor their cardiograms routinely. Elevations of serum aspartate transaminase (AST) concentration closely parallel the intensity of myocarditis and so may be used to monitor its course. From a prognostic standpoint, patients with ECG changes of myocarditis have a mortality rate 3 to 4 times higher than those with normal tracings. In particular, AV and left bundle-branch blocks carry a mortality rate of 60% to 90%. Patients with prolonged P-R interval and minor T-wave changes generally do well, and these abnormalities ordinarily resolve with time. Patients with bundle-branch blocks and complete AV dissociation have a much higher incidence of death, and survivors may be left with permanent conduction defects.[51]

Neurologic Toxicity. This complication is also proportional to the severity of the primary infection: mild disease only occasionally produces neurotoxicity, but up to three fourths of patients with severe disease can develop neuropathy. Within the first few days of disease, local paralysis of the soft palate and posterior pharyngeal wall occurs commonly, manifested by regurgitation of swallowed fluids through the nose. Thereafter, cranial neuropathies causing oculomotor and ciliary paralysis are also common, and dysfunction of facial, pharyngeal, or laryngeal nerves, although rare, can contribute to the risk for aspiration. Peripheral neuritis develops later, from 10 days to 3 months after the onset of disease in the throat.[52] Principally a motor defect, it begins with proximal muscle groups in the extremities and extends distally, particularly affecting the dorsiflexors of the feet. Dysfunction varies from mild weakness with diminished tendon reflexes to total paralysis. Occasionally motor nerves of the trunk, neck, and upper extremity are involved, as are sensory nerves, resulting in a glove-and-stocking neuropathy. Microscopic examination of affected nerves shows degeneration of myelin sheaths and axon cylinders. Although slow, total resolution of all diphtheritic nerve damage is the rule.

Other Complications. Renal failure from direct toxin action or hypotension and pneumonia are common in severe cases. Rarely, encephalitis and cerebral infarction have been described.

Several excellent clinical descriptions of endemic and epidemic diphtheria in the United States indicate that both the frequency of various symptoms and the severity of disease are inversely proportional to the patient's immunization history.[52-56] Roughly half of these

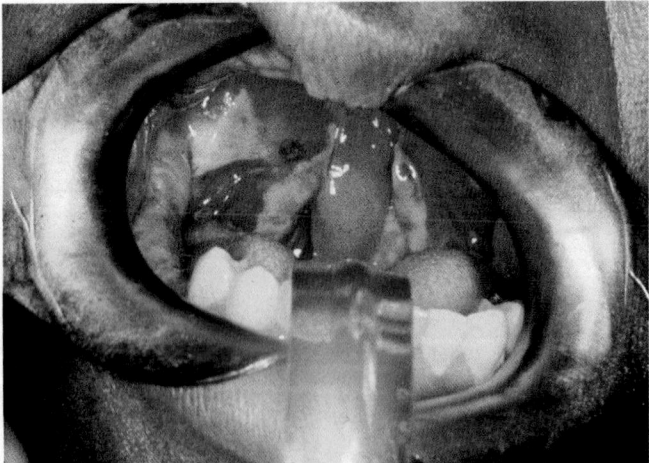

Figure 205-4 **Pharynx of a 39-year-old woman with bacteriologically confirmed diphtheria.** Photograph taken 4 days after the onset of fever, malaise, and sore throat. Hemorrhage due to removal of the membrane by swabbing appears as *dark area* on the left.

reported cases were categorized as mild, often without a membrane. Mortality rates vary from 3.5% to 12% and have not changed in the past 50 years. Rates are highest in the very young and very old. Most deaths occur in the first 3 to 4 days from asphyxia or myocarditis; fatal outcome is rare in a fully immunized individual. Sore throat (85% to 90%), fever (50% to 85%), and dysphagia (26% to 40%) are the most common symptoms, and membranes and cervical adenopathy are seen in about half of cases. The recent experience in Russia has been similar.[42] The frequency of complications such as myocarditis and neuritis is directly related to the time between onset of symptoms and administration of antitoxin and to the extent of membrane formation.

CUTANEOUS DIPHTHERIA

It has long been recognized that, particularly in the tropics, *C. diphtheriae* can cause clinical skin infections characterized by chronic nonhealing ulcers with a dirty gray membrane and often associated with *Staphylococcus aureus* and group A streptococci. More recently, the significance of this infection in the United States has been emphasized by several outbreaks among alcoholic homeless men and impoverished groups such as Native Americans.[13-16] The presentation is indolent and nonprogressive and is only rarely associated with signs of intoxication. Nonetheless, these infections can induce high antitoxin levels and thus appear to act as natural immunizing events.[57,58] They also serve as a reservoir for the organism under conditions of both endemic and epidemic respiratory tract diphtheria: cutaneous sites of *C. diphtheriae* have been shown both to contaminate the inanimate environment and to induce throat infections more efficiently than does pharyngeal colonization, and bacterial shedding from cutaneous infections continues longer than from the respiratory tract.[15,26,59] Despite these facts, the clinical significance of isolating the organism from an individual skin lesion is often unclear. Most lesions from which *C. diphtheriae* is isolated are indistinguishable from other chronic dermatologic conditions (e.g., eczema, psoriasis), and only about 15% fit the classic description of diphtheritic ulcers given previously.[60] Moreover, because *C. diphtheriae* is usually isolated in association with other known skin pathogens, and because the ulcers do not respond to antitoxin therapy, there is debate about whether the isolates are actually causing clinical disease. By 1975, cutaneous diphtheria accounted for 56% of total *C. diphtheriae* isolates reported in the United States, and in 1980, the Centers for Disease Control and Prevention (CDC), in an effort to focus attention on respiratory tract diphtheria, removed nontoxigenic skin isolates from its list of reportable diseases. Of note, *C. ulcerans* is named for its ability to cause chronic skin ulcers, but like *C. diphtheriae*, toxin-induced disease is uncommon with *C. ulcerans* skin lesions.[61]

INVASIVE DISEASE

Endocarditis, mycotic aneurysms, osteomyelitis, and septic arthritis have been described recently in clusters of drug addicts, alcoholics, Australian aboriginals, and young adults[13,29-34]—all caused by nontoxigenic *C. diphtheriae*. Ribotyping has indicated that these outbreaks have been caused by unique epidemic strains, and both skin and throat colonization have been implicated as portals of entry. These illnesses have been characterized by aggressive course, a high proportion of bacteremia, endocarditis, arterial embolization, metastatic sites of infection (joints, spleen, central nervous system), and high mortality. Why these nontoxigenic strains are so virulent remains a mystery. Coincident with these outbreaks of invasive disease, examples of non–toxin-producing strains causing clinical pharyngitis[35-37] and even fatal respiratory tract diphtheria[38] have been published since 1990.

OTHER SITES

On rare occasions, clinical infection with *C. diphtheriae* can be seen in other sites such as the ear, conjunctivae, or vagina.

Diagnosis

The clinical outcome in diphtheria is improved by the prompt initiation of treatment. Therefore, physicians must act on a presumptive diagnosis, based on several clinical clues: (1) mildly painful tonsillitis or pharyngitis with associated membrane, especially if the membrane extends to the uvula and soft palate; (2) adenopathy and cervical swelling, especially if associated with membranous pharyngitis and signs of systemic toxicity; (3) hoarseness and stridor; (4) palatal paralysis; (5) serosanguineous nasal discharge with associated mucosal membrane; (6) temperature elevation rarely in excess of 102.5° F; and (7) history of recent travel to a country where diphtheria is endemic. Moderate elevation of white blood cell count and transient proteinuria are common, but nonspecific. In former times when the disease was common, skilled practitioners could often make the diagnosis on examination of methylene blue–stained smears of the membrane or of throat swabs. Definitive identification of *C. diphtheriae* is made on the basis of colonial morphology, microscopic appearance, and fermentation reactions of isolates from bits of membrane or submembrane swabs cultured on tellurite-selective media such as Tinsdale agar. Although Tinsdale medium requires inoculation within 24 hours of preparation, it has an advantage in that a brown-black colony with a surrounding gray-brown halo is suggestive of the diagnosis. The combination of "Chinese characters" as seen on Gram stain, distinctive colonies with halos on Tinsdale medium, and the presence of metachromatic granules with methylene blue stain allows a presumptive identification of *C. diphtheriae*. Final identification requires biochemical tests. Toxin production is normally demonstrated by an in vitro test available at CDC, which detects the development of an immunoprecipitin band on antitoxin-impregnated filter paper that has been laid over an agar culture of the organism in question (Elek test). Recently, polymerase chain reaction probing of suspect organisms for DNA sequences coding for the toxin's A subunit has proved to be sensitive and accurate in rapid identification of *tox*+ strains.[62,63] Nonetheless, because a strain can be *tox*+ but not be toxigenic, a confirmatory Elek test is necessary to demonstrate the presence of toxin. Although an immunochromatographic strip test has been developed that has shown excellent correlation with the Elek test,[64] it is not commercially available. Because routine methods of throat culture do not promote the isolation and identification of *C. diphtheriae*, the laboratory must be alerted to use selective media when the disease is suspected.

The differential diagnosis includes faucial mononucleosis, streptococcal or viral pharyngitis and tonsillitis, Vincent angina, and acute epiglottitis. The membrane of mononucleosis characteristically remains on the tonsils, rarely loses its creamy-white appearance, and does not cause bleeding when removed. Streptococcal infection usually produces a more intense local pharyngitis, higher fever, and more pronounced dysphagia. Vincent's angina often involves the gums, and Gram stain of the exudate from the necrotic ulcerative pharyngeal lesions shows characteristic fusobacteria and spirochetes. Bacterial epiglottitis secondary to *Haemophilus influenzae* often develops more acutely, and indirect laryngoscopy shows a bright-red epiglottis without associated membrane. Finally, toxin-producing *C. ulcerans* can cause typical respiratory diphtheria, requiring the same treatment.[39,40]

Treatment

Diphtheria antitoxin (DAT), hyperimmune antiserum produced in horses, has been the cornerstone of therapy for diphtheria since it was first shown to reduce mortality from 7% to 2.5% in a controlled trial published in 1898. The antibodies only neutralize toxin before its entry into cells, so it is critical that DAT be administered as soon as a presumptive clinical diagnosis has been made, before laboratory confirmation. The degree of protection is inversely related to the duration of clinical illness preceding its administration.[53] Although the minimal therapeutic dose has never been determined, traditional (empirical) dosage recommendations assume that the duration of disease and extent of membrane formation roughly indicate the patient's toxin burden. The Committee on Infectious Diseases of the American Academy of Pediatrics recommends 20,000 to 40,000 units of antitoxin for pharyngeal or laryngeal disease of 48 hours' duration or less; 40,000 to 60,000 units for nasopharyngeal lesions; and 80,000 to 120,000 units for extensive disease of 3 or more days' duration and for anyone with brawny swelling of the neck.[65] It recommends administration by intravenous infusion over 60 minutes to inactivate toxin as rapidly as possible, but other experts suggest intramuscular injection of antitoxin for moderate disease and combined intramuscular and intravenous administration for severe disease. Repeated injections are of no additional benefit. Because 5% to 20% of individuals may show some hypersensitivity to horse protein, even very sick patients must be questioned first concerning known allergy and evaluated first with a scratch test (a drop of 1:1000 dilution of serum applied to a superficial scratch on the forearm), followed in 15 minutes if no wheal develops with 0.02 mL of a 1:1000 dilution injected intracutaneously, with epinephrine available for immediate administration.[65] If an immediate reaction occurs, the patient should be desensitized with progressively higher doses of antiserum. The incidence of serum sickness of about 10% is acceptable in light of the pronounced reduction in mortality resulting from antitoxin administration. Diphtheria antitoxin is no longer licensed in the United States, but a foreign-licensed product is available from the CDC Director's Emergency Operations Center by calling 770-488-7100.

Antibiotic therapy, by killing the organism, has three benefits: (1) termination of toxin production; (2) amelioration of the local infection; and (3) prevention of spread of the organism to uninfected contacts. Although several antibiotics, including penicillin, erythromycin, clindamycin, rifampin, and tetracycline, are effective, only penicillin and erythromycin are generally recommended. Intramuscular administration of procaine penicillin G (300,000 units for patients weighing less than 20 lb; 600,000 units for those weighing more than 20 lb) at 12-hour intervals is recommended until the patient is able to swallow comfortably, when oral penicillin V (125 to 250 mg 4 times daily) or erythromycin estolate or succinate (125 to 500 mg 4 times daily) may be substituted for a recommended total treatment period of 14 days. Both drugs are equally effective in resolving fever and local symptoms and in time to disappearance of membrane. Because erythromycin is marginally superior to penicillin in eradicating the carrier state, some authorities prefer it for initial treatment despite a significant incidence of thrombophlebitis when it is given intravenously and of gastrointestinal irritation when given orally. Patients should be maintained in strict isolation throughout therapy and, after therapy, should have two consecutive negative cultures at 24-hour intervals to document eradication of the organism.[65] The carrier state has a slow rate of spontaneous resolution (12% after 1 month in one study)[66] and so should be treated to prevent spread of infection. Erythromycin orally for 10 to 14 days is the treatment of choice because of several reports demonstrating its greater efficacy in comparison with penicillin.[55,56] However, the issue is clouded by a report showing that 21% of cultures taken 2 weeks after completion of erythromycin treatment were again positive for C. diphtheriae.[67] Therefore, it is necessary to obtain cultures at least 2 weeks after completing therapy to ensure eradication of the organism. A single intramuscular dose of benzathine penicillin G (600,000 to 1,200,000 units) is prudent when compliance with oral therapy is uncertain.[65]

Supportive care is also important. Bed rest is recommended during the acute illness, but proof of its benefit when the patient feels able to ambulate is lacking. Early in the disease, respiratory and cardiac complications are the biggest threats: airway obstruction can result from aspiration of dislodged pharyngeal membrane, its direct extension into the larynx, or from external compression by enlarged nodes and edema. For this reason, many experts recommend tracheostomy or intubation as an early measure, particularly when the larynx is involved, thereby providing access for mechanical removal of tracheobronchial membranes and avoiding the risk for sudden asphyxia. Vigilance must

be maintained to detect the development of primary or secondary bacterial pneumonia. Cardiac complications can be minimized by close electrocardiographic monitoring and prompt initiation of electrical pacing for conduction disturbances, drugs for arrhythmias, or digitalis for heart failure. Physical therapy can preserve range of motion in paretic extremities while awaiting return of neurologic function. A recent study has shown that treatment of acute diphtheria with prednisone did not reduce the incidence of carditis or neuritis.[68]

Treatment of systemic infection such as endocarditis and arthritis has not been studied systematically, but most reports describe administration of intravenous penicillin or ampicillin, usually with an aminoglycoside, for 4 to 6 weeks.[34] Mortality rates of 30% to 40% occur with bacteremic disease, and valve replacement is often necessary in cases of endocarditis.[31,32]

Prevention

The major manifestations of diphtheria can be prevented in individual patients by immunization with formalin-inactivated toxin ("toxoid"). Therefore, documentation of inadequate levels of antitoxin in a large proportion of the adult population in North America and Western Europe has caused great concern that a toxigenic strain introduced into these populations could cause an outbreak of disease similar to that in the former Soviet Union. Historically, the presence of immunity against diphtheria toxin was determined by the response to intradermal injection of small amounts of toxin (the Schick test). Currently, serum antitoxin levels can be measured by toxin neutralization tests in rabbit or guinea pig skin or by protection against cytopathic effect in Vero cell culture, with roughly equivalent results. Hemagglutination and enzyme-linked immunosorbent assays are less sensitive at the lower levels of antitoxin. Concentrations of 0.1 to 0.01 IU generally are thought to confer protection. For example, data from a recent outbreak showed that 90% of clinical cases had antitoxin levels below 0.01 IU/mL, whereas 92% of asymptomatic carriers had titers above 0.1 IU/mL.[69] After immunization, antitoxin levels decline slowly over time so that as many as 50% of individuals older than 60 years have serum titers below 0.01 IU/mL.[21,66,67] For this reason, booster doses of toxoid should be administered at 10-year intervals, to maintain antitoxin levels in the protective range.

Recommendations from the Advisory Committee on Immunization Practices were updated in 2006 and 2008, and published by CDC[70-72]:

For children from 6 weeks to 7 years of age: three 0.5-mL intramuscular injections of DTaP vaccine should be given at 4- to 8-week intervals, beginning at 6 to 8 weeks of age, followed by a fourth dose 6 to 12 months after the third. A fifth dose is given at age 4 to 6 years.

For children 7 to 10 years old: 0.5 mL Td (toxoid-adult) is given twice at a 4- to 8-week interval, with a third dose 6 to 12 months later. Because the pertussis component of DPT is responsible for most of its side effects, and the risk for pertussis is much less after age 6 years, that component of the vaccine is omitted and is no longer available in the United States. Moreover, because subjects older than 7 years have a higher incidence of local and systemic reactions to the concentration of diphtheria toxoid in pediatric DTaP vaccine (7 to 25 limit flocculation [Lf] units) and because a lower dose of toxoid has been shown to induce protective levels of antitoxin,[73] the Td formulation of vaccine contains a maximal concentration of 2 Lf units of diphtheria toxoid. If the recommended sequence of primary immunizations is interrupted, normal levels of immunity can be achieved simply by administering the remaining doses without need to restart the series.

For persons 11 or more years old: a single 0.5 mL Tdap is followed 4 to 8 weeks later by 0.5 mL Td, with a second dose of Td 6 to 12 months after the first

Booster immunizations: persons 11 to 18 years old should receive one dose of Tdap and then receive the standard Td booster at 10-year intervals (or Tdap, pending U.S. Food and Drug Administration approval). Those 19 to 64 years old should also have their next booster as Tdap, to reduce carriage, clinical illness, and transmission of pertussis.[71,72] As a help to memory, this should be done at decade or mid-decade intervals (e.g., ages 15, 25, 35, etc., or 20, 30, 40, etc.). Careful attention to this adult booster strategy is important to ensure population protection in areas with excellent childhood immunization programs. Travelers to areas where diphtheria is still endemic should be particularly careful to be sure their immunization is current. Although the recommended booster dose of 1.5 to 2.0 Lf units will increase antitoxin levels to above 0.01 IU in 90% to 100% of previously immunized individuals,[74,75] some authorities have recommended using 5 Lf units because antitoxin levels remain above 0.01 IU/mL for a longer period than with 2 Lf units.[74]

Patients should receive toxoid immunization in the convalescent stage of their disease because clinical infection does not always induce adequate levels of antitoxin. Close contacts whose immunization status is incomplete or unclear should promptly receive a dose of toxoid appropriate for their age and complete the proper series of immunizations. In addition, they should receive prophylactic treatment with erythromycin or penicillin, pending the results of pretreatment cultures. Given these preventive measures, the prophylactic use of antitoxin is considered unwarranted.

REFERENCES

1. English PC. Diphtheria and theories of infectious disease: Centennial appreciation of the critical role of diphtheria in the history of medicine. *Pediatrics.* 1985;76:1-9.
2. Hammond EM. *Childhood's Deadly Scourge.* Baltimore: Johns Hopkins University Press; 1999.
3. Loeffler F. Untersuchugen uber die Bedeutung der Mikroorganismen fur die Entstehung der Diphtherie. *Mitt Kaiserlichen Gesundheitsamt.* 1884;2:421-499.
4. Groman NB. Conversion by corynephages and its role in the natural history of diphtheria. *J Hyg (Camb).* 1984;93:405-417.
5. Pappenheimer AM. Diphtheria studies on the biology of an infectious disease. *Harvey Lect.* 1982;76:45-73.
6. Freeman VJ. Studies on the virulence of bacteriophage-infected strains of *Corynebacterium diphtheriae*. *J Bacteriol.* 1951;61: 675-688.
7. Golaz A, Hardy IR, Strebel P, et al. Epidemic diphtheria in the Newly Independent States of the former Soviet Union: implications for diphtheria control in the United States. *J Infect Dis.* 2000;181(suppl 1):S237-S243.
8. DeZoysa A, Efstratiou A, George RC, et al. Molecular epidemiology of *C. diphtheriae* from Northwestern Russia and surrounding countries studied by using ribotyping and pulsed-field gel electrophoresis. *J Clin Microbiol.* 1995;33:1080-1083.
9. Popovic T, Kombarova SY, Reeves MW, et al. Molecular epidemiology of diphtheria in Russia, 1985-1994. *J Infect Dis.* 1996; 174:1064-1072.
10. Grimont F, Lelay-Collin M, Grimond PAD. Adaptation of the International *Corynebacterium diphtheriae* Ribotypes Database to RiboPrinter, 7th International Meeting of the European Laboratory Working Group on Diphtheria. Vienna, Austria, 2002: 82-83.
11. Pappenheimer AM, Murphy JR. Studies on the molecular epidemiology of diphtheria. *Lancet.* 1983;2:923-926.
12. Kalapothaki V, Sapounas T, Xirouchaki E, et al. Prevalence of diphtheria carriers in a population with disappearing clinical diphtheria. *Infection.* 1984;12:387-389.
13. Romney MG, Roscoe DL, Bernard K, et al. Emergence of an invasive clone of nontoxigenic *Corynebacterium diphtheriae* in the urban poor population of Vancouver, Canada. *J Clin Micro.* 2006;44:1625-1629.
14. Harnisch JP, Tronca E, Nolan CM, et al. Diphtheria among alcoholic urban adults. A decade of experience in Seattle. *Ann Intern Med.* 1989;111:71-82.
15. Koopman JS, Campbell J. The role of cutaneous diphtheria infections in a diphtheria epidemic. *J Infect Dis.* 1975;131:239-244.
16. Belsey MA, Sinclair M, Roder MR, et al. *Corynebacterium diphtheriae* skin infections in Alabama and Louisiana. *N Engl J Med.* 1969;280:135-141.
17. Bisgard KM, Hardy IRB, Popovic T, et al. Respiratory diphtheria in the United States, 1980-1995. *Am J Pub Health.* 1998;88:787-791.
18. World Health Organization. WHO vaccine-preventable diseases: monitoring system 2006 global summary. Available at: <http://www.who.int/vaccines-documents/GlobalSummary/GlobalSummary.pdf>.
19. Dixon JMS. Diphtheria in North America. *J Hyg (Camb).* 1984;93:419-432.
20. Kwantes W. Diphtheria in Europe. *J Hyg (Camb).* 1984;93: 433-437.
21. World Health Organization. *Expanded Programme on Immunization (EPI) Information System.* Geneva: WHO; April 1993.
22. Galazka AM, Robertson SE. Diphtheria: changing patterns in the developing world and the industrialized world. *Eur J Epidemiol.* 1995;11:107-117.
23. Dittmann S, Wharton M, Vitek C, et al. Successful control of epidemic diphtheria in the states of the former Union of Soviet Socialist Republics: lessons learned. *J Infect Dis.* 2000;181 (suppl 1):S10-22.
24. Diphtheria Morbidity in the Russian Federation, 1999-2003. Public Health and Environment Bulletin, Issues #1-3 (2001, 2002, 2003). Federal Center of the State Sanitary and Epidemiological Surveillance of the Public Health Ministry of the Russian Federation (Moscow, RF). Available at: <http://www.fcgsen.ru>.
25. Hardy IRB, Dittmann S, Sutter RW. Current situation and control strategies for resurgence of diphtheria in newly independent states of the former Soviet Union. *Lancet.* 1996;347:1739-1744.
26. Vitek CR, Wharton M. Diphtheria in the former Soviet Union: re-emergence of a pandemic disease. *Emerg Infect Dis.* 1998;4: 539-550.
27. Popovic T, Kim C, Reiss J, et al. Use of molecular subtyping to document long-term persistence of *Corynebacterium diphtheriae* in South Dakota. *J Clin Microbiol.* 1999;37:1092-1099.
28. Centers for Disease Control and Prevention. Toxigenic *Corynebacterium diphtheriae*: Northern Plains Indian community, August-October 1996. *MMWR Morb Mortal Wkly Rep.* 1997;46: 506-510.
29. Wilson APR, Efstratiou A, Weaver E, et al. Unusual non-toxigenic *Corynebacterium diphtheriae* in homosexual men. *Lancet.* 1992; 339:998.
30. Millar OS, Cooper ON, Kakkar VV, et al. Invasive infection with *Corynebacterium diphtheriae* among drug users. *Lancet.* 1992;339: 1359.
31. Lortholary O, Buu-Hoi A, Gutmann L, et al. *Corynebacterium diphtheriae* endocarditis in France. *Clin Infect Dis.* 1993;17:1072-1074.
32. Tiley SM, Kociuba KR, Heron LG, et al. Infective endocarditis due to nontoxigenic *Corynebacterium diphtheriae*: report of seven cases and review. *Clin Infect Dis.* 1993;16:271-275.
33. Gruner E, Opravil M, Altwegg M, et al. Nontoxigenic *Corynebacterium diphtheriae* isolated from intravenous drug users. *Clin Infect Dis.* 1994;18:94-96.
34. Patey O, Bimet F, Riegel P, et al. clinical and molecular study of *Corynebacterium diphtheriae* systemic infections in France. *J Clin Microbiol.* 1997;35:441-445.
35. Wilson APR. The return of *Corynebacterium diphtheriae*: the rise of non-toxigenic strains. *J Hosp Infect.* 1995;30(Suppl): 306-312.
36. Efstratiou A, George RC, Begg NT. Non-toxigenic *Corynebacterium diphtheriae* var gravis in England. *Lancet.* 1993;341:1592-1593.
37. Reacher M, Ramsay M, White J, et al. Nontoxigenic *Corynebacterium diphtheriae*: an emerging pathogen in England and Wales? *Emerg Infect Dis.* 2000;6:640-645.
38. Rakhmanova AG, Lumio J, Groundstroem KWE, et al. Fatal respiratory tract diphtheria apparently caused by nontoxigenic strains of *Corynebacterium diphtheriae*. *Eur J Clin Microbiol Infect Dis.* 1997;16:816-820.
39. Kelly C, Efstratiou A. Seventh international meeting of the European laboratory working group in diphtheria—Vienna, June 2002. *Euro Surveill.* 2003;8:189-195.
40. Tiwari TSP, Golaz A, Yu DT, et al. Investigations of 2 cases of diphtheria-like illness due to toxigenic *Corynebacterium ulcerans*. *CID.* 2008;46:395-401.
41. Brooks GF, Bennett JV, Feldman RA. Diphtheria in the United States, 1959-1970. *J Infect Dis.* 1974;129:172-178.
42. Rakhmanova AG, Lumio J, Groundstroem K, et al. Diphtheria outbreak in St. Petersburg: Clinical characteristics of 1,860 adult patients. *Scand J Infect Dis.* 1996;28:37-40.
43. Galazka A. The changing epidemiology of diphtheria in the vaccine era. *J Infect Dis.* 2000;181(suppl 1):S2-S9.
44. McQuillan GM, Kruszon-Moran D, Deforest A, et al. Serologic immunity to diphtheria and tetanus in the United States. *Ann Intern Med.* 2002;136:660-666.
45. Williams BC. Immunization coverage among preschool children: The United States and selected European countries. *Pediatrics.* 1990;86:1052-1056.
46. National, state, and urban area vaccination coverage among children aged 19-35 months—United States 2003. *MMWR Morb Mortal Wkly Rep.* 2004;53;658-661.
47. Rappuoli R, Perugini M, Falsen E. Molecular epidemiology of the 1984-86 outbreak of diphtheria in Sweden. *N Engl J Med.* 1988;318:12-14.
48. Pappenheimer AM. The diphtheria bacillus and its toxin: A model system. *J Hyg (Camb).* 1984;93:397-440.
49. Boyer NH, Weinstein L. Diphtheritic myocarditis. *N Engl J Med.* 1948;239:913.
50. Morgan BC. Cardiac complications of diphtheria. *Pediatrics.* 1963;32:549-557.
51. Ledbetter MK, Cannon AB, Costa AF. The electrocardiogram in diphtheritic myocarditis. *Am Heart J.* 1964;68:599-611.
52. Dobie RA, Tobey DN. Clinical features of diphtheria in the respiratory tract. *JAMA.* 1979;242:2197-2201.
53. Naiditch MJ, Bower AG. Diphtheria. A study of 1433 cases observed during a ten year period at the Los Angeles County Hospital. *Am J Med.* 1954;17:229-245.
54. Kallick CA, Brooks GF, Dover AS, et al. A diphtheria outbreak in Chicago. *Ill Med J.* 1970;137:505-512.
55. Zalma VM, Older JJ, Brooks GF. The Austin, Texas, diphtheria outbreak. *JAMA.* 1970;211:2125-2129.
56. McCloskey RV, Eller JJ, Green M, et al. The 1970 epidemic of diphtheria in San Antonio. *Ann Intern Med.* 1971;75:495-503.
57. Bray JP, Burt EG, Potter EV, et al. Epidemic diphtheria and skin infections in Trinidad. *J Infect Dis.* 1972;126:34-40.
58. Hewlett EL. Selective primary health care: Strategies for control of disease in the developing world. XVIII. Pertussis and diphtheria. *Rev Infect Dis.* 1985;7:426-433.
59. Belsey MA, LeBlanc DR. Skin infections and the epidemiology of diphtheria: Acquisition and persistence of *C. diphtheriae* infections. *Am J Epidemiol.* 1975;102:179-184.
60. Jellard CH. Diphtheria infection in Northwest Canada, 1969, 1970, and 1971. *J Hyg.* 1972;70:503-510.
61. Wagner J, Ignatus R, Voss S, et al. Infection of the skin caused by *Corynebacterium ulcerans* and mimicking classical cutaneous diphtheria. *Clin Infect Dis.* 2001; 33: 1598-1600
62. Mikhailovich VM, Melnikov VG, Mazurova IK, et al. Application of PCR for detection of toxigenic *Corynebacterium diphtheriae* strains isolated during the Russian diphtheria epidemic, 1990 through 1994. *J Clin Microbiol.* 1995;33:3061-3063.
63. Mothershed EA, Cassiday PK, Pierson K, et al. Development of a real-time fluorescence PCR assay for rapid detection of the diphtheria toxin gene. *J Clin Microbiol.* 2002;40:4713-4719.
64. Engler KH, Efstratiou A, Norn D, et al. Immunochromatographic strip test for rapid detection of diphtheria toxin: description and multicenter evaluation in areas of low and high prevalence of diphtheria. *J Clin Microbiol.* 2002;40:80-83.
65. American Academy of Pediatrics. Diphtheria. In: Pickering LK, Baker CJ, Long SS, McMillan JA, eds. *Red Book: 2006 Report of the Committee on Infectious Diseases.* 27th ed. Elk Grove Village, IL: American Academy of Pediatrics; 2006:277-281.
66. Kiselev VI. The use of various antibiotic combinations in the control of diphtheria bacilli carrier state. *Antibiotiki.* 1964;9: 361-363.
67. Miller LW, Bickham S, Jones WL, et al. Diphtheria carriers and the effect of erythromycin therapy. *Antimicrob Agents Chemother.* 1974;6:166-169.
68. Thisyakorn USA, Wongvanich J, Kumpeng V. Failure of corticosteroid therapy to prevent diphtheritic myocarditis or neuritis. *Pediatr Infect Dis.* 1984;3:126-128.
69. Bjorkholm B, Bottiger M, Christenson B, et al. Antitoxin antibody levels and the outcome of illness during an outbreak of diphtheria among alcoholics. *Scand J Infect Dis.* 1986;18: 235-239.
70. Centers for Disease Control and Prevention. Preventing Tetanus, Diphtheria, and Pertussis Among Adults: Use of Tetanus Toxoid, Reduced Diphtheria Toxoid and Acellular Pertussis Vaccine. Recommendations of the Advisory Committee on Immunization Practices and Recommendation of ACIP, supported by the Healthcare Infection Control Practices Advisory Committee (HICPAC), for Use of Tdap Among Health-Care Personnel. *MMWR Morb Mortal Wkly Rep.* 2006;55:RR17.
71. Centers for Disease Control and Prevention. Recommended Immunization Schedules for Persons Aged 0-18 years—United States, 2008. *MMWR Morb Mortal Wkly Rep.* 2007;56(51-52): Q1-Q4.
72. Centers for Disease Control and Prevention. Health Information for International Travel 2008. Paul Arguin, Phyllis Kozarsky, Christie Reed, eds. Atlanta, Ga: US Department of Health and Human Services; 2008:142-145.
73. Myers MG, Beckman CW, Vosdingh RA, et al. Primary immunization with tetanus and diphtheria toxoids. *JAMA.* 1982;248:2478-2480.
74. Simonsen O, Klaerke M, Klaerke A, et al. Revaccination of adults against diphtheria II: Combined diphtheria and tetanus revaccination with different doses of diphtheria toxoid 20 years after primary vaccination. *Acta Pathol Microbiol Immunol Scand [C].* 1986;94:219-225.
75. Ruben RL, Nagel J, Fireman P. Antitoxin responses in the elderly to tetanus-diphtheria immunization. *Am J Epidemiol.* 1978;108: 145-149.

206

Other Coryneform Bacteria and Rhodococci

DANIEL K. MEYER | ANNETTE C. REBOLI

Coryneform Bacteria Other than Corynebacterium diphtheriae

Corynebacterium was proposed as a genus by Lehmann and Neumann in 1896, who derived the name from the Greek *koryne*, which means "club," and *bacterion*, meaning "little rod."[1] *Corynebacterium diphtheriae* serves as the type species, leading to the term *diphtheroids* to describe other bacteria sharing similar morphology. Also known as *coryneform bacteria*, bacteria demonstrating morphology similar to that of corynebacteria include the genera *Corynebacterium, Arcanobacterium, Brevibacterium, Dermabacter, Microbacterium, Rothia, Turicella, Arthrobacter,* and *Oerskovia*.[2]

Coryneform bacteria are widely distributed in the environment as normal inhabitants of soil and water. They are commensals colonizing the skin and mucous membranes of humans and other animals.[3-5] In the hospital setting, coryneform may be cultured from the hospital environment, including surfaces and medical equipment.[6] Coryneform bacteria other than *C. diphtheriae* have been isolated frequently in clinical specimens and were commonly considered contaminants without clinical significance. There is an increasing body of evidence of the pathogenicity of the coryneform bacteria, particularly as a cause of nosocomial infection in hospitalized and immunocompromised patients.[7,8] Several of the members of the genus *Corynebacterium* are better known as pathogens in animals and only incidentally cause infection in humans as zoonoses.

The coryneform bacteria are pleomorphic, demonstrating different forms at various stages of the life cycle, irregularly shaped gram-positive rods that are aerobically cultured, not spore forming, and not partially acid-fast.[2] A history of misidentification of coryneform bacteria has made interpretation of the medical literature difficult. Initial identification is aided by observation of colony size and appearance and the presence or absence of hemolysis on sheep blood agar. Odor production by colonies assists in identification, particularly of *Brevibacterium casei* and *Corynebacterium urealyticum*. Several of the medically relevant coryneform bacteria are lipophilic, demonstrating enhanced growth with the addition of Tween 80 to the culture medium.

True corynebacteria demonstrate club-shaped gram-positive rods on Gram stain, whereas other coryneform bacteria may not appear distinctly club shaped. Cells demonstrate variable sizes and appearance, from coccoid to bacillary forms depending on the stage of the life cycle, and Gram stain results may be uneven. Coryneform bacteria typically form arrangements such as "Chinese letters" or picket-fence configurations as a result of "snapping" after the cells divide. Lack of spore formation helps distinguish them from *Bacillus* species.[2]

The spectrum of human infections attributed to the coryneform bacteria is broad but can be understood in two general categories: community-acquired infections and nosocomial infections. Community-acquired infections include pharyngitis, native valve endocarditis, genitourinary tract infections, acute and chronic prostatitis, and periodontal infections (Table 206-1).[9] Many case reports of nosocomial infections attributed to coryneform bacteria are in the medical literature and include intravascular catheter-associated septicemia, native and prosthetic valve endocarditis, device-related infections, and postoperative surgical site infections. Common nosocomial pathogens

include *Corynebacterium jeikeium, C. urealyticum, Corynebacterium amycolatum,* and *Corynebacterium striatum* (Table 206-2).[10] It is expected that nosocomial infections with the coryneform bacteria will continue to increase, reflecting the increased numbers of severely ill patients with extended stays in intensive care units and multiple antibiotic exposures.

TAXONOMY

The taxonomy of the coryneform bacteria has evolved extensively over the past 20 years and continues to be refined. Hollis and Weaver at the Special Bacteriology Laboratory, Centers for Disease Control and Prevention (CDC) in Atlanta, completed the first extensive compilation of coryneform bacteria isolated from clinical specimens.[11] Coryneform bacteria were grouped based on colony and biochemical characteristics. Since then, further work has been done to analyze these groups and define species. Table 206-3 lists the significant coryneform bacteria and the CDC group to which they previously belonged. New species continue to be identified yearly, not all of which appear to be clinically relevant.

Analysis of cell wall composition and cellular fatty acid patterns is performed in reference laboratories to confirm species identification.[2,12] In addition, the use of molecular genetics has resulted in continued revision of the taxonomy of the coryneform bacteria and provides useful information on the epidemiology and pathogenicity of the genera. Molecular genetic studies such as restriction analysis of 16S recombinant DNA and repetitive extragenic palindromic polymerase chain reaction (PCR) typing are used in reference laboratories to confirm identification at the species level.[2,13]

MICROBIOLOGY

Because the coryneforms are frequently cultured in polymicrobial infections and may be contaminants in cultures collected with poor sterile technique, clinician communication with the microbiology laboratory is essential to determine when species identification is appropriate. The decision to identify the coryneform bacteria to the species level is recommended when the bacteria are cultured from normally sterile sites such as blood or cerebrospinal fluid (CSF), if the bacteria appear in significant numbers on Gram stains of clinical material, if they are obtained in pure culture, or if they are cultured in large numbers from the specimen.[2]

Media used for initial specimen processing are standard blood agar plates for most specimens, thioglycollate broth for wound cultures, and standard blood culturing systems using continuous monitoring for CO_2 production. Special media used for species identification include tryptic soy agar with and without 1% Tween 80 to assess lipid-enhanced growth.[2]

Identification to the species level in the microbiology laboratory is confirmed by biochemical testing. Initial testing includes the catalase test with 3% H_2O_2. Additional tests include nitrate reduction; urea production; and hydrolysis patterns from glucose, maltose, sucrose, mannitol, and xylose. A frequently used system of biochemical testing for medically relevant coryneform bacteria is the API CORYNE system,

TABLE 206-1	Community-Acquired Coryneform Infections
Conjunctivitis	*Corynebacterium macginleyi*
Pharyngitis	*Arcanobacterium haemolyticum*
	Corynebacterium ulcerans
	Corynebacterium pseudodiphtheriticum
Peritonsillar and pharyngeal abscess	*A. haemolyticum*
Odontogenic infections	*A. haemolyticum*
	Rothia dentocariosa
Lymphadenitis	*Corynebacterium pseudotuberculosis*
Genitourinary tract infection	*Corynebacterium glucuronolyticum*
	Corynebacterium riegelii
Chronic prostatitis	*Corynebacterium glucuronolyticum*
Skin and soft tissue infections	*Arcanobacterium haemolyticum*
	Arcanobacterium pyogenes
	Corynebacterium minutissimum
	Corynebacterium pseudotuberculosis
	Corynebacterium confusum
Breast abscess	*Corynebacterium kroppenstedtii*
	Corynebacterium tuberculostearicum
	C. minutissimum
Native valve endocarditis	*A. haemolyticum*
	R. dentocariosa
	Corynebacterium pseudodiphtheriticum

TABLE 206-2	Nosocomial Infections Caused by Coryneform Bacteria
Cerebrospinal fluid shunt infections	*C. jeikeium*
Meningitis	*C. jeikeium*
	Brevibacterium spp.
Pneumonia	*C. amycolatum (C. xerosis)*
	C. striatum
	C. urealyticum
Intravenous catheter–related bloodstream infection	*C. jeikeium*
	C. amycolatum
	C. striatum
	C. urealyticum
	Brevibacterium casei
	C. macginleyi
	C. minutissimum
	C. afermentans afermentans
	Arcanobacterium bernardiae
	Arcanobacterium pyogenes
	Oerskovia spp.
	Microbacterium spp.
Native valve endocarditis	*C. amycolatum*
	C. jeikeium
	C. striatum
	C. urealyticum
Prosthetic valve endocarditis	*C. jeikeium*
	C. amycolatum
	C. striatum
	Brevibacterium casei
Skin and soft tissue infection	*C. amycolatum*
	C. minutissimum
	C. urealyticum
Postsurgical infections	*C. jeikeium*
	C. urealyticum
	C. striatum
Prosthetic joint infections	*C. jeikeium*
Urinary tract infections and encrusted cystitis	*C. urealyticum*
Continuous ambulatory peritoneal dialysis–related peritonitis	*C. jeikeium*
	Brevibacterium spp.
	C. urealyticum
	Dermabacter
	Rothia dentocariosa

which includes 20 biochemical tests and will identify many of the important corynebacteria and other coryneform bacteria, including *Arcanobacterium* species and *Brevibacterium* species, as well as *Rhodococcus equi*, *Listeria monocytogenes*, *Erysipelothrix rhusiopathiae,* and *Gardnerella vaginalis*.[14] An evaluation of the updated CORYNE database 2.0 gave correct identification for 90.5% of the coryneforms tested.[15] The RapID CB Plus system correctly identifies 80.9% strains to the species level and an additional 12.2% to the genus level. It has the advantage of requiring only 4 hours to perform, compared with 24 hours for the CORYNE system.[16]

In a few cases the CAMP test, named for the initial investigators Christie, Atkins, and Munch-Petersen, helps to identify the organism to the species level.[2] A streak of a β-lysin–producing strain of *Staphylococcus aureus* is plated on sheep blood agar, and a streak of the test strain is plated perpendicular to it. A positive CAMP reaction is noted if the CAMP factor, a cohemolysin secreted by the tested coryneform, enhances hemolysis in a synergistic fashion. Although most coryneform bacteria are CAMP negative, a few species such as *Corynebacterium auris* and *Corynebacterium gluronolyticum* have been shown to produce CAMP factor.

Susceptibility testing has historically been problematic in the coryneforms.[17] The Clinical and Laboratory Standards Institute (CLSI) released standards for susceptibility testing of coryneform bacteria in 2006.[18] Isolates uniformly show susceptibility to the glycopeptides, vancomycin and teicoplanin, and the lipopeptide, daptomycin.[19] The *vanA* gene has been identified in *Oerskovia turbata* and *Arcanobacterium haemolyticum,* but no documented infections with vanocmycin-resistant coryneforms have appeared in the literature.[20] When a clinically important isolate is obtained, susceptibility testing is recommended to ensure antimicrobial activity.

For consistency, the coryneform bacteria are reviewed here within groups identified by the presence or absence of lipid-enhanced culture (lipophilic or nonlipophilic) and fermentation activity.

NONLIPOPHILIC, FERMENTATIVE CORYNEBACTERIA

Advances made in the identification of species in the nonlipophilic fermentative group have resulted in a revision of thinking of the pathogenic role of several species, particularly for *Corynebacterium xerosis*

and *C. amycolatum.*[21] Interpretation of the literature that does not include detailed information on laboratory identification is difficult because recent reviews have found a great deal of misidentification in the nonlipophilic fermentative group. As laboratories implement improved strategies for identification of coryneform bacteria in clinical specimens from normally sterile sites, one hopes the pathogenic role of the nonlipophilic fermentative corynebacteria will be clarified.[2]

Corynebacterium ulcerans and Corynebacterium pseudotuberculosis

C. ulcerans and *C. pseudotuberculosis* are members of the *C. diphtheriae* group and are known primarily as animal pathogens, although disease in humans has been reported as a zoonotic infection. Both *C. ulcerans* and *C. pseudotuberculosis* may elaborate diphtheria toxin.

C. ulcerans is known primarily as a cause of bovine mastitis but has the potential to elaborate diphtheria toxin and cause an exudative pharyngitis in humans indistinguishable from diphtheria.[22,23] Several

TABLE 206-3	Medically Relevant Coryneform Bacteria	
Classification	**CDC Coryneform Group**	
Nonlipophilic, Fermentative Corynebacteria		
C. ulcerans	C. diphtheriae group	
C. pseudotuberculosis	C. diphtheriae group	
C. xerosis	F-2, I-2	
C. striatum	I-1	
C. minutissimum		
C. amycolatum	F-2, I-2	
C. glucuronolyticum		
Others: C. argentoratense, C. matruchotii, C. riegelii, C. confusum, C. simulans, C. sundvallense, C. thomssensii, C. freneyi, C. aurimucosum		
Nonlipophilic, Nonfermentative Corynebacteria		
C. afermentans afermentans	ANF-1	
C. auris		
C. pseudodiphtheriticum		
C. propinquum	ANF-3	
Lipophilic Corynebacteria		
C. jeikeium	JK	
C. urealyticum	D-2	
Others: C. afermentans lipophilum, C. accolens, C. macginleyi, C. tuberculostearum, C. kroppenstedtii, C. bovis, CDC coryneform groups F-1 and G, C. lipophiloflavum		
Arcanobacteria		
A. haemolyticum		
A. pyogenes (Actinomyces pyogenes)		
A. bernardiae		
Other coryneform bacterial genera: Turicella, Arthrobacter, Brevibacterium, Dermabacter, Rothia, Oerskovia, Microbacterium, Leifsonia aquatica		
Rhodococci		

reported outbreaks of diphtheria have been found to be caused by C. ulcerans rather than C. diphtheriae. This has made the identification of the causative organism important for epidemiology, and guidelines for laboratory diagnosis of diphtheria cases have been published.[24] The spectrum of illness with C. ulcerans is similar to C. diphtheriae.[25,26] Fatalities have been reported, including sudden death from toxin-induced cardiac injury and a case of fatal necrotizing sinusitis.[27] Skin infection by C. ulcerans mimics that of C. diphtheriae.[28] Infection of the lower respiratory tract may occur, causing pneumonia and pulmonary nodules.[29,30] Treatment of pharyngitis caused by C. ulcerans is similar to treatment of diphtheria, including the use of antibiotics such as erythromycin and diphtheria antitoxin when appropriate.

C. pseudotuberculosis is a significant pathogen in animals, particularly sheep, in which it causes caseous lymphadenitis. Human disease is rare, manifesting as granulomatous lymphadenitis, found mainly in farm workers and veterinarians who have had exposure to infected animals.[31,32] It has been reported to be a cause of eosinophilic pneumonia and has also been isolated from soft tissue abscesses in a young butcher.[33,34] Management of C. pseudotuberculosis infection includes excision of affected lymph nodes and treatment with β-lactam antibiotics, macrolides, or tetracyclines. A vaccine for caseous lymphadenitis in sheep is in use that may reduce the incidence of human disease.

Corynebacterium xerosis

C. xerosis is a colonizer of the human nasopharynx, conjunctiva, and skin.[35] C. xerosis has been described in the literature as a pathogen causing serious human disease, especially in immunocompromised hosts, including sepsis, endocarditis, pneumonia, peritonitis, ventriculoperitoneal shunt infection, and postoperative sternal wound infection. Recent investigations have questioned the reliability of C. xerosis identification in the microbiology laboratory.[36,37] In one study, all iso-

lates originally identified as C. xerosis were in actuality C. amycolatum.[37] This calls into question preceding case reports attributing disease to C. xerosis because true C. xerosis isolates apparently are quite rare. Recent reports have included C. xerosis isolated from a brain abscess and a case of sepsis in a pediatric patient with sickle cell disease.[38,39] Future case reports that include methods of identification used to identify the organism may help to clarify the role of C. xerosis in human disease. True C. xerosis strains are susceptible to most antibiotics, which helps to distinguish them from C. amycolatum, which demonstrates multiple antibiotic resistances.

Corynebacterium striatum

C. striatum has been one of the more commonly isolated coryneform bacteria in the clinical microbiology laboratory.[2] As in the case of other nonlipophilic fermentative corynebacteria, a high degree of misidentification of C. striatum has occurred in the past in microbiology laboratories, and investigators have found many isolates to be C. amycolatum on detailed retesting.[36,40]

C. striatum is ubiquitous and colonizes the skin and mucous membranes of normal hosts and hospitalized patients.[41,42] Although it is isolated frequently in polymicrobial infections, its degree of pathogenicity has been unclear, and differentiation of colonization from pathogen-causing infection has been difficult.[7,8] In a large recent series of 150 clinical specimens from which coryneform bacteria had been isolated, C. striatum was identified in 11 isolates, only one of which was considered to be related to an infectious process.[7] There is evidence for patient-to-patient transmission of C. striatum in hospital settings, which may account for the frequency with which it is isolated in hospitalized patients.[43,44]

Reports of true infection confirmed by isolation of C. striatum from a sterile site are rare and have been reported mainly for patients with indwelling devices or immunosuppression. Recent case reports in the literature include native and prosthetic valve endocarditis, pacemaker-related endocarditis, meningitis, pulmonary abscess, septic arthritis, and vertebral osteomyelitis. A nosocomial outbreak of C. striatum has been reported in patients with chronic obstructive pulmonary disease.[45] Nosocomial endocarditis has been reported in a patient with vascular access for dialysis that was successfully treated with vancomycin and rifampicin.[46] C. striatum may be resistant to penicillin but is susceptible to other β-lactams and vancomycin. Resistance has been demonstrated to ciprofloxacin, erythromycin, rifampin, and tetracyclines; there is variable susceptibility to aminoglycosides.[47]

Corynebacterium minutissimum

Defined in 1983 by Collins, C. minutissimum is a colonizer of human skin, particularly moist intertriginous areas.[48,49] As with other members of this group, C. amycolatum has been misidentified as C. minutissimum in the past.[50] Although historically C. minutissimum has been considered the causative agent in erythrasma, that association has been questioned because cultures tend to show polymicrobial infection.[2] Erythrasma is a superficial skin infection occurring in intertriginous areas between skin folds, axillae, groin, and fingers and toes. It presents as reddened scaling patches that may be accompanied by pruritus. Skin patches glow coral-red under Wood lamp. Diagnosis is made by clinical appearance and symptoms and by culture of skin scrapings. Colonies also appear coral-red under ultraviolet light. Treatment includes topical and oral antibiotics. Recurrences are frequent.

Other rare infections attributed to C. minutissimum include septicemia and endocarditis in immunocompromised patients and patients with indwelling central venous catheters, peritonitis in patients undergoing continuous ambulatory peritoneal dialysis (CAPD), and pyelonephritis[51] A recent case of bacteremia and meningitis has been reported.[52] It has been reported to cause cutaneous granulomas and costochondral abscess in patients with acquired immunodeficiency virus (AIDS) and been implicated as a cause of recurrent breast abscesses. Supporting evidence for the microbiologic diagnosis in several case reports is slim, and these infections may actually have been caused by other members of the nonlipophilic fermentative group.

Corynebacterium amycolatum

Defined as a new species in 1988 by Collins, *C. amycolatum* was first isolated from the skin of healthy humans.[53] Noted for its lack of mycolic acids, the species corresponds to the CDC coryneform groups F-2 and I-2. *C. amycolatum* forms small dry nonhemolytic colonies of 1 mm to 1.5 mm when cultured at 37° C.[3] The organisms are pleomorphic and vary from single organisms to an array of Chinese letters. *C. minutissimum* and *C. amycolatum* may not be correctly identified on the API CORYNE system but can be distinguished on the basis of colony morphology.[2,21] New techniques to identify corynebacteria to the species level have increased the reporting of isolates identified as *C. amycolatum*. By recent identification techniques, it is the nonlipophilic coryneform bacteria most frequently isolated from clinical specimens.[7,8]

Although case reports of infections attributed to *C. amycolatum* are rare, many previously reported infections by other members of the nonlipophilic fermentative group were most likely caused by *C. amycolatum*. Recent reports with reliable information on organism identification include nosocomial endocarditis following intravenous catheter–related infection, septic arthritis, a case of native valve endocarditis with aorta-to–left atrial fistula, and neonatal sepsis.[54-57] Susceptibility testing has shown resistance to penicillins, cephalosporins, macrolides, fluoroquinolones, and rifampin, and susceptibility to vancomycin, daptomycin, linezolid, and teicoplanin.[58] There is variable resistance to aminoglycosides and tetracyclines.[19] Reports of successful treatment include the use of vancomycin and rifampin.

Corynebacterium glucuronolyticum

C. glucuronolyticum was defined in 1995, and since 2000, the species has included those isolates previously identified as *Corynebacterium seminale* that had been defined by Riegel and co-workers in 1996.[59,60] Although it has been isolated from the genitourinary tract of animals, in humans, it may be included in the normal flora of the genitourinary tract. It is commonly isolated from males with genitourinary tract infections and is associated with chronic prostatitis.[61] *C. glucuronolyticum* strains are susceptible to β-lactam antibiotics, gentamicin, rifampin, and vancomycin, but demonstrate resistance to fluoroquinolones, macrolides, and tetracyclines.

Other Nonlipophilic, Fermentative Corynebacteria

Corynebacterium argentoratense has been isolated from the throats of healthy volunteers and from mucosal biofilms on adenoid tissue from children with chronic or recurrent otitis media. The clinical significance of this finding is unclear.[3,62,63] *Corynebacterium matruchotii* is identified by its characteristic "whip handle" appearance on Gram stain.[2] It was previously identified as *Bacterionema matruchotii* until 1983, when it was reclassified as a *Corynebacterium* species by Collins. Mainly an inhabitant of the oral cavity of humans and animals, *C. matruchotii* has been rarely associated with human disease.

In 1998 Funke and colleagues identified a new species of *Corynebacterium* isolated from female patients with symptomatic urinary tract infections.[64] Given the name *Corynebacterium riegelii*, it is nonlipophilic, weakly fermentative, and facultatively anaerobic. Similar to the lipophilic *Corynebacterium urealyticum*, it demonstrates strong urease activity. It is susceptible to penicillins, cephalosporins, gentamicin, fluoroquinolones, rifampin, and tetracyclines.

Corynebacterium confusum was defined in 1998 by Funke and colleagues from three human clinical specimens.[65] It is nonlipophilic and very slowly fermentative. Two of the specimen sources were from foot infections, and the third from a bloodstream isolate. No further reports have been published. Additional nonlipophilic fermentative *Corynebacterium* species identified recently from human clinical specimens include *Corynebacterium simulans*, *Corynebacterium sundvallense*, *Corynebacterium thomssenii*, *Corynebacterium freneyi*, *Corynebacterium aurimucosum*, *Corynebacterium tuscaniae*, and *Corynebacterium coyleae*.[66-71] Further information from case reports is needed to determine the medical relevance of these isolates.

NONLIPOPHILIC, NONFERMENTATIVE CORYNEBACTERIA

The nonlipophilic, nonfermentative corynebacteria do not produce acid from any sugars and were designated as absolute nonfermenters (ANF) by Hollis and Weaver.[11] They are colonizers of the human respiratory tract and ear canal and infrequent pathogens.

Corynebacterium afermentans *Subspecies* afermentans

C. afermentans subsp. *afermentans* was included in the CDC coryneform group ANF-1 until 1993, when Riegel and co-workers defined the species as *C. afermentans* with two subspecies: *C. afermentans* subsp. *afermentans* and *C. afermentans* subsp. *lipophilum*.[72] *C. afermentans* subsp. *afermentans* is a rare human pathogen but has been reported to cause septicemia in immunocompromised patients.[73]

Corynebacterium auris

As in the case of *Turicella otitidis*, *C. auris* was initially isolated from middle ear fluid of pediatric patients with otitis media and was presumed to be among the pathogens causing otitis media. Subsequent studies have cultured *C. auris* from the external ear canal and cerumen of healthy subjects, both children and adults, and its role as a pathogen has been discounted.[4,74] *C. auris* is resistant to penicillins, clindamycin, and erythromycin and susceptible to fluoroquinolones, gentamicin, rifampin, tetracyclines, and vancomycin.[17]

Corynebacterium pseudodiphtheriticum

C. pseudodiphtheriticum is included in the normal bacterial flora of the human upper respiratory tract. Lehmann and Neumann described the organism in 1896, giving it the name *Bacillus pseudodiphtheriticum*.[1] Since 1925, it has been known as *Corynebacterium pseudodiphtheriticum*. Historically, *C. pseudodiphtheriticum* was associated with endocarditis of native and prosthetic valves.[75] The first cases of infections at other sites attributable to *C. pseudodiphtheriticum* became known in 1982, and since then, *C. pseudodiphtheriticum* has been associated primarily with respiratory infections, particularly in immunocompromised hosts.[76,77] It has been isolated from patients with pneumonia and advanced AIDS.[78] Other sites of infections have been the eye, intervertebral disk, and lymph nodes. Although *C. pseudodiphtheriticum* does not elaborate toxins, it has been isolated from three patients with exudative pharyngitis with pseudomembrane formation, not unlike *C. diphtheriae*.[79] In one case, colonization of close contacts was demonstrated. Recent reports include *C. diphtheriticum* as a cause of skin ulcer and infectious arthritis.[80,81] Some isolates of *C. pseudodiphtheriticum* have demonstrated resistance to macrolide antibiotics but have maintained susceptibility to penicillins, cephalosporins, doxycycline, and glycopeptides.

Corynebacterium propinquum

Before 1994, *C. propinquum* was known as CDC coryneform group ANF-3.[82] Primarily isolated from the human respiratory tract, its role as a pathogen is yet to be defined. There are reports of isolation of *C. propinquum* from blood specimens that lack clinical information necessary to interpret the finding and one case of endocarditis. One report of *C. propinquum* isolated from a pulmonary pleural effusion has been published.

LIPOPHILIC CORYNEBACTERIA

Lipophilic corynebacteria are fastidious, slow-growing bacteria that form tiny nonhemolytic colonies on standard media but demonstrate enhanced growth with the addition of lipids to the culture medium.[2] The group includes the significant human pathogens *C. jeikeium* and *C. urealyticum*.

Corynebacterium jeikeium

C. jeikeium was initially described in 1976 as a highly resistant coryneform bacteria causing severe sepsis in patients with hematologic malignancies and profound neutropenia and in one patient with ventricular CSF shunt.[83] In 1979, it was designated as CDC group JK, and in 1988, the designation was revised to *C. jeikeium*.[84] *C. jeikeium* colonizes the skin of hospitalized patients, especially those treated with multiple antibiotics, and can also be isolated from the hospital environment.[85] There is some evidence that patient-to-patient transmission occurs in the hospital.[6,86] It is the most frequently isolated corynebacterium in the acute care setting and is the most important pathogen of the lipophilic corynebacteria.[7]

Microbiology. *C. jeikeium* is a pleomorphic gram-positive rod, which varies in form from coccobacillary to bacillary; some appear club shaped. It is nonhemolytic on standard media and forms small gray-white colonies on routine culture.[2] It is lipophilic, forming large colonies on sheep blood agar supplemented with 1% Tween 80. *C. jeikeium* produces urease, reduces nitrate, and ferments glucose. It has variable fermentation of galactose and maltose.[87]

Pathogenicity. *C. jeikeium* is a cause of severe infections in the hospitalized patient.[6] Predisposing factors for infection include immunocompromised states such as malignancy, neutropenia, and AIDS.[6,88] Other risk factors include the presence of indwelling medical devices such as central venous catheters, peritoneal dialysis catheters, prosthetic valves, and CSF shunts. Prolonged hospital stay, treatment with broad-spectrum antibiotics, and impaired skin integrity are well-described risk factors for development of infection with *C. jeikeium*.

Infectious processes include septicemia from infected intravascular devices, native and prosthetic valve endocarditis, CSF shunt infections, meningitis and transverse myelitis, and prosthetic joint infections.[89-91] It has been reported to cause postsurgical infections, peritonitis in patients undergoing CAPD, liver abscess, otitis media, and osteomyelitis of the foot. Skin findings with *C. jeikeium* infection are common: half of neutropenic patients with *C. jeikeium* septicemia have reported skin findings, including rash and subcutaneous nodules.[92] Palpable purpura has been reported in patients with *C. jeikeium* endocarditis.[93]

Treatment. *C. jeikeium* is resistant to many antibiotics, including penicillins, cephalosporins, and aminoglycosides, and there is inducible resistance to macrolides.[94,95] It remains susceptible to vancomycin, which is the recommended treatment. Although catheter removal has been routinely recommended in the setting of intravascular catheter-related infection, recent experience has shown a high success rate in catheter salvage with appropriate antimicrobial therapy.[96]

Corynebacterium urealyticum

First described in 1974, this bacterium was designated as CDC group D2 until 1992, when the name *Corynebacterium urealyticum* was proposed.[97] *C. urealyticum* colonizes the skin of 25% to 37% of hospitalized patients. Because of its ability to adhere to uroepithelial cells, it is most commonly associated with urinary tract infections, especially in cases of abnormal anatomy, and has been implicated as the cause of encrusted cystitis and encrusted pyelitis.[98,99]

Microbiology. Colonies of *C. urealyticum* are slow growing and lipophilic and appear nonhemolytic and pinpoint when cultured on sheep blood agar under CO_2 for 48 hours.[2] It is a strict aerobe, with no growth under anaerobic conditions. On Gram stain, organisms are palisading, non–spore-forming coccobacilli. They are catalase positive and oxidase negative, with a rapid production of urease. Laboratories should be made aware of the need for further investigation of diphtheroid bacilli from urinary tract specimens in the proper clinical setting because *C. urealyticum* may not grow in standard urine culture.[2]

Pathogenicity. *C. urealyticum* is primarily a cause of chronic and recurrent urinary tract infections, occurring mainly in elderly people and those with debilitation or immunosuppression. Additional risk factors include prolonged hospitalization, the use of bladder drainage catheters, and urinary tract procedures. It has been reported to cause infections in renal transplant recipients.[98] Clues to diagnosis of *C. urealyticum* infection include sterile pyuria, alkaline urine, and the presence of white blood cells and struvite crystals.[100] *C. urealyticum* causes encrusted cystitis, which appears as chronic inflammation of the bladder mucosa with crystal deposits on the bladder mucosa surrounded by erythema. Encrusted pyelitis may occur if there are abnormalities of the upper urinary tract. In rare cases, *C. urealyticum* has been reported as a causative agent in peritonitis, endocarditis, pneumonia, septicemia, osteomyelitis, soft tissue infections, and superinfection of wounds.[101,102]

Treatment. In general, *C. urealyticum* is resistant to β-lactams, aminoglycosides, and trimethoprim-sulfamethoxazole. There is variable susceptibility to fluoroquinolones, macrolides, and tetracycline.[7,101] The treatment of choice is vancomycin, to which it remains susceptible. For urinary tract infections, in addition to vancomycin, endoscopic removal of bladder mucosa encrustations or acidification of urine by instilling acid into the bladder in cases of encrusted cystitis may be required, and urologic consultation is recommended. Percutaneous nephrostomy tube placement and irrigation of upper urinary tract with Thomas' acid solution in cases of upper tract disease has been described.[103]

Other Lipophilic Corynebacteria

Corynebacterium afermentans subsp. *lipophilum* is a rarely reported human pathogen.[72] It has been reported to cause intravascular catheter–related septicemia, prosthetic valve endocarditis, lung abscess, empyema, and brain abscess. *Corynebacterium accolens* was previously known as CDC coryneform group 6. There were discrepancies in the definition until 1991, when it was defined further by Neubauer and associates and given the name *Corynebacterium accolens*.[103a] Known to colonize the human upper respiratory tract, *C. accolens* is a rarely reported human pathogen but has been reported to cause septicemia, endocarditis, and breast abscess.[104,105] *Corynebacterium macginleyi* was initially isolated solely from the human eye as a cause of conjunctivitis.[106] There has been one report of intravascular catheter–associated bloodstream infection by *C. macginleyi*, one report of urinary tract infection associated with a bladder drainage catheter, and one report of septicemia in an immunocompromised patient.[107] Other lipophilic corynebacteria including *Corynebacterium tuberculostearicum* and *Corynebacterium kroppenstedtii* have been cultured from inflammatory breast tissue in cases of granulomatous mastitis.[108,109] *Corynebacterium bovis* is a cause of bovine mastitis but in humans has been described as a cause of endocarditis, chronic otitis media, central nervous system (CNS) infection, and line-related septicemia.[110,111] CDC coryneform group F1 may be a cause of urinary tract infection; it is similar to *C. urealyticum* in its very rapid urease reaction and differs from the latter in its very high susceptibility on antimicrobial testing. CDC coryneform group G has been a cause of endocarditis and septic arthritis and shows multiple antibiotic resistances. *Corynebacterium lipophiloflavum* has been isolated from a patient with bacterial vaginosis. *Corynebacterium kutscheri*, an oral commensal of mice and rats, has been isolated from a human after a rat bite.[112] New species of coryneform bacteria continue to be defined. *Corynebacterium resistens* is a recently described multidrug-resistant coryneform bacteria isolated from blood, bronchial aspirate, and abscess specimens.[113] *Corynebacterium ureicelerivorans* has been isolated from a blood culture.[114]

ARCANOBACTERIA

Collins defined the genus *Arcanobacterium* in 1982, from "arcane," meaning "mysterious or secret" and "bacterium."[115] For many years, *Arcanobacterium haemolyticum* was the only species in this genus. However, in 1997, further investigation of several *Actinomyces* species resulted in the reclassification of *Actinomyces pyogenes* and *Actinomyces bernardiae* as *Arcanobacterium* species and defined two additional new species of arcanobacteria.[116]

Arcanobacterium haemolyticum

A. haemolyticum was first isolated by MacLean and co-workers in 1946 from American soldiers and Pacific Islanders with pharyngeal and skin infections in the South Pacific.[117] The initial classification as *Corynebacterium haemolyticum* endured until 1982, when the genus *Arcanobacterium* was defined by Collins.

Microbiology. *A. haemolyticum* is a catalase-negative, gram-positive to gram-variable rod that does not form spores and is nonmotile.[2] It is β-hemolytic, but expression can vary by culture media and conditions, with hemolysis best observed on human blood agar.[118] Growth is enhanced in the presence of CO_2. It is known for forming dark pits under the colonies. Poor growth on tellurite helps to differentiate it from *C. diphtheriae*.

Colony morphology has been described as either rough or smooth type.[119] Rough-type colonies are rough appearing, nonhemolytic, and β-glucuronidase positive, and they do not ferment sucrose and trehalose. Smooth-type colonies are smooth appearing, β-hemolytic, and β-glucuronidase negative, and they ferment sucrose or trehalose. Both types ferment glucose and maltose. Rough-type colonies are most frequently associated with respiratory isolates; smooth biotypes are most frequently associated with wound isolates. *A. haemolyticum* does not ferment xylose, which differentiates it from *Arcanobacterium (Actinomyces) pyogenes*. A positive α-mannosidase test identifies *A. haemolyticum* and differentiates it from *A. pyogenes* and other coryneform-like bacteria, including *R. equi* and *E. rhusiopathiae*. Because of the presence of phospholipase D activity similar to *C. ulcerans* and *C. pseudotuberculosis*, the reverse CAMP test will be positive, with inhibition of the hemolytic zone of a β-lysin–producing strain of *S. aureus*. Other secreted toxins include neuraminidase and a hemolysin.

Infections in Humans. *A. haemolyticum* is a well-recognized cause of pharyngitis in humans, with a spectrum of illness from mild to diphtheria-like.[120-122] It accounts for about 0.5% of pharyngeal infections overall and 2.5% in individuals in the 15- to 25-year–old age range. In studies, *A. haemolyticum* has not been isolated from healthy control populations but has been isolated from 2.5% of a symptomatic young adult population.[122-124] It is indistinguishable from streptococcal pharyngitis in clinical appearance, and about 50% of cases of pharyngitis are exudative. Cervical adenopathy is usually present. *A. haemolyticum* pharyngitis is accompanied with an exanthem in about 50% of cases. The rash generally appears after the onset of the pharyngitis and has a variable appearance, often described as an erythematous morbilliform or scarlatiniform rash, appearing on the trunk, neck, and extremities (Fig. 206-1). It may also present as an erythematous urticarial rash with an appearance similar to that of erythema multiforme. Complications of *A. haemolyticum* pharyngitis include peritonsillar and pharyngeal abscesses, with *A. hemolyticum* the sole pathogen in 50% of cases in adolescents and young adults, and the remaining 50% coinfected with β-hemolytic streptococci.[123]

A. haemolyticum has been isolated from soft tissue infections, including chronic ulcers, wound infections, cellulitis, and paronychia. It is frequently a component of polymicrobial infection in this setting but has been isolated as the sole pathogen as well. Underlying conditions in polymicobial chronic ulcers include diabetes and peripheral vascular disease. Post-traumatic wound infections have been reported, as has coinfection or superinfection with leprosy ulcers.[125]

Lemierre disease with *Fusobacterium necrophorum* and *A. haemolyticum* has been reported, accompanied by a skin rash typical for *A. haemolyticum* infection.[126] Sepsis syndrome from *A. haemolyticum* has been described, occurring in all age groups and without predisposing factors.[127] Other infections reported include sinusitis, orbital cellulitis, brain abscess, endocarditis, cavitary pneumonia, and vertebral osteo-

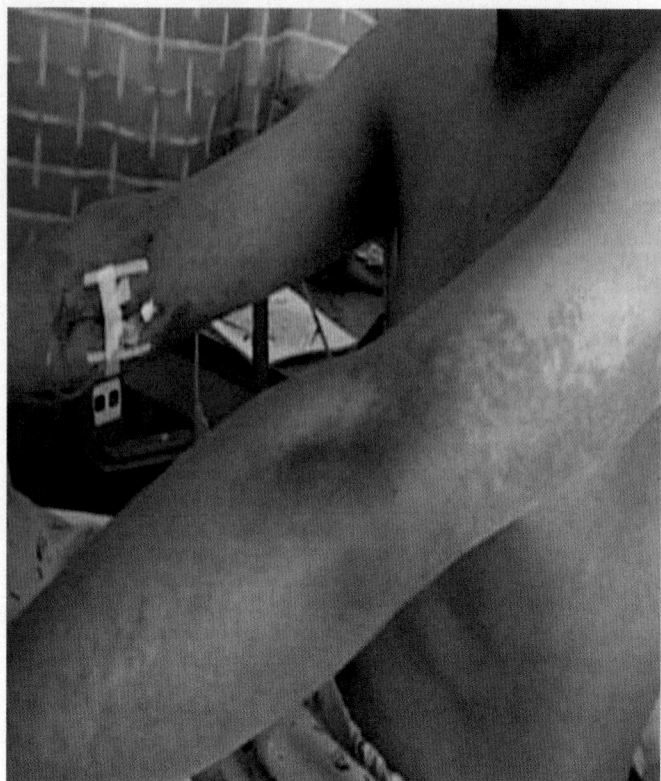

Figure 206-1   **Skin rash in a patient with *Arcanobacterium haemolyticum* pharyngitis.**

myelitis. *A. haemolyticum* may be present in subperiosteal abscesses in periodontal disease.[125,128]

Treatment. Susceptibility information for *A. haemolyticum* has been reviewed extensively.[129] Although in vitro studies show most strains to be penicillin susceptible, treatment failures may occur because of tolerance and poor penetration into the intracellular space. Other β-lactams have shown in vitro activity as well. The most reliable clinical data have shown efficacy of the macrolides, and erythromycin and azithromycin have been proposed as drugs of choice.[129] Clindamycin and doxycycline are also efficacious, as are ciprofloxacin and vancomycin. Resistance to trimethoprim-sulfamethoxazole is well documented. Three vancomycin-resistant strains of *A. haemolyticum* expressing the *vanA* gene were recovered in a surveillance study, but no vancomycin-resistant infections have been reported. Surgical management of wound infections and drainage of soft tissue abscesses are recommended.

Arcanobacterium (Actinomyces) pyogenes

Initially described by Glage in 1903, this organism was initially named *Bacillus pyogenes*. It was known as *Corynebacterium pyogenes* until 1982, when it was reassigned to the genus *Actinomyces*. Since 1997, it has been known as *Arcanobacterium pyogenes*.[116] *A. pyogenes* is primarily an animal pathogen causing pyogenic infections in cattle, including pneumonia, endometritis, endocarditis, wound infections, and mastitis. Abscess formation is aided by neuraminidases, which facilitate adhesion to host epithelial cells.[130] Transmission of *A. pyogenes* by flies has been proposed. *A. pyogenes* has not been isolated as normal human flora. Most human cases are acquired in rural settings and include annual outbreaks of leg ulcers in Thai children, septicemia in a patient with colon carcinoma, polymicrobial-infected diabetic foot ulcers, spondylodiscitis and psoas abscess, subcutaneous abscesses, and intra-abdominal infections.[131] A case of fatal endocarditis in a patient with no animal contact has been reported.[132] *A. pyogenes* is cultured on sheep blood agar under CO_2 enrichment. Colonies are weakly hemolytic at 24 hours and become more strongly hemolytic at 48 hours.[2] Differentiation from *A. haemolyticum* is made by observation of the CAMP reaction, by fermentation of xylose, and by the α-mannosidase test. *A. pyogenes* is susceptible to most antibiotics, including penicillins, cephalosporins, macrolides, tetracyclines, and aminoglycosides.

Arcanobacterium bernardiae

Originally described as CDC coryneform group 2 in 1987, it was assigned the species name *Actinomyces bernardiae* in 1995. In 1997, it was transferred to the genus *Arcanobacterium* as *Arcanobacterium bernardiae*.[116] On Gram stain, it appears as short gram-positive rods without branching. It is identified by the ability to ferment maltose more rapidly than glucose, which separates it from other coryneform bacteria. It is distinguished from *A. pyogenes* by the inability to ferment sucrose, mannitol, and xylose.[2] *A. bernardiae* is a rare human pathogen, with recovery of the organism from the bloodstream, abscesses, urinary tract, the eye, and wounds.[133-135]

MISCELLANEOUS CORYNEFORM BACTERIA

Turicella otitidis

Initially isolated from patients with otitis media, *Turicella otitidis* is believed to be a colonizer of the human auditory canal and not a true pathogen in this setting because it has been isolated in the same frequency from an asymptomatic control population.[4,74,136] It has been reported as a cause of mastoiditis and posterior auricular abscess in immunocompetent children and septicemia in a neutropenic child. *T. otitidis* is resistant to clindamycin and erythromycin but susceptible to penicillins, cephalosporins, tetracyclines, fluoroquinolones, rifampin, and vancomycin.[17]

Arthrobacter *Species*

An environmental coryneform found in animal sheds, schools, and daycare centers, *Arthrobacter* has rarely been isolated from human clinical specimens. Identified species include *Arthrobacter cumminsii*, *Arthrobacter oxydans*, *Arthrobacter luteolus*, and *Arthrobacter albus*.[137,138] There are reports of septicemia in immunocompromised patients and isolation of *Arthrobacter* from human urine specimens. One unusual case report was of Whipple syndrome caused by *Arthrobacter*.

Brevibacterium *Species*

Brevibacterium species are short coryneforms isolated from milk and dairy products and are known colonizers of human skin.[8] They have been identified in environmental dust in schools, daycare centers, and animal sheds. Brevibacteria show a biphasic morphology on culture, with young colonies demonstrating typical coryneform features. As colonies age, the organisms mature into cocci or a coccobacillary appearance.[2] Brevibacteria have been implicated in causing human foot odor when confining footwear results in a moist environment. Although seven species of *Brevibacterium* exist, only four species have been associated with human infection: *Brevibacterium casei*, *Brevibacterium epidermidis*, *Brevibacterium mcbrellneri*, and *Brevibacterium otitidis*.[139]

B. casei is the species of this genus that is most frequently isolated from human clinical specimens. On culture, it forms white-gray colonies with a distinctive cheese odor. On Gram stain, it is a short, club-shaped rod that is catalase positive and non–spore-forming.[2,139] Human infections with brevibacteria have most frequently been intravascular catheter–related bloodstream infections, particularly in immunocompromised patients and patients with AIDS. There have been additional reports of meningitis, cholangitis, salpingitis, and peritonitis in patients undergoing CAPD. In addition, there is one report each of prosthetic valve endocarditis and osteomyelitis of the sternum in a neonate following an episode of mastitis in the mother.[140] Susceptibility testing shows some resistance to β-lactam antibiotics, fluoroquinolones, clindamycin, and macrolides. Vancomycin is the treatment of choice for serious infections.[17,141] *Brevibacterium sanguinis* is a recently described organism isolated from six patients, five of whom had septicemia.[142]

Dermabacter hominis

Dermabacter species were previously identified as CDC group 3 and group 5 coryneform bacteria and are skin colonizers of humans.[143] They have been a cause of bacteremia in patients with prolonged hospitalizations and in those undergoing CAPD who have immune compromise and peritonitis. *Dermabacter* has been isolated from a cerebral abscess in a renal transplant recipient and from a patient with chronic osteomyelitis with *Actinomyces neuii* as copathogen.[144] *D. hominis* exhibits variable resistance to many antibiotics, including penicillins, fluoroquinolones, macrolides, chloramphenicol, and tetracyclines, and susceptibility to vancomycin and teicoplanin.[17]

Rothia dentocariosa *and* Rothia mucilaginosa

Rothia are found as colonizers of the human oral cavity and have been isolated from dental plaque and in cases of periodontal disease.[145] *Rothia dentocariosa* has the potential for misidentification as *Dermabacter* or *Actinomyces* species in the microbiology laboratory.[2]

Case reports with reliable information on identification of the organisms have found it to be a pathogen in several cases of native and prosthetic valve endocarditis, including presentations with abscesses, mycotic aneurysms, and vertebral osteomyelitis.[146-148] It has also been isolated as a cause of bacteremia without endocarditis. It has been found in cases of pneumonia in patients with leukemia and lung cancer and has caused peritonitis in a patient undergoing CAPD.

Rothia mucilaginosa, formerly *Stomatococcus mucilaginosus*, is a normal resident of the human mouth and nasopharynx. On culture, it usually appears as gram-positive cocci in clusters—hence the previous classification as a *Stomatococcus*. *R. mucilaginosa* is a rare cause of sepsis from an oral source, but cases of meningitis and spondylodiscitis have also been reported.[149] Most isolates are susceptible to ampicillin.

Oerskovia *Species*

Included in CDC group A-1 and A-2, *Oerskovia* species are rare human pathogens but have been reported to cause infection in immunocompromised hosts, patients with implanted devices, and those with indwelling central venous catheters.[2] The spectrum of infections has ranged from bacteremia, endocarditis, meningitis associated with CSF shunt infection, soft tissue infection, prosthetic joint infection, and peritonitis in a patient undergoing CAPD.[150-152] One report of endophthalmitis following eye injury with a metallic foreign body exists in the literature.

Microbacterium *Species*

CDC coryneform group A-4 and A-5 bacteria were defined as *Microbacterium* species, and since 1998, the genus *Aureobacterium* has been included in the genus *Microbacterium*.[153-154] *Microbacterium* species have been found as a cause of bacteremia in patients on an oncology ward and in specimens from patients with endophthalmitis. Most commonly, it has been a nosocomial pathogen in debilitated and immunocompromised patients.[155]

Leifsonia aquatica

Corynebacterium aquaticum was reclassified in 2000 as *Leifsonia aquatica*.[156] Because of inconsistencies of identification and confusion with *Aureobacterium* in previous reports, it has been difficult to determine the pathogenicity of this species. It is expected that future case reports will help to clarify this. Case reports for *Leifsonia aquatica* are rare, although *C. aquaticum* had been reported to cause septicemia in immunocompromised hosts, peritonitis in patients on CAPD, and bacteremia in a hemodialysis patient. In addition, urinary tract infection in a neonate and meningitis in an infant have been reported.

Although strains of *Exiguobacterium*, *Cellulomonas*, and *Sanguibacter* have been isolated from human clinical specimens, no reports of human disease attributed to them exist in the literature.[2,157]

Rhodococci

Rhodococcus (red coccus) belongs to the family Nocardioform, order Actinomycetes, which includes *Nocardia, Corynebacterium, Mycobacterium,* and *Gordonia* species. *R. equi* is the most commonly isolated species causing human infection, especially among immunocompromised hosts with defective cell-mediated immunity. Other members of this genus that are human pathogens include *Rhodococcus rhodochrous, Rhodococcus fascians (Rhodococcus luteus),* and *Rhodococcus erythropolis.*

RHODOCOCCUS EQUI

R. equi (formerly *Corynebacterium equi*) was first identified as a pathogen in 1923 when it was isolated from the lungs of foals with pyogranulomatous pneumonia. It has subsequently been identified in a variety of animals, including cattle, swine, sheep, goats, deer, bears, wild birds, seals, dogs, and cats.[158] The first case of human infection was reported in 1967 when *R. equi* was cultured from lung specimens of a young man working in a stockyard who was being treated with corticosteroids and 6-mercaptopurine for autoimmune hepatitis and presented with fever and cavitary pneumonia. During the next decade, sporadic cases of infection in humans were reported. Beginning in the early 1980s, the incidence of *R. equi* infection increased markedly. This increase has been attributed to the human immunodeficiency virus (HIV) infection epidemic, advances in chemotherapy for malignancies, and organ transplantation. In addition, improvements in microbiology laboratory identification techniques and increasing recognition of *R. equi* as a pathogen may also explain part of the increase in incidence.[159] The frequency of *R. equi* infections in HIV-infected patients seems to have decreased in recent years, largely related to highly active antiretroviral therapy (HAART) and possibly to prophylaxis with azithromycin. More than 180 cases of infection caused by *R. equi* have been published. *R. equi* has been isolated from water and soil worldwide and from the manure of herbivores.[158] Infection in both animals and humans is thought to be acquired through inhalation or ingestion of the organism. Inoculation into a wound can also lead to infection. Exposure to farm soil, animals, or manure has been reported in many human cases, although it is less common in HIV-positive patients.[160,161] *R. equi* has been rarely isolated from healthy persons.[162] Most infected individuals have had defective cell-mediated immunity, with or without a history of animal exposure. Health care–associated cases of *R. equi* have been reported.[163] Human-to-human transmission has been suspected in cases of *R. equi* pneumonia acquired by HIV-infected patients who were roommates of patients infected with *R. equi.*[164] Occupational acquisition of *R. equi* by a healthy laboratory worker who developed pneumonia has been reported. *Rhodococcus* species with properties very similar to those of *R. equi* have been isolated as nasal flora in adults.[165]

R. equi is a gram-positive obligate aerobe that is asporogenous and nonmotile. It may appear coccoid or bacillary depending on growth conditions. Its bacillary appearance varies from long, curved, clubbed forms to short filaments with branching. *R. equi* can grow at a variety of temperatures but grows optimally at 30° C. Colonies on solid media appear large, irregular, smooth, and mucoid. They are pale salmon-pink in color; however, this characteristic color may not appear until days 4 to 7 of incubation. Although it grows well on ordinary media, if cultured in this manner, the organism may be overlooked or discarded as a nonpathogenic coryneform, or misidentified as *Nocardia* or *Micrococcus*. Isolation of *R. equi* from contaminated specimens is facilitated by the use of selective media such as colistin-nalidixic agar (CNA), phenyl-ethanol agar (PEA), or ceftazidime-novobiocin agar. *R. equi* is catalase, lipase, urease, and phosphatase positive. It is oxidase, elastase, deoxyribonuclease, and protease negative. Differentiation from other pathogenic coryneforms is based on a lack of ability to ferment carbohydrates or liquefy gelatin.[2] Because it is sometimes acid fast, it may be mistaken for a *Mycobacterium*.[158] It can be distinguished from some mycobacterial species by the 14-day arylsulfatase test because *Rhodococcus* is negative for this reaction. Two special features of *R. equi* help distinguish it from other similar organisms: (1) when *R. equi* is cultured on sheep blood agar that is cross-streaked with other bacteria, such as *Staphylococcus aureus, Corynebacterium pseudotuberculosis,* or *Listeria monocytogenes,* synergistic hemolysis occurs; and (2) in vitro antagonism between imipenem and other β-lactams is widespread among *R. equi* isolates.[166] Generally, the identification of *Rhodococcus* species using traditional tests may be difficult. There is no simple, reproducible method for rapid identification and differentiation. Ribotyping, PCR restriction fragment length polymorphism (RFLP), and an *R. equi*-specific PCR may prove to be rapid, useful adjuncts.[167,168]

R. equi is a facultative, intracellular pathogen. It infects macrophages and survives inside the lysosomes. Its ability to cause chronic infection may be based on its complex cell wall, which is thought to prevent phagosome-lysosome fusion, resists the oxidative burst, and causes a nonspecific degranulation of lysosomes, which permits intrahistiocytic survival.[169] Although virulence factors associated with *R. equi* infections in animals have been defined and include plasmid-associated surface proteins, they may not be important in infection in humans.[170,171] Histopathology usually reveals a necrotizing granulomatous reaction. Endobronchial granulomas have been reported.[172] Multiple microabscesses may be seen. Malakoplakia is a rare, chronic, granulomatous inflammatory process that is associated with an impaired ability to process microorganisms within histiocytes. It is characterized by accumulations of benign macrophages associated with intracellular and extracellular aggregates of periodic acid–Schiff stain–positive histiocytes that contain lamellated iron and calcium inclusions and are termed *Michaelis-Guttman bodies*.[169] Lung malakoplakia is a rare condition; most of the reported patients had *R. equi* pneumonia.[173]

R. equi has been cultured from a variety of human tissues and fluids, including sputum, bronchial washings, lung tissue, pleural fluid, blood, cerebrospinal fluid (CSF), brain, skin, lymph nodes, peritoneal fluid, bone, stool, pharyngeal exudates, and wounds.[160,174-186] It has been recovered from peritoneal dialysate, intravenous catheters, and CSF after ventriculoperitoneal shunt insertion.[160,187,188] Pneumonia accounts for about 80% of human cases of infection reported in the literature.[159,189] Most published cases of pulmonary infection have occurred in immunocompromised hosts.[189] The lung was the only site of infection in more than 80% of cases; a concurrent extrapulmonary site was reported in about 20% of cases of pulmonary infection.[160] Typically, the presentation is subacute in onset. Common symptoms include fever, productive or nonproductive cough, and fatigue.[160] Pleuritic chest pain is also common. Hemoptysis has been reported in about 15% of patients. *R. equi* bacteremia frequently complicates pneumonia. Other complications include the development of lung abscess, pleural effusion, empyema, pneumothorax, endobronchial lesions, pericarditis, cardiac tamponade, and mediastinitis.[160,185,189,190] Chest radiographs reveal nodules, cavities (single or multiple), infiltrates, and pleural effusions.[164,185] More than one type of lesion may be present. In a case series of pulmonary cavitary lesions in HIV-infected persons, *R. equi* was the fifth most common microbiologically proven cause, accounting for about 9% of cases.[191] It followed *Mycobacterium tuberculosis, Pneumocystis jirovecii, Pseudomonas aeruginosa,* and *S. aureus* in frequency. The cavities have been described as thick walled and sometimes have an air-fluid level.[160] Necrotizing pneumonia due to *R. equi* closely resembles tuberculosis or nocardiosis. Nodules or cavities of the upper lung lobes, or both, may be seen. Air-fluid levels are seen in cavitary lesions caused by *R. equi*, but not in those seen with tuberculosis. Mediastinal enlargement has been noted. The most common computed tomography finding is consolidation with cavitation.[192] Although a good-quality sputum specimen can yield a microbiologic diagnosis, in many instances, invasive techniques such as bronchoscopy, thoracentesis, or surgical resection are required to make a microbiologic diagnosis. Blood cultures are positive in about 50%

of HIV-infected individuals and in 25% of solid organ transplant recipients who are infected with *R. equi*. Up to 30% of immunocompetent hosts are bacteremic.[162,174,176]

Extrapulmonary infection with *R. equi* occurs in about 20% of cases with pulmonary infection; infection of extrapulmonary sites occurs in about 25% of cases without evidence of pulmonary involvement. Most common extrapulmonary sites reported were brain and subcutaneous abscesses.[160,193,194] Extrapulmonary infection is frequently a late manifestation of the initial pulmonary infection. Abscesses in the liver, spleen, thyroid, kidney, psoas muscle, bone, prostate, intra-abdominal cavity, and paraspinous tissue have occurred.[189,193] Extrapulmonary infections not associated with pulmonary disease have been noted to present in three distinct patterns.[160] The first pattern includes wound infections, traumatic septic arthritis, and endophthalmitis following ocular injury. In these cases, infection remains localized at the primary site and drainage procedures appear to hasten recovery. The second group consists of cases of isolated bacteremia that manifested with fever. Most of these patients had malignancies and were neutropenic or had recently received chemotherapy. Central venous catheters were present in most of these cases. The third pattern may have resulted from inoculation of the gastrointestinal tract with dissemination to regional lymph nodes. Conditions in this group included peritonitis, pelvic masses, and mesenteric adenitis. Other reported types of infection include otitis media with mastoiditis; colonic polyps infiltrated with *R. equi;* and osteomyelitis of the vertebrae, long bones, and mandible.[160]

More than 85% of cases of *R. equi* infection described in the literature have occurred in immunocompromised hosts, particularly those with HIV infection. HIV-infected patients account for two thirds of cases.[159] Other immunocompromised hosts reported to be infected with *R. equi* include recipients of organ transplants, diabetics, alcoholics, those with chronic renal failure, leukemia, lymphomas, lung cancer, sarcoidosis, and preterm infants. Infection has occurred as a complication of chemotherapy, corticosteroid use, and treatment with monoclonal antibodies.[195] Infection of immunocompetent persons with *R. equi,* however, may be more common than previously assumed because in a recent series, immunocompetent hosts accounted for 42% of cases.[162] Clearance of *R. equi* is impaired in the immunocompromised host, and relapses are common despite maintenance antibiotic therapy.[196] In the pre-HAART era, relapses of pneumonia were described in up to 80% of HIV-infected patients. Infection occurs primarily in patients with CD4 counts of fewer than 100 cells/µL.[159] About 10% of *R. equi* infections occur in transplant recipients receiving immunosuppressive therapy and are generally a late complication.[159,178,184,197-199] Most of these patients were solid organ transplant recipients. The primary site of infection was the lung. Findings included both nodular lesions and infiltrates. Cavitary lesions were frequent. Pseudotumor has been reported.[198] In about half of transplant recipients, extrapulmonary infection was present and included brain abscesses, paravertebral abscess, purulent pericarditis, subcutaneous nodules, and osteomyelitis of the femur. Among immunocompetent hosts, localized infections account for nearly 50%.[162] Pulmonary infection was present in more than 40%. Disseminated infection also occurred.[182,183,193] Recurrent infection has been reported.[200] The mortality rate is greatest among patients with HIV and has been reported to be as high as 58%.[160,174,176] In a study from Thailand, HIV-infected persons with community-acquired pneumonia caused by *R. equi* were more likely to die than those infected with other organisms.[201] Mortality in immunocompetent hosts has been reported to be 11%; it is about 20% for non–HIV-infected immunocompromised hosts.[159,178]

For several reasons, including the small number of reported cases, standards for treatments of *R. equi* infection have not been established. *R. equi* is usually susceptible in vitro to vancomycin, erythromycin, fluoroquinolones, rifampin, glycopeptides, carbapenems, aminoglycosides, and linezolid.[159,160,202-204] Of the quinolones, moxifloxacin and gatifloxacin are the most active in vitro.[205,206] Gatifloxacin is no longer available in the United States. Susceptibility to clinda-

mycin, tetracycline, chloramphenicol, and cephalosporins is variable; *R. equi* is usually resistant to penicillins, and even if susceptible in vitro, the use of penicillins is not recommended because resistance can develop.[160,162] In an animal model, the most effective agents were vancomycin, imipenem, and rifampin.[207] Rifampin-resistant isolates have been reported.[208] Monotherapy has been ineffective in a number of cases and is not recommended. Combinations of two or three antimicrobial agents have generally yielded partial or complete therapeutic responses. Localized, non-CNS infections in immunocompetent hosts can usually be treated with oral agents.[162] Two-drug regimens that include a macrolide, rifampin, fluoroquinolone, or a combination can be started empirically and should be adjusted based on the results of susceptibility testing.[159] Immunocompromised hosts and those with serious infections should be treated with two- or three-drug regimens that include vancomycin or a carbapenem (imipenem, ertapenem, or meropenem), rifampin, a fluoroquinolone, an aminoglycoside, or a macrolide.[199,209] Linezolid has been used successfully to treat relapsing infection.[196] It has been suggested that intravenous antibiotics be continued until clinical improvement occurs or for a minimum of 2 to 3 weeks.[159] Oral agents should then be given until cultures are negative and signs and symptoms have resolved. A minimum of 2 to 6 months of antimicrobial therapy is advised for immunocompromised hosts and those with pulmonary, bone, joint, or CNS infections. Brain abscess has been successfully treated with 8 weeks of intravenous therapy.[193] Because the CNS is a frequent secondary site of infection, agents that penetrate this site should be administered.[160] Drainage of localized abscesses, empyemas, and large cavities may be beneficial.[210] Lung lobectomy has been performed when poor clinical response was noted with antimicrobial therapy. It is generally recommended that after the treatment course is completed, HIV-infected individuals and persons with ongoing immunosuppression receive long-term suppressive therapy with a macrolide plus rifampin or a quinolone or doxycycline with rifampin. For HIV-positive patients, oral suppressive therapy should be continued until immune reconstitution occurs. Infection may develop or become manifest at other sites during therapy. Relapses are common. They can occur at the initial site of infection or at other sites.

OTHER *RHODOCOCCUS* SPECIES AND RELATED GENERA

Infections caused by other *Rhodococcus* species and related genera such as *Gordonia* and *Tsukamurella* have generally been associated with medical procedures or devices. *Gordonia* species, previously classified as *Rhodococcus* species, have caused bacteremia, endocarditis, and CNS infections in both immunocompromised and immunocompetent hosts.[211-215] *Gordonia bronchialis* (formerly *Rhodococcus bronchialis*) has been reported to cause sternal wound infection after coronary artery bypass surgery, bacteremia, and recurrent breast abscess.[216-218] Pulmonary infection resembling tuberculosis has been reported to be caused by *Gordonia rubripertinctus* (formerly *Rhodococcus rubropertinctus*) in a patient who was not immunosuppressed.[219] Speciation is best accomplished by I6S rRNA sequencing.[217,218] *Tsukamurella* species, including *Tsukamurella paurometabola* (formerly *Rhodococcus aurantiacus* and *Corynebacterium paurometabolum*), have caused central venous catheter–related bacteremia in patients with malignancies, patients who were receiving parenteral nutrition, and those with infection of an implantable cardioverter defibrillator, pneumonia, meningitis, conjunctivitis, and soft tissue abscesses and necrotizing tenosynovitis.[219-226] Underreporting of cases has probably occurred as a result of misidentification as atypical *Mycobacterium* species.[227] Effective therapy has include the combination of a β-lactam and an aminoglycoside or a fluoroquinolone and rifampin.[224] *Rhodococcus fasciens (Rhodococcus luteus)* and *Rhodococcus erythropolis* have been associated with chronic endophthalmitis after lens implantation.[228] *R. erythropolis* has been isolated from patients with peritonitis who were undergoing ambulatory peritoneal dialysis, from subcutaneous nodules in a patient with

AIDS, and from sputum in a patient with pneumonia.[229,230] *Rhodococcus rhodochrous* has caused pneumonia, bacteremia, pericarditis, skin lesions, meningoencephalitis, ventriculoperitoneal shunt infection, and chronic corneal ulceration.[231,232] Meningitis due to non-*equi Rhodococcus* has been reported in an immunocompetent host.[233] Antimicrobial therapy for these infections should be based on susceptibility testing. When *Rhodococcus* infection occurs in association with a medical device, the device should be removed.

REFERENCES

1. Lehmann KB, Neumann R. *Atlas und Grundriss der bakteriologie und Lehrbuch der speziellen bacteriologischen Diagnostik*. 1st ed. Munich: JF Lehmann; 1896.
2. Funke G, von Graevenitz A, Clarridge J III, et al. Clinical microbiology of coryneform bacteria. *Clin Microbiol Rev*. 1997;10:125-159.
3. von Graevenitz A, Punter-Streit V, Riegel P, et al. Coryneform bacteria in throat cultures of healthy individuals. *J Clin Microbiol*. 1998;36:2087-2088.
4. Stroman DW, Roland PS, Dohar J, et al. Microbiology of normal external auditory canal. *Laryngoscope*. 2001;111:2054-2059.
5. Shapiro M, Smith KJ, James WD, et al. Cutaneous microenvironment of human immunodeficiency virus (HIV)-seropositive and HIV-seronegative individuals, with special reference to *Staphylococcus aureus* colonization. *J Clin Microbiol*. 2000; 38:3174-3178.
6. Young VM, Meyers WF, Moody MR, et al. The emergence of coryneform bacteria as a cause of nosocomial infections in compromised hosts. *Am J Med*. 1981;70:646-650.
7. Lagrou K, Verhaegen J, Janssens M, et al. Prospective study of catalase-positive coryneform organisms in clinical specimens: Identification of clinical relevance and antibiotic susceptibility. *Diagn Microbiol Infect Dis*. 1998;30:7-15.
8. Bernard KA, Munro C, Wiebe D, et al. Characteristics of rare or recently described *Corynebacterium* species recovered from human clinical material in Canada. *J Clin Microbiol*. 2002; 40:4375-4381.
9. Belmares J, Detterline S, Pak JB, et al. *Corynebacterium* endocarditis species-specific risk factors and outcomes. *BMC Infect Dis* 2007;7:4.
10. Riegel P, Ruimy R, Christen R, et al. Species identities and antimicrobial susceptibilities of *Corynebacteria* isolated from various clinical sources. *Eur J Clin Micrbiol Infect Dis*. 1996; 15:657-662.
11. Hollis DG, Weaver RE. *Gram-positive organisms: A guide to identification. Special Bacteriology Section*. Atlanta, Georgia: Centers for Disease Control and Prevention; 1981.
12. Bernard KA, Bellefeuille M, Ewan EP. Cellular fatty acid composition as an adjunct to identification of asporogenous, aerobic gram-positive rods. *J Clin Microbiol*. 1991;29:83-89.
13. Tang Y, von Graevenitz A, Waddington M, et al. Identification of coryneform bacterial isolates by ribosomal DNA sequence analysis. *J Clin Microbiol*. 2000;38:1676-1678.
14. Soto A, Zapardiel J, Soriano F. Evaluation of API CORYNE system for identifying coryneform bacteria. *J Clin Pathol*. 1994;47:756-759.
15. Funke G, Renaud FN, Freney J, et al. Multicenter evaluation of the updated and extended API (RAPID) Coryne database 2.0. *J Clin Microbiol*. 1997;35:3122-3126.
16. Funke G, Peters K, Aravena-Roman M. Evaluation of the RapID CB plus system for identification of coryneform bacteria in *Listeria* spp. *J Clin Microbiol*. 1998;36:2439-2442.
17. Funke G, Punter V, von Graevenitz A. Antimicrobial susceptibility patterns of some recently established coryneform bacteria. *Antimicrob Agents Chemother*. 1996;40:2874-2878.
18. *Methods for antimicrobial dilution and disk susceptibility testing of infrequently isolated or fastidious bacteria. Approved standard M45-A*. Wayne, PA: Clinical and Laboratory Standards Institute; 2006.
19. Goldstein EJ, Citron DM, Merriam CV, et al. In vitro activities of daptomycin, vancomycin, quinupristin-dalfopristin, linezolid, and five other antimicrobials against 307 gram-positive anaerobic and 31 *Corynebacterium* clinical isolates. *Antimicrob Agents Chemother*. 2003;47:337-341.
20. Power EG, Abdulla YH, Talsania H, et al. vanA genes in vancomycin-resistant clinical isolates of *Oerskovia turbata* and *Arcanobacterium (Corynebacterium) haemolyticum*. *J Antimicrob Chemother*. 1995;36:595-606.
21. Wauters G, Van Bosterhaut B, Janssens M, et al. Identification of *Corynebacterium amycolatum* and other nonlipophilic fermentative corynebacteria of human origin. *J Clin Microbiol*. 1998; 36:1430-1432.
22. Efstratiou A, Engler KH, Dawes CS, et al. Comparison of phenotypic and genotypic methods for detection of diphtheria toxin among isolates of pathogenic corynebacteria. *J Clin Microbiol*. 1998;36:3173-3177.
23. von Hunolstein C, Alfarone G, Scopetti F, et al. Molecular epidemiology and characteristics of *Corynebacterium diphtheriae* and *Corynebacterium ulcerans* strains isolated in Italy during the 1990's. *J Med Microbiol*. 2003;52:181-188.
24. Efstratiou A, George RC. Laboratory guidelines for the diagnosis of infections caused by *Corynebacterium diphtheriae* and *C. ulcerans*. *Commun Dis Publ Health*. 1999;2:250-257.
25. Mann PG. *Corynebacterium ulcerans* infections. *Lancet*. 1970; 1:839.
26. Kaufmann D, Ott P, Zbinden R. Laryngopharyngitis by *Corynebacterium ulcerans*. *Infection*. 2002;30:168-170.
27. Wellinghausen N, Sing A, Kern WV, et al. A fatal case of necrotizing sinusitis due to toxigenic *Corynebacterium ulcerans*. *Int J Med Microbiol*. 2002;292:59-63.
28. Wagner J, Ignatius R, Voss S, et al. Infection of the skin caused by *Corynebacterium ulcerans* and mimicking classical cutaneous diphtheria. *Clin Infect Dis*. 2001;33:1598-1600.
29. Dessau RB, Brandt-Christensen M, Jensen OJ, et al. Pulmonary nodules due to *Corynebacterium ulcerans*. *Eur Respir J*. 1995; 8:651-653.
30. Nureki S, Miyazaki E, Metsuno O, et al. *Corynebacterium ulcerans* infection of the lung mimicking the histology of Churg-Strauss syndrome. *Chest*. 2007;131:1237-1239.
31. Mills AE, Mitchell RD, Lim EK. *Corynebacterium pseudotuberculosis* is a cause of human necrotising granulomatous. *Pathology*. 1997;29:231-233.
32. Peel MM, Palmer GG, Stacpoole AM, et al. Human lymphadenitis due to *Corynebacterium pseudotuberculosis*: Report of ten cases from Australia and review. *Clin Infect Dis*. 1997; 24:185-191.
33. Keslin MH, McCoy EL, McCusker JJ, et al. *Corynebacterium pseudotuberculosis*. A new cause of infectious and eosinophilic pneumonia. *Am J Med*. 1979;67:228-231.
34. Richards M, Hurse A. *Corynebacterium pseudotuberculosis* abscesses in a young butcher. *Aust N Z J Med*. 1985;15:85-86.
35. Porschen RK, Goodman Z, Rafai B. Isolation of *Corynebacterium xerosis* from clinical specimens: Infection and colonization. *Am J Clin Pathol*. 1977;68:290-293.
36. Esteban J, Nieto E, Calvo R, et al. Microbiological characterization and clinical significance of *Corynebacterium amycolatum* strains. *Eur J Clin Microbiol Infect Dis*. 1999;18:518-521.
37. Funke G, Lawson PA, Bernard KA, et al. Most *Corynebacterium xerosis* strains identified in the routine clinical laboratory correspond to *Corynebacterium amycolatum*. *J Clin Microbiol*. 1996;34:1124-1128.
38. Wooster SL, Qamruddin A, Clarke R, et al. Brain abscess due to *Corynebacterium xerosis*. *J Infect*. 1999;38:55-56.
39. Robins E, Haile-Selassie T. *Corynebacterium xerosis* sepsis in a pediatric patient with sickle cell disease (as case report). *Clin Pediatr*. 2001;40:181-182.
40. Voisin S, Deruaz D, Freney J, et al. Differentiation of *Corynebacterium amycolatum*, C. minutissimum, *C. striatum* and related species by pyrolysis-gas-liquid chromatography with atomic emission detection. *Res Microbiol*. 2002;153:307-311.
41. Watkins DA, Chahine A, Creger RJ, et al. *Corynebacterium striatum*: A diphtheroid with pathogenic potential. *Clin Infect Dis*. 1993;17:21-25.
42. Martinez-Martinez L, Suarez AI, Winstanley J, et al. Phenotypic characteristics of 31 strains of *Corynebacterium striatum* isolated from clinical samples. *J Clin Microbiol*. 1995;33:2458-2461.
43. Brandenburg AH, van Belkum A, van Pelt C, et al. Patient-to-patient spread of a single strain of *Corynebacterium striatum* causing infections in a surgical intensive care unit. *J Clin Microbiol*. 1996;34:2089-2094.
44. Leonard RB, Nowowiejski DJ, Warren JJ, et al. Molecular evidence of person-to-person transmission of a pigmented strain of *Corynebacterium striatum* in intensive care units. *J Clin Microbiol*. 1994;32:164-169.
45. Remom F, Garau M, Rubi M, et al. Nosocomial outbreak of *Corynebacterium striatum* infection in patients with chronic obstructive pulmonary disease. *J Clin Microbiol*. 2007;45(6): 2064-2067.
46. Knox KL, Holmes AH. Nosocomial endocarditis caused by *Corynebacterium amycolatum* and other nondiphtheriae *Corynebacteria*. *Emerg Infect Dis*. 2002;8:97-99.
47. Martinez-Martinez L, Pascual A, Bernard K, et al. Antimicrobial susceptibility pattern of *Corynebacterium striatum*. *Antimicrob Agents Chemother*. 1996;40:2671-2672.
48. Collins MD, Jones D. *Corynebacterium minutissimum* sp. nov., nom. rev. *Int J Syst Bacteriol*. 1983;33:870-871.
49. Yassin AF, Steiner U, Ludwig W. *Corynebacterium aurimucosum* sp. nov. and emended description of *Corynebacterium minutissimum* Collins and Jones (1983). *Int J Systemat Evol Microbiol*. 2002;52:1001-1005.
50. Zinkernagel AS, von Graevenitz A, Funke G. Heterogeneity within *Corynebacterium minutissimum* strains is explained by misidentified *Corynebacterium amycolatum* strains. *Am J Clin Pathol*. 1996;106:378-383.
51. Aperis G, Moyssakis I. *Corynebacterium minutissimum* endocarditis: a case report and review. *J Infect*. 2007;54:e79-e81.
52. Dalal A, Likhi R. *Corynebacterium minutissimum* bacteremia and meningitis: a case report and review of literature. *J Infect*. 2008;56:77-79.
53. Collins MD, Burton RA, Jones D. *Corynebacterium amycolatum* sp. nov., a new mycolic acid-less *Corynebacterium* species from human skin. *FEMS Microbiol Lett*. 1988;49:349-352.
54. von Graevenitz A, Frommelt L, Punter-Streit V, et al. Diversity of coryneforms found in infections following prosthetic joint insertion and open fractures. *Infection*. 1998;26:36-38.
55. Clarke R, Qamruddin A, Taylor M, et al. Septic arthritis caused by *Corynebacterium amycolatum* following vascular graft sepsis. *J Infect*. 1999;38:126-127.
56. Daniels C, Schoors D, van Camp G. Native valve endocarditis with aorta-to-left atrial fistula due to *Corynebacterium amycolatum*. *Eur J Echocardiogr*. 2003;4:68-70.
57. Adderson EE, Boudreaux JW, Hayden RT. Infections caused by coryneform bacteria in pediatric oncology patients. *Pediatr Infect Dis J*. 2008;27(2):136-141.
58. Goldstein EJ, Citron DM, Merriam CV, et al. In vitro activities of the new semisynthetic glycopeptide telavancin (TD-6424), vancomycin, daptomycin, linezolid, and four comparator agents against anaerobic gram-positive species and *Corynebacterium* spp. *Antimicrob Agents Chemother*. 2004;48(6):2149-2152.
59. Funke G, Bernard KA, Bucher C, et al. *Corynebacterium glucuronolyticum* sp. nov., isolated from male patients with genitourinary tract infections. *Med Microbiol Lett*. 1995;4:204-215.
60. Devriese LA, Riegel P, Hommez J, et al. Identification of *Corynebacterium glucuronolyticum* strains from the urogenital tract of humans and pigs. *J Clin Microbiol*. 2000;38:4657-4659.
61. Tanner MA, Shoskes D, Shahed A, et al. Prevalence of corynebacterial 16S rRNA sequences in patients with bacterial and "nonbacterial" prostatitis. *J Clin Microbiol*. 1999;37:1863-1870.
62. Riegel P, Ruimy R, De Briel D, et al. *Corynebacterium argentoratense* sp. nov., from the human throat. *Int J Syst Bacteriol*. 1995;45:533-537.
63. Kania RE, Lamers GE, Vonk MJ, et al. Characterization of mucosal biofilms on human adenoid tissues. *Laryngoscope*. 2008;118(1):128-134.
64. Funke G, Lawson PA, Collins MD. *Corynebacterium riegelii* sp. nov.: An unusual species is isolated from female patients with urinary tract infections. *J Clin Microbiol*. 1998;36:624-627.
65. Funke G, Osorio CR, Frei R, et al. *Corynebacterium confusum* sp. nov., isolated from human clinical specimens. *Int J Syst Bacteriol*. 1998;48:1291-1296.
66. Wattiau P, Janssens M, Wauters G. *Corynebacterium simulans* sp. nov., a non-lipophilic, fermentative *Corynebacterium*. *Int J Syst Evol Microbiol*. 2000;50:347-353.
67. Collins MD, Bernard KA, Hutson RA, et al. *Corynebacterium sundsvallense* sp. nov., from human clinical specimens. *Int J Syst Bacteriol*. 1999;49:361-366.
68. Zimmermann O, Sproer C, Kroppenstedt RM, et al. *Corynebacterium thomssenii* sp. nov., a *Corynebacterium* with N-acetyl-beta-glucosaminidase activity from human clinical specimens. *Int J Syst Bacteriol*. 1998;48:489-494.
69. Renaud FN, Aubel D, Riegel P, et al. *Corynebacterium freneyi* sp. nov., alpha-glucosidase-positive strains related to *Corynebacterium xerosis*. *Int J Syst Evol Microbiol*. 2001;51:1723-1728.
70. Fernandez-Natal MI, Saez-Nieto A, Fernandez-Roblas R, et al. The isolation of *Corynebacterium coyleae* from clinical samples: clinical and microbiological data. *Eur J Clin Micro Infect Dis*. 2008;27:177-184.
71. Riegel P, Creti R, Mattei R, et al. Isolation of *Corynebacterium tuscaniae* sp. nov. from blood cultures of a patient with endocarditis. *J Clin Microbiol*. 2006;44(2):307-312.
72. Riegel P, de Briel D, Prevost G, et al. Taxonomic study of *Corynebacterium* group ANF-1 strains: Proposal of *Corynebacterium afermentans* sp. nov. containing subspecies *C. afermentans* subsp. afermentans subsp. nov. and afermentans subsp. lipophilum subsp. nov. *Int J Syst Bacteriol*. 1993;43:287-292.
73. Kumari P, Tyagi A, Marks P, et al. *Corynebacterium afermentans* spp. afermentans sepsis in a neurosurgical patient. *J Infect*. 1997;35:201-202.
74. Holzmann D, Funke G, Linder T, et al. Turicella otitidis and *Corynebacterium auris* do not cause otitis media with effusion in children. *Pediatr Infect Dis J*. 2002;21:1124-1126.
75. Wilson ME, Shapiro DS. Native valve endocarditis due to *Corynebacterium pseudodiphtheriticum*. *Clin Infect Dis*. 1992;15: 1059-1060.
76. Manzella JP, Kellogg JA, Parsey KS. *Corynebacterium pseudodiphtheriticum*: A respiratory tract pathogen in adults. *Clin Infect Dis*. 1995;20:37-40.
77. Ahmed K, Kawakami K, Watanabe K, et al. *Corynebacterium pseudodiphtheriticum*: A respiratory tract pathogen. *Clin Infect Dis*. 1995;20:41-46.
78. Gutierrez-Rodero F, Ortiz de la Tabla V, Martinez C, et al. *Corynebacterium pseudodiphtheriticum*: An easily missed respiratory pathogen in HIV-infected patients. *Diagn Microbiol Infect Dis*. 1999;33:209-216.

79. Izurieta HS, Strebel PM, Youngblood T, et al. Exudative pharyngitis possibly due to *Corynebacterium pseudodiphtheriticum*, a new challenge in the differential diagnosis of diphtheria. *Emerg Infect Dis.* 1997;3:65-68.
80. Cantarelli VV, Brodt TC, Secchi C, et al. Cutaneous infection caused by *Corynebacterium pseudodiphtheriticum*. A microbiological report. *Rev Inst Med Trop S Paulo.* 2008;50(1):51-52.
81. Kemp M, Holtz K, Andresen K, et al. Demonstration by PCR and DNA sequencing of *Corynebacterium pseudodiphtheriticum* as a cause of joint infection and isolation of the same organism from a surface swab specimen from a patient. *J Med Microbiol.* 2005;54:689-691.
82. Riegel P, De Briel D, Prevost G, et al. Proposal of *Corynebacterium propinquum* sp. nov. for *Corynebacterium* group ANF-3 strains. *FEMS Microbiol.* 1993;113:229-234.
83. Hande KR, Witebsky FG, Brown MS, et al. Sepsis with a new species of *Corynebacterium*. *Ann Intern Med.* 1976;85:423-426.
84. Jackman PJ, Pitcher DG, Pelczynska S, et al. Classification of corynebacteria associated with endocarditis (group JK) as *Corynebacterium jeikeium* sp. nov. *Syst Appl Microbiol.* 1987; 9:83-90.
85. Soriano F, Rodriguez-Tudela JL, Fernandez-Roblas R, et al. Skin colonization by *Corynebacterium* groups D2 and JK in hospitalized patients. *J Clin Microbiol.* 1988;26:1878-1880.
86. Pitcher D, Johnson A, Allerberger F, et al. An investigation of nosocomial infection with *Corynebacterium jeikeium* in surgical patients using a ribosomal RNA gene probe. *Eur J Clin Microbiol Infect Dis.* 1990;9:643-648.
87. Ersgaard H, Justesen T. Multiresistant lipophilic corynebacteria from clinical specimens. Biochemical reactions and antimicrobial agents susceptibility. *Acta Pathol Microbiol Scand.* 1984;92:39-43.
88. van der Lelie H, Leverstein-Van Hall M, Mertens M, et al. *Corynebacterium* CDC group JK (*Corynebacterium jeikeium*) sepsis in haemotologic patients: A report of three cases and a systematic literature review. *Scand J Infect Dis.* 1995;27:581-584.
89. Vanbosterhaut B, Surmont I, Vandeven J, et al. *Corynebacterium jeikeium* (group JK diphtheroid) endocarditis. A report of five cases. *Diagn Microbiol Infect Dis.* 1989;12:265-268.
90. Mookadam F, Cikes M, Baddour LM, et al. *Corynebacterium jeikeium* endocarditis: a systematic overview spanning four decades. *Eur J Clin Microbiol Infect Dis.* 2006;25:349-353.
91. Greene KA, Clark RJ, Zabramski JM. Ventricular CSF shunt infections associated with *Corynebacterium jeikeium*: Report of three cases and review. *Clin Infect Dis.* 1993;16:139-141.
92. Dan M, Somer I, Knobel B, Gutman R. Cutaneous manifestations of infection with *Corynebacterium* group JK. *Rev Infect Dis.* 1988;10:1204-1207.
93. Spach DH, Celum CL, Collier AC, et al. Palpable purpura associated with *Corynebacterium jeikeium* endocarditis. *Arch Dermatol.* 1991;127:1071-1072.
94. Traub WH, Geipel U, Leonhard B, et al. Antibiotic susceptibility of testing (agar disk diffusion and agar dilution) of clinical isolates of *Corynebacterium jeikeium*. *Chemotherapy.* 1998;44: 230-237.
95. Rosato AE, Lee BS, Nash KA. Inducible macrolide resistance in *Corynebacterium jeikeium*. *Antimicrob Agents Chemother.* 2001;45:1982-1989.
96. Wang CC, Mattson D, Wald A. *Corynebacterium jeikeium* bacteremia in bone marrow transplant patients with Hickman catheters. *Bone Marrow Transplant.* 2001;27:445-449.
97. Pitcher D, Soto A, Soriano F, et al. Classification of coryneform bacteria associated with human urinary tract infection (group D2) as *Corynebacterium urealyticum* sp. nov. *Int J Syst Bacteriol.* 1992;42:178-181.
98. Lopez-Medrano F, Garcia-Bravo M, Morales JM, et al. Urinary tract infection due to *Corynebacterium urealyticum* in kidney transplant recipients: an underdiagnosed etiology for obstructive uropathy and graft dysfunction-results of a prospective cohort study. *Clin Infect Dis.* 2008;46(6):825-830.
99. Soriano F, Ponte C, Santamaria M, et al. *Corynebacterium* group D2 as a cause of alkaline-encrusted cystitis: Report of four cases and characterizations of the organisms. *J Clin Microbiol.* 1985;21;788-792.
100. Soriano F, Ponte C, Santamaria M, et al. In vitro and in vivo study of stone formation by Corynebacterium group D2 (*Corynebacterium urealyticum*). *J Clin Microbiol.* 1986;23:691-694.
101. Natal IF, Garcia FC, Laso JG, et al. Brief reports: Bacteremia caused by multiply resistant *Corynebacterium urealyticum*: Six case reports and review. *Eur J Clin Microbiol Infect Dis.* 2001; 20:514-517.
102. Soriano F, Ponte C, Ruiz P, et al. Non-urinary tract infections caused by multiply antibiotic-resistant *Corynebacterium urealyticum*. *Clin Infect Dis.* 1993;17:890-891.
103. Meria P, Desgrippes A, Fournier R, et al. The conservative management of *Corynebacterium* group D2 encrusted pyelitis. *BJU Int.* 1999;84:270-275.
103a. Neubauer M, Sourek J, Ryc M, et al. *Corynebacterium accolens* sp. nov., a gram-positive rod exhibiting satellitism, from clinical material. *Syst Appl Microbiol.* 1991;14:46-51.
104. Claeys G, Vanhouteghem H, Riegel P, et al. Endocarditis of native aortic and mitral valves due to *Corynebacterium accolens*: Report of a case and application of phenotypic and genotypic techniques for identification. *J Clin Microbiol.* 1996;34:1290-1292.
105. Ang L, Brown H. *Corynebacterium accolens* isolated from breast abscess: possible association with granulomatous mastitis. *J Clin Microbiol.* 2007;45(5):1666-1668.
106. Funke G, Pagano-Niederer M, Bernauer W. *Corynebacterium macginleyi* has to date been isolated exclusively from conjunctival swabs. *J Clin Microbiol.* 1998;36:3670-3673.
107. Villamil-Cajoto I, Rodriguez-Otero L, Garcia-Zabarte MA, et al. Septicemia caused by *Corynebacterium macginleyi*: a rare form of extraocular infection. *Int J Infect Dis.* 2008;12:333-335.
108. Taylor G, Paviour S. Musaad S, et al. A clinicopathological review of 34 cases of inflammatory breast disease showing an association between corynebacteria infection and granulomatous mastitis. *Pathology* 2003;34:109-119.
109. Paviour S, Musaad S, Roberts S, et al. *Corynebacterium* species isolated from patients with mastitis. *Clin Infect Dis.* 2002; 35:1434-1440.
110. Vale JA, Scott GW. *Corynebacterium bovis* as a cause of human disease. *Lancet* 1977;2:682-684.
111. Dalal A, Urban C, Ahluwalia M, et al. *Corynebacterium bovis* line related septicemia: a case report and review of the literature. *Scandinavian J Infect Dis.* 2008;40(6):575-577.
112. Holmes NE, Korman TM. *Corynebacterium kutscheri* infection of skin and soft tissue following rat bite. *J Clin Microbiol.* 2007;45:3468-3469.
113. Otsuka Y, Kawamura Y, Koyama T, et al. *Corynebacterium resistens* sp. nov., a new multidrug-resistant coryneform bacterium isolated from human infections. *J Clin Microbiol.* 2005;43:3713-3717.
114. Yassin AF. *Corynebacterium ureicelerivorans* sp. nov., a lipophilic bacterium isolated from blood culture. *Int J System Evol Microbiol.* 2007;57:1200-1203.
115. Collins MD, Jones D, Schofield GM. Reclassification of "*Corynebacterium haemolyticum*" (MacLean Liebow & Rosenberg) in the genus Arcanobacterium gen.nov. *Arcanobacterium haemolyticum* nom.rev., comb.nov. *J Gen Microbiol.* 1982;128:1279-1281.
116. Ramos CP, Foster G, Collins MD. Phylogentic analysis of the genus *Actinomyces* based on 16S rRNA gene sequences: description of *Arcanobacterium phocase* sp. nov., *Arcanobacterium bernardiae* comb. nov., and *Arcanobacterium pyogenes* comb. nov. *Int J Syst Bacteriol.* 1997;47:46-53.
117. MacLean PD, Liebow AA, Rosenberg A. Haemolytic corynebacterium resembling *Corynebacterium ovis* and *C. pyogenes* in man. *J Infect Dis.* 1946;79:69-90.
118. Cummings LA, Wu WK, Larson AM, et al. Effects of media, atmosphere, and incubation time on colonial morphology of *Arcanobacterium haemolyticum*. *J Clin Microbiol.* 1993;31: 3223-3226.
119. Carlson P, Lounatmaa K, Kontiainen S. Biotypes of *Arcanobacterium haemolyticum*. *J Clin Microbiol.* 1994;32:1654-1657.
120. Ryan WJ. Throat infection and rash associated with an unusual *Corynebacterium*. *Lancet.* 1972;2:1345-1347.
121. Miller RA, Brancato F, Holmes KK. *Corynebacterium hemolyticum* as a cause of pharyngitis and scarlatiniform rash in young adolescents. *Ann Intern Med.* 1986;105:867-872.
122. Banck G, Nyman M. Tonsillitis and rash associated with *Corynebacterium haemolyticum*. *J Infect Dis.* 1986;154:1037-1040.
123. Carlson P, Renkonen OV, Kontiainen S. *Arcanobacterium haemolyticum* and streptococcal pharyngitis. *Scand J Infect Dis.* 1994;26:283-287.
124. Mackenzie A, Fuite LA, Chan FT, et al. Incidence and pathogenicity of *Arcanobacterium haemolyticum* during a 2-year study in Ottawa. *Clin Infect Dis.* 1995;21:177-181.
125. Skov RL, Sanden AK, Danchell VH, et al. Note: Systemic and deep-seated infections caused by *Arcanobacterium haemolyticum*. *Eur J Clin Microbiol Infect Dis.* 1998;17:578-582.
126. Younus F, Chua A, Tortora G, et al. Lemierre's disease caused by co-infection of *Arcanobacterium haemolyticum* and *Fusobacterium necrophorum*: A case report. *J Infect.* 2002;45:114-117.
127. Tan TY, Ng SY, Thomas H, et al. *Arcanobacterium haemolyticum* bacteraemia and soft-tissue infections: case report and review of the literature. *J Infect.* 2006;53:e69-e74.
128. Ford JG, Yeatts RP, Givner LB. Orbital cellulitis, subperiosteal abscess, sinusitis, and septicemia caused by *Arcanobacterium haemolyticum*. *Am J Ophthalmol.* 1995;120:261-262.
129. Carlson P, Kontiainen S, Renkonen OV. Antimicrobial susceptibility of *Arcanobacterium haemolyticum*. *Antimicrob Agents Chemother.* 1994;38:142-143.
130. Jost BH, Songer JG, Billington SJ. Identification of a second *Arcanobacterium pyogenes* neuraminidase and involvement of neuraminidase activity in host cell adhesion. *Infect Immun.* 2002;70:1106-1112.
131. Gahrn-Hansen B, Frederiksen W. Human infections with *Actinomyces pyogenes* (*Corynebacterium pyogenes*). *Diagn Microbiol Infect Dis.* 1992;15:349-354.
132. Plamondon M, Martinez G, Raynal L, et al. A fatal case of *Arcanobacterium pyogenes* endocarditis in a man with no identified animal contact: case report and review of the literature. *Eur J Clin Microbiol Infect Dis.* 2007;26:663-666.
133. Lepargneur JP, Heller R, Soulie R, et al. Urinary tract infection due to *Arcanobacterium bernardiae* in a patient with a urinary tract diversion. *Eur J Clin Microbiol Infect Dis.* 1998;17: 399-401.
134. Adderson EE, Croft A, Leonard R, et al. Septic arthritis due to *Arcanobacterium bernardiae* in an immunocompromised patient. *Clin Infect Dis.* 1998;27:211-212.
135. Ieven M, Verhoeven J, Gentens P, et al. Severe infection due to *Actinomyces bernardiae*: Case report. *Clin Infect Dis.* 1996;22: 157-158.
136. Funke G, Stubbs S, Altwegg M, et al. *Turicella otitidis* gen. nov., sp. nov. a coryneform bacterium isolated from patients with otitis media. *Int J Syst Bacteriol.* 1994;44:270-273.
137. Funke G, Pagano-Niederer M, Sjoden B, et al. Characteristics of *Arthrobacter cumminsii*, the most frequently encountered *Arthrobacter* species in human clinical specimens. *J Clin Microbiol.* 1998;36:1539-1543.
138. Wauters G, Charlier J, Janssens M, et al. Identification of *Arthrobacter oxydans, Arthrobacter luteolus* sp. nov., and *Arthrobacter albus* sp. nov., isolated from human clinical specimens. *J Clin Microbiol.* 2000;38:2412-2415.
139. Funke G, Carlotti A. Differentiation of *Brevibacterium* spp. encountered in clinical specimens. *J Clin Microbiol.* 1994; 32:1729-1732.
140. Gruner E, Steigerwalt AG, Hollis DG, et al. Human infections caused by *Brevibacterium casei*, formerly CDC groups B-1 and B-3. *J Clin Microbiol.* 1994;32:1511-1518.
141. Troxler R, Funke G, von Graevenitz A, et al. Natural antibiotic susceptibility of recently established coryneform bacteria. *Eur J Clin Microbiol Infect Dis.* 2001;20:315-323.
142. Wauters G, Haase G, Avesani V, et al. Identification of a novel *Brevibacterium* species isolated from humans and description of *Brevibacterium sanguinis* sp. nov. *J Clin Microbiol.* 2004;42:2829-2832.
143. Funke G, Stubbs S, Pfyffer GE, et al. Characteristics of CDC group 3 and group 5 coryneform bacteria isolated from clinical specimens and assignment to the genus *Dermabacter*. *J Clin Microbiol.* 1994;32:1223-1228.
144. Gruner E, Steigerwalt AG, Hollis DG, et al. Recognition of *Dermabacter hominis*, formerly CDC fermentative coryneform group 3 and group 5, as a potential human pathogen. *J Clin Microbiol.* 1994;32:1918-1922.
145. Lesher RJ, Gerencser VF, Morrison DJ. Presence of Rothia dentocariosa strain 477 serotype 2 in gingiva of patients with inflammatory periodontal disease. *J Dent Res.* 1977;56:189.
146. Binder D, Zbinden R, Widmer U, et al. Native and prosthetic valve endocarditis caused by *Rothia dentocariosa*: Diagnostic and therapeutic considerations. *Infection.* 1997;25:22-26.
147. Boudewijns M, Magerman K, Verhaegen J, et al. *Rothia dentocariosa*, endocarditis and mycotic aneurysms: case report and review of the literature. *Clin Microbiol Infect.* 2003;9: 222-229.
148. Anderson MD, Kennedy CA, Walsh TP, et al. Prosthetic valve endocarditis due to *Rothia dentocariosa*. *Clin Infect Dis.* 1994;17:945-946.
149. Lee AB, Harker-Murray P, Ferrieri O, et al. Bacterial meningitis in patients with malignancy or undergoing hematopoietic stem cell transplantation. *Pediatr Blood Cancer.* 2008;50:673-676.
150. Reller LB, Maddoux GL, Eckman MR, et al. Bacterial endocarditis caused by *Oerskovia turbata*. *Ann Intern Med.* 1975; 83:664-666.
151. Maguire JD, McCarthy MC, Decker CF. *Oerskovia xanthineolytica* bacteremia in an immunocompromised host: Case report and review. *Clin Infect Dis.* 1996;22:554-556.
152. Rihs JD, McNeil MM, Brown JM, et al. *Oerskovia xanthineolytica* implicated in peritonitis associated with peritoneal dialysis: Case report and review of *Oerskovia* infections in humans. *J Clin Microbiol.* 1990;28:1924-1937.
153. Funke G, Falsen E, Barreau C. Primary identification of *Microbacterium* spp. encountered in clinical specimens as CDC coryneform group A-4 and A-5 bacteria. *J Clin Microbiol.* 1995;33:188-192.
154. Takeuchi M, Hatano K. Union of the genera *Microbacterium* Orla-Jensen and *Aureobacterium* Collins et al. in a redefined genus Microbacterium. *Int J Syst Bacteriol.* 1998;48:739-747.
155. Funke G, Haase G, Schnitzler N, et al. Endophthalmitis due to *Microbacterium* species: Case report and review of *Microbacterium* infections. *Clin Infect Dis.* 1997;24:713-716.
156. Evtushenko LI, Dorofeeva LV, Subbotin SA, et al. *Leifsonia poae* gen. nov., sp. nov., isolated from nematode galls on *Poa annua*, and reclassification of "*Corynebacterium aquaticum*" Leifson 1962 as Leifsonia aquatica (ex Leifson 1962) gen. nov., nom. rev., comb. nov. and *Clavibacter xyli Davis* et al. 1984 with two subspecies as *Leifsonia xyli* (Davis et al. 1984) gen. nov., comb. nov. *Int J Syst Evol Microbiol.* 2000;50:371-380.
157. Funke G, Ramos CP, Collins MD. Identification of some clinical strains of CDC coryneform group A-3 and A-4 bacteria as *Cellulomonas* species and proposal of *Cellulomonas hominis* sp. nov. for some group A-3 strains. *J Clin Microbiol.* 1995;33: 2091-2097.
158. Walsh RD, Schoch PE, Cunha BA. *Rhodococcus*. *Infect Contr Hosp Epidemiol.* 1993;14:282-287.
159. Weinstock DM, Brown AE. *Rhodoccus equi*: An emerging pathogen. *Clin Infect Dis.* 2002;34:1379-1385.
160. Verville TD, Huycke MM, Greenfield RA, et al. *Rhodococcus equi* infections in humans: 12 cases and a review of the literature. *Medicine.* 1994;73:119-132.
161. Takai S, Ohbushi S, Koike K, et al. Prevalence of virulent *Rhodococcus equi* in isolates from soil and feces of horses from horse-breeding farms with and without endemic infections. *J Clin Microbiol.* 1991;29:2887-2889.
162. Kedlaya I, Ing MB, Wong SS. *Rhodococcus equi* infections in immunocompetent hosts: Case report and review. *Clin Infect Dis.* 2001;32:39-46.
163. Scotton PG, Tonon E, Giobbia M, et al. *Rhodococcus equi* nosocomial meningitis cured by levofloxacin and shunt removal. *Clin Infect Dis.* 2000;30:223-224.

164. Arlotti M, Zoboli G, Moscatelli GL, et al. *Rhodococcus equi* infection in HIV-positive subjects: A retrospective analysis of 24 cases. *Scand J Infect Dis.* 1996;28:463-467.
165. Rasmussen TT, Kirkeby LP, Poulsen K, et al. Resident aerobic microbiota of the adult human nasal cavity. *APMIS.* 2000;108:663-675.
166. Nordmann P, Nicolas MH, Gutmann L. Pencillin-binding proteins of *Rhodococcus equi*: potential role in resistance to imipenem. *Antimicrob Agents Chemother.* 1993;37:1406-1409.
167. Lasker BA, Brown JM, McNeil MM. Identification and epidemiological typing of clinical and environmental isolates of the genus *Rhodococcus* with use of a digoxigenin-labeled rDNA gene probe. *Clin Infect Dis.* 1992;15:223-233.
168. Steingrube VA, Wilson RW, Brown BA, et al. Rapid identification of clinically significant species and taxa of aerobic actinomycetes, including *Actinomadura, Gordona, Nocardia, Rhodococcus, Streptomyces*, and *Tsukamurella* isolates, by DNA amplification and restriction endonuclease analysis. *J Clin Microbiol.* 1997; 35:817-822.
169. Drancourt M, Bonnet E, Gallais H, et al. *Rhodococcus equi* infection in patients with AIDS. *J Infect.* 1992;24:123-131.
170. Giguere S, Hondalus MK, Yager JA, et al. Role of the 85-kilobase plasmid and plasmid-encoded virulence-associated protein A in intracellular survival and virulence of *Rhodococcus equi. Infect Immun.* 1999;67:3548-3557.
171. Takai S, Imai Y, Fukunaga N, et al. Identification of virulence associated antigens and plasmids in *Rhodococcus equi* from patients with AIDS. *J Infect Dis.* 1995;172:1306-1311.
172. Fidvi SA, Brudnicki AR, Chowdhury MI, et al. Cavitary *Rhodococcus equi* pneumonia with endobronchial granulomas: report of an unusual case. *Pediatr Radiol.* 2003;33(2):140-142.
173. Guerrero MF, Ramos JM, Renedo G, et al. Pulmonary malacoplakia associated with *Rhodococcus equi* infection in patients with AIDS: Case report and review. *Clin Infect Dis.* 1999; 28:1334-1336.
174. Harvey RL, Sunstrum JC. *Rhodococcus equi* infection in patients with and without human immunodeficiency virus infection. *Rev Infect Dis.* 1991;13:139-145.
175. Lasky JA, Pulkingham N, Powers MA, et al. *Rhodococcus equi* causing human pulmonary infection: Review of 29 cases. *South Med J.* 1991;84:1217-1220.
176. Donisi A, Suardi MG, Casari S, et al. *Rhodococcus equi* infection in HIV-infected patients. *AIDS.* 1996;10:359-362.
177. Hsueh P-R, Hung C-C, Teng L-J, et al. Report of invasive *Rhodococcus equi* infections in Taiwan, with an emphasis on the emergence of multidrug-resistant strains. *Clin Infect Dis.* 1998;27:370-375.
178. Munoz P, Burillo A, Palomo J, et al. *Rhodococcus equi* infection in transplant recipients: Case report and review of the literature. *Transplantation.* 1998;65:449-453.
179. Linder R. *Rhodococcus equi* and *Arcanobacterium haemolyticum*: Two "coryneform" bacteria increasingly recognized as agents of human infection. *Emerg Infect Dis.* 1997;3:145-153.
180. Ferruzzi S, Mamprim F, Vailati F. *Rhodococcus equi* infection in non-HIV-infected patients: Two case reports and review. *Clin Microbiol Infect.* 1997;3:12-18.
181. Akan H, Akova M, Ataoglu H, et al. *Rhodococcus equi* and *Nocardia brasiliensis* infection of the brain and liver in a patient with acute nonlymphoblastic leukemia. *Eur J Clin Microbiol Infect Dis.* 1998;17:737-739.
182. Sigler E, Miskin A, Shtlarid M, et al. Fever of unknown origin and anemia with *Rhodococcus equi* infection in an immunocompetent patient. *Am J Med.* 1998;104:510.
183. Linares MJ, Lopez-Encuentra A, Perea S. Chronic pneumonia caused by *Rhodococcus equi* in a patient without impaired immunity. *Eur Respir J.* 1997;10:248-250.
184. Munoz P, Palomo J, Guembe P, et al. Lung nodular lesions in heart transplant recipients. *J Heart Lung Transplant.* 2000; 19:660-667.
185. Torres-Tortosa M, Arrizabalaga J, Villanueva JL, et al. Prognosis and clinical evaluation of infection caused by *Rhodococcus equi* in HIV-infected patients: A multicenter study of 67 cases. *Chest.* 2003;123:1970-1976.
186. Antinori S, Esposito R, Cernuschi M, et al. Disseminated *Rhodococcus equi* infection initially presenting as foot mycetoma in an HIV-positive patient. *AIDS.* 1992;6:740-742.
187. Chow KM, Szeto CC, Chow VC, et al. *Rhodococcus equi* peritonitis in continuous ambulatory peritoneal dialysis. *Nephrology* 2003;16(5):736-739.
188. Strunk T, Gardiner K, Simmer K, et al. *Rhodococcus equi* meningitis after ventriculoperitoneal shunt insertion in a preterm infant. *Pediatr Infect Dis J.* 2007;26:1076-1077.
189. Cornish N, Washington JA. *Rhodococcus equi* infections: Clinical features and laboratory diagnosis. *Curr Clin Top Infect Dis.* 1999;19:198-215.
190. Tuon FF, Sicilliano RF, Al-Musawi T, et al. *Rhodococcus equi* bacteremia with lung absess misdiagnosed as corynebacterium: a report of 2 cases. *Clinics.* 2007;62:795-798.
191. Rodriguez Arrondo F, von Wichmann MA, Arrizabalago J, et al. Pulmonary cavitation lesions in patients with the human immunodeficiency virus: An analysis of a series of 78 cases. *Med Clin (Barcelona).* 1998;111:725-730.
192. Marchiori E, Müller NL, de Mendonça RG, et al. *Rhodococcus equi* pneumonia in AIDS: high-resolution CT findings in five patients. *Br J Radiol.* 2005;78:783-786.
193. Kamboj M, Kalra A, Kak V. *Rhodococcus equi* brain abscess in patients without HIV. *J Clin Pathol.* 2005;58:423-425.
194. Ulivieri S, Oliveri G. Cerebellar abscess due to *Rhodococcus equi* in an immunocompetent patient: case report and literature review. *J Neurosurg Sci.* 2006;50:127-129.
195. Meeuse JJ, Sprenger HG, van Assen S, et al. *Rhodococcus equi* infection after alemtuzumab therapy for T-cell prolymphocytic leukemia. *Emerg Infec Dis.* 2007;13:1942-1943.
196. Munoz P, Palomo J, Guinea J, et al. Relapsing *Rhodococcus equi* infection in a heart transplant recipient successfully treated with long-term linezolid. *Diagn Microbiol Infect Dis.* 2008;60: 197-199.
197. Arya B, Hussian S, Hariharan S. *Rhodococcus equi* pneumonia in a renal transplant patient: a case report and review of literature. *Clin Transplant.* 2004;18:748-752.
198. Speck D, Koneth I, Diethelm M, et al; Medscape. A pulmonary mass caused by *Rhodococcus equi* infection in a renal transplant recipient. *Nat Clin Pract Nephrol.* 2008;4:398-403.
199. Cronin SM, Abidi MH, Shearer CJ, et al. *Rhodococcus equi* lung infection in an allogeneic hematopoietic stem cell transplant recipient. *Transpl Infect Dis.* 2008;10:48-51.
200. Gabriels P, Joosen H, Put E, et al. Recurrent *Rhodococcus equi* infection with fatal outcome in an immunocompetent patient. *Eur J Clin Microbiol Infect Dis.* 2006;25:46-48.
201. Watanabe H, Asoh N, Kobayashi S, et al. Clinical and microbiological characteristics of community-acquired pneumonia among human immunodeficiency virus-infected patients in northern Thailand. *J Infect Chemother.* 2008;14:105-109.
202. Bowersock TL, Salmon SA, Portis ES, et al. MICs of oxazolidinones for *Rhodococcus equi* strains isolated from humans and animals. *Antimicrob Agents Chemother.* 2000;44:1367-1369.
203. Jacks SS, Giguere S, Nguyen A. In vitro susceptibilities of *Rhodococcus equi* and other common equine pathogens to azithromycin, clarithromycin, and 20 other antimicrobials. *Antimicrob Agents Chemother.* 2003;47:1742-1745.
204. Puthucheary SD, Sangkar V, Hafeez A, et al. *Rhodococcus equi*-an emerging human pathogen in immunocompromized hosts: a report of four cases from Malaysia. *Southeast Asian J Trop Med Public Health.* 2006;37:157-161.
205. Rolston KV, Frisbee-Hume S, LeBlanc B, et al. In vitro antimicrobial activity of moxifloxacin compared to other quinolones against recent clinical bacterial isolates from hospitalized and community-based cancer patients. *Diagn Microbiol Infect Dis.* 2003;47:441-449.
206. Rolston KV, Vaziri I, Frisbee-Hume S, et al. In vitro antimicrobial activity of gatifloxacin compared with other quinolones against clinical isolates from cancer patients. *Chemotherapy.* 2004; 50:214-220.
207. Nordmann P, Kerestedjian JJ, Ronco E. Therapy of *Rhodococcus equi* disseminated infections in nude mice. *Antimicrob Agents Chemother.* 1992;36:1244-1248.
208. Asoh N, Watanabe H, Fines-Guyon M, et al. Emergence of rifampin-resistant *Rhodococcus equi* with several types of mutations in the rpoB gene among AIDS patients in northern Thailand. *J Clin Microbiol.* 2003;41:2337-2340.
209. Tse KC, Tang SC, Chan TM, et al. *Rhodococcus* lung abscess complicating kidney transplantation: successful management by combination antibiotic therapy. *Transpl Infect Dis.* 2008; 10:44-47.
210. Napoleao F, Damasco PV, Camello TC, et al. Pyogenic liver abscess due to *Rhodococcus equi* in an immunocompetent host. *J Clin Microbiol.* 2005;43:1002-1004.
211. Buchman AL, McNeil MM, Brown JM, et al. Central venous catheter sepsis caused by unusual *Gordona (Rhodococcus)* species: identification with a digoxigenin-labeled rDNA probe. *Clin Infect Dis.* 1992;15:694-697.
212. Drancourt M, McNeill MM, Brown JM, et al. Brain abscess due to Gordona terrae in an immunocompromised child: case report and review of infections caused by *G. terrae. Clin Infect Dis.* 1994;19:258-262.
213. Drancourt M, Pelletier J, Cherif AA, et al. *Gordona terrae* central nervous systems infection in an immunocompetent patient. *J Clin Microbiol.* 1997;35:379-382.
214. Lesens O, Hansmann Y, Riegel P, et al. Bacteremia and endocarditis caused by a *Gordonia* species in a patient with a central venous catheter. *Emerg Infect Dis.* 2000;6:382-385.
215. Pham AS, Dé I, Rolston V, et al. Catheter-related bacteremia caused by the nocardioform actinomycete *Gordonia terrae. Clin Infect Dis.* 2003;36:524-527.
216. Richet HM, Craven PC, Brown JM, et al. A cluster of *Rhodococcus (Gordona)* bronchialitis sternal-wound infections after coronary-artery bypass surgery. *N Engl J Med.* 1991;324:104-109.
217. Sng LH, Koh TH, Toney SR, et al. Bacteremia caused by *Gordonia bronchialis* in a patient with sequestrated lung. *J Clin Microbiol.* 2004;42:2870-2871.
218. Werno AM, Anderson TP, Chambers ST, et al. Recurrent breast abscess caused by *Gordonia bronchialis* in an immunocompetent patient. *J Clin Microbiol.* 2005;43:3009-3010.
219. Osoagbaka OU. Evidence for the pathogenic role of *Rhodococcus* species in pulmonary disease. *J Appl Bacteriol.* 1989;66: 497-506.
220. Shapiro CL, Haft RF, Gantz NM, et al. *Tsukamurella paurometabolum*: A novel pathogen causing catheter-related bacteremia in patients with cancer. *Clin Infect Dis.* 1992;14:200-203.
221. Almehmi A, Pfister AK, McCowan R, et al. Implantable cardioverter-defibrillator infection caused by *Tsukamurella. W V Med J.* 2004;1100:185-186.
222. Woo PC, Ngan AH, Lau SK, et al. *Tsukamurella* conjunctivitis: a novel clinical syndrome. *J Clin Microbiol.* 2003;41:3368-3371.
223. Elshibly S, Doherty J, Xu J, et al. Central line-related bacteraemia due to *Tsukamurella tyrosinosolvens* in a haematology patient. *Ulster Med J.* 2005;74:43-46.
224. Alcaide ML, Espinoza L, Abbo L. Cavitary pneumonia secondary to *Tsukamurella* in AIDS patient. First case and review of the literature. *J Infect.* 2004;49:17-19.
225. Tsukamura M, Hikosaka K, Nishimura K, et al. Severe progressive subcutaneous abscesses and necrotizing tenosynovitis caused by *Rhodococcus aurantiacus. J Clin Microbiol.* 1988; 26:201-205.
226. Prinz G, Ban E, Fekete S, et al. Meningitis caused by *Gordona aurantiaca (Rhodococcus aurantiacus). J Clin Microbiol.* 1985; 22:472-474.
227. Stanley T, Crothers L, McCalmont M, et al. The potential misidentification of *Tsukamurella pulmonis* as an atypical *Mycobacterium* species: a cautionary tale. *J Med Microbiol.* 2006; 55:475-478.
228. von Below H, Wilk CM, Schaal KP, et al. *Rhodococcus* luteus and *Rhodococcus erythropolis* chronic endophthalmitis after lens implantation. *Am J Ophthalmol.* 1991;112:596-597.
229. Brown E, Hendler E. *Rhodococcus peritonitis* in a patient treated with peritoneal dialysis. *Am J Kidney Dis.* 1989;14:417-418.
230. Vernazza PL, Bodmer T, Galeazzi RL. *Rhodococcus erythropolis* infection in HIV-associated immunodeficiency. *Schweiz Med Wochenschr.* 1991;121:1095-1098.
231. Haburchak DR, Jeffrey B, Higbee JW, et al. Infections by *Rhodachrous. Am J Med.* 1978;65:298-302.
232. Gopaul D, Ellis C, Maki A Jr, et al. Isolation of *Rhodococcus rhodochrous* from a chronic corneal ulcer. *Diagn Microbiol Infect Dis.* 1988;10:185-190.
233. DeMarais PL, Kocka FE. *Rhodococcus* meningitis in an immunocompetent host. *Clin Infect Dis.* 1995;20:167-169.

Listeria monocytogenes

BENNETT LORBER

Listeria monocytogenes is an uncommon cause of illness in the general population. However, in some groups, including neonates, pregnant women, elderly persons, immunosuppressed transplant recipients, and others with impaired cell-mediated immunity, it is an important cause of life-threatening bacteremia and meningoencephalitis.[1,2] Growing interest in this organism has resulted from foodborne outbreaks and concerns about food safety. Separate from its clinical and public health relevance, the study of listeriosis has provided insights into bacterial pathogenesis and the role of cell-mediated immunity in resistance to infection with intracellular pathogens.

Microbiology

L. monocytogenes is a facultatively anaerobic, nonsporulating, catalase-positive, oxidase-negative, short, nonbranching, gram-positive rod that grows readily on blood agar, producing incomplete β-hemolysis.[3] The bacterium possesses one to five polar flagellae and exhibits a characteristic tumbling motility at 25° C. Optimal growth occurs at 30 to 37° C, but *L. monocytogenes* grows better than other bacteria at refrigerator temperatures (4 to 10° C), and by so-called cold enrichment can be separated from other contaminating bacteria by long incubation in this temperature range. Selective media have been developed to isolate the organism from specimens containing multiple species (food, stool) and appear superior to cold enrichment.[3,4] When grown on blood-free agar and viewed with light transmitted at a 45-degree angle (Henry's illumination), colonies of *L. monocytogenes* appear blue-gray, whereas other bacterial colonies appear yellowish or orange.

Routine media are effective for isolating *L. monocytogenes* from specimens obtained from normally sterile sites (cerebrospinal fluid [CSF], blood, joint fluid), but media typically used to isolate diarrhea-causing bacteria from stool cultures inhibit listerial growth. *L. monocytogenes* grows best at neutral to slightly alkaline pH and dies at pH below 5.5.

In clinical specimens, the organisms may be gram-variable and look like diphtheroids, cocci, or diplococci. Laboratory misidentification as diphtheroids, streptococci, or enterococci is not uncommon,[1,5] and the isolation of a "diphtheroid" from blood or CSF always should alert one to the possibility that the organism is really *L. monocytogenes*.

Of the six species of *Listeria*, *L. monocytogenes*, *L. seeligeri*, *L. welshimeri*, *L. innocua*, *L. ivanovii*, and *L. grayi* (Table 207-1), only *L. monocytogenes* is pathogenic for humans. There are at least 13 serovars of *L. monocytogenes*, based on cellular O and flagellar H antigens, but almost all disease is due to types 4b, 1/2a, and 1/2b,[6] limiting the value of serotyping for epidemiologic investigations. Phage typing can be accomplished for 60% to 80% of clinical isolates. A number of molecular techniques, including pulsed-field gel electrophoresis (PFGE), ribotyping, and multilocus enzyme electrophoresis, have been employed to separate isolates into distinct groups for epidemiologic purposes.[3,6] Multilocus enzyme electrophoresis and PFGE can separate *L. monocytogenes* serovars into many unique types and have proved useful in investigating outbreaks.[7]

Epidemiology

L. monocytogenes is an important cause of zoonoses, especially in herd animals. It is widespread in nature, being found commonly in soil, decaying vegetation, and water and as part of the fecal flora of many mammals.[6] The organism has been isolated from the stool of approximately 5% of healthy adults,[6,8] with higher rates of recovery reported from household contacts of patients with clinical infection.[9] In three healthy, asymptomatic adults followed for one year, *L. monocytogenes* was transiently present in 3.5% of stool specimens.[10] Many foods are contaminated with *L. monocytogenes*, and recovery rates of 15% to 70% are common from raw vegetables, raw milk, cheese, and meats, including fresh, frozen, and processed chicken and beef available at supermarkets or delicatessen counters.[11] Ingestion of *L. monocytogenes* must be an exceedingly common occurrence.

Listeriosis was not made a nationally reportable disease until 2000. Data from two active surveillance studies performed from 1980 to 1982 and in 1986 by the Centers for Disease Control and Prevention (CDC) indicated annual infection rates of 7.4 per million population, accounting for approximately 1850 cases per year in the United States with 425 deaths.[12] By 1993, following food industry regulations instituted to minimize the risk of foodborne listeriosis, the annual incidence had declined to 4.4 cases per million, or 1092 cases with 248 deaths.[13] From 1996 through 2003 the crude incidence decreased 26% from 4.1 cases per million population to 3.1 cases per million; estimated cases in the United States were 2228 and 1803 in 1996 and 2003, respectively, and deaths were 462 and 378.[14] The highest infection rates are seen in infants younger than 1 month and adults older than 60 years.[6,12] Pregnant women account for about 30% of all cases and 60% of cases in the 10- to 40-year age group. Almost 70% of nonperinatal infections occur in those with hematologic malignancy or acquired immunodeficiency syndrome (AIDS), organ transplantation recipients, and those receiving corticosteroid therapy, but seemingly normal persons may develop invasive disease, particularly those older than 60 years.[6,15-19]

Subsequent to the 1983 report of a widespread outbreak of foodborne human listerial infection caused by contaminated coleslaw,[9] a number of other foodborne outbreaks have been documented[2,6] with vehicles including milk, soft cheeses, butter, pâté, ready-to-eat pork products, gravad or cold-smoked trout, hot dogs, and deli-ready turkey. In 2002, *L. monocytogenes* was found in sliced deli-style turkey meat, the ingestion of which produced illness in 54 patients in 9 states, resulting in the largest recall of meat ever in the United States (>30 million pounds of food products).[20] Sporadic cases have been traced to contaminated cheese, turkey frankfurters, and alfalfa tablets.[1,2] The importance of food as a source for sporadic listeriosis is illustrated by two CDC studies in which 11% of all refrigerator food samples were contaminated and 64% of patients had at least one contaminated food, and, in 33% of instances, both the patient and the food isolates had the same multilocus enzyme electrophoresis type (much higher than would be predicted by chance).[21,22] Delicatessen ready-to-eat meats, especially chicken, had the highest rates of contamination. Patients were more likely than controls to have eaten soft cheeses or delicatessen counter meats, and 32% of sporadic cases could be attributed to these foods.

Although most human listeriosis appears to be foodborne, other modes of transmission occur, including from mother to child transplacentally or through an infected birth canal, from cross-infection in neonatal nurseries,[23,24] and in one common-source outbreak traced to contaminated mineral oil used for bathing infants.[25] Localized cutaneous infections have occurred in veterinarians and farmers after direct contact with aborted calves and infected poultry.

The CDC has established PulseNet (*http://www.cdc.gov/pulsenet/*), a network of public health and food regulatory laboratories that use pulsed-field gel electrophoresis to subtype foodborne pathogens in order to quickly detect disease clusters that may have a common

| TABLE 207-1 | Laboratory Differentiation of Species in the Genus *Listeria** | | | | | | | |

Characteristic	L. monocytogenes	L. grayi	L. innocua	L. ivanovii subsp. ivanovii	L. ivanovii subsp. londoniensis	L. seeligeri	L. welshimeri
β-hemolysis	+	−	−	++†	++	+	−
CAMP test reaction for							
Staphylococcus aureus	+	−	−	−	−	+	−
Rhodococcus equi	V	−	−	+	+	−	−
Acid production from							
Mannitol	−	+	−	−	−	−	−
α-Methyl-D-mannoside	+	+	+	−	−	−	+
L-Rhamnose	+	V	V	−	−	−	V
Soluble starch	−	+	−	−	−	ND	ND
D-Xylose	−	−	−	+	+	+	+
Ribose	−	V	−	+	−	−	−
N-Acetyl-β-D-mannosamine	ND	ND	ND	V	+	ND	ND
Hippurate hydrolysis	+	−	+	+	+	ND	ND
Reduction of nitrate	−	V	−	−	−	ND	ND
Pathogenicity for mice	+	−	−	+	?	−	−
Associated serovar(s)	1/2a, 1/2b, 1/2c, 3a, 3b, 3c, 4ab, 4b, 4c, 4d, 4e, 7	S	4ab, US, 6a, 6b	5	5	1/2a, 1/2b, 1/2c, US, 4b, 4d, 6b	1/2b, 4c, 6a, 6b, US

*From Bille J. *Listeria* and *Erysipelothrix*. In: Murray PR, Baron EJ, Jorgensen JH, et al, eds. *Manual of Clinical Microbiology*. 9th ed. Washington, DC: American Society for Microbiology Press; 2007:474–484.
†Usually a wide zone or multiple zones.
Abbreviations: +, ≥90% of strains are positive; −, ≥90% of strains are negative; ND, not determined; S, specific; US, undesignated serotype; V, variable.

source.[26] *L. monocytogenes* was added to PulseNet in 1998; this system has proved effective in the early detection of outbreaks of listeriosis.[6,27]

Pathogenesis

Except for vertical transmission from mother to fetus and rare instances of cross-contamination in the delivery suite or newborn nursery, human-to-human infection has not been documented.

Most often, *Listeria* are transmitted via the ingestion of contaminated food. The oral inoculum required to produce clinical infection is unknown; experiments in healthy mammals indicate that 10[9] organisms or more are required.[28] Alkalinization of the stomach by antacids, H$_2$ blockers, proton pump inhibitors, ulcer surgery, or the achlorhydria associated with advanced age may promote infection.[29] The incubation period for invasive illness is not well established, but evidence from a few cases related to specific ingestions points to incubation periods ranging from 11 to 70 days, with a mean of 31 days. In one report, two pregnant women whose only common exposure was attendance at a party developed listerial bacteremia with the same uncommon enzyme type; incubation periods for illness were 19 and 23 days.[30]

Virulent *L. monocytogenes* is probably sufficient to cause disease without promoter organisms, but one outbreak that could not be traced to a particular source suggested that intercurrent gastrointestinal infection with another pathogen may enhance invasion in individuals colonized with *L. monocytogenes*.[31] Evidence for this is found in the common history of antecedent gastrointestinal symptoms in patients and household contacts, the long incubation period from ingestion to clinical illness, and two instances in which invasive listeriosis closely followed shigellosis.[32] Both listerial meningitis and bacteremia have occurred shortly after colonoscopy or sigmoidoscopy.[33,34]

In the intestine, *L. monocytogenes* crosses the mucosal barrier aided by active endocytosis of organisms by endothelial cells.[11,35] Once it is in the bloodstream, hematogenous dissemination may occur to any site; *L. monocytogenes* has a particular predilection for the central nervous system (CNS) and the placenta. Experimental data indicate that *L. monocytogenes* can use several different mechanisms to invade the CNS: (1) via direct invasion of endothelial cells of the blood-brain barrier by blood-borne bacteria, (2) transportation of bacteria to the

CNS within circulating leukocytes in a phagocyte-facilitated ("Trojan horse") mechanism, and (3) via a neural route whereby bacteria are inoculated into oral tissues when abrasive food is chewed, followed by tissue macrophage phagocytosis of the bacteria making possible the invasion of cranial nerves.[36,37] In the last instance, bacteria move in a retrograde direction through the nerve axons, eventually reaching the CNS, where they continue to spread intercellularly to the parenchyma. Intra-axonal spread may be particularly important in the development of rhombencephalitis.[36-38]

The intracellular, molecular pathogenesis of listeriosis has been reviewed in detail.[39-41] Obviously, it is advantageous for an intracellular organism such as *L. monocytogenes* to get inside mammalian cells as efficiently as possible. *Listeria* possess the cell surface protein internalin,[42] which interacts with E-cadherin, a receptor on epithelial cells and macrophages, resulting in the induction of phagocytosis. Once phagocytosed, listeriolysin O, the major virulence factor, along with phospholipases, enables *Listeria* to escape from phagosomes and avoid intracellular killing.[43] Now free in the cytoplasm, the bacteria can divide (doubling time about 1 hour) and, by inducing host cell actin polymerization, propel themselves to the cell membrane. Subsequently, by pushing against the host cell membrane, they form elongated pseudopod-like projections (filopods) that can be ingested by adjacent cells such as macrophages, enterocytes, and hepatocytes. The bacterial surface protein Act A is necessary for the induction of actin filament assembly and cell-to-cell spread and, therefore, is a major virulence factor.

Thus, through this novel life cycle, *L. monocytogenes* can move from cell to cell without being exposed to antibodies, complement, or neutrophils.

Iron, essential for the life of most microorganisms, appears to be an important virulence factor for *L. monocytogenes*. *L. monocytogenes* siderophores enable it to take iron from transferrin.[11] In vitro, iron enhances organism growth. In animal models of listerial infection, iron overload is associated with enhanced susceptibility to infection, whereas iron depletion results in prolonged survival and iron supplementation in enhanced lethality.[44] The clinical associations of sporadic listerial infection with hemochromatosis[5] and outbreaks with transfusion-induced iron overload in dialysis patients[45] attest to the importance of iron as a virulence factor in humans.

Immunity

Resistance to infection with the intracellular bacterium *L. monocytogenes* involves both innate and adaptive immune responses.[46] The adaptive response is predominantly cell mediated, as evidenced by the experiments of Mackaness showing that immunity could be transferred by sensitized lymphocytes but not by serum that contained antibodies. Further evidence is provided by the overwhelming clinical association between listerial infection and conditions of impaired cellular immunity including lymphomas, pregnancy, AIDS, and corticosteroid immunosuppression, particularly, but not exclusively, in transplant recipients.[1,2,5,6,15-18,47] Combined treatment with fludarabine and prednisone in patients with chronic lymphocytic leukemia decreased their CD4+ T-lymphocyte counts and increased their incidence of listeriosis; fludarabine alone was not associated with listeriosis.[48] Tumor necrosis factor–α (TNFα) neutralizing agents (e.g., infliximab, etanercept) are increasingly used to treat rheumatoid arthritis and Crohn's disease; invasive listeriosis has complicated use of these immune modulating agents.[49-51] An interesting correlate of these clinical events is the observation that, in a murine model, TNF was found to play a crucial role in the intracerebral control of *L. monocytogenes* infection.[52] Toll-like receptor 2 contributes to the recognition and control of listerial infection,[53] and the production of nitric oxide by activated macrophages may play a role in natural immunity to listeriosis independent of T-cell function.[54,55] The role of humoral immunity is unknown, although both immunoglobulin M (absent in newborns) and classic complement activity (low in newborns) have been shown to be necessary for efficient opsonization of *L. monocytogenes*,[56] and protein 60–specific antibodies, present in most immune-competent adults, opsonize *L. monocytogenes* and enhance their uptake by monocyte-derived dendritic cells, which are active in killing the organism.[57]

Although listeriosis is 100 to 1000 times more common in patients with AIDS than in an age-matched population,[2,58,59] it is somewhat surprising that it is not seen more commonly given the ubiquity of the organism. It is likely that many cases are prevented by routine *Pneumocystis* prophylaxis with trimethoprim-sulfamethoxazole. Most cases have occurred in those with advanced disease, that is, CD4 lymphocyte counts of less than 100/mm³.

There is no increased frequency of listeriosis in those with deficiencies in neutrophil numbers or function, splenectomy, complement deficiency, or immune globulin disorders, the latter not surprising given that *L. monocytogenes* can be passed from cell to cell without being exposed to antibody.

Clinical Syndromes

The species name derives from the fact that an extract of the *L. monocytogenes* cell membrane has potent monocytosis-producing activity in rabbits,[60] but monocytosis is a very uncommon feature of human infection.

INFECTION IN PREGNANCY

During gestation, there is mild impairment of cell-mediated immunity,[61] and pregnant women are prone to develop listerial bacteremia with an estimated 17-fold increase in risk.[62] *Listeria* proliferate in the placenta in areas that appear to be unreachable by usual defense mechanisms,[63] and cell-to-cell spread facilitates maternal-fetal transmission.[64] For unexplained reasons, CNS infection, a commonly recognized form of listeriosis in other groups, is extremely rare during pregnancy in the absence of other risk factors.[12,62] Bacteremia is manifested clinically as an acute febrile illness, often accompanied by myalgias, arthralgias, headache, and backache. Illness usually occurs in the third trimester, probably related to the major decline in cell-mediated immunity seen at 26 to 30 weeks of gestation.[61] Twenty-two percent of human perinatal infections result in stillbirth or neonatal death; spontaneous abortion is common. Untreated bacteremia is generally self-limited, although if there is a complicating amnionitis, fever in the mother may persist until the fetus is spontaneously or therapeutically aborted. Among women who have listeriosis during pregnancy, two thirds of surviving infants develop clinical neonatal listeriosis. Early diagnosis and antimicrobial treatment of the infected woman can result in the birth of a healthy infant.[1,62]

There is no convincing evidence that listeriosis is a cause of habitual abortion in humans.

NEONATAL INFECTION

In a pregnant primate model, oral administration of *L. monocytogenes* resulted in stillbirth with isolation of the bacterium from placental and fetal tissues.[65] When human in utero infection occurs, it may precipitate spontaneous abortion and the fetus may be stillborn or die within hours of a disseminated form of listerial infection known as *granulomatosis infantiseptica*, characterized by widespread microabscesses and granulomas, particularly prevalent in the liver and spleen. In this entity, abundant bacteria are often visible on Gram stain of meconium.[66]

More commonly, neonatal infection manifests like group B streptococcal disease in one of two forms[1]: (1) an early-onset sepsis syndrome usually associated with prematurity and probably acquired in utero, and (2) a late-onset meningitis occurring about 2 weeks postpartum in term babies most likely infected by organisms present in the maternal vagina at parturition, although cases have occurred after cesarean section, and nosocomial transmission has been suggested. In early-onset disease, *L. monocytogenes* can be isolated from the conjunctivae, external ear, nose, throat, meconium, amniotic fluid, placenta, blood, and sometimes CSF; Gram stain of meconium may show gram-positive rods and provide early diagnosis. Highest concentrations of bacteria are found in the neonatal lung and gut, suggesting that infection is acquired in utero by inhalation of infected amniotic fluid rather than via a hematogenous route.[67] Purulent conjunctivitis and a disseminated papular rash rarely have been described in newborns with early-onset disease, but clinical infection is otherwise similar to that due to other bacterial pathogens.

BACTEREMIA

Bacteremia without an evident focus is the most common manifestation of listeriosis after the neonatal period.[2,6] Clinical manifestations are similar to those seen in bacteremia due to other causes and typically include fever and myalgias; a prodromal illness with diarrhea and nausea may occur. Because immunocompromised patients are more likely than healthy persons to have blood cultured during febrile illnesses, transient bacteremias in healthy persons may go undetected.

CENTRAL NERVOUS SYSTEM INFECTION

The organisms that cause bacterial meningitis most frequently (*Streptococcus pneumoniae, Neisseria meningitidis, Haemophilus influenzae*) rarely cause parenchymal brain infections such as cerebritis and brain abscess. In contrast, *L. monocytogenes* has tropism for the brain itself, particularly the brain stem, as well as for the meninges.[1,2,5] Many patients with meningitis have altered consciousness, seizures, or movement disorders, or all of these, and truly have a meningoencephalitis.

Meningitis

In an active surveillance study of bacterial meningitis reported by the CDC in 1990, *L. monocytogenes* was the fifth most common cause behind *H. influenzae, S. pneumoniae, N. meningitidis,* and group B streptococcus but had the highest mortality at 22%.[68] In 1995, 5 years after the introduction of *H. influenzae* conjugate vaccines, a survey of bacterial meningitis showed that *H. influenzae* had become less common than *L. monocytogenes,* which accounted for 20% of cases in neonates and 20% in those older than 60 years.[69]

TABLE 207-2	Features Particular to Listerial Meningitis*	
Feature		**Frequency (%)**
Presentation can be subacute > 24 hours[†]		~60
Stiff neck		75
Movement disorders (ataxia, tremors, myoclonus)		15-20
Seizures		10-25
Fluctuating mental status		~75
Focal neurologic findings		35-40
Positive blood culture		50-75
Cerebrospinal fluid (CSF)		
Positive Gram stain		30-40
Normal CSF glucose		>60
Neutrophil predominance		~70

*Adapted from references 1, 15, 72.
[†]May be several days or more and mimic tuberculous meningitis in ~10% to 30%.

Worldwide, *L. monocytogenes* is one of the three major causes of neonatal meningitis; is second only to pneumococcus as a cause of bacterial meningitis in adults older than 50 years; and is the most common cause of bacterial meningitis in patients with lymphomas,[70] organ transplant recipients, and those receiving corticosteroid immunosuppression for any reason.[1]

Clinically, meningitis caused by *L. monocytogenes* is usually similar to that due to more common causes[1,15,71]; features particular to listerial meningitis are summarized in Table 207-2. Despite the name *monocytogenes,* 67% of patients present with a predominance of neutrophils in their CSF.[15]

In a comprehensive review[15] of 33 years' experience at Massachusetts General Hospital with CNS listeriosis outside of the neonatal period and pregnancy, including their case series of 41 patients and 776 episodes from the literature, the most common predisposing factor for developing listerial meningitis was malignancy (both solid tumor and hematologic), occurring in 24% of patients. The next most common predisposing factor was transplantation (21%), followed by alcoholism/liver disease (13%), immunosuppression/steroid treatment for miscellaneous reasons (11%), diabetes mellitus (8%), and HIV/AIDS (7%). In 36% of meningitis cases no risk factor was identified.

The first prospective study of meningitis due to *L. monocytogenes* was recently reported from the Netherlands.[72] In this nationwide cohort study of 30 adults, notable clinical features of listerial meningitis included headache in 88%, nausea in 83%, and fever in 90%; but only 75% of patients had a stiff neck at the time of presentation. A focal neurologic deficit was present in 37% (many patients with meningitis have simultaneous infection of the brain parenchyma and truly have a meningoencephalitis). Only 43% had the classic meningitis triad of fever, neck stiffness, and change in mental status. At the time of presentation, 19 of 30 patients had symptoms persisting for greater than 24 hours and 8 had symptoms for 4 days or longer. Remarkable CSF findings included a median white blood cell count of 620 (range 24-16,003) and protein of 2.52 g/L. Spinal fluid Gram stain revealed a gram-positive rod in only 28% of patients while blood cultures were positive for *L. monocytogenes* in 46% of patients. These data illustrate how difficult it can be to make a definitive diagnosis of listerial meningitis at initial presentation.

In the Netherlands study,[72] sequelae in survivors included hemiparesis in two patients and cranial nerve palsies in two others. Mortality from listerial meningitis has variously been reported at 15% in the CDC active surveillance study,[69] 27% in the Massachusetts General Hospital review,[15] and 17% in the prospective study from the Nether-

lands.[72] In the last report, all deaths occurred within 3 days of admission to the hospital. Mortality is low (zero to 13%) for adults without serious underlying disease or immunosuppressive treatment.[5]

Encephalitis (Cerebritis)

This rare form of CNS listeriosis probably represents early, localized parenchymal infection of the brain cortex before a continuing suppurative process leads to abscess formation. In these cases, the clinical picture is dominated by altered consciousness or cognitive dysfunction. Spinal fluid cultures are positive in about one-half of cases; the same is true of blood cultures. Case reports indicate that encephalitis due to *L. monocytogenes* may mimic herpes encephalitis.[73]

Brain Stem Encephalitis (Rhombencephalitis)

An unusual form of listerial encephalitis involves the brain stem[74] and is similar to the unique zoonotic listerial infection known as circling disease of sheep. In contrast to other listerial CNS infections, this illness usually occurs in healthy adults; neonatal cases have not been reported. The typical clinical picture is one of a biphasic illness with a prodrome of fever, headache, nausea, and vomiting lasting about 4 days followed by the abrupt onset of asymmetrical cranial nerve deficits, cerebellar signs, and hemiparesis or hemisensory deficits, or both. About 40% of patients develop respiratory failure. Nuchal rigidity is present in about one-half, and CSF findings are only mildly abnormal with a positive CSF culture in about one-third. Almost two-thirds of patients are bacteremic. Magnetic resonance imaging is superior to computed tomography for demonstrating brain stem encephalitis (Fig. 207-1).[75] Mortality is high, and serious sequelae are common in survivors.

Brain Abscess

Macroscopic brain abscesses account for about 10% of CNS listerial infections. Bacteremia is almost always present, and concomitant meningitis with isolation of *L. monocytogenes* from the CSF is found in 25% to 40%; both these features are rare in other forms of bacterial brain abscess.[76] Most cases occur in groups at known risk for listerial infection.[77] Subcortical abscesses located in the thalamus, pons, and medulla are common; these sites are exceedingly rare when abscesses are caused by other bacteria. Mortality is high, and survivors usually have serious sequelae.

Spinal Cord Infection

Rare instances of spinal cord infection have been reported.[15,71] Most cases were diagnosed when paraparesis developed during treatment for known listerial meningitis/meningoencephalitis. If spinal symptoms develop in the setting of acute bacterial meningitis of uncertain etiology, *L. monocytogenes* infection should be considered.

ENDOCARDITIS

Listerial endocarditis accounts for about 7.5% of adult listerial infections,[5] affects the population at risk for viridans streptococcal endocarditis, produces both native valve and prosthetic valve disease, and has a high rate of septic complications and a mortality of 48%.[78] Listerial endocarditis, but not bacteremia per se, may be an indicator of underlying gastrointestinal tract abnormality, including cancer.[1] Cases in children are rare.

LOCALIZED INFECTION

Rare reports of focal infections from which *L. monocytogenes* has been isolated include direct inoculation resulting in conjunctivitis, skin infection, and lymphadenitis.[1,2] Bacteremia can lead to hepatitis and hepatic abscess, cholecystitis, peritonitis, splenic abscess, pleuropulmonary infection, joint infection, osteomyelitis, pericarditis, myocarditis, arteritis, and endophthalmitis.[1,2] There is nothing clinically unique about these localized infections; many, but not all, have occurred in those known to be at risk for listeriosis.

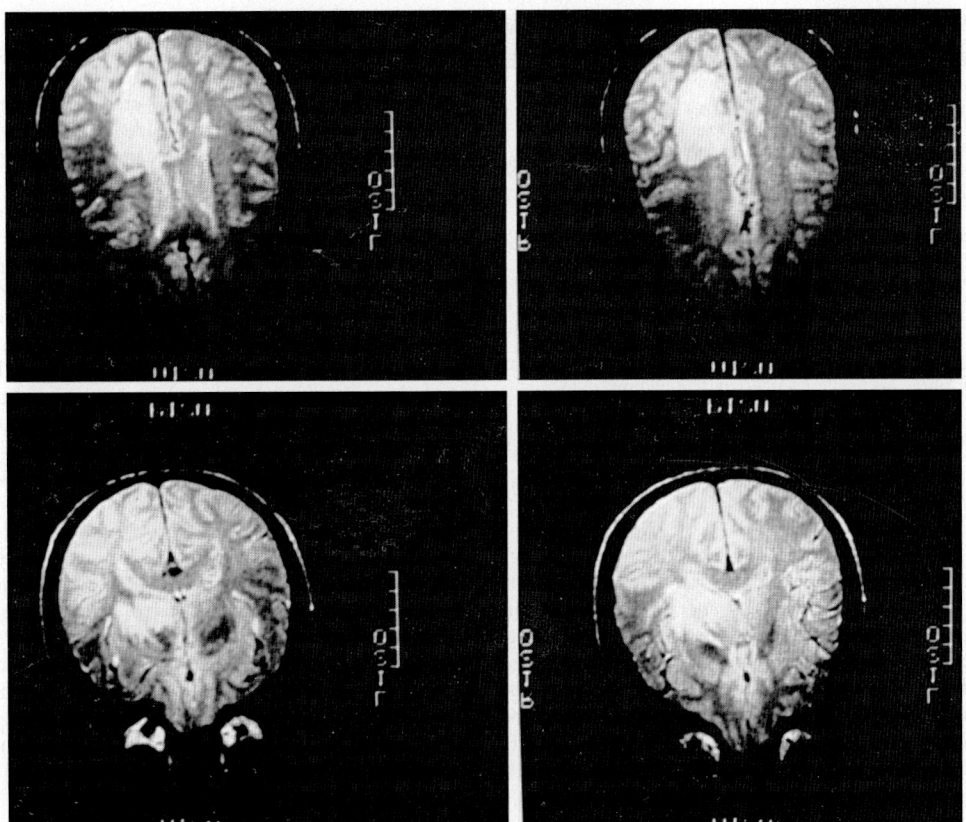

Figure 207-1 **Magnetic resonance imaging scan of the brain of a patient with chronic lymphocytic leukemia, cerebritis, hemiparesis, *Listeria monocytogenes* in blood cultures, and a negative result on spinal fluid examination.** Six weeks of ampicillin and gentamicin resulted in a complete recovery.

FEBRILE GASTROENTERITIS

Many patients with listerial bacteremia or CNS infection give a history of antecedent gastrointestinal symptoms including diarrhea, nausea, and vomiting, often accompanied by fever.[5,31] Large inocula of orally administered *L. monocytogenes* produce diarrheal disease in primates.[28] Investigation of a point-source foodborne listeriosis outbreak, which resulted in bacteremia in two pregnant women, strongly suggested that ingestion of contaminated food by healthy, nonpregnant individuals produced a self-limited, febrile gastroenteritis.[30]

Convincing evidence that *L. monocytogenes* can cause foodborne noninvasive disease in healthy persons was provided by the report of an outbreak of diarrhea and fever among attendees at a Holstein cow show in Illinois that was traced to ingestion of contaminated chocolate milk.[79] The contamination level in the milk was exceedingly high, and the median dose of ingested *Listeria* may have been as high as 2.9×10^{11} colony-forming units per person. The epidemic appeared to be caused by postpasteurization contamination. In this outbreak, serologic testing for antibodies to listeriolysin O was shown to be a useful tool for retrospectively identifying infected ill persons. Active surveillance identified three persons with invasive disease (bacteremia, brain abscess) related to ingestion of chocolate milk from the implicated dairy, providing further evidence that many cases of seemingly sporadic invasive disease are, in fact, part of foodborne outbreaks.

At least six other outbreaks of foodborne gastroenteritis have been described.[80] In the largest outbreak,[7] illness occurred in more than 1500 school children who ingested a corn salad as part of a catered school lunch program; 19% were hospitalized, 87% of stool cultures were positive, and one of 40 blood cultures grew *L. monocytogenes.*

Illness typically has occurred 24 hours (range 6 hours to 10 days) after ingestion of a large inoculum of bacteria and usually lasts 1-3 days (range 1-7 days); attack rates have been quite high (52% to 100%).

Common symptoms include fever, watery diarrhea, nausea, headache, and pains in joints and muscles. Vehicles of infection have included chocolate milk, cold corn and tuna salad, cold smoked trout, and delicatessen meat. *L. monocytogenes* should be considered as a possible cause of foodborne outbreaks of febrile gastroenteritis when routine stool cultures fail to identify a pathogen.

COMPLICATIONS

Complications of invasive disease including disseminated intravascular coagulation, adult respiratory distress syndrome, and rhabdomyolysis with acute renal failure have been documented. Rare episodes of reinfection have occurred.[81]

█ Diagnosis

Clinical settings in which listeriosis should be given strong consideration as part of the differential diagnosis are listed in Table 207-3.

Diagnosis requires isolation of *L. monocytogenes* from normally sterile clinical specimens (CSF, blood, joint fluid, and so forth) and identification through standard microbiologic techniques. Antibodies to listeriolysin O have not proved useful for acute diagnosis of invasive disease, nor yet have polymerase chain reaction probes. Serodiagnosis of listeriosis employing measurement of antibodies to listeriolysin O has proved useful for identifying infected individuals with noninvasive disease (asymptomatic infection, gastroenteritis) during foodborne outbreaks.[79] A polypeptide limited to an amino-terminal residue of listeriolysin O appears to be a more specific antigen for use in serologic tests than those previously employed.[82]

Magnetic resonance imaging is superior to computerized tomography for demonstrating parenchymal brain involvement, especially in the brain stem.[74,75,83]

TABLE 207-3	Clinical Settings in Which Listeriosis Should be Considered Strongly in the Differential Diagnosis

Neonatal sepsis or meningitis
Meningitis or parenchymal brain infection in
  • Patients with hematologic malignancies, AIDS, organ transplantation, corticosteroid immunosuppression, and those receiving anti–tumor necrosis factor (anti-TNF) agents
  • Patients with a subacute presentation of meningitis
  • Adults older than 50 years of age
Simultaneous infection of the meninges and brain parenchyma
Subcortical brain abscess
Spinal symptoms in the setting of acute bacterial meningitis of uncertain etiology
Fever during pregnancy, particularly in the third trimester
Blood, CSF, or other normally sterile specimen reported to have "diphtheroids" on Gram stain or culture
Foodborne outbreak of febrile gastroenteritis when routine cultures fail to identify a pathogen

Treatment

There have been no controlled trials to establish a drug of choice or the duration of therapy for listerial infection. Comprehensive reviews of antimicrobial activity against *L. monocytogenes* and treatment of listeriosis have been published.[84,85] Recommendations regarding therapy are based on data obtained from in vitro susceptibility testing, animal models, and clinical experience with small numbers of patients compared with historical controls and, therefore, are subject to interpretation and individual preferences. In the absence of a positive CSF Gram stain, initial therapy for bacterial meningitis in all adults older than 50 years should include either ampicillin or trimethoprim-sulfamethoxazole, especially if there is no associated pneumonia, otitis, sinusitis, or endocarditis that would point to causes other than *L. monocytogenes*.

Ampicillin is generally considered the preferred agent, although its superiority to penicillin is questionable. The β-lactam antibiotics are often described as being bacteriostatic for *Listeria*. In fact, they demonstrate delayed in vitro bactericidal activity (48 hours) at levels that are obtainable in the CSF. The same phenomenon has been shown with imipenem and vancomycin. Based on synergy in vitro and in animal models, most authorities suggest adding gentamicin to ampicillin for the treatment of bacteremia in those with severely impaired T-cell function and in all cases of meningitis and endocarditis.

For those intolerant of penicillins, trimethoprim-sulfamethoxazole as a single agent is thought to be the best alternative. Although data are limited, this combination is bactericidal for *Listeria*, and outcomes appear at least comparable to those achieved with ampicillin and gentamicin. In a non-randomized study of patients with severe listerial meningoencephalitis, the combination of trimethoprim-sulfamethoxazole plus ampicillin was associated with a much lower failure rate and fewer neurologic sequelae than ampicillin combined with an aminoglycoside.[86] In the absence of underlying immunosuppressive illness or treatment, pregnant women virtually never develop CNS infection. Therefore, a penicillin-allergic pregnant woman, at a time in the pregnancy when sulfonamides should be avoided, reasonably could be treated with a macrolide or vancomycin.

Chloramphenicol should not be used to treat listerial infection because of unacceptable failure and relapse rates. No currently available cephalosporin should be used; they have limited activity, and meningitis has developed in patients while receiving cephalosporins. Reports have documented the utility of erythromycin and tetracycline in isolated cases, but these agents are unreliable and should be avoided. One center has reported a clindamycin resistance rate of more than 95%.[87] Several quinolones have good in vitro activity,[88,89] but clinical experience is minimal, and listerial meningitis may have developed, or at the very least progressed, during ciprofloxacin treatment.[90]

Vancomycin has been used successfully in a few penicillin-allergic patients, but others have developed listerial meningitis while receiving the drug. Rifampin is quite active in vitro and is known to penetrate

phagocytic cells; however, clinical experience is minimal, and in animal models the addition of rifampin to ampicillin was not more effective than ampicillin alone. Both imipenem and meropenem have been used successfully to treat listeriosis, but caution is advised because both drugs lower the seizure threshold, imipenem was less effective than ampicillin in a mouse model,[91] and meropenem clinical failure has been documented.[92]

Meningitis doses should be used for all patients, even in the absence of CNS or CSF abnormalities, because of the high affinity of this organism for the CNS. Relapses and treatment failures are reported in those with meningitis treated for less than 2 weeks; therefore, treatment for 3 weeks is recommended for all cases of meningitis.[1,15] Bacteremic patients without CSF abnormalities can be treated for 2 weeks. Patients with rhombencephalitis or brain abscess should be treated for at least 6 weeks and followed with serial magnetic resonance imaging studies (or computed tomography scans). Endocarditis should be treated for 4 to 6 weeks.

No data exist concerning antimicrobial efficacy in listerial gastroenteritis; the illness is self-limited, and treatment is not warranted.

Clinically significant antimicrobial resistance has not been encountered, but vigilance is warranted because transfer of resistance from enterococci to *L. monocytogenes* has been documented.[93]

Iron is a virulence factor for *L. monocytogenes*, and clinically, iron-overload states are risk factors for listerial infection. Therefore, in patients with iron deficiency, it seems prudent to withhold iron replacement until treatment for listerial infection is completed. Corticosteroids appear to be important adjunctive agents in treating the most common forms of bacterial meningitis; their role in the treatment of listerial CNS infections is unknown.

Prevention

Recommendations for consumer prevention of listeriosis from a foodborne source were developed by the CDC in 1992 and are presented in Table 207-4. People at high risk for listeriosis may choose to avoid soft cheeses. It is best to avoid foods from deli counters, such as prepared salads, meats, and cheeses. Those at risk who choose to eat these high-risk foods should be instructed to thoroughly cook them, avoid cross-contamination, and only refrigerate cooked perishable foods for short periods of time.[94]

In 1989, following documentation of listeriosis after the ingestion of contaminated turkey frankfurters, the U.S. Department of Agriculture began a surveillance program for *L. monocytogenes* in ready-to-eat processed meats and enforced regulations prohibiting the sale of contaminated meat (so-called zero-tolerance policy).[13] Active surveillance of listeriosis in the United States suggests that industry cleanup efforts combined with the 1992 dietary recommendations for persons at

TABLE 207-4	Dietary Recommendations for Preventing Foodborne Listeriosis

For all persons:
Thoroughly cook raw food from animal sources (e.g., beef, pork, poultry)
Thoroughly wash raw vegetables before eating
Keep uncooked meats separate from vegetables, cooked foods, and ready-to-eat foods
Avoid consumption of raw (unpasteurized) milk or foods made from raw milk
Wash hands, knives, and cutting boards after handling uncooked foods
Additional recommendations for persons at high risk (those immunocompromised by illness or medications, pregnant women, and the elderly):
Avoid soft cheeses, e.g., Mexican-style, feta, Brie, Camembert, and blue-veined cheese (no need to avoid hard cheeses, cream cheese, cottage cheese, or yogurt)
Leftover foods or ready-to-eat foods (e.g., hot dogs) should be reheated until steaming hot before eating
Although the risk for listeriosis associated with foods from delicatessen counters is relatively low, pregnant women and immunosuppressed persons may choose to avoid these foods or to thoroughly reheat cold cuts before eating

increased risk were effective measures. From 1989 through 1993 there was a 44% reduction in invasive listerial illness and a 48% reduction in deaths.[13] A similar decline in incidence of human listeriosis was seen in France following control measures to decrease food contamination.[95] Following more recent risk assessment for *L. monocytogenes* in deli meats, regulatory and industry changes have been designed to prevent future contamination of ready-to-eat meat and poultry.[20]

Except from infected mother to fetus, human-to-human transmission of listeriosis does not occur; therefore, patients do not need to be isolated. Neonatal listerial infection complicating successive pregnancies is virtually unheard of, and intrapartum antibiotics are not recommended for mothers with a history of perinatal listeriosis. There is no vaccine.

Listerial infections are effectively prevented by trimethoprim-sulfamethoxazole given as *Pneumocystis* prophylaxis to organ transplant recipients or individuals with human immunodeficiency virus infection.[96] In areas with a high prevalence of AIDS, the widespread use of trimethoprim-sulfamethoxazole prophylaxis against *Pneumocystis* pneumonia appears to have resulted in a marked decline in nonperinatal listeriosis.

The utility, or even the feasibility, of eradicating gastrointestinal colonization as a means to prevent invasive disease is unknown. However, asymptomatic people at high risk for listeriosis, known to have ingested a food implicated in an outbreak, reasonably could be given oral ampicillin or trimethoprim-sulfamethoxazole for several days.

REFERENCES

1. Lorber B. Listeriosis. *Clin Infect Dis.* 1997;24:1-11.
2. Painter J, Slutsker L. Listeriosis in humans. In: Ryser ET, Marth EH, eds. *Listeria, Listeriosis and Food Safety.* 3rd ed. Boca Raton, Florida: CRC Press; 2007:85-109.
3. Bille J. *Listeria* and *Erysipelothrix.* In: Murray PR, Baron EJ, Jorgensen JH, et al, eds. *Manual of Clinical Microbiology.* 9th ed. Washington, DC: American Society for Microbiology Press; 2007:474-484.
4. Hayes PS, Graves LM, Ajello GW, et al. Comparison of cold enrichment and US Department of Agriculture methods for isolating *Listeria monocytogenes* from naturally contaminated foods. *Appl Environ Microbiol.* 1991;57:2109-2113.
5. Nieman RE, Lorber B. Listeriosis in adults: a changing pattern: report of eight cases and review of the literature, 1968-1978. *Rev Infect Dis.* 1980;2:207-227.
6. Swaminathan B, Gerner-Smidt P. The epidemiology of human listeriosis. *Microbes Infect.* 2007;9:1236-1243.
7. Aureli P, Fiorucci GC, Caroli D, et al. An outbreak of febrile gastroenteritis associated with corn contaminated by *Listeria monocytogenes*. *N Engl J Med.* 2000;342:1235-1241.
8. Schlech WF III, Lavigne PM, Bortolussi RA, et al. Epidemic listeriosis—evidence for transmission by food. *N Engl J Med.* 1983;308:203-206.
9. Schuchat A, Deaver K, Hayes PS, et al. Gastrointestinal carriage of *Listeria monocytogenes* in household contacts of patients with listeriosis. *J Infect Dis.* 1993;167:1261-1262.
10. Grif K, Patscheider G, Dierich MP, et al. Incidence of fecal carriage of *Listeria monocytogenes* in three healthy volunteers: a one-year prospective stool survey. *Eur J Clin Microbiol Infect Dis.* 2003;22:16-20.
11. Farber JM, Peterkin PI. *Listeria monocytogenes,* a food-borne pathogen. *Microbiol Rev.* 1991;55:476-511.
12. Ciesielski CA, Hightower AW, Parsons SK, et al. Listeriosis in the United States: 1980-1982. *Arch Intern Med.* 1988;148:1416-1419.
13. Tappero JW, Schuchat A, Deaver KA, et al. Reduction in the incidence of human listeriosis in the United States: effectiveness of prevention efforts? *JAMA.* 1995;273:1118-1122.
14. Voetsch AC, Angulo FJ, Jones TF, et al. Reduction in the incidence of invasive listeriosis in foodborne diseases active surveillance network sites, 1996-2003. *Clin Infect Dis.* 2007;44:513-520.
15. Mylonakis E, Hohmann EL, Calderwood SB. Central nervous system infection with *Listeria monocytogenes:* 33 years' experience at a general hospital and review of 776 episodes from the literature. *Medicine.* 1998;77:313-336.
16. Siegman-Igra Y, Levin R, Weinberger M, et al. *Listeria monocytogenes* infection in Israel and review of cases worldwide. *Emerg Infect Dis.* 2002;8:305-310.
17. Buchholz U, Mascola L. Transmission, pathogenesis, and epidemiology of *Listeria monocytogenes. Infect Dis Clin Pract.* 2001;10:34-41.
18. Safdar A, Papadopoulous EB, Armstrong D. Listeriosis in recipients of allogeneic blood and marrow transplantation: thirteen year review of disease characteristics, treatment outcomes and a new association with human cytomegalovirus infection. *Bone Marrow Transplant.* 2002;29:913-916.
19. Goulet V, Hedberg C, Le Monnier A, et al. Increasing incidence of listeriosis in France and other European countries. *Emerg Infect Dis.* 2008;14:734-740.
20. Gottlieb SL, Newbern EC, Griffin PM, et al. Multistate outbreak of listeriosis linked to turkey deli meat and subsequent changes in US regulatory policy. *Clin Infect Dis.* 2006;42:29-36.
21. Schuchat A, Deaver KA, Wenger JD, et al. Role of foods in sporadic listeriosis. 1. Case-control study of dietary risk factors. *JAMA.* 1992;267:2041-2045.
22. Pinner RW, Schuchat A, Swaminathan B, et al. Role of foods in sporadic listeriosis. 2. Microbiologic and epidemiologic investigation. *JAMA.* 1992;267:2046-2050.
23. Farber JM, Peterkin PI, Carter AO, et al. Neonatal listeriosis due to cross-infection confirmed by isoenzyme typing and DNA fingerprinting. *J Infect Dis.* 1991;163:927-928.
24. Colodner R, Sakran W, Miron D, et al. *Listeria monocytogenes* cross-contamination in a nursery. *Am J Infect Control.* 2003;31:322-324.
25. Schuchat A, Lizano C, Broome CV, et al. Outbreak of neonatal listeriosis associated with mineral oil. *Pediatr Infect Dis.* 1991;10:183-189.
26. Swaminathan B, Barrett TJ, Hunter SB, et al. PulseNet: the molecular subtyping network for foodborne bacterial disease surveillance, United States. *Emerg Infect Dis.* 2001;7:382-389.
27. Sauders BD, Fortes ED, Morse DL, et al. Molecular subtyping to detect human listeriosis clusters. *Emerg Infect Dis.* 2003;9:672-680.
28. Farber JM, Daley E, Coates F, et al. Feeding trials of *Listeria monocytogenes* with a nonhuman primate model. *J Clin Microbiol.* 1991;29:2606-2608.
29. Schlech WF III, Chase DP, Badley A. A model of food-borne *Listeria monocytogenes* infection in the Sprague-Dawley rat using gastric inoculation: development and effect of gastric acidity on infective dose. *Int J Food Microbiol.* 1993;18:15-24.
30. Riedo FX, Pinner RW, Tosca ML, et al. A point-source foodborne listeriosis outbreak: documented incubation period and possible mild illness. *J Infect Dis.* 1994;170:693-696.
31. Schwartz B, Hexter D, Broome CV, et al. Investigation of an outbreak of listeriosis: new hypotheses for the etiology of epidemic *Listeria monocytogenes* infections. *J Infect Dis.* 1989;159:680-685.
32. Lorber B. Listeriosis following shigellosis. *Rev Infect Dis.* 1991; 13:865-866.
33. Witlox MA, Klinkenberg-Knol EC, Meuwissen SGM. *Listeria* sepsis as a complication of endoscopy. *Gastrointest Endosc.* 2000;51:235-236.
34. Minami M, Hasegawa T, Ando T, et al. Post-colonoscopic *Listeria* septicemia in ulcerative colitis during immunosuppressive therapy. *Intern Med.* 2007;46:2023-2027.
35. Lecuit M, Vandormael-Pournin S, Lefort J, et al. A transgenic model for listeriosis: role of internalin in crossing the intestinal barrier. *Science.* 2001;292:1722-1725.
36. Drevets DA, Leenen PJ, Greenfield RA. Invasion of the central nervous system by intracellular bacteria. *Clin Microbiol Rev.* 2004;17:323-347.
37. Drevets DA, Bronze MS. *Listeria monocytogenes:* epidemiology, human disease, and mechanisms of brain invasion. *FEMS Immunol Med Microbiol.* 2008;53:151-165.
38. Antal E-A, Leberg EM, Bracht P, et al. Evidence for intraaxonal spread of *Listeria monocytogenes* from the periphery to the central nervous system. *Brain Pathol.* 2001;11:432-438.
39. Wing EJ, Gregory SH. *Listeria monocytogenes:* clinical and experimental update. *J Infect Dis.* 2002;185(suppl 1):S18-S24.
40. Hamon M, Bierne H, Cossart P. *Listeria monocytogenes:* a multifaceted model. *Nat Rev Microbiol.* 2006;4:423-434.
41. Seveau S, Pizarro-Cerda J, Cossart P. Molecular mechanism exploited by *Listeria monocytogenes* during host cell invasion. *Microbes Infect.* 2007;9:1167-1175.
42. Bierne H, Sabet C, Personnic N, et al. Internalins: a complex family of leucine-rich repeat-containing proteins in *Listeria monocytogenes. Microbes Infect.* 2007;9:1156-1166.
43. Schnupf P, Portnoy DA. Listeriolysin O: a phagosome-specific lysin. *Microbes Infect.* 2007;9:1176-1187.
44. Ampel NM, Bejarano GC, Saavedra Jr M. Deferoxamine increases the susceptibility of beta-thalassemic, iron-overloaded mice to infection with *Listeria monocytogenes. Life Sci.* 1992;50:1327-1332.
45. Mossey RT, Sondheimer J. Listeriosis in patients with long-term hemodialysis and transfusional iron overload. *Am J Med.* 1985;79:379-400.
46. Zenewicz LA, Shen H. Innate and adaptive responses to *Listeria monocytogenes:* a short overview. *Microbes Infect.* 2007;9:1208-1215.
47. Mizuno S, Zendejas IR, Reed AI, et al. *Listeria monocytogenes* following orthotopic liver transplantation: central nervous system involvement and review of the literature. *World J Gastroenterol.* 2007;13:4391-4393.
48. Anaissie E, Kontoyiannis DP, Kantarjian H, et al. Listeriosis in patients with chronic lymphocytic leukemia who were treated with fludarabine and prednisone. *Ann Intern Med.* 1992;117:466-469.
49. Slifman NR, Gershon SK, Lee JH, et al. *Listeria monocytogenes* infection as a complication of treatment with tumor necrosis factor alpha–neutralizing agents. *Arthritis Rheum.* 2003; 48:319-324.
50. La Montagna G, Valentini G. *Listeria monocytogenes* meningitis in a patient receiving etanercept for Still's disease. *Clin Exp Rheumatol.* 2005;23:121.
51. Schett G, Herak P, Graninger W, et al. *Listeria*-associated arthritis in a patient undergoing etanercept therapy: case report and review of the literature. *J Clin Microbiol.* 2005;43:2537-2541.
52. Virna S, Deckert M, Lutjen S, et al. TNF is important for pathogen control and limits brain damage in murine cerebral listeriosis. *J Immunol.* 2006;177:3972-3982.
53. Janot L, Secher T, Torres D, et al. CD14 works with Toll-like receptor 2 to contribute to recognition and control of *Listeria monocytogenes* infection. *J Infect Dis.* 2008;198:115-124.
54. Hibbs Jr JB. Infection and nitric oxide. *J Infect Dis.* 2002;185(Suppl):S9-S17.
55. Carryn S, Van de Velde S, Van Bambeke F, et al. Impairment of growth of *Listeria monocytogenes* in THP-1 macrophages by granulocyte macrophage colony-stimulating factor: release of tumor necrosis factor-α and nitric oxide. *J Infect Dis.* 2004;189:2101-2109.
56. Bortolussi R, Issekutz A, Faulkner G. Opsonization of *Listeria monocytogenes* type 4b by human adult and newborn sera. *Infect Immun.* 1986;52:493-498.
57. Kolb-Maurer A, Pilgrim S, Kampgen E, et al. Antibodies against listerial protein 60 act as an opsonin for phagocytosis of *Listeria monocytogenes* by human dendritic cells. *Infect Immun.* 2001;69:3100-3109.
58. Ewert DP, Lieb L, Hayes PS, et al. *Listeria monocytogenes* infection and serotype distribution among HIV-infected persons in Los Angeles County, 1985-92. *J Acquir Immune Defic Syndr Hum Retrovirol.* 1995;8:461-465.
59. Decker CF, Simon GL, DiGioia RA, et al. *Listeria monocytogenes* infections in patients with AIDS: report of five cases and review. *Rev Infect Dis.* 1991;13:413-417.
60. Stanley NF. Studies of *Listeria monocytogenes.* 1. Isolation of a monocytosis-producing agent (MPA). *Aust J Exp Biol Med Sci.* 1949;27:123-131.
61. Weinberg ED. Pregnancy-associated depression of cell-mediated immunity. *Rev Infect Dis.* 1984;6:814-831.
62. Mylonakis E, Paliou M, Hohmann EL, et al. Listeriosis during pregnancy: a case series and review of 222 cases. *Medicine.* 2002;81:260-269.
63. Bakardjiev AI, Theriot JA, Portnoy D. *Listeria monocytogenes* traffics from maternal organs to the placenta and back. *PLoS Pathog.* 2006;2:e66.
64. Bakardjiev AI, Stacy BA, Portnoy DA. Growth of *Listeria monocytogenes* in the guinea pig placenta and role of cell-to-cell spread in fetal infection. *J Infect Dis.* 2005;191:1889-1897.
65. Smith MA, Takeuchi K, Brackett RE, et al. Nonhuman primate model for *Listeria monocytogenes*–induced stillbirths. *Infect Immun.* 2003;71:1574-1579.
66. Larsson S, Linell F. Correlations between clinical and postmortem findings in listeriosis. *Scand J Infect Dis.* 1979;11:55-58.
67. Becroft DMO, Farmer K, Seddon RJ, et al. Epidemic listeriosis in the newborn. *Br Med J.* 1971;3:747-751.
68. Wenger JD, Hightower AW, Facklam RR, et al. Bacterial meningitis in the United States, 1986: report of a multistate surveillance study. *J Infect Dis.* 1990;162:1316-1623.
69. Schuchat A, Robinson K, Wenger JD, et al. Bacterial meningitis in the United States in 1995. *N Engl J Med.* 1997;337:970-976.
70. Safdar A, Armstrong D. Listeriosis in patients at a comprehensive cancer center, 1955-1997. *Clin Infect Dis.* 2003;37:359-364.
71. Clauss HE, Lorber B. CNS infection with *Listeria monocytogenes. Curr Infect Dis Rep.* 2008;10:300-306.
72. Brouwer MC, van de Beek D, Heckenberg SG, et al. Community-acquired *Listeria monocytogenes* meningitis in adults. *Clin Infect Dis.* 2006;43:1233-1238.
73. Cunha BA, Fatehpuria R, Eisenstein LE. *Listeria monocytogenes* encephalitis mimicking Herpes Simplex virus encephalitis: the differential diagnostic importance of cerebrospinal fluid lactic acid levels. *Heart Lung.* 2007;36:226-231.

74. Armstrong RW, Fung PC. Brainstem encephalitis (rhombencephalitis) due to *Listeria monocytogenes:* case report and review. *Clin Infect Dis.* 1993;16:689-702.

75. Alper G, Knepper L, Kanal E. MR findings in listerial rhombencephalitis. *AJNR Am J Neuroradiol.* 1996;17:593-596.

76. Eckburg PB, Montoya JG, Vosti KL. Brain abscess due to *Listeria monocytogenes:* five cases and a review of the literature. *Medicine.* 2001;80:223-235.

77. Cone LA, Leung MM, Byrd RG, et al. Multiple cerebral abscesses because of *Listeria monocytogenes:* three case reports and a literature review of supratentorial listerial brain abscess(es). *Surg Neurol.* 2003;59:320-328.

78. Carvajal A, Frederiksen W. Fatal endocarditis due to *Listeria monocytogenes. Rev Infect Dis.* 1988;10:616-623.

79. Dalton CB, Austin CC, Sobel J, et al. An outbreak of gastroenteritis and fever due to *Listeria monocytogenes* in milk. *N Engl J Med.* 1997;336:100-105.

80. Ooi ST, Lorber B. Gastroenteritis due to *Listeria monocytogenes. Clin Infect Dis.* 2005;40:1327-1332.

81. Van J-C N, Nguyen L, Guillemam R, et al. Relapse of infection or reinfection by *Listeria monocytogenes* in a patient with heart transplant: usefulness of pulsed-field gel electrophoresis for diagnosis. *Clin Infect Dis.* 1994;19:208-209.

82. Gholizadeh Y, Poyart C, Jovin M, et al. Serodiagnosis of listeriosis based on detection of antibodies against recombinant truncated forms of listeriolysin O. *J Clin Microbiol.* 1996;34:1391-1395.

83. Faidas A, Shepard DL, Lim J, et al. Magnetic resonance imaging in listerial brain stem encephalitis. *Clin Infect Dis.* 1993; 16:186-187.

84. Hof H, Nichterlein T, Kretschmar M. Management of listeriosis. *Clin Microbiol Rev.* 1997;10:345-357.

85. Lorber B. *Listeria monocytogenes.* In: Yu VL, Weber R, Raoult D, eds. *Antimicrobial Therapy and Vaccines.* 2nd ed. New York: Apple Trees Productions; 2002:429-436.

86. Merle-Melet M, Dossou-Gbete L, Meyer P, et al. Is amoxicillin-cotrimoxazole the most appropriate antibiotic regimen for listeria meningoencephalitis? Review of 22 cases and the literature. *J Infect.* 1996;33:79-85.

87. Safdar A, Armstrong D. Antimicrobial activities against 84 *Listeria monocytogenes* isolates from patients with systemic listeriosis at a comprehensive cancer center (1955-1997). *J Clin Microbiol.* 2003;41:483-485.

88. Viale P, Furlanut M, Cristini F, et al. Major role of levofloxacin in the treatment of a case of *Listeria monocytogenes* meningitis. *Diagn Microbiol Infect Dis.* 2007;58:137-139.

89. Grayo S, Join-Lambert O, Desroches MC, et al. Comparison of the in vitro efficacies of moxifloxacin and amoxicillin against *Listeria monocytogenes. Antimicrob Agents Chemother.* 2008; 52:1697-1702.

90. Grumbach NM, Mylonakis E, Wing EJ. Development of listerial meningitis during ciprofloxacin treatment. *Clin Infect Dis.* 1999;29:1340-1341.

91. Kim KS. In vitro and in vivo studies of imipenem—cilastatin alone and in combination with gentamicin against *Listeria monocytogenes. Antimicrob Agents Chemother.* 1986;29:289-293.

92. Stepanović S, Lazarević G, Ješić M, et al. Meropenem therapy failure in *Listeria monocytogenes* infection. *Eur J Clin Microbiol Infect Dis.* 2004;23:484-486.

93. Charpentier E, Courvalin P. Antibiotic resistance in *Listeria* spp. *Antimicrob Agents Chemother.* 1999;43:2103-2108.

94. Goulet V. What can we do to prevent listeriosis in 2006? *Clin Infect Dis.* 2007;44:529-530.

95. Goulet V, de Valk H, Pierre O, et al. Effect of prevention measures on incidence of human listeriosis, France, 1987-1997. *Emerg Infect Dis.* 2001;7:983-989.

96. Dworkin MS, Williamson J, Jones JL, et al. Prophylaxis with trimethoprim-sulfamethoxasole for human immunodeficiency virus-infected patients: impact on risk for infectious diseases. *Clin Infect Dis.* 2001;33:393-398.

ADDITIONAL READING

Goldfine H, Shen H, eds. *Listeria monocytogenes: Pathogenesis and Host Response.* New York: Springer; 2007.

Ryser ET, Marth EH, eds. *Listeria, Listeriosis and Food Safety.* 3rd ed. Boca Raton, Fla: CRC Press; 2007.

208

Bacillus anthracis (Anthrax)

GREGORY J. MARTIN | ARTHUR M. FRIEDLANDER

Anthrax has never been a cause of the massive number of human deaths associated with cholera, plague, or smallpox but has played a prominent role in the history of infectious diseases. While much of the industrialized world is focused on anthrax as an agent of bioterrorism, anthrax remains a significant cause of animal deaths, as well as more limited numbers of human cases, in much of the developing world. This chapter focuses on naturally occurring anthrax disease and Chapter 325 on anthrax as an agent of bioterrorism.

There are references to a disease that likely was anthrax in the Christian Bible as well as descriptions of inflamed papules from exposure to tainted wool in Virgil's writings.[1] Anthrax was the first disease definitively attributed to a bacterium by Robert Koch in 1877 and fulfilled what became known as Koch's postulates. Louis Pasteur established the concept of attenuating a bacterial pathogen by serial passage and used this approach in 1881 to develop an anthrax vaccine shown to be protective in a field trial in domesticated animals.[2] With the initiation of the factory processing of hides and wool in the industrial age, deaths from inhalational anthrax among 19th century British and German woolsorters and ragpickers introduced the concept of occupational infectious disease risk and the need to protect workers from these risks.[3] In 1979, an accidental release of anthrax spores from a Soviet military microbiology facility in Sverdlovsk, Russia, was responsible for approximately 70 cases of inhalational anthrax that were originally said to be gastrointestinal anthrax until details were finally published years later.[4] This outbreak and the revelations that Iraq had produced anthrax spores in 1991[5] raised the possibility of anthrax being used as a weapon. This was unfortunately realized with the dissemination of anthrax spores from letters sent through the U.S. Postal Service in 2001, leading to 22 cases of human anthrax and five deaths and made what had been nearly a forgotten disease in Europe and North America the subject of intense public attention and renewed scientific and medical interest.

Microbiology

Bacillus anthracis, the causative agent of anthrax, is a large (1-1.5 × 3-8 μm), gram-positive bacillus with rapid, non-hemolytic growth on blood agar that readily forms spores in the presence of oxygen. Colonies have a characteristic "Medusa's head appearance," sometimes also referred to as a "comet tail," appearing slightly curled at the periphery (Fig. 208-1). The white or gray-white colonies are tenacious when attempts are made to remove them from agar, and this is often described as "a whipped egg white appearance" when a loop is passed through a colony (see Fig. 208-1). In culture the bacilli may form long chains with prominent central or paracentral oval spores that do not cause swelling of the bacilli (Fig. 208-2). In infected tissue, bacteria occur singly, or in short chains of two to three bacilli without spores. In the presence of CO_2 in the laboratory, or of bicarbonate in tissue, *B. anthracis* forms a prominent poly-D-γ-glutamic acid (PGA) capsule important in the inhibition of phagocytosis of the vegetative bacilli. Catalase positivity and non-motility of organisms are further characteristics that differentiate *B. anthracis* from other *Bacillus* species.

These basic identification techniques can typically be performed in nearly all microbiology laboratories, but definitive identification of *B. anthracis* requires further demonstration of lysis by γ-phage, detection of the capsule by fluorescent antibody, and identification of toxin genes by polymerase chain reaction (PCR), usually best performed at a reference laboratory.

In contrast to growth during in vitro cultivation, *B. anthracis* sporulation does not occur in viable tissues until they are exposed to atmospheric levels of oxygen, typically after an infected animal has died and the carcass is opened. The spores, although sensitive to prolonged ultraviolet radiation, are extremely hardy and may survive in certain soil conditions for decades. In the interior of buildings, typically shielded from utter volet light, spores may remain viable for years. Although spores have demonstrated viability in soil for decades, in a terrorist's vial for 80 years,[6] and even longer in bones from an archeological site, in most environments, where the organism must compete with other soil-dwelling bacteria, they typically survive only for months and rarely more than 4 years. Spores may also remain dormant, but viable, in animals for a period of at least 100 days as demonstrated by primate studies in which viable organisms were recovered at necropsy from the lungs of apparently healthy animals,[7-9] a finding that has important therapeutic implications, as discussed below.

The two major virulence factors are the anti-phagocytic PGA capsule encoded on the pX02 plasmid, and two exotoxins encoded on a separate plasmid, pX01. The anthrax toxins have been intensively studied, and components of the toxins have important use in vaccines, in diagnostics, and as targets for new adjunctive therapeutics.

The pX01 plasmid encodes three components, known as protective antigen (PA), edema factor (EF), and lethal factor (LF), each of which individually is biologically inactive. Studies in the 1950s and 1960s established that edema toxin, composed of PA combined with EF, produces local skin edema and that lethal toxin, composed of the same PA together with LF, was highly lethal for experimental animals. The combination of all three components was the most lethal and produced many characteristics of an actual anthrax infection.[10]

PA, which was originally identified as an antigen able to protect animals from experimental anthrax, attaches to the anthrax toxin receptors—tumor endothelial marker 8 and capillary morphogenesis gene 2—on the cell surface and is cleaved by a cell-surface protease into PA_{63}, which forms a heptamer to which up to three EF and/or LF molecules may attach.[11] PA may also be cleaved by a serum protease with formation of toxins in the circulation. When the PA heptamer complexes with EF, it forms edema toxin, and with LF it forms lethal toxin. The toxins are then taken into the cytosol, where they mediate cellular damage. LF is a calmodulin-dependent zinc metalloprotease that cleaves and inactivates multiple mitogen-activated protein kinases and interferes with signal transduction, whereas EF is an adenylate cyclase that increases intracellular cyclic AMP concentrations and interferes with cell function. The toxins have been shown in vitro to impair cell functions associated with innate immunity, including neutrophil chemotaxis, phagocytosis, and superoxide production, and macrophage, T and B lymphocyte, and dendritic cell function,[12-15] and likely affect many other cells possessing toxin receptors. Studies with isolated toxins suggest they both cause hypotension in experimental animals and are additive, but shock has not been a prominent finding in patients presenting with inhalational anthrax. Edema toxin was so named because of its ability to cause edema in experimental animals, and lethal toxin has also recently been shown to increase vascular

---

*The opinions and assertions herein are those of the authors and should not be construed as official or representing the views of the Department of the Navy, the Department of the Army, the Department of Defense, or the U.S. government.

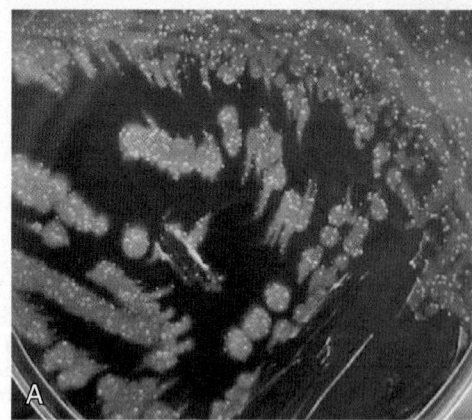
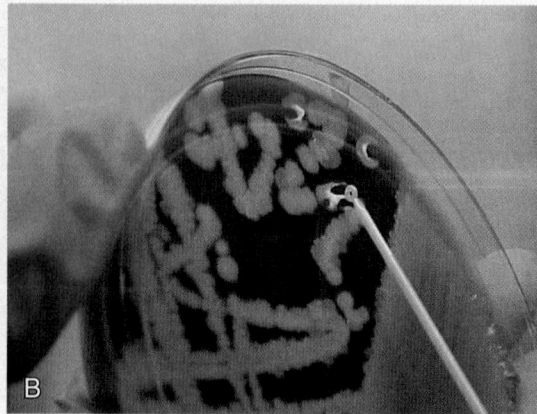

Figure 208-1 **A,** Colonies of *B. anthracis* on sheep blood agar demonstrating white-gray colonies and "comet trail" or "Medusa head" outgrowths from colony margins. **B,** "Whipped egg white" appearance of tenacious *B. anthracis* colonies while being removed from sheep blood agar. *(Courtesy of Robert Paolucci, National Naval Medical Center, Bethesda, Maryland.)*

permeability.[16] However, there are discrepancies between effects of toxins observed on cells in vitro and in vivo and the findings observed in experimental infections. The cell targets and exact role and mechanisms of toxin-induced host dysfunction during infection remain under investigation. Other recently identified bacterial factors contributing to virulence, although of less importance than the capsule and toxins, include a siderophore,[17] a manganese ATP Binding Cassette transporter,[18] phospholipases C and a cholesterol-dependent cytolysin,[19] and nitric oxide synthase.[20]

Epidemiology

Anthrax is a worldwide disease of domesticated and wild animals that secondarily may occur in humans. Estimates of worldwide cases vary widely, but it is estimated by the World Health Organization (WHO) that there are between 2000 and 20,000 human cases per year (Fig. 208-3).[21] Although cases occur worldwide, there is little genetic diversity among isolates. Examination of variable-number tandem repeats (VNTRs) loci identifies six major clones among two branches. Based on identification of VNTRs in different geographic areas, it appears that southern Africa has the greatest diversity of strains and is believed to be the geographic origin of *B. anthracis*.[22,23] The actual number of anthrax cases worldwide has been difficult to ascertain owing to poor reporting, but anthrax in animals has been reported from 82 nations. It is significantly more common among grazing herbivores in some areas of the Middle East, Africa, and Latin America than in more developed countries. The enormous areas of savannah and large populations of ungulate herbivores in southern Africa are ideal for anthrax. In 1923 in South Africa it was estimated that 30,000 to 60,000 animals died of anthrax.[24]

The largest human outbreak of anthrax occurred in Zimbabwe from 1979 to 1985 with some 10,000 reported cases and 182 deaths. These cases, almost all cutaneous, were associated with cattle ranching and lapsed veterinary control practices during the civil war that established Zimbabwe.[25,26] Anthrax remains enzootic in Zimbabwe with continued cases in wildlife and livestock and more cases in humans than in most other nations combined.[27]

In most of Europe and North America, human cases are rare and animal cases are sporadic and uncommon. A single animal death usually is met with an intense veterinary public health response that mandates proper disposal of carcasses, decontamination of fields, and immunization of surviving, potentially exposed animals.

Animals are infected when they graze on fields or grain contaminated with spores or through the bites of flies that have fed on infected carcasses. Seasonal variations have been noted for decades. Heavy spring rains may serve to concentrate spores into low-lying area, and if this is followed by a hot, dry period, animals grazing on these areas

with high spore burdens may become infected. Additionally, in periods of drought, animals grazing on dried grasses close to the soil surface have increased oral abrasions from the dry vegetation. This trauma provides areas for spore entry and germination and a subsequent increase in animal cases of anthrax.[28]

Human cases usually are associated with exposure to infected animals or contaminated animal products. Numerous products have been implicated in transmission to humans including wool, hair, bone and bone meal, meat, horns, and hides. The source may not be readily evident as the animal product may have been processed, e.g., goat-skin drums, wool-based tapestries, and bone meal–based fertilizers.[29,30] Transmission from flies has also been documented; biting flies may carry spores or vegetative forms from a carcass to another animal or human, and even non-biting flies have been shown to carry *B. anthracis* in feces or vomit that they deposit onto vegetation. Birds such as vultures shed anthrax spores in their feces for up to 2 weeks after they ingest infected meat.[31]

Spores are the usual infecting form of anthrax although ingestion of either spore or vegetative forms of *B. anthracis* in contaminated meat may lead to gastrointestinal infection.

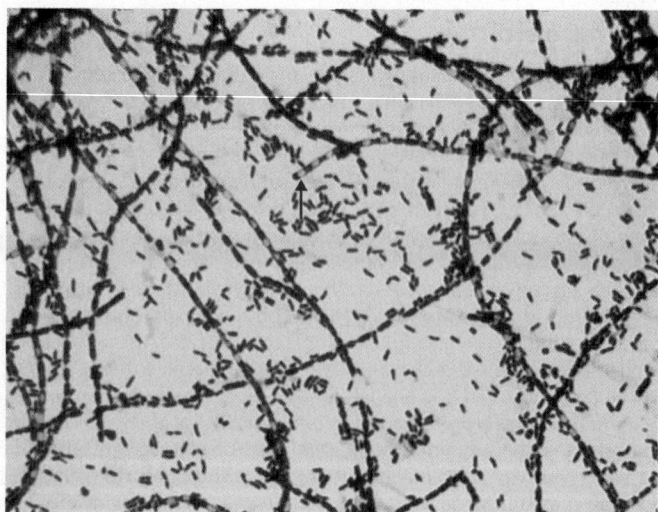

Figure 208-2 **Gram stain of *B. anthracis* demonstrating long chains of bacilli that form when grown in culture.** The prominent central or paracentral spores do not stain with gram staining and appear as clear areas in many of the bacilli in chains (example shown at red arrow). *(Courtesy of Robert Paolucci, National Naval Medical Center, Bethesda, Maryland.)*

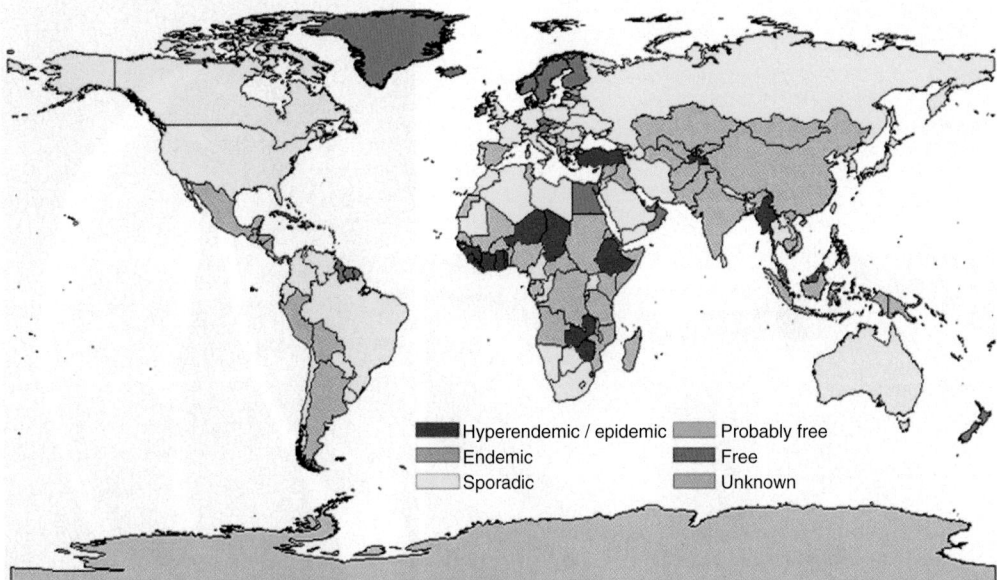

Figure 208-3 **World distribution of anthrax cases as compiled by the World Health Organization (WHO).** Available at: http://www.vetmed. lsu.edu/whocc/mp_world.htm.

The world distribution of anthrax cases in humans and animals is tracked via a geographic information system and remote sensing by the WHO as part of the World Anthrax Data Site and is available on-line at http://www.vetmed.lsu.edu/whocc/mp_world.htm. This includes an updated nation-by-nation breakdown of cases by species and year.[21]

Clinical Manifestations and Diagnosis

The clinical manifestations of anthrax in animals and humans have been well described since the 1800s when cases were relatively common in many areas of the world. The three primary forms of anthrax are dependent on the route of exposure: cutaneous, gastrointestinal, and inhalational. Bacteremia secondary to any of the primary forms of anthrax may lead to seeding of any site, including the central nervous system (CNS) with the resulting hemorrhagic meningoencephalitis being nearly always fatal.

Online resources for clinicians considering a diagnosis of anthrax are currently plentiful. The Infectious Diseases Society of America (IDSA) and the Center for Infectious Disease Research and Policy (CIDRAP) at the University of Minnesota share a frequently updated and extensively referenced anthrax Web site for both naturally occurring and bioterrorism-associated disease: http://www.cidrap.umn.edu/idsa/bt/anthrax/biofacts/anthraxfactsheet.html. The American College of Physicians (ACP) *Physician's Information and Education Resource* (PIER) offers a helpful online anthrax resource that includes skin lesions, radiographs, and differential diagnosis considerations for all forms of anthrax at http://pier.acponline.org/physicians/public/d892/diagnosis/d892-s3.html. Additional resources are available from the Centers for Disease Control and Prevention (CDC) at http://emergency.cdc.gov/agent/anthrax/index.asp and from the WHO at http://www.who.int/topics/anthrax/en. The WHO site features a comprehensive handbook of WHO guidelines for anthrax in animals and humans including handling of carcasses, disinfection, and control of infections.[32]

CUTANEOUS ANTHRAX

Naturally occurring anthrax infections in humans are, in more than 95% of cases, cutaneous disease. In an interesting series from 1955, Gold carefully reported the findings of 117 cases of anthrax he had followed near a Philadelphia goat-hair mill over 20 years. All but one case was cutaneous anthrax, and the only fatalities were the single pulmonary case and one cutaneous case.[33]

As described earlier, a multitude of contaminated animal sources have been implicated in naturally acquired cutaneous anthrax in humans. After the introduction of anthrax spores into the skin, often with just trivial trauma, there is an incubation period of 1-7 (more commonly 2-5) days, leading to the development of a small, pruritic papule at the inoculation site. The majority of lesions are on exposed areas of the head, neck, and extremities. Owing to the associated pruritus, patients (and clinicians) often attribute these painless lesions to an insect or spider bite and ignore them.

A day or two after the formation of the papule, vesicles form around the lesion and may become quite large, 1-2 cm in diameter. The vesicles contain a clear to serosanguineous fluid, and Gram stain reveals numerous bacilli but a paucity of leukocytes. Culture of vesicular fluid will readily yield *B. anthracis* in most cases in which antibiotics have not been given. There is no purulence, and the lesions remain painless. The vesicles are thin roofed and easily rupture, leading to formation of a dark brown, turning to black, eschar at the base of a shallow ulcer. The ulcer is typically surrounded by an area of induration, and in some cases non-pitting edema may be marked[34] (Fig. 208-4). Most other organisms that cause skin infections usually are not associated with extensive induration around a skin lesion or with frank edema, so these findings may be the first clue to the diagnosis of anthrax.

As the ulcer matures, its base becomes characteristically black and is the source of the name anthrax, which derives from the Greek word *anthrakis,* "coal."

In uncomplicated cases (i.e., without secondary spread) lesions slowly heal over a period of 1-3 weeks and the eschar loosens and falls off, typically without leaving a scar. Antibiotics do not affect the evolution of the skin lesions. In most cases, patients report associated headache, malaise. and low-grade fever even if the infection does not progress to bacteremia.

Multiple lesions may occur in some cases, probably representing multiple inoculation sites, but at other times, small satellite lesions may appear around an initial isolated lesion. Serious cutaneous disease may be marked by extensive edema that involves an entire extremity or the trunk from neck to groin. This has been described as "malignant edema" and may be associated with inflammation of the overlying skin

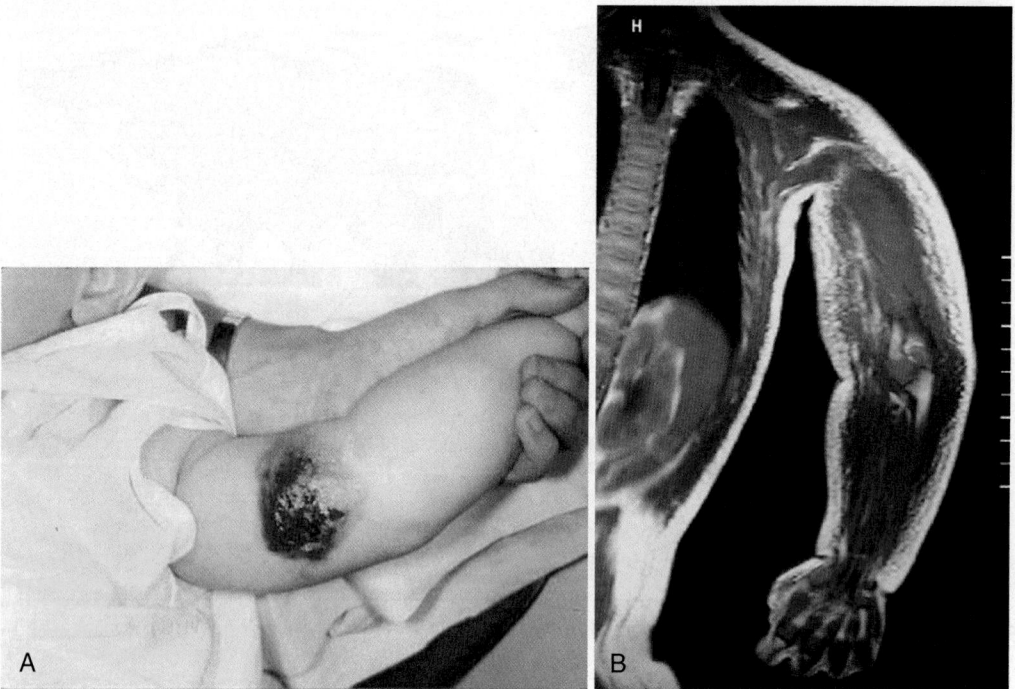

Figure 208-4 **A,** Cutaneous anthrax with extensive nontender swelling and erythema in a 7-month-old child in New York in 2001. **B,** MRI demonstrates extensive subcutaneous edema from shoulder to hand. *(From Roche KJ, Chang MW, Lazarus H. Cutaneous anthrax infection: images in clinical medicine. N Engl J Med. 2001;345:1611. Copyright © 2001 Massachusetts Medical Society. All rights reserved.)*

with pain, signs of toxemia, and subsequent secondary seeding of other sites as bacteremia develops.

Untreated cutaneous disease in humans has been associated with a fatality rate of 10% to 20%, while treated cutaneous disease (before the onset of secondary bacteremic spread) is rarely fatal. Repeat infections are rarely reported and tend to be milder, implying some degree of acquired immunity.[33]

Clinical characteristics that should place cutaneous anthrax high in the differential diagnosis include a painless lesion (during initial stages), the presence of edema out of proportion to the size of the lesion, and a Gram stain of vesicular fluid or ulcer swab with gram-positive rods but rare white blood cells.

The differential diagnosis of the unusual skin lesions associated with cutaneous anthrax includes many diseases seldom encountered by most clinicians. Brown recluse spider bites, which may also cause a black eschar and some associated edema, may be confused with cutaneous anthrax lesions. The key difference is the significant pain associated with a recluse spider bite and the absence of pain in anthrax lesions (although there may be tender adenopathy in association with a skin lesion).

The differential diagnosis of cutaneous anthrax includes tularemia, scrub typhus, rat bite fever, blastomycosis, ringworm acquired from animals, and mycobacterial infection with *Mycobacterium marinum*.[35]

Diagnostic procedures for cutaneous anthrax should preferably be performed prior to initiation of antibiotics, as vesicular fluid and biopsy material are quickly rendered noninfectious after initiation of antibiotics. Appropriate samples for Gram stain and culture include vesicle fluid, either in a syringe or on a swab; a specimen from swabbing the edge of the base of an eschar; and material from a full-thickness punch biopsy of the edge of a vesicle and/or the center of an eschar. In patients already taking antibiotics, samples may be sent for PCR analysis and for silver staining and immunohistology, but these are usually only available at reference laboratories. Since the anthrax attacks in the United States in 2001, a number of rapid PCR assays have been developed. Some of these can be used on either clinical or environmental samples and may be available in some hospitals or to

hazardous material teams. Caution must be used in interpreting these results, as false-positive and -negative results may occur.

As blood cultures are frequently positive in cases that have progressed to sepsis, consideration should be given to obtaining blood cultures early in the evaluation, especially if there are any systemic symptoms. Automated blood culture systems commonly used in hospitals will readily support growth of *B. anthracis*.

In general, culture of *B. anthracis* remains the gold standard for the diagnosis of anthrax infections. Table 208-1 outlines diagnostic specimen preparation, handling, and testing.

Acute and convalescent serum samples should be obtained for serology at 0-7 days of illness and at 14-28 days. Three of the cutaneous cases in 2001 had no culture or PCR evidence of disease, but acute and convalescent serology demonstrated an anti-PA antibody response that confirmed the diagnosis. A rapid enzyme-linked immunosorbent assay (ELISA) that measures total antibody to PA has been approved. The Immunetics QuickELISA Anthrax-PA kit can be used on serum to diagnose all types of anthrax or to demonstrate seroconversion after immunization. Retrospectively, it was positive in 100% of both cutaneous and inhalation cases from 2001. Unfortunately, it is not positive early in disease, taking approximately a week after symptoms begin before detecting PA antibody.[36,37]

INHALATIONAL OR PULMONARY ANTHRAX

Even a single case of inhalational anthrax should raise the possibility of a deliberate spread of spores, as naturally occurring inhalation disease is currently extraordinarily rare. Chapter 325 addresses the use of anthrax as an agent of bioterrorism and more fully addresses this route of exposure.

Inhalational anthrax is an exceptionally dangerous type of *B. anthracis* infection that in the preantibiotic era was nearly uniformly fatal. In a review of 82 reported cases of inhalational anthrax from 1900 to 2005, there was an overall 92% mortality rate despite treatment with anthrax antiserum and/or antibiotics in the majority of cases.[38] During the 2001 anthrax attacks in the United States, 5 of the 11, or 45%, of

Collection and Transport of Laboratory Specimens for the Diagnosis of Anthrax

Type of Illness	Specimen Collection and Transport	Comments
Cutaneous anthrax	All stages: Collect two swabs, one for Gram stain and culture, and one for PCR. Vesicular stage: Perform Gram stain, culture, and PCR of fluids from unroofed vesicle (soak two dry sterile swabs in vesicular fluid). Note: Gram stain is most sensitive during vesicular stage. Eschar stage: Perform Gram stain, culture, and PCR of ulcer base or edge of eschar without removing it. Ulcer (no vesicle or eschar present): Swab base of ulcer with pre-moistened sterile saline. A punch biopsy for IHC testing and a second biopsy for culture, Gram stain, PCR, and frozen-tissue IHC if patient has not received antibiotics should be obtained on all patients with suspected cutaneous anthrax. Include skin adjacent to papule or vesicle. If vesicles and eschars are both present, separate biopsies should be obtained. Serum: Collect acute serum within first 7 days of symptom onset, and convalescent serum 14-35 days after symptom onset. Collect blood for culture and PCR with evidence of systemic involvement.	Swabs: Moisten with sterile saline or water; transport in sterile tube at at 2-8° C. Transport swabs for PCR only at −70° C. Do not use transport medium. Tissue, fresh: ≥5 mm³; store and transport at 2-8°C (≤2 hr) or frozen at −70°C (>2 hr). Tissue, preserved in 10% buffered formalin: 1.0 cm³; store and transport at room temperature. Take biopsy of lesions for histopathology, preserved in 10% buffered formalin: 0.3 mm diameter; store and transport at room temperature. Freeze serum after separation at −20°C or colder, ship on dry ice. Ship part of sample (>1.0 mL) and retain part in case of shipping problems. Obtain blood for culture per local protocol. Collect blood for PCR in EDTA (purple top) tube. Ship at room temperature (≤2 hr transport) or 2-8°C (>2 hr transport).
Inhalational anthrax	If sputum is being produced, collect sputum specimen for Gram stain and culture (*note:* inhalational anthrax does not usually result in sputum production). Obtain blood for smear, culture, and PCR. If a pleural effusion is present, collect a specimen for culture, Gram stain, and PCR. Collect CSF if meningeal signs are present or meningitis is suspected for culture, Gram stain, and PCR. Serum: Collect acute serum within first 7 days of symptom onset, and convalescent serum 14-35 days after symptom onset. Biopsy material: Bronchial or pleural biopsy material can be evaluated if available.	Sputum: Transport at room temperature in sterile, screw-capped container (<1 hr transport time) or at 2-8°C (>1 hr transport time). Blood cultures: Obtain appropriate blood volume, number, and timing of sets per laboratory protocol; transport at room temperature. Blood for PCR: 10 mL in EDTA (for pediatric patients collect volumes allowable). Transport directly to laboratory at room temperature (2-8°C if transport ≥2 hr). Pleural fluid: Collect >1 mL in sterile container. Store and transport at 2-8°C. CSF: Transport directly to laboratory at room temperature, or 2-8°C if transport ≥2 hr. Transport serum or citrated plasma (separated and removed from clot) at 2-8°C (transport <2 hr) or freeze at −20°C or colder (transport ≥2 hr); ship on dry ice. Ship part of sample (>1.0 mL) and retain part in case of shipping problems. Preserve biopsies in 10% buffered formalin, and transport at room temperature.
Gastrointestinal anthrax	Obtain stool specimen for culture (>5 g). Obtain rectal swab from patients unable to produce stool (insert swab 1 in. beyond anal sphincter). Obtain blood for smear and culture (and possibly PCR testing). Blood cultures most likely to yield *B. anthracis* if taken 2-8 days postexposure and prior to administration of antibiotics. If ascites is present, obtain a specimen for Gram stain and culture (and possibly PCR testing).	Stool: Transport in sterile container unpreserved (≤1 hr transport time) or at 2-8°C in Cary-Blair medium or equivalent (>1 hr transport time); specimen >5.0 g. Blood: Transport at room temperature.
Anthrax meningitis	Obtain CSF specimen for Gram stain, culture, and PCR. Obtain blood for Gram stain, culture, and PCR.	See comments above for collection and transport of blood and CSF for Gram stain, culture, and PCR.

CSF, cerebrospinal fluid; EDTA, ethylenediaminetetraacetic acid; IHC, immunohistochemistry; PCR, polymerase chain reaction.
Modified from Infectious Diseases Society of America. Anthrax: current, comprehensive information on pathogenesis, microbiology, epidemiology, diagnosis, treatment, and prophylaxis. Available at http://www.cidrap.umn.edu/idsa/bt/anthrax/biofacts/anthraxfactsheet.html#_Specimen_Collection.[37]

those with inhalational anthrax succumbed to the disease despite aggressive intensive care unit (ICU) management. Early diagnosis, initiation of antibiotics, and aggressive management are critical to survival in inhalational anthrax.

During the 19th century, inhalational anthrax ("woolsorter's disease") occurred frequently among factory workers handling hair, wool, or hides contaminated with anthrax spores, with studies demonstrating that as many as 50% of samples of raw materials were contaminated with spores. In the Bradford district of England, 23 cases of inhalational anthrax were reported during the year 1880. Much of our experience with naturally acquired inhalational anthrax was gained in the preantibiotic era.[39,40] Studies in the 1950s revealed that during an 8-hour period, mill workers inhaled hundreds of spores smaller than 5 μm in size and some had positive nasal or pharyngeal cultures and yet inhalational anthrax remained extraordinarily uncommon.[9,21] In a serologic study of unvaccinated mill employees, nearly 15% had antibodies to anthrax.[41] It is evident that there is some threshold number of spores that even in the absence of prior immunization can be destroyed through the innate immune response.[42,43] As safeguards were built into the process so that wool was decontaminated prior to handling by workers and ventilation was improved in factories, the number of annual cases in developed countries in the second half of

the 19th century dropped significantly, and with the addition of vaccines and respirators in the 1950s and 1960s, cases dropped nearly to zero. In 2005 Lucey[44] proposed a modified staging system for inhalational anthrax that has generally become accepted as reflecting the course of both the terrorist-associated and recent naturally occurring inhalational anthrax and is utilized here.

As spores are inhaled, those larger than 5 μm are captured in the upper airways and transported out of the airways via the mucociliary elevator to the mouth. Spores in particles smaller than 5 μm may reach the terminal bronchioles and alveoli where they are quickly phagocytized by alveolar phagocytic cells and transported to draining lymph nodes and then to mediastinal lymph nodes. This clinically silent incubation is the symptomatic stage of inhalational anthrax and lasts 1-6 days after initial exposure. While it has been extremely rare to see inhalational cases develop more than 1 week after natural exposure, significant controversy exists about potential incubation periods of 60 days or longer following very low dose exposure.[45] This is further discussed in Chapter 325.

The first symptoms occur in the early prodromal stage with a "flu-like" illness characterized by low-grade fever, malaise, fatigue, and myalgias. Headache may be prominent, the fatigue may be profound, and blurred vision and photophobia occur in some cases. Dry cough and mild precordial discomfort are also seen in some patients. Patients may experience a biphasic illness during which they feel somewhat improved after the 2-3 days of the prodromal illness, while others progress directly to the intermediate-progressive stage associated with high fever, declining pulmonary status, respiratory distress, dyspnea, marked diaphoresis, pleuritic chest pain, and confusion or syncope. Blood cultures are typically positive in this stage, and mediastinal widening and pleural effusions are noted radiographically. Diagnosis during this stage and treatment with appropriate antibiotics and support are associated with survival in most cases.

With or without therapy patients may progress to the late-fulminant stage (often referred to in older literature as the fulminant acute phase). These patients have some combination of respiratory failure requiring intubation, sepsis, meningitis, and multi-organ failure associated with overwhelming bacteremia/toxemia. Death frequently occurs within 24 hours. In addition to aggressive antibiotics and intensive care management, these patients may be candidates for immunotherapeutics that currently remain investigational.

Inhalational anthrax is generally regarded as a mediastinal process and not a primary airspace disease. While the majority of inhaled spores are ingested by alveolar phagocytes and believed to germinate into vegetative organisms while being carried to (or after arrival in) the mediastinal lymph nodes, studies in nonhuman primates have demonstrated that some spores remain dormant for weeks to months.[9] As the vegetative bacilli destroy the macrophage and burst out of the cell, they infect other leukocytes and are released into the systemic circulation, leading to seeding of multiple organs including the meninges. Vegetative bacteria reach high levels in the blood and may be visible on staining of the buffy coat. Levels of the lethal toxin may become high enough terminally that a bacteria-free serum sample may contain enough toxin to kill another animal. The associated signs and symptoms of inhalational anthrax are not very specific, and discriminating between early inhalational anthrax and influenza can be quite difficult although the characteristic upper respiratory symptoms seen with influenza are usually absent in anthrax.[38,46]

Chest radiographs (CXR), or now more commonly CT scans, reveal a widened mediastinum and often bilateral pleural effusions. The progression of inhalational anthrax with CT from a 2001 bioterrorism case scan is seen in Figure 325-3.[47] Prior to the bioterrorist-associated anthrax cases in 2001, it was generally accepted that pulmonary infiltrates or consolidation were not typically prominent in inhalational anthrax (as it is not a primary parenchymal lung disease), but 7 of 10 inhalational cases in the 2001 attacks were noted to have pulmonary infiltrates. However, it was found that areas of pulmonary infiltrate on CXR actually corresponded to pulmonary edema and hyaline membrane formation at necropsy, not pneumonia with bacterial infiltration of the alveoli.[48,49] Pleural effusions are seen in most cases and are typically serosanguineous or hemorrhagic. They may rapidly reaccumulate after thoracentesis requiring placement of thoracostomy drainage tubes. Adequate pleural fluid drainage is important to achieve, as it was associated with a significant survival advantage in the meta-analysis of 82 inhalational cases.[38]

Table 208-1 outlines diagnostic specimen preparation, handling, and testing. Although inhalational anthrax is typically not associated with production of sputum, if it is produced sputum should be sent for Gram stain, culture, and PCR analysis. Pleural fluid is more frequently present and should be sent for diagnostic testing, as it is much more likely to yield bacilli on staining, culture, or PCR. Much more frequently than in cutaneous anthrax, the diagnosis of inhalational anthrax is made by finding positive blood cultures, and these should be obtained before any antibiotics are administered. Especially in cases that have received antibiotics, blood samples should be sent for PCR. Additionally, buffy coat smears can also be examined for the presence of bacilli, an ominous sign that the patient has entered the late fulminant stage of anthrax. It should be emphasized that immunohistologic studies of tissue specimens for the presence of bacillus cell wall and capsule antigens may be of particular value in treated patients because it may be positive when culture, Gram stain, and PCR are negative.[36]

GASTROINTESTINAL ANTHRAX

Oropharyngeal or intestinal infections with *B. anthracis* comprise gastrointestinal anthrax. This form of the disease is quite common in the grazing herbivores that are the usual hosts for anthrax infections but is uncommon in humans, responsible for approximately 1% of cases almost exclusively in rural areas of the developing world. It is generally felt to be under-reported.[50] Like inhalational anthrax, gastrointestinal anthrax is more likely to be associated with bacteremia, sepsis, and seeding of other sites and, without antibiotics, is associated with a mortality rate of approximately 40%. Recognition and early treatment are crucial to survival, but since many victims are impoverished inhabitants in remote regions, antibiotics are often delayed until the disease has progressed to later stages.

Most human cases are associated with the ingestion of undercooked meat (or uncooked dried meat) from an animal infected with anthrax. Large outbreaks in communities that have shared meat from dead animals have occurred, especially in Africa and Asia. In these settings, gastrointestinal anthrax cases may exceed the number of cutaneous cases.[50,51] Anthrax typically halts milk production in infected cows but even those still producing have not been demonstrated to shed bacilli or spores in their milk. Furthermore, pasteurization kills vegetative *B. anthracis* but not spores.[51] There have been no documented cases of natural infection from milk.

Typically symptoms develop 1-5 days after exposure for either oropharyngeal or intestinal disease, which may also be present concomitantly.

Oropharyngeal anthrax demonstrates symptoms and signs at the site of inoculation in the mouth or pharynx of swelling, severe pharyngitis, dysphagia, odynophagia, fever, and in some cases, respiratory distress due to marked edema and lymphadenitis. An ulcer may be observed in the mouth or pharynx, and in one Turkish series, it was localized to the tonsil in five of six patients and to the tongue in the sixth patient.[52] Pseudomembranes often form over the ulcer after the first week, bringing diphtheria into the differential diagnosis. Although significant neck swelling is seen in all oropharyngeal cases, massive facial and neck edema is occasionally seen. Consideration of a peritonsillar abscess often arises, but incision never yields purulent drainage. A swab of the base of oropharyngeal lesions typically reveals gram-positive bacilli and yields a positive culture.[53]

Intestinal disease occurs with infection of the stomach or bowel wall. The patient presents with nausea, vomiting, and fever, followed by severe abdominal pain often manifested as a surgical abdomen. Many cases will be associated with hematemesis, massive ascites, and bloody diarrhea. Secondary meningitis is also common.

Table 208-1 outlines diagnostic specimen preparation, handling, and testing. Blood, stool, and ascites samples should all be considered for culture and PCR testing.

ANTHRAX MENINGITIS

The frequency of anthrax meningitis is difficult to ascertain from published reports. Meningitis is an uncommon sequela of cutaneous anthrax but a frequent complication of the rarer inhalational or gastrointestinal disease, occurring in up to 50% of cases of the former. Although meningitis may rarely be the presenting symptom in some anthrax cases, it does not represent the initial site of infection (with the exception of a few case reports).[54,55]

As anthrax bacilli are released from macrophages into the bloodstream, the high-level bacteremia that ensues leads to seeding of other sites. The lethal and edema toxins have also been demonstrated to inhibit the innate immune responses of the blood-brain barrier in experimental infection, which may thus allow for easier access of the vegetative bacilli to the CNS.[56] Spread to the CNS may result from a focus of hemorrhagic necrosis that permits bacilli to pass to the meninges, cerebrospinal fluid (CSF), and brain parenchyma. The hallmark of anthrax meningitis is its hemorrhagic component associated with large gram-positive bacilli. CNS involvement may also include parenchymal brain hemorrhage and subarachnoid hemorrhage possibly owing to a diffuse cerebral arteritis or necrotizing vasculitis. As might be expected from anthrax infections in other sites, cerebral edema may also be prominent.

Symptoms of meningitis usually occur in the face of fulminant disease and are followed by death within 24 hours in 75% of cases. Initial symptoms include abrupt onset of severe headache, malaise, fever, chills, nausea, and vomiting. Meningeal signs such as nuchal rigidity may be absent early in the course but develop as the patient deteriorates. Seizures, delirium, and coma usually follow within hours. Death was inevitable in the preantibiotic era but is currently estimated at approximately 95% of cases.[57] Only with early and aggressive antibiotic therapy focused on CNS penetration is there potential for survival. Table 208-1 outlines diagnostic specimen preparation, handling, and testing for anthrax meningitis. Blood and CSF should be obtained for stains, culture, and PCR testing.

Treatment

Rapid initiation of appropriate antibiotic therapy is critical in the treatment of anthrax, especially in the more severe non-cutaneous cases. Table 208-2 outlines initial consideration for treatment of anthrax in each of its clinical presentations.

Penicillin had been the drug of choice for all types of anthrax since the 1940s, but naturally occurring strains are increasingly reported to be resistant. Fortunately, *B. anthracis* is sensitive to a broad range of antibiotics including tetracyclines, macrolides, aminoglycosides, fluoroquinolones, carbapenems, clindamycin, rifampin, chloramphenicol, and first-generation (but not second- or third-generation) cephalosporins.[58] In a study of 96 French anthrax isolates collected from the environment, animals, and one human case between 1994 and 2000,

there was uniform resistance to third-generation cephalosporins, aztreonam, and trimethoprim-sulfamethoxazole. Of the strains 11.5% demonstrated penicillin and amoxicillin resistance as well as decreased sensitivity to second-generation cephalosporins, but there was nearly 100% sensitivity to the other 16 antibiotics tested.[59] The minimum inhibitory concentrations (MICs) for many antibiotics from four recent studies have been summarized by CIDRAP-IDSA (Table 208-3).[37,58-61]

Most strains of naturally occurring *B. anthracis* have a chromosomally mediated, weak, inducible β-lactamase and cephalosporinase, and there have been rare reports of the development of resistance during therapy with penicillin. However, it must be emphasized that it is relatively easy to select for antibiotic-resistant strains of *B. anthracis* in the laboratory, and the resistance pattern of bioterrorist strains must be carefully assessed and therapy modified accordingly.[62,63] The guidelines for bioterrorism-associated anthrax recommend use of fluoroquinolones and doxycycline until resistance testing is available, as β-lactam resistance in such strains is presumed to be likely.[14]

CUTANEOUS ANTHRAX

Naturally acquired (i.e., with no possibility of intentional release of spores) cutaneous anthrax with no evidence of systemic symptoms has been traditionally treated with oral penicillin for 7-10 days (amoxicillin 500 mg every 8 hours, or 80 mg/kg/day in divided doses every 8 hours in children, not to exceed 500 mg every 8 hours). Although penicillin resistance appears in approximately 10% of strains of *B. anthracis*, the consensus of authorities convened by the CDC recommended continued use of penicillin for naturally acquired cutaneous disease coupled with sensitivity testing of the isolate and close follow-up of the patient.[64]

TABLE 208-2	Treatment Recommendations for Inhalational, Gastrointestinal, and Oropharyngeal Anthrax*	
Patient Category	*Initial IV Therapy*[††]	*Oral Regimens (continue therapy for 60 days [IV and PO combined])*
Adults	Ciprofloxacin, 400 mg every 12 hr *or* Doxycycline, 100 mg every 12 hr[¶] *and* One or two additional antimicrobials (agents with in vitro activity include rifampin, vancomycin, penicillin, ampicillin, chloramphenicol, imipenem, clindamycin, and clarithromycin)[¶]	Patients should be treated with IV therapy initially.[††] Treatment can be switched to oral therapy when clinically appropriate: Ciprofloxacin, 500 mg PO twice daily *or* Doxycycline, 100 mg PO twice daily
Children	Ciprofloxacin, 10-15 mg/kg every 12 hr not to exceed 1 g/day[#] *or* Doxycycline[¶**]: >8 yr and >45 kg: 100 mg every 12 hr not to exceed 200 mg/day >8 yr and ≤45 kg: 2.2 mg/kg every 12 hr not to exceed 200 mg/day ≤8 yr: 2.2 mg/kg every 12 hr *and* One or two additional antimicrobials (see agents listed under therapy for adults)[¶]	Patients should be treated with IV therapy initially.[††] Treatment can be switched to oral therapy when clinically appropriate: Ciprofloxacin, 10-15 mg/kg PO every 12 hr not to exceed 1 g/day *or* Doxycycline**: >8 yr and >45 kg: 100 mg PO every 12 hr >8 yr and ≤45 kg: 2.2 mg/kg PO every 12 hr not to exceed 20 mg/day ≤8 yr: 2.2 mg/kg PO every 12 hr not to exceed 200 mg/day
Pregnant women[§]	Same as for nonpregnant adults (high death rate from the infection outweighs risk posed by antimicrobial agent)	Patients should be treated with IV therapy initially.[††] Treatment can be switched to PO when clinically appropriate. Oral therapy regimens are the same as for nonpregnant adults.
Immunocompromised persons	Same as for nonimmunocompromised persons and children	Same as for nonimmunocompromised persons and children.

*Meningitis involvement must be assumed in all systemic infections. Antibiotic selection must consider penetration across blood-brain barrier. These treatment recommendations were made during U.S. 2001 anthrax outbreak. In other situations, antimicrobial susceptibility testing should be used to guide therapy decisions.

[†]Ciprofloxacin or doxycycline should be considered an essential part of first-line therapy for inhalational anthrax.

[‡]Steroids may be considered an adjunct therapy for patients with severe edema and for meningitis based on experience with bacterial meningitis of other etiologies.

[§]Although tetracyclines are not recommended for pregnant women, their use may be indicated for life-threatening illness. Adverse effects on developing teeth and bones are dose-related; therefore, doxycycline might be used for a short time (7-14 days) before 6 months of gestation.

[¶]If meningitis is suspected, doxycycline may be less optimal because of poor central nervous system penetration.

[¶]Because of concerns of constitutive and inducible beta-lactamases in *B. anthracis* isolates, penicillin and ampicillin should not be used alone. Consultation with an infectious disease specialist is advised. Other agents with in vitro activity include tetracycline, linezolid, macrolides, aminoglycosides, and cefazolin. *B. anthracis* strains are naturally resistant to sulfamethoxazole, trimethoprim, cefuroxime, cefotaxime sodium, aztreonam, and ceftazidime.

[#]If intravenous ciprofloxacin is not available, oral ciprofloxacin may be acceptable because it is rapidly and well absorbed from gastrointestinal tract with no substantial loss by first-pass metabolism. Maximum serum concentrations are attained 1-2 hr after oral dosing but may not be achieved if vomiting or ileus is present.

**American Academy of Pediatrics recommends treatment of young children with tetracyclines for serious infections (e.g., Rocky Mountain Spotted Fever). Dose should not exceed 200 mg/day.

[††]Initial therapy may be altered based on clinical course of patient; one or two antimicrobial agents (e.g., ciprofloxacin or doxycycline) may be adequate as patient improves.

IV, intravenously; PO, orally.

Adapted from Centers for Disease Control and Prevention (CDC). Update: investigation of bioterrorism-related anthrax and interim guidelines for exposure management and antimicrobial therapy, October 2001. *MMWR Morb Mortal Wkly Rep.* 2001;26;50:909-919 (erratum in: *MMWR Morb Mortal Wkly Rep.* 2001;50:962); and Stern E, Uhde K, Shadomy S, et al. Conference report on public health and clinical guidelines for anthrax. *Emerg Infect Dis.* 2008;14:pii:07-0969.

TABLE 208-3	Minimum Inhibitory Concentrations (MICs) of Various Antibiotics for *Bacillus anthracis* Isolates as Identified in Four Studies[58-61]							
	Study							
	Mohammed[60] 2002		**Coker[58] 2002**		**Cavallo[59] 2002**		**Turnbull[61] 2004**	
Antibiotic	MIC range*	S-I-R (%)†	MIC range*	S-I-R (#)†	MIC range*	S-I-R (%)†	MIC range*‡	S-I-R (%)†
Amoxicillin					0.125-16	88.5-0-11.5		
Amoxicillin-clavulanic acid							0.016-0.5	100-0-0
Azithromycin							1-12	26-64-10
Aztreonam					1≥128	0-0-100		
Cefaclor			0.125-0.75	25-0-0				
Cefotaxime							3-32	1-0-99
Cefoxitin					1-64	74-15.3-10.7		
Ceftriaxone	4-32	22-78-0			4-64	1-100-0		
Cefuroxime			6-48	1-19-5				
Cephalexin			0.38-2	25-0-0				
Cephalothin					0.125-32	83.2-12.2-24.6		
Chloramphenicol	2-8	100-0-0			1-4	100-0-0		
Ciprofloxacin	0.03-0.12§	100-0-0§	0.032-0.38	25-0-0	0.03-0.5	100-0-0	0.032-0.094	100-0-0
Clindamycin	≤0.5-1	94-6-0			0.125-1	100-0-0		
Doxycycline			0.094-0.38	25-0-0	0.125-0.25	100-0-0		
Erythromycin	0.5-1¶	3.97-0¶			0.5-4	95.4-4.6-0	0.5-4	15-85-0
Gatifloxacin					0.125-0.125	100-0-0		
Gentamicin					0.125-0.5	100-0-0	0.064-0.5	100-0-0
Imipenem					0.125-2	100-0-0		
Levofloxacin					0.03-1	100-0-0		
Nalidixic acid					0.125-32	94.8-4.2-1		
Ofloxacin					0.06-2	99-1-0		
Penicillin	≤0.06-128	97-0-3	<0.016-0.5	22-0-3	0.125-16	88.5-0-11.5	<0.016≥32	97-0-3
Pefloxacin					0.03-1	100-0-0		
Piperacillin					0.25-32	99-1-0		
Rifampin	≤0.25-0.5	100-0-0			0.125-0.5	100-0-0		
Streptomycin					0.5-2	100-0-0		
Teicoplanin					0.125-0.5	100-0-0		
Tetracycline	0.03-0.06	100-0-0					0.016-0.094	100-0-0
Tobramycin			0.25-1.5	25-0-0				
Vancomycin	0.5-2	100-0-0			0.25-2	100-0-0	0.75-5	99-1-0

*MIC values in µg/mL.

†Categorical interpretation: susceptible (S), intermediate (I), and resistant (R); expressed as percent of isolates (%) or number of isolates (#), per author preference. (*Note*: Standard interpretive criteria for *B. anthracis* have not been established.)

‡MIC determination by Etest.

§A subset of 20 isolates were tested and found to be susceptible to clinafloxacin, gatifloxacin, gemifloxacin, levofloxacin, moxifloxacin, ofloxacin, sparfloxacin, and trovafloxacin.

¶A subset of 20 isolates were also tested to clarithromycin (MIC range: 0.12-0.25 µg/mL), azithromycin (MIC range: 1-2 µg/mL), and doxycycline (MICs ≤ 0.015 µg/mL).

Available at: http://www.cidrap.umn.edu/idsa/bt/anthrax/biofacts/anthraxfactsheet.html.[37]

Unless there is clear evidence that an infection was naturally acquired, it should be considered to result from an intentional release with presumed concomitant inhalation of spores, and 60 days of treatment with a fluoroquinolone or doxycycline is recommended as first-line therapy (ciprofloxacin 500 mg orally twice daily, or levofloxacin 500 mg daily, or doxycycline 100 mg orally twice daily). If cultures were obtained from the lesions, modifications of the regimen may be made in response to the resistance profile seen. If systemic symptoms have developed, the patient should be treated with intravenous antibiotics as described below for inhalational anthrax.

INHALATIONAL, GASTROINTESTINAL, AND MENINGEAL ANTHRAX

These frequently lethal forms of anthrax require aggressive management with intravenous antibiotics, a vasopressor, a ventilator, and ICU support. The use of additional modalities such as anthrax immune globulin (AIG) or anthrax monoclonal antibodies should be considered in consultation with the CDC and other experts. Patients frequently demonstrate an acute, rapid deterioration as the anthrax progresses to the fulminant stages of bacteremia and, when possible, should be closely monitored in the ICU, even if they initially appear clinically stable.

Initial therapy should include an intravenous fluoroquinolone or doxycycline in combination with one or two additional antibiotics such as rifampin, clindamycin, vancomycin, a carbapenem, penicillin, ampicillin, chloramphenicol, linezolid, aminoglycosides, or clarithromycin. If meningitis is suspected, a quinolone and not doxycycline should be utilized because of the poor CNS penetration of doxycycline. The choice of the second and third antibiotics is somewhat arbitrary and may be made out of concern for concomitant meningitis and the necessity of improved CNS penetration seen with penicillin, carbapenems, rifampin, vancomycin, and chloramphenicol or the possibility of diminishing bacterial toxin synthesis with rifampin, clindamycin, doxycycline, and clarithromycin.[65]

Owing to the critical need to use the most effective antimicrobial agents, the usual avoidance of quinolones and tetracyclines in children and pregnancy is superseded. As the resistance profile of the anthrax strain is determined and clinical improvement has been demonstrated, modifications of regimens can be made to diminish possible toxicity.

Patients may also be transitioned to oral therapy as improvement occurs. Since the 2001 anthrax attacks, the recommendations for duration of therapy have been for a total of 60 days out of concern for delayed germination of inhaled spores. In most cases, a minimum of 10-14 days of intravenous therapy are required, followed by oral therapy. Recent data from studies in nonhuman primates with bacteremic inhalational anthrax showed that after a short course of antibiotic therapy animals developed an immune response and were protected against death from the delayed germination of retained spores after discontinuance of antibiotics.[66]

MANAGEMENT OF PLEURAL EFFUSION

Inhalational anthrax is associated with significant lymphatic obstruction leading to pulmonary edema and rapid accumulation of pleural fluid. Pleural fluid in the 2001 cases demonstrated the highest levels of anthrax bacilli as well as bacterial cell wall and capsular antigens.[49] PCR for *B. anthracis* was most often positive from the pleural fluid.[67] After review of the cases of inhalational anthrax in 2001 and 2006, as well as the statistically significant decrease in mortality seen in the series of cases from 1990 to 2005, the consensus of experts is that early and aggressive management of pleural effusions with repeated thoracentesis or thoracostomy drainage is associated with increased survival.[29,38,48,49] In addition to the improved oxygenation afforded by minimizing loss of lung volume, study of toxin levels in the 2006 case demonstrated that pleural fluid has very high levels of LF.[68] This is essentially subjecting inhalational anthrax to the same standard of care as for an empyema or a complicated parapneumonic effusion.

ROLE OF STEROIDS AND MANAGEMENT OF SEVERE EDEMA

The addition of corticosteroids has been advocated for treatment of cerebral edema and increased intracranial pressure in anthrax meningitis, based upon its effect in improving outcomes in pneumococcal meningitis, although no controlled studies have been reported for anthrax. In addition, most recommendations for treatment of increased intracranial pressure include the use of hyperventilation and mannitol. Steroid treatment has also been considered for the severe edema often associated with cutaneous, inhalational, and gastrointestinal cases resulting in life-threatening obstruction, massive pleural effusions, and ascites despite any controlled studies demonstrating efficacy.[69] Further animal studies with steroids and elucidation of the pathogenesis of fluid accumulation and meningitis will give more objective evidence to support the use of steroids in human anthrax.

ANTHRAX IMMUNOTHERAPEUTICS

In the preantibiotic era, treatment of anthrax included incision, cautery, and application of acid. In the late 1890s, French and Italian researchers developed animal-derived hyperimmune serum that eventually became the standard of care in North America by the 1920s and was used well into the 1950s. Antiserum was used to treat all forms of anthrax and was reported to have decreased the overall mortality rate of cutaneous cases from 24% to 6% in uncontrolled studies.[70] Serum preparations used and quantity and routes of administration were almost arbitrarily determined, but case reports of survival of even bacteremic patients and lack of other effective treatments established antiserum as the treatment of choice. With the development of effective antibiotics, the use of antiserum gradually fell out of favor in most of the world, and it is no longer available in most countries. Anthrax antiserum is still available in some countries of the former Soviet Union and China, although it is seldom used.

Since the 2001 anthrax attacks, because of the high mortality associated with inhalational anthrax and the renewed appreciation of the role of the toxins in pathogenesis, there has been renewed interest in the development of adjunctive therapies including antibodies.

Currently, anthrax immunoglobulin (AIG) is produced from plasmaphoresis of individuals recently immunized with the licensed vaccine that consists mainly of PA. It is produced as an Investigational New Drug (IND) under contract to the U.S. government by Cangene Corporation in Canada. It was used in conjunction with antibiotics and ICU management for a single naturally acquired inhalation case in Pennsylvania in 2006.[68]

Human monoclonal antibodies (MAbs) with high affinity for PA, raxibacumab (ABthrax) and MDX-1303 (Valortim) are currently in production for stockpiling by the U.S. Department of Homeland Security (but also remain in the final stages of approval from the U.S. Food and Drug Administration [FDA]). MDX-1303 has demonstrated efficacy in the rabbit and nonhuman primate model in which 90% to 100% of the animals given intramuscular MAbs at the time of aerosol challenge with 200 times the LD_{50} survived while all control animals died within 1 week.[71] Phase 1 human studies suggest that a single intramuscular dose could give antibody levels comparable to those seen in vaccinated animals for up to 2 months.[72] The role of anthrax MAb in treatment of anthrax cases remains undefined but will likely be used on a compassionate use, emergency IND basis while studies are ongoing.

Potential use of anthrax immunotherapeutics can be considered in the United States after consultation with the CDC.

VACCINATION

Vaccines against anthrax for both animals and humans have been used for over 100 years, and effective use of live attenuated veterinary vaccines has been associated with the decrease in animal and human cases in many regions of the world. Although there is some anecdotal evidence that immunity develops after infection based upon the observation that human anthrax reinfections are rare and less severe, the best data are from studies in nonhuman primates demonstrating resistance to reinfection after recovery from inhalational anthrax.[73] Humoral immunity plays the critical role in the response to anthrax. Anti-PA antibody is the most important antibody, and PA is the protective immunogen and the basis of the protection afforded by the human vaccines currently available. The role of the immune response to the other toxin components, EF and LF, in protection from anthrax infection is controversial with conflicting studies demonstrating either additional or no added protection benefit when used to vaccinate animals despite adequate antibody responses.[74-76]

The currently approved U.S. human vaccine, anthrax vaccine adsorbed (AVA) or AVA BioThrax, is a cell-free culture supernatant containing PA, derived from an unencapsulated, toxin-producing strain of *B. anthracis,* that has been adsorbed to an aluminum hydroxide gel. The vaccine, developed by Wright and co-workers in the early 1950s, was licensed in 1970 and has been used for preexposure prophylaxis by veterinarians; laboratory, textile, and other workers who may be occupationally exposed; and the U.S. military. Vaccination, although currently not approved by the FDA for postexposure, should also be used (under IND) in conjunction with antibiotics for the optimal management of postexposure prophylaxis of inhalational anthrax.[65]

The FDA approved a new five-dose regimen and administration route for the AVA in December 2008. The change from subcutaneous to intramuscular administration decreased local side effects and dropping the two-week dose simplifies the regimen with no significant decrease in immunogenicity at 7 months.[76a] At 0 and 4 weeks 0.5 mL of AVA is administered intramuscularly followed by subsequent injections at 6, 12, and 18 months as well as yearly boosters. The vaccine approved in the U.K., anthrax vaccine precipitated (AVP), is similar to AVA but is given as a four-dose series at 0, 3, and 6 weeks and 6 months, followed by annual boosters. Mild local side effects are as common with AVA as with other common adult vaccines, as are rare, idiosyncratic, serious side effects.[77] In a U.S. Army study of 601 AVA recipients, 20% reported symptoms that they personally judged as so mild that they could be ignored, 15% reported symptoms that affected their activity for a short time but did not limit their work duties, 8% reported short-term symptoms that were relieved with nonprescription medication, and only 2% reported symptoms unrelieved with medication with short-term limitation of their work duties. Itching, subcutaneous nodules, and erythema were the most commonly reported symptoms, and reported symptoms were more common in women than in men.[78]

The safety of AVA vaccine has been the object of considerable controversy in relation to its mandatory use in the U.S. military and objections to its side effects and purported long-term effects. However, the safety and efficacy of AVA were confirmed in an extensive review by the Institute of Medicine of the National Academy of Sciences in 2002[79] and additional safety studies since then.[5] In a review by the CDC of those given the vaccine as postexposure prophylaxis after the 2001 anthrax events, no serious adverse events were noted.[80] As a cell-free filtrate, AVA cannot cause anthrax, it has not been associated with birth defects, and a possible association with optic neuritis and multiple sclerosis was shown not to be statistically significant.[79,81]

A live attenuated vaccine consisting of spores from an unencapsulated toxigenic strain of B. anthracis has been used in the former Soviet Union since 1953. The vaccine given via scarification or subcutaneously is said to be reasonably well tolerated and is reported to afford some degree of protection against cutaneous anthrax.[78] The Chinese developed a similar live spore vaccine in the 1960s.

Since the 2001 anthrax attacks there has been an intense effort to produce newer anthrax vaccines with a less cumbersome dosing schedule and less local reactogenicity. A highly purified, recombinant PA-based vaccine adjuvanted with aluminum hydroxide has been shown to protect nonhuman primates against inhalational anthrax with only one or two doses and is undergoing clinical trials.[82] Additional efforts to improve PA-based vaccines include using PA with other adjuvants and delivery systems and given by different routes. Research has also identified additional antigens as potential future vaccine candidates, such as the anthrax capsule[83,84] and spore proteins[85] that have been shown to be protective in experimental animals.

REFERENCES

1. Dirckx J. Virgil on anthrax. Am J Dermatopathol. 1981;3:191-195.
2. Jay V. The legacy of Robert Koch. Arch Pathol Lab Med. 2001;125:1148-1149.
3. Carter T. The dissemination of anthrax from imported wool: Kidderminster 1900-1914. Occup Environ Med. 2004;61:103-107.
4. Abramova F, Grinberg L, Yampolskaya O, et al. Pathology of inhalational anthrax in 42 cases from the Sverdlovsk outbreak of 1979. Proc Natl Acad Sci U S A. 1993;90:2291-2294.
5. Stone R. Peering into the shadows: Iraq's bioweapons program. Science. 2002;297:1110-1112.
6. Redmond C, Pearce MJ, Manchee RJ, et al. Deadly relic of the Great War. Nature. 1998;393:747-748.
7. Glassman H. Industrial inhalation anthrax (discussion). Bacteriol Rev. 1966;30:657-659.
8. Gochenour W, Sawyer W, Henderson J, et al. On the recognition and therapy of Simian woolsorter's disease. J Hyg. 1963;61:317-322.
9. Henderson D, Peacock S, Belton F. Observations on the prophylaxis of experimental pulmonary anthrax in the monkey. J Hyg. 1956;54:28-36.
10. Stanley J, Smith H. Purification of factor I and recognition of a third factor of the anthrax toxin. J Gen Microbiol. 1961;26:49-66.
11. Young J, Collier R. Anthrax toxin: receptor binding, internalization, pore formation, and translocation. Annu Rev Biochem. 2007;76:243-265.
12. Baldari C, Tonello F, Paccani S, et al. Anthrax toxins: a paradigm of bacterial immune suppression. Trends Immunol. 2006;27:434-440.
13. Tournier J, Quesnel Hellmann A, Cleret A. Contribution of toxins to the pathogenesis of inhalational anthrax. Cell Microbiol. 2007;9:555-565.
14. Inglesby T, O'Toole T, Henderson D, et al. Anthrax as a biological weapon, 2002: updated recommendations for management. JAMA. 2002;287:2236-2252.
15. Sherer K, Li Y, Cui X. Lethal and edema toxins in the pathogenesis of Bacillus anthracis septic shock. Am J Respir Crit Care Med. 2007;175:211-221.
16. Bolcome R, Sullivan S, Zeller R, et al. Anthrax lethal toxin induces cell death-independent permeability in zebrafish vasculature. Proc Natl Acad Sci U S A. 2008;105:2439-2444.
17. Cendrowski S, MacArthur W, Hanna P. Bacillus anthracis requires siderophore biosynthesis for growth in macrophages and mouse virulence. Mol Microbiol. 2004;51:407-417.
18. Gat O, Mendelson I, Chitlaru T, et al. The solute-binding component of a putative Mn(II) ABC transporter (MntA) is a novel Bacillus anthracis virulence determinant. Mol Microbiol. 2005;58:533-551.
19. Heffernan B, Thomason B, Herring-Palmer A, et al. Bacillus anthracis anthrolysin O and three phospholipases C are functionally redundant in a murine model of inhalation anthrax. FEMS Microbiol Lett. 2007;271:98-105.
20. Shatalin K, Gusarov I, Avetissova E, et al. Bacillus anthracis-derived nitric oxide is essential for pathogen virulence and survival in macrophages. Proc Natl Acad Sci U S A. 2008;105:1009-1013.
21. World Health Organization (WHO). World Anthrax Data Site, 2003. Available at: <http://www.vetmed.lsu.edu/whocc/mp_world.htm>; Accessed March 19, 2009.
22. Smith KL, deVos V, Bryden H, et al. Bacillus anthracis diversity in Kruger National Park. J Clin Microbiol. 2000;38:3780-3784.
23. Smith KL, deVos V, Bryden HB, et al. Meso-scale ecology of anthrax in southern Africa: a pilot study of diversity and clustering. J Appl Microbiol. 1999;87:204-207.
24. Sterne M. Distribution and economic importance of anthrax. Fed Proc. 1967;26:1493-1495.
25. Davies J. A major epidemic of anthrax in Zimbabwe. Cent Afr J Med. 1982;28:291-298.
26. Davies J. A major epidemic of anthrax in Zimbabwe: the experience at the Beatrice Road Infectious Diseases Hospital, Harare. Cent Afr J Med. 1985;31:176-180.
27. Clegg SB, Turnbull PC, Foggin CM, et al. Massive outbreak of anthrax in wildlife in the Malilangwe Wildlife Reserve, Zimbabwe. Vet Rec. 2007;160:113-118.
28. Hugh-Jones ME, deVos V. Anthrax and wildlife. Rev Sci Tech. 2002;21:359-383.
29. Centers for Disease Control (CDC). Inhalation anthrax associated with dried animal hides—Pennsylvania and New York City, 2006. MMWR Morb Mortal Wkly Rep. 2006;55:280-282.
30. Centers for Disease Control (CDC). Cutaneous anthrax associated with drum making using goat hides from West Africa—Connecticut, 2007. MMWR Morb Mortal Wkly Rep. 2008;57:628-631.
31. de Vos V. The ecology of anthrax in the Kruger National Park, South Africa. Salisbury Med Bull. 1990;68(Spec Suppl):19-23.
32. Turnbull PCB. Guidelines for the Surveillance and Control of Anthrax in Human and Animals. 3rd ed. Geneva: WHO; 1998. Available at: <http://www.who.int/csr/resources/publications/anthrax/whoemczdi986text.pdf>; Accessed March 19, 2009.
33. Gold H. Anthrax: a report of one hundred seventeen cases. AMA Arch Intern Med. 1955;96:387-396.
34. Roche K, Chang M, Lazarus H. Cutaneous anthrax infection. N Engl J Med. 2001;345:1611.
35. Cinti S, Robinson-Dunn B, Mackler N. Anthrax. Available at: <http://pier.acponline.org/physicians/public/d892/primary.prevention/d892-s1.html>; Accessed March 19, 2009.
36. Quinn C, Dull P, Semenova V, et al. Immune responses to Bacillus anthracis protective antigen in patients with bioterrorism-related cutaneous or inhalation anthrax. J Infect Dis. 2004;190:1228-1236.
37. Infectious Diseases Society of America. Anthrax: current, comprehensive information on pathogenesis, microbiology, epidemiology, diagnosis, treatment, and prophylaxis. Available at: <http://www.cidrap.umn.edu/idsa/bt/anthrax/biofacts/anthraxfactsheet.html>; Accessed March 19, 2009.
38. Holty J, Bravata D, Liu H, et al. Systematic review: a century of inhalational anthrax cases from 1900 to 2005. Ann Intern Med. 2006;144:270-280.
39. Plotkin S, Brachman P, Utell M, et al. An epidemic of inhalation anthrax, the first in the twentieth century. 1. Clinical features. Am J Med. 1960;29:992-1001.
40. Macher A. Industry-related outbreak of human anthrax, Massachusetts, 1868. Emerg Infect Dis. 2002;8:1182.
41. Norman P, Ray J, Brachman P, et al. Serological testing for anthrax antibodies in workers in a goat hair processing mill. Am J Hyg. 1960;72:32-37.
42. Chakrabarty K, Wu W, Leland Booth J, et al. Human lung innate immune response to Bacillus anthracis spore infection. Infect Immun. 2007;75:3729-3738.
43. Coleman M, Thran B, Morse S, et al. Inhalation anthrax: dose response and risk analysis. Biosecur Bioterr. 2008;6:147-159.
44. Lucey D. Anthrax. In: Mandell G, Bennett J, Dolin R, eds. Principles and Practice of Infectious Diseases. 6th ed. Philadelphia: Elsevier Churchill Livingstone; 2005:3620.
45. Brookmeyer R, Johnson E, Bollinger R. Modeling the optimum duration of antibiotic prophylaxis in an anthrax outbreak. Proc Natl Acad Sci U S A. 2003;100:10129-10132.
46. Fine A, Wong J, Fraser H, et al. Is it influenza or anthrax? A decision analytic approach to the treatment of patients with influenza-like illnesses. Ann Emerg Med. 2004;43:318-328.
47. Wood B, DeFranco B, Ripple M, et al. Inhalational anthrax: radiologic and pathologic findings in two cases. Am J Roentgenol. 2003;181:1071-1078.
48. Jernigan J, Stephens D, Ashford D, et al. Bioterrorism-related inhalational anthrax: the first 10 cases reported in the United States. Emerg Infect Dis. 2001;7:933-943.
49. Guarner J, Jernigan J, Shieh W. Pathology and pathogenesis of bioterrorism-related inhalational anthrax. Am J Pathol. 2003;163:701-709.
50. Sirisanthana T, Brown A. Anthrax of the gastrointestinal tract. Emerg Infect Dis. 2002;8:649-651.
51. Beatty M, Ashford D, Griffin P, et al. Gastrointestinal anthrax. Arch Intern Med. 2003;163:2527-2531.
52. Doganay M, Almac A, Hanagasi R. Primary throat anthrax. Scand J Infect Dis. 1986;18:415-419.
53. Sirisanthana T, Navachareon N, Tharavichitkul P, et al. Outbreak of oral-pharyngeal anthrax: an unusual manifestation of human infection with Bacillus anthracis. Am J Trop Med Hyg. 1984;33:144-150.
54. Haight T. Anthrax meningitis: review of the literature and report of two cases with autopsies. Am J Med Sci. 1952;224:57-69.
55. Sejvar J, Tenover F, Stephens D. Management of anthrax meningitis. Lancet Infect Dis. 2005;5:287-295.
56. van Sorge NM, Ebrahimi CM, McGillivray SM, et al. Anthrax toxins inhibit neutrophil signaling pathways in brain endothelium and contribute to the pathogenesis of meningitis. PLoS ONE. 2008;3:e2964.
57. Lanska D. Anthrax meningoencephalitis. Neurology. 2002;59:327-334.
58. Coker P, Smith K, Hugh-Jones M. Antimicrobial susceptibilities of diverse Bacillus anthracis isolates. Antimicrob Agents Chemother. 2002;46:3843-3845.
59. Cavallo J, Ramisse F, Girardet M, et al. Antibiotic susceptibilities of 96 isolates of Bacillus anthracis isolated in France between 1994 and 2000. Antimicrob Agents Chemother. 2002;46:2307-2309.
60. Mohammed M, Marston C, Popovic T, et al. Antimicrobial susceptibility testing of Bacillus anthracis: comparison of results obtained by using the National Committee for Clinical Laboratory Standards broth microdilution reference and Etest agar gradient diffusion methods. J Clin Microbiol. 2002;40:1902-1907.
61. Turnbull P, Sirianni N, LeBron C. MICs of selected antibiotics for Bacillus anthracis, Bacillus cereus, Bacillus thuringiensis, and Bacillus mycoides from a range of clinical and environmental sources as determined by the Etest. J Clin Microbiol. 2004;42:3626-3634.
62. Brook I, Elliott T, Pryor II H, et al. In vitro resistance of Bacillus anthracis Sterne to doxycycline, macrolides and quinolones. Int J Antimicrob Agents. 2001;18:559-562.
63. Athamna A, Athamna M, Abu-Rashed N, et al. Selection of Bacillus anthracis isolates resistant to antibiotics. J Antimicrob Chemother. 2004;54:424-428.
64. Stern E, Uhde K, Shadomy S, et al. Conference report on public health and clinical guidelines for anthrax. Emerg Infect Dis. 2008;14:07-0969.
65. Bartlett J, Inglesby Jr T, Borio L. Management of anthrax. Clin Infect Dis. 2002;35:851-858.
66. Vietri N, Purcell B, Tobery S, et al. A short course of antibiotic treatment is effective in preventing death from experimental inhalational anthrax. J Infect Dis. 2009;199:336-341.
67. Hoffmaster A, Meyer R, Bowen M, et al. Evaluation and validation of real-time polymerase chain reaction assay for rapid iden-

tification of *Bacillus anthracis*. *Emerg Infect Dis*. 2002;8:1178-1181.
68. Walsh J, Pesik N, Quinn C, et al. A case of naturally acquired inhalation anthrax: clinical care and analyses of anti–protective antigen immunoglobulin G and lethal factor. *Clin Infect Dis*. 2007;44:968-971.
69. Doust J, Sarkarzadeh A, Kavoossi K. Corticosteroid in treatment of malignant edema of chest wall and neck (anthrax). *Dis Chest*. 1968;53:773-774.
70. Regan J. The advantage of serum therapy as shown by comparison of carious methods of treatment of anthrax. *Am J Med Sci*. 1921;162:406-423.
71. Vitale L, Blanset D, Lowy I, et al. Prophylaxis and therapy of inhalational anthrax by a novel monoclonal antibody to protective antigen that mimics vaccine-induced immunity. *Infect Immun*. 2006;74:5840-5847.
72. Subramanian G, Cronin P, Poley G, et al. A phase 1 study of PAmAb, a fully human monoclonal antibody against *Bacillus anthracis* protective antigen, in healthy volunteers. *Clin Infect Dis*. 2005;41:1220.
73. Vietri N, Purcell B, Lawler J, et al. Short-course postexposure antibiotic prophylaxis combined with vaccination protects against experimental inhalational anthrax. *Proc Natl Acad Sci U S A*. 2006;102:7813-7816.
74. Mahlandt B, Klein F, Lincoln R, et al. Immunologic studies of anthrax. 4. Evaluation of the immunogenicity of three components of anthrax toxin. *J Immunol*. 1966;96:727-733.
75. Wright G, Green T, Kanode RJ. Studies on immunity in anthrax. 5. Immunizing activity of alum-precipitated protective antigen. *J Immunol*. 1954;73:387-391.
76. Little S, Knudson G. Comparative efficacy of *Bacillus anthracis* live spore vaccine and protective antigen vaccine against anthrax in the guinea pig. *Infect Immun*. 1986;52:509-512.
76a. BioThrax [package insert]. Lansing, MI, Emergent BioDefense Operations Lansing Inc; 2009.
77. Grabenstein J. Vaccines: Countering anthrax—vaccines and immunoglobulins. *Clin Infect Dis*. 2008;46:129-136.
78. Brachman P, Friedlander A, Grabenstein J. Anthrax vaccines. In: Plotkin S, Orenstein W, Offit P, eds. *Vaccines*. Philadelphia: Saunders Elsevier; 2008:111-126.
79. Committee to Assess the Safety and Efficacy of the Anthrax Vaccine MFA. *The Anthrax Vaccine: Is It Safe? Does It Work?* Washington, DC: Institute of Medicine (IOM); 2002.
80. Tierney B, Martin S, Franzke L, et al. Serious adverse events among participants in the Centers for Disease Control and Prevention's Anthrax Vaccine and Antimicrobial Availability Program for persons at risk for bioterrorism-related inhalational anthrax. *Clin Infect Dis*. 2003;37:905-911.
81. Payne D, Rose C, Kerrison J, et al. Anthrax vaccination and risk of optic neuritis in the United States military, 1998-2003. *Arch Neurol*. 2006;63:871-875.
82. Gorse G, Keitel W, Keyserling H, et al. Immunogenicity and tolerance of ascending doses of a recombinant protective antigen (rPA 102) anthrax vaccine: a randomized, double-blinded, controlled, multicenter trial. *Vaccine*. 2006;24:5950-5959.
83. Chabot D, Scorpio A, Tobery S, et al. Anthrax capsule vaccine protects against experimental infection. *Vaccine*. 2004;23:43-47.
84. Joyce J, Cook J, Chabot D, et al. Immunogenicity and protective efficacy of *Bacillus anthracis* poly-gamma-D-glutamic acid capsule covalently coupled to a protein carrier using a novel triazine-based conjugation strategy. *J Biol Chem*. 2006;281:4831-4843.
85. Brossier F, Levy M, Mock M. Anthrax spores make an essential contribution to vaccine efficacy. *Infect Immun*. 2002;70:661-664.

209

Bacillus Species and Related Genera Other than Bacillus anthracis

THOMAS FEKETE

Microbiology

Bacteria of the genus *Bacillus* are well adapted to their normal environment of soil. This includes *Bacillus anthracis*, discussed elsewhere in this text (Chapter 208). These gram-positive or gram-variable, aerobic or facultatively anaerobic rod-shaped bacilli have rounded or squared-off ends, form endospores, tolerate extremes of temperature and moisture, and are ubiquitous. They are found in superficial lake and ocean sediment, even in deep water. Their hardiness under conditions of desiccation and heat has been used to determine the efficacy of heat sterilization *(B. stearothermophilus)* and fumigation procedures *(B. subtilis)*. For many members of the genus *Bacillus*, an association with animals (either saprophytic or pathogenic) has also been noted. These animals range from small insects to large mammals, including humans.

Changes in the taxonomy of *Bacillus* species include the movement of *B. alvei* into the genus *Paenibacillus* and placement of both *B. brevis* and *B. laterosporus* into the genus *Brevibacillus.*[1] *B. cereus*, *B. anthracis*, *B. thuringiensis*, *B. pseudomycoides*, *B. weihenstephanensis*, and *B. mycoides* have been placed into a single group, known as the *B. cereus* group based on their close similarity.[2] More sophisticated genetic typing and a discovery of new strains in different environmental niches, particularly at extremes of environmental temperatures, has shown a great divergence of strain types within the species.[3] Much of this relatedness has to do with the substantial amount of genetic and enzymatic heterogeneity within *B. cereus*. In fact, different strains within a species of the *B. cereus* group may be more closely related to other species in the group than to other strains within their own species.[4] On the other hand, there is a very narrow range of diversity within *B. anthracis*, whose isolates occupy a tight band within the breadth of *B. cereus*, suggesting that *B. anthracis* is a newer species derived from *B. cereus*. This similarity of DNA and various enzymes may seem surprising insofar as there are great clinical differences between *B. cereus* and *B. anthracis* disease, but it should serve as a reminder of how little need change to convert a fairly innocuous organism into a serious pathogen. Detailed chromosomal DNA sequencing shows subtle distinctions within the group and indicates substantial lateral gene transfer, most likely through the acquisition of stable, integrated phages.[4] Less related species of *Bacillus* that may be encountered less commonly in the human clinical microbiology laboratory are *B. subtilis*, *B. licheniformis*, *B. megaterium*, *B. pumilus*, and *B. sphaericus*. *Bacillus* species are easy to grow on the usual culture media of the clinical laboratory. Most strains grow best at environmental temperatures (25° to 37°C). All have the capacity to form spores—this is part of the definition of the genus—but they vary widely in motility, colony morphology, and nutritional requirements. They are fairly large bacteria, with dimensions ranging from 3 by 0.4 to 9 by 2 μm. Although they are usually gram-positive in early growth, old cultures can be gram-variable or even gram-negative.[5] In most clinical laboratories, the first and most urgent task is to distinguish *B. anthracis* from other *Bacillus* species. *B. anthracis* is nonhemolytic on sheep or horse blood agar and nonmotile, whereas most other clinical isolates are motile and β-hemolytic. Strains of *B. anthracis* that are slightly hemolytic have been reported, and some of the less frequently isolated non-*anthracis* strains are nonmotile and nonhemolytic. For the latter strains, detailed biochemical analysis and toxin testing may

be required. Automated diagnostic kits for gram-positive bacteria are usually able to distinguish *B. anthracis* from other *Bacillus* species. It is perhaps surprising, yet fortunate, that the commercial tests to distinguish *B. anthracis* from its near relatives generally are easily carried out. Some species such as *B. sphaericus* and *B. badius* are biochemically unreactive and difficult to identify using commercial biochemical kits. Identification and characterization of individual strains can be made in reference laboratories with various tests, including flagellar antigens, phage typing, gas-liquid chromatography, and mass spectroscopy.[5]

Epidemiology

The widespread distribution in nature of *Bacillus* species explains its frequent isolation in the laboratory. In many cases, the isolation of *Bacillus* species from a clinical specimen raises the possibility of contamination, because environmental spores can germinate quickly on various laboratory media. *Bacillus* species is a transient but normal part of the fecal flora.[6] Children and adults were tested for the presence of *B. cereus* in the stool, and rates of recovery from 0% to 43% were found in the absence of diarrhea. The density of *B. cereus* in stool is usually low (about 100 viable organisms/g), but can be considerably higher. Strains of *B. cereus* in the stool are the same as those found in the food supply, and the ubiquity of *B. cereus* is reflected in a large number of different strains in fecal cultures of healthy people. However, during outbreaks, it can be shown that the strain of *B. cereus* causing food poisoning is consistent by biotype, serotype, toxin production, and phage type among patients.[7]

Hospital outbreaks of *Bacillus* species infection have occasionally been reported.[6] In one medical center, *B. cereus* was an ongoing cause of positive respiratory cultures and morbidity (including two cases of true bacteremia and one fatal pneumonia) in an intensive care unit.[8] This epidemic was the consequence of inadequate sterilization of respiratory circuits. No other bacterial infections occurred at higher than usual rates during the epidemic period because the degree of sterilization was sufficient to eradicate non–spore-forming bacteria but not *B. cereus*. Other species of *Bacillus* can persist for a long period and then can cause intermittent medical problems, such as 12 cases in 10 years of *B. sphaericus* bacteremia in a children's cancer hospital in Italy.[9]

Pseudoinfection and Contamination

More common than true outbreaks are pseudoepidemics, in which a strain or strains of *Bacillus* species are recovered from patients with a common source of contamination.[10,11] In these settings, biochemical and molecular studies can show that a single strain is found, even though it was not actually causing disease. Conversely, clusters of *Bacillus* spp. infection may look like point source outbreaks when they represent a higher than expected rate of infection by environmental organisms. One small cluster of serious *Bacillus* spp. infections, all of which were accompanied by bacteremia, occurring over 10 days in a children's cancer ward showed that the strains recovered were different from one another and from other isolates submitted for analysis.[12]

Bacillus spp. contamination has resulted in false-positive rates of up to 0.1% to 0.9% of all blood cultures submitted.[13] Because *Bacillus* spp.

is such a common contaminant and such a rare cause of disease, many laboratories do not identify *Bacillus* to the species level, except to exclude the possibility of *B. anthracis. Bacillus* spp. can survive in high concentrations of ethyl alcohol, up to 95%, including the sprays of 70% ethanol that are sometimes used for hand hygiene.[10] In one pseudo-epidemic, construction on a hospital driveway resulted in a 13-fold increase in the number of blood cultures that tested positive for *Bacillus* species.[11] The problem was related to direct contamination of stored blood culture bottles and inadequate cleaning of the bottles before introduction of the specimen. Even in the absence of a pseudo-epidemic, it can be difficult to separate true *Bacillus* spp. infection from contamination. The best indicator of true bacteremia, for example, is the presence of multiple positive cultures or recurrent bacteremia. In one study that compared patients for whom both bottles were positive in a set with *Bacillus* species against patients with only a single bottle positive, 29% (5/17) of episodes with both bottles positive were associated with a subsequent positive blood culture, as opposed to 3% (2/59) in patients with only a single bottle positive.[14] This suggests that skin preparation may be less important than specimen handling in false-positive blood cultures for *Bacillus* spp. In a Japanese hospital, 29 patients were noted to have *Bacillus* spp. bacteremia (more than half of these were *B. cereus*).[15] However, these patients were not treated for *Bacillus* spp. and did well clinically. Review of infection control policies showed suboptimal approaches to handling the catheters—wrong disinfectant, pauses during infusion, and reuse of caps on stopcocks. When these shortcomings were corrected, the *Bacillus* spp. bacteremia pseudoepidemic ceased. False-positive cultures of cerebrospinal fluid (CSF) for *Bacillus* spp. have also been reported.[16]

Commercial Uses of *Bacillus* Species

The toxins of the insect pathogen *B. thuringiensis* (Bt) have been purified and are among the most widely used "natural" control agents in agriculture. *B. thuringiensis* organisms or their purified toxins can be applied to commercially important plants to reduce damage from insect pests, and these can be easily purchased in garden centers to spray or dust in areas of insect activity. Genetic engineering has allowed the insertion of the toxin gene from Bt into other bacteria that can live closely with plants (e.g., among their roots or even between their cells) and protect them. Bt toxin genes have been inserted into commercially farmed plants such as tobacco, tomato, and cotton, making them naturally resistant to insects. *Bacillus* spp. spores have been marketed in nonchemical drain cleaners that work when the spores germinate and enzymatically digest part of the clog.[17] *B. subtilis* has been sold as a probiotic for ingestion, resulting in infection of at least one immunocompromised patient.[18]

Adherence Properties

Adherence of some *Bacillus* species to plastic intravascular catheters may help account for the frequency with which *Bacillus* spp. infection presents as bacteremia, accounting for 26 of 38 patients in one series.[19] Scanning electron microscopy of a Hickman catheter removed from a cancer patient with persistent *Bacillus* spp. bacteremia showed organisms embedded in a layer of glycocalyx.[20] *B. licheniformis* is often mucoid in colonial morphology, which may account in part for its ability to cause somewhat indolent but difficult to treat infections in patients with long-term indwelling vascular catheters.[21]

Clinical Manifestations

FOOD POISONING

Intoxication from the ingestion of *Bacillus* species–derived toxins is an uncommon but well described form of food poisoning. A report from England and Wales in the mid-1980s showed that there was one food poisoning from *Bacillus* spp. for every 129 of *Campylobacter,* 95 of other bacteria (e.g., *Salmonella, Shigella*), and 5.6 of *Clostridium per-*

fringens.[22] Like other toxin-mediated food poisonings, *Bacillus* spp. food poisoning occurs within 24 hours of eating, often within a few hours of the offending meal. *Bacillus* spp. toxins can produce one of two distinct syndromes, diarrheal and emetic. The diarrheal syndrome is characterized by profuse diarrhea and cramping but rarely vomiting or fever. The onset is about 8 to 16 hours after the ingestion of contaminated food, and the illness is brief (median duration, 24 hours). The emetic form (similar to *Staphylococcus aureus* food enterotoxin) has an even faster onset (1 to 5 hours) and is characterized by nausea, vomiting, and cramps, although diarrhea can occur in about one third of cases. It also resolves within 24 hours. The toxins responsible for these two clinical syndromes have been shown to differ in a number of ways. The diarrheal toxin is actually a mixture of two or more proteins with molecular weights of 36 to 45 kDa. The precise mode of action is unknown, although in animal models the toxins disrupt cell membranes and may have sphingomyelinase activity. The diarrheal toxin is heat-labile and can be reduced or eliminated by heating food to a high enough temperature to kill the vegetative phase of the organism. This is important because it is believed that the ingestion of toxin-producing *Bacillus* spp. can lead to diarrheal food poisoning by elaboration of toxin in the upper gastrointestinal tract. Foods most commonly associated with *Bacillus* spp. diarrheal food poisoning include meats, vegetables, and sauces.[22] Although most isolates of the diarrheal form of *Bacillus* spp. food poisoning are *B. cereus*, there have been outbreaks related to *B. licheniformis* and *B. pumilus.*[23]

The emetic toxin is a small peptide of about 10 kDa. It is heat-stable and associated with starchy foods, such as rice. This problem is worsened when rice is kept at room temperature overnight (to prevent clumping during refrigeration) and reheated the next day (e.g., fried rice). Heating or reheating food may eliminate viable *Bacillus* spp. organisms and the diarrheal toxin, but not the emetic toxin. Strains of *Bacillus* may produce one toxin or the other, but they almost never produce both. Genetic studies of strains that produce emetic toxin show that they belong to a single *B. cereus* genetic group (III) and subgroup (BC05), whereas strains producing diarrheal toxin may belong to any one of five of the seven *B. cereus* genetic groups.[24] Another member of the *B. cereus* group has been associated with rare but severe food-borne illness. This strain is not yet named, but it is genetically distinguished by a 25% smaller genome than most *B. cereus.*[4] At least one outbreak of *B. licheniformis* food poisoning was clinically comparable with the emetic syndrome of *B. cereus*, but the polypeptide toxin of *B. licheniformis* differs from that found in *B. cereus.*[25] On rare occasions, emetic toxin can lead to significant liver disease, including fulminant hepatic failure.[26] This is thought to be the result of inhibition of mitochondrial fatty acid oxidation.

Both these types of food poisoning can be diagnosed by culturing food, diarrheal fluid, or vomitus. Although cultivation of the *Bacillus* spp. organisms is easily done, it is not routinely done in the evaluation of diarrhea when stool cultures are submitted. Testing for the toxins themselves is difficult because commercial assays are not widely available. Sometimes, the cause of food poisoning is inferred rather than documented. Large studies of restaurant-associated outbreaks have allowed for a probabilistic determination of the cause of food-borne illness based on the relative contributions of poor hygiene, poor cooking, poor holding, or contaminated equipment.[27] Improper food holding is the most likely culprit for *B. cereus*–associated disease, as is the case for *C. perfringens* and *S. aureus* toxin-related vomiting and diarrhea. Although *Bacillus* spp. food poisoning often occurs in point source epidemics, the exact infective or toxic dose of *Bacillus* spp. in food is not known. Food screening that finds concentrations of *B. cereus* that are higher than 10^5/g of food is worrisome and should lead to a careful assessment of food handling and storage, even in the absence of known food poisoning.[28] In one outbreak in which *B. cereus* food poisoning was associated with mayonnaise in potato salad, only 10^3 bacteria were recovered per gram of mayonnaise.[29] The concentration of *B. cereus* in the food actually served may have been higher, because the potato salad was prepared by an inexperienced caterer and left at room temperature. Some *Bacillus* spp. food poisoning epidemics have been large. In London, diarrheal *B. cereus* food poisoning involved at least 139 out of almost 1000 people who ate together at a university field event where a barbeque meal was served.[30] Of the responders with food poisoning, one fifth had fever (low-grade), and one third developed symptoms outside the usual 6- to 24-hour window (mostly 6 hours) after exposure. Some people were ill for up to 20 days after the start of symptoms, although the median duration was 2 days. The vehicle was pork with more than 10^5/g *Bacillus cereus*, as determined from leftovers after the actual food poisoning; the concentration at the time of the event is unknown.

Attack rates with *Bacillus* spp. food poisoning can be high. In an outbreak from a hospital cafeteria, 160 of 249 (64%) employees reported an illness compatible with the diarrheal form of *Bacillus* spp. food poisoning related to rice or chicken, both of which cultured positive for *B. cereus*.[31]

A distinct form of food poisoning has been associated with *B. subtilis*. This syndrome is characterized by a short incubation period (median, 2.5 hours), vomiting, diarrhea (in about 50% of cases), and various other manifestations such as flushing, sweating, and headaches in about 10% of patients.[22] Large amounts of *B. subtilis* are required to cause this syndrome; cultures of vomitus and food show 10^7 to 10^9 organisms/g.

SYSTEMIC INFECTIONS

The rare but definite association between *Bacillus* spp. and deep infection have been recognized for over 4 decades (Table 209-1). Bacteremia has been the most common presentation, but distinguishing infection from contamination may be difficult.[8,15,32] In a review of positive blood cultures for *Bacillus* spp. in a North Carolina hospital in the 1980s, 5 of 78 isolates were thought to represent true infection.[33] All the definite infections were caused by *B. cereus*, whereas 70% of the possible and only 45% of the nonsignificant isolates were *B. cereus*. The most common feature in true *Bacillus* spp. bacteremia is the presence of an intravascular catheter, particularly a surgically implanted catheter.[21] The largest number of the bloodstream isolates of *Bacillus* are *B. cereus*, but other species such as *B. licheniformis* have also been reported.[21]

TABLE 209-1	Bacillus Species and Related Genera with Their Reported Clinical Syndromes, Other than Anthrax
Species	**Clinical Syndromes**
B. cereus	Bacteremia, pneumonia, ophthalmitis, keratitis, osteomyelitis, endocarditis, soft tissue infections, nosocomial infections, meningoencephalitis, fulminant hepatitis, diarrheal food poisoning, emetic food poisoning
B. circulans	Meningitis, CSF shunt infection, endocarditis, wound infection, endophthalmitis
B. licheniformis	Bacteremia, catheter-related sepsis, food poisoning, CNS infections after surgery or trauma
B. megaterium	Meningitis, bacteremia
B. pumilus	Meningitis, bacteremia, soft tissue infection
B. sphaericus	Peritonitis, pleuritis, pericarditis, pseudotumor of the lung, meningitis, bacteremia
B. subtilis	Meningitis after lumbar puncture or head trauma, otitis, mastoiditis, wound infection, bacteremia, pneumonia, endocarditis, shunt infection, emetic food poisoning
Brevibacillus brevis	Keratitis, food poisoning
Brevibacillus laterosporus	Bacteremia
Paenibacillus alvei	Sepsis, meningitis, prosthetic joint infection, wound infection

Disseminated *Bacillus* spp. infections in neonates and young children have been described. These infections can cause multisystem involvement, and in neonates they seem to be acquired perinatally.[34] A case of probable maternal-fetal infection has been reported in an injection drug user.[35]

Bacillus spp. infections can be serious and even fatal, especially when the patient has major immune compromise, such as neutropenia.[32,36] Injection drug users also seem to be at higher risk of *Bacillus* spp. Infection, presumably from direct injection of the organism from the drugs themselves or the injection paraphernalia,[37] although these infections are rarely fatal. Bacteremia from *Bacillus* spp. can be disseminated to other body sites such as the bones or eyes. *Bacillus* species are rarely the cause of native valve endocarditis and, when this occurs, it is almost always in injection drug users.[37,38]

CENTRAL NERVOUS SYSTEM INFECTIONS

Bacillus spp. usually enters the neuraxis through trauma or surgery, particularly implantation of a CSF shunt.[39] Removal of the hardware is usually required to achieve a cure. Lumbar puncture for diagnostic or therapeutic purposes can also lead to *Bacillus* spp. meningitis.[40] Brain abscess or encephalitis can be found alone or in combination with meningitis.[41]

RESPIRATORY INFECTIONS

Bacillus species are rarely the cause of pneumonia, but there have been sporadic cases of severe pneumonia associated with *B. cereus*.[42-44] Detailed evaluation of these strains has shown that they differ from typical *B. cereus* strains by virtue of capsule production and close genetic relatedness to *B. anthracis*. The phylogenetic similarities within the *B. cereus* group make it hard to tell if these should properly be considered to be downgraded variants of *B. anthracis* or are actually members of *B. cereus* recently diverged from *B. anthracis*.

EYE INFECTIONS

Bacillus species, usually *B. cereus*, can cause a rapidly destructive endophthalmitis, resulting from ocular trauma, therapeutic injection or surgery, or hematogenous dissemination.[45-48] The latter route is usually in an injection drug user. In animal models, the presence of toxins accounts for a significant amount of tissue ocular destruction.[49] A large case series of *Bacillus* spp. endophthalmitis from India, mostly but not entirely the result of trauma, has shown that aggressive therapy combining vitrectomy, topical and systemic antibiotics, and occasionally steroids could result in a surprisingly good outcome.[50] In a similar collection from the United States, 22 patients with *Bacillus* spp. endophthalmitis were treated with vitrectomy and antibiotics (intraocular vancomycin plus a cephalosporin or aminoglycoside), and 18% had a visual acuity of 20/60 in the affected eye.[51]

Bacillus spp. keratitis is an uncommon sequela to eye trauma or other conditions that affect the cornea. Scrapings of the cornea can reveal characteristic gram-positive or gram-variable rods that grow easily in culture.[52] The eye complaints usually begin soon after injury but may be delayed for weeks or even months. Conservative treatment is often successful in curing the infection with reasonable visual acuity after therapy. There have also been reports of *B. cereus* keratitis as a result of contact lens wear.[53] In this study, normal disinfection methods for the contact lens case were insufficient to eliminate *B. cereus*. One of the rare infectious complications of refractive surgery is keratitis from *Bacillus* sp. This was seen in a case of delayed lamellar keratitis caused by *B. megaterium* in a healthy adult despite aseptic surgical technique and perioperative antibiotics.[54]

SOFT TISSUE, SKIN, AND MUSCLE INFECTION

Bacillus spp. soft tissue and bone infection has been associated with injuries and wounds, notably including those received in motor vehicle accidents.[55] In one series of Swedish orthopedic patients with postoperative or post-traumatic wounds, about one patient per month had *Bacillus* spp. obtained from wounds, of which half were considered to represent moderate to severe infections.[56] *Bacillus* spp. was isolated from 25% of patients with wound complications following total hip arthroplasty, and these patients had a longer hospital stay than other patients. A large outbreak ($N = 94$) of scalp infections occurred among 660 university military cadets in the summer of 2004.[57] Three cadets had scalp cultures with indistinguishable strains of *B. cereus*, whereas numerous environmental *B. cereus* strains (including from barber clippers) were distinct from one another and from the clinical isolates. The timing of the lesions suggested a point source outbreak abetted by microabrasions caused by the recent haircut. In a case series from Costa Rica, *B. cereus* was found in 14 of 18 patients with traumatic wounds acquired in the rain forest.[58] These isolates were toxin producers, and in most cases wound cultures showed *B. cereus* to be present in pure cultures and in large numbers. A drug abuser with *Bacillus* spp. crepitant cellulitis had the same isolate obtained from his heroin.[59]

Prevention of *Bacillus* Species Infection

Guidelines for the safe preparation and handling of food are available at www.cfsan.fda.gov/list.html. Education of commercial food vendors is of obvious importance.[28] The best way to avoid both forms of food poisoning is to cook foods adequately and eat them immediately. Cooking will kill vegetative *Bacillus* spp. and destroy preformed diarrheal toxin, although not emetic toxin. If food cannot be consumed immediately, it should be refrigerated as soon as possible, because *Bacillus* spp. metabolism and toxin production are inhibited by cold temperature. Cooked rice should not be held at room temperature for prolonged periods before preparation of fried rice. Education of contact lens wearers about proper decontamination is important in preventing keratitis.[53]

Treatment

There is no specific treatment for the food poisoning syndromes other than symptomatic measures. For deep tissue infections, removal of prosthetic material, including infected intravascular catheters, is vital to achieve cure.[14] Most *Bacillus* spp. isolates are susceptible to vancomycin, clindamycin, fluoroquinolones, aminoglycosides, carbapenems and, variably, penicillins and cephalosporins.[60-62] *B. cereus* is often resistant to all β-lactams (other than carbapenems), and serious infections are best treated with vancomycin or clindamycin, with or without an aminoglycoside.[61,62]

Ciprofloxacin was the only drug uniformly active in vitro and was effective in vivo in a series of children with *B. sphaericus* bacteremia.[13] The β-lactamase of *B. cereus* and several other species of *Bacillus* spp. is a zinc-based enzyme that is evolutionarily different from β-lactamases in other gram-positive bacteria. Imipenem and some extended-spectrum β-lactams such as mezlocillin seem to be active against almost all *Bacillus* spp., despite the presence of a β-lactamase enzyme in *B. cereus* and *B. thuringiensis*. For strains other than *B. cereus*, various β-lactams are active in vitro but clindamycin is less reliably active. Vancomycin appears to be active in vitro against most *Bacillus* strains, but resistance via the *VanA* gene cluster has been reported.[63]

For native valve endocarditis, a long course of therapy has been reported to be successful,[36] and clindamycin has been surprisingly effective in a few cases, despite its bacteriostatic activity. For prosthetic valve disease, valve replacement is usually performed.[37] In some patients with deep infection, removal of a device can be effective without antimicrobial therapy and, in a small number of cases, no intervention was needed to achieve a good outcome.[16] Surgical drainage and removal of necrotic debris or implanted devices is important. In endophthalmitis, pars plana vitrectomy and intravitreal antibiotics have been advocated. *Bacillus* spp. keratitis is treated topically—for example, with a fluoroquinolone. A good visual outcome is most likely when the lesion is treated early and does not involve the central part of the cornea.[47]

REFERENCES

1. Logan NA, Turnbull PCB. Bacillus and other aerobic endospore-forming bacteria. In: Murray PR, Baron EJ, Jorgensen JH, et al, eds. *Manual of Clinical Microbiology*. Washington, DC: American Society for Microbiology Press; 2003:445-460.
2. Helgason E, Okstad OA, Caugant DA, et al. *Bacillus anthracis*, *Bacillus cereus*, and *Bacillus thuringiensis*—one species on the basis of genetic evidence. *Appl Environm Microbiol*. 2000;66:2627-2630.
3. Guinebretiere M-H, Thompson FL, Sorokin A, et al. Ecological diversification in the *Bacillus cereus* group. *Environmental Microbiol*. 2008;10:851-865.
4. Vilas-Boas GT, Peruca APS, Arantes OMN. Biology and taxonomy of *Bacillus cereus*, *Bacillus anthracis*, and *Bacillus thuringiensis*. *Can J Microbiol*. 2007;53:673-687.
5. Drobniewski FA. *Bacillus cereus* and related species. *Clin Microbiol Rev*. 1993;6:324-338.
6. Turnbull PC, Kramer JM. Intestinal carriage of *Bacillus cereus*: Faecal isolation in three population groups. *J Hyg*. 1985;95:629-638.
7. DeBuono BA, Brondum J, Kramer JM, et al. Plasmid, serotypic and enterotoxin analysis of *Bacillus cereus* in an outbreak setting. *J Clin Microbiol*. 1988;26:1571-1574.
8. Bryce EA, Smith JA, Tweeddale M, et al. Dissemination of *Bacillus cereus* in an intensive care unit. *Infect Contr Hosp Epidemiol*. 1993;14:459-462.
9. Castagnola E, Fioredda F, Barretta MA, et al. *Bacillus sphaericus* bacteraemia in children with cancer: Case reports and literature review. *J Hosp Infect*. 2001;48:142-145.
10. Hsueh PR, Teng LJ, Yang PC, et al. Nosocomial pseudoepidemic caused by *Bacillus cereus* traced to contaminated ethyl alcohol from a liquor factory. *J Clin Microbiol*. 1999;37:2280-2284.
11. Loeb M, Wilcox L, Thornley D, et al. *Bacillus* species pseudobacteremia following hospital construction. *Can J Infect Contr*. 1995;10:37-40.
12. Christenson JD, Byington C, Korgensi EK, et al. *Bacillus cereus* infections among oncology patients at a children's hospital. *Am J Infect Contr*. 1999;27:543-546.
13. Pearson HE. Human infections caused by organisms of the bacillus species. *Am J Clinic Pathol*. 1970;53:506-515.
14. Cotton DJ, Gill VJ, Marshall DJ, et al. Clinical features and therapeutic interventions in 17 cases of *Bacillus* bacteremia in

an immunosuppressed patient population. *J Clin Microbiol*. 1987;25:672-674.
15. Matsumoto S, Suenaga H, Naito K, et al. Management of suspected nosocomial infection: An audit of 19 hospitalized patients with septicemia caused by *Bacillus* species. *Jpn J Infect Dis*. 2000;53:196-202.
16. Cunha BA, Schoch PE, Bonoan JT. *Bacillus* species pseudomeningitis. *Heart Lung*. 1997;26:249-251.
17. Hannah WN, Ender PT. Persistent *Bacillus licheniformis* bacteremia associated with an intentional injection of organic drain cleaner. *Clin Infect Dis*. 1999;29:659-661.
18. Oggioni MR, Pozzi G, Valensin PE, et al. Recurrent septicemia in an immunocompromised patient due to probiotic strains of *Bacillus subtilis*. *J Clin Microbiol*. 1998;36:325-326.
19. Sliman R, Rehm S, Schlaes DM. Serious infections caused by *Bacillus* species. *Medicine*. 1987;66:218-223.
20. Banerjee C, Bustamante CI, Wharton R, et al. *Bacillus* infections in patients with cancer. *Arch Intern Med*. 1988;148:1769-1774.
21. Blue SR, Singh VR, Saubolle MA. *Bacillus licheniformis* bacteremia: Five cases associated with indwelling central venous catheters. *Clin Infect Dis*. 1995;20:629-633.
22. Lund BM. Foodborne disease due to *Bacillus* and *Clostridium* species. *Lancet*. 1990;336:982-986.
23. Mikkola R, Kolari M, Andersson MA, et al. Toxic lactonic lipopeptide from food poisoning isolates of *Bacillus licheniformis*. *Eur J Biochem*. 2000;267:4068-4074.
24. Lapidus A, Goltsman E, Auger S, et al. Extending the *Bacillus cereus* group to putative food-borne pathogens of different toxicity. *Chem Biol Interact*. 2008;171:236-249.
25. Salkinoja-Salonen MS, Vuorio R, Andersson MA, et al. Toxigenic strains of *Bacillus licheniformis* related to food poisoning. *Appl Environm Microbiol*. 1999;65:4637-4645.
26. Mahler H, Pasi A, Kramer JM, et al. Fulminant liver failure in association with the emetic toxin of *Bacillus cereus*. *N Engl J Med*. 1997;336:1142-1148.
27. Hedberg CW, Palazzi-Churas KL, Radke VJ, et al. The use of clinical profiles in the investigation of foodborne outbreaks in restaurants: United States, 1982-1997. *Epidemiol Infect*. 2008;136:65-72.
28. Little CL, Barnes J, Mitchell RT. Microbiological quality of takeaway cooked rice and chicken sandwiches: Effectiveness of food

hygiene training of the management. *Commun Dis Publ Hlth*. 2002;5:289-298.
29. Gaulin C, Viger YB, Fillion L. An outbreak of *Bacillus cereus* implicating a part-time banquet caterer. *Can J Publ Hlth*. 2002;93:353-355.
30. Luby S, Jones J, Dowda H, et al. A large outbreak of gastroenteritis caused by diarrheal toxin-producing *Bacillus cereus*. *J Infect Dis*. 1993;167:1452-1455.
31. Baddour LM, Gaia SM, Griffin R, et al. A hospital cafeteria-related food-borne outbreak due to *Bacillus cereus*: Unique features. *Infect Contr*. 1986;7:462-465.
32. Ihde DC, Armstrong D. Clinical spectrum of infection due to *Bacillus* species. *Am J Med*. 1973;55:839-845.
33. Weber DJ, Saviteer SM, Rutala WA, et al. Clinical significance of *Bacillus* species isolated from blood cultures. *South Med J*. 1989;82:705-709.
34. Patrick CC, Langston C, Baker CJ. *Bacillus* species infections in neonates. *Rev Infect Dis*. 1989;4:612-615.
35. Workowski KA, Flaherty JP. Systemic *Bacillus* species infection mimicking listeriosis of pregnancy. *Clin Infect Dis*. 1992;14:694-696.
36. Guioit HFL, de Planque MM, Richel DJ, et al. *Bacillus cereus*: A snake in the grass for granulocytopenic patients. *J Infect Dis*. 1986;153:1186.
37. Tuazon CU, Murray HW, Levy C, et al. Serious infections from *Bacillus* sp. *JAMA*. 1979;241:1137-1140.
38. Steen MK, Bruno-Murtha LA, Chaux G, et al. *Bacillus cereus* endocarditis: Report of a case and review. *Clin Infect Dis*. 1992;14:945-946.
39. Berner R, Heinen F, Pelz K, et al. Ventricular shunt infection and meningitis due to *Bacillus cereus*. *Neuropediatrics*. 1997;28:333-334.
40. Gaur AH, Patrick CC, McCullers JA, et al. *Bacillus cereus* bacteremia and meningitis in immunocompromised children. *Clin Infect Dis*. 2001;32:1456-1462.
41. Weisse ME, Bass JW, Jarrett RV, et al. Nonanthrax *Bacillus* infections of the central nervous system. *Pediatr Infect Dis J*. 1991;10:243-246.
42. Sue D, Hoffmaster AR, Popovic T, et al. Capsule production in *Bacillus cereus* strains associated with severe pneumonia. *J Clin Microbiol*. 2006;44:3426-3428.

43. Hoffmaster AR, Hill KK, Gee JE, et al. Characterization of *Bacillus cereus* isolates associated with fatal pneumonias: strains are closely related to *Bacillus anthracis* and harbor *B. anthracis* virulence genes. *J Clin Microbiol.* 2006;44:3352-3360.

44. Vassileva M, Torii K, Oshimoto M, et al. Phylogenetic analysis of *Bacillus cereus* isolates from severe systemic infections using multilocus sequence typing scheme. *Microbiol Immunol.* 2006;50:743-749.

45. Davey TF, Tauber WB. Posttraumatic endophthalmitis: The emerging role of *Bacillus cereus* infection. *Rev Infect Dis.* 1987;9:110-123.

46. Shamsuddin D, Tuazon CU, Levy C, et al. *Bacillus cereus* panophthalmitis: Source of the organism. *Rev Infect Dis.* 1982;4:97-103.

47. Shrader SK, Band JD, Lauter CB, et al. The clinical spectrum of endophthalmitis: Incidence, predisposing factors, and features influencing outcome. *J Infect Dis.* 1990;162:115-120.

48. Kopel AC, Carvounis PE, Holz ER. Bacillus cereus endophthalmitis following intravitreal bevacizumab injection. *Ophthalm Surg Lasers Imaging.* 2008;39:153-154.

49. Beecher DJ, Pulido JS, Barney NP, et al. Extracellular virulence factors in *Bacillus cereus* endophthalmitis: Methods and implica-tion of involvement of hemolysin BL. *Infect Immun.* 1995;63:632-639.

50. Das T, Choudhury K, Sharma S, et al. Clinical profile and outcome in *Bacillus* endophthalmitis. *Ophthalmology.* 2001;108:1819-1825.

51. Miller JJ, Scott IU, Flynn HW, et al. Endophthalmitis caused by Bacillus species. *Am J Ophthalmol.* 2008;145:883-888.

52. Choudhuri KK, Sharma S, Garg P, et al. Clinical and microbio-logical profile of Bacillus keratitis. *Cornea.* 2000;19:301-306.

53. Pinna A, Sechi LA, Zanetti S, et al. *Bacillus cereus* keratitis associ-ated with contact lens wear. *Ophthalmology.* 2001;108:1830-1834.

54. Ramos-Esteban JC, Servat JJ, Tauber S, et al. Bacillus megaterium delayed onset lamellar keratitis after LASIK. *J Refractive Surg.* 2006;22:309-312.

55. Wong MT, Dolan MJ. Significant infections due to *Bacillus* species following abrasions associated with motor vehicle-related trauma. *Clin Infect Dis.* 1992;15:855-857.

56. Akesson A, Hedstrom SA, Ripa T. *Bacillus cereus:* A significant pathogen in postoperative and post-traumatic wounds on ortho-paedic wards. *Scand J Infect Dis.* 1991;23:71-77.

57. Centers for Disease Control and Prevention (CDC). Outbreak of cutaneous Bacillus cereus infections among cadets in a university military program—Georgia, August 2004. *MMWR Morb Mortal Wkly Rep.* 2005;54:1233-1235.

58. Dryden MS, Kramer JM. Toxigenic *Bacillus cereus* as a cause of wound infections in the tropics. *J Infect.* 1987;15:207-212.

59. Dancer SJ, McNair D, Finn P, et al. *Bacillus cereus* cellulitis from contaminated heroin. *J Med Microbiol.* 2002;51:278-281.

60. Andrews JM, Wise R. Susceptibility testing of *Bacillus* species. *J Antimicrob Chemother.* 2002;49:1039-1046.

61. Krause A, Freeman R, Sisson PR, et al. Infection with *Bacillus cereus* after close-range gunshot injuries. *J Trauma.* 1996;41:546-548.

62. Weber DJ, Saviteer SM, Rutala WA, et al. In vitro susceptibility of *Bacillus* spp. to selected antimicrobial agents. *Antimicrob Agents Chemother.* 1988;32:642-645.

63. Ligozzi M, Cascio GL, Fontana R. *vanA* gene cluster in a vanco-mycin-resistant clinical isolate of *Bacillus circulans. Antimicrob Agents Chemother.* 1998;42:2055-2059.

210

Erysipelothrix rhusiopathiae

ANNETTE C. REBOLI

Erysipelothrix rhusiopathiae, formerly known as *Erysipelothrix insidiosa*, is a thin, pleomorphic, nonsporulating, gram-positive rod. First isolated from mice by Robert Koch in 1878 and from swine by Louis Pasteur in 1882, it was established as the etiologic agent of swine erysipelas in 1886 by Löffler and as a human pathogen in 1909 when Rosenbach isolated it from a patient with localized cutaneous lesions.[1] Rosenbach coined the term *erysipeloid* to avoid confusion with *erysipelas*, a superficial cellulitis with prominent lymphatic involvement that is almost always caused by group A streptococci.[2]

Microbiology

E. rhusiopathiae is a straight or slightly curved aerobic or facultatively anaerobic bacillary organism; it is 0.2 to 0.4 μm in diameter and 0.8 to 2.5 μm in length. It is gram-positive but may appear gram-negative because it decolorizes readily. Organisms may be arranged singly, in short chains, in pairs in a V configuration, or grouped randomly. Nonbranching filaments, which can be longer than 60 μm, are sometimes seen. Colonial and microscopic appearance varies with the medium, pH, and temperature of incubation.[1] After growing for 24 hours at 37°C, colonies are small and transparent, with a smooth, glistening surface. On blood agar, it may be α-hemolytic. *E. rhusiopathiae* is catalase-, oxidase-, indole-, Voges-Proskauer–, and methyl red–negative.[2] Acid without gas is produced from the fermentation of glucose, fructose, lactose, and galactose. Most strains produce hydrogen sulfide, a diagnostically important reaction. On triple sugar iron (TSI) agar slants, hydrogen sulfide causes a blackened butt. *E. rhusiopathiae* is sometimes confused with other gram-positive bacilli—in particular, *Listeria monocytogenes*, *Actinomyces (Arcanobacterium) pyogenes*, and *Arcanobacterium (Corynebacterium) haemolyticum*, but these three species are β-hemolytic on blood agar and do not produce hydrogen sulfide in the butt on TSI agar slants. Furthermore, *L. monocytogenes* is catalase-positive and motile.[1]

Epidemiology

E. rhusiopathiae is found worldwide. It has been reported as a commensal or a pathogen in a wide variety of vertebrate and invertebrate species, but the major reservoir is believed to be domestic swine.[2] Mites may serve as a vector of the organism, allowing it to persist in coops and pens.[3] It does not appear to cause disease in fish but can persist for long periods in the mucoid exterior slime of these animals. It may live long enough in soil to cause infection weeks or months after initial contamination. The greatest commercial impact of *E. rhusiopathiae* infection is the result of disease in swine, but infection of poultry and sheep is also important. The organism is communicable from animals to humans by direct cutaneous contact. There have been reports of bacteremia, one with endocarditis, which occurred after ingestion of undercooked pork. There was an outbreak of *E. rhusiopathiae* in racing pigeons following ingestion of compost.[4] The risk of human infection with *Erysipelothrix* is closely related to the opportunity for exposure to the organism; accordingly, most human cases are related to occupational exposure. Although infection with *Erysipelothrix* has been associated with many occupations, persons at greatest risk include fishermen, fish handlers, butchers, farmers, slaughterhouse workers, veterinarians, and homemakers.[2] Infection is especially common among persons who handle fish. Of the 329 cases of erysipeloid described by Gilchrist, 323 were associated with injuries from crabs.[5]

"Whale finger" is erysipeloid seen in persons who sustain cuts to the fingers and hands while engaged in whaling. Human-to-human transmission of infection has not been reported. Cases of infection that do not have an occupational link have occurred mainly in immunocompromised hosts and suggest that colonization of the oropharynx or gastrointestinal tract may occur.[6] Chronic alcoholism is a common underlying condition. There have been a few reports of erysipeloid following cat and dog bites.[7]

Pathogenesis

Abrasions or puncture wounds of the skin probably serve as the portal of entry of *Erysipelothrix* organisms in most cases of infection in humans and animals. Virulence factors include a capsule, enzymes (neuraminidase and hyaluronidase), and surface proteins.[8] In the absence of specific antibodies, *E. rhusiopathiae* evades phagocytosis but, even if phagocytized, it is capable of intracellular replication.[8]

Clinical Manifestations

Three well-defined clinical categories of human disease have been described: (1) erysipeloid, a localized skin lesion; (2) a diffuse cutaneous eruption with systemic symptoms; and (3) bacteremia, which is often associated with endocarditis.

The localized cutaneous form—the "erysipeloid" of Rosenbach—is a subacute cellulitis and is the most common type of *Erysipelothrix* infection seen in humans. Because the organism is acquired through contact with infected animals or fish, or with products made from them, gaining entrance via cuts or abrasions on the skin, most lesions are on the fingers. Following an incubation period of 2 to 7 days, pain, which is often severe and described as burning, itching, or throbbing, and swelling of the involved digit or part of the hand develop. The lesion is well defined, slightly raised, and violaceous (Fig. 210-1).[2,5] As it spreads peripherally, the central area fades. Vesiculation may occur. Regional lymphadenopathy and lymphangitis occur in approximately one third of cases.[9] There may be inflammation of an adjacent joint. Systemic symptoms are uncommon. Approximately 10% of the patients have low-grade fever and arthralgias.[9] Clinically, erysipeloid resembles staphylococcal or streptococcal cellulitis, but a history of occupational exposure, lesions on the hands, subacute course, absence of suppuration, lack of pitting edema, violaceous color, and the disproportionate pain should suggest the possibility of erysipeloid.[10] Because organisms are located only in deeper parts of the skin in erysipeloid, aspirates or biopsy specimens should incorporate the entire thickness of the dermis, as well as tissue from the periphery of the lesion, to maximize the chance of recovery of the organism. Erysipeloid usually resolves without treatment within 3 or 4 weeks.

The diffuse cutaneous form, which is rare, occurs when the violaceous cutaneous lesion progresses proximally from the site of inoculation or appears at remote areas.[1,2] Lesions may appear urticarial, with the rhomboid pattern characteristic of swine erysipelas.[2] Fever and arthralgias are common. Blood cultures are negative. The course is more protracted than in the localized form, and recurrence is common.

Systemic infection with *E. rhusiopathiae* is unusual. More than 90 cases of bacteremia have been reported, most complicated by endocarditis.[11-19] Although this organism has caused prosthetic valve endocarditis, most reported cases of endocarditis have involved native valves. There was a history of an antecedent or concurrent skin lesion of

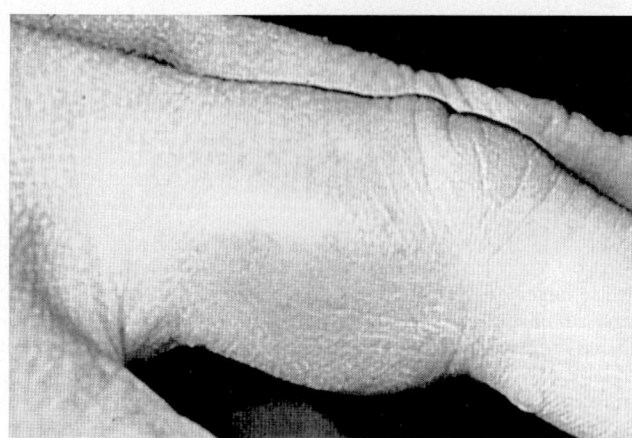

Figure 210-1 Lesion of erysipeloid. *(From Lambert HP, Farrar WE. Cutaneous manifestations of infection. II: Bacterial infections. In: Lambert HP, Farrar WE, eds. Infectious Diseases Illustrated. London: Gower Medical Publishing; 1982:Section 5.10. By permission of Mosby International.)*

body fluid. Standard methods for culturing blood or biopsy tissue should suffice if incubation is continued up to 7 days. Erysipelothrix grows best at 35°C in 5% CO_2. Culture-based methods can be problematic and may lead to an incorrect diagnosis.[22] Despite the use of selective media to improve isolation from contaminated specimens, it is difficult to isolate *E. rhusiopathiae* from heavily contaminated specimens because of its small colony size, slow growth rate, and the inability to inhibit all contaminants.. There are no reliable serologic tests for the diagnosis of infection in humans. The polymerase chain reaction (PCR) assay has been used for rapid diagnosis in swine and has been applied successfully to human and environmental samples.[31]

Treatment and Prevention

Susceptibility data for *E. rhusiopathiae* are limited. Most strains are highly susceptible to penicillins, cephalosporins, clindamycin, imipenem, and ciprofloxacin.[32,33] Penicillin and imipenem are the most active agents in vitro. Susceptibility to chloramphenicol, erythromycin, and tetracycline is variable. Most strains are resistant to vancomycin, sulfonamides, trimethoprim-sulfamethoxazole, novobiocin, teicoplanin, and aminoglycosides. Resistance to vancomycin is important because this agent is often used empirically to treat bacteremia caused by gram-positive organisms. Because minimum inhibitory concentrations (MICs) of penicillin range from 0.0025 to 0.06 µg/mL, and minimum bactericidal concentrations (MBCs) have been reported in the range of 0.0025 to 0.75 µg/mL, penicillin G (12 to 20 million units/day) is the drug of choice for serious infections caused by *E. rhusiopathiae*. Ampicillin and ceftriaxone have also been used successfully. Ciprofloxacin has MIC and MBC values similar to those obtained with β-lactam antibiotics.[32,33] Daptomycin has demonstrated in vitro activity against clinical isolates of *E. rhusiopathiae*.[34] Use of fluoroquinolones or daptomycin may be considered in *Erysipelothrix* infections when β-lactams are contraindicated. In cases of endocarditis, the duration of IV antibiotic therapy should be 4 to 6 weeks, although shorter courses (2 weeks of IV therapy followed by 2 to 4 weeks of oral therapy) have been successful.[2] Although erysipeloid usually resolves spontaneously, healing is hastened by antibiotic therapy. Oral therapy with amoxicillin or a quinolone can be used.

Prevention of infection for persons in high-risk occupations depends on adequate hand washing, the use of protective attire such as gloves, and disinfection of contaminated surfaces. Unprotected direct contact with animal body tissues and secretions should be avoided. Although commercial vaccines are available for veterinary use, research to develop more immunogenic and safer vaccines continues.[35] Use of vaccination along with other measures, such as improved waste disposal, have helped control swine erysipelas.

erysipeloid in 36% of patients.[12] When clinical features of *E. rhusiopathiae* endocarditis were compared with those of endocarditis caused by other bacteria, there was a higher male-to-female ratio (which probably reflects occupational exposure), a greater propensity for involvement of the aortic valve, and a much higher mortality rate among patients with *E. rhusiopathiae* endocarditis (38% vs. 20% in endocarditis caused by other organisms).[18] In approximately 60% of patients, *E. rhusiopathiae* endocarditis developed in previously normal heart valves. In patients with bacteremia, endocarditis, or both, routine blood culture techniques are adequate for recovery of the organism.[1] Complications of *Erysipelothrix* endocarditis include congestive heart failure, myocardial abscess, aortic valve perforation, meningitis, brain infarctions, glomerulonephritis, septic arthritis, and osteomyelitis.[11-16,18,19] More than one third of the patients require valve replacement.[12]

Bacteremia without endocarditis has been reported with increasing frequency. It has occurred primarily in immunocompromised hosts.[20,21] Brain abscess, necrotizing fasciitis, meningitis, peritonitis (including peritoneal dialysis–related peritonitis), osteomyelitis, and septic arthritis (including infection of an arthroplasty and a reconstructed ligament) have also been reported.[2,22-30]

Definitive diagnosis of infection with *Erysipelothrix* requires isolation of the organism from a biopsy specimen, blood, or other sterile

REFERENCES

1. Reboli AC, Farrar WE. The genus *Erysipelothrix*. In: Balows A, Truper HG, Dworkin M, et al, eds. The Prokaryotes. *A Handbook on the Biology of Bacteria: Ecophysiology, Isolation, Identification, Applications.* 2nd ed. New York: Springer-Verlag; 1992: 1629-1642.
2. Reboli AC, Farrar WE. *Erysipelothrix rhusiopathiae*: An occupational pathogen. *Clin Microbiol Rev.* 1989;2:354-359.
3. Chirico J, Eriksson H, Fossum O, et al. The poultry red mite, Dermanyssus gallinae, a potential vector of *Erysipelothrix rhusiopathiae* causing erysipelas in hens. *Med Vet Entomol.* 2003;17:232-234.
4. Cousquer G. *Erysipelas* outbreak in racing pigeons following ingestion of compost. *Vet Rec.* 2005;156:656.
5. Gilchrist TC. Erysipeloid, with a record of 329 cases, of which 323 were caused by crab bites, or lesions produced by crabs. *J Cutan Dis.* 1904;22:507-519.
6. Schuster MG, Brennan PJ, Edelstein P. Persistent bacteremia with *Erysipelothrix rhusiopathiae* in a hospitalized patient. *Clin Infect Dis.* 1993;17:783-784.
7. Talan DA, Citron DM, Abrahamian FM, et al. Bacteriologic analysis of infected dog and cat bites. Emergency Medicine Animal Bite Infection Study Group. *N Engl J Med.* 1999; 340:85-92.
8. Shimoji Y. Pathogenicity of *Erysipelothrix rhusiopathiae*: Virulence factors and protective immunity. *Microbes Infect.* 2000; 2:965-972.

9. Nelson E. Five hundred cases of erysipeloid. *Rocky Mtn Med J.* 1955;52:40-42.
10. Robson JM, McDougall R, van der Valk S, et al. *Erysipelothrix rhusiopathiae*: An uncommon but ever present zoonosis. *Pathology.* 1998;30:391-394.
11. Hill DC, Ghassemian JN. *Erysipelothrix rhusiopathiae* endocarditis. Clinical features of an occupational disease. *South Med J.* 1997;90:1147-1148.
12. Gorby GL, Peacock JE. *Erysipelothrix rhusiopathiae* endocarditis: Microbiologic, epidemiologic and clinical features of an occupational disease. *Rev Infect Dis.* 1988;10:317-325.
13. Artz AL, Szabo S, Zabel LT, et al. Aortic valve endocarditis with paravalvular abscesses caused by *Erysipelothrix rhusiopathiae*. *Eur J Clin Microbiol Infect Dis.* 2001;20:587-588.
14. Nandish S, Khardori N. Valvular and myocardial abscesses due to *Erysipelothrix rhusiopathiae*. *Clin Infect Dis.* 1999;29: 1351-1352.
15. Ko SB, Kim DE, Kwon HM, et al. A case of multiple brain infarctions associated with *Erysipelothrix rhusiopathiae* endocarditis. *Arch Neurol.* 2003;60:434-436.
16. Romney M, Cheung S, Montessori V. *Erysipelothrix rhusiopathiae* endocarditis and presumed osteomyelitis. *Can J Infect Dis.* 2001;12:254-256.
17. Boo TW, Hone R, Hurley J. *Erysipelothrix rhusiopathiae* endocarditis: a preventable zoonosis? *Ir J Med Sci.* 2003;172: 81-82.

18. Nassar IM, de la Llana R, Garrido P, et al. Mitro-aortic infective endocarditis produced by *Erysipelothrix rhusiopathiae*: case report and review of the literature. *J Heart Valve Dis.* 2005;14:320-324.
19. Yamamoto Y, Shioshita K, Takazono T, et al. An autopsy case of *Erysipelothrix rhusiopathiae* endocarditis. *Intern Med.* 2008;47:1437-1440.
20. Surrun SK, Jaufeerally FR, Sim HC. *Erysipelothrix rhuseopathiae* septicaemia with prolonged hypotension: a case report. *Ann Acad Med Singapore.* 2008;37:251-252.
21. Cooke LJ, Bowles KM, Craig JI, et al. Occupational injury in a fishmonger with a macular rash, hepatosplenomegaly and pancytopenia. *J Clin Pathol.* 2006;59:993-994.
22. Dunbar SA, Clarridge JE 3rd. Potential errors in recognition of *Erysipelothrix rhusiopathiae*. *J Clin Microbiol.* 2000;38:1302-1304.
23. Ruiz ME, Richards JS, Kerr GS, et al. *Erysipelothrix rhusiopathiae* septic arthritis. *Arthritis Rheum.* 2003;48:1156-1157.
24. Wong RC, Kong KO, Lin RV, et al. Chronic monoarthritis of the knee in systemic lupus erythematosus. *Lupus.* 2003;12:324-326.
25. Allianatos PG, Tilentzoglou AC, Koutsoukou AD. Septic arthritis caused by *Erysipelothrix rhusiopathiae* infection after arthroscopically assisted anterior cruciate ligament reconstruction. *Arthroscopy.* 2003;19:26E.
26. Traer EA, Williams MR, Keenan JN. *Erysipelothrix rhusiopathiae* infection of a total knee arthroplasty: an occupational hazard. *J Arthroplasty.* 2008;23:609-611.

27. Kim SR, Kwon MJ, Lee JH, et al. Chronic meningitis caused by *Erysipelothrix rhusiopathiae*. *J Med Microbiol*. 2007;56(Pt 10):1405-1406.

28. Hardman SC, Carr SJ, Swann RA. Peritoneal dialysis-related peritonitis with bacteraemia due to *Erysipelothrix rhusiopathiae*. *Nephrol Dial Transplant*. 2004;19:1340-1341.

29. Simionescu R, Grover S, Shekar R, et al. Necrotizing fasciitis caused by *Erysipelothrix rhusiopathiae*. *South Med J*. 2003;96: 937-939.

30. Brook CJ, Riley TV. *Erysipelothrix rhusiopathiae*: Bacteriology, epidemiology and clinical manifestations of an occupational pathogen. *J Med Microbiol*. 1999;48:789-799.

31. Fidalgo SG, Riley TV. Detection of *Erysipelothrix rhusiopathiae* in clinical and environmental samples. *Methods Mol Biol*. 2004;268:199-205.

32. Venditti M, Gelfusa V, Tarasi A, et al. Antimicrobial susceptibilities of *Erysipelothrix rhusiopathiae*. *Antimicrob Agents Chemother*. 1990;34:2038-2040.

33. Fidalgo SG, Longbottom CJ, Riley TV. Susceptibility of *Erysipelothrix rhusiopathiae* to antimicrobial agents and home disinfectants. *Pathology*. 2002;34:462-465.

34. Piper KE, Steckelberg JM, Patel R. In vitro activity of daptomycin against clinical isolates of Gram-positive bacteria. *J Infect Chemother*. 2005; 11:207-209.

35. To H, Nagai S. Genetic and antigenic diversity of the surface protective antigen proteins of *Erysipelothrix rhusiopathiae*. *Clin Vaccine Immunol*. 2007; 14:813-820.

211

Neisseria meningitidis

MICHAEL A. APICELLA

Epidemic cerebrospinal fever (meningococcal meningitis) was first described in Geneva by Vieusseaux in 1805.[1] Subsequent reports throughout the 19th century confirmed its episodic, epidemic nature with a propensity for afflicting young children and military recruits assembled in stationary barracks situations.[2] In 1887, Weichselbaum isolated the meningococcus from cerebrospinal fluid (CSF), and the etiologic relationship between this organism and epidemic meningitis was firmly established.[3] Kiefer in 1896[4] and Albrecht and Ghon in 1901[5] found that healthy persons could become carriers of the meningococcus. Serotypes of the meningococcus were first recognized by Dopter in 1909.[6] This finding laid the basis for serum therapy in the treatment of meningococcal infection by Flexner in 1913.[7] Glover was the first to note that carrier rates in military recruit camps rose with periods of crowding, and he believed that they were associated with an increased incidence of cases.[8] In 1928 to 1930[9,10] and in 1941,[11] significant national and worldwide epidemics occurred. In 1937, sulfonamide therapy radically altered the outcome of meningococcal infection and replaced serum in its treatment.[12] Prophylaxis with sulfonamides eradicated the carrier state[13] and provided a simple and safe method for the prevention of epidemics, particularly in the crowded environments of military barracks. With the advent of antibiotic agents, treatment of meningococcal infection became more effective, and mortality declined. Increasing sulfonamide resistance among meningococci was recognized by Schoenback and Phair[14] in 1941 to 1943 but did not become a clinically significant problem until meningococcal epidemics in 1963 in two military bases in California.[15,16] With the subsequent worldwide emergence of resistant strains and the absence of effective chemoprophylaxis, renewed interest in immunoprevention led to the development of safe and effective vaccines against serogroup A and C meningococcal infection.[17]

Many problems still exist in the understanding, prevention, and treatment of meningococcal infection, including the susceptibilities of certain populations to this infection, its sporadic epidemic nature, the mechanisms responsible for carrier eradication by antibiotics, the reasons for the fulminant nature of the infection, and the inability of humans to develop antibody to the group B polysaccharide vaccine. Until these and many other questions are answered, meningococcal infections will continue to be a scourge among human populations.

▣ Etiologic Agent and Morphologic, Cultural, and Biochemical Characteristics

N. meningitidis is a gram-negative diplococcus (0.6 × 0.8 μm). The adjacent sides are flattened to produce the typical biscuit shape. Because the organism tends to readily undergo autolysis, considerable size and shape variation can be seen in older cultures. The organism produces a polysaccharide capsule, which is the basis of the serogroup typing system. Because the organism is considered fastidious in its growth conditions, appropriate media and growth conditions are necessary. On solid media, the meningococcus grows as a transparent, nonpigmented, nonhemolytic colony about 1 to 5 mm in diameter. Colonies are convex and, if large amounts of polysaccharide are present, will appear mucoid rather than smooth. Optimal growth conditions are achieved in a moist environment at 35° to 37°C under an atmosphere of 5% to 10% carbon dioxide. The organism will grow well on a number of medium bases, including blood agar base, trypticase soy agar, supplemented chocolate agar, and Mueller-Hinton agar. Confirmation of the presence of this organism in clinical specimens is

dependent on a series of carbohydrate fermentations. The meningococcus will metabolize glucose and maltose to acid without gas formation and fails to metabolize sucrose or lactose. In addition, the organism contains cytochrome oxidase in its cell wall. This enzyme will oxidize the dye tetramethyl phenylenediamine from colorless to deep pink. This latter test was initially considered specific for *Neisseria*, but subsequent studies have shown that other genera also exhibit high tetramethyl phenylenediamine oxidase activities, including *Pseudomonas, Aeromonas,* and *Moraxella*. Use of molecular methods based on a variety of polymerase chain reaction (PCR) techniques has supplemented culture in confirmation of patients infected with the meningococcus. This is particularly true in patients treated with antibiotics before being cultured.

The meningococcus has a rapid autolytic rate. Hebeler and Young have demonstrated the presence of an autolysin, an amidase, that acts on the peptidoglycan layer of the gonococcus.[18] Whether the mechanism of autolysis is similar in the meningococcus is uncertain. The process appears to be enzymatic because autolysis can be stopped by the addition of potassium cyanide or formalin or by heating cultures to 65°C for 30 minutes.

The importance of iron in the survival of microbes has stimulated interest in the mechanisms that *Neisseria* organisms use for iron acquisition. It has been shown that iron-loaded animals are more susceptible to fatal meningococcal infection.[19] The meningococcus does not produce a soluble siderophore but possesses a series of membrane proteins that selectively scavenge iron from hemoglobin, transferrin, and lactoferrin.[20,21]

ANTIGENIC STRUCTURE OF THE MENINGOCOCCUS

Capsular Polysaccharides

Shortly after identification of the meningococcus as the etiologic agent in epidemic meningitis and after recognition of healthy nasopharyngeal carriers of the organism, investigations into the application of immunologic methods for the detection and differentiation of meningococci were performed. It became apparent that antigenically diverse meningococci existed, and spurred on by the introduction of serum therapy,[7] English workers identified four antigenically distinct types of meningococci.[22] The relationship between this antigenic polysaccharide[23] and the capsule of the meningococcus was established through the Quellung reaction by Clapp and associates in group A strains.[24] Branham and Carlin, using group C strains, were able to demonstrate that these antigens elicited antibodies that conferred specific protection in mice.[25] Meningococci can now be segregated by seroagglutination into at least 13 serogroups: A, B, C, D[26,27]; X, Y, Z[28,29]; E, W-135[29]; H, I, K[30]; and L.[31] Table 211-1 gives the chemical composition of the capsular polysaccharide of the eight most common capsular serogroups causing human disease. Capsular polysaccharides responsible for the serogrouping specificity of groups A, B, C, X, Y, Z, W-135, and L have been purified. These polysaccharides have been isolated from the broth supernatant of overnight cultures, and a number of effective methods using either detergent precipitation or molecular sieve and ion-exchange chromatography have been used in their separation.[32-34] Group C polysaccharides can be biochemically divided into neuraminidase-sensitive and neuraminidase-resistant polysaccharides.[35,36]

After the introduction of antibiotics, interest in the development of serogroup-specific antigens for use as vaccines diminished greatly, but Watson and colleagues continued their efforts and identified the specific soluble substance from the group C meningococcus and showed

TABLE 211-1	Chemical Composition of Meningococcal Capsular Polysaccharides
Capsular Serogroup Antigen	**Chemical Composition of Capsular Polymer**
A	Partially O-acetylated 2-acetamido-2-deoxy-D-mannose-6-phosphate
B	(2 → 8)-Linked N-acetylneuraminic acid
C_{1+}	O-acetylated (2 → 9)-linked N-acetylneuraminic acid
C_1	(2 → 9)-Linked N-acetylneuraminic acid
X	2-Acetamido-2-deoxy-D-glucose-4-phosphate
Y	Partially O-acetylated alternating sequence of D-glucose and N-acetylneuraminic acid
W-135	Alternating sequence of D-galactose and N-acetylneuraminic acid
L	N-acetylglucosamine phosphate

its sialic acid nature.[37] A major impetus that renewed interest in meningococcal immunobiology was the emergence of sulfonamide-resistant meningococci as a clinical problem. This development made antibiotic prophylaxis ineffective, and persistent epidemics of serogroup B and C strains on military recruit reservations during the 1960s prompted reinvestigations into the feasibility of using capsular polysaccharide antigens as vaccine materials.

The immunogenicity of group A and C polysaccharide in humans appears to be a function of their molecular size.[38] In addition, studies have indicated that group C vaccine is stable and immunogenic after up to 4 years of storage. Group B polysaccharide has been purified and described immunochemically,[39,40] but it has proved to be a very poor immunogen in humans. At the present time, no effective vaccine preparation exists for this serogroup.[41] With the increasing frequency of clinical cases caused by group Y meningococci, interest in capsular polysaccharide strains from this serogroup has renewed,[42] and studies by Griffiss and co-workers have demonstrated the safety and immunogenicity of group Y and W-135 capsular polysaccharides in humans.[43]

Noncapsular Cell Wall Antigens

The meningococcal outer membrane is similar in structure to that of other gram-negative bacteria. It contains a number of somatic antigens that are important in pathogenesis and immunobiology. The principal antigens that have been studied include lipo-oligosaccharide, which is analogous to the lipopolysaccharide of enteric gram-negative bacilli and the outer membrane proteins. Lipo-oligosaccharide is serologically diverse, and Mandrell and Zollinger have demonstrated at least 12 different serotypes.[44] The chemical structure of the oligosaccharide portion of meningococcal lipo-oligosaccharide from all L types has been studied by Jennings and co-workers.[45,46] Several of these structures are immunochemically similar to human glycosphingolipid antigens. An association between lipo-oligosaccharide immunotype expression and invasive disease has been found.[47] Ninety-seven percent of isolates from epidemics in England expressed the L3, 7, 9 immunotype. The lipo-oligosaccharide immunotypes of carriers were more heterogeneous. Studies have suggested that specific lipo-oligosaccharide epitopes of oligosaccharide may be effective vaccines.[48,49]

Interest in the meningococcal outer membrane proteins was stimulated by the work of Gold and associates, who showed that a noncapsular typing system could be derived by using bactericidal techniques.[50,51] Using similar methods, Frasch and Chapman succeeded in identifying 11 distinct serotypes of group B meningococci.[52] Frasch and Gotschlich have shown that the antigens responsible for this serotyping system are protein in nature and reside in the outer membrane as part of a lipoprotein–lipo-oligosaccharide complex. Serogroup B and C meningococci can be subdivided into at least 15 protein serotypes based on antigenically different outer membrane proteins.[53] Studies by Broud and co-workers indicate that endemic meningococcal disease appears to be caused by a broad, heterogeneous distribution of serotypes.[54] This observation is in contrast to epidemics that appear to be caused

by a single serotype. The successful application of molecular techniques has resulted in the cloning of a number of important outer membrane protein antigens of the meningococcus.[55,56] Frasch and co-workers[57] suggested revising the classification system for the somatic antigen serotypes of the meningococcus. These investigators proposed a schema based on the major class 2 (41,000 kDa) and class 3 (38,000 kDa) outer membrane proteins and the lipo-oligosaccharides. In their example, a meningococcal strain would be identified by serogroup, protein serotype, and lipo-oligosaccharide serotype. Addition of the class 1 protein (46,000 kDa) characteristics could be also used to further define the strain. This system has worked well in identifying epidemic strains of serogroup B.

The lack of a serogroup B vaccine combined with the availability of the sequence of the meningococcal genome has spurred interest in using this database to identify new noncapsular vaccine targets in an approach designated *reverse vaccinology*.[58]

Using analysis of multilocus enzyme genotypes, Selander and co-workers have developed a system for defining the clonal distribution of bacterial isolates.[59] Applying this method to studies of the meningococcus, Olyhoek and colleagues have shown that epidemics caused on a worldwide basis by a strain of serogroup A meningococcus are derived from a single clonotype.[60] Caugant and co-workers have studied 650 meningococcal strains of different capsular serogroups and have shown that over periods of many years the genetic structure of *N. meningitidis* is basically clonal as a result of low rates of recombination of chromosomal genes.[61]

Meningococci have been shown to have pili.[62,63] Meningococcal pili undergo both phase and antigenic variation. These structures can be maintained under special cultural conditions in vitro, and their role as ligands in attachment to human cells has been studied.[64] Piliate meningococci attach to human nasopharyngeal cells in greater numbers than do meningococci devoid of pili. Trypsin or mechanical shearing causes loss of pili and decreased attachment. Meningococci appear to have wide differences in attachment capability that depend on the site of isolation of the epithelial cell.[65]

PATHOGENESIS OF INFECTION

The pathogenesis of *N. meningitidis* begins on the nasopharyngeal surface. The nasopharynx is a mixed epithelial surface containing ciliated secretory and nonciliated nonsecretory cells. The airway epithelial surface is covered with a mucus layer that the organism must penetrate. How penetration occurs is not clearly understood. The meningococcus uses bacterial surface factors to adhere to nonciliated cells on the airway surface. Pili enhance attachment but are not necessary for attachment.[65] They act as long-range attachment organelles. It has been shown that purified pili bind to a human cell surface protein CD46 that is widely distributed and involved in regulation of complement activation.[66] Transgenic mice expressing this human protein become susceptible to meningococcal disease because bacteria cross the blood-brain barrier.[67] Attachment of the bacteria to epithelial cells is blocked by polyclonal and monoclonal antibodies directed against membrane cofactor protein, which suggests that this complement regulator is a receptor for piliate *Neisseria*. Recombinant membrane cofactor protein produced in *Escherichia coli* inhibits attachment of the bacteria to target cells. As the organism draws closer to the cell, outer membrane surface proteins such as the class V proteins (Opa and Opc) play a role in attachment and may be important in defining the tissue specificity of the organism.[68]

The hydrophilic, highly charged nature of the capsular polysaccharide prevent interactions with the epithelial cell surface. Only unencapsulated meningococci enter epithelial cells, and capsular biosynthesis has been shown to stop as the meningococcus enters the epithelial cell.[69,70] This is the result of a mechanism designated *slip-strand mispairing*, which results in the termination of translation of one of the sialyltransferases involved in capsular biosynthesis.[69] This "molecular switch" varies capsular expression at a frequency of 10^{-3}. Bloodstream encapsulated meningococcal isolates were universally found to have the "switch" in the "on" position, whereas nasopharyngeal unencapsulated carrier isolates had the switch in the "off" position. This suggested that there is a correlation between capsular phase variation, bacterial invasion, and the outbreak of meningococcal disease.[69] On contact with epithelial and endothelial cells, the meningococcus initiates cytoskeletal changes within these cell types. It appears that either Opc- or OpaA-mediated adhesion can trigger cortical actin rearrangements.[71,72] These rearrangements are not triggered by nonadherent meningococcal strains, by heat-killed or chloramphenicol-treated organisms, or by *Escherichia coli* recombinants that adhere to cells through OpaA or Opa1 fusion proteins. These observations suggest that additional neisserial components are involved. Studies have indicated that neisserial porin, which can translocate into eukaryotic membranes, might be the factor responsible for actin rearrangement. The bacteria are incorporated into vacuoles and are transported to the basolateral surface of the cell. Factors allowing survival of the organism within the epithelial cell are now being elucidated. So and co-workers have shown that the *Neisseria* type 2 immunoglobulin A_1 (IgA_1) protease cleaves LAMP1 and promotes the survival of bacteria within epithelial cells. Infection of human epithelial cells by *N. meningitidis* and *Neisseria gonorrhoeae* increases the rate of degradation of LAMP1, a major integral membrane glycoprotein of late endosomes and lysosomes.[73] Nassif and colleagues have suggested that meningococcal *pilC* is upregulated and that pilus-mediated attachment may be important in crossing of the blood-brain barrier.[74]

HUMAN IMMUNOLOGIC RESPONSE TO MENINGOCOCCAL ANTIGENS

Goldschneider and associates have demonstrated that the percentage of people with bactericidal activity against *N. meningitidis* in their serum is inversely proportional to the incidence of meningococcal meningitis during the first 12 years of life.[75,76] At birth, as a result of maternal transfer of antibodies, about half of infants have bactericidal antibody titers. The prevalence of bactericidal antibody decreases after birth and reaches its nadir between 6 and 24 months of age. Thereafter, a linear increase in antibody occurs until age 12 years. In early adulthood, the prevalence of bactericidal antibody varies with the serogroup but ranges from 67% for group A to 86% for group B. These same investigators demonstrated the protective nature of bactericidal antibody against homologous serogroups during an epidemic situation. Only 3 of 54 sera from patients contained bactericidal antibody in prebleed specimens against the ultimately infecting serogroup, whereas 444 of 550 prebleed sera from matched control subjects who did not become infected contained homologous bactericidal antibody. Goldschneider and colleagues observed that systemic meningococcal disease developed in 38.5% of persons who lacked bactericidal antibody and acquired the epidemic strain in their nasopharynx in the military recruit environment. Their conclusion was that in the presence of nasopharyngeal colonization with a disease-causing strain, deficiency of circulating antimeningococcal antibodies is firmly associated with the establishment of meningococcemia. It appears that bactericidal antibodies are directed against both the capsular polysaccharide and other cell wall antigens, which may cross react within the family Neisseriaceae and with other bacterial genera. Goldschneider and associates demonstrated that the meningococcal carrier state is an immunizing process and that production of antibodies to meningococci can be identified within 2 weeks of colonization.[75,76] Nontypable meningococcal strains, which are seen in carrier studies in children, contain antigens that cross react with the encapsulated strains, and bactericidal antibody to these strains develops after nasopharyngeal colonization. Goldschneider and co-workers also showed that serogroup-specific antibodies arise during the carrier state.

Studies of Robbins and associates indicate that serologic cross-reactions occur between meningococcal group A polysaccharide and *Bacillus pumilis* and that *E. coli* K1 antigen is immunologically and chemically identical to group B capsular polysaccharide.[77,78] These unrelated yet immunologically similar antigens may play an important role in the development of natural immunity to the meningococcus and ultimately in protection against virulent meningococci. Cross-reactivity has now been clearly demonstrated between neonatal tissue and group B capsular polysaccharide. Monoclonal antibodies specific for this capsule have been used to show that cross-reactivity exists between central nervous system, cardiac, liver, and renal glycoproteins[79] in the infant rat and group B polysaccharide. As the animal matures, the cross-reacting antigens persist in the central nervous system. These studies suggest that the poor immunogenicity of this polysaccharide may be due to the fact that it resembles host antigens.

It should be stressed that although specific antibody is generally protective, this immunity is not absolute. Greenwood and co-workers and Kayhty and associates documented illness in individuals with pre-existing antibody titers that are considered protective.[80,81]

The exact role of local IgA antibody in protection or modulation of the carrier state is unknown. Plaut and colleagues have shown that the meningococcus produces a protease that cleaves the Fc fragment of secretory and serum IgA from the Fab portion of the molecule.[82] The impact of this enzyme on carriage is not known. However, production of this enzyme in *Neisseria* organisms is confined to the pathogenic members, the meningococcus and the gonococcus.[83]

THE MENINGOCOCCAL CARRIER STATE

Carriage of *N. meningitidis* in the nasopharynx in otherwise healthy humans has been recognized since 1896. Like the carrier states seen with cholera, diphtheria, and typhoid, the dichotomy between the presence of these dreaded organisms and absence of the associated disease process seemed a paradox to early investigators. Dopter, before the elucidation of distinct meningococcal serogroups, found organisms in the nasopharynx that had all the characteristics of meningococci but failed to agglutinate with antimeningococcic serum prepared from strains isolated from spinal fluid. He labeled these organisms parameningococci.[6] Considerable confusion arose, but subsequent investigators demonstrated that all four of the known serotypes, including the parameningococci of Dopter, could cause meningitis.

In 1908, Bruns and Hohn noted a close relationship between the carrier rate in a population and the onset, rise, and decline of an epidemic.[84] Glover noted the same association in the British Army military camps of World War I and believed that when the carrier rate exceeded 20%, the community was in danger of an epidemic, usually caused by the predominant carrier serotype.[8]

Transmission of meningococci from carrier to carrier is probably through the respiratory route. The rate of spread of the carrier state through a population has been the subject of a number of studies. During epidemics in military camps, the rate of new carrier acquisition can be very rapid, whereas in nonepidemic situations, both military and civilian, the rate of new carrier acquisition can be considerably slower, and the state of carriage can exist for prolonged periods. Rake demonstrated that carriers fall into three groups—chronic, intermittent, and transient—and that chronic carriers could be constantly affected for up to 2 years.[85] He also demonstrated that such factors as coryza unassociated with concomitant rises in other bacterial flora had no effect on the population of meningococci, whereas streptococcal pharyngitis or any other condition that increases other members of the resident flora of the nasopharynx causes a concomitant decrease in the number of meningococci present. Greenfield and colleagues studied carrier rates in families not exposed to clinically important meningococcal infection during a nonepidemic period. Eighty-eight percent of the strains isolated were groupable, with group B being the most common serogroup isolated.[86] During the 32-month observation period, 18% of the population were carriers at least once. The median duration of carriage was 9.6 months, and in 38%, it exceeded 16 months. Adult men had the highest incidence of carriage, from 19% to 39%. The adult male introduced the organism into the household 50% of the time, and when such a pattern occurred, the carrier rate in the children and women in the family increased to levels comparable to those for adult men. The rate of transmission in these circumstances was considered low in comparison to most communicable pathogens, and it was estimated that at this level a susceptible person would have more than a 50% chance of escaping carriage even if continually exposed to household carriers for a 5-year period.

A combination of factors is probably responsible for the transition from nasopharyngeal carriage to invasive disease. We previously pointed out the role of the encapsulation switching. Interestingly, organisms from healthy meningococcal carriers lacked the operons necessary for the synthesis, lipid modification, and transport of capsular polysaccharide.[87] Invasive meningococcal disease occurs primarily in persons who become newly infected with the organism.[88] Edwards and co-workers found that 31 of 36 patients had negative nasopharyngeal cultures during the 2 weeks before becoming ill and that 4 of these patients were culture negative the day before the development of disease.[88] The remaining 5 of 36 patients had positive cultures less than 4 days before the onset of illness. Other studies have shown that meningococcal epidemics occur not at times of high pharyngeal carriage but when the rates of acquisition of infection are increasing.[89] Coincident viral infection may affect the acquisition of meningococcal nasopharyngeal carriage. It has been noted that in a study of household contacts, individuals who had a recent history of symptoms of upper respiratory infection had a significantly higher carriage rate than did household members without such symptoms.[90] Moore and co-workers have shown that preceding *Mycoplasma* infection may be a cofactor in meningococcal meningitis in Chad.[91]

The carrier state is an immunizing process. Indirect evidence for this phenomenon is the fact that although military recruits have a high frequency of meningococcal carriage and disease, seasoned veterans have a much lower carriage rate and a disease incidence no different from that of the civilian population. In military recruits, antimeningococcal antibodies have been shown to persist for a minimum of 4 to 6 months after exposure. These antibodies are of the three major immunoglobulin classes and combine with group-specific and cross-reactive antigens.[75,76] Reller and associates demonstrated the development of bactericidal antibodies to the meningococcus in 38 military recruits who became colonized with nongroupable meningococcal strains. Thirty-nine percent of these men had bactericidal antibody to the homologous strains, and in addition, antibodies directed against groupable strains developed in 7% to 52%.[92] These same investigators found greatly enhanced (10- to 100-fold increase) bactericidal activity to known pathogenic strains of groups A, B, C, and Y after colonization with nongroupable meningococci, which suggests that these organisms may be at least as capable of stimulating cross-reactive antibody as groupable meningococci through either an initial or anamnestic response. A review of the meningococcal carrier state has been provided by Broome.[93]

Epidemiology of Meningococcal Disease

Epidemics in Africa, New Zealand, and Singapore indicate that this infection is still a worldwide major public health problem.[94-96] Children previously and presently account for the greatest percentage of these cases. Meningococcal disease is still a major worldwide health problem. Feldman estimates that during the period 1939 to 1962, almost 600,000 cases of meningococcal disease developed around the world, more than 100,000 of which were fatal.[97]

The case rate during endemic situations varies widely and has increased in the United States over a 5-year period (1991 to 1996) from 0.84 to 1.3 per 100,000 population. In 2001, 2333 cases were reported to the Centers for Disease Control and Prevention (CDC).[98] Serogroup Y accounted for 33% of the typed isolates. Peltola and co-workers have pointed out that shifts in this age distribution of meningococcal disease in a population can forecast an epidemic situation. Relatively more cases arise in the 5- through 19-year-old group during epidemic than during nonepidemic circumstances.[99,100] Careful surveillance of age

distribution patterns may be valuable in recognizing an epidemic during its inception.

Outbreaks of meningococcal infection account for less than 5% of reported cases in the United States but continue to occur in semiclosed populations, such as child care centers, military recruit camps, colleges, and schools.

The case-fatality rate varies depending on the prevalence of disease, the nature of the infection, and the socioeconomic conditions of the society in which the infections occur. During endemic situations in industrialized countries, case-fatality rates can be as low as 7% for meningitis and as high as 19% for septicemia without meningeal involvement.[101] During epidemic situations in some Third World countries, mortality for meningitis can vary from 2% to 10%, and mortality for septicemia can be as high as 70%.[102,103] In the United States, an 8% case-fatality rate has been reported from major medical centers during endemic periods.[104]

The dramatic effect of antibiotics on the case-fatality rate can be seen by comparing two epidemics. Norton and Gordon described an epidemic in Detroit from 1929 to 1931 that involved 1272 patients. The overall case-fatality rate was 50%, with the highest mortality occurring in infants (84%) and in adults older than 40 years (72%).[9] During an epidemic in Chile in 1940 to 1943,[11] the case rate in the province of Valparaiso during 1942 was 188.1 per 100,000 population. In Santiago at the peak of the same epidemic, the case rate in infants was 838.1 per 100,000 population. The meningococcal serotype responsible for this epidemic was group A. Sulfonamides were used for treatment, and the case-fatality rate was 16%.

It is clear that serogroup A, B, and C strains have different epidemic potential.[105] Serogroup B strains cause epidemics usually in developed nations with attack rates of 50 to 100 cases per 10^5 population. Serogroup C disease occurs in both developed and less developed nations and can have attack rates as high as 500 cases per 10^5 population. Serogroup A epidemics occur in less developed nations and have attack rates usually as high as 500 cases per 10^5 population. In all instances, epidemics occur among the poorest groups, where crowding and lack of sanitation are common.

During the past decade, areas of the world that have experienced epidemic meningococcal disease are Australia, Norway, the Netherlands, China, Egypt, Saudi Arabia, Kenya, and eastern Canada. Epidemics have occurred in school-aged children in northern Georgia and Los Angeles County. Several reviews about the problems of meningococcal epidemics in Africa have been written.[106,107] An epidemic of meningococcal disease has been occurring in New Zealand since 1991. The case rate has gone from 1.6 per 100,000 population in 1990 to 16.9 per 100,000 population in 1997. The predominate strain has had the phenotype B:4:P1.7b.4, which accounted for 84% of the cases by year 2000.[96] The case-fatality rate has been 4.5%, and the disease has disproportionately effected Maori and Pacific Island children in the northern part of North Island New Zealand.

An international outbreak of meningococcal disease caused by *N. meningitidis* W-135 occurred in association with the Hajj pilgrimage in 2000 and 2001,[94] with a high attack rate not only among the pilgrims but also among household contacts of returning pilgrims.[95] Although vaccination may protect the pilgrims from invasive disease, the data show that returning pilgrims represent a sizeable reservoir of a highly transmissible and persistent W-135 clone, which places their unvaccinated family contacts (and possibly the community at large) at risk for invasive disease.[95] *N. meningitidis* W-135 cases related to the ET-37 clone associated with the Haji outbreak have been reported since 2000 in countries in Europe, Africa, and Asia.

Epidemic meningococcal disease occurs during the dry season in the sub-Sahara regions of Africa with regularity. Because of the poor economic conditions of the countries involved, the inaccessibility of some of the regions, the paucity of the infrastructure, and the lack of funds available to international agencies, little has been done in terms of prevention until these epidemics begin. By that time, thousands of cases with a very high mortality have occurred, primarily in small children. Studies indicate that the development of meningococcal protein-capsular conjugate vaccine can overcome this problem if costs can be kept to a level that the less well-developed countries can afford.[108]

Clinical Manifestations

The difficulty in identifying meningococcal disease is due, in part, to the fact that clinicians in the community see so few cases in their lifetime and that the classic clinical features of meningococcal disease (e.g., hemorrhagic rash, meningismus, and impaired consciousness) appear late in the illness. The critical need for diagnosis as early as possible, because of the narrow time-window between progression from initial symptoms to death, prompted a systematic study of the occurrence of symptoms before admission to the hospital in children and adolescents (aged 16 years or younger) with meningococcal disease.[109] Nonspecific symptoms occurred for the first 4 to 6 hours, with more severe symptoms developing by 8 hours, such as leg pains, cold hands, cold feet, and abnormal skin color. Median time to hospital admission was 19 hours. By 24 hours, children were close to death.[109]

Studies in Boston describing a 20-year experience have shown that *N. meningitidis* is the second most common cause of community-acquired adult bacterial meningitis in the United States.[110] The successful use of *Haemophilus influenzae* type B capsular conjugate vaccine and the pneumococcal conjugate vaccines have made *N. meningitis* the leading cause of bacterial meningitis in children and young adults in the United States, with an overall mortality rate of 13% for meningitic disease. The clinical manifestations of meningococcal disease can be quite varied and can range from transient fever and bacteremia to fulminant disease with death ensuing within hours of the onset of clinical symptoms. Wolfe and Birbara[111] have described four clinical situations:

1. *Bacteremia without sepsis.* Admission is for an upper respiratory illness or viral exanthem. After recovery and frequently after discharge without specific antimicrobial therapy, the results of blood cultures are reported as positive for *N. meningitidis.* Sullivan and LaScolea reported three children with such occult bacteremia who recovered from meningococcal sepsis spontaneously without antibiotics. The serum level of bacteremia in these children was low, from 22 to 325 organisms per milliliter of blood.[112]
2. *Meningococcemia without meningitis.* In these cases, the patient's condition is septic, and signs of leukocytosis, skin rash, generalized malaise, weakness, headache, and hypotension develop on admission or shortly thereafter.
3. *Meningitis with or without meningococcemia.* In these patients, headache, fever, and meningeal signs are present with a cloudy spinal fluid. The state of the sensorium may vary widely from fully alert to completely depressed. Deep tendon and superficial reflexes are present. No pathologic reflexes are seen.
4. *The meningoencephalitic manifestation.* These patients are profoundly obtunded with meningeal signs and septic spinal fluid. The deep tendon and superficial reflexes are altered (either absent or rarely hyperactive). Pathologic reflexes are frequently present.

Variations of these manifestations can occur, and the patient can progress from one to the other during the course of disease.

The wide range of clinical expression requires a high index of suspicion and a careful search for clues of disease, particularly in an endemic situation in which a sporadic case is involved. Carpenter and Petersdorf in 53 such cases of meningococcal meningitis reported that headache, confusion, and stiff neck occurred as symptoms in less than half the patients.[113] In infants and small children, fever and vomiting are often the only complaints, and children are frequently not brought to the hospital until an insidious impairment in consciousness or convulsions occurs. In a multicenter surveillance study of invasive meningococcal infection in children that identified 159 cases between January 2001 and March 2005, meningitis accounted for 112 cases (70%) and bacteremia without meningitis for 43 cases (27%).[114]

The typical initial presentation of meningitis due to *N. meningitidis* consists of the sudden onset of fever, nausea, vomiting, headache, decreased ability to concentrate, and myalgias in an otherwise healthy patient. In a prospective observational cohort study, the classic meningitis triad of fever, neck stiffness, and altered mental status was present in 70 of the 258 patients (27%) with meningococcal meningitis; when rash was added, 89% of patients had at least two of these four signs.[115] The classic triad is much more common in pneumococcal meningitis (58% in the same cohort study).[116]

The signs of meningococcal disease can vary widely. Petechial lesions are a common harbinger of this infection, but occasionally if the patient is not completely undressed when examined or if examination of mucous surfaces such as the palpebral conjunctiva is omitted, important telltale lesions can be missed (Fig. 211-1). The petechial rash is manifested as discrete lesions 1 to 2 mm in diameter, most frequently on the trunk and lower portions of the body (Figs. 211-2 and 211-3). These lesions are commonly seen in clusters in areas where pressure

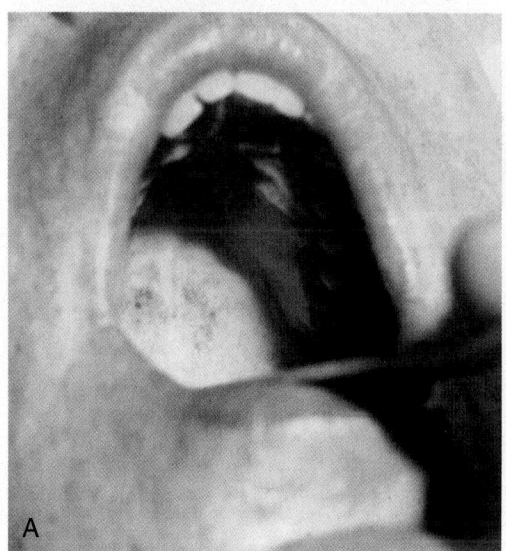

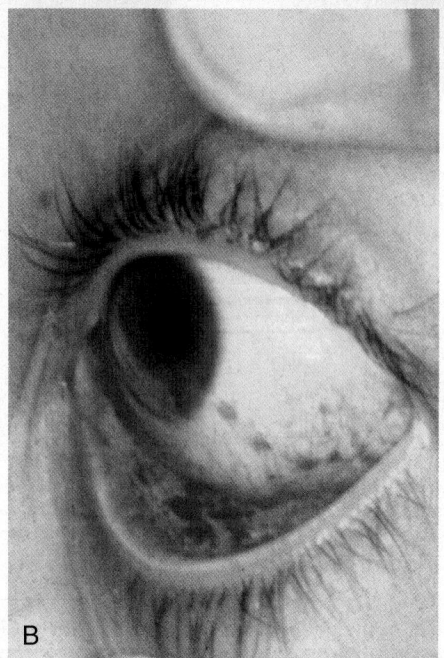

Figure 211-1 **Petechiae. A,** Petechial rash on the hard palate in a patient with meningococcemia. **B,** Palpebral and conjunctival petechiae resulting from meningococcal sepsis.

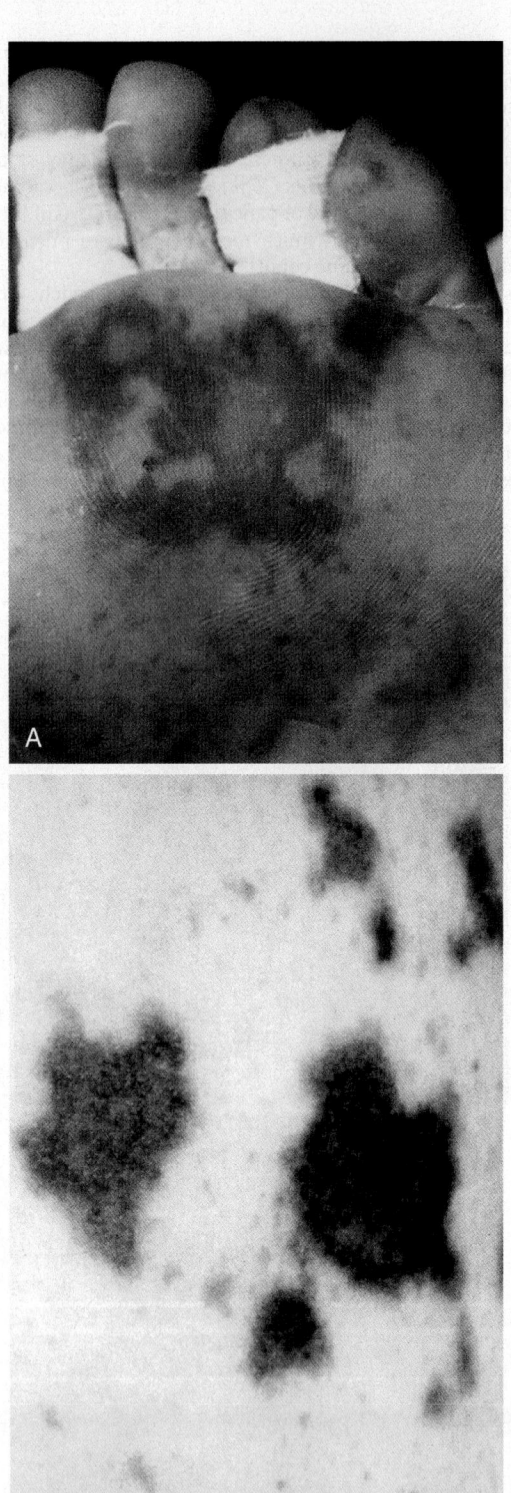

Figure 211-2 Subcutaneous ecchymoses. A, Subcutaneous ecchymoses on a sole resulting from meningococcal sepsis. **B,** Subcutaneous ecchymoses on the back resulting from meningococcal sepsis. *(Courtesy of Dr. Peter Densen.)*

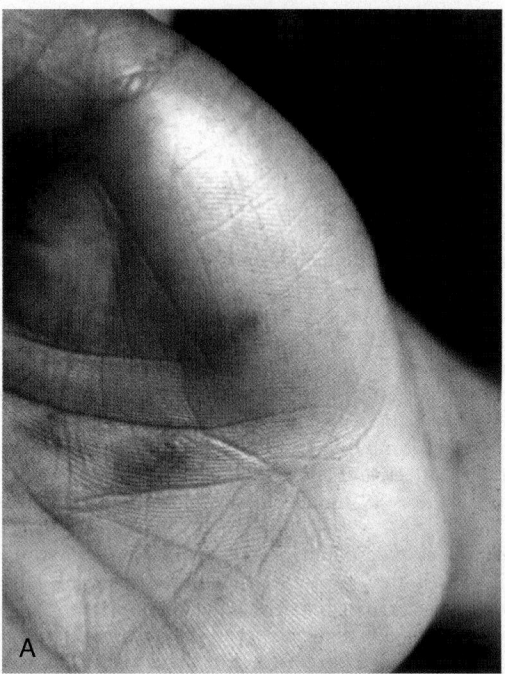

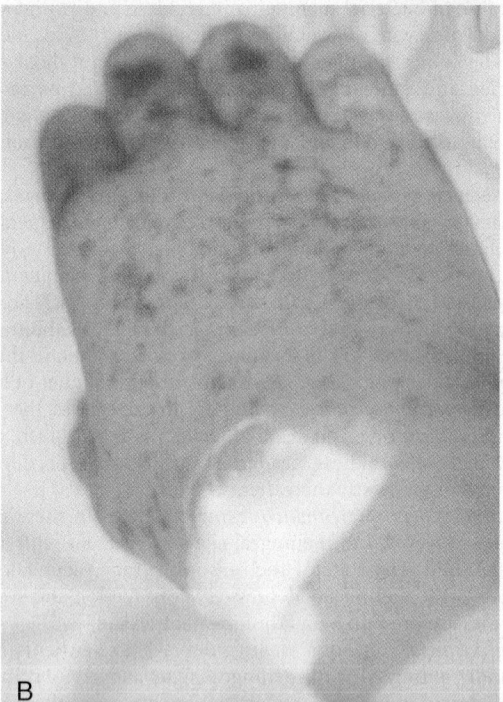

Figure 211-3 Embolic lesions and petechiae on the hand. A, Embolic lesions on a palm secondary to meningococcal sepsis. **B,** Petechiae on the dorsum of a hand resulting from meningococcal sepsis. *(Courtesy of Dr. Peter Densen.)*

may be applied to the skin by elastic in underwear or stockings, thus demonstrating the importance of completely disrobing the patient for an adequate examination. The petechial lesions can coalesce and form larger lesions that appear ecchymotic. These lesions may actually be secondary to subcutaneous hemorrhage, can occasionally be vesicular,

and frequently desquamate as the patients recover. The petechiae correlate with the degree of thrombocytopenia and are clinically important as an indicator in the evolution of bleeding complications secondary to the disseminated intravascular coagulopathy (DIC) that ensues. Early and aggressive intervention with antimicrobials and support of vascular perfusion are keys to prevention of this complication. Studies with activated protein C concentrate have shown promising results in reversing purpura fulminans once the process has begun. The drug is safe, although extremely expensive, and has been shown to lead to dose-related increases of plasma-activated protein C and

Figure 211-4 Rubella-like rash seen early in meningococcal sepsis.

resolution of coagulation imbalances.[117] At times, surgical débridement of lesions and skin grafting may be necessary. Deep necrosis of limbs or digits may call for amputation.[117]

A number of authors have described another type of rash associated with meningococcal infection.[97,111] This rash is a maculopapular eruption that can vary somewhat in hue and can be mistaken for a wide variety of viral exanthems, particularly rubella (Fig. 211-4). This eruption is not purpuric or pruritic and is transient; it usually does not last more than 2 days and is frequently gone hours after first observation. Generalized muscle tenderness may also be an important differential sign. Occasionally, the pain from these myalgias is quite intense and causes the patient considerable discomfort.

The neurologic problems seen with meningococcal meningitis are somewhat different from those seen with other forms of purulent meningitis. Evidence of meningeal irritation is common except in the very young and old. Feigin and Dodge showed that focal neurologic signs and seizures were less common in meningococcal meningitis than in pneumococcal meningitis or in meningitis caused by *Haemophilus,* whereas levels of unconsciousness were very similar in the three diseases.[118] This observation correlates with postmortem findings described by Thomas in which focal cerebral involvement in meningococcal meningitis was rare. The cause of death was related to toxins produced by the agent or by cerebral edema and to secondary effects on the vital centers in the midbrain region.[119] Ducker and Simmons supported these clinical findings by observing that doses of meningococcal endotoxin that produced no effect intravenously when introduced into the ventricular system of dogs produced massive hemorrhagic pulmonary edema, subendocardial hemorrhage, hemorrhage and edema of both the mitral and tricuspid valves, visceral congestion, and adrenal hemorrhage.[120] These lesions are similar to those seen outside the central nervous system in soldiers dying of meningococcal meningitis and bacteremia.[121]

Brandtzaeg and co-workers have made major contributions to our understanding of the physiologic effects of lipo-oligosaccharide during sepsis and meningitis caused by *N. meningitidis.* Their studies have placed a pathogenetic rationale for the clinical states of infection described by Wolfe and Birbara.[111,122-127] Brandtzaeg and colleagues have demonstrated the ability to measure lipo-oligosaccharide in the plasma and CSF of infected patients and have shown a close correlation between plasma lipo-oligosaccharide levels and prognosis. They have demonstrated that compartmentalization of lipo-oligosaccharide production correlates with the clinical findings in meningococcal infec-

tion.[124] Lipo-oligosaccharide levels in patients defined as having septicemia were high in plasma (median, 3500 ng) and low in CSF, whereas in patients with meningitis, lipo-oligosaccharide was detectable in the plasma of 3 of 19 patients and in the CSF of 18 of 19 patients with median levels of 2500 ng. Physiologic studies of meningococcal lipo-oligosaccharide in the plasma of infected patients revealed that it has a high sedimentation coefficient. Bacterial outer membrane fragments were found in the plasma of three patients. The plasma of one of these patients contained a bacterium covered with multiple, long membrane protrusions, thus indicating that surplus outer membrane (blebbing) does occur in vivo.[123] Mass spectrometric analysis of the endotoxin from patients with meningococcal sepsis indicated that it was of meningococcal origin rather than arising from the gastrointestinal tract as a result of increased permeability during infection.[127] Sedimentation analysis indicated that most of the lipo-oligosaccharide in these patients was not associated with high-density or low-density lipoproteins.

Outer membrane bleb formation by the group A meningococcus was first demonstrated by Cesarini and co-workers.[128] DeVoe and Gilchrist found that strains of meningococcal serogroups A, B, and C released membrane blebs in the log phase of growth but not in the lag phase.[129] The release of lipo-oligosaccharide from the surface of the meningococcus in the form of membrane blebs is now considered to be the principal factor associated with the high endotoxin levels in meningococcal sepsis.

The myocardial problems associated with this infection have been described.[130] Evidence of myocardial failure as manifested by a gallop rhythm, by congestive heart failure with pulmonary edema, and by high central venous pressure in the face of poor peripheral perfusion has been reported.[130] Treatment of the myocardial failure with cardiac glycosides has resulted in reversing this constellation of problems. Postmortem studies by Hardman[121] and by Gore and Saphir[131] have indicated that myocarditis of varying degrees of severity is present in more than half the patients who die of meningococcal disease. Studies have also shown myocardial dysfunction in children with acute meningococcemia.[132] Acute meningococcemia was not fatal in children without evidence of myocardial dysfunction. In contrast, three of seven children with evidence of myocardial dysfunction died.

The shock state all too frequently dominates the clinical picture. The patient is poorly responsive, and peripheral vasoconstriction is maximum, with cyanotic, poorly perfused extremities. Arterial blood gas analysis demonstrates evidence of acidosis in the range of pH 7.25 to 7.3, and depending on the degree of shock, anoxia may be manifested by an arterial Po_2 below 70 mm Hg. Probably the most dramatic consequence of this clinical problem is the presence of DIC. Clinical evidence of its occurrence can be obtained by documenting increasing petechiae within prescribed areas, gastric or gingival bleeding, or oozing at sites of venipuncture or intravenous infusions.

Either concomitant with the initial evaluation of the patient or later in the recovery phase of the illness, a number of unusual complications have been reported, including arthritis, pericarditis, conus medullaris syndrome, and cranial nerve dysfunction, particularly of the sixth, seventh, and eighth cranial nerves.[117,133-137] The pericarditis can cause massive tamponade. It is of interest that this complication may be unrelated to organism invasion of the pericardium but rather be due to an immunologic reaction or toxin. In the report of Pierce and Cooper, evidence of pericardial involvement occurred after two of the patients were in the recovery phase of their disease.[135] In one of these patients, the first symptoms of pericarditis occurred on the 20th day after the institution of therapy with penicillin. In the other patient, the first symptoms occurred 5 days after therapy began and recurred after pericardiocentesis and prednisone therapy on the 34th hospital day. This patient had a friction rub until the 49th hospital day and was not discharged until almost 3 months after admission. The incidence of this complication is about 19%. Cases of pericarditis occurred in the convalescent phase of the disease and in disease caused by the group C meningococcus. A report described serogroup W-135 in a patient with meningococcal myopericarditis.[135]

CHRONIC MENINGOCOCCEMIA

Persistent meningococcal bacteremia associated with low-grade fever, rash, and arthritis has been reported.[138-140] The distribution and appearance of the cutaneous lesions are identical to those seen in chronic gonococcemia, for which it is mistaken. Feldman has commented on a patient with chronic meningococcemia who appeared normal in every respect, including the ability to produce antibodies against the capsular polysaccharide of the infecting organism.[97] The frequency of meningococcus in the acute arthritis-dermatitis syndrome appears to be increasing.[139] Rompalo and co-workers compared the isolation of gonococcus and meningococcus from blood or synovial fluid from 1970 to 1972 with isolation of these organisms from 1980 to 1983.[140] The ratio of gonococcal to meningococcal isolates changed from 15:1 in 1970 to 1972 to 9:5 in 1980 to 1983. These authors believe that systemic meningococcal infection should figure more prominently in the differential diagnosis of the acute arthritis-dermatitis syndrome.

COMPLEMENT DEFICIENCY AND MENINGOCOCCEMIA

The syndrome of chronic meningococcemia must be distinguished from the problem of recurrent episodes of meningococcal meningitis. Studies by Lim and co-workers have demonstrated an absence of the sixth complement component in such a patient.[141] In addition, at least one of the patients with recurrent meningococcal disease studied by Alper and colleagues lacked C3.[142] Studies by Petersen and associates indicated that human deficiency of C8 has been found in some persons with disseminated gonococcal infection and that this complement component is required for serum bactericidal activity against the gonococcus.[143] Ellison and co-workers have evaluated the complement system in 20 patients with first episodes of serious systemic meningococcal infection. Six of 20 had a complement deficiency. Three had deficiencies in a terminal complement protein or proteins, and three had deficiencies of multiple factors associated with underlying disease states.[144] Densen and co-workers have studied a family with properdin deficiency whose members had a high rate of fatal meningococcal disease.[145] These investigators demonstrated that the bactericidal defect could be corrected by vaccination of this population. Studies by Ross and co-workers suggest that vaccinating individuals deficient in late-complement components may shift the burden of host defense from serum bactericidal activity to phagocytosis.[146] These studies would stress the previously unrecognized importance of the complement system in protection against neisserial infections. The role of complement in meningococcal infection has been reviewed by Densen.[147]

RESPIRATORY INFECTIONS WITH THE MENINGOCOCCUS

Meningococcal pneumonia has been recognized as a clinical syndrome for more than 80 years. Because of nasopharyngeal carriage of the meningococcus, establishing the diagnosis by sputum culture alone is hazardous. The incidence of sepsis associated with this type of meningococcal infection appears to be quite low.[148] Therefore, blood cultures may not be of value. Koppes and associates used transtracheal cultures to establish the diagnosis in 68 Air Force recruits with group Y meningococcal pneumonia.[148] In this series, a history of cough, chest pain, chills, and previous upper respiratory infection occurred in more than half the patients. Rales and fever occurred in almost all patients, and evidence of pharyngitis was present in more than 80%. The disease involved more than one lobe in 40%, with the right lower and middle lobes involved most frequently. The prognosis was good, with no deaths occurring in the 68 patients with pneumonia. The association of meningococcal infection with preceding viral respiratory infection has been reported. Young and co-workers investigated an outbreak of meningococcal infection in an aged population, most of whom had serologic evidence of influenza.[149] Goldstein and associ-

ates have shown that pulmonary clearance of meningococci is diminished in animals previously exposed to an avirulent encephalomyocarditis virus.[150] In a study of the etiology of community-acquired pneumonia in Finland, *N. meningitidis* was implicated as the etiologic agent in 6 of 162 cases.[151]

A review of 58 cases of meningococcal pneumonia over a 25-year period revealed both marked changes in antibiotic therapy and variation of serogroups causing disease.[152] Antibiotic therapy had shifted from primarily penicillin to cephalosporins over the past decade. In patients from whom organisms were isolated, serogroup Y was the most prevalent single serogroup causing disease (44%), followed by serogroups B (18%), W-135 (16%), and C (14%). There were five fatalities (8.6%) in this study.

Meningococcal upper respiratory tract infection (pharyngitis) associated with contacts of cases and as a prior symptom and sign in cases of serious meningococcal disease has been described.[153] Suggestions that pharyngeal inflammation is the predecessors to bacteremic dissemination have been made but are unsubstantiated.

FULMINANT MENINGOCOCCAL SUPRAGLOTTIS

Fulminant meningococcal supraglottis is a rare presentation of meningococcal infection. It was first reported as a syndrome in 1995, and since then, five reports have been published. The diagnosis should be considered with the patient's clinical picture of sore throat, dysphagia, fever, muffled voice, and swollen supraglottic tissues, as seen on plain films, fiberoptic laryngoscopy, and cervical CT scan.[154]

MENINGOCOCCAL URETHRITIS

Meningococci have been isolated from the urethra and can be the etiologic agent in urethritis. An association between orogenital sex and acquisition of the organism has been suggested.[155] In a population of homosexual males, the organism was isolated from the oropharynx (93% of isolates), rectum (6% of isolates), and urethra (1% of isolates).[155]

▣ Laboratory Diagnosis of Meningococcal Infection

Definitive diagnosis of serious meningococcal infection has as a prerequisite the bacteriologic isolation of *N. meningitidis* from a usually sterile body fluid such as blood, CSF, or synovial, pleural, or pericardial fluid. CSF and blood are the most fruitful sources of positive cultures.[156,157] It is important to isolate the organism not only to confirm an etiology of infection but also to perform antibiotic susceptibility testing. Meningococci with increasing resistance to the penicillins, chloramphenicol, and cephalosporins have been reported.[158-162] In an analysis of 727 cases of meningococcal disease, Hoyne and Brown described the results of 400 blood cultures, of which 51.4% were positive for meningococci.[163] Spinal fluid examination of 423 patients from the same series indicated that 94% were positive for gram-negative diplococci by either smear or culture for the meningococci. Carpenter and Petersdorf indicated that 46% of their cases of meningococcal meningitis were positive by CSF culture.[113] In an additional 12% of the cases, the diagnosis was made by smear of the spinal fluid and by the clinical manifestations. Levin and Painter studied 28 patients with culture-proven meningococcal disease, and in 22 of 27 patients tested, the spinal fluid was positive, whereas 15 of 28 had positive blood cultures.[130] It is of interest that in 8 of 12 patients considered to have meningococcemia without clinical evidence of meningitis, spinal fluid cultures were positive. Feldman has quantitated the bacterial counts of meningococcal meningitis in CSF and reported a mean of 1.27×10^5 (1.5×10^2 to 6×10^7) organisms per milliliter.[164] The ability to see or to culture meningococci in petechial skin and mucosal lesions varies widely. Hoyne and Brown reported identification in 69.8% of the petechial smears examined.[163] Skin biopsy may play a role in the diagnosis of meningococcal infection. This issue was addressed in a prospective study of the use of Gram stain and culture from biopsies of skin lesions in 31 patients with suspected meningococcal infection and 12 controls.[165] The sensitivities of cultures of blood, CSF, and skin biopsies were 56%, 50%, and 36%, respectively. When culture and Gram stain were combined, the sensitivities were 56%, 64%, and 56%, respectively. In three patients, the diagnosis of meningococcal infection was based solely on positive skin biopsy results. Thus, Gram stain and culture of a skin lesion can increase the diagnostic yield. Care should be taken with these specimens because of difficulty in interpretation, and negative results do *not* exclude the diagnosis of meningococcal infection.

Studies of pericardial fluid have failed to demonstrate the organism by smear or culture.[134] Chemical and cytologic examination of spinal fluid in meningococcal infection can yield variable results. Carpenter and Petersdorf examined the spinal fluid of 58 patients with meningococcal meningitis.[113] The median leukocyte count was about 1200, with a range of less than 10 to 65,000/mm^3. About 75% had CSF glucose levels below 40 mg/dL. Unfortunately, spinal fluid–to–serum glucose ratios were not given. CSF protein levels ranged from 25 to more than 800 mg/dL, with the median value of about 150 mg/dL. Although not commented on specifically by these authors, the cell type in untreated cases is almost always polymorphonuclear. Partially treated patients may have a pleomorphic spinal fluid.

PCR, which detects small quantities of bacterial DNA, has the potential to be an important tool in the rapid diagnosis of meningococcal infection. PCR has been used in the diagnosis of meningococcal meningitis by examination of CSF. The sensitivity and specificity of PCR for the diagnosis of meningococcal meningitis are more than 90%. This technique has proved to be particularly useful in confirmation of the diagnosis in situations in which culture has little value because of prior antibiotic administration. Studies in Great Britain have shown the usefulness of multiplex PCR in establishing the diagnosis of meningococcal disease.[166-169] PCR also has the capability of rapidly typing strains, a useful adjunct in situations that appear to be an evolving epidemic.[166]

PCR has a number of advantages compared with culture for the diagnosis of meningococcal infection.[170] It can establish the diagnosis more rapidly if available as an in-hospital test. PCR results are often available on the day of presentation, compared with 1 or 2 days or more for culture confirmation.[170] Because viable bacteria are not required, sensitivity is not affected by prior antibiotic administration, which can sterilize the CSF within 1 to 2 hours[171]; it can rapidly type strains, a useful adjunct in situations that appear to be an epidemic in evolution[172,173]; and multiplex PCR permits simultaneous testing for meningococcal, pneumococcal, and *H. influenzae* infection.[174]

The performance of real-time PCR was assessed in a report of 24 patients with meningococcal infection[170] The sensitivity and specificity were 96% and 100%, respectively; in contrast, the sensitivity of CSF or blood culture was only 63%. In all nine patients in whom blood was tested more than once, PCR remained positive longer than culture after the initiation of antibiotic therapy; in three patients, more than 72 hours longer.

Despite these benefits, PCR has not replaced traditional culture methods because it cannot be used to determine antimicrobial susceptibility and is not routinely performed by most hospital laboratories. Nonetheless, PCR has now established itself as an important tool in the rapid diagnosis of meningococcal infection.

▓ Treatment of Meningococcal Infections

The introduction of antibiotics has dramatically altered the prognosis of meningococcal disease. Today, the expected mortality under optimal conditions should not exceed 8% to 10%.[101,111] Random cases frequently fare poorer than those in an epidemic because medical personnel are not alerted to the diagnosis and may overlook the early signs and symptoms. The value of early diagnosis in lowering the mortality rate is exemplified by the results at Fort Dix, where an intense surveillance program was established between 1968 and 1969 and the mortality was less than 5%. Mortality rates in patients with meningococcal meningitis are about 10% to 15% despite antibiotic treatment.[114] A retrospective population-based analysis of meningococcal disease mortality in the United States from 1990 to 2002 identified 3335 meningococcal deaths. The following findings were noted:

- The crude and age-adjusted mortality rates were 0.10 deaths per 100,000 population per year; most deaths occurred among persons younger than 25 years (58%).
- Mortality was highest in infants (crude mortality rate, 0.95 per 100,000 population).
- Age-adjusted mortality rates were significantly higher among African Americans (0.13 per 100,000 population) compared with other racial or ethnic groups.
- Mortality rates were higher in winter than summer months.
- Mortality rates increased from 1990 to 1997 and decreased from 1998 to 2002 (primarily due to declining mortality in children younger than 5 years and infants).
- In the multicenter surveillance study of invasive meningococcal infection in children noted above, mortality was greatest for children 11 years of age and older (21%, compared with 5% in those younger than 11 years).[109]
- In the multicenter surveillance study of invasive meningococcal infection in children noted above, mortality was greatest for children 11 years and older (21%, compared with 5% in those younger than 11 years)[109] (refer to the Meningococcal Vaccine Information Statement, National Immunization Program Webpage, at http://www.cdc.gov/vaccines/pubs/vis/downloads/vis-mening.pdf).

In addition to the use of antibiotics, the application of supportive care to treat the problems of DIC, shock, heart failure, prolonged mental obtundation, pericarditis, and pneumonia, which complicate this infection, has had a decided impact on prognosis.

ANTIBIOTIC THERAPY

The era of chemotherapy for meningococcal infection began with a report of Schwentker and associates in 1937 that demonstrated that sulfonamides could be successfully used in the treatment of meningococcal meningitis and meningococcemia.[12] Feldman and co-workers confirmed these observations. A dramatic change occurred in the prognosis of epidemic meningitis.[175] As new antibiotics were introduced through the 1940s and 1950s, reports appeared that documented the efficacy of several agents used alone and in combination. Early studies of penicillin given in relatively low doses (120,000 units/day intramuscularly) indicated that it was not as effective as sulfonamides.[176] Using larger amounts of the drug (360,000 units/day intramuscularly), Kinsman and D'Alonzo demonstrated that treatment results with penicillin were identical to those with sulfonamides.[177] The efficacy of chloramphenicol as a therapeutic agent was demonstrated by McCrumb and co-workers.[178] In 15 patients treated with this drug, all survived, and only 1 patient had a complication secondary to the infection, ophthalmoplegia, which subsequently cleared.

The therapeutic efficacy of first-generation cephalosporins was studied in the 1960s. These agents produced variable results, and their use is now contraindicated in treating meningococcal infection.[179] Third-generation cephalosporins demonstrate excellent in vitro effectiveness against the meningococcus[180] and achieve central nervous system concentrations adequate to treat meningococcal meningeal infection (Table 211-2).

Sulfonamides now have a very limited role in the treatment of meningococcal infection. Studies by Schoenback and Phair[14] and by Love and Finland[181] revealed small populations of sulfonamide-resistant meningococci. In 1963, an epidemic of group B meningococcal infection occurred at Ford Ord, California, in which the infecting strain was resistant to sulfonamides.[18,182] Since that time, most isolates,

TABLE 211-2	Treatment and Prevention of Serious Meningococcal Infection	
Problem	**Treatment**
Meningococcal meningitis and meningococcemia	Ceftriaxone, in children 25 mg/kg q12h IV up to 1 g. Adult dose, 1 g IV q12h.[193] Or penicillin G, 50,000 U/kg q4h IV, up to 4 million U q4h. If penicillin and cephalosporin allergic, chloramphenicol, 25 mg/kg q6h IV up to 1 g q6h.[189]
Antibiotic chemoprophylaxis for household or intimate contacts*	Rifampin: adults, 600 mg q12h for 2 days; children < 1 mo, 5 mg/kg q12h for 2 days; children > 1 mo, 10 mg/kg q12h (maximum, 600 mg) orally for 2 days. Ciprofloxacin: adults, 500 mg, single dose.† Ceftriaxone: children < 15 yr, 125 mg, single IM dose; adults, 250 mg, single dose[187,205]
Immunoprophylaxis	Meningococcal conjugate vaccine (MCV4) is administered once by volume according to the manufacturer's instructions. A single dose contains 4 micrograms of each capsular polysaccharide (A, C, Y, W135) conjugated to 48 micrograms of diphtheria toxoid.[248,251,258,259] Vaccination should be considered an adjunct to antibiotic chemoprophylaxis for household or intimate contacts of patients with meningococcal disease when appropriate serogroups are causing disease.[251,258]

*Recommended groups for chemoprophylaxis, based on exposure to the case in the week before onset of illness:
- Household contacts and persons sharing the same living quarters, particularly young children
- Daycare center or child care contacts, frequent playmates of young children
- Close social contacts who were exposed to oral secretions in week before onset, such as by kissing, sharing eating utensils or toothbrushes

†Cases of ciprofloxacin resistance have been reported, and use for prophylaxis should be based on local sensitivity of the meningococcus to the drug.[234]

primarily serogroups B and C in the United States and group A from worldwide locations, have been resistant to sulfadiazine.[183-185]

Penicillin therapy for meningococcal infections is safe and effective. Almost all US strains remain sensitive to this antibiotic.[186] A goal of antibiotic therapy for meningitis is to establish concentrations of antibiotics in the spinal fluid that approximate 10 times the minimal inhibitory concentration of the organism for that agent.[187] A dose of 300,000 units/kg/day is recommended, with an upper limit of 24 million units/day as 2 million units every 2 hours.[188] Reports of penicillin-insensitive N. meningitidis have come from Great Britain, Spain, and less commonly, the United States.[189,190] In these cases, penicillin should never be used, and third-generation cephalosporins would be the agents of choice (care should be taken to choose an active cephalosporin[190]). Relative resistance to penicillin is due to a reduced affinity of penicillin-binding proteins 2 and 3.[190] Spinal fluid levels of penicillin averaged 0.8 μg/mL on the first day of therapy. This concentration approximated the minimal inhibitory concentration for penicillin G for the most resistant isolate studied by this group. These strains were also relatively resistant to cefuroxime, but cefotaxime and ceftriaxone appear to be active against these strains in vitro. High-level resistance in β-lactamase–producing strains has also been reported. Although resistant meningococcal strains have been infrequently reported to date, clinicians should be alerted to the possibility of their occurrence in unexplained treatment failures or in cases of slowly resolving, documented meningococcal central nervous system infections. Chloramphenicol is an effective substitute in penicillin-allergic patients and should be administered intravenously in a dose of 100 mg/kg/day up to a maximum of 4 g/day in total dose.[188] Chloramphenicol-resistant strains have been reported but remain rare in the United States.[191] Third-generation cephalosporins, including cefotaxime, ceftriaxone, ceftizoxime, and ceftazidime, have been used successfully in the treatment of pediatric cases of meningococcal meningitis, and treatment with ceftriaxone is the treatment of choice in the United States.[192] Penetration of second- and third-generation agents into spinal fluid has been studied (Table 211-3).[193] Ceftriaxone, cefotaxime, and ceftazidime achieve levels in CSF several orders of magnitude greater than the susceptibility of the meningococcus to these agents. The ability to

administer ceftriaxone once daily makes this drug particularly attractive. The duration of antibiotic therapy will vary somewhat with the manifestation of the disease and with the response of the patient. At present, when the meningococcus is sensitive to the agents just mentioned, 10 to 14 days of therapy is usually sufficient. A prospective study in 58 patients (44 confirmed and 14 probable) during an epidemic of serogroup B meningococcal disease indicated that benzyl penicillin G (8 to 12 million units/day) could be used for 3 days with an 8.6% mortality rate. Three of the five patients who died in this study did so within 24 hours of admission. None of the surviving patients relapsed (mean follow-up was 23.9 months ± 14.7 months).[194] This study was performed during an epidemic situation when awareness of the illness was high, and such therapy should be reserved for epidemic situations, in which cost of treatment may be a major factor and the antibiotic sensitivity is known.

Studies in England have suggested that administration of parenteral penicillin by practitioners as soon as the diagnosis was suspected led to a significantly more favorable outcome.[195,196] The doses given in the studies were not provided. Studies have confirmed the value of early treatment of invasive meningococcal infection to a favorable outcome.[197] Studies by Barquet and co-workers have shown that receipt of antibiotic therapy before hospital admission was associated with a reduced likelihood of death.[197] In the patient group defined as having acute clinical infection, a single death occurred in 119 patients treated with antibiotics before admission, compared with 15 deaths in 329 similar patients (P = .04) who were not given prehospitalization therapy.

SUPPORTIVE CARE

Common complications of meningococcal disease are vascular collapse and shock, primarily caused by the effects of meningococcal lipo-oligosaccharide, which is a potent toxin. The cytokine tumor necrosis factor-α (TNF-α) may be a mediator of endotoxic shock because when it is injected into animals, it induces hypotension, metabolic acidosis, and death.[198-201] Studies in animals suggest that treatment or pretreatment with polyclonal[200] or monoclonal[202] antibodies against TNF-α could be beneficial in purpura fulminans. Girardin and co-workers have demonstrated that serum levels of TNF-α, interleukin-1 (IL-1), and interferon-γ correlated with the severity of meningococcemia in children.[203] At the present time, it is not known whether these cytokines play a deleterious or protective role in shock secondary to meningococcal sepsis. Brandtzaeg and co-workers have extensively studied this question during an epidemic in Norway.[122-127,198] These investigators showed that IL-6 and IL-1 are released into the serum and coexist with TNF-α and lipopolysaccharide in the systemic circulation during the initial phase of meningococcal septic shock. High levels of IL-6 and IL-1 are associated with a fatal outcome, and IL-1 was detected exclusively in patients who had high levels of IL-6, TNF-α, and lipopolysaccharide and a rapid fatal outcome. These investigators also showed that lipopolysaccharide was compartmentalized primarily in the plasma in patients with meningococcemia, whereas patients with meningitis had high levels in CSF and low or undetectable levels in plasma. In other studies, this group has shown that extensive complement activation occurs in fulminant cases of meningococcemia.[125] The results in these studies suggested that the lipopolysaccharide was an important activator of complement in systemic

TABLE 211-3	Susceptibilities of Meningococci, Kinetics, and Cerebrospinal Fluid Penetration of Selected Second- and Third-Generation Cephalosporins		
Cephalosporin	**Susceptibility (μg/mL)**	**CSF Concentration (μg/mL)**	**CSF Penetration (%)**
Cefuroxime	<0.2-1.6	1.1-17.1	11.6-13.7
Ceftriaxone	<0.001	2.1-7.2	1.5-7.4
Cefotaxime	<0.008	1.2-83 (mean, 6.3)	4-54 (mean, 22.7)
Ceftazidime	0.007-0.5	2.5-30 (mean, 9.8)	14

Data from references 177-183.

meningococcal disease and that complement-activating products in concert with other mediators may contribute to the multiple-organ failure and death occurring in the most severe cases.[125] New therapies are emerging that may have a significant impact on the management of meningococcal sepsis. Preliminary evaluation of the administration of a recombinant protein composed of the *N*-terminal fragment of human bactericidal and permeability-increasing protein in children with meningococcal sepsis has been encouraging. Data from the phase III, randomized, placebo-controlled trial indicate that administration of recombinant bactericidal permeability-increasing protein (rBPI 21) reduces clinically significant morbidities and improves the functional outcome of children with severe meningococcemia.[204] No statistically significant benefit in mortality was demonstrated. Because of the rare incidence of disease and the rapidity of death in this study, the trial was substantially underpowered to detect a statistically significant mortality advantage. Before the completion of the trial, the probability that the study might have been underpowered to detect a significant reduction in mortality was recognized. An attempt at selecting a previously unvalidated composite end point to increase the meaningful event rate for the primary end point proved unsuccessful. Significant improvements were seen in other prospectively defined outcome variables that suggest an overall substantial benefit of therapy with rBPI21 in children with severe meningococcemia.

Clinical studies in patients with septic shock treated with recombinant activated protein C substitution (Xigris, drotrecogin alfa) have demonstrated its safety and efficacy. The incidence of serious bleeding was increased in the drotrecogin alfa–treated group.[205] A study of recombinant activated protein C substitution on imminent peripheral necroses and outcome was performed on 12 patients, 5 of whom had meningococcal sepsis. This study concluded that protein C limited the extent of tissue necrosis but was too small to make any recommendations on the use of protein C in sepsis-related purpura fulminans and shock.[206] Whenever a patient with meningococcal sepsis and shock is being considered for drotrecogin alfa therapy, the exclusion criteria used in the PROWESS trial should be reviewed and applied.[205,207] Meningococcal shock patients who evidence bleeding should be excluded.

In every case of systemic meningococcal infection, the potential for shock must be always considered. Observation for shock and its therapy[208-211] are best accomplished in an intensive care unit. The use of steroids, particularly in patients with evidence of purpura fulminans and concomitant adrenal hemorrhage (Waterhouse-Friderichsen syndrome), is still controversial. In the 1950s, several investigators recommended the use of corticosteroid replacement therapy. However, the studies of Belsey and colleagues were inconclusive in demonstrating a beneficial effect of the application of low-dose steroid in meningococcal infection.[212] In a study of the clinical effect of early adjunctive dexamethasone therapy in management of adults with bacterial meningitis, Thomas and co-workers could not demonstrate differences in outcome as measured by neurologic sequelae. They did demonstrate that antibiotic penetration into the CSF was impaired and cautioned about the effect this might have on outcomes in patients with borderline sensitive organisms.[213]

As pointed out earlier, the problem of DIC is ominous. Petechiae are frequent accompaniments of meningococcal sepsis. The development of increasing petechial lesions, confluent ecchymoses, persistently bleeding venipuncture sites, and bleeding gums despite adequate antimicrobial therapy and supportive care is indicative of DIC. Heparin treatment of this complication of meningococcal disease is probably not indicated.[214] As many patients can be harmed by the inappropriate treatment of DIC as by DIC itself. To complicate matters, in severe DIC, the problem of plasmin activation with fibrinolysis becomes a clinical reality. It appears that impairment of the protein C anticoagulation pathway is critical to the thrombosis associated with sepsis and to the development of purpura fulminans in meningococcemia. This occurs because protein C activation is impaired, a finding consistent with the downregulation of the thrombomodulin-endothelial protein C receptor pathway.[215]

Other major life-threatening complications necessitating therapy include adult respiratory distress syndrome, neurologic sequelae ranging from coma to diabetes insipidus, pneumonia that is not necessarily meningococcal but may be secondary to aspiration during the obtunded state, and pericarditis. This last problem can be insidious and can appear in the convalescent stage of disease. Awareness that it can occur will readily lead to its diagnosis and treatment.

The ability to define the outcome of meningococcal sepsis based on a number of indicators has been studied extensively.[216-218] Kornelisse and co-workers have used a set of objective indicators, including the C-reactive protein level, base excess, serum potassium level, and platelet count. This system was predictive of death or survival in 86% of the patients studied.[216]

Studies have shown that children with meningococcal sepsis have higher than normal concentrations of plasminogen activator inhibitor-1 (PAI-1) in plasma. It has been found that children with the functional deletion/insertion (4G/5G) polymorphism in the promoter region of PA-1 produce higher concentrations of PAI-1, develop more severe coagulopathy, and are at greater risk for death during meningococcal sepsis.[219]

CHEMOPROPHYLAXIS OF THE MENINGOCOCCAL CARRIER

Shortly after the clinical use of sulfonamides for the treatment of serious meningococcal disease, it became apparent that short courses of the sulfadiazine resulted in the disappearance of meningococcal carriage for prolonged periods.[220,221] As Feldman pointed out, despite the arguments about the relationship "if there are no carriers, there are no cases," the use of sulfonamides to reduce carrier rates did decrease the number of cases.[97]

Treatment of the meningococcal carrier state with sulfonamides eradicated carriage quickly and for prolonged periods.[222] The length of time was a function of the initial dose of sulfonamides, and with doses as high as 8 g, the carrier rate was reduced from about 45% to less than 10% at 16 weeks. Cheever demonstrated that after two doses of 3 and 2 g of sulfadiazine, the carrier rate dropped from 79% to 0% in 72 hours.[223] On military bases and in closed environments such as boarding schools, institutions, and family units in which cases arose, this form of chemoprophylaxis was effective in disrupting the spread of meningococcal infection.

With the recognition of widespread sulfonamide-resistant meningococci and the failure of sulfadiazine to have an impact on the epidemic at Fort Ord,[15,16,182] these agents have been abandoned for meningococcal chemoprophylaxis except in instances in which the meningococcal case strains are known to be sulfa sensitive.

The search for new agents for chemoprophylaxis has been extensive. Penicillin has proved ineffective for several reasons: long-acting mixtures do not eradicate nasopharyngeal carriage, and although massive doses cause people to become noncarriers, the carrier state recurs promptly after discontinuation of use of the drug.[97,224] Minocycline and rifampin have been shown to eradicate the carrier state rapidly, and this eradication persists for up to 6 to 10 weeks after treatment.[225,226] Problems occur with both drugs. Minocycline has been shown to cause vertigo, probably secondary to an effect on the vestibular system.[227] Rifampin treatment can result in the emergence of rifampin-resistant meningococci in 10% to 27% of patients treated.[228] In addition, rifampin causes red urine in almost all patients, which can be quite disconcerting unless some forewarning is given. Rifampin should be avoided in pregnant women and may reduce efficacy of oral contraceptives. Studies by Pugsley and co-workers have demonstrated in 21 persistent meningococcal nasopharyngeal carriers that ciprofloxacin, 500 mg every 12 hours for 5 days, eradicated the meningococcus from the nasopharynx in 100% of individuals for up to 13 days after the completion of therapy. An untreated comparative control group had a carriage rate of 85% at that time.[229] Gilja and co-workers used a single dose of 400 mg of ofloxacin in a controlled study and showed that it can eradicate nasopharyngeal carriage for up to 33 days in 97% of subjects.[230] A single dose of ceftriaxone (250 mg intramuscularly for adults and 125 mg for children younger than 15 years) has also been shown to eradicate nasopharyngeal carriage for 14 days.[230] A single 500-mg dose of azithromycin has been found to be as effective as rifampin in eradicating meningococci from the nasopharynx of asymptomatic carriers.[231]

The recommended therapy for meningococcal prophylaxis has been expanded to include either rifampin, ciprofloxacin, or ceftriaxone[186] (see Table 211-2).

A number of other agents active against meningococci in vitro have been tested but have failed to provide prophylaxis. These agents include erythromycin, trimethoprim, cephalexin, oxytetracycline, and nalidixic acid. Hoeprich has studied a number of these drugs and speculates that the primary factor determining effectiveness as a meningococcal prophylactic agent is the ability to achieve bactericidal levels in tears and saliva.[232] Cases of fluoroquinolone-resistant meningococci have been reported worldwide.[233]

The question of who should receive prophylaxis has concerned public health officials since the advent of effective chemoprophylaxis. Initially with sulfonamides, little discrimination between high-risk and low-risk populations was attempted, and the drug was administered very widely to people without the remotest increased risk for disease. Since the clinical emergence of sulfa resistance and the problem in finding agents that are safe and effective, more attention has been paid to the populations at greatest risk who need chemoprophylaxis. During epidemics and in endemic situations in civilian populations, household contacts have been shown to be at increased risk for infection.[9,11,104] Analysis by the CDC meningococcal surveillance group showed that the attack rate in this group was 500 to 800 times greater than that determined for the general population studied.[103] Similar high-risk situations exist in closed populations such as in some college dormitories, long-term care hospitals, nursery schools,[234] and military barracks. In the community, chemoprophylaxis is recommended for household contacts, daycare center members, and anyone exposed to the patient's oral secretions, but not school, transportation, or office contacts. Secondary cases usually occur within 10 days of the primary case, but longer intervals have been described. Close surveillance of this group for at least 10 days would ensure prompt treatment of any secondary cases that might arise in the absence of effective chemoprophylaxis. Beginning chemoprophylaxis more than 2 weeks after exposure to the index case would be too late to prevent secondary cases. Hospital personnel are not at increased risk and in general should not receive chemoprophylaxis[235]; however, medical staff who have an intimate exposure such as mouth-to-mouth resuscitation or endotracheal intubation should receive prophylaxis.[97,236] The index case should also be treated before leaving the hospital if penicillin or ampicillin was used because these antibiotics do not reliably end the carrier state.

IMMUNOPROPHYLAXIS OF MENINGOCOCCAL INFECTION

An intense effort was directed at the development of a vaccine for prevention of meningococcal infections in this high-risk population after the emergence of sulfa-resistant meningococci in the 1960s. The result was the development of vaccines derived from the capsular polysaccharide of groups A and C meningococci. Artenstein and co-workers demonstrated the effectiveness of the group C vaccine in studies of US Army recruits.[17] Only 1 case of meningococcal disease occurred among 13,763 vaccinees, whereas 38 bacteriologically proven cases occurred in a control group of 68,072. This vaccine resulted in an 87% reduction in disease, which was statistically significant. Makela and associates showed that administration of group A polysaccharide to Finnish military recruits significantly lowered the incidence of disease caused by this serogroup when compared with an unvaccinated control population.[237] Studies from Finland during a group A epidemic demonstrated the effectiveness of this vaccine in children 3 months to 5 years of age.[16] Studies from Africa by Reingold and colleagues indi-

cate that efficacy in this population 1 year after serogroup A vaccination is less than 30% in children younger than 4 years.[238]

After the initial development of the meningococcal vaccine for use in military recruits, the vaccine was introduced for use in civilian populations. The polysaccharide vaccine was expanded to other serogroups, resulting in a tetravalent serogroup A, C, Y, and W-135 capsular polysaccharide vaccine (MPSV4).[239] No vaccine has been developed that will prevent infections caused by N. meningitidis serogroup B. MPSV4 has been shown to have clinical efficacies of less than 85% among school-aged children and adults and to be useful in controlling outbreaks of disease. The vaccine is safe.[239,240] Reactions appear to be limited to local erythema at the site of injection in about 4% and some increased irritability in young children in about 6% of the vaccine recipients. Multiple doses of the polysaccharide A and C vaccine might cause immunologic hyporesponsiveness to group A and group C polysaccharide. The clinical relevance of such hyporesponsiveness is unclear.

The immunologic response of the group C vaccine in children younger than 2 years is poor, however, and studies from Brazil indicate that group C vaccine is not protective in children younger than 24 months.[241] Studies of the immune response to the A and C vaccine by Gold and co-workers in infants have demonstrated that detectable levels of antibody are generated but that these levels are significantly lower than the levels in older children.[242] In adults, the duration of group C antibody titer persisted for 2 to 4 years after vaccination, and in children studied in Egypt who were vaccinated with group A polysaccharide, protection lasted at least 2 years.[243,244] With the development of a meningococcal conjugate vaccine, successful immunization of infants is now possible. A monovalent meningococcal serogroup C conjugate vaccine was developed in 1999 in Great Britain in response to a nationwide outbreak of infection.[245] The vaccine proved very effective in children 3 months of age and older.[246] The effectiveness ranged from 88% to 98% among school-aged children in the first year after vaccination. However, in infants, efficacy declined substantially 1 year after vaccination. The number of cases in vaccinated children remained low, but questions remain as to the need for booster vaccinations in infants. During the period of vaccination, serogroup C carriage rates declined in the population 66%. In addition, studies suggested that disease rates in nonvaccinated populations declined as a result of herd immunity conferred by the vaccine.[247]

A tetravalent vaccine conjugate vaccine (MCV4; A, C, Y, W-135) was approved for use in the United States in 2005.[246] No vaccine is currently available that will prevent infection caused by N. meningitidis serogroup B. The MCV4 results in generation of immune responses correlating with protection between 80% and 90% of the population vaccinated. The polysaccharides are conjugated to diphtheria toxoid, and studies have demonstrated that concomitant administration with other vaccines, including tetanus-diphtheria toxoid, is safe and that both vaccines are immunogenic. Reports suggested that this vaccine may be associated with increased risk for Guillain-Barré syndrome.[248] The background incidence rate of Guillain-Barré syndrome in patients 11 to 19 years of age was estimated at 0.11 case per 100,000 person-months. Subsequent analysis of MCV4 use based on the Vaccine Safety Datalink data revealed that during an 18-month interval, a total of 126,506 doses of MCV4 were delivered, and no cases of Guillain-Barré syndrome were observed among vaccine recipients within 6 weeks of vaccination. During the same period, two cases were reported among an equal number of persons aged 11 to 19 years from a matched comparison group who had not received the vaccination.[248]

The costs of vaccination with conjugate vaccines are substantial and until recently have been beyond the budgets of a number of less well-developed countries with the highest incidence of meningococcal disease. In these areas, factors such as underlying parasitic infections, the state of nutrition, and age of the vaccine recipient play a role in the response to vaccination.[249] There is considerable support for the development of an inexpensive conjugate meningococcal serogroup A conjugate vaccine for mass vaccination in African countries.[250] In June

2008, a phase 2 study was completed that demonstrated the vaccine was safe and generated antibody levels indicative of protection (see http://www.meningvax.org/files/press-0706-improved-phase2.html).

VACCINE RECOMMENDATIONS

The Advisory Committee on Immunization Practices (ACIP) has made the following recommendations on vaccination with MCV4 and MPSV4.[246,251] Routine vaccination of children 2 to 10 years of age is not recommended. The ACIP recommends vaccination for children aged 2 to 10 years who are at increased risk for meningococcal disease. These children include travelers to or residents of countries in which meningococcal disease is hyperendemic or epidemic, children who have terminal complement deficiencies, and children with anatomic or functional asplenia. Health care workers may elect to immunize children aged 2 to 10 years who are infected with HIV type 1. MCV4 is preferred to the polysaccharide vaccine, MPSV4, for such children at risk. If individuals have not been vaccinated previously with MCV4, the ACIP recommends vaccination of persons before high school entry (11 to 12 years of age) with MCV4 as an effective strategy to reduce meningococcal disease among adolescents and young adults. Routine vaccination is also recommended for persons at risk for meningococcal disease. Use of MCV4 is preferred among persons aged 11 to 55 years. If MCV4 is unavailable, MPSV4 is an acceptable alternative. The following populations are at risk for meningococcal disease: college freshmen living in dormitories; microbiologists who are routinely exposed to *N. meningitidis*; military recruits; persons who travel to or reside in countries in which *N. meningitidis* is hyperendemic or epidemic; persons who have terminal complement component deficiencies; and persons who have functional or anatomic asplenia. Individuals who have HIV type 1 infection are likely at increased risk for meningococcal infection, and vaccination should be considered in this group. Vaccination is not recommended for those older than 55 years who are not identified as being at risk for meningococcal disease. MCV4 is administered as a single 0.5-mL intramuscular dose, and MPSV4 is administered as a single 0.5-mL subcutaneous dose. Revaccination with MCV4 of individuals initially vaccinated with MPSV4 may be indicated 2 to 3 years after the initial vaccine if the risk for meningococcal infection still persists. Persons with a history of Guillain-Barré syndrome might be at increased risk after MCV4 vaccination; therefore, a history of Guillain-Barré syndrome is a precaution to administration of MCV4.

REFERENCES

1. Vieusseaux M. Memoire sur le maladie qui a regne a Geneve au printemps de 1805. *J Med Chir Pharmacol.* 1805;11:163.
2. Hedrich AW. The movements of epidemic meningitis, 1915-1930. *Public Health Rep.* 1931;46:2709.
3. Weichselbaum A. Ueber die Aetiologie der akuten Meningitis cerebrospinalis. *Fortschr Med.* 1887;5:573.
4. Kiefer F. Zur differential Diagnose des Erregers der epidemischen Cerebrospinalmeningitis und der Gonorrhoea. *Berl Klin Wochenschr.* 1896;33:628.
5. Albrecht H, Ghon A. Uber die Aetiologie und pathologische Anatomie der Meningitis cerebro spinalis epidemica. *Wien Klin Wochenschr.* 1901;14:984.
6. Dopter C. Etude de quelques germes isoles du rhino-pharynx, voisans du meningocoque (parameningocoques). *C R Soc Biol (Paris).* 1909;67:74.
7. Flexner S. The results of the serum treatment in thirteen hundred cases of epidemic meningitis. *J Exp Med.* 1913;17:553.
8. Glover JA. The cerebrospinal fever epidemic of 1917 at "X" depot. *J R Army Med Corps.* 1918;30:23.
9. Norton JF, Gordon JE. Meningococcus meningitis in Detroit in 1928-1929. *I Epidemiology J Prev Med.* 1930;4:207.
10. French MR. Epidemiological study of 383 cases of meningococcus meningitis in the city of Milwaukee, 1927-1928 and 1929. *Am J Public Health.* 1931;21:130.
11. Pizzi M. A severe epidemic of meningococcus meningitis in Chile, 1941 and 1942. *Am J Public Health.* 1944;34:231-238.
12. Schwentker FF, Gelman S, Long PH. The treatment of meningococcic meningitis with sulfonamide. Preliminary report. *JAMA.* 1937;108:1407.
13. Kuhns DM, Nelson CT, Feldman HA, et al. The prophylactic value of sulfadiazine in the control of meningococcic meningitis. *JAMA.* 1943;123:335-339.
14. Schoenback EB, Phair JJ. The sensitivity of meningococci to sulfadiazine. *Am J Hyg.* 1948;47:177-186.
15. Gauld JR, Nitz RE, Hunter DH, et al. Epidemiology of meningococcal meningitis at Fort Ord. *Am J Epidemiol.* 1965;82:56-72.
16. Bristow MW, Van Peenen PFD, Volk R. Epidemic meningitis in naval recruits. *Am J Public Health.* 1965;55:1039-1045.
17. Artenstein MS, Gold R, Zimmerly JG, et al. Prevention of meningococcal disease by group C polysaccharide vaccine. *N Engl J Med.* 1970;282:417-420.
18. Hebeler BH, Young FE. Autolysis of *Neisseria gonorrhoeae. J Bacteriol.* 1976;122:385-392.
19. Holbein BE. Enhancement of *Neisseria meningitidis* infection in mice by addition of iron bound to transferrin. *Infect Immun.* 1981;34:120-125.
20. West WF, Sparling PF. The response of *Neisseria gonorrhoeae* to iron limitation: Alterations in expression of membrane proteins without apparent siderophore production. *Infect Immun.* 1985;47:388-394.
21. Dyer D, West EP, Sparling PF. Effects of seven carrier proteins on the growth of pathogenic *Neisseria* with heme-bound iron. *Infect Immun.* 1987;55:2171.
22. Gorden MH, Murray EG. Identification of the meningococcus. *J R Army Med Corps.* 1915;5:411.
23. Scherp HW, Rake GJ. Studies on the meningococcus. VIII. The type I specific substance. *J Exp Med.* 1935;61:753.
24. Clapp FL, Phillips SW, Stahl HJ. Quantitative use of Neufeld reaction with special reference to titration of type III antipneumococcic sera. *Proc Soc Exp Biol Med.* 1935;33:302.
25. Branham SE, Carlin SA. Comments on a newly recognized group of the meningococcus. *Proc Soc Exp Biol Med.* 1942;49:141-144.
26. Branham SE. Serological relationship among meningococci. *Bacteriol Rev.* 1953;17:175-188.
27. Branham SE. Reference strains for the serologic groups of meningococcus (*Neisseria meningitidis*). *Int Bull Bacteriol Nomenclature Taxonomy.* 1958;8:1-15.
28. Slaterus K. Serological typing of meningococci by means of microprecipitation. *Antonie Van Leeuwenhoek.* 1961;27:304-315.
29. Evans JR, Artenstein MS, Hunter DH. Prevalence of meningococcal serogroups and a description of new groups. *Am J Epidemiol.* 1968;87:643-646.
30. Ding S, Ye R, Zhang H. Three new serogroups of *Neisseria meningitidis. J Biol Stand.* 1981;9:305-315.
31. Ashton FE, Ryan A, Diena B, et al. A new serogroup (L) of *Neisseria meningitidis. J Clin Microbiol.* 1983;17:722-727.
32. Gotschlich EC, Liu TY, Artenstein MS. Preparation and immunochemical properties of the group A, group B, and group C meningococcal polysaccharides. *J Exp Med.* 1969;129:1349-1365.
33. Bundle DR, Jennings JH, Kenny CP. Studies on the group specific polysaccharide of *Neisseria meningitidis* serogroup X and an improved procedure for its isolation. *J Biol Chem.* 1974;249:4797-4801.
34. Robinson JA, Apicella MA. Isolation and characterization of *Neisseria meningitidis* groups A, C, X and Y polysaccharide antigens. *Infect Immun.* 1970;1:8-14.
35. Apicella MA. Identification of a subgroup antigen on the *Neisseria meningitidis* group C capsular polysaccharide. *J Infect Dis.* 1974;129:147-153.
36. Apicella MA. Immunological and biochemical studies of meningococcal C polysaccharide isolated by diethylaminoethyl chromatography. *Infect Immun.* 1976;14:106-113.
37. Watson RG, Marinetti GV, Scherp HW. The specific hapten of group C (group II) meningococcus. II. Chemical nature. *J Immunol.* 1958;81:337-344.
38. Brandt BL, Artenstein MS, Smith CD. Antibody response to meningococcal polysaccharide vaccines. *Infect Immun.* 1973;8:590-596.
39. Bhattacharjee AK, Jennings HJ, Kenny CP, et al. Structural determination of the sialic acid polysaccharide antigens of *Neisseria meningitidis* serogroup B and C with carbon 13 nuclear magnetic resonance. *J Biol Chem.* 1975;250:1926-1932.
40. Maloney PC, Schneider H, Brandt BL. Production and degrading of serogroup B *Neisseria meningitidis* polysaccharide. *Infect Immun.* 1972;6:657-661.
41. Wyle FA, Artenstein MS, Brandt BL, et al. Immunologic response of man to group B meningococcal polysaccharide vaccines. *J Infect Dis.* 1972;126:514-522.
42. Bhattacharjee AK, Jennings JH, Kenny CP. Characterization of 3-deoxy-D-manno-octulosonic acid as a component of the capsular polysaccharide antigen from *Neisseria meningitidis* serogroup 29E. *Biochem Biophys Res Commun.* 1974;61:489-493.
43. Griffiss JM, Brandt BL, Broud DO. Human immune response to various doses of group Y and W135 meningococcal polysaccharide vaccines. *Infect Immun.* 1982;37:205-208.
44. Mandrell RE, Zollinger WD. Lipopolysaccharide serotyping of *Neisseria meningitidis* by hemagglutination inhibition. *Infect Immun.* 1977;16:471-475.
45. Jennings HL, Johnson KG, Kenne L. The structure of the R-type oligosaccharide core obtained from some lipopolysaccharides of *Neisseria meningitidis. Carbohydr Res.* 1983;121:233-241.
46. Gamian A, Beurret M, Michon F, et al. Structure of the L2 lipopolysaccharide core oligosaccharides of *Neisseria meningitidis. J Biol Chem.* 1992;267:922-925.
47. Jones DM, Borrow R, Fox AJ, et al. The lipooligosaccharide immunotype as a virulence determinant in *Neisseria meningitidis. Microbiol Pathol.* 1992;13:219-224.
48. Verheul AFM, Snippe H, Poolman JT. Meningococcal lipopolysaccharides: Virulence factor and potential vaccine component. *Microbiol Rev.* 1993;57:34-49.
49. Estabrook MM, Baker CJ, Griffiss JM. The immune response of children to meningococcal lipooligosaccharides during disseminated disease is directed primarily against two monoclonal antibody-defined epitopes. *J Infect Dis.* 1993;167:966-970.
50. Gold R, Wyle FA. New classification of *Neisseria meningitidis* by means of bactericidal reactions. *Infect Immun.* 1970;1:479-484.
51. Gold R, Winklehake JL, Mars RS, et al. Identification of epidemic strain of group C *Neisseria meningitidis* by bactericidal serotyping. *J Infect Dis.* 1971;124:593-597.
52. Frasch CE, Chapman SS. Classification of *Neisseria meningitidis* group B into distinct serotypes. III. Application of a new bactericidal-inhibition technique to distribution of serotypes among cases and carriers. *J Infect Dis.* 1973;127:149-154.
53. Frasch CE, Golschlich EC. Noncapsular surface antigens of *Neisseria meningitidis.* In: Weinstein L, Fields BN, eds. *Seminars in Infectious Diseases.* New York: Stratton; 1979:304-337.
54. Broud DD, Griffiss JM, Baker CJ. Heterogeneity of serotypes of *Neisseria meningitidis* that cause endemic disease. *J Infect Dis.* 1979;140:465-470.
55. Kawula TH, Spinola SM, Klapper DG, et al. Localization of a conserved epitope and an azurin-like domain in the H.8 protein of pathogenic *Neisseria. Mol Microbiol.* 1987;1:179-185.
56. Barlow AK, Heckels JE, Clarke IN. Molecular cloning and expression of *Neisseria meningitidis* class 1 outer membrane protein in *Escherichia coli* K-12. *Infect Immun.* 1987;55:2734-2740.
57. Frasch CE, Zollinger WD, Poolman JT. Proposed schema for identification of serotypes of *Neisseria meningitidis.* In: Schoolnik GK, ed. *The Pathogenic Neisseria.* Washington, DC: American Society for Microbiology; 1985:519-524.
58. Rappuoli R. Reverse vaccinology, a genome-based approach to vaccine development. *Vaccine.* 2001;19:2688-2691.
59. Selander RK, Caugant DA, Ochman H, et al. Methods of multilocus enzyme electrophoresis for bacterial populations genetics and systematics. *Appl Environ Microbiol.* 1986;132:2855-2861.
60. Olyhoek T, Crowe B, Achtman M. Epidemiological analysis and geographic distribution of *Neisseria meningitidis* group A. In: Schoolnik GK, ed. *The Pathogenic Neisseria.* Washington, DC: American Society for Microbiology; 1985:530-535.
61. Caugant DA, Mocca IF, Frasch CE, et al. Genetic structure of *Neisseria meningitidis* populations in relation to serogroup, serotype, and outer membrane protein pattern. *J Bacteriol.* 1987;169:2781-2792.
62. Pinner R, Spellmam P, Stephens DS. Evidence for functionally distinct pili expressed by *Neisseria meningitidis. Infect Immun.* 1991;59:3169-3175.
63. DeVoe IW, Gilchrist JE. Piliation and colonial morphology among laboratory strains of meningococci. *J Clin Microbiol.* 1978;7:379-384.

64. DeVoe IW, Gilchrist JE. Pili on meningococci from primary culture of nasopharyngeal carriers and cerebrospinal fluid of patients with acute disease. *J Exp Med.* 1975;141:297-305.
65. Stephens DS, McGee ZA. Attachment of *Neisseria meningitidis* to human mucosal surfaces: Influence of pili and type of receptor cell. *J Infect Dis.* 1981;143:525-532.
66. Kallstrom H, Liszewski MK, Atkinson JP, et al. Membrane cofactor protein (MCP or CD46) is a cellular pilus receptor for pathogenic *Neisseria. Mol Microbiol.* 1997;25:639-647.
67. Johnson L, Rytknen A, Bergman P, et al. CD46 in meningococcal disease. *Science.* 2003;301:373-375.
68. Virji M, Makepeace K, Ferguson DJ, et al. Meningococcal Opa and Opc proteins: Their role in colonization and invasion of human epithelial and endothelial cells. *Mol Microbiol.* 1993;10:499-510.
69. Hammerschmidt S, Muller A, Sillmann H, et al. Capsule phase variation in *Neisseria meningitidis* serogroup B by slipped-strand mispairing in the polysialyltransferase gene (siaD): correlation with bacterial invasion and the outbreak of meningococcal disease. *Mol Microbiol.* 1996;20:1211-1220.
70. Hammerschmidt S, Hilse R, van Putten JPM, et al. Modulation of cell surface sialic acid expression in *Neisseria meningitidis* via a transposable genetic element. *EMBO J.* 1996;15:192-198.
71. Virji M, Makepeace K, Peak IR, et al. Pathogenic mechanisms of pathogenic *Neisseria. Ann N Y Acad Sci.* 1995;797:273-276.
72. Lin L, Ayala P, Larson J, et al. The *Neisseria* type 2 IgA1 protease cleaves LAMP1 and promotes survival of bacteria within epithelial cells. *Mol Microbiol.* 1997;24:1083-1094.
73. Lin L, Ayala P, Larson J, et al. The *Neisseria* IgA1 protease cleaves LAMP1 and promotes survival of bacteria within epithelial cells. *Mol Microbiol.* 1997;24:1083-1094.
74. Nassif X, Marceau M, Pujol C, et al. Type-4 pili and meningococcal adhesiveness. *Gene.* 1997;192:149-153.
75. Goldschneider I, Gotschlich EC, Artenstein MS. Human immunity to the meningococcus. I. The role of humoral antibody. *J Exp Med.* 1969;129:1307-1326.
76. Goldschneider I, Gotschlich EC, Artenstein MS. Human immunity to the meningococcus. II. Development of natural immunity. *J Exp Med.* 1969;129:1327-1328.
77. Robbins JB, Myerowitz RL, Whesnant JK, et al. Enteric bacteria cross-reactive with *Neisseria meningitidis* groups A and C and *Diplococcus pneumoniae* types I and II. *Infect Immun.* 1972;6: 651-656.
78. Grados O, Ewing WH. Antigenic relationship between *Escherichia coli* and *Neisseria meningitidis. J Infect Dis.* 1970;122: 100-103.
79. Finne J, Bitter-Suermann D, Goudis C, et al. An IgG monoclonal antibody to group B meningococci cross reacts with developmentally regulated polysialic acid units of glycoproteins in neural and extraneural tissue. *J Immunol.* 1987;138:4402-4407.
80. Greenwood BM, Greenwood AM, Bradley AK, et al. Factors influencing the susceptibility to meningococcal disease during an epidemic in The Gambia, West Africa. *J Infect.* 1987;14: 167-184.
81. Kayhty H, Jousimies-Somer H, Peltola H, et al. Antibody response to capsular polysaccharides of groups A and C *Neisseria meningitidis* and *Haemophilus influenzae* type b during bacteremic disease. *J Infect Dis.* 1981;143:32-41.
82. Plaut AG, Gilbert JV, Artenstein MS, et al. *Neisseria gonorrhoeae* and *Neisseria meningitidis*: Extracellular enzyme cleaves human immunoglobulin A. *Science.* 1975;190:1103-1105.
83. Mulks M, Plaut AG. IgA protease production as a characteristic distinguishing pathogenic from harmless Neisseriaceae. *N Engl J Med.* 1978;299:973-976.
84. Bruns H, Hohn J. Meningokokken im Nasenrachenraum. *Klin Jahrb Jena.* 1908;28:285.
85. Rake G. Studies on meningococcus infection. VI. The carrier problem. *J Exp Med.* 1934;59:553.
86. Greenfield S, Sheede PR, Feldman HA. Meningococcal carriage in a population of "normal" families. *J Infect Dis.* 1971;123: 67-73.
87. Claus H, Maiden MC, Maag R, et al. Many carried meningococci lack the genes required for capsule synthesis and transport. *Microbiology.* 2002;148:1813-1819.
88. Edwards EA, Devine LF, Sengbusch CH, et al. Immunological investigations of meningococcal disease. III. Brevity of group C acquisition prior to disease occurrence. *Scand J Infect Dis.* 1987;9:105-110.
89. Wenzel RP, Davies JA, Mitzel JR, et al. Nonusefulness of meningococcal carriage rates. *Lancet.* 1973;2:205.
90. Olcen P, Kellander J, Danielsson D, et al. Epidemiology of *Neisseria meningitidis* prevalence and symptoms from the upper respiratory tract in family members to patients with meningococcal disease. *Scand J Infect Dis.* 1981;13:105-109.
91. Moore PS, Hierholzer J, DeWitt W, et al. Respiratory viruses and mycoplasma as cofactors for epidemic group A meningococcal meningitis. *JAMA.* 1990;264:1271-1275.
92. Reller BL, MacGregor RR, Beaty HN. Bactericidal antibody after colonization with *Neisseria meningitidis. J Infect Dis.* 1973; 127:56-62.
93. Broome CV. The carrier state: *Neisseria meningitidis. J Antimicrob Chemother.* 1986;18(Suppl A):S25-S34.
94. Meningococcal disease, serogroup W135. *Wkly Epidemiol Rec.* 2001;76:141-142.
95. Wilder-Smith A, Barkham TM, Ravindran S, et al. Persistence of W135 Neisseria meningitidis carriage in returning Hajj pilgrims: risk for early and late transmission to household contacts. *Emerg Infect Dis.* 2003;9:123-126.
96. Martin DR, Walker SJ, Baker MG, et al. New Zealand epidemic of meningococcal disease identified by a strain with phenotype B:4:P1.4. *J Infect Dis.* 1998;177:497-500.
97. Feldman HA. Meningococcal infections. *Adv Intern Med.* 1972;18:117-140.
98. Centers for Disease Control and Prevention. Summary of notifiable diseases, United States-2001. *MMWR Morb Mortal Wkly Rep.* 2003;50:1-136.
99. Peltola H. Meningococcal disease: Still with us. *Rev Infect Dis.* 1983;5:71-91.
100. Peltola H, Kataja JM, Makela PH. Shift in the age distribution of meningococcal disease as predictor of an epidemic. *Lancet.* 1982;2:595-597.
101. Andersen BM. Mortality in meningococcal infections. *Scand J Infect Dis.* 1978;10:277-282.
102. deMorais JS, Munford RS, Risi JB, et al. Epidemic disease due to serogroup C *Neisseria meningitidis* in Sao Paulo, Brazil. *J Infect Dis.* 1974;129:568-571.
103. Oberli J, Hoi NT, Caravano R, et al. Etude d'une epidemie de meningococcie au Viet Nam (provinces du Sud). *Bull World Health Organ.* 1981;59:585-590.
104. The Meningococcal Disease Surveillance Group. Analysis of endemic meningococcal disease by serogroup and evaluation of chemoprophylaxis. *J Infect Dis.* 1976;134:201.
105. Schwartz B, Moore P, Broome CV. Global epidemiology of meningococcal disease. *Clin Rev Microbiol.* 1989;2(Suppl): S118-S124.
106. Greenwood BM. The epidemiology of acute bacterial meningitis in tropical Africa. In: Williams JD, Burnet J, eds. *Bacterial Meningitis.* New York: Academic Press; 1987:61-92.
107. Tikhomirov E, Santamaria M, Esteves K. Meningococcal disease: Public health burden and control. *World Health Stat Q.* 1997;50:170-177.
108. Ramsay ME, Andrews N, Kaczmarski EB, et al. Efficacy of meningococcal serogroup C conjugate vaccine in teenagers and toddlers in England. *Lancet.* 2001;357:195-196.
109. Thompson MJ, Ninis N, Perera R, et al. Clinical recognition of meningococcal disease in children and adolescents. *Lancet.* 2006;367:397.
110. Durand ML, Calderwood SB, Weber DJ, et al. Acute bacterial meningitis in adults. *N Engl J Med.* 1993;328:21-28.
111. Wolfe RE, Birbara CA. Meningococcal infections at an army training center. *Am J Med.* 1968;44:243-255.
112. Sullivan TD, LaScolea LJ. *Neisseria meningitidis* bacteremia in children: Quantitation of bacteremia and spontaneous clinical recovery without antibiotic therapy. *Pediatrics.* 1987;80:63-87.
113. Carpenter RR, Petersdorf RG. The clinical spectrum of bacterial meningitis. *Am J Med.* 1962;33:262-275.
114. Kaplan SL, Schutze GE, Leake JA, et al. Multicenter surveillance of invasive meningococcal infections in children. *Pediatrics.* 2006;118:e979-e984.
115. Heckenberg SG, de Gans J, Brouwer MC, et al. Clinical features, outcome, and meningococcal genotype in 258 adults with meningococcal meningitis: a prospective cohort study. *Medicine (Baltimore)* 2008;87:185.
116. van de Beek D, de Gans J, Spanjaard L, et al. Clinical features and prognostic factors in adults with bacterial meningitis. *N Engl J Med.* 2004;351:1849.
117. Feigin RD, Dodge PR. Bacterial meningitis: Newer concepts of pathophysiology and neurologic sequelae. *Pediatr Clin North Am.* 1976;23:541-556.
118. Wheeler JS, Anderson BJ, De Chalain TM. Surgical interventions in children with meningococcal purpura fulminans: a review of 117 procedures in 21 children. *J Pediatr Surg.* 2003;38:597.
119. Thomas HM. Meningococcic meningitis and septicemia. Report of an outbreak in the fourth service command during the winter and spring of 1942-1943. *JAMA.* 1943;123:264-272.
120. Ducker TB, Simmons RL. The pathogenesis of meningitis. Systemic effects of meningococcal endotoxin within the cerebrospinal fluid. *Arch Neurol.* 1968;18:123-128.
121. Hardman JM. Fatal meningococcal infections: The changing pathologic picture in the '60's. *Mil Med.* 1968;133:951-964.
122. Brandtzaeg P, Oktedalen O, Kierulf P, et al. Elevated VIP and endotoxin plasma levels in human gram-negative septic shock. *Regul Pept.* 1989;24:37-44.
123. Brandtzaeg P, Kierulf P, Gaustad P, et al. Plasma endotoxin as a predictor of multiple organ failure and death in systemic meningococcal disease. *J Infect Dis.* 1989;159:195-204.
124. Brandtzaeg P, Ovsteboo R, Kierulf P. Compartmentalization of lipopolysaccharide production correlates with clinical presentation in meningococcal disease. *J Infect Dis.* 1992;166: 650-652.
125. Brandtzaeg P, Mollnes TE, Kierulf P. Complement activation and endotoxin levels in systemic meningococcal disease. *J Infect Dis.* 1989;160:58-65.
126. Brandtzaeg P, Sandset PM, Joo GB, et al. The quantitative association of plasma endotoxin, antithrombin, protein C, extrinsic pathway inhibitor and fibrinopeptide A in systemic meningococcal disease. *Thromb Res.* 1989;55:459-470.
127. Brandtzaeg PK, Bryn P, Kierulf P, et al. Meningococcal endotoxin in lethal septic shock plasma studied by gas chromatography, mass-spectrometry, ultracentrifugation, and electron microscopy. *J Clin Invest.* 1992;89:816-823.
128. Cesarini JP, Vandekerkove M, Faucon R, et al. Ultrastructure of the wall of *Neisseria meningitidis* (in French). *Ann Inst Pasteur.* 1967;113:833-841.
129. Devoe IW, Gilchrist JE. Release of endotoxin in the form of cell wall blebs during in vitro growth of *Neisseria meningitidis. J Exp Med.* 1973;138:1156-1167.
130. Levin S, Painter MB. The treatment of acute meningococcal infection in adults. *Ann Intern Med.* 1966;64:1049-1056.
131. Gore I, Saphir Q. Myocarditis, a classification of 1402 cases. *Am Heart J.* 1947;34:827-831.
132. Boucek MM, Boerth RC, Artman M, et al. Myocardial dysfunction in children with acute meningococcemia. *J Pediatr.* 1984;105:538-542.
133. Gotschall RA. Conus medullaris syndrome after meningococcal meningitis. *N Engl J Med.* 1972;286:882-883.
134. Herman RA, Rubin HA. Meningococcal pericarditis without meningitis presenting as tamponade. *N Engl J Med.* 1974;290: 143-144.
135. Pierce I, Cooper E. Meningococcal pericarditis, clinical features and therapy in five patients. *Arch Intern Med.* 1972;129: 918-922.
136. Maron BJ, Macoul KL, Benaron P. Unusual complications of meningococcal meningitis. *Johns Hopkins Med J.* 1972;131: 64-68.
137. Brasier AR, Macklis JD, Vaughn D, et al. Myopericarditis as an initial presentation of meningococcemia. Unusual manifestations of infection with serotype W135. *Am J Med.* 1987;82: 641-644.
138. Frank ST, Gomez RM. Chronic meningococcemia. *Mil Med.* 1968;133:918-920.
139. Saslaw S. Chronic meningococcemia: Report of a case. *N Engl J Med.* 1962;266:605-607.
140. Rompalo AM, Hood EW, Roberts PL, et al. The acute arthritis dermatitis syndrome. The changing importance of *Neisseria gonorrhoeae* and *Neisseria meningitidis. Arch Intern Med.* 1987;147:281-283.
141. Lim D, Gewurz A, Lint TF, et al. Absence of the sixth component of complement in a patient with repeated episodes of meningococcal meningitis. *J Pediatr.* 1976;89:42.
142. Alper CA, Abramson N, Johnston RB Jr. Increased susceptibility to infection associated with abnormalities of complement-mediated functions and of the third component of complement (C3). *N Engl J Med.* 1970;282:349-354.
143. Petersen BH, Graham JA, Brooks GF. Human deficiency of the eighth component of complement. The requirement of C8 for serum *Neisseria gonorrhoeae* bactericidal activity. *J Clin Invest.* 1976;57:283-290.
144. Ellison RT, Kohler PF, Curd JG, et al. Prevalence of congenital or acquired complement deficiency in patients with sporadic meningococcal disease. *N Engl J Med.* 1983;308:913-916.
145. Densen P, Weiler JM, Griffiss JM, et al. Familial properdin deficiency and fatal bacteremia. Correction of the bactericidal defect by vaccination. *N Engl J Med.* 1987;316:922-926.
146. Ross SC, Rosenthal PJ, Berberich HM, et al. Killing of *Neisseria meningitidis* by human neutrophils: Implications for normal and complement deficient individuals. *J Infect Dis.* 1987;155: 1266-1275.
147. Densen P. Complement deficiencies and meningococcal disease. *Clin Exp Immunol.* 1991;86(Suppl 1):S57-S62.
148. Koppes GM, Ellenbogen C, Gebhart RJ. Group Y meningococcal disease in United States Air Force recruits. *Am J Med.* 1977;62:661-666.
149. Young LS, LaForce FM, Head JJ, et al. A simultaneous outbreak of meningococcal and influenza infections. *N Engl J Med.* 1972;287:5-9.
150. Goldstein E, Buhlers WC, Akers TC, et al. Murine resistance to inhaled *Neisseria meningitidis* after infection with an encephalomyocarditis virus. *Infect Immun.* 1972;6:398-402.
151. Kerttula Y, Leinonen M, Koskela M, et al. The etiology of pneumonia, application of bacterial serology and basic laboratory methods. *J Infect.* 1987;14:21-30.
152. Winstead JM, McKinsey DS, Tasker S, et al. Meningococcal pneumonia: characterization and review of cases seen over the past 25 years. *Clin Infect Dis.* 2000;30:87-94.
153. McCracken GH. Rapid identification of specific etiology in meningitis. *J Pediatr.* 1976;88:706-708.
154. Schwam E, Cox J. Fulminant meningococcal supraglottitis: An emerging infectious syndrome? *Emerg Infect Dis.* 1999;5: 464-467.
155. Salet IE, Frasch CE. Seroepidemiologic aspects of *Neisseria meningitidis* in homosexual men. *Can Med Assoc J.* 1982;126: 38-41.
156. Rosenstein NE, Perkins BA, Stephens DS, et al. Meningococcal disease. *N Engl J Med.* 2001;344:1378.
157. Gardner P. Clinical practice. Prevention of meningococcal disease. *N Engl J Med.* 2006;355:1466.
158. Fangio P, Desbouchages L, Lacherade JC, et al. Neisseria meningitidis C:2b:P1.2,5 with decreased susceptibility to penicillin isolated from a patient with meningitis and purpura fulminans. *Eur J Clin Microbiol Infect Dis.* 2005;24:140.
159. Angyo IA, Okpeh ES. Changing patterns of antibiotic sensitivity and resistance during an outbreak of meningococcal infection in Jos, Nigeria. *J Trop Pediatr.* 1998;44:263.
160. Sprott MS, Kearns AM, Field JM. Penicillin insensitive *Neisseria meningitis. Lancet.* 1988;1:1167.
161. Mendelman PM, Campos J, Chaffin DO, et al. Relative penicillin G resistance in *Neisseria meningitidis* and reduced affinity of

penicillin binding protein 3. *Antimicrob Agents Chemother.* 1988;32:706.

162. Saez-Nieto JA, Lujan R, Berron S, et al. Epidemiology and molecular basis of penicillin-resistant Neisseria meningitidis in Spain: A five-year history (1985 to 1989). *Clin Infect Dis.* 1992; 14:394.

163. Hoyne AL, Brown RH. 727 Meningococcic cases, an analysis. *Ann Intern Med.* 1948;28:248-259.

164. Feldman WE. Concentrations of bacteria in cerebrospinal fluid of patients with bacterial meningitis. *J Pediatr.* 1976; 88:549-552.

165. Arend SM, Lavrijsen AP, Kuijken I, et al. Prospective controlled study of the diagnostic value of skin biopsy in patients with presumed meningococcal disease. *Eur J Clin Microbiol Infect Dis.* 2006;25:643.

166. Borrow R, Claus H, Chaudhry U, et al. siaD PCR ELISA for confirmation and identification of serogroup Y and W135 meningococcal infections. *FEMS Microbiol Lett.* 1998;159: 209-214.

167. Seward RJ, Towner KJ. Evaluation of a PCR-immunoassay technique for detection of Neisseria meningitidis in cerebrospinal fluid and peripheral blood. *J Med Microbiol.* 2000;49:451-456.

168. Corless CE, Guiver M, Borrow R, et al. Simultaneous detection of Neisseria meningitidis, Haemophilus influenzae, and Streptococcus pneumoniae in suspected cases of meningitis and septicemia using real-time PCR. *J Clin Microbiol.* 2001;39:1553-1558.

169. Diggle MA, Clarke SC. Detection and genotyping of meningococci using a nested PCR approach. *J Med Microbiol.* 2003;52:51-57.

170. Bryant PA, Li HY, Zaia A, et al. Prospective study of a real-time PCR that is highly sensitive, specific, and clinically useful for diagnosis of meningococcal disease in children. *J Clin Microbiol.* 2004;42:2919.

171. Tunkel AR, Scheld WM. Acute meningitis. In: Mandell GL, Bennett JE, Dolin R, eds. *Principles and Practice of Infectious Diseases.* 6th ed. Churchill Livingstone: Philadelphia; 2005:1083.

172. Diggle MA, Clarke SC. Molecular methods for the detection and characterization of Neisseria meningitidis. *Expert Rev Mol Diagn.* 2006;6:79.

173. Gray SJ, Trotter CL, Ramsay ME, et al. Epidemiology of meningococcal disease in England and Wales 1993/94 to 2003/04: contribution and experiences of the Meningococcal Reference Unit. *J Med Microbiol.* 2006;55:887.

174. Corless CE, Guiver M, Borrow R, et al. Simultaneous detection of Neisseria meningitidis, Haemophilus influenzae, and Streptococcus pneumoniae in suspected cases of meningitis and septicemia using real-time PCR. *J Clin Microbiol.* 2001;39:1553.

175. Feldman HA, Sweet LA, Dowling HF. Sulfadiazine therapy of purulent meningitis. *War Med.* 1942;2:995-1007.

176. Mead M, Harris W, Samper BA, et al. Treatment of meningococcal meningitis with penicillin. *N Engl J Med.* 1944;231:509-517.

177. Kinsman JM, D'Alonzo CA. Meningococcemia: A description of the clinical picture and a comparison of the efficacy of sulfadiazine and penicillin in the treatment of thirty cases. *Ann Intern Med.* 1946;24:606-617.

178. McCrumb FR, Hall HE, Meridith AM, et al. Chloramphenicol in the treatment of meningococcal meningitis. *Am J Med.* 1951;10:696-703.

179. Brown JD, Mathies AW, Ivler D, et al. Variable results of cephalothin therapy for meningococcal meningitis. In: Hobby G, ed. *Antimicrobial Agents and Chemotherapy.* 1969. Bethesda, Md: American Society for Microbiology; 1970:432.

180. Schribner RK, Wedro BC, Weber AH, et al. Activities of eight new beta-lactam and seven antibiotic combinations against Neisseria meningitidis. *Antimicrob Agents Chemother.* 1982;21: 678-680.

181. Love BD, Finland M. In vitro susceptibility of meningococcus to 11 antibiotics and sulfadiazine. *Am J Med.* 1954;228: 534-539.

182. Brown JW, Condit PK. Meningococcal infections: Fort Ord and California. *Calif Med.* 1965;102:171-180.

183. Eickhoff TC, Finland M. Changing susceptibility of meningococci to antimicrobial agents. *N Engl J Med.* 1965;272:395-398.

184. Feldman HA. Sulfonamide resistant meningococci. *Annu Rev Med.* 1967;18:495-506.

185. Alexander CE, Sanborn WR, Cherriere G, et al. Sulfadiazine resistant group A Neisseria meningitidis. *Science.* 1968;161:1019.

186. Centers for Disease Control and Prevention. Control and prevention of meningococcal disease and control and prevention of serogroup C meningococcal diseases: Evaluation and management of suspected outbreaks. *MMWR Morb Mortal Wkly Rep.* 1997;46(RR-5):1-22.

187. Scheld WM, Sande M. Bactericidal versus bacteriostatic antibiotic therapy of experimental pneumococcal meningitis in rabbits. *J Clin Invest.* 1983;71:411-419.

188. Berkow R, ed. *The Merck Manual of Diagnosis and Therapy.* Rahway, NJ: Merck Sharp & Dohme; 1977:1432.

189. Sprott MS, Kearns AM, Field JM. Penicillin insensitive Neisseria meningitidis (Letter). *Lancet.* 1988;1:1167.

190. Saez-Nieto JA, Lujan R, Berron S, et al. Epidemiology and molecular basis of penicillin-resistant Neisseria meningitidis in Spain: A 5-year history (1985-1989). *Clin Infect Dis.* 1992; 14:394-402.

191. Galimand M, Gerbaud G, Guibourdenche M, et al. High level chloramphenicol resistance in Neisseria meningitidis. *N Engl J Med.* 1998;339:868-874.

192. Neu HC. Cephalosporins in the treatment of meningitis. *Drugs.* 1987;34(Suppl 2):S135-S153.

193. Cherubin CE, Eng RK, Noorby R, et al. Penetration of newer cephalosporins into spinal fluid. *Rev Infect Dis.* 1989;11: 526-548.

194. Ellis-Pegler R, Galler L, Roberts S, et al. Three days of intravenous benzyl penicillin therapy for meningococcal disease in adults. *Clin Infect Dis.* 2003;37:658-662.

195. Cartwright K, Reilly S, White D, et al. Early treatment with parenteral penicillin in meningococcal disease. *BMJ.* 1992; 305:143-147.

196. Strang JR, Pugh EJ. Meningococcal infections: Reducing the case fatality rate by giving penicillin before admission to hospital. *BMJ.* 1992;305:141-143.

197. Barquet N, Domingo P, Cayla JA, et al. Prognostic factors of a bedside predictive model and scoring system. *JAMA.* 1997; 278:491-496.

198. Waage A, Brandtzaeg P, Halstensen A, et al. The complex pattern of cytokines in serum from patients with meningococcal septic shock. *J Exp Med.* 1989;169:333-338.

199. Beutler B, Milsark IW, Cerami AC. Passive immunization against cachectin/tumor necrosis factor protects mice from the lethal effects of endotoxin. *Science.* 1985;229:869-871.

200. Beutler B, Cerami A. Cachectin: More than a tumor necrosis factor. *N Engl J Med.* 1987;316:379-385.

201. Tracey KJ, Beutler B, Lowry SF, et al. Shock and tissue injury induced by recombinant human cachectin. *Science.* 1986;234: 470-474.

202. Tracey KJ, Fong Y, Hesse DG, et al. Anti-cachectin/TNF monoclonal antibodies prevent septic shock during lethal bacteremia. *Nature.* 1987;330:662-664.

203. Girardin E, Grau GE, Dayr JM, et al. Tumor necrosis factor and interleukin-1 in the serum of children with severe infectious purpura. *N Engl J Med.* 1988;319:397-400.

204. Giroir BP, Scannon PJ, Levin M. Bactericidal/permeability-increasing protein: lessons learned from the phase III, randomized, clinical trial of rBPI21 for adjunctive treatment of children with severe meningococcemia. *Crit Care Med.* 2001;29(7 Suppl): S130-S135.

205. Bernard Gr, Vincent JL, Laterre PF, et al. Efficacy and safety of recombinant human activated protein C for severe sepsis. *N Engl J Med.* 2001;344,699-709.

206. Rintala E, Kauppila M, Seppala OP, et al. Protein C substitution in sepsis-associated purpura fulminans. *Crit Care Med.* 2000;28:2373-2378.

207. Morris PE, Light RB, Garber GE, Identifying patients with severe sepsis who should be not be treated with drotrecogin alfa (activated). *Am J Surg.* 2002;184(Suppl 1):19S-24S.

208. Monsalve F, Rucabado L, Salvador A, et al. Myocardial depression in septic shock caused by meningococcal infection. *Crit Care Med.* 1984;12:1021-1032.

209. de la Cal MA, Miravalles E, Pascual T, et al. Dose-related hemodynamic and renal effects of dopamine in septic shock. *Crit Care Med.* 1984;12:22-25.

210. Fisher CJ, Horowilx BZ, Albertson TE. Cardiorespiratory failure in toxic shock syndrome: Effect of dobutamine. *Crit Care Med.* 1985;13:160-165.

211. Duff P. Pathophysiology and management of septic shock. *J Reprod Med.* 1980;24:109-117.

212. Belsey MA, Hoffpauir CW, Smith MHD. Dexamethasone in the treatment of acute bacterial meningitis: The effect of study design on the interpretation of results. *Pediatrics.* 1969;44: 503-513.

213. Thomas R, Le Tulzo Y, Bouget J, et al. Trial of dexamethasone treatment for severe bacterial meningitis in adults. Adult Meningitis Steroid Group. *Intens Care Med.* 1999;25:475-480.

214. Corrigan JJ Jr, Jordan CM. Heparin therapy in septicemia with disseminated intravascular coagulation. Effect on mortality and on correction of hemostatic defects. *N Engl J Med.* 1970; 283:778-782.

215. Faust SN, Levin M, Harrison OB, et al. Dysfunction of endothelial protein C activation in severe meningococcal sepsis. *N Engl J Med.* 2001;345:408-416.

216. Kornelisse RF, Hazelzet JA, Hop WCJ, et al. Meningococcal septic shock in children: Clinical and laboratory features, outcome, and development of a prognostic score. *Clin Infect Dis.* 1997;25:640-646.

217. LeClerc F, Chenaud M, Delepoulle F, et al. Prognostic value of C-reactive protein level in severe infectious purpura: A comparison with eight other scores. *Crit Care Med.* 1991;19: 430-432.

218. Pollack MM, Ruttimann UE, Getson PR. Pediatric risk of mortality (PRISM) score. *Crit Care Med.* 1988;16:1-25.

219. Hermans PWM, Hibbard ML, Booy R, et al. For the Meningococcal Research Group. 4G/5G promoter polymorphism in the plasminogen-activator-inhibitor-1 gene and outcome of meningococcal disease. *Lancet.* 1999;354:556-560.

220. Fairbrother RW. Cerebrospinal meningitis: The use of sulphonamide derivatives in prophylaxis. *BMJ.* 1940;2: 859-862.

221. Gray FC, Gear J. Sulphapyridine, M and B 693 as a prophylactic against cerebrospinal meningitis. *S Afr Med J.* 1941;15:139.

222. Aycock WL, Mueller JH. Meningococcus carrier rates and meningitis incidence. *Bacteriol Rev.* 1950;14:115-160.

223. Cheever FS. The control of meningococcal meningitis by mass chemoprophylaxis with sulfadiazine. *Am J Med Sci.* 1945; 209:74-75.

224. Artenstein MS, Lamson TH, Evans JR. Attempted prophylaxis against meningococcal infection using intramuscular penicillin. *Mil Med.* 1967;132:1009-1011.

225. Guttler RB, Counts GW, Avent CK, et al. Effect of rifampin and minocycline on meningococcal carrier rates. *J Infect Dis.* 1971;124:199-205.

226. Devine LF, Johnson DP, Rhode SL, et al. Rifampin: Effect of two day treatment on meningococcal carrier state and the relationship of the levels of drug in sera and saliva. *Am J Med Sci.* 1971;261:79-83.

227. Jacobson JA, Daniel B. Vestibular reactions associated with minocycline. *Antimicrob Agents Chemother.* 1975;8:453-456.

228. Weidner CE, Dunkel TB, Pettyjohn FS, et al. Effectiveness of rifampin in eradicating the meningococcal carrier state in a relatively closed population: Emergence of resistant strains. *J Infect Dis.* 1971;124:172-178.

229. Pugsley MP, Dworzack DI, Horowitz EA, et al. Efficacy of ciprofloxacin in treatment of nasopharyngeal carriers of Neisseria meningitidis. *J Infect Dis.* 1987;156:211-213.

230. Gilja HO, Halstensen A, Digranes A, et al. Single-dose ofloxacin to eradicate tonsillopharyngeal carriage of Neisseria meningitidis. *Antimicrob Agents Chemother.* 1993;37:2024-2026.

231. Girgis N, Sultan Y, Frenck RW Jr, et al. Azithromycin compared with rifampin for eradication of nasopharyngeal colonization by Neisseria meningitidis. *Pediatr Infect Dis J.* 1998;17:816-819.

232. Hoeprich PD. Prediction of antimeningococcic chemoprophylactic efficacy. *J Infect Dis.* 1971;123:125-133.

233. Rainbow J, Boxrud D, Glennen A, et al. Emergence of fluoroquinolone resistant Neisseria meningitidis: Minnesota and North Dakota, 2007-2008. *MMWR Morb Mortal Wkly Rep.* 2008;57:173-175.

234. DeWals P, Herlozhe L, Borlee-Grimee I, et al. Meningococcal disease in Belgium. Secondary attack rate among household day-care nursery and pre-elementary school contacts. *J Infect.* 1983;1(Suppl 1):S53-S61.

235. Artenstein MS, Ellis RE. The risk of exposure to a patient with meningococcal meningitis. *Mil Med.* 1968;133:474-477.

236. Centers for Disease Control and Prevention. Meningococcal infections—United States, 1981. *MMWR Morb Mortal Wkly Rep.* 1981;30:113-115.

237. Makela PH, Kayhty H, Weekstrom P, et al. Effect of group A meningococcal vaccine in army recruits in Finland. *Lancet.* 1975;2:883-886.

238. Reingold AL, Hightower AW, Bolan GA, et al. Age specific differences in duration of clinical protection after vaccination with meningococcal polysaccharide vaccine. *Lancet.* 1985;2: 114-118.

239. Lepow ML, Beeler J, Randolph M, et al. Reactogenicity and immunogenicity of a quadrivalent combined meningococcal vaccine in children. *J Infect Dis.* 1986;154:1033-1036.

240. Advisory Committee on Immunization Practices. Meningococcal polysaccharide vaccines. *Ann Intern Med.* 1976;84:179-180.

241. Taunay A de E, Galvao PA, de Morais JS, et al. Disease prevention by meningococcal serogroup C polysaccharide vaccine in pre-school: Results after eleven months in Sao Paulo, Brazil (Abstract). *Pediatr Res.* 1974;8:429.

242. Gold R, Lepow ML, Goldschneider I, et al. Clinical evaluation of group A and group C meningococcal polysaccharide vaccines in infants. *J Clin Invest.* 1975;56:1536-1547.

243. Wahdan MH, Rizh F, El-Akkad AM, et al. A controlled field trial of a serogroup A meningococcal polysaccharide vaccine. *Bull World Health Organ.* 1973;48:667-673.

244. Brandt B, Artenstein MS. Duration of antibody responses after vaccination with group C Neisseria meningitidis polysaccharide. *J Infect Dis.* 1975;131:569.

245. Salisbury D. Introduction of a conjugate meningococcal type C vaccine programme in the UK. *J Paediatr Child Health.* 2001;37:S34-36.

246. Recommendations of the Advisory Committee on Immunization Practices (ACIP) for use of quadrivalent meningococcal conjugate vaccine (MCV4) in children aged 2-10 years at increased risk for invasive meningococcal disease. *MMWR Morb Mortal Wkly Rep.* 2007;56:1265-1266.

247. Ramsay ME, Andrews NJ, Trotter CL, et al. Herd immunity from meningococcal serogroup C conjugate vaccination in England: database analysis. *BMJ.* 2003;326:365-366.

248. Update: Guillian-Barre syndrome among recipients of Menactra meningococcal conjugate vaccine—United States, June 2005-September 2006. *MMWR Morb Mortal Wkly Rep.* 2006;55:1120-1124.

249. Greenwood BM, Bradley AK, Blakebrough IS, et al. The immune response to a meningococcal polysaccharide in an African village. *Trans R Soc Trop Med Hyg.* 1980;74:340-346.

250. LaForce MF, Konda K, Viviani S, et al. The meningitis vaccine project. *Vaccine.* 2007;25(Suppl 1):A97-A100.

251. Report from the advisory committee on immunization practices (ACIP): Decision not to recommend routine vaccination of all children aged 2 -10 years with quadrivalent meningococcal conjugate vaccine (MCV4). *MMWR Morb Mortal Wkly Rep.* 2008;57:462-464.

252. Humbert G, Leroy A, Nair SR, et al. Concentration of cefotaxime and the desacetyl metabolite in serum and CSF of patients with meningitis. *J Antimicrob Chemother.* 1984; 13:487-494.

253. Latif R, Dajani AS. Ceftriaxone diffusion into cerebrospinal fluid of children with meningitis. *Antimicrob Agents Chemother.* 1983;23:46-48.

254. Modai J, Vittecoq D, Decazes JM, et al. Penetration of ceftazidime into cerebrospinal fluid of patients with bacterial meningitis. *Antimicrob Agents Chemother*. 1983;24: 126-128.

255. Fu KP, Neu H. Anitimicrobial activity of ceftizoxime, a beta lactamase–stable cephalosporin. *Antimicrob Agents Chemother*. 1980;17:583-590.

256. Jones RN, Barry AL, Thornsberry C. Ceftriaxone: a summary of in vitro antibacterial susceptibility tests with 30 μg disks. *Diagn Microbiol Infect Dis*. 1983;1:295-311.

257. Phillips I, Warren C, Shannon K, et al. Ceftazidime: in vitro antibacterial activity and susceptibility to beta-lactamases compared with that of cefotaxime, moxalactam and other beta-lactam antibiotics. *J Antimicrob Chemother*. 1981;8(Suppl. B):S23-S31.

258. Bilukha OO, Rosenstein N. Prevention and control of meningococcal disease: Recommendations of the Advisory Committee on Immunization Practices (ACIP). *MMWR Morbid Mortal Weekly Rep*. 2005;54(RR-07):1-2.

259. Anonymous. Statement on conjugate meningococcal vaccine for serogroups A, C, Y and W135. *Canada Comm Dis Rep*. 2007;33(ACS-3).

212

Neisseria gonorrhoeae

JEANNE M. MARRAZZO | H. HUNTER HANDSFIELD | P. FREDERICK SPARLING

Gonorrhea is a common bacterial infection that is transmitted almost exclusively by sexual contact or perinatally and primarily affects the mucous membranes of the urethra and cervix and, less frequently, those of the rectum, oropharynx, and conjunctivae. Ascending genital infection in women leads to endometritis and salpingitis—collectively called pelvic inflammatory disease (PID), the predominant complication and one of the most common causes of female infertility. Other complications include acute epididymitis; ophthalmitis; disseminated infection with arthritis, dermatitis, and sometimes endocarditis; and transmission to the neonate with attendant conjunctivitis (ophthalmia neonatorum).

Gonorrhea is one of the oldest known human illnesses, and references to sexually acquired urethritis can be found in ancient Chinese writings, the biblical Old Testament (Leviticus), and other works of antiquity. Galen (AD 130) introduced the term *gonorrhea* ("flow of seed"), implying interpretation of urethral exudate as semen. The causative organism was described by Neisser in 1879 and was first cultivated in 1882 by Leistikow and Löffler. Untreated infections were understood to resolve spontaneously over several weeks or months, but reinfection was recognized. Many therapies were tried, but not until the advent of the sulfonamides in the 1930s and penicillin in 1943 was truly effective treatment available. Growth of fundamental knowledge about the organism and the host response to infection was slow for 80 years, but a remarkable surge of new information began in the 1970s, and the molecular biology of the gonococcus and the pathogenesis of gonorrhea have been well elucidated. Public health control efforts have met with variable success, and gonorrhea remains the second most common reportable disease in the United States (following sexually transmitted chlamydial infection), a prime example of the influence that social, behavioral, and demographic factors can have on the epidemiology of an infectious disease despite highly effective antimicrobial therapy.

The Organism

DESCRIPTION

Neisseria gonorrhoeae is a nonmotile, non–spore-forming, gram-negative coccus that characteristically grows in pairs (diplococci) with adjacent sides flattened. It closely resembles the related pathogen *Neisseria meningitidis*, as well as several species of nonpathogenic *Neisseria*. All *Neisseria* spp. rapidly oxidize dimethylparaphenylene diamine or tetramethylparaphenylene diamine, the basis of the diagnostic oxidase test. Traditionally, gonococci are differentiated from other *Neisseria* by their ability to grow on selective media; to use glucose but not maltose, sucrose, or lactose; to reduce nitrites; and by their inability to grow well at reduced temperature or on simple nutrient agar.[1]

GROWTH AND CULTIVATION

Gonococci do not tolerate drying, and patient samples to be used for cultivation should be inoculated immediately onto an appropriate growth or transport medium. Growth is best for most strains at 35°C to 37°C, and many freshly isolated strains have a relative or absolute requirement for atmospheric CO_2 in concentrations of approximately 5%. All strains are strictly aerobic under usual growth conditions, but the organism grows anaerobically when nitrite is provided as an electron acceptor. Colonies appear in 24 to 48 hours, but on most media viability is rapidly lost after 48 hours because of autolysis.[1]

Gonococci are inhibited by many fatty acids, and it is necessary to incorporate starch or other substances that absorb fatty acids into most growth media. All strains have complex growth requirements, including requirements for several vitamins, amino acids, iron, and other factors. For clinical purposes, a satisfactory medium is chocolate agar enriched with glucose and other defined supplements. Isolation of gonococci from sites that normally contain high concentrations of saprophytic microorganisms, especially the pharynx, rectum, and cervix, may be difficult because of overgrowth of the hardier normal flora—a problem that is largely overcome by use of media containing antimicrobial agents that inhibit most nonpathogenic *Neisseria* and other species but permit growth of most strains of *N. gonorrhoeae* and *N. meningitidis*. Chocolate agar that contains vancomycin, colistin, nystatin, and trimethoprim (modified Thayer-Martin medium) is widely used for this purpose in the United States; a similarly constituted translucent selective medium (New York City medium) is also commonly used.[1] Specimens from sites that usually do not harbor indigenous flora (e.g., blood, synovial fluid, and cerebrospinal fluid) should be cultured on antibiotic-free medium.

SURFACE STRUCTURES

The envelope of *N. gonorrhoeae* is similar in basic structure to that of other gram-negative bacteria. As the interface between the gonococcus and host, the cell surface has been intensively studied (Fig. 212-1), and specific surface components have been related to adherence, tissue and cellular penetration, cytotoxicity, and evasion of host defenses both systemically and at the mucosal level.

Pili

Varied colonial forms can be distinguished when *N. gonorrhoeae* is grown on translucent agar.[2] Fresh clinical isolates initially form colony types P^+ and P^{++} (formerly called T1 and T2), and the organisms have numerous pili extending from the cell surface (Fig. 212-2); P^- colonies (formerly T3 and T4) lack pili. Piliated gonococci are better able to attach to human mucosal surfaces and are more virulent in animal and organ culture models and in human inoculation experiments than nonpiliated variants.[2-5] Expression of pili is a function of the *pil* gene complex. A spontaneous shift between P^+ or P^{++} colonies to P^- colony types, known as phase variation, occurs after 20 to 24 hours of growth in vitro and is mediated principally by recombination between incomplete (silent) loci that contain slightly variant copies of *pil* DNA and loci with the complete *pil* structural gene, *pilE*.[6]

Pili traverse the outer membrane of the gonococcus through an integral outer membrane protein known as PilQ.[7] Mature pili are composed of repeating protein subunits (pilin) with a molecular weight of 19 + 2.5 kDa.[5] Pilin has regions of considerable interstrain antigenic similarity, especially near the amino terminus, but areas of extreme antigenic variability are also present.[5,6] A single strain of *N. gonorrhoeae* is capable of producing pili with differing antigenic compositions, compromising the utility of pilus-based vaccines against gonorrhea. In addition to mediating attachment, pili contribute to resistance to killing by neutrophils. In the fallopian tube mucosa model (Fig. 212-3), pili facilitate attachment to nonciliated epithelial cells, which initiates a process of entry and transport through these

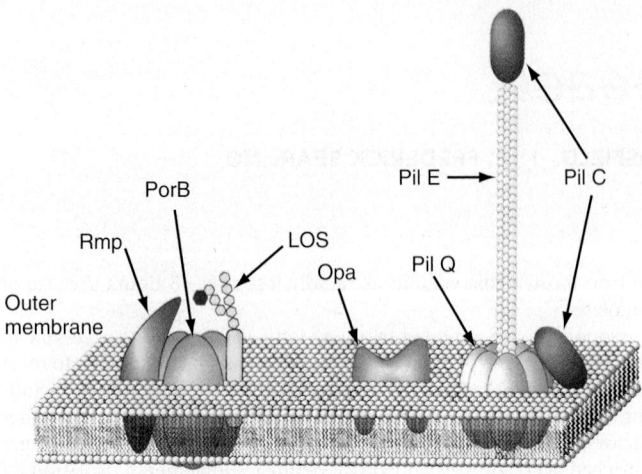

Figure 212-1 Illustration of gonococcal outer membrane depicting many of the antigens described in the text. Rmp, reduction modifiable protein; Por B, porin protein; LOS, lipo-oligosaccharide: the branched and phase variable LOS polysaccharide chain is shown as being bound by sialic acid, designated by a red hexagon; Opa, opacity protein; PilQ, pilin accessory protein Q, a secretin through which the assembled pilus extrudes; PilE, pilin, the subunits that are assembled into the α-helical pilus fibril; PilC, the outer membrane protein PilC, which is proposed to be presented by the pilus fibril as a tip adhesin. *(Courtesy of C. E. Thomas, University of North Carolina School of Medicine, Chapel Hill, NC.)*

cells into intercellular spaces near the basement membrane or directly into the subepithelial space while concurrently nearby ciliated mucosal cells lose their cilia and are sloughed.[4] CD46 was considered to be the main pilin receptor,[6] but the issue is currently uncertain and the identity of the pilus receptor is an area of active study. Other pilus-associated proteins are likely to be important to adhesion to host cells, particularly PilC.[8,9] Other factors also mediate attachment, notably opacity proteins (Opa), discussed later.

Outer Membrane

Like all gram-negative bacteria, the gonococcus possesses a cell envelope composed of three distinct layers: an inner cytoplasmic membrane, a middle peptidoglycan cell wall, and an outer membrane. The outer membrane contains lipo-oligosaccharide (LOS), phospholipid, and a variety of proteins (see Fig. 212-1). Porin, formerly designated protein I, has a molecular weight of 32 to 36 kDa and is closely associated in the membrane with LOS. Porin provides channels that allow aqueous solutes to pass through the otherwise hydrophobic outer membrane and is believed to play an important role in pathogenesis.[10] Porin is the product of a gene designated *porB*. It was formerly designated as protein 1. Porin proteins occur in two major antigenic classes, designated PorB1A and PorB1B, each of which is composed of many distinct genetic variants. Variations in Por sequence or antigenic types form the basis for the most commonly used gonococcal typing systems.[11] Strains expressing PorB1A and occasionally PorB1B are associated with genotypic resistance of *N. gonorrhoeae* to the bactericidal effect of normal (nonimmune) human serum and, perhaps as a direct result, with an enhanced propensity to cause bacteremia.[11] Porin-related serum resistance is due to binding to loops on porin protein of the complement downregulatory components C4bp or factor H.[12,13] PorB1A also appears to directly promote invasion of epithelial cells,[14] which also helps explain the propensity for bacteremic dissemination. Porin is the focus of extensive investigation directed toward the development of a gonococcal vaccine.[15]

Opa proteins are outer membrane proteins with molecular weights of 20 to 28 kDa. They are members of a family of proteins, each produced from its own *opa* gene. The amino acid sequence of the Opa proteins varies somewhat, primarily because of differences in two

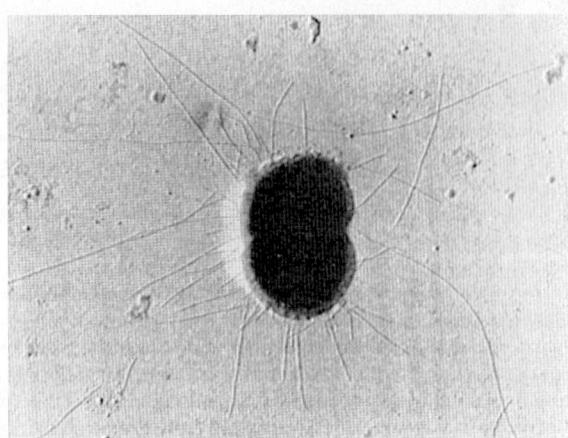

Figure 212-2 *Neisseria gonorrhoeae* with numerous pili extending from the cell surface. *(Courtesy of Dr. Gour Biswas, University of North Carolina School of Medicine, Chapel Hill, NC.)*

hypervariable regions in each protein.[16] Expression of Opa varies because of high-frequency variations in *opa* DNA that result in translational frame shifting. An individual strain of *N. gonorrhoeae* can express none or up to 11 Opa variants but usually not more than 3 at a time.[16] Gonococci isolated from mucosal sites usually express Opa and their colonies are opaque, but most isolates obtained from the cervix during menstruation and isolates from normally sterile sites, such as fallopian tubes, blood, and synovial fluid, generally lack Opa and form translucent colonies.[17] Many Opa proteins increase adherence between gonococci and to a variety of eukaryotic cells, including phagocytes.[17] Certain Opa variants appear to promote invasion of epithelial cells. Two classes of Opa receptor on eukaryotic cells have been identified: heparin-related compounds[18] and CD66, or carcinoembryonic antigen-related cell adhesion molecules (CEACAM).[19] Certain Opa proteins are able to bind to CEACAM receptors on B and T cells, resulting in downregulation of immune responses.[20] This may help account for the poor immune response to natural infection.[21]

Reduction-modifiable protein (Rmp) has a molecular weight of 30 to 31 kDa; is present in all gonococci in close association with porin and LOS; and shows little, if any, interstrain antigenic variation.[10] Rmp can stimulate blocking antibodies that reduce serum bactericidal

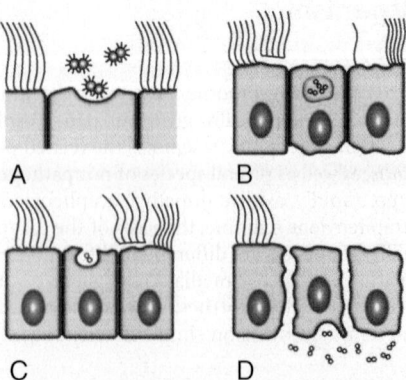

Figure 212-3 Schematic representation of the interaction between fallopian tube explant epithelial cells and *Neisseria gonorrhoeae*. **A,** Attachment of the piliated gonococci to the surface of a nonciliated host cell. **B,** Endocytosis of gonococci and loss of cilia on adjacent cells, mediated by lipo-oligosaccharide (LOS). **C,** Transport of gonococci through an epithelial cell in an endocytotic vacuole, in which the organism may replicate; progression of LOS-associated cytotoxicity. **D,** Release of organisms into subepithelial space. *(From Dallabetta G, Hook EW III. Gonococcal infections. Infect Dis Clin North Am. 1987;1:25-54.)*

activity against *N. gonorrhoeae*, which may potentiate infection after sexual exposure to an infected partner.[22] Several other outer membrane proteins have been identified, including multiple iron-repressible proteins, some of which are shared with *N. meningitidis*. Two of the iron-repressible proteins (85 and 110 kDa) constitute a specific receptor for transferrin,[23] and two others form a receptor for human lactoferrin.[24] The transferrin receptor is required for successful experimental urethral infection, but the role of the lactoferrin receptor is unclear; it does not influence infectivity.[25,26] Two additional proteins constitute a receptor for hemoglobin.[25] Other proteins are expressed only during anaerobic growth.[27] The ability of *N. gonorrhoeae* to grow anaerobically after removing available oxygen from the microenvironment may contribute to secondary invasion of fallopian tubes by strict anaerobes and thus to the pathogenesis of salpingitis. IgA₁ proteases, present in *N. gonorrhoeae* and *N. meningitidis* but not in nonpathogenic *Neisseria*, are assumed to protect the organism from secretory IgA antibody at mucosal surfaces, but this role has not been proved.

Gonococcal LOS is composed of lipid A and a core oligosaccharide that, in contrast with the polysaccharide of most gram-negative bacteria, lacks O-antigenic side chains. Sialylation of LOS core sugars in vitro or in vivo[28] masks epitopes on both LOS and porin and contributes to resistance to bactericidal antibodies.[29] LOS possesses endotoxic activity and contributes to ciliary loss and the death of mucosal cells in the fallopian tube explant model (see Fig. 212-3).[4] LOS core sugars undergo high-frequency phase and antigenic variation in vitro and in vivo,[28] which may contribute to the pathogenesis of infection, including resistance to bacterial anti-LOS antibodies present in normal serum and invasion of epithelial cells.[30]

The peptidoglycan layer of *N. gonorrhoeae* may also contribute to the inflammatory response. Peptidoglycan fragments are toxic in the fallopian tube explant system and cause complement consumption in vitro. In addition, peptidoglycan fragments have been found in the apparently sterile synovial fluid of patients with gonococcal arthritis-dermatitis syndrome.[31] Gonococci produce a surface polyphosphate that may have capsule-like functions, such as creating a hydrophilic, negatively charged cell surface. However, a carbohydrate capsule analogous to that of *N. meningitidis* or *Streptococcus pneumoniae* is not produced.

STRAIN TYPING

Studies of the clinical manifestations and epidemiology of gonorrhea have been greatly enhanced by the development of reproducible methods for typing *N. gonorrhoeae*. Characterization of gonococcal strains was formerly based on two primary methodologies, auxotyping and serotyping, and results from those now generally outdated methods are still instructive.[11,32] Auxotyping relied on the genetically stable requirements of strains for specific nutrients or cofactors, as defined by isolates' ability to grow on chemically defined media that lack selected factors.[32] Examples of common auxotypes, among more than 30 that were identified, include prototrophic, also known as "zero" or "wild type"; proline-requiring (pro⁻); and strains that require arginine, either hypoxanthine or proline, and uracil (AHU⁻ and PAU⁻).

The most widely used serotyping system was based on porin, which was antigenically classified into two groups, IA (current PorB1A) and IB (current PorB1B).[11] Subdivision of these groups into serovars was in turn based on patterns of coagglutination reactions with panels of monoclonal antibodies that reacted with various epitopes of Por IA (e.g., serovar IA-4) or IB (e.g., serovar IB-12).[11] In practice, auxotyping and porin serotyping were often used together to provide enhanced discrimination of strains. This system was instrumental in mapping the geographic and temporal occurrence of gonorrhea in communities, in analyzing patterns of antibiotic resistance, and in studies of sexual transmission dynamics.[11,33] Currently, these strain typing methods are used infrequently because auxotyping is cumbersome and serotyping monoclonal antibodies are no longer generally available. Typing based on differences in PorB structure is now done mostly by

patterns of hybridization to *porB*-based oligonucleotides or by rapid DNA sequencing of *porB*. The results are even more discriminative than those of auxotyping and serotyping and can be obtained rapidly in labs set up for this purpose.[34-36] These methods are not widely available in clinical laboratories, however.

Patterns of susceptibility to various antimicrobial agents, antigenic variations in LOS, and the plasmid content of isolates have also been analyzed to distinguish gonococcal strains, but with less success and reproducibility because these characteristics are not genetically stable. Analysis of DNA sequence variations, either by the method of Opa typing[37] or by automated DNA sequencing of particular genes (e.g., *por*), can also play an important role in strain typing.[38] Pulsed-field gel electrophoresis of selected gonococcal DNA sequences can rapidly differentiate genetically distinct strains of *N. gonorrhoeae*, often within auxotype/serovar classes.[39] Multilocus sequence typing[40] is a new tool that can rapidly differentiate between strains of several organisms and has been useful in epidemiologic studies of gonorrhea.

GENETICS

Plasmids

Many gonococci possess a 24.5-mDa conjugative plasmid and can thereby conjugally transfer other non–self-transferable plasmids with high efficiency; chromosomal genes are not mobilized. Many gonococci carry a plasmid (Pcʳ) that specifies production of a TEM-1 type of β-lactamase (penicillinase). The two most common Pcʳ plasmids have molecular weights of 3.2 and 4.4 mDa and are closely related to each other and to similar plasmids found in certain *Haemophilus* spp., including *Haemophilus ducreyi*.[41] In fact, it is suspected that gonococci first acquired Pcʳ plasmids from *H. ducreyi*.[41] Pcʳ plasmids are commonly mobilized to other gonococci by the conjugative plasmid.

Gonococci with plasmid-mediated high-level resistance to tetracycline, with minimal inhibitory concentrations (MICs) of 16 mg/L or greater, carry the 24.5-mDa conjugative plasmid into which the *tetM* transposon has been inserted.[42] The *tetM* determinant also confers tetracycline resistance to a variety of other bacteria, including some *Streptococcus* and *Mycoplasma* spp. and various genital organisms such as *Gardnerella vaginalis* and *Ureaplasma urealyticum*. Because of its location on the conjugative plasmid, high-level tetracycline resistance is readily transferred among gonococci.[42] The *tetM* determinant functions by encoding a protein that protects ribosomes from the effect of tetracycline. Finally, all gonococci contain a small (2.6 mDa) cryptic plasmid of unknown function.

Chromosomal Mutations and Transformation

Mutations in biosynthetic pathways are common, presumably reflecting the ready availability in vivo of essential nutrients such as amino acids, purines, and pyrimidines at infected mucosal sites. Nevertheless, *N. gonorrhoeae* is not highly mutable in that it lacks error-prone repair systems and is relatively resistant to external mutagenic stimuli such as ultraviolet light. Instead, gonococci have evolved efficient systems for phase and antigenic variation of surface components (pili, Opa, and LOS) that do not depend on such mutagenic pathways.

Gonococci also use transfer of naked DNA between cells (transformation) to promote genetic variability. The piliated variants of virtually all clinical isolates of *N. gonorrhoeae* are highly competent in transformation, but loss of the ability to express pili is always accompanied by a dramatic reduction in transformation competence. Uptake of transforming DNA is limited to homologous (i.e., gonococcal) DNA, which reflects recognition of a unique nucleotide sequence by a surface receptor.[43] No bacteriophages have been found in *N. gonorrhoeae*.

Chromosomal resistance of *N. gonorrhoeae* to β-lactam antibiotics and the tetracyclines results from interactions between a series of individual mutations, some of which (e.g., the *mtr* determinant) alter the net accumulation of antimicrobials inside the cell. The *mtr* locus has been shown to be an efflux pump similar to other membrane transporters.[44] The *penA* locus alters penicillin-binding protein 2 to reduce its affinity for penicillin.[45] For epidemiologic purposes, chromosomal resistance is defined when the MIC is such that clinical failures are common with the maximum practical therapeutic dose, which corresponds to MICs of 2 mg/L or greater for both tetracycline and penicillin G.[46] Clinically significant resistance to the fluoroquinolones, indicated by MICs of ciprofloxacin of 1 mg/L or higher (up to 16 mg/L),[46] result from the additive effects of multiple chromosomal mutations involving the genes *gyrA* and *gyrB*, which code for DNA gyrases, and *parC* and *parE*, which code for topoisomerases.[47,48]

Pathology

N. gonorrhoeae primarily infects columnar or cuboidal epithelium. The histopathology of gonorrhea is not materially different from that of most mucosal pyogenic infections. Attachment to mucosal epithelium, mediated in part by pili and Opa, is followed within 24 to 48 hours by penetration of the organism between and through epithelial cells to the submucosal tissues (see Fig. 212-3).[4] Of note, certain *Lactobacillus* species that predominate in the healthy vagina, including *Lactobacillus jensenii*, reduce gonococcal adherence to and invasion of human endometrial epithelial cells in a cell culture model,[49] providing insight into the clinical observation that bacterial vaginosis, with concomitant loss of hydrogen peroxide-producing lactobacilli, is a risk for acquisition of gonorrhea.[50,51] After epithelial invasion, a vigorous response by neutrophils ensues, with sloughing of the epithelium, development of submucosal microabscesses, and exudation of pus. Stained smears usually reveal large numbers of gonococci within a few neutrophils, whereas most cells contain no organisms (Fig. 212-4). The explanation for this phenomenon may involve stimulation or production of cellular receptors for gonococci after initial contact with the first organism, or other alterations of the host cell cytoskeleton[52] might stimulate efficient phagocytosis of additional organisms. In addition, some gonococci may evade killing mechanisms and continue to multiply intracellularly. In untreated infections, neutrophils are gradually replaced by macrophages and lymphocytes. Lymphocytic and mononuclear infiltration persists in tissue for up to several weeks after *N. gonorrhoeae* can no longer be identified histologically or recovered by culture.

Epidemiology

INCIDENCE

Many industrialized countries but few developing ones possess reporting systems that permit reliable estimates of the incidence of gonorrhea. The number of reported cases in the United States increased from

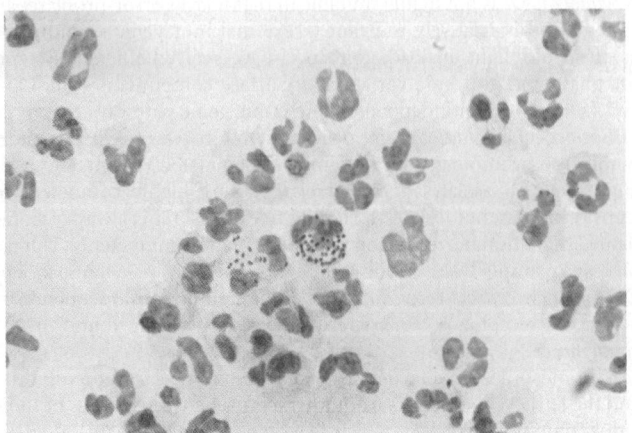

Figure 212-4 Gram-stained smear of urethral exudates showing intracellular gram-negative diplococci that are characteristic of gonorrhea.

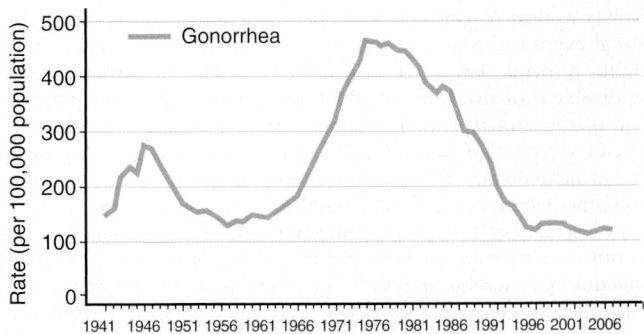

Figure 212-5 **Incidence of reported gonorrhea per 100,000 residents, United States, 1941 to 2007.** *(From Centers for Disease Control and Prevention. Sexually Transmitted Disease Surveillance, 2007. Atlanta, GA: U.S. Department of Health and Human Services, 2008.)*

approximately 250,000 cases in the early 1960s to a high of 1.01 million cases in 1978. The peak incidence of reported infection in modern times, 468 cases per 100,000 population, occurred in 1975 (Fig. 212-5).[53] The incidence then declined rapidly, largely the result of systematic public health prevention measures implemented in the 1970s. The decline ceased in the mid-1990s, and the incidence remained relatively stable at 128 to 130 cases per 100,000 from 1998 through 2006. The rate may be declining once again, with 355,991 reported cases (118.9 cases per 100,000) in 2007.[46] Although overall trends remain stable, regional variation occurs; the rate in the western United States decreased slightly in 2007 after a 29% increase between 2003 and 2006.[54] These statistics likely represent a significant underestimate of the true burden of disease; in 2000, for example, the true incidence was estimated to be approximately 718,000 incident cases, roughly double the reported rate.[55]

The incidence of gonorrhea is substantially lower in all countries of western Europe than in the United States, but high and rising rates have been documented in eastern Europe. In the past, the highest incidences of gonorrhea and its complications have occurred in developing countries, and this likely remains true in some areas of the world, with particularly devastating consequences for women and their reproductive health.[56] However, extensive use of antibiotic regimens for syndromic management of genital complaints, including urethral and vaginal discharge and PID, has apparently effected a decline in gonorrhea prevalence in many countries.[57]

In the United States, the highest attack rates occur in 15- to 24-year-old women and men, but after adjustment for sexual experience, the highest rates are seen in sexually active 15- to 19-year-old women (Fig. 212-6).[53,58,59] According to the population-based National Health and Nutrition Examination Survey, from 1999 to 2002, the prevalence was higher among non-Hispanic blacks relative to whites (1.2%; 95% confidence interval [CI], 0.7% to 1.9%), and 46% of those infected with gonorrhea also had *Chlamydia trachomatis* detected.[60] The Ad Health study of young adults showed similar results in 2001 and 2002. Among 12,548 adults aged 18 to 26 years, the prevalence of gonorrhea was 0.43% (95% CI, 0.29% to 0.63%), and it was strikingly higher in blacks than in whites (2.13%; 95% CI, 1.46% to 3.10%).[61]

Overall, more cases of gonorrhea are reported in men than in women, which probably reflects both a greater ease of diagnosis in men and a substantially higher rate of infection in men who have sex with men (MSM) than in heterosexual men and women. The incidence of gonorrhea among MSM in industrialized countries has been relentlessly increasing in the past several years, the result of behavioral disinhibition in response to improved therapy and survival of people with human immunodeficiency virus (HIV) infection.[62] These trends are evidenced in data from the Centers for Disease Control and Prevention's (CDC) MSM Prevalence Monitoring Project, in which eight U.S. cities submitted gonorrhea test data from 120,164 MSM visits to public clinics from 1999 through 2007 (Fig. 212-7). In 2007, median clinic

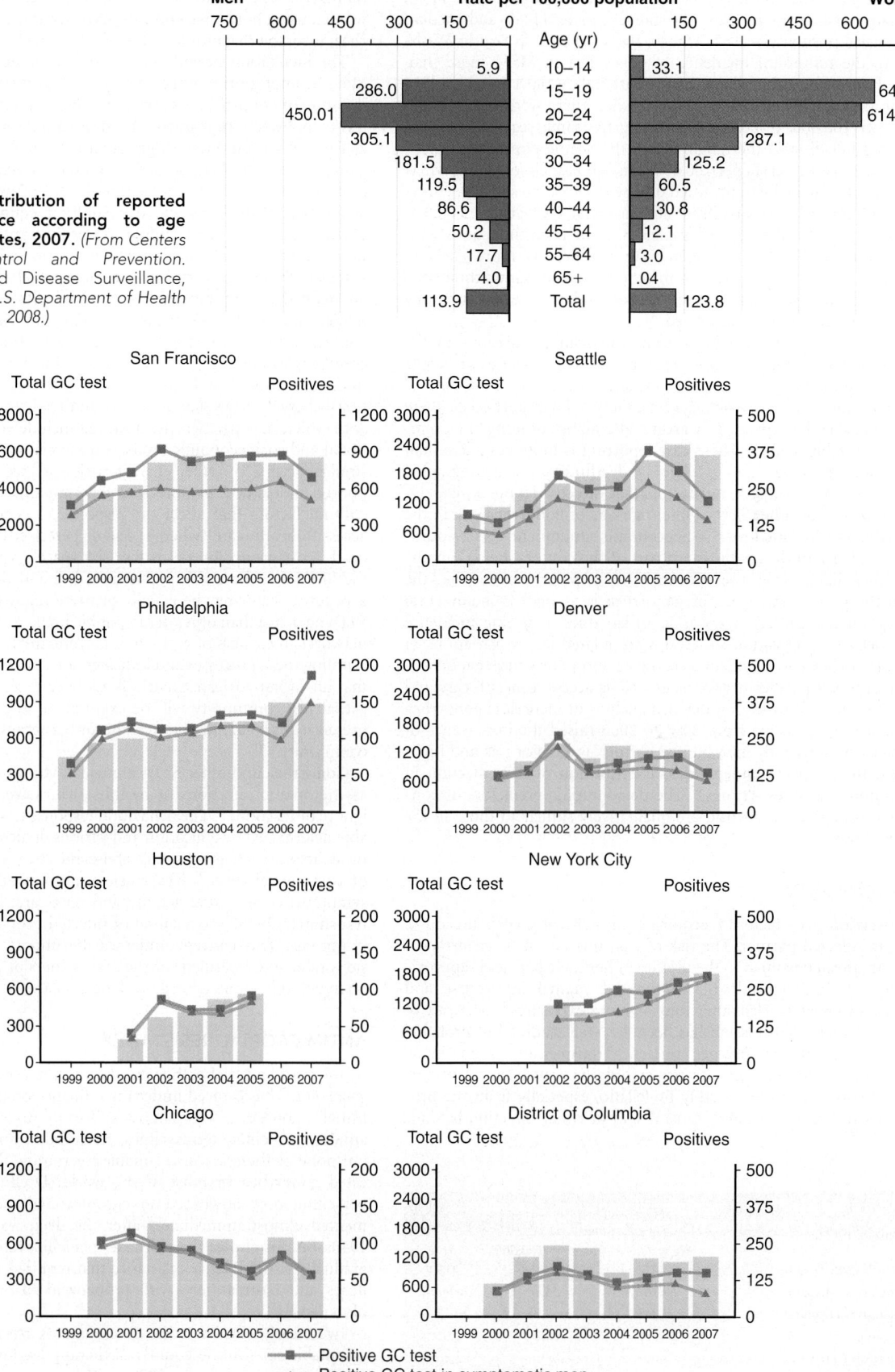

Figure 212-6 Distribution of reported gonorrhea incidence according to age and sex, United States, 2007. *(From Centers for Disease Control and Prevention. Sexually Transmitted Disease Surveillance, 2007. Atlanta, GA: U.S. Department of Health and Human Services, 2008.)*

Figure 212-7 **Number of gonorrhea tests and number of positive tests in men who have sex with men, STD clinics, 1999 to 2007.** *(From Centers for Disease Control and Prevention. Sexually Transmitted Disease Surveillance, 2007. Atlanta, GA: U.S. Department of Health and Human Services, 2008.)*

urethral gonorrhea positivity in MSM was 8% (range, 5% to 15%), median rectal positivity was 7% (range, 3% to 11%), and median pharyngeal positivity was 6% (range, 1% to 13%).[53] In Seattle, Washington, the minimum incidence of gonorrhea in MSM more than tripled from 1995, when there were at least 209 cases per 100,000 MSM in the population, to 2002 and 2003, when there were 725 and 645 cases per 100,000, respectively.[63] During the same years, the rate of reported infection in the remainder of the Seattle population varied between 74 and 97 cases per 100,000.[63] In San Francisco, among MSM attending two sexually transmitted disease (STD) clinics in 2003, prevalence of gonorrhea by anatomic site was rectal, 6.9%; urethral, 6.0%; and pharyngeal, 9.2%. Approximately 85% of rectal infections were asymptomatic. HIV-positive men were significantly more likely to have gonorrhea. Because 64% of infections were at nonurethral sites, these infections would have been missed and not treated had only urethral screening been performed.[64]

The rate of gonorrhea in African American populations in the United States is almost 25 times higher than that in whites or people of Asian ancestry; Latino populations and Native Americans experience intermediate rates (Table 212-1). Only a small portion of these differences can be explained by greater attendance of nonwhite populations at public clinics, where case reporting is more complete than in private health facilities.[58,59] Race and ethnicity are demographic markers of increased risk, not factors that directly denote a high risk for gonorrhea or other STDs. Other markers of gonorrhea risk in the United States include lower socioeconomic attainment, lesser education, residence in the southeastern part of the country, being unmarried, and illicit drug use. Contrary to popular perceptions, the population-based incidence of gonorrhea is as high in many rural settings in the United States as in urban ones. Differing incidence rates between population subgroups are related less to variations in numbers of sex partners than to complex and poorly understood differences in sex partner networks, as well as access to health care and related societal factors.[65,66] A detailed analysis of increasing gonorrhea incidence in California from 2003 to 2005 raised the importance of contact with a recently incarcerated partner as a major risk and highlighted the relatively understudied contribution of this infection in correctional facilities settings.[67] The demographic predictors of gonorrhea throughout the world are qualitatively similar to those in the United States.[68]

TRANSMISSION

The overriding risk factor for acquiring gonorrhea is sexual intercourse with an infected partner. The risk of transmission of *N. gonorrhoeae* from an infected woman to the urethra of her male partner is approximately 20% per episode of unprotected vaginal intercourse and increases to 60% to 80% after four or more exposures.[69] The risk of male-to-female transmission has been less well studied but probably approximates 50% to 70% per contact.[70] Transmission by anal intercourse is efficient, but the risk per episode has not been quantified. Transmission occurs less readily by fellatio, especially from the oropharynx to the urethra, and transmission in either direction by cunnilingus is believed to be rare.[71] Data are conflicting as to whether women using hormonal contraception are at increased risk for gonorrhea; if so, the magnitude of the effect is small.[72,73]

The incubation period is brief, and prominent genital symptoms often promptly bring infected people to treatment so that the mean duration of gonorrhea is short, typically several days in men and often less than 2 weeks in women. The approximate 50% transmission efficiency of uncomplicated gonorrhea through heterosexual intercourse[69,70] dictates that especially high rates of sex partner change—an average of two new partners within the 1- or 2-week interval between acquisition of infection and its resolution, equivalent to 50 or more partners per year—are required to sustain transmission in a population. People who have unprotected intercourse with new partners with sufficient frequency to maintain a stable prevalence in the community are defined as core transmitters.[74,75] Originally developed as a mathematical model,[75] the core transmission hypothesis has been empirically confirmed by several studies,[33,59,74] and a central focus of gonorrhea control is to identify the core group and to target members for case finding, treatment, and other prevention strategies. Demographic and social characteristics that directly or indirectly influence the frequency with which new partners are acquired include young age, low educational and socioeconomic levels, commercial sex, illicit drug use, and similar factors.[74,75] Other characteristics of core transmitters include poorly understood psychosocial determinants of partner selection, cultural factors that affect the response to symptoms, and reduced access to health care (whether real or perceived).[66] A recent variation on the core group concept is the "risk space" hypothesis, namely, that the locations where risk populations live and the sites where sexual exposures occur may be equally or more important determinants of STD incidence than other demographic predictors.[76] Analysis of sexual networks in clusters of gonorrhea is increasingly important in understanding these processes and indicates, for example, that the likelihood that an urban African American adolescent residing in a high STD prevalence community will be exposed to an STD is related to the presence of sexual links between his or her recent sex partners and the community.[77,78]

Gonorrhea and other STDs are usually transmitted by people with asymptomatic infections or by those who have symptoms that they ignore or discount.[79] The behavioral response to symptoms is presumably determined by education and various demographic and sociocultural factors, such as substance abuse and the economic determinants of commercial sex.[59,74] Nevertheless, most people with new genital symptoms cease sexual activity and seek care. It follows that many transmitters belong to a subset of infected people who lack or ignore symptoms. This concept underlies the importance of taking active steps to ensure treatment of the sex partners of infected people, who often will not spontaneously seek health care.

ANTIMICROBIAL RESISTANCE

As for most bacterial pathogens, the antimicrobial susceptibility of *N. gonorrhoeae* has evolved under the influence of antimicrobial therapy. Initially, gonococci were almost uniformly susceptible to the sulfonamides, penicillin, tetracyclines, macrolides, and fluoroquinolones, but none of these are now suitable for routine therapy of uncomplicated gonorrhea in most of the world. Declining susceptibility to penicillin, now attributed to chromosomal mutations, was documented almost immediately after the drug was introduced in the 1940s, but for almost three decades penicillin remained useful despite gradually rising relative resistance that required incrementally higher doses and co-treatment with probenecid to enhance and prolong blood levels.

Two nearly simultaneous developments rendered the penicillins unsuitable for routine gonorrhea therapy worldwide. Most dramatic was the appearance in the 1970s of β-lactamase–producing strains of *N. gonorrhoeae* bearing plasmids with the Pc^r determinant, followed by worldwide dissemination within a decade. Several plasmid variants now carry the Pc^r determinant, including the still dominant 4.4- and

TABLE 212-1	Reported Cases and Rates of Gonorrhea According to Race and Ethnicity, United States, 2007		
Racial/Ethnic Group	*Reported Cases*	*Cases per 100,000 Population*	*Rate Ratio*
White, non-Hispanic	69,767	34.7	Referent
Black, non-Hispanic	250,245	662.9	19.1
Hispanic	30,680	69.2	2.0
American Indian/Alaska Native	2,657	107.1	3.1
Asian/Pacific Islander	2,643	18.8	0.5
Total	355,992	118.9	

From Centers for Disease Control and Prevention. *Sexually Transmitted Disease Surveillance, 2007*. Atlanta, GA: U.S. Department of Health and Human Services, 2008.

3.2-mDa plasmids originally associated with Asia and Africa, respectively.[33,80] Second, in the 1970s and 1980s, chromosomal resistance progressed to the point that treatment failures became common with the maximum practical single-dose regimens of procaine penicillin, ampicillin, or amoxicillin. Although the proportion of gonococcal infections in the United States due to β-lactamase–producing strains declined from a peak of 11% in 1991 to only 0.4% of isolates in 2006, an additional 9% of infections are due to gonococci with high-level chromosomal penicillin resistance.[46]

Strains of *N. gonorrhoeae* with plasmid-mediated high-level tetracycline resistance were first documented in the United States in 1985. The location of the responsible *tetM* gene on the conjugative plasmid probably contributed to especially rapid worldwide spread of such strains. The prevalence of tetracycline-resistant *N. gonorrhoeae* (TRNG) peaked in 1997 at 7.3% and decreased for several years. It increased from 4.5% in 2005 to 4.6% in 2006.[46] Fortunately, the tetracyclines are no longer recommended and are little used as sole therapy for gonorrhea.

The mutations responsible for chromosomal resistance include *mtr*, which results in increased efflux of several antibiotics and other toxic compounds, such as fatty acids and bile salts; *penA*, which modifies the affinity of penicillin-binding proteins to β-lactam antibiotics; and *penB*, which alters the ability of antibiotics to transit the cell membrane through the porin protein.[44,45] Simultaneous mutations are common, with additive effects that result in resistance to several antibiotics and to all or most members of each affected drug class. Thus, simultaneous chromosomal resistance to penicillin, the tetracyclines, and macrolides is common. The cephalosporins are also affected, but MICs in strains tested throughout most of the world have remained within ranges that do not typically affect treatment efficacy. For example, the MICs of ceftriaxone for strains with chromosomal resistance are many times higher (e.g., 0.015 to 0.125 mg/L) than those for fully susceptible gonococci (usually 0.0001 to 0.008 mg/L), but even these higher levels are greatly exceeded by the blood levels achieved with routinely recommended regimens so that therapeutic efficacy is not affected.[80] Infection with chromosomally resistant *N. gonorrhoeae* is especially common in MSM.[46,81] This occurs because rectal infection is required for propagation of gonorrhea in MSM, and fecal bile salts and fatty acids confer selection pressure for *mtr*.[82]

The most important recent development in gonorrhea therapeutics is the spread of strains resistant to the fluoroquinolones and their progressive increase in numbers in North America and Europe. As for penicillin and other drugs, low-level resistance to the fluoroquinolones began to appear in *N. gonorrhoeae* almost immediately after they were introduced and soon was observed sporadically throughout the world.[83,84] Clinically significant resistance, with ciprofloxacin MICs of 1 to 16 mg/L, began to evolve soon thereafter due to the additive effects of multiple chromosomal mutations, particularly in the DNA gyrase complex (*gyrA* and *gyrB*) and topoisomerases (*parC* and *parE*).[47] Ciprofloxacin MICs of 4 mg/L or greater are associated with at least 50% rates of treatment failure with the recommended regimens of ciprofloxacin or other fluoroquinolones.[85] In the Philippines, the prevalence of high-level resistance to the fluoroquinolones among people with gonorrhea increased from 12% in 1994 to more than 70% in 1996 and 1997,[85] and similar prevalences are now the norm throughout Asia and the Pacific.[84-86] Such strains caused approximately 20% of all gonorrhea cases in Hawaii by 2001 and 10% of all gonorrhea cases in California in 2002, and by late 2003 they had appeared in substantial numbers in Washington State and Massachusetts, especially among MSM.[84,86] The proportion of fluoroquinolone-resistant isolates from MSM nationally increased to 23.8% by 2004, compared to only 2.9% in heterosexuals. Overall, prevalence of fluoroquinolone-resistant strains, which was less than 1% from 1990 to 2001, increased to 4.1% in 2003 and 13.8% in 2006.[46] Gonococci with high-level fluoroquinolone resistance also have appeared in areas of Canada and are now common in India, Israel, and areas of Europe. Such increases prompted the CDC to recommend in 2007 that fluoroquinolones no longer be used to treat gonorrhea in the United States.[87]

Clinical Manifestations

GENITAL INFECTION IN MEN

Uncomplicated Infection

Acute urethritis is the predominant manifestation of gonorrhea in men (see Chapter 106). The incubation period is typically 2 to 5 days but ranges from 1 to 10 days or longer (Fig. 212-8). Urethral discharge and dysuria, usually without urinary frequency or urgency, are the major symptoms. The discharge may initially be scant and mucoid, but within 1 or 2 days it becomes overtly purulent. These observations have been confirmed in studies of experimental gonococcal urethritis in humans.[3] Compared with nongonococcal urethritis, the incubation period of gonorrhea is shorter, dysuria is usually more prominent, and the discharge is generally more profuse and purulent (Fig. 212-9). However, exceptions are common and a small proportion of men with urethral gonorrhea remain asymptomatic and lack signs of urethritis.[79] The symptomatology of urethral gonorrhea depends in part on the infecting organism. Some Por IA serovars and the AHU⁻ and related auxotypes of *N. gonorrhoeae* are more frequently associated with asymptomatic urethral infection in men than are other gonococcal types.[11,88] The decline in the prevalence of such strains in North America probably has been accompanied by a decreasing frequency of asymptomatic gonorrhea in men. Most cases of untreated gonococcal urethritis resolve spontaneously over several weeks.

Localized Complications

Acute epididymitis is the most common complication of urethral gonorrhea but now is uncommon in industrialized countries; most cases of epididymitis in young men are due to *C. trachomatis* (see Chapter 109).[89] Penile edema without other overt inflammatory signs ("bull-headed clap") is occasionally seen in gonococcal or nongonococcal urethritis. Penile lymphangitis, periurethral abscess, acute prostatitis, seminal vesiculitis, and infections of Tyson's and Cowper's glands are uncommon complications. Urethral stricture as a result of gonorrhea is also uncommon. Although once considered a common consequence of gonococcal urethritis, many strictures in the preantibiotic era might have resulted primarily from treatment by urethral irrigation with caustic solutions, such as silver nitrate or potassium permanganate, rather than from gonorrhea.

UNCOMPLICATED UROGENITAL INFECTION IN WOMEN

The primary loci of genital infection in women are the columnar epithelial cells that line the endocervix (see Chapter 107). *N. gonorrhoeae* can often be recovered from the urethra or rectum and occasionally from the periurethral (Skene's) glands and the ducts of Bartholin's

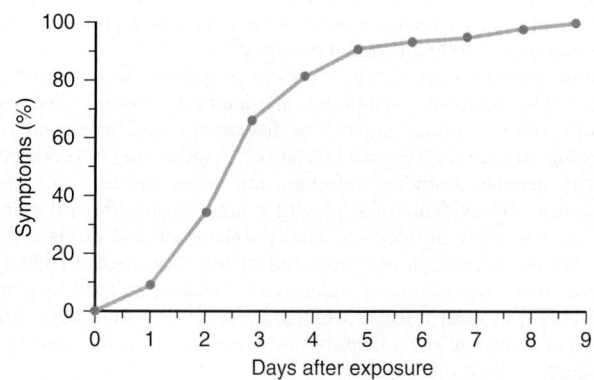

Figure 212-8 Incubation period in 44 men with gonococcal urethritis. *(From Harrison WO, Hooper RR, Weisner PJ, et al. A trial of minocycline given after exposure to prevent gonorrhea. N Engl J Med. 1979;300:1074-1078.)*

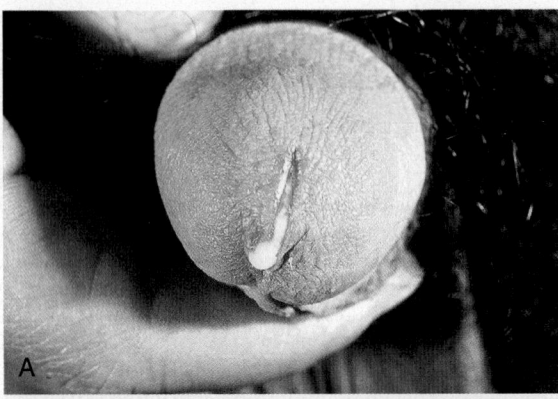
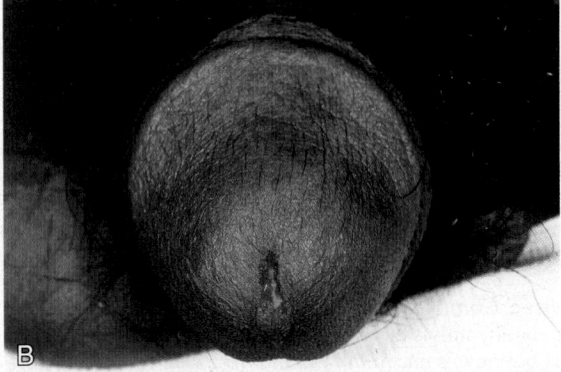

Figure 212-9 Gonococcal urethritis. A, Purulent exudates due to gonorrhea. **B,** Mucopurulent discharge mimicking the usual appearance of nongonococcal urethritis due to *Chlamydia trachomatis* and other pathogens.

glands, but these are rarely the sole infected sites except in women who have undergone hysterectomy. The vagina per se is not infected in sexually mature women because under the influence of estrogen the squamous epithelium of the vaginal mucosa is not susceptible to gonococcal infection.

The natural course of gonorrhea is less well understood in women than in men. Symptoms probably develop in most infected women,[90] but many remain asymptomatic or have only minor symptoms and do not seek medical care.[91] Thus, women with subclinical infection accumulate in the population, and in settings in which sexually active women are routinely screened for subclinical infection, up to 80% of women with gonorrhea are asymptomatic.[91] By contrast, in settings that attract symptomatic patients, such as urgent care clinics and hospital emergency departments, most women with gonorrhea are overtly symptomatic.[91] Women infected with AHU⁻ and related auxotypes of *N. gonorrhoeae*, like men, are more likely to have asymptomatic infection and more subtle inflammatory signs.[88]

Most infected women who develop symptoms do so within 10 days.[90] The dominant symptoms are increased vaginal discharge, dysuria (often without urgency or frequency), and intermenstrual bleeding, sometimes triggered by coitus.[91,92] Abdominal or pelvic pain usually denotes ascending infection, but some women with these symptoms lack evidence of salpingitis at laparoscopy. Physical examination may show purulent or mucopurulent cervical exudate (Fig. 212-10) and other signs of mucopurulent cervicitis, such as edema in a zone of cervical ectopy or endocervical bleeding induced by gentle swabbing[92]; in most infected women, these cervical signs are absent. Purulent discharge can sometimes be expressed from the urethra or the ducts of Bartholin's glands.

Rectal Gonococcal Infection

N. gonorrhoeae can be isolated from the rectum in up to 40% of women and a similar proportion of MSM with uncomplicated gonorrhea. The rectum is often the only infected site in MSM, whereas isolated rectal infection is found in approximately 5% of women with gonorrhea.[81,91,93,94] Rectal infection is acquired both through receptive anal intercourse, which accounts for virtually all cases in men, and perineal contamination with cervicovaginal secretions, which is believed to be responsible for many infections in women. Rectal gonococcal infection is usually asymptomatic, but some patients have acute proctitis manifested by anal pruritus, tenesmus, purulent discharge, or rectal bleeding.[95] Gonorrhea was the most common identified etiology of proctitis among 101 men seen in the San Francisco STD Clinic (2001 and 2002), accounting for 30% of cases.[96] The apparently higher rate of clinically apparent proctitis in men than in women suggests that inoculum size or trauma during anal intercourse may influence the development of symptoms. Anoscopy sometimes reveals mucopurulent exudate and inflammatory changes in the rectal mucosa, but infection with *C. trachomatis*, herpes simplex virus, or other sexually transmitted pathogens can produce the same findings.[95]

Pharyngeal Infection

Pharyngeal gonococcal infection is acquired by receptive oral sex but probably rarely, if ever, by kissing. Acquired more efficiently by fellatio than by cunnilingus,[71] pharyngeal infection can be found in 10% to 20% of heterosexual women with gonorrhea and 10% to 25% of infected MSM, but it is present in only 3% to 7% of heterosexual men with gonorrhea.[71,81,93] Almost all pharyngeal infections are asymptomatic, but rare cases may cause overt pharyngitis.[71]

The importance of documenting pharyngeal gonorrhea is debated, and several factors argue against routine screening or diagnostic testing in the general sexually active adult population. Most cases are asymptomatic and resolve spontaneously, pharyngeal infection is probably less transmissible than rectal or genital gonorrhea, and the pharynx is rarely the only infected site. Furthermore, identification of *N. gonorrhoeae* in pharyngeal cultures is more expensive than identification in anogenital cultures, and nonculture diagnostic assays have not been cleared by the Food and Drug Administration (FDA) (although they have been validated by some health department laboratories).[97] On the other hand, pharyngeal infection can be symptomatic and is sometimes the source of transmission to sex partners, especially among MSM,[98] or of systemic dissemination of *N. gonorrhoeae*. In addition, some regimens recommended for treatment of genital or rectal gonorrhea are less effective in eradicating pharyngeal infection, although ceftriaxone and cefixime are usually effective.[71,99] Current recommendations are to routinely test for pharyngeal infection in HIV-infected people who report receptive oral sex,[100] and many experts recommend routine pharyngeal screening in MSM given the continued high incidence of disease in this group.[53]

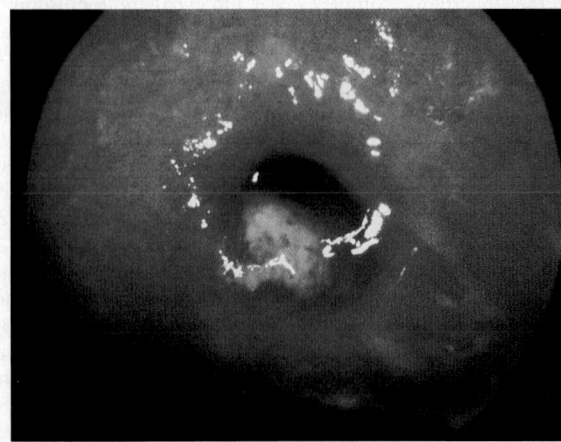

Figure 212-10 Purulent endocervical exudate in gonococcal cervicitis. *(From Handsfield HH.* Color Atlas and Synopsis of Sexually Transmitted Diseases. *2nd ed. New York, McGraw-Hill, 2001; courtesy of King K. Holmes.)*

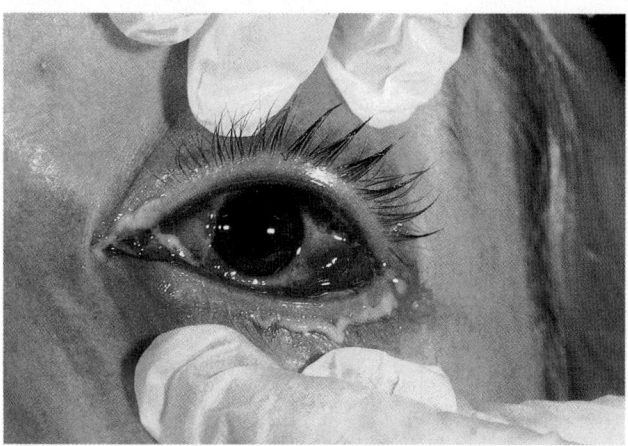

Figure 212-11 **Acute gonococcal conjunctivitis in an adult.** *(From Handsfield HH.* Color Atlas and Synopsis of Sexually Transmitted Diseases, *2nd ed. New York, McGraw-Hill, 2001.)*

Other Local Manifestations

Gonococcal conjunctivitis in adults is usually seen in people with genital gonorrhea, and most cases probably result from autoinoculation, but some cases may be acquired by other routes, such as orogenital exposure. Gonococcal conjunctivitis is usually painful, with prominent photophobia and copious, purulent exudate (Fig. 212-11), and corneal ulceration can supervene rapidly in the absence of prompt antibiotic therapy. However, some infections are mild, perhaps related to specific gonococcal strains. *N. gonorrhoeae* has been isolated in cases of acute gingivitis, otherwise unexplained oral ulcerations, and intra-oral abscesses. Cutaneous abscesses have been described, typically involving the finger or the penile shaft, and probably result from inoculation of preexisting lesions. For example, gonococcal abscess is sometimes the first clinical presentation of a congenitally patent median raphe duct of the penis.

Pelvic Inflammatory Disease

Pelvic inflammatory disease (PID) (see Chapter 108) refers to a spectrum of upper genital tract infections and may occur with or without overt symptoms. When symptomatic, PID is manifested by various combinations of endometritis, salpingitis, tuboovarian abscess, pelvic peritonitis, and perihepatitis.[91,101] The immediate and long-term sequelae are a primary impetus for prevention strategies against gonorrhea and chlamydial infection. Infection with *N. gonorrhoeae, C. trachomatis,* perhaps *Mycoplasma genitalium,* and vaginal anaerobes associated with bacterial vaginosis may be involved, often in combination.[102] Teen girls are at higher risk than older women probably because of both innate susceptibility, perhaps due to a high prevalence of cervical ectopy that may facilitate ascending infection, and sexual network factors that confer a higher likelihood of exposure to infected sex partners. Women using anovulatory hormones have been shown to have a lower risk of chlamydial salpingitis but not of gonococcal PID in some studies[103,104]; however, other analyses have not reported this association.[105] Case-control studies have suggested that vaginal douching, whether for perceived infection or as a hygienic measure, is a potent risk factor for clinical PID, cervicitis, endometritis, and ectopic pregnancy.[106-108] Bacterial vaginosis, which is characterized by a marked increase in the vaginal concentration of potentially pathogenic anaerobic and facultative bacteria, is strongly associated with the occurrence of PID.[109]

PID is estimated to occur in 10% to 20% of women with gonorrhea detected at the cervix. Among 57 women with gonorrhea but with no clinical signs or symptoms of PID, endometrial biopsies revealed histologic endometritis (termed "subclinical PID" by the authors) in 15 (26%); this was a significantly higher percentage than that seen among women without gonorrhea (11%; *P* < .001).[110]

The most consistent symptom of PID is low abdominal pain, and most women also have symptoms of lower genital tract infection.[101] Gonococcal PID often follows the onset of menses by a few days.[91] Fever, chills, nausea, and vomiting may occur, but most patients lack these manifestations. The primary finding on physical examination is pelvic adnexal tenderness, usually bilateral. Other common findings are uterine fundal tenderness, pain elicited on moving the cervix, and one or more tender adnexal masses. Abdominal examination usually elicits tenderness over the lower quadrants, and signs of peritoneal inflammation are common in severe cases. Many women with PID have bacterial vaginosis, and many have signs of mucopurulent cervicitis. Fever, leukocytosis, and an elevated erythrocyte sedimentation rate or C-reactive protein level are common, but they are absent in approximately one third of patients with laparoscopically documented PID. In practice, the clinical diagnosis of PID is imprecise.

The proportion of PID cases associated with gonorrhea varies greatly across population groups and with the background rates of gonorrhea and chlamydial infection. In the 1980s, 20% to 40% of cases of PID in most urban areas of the United States were associated with gonorrhea. The presence of cervical gonococcal or chlamydial infection does not exclude fallopian tube infection with other organisms, nor does failure to isolate *N. gonorrhoeae* or *C. trachomatis* definitively exclude their contribution to salpingitis. Facultative and anaerobic bacterial flora of the vagina may also contribute to acute PID, especially in patients with pelvic abscess or otherwise severe infections.[109]

Infertility resulting from fallopian tube obstruction is the most common serious consequence of PID and occurs in 15% to 20% of women after a single episode and 50% to 80% of those who experience three or more episodes.[111] Infertility may be more common after chlamydial than after gonococcal PID, perhaps because the more acute inflammatory signs associated with gonorrhea bring women to diagnosis and treatment sooner. This pattern was evident in the PID Evaluation and Clinical Health study, which enrolled more than 800 women aged 14 to 37 years with symptomatic PID.[112] Despite clinical cure and apparent microbiologic eradication of gonorrhea, as evidenced by lower tract cultures, infertility rates were 13% for women with *N. gonorrhoeae* identified, 19% for those with *C. trachomatis,* and 22% for those with anaerobic bacteria during a median follow-up of 35 months.[113] Rates of chronic pelvic pain were 27% among women with gonococcal infection.[114]

Perihepatitis

Acute perihepatitis, or Fitz-Hugh-Curtis syndrome, occurs primarily by direct extension of *N. gonorrhoeae* or *C. trachomatis* from the fallopian tube to the liver capsule and overlying peritoneum. Some cases may result from lymphangitic spread or bacteremic dissemination, which may explain rare cases of apparent perihepatitis in men. Perihepatitis results in abdominal pain, hepatic tenderness, and right upper quadrant peritoneal inflammatory signs. Most cases occur in association with overt PID, but many women lack pelvic symptoms or signs. Perihepatitis should be considered in the differential diagnosis of right upper quadrant pain in young, sexually active women; it is commonly mistaken for acute cholecystitis or viral hepatitis. Laparoscopy may show "violin string" adhesions between the liver capsule and the parietal peritoneum.

Gonorrhea in Pregnancy

Gonorrhea during pregnancy is associated with spontaneous abortion, premature labor, early rupture of fetal membranes, and perinatal infant mortality.[115,116] The clinical manifestations of gonorrhea are unchanged in pregnant women, except that PID and perihepatitis are uncommon after the first trimester, when the products of conception obliterate the uterine cavity. A higher prevalence of pharyngeal infection has been reported in pregnant than in nonpregnant women with gonorrhea,[117] perhaps because the frequency of fellatio increases in lieu of vaginal intercourse as pregnancy progresses. However, the anatomic sites of gonococcal infection in pregnant women have not been studied in recent decades. Reports are conflicting as to whether pregnancy is a risk factor for gonococcal bacteremia.

Disseminated Gonococcal Infection

Disseminated gonococcal infection (DGI) results from bacteremic dissemination of *N. gonorrhoeae*, although immune complexes or other indirect immunologic mechanisms may contribute to pathogenesis and symptoms in some cases. Although once estimated to occur in 0.5% to 3% of infected patients,[118,119] the rate undoubtedly is lower at present because of declining prevalences of gonococcal strains prone to disseminate.[120] However, discrete outbreaks of DGI have recently been documented.[121] Septic arthritis and a characteristic syndrome of polyarthritis and dermatitis are the predominant manifestations, and DGI is a relatively common cause of infective arthritis in young adults.[118,119,122,123] Gonococcal endocarditis was common in the preantibiotic era but now is rare.[124] Meningitis, osteomyelitis, septic shock, and acute respiratory distress syndrome are rare manifestations.[125-128]

Properties of *N. gonorrhoeae* classically associated with dissemination include resistance to the bactericidal action of nonimmune human serum, the AHU⁻ auxotype, specific Por IA serovars, and marked susceptibility to penicillin—characteristics also associated with asymptomatic genital gonorrhea.[11,120] However, an increasing proportion of DGI cases have been associated with other auxotype/serovar classes as the prevalence of Por IA/AHU⁻ gonococci has declined, and antibiotic-resistant strains have caused DGI.[119,120] According to one report, as the frequency of DGI has declined, more apparent cases in fact are due to meningococcemia.[129]

Complement deficiency predisposes to gonococcal and meningococcal bacteremia.[130] Up to 13% of patients with DGI have been reported to have complement deficiencies, and patients with repeated episodes of neisserial bacteremia should be tested with an assay for total hemolytic complement activity. Other host factors associated with dissemination include female sex, menstruation, and perhaps pharyngeal gonococcal infection and pregnancy.[118,119,130] In approximately half of affected women, symptoms of DGI begin within 7 days of the onset of menses.[118]

The most common presentation of DGI is the arthritis-dermatitis syndrome.[122] During the first few days, most patients experience polyarthralgias that primarily involve the knees, elbows, and more distal joints; the axial skeleton is usually not involved. Physical examination usually shows objective signs of arthritis or tenosynovitis in at least two joints.[118,119] Asymmetrical involvement of only a few joints helps distinguish DGI from polyarthritis caused by most immune complex–mediated disorders, which typically are manifested by symmetrical involvement of many joints. A characteristic dermatitis (Fig. 212-12) is present in approximately 75% of patients and consists of discrete papules and pustules, often with a hemorrhagic component. Hemorrhagic bullae or overtly necrotic lesions that mimic ecthyma gangrenosum are sometimes seen. The lesions usually number 5 to 40 and occur predominantly on the extremities. Fever, systemic toxicity, and polymorphonuclear leukocytosis are common, but they are usually mild and are often absent.

Untreated, inflammation regresses in most joints and the dermatitis resolves, but overt septic arthritis supervenes in one or two joints, most commonly the knee, ankle, elbow, or wrist, although any joint may be involved. Septic gonococcal arthritis develops in some patients without prior polyarthritis or dermatitis, and in the absence of the characteristic dermatitis or overt genital infection, it is clinically indistinguishable from septic arthritis of any etiology.[118,119]

During the arthritis-dermatitis stage, gonococci often can be recovered by blood culture, but synovial fluid, if it can be obtained, usually contains fewer than 20,000 leukocytes/mm³ and is sterile. Gonococci can often be seen by immunochemical methods in biopsy specimens of skin lesions, but cultures are generally sterile. In septic gonococcal arthritis, synovial fluid usually contains more than 50,000 leukocytes/mm³ and culture is often positive, but at this stage blood cultures are usually negative.[118,119]

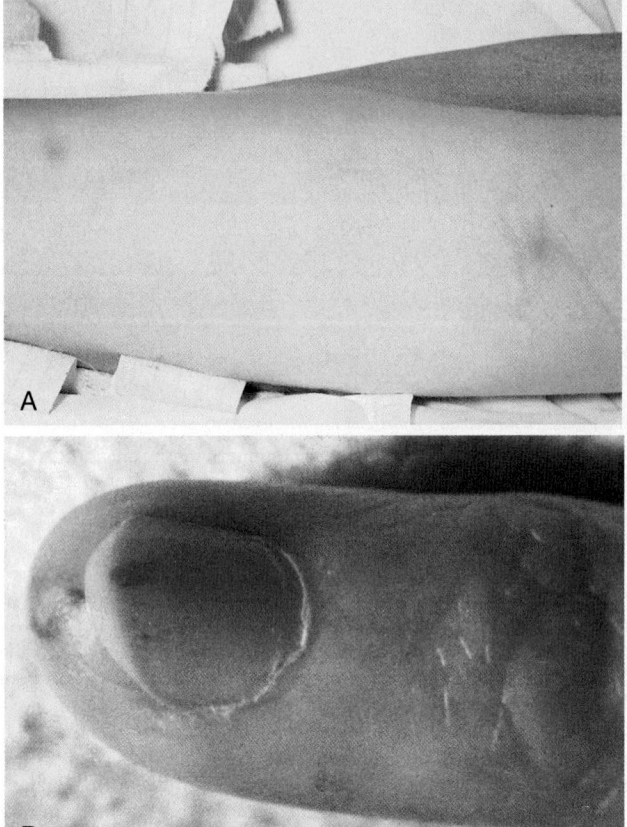

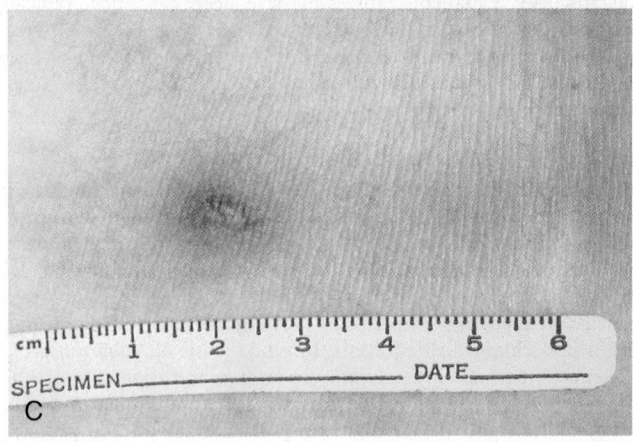

Figure 212-12 Cutaneous lesions in disseminated gonococcal infection. A, Early papular lesions. **B,** Pustular lesion associated with subungual hemorrhage. **C,** Ulcerated pustular lesion.

Gonococcal bacteremia is often intermittent, so a minimum of three blood cultures should be obtained when DGI is suspected. Synovial fluid should be cultured if a specimen can be obtained. However, only approximately half of patients with DGI have positive cultures of blood or synovial fluid. Although uncommonly positive, gram-stained smears and cultures of pustular skin lesions are simple to perform and should be obtained. *N. gonorrhoeae* can be recovered from a mucosal site in at least 80% of patients,[118,119] so the urethra or endocervix, the rectum, and the pharynx should be tested regardless of symptoms or exposure history, and patients' sex partners should be examined and tested. Nucleic acid amplification tests (NAATs), including polymerase chain reaction, appear to be more sensitive than culture in detecting gonococci in synovial fluid,[131] and they have recently been applied to skin lesions of DGI with success.[132,133] The diagnosis of DGI is confirmed if *N. gonorrhoeae* is identified in a nonmucosal specimen such as blood, synovial fluid, or a skin lesion, and the diagnosis is probable if infection is documented at a mucosal site or in a sex partner of a patient with a typical clinical syndrome.

The differential diagnosis of the gonococcal arthritis-dermatitis syndrome includes meningococcemia,[129] septic arthritis due to other pyogenic bacteria, and the entire range of inflammatory arthritis. Reactive arthritis is easily confused with DGI because it is common in sexually active young adults and is associated with urethritis, cervicitis, and skin lesions that sometimes have a pustular component. Usually, careful clinical and microbiologic assessment readily differentiates these disorders, but a trial of antibiotic therapy may be required.[87,88,118,119,122]

Gonococcal endocarditis, which usually involves the aortic valve, is a rare but serious manifestation that occurs in an estimated 1% or 2% of patients with DGI.[118,124] Although often associated with the arthritis-dermatitis syndrome, endocarditis may be the sole manifestation of DGI.[124] In the preantibiotic era, median survival was 6 to 8 weeks, reflecting a typical rate of valve destruction between that of acute staphylococcal or pneumococcal endocarditis and subacute endocarditis caused by viridans streptococci.

Neonatal and Pediatric Infections

Gonococcal conjunctivitis of the newborn (ophthalmia neonatorum) is the most common clinically recognized manifestation of neonatal infection[134-137]; it was once a common cause of blindness in the United States and may remain so in some developing countries. Prophylaxis by instillation of antibiotics or a 1% aqueous solution of silver nitrate into the conjunctivae soon after delivery is highly effective, although occasional failures occur. The most important preventive measure is routine screening and treatment of pregnant women for gonorrhea before term. The diagnosis of gonococcal ophthalmia should be suspected clinically when acute conjunctivitis develops within a few days of delivery and is confirmed by identification of gonococci in conjunctival secretions. Systemic illness with septicemia and arthritis can also develop in newborns exposed to gonorrhea, but these are rare. *N. gonorrhoeae* can often be recovered from the gastric aspirates of infants born to infected mothers, but many cases probably reflect transient colonization rather than clinically important infection.[135]

Rectal gonococcal infection is sometimes seen in newborns, but vaginal infection is uncommon because the neonatal vaginal mucosa is well estrogenized by circulating maternal hormone. Purulent vaginitis is the primary manifestation of gonorrhea in prepubertal girls after the neonatal period,[135,137] but otherwise the clinical manifestations of gonorrhea in children are not materially different from those in adults. After the neonatal period until 1 year of age, most cases in children appear to be acquired nonsexually from an infected parent, usually in a setting of poor hygiene.[137] After 1 year of age, most cases are acquired by sexual abuse, most commonly by a male relative or the mother's nonmarital sex partner, other than the child's biologic father.[135,137] Nonsexual transmission of ocular infection occasionally occurs among young children in tropical settings.

Diagnosis

Isolation of *N. gonorrhoeae* is the historical standard for diagnosis. Culture is inexpensive and reasonably sensitive, the only widely validated diagnostic test for rectal and pharyngeal infection, and preserves an isolate for antimicrobial susceptibility testing when clinically indicated or for surveillance. Culture is widely considered the only appropriate test in forensic settings, as in testing people who have been sexually assaulted or children with suspected gonorrhea. Nevertheless, NAATs have supplanted culture in most settings, due to convenient specimen management and their utility in testing urine and self-obtained vaginal swabs. Nonamplified DNA probe tests remain in common use despite their lower sensitivity compared with culture or NAATs. Microscopy of Gram-stained smears is effective in the diag-

nosis of symptomatic urethritis in men but has marginal utility in other settings. There is no clinically useful serologic test.

CULTURE

A single culture on antibiotic-containing selective medium, such as modified Thayer-Martin agar, has a sensitivity of 95% or more for urethral specimens from men with symptomatic urethritis and 80% to 90% for endocervical infection in women. Results may vary depending on the quality of the medium and the adequacy of the clinical specimen.[1,138,139] Simultaneous inoculation of both selective and nonselective media maximizes sensitivity for cervical infection[1,139] but is impractical in most settings. Normally sterile clinical specimens, such as blood, synovial fluid, and cerebrospinal fluid, should be inoculated onto enriched chocolate agar or another nonselective medium as well as broth medium[87] and should also be tested by NAAT, but no published studies have systematically analyzed the detection of *N. gonorrhoeae* in broth cultures with the automated techniques now used by most clinical laboratories.

Up to 5% of gram-negative, oxidase-positive diplococci isolated from the genital tract and substantially greater proportions of those from the rectum and pharynx are in fact *N. meningitidis*.[71,93,140,141] Some of these cases are associated with urethritis, cervicitis, or proctitis that is clinically indistinguishable from gonorrhea.[93,142] Therefore, speciation of *Neisseria* isolates is desirable for positive genital cultures and should be routine for pharyngeal and rectal specimens. The NAATs for *N. gonorrhoeae* are believed to reliably exclude meningococcal infection.[143,144] Antimicrobial susceptibility testing of *N. gonorrhoeae* is not generally recommended except when conducting surveillance for antimicrobial resistance, but it should be routine following treatment failure and in cases of disseminated infection.

NUCLEIC ACID AMPLIFICATION TESTS

Currently available NAATs for *N. gonorrhoeae* utilize several related technologies, including transcription-mediated amplification (e.g., APTIMA; Gen-Probe, San Diego, CA), polymerase chain reaction (e.g., Amplicor; Roche, Nutley, NJ), and the DNA strand displacement assay (e.g., Probe-Tec; Becton Dickinson, Franklin Lakes, NJ). An assay based on ligase chain reaction (LCx; Abbott, Abbott Park, IL) is no longer commercially available in the United States. The NAATs have largely replaced culture in most settings in which people are screened for asymptomatic genital infection and, in particular, in which assays with combined targets for gonorrhea and chlamydial infection, such as the APTIMA Combo 2 assay (Gen-Probe), are used to screen for *C. trachomatis*.[143-145] These tests are not significantly more sensitive than culture for detecting *N. gonorrhoeae* in cervical or urethral specimens (unlike the diagnosis of *C. trachomatis*, for which the NAATs are more sensitive than all other tests). However, the NAATs for *N. gonorrhoeae* appear to have specificities greater than 99%, offer important advantages in specimen management, and retain sensitivity when used to test voided urine or self-collected vaginal swabs, an important advantage for laboratory screening in many settings.[143,145,146] The transcription-mediated amplification test has a positive predictive value of at least 95% in women in settings in which gonorrhea prevalence is as low as 0.5%, indicating that false-positive results are rare even when screening low-prevalence populations.[147] Concern has been expressed that persisting DNA may cause false-positive results when NAATs are used to test patients soon after treatment, but NAATs for *N. gonorrhoeae* become negative within 2 weeks of successful treatment.[148] Data suggest that the APTIMA test for *N. gonorrhoeae* and *C. trachomatis* is reliable for diagnosis of rectal and pharyngeal infection,[149] but these assays remain uncleared by the FDA for routine use; thus, they may be used if validation by local laboratories has been documented. These observations may not extend to other NAATs because the Probe-Tec assay evidenced low positive predictive value when applied to pharyngeal and rectal specimens in a community-based sample of MSM in one study.[150]

GRAM-STAINED SMEARS

The Gram stain has been used for more than a century to identify gonococci in clinical specimens; methylene blue and other dyes have been used as well. Microscopy of Gram-stained smears is positive if gram-negative diplococci of typical morphology are observed in association with neutrophils (see Fig. 212-4), negative if no such organisms are seen, and equivocal if typical morphotypes are not associated with neutrophils or morphologically atypical organisms are seen.[139] Nonpathogenic Neisseraceae are not usually associated with leukocytes. In men with symptomatic urethritis, microscopy is at least 95% sensitive and is highly specific for diagnosis of gonorrhea, but microscopy is less useful for other anatomic sites. The sensitivity approximates 50% for asymptomatic urethral infection in men and for cervical or rectal infection[139]; the specificity is said to be high, but this likely is true only for highly experienced observers. Microscopy is both insensitive and nonspecific for detection of pharyngeal gonococcal infection and is not recommended.

OTHER DIAGNOSTIC METHODS

Nonamplified DNA probe tests are somewhat less sensitive than culture or NAATs, and they are not useful in the diagnosis of rectal or pharyngeal infection or for testing urine. However, these assays are inexpensive and are offered by many laboratories in combination with assays for *C. trachomatis*. Immunochemical detection of gonococcal antigens, such as enzyme immunoassays with polyclonal antigonococcal antibodies and fluorescein-conjugated monoclonal antibodies for direct fluorescence microscopy, had modest usage in the 1980s, but these tests were relatively insensitive and now are little used.

Treatment

The antimicrobial susceptibility of *N. gonorrhoeae* is labile, varies greatly across geographic areas and populations, and fluctuates over time.[151] Clinical treatment decisions almost invariably are made without knowledge of the antimicrobial susceptibility of the infecting strain. Therefore, when possible, the regimens for routine treatment of gonorrhea should have efficacies that approach 100%, regardless of the distribution of sensitive and resistant strains of *N. gonorrhoeae* in the community, and treatments with efficacies less than 95% should be avoided.[87,152] Other factors that influence therapeutic decisions for gonorrhea are the pharmacokinetic characteristics of the agent, its efficacy in complicated versus uncomplicated infection, differential efficacy at various anatomic sites of infection, toxicity, availability, convenience of administration, and cost. An additional consideration is the potential efficacy of an agent for concurrent infection. Historically, this concern focused on syphilis, but even in settings with high prevalences of both gonorrhea and syphilis, the occurrence of syphilis in people with gonorrhea is not measurably affected by use of treatment regimens with or without activity against *Treponema pallidum*.[153] The most common coexisting pathogen in people with gonorrhea is *C. trachomatis*, and many studies during three decades have given remarkably consistent results: 15% to 25% of heterosexual men, 10% to 15% of MSM, and 35% to 50% of women with gonorrhea have concurrent chlamydial infections.[58,60] The treatment of gonorrhea has been greatly facilitated by the excellent efficacy of single-dose regimens; however, with increasing resistance to several classes of antibiotics (detailed later), this approach may eventually need to be reevaluated. Gonorrhea in pregnant women responds to the recommended regimens.[97,154]

UNCOMPLICATED GONORRHEA IN ADULTS

Initial Single-Dose Treatment

Recommendations for the treatment of uncomplicated gonorrhea, modified from those published in the 2006 Sexually Transmitted Diseases Treatment Guidelines from the CDC, are summarized in Table 212-2.[97,152] Either a single 125-mg intramuscular dose of ceftriaxone or a single 400-mg oral dose of cefixime is effective for infection of all mucosal sites, with cure rates that exceed 98% for urethral, cervical, and rectal gonorrhea and 90% for pharyngeal infection, and both regimens are safe and effective in pregnant women.[155,156] Cefixime recently became available again in the United States after several years of unavailability. Cefpodoxime, in a single oral dose of 400 mg, has favorable pharmacokinetics, performed favorably in a dose-ranging trial and a clinical trial,[99,157] and is approved for treatment of gonorrhea by the FDA. Nevertheless, few comparative clinical trials support its therapeutic efficacy, and cefpodoxime is designated by the CDC as an alternative therapy. In a randomized clinical trial of 331 people with confirmed gonorrhea, 400 mg of cefpodoxime effected cure among men and women infected at any urogenital or rectal site in 96.5% (lower bound of 95% CI, 93.9%).[99] Among 281 males with urethral gonorrhea, 96.1% were cured (lower bound of 95% CI, 93.1%), and of 35 people with pharyngeal gonorrhea, 74.0% were cured. Cefuroxime, 1 g orally, appears to be effective in women, with a reported cure rate of 97%, but it was only 93% effective against gonococcal urethritis in men.[158] Of note, allergic cross-reactions between penicillin and the cephalosporins appear to be uncommon, and penicillin-allergic people can often be treated for gonorrhea with a cephalosporin.[159] Finally, strains resistant to oral third-generation cephalosporins have been reported from Japan.[160,161] Although these strains were still susceptible to ceftriaxone, some data suggest that the MICs to this drug may be on the rise.[162]

As a class, the fluoroquinolones were an important advance in gonorrhea therapy, with many members of the class demonstrated to be highly effective in single doses against infection due to susceptible gonococci, with cure rates at least 98% for all anatomic sites.[152] Unfortunately, due to the relentless worldwide increase in the resistance of *N. gonorrhoeae* strains to fluoroquinolones, they now have limited clinical utility. Increasingly widespread fluoroquinolone resistance in the United States led the CDC to recommend against their use to treat

TABLE 212-2	Options for the Treatment of Gonorrhea*

Uncomplicated Infection of the Cervix, Urethra, and Rectum†
Cefixime 400 mg PO single dose
Ceftriaxone 125 mg IM single dose
Infection of the Pharynx
Ceftriaxone 250 mg IM single dose
Conjunctivitis (Not Ophthalmia Neonatorum)
Ceftriaxone 1 g IM single dose
Disseminated Gonococcal Infection
Ceftriaxone 1 g IM or IV every 24 hr for 24-48 hr‡ after improvement, with switch to oral therapy for completion of 1 week total antibiotic therapy, including cefixime 400 mg PO twice daily
Meningitis and Endocarditis
Ceftriaxone 1-2 g IV every 12 hr for 10-14 days (meningitis) or ≥4 weeks (endocarditis)
Ophthalmia Neonatorum
Ceftriaxone 25-50 mg/kg IV or IM in a single dose, not to exceed 125 mg§

*Treatment of gonorrhea in the adult should always be accompanied by treatment for chlamydial infection, and patients should abstain from sex during treatment. Test of cure is not routinely recommended.

†All regimens for uncomplicated genital and conjunctival infection are given as a single dose. Cefixime is the recommended cephalosporin for oral treatment, and it only recently became available again in the United States. Limited data support the use of cefpodoxime as an oral alternative. For other cephalosporin options, see www.cdc.gov/std/treatment. Spectinomycin can be used in people intolerant to cephalosporins and quinolines; however, its availability is uncertain.

‡Ceftriaxone administered IM may be reconstituted in 1% lidocaine solution to minimize injection pain. Alternative parenteral regimens include cefotaxime, ceftizoxime, and spectinomycin. See www.cdc.gov/std/treatment for specific regimens.

§Topical antibiotic therapy alone is inadequate for treatment of ophthalmia neonatorum.

Modified from Centers for Disease Control and Prevention. Sexually transmitted diseases treatment guidelines, 2006. *MMWR Morb Mortal Wkly Rep.* 2006;51(RR-11); and relevant updates, including *MMWR Morb Mortal Wkly Rep.* 2007;56(RR-14).

gonorrhea in MSM in 2004 and, in August 2007, against routine use for all cases of gonorrhea.[163,164] Nonetheless, fluoroquinolones are highly effective against infection due to susceptible gonococci, with cure rates at least 98% for all anatomic sites.[152] Although their general use should be discouraged, these drugs retain a useful role in patients in whom no other option is feasible, such as those with absolute contraindications to cephalosporin; however, as noted previously, allergic cross-reactions between penicillin and the cephalosporins appear to be uncommon, and penicillin-allergic people often can be treated for gonorrhea with a cephalosporin.[159] When a fluoroquinolone is the only feasible option for gonorrhea treatment, it is prudent to obtain a culture isolate so that susceptibility testing can be performed and for reference in the event of treatment failure. For geographic areas in which rates of fluoroquinolone resistance remain sufficiently low to continue routine use in the treatment of gonorrhea, active surveillance for evolution of fluoroquinolone resistance is critical.

Single-dose regimens with several other cephalosporins, quinolones, or other antibiotics may be used, but they have no advantages over the recommended regimens.[97,152] In small trials, a single dose of 2 g of azithromycin has been effective against both gonorrhea and chlamydial infection, and it may be considered an alternative treatment at this dose in some situations. However, cost and gastrointestinal intolerance limit its utility, and increasing resistance is an emerging concern to the point where some authors, notably in the United Kingdom, recommend against its use for this purpose. A sentinel surveillance project using gonococcal isolates in Europe documented a rate of azithromycin resistance higher than 5% for the first time in 2004.[165-170] Azithromycin resistance in the United States remains relatively low,[164] but familiar trends in other countries suggest that it will not remain a viable option for very long.

Spectinomycin, 2 g intramuscularly, is effective for genital and rectal gonorrhea in the United States despite the occasional occurrence of spectinomycin-resistant gonococci, but it is ineffective for pharyngeal infection and is currently not available in the United States; its eventual availability is uncertain.[87] Its sole indication is the treatment of pregnant women with histories of rapid-onset allergic reactions to penicillin or documented cephalosporin allergy—a rare confluence of events. Other options to treat such women are limited and have not been studied; these include desensitization to recommended agents or use of alternative drugs with test of cure, such as azithromycin. However, resistance to most alternative drugs, including azithromycin, has been reported.

Co-treatment for Chlamydial Infection

Regardless of the single-dose regimen used, treatment of gonorrhea should be accompanied by a regimen active against *C. trachomatis.*[87] In addition to treating chlamydial infection, with attendant reduction in the risk of postgonococcal urethritis and salpingitis,[171] giving a second drug with a different mechanism of action than the primary treatment may reduce selection pressure for antimicrobial resistance in *N. gonorrhoeae.* Hypothetically, the worldwide spread of fluoroquinolone-resistant gonococci may have been slower than the dissemination of penicillinase-producing strains 25 years earlier in part because penicillin monotherapy was the rule in the 1970s, whereas antichlamydial co-therapy was the norm in the 1990s. The recommended regimens are a single oral dose of azithromycin, 1 g, or doxycycline, 100 mg orally twice daily for 7 days.[97] Erythromycin, in a divided-dose regimen totaling 2 g/day orally, is acceptable as follow-up therapy if neither azithromycin nor a tetracycline can be given, and ofloxacin or levofloxacin (but not ciprofloxacin) is effective (but requires a 7-day course).

FOLLOW-UP OF PATIENTS TREATED FOR UNCOMPLICATED GONORRHEA

Treatment failure is uncommon, and retesting to document cure is not recommended unless therapeutic compliance is in question or symptoms persist.[152] However, most patients with gonorrhea remain at con-tinuing risk, and studies have found recurrent gonorrhea in 10% to 15% of people retested 1 to 4 months after treatment.[52,172-175] Accordingly, retesting for recurrent or persistent infection, or rescreening, should be done routinely 3 or 4 months after treatment. Rescreening is also indicated for men and women with chlamydial infection.[97] Testing urine or self-collected vaginal specimens by NAAT can be accomplished in asymptomatic patients without a clinical examination or, if using mailed specimens, without a clinic visit.

PELVIC INFLAMMATORY DISEASE

The treatment of PID is addressed in detail in Chapter 108. In individual patients, the specific pathogens responsible for ascending genital infection usually are not known, and the recommendations for initial treatment of acute PID are similar regardless of whether the initial infection is due to *N. gonorrhoeae, C. trachomatis,* or other pathogens. Guidelines for the treatment of PID are summarized in Table 212-3.[87,97,102] The main regimen for outpatient therapy is single-dose treatment with ceftriaxone or with cefoxitin plus probenecid, followed by oral therapy with doxycycline, 100 mg twice a day orally, and metronidazole, 500 mg twice a day orally. In a well-designed study, this regimen (without metronidazole) was equally effective as the equivalent inpatient, parenteral regimen both in short-term resolution and in preservation of fertility after a 3-year follow-up.[113] The use of azithromycin for treatment of PID has been controversial and is not currently recommended.[102,176-178] The CDC guidelines stipulate that fluoroquinolone use may be considered as the antibiotic for gonorrhea coverage in PID if the community prevalence and individual risk for fluoroquinolone-resistant gonorrhea are low, and the guidelines recommend performing diagnostic testing with appropriate management according to the result. In addition, in many communities gonorrhea is now a relatively uncommon cause of PID, reducing concern about fluoroquinolone resistance.

In addition to providing treatment aimed at gonorrhea and chlamydial infection, the importance of routinely providing treatment

TABLE 212-3	Recommended Treatment of Acute Pelvic Inflammatory Disease
Hospitalized Patients	
Regimen A	
Cefotetan, 2 g IV q12h, or cefoxitin, 2 g IV q6h	
plus	
Doxycycline, 100 mg IV or PO q12h	
Continue both drugs IV for 24 hr after the patient substantially improves, then continue doxycycline, 100 mg PO bid, to complete 14 days total therapy. Either clindamycin or metronidazole may be added to the oral regimen if tuboovarian abscess is suspected.	
or	
Regimen B	
Clindamycin, 900 mg IV q8h	
plus	
Gentamicin, 2 mg/kg IV once, followed by 1.5 mg/kg q8h*	
Continue both drugs IV for 24 hr after the patient substantially improves, then continue doxycycline, 100 mg PO twice daily, or clindamycin, 450 mg PO four times daily, to complete 14 days total therapy. Clindamycin may be preferable when tuboovarian abscess is suspected.	
Outpatients	
Single-dose cefoxitin, 2 g IM, plus probenecid, 1 g PO; or ceftriaxone, 250 mg IM; or other parenteral third-generation cephalosporin (e.g., ceftizoxime or cefotaxime)	
plus	
Doxycycline, 100 mg PO bid for 14 days	
with or without	
Metronidazole 500 mg PO bid for 14 days	

*Single daily dosing may be substituted.

Modified from Centers for Disease Control and Prevention. Sexually transmitted diseases treatment guidelines, 2006. *MMWR Morb Mortal Wkly Rep.* 2006;51(RR-11); and relevant updates, including *MMWR Morb Mortal Wkly Rep.* 2007;56(RR-14) and www.cdc.gov/std/treatment.

active against anaerobic bacteria for the entire 2-week treatment period is debated.[102] Anaerobes can often be isolated from intra-abdominal specimens obtained from women with PID, but clinical resolution appears to be equally rapid and complete for women treated only with ofloxacin[179] or doxycycline,[113] neither of which inhibits most anaerobes associated with PID. Nevertheless, because direct comparative trials have not been undertaken and no published data address long-term efficacy in preventing infertility, ectopic pregnancy, or chronic pelvic pain, the CDC and most experts recommend routine provision of anaerobic coverage.[87,97,102]

Regardless of the initial treatment, close follow-up is indicated. Clinical progression or failure of the patient to improve within 3 days is an indication for diagnostic imaging and to hospitalize the patient for parenteral therapy and possible laparoscopy to confirm the diagnosis and obtain intra-abdominal culture specimens to facilitate selection of improved, parenteral antimicrobial therapy.[97] The patient's sex partner(s) should be tested and treated for chlamydial infection and gonorrhea, unless both infections can be reliably excluded in the index patient.

ACUTE EPIDIDYMITIS

The treatment of acute epididymitis is addressed in Chapter 109. Most cases in young adults are due to *C. trachomatis* or *N. gonorrhoeae*, but coliforms and other urinary tract pathogens are common causes in older men or after urinary tract instrumentation, and perhaps in men who participate in unprotected insertive anal intercourse. Most cases can be managed on an outpatient basis with ceftriaxone, 250 mg intramuscularly, plus 10 days of treatment with doxycycline, 100 mg twice daily.[87] Ofloxacin, 400 mg orally twice daily, or levofloxacin, 500 mg daily, for 10 days, provides better coverage for coliforms and nonsexually transmitted pathogens and is effective against chlamydial infection but should be avoided if gonorrhea is suspected.

DISSEMINATED GONOCOCCAL INFECTION

Few data are available on the treatment of patients with DGI since the evolution and spread of gonococci with high levels of antibiotic resistance, and all recommendations are empirical. Antimicrobial susceptibility testing should be routinely employed to guide therapy in case the initial response to empirical treatment is suboptimal. Patients with the gonococcal arthritis-dermatitis syndrome should be treated initially with ceftriaxone, 1 g once daily, either intramuscularly or intravenously.[97,122,180] Most patients without complications can be treated as outpatients. Equivalent doses of other third-generation cephalosporins undoubtedly would be effective and are recommended as options.[87] No reported studies have systematically evaluated the fluoroquinolones, but these drugs undoubtedly are effective if the organism is susceptible. After clinical improvement begins, treatment of patients without septic arthritis or other complications may be switched to an oral cephalosporin (e.g., cefixime 400 mg twice daily) or a fluoroquinolone (e.g., levofloxacin 500 mg daily) to complete 7 to 10 days of total therapy.[97] The penicillins or tetracyclines may be used if the infecting organism is documented to be susceptible. Patients with gonococcal endocarditis should receive 4 weeks of parenteral therapy, usually starting with ceftriaxone or an equivalent cephalosporin and later modifying the regimen if dictated by the results of antimicrobial susceptibility testing.[97] Meningitis should be treated with a 10- to 14-day course of ceftriaxone.[97]

GONORRHEA IN CHILDREN

Relatively few cases of gonorrhea are seen in children, and treatment has not been well studied; most treatment recommendations are extrapolated from those for adults. Uncomplicated infections in neonates and older children should normally be treated with ceftriaxone in a single intramuscular dose of 25 to 50 mg/kg body weight, up to 125 mg.[87] Little is known about the prevalence of chlamydial infection in pediatric patients with gonorrhea, and the usual practice is to perform a test for *C. trachomatis* and withhold specific treatment unless infection is diagnosed.[181] DGI and gonococcal conjunctivitis in children are treated with 7 to 10 days of ceftriaxone, 25 to 50 mg/kg body weight per day intramuscularly or intravenously, or with an equivalent regimen of another third-generation cephalosporin. Continuous irrigation of the conjunctivae with physiologic saline solution is often used in gonococcal conjunctivitis, but topical antibiotics probably offer no additional benefit.[87]

MANAGEMENT OF SEX PARTNERS

Management of sex partners is an integral part of treating patients with gonorrhea and other STDs because failure to ensure that the partner is treated risks reinfection of the patient and fosters continued transmission. Few state or local health departments in the United States provide direct assistance in contacting or managing the partners of people with gonorrhea or chlamydial infection diagnosed outside public clinics (and often not there)[182]; the physician and patient should work together to this end.

Ideally, the sex partners of people with gonorrhea or chlamydial infection should be examined, tested for both infections and other common STDs, and counseled on prevention. Unfortunately, success in bringing partners to clinical care is low, and in most settings treatment can be documented for less than half the partners of infected people.[182] Studies suggest that this proportion can be increased and the rate of reinfection in index patients reduced by arranging for treatment without examination—that is, by giving the index patient an antibiotic for the partner or a prescription in the partner's name, or calling in a prescription directly for the partner. Collectively, these strategies have been termed *expedited partner therapy* (EPT).[173,183] Although EPT has uncertain legal underpinnings in some states, surveys indicate that many clinicians frequently pursue the practice in managing their patients with STDs.[184,185] Furthermore, several states with formerly restrictive laws or regulations have modified them to permit EPT, and others reportedly are considering such steps. The CDC provides up-to-date reports of the legal status of EPT throughout the United States at www.cdc.gov/std/ept. Clinicians should routinely employ EPT for the partners of people with gonorrhea or chlamydial infection, to the extent permitted by regional laws and regulations, whenever success is not ensured in personal evaluation of the partners. EPT for gonorrhea can be accomplished with single-dose oral therapy active against both *N. gonorrhoeae* (e.g., cefixime) and *C. trachomatis* (azithromycin); for the partners of patients with chlamydial infection alone, azithromycin is appropriate.

Prevention and Control

PUBLIC HEALTH STRATEGIES

Screening of sexually active people is a mainstay of public health strategies to prevent gonorrhea and the other treatable bacterial STDs, and it is largely responsible for the dramatic declines observed in the incidence of gonorrhea nationwide after the mid-1970s (see Fig. 212-5). Women at risk who undergo routine pelvic examinations should be tested for *N. gonorrhoeae* and *C. trachomatis* using published guidelines where available. The U.S. Preventive Services Task Force recommends routine annual testing for gonorrhea in sexually active women younger than the age of 25 years and for older women with specific risks.[186] Some authors have used more refined epidemiologic analyses to help narrow these relatively broad recommendations for screening and have suggested that using local gonorrhea prevalence rates may be especially useful.[187] When pelvic examination is otherwise not indicated, urine or a self-collected vaginal swab can be tested by NAAT. Universal screening of all heterosexual men and women usually is not cost-effective except in special settings, such as public STD clinics. In screening women or heterosexual men, a pharyngeal culture should be obtained if symptoms of pharyngitis are present, and it may be warranted if the patient has performed fellatio on a person known to have genital gonorrhea.

Although asymptomatic cervical gonorrhea has been recognized for some time, of increasing concern is the underappreciated prevalence of asymptomatic gonorrhea in some populations, particularly rectal and pharyngeal infection in MSM. Sexually active MSM should be tested routinely for both gonococcal and chlamydial infection, depending on the anatomic sites exposed.[188] Furthermore, it was shown more than a decade ago that urethritis increases HIV viral load in semen, and treatment concomitantly lowers levels of HIV RNA.[189] Thus, prompt diagnosis and treatment of urethritis along with routine, periodic screening at all exposed anatomic sites is recommended for all HIV-infected people at initial evaluation and thereafter at least every 12 months and more frequently for those at higher risk.[190] Among asymptomatic MSM, the highest yield will be achieved by culturing the rectum if the patient practices receptive anal intercourse. Some experts recommend screening for urethral infection as well, although asymptomatic urethral gonorrhea is uncommon in this population.[81,93] Pharyngeal testing should be strongly considered when screening asymptomatic MSM.[97]

Public health control measures for gonorrhea and chlamydial infection also include routine rescreening and treatment of patients' sex partners, both discussed previously. Other elements include appropriate diagnostic testing in people with compatible clinical syndromes, adherence to recommended treatment regimens, and periodic testing of gonococcal isolates to monitor trends in antimicrobial resistance. Reporting of cases by health care providers, preferably supplemented by direct reporting by laboratories of people with positive test results, is important for epidemiologic monitoring and to facilitate targeted control efforts. Public education and personal counseling, in an effort to encourage healthy sexual behavior and the use of barrier contraceptives, is central to the control of gonorrhea and all STDs. Finally, all people with a newly acquired STD should routinely be tested for other common infections. For example, screening tests for gonorrhea, chlamydial infection, syphilis, and HIV should be undertaken in people diagnosed with any STD; women with STDs should have cervical cytology and diagnostic testing for vaginal infections.[87,191]

CONDOMS AND MICROBICIDES

Properly used male condoms provide a high degree of protection against transmission or acquisition of gonorrhea, chlamydial infection, HIV, and other STDs transmitted by infected secretions.[192-194] Methodologic limitations of most studies that have attempted to esti-

mate the magnitude of condom effectiveness tend to result in an underestimate of protection. Nevertheless, a well-designed systematic review reported that most studies found condom use to be associated with reduced risk of both gonorrhea and chlamydia.[194] The female condom likely provides comparable protection against gonococcal infection.[195] Logically, diaphragms and cervical caps might be expected to offer some protection against gonorrhea. Although a randomized controlled cohort study in South Africa failed to show a protective effect against HIV, a subset analysis revealed that women who reported consistent diaphragm use experienced a significant reduction in incident gonococcal infection (relative hazard, 0.61; 95% CI, 0.41 to 0.91).[196] The spermicide nonoxynol-9 provides no significant protection against gonorrhea or chlamydial infection and is associated with increased risk of vulvovaginal candidiasis and bacterial urinary tract infection, and increased risk of HIV acquisition in a large trial.[197,198] Although spermicidal preparations with nonoxynol-9 enhance the contraceptive efficacy of barrier methods, they should be avoided by people at high risk for STD, as should condoms packaged with lubricant containing nonoxynol-9.[97] Research is under way to identify alternative microbicides for vaginal or rectal use. No evidence has been presented that such time-honored measures as washing, urinating, or douching after exposure materially reduce the risk of gonorrhea or any other STD.

OTHER PREVENTION STRATEGIES

Administration of systemic antibiotics immediately before or soon after sexual exposure can reduce the risk of gonorrhea,[199] and mass treatment of populations with high rates of syphilis and other treponematoses has been effective in reducing morbidity. At best, however, such approaches have had transient, minor influences on the incidence of gonorrhea in treated populations, and they may carry a risk of fostering the spread of resistant gonococci.

The development of a vaccine to prevent gonorrhea is a high research priority, but an experimental vaccine containing purified gonococcal pili conferred only partial protection against experimental infection with the homologous strain of *N. gonorrhoeae* and no protection from heterologous challenge.[200] The extraordinary degree of antigenic variability in pili, Opa, and LOS, both at the community level and during the course of each infection, presents formidable barriers to developing a gonorrhea vaccine based on these antigens.[3,15] Other more antigenically stable proteins, including porin, are under investigation as possible vaccine candidates, but success probably lies in the distant future.[15,200]

REFERENCES

1. Janda W, Gaydos C. Neisseria. In: Murray PR, Baron EJ, Jorgensen JH, et al, eds. *Manual of Clinical Microbiology*. 9th ed. Washington, DC: American Society of Microbiology; 2007.
2. Kellogg DS Jr, Peacock WL Jr, Deacon WE, et al. *Neisseria gonorrhoeae*: I. Virulence genetically linked to clonal variation. *J Bacteriol*. 1963;85:1274-1279.
3. Cohen MS, Cannon JG. Human experimentation with *Neisseria gonorrhoeae*: progress and goals. *J Infect Dis*. 1999;179: S375-S379.
4. McGee ZA, Johnson AP, Taylor-Robinson D. Pathogenic mechanisms of *Neisseria gonorrhoeae*: observations on damage to human fallopian tubes in organ culture by gonococci of colony type 1 or type 4. *J Infect Dis*. 1981;143:413-422.
5. Schoolnik GK, Fernandez R, Tai JY, et al. Gonococcal pili: primary structure and receptor binding domain. *J Exp Med*. 1984;159:1351-1370.
6. Forest KT, Bernstein SL, Getzoff ED, et al. Assembly and antigenicity of the *Neisseria gonorrhoeae* pilus mapped with antibodies. *Infect Immun*. 1996;64:644-652.
7. Chen CJ, Tobiason DM, Thomas CE, et al. A mutant form of the *Neisseria gonorrhoeae* pilus secretin protein PilQ allows increased entry of heme and antimicrobial compounds. *J Bacteriol*. 2004;186:730-739.
8. Kirchner M, Heuer D, Meyer TF. CD46-independent binding of neisserial type IV pili and the major pilus adhesin, PilC, to human epithelial cells. *Infect Immun*. 2005;73:3072-3082.
9. Rudel T, van Putten JP, Gibbs CP, et al. Interaction of two variable proteins (PilE and PilC) required for pilus-mediated adher-

ence of *Neisseria gonorrhoeae* to human epithelial cells. *Mol Microbiol*. 1992;6:3439-3450.
10. Blake MS, Gotschlich EC. Gonococcal membrane proteins: speculation on their role in pathogenesis. *Prog Allergy*. 1983;33:298-313.
11. Knapp JS, Tam MR, Nowinski RC, et al. Serological classification of *Neisseria gonorrhoeae* with use of monoclonal antibodies to gonococcal outer membrane protein I. *J Infect Dis*. 1984; 150:44-48.
12. Ram S, Cullinane M, Blom AM, et al. C4bp binding to porin mediates stable serum resistance of *Neisseria gonorrhoeae*. *Int Immunopharmacol*. 2001;1:423-432.
13. Ram S, McQuillen DP, Gulati S, et al. Binding of complement factor H to loop 5 of porin protein 1A: a molecular mechanism of serum resistance of nonsialylated *Neisseria gonorrhoeae*. *J Exp Med*. 1998;188:671-680.
14. Van Putten JPM. Gonococcal invasion of epithelial cells driven by the P.IA porin. In: Nassif X, Quentin-Millet M-J, Taha M-K, eds. *Proceedings of the Eleventh International Pathogenic Neisseria Conference, Nice, France*. Paris: Editions E.D.K.; 1998:35.
15. Blake MS, Wetzler LM. Vaccines for gonorrhea: where are we on the curve? *Trends Microbiol*. 1995;3:469-474.
16. Connell TD, Shaffer D, Cannon JG. Characterization of the repertoire of hypervariable regions in the protein II (opa) gene family of *Neisseria gonorrhoeae*. *Mol Microbiol*. 1990;4: 439-449.
17. Fischer SH, Rest RF. Gonococci possessing only certain P.II outer membrane proteins interact with human neutrophils. *Infect Immun*. 1988;56:1574-1579.

18. Van Putten JP, Duensing TD, Cole RL. Entry of OpaA+ gonococci into HEp-2 cells requires concerted action of glycosaminoglycans, fibronectin and integrin receptors. *Mol Microbiol*. 1998;29:369-379.
19. Wang J, Gray-Owen SD, Knorre A, et al. Opa binding to cellular CD66 receptors mediates the transcellular traversal of *Neisseria gonorrhoeae* across polarized T84 epithelial cell monolayers. *Mol Microbiol*. 1998;30:657-671.
20. Boulton IC, Gray-Owen SD. Neisserial binding to CEACAM1 arrests the activation and proliferation of CD4+ T lymphocytes. *Nat Immunol*. 2002;3:229-236.
21. Hedges SR, Mayo MS, Mestecky J, et al. Limited local and systemic antibody responses to *Neisseria gonorrhoeae* during uncomplicated genital infections. *Infect Immun*. 1999;67: 3937-3946.
22. Plummer FA, Chubb H, Simonsen JN, et al. Antibody to Rmp (outer membrane protein 3) increases susceptibility to gonococcal infection. *J Clin Invest*. 1993;91:339-343.
23. Cornelissen CN, Sparling PF. Iron piracy: acquisition of transferrin-bound iron by bacterial pathogens. *Mol Microbiol*. 1994;14:843-850.
24. Biswas GD, Sparling PF. Characterization of lbpA, the structural gene for a lactoferrin receptor in *Neisseria gonorrhoeae*. *Infect Immun*. 1995;63:2958-2967.
25. Chen CJ, Sparling PF, Lewis LA, et al. Identification and purification of a hemoglobin-binding outer membrane protein from *Neisseria gonorrhoeae*. *Infect Immun*. 1996;64:5008-5014.
26. Cornelissen CN, Kelley M, Hobbs MM, et al. The transferrin receptor expressed by gonococcal strain FA1090 is required for

the experimental infection of human male volunteers. *Mol Microbiol.* 1998;27:611-616.

27. Clark VL, Campbell LA, Palermo DA, et al. Induction and repression of outer membrane proteins by anaerobic growth of *Neisseria gonorrhoeae. Infect Immun.* 1987;55:1359-1364.

28. Mandrell RE, Lesse AJ, Sugai JV, et al. In vitro and in vivo modification of *Neisseria gonorrhoeae* lipooligosaccharide epitope structure by sialylation. *J Exp Med.* 1990;171:1649-1664.

29. Elkins C, Carbonetti NH, Varela VA, et al. Antibodies to N-terminal peptides of gonococcal porin are bactericidal when gonococcal lipopolysaccharide is not sialylated. *Mol Microbiol.* 1992;6:2617-2628.

30. Van Putten JP, Robertson BD. Molecular mechanisms and implications for infection of lipopolysaccharide variation in *Neisseria. Mol Microbiol.* 1995;16:847-853.

31. Fleming TJ, Wallsmith DE, Rosenthal RS. Arthropathic properties of gonococcal peptidoglycan fragments: implications for the pathogenesis of disseminated gonococcal disease. *Infect Immun.* 1986;52:600-608.

32. Catlin BW. Nutritional profiles of *Neisseria gonorrhoeae, Neisseria meningitidis,* and *Neisseria lactamica* in chemically defined media and the use of growth requirements for gonococcal typing. *J Infect Dis.* 1973;128:178-194.

33. Handsfield HH, Rice RJ, Roberts MC, et al. Localized outbreak of penicillinase-producing *Neisseria gonorrhoeae*: paradigm for introduction and spread of gonorrhea in a community. *JAMA.* 28 1989;261:2357-2361.

34. Bash MC, Zhu P, Gulati S, et al. por Variable-region typing by DNA probe hybridization is broadly applicable to epidemiologic studies of *Neisseria gonorrhoeae. J Clin Microbiol.* 2005;43:1522-1530.

35. Lynn F, Hobbs MM, Zenilman JM, et al. Genetic typing of the porin protein of *Neisseria gonorrhoeae* from clinical noncultured samples for strain characterization and identification of mixed gonococcal infections. *J Clin Microbiol.* 2005;43:368-375.

36. Perez-Losada M, Viscidi RP, Demma JC, et al. Population genetics of *Neisseria gonorrhoeae* in a high-prevalence community using a hypervariable outer membrane porB and 13 slowly evolving housekeeping genes. *Mol Biol Evol.* 2005;22:1887-1902.

37. O'Rourke M, Ison CA, Renton AM, et al. Opa-typing: a high-resolution tool for studying the epidemiology of gonorrhoea. *Mol Microbiol.* 1995;17:865-875.

38. McKnew DL, Lynn F, Zenilman JM, et al. Porin variation among clinical isolates of *Neisseria gonorrhoeae* over a 10-year period, as determined by Por variable region typing. *J Infect Dis.* 2003;187:1213-1222.

39. Unemo M, Berglund T, Olcen P, et al. Pulsed-field gel electrophoresis as an epidemiologic tool for *Neisseria gonorrhoeae*: identification of clusters within serovars. *Sex Transm Dis.* 2002;29:25-31.

40. Meats E, Feil EJ, Stringer S, et al. Characterization of encapsulated and noncapsulated *Haemophilus influenzae* and determination of phylogenetic relationships by multilocus sequence typing. *J Clin Microbiol.* 2003;41:1623-1636.

41. Anderson B, Albritton WL, Biddle J, et al. Common beta-lactamase-specifying plasmid in *Haemophilus ducreyi* and *Neisseria gonorrhoeae. Antimicrob Agents Chemother.* 1984;25:296-297.

42. Morse SA, Johnson SR, Biddle JW, et al. High-level tetracycline resistance in *Neisseria gonorrhoeae* is result of acquisition of streptococcal *tetM* determinant. *Antimicrob Agents Chemother.* 1986;30:664-670.

43. Elkins C, Thomas CE, Seifert HS, et al. Species-specific uptake of DNA by gonococci is mediated by a 10-base-pair sequence. *J Bacteriol.* 1991;173:3911-3913.

44. Shafer WM, Balthazar JT, Hagman KE, et al. Missense mutations that alter the DNA-binding domain of the MtrR protein occur frequently in rectal isolates of *Neisseria gonorrhoeae* that are resistant to faecal lipids. *Microbiology.* 1995;141:907-911.

45. Spratt BG. Hybrid penicillin-binding proteins in penicillin-resistant strains of *Neisseria gonorrhoeae. Nature.* 1988;332:173-176.

46. Centers for Disease Control and Prevention. *Sexually Transmitted Disease Surveillance 2006 Supplement: Gonococcal Isolate Surveillance Project (GISP) Annual Report 2006.* Atlanta, Ga: U.S. Department of Health and Human Services, Centers for Disease Control and Prevention; 2008.

47. Deguchi T, Yasuda M, Nakano M, et al. Quinolone-resistant *Neisseria gonorrhoeae*: correlation of alterations in the GyrA subunit of DNA gyrase and the ParC subunit of topoisomerase IV with antimicrobial susceptibility profiles. *Antimicrob Agents Chemother.* 1996;40:1020-1023.

48. Lindback E, Rahman M, Jalal S, et al. Mutations in *gyrA, gyrB, parC,* and *parE* in quinolone-resistant strains of *Neisseria gonorrhoeae. Apmis.* 2002;110:651-657.

49. Spurbeck RR, Arvidson CG. Inhibition of *Neisseria gonorrhoeae* epithelial cell interactions by vaginal *Lactobacillus* species. *Infect Immun.* 2008;76:3124-3130.

50. Martin HL, Richardson BA, Nyange PM, et al. Vaginal lactobacilli, microbial flora, and risk of human immunodeficiency virus type 1 and sexually transmitted disease acquisition. *J Infect Dis.* 1999;180:1863-1868.

51. Wiesenfeld HC, Hillier SL, Krohn MA, et al. Bacterial vaginosis is a strong predictor of *Neisseria gonorrhoeae* and *Chlamydia trachomatis* infection. *Clin Infect Dis.* 2003;36:663-668.

52. Giardina PC, Williams R, Lubaroff D, et al. *Neisseria gonorrhoeae* induces focal polymerization of actin in primary human urethral epithelium. *Infect Immun.* 1998;66:3416-3419.

53. Centers for Disease Control and Prevention. *Sexually Transmitted Disease Surveillance, 2006.* Atlanta, Ga: U.S. Department of Health and Human Services; 2007.

54. Centers for Disease Control and Prevention. Increases in gonorrhea—eight western states, 2000-2005. *MMWR Morb Mortal Wkly Rep.* 2007;56:222-225.

55. Weinstock H, Berman S, Cates W Jr. Sexually transmitted diseases among American youth: incidence and prevalence estimates, 2000. *Perspect Sex Reprod Health.* 2004;36:6-10.

56. Glasier A, Gulmezoglu AM, Schmid GP, et al. Sexual and reproductive health: a matter of life and death. *Lancet.* 2006;368:1595-1607.

57. Paz-Bailey G, Rahman M, Chen C, et al. Changes in the etiology of sexually transmitted diseases in Botswana between 1993 and 2002: implications for the clinical management of genital ulcer disease. *Clin Infect Dis.* 2005;41:1304-1312.

58. Dicker LW, Mosure DJ, Berman SM, et al. Gonorrhea prevalence and coinfection with chlamydia in women in the United States, 2000. *Sex Transm Dis.* 2003;30:472-476.

59. Rice RJ, Roberts PL, Handsfield HH, et al. Sociodemographic distribution of gonorrhea incidence: implications for prevention and behavioral research. *Am J Public Health.* 1991;81:1252-1258.

60. Datta SD, Sternberg M, Johnson RE, et al. Gonorrhea and chlamydia in the United States among persons 14 to 39 years of age, 1999 to 2002. *Ann Intern Med.* 2007;147:89-96.

61. Miller WC, Ford CA, Morris M, et al. Prevalence of chlamydial and gonococcal infections among young adults in the United States. *JAMA.* 2004;291:2229-2236.

62. Fenton KA, Imrie J. Increasing rates of sexually transmitted diseases in homosexual men in Western Europe and the United States: why? *Infect Dis Clin North Am.* 2005;19:311-331.

63. Kerani RP, Handcock MS, Handsfield HH, et al. Comparative geographic concentrations of 4 sexually transmitted infections. *Am J Public Health.* 2005;95:324-330.

64. Kent CK, Chaw JK, Wong W, et al. Prevalence of rectal, urethral, and pharyngeal chlamydia and gonorrhea detected in 2 clinical settings among men who have sex with men: San Francisco, California, 2003. *Clin Infect Dis.* 2005;41:67-74.

65. Farley TA. Sexually transmitted diseases in the southeastern United States: location, race, and social context. *Sex Transm Dis.* 2006;33(Suppl):S58-S64.

66. Stoner BP, Whittington WL, Hughes JP, et al. Comparative epidemiology of heterosexual gonococcal and chlamydial networks: implications for transmission patterns. *Sex Transm Dis.* 2000;27:215-223.

67. Barry PM, Kent CK, Klausner JD. Risk factors for gonorrhea among heterosexuals—San Francisco, 2006. *Sex Transm Dis.* 2009;36(Suppl):S62-S65.

68. Franceschi S, Smith JS, van den Brule A, et al. Cervical infection with *Chlamydia trachomatis* and *Neisseria gonorrhoeae* in women from ten areas in four continents: a cross-sectional study. *Sex Transm Dis.* 2007;34:563-569.

69. Hooper RR, Reynolds GH, Jones OG, et al. Cohort study of venereal disease. I: The risk of gonorrhea transmission from infected women to men. *Am J Epidemiol.* 1978;108:136-144.

70. Lin JS, Donegan SP, Heeren TC, et al. Transmission of *Chlamydia trachomatis* and *Neisseria gonorrhoeae* among men with urethritis and their female sex partners. *J Infect Dis.* 1998;178:1707-1712.

71. Wiesner PJ, Tronca E, Bonin P, et al. Clinical spectrum of pharyngeal gonococcal infection. *N Engl J Med.* 1973;288:181-185.

72. McCormack WM, Reynolds GH. Effect of menstrual cycle and method of contraception on recovery of *Neisseria gonorrhoeae. JAMA.* 1982;247:1292-1294.

73. Mohllajee AP, Curtis KM, Martins SL, et al. Hormonal contraceptive use and risk of sexually transmitted infections: a systematic review. *Contraception.* 2006;73:154-165.

74. Wasserheit JN, Aral SO. The dynamic topology of sexually transmitted disease epidemics: implications for prevention strategies. *J Infect Dis.* 1996;174:S201-S213.

75. Yorke JA, Hethcote HW, Nold A. Dynamics and control of the transmission of gonorrhea. *Sex Transm Dis.* 1978;5:51-56.

76. Jennings JM, Curriero FC, Celentano D, et al. Geographic identification of high gonorrhea transmission areas in Baltimore, Maryland. *Am J Epidemiol.* 2005;161:73-80.

77. Ellen JM, Brown BA, Chung SE, et al. Impact of sexual networks on risk for gonorrhea and chlamydia among low-income urban African American adolescents. *J Pediatr.* 2005;146:518-522.

78. Fichtenberg CM, Muth SQ, Brown B, et al. Sexual network structure among a household sample of urban African American adolescents in an endemic sexually transmitted infection setting. *Sex Transm Dis.* 2008;36:41-48.

79. Handsfield HH, Lipman TO, Harnisch JP, et al. Asymptomatic gonorrhea in men: diagnosis, natural course, prevalence and significance. *N Engl J Med.* 1974;290:117-123.

80. Dillon JA, Yeung KH. Beta-lactamase plasmids and chromosomally mediated antibiotic resistance in pathogenic *Neisseria* species. *Clin Microbiol Rev.* 1989;2:S125-S133.

81. Handsfield HH, Knapp JS, Diehr PK, et al. Correlation of auxotype and penicillin susceptibility of *Neisseria gonorrhoeae* with sexual preference and clinical manifestations of gonorrhea. *Sex Transm Dis.* 1980;7:1-5.

82. Morse SA, Lysko PG, McFarland L, et al. Gonococcal strains from homosexual men have outer membranes with reduced permeability to hydrophobic molecules. *Infect Immun.* 1982;37:432-438.

83. Fox KK, Knapp JS, Holmes KK, et al. Antimicrobial resistance in *Neisseria gonorrhoeae* in the United States, 1988-1994: the emergence of decreased susceptibility to the fluoroquinolones. *J Infect Dis.* 1997;175:1396-1403.

84. Zenilman JM. Update on quinolone resistance in *Neisseria gonorrhoeae. Curr Infect Dis Rep.* 2002;4:144-147.

85. Aplasca De Los Reyes MR, Pato-Mesola V, Klausner JD, et al. A randomized trial of ciprofloxacin versus cefixime for treatment of gonorrhea after rapid emergence of gonococcal ciprofloxacin resistance in the Philippines. *Clin Infect Dis.* 2001;32:1313-1318.

86. Centers for Disease Control and Prevention. Increases in fluoroquinolone-resistant *Neisseria gonorrhoeae*—Hawaii and California, 2001. *MMWR Morb Mortal Wkly Rep.* 2002;51:1041-1044.

87. Centers for Disease Control and Prevention. Update to CDC's sexually transmitted diseases treatment guidelines, 2006: fluoroquinolones no longer recommended for treatment of gonococcal infections. *MMWR Morb Mortal Wkly Rep.* 2007;56:332-336.

88. Brunham RC, Plummer F, Slaney L, et al. Correlation of auxotype and protein I type with expression of disease due to *Neisseria gonorrhoeae. J Infect Dis.* 1985;152:339-343.

89. Berger RE, Alexander ER, Harnisch JP, et al. Etiology, manifestations and therapy of acute epididymitis: prospective study of 50 cases. *J Urol.* 1979;121:750-754.

90. Platt R, Rice PA, McCormack WM. Risk of acquiring gonorrhea and prevalence of abnormal adnexal findings among women recently exposed to gonorrhea. *JAMA.* 1983;250:3205-3209.

91. McCormack WM, Stumacher RJ, Johnson K, et al. Clinical spectrum of gonococcal infection in women. *Lancet.* 1977;1:1182-1185.

92. Brunham RC, Paavonen J, Stevens CE, et al. Mucopurulent cervicitis—the ignored counterpart in women of urethritis in men. *N Engl J Med.* 1984;311:1-6.

93. Janda WM, Bohnoff M, Morello JA, et al. Prevalence and site-pathogen studies of *Neisseria meningitidis* and *N gonorrhoeae* in homosexual men. *JAMA.* 1980;244:2060-2064.

94. Gunn RA, O'Brien CJ, Lee MA, et al. Gonorrhea screening among men who have sex with men: value of multiple anatomic site testing, San Diego, California, 1997-2003. *Sex Transm Dis.* 2008;35:845-848.

95. Quinn TC, Stamm WE, Goodell SE, et al. The polymicrobial origin of intestinal infections in homosexual men. *N Engl J Med.* 1983;309:576-582.

96. Klausner JD, Kohn R, Kent C. Etiology of clinical proctitis among men who have sex with men. *Clin Infect Dis.* 2004;38:300-302.

97. Centers for Disease Control and Prevention. Sexually transmitted disease treatment guidelines, 2006. *MMWR Morb Mortal Wkly Rep.* 2006;51(RR-11:42-49.

98. Lafferty WE, Hughes JP, Handsfield HH. Sexually transmitted diseases in men who have sex with men: acquisition of gonorrhea and nongonococcal urethritis by fellatio and implications for STD/HIV prevention. *Sex Transm Dis.* 1997;24:272-278.

99. Hall CS, McElroy MD, Samuel MC, et al. Single-dose, oral cefpodoxime proxetil is effective for treatment of uncomplicated urogenital and rectal gonorrhea [abstract No. P-459]. Paper presented at the 17th Biennial Meeting of the International Society for Sexually Transmitted Diseases Research. Seattle, Wash., 2007.

100. Aberg JA, Gallant JE, Anderson J, et al. Primary care guidelines for the management of persons infected with human immunodeficiency virus: recommendations of the HIV Medicine Association of the Infectious Diseases Society of America. *Clin Infect Dis.* 2004;39:609-629.

101. Paavonen J, Westrom L, Eschenbach D. Pelvic inflammatory disease. In: Holmes KK, Sparling PF, Stamm WE, et al, eds. *Sexually Transmitted Diseases.* 4th ed. New York: McGraw-Hill; 2008:1017-1050.

102. Walker CK, Wiesenfeld HC. Antibiotic therapy for acute pelvic inflammatory disease: the 2006 Centers for Disease Control and Prevention sexually transmitted diseases treatment guidelines. *Clin Infect Dis.* 2007;44(Suppl 3):S111-S122.

103. Wolner-Hanssen P, Eschenbach DA, Paavonen J, et al. Decreased risk of symptomatic chlamydial pelvic inflammatory disease associated with oral contraceptive use. *JAMA.* 1990;263:54-59.

104. Baeten JM, Nyange PM, Richardson BA, et al. Hormonal contraception and risk of sexually transmitted disease acquisition: results from a prospective study. *Am J Obstet Gynecol.* 2001;185:380-385.

105. Ness RB, Soper DE, Holley RL, et al; PID Evaluation and Clinical Health PEAC. Hormonal and barrier contraception and risk of upper genital tract disease in the PID Evaluation and Clinical Health (PEACH) study. *Am J Obstet Gynecol.* 2001;185:121-127.

106. Wolner-Hanssen P, Eschenbach DA, Paavonen J, et al. Association between vaginal douching and acute pelvic inflammatory disease. *JAMA.* 1990;263:1936-1941.

107. Ness RB, Hillier SL, Kip KE, et al. Douching, pelvic inflammatory disease, and incident gonococcal and chlamydial genital

infection in a cohort of high-risk women. *Am J Epidemiol.* 2005;161:186-195.
108. Scholes D, Daling JR, Stergachis A, et al. Vaginal douching as a risk factor for acute pelvic inflammatory disease. *Obstet Gynecol.* 1993;81:601-606.
109. Ness RB, Kip KE, Hillier SL, et al. A cluster analysis of bacterial vaginosis-associated microflora and pelvic inflammatory disease. *Am J Epidemiol.* 2005;162:585-590.
110. Wiesenfeld HC, Hillier SL, Krohn MA, et al. Lower genital tract infection and endometritis: insight into subclinical pelvic inflammatory disease. *Obstet Gynecol.* 2002;100:456-463.
111. Westrom L, Joesoef R, Reynolds G, et al. Pelvic inflammatory disease and fertility: a cohort study of 1844 women with laparoscopically verified disease and 657 control women with normal laparoscopic results. *Sex Transm Dis.* 1992;19:185-192.
112. Ness RB, Soper DE, Peipert J, et al. Design of the PID Evaluation and Clinical Health (PEACH) study. *Control Clin Trials.* 1998;19:499-514.
113. Ness RB, Soper DE, Holley RL, et al. Effectiveness of inpatient and outpatient treatment strategies for women with pelvic inflammatory disease: results from the Pelvic Inflammatory Disease Evaluation and Clinical Health (PEACH) randomized trial. *Am J Obstet Gynecol.* 2002;186:929-937.
114. Haggerty CL, Schulz R, Ness RB. Lower quality of life among women with chronic pelvic pain after pelvic inflammatory disease. *Obstet Gynecol.* 2003;102(Pt 1):934-939.
115. Wendel PJ, Wendel GDJ. Sexually transmitted diseases in pregnancy. *Semin Perinatol.* 1993;17:443-451.
116. Burgis JT, Nawaz H 3rd. Disseminated gonococcal infection in pregnancy presenting as meningitis and dermatitis. *Obstet Gynecol.* 2006;108(Pt 2):798-801.
117. Corman LC, Levison ME, Knight R, et al. The high frequency of pharyngeal gonococcal infection in a prenatal clinic population. *JAMA.* 1974;230:568-570.
118. Holmes KK, Counts GW, Beaty HN. Disseminated gonococcal infection. *Ann Intern Med.* 1971;74:979-993.
119. Wise CM, Morris CR, Wasilauskas BL, et al. Gonococcal arthritis in an era of increasing penicillin resistance: presentations and outcomes in 41 recent cases (1985-1991). *Arch Intern Med.* 1994;154:2690-2695.
120. Tapsall JW, Phillips EA, Shultz TR, et al. Strain characteristics and antibiotic susceptibility of isolates of *Neisseria gonorrhoeae* causing disseminated gonococcal infection in Australia. Members of the Australian Gonococcal Surveillance Programme. *Int J STD AIDS.* 1992;3:273-277.
121. Golden MR, Public Health, Seattle and King County, personal communication, 2008.
122. Rice PA. Gonococcal arthritis (disseminated gonococcal infection). *Infect Dis Clin North Am.* 2005;19:853-861.
123. Rice P, Handsfield HH. Arthritis associated with sexually transmitted diseases. In: Holmes KK, Sparling PF, Mardh P-A, et al, eds. *Sexually Transmitted Diseases.* 4th ed. New York: McGraw-Hill; 2008.
124. Jackman JD Jr, Glamann DB. Gonococcal endocarditis: twenty-five year experience. *Am J Med Sci.* 1991;301:221-230.
125. Belding ME, Carbone J. Gonococcemia associated with adult respiratory distress syndrome. *Rev Infect Dis.* 1991;13:1105-1107.
126. Billings FT 3rd, Evans VA, Wittlinger PS, et al. "Primary" gonococcal meningitis. *Sex Transm Dis.* 1991;18:129-130.
127. Ingram CW, Nichole B, Martinez S, et al. Gonococcal osteomyelitis: case report and review of the literature. *Arch Intern Med.* 1991;151:177-179.
128. Thiery G, Tankovic J, Brun-Buisson C, et al. Gonococcemia associated with fatal septic shock. *Clin Infect Dis.* 2001;32:E92-E93.
129. Rompalo AM, Hook EW 3rd, Roberts PL, et al. The acute arthritis-dermatitis syndrome: the changing importance of *Neisseria gonorrhoeae* and *Neisseria meningitidis*. *Arch Intern Med.* 1987;147:281-283.
130. Ellison RT 3rd, Curd JG, Kohler PF, et al. Underlying complement deficiency in patients with disseminated gonococcal infection. *Sex Transm Dis.* 1987;14:201-204.
131. Liebling MR, Arkfeld DG, Michelini GA, et al. Identification of *Neisseria gonorrhoeae* in synovial fluid using the polymerase chain reaction. *Arthritis Rheum.* 1994;37:702-709.
132. Kimmitt PT, Kirby A, Perera N, et al. Identification of *Neisseria gonorrhoeae* as the causative agent in a case of culture-negative dermatitis-arthritis syndrome using real-time PCR. *J Travel Med.* 2008;15:369-371.
133. Read P, Abbott R, Pantelidis P, et al. Disseminated gonococcal infection in a homosexual man diagnosed by nucleic acid amplification testing from a skin lesion swab. *Sex Transm Infect.* 2008;84:348-349.
134. Desenclos JC, Garrity D, Scaggs M, et al. Gonococcal infection of the newborn in Florida, 1984-1989. *Sex Transm Dis.* 1992;19:105-110.
135. Ingram DL. *Neisseria gonorrhoeae* in children. *Pediatr Ann.* 1994;23:341-345.
136. Woods CR. Gonococcal infections in neonates and young children. *Semin Pediatr Infect Dis.* 2005;16:258-270.
137. Rawstron SA, Bromberg K, Hammerschlag MR. STD in children: syphilis and gonorrhoea. *Genitourin Med.* 1993;69:66-75.
138. Bonin P, Tanino TT, Handsfield HH. Isolation of *Neisseria gonorrhoeae* on selective and nonselective media in a sexually transmitted disease clinic. *J Clin Microbiol.* 1984;19:218-220.
139. Ison CA. Laboratory methods in genitourinary medicine: methods of diagnosing gonorrhoea. *Genitourin Med.* 1990;66:453-459.
140. McKenna JG, Fallon RJ, Moyes A, et al. Anogenital non-gonococcal neisseriae: prevalence and clinical significance. *Int J STD AIDS.* 1993;4:8-12.
141. Russell JM, Azadian BS, Roberts AP, et al. Pharyngeal flora in a sexually active population. *Int J STD AIDS.* 1995;6:211-215.
142. Maini M, French P, Prince M, et al. Urethritis due to *Neisseria meningitidis* in a London genitourinary medicine clinic population. *Int J STD AIDS.* 1992;3:423-425.
143. Koumans EH, Johnson RE, Knapp JS, et al. Laboratory testing for *Neisseria gonorrhoeae* by recently introduced nonculture tests: a performance review with clinical and public health considerations. *Clin Infect Dis.* 1998;27:1171-1180.
144. Koumans EH, Black CM, Markowitz LE, et al. Comparison of methods for detection of *Chlamydia trachomatis* and *Neisseria gonorrhoeae* using commercially available nucleic acid amplification tests and a liquid pap smear medium. *J Clin Microbiol.* 2003;41:1507-1511.
145. Cosentino LA, Landers DV, Hillier SL. Detection of *Chlamydia trachomatis* and *Neisseria gonorrhoeae* by strand displacement amplification and relevance of the amplification control for use with vaginal swab specimens. *J Clin Microbiol.* 2003;41:3592-3596.
146. Cook RL, Hutchison SL, Ostergaard L, et al. Systematic review: noninvasive testing for *Chlamydia trachomatis* and *Neisseria gonorrhoeae*. *Ann Intern Med.* 2005;142:914-925.
147. Golden MR, Hughes JP, Cles LE, et al. Positive predictive value of Gen-Probe APTIMA Combo 2 testing for *Neisseria gonorrhoeae* in a population of women with low prevalence of *N. gonorrhoeae* infection. *Clin Infect Dis.* 2004;39:1387-1390.
148. Bachmann LH, Desmond RA, Stephens J, et al. Duration of persistence of gonococcal DNA detected by ligase chain reaction in men and women following recommended therapy for uncomplicated gonorrhea. *J Clin Microbiol.* 2002;40:3596-3601.
149. Schachter J, Moncada J, Liska S, et al. Nucleic acid amplification tests in the diagnosis of chlamydial and gonococcal infections of the oropharynx and rectum in men who have sex with men. *Sex Transm Dis.* 2008;35:637-642.
150. McNally LP, Templeton DJ, Jin F, et al. Low positive predictive value of a nucleic acid amplification test for nongenital *Neisseria gonorrhoeae* infection in homosexual men. *Clin Infect Dis.* 2008;47:e25-e27.
151. Workowski KA, Berman SM, Douglas JM Jr. Emerging antimicrobial resistance in *Neisseria gonorrhoeae*: urgent need to strengthen prevention strategies. *Ann Intern Med.* 2008;148:606-613.
152. Newman LM, Moran JS, Workowski KA. Update on the management of gonorrhea in adults in the United States. *Clin Infect Dis.* 2007;44(Suppl 3):S84-S101.
153. Peterman TA, Zaidi AA, Lieb S, et al. Incubating syphilis in patients treated for gonorrhea: a comparison of treatment regimens. *J Infect Dis.* 1994;170:689-692.
154. Ramus RM, Sheffield JS, Mayfield JA, et al. A randomized trial that compared oral cefixime and intramuscular ceftriaxone for the treatment of gonorrhea in pregnancy. *Am J Obstet Gynecol.* 2001;185:629-632.
155. Handsfield HH, Hook EW 3rd. Ceftriaxone for treatment of uncomplicated gonorrhea: routine use of a single 125-mg dose in a sexually transmitted disease clinic. *Sex Transm Dis.* 1987;14:227-230.
156. Handsfield HH, McCormack WM, Hook EW 3rd, et al. A comparison of single-dose cefixime with ceftriaxone as treatment for uncomplicated gonorrhea. The Gonorrhea Treatment Study Group. *N Engl J Med.* 1991;325:1337-1341.
157. Novak E, Paxton LM, Tubbs HJ, et al. Orally administered cefpodoxime proxetil for treatment of uncomplicated gonococcal urethritis in males: a dose-response study. *Antimicrob Agents Chemother.* 1992;36:1764-1765.
158. Thorpe EM, Schwebke JR, Hook EW, et al. Comparison of single-dose cefuroxime axetil with ciprofloxacin in treatment of uncomplicated gonorrhea caused by penicillinase-producing and non-penicillinase-producing *Neisseria gonorrhoeae* strains. *Antimicrob Agents Chemother.* 1996;40:2775-2780.
159. DePestel DD, Benninger MS, Danziger L, et al. Cephalosporin use in treatment of patients with penicillin allergies. *J Am Pharm Assoc.* 2008;48:530-540.
160. Ito M, Deguchi T, Mizutani KS, et al. Emergence and spread of *Neisseria gonorrhoeae* clinical isolates harboring mosaic-like structure of penicillin-binding protein 2 in central Japan. *Antimicrob Agents Chemother.* 2005;49:137-143.
161. Ito M, Yasuda M, Yokoi S, et al. Remarkable increase in central Japan in 2001-2002 of *Neisseria gonorrhoeae* isolates with decreased susceptibility to penicillin, tetracycline, oral cephalosporins, and fluoroquinolones. *Antimicrob Agents Chemother.* 2004;48:3185-3187.
162. Matsumoto T. Trends of sexually transmitted diseases and antimicrobial resistance in *Neisseria gonorrhoeae*. *Int J Antimicrob Agents.* 2008;31:S35-S39.
163. Centers for Disease Control and Prevention. Increases in fluoroquinolone-resistant *Neisseria gonorrhoeae* among men who have sex with men—United States, 2003, and revised recommendations for gonorrhea treatment, 2004. *MMWR Morb Mortal Wkly Rep.* 2004;53:335-338.
164. Wang SA, Harvey AB, Conner SM, et al. Antimicrobial resistance for *Neisseria gonorrhoeae* in the United States, 1988 to 2003: the spread of fluoroquinolone resistance. *Ann Intern Med.* 2007;147:81-88.
165. Cousin SL Jr, Whittington WL, Roberts MC. Acquired macrolide resistance genes and the 1 bp deletion in the mtrR promoter in *Neisseria gonorrhoeae*. *J Antimicrob Chemother.* 2003;51:131-133.
166. Tapsall JW, Shultz TR, Limnios EA, et al. Failure of azithromycin therapy in gonorrhea and discorrelation with laboratory test parameters. *Sex Transm Dis.* 1998;25:505-508.
167. Chisholm SA, Ison C. Emergence of high-level azithromycin resistance in *Neisseria gonorrhoeae* in England and Wales. *Eur Surveill.* 2008;13(15):pii-18832.
168. Palmer HM, Young H, Winter A, et al. Emergence and spread of azithromycin-resistant *Neisseria gonorrhoeae* in Scotland. *J Antimicrob Chemother.* 2008;62:490-494.
169. Vorobieva V, Firsova N, Ababkova T, et al. Antibiotic susceptibility of *Neisseria gonorrhoeae* in Arkhangelsk, Russia. *Sex Transm Infect.* 2007;83:133-135.
170. Martin IM, Hoffmann S, Ison CA. European Surveillance of Sexually Transmitted Infections (ESSTI): the first combined antimicrobial susceptibility data for *Neisseria gonorrhoeae* in Western Europe. *J Antimicrob Chemother.* 2006;58:587-593.
171. Stamm WE, Guinan ME, Johnson C, et al. Effect of treatment regimens for *Neisseria gonorrhoeae* on simultaneous infection with *Chlamydia trachomatis*. *N Engl J Med.* 1984;310:545-549.
172. Sparks R, Helmers JR, Handsfield HH, et al. Rescreening for gonorrhea and chlamydial infection through the mail: a randomized trial. *Sex Transm Dis.* 2004;31:113-116.
173. Golden MR, Whittington WL, Handsfield HH, et al. Effect of expedited treatment of sex partners on recurrent or persistent gonorrhea or chlamydial infection. *N Engl J Med.* 2005;352:676-685.
174. Peterman TA, Tian LH, Metcalf CA, et al. High incidence of new sexually transmitted infections in the year following a sexually transmitted infection: a case for rescreening. *Ann Intern Med.* 2006;145:564-572.
175. Bernstein KT, Zenilman J, Olthoff G, et al. Gonorrhea reinfection among sexually transmitted disease clinic attendees in Baltimore, Maryland. *Sex Transm Dis.* 2006;33:80-86.
176. Bevan CD, Ridgway GL, Rothermel CD. Efficacy and safety of azithromycin as monotherapy or combined with metronidazole compared with two standard multidrug regimens for the treatment of acute pelvic inflammatory disease. *J Int Med Res.* 2003;31:45-54.
177. Haggerty CL, Ness RB. Newest approaches to treatment of pelvic inflammatory disease: a review of recent randomized clinical trials. *Clin Infect Dis.* 2007;44:953-960.
178. Savaris RF, Teixeira LM, Torres TG, et al. Comparing ceftriaxone plus azithromycin or doxycycline for pelvic inflammatory disease: a randomized controlled trial. *Obstet Gynecol.* 2007;110:53-60.
179. Peipert JF, Sweet RL, Walker CK, et al. Evaluation of ofloxacin in the treatment of laparoscopically documented acute pelvic inflammatory disease (salpingitis). *Infect Dis Obstet Gynecol.* 1999;7:138-144.
180. Handsfield HH, Wiesner PJ, Holmes KK. Treatment of the gonococcal arthritis-dermatitis syndrome. *Ann Intern Med.* 1976;84:661-667.
181. Rawstron SA, Bromberg K, Hammerschlag MR. STD in children: syphilis and gonorrhoea. *Genitourin Med.* 1993;69:66-75.
182. Golden MR, Hogben M, Handsfield HH, et al. Partner notification for HIV and STD in the United States: low coverage for gonorrhea, chlamydial infection, and HIV. *Sex Transm Dis.* 2003;30:490-496.
183. Hogben M. Partner notification for sexually transmitted diseases. *Clin Infect Dis.* 2007;44(Suppl 3):S160-S174.
184. Hogben M, McCree DH, Golden MR. Patient-delivered partner therapy for sexually transmitted diseases as practiced by U.S. physicians. *Sex Transm Dis.* 2005;32:101-105.
185. Packel LJ, Guerry S, Bauer HM, et al. Patient-delivered partner therapy for chlamydial infections: attitudes and practices of California physicians and nurse practitioners. *Sex Transm Dis.* 2006;33:458-463.
186. U.S. Preventive Services Task Force. Screening for gonorrhea: recommendation statement. *Ann Fam Med.* 2005;3:263-267.
187. Manhart LE, Marrazzo JM, Fine DN, et al. Selective testing criteria for gonorrhea among young women screened for chlamydial infection: contribution of race and geographic prevalence. *J Infect Dis.* 2007;196:731-737.
188. Mayer KH, Klausner JD, Handsfield HH. Intersecting epidemics and educable moments: sexually transmitted disease risk assessment and screening in men who have sex with men. *Sex Transm Dis.* 2001;28:464-467.
189. Cohen MS, Hoffman IF, Royce RA, et al. Reduction of concentration of HIV-1 in semen after treatment of urethritis: implications for prevention of sexual transmission of HIV-1. AIDSCAP Malawi Research Group. *Lancet.* 1997;349:1868-1873.
190. Centers for Disease Control and Prevention; Health Resources and Services Administration; National Institutes of Health; HIV Medicine Association of the Infectious Diseases Society of America; HIV Prevention in Clinical Care Working Group.

Recommendations for incorporating human immunodeficiency virus (HIV) prevention into the medical care of persons living with HIV. *Clin Infect Dis.* 2004;38:104-121.

191. Branson BM, Handsfield HH, Lampe MA, et al. Revised recommendations for HIV testing of adults, adolescents, and pregnant women in health-care settings. *MMWR Recomm Rep.* 2006;55: 1-17; quiz CE11-14.

192. Holmes KK, Levine R, Weaver M. Effectiveness of condoms in preventing sexually transmitted infections. *Bull World Health Organ.* 2004;82:454-461.

193. Cates W Jr. The NIH condom report: the glass is 90% full. *Fam Plann Perspect.* 2001;33:231-233.

194. Warner L, Stone KM, Macaluso M, et al. Condom use and risk of gonorrhea and chlamydia: a systematic review of design and measurement factors assessed in epidemiologic studies. *Sex Transm Dis.* 2006;33:36-51.

195. French PP, Latka M, Gollub EL, et al. Use-effectiveness of the female versus male condom in preventing sexually transmitted disease in women. *Sex Transm Dis.* 2003;30: 433-439.

196. Ramjee G, van der Straten A, Chipato T, et al. The diaphragm and lubricant gel for prevention of cervical sexually transmitted infections: results of a randomized controlled trial. *PLoS ONE.* 2008;3:e3488.

197. Richardson BA. Nonoxynol-9 as a vaginal microbicide for prevention of sexually transmitted infections: it's time to move on. *JAMA.* 2002;287:1171-1172.

198. Roddy RE, Zekeng L, Ryan KA, et al. Effect of nonoxynol-9 gel on urogenital gonorrhea and chlamydial infection: a randomized controlled trial. *JAMA.* 2002;287:1117-1122.

199. Harrison WO, Hooper RR, Wiesner PJ, et al. A trial of minocycline given after exposure to prevent gonorrhea. *N Engl J Med.* 1979;300:1074-1078.

200. Boslego JW, Tramont EC, Chung RC, et al. Efficacy trial of a parenteral gonococcal pilus vaccine in men. *Vaccine.* 1991;9:154-162.

213

Moraxella catarrhalis, Kingella, and Other Gram-Negative Cocci

TIMOTHY F. MURPHY

Over the past 3 decades, *Moraxella (Branhamella) catarrhalis* has emerged as an important and common human respiratory tract pathogen. In this chapter, *M. catarrhalis* is discussed. In addition, *Kingella* and other gram-negative cocci, including *Neisseria* other than *N. meningitidis* and *N. gonorrhoeae*, and other *Moraxella*, which are less common causes of human infection, are considered. *Acinetobacter* is discussed in Chapter 222 and *Oligella* is discussed in Chapter 237. *N. meningitidis* and *N. gonorrhoeae* are discussed in Chapters 211 and 212, respectively.

🔲 Moraxella catarrhalis

HISTORY

M. catarrhalis has an interesting and checkered taxonomic history. The bacterium was first described a century ago and was suspected by Sir William Osler to be the cause of his own terminal pneumonia.[1] After having been initially named *Micrococcus catarrhalis*, the organism's name was subsequently changed to *Neisseria catarrhalis* because of its similarities in phenotype and ecologic niche to *Neisseria* species. In 1970, it was transferred to the new genus *Branhamella* on the basis of differences in fatty acid content and DNA hybridization studies compared with other *Neisseriaceae*.[2] The name *Moraxella catarrhalis* was subsequently proposed and this is the most widely accepted name at this time.

For most of the last century, *M. catarrhalis* was regarded as an upper respiratory tract commensal. However, since the late 1970s, investigators from many centers have accumulated compelling evidence that *M. catarrhalis* is an important and common respiratory tract pathogen in humans.[3-5]

MICROBIOLOGY

Current taxonomic claasification schemes include three genera in the family *Moraxellaceae*—*Moraxella*, *Acinetobacter*, and *Psychrobacter*. *M. catarrhalis* is a gram-negative diplococcus that is indistinguishable from *Neisseria* by Gram stain. The organism grows well on blood agar, chocolate agar, and a variety of media. *M. catarrhalis* are difficult to distinguish from *Neisseria* by colony morphology, particularly after overnight growth on agar plates. After 48 hours of growth, *M. catarrhalis* colonies tend to be larger than *Neisseria* and take on a pink color. In addition, colonies display the hockey puck sign by sliding along the surface of the agar when pushed. Because samples from the respiratory tract frequently contain *Neisseria*, suspicious colonies should be tested for the possibility that they are *M. catarrhalis*. The similarity in colony morphology between commensal *Neisseria* and *M. catarrhalis* results in the underestimation of *M. catarrhalis* in cultures of human respiratory tract samples. *M. catarrhalis* produces oxidase, catalase and DNase. Several kits to speciate *M. catarrhalis* are commercially available.[6,7]

EPIDEMIOLOGY AND RESPIRATORY TRACT COLONIZATION

M. catarrhalis has been recovered exclusively from humans. The prevalence of colonization is highly dependent on age. The upper respiratory tract of approximately 1% to 5% of healthy adults is colonized by *M. catarrhalis*.[8,9] By contrast, nasopharyngeal colonization with *M. catarrhalis* is common throughout infancy. Some published studies have shown a higher rate of colonization during winter months; this higher rate may be a result of the appearance of respiratory viral illnesses during colder months. Substantial regional differences in colonization rates are observed. For example, 66% of infants in a study in Buffalo, New York, were colonized during the first year of life,[10] whereas a similar study in Goteborg, Sweden, showed a colonization rate of approximately half of that level.[11] A study of rural Aboriginal infants near Darwin, Australia, revealed that 100% of infants were colonized by *M. catarrhalis* by the age of 3 months.[12] The explanation for the marked differences in rates of colonization is not yet defined. One study showed a higher rate of colonization with *M. catarrhalis* in children who attend daycare centers compared with those who do not.[13] Several factors, including living conditions, hygiene, environmental factors (e.g., household smoking), genetic characteristics of the populations, and host factors, may play a role. The widespread use of pneumococcal conjugate vaccines has caused changes in patterns of nasopharyngeal colonization by reducing colonization with vaccine serotypes of *Streptococcus pneumoniae*. This effect has resulted in "replacement" of vaccine serotypes of *S. pneumoniae* by nonvaccine pneumococcal serotypes, nontypeable *H. influenzae*, and *M. catarrhalis*.[14]

Nasopharyngeal colonization with middle ear pathogens, including *M. catarrhalis*, is associated with otitis media. Early colonization is a risk factor for recurrent otitis media.[10,15] Otitis-prone children are colonized with *M. catarrhalis* at a higher rate compared with healthy children.[10,16,17]

M. catarrhalis is isolated from the sputum of adults with chronic obstructive pulmonary disease (COPD). Approximately 50% of episodes of acquisition of *M. catarrhalis* are associated with acute exacerbations of COPD.[18] Adults with COPD develop systemic and mucosal immune responses and clear *M. catarrhalis* from the respiratory tract efficiently after a relatively short duration (less than 1 month).[19,20] Acquisition and clearance of the organism results in strain-specific protection.

PATHOGENESIS

M. catarrhalis causes mucosal infections in children and adults. The pathogenesis of infection appears to involve contiguous spread of the bacterium from its colonizing position in the respiratory tract to cause clinical signs of infection. In the case of otitis media, the isolates recovered from the middle ear are present in the nasopharynx, indicating that the middle ear isolate came from the nasopharynx via the eustachian tube. Current data suggest that colonization of the upper respiratory tract with middle ear pathogens, including *M. catarrhalis*, is a necessary first step in the pathogenesis of otitis media. However, colonization alone is not sufficient to cause disease. An inciting event, such as a viral infection, in a child colonized with a middle ear pathogen is probably necessary for bacteria to move to the middle ear and cause otitis media. In the case of infection in adults with COPD, the acquisition of a new strain is critical in the pathogenesis of infection.[18,21]

A key step in the initiation of infection is adherence of *M. catarrhalis* to the human respiratory epithelium. Several adhesins with varying

TABLE 213-1	Adhesins and Putative Adhesins of *Moraxella catarrhalis*	
Adhesin	Molecular Mass (kDa)	Observation
UspA1	88 (oligomer)	Adhesin for respiratory epithelial cells, binds laminin
MID/Hag	200	Hemagglutinin, binds IgD
OMP CD	45	Adhesin for respiratory epithelial cells; binds mucin; OMPA-like protein
McmA	110,000	Metallopeptidase-like adhesin
MchA1 (MhaB1)	184	Homology with filamentous
MchA2 (MhaB2)	201	hemagglutinin of *Bordetella pertussis*
McaP	66	Adhesin and phospholipase B
OlpA	24	Putative adhesin based on homology with Opa proteins
OMP J	19 16	Exists in two forms; putative adhesins based on homology with Opa proteins
Type 4 pili	16	Also essential for transformation; involved in biofilm formation

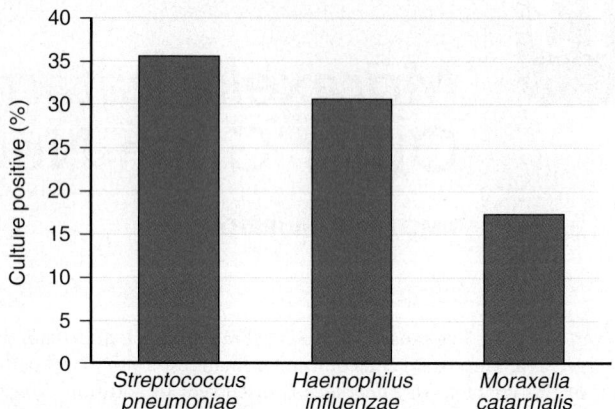

Figure 213-1 Causes of otitis media. These are the results of bacterial cultures of middle ear fluids obtained from children with otitis media (averages from seven studies).

specificities for host cells have been identified (Table 213-1). Some of these surface antigens and others are being evaluated as potential vaccine antigens.[5,22] In addition to adherence to the epithelial surface, *M. catarrhalis* also resides within and beneath the epithelium and invades host cells.[23,24] Indeed, colonization of the nasopharynx by *M. catarrhalis* is more frequent than is revealed by surface culture.

The outer membrane of *M. catarrhalis* contains lipo-oligosaccharide (LOS). LOS consists of a lipid A core coupled to oligosaccharides. The structure of the LOS resembles that of other nonenteric gram-negative bacteria in that the molecule lacks the long polysaccharide side chains observed in enteric gram-negative bacteria. Three major antigenic types of LOS can be distinguished, accounting for 95% of all strains.[25] The different serotypes are based on differences in terminal sugars in the LOS molecule.

The interaction of selected surface antigens with receptors of various host cells in the respiratory tract have important effects in mediating host responses to *M. catarrhalis*. For example *M. catarrhalis* is mitogenic for B lymphocytes through interaction with the MID/Hag protein.[26,27] The surface protein UspA2 regulates nuclear factor kappa B (NF-κB) and subsequent interleukin-8 (IL-8) release by human respiratory epithelial cells.[28] Lipo-oligosaccharide stimulates human monocytes to produce proinflammatory cytokines in both TLR4- and CD14-dependent pathways.[29] Host inflammatory responses in the middle ear and in the airways are likely mediated by these and other interactions.

A reliable animal model that parallels human infection has not yet been developed for *M. catarrhalis*. The specificity of *M. catarrhalis* for humans creates challenges for the development of a useful model to study pathogenesis. The chinchilla model of otitis media, which is used widely to study otitis media caused by other bacteria, is not useful because chinchillas readily clear *M. catarrhalis* from the middle ear. However, *M. catarrhalis* colonizes the nasopharynx of the chinchilla, so this model may prove useful.[30] The most widely used model is a mouse pulmonary clearance model that measures the rate of clearance of *M. catarrhalis* from the lungs following intratracheal challenge. This model does not parallel human infection but has been used as a guide to identify and study potential vaccine antigens.

CLINICAL MANIFESTATIONS

Otitis Media
Approximately 80% of children experience at least one episode of acute otitis media by the age of 3 years. A subset of children experiences recurrent otitis media, which is associated with a delay in speech and language development. Careful studies from many centers have defined the cause of acute otitis media by culturing middle ear fluid obtained

by tympanocentesis. Culture of middle ear fluid is the most reliable method for determining the cause of otitis media. Although some differences among studies are observed, the results from centers in the United States and Europe are remarkably consistent in showing that *Streptococcus pneumoniae*, nontypeable *Haemophilus influenzae*, and *M. catarrhalis* are the predominant bacterial causes of acute otitis media. Overall, based on cultures of middle ear fluid, approximately 15% to 20% of cases of acute otitis media are caused by *M. catarrhalis* (Fig. 213-1).[31-37]

Otitis media with effusion is defined as the presence of middle ear fluid in the absence of signs and symptoms of acute otitis media. Bacterial cultures are negative in most middle ear fluids from children with otitis media with effusion. Analysis of middle ear fluids by polymerase chain reaction (PCR) assay reveals that a substantial proportion contain bacterial DNA, particularly from *M. catarrhalis* and *H. influenzae*, suggesting a bacterial cause.[38-40]

Lower Respiratory Tract Infections in Chronic Obstructive Pulmonary Disease
M. catarrhalis causes lower respiratory tract infections in adults, particularly in the setting of COPD. The recognition of *M. catarrhalis* as a pathogen in this setting was delayed until the past 20 years because *M. catarrhalis* is indistinguishable from commensal *Neisseria* by Gram stain and difficult to distinguish by colony morphology. Therefore, unless clinical microbiology laboratories specifically test colonies that appear to be *Neisseria*, *M. catarrhalis* will be missed as a potential pathogen in sputum.

Several lines of evidence have established that *M. catarrhalis* causes exacerbations of COPD[41,42]:

- Analysis of sputum samples of a subset of patients with exacerbations of COPD demonstrates a predominance of gram-negative diplococci on Gram stain and almost pure cultures of *M. catarrhalis*.
- Studies using transtracheal aspiration and bronchoscopy with the protected specimen brush to sample the lower airways have revealed pure cultures of *M. catarrhalis* in some patients with exacerbations of COPD.
- The levels of inflammatory markers in the sputum of patients with exacerbations with positive cultures for *M. catarrhalis* are higher than the level in sputum of culture-negative exacerbations.[43]
- A specific immune response has been observed following exacerbations of COPD associated with *M. catarrhalis* in the sputum.[18-20]
- Acquisition of a new strain of *M. catarrhalis* is associated with clinical exacerbation.[18,21]

M. catarrhalis causes approximately 10% of exacerbations of COPD, making the bacterium the second most common bacterial cause of exacerbations after nontypeable *H. influenzae*.

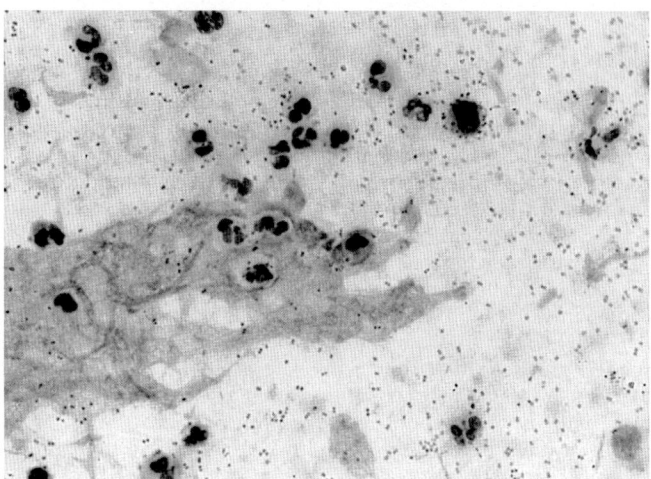

Figure 213-2 **Sputum sample from a patient with chronic obstructive pulmonary disease experiencing an exacerbation caused by *Moraxella catarrhalis*.** Note the abundance of leukocytes, the presence of large numbers of gram-negative diplococci as the exclusive bacterial form, and the presence of intracellular bacteria in leukocytes (Gram stain; ×1000).

The clinical manifestations of exacerbations of COPD caused by *M. catarrhalis* are similar to those of exacerbations caused by other bacteria, such as nontypeable *H. influenzae*. Patients experience increased cough and sputum production, increased sputum purulence, and increased dyspnea compared to baseline symptoms. Sputum Gram staining shows intracellular and extracellular gram-negative diplococci as the exclusive or predominant bacterial form (Fig. 213-2), and cultures grow predominantly *M. catarrhalis*.

Pneumonia in Older Adults
M. catarrhalis causes pneumonia in older adults, but it is difficult to state the precise proportion. One prospective study has estimated that *M. catarrhalis* caused 10% of community-acquired pneumonia in older adults.[44] Most older patients who experience pneumonia caused by *M. catarrhalis* have underlying illnesses, including COPD, congestive heart failure, and diabetes. Although *M. catarrhalis* causes a significant illness in older adults, fulminant pneumonia is uncommon.

Nosocomial Respiratory Tract Infections
Nosocomial lower respiratory tract infections caused by *M. catarrhalis* have been observed in respiratory units in health care facilities. The presence of a susceptible population of adults with underlying cardiopulmonary disease may be important in these apparent outbreaks. Analysis of isolates by various typing methods has indicated that some of these clusters involved multiple strains of *M. catarrhalis* and some were caused by a single strain, indicating person-to-person spread of the organism.

Sinusitis
The cause of sinusitis is determined by culture of sinus aspirates, a relatively invasive procedure that is not performed routinely. Studies that have used sinus aspiration to determine the cause of sinusitis have shown that *M. catarrhalis* is the third most common cause of sinusitis in adults and children after nontypeable *H. influenzae* and *S. pneumoniae*.

Bacteremia
Published reports have documented the occurrence of bacteremia caused by *M. catarrhalis*.[45-47] Bacteremia is an infrequent manifestation of *M. catarrhalis* infection. The severity of clinical manifestations ranges from mild to life-threatening. Bacteremia has been reported in those of all ages, from neonates to older adults. Most patients have clinical evidence of respiratory tract infection. Whereas many infants with bacteremia caused by *M. catarrhalis* are immunocompetent, most adults have underlying illnesses, including cardiopulmonary disease, malignancy, immunodeficiency, and chronic debilitation. A review of *M. catarrhalis* bacteremia has noted a mortality of 21%.[47] The underlying illness is an important determinant of outcome.

TREATMENT

A rapid increase in the proportion of strains that produce β-lactamase occurred simultaneously in the United States and Europe, beginning in the late 1970s.[48] This is one of the most dramatic examples of a rapid increase in antimicrobial resistance by a bacterial species. Currently, almost all strains of *M. catarrhalis* produce β-lactamase. Three different β-lactamases (BRO-1, BRO-2, and BRO-3) have been identified and characterized.[49,50] The β-lactamase of *M. catarrhalis* is inducible and cell-associated. Because an inoculum-dependent susceptibility to ampicillin is observed, ampicillin should not be used for β-lactamase–producing strains, regardless of the results of susceptibility testing.

Many infections caused by *M. catarrhalis* can be treated with oral antibiotics. The organism is generally susceptible to amoxicillin-clavulanate, trimethoprim-sulfamethoxazole, tetracyclines, oral cephalosporins (e.g., cefixime, cefpodoxime, cefaclor, loracarbef, cefuroxime), macrolides (e.g., azithromycin, clarithromycin), and fluoroquinolones. *M. catarrhalis* is also uniformly susceptible to ticarcillin, piperacillin, second- and third-generation cephalosporins, and aminoglycosides. *M. catarrhalis* is resistant to penicillin, ampicillin, vancomycin, and clindamycin.

Other *Neisseria*

N. meningitidis and *N. gonorrhoeae* have long been recognized as the pathogenic *Neisseria*. Other *Neisseria* species are common components of the normal flora of the upper respiratory tract of humans and are often called commensal *Neisseria*. Table 213-2 lists several biochemical and growth characteristics used to distinguish among various *Neisseria* species and *M. catarrhalis*. Commensal *Neisseria* species lack several virulence factors, including pili, Opa, and the H8 antigen, that are expressed by meningococci and gonococci.[51] However, commensal *Neisseria* express a variety of surface antigens that share homology with antigens of *N. meningitidis* and *N. gonorrhoeae*.[52,53] Immune responses to cross-reactive antigens on commensal *Neisseria*, particularly *N. lactamica*, may contribute to acquisition of natural immunity to *N. meningitidis*.[54]

Neisseria species such as *N. sicca*, *N. subflava*, *N. cinerea*, *N. lactamica*, and others occasionally cause invasive infections in humans. These infections, documented primarily by individual case reports, include meningitis, endocarditis, bacteremia, ocular infections, pericarditis, empyema, peritonitis, septic arthritis, bursitis, and osteomyelitis. *N. cinerea* appears to have a propensity to cause ocular infections in young children.

N. weaveri (formerly Centers for Disease Control and Prevention [CDC] group M5) is a component of the normal oropharyngeal flora of dogs and is an important cause of infection in dog bite wounds in humans. These infections are occasionally associated with bacteremia.

Many of these infections have been treated successfully with penicillin and ampicillin. However, isolates of *Neisseria* species have shown increased resistance to penicillin, so susceptibility testing should be performed on isolates that cause invasive infections and the results should be used to guide antimicrobial therapy.

Neisseria are naturally competent for uptake of DNA. Genetic recombination occurs among bacteria that make up the complex flora of the upper respiratory tract. Virulence determinants are exchanged with pathogenic *Neisseria*, genes encoding altered penicillin-binding proteins are passed between species, and extensive interspecies recombination of a variety of genes occurs in vivo.[55-57] These observations have important implications in the role of acquisition of antibiotic resistance and evolution of pathogens in the human respiratory tract. Indeed, interspecies transfer of *penA* genes from commensal *Neisseria* is an important mechanism of acquisition of penicillin resistance of *N. gonorrhoeae* and *N. meningitidis*.[55]

Other *Moraxella*

Bacteria of the genus *Moraxella* are normal commensals of the human upper respiratory tract and are occasionally recovered from the skin and urogenital tract. Species are generally differentiated biochemically. Table 213-3 shows biochemical reactions and growth characteristics used to distinguish among several *Moraxella* species.

Moraxella species other than *M. catarrhalis* are unusual pathogens in humans. Several reports have emphasized the role of other *Moraxella* as ocular pathogens. These bacteria cause conjunctivitis, keratitis and, rarely, endophthalmitis.[58-60] Most episodes of *Moraxella* keratitis have predisposing local ocular pathology. Healing may take weeks to months. *Moraxella* species are susceptible to all conventional topical ocular antibiotics.

Case reports have established *Moraxella* species as unusual causes of invasive infections in humans, including endocarditis, bacteremia, septic arthritis, purulent pericarditis, cellulitis, and meningitis. Patients who experience meningitis caused by *Moraxella* species have a high frequency of inherited and acquired complement deficiencies, and these should be investigated following recovery.[61]

Antimicrobial susceptibility should be performed on isolates recovered from normally sterile sites, but *Moraxella* species are generally susceptible to penicillins and cephalosporins.

Kingella

HISTORY AND MICROBIOLOGY

Current taxonomic classification schemes place *Kingella* in the family Neisseriaceae. *Kingella* are short gram-negative coccoids to medium-sized rods with tapered ends. Four species have been identified—*K. kingae*, *K. indologenes*, *K. denitrificans*, and *K. oralis*. *Kingella* species are recovered from the human respiratory tract and have previously been recognized as rare causes of human disease. However, in the past 2 decades, infections caused by *Kingella* have been recognized with surprising frequency in reports from the United States, Europe, and Israel.

The increase in the recognition of *Kingella* infections may be a result of several factors. Because the bacterium is slow-growing and fastidious, special attention by the microbiology laboratory is often required to isolate the organism. For example, *K. kingae* in joint fluid will often fail to grow when plated directly onto solid media, but will grow when the joint fluid is inoculated into blood culture bottles.[62,63] Another factor accounting for the increased recognition of *Kingella* as a human pathogen is that the bacterium has likely been misidentified as *Moraxella* and other *Neisseria* by many laboratories. Finally, in the past, *Kingella* was unfamiliar to most personnel in clinical microbiology laboratories and was likely frequently dismissed as a contaminant.

K. kingae, the most common human pathogen of the *Kingella* species, grows on blood and chocolate agar but fails to grow on MacConkey agar. The bacterium has a tendency to resist decolorization and may therefore sometimes be mistaken for a gram-positive organism. It is oxidase-positive, produces acid from glucose and maltose, and lacks catalase, urease, and indole. Table 213-3 lists several characteristics that distinguish *Kingella* from related bacteria.

Little is known about the pathogenesis of *K. kingae* infections. Analysis of DNA sequences has suggested that considerable variability is present among strains and that different strains may demonstrate varying degrees of virulence.[64] An RTX toxin with wide cellular specificity has recently been identified in *K. kingae*.[65]

EPIDEMIOLOGY AND RESPIRATORY TRACT COLONIZATION

K. kingae frequently colonizes the throats of young children. In one prospective study in which cultures were performed every 2 weeks for 11 months, 73% of all children had at least one positive throat culture for *K. kingae*.[66] The organism has not been recovered from cultures of the nasopharynx. The highest rate of colonization is observed in children ages 6 months to 4 years, which corresponds to the peak age incidence of invasive disease. Infants younger than 6 months are not colonized. This pattern of colonization parallels that of other respiratory tract pathogens such as *M. catarrhalis* and *S. pneumoniae*, which show low rates of colonization in the neonatal period (presumably as a result of maternal antibodies), followed by higher rates of colonization and infection in infancy and childhood, with a declining incidence of infection in adulthood. *K. kingae* is transmitted person to person

TABLE 213-2	Biochemical and Growth Characteristics of *Neisseria* and *Moraxella catarrhalis*										
	Production of Acid from										
Species	Glucose	Maltose	Sucrose	Lactose (ONPG)	Fructose	H₂S*	Oxidase	Extra CO₂	Growth at 22°C	Polysaccharide†	Pigment‡
N. gonorrhoeae	+	−	−	−	−	−	+	VI	−	NG	−
N. meningitidis	+	+	−	−	−	−	+	I	−	NG	−
N. lactamica	+	+	−	+	−	+	+	v	v	−	+Y
N. sicca	+	+	+	−	+	+	+	−	+	+	−(slY)
N. subflava	+	+	v	−	v	+	+	−	+	v	+Y
N. mucosa	+	+	+	−	+	+	+	−	+	+	−(slY)
N. flavescens	−	−	−	−	−	+	+	−	+	+	+Y
N. cinerea	−	−	−	−	−	−	+	−	v	−	Grayish
N. polysaccharea	+	+	−	−	−	−	+	−	−	+	−(slY)
N. elongata	−	−	−	−	−	−	+	−	+	−	Grayish/slY
N. weaveri	−	−	−	−	−	+	+	−	+	−	−(slY)
M. catarrhalis	−	−	+	−	−	+	+	−	v	−	Grayish

*With lead acetate paper.
†Synthesis of polysaccharide from 5% sucrose.
‡On Loeffler slant.
I, important for growth; NG, no growth; ONPG, O-nitrophenol-β-D-galactopyranoside; sl, slightly; VI, very important for growth; v, variable; Y, yellow.
From Gröschel DM. *Moraxella catarrhalis* and other gram-negative cocci. In: Mandell GL, Bennett JE, Dolin R, eds. *Principles and Practice of Infectious Diseases*. 4th ed. New York: Churchill Livingstone; 1995:1926.

TABLE 213-3 Laboratory Procedures Useful for Identification of Moraxella, Oligella, Moraxella-like Organisms, and Kingella

Species	Motility	Oxidase	Catalase	OF Glucose	Serum Required	Urease	Indole	Nitrate	Phenylalanine	Gelatin	Assimilation of Acetate	Growth on MacConkey Agar
M. catarrhalis	−	+	+	−	−	−	−	−	−	−	v	v
M. lacunata	−	+	+	−	+	−	−	+	v	v	−	−
M. nonliquefaciens	−	+	+	−	v	−	−	+	−	−	−	−
M. osloensis	−	+	+	−	−	−	−	v	v	−	+	v
M. phenylpyruvica	−	+	+	−	−	+	−	v	+	−	v	v
M. atlantae	−	+	+	−	+	−	−	−	−	−	v	+
O. urethralis	−	+	+	−	−	−	−	−	+	−	v	+
N. weaveri (M-5)	−	1	+	−	−	−	−	−	+	−	−	−
N. elongata (M-6)	−	+	−	−	−	−	−	1	−	−	v	v
K. kingae*	−	+	−	F†	−	−	−	−	−	−	−	v
K. indologenes	−	+	−	F	−	−	+	−	−	−	−	
K. denitrificans	−	+	−	F	−	−	−	1	−	−	−	−

*Most strains hemolytic on blood agar.
†May take 3 or more days; some strains require serum supplement.
OF, oxidation or fermentation; v, variable.
From Gröschel DM. *Moraxella catarrhalis* and other gram-negative cocci. In: Mandell GL, Bennett JE, Dolin R, eds. *Principles and Practice of Infectious Diseases.* 4th ed. New York: Churchill Livingstone; 1995:1926.

and outbreaks of invasive infection have been observed in daycare centers.[64,67]

In studies of the microbiology of the human oral cavity, a bacterium that resembled *Eikenella corrodens* was recovered frequently from dental plaque.[68] On the basis of 16S ribosomal sequences, these organisms were designated as the new species *K. oralis*.[69] *K. oralis* is present in plaque or on the tooth surface in most people with or without periodontal disease.[70] The role of *K. oralis* in periodontal disease is not known at this time.

CLINICAL MANIFESTATIONS

K. kingae is the most frequent human pathogen of the *Kingella* species. Approximately 90% of invasive disease caused by *K. kingae* occurs in children younger than the age of 4 years, with most occurring between the ages of 6 months and 2 years.[71] Invasive infections have not been reported in infants younger than 6 months. Infection shows a seasonal distribution, with the rate of cases being higher in the autumn and winter months.[72] The most common clinical manifestation of *K. kingae* disease are skeletal infections, endocarditis, and bacteremia.

Skeletal Infections

K. kingae has a remarkable propensity to cause infections of the skeletal system in young children.[73-76] The most common such infection is septic arthritis. The disease most frequently affects large weight-bearing joints, especially the knee and ankle. Gram staining of the joint fluid is usually negative. The diagnosis is made by recovering the organism from culture of joint fluid. Inoculating blood culture bottles with joint fluid substantially enhances the likelihood of recovering the organism compared to direct inoculation of agar plates.[62,63] PCR-based assays have revealed that *K. kingae* is a more common cause of osteoarticular infection than is revealed by culture.[77,78] Osteomyelitis caused by *K. kingae* most frequently involves the bones of the lower extremity. The onset is insidious and the diagnosis is often delayed. Hematogenous invasion of the intervertebral disk by *K. kingae* is observed most commonly in the lumbar intervertebral spaces but can occur at any level.[76,79]

Endocarditis

In contrast to other clinical manifestations of *Kingella* infections, endocarditis can be seen at all ages, including school-aged children and adults. Endocarditis has involved native and prosthetic valves. Although

many cases of endocarditis occur in those who have preexisting valvular disease, *Kingella* can cause endocarditis on normal valves as well. Cases of endocarditis can be caused by *K. denitrificans* and *K. indologenes* as well as *K. kingae*. *Kingella* sp. are one of the so-called HACEK group of organisms, which include fastidious bacteria capable of causing endocarditis. The HACEK group consists of the following: *Haemophilus parainfluenzae*; three *Aggregatibacter* species—*A. (Haemophilus) aphrophilus*, *A. (Haemophilus) paraphrophilus*, and *A. (Actinobacillus) actinomycetemcomitans*; *Cardiobacterium hominis*, *Eikenella corrodens*, and *K. kingae*. The difficulty in recovering and identifying *K. kingae* in blood cultures frequently results in a delay in the diagnosis, which may account for the relatively high rate of morbidity seen with *Kingella* endocarditis. Because of the serious nature of *Kingella* endocarditis, all patients with *Kingella* bacteremia should be carefully evaluated for the presence of endocarditis.

Bacteremia

Approximately 50% of children with *K. kingae* bacteremia have a concomitant focal source such as the skeletal system. The remainder have occult bacteremia. The presumed source of the bacteremia is the respiratory tract.

Other Infections

Kingella species have been documented by case reports to cause infections in a variety of sites, including pneumonia, epiglottitis, meningitis, soft tissue infections, and ocular infections.

TREATMENT

The antimicrobial susceptibility of isolates of *Kingella* has not been well studied. *Kingella* species appear to be susceptible to a wide variety of penicillins and cephalosporins, although a single isolate of β-lactamase producing *K. kingae* has been identified.[80-82] Disease-associated isolates should be tested for antimicrobial susceptibility; if the isolate is susceptible, a penicillin or cephalosporin should be used. Other agents with in vitro activity include aminoglycosides, trimethoprim-sulfamethoxazole, tetracycline, erythromycin, and fluoroquinolones.

The drugs of choice for the treatment of endocarditis caused by *Kingella* species (and other HACEK organisms) are the third-generation cephalosporins cefotaxime or ceftriaxone.[83] The duration of treatment for native valve endocarditis should be 3 to 4 weeks and the duration of treatment for prosthetic valve endocarditis should be 6 weeks.

REFERENCES

1. Berk SL. From *Micrococcus* to *Moraxella*—the reemergence of *Branhamella catarrhalis*. *Arch Intern Med.* 1990;150:2254-2257.
2. Catlin BW. Transfer of the organism named *Neisseria catarrhalis* to *Branhamella* genus. *Int J Syst Bacteriol.* 1970;20:155-159.
3. Murphy TF. *Branhamella catarrhalis*: Epidemiology, surface antigenic structure, and immune response. *Microbiol Rev.* 1996;60:267-279.
4. Karalus R, Campagnari A. *Moraxella catarrhalis*: A review of an important human mucosal pathogen. *Microbes Infect.* 2000;2:547-559.
5. Murphy TF. Vaccine development for non-typeable *Haemophilus influenzae* and *Moraxella catarrhalis*: Progress and challenges. *Expert Rev Vaccines.* 2005;4:843-853.
6. Speeleveld E, Fossepre J-M, Gordts B, et al. Comparison of three rapid methods, tributyrine, 4-methylumbelliferyl butyrate, and indoxyl acetate, for rapid identification of *Moraxella catarrhalis*. *J Clin Microbiol.* 1994;32:1362-1363.
7. Janda WM, Montero MC, Wilcoski LM. Evaluation of the Bacti-Card *Neisseria* for identification of pathogenic *Neisseria* species and *Moraxella catarrhalis*. *Eur J Clin Microbiol Infect Dis.* 2002;21:875-879.
8. Ejlertsen T, Thisted E, Ebbesen F, et al. *Branhamella catarrhalis* in children and adults. A study of prevalence, time of colonisation, and association with upper and lower respiratory tract infections. *J Infect.* 1994;29:23-31.
9. Vaneechoutte M, Verschraegen G, Claeys G, et al. Respiratory tract carrier rates of *Moraxella (Branhamella) catarrhalis* in adults and children and interpretation of the isolation of *M. catarrhalis* from sputum. *J Clin Microbiol.* 1990;28:2674-2680.
10. Faden H, Harabuchi Y, Hong JJ, et al. Epidemiology of *Moraxella catarrhalis* in children during the first 2 years of life: relationship to otitis media. *J Infect Dis.* 1994;169:1312-1317.
11. Aniansson G, Alm B, Andersson B, et al. Nasopharyngeal colonization during the first year of life. *J Infect Dis.* 1992; 165(S1):S38-S42.
12. Leach AJ, Boswell JB, Asche V, et al. Bacterial colonization of the nasopharynx predicts very early onset and persistence of otitis media in Australian Aboriginal infants. *Pediatr Infect Dis J.* 1994;13:983-989.
13. Peerbooms PG, Engelen MN, Stokman DA, et al. Nasopharyngeal carriage of potential bacterial pathogens related to day care attendance, with special reference to the molecular epidemiology of *Haemophilus influenzae*. *J Clin Microbiol.* 2002;40: 2832-2836.
14. Revai K, McCormick DP, Patel J, et al. Effect of pneumococcal conjugate vaccine on nasopharyngeal bacterial colonization during acute otitis media. *Pediatrics.* 2006;117:1823-1829.
15. Faden H, Duffy L, Wasielewski R, et al. Relationship between nasopharyngeal colonization and the development of otitis media in children. *J Infect Dis.* 1997;175:1440-1445.
16. Dhooge I, Van Damme D, Vaneechoutte M, et al. Role of nasopharyngeal bacterial flora in the evaluation of recurrent middle ear infections in children. *Clin Microbiol Infect.* 1999;5: 530-534.
17. Prellner K, Christensen P, Hovelius B, et al. Nasopharyngeal carriage of bacteria in otitis-prone and non–otitis-prone children in day-care centres. *Acta Otolaryngol.* 1984;98:343-350.
18. Murphy TF, Brauer AL, Grant BJ, et al. *Moraxella catarrhalis* in chronic obstructive pulmonary disease. Burden of disease and immune response. *Am J Respir Crit Care Med.* 2005;172: 195-199.
19. Murphy TF, Brauer AL, Aebi C, et al. Identification of surface antigens of *Moraxella catarrhalis* as targets of human serum antibody responses in chronic obstructive pulmonary disease. *Infect Immun.* 2005;73:3471-3478.
20. Murphy TF, Brauer AL, Aebi C, et al. Antigenic specificity of the mucosal antibody response to *Moraxella catarrhalis* in chronic obstructive pulmonary disease. *Infect Immun.* 2005;73: 8161-8166.
21. Sethi S, Evans N, Grant BJB, et al. New strains of bacteria and exacerbations of chronic obstructive pulmonary disease. *N Engl J Med.* 2002;347:465-471.
22. Ruckdeschel EA, Kirkham C, Lesse AJ, et al. Mining the *Moraxella catarrhalis* genome: Identification of potential vaccine antigens expressed during human infection. *Infect Immun.* 2008;76:1599-1607.
23. Heiniger N, Spaniol V, Troller R, et al. A reservoir of *Moraxella catarrhalis* in human pharyngeal lymphoid tissue. *J Infect Dis.* 2007;196:1080-1107.
24. Slevogt H, Seybold J, Tiwari KN, et al. *Moraxella catarrhalis* is internalized in respiratory epithelial cells by a trigger-like mechanism and initiates a TLR2- and partly NOD1-dependent inflammatory immune response. *Cell Microbiol.* 2007;9: 694-707.
25. Edwards KJ, Schwingel JM, Datta AK, et al. Multiplex PCR assay that identifies the major lipooligosaccharide serotype expressed by *Moraxella catarrhalis* clinical isolates. *J Clin Microbiol.* 2005;43:6139-6143.
26. Gjorloff Wingren A, Hadzic R, Forsgren A, et al. The novel IgD binding protein from *Moraxella catarrhalis* induces human B lymphocyte activation and Ig secretion in the presence of Th2 cytokines. *J Immunol.* 2002;168:5582-5588.
27. Jendholm J, Samuelsson M, Cardell LO, et al. *Moraxella catarrhalis*–dependent tonsillar B cell activation does not lead to apoptosis but to vigorous proliferation resulting in nonspecific IgM production. *J Leukoc Biol.* 2008;83:1370-1378.
28. Slevogt H, Maqami L, Vardarowa K, et al. Differental regulation of *Moraxella catarrhalis*-induced IL-8 response by PKC isoforms. *Eur Respir J.* 2008;31:725-735.
29. Xie H, Gu XX. *Moraxella catarrhalis* lipooligosaccharide selectively upregulates ICAM-1 expression on human monocytes and stimulates adjacent naive monocytes to produce TNF-alpha through cellular cross-talk. *Cell Microbiol.* 2008;10: 1453-1467.
30. Luke NR, Jurcisek JA, Bakaletz LO, et al. Contribution of *Moraxella catarrhalis* type IV pili to nasopharyngeal colonization and biofilm formation. *Infect Immun.* 2007;75:5559-5564.
31. Ruohola A, Meurman O, Nikkari S, et al. Microbiology of acute otitis media in children with tympanostomy tubes: Prevalences of bacteria and viruses. *Clin Infect Dis.* 2006;43:1417-1422.
32. Arguedas A, Dagan R, Leibovitz E, et al. A multicenter, open label, double tympanocentesis study of high dose cefdinir in children with acute otitis media at high risk of persistent or recurrent infection. *Pediatr Infect Dis J.* 2006;25:211-218.
33. Kilpi T, Herva E, Kaijalainen T, et al. Bacteriology of acute otitis media in a cohort of Finnish children followed for the first two years of life. *Pediatr Infect Dis J.* 2001;20:654-662.
34. Aspin MM, Hoberman A, McCarty J, et al. Comparative study of the safety and efficacy of clarithromycin and amoxicillin-clavulanate in the treatment of acute otitis media in children. *J Pediatr.* 1994;125:135-141.
35. Chonmaitree T, Owen MJ, Patel JA, et al. Effect of viral respiratory tract infection on outcome of acute otitis media. *J Pediatr.* 1992;120:856-862.
36. DelBeccaro MA, Mendelman PM, Inglis AF, et al. Bacteriology of acute otitis media: A new perspective. *J Pediatr.* 1992; 120:81-84.
37. Faden H, Bernstein J, Stanievich J, et al. Effect of prior antibiotic treatment on middle ear disease in children. *Ann Otol Rhinol Laryngol.* 1992;101:87-91.
38. Post JC, Preston RA, Aul JJ, et al. Molecular analysis of bacterial pathogens in otitis media with effusion. *JAMA.* 1995;273: 1598-1604.
39. Hendolin PH, Markkanen A, Ylikoski J, et al. Use of multiplex PCR for simultaneous detection of four bacterial species in middle ear effusions. *J Clin Microbiol.* 1997;35:2854-2858.
40. Hendolin PH, Paulin L, Ylikoski J. Clinically applicable multiplex PCR for four middle ear pathogens. *J Clin Microbiol.* 2000;38:125-132.
41. Sethi S, Murphy TF. Bacterial infection in chronic obstructive pulmonary disease in 2000. A state of the art review. *Clin Microbiol Rev.* 2001;14:336-363.
42. Sethi S, Murphy TF. Infection in the course and pathogenesis of chronic obstructive pulmonary disease. *N Engl J Med.* 2008;359:2355-2365.
43. Sethi S, Muscarella K, Evans N, et al. Airway inflammation and etiology of acute exacerbations of chronic bronchitis. *Chest.* 2000;118:1557-1565.
44. Carr B, Walsh JB, Coakley D, et al. Prospective hospital study of community acquired lower respiratory tract infection in the elderly. *Respir Med.* 1991;85:185-187.
45. Ahmed A, Broides A, Givon-Lavi N, et al. Clinical and laboratory aspects of *Moraxella catarrhalis* bacteremia in children. *Pediatr Infect Dis J.* 2008;27:459-461.
46. Meyer GA, Shope TR, Waecker NJ Jr, et al. *Moraxella (Branhamella) catarrhalis* bacteremia in children. *Clin Pediatr (Phila).* 1995:146-150.
47. Ioannidis JPA, Worthington M, Griffiths JK, et al. Spectrum and significance of bacteremia due to *Moraxella catarrhalis*. *Clin Infect Dis.* 1995;21:390-397.
48. Nissinen A, Gronroos P, Huovinen P, et al. Development of β-lactamase–mediated resistance to penicillin in middle-ear isolates of *Moraxella catarrhalis* in Finnish children, 1978-1993. *Clin Infect Dis.* 1995;21:1193-1196.
49. Bootsma HJ, van Dijk H, Vauterin P, et al. Genesis of β-lactamase-producing *Moraxella catarrhalis*: Evidence for transformation-mediated horizontal transfer. *Mol Microbiol.* 2000;36:93-104.
50. Schmitz FJ, Beeck A, Perdikouli M, et al. Production of BRO beta-lactamases and resistance to complement in European *Moraxella catarrhalis* isolates. *J Clin Microbiol.* 2002;40: 1546-1548.
51. Aho EL, Murphy GL, Cannon JG. Distribution of specific DNA sequences among pathogenic and commensal *Neisseria* species. *Infect Immun.* 1987;55:1009-1013.
52. Serino L, Virji M. Phosphorylcholine decoration of lipopolysaccharide differentiates commensal *Neisseriae* from pathogenic strains: Identification of licA-type genes in commensal *Neisseriae*. *Mol Microbiol.* 2000;35:1550-1559.
53. Snyder LA, Saunders NJ. The majority of genes in the pathogenic *Neisseria* species are present in non-pathogenic *Neisseria lactamica*, including those designated as "virulence genes". *BMC Genomics.* 2006;7:128.
54. Troncoso G, Sanchez S, Criado MT, et al. Analysis of *Neisseria lactamica* antigens putatively implicated in acquisition of natural immunity to *Neisseria meningitidis*. *FEMS Immunol Med Microbiol.* 2002;34:9-15.
55. Bowler LD, Zhang Q-Y, Riou J-Y, et al. Interspecies recombination between the *penA* genes of *Neisseria meningitidis* and commensal *Neisseria* species during the emergence of penicillin resistance of *N. meningitidis*: Natural events and laboratory simulation. *J Bacteriol.* 1994;176:333-337.
56. Feil E, Zhou J, Smith JM, et al. A comparison of the nucleotide sequences of the *adk* and *recA* genes of pathogenic and commensal *Neisseria* species: Evidence for extensive interspecies recombination within *adk*. *J Mol Evol.* 1996;43:631-640.
57. Snyder LA, McGowan S, Rogers M, et al. The repertoire of minimal mobile elements in the *Neisseria* species and evidence that these are involved in horizontal gene transfer in other bacteria. *Mol Biol Evol.* 2007;24:2802-2815.
58. Schaefer F, Bruttin O, Zografos L, et al. Bacterial keratitis: A prospective clinical and microbiological study. *Br J Ophthalmol.* 2001;85:842-847.
59. Laukeland H, Bergh K, Bevanger L. Posttrabeculectomy endophthalmitis caused by *Moraxella nonliquefaciens*. *J Clin Microbiol.* 2002;40:2668-2770.
60. Das S, Constantinou M, Daniell M, et al. *Moraxella* keratitis: Predisposing factors and clinical review of 95 cases. *Br J Ophthalmol.* 2006;90:1236-1238.
61. Fijen CAP, Kuijper EJ, Tjia HG, et al. Complement deficiency predisposes for meningitis due to nongroupable meningococci and *Neisseria*-related bacteria. *Clin Infect Dis.* 1994;18:780-784.
62. Host B, Schumacher H, Prag J, et al. Isolation of *Kingella kingae* from synovial fluids using four commercial blood culture bottles. *Eur J Clin Microbiol Infect Dis.* 2000;19:608-611.
63. Yagupsky P, Dagan R, Howard CW, et al. High prevalence of *Kingella kingae* in joint fluid from children with septic arthritis revealed by the BACTEC blood culture system. *J Clin Microbiol.* 1992;30:1278-1281.
64. Kiang KM, Ogunmodede F, Juni BA, et al. Outbreak of osteomyelitis/septic arthritis caused by *Kingella kingae* among child care center attendees. *Pediatrics.* 2005;116:e206-e213.
65. Kehl-Fie TE, St. Geme JW 3rd. Identification and characterization of an RTX toxin in the emerging pathogen *Kingella kingae*. *J Bacteriol.* 2007;189:430-436.
66. Yagupsky P, Dagan D, Prajgrod F, et al. Respiratory carriage of *Kingella kingae* among healthy children. *Pediatr Infect Dis J.* 1995;14:673-678.
67. Yagupsky P, Erlich Y, Ariela S, et al. Outbreak of *Kingella kingae* skeletal system infections in children in daycare. *Pediatr Infect Dis J.* 2006;25:526-532.
68. Chen C-KC, Dunford RG, Reynolds HS, et al. *Eikenella corrodens* in the human oral cavity. *J Periodontol.* 1989;60:611-616.
69. Dewhirst FE, Chen C-KC, Paster BJ, et al. Phylogeny of species in the family *Neisseriaceae* isolated from human dental plaque and description of *Kingella oralis* sp. nov. *Int J Syst Bacteriol.* 1993;43:490-499.
70. Chen C. Distribution of a newly described species, *Kingella oralis*, in the human oral cavity. *Oral Microbiol Immunol.* 1996;11: 425-427.
71. Slonim A, Steiner M, Yagupsky P. Immune response to invasive *Kingella kingae* infections, age-related incidence of disease, and levels of antibody to outer-membrane proteins. *Clin Infect Dis.* 2003;37:521-527.
72. Yagupsky P, Peled N, Katz O. Epidemiological features of invasive *Kingella kingae* infections and respiratory carriage of the organism. *J Clin Microbiol.* 2002;40:4180-4184.
73. Dodman T, Robson J, Pincus D. *Kingella kingae* infections in children. *J Paediatr Child Health.* 2000;36:87-90.
74. Moylett EH, Rossmann SN, Epps HR, et al. Importance of *Kingella kingae* as a pediatric pathogen in the United States. *Pediatr Infect Dis J.* 2000;19:263-265.
75. Birgisson H, Steingrimsson O, Gudnason T. *Kingella kingae* infections in paediatric patients: 5 cases of septic arthritis, osteomyelitis and bacteraemia. *Scand J Infect Dis.* 1997;29:495-498.
76. Garron E, Viehweger E, Launay F, et al. Nontuberculous spondylodiscitis in children. *J Pediatr Orthop.* 2002;22:321-328.
77. Verdier I, Gayet-Ageron A, Ploton C, et al. Contribution of a broad range polymerase chain reaction to the diagnosis of osteoarticular infections caused by *Kingella kingae*: description of twenty-four recent pediatric diagnoses. *Pediatr Infect Dis J.* 2005;24:692-696.
78. Chometon S, Benito Y, Chaker M, et al. Specific real-time polymerase chain reaction places *Kingella kingae* as the most common cause of osteoarticular infections in young children. *Pediatr Infect Dis J.* 2007;26:377-381.
79. Amir J, Schockelford PG. *Kingella kingae* intervertebral disk infection. *J Clin Microbiol.* 1991;29:1083-1086.
80. Yagupsky P, Katz O, Peled N. Antibiotic susceptibility of *Kingella kingae* isolates from respiratory carriers and patients with invasive infections. *J Antimicrob Chemother.* 2001;47:191-193.
81. Kugler KC, Biedenbach DJ, Jones RN. Determination of the antimicrobial activity of 29 clinically important compounds tested against fastidious HACEK group organisms. *Diagn Microbiol Infect Dis.* 1999;34:73-76.
82. Sordillo EM, Rendel M, Sood R, et al. Septicemia due to β-lactamase-positive *Kingella kingae*. *Clin Infect Dis.* 1993; 17:818-819.
83. Wilson WR, Karchmer AW, Dajani AS, et al. Antibiotic treatment of adults with infective endocarditis due to streptococci, enterococci, staphylococci, and HACEK microorganisms. *JAMA.* 1995;274:1706-1713.

214

Vibrio cholerae

CARLOS SEAS | EDUARDO GOTUZZO

Cholera is a historically feared epidemic diarrheal disease that still affects different regions of the world, imposing significant economic constraints on already impoverished developing countries. More recent epidemics are the Latin American extension of the seventh pandemic of cholera at the beginning of 1991, the epidemic of cholera in Zaire in 1994, and the epidemic of cholera caused by *Vibrio cholerae* O139 in 1992 in Asia (Fig. 214-1). These epidemics show that it is still not possible to predict when and where a new epidemic of cholera will start, that appropriate therapy may reduce the mortality to values below 1%, and that changes in the cause of this ancient disease are still taking place.

The term *cholera* has ancient origins and is derived from Greek words meaning "a flow of bile."[1] Thomas Sydenham was the first to distinguish cholera, the disease, from cholera, the state of anger.[1] He proposed the term *cholera morbus* for the disease. Because earlier descriptions of the disease confused cholera with other diarrheal diseases, the modern history of cholera began with Sydenham's description in 1817.

The modern era of cholera is characterized by seven pandemics. The first six occurred between 1817 and 1923. These pandemics were most likely caused by *V. cholerae* O1 of the classic biotype and largely originated in Asia, usually the Indian subcontinent, with subsequent extension to Europe and the Americas. Filippo Pacini published his observations on the discovery of a curved bacillus in the stools of victims of cholera in Italy in 1854. He coined the name *Vibrio cholerae*.[2] In 1883, Robert Koch made the same discovery. Transmission of the disease was recognized only after the brilliant work of John Snow during the second pandemic affecting London in 1849, even before knowing the cause of the disease. He reduced the transmission of cholera by blocking access to contaminated water in one area of London.

The seventh pandemic of cholera differed from the prior six. This pandemic was caused by the biotype El Tor of *V. cholerae* O1, a biotype that had been isolated for the first time in Egypt at the beginning of the century and was associated with sporadic cases until 1961. In 1961, the pandemic originated in the Celebes Islands, Indonesia, instead of the Indian subcontinent. This pandemic has been the longest lasting and has affected more countries and continents than the other six. The last extension of this pandemic in Latin America occurred in 1991, where it caused higher attack rates than those seen during the last century but the lowest case-fatality rates.[3] The pandemic is still going on in many countries—for example, 632 outbreaks were reported to ProMED between 1995 and 2005, and 66% of them were reported from Africa.[4] Fifty-three countries officially reported 177,963 cases to the World Health Organization in 2007, with 4031 deaths; 94% of these cases were reported from Africa. However, it is estimated that only 1% of the actual number of cases is officially reported.[5] Epidemic cholera was mostly restricted to Africa during 2007, with 34 reporting countries and five countries (Angola, Ethiopia, Democratic Republic of the Congo, Somalia, and Sudan) accounting for 76% of the total number of cases and fatalities. Social disruption, poverty, poor sanitary and hygienic conditions, and poor access to health care explain the high prevalence and mortality rates still observed in Africa.[6]

Finally, in October 1992, a totally unexpected epidemic of a cholera-like disease was observed in Madras, India, with subsequent cases being reported along the Bay of Bengal.[7] *V. cholerae* of the new serogroup O139 was responsible for this epidemic, the first non–O1 *Vibrio* to do so. The epidemic was widespread in the Asiatic continent, with imported cases reported from developed countries.[8-10] Some regarded this as the eighth cholera pandemic,[11] although the epidemic has remained confined to Bangladesh and India. The O139 serogroup today coexists with O1 *V. cholerae*, being responsible for continuous epidemics in Bangladesh.[12]

Microbiology

V. cholerae is a curved gram-negative bacillus varying in size from 1 to 3 µm in length by 0.5 to 0.8 µm in diameter. It belongs to the family Vibrionaceae and shares common characteristics with the family Enterobacteriaceae. The bacterium has a single polar flagellum that confers the erratic movement on microscopy. The antigenic structure of *V. cholerae* is similar to that of other members of the family Enterobacteriaceae, with a flagellar H antigen and a somatic O antigen. The O antigen is used to classify *V. cholerae* further, into serogroups O1 and non-O1. Approximately 206 serogroups of *V. cholerae* have been identified to date, but only the serogroups O1 and O139 are associated with clinical cholera and have pandemic potential.

V. cholerae O1 can be classified into three serotypes according to the presence of somatic antigens and into two biotypes according to specific phenotypic characteristics. Serotype Inaba carries the O antigens A and C, serotype Ogawa carries the antigens A and B, and serotype Hikojima carries the three antigens A, B, and C. No evidence of different clinical spectra among these three serotypes of *V. cholerae* has ever been presented. During epidemics, a shift from one serotype to another may occur.[13,14] A serotype-cycling behavior has been reported from Bangladesh; the predominance of one serotype over others depends on the immunity level of the population.[15] The differences between the two biotypes of *V. cholerae* O1 are remarkable. The classic biotype, probably responsible for the first six pandemics of cholera, causes an approximately equal number of symptomatic and asymptomatic cases. In contrast, the El Tor biotype causes more asymptomatic infections, with a ratio between 20 and 100 asymptomatic infections to 1 symptomatic case. The classic biotype is confined to the south of Bangladesh, whereas the El Tor biotype is responsible for the current pandemic. These two biotypes are not derived from each other, but rather from environmental nontoxigenic strains.[16] They have coexisted for decades in their natural environment, possibly interacting genetically to produce hybrids, as has been reported recently from patients in Bangladesh and Mozambique.[17] The persistence of the classic biotype has suggested the possible need for the development of multivalent vaccines. The O139 serogroup is composed of a variety of genetically diverse strains, both toxigenic and nontoxigenic, with at least nine different ribotypes identified.[18] This novel serogroup is genetically closer to El Tor *V. cholerae*, and might have been originated from it, acquiring distinctive features from a nonidentified donor, likely a non-O1 vibrio, through recombination of genetic material.[18]

ISOLATION AND IDENTIFICATION

V. cholerae O1 or O139 can easily be observed under darkfield examination. The chaotic movements and high numbers of bacteria seen in a stool sample from patients with clinical disease are characteristic of

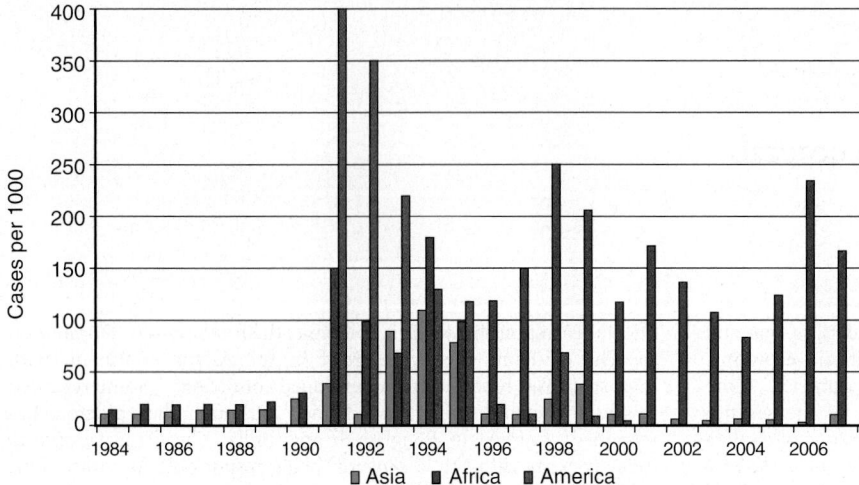

Figure 214-1 **Cholera cases reported to the World Health Organization from 1984 to 2007.** A substantial increase in the number of cases has been observed since 1990. This is the result of large epidemics of cholera caused by *V. cholerae* O1 in America and Africa, and the appearance of a new serogroup, O139, in Asia. At present, cholera is restricted to Africa. *(Adapted from World Health Organization. Cholera. Wkly Epidemiol Rec. 2008;83:269-284.)*

V. cholerae infection. The use of specific antisera against the serotype blocks the movement of these vibrios and allows confirmation of the diagnosis. However, under epidemic conditions, the presence of bacteria with darting movements under darkfield microscopy in a stool sample from patients highly suspected of having cholera is sufficient to make the diagnosis, but definitive confirmation still requires isolation of the bacteria in culture. A specific medium is needed to isolate *V. cholerae* from stool. The two media most commonly used are thiosulfate citrate bile salts sucrose agar and tellurite taurocholate gelatin agar. These two media are equally sensitive to isolate either O1 or O139 *V. cholerae*. Enrichment media or the addition of antibiotics to culture medium may be used when the number of bacteria in the stool is small or when environmental samples are evaluated for the presence of *Vibrio*.[19] High sensitivity and specificity have been reported more recently using polymerase chain reaction (PCR) assay and real-time nucleic acid sequence-based amplification assays for detecting vibrios in stool and environmental samples.[20-22] A rapid diagnosis of cholera can be made in the field using a highly sensitive and specific immunochromatographic dipstick test applied to fresh stools.[23]

Pathophysiology

V. cholerae O1 and O139 cause clinical disease by secreting an enterotoxin that promotes secretion of fluids and electrolytes by the small intestine. The infectious dose of bacteria varies with the vehicle. When water is the vehicle, more bacteria (10^3 to 10^6) are needed to cause disease, but when the vehicle is food, the amount needed is lower (10^2 to 10^4).[24] Conditions that reduce gastric acidity, such as the use of antacids or histamine receptor blockers, gastrectomy, or chronic gastritis induced by *Helicobacter pylori*, increase the risk of getting the disease and predispose the patient to more severe clinical forms. Toxin is produced, but *V. cholerae* does not invade the intestinal wall and few neutrophils are found in the stool. The incubation period varies with the infectious dose and gastric acidity and lasts 12 to 72 hours.

Both Koch and Snow suspected that a toxin was responsible for some of the disease manifestations, but it was not until 1959 that De and Dutta and colleagues, working in different laboratories, showed that *V. cholerae* promoted intestinal secretion in animal models.[25,26] The toxin was finally purified by Finkelstein and LoSpalluto in 1969.[27] The toxin has five B subunits and two A subunits. The B subunits allow binding of the toxin to a specific receptor, a ganglioside (GM_1) located on the surface of the cells lining the mucosa along the intestine of humans and certain suckling mammals. The active, or A, subunit has two components, A1 and A2, linked by a disulfide bond. Activation of the A1 component by adenylate cyclase results in a net increase in cyclic adenosine monophosphate, which blocks the absorption of sodium and chloride by microvilli and promotes the secretion of chloride and

water by crypt cells. The result of these events is the production of watery diarrhea with electrolyte concentrations similar to those of plasma, as shown in Table 214-1.

The complete genomic sequence of *V. cholerae* O1 El Tor is well known today. The genetic material consists of two circular chromosomes, with the larger containing 3 megabases, and the smaller containing 1.07 megabases.[28] The main virulence genes are *ctx*A and *ctx*B, which encode for cholera toxin subunits A and B, respectively, and *tcp*A, which codes for toxin-coregulated pilus. The regulation of the expression of these genes is complex. Environmental factors, such as sunlight and possibly others, may influence the expression of genes encoding for cholera toxin.[29]

Epidemiology

Cholera has unique epidemiologic features. Perhaps the most intriguing are the predisposition to cause epidemics with pandemic potential and the ability to remain endemic in all affected areas.[30] These two epidemiologic patterns, the epidemic and endemic patterns, are summarized in Table 214-2. Recognizing the different age groups at risk, depending on the epidemiologic pattern, is useful in designing preventive measures.

New insights into the life cycle of *V. cholerae* have allowed a better understanding of cholera transmission. *V. cholerae* lives in aquatic environments, which are their natural reservoirs.[31] Both O1 and non-O1 strains coexist in these environments, with non-O1 and non-

TABLE 214-1	Electrolyte Concentration of Cholera Stools and Common Solutions Used for Treatment				
	Electrolyte and Glucose Concentration (mmol/L)				
	Na+	*Cl−*	*K+*	*HCO3−*	*Glucose*
Cholera stool					
Adults	130	100	20	44	
Children	100	90	33	30	
Intravenous solutions					
Ringer's lactate	130	109	4	28*	0
Dhaka	133	98	13	48	0
Normal saline	154	154	0	0	0
Peru polyelectrolyte	90	80	20	30	111
Reduced osmolarity WHO ORS	75	65	20	10†	75

*Ringer's lactate solution does not contain HCO_3^-; it contains lactate instead.
†Bicarbonate is replaced by trisodium citrate, which persists longer than bicarbonate in sachets.
WHO ORS, World Health Organization oral rehydration solution.

TABLE 214-2	Epidemiologic Patterns of Cholera	
Epidemiologic Features	**Epidemic Pattern**	**Endemic Pattern**
Age at greatest risk	All ages	Children, 2-15 yr
Modes of transmission	Single introduction with fecal-oral spread	Multiple modes of introduction—water, food, fecal-oral spread
Reservoir	None	Aquatic reservoir
Asymptomatic infections	Less common	Asymptomatic people more common
Immune status of the population	No preexisting immunity	Preexisting immunity; evidence of infection increases with age
Secondary spread	High	Variable

Adapted from Glass RI, Black RE. The epidemiology of cholera. In: Barua D, Greenough WB III. eds. *Cholera*. New York: Plenum Press; 1992:129-154.

toxigenic O1 strains predominating over toxigenic O1 strains.[32] In its natural environment, *V. cholerae* lives attached to a particular type of algae or attached to crustacean shells and copepods (zooplankton), which coexist in a symbiotic manner (Fig. 214-2).[33,34] When conditions in the environment such as temperature, salinity, and availability of nutrients are suitable, *V. cholerae* multiplies and can survive for years in a free-living cycle without the intervention of humans. Otherwise, when conditions are not suitable for its growth, *V. cholerae* switches from a metabolically active state to a dormant state.[32] In this dormant state, *V. cholerae* cannot be cultured from the water on standard or enrichment media but appears to survive under difficult environmental conditions. Immunofluorescent techniques using monoclonal antibodies have been used to detect dormant *V. cholerae*.[35] Experimentally, the switch from a nonculturable to culturable state has been attained in the laboratory, as well as in human volunteers.[36] *V. cholerae* may also persist in the environment and adopts a rugose form visible on a special agar, Luria agar.[37] Recently, it has been shown that *V. cholerae* can form biofilms, surface-associated communities of bacteria with enhanced survival under negative conditions, that can switch to active bacteria and induce epidemics.[38] Humans infected by *V. cholerae* may shed the bacteria for a long time, sometimes for months or years. Recent evidence has suggested that *V. cholerae* can upregulate certain genes in the intestine of humans, resulting in a short-time hyperinfectious state.[39] Interestingly, households in contact with acutely ill patients who shed large amounts of *V. cholerae* O1 Inaba El Tor in their stools are more likely to develop cholera than those in contact with

environmental strains. Also, the abundance of *V. cholerae* O1 in the intestine of cholera patients is in part determined by the presence of lytic phages.[40]

From its aquatic environment, *V. cholerae* is introduced to humans through contamination of water sources and contamination of food. The cycle of transmission is closed when infected humans shed the bacteria into the environment and contaminate water sources and food. Once humans are infected, incredibly high attack rates may ensue, especially in previously nonexposed populations. Additional evidence of very high household transmission rates exists, as occurred during the last Latin American epidemic or, more recently, during the epidemic in Zaire in 1994.[41,42] Transmission via contaminated water and food has been recognized for years.[43] During the Latin American epidemic and more recent epidemics in Africa, acquisition of the disease by drinking contaminated water from rivers, ponds, lakes, and even tube well sources has been documented.[6,44,45] Contamination of municipal water was the main route of transmission of cholera in Trujillo, Peru, during the epidemic of 1991.[46] Drinking unboiled water, introducing hands into containers used to store drinking water, drinking beverages from street vendors, drinking beverages when contaminated ice had been added, and drinking water outside the home are recognized risk factors to acquire cholera. On the other hand, drinking boiled water, acidic beverages, and carbonated water, as well as using narrow-necked vessels for storing water, are protective.[47] *V. cholerae* survives for up to 14 days in some foods, especially when contamination occurs after preparation of the food.[48] Cooking and heating the food eliminate the bacteria. Epidemics of cholera associated with the ingestion of leftover rice, raw fish, cooked crabs, seafood, raw oysters, and fresh vegetables and fruits have been documented.

Transmission of cholera during funerals in Africa has been reported. Risk factors identified included eating at the funeral with a nondisinfected corpse and touching the body.[49] Eating rice at the funeral was the main risk factor for the acquisition of cholera in one study.[50] Person-to-person transmission is less likely to occur because a large inoculum is necessary to transmit disease. However, anecdotal reports exist in the literature.[51-53] Careful evaluation of these reports shows that other potential risk factors might have been implicated in the transmission. Other vehicles of transmission such as insects and fomites have been incriminated, but are less likely to be important in epidemic situations.

Seasonality is another typical characteristic of cholera. Epidemics tend to occur during the hot seasons, and countries with more than one hot season per year may also have more than one epidemic, such as seen in Bangladesh.[54] Data from the epidemic of cholera in Peru from 1991 to 1995 also confirmed that outbreaks are associated with the warmest months of the year.[55] A recent evaluation of data reported to the World Health Organization has suggested that countries located near the equator have more constant outbreaks not related to seasonal variations; in contrast, countries far from the equator have less intense outbreaks clearly associated to seasonal variations.[56] Climate change and climate variability may affect the incidence of certain infectious diseases.[57] The El Niño–Southern Oscillation (ENSO), a periodic phenomenon representative of global climate variability, has been studied in relation to its effect on the transmission of cholera and vector-borne diseases. A strong association between ENSO and cholera has been observed in Bangladesh and also proposed for Latin America, with studies suggesting that this relationship may be even more intense in future years.[58-61] ENSO causes warming of normally cool waters on the Pacific coastline of Peru, promoting phytoplankton bloom, which in turn promotes zooplankton bloom and *V. cholerae* proliferation. Lipp and associates[57] have elegantly described the complex associations among various climatic, seasonal, bacterial, and human factors acting on cholera transmission in a hierarchical model (Fig. 214-3). Interestingly, as noted previously, environmental conditions modulate vibrio abundance and may affect the expression of virulence genes of *V. cholerae*,[29,57,62,63] thus promoting the beginning of epidemics, as might have been the situation in Peru during 1991.[64] In addition, abundance of lytic phages in the environment inversely correlate with the burden

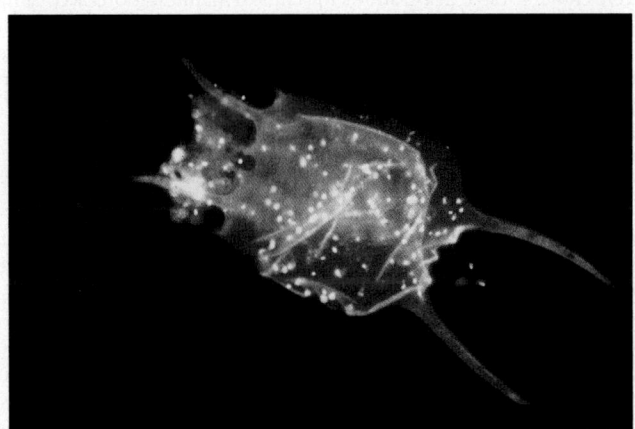

Figure 214-2 *Vibrio cholerae* **attached to a copepod (stained with fluorescent techniques).** *(Courtesy of Dr. Rita Colwell and Dr. Anwarul Huq, University of Maryland, College Park, Md.)*

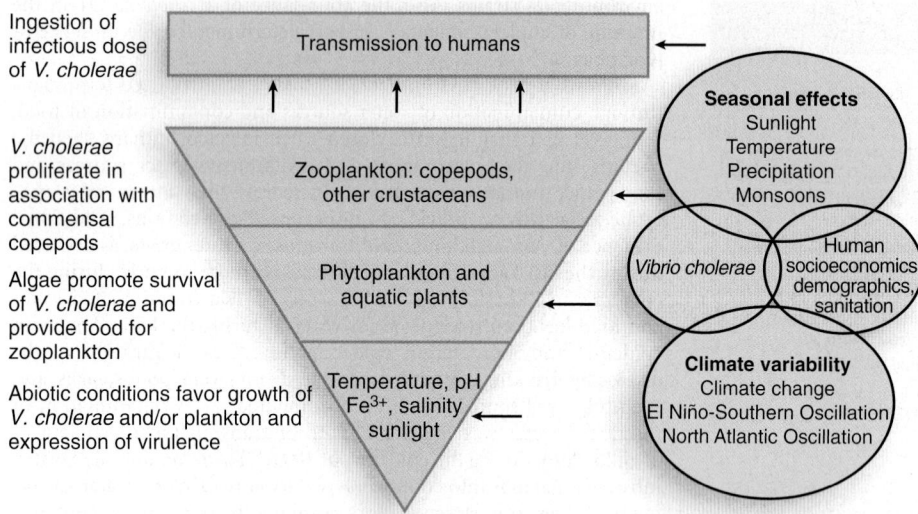

Figure 214-3 A hierarchical model for cholera transmission. (From Lipp EK, Huq A, Colwell RR. Effects of global climate on infectious disease: The cholera model. Clin Microbiol Rev. 2002;15:757-770.)

of vibrio and may influence transmission to humans.[65] Drastic climatic events such as floods and droughts also influence cholera transmission.[66]

Some host factors are important in the transmission of cholera. Among them, infection by *H. pylori,* the effect of the O blood group, and the protective effect of breast milk deserve special consideration. Data from Bangladesh have shown that people infected by *H. pylori* are at higher risk of acquiring cholera than those not infected by *H. pylori.*[67] Additionally, the risk of acquiring severe cholera in people infected by *H. pylori* was higher in patients without previous contact with *V. cholerae,* as measured by the absence of vibriocidal antibodies in the serum.[68] *H. pylori* causes a chronic gastritis that induces hypochlorhydria, which in turn reduces the ability of the stomach to contain the *Vibrio* invasion. The impact of the association of these two infections is particularly interesting because *H. pylori* infection is very common in persons of all ages in developing countries.[68] In support of these previous observations, endoscopic findings in patients with severe cholera and mixed infection with *H. pylori* in Peru have revealed hypochlorhydria, chronic atrophic gastritis, and intestinal metaplasia.[69] Patients carrying the O blood group have a higher risk of developing severe cholera caused by O1 or O139 *V. cholerae* and disclose higher purging volumes of diarrhea, but have a lower risk of acquiring infection by *V. cholerae* O1.[70] Higher affinity of the cholera toxin to the ganglioside receptor in patients with O blood group and lower affinity in patients of A, B, and AB blood groups explains this association. Finally, the protective effect of breast milk has been reported, and it is linked to higher concentrations of IgA anti–cholera toxin.[71]

Although mainly countries with poor sanitary conditions are affected by cholera, a few developed countries such as the United States, Canada, and Australia have reported indigenous cases. Two different *V. cholerae* O1 strains have been isolated from these regions, and these vibrios differ from the strain responsible for the seventh pandemic.[72-74] Sporadic cases are reported periodically from these areas. Surveillance of cholera is needed to detect future epidemics and to identify current trends in serogroup predominance and susceptibility to antimicrobial agents in endemic areas. A 4-year surveillance study in four rural areas of Bangladesh has shown that noncholera pathogens predominated as a cause of diarrhea in children younger than 2 years, O1 *V. cholerae* predominated in young children, and O139 *V. cholerae* was observed in people of all ages but especially in older adults, suggesting that this new serogroup is still not endemic in the area.[75] Identifying areas of high transmission is desirable to focus prevention on a more local level. Integration of socioeconomic, behavioral, and biologic factors is needed to achieve that goal.[76]

Clinical Manifestations and Laboratory Abnormalities

The hallmark of cholera is the production of watery diarrhea, with varying degrees of dehydration ranging from none to severe and life-threatening diarrhea. Patients with mild to moderate dehydration secondary to cholera are difficult to differentiate from those infected by other enteric pathogens, such as enterotoxigenic *Escherichia coli* or rotavirus. Patients with severe dehydration from cholera are easy to identify because no other clinical illness produces such severe dehydration in a matter of a few hours as cholera. Onset of the disease is abrupt and characterized by the production of watery diarrhea without strain, tenesmus, or prominent abdominal pain, rapidly followed or sometimes preceded by vomiting. As the diarrhea continues, other symptoms of severe dehydration are manifest, such as generalized cramps and oliguria. Physical examination will show an alert patient most of the time, despite the fact that the pulse is nonpalpable and blood pressure cannot be measured. Fever is observed in less than 5% of cases. Patients look anxious and restless or sometimes obtunded, the eyes are very sunken, mucous membranes are dry, the skin has lost its elasticity and when pinched retracts very slowly, the voice is almost nonaudible, and the intestinal sounds are prominent. Patients in this condition are difficult to confuse with patients with other medical conditions. Figure 214-4 shows a typical patient with severe cholera. Table 214-3 shows the clinical manifestations according to the degree of dehydration as a guide to the proper administration of fluids. Although watery diarrhea is the hallmark of cholera, some patients do not have diarrhea but instead have abdominal distention and ileus, a relatively rare type of cholera called cholera "sicca."[77] Management of these patients is particularly difficult because evaluation of the degree of dehydration is overshadowed by the accumulation of fluid in the intestinal lumen.

Laboratory abnormalities reflect the isotonic dehydration characteristic of cholera. Increases in packed cell volume, serum specific gravity, and total protein are typically seen in patients with moderate to severe dehydration. Although abnormal results of these tests correlate with the degree of dehydration on arrival at a health center, they are less useful for monitoring rehydration status. Biochemical and acid-base laboratory abnormalities typical of severe dehydration are prerenal azotemia, metabolic acidosis with a high anion gap, normal or low serum potassium levels, and normal or slightly low sodium and chloride levels. The calcium and magnesium content in plasma is also high as a result of hemoconcentration. The white blood cell count is high in patients with severe cholera. Hyperglycemia caused by high concen-

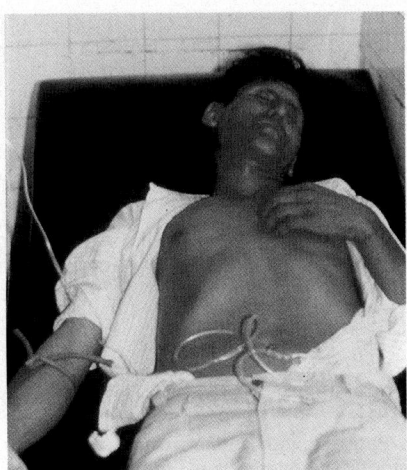

Figure 214-4   A Peruvian patient with severe cholera. Sunken eyes and washer woman's hands are typical of patients with severe dehydration.

trations of epinephrine, glucagon, and cortisol stimulated by hypovolemia is more commonly seen than hypoglycemia, but hypoglycemic children have a higher risk of dying than nonhypoglycemic children.[78] Acute renal failure is the most severe complication of cholera. Incidence rates of 10.6 cases/1000 were reported in Peru during the first months of the epidemic in 1991.[41] Patients with acute renal failure had a history of improper rehydration. All age groups were equally affected, and the mortality rate in this group of patients was extremely high (18%), particularly in older patients.[41]

The clinical manifestation of cholera in children is similar to that in adults. However, hypoglycemia, seizures, fever, and mental alteration are more common in children.[79] Cholera in pregnant women carries a bad prognosis and portends more severe clinical illness, especially when the disease is acquired at the end of the pregnancy.[80] Fetal loss occurs in as many as 50% of these pregnancies. Cholera in older patients also carries a bad prognosis because of more complications, particularly acute renal failure, severe metabolic acidosis, and pulmonary edema.[41] Proper hydration may correct all electrolyte and acid-base abnormalities in older patients.[81] Recent observations have suggested that HIV infection in Africa is associated with an increased risk for cholera.[82]

Treatment

The goal of therapy is to restore the fluid losses caused by diarrhea and vomiting. Although treatment of patients without severe dehydration is easy, treatment of patients with severe dehydration requires experience and proper training. Basic training in how to recognize the degree of dehydration, select the proper intravenous solution, and rapidly rehydrate the patient is crucial. Recent experience during the epidemic in Zaire, in which untrained people played a negative role, cannot be overemphasized. Conversely, well-trained staff provided with adequate supplies can successfully treat patients, even under epidemic situations.[42,83,84] Guidelines to rehydrate cholera patients have been written and reviewed elsewhere.[85-87] The IV route should be restricted to patients with moderate dehydration who do not tolerate the oral route, those who purge more than 10 to 20 mL/kg/hr, and patients with severe dehydration. Rehydration should be accomplished in two phases, the rehydration phase and the maintenance phase. The purpose of the rehydration phase is to restore normal hydration status, and it should last no longer than 4 hours. IV fluids should be infused at a rate of 50 to 100 mL/kg/hr in severely dehydrated patients. Ringer's lactate solution is the most frequently recommended solution, but other solutions may also be used, as shown in Table 214-1. Normal saline solution is not recommended because it does not correct the metabolic acidosis. When IV access proves difficult, nasogastric tubes or intraosseous catheters can be used, although problems with IV access were not common during the last cholera epidemic in Peru.[55]

After finishing the rehydration phase, all signs of dehydration should have abated and the patient should pass urine at a rate of 0.5 mL/kg/hr or higher. The maintenance phase then begins. During this phase, the objective is to maintain normal hydration status by replacing ongoing losses. The oral route is preferred during this phase, and the use of oral rehydration solutions at a rate of 500 to 1000 mL/hr is highly recommended. Oral rehydration therapy uses the principle of common transportation of solutes, electrolytes, and water by the portion of the intestine not affected by the cholera toxin. People with diarrhea can undergo successful rehydration with simple solutions containing glucose and electrolytes that may be prepared at home. In 2002, the World Health Organization recommended the use of oral rehydration solutions with lower osmolarity (250 mOsm/L) than previously recommended in 1978 (311 mOsm/L).[88] The recommendation was based on a meta-analysis showing a lesser need to use IV fluids during treatment, and lower volumes of diarrhea and vomiting in children treated with the reduced osmolarity solution compared with the standard solution.[89] These results are also applicable to adults. Symptomatic hyponatremia in children in Bangladesh was lower with the reduced osmolarity solution compared with the standard rehydration solution.[90] Substitution of glucose for rice, amino acids, or amylase-resistant starch seems to improve the efficacy of the oral salts reducing further the volume and duration of diarrhea.[91,92] Evaluation of rehydration status and accurate recording of intake and output volumes are essential. Patients without severe dehydration who tolerate the oral route can be rehydrated with oral rehydration solutions exclusively and discharged promptly from the health center. Practical guidelines[87] are summarized in Table 214-4.

Discharging patients from health centers, particularly those with severe dehydration, is a critical issue, especially during epidemics. No significant readmission of patients was observed in Peru during the epidemic in 1991 when the following criteria were used to discharge patients: urine volume higher than 40 mL/hr, diarrhea output below 400 mL/hr, and oral ingestion of rehydration solutions between 600 and 800 mL/hr.[41] Adequate organization of health centers to accommodate and properly treat hundreds of patients, and proper allocation of available resources are critical under epidemic situations. Examples of successful use of resources during the O139 cholera epidemic of 1993 in Dhaka, Bangladesh, and during the O1 epidemic in Peru of 1991 are shown in Figures 214-5 and 214-6, respectively. The case-fatality rate during epidemics may be reduced to below 1%, even in disaster situations, provided that adequate access to health care centers

TABLE 214-3	Clinical Findings According to Degree of Dehydration		
	Degree of Dehydration		
Finding	*Mild*	*Moderate*	*Severe*
Loss of fluid*	<5%	5%-10%	>10%
Mentation	Alert	Restless	Drowsy or comatose
Radial pulse			
Rate	Normal	Rapid	Very rapid
Intensity	Normal	Weak	Feeble or impalpable
Respiration	Normal	Deep	Deep and rapid
Systolic blood pressure	Normal	Low	Very low or unrecordable
Skin elasticity	Retracts rapidly	Retracts slowly	Retracts very slowly
Eyes	Normal	Sunken	Very sunken
Voice	Normal	Hoarse	Not audible
Urine production	Normal	Scant	Oliguria

*Percentage of body weight.

From Bennish ML. Cholera: Pathophysiology, clinical features, and treatment. In: Wachsmuth IK, Blake PA, Olsvik O, eds. *Vibrio cholerae and Cholera: Molecular to Global Perspectives.* Washington, DC: ASM Press; 1994:229-255.

TABLE 214-4	Practical Guidelines for the Treatment of Cholera

1. Evaluate the degree of dehydration on arrival.
2. Rehydrate the patients in two phases:
   Rehydration phase: Lasts 2-4 hr
   Maintenance phase: Lasts until diarrhea abates
3. Register output and intake volumes in predesigned charts and periodically review the data.
4. Use the intravenous route only for:
   Severely dehydrated patients during the rehydration phase, in whom an infusion rate of 50-100 mL/kg/hr is advised
   Moderately dehydrated patients who do not tolerate the oral route
   High stool volume (>10 mL/kg/hr) during the maintenance phase
5. Use ORS for patients during the maintenance phase at a rate of 800-1000 mL/hr, matching ongoing losses with ORS.
6. Discharge patients to the treatment center if the following conditions are fulfilled:
   Oral tolerance ≥1000 mL/hr
   Urine volume ≥40 mL/hr
   Stool volume ≤400 mL/hr

ORS, Oral rehydration solution.
From Seas C, Dupont HL, Valdez LM, et al. Practical guidelines for the treatment of cholera. *Drugs*. 1996;51:966-973.

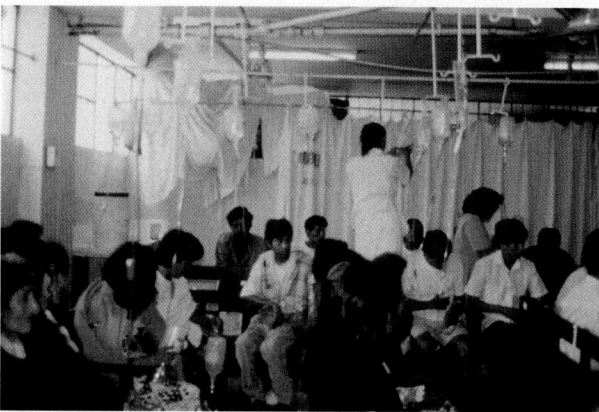

Figure 214-6 Patients with cholera caused by El Tor *V. cholerae* O1. In this photograph, patients were being treated in the Rehydration Unit at Hospital Nacional Cayetano Heredia, Lima, Peru. Cholera chairs instead of cholera cots were successfully used during the large epidemic of 1991. *(Courtesy of Dr. Eduardo Salazar, Department of Pediatrics, Hospital Nacional Cayetano Heredia, Lima, Peru.)*

and proper management of patients can be ensured.[41,84] A case-fatality rate of 3.7% among hospitalized patients was reported from a specialized center in Dhaka, Bangladesh, in 1996.[93] In this setting, the overall case-fatality rate was 0.14%, and pneumonia was the leading cause of death. In contrast, figures as high as 10% have been reported in epidemic settings when patients had no access to health care or received improper treatment.[94] Treatment of cholera caused by O139 *V. cholerae* is the same. No significant differences in clinical manifestations of the disease caused by these two agents have been found.[95]

Antimicrobial agents play a secondary role in the treatment of cholera. Clinical trials have shown that when patients with severe dehydration are given antibiotics, the duration of diarrhea is decreased and the volume of stool is reduced by almost 50%.[96] Early discharge and lessened hydration decrease hospital expense. These benefits are critical in epidemic conditions. Oral tetracycline and doxycycline are the agents of choice in areas of the globe where sensitive strains predominate. A single dose of doxycycline (300 mg) is the preferred regimen.[97] Tetracyclines are not safe in children younger than 7 years, and alternatives such as trimethoprim-sulfamethoxazole, erythromycin, and furazolidone are preferred over tetracyclines. Pregnant women can be treated with erythromycin or furazolidone. Currently recommended regimens are presented in Table 214-5.

Selection of an adequate antimicrobial in certain parts of the world has been complicated by the appearance of strains resistant to tetracyclines and other antimicrobial agents.[98,99] New agents have been tested in endemic and epidemic areas, with quinolones being the most effective.[100] Ciprofloxacin has been more extensively studied than other quinolones, showing at least similar if not better results than comparators in adults and children with severe cholera caused by O1 or O139 *V. cholerae* in single- or multiple-dose oral regimens.[101-103] However, single-dose regimens have shown lower clearance of the pathogen in the stools. More recently, strains resistant to quinolones have been reported from India.[104,105] The high cost and concern about cartilage damage in young children are drawbacks to large-scale quinolone use. Azithromycin has arisen as an alternative for the treatment of certain diarrheal diseases of bacterial origin. A single dose of azithromycin (20 mg/kg) in children with severe cholera in Bangladesh has shown clinical and bacteriologic results comparable to a 3-day regimen with erythromycin.[106] Better clinical and bacteriologic results were observed with single-dose azithromycin in adult patients with severe cholera compared with single-dose ciprofloxacin at the same institution.[107] Advantages of single-dose regimens like this are not only assurance of

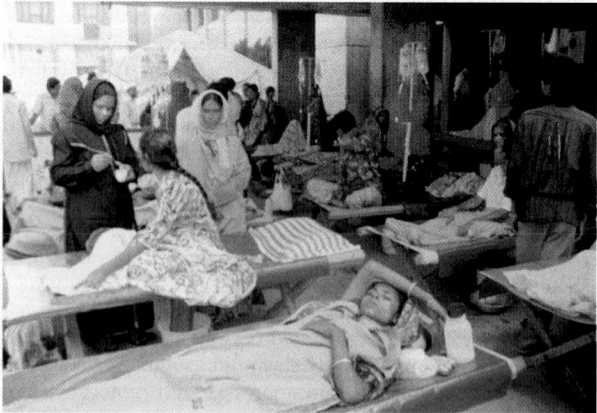

Figure 214-5 Patients with cholera caused by the O139 serogroup of *V. cholerae*. In this photograph, patients were being treated in the parking lot of the International Center for Diarrhoeal Disease Research, Dhaka, Bangladesh. Use of cholera cots, rehydration by the intravenous route of severely dehydrated patients, and rehydration by the oral route with oral rehydration therapy are shown. *(Courtesy of Dr. Wasif Ali Khan, International Center for Diarrhoeal Disease Research, Dhaka, Bangladesh.)*

TABLE 214-5	Antimicrobial Regimens for the Treatment of Cholera	
	Dose	
Drug	*Adult*	*Children*
Tetracycline	500 mg qid for 3 days	50 mg/kg of body weight qid for 3 days
Doxycycline	300 mg as a single dose	Not evaluated
Furazolidone	100 mg qid for 3 days	5 mg/kg/day in four divided doses for 3 days or 7 mg/kg as a single dose
Cotrimoxazole	160 mg of trimethoprim/800 mg of sulfamethoxazole bid for 3 days	8 mg of trimethoprim/40 mg of sulfamethoxazole/kg divided in two doses for 3 days
Norfloxacin	400 mg bid for 3 days	Not recommended
Ciprofloxacin	1 g as a single dose	20 mg/kg of body weight as a single dose
	250 mg/day for 3 days	Dosing regimen not evaluated in children
Azithromycin	1 g as a single dose	20 mg/kg of body weight as a single dose

From Seas C, DuPont HL, Valdez LM, et al. Practical guidelines for the treatment of cholera. *Drugs*. 1996;51:966-973.

compliance, but also the potential reduction of resistance and the appeal for using them under extreme epidemic situations. The use of other drugs, such as antimotility agents (e.g., loperamide, diphenoxylate), adsorbents, analgesics, and antiemetics, is not recommended. The addition of oral zinc (30 mg/day) to an erythromycin regimen in children with cholera in Bangladesh resulted in a 12% reduction in the duration of diarrhea and an 11% decrease in the volume of stools compared with placebo; its incorporation into daily practice was recommended.[108] Chemoprophylaxis of household contacts of cholera cases has been proposed. However, published data do not support this concept.[5,109,110] Moreover, when transmission of the disease is low, as occurs in endemic areas, the usefulness of chemoprophylaxis is not significant.[111] Prophylaxis with antibiotics might be considered in situations in which the rate of transmission of the disease is high, along with other measures to curtail transmission.

Prevention and the Role of Vaccines

John Snow was the first scientist to show that transmission of cholera may be significantly reduced when uncontaminated water is provided to the population. Providing potable water and ensuring proper management of excreta to avoid contamination of other water sources are important measures to reduce cholera transmission. The limited number of indigenous cases reported from the United States and Australia, despite the fact that *Vibrio* is isolated from the environment in these countries, provides further evidence that hygiene and sanitation contain cholera transmission. However, the experience with continuing epidemics in developing countries shows that these simple measures are almost impossible to implement.

Alternative ways to prevent cholera transmission are necessary. Water can be made safer to drink by boiling or adding chlorine. Both methods are expensive and difficult to implement under epidemic situations. Exposing water to sunlight has also been considered, but its implementation is again not feasible in developing countries. Education of the population at risk about appropriate hygienic practices is always recommended, but the impact of massive educational campaigns on the reduction of cholera transmission is questionable. Identification of local customs that place people at risk may help in eliminating such practices. A simple preventive measure derived from better knowledge of the ecologic basis for disease transmission has been proposed by Colwell and colleagues.[112] Sari cloth, a traditional cloth of India and Bangladesh made of cotton, was folded eight times to retain particles larger than 20 μm, including copepods to which *V. cholerae* is attached, and was used to filter water for drinking purposes in the field. A marked reduction in cholera incidence in rural Bangladesh was observed by using this method. Simple measures such as this may be implemented in developing countries, with potential impact on transmission. Predicting the onset of an epidemic may have a tremendous impact on prevention. Searching for *V. cholerae* O1 from municipal sewage and environmental samples in endemic areas is a warning signal of future epidemics, because its detection precedes the occurrence of human cases.[113] The possibility of predicting an epidemic by monitoring the movement of plankton by satellite seems attractive, but more data are needed to support this method.

An inability to implement these measures to curtail cholera transmission has necessitated a search for vaccines. An ideal vaccine against cholera should elicit a fast and long-lasting immune response, with minimal side effects. Additionally, the vaccine should be locally produced and, to increase compliance, a single dose is highly desirable.

The parenteral vaccine once available in the United States had poor efficacy and required boosting every 6 months. That vaccine is no longer available. The disappointing experience with parenteral vaccines and the improved knowledge of the immune response to natural infection that has accumulated during recent years clearly show that an oral route for administering the vaccine is preferred. The ideal vaccine is still not available, but significant progress has been made. Two oral vaccines have been studied in epidemic and endemic settings. The oral inactivated vaccine WC-BS (whole cell plus B subunit) has been more extensively evaluated. Short- and long-term data from a large field trial conducted in Matlab, Bangladesh, have shown protective efficacy of 85% after 6 months, declining to 50% after 3 and 5 years.[114,115] Significant drawbacks were the need of two doses to confer protection, less protection against the El Tor biotype, less protection in children, and less protection in persons with blood group O. Benefits of THS vaccine, apart from its moderate direct protection, are indirect protection (herd immunity) of young infants and other residents in endemic areas,[116-118] and excellent protective efficacy (estimated to be 78%) after mass vaccination in field conditions in Africa, including refugee settings.[119,120] A vaccine with inactivated whole cells of four strains plus recombinant B subunit is available in some countries for adults and children 2 years of age or older, marketed as Dukoral. It is given as two doses 10 to 14 days apart. The vaccine does not reach maximal efficacy until 10 days after the second dose. A killed oral whole-cell cholera vaccine (without the B-subunit component), containing initially only O1 and more recently a reformulated bivalent vaccine (containing both O1 and O139 serogroups, biv-WC), has been produced and used in a national vaccination program in Vietnam[121,122] and has been tested in Kolkata, India.[123]

Another group of oral cholera vaccines is the live attenuated vaccines, especially the third-generation CVD 103–HgR. A live attenuated vaccine derived from reference strain 569B (classic O1, Inaba) is licensed in several countries as Orochol-E. Protective efficacy was achieved after 8 days in a volunteer study. Promising results with this vaccine, even in those with O blood group, were not confirmed when a large field trial was conducted in Jakarta, Indonesia.[124] The field trial showed no benefit from administration of the vaccine.

New vaccine candidates are currently being evaluated, including the live attenuated vaccine Peru-15, which contains El Tor vibrio.[116,125] Potential usefulness of cholera vaccines include use for high-risk persons in endemic areas, vulnerable populations under emergency situations, outbreaks if rapid implementation is feasible, and travelers.[126] A mathematical model has shown that by using the killed whole-cell vaccine, WC-BS, and covering 50% to 70% of the population, it is possible to achieve 89% reduction in cholera incidence in an endemic area.[127] An expert panel convened by the World Health Organization in 2005 recommended the use of oral cholera vaccines for certain endemic situations.[128] More recent statements consider the vaccines as promising strategies, in addition to known public health measures.[5] Current challenges are how to predict new epidemics, detect the appearance of new strains in the environment that may cause epidemics early, and induce lasting protective immunity, irrespective of age and blood group, with a single dose of an oral vaccine. Our understanding of this ancient scourge has improved significantly since the time of John Snow, but the solution remains the same.[129]

REFERENCES

1. Barua D. History of cholera. In: Barua D, Greenough WB, eds. *Cholera.* New York: Plenum Press; 1992:1-36.
2. Barua D. Cholera during the last hundred years (1884-1983). In: Takeda Y, ed. *Vibrio cholerae and Cholera.* Tokyo: KTK Scientific; 1988:9-14.
3. Centers for Disease Control (CDC). Cholera—Peru, 1991. *MMWR Morb Mortal Wkly Rep.* 1991;40:108-110.
4. Griffith DC, Kelly-Hope LA, Miller MA. Review of reported cholera outbreaks worldwide, 1995-2005. *Am J Trop Med Hyg.* 2006;75:973-977.
5. World Health Organization. Cholera. *Wkly Epidemiol Rec.* 2008;83:269-284.
6. Gaffga NH, Tauxe RV, Mintz ED. Cholera: A new homeland in Africa. *Am J Trop Med Hyg.* 2007;77:705-713.
7. Cholera Working Group. International Centre for Diarrhoeal Disease Research, Bangladesh. Large epidemic of cholera-like disease in Bangladesh caused by *Vibrio cholerae* O139 synonym Bengal. *Lancet.* 1993;342:387-390.
8. Hoge CW, Bodhidatta L, Echeverria P, et al. Epidemiologic study of O1 and O139 in Thailand: At the advancing edge of the eighth pandemic. *Am J Epidemiol.* 1996;143:263-268.
9. Boyce TG, Mintz DE, Greene KD, et al. *Vibrio cholerae* O139 Bengal infections among tourists to Southeast Asia: An intercontinental foodborne outbreak. *J Infect Dis.* 1995;172:1401-1404.
10. Cheasty R, Rowe B, Said B, Frost J. *Vibrio cholerae* serogroup O139 in England and Wales. *BMJ.* 1993;307:1007.
11. Swerdlow DL, Ries AA. *Vibrio cholerae* non-O1—the eighth pandemic? *Lancet.* 1993;342:382-383.
12. Alam M, Hasan NA, Sadique A, et al. Seasonal cholera caused by *Vibrio cholerae* serogroup O1 and O139 in the coastal aquatic environment of Bangladesh. *Appl Environ Microbiol.* 2006;72:4096-4104.
13. Stroeher UH, Karageogos LE, Morona R, et al. Serotype conversion in *Vibrio cholerae* O1. *Proc Natl Acad Sci U S A.* 1992;89:2566-2570.

14. Vugia DJ, Rodriguez M, Vargas M, et al. Epidemic cholera in Trujillo, Peru 1992: Utility of a clinical case definition and shift in *Vibrio cholerae* O1 serotype. *Am J Trop Med Hyg.* 1994; 50:566-569.
15. Koelle K, Pascual M, Yunus M. Serotype cycles in cholera dynamics. *Proc Biol Sci.* 2006;273:2879-2886.
16. Karaolis DK, Lan R, Reeves PR. The sixth and seventh cholera pandemics are due to independent clones separately derived from environmental nontoxigenic non-O1 *Vibrio cholerae. J Bacteriol.* 1995;177:3191-3198.
17. Ansaruzzaman M, Bhuiyan NA, Safa A, et al. Genetic diversity of El Tor strains of *Vibrio cholerae* O1 with hybrid traits isolated from Bangladesh and Mozambique. *Int J Med Microbiol.* 2007;297:443-449.
18. Faruque SM, Sack DA, Sack RB, et al. Emergence and evolution of *Vibrio cholerae* O139. *Proc Natl Acad Sci U S A.* 2003;100: 1304-1309.
19. Faruque SM, Islam MJ, Ahmed QS, et al. An improved technique for isolation of environmental *Vibrio cholerae* with epidemic potential: Monitoring the emergence of a multiple antibiotic-resistant epidemic strain in Bangladesh. *J Infect Dis.* 2006; 193:1029-1036.
20. Khuntia HK, Pal BB, Chhotray GP. Quadruplex PCR for simultaneous detection of serotype, biotype, toxigenic potential, and central regulating factor of *Vibrio cholerae. J Clin Microbiol.* 2008;46:2399-2401.
21. Tarr CL, Patel JS, Puhr ND, et al. Identification of *Vibrio* isolates by multiplex PCR assay and *rpo*B sequence determination. *J Clin Microbiol.* 2007;45:134-140.
22. Fykse EM, Skogan G, Davies W, et al. Detection of *Vibrio cholerae* by real-time nucleic acid sequence-based amplification. *Appl Environ Microbiol.* 2007;73:1457-1466.
23. Wang XY, Ansaruzzaman M, Vaz R, et al. Field evaluation of a rapid immunochromatographic dipstick test for the diagnosis of cholera in a high-risk population. *BMC Infect Dis.* 2006; 6:17.
24. Cash RA, Music SI, Libonati JP, et al. Response of man to infection with *Vibrio cholerae.* 1. Clinical, serologic, and bacteriologic responses to a known inoculum. *J Infect Dis.* 1974;129:45-52.
25. De SN. Enterotoxicity of bacteria-free culture filtrate of *Vibrio cholerae. Nature.* 1959;183:1533-1534.
26. Dutta NK, Panse MW, Kulkarni DR. Role of cholera toxin in experimental cholera. *J Bacteriol.* 1959;78:594-595.
27. Finkelstein RA, LoSpalluto JJ. Pathogenesis of experimental cholera: Preparation and isolation of choleragen and choleragenoid. *J Exp Med.* 1969;130:185-202.
28. Heidelberg JF, Eisen JA, Nelson WC, et al. DNA sequence of both chromosomes of the cholera pathogen *Vibrio cholerae. Nature.* 2000;406:477-483.
29. Faruque SM, Rahman MM, Waldor MK, et al. Sunlight-induced propagation of the lysogenic phage encoding cholera toxin. *Infect Immun.* 2000;68:4795-4801.
30. Zuckerman JN, Rombo L, Fisch A. The true burden and risk of cholera: Implications for prevention and control. *Lancet Infect Dis.* 2007;7:521-530.
31. Kaper JB, Morris JG, Levine MM. Cholera. *J Clin Microbiol Rev.* 1995;8:48-86.
32. Colwell RR, Huq A: Vibrios in the environment: Viable but nonculturable *Vibrio cholerae.* In: Wachsmuth IK, Blake PA, Olsvik O, eds. *Vibrio cholerae and Cholera: Molecular to Global Perspectives.* Washington DC: ASM Press; 1994:117-134.
33. Huq A, Small EB, West PA, et al. Ecology of *Vibrio cholerae* O1 with special reference to planktonic crustacean copepods. *Appl Environ Microbiol.* 1983;45:275-283.
34. Huq A, West PA, Small EB, et al. Influence of water temperature, salinity, and pH on survival and growth of toxigenic *Vibrio cholerae* serovar O1 associated with live copepods in laboratory microcosms. *Appl Environ Microbiol.* 1983;48:420-424.
35. Huq A, Colwell RR, Rahman R, et al. Detection of *Vibrio cholerae* O1 in the aquatic environment by fluorescent-monoclonal antibody and culture methods. *Appl Environm Microbiol.* 1990;56:2370-2373.
36. Colwell RR, Tamplin ML, Brayton PR, et al. Environmental aspects of *Vibrio cholerae* in transmission of cholera. In: Sack RB, Zinnaka Y, eds. *Advances in Research on Cholera and Related Diarrheas.* Vol. 7. Tokyo: KTK Scientific; 1990:327-333.
37. Rice EW, Johnson CJ, Clark RM, et al. Chlorine and survival of rugose *Vibrio cholerae. Lancet.* 1992;340:740.
38. Faruque SM, Biswas K, Udden SM, et al. Transmissibility of cholera: In vivo formed biofilms and their realtionship to infectivity and persistence in the environment. *Proc Natl Acad Sci U S A.* 2008;103:6350-6355.
39. Hartley DM, Morris JG, Smith D. Hyperinfectivity: A critical element in the ability of *V. cholerae* to cause epidemics? *PLoS Med.* 2006;3:e7.
40. Nelson EJ, Chowdhury A, Harris JB, et al. Complexity of rice-water stool from patients with Vibrio cholerae plays a role in the transmission of infectious diarrhea. *Proc Natl Acad Sci U S A.* 2007;104:19091-19096.
41. Gotuzzo E, Cieza J, Estremadoyro L, et al. Cholera: Lessons from the epidemic in Peru. *Infect Dis Clin North Am.* 1994;8: 183-205.
42. Goma Epidemiology Group. Public health impact of Rwandan refugee crisis: What happened in Goma, Zaire, in July 1994? *Lancet.* 1995;345:339-344.
43. Ries AA, Vugia DJ, Beingolea L, et al. Cholera in Piura, Peru: A modern urban epidemic. *J Infect Dis.* 1992;166:1429-1433.
44. Bompangue D, Giraudoux P, Handschumacher P, et al. Lakes as source of cholera outbreaks, Democratic Republic of Congo. *Emerg Infect Dis.* 2008;14:798-800.
45. Swerdlow DL, Malenga G, Begkoyian G, et al. Epidemic cholera among refugees in Malawi Africa: Treatment and transmission. *Epidemiol Infect.* 1997;118:207-214.
46. Swerdlow DL, Mintz ED, Rodriguez M, et al. Waterborne transmission of epidemic cholera in Trujillo, Peru: Lessons for a continent at risk. *Lancet.* 1992;340:28-33.
47. Deb BC, Sircar BK, Sengupta PG, et al. Studies on intervention to prevent El Tor cholera transmission in urban slums. *Bull World Health Organ.* 1986;64:127-131.
48. Kolvin JL, Roberts D. Studies on the growth of *Vibrio cholerae* biotype El Tor and biotype classical in foods. *J Hyg.* 1982; 89:243-252.
49. Gunnlaugsson G, Einarsdottir J, Angulo FJ, et al. Funerals during the 1994 cholera epidemic in Guinea-Bissau, West Africa: The need for disinfection of bodies of persons dying of cholera. *Epidemiol Infect.* 1998;120:7-15.
50. St Louis ME, Porter JD, Helal A, et al. Epidemic cholera in West Africa: The role of food handling and high-risk foods. *Am J Epidemiol.* 1990;131:719-728.
51. Mhalu FS, Mtango EDE, Msengi AE. Hospital outbreaks of cholera transmitted through close person-to-person contact. *Lancet.* 1984;2:82-84.
52. Cliff JL, Zinkin P, Martelli A. A hospital outbreak of cholera in Maputo, Mozambique. *Trans R Soc Trop Med Hyg.* 1986; 80:473-476.
53. Mosley WH, Alvero MG, Joseph PR, et al. Studies of cholera El Tor in the Philippines. 4. Transmission of infection among neighborhood and community contacts of cholera patients. *Bull World Health Organ.* 1965;33:651-660.
54. Glass RI, Becker S, Huq MI, et al. Endemic cholera in rural Bangladesh, 1966-1980. *Am J Epidemiol.* 1982;116:959-970.
55. Seas C, Gotuzzo E. Cholera: Overview of epidemiologic, therapeutic, and preventive issues learned from recent epidemics. *Int J Infect Dis.* 1996;1:37-40.
56. Emch M, Feldacker C, Islam MS, et al. Seasonality of cholera from 1974 to 2005: A review of global patterns. *Int J Health Geogr.* 2008;7:31.
57. Lipp EK, Huq A, Colwell RR. Effects of global climate on infectious disease: The cholera model. *Clin Microbiol Rev.* 2002; 15:757-770.
58. Pascual M, Rodó X, Ellner SP, et al. Cholera dynamics and El Niño-Southern Oscillation. *Science.* 2000;289:1766-1769.
59. Rodó X, Pascual M, Fuchs G, et al. ENSO and cholera: A non-stationary link related to climate change? *Proc Natl Acad Sci U S A.* 2002;99:12901-12906.
60. Koelle K, Rodó X, Pacual M, et al. Refractory periods and climate forcing in cholera dynamics. *Nature.* 2005;436:696-700.
61. Salazar-Lindo E, Seas C, Gutierrez D. The ENSO and cholera in South America: What we can learn about it from the 1991 cholera outbreak. *Int J Environ Health.* 2008;2:30-36.
62. Emch M, Feldacker C, Yunus M, et al. Local environmental predictors of cholera in Bangladesh and Vietnam. *Am J Trop Med Hyg.* 2008;78:823-832.
63. Constantin de Magny G, Guegan JF, Petit M, et al. Regional-scale climate-variability synchrony of cholera epidemics in West Africa. *BMC Infect Dis.* 2007;7:20.
64. Seas C, Miranda J, Gil AI, et al. New insights on the emergence of cholera in Latin America during 1991: The Peruvian experience. *Am J Trop Med Hyg.* 2000;62:513-517.
65. Jensen MA, Faruque SM, Mekalanos JJ, et al. Modeling the role of bacteriophage in the control of cholera outbreaks. *Proc Natl Acad Sci U S A.* 2006;103:4652-4657.
66. Schwartz BS, Harris JB, Khan AI, et al. Diarrheal epidemics in Dhaka, Bangladesh, during three consecutive floods: 1988, 1998 and 2004. *Am J Trop Med Hyg.* 2006:74:1067-1073.
67. Clemens J, Albert MJ, Rao M, et al. Impact of infection by *Helicobacter pylori* on the risk and severity of endemic cholera. *J Infect Dis.* 1995;171:1653-1656.
68. Taylor DN, Blaser MJ. The epidemiology of *Helicobacter pylori* infection. *Epidemiol Rev.* 1991;13:42-59.
69. León-Barúa R, Recavarren-Arce S, Chinga-Alayo E, et al. *Helicobacter pylori*-associated chronic atrophic gastritis involving the gastric body and severe disease by *Vibrio cholerae. Trans R Soc Trop Med Hyg.* 2006;100:567-572.
70. Harris JB, Khan AI, LaRocque RC, et al. Blood group, immunity, and risk of infection with Vibrio cholerae in an area of endemicity. *Infect Immun.* 2005;73:7422-7427.
71. Qureshi K, Molbak K, Sandstrom A, et al. Breast milk reduces the risk of illness in children of mothers with cholera. *Pedaitr Infect Dis J.* 2006;25:1163-1166.
72. Rogers RC, Cuffe RG, Cossins YM, et al. The Queensland cholera incident of 1977. 2. The epidemiological investigation. *Bull World Health Organ.* 1980;58:665-669.
73. Johnston JM, Martin DL, Perdue J, et al. Cholera on a Gulf Coast oil rig. *N Engl J Med.* 1983;309:523-526.
74. Blake PA, Allegra DT, Snyder JD, et al. Cholera—a possible endemic focus in the United States. *N Engl J Med.* 1980; 302:305-309.
75. Sack RB, Siddique AK, Longini IM, et al. A 4-year study of the epidemiology of Vibrio cholerae in four rural areas of Bangladesh. *J Infect Dis.* 2003;187:96-101.
76. Emch M. Diarrhoeal disease risk in Matlab, Bangladesh. *Soc Sci Med.* 1999;49:519-530.
77. Greenough WB III. *Vibrio cholerae* and cholera. In: Mandell GL, Douglas JE, Dolin R, eds. *Principles and Practice of Infectious Diseases.* 4th ed. New York: Churchill Livingstone; 1995: 1934-1945.
78. Bennish ML, Azad AK, Rahman O, et al. Hypoglycemia during diarrhea: Prevalence, pathophysiology and therapy in Asiatic cholera. *N Engl J Med.* 1990;322:1357-1363.
79. Mahalanabis D, Wallace CK, Kallen RJ, et al. Water and electrolyte losses due to cholera in infants and small children: A recovery balance study. *Pediatrics.* 1970;45:374-385.
80. Hirschhorn N, Chowdhury AK, Lindenbaum J. Cholera in pregnant women. *Lancet.* 1969;1:1230-1232.
81. Cieza J, Sovero Y, Estremadoyro L, et al. Electrolyte disturbances in elderly patients with severe diarrhea due to cholera. *J Am Soc Nephrol.* 1995;6:1463-1467.
82. von Seidlien L, Wang XY, Macuamule A, et al. Is HIV infection associated with an increased risk for cholera? Findings from a case-control study in Mozambique. *Trop Med Int Health.* 2008;13:683-688.
83. Piarroux R. Management of cholera epidemic by a humanitarian organization. *Med Trop.* 2002;62:361-367.
84. Kakar F, Ahmadzai AH, Habib N, et al. A successful response to an aoutbreak of cholera in Afghanistan. *Trop Doct.* 2008; 38:17-20.
85. World Health Organization. *Guidelines for Cholera Control.* Geneva: World Health Organization; 1992.
86. Bennish ML: Cholera: Pathophysiology, clinical features, and treatment. In: Wachsmuth IK, Blake PA, Olsvik O, eds. *Vibrio cholerae and Cholera: Molecular to Global Perspectives.* Washington, DC: ASM Press; 1994:229-255.
87. Seas C, DuPont HL, Valdez LM, et al. Practical guidelines for the treatment of cholera. *Drugs.* 1996;51:966-973.
88. World Health Organization. *Reduced Osmolarity Rehydration Salts (ORS) Formulation.* New York: UNICEF House; 2001.
89. Hahn S, Kim Y, Garner P. Reduced osmolarity oral rehydration solution for treating dehydration due to diarrhoea in children: Systematic review. *BMJ.* 2001;323:81-85.
90. Alam NH, Yunus M, Faruque ASG, et al. Symptomatic hyponatremia during treatment of dehydrating diarrheal disease with reduced osmolarity oral rehydration solution. *JAMA.* 2006; 296:567-573.
91. Rabbani GH, Sack DA, Ahmed S, et al. Antidiarrheal effects of L-histidine–supplemented rice-based oral rehydration solution in the treatment of male adults with severe cholera in Bangladesh: A double-blind, randomized trial. *J Infect Dis.* 2005; 191:1507-1514.
92. Ramakrishna BS, Subramanian V, Mohan V, et al. A randomized controlled trial of glucose versus amylase-resistant starch hypo-osmolar oral rehydration solution for adult acute dehydrating diarrhea. *PLoS ONE.* 2008;3:e1587.
93. Ryan ET, Dhar U, Khan WA, et al. Mortality, morbidity, and microbiology of endemic cholera among hospitalized patients in Dhaka, Bangladesh. *Am J Trop Med Hyg.* 2000; 63:12-20.
94. Quick RE, Vargas R, Moreno D, et al. Epidemic cholera in the Amazon: The challenge of preventing death. *Am J Trop Med Hyg.* 1993;48:597-602.
95. Dhar U, Bennish ML, Khan WA, et al. Clinical features, antimicrobial susceptibility and toxin production in *Vibrio cholerae* O139 infection: Comparison with *Vibrio cholerae* O1 infection. *Trans R Soc Trop Med Hyg.* 1996;90:402-405.
96. Greenough WB III, Gordon RS, Rosenberg IS, et al. Tetracycline in the treatment of cholera. *Lancet.* 1964;1:355-377.
97. Alam AN, Alam NH, Ahmed T, et al. Randomized double-blind trial of single dose doxycycline for treating cholera in adults. *BMJ.* 1990;300:1619-1621.
98. Faruque ASG, Alam K, Malek MA, et al. Emergence of multi-drug-resistant strain of *Vibrio cholerae* O1 in Bangladesh and reversal of their susceptibility after two years. *J Health Popul Nutr.* 2007;25:241-243.
99. Okeke IN, Aboderin OA, Byarugaba DK, et al. Growing problem of multidrug-resistant enteric pathogens in Africa. *Emerg Infect Dis.* 2007;13:1640-1646.
100. Seas C, Gotuzzo E. Recent advances in the treatment and prophylaxis of cholera. *Curr Opin Infect Dis.* 1996;9:380-384.
101. Gotuzzo E, Seas C, Echevarriá J, et al. Ciprofloxacin for the treatment of cholera: A randomized, double-blind, controlled trial of a single daily dose in Peruvian adults. *Clin Infect Dis.* 1995;20:1485-1490.
102. Khan WA, Bennish ML, Seas C, et al. Randomized controlled comparison of single-dose ciprofloxacin and doxycycline for cholera caused by *Vibrio cholerae* O1 or O139. *Lancet.* 1996;348:296-300.
103. Saha D, Khan WA, Karim MM, et al. Single-dose cirprofloxacin versus 12-dose erythromycin for childhood cholera: A randomized controlled trial. *Lancet.* 2005;366:1085-1093.
104. Jesudason MV, Balaji V, Thomson CJ. Quinolone susceptibility of *Vibrio cholerae* O1 and O1139 isolates from Vellore. *Ind J Med Res.* 2002;116:96-98.
105. Krisna BVS, Patl AB, Chandrasekhar MR. Fluoroquinolone-resistant *Vibrio cholerae* isoalted during a cholera outbreak in India. *Trans R Soc Trop Med Hyg.* 2006;100:224-226.
106. Khan WA, Saha D, Rahman A, et al. Comparison of single-dose azithromycin and 12-dose, 3-day erythromycin for childhood cholera: A randomized, double-blind trial. *Lancet.* 2002; 360:1722-1727.

107. Saha D, Karim MM, Khan WA, et al. Single-dose azithromycin for the treatment of cholera in adults. *N Eng J Med.* 2006; 354:2452-2462.

108. Roy SK, Hossain MJ, Khatun W, et al. Zinc supplementation in children with cholera in Bangladesh: Randomised controlled trial. *BMJ.* 2008;336:266-268.

109. Ghosh S, Sengupta PG, Gupta DN, et al. Chemoprophylaxis studies in cholera: A review of selective works. *J Commun Dis.* 1992;24:55-57.

110. Sack DA, Sack RB, Chaignat CL. Getting serious about cholera. *N Eng J Med.* 2006;355:649-651.

111. Echevarria J, Seas C, Carrillo C, et al. Efficacy and tolerability of ciprofloxacin prophylaxis in adult household contacts of patients with cholera. *Clin Infect Dis.* 1995;20:1480-1484.

112. Colwell RR, Huq A, Islam MS, et al. Reduction of cholera in Bangladeshi villages by simple filtration. *Proc Natl Acad Sci U S A.* 2003;100:1051-1055.

113. Franco AA, Fix AD, Prada A, et al. Cholera in Lima, Peru, correlates with prior isolation of *Vibrio cholerae* from the environment. *Am J Epidemiol.* 1997;146:1067-1075.

114. Clemens JD, Sack DA, Harris JR, et al. Field trial of oral cholera vaccines in Bangladesh: Results from three-year follow-up. *Lancet.* 1990;335:270-273.

115. Van Loon FP, Clemens JD, Chakraborty J, et al. Field trial of inactivated oral cholera vaccines in Bangladesh: Results from 5 years of follow-up. *Vaccine.* 1996;14:162-166.

116. Lopez Al, Clemens JD, Deen J, et al. Cholera vaccines for the developing countries. *Hum Vaccin.* 2008;4:165-169.

117. Ali M, Emch M, von Seidlein L, et al. Herd immunity conferred by killed oral cholera vaccines in Bangladesh: A reanalysis. *Lancet.* 2005;366:44-49.

118. Ali M, Emch M, Yunus M, et al. Vaccine protection of Bangladeshi infants and young children against cholera. *Pediatr Infect Dis J.* 2008;27:33-37.

119. Lucas ME, Deen JL, von Seidlein L, et al. Effectivenes of mass cholera vaccination in Beira, Mozambique. *N Engl J Med.* 2005;352:757-767.

120. von Seidlein L. Vaccines for cholera control: Does herd immunity play a role? *PLoS Med.* 2007;4:e331.

121. Thiem VD, Deen JL, von Seidlein L, et al. Long-term effectiveness against cholera of oral killed whole-cell vaccine produced in Vietnam. *Vaccine.* 2006;24:4297-4303.

122. Anh DD, Canh DG, Lopez AL, et al. Safety and immunogenicity of a reformulated Vietnamese bivalent killed, whole cell, oral cholera vaccine in adults. *Vaccine.* 2007;25:1149-1155.

123. Mahalanabis D, Lopez AL, Sur D, et al. A randomized, placebo-controlled trial of bivalent killed, whole-cell, oral cholera vaccine in adults and children in a cholera endemic area in Kolkata, India. *PLoS ONE.* 2008;3:e2323.

124. Richie EE, Punjabi NH, Sidharta YY, et al. Efficacy trial of a single-dose live oral cholera vaccine CVD 103-HgR in North Jakarta, Indonesia, a cholera-endemic area. *Vaccine.* 2000;18:2399-2410.

125. Qadri F, Chowdhury MI, Faruque SM, et al. Peru-15, a live attenuated oral cholera vaccine, is safe and immunogenic in Bangladeshi todlers and infants. *Vaccine.* 2007;25:231-238.

126. Calain P, Chaine JP, Johnson E, et al. Can oral cholera vaccination play a role in controlling a cholera outbreak? *Vaccine.* 2004;22:2444-2451.

127. Longini IM, Nizam A, Ali M, et al. Controlling endemic holera with oral vaccines. *PLoS Med.* 2007;4:e336.

128. World Health Organization. Global Task Force on Cholera Control. Oral Cholera Vaccines Use in Complex Emergencies. What Next? Report: Who Meeting, 14-16 December 2005, Cairo, Egypt. Available at <http://www.who.int/cholera/publications/cholera_vaccines_ emergencies_2005.pdf>.

129. Seas C, Gotuzzo E. *Vibrio cholerae* (cholera). In: Yu VL, Rainer W, Raoult D, eds. *Antimicrobial Therapy and Vaccines. vol 1: Microbes.* New York: Apple Trees Productions; 2002:763-772.

215

Other Pathogenic Vibrios

MARGUERITE A. NEILL | CHARLES C. J. CARPENTER

In addition to *Vibrio cholerae* O1 and *Campylobacter fetus* (formerly known as *Vibrio fetus*), three additional major groups of vibrios have been clearly associated with human disease. These include the following: the halophilic vibrios *V. parahaemolyticus* and *V. vulnificus*, of which the epidemiologic and clinical features are well delineated; other halophilic vibrios, including *V. alginolyticus*, *V. fluvialis*, *V. hollisae* (now *Grimontia hollisae*), *V. damsela* (now *Photobacterium damsela*), *V. furnissii*, *V. metschnikovii*, and *V. cincinnatiensis*, which are less common causes of human disease; and the nonhalophilic non-O1 *V. cholerae* and *V. mimicus*, which are worldwide in distribution and have frequently been incriminated in human illness.

Vibrio species are ubiquitous in estuarine waters in the temperate zones. Plankton blooms and temperature upshifting in the spring are followed by rapid outgrowth of most vibrios. Molluscan shellfish, which are filter feeders, acquire vibrios as part of their normal microflora during the warmer months. Shellfish contamination thus occurs as a consequence of the normal climate-associated changes in vibrio prevalence in coastal waters rather than as a result of sewage contamination of shellfish beds.

In the United States, illnesses caused by the commonly isolated pathogenic vibrios have a marked seasonal peak, with more than 90% of cases occurring between April and October. This presumably reflects both foodborne and non-foodborne acquisition of infection as a result of seasonal changes in shellfish consumption, recreational water exposure, and the increase in densities of vibrios in marine waters during the warmer months.

Vibrio parahaemolyticus

Vibrio parahaemolyticus, a halophilic (salt-requiring) vibrio, has long been recognized as a major cause of acute diarrheal disease in Japan.[1] In the United States, *V. parahaemolyticus* was the most commonly isolated vibrio species over a 13-year period in Florida[2] and the most common of the speciated vibrios reported over 25 years in Louisiana.[3] This pathogen was the most common bacterial cause of foodborne disease in Taiwan, accounting for 35% of all outbreaks[4] and, in less developed countries, it has been incriminated in up to 20% of acute diarrheal illnesses. A specific serotype, *V. parahaemolyticus* O3:K6, emerged as an important cause of human illness in southeast Asia[5] and, since 1996, has become established globally by a pandemic clone.[6] In 1998, this serotype first appeared in the United States,[7] causing a large multistate outbreak that prompted regulatory changes in programs for bacteriologic monitoring of shellfish.[8] In 2004, an outbreak of gastroenteritis caused by serotype O6:K18 was traced to raw oysters from the Gulf of Alaska, harvested when the water temperature was higher than 15°C.[9] Whether global warming trends will portend locally acquired *V. parahaemolyticus* infection, even at high northern latitudes, emphasizes the need for surveillance and appropriate diagnostics, a recurring theme in emerging infectious diseases.

Enteric illness caused by *V. parahaemolyticus* comprises a broad spectrum of clinical manifestations ranging from mild watery diarrhea to a frank, dysentery-like syndrome. As suggested by the clinical disease as well as by experimental studies in animals, *V. parahaemolyticus* has the capacities both to produce an enterotoxin and to cause an inflammatory reaction in the small bowel mucosa. Major degrees of intestinal fluid loss are seldom seen, and the tissue damage caused by this halophilic vibrio is generally less extensive than that observed in shigellosis. Two hemolysins, thermostable direct hemolysin (TDH) and TDH-related hemolysin (TRH), have been characterized and have enterotoxin activity; strains negative for TDH and TRH are usually nonvirulent.

The genome of *V. parahaemolyticus* has been sequenced.[10] Like *V. cholerae*, *V. parahaemolyticus* has two circular chromosomes, but unlike *V. cholerae*, a type III secretion system has been found on each of the two chromosomes of *V. parahaemolyticus*.[11] Type III secretion systems permit direct injection of bacterial proteins into the cytoplasm of host cells, a feature shared by enteropathogenic *E. coli*, shigellae, and salmonellae. This finding likely underlies the inflammatory diarrhea seen in *V. parahaemolyticus*, but not *V. cholerae*, infection, and suggests distinctly different mechanisms for diarrhea from these two pathogenic vibrios.

EPIDEMIOLOGY

Because of lack of specificity of the clinical features of the illness, the epidemiologic history usually provides the most important clue to diagnosis. The halophilic *V. parahaemolyticus* is ubiquitous in coastal waters,[1] although this pathogen typically is not recovered from estuarine waters during winter months in temperate zones. During periods of low temperature or nutrient deprivation, it enters a viable but nonculturable state.[12] *Acanthamoeba castellanii* has been noted to support the survival of *V. parahaemolyticus* but this protozoan does not internalize the pathogen and apparently secretes a factor that supports a dormant phase.[13]

Consumption of raw or undercooked shellfish is the most common means of acquiring *V. parahaemolyticus* infection. In the United States, raw oysters are the most common vehicle.[14] In a microbiologic survey of oysters harvested from U.S. waters, the frequency of *V. parahaemolyticus* contamination was consistently greater than that for *V. vulnificus*.[15] Inadequately cooked seafood can harbor small numbers of surviving vibrios, as can food contaminated by seawater on ships. *V. parahaemolyticus* can proliferate rapidly to reach high colony counts in contaminated foods held at ambient temperature for a few hours. This presumably contributes to the high attack rate seen in common source outbreaks.

Person-to-person transmission has not been documented, suggesting that the infective dose for normal persons is relatively high. *Vibrio parahaemolyticus* has rarely been cultured from asymptomatic people, and no carrier state has been identified. There is no known mammalian reservoir of infection.

CLINICAL MANIFESTATIONS

Gastroenteritis is the most common clinical illness associated with *V. parahaemolyticus* infection; wound infections and septicemia may be seen, but much less frequently.[2,3] Enteric illness commonly begins with the acute onset of explosive watery diarrhea generally within 24 to 72 hours of ingestion of the contaminated seafood. Often, the diarrhea is accompanied by mild to moderately severe cramping and abdominal pain; low-grade fever, mild chills, and headache occur in less than half of cases. The fluid loss is rarely severe enough to cause decreased skin turgor or postural hypotension. Deaths caused by *V. parahaemolyticus* are rare, usually occurring in very young children, older adults, or persons with underlying disease.

LABORATORY FINDINGS

The diarrheal fluid is characteristically watery, sometimes mucoid, and occasionally bloody (less than 15%). Fecal leukocytes are often present. *Vibrio parahaemolyticus* is a pleomorphic gram-negative rod that is a facultative anaerobe. It grows poorly on the standard desoxycholate culture plates but is readily identified on the selective thiosulfate citrate bile salts sucrose (TCBS) agar, on which it appears as a distinct opaque green colony. Final identification is made by standard biochemical tests.[15] Enrichment cultures of fecal specimens using hypertonic saline media can be especially useful for epidemiologic investigation. Almost all clinical isolates of *V. parahaemolyticus* cause β-hemolysis of human erythrocytes (the Kanagawa reaction), which is caused by the production of TDH, noted earlier as also having enterotoxin activity.[16] Interestingly, growth in a bile salt–containing environment has been shown to enhance the expression of several virulence traits in *V. parahaemolyticus*.[17]

The immune response in patients with *V. parahaemolyticus* enteric infection has been described.[18] Both serum and coproantibody responses to lipopolysaccharide and to TDH were detected. Mucosal biopsies from the duodenum and rectum showed inflammatory changes in both, suggesting that the small and large intestines are affected. Tumor necrosis factor-α (TNF-α) levels were noted to be elevated acutely in *V. parahaemolyticus* infection, similar to what has been observed in shigellosis and in contrast to cholera infections, in which TNF-α is not elevated.

DIFFERENTIAL DIAGNOSIS

Because *V. parahaemolyticus* is ubiquitous in coastal waters throughout the temperate and tropical zones of the world, this pathogen must be considered in the differential diagnosis of all acute diarrheal illnesses that follow the ingestion of seafood. There are no clinical features that, in the individual case, reliably distinguish diarrhea caused by *V. parahaemolyticus* from that caused by enterotoxigenic *Escherichia coli* or from milder cases of shigellosis or salmonellosis. Vomiting is characteristically less prominent than in disease caused by staphylococcal enterotoxin, and the cramping abdominal pain is generally less severe than that typical of food poisoning caused by *Clostridium perfringens*.

TREATMENT

No treatment is required by most patients because the gastroenteritis is usually self-limited. However, antimicrobial therapy could be considered for those patients with diarrhea lasting longer than 5 days[19] Therapy with a tetracycline or quinolone would be expected to shorten the clinical course and duration of pathogen excretion. Antiperistaltic agents are of no clear-cut benefit. Occasional patients, usually at the extremes of age, may lose sufficient quantities of fluid to require oral or intravenous electrolyte therapy. In such cases, therapy is guided by the same principles used for the treatment of cholera.

PREVENTION

Because the illness usually results from the ingestion of raw or inadequately cooked seafood or food that has been rinsed with contaminated seawater, simple means of prevention are available. *Vibrio parahaemolyticus* can remain viable in shrimp or crab meat for several minutes at temperatures as high as 80°C, and it is especially important when cooking large quantities of such foods to ensure that all portions of the seafood are exposed to cooking temperatures adequate to kill the microorganism. Of only slightly less importance is the necessity of refrigerating cooked seafood if it is not to be eaten immediately after cooking. Shipboard outbreaks can obviously be prevented by avoiding the use of untreated seawater in galleys or by adequate refrigeration of cooked seafood until it is served. The use of irradiation at a dose of 3.0 kGy can reduce *V. parahaemolyticus* levels by 6 logs without killing the oysters or adversely affecting their organoleptic qualities[20]; however, lower doses may not inactivate viruses.

Prevention of disease caused by *V. parahaemolyticus* in Japan remains a problem because of the popularity of uncooked seafood in that nation. In delta areas such as Bangladesh, in which people have daily contact with contaminated water, there is little likelihood of altering the incidence of *V. parahaemolyticus* infections in the foreseeable future.

It is not known whether protective immunity is conferred by clinical infection. No effective vaccine is currently available.

Vibrio vulnificus

Like other potentially pathogenic halophilic vibrios, *V. vulnificus* is part of the normal marine flora and, in the temperate zones, reaches sufficient concentrations to cause clinical illness only in the warmer months of the year. Almost all oysters harvested in the summer from the Chesapeake Bay contain this pathogen, as do 10% of crabs. This pathogen was the most common *Vibrio* species isolated from human cases in Louisiana over 25 years; the annual number of cases tripled while those caused by *V. parahaemolyticus* stayed the same.[3] In the United States, 25% of all vibrio infections were from a nonfoodborne source and *V. vulnificus* was the most common species isolated in this setting; almost half of all *V. vulnificus* infections were non-foodborne.[21] Following Hurricane Katrina in 2005, 18 cases of wound infection caused by vibrios were reported, 14 (82%) caused by *V. vulnificus*, with 3 deaths.[22] Infections from *V. vulnificus* may be increasing in the United States, particularly in association with Gulf Coast oyster consumption,[23] and warmer water temperatures (higher than 22°C) in the Gulf of Mexico may be contributing in part to the increase. The case-fatality rate of 25% is the highest among infections caused by the *Vibrio* species and *V. vulnificus* is estimated to account for 90% of all seafood-related deaths in the United States. Hippocrates may have provided the first description of a *V. vulnificus* infection in the 5th century BC; he described the rapid progression of a severe foot cellulitis with black blisters in Criton of Thasos, which was fatal in 48 hours.[24]

CLINICAL MANIFESTATIONS

Vibrio vulnificus is the most virulent of the noncholera vibrios. It is primarily associated with a severe, distinctive soft tissue infection and/or septicemia, rather than diarrheal illness.[25,26] In compromised hosts, especially patients with cirrhosis, *V. vulnificus* has the ability to invade the bloodstream without causing gastrointestinal symptoms. The clinical picture is one of abrupt onset of chills and fever, often (in 33% of cases) followed by hypotension, usually (in 75%) followed by the development of metastatic cutaneous lesions within 36 hours after onset. These begin as erythematous lesions and rapidly evolve to hemorrhagic bullae or vesicles and then to necrotic ulcers (Fig. 215-1). *V. vulnificus* bacteremia has been fatal in over 50% of patients in whom this syndrome has been identified, including all patients in whom hypotension developed.[26] More than 90% of such patients had a history of having consumed raw oysters in the 7 days prior to illness onset; concentrations of *V. vulnificus* of 10^3 colony-forming units (CFU)/g of oysters have produced illness. Although oysters harbor genetically heterogeneous populations of *V. vulnificus*, only one strain type has been recovered from human tissues in invasive infections.[27] In addition to cirrhosis, other risk factors for the septicemic form of *V. vulnificus* infection include liver disease, iron overload states such as hemochromatosis, hemolytic anemia or chronic renal failure, malignancy, human immunodeficiency virus (HIV) infection, and immunosuppressive medications. In chronic alcoholics undergoing treatment for substance abuse, reduced levels of glutathione correlated with decreased cytokine production by peripheral blood mononuclear cells after exposure in vitro to *V. vulnificus*.[28] Such a weak cytokine response likely contributes to the poor bloodstream clearance and resulting high frequency of bacteremia in *V. vulnificus* infections.

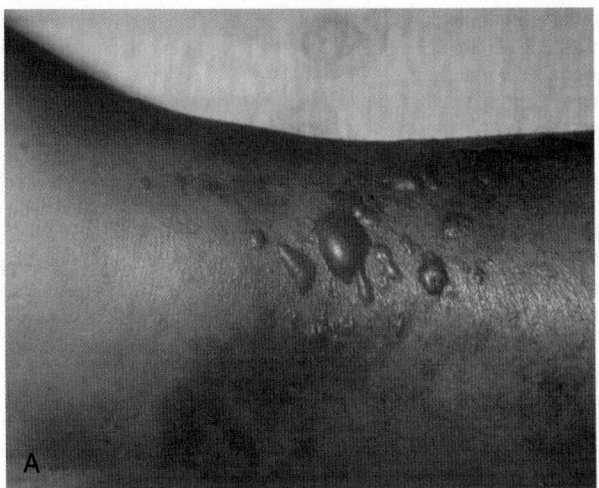
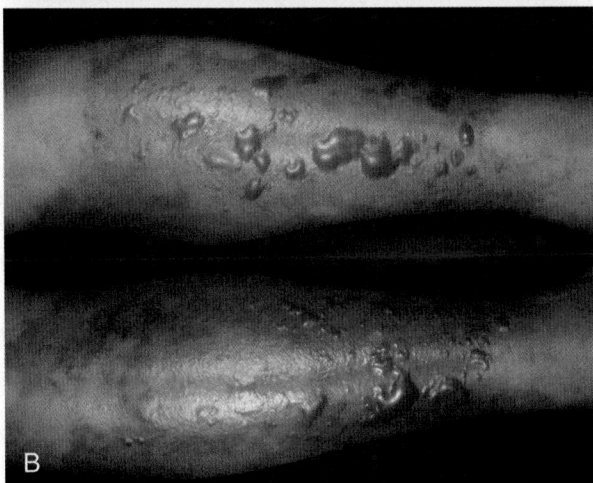

Figure 215-1 Cellulitis (A) and hemorrhagic bullae (B) in *Vibrio vulnificus* infection. *(From Centers for Disease Control and Prevention [CDC]. Vibrio illnesses after Hurricane Katrina—multiple states, August-September, 2005. MMWR Morb Mortal Wkly Rep. 2005;54:928-931; reprinted with permission from Logical Images.)*

After contamination of a superficial wound by warm seawater, *V. vulnificus* can cause a rapidly developing, intense cellulitis, necrotizing vasculitis, and ulcer formation in both healthy persons and compromised hosts, and bacteremia is frequent. In one case, *V. vulnificus* apparently survived on intact skin for more than 24 hours after handling tilapia fish, with the subsequent development of a necrotic cellulitis following a traumatic injury to the hand while the patient was working on a motor vehicle engine.[29] *Vibrio vulnificus* is an infrequent cause of acute, self-limited diarrheal illness in persons receiving gastric acid suppression therapy,[30] ocular infections usually following an injury from molluscan shell fragments[31] and, rarely, septic arthritis.[32]

The major determinant of virulence in *V. vulnificus* is its polysaccharide capsule, which renders the bacterium resistant to serum killing and directly stimulates release of inflammatory cytokines such as TNF-α.[33] Other contributors to pathogenicity include a variety of extracellular proteins and cell wall lipopolysaccharide. Host-derived factors that contribute to the pathogen's virulence include the availability of iron and at least one inflammatory mediator. *V. vulnificus* can alter expression of several genes differentially in response to low-iron and iron-rich conditions and, in the latter, can multiply rapidly.[34] The predilection of this vibrio to cause disease in patients with iron overload states can be explained by its ability to sequester iron from hemoglobin and 100% saturated (but not 30%, or normally saturated)

transferrin. Elevated levels of several proinflammatory cytokines, including TNF-α, interleukin-1β, and interleukin-6, have been noted in septicemic patients with *V. vulnificus* infection.[35]

DIFFERENTIAL DIAGNOSIS

Vibrio vulnificus should be suspected in any immunocompromised host (but especially with cirrhosis or underlying liver disease) who develops a septicemic illness associated with necrotizing cutaneous lesions within 1 to 3 days after the ingestion of oysters. Although rare, the clinical syndrome is distinct and should suggest this diagnosis.

Similarly, the development of cellulitis in persons occupationally or recreationally exposed to seawater should suggest *V. vulnificus* (especially in the presence of severe, necrotizing cellulitis). Other *Vibrio* species may cause soft tissue infections but these are usually less severe.

Vibrio vulnificus grows readily on MacConkey agar and the more selective TCBS medium; final identification is made by standard biochemical tests. Because *V. vulnificus* ferments lactose, it can be overlooked in cultures grown on MacConkey agar in a routine diagnostic laboratory unless the technician is advised to look specifically for this microorganism. Clinicians cannot assume that routine diagnostic practice in the laboratory includes media for detection of *Vibrio* infections, even in endemic areas, because only 25% of laboratories in Gulf Coast states routinely culture all stools for *Vibrio* species.[36] Thus, communication between the clinician and microbiology laboratory personnel is key to ensure diagnosis.

The severity of infection, the rapidity of progression, and the high fatality rate in *V. vulnificus* infection together exert pressure to make a correct diagnosis rapidly to guide antimicrobial adjustment and inform surgical consultation. A real-time quantitative polymerase chain reaction (PCR) assay to detect the *ToxR* of *V. vulnificus* has been developed and shown to be capable of detecting five copies/μL in serum in 2 hours (start to finish); positive real-time (RT)–PCR results were obtained in 5 of 22 patients in whom blood cultures were negative but in whom *V. vulnificus* was isolated from soft tissue.[37]

TREATMENT

Cellulitis caused by *V. vulnificus* generally responds well to appropriate antibiotics but early administration is critical because the cellulitis can advance very rapidly. Early surgical consultation should be obtained; débridement of all devitalized tissue or even amputation may be lifesaving. Bacteremic *V. vulnificus* infections in compromised hosts respond less well to therapy. Fluoroquinolones, third-generation cephalosporins and doxycycline are highly active against *V. vulnificus* and the combination of ciprofloxacin and cefotaxime exhibited synergy.[15] Reported mortality was lowest for bacteremic patients begun on antibiotics within 24 hours of onset of illness but was still unacceptably high at 33%.[26]

PREVENTION

Although patients with underlying liver disease and other chronic illnesses should be warned of the hazards of eating raw oysters, this has not been accomplished effectively in the United States, even when required by law.[38] A capsular polysaccharide conjugate vaccine has been developed, but studies indicate that polyclonal immunoglobulin, actively or passively derived, was necessary for cross-protection among capsular types of *V. vulnificus*.[39] At present, thorough cooking of seafood remains the only effective means of prevention.

Vibrio alginolyticus

Vibrio alginolyticus has been predominantly associated with cellulitis and acute otitis media or externa rather than gastroenteritis.[3,21] These infections generally occurred after local trauma in otherwise healthy seawater swimmers or fishermen and responded well to appropriate antibiotics.[3,40,41] Necrotizing fasciitis has developed following a soft tissue injury from a coral reef to the leg of an apparently immunocompetent individual.[42] *V. alginolyticus* caused a pacemaker pocket infection in a man who swam off the Atlantic coast of France,[43] showing that *Vibrio* infections also can be diseases of medical progress. Isolation is similar to that for *V. vulnificus;* however, *V. alginolyticus* does not ferment lactose.

Halophilic Vibrios

Several other *Vibrio* species are recognized as causative agents of human disease acquired through ingestion of contaminated seafood or contact of traumatized skin with seawater or brackish water. *G. hollisae* (*V. hollisae*) primarily causes a moderate to severe diarrheal illness, often requiring hospital admission.[44,45] *P. damsela* (*V. damsela*) causes serious wound infections, with findings reminiscent of the clinical picture of *V. vulnificus.*[46,47] *V. fluvialis* previously was primarily associated with sporadic gastroenteritis; more recently it has caused peritonitis (one of which was in association with continuous ambulatory peritoneal dialysis [CAPD])[48,49] and a severe hemorrhagic cellulitis.[50] *V. furnissii* has been rarely isolated in sporadic cases of diarrhea.[15] *V. metschnikovii* has been a rare cause of severe infections, including pneumonia, cellulitis, and bacteremia[51-53] and *V. cincinnatiensis* has caused bacteremia and meningitis.[54] *V. harveyi* (*Vibrio carchariae*) has caused cellulitis following a shark bite[55] and sepsis in a pediatric patient with a central venous catheter.[56]

Nonhalophilic Vibrios: Non-O1 *Vibrio cholerae* and *Vibrio mimicus*

Vibrios that are biochemically similar to *V. cholerae* but that do not agglutinate in *V. cholerae* O1 or O139 antiserum are taxonomically included in the species *V. cholerae* and are referred to as non-O1 *V. cholerae*. *V. mimicus* is closely related to non-O1 *V. cholerae*, but differs biochemically in being sucrose negative and Voges-Proskauer reaction–negative. These nonhalophilic vibrios require only trace amounts of sodium chloride for growth in culture medium; this characteristic distinguishes them from the true halophilic vibrios *V. parahaemolyticus*, *V. vulnificus*, and *V. alginolyticus*, which require larger concentrations of sodium chloride in culture media and have the remarkable ability to grow in 10% sodium chloride.

EPIDEMIOLOGY

Non-O1 *V. cholerae* organisms are worldwide in distribution and ubiquitous in seawater and estuarine water sources. The burden of disease from these strains has been in the severity of illness in individual patients. They have not been observed to cause sweeping epidemics, as have *V. cholerae* O1 and O139, although a few non-O1 strains have caused explosive outbreaks. The molecular basis for this epidemiologic behavioral difference resides in a large (39.5-kb) vibrio pathogenicity island (VPI) that contains gene clusters responsible for cholera toxin acquisition and expression as well as sequences involved in colonization.[57] The group of virulence genes within the VPI is strongly tied to epidemic ability. The VPI is present in epidemic and pandemic *V. cholerae* O1 strains, in Bengal O139, and in two non-O1 *V. cholerae* strains that caused outbreaks. The VPI was absent in sporadic diarrheal and nontoxigenic environmental isolates of non-O1 *V. cholerae*.[57] Horizontal gene transfer of this pathogenicity island may be an initial

step for the acquisition of epidemic capability by non-O1 *V. cholerae* strains. Rather than being regarded as a heterogeneous group of lesser consequence, the non-O1 *V. cholerae* are perhaps more properly viewed as strains with the underlying potential to cause epidemic disease if the appropriate complement of virulence genes is acquired.

In every carefully studied major outbreak of cholera, non-O1 vibrios have been isolated from a small proportion of patients (1% to 5%) with illnesses indistinguishable from those caused by *V. cholerae*. Possible explanations for this observation include the loss by certain classic *V. cholerae* of the relevant agglutinating surface antigens and the acquisition by non-O1 *V. cholerae* of the gene coding for the production of cholera enterotoxin.

CLINICAL MANIFESTATIONS

Non-O1 *V. cholerae* organisms produce a wide spectrum of diarrheal illness, ranging from severe watery diarrhea indistinguishable from cholera to the milder traveler's diarrhea of the type commonly associated with enterotoxigenic *Escherichia coli*. Some clinical isolates of non-O1 *V. cholerae* produce cholera toxin but most are nontoxigenic. No clinical features distinguish the severe diarrheal illnesses caused by enterotoxin-producing non-O1 *V. cholerae* from those caused by classic *V. cholerae*. This was aptly illustrated in a recent report of eight sporadic cases of severe diarrhea with dehydration in the southeastern United States; *V. cholerae* serotype O75 was isolated from the patients and environmental samples, and all isolates produced cholera toxin.[58] Non-O1 *V. cholerae* strains can rarely cause bacteremia, almost invariably in patients with liver disease,[59,60] but occasionally in normal persons also.

V. mimicus has caused sporadic cases of acute diarrheal illness in the United States and the tropics. Illness was associated with ingestion of raw seafood, including the unusual vehicle of turtle eggs.[61]

LABORATORY FINDINGS

With intestinal infections caused by both non-O1 *V. cholerae* and *V. mimicus*, the diarrheal fluid varies from the watery isotonic fluid characteristic of cholera gravis to loose stools in which small numbers of leukocytes and erythrocytes may be seen. The organisms are readily identified on TCBS agar, on which *V. cholerae* appears as opaque yellow colonies and *V. mimicus* as green; final speciation is made by biochemical tests and lack of agglutination in O1 antisera.

TREATMENT

No treatment is required by the large majority of patients with diarrheal disease, and antimicrobials have not been shown to shorten the clinical course. In occasional patients, especially those in the developing world, the intestinal fluid loss is sufficient to require oral or intravenous electrolyte therapy. In this situation, therapy is guided by the same principles used for the treatment of cholera.

PREVENTION

Because non-O1 *V. cholerae* organisms exist in a variety of water sources, ranging from freshwater rivers to the oceans, purification of water sources and adequate cooking of fish and other seafood provide the only certain protection against these occasional pathogens.

REFERENCES

1. Zen-Yoji H, Sakai S, Terayama T, et al. Epidemiology, enteropathogenicity, and classification of *Vibrio parahaemolyticus*. J Infect Dis. 1965;115:436-444.
2. Hlady WG, Klontz KC. The epidemiology of *Vibrio* infections in Florida, 1981-1993. J Infect Dis. 1996;173:1176-1183.
3. Thomas A, Straif-Bourgeois S, Sokol TM, et al. Vibrio infections in Louisiana: Twenty-five years of surveillance 1980-2005. J La State Med Soc. 2007;159:205-211.
4. Pan T-M, Wang T-K, Lee C-L, et al. Food-borne disease outbreaks due to bacteria in Taiwan, 1986 to 1995. J Clin Microbiol. 1997;35:1260-1262.
5. Okuda J, Ishibashi M, Hayakawa E, et al. Emergence of a unique O3:K6 clone of *Vibrio parahaemolyticus* in Calcutta, India, and isolation of strains from the same clonal group from Southeast Asian travelers arriving in Japan. J Clin Microbiol. 1997;35:3150-3155.
6. Nair GB, Ramamurthy T, Bhattacharya SK, et al. Global dissemination of *Vibrio parahaemolyticus* serotype O3:K6 and its serovariants. Clin Microbiol Rev. 2007;20:39-48.
7. Daniels NA, Ray B, Easton A, et al. Emergence of a new *Vibrio parahaemolyticus* serotype in raw oysters. JAMA. 2000;284:1541-1545.
8. Oliver JF, Ostroff SM. Preventing *Vibrio parahaemolyticus* infection. JAMA. 2001;285:42-43.

9. McLaughlin JB, Depaola A, Bopp CA, et al. Outbreak of *Vibrio parahaemolyticus* gastroenteritis associated with Alaskan oysters. *N Engl J Med*. 2005;353:1463-1470.

10. Makino K, Oshima K, Kurokawa K, et al. Genome sequence of *Vibrio parahaemolyticus*: A pathogenic mechanism distinct from that of *V. cholerae*. *Lancet*. 2003;361:743-749.

11. Honda T, Ilida T, Akeda Y, et al. Sixty years of *Vibrio parahaemolyticus* research. *Microbe*. 2008;3:462-466.

12. Jiang X, Chai T-J. Survival of *Vibrio parahaemolyticus* at low temperatures under starvation conditions and subsequent resuscitation of viable, nonculturable cells. *Appl Environ Microbiol*. 1996;62:1300-1305.

13. Laskowski-Arce MA, Orth K. *Acanthamoeba castellanii* promotes the survival of *Vibrio parahaemolyticus*. *Appl Environ Microbiol*. 2008;74:7183-7188.

14. Daniels NA, MacKinnon L, Bishop R, et al. *Vibrio parahaemolyticus* infections in the United States, 1973-1998. *J Infect Dis*. 2000;181:1661-1666.

15. Cook DW, O'Leary P, Hunsucker JC, et al. *Vibrio vulnificus* and *Vibrio parahaemolyticus* in U.S. retail shell oysters: A national survey from June 1998 to July 1999. *J Food Prot*. 2002;65:79-87.

16. Nishibuchi M, Kaper JB. Thermostable direct hemolysin gene of *Vibrio parahaemolyticus*: A virulence gene acquired by a marine bacterium. *Infect Immun*. 1995;63:2093-2099.

17. Pace JL, Chai T-J, Rossi HA, et al. Effect of bile on *Vibrio parahaemolyticus*. *Appl Environ Microbiol*. 1997;63:2372-2377.

18. Qadri F, Alam MS, Nishibuchi M, et al. Adaptive and inflammatory immune responses in patients infected with strains of *Vibrio parahaemolyticus*. *J Infect Dis*. 2003;187:1085-1096.

19. Morris JG. Cholera and other types of vibriosis: A story of human pandemics and oysters on the half shell. *Clin Infect Dis*. 2003;37:272-280.

20. Jakabi M, Gelli DS, Torre J. Inactivation by ionizing radiation of *Salmonella enteritidis*, *Salmonella infantis*, and *Vibrio parahaemolyticus* in oysters (*Crassostrea brasiliana*). *J Food Prot*. 2003;66:1025-1029.

21. Dechet AM, Yu PA, Koram N, et al. Nonfoodborne *Vibrio* Infections: An important cause of morbidity and mortality in the United States, 1997-2006. *Clin Infect Dis*. 2008;46:970-976.

22. Centers for Disease Control and Prevention (CDC). Vibrio illnesses after Hurricane Katrina—multiple states, August-September, 2005. *Morb Mortal Wkly Rep MMWR*. 2005;54:928-931.

23. Shapiro RL, Altekruse S, Hutwagner L, et al. The role of Gulf Coast oysters harvested in warmer months in *Vibrio vulnificus* infections in the United States, 1988-1996. *J Infect Dis*. 1998;178:752-759.

24. Baethge BA, West BC. *Vibrio vulnificus*: Did Hippocrates describe a fatal case? *Rev Infect Dis*. 1988;10:614-615.

25. Tacket CO, Brenner F, Blake PA. Clinical features and an epidemiologic study of *Vibrio vulnificus* infections. *J Infect Dis*. 1984;149:558-561.

26. Klontz KC, Lieb S, Schreiber M, et al. Syndromes of *Vibrio vulnificus* infections: Clinical and epidemiologic features in Florida cases, 1981-1987. *Ann Intern Med*. 1988;109:318-323.

27. Jackson JK, Murphree RL, Tamplin ML. Evidence that mortality from *Vibrio vulnificus* infection results from single strains among heterogeneous populations in shellfish. *J Clin Microbiol*. 1997;35:2098-2101.

28. Powell JL, Strauss KA, Wiley C, et al. Inflammatory cytokine response to *Vibrio vulnificus* elicited by peripheral blood mononuclear cells from chronic alcohol users is associated with biomarkers of cellular oxidative stress. *Infect Immun*. 2003;71:4212-4216.

29. Colondner R, Chazan B, Kopelowitz J, et al. Unusual portal of entry of *Vibrio vulnificus*: Evidence of its prolonged survival on the skin. *Clin Infect Dis*. 2002;34:714-715.

30. Johnston JM, Becker SF, McFarland LM. Gastroenteritis in patients with stool isolates of *Vibrio vulnificus*. *Am J Med*. 1986;80:336-338.

31. Penland RL, Boniuk M, Wilhelmus KR. *Vibrio* ocular infections on the U.S. Gulf Coast. *Cornea*. 2000;19:26-29.

32. Johnson RW, Arnett FC. A fatal case of *Vibrio vulnificus* presenting as septic arthritis. *Arch Intern Med*. 2002;161:2616-2618.

33. Powell JL, Wright AC, Wasserman SS, et al. Release of tumor necrosis factor alpha in response to *Vibrio vulnificus* capsular polysaccharide in in vivo and in vitro models. *Infect Immun*. 1997;65:3713-3718.

34. Alice AF, Naka H, Crosa JH. Global gene expression as a function of the iron status of the bacterial cell: Influence of differentially expressed genes in the virulence of the human pathogen *Vibrio vulnificus*. *Infect Immun*. 2008;76:4019-4037.

35. Shin SH, Shin DH, Ryu PY, et al. Proinflammatory cytokine profile in *Vibrio vulnificus* septicemic patients' sera. *FEMS Immunol Med Microbiol*. 2002;33:133-138.

36. Marano NN, Daniels NA, Easton AN, et al. A survey of stool culturing practices for *Vibrio* species at clinical laboratories in Gulf Coast states. *J Clin Microbiol*. 2000;38:2267-2270.

37. Kim HS, Kim DM, Neupane GP, et al. Comparison of conventional, nested, and real-time PCR assays for rapid and accurate detection of *Vibrio vulnificus*. *J Clin Microbiol*. 2008;46:2992-2998.

38. Mouzin E, Mascola L, Tormey M, et al. Prevention of *Vibrio vulnificus* infections: Assessment of regulatory educational strategies. *JAMA*. 1997;278:576-578.

39. Devi SJN, Hayat U, Powell JL, et al. Preclinical immunoprophylactic and immunotherapeutic efficacy of antisera to capsular polysaccharide-tetanus toxoid conjugate vaccines of *Vibrio vulnificus*. *Infect Immun*. 1996;64:2220-2224.

40. Schmidt U, Chmel H, Cobbs C. *Vibrio alginolyticus* infections in humans. *J Clin Microbiol*. 1979;10:666-668.

41. Opal SM, Saxon JR. Intracranial infection by *Vibrio alginolyticus* following injury in salt water. *J Clin Microbiol*. 1986;23:373-374.

42. Gomez JM, Fajardo R, Patino JF, et al. Necrotizing fasciitis due to *Vibrio alginolyticus* in an immunocompetent patient. *J Clin Microbiol*. 2003;41:3427-3429.

43. Flock F, Boutille D. Pacemaker infection due to *Vibrio alginolyticus*. *Eur J Intern Med*. 2008;19:e109-e110.

44. Morris JG, Miller HG, Wilson R, et al. Illness caused by *Vibrio damsela* and *Vibrio hollisae*. *Lancet*. 1982;1:1294-1297.

45. Hinestrosa F, Madeira RG, Bourbeau PP. Severe gastroenteritis and hypovolemic shock caused by *Grimontia* (*Vibrio*) *hollisae* infection. *J Clin Microbiol*. 2007;45:3462-3463.

46. Fraser SL, Purcell BK, Delgado B, et al. Rapidly fatal infection due to *Photobacterium* (*Vibrio*) *damsela*. *Clin Infect Dis*. 1997;25:935-936.

47. Yamane K, Asato J, Kawade N, et al. Two cases of fatal necrotizing fasciitis caused by *Photobacterium damsela* in Japan. *J Clin Microbiol*. 2004;42:1370-1372.

48. Lee JY, Park JS, Oh SH, et al. Acute infectious peritonitis caused by *Vibrio fluvialis*. *Diagn Microbiol Infect Dis*. 2008;62:216-218.

49. Ratnaraja N, Blackmore T, Byrne J, et al. *Vibrio fluvialis* peritonitis in a patient receiving continuous ambulatory peritoneal dialysis. *J Clin Microbiol*. 2005;43:514-515.

50. Huang KC, Hsu RWW. *Vibrio fluvialis* hemorrhagic cellulitis and cerebritis. *Clin Infect Dis*. 2005;40:e75-e77.

51. Jean-Jacques W, Rajashekaraiah KR, Farmer JJ 3rd. *Vibrio metschnikovii* bacteremia in a patient with cholecystitis. *J Clin Microbiol*. 1981;14:711-712.

52. Hansen W, Freney J, Benyagoub H, et al. Severe human infections caused by *Vibrio metschnikovii*. *J Clin Microbiol*. 1993;31:2529-2530.

53. Wallet F, Tachon M, Nseir S, et al. *Vibrio metschnikovii* pneumonia. *Emerg Infect Dis*. 2005;10:1641-1642.

54. Bode RB, Brayton PR, Colwell RR, et al. A new *Vibrio* species, *Vibrio cincinnatiensis*, causing meningitis: Successful treatment in an adult. *Ann Intern Med*. 1986;104:55-56.

55. Pavia AT, Bryan JA, Maher KL, et al. *Vibrio carchariae* infection after a shark bite. *Ann Intern Med*. 1989;111:85-86.

56. Wilkins S, Millar M, Hemsworth S, et al. *Vibrio harveyi* sepsis in a child with cancer. *Pediatr Blood Cancer*. 2008;50:891-892.

57. Karaolis DK, Johnson JA, Bailey CC, et al. A *Vibrio cholerae* pathogenicity island associated with epidemic and pandemic strains. *Proc Natl Acad Sci U S A*. 1998;95:3134-3139.

58. Tobin-D'Angelo M, Smith AR, Bulens SN, et al. Severe diarrhea caused by cholera toxin–producing *Vibrio cholerae* serogroup O75 infections acquired in the southeastern United States. *Clin Infect Dis*. 2008;47:1035-1040.

59. Safrin S, Morris JG, Adams M, et al. Non-O1 *Vibrio cholerae* bacteremia: Case report and review. *Rev Infect Dis*. 1988;10:1012-1017.

60. Ko WC, Chuang YC, Huang GC, et al. Infections due to non-O1 *Vibrio cholerae* in southern Taiwan: Predominance in cirrhotic patients. *Clin Infect Dis*. 1998;27:774-780.

61. Campos E, Bolanos H, Acuna MT, et al. *Vibrio mimicus* diarrhea following ingestion of raw turtle eggs. *Appl Environ Microbiol*. 1996;62:1141-1144.

216

Campylobacter jejuni and Related Species

BAN MISHU ALLOS | MARTIN J. BLASER

Campylobacteriosis refers to the group of infections caused by gram-negative bacteria of the genus *Campylobacter*. Among the most common bacterial infections of humans in all areas of the world, campylobacters cause both diarrheal and systemic illnesses. Infection of domesticated animals with campylobacters is also widespread. *Campylobacter* is derived from the Greek *campylos*, meaning "curved," and *baktron*, meaning "rod." Following the recognition of *Campylobacter jejuni* as a major human pathogen, numerous related *Campylobacter*, *Arcobacter*, and *Helicobacter* species have been identified. The solving of the first *C. jejuni* genomic sequence in 2000 opened new doors in our understanding of these organisms.[1] Currently, the whole genome sequences for eight *Campylobacter* species have been determined and are available on various websites.[2]

Etiology

Campylobacter organisms are motile, non–spore-forming, comma-shaped, gram-negative rods.[3] Originally isolated from aborted sheep fetuses in 1909, these and similar organisms were considered subspecies of *Vibrio fetus*. However, because these organisms did not ferment carbohydrates and differed in their guanine plus cytosine (G + C) DNA content from true members of the genus *Vibrio*, a new genus, *Campylobacter*, was created. Fourteen species have been recognized within the genus; however, in recent years, taxonomic studies have indicated that splitting the genus is more appropriate.[4] The genus *Arcobacter* has been created, which now includes *Arcobacter butzleri* and *Arcobacter skirrowi*.[5] *Helicobacter cinaedi* and *Helicobacter fennelliae* had been named *Campylobacter cinaedi* and *Campylobacter fennelliae* when first discovered.[6] Although transfer to the genus *Helicobacter* is more appropriate on taxonomic grounds, because these two species cause intestinal rather than gastric illnesses, they are discussed in this chapter. *Helicobacter pylori*, previously named *Campylobacter pylori*, is discussed in Chapter 217. It is clear that new members of *Campylobacter* and related genera are being identified with regularity,[7-9] and that many of these will be found to be human pathogens.

Table 216-1 lists the *Campylobacter* and related species most commonly associated with human disease and indicates the differentiating characteristics. Certain species, such as *Campylobacter nitrofigilis*, *Arcobacter cryaerophila*, and *Campylobacter concisus*, have not yet been associated with human illness. In contrast, the "nitrate-negative" campylobacters are associated with diarrheal illnesses, but the appropriate nomenclature for the organisms has not been determined. Two types of illnesses are associated with *Campylobacter* spp.: enteric and extraintestinal. For each of these illnesses, one *Campylobacter* species predominates, and other species are less commonly present. The prototype for enteric infection is *C. jejuni*; for extraintestinal infection it is *Campylobacter fetus* (Table 216-2). Because the organisms causing enteric and extraintestinal illnesses are generally the same, they are considered together in the following discussion.

Campylobacters and related organisms grow best in an atmosphere containing 5% to 10% oxygen and are thus considered microaerophilic.[3,4] Although most of these organisms will not grow under aerobic or anaerobic conditions, *C. jejuni* can grow in candle jars, which permits isolation when the optimal atmosphere cannot be achieved. All campylobacters grow at 37°C; however, *C. jejuni* grows best at 42°C. Because *C. jejuni* is the most common enteric pathogen of humans, many laboratories have used incubation at 42°C for optimal isolation; however, use of this temperature will not permit detection of infections by many of the related species. In particular, *Campylobacter upsaliensis* may be missed.

Campylobacters multiply more slowly than do the usual bacteria of the enteric flora and therefore cannot be isolated from fecal specimens unless selective techniques are used. The most common isolation methods use blood-based, antibiotic-containing media. Three such media—Skirrow's, Butzler's, and Campy-BAP—or variations of these have been in wide use.[4] The last two media contain cephalothin, which inhibits *C. fetus* and several other *Campylobacter* subspecies, but are best suited for isolating *C. jejuni*. Several enrichment broths have been developed, but because ill humans usually excrete 10^6 to 10^9 *C. jejuni* colony-forming units per gram of stool, enrichment usually is not necessary. Blood-free media can also be used.[10] Due to their small size (0.3 to 0.6 μm in diameter) and motility, campylobacters and related organisms pass through 0.45- or 0.65-μm filters that retard the usual enteric flora. Filtration methods permit isolation without use of antibiotic-containing media. It is now clear that use of filtration techniques and nonselective rich media such as chocolate agar, with incubation of plates at 37°C, improves stool culture yields of both *C. jejuni* and the "atypical" enteric campylobacters.[11,12] The development of filtration techniques represents a significant advance over the use of selective media, and such techniques are now recommended for primary isolation of campylobacters from fecal specimens or swabs.

Visible colonies usually appear on the plating media within 24 to 48 hours. Occasionally, growth takes place after 72 to 96 hours of incubation, especially for the "atypical" species. The campylobacters can be distinguished from other microorganisms on the basis of several standard criteria and can be distinguished from one another on the basis of biochemical testing.[4,13] Organisms from young cultures have a typical vibrioid appearance (Fig. 216-1), but after 48 hours of incubation, organisms appear coccoid. The ability to hydrolyze hippurate distinguishes *C. jejuni* from most other members of the genus, but hippurate-negative *C. jejuni* isolates also occur. State-of-the-art identification to the species level should include polymerase chain reaction (PCR) studies of 16S recombinant RNA or other targets for comparison with known species.[14,15] Isolation of campylobacters from sites without a normal flora, such as the bloodstream, is not difficult, although when this organism is the suspected pathogen, incubation of cultures should be extended to 2 weeks. With radiometric detection systems, turbidity of the medium may not be present, and the increase in released radiolabel may be less than usually specified thresholds, reflecting suboptimal conditions for certain of these organisms.[16] PCR-based techniques have been developed for culture confirmation and for typing of strains.[17-19]

As with other bacteria whose ecologic niche is the gastrointestinal tract of mammals, the serotypic diversity of *C. jejuni* is enormous. More than 90 different serotypes based on somatic (O) antigens and 50 different serotypes based on heat-labile (capsular and flagellar) antigens have been identified[4]; phase variation of flagellar antigens occurs. O-antigen variation reflects the presence of differing genetic cassettes that contain the enzymes for O-antigen formation. No group somatic or flagellar antigen has been identified; however, several

TABLE 216-1 Differential Characteristics of *Campylobacter* and Related Species Most Commonly Associated with Pathogenicity in Humans										
	Growth				H₂S Production			Susceptibility to 30-µg Disk		
Species	25°C	37°C	42°C	Nitrate Reduction	On TSI	On Lead Acetate Paper	Hippurate Hydrolysis	Cephalothin	Nalidixic Acid	C-19 Fatty Acid Reduction
Campylobacter jejuni	–	+	+	+	–	+	+*	R	S	+
Campylobacter coli	–	+	+	+	v	+	–	R	S	+
Campylobacter lari	–	+	+	+	–	+	–	R	R	+
Campylobacter fetus subsp. *fetus*	+	+	v	+	–	v	–	S	R	–
Campylobacter hyointestinalis	v	+	v	+	+	+	–	S	R	+
Helicobacter cinaedi	–	+	–	+	–	+	–	S	S	–
Campylobacter upsaliensis†	–	+	+‡	+	–	+	–	S	S	–
Helicobacter fennelliae	–	+	–	–	–	+	–	S	S	–

*Approximately 5% to 10% of *C. jejuni* strains are hippurate negative.
†Catalase negative or weak.
‡Occasional isolates fail to grow at 42°C.
–, Does not have the characteristic; +, has the characteristic; R, resistant; S, susceptible; TSI, triple sugar iron agar slant; v, variable (some strains show the characteristic).

superficial proteins appear to have broad serotypic specificity, a factor that may aid in the development of a broadly specific vaccine.

C. jejuni cannot long withstand drying or freezing temperatures, which are characteristics that limit its transmission.[20] However, *C. jejuni* survives in milk or other foods or in water kept at 4°C for several weeks. Pasteurization effectively destroys the organism, as does chlorine at concentrations in standard use for water disinfection.

Epidemiology

Campylobacteriosis is a worldwide zoonosis. Campylobacters are commonly found as commensals of the gastrointestinal tract in wild or domesticated cattle, sheep, swine, goats, dogs, cats, rodents, and all varieties of fowl.[3,20] *C. jejuni* has a very varied reservoir, but *Campylobacter coli* and *Campylobacter hyointestinalis* are most commonly isolated from swine, and *C. upsaliensis* is most commonly isolated from dogs.[21,173] *C. fetus* subsp. *fetus* has been isolated from sheep, cattle, poultry, reptiles, and swine.[3] Primary acquisition of *Campylobacter* species by animals often occurs early in life and may lead to morbidity or mortality, but in most colonized animals, a lifelong carrier state develops. The vast reservoir in animals is probably the ultimate source for most enteric *Campylobacter* infections in humans. Meats originating from infected animals frequently become contaminated with intestinal contents during the slaughtering process.[20] In particular, commercially raised poultry is nearly always colonized with *C. jejuni*,

slaughterhouse procedures amplify contamination, and chicken and turkey in supermarkets, ready for consumers to take home, frequently is contaminated.[20,22] Excreta from infected animals may contaminate soil or water. Most infections in humans probably result from consumption of contaminated food and water. Investigations of more than 50 outbreaks indicate that unpasteurized (raw) milk is such a vehicle.[20] Similarly, untreated surface water has been responsible for both endemic and epidemic campylobacteriosis. Backpackers in Wyoming who drank untreated water and developed acute diarrheal illnesses had three times more *Campylobacter* infections than *Giardia* infections.[23] Several large outbreaks have been traced to defects in municipal water systems.[24,25] Undercooked meats, especially poultry, have been associated with infection.[26-29] Other vehicles include raw clams, raw or undercooked beef, and unpasteurized cheeses and goat's milk. In one study, infants in the United States riding in shopping carts next to raw meat or poultry in grocery stores had higher rates of *Campylobacter* infections than controls.[30] Nevertheless, consumption of undercooked poultry is estimated to be responsible for 50% to 70% of sporadic *Campylobacter* infections in developed countries. Increases in the isolation of *Campylobacter* spp. reflect both improved recognition and increased consumption of poultry in recent years.

Direct contact with infected animals may result in transmission. Household pets, especially young dogs and cats with diarrhea, have been implicated as vectors for campylobacteriosis.[18,21,30,31] Because healthy dogs, cats, rodents, and birds may excrete campylobacters and

TABLE 216-2 *Campylobacter, Helicobacter,* and *Arcobacter* Species Associated with Different Clinical Manifestations of Infection	
Disease Syndrome	
Enteric	Extraintestinal
Major Pathogen	
Campylobacter jejuni	*Campylobacter fetus*
Minor Pathogens	
Campylobacter coli	*Campylobacter jejuni*
Campylobacter lari	*Campylobacter coli*
Campylobacter fetus	*Campylobacter lari*
Helicobacter fennelliae	*Helicobacter fennelliae*
Helicobacter cinaedi	*Helicobacter cinaedi*
Campylobacter upsaliensis	*Campylobacter sputorum*
Arcobacter butzleri	*Campylobacter hyointestinalis*
Arcobacter skirrowi	*Helicobacter rappini*
Arcobacter cryaeophila	

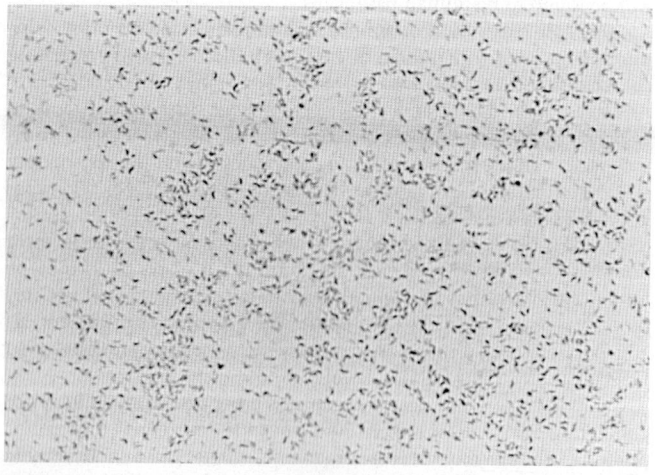

Figure 216-1 Fine curved, S-shaped, or spiral, lightly staining gram-negative appearance of *Campylobacter jejuni* in pure culture (×1000).

related organisms, it is not surprising that human infections associated with these animals also have been reported. People with occupational exposure to cattle, sheep, and other farm animals are at increased risk for infection, and laboratory-acquired infections have been reported. *C. fetus* strains in reptiles and mammals probably diverged 200 million years ago[32]; however, humans may become infected with reptile strains, possibly due to consuming a food of reptile origin. Most reported strains in the United States have been from Asian Americans.[33]

As with other enteric pathogens, fecal-oral person-to-person transmission of *C. jejuni* has been reported. Persons in contact with the excreta of infected persons who are not feces continent (e.g., infants) are at risk of infection. Infected school-age children rarely may transmit *Campylobacter* infection. Transmission from infected food handlers who are asymptomatic is at best uncommon. Perinatal transmission from a mother who may not have been symptomatic may be due to exposure in utero, during passage through the birth canal, or during the first days of life.[34] Infection has been associated with blood transfusion from an infected patient.[35] Because of a variety of sexual practices, homosexual men appear to be at increased risk for infection caused by *H. cinaedi*, *H. fennelliae*, and other "atypical" campylobacters.[36] Human immunodeficiency virus (HIV)-infected patients are at substantially increased risk of infection.[37] The standardization of serotyping methods[38] and the development of molecular methods for identification and typing of *C. jejuni* and related organisms[14,15,17-19,39,40] should improve our understanding of transmission.

C. jejuni infections occur year-round in the United States and other developed countries but with a sharp peak in summer and early fall. *C. fetus* infections show the same seasonal variation, but the peak is less marked. The reason for this seasonal variation is unclear. In developed countries, the incidence of infection is higher when air temperatures rise.[41] Flies also have been suggested as a potential source of transmission to humans.[42] In tropical countries, the seasonal variation of *C. jejuni* infection appears to be influenced by rainfall.

For many years, the incidence of *C. jejuni* infections continued to rise in the United States and Europe and exceeded rates of *Salmonella* and *Shigella* infections combined.[43,44] However, between 1996 and 2005, *Campylobacter* infections in the United States declined so much that they are now exceeded in frequency by *Salmonella*.[45] Improved hygienic practices on farms and especially poultry slaughterhouses may have contributed to this decline. Based on estimates of the number of *Salmonella* infections, there are probably more than 2 million *Campylobacter* infections annually in the United States. Population-based studies show peak incidence in children younger than age 1 year and in people 15 to 29 years old[46]; however, cases have been reported in patients of all ages. The incidence in males may be higher. The prevalence of infection in healthy people is very low (<1%).

The epidemiology of infection in developing countries is markedly different. *C. jejuni* is often isolated from healthy persons, and the infection is especially common during the first 5 years of life.[47,48] During the first 2 years of life, most children have numerous *Campylobacter* infections, but those occurring early in life frequently are symptomatic, whereas later infections are mostly asymptomatic.[48] The source of these frequent infections has not been defined, but preliminary evidence suggests that human-to-human transmission may be more common than in developed countries. The substantial age-related difference in the infection-to-illness ratios in developed and developing countries appears primarily to be due to differences in age- or exposure-related immunity of the populations rather than to differences in the isolates.[49,50] Interestingly, even in developed nations, the incidence of infection in rural areas is higher, similar to patterns observed in developing nations.[51] *C. jejuni* and other campylobacters are important causes for the acute diarrheal illnesses suffered by travelers.[52]

Pathogenesis and Pathologic Characteristics

Not all *Campylobacter* infections produce illness. Although all factors responsible for this phenomenon are not known, three of the most

important appear to be the dose of organisms reaching the small intestine, the virulence of the infecting strain, and the specific immunity of the host to the pathogen ingested. Among exposed persons who become ill, the incubation period varies from 1 to 7 days, a characteristic that is probably inversely related to the dose ingested. Most infections occur 2 to 4 days after exposure. In one study, volunteers became ill after ingesting as few as 500 organisms, but with a dose of less than 10^4 organisms, illness was infrequent.[53] *C. jejuni*, like *Salmonella typhimurium*, is susceptible to hydrochloric acid.[54] Taken together, these data suggest that the infectious dose for *C. jejuni* is similar to that for *Salmonella*. Vehicles such as milk, fatty foods, and water that favor passage through the gastric acid barrier may permit some infections to occur at relatively low doses. The acidic milieu of the stomach provides an effective barrier against *Campylobacter* infection. Patients who use proton pump inhibitors or H2 blockers are more susceptible to infection.[55,56] Some campylobacters appear to be well adapted to survival outside animal hosts and are more resilient to physical stresses[57]; these strains may be more available to infect humans.

C. jejuni multiplies in human bile,[54] a characteristic that aids colonization of the bile-rich upper small intestine early in infection. The sites of tissue injury include the jejunum, ileum, and colon, with similar pathologic features in each. Inspection of affected tissues may reveal a diffuse, bloody, edematous, and exudative enteritis,[58] but pathologic examinations are generally performed on specimens from patients with the most severe cases. Microscopic examination of rectal biopsy specimens has shown a nonspecific colitis with an inflammatory infiltrate of neutrophils, mononuclear cells, and eosinophils in the lamina propria; degeneration, atrophy, loss of mucus, and crypt abscesses in the epithelial glands; and ulceration of the mucosal epithelium.[59,60] Rectal biopsy samples with these nonspecific features have been interpreted as showing acute ulcerative colitis or Crohn's disease. In other cases, the appearance of the rectal biopsy sample has been similar to that of specimens obtained in *Salmonella* or *Shigella* infections. In a series of 124 patients with *C. jejuni* infection, 18 of the most severely ill patients underwent sigmoidoscopic examination or rectal biopsy; 17 of these procedures showed colonic involvement.[61] Some patients have terminal ileitis as well as colitis. Host factors are also clearly important; in volunteers, a single strain produced a wide spectrum of clinical manifestations.[53]

The absence of a nonprimate animal model that is closely analogous to human infection makes understanding *Campylobacter* pathogenesis more difficult. Experimental challenges both in monkeys[62] and in vitro[63-66] confirm the invasiveness of *C. jejuni*. The presence of bacteremia in some patients, the finding of cellular infiltration in biopsy specimens, and the presence of blood in stools from patients with *Campylobacter* colitis also suggest that tissue invasion occurs. The process of *C. jejuni* invasion is multifactorial. Some evidence suggests *C. jejuni* breeches epithelial cell barriers by disrupting the tight junctions of epithelial cells.[67] After invasion, cellular architecture is altered. Microtubule-dependent mechanisms may be important in the organism's ability to invade the intestinal epithelium.[68]

The bacteria's flagellae are also important virulence factors because they promote the motility and chemotaxis needed for *C. jejuni* to colonize the intestinal tract[63,69] and because the flagellar export apparatus is involved in the secretion of a number of proteins that affect invasion.[70] In vivo passage favors flagellated cells[71]; intact flagellar synthesis genes are required for maximal *C. jejuni* invasiveness.[72,73] Some secreted proteins produce rapid apoptotic death of cell cultures[74]; however, the role of these proteins in causing diarrhea is not known. A cytolethal distending toxin may affect cell cycle kinetics.[75,76] This toxin's role in pathogenesis also remains unknown, but it may play a role in suppressing innate immunity by inducing death of macrophages.[77,78] A high-molecular-weight plasmid also enhances the invasive capabilities of *C. jejuni* virulence.[79-81] The plasmid, pVir, has been identified in some clinical *Campylobacter* isolates and was significantly associated with bloody stools.[82] *C. jejuni* may adhere to epithelial cells,[83] which favors gut colonization. A superficial antigen (PEB1) that appears to be the major adhesin[84] is conserved among *C. jejuni* strains, is a target of the immune response,[85] and may represent a vaccine candidate.[86,87] Other important adhesins include JlpA, a surface-exposed lipoprotein,[88] and CadF, which mediates adhesion by binding to fibronectin.[89] Chemotaxis[90] and production of fimbriae[91] are also important in virulence. Acquisition of ferrous and ferric iron in the gut is critical for colonization by *C. jejuni*.[92]

Campylobacter outer membranes contain lipopolysaccharides (LPSs) with typical endotoxic activity.[93] The structure of the LPS O-antigen is highly variable.[38] Many *C. jejuni* O-antigens possess sialic acid-containing structures.[94] Their close resemblance to those seen in human gangliosides such as GM_1, GD_{1a}, GD_3, and GT_{1a} and their presence in strains isolated from patients who developed the Guillain-Barré syndrome (GBS) suggest a role in the pathogenesis of this disorder.[94-96]

Extracellular toxins with cytopathic activities have been found, and classic enterotoxins have also been demonstrated, although generally at low concentrations.[97-99] However, the *C. jejuni* genome does not contain any of the known enterotoxins. Two strains lacking detectable enterotoxin production and with low-level in vitro cytotoxin production were found to be fully virulent in volunteers.[53] Infected persons do not develop neutralizing antibodies to these toxins, casting further doubt on their in vivo significance.

Patients in developed countries with *Campylobacter* infection excrete the organism in feces for an average of 2 or 3 weeks. By 3 months after infection, convalescent excretion is rare. In developing countries, the period of convalescent excretion is even briefer, probably reflecting high levels of immunity in the population.[49]

Bacteremia can sometimes be detected in patients with *Campylobacter* infections, whether or not they show signs of systemic illness. Most bacteremias reported to the Centers for Disease Control and Prevention have been due to *C. fetus* subsp. *fetus*, whereas *C. jejuni* is by far the more common pathogen. One explanation for the apparently greater tendency of *C. fetus* to cause bacteremia is that it is usually resistant, whereas *C. jejuni* is susceptible to the bactericidal activity present in normal human serum.[100] After oral ingestion and intestinal colonization with or without acute diarrheal disease, *C. fetus* bacteremia may occur.[101]

C. fetus is covered with a surface (S)-layer protein that functions as a capsule.[102,103] Virtually all human isolates of *C. fetus* possess an S-layer protein that completely disrupts C3b binding to these organisms.[104] Lack of C3b binding explains both serum and phagocytosis resistance. In a mouse model, after oral inoculation, strains carrying the S-layer protein develop bacteremia, whereas strains without the S-layer protein do not.[105] *C. fetus* also has the ability to change the major S-layer protein expressed. This results in antigenic variation[106] and is facilitated by recombination among several highly homologous genes encoding full-length proteins.[107,108] The S-layer protein of *C. fetus* is the major virulence factor explaining its extraintestinal spread (Fig. 216-2).

Immunity

Host immune responses to *Campylobacter* infection play a critical role in curtailing disease severity and pathologic outcomes.[2] Volunteers rechallenged with the homologous *C. jejuni* organism developed infection but were protected from illness.[53,109] In developing countries, where *C. jejuni* infection is hyperendemic, the decreasing case-to-infection ratio with age suggests acquisition of immunity. Patients infected with campylobacters develop specific immunoglobulin (Ig) G, IgM, and IgA antibodies in serum[98,109] and IgA antibodies in intestinal secretions.[109]

In developing countries, specific serum IgA levels rise progressively with age, reflecting recurring exposure to *C. jejuni*. In volunteers, increasing levels of specific serum IgA have been correlated with increasing specific intestinal levels as well.[53,109] Supporting the notion that humoral immunity is protective against *C. jejuni* infections have been the numerous reports of severe and recurrent *C. jejuni* infection in patients with congenital or acquired hypogammaglobulinemia.[110,111]

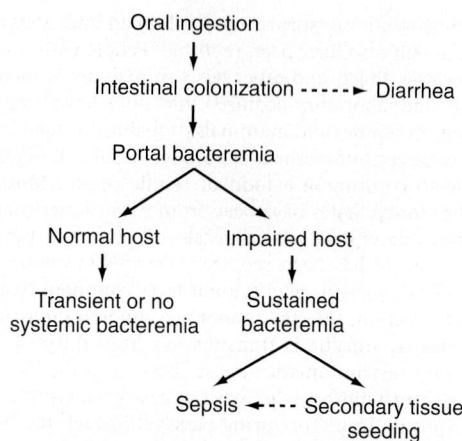

Figure 216-2 Pathogenesis of *Campylobacter fetus* infections. *(From Blaser MJ. Campylobacter fetus: emerging infection and model system for bacterial pathogenesis at mucosal surfaces. Clin Infect Dis. 1998;27:256-258.)*

In HIV-infected patients as well, failure of *C. jejuni* infection to respond to antimicrobial therapy has been correlated with failure to produce a humoral response to infection.[112] Nevertheless, the markedly increased incidence of *C. jejuni* infection in patients with acquired immunodeficiency syndrome (AIDS)[37,113] in both industrialized and developing nations demonstrates that cell-mediated immunity is also important in preventing and terminating infection. Studies have shown that campylobacters induce maturation and cytokine production in dendritic cells, indicating that these bacteria elicit innate immune responses.[114]

Despite these exceptions, most patients who become infected with *C. jejuni* were previously healthy and recover rapidly from infection. In contrast, patients with *C. fetus* infections much more frequently have evidence of impaired immunity, including conditions such as chronic alcoholism, liver disease, old age, diabetes mellitus, and malignancies.[115,116] *C. fetus* infections may produce diarrheal illnesses in healthy people or opportunistic infections in debilitated people.[101]

Clinical Manifestations

CAMPYLOBACTER JEJUNI INFECTIONS

The clinical manifestations of infections caused by all of the *Campylobacter* spp. that cause enteric illnesses appear identical; *C. jejuni* infection may be regarded as the prototype. Acute enteritis is the most common presentation of *C. jejuni* infection. Symptoms may last from 1 day to 1 week or longer. Often, there is a prodrome with fever, headache, myalgia, and malaise 12 to 24 hours before the onset of intestinal symptoms.[117] In some patients, the constitutional symptoms may coincide with the intestinal phase or, less often, may follow it. The most common symptoms are diarrhea, malaise, fever, and abdominal pain.[117-119] Diarrhea may range in severity from loose stools to massive watery or grossly bloody stools. In any patient, the entire spectrum of diarrhea may be seen. For most patients, there are 10 or more bowel movements on the worst day of the illness. Abdominal pain is usually cramping in nature and is relieved by defecation; it may be the predominant manifestation of illness. *Campylobacter* enteritis is frequently self-limiting, with a gradual resolution of symptoms over several days; however, illness lasting longer than 1 week occurs in approximately 10% to 20% of patients seeking medical attention, and relapse may be seen in another 5% to 10% of patients who do not receive treatment.[39,117,118]

Infection also may be manifested as an acute colitis, with symptoms of fever, abdominal cramps, and bloody diarrhea persisting for 1 week or longer.[59,119] Fever may be low grade or consist of daily peaks above

40°C. Initially, stools may be watery, but as the illness progresses they may become frankly bloody; tenesmus is a common symptom. In the most severe forms, patients appear very ill, and toxic megacolon has been reported.[120] Because of the propensity of *Campylobacter* infection to affect young adults and the characteristic clinical presentation, it may be readily confused with ulcerative colitis or Crohn's disease.[59,117] The pathologic findings on rectal biopsy are nonspecific, and the clinical features and radiographic findings are also nondiagnostic. Therefore, the clinician should have a high index of suspicion for *Campylobacter* infection in a patient who presents with this symptom complex. Because of the often fastidious nature of these organisms,[121,122] a single negative culture does not rule out infection, especially if optimal filtration methods are not used for primary isolation of a pathogen.

Occasionally, acute abdominal pain may be the major or only symptom of infection.[123] Although any quadrant of the abdomen may be affected, patients most often complain of pain in the right lower quadrant. As with *Yersinia enterocolitica* and *Salmonella enteritidis*, *C. jejuni* may cause pseudoappendicitis.[39,117] In most cases, the removed appendix has shown minimal or no inflammation. Enlarged mesenteric nodes (mesenteric adenitis) and terminal ileitis[39] also may be responsible for symptoms. Diagnosis is often made during the postoperative period, when diarrhea ensues. *Campylobacter* infection occasionally may present solely as a gastrointestinal hemorrhage.[124] Among neonates, *C. jejuni* infection may be manifested as one or more grossly bloody stools and no other symptoms, with findings suggesting intussusception,[125] or with extraintestinal foci.[126] Fever also may be the sole manifestation of *C. jejuni* infection. Temperature elevation may be so severe and persistent that typhoid fever is the initial diagnosis until *C. jejuni* is isolated from stools. Febrile convulsions in young children before the onset of the enteric phase of illness may also occur.[127]

Bacteremia has been noted in less than 1% of patients with *C. jejuni* infection. In part, this low frequency reflects the fact that physicians rarely perceive diarrheal illness as an indication for blood culture, even when fever is present. Nevertheless, bacteremia appears to be more common in infections in people at the extremes of age.[46,128] Meningitis and endocarditis are rare manifestations of *C. jejuni* infection. In general, three patterns of extraintestinal *C. jejuni* infection have been noted.[129] First, there may be a transient bacteremia in a normal host with acute *Campylobacter* enteritis. The bacteremia may be discovered several days after blood cultures are obtained, by which time the patient usually has completely recovered. The course is benign, and no specific treatment based on the positive blood culture result is usually indicated. Second, there may be a sustained bacteremia or deep focus of infection in a previously normal host; usually the patient has an acute enteritis as well. The *C. jejuni* isolates are generally relatively or absolutely serum resistant.[129] Bacteremia usually has its origin in the intestinal tract inflammation and responds to antimicrobial therapy. Third, sustained bacteremia or deep infection may occur in a compromised host; many such patients do not have an acute enteritis. *C. jejuni* isolates are usually serum sensitive.[129] Antimicrobial therapy, which may need to be prolonged, is required for elimination or suppression of this infection.

C. jejuni may cause septic abortion,[130] but sustained bacteremia in a pregnant patient does not necessarily imply fetal infection or a bad outcome.[129] There have been infrequent reports of *C. jejuni* infections manifesting as acute cholecystitis,[131] pancreatitis,[132,133] and cystitis.[133-135] These manifestations probably reflect local extension rather than hematogenous (metastatic) spread of infection. People with immunoglobulin deficiencies often develop prolonged, severe, and recurrent *C. jejuni* infections,[110,111] often with bacteremia and other extraintestinal manifestations such as erysipelas-like skin lesions or osteomyelitis.[136] *C. jejuni* has been associated with immunoproliferative small intestinal disease. The organism was detected by PCR in small intestinal biopsies from patients with mucosa-associated lymphoid tissue (MALT).[137] This is analogous to the role of *Helicobacter pylori* in gastric MALT lymphomas. A reactive arthritis may occur up to several weeks after infection, and prolonged rheumatic symptoms have also been reported.

The relation of this phenomenon to the presence of HLA-B27 histocompatibility antigens is not clear.[138-140,219] Myopericarditis,[141,142] hepatitis,[143] cellulitis,[144] interstitial nephritis, the hemolytic uremic syndrome, and IgA nephropathy[145] are other reported complications.

GBS is an uncommon consequence of *C. jejuni* infection (estimated at 1 case per 2000 infections) that usually occurs 2 or 3 weeks after the diarrheal illness.[146,147] From 20% to 50% of Guillain-Barré cases follow *C. jejuni* infections, reflecting in part the high incidence of these infections.[146-150] A particular *C. jejuni* clone marked by LPS(O) type 19 is overrepresented among people who develop GBS.[150-152] O-type 41 has also been implicated, and other sporadic cases may be due to specific *C. jejuni* strains with sialylation of their LPS molecules.[94-96]

CAMPYLOBACTER FETUS INFECTIONS

In contrast to *C. jejuni*, *C. fetus* subsp. *fetus* less frequently causes diarrheal illness. As summarized in Table 216-3, the clinical, laboratory, and epidemiologic characteristics of *C. jejuni* infections differ significantly from those of *C. fetus* subsp. *fetus*, which often produce systemic manifestations. *C. fetus* infections may cause intermittent diarrhea or nonspecific abdominal pain without localizing signs. The diarrheal illness may manifest exactly like *C. jejuni* infection and is more common than was suspected several years ago. Clinical manifestations are similar and sequelae uncommon. Nearly all affected patients survive the infections when appropriate antibiotic treatment is given and usually do well without antibiotic treatment. *C. fetus* also may cause a prolonged relapsing illness characterized by fever, chills, and myalgias in which a source of infection cannot be demonstrated.[115,116,153,154] Occasionally, secondary seeding of an organ will occur, leading to a more complicated infection[153-157] and sometimes to a fulminant, fatal course.

C. fetus infections appear to have a predilection for vascular sites; vascular necrosis occurs in patients with endocarditis and pericarditis resulting from this organism.[158,159] Mycotic aneurysms of the abdominal aorta also occur. Thrombophlebitis may be associated with *C. fetus* bacteremia,[160] but whether it is the primary event or a secondary manifestation of the infection is uncertain. Patients with a bacteremic illness without localization should be carefully evaluated for the presence of septic thrombophlebitis because when this condition is treated with appropriate antibiotics, the response is good. Infections during pregnancy primarily have been manifested as upper respiratory symptoms, pneumonitis, fever, and bacteremia. However, four of five *C.*

TABLE 216-3	Biologic and Clinical Characteristics of *Campylobacter jejuni* and *Campylobacter fetus* Subsp. *fetus*	
Feature	**Campylobacter jejuni**	**Campylobacter fetus Subsp. fetus**
Epidemiologic Characteristics		
Major reservoir	Avian species, food animals	Cattle and sheep (reptiles)
Affected hosts	Normal hosts; all ages affected; often in clusters of cases	Opportunistic agent in debilitated hosts; clustering rare; healthy hosts may be affected
Laboratory Characteristics		
Range of growth temperatures	32-42° C	25-37° C*
Usual source of isolation	Feces	Bloodstream
Clinical Characteristics		
As a cause for diarrheal illness	Common	Uncommon
Clinical manifestations	Acute gastroenteritis, colitis	Systemic illness with bacteremia, meningitis, vascular infections, abscesses; gastroenteritis
Outcome of infection	Usually self-limited	May be fatal in debilitated hosts

*Occasionally grows at 42° C.

fetus-infected second-trimester patients delivered dead infants despite antibiotic therapy. One patient received antibiotic therapy and delivered a normal term infant. All the mothers survived their infection.[161]

Central nervous system (CNS) infections with *C. fetus* occur in neonates and adults. The prognosis is poor for premature infants, but five of six full-term neonates in one series survived infection. Infection is manifested as a meningoencephalitis with a cerebrospinal fluid polymorphonuclear pleocytosis. Subdural effusion may complicate infection. Meningoencephalitis is also the most common CNS manifestation of *C. fetus* infection in adults.[162] Cerebrovascular accidents, subarachnoid hemorrhages, and brain abscesses also occur. The prognosis is better in adults than in neonates, with a survival rate of approximately 67%, although neurologic sequelae are frequent.[153] *C. fetus* has been shown to cause a variety of other types of localized infections, including septic arthritis, spontaneous bacterial peritonitis, salpingitis, lung abscess, empyema, cellulitis, urinary tract infection, vertebral osteomyelitis, and cholecystitis.[153,163,164] Although most patients with these illnesses recovered with appropriate antibiotics and drainage procedures, the clinical course was frequently prolonged and relapsing. Antibiotic resistance to fluoroquinolones may develop in immunocompromised patients who receive monotherapy regimens.[165] Nevertheless, in other patients, self-limiting bacteremia without any sequelae has been observed. Hypogammaglobulinemic patients may have persistent bacteremia and local symptoms unless given chronic suppressive therapy with antibiotics.

INFECTION CAUSED BY OTHER ENTERIC CAMPYLOBACTER SPECIES

The clinical manifestations of infection caused by other enteric campylobacters overlap substantially with those of *C. jejuni* infection.[122,166,167] On average, *C. coli* may produce more mild disease.[49] In one series of homosexual men, *H. cinaedi* and *H. fennelliae* infections were more often asymptomatic than were those caused by *C. jejuni*.[168] Among immunocompromised patients, especially those with AIDS, bacteremia from the "atypical" campylobacters appears relatively commonly.[169-171] As with *C. fetus*, *C. upsaliensis* mostly causes diarrheal diseases in previously normal people[21,172,173] and bacteremia in compromised hosts; most strains of the latter species are serum resistant.[138] Other extraintestinal manifestations such as breast abscess have been observed.[174] Although dogs have long been considered an important source of human *C. upsaliensis* infections, genetic studies have shown that human and canine strains are distinct.[175] Cellulitis may occur in compromised hosts infected with any of a variety of these "atypical" species.[171] *C. hyointestinalis*, which resembles *C. fetus* in its biochemical characteristics,[176] also may cause bacteremia in compromised hosts. *A. butzleri* may cause abdominal cramps without diarrheal illness.[177] *Helicobacter* (*Flexispira*) *rappini* has been reported to cause bacteremia in compromised hosts.[178]

C. fetus subsp. *venerealis*, which had never been considered a human pathogen, was reported to have been isolated from stools from two homosexual men in Australia and from two women with bacterial vaginosis. *C. fetus* subsp. *fetus* has been isolated from two other patients with vaginosis. *Campylobacter curvus* has caused septicemia, liver abscess, and possibly chronic (Brainerd) diarrhea.[179,180] *Campylobacter sputorum* subsp. *sputorum*, which is indigenous to the human mouth and intestine, has been isolated from perianal boils and lung abscesses. *C. sputorum* subsp. *bubulus*, a commensal of sheep and cattle, has been isolated from boils and skin abscesses from humans. *Campylobacter insulaenigrae*, a recently identified species seen primarily in marine mammals, has been isolated from the stool and blood of a patient with end-stage renal and hepatic disease.[181]

Diagnosis

Clinical diagnosis of enteric campylobacteriosis may be established by demonstration of the organisms by direct examination of feces or by

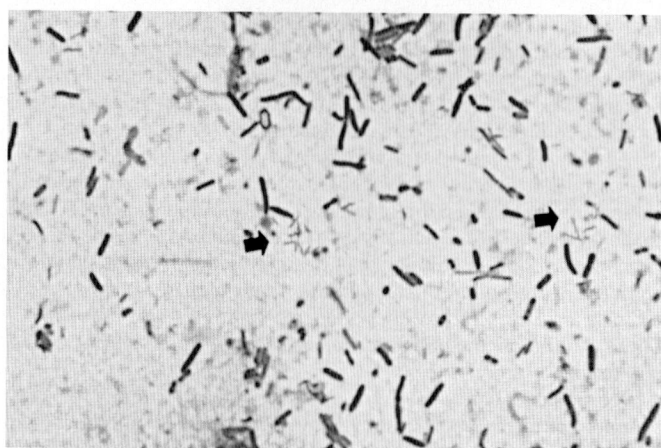

Figure 216-3 **Gram stain of fecal specimen from a patient with** *Campylobacter* **enteritis.** Arrows point to typical gram-negative fine, small, spiral, and *Vibrio*-like organisms (×1024).

isolation of the organisms. The use of serologic methods for diagnosis is currently a research tool only.

DIRECT EXAMINATION OF FECES

Examination of diarrheal fecal specimens by darkfield or phase-contrast microscopy within 2 hours of passage can permit a rapid presumptive diagnosis of *Campylobacter* enteritis if the characteristic darting motility of the *Campylobacter* organism is seen.[119,182] This test is particularly useful in the acute phase of the illness. Similarly, the presence of vibrio forms in Gram-stained stool specimens is a very specific diagnostic feature, although the sensitivity of this finding is 50% to 75% (Fig. 216-3).[183] Direct microscopy is also of value for detecting red blood cells and neutrophils, which are present in the feces of 75% of patients with *Campylobacter* enteritis.[53,117] Use of PCR techniques for direct detection of organisms has been successful in research studies but has not yet been applied to the clinical setting. Fluorescence in situ hybridization (FISH), a microscopic method that uses fluorescently labeled DNA probes that bind to unique target sites on ribosomal RNA in several *Camplylobacter* species, may provide another means for rapid identification of *Campylobacter* isolates.[184]

BACTERIOLOGIC STUDIES

Confirmation of the diagnosis of *C. jejuni* infection is based on a positive result on stool culture or, occasionally, blood culture. Because blood cultures are not often performed in the evaluation of patients presenting with diarrheal symptoms, the frequency of bacteremia is not known. Results with use of radiometric blood culture detection systems may be falsely negative for some *Campylobacter* and related species using standard procedures.[16] Campylobacters cannot be isolated from fecal specimens unless microaerobic incubation conditions and selective techniques that reduce the growth of competing microorganisms are used.[4,38] *C. fetus* is usually isolated from blood cultures 4 to 14 days after the specimen has been obtained.[116] Occasionally, *C. fetus* may be isolated from feces of patients with either diarrheal or systemic infections.[101] If *C. fetus* or another of the atypical species is suspected, incubation at 37°C and use of media without cephalosporins are necessary. The use of filtration techniques will eliminate such difficulties.

Therapy

Fluid and electrolyte replacement constitutes the cornerstone of treatment of diarrheal illnesses. Patients with *Campylobacter* infections who are severely dehydrated should undergo rapid volume expansion using intravenous solutions of electrolytes in water. For patients with less serious volume depletion, oral rehydration using glucose and electrolyte solutions is indicated. People infected with *C. jejuni* who are ill enough to seek medical attention and from whom a fecal culture is obtained represent only a subset of all those infected. Nevertheless, even among these patients, less than half are candidates for specific antimicrobial therapy.[117] In a meta-analysis of 11 small randomized trials, antimicrobial agents reduced the duration of intestinal symptoms by approximately 1.3 days.[185] Because the greatest therapeutic benefit occurs when antimicrobial therapy is started early, the rapid presumptive diagnosis of *Campylobacter* infection by means of direct visualization of the organisms in stool is clinically relevant. Treatment with antibiotics seems prudent in those patients with high fever, bloody diarrhea, or more than eight stools per day; in patients whose symptoms have not lessened or are worsening at the time the diagnosis is made; or in those in whom symptoms have persisted for more than 1 week.[186]

In vitro, *C. jejuni* is susceptible to a wide variety of antimicrobial agents, including erythromycin, the tetracyclines, the aminoglycosides, chloramphenicol, the quinolones, the nitrofurans, and clindamycin.[187-193] Because of ease of administration, lack of serious toxicity, and apparent efficacy, erythromycin has been the agent of choice.[119,194,195] The recommended dosage for adults is 250 mg PO four times daily for 5 to 7 days; the recommended dosage for children is 30 to 50 mg/kg/day in divided doses for the same period. One concern with erythromycin, which is primarily metabolized by CYP3A4, is the very slight risk of sudden cardiac death. The risk is increased fivefold when erythromycin is given with medications that inhibit CYP3A4, especially calcium channel blocking agents.[196,197] In patients taking one or more of these medications, we suggest using azithromycin in place of erythromycin. Therapy with extended-spectrum macrolides such as clarithromycin or azithromycin should be equally effective. In a trial involving U.S. military personnel in Thailand, azithromycin was effective in shortening duration of illness and *Campylobacter* excretion.[197] Macrolide resistance, based on mutations in 23S ribosomal DNA, is increasing in some areas of the world[198] but has remained under 5% in most places.[199] Rapid techniques for identification of macrolide resistance using FISH have been developed and may speed identification of appropriate drugs.[200]

An alternative agent is ciprofloxacin, 500 mg PO twice daily for 5 to 7 days, which has activity across a broad spectrum of bacteria causing diarrheal illness, including campylobacters. However, fluoroquinolones should be used with caution because rising rates of resistance to these agents have limited their usefulness in treating *Campylobacter* infections.[201-204] Resistance rates of 10% to 20% are common in much of Europe and exceed 50% in Spain, Hungary, and many developing countries.[205-206] In the United States as in other areas of the world, resistance rates have increased rapidly in recent decades.[199,207] The impact on human health becomes apparent when outcomes of infection with resistant strains are examined: Infection with *C. jejuni* strains resistant to erythromycin or fluoroquinolones is more likely to result in prolonged or invasive illness or death.[208,209] The rapid rise in fluoroquinolone resistance among human *Campylobacter* isolates has paralleled the resistance observed in isolates from commercially raised poultry. The use of fluoroquinolones in poultry in the United States in the mid-1990s fueled escalating resistance rates.[207,210] Faced with mounting evidence of an adverse impact on human health, the Food and Drug Administration banned use of fluoroquinolones to poultry flocks in 2005[211]; however, high rates of resistance are likely to persist before declining because of continued circulation of such strains in poultry flocks.

Another alternative agent is tetracycline, except in children younger than age 9 years; in such patients, clindamycin may be used. Most *C. jejuni* and *C. coli* isolates are not susceptible to most cephalosporins or penicillin, and these agents should not be used. However, amoxicillin or ticarcillin plus clavulanic acid appears to be universally effective.[212] Susceptibility to sulfonamides and metronidazole is variable. Unlike in *Salmonella* infections, treatment with antimicrobial agents does not prolong carriage of *C. jejuni*; on the contrary, erythromycin eliminates carriage within 72 hours in most patients.[188]

H. cinaedi and those *Campylobacter* strains acquired in developing countries, especially *C. coli*, are more likely to be resistant to erythromycin and tetracycline.[213] In such cases, when treatment is indicated, alternative agents should be used until susceptibility is known. Use of an antimotility agent appears to prolong duration of symptoms and has been associated with fatalities.[214] The necessity for treating septic or bacteremic episodes with agents other than erythromycin has not been established. For those patients who appear very ill, treatment with gentamicin, imipenem, or chloramphenicol is indicated, but susceptibility tests should be performed. In hypogammaglobulinemic patients with recurrent *C. jejuni* bacteremias, fresh-frozen plasma with appropriate antibiotics may eradicate the infection[136]; oral immune globulin therapy may have some value as well for recurrent diarrheal illness.[215] Systemic *C. fetus* infections should be treated parenterally, but erythromycin should not be used.[216,217] Occasionally, systemic infections diagnosed only retrospectively by positive results on blood culture resolve after empirical oral therapy. In these cases, follow-up cultures are recommended; if results are no longer positive, further treatment is not required. If necessary, ampicillin treatment has been associated with good results. Patients with endovascular infections caused by *C. fetus* require at least 4 weeks of therapy, and gentamicin or ampicillin is probably the agent of choice.[217] Treatment with imipenem or meropenem constitutes another alternative. Infections of the CNS should be treated with ampicillin, imipenem, or chloramphenicol for 2 or 3 weeks. Patients with other serious infections should also receive parenteral gentamicin or another aminoglycoside, ampicillin, or imipenem for at least 2 weeks. Because antibodies to *C. fetus* are not usually present in serum from normal people, intravenous immune globulin is not helpful for this infection in immunodeficient patients.[157] For *C. fetus*-infected patients with diarrheal illness or other less severe infections, treatment need not be as intense or as prolonged.

Prognosis

The vast majority of patients recover fully after *C. jejuni* infections, either spontaneously or after appropriate antimicrobial therapy. The "reactive arthritis," or Reiter's syndrome, occurring in HLA-B27-positive people closely resembles that seen after *Yersinia*, *Salmonella*, or *Shigella* infections and should not be considered a specific consequence of *C. jejuni* infection. However, rheumatologic symptoms may persist for several months or possibly for years in a few affected people.[218] GBS is an uncommon sequela of *Campylobacter* enteritis, but because of their high prevalence, *Campylobacter* infections are the most important recognized antecedent of this disorder.[146,147] Occasional deaths after *C. jejuni* infections have been reported in developed countries[214]; in most cases, the victim was an elderly person or a compromised host. However, fatalities in previously healthy young adults may occur, probably as a result of volume depletion. Some of the deaths that occur in Guillain-Barré patients can be attributed to the consequences of *C. jejuni* infection. Because in developing countries most symptomatic *Campylobacter* infections occur in children younger than 2 years of age[48] and frequently produce a dysenteric picture, it is reasonable to conclude that *C. jejuni* infection may play a role in the dehydration and malnutrition that often accompany infantile diarrhea in these geographic areas. The outcome of infections caused by newly discovered *Campylobacter*-like organisms[7,178] remains to be determined.

C. fetus infection may be lethal to patients with chronic compensated diseases such as cirrhosis or diabetes mellitus or may hasten the demise of seriously compromised patients. For compromised hosts with systemic *C. fetus* infections, prognosis is most dependent on the rapidity with which appropriate antimicrobial therapy is begun. Previously healthy people infected with *C. fetus* usually survive the illness without permanent sequelae.

Because *C. jejuni* infections are "accidentally" acquired by humans, and because there is evidence for the natural development of immunity among people in developing countries, the goal of producing a vaccine is probably achievable.

REFERENCES

1. Parkhill J, Wren BW, Mungall K, et al. The genome sequence of the food-borne pathogen *Campylobacter jejuni* reveals hypervariable sequences. *Nature.* 2000;403:665-668.
2. Poly F, Guerry P. Pathogenesis of *Campylobacter. Curr Opin Gastroenterol.* 2008;24:27-31.
3. Smibert RM. Genus *Campylobacter*. In: Krieg NR, Holt HG, eds. *Bergey's Manual of Systematic Bacteriology*. Baltimore: Williams & Wilkins; 1984:111-118.
4. Nachamkin I. *Campylobacter, Helicobacter*, and related spiral bacteria. In: Murray PR, ed. *Manual of Clinical Microbiology*. 6th ed. Washington, DC: American Society for Microbiology; 1996:402-409.
5. Vandamme P, Vancanneyt M, Pot B, et al. Polyphasic taxonomic study of the emended genus *Arcobacter* with *Arcobacter butzleri* comb. nov. and *Arcobacter skirrowi* sp. nov., an aerotolerant bacterium isolated from veterinary specimens. *Int J Syst Bacteriol.* 1992;42:344-356.
6. Fennell CL, Totten PA, Quinn TC, et al. Characterization of *Campylobacter*-like organisms isolated from homosexual men. *J Infect Dis.* 1984;149:58-66.
7. Burnens AP, Stanley J, Schaad UB, et al. Novel *Campylobacter*-like organism resembling *Helicobacter fennelliae* isolated from a boy with gastroenteritis and from dogs. *J Clin Microbiol.* 1993;31:1916-1917.
8. Foley JE, Solnick JV, LaPointe J-M, et al. Identification of a novel enteric *Helicobacter* species in a kitten with severe diarrhea. *J Clin Microbiol.* 1998;36:908-912.
9. Husman M, Gries C, Jehnichen P, et al. *Helicobacter* sp. strain *Mainz* isolated from an AIDS patient with septic arthritis: case report and nonradioactive analysis of 16S rRNA sequence. *J Clin Microbiol.* 1994;32:3037-3039.
10. Bolton GJ, Hutchinson DN, Coates D. Blood-free selective medium for isolation of *Campylobacter jejuni* from feces. *J Clin Microbiol.* 1984;19:169-171.
11. Steele TW, McDermott JN. Technical note: the use of membrane filters applied directly to the surface of agar plates for the isolation of *Campylobacter jejuni* from feces. *Pathology.* 1984;16:263-265.
12. Lastovica AJ, LeRoux E. Efficient isolation of *Campylobacter upsaliensis* from stools. *J Clin Microbiol.* 2001;39:4222-4223.
13. Burnens AP, Nicolet J. Three supplementary diagnostic tests for *Campylobacter* species and related organisms. *J Clin Microbiol.* 1993;31:708-710.
14. van Camp G, Fierens H, Vandamme P, et al. Identification of enteropathogenic *Campylobacter* species by oligonucleotide probes and polymerase chain reaction based on 16S rRNA genes. *Syst Appl Microbiol.* 1993;16:30-36.
15. Ng L-K, Kingombe CIB, Yan W, et al. Specific detection and confirmation of *Campylobacter jejuni* by DNA hybridization and PCR. *Appl Environ Microbiol.* 1997;63:4558-4563.
16. Wang WLL, Blaser MJ. Detection of pathogenic *Campylobacter* species in blood culture systems. *J Clin Microbiol.* 1986;23:709.
17. Giesendorf BAJ, Quint WGV, Henkens MHC, et al. Rapid and sensitive detection of *Campylobacter* spp. in chicken products by using the polymerase chain reaction. *Appl Environ Microbiol.* 1992;58:3804-3808.
18. Giesendorf BAJ, van Belkum A, Koeken A, et al. Development of species-specific DNA probes for *Campylobacter jejuni, Campylobacter coli,* and *Campylobacter lari* by polymerase chain reaction fingerprinting. *J Clin Microbiol.* 1993;31:1541-1546.
19. Oyofo BA, Thornton SA, Burr DH, et al. Specific detection of *Campylobacter jejuni* and *Campylobacter coli* by using polymerase chain reaction. *J Clin Microbiol.* 1992;30:2613-2619.
20. Blaser MJ, Taylor DN, Feldman RA. Epidemiology of *Campylobacter jejuni* infections. *Epidemiol Rev.* 1983;5:157.
21. Labarca JA, Sturgen J, Borenstein L, et al. *Campylobacter upsaliensis*: another pathogen for consideration in the United States. *Clin Infect Dis.* 2002;34:e59-e60.
22. Atabay HI, Corry JEL. The prevalence of campylobacters and arcobacters in broiler chickens. *J Appl Microbiol.* 1997;83:619-626.
23. Taylor DN, McDermott KT, Little JR, et al. *Campylobacter* enteritis associated with drinking untreated water in backcountry areas of the Rocky Mountains. *Ann Intern Med.* 1983;99:38.
24. Mentzing L-O. Waterborne outbreaks of *Campylobacter* enteritis in central Sweden. *Lancet.* 1981;2:352.
25. Richardson G, Thomas DR, Smith RM, et al. A community outbreak of *Campylobacter jejuni* infection from a chlorinated public water supply. *Epidemiol Infect.* 2007;135:1151-1158.
26. Friedman CR, Hoekstra RM, Samuel M, et al. Risk factors for sporadic *Campylobacter* infection in the United States: a case-control study in FoodNet sites. *Clin Infect Dis.* 2004;38(suppl 3):S285-S296.
27. Gallay A, Bosquet V, Siret V, et al. Risk factors for acquiring sporadic *Campylobacter* infection in France: results from a national case-control study. *J Infect Dis.* 2008;197:1477-1484.
28. Stafford RJ, Schluter PJ, Wilson AJ, et al. OzFoodNet Working Group. Population-attributable risk estimates for risk factors associated with *Campylobacter* infection, Australia. *Emerg Infect Dis.* 2008;14:895-901.
29. Deming MS, Tauxe RV, Blake PA, et al. *Campylobacter* enteritis at a university: transmission from eating chicken and from cats. *Am J Epidemiol.* 1987;126:526-534.
30. Fullerton KE, Ingram LA, Jones TF, et al. Sporadic *Campylobacter* infection in infants: a population-based surveillance case-control study. *Pediatr Infect Dis J.* 2007;26:19-24.
31. Skirrow MB. *Campylobacter* enteritis in dogs and cats: a "new" zoonosis. *Vet Res Commun.* 1981;5:13.
32. Tu Z-C, Dewhirst FE, Blaser MJ. Evidence that the *Campylobacter fetus sap* locus is an ancient genomic constituent with origins before mammals and reptiles diverged. *Infect Immun.* 2001;69:2237-2244.
33. Tu Z, Zeitlin G, Gagner J-P, et al. *Campylobacter fetus* of reptile origin as a human pathogen. *J Clin Microbiol.* 2004;42:4405-4407.
34. Vesikari T, Huttunen L, Maki R. Perinatal *Campylobacter fetus* ss. *jejuni* enteritis. *Acta Paediatr Scand.* 1981;70:261.
35. Pepersack F, Prigogyne T, Butzler JP, et al. *Campylobacter jejuni* posttransfusional septicemia. *Lancet.* 1979;2:911.
36. Totten PA, Fennell CL, Tenover FC, et al. *Campylobacter cinaedi* (sp. nov.) and *Campylobacter fennelliae* (sp. nov.): two new *Campylobacter* species associated with enteric disease in homosexual men. *J Infect Dis.* 1985;151:131.
37. Sorvillo FJ, Lieb LE, Waterman SH. Incidence of campylobacteriosis among patients with AIDS in Los Angeles County. *J Acquir Immune Defic Syndr.* 1991;4:598-602.
38. Penner JL. The genus *Campylobacter*: a decade of progress. *Clin Microbiol Rev.* 1988;1:157-172.
39. Nachamkin I, Blaser MJ, Szymanski C, eds. *Campylobacter jejuni*. 3rd ed. Washington, DC: American Society for Microbiology; 2008.
40. Champion OL, Gaunt MW, Gundogdu O, et al. Comparative phylogenomics of the food-borne pathogen *Campylobacter jejuni* reveals genetic markers predictive of infection source. *Proc Natl Acad Sci U S A.* 2005;102:16043-16048.
41. Louis VR, Gillespie IA, O'Brien SJ, et al. Temperature-driven *Campylobacter* seasonality in England and Wales. *Appl Environ Microbiol.* 2005;71:85-92.
42. Nichols GL. Fly transmission of *Campylobacter. Emerg Infect Dis.* 2005;11:361-364.
43. Blaser MJ, Wells JF, Feldman RA, et al. *Campylobacter* enteritis in the United States: a multicenter study. *Ann Intern Med.* 1983;98:360.
44. Mead PS, Slutsker L, Dietz V, et al. Food-related illness and death in the United States. *Emerg Infect Dis.* 1999;5:607-625.
45. Centers for Disease Control and Prevention. Preliminary FoodNet data on the incidence of infection with pathogens transmitted commonly through food—10 states, United States, 2005. *MMWR Morb Mortal Wkly Rep.* 2006;55:392.
46. Tauxe RV. Epidemiology of *Campylobacter jejuni* infections in the United States and other industrialized nations. In: Nachamkin I, Blaser MJ, Tompkins LS, eds. *Campylobacter jejuni: Current Status and Future Trends*. Washington, DC: American Society for Microbiology; 1992:9-19.
47. Glass RI, Stoll BJ, Huq MI, et al. Epidemiologic and clinical features of endemic *Campylobacter jejuni* infection in Bangladesh. *J Infect Dis.* 1983;148:292.
48. Calva JJ, Ruiz-Pallacios GM, Lopez-Vidal AB, et al. Cohort study of intestinal infection with *Campylobacter* in Mexican children. *Lancet.* 1988;1:503-506.
49. Taylor DN, Echeverria P, Pitarangsi C, et al. The influence of immunity and strain characteristics on the epidemiology of campylobacteriosis. *J Clin Microbiol.* 1988;26:863.
50. Taylor DN, Perlman D, Echeverria PD, et al. *Campylobacter* immunity and quantitative excretion rates in Thai children. *J Infect Dis.* 1993;168:754-758.
51. Ethelberg S, Simonsen J, Gerner-Smidt P, et al. Spatial distribution and registry-based case-control analysis of *Campylobacter* infections in Denmark, 1991-2001. *Am J Epidemiol.* 2005;162:1008-1015.
52. Speelman P, Struelens MJ, Sanyal SC, et al. Detection of *Campylobacter jejuni* and other potential pathogens in traveler's diarrhea in Bangladesh. *Scand J Gastroenterol.* 1983;84(Suppl):19-23.
53. Black RE, Levine MM, Clements ML, et al. Experimental *Campylobacter jejuni* infection in humans. *J Infect Dis.* 1988;157:472.
54. Blaser MJ, Hardesty HL, Powers B, et al. Survival of *Campylobacter fetus* subsp. *jejuni* in biological milieus. *J Clin Microbiol.* 1980;11:309.
55. Doorduyn Y, Van Pelt W, Siezen CL, et al. Novel insight in the association between salmonellosis or campylobacteriosis and chronic illness, and the role of host genetics in susceptibility to these diseases. *Epidemiol Infect.* 2008;136:1225-1234.
56. Neal KR, Scott HM, Slack RC, et al. Omeprazole as a risk factor for campylobacter gastroenteritis: case-control study. *BMJ.* 1996;312:414-415.
57. Sopwith W, Birtles A, Matthews M, et al. Identification of potential environmentally adapted *Campylobacter jejuni* strain, United Kingdom. *Emerg Infect Dis.* 2008;14:1769-1773.
58. King EO. The laboratory recognition of *Vibrio fetus* and a closely related vibrio isolated from cases of human vibriosis. *Ann N Y Acad Sci.* 1962;90:700.
59. Lambert ME, Schofield PF, Ironside AG, et al. *Campylobacter* colitis. *BMJ.* 1979;1:857.
60. Van Spreeuwel JP, Duursma GC, Meijer CJLM, et al. *Campylobacter* colitis: histologic, immunohistochemical and ultrastructural findings. *Gut.* 1985;26:945-951.
61. Blaser MJ, Reller LB, Luechtefeld NW, et al. *Campylobacter* enteritis in Denver. *West J Med.* 1982;136:287.
62. Russell RG, O'Donnoghue M, Blake Jr DC, et al. Early colonic damage and invasion of *Campylobacter jejuni* in experimentally challenged infant *Macaca mulatta*. *J Infect Dis.* 1993; 168:210-215.
63. Grant CCR, Konkel ME, Cieplak W, et al. Role of flagella in adherence, internalization, and translocation of *Campylobacter jejuni* in nonpolarized and polarized epithelial cell cultures. *Infect Immun.* 1993;61:1764-1771.
64. Babakhani FK, Joens LA. Primary swine intestinal cells as a model for studying *Campylobacter jejuni* invasiveness. *Infect Immun.* 1993;61:2723-2726.
65. Konkel ME, Hays SF, Joens LA, et al. Characteristics of the internalization and intracellular survival of *Campylobacter jejuni* in human epithelial cell cultures. *Microb Pathog.* 1992; 13:357-370.
66. Hu L, Kopecko J. *Campylobacter jejuni* 81-176 associates with microtubules and dynein during invasion of human intestinal cells. *Infect Immun.* 1999;67:4171-4182.
67. Chen ML, Ge Z, Fox JG, et al. Disruption of tight junctions and induction of proinflammatory cytokine responses in colonic epithelial cells by *Campylobacter jejuni*. *Infect Immun.* 2006;74: 6581-6589.
68. Kopecko DJ, Hu L, Zaal KJM. *Campylobacter jejuni*-microtubule-dependent invasion. *Trends Microbiol.* 2001;9: 389-396.
69. Yao R, Burr DH, Doig P, et al. Isolation of motile and non-motile insertional mutants of *Campylobacter jejuni*: the role of motility in adherence and invasion of eukaryotic cells. *Mol Microbiol.* 1994;14:883-893.
70. Konkel ME, Klena JD, Rivera-Amill V, et al. Secretion of virulence proteins from *Campylobacter jejuni* is dependent on a functional flagellar export apparatus. *J Bacteriol* 2004;186: 3296-3303.
71. Caldwell MB, Guerry P, Lee EC, et al. Reversible expression of flagella in *Campylobacter jejuni*. *Infect Immun.* 1985;50: 941-943.
72. Rivera-Amill V, Konkel ME. Secretion of *Campylobacter jejuni* Cia proteins is contact dependent. In: Paul PS, Francis DH, eds. *Mechanisms in the Pathogenesis of Enteric Diseases 2*. New York: Plenum; 1999:225-229.
73. Konkel ME, Kim BJ, Rivera-Amill V, et al. Bacterial secreted proteins are required for the internalization of *Campylobacter jejuni* into cultured mammalian cells. *Mol Microbiol.* 1999;32: 691-701.
74. Poly F, Ewing C, Goon S, et al. Heterogeneity of a *Campylobacter jejuni* protein that is secreted through the flagella filament. *Infect Immun.* 2007;75:3859-3867.
75. Whitehouse CA, Balbo PB, Pesci EC, et al. *Campylobacter jejuni* cytolethal distending toxin causes a G_2-phase cell cycle block. *Infect Immun.* 1998;66:1934-1940.
76. Pickett CL, Pesci EC, Cottle DL, et al. Prevalence of cytolethal distending toxin production in *Campylobacter jejuni* and relatedness of *Campylobacter* sp *cdtB* genes. *Infect Immun.* 1996;64: 2070-2078.
77. Hickey TE, Majam G, Guerry P. Intracellular survival of *Campylobacter jejuni* in human monocytic cells and induction of apoptotic death by cytholethal distending toxin. *Infect Immun.* 2005;73:5194-5197.
78. Shenker BJ, Besack D, McKay T, et al. Induction of cell cycle arrest in lymphocytes by *Actinobacillus actinomycetemcomitans* cytolethal distending toxin requires three subunits for maximum activity. *J Immunol.* 2005;174:2228-2234.
79. Bacon DJ, Alm RA, Burr DH, et al. Involvement of a plasmid in virulence of *Campylobacter jejuni* 81-176. *Infect Immun.* 2000;68:4384-4390.
80. Bacon DJ, Alm RA, Hu L, et al. DNA sequence and mutational analyses of the pVir plasmid of *Campylobacter jejuni* 81-176. *Infect Immun.* 2002;70:6242-6250.
81. Bacon DJ, Alm RA, Burr DH, et al. Involvement of a plasmid in virulence of *Campylobacter jejuni* 81-176. *Infect Immun.* 2002;68:4384-4390.
82. Tracz DM, Keelan M, Ahmed-Bentley J, et al. pVir and bloody diarrhea in *Campylobacter jejuni* enteritis. *Emerg Infect Dis.* 2005;11838-11843.
83. Fauchere JL, Rosenau A, Veron M, et al. Association with HeLa cells of *Campylobacter jejuni* and *Campylobacter coli* isolated from human feces. *Infect Immun.* 1986;54:283-287.
84. Kervella M, Pages J-M, Pei Z, et al. Isolation and characterization of two *Campylobacter* glycine-extracted proteins that bind to HeLa cell membranes. *Infect Immun.* 1993;61: 3440-3448.
85. Pei Z, Ellison RT III, Blaser MJ. Identification, purification and characterization of major antigenic proteins of *Campylobacter jejuni*. *J Biol Chem.* 1991;266:16363-16369.
86. Pei Z, Blaser MJ. PEB1, the major cell-binding factor of *Campylobacter jejuni*, is a homolog of the binding component in gram negative nutrient transport systems. *J Biol Chem.* 1993; 267:18717-18725.
87. Pei Z, Burucoa C, Grignon B, et al. Mutation in the *peb1A* locus of *Campylobacter jejuni* reduces interactions with epithelial cells and intestinal colonization of mice. *Infect Immun.* 1998; 66:938-943.

88. Jin S, Song YC, Emili A, et al. JlpA of *Campylobacter jejuni* interacts with surface-exposed heat shock protein 90 alpha and triggers signalling pathways leading to the activation of NF-kappaB and p38 MAP kinase in epithelial cells. *Cell Microbiol.* 2003;5:165-174.
89. Konkel ME, Garvis SG, Tipton SL, et al. Identification and molecular cloning of a gene encoding a fibronectin-binding protein (CadF) from *Campylobacter jejuni. Mol Microbiol.* 1997;24:953-963.
90. Yao R, Burr DH, Guerry P. Che Y-mediated modulation of *Campylobacter jejuni* virulence. *Mol Microbiol.* 1997; 23:1021-1031.
91. Doig P, Yao R, Burt DH, et al. An environmentally regulated pilus-like appendage involved in *Campylobacter* pathogenesis. *Mol Microbiol.* 1996;20:885-894.
92. Naikare H, Palyada K, Panciera R, et al. Major role for FeoB in *Campylobacter jejuni* ferrous iron acquisition, gut colonization, and intracellular survival. *Infect Immun.* 2006;74:5433-5444.
93. Pérez-Pérez GI, Blaser MJ. Lipopolysaccharide characteristics of pathogenic campylobacters. *Infect Immun.* 1985;47:353-359.
94. Aspinall GO, Fujimoto S, McDonald AG, et al. Lipopolysaccharides from *Campylobacter jejuni* associated with Guillain-Barré syndrome patients mimic human gangliosides in structure. *Infect Immun.* 1994;62:2122-2125.
95. Ang CW, De Klerk MA, Endtz HP, et al. Guillain-Barre syndrome- and Miller Fisher syndrome-associated *Campylobacter jejuni* lipopolysaccharides induce anti-GM1 and GQ1b antibodies in rabbits. *Infect Immun.* 2001;69:2462-2469.
96. Goodyear CS, O'Hanlon GM, Plomp JJ, et al. Monoclonal antibodies raised against Guillain-Barre syndrome-associated *Campylobacter jejuni* lipopolysaccharides react with neuronal gangliosides and paralyze muscle-nerve preparations. *J Clin Invest.* 1999;104:697-708.
97. Johnson WM, Lior H. Cytotoxic and cytotonic factors produced by *Campylobacter jejuni, Campylobacter coli*, and *Campylobacter laridis. J Clin Microbiol.* 1986;24:275-281.
98. Walker RI, Caldwell MB, Lee EC, et al. Pathophysiology of *Campylobacter* enteritis. *Microbiol Rev.* 1985;50:81-94.
99. Wassenaar T. Toxin production by *Campylobacter* spp. *Rev Clin Microbiol.* 1997;10:466-476.
100. Blaser MJ, Smith PF, Kohler PA. Susceptibility of *Campylobacter* isolates to the bactericidal activity in human serum. *J Infect Dis.* 1985;151:227.
101. Blaser MJ. *Campylobacter fetus*: emerging infection and model system for bacterial pathogenesis at mucosal surfaces. *Clin Infect Dis.* 1998;27:256-258.
102. Blaser MJ, Smith PF, Hopkins JA, et al. Pathogenesis of *Campylobacter fetus* infections: serum resistance associated with high molecular weight surface proteins. *J Infect Dis.* 1987;155: 696.
103. Dworkin J, Blaser MJ. Molecular mechanisms of *Campylobacter fetus* surface layer protein expression. *Mol Microbiol.* 1997;26:433-440.
104. Blaser MJ, Smith PF, Repine JE, et al. Pathogenesis of *Campylobacter fetus* infections: failure of C3b to bind explains serum and phagocytosis resistance. *J Clin Invest.* 1988;81:1434-1444.
105. Pei Z, Blaser MJ. Pathogenesis of *Campylobacter fetus* infections: role of surface array proteins in virulence in a mouse model. *J Clin Invest.* 1990;85:1036-1043.
106. Wang E, Garcia MM, Blake MS, et al. Shift in S-layer protein expression responsible for antigenic variation in *Campylobacter fetus. J Bacteriol.* 1993;175:4979-4984.
107. Tummuru MKR, Blaser MJ. Rearrangement of *sapA* homologs with conserved and variable regions in *Campylobacter fetus. Proc Natl Acad Sci U S A.* 1993;90:7265-7269.
108. Tu Z-C, Gaudreau C, Blaser MJ. Mechanisms underlying *Campylobacter fetus* pathogenesis in humans: surface-layer protein variation in relapsing infections. *J Infect Dis.* 2005;191:2082-2089.
109. Black RF, Perlman D, Clements ML, et al. Human volunteer studies with *C. jejuni.* In: Nachamkin I, Blaser MJ, Tompkins LS, eds. *Campylobacter jejuni: Current Status and Future Trends.* Washington, DC: American Society for Microbiology; 1992:207-215.
110. Johnson RJ, Wang SP, Shelton WR, et al. Persistent *Campylobacter jejuni* infection in an immunocompromised host. *Ann Intern Med.* 1984;100:832-834.
111. Melamed I, Bujanover Y, Igra YS, et al. *Campylobacter* enteritis in normal and immunodeficient children. *Am J Dis Child.* 1983;137:752-753.
112. Perlman DM, Ampel NM, Schiffman RB, et al. Persistent *Campylobacter jejuni* infections in patients infected with the human immunodeficiency virus: association with abnormal serological response to *C. jejuni* and emergence of erythromycin resistance during therapy. *Ann Intern Med.* 1988;108:540-546.
113. Coker AO, Isokpehi RD, Thomas BN, et al. Human campylobacteriosis in developing countries. *Emerg Infect Dis.* 2002;8:237-244.
114. Hu L, Bray MD, Osorio M, et al. *Campylobacter jejuni* induces maturation and cytokine production in human dendritic cells. *Infect Immun.* 2006;74:2697-2705.
115. Bokkenheuser V. *Vibrio fetus* infection in man: I. Ten new cases and some epidemiologic observations. *Am J Epidemiol.* 1970;91:400.
116. Guerrant RL, Lahita RG, Winn Jr EC, et al. Campylobacteriosis in man: pathogenic mechanisms and review of 91 bloodstream infections. *Am J Med.* 1978;65:484.
117. Blaser MJ, Berkowitz ID, LaForce FM, et al. *Campylobacter* enteritis: clinical and epidemiologic features. *Ann Intern Med.* 1979;91:179.
118. Skirrow MB. *Campylobacter* enteritis: a "new" disease. *BMJ.* 1977;2:9.
119. Karmali MA, Fleming PC. *Campylobacter* enteritis in children. *J Pediatr.* 1979;94:527.
120. McKinley MJ, Taylor M, Sangree MH. Toxic megacolon with *Campylobacter* colitis. *Conn Med.* 1980;44:496.
121. Tee W, Anderson BN, Ross BC, et al. Atypical campylobacters associated with gastroenteritis. *J Clin Microbiol.* 1987; 25:1248-1252.
122. Steele TW, Sangster N, Lanser JA. DNA relatedness and biochemical features of *Campylobacter* spp. isolated in central and south Australia. *J Clin Microbiol.* 1985;22:71-74.
123. Drake AA, Gilchrist MJR, Washington JA II, et al. Diarrhea due to *Campylobacter fetus* subspecies *jejuni*: a clinical review of 73 cases. *Mayo Clin Proc.* 1981;56:414.
124. Michalak DM, Perrault J, Gilchrist MJ, et al. *Campylobacter fetus* ss. *jejuni*: a cause of massive lower gastrointestinal hemorrhage. *Gastroenterology.* 1980;79:742.
125. Anders BJ, Lauer BA, Paisley JW. *Campylobacter* gastroenteritis in neonates. *Am J Dis Child.* 1981;135:900.
126. Goossens H, Henocque G, Kremp L, et al. Nosocomial outbreak of *Campylobacter jejuni* meningitis in newborn infants. *Lancet.* 1986;2:146-149.
127. Wright EP, Seager J. Convulsions associated with *Campylobacter* enteritis. *BMJ.* 1980;281:454.
128. Orlicek SL, Welch DF, Kuhls TL. Septicemia and meningitis caused by *Helicobacter cinaedi* in a neonate. *J Clin Microbiol.* 1993;31:569-571.
129. Blaser MJ, Perez GP, Smith PF, et al. Extraintestinal *Campylobacter jejuni* and *Campylobacter coli* infections: host factors and strain characteristics. *J Infect Dis.* 1986;153:552.
130. Gilbert GL, Davoren RA, Cole ME, et al. Midtrimester abortion associated with septicaemia caused by *Campylobacter jejuni. Med J Aust.* 1981;1:585.
131. Mertens A, DeSmet M. *Campylobacter* cholecystitis. *Lancet.* 1979;1:1092.
132. Gallagher P, Chadwick P, Jones DM, et al. Acute pancreatitis associated with *Campylobacter* infection. *Br J Surg.* 1981;68:383.
133. Ezpeleta C, Rojo de Ursua P, Obregon F, et al. Acute pancreatitis associated with *Campylobacter jejuni* bacteremia. *Clin Infect Dis.* 1992;15:1050.
134. Davies JS, Penfold JB. *Campylobacter* urinary infection. *Lancet.* 1979;1:1091.
135. Feder HM, Rasoulpour M, Rodriquez AJ. *Campylobacter* urinary tract infection: value of the urine gram stain. *JAMA.* 1986;256:2389.
136. Kersten PJSM, Endtz HP, Meis JFGM, et al. Erysipelas-like skin lesions associated with *Campylobacter jejuni* septicemia in patients with hypogammaglobulinemia. *Eur J Clin Microbiol Infect Dis.* 1992;11:842-847.
137. Lecuit M, Abachin E, Martin A, et al. Immunoproliferative small intestinal disease associated with *Campylobacter jejuni. N Engl J Med.* 2004;350:239-248.
138. Kosunen TU, Kauranen O, Martio J, et al. Reactive arthritis after *Campylobacter jejuni* enteritis in patients with HLA-B27. *Lancet.* 1980;1:1312.
139. Hannu T, Kauppi M, Tuomala M, et al. Reactive arthritis following an outbreak of *Campylobacter jejuni* infection. *J Rheum.* 2004;31:528-530.
140. Pope JE, Krizova A, Garg AX, et al. *Campylobacter* reactive arthritis: a systematic review. *Semin Arthritis Rheum.* 2007;37:48-55.
141. Uzoigwe C. *Campylobacter* infections of the pericardium and myocardium. *Clin Microbiol Infect.* 2005;11:253-255.
142. Kotilainen P, Lehtopolku M, Hakanen AJ. Myopericarditis in a patient with *Campylobacter* enteritis: a case-report and literature review. *Scand J Infect Dis.* 2006;38:549-552.
143. Humphrey KS. *Campylobacter* infection and hepatocellular injury. *Lancet.* 1993;341:49.
144. Monselise A, Blickstein D, Ostfeld I, et al. A case of cellulitis complicating *Campylobacter jejuni* subspecies *jejuni* bacteremia and review of the literature. *Eur J Clin Microbiol Infect Dis.* 2004;23:718-721.
145. Carter JE, Cimolai N. IgA nephropathy associated with *Campylobacter jejuni* enteritis. *Nephron.* 1991;58:101-102.
146. Mishu B, Blaser MJ. The role of *Campylobacter jejuni* infection in the initiation of Guillain-Barré syndrome. *Clin Infect Dis.* 1993;17:104-108.
147. Rees JH, Soudain SE, Gregory NA, et al. *Campylobacter jejuni* infection and Guillain-Barré syndrome. *N Engl J Med.* 1995;333:1374-1379.
148. Kaldor J, Speed BR. Guillain-Barré syndrome and *Campylobacter jejuni*: a serological study. *BMJ (Clin Res Ed).* 1984;288:1867-1870.
149. Mishu B, Ilyas AA, Koski CL, et al. Serologic evidence of *Campylobacter jejuni* infection preceding Guillain-Barré syndrome. *Ann Intern Med.* 1993;118:947-953.
150. Kuroki S, Saida T, Nukina M, et al. *Campylobacter jejuni* strains from patients with Guillain-Barré syndrome belong mostly to Penner serogroup 19 and contain β-*N*-acetylglucosamine residues. *Ann Neurol.* 1993;33:243-247.
151. Fujimoto S, Allos BM, Misawa N, et al. Restriction fragment length polymorphism analysis and random amplified polymorphic DNA analysis of *Campylobacter jejuni* strains isolated from patients with Guillain-Barré syndrome. *J Infect Dis.* 1997;176: 1105-1108.
152. Allos BM, Lippy FT, Carlsen A, et al. *Campylobacter jejuni* strains from patients with Guillain-Barré syndrome. *Emerg Infect Dis.* 1998;4:263-268.
153. Franklin B, Ulmer DD. Human infection with *Vibrio fetus. West J Med.* 1974;120:200.
154. Gazaigne L, Legrand P, Renaud B, et al. *Campylobacter fetus* bloodstream infection: risk factors and clinical features. *Eur J Clin Microbiol Infect Dis.* 2008;27:185-189.
155. Collins HS, Blevins A, Baxter E. Protracted bacteremia and meningitis due to *Vibrio fetus. Arch Intern Med.* 1964;113:361.
156. Park CH, McDonald F, Twohig AM, et al. Septicemia and gastroenteritis due to *Vibrio fetus. South Med J.* 1973;66:531.
157. Neuzil KM, Wang E, Haas D, et al. Persistence of *Campylobacter fetus* bacteremia associated with absence of opsonizing antibodies. *J Clin Microbiol.* 1994;32:1718-1720.
158. Loeb H, Bettag JL, Yantz NK, et al. *Vibrio fetus* endocarditis. *Am Heart J.* 1966;71:381.
159. Killiam HA, Crowder JG, White AC, et al. Pericarditis due to *Vibrio fetus. Am J Cardiol.* 1966;17:723.
160. Vesely D, MacIntyre S, Ratzan KR. Bilateral deep brachial vein thrombophlebitis due to *Vibrio fetus. Arch Intern Med.* 1975;135:994.
161. Eden AH. Perinatal mortality caused by *Vibrio fetus*: review and analysis. *J Pediatr.* 1966;68:297.
162. Gunderson CH, Sack GE. Neurology of *Vibrio fetus. Neurology.* 1971;21:307.
163. Kilo C, Hagemann PO, Maryi J. Septic arthritis and bacteremia due to *Vibrio fetus. Am J Med.* 1965;38:962.
164. Lawrence R, Nibbe AF, Levin S. Lung abscess secondary to *Vibrio fetus* malabsorption syndrome and acquired agammaglobulinemia. *Chest.* 1971;60:191.
165. Meier PA, Dooley DP, Jorgensen JH, et al. Development of quinolone-resistant *Campylobacter fetus* bacteremia in human immunodeficiency virus-infected patients. *J Infect Dis.* 1998;177:951-954.
166. Benjamin JS, Leaper S, Owen RJ, et al. Description of *Campylobacter laridis*, a new species comprising the nalidixic acid resistant thermophilic *Campylobacter* (NARTC group). *Curr Microbiol.* 1983;8:231-238.
167. Simor AE, Wilcox L. Enteritis associated with *Campylobacter laridis. J Clin Microbiol.* 1987;25:10-12.
168. Quinn TC, Goodell SE, Fennell C, et al. Infections with *Campylobacter jejuni* and *Campylobacter*-like organisms in homosexual men. *Ann Intern Med.* 1984;101:187-192.
169. Kemper CA, Mickelsen P, Morton A, et al. *Helicobacter* (*Campylobacter*) *fennelliae*-like organisms as an important but occult cause of bacteremia in a patient with AIDS. *J Infect.* 1993;26:97-101.
170. Fleisch F, Burnens A, Weber R, et al. *Helicobacter* species strain *Mainz* isolated from cultures of blood from two patients with AIDS. *Clin Infect Dis.* 1998;26:526-527.
171. Kiehlbauch JA, Tauxe RV, Baker CN, et al. *Helicobacter cinaedi*-associated bacteremia and cellulitis in immunocompromised patients. *Ann Intern Med.* 1994;121:90-93.
172. Goosens H, Pot B, Vlaes L, et al. Characterization and description of "*Campylobacter upsaliensis*" isolated from human feces. *J Clin Microbiol.* 1990;28:1039-1046.
173. Patton CM, Shaffer N, Edmonds P, et al. Human disease associated with "*Campylobacter upsaliensis*" (catalase-negative or weakly positive *Campylobacter* species) in the United States. *J Clin Microbiol.* 1989;27:66-73.
174. Gaudreau C, Lamothe F. *Campylobacter upsaliensis* isolated from a breast abscess. *J Clin Microbiol.* 1992;30:1354-1356.
175. Damborg P, Guardabassi L, Pedersen K, et al. Comparative analysis of human and canine *Campylobacter upsaliensis* isolates by amplified fragment length polymorphism. *J Clin Microbiol.* 2008;46:1504-1506.
176. Edmonds P, Patton CM, Griffin PM, et al. *Campylobacter hyointestinalis* associated with human gastrointestinal disease in the United States. *J Clin Microbiol.* 1987;25:685-691.
177. Vandamme P, Pugina P, Benzi G, et al. Outbreak of recurrent abdominal cramps associated with *Arcobacter butzleri* in an Italian school. *J Clin Microbiol.* 1992;30:2335-2337.
178. Sorlin P, van Damme P, Nortier J, et al. Recurrent "*Flexispira rappini*" bacteremia in an adult patient undergoing hemodialysis: case report. *J Clin Microbiol.* 1999;37:1319-1323.
179. Abbott SL, Waddington M, Lindquist D, et al. Description of *Campylobacter curvus* and *C. curvus*-like strains associated with sporadic episodes of bloody gastroenteritis and Brainerd's diarrhea. *J Clin Microbiol.* 2005;43:585-588.
180. Wetsch NM, Somani K, Tyrrell GJ, et al. *Campylobacter curvus*-associated hepatic abscess: a case-report. *J Clin Microbiol.* 2006;44:1909-1911.
181. Chua K, Gurtler V, Montgomery J, et al. *Campylobacter insulaenigrae* causing septicaemia and enteritis. *J Med Microbiol.* 2007;56(Pt 11):1565-1567.
182. Paisley JW, Mirrett S, Lauer BA, et al. Darkfield microscopy of human feces for the presumptive diagnosis of *Campylobacter* enteritis. *J Clin Microbiol.* 1982;15:61.
183. Sazie ESM, Titus AE. Rapid diagnosis of *Campylobacter* enteritis. *Ann Intern Med.* 1982;96:62.
184. Poppert S, Haas M, Yildiz T, et al. Identification of thermotolerant *Campylobacter* species by fluorescence in situ hybridization. *J Clin Microbiol.* 2008;46:2133-2136.

185. Ternhag A, Asikainen T, Giesecke J, et al. A meta-analysis on the effects of antibiotic treatment on duration of symptoms caused by infection with *Campylobacter* species. *Clin Infect Dis.* 2007;44:696.

186. Ruiz-Palacios GM. The health burden of *Campylobacter* infection and the impact of antimicrobial resistance: playing chicken. *Clin Infect Dis.* 2007;44:701.

187. Salazar-Lindo E, Sack RB, Chea-Woo E, et al. Early treatment with erythromycin of *Campylobacter jejuni*-associated dysentery in children. *J Pediatr.* 1986;109:355.

188. Anders BJ, Lauer BA, Paisley JW, et al. Double-blind placebo controlled trial of erythromycin for treatment of *Campylobacter* enteritis. *Lancet.* 1982;1:131.

189. Vanhoof R, Vanderlinden MP, Dierickx R, et al. Susceptibility of *Campylobacter fetus* subsp. *jejuni* to twenty-nine antimicrobial agents. *Antimicrob Agents Chemother.* 1978;14:553.

190. Walder M. Susceptibility of *Campylobacter fetus* subsp. *jejuni* to twenty antimicrobial agents. *Antimicrob Agents Chemother.* 1979;16:37.

191. Vanhoof R, Gordts B, Dierickx R, et al. Bacteriostatic and bactericidal activities of 24 antimicrobial agents against *Campylobacter fetus* subsp. *jejuni*. *Antimicrob Agents Chemother.* 1980;18:118.

192. Huang MB, Baker CN, Banerjee S, et al. Accuracy of the E test for determining antimicrobial susceptibilities of staphylococci, enterococci, *Campylobacter jejuni*, and gram-negative bacteria resistant to antimicrobial agents. *J Clin Microbiol.* 1992;30:3243-3248.

193. Sjögren E, Kaijser B, Werner M. Antimicrobial susceptibilities of *Campylobacter jejuni* and *Campylobacter coli* isolated in Sweden: a 10-year follow-up report. *Antimicrob Agents Chemother.* 1992;36:2847-2849.

194. Blaser MJ, Reller LB. *Campylobacter* enteritis. *N Engl J Med.* 1981;305:1444.

195. Skirrow MB, Blaser MJ. *Campylobacter jejuni.* In: Blaser MJ, Smith PD, Ravdin J, et al, eds. *Infections of the Gastrointestinal Tract.* 2nd ed. Philadelphia: Lippincott-Raven; 2002:825-848.

196. Ray WA, Murray KT, Meredith S, et al. Oral erythromycin and the risk of sudden death from cardiac causes. *N Engl J Med.* 2004;351:1089.

197. Kuschner RA, Trofa AF, Thomas RJ, et al. Use of azithromycin for the treatment of *Campylobacter* enteritis in travelers to Thailand, an area where ciprofloxacin resistance is prevalent. *Clin Infect Dis.* 1995;21:536-541.

198. Engberg J, Aarestrup FM, Taylor DE, et al. Quinolone and macrolide resistance in *Campylobacter jejuni* and *C. coli:* resistance mechanisms and trends in human isolates. *Emerg Infect Dis.* 2001;7:24-34.

199. Gupta A, Nelson JM, Barrett TJ, et al. Antimicrobial resistance among *Campylobacter* strains, United States, 1997-2001. *Emerg Infect Dis.* 2004;10:1102.

200. Haas M, Essig A, Bartelt E, et al. Detection of resistance to macrolides in thermotolerant *Campylobacter* species by fluorescence in situ hybridization. *J Clin Microbiol.* 2008;46:3842-3844.

201. Segreti J, Gootz TD, Goodman LJ, et al. High-level quinolone resistance in clinical isolates of *Campylobacter jejuni.* *J Infect Dis.* 1992;165:667-670.

202. Reina J, Borrell N, Serra A. Emergence of resistance to erythromycin and fluoroquinolone in thermotolerant *Campylobacter* strains isolated from feces 1987-1991. *Eur J Clin Microbiol Infect Dis.* 1992;11:1163-1166.

203. Smith KE, Besser JM, Hedberg CW, et al. Quinolone-resistant *Campylobacter jejuni* infections in Minnesota, 1992-1998. *N Engl J Med.* 1999;340:1525-1532.

204. Wistrom J, Jertborn M, Ekwall E, et al. Empiric treatment of acute diarrheal disease with norfloxacin: a randomized, placebo-controlled study. *Ann Intern Med.* 1992;117:202-208.

205. Gaunt PN, Piddock LJ. Ciprofloxacin resistant *Campylobacter* spp. in humans: an epidemiological and laboratory study. *J Antimicrob Chemother.* 1996;37:747.

206. The Campylobacter Sentinel Surveillance. Ciprofloxacin resistance in *Campylobacter jejuni:* case-case analysis as a tool for elucidating risks at home and abroad. *J Antimicrob Chemother.* 2002;50:561.

207. Smith KE, Besser JM, Hedberg CW, et al. Quinolone-resistant *Campylobacter jejuni* infections in Minnesota, 1992-1998. *N Engl J Med.* 1999;340:1525.

208. Nelson JM, Smith KE, Vugia DJ, et al. Prolonged diarrhea due to ciprofloxacin-resistant *Campylobacter* infection. *J Infect Dis.* 2004;190:1565-1566.

209. Helms M, Simonsen J, Olsen KE, et al. Adverse health events associated with antimicrobial drug resistance in *Campylobacter* species: a registry-based cohort study. *J Infect Dis.* 2005;191:1050-1055.

210. Unicomb LE, Ferguson J, Stafford RJ, et al. Low-level fluoroquinolone resistance among *Campylobacter jejuni* isolates in Australia. *Clin Infect Dis.* 2006;42:1368.

211. Nelson JM, Chiller TM, Powers JH, et al. Fluoroquinolone-resistant *Campylobacter* species and the withdrawal of fluoroquinolones from use in poultry: a public health success story. *Clin Infect Dis.* 2007;44:977.

212. Lachance N, Gaudreau C, Lamothe F, et al. Susceptibilities of β-lactamase-positive and -negative strains of *Campylobacter coli* to β-lactam agents. *Antimicrob Agents Chemother.* 1993;37:1174-1176.

213. Taylor DN, Blaser MJ, Echeverria P, et al. Erythromycin-resistant *Campylobacter* infections in Thailand. *Antimicrob Agents Chemother.* 1987;31:438-442.

214. Smith GS, Blaser MJ. Fatalities associated with *Campylobacter jejuni* infections. *JAMA.* 1985;253:2873.

215. Hammarström V, Smith CIE, Hammarström L. Oral immunoglobulin treatment in *Campylobacter jejuni* enteritis. *Lancet.* 1993;341:1036.

216. Francioli P, Herzstein J, Grob J-P, et al. *Campylobacter fetus* subspecies *fetus* bacteremia. *Arch Intern Med.* 1985;145:289-292.

217. Tremblay C, Gaudreau C, Lorange M. Epidemiology and antimicrobial susceptibilities of 111 *Campylobacter fetus* subsp. *fetus* strains isolated in Quebec, Canada from 1983 to 2000. *J Clin Microbiol.* 2003;41:463-466.

218. Bremell T, Bjelle A, Svedhem A. Rheumatic symptoms following an attack of *Campylobacter* enteritis: a five year follow up. *Ann Rheum Dis.* 1991;50:934-948.

219. CYP3A and drug interactions. *The Medical Letter.* 2005;47(1212):54.

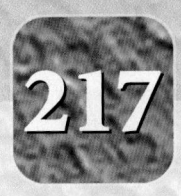

217

Helicobacter pylori and Other Gastric *Helicobacter* Species

MARTIN J. BLASER

Helicobacter pylori (formerly known as *Campylobacter pylori* or *pyloridis*) was first isolated from humans in 1982.[1] This highly motile, curved, gram-negative rod lives within the mucus layer overlying the gastric and occasionally the duodenal or esophageal mucosal epithelium.[2] *H. pylori* is commonly found in the human stomach, when present, as the single dominant species; essentially all persons colonized with *H. pylori* have a cellular infiltrate in the lamina propria of the gastric antrum and fundus.[3] Of special significance is that *H. pylori* is present in most persons with "idiopathic" peptic ulcer disease. The first isolation of *H. pylori* in pure culture and its association with gastritis and peptic ulcer disease led to the awarding of the Nobel Prize in Medicine in 2005 to Barry Marshall and Robin Warren, two physicians in Australia. The presence of *H. pylori* increases the risk of peptic ulcer disease[4] and gastric cancer,[5,6] but decreases the risk of esophageal reflux and its consequences[7] and may protect against childhood asthma and related disorders.[8-11] With the development of effective therapies to eradicate *H. pylori*, physicians are faced with the challenge of determining which patients will benefit from therapy and which may be harmed. This view of the role of *H. pylori* in human disease represents a major departure from the previous decade's assessment of gastroduodenal pathophysiology. Other *Helicobacter* species and related organisms are increasingly being recognized in clinical materials; however, their role in disease is largely uncertain.

Microbiology

H. pylori organisms are small (0.5 to 1.0 μm in width and 2.5 to 4.0 μm in length), curved, microaerophilic gram-negative rods.[12,13] Because they closely resemble members of the genus *Campylobacter*, they were initially considered to belong to that genus. However, multiple genotypic and phenotypic characteristics are different from those of campylobacters, and a new genus, *Helicobacter*, was established.[13] Other newly recognized organisms include *Helicobacter mustelae* in ferrets,[13,14] *Helicobacter felis* in dogs and cats,[14] *Helicobacter muridarum* in mice, *Helicobacter nemestrinae* in nonhuman primates, and *Helicobacter acinonyx* in cheetahs.[15] Essentially every mammal studied to date has gastric colonization with one or more *Helicobacter* species. These seem largely species specific and indicate that the mammalian stomach is a major niche for these organisms.

Helicobacter heilmannii is a gastric spirochete of humans and is considered in a separate section of this chapter. *Helicobacter fennelliae* and *Helicobacter cinaedi* are intestinal organisms causing diarrheal illnesses; because the clinical features of these infections resemble those of *Campylobacter* spp., they are discussed in Chapter 216. Based on the recent and intense interest of microbiologists in gastric bacteria, it is likely that the genus *Helicobacter* will continue to expand. Nevertheless, *H. pylori* is the most important human organism and may be considered the prototype for these organisms. *Helicobacter* spp. (such as *Helicobacter hepaticus*, *Helicobacter bilis*, and *Helicobacter rappini*) have also been identified in the colon and biliary tract of rodents, and there is human carriage as well.[15-17] Preliminary evidence suggests that they might colonize the diseased human biliary tract,[18,19] but whether they participate in the pathophysiologic process is uncertain.[20] They have caused chronic bacteremia and indolent cellulitis in patients with X-linked hypogammaglobulinemia and common variable immunode-ficiency. Thus, there are both gastric and intestinal residential *Helicobacter* spp. in humans, but the role, if any, of the intestinal species in human mucosal disease has not been defined.

H. pylori cells are highly motile, with a rapid corkscrew motion, and have multiple polar sheathed flagella.[13] Although these cells are classically curved or spiral in fresh cultures, spherical (coccoid) forms are present in older cultures. The major biochemical properties of *H. pylori* and several related bacteria are shown in Table 217-1. The outstanding biochemical characteristic of helicobacters is their high production of urease. *H. pylori* urease is a hexadimer consisting of 61- and 28-kDa subunits, both of which are essential for activity.[21] Regulation of urease is complex, and multiple other genes are necessary for full activity.[22] All clinical isolates are urease positive, but urease-negative strains have been derived in the laboratory.

The nucleotide sequence of the chromosome from several *H. pylori* strains (26695 and J99) has been determined.[23-26] Comparison of these sequences has opened new avenues for the study of *H. pylori* microbiology. A core genome has been defined[27]; the strains share many but not all genes, and even conserved genes show polymorphisms, strain-specific genes that include restriction-modification enzymes,[28] and others concerned with cell surface structures.[29,30] *H. pylori* has few two-component regulatory proteins, but frameshifts are common within open reading frames encoding certain *H. pylori* proteins. This suggests that *H. pylori* may use mutation to control phenotype, with the host selecting for the "most fit" organism within a particular environmental niche.[31,32]

Although *H. pylori* is highly homogeneous in the biochemical characteristics used in clinical microbiology, including urease, oxidase, and catalase positivity, wide variation is noted at a genetic level.[32-34] Humans may be simultaneously colonized with more than one strain of *H. pylori*.[35-37] Plasmids are present in most *H. pylori* isolates; they vary in size and mostly are cryptic at present. *H. pylori* strains are naturally competent, that is, able to take up heterologous DNA; studies of individual *H. pylori* isolates and of populations of strains indicate that recombination is an important characteristic.[34,37,38] Through point mutation and intergenomic and intragenomic recombination, *H. pylori* are among the most varied of all species in the human biosphere.[39-41] The strain-specific restriction-modification systems[28] diminish recombination and may permit different strains to simultaneously colonize a host.[42]

The most important dichotomy among *H. pylori* strains is the presence of the *cag* pathogenicity island, a 35- to 40-kilobase chromosomal region encoding *cagA* and a number of type IV secretion system genes.[43-46] Both *cagA*+ and *cagA*− strains are present in *H. pylori* populations in most parts of the world,[47] which suggests that the acquisition of this region by *H. pylori* is ancient. It now is known that the type IV secretion system injects its substrate, the CagA protein, into host epithelial cells.[48,49] The 3′ region of *cagA* contains DNA repeats flanking sites that encode tyrosine phosphorylation motifs. By intragenomic recombination, *H. pylori* populations include individual cells with 0, 1, 2, or more tyrosine phosphorylation motifs in its CagA product.[50] Once injected into the epithelium by the type IV secretion system, Src-kinases phosphorylate these tyrosine residues,[51] and the phospho-CagA interacts with SHP-2[52] and other regulatory molecules that affect mitogen-activated protein kinases and the actin cytoskeleton; these

TABLE 217-1	Biochemical Characteristics of *Helicobacter pylori* and Related Bacteria			
Characteristic	*Helicobacter pylori*	*Helicobacter mustelae*	*Helicobacter felis*	*Campylobacter jejuni*
Urease	+	+	+	−
Catalase	+	+	+	+
Oxidase	+	+	+	+
H₂S production	−	−	−	+
Guanosine plus cytosine content	35-38	36	42.5	33-36
Hippurate hydrolysis	−	−	−	+
Nitrate reduction	−	+	+	+
Resistance to nalidixic acid (30-μg disk)	+	−	+	−
Cephalothin (30-μg disk)	−	+	+	−
Growth at 42°C	−	+	−	+
Growth at 37°C	−	+	+	+
Growth at 25°C	+	+	+	−

Data from references 13 to 16.

pathways affect cell shape and cycle events and cytokine production.[53-55] Thus, CagA is an important *H. pylori* molecule that signals the host. The type IV secretion system also injects peptidoglycan into epithelial cells, which affects Nod1 signaling.[56] The *cag* island is metastable, and isolates in individual patients may vary in the presence of the island, specific genes or regions, or subgenic sequences,[57,58] as in the case of the 3′ region of *cagA*.[50] This instability creates a population of variants that can interact with the host in a myriad of ways. Although important in their own right, the cag polymorphisms are indicative of similar phenomena at other *H. pylori* loci.[59] The *cag* status of an *H. pylori* strain is relevant to the risk of a number of clinical outcomes (see later).

Another heterogeneous locus affects *vacA,* a conserved gene that encodes a secreted protein (vacuolating cytotoxin) that interacts with epithelial cells.[60] Three parts of *vacA* have major polymorphisms: the *s* region (with alleles s1a, s1b, s1c, and s2), the *m* region (with alleles m1, m2a, and m2b), and the *i* region (i1 and i2).[61-63] Because s1 genotypes are strongly linked to *cag* positivity, many of the same clinical associations with *cag* are also present.[64] Effects of the *vacA* product on pore formation[65,67] affect immune function.[67,68] It now is clear that *vacA* is an immunosuppressing molecule, analogous to FK-506, that downregulates T-cell activity.[69] Both *cagA* and *vacA* are human-specific adaptations that favor persistent colonization.

☐ Epidemiology

H. pylori has been isolated from persons in all parts of the world[70-72] (Fig. 217-1). Similar organisms have been isolated from primates, but other animal sources for *H. pylori* have not been identified, nor have reservoirs been found in food, soil, or water. It now appears likely that humans are the major, if not sole, reservoir for *H. pylori.* Genetic loci with phylogeographic affinities indicate that *H. pylori* has been present in humans for at least 50,000 years, if not longer; the current geographic distribution of *H. pylori* alleles reflects ancient migrations of human populations.[71-73] These data support the notion that *H. pylori* is indigenous to humans, as its relatives are to other mammals, but that they are disappearing as a result of modernization.[9,74,75] On occasion, transmission occurs from person to person via improperly cleaned endoscopes.[76]

The high prevalence and incidence of colonization among persons in settings where sanitary conditions are suboptimal, including institutions for the mentally retarded and orphanages, and in developing countries do not reflect modern standards, suggesting that fecal-oral transmission occurs.[70,77] *H. pylori* has occasionally been isolated from feces, especially from children.[78] *H. pylori* has been isolated from dental plaque,[35] and DNA products may be detected in saliva by polymerase chain reaction, which raises the possibility of oral-oral transmission as well. However, studies of persons attending clinics for either sexually

transmitted diseases or infertility indicate that sexual transmission does not occur very frequently, if at all.[79] The relative contribution of fecal-oral, oral-oral, or vomitus-oral[80] transmission of *H. pylori* is not known. *H. pylori* infection clusters in families,[81] and the presence of a colonized child is highly associated with large family size and older siblings.[82,83]

The prevalence of *H. pylori* colonization is chiefly related to age[77,84] and geographic location. Males and females have essentially equal rates of colonization (slight male predominance). In developing countries, by age 10, more than 70% carry *H. pylori,* and by age 20, carriage is nearly universal. In the United States, among non-Hispanic whites, little colonization occurs during childhood, and rates gradually increase during adulthood and reach a prevalence of 50% among persons older than 60 years.[85] Among blacks and Hispanics, a higher prevalence is seen at all ages.[86-88] The annual incidence of acquisition has ranged from 0.5% among epidemiologists in the United States to 7.4% among persons at an institution for the mentally retarded in Australia.[89] In most populations, *H. pylori* appears to be mainly acquired during childhood,[70,90] but not in the first year of life.[91] The incidence of *H. pylori* has been progressively declining in the United States and other developed countries,[89,92] probably as a result of smaller

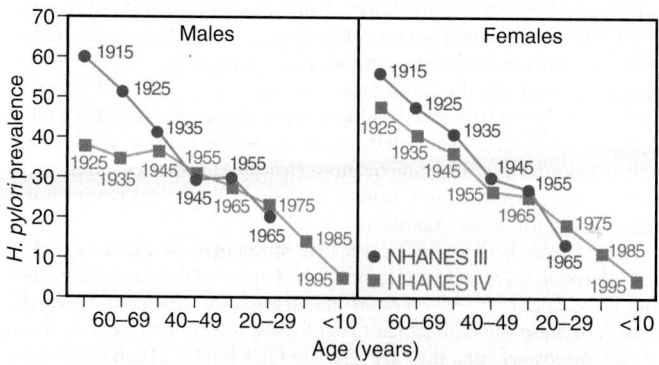

Figure 217-1 **Age-specific prevalence of *Helicobacter pylori* positivity among men and women in the National Health and Nutrition Examination Survey (NHANES) III phase I (1988 to 1991; *red squares*) and NHANES 1999 to 2000 (*blue squares*), by age and year of birth.** Year of birth is shown at the midpoint of decade birth categories. Prevalence data for participants 19 years of age or younger were not available in NHANES III. For consistency, we did not consider the *H. pylori* cagA immunoglobulin G enzyme-linked immunosorbent assay results in NHANES III and in participants with an immune status ratio of 0.91 to 1.09 in NHANES 1999 to 2000. (*From Chen Y, Blaser MJ. Helicobacter pylori colonization is inversely associated with childhood asthma. J Infect Dis. 2008;198:553-560.*)

family sizes, decreased crowding, improved sanitation, and now more than 60 years of widespread antibiotic use.[74,93,94] Thus, the age-related increase in prevalence reflects both a birth cohort phenomenon (with persons born earlier having higher acquisition rates in childhood) and continuing exposure and low-level new colonization into adulthood. The birth cohort effect predominates. Being an immigrant and of lower socioeconomic status are risk factors for *H. pylori* presence.[84,86,88] In total, in less than one century in the United States, colonization has gone from being ubiquitous to being present in 5% of children[9]; this is a change in human microecology of major proportion.

Pathology and Pathogenesis

H. pylori is able to survive and multiply in the gastric environment, which is hostile to the growth of most bacteria.[31] When intraluminal acidity diminishes as a result of gastric atrophy, *H. pylori* is no longer able to colonize, possibly because of competing organisms. Outstanding *H. pylori* characteristics that permit gastric colonization include microaerophilism for survival within the mucus gel, spiral shape and flagella for motility within this viscous layer, and urease activity, which generates ammonium ions that buffer gastric acidity.[95] Numerous adaptations permit survival of *H. pylori* in the acidic milieu of the stomach.[96-100] Although most organisms appear to be free living in the mucus layer, smaller numbers appear to be adherent to the mucosal epithelial cells and form adherence pedestals resembling those produced by enteropathogenic *Escherichia coli*[101]; several important adhesins have been identified.[102-104]

H. pylori overlies only gastric-type, but not intestinal-type, epithelial cells. Affected gastric epithelial cells may be in the gastric antrum or fundus[105] or may be ectopic in the duodenum or in the esophagus.[3,106,107] In contrast, *H. pylori* does not colonize intestinal epithelium, even when present in the stomach.[3] The gastric tissue underneath *H. pylori* colonization virtually always has a cellular infiltrate. The lamina propria most commonly contains mononuclear cells, including lymphocytes, monocytes, and plasma cells. Neutrophils and, to a lesser extent, eosinophils may be present in the lamina propria and epithelium. The epithelial glands have a more complex architecture and less mucus than when *H. pylori* is absent.[3,108] In children, a follicular lymphoid pattern is common. The presence of *H. pylori* induces these changes and the bacterium is not just a secondary colonizer; the T-cell responses may have systemic regulatory functions.[109-111]

The mechanisms of tissue injury are not clearly established, and both bacterial and host factors may be determinants of outcome.[112-116] *H. pylori* does not appear to invade tissues, except as an incidental finding. Thus, the lesions are likely to reflect a response to extracellular products or to contact from the organism. Ammonia, produced by urease and by deaminases, may potentiate neutrophil-induced mucosal injury.[117] Both the CagA and VacA proteins are important signaling molecules elaborated by *H. pylori*[118,119] (see previously), and the host mounts antibody responses to both.[120,121] Strains from patients with ulcers produce higher levels of VacA in vitro than do strains from patients without ulcers.[60,61,122] Similarly, strains from patients with ulcers or stomach cancer more commonly express CagA compared with controls.[4,107,123] Urease may be shed by *H. pylori* cells, has been observed in affected tissues, and is a chemoattractant and activator of host phagocytic cells.[124,125]

Bacterial lipopolysaccharide usually has proinflammatory activities, but *H. pylori* lipopolysaccharide has remarkably little.[126] *H. pylori* lipopolysaccharide may express the type II Lewis (Lewis[x], Lewis[y]), neither, or both of these antigens,[29,30,127] as well as type I antigens (Le[a], Le[b]). This observation is significant because these antigens are present on gastric epithelial cells, and there is evidence that the host Lewis phenotype selects for the particular Lewis expression of the *H. pylori* population.[128] The presence of *H. pylori* overlying the gastric mucosa activates epithelial cells to produce proinflammatory cytokines[129-132] and activates mononuclear and polymorphonuclear cells to produce cytokines, superoxide, tumor necrosis factor-α, and other proinflammatory molecules.[125,133,134] Because *H. pylori* can persist in the stomach

for many decades, these proinflammatory activities must be downregulated to permit this universally stable colonization.[31,135] *H. pylori*–positive persons have different T-cell populations in the gastric mucosa, with increased numbers of T-reg and T_H17 cells.[109,110] These may be downregulating the local inflammatory responses but also may have systemic consequences (see later).

Humans are polymorphic in the genetic loci involved in regulating proinflammatory cytokine production. Proinflammatory alleles regulating interleukin-1β and interleukin-10 affect risk of gastric cancer in *H. pylori*–positive persons.[136-138] Virtually all patients with duodenal ulceration are colonized by strains possessing *cagA* (and thus the *cag* pathogenicity island).[139] Thus *cagA*, the first gene described to not be conserved among all *H. pylori* strains, is highly associated with both peptic ulcer disease and gastric cancer.[6,71] In East Asia, most *H. pylori* strains are *cagA*+.

Persons colonized with *H. pylori* have different gastric secretory physiology than do those who are not colonized. On average, colonized persons have higher gastrin levels, which are reduced by eradication of the organism.[140,141] The mechanism for increased gastrin production appears to be related to low gastric somatostatin levels,[142,143] which may reflect cytokine production in the colonized antrum.[135,144] Increased gastrin may contribute to the increase in parietal cell mass observed in many patients with duodenal ulceration. In contrast, *H. pylori* products may directly affect parietal cells,[145] which may diminish acid production. That *H. pylori* involves gastric tissues concerned with both acid production (fundus) and its regulation (antrum) may in part be responsible for the multiplicity of potential outcomes of its colonization.[107,135,146] Differences among colonized hosts in cell-mediated immunity and cytokine responses to *H. pylori* are other possible determinants of outcome variability.[147-150] Findings similar to those observed in humans develop in nonhuman primates colonized with *H. pylori*.[151,152] The development of experimental *H. pylori* infections in conventional rodents and in human volunteers[153] has allowed new avenues for exploring host-microbe interactions.[154-157]

Clinical Consequences Associated with *H. pylori* Colonization

Although *H. pylori* is commonly isolated from the human stomach, colonization is associated with certain types of upper gastrointestinal pathology, appears to protect against other diseases, and is neutral for still others (Table 217-2). From a clinical standpoint, the major consequences of *H. pylori* colonization are as follows.

ACUTE ACQUISITION

Natural, voluntary, or accidental *H. pylori* acquisition may cause an acute upper gastrointestinal illness with nausea and upper abdominal pain.[76,182,183] Vomiting, burping, and fever may also be present. Symptoms last from 3 to 14 days, with most illnesses persisting less than 1 week. A diagnosis of food poisoning may be made in persons seeking medical attention. For many individuals, the acquisition of *H. pylori* is clinically silent.[183] Most data suggesting symptomatic acquisition relate to adults, but worldwide, most acquisition actually occurs in children; the relative proportion of symptomatic and asymptomatic acute acquisition at any age is not known. In the weeks after acquisition, intense gastritis develops; hypochlorhydria ensues and may persist for as long as 1 year. In children, there is a transient increase in serum pepsinogen I levels.[91] One adult volunteer who ingested *H. pylori* seemed to have had an acute self-limited infection[182]; the frequency of this phenomenon is not known.

PERSISTENT COLONIZATION

It now is clear that, after acquisition, *H. pylori* persists for years, if not decades, in most persons[183,184] (Fig. 217-2). Not every exposure to *H. pylori* leads to persistent colonization, either due to lack of adaptation to the particular host[185] or to coincident or proximate use of antibiot-

TABLE 217-2
Association of *Helicobacter pylori* with Common Pathologic Lesions of the Upper Gastrointestinal Tract and with Nongastrointestinal Diseases

Lesion	Association with *H. pylori*
Chronic diffuse superficial gastritis	Nearly always associated[3,84]
Type A (pernicious anemia) gastritis	Negative association[158,159]
NSAID gastropathy	Negative or no association[160]
Acute erosive gastritis (e.g., alcohol, aspirin)	No association[3]
Gastric ulceration	Commonly observed in patients who are not ingesting NSAIDs or aspirin[4,159,161,162]
Duodenal ulceration	Usually associated with idiopathic lesions (non–drug induced, non–Zollinger-Ellison syndrome)[4,162-164]
Gastric adenocarcinoma	Positively associated with (noncardia) cancers of the body and antrum[6,7,98,100,107,165-167]
Gastric lymphoma	Strongly associated with MALT-type B-cell lymphomas[168,169]
Idiopathic thrombocytopenic purpura	Often associated[170-172]
Nonulcer dyspepsia	Little or no association[173-177]
Gastroesophageal reflux disease	Presence of *cag*⁺ strains has protective association[178,179]
Barrett's esophagus	May colonize distalmost gastric epithelium in patients with gastric colonization[3]; presence of *cag*⁺ strains has protective association[179]
Adenocarcinoma of the esophagus	Presence of *cag*⁺ strains has protective association[107,180,181]
Childhood asthma and related allergic disorders (allergic rhinitis, eczema and skin sensitization)	Presence of *cag*⁺ strains has protective association[8-11]

MALT, mucosa-associated lymphoid tumor; NSAID, nonsteroidal anti-inflammatory drug.

ics. Tissue and serologic responses to colonization develop in essentially all persistently colonized persons.[84] The acute *H. pylori*–induced upper gastrointestinal symptoms do not return in most persons; most with persistent *H. pylori* colonization are asymptomatic. However, studies of patients with nonulcer dyspepsia indicate that *H. pylori* may be slightly more common in cases than in age-matched controls[173] and that *H. pylori* colonization may be one of the causes of this common but poorly defined and heterogeneous group of disorders. Supporting this hypothesis are the results of some studies indicating that some patients with nonulcer dyspepsia who are colonized with *H. pylori* show better responses to antimicrobial therapy than to placebo,[174] an

effect not seen in patients with nonulcer dyspepsia who do not have *H. pylori* colonization.[175] However, in other studies, no difference between *H. pylori* treatment and placebo was found.[176,177] In total, *H. pylori* is unlikely to be responsible for any more than 5% to 10% of cases of nonulcer dyspepsia and possibly for far fewer. Even if such an association exists, no markers are available that would indicate those patients with nonulcer dyspepsia in whom a real effect occurs. Better definition of nonulcer dyspepsia and ascertainment of both *H. pylori* and host genotypes in individual patients should permit elucidation of the question of whether *H. pylori* persistence is associated with symptoms in particular patients in the absence of ulceration or neoplasia.

DUODENAL ULCERATION

In the absence of medication-associated ulceration, more than 90% of patients with duodenal ulceration carry *H. pylori*,[161] an occurrence that is significantly more common than in age-matched controls.[159] Conversely, duodenal ulceration in the absence of aspirin or nonsteroidal anti-inflammatory drug use or Zollinger-Ellison syndrome usually is associated with *H. pylori* colonization. *H. pylori* may colonize the duodenum but only overlies metaplastic islands of gastric-type epithelium (gastric metaplasia).[3,164] The occurrence of *H. pylori* colonization and gastric metaplasia is highly associated with active duodenitis, a precursor lesion to ulceration,[186] and the presence of *H. pylori* in the duodenum is associated with a markedly increased risk of duodenal ulceration.[164] Previous *H. pylori* colonization is associated with a three- to fourfold increased risk of development of either gastric or duodenal ulceration[161] and that risk is enhanced with *cagA*⁺ strains.[4] In total, a significant body of evidence associating *H. pylori* colonization with idiopathic duodenal ulceration has accumulated. A causative role of *H. pylori* in ulcer disease is unproven; none of the experimental human studies have shown progression to ulceration, and why peptic ulcer disease has a remitting and relapsing course in the face of persistent colonization has never been resolved.[74] However, a large number of treatment studies using antimicrobial agents have helped define the natural history of ulcer disease. First, the use of antimicrobial agents (in the absence of acid-suppressive therapy) can heal duodenal ulcers at a rate similar to that observed with acid-suppressive therapy alone.[187,188] Second, after ulcer healing, eradication of *H. pylori* is associated with significantly lower recurrence rates than if the organism remains present.[187-190] When antimicrobial therapy that eradicates *H. pylori* is added to short-term acid-suppressive treatment, long-term ulcer relapse rates are markedly reduced, although not completely eliminated.[189,190]

Altogether, these findings implicate *H. pylori* as playing a role in ulcer pathogenesis and demonstrate that antimicrobial therapy rather

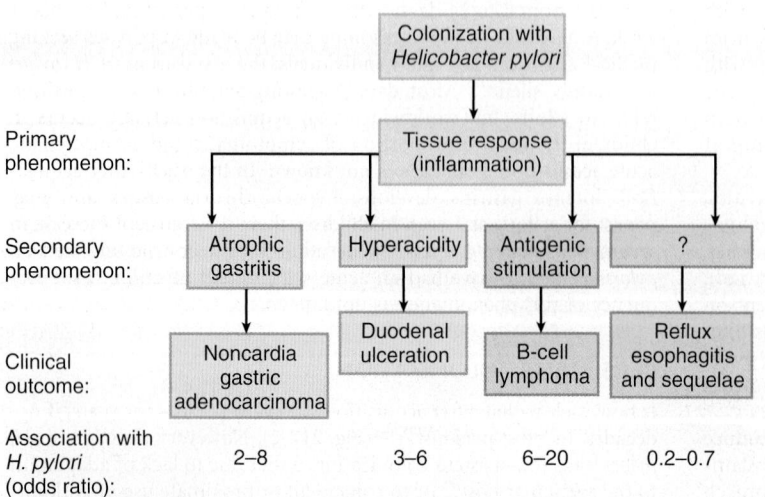

Figure 217-2 Association of *Helicobacter pylori* colonization and disease states. After *H. pylori* acquisition, virtually all persons develop persistent colonization that lasts for life. Colonization induces tissue responses termed chronic gastritis. This process affects gastric physiology, including glandular structure, acid secretion, and antigen processing, which in turn affect disease risk. Colonization with *H. pylori* increases the risk of certain diseases (duodenal ulcer, gastric ulcer, noncardia gastric adenocarcinoma, and B-cell lymphomas and possibly idiopathic thrombocytopenic purpura) but decreases the risk of gastroesophageal reflux disease and its complications, including Barrett's esophagus, and adenocarcinoma of the esophagus or gastric cardia, and possibly childhood asthma and related allergic disorders.

than long-term acid-suppressive therapy is indicated for most patients[162] because it changes the natural history of idiopathic ulcer disease. However, recent studies have provided evidence that, after *H. pylori* eradication, the incidence of reflux esophagitis doubled compared with failed eradication.[191] Thus, removal of *H. pylori* from the stomach of patients with duodenal ulceration has both benefits and costs. As more studies become available, physicians will need to develop criteria for treatment to optimize the therapeutic-to-toxic ratio.

GASTRIC ULCERATION

A smaller (50% to 80%) proportion of patients with benign gastric ulcers than with duodenal ulceration are colonized by *H. pylori*. The major reason is that a much higher proportion of gastric ulcers are due to nonsteroidal anti-inflammatory drug or aspirin use. When such use is excluded, most of the remaining patients with benign gastric ulcers are colonized with *H. pylori*, which is significantly more common than in age-matched controls.[159,161] The results of treatment of gastric ulceration with antimicrobial agents parallel the results of treatment of duodenal ulceration,[192] changing its natural history.

GASTRIC CARCINOMA

Because *H. pylori* colonization induces a tissue response (termed chronic gastritis) and because chronic gastritis is well-known as a risk factor for the development of gastric carcinoma,[193] a role for this organism in carcinogenesis has been advanced.[107] The decreasing incidence of gastric carcinoma in developed countries is consistent with an older age[194,195] and decreasing frequency of acquiring *H. pylori* as industrialization has proceeded.[9,196] The epidemiologic characteristics of *H. pylori* colonization, including increasing prevalence at an older age; higher prevalence in blacks, Hispanics, and Asians; association with lower socioeconomic status; and early-life crowding, are all similar to the characteristics associated with gastric cancer.[70] In addition, the development of intestinal metaplasia and atrophic gastritis, two pathologic entities that are risk factors for gastric cancer, is associated with *H. pylori*.[197,198] Thus, a direct role of this organism in gastric cancer is biologically plausible, and countries with high *H. pylori* prevalence rates have high gastric cancer rates.[199,200] Prospective studies of gastric cancer conducted in Hawaii, California, and England[165-167] and several retrospective and prospective studies each indicate that *H. pylori* is a risk factor for gastric cancer.[107] This association involves adenocarcinoma of the antrum and body of the stomach of both the intestinal and diffuse histologic types.[7,165-167] Odds ratios range from approximately 2.7 to 6.0, and the risk of gastric cancer attributable to *H. pylori* infection is approximately 60% to 80%.[166,167,200] The presumed mechanism for adenocarcinoma involves the chronicity of *H. pylori*–induced tissue responses (inflammation), with progression to atrophic and subsequently metaplastic histology as important pathogenetic steps.[201] The relationship between epithelial cell proliferation and apoptosis is probably also important.[201-203] However, this process probably requires decades on average, and *H. pylori* colonization is neither necessary nor sufficient for oncogenesis. No positive association has been observed with cancers at the cardia,[7,165-167] and increasing data indicate that *H. pylori* carriage may have a protective effect.[180,181] Further understanding of the role of *H. pylori* in carcinogenesis could lead to reevaluation of the clinical approach to asymptomatic colonization. *H. pylori* alteration of signal transduction and cell cycle kinetics in epithelial cells also may predispose to neoplasia,[204-206] and intracellular effects are most marked for *cag+* strains, which are associated with highest cancer risk.[107] Definition of additional host and bacterial factors that increase the risk of cancer development (or protection; see later) is an important research priority. Nevertheless, in Japan, treatment of high-risk persons to eradicate *H. pylori* lowered subsequent gastric cancer risk.[207] An important question is whether eradication of the organism from persons with more moderate risk can lower gastric cancer risk appreciably; studies to date have not been encouraging.[208,209]

This means that we must find better markers for risk so that preventive regimens target those with greatest need.

Reflecting the decline in *H. pylori* acquisition in developed countries, the incidence of adenocarcinomas of the gastric antrum and body has decreased. In contrast, the incidence of adenocarcinoma of the gastric cardia (and lower portion of the esophagus) has risen dramatically.[210] This temporal relationship suggests that *H. pylori* loss may play a role in the increase of these cancers, and substantial evidence supports this hypothesis.[180,181]

GASTRIC LYMPHOMA

Most gastric lymphomas arise from B lymphocytes and are termed mucosa-associated lymphoid tumors (MALTomas). *H. pylori* colonization is strongly associated with these tumors,[168,169] and eradication of *H. pylori* often leads to improvement in tumor histology.[211] Whether *H. pylori* eradication improves true malignancies, which are rare,[212] in contrast to the more common and more benign monoclonal lymphoid proliferation in response to *H. pylori* is unknown. The pathogenesis of these disorders may involve chronic antigenic stimulation by *H. pylori* and subsequent induction of a polyclonal lymphoid response, a single clone of which proliferates and then undergoes neoplastic transformation.

ESOPHAGEAL DISEASES

Much evidence has accumulated that the incidence of *H. pylori* colonization progressively decreased in developed countries during the 20th century,[196] especially *cagA+* strains.[75] During this time, the occurrence of three related diseases, gastroesophageal reflux disease, Barrett's esophagus, and adenocarcinoma of the esophagus, has been increasing dramatically.[213] It is generally believed that Barrett's esophagus will develop in a proportion of patients with gastroesophageal reflux disease and that adenocarcinoma will develop in some of these patients. An extremely important question is whether the loss of *H. pylori* from populations in developed countries may in some way predispose to this pathogenetic sequence. Patients with gastroesophageal reflux disease are less likely to be colonized with *H. pylori* (especially *cagA* strains) than are controls,[178] and eradication of *H. pylori* in patients with duodenal ulceration doubled the rate of gastroesophageal reflux disease development.[191] The presence of *cagA+ H. pylori* strains is inversely associated with Barrett's esophagus and esophageal adenocarcinomas.[214-216] There is a clear and consistent inverse relationship between colonization with *H. pylori* (especially *cag+*) strains, and each of the disorders in the gastroesophageal reflux disease → adenocarcinoma pathway.[181] These findings suggest that *H. pylori* in the stomach protects the esophagus. The presence of decreased gastric acidity induced by long-term *H. pylori* persistence may be partially responsible.[216-219] Other potential mechanisms include *H. pylori* effects on gastric hormones such as leptin[220] or on the microbiota colonizing the stomach and esophagus.[221,222] Research is ongoing in this area, but these findings substantially alter clinical approaches to *H. pylori*.

Asthma and Related Disorders

In recent years, asthma and related allergic disorders, including allergic rhinitis, eczema (atopic dermatitis), and skin allergies, have become markedly more prevalent, just as *H. pylori* colonization has been becoming less common; today, less than 6% of U.S. children are colonized with *H. pylori*,[9] a progressive decrease from the presumed near universality a century ago. Increasing evidence is showing specific inverse relationships between *H. pylori* and these disorders (reviewed by Reibman and colleagues[10]). Several points have emerged about the inverse relationships. First, they are essentially entirely associated with childhood-onset asthma.[8,9] Second, the effects for allergic rhinitis, eczema, and skin sensitization parallel those for asthma.[8-11] Third, the relationships have been observed not only in the United States but in other developed countries.[11] Fourth, the strongest effect is with the (more interactive) *cag*⁺ strains.

These findings are consistent with the hypothesis that *H. pylori* protects against these disorders or is a marker for other changes in microecology that actually are the protective factors. In favor of the former possibility is that the *H. pylori*–positive stomach includes a rich compartment of T-reg cells that is much better developed than in *H. pylori*–negative persons,[109,110] which could influence system immunity. The work in this area is in the early stages, but if *H. pylori* contributes to the protection against childhood asthma, that markedly affects the goals of mass eradication.

Metabolic Disorders

In recent years, it has become clear that the stomach produces hormones related to satiety and energy homeostasis, leptin,[223,224] and, to a greater extent, ghrelin, which has opposing effects.[225] A growing body of studies indicate that *H. pylori* status affects the levels of these hormones,[226] and, in particular, *H. pylori* eradication leads to an increase in ghrelin.[225] The data indicate that *H. pylori* colonization, by its effects on epithelial and immune cells, is involved in the regulation of these hormones.[226] It is now also clear that a generation of children in developed countries is growing up with *H. pylori* in their stomachs regulating these hormones.[227] The full consequences of this change are unknown, but at the least, *H. pylori*–positive persons are taller.[228] Large cross-sectional studies of healthy adults have found no relationships of *H. pylori* with body mass index,[229,230] but several focused studies have.[231] This will be an important area to consider in future years.

Idiopathic Thrombocytopenic Purpura

In the past 10 years, there has been an increasing number of reports, chiefly from East Asia, showing an epidemiologic association between the presence of *H. pylori* and the diagnosis of idiopathic thrombocytopenic purpura (ITP).[170-172] *H. pylori* eradication has been attempted as a therapy for ITP, and although not conclusive, results are promising.[172] At present, for patients diagnosed with ITP, physicians should assess *H. pylori* status, and, if positive, should consider eradicating colonization of *H. pylori* as one therapeutic approach.[172]

Diagnosis

Ascertainment of *H. pylori* colonization can be made either invasively by endoscopy and biopsy or noninvasively by serologic analysis, breath test, or fecal antigen analysis. Properly done, each of these methodologies has a diagnostic accuracy exceeding 95%; each has advantages and disadvantages (Table 217-3).

Endoscopy with biopsy involves the most expense and invasion of the patient, but it may be used to yield a great deal of information.[232] Biopsy specimens may be cultured for *H. pylori* on antibiotic-containing media (to diminish overgrowth by any competing flora) such as Skirrow's medium, as well as with a nonselective medium such as chocolate agar.[232] Use of two media increases the yield. Plates should be incubated for 2 to 5 days at 35°C to 37°C in a moist microaerobic atmosphere (with 5% oxygen). Comma- or S-shaped motile organisms with catalase, oxidase, and urease activity may be identified as *H. pylori*.[232] Culture enables a determination of antimicrobial susceptibilities, which may be increasingly important as antimicrobial resistance broadens. Alternatively, the organisms may be visualized on histologic sections prepared with Gram, silver, Giemsa, or acridine orange stain or by immunofluorescence or immunoperoxidase methods.[232] DNA probe and polymerase chain reaction methodologies have been developed as well, but they have no current clinical justification unless genotyping of strains becomes more clinically important.[138] For rapid detection of *H. pylori*, biopsy samples may be incubated at 37°C to examine for preformed urease activity.[136] After incubation for 1 hour, the assay has a sensitivity of approximately 60%, and by 24 hours, more than 90%; bacterial overgrowth of the stomach may reduce the

TABLE 217-3	Modalities for *Helicobacter pylori* Diagnosis	
Modality	*Advantages*	*Disadvantages*
Endoscopy with biopsy	Permits inspection of pathology, allows detection of ulcers, neoplasms	Invasive, expensive, time-consuming
Culture	Permits determination of antimicrobial susceptibilities and pathogenic features of isolates	Not optimally sensitive in most laboratories. Requires several days for results
Histology	Generally more sensitive than culture. Allows direct visualization of organism and extent and nature of tissue involvement	Gastritis may be patchy and biopsy may be performed on wrong area. Insensitivity to detect small numbers of organisms. Requires several days for results
Urease detection	Rapid; most positive results seen within 2 hours	Increased sensitivity requires longer incubation. May be false-positive results with bacterial overgrowth
Serology	Noninvasive, rapid, quantitative, inexpensive	No determination of lesions or pathology, no antimicrobial susceptibility. Not rapidly responsive to therapy
Urea breath tests	Relatively noninvasive, relatively rapid, quantitative, rapidly responsive to therapy. Most valuable for assessing response to eradication therapy after 4 to 8 weeks	Involves expensive instrumentation or administration of radioisotopes. More invasive and less convenient than serology. No determination of lesions or pathology, no antimicrobial susceptibility
Stool antigen tests	Relatively noninvasive, relatively rapid, rapidly responsive to therapy. Most valuable for assessing response to eradication therapy after 6 to 8 weeks	Not quantitative. Requires stool specimen, relatively expensive for developing countries. No determination of lesions or pathology, no antimicrobial susceptibility

test's specificity, especially for longer incubations and in older patients. Endoscopy also permits assessment of structural lesions such as ulcers, masses, and strictures.

High-titer, stable serum immunoglobulin G responses and, less frequently, immunoglobulin A responses nearly universally develop in *H. pylori*–colonized persons.[172,233,234] Because serology in essence samples the entire stomach, whereas biopsy only samples a small region and the inflammatory process may be patchy, serologic analysis may be more sensitive than diagnostic methods involving biopsies.[234] With successful antimicrobial therapy, antibody levels decrease, although 3 to 6 months may be required for a noticeable effect; after ineffective therapy, high antibody levels persist.[235,236] Soon after the initial acquisition of *H. pylori*, immunoglobulin M seroconversion is noted, but levels return to baseline; with recurrence after inadequate therapy, immunoglobulin M seroconversion may again be observed.[184] A number of testing services and kits are commercially available that allow physicians to detect *H. pylori* in individual patients; the serologic assays have generally been standardized for adults, and thus interpretation of results in children requires caution.[237] Office-based rapid serologic tests have lower sensitivity and specificity for both adults and children. *H. pylori*–positive persons also shed *H. pylori* antigens in their stools. Stool assay is a relatively noninvasive means to detect positivity and to monitor therapeutic responses 1 month after ending treatment.

The high urease activity of *H. pylori* has also facilitated the development of urease breath tests. Subjects fast and are then given a meal containing ^{13}C- or ^{14}C-urea; over the next hour, their breath is correspondingly examined for $^{13}CO_2$ or $^{14}CO_2$.[238,239] Results of these assays correlate with numbers of urease-producing *H. pylori* organisms and can be falsely negative after therapy that suppresses but does not eradicate the organism. However, negativity 1 to 3 months after therapy has ceased usually indicates eradication of the organism. Urea breath testing services also are commercially available.

Treatment

INDICATIONS

At present, several indications have emerged for considering therapy directed against *H. pylori*. For patients with peptic ulceration who are colonized with *H. pylori*, antimicrobial therapies that eradicate *H. pylori* are associated with substantially lower ulcer recurrence rates than are short-course therapies directed exclusively against gastric acidity.[189,190] Thus, antimicrobial therapy now is included in the primary therapy for essentially all cases of duodenal ulceration.[162] Gastric ulcers associated with *H. pylori* can be treated in the same manner as for duodenal ulceration.[192] In patients with gastric MALTomas, antimicrobial therapy directed against *H. pylori* seems to cause tumor regression in most patients.[169] For patients with ITP who are *H. pylori* positive, eradication therapy also should be considered.[172] However for most cases of *H. pylori*–associated nonulcer dysplasia, data concerning the efficacy of antimicrobial therapy are not clear-cut.[174,177,186] Because of the risk of developing or worsening esophageal disease, treatment is not recommended in asymptomatic persons who are *H. pylori* positive; a possible exception would be a patient with a strong family history of gastric cancer. Similarly, the persistence of antibiotic resistance of *H. pylori* and commensal bacteria after treatment argues against widespread eradication campaigns.[240] Similarly, if *H. pylori* protects against diarrheal diseases, as some evidence suggests,[241-243] eradication of *H. pylori* among children in developing countries could increase the risk of morbidity and mortality in childhood. Finally, if the data showing an inverse association of *H. pylori* with childhood asthma and allergic conditions and possible metabolic syndromes reflect an actual protective effect, then there should be great caution about treating young children to eradicate *H. pylori*.[227]

THERAPIES

Virtually all *H. pylori* isolates are susceptible in vitro to a variety of antimicrobial agents, including bismuth salts, amoxicillin, macrolides, nitrofurans, tetracyclines, and aminoglycosides.[219,244,245] However, in vitro susceptibility is no guarantee of in vivo effectiveness. Primary resistance to imidazoles (such as metronidazole and tinidazole) occurs in 20% to 40% of isolates[245,246] and is most common in young women who may have received this agent for gynecologic infections or in persons from developing countries treated for parasitic infections. However, primary resistance is present in isolates from both men and women in all age groups[247] and is associated with previous exposure to a nitroimidazole, even decades earlier.[248] Primary resistance to macrolides is less common but increasing,[245] and resistance to amoxicillin and fluoroquinolones also has been reported.

Several principles of chemotherapy have emerged. First, treatment with a single agent results in apparent eradication of organisms in only a minority of cases. The cumulative effects of multiple monotherapy antibiotic courses may have hastened the disappearance of *H. pylori* from the general population, but because of its unreliability for eradication, all current treatments use combination therapy.[249] Second, some agents that are effective in vitro may be ineffective in vivo, even in combination with other agents. Erythromycin is a good example of this phenomenon.[250] The ineffectiveness of many antibiotics at an acidic pH may be responsible for the lack of activity in vivo. Third, acquired resistance frequently develops after therapy with some agents but not others. To date, no confirmed resistance to bismuth salts and tetracycline has been reported. In contrast, acquired resistance to quinolones is so frequent that it appears to preclude their general use. Secondary resistance to imidazoles occurs in 10% to 30% of cases, even when used in combination with other agents.[251] The development of resistance to macrolides and rifampin has also been reported. Fourth, to determine true eradication of the organism and not just temporary

TABLE 217-4	Treatment Regimens for *Helicobacter pylori*
Proton pump inhibitor (PPI) triple therapy: PPI (standard dose twice daily) + amoxicillin (1 g twice daily) + clarithromycin (500 mg twice daily) for 7 to 10 days
Quadruple therapy: PPI (standard dose twice daily) + metronidazole (500 mg 3 times daily) + tetracycline (500 mg 3 times daily) + bismuth (dose depends on preparation) for 10 days
Sequential therapy: PPI (standard dose twice daily) + amoxicillin (1 g twice daily) for 5 days followed by PPI (standard dose twice daily) + clarithromycin (500 mg twice daily) + tinidazole (500 mg twice daily) for 5 days
Levofloxacin triple therapy: PPI (standard dose twice daily) + amoxicillin (1 g twice daily) + levofloxacin (500 mg twice daily) for 10 days
Rifabutin triple therapy: PPI (standard dose twice daily) + amoxicillin (1 g twice daily) + rifabutin (150-300 mg/day) for 10 days

From Vakil N, Vaira D. Sequential therapy for *Helicobacter pylori*: time to consider making the switch? *JAMA* 2008;300:1346-1347.

suppression, the patient must be shown to be free of the organism at least 1 month after the cessation of therapy if biopsy, breath test, or stool antigen test is used and at least 6 months if serologic examination is used. Better definition of these end points is currently under investigation.

The most commonly used therapies include proton pump inhibitors, such as omeprazole and lansoprazole, and are used as parts of triple, quadruple, and sequential therapies (Table 217-4).[252-254] These agents are directly inhibitory to *H. pylori*[255] and seem to be potent urease inhibitors,[256] in contrast to H_2 receptor antagonists, and are also more effective for inducing pH neutrality, which may permit better antimicrobial efficacy. Seven to 10 days of twice-daily therapy with a proton pump inhibitor plus amoxicillin and clarithromycin or the combination of a proton pump inhibitor, amoxicillin, and metronidazole also is highly effective.[257] Quadruple therapy with a proton pump inhibitor (for 10 days) and bismuth-based triple therapy (for days 4 to 10) seems to be most effective.[258] Bismuth salts appear to be particularly useful against slowly growing bacteria.[253] Although bismuth salts vary in their particular minimal inhibitory concentrations toward *H. pylori* and in their pharmacokinetics, the levels achieved in the gastric lumen after oral administration are so high that no difference among the salts is apparent. Triple therapy with bismuth salts, metronidazole, and amoxicillin has resulted in eradication rates of 60% to 90%. Tetracycline seems to be at least as beneficial as amoxicillin.[189,251] Both poor patient compliance[254] and primary and secondary resistance to metronidazole appear to be important factors limiting eradication. The optimal therapeutic regimen has not been defined. In studies of patients with duodenal ulceration, combination therapies decreased 1-year recurrence rates from 80% to less than 30%.[187-189] For ulcer healing, several excellent regimens have been described in which an acid-suppressing agent is used for 4 to 6 weeks and antimicrobial therapy for the first 10 to 14 days. One standard is ranitidine plus triple therapy[187]; similarly, ranitidine bismuth citrate plus two antibiotics is also highly effective. No evidence has shown any one histamine type 2 antagonist to be superior to the others, but patient compliance is an important variable.[254] However, use of proton pump inhibitors has largely supplanted the use of H_2 antagonists. One other approach that is gaining favor is sequential therapy[259] (see Table 217-4). From limited trials, eradication rates seem best.[259]

Physicians must balance the use of these particular regimens with possible adverse consequences, which include medication-induced upper gastrointestinal symptoms and uncommon complications such as antibiotic-associated colitis and candidiasis, and development of antimicrobial resistance. Determination of optimal therapy must await head-to-head clinical trials. Because there is evidence that eradication of *H. pylori* affects the gastric hormones leptin and ghrelin,[260-262] which affect appetite and satiety,[262,263] weight gain after eradication may reflect disruption of this physiologic axis.[260,261]

In patients in whom *H. pylori* is again isolated after therapy, the organisms usually are identical to the initial isolates, thus indicating that recurrence reflects relapse rather than the acquisition of a new agent. When imidazoles or macrolides are used and fail, virtually all the recurrent organisms are resistant. After treatment failure, a second course of triple therapy (containing metronidazole) may nevertheless be effective; alternatively, a regimen not including imidazoles may be used[257] (see Table 217-4).

Other Gastric Helicobacters

In addition to *H. pylori*, other spiral organisms may occasionally be present in the human stomach. The predominant organisms, origi-nally called *Gastrospirillum hominis*, are spirochetal in morphology and also are strongly urease positive.[264-266] Taxonomic study based on ribosomal RNA homologies indicates that this organism is a member of the genus *Helicobacter*, and the name *Helicobacter heilmanii* has been used.[267] *H. heilmanii* is much less commonly observed in the gastric mucosa than *H. pylori* and occurs in perhaps 1% of persons.[266] This organism rarely has been cultivated in vitro, which limits studies of its clinical role. However, these 0.5- to 1.0-μm by 4- to 8-μm spi-rochetes are easily visualized in specimens from colonized persons. Both *H. pylori* and *H. heilmanii* may be present in the same person. In monkeys, these organisms appear to not be pathogens, and their role in humans is uncertain.

REFERENCES

1. Marshall BJ. History of the discovery of *Campylobacter pylori*. In: Blaser MJ, ed. *Campylobacter pylori in Gastritis and Peptic Ulcer Disease*. New York: Igaku Shoin; 1989:7-23.
2. Hazell SL, Lee A, Brady L, et al. *Campylobacter pyloridis* and gastritis: association with intracellular spaces and adaptation to an environment of mucus as important factors in colonization of the gastric epithelium. *J Infect Dis*. 1986;153:658-663.
3. Tham KT, Peek RM, Atherton JC, et al. *Helicobacter pylori* geno-types, host factors, and gastric mucosal histopathology in peptic ulcer disease. *Hum Pathol*. 2001;32:264-273.
4. Nomura AMY, Perez-Perez GI, Lee J, et al. Relationship between *H. pylori cagA* status and risk of peptic ulcer disease. *Am J Epi-demiol*. 2002;155:1054-1059.
5. Blaser MJ. The changing relationships of *Helicobacter pylori* and humans: implications for health and disease. *J Infect Dis*. 1999;179:1523-1530.
6. Nomura AMY, Lee J, Stemmerman G, et al. *Helicobacter pylori cagA* seropositivity and gastric carcinoma risk in a Japanese American population. *J Infect Dis*. 2002;186:1138-1144.
7. *Helicobacter* and Cancer Collaborative Group. Gastric cancer and *Helicobacter pylori*: a combined analysis of twelve case-control studies nested within prospective cohorts. *Gut*. 2001;49:347-353.
8. Chen Y, Blaser MJ. Inverse associations of *Helicobacter pylori* with asthma and allergy. *Arch Intern Med*. 2007;167:821-827.
9. Chen Y, Blaser MJ. *Helicobacter pylori* colonization is inversely associated with childhood asthma. *J Infect Dis*. 2008; 198:553-560.
10. Reibman J, Marmor M, Filner J, et al. Asthma is inversely associ-ated with *Helicobacter pylori* status in an urban population. *PLoS ONE*. 2008;3:e4060.
11. Blaser MJ, Chen Y, Reibman J. Does *Helicobacter pylori* protect against asthma and allergy? *Gut*. 2008;57:561-567.
12. Marshall BJ, Warren JR. Unidentified curved bacilli in the stomach of patients with gastritis and peptic ulceration. *Lancet*. 1984;1:1311-1313.
13. Goodwin CS, Armstrong JA, Chilvers T, et al. Transfer of *Cam-pylobacter pylori* and *Campylobacter mustelae* to *Helicobacter* gen. nov. as *Helicobacter pylori* comb. nov. and *Helicobacter mustelae* comb. nov., respectively. *Int J Syst Bacteriol*. 1989;39:397-405.
14. Paster BJ, Lee A, Fox JG, et al. Phylogeny of *Helicobacter felis* sp. nov, *Helicobacter mustelae*, and related bacteria. *Int J Syst Bacte-riol*. 1991;41:31-38.
15. Eaton KA, Dewhirst FE, Radin MJ, et al. *Helicobacter acinonyx* sp. nov., isolated from cheetahs with gastritis. *Int J Syst Bacteriol*. 1993;43:99-106.
16. Fox JG, Dewhirst FE, Tully JG, et al. *Helicobacter hepaticus* sp nov, a microaerophilic bacterium isolated from livers and intes-tinal mucosal scrapings from mice. *J Clin Microbiol*. 1994; 32:1238-1245.
17. Fox JG, Drolet R, Higgins R, et al. *Helicobacter canis* isolated from a dog liver with multifocal necrotizing hepatitis. *J Clin Microbiol*. 1996;34:2479-2482.
18. Fox JG, Dewhirst FE, Shen Z, et al. Hepatic *Helicobacter* species identified in bile and gallbladder tissue from Chileans with chronic cholecystitis. *Gastroenterology*. 1998;114:755-763.
19. Matsukura N, Yokomuro S, Yamada S, et al. Association between *Helicobacter bilis* in bile and biliary tract malignancies: *H. bilis* in bile from Japanese and Thai patients with benign and malignant diseases in the biliary tract. *J Cancer Res*. 2002; 93:842-847.
20. Blaser MJ. Helicobacters and biliary tract disease. *Gastroenterol-ogy*. 1998;114:840-842.
21. Dunn BE, Campbell GP, Pérez-Pérez GI, et al. Purification and characterization of *Helicobacter pylori* urease. *J Biol Chem*. 1990;265:9464-9469.
22. Cussac V, Ferrero RL, Labigne A. Expression of *Helicobacter pylori* urease genes in *Escherichia coli* grown under nitrogen-limiting conditions. *J Bacteriol*. 1992;174:2466-2473.
23. Tomb J-F, White O, Kerlavage AR, et al. The complete genome sequence of the gastric pathogen *Helicobacter pylori*. *Nature*. 1997;388:539-547.
24. Alm RA, Ling LL, Moir DT, et al. Genomic-sequence compari-son of two unrelated isolates of the human gastric pathogen *Helicobacter pylori*. *Nature*. 1999;397:176-180.
25. Oh JD, Kling-Bäckhed H, Giannakis M, et al. The complete genome sequence of a chronic atrophic gastritis *Helicobacter pylori* strain: evolution during disease progression. *Proc Natl Acad Sci U S A*. 2006;103:9999-10004.
26. McClain MS, Shaffer CL, Israel DA, et al. Genome sequence analysis of *Helicobacter pylori* strains associated with gastric ulceration and gastric cancer. *BMC Genomics*. 2009;10:3.
27. de Reuse H, Bereswill S. Ten years after the first *Helicobacter pylori* genome: comparative and functional genomics provide new insights in the variability and adaptability of a persistent pathogen. *FEMS Immunol Med Microbiol*. 2007;50:165-176.
28. Xu Q, Morgan RD, Roberts RJ, et al. Identification of type II restriction and modification systems in *Helicobacter pylori* reveals their substantial diversity among strains. *Proc Natl Acad Sci U S A*. 2000;97:9671-9676.
29. Appelmelk BJ, Martino MC, Veenhof E, et al. Phase variation in H type I and Lewis a epitopes of *Helicobacter pylori* lipopolysac-charide. *Infect Immun*. 2000;68:5928-5932.
30. Wang G, Ge Z, Rasko DA, et al. Lewis antigens in *Helicobacter pylori*: biosynthesis and phase variation. *Mol Microbiol*. 2000;36:1187-1196.
31. Blaser MJ, Atherton JC. *Helicobacter pylori* persistence: biology and disease. *J Clin Invest*. 2004;113:321-333.
32. Webb GF, Blaser MJ. Dynamics of bacterial phenotype selection in a colonized host. *Proc Natl Acad Sci U S A*. 2002;99: 3135-3140.
33. Akopyanz N, Bukanov NO, Westblom TU, et al. DNA diversity among clinical isolates of *Helicobacter pylori* detected by PCR-based RAPD fingerprinting. *Nucleic Acids Res*. 1992;20:5137-5142.
34. Achtman M, Azuma T, Berg DE, et al. Recombination and clonal groupings within *Helicobacter pylori* from different geo-graphical regions. *Mol Microbiol*. 1999;32:459-470.
35. Shames B, Krajden S, Fuksa M, et al. Evidence for the occurrence of the same strain of *Campylobacter pylori* in the stomach and dental plaque. *J Clin Microbiol*. 1989;27:2849-2850.
36. Kersulyte D, Chalkauskas H, Berg DE. Emergence of recombi-nant strains of *Helicobacter pylori* during human infection. *Mol Microbiol*. 1999;31:31-43.
37. Suerbaum S, Smith JM, Bapumia K, et al. Free recombination with *Helicobacter pylori*. *Proc Natl Acad Sci U S A*. 1998; 95:12619-12624.
38. Falush D, Kraft C, Taylor NS, et al. Recombination and muta-tion during long-term gastric colonization by *Helicobacter pylori*: estimates of clock rates, recombination size, and minimal age. *Proc Natl Acad Sci U S A*. 2001;98:15056-15061.
39. Bjorkholm B, Sjolund M, Falk PG, et al. Mutation frequency and biological cost of antibiotic resistance in *Helicobacter pylori*. *Proc Natl Acad Sci U S A*. 2001;98:14607-14612.
40. Israel DA, Salama N, Krishna U, et al. *Helicobacter pylori* genetic diversity within the gastric niche of a single human host. *Proc Natl Acad Sci U S A*. 2001;98:14625-14630.
41. Aras RA, Kang J, Tschumi A, et al. Extensive repetitive DNA facilitates prokaryotic genome plasticity. *Proc Natl Acad Sci U S A*. 2003;100:13579-13584.
42. Ando T, Xu Q, Torres M, et al. Restriction-modification system differences in *Helicobacter pylori* are a barrier to interstrain plasmid transfer. *Mol Microbiol*. 2000;7:1052-1065.
43. Censini S, Lange C, Xiang J, et al. *cag*, a pathogenicity island of *Helicobacter pylori* encodes type I-specific and disease-associated virulence factors. *Proc Natl Acad Sci U S A*. 1996;93: 14648-14653.
44. Akopyanz NS, Clifton SW, Kersulyte D, et al. Analyses of the *cag* pathogenicity island of *Helicobacter pylori*. *Mol Microbiol*. 1998;28:37-53.
45. Tummuru MKR, Sharma SA, Blaser MJ. *Helicobacter pylori picB*, a homologue of the *Bordetella pertussis* toxin secretion protein, is required for induction of IL-8 in gastric epithelial cells. *Mol Microbiol*. 1995;18:867-876.
46. Tammer I, Brandt S, Hartig R, et al. Activation of Abl by *Heli-cobacter pylori*: a novel kinase for CagA and crucial mediator of host cell scattering. *Gastroenterology*. 2007;132:1309-1319.
47. Pérez-Pérez GI, Bhat N, Gaensbauer J, et al. Country-specific constancy by age in *cagA*$^+$ proportion of *Helicobacter pylori* infections. *Int J Cancer*. 1997;72:453-456.
48. Odenbreit S, Puls J, Sedlmaier B, et al. Translocation of *Helico-bacter pylori* CagA into gastric epithelial cells by type IV secre-tion. *Science*. 2000;287:1497-1500.
49. Segal ED, Cha J, Lo J, et al. Altered states: involvement of phos-phorylated CagA in the induction of host cellular growth changes by *Helicobacter pylori*. *Proc Natl Acad Sci U S A*. 1999;96:14559-14564.
50. Aras RA, Lee Y, Kim S-K, et al. Natural variation in populations of persistently colonizing bacteria affect human host cell pheno-type. *J Infect Dis*. 2003;188:486-496.
51. Selbach M, Moese S, Hauck CR, et al. Src is the kinase of *Heli-cobacter pylori* CagA protein in vitro and in vivo. *J Biol Chem*. 2002;277:6775-6778.
52. Higashi H, Tsutsumi R, Muto S, et al. SHP-2 tyrosine phospha-tase as an intracellular target of *Helicobacter pylori* CagA protein. *Science*. 2002;295:683-686.
53. Mimuro H, Suzuki T, Tanaka J, et al. Grb2 is a key mediator of *Helicobacter pylori* CagA protein activities. *Mol Cell*. 2002;10:745-755.
54. Tsutsumi R, Higashi H, Higuchi M, et al. Attenuation of *Heli-cobacter pylori* CagA x SHP-2 signaling by interaction between CagA and C-terminal Src kinase. *J Biol Chem*. 2003;278: 3664-3670.
55. Selbach M, Moese S, Hurwitz R, et al. The *Helicobacter pylori* CagA protein induces cortactin dephosphorylation and actin rearrangement by c-Src inactivation. *EMBO J*. 2003;22: 515-528.
56. Viala J, Chaput C, Boneca IG, et al. Nod1 responds to peptido-glycan delivered by the *Helicobacter pylori* cag pathogenicity island. *Nat Immunol*. 2004;5:1166-1174.
57. Sozzi M, Crosarri M, Kim S-K, et al. Heterogeneity of *Helico-bacter pylori cag* genotypes in experimentally infected mice. *FEMS Microbiol Lett*. 2001;203:109-114.
58. Ko JS, Seo JK. cag pathogenicity island of *Helicobacter pylori* in Korean children. *Helicobacter*. 2002;7:232-236.
59. Aras RA, Takata T, Ando T, et al. Regulation of the HpyII restriction-modification system of *Helicobacter pylori* by gene deletion and horizontal reconstitution. *Mol Microbiol*. 2001;42:369-382.
60. Cover TL, Blanke SR. *Helicobacter pylori* VacA, a paradigm for toxin multifunctionality. *Nat Rev Microbiol*. 2005;3: 320-332.
61. Atherton J, Cao P, Peek RM, et al. Mosaicism in vacuolating cytotoxin alleles of *Helicobacter pylori*: association of specific *vacA* types with cytotoxin production and peptic ulceration. *J Biol Chem*. 1995;270:1771-1777.
62. van Doorn L-J, Figueiredo C, Sanna R, et al. Expanding allelic diversity of *Helicobacter pylori vacA*. *J Clin Microbiol*. 1998;36:2597-2603.
63. Rhead JL, Letley DP, Mohammadi M, et al. A new *Helicobacter pylori* vacuolating cytotoxin determinant, the intermediate region, is associated with gastric cancer. *Gastroenterology*. 2007;133:926-936.
64. Atherton JC, Peek RM, Tham KT, et al. The clinical and patho-logical importance of heterogeneity in *vacA*, encoding the vacu-olating cytotoxin of *Helicobacter pylori*. *Gastroenterology*. 1997;112:92-99.
65. Papini E, Satin B, Norais N, et al. Selective increase of the perme-ability of polarized epithelial cell monolayers by *Helicobacter pylori* vacuolating toxin. *J Clin Invest*. 1998;102:813-820.
66. Iwamoto H, Czajkowsky DM, Cover TL, et al. VacA from *Heli-cobacter pylori*: a hexameric chloride channel. *FEBS Lett*. 1999;450:101-104.
67. Molinari M, Salio M, Galli C, et al. Selective inhibition of Ii-dependent antigen presentation by *Helicobacter pylori* toxin VacA. *J Exp Med*. 1998;187:135-140.
68. Zheng PY, Jones NL. *Helicobacter pylori* strains expressing the vacuolating cytotoxin interrupt phagosome maturation in mac-rophages by recruiting and retaining TACO (coronin 1) protein. *Cell Microbiol*. 2003;5:25-40.
69. Gebert B, Fischer W, Weiss E, et al. *Helicobacter pylori* vacuolat-ing cytotoxin inhibits T lymphocyte activation. *Science*. 2003;301:1099-1102.
70. Taylor DN, Blaser MJ. The epidemiology of *Helicobacter pylori* infections. *Epidemiol Rev*. 1991;13:42-59.

71. Falush D, Wirth T, Linz B, et al. Traces of human migration in *Helicobacter pylori* populations. *Science*. 2003;299:1582-1585.
72. Linz B, Balloux F, Moodley Y, et al. An African origin for the intimate association between humans and *Helicobacter pylori*. *Nature*. 2007;445:915-918.
73. Ghose C, Perez-Perez GI, Dominguez-Bello MG, et al. East Asian genotypes of *Helicobacter pylori*: strains in Amerindians provide evidence for its ancient human carriage. *Proc Natl Acad Sci U S A*. 2002;99:15107-15111.
74. Blaser MJ. Helicobacters are indigenous to the human stomach: duodenal ulceration is due to changes in gastric microecology in the modern era. *Gut*. 1998;43:721-727.
75. Perez-Perez GI, Salomaa A, Kosunen TU, et al. Evidence that *cagA*⁺ *Helicobacter pylori* strains are disappearing more rapidly than *cagA*⁻ strains. *Gut*. 2002;50:295-298.
76. Graham DY, Alpert LC, Smith JL, et al. Iatrogenic *Campylobacter pylori* infection is a cause of epidemic achlorhydria. *Am J Gastroenterol*. 1988;83:974-980.
77. Pérez-Pérez GI, Bodhidatta L, Wongsrichanalai J, et al. Seroprevalence of *Helicobacter pylori* infections in Thailand. *J Infect Dis*. 1990;161:1237-1241.
78. Thomas JE, Gibson GR, Darboe MK, et al. Isolation of *Helicobacter pylori* from human faeces. *Lancet*. 1992;340:1194-1195.
79. Polish LB, Douglas JM, Davidson AJ, et al. Characterization of risk factors for *Helicobacter pylori* infection among men attending an STD clinic: lack of evidence for sexual transmission. *J Clin Microbiol*. 1991;29:2139-2143.
80. Parsonnet J, Shmuely H, Haggerty T. Fecal and oral shedding of *Helicobacter pylori* from healthy infected adults. *JAMA*. 1999;282:2240-2245.
81. Drumm B, Pérez-Pérez GI, Blaser MJ, et al. Intrafamilial clustering of *Helicobacter pylori* infection. *N Engl J Med*. 1990;322:359-363.
82. Goodman KJ, Correa P, Tengana Aux HJ, et al. *Helicobacter pylori* infection in the Colombian Andes: a population-based study of transmission pathways. *Am J Epidemiol*. 1996;144:290-299.
83. Goodman KJ, Correa P. Transmission of *Helicobacter pylori* among siblings. *Lancet*. 2000;355:358-362.
84. Dooley CP, Fitzgibbons PL, Cohen H, et al. Prevalence of *Helicobacter pylori* infection and histologic gastritis in asymptomatic persons. *N Engl J Med*. 1989;321:1562-1566.
85. Everhart JE, Kruszon-Moran D, Perez-Perez GI, et al. Seroprevalence and ethnic differences in *Helicobacter pylori* infection among adults in the United States. *J Infect Dis*. 2000;181:1359-1363.
86. Graham DY, Malaty HM, Evans DG, et al. Epidemiology of *Helicobacter pylori* in an asymptomatic population in the United States: effect of age, race and socioeconomic status. *Gastroenterology*. 1991;100:1495-1501.
87. Dehesa M, Dooley CP, Cohen HA, et al. High prevalence of *Helicobacter pylori* in an asymptomatic Hispanic population. *J Clin Microbiol*. 1991;29:1128-1131.
88. Everhart JE, Kruszon-Moran D, Perez-Perez G. Reliability of *Helicobacter pylori* and CagA serological assays. *Clin Diagn Lab Immunol*. 2002;9:412-416.
89. Parsonnet J. The incidence of *Helicobacter pylori* infection. *Aliment Pharmacol Ther*. 1995;9:45-51.
90. Mitchell HM, Li YY, Hu PJ, et al. Epidemiology of *Helicobacter pylori* in southern China: identification of early childhood as the critical period for acquisition. *J Infect Dis*. 1992;166:149-153.
91. Perez-Perez GI, Sack RB, Reid R, et al. Transient and persistent *Helicobacter pylori* colonization in Native American children. *J Clin Microbiol*. 2003;41:2401-2407.
92. Banatvala N, Mayo K, Megraud F, et al. The cohort effect and *Helicobacter pylori*. *J Infect Dis*. 1993;168:219-221.
93. Mendall MA, Googin PM, Molineaux N, et al. Childhood living conditions and *Helicobacter pylori* seropositivity in adult life. *Lancet*. 1992;339:896.
94. Sitas F, Forman D, Yarnell JWG, et al. *Helicobacter pylori* infection rates in relation to age and social class in a Welsh male population. *Gut*. 1941;32:25-28.
95. Scott DR, Weeks D, Hong C, et al. The role of internal urease in acid resistance of *Helicobacter pylori*. *Gastroenterology*. 1998;114:58-70.
96. Amieva MR, Vogelmann R, Covacci A, et al. Disruption of the epithelial apical-junctional complex by *Helicobacter pylori* CagA. *Science*. 2003;300:1430-1434.
97. McGowan CC, Necheva AS, Forsyth MH, et al. Promoter analysis of *Helicobacter pylori* genes whose expression is enhanced at low pH. *Mol Microbiol*. 2003;48:1225-1239.
98. Wirth H-P, Yang M, Peek RM, et al. Phenotypic diversity in Lewis expression of *Helicobacter pylori* isolates from the same host. *J Lab Clin Med*. 1999;133:488-500.
99. Mimuro H, Suzuki T, Tanaka J, et al. Grb2 is a key mediator of *Helicobacter pylori* CagA protein activities. *Mol Cell*. 2002;295:683-686.
100. Selbach M, Moese S, Hurwitz R, et al. The *Helicobacter pylori* CagA protein induces cortactin dephosphorylation and actin rearrangement by c-Src inactivation. *EMBO J*. 2003;22:515-528.
101. Smoot DT, Resau JH, Naab T, et al. Adherence of *Helicobacter pylori* to cultured human gastric epithelial cells. *Infect Immun*. 1993;61:350-355.
102. Ilver D, Arnqvist A, Ogren J, et al. *Helicobacter pylori* adhesion binding fucosylated histo-blood group antigens revealed by retagging. *Science*. 1998;279:373-377.
103. Mahdavi J, Sonden B, Hurtig M, et al. *Helicobacter pylori* SabA adhesin in persistent infection and chronic inflammation. *Science*. 2002;297:573-578.
104. Pride DT, Blaser MJ. Concerted evolution between duplicated genetic elements in *Helicobacter pylori*. *J Mol Biol*. 2002;316:627-640.
105. Morris A, Maher K, Thomsen L, et al. Distribution of *Campylobacter pylori* in the human stomach obtained at postmortem. *Scand J Gastroenterol*. 1988;23:257-264.
106. Price AB. Histological aspects of *Campylobacter pylori* colonization and infection of gastric and duodenal mucosa. *Scand J Gastroenterol*. 1988;23:21-24.
107. Peek RM, Blaser MJ. *Helicobacter pylori* and gastrointestinal tract adenocarcinomas. *Nat Rev Cancer*. 2002;2:28-37.
108. Gilman RJ, Leon-Barua R, Koch J, et al. Rapid identification of pylori campylobacter in Peruvians with gastritis. *Dig Dis Sci*. 1986;31:1089-1094.
109. Lundgren A, Stromberg E, Sjoling A, et al. Mucosal FOXP3-expressing CD4+ CD25 high regulatory T cells in *Helicobacter pylori*-infected patients. *Infect Immun*. 2005;73:523-531.
110. Robinson K, Kenefeck R, Pidgeon EL, et al. *Helicobacter pylori*-induced peptic ulcer disease is associated with inadequate regulatory T cell responses. *Gut*. 2008;57:1375-1385.
111. Wunder C, Churin Y, Winau F, et al. Cholesterol glucosylation promotes immune evasion by *Helicobacter pylori*. *Nat Med*. 2006;12:1030-1038.
112. Letley DP, Rhead JL, Twells RJ, et al. Determinants of nontoxicity in the gastric pathogen *Helicobacter pylori*. *J Biol Chem*. 2003;278:26734-26741.
113. D'Elios MM, Manghetti M, De Carli M, et al. T helper 1 effector cells specific for *Helicobacter pylori* in the gastric antrum of patients with peptic ulcer disease. *J Immunol*. 1997;158:962-967.
114. Wang J, Brooks EG, Bamford KB, et al. Negative selection of T cells by *Helicobacter pylori* as a model for bacterial strain selection by immune evasion. *J Immunol*. 2001;167:926-934.
115. Allen LA, Schlesinger LS, Kang B. Virulent strains of *Helicobacter pylori* demonstrate delayed phagocytosis and stimulate homotypic phagosome fusion in macrophages. *J Exp Med*. 2000;191:115-128.
116. Mohammadi M, Nedrud J, Redline R, et al. Murine CD4 T-cell response to *Helicobacter* infection: TH1 cells enhance gastritis and TH2 cells reduce bacterial load. *Gastroenterology*. 1997;113:1848-1857.
117. Suzuki M, Miura S, Suematsu M, et al. *Helicobacter pylori*-associated ammonia production enhances neutrophil-dependent gastric mucosal cell injury. *Am J Physiol*. 1992;263:G719-G725.
118. Yamazaki S, Yamakawa A, Yoshiuki I, et al. The CagA protein of *Helicobacter pylori* is translocated into epithelial cells and binds to SHP-2 in human gastric mucosa. *J Infect Dis*. 2003;187:334-337.
119. McClain MS, Cao P, Iwamoto H, et al. A 12-amino-acid segment, present in type s2 but not type s1 *Helicobacter pylori* VacA proteins, abolishes cytotoxin activity and alters membrane channel formation. *J Bacteriol*. 2001;183:6499-6508.
120. Cover TC, Cao P, Murthy UK, et al. Serum neutralizing antibody response to the vacuolating cytotoxin of *Helicobacter pylori*. *J Clin Invest*. 1992;90:913-918.
121. Aras RA, Fischer W, Perez-Perez GI, et al. Plasticity of repetitive DNA sequences within a bacterial (type IV) secretion system component. *J Exp Med*. 2003;198:1349-1360.
122. Figura N, Guglielmetti P, Rossolini A, et al. Cytotoxin production by *Campylobacter pylori* strains isolated from patients with peptic ulcers and from patients with chronic gastritis only. *J Clin Microbiol*. 1989;27:225-226.
123. Atherton JC. The pathogenesis of *Helicobacter pylori*-induced gastroduodenal disease. *Annu Rev Pathol Mech Dis*. 2006;1:63-96.
124. Mai UE, Pérez-Pérez GI, Allen JB, et al. Surface proteins from *Helicobacter pylori* exhibit chemotactic activity for human leukocytes and are present in gastric mucosa. *J Exp Med*. 1992;175:517-525.
125. Mai UEH, Pérez-Pérez GI, Wahl LM, et al. Soluble surface proteins from *Helicobacter pylori* activate monocytes/macrophages by lipopolysaccharide-independent mechanism. *J Clin Invest*. 1991;87:894-900.
126. Pérez-Pérez GI, Shepherd VL, Morrow JD, Blaser MJ. Activation of human THP-1 and rat bone marrow-derived macrophages by *Helicobacter pylori* lipopolysaccharide. *Infect Immun*. 1995;63:1183-1187.
127. Aspinall GO, Monteiro MA, Pang H, et al. Lipopolysaccharide of the *Helicobacter pylori* type strain NCTC 11637 (ATCC 43504): Structure of the O antigen and core oligosaccharide regions. *Biochemistry*. 1996;35:2489-2497.
128. Wirth HP, Yang M, Peek RM, et al. *Helicobacter pylori* Lewis expression is related to the host Lewis phenotype. *Gastroenterology*. 1997;113:1091-1098.
129. Sharma SA, Tummuru MKR, Miller GG, et al. Interleukin-8 response of gastric epithelial cell lines to *Helicobacter pylori* stimulation in vitro. *Infect Immun*. 1995;63:1681-1687.
130. Isomoto H, Miyazaki M, Mizuta Y, et al. Expression of nuclear factor kappa B in *Helicobacter pylori*-infected gastric mucosa detected with Southwestern histochemistry. *Scand J Gastroenterol*. 2000;35:247-254.
131. Su B, Ceponis PJ, Lebel S, et al. *Helicobacter pylori* activates Toll-like receptor 4 expression in gastrointestinal epithelial cells. *Infect Immun*. 2003;71:3496-3502.
132. Backhed F, Rokbi B, Torstensson E, et al. Gastric mucosal recognition of *Helicobacter pylori* is independent of Toll-like receptor 4. *J Infect Dis*. 2003;187:829-836.
133. Foryst-Ludwig A, Naumann M. p21-activated kinase 1 activates the nuclear factor kappa B (NF-kappa B)-inducing kinase-I kappa B kinases NF-kappa B pathway and proinflammatory cytokines in *Helicobacter pylori* infection. *J Biol Chem*. 2000;275:39779-39785.
134. Crabtree JE, Shallcross T, Wyatt JI, et al. Tumour necrosis factor alpha secretion by *Helicobacter pylori* colonized gastric mucosa. *Gut*. 1991;32:1473-1477.
135. Blaser MJ. Hypotheses on the pathogenesis and natural history of *Helicobacter pylori*-induced inflammation. *Gastroenterology*. 1992;102:720-727.
136. El-Omar EM, Carrington M, Chow WH, et al. Interleukin-1 polymorphisms associated with increased risk of gastric cancer. *Nature*. 2000;404:398-402.
137. El-Omar EM, Rabkin CS, Gammon MD, et al. Increased risk of noncardia gastric cancer associated with proinflammatory cytokine gene polymorphisms. *Gastroenterology*. 2003;124:1193-1201.
138. Figueiredo C, Machado JC, Pharoah P, et al. *Helicobacter pylori* and interleukin 1 genotyping: an opportunity to identify high-risk individuals for gastric carcinoma. *J Natl Cancer Inst*. 2002;94:1680-1687.
139. Blaser MJ, Crabtree JE. CagA and the outcome of *Helicobacter pylori* infection. *Am J Clin Pathol*. 1996;106:565-567.
140. Smith JTL, Pounder RF, Nwokolo CU, et al. Inappropriate hypergastrinaemia in asymptomatic healthy subjects with *Helicobacter pylori*. *Gut*. 1990;31:522-525.
141. McColl KEL, Fullarton GM, Nujumi AM, et al. Lowered gastrin and gastric activity after eradication of *Campylobacter pylori* in duodenal ulcer. *Lancet*. 1989;2:499-500.
142. Moss SF, Legon S, Bishop AE, et al. Effect of *Helicobacter pylori* on gastric somatostatin in duodenal ulcer disease. *Lancet*. 1992;340:930-932.
143. Tham TCK, Chen L, Dennison N, et al. Effect of *Helicobacter pylori* eradication on antral somatostatin cell density in humans. *Eur J Gastroenterol Hepatol*. 1998;10:289-291.
144. Yamamoto S, Kaneko H, Konagaya T, et al. Interactions among gastric somatostatin, interleukin-8, and mucosal inflammation in *Helicobacter pylori*-positive peptic ulcer patients. *Helicobacter*. 2001;6:136-145.
145. Cave DR, Vargas M. Effect of a *Campylobacter pylori* protein on acid secretion by parietal cells. *Lancet*. 1989;2:187-189.
146. Blaser MJ. Ecology of *Helicobacter pylori* in the human stomach. *J Clin Invest*. 1997;100:759-762.
147. Karttunen R. Blood lymphocyte proliferation, cytokine secretion and appearance of T cells with activation surface markers in cultures with *Helicobacter pylori*: comparison of the responses of subjects with and without antibodies to *H. pylori*. *Clin Exp Immunol*. 1991;83:396-400.
148. Fox JG, Beck P, Dangler CA, et al. Concurrent enteric helminth infection modulates inflammation and gastric immune responses and reduces *Helicobacter*-induced gastric atrophy. *Nat Med*. 2000;6:536-542.
149. El-Omar EM, Rabkin CS, Gammon MD, et al. Increased risk of noncardia gastric cancer associated with proinflammatory cytokine gene polymorphisms. *Gastroenterology*. 2003;24:1193-1201.
150. Machado JC, Pharoah P, Sousa S, et al. Interleukin 1B and interleukin 1RN polymorphisms are associated with increased risk of gastric carcinoma. *Gastroenterology*. 2001;121:823-829.
151. Hazell SL, Eichberg JW, Lee DR, et al. Selection of the chimpanzee over the baboon as a model for *Helicobacter pylori* infection. *Gastroenterology*. 1992;103:848-854.
152. Dubois A, Berg DE, Incecik ET, et al. Transient and persistent experimental infection of non-human primates with *Helicobacter pylori*: implications for human disease. *Infect Immun*. 1996; 64:2885-2891.
153. Aebischer T, Bumann D, Epple HJ, et al. Correlation of T cell response and bacterial clearance in human volunteers challenged with *Helicobacter pylori* revealed by randomised controlled vaccination with Ty21a-based *Salmonella* vaccines. *Gut*. 2008;57:1065-1072.
154. Marchetti M, Arico B, Burroni D, et al. Development of a mouse model of *Helicobacter pylori* infection that mimics human disease. *Science*. 1995;267:1655-1658.
155. Wirth H-P, Beins MH, Yang M, et al. Experimental infection of Mongolian gerbils with wild-type and mutant *Helicobacter pylori* strains. *Infect Immun*. 1998;66:4856-4866.
156. Sakagami T, Dixon M, O'Rourke J, et al. Atrophic gastric changes in both *Helicobacter felis* and *Helicobacter pylori* infected mice are host dependent and separate from antral gastritis. *Gut*. 1996;39:639-648.
157. Peek RM Jr, Wirth HP, Moss SF, et al. *Helicobacter pylori* alters gastric epithelial cell cycle events and gastrin secretion in Mongolian gerbils. *Gastroenterology*. 2000;118:48-59.
158. Fong T-L, Dooley CP, Dehesa M, et al. *Helicobacter pylori* infection in pernicious anemia: a prospective controlled study. *Gastroenterology*. 1991;100:328-332.
159. Blaser MJ, Pérez-Pérez GI, Lindenbaum J, et al. Association of infection due to *Helicobacter pylori* with specific upper gastrointestinal pathology. *Rev Infect Dis*. 1991;13(Suppl):S704-S708.

160. Inglehart LW, Edlow DW, Mills L, et al. The presence of *Campylobacter pylori* in nonsteroidal antiinflammatory drug associated gastritis. *J Rheumatol.* 1989;16:599-603.

161. Nomura A, Stemmerman GN, Chyou PH, et al. *Helicobacter pylori* infection and the risk for duodenal and gastric ulceration. *Ann Intern Med.* 1994;120:977-981.

162. NIH Consensus Conference. *Helicobacter pylori* in peptic ulcer disease. *JAMA.* 1994;272:65-69.

163. Johnston BJ, Reed PI, Ali MH. *Campylobacter*-like organisms in duodenal and antral endoscopic biopsies: relationship to inflammation. *Gut.* 1986;27:1132-1137.

164. Carrick J, Lee A, Hazell S, et al. *Campylobacter pylori*, duodenal ulcer and gastric metaplasia: possible role of functional heterotrophic tissue in ulcerogenesis. *Gut.* 1989;30:790-797.

165. Forman D, Newell DG, Fullerton F, et al. Association between infection with *Helicobacter pylori* and risk of gastric cancer: evidence from a prospective investigation. *Br Med J.* 1991;302:1302-1305.

166. Nomura A, Stemmerman GN, Chyou P-H, et al. *Helicobacter pylori* infection and gastric carcinoma in a population of Japanese-Americans in Hawaii. *N Engl J Med.* 1991;325:1132-1136.

167. Parsonnet J, Friedman GD, Vandersteen DP, et al. *Helicobacter pylori* infection and the risk of gastric carcinoma. *N Engl J Med.* 1991;325:1127-1131.

168. Parsonnet J, Hansen S, Rodriguez L, et al. *Helicobacter pylori* infection and gastric lymphoma. *N Engl J Med.* 1994;330:1267-1271.

169. Wotherspoon AC, Ortiz Hidalgo C, Falzon MR, et al. *Helicobacter pylori*-associated gastritis and primary B-cell gastric lymphoma. *Lancet.* 1991;338:1175-1176.

170. Franchini M, Veneri D. *Helicobacter pylori* infection and immune thrombocytopenic purpura: an update. *Helicobacter.* 2004;9:342-346.

171. Rostami N, Keshtkar-Jahromi M, Rahnavardi M, et al. Effect of eradication of *Helicobacter pylori* on platelet recovery in patients with chronic idiopathic thrombocytopenic purpura: a controlled trial. *Am J Hematol.* 2008;83:376-381.

172. Satake M, Nishikawa J, Fukagawa Y, et al. The long-term efficacy of *Helicobacter pylori* eradication therapy in patients with idiopathic thrombocytopenic purpura. *J Gastroenterol Hepatol.* 2007;22:2233-2237.

173. Shallcross TM, Rathbone BJ, Heatley RV. *Campylobacter pylori* and non-ulcer dyspepsia. In: Rathbone BJ, Heatley RV, eds. *Campylobacter pylori and Gastroduodenal Disease.* Oxford: Blackwell; 1989:155-166.

174. McColl K, Murray L, El-Omar E, et al. Symptomatic benefit from eradicating *Helicobacter pylori* infection in patients with nonulcer dyspepsia. *N Engl J Med.* 1998;339:1869-1874.

175. Kang JY, Tay HH, Wee A, et al. Effect of colloidal bismuth subcitrate on symptoms and gastric histology in non-ulcer dyspepsia: a double blind placebo controlled study. *Gut.* 1990;31:476-480.

176. Talley NJ, Vakil N, Ballard ED 2nd, et al. Absence of benefit of eradicating *Helicobacter pylori* in patients with nonulcer dyspepsia. *N Engl J Med.* 1999;341:1106-1111.

177. Blum AL, Talley NJ, O'Moráin C, et al. Lack of effect of treating *Helicobacter pylori* infection in patients with nonulcer dyspepsia. *N Engl J Med.* 1998;339:1875-1881.

178. Loffeld RJLF, Werdmuller BFM, Kusters JG, et al. Colonization with *cagA*-positive *H. pylori* strains inversely associated with reflux oesophagitis and Barrett's oesophagitis. *Digestion.* 2000;62:95-99.

179. Vicari JJ, Peek RM, Falk GW, et al. The seroprevalence of *cagA* positive *Helicobacter pylori* strains in the spectrum of gastroesophageal reflux disease. *Gastroenterology.* 1998;115:50-57.

180. Chow W-H, Blaser MJ, Blot WJ, et al. An inverse relation between *cagA*⁺ strains of *Helicobacter pylori* infection and risk of esophageal and gastric cardia adenocarcinoma. *Cancer Res.* 1998;58:588-590.

181. Islami F, Kamangar F. *Helicobacter pylori* and esophageal cancer risk: a meta-analysis. *Cancer Prev Res.* 2008;1:329-338.

182. Morris A, Nicholson G. Experimental and accidental *C. pylori* infection of humans. In: Blaser MJ, ed. *Campylobacter pylori in Gastritis and Peptic Ulcer Disease.* New York: Igaku Shoin; 1989:61-72.

183. Harford WV, Barnett C, Lee E, et al. Acute gastritis with hypochlorhydria: report of 35 cases with long-term follow-up. *Gut.* 2000;47:467-472.

184. Morris AJ, Ali MR, Nicholson GI, et al. Long term follow-up of voluntary ingestion of *Helicobacter pylori*. *Ann Intern Med.* 1991;114:662-663.

185. Kang J, Blaser MJ. Bacterial populations as perfect gases: genomic integrity and diversification tensions in *Helicobacter pylori*. *Nat Rev Microbiol.* 2006;4:826-836.

186. Wyatt JI, Rathbone BJ, Dixon MF, et al. *Campylobacter pyloridis* and acid-induced gastric metaplasia in the pathogenesis of duodenitis. *J Clin Pathol.* 1987;40:841-848.

187. Coghlan JG, Gilligan D, Humphreys H, et al. *Campylobacter pylori* and recurrence of duodenal ulcers—a 12-month follow-up study. *Lancet.* 1987;2:1109-1111.

188. Marshall BJ, Goodwin CS, Warren JR, et al. Prospective double-blind trial of duodenal ulcer relapse after eradication of *Campylobacter pylori*. *Lancet.* 1988;2:1437-1445.

189. Graham DY, Lew GM, Klein PD, et al. Effect of treatment of *Helicobacter pylori* infection on the long-term recurrence of gastric or duodenal ulcer: a randomized, controlled study. *Ann Intern Med.* 1992;116:705-708.

190. Hentschel E, Brandstatter G, Dragoisics B, et al. Effect of ranitidine and amoxicillin plus metronidazole on the eradication of *Helicobacter pylori* and the recurrence of duodenal ulcer. *N Engl J Med.* 1993;328:308-312.

191. Labenz J, Blum AL, Bayerdörffer E, et al. Curing *Helicobacter pylori* infection in patients with duodenal ulcer may provoke reflux esophagitis. *Gastroenterology.* 1997;112:1442-1447.

192. Sung JJ, Chung SC, Ling TK, et al. Antibacterial treatment of gastric ulcers associated with *Helicobacter pylori*. *N Engl J Med.* 1995;332:139-142.

193. Correa P. Human gastric carcinogenesis: a multistep and multifactorial process—first American Cancer Society Award lecture on cancer epidemiology and prevention. *Cancer Res.* 1992;52:6735-6740.

194. Blaser MJ, Chyou PH, Nomura A. Age at establishment of *Helicobacter pylori* infection and gastric carcinoma, gastric ulcer, and duodenal ulcer risk. *Cancer Res.* 1995;55:562-565.

195. Blaser MJ, Nomura A, Lee J, et al. Early life family structure and microbially-induced cancer risk. *PLOS Med.* 2007;4:53-58.

196. Kosunen TU, Aromaa A, Knekt P, et al. *Helicobacter* antibodies in 1973 and 1994 in the adult population of Vammala, Finland. *Epidemiol Infect.* 1997;119:29-34.

197. Craanen ME, Dekker W, Blok P, et al. Intestinal metaplasia and *Helicobacter pylori*: an endoscopic bioptic study of the gastric antrum. *Gut.* 1992;33:16-20.

198. Kuipers EJ, Uyterlinde AM, Pena AS, et al. Long-term sequelae to *Helicobacter pylori* gastritis. *Lancet.* 1995;345:1525-1528.

199. Forman D, Sitas F, Newell DG, et al. Geographic association of *Helicobacter pylori* antibody prevalence and gastric cancer mortality in rural China. *Int J Cancer.* 1990;46:608-611.

200. The Eurogast Study Group. An international association between *Helicobacter pylori* infection and gastric cancer. *Lancet.* 1993;341:1359-1362.

201. Peek RM Jr, Moss SF, Tham KT, et al. *Helicobacter pylori* cagA+ strains and dissociation of gastric epithelial cell proliferation from apoptosis. *J Natl Cancer Inst.* 1997;89:863-868.

202. Moss SF, Calam J, Agarwal B, et al. Induction of gastric epithelial apoptosis by *Helicobacter pylori*. *Gut.* 1996;38:498-501.

203. Hoshi T, Sasano H, Kato K, et al. Cell damage and proliferation in human gastric mucosa infected by *Helicobacter pylori*—a comparison before and after *H. pylori* eradication in non-atrophic gastritis. *Hum Pathol.* 1999;30:1412-1417.

204. Smoot DT, Wynn Z, Elliott TB, et al. Effects of *Helicobacter pylori* on proliferation of gastric epithelial cells in vitro. *Am J Gastroenterol.* 1999;94:1508-1511.

205. Meyer-ter-Vehn T, Covacci A, Kist M, et al. *Helicobacter pylori* activates mitogen-activated protein kinase cascades and induces expression of the proto-oncogenes c-fos and c-jun. *J Biol Chem.* 2000;275:16064-16072.

206. Maeda S, Yoshida H, Mitsuno Y, et al. Analysis of apoptotic and antiapoptotic signaling pathways induced by *Helicobacter pylori*. *Mol Pathol.* 2002;55:286-293.

207. Uemura N, Okamoto S, Yamamoto S, et al. *Helicobacter pylori* infection and the development of gastric cancer. *N Engl J Med.* 2001;345:784-789.

208. Wong BC, Lam SK, Wong WM, et al. *Helicobacter pylori* eradication to prevent gastric cancer in a high-risk region of China: a randomized controlled trial. *JAMA.* 2004;291:187-194.

209. Fukase K, Kato M, Kikuchi S, et al. Effect of eradication of *Helicobacter pylori* on incidence of metachronous gastric carcinoma after endoscopic resection of early gastric cancer: an open-label, randomised controlled trial. *Lancet.* 2008;372:392-397.

210. Devesa SS, Blot WJ, Fraumeni JF Jr. Changing patterns in the incidence of esophageal and gastric carcinoma in the United States. *Cancer.* 1998;83:2049-2053.

211. Neubauer A, Thiede C, Morgner A, et al. Cure of *Helicobacter pylori* infection and duration of remission of low-grade gastric mucosa-associated lymphoid tissue lymphoma. *J Natl Cancer Inst.* 1997;89:1350-1353.

212. Pinotti G, Zucca E, Roggero E, et al. Clinical features, treatment and outcome in a series of 93 patients with low-grade gastric MALT lymphoma. *Leuk Lymphoma.* 1997;26:527-537.

213. El-Serag HB, Sonnenberg A. Opposing time trends of peptic ulcer and reflux disease. *Gut.* 1998;43:327-333.

214. Vaezi MF, Falk GW, Peek RM, et al. CagA-positive strains of *Helicobacter pylori* may protect against Barrett's esophagus. *Am J Gastroenterol.* 2000;95:2206-2211.

215. Warburton-Timms VJ, Charlett A, Valori RM, et al. The significance of cagA(+) *Helicobacter pylori* in reflux oesophagitis. *Gut.* 2001;49:341-346.

216. Roulton-Jones J, Logan R. An inverse relation between cagA-positive strains of *Helicobacter pylori* infection and risk of esophageal and gastric cardia adenocarcinoma. *Helicobacter.* 1999;4:281-283.

217. Yamaji Y, Mitsushima T, Ikuma H, et al. Inverse background of *Helicobacter pylori* antibody and pepsinogen in reflux oesophagitis compared with gastric cancer: analysis of 5732 Japanese subjects. *Gut.* 2001;49:335-340.

218. Quieroz DMM, Rocha GA, de Oliveira CA, et al. Role of corpus gastritis and cagA-positive *Helicobacter pylori* infection in reflux esophagitis. *J Clin Microbiol.* 2002;40:2849-2853.

219. Koike T, Ohara S, Sekine H, et al. *Helicobacter pylori* infection prevents erosive reflux oesophagitis by decreasing gastric acid secretion. *Gut.* 2001;49:330-334.

220. Francois F, Roper J, Goodman AJ, et al. The association of gastric leptin with oesophageal inflammation and metaplasia. *Gut.* 2008;57:16-24.

221. Bik EM, Eckburg PB, Gill SR, et al. Molecular analysis of the bacterial microbiota in the human stomach. *Proc Natl Acad Sci U S A.* 2006;103:732-737.

222. Pei Z, Bini EJ, Yang L, et al. Bacterial biota in the human distal esophagus. *Proc Natl Acad Sci U S A.* 2004;101:4250-4255.

223. Breidert M, Miehlke S, Glasow A, et al. Leptin and its receptor in normal human gastric mucosa and in *Helicobacter pylori*-associated gastritis. *Scand J Gastroenterol.* 1999; 34:954-961.

224. Sobhani I, Bado A, Vissuzaine C, et al. Leptin secretion and leptin receptor in the human stomach. *Gut.* 2000;47:178-183.

225. Nwokolo CU, Freshwater DA, O'Hare P, et al. Plasma ghrelin following cure of *Helicobacter pylori*. *Gut.* 2003;52:637-640.

226. Roper J, Francois F, Shue PL, et al. Leptin and ghrelin in relation to *Helicobacter pylori* status in adult males. *J Clin Endocrinol Metab.* 2008;93:2350-2357.

227. Blaser MJ. Who are we? Indigenous microbes and the ecology of human diseases. *EMBO Rep.* 2006;7:956-960.

228. Richter T, Richter T, List S, et al. Five- to 7-year-old children with *Helicobacter pylori* infection are smaller than *Helicobacter*-negative children: a cross-sectional population-based study of 3,315 children. *J Pediatr Gastroenterol Nutr.* 2001;33:472-475.

229. Ioannou GN, Weiss NS, Kearney DJ. Is *Helicobacter pylori* seropositivity related to body mass index in the United States? *Aliment Pharmacol Ther.* 2005;21:765-772.

230. Cho I, Blaser MJ, Francois F, et al. *Helicobacter pylori* and overweight status in the United States: data from the Third National Health and Nutrition Examination Survey. *Am J Epidemiol.* 2005;162:579-584.

231. Wu MS, Lee WJ, Wang HH, et al. A case-control study of association of *Helicobacter pylori* infection with morbid obesity in Taiwan. *Arch Intern Med.* 2005;165:1552-1555.

232. Dunn BE, Cohen H, Blaser MJ. *Helicobacter pylori*. *Clin Microbiol Rev.* 1997;10:720-741.

233. Evans DJ Jr, Evans DG, Graham DY, et al. A sensitive and specific serologic test for detection of *Campylobacter pylori* infection. *Gastroenterology.* 1989;96:1004-1008.

234. Romero-Gallo J, Perez-Perez GI, Novick RP, et al. Responses to *Helicobacter pylori* whole cell and CagA antigens amongst Ladakh patients undergoing endoscopy. *Clin Diagn Lab Immunol.* 2002;9:1313-1317.

235. Kosunen TU, Seppala K, Sarna S, et al. Diagnostic value of decreased IgG, IgA, and IgM antibody titres after eradication of *Helicobacter pylori*. *Lancet.* 1992;339:893-895.

236. Pérez-Pérez GI, Cutler AF, Blaser MJ. Value of serology as a non-invasive method to evaluate the efficacy of treatment in *Helicobacter pylori* infection. *Clin Infect Dis.* 1997;25:1038-1043.

237. Khanna B, Cutler A, Israel NR, et al. Use caution with serologic testing for *Helicobacter pylori* infection in children. *J Infect Dis.* 1998;178:460-465.

238. Graham DY, Evans DJ, Alpert LC, et al. *Campylobacter pylori* detected non-invasively by the ¹³C-urea breath test. *Lancet.* 1987;1:1174-1177.

239. Marshall BJ, Surveyor I. Carbon-14 urea breath test for the diagnosis of *Campylobacter pyloridis*-associated gastritis. *J Nucl Med.* 1988;29:11-16.

240. Sjolund M, Wreiber K, Andersson DI, et al. Long-term persistence of resistant *Enterococcus* species after antibiotics to eradicate *Helicobacter pylori*. *Ann Intern Med.* 2003;139:483-487.

241. Rothenbacher D, Blaser MJ, Bode G, et al. An inverse relationship between gastric colonization by *Helicobacter pylori* and diarrheal illnesses in children: results of a population-based cross-sectional study. *Infect Dis.* 2000;182:1446-1449.

242. Putsep K, Branden CI, Boman HG, et al. Antibacterial peptide from *H. pylori*. *Nature.* 1999;398:671-672.

243. Mattsson A, Lonroth H, Quiding-Jarbrink M, et al. Induction of B cell responses in the stomach of *Helicobacter pylori*-infected subjects after oral cholera vaccination. *J Clin Invest.* 1998;102:51-56.

244. Goodwin CS, Blake P, Blincow E. The minimum inhibitory and bactericidal concentrations of antibiotics and anti-ulcer agents against *Campylobacter pyloridis*. *J Antimicrob Chemother.* 1986;17:309-314.

245. Megraud F. Resistance of *Helicobacter pylori* to antibiotics. *Aliment Pharmacol Ther.* 1997;11:43-53.

246. Xia HX, Daw MA, Beattie S, et al. Prevalence of metronidazole-resistant *Helicobacter pylori* in dyspeptic patients. *Ir J Med Sci.* 1993;162:91-94.

247. Rautelin H, Seppala K, Renkonen OV, et al. Role of metronidazole resistance in therapy of *Helicobacter pylori* infections. *Antimicrob Agents Chemother.* 1992;36:163-166.

248. European Study Group on Antibiotic Susceptibility of *Helicobacter pylori*. Results of a multicentre European survey in 1991 of metronidazole in *Helicobacter pylori*. *Eur J Clin Microbiol Infect Dis.* 1992;11:777-781.

249. Pavicic MJ, Namavar F, Verboom T, et al. In vitro susceptibility of *Helicobacter pylori* to several antimicrobial combinations. *Antimicrob Agents Chemother.* 1993;37:1184-1186.

250. McNulty CAM, Gearty JC, Crump B, et al. *Campylobacter pyloridis* and associated gastritis: investigator blind, placebo controlled trial of bismuth salicylate and erythromycin ethylsuccinate. *Br Med J.* 1986;293:645-649.

251. Logan RPH, Gummett PA, Misiewicz JJ, et al. One week eradication regimen for *Helicobacter pylori*. *Lancet.* 1991;338:1249-1252.

252. Vakil N, Vaira D. Sequential therapy for *Helicobacter pylori*: time to consider making the switch? *JAMA.* 2008;300:1346-1347.

253. Millar MR, Pike J. Bactericidal activity of antimicrobial agents against slowly growing *Helicobacter pylori*. *Antimicrob Agents Chemother*. 1992;36:185-187.
254. Graham DY, Lew GM, Malaty HM, et al. Factors influencing the eradication of *Helicobacter pylori* with triple therapy. *Gastroenterology*. 1992;102:493-496.
255. Iwahi T, Satoh H, Nakao M, et al. Lansoprazole, a novel benzimidazole proton pump inhibitor, and its related compounds have selective activity against *Helicobacter pylori*. *Antimicrob Agents Chemother*. 1991;35:490-496.
256. Nagata K, Satoh H, Iwahi T, et al. Potent inhibitory action of the gastric proton pump inhibitor lansoprazole against urease activity of *Helicobacter pylori*: unique action selective for *H. pylori* cells. *Antimicrob Agents Chemother*. 1993;37:769-774.
257. Vakil N, Megraud F. Eradication therapy for *Helicobacter pylori*. *Gastroenterology*. 2007;133:985-1001.
258. de Boer W, Driessen W, Jansz A, et al. Effect of acid suppression on efficacy of treatment for *Helicobacter pylori* infection. *Lancet*. 1995;345:817-820.
259. Vaira D, Zullo A, Vakil N, et al. Sequential therapy versus standard triple-drug therapy for *Helicobacter pylori* eradication: a randomized trial. *Ann Intern Med*. 2007;146:556-563.
260. Blaser MJ, Kirschner D. The equilibria that allow bacterial persistence in human hosts. *Nature*. 2007;449:843-849.
261. Azuma T, Suto H, Ito Y, et al. Gastric leptin and *Helicobacter pylori* infection. *Gut*. 2001;49:324-329.
262. Blaser MJ. Who are we? Indigenous microbes and the ecology of human diseases. *EMBO Rep*. 2006;7:956-960.
263. Konturek JW, Konturek SJ, Kwiecien N, et al. Leptin in the control of gastric secretion and gut hormones in humans infected with *Helicobacter pylori*. *Scand J Gastroenterol*. 2001;36:1148-1154.
264. Dent JC, McNulty CAM, Ulff JS, et al. Spiral organisms in the gastric antrum. *Lancet*. 1987;2:96.
265. McNulty CAM, Dent JC, Curry A, et al. New spiral bacterium in gastric mucosa. *J Clin Pathol*. 1989;42:585-591.
266. Heilmann KL, Borchard F. Gastritis due to spiral shaped bacteria other than *Helicobacter pylori*: clinical, histological, and ultrastructural findings. *Gut*. 1991;32:137-140.
267. Solnick JV, O'Rourke J, Lee A, et al. An uncultured gastric spiral organism is a newly identified *Helicobacter* in humans. *J Infect Dis*. 1993;168:379-385.

218

Enterobacteriaceae

MICHAEL S. DONNENBERG

The family Enterobacteriaceae falls within the domain Bacteria, phylum Proteobacteria, class Gammaproteobacteria, and order Enterobacteriales (dx.doi.org/10.1007/bergeysoutline200210) and includes the medically important genera and species listed in Table 218-1. Of these genera, *Salmonella, Shigella* (actually not a true genus, but in fact a pathotype of *Escherichia coli*),[1] and *Yersinia* have distinctive features and particular medical importance that merit separate discussions found elsewhere in this volume (see Chapters 223, 224, and 229). Members of the family Enterobacteriaceae are gram-negative, non–spore-forming, facultative anaerobes that ferment glucose and other sugars, reduce nitrate to nitrite, and produce catalase, but (with the exception of *Plesiomonas*) do not produce oxidase. Most are motile by virtue of peritrichous (as opposed to polar) flagellae. Members of the family Enterobacteriaceae are often referred to as enterics because the principal habitat of many of these organisms is the lower gastrointestinal tract of various animals. However, these terms are not synonymous because several species do not typically inhabit the gastrointestinal tract, and other intestinal pathogens that do not fall within the family, such as *Vibrio* spp., are also referred to as enteric bacteria. Furthermore, the designation belies the fact that members of the family Enterobacteriaceae are widely distributed and are commonly found in the environment. This chapter includes a discussion of the general properties of the group, including common pathogenic features, followed by sections on individual pathogens and the diseases that they cause.

General Properties

EPIDEMIOLOGY

Although the natural habitat of many medically important members of the family Enterobacteriaceae is the lower gastrointestinal tract of humans and other animals, these organisms are actually quite widespread in nature and may be found, for example, in water and soil. Furthermore, certain individuals, including alcoholics and those with diabetes mellitus, have high rates of oropharyngeal colonization with members of this family.[2] Moreover, enterobacterial species rapidly colonize the oropharynx of many hospitalized patients regardless of whether they receive antimicrobials.[3] In addition, women who use diaphragms and/or spermicidal agents for contraception and postmenopausal women have increased rates of vaginal colonization with *E. coli* and other members of the family.[4,5] The extended niche that Enterobacteriaceae may occupy under these circumstances is an important predisposing factor that allows subsequent extraintestinal infections to occur.

Members of the family Enterobacteriaceae cause a wide variety of infections in both the community and the hospital setting, affecting normal hosts and those with preexisting illnesses. They comprise the most common gram-negative isolates in microbiology laboratories, including the vast majority of urinary isolates and a large proportion of isolates from the blood, the peritoneal cavity, and the respiratory tract. They may be isolated from numerous other sites, including cerebrospinal fluid, synovial fluid, and abscesses. The proportion of multiple antimicrobe-resistant isolates, including those producing extended-spectrum β-lactamases and those resistant to fluoroquinolones, has increased steadily so that the majority of nosocomial and many community-acquired isolates are now resistant to several important antimicrobial classes.

Infections caused by members of the family Enterobacteriaceae may be sporadic or occur in outbreaks. The recognition of community-acquired or nosocomial outbreaks of these infections is facilitated by molecular diagnostic techniques that indicate whether strains isolated from different patients arose from a recent common ancestor (i.e., belong to the same clone). Among these techniques are pulsed-field gel electrophoresis, ribotyping, random-primed polymerase chain reaction (PCR), and multilocus sequence typing. Databases containing archived electrophoresis patterns resulting from applying these techniques to previously isolated strains under standard conditions have greatly facilitated outbreak recognition.[6]

STRUCTURAL AND SURFACE ANTIGENIC FEATURES

Members of the family Enterobacteriaceae are rod-shaped organisms, generally 1 to 3 μm in length and 0.5 μm in diameter. Surface appendages, including pili and flagellae, are common and may be numerous. The cytoplasm of enterobacterial organisms, like that of other bacteria, does not have membrane-enclosed organelles, as do eukaryotic cells. Therefore, there is no nucleus, and the genome, which usually consists of a single circular chromosome and may include multiple plasmids of various sizes, is dispersed within the cytoplasm. Likewise, there is no endoplasmic reticulum and so ribosomes are not membrane associated, and respiration takes place at the cytoplasmic membrane rather than in mitochondria. As gram-negative organisms, enterobacteria have both inner and outer phospholipid membranes, which enclose a periplasmic space that contains the peptidoglycan cell wall (Fig. 218-1). Much of the specific information in the following sections comes from studies of *E. coli*, but may be assumed to apply to the entire family.

Inner Membrane

The inner or cytoplasmic membrane, impermeable to polar molecules, regulates the passage of nutrients, metabolites, macromolecules, and information in and out of the cytoplasm and maintains the proton motive force required for energy storage. More than 100 different proteins are associated with the inner membrane of *E. coli*,[7] including integral membrane proteins that have one or more transmembrane domains that traverse the phospholipid bilayer, lipoproteins inserted into the outer leaflet of the membrane, and peripheral membrane proteins that may be associated with the inner or outer leaflet or may be components of protein complexes that include integral membrane proteins. Among these inner membrane proteins are those involved in electron transfer and oxidative phosphorylation, the F_1F_0 adenosine triphosphatase that couples proton transport to adenosine triphosphate synthesis, efflux pumps that export toxins and antimicrobials, numerous specific solute transporters, various protein translocation systems, polysaccharide export systems, and a large number of two-component histidine kinase signaling proteins that link external stimuli to changes in gene transcription.[8]

Periplasmic Space

Between the inner and outer membranes is the periplasm, an aqueous environment containing a high concentration of proteins and the peptidoglycan, which probably forms a hydrated gel.[9] In contrast to the reducing environment of the cytoplasm, the periplasm is an oxidizing environment and thus the cysteine residues of periplasmic proteins are frequently involved in disulfide bonds. A variety of functional catego-

TABLE 218-1	Medically Important Genera and Species of the Family Enterobacteriaceae
Genus	**Species**
Citrobacter	freundii
	koseri
	amalonaticus
Edwardsiella	tarda
Enterobacter	cloacae
	aerogenes
	sakasakii
Escherichia	coli
	albertii
Hafnia	alvei
Klebsiella	pneumoniae
	oxytoca
	granulomatis
Morganella	morganii
Pantoea (formerly Enterobacter)	agglomerans
Plesiomonas	shigelloides
Proteus	mirabilis
	vulgaris
Providencia	stuartii
	rettgeri
Salmonella	enterica
Serratia	marcescens
Shigella (belongs within the E. coli species)	dysenterii
	flexneri
	sonnei
	boydii
Yersinia	pestis
	enterocolitica
	pseudotuberculosis

ries of protein are found in the periplasm, including disulfide oxidoreductases, peptidyl-prolyl isomerases, chaperones, and proteases involved in protein folding and degradation; solute-binding proteins that ferry sugars, amino acids, ions, and vitamins across the space; lipoprotein-sorting proteins; detoxifying enzymes; and enzymes involved in the biogenesis of peptidoglycan, lipopolysaccharide (LPS), and capsule.

Peptidoglycan Cell Wall

The gram-negative cell wall is composed of a thin layer of peptidoglycan (also known as murein), which consists of alternating N-acetylglucosamine and N-acetylmuramic acid amino sugars joined by β-1,4 linkages, with a short peptide composed of L-alanine, D-glutamic acid, L-meso-diaminopalmelic acid, and D-alanine attached to the carboxyl group of the muramic acid.[10] Strands of the linear peptidoglycan molecules are covalently linked principally through an amide bond between the carboxyl group of the D-alanine residue at position 4 and the free amino group of the diaminopalmelic acid in an adjacent strand. Murein lipoprotein is also covalently attached to the peptide, which anchors the layer to the inner leaflet of the outer membrane in which the lipoprotein is embedded. The peptidoglycan layer of each bacterium is thought to comprise a single contiguous molecule enveloping the organism. In contrast to that of gram-positive organisms, this murein sacculus of gram-negative organisms is predominantly one layer thick. This thin envelope is responsible for the shape and osmotic stability of the organism, but it is constantly being remodeled as the bacterium elongates and divides.

Outer Membrane

The outer membrane of gram-negative bacteria is an asymmetrical lipid bilayer. Phospholipids occur almost exclusively in the inner leaflet, whereas the outer lipid is mostly composed of LPS. The polar nature of the LPS protruding from the outer membrane poses a significant barrier to the penetration of lipophilic molecules and thus plays a major role in protecting the bacteria from various detergents

(including bile salts), dyes (including methylene blue), and hydrophobic antibiotics.[11] These features are exploited in the microbiology laboratory on selective media for gram-negative organisms. In addition to containing lipoproteins, the outer membrane features porin proteins that regulate the passage of hydrophilic molecules. Porins, like other integral outer membrane proteins, have a conserved β-barrel fold that encloses a central aqueous channel.[12]

Lipopolysaccharide

The enterobacterial LPS is an extremely potent virulence factor, as discussed later. LPS has three major domains, the lipid A backbone, the core phosphorylated oligosaccharide, and the repeating oligosaccharide side chains.[13] Lipid A, also known as endotoxin, is the biologically active portion of the molecule that is recognized by host pattern recognition receptors. It is composed of a β-1,6 disaccharide of glucosamine, which is phosphorylated and substituted with saturated hydroxylated acyl chains. The acyl groups of lipid A are inserted into the outer leaflet of the outer membrane. The core oligosaccharide is composed of a pair of 8-carbon sugars known as Kdo linked to lipid A, which are in turn linked to 6 to 10 additional sugars, forming a branched chain. Core oligosaccharides are heterogeneous and differ within and between species. The repeating oligosaccharide attached to the LPS core is known as the O antigen. There may be 1 to 60 repeats of the oligosaccharide unit. The O antigen is the basis for serogroup classification. There are more than 170 different O-antigen serogroups in E. coli alone.[14] The genes encoding the enzymes that synthesize the O antigen are quite variable and show evidence of interspecies lateral gene transfer. Mutants lacking the ability to synthesize O antigen, including the venerable K-12 laboratory strain of E. coli and its many derivatives, have rough colony morphologies.

Capsule and Other Surface Polysaccharides

In addition to the O-antigen component of LPS, members of the family Enterobacteriaceae produce additional surface polysaccharides including enterobacterial common antigen, colanic acid, and an envelope of surface polysaccharide known as capsule. Enterobacterial common antigen is a repeating trisaccharide covalently linked to phosphoglyceride and, in some strains also to LPS, which is embedded in the outer leaflet of the outer membrane.[15] The role of enterobacterial common antigen in the biology of the bacteria is not known, but its remarkable conservation in all members of the family favors an important function. Many strains of E. coli and related organisms produce a surface layer of another polysaccharide termed colanic acid, which resembles in many ways a subset of capsule types. True capsules fall into several types, depending on genetic and biochemical features including whether they are linked to LPS or α-glycerol phosphate.[16] In some genera, such as Klebsiella and Enterobacter, the capsules can be quite luxuriant, imparting to the bacteria a highly mucoid colonial morphology. Early on, capsules were characterized based on their ability to mask the O antigen from agglutinating antibody, in a manner that was sensitive to heating. Capsules vary widely in chemical structure and are the basis of the K-antigen serotyping scheme. There are more than 80 K-antigen types in E. coli alone.[14]

Flagellae

Most members of the enterobacterial family are motile, and even those that are not often possess the genes that specify the expression of flagellae and may retain the capacity for motility under certain conditions.[17] Flagellae are flexible surface appendages that rotate and propel the bacteria through liquid environments. In most enterobacteria, they emanate from all sides of the microorganisms (Fig. 218-2A). The biogenesis of flagellae is quite complex, proceeds in a specific order from the base to the tip of the organelle, and involves an intricate secretion machinery that resembles that of the type III secretion systems[18] (see later). Flagellar assembly and motility are under the control of a complex regulatory network that responds to a variety of extracellular signals. The flagellar filament is composed of a hollow helical array of a single protein, flagellin. The amino and carboxyl termini of flagellin

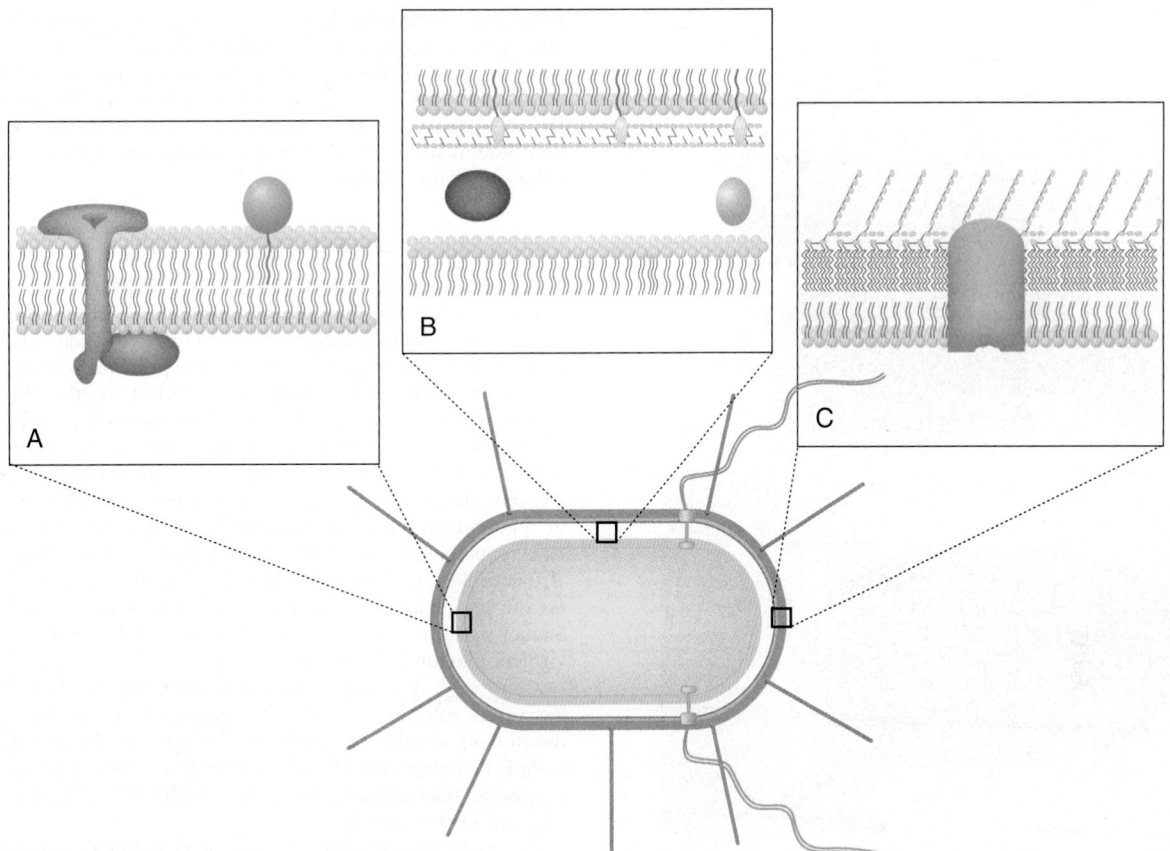

Figure 218-1 Cartoon of the architecture of an enterobacterial cell. Cartoon of the architecture of an enterobacterial cell. The cytoplasm is depicted in blue, the inner (cytoplasmic) membrane in yellow, the periplasmic space in white, the peptidoglycan layer in purple, and the outer membrane in orange. Pili (also known as fimbriae) are depicted in black as linear organelles extending from the outer membrane, and flagellae are shown in green as hollow, flexible organelles emanating from an assembly and secretion apparatus that spans both membranes and the periplasmic space. *Insets* show closer views of the envelope. **A,** The cytoplasmic membrane has a phospholipid bilayer, transmembrane (red) proteins, peripheral membrane (blue) proteins, and lipoproteins (green). **B,** The periplasmic space is surrounded by the inner and outer membranes and includes soluble proteins (purple and blue). The peptidoglycan layer, composed of disaccharide and peptide cross-linkages, is associated with the inner leaflet of the outer membrane through covalent attachment to lipoprotein (yellow). **C,** The outer membrane layer has an inner phospholipid leaflet and an outer lipopolysaccharide leaflet. Traversing the membrane are porin proteins that regulate the passage of molecules (green).

are highly conserved within and across species of the family. However, the middle of the molecule, which is surface exposed, is highly variable in amino acid composition, apparently as a result of both recombination following horizontal gene transfer and selection for diversifying mutations.[19] This diversity is represented in the H-antigen typing scheme, the third component of O:K:H serotyping. There are at least 54 flagellin H-antigen types in *E. coli* alone. Like LPS, flagellin is recognized by the host innate immune system pattern recognition receptors, which can lead to neutrophil recruitment and initiation of a proinflammatory response.[20-22]

Fimbriae

Most enterobacterial species produce additional surface appendages referred to as either *fimbriae* (from the Latin for "thread") or *pili* (from the Latin for "hair"). These appendages are thinner than flagellae, ranging in diameter from 2 to 7 nm and extending several micrometers from the surface.[23] Fimbriae can serve roles in adhesion to host cells, in autoaggregation, and in genetic exchange through conjugation. There are several types of fimbriae, which differ in morphology, biosynthetic pathways, and function.

The chaperone-usher group of fimbriae is widespread among the Enterobacteriaceae and includes the ubiquitous type 1 pili, produced by most members of the family (see Fig. 218-2*B*). Individual strains may have the genes required to produce 10 or more different chaperone-usher type pili.[24-26] Many of these pili are composite fibers, with a

rigid rod composed of a helical array of the major structural subunit pilin protein joined end-to-end to a thinner, more flexible tip.[27,28] The adhesin may be at the distal end of the tip. Other members of the family, sometimes referred to as fibrillae, have a uniform wiry appearance that resembles that of the tip of the composite fibers. Assembly of the chaperone-usher type of fimbria proceeds by a dedicated pathway in which the subunits are exported by the general secretion machinery to the periplasm, where they bind to specific chaperones that prevent premature interactions between subunits. The pilin-chaperone complexes are delivered to an outer membrane channel protein known as the usher, to which the proximal end of the pilus remains attached and which exports the subunits across the outer membrane in a specific order starting with the tip protein.[29,30]

Type IV fimbriae are also widespread among the Enterobacteriaceae, produced by certain pathotypes of *E. coli*[31-33]; certain strains of *Salmonella enterica,* including serovar Typhi[34]; and some strains of *Yersinia pseudotuberculosis.*[35] In many cases, type IV pili are expressed exclusively at the poles of the bacteria and often aggregate laterally to form ropelike bundles (see Fig. 218-2*C*). Type IV pili are retractable, and this retraction can be harnessed for a type of bacterial locomotion called "twitching motility."[36] The ability of the fimbriae to bundle and retract is associated with bacterial aggregation and disaggregation. Type IV pili are generally formed of a single pilin protein, which is processed to its mature form by a dedicated pre-pilin peptidase that also *N*-methylates the amino-terminal residue. A complex and poorly

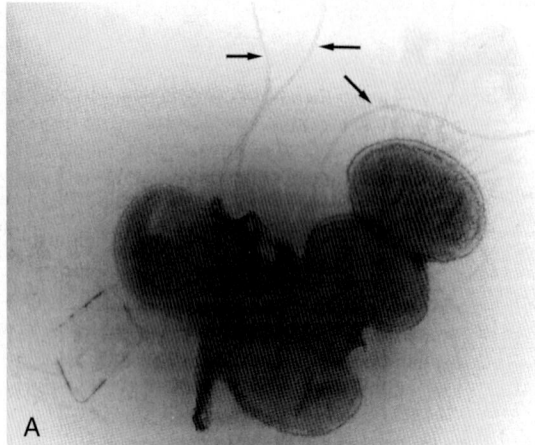

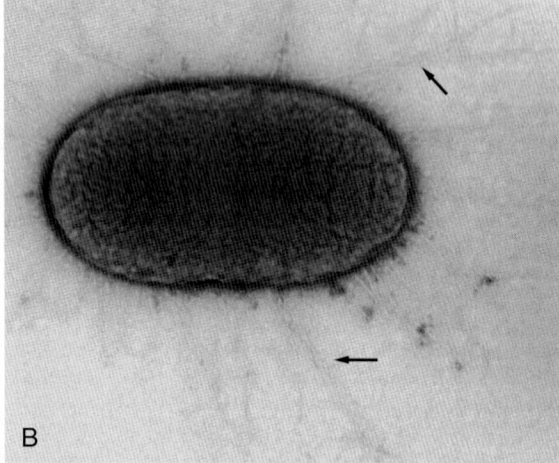

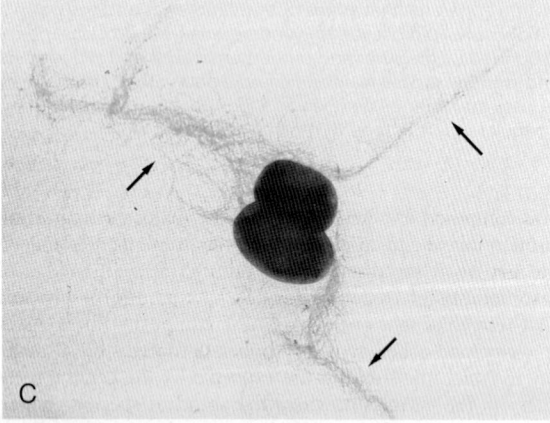

Figure 218-2 **Transmission electron micrographs of negatively stained _Escherichia coli_ cells. A** and **B,** An extraintestinal pathogenic _E. coli_ strain grown under conditions favoring the expression of type 1 pili demonstrates both flagellae (_arrows_ in **A**) and pili (_arrows_ in **B**). **C,** An enteropathogenic _E. coli_ strain grown under conditions favoring expression of bundle-forming type IV pili (_arrows_). _(Courtesy of Eric Buckles and Paula J. Fernandes.)_

understood molecular machine responsible for pilin export and pilus formation is composed of approximately 10 proteins localized to the cytoplasm, inner membrane, periplasm, and outer membrane.[37] Some of the components of this machine are related to components of the type II secretion apparatus (see later).

Self-transmissible plasmids that allow DNA transfer via conjugation are ubiquitous in the family Enterobacteriaceae. These plasmids, which often harbor virulence genes, transposons, and antibiotic resistance genes, encode pili that mediate intercellular contact and DNA transfer. Some of these plasmids are host restricted, but others are capable of transfer among distantly related species. The pili and transfer mechanisms encoded by such plasmids are related to type IV secretion systems such as those that export virulence factors in _Helicobacter pylori_ and _Bordetella pertussis_.[38]

VIRULENCE AND VIRULENCE FACTORS

The ability of members of the family Enterobacteriaceae to cause disease is quite variable, encompassing rarely harmful commensal flora, opportunistic pathogens that can inflict considerable morbidity and mortality on compromised hosts, and principal pathogens capable of initiating illness in individuals in perfect health. This range of pathogenic potential is a reflection of the expression, or lack thereof, of specific virulence factors that play roles in the disease process. The precise definition of a virulence factor is often the subject of vigorous debate. Researchers do not agree as to whether structures or functions that are indispensable for disease but that are not specific to pathogens or to the disease process should be considered virulence factors. However, there is general conceptual agreement on the principle of "molecular Koch's postulates," as articulated by Stanley Falkow.[39] By this definition, a trait is considered to be a virulence factor if it is found specifically in strains of a microbe that cause disease; if mutation of a gene encoding the factor results in less severe infection in a suitable model of the disease; and if restoration of a wild-type allele of the gene to the mutant (genetic complementation, usually achieved by transforming the mutant with a plasmid that contains the gene) results in reinstatement of the original disease severity.

In considering virulence factors, it is useful to contemplate the phases of the infectious cycle implemented by most pathogenic microorganisms. These phases include entry, establishment and multiplication, avoidance of host defense mechanisms, tissue damage, and exit.[40] The following sections review the established and proposed virulence factors common to many members of the enterobacterial family. Specific factors are also considered during the discussions of individual microorganisms.

ADHESINS

Part of the accepted dogma of microbial pathogenesis holds that initial adherence of pathogen to host cells is an absolute prerequisite for disease. Furthermore, adherence is not the result of nonspecific "stickiness," but rather requires particular microbial adhesins that bind selectively and avidly to cognate receptors on host surfaces to overcome the electrostatic repulsion resulting from the net negative charge on both cells. Enterobacterial pathogens may produce a variety of adhesins, including fimbriae and outer membrane proteins. In some cases, surface carbohydrates can also have adhesive properties. The bacteria may simultaneously produce many different adhesins or produce various adhesins in sequence, as a result of random phase variation or in response to environmental cues.

Type 1 fimbriae are ubiquitous among the Enterobacteriaceae. These organelles belong to the chaperone-usher family of pili and are composed of a rigid rod formed by repeating subunits of the FimA (also known as PilA) protein arranged in a tight helical array. The tips of these pili contain a short fiber, which is composed of the FimG and FimH subunits, joined end to end to the FimA rod.[27] FimH, the type 1 fimbrial adhesin, binds to mannose residues found in glycoproteins and glycolipids on host cell surfaces.[41,42] Adhesion via type 1 fimbriae is enhanced under flow conditions, such as may be found in the urinary tract.[43] The expression of type 1 fimbriae is subject to phase variation because of the presence of an invertible DNA element that flanks the promoter for the _fim_ operon encoding the pili.[44] This invertible element allows the orientation of the promoter to oscillate so that it either faces toward or away from the operon, allowing or precluding pilus expression. Thus, bacteria that produce the pili arise at random from populations of bacteria that do not and vice versa. Under conditions in which type 1 pili are useful, bacteria expressing them predominate, whereas under conditions in which type 1 pili are detrimental, selection favors those lacking them. In a murine model of *E. coli* urinary tract infections (UTIs), type 1 pili have been proven to be critical for colonization and disease.[45] Type 1 pili have also been demonstrated to play an important role in transmission of bacteria from neonatal rats that have *E. coli* colonization of the intestine to the oropharynx and subsequently the gastrointestinal tract and blood of littermates.[46,47]

In addition to type 1 fimbriae, individual strains may produce multiple additional chaperone-usher type pili and may produce one or more type IV fimbriae. Together members of the enterobacterial family undoubtedly produce a vast number of distinct fimbrial types. Characterized pili bind to a wide variety of different receptors. Thus, the entire repertoire of adhesive pili and their receptors is extraordinarily extensive. Additional pili that play roles in the pathogenesis of particular strains within the enterobacterial family are discussed in sections devoted to these bacteria.

Pili are not the only adhesins produced by bacteria. A variety of outer membrane proteins also serve as adhesins. Among the best characterized of these is the invasin-intimin family of proteins. These proteins share a common structure and have detectable amino acid sequence similarities, especially in their amino-terminal and central domains. They are inserted into the outer membrane via their amino termini, which are predicted to form the β-barrel structure typical of outer membrane proteins. The membrane portion of these molecules is connected via a flexible hinge region to a rigid rod composed of repeating units, each similar in structure to portions of immunoglobulin molecules. The carboxyl-terminal adhesin domain bears similarities to calcium-binding lectin molecules.[48-50] In the case of the invasin molecule of *Y. pseudotuberculosis,* this portion of the molecule binds to β-integrins in the host cell membrane with an affinity more than 100-fold greater than does their natural ligand fibronectin.[51] In the case of intimin from enteropathogenic strains of *E. coli,* the primary receptor is a protein produced by the bacteria and injected into the host cell membrane.[52]

SECRETION SYSTEMS AND TOXINS

Toxins were the first and arguably remain the best studied virulence factors. Toxins are released by bacteria into the environment or directed to host cells. Toxins have physiologically relevant activity when administered in purified form into animals or applied to tissue culture cells. However, many enterobacterial toxins do not fully reproduce the disease in the absence of the bacteria that produce them. Thus, toxins often play ancillary or unknown roles in pathogenesis. Toxins are numerous and may be categorized in various schemes, such as by function, target, activity, and structural similarity.

The inner and outer membranes of gram-negative bacteria together pose a formidable barrier against the diffusion of macromolecules. Thus, many toxins require specific secretion machineries for their export.[53] The simplest of these export strategies is exemplified by the autotransported proteases produced by many gram-negative species.[54] These proteins are produced with typical signal sequences at their amino termini, which are cleaved as the proteins are exported across the inner membrane by the general secretion machinery. The proteins are then inserted into the outer membrane via the β-barrel structure of their mature amino termini. The so-called passenger domain at the carboxyl terminus, which possesses the enzymatic activity, may then be cleaved off and released into the media via either its own protease activity or that of other bacterial proteases. A subset of these proteins has been termed the SPATE family (serine protease autotransporters of the Enterobacteriaceae). Several SPATE family members have been characterized from various pathotypes of *E. coli* and *Shigella.* These proteins include several toxins categorized as having cytopathic effects and toxins that elicit fluid secretion from intestinal epithelia.[55] The

precise roles of these proteins in disease and the relevant host cell targets are largely unknown.

Many members of the family Enterobacteriaceae produce toxins capable of inducing lysis of host cells. Strains that produce these factors often induce zones of clearing on blood agar plates, so the toxins are often termed *hemolysins.* One of the best studied hemolysins is that of *E. coli.* This protein is secreted in a single step across both inner and outer membranes by a three-protein apparatus known as a type I secretion system. The type I secretion system is composed of an integral inner membrane adenosine triphosphatase (HlyD) and another integral inner membrane protein (HlyB), both of which are able to recognize a carboxyl-terminal secretion signal and bind the hemolysin protein. The HlyD-HlyB-hemolysin complex is then able to engage a remarkable tunnel-channel protein called TolC, which spans the periplasmic space and outer membrane, opens up to allow passage of hemolysin through the outer membrane, and then disengages from the HlyD-HlyB complex.[56,57] TolC interacts with different substrate-specific inner membrane proteins to serve the same function for a variety of other substrates, including other toxins such as *E. coli* heat-stable enterotoxin,[58] and antibiotics. The precise mechanism by which hemolysin induces cell lysis is still under investigation. It is clear that hemolysin inserts into host cell membranes, but it is not clear whether it forms a transmembrane channel that leads to osmotic lysis or it inserts only into the outer leaflet of the host cell membrane and induces lysis by another mechanism.[59] Furthermore, low concentrations of hemolysin, which may be relevant in vivo, lead to oscillations in intracellular calcium concentrations and signaling through nuclear factor kappa B.[60] Hemolysin is found in a higher proportion of extraintestinal pathogenic *E. coli* than in fecal strains or strains associated with diarrhea and seems to contribute to submucosal hemorrhage and epithelial cell destruction early in the course of experimental UTI.[61]

E. coli; most, if not all, members of the enterobacterial family; and many other gram-negative organisms contain an additional secretion machine known as the main terminal branch of the general secretory pathway or the type II secretion system (T2SS).[62] A variety of enzymes, including some toxins, are exported first by the general secretion system to the periplasmic space and then by the T2SS to the external environment. For example, the *E. coli* chromosome encodes a T2SS that secretes chitinase, whereas the O157:H7 clone of enterohemorrhagic *E. coli* expresses an additional, plasmid-encoded T2SS that secretes a metalloprotease capable of degrading C1 esterase inhibitor.[63] T2SSs are composed of approximately 12 proteins, including an outer membrane gated channel and several inner membrane proteins. It is proposed that these proteins are the components of a piston-like machine that exports the proteins across the outer membrane. T2SSs are related to systems required for the biogenesis of type IV pili and filamentous bacteriophages.

Many gram-negative organisms that interact directly with eukaryotic cells, including several important enterobacterial pathogens, have a type III secretion system (T3SS) that not only exports proteins through the inner and outer bacterial membranes but also injects them into or through the host cell membrane.[64,65] More than 20 proteins make up this remarkably complex secretion machine, which resembles both morphologically and evolutionarily the apparatus responsible for assembly of flagella. The T3SS apparatus has been likened to a molecular syringe that spans both inner and outer membranes, with a needle that extends from the outer membrane toward the host cell. Specific "translocator" proteins secreted through this needle are thought to form a pore in the host cell membrane through which other secreted "effector" proteins pass. Translocation of effector proteins requires direct contact between the bacterium and the host cell. A wide variety of such effector proteins exists, many of which subvert host cell pathways through structural mimicry to serve diverse functions for the bacterium.[66] Among these effector proteins are bacterial adhesin receptors, protein tyrosine phosphatases, serine kinases, and proteins that either activate the guanosine triphosphatase activity or catalyze the exchange of guanosine triphosphate for guanosine diphosphate in small regulatory G proteins. These effector proteins may be considered a newly discovered class of toxins, which are delivered by pathogens directly to target cells.

IRON ACQUISITION

Iron is an essential element, required by virtually all organisms as a cofactor for several indispensable enzymes. Microorganisms that colonize the surfaces or invade the tissues of mammals must compete with their hosts to acquire free iron, which the host maintains at extremely low concentrations ($\sim 10^{-24}$ M) through the use of iron-binding proteins such as transferrin and lactoferrin. Thus, enterobacterial pathogens have developed several highly efficient systems that scavenge iron. These systems are under the control of a ubiquitous regulator protein called Fur, which activates gene transcription at low iron concentrations.[67] Many members of the family Enterobacteriaceae produce a chromosomally encoded siderophore known as enterobactin.[68] Siderophores are low-molecular-weight iron-chelating molecules that are synthesized, secreted, and recaptured by microorganisms. Humans appear to have countered enterobactin by producing a protein that has even higher affinity for the siderophore than does the bacterial enterobactin outer membrane receptor protein. Thus, enterobacterial species produce other siderophores in addition to enterobactin. For example, many strains of *E. coli* isolated from extraintestinal infections produce a plasmid-encoded siderophore called aerobactin.[69,70] Some strains are also able to bind and transport heme. Common to all these iron uptake systems and to systems for the transport of nutrients such as vitamin B_{12} is a cytoplasmic membrane protein called TonB.[71] TonB spans the periplasm and contacts siderophore receptors and other gated porins in the outer membrane to allow them to open upon ligand binding.[72] Thus TonB is a point of convergence in enterobacterial iron uptake pathways and a potential drug target. The role of iron-scavenging systems in enterobacterial virulence is well established. Early studies showed that the minimum lethal dose of *E. coli* is reduced substantially when iron is delivered by vein along with the inoculum. More recently, molecular Koch's postulates were fulfilled for TonB, and evidence implicating the importance of aerobactin and heme uptake was provided using a murine model of ascending *E. coli* UTI.[71]

LIPOPOLYSACCHARIDE AND CAPSULES

Lipopolysaccharide is an essential component of the outer membrane of all gram-negative bacteria. Therefore, some would argue that LPS is not a true virulence factor. However, LPS molecules from different organisms have different chemical compositions and different biologic activities and potency, and, therefore, the effects of LPS on the host differ depending on its source and chemical composition.[73] Moreover, the highly variable O-antigen component of LPS has biologic properties that may influence virulence as well. Thus, it is appropriate to consider LPS in any discussion of the virulence of gram-negative organisms.

The extraordinary potency of enterobacterial LPS as an inducer of the innate immune response is due to signaling through Toll-like receptor 4.[74] LPS, often in complex with LPS binding protein, binds to CD14, a glycerophosphatidylinositol-linked nontransmembrane receptor. This complex interacts with Toll-like receptor 4 and MD2, which through MyD88 and other intermediates activates nuclear factor kappa B to initiate transcription of a variety of proinflammatory mediators, including cytokines such as tumor necrosis factor, chemokines, and major histocompatibility complex receptors. The host response to LPS through Toll-like receptor 4 is a key factor in determining outcome to infections with gram-negative bacteria. Mice deficient in Toll-like receptor 4 are highly susceptible to bacteremia with enterobacterial organisms and fail to recruit neutrophils to clear *E. coli* UTIs.[75,76] Furthermore, there appears to be an association between Toll-like receptor 4 polymorphisms and susceptibility to severe gram-negative infections in humans.[77,78]

In addition to the important biologic effects of lipid A, the highly variable O antigen of LPS is also important for pathogenesis and immunity to enterobacterial infections. For example, some *E. coli* mutants lacking the ability to synthesize O antigen are highly sensitive to serum.[79] There also appears to be a relationship between the presence of antibodies against LPS and against specific O antigens and susceptibility to disease with several enterobacterial pathogens.[80-83] However, these studies are not able to distinguish whether the anti-LPS antibodies are themselves protective or merely a marker for protective responses.

Capsules are common among members of the family Enterobacteriaceae. Some capsules appear to endow the bacteria with the ability to avoid phagocytosis and to avoid killing by human serum.[84-86] In some cases, animal models have suggested a role of capsule in the pathogenesis of particular infections. For example, the K1 capsule produced by many *E. coli* strains isolated from patients with neonatal sepsis and meningitis has been implicated in bacterial survival while passing through the blood-brain barrier.[87] The K2 and K15 capsules of *E. coli* and the capsule of *Klebsiella pneumoniae* are important for colonization of the urinary tract,[88-90] and the K54 capsule of *E. coli* is important for systemic infections.[91]

PLASMIDS

Plasmids, extrachromosomal autonomously replicating DNA elements, are not virulence factors per se. However, the genes encoded on plasmids may play major roles in pathogenesis. As examples, the entire T3SS that endows enteroinvasive *E. coli* and *Shigella* strains with the ability to invade epithelial cells is encoded on similar large plasmids,[92] the type IV pilus of enteropathogenic *E. coli* strains is encoded on a large plasmid that is required for full virulence,[93,94] and the large plasmids of enterohemorrhagic *E. coli* strains encode a T2SS, a protease, and a hemolysin that are potential virulence factors.[63,95,96] In addition, plasmids may be self-transmissible, encoding elaborate systems specifying the production of pili for DNA transfer.[38] Many of these plasmids are very promiscuous with regard to their ability to transfer between disparate genera. The emergence and dissemination of broad host range R plasmids containing antimicrobial resistance genes have been major factors in the global spread of bacteria resistant to multiple antibiotics. These resistance genes may be present on transposons, allowing them to jump to other plasmids or chromosomes, or they may be found on integrons, which have loci downstream of strong promoters at which resistance genes may insert by site-specific recombination to be expressed at high levels. Such mobile genetic elements are important factors contributing to the rapid evolution of highly antibiotic-resistant isolates and subsequent dissemination within the enterobacterial family.[97]

The Specific Pathogens

ESCHERICHIA

E. coli is the type species of the genus *Escherichia*, which in turn is the type genus of the family Enterobacteriaceae. The genus is named for Theodore Escherich, who performed pioneering studies on the fecal flora of neonates and described the organism in 1885.[98] *E. coli* is both the most common species of facultative anaerobe found in the human gastrointestinal tract and the most commonly encountered pathogen from the enterobacterial family. An enormous amount of information is available regarding the genetics, structure, and physiology of this organism, and an effort is under way to fully characterize the biochemistry and cell biology of the nonpathogenic K-12 strain of this species (http://ecocyc.org/). *E. coli* is usually distinguished from other members of the family by the ability of most strains to ferment lactose and other sugars and to produce indole from tryptophan. In addition, most strains are motile.

Although most strains of *E. coli* reside harmlessly in the lumen of the colon and seem to be poorly adapted to cause disease in healthy individuals, there exists a plethora of pathotypes that can cause specific types of illness in both normal hosts and those with compromised nonspecific defense mechanisms (Table 218-2). *E. coli* exhibits tremendous versatility in its ability to cause disease and the mechanisms by which it does so. Pathogenic strains differ from commensal organisms in that they produce virulence factors specific for each pathotype, which may be encoded by bacteriophages, on plasmids, or on stretches of the chromosome known as pathogenicity islands. Comparisons among the fully sequenced genomes of nonpathogenic and pathogenic strains have revealed an average genome size of approximately 5000 genes, but only approximately 2200 of these are shared among all *E. coli* strains. Most of the pathogens have larger genomes than do the nonpathogenic strains.[26,99] Furthermore, many of the genes that are not found in the nonpathogenic strain are specific to particular strains or pathotypes. It is estimated that the total "pangenome" of *E. coli* consists of more than 13,000 genes.[99]

Despite the vast repertoire of virulence factors that may be produced by various pathotypes, there are some common features of pathogenic *E. coli* strains. These include fimbrial adhesins, secretion systems to export proteins involved in pathogenesis, and toxins.

Extraintestinal Pathogenic E. coli

E. coli is the most common cause of UTIs, is a leading cause of neonatal meningitis, and can cause a wide variety of other extraintestinal infections, such as nosocomial pneumonia, cholecystitis and cholangitis, peritonitis, cellulitis, osteomyelitis, and infectious arthritis. It has been appreciated for some time that strains of *E. coli* isolated from the urine or blood of patients with UTIs differ from those cultured from the feces of healthy individuals and from those that cause diarrhea.[100,101]

Thus, the term *uropathogenic E. coli* was coined to refer to such strains. Furthermore, reports of community outbreaks and geographically widespread clones causing UTI lend credence to the notion that some strains are particularly capable of causing these infections.[102-108] Uropathogenic *E. coli* strains are more likely than fecal strains to produce P fimbriae, which bind to glycolipid receptors on the surface of host cells, to be encapsulated, to produce the cytolytic toxin hemolysin, and to have multiple systems for the acquisition of iron. Similarly, strains isolated from patients with neonatal meningitis are more likely than fecal strains to produce the K1 capsule and to produce S fimbriae.[109] However, many of these same factors are found in strains isolated from a wide variety of extraintestinal infections.[110] Furthermore, strains representing a clonal group that commonly causes neonatal meningitis are also frequently isolated from UTIs.[102] Therefore, the term *extraintestinal pathogenic E. coli* (ExPEC) was coined to describe strains that have the potential to cause a number of infections outside the gut.[111] Nevertheless, there is evidence to suggest that some strains are more likely to cause meningitis than urosepsis in neonates and vice versa.[112] It should also be noted that *E. coli* strains isolated from individuals with compromised defenses against infection are less likely to resemble ExPEC and more likely to resemble strains isolated from the fecal flora. This observation holds both for strains that cause UTI in patients with abnormal urinary tracts (e.g., those with stones, disorders of bladder function, anatomic abnormalities, and foreign bodies)[113-115] and for infections elsewhere (e.g., cholangitis in patients with biliary tract obstruction).[116]

Efforts to elucidate the molecular pathogenesis of *E. coli* UTI have begun to bear fruit. A murine model of ascending infection has been useful because it distinguishes between ExPEC strains and control

TABLE 218-2	Summary of Epidemiology, Clinical Features, Pathogenesis, Diagnosis, and Therapy of *Escherichia coli* Pathotypes That Cause Diarrhea				
Pathotype	**Epidemiology**	**Clinical Features**	**Pathogenesis**	**Diagnosis**	**Adjunctive Therapy***
ETEC	Contaminated water and food. Major cause of childhood diarrhea in developing countries; leading cause of travelers' diarrhea	Acute watery diarrhea, occasionally severe	Large number of fimbrial adhesins; heat-stable and heat-labile enterotoxins	PCR or DNA probes for enterotoxins	Loperamide (may be combined with fluoroquinolones), azithromycin, or rifaximin for travelers
EPEC	Person-to-person transmission. Leading cause of infantile diarrhea in developing countries	Severe acute diarrhea and vomiting, may be persistent	Localized adherence via bundle-forming pilus; attaching and effacing via intimin-Tir	PCR or DNA probes for *bfp*† or *eae* genes or tissue culture assay for localized adherence†	Antibiotics guided by susceptibility testing for severe or protracted cases
EHEC and other STEC	Food, water, and person-to-person spread. Major cause of bloody diarrhea in developed countries	Watery and bloody diarrhea, may be complicated by hemolytic uremic syndrome	Shiga toxins; intimin-Tir–mediated attaching and effacing in EHEC strains	Sorbitol-MacConkey agar,‡ immunoassay for Shiga toxin, PCR or DNA probes for *stx* genes	Supportive care. Antibiotics and antimotility agents contraindicated
EAEC	Mode of transmission unknown. Important cause of chronic diarrhea in developing countries; emerging cause of acute, chronic, and travelers' diarrhea	Mucoid diarrhea, often persistent	Aggregative adherence via several fimbriae; Pet and other toxins	Tissue culture assay for aggregative adherence or PCR for *aggR* gene	Fluoroquinolones may be of benefit for travelers and HIV patients
EIEC	Contaminated food. Outbreaks in developed countries	Watery diarrhea or dysentery	Cellular invasion, intracellular motility, and cell-to-cell spread	PCR or DNA probes for *inv* genes	Unknown
DAEC	Mode of transmission unknown. Diarrhea in older children in developing countries	Poorly described	Unknown	Tissue culture assay for diffuse adherence	

DAEC, diffuse adhering *E. coli*; EAEC, enteroaggregative *E. coli*; EHEC, enterohemorrhagic *E. coli*; EIEC, enteroinvasive *E. coli*; EPEC, enteropathogenic *E. coli*; ETEC, enterotoxigenic *E. coli*; HIV, human immunodeficiency virus; PCR, polymerase chain reaction; Pet, plasma-encoded enterotoxin; STEC, Shiga toxin–producing *E. coli*; Tir, translocated intimin receptor.

*The cornerstone of therapy for all diarrheal disease is rehydration, preferably via the oral route.

†Detects typical strains only.

‡Detects O157:H7 strains only.

strains from the feces of healthy volunteers and, among ExPEC strains, between strains isolated from patients with cystitis and those from patients with pyelonephritis.[117-119] A primate model has also been extremely valuable, but at considerable cost.[120,121] Using these models, it has been firmly established that type 1 fimbriae are essential virulence determinants in *E. coli* UTI.[45,120] Type 1 fimbriae appear to be especially important in colonization of the bladder,[122] where potential mannose-containing receptors include uroplakin.[123] Apparent binding of *E. coli* to uroplakin in superficial bladder epithelial cells via type 1 pili has been observed by electron microscopy, and this binding appears to lead to exfoliation of the cells and invasion of deeper cell layers.[124] As mentioned earlier, the expression of type 1 pili is subject to phase variation under the control of an invertible DNA element that includes the promoter for the operon.[44] Thus, *E. coli* can produce the pili when it is most advantageous to do so, such as early in the course of UTI, and not when it may be detrimental to the bacteria.[125,126] Despite the importance of type 1 pili in the pathogenesis of UTI, the ability to express these fimbriae does not explain the relative virulence of ExPEC strains because essentially all *E. coli* and other members of the enterobacterial family are able to do so. Among other potential adhesins relevant to the pathogenesis of UTI, P fimbriae stand out as being particularly associated with ExPEC strains, especially those isolated from patients with pyelonephritis.[100,101] These chaperone-usher pili bind to glycosphingolipids containing the disaccharide galactose(α1-4)galactose, which are found on the surface of epithelial cells in the human kidney.[127,128] A role for P fimbriae in the pathogenesis of UTI has been substantiated by the fact that a strain with a mutation in *papG*, the gene encoding the P fimbrial tip adhesin, colonized the kidney of cynomolgus monkeys for a shorter period and did less damage than did the wild-type strain from which it was derived.[129] However, molecular Koch's postulates remain unfulfilled for P fimbriae because complementation studies were not performed. In addition to type 1 and P fimbriae, ExPEC may express many other types of pilus and nonpilus adhesins.[26,130-132] The roles played by these factors in the establishment of *E. coli* UTI have not been sufficiently studied. In addition to adhesion, other attributes that have been implicated in the pathogenesis of *E. coli* UTI include the production of the toxins hemolysin[61] and cytotoxic necrotizing factor (discussed later)[133]; the ability to sequester iron[71]; the production of O antigen, capsule, and other extracellular polysaccharides[88,134,135]; and the expression of regulatory genes.[136,137] Further details on clinical aspects of *E. coli* UTI can be found elsewhere (see Chapter 69).

E. coli is one of the leading causes of neonatal bacteremia, sepsis, and meningitis, historically second only to *Streptococcus agalactiae* in this regard. However, with improved strategies to prevent infections caused by the latter species, its relative importance has increased. Studies of newborns with *E. coli* bacteremia and experiments in neonatal rats have shown that meningitis is much more likely when the level of *E. coli* bacteremia exceeds 10^3 colony-forming units/mL of blood.[138] The *E. coli* strains that cause neonatal meningitis frequently express the K1 capsule, which may facilitate this high level of bacteremia. Although this polysialic acid capsule, indistinguishable from that of *Neisseria meningitidis* group B strains, is one of the most common types produced by *E. coli*, it is expressed by a disproportionate percentage of neonatal meningitis isolates.[109,139] In addition to its role in serum resistance, it appears that K1 capsule facilitates survival of the bacteria as they traverse the blood-brain barrier.[87] Many strains isolated from neonates with sepsis or meningitis express S fimbriae, members of the chaperone-usher fimbrial family that bind to oligosaccharides containing sialic acid, which can be found on brain endothelial cells and human kidney cells.[140-142] P fimbrial expression is also common among these strains.[109] Strains isolated from neonatal sepsis and meningitis frequently express toxins such as hemolysin, cytotoxic necrotizing factor, and cytolethal distending toxin.[109,143] Cytotoxic necrotizing factor, which is found almost exclusively in strains that produce hemolysin and is frequently encoded adjacent to the hemolysin operon,[144,145] affects the host cell cytoskeleton by deamidating members of the Rho family of small guanosine triphosphatases, which regulate actin fila-

ment formation.[146] Mutants with disruptions in the *cnf* gene are less able to invade human brain endothelial cells in vitro and less able to enter the cerebrospinal fluid in vivo. This ability to invade human brain endothelial cells has been exploited to identify other genes that may play a role in traversal of the blood-brain barrier.[147,148] Among *E. coli* strains that cause neonatal meningitis, the serotype O18:K1:H7 is particularly common, and strains belonging to this clone have been used as prototypes in research. Interestingly, strains of the same serotype are often found in cases of cystitis and belong to the same clone, a finding that supports the concept that ExPEC may cause different types of infections.[149]

Very little is known about the pathogenesis of extraintestinal *E. coli* infections other than UTI and neonatal meningitis.

Enterotoxigenic *E. coli*

E. coli can cause diarrhea by no less than six different mechanisms, each displayed by a pathotype with characteristic virulence determinants that contribute to its pathogenic mechanisms.[150] Five of these pathotypes, for which at least some information on pathogenic mechanisms is available, are included in the discussion in this chapter. The first pathotype of diarrheogenic *E. coli* for which the broad outlines of pathogenesis were elucidated was enterotoxigenic *E. coli* (ETEC).

ETEC strains are a common and important cause of childhood diarrhea throughout the developing world and a leading cause of diarrhea in travelers who visit these countries.[150,151] Outbreaks may also occur in developed countries.[152] ETEC infections are acquired through ingestion of heavily contaminated water or food and thus result from a failure of sanitation. Infections caused by ETEC range from asymptomatic carriage to severe cholera-like illness. The predominant symptom is watery diarrhea, which may be accompanied by nausea and cramps. Vomiting, severe cramps, and fever are not prominent, and the stool does not contain blood, mucus, or fecal leukocytes. The incubation period ranges from a few hours to 2 days, and symptoms usually last less than 5 days.

The pathogenesis of ETEC infection as it is currently understood involves mucosal adherence and toxin-mediated fluid secretion. The genes encoding the toxins and many of the genes encoding the adhesins are found on plasmids. However, recent research has focused on chromosomal loci that may be involved in adherence and toxin secretion.[153-156]

For historical reasons, the pili of ETEC are known as colonization factor antigens (e.g., CFAI, CFAIII) or coli surface antigens (e.g., CS3, CS6). These appendages include classic chaperone-usher type pili; thinner, more wiry chaperone-usher type fibrillae; and type IV pili. Some strains express afimbrial factors that are not associated with detectable organelles. More than 20 of these pilus-related factors have been described.[157] Strains of ETEC that produce several such factors at a time and strains that produce none of the known factors are common.[158] The ETEC colonization factors are presumed to mediate attachment to the small intestinal mucosa. Experiments involving strains of ETEC that naturally infect animals have demonstrated that expression of these pili is required for colonization and signs of disease. In adult volunteer experiments, immunity against ETEC disease can be demonstrated upon rechallenge with the same strain, but not with a heterologous strain.[159] The diversity of colonization factors that may be expressed by ETEC strains is thought to be a major factor that allows children in developing countries to have multiple bouts of ETEC diarrhea. According to this theory, adults in developing countries are protected from illness after repeated exposure to multiple ETEC strains during their lifetime, whereas travelers to such countries are susceptible. Recently, a secreted protein, EtpA, produced by many but not all ETEC strains, was demonstrated to be important for colonization in a murine model, to bind to the tips of flagellae, and to promote adherence to intestinal cells.[160,161]

ETEC strains may express either or both of two enterotoxins, known as heat-labile enterotoxin and heat-stable enterotoxin, that are responsible for the secretory diarrhea seen in symptomatic patients. Heat-labile enterotoxin is closely related to cholera toxin, has an almost identical quaternary structure,[162] and has an identical mechanism of action. Like cholera toxin, heat-labile enterotoxin is composed of a single catalytic A subunit and a pentamer of identical receptor-binding B subunits, which are secreted as the holotoxin via a T2SS.[156] The B subunits bind to the glycolipid asialo-GM$_1$ in the apical membrane of enterocytes. After endocytosis and passage through the Golgi apparatus, the A subunit makes its way to its target in the basolateral membrane, the regulatory subunit of a heterotrimeric G protein, Gα_S. The A subunit is an adenosine diphosphate ribosyltransferase that cleaves nicotinamide adenine dinucleotide and covalently attaches adenosine diphosphate-ribose to Gα_S, thereby locking the protein in its active form so that it, in turn, constitutively activates its target, adenylyl cyclase. The elevated levels of cyclic adenosine monophosphate that ensue lead to activation of protein kinase A, which phosphorylates and activates the cystic fibrosis transmembrane conductance regulator. Thus, a complex cascade leads to active secretion of chloride and, when sodium and water passively follow, copious fluid secretion into the small intestinal lumen. Heat-stable enterotoxin is a very different molecule than heat-labile enterotoxin. Heat-stable enterotoxin is a small peptide that contains six cysteine residues involved in three intramolecular disulfide bonds. It resembles a mammalian peptide hormone, guanylin, and binds to the guanylin receptor, a guanosine triphosphatase found in the apical membrane.[163] The resulting elevated cyclic guanosine monophosphate levels lead to activation of protein kinase G, phosphorylation of cystic fibrosis transmembrane conductance regulator, and chloride secretion.[164]

The diagnosis of ETEC infection is not usually confirmed because it rests on detection of the genes encoding heat-labile enterotoxin and heat-stable enterotoxin by PCR or DNA probes or on assays for the biologic activity of these toxins.

Travelers to endemic areas can reduce the risk of ETEC infection by strict adherence to advice regarding the ingestion of safe food and water.[151] Those wishing to avoid travelers' diarrhea should drink only bottled beverages, avoid ice, eschew meat and vegetables that are not served steaming hot, and shun fruit that they do not peel themselves. Dry packaged or canned foods carry no risk. The prophylactic use of bismuth subsalicylate tablets can also reduce the risk of travelers' diarrhea, but conveys some inconvenience.[165] The development of a safe and effective ETEC vaccine has been the goal of numerous laboratories for many years, but is hampered by the heterogeneity of antigenic determinants required for protective immunity.

Treatment of all diarrheal disease rests first and foremost on providing adequate fluid replacement via the oral or, if necessary, parenteral route. Further information on treatment of ETEC infections can be inferred from trials enrolling patients with travelers' diarrhea, much of which is caused by ETEC. Prompt therapy with an antimotility agent such as loperamide can reduce symptoms. Combination therapy with a fluoroquinolone and loperamide seems to provide the most rapid response.[166] Alternatives to fluoroquinolones include azithromycin and rifaximin.[167,168] These medications can be provided to travelers for use should diarrhea develop during a trip to an endemic country.

Enteropathogenic E. coli

Enteropathogenic *E. coli* (EPEC) strains are defined by the characteristic attaching and effacing effect that they elicit on interaction with epithelial cells (Fig. 218-3) and by the fact that they do not produce Shiga toxins.[169] Typical EPEC strains carry a large EPEC adherence factor plasmid that encodes bundle-forming pili (BFP)[93] and the ability to form microcolonies on tissue culture cells, a pattern called localized adherence (Fig. 218-4A).[170,171] EPEC strains were first identified as the cause of devastating outbreaks of nosocomial and community-acquired neonatal diarrhea in the 1940s,[172] but such outbreaks are now rare in the developed world. However, EPEC remains a leading cause of severe diarrhea among infants in developing countries.[173-178] Furthermore, atypical EPEC strains lacking BFP are emerging as an important cause of diarrhea among children in developed countries.[179-181] EPEC infections appear to be acquired principally by person-to-person spread and hospitals continue to be a source of

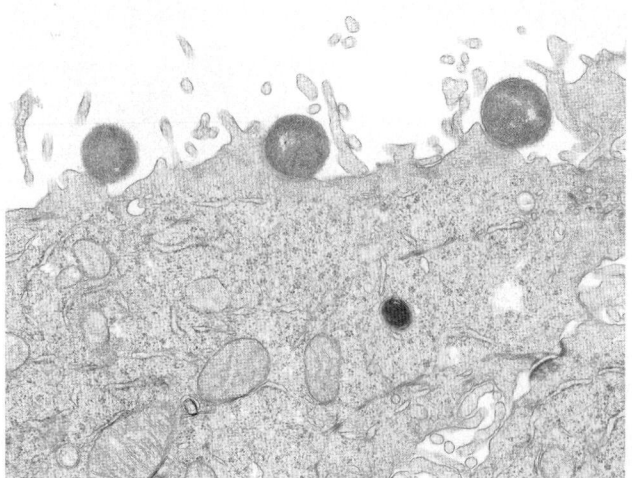

Figure 218-3 Transmission electron micrograph of enteropathogenic *Escherichia coli* infecting a tissue culture cell demonstrating the attaching and effacing effect. Note the loss of microvilli, the intimate attachment of bacteria to the cell, and the cuplike pedestal composed of cytoskeletal proteins to which the bacteria are attached. Attaching and effacing effects are also seen with enterohemorrhagic *E. coli* strains and *Escherichia albertii* strains.

infection.[182-184] Infections caused by EPEC are difficult to differentiate from those with other causes; symptoms include watery diarrhea sometimes accompanied by low-grade fever and vomiting.[185] However, EPEC infection may be severe, vomiting may make oral rehydration difficult, and life-threatening dehydration may ensue.[174,186,187] Furthermore, disease caused by EPEC may be protracted, resulting in weight loss, malnutrition, and death.[188]

The histopathologic hallmark of EPEC infection, the attaching and effacing effect, involves the intimate attachment of the bacteria to the apical surface of intestinal epithelial cells accompanied by the loss (effacement) of microvilli and the formation of a cuplike pedestal composed of actin and other cytoskeletal proteins upon which the bacteria rest.[189,190] The attaching and effacing effect is directed by a 41-gene pathogenicity island known as the locus of enterocyte effacement that encodes a T3SS (see "Secretion Systems and Toxins"), the outer membrane adhesin intimin, the translocated intimin receptor, regulators, and effector proteins.[191-193] Additional effectors translocated into host cells by the T3SS are encoded outside the locus of enterocyte effacement.[194] The EPEC T3SS has an unusual translocation protein known as EspA that forms a filamentous extension of the needle and connects the bacteria to the host cells.[195] Translocated intimin receptor is believed to transit a central canal in the EspA filament, pass through a putative pore in the host cell membrane formed by the EspB and EspD proteins, and then insert in the host cell membrane, where it serves as the receptor for intimin.[52] EspB has been proven in volunteers to be required for virulence.[196] Intimin, another proven EPEC virulence factor,[197] protrudes from the surface of the bacteria and binds to translocated intimin receptor in a ratio of two intimin molecules to one translocated intimin receptor dimer.[49] When EPEC translocated intimin receptor binds intimin, it becomes phosphorylated by host tyrosine kinases, and then a cascade of events leads to the activation of the N-WASP and Arp2/3 actin-nucleating and filament formation machinery and pedestal formation.[198-200] Thus, EPEC carries around its own receptor, injects it into host cells, binds to it, and uses it to modify host cell architecture.

Typical EPEC strains, which possess an EPEC adherence factor plasmid that encodes BFP, may be more pathogenic than atypical EPEC strains.[201,202] Both the EPEC adherence factor plasmid and BFP have been demonstrated to be virulence factors.[94,203] Because BFP aggregate into ropelike bundles (see Fig. 218-2C) and expression of BFP is associated with reversible autoaggregation of the bacteria in

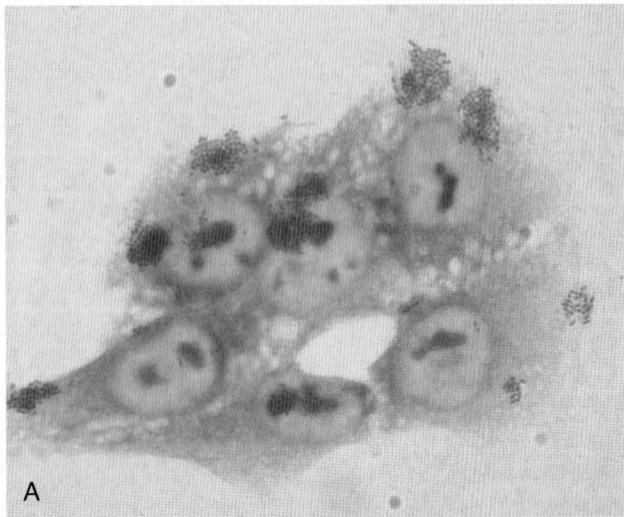

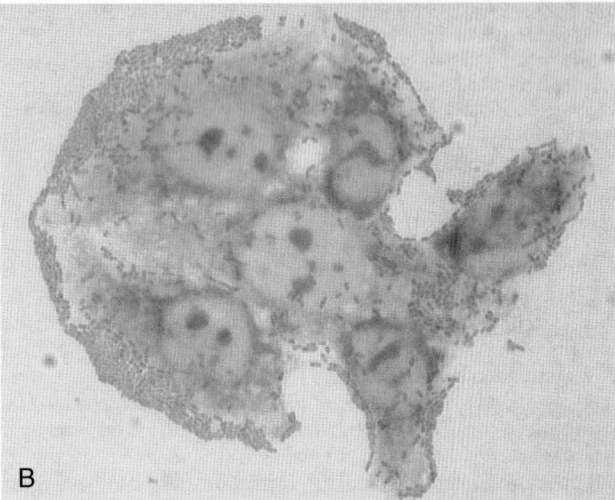

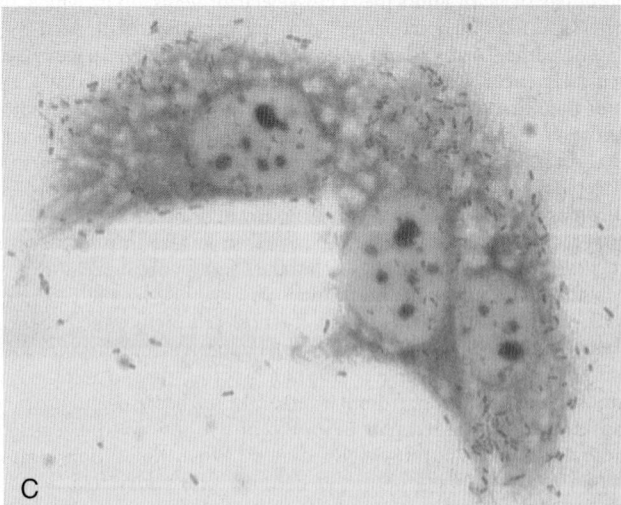

Figure 218-4 **Patterns of cellular adherence displayed by various** *Escherichia coli* **pathotypes that cause diarrhea. A,** The localized adherence pattern exhibited by typical strains of enteropathogenic *E. coli* is characterized by discrete three-dimensional microcolonies of bacteria. **B,** The aggregative adherence pattern exhibited by enteroaggregative *E. coli* strains is characterized by two-dimensional "stacked brick" aggregates associated with both host cells and the glass or plastic substratum. **C,** Diffuse adherent *E. coli* strains adhere individually at random to tissue culture cells.

culture and localized adherence, BFPs are believed to mediate the initial adherence to and subsequent dispersal of bacteria from the intestinal surface. Additionally, some BFP also bind to host cell glycoconjugates containing *N*-acetyllactosamine.[204] The relative importance of BFP, EspA, and intimin in binding to the intestinal epithelium is a matter of some debate, but a triple-mutant strain unable to express any of these three adhesins does not adhere in detectable numbers to cells.[205]

The mechanism by which EPEC strains cause diarrhea is not fully understood. In fact, there is evidence that several factors may be involved, including loss of microvillous surface area, loosening of tight junctions, and direct fluid secretion.

The diagnosis of EPEC infection rests on detection of the genes encoding specific virulence factors using DNA probes or PCR with targets such as the *eae* gene that encodes intimin, the *bfpA* gene that encodes the structural subunit of BFP, and the *stx* genes that encode Shiga toxins (which are absent in EPEC strains).[206] Alternatively, tissue culture assays for the localized adherence pattern are highly specific for EPEC but do not detect atypical strains.

It was appreciated from the 1940s that breast-feeding is highly protective against EPEC infection, and more recent studies confirm this finding.[184,207-209] Breast milk contains factors found in both the lipid and the immunoglobulin fractions that inhibit EPEC adherence, including in women from endemic areas antibodies against intimin, BFP, EspA, and EspB.[210-214] There is at present no vaccine to prevent EPEC. Treatment of EPEC infection rests first on fluid replacement, which may require parenteral routes of administration in children who have profuse vomiting. Mild EPEC illness does not require antimicrobial therapy, but antibiotics can shorten the duration of illness in those with more severe disease.[215,216] Unfortunately, strains of EPEC are often resistant to multiple antibiotics.[217-219]

Enterohemorrhagic E. coli and Other Shiga Toxin–Producing E. coli Strains

Shiga toxins (also called verotoxins) are related bacteriophage-encoded cytotoxins that block protein synthesis and induce host cell death. Strains that produce Shiga toxins can cause disease of varying severity, including watery diarrhea, bloody diarrhea, hemorrhagic colitis, hemolytic-uremic syndrome (HUS), and death.[220] Among Shiga toxin–producing *E. coli* (STEC) strains, those that share with EPEC strains the ability to induce the attaching and effacing effect encoded by the locus of enterocyte effacement pathogenicity island are known as enterohemorrhagic *E. coli* (EHEC) (Fig. 218-5). EHEC strains, especially those belonging to serotype O157:H7, have been responsible for larger outbreaks of infection, have higher rates of complications, and seem to be more pathogenic than non-EHEC STEC strains. The reservoir of EHEC strains is the gastrointestinal tract of young cattle and other large herbivorous mammals, but these strains can survive for long periods in the environment even at very low pH and can proliferate in vegetables and other foods and beverages. Outbreaks are often linked to the consumption of undercooked ground beef or from produce, but can arise from a wide variety of other food sources, drinking and recreational water, or petting zoos and by direct person-to-person contact.[221-225] The low infectious dose of EHEC strains, estimated to be fewer than 100 organisms,[226] no doubt facilitates the transmission of the organism. EHEC infections are manifest by the onset of severe abdominal cramping, which may progress to watery and bloody diarrhea. The frequent absence of fever and the appearance of frank hematochezia can divert the clinician toward considering noninfectious diagnoses such as intussusception in children, inflammatory bowel disease in young adults, and ischemic bowel in the elderly.[227] EHEC infection is the primary cause of HUS and the leading cause of renal insufficiency in children, which may occur in 5% to 10% of individuals during EHEC outbreaks and is often heralded by high leukocytosis. Children younger than the age of 5 and the elderly are more likely than those between the age extremes to develop HUS. HUS is a microangiopathic hemolytic anemia marked by the appearance of schistocytes, thrombocytopenia, and azotemia. Although the kidneys are the most

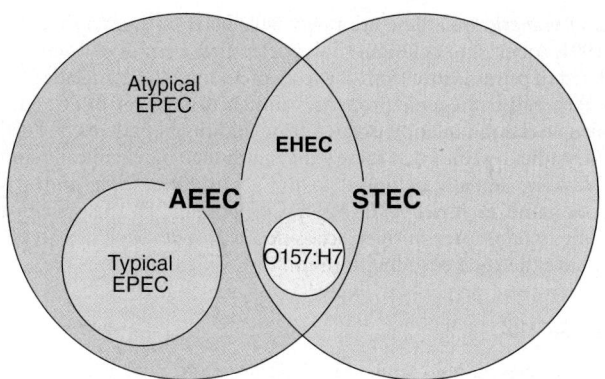

Figure 218-5 **Venn diagram illustrating the relationship between enteropathogenic** *Escherichia coli* **(EPEC) and Shiga toxin–producing** *E. coli* **(STEC) strains.** Both the EPEC and the enterohemorrhagic *E. coli* (EHEC) subsets of STEC strains are capable of the attaching and effacing effect and are sometimes referred to as attaching and effacing *E. coli* (AEEC). The O157:H7 serotype is the most important clone of EHEC. EPEC can be divided into typical strains that produce bundle-forming pili and exhibit localized adherence and atypical strains with neither of these properties. *(Adapted from Donnenberg MS, Whittam TS. Pathogenesis and evolution of virulence in enteropathogenic and enterohemorrhagic* Escherichia coli. *J Clin Invest. 2001;107:539-548.)*

vulnerable target organs, any tissue can become ischemic from capillary and larger vessel thrombosis. The brain (strokes), eyes (blindness), and colon (ischemic bowel) are other organs commonly affected. In adults, the involvement of the brain and other organs often leads to the diagnosis of thrombotic thrombocytopenic purpura. HUS carries a 12% risk of death or end-stage renal disease, and 25% of survivors experience long-term renal sequelae such as hypertension, proteinuria, and renal insufficiency.[228]

The principal virulence factors of STEC strains are a group of related cytotoxins called Shiga toxins. Stx1 is virtually identical to the toxin produced by *Shigella dysenteriae* type 1, and Stx2 shares a high degree of sequence similarity and identical functional features. Shiga toxins are encoded on temperate bacteriophages.[229] Importantly, these bacteriophages are induced and lyse the *E. coli* strains that harbor them when the cells are stressed by various conditions, including exposure to certain antibiotics.[230] As a result, high levels of Shiga toxins are released. Shiga toxins have five identical B subunits that bind to globotriaosylceramide and related glycosphingolipids (the same receptor used by P fimbriae and parvovirus B19).[231] The single catalytic A subunit, after endocytosis and retrograde transport to the endoplasmic reticulum,[232] catalyzes the depurination of a specific adenine residue in the 28S ribosomal RNA, rendering the ribosome nonfunctional. Dissemination of the toxin from the gastrointestinal tract throughout the bloodstream may be facilitated by binding to leukocytes.[233] Endothelial cells are susceptible to intoxication and may be the most relevant target cells in EHEC-induced HUS.[234] Endothelial cell intoxication is believed to result in increased expression of procoagulants and subsequent microvascular thrombosis.[235]

In addition to Shiga toxins, EHEC strains (but not non-EHEC STEC strains) harbor the locus of enterocyte effacement pathogenicity island and are capable of inducing the attaching and effacing effect.[236] Mutation of the gene encoding intimin from an O157:H7 EHEC strain resulted in reduced colonization of neonatal piglets[237] but did not affect neurologic complications, which are manifestations of Shiga toxin.[238]

STEC infection should be suspected in any patient with grossly bloody diarrhea and should be considered in any individual with diarrhea and cramps. The diagnosis of infection with STEC is vital because of the importance of recognizing potential outbreaks and of taking action to prevent further infections.[227] The laboratory should be notified that STEC infection is suspected because many laboratories do not routinely test for these strains. Sorbitol-MacConkey agar plates can be used to detect O157:H7 colonies, but confirmatory testing is required and these plates will not identify STEC strains of other serotypes. This can be accomplished using immunoassays for Shiga toxin or PCR to detect *stx* genes.

Treatment of EHEC infection is entirely supportive. Antibiotics are currently contraindicated because they can induce the expression and release of Shiga toxins and because some studies have indicated that their use is associated with a higher risk of HUS in children with EHEC infection.[239] Whether any antibiotics are safe is a matter not yet settled. Studies of alternative treatment modalities, including soluble toxin receptors and humanized monoclonal antitoxin antibodies, are ongoing.[240-243] In one randomized, double-blind clinical study, an oral toxin receptor analogue was not beneficial in patients with HUS; however, this approach has not been tried in patients before the onset of HUS.[244]

The risk of STEC infection can be reduced by following safe practices in food handling and preparation and in other areas of hygiene. Ground beef should be cooked to 155°F (68.3°C)[225] or until "the juices run clear," caution should be applied to prevent cross-contamination between uncooked meat and foods to be served without further cooking, unpasteurized juices and milk should be avoided, care should be taken to prevent infants and children who are not toilet trained from defecating in public swimming areas, and hands should be washed after touching animals in farms and petting zoos. Investigators are taking several approaches to vaccine development, including an O157 polysaccharide-protein conjugate vaccine, Shiga toxoid vaccines, proteins secreted by the T3SS, cell envelopes, and intimin vaccines.[245-249] Such vaccines and other preventive strategies may be targeted either to cattle or humans.

Enteroaggregative E. coli

Enteroaggregative *E. coli* (EAEC) may be considered a true emerging infection, both because of its relatively recent recognition and because of apparent increases in its importance in some settings. EAEC strains, first recognized as a cause of diarrhea in 1987,[250] are defined by their aggregative pattern of adherence to tissue culture cells (see Fig. 218-4*B*). These bacteria form two-dimensional clusters when they adhere to cells in vitro, to glass slides, to plastic, or to the intestinal mucosa.[251,252] Several case-control studies and a meta-analysis have confirmed that *E. coli* strains with this pattern of adherence are isolated with increased frequency from children with acute diarrhea in both developing and developed countries.[253] Additionally, volunteer studies have confirmed the pathogenicity of one EAEC strain but not others.[254] This and other evidence indicates that EAEC strains are heterogeneous, and some may be more pathogenic than others.[255,256] Importantly, studies have linked EAEC strains to chronic diarrhea.[257-259] EAEC has also been associated with travelers' diarrhea at frequencies rivaling those recorded for ETEC.[260,261] EAEC strains have also been implicated as a cause of persistent diarrhea in human immunodeficiency virus–infected patients.[262-264] Clinical descriptions of EAEC infection are sparse, but infection has been associated with intestinal colic, hematochezia, and mucus.[254,265-267] Infection with EAEC, whether symptomatic or not, has also been correlated with intestinal interleukin-8 production and growth retardation.[268]

The pathogenesis of EAEC disease is not well understood. EAEC strains cause mucosal damage with loss of microvilli and cell death when they adhere to polarized colonic epithelial cells or to explanted human colonic mucosa.[252] Aggregative adherence has been linked to the expression of several plasmid-encoded chaperone-usher type adhesins known as aggregative adherence fimbriae (e.g., AAF/I, AAF/II) that are related to the Dr family of adhesins also found in diffuse-adhering and some uropathogenic *E. coli* strains.[269-271] However, many strains that display aggregative adherence express none of these fimbrial types. AggR, a positive regulator of expression of aggregative adherence fimbrial operons, is present in a majority of EAEC strains and seems to be specific for this pathotype. Dispersin, a surface protein secreted by EAEC strains that is recognized by antibodies from volunteers after experimental infection, seems to play a role in limiting the aggregation of the strains.[272] Several toxins have been described that are expressed by some, but not all, EAEC strains. Enteroaggregative heat-stable enterotoxin (EAST) is similar to heat-stable enterotoxin and seems to act by a similar mechanism, but is found in many non–EAEC *E. coli* strains.[273] Plasmid-encoded enterotoxin is a member of the SPATE family (see "Secretion Systems and Toxins"). It causes cell rounding and detachment in tissue culture and crypt dilatation and cell damage in human intestinal explants.[274,275]

A diagnosis of EAEC infection can be suspected in the appropriate setting (acute diarrhea in children or recent travelers, persistent diarrhea in children or human immunodeficiency virus–infected patients), but confirmation requires performing tissue culture adhesion assays.[250] A simple test for identifying EAEC involving clump formation in Mueller-Hinton broth has been reported but may require confirmation.[276,277] DNA probes and PCR tests, particularly for the AggR regulator, may be useful but are not commercially available. Because strains that display aggregative adherence are extremely heterogeneous and may vary in pathogenicity and because EAEC organisms are often isolated from asymptomatic individuals, it is difficult to be certain that an EAEC strain isolated from an individual patient with diarrhea is the cause of his or her symptoms.

Data regarding the prevention and treatment of EAEC infections are sparse. One might assume that nonspecific methods for preventing other *E. coli* enteric infections would be effective for EAEC as well. There is no vaccine. There are reports that human immunodeficiency virus–infected individuals and travelers may benefit from treatment of EAEC infections with fluoroquinolones, but neither study had a prospective, randomized, placebo-controlled, noncrossover design.[267,278] Like EPEC strains, EAEC strains are often resistant to multiple antibiotics.[279]

Enteroinvasive E. coli

Because enteroinvasive *E. coli* (EIEC) strains are very similar to *Shigella* strains in terms of clinical features and pathogenesis, they are discussed only briefly here. Like *Shigella*, EIEC strains have a large invasion plasmid that encodes a T3SS enabling the bacteria to invade epithelial cells, escape from the phagosome, multiply in the cytoplasm, usurp the host actin-filament assembly machine, and spread directly from cell to cell. In fact, unlike most *E. coli* organisms, both EIEC and *Shigella* strains are usually nonmotile, cannot ferment lactose, and, because of a chromosomal deletion, are lysine decarboxylase negative.[280] They are differentiated from *Shigella* principally by the fact that EIEC strains ferment glucose and xylose.[92] The pathophenotype of EIEC and *Shigella* strains is an example of convergent evolution involving the gain of similar plasmids and the gain and loss of chromosomal loci because EIEC and *Shigella* strains each represent several distinct evolutionary lineages within the genus *Escherichia*.[1,281,282] Like *Shigella*, EIEC can cause watery diarrhea, which may progress to dysentery characterized by severe abdominal cramps, fever, tenesmus, and frequent passage of small-volume stools that may contain mucus and blood. Based on a volunteer study, it has been estimated that the infectious dose of EIEC is approximately 10^8 bacteria, considerably higher than that of *Shigella*.[283] EIEC strains are detected in culture as lactose-negative colonies and confirmed either by DNA probes or PCR for virulence-associated genes. By analogy with *Shigella* infections, it is assumed that antibiotic treatment of EIEC infection may shorten the duration of illness, but care must be taken to exclude infection with STEC before initiating therapy.

Other Pathotypes of E. coli and Species of Escherichia

Several epidemiologic studies have provided evidence that *E. coli* strains that adhere to tissue culture cells in a diffuse pattern (see Fig. 218-4C) are associated with diarrhea, especially in older children.[177,284-286] However, Koch's postulates have not been fulfilled in volunteer studies.[287] It is clear that these strains, like EAEC, are quite heterogeneous, and perhaps some are more pathogenic than others.[256]

In addition to *E. coli*, the genus *Escherichia* contains several other species including *Escherichia blattae*, *Escherichia fergusonii*, and *Esch-*

erichia vulneris, but these are rarely isolated from human infections. In 1991, Albert and colleagues[288] reported that a strain of *Hafnia alvei* isolated in pure culture from the feces of an infant in Bangladesh with diarrhea had pathogenic properties similar to those of EPEC. Similar strains were subsequently isolated from additional patients.[289] Further DNA studies revealed that these strains, although biochemically similar to *H. alvei*, actually belonged to the genus *Escherichia*, and a new species name, *Escherichia albertii*, was proposed.[290,291] This species also includes strains, previously misclassified as *Shigella boydii* serotype 13, that have the gene encoding intimin.[292]

KLEBSIELLA

Three species in the genus *Klebsiella* are associated with illness in humans: *Klebsiella pneumoniae*, *Klebsiella oxytoca*, and *Klebsiella granulomatis*. Organisms previously known as *Klebsiella ozaenae* and *Klebsiella rhinoscleromatis* are considered nonfermenting subspecies of *K. pneumoniae* that have characteristic clinical manifestations. With those exceptions, strains within this genus ferment lactose, most produce highly mucoid colonies on plates because of the production of a luxuriant polysaccharide capsule, and all are nonmotile.

K. pneumoniae is a primary pathogen capable of causing UTIs, liver abscess, and pneumonia in otherwise healthy people. However, most infections caused by *K. pneumoniae* are acquired in the hospital and/or occur in those who are debilitated by various underlying conditions.[293] In addition to pneumonia and UTIs, nosocomial infections caused by *K. pneumoniae* include wound infections, infections of intravascular and other invasive devices, biliary tract infections, peritonitis, and meningitis. *K. pneumoniae* can cause UTIs in individuals with normal as well as abnormal urinary tracts and is second only to *E. coli* as a cause of bacteremia resulting from UTI and of gram-negative bacteremia.[294-296] UTIs caused by *K. pneumoniae* do not have clinical features that distinguish them from those caused by other bacterial species. Pneumonia caused by *K. pneumoniae* has classically been described as having particular distinguishing features, warranting the eponym Friedländer's disease. Among these classic features are its severity, its frequency in alcoholics, its propensity to affect the upper lobes, the production of "currant jelly" sputum resulting from hemoptysis (see Fig. 6-1 in Chapter 6), the bulging fissure sign on radiography caused by edematous lobar consolidation, and its tendency for abscess formation. Despite these compelling descriptions, pneumonia caused by *K. pneumoniae* cannot be distinguished on clinical grounds from that caused by other organisms, and many of the described features are likely the result of misdiagnosis, caused by culture of expectorated sputum, of anaerobic pulmonary infections.[297]

The principal virulence factor that has been described for *K. pneumoniae* is its polysaccharide capsule, which comes in more than 70 antigenic varieties and is responsible for its mucoid colony phenotype.[293] Some capsule types, such as K1 and K2, may be more important than others. The mechanism by which capsule promotes virulence is thought to be due to inhibition of phagocytosis (see earlier). Animal models have revealed a role for the capsule in infection of the urinary tract and pneumonia.[90,298] *K. pneumoniae* can produce a variety of fimbrial types, including type 1 pili that are involved in adherence to host cells.[293,299,300] As with other enterobacterial species that cause systemic infections, *K. pneumoniae* seems to require LPS and iron uptake mechanisms to cause disease.[298,301]

All strains of *K. pneumoniae* are resistant to ampicillin as a result of the presence of a chromosomal gene encoding a penicillin-specific β-lactamase.[302] In addition, nosocomial isolates are frequently resistant to numerous other antibiotics as a result of the acquisition of multidrug-resistant plasmids. For example, *K. pneumoniae* is one of the most common organisms to carry plasmids encoding extended-spectrum β-lactamases and bacteremia with such strains is associated with higher rates of treatment failure and death.[303] Therapeutic options for infections caused by non–multidrug-resistant strains include first-generation cephalosporins, penicillin/β-lactamase inhibi-

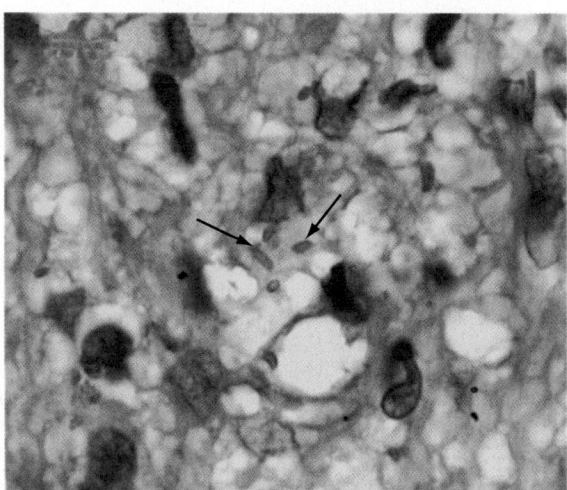

Figure 218-6 **Photomicrograph of Mikulicz cells in a patient with rhinoscleroma.** The periodic-acid-Schiff–positive structures within the macrophage are the causative organism, *Klebsiella rhinoscleromatis*. (From ID Images. © The Infectious Disease Society of America [IDSA]. Case presented by Danielle Osterholzer, Tom E. Davis, and Stephen D. Allen.)

tor combinations, trimethoprim-sulfamethoxazole, fluoroquinolones, and aminoglycosides. For multidrug-resistant strains, especially those expressing extended-spectrum β-lactamases, treatment options are often limited to fourth-generation cephalosporins or carbapenems.

The *K. pneumoniae* subspecies *rhinoscleromatis* is the causative agent of respiratory scleroma, also known as rhinoscleroma, a chronic granulomatous infection of the nasal passages and other parts of the respiratory tract.[304] The disease is found primarily in impoverished areas of Central and South America, Africa, and Asia or in immigrants from these areas[304,305] and is transmitted by close contact. Respiratory scleroma is characterized by nodules and masses that often involve the nasal passages, but may be found in the sinuses, palate, glottis, and lower respiratory tract. Occasionally, the infection can erode through bone and invade the central nervous system. The differential diagnosis includes tuberculosis, leprosy, fungal infections, Wegener's granulomatosis, malignancies, and sarcoidosis. Biopsies show granulomatous inflammation with foamy macrophages (Mikulicz cells) containing intracellular organisms (Fig. 218-6).[306]

The bacteria can be grown on ordinary laboratory media. Antibiotic therapy for 6 to 8 weeks is required for cure, but relapses are common. Traditionally, streptomycin or tetracycline has been used, but more recent reports indicate success and perhaps less risk of adverse effects with trimethoprim-sulfamethoxazole or fluoroquinolones.[305]

The *K. pneumoniae* subspecies *ozaenae* can colonize the nasopharynx of healthy individuals. Its association with chronic atrophic rhinitis (ozena) has been noted, but its etiologic role in this syndrome is controversial. The organism has only rarely been isolated from patients with a variety of infections, including otitis media and mastoiditis, cystitis and pyelonephritis, soft tissue infections, bacteremia associated with neutropenia, pneumonia, and meningitis.[307,308] It is usually susceptible to multiple antibiotics except when isolated from hospitalized patients who had received previous antimicrobial therapy.

K. oxytoca, like *K. pneumoniae*, can cause a variety of nosocomial infections. It is distinguished from *K. pneumoniae* based on its ability to produce indole from tryptophan. It may also be resistant to multiple antibiotics. There is evidence that *K. oxytoca* can cause hemorrhagic colitis associated with antibiotic use.[309]

K. granulomatis (formerly *Calymmatobacterium granulomatis*) is a fastidious member of the genus that causes chronic genital ulcerative disease (see Chapter 236).

ENTEROBACTER, PANTOEA, SERRATIA, CITROBACTER, AND HAFNIA

Microorganisms belonging to the genera *Enterobacter, Pantoea, Serratia,* and *Citrobacter* rarely cause infections in normal hosts, but are common nosocomial isolates. *Hafnia* is not as common, but is included in this section because of its close phylogenic relationship to the group.

ENTEROBACTER SPECIES AND *PANTOEA* (ENTEROBACTER) AGGLOMERANS

Three species of *Enterobacter, Enterobacter cloacae, Enterobacter aerogenes,* and *Enterobacter sakazakii,* are responsible for the vast majority of *Enterobacter* infections. *Pantoea agglomerans,* until recently known as *Enterobacter agglomerans,* is also a common isolate and, because its new nomenclature is not yet widely in use, is grouped with the *Enterobacter* spp. here. These bacteria ferment lactose, are motile, and form mucoid colonies. *Enterobacter* strains commonly arise from the endogenous intestinal flora of hospitalized patients, but can occur in common source outbreaks or are spread from patient to patient. Infections are especially common in patients who have received antimicrobial therapy and in those in intensive care units.[310] *Enterobacter* spp. may cause a wide variety of nosocomial infections, including pneumonia, UTIs, wound and burn infections, infections of intravascular and other prosthetic devices, and meningitis. There do not seem to be distinguishing characteristics among infections caused by *E. cloacae* and *E. aerogenes*. *E. sakazakii* causes bacteremia and meningitis primarily in neonates and is associated with consumption of powdered milk formula.[311] *P. agglomerans,* a plant pathogen, is often associated with contaminated catheters or penetrating trauma.[312]

Little is known regarding potential virulence characteristics of these bacteria. In addition to their capsule, which may contribute to serum resistance and resistance to phagocytosis, strains of *E. cloacae* frequently produce aerobactin, adhere to tissue culture cells, and exhibit mannose-sensitive hemagglutination, possibly the result of type 1 fimbriae expression.[313] *E. sakazakii* can adhere to and invade brain microvascular endothelial cells, a trait that it shares with strains of ExPEC that produce K1 capsule and cause neonatal meningitis.[314] *E. cloacae, E. aerogenes,* and most strains of *E. sakazakii* are intrinsically resistant to ampicillin and first- and second-generation cephalosporins as a result of an inducible *ampC* chromosomal β-lactamase that is controlled by both positive and negative regulators.[315] Furthermore, mutants that constitutively produce high levels of β-lactamase, conferring resistance to third-generation cephalosporins, arise at frequencies of 10^{-4} to 10^{-7}, usually as a result of mutations in the regulatory loci, such that resistant mutants are already present in most patients with *Enterobacter* infections before initiation of therapy. In addition, like other members of the family Enterobacteriaceae, members of the genus *Enterobacter* may carry plasmids encoding resistance to multiple antimicrobial agents. Therapy for *Enterobacter* infections must therefore be tailored to individual isolates and based on antimicrobial susceptibility testing. However, clinicians must be aware that emergence of stably derepressed resistant mutants may lead to treatment failure when third-generation cephalosporins are chosen, even if the isolates appear susceptible on initial testing.[316] Therefore, fourth-generation cephalosporins, carbapenems, or other agents may be better choices than other β-lactam antibiotics for serious infections involving large numbers of bacteria.

SERRATIA SPECIES

Of the many species in the genus *Serratia, Serratia marcescens* is the one most commonly isolated from human infections, and *Serratia liquefaciens* is occasionally grown. *Serratia* strains are motile, rarely ferment lactose, and produce an extracellular DNase. The organism is widespread in the environment but not a common component of the human fecal flora. Thus, most infections are acquired exogenously. Many environmental and some clinical strains of *S. marcescens* produce a red pigment, prodigiosin. In fact, in one of the first instances in which an artificial medium was used to cultivate a microorganism, an Italian pharmacist named Bartolemeo Bizio first described the organism in 1819 as the cause of red discoloration of polenta (corn meal mush), thereby discrediting the claim that the growth was due to the miraculous appearance of blood. He gave the bacterium its genus name to honor Serafino Serrati, whom he believed had not received proper credit for the invention of the steamboat, and its species name for the Latin word for "to decay" because of the tendency of the pigment to change color as the colonies age.[317] The production of prodigiosin and the belief that the bacterium was harmless led to its frequent use as a biologic marker to study, among other things, the transmission of bacteria through speech and contact, ascending colonization of the bladder in patients with urinary catheters, and the dissemination of aerosolized bacteria after experimental release in models of biologic warfare.[318] It is now appreciated that *S. marcescens* can cause a wide variety of nosocomial infections. In addition, the bacterium has a particular association with infections in injecting drug users.

Potential virulence factors of *Serratia* have not received a great deal of attention, but strains may be capable of both mannose-sensitive (presumably as a result of type 1 fimbriae) and mannose-resistant hemagglutination, as well as adherence to uroepithelial cells, and may be cytotoxic to tissue culture cells.[299,319,320] The organism can survive under harsh conditions, including in a variety of disinfectants, some of which have been the sources of outbreaks.[321] Infections caused by *S. marcescens* may begin with exogenous contamination and spread within or among hospitals on the hands of personnel.[322] The most common site of infection is the urinary tract, but the organism is frequently isolated from the respiratory tract and from wounds.[322] Cases of osteomyelitis, infectious arthritis, and endophthalmitis may follow hematogenous dissemination, whereas meningitis may occur after neurologic procedures. As previously noted, injection drug users are at particular risk of *S. marcescens* infections, including endocarditis, which is frequently left sided,[323] and infections at other sites after hematogenous spread.[318] *Serratia* isolates are resistant to ampicillin and first-generation cephalosporins because of an inducible, chromosomal AmpC β-lactamase similar to that of *Enterobacter*.[324] Mutants that produce high levels of these enzymes as a result of stable derepression may arise during therapy. In addition, many isolates possess plasmids encoding resistance to other cephalosporins, penicillins, carbapenems, and aminoglycosides.[321,322] Fluoroquinolone resistance and resistance to trimethoprim-sulfamethoxazole are also encountered. Thus, treatment of infections caused by *S. marcescens* can be quite difficult, and every effort should be made to identify point sources of outbreaks and control the spread of the organism.

CITROBACTER SPECIES

Members of the genus *Citrobacter* are named for their ability to use citrate as their sole carbon source. Of the dozen species, *Citrobacter freundii*, *Citrobacter koseri* (formerly *Citrobacter diversus*), and *Citrobacter amalonaticus* are linked to human disease. They are differentiated by their ability to convert tryptophan to indole, ferment lactose, and use malonate.[325] *C. freundii* produces H_2S and hence can be confused with *Salmonella*, with which it was classified at one time. The urinary tract is the most frequent site from which *Citrobacter* is cultured, often in association with an indwelling catheter. These bacteria may also be cultured from the respiratory tract, a finding that more often represents colonization than symptomatic infection. *Citrobacter* strains are also involved in intra-abdominal infections and can cause soft tissue infections and osteomyelitis.[326,327] Invasive procedures may play a role in *Citrobacter* bacteremia.[328] *C. koseri* has caused frequent nosocomial outbreaks of neonatal meningitis. In several instances, the outbreaks have been accompanied by high rates of intestinal colonization in infants by the organism and by carriage of the bacteria on the hands of health care workers.[329] *C. freundii* strains, like strains

of *Enterobacter* and *Serratia*, have inducible *ampC* genes encoding resistance to ampicillin and first-generation cephalosporins that can be produced constitutively at high levels after mutations. In addition, like members of these other genera, isolates of *Citrobacter* may be resistant to multiple other antibiotics as a result of plasmid-encoded resistance genes.

HAFNIA ALVEI

H. alvei (formerly *Enterobacter hafniae*) is currently the sole species in the genus *Hafnia*. It resides in the gastrointestinal tract of humans and many animal species.[330] These microorganisms are motile, but do not ferment lactose. Although *H. alvei* may be cultured from various sites, it is frequently isolated along with other organisms.[331] Thus, in many cases, the role of the organism in disease is not clear. Most infections with *H. alvei* occur in patients with severe underlying illness, including malignancies, those with trauma, and postoperative patients. There have been numerous reports linking diarrhea to the isolation of *H. alvei* from stool specimens. Because the organism is part of the normal fecal flora, these reports must be interpreted with caution. Furthermore, those strains initially reported to produce attaching and effacing lesions via a mechanism similar to that used by EPEC are now recognized as belonging to a new species, *Escherichia albertii*.[290] However, in a case-control study of Finnish tourists returning from Morocco, the prevalence of *H. alvei* in those with diarrhea was significantly greater than in those without diarrhea, substantiating a possible etiologic role.[332] Furthermore, these strains were all negative in PCR testing for the *eae* gene encoding intimin, which is found in EPEC and *E. albertii*. Treatment of serious *H. alvei* infections is guided by antimicrobial susceptibility testing.

PROTEUS, PROVIDENCIA, AND MORGANELLA

The genera *Proteus*, *Providencia*, and *Morganella* are related members of the family Enterobacteriaceae that are lactose negative and motile and produce phenylalanine deaminase. There are several species of *Proteus*, but *Proteus mirabilis* and *Proteus vulgaris* account for the vast majority of clinical isolates in this genus. Both produce urease, and the latter is indole positive. Members of this genus also produce H_2S. These bacteria are capable of swarming motility as they differentiate from typical enterobacterial bacilli expressing fimbriae and flagellae into highly elongated rods with thousands of flagellae that translocate rapidly across the surface of agar plates. In fact, the name *Proteus* was chosen from a character in Homer's *Odyssey*, who was capable of changing form. *Providencia stuartii* is the most common species of its genus isolated from clinical specimens, but *Providencia rettgeri* is occasionally grown. These bacteria can be differentiated from *Proteus* and *Morganella* based on their ability to use citrate and ferment D-mannitol.[333] *Morganella morganii* is at present the only member of its genus. It is citrate negative.

Proteus spp. are common causes of UTIs, occasionally in normal hosts and very commonly in those with indwelling catheters or anatomic or functional abnormalities of the urinary tract. UTIs caused by *Proteus* spp. tend to be more severe than those caused by *E. coli*, with a higher proportion representing pyelonephritis.[334] *Proteus* spp. are commonly isolated from the bloodstream, the vast majority secondary to UTI, often associated with urinary catheters.[294] *P. mirabilis* may be second only to *E. coli* as a cause of bacteremia from a urinary source.[294,335] In addition to UTI, *Proteus* spp. may cause miscellaneous other infections, particularly in hospitalized patients. There is some suspicion, based on anecdotal reports and case-control studies, that some strains of *P. mirabilis* can cause diarrhea.[336] The pathogenesis of UTI caused by *P. mirabilis* has received considerable attention. These microorganisms may produce several types of pili, the most important of which, known as MR/P fimbriae, is subject to phase variation as a result of an invertible element similar to that which controls type 1 pili in *E. coli*.[337,338] MR/P fimbriae have been shown to contribute to bladder colonization in a murine model of UTI.[339] The ability of

P. mirabilis to produce a potent urease has also been confirmed to be a virulence factor in this murine model,[340] contributing to both colonization and stone formation. Indeed, the enzyme, by hydrolyzing urea to form CO_2 and ammonia, alkalinizes the urine, which leads to the precipitation of struvite, formation of calculi, and obstruction of urinary catheters. The kidney stones serve as foreign bodies in which the bacteria are embedded and from which they emerge to cause recurrent infections. Treatment of infections caused by *P. mirabilis* is usually straightforward because most strains are susceptible to commonly used antibiotics, except for tetracycline.[333] Of course, multiply resistant strains are sometimes encountered, and strains of *P. vulgaris* are generally more resistant.

P. stuartii is a rather uncommon clinical isolate, except from the urine of nursing home patients with long-term indwelling urinary catheters. In that setting, *P. stuartii* is found as commonly as more familiar urinary tract isolates.[341] These infections are sometimes complicated by bacteremia and death.[342] *P. stuartii* and *P. rettgeri* are often resistant to multiple antibiotics, including gentamicin, first-generation cephalosporins, and ampicillin. Therapy is guided by susceptibility testing.

M. morganii is an infrequent nosocomial isolate, usually isolated from urine or wounds.[333,343,344] A potential role in diarrhea remains controversial.[333,336,345] In one study from Korea, *M. morganii* bacteremia was frequently associated with biliary tract disease and biliary drainage catheters and previous surgery or procedures.[346] As with other members of this group, *M. morganii* may cause nosocomial outbreaks.[343] *M. morganii* strains possess inducible AmpC β-lactamases and therefore are intrinsically resistant to ampicillin and first-generation cephalosporins; spontaneous derepressed mutants resistant to extended-spectrum β-lactamases similar to those described previously for *Enterobacter* spp. may arise.[347]

MISCELLANEOUS GENERA

There are a number of other genera within the family Enterobacteriaceae that have been associated with human disease.

Edwardsiella tarda is found in freshwater environments. It has been associated in case-control studies with diarrhea and can cause wound infections, abscesses. and bacteremia, sometimes in association with marine exposure.[348] Mortality may be high in patients with liver disease and iron overload.[349]

Plesiomonas shigelloides is another organism found in water that has been associated with diarrhea and rarely with extraintestinal infections.[350] *P. shigelloides* was previously grouped with vibrios because of a number of shared features, including oxidase production and polar flagellae, but was reassigned to the enterobacterial family based on phylogeny as assessed by ribosomal DNA sequencing.[351] It is an infrequent isolate from patients with gastroenteritis, but case-control studies reveal a significant association with diarrhea. Furthermore, there have been reports of outbreaks of gastroenteritis in which the organism was the only potential pathogen cultured from patients. Patients in the United States with *P. shigelloides*–associated diarrhea frequently have gross blood in the stool and are more likely than controls to have recently ingested raw shellfish or to have traveled outside the United States.[352] Despite these compelling associations, volunteer experiments have not confirmed that this organism can cause diarrhea.[353]

Ewingella americana, named after William Ewing, who made many contributions to our understanding of the microbiology of the Enterobacteriaceae, is an extremely rare cause of nosocomial bacteremia, peritonitis associated with peritoneal dialysis, and conjunctivitis.[354-356] Most isolates have been highly sensitive to antibiotics.

Infections caused by organisms belonging to the genus *Kluyvera*, which closely resembles *E. coli*, are rare. These bacteria have been recovered from urine, sputum, or wounds, and in many cases, the pathologic significance of their presence is unclear. However, pyelonephritis, bacteremia, and soft tissue infections caused by *Kluyvera* spp. have occurred, and some infections have been fatal.[357-359]

Bacteria belonging to the genus *Photorhabdus* are fascinating bioluminescent symbionts of nematodes that are parasites of certain insect larvae. Recently there have been a few case reports from Australia and the United States of soft tissue infections and bacteremia caused by members of a new, nonluminescent species *Photorhabdus asymbiotica*.[360,361]

Most reported human infections caused by bacteria described as *Erwinia* were caused by the organism now known as *P. agglomerans* (see earlier). Current members of the genus *Erwinia* are primarily pathogens of plants rather than humans.

REFERENCES

1. Pupo GM, Karaolis DKR, Lan RT, et al. Evolutionary relationships among pathogenic and nonpathogenic *Escherichia coli* strains inferred from multilocus enzyme electrophoresis and *mdh* sequence studies. *Infect Immun.* 1997;65:2685-2692.
2. Mackowiak PA, Martin RM, Jones SR, et al. Pharyngeal colonization by gram-negative bacilli in aspiration-prone persons. *Arch Intern Med.* 1978;138:1224-1227.
3. Johanson WG, Pierce AK, Sanford JP. Changing pharyngeal bacterial flora of hospitalized patients: emergence of gram-negative bacilli. *N Engl J Med.* 1969;281:1137-1140.
4. Raz R, Stamm WE. A controlled trial of intravaginal estriol in postmenopausal women with recurrent urinary tract infections. *N Engl J Med.* 1993;329:753-756.
5. Gupta K, Hillier SL, Hooton TM, et al. Effects of contraceptive method on the vaginal microbial flora: a prospective evaluation. *J Infect Dis.* 2000;181:595-601.
6. Allos BM, Moore MR, Griffin PM, et al. Surveillance for sporadic foodborne disease in the 21st century: the FoodNet perspective. *Clin Infect Dis.* 2004;38(Suppl 3):S115-S120.
7. Kadner RJ. Inner Membrane. In: Neidhardt FC, ed. *Escherichia coli and Salmonella: Cellular and Molecular Biology.* Washington, DC: ASM Press; 1996:58-87.
8. Blattner FR, Plunkett G III, Bloch CA, et al. The complete genome sequence of *Escherichia coli* K-12. *Science.* 1997;277:1453-1462.
9. Oliver DB. Periplasm. In: Neidhardt FC, ed. *Escherichia coli and Salmonella: Cellular and Molecular Biology.* Washington, DC: ASM Press; 1996:88-103.
10. Park JT. The murein sacculus. In: Neidhardt FC, ed. *Escherichia coli and Salmonella: Cellular and Molecular Biology.* Washington, DC: ASM Press; 1996:48-57.
11. Nikaido H. Outer membrane. In: Neidhardt FC, ed. *Escherichia coli and Salmonella: Cellular and Molecular Biology.* Washington, DC: ASM Press; 1996:29-47.
12. Koebnik R, Locher KP, Van Gelder P. Structure and function of bacterial outer membrane proteins: barrels in a nutshell. *Mol Microbiol.* 2000;37:239-253.
13. Raetz CRH. Bacterial lipopolysaccharides: a remarkable family of bioactive macroamphiphiles. In: Neidhardt FC, ed. *Escherichia coli and Salmonella: Cellular and Molecular Biology.* Washington, DC: ASM Press; 1996:1035-1063.
14. Ørskov F, Ørskov I. *Escherichia coli* serotyping and disease in man and animals. *Can J Microbiol.* 1992;38:699-674.
15. Rick PD, Silver RP. Enterobacterial common antigen and capsular polysaccharides. In: Neidhardt FC, ed. *Escherichia coli and Salmonella: Cellular and Molecular Biology.* Washington, DC: ASM Press; 1996:104-122.
16. Whitfield C, Roberts IS. Structure, assembly and regulation of expression of capsules in *Escherichia coli. Mol Microbiol.* 1999;31:1307-1319.
17. Girón JA. Expression of flagella and motility by *Shigella. Mol Microbiol.* 1995;18:63-75.
18. Kubori T, Matsushima Y, Nakamura D, et al. Supramolecular structure of the *Salmonella typhimurium* type III protein secretion system. *Science.* 1998;280:602-605.
19. Wang L, Rothemund D, Curd H, et al. Species-wide variation in the *Escherichia coli* flagellin (H-antigen) gene. *J Bacteriol.* 2003;185:2936-2943.
20. Hayashi F, Smith KD, Ozinsky A, et al. The innate immune response to bacterial flagellin is mediated by Toll-like receptor 5. *Nature.* 2001;410:1099-1103.
21. Gewirtz AT, Simon Jr PO, Schmitt CK, et al. *Salmonella typhimurium* translocates flagellin across intestinal epithelia, inducing a proinflammatory response. *J Clin Invest.* 2001;107:99-109.
22. Steiner TS, Nataro JP, Poteet-Smith CE, et al. Enteroaggregative *Escherichia coli* expresses a novel flagellin that causes IL-8 release from intestinal epithelial cells. *J Clin Invest.* 2000;105:1769-1777.
23. Ottow JC. Ecology, physiology, and genetics of fimbriae and pili. *Annu Rev Microbiol.* 1975;29:79-108.
24. McClelland M, Sanderson KE, Spieth J, et al. Complete genome sequence of *Salmonella enterica* serovar Typhimurium LT2. *Nature.* 2001;413:852-856.
25. Parkhill J, Dougan G, James KD, et al. Complete genome sequence of a multiple drug resistant *Salmonella enterica* serovar Typhi CT18. *Nature.* 2001;413:848-852.
26. Welch RA, Burland V, Plunkett III G, et al. Extensive mosaic structure revealed by the complete genome sequence of uropathogenic *Escherichia coli. Proc Natl Acad Sci U S A.* 2002;99:17020-17024.
27. Jones CH, Pinkner JS, Roth R, et al. FimH adhesin of type 1 pili is assembled into a fibrillar tip structure in the Enterobacteriaceae. *Proc Natl Acad Sci U S A.* 1995;92:2081-2085.
28. Kuehn MJ, Heuser J, Normark S, et al. P pili in uropathogenic *E. coli* are composite fibres with distinct fibrillar adhesive tips. *Nature.* 1992;356:252-255.
29. Thanassi DG, Saulino ET, Lombardo MJ, et al. The PapC usher forms an oligomeric channel: implications for pilus biogenesis across the outer membrane. *Proc Natl Acad Sci U S A.* 1998;95:3146-3151.
30. Dodson KW, Jacob-Dubuisson F, Striker RT, et al. Outer-membrane PapC molecular usher discriminately recognizes periplasmic chaperone-pilus subunit complexes. *Proc Natl Acad Sci U S A.* 1993;90:3670-3674.
31. Girón JA, Ho ASY, Schoolnik GK. An inducible bundle-forming pilus of enteropathogenic *Escherichia coli. Science.* 1991;254:710-713.
32. Girón JA, Levine MM, Kaper JB. Longus: a long pilus ultrastructure produced by human enterotoxigenic *Escherichia coli. Mol Microbiol.* 1994;12:71-82.
33. Xicohtencatl-Cortes J, Monteiro-Neto V, Ledesma MA, et al. Intestinal adherence associated with type IV pili of enterohem-

orrhagic *Escherichia coli* O157:H7. *J Clin Invest.* 2007;117: 3519-3529.

34. Zhang XL, Tsui IS, Yip CM, et al. *Salmonella enterica* serovar Typhi uses type IVB pili to enter human intestinal epithelial cells. *Infect Immun.* 2000;68:3067-3073.

35. Collyn F, Lety MA, Nair S, et al. *Yersinia pseudotuberculosis* harbors a type IV pilus gene cluster that contributes to pathogenicity. *Infect Immun.* 2002;70:6196-6205.

36. Merz AJ, So M, Sheetz MP. Pilus retraction powers bacterial twitching motility. *Nature.* 2000;407:98-102.

37. Craig L, Pique ME, Tainer JA. Type IV pilus structure and bacterial pathogenicity. *Nat Rev Microbiol.* 2004;2:363-378.

38. Lessl M, Lanka E. Common mechanisms in bacterial conjugation and Ti-mediated T-DNA transfer to plant cells. *Cell.* 1994;77:321-324.

39. Falkow S. Molecular Koch's postulates applied to microbial pathogenicity. *Rev Infect Dis.* 1988;10(Suppl 2):S274-S276.

40. Finlay BB, Falkow S. Common themes in microbial pathogenicity revisited. *Microbiol Rev.* 1997;61:136-169.

41. Hung CS, Bouckaert J, Hung D, et al. Structural basis of tropism of *Escherichia coli* to the bladder during urinary tract infection. *Mol Microbiol.* 2002;44:903-915.

42. Ofek I, Mirelman D, Sharon N. Adherence of *Escherichia coli* to human mucosal cells mediated by mannose receptors. *Nature.* 1977;265:623-625.

43. Thomas WE, Trintchina E, Forero M, et al. Bacterial adhesion to target cells enhanced by shear force. *Cell.* 2002;109:913-923.

44. Abraham JM, Freitag CS, Clements JR, et al. An invertible element of DNA controls phase variation of type 1 fimbriae of *Escherichia coli. Proc Natl Acad Sci U S A.* 1985;82:5724-5727.

45. Connell H, Agace W, Klemm P, et al. Type 1 fimbrial expression enhances *Escherichia coli* virulence for the urinary tract. *Proc Natl Acad Sci U S A.* 1996;93:9827-9832.

46. Bloch CA, Stocker BAD, Orndorff PE. A key role for type 1 pili in enterobacterial communicability. *Mol Microbiol.* 1992;6: 697-701.

47. Bloch CA, Orndorff PE. Impaired colonization by and full invasiveness of *Escherichia coli* K1 bearing a site-directed mutation in the type 1 pilin gene. *Infect Immun.* 1990;58:275-278.

48. Hamburger ZA, Brown MS, Isberg RR, et al. Crystal structure of invasin: a bacterial integrin-binding protein. *Science.* 1999;286:291-295.

49. Luo Y, Frey EA, Pfuetzner RA, et al. Crystal structure of enteropathogenic *Escherichia coli* intimin-receptor complex. *Nature.* 2000;405:1073-1077.

50. Kelly G, Prasannan S, Daniell S, et al. Structure of the cell-adhesion fragment of intimin from enteropathogenic *Escherichia coli. Nature Struct Biol.* 1999;6:313-318.

51. Tran Van Nhieu G, Isberg RR. The *Yersinia pseudotuberculosis* invasin protein and human fibronectin bind to mutually exclusive sites on the $\alpha_5\beta_1$ integrin receptor. *J Biol Chem.* 1991;266:24367-24375.

52. Kenny B, DeVinney R, Stein M, et al. Enteropathogenic *E. coli* (EPEC) transfers its receptor for intimate adherence into mammalian cells. *Cell.* 1997;91:511-520.

53. Economou A, Christie PJ, Fernandez RC, et al. Secretion by numbers: protein traffic in prokaryotes. *Mol Microbiol.* 2006;62:308-319.

54. Henderson IR, Nataro JP. Virulence functions of autotransporter proteins. *Infect Immun.* 2001;69:1231-1243.

55. Dutta PR, Cappello R, Navarro-Garcia F, et al. Functional comparison of serine protease autotransporters of Enterobacteriaceae. *Infect Immun.* 2002;70:7105-7113.

56. Koronakis V, Sharff A, Koronakis E, et al. Crystal structure of the bacterial membrane protein TolC central to multidrug efflux and protein export. *Nature.* 2000;405:914-919.

57. Thanabalu T, Koronakis E, Hughes C, et al. Substrate-induced assembly of a contiguous channel for protein export from *E. coli*: reversible bridging of an inner-membrane translocase to an outer membrane exit pore. *EMBO J.* 1998;17:6487-6496.

58. Foreman DT, Martinez Y, Coombs G, et al. TolC and DsbA are needed for the secretion of ST_b, a heat-stable enterotoxin of *Escherichia coli. Mol Microbiol.* 1995;18:237-245.

59. Soloaga A, Veiga MP, García-Segura LM, et al. Insertion of *Escherichia coli* α-haemolysin in lipid bilayers as a non-transmembrane integral protein: prediction and experiment. *Mol Microbiol.* 1999;31:1013-1024.

60. Uhlén P, Laestadius Å, Jahnukainen T, et al. α-haemolysin of uropathogenic *E. coli* induces Ca^{2+} oscillations in renal epithelial cells. *Nature.* 2000;405:694-697.

61. Smith YC, Rasmussen SB, Grande KK, et al. Hemolysin of uropathogenic *Escherichia coli* evokes extensive shedding of the uroepithelium and hemorrhage in bladder tissue within the first 24 hours after intraurethral inoculation of mice. *Infect Immun.* 2008;76:2978-2990.

62. Sandkvist M. Biology of type II secretion. *Mol Microbiol.* 2001;40:271-283.

63. Lathem WW, Grys TE, Witowski SE, et al. StcE, a metalloprotease secreted by *Escherichia coli* O157:H7, specifically cleaves C1 esterase inhibitor. *Mol Microbiol.* 2002;45:277-288.

64. Galán JE, Collmer A. Type III secretion machines: bacterial devices for protein delivery into host cells. *Science.* 1999;284:1322-1328.

65. Cornelis GR. The type III secretion injectisome. *Nat Rev Microbiol.* 2006;4:811-825.

66. Stebbins CE, Galán JE. Structural mimicry in bacterial virulence. *Nature.* 2001;412:701-705.

67. Escolar L, Pérez-Martín J, De Lorenzo V. Opening the iron box: transcriptional metalloregulation by the Fur protein. *J Bacteriol.* 1999;181:6223-6229.

68. Raymond KN, Dertz EA, Kim SS. Enterobactin: an archetype for microbial iron transport. *Proc Natl Acad Sci U S A.* 2003; 100:3584-3588.

69. Carbonetti NH, Boonchai S, Parry SH, et al. Aerobactin-mediated iron uptake by *Escherichia coli* isolates from human extraintestinal infections. *Infect Immun.* 1986;51:966-968.

70. Johnson JR, Moseley SL, Roberts PL, et al. Aerobactin and other virulence factor genes among strains of *Escherichia coli* causing urosepsis: association with patient characteristics. *Infect Immun.* 1988;56:405-412.

71. Torres AG, Redford P, Welch RA, et al. TonB-dependent systems of uropathogenic *Escherichia coli*: aerobactin and heme transport and TonB are required for virulence in the mouse. *Infect Immun.* 2001;69:6179-6185.

72. Jiang XQ, Payne MA, Cao ZH, et al. Ligand-specific opening of a gated-porin channel in the outer membrane of living bacteria. *Science.* 1997;276:1261-1264.

73. Reife RA, Shapiro RA, Bamber BA, et al. *Porphyromonas gingivalis* lipopolysaccharide is poorly recognized by molecular components of innate host defense in a mouse model of early inflammation. *Infect Immun.* 1995;63:4686-4694.

74. Miller SI, Ernst RK, Bader MW. LPS, TLR4 and infectious disease diversity. *Nat Rev Microbiol.* 2005;3:36-46.

75. Poltorak A, He X, Smirnova I, et al. Defective LPS signaling in C3H/HeJ and C57BL/10ScCr mice: mutations in Tlr4 gene. *Science.* 1998;282:2085-2088.

76. Ashkar AA, Mossman KL, Coombes BK, et al. FimH adhesin of type 1 fimbriae is a potent inducer of innate antimicrobial responses which requires TLR4 and type 1 interferon signalling. *PLoS Pathog.* 2008;4:e1000233.

77. Agnese DM, Calvano JE, Hahm SJ, et al. Human toll-like receptor 4 mutations but not CD14 polymorphisms are associated with an increased risk of gram-negative infections. *J Infect Dis.* 2002;186:1522-1525.

78. Faber J, Henninger N, Finn A, et al. A Toll-like receptor 4 variant is associated with fatal outcome in children with invasive meningococcal disease. *Acta Paediatr.* 2008.

79. Pluschke G, Mayden J, Achtman M, et al. Role of the capsule and the O antigen in resistance of O18:K1 *Escherichia coli* to complement-mediated killing. *Infect Immun.* 1983;42: 907-913.

80. Zinner SH, McCabe WR. Effects of IgM and IgG antibody in patients with bacteremia due to gram-negative bacilli. *J Infect Dis.* 1976;133:37-45.

81. Neter E, Westphal O, Lüderitz O, et al. Demonstration of antibodies against enteropathogenic *Escherichia coli* in sera of children of various ages. *Pediatrics.* 1955;16:801-808.

82. Cohen D, Green MS, Block C, et al. Prospective-study of the association between serum antibodies to lipopolysaccharide O-antigen and the attack rate of shigellosis. *J Clin Microbiol.* 1991;29:386-389.

83. Cohen D, Green MS, Block C, et al. Serum antibodies to lipopolysaccharide and natural immunity to shigellosis in an Israeli military population. *J Infect Dis.* 1988;157:1068-1071.

84. Horwitz MA, Silverstein SC. Influence of the *Escherichia coli* capsule on complement fixation and on phagocytosis and killing by human phagocytes. *J Clin Invest.* 1980;65:82-94.

85. Cross AS, Kim KS, Wright DC, et al. Role of lipopolysaccharide and capsule in the serum resistance of bacteremic strains of *Escherichia coli. J Infect Dis.* 1986;154:497-503.

86. Russo TA, Moffitt MC, Hammer CH, et al. TnphoA-mediated disruption of K54 capsular polysaccharide genes in *Escherichia coli* confers serum sensitivity. *Infect Immun.* 1993;61: 3578-3582.

87. Hoffman JA, Wass C, Stins MF, et al. The capsule supports survival but not traversal of *Escherichia coli* K1 across the blood-brain barrier. *Infect Immun.* 1999;67:3566-3570.

88. Buckles EL, Wang X, Lane MC, et al. The role of K2 capsule in *Escherichia coli* urinary tract infection and serum resistance. *J Infect Dis.* 2009; In Press.

89. Schneider G, Dobrindt U, Bruggemann H, et al. The pathogenicity island-associated K15 capsule determinant exhibits a novel genetic structure and correlates with virulence in uropathogenic *Escherichia coli* strain 536. *Infect Immun.* 2004;72: 5993-6001.

90. Struve C, Krogfelt KA. Role of capsule in *Klebsiella pneumoniae* virulence: lack of correlation between in vitro and in vivo studies. *FEMS Microbiol Lett.* 2003;218:149-154.

91. Russo TA, Liang Y, Cross AS. The presence of K54 capsular polysaccharide increases the pathogenicity of *Escherichia coli* in vivo. *J Infect Dis.* 1994;169:112-118.

92. Day WA, Maurelli AT. *Shigella* and enteroinvasive *Escherichia coli*: paradigms for pathogen evolution and host-parasite interactions. In: Donnenberg MS, ed. Escherichia coli: *Virulence Mechanisms of a Versatile Pathogen.* San Diego: Academic Press; 2002:209-237.

93. Girón JA, Donnenberg MS, Martin WC, et al. Distribution of the bundle-forming pilus structural gene (*bfpA*) among enteropathogenic *Escherichia coli. J Infect Dis.* 1993;168:1037-1041.

94. Levine MM, Nataro JP, Karch H, et al. The diarrheal response of humans to some classic serotypes of enteropathogenic *Escherichia coli* is dependent on a plasmid encoding an enteroadhesiveness factor. *J Infect Dis.* 1985;152:550-559.

95. Bauer ME, Welch RA. Characterization of an RTX toxin from enterohemorrhagic *Escherichia coli* O157:H7. *Infect Immun.* 1996;64:167-175.

96. Schmidt H, Kernbach C, Karch H. Analysis of the EHEC *hly* operon and its location in the physical map of the large plasmid of enterohaemorrhagic *Escherichia coli* O157:H7. *Microbiology.* 1996;142:907-914.

97. Leverstein-van Hall MA, Blok HEM, Donders AR, et al. Multidrug resistance among Enterobacteriaceae is strongly associated with the presence of integrins and is independent of species or isolate origin. *J Infect Dis.* 2003;187:251-259.

98. Shulman ST, Friedmann HC, Sims RH. Theodor Escherich: the first pediatric infectious diseases physician? *Clin Infect Dis.* 2007;45:1025-1029.

99. Rasko DA, Rosovitz MJ, Myers GS, et al. The pangenome structure of *Escherichia coli*: comparative genomic analysis of *E. coli* commensal and pathogenic isolates. *J Bacteriol.* 2008;190: 6881-6893.

100. Johnson JR. Virulence factors in *Escherichia coli* urinary tract infection. *Clin Microbiol Rev.* 1991;4:80-128.

101. Donnenberg MS, Welch RA. Virulence determinants of uropathogenic *Escherichia coli.* In: Mobley HLT, Warren JW, eds. *Urinary Tract Infections: Molecular Pathogenesis and Clinical Management.* Washington, DC: ASM Press; 1996:135-174.

102. Kunin CM, Hua TH, Krishnan C, et al. Isolation of a nicotinamide-requiring clone of *Escherichia coli* O18:K1:H7 from women with acute cystitis: resemblance to strains found in neonatal meningitis. *Clin Infect Dis.* 1993;16:412-416.

103. Manges AR, Johnson JR, Foxman B, et al. Widespread distribution of urinary tract infections caused by a multidrug-resistant *Escherichia coli* clonal group. *N Engl J Med.* 2001;345: 1007-1013.

104. Phillips I, Eykyn S, King A, et al. Epidemic multiresistant *Escherichia coli* infection in West Lambeth health district. *Lancet.* 1988;1:1038-1041.

105. Tullus K, Hörlin K, Svenson SB, et al. Epidemic outbreaks of acute pyelonephritis caused by nosocomial spread of P fimbriated *Escherichia coli* in children. *J Infect Dis.* 1984;150:728-736.

106. Johnson JR, Stapleton AE, Russo TA, et al. Characteristics and prevalence within serogroup O4 of a J96-like clonal group of uropathogenic *Escherichia coli* O4:H5 containing the class I and class III alleles of *papG. Infect Immun.* 1997;65:2153-2159.

107. Johnson JR, O'Bryan TT, Delavari P, et al. Clonal relationships and extended virulence genotypes among *Escherichia coli* isolates from women with a first or recurrent episode of cystitis. *J Infect Dis.* 2001;183:1508-1517.

108. Zhang LX, Foxman B, Tallman P, et al. Distribution of *drb* genes coding for Dr binding adhesins among uropathogenic and fecal *Escherichia coli* isolates and identification of new subtypes. *Infect Immun.* 1997;65:2011-2018.

109. Korhonen TK, Valtonen MV, Parkkinen J, et al. Serotypes, hemolysin production, and receptor recognition of *Escherichia coli* strains associated with neonatal sepsis and meningitis. *Infect Immun.* 1985;48:486-491.

110. Johnson JR, Russo TA. Uropathogenic *Escherichia coli* as agents of diverse non-urinary tract extraintestinal infections. *J Infect Dis.* 2002;186:859-864.

111. Russo TA, Johnson JR. Proposal for a new inclusive designation for extraintestinal pathogenic isolates of *Escherichia coli*: ExPEC. *J Infect Dis.* 2000;181:1753-1754.

112. Bidet P, Mahjoub-Messai F, Blanco J, et al. Combined multilocus sequence typing and O serogrouping distinguishes *Escherichia coli* subtypes associated with infant urosepsis and/or meningitis. *J Infect Dis.* 2007;196:297-303.

113. Benton J, Chawla J, Parry S, et al. Virulence factors in *Escherichia coli* from urinary tract infections in patients with spinal injuries. *J Hosp Infect.* 1992;22:117-127.

114. Johnson JR, Roberts PL, Stamm WE. P fimbriae and other virulence factors in *Escherichia coli* urosepsis: association with patients' characteristics. *J Infect Dis.* 1987;156:225-229.

115. Warren JW. Clinical presentations and epidemiology of urinary tract infections. In: Mobley HLT, Warren JW, eds. *Urinary Tract Infections: Molecular Pathogenesis and Clinical Management.* Washington, DC: ASM Press; 1996:3-27.

116. Wang MC, Tseng CC, Chen CY, et al. The role of bacterial virulence and host factors in patients with *Escherichia coli* bacteremia who have acute cholangitis or upper urinary tract infection. *Clin Infect Dis.* 2002;35:1161-1166.

117. Mobley HLT, Green DM, Trifillis AL, et al. Pyelonephritogenic *Escherichia coli* and killing of cultured human renal proximal tubular epithelial cells: role of hemolysin in some strains. *Infect Immun.* 1990;58:1281-1289.

118. Johnson DE, Russell RG. Animal models of urinary tract infection. In: Mobley HLT, Warren JW, eds. *Urinary Tract Infections: Molecular Pathogenesis and Clinical Management.* Washington, DC: ASM Press; 1996:377-403.

119. Johnson DE, Lockatell CV, Russell RG, et al. Comparison of *Escherichia coli* strains recovered from human cystitis and pyelonephritis infections in transurethrally challenged mice. *Infect Immun.* 1998;66:3059-3065.

120. Langermann S, Mollby R, Burlein JE, et al. Vaccination with FimH adhesin protects cynomolgus monkeys from colonization and infection by uropathogenic *Escherichia coli. J Infect Dis.* 2000;181:774-778.

121. Roberts JA, Kaack B, Källenius G, et al. Receptors for pyelonephritogenic *Escherichia coli* in primates. *J Urol.* 1984;131: 163-168.

122. Gunther NW, Snyder JA, Lockatell V, et al. Assessment of virulence of uropathogenic *Escherichia coli* type 1 fimbrial mutants in which the invertible element is phase-locked on or off. *Infect Immun.* 2002;70:3344-3354.
123. Wu XR, Sun TT, Medina JJ. In vitro binding of type 1-fimbriated *Escherichia coli* to uroplakins Ia and Ib: relation to urinary tract infections. *Proc Natl Acad Sci U S A.* 1996;93:9630-9635.
124. Mulvey MA, Lopez-Boado YS, Wilson CL, et al. Induction and evasion of host defenses by type 1-piliated uropathogenic *Escherichia coli. Science.* 1998;282:1494-1497.
125. Gunther NW, Lockatell V, Johnson DE, et al. In vivo dynamics of type 1 fimbria regulation in uropathogenic *Escherichia coli* during experimental urinary tract infection. *Infect Immun.* 2001;69:2838-2846.
126. Lim JK, Gunther NW, Zhao H, et al. In vivo phase variation of *Escherichia coli* type 1 fimbrial genes in women with urinary tract infection. *Infect Immun.* 1998;66:3303-3310.
127. Johanson I, Lindstedt R, Svanborg C. Roles of the *pap*- and *prs*-encoded adhesins in *Escherichia coli* adherence to human uroepithelial cells. *Infect Immun.* 1992;60:3416-3422.
128. Korhonen TK, Virkola R, Holthofer H. Localization of binding sites for purified *Escherichia coli* P fimbriae in the human kidney. *Infect Immun.* 1986;54:328-332.
129. Roberts JA, Marklund B-I, Ilver D, et al. The Gal(α1-4)Gal-specific tip adhesin of *Escherichia coli* P-fimbriae is needed for pyelonephritis to occur in the normal urinary tract. *Proc Natl Acad Sci U S A.* 1994;91:11889-11893.
130. Buckles EL, Bahrani-Mougeot FK, Molina A, et al. Identification and characterization of a novel uropathogenic *Escherichia coli*-associated fimbrial gene cluster. *Infect Immun.* 2004;72:3890-3901.
131. Brzuszkiewicz E, Brüggemann H, Liesegang H, et al. How to become a uropathogen: comparative genomic analysis of extraintestinal pathogenic *Escherichia coli* strains. *Proc Natl Acad Sci U S A.* 2006;103:12879-12884.
132. Rendón MA, Saldaña Z, Erdem AL, et al. Commensal and pathogenic *Escherichia coli* use a common pilus adherence factor for epithelial cell colonization. *Proc Natl Acad Sci U S A.* 2007;104:10637-10642.
133. Rippere-Lampe KE, O'Brien AD, Conran R, et al. Mutation of the gene encoding cytotoxic necrotizing factor type 1 (cnf_1) attenuates the virulence of uropathogenic *Escherichia coli. Infect Immun.* 2001;69:3954-3964.
134. Russo TA, Brown JJ, Jodush ST, et al. The O4 specific antigen moiety of lipopolysaccharide but not the K54 group 2 capsule is important for urovirulence of an extraintestinal isolate of *Escherichia coli. Infect Immun.* 1996;64:2343-2348.
135. Bahrani-Mougeot FK, Buckles EL, Lockatell CV, et al. Type-1 fimbriae and extracellular polysaccharides are preeminent uropathogenic *Escherichia coli* virulence determinants in the murine urinary tract. *Mol Microbiol.* 2002;45:1079-1093.
136. Nagy G, Dobrindt U, Schneider G, et al. Loss of regulatory protein RfaH attenuates virulence of uropathogenic *Escherichia coli. Infect Immun.* 2002;70:4406-4413.
137. Buckles EL, Wang X, Lockatell CV, et al. PhoU enhances the ability of extraintestinal pathogenic *Escherichia coli* strain CFT073 to colonize the murine urinary tract. *Microbiology.* 2006;152:153-160.
138. Kim KS, Itabashi H, Gemski P, et al. The K1 capsule is the critical determinant in the development of *Escherichia coli* meningitis in the rat. *J Clin Invest.* 1992;90:897-905.
139. Siitonen A, Takala A, Ratiner YA, et al. Invasive *Escherichia coli* infections in children: bacterial characteristics in different age groups and clinical entities. *Pediatr Infect Dis J.* 1993;12:606-612.
140. Korhonen TK, Parkkinen J, Hacker J, et al. Binding of *Escherichia coli* S fimbriae to human kidney epithelium. *Infect Immun.* 1986;54:322-327.
141. Parkkinen J, Rogers GN, Korhonen T, et al. Identification of the O-linked sialyloligosaccharides of glycophorin A as the erythrocyte receptors for S-fimbriated *Escherichia coli. Infect Immun.* 1986;54:37-42.
142. Parkkinen J, Korhonen TK, Pere A, et al. Binding sites in the rat brain for *Escherichia coli* S fimbriae associated with neonatal meningitis. *J Clin Invest.* 1988;81:860-865.
143. Johnson JR, Oswald E, O'Bryan TT, et al. Phylogenetic distribution of virulence-associated genes among *Escherichia coli* isolates associated with neonatal bacterial meningitis in the Netherlands. *J Infect Dis.* 2002;185:774-784.
144. Blum G, Falbo V, Caprioli A, et al. Gene clusters encoding the cytotoxic necrotizing factor type 1, Prs-fimbriae and α-hemolysin form the pathogenicity island II of the uropathogenic *Escherichia coli* strain J96. *FEMS Microbiol Lett.* 1995;126:189-196.
145. Falbo V, Famiglietti M, Caprioli A. Gene block encoding production of cytotoxic necrotizing factor 1 and hemolysin in *Escherichia coli* isolates from extraintestinal infections. *Infect Immun.* 1992;60:2182-2187.
146. Schmidt G, Sehr P, Wilm M, et al. Gln 63 of Rho is deamidated by *Escherichia coli* cytotoxic necrotizing factor-1. *Nature.* 1997;387:725-729.
147. Badger JL, Wass CA, Weissman SJ, et al. Application of signature-tagged mutagenesis for identification of *Escherichia coli* K1 genes that contribute to invasion of human brain microvascular endothelial cells. *Infect Immun.* 2000;68:5056-5061.
148. Badger JL, Wass CA, Kim KS. Identification of *Escherichia coli* K1 genes contributing to human brain microvascular endothelial cell invasion by differential fluorescence induction. *Mol Microbiol.* 2000;36:174-182.
149. Johnson JR, Delavari P, O'Bryan TT. *Escherichia coli* O18:K1:H7 isolates from patients with acute cystitis and neonatal meningitis exhibit common phylogenetic origins and virulence factor profiles. *J Infect Dis.* 2001;183:425-434.
150. Nataro JP, Kaper JB. Diarrheagenic *Escherichia coli. Clin Microbiol Rev.* 1998;11:142-201.
151. Ericsson CD, DuPont HL. Travelers' diarrhea: approaches to prevention and treatment. *Clin Infect Dis.* 1993;16:616-626.
152. Beatty ME, Adcock PM, Smith SW, et al. Epidemic diarrhea due to enterotoxigenic *Escherichia coli. Clin Infect Dis.* 2006;42:329-334.
153. Elsinghorst EA, Weitz JA. Epithelial cell invasion and adherence directed by the enterotoxigenic *Escherichia coli tib* locus is associated with a 104-kilodalton outer membrane protein. *Infect Immun.* 1994;62:3463-3471.
154. Fleckenstein JM, Lindler LE, Elsinghorst EA, et al. Identification of a gene within a pathogenicity island of enterotoxigenic *Escherichia coli* H10407 required for maximal secretion of the heat-labile enterotoxin. *Infect Immun.* 2000;68:2766-2774.
155. Mammarappallil JG, Elsinghorst EA. Epithelial cell adherence mediated by the enterotoxigenic *Escherichia coli* tia protein. *Infect Immun.* 2000;68:6595-6601.
156. Tauschek M, Gorrell RJ, Strugnell RA, et al. Identification of a protein secretory pathway for the secretion of heat-labile enterotoxin by an enterotoxigenic strain of *Escherichia coli. Proc Natl Acad Sci U S A.* 2002;99:7066-7071.
157. Elsinghorst EA. Enterotoxigenic *Escherichia coli.* In: Donnenberg MS, ed. *Escherichia coli: Virulence Mechanisms of a Versatile Pathogen.* San Diego: Academic Press; 2002:155-187.
158. Steinsland H, Valentiner-Branth P, Perch M, et al. Enterotoxigenic *Escherichia coli* infections and diarrhea in a cohort of young children in Guinea-Bissau. *J Infect Dis.* 2002;186:1740-1747.
159. Levine MM, Nalin DR, Hoover DL, et al. Immunity to enterotoxigenic *Escherichia coli. Infect Immun.* 1979;23:729-736.
160. Roy K, Hilliard GM, Hamilton DJ, et al. Enterotoxigenic *Escherichia coli* EtpA mediates adhesion between flagella and host cells. *Nature.* 2008.
161. Roy K, Hamilton D, Allen KP, et al. The EtpA exoprotein of enterotoxigenic *Escherichia coli* promotes intestinal colonization and is a protective antigen in an experimental model of murine infection. *Infect Immun.* 2008;76:2106-2112.
162. Sixma TK, Pronk SE, Kalk KH, et al. Crystal structure of a cholera toxin-related heat-labile enterotoxin from *E. coli. Nature.* 1991;351:371-377.
163. Forte LR, Eber SL, Turner JT, et al. Guanylin stimulation of Cl^- secretion in human intestinal T_{84} cells via cyclic guanosine monophosphate. *J Clin Invest.* 1993;91:2423-2428.
164. Field M. Intestinal ion transport and the pathophysiology of diarrhea. *J Clin Invest.* 2003;111:931-943.
165. DuPont HL, Ericsson CD. Drug therapy: prevention and treatment of traveler's diarrhea. *N Engl J Med.* 1993;328:1821-1827.
166. Adachi JA, Ostrosky-Zeichner L, DuPont HL, et al. Empirical antimicrobial therapy for traveler's diarrhea. *Clin Infect Dis.* 2000;31:1079-1083.
167. Adachi JA, Ericsson CD, Jiang ZD, et al. Azithromycin found to be comparable to levofloxacin for the treatment of US travelers with acute diarrhea acquired in Mexico. *Clin Infect Dis.* 2003;37:1165-1171.
168. DuPont HL, Jiang ZD, Ericsson CD, et al. Rifaximin versus ciprofloxacin for the treatment of traveler's diarrhea: a randomized, double-blind clinical trial. *Clin Infect Dis.* 2001;33:1807-1815.
169. Kaper JB. Defining EPEC. *Rev Microbiol Sao Paulo.* 1996;27(Suppl 1):130-133.
170. Cravioto A, Gross RJ, Scotland SM, et al. An adhesive factor found in strains of *Escherichia coli* belonging to the traditional infantile enteropathogenic serotypes. *Curr Microbiol.* 1979;3:95-99.
171. Scaletsky ICA, Silva MLM, Trabulsi LR. Distinctive patterns of adherence of enteropathogenic *Escherichia coli* to HeLa cells. *Infect Immun.* 1984;45:534-536.
172. Bray J. Isolation of antigenically homogeneous strains of *Bact. coli neapolitanum* from summer diarrhoea of infants. *J Pathol Bacteriol.* 1945;57:239-247.
173. Kain KC, Barteluk RL, Kelly MT, et al. Etiology of childhood diarrhea in Beijing, China. *J Clin Microbiol.* 1991;29:90-95.
174. Gomes TAT, Rassi V, Macdonald KL, et al. Enteropathogens associated with acute diarrheal disease in urban infants in São Paulo, Brazil. *J Infect Dis.* 1991;164:331-337.
175. Gunzburg ST, Chang BJ, Burke V, et al. Virulence factors of enteric *Escherichia coli* in young Aboriginal children in north-west Australia. *Epidemiol Infect.* 1992;109:283-289.
176. Valentiner-Branth P, Steinsland H, Fischer TK, et al. Cohort study of Guinean children: incidence, pathogenicity, conferred protection, and attributable risk for enteropathogens during the first 2 years of life. *J Clin Microbiol.* 2003;41:4238-4245.
177. Germani Y, Begaud E, Duval P, et al. Prevalence of enteropathogenic, enteroaggregative, and diffusely adherent *Escherichia coli* among isolates from children with diarrhea in New Caledonia. *J Infect Dis.* 1996;174:1124-1126.
178. Albert MJ, Faruque SM, Faruque ASG, et al. Controlled study of *Escherichia coli* diarrheal infections in Bangladeshi children. *J Clin Microbiol.* 1995;33:973-977.
179. Afset JE, Bevanger L, Romundstad P, et al. Association of atypical enteropathogenic *Escherichia coli* (EPEC) with prolonged diarrhoea. *J Med Microbiol.* 2004;53:1137-1144.
180. Cohen MB, Nataro JP, Bernstein DI, et al. Prevalence of diarrheagenic *Escherichia coli* in acute childhood enteritis: a prospective controlled study. *J Pediatr.* 2005;146:54-61.
181. Robins-Browne RM, Bordun AM, Tauschek M, et al. *Escherichia coli* and community-acquired gastroenteritis, Melbourne, Australia. *Emerg Infect Dis.* 2004;10:1797-1805.
182. Paulozzi LJ, Johnson KE, Kamahele LM, et al. Diarrhea associated with adherent enteropathogenic *Escherichia coli* in an infant and toddler center, Seattle, Washington. *Pediatrics.* 1986;77:296-300.
183. Wu S-X, Peng R-Q. Studies on an outbreak of neonatal diarrhea caused by EPEC 0127:H6 with plasmid analysis restriction analysis and outer membrane protein determination. *Acta Paediatr Scand.* 1992;81:217-221.
184. Blake PA, Ramos S, Macdonald KL, et al. Pathogen-specific risk factors and protective factors for acute diarrheal disease in urban Brazilian infants. *J Infect Dis.* 1993;167:627-632.
185. Thorén A, Stintzing G, Tufvesson B, et al. Aetiology and clinical features of severe infantile diarrhoea in Addis Ababa, Ethiopia. *J Trop Pediatr.* 1982;28:127-131.
186. Bower JR, Congeni BL, Cleary TG, et al. *Escherichia coli* O114: nonmotile as a pathogen in an outbreak of severe diarrhea associated with a day care center. *J Infect Dis.* 1989;160:243-247.
187. Clausen CR, Christie DL. Chronic diarrhea in infants caused by adherent enteropathogenic *Escherichia coli. J Pediatr.* 1982;100:358-361.
188. Rothbaum R, McAdams AJ, Giannella R, et al. A clinicopathological study of enterocyte-adherent *Escherichia coli*: a cause of protracted diarrhea in infants. *Gastroenterol.* 1982;83:441-454.
189. Staley TE, Jones EW, Corley LD. Attachment and penetration of *Escherichia coli* into intestinal epithelium of the ileum in newborn pigs. *Am J Pathol.* 1969;56:371-392.
190. Moon HW, Whipp SC, Argenzio RA, et al. Attaching and effacing activities of rabbit and human enteropathogenic *Escherichia coli* in pig and rabbit intestines. *Infect Immun.* 1983;41:1340-1351.
191. McDaniel TK, Jarvis KG, Donnenberg MS, et al. A genetic locus of enterocyte effacement conserved among diverse enterobacterial pathogens. *Proc Natl Acad Sci U S A.* 1995;92:1664-1668.
192. McDaniel TK, Kaper JB. A cloned pathogenicity island from enteropathogenic *Escherichia coli* confers the attaching and effacing phenotype on K-12 *E. coli. Mol Microbiol.* 1997;23:399-407.
193. Deng W, Puente JL, Gruenheid S, et al. Dissecting virulence: systematic and functional analyses of a pathogenicity island. *Proc Natl Acad Sci U S A.* 2004;101:3597-3602.
194. Iguchi A, Thomson NR, Ogura Y, et al. Complete genome sequence and comparative genome analysis of enteropathogenic *Escherichia coli* O127:H6 strain E2348/69. *J Bacteriol.* 2009;191:347-354.
195. Knutton S, Rosenshine I, Pallen MJ, et al. A novel EspA-associated surface organelle of enteropathogenic *Escherichia coli* involved in protein translocation into epithelial cells. *EMBO J.* 1998;17:2166-2176.
196. Tacket CO, Sztein MB, Losonsky G, et al. Role of EspB in experimental human enteropathogenic *Escherichia coli* infection. *Infect Immun.* 2000;68:3689-3695.
197. Donnenberg MS, Tacket CO, James SP, et al. The role of the *eaeA* gene in experimental enteropathogenic *Escherichia coli* infection. *J Clin Invest.* 1993;92:1412-1417.
198. Kalman D, Weiner OD, Goosney DL, et al. Enteropathogenic *E. coli* acts through WASP and Arp2/3 complex to form actin pedestals. *Nat Cell Biol.* 1999;1:389-391.
199. Campellone KG, Giese A, Tipper DJ, et al. A tyrosine-phosphorylated 12-amino-acid sequence of enteropathogenic *Escherichia coli* Tir binds the host adaptor protein Nck and is required for Nck localization to actin pedestals. *Mol Microbiol.* 2002;43:1227-1241.
200. Gruenheid S, DeVinney R, Bladt F, et al. Enteropathogenic *E. coli* Tir binds Nck to initiate actin pedestal formation in host cells. *Nat Cell Biol.* 2001;3:856-859.
201. Gomes TAT, Vieira MAM, Wachsmuth IK, et al. Serotype-specific prevalence of *Escherichia coli* strains with EPEC adherence factor genes in infants with and without diarrhea in São Paulo, Brazil. *J Infect Dis.* 1989;160:131-135.
202. Trabulsi LR, Keller R, Gomes TAT. Typical and atypical enteropathogenic *Escherichia coli. Emerg Infect Dis.* 2002;8:508-513.
203. Bieber D, Ramer SW, Wu CY, et al. Type IV pili, transient bacterial aggregates, and virulence of enteropathogenic *Escherichia coli. Science.* 1998;280:2114-2118.
204. Hyland RM, Sun J, Griener TP, et al. The bundling pilin protein of enteropathogenic *Escherichia coli* is an N-acetyllactosamine-specific lectin. *Cell Microbiol.* 2008;10:177-187.
205. Cleary J, Lai L-C, Donnenberg MS, et al. Enteropathogenic *E. coli* (EPEC) adhesion to intestinal epithelial cells: role of bundle-forming pili (BFP), EspA filaments and intimin. *Microbiology.* 2004;150:527-538.
206. Aranda KR, Fagundes-Neto U, Scaletsky IC. Evaluation of multiplex PCRs for diagnosis of infection with diarrheagenic *Escherichia coli* and *Shigella* spp. *J Clin Microbiol.* 2004;42:5849-5853.
207. Giles C, Sangster G, Smith J. Epidemic gastroenteritis of infants in Aberdeen during 1947. *Arch Dis Child.* 1949;24:45-53.

208. Robins-Browne R, Still CS, Miliotis MD, et al. Summer diarrhoea in African infants and children. *Arch Dis Child.* 1980;55:923-928.
209. Taylor J, Powell BW, Wright J. Infantile diarrhea and vomiting: a clinical and bacteriological investigation. *Br Med J.* 1949;2:117-141.
210. Camara LM, Carbonare SB, Silva MLM, et al. Inhibition of enteropathogenic *Escherichia coli* (EPEC) adhesion to HeLa cells by human colostrum: detection of specific sIgA related to EPEC outer-membrane proteins. *Int Arch Allergy Immunol.* 1994; 103:307-310.
211. Cravioto A, Tello A, Villafán H, et al. Inhibition of localized adhesion of enteropathogenic *Escherichia coli* to HEp-2 cells by immunoglobulin and oligosaccharide fractions of human colostrum and breast milk. *J Infect Dis.* 1991;163:1247-1255.
212. Loureiro I, Frankel G, Adu-Bobie J, et al. Human colostrum contains IgA antibodies reactive to enteropathogenic *Escherichia coli* virulence-associated proteins: intimin, BfpA, EspA, and EspB. *J Pediatr Gastroenterol Nutr.* 1998;27:166-171.
213. Noguera-Obenza M, Ochoa TJ, Gomez HF, et al. Human milk secretory antibodies against attaching and effacing *Escherichia coli* antigens. *Emerg Infect Dis.* 2003;9:545-551.
214. Parissi-Crivelli A, Parissi-Crivelli JM, Girón JA. Recognition of enteropathogenic *Escherichia coli* virulence determinants by human colostrum and serum antibodies. *J Clin Microbiol.* 2000;38:2696-2700.
215. Senerwa D, Mutanda LN, Gathuma JM, et al. Antimicrobial resistance of enteropathogenic *Escherichia coli* strains from a nosocomial outbreak in Kenya. *APMIS.* 1991;99:728-734.
216. Thorén A, Wolde-Mariam T, Stintzing G, et al. Antibiotics in the treatment of gastroenteritis caused by enteropathogenic *Escherichia coli. J Infect Dis.* 1980;141:27-31.
217. Antai SP, Anozie SO. Incidence of infantile diarrhoea due to enteropathogenic *Escherichia coli* in Port Harcourt metropolis. *J Appl Bacteriol.* 1987;62:227-229.
218. Vila J, Vargas M, Casals C, et al. Antimicrobial resistance of diarrheagenic *Escherichia coli* isolated from children under the age of 5 years from Ifakara, Tanzania. *Antimicrob Agents Chemother.* 1999;43:3022-3024.
219. Lim YS, Ngan CCL, Tay L. Enteropathogenic *Escherichia coli* as a cause of diarrhoea among children in Singapore. *J Trop Med Hyg.* 1992;95:339-342.
220. Griffin PM, Ostroff SM, Tauxe RV, et al. Illnesses associated with *Escherichia coli* O157:H7 infections: a broad clinical spectrum. *Ann Intern Med.* 1988;109:705-712.
221. Jay MT, Cooley M, Carychao D, et al. *Escherichia coli* O157:H7 in feral swine near spinach fields and cattle, central California coast. *Emerg Infect Dis.* 2007;13:1908-1911.
222. Olsen SJ, Miller G, Breuer T, et al. A waterborne outbreak of *Escherichia coli* O157:H7 infections and hemolytic uremic syndrome: implications for rural water systems. *Emerg Infect Dis.* 2002;8:370-375.
223. Crump JA, Sulka AC, Langer AJ, et al. An outbreak of *Escherichia coli* O157:H7 infections among visitors to a dairy farm. *N Engl J Med.* 2002;347:555-560.
224. Michino H, Araki K, Minami S, et al. Massive outbreak of *Escherichia coli* O157:H7 infection in schoolchildren in Sakai City, Japan, associated with consumption of white radish sprouts. *Am J Epidemiol.* 1999;150:787-796.
225. Bell BP, Goldoft M, Griffin PM, et al. A multistate outbreak of *Escherichia coli* O157:H7-associated bloody diarrhea and hemolytic uremic syndrome from hamburgers: the Washington experience. *JAMA.* 1994;272:1349-1353.
226. Tilden Jr J, Young W, McNamara AM, et al. A new route of transmission for *Escherichia coli*: infection from dry fermented salami. *Am J Public Health.* 1996;86:1142-1145.
227. Griffin PM, Tauxe RV. The epidemiology of infections caused by *Escherichia coli* O157:H7, other enterohemorrhagic *E. coli*, and the associated hemolytic uremic syndrome. *Epidemiol Rev.* 1991;13:60-98.
228. Garg AX, Suri RS, Barrowman N, et al. Long-term renal prognosis of diarrhea-associated hemolytic uremic syndrome—a systematic review, meta-analysis, and meta-regression. *JAMA.* 2003;290:1360-1370.
229. O'Brien AD, Newland JW, Miller SF, et al. Shiga-like toxin-converting phages from *Escherichia coli* strains that cause hemorrhagic colitis or infantile diarrhea. *Science.* 1984;226:694-696.
230. Zhang XP, McDaniel AD, Wolf LE, et al. Quinolone antibiotics induce shiga toxin-encoding bacteriophages, toxin production, and death in mice. *J Infect Dis.* 2000;181:664-670.
231. Jacewicz MS, Mobassaleh M, Gross SK, et al. Pathogenesis of *Shigella* diarrhea: XVII. A mammalian cell membrane glycolipid, Gb3, is required but not sufficient to confer sensitivity to Shiga toxin. *J Infect Dis.* 1994;169:538-546.
232. Sandvig K, Garred O, Prydz K, et al. Retrograde transport of endocytosed Shiga toxin to the endoplasmic reticulum. *Nature.* 1992;358:510-512.
233. Te Loo DM, van Hinsbergh VW, van den Heuvel LP, et al. Detection of verocytotoxin bound to circulating polymorphonuclear leukocytes of patients with hemolytic uremic syndrome. *J Am Soc Nephrol.* 2001;12:800-806.
234. Yoshida T, Fukada M, Koide N, et al. Primary cultures of human endothelial cells are susceptible to low doses of Shiga toxins and undergo apoptosis. *J Infect Dis.* 1999;180:2048-2052.
235. Chandler WL, Jelacic S, Boster DR, et al. Prothrombotic coagulation abnormalities preceding the hemolytic-uremic syndrome. *N Engl J Med.* 2002;346:23-32.
236. Perna NT, Mayhew GF, Pósfai G, et al. Molecular evolution of a pathogenicity island from enterohemorrhagic *Escherichia coli* O157:H7. *Infect Immun.* 1998;66:3810-3817.
237. Donnenberg MS, Tzipori S, McKee M, et al. The role of the *eae* gene of enterohemorrhagic *Escherichia coli* in intimate attachment in vitro and in a porcine model. *J Clin Invest.* 1993;92:1418-1424.
238. Tzipori S, Gunzer F, Donnenberg MS, et al. The role of the *eaeA* gene in diarrhea and neurological complications in a gnotobiotic piglet model of enterohemorrhagic *Escherichia coli* infection. *Infect Immun.* 1995;63:3621-3627.
239. Wong CS, Jelacic S, Habeeb RL, et al. The risk of the hemolytic-uremic syndrome after antibiotic treatment of *Escherichia coli* O157:H7 infections. *N Engl J Med.* 2000;342:1930-1936.
240. Mukherjee J, Chios K, Fishwild D, et al. Human Stx2-specific monoclonal antibodies prevent systemic complications of *Escherichia coli* O157:H7 infection. *Infect Immun.* 2002;70:612-619.
241. Nishikawa K, Matsuoka K, Kita E, et al. A therapeutic agent with oriented carbohydrates for treatment of infections by Shiga toxin-producing *Escherichia coli* O157:H7. *Proc Natl Acad Sci U S A.* 2002;99:7669-7674.
242. Armstrong GD, Rowe PC, Goodyer P, et al. A phase I study of chemically synthesized verotoxin (Shiga-like toxin) Pk-trisaccharide receptors attached to chromosorb for preventing hemolytic-uremic syndrome. *J Infect Dis.* 1995;171:1042-1045.
243. Mulvey GL, Marcato P, Kitov PI, et al. Assessment in mice of the therapeutic potential of tailored, multivalent Shiga toxin carbohydrate ligands. *J Infect Dis.* 2003;187:640-649.
244. Trachtman H, Cnaan A, Christen E, et al. Effect of an oral Shiga toxin-binding agent on diarrhea-associated hemolytic uremic syndrome in children—a randomized controlled trial. *JAMA.* 2003;290:1337-1344.
245. Ahmed A, Li J, Shiloach Y, et al. Safety and immunogenicity of *Escherichia coli* O157 O-specific polysaccharide conjugate vaccine in 2-5-year-old children. *J Infect Dis.* 2006;193:515-521.
246. Mayr UB, Haller C, Haidinger W, et al. Bacterial ghosts as an oral vaccine: a single dose of *Escherichia coli* O157:H7 bacterial ghosts protects mice against lethal challenge. *Infect Immun.* 2005;73:4810-4817.
247. Potter AA, Klashinsky S, Li Y, et al. Decreased shedding of *Escherichia coli* O157:H7 by cattle following vaccination with type III secreted proteins. *Vaccine.* 2004;22:362-369.
248. Dean-Nystrom EA, Gansheroff LJ, Mills M, et al. Vaccination of pregnant dams with intimin O157 protects suckling piglets from *Escherichia coli* O157:H7 infection. *Infect Immun.* 2002;70:2414-2418.
249. Konadu E, Donohue-Rolfe A, Calderwood SB, et al. Syntheses and immunologic properties of *Escherichia coli* O157 O-specific polysaccharide and Shiga toxin 1 B subunit conjugates in mice. *Infect Immun.* 1999;67:6191-6193.
250. Nataro JP, Kaper JB, Robins-Browne R, et al. Patterns of adherence of diarrheagenic *Escherichia coli* to HEp-2 cells. *Pediatr Infect Dis J.* 1987;6:829-831.
251. Yamamoto T, Koyama Y, Matsumoto M, et al. Localized, aggregative, and diffuse adherence to HeLa cells, plastic, and human small intestines by *Escherichia coli* isolated from patients with diarrhea. *J Infect Dis.* 1992;166:1295-1310.
252. Nataro JP, Hicks S, Phillips AD, et al. T84 cells in culture as a model for enteroaggregative *Escherichia coli* pathogenesis. *Infect Immun.* 1996;64:4761-4768.
253. Huang DB, Nataro JP, DuPont HL, et al. Enteroaggregative *Escherichia coli* is a cause of acute diarrheal illness: a meta-analysis. *Clin Infect Dis.* 2006;43:556-563.
254. Nataro JP, Yikang D, Cookson S, et al. Heterogeneity of enteroaggregative *Escherichia coli* virulence demonstrated in volunteers. *J Infect Dis.* 1995;171:465-468.
255. Okeke IN, Lamikanra A, Czeczulin J, et al. Heterogeneous virulence of enteroaggregative *Escherichia coli* strains isolated from children in southwest Nigeria. *J Infect Dis.* 2000;181:252-260.
256. Czeczulin JR, Whittam TS, Henderson IR, et al. Phylogenetic analysis of enteroaggregative and diffusely adherent *Escherichia coli. Infect Immun.* 1999;67:2692-2699.
257. Bhatnagar S, Bhan MK, Sommerfelt H, et al. Enteroaggregative *Escherichia coli* may be a new pathogen causing acute and persistent diarrhea. *Scand J Infect Dis.* 1993;25:579-583.
258. Wanke CA, Schorling JB, Barrett LJ, et al. Potential role of adherence traits of *Escherichia coli* in persistent diarrhea in an urban Brazilian slum. *Pediatr Infect Dis J.* 1991;10:746-751.
259. Bhan MK, Raj P, Levine MM, et al. Enteroaggregative *Escherichia coli* associated with persistent diarrhea in a cohort of rural children in India. *J Infect Dis.* 1989;159:1061-1064.
260. Adachi JA, Ericsson CD, Jiang ZD, et al. Natural history of enteroaggregative and enterotoxigenic *Escherichia coli* infection among US travelers to Guadalajara, Mexico. *J Infect Dis.* 2002;185:1681-1683.
261. Adachi JA, Jiang ZD, Mathewson JJ, et al. Enteroaggregative *Escherichia coli* as a major etiologic agent in traveler's diarrhea in 3 regions of the world. *Clin Infect Dis.* 2001;32:1706-1709.
262. Gassama-Sow A, Sow PS, Guèye M, et al. Characterization of pathogenic *Escherichia coli* in human immunodeficiency virus-related diarrhea in Senegal. *J Infect Dis.* 2004;189:75-78.
263. Durrer P, Zbinden R, Fleisch F, et al. Intestinal infection due to enteroaggregative *Escherichia coli* among human immunodeficiency virus-infected persons. *J Infect Dis.* 2000;182:1540-1544.
264. Wanke CA, Mayer H, Weber R, et al. Enteroaggregative *Escherichia coli* as a potential cause of diarrheal disease in adults infected with human immunodeficiency virus. *J Infect Dis.* 1998;178:185-190.
265. Huppertz HI, Rutkowski S, Aleksic S, et al. Acute and chronic diarrhoea and abdominal colic associated with enteroaggregative *Escherichia coli* in young children living in western Europe. *Lancet.* 1997;349:1660-1662.
266. Cravioto A, Tello A, Navarro A, et al. Association of *Escherichia coli* HEp-2 adherence patterns with type and duration of diarrhoea. *Lancet.* 1991;337:262-264.
267. Glandt M, Adachi JA, Mathewson JJ, et al. Enteroaggregative *Escherichia coli* as a cause of traveler's diarrhea: clinical response to ciprofloxacin. *Clin Infect Dis.* 1999;29:335-338.
268. Steiner TS, Lima AAM, Nataro JP, et al. Enteroaggregative *Escherichia coli* produce intestinal inflammation and growth impairment and cause interleukin-8 release from intestinal epithelial cells. *J Infect Dis.* 1998;177:88-96.
269. Nataro JP, Deng Y, Maneval DR, et al. Aggregative adherence fimbriae I of enteroaggregative *Escherichia coli* mediate adherence to HEp-2 cells and hemagglutination of human erythrocytes. *Infect Immun.* 1992;60:2297-2304.
270. Czeczulin JR, Balepur S, Hicks S, et al. Aggregative adherence fimbria II, a second fimbrial antigen mediating aggregative adherence in enteroaggregative *Escherichia coli. Infect Immun.* 1997;65:4135-4145.
271. Boisen N, Struve C, Scheutz F, et al. New adhesin of enteroaggregative *Escherichia coli* related to the Afa/Dr/AAF family. *Infect Immun.* 2008;76:3281-3292.
272. Sheikh J, Czeczulin JR, Harrington S, et al. A novel dispersin protein in enteroaggregative *Escherichia coli. J Clin Invest.* 2002;110:1329-1337.
273. Savarino SJ, Fasano A, Watson J, et al. Enteroaggregative *Escherichia coli* heat-stable enterotoxin 1 represents another subfamily of *E. coli* heat-stable toxin. *Proc Natl Acad Sci U S A.* 1993;90:3093-3097.
274. Eslava C, Navarro-García F, Czeczulin JR, et al. Pet, an autotransporter enterotoxin from enteroaggregative *Escherichia coli. Infect Immun.* 1998;66:3155-3163.
275. Henderson IR, Hicks S, Navarro-Garcia F, et al. Involvement of the enteroaggregative *Escherichia coli* plasmid-encoded toxin in causing human intestinal damage. *Infect Immun.* 1999;67:5338-5344.
276. Iwanaga M, Song T, Higa N, et al. Enteroaggregative *Escherichia coli*: incidence in Japan and usefulness of the clump-formation test. *J Infect Chemother.* 2002;8:345-348.
277. Albert MJ, Qadri F, Haque A, et al. Bacterial clump formation at the surface of liquid culture as a rapid test for identification of enteroaggregative *Escherichia coli. J Clin Microbiol.* 1993;31:1397-1399.
278. Wanke CA, Gerrior J, Blais V, et al. Successful treatment of diarrheal disease associated with enteroaggregative *Escherichia coli* in adults infected with human immunodeficiency virus. *J Infect Dis.* 1998;178:1369-1372.
279. Yamamoto T, Echeverria P, Yokota T. Drug resistance and adherence to human intestines of enteroaggregative *Escherichia coli. J Infect Dis.* 1992;165:744-749.
280. Maurelli AT, Fernandez RE, Bloch CA, et al. "Black holes" and bacterial pathogenicity: a large genomic deletion that enhances the virulence of *Shigella* spp. and enteroinvasive *Escherichia coli. Proc Natl Acad Sci U S A.* 1998;95:3943-3948.
281. Wirth T, Falush D, Lan R, et al. Sex and virulence in *Escherichia coli*: an evolutionary perspective. *Mol Microbiol.* 2006;60:1136-1151.
282. Martinez MB, Whittam TS, McGraw EA, et al. Clonal relationship among invasive and non-invasive strains of enteroinvasive *Escherichia coli* serogroups. *FEMS Microbiol Lett.* 1999;172:145-151.
283. DuPont HL, Formal SB, Hornick RB, et al. Pathogenesis of *Escherichia coli* diarrhea. *N Engl J Med.* 1971;285:1-9.
284. Gunzburg ST, Chang BJ, Elliott SJ, et al. Diffuse and enteroaggregative patterns of adherence of enteric *Escherichia coli* isolated from aboriginal children from the Kimberley region of Western Australia. *J Infect Dis.* 1993;167:755-758.
285. Levine MM, Ferreccio C, Prado V, et al. Epidemiologic studies of *Escherichia coli* diarrheal infections in a low socioeconomic level peri-urban community in Santiago, Chile. *Am J Epidemiol.* 1993;138:849-869.
286. Girón JA, Jones T, Millán-Velasco F, et al. Diffuse-adhering *Escherichia coli* (DAEC) as a putative cause of diarrhea in Mayan children in Mexico. *J Infect Dis.* 1991;163:507-513.
287. Tacket CO, Moseley SL, Kay B, et al. Challenge studies in volunteers using *Escherichia coli* strains with diffuse adherence to HEp-2 cells. *J Infect Dis.* 1990;162:550-552.
288. Albert MJ, Alam K, Islam M, et al. *Hafnia alvei*, a probable cause of diarrhea in humans. *Infect Immun.* 1991;59:1507-1513.
289. Albert MJ, Faruque SM, Ansaruzzaman M, et al. Sharing of virulence-associated properties at the phenotypic and genetic levels between enteropathogenic *Escherichia coli* and *Hafnia alvei. J Med Microbiol.* 1992;37:310-314.
290. Huys G, Cnockaert M, Janda JM, et al. *Escherichia albertii* sp. nov., a diarrhoeagenic species isolated from stool specimens of Bangladeshi children. *Int J Syst Evol Microbiol.* 2003;53:807-810.
291. Janda JM, Abbott SL, Albert MJ. Prototypal diarrheagenic strains of *Hafnia alvei* are actually members of the genus *Escherichia. J Clin Microbiol.* 1999;37:2399-2401.
292. Hyma KE, Lacher DW, Nelson AM, et al. Evolutionary genetics of a new pathogenic *Escherichia* species: *Escherichia albertii*

and related *Shigella boydii* strains. *J Bacteriol.* 2005;187:619-628.

293. Podschun R, Ullmann U. *Klebsiella spp.* as nosocomial pathogens: epidemiology, taxonomy, typing methods, and pathogenicity factors. *Clin Microbiol Rev.* 1998;11:589-603.

294. Bishara J, Leibovici L, Huminer D, et al. Five-year prospective study of bacteraemic urinary tract infection in a single institution. *Eur J Clin Microbiol Infect Dis.* 1997;16:563-567.

295. Garcia de la Torre M, Romero-Vivas J, Martinez-Beltrán J, et al. *Klebsiella* bacteremia: an analysis of 100 episodes. *Rev Infect Dis.* 1985;7:143-150.

296. Geerdes HF, Ziegler D, Lode H, et al. Septicemia in 980 patients at a University Hospital in Berlin: prospective studies during 4 selected years between 1979 and 1989. *Clin Infect Dis.* 1992;15:991-1002.

297. Carpenter JL. *Klebsiella* pulmonary infections: occurrence at one medical center and review. *Rev Infect Dis.* 1990;12:672-682.

298. Lawlor MS, Hsu J, Rick PD, et al. Identification of *Klebsiella pneumoniae* virulence determinants using an intranasal infection model. *Mol Microbiol.* 2005;58:1054-1073.

299. Livrelli V, De Champs C, Di Martino P, et al. Adhesive properties and antibiotic resistance of *Klebsiella*, *Enterobacter*, and *Serratia* clinical isolates involved in nosocomial infections. *J Clin Microbiol.* 1996;34:1963-1969.

300. Sahly H, Podschun R, Oelschlaeger TA, et al. Capsule impedes adhesion to and invasion of epithelial cells by *Klebsiella pneumoniae*. *Infect Immun.* 2000;68:6744-6749.

301. Lawlor MS, O'Connor C, Miller VL. *Yersinia* bactin is a virulence factor for *Klebsiella pneumoniae* during pulmonary infection. *Infect Immun.* 2007;75:1463-1472.

302. Hæggman S, Löfdahl S, Burman LG. An allelic variant of the chromosomal gene for class A beta-lactamase K2, specific for *Klebsiella pneumoniae*, is the ancestor of SHV-1. *Antimicrob Agents Chemother.* 1997;41:2705-2709.

303. Tumbarello M, Spanu T, Sanguinetti M, et al. Bloodstream infections caused by extended-spectrum-beta-lactamase-producing *Klebsiella pneumoniae*: risk factors, molecular epidemiology, and clinical outcome. *Antimicrob Agents Chemother.* 2006;50:498-504.

304. Andraca R, Edson RS, Kern EB. Rhinoscleroma: a growing concern in the United States? Mayo Clinic experience. *Mayo Clin Proc.* 1993;68:1151-1157.

305. de Pontual L, Ovetchkine P, Rodriguez D, et al. Rhinoscleroma: a French national retrospective study of epidemiological and clinical features. *Clin Infect Dis.* 2008;47:1396-1402.

306. Lenis A, Ruff T, Diaz JA, et al. Rhinoscleroma. *South Med J.* 1988;81:1580-1582.

307. Goldstein EJ, Lewis RP, Martin WJ, et al. Infections caused by *Klebsiella ozaenae*: a changing disease spectrum. *J Clin Microbiol.* 1978;8:413-418.

308. Tang LM, Chen ST. *Klebsiella ozaenae* meningitis: report of two cases and review of the literature. *Infection.* 1994;22:58-61.

309. Högenauer C, Langner C, Beubler E, et al. *Klebsiella oxytoca* as a causative organism of antibiotic-associated hemorrhagic colitis. *N Engl J Med.* 2006;355:2418-2426.

310. Sanders Jr WE, Sanders CC. *Enterobacter* spp.: pathogens poised to flourish at the turn of the century. *Clin Microbiol Rev.* 1997;10:220-241.

311. Bowen AB, Braden CR. Invasive *Enterobacter sakazakii* disease in infants. *Emerg Infect Dis.* 2006;12:1185-1189.

312. Cruz AT, Cazacu AC, Allen CH. *Pantoea agglomerans*, a plant pathogen causing human disease. *J Clin Microbiol.* 2007;45:1989-1992.

313. Keller R, Pedroso MZ, Ritchmann R, et al. Occurrence of virulence-associated properties in *Enterobacter cloacae*. *Infect Immun.* 1998;66:645-649.

314. Townsend S, Hurrell E, Forsythe S. Virulence studies of *Enterobacter sakazakii* isolates associated with a neonatal intensive care unit outbreak. *BMC Microbiol.* 2008;8:64.

315. Korfmann G, Wiedemann B. Genetic control of beta-lactamase production in *Enterobacter cloacae*. *Rev Infect Dis.* 1988;10:793-799.

316. Chow JW, Fine MJ, Shlaes DM, et al. *Enterobacter* bacteremia: clinical features and emergence of antibiotic resistance during therapy [see comments]. *Ann Intern Med.* 1991;115:585-590.

317. Sehdev PS, Donnenberg MS. Arcanum: the 19th-century Italian pharmacist pictured here was the first to characterize what are now known to be bacteria of the genus *Serratia*. *Clin Infect Dis.* 1999;29:770, 925.

318. Yu VL. *Serratia marcescens*: historical perspective and clinical review. *N Engl J Med.* 1979;300:887-893.

319. Hertle R, Schwarz H. *Serratia marcescens* internalization and replication in human bladder epithelial cells. *BMC Infect Dis.* 2004;4:16.

320. Parment PA, Svanborg-Edén C, Chaknis MJ, et al. Hemagglutination (fimbriae) and hydrophobicity in adherence of *Serratia marcescens* to urinary tract epithelium and contact lenses. *Curr Microbiol.* 1992;25:113-118.

321. Hejazi A, Falkiner FR. *Serratia marcescens*. *J Med Microbiol.* 1997;46:903-912.

322. Acar JF. *Serratia marcescens* infections. *Infect Control.* 1986;7:273-278.

323. Mills J, Drew D. *Serratia marcescens* endocarditis: a regional illness associated with intravenous drug abuse. *Ann Intern Med.* 1976;84:29-35.

324. Mahlen SD, Morrow SS, Abdalhamid B, et al. Analyses of *ampC* gene expression in *Serratia marcescens* reveal new regulatory properties. *J Antimicrob Chemother.* 2003;51:791-802.

325. Lipsky BA, Hook EW III, Smith AA, et al. *Citrobacter* infections in humans: experience at the Seattle Veterans Administration Medical Center and a review of the literature. *Rev Infect Dis.* 1980;2:746-760.

326. Shih CC, Chen YC, Chang SC, et al. Bacteremia due to *Citrobacter* species: significance of primary intraabdominal infection. *Clin Infect Dis.* 1996;23:543-549.

327. Samonis G, Karageorgopoulos DE, Kofteridis DP, et al. *Citrobacter* infections in a general hospital: characteristics and outcomes. *Eur J Clin Microbiol Infect Dis.* 2009;28:61-68.

328. Drelichman V, Band JD. Bacteremias due to *Citrobacter diversus* and *Citrobacter freundii*: incidence, risk factors, and clinical outcome. *Arch Intern Med.* 1985;145:1808-1810.

329. Williams WW, Mariano J, Spurrier M, et al. Nosocomial meningitis due to *Citrobacter diversus* in neonates: new aspects of the epidemiology. *J Infect Dis.* 1984;150:229-235.

330. Janda JM, Abbott SL. The genus *Hafnia*: from soup to nuts. *Clin Microbiol Rev.* 2006;19:12-18.

331. Günthard H, Pennekamp A. Clinical significance of extraintestinal *Hafnia alvei* isolates from 61 patients and review of the literature. *Clin Infect Dis.* 1996;22:1040-1045.

332. Ridell J, Siitonen A, Paulin L, et al. *Hafnia alvei* in stool specimens from patients with diarrhea and healthy controls. *J Clin Microbiol.* 1994;32:2335-2337.

333. O'Hara CM, Brenner FW, Miller JM. Classification, identification, and clinical significance of *Proteus*, *Providencia*, and *Morganella*. *Clin Microbiol Rev.* 2000;13:534-546.

334. Fairley KF, Carson NE, Gutch RC, et al. Site of infection in acute urinary-tract infection in general practice. *Lancet.* 1971;2:615-618.

335. Bryan CS, Reynolds KL. Community-acquired bacteremic urinary tract infection: epidemiology and outcome. *J Urol.* 1984;132:490-493.

336. Müller HE. Occurrence and pathogenic role of *Morganella-Proteus-Providencia* group bacteria in human feces. *J Clin Microbiol.* 1986;23:404-405.

337. Li X, Lockatell CV, Johnson DE, et al. Identification of MrpI as the sole recombinase that regulates the phase variation of MR/P fimbria, a bladder colonization factor of uropathogenic *Proteus mirabilis*. *Mol Microbiol.* 2002;45:865-874.

338. Zhao H, Li X, Johnson DE, et al. In vivo phase variation of MR/P fimbrial gene expression in *Proteus mirabilis* infecting the urinary tract. *Mol Microbiol.* 1997;23:1009-1019.

339. Bahrani FK, Massad G, Lockatell CV, et al. Construction of an MR/P fimbrial mutant of *Proteus mirabilis*: role in virulence in a mouse model of ascending urinary tract infection. *Infect Immun.* 1994;62:3363-3371.

340. Johnson DE, Russell RG, Lockatell CV, et al. Contribution of *Proteus mirabilis* urease to persistence, urolithiasis, and acute pyelonephritis in a mouse model of ascending urinary tract infection. *Infect Immun.* 1993;61:2748-2754.

341. Warren JW. *Providencia stuartii*: a common cause of antibiotic-resistant bacteriuria in patients with long-term indwelling catheters. *Rev Infect Dis.* 1986;8:61-67.

342. Muder RR, Brennen C, Wagener MM, et al. Bacteremia in a long-term-care facility: a five-year prospective study of 163 consecutive episodes. *Clin Infect Dis.* 1992;14:647-654.

343. McDermott C, Mylotte JM. *Morganella morganii*: epidemiology of bacteremic disease. *Infect Control.* 1984;5:131-137.

344. Falagas ME, Kavvadia PK, Mantadakis E, et al. *Morganella morganii* infections in a general tertiary hospital. *Infection.* 2006;34:315-321.

345. Ikeobi CC, Ogunsanya TO, Rotimi VO. Prevalence of pathogenic role of *Morganella-Proteus-Providencia* group of bacteria in human faeces. *Afr J Med Med Sci.* 1996;25:7-12.

346. Kim BN, Kim NJ, Kim MN, et al. Bacteraemia due to tribe Proteeae: a review of 132 cases during a decade (1991-2000). *Scand J Infect Dis.* 2003;35:98-103.

347. Poirel L, Guibert M, Girlich D, et al. Cloning, sequence analyses, expression, and distribution of *ampC-ampR* from *Morganella morganii* clinical isolates. *Antimicrob Agents Chemother.* 1999;43:769-776.

348. Slaven EM, Lopez FA, Hart SM, et al. Myonecrosis caused by *Edwardsiella tarda*: a case report and case series of extraintestinal *E. tarda* infections. *Clin Infect Dis.* 2001;32:1430-1433.

349. Janda JM, Abbott SL. Infections associated with the genus *Edwardsiella*: the role of *Edwardsiella tarda* in human disease. *Clin Infect Dis.* 1993;17:742-748.

350. Brenden RA, Miller MA, Janda JM. Clinical disease spectrum and pathogenic factors associated with *Plesiomonas shigelloides* infections in humans. *Rev Infect Dis.* 1988;10:303-316.

351. Ruimy R, Breittmayer V, Elbaze P, et al. Phylogenetic analysis and assessment of the genera *Vibrio*, *Photobacterium*, *Aeromonas*, and *Plesiomonas* deduced from small-subunit rRNA sequences. *Int J Syst Bacteriol.* 1994;44:416-426.

352. Holmberg SD, Wachsmuth IK, Hickman-Brenner FW, et al. *Plesiomonas* enteric infections in the United States. *Ann Intern Med.* 1986;105:690-694.

353. Herrington DA, Tzipori S, Robins-Browne RM, et al. In vitro and in vivo pathogenicity of *Plesiomonas shigelloides*. *Infect Immun.* 1987;55:979-985.

354. Devreese K, Claeys G, Verschraegen G. Septicemia with *Ewingella americana*. *J Clin Microbiol.* 1992;30:2746-2747.

355. Kati C, Bibashi E, Kokolina E, et al. Case of peritonitis caused by *Ewingella americana* in a patient undergoing continuous ambulatory peritoneal dialysis. *J Clin Microbiol.* 1999;37:3733-3734.

356. Pien FD, Bruce AE. Nosocomial *Ewingella americana* bacteremia in an intensive care unit. *Arch Intern Med.* 1986;146:111-112.

357. Carter JE, Evans TN. Clinically significant *Kluyvera* infections: a report of seven cases. *Am J Clin Pathol.* 2005;123:334-338.

358. Luttrell RE, Rannick GA, Soto-Hernandez JL, et al. *Kluyvera* species soft tissue infection: case report and review. *J Clin Microbiol.* 1988;26:2650-2651.

359. Sarria JC, Vidal AM, Kimbrough RC III. Infections caused by *Kluyvera* species in humans. *Clin Infect Dis.* 2001;33:E69-E74.

360. Akhurst RJ, Boemare NE, Janssen PH, et al. Taxonomy of Australian clinical isolates of the genus *Photorhabdus* and proposal of *Photorhabdus asymbiotica* subsp. *asymbiotica* subsp. nov. and *P. asymbiotica* subsp. *australis* subsp. nov. *Int J Syst Evol Microbiol.* 2004;54:1301-1310.

361. Gerrard JG, McNevin S, Alfredson D, et al. *Photorhabdus* species: bioluminescent bacteria as emerging human pathogens? *Emerg Infect Dis.* 2003;9:251-254.

219

Pseudomonas aeruginosa

GERALD B. PIER | REUBEN RAMPHAL

Microbiology

Pseudomonas aeruginosa is the major pathogenic species in the family Pseudomonadaceae and is readily identified as a gram-negative straight or slightly curved rod with a length ranging from 1 to 3 µm and a width of 0.5 to 1.0 µm. Major morphologic characteristics on laboratory media include production of pigments, notably a soluble blue-colored phenazine pigment called pyocyanin. Some strains produce red or black colonies because of synthesis of pigments termed pyorubin and pyomelanin, respectively. Another diffusible yellow-green to yellow-brown pigment produced by *P. aeruginosa* is pyoverdin, which, when produced along with pyocyanin, gives rise to a typical green to green-blue colony on solid media. The name *aeruginosa* stems from the green-blue hue seen within colonies of many clinical isolates. Colonies of *P. aeruginosa* can have a highly varied morphology, with typical colonies appearing to spread over the plate, lie flat with a metallic sheen, and frequently produce a gelatinous or "slimy" appearance, particularly in areas of heavy growth. However, colonial variants including dwarf, coliform, and mucoid morphotypes are seen, the last morphology particularly frequent when cultures from the respiratory tract and secretions of patients with cystic fibrosis (CF) are observed (Fig. 219-1). A characteristic "grapelike" or "corn taco-like" odor is produced by most strains as well.

P. aeruginosa is able to grow on a wide variety of media, ranging from minimal to complex, and can metabolize a large array of carbon sources. It grows best aerobically but can be grown anaerobically in the presence of nitrate as a terminal electron acceptor. *P. aeruginosa* does not ferment carbohydrates but produces acid from sugars such as glucose, fructose, and xylose, but not lactose or sucrose. It is strongly positive in an indophenol oxidase test and can grow at 42° C, which differentiates this species from the rarely pathogenic *Pseudomonas fluorescens* and *Pseudomonas putida*. A commonly used selective medium is cetrimide agar, which contains a detergent that inhibits growth of many other organisms, although with some exceptions. On triple sugar iron agar, the organism has a reaction of alkaline over no change in growth, and it is Simmons' citrate positive and L-arginine dehydrolase positive. *P. aeruginosa* gives negative reactions for L-lysine decarboxylase and L-ornithine decarboxylase, and it does not produce hydrogen sulfide.

At the ultrastructural level, *P. aeruginosa* produces a single or monotrichous polar flagellum and many cell surface fimbriae or pili (Fig. 219-2). Almost all strains carry the biosynthetic genes to produce an extracellular polysaccharide known as alginate because of its chemical similarity to seaweed alginate. This material has also been referred to as mucoid exopolysaccharide in the literature,[1] and its overproduction is the basis for the mucoid colony phenotype associated with isolates from CF patients as well as occasional isolates from other patients with chronic *P. aeruginosa* infections, such as chronic obstructive pulmonary disease, or chronic infections in patients with indwelling urinary catheters. In general, strains of *P. aeruginosa* isolated from the environment and nosocomial infections are considered nonmucoid, but in reality most nonmucoid strains can express low levels of the alginate polysaccharide when grown in vitro.[2,3] Recently identified extracellular polysaccharides involved in the formation of pellicles and

biofilms, termed Pel and Psl, also appear to be important factors involved in pathogenesis.[4]

Environmental and nosocomial isolates also produce a smooth lipopolysaccharide (LPS) substituted with long (5 to 100 kDa) polysaccharide O side chains, but only approximately 10% to 30% of the LPS molecules contain O side chains. The rest of the LPS molecules are in the form of LPS rough molecules containing lipid A, inner- and outer-core regions (Fig. 219-3) but lacking O side chains. Studies have shown that the outer-core region of the LPS containing O side chains differs structurally from that of molecules lacking O side chains (see Fig. 219-3). The outer membrane is typical of those for gram-negative bacteria and contains a large array of outer membrane proteins (OMPs) with a variety of functions critical for cellular growth and metabolism. From the sequences of the genomes of *P. aeruginosa* strains,[5-7] it is estimated that there may be more than 300 potential OMPs, and it is clear that their expression varies dramatically depending on growth conditions or phenotype of strains used for analysis of the OMPs.[8-10]

History

Before the advent of modern medical microbiology there was evidence that *P. aeruginosa* was a cause of serious wound and surgical infections, as elaborated by Doggett.[11] In 1850, it was noted by Sédillot that there were sometimes blue-green discharges on surgical dressings that were associated with infection, and in 1862 Luke noted rod-shaped microscopic entities within the blue-green pus. In 1882, Gessard isolated the organisms and originally designated them as *Bacillus pyocyaneus*, and other early microbiologists also isolated the organism from infected sites. Osler in 1925 thought the organism to be more of a secondary or opportunistic invader of damaged tissues as opposed to a primary cause of infection in healthy tissues—an observation well borne out since his time. *P. aeruginosa* emerged as a major human pathogen in the 1960s because of its ability to cause infections in immunocompromised and burned hosts as well as CF patients, all of whom were surviving much longer with modern medical treatments. Since that time, *P. aeruginosa* has become one of the most serious causes of nosocomial bacterial infections, notably in the lung, blood, and urinary tract. Furthermore, as a result of its considerable potential to become resistant to many antibiotics, increasingly more multiply antibiotic-resistant strains are being encountered as clinical isolates, leaving physicians with a decreasing armamentarium of effective drugs for treatment.

Epidemiology

In adult clinical medicine, *P. aeruginosa* is primarily encountered as a nosocomial pathogen, which reflects its great propensity to grow in a variety of environments with minimal nutritional components.[12] However, as CF patients survive longer and their medical care as adults is increasingly shifted away from pediatric providers, treatment of CF lung disease by adult practitioners is becoming more common.[13] Outside the hospital, *P. aeruginosa* is commonly found in soil, water, and plants and can occasionally be associated with colonization of

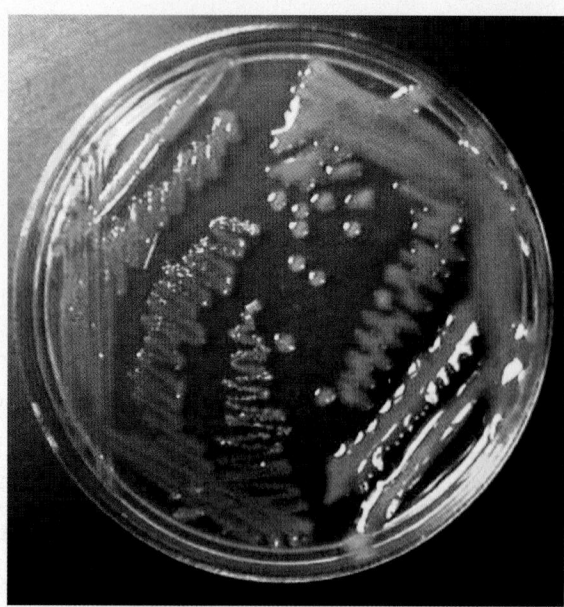

Figure 219-1 Phenotypic appearance of nonmucoid, generally lipopolysaccharide (LPS)-smooth *(left)* and mucoid, LPS-rough *(right)* colonies of *Pseudomonas aeruginosa.*

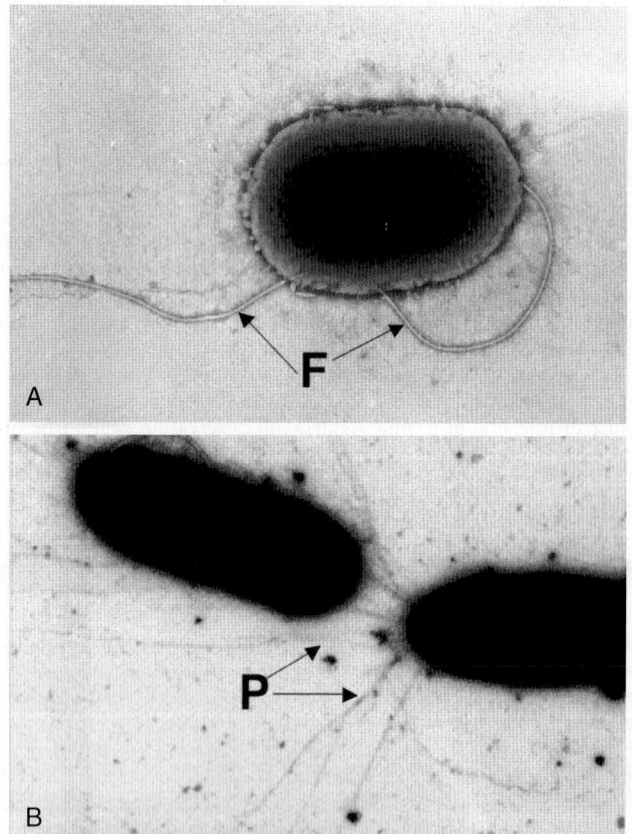

Figure 219-2 Electron micrographs of *Pseudomonas aeruginosa* cell showing ultrastructural features. **A,** Single cell with polar flagellum (F) with part of the flagellum running under the cell body. **B,** Two cells showing thin, hairlike pili (P). *(A, Courtesy of Dr. Steven Lory; B, from Pier GB. Molecular mechanisms of bacterial pathogenesis. In: Kasper DL, Braunwald E, Hauser S, et al, eds. Harrison's Principles of Internal Medicine. 16th ed. New York: McGraw-Hill; 2004.)*

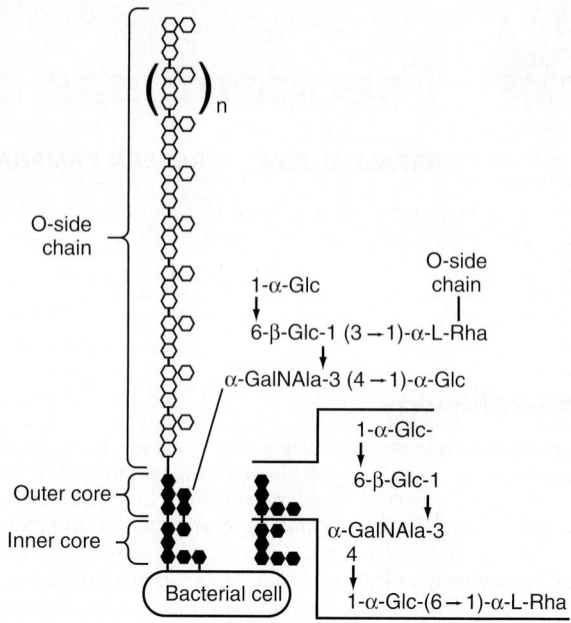

Figure 219-3 Structure of the two isoforms (glycoforms) of the *Pseudomonas aeruginosa* lipopolysaccharide. **Left,** Structure of the glycoform that accepts the long O side chains. **Right,** Structure of the glycoform that is not substituted with O side chains. GalNAla, *N*-alanylgalactosamine; Glc, glucose; Rha, rhamnose.

otherwise healthy humans and animals. The organism is tolerant to temperatures as high as 45° C to 50° C and can grow in distilled water using dissolved carbon dioxide and residual sulfur, phosphorus, iron, and divalent cations as carbon and essential nutritional substrates. However, water buffered to a pH of 4.5 or lower does not support survival of *P. aeruginosa.* Within the hospital, *P. aeruginosa* can colonize moist surfaces of patients on the axilla, ear, and perineum and is also isolated from other moist, inanimate environments including water in sinks and drains, toilets, and showers. Pathogenic strains have also been isolated from the water used for flowers in patients' rooms. Hospital equipment that comes in contact with water, such as mops, respiratory ventilators, cleaning solutions, and food and food processing machines, can be sources of *P. aeruginosa.*

Although much less a problem than nosocomial infection, community-acquired *P. aeruginosa* infection does occur in certain settings,[14] and infection is often associated with exposure to moist environments. *P. aeruginosa* skin infections related to use of hot tubs, whirlpools, swimming pools, and other types of baths are well-recognized clinical presentations of community-acquired infection.[15] Individuals who use contact lenses, particularly of the extended-wear variety that can be kept in the eyes for several weeks, have a greatly increased risk of *P. aeruginosa* ulcerative keratitis associated with the presence of the bacteria in their contact lens solutions.[16,17] Otitis externa is frequently caused by *P. aeruginosa.*[18] Puncture wounds through tennis shoes can give rise to serious *P. aeruginosa* infection,[19] although this condition is found primarily in children. Infections of the interdigital webs of the toes are associated with maceration from topical antibiotic ointment. Perinychia is associated with constant exposure of the extremities to water, detergents, or mechanical stress. *P. aeruginosa* endophthalmitis after surgery or eye trauma can result in serious compromise of vision,[20] and *P. aeruginosa* endocarditis can occur in injection drug users.[21]

P. aeruginosa nosocomial infections are usually attributed to acquisition of the organism in the hospital, particularly in patients undergoing mechanical ventilation, antibiotic treatment, chemotherapy, or surgery.[22] However, *P. aeruginosa* can be found among normal microorganisms carried by a small proportion of humans. It has been suggested that endogenous *P. aeruginosa* brought into intensive care units (ICUs) by patients from the community can serve as sources of serious infection.[23,24] Patients with significant burn wounds are at high risk for *P. aeruginosa* infection, but in the most modern burn trauma centers, effective topical antimicrobial therapy and burn wound excision have greatly reduced the incidence of *P. aeruginosa* infection.[25] Up to 7% of healthy humans carry *P. aeruginosa* in the throat, nasal mucosa, or on the skin, and carriage rates as high as 24% in the stool have been reported.[24]

A prior period of colonization frequently precedes invasive *P. aeruginosa* infection and can occur in as many as 50% of infected patients with an underlying risk factor for infection. Yet it has been difficult to identify precisely which patients with colonization will go on to have invasive disease or to identify with any assurance the initial source or mode of transmission of the infecting strain. In the absence of an identifiable hospital outbreak, usually associated with a particular source, *P. aeruginosa* infection can start from any of the moist reservoirs patients come in contact with, including showers, sinks, flower vases, and uncooked vegetables. Many patients, particularly those receiving mechanical ventilation, become colonized with *P. aeruginosa* in the upper airways, but only a minority go on to develop pneumonia.[26] Gastrointestinal (GI) colonization with *P. aeruginosa*, usually secondary to antibiotic use that disrupts the normal microbial populations of the GI tract, can lead to aspiration, respiratory tract colonization, and sometimes pneumonia. Selective decontamination of the GI tract with orally nonabsorbable antibiotics along with a course of intravenous antibiotics for prevention of infection and associated mortality in the ICU had strong advocates, and several studies showed efficacy in reducing mortality, including that from *P. aeruginosa* ventilator-associated pneumonia (VAP), with use of this treatment.[27-29] However, a meta-analysis of this practice failed to confirm a consistent effect in clinical trials.[30] This analysis indicated that oral chlorhexidine reduced VAP but not mortality. Selective GI decontamination with antibiotics has not gained widespread acceptance particularly in North America, and significant questions about its efficacy remain.

Determining the source and prevalence of *P. aeruginosa* in the hospital environment is essential for effective epidemiologic control of infection, and many newer techniques are available to carry out effective investigations using modern molecular typing techniques.[31] Typing by colonial morphology or phenotype, antibiogram, serology of variant LPS antigens, bacteriophages, bacteriocins known as pyocins, or biochemical profiles using standard clinical microbiologic analysis is fairly limited and generally has insufficient discriminatory power. Preferred techniques target genomic sequences and include DNA size analysis by pulsed-field gel electrophoresis (PFGE), analysis of DNA restriction enzyme-based fragment polymorphisms (RFLPs), use of randomly amplified pieces of DNA showing a high degree of polymorphism among strains (termed RAPD for randomly amplified polymorphic DNA or AFLP for amplified fragment length polymorphism), use of multilocus sequence typing (MLST) wherein short DNA sequences in defined genes known to be variable among strains are determined and used for strain classification, and use of polymerase chain reaction (PCR)-RFLP to discriminate strains on the basis of DNA sequence variations found in the small subunit ribosomal RNA genes (ribotyping or riboprinting). Each of these techniques has strengths and some weaknesses with regard to its discriminatory power, with one common limitation being their availability primarily in specialty or research laboratories. A study comparing PFGE and MLST showed strengths and limitations of both techniques.[32] PFGE was more discriminatory, and thus better able to find differences in *P. aeruginosa* clones, whereas MLST was better for detecting relatedness among clones. However, the differences were small, indicating that both techniques are highly useful for typing of *P. aeruginosa* strains. Changes in the epidemiology and incidence of various nosocomial infections are frequent, and many of the problems seem to occur in local environments or as sporadic, epidemic outbreaks. However, infections with *P. aeruginosa* have remained relatively constant in terms of incidence and tissue sites of occurrence during the past 30 to 40 years, and relative frequencies of hospital-acquired pneumonia and VAP can vary significantly among health care settings in different countries. In 2003, in ICUs in the

United States, *P. aeruginosa* accounted for 18.1% of hospital-acquired pneumonias and a significant percentage of urinary tract infections (16.3%), surgical site infections (9.5%), and bloodstream infections (3.4%).[33] With increasing problems due to infections with strains of *P. aeruginosa* resistant to multiple antibiotics, it can be anticipated that therapeutic problems with this organism will remain a major cause of morbidity and mortality for some time.[34]

Pathogenesis

The bacterial virulence factors brought to bear on the pathologic process associated with *P. aeruginosa* infection are large and varied in both form and function. Multiple pathogenic factors with redundant functions are expressed by *P. aeruginosa* clinical isolates, often making it difficult to determine experimentally whether a specific factor plays a significant role in pathogenesis. The role and importance of different virulence factors are affected by the host in significant ways; innate and acquired immune function, site of infection, and comorbid conditions, to name a few, determine whether a given bacterial virulence factor plays a major or minor role in pathogenesis. There is a fine balance between effective, innate immunity that controls the spread of the organism and pathologic inflammation associated with bacterial growth and poor control of the organism. Because both of these states rely on the same general host effector and signaling molecules for their manifestations, tipping the balance one way or the other could be the difference between benign and serious *P. aeruginosa* infection. Nonetheless, during the past several decades a number of specific factors involved in various aspects of *P. aeruginosa* virulence have been identified through molecular, cellular, and animal studies that provide some important insights into the basis for *P. aeruginosa* disease.

HOST FACTORS IN PATHOGENESIS

Because the major manifestations of *P. aeruginosa* infection are nosocomial infection, chronic lung infection in CF, and contact lens-associated keratitis, it is clear that the primary determinant of the pathogenic potential of *P. aeruginosa* virulence factors is the health status of the human host. Because healthy humans are generally highly resistant to *P. aeruginosa* infection, some compromise in host health status underlies most of the serious problems with *P. aeruginosa* infection. Although many factors contribute to host susceptibility to *P. aeruginosa* infection, one overarching factor for community-acquired and nosocomial *P. aeruginosa* infection appears to be neutropenia. Animal studies clearly show that in the absence of functional polymorphonuclear neutrophil (PMN) there is virtually no host resistance to very low inocula of *P. aeruginosa* into the lung[35] or other sites.[36] Innate immune resistance to infection starts with the anatomic barrier functions of the skin and mucosal surfaces, and any disruption to the integrity of these barriers establishes a situation in which *P. aeruginosa* can become invasive. Typical problems are associated with burn wounds and somewhat less frequently with other types of wounds to the skin, use of intravenous or urinary catheters, and particularly use of endotracheal tubes. Because of its ubiquity in the environment, *P. aeruginosa* is the preeminent opportunistic pathogen taking advantage of compromises to the integrity of physical and mucosal barriers to infection.

Molecular and Cellular Basis for Loss of Host Resistance to Pseudomonas aeruginosa *Infection*

Anatomic and Physiologic Barriers. With regard to the specific molecular and cellular events that ensue when a patient enters a state of increased risk for *P. aeruginosa* infection, many of what are thought to be critical factors have been identified from studies on animals as well as studies focusing on *P. aeruginosa* and CF lung disease. In the simplest sense, for burn and wound infections, *P. aeruginosa* is able to take advantage of the dead or poorly perfused tissue, grow in this site, and eventually achieve a density in the wound sufficient to allow it to seed the blood at levels that overwhelm the host's innate immunity. Usually, infection of intact skin with *P. aeruginosa* is uncommon,[37] and when it is seen, it is generally confined to localized epidermal infections of the nail beds (green nail syndrome) or web-space infection and sometimes somewhat more serious cutaneous folliculitis and otitis externa.

In burned or wounded skin, the situation is different. In the development of the burned mouse model used extensively in research on *P. aeruginosa* pathogenesis, Stieritz and Holder[38] showed that *P. aeruginosa* grew to high levels in burned skin after inoculation of as few as 10 organisms, after which there was systemic dissemination and lethality. Healthy skin required five to six logs more organisms to achieve a comparable effect. However, by 3 days after the burn, the mouse skin had recovered sufficiently that it was actually more resistant than normal skin to *P. aeruginosa* growth. In wounded tissue, it appears *P. aeruginosa* can find a haven safe from host immune effectors and grow to sufficient levels to elaborate a multitude of toxins that break down such host factors as complement, fibrin, and antiproteinases. One of the major bacterial factors implicated in pathogenesis is elastase.[39] The healthy eye is highly resistant to *P. aeruginosa* infection, but when the physical integrity of the corneal epithelium is breached, *P. aeruginosa* becomes a major pathogen.[20,40,41] In these situations, it is likely that the major underlying cellular mechanism related to increased host susceptibility to infection is loss of tissue integrity.

Loss of mucosal barrier function is another host condition that allows *P. aeruginosa* to be a major pathogen. Mucous membranes protect against pathogens by a variety of mechanisms that, when compromised, give rise to dramatically increased susceptibility to infection. In the GI tract and oropharynx, the normal bacterial flora provides stiff competition for pathogens to colonize and grow. Mucus entraps foreign organisms, which are cleared by peristalsis in the GI tract, mucociliary clearance in the respiratory tract, and urination in the genitourinary tract. Within the mucus are antimicrobial factors such as lysozyme, lactoferrin, and defensins,[42] the last being small peptides that insert themselves into bacterial membranes and disrupt their integrity, leading to microbial death. The propensity of this organism to colonize the GI tract in the setting of cancer chemotherapy and antibiotic use and the frequent colonization of the upper respiratory tract in patients with endotracheal tubes result from disruption of the normal resistance mechanisms present on these surfaces.

Soluble Factors on Mucosal Surfaces and in Blood

Complement. Soluble host factors present on mucosal surfaces that have been implicated in high-level resistance to *P. aeruginosa* infection include complement proteins, lung surfactants and similar members of the collectin family, and a variety of cytokines and chemokines. Complement has two major roles in modulating *P. aeruginosa* infection: The major opsonins derived from complement component 3 (C3), C3b and iC3b, effectively promote phagocytosis and killing of *P. aeruginosa*,[43] and the so-called anaphylatoxins, derived from C3 and C5, C3a and C5a, promote neutrophil recruitment and activation needed for effective phagocytosis. Complement-deficient mice are more susceptible to *P. aeruginosa* infection,[44] and failure to produce C3a in C3-deficient mice and C5a in C5-deficient mice resulted in increased *P. aeruginosa* lung burdens and mortality rates. Interestingly, the functions of C3a and C5a were not in PMN recruitment, because both C3- and C5-deficient mice infected with *P. aeruginosa* had higher levels of these inflammatory cells in the lungs than wild-type animals,[44] but the ability of the neutrophils to phagocytose and kill *P. aeruginosa* was clearly compromised in complement-deficient animals. However, *P. aeruginosa* infection is not reported to be a complication of congenital complement deficiency in humans, suggesting that in this setting other effectors of immunity can compensate for loss of complement function.

Collectins. The collectins are soluble molecules involved in innate resistance to *P. aeruginosa* infection and include the surfactant proteins A (SP-A) and D (SP-D) and mannose (or mannan)-binding lectin (MBL).[45] Collectins are composed of multiple subunits and include a carbohydrate recognition domain that binds to conserved pattern recognition molecules on the bacterial surface attached to a collagen-like stalk that can bind to the collectin receptor on phagocytes. In addition, the collectins activate complement through the lectin-binding pathway, a pathway that leads to generation of complement opsonins and anaphylatoxins. Mice deficient in SP-A are more susceptible to the mucoid *P. aeruginosa* strains that cause chronic lung infections in CF patients. SP-D promotes opsonization of *P. aeruginosa* by alveolar macrophages,[46] which may be important in the early handling of *P. aeruginosa* lung infection. SP-D in human corneal tear fluid inhibits *P. aeruginosa* uptake by corneal epithelial cells, possibly important in the pathogenesis of keratitis.[47]

Variant alleles of MBL that code for MBL deficiency have been associated with more severe lung disease in *P. aeruginosa*-infected CF patients.[48] Lack of MBL in mice increases susceptibility to *P. aeruginosa* burn wound infection.[49] However, others were unable to find evidence of MBL binding to *P. aeruginosa*,[50] raising questions about the mechanisms whereby MBL deficiency led to enhanced *Pseudomonas* lung disease in CF patients.

Cytokines, Chemokines, and Related Factors of Innate Immunity. The panoply of cytokines and chemokines that humans can produce in response to infection, with their additive, synergistic, and complementary as well as antagonistic effects, makes it difficult to ascribe a role in resistance to *P. aeruginosa* infection to a single cytokine. Even more problematic is the likelihood that a particular cytokine or set of cytokines may be protective at one point in the infectious cycle and contribute to inflammation-induced pathology at a later time point. As noted by Alexander and Rietschel,[51] the same cytokine or chemokine mediators of inflammation that provide effective antimicrobial immunity when produced in a controlled, physiologic manner also mediate the pathology associated with highly consequential inflammation, including tissue destruction, the sepsis syndrome, and death. Consistent with these observations are the numerous reports, mostly from studies in transgenic mice, implicating some cytokines and chemokines as key elements in both resistance and enhancement of pathology related to *P. aeruginosa* infection.

Interleukin-1 (IL-1) is a factor involved in both resistance to infection and succumbing to the pathologic effects of overwhelming infection. Early studies showed that pretreatment of mice with IL-1 protected against infection with *P. aeruginosa* and other gram-negative pathogens. *P. aeruginosa* binding to the cystic fibrosis transmembrane conductance regulator (CFTR) induces rapid IL-1 release, and lack of a functional IL-1 receptor in mice allows for establishment of a chronic *P. aeruginosa* lung infection not unlike that achieved in CF patients.[52] Proposed mechanisms for the protective effects of IL-1 against *P. aeruginosa* infection include activation of nuclear factor kappa B (NF-κB)–dependent induction or protective cytokines,[52] induction of antibacterial T cells, inhibition of bacterial growth,[53] induction of defensins,[54] and activation and modulation of phagocytic cell activity.[55] However, severe *P. aeruginosa* infections were associated with highly elevated levels of IL-1 in both local tissues and blood and the level of IL-1β was a marker for alveolar inflammation in mechanically ventilated patients with community-acquired pneumonia.[56] In mice given a sufficient dose of *P. aeruginosa* to cause a lethal infection, IL-1 contributed significantly to pathology because there was a better outcome in animals after neutralization of IL-1 or in mice unable to respond to IL-1 due to loss of the IL-1 receptor.[57,58] It appears that pretreatment with IL-1 or the levels of IL-1 produced in response to low infectious doses of *P. aeruginosa* augment host resistance to infection, whereas when high infectious doses are given or *P. aeruginosa* grows to high levels in compromised hosts, the continued production of IL-1 and signaling through the IL-1 receptor increase inflammation to the point at which it contributes to pathology.

Tumor necrosis factor-α (TNF-α) has also been implicated as a cytokine affecting *P. aeruginosa* infection in both a positive and a pathologic manner. BALB/c mice, reported by some to be more resistant to *P. aeruginosa* pulmonary infection, had higher levels of TNF-α gene expression and protein secretion in the alveoli in response to this organism, and malnourished mice were more susceptible to *P. aeruginosa* pulmonary infection, in part because of diminished TNF-α production.[59] TNF-α knockout mice had a diminished capacity to clear *P. aeruginosa*.[59] TNF-α modulation of inflammation has been associated with differences in outcome in experimental *P. aeruginosa* pulmonary infection, with protection associated with enhanced alveolar macrophage presence and activity and pathology associated with sustained PMN infiltration in the lungs. TNF-α levels are well-known to be elevated in the blood of patients infected with a variety of bacterial agents, and TNF-α is thought to be a major mediator of the pathogenesis of sepsis, but attempts to blockade its activity in a therapeutic manner have been unsuccessful.[60] Indeed, in some clinical trials, patients treated with high doses of anti-TNF molecules had a worse outcome.[61] TNF-α levels in the lungs and serum of chronically infected CF patients are elevated in comparison with those in healthy individuals, but they do not generally appear to change during exacerbation of infection.[62] Similarly to IL-1, TNF-α probably augments innate immunity in situations of low-level exposure to *P. aeruginosa*, but if innate immunity fails, continued attempts to reestablish tissue sterility by production of TNF-α lead to inflammation-associated pathology.

Other cytokines, chemokines, and small molecular effectors of innate immunity found in experimental studies to affect *P. aeruginosa* infection include IL-4, IL-6,[41,63] IL-9,[64] IL-10, IL-17, IL-18,[64,65] IL-23,[66,67] transforming growth factor-β, and nitric oxide.[59,68] As is often found in such studies, both positive and negative effects of these factors have been noted. Again, context is probably highly important, with positive effects of inflammatory cytokines such as IL-4, IL-6, and IL-18 important in innate immunity at low doses of *P. aeruginosa*, whereas high levels of these factors exacerbate illness when *P. aeruginosa* levels become elevated in infected tissues. Recently there has been much interest in the pathogenesis of *P. aeruginosa* infection related to the role of a type of T cell noted for its ability to secrete IL-17 (Th17) following stimulation by IL-23. Th17 cells secrete cytokines that drive neutrophil recruitment to tissues, and IL-17 and IL-23 levels are elevated in the PMN-dominated, chronically infected lungs of CF patients.[66,69] Similarly, anti-inflammatory factors such as IL-9, IL-10, and nitric oxide are found to be deficient during *P. aeruginosa*-induced disease because of high levels of bacteria, and increasing the anti-inflammatory activity in this situation brings about salutary effects. However, the potential of any of these factors, or inducers of their production, to be clinically efficacious remains low because of many problems, including pharmacokinetics; costs; the ability to induce or inhibit the factor at the correct time during infection in the correct tissue at a therapeutic, nontoxic dose; and the complexity of the interactions among cytokines, chemokines, and related molecules that cannot be readily controlled to bring about a clinical benefit.

Cellular Mediators of Resistance to Pseudomonas aeruginosa Infection

Leukocytes. Although all known monocytic, granulocytic, and lymphocytic cell types have shown some effect on *P. aeruginosa* infections in both humans and experimental animals, it is overwhelmingly clear that the major cellular mediator of resistance to *P. aeruginosa* infection is the PMN. Although the incidence of serious nosocomial *P. aeruginosa* infections seems to have declined in some hospitals in the past two decades compared with that in the 1970s,[70] neutropenia in humans is still a major risk factor for *P. aeruginosa* infection.[71] Also, even though it is appreciated that advanced acquired immunodeficiency syndrome (AIDS) predisposes to *P. aeruginosa* infection, these patients usually have neutropenia as a complication of their disease, which contributes, along with other factors such as indwelling urinary or vascular catheters, to severe *P. aeruginosa* infection. Animal studies completely confirm that neutropenia dramatically increases susceptibility to *P. aeruginosa* infection. For example, a minimal dose of *P. aeruginosa* lethal to nearly 100% of mice when delivered to the lungs usually ranges from 10^7 to 5×10^8 colony-forming units (CFUs) per animal, whereas after three doses of cyclophosphamide of 150 mg/kg, which results in absolute neutrophil counts close to zero, most wild-

type *P. aeruginosa* strains are lethal to the animals after inoculation with as few as 1 to 50 CFUs per animal. Indeed, it could be persuasively argued that the PMNs are the only critical mediators of innate immunity to *P. aeruginosa* infection because their absence so dramatically affects susceptibility to infection.

Regarding non-PMN leukocytes, numerous papers have reported the ability of blood and alveolar macrophages to phagocytose *P. aeruginosa*, suggesting a role in resistance to infection. However, in animal studies, depletion of alveolar macrophages in mice with liposome-encapsulated clodronate disodium or liposome-encapsulated dichloromethylene diphosphonate failed to alter the outcome of *P. aeruginosa* infection, although changes in production of some cytokines were noted. These studies suggest no essential role for macrophages in innate immunity to *P. aeruginosa* infection, but local macrophages may affect production of soluble factors that contribute to host resistance because of effects, for example, on PMN recruitment and activation. However, these soluble factors are probably produced by multiple cell types in addition to macrophages, making the loss of the macrophage overshadowed by compensatory production of soluble factors from other cell types. Similarly, eosinophils do not appear to play a role in host resistance to *P. aeruginosa* infection, but either the cells themselves or released granule contents such as major basic protein may contribute to the atopic-like pathology found in chronically infected CF patients. Basophils, particularly tissue mast cells, are important producers of mediators of inflammation in response to infection, and several studies have shown the importance of mast cell mediator release in recruitment of PMNs to sites of *P. aeruginosa* infection.[72-75] Again, the major effector called into play is the PMN.

Numerous studies have indicated a role of T-cell–mediated immunity in development of resistance to *P. aeruginosa* infection after vaccination with a variety of immunogens, and some have suggested that differences in susceptibility to experimental infection in mice correlate with innate delayed-type hypersensitivity responses to *P. aeruginosa*. The occurrence of *P. aeruginosa* infection in severely ill AIDS patients also suggests a role for CD4+ T cells in resistance to infection,[76] but there are other associated risk factors for infection in this population. An established paradigm of modern immunology indicates that T cells can be divided into at least two populations, known as helper T 1 (Th1) and Th2 subsets, that differ in their ability to activate cell-mediated or antibody-mediated immune responses through production of IL-12 and interferon-γ (IFN-γ) (Th1 cells activate cell-mediated immunity) or production of IL-4, IL-5, and IL-10 (leading to antibody production). Some studies have suggested that a Th1 response results in better outcomes in mice chronically infected with *P. aeruginosa*, but these studies found opposite results with regard to mouse strains producing Th1 versus Th2 responses to *P. aeruginosa*. This immunologic paradigm probably does not readily apply to most *P. aeruginosa* infections because the organism produces so many factors capable of eliciting either Th1 or Th2 responses that both subsets are activated in infected patients. Other lymphocytic subsets, such as CD1-restricted T cells,[77] have been reported to contribute to murine clearance of *P. aeruginosa* lung infection, and γδ T cells[78] from CF patients and healthy humans have been shown to produce cytokines in response to *P. aeruginosa*. However, the significance of these findings for the overall contribution of host factors to *P. aeruginosa* pathogenesis is unclear.

Leukocytes with specific markers or properties have also been implicated, via mouse infection studies, as important components of resistance and susceptibility to *P. aeruginosa* infection. As noted previously, activation of Th17 cells to promote PMN recruitment to the lung is associated with chronic inflammation in the setting of CF. However, it has also been reported that IL-17 production was critical for mediating adaptive immune resistance to lung infection in mice immunized with a live, attenuated *P. aeruginosa* vaccine, indicating that in this setting recruitment of PMN effector phagocytes via Th17 cells was a major factor in the vaccine's efficacy. Earlier studies had indicated that generation of the chemotactic fragment of complement component 5, referred to as C5a, was needed for full resistance to lung infection due to promotion of bacterial clearance. Another finding is that C5a promotes expression of the immunoglobulin Fc receptor (FcR) isoform known as FcγRIII, a stimulatory receptor that promotes bacterial clearance. In the absence of FcγRIII, mice were more susceptible to *P. aeruginosa* lung infection.[79]

Epithelial Cells. Epithelial cells are among the first cell types to encounter *P. aeruginosa* after exposure. Principally through studies directed at elucidating why CF patients are so commonly infected with *P. aeruginosa* (more than 80% of patients are infected by 15 to 20 years of age), a great deal has been learned about the role of epithelial cells in orchestrating innate immunity to *P. aeruginosa* infection. The major challenge has been to correlate the genetic defect leading to synthesis of either no CFTR protein or dysfunctional CFTR to the pathogenesis of *P. aeruginosa* infection. CFTR is known principally as a channel conducting chloride and bicarbonate across cell membranes,[80,81] but how this is related to hypersusceptibility to *P. aeruginosa* infection is not fully understood.

Four major hypotheses have been proposed for the basis for the susceptibility of CF patients to *P. aeruginosa*.[82] A long-standing proposal has been that epithelial cells in the lung in CF express higher levels of a receptor for *P. aeruginosa*, asialo GM1,[83] and the bacteria have higher binding to epithelial cells, increasing their ability to withstand host clearance. Although several investigators have confirmed the observations of increased bacterial adherence to epithelial cells in culture,[84] the hypothesis has been challenged by other investigators.[85] The basis for the challenge includes inconsistent findings of increased adherence of *P. aeruginosa* to CF airway epithelial cells, findings of increased adherence only to epithelial cells from the subset of CF patients homozygous for the ΔF508 allele of *CFTR* (50% of patients) whereas many patients with other *CFTR* genotypes contract a comparable lung disease from *P. aeruginosa*, and the use of only a few laboratory strains to study adherence in most of the studies[84] whereas studies with clinical isolates failed to show that asialo GM1 was a significant receptor for *P. aeruginosa*.[85] In addition, although an antiserum raised to asialo GM1 has been shown in several studies to reduce *P. aeruginosa* binding to epithelial cells,[84] this antiserum was found to have high titers of antibodies to *P. aeruginosa* because of use of complete Freund's adjuvant, which contains mycobacteria expressing antigens cross-reactive with those of *P. aeruginosa*. It is likely that apparent reductions in bacterial binding observed in the presence of this antiserum are, in fact, due to agglutination of *P. aeruginosa* cells in the experimental tubes, which leads to reduced colony counts when agglutinated organisms are plated on agar media. More important, in none of the studies could inhibition of binding of *P. aeruginosa* to asialo GM1 on cell surfaces be ascribed to the anti-asialo GM1 activity of the serum.

It has also been proposed that the chloride ion conductance defect of CFTR leads to increased salt concentrations in the thin airway surface liquid (ASL) that overlies the bronchial epithelium between the apical surface of the cell and the more viscous mucous layer.[86] This high salt concentration has been proposed to interfere with the activity of antimicrobial peptides.[86] However, most studies failed to find a difference in salt concentration between normal and CF ASL, and this hypothesis fails to account for the high frequency of *P. aeruginosa* in the setting of CF. A third hypothesis is that lack of functional CFTR also leads to dehydration of the ASL, producing a more viscous pericellular ASL layer that cannot be readily cleared by mucociliary activity of the respiratory epithelium.[87,88] This leads to formation of mucus plugs, which harbor mucin receptors for *P. aeruginosa*, and also produces an anaerobic environment that has been proposed to augment synthesis of the bacterial alginate associated with infection.[89,90] Although mucus plugs loaded with *P. aeruginosa* can be clearly seen in lung sections obtained at autopsy or at transplantation from CF patients, the depleted ASL hypothesis also fails to account for the specificity of CF lung disease for *P. aeruginosa*, and there is no evidence that the initial *P. aeruginosa* infection relies on mucus plugs for bacterial adherence.

The fourth proposed hypothesis directly addresses the issue of the role of epithelial cells in susceptibility to *P. aeruginosa* lung infection, makes a direct link to CFTR, and involves the PMN, which is critically important in innate immunity to this pathogen.[91] It has been shown that cells lacking functional CFTR are less able to internalize *P. aeruginosa* and high levels of bacterial internalization correlate with host resistance to infection. CFTR was shown to be an epithelial cell receptor for binding and internalization of *P. aeruginosa* (Fig. 219-4), and the bacterial ligand is the outer-core oligosaccharide of the LPS. Inhibiting the ability of epithelial cells to interact with *P. aeruginosa* by adding to an infectious inoculum of *P. aeruginosa* either a purified outer-core oligosaccharide or a CFTR peptide that blocks bacterial binding to this protein resulted in decreased epithelial cell uptake and increased bacterial levels in the lungs. Transgenic CF mice lacking functional CFTR also had lowered epithelial cell uptake of *P. aeruginosa* and higher total lung burdens after experimental challenge in an acute infection model.[92]

Perhaps more important than epithelial cell ingestion of *P. aeruginosa* is the CFTR-dependent activation of inflammatory gene transcription related to nuclear translocation of the NF-κB transcription factor that centrally orchestrates cellular responses to many pathogens.[93] In this regard, it was shown that CFTR recognition of *P. aeruginosa* leads to actual extraction of the LPS from the bacterial outer membrane, and this is essential for NF-κB nuclear translocation in both cultured human airway epithelial cells and lungs of infected normal mice (see Fig. 219-4). NF-κB translocation causes increases in transcription of genes involved in PMN recruitment and activation: IL-6, IL-8, GRO1, and intercellular adhesion molecule 1.[94] These CFTR-dependent innate immune responses of the lung epithelium are dependent on the formation of cholesterol-rich membrane microdomains, or lipid rafts, containing CFTR.[95,96]

A prominent protein in these rafts is the major vault protein (MVP), a component of large, barrel-shaped cellular structures known as vaults.[97] MVP's function remained unidentified for almost 20 years after its discovery until it was found to be needed for epithelial cell ingestion of *P. aeruginosa* and promotion of complete clearance from the lung.[98]

CFTR-mediated recognition of *P. aeruginosa* also facilities apoptosis of epithelial cells,[99] a process critical for resolution of the inflammatory response. Delay in this response could underlie the expanded inflammatory state observed in CF lungs, and proper apoptosis of epithelial cells in *P. aeruginosa*-infected mice has been shown to be critical for resistance to infection.[100-102]

In addition, *P. aeruginosa* infection activates tyrosine kinase signaling molecules in infected epithelial cells, an activation that is dependent on bacterial binding to CFTR,[103] and such signaling is clearly important in orchestrating effective host resistance to infection. Interestingly, CFTR–*P. aeruginosa* interactions have been shown to be critical components of the pathogenesis of experimental corneal keratitis in a wounded-cornea model of infection.[104] However, in this model the injury allows *P. aeruginosa* to penetrate through a layer of corneal epithelium that is five or six cells thick to the underlying stroma, where the bacteria use CFTR to enter the epithelial cells and avoid the host's PMN-based defenses. Disruption of the membrane-raft entry site of *P. aeruginosa* into the corneal epithelial cells by extracting cholesterol from the membrane with β-cyclodextrin decreases pathology and bacterial levels in the eyes of mice with experimental ulcerative keratitis.[104] Thus, in contrast to the lung, where the infected epithelial cells are on the airway surface and can desquamate into the lumen to remove ingested *P. aeruginosa*, in the wounded eye the subsurface epithelial cells provide a safe haven for the microbe. Overall, there are now considerable data from numerous studies and independent groups to conclude that *P. aeruginosa*–CFTR interactions at the epithelial surface of the lung comprise a key molecular component of host resistance to pulmonary infection, and loss of this component of innate immunity dramatically increases susceptibility to *P. aeruginosa* infection, as seen in CF.

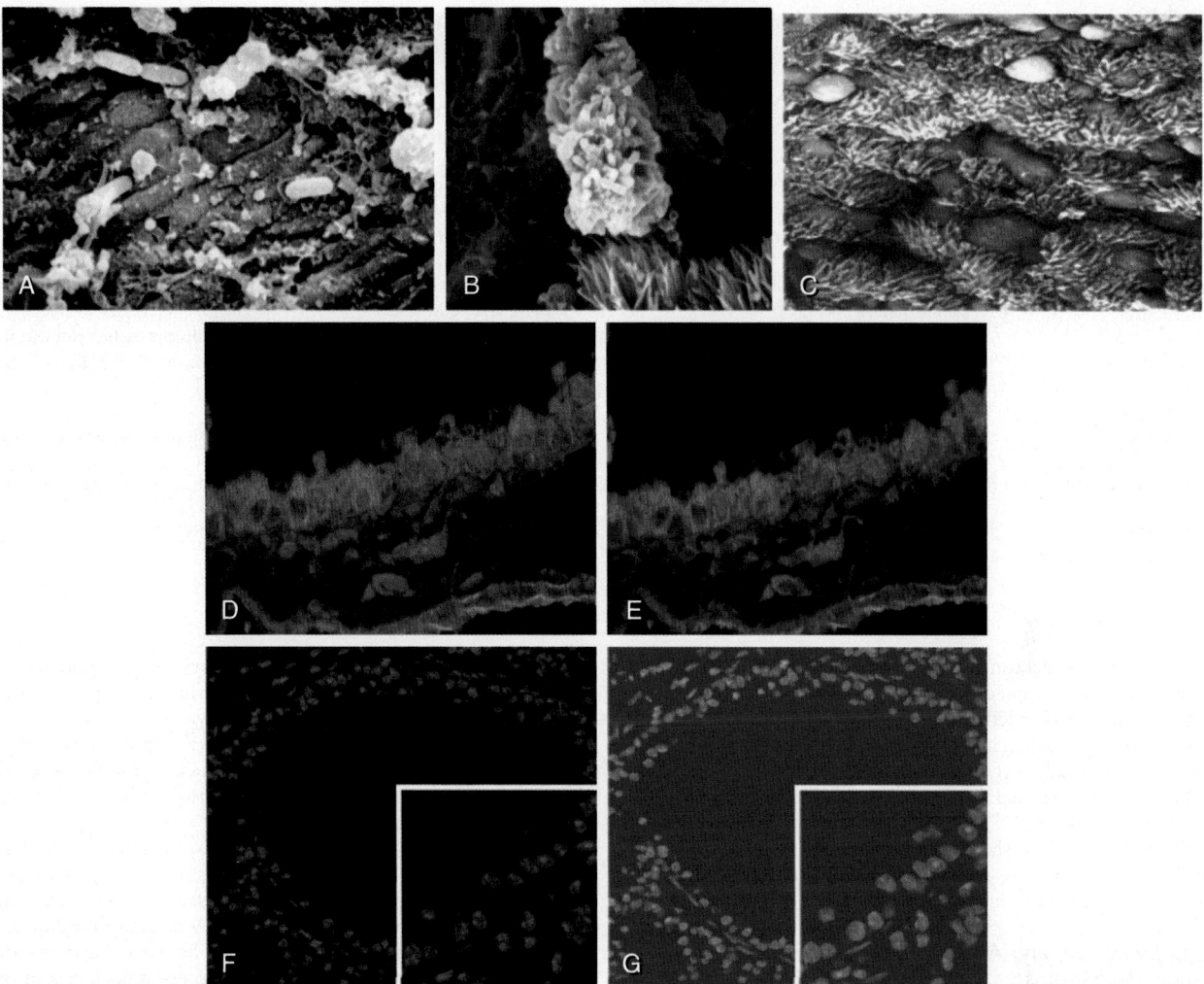

Figure 219-4 Entry of *Pseudomonas aeruginosa* into airway epithelial cells and activation of nuclear factor kappa B (NF-κB) nuclear translocation in wild-type and transgenic cystic fibrosis (CF) mice. **A,** Scanning electron micrograph (SEM) of *P. aeruginosa* entering mouse tracheal epithelial cells 4 hours after intranasal infection with bacteria. **B,** SEM of desquamating tracheal epithelial cell with internalized and attached *P. aeruginosa* cells. **C,** SEM of tracheal epithelium of a transgenic CF mouse 4 hours after intranasal infection with bacteria showing intact epithelium and no bacterial binding or entry to the CF transmembrane conductance regulator (CFTR)-deficient cells. **D** through **G,** Confocal laser scanning micrographs of NF-κB nuclear translocation in bronchial epithelial cells of a wild-type mouse (D and E) or transgenic CF mouse (F and G). Sections were stained for NF-κB (red), CFTR (green), and DNA in the nucleus (blue). Co-localization of NF-κB and CFTR in the cytoplasm of the cells from the wild-type mouse (D) appears as an orange-red color. Nuclear translocation of NF-κB is represented by pseudocolored magenta (co-localization of red and blue colors) in E and G. No CFTR is present in the transgenic CF mouse bronchial epithelium (F, only the red NF-κB is seen), and no NF-κB migrates to the nucleus in the transgenic CF mouse (G). D through G, ×400; insets in F and G, ×800. (*B, From Schroeder TH, Reiniger N, Meluleni G, et al. Transgenic cystic fibrosis mice exhibit reduced early clearance of* Pseudomonas aeruginosa *from the respiratory tract. J Immunol. 2001;166:7410-7418, copyright 2001, The American Association of Immunologists, Inc. and used with permission; D through G, from Schroeder TH, Lee MM, Yacono PW, et al. CFTR is a pattern recognition molecule that extracts* Pseudomonas aeruginosa *LPS from the outer membrane into epithelial cells and activates NF-kappa B translocation. Proc Natl Acad Sci U S A. 2002;99:6907-6912.*)

BACTERIAL FACTORS IN PATHOGENESIS

P. aeruginosa is a fascinating bacterial pathogen to study and a formidable pathogen for humans because of the multitude, diversity, and complexity of its virulence factors. The organism has a large genome more than 6 megabases in size[5] that is highly plastic in terms of ability to incorporate and modify DNA. Virtually all major classes of bacterial virulence systems are found in this organism (Table 219-1), including exotoxins, endotoxins, type III secreted toxins, pili, flagella, proteases, phospholipases, iron-binding proteins, exopolysaccharides, the ability to form biofilms, and elaboration of pyocyanins. The potential of *P. aeruginosa* to cause infection in virtually any body site is probably due to the array of factors it can call on from its large genome to establish itself at a specific site and utilize a wide variety of nutrients for growth

along with the ability to produce a panoply of factors to counteract host defenses. The organism can grow anaerobically if a source of nitrate is present. *P. aeruginosa* is a significant pathogen in part because of modern medical practices that utilize an extensive array of implanted medical devices ranging from venous catheters to orthopedic implants on which the organism can colonize and form a biofilm and then disseminate systemically.

Understanding of the array of *P. aeruginosa* pathogenic factors and how they affect infection, growth, and disease has increased dramatically, but because of the redundancy of these factors in terms of their effects on the host, along with other issues such as tissue-specific sites of expression of virulence factors, there is no straightforward picture of *P. aeruginosa* pathogenesis at the molecular level. Indeed, although

TABLE 219-1	Virulence Factors of *Pseudomonas aeruginosa*	
Location or Class	*Example(s)*	*Activity/Effects on Host*
Cell surface	Alginate	Antiphagocytic/resist opsonic killing
	LPS	Endotoxic/antiphagocytic/avoid preformed antibody to previously encountered O-antigens
	Pili	Twitching motility; biofilm formation; adherence to host tissues
	Flagella	Motility; biofilm formation; adherence to host tissues and mucin components
	Injection of type III secretion factors	PcrG, PcrV, PcrH, PopB, and PopD proteins form injection bridge for type III effectors
Outer membrane	Siderophore receptors	Provides iron for microbial growth and survival
	Efflux pumps	Remove antibiotics
Type III secretion	ExoS; ExoT; ExoU; ExoY	Intoxicates cells (ExoS/ExoT); cytotoxic (ExoU); disrupts actin cytoskeleton
Secreted proteases	LasA protease; LasB elastase; alkaline protease; protease IV	Degrades host immune effectors (antibody, complement, etc.); degrades matrix proteins
Iron acquisition	Pyoverdin; pyochelin	Scavenge iron from the host for bacterial use
Secreted toxins	Exotoxin A; leukocidin phospholipases; hemolysins; rhamnolipid	Inhibit protein synthesis; kill leukocytes; hemolysis of red blood cells; degrade host cell surface glycolipids
Secreted oxidative factors	Pyocyanin; ferripyochelin	Produces reactive oxygen species: H_2O_2; O_2 inflammatory; disrupts epithelial cell function
Quorum sensing	LasR/LasI;RhlR/RhlI PQS	Biofilm formation; regulation of virulence factor secretion

LPS, lipopolysaccharide; PQS, *Pseudomonas* quinolone system.

many of the factors demonstrated in laboratory studies to affect pathogenesis are well-accepted contributors to the pathogenic process, laboratory studies are limited by use of a few, often highly selected, strains for study. Thus, when investigators examine large sets of clinical isolates, they can usually recover strains from patients that lack some of the factors demonstrated in laboratory studies to be important contributors to virulence.[105,106] Nonetheless, some general features of *P. aeruginosa* pathogenesis shared by the majority of strains are now very well studied, and these studies have contributed greatly to our understanding of the molecular basis for virulence of *P. aeruginosa*.

Entry, Colonization, and Avoidance of Innate Clearance Mechanisms

It is often written that bacteria must first adhere to a host tissue to initiate infection, and although this basically obvious statement must hold true, otherwise the organism would be expelled from a mucosal surface, it is naïve to consider that bacterial adherence to host tissues is necessarily going to promote establishment of colonization. Adherence of many pathogens, including *P. aeruginosa*, to epithelial cells initiates vigorous host innate immune responses that much more often than not promote bacterial clearance. Thus, establishing early colonization is a combination of use of bacterial factors that allow the organism to find a niche in which to grow and factors that overcome innate immune clearance.

Entry of *P. aeruginosa* into most humans occurs by the oral or respiratory route. *P. aeruginosa* has virtually no pathogenic capacity in the normal GI tract, although there are occasional reports of isolation of *P. aeruginosa* from fecal or stool cultures in patients with severe diarrhea, but no clear basis for *P. aeruginosa* contributing to this has been established. In the respiratory tract, however, establishment of *P. aeruginosa* infection can have serious consequences, particularly for those with underlying comorbidities or a genetic predisposition such as in CF. Generally, the two major adhesins considered to play a role here are pili and flagella (see Fig. 219-2), which have several functions, including both motility and binding to receptors.

Pili. *P. aeruginosa* pili are formed from a 15-kDa pilin monomer encoded by the *pilA* gene and are located at the poles of the rod, forming typical polar pili. More than 50 genetic loci have been identified that control pilin synthesis and pili production.[107] Five distinct *pilA* alleles (groups I to V) have been identified in *P. aeruginosa*.[108] Group I PilA proteins are glycosylated with an LPS O-antigen subunit, and these can elicit protective immunity to O-antigen homologous

strains,[109] whereas group IV pili are glycosylated by a polymer of one sugar, D-arabinofuranose. This polysaccharide is also part of the lipo-arabinomannan and arabinogalactan cell wall polymers of *Mycobacterium tuberculosis* and *Mycobacterium leprae*.[110] Transcription of *pilA* is regulated by the alternative RNA polymerase sigma factor known as RpoN or σ^{54} and by classic bacterial two-component regulators encoded by the *pilS* and *pilR* genes.

Functionally, pili have been proposed as mediators of local adherence to host tissues, and although mutants of *P. aeruginosa* unable to make pili have been reported to be less virulent in some animal models of infection, this cannot be ascribed to any defect in binding to host tissues because this specific function of pili has never been investigated in vivo. Also, in the corneal scratch-injured eye model, lack of pili on strain PAK did not compromise virulence. Pili have also been proposed to bind to asialo GM1 and GM1 on target tissues, but again this conclusion is mostly derived from in vitro studies with little in the way of in vivo correlates. Surprisingly, and problematically, the portion of the pilus that has been identified as binding to these glycolipid receptors, formed by a critical disulfide bond in the carboxyl-terminal loop of the pilin monomer, has been shown by x-ray crystallographic studies to be buried within the pilus and not surface exposed at the pilus tip, where it could mediate adhesion to host cells.[111,112] Although it is possible that the receptor-binding disulfide loop becomes exposed upon bacterial contact with glycolipid receptors on host tissues, this idea is speculative. Pilin sequences, and hence serologic relatedness, vary among *P. aeruginosa* strains, although it has been proposed that a conserved binding architecture can be identified in all *P. aeruginosa* pili that bind to the target glycolipid receptors.[113]

Pili also mediate twitching motility of *P. aeruginosa*, a factor found to be important in formation of in vitro biofilms on abiotic surfaces.[114] Twitching motility may also be important in avoidance of host phagocytes. Pili have other roles that may be important in helping the organism to survive in vivo, such as natural DNA uptake, autoaggregation of cells, and development of microbial communities. Because studies with mutants of *P. aeruginosa* unable to make pili compromise all of the functions of this structure, one can never know which of the pili-mediated functions are essential to virulence until such times as mutants producing pili with compromises only in specific functions can be made and tested.

Flagella. The flagella of *P. aeruginosa* are one of its more prominent virulence factors as assessed by laboratory studies dating back more than 25 years. *P. aeruginosa* makes a single polar flagellum that imparts a number of properties to the cell, including motility and ability to bind to host tissues. Synthesis of the flagella is quite complex, with more than 40 known genes involved in regulation of transcription and production of the complex structure that makes up the entire flagellar unit, including the flagellar basal body, circular structures designated as the MS and P rings, and a motor switch complex. The key structural components of the flagella are the flagellin subunit protein, encoded by the *fliC* gene, and a protein that caps off the flagella, FliD, encoded by the *fliD* gene. There are two major types of flagella in *P. aeruginosa*, the a type and the b type, each produced by allelic variants in the *fliC* and *fliD* genes that are coinherited.[115] Flagella are produced by most environmental and nosocomial isolates of *P. aeruginosa*, but production is often lost by the mucoid, chronically infecting variants isolated from CF patients.

Although flagella-mediated motility is thought to be a key component of *P. aeruginosa* pathogenesis, work in a mouse model of acute pneumonia indicates that an engineered strain that produces a non-motile flagella is actually somewhat more virulent than the wild-type, fully motile strain.[116] At another level, flagella may promote bacterial adherence to host possibly by binding to asialo GM1 as well as glycolipids GM1 and GD1a, but flagella-mediated binding to epithelial cells is apparently a rare event. The FliD cap protein binds avidly to the carbohydrate portion of mucins, including a variety of neutral and acidic oligosaccharides.[117] Increased mucin production occurs in response to infection, and normally this would promote removal of the organism from the host tissue and prevent bacterial access to more vulnerable epithelial surfaces. However, in pulmonary and ocular infections, *P. aeruginosa* can take advantage of mucin binding to anchor itself to host tissues, which, when combined with such factors as reduced mucociliary clearance in the lung or entrapment of mucus under an extended-wear contact lens, results in an enhanced ability to cause disease. Of note, flagella may only be produced in the early phases of lung infection because neutrophil elastase in inflammatory secretions can cleave the flagella hook protein, FlgE, preventing formation of the flagella basal body in the outer membrane, and thus secretion of flagella. This then induces a repressor of FliC synthesis, FlgM, to accumulate inside the *P. aeruginosa* cells living in inflammatory mucus, thus accounting for loss of flagella production.

Significant interest in the ability of the *P. aeruginosa* flagellin monomer to interact with TLR5 and stimulate inflammatory responses has emerged. Of note, the TLR5 activating site is not exposed on the multimeric flagella on the bacterial surface but, rather, on the flagellin monomer, indicating that this structure has to be produced or released from the flagella in order to activate TLR5. A precise mechanism for this has not been elucidated, and evidence is against monomeric flagellin being secreted in large quantities by the bacterium.[116] When strains of *P. aeruginosa* were engineered to secrete excess monomeric flagellin, they were more virulent in a mouse lung infection model, which was attributed to their excess activation of proinflammatory cytokines via activation of TLR5. Transgenic mice lacking TLR-5 were no different than wild-type mice with regard to their susceptibility to *P. aeruginosa* lung infection,[118] but double transgenic mice lacking both TLR5 and the LPS-activated TLR4 died much sooner than wild-type or single trangenic mice, indicating in this setting that activation of both TLR4 and TLR5 contributed to innate immune resistance to *P. aeruginosa* lung infection. Similarly, mice unable to produce both TLR2 and TLR4 were more susceptible to lung infection with a nonflagellated variant of *P. aeruginosa* that could not activate TLR5, again indicating that early in infection responses of multiple TLRs to *P. aeruginosa* are needed for optimal resistance. Additional studies have shown that corneal and conjunctival cells in the eye express TLR5 and can respond to bacterial flagellin by synthesizing inflammatory cytokines.[119,120] Pretreatment of mice with *P. aeruginosa* flagellin by either the intraperitoneal or the subconjunctival route enhanced resistance to corneal infection.[120] Overall, the *P. aeruginosa* flagella via their flagellin subunits appear to initially activate host innate immunity via TLR5, but if infection is not controlled or excess flagellin is made, then harmful effects from the enhanced activation of inflammation ensue. Although

it has been suggested that TLR5-mediated inflammation could play a role in chronic lung infection in CF,[121,122] and that *P. aeruginosa* isolates from these patients do produce TLR5-activating antigens,[122] it does not appear that flagella or flagellin are being made in the inflammatory milieu of the CF lung. Thus, it remains to be seen if reported increases in TLR5 on cells within the CF lung are of consequence for infection or pathology.

Other Adhesins Potentially Involved in Colonization

A number of other *P. aeruginosa* molecules have been reported to mediate adherence of the organism to host tissues and cells. As noted previously, the outer-core oligosaccharide of *P. aeruginosa* binds to CFTR, a process important in resistance to infection in humans with normal CFTR, and LPS has also been reported to bind to asialo GM1 and the galectin-3 protein on epithelial cell surfaces. *P. aeruginosa* produces some lectin-like molecules known as PA-IL and PA-IIL that appear to promote binding to sugar molecules on tissues.[123] Also, *P. aeruginosa* OMPs, notably ompF,[124] have been shown to mediate adherence to mammalian cells as well, with one proposal that the targets on host tissues are cell surface heparin proteoglycans.[125] Overall, the adherence of *P. aeruginosa* to mucins, tissues, cells, and so forth is clearly complex and a variety of microbial products and host targets are involved, with the different interactions probably contributing to pathogenesis, but no one interaction is dominant in the context of establishing early colonization in and on host tissues.

Avoidance of Host Defenses

P. aeruginosa, like every other pathogen, encounters a rich array of innate and acquired immune factors that usually mediate high-level resistance to infection. Thus, in the settings in which colonization succeeds, it must be due to avoidance of host defenses. Host factors involved in resistance to infection were noted previously. Counteracting these are a variety of bacterial factors.

Lipopolysaccharide. *P. aeruginosa* LPS plays a key role in resisting host innate defenses. Expression of long O side chains by environmental and nosocomial strains prevents lysis by complement. The LPS O side chain structure in *P. aeruginosa* can have significant variation that affects resistance to antimicrobial peptides. In CF, the lipid A portion of *P. aeruginosa* is structurally altered, leading to changes in host inflammatory responses that promote pathogenesis.

Proteases. *P. aeruginosa* produces a variety of proteases that can inactivate host immune effectors, are cytotoxic to cells, and can degrade tissue components, allowing the organism to advance the infectious process. The best studied proteases of *P. aeruginosa* are elastolytic proteases encoded by the *lasA* (LasA protease) and *lasB* (elastase) genes, alkaline protease, and protease IV. These proteins have a broad range of substrate specificities and are thought to contribute to pathogenesis by their diverse ability to degrade host proteins. However, it is not always easy to show that the various proteases produced by *P. aeruginosa* play a role in pathogenesis because of redundancy and overlap in production of related but distinct proteases. LasA enhances the elastolytic activity of elastase and can also degrade cell walls of *Staphylococcus aureus* by digesting the pentaglycine peptidoglycan bridge. Elastase is well studied, has been crystallized, and has a variety of substrates, but loss of elastase activity generally does not always affect virulence in animal models. Nonetheless, it is of considerable interest that the LasA protease causes shedding of the ectodomain of syndecan-1, a heparin sulfate proteoglycan produced abundantly on respiratory mucosal surfaces. Although it was initially hypothesized that syndecans function in host defense, it was found that shedding of syndecan-1 enhanced *P. aeruginosa* infection in newborn mice and mice genetically deficient in syndecan-1 had increased resistance to infection. Treating the syndecan-1–deficient mice with syndecan-1 at the time of infection restored their level of susceptibility to *P. aeruginosa* infection. This surprising finding indicates that *P. aeruginosa* utilizes the shed ectodomain of syndecan-1 to protect itself from host defenses, possibly by interfering with the ingestion or killing capability of local phagocytes or by interfering with the activity of antimicrobial peptides.

Another major *P. aeruginosa* protease, alkaline protease, has high proteolytic activity but no clear role in virulence. A different protease, protease IV, has been reported to contribute significantly to experimental ulcerative keratitis in mice and also degrades a variety of substrates, but these studies have been conducted using only one strain of *P. aeruginosa* and complementation studies wherein the mutant phenotype is changed back to the wild-type phenotype have not been reported. Numerous other proteases and potential proteases have been identified both phenotypically by activity assays and genomically by homology searches of the *P. aeruginosa* genome with those of other microbes, but to date no one protease stands out as a major contributor to pathogenesis.

The Role of Iron Acquisition, Intoxication, and Local Pathologic Effects in Virulence

For infection to proceed, *P. aeruginosa* must grow initially at the local site of infection and exert pathologic effects while still avoiding host defenses. Mammalian tissues provide a stressed environment for most microbes, with reduced availability of nutrients, oxygen, and other essential factors making growth suboptimal. Microbes counteract by producing factors for acquiring limited nutrients or using alternative metabolic pathways to survive in the stressed environment. The host environment triggers a plethora of transcriptional and regulatory responses in the microbe, and these often lead to intoxication of host antibacterial effector cells that reduces bacterial killing and also probably leads to liberation of nutrients. The balance between the microbe's ability to respond to the in vivo environment and the host's antimicrobial responses determines to a large degree the progression from colonization to infection and disease-defining pathology.

Iron Acquisition and Role in Virulence. As a nutritionally versatile organism, *P. aeruginosa* can usually grow well with a minimal amount of basic inorganic and organic nutrients. Simple sources of carbon, nitrogen, phosphorous, sulfate, and magnesium appear to be all the organism needs for growth, along with a further essential requirement for iron. Obtaining iron within an infected mammal is difficult because of sequestration in hemoglobin, transferrin, and so forth, and *P. aeruginosa*, like all microbes, has evolved sophisticated means to acquire iron and to respond to the level of iron it encounters. Iron acquisition affects a number of important *P. aeruginosa* functions, including transcription of genes involved in regulating other systems, genes that affect basic metabolic processes such as the Krebs cycle, genes required to survive oxidative stress, genes necessary for scavenging iron, and genes that contribute to virulence. Notably, iron levels regulate *P. aeruginosa*'s ability to produce exotoxin A, one of the bacterial exoproteins that probably plays an important role in pathogenesis.

P. aeruginosa uses typical siderophore systems to acquire iron. There are two well-studied iron acquisition systems in *P. aeruginosa* involving the pigments pyoverdin and pyochelin. Pyoverdin synthesis depends on genes located in the *pvc* and *pvd* loci, whereas pyochelin is produced as a nonribosomal peptide from a number of precursor biosynthetic proteins. When iron is high, the master regulator of the system, a repressor protein called Fur, negatively regulates transcription of the genes encoding proteins needed for iron acquisition, including a second-tier regulatory gene, *pvdS*. When iron is low, Fur inhibition is relieved and PvdS protein is produced, which directs transcription of the *pvd* genes and also induces synthesis of the PtxR protein, which is needed for transcription of the *pvc* genes. Pyoverdin is secreted, scavenges iron from mammalian sources, and brings it back to the cell in the form of ferripyoverdin by binding to the FpvA membrane receptor. Production of FpvA is regulated by the signaling protein FpvR and an alternative sigma factor, FpvI. The FpvR protein also affects the activity of the PvdS regulatory factor. Pyochelin binds to the ferric pyochelin receptor encoded by the *fptA* gene.

Recent work has also identified other factors involved in iron-regulated responses of *P. aeruginosa*. Small regulatory RNAs have been recognized whose expression is also controlled by Fur, and these regulatory RNAs control production of factors known as quorum sensors that tell *P. aeruginosa* how to respond to its environment.[126] Another factor, the twin-arginine translocase (Tat) system, is needed for production of pyoverdin because Tat allows for an essential component of pyoverdin synthesis, PvdN, to end up in the periplasm.[127]

There is evidence suggesting that *P. aeruginosa* can also use siderophores produced by a variety of organisms to acquire iron,[128] and, interestingly, human neutrophils can bind *P. aeruginosa* siderophores and thus sequester iron from the microbe.[129] Limited virulence studies using only a few *P. aeruginosa* strains indicate that disruption of either the pyoverdin or the pyochelin system reduces pathogenicity of *P. aeruginosa*, but in general, because of the redundancy of these systems along with the availability of other potential means to acquire iron,[128] an essential role in virulence for either pyoverdin or pyochelin has not been demonstrated. Nonetheless, acquiring iron is indispensable for the organism's survival and growth, and hence iron acquisition is a vital virulence factor.

In addition to its role in iron acquisition, ferripyochelin damages pulmonary artery endothelial cells by catalyzing hydroxyl radical formation that enhances oxidant-mediated injury to the cells and also damages respiratory epithelial cells. It has also been reported that ferripyochelin can use superoxide (O_2^-) and hydrogen peroxide (H_2O_2) generated by neutrophils to enhance damage of endothelial cells. Pyochelin in the absence of bound iron does not appear to be toxic to mammalian cells. Thus, the iron-bound *P. aeruginosa* siderophore ferripyochelin contributes to local pathology by being toxic to cells.

Toxin Production: Exotoxin A, Leukocidin, Phospholipases, and Hemolysins. The major cellular toxin produced by *P. aeruginosa* is exotoxin A, an adenosine diphosphate (ADP)-ribosylating toxin with activity very similar to that of diphtheria toxin. Purified exotoxin A is lethal to experimental animals in small doses, its production is affected by iron levels, and it has been used in a variety of settings as a chimeric protein fused to growth factors or targeting antibodies to effect potential clinical benefits in settings such as autoimmune disease and cancer.[130] Exotoxin A inhibits protein synthesis by ADP-ribosylating and thus inactivating elongation factor-2 involved in moving the nascent growing peptide produced on the ribosome. Although exotoxin A has been widely studied for its part in pathogenesis, it has been difficult to define a clear role for it in *P. aeruginosa* virulence. Animal studies with a limited number of strains showed some loss of virulence when the *toxA* gene encoding exotoxin A was interrupted, but this has not been a generally applicable finding for a majority of strains. Along the same lines, immunization studies with exotoxin A toxoids have shown only a limited effect, either when used against specific strains or in combination with other immunogens. Thus, although a primary or critical role for exotoxin A in virulence has not been established, its high toxicity for cells, particularly in the liver, and production by the majority of clinical isolates suggest that it certainly contributes to both local and systemic pathology.

Another *P. aeruginosa* toxin-like factor is referred to as a cytotoxin or leukocidin and is produced from the genome of a temperate phage integrated into the chromosome of *P. aeruginosa* strain 158. Despite extensive study of this toxin, it appears to be found in only a few *P. aeruginosa* strains, although one cannot totally discount the potential of the phage genome encoding this toxin to be introduced into other strains.

Strains of *P. aeruginosa* can induce hemolysis of red blood cells by production of a hemolytic phospholipase C, PlcHR. A second, nonhemolytic phospholipase C is also made by *P. aeruginosa* strains—PlcN. PlcHR hydrolyzes phosphatidylcholine and sphingomyelin, and PlcN hydrolyzes phosphatidylcholine and phosphatidylserine. PlcHR also has an unusual property for a bacterial protein in that it can synthesize sphingomyelin by transferring the phosphoryl choline moiety from phosphatidylcholine onto the primary hydroxyl of ceramide, which results in sphingomyelin and diacylglycerol production. PlcHR has been shown to modulate virulence in several animal models and in vitro systems, whereas a contribution to virulence from PlcN has not been demonstrated.

An additional hemolysin made by *P. aeruginosa* is a rhamnolipid molecule that has multiple properties in addition to being hemolytic. Rhamnolipids function as surfactants, making them able to disrupt cell membranes, and studies in nonmammalian model hosts indicate a role for rhamnolipids in virulence. Rhamnolipid synthesis is controlled by the quorum-sensing systems of *P. aeruginosa*, and inhibition of rhamnolipid production has effects on multiple *P. aeruginosa* virulence factors, making it difficult to ascribe a singular role in virulence to rhamnolipids.

Intoxication by Type III Secretion Factors. Type III secretion systems are highly conserved features of bacterial pathogens, including *P. aeruginosa*. This system allows direct injection of bacterial toxins into eukaryotic cells, causing disruptions in cellular trafficking by inhibiting the actin cytoskeleton and also by affecting protein synthesis. For *P. aeruginosa*, expression of type III toxins is significantly associated with poor clinical outcomes, including increased mortality in acutely infected patients.[105,131] Four major effector proteins are known: exoenzyme (Exo) S, ExoT, ExoU, and ExoY. The apparatus for injection is formed as a complex structure on the bacterial surface composed of five proteins—PcrG, PcrV, PcrH, PopB, and PopD—encoded in the chromosomal pcrGVH-popBD operon. The PcrV protein, in conjunction with the PopB and PopD proteins, forms the pore bridging the bacterial and eukaryotic cells through which the effector proteins are injected. PcrG and PcrH appear to be involved in regulating this apparatus, and it has been found that PcrG binds to PcrV and PcrH binds to PopB and PopD. PcrV expression by clinical isolates has been associated with enhanced mortality of patients.[105]

ExoS and ExoT have multiple enzymatic and chemical functions. Both can ADP-ribosylate target proteins, although the activity of the ExoT protein is much lower than that of ExoS. ExoS has an amino-terminal Rho guanosine triphosphatase (GTPase)-activating protein (GAP) activity and a carboxyl-terminal ADP-ribosyltransferase domain and requires the eukaryotic cellular protein known as factor-activating ExoS (FAS) for its ADP-ribosyltransferase activity. ExoS inactivates low-molecular-weight G proteins in the Ras family, which leads to cytoskeletal changes, changes in cellular morphology and adherence, and inhibition of DNA synthesis, thus affecting target cell growth. ExoS is also required for cellular apoptosis and can ADP-ribosylate itself, leading to decreases in the Rho GTPase activity of the protein.

ExoT is composed of an amino-terminal RhoGAP domain and a carboxyl-terminal ADP-ribosyltransferase domain. ExoT interferes with internalization of *P. aeruginosa* by epithelial cells and macrophages, two processes of importance in the innate immune resistance to infection. The RhoGAP domain of ExoT inactivates proteins that regulate the cytoskeleton, including Rho, Rac, and Cdc42, and the ADP-ribosylation domain targets the eukaryotic cellular proteins Crk-I and Crk-II, two Src homology adaptor proteins that affect signal transduction important for cellular adhesion and phagocytosis. Definitive evidence for an essential role of ExoT in pathogenesis has not been produced. However, in a mouse model of *P. aeruginosa* keratitis, deletion of both ExoT and another type III effector, ExoU, reduced virulence of a strain with cytotoxic properties, and virulence was recovered with restoration of production of either ExoT or ExoU proteins.

ExoU is a potent cytotoxin, described as a phospholipase with phospholipase A_2-like activity, that readily lyses a variety of target cells. Mammalian cytoplasmic superoxide dismutases have been identified as co-factors for ExoU enzymatic lysis of target cells.[132] ExoU was first identified among *P. aeruginosa* strains shown to be cytotoxic to cultured mammalian cells, and, interestingly, carriage of the *exoS* and *exoU* genes by *P. aeruginosa* strains is virtually a mutually exclusive phenomenon. Approximately 20% to 30% of *P. aeruginosa* strains

produce ExoU, mostly isolates from eye infections and acute pneumonia. Interestingly, isolates from patients with CF rarely produce ExoU.[105] ExoU is a clear virulence factor in animal studies for the strains of *P. aeruginosa* that produce this toxin, and ExoU appears to be a marker for highly virulent clinical isolates.[106] Strains secreting ExoU are almost always more virulent in a variety of animal models, and loss of ExoU production is associated with significant decreases in virulence in animal studies. ExoU has been shown to modulate gene expression in airway epithelial cells and to increase the release of Ca^{2+} from the endoplasmic reticulum, leading to the activation of Ca channels in membranes of epithelial cells. Strains carrying *exoU* appear to be clonally derived, with evidence that the *exoU* gene and associated genetic material have been obtained through horizontal gene transfer and expansion of an original clone.

ExoY is the fourth known type III effector protein of *P. aeruginosa*, and it has adenyl cyclase activity similar to that of the extracellular adenyl cyclases of *Bordetella pertussis* and *Bacillus anthracis*. Results from animal virulence studies with mutants lacking ExoY have not been published.

Numerous environmental and genetic factors regulating expression of type III secreted toxins have been found.[133] Expression is regulated by contact with eukaryotic cells along with the presence of serum and low calcium levels. These conditions lead to transcription of four operons (*exsD-pscL*, *pscG-popD*, *pcrD-pcrR*, and *pscN-pscU*) needed to produce the type III proteins and translocate them. Control of transcription is by a master regulator encoded by the *exsA* gene. In addition, a membrane-bound adenyl cyclase distinct from ExoY regulates transcription of type III secretion genes, and a global regulator of virulence in *P. aeruginosa*, Vfr, is also involved in regulation because it is a receptor for cyclic adenosine monophosphate (cAMP). Insight into the regulators of type III secretion provides opportunities for development of possible therapeutic agents, given the clear role these molecules have in the pathogenesis of *P. aeruginosa* infection.

Toxic Effects of Pyocyanin and Role of Reactive Oxygen Species in Virulence. Extensive cellular injury occurs during *P. aeruginosa* infection, particularly in the lung, involving both epithelial and endothelial cells. Some of this damage is mediated by pyocyanin, the blue phenazine pigment partly responsible for the color of *P. aeruginosa* on agar plates, which is also detectable in the sputum of CF patients, indicating in vivo production. Pyocyanin damages cells by producing reactive oxygen species such as hydrogen peroxide and superoxide, much as ferripyochelin does. Numerous effects of pyocyanin on host cells and tissue responses have been reported, including disruption of nasal ciliary function, induction of proinflammatory effects by augmenting IL-8 production, inactivation of α_1-proteinase inhibitor, and inhibition of prostacyclin release. Mammalian cells counteract the reactive oxygen species generated by pyocyanin by producing superoxide dismutases and catalase enzymes. Pyocyanin has been reported to decrease the activity of catalase, but not the superoxide dismutases, by both transcriptional inhibition and inactivation of the enzyme. In a rat model of infection, oxidant-induced stress correlated directly with the degree of pathology from *P. aeruginosa* infection.

Because reactive oxygen species (also called reactive oxygen intermediates) are also deleterious to *P. aeruginosa*, the organism must protect itself from the effects of pyocyanin along with reactive oxygen species produced by aerobic respiration and by host phagocytic cells. *P. aeruginosa* accomplishes this, in part, by limiting the redox cycling of pyocyanin and producing three catalases (KatA, KatB, and KatC) and two superoxide dismutases—one using manganese as a cofactor and the other using iron. Production of these detoxifying enzymes requires the Fur protein that regulates *P. aeruginosa* responses to iron. Additional factors modulating the effects of reactive oxygen species include iron sequestration, agents that scavenge free radicals, DNA-binding proteins, and DNA repair enzymes. *P. aeruginosa* also synthesizes four alkyl hydroperoxide reductases. Sensing of O_2^- by the SoxR protein leads to changes in this protein that activate its ability to function as a transcription factor for genes involved in modulating potential oxidative stress. An additional regulator is the OxyR protein, which modulates transcriptional responses to H_2O_2.

Growth, Establishment of Infectious Foci, Local Tissue Spread, and Systemic Dissemination

For most *P. aeruginosa* infections, a period of growth at a local site of infection precedes dissemination or translocation to additional areas of the initially infected tissue, to another tissue, or systemically through the blood, wherein clear manifestations and clinical presentations of severe infection occur. The establishment of these local foci of infection may or may not result in clinically significant disease, and the local foci of infection often present a diagnostic challenge related to the likelihood of more significant disease occurring. Examples include GI colonization that can lead to bacteremia or to aspiration to the respiratory tract, catheter colonization that can lead to local or systemic infection, growth in burned or wounded skin, and colonization of endobronchial or endotracheal tubes that can lead to serious pneumonia. All of the microbial factors noted previously continue to play important roles in maintaining the colonization phase of the pathogenic process, with additional virulence factors coming into play at the stage at which further infection occurs, resulting in disease progression.

Quorum Sensing and Virulence Factor Production. As bacterial counts increase in a tissue, the organisms reach a critical mass that is thought to allow them to communicate effectively with each other through the system of quorum sensing (QS). At critical bacterial masses, low-molecular-weight mediators of the QS response are synthesized and secreted, diffusing through the cells of the bacterial community to influence gene transcription and virulence factor production. For *P. aeruginosa*, three major, interrelated QS systems are known, designated the las, rhl, and *Pseudomonas* quinolone system (PQS). The molecular mediators of the QS are known as autoinducers (AIs) because of their self-regulatory effects on bacterial responses to the environment. The AI mediator of the las QS system is an acyl-homoserine lactone known as *N*-(3-oxododecanoyl)-L-homoserine lactone (C12-HSL); for the rhl system, the AI mediator is *N*-butyryl-L-homoserine lactone (C4-HSL). The PQS system uses 2-heptyl-3-hydroxy-4-quinolone for signaling. These three systems, along with some other regulatory factors, have a complex interaction in the context of regulation of gene transcription and virulence factor production.

For the las and rhl QS systems, the synthetic enzymes for producing the AIs are encoded by the *lasI* and *rhlI* genes, respectively. The AIs act on a second component, the LasR or RhlR proteins, which are transcriptional regulators of the genes affected by the QS systems. When LasR complexes with C12-HSL, it forms multimers that bind to transcriptional activation sites on QS-regulated genes. Similarly, when RhlR is complexed with C4-HSL, it can act as a transcriptional regulator, but whether this involves multimers is not known. A regulator of the transcription of the AI synthetic genes is QscR, which appears to inhibit the transcription of *lasI* and production of C12-HSL, and it appears to act to ensure that QS responses are made under proper environmental conditions of high bacterial density. The PQS system also controls transcription of the *rhlI* gene, providing an additional level of regulation. Finally, another regulator of this system is the cAMP receptor protein encoded by *vfr*, which binds to the promoter region or *lasR*.

The genes whose transcription is regulated by the QS molecule are large in number, but the exact ones are not clearly known despite published reports addressing this question using modern DNA microarray analysis.[134,135] Because of differences in strains, conditions of analysis, and methodologies used to identify QS-regulated genes, the studies agreed only on 97 QS-regulated genes being present in the *P. aeruginosa* PAO1 chromosome, but each study found between 163 and 388 genes so affected. Many of these genes did not have promoter binding sites for LasR or RhlR, indicating secondary regulation through QS intermediates. The actual number probably varies from strain to strain but overall can be considered large. Notably, the majority of QS-regulated genes identified in the microarray studies have an unknown function. Genes that could be identified as being regulated by QS include membrane proteins, secreted enzymes with a variety of functions, transcription factors for regulating other genes, genes that are parts of two-component regulatory systems, genes for energy metabolism, and genes involved in movement of small molecules in and out of the cell.

Our knowledge about the importance of the QS response in the pathogenesis of *P. aeruginosa* infection is currently limited by lack of clear data concerning the extent to which it is important among clinical isolates. Virtually all of the studies of *P. aeruginosa* QS have used the PAO1 or PA14 strains to identify the factors, the regulated genetic targets, and the effect of loss of QS on virulence. Dual *las* and *rhl* system mutants of strain PAO1 have reduced virulence in animal models of burn wound infection[136] and acute[137] and chronic[138] lung infection, but studies with other strains are lacking. Of note, Cabrol and colleagues[139] studied the QS response of 35 clinical and environmental isolates and found that only one half showed a correlation between transcription of the *lasR* gene and transcription of two QS-controlled genes, *lasB* and *aprA*. Whether this indicates that only approximately 50% of *P. aeruginosa* clinical isolates regulate virulence factor production through the las QS system or whether the analysis of these systems by transcriptional responses is too limited to determine the extent of use of QS among *P. aeruginosa* clinical isolates is not known. However, the study of Cabrol and colleagues does raise the issue that the las and rhl QS systems may not be critical for the virulence of many clinical isolates. Thus, calls for development of inhibitors of QS as potential therapeutic agents for *P. aeruginosa* infections[140] need to be tempered by the current lack of knowledge of the extent of the use of these systems by clinical isolates.

Data indicate that the AIs are made during infection, although these findings have all come from studies of sputum samples from CF patients. Notably, the animal models for which there are the most robust data showing an important role for QS in *P. aeruginosa* virulence are models of acute, not chronic, infection, whereas one might predict that it is in chronic infection that the effects of QS might be more pronounced. Nonetheless, correlations between levels of transcripts for the QS genes and the QS-regulated genes in CF sputum have been found, and AIs have also been detected in CF sputum samples.[141-143] These results must be interpreted with caution because the presence of AIs and correlations with transcription do not establish that QS-mediated virulence factor production is a critical component of the pathogenesis of CF lung infection. Notably, some patients did not have detectable AIs in sputum.[141,142] Also, because the progression of CF lung disease is slow, a case could be made that AI production and QS regulation of virulence factors could actually be beneficial to the patient, preventing a more acute, rapid, and life-threatening infection from occurring in the CF lung. Further indications are that QS may not be a major factor in chronic infection. Smith and co-workers[144] found that a large number of *P. aeruginosa* isolates from long-term infected CF patients had mutations in the *lasR* gene needed for QS signaling molecules to be synthesized. Overall, it is still far from clear whether AI production and QS control of virulence contribute to the pathogenesis of either acute or chronic *P. aeruginosa* infection in humans.

Quorum Sensing and Biofilm Formation. Another major bacterial phenotype regulated by the QS system is the formation of *P. aeruginosa* biofilms, a well-studied area but with some important limitations in terms of applicability to clinical infection and disease. The extensive use of implantable devices in modern medicine has led to the appreciation that structured bacterial communities known as biofilms can form on these devices and contribute to infection.[145] In addition, in chronic infections such as osteomyelitis or CF lung infection, it is thought that biofilms play an important role in pathogenesis.[146] *P. aeruginosa* is the most studied pathogen in terms of the molecular aspects of biofilm formation,[146,147] but almost all of these studies have been done in vitro using abiotic surfaces such as polycarbonate plastic or plastic or glass flow cells. The major components of a biofilm reside in an extracellular matrix sometimes called a glycocalyx, which is thought to be heavily composed of polysaccharide for most bacterial species studied.[148] In *P. aeruginosa*, a major component of the glycocalyx is actually extracellular DNA,[149] perhaps because *P. aeruginosa* does not produce an extracellular nuclease. Two other components are polysaccharides termed Pel and Psl. Pel is a glucose-rich polymer synthesized by 7 genes in the *pel* locus,[150] whereas Psl synthesis is controlled by 15 genes in the *psl* locus.[151] The Psl polysaccharide is a galactose- and mannose-rich polymer.[152] Although impressive microscopic and artistic renditions of *P. aeruginosa* biofilms have been published,[153] these structured communities are not really observed in infected tissues, notably the CF lung.[141,153] Rather, microcolonies of aggregates of bacteria are present, and these microcolonies contain not only bacterial factors but also host factors, including host DNA, mucus, actin, and probably other products from dead and dying bacterial and host cells. How these in vivo microcolonies are related to the QS-controlled biofilms studied in vitro on abiotic surfaces is unclear, and the relationship is doubtful in many investigators' minds.

Using the in vitro systems, it has been shown that QS molecules are needed for the production of structured *P. aeruginosa* biofilms.[147] These structures are also produced under conditions of flow of nutrient media over a solid surface where the biofilm is forming, but such conditions are unlikely to be present in the lung or bone but may be present in vascular tissues. *P. aeruginosa* endocarditis and arterial graft infections are not uncommon, but no studies of the role of QS or biofilms in these diseases have been published. Within the chronically infected CF lung, where the biofilm mode of growth is most often invoked as representative of the importance of this bacterial lifestyle in pathogenesis, the establishment of chronic infection, the onset of accelerated deterioration in lung function, and the worsening of the patient's clinical condition are clearly associated with the emergence of the alginate-overproducing, mucoid phenotype of *P. aeruginosa*.[154] Yet alginate is not a component of the QS-dependent biofilms formed on abiotic surfaces under conditions of media flow,[148] further raising questions about the role of QS in biofilm formation in the CF lung. Overall, it will be a while before definitive studies linking QS, biofilm formation, and virulence in the multitude of infections *P. aeruginosa* is capable of causing will emerge. Until then, caution in ascribing a critical role for QS in virulence of *P. aeruginosa* disease, and in particular in virulence-related biofilm formation, is needed.

Local Tissue Spread. The most serious consequences of *P. aeruginosa* infection are spread throughout a susceptible tissue and vascular dissemination. Serious pneumonia is the most common manifestation of *P. aeruginosa* infection, with an attributable mortality rate approaching 40%.[155,156] No specific bacterial virulence factors in addition to those noted previously have been implicated in the development of *P. aeruginosa* pneumonia, but it is of note that this clinical presentation is rarely accompanied by systemic spread. For *P. aeruginosa* bacteremia to occur, the organism needs to produce a smooth LPS substituted with O side chains; otherwise, the bactericidal activity of serum complement would readily kill the organism in the blood. Interestingly, isolates from chronically infected CF patients do not produce a smooth LPS, indicating that in the infected lung complement levels are insufficient to be bactericidal. In addition, respiratory isolates from *P. aeruginosa* pneumonia are less likely to produce a smooth LPS than bloodstream isolates, suggesting that even in acute pneumonia a smooth LPS is not a requirement.

As increasingly more CF patients live into adulthood, their care is being assumed by specialists in adult medicine and they are increasingly managed in nonpediatric settings. Thus, the understanding of the pathogenesis of this disease is now relevant to adult infectious disease practices. Because most CF patients are chronically colonized by their 18th birthday with mucoid strains of *P. aeruginosa*, they usually have significant progression of their lung disease in adulthood. The major factors considered to be relevant to pathogenesis in this setting are overproduction of alginate[157] and the host inflammatory response,

the former protecting the organism from host defenses and the latter causing significant tissue damage. The molecular genetic basis for increased alginate production is well understood,[157] although whether there is a common or unifying genetic or environmental event that initiates or sustains alginate overproduction by CF isolates of *P. aeruginosa* is not clear. Alginate clearly protects the organism from phagocytosis, and it appears that the O-acetyl substituents on the alginate molecule are critical for manifestation of this phenotype. In addition, alginate has been shown to be a key bacterial factor needed for establishing chronic *P. aeruginosa* oropharyngeal colonization in transgenic CF mice.[158]

Interestingly, CF patients produce high titers of antibodies to alginate and other *P. aeruginosa* antigens during infection, but these antibodies obviously fail to mediate protection from infection.[157] It has been proposed that the antibodies to alginate are deficient in opsonic killing activity, a clear in vitro correlate of protective antibody activity, because of an inability to deposit the critical complement opsonin iC3b onto the bacterial surface.[43] In animal models, alginate-specific opsonic antibodies mediate protection against infection. Of interest, because *P. aeruginosa* is thought to grow as some sort of biofilm in the CF lung, Meluleni and colleagues[159] showed that the antibodies CF patients make to *P. aeruginosa* are able to mediate opsonic killing of suspended or planktonic *P. aeruginosa* but not of bacterial cells growing in a biofilm. Opsonic antibodies to alginate did, however, promote killing of biofilm cells of *P. aeruginosa*. As the bacteria in the CF lung spread and fail to be cleared, the associated inflammatory response contributes significantly to tissue destruction, with the neutrophil-dominated infiltrate causing damage by a variety of molecular mechanisms emanating mostly from contents in spilled neutrophil granules.[160] However, it is important to keep in mind that CF is a chronic, progressive disease associated with high bacterial burdens for many years; probably, the immune-inflammatory response in this setting is mediating important, positive outcomes that limit the kinetics and magnitude of bacterial spread and turn what otherwise would be an acute, potentially lethal situation into one in which the patient's survival is much longer.

Spread of *P. aeruginosa* throughout the cornea can cause severe tissue damage, with loss of sight a distinct possibility. In this tissue, ExoU and ExoT are also clear virulence factors for cytotoxic strains of *P. aeruginosa* (i.e., those able to kill eukaryotic cells readily in vitro), as determined in experimental models of ulcerative keratitis, and *exoU*-positive strains of *P. aeruginosa* are also frequently isolated from contact lens-associated keratitis. Concurrent with tissue spread is a vigorous host inflammatory response in the eye, despite the fact that the cornea is avascular. It appears that the inflammation that ensues is the primary cause of corneal damage because pathology seems to continue to develop long after bacterial numbers subside in the tissue. The ongoing inflammation may be due to residual bacterial factors known to activate inflammation, including LPS, flagella, and toxins.

Aside from the lung and the eye, *P. aeruginosa* spread in other tissues resulting in damage and physiologic compromise is much less studied, although this highly versatile organism is capable of causing serious disease in any otherwise sterile tissue that it infects. It is likely that the same factors involved in lung and eye infections dictate the magnitude and kinetics of spread of *P. aeruginosa* in other tissues.

Bloodstream Dissemination. *P. aeruginosa* is among the top five causes of nosocomial bacteremia, and severe infection can lead to sepsis. Because of the multitude of virulence factors the organism elaborates, coupled with increasing antibiotic resistance, *P. aeruginosa* continues to be a problematic pathogen in this setting. When *P. aeruginosa* spreads from a tissue source, it probably does so by breaking down epithelial and endothelial barriers to gain access to the blood.[161] Breakdown of the epithelial barrier of the lung in an experimental model of *P. aeruginosa* sepsis in rabbits was associated with release of proinflammatory mediators into the blood, leading to sepsis.[161] Provision of antibodies to TNF-α or of the counterinflammatory cytokine IL-10 improved both the signs of septic shock and the levels of bacteremia in the experimental animals. Thus, the bacterial factors that promote release of TNF-α and probably IL-1, which also contributes to cytokine-mediated sepsis and death in experimental animals,[57,58] represent major virulence traits promoting pathology in *P. aeruginosa* bloodstream infection. Of note, in mice whose normal GI microbial flora was disrupted by oral antibiotics and whose GI tracts were subsequently colonized by *P. aeruginosa* that had been inoculated into the drinking water, systemic spread and death were induced by merely making the mice neutropenic with a neutrophil-depleting monoclonal antibody.[162] In this setting, the organism appeared to be able to induce tissue damage to allow for submucosal translocation and eventual systemic dissemination.

Vaccines and Immunotherapies

A variety of antigenic targets expressed by *P. aeruginosa* are being evaluated for development of active and passive immunotherapies (Table 219-2). Active vaccination would be indicated in young CF patients, although they represent a small target population. Potential additional targets include police, firefighters, soldiers, and similar individuals at risk for burn or wound infection. Whether individuals undergoing elective surgery would be a reasonable target for immunization will probably depend on future trends in infection rates, antimicrobial resistance, cost-benefit analysis, and so forth. An effective passive immunotherapy, consisting of either immunoglobulin G (IgG) derived from donors given a vaccine or an individual or set of human monoclonal antibodies, can be reasonably envisioned as a useful adjunct to antibiotic therapy or perhaps as a prophylactic measure in an ICU or similar setting of high risk for *P. aeruginosa* infection.

The highly variable O-antigen component of the LPS is clearly the most effective target for preventing *P. aeruginosa* infection, but with 20 to 30 potential O-antigen variants that need to be incorporated into an effective vaccine or passive immunotherapeutic agent, producing an effective vaccine or immunotherapy using these antigens is daunting. OMPs have shown success as candidate vaccines in animal models, and some OMPs are already in clinical trials.[163] The bacterial flagella have shown excellent promise as a vaccine in animal models,[164] and a clinical trial in European CF patients[165,166] has shown efficacy in reduc-

ing new-onset infection but not the development of chronic infection due to an inadequate number of controls becoming chronically infected during the course of the study. Pili have been promoted as potential vaccines, but preclinical data from animals are limited and there is significant variability in pilin monomers, which may form some of the antigenic targets in a vaccine. A promising approach has been to target the PcrV protein that is part of the type III secretion complex,[167-169] but to date this PcrV vaccination has shown efficacy with only a limited number of ExoU-producing cytotoxic strains using two different pneumonia models and a burn wound infection model. Protection against death by one of the three strains used in the burn wound model required additional immunization against exotoxin A. Alginate has shown efficacy in animal models of chronic *P. aeruginosa* infection, and a fully human IgG1 monoclonal antibody to alginate protected mice against lung infection by both mucoid and nonmucoid strains that made small, but not zero, amounts of alginate.[170] Antibody to alginate also reduced bacterial levels and tissue pathology in an experimental keratitis model.[171] Antitoxic immunity to such factors as exotoxin A and proteases seems to be effective only in limited situations or with special strains and does not appear to be a generally useful strategy.

Live, attenuated vaccine strains of *P. aeruginosa* have shown efficacy in animal models of pneumonia after intranasal immunization[172,173] and could potentially deliver a variety of antigens to the immune system resulting in broad-based immunity. Protection across LPS serotypes was found to require activation of the Th17 cell that augments PMN recruitment to the site of infection—in this setting, the lung.[174] Of note, the finding that *P. aeruginosa* enters epithelial cells by CFTR-based endocytosis[91,93] indicates that a portion of the organisms have an intracellular phase and, thus, cell-mediated immunity may be an important component of host resistance to *P. aeruginosa* infection. The live, attenuated vaccine has the potential to elicit cell-mediated immune effectors, and a combination of both humoral and cellular immunity may be needed for full-fledged host resistance to infection. Overall, a *P. aeruginosa* vaccine or passive immunotherapeutic agent could be of tremendous benefit in a variety of infectious situations caused by this pathogen if the proper immune factors, benefits to patients, and costs appropriate to the situation are identified and evaluated.

Clinical Characteristics of *Pseudomonas aeruginosa* Infections

P. aeruginosa has been reported to cause infections at almost all sites of the body or to colonize almost any site subjected to injury. Thus, this organism has a wide potential for disease causation that is determined by development of host susceptibility leading to predisposition to infection and by the possession of a wide range of virulence factors as already described. That *P. aeruginosa* is particularly adapted to the respiratory tract of humans is suggested by the fact that it is the most prominent cause of lung disease in patients with CF[82] and ranks as number one or two as a cause of VAPs.[155] It also has potential as a chronic airway colonizer of individuals with chronic lung diseases such as bronchiectasis[175] and panbronchiolitis, a disease that is seen primarily in Japan.[176] Thus, the role of this organism as measured in both disease and the potential for disease by colonizing and infecting the airways is unmatched by most other bacteria except those traditionally associated with lung disease, such as *Streptococcus pneumoniae* and *Haemophilus influenzae*. However, the disease-producing potential of *P. aeruginosa* goes far beyond this primary site of tropism, resulting in a number of different clinical syndromes that are often manifestations of its opportunism.

SITE-SPECIFIC *PSEUDOMONAS* INFECTIONS

Bacteremia

P. aeruginosa remains one of the most feared organisms that cause bacteremia. In older studies of this infection, there were reports of

TABLE 219-2	Antigenic Targets for Vaccines
Antigen	*Mechanism of Immunity, Utility, and Problems*
LPS O side chain	Opsonic killing by phagocytes; most effective vaccine target but extensive serologic variation and problems with immunodominance of protective epitopes
Outer membrane proteins	Opsonic killing by phagocytes (not clear); antigenically conserved; effective in animals; produce recombinant forms; no effective human vaccine based on these antigens produced to date; opsonins binding to OMPs can be masked by LPS O side chains or alginate
PcrV antigen	Mechanism not clear; produced by many strains; antigenically conserved; utility for many strains not demonstrated; some strains do not produce PcrV
Alginate	Opsonic killing by phagocytes; antigenically conserved; utility for mucoid strains demonstrated, not clear if useful for nonmucoid strains; problems with immunodominance of protective epitopes
Exotoxins	Neutralization; antigenically conserved; utility in animal models is minimal and mostly effective against purified toxin, not against whole bacterial infections
Live, attenuated bacteria	Opsonization and other effects; immunity to variety of antigens induced; both humoral and cellular immunity can be induced; number of strains needed unknown; safety unknown; antigenic specificity of immunity not known

LPS, lipopolysaccharide; OMP, outer membrane protein.

mortality rates exceeding 50%[177-179] when crude mortality was used as the end point. In neutropenic patients, mortality was as high as 70% in an era when aminoglycosides and polymyxins were the primary antimicrobial therapies. Consequently, *P. aeruginosa* bacteremia became a dreaded clinical syndrome, resulting in attempts to manage this disease by the administration of multiple antibiotics. However, since the introduction of β-lactam antibiotics with specific antipseudomonal activity, there have been no populations of patients in which such a high mortality is directly a consequence of a *P. aeruginosa* infection.[180] Examination of published mortality data over an 8-year period showed widely varying mortality rates,[180] but recent publications show attributable mortality rates of 28% to 44%,[181] depending on the adequacy of treatment and the seriousness of the underlying diseases. Remarkably, in a matched cohort of non-neutropenic patients, mortality attributable to *P. aeruginosa* infection was reported to be as low as 15%.[182] Whether such low rates are a reflection of early appropriate therapy or differences in the populations examined is not known. Undoubtedly, the population most at risk for *P. aeruginosa* bacteremia includes the sickest and most compromised group of hospitalized individuals. Thus, their risk for death during bacteremia is likely to remain high.

It is difficult to obtain up-to-date estimates of the true incidence of *P. aeruginosa* bacteremia in North America or anywhere else. However, cross-sectional studies, which tend to be concentrated in academic centers, were published by the SENTRY Antimicrobial Surveillance Program. Between 1997 and 1999, 4.4% of bacteremias occurring in the United States were due to *P. aeruginosa*, with even higher rates in Europe and Latin America.[183] Therefore, the occurrence of *P. aeruginosa* bacteremia may be influenced by national or regional factors or may even be related to climatic conditions. The sources of *P. aeruginosa* bacteremia have also undergone changes. The classic patient with *P. aeruginosa* bacteremia was considered to be the neutropenic or burned patient, implicating the gut and skin as the portals of entry, but a minority of patients with burn wound infections now suffer from bacteremic *P. aeruginosa* infections,[184] although it remains a common organism isolated from the burn wound.[185] *P. aeruginosa* bacteremia is still seen in neutropenic patients, but this organism plays a much smaller role in infections in these patients, occurring on average in less than 10% of severely neutropenic patients who have documented bacterial infections.[180] The most frequently documented sources are now the respiratory and urinary tracts, probably because of changes in the management of patients in hospitals related to more prolonged supportive care utilizing ventilators and urinary catheters.

Clinical Presentation. The clinical presentation of *P. aeruginosa* bacteremia is rarely different from that of sepsis in general. Patients are usually febrile, but more severely ill patients in shock may be hypothermic. The only point differentiating this entity from other causes of gram-negative sepsis may be the occurrence of distinctive infarcted skin lesions known as ecthyma gangrenosa, which occur almost exclusively in markedly neutropenic patients. The source may be hematogenous spread or inoculation at the site of minor trauma, such as a vascular catheter access site or even a shaving nick. These are small, painful, reddish, maculopapular, well-circumscribed lesions that have a geographic margin and begin as pink, darken to purple, and finally become black and necrotic (Fig. 219-5). Histopathology indicates that the lesions are due to vascular invasion after bacteremia and are teeming with bacteria. Similar lesions do occur with other infections, particularly aspergillosis and mucormycosis, but their presence should suggest *P. aeruginosa* bacteremia as the most likely cause, requiring the appropriate empirical antibiotic therapy.

Treatment of Bacteremia. Antimicrobial therapy is the mainstay in the treatment of bacteremia, but removal of an infected vascular catheter may be needed to control device-related bacteremia.

At least four studies—none of them prospective, double-blind studies—have indicated that *P. aeruginosa* bacteremia has the same outcome when treated with a single antipseudomonal β-lactam or

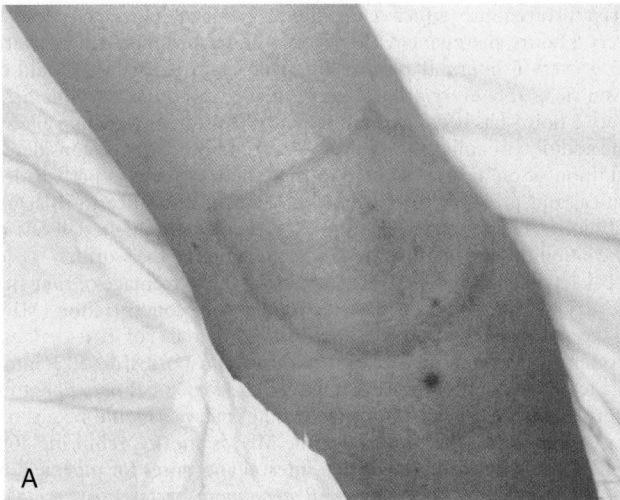

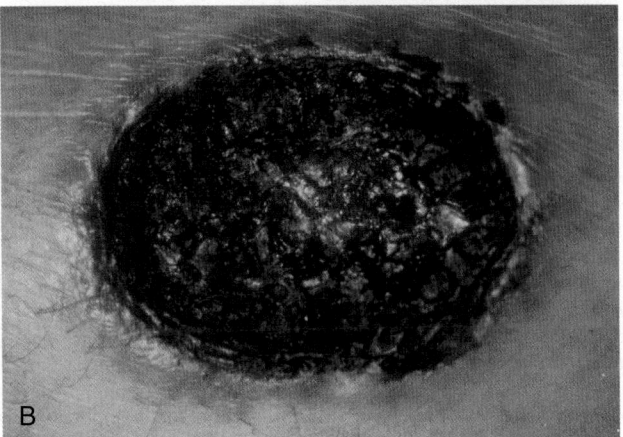

Figure 219-5 **Ecthyma gangrenosa from *Pseudomonas aeruginosa* bacteremia in neutropenic patients. A,** Lesion 72 hours after onset. **B,** Lesion late in the course with typical well-defined area of necrosis.

such an agent combined with an aminoglycoside.[70,186-188] The latest study on this subject suggests that there is marginally higher mortality after 30 days when patients are treated with adequate empirical monotherapy compared with adequate empirical combination therapy, but no difference in mortality was found when patients were treated with an adequate definitive monotherapy or an adequate combination therapy.[189] Thus, none of the dogmas concerning the appropriate therapy for *P. aeruginosa* bacteremia can be considered to be established by blinded, controlled clinical studies. One firm conclusion appears to be that monotherapy with an aminoglycoside dosed in the approved way should not be the primary choice for antibiotic treatment. Unquestionably, the majority of infectious disease experts still favor the use of combination therapy for *P. aeruginosa* bacteremia. However, it is difficult to indict the use of a single modern antipseudomonal β-lactam antibiotic as being inadequate therapy. Even in the patients most at risk for dying rapidly from *P. aeruginosa* bacteremia (i.e., high-risk patients with fever and neutropenia), empirical monotherapy designed to treat *P. aeruginosa* is considered to be as efficacious as empirical combination therapy in the Practice Guidelines of the Infectious Diseases Society of America (IDSA).[190]

Adequate empirical therapy to cover this organism should include the agents against which there are the lowest levels of antibiotic resistance within an institution and which are predictably most stably effective against *P. aeruginosa*. Depending on the antibiotic susceptibility of *P. aeruginosa* isolates in the institution, one of the following regimens would be appropriate for *P. aeruginosa* bacteremia, pending return of susceptibility results: Adult, nonazotemic patients may be given intravenously either ceftazidime 2 g every 8 hours, cefepime 2 g every 8 hours, meropenem 1.0 g every 8 hours, or imipenem-cilastatin 0.5 g every 6 hours. If piperacillin-tazobactam is used, it should be given as 3.375 g every 4 hours or 4.5 g every 6 hours. Aztreonam 2 g every 8 hours has been used for patients with serious β-lactam allergy. The addition of amikacin 15 mg/kg every 24 hours may be considered. Addition of an aminoglycoside to the other regimens is perhaps less critical and probably depends on the level of resistance to β-lactam antibiotics in any given institution. Currently, the highest levels of susceptibilities are to amikacin in most regions of the world.[183]

β-Lactam efficacy is best correlated with the percentage of time that the active drug is above the minimal inhibitory concentration (MIC) of the pathogen in regard to the dosing interval. For *P. aeruginosa*, enough antipseudomonal penicillins or cephalosporins, dosed at intervals to achieve serum levels that exceed the MIC of *P. aeruginosa* for approximately 60% to 70% of the dosing interval, should be given.[74] For carbapenems, the time above the MIC is shorter, requiring 40% of the dosing interval. The dosing interval and doses for piperacillin-tazobactam for the treatment of *P. aeruginosa* bacteremia have also been evaluated on the basis of pharmacodynamic behaviors.[191] It is suggested that these agents be given by continuous infusion to achieve the pharmacokinetic and pharmacodynamic parameters that predict efficacy, although there is no clinical confirmation of this recommendation. Indications for aminoglycoside dosing have also undergone changes in the past decade. Because their ability to kill is concentration dependent, a single total daily dose of an aminoglycoside is predicted to achieve better results. In addition, this approach has not increased toxicity.[192] Whether aminoglycosides given as a single daily dose would result in better outcomes in *P. aeruginosa* bacteremia has not been examined prospectively. The interval from the time a subsequently positive blood culture is taken to the time appropriate therapy is administered has been found to be as critical as the drugs chosen. Studies suggest that 30-day mortality from *P. aeruginosa* bacteremia may at least double if there is a delay of more than 52 hours in administering the appropriate drug from the time the blood culture is taken.[193] Thus, the timely administration of appropriate empirical therapy is essential.

Besides the issue of outcomes, combination therapy for *P. aeruginosa* bacteremia utilizing a β-lactam antibiotic plus an aminoglycoside has been espoused to prevent the development of resistance. Development of resistance is a legitimate concern and was demonstrated in in vitro and animal studies. However, clinical data from human studies have not definitely substantiated this assumption. In addition, it has been convincingly demonstrated that the addition of an aminoglycoside to a carbapenem for *P. aeruginosa* infection of the respiratory tract does not prevent the development of resistance to the carbapenem.

In some institutions and countries, the susceptibilities of *P. aeruginosa* to the first-line antibiotic agents are less than 80%. In such settings, combination empirical therapy for a patient with bacteremia or sepsis who has a significant chance of a *P. aeruginosa* infection should be started until pathogen identification and antibiotic susceptibilities are available. Whether one or two agents should be continued is usually left to individual preferences. The length of therapy for *P. aeruginosa* bacteremia has not undergone careful scrutiny. It is generally recommended that neutropenic patients be treated until recovery of their neutrophil levels. Relatively simple bacteremias in non-neutropenic patients may be treated with shorter courses of therapy, assuming that any devices that may have predisposed to the bacteremia have been removed. On the other hand, the management of some other forms of *P. aeruginosa* bacteremia is not so straightforward. Complex bacteremias that also involve infections in tissues such as the lung, kidney, and skin may be more difficult to treat, especially in neutropenic patients. It is therefore recommended that such patients receive longer courses of therapy.

Acute Pneumonia
The respiratory tract remains the most frequent site of infection caused by *P. aeruginosa*. This organism ranks either first or second in most

lists as the causative pathogen in VAP.[155,194] However, much debate centers on the actual role of the organism in VAP because the conclusion that *P. aeruginosa* plays a major role is based on results of cultures of sputum and endotracheal tube aspirates, which can frequently represent nothing more than nonpathogenic colonization of the tracheobronchial tree, formation of an innocuous biofilm on the endotracheal tube, or simple tracheobronchitis. In the absence of radiologic evidence of pneumonia, the question remains whether *P. aeruginosa* is the cause of purulence in the tracheobronchial secretions (i.e., tracheobronchitis).[195]

Although the incidence of *P. aeruginosa* pneumonia may not be as high as has been assumed on the basis of results of cultures from the upper respiratory tract, many studies using bronchoscopic techniques have supported an important role for *P. aeruginosa* in acute lung infections in the hospitalized patient on a ventilator.[194] *P. aeruginosa* was once thought to have a significant role in pneumonia in febrile neutropenic patients, but its occurrence at this site in these patients is now relatively uncommon. There have been increasing reports of community-acquired *P. aeruginosa* pneumonia at opposite ends of the spectrum of host compromise, including the AIDS patient with low CD4 counts[195] and the relatively healthy patient with or without underlying lung disease.[196] Reports of community-acquired pneumonia related to *P. aeruginosa* have been rare in the past, and recent reports that 7% of patients admitted for community-acquired pneumonia have *P. aeruginosa* are troubling.[197]

Older reports of *P. aeruginosa* pneumonia describe patients with an acute clinical syndrome of fever, chills, cough, and a necrotizing pneumonia not very different from acute staphylococcal pneumonia. The pathogenesis of this disease is believed to be direct inoculation of large numbers of the organism into the lungs by aspiration or inhalation. Most of these cases occurred in hospitalized patients who had received antibiotics. The traditional accounts describe a fulminant infection, with cyanosis, tachypnea, copious sputum, and systemic toxicity. Chest radiographs demonstrated bilateral pneumonia, often with nodular densities. This picture is now remarkably rare. Today, the typical patient is being mechanically ventilated, has a slowly progressive lung infiltrate, and has been colonized with *P. aeruginosa* for days. Although some cases may progress rapidly over a 48- to 72-hour period, this form of presentation is the exception and nodular densities are generally not seen. However, the infiltrates may go on to necrosis. This form of the disease has also been seen in the community, for example, after the inhalation of hot tub water contaminated by *P. aeruginosa*.[198] The typical patient is febrile and has a leukocytosis and purulent sputum, and the chest radiograph shows a new infiltrate or an increase in a preexisting infiltrate. Chest examination generally demonstrates rales or dullness. Such findings are quite common in ventilated ICU patients, making the diagnosis somewhat difficult without an invasive procedure.

There is an emerging consensus that an invasive procedure such as bronchoalveolar lavage or protective brush sampling of the distal airways should be used to obtain quantitative cultures of the lung to substantiate the occurrence of *P. aeruginosa* pneumonia[194] (Chapter 303). In a ventilated patient, however, the diagnostic accuracy using endotracheal aspirates appears to be just as good as in patients who had bronchoalveolar lavage done as the diagnostic procedure.[199] Therapy for *P. aeruginosa* pneumonia has been unsatisfactory. The disease has an appreciable mortality rate when the organism remains confined to the lungs. Reports suggest up to 70% to 80% mortality,[194] but the question remains how much of this mortality is attributable to the underlying lung disease. Some studies suggest a mortality attributable to *P. aeruginosa* infection of approximately 40%. However, when complicated by bacteremia, *P. aeruginosa* pneumonia in neutropenic patients or in the ventilated patient has a considerably worse prognosis with higher mortality rates, approaching 90%.[181,200]

Treatment of Pneumonia. The therapy for *P. aeruginosa* pneumonia has not been determined by rigorous studies. Some of the issues involve the differentiation of colonization from infection and the question of attributable mortality. High failure rates were seen when aminoglycosides were used as single agents. The failure was subsequently attributed to several factors, including low antibiotic levels achieved in the airways, inactivation of aminoglycosides in the acidic environment of the lungs, and binding of drugs to human mucus. Another factor may be the lack of an appreciation of the concentration-dependent killing mediated by aminoglycosides, which suggests that single high doses may be more effective than twice- or thrice-daily dosing at low levels. The drugs of choice for *P. aeruginosa* pneumonia appear to be similar to those discussed previously for bacteremia. A strong case cannot be made for the inclusion of the aminoglycoside component for fully susceptible organisms, given the evidence that aminoglycosides are not optimally active in the lungs at concentrations normally used with intravenous administration. Aerosolized aminoglycosides might provide adequate drug levels in the tracheobronchial tree, but there is no reason to believe that the drug would penetrate into the consolidated lung. Densities of *P. aeruginosa* are reduced[201,202] and inflammatory markers are diminished with inhaled aminoglycosides, but efficacy in the treatment of acute *P. aeruginosa* pneumonia has not been demonstrated in a controlled trial. The usually recommended drug is tobramycin, 300 mg inhaled daily. Patients with nosocomial pneumonia may have *P. aeruginosa* isolates resistant to many of the usual drugs, a problem that appears to be becoming progressively worse.

Chronic Respiratory Tract Infections

P. aeruginosa is responsible for chronic infections of the airways associated with a number of underlying or predisposing conditions, the most prevalent being CF, found mostly in white populations. The description and management of *P. aeruginosa* infection in this entity can be found in Chapter 68. A somewhat similar state of chronic colonization beginning early in childhood is seen in some Asian populations in a disease of unknown etiology called chronic or diffuse panbronchiolitis.[176] The disease is most often described in Japan but is not restricted to that country. In this disease, not unlike CF, there is a chronic relapsing infection by *P. aeruginosa*, characterized by increased sputum production, fever, and focal lung infiltrates. Strains of *P. aeruginosa* isolated from these patients undergo the same type of mucoid conversion as strains from patients with CF. Patients with diffuse panbronchiolitis respond clinically to antipseudomonal therapy, but the organism is not eradicated. However, significant advances have been made in its management with the long-term use of macrolides,[203] a class of drugs that have no antibacterial activity against *P. aeruginosa* but are thought to suppress the inflammatory response[204] and perhaps suppress production of *P. aeruginosa* virulence factors.[205] The most commonly used agents have been clarithromycin and azithromycin.

P. aeruginosa is one of the organisms that colonizes damaged bronchi in bronchiectasis, a disease secondary to multiple causes in which there are profound structural abnormalities of the airways resulting in the stasis of mucus. The issues concerning the management of *P. aeruginosa* in this setting are less clear. The organism establishes a state of chronic colonization and is not eradicated by antibiotics. The behavior of the organism is not unlike that in CF. Treatment is given during exacerbations, but its role has not been examined objectively in terms of the effect of treatment on decline of lung function. Aerosolized tobramycin results in a reduction of the bacterial load.[202] Patients may also be given an injectable antipseudomonal β-lactam antibiotic.

Bone and Joint Infections

P. aeruginosa is not a frequent cause of bone or joint infections. Such infections result from at least three different mechanisms: bacteremia, direct inoculation into bone, and spread from contiguous infection. Bacteremia caused by the injection of contaminated illicit drugs or resulting from infective endocarditis in the addict population has been well documented to cause vertebral oseomyelitis[206] and sternoclavicular joint arthritis.[207] However, *P. aeruginosa* bacteremia from the lungs, urinary tract, or other tissues rarely leads to seeding of bone sites, such as the vertebral disks or the axial skeleton, compared with the frequency noted for *S. aureus*.

The clinical presentation of vertebral *P. aeruginosa* osteomyelitis is more indolent than that of staphylococcal osteomyelitis. The duration of symptoms in the addict population with vertebral osteomyelitis is weeks to months. Fever is not uniformly present and, when present, it tends to be low grade.[206] There may be mild tenderness at the site of involvement. Leukocytosis may or may not be present, but the erythrocyte sedimentation rate (ESR) is invariably elevated. Blood cultures are usually negative unless there is concomitant endocarditis. Plain radiographs have been reported to be normal on admission. Therefore, when radiographs are negative, magnetic resonance imaging (MRI) should be obtained for possible drug addicts with symptoms suggesting osteomyelitis. The appropriate diagnostic procedure once the site is located is a computed tomography guided needle biopsy or aspiration in cases in which blood cultures are negative. Open biopsy may be needed in some cases because other causes of osteomyelitis must be considered in indolent disease in addicts whose blood cultures and needle aspirates are culture negative. Although unusual, vertebral osteomyelitis due to *P. aeruginosa* has also been reported in elderly people, originating from urinary tract infections,[208] the infection generally involves the lumbosacral area because of a shared venous drainage (Batson's plexus) between the lumbosacral spine and pelvis.

Sternoclavicular septic arthritis caused by *P. aeruginosa* is seen almost exclusively in intravenous drug addicts.[207] It may occur with or without endocarditis, but a primary site of infection is often not found. The disease is most often monoarticular. Sometimes there is sternochondral joint involvement. Patients generally complain of anterior chest pain over the involved joint and restriction of movement of the ipsilateral shoulder. There is often swelling over the affected joint. Laboratory findings are usually mild, but the ESR is almost always elevated. Plain radiographs show joint or bone involvement. Biopsies may be needed for diagnosis, at which time drainage and débridement may be done because there may be abscess formation and necrotic cartilage, requiring excision or débridement for cure.

P. aeruginosa may also involve the pubic symphysis in addicts, but involvement at that site is not limited to this population.[209] It has been seen after pelvic surgery and as a complication of femoral artery catheterization. Patients present with a variety of ill-defined painful syndromes that may involve the lower abdomen, hips, groin, or thighs, and symptoms are exacerbated by walking. There is generally exquisite tenderness of the pubic symphysis. Radiographs may be normal or abnormal, but bone scans are usually diagnostic. If there is no concomitant bacteremia, needle aspiration or biopsy should be done in these cases.

Pseudomonas osteomyelitis of the foot most often follows puncture wounds through sneakers. The organism has been found between the layers of the rubber soles of sneakers in many cases.[210,211] Most of these cases are reported in children, but the disease is also seen in adults.[212] The main manifestation is pain in the foot, and there may be a superficial cellulitis around the puncture wound and tenderness on deep palpation of the wound. Multiple joints or bones of the foot may be involved. Systemic symptoms are generally absent. Blood cultures are usually negative, but the ESR tends to be elevated. Radiographs may or may not be abnormal, but the bone scan is usually positive, as are MRI studies.[213] Needle aspiration usually yields a diagnosis. Prompt surgery, with exploration of the nail puncture tract and débridement of the involved bones and cartilage, is generally recommended for the treatment of this disease, in addition to antibiotic therapy. This entity is perhaps the only form of *P. aeruginosa* osteomyelitis wherein short courses of therapy for 2 weeks have been successful.[214] However, it is advisable to monitor therapy with ESR or C-reactive protein measurements, which may predict treatment failure.

Another form of *P. aeruginosa* osteomyelitis, often referred to as chronic contiguous osteomyelitis, is probably a mixture of different entities that have in common infection of bone extending from an infected, contiguous area.[206] It may involve infection of an open fracture or even a closed fracture after a surgical procedure contiguous to the site of the fracture. Some of the more frequent occurrences are in the setting of decubitus ulcers, the diabetic foot, and ischemic ulcers secondary to peripheral vascular disease. In the latter situations in which the ulcer has been chronic, there is often a mixed flora, making it difficult to ascertain the role of *P. aeruginosa*. Deep bone biopsies, considered the "gold standard" for making a microbiologic diagnosis,[215] have been recommended to ascertain the cause of osteomyelitis but are not routinely done. A pure culture of *P. aeruginosa* would be indicative of a true *P. aeruginosa* infection given its ability to infect bone, but that is uncommon from wound cultures. MRI scans to implicate bone rather than simple soft tissue involvement followed by a bone biopsy, histology studies, and culture may be a means of making a more certain diagnosis. ESR determinations are of considerable help in diagnosis and therapy of most acute bone infections; however, in chronic contiguous osteomyelitis these measurements have been less reliable. If the ESR is elevated, it may be useful to observe the patient for bone involvement, but this is not seen in the majority of cases. Therapy of contiguous osteomyelitis almost always requires or involves surgery to débride overlying infected or colonized tissue and to remove dead bone.

Treatment of Bone Infections. With the exception of the osteomyelitis after puncture wounds that occurs mainly in children, antibiotic therapy of *P. aeruginosa* osteomyelitis is difficult. The choices are single-drug therapy with an antipseudomonal β-lactam antibiotic[216] or ciprofloxacin.[217,218] The success of ciprofloxacin in many forms of *P. aeruginosa* osteomyelitis, despite relatively low peak serum levels with the usual doses used to treat osteomyelitis (500 or 750 mg PO twice daily) and low ratios of the area under the curve to the MIC, suggests that there may be specific factors that allow effective therapy. Some reasons may be a low density of organisms in osteomyelitis and perhaps slow multiplication rates allowing less selection of resistant mutants, but most important may be the good penetration of this agent into bone. Vertebral disease in drug addicts has been treated with single-drug therapy, including aminoglycosides.[206] However, it is suggested that nonaminoglycosides in maximal recommended doses be used as first-line agents for at least 4 weeks of therapy, as long as the isolate is sensitive to the antibiotic. Whether *P. aeruginosa* bone infections require combination therapy has not been evaluated in clinical trials in humans. If, however, there is accompanying endocarditis, therapy should be directed to that disease, and this may change the management approach in terms of length of therapy and whether a single agent should be used. Most other acute forms of *P. aeruginosa* osteomyelitis may be managed similarly. There are no guidelines that have been subjected to scrutiny. Therapy with single β-lactam antibiotics may be started and the clinical response followed by ESR. If the patient is not responding, a second agent such as an aminoglycoside may be added. Alternatively, therapy may be started with ciprofloxacin at the higher end of the dosing range. Therapy is generally for 4 to 6 weeks, but foot infections have been treated successfully with 750 mg twice daily of ciprofloxacin taken orally for 14 days. Most of the published information for significant bone infection recommends up to 6 months of ciprofloxacin if this agent is being used.

The antibiotic therapy for chronic osteomyelitis related to *P. aeruginosa* is difficult, not unlike therapy for all forms of chronic osteomyelitis. The suggestions for acute therapy may not be appropriate in this setting. Surgery plays a much greater role in chronic osteomyelitis in order to remove dead and scarred areas where antibiotic penetration may be poor. The history of treatment of this entity is one of relapsing infection. The success of fluoroquinolones in managing a number of acute and chronic *P. aeruginosa* bone infections suggests that they may be useful alone or in conjunction with other agents. One approach, therefore, may be to begin therapy in cases of chronic osteomyelitis with a β-lactam antibiotic that is given for 4 weeks followed by 4 to 6 months of ciprofloxacin if the organism is sensitive. However, *Pseudomonas* resistance to ciprofloxacin has increased dramatically worldwide, which may preclude its use in many cases. In such cases, more aggressive initial therapy with 2 weeks of a combination of a β-lactam

and an aminoglycoside antibiotic followed by 2 months of the β-lactam alone is suggested. If an elevated ESR is present after débridement, it may be a useful measurement for following the patient in order to determine the approximate length of therapy. Note, however, that regardless of whether injectable or oral antibiotics are given, there is a high failure rate in chronic bone infections and many require re-treatment.

Central Nervous System Infections

Primary central nervous system infections with *P. aeruginosa* are a relative rarity. Involvement is almost always secondary to a surgical procedure or head trauma and occasionally bacteremia.[219] The entities seen most often are postoperative or post-traumatic meningitis and occasionally subdural or epidural infections that result from contamination of these areas. Embolic disease from endocarditis in intravenous drug addicts leading to brain abscesses has also been described. The cerebrospinal fluid (CSF) profile of *P. aeruginosa* meningitis is no different from that of a pyogenic meningitis. Treatment of this entity is difficult; little published information is available,[220-222] and no controlled trials in humans have been undertaken as they have for other forms of meningitis. However, the general principles involved in the treatment of meningitis apply—that is, the need for high doses of bactericidal agents to attain high levels within the CSF.

The agent with which there is some published experience for *P. aeruginosa* meningitis is ceftazidime,[220-222] but other antipseudomonal β-lactam agents that achieve high CSF concentrations, such as cefepime and meropenem, have also been used successfully. The tendency for easy development of resistance to imipenem and its neurotoxicity at high doses would preclude the use of this agent as first-line therapy. Aztreonam, which has been used successfully in the treatment of gram-negative meningitis, could also be considered if the isolate is sensitive. Ciprofloxacin has also been used in isolated cases,[223] but there is little clinical experience to suggest that it can be used as a first-line agent considering the limited CSF penetration and possible development of resistance. Some studies have used aminoglycosides in combination with β-lactam agents, but their necessity is unproved unless one is dealing with a β-lactam-resistant organism, in which case intrathecal or intraventricular administration of aminoglycosides may be required for optimal activity (see Chapter 84).

The length of therapy for *Pseudomonas* meningitis has been described as a minimum of 2 weeks. Relapse even after 2 weeks of maximal doses of ceftazidime and meropenem has been seen. The best guide to length of therapy may be an early trend to normalization of the CSF profile. Removal of any foreign bodies, such as ventriculostomy tubes and dural grafts, is mandatory for successful treatment. Even apparently successfully treated cases may relapse, requiring re-treatment. It is also mandatory in such cases that the isolates be reexamined by the microbiology laboratory to ascertain that they remain susceptible to the antibiotic being used because relapse may be due to the development of drug resistance.

Other forms of *P. aeruginosa* central nervous system infection, such as brain abscesses and epidural and subdural empyema, generally require surgical drainage in addition to antibiotics. The length of therapy for these closed space infections depends on a variety of factors, including adequacy of drainage. The time is left to clinical judgment, but they require at least 2 weeks of therapy.

Eye Infections

Eye infections with *P. aeruginosa* result from direct inoculation into the tissue related to trauma or surface injury caused by contact lenses. Bacteremia is also a rare cause of endophthalmitis. *P. aeruginosa* eye infections may be extremely devastating, rapidly leading to loss of sight. Keratitis is the most frequent type of disease seen, and its association with contact lens wear, especially extended-wear lenses, is well established (see Chapter 111).[224,225] However, any form of trauma may predispose to this type of infection, including surgery and burns. Cases have also occurred in intubated patients,[226] whose eyes were probably dried out and ulcerated and then contaminated by *P. aeruginosa* from the environment. The requirement for injury to the surface of the cornea leading to adhesion of the organism appears to be absolute because the disease cannot be produced in animals without injury to the cornea and human cases always occur in the setting of injury to the cornea. Keratitis can be slowly or rapidly progressive, but the classic description is that of disease progressing over 48 hours leading to involvement of the entire cornea, with opacification and sometimes perforation. *P. aeruginosa* keratitis should be considered a medical emergency because of the rapidity with which it can progress, leading to loss of sight. The eye lesions should be scraped and the scrapings Gram stained and cultured. If gram-negative rods are seen, the patient should be treated as though *P. aeruginosa* is present until culture results are reported. The usual therapy for keratitis is topical antibiotics. Fortified aminoglycoside preparations or fluoroquinolones are recommended. In cases in which the involvement is extensive, ceftazidime or gentamicin may be given by subconjunctival injection.

P. aeruginosa endophthalmitis is one of the most feared *P. aeruginosa* infections. Loss of sight and very much reduced visual acuity are the most common outcomes of these infections.[20] This entity may result from penetrating injuries, surgery, perforation of a corneal ulcer, or seeding from bacteremia. The disease is fulminant, with severe pain, chemosis, decreased visual acuity, anterior uveitis, vitreous involvement, and panophthalmitis. Therapy for such infections includes systemic antibiotics at high doses to achieve better concentrations in the eye as well as intravitreal antibiotics. Ceftazidime has been the most frequently used antibiotic for this entity, but little is written about outcomes. Its penetration into the vitreous is excellent.[227] Aminoglycosides are also injected subconjunctivally and by the intraocular route and sometimes given intravenously. Adjunctive surgery is generally done to remove infected vitreous.

P. aeruginosa also causes a number of uncommon eye infections, including orbital cellulitis in neutropenic patients[228] and gangrene necrosis of the eyelids,[229] both of which result from bacteremia.

Ear Infections

P. aeruginosa infections of the ears vary from the mild swimmer's ear that is seen in children to chronic persistent draining ears and serious life-threatening infections that lead to neurologic sequelae or even death. Swimmer's ear is commonly seen in children and results from infection of moist macerated skin of the external ear canal. The source of the organism is likely to be the swimming pool if underchlorinated.[230] The natural history of most of these cases is resolution without sequelae, but in some patients chronic drainage occurs. The pinna may be tender when pulled, and the ear canal may be tender with an exudate present. The management of this entity utilizes topical antibiotic agents (otic solutions). Aminoglycoside-containing solutions are most frequently used. Recurrences are frequent and may lead to chronically draining ears that can require more intensive topical therapy. The management of such cases is described in Chapter 57.

The most dreaded form of *Pseudomonas* infection involving the ear has been given various names, two of which, malignant otitis externa and necrotizing otitis externa, are now used for the same entity. This disease was originally described in elderly diabetic patients,[231] in whom the majority of cases still occur. However, the disease is not restricted to this population and has been described in AIDS patients[232,233] and elderly patients without underlying diabetes or immunocompromise. The pathogenesis is believed to start with infection of the ear canal with penetration to the cartilage surrounding the external auditory canal and eventual extension to the middle ear, mastoid air cells, and temporal bone.[234] Facial paralysis occurs when the seventh cranial nerve is involved as it courses through the medial wall of the middle ear. Temporomandibular joint extension can cause pain on mastication. Extension to the petrous pyramid can cause Gradenigo's syndrome, with fifth- and sixth-nerve cranial palsies. The most serious complications occur with further extension of the infection, resulting in thrombosis of the venous sinuses of the brain, including the sigmoid (transverse) sinus, contiguous to the mastoid air cells, and the cavernous sinus, contiguous to the petrous pyramid. It may also result in thrombosis of the carotid artery with subsequent brain infarction. The infection may cross to the other side of the skull and even involve the contralateral cranial nerves.

The clinical presentation is usually decreased hearing and ear pain, which may be severe and lancinating without drainage.[234] Some patients have an exudate. These symptoms in an elderly diabetic patient must raise the specter of malignant external otitis until proved otherwise. Facial palsy may appear early. The pinna is usually painful when pulled on, and the external canal may be tender on pressure. The ear canal almost always shows signs of inflammation with erythema, granulation tissue, and exudate. The tympanic membrane, if visualized, may be normal or ruptured. There may also be tenderness on pressure anterior to the tragus, extending even to the temporomandibular joint and mastoid process. Systemic symptoms such as fever occur in a small minority of patients.

Diagnosis is made easily as long as there is a high index of suspicion in diabetic patients and patients with AIDS. In less severe cases in noncompromised individuals, the distinction between ordinary otitis externa and malignant otitis externa needs to be made because the former is much more frequent. *P. aeruginosa* is often found in the ear canal if patients have not received prolonged topical or parenteral therapy. For practical purposes, this disease can be considered specific to *P. aeruginosa*, but it has been described as rarely caused by fungi[235] and *Staphylococcus aureus*. The ESR is invariably elevated in the range of 100 mm/hour or greater. The diagnosis is easily made on clinical grounds in the more severe cases, but the gold standard may be a positive technetium 99 bone scan[236] in a patient with otitis externa along with *P. aeruginosa* grown from the ear exudate. Even in diabetic patients who fail to grow *P. aeruginosa*, a positive technetium 99 bone scan would be presumptive evidence for the existence of this condition and for a biopsy or empirical therapy to be initiated. MRI may demonstrate inflammation of the temporal bone. Both MRI and computed tomography scans may show fluid in the middle ear and mastoid cells.[237]

Another poorly understood form of *P. aeruginosa* ear infection is chronic middle ear drainage, called chronic suppurative otitis media. *P. aeruginosa* is isolated from a large percentage of these draining middle ears. Often, it is in mixed culture, but in approximately 30% of cases it is the sole organism isolated from aerobic cultures. The pathogenesis of this condition is unclear. It is possible that it begins with external otitis similar to swimmer's ear and then there is middle ear involvement followed by chronic mastoiditis. Topical antibiotics[238-240] have been used with success early in the disease course. Very high success rates have also been reported with intravenous ceftazidime.[240] The management is now mainly medical in the absence of cholesteatomas.

Pseudomonal infection of the ear has resulted from ear piercing of the ear cartilage (not the earlobe) when contaminated cleansing solutions were used. Infection has resulted in severe cosmetic damage to the pinna when antipseudomonal therapy was delayed.

Treatment of Ear Infections. The treatment of malignant external otitis has undergone significant changes since it was first described by Chandler in 1968.[231] Extensive surgery was deemed necessary. Currently, the approach appears to be débridement of the ear canal, including any necrotic tissue cartilage and adjacent bone, rather than extensive bone débridement or facial nerve decompression. This change may be due to earlier recognition of this disease before there is more extensive involvement.[240] Treatment with a single agent, usually ceftazidime[241] or ciprofloxacin,[242] has been successful. However, cefepime may also be used in place of ceftazidime. The generally recommended length of therapy is 6 weeks when β-lactams are used. Oral ciprofloxacin has been used for varying periods of time from 8 weeks to 6 months. There are no comparative data on relapse rates between treatment with β-lactams and treatment with ciprofloxacin, but relapses can occur up to 1 year after completion of therapy, typically heralded by the return of pain. Serial ESR measurements have been used to follow the progress of treatment and in selecting an end point for the length of therapy. One caveat is the increasing resistance to ciprofloxacin, which suggests that empirical ciprofloxacin may be losing its efficacy.[243]

Urinary Tract Infections

P. aeruginosa urinary tract infections generally occur as a complication of the presence of a foreign body such as a stone, stent, or catheter in the urinary tract or the presence of an obstruction within the genitourinary system or after instrumentation or surgery on the urinary tract. Paraplegic patients are at high risk for *P. aeruginosa* urinary tract infections (see Chapter 304), and frequent use of antibiotics in this setting may select for *P. aeruginosa*. Notwithstanding the relationship between obstructive lesions and *P. aeruginosa* urinary tract infections, there have been descriptions of *P. aeruginosa* urinary tract infections in outpatient children[244] without stones or evident obstruction. One of the most important aspects of *P. aeruginosa* urinary tract infections is that they frequently serve as the nidus for *P. aeruginosa* bacteremia by ascending infection.

Most *P. aeruginosa* urinary tract infections fit into the category of complicated urinary tract infections, in which therapy is more prolonged than the usual course recommended for cystitis. There are no real comparative data on proper therapies because such cases are lumped in with other cases of complicated urinary tract infections in clinical trials. However, certain guidelines to prevent relapses may be inferred from clinical experience. Foley catheters, stents, or stones should be removed if possible to prevent relapse. Intermittent catheterization is preferred to retaining a Foley catheter. Generally, 7 to 10 days of antibiotic treatment suffice, with up to 2 weeks for pyelonephritis. Renal abscess or bacteremia caused by *P. aeruginosa* requires a longer course of therapy. Antipseudomonal β-lactams, ciprofloxacin, levofloxacin, and aminoglycosides given once daily are all equally acceptable, given their normally high levels of urinary excretion. Alternative antibiotics that may be used for oral treatment of *P. aeruginosa* urinary tract infections include doxycycline, to which many strains are sensitive, and in cases of multiple antibiotic resistance or in patients with very low urinary output, bladder irrigation with 0.25% acetic acid may be useful. Relapse is common and may be due not to antibiotic resistance but to host factors.

Skin and Soft Tissue Infections, Including Burns

P. aeruginosa causes ecthyma gangrenosum in neutropenic patients, an entity described previously in this chapter.[245,246] Secondary infection of chronic skin ulcers or burns (see later) can also occur. Maceration of normal skin, such as from soaking in a hot tub, can lead to superficial infection.[37,247]

Folliculitis and other papular or vesicular lesions related to *P. aeruginosa*, collectively called dermatitis, have been extensively described.[248,249] Multiple outbreaks have been linked to whirlpools, spas, and swimming pools. One nosocomial outbreak was linked to a contaminated hydrotherapy pool in a hospital and another to a contaminated water supply in a hospital. Thus, control of growth of this organism in the home or recreational environment by proper chlorination of water is essential, comparable to the control commonly practiced in hospitals. Besides the dermatitis syndromes, contaminated water has resulted in necrotizing pneumonia[198] and even ecthyma gangrenosum in neutropenic patients[250] and in two ostensibly healthy children.[251] However, most cases of hot tub folliculitis are self-limited, requiring no specific form of therapy besides avoidance of exposure to the contaminated source of water.

Burn wound infections with *P. aeruginosa* constituted one of the most significant problems caused by this organism during the 1960s and 1970s (see Chapter 318). A specific clinical picture of sepsis, with high colony counts of *P. aeruginosa* exceeding 10^5 organisms per gram of tissue, was the defining feature. Patients generally had progressive formation of a black necrotic eschar, with a sepsis picture, with or without bacteremia. The occurrence of *P. aeruginosa* burn wound sepsis does not appear to be as frequent as reported in the past,[252] when as many as 10% of burn patients had *P. aeruginosa* sepsis. In a more recent large study of more than 1400 burn patients, *P.*

aeruginosa sepsis occurred in only approximately 1% of patients.[184] However, the organism still remains a prominent isolate from burn wounds.[185] Early surgical treatment and the recognition that hydrotherapy[185] can commonly be a source of infection may have contributed to reductions in the occurrence of burn wound sepsis, at least in developed nations. Typically, burn wound sepsis caused by *P. aeruginosa* followed invasion of the burn eschar,[253] with bacterial growth achieving high densities followed by invasion into subcutaneous tissues. From here, the bacteria spread along fibrous septa into the lymphatics and also invaded blood vessels, resulting in bacteremia. Patients show all the typical manifestations of sepsis, which must be recognized as such and differentiated from the "systemic inflammatory response syndrome" that occurs as a result of thermal injury. Diagnosis may be made by blood cultures or by the pathognomonic clinical picture of an expanding burn lesion related to infection by *P. aeruginosa*. Systemic manifestations of sepsis related most likely to liberated cytokines may be present before bacteremia. Quantitative wound cultures showing more than 10^5 *P. aeruginosa* organisms per gram of burn tissue[185] had been reported to be correlated with the presence of burn wound sepsis, but the imprecision of such cultures has led to less reliance on quantitative cultures as a means of diagnosis. Clinicians now rely on the isolation of *P. aeruginosa* from wounds or blood in the presence of a sepsis picture in diagnosing burn wound sepsis caused by *P. aeruginosa*.

Treatment of *Pseudomonas aeruginosa*–Infected Burn Wounds. The management of *P. aeruginosa*-infected burn wounds is both surgical and medical. Extensive débridement of colonized eschar or necrotic tissue is required. The general principle is to reduce the organism count, which would probably diminish the sepsis response but would also reduce the risk of resistance developing during therapy given the extremely high microbial burden of such wounds. Currently, true burn wound sepsis related to *P. aeruginosa* is probably best managed with a combination of antibiotics. There is scant literature on ceftazidime monotherapy, but the recommended dose is 6 g/day.[254] The same dose might apply to cefepime. The use of imipenem as monotherapy may not be advisable on the basis of a single study on burns in which rapid development of resistance occurred[255] and what is known about resistance developing against this agent in areas where there is a high count of *P. aeruginosa*. Early *P. aeruginosa* colonization of burn wounds has been managed by the application of topical agents such as silver sulfadiazine and mafenide acetate.[256] This is done to attempt to reduce the organism count in the burn eschar and to treat local infection.

Endovascular Infections

P. aeruginosa may cause endovascular infections, including infective endocarditis.[21,257] In intravenous drug addicts, the source is usually contaminated paraphernalia or the illicit drugs.[258] This organism has also been reported to cause prosthetic valve endocarditis. *P. aeruginosa* endocarditis on native heart valves has been described in particular cities, probably resulting from local contamination of illicit drugs. One specific outbreak caused by serotype O11 among pentazocine[259] and tripelennamine abusers was probably due to a common source of contamination either in the agents or in their preparation for injection. There have not been reported outbreaks since the 1980s, although they undoubtedly occur. The pathogenesis of this disease is not thought to be different from that of other forms of endocarditis. Prior injury to native valves caused by the injection of foreign material such as talc or fibers probably serves as a nidus for bacterial attachment to the heart valve. This organism appears to have strong affinity for the endocardium, and the affinity is augmented after injury.

The manifestations of *P. aeruginosa* endocarditis resemble those of other forms of acute endocarditis in addicts except that they appear to be more indolent than those of *S. aureus*. Most cases occur as right-sided disease, as would be expected from the postulated etiology of injury of the right side of the heart caused by inoculation of the venous circulation, followed by bacterial adhesion. Although most disease involves the right side of the heart, left-sided involvement is not rare and multivalvular disease is common. Fever is a frequent manifestation, and pulmonary involvement occurs with septic embolization to the lungs. Hence, patients may also complain of chest pain and have hemoptysis. Involvement of the left side of the heart may lead to signs of cardiac failure, systemic embolization, and local cardiac involvement with sinus of Valsalva abscesses and conduction defects. Skin manifestations are rare in this disease, and ecthyma gangrenosum is not seen in *P. aeruginosa* endocarditis.

There are no pathognomonic symptoms or signs of endocarditis caused by *P. aeruginosa*. The diagnosis is made by blood cultures along with clinical signs of endocarditis. Other causes of *P. aeruginosa* bacteremia must be excluded; rarely, an infected prosthesis or indwelling vascular catheter leading to endocarditis may be found. *P. aeruginosa* bacteremia or osteomyelitis in an addict or healthy individual in the absence of surgery, trauma, or a chronic ulcer should trigger a search for an endovascular focus. It has been unusual to find *P. aeruginosa* endocarditis as a complication of nosocomial bacteremia despite the reported predilection of this organism for the heart valves.

Treatment of Endovascular Infections. The therapy for *P. aeruginosa* endocarditis has never been subjected to a controlled trial. It has been customary to use synergistic combinations of antibiotics against *P. aeruginosa* for a number of reasons, including the role that synergy has been shown to play in the treatment of some forms of endocarditis and the development of resistance during therapy with a single antipseudomonal β-lactam agent during therapy of *P. aeruginosa* endocarditis. In animal models, resistance developed to both aminoglycosides and ceftazidime,[260] but nevertheless this is the standard of care.

It is unclear which combination therapy is best because all combinations have resulted in failures with rare exceptions.[261] A triple-drug combination of a β-lactam, aminoglycoside, and rifampin was reported to salvage some of the failures that occurred with combination therapy, but no further studies have been published. A combination of meropenem and tobramycin[262] was successful in treating a case of left-sided *P. aeruginosa* endocarditis and is worthy of consideration because meropenem is not susceptible to the chromosomal β-lactamase of *P. aeruginosa* and does not enter through the same porin protein that results in the rapid development of resistance to imipenem. There is no published information about the efficacy of the antipseudomonal cephalosporin cefepime in endovascular infections. A possible difference between this agent and older cephalosporin drugs may be the lack of selection of *P. aeruginosa ampC* mutants. However, given the high density of this organism in vegetations, other mutants may still arise, leading to drug resistance. Other antibacterial agents that have shown promise in animal models include ciprofloxacin, but human data are lacking. Ciprofloxacin has been used successfully for long-term suppression of *P. aeruginosa* infection of a prosthetic heart valve.[263] The one common theme of all antibiotic therapy for *P. aeruginosa* endocarditis is the likelihood of the patient's organism becoming resistant to therapy even if there is initially bloodstream sterilization. Resistance occurs for a variety of reasons that are specific to this organism and to the nature of the disease, with very high microbial densities in vegetations that allow the selection of naturally occurring resistant mutants from this large population of bacteria.

Cases of *P. aeruginosa* endocarditis may relapse, often with resistant organisms, suggesting the need for adjunctive surgical therapy. The timing of surgical therapy is probably governed by the location of the involved cardiac valves. The average young male with right-sided endocarditis is able to survive an incompetent tricuspid valve in cases of failure of therapy or valve destruction; therefore, the case for very early surgery is not strong unless complications such as embolic disease to the lungs continue during therapy. When surgery is done, the choice of surgical procedure is critical because prosthetic valve insertion has not been successful. For tricuspid endocarditis, valvectomy may be the surgery of choice.[264] Disease on the left side of the heart,[265] either primary or relapsed, may require early surgery because

of the threat of cardiac decompensation, particularly given the high failure rate of antibiotic therapy. Guidelines for the timing of surgery for the latter group are based on the behavior of other forms of endocarditis. Failure to sterilize the bloodstream after 1 or 2 weeks of antibiotics, the continuing occurrence of major emboli, and increasing cardiac failure, as with other forms of endocarditis, would be some of the considerations. Patients whose primary therapy was apparently successful but who have relapses of infection should also have a valve replacement because of the high likelihood of bacterial resistance to the antibiotics used.

Pseudomonas aeruginosa *Infections in Febrile Neutropenia*

P. aeruginosa occupies a historical place in febrile neutropenia as the organism against which empirical coverage must always be included. This dogma results from observations in the 1960s and early 1970s that showed high mortality caused by this organism as well as its common occurrence in these patients. Currently, the organism does not appear to be as common in neutropenic patients as it once was. However, the importance of *P. aeruginosa* infection in neutropenic patients has not diminished, because when it causes bacteremia mortality is likely to be high if the infection is not appropriately treated by empirical therapy. In some areas of the world, *P. aeruginosa* continues to be a significant problem in neutropenic patients, responsible for the largest proportion of infections caused by a single organism. For example, in studies from the Indian subcontinent, *P. aeruginosa* was responsible for 28% of documented infections in 499 neutropenic patients[266] and constituted 31% of pathogens in another study.[267] In a large study from Japan of infections in leukemia patients, *P. aeruginosa* was the most frequently documented cause of bacterial infection.[268] In studies in North America, northern Europe, and Australia, the occurrence of *P. aeruginosa* bacteremia in the setting of febrile neutropenia is quite variable. In a review of 97 reports from 1987 to 1994, the incidence was reported to be 1% to 2.5% among febrile neutropenic patients given empirical therapy and 5% to 12% among microbiologically documented infections. Thus, the occurrence of *P. aeruginosa* bacteremia may be influenced by geography and perhaps climate and certainly by whether antibiotic prophylaxis is used.

The historical clinical syndromes in febrile neutropenic patients were bacteremia, pneumonia, and soft tissue infections that were mainly manifested as ecthyma gangrenosum. For reasons that are unclear, the occurrence of *P. aeruginosa* pneumonia in these patients has greatly diminished. Whether this is due to the use of antibiotic prophylaxis or to better methods of infection control in hematology units has not been studied. *P. aeruginosa* is still believed to cause the most deaths among bacterial infections in febrile neutropenic patients, but the mortality data reported show wide variability—as low as 5% in single-agent bacteremia and up to 50% as part of a polymicrobial bacteremia. Improvements in the response rate to antibiotic therapy have been reported in many studies. Studies from the M. D. Anderson Cancer Center involving a large number of cases of *P. aeruginosa* bacteremia showed an improvement from a historical response rate of 60% to 80%.[70] Another study of 127 patients demonstrated a reduction in mortality from 71% to 25% with the introduction of ceftazidime and imipenem.

Treatment of *Pseudomonas aeruginosa* Infections in Febrile, Neutropenic Patients. The IDSA guidelines on the management of fever and neutropenia[190] recommend that modern antipseudomonal β-lactams such as cefepime, ceftazidime, or a carbapenem be used either alone or in combination with an aminoglycoside. Alternatively, an antipseudomonal penicillin, such as piperacillin, in combination with an aminoglycoside can be used if preferred. The length of therapy required has not been rigorously examined; therefore, therapy is recommended for the duration of the neutropenic episode. Maximal doses of antipseudomonal β-lactam antibiotics should be used for the management of *P. aeruginosa* bacteremia in febrile neutropenia because the normal host defenses against this organism, neutrophils, are absent. Whether the relatively low incidence of *P. aeruginosa* bacteremia in the developed world will continue is likely to depend at least in part on the extent and choice of prophylactic antibiotics.

Pseudomonas aeruginosa *Infections in Acquired Immunodeficiency Syndrome*

P. aeruginosa infections in AIDS were noted before the introduction of highly active antiretroviral therapy (HAART). These infections are both community and nosocomially acquired, but since the advent of HAART the majority appear to be community acquired. Since the introduction of protease inhibitors, *P. aeruginosa* infections in AIDS patients have been seen infrequently, but they still do occur, particularly sinusitis. They are most likely to occur in patients whose disease is not under control by antiretroviral agents or whose therapy has failed and can even be the initial presentation of human immunodeficiency virus infection. It was originally thought that the occurrence of *P. aeruginosa* infections in AIDS patients was due to neutropenia, but many of these patients were not quantitatively neutropenic,[269] suggesting a role of T cells in defense against this organism. This observation also suggests that qualitative defects may be present in neutrophils from AIDS patients. The risk factors for these infections in the nosocomial setting are no different from those for other patients, but low CD4 counts play a role in the ability of AIDS patients to contain *P. aeruginosa* infections. Bacteremia,[270] generally complicating pneumonia or sinusitis, is seen. A variety of other *P. aeruginosa* infections have also been seen in AIDS patients, including catheter-associated infections in the nosocomial setting, skin infections including ecthyma gangrenosum, unusual abscesses in different locations,[271] externa including malignant external otitis (see Chapter 57),[232,233] and orbital cellulitis.[272]

The clinical presentation of the AIDS patient with *Pseudomonas* infection is remarkable for its "nonseverity," although infection may nonetheless be fatal. This is particularly true for pneumonia and bacteremia. Patients with bacteremia may have only a low-grade fever and rarely present with ecthyma gangrenosum. The occurrence of bacteremia may be a herald of underlying disease elsewhere, often pneumonia or sinusitis.[273] Isolated bacteremia may occur, and its origin has been surmised to be the skin, with folliculitis or cellulitis possibly related to exposure to contaminated water sources such as a hot tub. Pneumonia with or without bacteremia is perhaps the most common type of *P. aeruginosa* infection seen in AIDS patients.[270,273] Patients with pneumonia may present with classic clinical signs and symptoms of pneumonia, such as fever, productive cough, and chest pain. The infections may be lobar or multilobar without predisposition for any particular location. The most striking feature, however, is the frequency with which cavitary disease occurs. *P. aeruginosa*, *Nocardia asteroides*, and *Rhodococcus equi* are among the most frequent bacterial causes of cavitary lung disease in AIDS.[274]

Therapy of such infections is plagued by a relatively high incidence of relapse. Most patients with pulmonary disease have relapses after therapy unless suppressive antibiotic therapy is administered. The same holds for *P. aeruginosa* bacteremia and sinusitis. Although this relapsing behavior has been described commonly in the North American literature,[269] a European study indicates that it is being seen less frequently.[270] Therapy for any of these conditions in AIDS is no different from that in other patients except that relapse can be considered a rule unless the patient's CD4 count rises above 50 cells/μL or suppressive antibiotic therapy is given. In attempts to achieve cures and prevent relapses, therapy tends to be more prolonged than in other patients.

Uncommon Pseudomonas aeruginosa *Infections*

In addition to the entities that have been described in greater detail, *P. aeruginosa* can cause a number of infrequently seen syndromes, including noma neonatorum,[275] a necrotizing mucosal and perianal infection of newborns; toe web infections, especially in the tropics; and the "green nail syndrome" caused by *P. aeruginosa* paronychia,[37] which results from frequent submersion of the hands in water. In the last

entity, the green discoloration results from diffusion of pyocyanin into the nail bed.

ANTIBIOTIC RESISTANCE AND ANTIBIOTIC THERAPY OF MULTIRESISTANT *PSEUDOMONAS* INFECTIONS

After the introduction of carbenicillin, there were continuous improvements in the development of antipseudomonal agents that more or less ceased after the release of the fourth-generation agent cefepime and the carbapenem meropenem. Doripenem might be less susceptible to the development of resistance compared with older carbapenems and is often active against imipenem-resistant isolates. There is a paucity of clinical data on the use of this agent, but it appears to be as efficacious and as safe as the older carbapenems and other antipseudomonal agents.[276] Although the availability of these agents and a variety of other older agents provided the medical community with a certain degree of security, the situation has changed because of the selection of strains of *P. aeruginosa*, literally occurring worldwide, carrying multiple resistance determinants that mediate β-lactam multiresistance along with fluoroquinolone and aminoglycoside resistance.[277-280] The medical community is now turning to drugs such as colistin and polymyxin, which were discarded decades ago but are now being considered as "antimicrobials for the 21st century" (see Chapter 32).[281]

P. aeruginosa now carries multiple genetically based resistance determinants, which may act independently or in concert with others.[282] Among those of greatest concern are the chromosomal β-lactamases belonging to the Bush group 1 class of β-lactamases and extended-spectrum β-lactamases belonging to the OXA, PER, IMP, GES, and VIM families, some of which actually degrade carbapenems. The possession of such enzymes, combined with mutations that increase the levels of a number of efflux systems that pump out β-lactam antibiotics, may result in even higher MICs against β-lactam drugs, resulting in the inability to use such drugs even if they are only minimally degraded by β-lactamases.[283] Mutations leading to lack of expression of OprD or its decreased production may further compromise the efficacy of drugs such as imipenem by limiting the amount that enters the bacterial periplasmic space. Thus, multiresistance to β-lactam antibiotics has become a reality.

The reason why high-level antibiotic resistance in *P. aeruginosa* is occurring worldwide is of considerable importance, but the problem has not reached such levels that serious debate has begun to take place. There is evidence that the emergence of resistance may be driven by use of carbapenems[284,285] because there is substantial resistance to all β-lactam antibiotics whenever there is imipenem resistance. However, this does not explain why resistance to all β-lactam drugs, including those not degraded by the Bush group 1 chromosomal β-lactamases, also occurs. Unfortunately, such *P. aeruginosa* strains also show resistance to many aminoglycosides because of impermeability and possibly efflux. Some aminoglycoside resistance may also be encoded by genes that modify these agents,[282] especially in the case of gentamicin and tobramycin. Thus, multiple mechanisms of bacteria resistance also exist for these agents.

The last class of antibiotics with reasonable antipseudomonal activity consists of the fluoroquinolones, but the utility of these agents is now also compromised by mutational events in *P. aeruginosa* that result in loss of their activity combined with the increased production of one or more efflux pumps. That there should be a convergence of all these mechanisms on a global basis may be more than mere coincidence.

Alternative approaches to the management of multiresistant *P. aeruginosa* began some time ago because of the complexity of the management of such organisms in CF.[286,287] Colistin (polymyxin E) is used intravenously, notwithstanding its toxicity. This agent, or a related peptide antibiotic, polymyxin B, is rapidly becoming the therapeutic agent of last resort in non-CF patients infected with multiresistant *P. aeruginosa*.[288-292] Details of administration are given in Chapter 32.

The clinical outcome of multidrug-resistant *P. aeruginosa* infections treated with colistin is difficult to judge from the scant case reports and multiple drugs used in these complicated patients. However, a review of a large number of collected cases demonstrates a microbiologic eradication rate in excess of 50% and one approaching 100% in cases of meningitis requiring intrathecal usage.[293] Whereas the older literature found marginal efficacy and serious nephrotoxicity and neurotoxicity, recent reports have been more encouraging, particularly considering the limited alternative choices of drugs. Colistin does show synergy with other antimicrobials in vitro,[294,295] and it may be possible to reduce the dosage of colistin when combined with another agent if there is unacceptable toxicity from the colistin, but there are no human or animal studies to support this approach at this time. Another approach to the management of multidrug-resistant *P. aeruginosa* strains may be to use combinations of antibiotics to which the strain is resistant, such as aztreonam with amikacin[296,297] or other combinations. The need for new antimicrobials is urgent. Considering the 7- to 10-year time frame required for clinical development, multidrug-resistant *P. aeruginosa* strains are likely to be major pathogens of the 21st century.

REFERENCES

1. Theilacker C, Coleman F, Mueschenborn S, et al. Construction and characterization of a *Pseudomonas aeruginosa* mucoid exopolysaccharide/alginate conjugate vaccine. *Infect Immun*. 2003; 71:3875-3884.
2. Pier GB, DesJardins D, Aguilar T, et al. Polysaccharide surface antigens expressed by non-mucoid isolates of *Pseudomonas aeruginosa* from cystic fibrosis patients. *J Clin Microbiol*. 1986; 24:189-196.
3. Anastassiou ED, Mintzas AS, Kounavis C, et al. Alginate production by clinical nonmucoid *Pseudomonas aeruginosa*. *J Clin Microbiol*. 1987;25:656-659.
4. Ryder C, Byrd M, Wozniak DJ. Role of polysaccharides in *Pseudomonas aeruginosa* biofilm development. *Curr Opin Microbiol*. 2007;10:644-648.
5. Stover CK, Pham XQ, Erwin AL, et al. Complete genome sequence of *Pseudomonas aeruginosa* PA01, an opportunistic pathogen. *Nature*. 2000;406:959-964.
6. Lee DG, Urbach JM, Wu G, et al. Genomic analysis reveals that *Pseudomonas aeruginosa* virulence is combinatorial. *Genome Biol*. 2006;7:R90.
7. Mathee K, Narasimhan G, Valdes C, et al. Dynamics of *Pseudomonas aeruginosa* genome evolution. *Proc Natl Acad Sci U S A*. 2008;105:3100-3105.
8. Poole K, Hancock RE. Phosphate-starvation-induced outer membrane proteins of members of the families Enterobacteriaceae and Pseudomonadaceae: demonstration of immunological cross-reactivity with an antiserum specific for porin protein P of *Pseudomonas aeruginosa*. *J Bacteriol*. 1986;165:987-993.
9. Anwar H, Brown MRW, Day A, et al. Outer membrane antigens of mucoid *Pseudomonas aeruginosa* isolated directly from the sputum of a cystic fibrosis patient. *FEMS Microbiol Lett*. 1984;24:235-239.
10. Kelly NM, Macdonald MH, Martin N, et al. Comparison of the outer membrane protein and lipopolysaccharide profiles of mucoid and nonmucoid *Pseudomonas aeruginosa*. *J Clin Microbiol*. 1990;28:2017-2021.
11. Doggett RG. Microbiology of *Pseudomonas aeruginosa*. In: Doggett RG, ed. *Pseudomonas aeruginosa: Clinical Manifestations of Infection and Current Therapy*. New York: Academic Press; 1979:1-8.
12. National Nosocomial Infections Surveillance (NNIS) System Report, data summary from January 1992 to June 2002, issued August 2002. *Am J Infect Control*. 2002;30:458-475.
13. Wilmoth D, Walters PE, Tomlin R, et al. Caring for adults with cystic fibrosis. *Crit Care Nurse*. 2001;21:34-44.
14. Molina DN, Colon M, Bermudez RH, et al. Unusual presentation of *Pseudomonas aeruginosa* infections: a review. *Bol Asoc Med P R*. 1991;83:160-163.
15. *Pseudomonas* dermatitis/folliculitis associated with pools and hot tubs—Colorado and Maine, 1999-2000. *MMWR Morb Mortal Wkly Rep*. 2000;49:1087-1091.
16. Willcox MD. *Pseudomonas aeruginosa* infection and inflammation during contact lens wear: a review. *Optom Vis Sci*. 2007;84:273-278.
17. Robertson DM, Petroll WM, Jester JV, et al. Current concepts: contact lens related *Pseudomonas* keratitis. *Cont Lens Anterior Eye*. 2007;30:94-107.
18. Matar GM, Harakeh HS, Ramlawi F, et al. Comparative analysis between *Pseudomonas aeruginosa* genotypes and severity of symptoms in patients with unilateral or bilateral otitis externa. *Curr Microbiol*. 2001;42:190-193.
19. Niall DM, Murphy PG, Fogarty EE, et al. Puncture wound related *Pseudomonas* infections of the foot in children. *Ir J Med Sci*. 1997;166:98-101.
20. Eifrig CW, Scott IU, Flynn HW Jr, et al. Endophthalmitis caused by *Pseudomonas aeruginosa*. *Ophthalmology*. 2003;110:1714-1717.
21. Rajashekaraiah KR, Dhawan VK, Rice TW, et al. Increasing incidence of *Pseudomonas* endocarditis among parenteral drug abusers. *Drug Alcohol Depend*. 1980;6:227-230.
22. Agodi A, Barchitta M, Cipresso R, et al. *Pseudomonas aeruginosa* carriage, colonization, and infection in ICU patients. *Intensive Care Med*. 2007;33:1155-1161.
23. Kropec A, Huebner J, Riffel M, et al. Exogenous or endogenous reservoirs of nosocomial *Pseudomonas aeruginosa* and *Staphylococcus aureus* infections in a surgical intensive care unit. *Intensive Care Med*. 1993;19:161-165.
24. Berthelot P, Grattard F, Mahul P, et al. Prospective study of nosocomial colonization and infection due to *Pseudomonas aeruginosa* in mechanically ventilated patients. *Intensive Care Med*. 2001;27:503-512.
25. Edwards-Jones V, Greenwood JE. What's new in burn microbiology? James Laing Memorial Prize Essay 2000. *Burns*. 2003; 29:15-24.
26. Cardenosa Cendrero JA, Sole-Violan J, Bordes Benitez A, et al. Role of different routes of tracheal colonization in the development of pneumonia in patients receiving mechanical ventilation. *Chest*. 1999;116:462-470.
27. Krueger WA, Lenhart FP, Neeser G, et al. Influence of combined intravenous and topical antibiotic prophylaxis on the incidence of infections, organ dysfunctions, and mortality in critically ill surgical patients: a prospective, stratified, randomized, double-blind, placebo-controlled clinical trial. *Am J Respir Crit Care Med*. 2002;166:1029-1037.
28. Krueger WA, Unertl KE. Selective decontamination of the digestive tract. *Curr Opin Crit Care*. 2002;8:139-144.
29. de Jonge E, Schultz MJ, Spanjaard L, et al. Effects of selective decontamination of digestive tract on mortality and acquisition of resistant bacteria in intensive care: a randomised controlled trial. *Lancet*. 2003;362:1011-1016.
30. Chan EY, Ruest A, Meade MO, et al. Oral decontamination for prevention of pneumonia in mechanically ventilated adults: systematic review and meta-analysis. *BMJ*. 2007;334:889.
31. Speert DP. Molecular epidemiology of *Pseudomonas aeruginosa*. *Front Biosci*. 2002;7:e354-e361.
32. Johnson JK, Arduino SM, Stine OC, et al. Multilocus sequence typing compared to pulsed-field gel electrophoresis for molecular typing of *Pseudomonas aeruginosa*. *J Clin Microbiol*. 2007; 45:3707-3712.
33. Gaynes R, Edwards JR. Overview of nosocomial infections caused by gram-negative bacilli. *Clin Infect Dis*. 2005;41:848-854.
34. Klevens RM, Edwards JR, Gaynes RP. The impact of antimicrobial-resistant, health care-associated infections on mortality in the United States. *Clin Infect Dis*. 2008;47:927-930.
35. Scarff JM, Goldberg JB. Vaccination against *Pseudomonas aeruginosa* pneumonia in immunocompromised mice. *Clin Vaccine Immunol*. 2008;15:367-375.
36. Cryz SJ Jr, Furer E, Germanier R. Simple model for the study of *Pseudomonas aeruginosa* infections in leukopenic mice. *Infect Immun*. 1983;39:1067-1071.
37. Agger WA, Mardan A. *Pseudomonas aeruginosa* infections of intact skin. *Clin Infect Dis*. 1995;20:302-308.
38. Stieritz DD, Holder IA. Experimental studies of the pathogenesis of infections due to *Pseudomonas aeruginosa*: description of a burned mouse model. *J Infect Dis*. 1975;131:688-691.
39. Schmidtchen A, Holst E, Tapper H, et al. Elastase-producing *Pseudomonas aeruginosa* degrade plasma proteins and extracellular products of human skin and fibroblasts, and inhibit fibroblast growth. *Microb Pathog*. 2003;34:47-55.
40. Lawin-Brussel CA, Refojo MF, Leong FL, et al. Effect of *Pseudomonas aeruginosa* concentration in experimental contact lens-related microbial keratitis. *Cornea*. 1993;12:10-18.
41. Cole N, Krockenberger M, Bao S, et al. Effects of exogenous interleukin-6 during *Pseudomonas aeruginosa* corneal infection. *Infect Immun*. 2001;69:4116-4119.
42. Cole AM, Liao HI, Stuchlik O, et al. Cationic polypeptides are required for antibacterial activity of human airway fluid. *J Immunol*. 2002;169:6985-6991.
43. Pier GB, Grout M, DesJardins D. Complement deposition by antibodies to *Pseudomonas aeruginosa* mucoid exopolysaccharide (MEP) and by non-MEP specific opsonins. *J Immunol*. 1991;147:1869-1876.
44. Younger JG, Shankar-Sinha S, Mickiewicz M, et al. Murine complement interactions with *Pseudomonas aeruginosa* and their consequences during pneumonia. *Am J Respir Cell Mol Biol*. 2003;29:432-438.
45. Holmskov U, Thiel S, Jensenius JC. Collections and ficolins: humoral lectins of the innate immune defense. *Annu Rev Immunol*. 2003;21:547-578.
46. Bufler P, Schmidt B, Schikor D, et al. Surfactant protein A and D differently regulate the immune response to nonmucoid *Pseudomonas aeruginosa* and its lipopolysaccharide. *Am J Respir Cell Mol Biol*. 2003;28:249-256.
47. Ni M, Evans DJ, Hawgood S, et al. Surfactant protein D is present in human tear fluid and the cornea and inhibits epithelial cell invasion by *Pseudomonas aeruginosa*. *Infect Immun*. 2005;73:2147-2156.
48. Davies JC, Turner MW, Klein N. Impaired pulmonary status in cystic fibrosis adults with two mutated MBL-2 alleles. *Eur Respir J*. 2004;24:798-804.
49. Moller-Kristensen M, Ip WK, Shi L, et al. Deficiency of mannose-binding lectin greatly increases susceptibility to postburn infection with *Pseudomonas aeruginosa*. *J Immunol*. 2006;176: 1769-1775.
50. Davies J, Neth O, Alton E, et al. Differential binding of mannose-binding lectin to respiratory pathogens in cystic fibrosis. *Lancet*. 2000;355:1885-1886.
51. Alexander C, Rietschel ET. Bacterial lipopolysaccharides and innate immunity. *J Endotoxin Res*. 2001;7:167-202.
52. Reiniger N, Lee MM, Coleman FT, et al. Resistance to *Pseudomonas aeruginosa* chronic lung infection requires cystic fibrosis transmembrane conductance regulator-modulated interleukin-1 (IL-1) release and signaling through the IL-1 receptor. *Infect Immun*. 2007;75:1598-1608.
53. Meduri GU. Clinical review: a paradigm shift: the bidirectional effect of inflammation on bacterial growth: clinical implications for patients with acute respiratory distress syndrome. *Crit Care*. 2002;6:24-29.
54. Harder J, Meyer-Hoffert U, Teran LM, et al. Mucoid *Pseudomonas aeruginosa*, TNF-alpha, and IL-1beta, but not IL-6, induce human beta-defensin-2 in respiratory epithelia. *Am J Respir Cell Mol Biol*. 2000;22:714-721.
55. Lin TJ, Garduno R, Boudreau RT, et al. *Pseudomonas aeruginosa* activates human mast cells to induce neutrophil transendothelial migration via mast cell-derived IL-1 alpha and beta. *J Immunol*. 2002;169:4522-4530.
56. Wu CL, Lee YL, Chang KM, et al. Bronchoalveolar interleukin-1 beta: a marker of bacterial burden in mechanically ventilated patients with community-acquired pneumonia. *Crit Care Med*. 2003;31:812-817.
57. Schultz MJ, Rijneveld AW, Florquin S, et al. Role of interleukin-1 in the pulmonary immune response during *Pseudomonas aeruginosa* pneumonia. *Am J Physiol*. 2002;282: L285-L290.
58. Grassme H, Jendrossek V, Riehle A, et al. Host defense against *Pseudomonas aeruginosa* requires ceramide-rich membrane rafts. *Nat Med*. 2003;9:322-330.
59. Yu H, Nasr SZ, Deretic V. Innate lung defenses and compromised *Pseudomonas aeruginosa* clearance in the malnourished mouse model of respiratory infections in cystic fibrosis. *Infect Immun*. 2000;68:2142-2147.
60. Remick DG. Cytokine therapeutics for the treatment of sepsis: why has nothing worked? *Curr Pharm Des*. 2003;9:75-82.
61. Fisher CJ Jr, Agosti JM, Opal SM, et al. Treatment of septic shock with the tumor necrosis factor receptor:Fc fusion protein. The Soluble TNF Receptor Sepsis Study Group. *N Engl J Med*. 1996;334:1697-1702.
62. Jones AM, Martin L, Bright-Thomas RJ, et al. Inflammatory markers in cystic fibrosis patients with transmissible *Pseudomonas aeruginosa*. *Eur Respir J*. 2003;22:503-506.
63. Cole N, Bao S, Stapleton F, et al. *Pseudomonas aeruginosa* keratitis in IL-6-deficient mice. *Int Arch Allergy Immunol*. 2003;130:165-172.
64. Huang X, McClellan SA, Barrett RP, et al. IL-18 contributes to host resistance against infection with *Pseudomonas aeruginosa* through induction of IFN-gamma production. *J Immunol*. 2002;168:5756-5763.
65. Schultz MJ, Knapp S, Florquin S, et al. Interleukin-18 impairs the pulmonary host response to *Pseudomonas aeruginosa*. *Infect Immun*. 2003;71:1630-1634.
66. Dubin PJ, Kolls JK. IL-23 mediates inflammatory responses to mucoid *Pseudomonas aeruginosa* lung infection in mice. *Am J Physiol Lung Cell Mol Physiol*. 2007;292:L519-L528.
67. Lu Y-J, Gross J, Bogaert D, et al. Interleukin-17A mediates acquired immunity to pneumococcal colonization. *PLoS Pathog*. 2008;4:e1000159.

68. Davies JC. *Pseudomonas aeruginosa* in cystic fibrosis: pathogenesis and persistence. *Paediatr Respir Rev*. 2002;3:128-134.
69. McAllister F, Henry A, Kreindler JL, et al. Role of IL-17A, IL-17F, and the IL-17 receptor in regulating growth-related oncogene-alpha and granulocyte colony-stimulating factor in bronchial epithelium: implications for airway inflammation in cystic fibrosis. *J Immunol*. 2005;175:404-412.
70. Chatzinikolaou I, Abi-Said D, Bodey GP, et al. Recent experience with *Pseudomonas aeruginosa* bacteremia in patients with cancer: retrospective analysis of 245 episodes. *Arch Intern Med*. 2000;160:501-509.
71. Bodey GP. *Pseudomonas aeruginosa* infections in cancer patients: have they gone away? *Curr Opin Infect Dis*. 2001;14:403-407.
72. Lin TJ, Maher LH, Gomi K, et al. Selective early production of CCL20, or macrophage inflammatory protein 3alpha, by human mast cells in response to *Pseudomonas aeruginosa*. *Infect Immun*. 2003;71:365-373.
73. Boudreau RT, Garduno R, Lin TJ. Protein phosphatase 2A and protein kinase C-alpha are physically associated and are involved in *Pseudomonas aeruginosa*-induced interleukin 6 production by mast cells. *J Biol Chem*. 2002;277:5322-5329.
74. Ambrose PG, Owens RC Jr, Garvey MJ, et al. Pharmacodynamic considerations in the treatment of moderate to severe pseudomonal infections with cefepime. *J Antimicrob Chemother*. 2002;49:445-453.
75. Siebenhaar F, Syska W, Weller K, et al. Control of *Pseudomonas aeruginosa* skin infections in mice is mast cell-dependent. *Am J Pathol*. 2007;170:1910-1916.
76. Sorvillo F, Beall G, Turner PA, et al. Incidence and determinants of *Pseudomonas aeruginosa* infection among persons with HIV: association with hospital exposure. *Am J Infect Control*. 2001;29:79-84.
77. Nieuwenhuis EE, Matsumoto T, Exley M, et al. CD1d-dependent macrophage-mediated clearance of *Pseudomonas aeruginosa* from lung. *Nat Med*. 2002;8:588-593.
78. Raga S, Julia MR, Crespi C, et al. Gammadelta T lymphocytes from cystic fibrosis patients and healthy donors are high TNF-alpha and IFN-gamma-producers in response to *Pseudomonas aeruginosa*. *Respir Res*. 2003;4:1-9.
79. Rhein LM, Perkins M, Gerard NP, et al. FcgammaRIII is protective against *Pseudomonas aeruginosa* pneumonia. *Am J Respir Cell Mol Biol*. 2008;38:401-406.
80. Pitt BR. CFTR trafficking and signaling in respiratory epithelium. *Am J Physiol*. 2001;281:L13-L15.
81. Peters KW, Qi J, Watkins SC, et al. Mechanisms underlying regulated CFTR trafficking. *Med Clin North Am*. 2000;84:633-640.
82. Lyczak JB, Cannon CL, Pier GB. Lung infections associated with cystic fibrosis. *Clin Microbiol Rev*. 2002;15:194-222.
83. Prince A. The CFTR advantage—capitalizing on a quirk of fate. *Nat Med*. 1998;4:663-664.
84. Poschet JF, Boucher JC, Tatterson L, et al. Molecular basis for defective glycosylation and *Pseudomonas* pathogenesis in cystic fibrosis lung. *Proc Natl Acad Sci U S A*. 2001;98:13972-13977.
85. Schroeder TH, Zaidi TS, Pier GB. Lack of adherence of clinical isolates of *Pseudomonas aeruginosa* to asialo GM_1 on epithelial cells. *Infect Immun*. 2001;69:719-729.
86. Travis SM, Singh PK, Welsh MJ. Antimicrobial peptides and proteins in the innate defense of the airway surface. *Curr Opin Immunol*. 2001;13:89-95.
87. Boucher RC. An overview of the pathogenesis of cystic fibrosis lung disease. *Adv Drug Deliv Rev*. 2002;54:1359-1371.
88. Clunes MT, Boucher RC. Cystic fibrosis: the mechanisms of pathogenesis of an inherited lung disorder. *Drug Discov Today Dis Mech*. 2007;4:63-72.
89. Yoon SS, Hennigan RF, Hilliard GM, et al. *Pseudomonas aeruginosa* anaerobic respiration in biofilms: relationships to cystic fibrosis pathogenesis. *Dev Cell*. 2002;3:593-603.
90. Worlitzsch D, Tarran R, Ulrich M, et al. Effects of reduced mucus oxygen concentration in airway *Pseudomonas infections* of cystic fibrosis patients. *J Clin Invest*. 2002;109:317-325.
91. Pier GB. CFTR mutations and host susceptibility to *Pseudomonas aeruginosa* lung infection. *Curr Opin Microbiol*. 2002;5:81-86.
92. Schroeder TH, Reiniger N, Meluleni G, et al. Transgenic cystic fibrosis mice exhibit reduced early clearance of *Pseudomonas aeruginosa* from the respiratory tract. *J Immunol*. 2001;166:7410-7418.
93. Schroeder TH, Lee MM, Yacono PW, et al. CFTR is a pattern recognition molecule that extracts *Pseudomonas aeruginosa* LPS from the outer membrane into epithelial cells and activates NF-kappa B translocation. *Proc Natl Acad Sci U S A*. 2002;99:6907-6912.
94. Reiniger N, Ichikawa JK, Pier GB. Influence of cystic fibrosis transmembrane conductance regulator on gene expression in response to *Pseudomonas aeruginosa* infection of human bronchial epithelial cells. *Infect Immun*. 2005;73:6822-6830.
95. Kowalski MP, Pier GB. Localization of cystic fibrosis transmembrane conductance regulator to lipid rafts of epithelial cells is required for *Pseudomonas aeruginosa*-induced cellular activation. *J Immunol*. 2004;172:418-425.
96. Riethmuller J, Riehle A, Grassme H, et al. Membrane rafts in host-pathogen interactions. *Biochim Biophys Acta*. 2006;1758:2139-2147.
97. Mossink MH, van Zon A, Scheper RJ, et al. Vaults: a ribonucleoprotein particle involved in drug resistance? *Oncogene*. 2003;22:7458-7467.
98. Kowalski MP, Dubouix-Bourandy A, Bajmoczi M, et al. Host resistance to lung infection mediated by major vault protein in epithelial cells. *Science*. 2007;317:130-132.
99. Cannon CL, Kowalski MP, Stopak KS, et al. *Pseudomonas aeruginosa*-induced apoptosis is defective in respiratory epithelial cells expressing mutant cystic fibrosis transmembrane conductance regulator. *Am J Respir Cell Mol Biol*. 2003;29:188-197.
100. Grassme H, Kirschnek S, Riethmueller J, et al. CD95/CD95 ligand interactions on epithelial cells in host defense to *Pseudomonas aeruginosa*. *Science*. 2000;290:527-530.
101. Hotchkiss RS, Dunne WM, Swanson PE, et al. Role of apoptosis in *Pseudomonas aeruginosa* pneumonia. *Science*. 2001;294:1783.
102. Grassme H, Jin J, Wilker B, et al. Regulation of pulmonary *Pseudomonas aeruginosa* infection by the transcriptional repressor Gfi1. *Cell Microbiol*. 2006;8:1096-1105.
103. Esen M, Grassme H, Riethmuller J, et al. Invasion of human epithelial cells by *Pseudomonas aeruginosa* involves src-like tyrosine kinases p60Src and p59Fyn. *Infect Immun*. 2001;69:281-287.
104. Zaidi T, Bajmoczi M, Zaidi T, et al. Disruption of CFTR-dependent lipid rafts reduces bacterial levels and corneal pathology in a murine model of *Pseudomonas aeruginosa* keratitis. *Invest Ophthalmol Vis Sci*. 2008;49:1000-1009.
105. Roy-Burman A, Savel RH, Racine S, et al. Type III protein secretion is associated with death in lower respiratory and systemic *Pseudomonas aeruginosa* infections. *J Infect Dis*. 2001;183:1767-1774.
106. Schulert GS, Feltman H, Rabin SD, et al. Secretion of the toxin ExoU is a marker for highly virulent *Pseudomonas aeruginosa* isolates obtained from patients with hospital-acquired pneumonia. *J Infect Dis*. 2003;188:1695-1706.
107. Mattick JS. Type IV pili and twitching motility. *Annu Rev Microbiol*. 2002;56:289-314.
108. Kus JV, Tullis E, Cvitkovitch DG, et al. Significant differences in type IV pilin allele distribution among *Pseudomonas aeruginosa* isolates from cystic fibrosis (CF) versus non-CF patients. *Microbiology*. 2004;150:1315-1326.
109. Horzempa J, Held TK, Cross AS, et al. Immunization with *Pseudomonas aeruginosa* 1244 pilin provides O-antigen-specific protection. *Clin Vaccine Immunol*. 2008;15:590-597 .
110. Voisin S, Kus JV, Houliston S, et al. Glycosylation of *Pseudomonas aeruginosa* strain PA5196 type IV pilins with mycobacterium-like α-1,5-linked D-Ara*f* oligosaccharides. *J Bacteriol*. 2007;189:151-159.
111. Keizer DW, Slupsky CM, Kalisiak M, et al. Structure of a pilin monomer from *Pseudomonas aeruginosa*: implications for the assembly of pili. *J Biol Chem*. 2001;276:24186-24193.
112. Hazes B, Sastry PA, Hayakawa K, et al. Crystal structure of *Pseudomonas aeruginosa* PAK pilin suggests a main-chain-dominated mode of receptor binding. *J Mol Biol*. 2000;299:1005-1017.
113. Audette GF, Irvin RT, Hazes B. Crystallographic analysis of the *Pseudomonas aeruginosa* strain K122-4 monomeric pilin reveals a conserved receptor-binding architecture. *Biochemistry*. 2004;43:11427-11435.
114. Barken KB, Pamp SJ, Yang L, et al. Roles of type IV pili, flagellum-mediated motility and extracellular DNA in the formation of mature multicellular structures in *Pseudomonas aeruginosa* biofilms. *Environ Microbiol*. 2008;10:2331-2343.
115. Arora SK, Dasgupta N, Lory S, et al. Identification of two distinct types of flagellar cap proteins, FliD, in *Pseudomonas aeruginosa*. *Infect Immun*. 2000;68:1474-1479.
116. Balloy V, Verma A, Kuravi S, et al. The role of flagellin versus motility in acute lung disease caused by *Pseudomonas aeruginosa*. *J Infect Dis*. 2007;196:289-296.
117. Ramphal R, Arora SK. Recognition of mucin components by *Pseudomonas aeruginosa*. *Glycoconj J*. 2001;18:709-713.
118. Feuillet V, Medjane S, Mondor I, et al. Involvement of Toll-like receptor 5 in the recognition of flagellated bacteria. *Proc Natl Acad Sci U S A*. 2006;103:12487-12492.
119. Kojima K, Ueta M, Hamuro J, et al. Human conjunctival epithelial cells express functional Toll-like receptor 5. *Br J Ophthalmol*. 2008;92:411-416.
120. Kumar A, Hazlett LD, Yu FS. Flagellin suppresses the inflammatory response and enhances bacterial clearance in a murine model of *Pseudomonas aeruginosa* keratitis. *Infect Immun*. 2008;76:89-96.
121. Koller B, Kappler M, Latzin P, et al. TLR expression on neutrophils at the pulmonary site of infection: TLR1/TLR2-mediated up-regulation of TLR5 expression in cystic fibrosis lung disease. *J Immunol*. 2008;181:2753-2763.
122. Blohmke CJ, Victor RE, Hirschfeld AF, et al. Innate immunity mediated by TLR5 as a novel antiinflammatory target for cystic fibrosis lung disease. *J Immunol*. 2008;180:7764-7773.
123. Mitchell E, Houles C, Sudakevitz D, et al. Structural basis for oligosaccharide-mediated adhesion of *Pseudomonas aeruginosa* in the lungs of cystic fibrosis patients. *Nat Struct Biol*. 2002;9:918-921.
124. Azghani AO, Idell S, Bains M, et al. *Pseudomonas aeruginosa* outer membrane protein F is an adhesin in bacterial binding to lung epithelial cells in culture. *Microb Pathog*. 2002;33:109-114.
125. Plotkowski MC, Costa AO, Morandi V, et al. Role of heparan sulphate proteoglycans as potential receptors for non-piliated *Pseudomonas aeruginosa* adherence to non-polarised airway epithelial cells. *J Med Microbiol*. 2001;50:183-190.
126. Oglesby AG, Farrow JM 3rd, Lee JH, et al. The influence of iron on *Pseudomonas aeruginosa* physiology: a regulatory link between iron and quorum sensing. *J Biol Chem*. 2008;283:15558-15567.
127. Voulhoux R, Filloux A, Schalk IJ. Pyoverdine-mediated iron uptake in *Pseudomonas aeruginosa*: the Tat system is required for PvdN but not for FpvA transport. *J Bacteriol*. 2006;188:3317-3323.
128. Poole K, McKay GA. Iron acquisition and its control in *Pseudomonas aeruginosa*: many roads lead to Rome. *Front Biosci*. 2003;8:d661-d686.
129. Britigan BE, Rasmussen GT, Olakanmi O, et al. Iron acquisition from *Pseudomonas aeruginosa* siderophores by human phagocytes: an additional mechanism of host defense through iron sequestration? *Infect Immun*. 2000;68:1271-1275.
130. Pastan I. Immunotoxins containing *Pseudomonas* exotoxin A: a short history. *Cancer Immunol Immunother*. 2003;52:338-341.
131. Hauser AR, Cobb E, Bodi M, et al. Type III protein secretion is associated with poor clinical outcomes in patients with ventilator-associated pneumonia caused by *Pseudomonas aeruginosa*. *Crit Care Med*. 2002;30:521-528.
132. Sato H, Feix JB, Frank DW. Identification of superoxide dismutase as a cofactor for the pseudomonas type III toxin, ExoU. *Biochemistry*. 2006;45:10368-10375.
133. Yahr TL, Wolfgang MC. Transcriptional regulation of the *Pseudomonas aeruginosa* type III secretion system. *Mol Microbiol*. 2006;62:631-640.
134. Schuster M, Lostroh CP, Ogi T, et al. Identification, timing, and signal specificity of *Pseudomonas aeruginosa* quorum-controlled genes: a transcriptome analysis. *J Bacteriol*. 2003;185:2066-2079.
135. Hentzer M, Wu H, Andersen JB, et al. Attenuation of *Pseudomonas aeruginosa* virulence by quorum sensing inhibitors. *EMBO J*. 2003;22:3803-3815.
136. Rumbaugh KP, Griswold JA, Iglewski BH, et al. Contribution of quorum sensing to the virulence of *Pseudomonas aeruginosa* in burn wound infections. *Infect Immun*. 1999;67:5854-5862.
137. Pearson JP, Feldman M, Iglewski BH, et al. *Pseudomonas aeruginosa* cell-to-cell signaling is required for virulence in a model of acute pulmonary infection. *Infect Immun*. 2000;68:4331-4334.
138. Wu H, Song Z, Givskov M, et al. *Pseudomonas aeruginosa* mutations in lasI and rhlI quorum sensing systems result in milder chronic lung infection. *Microbiology*. 2001;147:1105-1113.
139. Cabrol S, Olliver A, Pier G, et al. Transcription of quorum-sensing system genes in clinical and environmental isolates of *Pseudomonas aeruginosa*. *J Bacteriol*. 2003;185:7222-7230.
140. Smith R, Iglewski B. *Pseudomonas aeruginosa* quorum sensing as a potential antimicrobial target. *J Clin Invest*. 2003;112:1460-1465.
141. Singh PK, Schaefer AL, Parsek MR, et al. Quorum-sensing signals indicate that cystic fibrosis lungs are infected with bacterial biofilms. *Nature*. 2000;407:762-764.
142. Geisenberger O, Givskov M, Riedel K, et al. Production of *N*-acyl-L-homoserine lactones by *P. aeruginosa* isolates from chronic lung infections associated with cystic fibrosis. *FEMS Microbiol Lett*. 2000;184:273-278.
143. Erickson DL, Endersby R, Kirkham A, et al. *Pseudomonas aeruginosa* quorum-sensing systems may control virulence factor expression in the lungs of patients with cystic fibrosis. *Infect Immun*. 2002;70:1783-1790.
144. Smith EE, Buckley DG, Wu Z, et al. Genetic adaptation by *Pseudomonas aeruginosa* to the airways of cystic fibrosis patients. *Proc Natl Acad Sci U S A*. 2006;103:8487-8492.
145. Donlan RM, Costerton JW. Biofilms: survival mechanisms of clinically relevant microorganisms. *Clin Microbiol Rev*. 2002;15:167-193.
146. Parsek MR, Singh PK. Bacterial biofilms: an emerging link to disease pathogenesis. *Annu Rev Microbiol*. 2003;57:677-701.
147. Davies DG, Parsek MR, Pearson JP, et al. The involvement of cell-to-cell signals in the development of a bacterial biofilm. *Science*. 1998;280:295-298.
148. Wozniak DJ, Wyckoff TJ, Starkey M, et al. Alginate is not a significant component of the extracellular polysaccharide matrix of PA14 and PAO1 *Pseudomonas aeruginosa* biofilms. *Proc Natl Acad Sci U S A*. 2003;100:7907-7912.
149. Whitchurch CB, Tolker-Nielsen T, Ragas PC, et al. Extracellular DNA required for bacterial biofilm formation. *Science*. 2002;295:1487.
150. Friedman L, Kolter R. Genes involved in matrix formation in *Pseudomonas aeruginosa* PA14 biofilms. *Mol Microbiol*. 2004;51:675-690.
151. Ma L, Jackson KD, Landry RM, et al. Analysis of *Pseudomonas aeruginosa* conditional psl variants reveals roles for the psl polysaccharide in adhesion and maintaining biofilm structure postattachment. *J Bacteriol*. 2006;188:8213-8221.
152. Ma L, Lu H, Sprinkle A, et al. *Pseudomonas aeruginosa* Psl is a galactose- and mannose-rich exopolysaccharide. *J Bacteriol*. 2007;189:8353-8356.
153. Costerton W, Veeh R, Shirtliff M, et al. The application of biofilm science to the study and control of chronic bacterial infections. *J Clin Invest*. 2003;112:1466-1477.
154. Parad RB, Gerard CJ, Zurakowski D, et al. Pulmonary outcome in cystic fibrosis is influenced primarily by mucoid *Pseudomonas*

aeruginosa infection and immune status and only modestly by genotype. *Infect Immun.* 1999;67:4744-4750.
155. Garau J, Gomez L. *Pseudomonas aeruginosa* pneumonia. *Curr Opin Infect Dis.* 2003;16:135-143.
156. Valles J, Mesalles E, Mariscal D, et al. A 7-year study of severe hospital-acquired pneumonia requiring ICU admission. *Intensive Care Med.* 2003;29:1981-1988.
157. Govan JRW, Deretic V. Microbial pathogenesis in cystic fibrosis: mucoid *Pseudomonas aeruginosa* and *Burkholderia cepacia*. *Microbiol Rev.* 1996;60:539-574.
158. Coleman FT, Mueschenborn S, Meluleni G, et al. Hypersusceptibility of cystic fibrosis mice to chronic *Pseudomonas aeruginosa* oropharyngeal colonization and lung infection. *Proc Natl Acad Sci U S A.* 2003;100:1949-1954.
159. Meluleni GJ, Grout M, Evans DJ, et al. Mucoid *Pseudomonas aeruginosa* growing in a biofilm in vitro are killed by opsonic antibodies to the mucoid exopolysaccharide capsule but not by antibodies produced during chronic lung infection in cystic fibrosis patients. *J Immunol.* 1995;155:2029-2038.
160. Johnson C, Butler SM, Konstan MW, et al. Factors influencing outcomes in cystic fibrosis: a center-based analysis. *Chest.* 2003;123:20-27.
161. Kurahashi K, Kajikawa O, Sawa T, et al. Pathogenesis of septic shock in *Pseudomonas aeruginosa* pneumonia. *J Clin Invest.* 1999;104:743-750.
162. Koh AY, Priebe GP, Pier GB. Virulence of *Pseudomonas aeruginosa* in a murine model of gastrointestinal colonization and dissemination in neutropenia. *Infect Immun.* 2005;73:2262-2272.
163. von Specht BU, Lucking HC, Blum B, et al. Safety and immunogenicity of a *Pseudomonas aeruginosa* outer membrane protein I vaccine in human volunteers. *Vaccine.* 1996;14:1111-1117.
164. Rotering H, Dorner F. Studies on a *Pseudomonas aeruginosa* flagella vaccine. *Antibiot Chemother.* 1989;42:218-228.
165. Doring G, Dorner F. A multicenter vaccine trial using the *Pseudomonas aeruginosa* flagella vaccine IMMUNO in patients with cystic fibrosis. *Behring Inst Mitt.* 1997:338-344.
166. Doring G, Meisner C, Stern M. A double-blind randomized placebo-controlled phase III study of a *Pseudomonas aeruginosa* flagella vaccine in cystic fibrosis patients. *Proc Natl Acad Sci U S A.* 2007;104:11020-11025.
167. Frank DW, Vallis A, Wiener-Kronish JP, et al. Generation and characterization of a protective monoclonal antibody to *Pseudomonas aeruginosa* PcrV. *J Infect Dis.* 2002;186:64-73.
168. Sawa T, Yahr TL, Ohara M, et al. Active and passive immunization with the *Pseudomonas* V antigen protects against type III intoxication and lung injury. *Nat Med.* 1999;5:392-398.
169. Imamura Y, Yanagihara K, Fukuda Y, et al. Effect of anti-PcrV antibody in a murine chronic airway *Pseudomonas aeruginosa* infection model. *Eur Respir J.* 2007;29:965-968.
170. Pier GB, Boyer D, Preston M, et al. Human monoclonal antibodies to *Pseudomonas aeruginosa* alginate that protect against infection by both mucoid and nonmucoid strains. *J Immunol.* 2004;173:5671-5678.
171. Zaidi T, Pier GB. Prophylactic and therapeutic efficacy of a fully human immunoglobulin G1 monoclonal antibody to *Pseudomonas aeruginosa* alginate in murine keratitis infection. *Infect Immun.* 2008;76:4720-4725.
172. Priebe GP, Meluleni GJ, Coleman FT, et al. Protection against fatal *Pseudomonas aeruginosa* pneumonia in mice after nasal immunization with a live, attenuated *aroA* deletion mutant. *Infect Immun.* 2003;71:1453-1461.
173. Priebe GP, Brinig MM, Hatano K, et al. Construction and characterization of a live, attenuated *aroA* deletion mutant of *Pseudomonas aeruginosa* as a candidate intranasal vaccine. *Infect Immun.* 2002;70:1507-1517.
174. Priebe GP, Walsh RL, Cederroth TA, et al. IL-17 is a critical component of vaccine-induced protection against lung infection by lipopolysaccharide-heterologous strains of *Pseudomonas aeruginosa*. *J Immunol.* 2008;181:4965-4975.
175. Nicotra MB, Rivera M, Dale AM, et al. Clinical, pathophysiologic, and microbiologic characterization of bronchiectasis in an aging cohort. *Chest.* 1995;108:955-961.
176. Yanagihara K, Kadoto J, Kohno S. Diffuse panbronchiolitis—pathophysiology and treatment mechanisms. *Int J Antimicrob Agents.* 2001;18(Suppl 1):S83-S87.
177. Whitecar JP Jr, Luna M, Bodey GP. *Pseudomonas* bacteremia in patients with malignant diseases. *Am J Med Sci.* 1970;60:216-223.
178. Fishman LS, Armstrong D. *Pseudomonas aeruginosa* bacteremia in patients with neoplastic disease. *Cancer.* 1972;30:764-773.
179. Gallagher PG, Watanakunakorn C. *Pseudomonas* bacteremia in a community teaching hospital, 1980-1984. *Rev Infect Dis.* 1989;11:846-852.
180. Maschmeyer G, Braveny I. Review of the incidence and prognosis of *Pseudomonas aeruginosa* infections in cancer patients in the 1990s. *Eur J Clin Microbiol Infect Dis.* 2000;19:915-925.
181. Kang CI, Kim SH, Kim HB, et al. *Pseudomonas aeruginosa* bacteremia: risk factors for mortality and influence of delayed receipt of effective antimicrobial therapy on clinical outcome. *Clin Infect Dis.* 2003;37:745-751.
182. Blot S, Vandewoude K, Hoste E, et al. Reappraisal of attributable mortality in critically ill patients with nosocomial bacteraemia involving *Pseudomonas aeruginosa*. *J Hosp Infect.* 2003;53:18-24.
183. Gales AC, Jones RN, Turnidge J, et al. Characterization of *Pseudomonas aeruginosa* isolates: occurrence rates, antimicrobial susceptibility patterns, and molecular typing in the global SENTRY Antimicrobial Surveillance Program, 1997-1999. *Clin Infect Dis.* 2001;32(Suppl 2):S146-S155.
184. Gang RK, Bang RL, Sanyal SC, et al. *Pseudomonas aeruginosa* septicaemia in burns. *Burns.* 1999;25:611-616.
185. Mayhall CG. The epidemiology of burn wound infections: then and now. *Clin Infect Dis.* 2003;37:543-550.
186. Vidal F, Mensa J, Almela M, et al. Epidemiology and outcome of *Pseudomonas aeruginosa* bacteremia, with special emphasis on the influence of antibiotic treatment: analysis of 189 episodes. *Arch Intern Med.* 1996;156:2121-2126.
187. Kuikka A, Valtonen VV. Factors associated with improved outcome of *Pseudomonas aeruginosa* bacteremia in a Finnish university hospital. *Eur J Clin Microbiol Infect Dis.* 1998;17:701-708.
188. Siegman-Igra Y, Ravona R, Primerman H, et al. *Pseudomonas aeruginosa* bacteremia: an analysis of 123 episodes, with particular emphasis on the effect of antibiotic therapy. *Int J Infect Dis.* 1998;2:211-215.
189. Chamot E, Boffi El Amari E, Rohner P, et al. Effectiveness of combination antimicrobial therapy for *Pseudomonas aeruginosa* bacteremia. *Antimicrob Agents Chemother.* 2003;47:2756-2764.
190. Hughes WT, Armstrong D, Bodey GP, et al. 2002 guidelines for the use of antimicrobial agents in neutropenic patients with cancer. *Clin Infect Dis.* 2002;34:730-751.
191. Kim MK, Capitano B, Mattoes HM, et al. Pharmacokinetic and pharmacodynamic evaluation of two dosing regimens for piperacillin-tazobactam. *Pharmacotherapy.* 2002;22:569-577.
192. Hansen M, Christrup LL, Jarlov JO, et al. Gentamicin dosing in critically ill patients. *Acta Anaesthesiol Scand.* 2001;45:734-740.
193. Lodise TP Jr, Patel N, Kwa A, et al. Predictors of 30-day mortality among patients with *Pseudomonas aeruginosa* bloodstream infections: impact of delayed appropriate antibiotic selection. *Antimicrob Agents Chemother.* 2007;51:3510-3515.
194. Chastre J, Fagon JY. Ventilator-associated pneumonia. *Am J Respir Crit Care Med.* 2002;165:867-903.
195. Schuster MG, Norris AH. Community-acquired *Pseudomonas aeruginosa* pneumonia in patients with HIV infection. *AIDS.* 1994;8:1437-1441.
196. Hatchette TF, Gupta R, Marrie TJ. *Pseudomonas aeruginosa* community-acquired pneumonia in previously healthy adults: case report and review of the literature. *Clin Infect Dis.* 2000;31:1349-1356.
197. Arancibia F, Bauer TT, Ewig S, et al. Community-acquired pneumonia due to gram-negative bacteria and *Pseudomonas aeruginosa*: incidence, risk, and prognosis. *Arch Intern Med.* 2002;162:1849-1858.
198. Crnich CJ, Gordon B, Andes D. Hot tub-associated necrotizing pneumonia due to *Pseudomonas aeruginosa*. *Clin Infect Dis.* 2003;36:e55-e57.
199. Canadian Critical Care Trials Group. A randomized trial of diagnostic techniques for ventilator-associated pneumonia. *N Engl J Med.* 2006;355:2619-2630.
200. Carratala J, Roson B, Fernandez-Sevilla A, et al. Bacteremic pneumonia in neutropenic patients with cancer: causes, empirical antibiotic therapy, and outcome. *Arch Intern Med.* 1998;158:868-872.
201. Palmer LB, Smaldone GC, Simon SR, et al. Aerosolized antibiotics in mechanically ventilated patients: delivery and response. *Crit Care Med.* 1998;26:31-39.
202. Barker AF, Couch L, Fiel SB, et al. Tobramycin solution for inhalation reduces sputum *Pseudomonas aeruginosa* density in bronchiectasis. *Am J Respir Crit Care Med.* 2000;162:481-485.
203. Kadota J, Mukae H, Ishii H, et al. Long-term efficacy and safety of clarithromycin treatment in patients with diffuse panbronchiolitis. *Respir Med.* 2003;97:844-850.
204. Jaffe A, Bush A. Anti-inflammatory effects of macrolides in lung disease. *Pediatr Pulmonol.* 2001;31:464-473.
205. Pechere JC. Azithromycin reduces the production of virulence factors in *Pseudomonas aeruginosa* by inhibiting quorum sensing. *Jpn J Antibiot.* 2001;54(Suppl C):87-89.
206. Sapico FL, Montgomerie JZ. Vertebral osteomyelitis in intravenous drug abusers: report of three cases and review of the literature. *Rev Infect Dis.* 1980;2:196-206.
207. Bayer AS, Chow AW, Louie JS, et al. Sternoarticular pyoarthrosis due to gram-negative bacilli: report of eight cases. *Arch Intern Med.* 1977;137:1036-1040.
208. Sapico FL. Microbiology and antimicrobial therapy of spinal infections. *Orthop Clin North Am.* 1996;27:9-13.
209. Ross JJ, Hu LT. Septic arthritis of the pubic symphysis: review of 100 cases. *Medicine (Baltimore).* 2003;82:340-345.
210. Lang AG, Peterson HA. Osteomyelitis following puncture wounds of the foot in children. *J Trauma.* 1976;16:993-999.
211. Fisher MC, Goldsmith JF, Gilligan PH. Sneakers as a source of *Pseudomonas aeruginosa* in children with osteomyelitis following puncture wounds. *J Pediatr.* 1985;106:607-609.
212. Siebert WT, Dewan S, Williams TW Jr. Case report: *Pseudomonas* puncture wound osteomyelitis in adults. *Am J Med Sci.* 1982;283:83-88.
213. Lau LS, Bin G, Jaovisidua S, et al. Cost effectiveness of magnetic resonance imaging in diagnosing *Pseudomonas aeruginosa* infection after puncture wound. *J Foot Ankle Surg.* 1997;36:36-43.
214. Crosby LA, Powell DA. The potential value of the sedimentation rate in monitoring treatment outcome in puncture-wound-related *Pseudomonas* osteomyelitis. *Clin Orthop.* 1984; September:168-172.
215. Livesley NJ, Chow AW. Infected pressure ulcers in elderly individuals. *Clin Infect Dis.* 2002;35:1390-1396.
216. Bach MC, Cocchetto DM. Ceftazidime as single-agent therapy for gram-negative aerobic bacillary osteomyelitis. *Antimicrob Agents Chemother.* 1987;31:1605-1608.
217. Hessen MT, Ingerman MJ, Kaufman DH, et al. Clinical efficacy of ciprofloxacin therapy for gram-negative bacillary osteomyelitis. *Am J Med.* 1987;82:262-265.
218. Norrby SR. Ciprofloxacin in the treatment of acute and chronic osteomyelitis: a review. *Scand J Infect Dis Suppl.* 1989;60:74-78.
219. Wise BL, Mathis JL, Jawetz E. Infections of the central nervous system due to *Pseudomonas aeruginosa*. *J Neurosurg.* 1969;31:432-434.
220. Marone P, Concia E, Maserati R, et al. Ceftazidime in the therapy of pseudomonal meningitis. *Chemioterapia.* 1985;4:289-292.
221. Fong IW, Tomkins KB. Review of *Pseudomonas aeruginosa* meningitis with special emphasis on treatment with ceftazidime. *Rev Infect Dis.* 1985;7:604-612.
222. Rodriguez WJ, Khan WN, Cocchetto DM, et al. Treatment of *Pseudomonas* meningitis with ceftazidime with or without concurrent therapy. *Pediatr Infect Dis J.* 1990;9:83-87.
223. Wong-Beringer A, Beringer P, Lovett MA. Successful treatment of multidrug-resistant *Pseudomonas aeruginosa* meningitis with high-dose ciprofloxacin. *Clin Infect Dis.* 1997;25:936-937.
224. Baum J, Barza M. *Pseudomonas* keratitis and extended-wear soft contact lenses. *Arch Ophthalmol.* 1990;108:663-664.
225. Wang AG, Wu CC, Liu JH. Bacterial corneal ulcer: a multivariate study. *Ophthalmologica.* 1998;212:126-132.
226. Smulders C, Brink H, Wanten G, et al. Conjunctival and corneal colonization by *Pseudomonas aeruginosa* in mechanically ventilated patients: a prospective study. *Neth J Med.* 1999;55:106-109.
227. Aguilar HE, Meredith TA, Shaarawy A, et al. Vitreous cavity penetration of ceftazidime after intravenous administration. *Retina.* 1995;15:154-159.
228. Atkins MC, Harrison GA, Lucas GS. *Pseudomonas aeruginosa* orbital cellulitis in four neutropenic patients. *J Hosp Infect.* 1990;16:343-349.
229. Lattman J, Massry GG, Hornblass A. Pseudomonal eyelid necrosis: clinical characteristics and review of the literature. *Ophthal Plast Reconstr Surg.* 1998;14:290-294.
230. Reid TM, Porter IA. An outbreak of otitis externa in competitive swimmers due to *Pseudomonas aeruginosa*. *J Hyg (London).* 1981;86:357-362.
231. Chandler JR. Malignant external otitis. *Laryngoscope.* 1968;78:1257-1294.
232. Hern JD, Almeyda J, Thomas DM, et al. Malignant otitis externa in HIV and AIDS. *J Laryngol Otol.* 1996;110:770-775.
233. Ress BD, Luntz M, Telischi FF, et al. Necrotizing external otitis in patients with AIDS. *Laryngoscope.* 1997;107:456-460.
234. Rubin J, Yu VL. Malignant external otitis: insights into pathogenesis, clinical manifestations, diagnosis, and therapy. *Am J Med.* 1988;85:391-398.
235. Bellini C, Antonini P, Ermanni S, et al. Malignant otitis externa due to *Aspergillus niger*. *Scand J Infect Dis.* 2003;35:284-288.
236. Parisier SC, Lucente FE, Som PM, et al. Nuclear scanning in necrotizing progressive "malignant" external otitis. *Laryngoscope.* 1982;92:1016-1019.
237. Lang R, Goshen S, Kitzes-Cohen R, et al. Successful treatment of malignant external otitis with oral ciprofloxacin: report of experience with 23 patients. *J Infect Dis.* 1990;161:537-540.
238. Fradis M, Brodsky A, Ben-David J, et al. Chronic otitis media treated topically with ciprofloxacin or tobramycin. *Arch Otolaryngol Head Neck Surg.* 1997;123:1057-1060.
239. Alper CM, Dohar JE, Gulhan M, et al. Treatment of chronic suppurative otitis media with topical tobramycin and dexamethasone. *Arch Otolaryngol Head Neck Surg.* 2000;126:165-173.
240. Miro N. Controlled multicenter study on chronic suppurative otitis media treated with topical applications of ciprofloxacin 0.2% solution in single-dose containers or combination of polymyxin B, neomycin, and hydrocortisone suspension. *Otolaryngol Head Neck Surg.* 2000;123:617-623.
241. Somekh E, Cordova Z. Ceftazidime versus aztreonam in the treatment of pseudomonal chronic suppurative otitis media in children. *Scand J Infect Dis.* 2000;32:197-199.
242. Johnson MP, Ramphal R. Malignant external otitis: report on therapy with ceftazidime and review of therapy and prognosis. *Rev Infect Dis.* 1990;12:173-180.
243. Berenholz L, Katzenell U, Harell M. Evolving resistant *Pseudomonas* to ciprofloxacin in malignant otitis externa. *Laryngoscope.* 2002;112:1619-1622.
244. Mocan H, Karaguzel G. Community-acquired *Pseudomonas aeruginosa* urinary tract infection in young children. *Pediatr Nephrol.* 1997;11:784-785.
245. Greene SL, Su WP, Muller SA. Ecthyma gangrenosum: report of clinical, histopathologic, and bacteriologic aspects of eight cases. *J Am Acad Dermatol.* 1984;11:781-787.
246. Huminer D, Siegman-Igra Y, Morduchowicz G, et al. Ecthyma gangrenosum without bacteremia: report of six cases and review of the literature. *Arch Intern Med.* 1987;147:299-301.

247. Greene SL, Su WP, Muller SA. *Pseudomonas aeruginosa* infections of the skin. *Am Fam Physician.* 1984;29:193-200.
248. Alomar A, Ausina V, Vernis J, et al. *Pseudomonas folliculitis. Cutis.* 1982;30:405-409.
249. Berger RS, Seifert MR. Whirlpool folliculitis: a review of its cause, treatment, and prevention. *Cutis.* 1990;45:97-98.
250. el Baze P, Thyss A, Caldani C, et al. *Pseudomonas aeruginosa* O-11 folliculitis: development into ecthyma gangrenosum in immunosuppressed patients. *Arch Dermatol.* 1985;121: 873-876.
251. Meislich D, Long SS. Invasive *Pseudomonas* infection in two healthy children following prolonged bathing. *Am J Dis Child.* 1993;147:18-20.
252. McManus AT, Mason AD Jr, McManus WF, et al. Twenty-five year review of *Pseudomonas aeruginosa* bacteremia in a burn center. *Eur J Clin Microbiol.* 1985;4:219-223.
253. Vistnes LM, Hogg GR. The burn eschar: a histopathological study. *Plast Reconstr Surg.* 1971;48:56-60.
254. Richard P, Le Floch R, Chamoux C, et al. *Pseudomonas aeruginosa* outbreak in a burn unit: role of antimicrobials in the emergence of multiply resistant strains. *J Infect Dis.* 1994;170:377-383.
255. Culbertson GR, McManus AT, Conarro PA, et al. Clinical trial of imipenem/cilastatin in severely burned and infected patients. *Surg Gynecol Obstet.* 1987;165:25-28.
256. Monafo WW, West MA. Current treatment recommendations for topical burn therapy. *Drugs.* 1990;40:364-373.
257. Reyes MP, Lerner AM. *Pseudomonas* endocarditis. *JAMA.* 1979;241:1576.
258. Rajashekaraiah KR, Rice TW, Kallick CA. Recovery of *Pseudomonas aeruginosa* from syringes of drug addicts with endocarditis. *J Infect Dis.* 1981;144:482.
259. Shekar R, Rice TW, Zierdt CH, et al. Outbreak of endocarditis caused by *Pseudomonas aeruginosa* serotype O11 among pentazocine and tripelennamine abusers in Chicago. *J Infect Dis.* 1985;151:203-208.
260. Bayer AS, Norman D, Kim KS. Efficacy of amikacin and ceftazidime in experimental aortic valve endocarditis due to *Pseudomonas aeruginosa. Antimicrob Agents Chemother.* 1985;28: 781-785.
261. Cabinian AE, Kaatz GW. Successful therapy of *Pseudomonas aeruginosa* endocarditis with ceftazidime and tobramycin. *Am J Med.* 1987;83:366-367.
262. Gavin PJ, Suseno MT, Cook FV, et al. Left-sided endocarditis caused by *Pseudomonas aeruginosa*: successful treatment with meropenem and tobramycin. *Diagn Microbiol Infect Dis.* 2003;47:427-430.
263. Uzun O, Akalin HE, Unal S, et al. Long-term oral ciprofloxacin in the treatment of prosthetic valve endocarditis due to *Pseudomonas aeruginosa. Scand J Infect Dis.* 1992;24:797-800.
264. Arbulu A, Holmes RJ, Asfaw I. Surgical treatment of intractable right-sided infective endocarditis in drug addicts: 25 years experience. *J Heart Valve Dis.* 1993;2:129-139.

265. Komshian SV, Tablan OC, Palutke W, et al. Characteristics of left-sided endocarditis due to *Pseudomonas aeruginosa* in the Detroit Medical Center. *Rev Infect Dis.* 1990;12:693-702.
266. Raje NS, Rao SR, Iyer RS, et al. Infection analysis in acute lymphoblastic leukemia: a report of 499 consecutive episodes in India. *Pediatr Hematol Oncol.* 1994;11:271-280.
267. Karim M, Khan W, Farooqi B, et al. Bacterial isolates in neutropenic febrile patients. *J Pak Med Assoc.* 1991;41:35-37.
268. Yoshida M, Tsubaki K, Kobayashi T, et al. Infectious complications during remission induction therapy in 577 patients with acute myeloid leukemia in the Japan Adult Leukemia Study Group studies between 1987 and 1991. *Int J Hematol.* 1999;70:261-267.
269. Mendelson MH, Gurtman A, Szabo S, et al. *Pseudomonas aeruginosa* bacteremia in patients with AIDS. *Clin Infect Dis.* 1994;18:886-895.
270. Manfredi R, Nanetti A, Ferri M, et al. *Pseudomonas* spp. complications in patients with HIV disease: an eight-year clinical and microbiological survey. *Eur J Epidemiol.* 2000;16:111-118.
271. Mevio E, Calabro P, De Paoli F, et al. Unusual extracranial complications of otitis media in a young HIV patient: retropharyngeal and Mouret's abscess. *Rev Laryngol Otol Rhinol (Bord).* 1998;119:199-201.
272. Cano-Parra J, Espana E, Esteban M, et al. *Pseudomonas* conjunctival and secondary orbital cellulitis in a patient with AIDS. *Br J Ophthalmol.* 1994;78:72-73.
273. Dropulic LK, Leslie JM, Eldred LJ, et al. Clinical manifestations and risk factors of *Pseudomonas aeruginosa* infection in patients with AIDS. *J Infect Dis.* 1995;171:930-937.
274. Gallant JE, Ko AH. Cavitary pulmonary lesions in patients infected with human immunodeficiency virus. *Clin Infect Dis.* 1996;22:671-682.
275. Freeman AF, Mancini AJ, Yogev R. Is noma neonatorum a presentation of ecthyma gangrenosum in the newborn? *Pediatr Infect Dis J.* 2002;21:83-85.
276. Keam SJ. Doripenem: a review of its use in the treatment of bacterial infections. *Drugs.* 2008;68:2021-2057.
277. Fluit AC, Verhoef J, Schmitz FJ. Antimicrobial resistance in European isolates of *Pseudomonas aeruginosa.* European SENTRY Participants. *Eur J Clin Microbiol Infect Dis.* 2000; 19:370-374.
278. Jones RN, Kirby JT, Beach ML, et al. Geographic variations in activity of broad-spectrum beta-lactams against *Pseudomonas aeruginosa*: summary of the worldwide SENTRY Antimicrobial Surveillance Program (1997-2000). *Diagn Microbiol Infect Dis.* 2002;43:239-243.
279. Goossens H. Susceptibility of multi-drug-resistant *Pseudomonas aeruginosa* in intensive care units: results from the European MYSTIC study group. *Clin Microbiol Infect.* 2003;9:980-983.
280. Andrade SS, Jones RN, Gales AC, et al. Increasing prevalence of antimicrobial resistance among *Pseudomonas aeruginosa* isolates in Latin American medical centres: 5 year report of the SENTRY Antimicrobial Surveillance Program (1997-2001). *J Antimicrob Chemother.* 2003;52:140-141.

281. Stein A, Raoult D. Colistin: an antimicrobial for the 21st century? *Clin Infect Dis.* 2002;35:901-902.
282. Livermore DM. Multiple mechanisms of antimicrobial resistance in *Pseudomonas aeruginosa*: our worst nightmare? *Clin Infect Dis.* 2002;34:634-640.
283. Livermore DM. Of *Pseudomonas*, porins, pumps and carbapenems. *J Antimicrob Chemother.* 2001;47:247-250.
284. Higgins PG, Fluit AC, Milatovic D, et al. Antimicrobial susceptibility of imipenem-resistant *Pseudomonas aeruginosa. J Antimicrob Chemother.* 2002;50:299-301.
285. Lepper PM, Grusa E, Reichl H, et al. Consumption of imipenem correlates with beta-lactam resistance in *Pseudomonas aeruginosa. Antimicrob Agents Chemother.* 2002;46:2920-2925.
286. Conway SP, Pond MN, Watson A, et al. Intravenous colistin sulphomethate in acute respiratory exacerbations in adult patients with cystic fibrosis. *Thorax.* 1997;52:987-993.
287. Beringer P. The clinical use of colistin in patients with cystic fibrosis. *Curr Opin Pulm Med.* 2001;7:434-440.
288. Linden PK, Kusne S, Coley K, et al. Use of parenteral colistin for the treatment of serious infection due to antimicrobial-resistant *Pseudomonas aeruginosa. Clin Infect Dis.* 2003;37:e154-e160.
289. Evans ME, Feola DJ, Rapp RP. Polymyxin B sulfate and colistin: old antibiotics for emerging multiresistant gram-negative bacteria. *Ann Pharmacother.* 1999;33:960-967.
290. Levin AS, Barone AA, Penco J, et al. Intravenous colistin as therapy for nosocomial infections caused by multidrug-resistant *Pseudomonas aeruginosa* and *Acinetobacter baumannii. Clin Infect Dis.* 1999;28:1008-1011.
291. Gunderson BW, Ibrahim KH, Hovde LB, et al. Synergistic activity of colistin and ceftazidime against multiantibiotic-resistant *Pseudomonas aeruginosa* in an in vitro pharmacodynamic model. *Antimicrob Agents Chemother.* 2003;47:905-909.
292. Markou N, Apostolakos H, Koumoudiou C, et al. Intravenous colistin in the treatment of sepsis from multiresistant gram-negative bacilli in critically ill patients. *Crit Care.* 2003;7: R78-R83.
293. Landmand D, Georgescu C, Martin DA, et al. Polymyxins revisited. *Clin Microbiol Rev.* 2008;21:449-465.
294. Rynn C, Wootton M, Bowker KE, et al. In vitro assessment of colistin's antipseudomonal antimicrobial interactions with other antibiotics. *Clin Microbiol Infect.* 1999;5:32-36.
295. Giamarellos-Bourboulis EJ, Sambatakou H, Galani I, et al. In vitro interaction of colistin and rifampin on multidrug-resistant *Pseudomonas aeruginosa. J Chemother.* 2003;15: 235-238.
296. Song W, Woo HJ, Kim JS, et al. In vitro activity of beta-lactams in combination with other antimicrobial agents against resistant strains of *Pseudomonas aeruginosa. Int J Antimicrob Agents.* 2003;21:8-12.
297. Oie S, Uematsu T, Sawa A, et al. In vitro effects of combinations of antipseudomonal agents against seven strains of multidrug-resistant *Pseudomonas aeruginosa. J Antimicrob Chemother.* 2003;52:911-914.

220

Stenotrophomonas maltophilia and Burkholderia cepacia Complex

GEORG MASCHMEYER | **ULF B. GÖBEL**

Stenotrophomonas maltophilia and species of the *Burkholderia cepacia* complex (Bcc) are important nosocomial pathogens in hospitalized patients, particularly those with prior broad-spectrum antibacterial therapy, primarily patients with cystic fibrosis (CF) (see Chapter 68). They are intrinsically resistant to most antimicrobial or disinfectant agents and are phenotypically unremarkable, and Bcc exhibits an extensive diversity of genotypes.

Microbiology, Taxonomy, and Identification

STENOTROPHOMONAS

S. maltophilia, formerly named *Pseudomonas* and then *Xanthomonas maltophilia,* is the only species in the genus. *S. maltophilia* bacteria are motile, free-living, glucose-nonfermentative, gram-negative aerobic bacilli with multitrichous polar flagella. *S. maltophilia* grows readily on most bacteriologic media, typically appearing pale-yellow, grayish, or lavender-green when grown on blood agar. Preliminary identification may be facilitated by its ammonia-like odor. Most clinical isolates are oxidase negative and use maltose and usually dextrose and xylose.[1] *S. maltophilia* may produce extracellular deoxyribonuclease on selected media, can hydrolyze esculin and orthonitrophenyl-β-D-galactopyranoside, and produces catalase and a strong acid reaction in oxidation-fermentation in maltose medium. Most strains require methionine for growth.[2] In vitro resistance patterns differ markedly between institutions, and testing results may not correctly predict clinical treatment response.

BURKHOLDERIA CEPACIA COMPLEX

B. cepacia, previously known as *Pseudomonas cepacia,* now represents genomovar I of the large and diverse Bcc. Like *Stenotrophomonas* species, Bcc bacteria are motile, free-living, glucose-nonfermentative, gram-negative aerobic bacilli with multitrichous polar flagella. The appearance of Bcc colonies is variable, depending on the strain and the culture medium used. Identification of highly treatment-resistant small-colony variants of Bcc on selective media may be of clinical importance.[3]

Based on phenotypic and genotypic analyses, Bcc has been divided into currently 10 genomic species (genomovars): *B. cepacia* (genomovar I); *B. multivorans* (genomovar II); *B. cenocepacia* (genomovar III, with four *recA* clusters, IIIA- IIID); *B. stabilis* (genomovar IV); *B. vietnamiensis* (genomovar V); *B. dolosa* (genomovar VI); *B. ambifaria* (genomovar VII); *B. anthina* (genomovar VIII), *B. pyrrocinia* (genomovar IX), and *B. ubonensis* (genomovar X).[4] Recently, five novel species, *B. latens, B. diffusa, B. aboris, B. seminalis,* and *B. metallica,* have been proposed as members of the Bcc using a polyphasic approach based on comparative 16S ribosomal RNA and *recA* sequencing, multilocus sequence typing (MLST), and intermediate DNA-DNA binding values.[5] At present, MLST represents the most promising way for identifying species and strains of the Bcc.[6]

To isolate Bcc organisms, selective media have been developed that usually contain sucrose with or without lactose, and antibiotics, such as polymyxin, gentamicin, or vancomycin. Three media are in use: the *Pseudomonas cepacia* agar (PCA), the oxidation-fermentation polymyxin bacitracin lactose agar (OFBL), and recently the *B. cepacia* selective agar (BCSA). The last is more selective by suppressing growth of non-Bcc bacteria, whereas Bcc members form visible pinpoint colonies within 24 hours. Colonies are smooth and slightly elevated. A comparison of all three media revealed a superior performance of the BCSA, achieving 43%, 93%, and 100% growth of Bcc organisms at 24, 48, and 72 hours, respectively.[7] It has, hence, been recommended to include the use of selective media and extended incubation for CF respiratory tract specimens. Meanwhile, these recommendations have been implemented in clinical microbiology laboratory protocols of most CF care sites reviewed recently.[8] Members of the Bcc can be identified by available commercial tests, such as API 20NE, Phoenix, MicroScan, or Vitek. However, misidentification occurs in a number of cases, and care should be taken to correctly differentiate *Burkholderia* species from *Achromobacter, Ralstonia,* and other nonfermenting, gram-negative rods. A large polyphasic analysis of 1051 isolates from 115 CF treatment centers in 91 US cities conducted in 2000 revealed an overall misidentification rate of 11% for isolates identified as Bcc by referring laboratories. This rate was even higher (36%) for isolates not specifically identified or identified as a species other than Bcc.[9] There is an increasing number of laboratories implementing semiautomated microbial identification systems. A recent comparison of the Phoenix automated microbiology system (BD Diagnostics, Sparks, Md) with the MicroScan WalkAway 96 system (Dade Behring, West Sacramento, Calif) revealed difficulties in correctly identifying at the species level five isolates representing *B. cenocepacia, B. multivorans,* and *B. gladioli.*[10] The evaluation of the new Vitek 2 colorimetric card (ID-GN; bioMérieux) for identification of nonfermentative, gram-negative rods revealed accurate identification of most Bcc isolates.[11]

Virulence Factors and Pathogenesis

Both *S. maltophilia* and members of the Bcc uncommonly cause community-acquired infections in previously healthy individuals. Their resistance to most antimicrobial agents selects them in specific patient populations. *S. maltophilia* is a nosocomial pathogen that occurs in many of the same types of hospitalized patients as Bcc. In most clinical situations, however, isolation of *S. maltophilia* will represent colonization or contamination rather than true infection, and it has been difficult in many instances to substantiate a causative role of *S. maltophilia* because of its rather limited pathogenicity and the lack of obvious virulence factors.[12] One candidate virulence factor may be a recently described alkaline serine protease, the StmPr1 protease, enabling *S. maltophilia* to degrade human serum and tissue proteins (e.g., the immunoglobulin G heavy chain).[13] The gene of another putative virulence factor has been identified in a clinical *S. maltophilia* isolate harboring a phage genome containing an open reading frame that exhibited significant sequence similarity to the *V. cholerae* zonula occludens toxin Zot.[14] A most remarkable property was its resistance to pan-protease inhibitors such as α_1-antitrypsin and α_2-macroglobulin. Biofilm formation contributes to succesful colonisation of abiotic surfaces, such as catheters and lung epithelia. A diffusible signal factor (DSF), methyl dodecenoic acid, regulates a number of virulence traits and antimicrobial resistance (e.g., motility, extracellular proteases, lipopolysaccharide (LPS) synthesis, microcolony formation, and tolerance toward antibiotics, and heavy metal ions).[15] DSF has been shown to influence *P. aeruginosa* in mixed *S. maltophilia*–*P. aeruginosa* biofilms, conferring increased bacterial stress tolerance (e.g., resistance to cationic antimicrobial peptides), an effect associated with increased tolerance to polymyxins.[16] In a neonatal mouse pneumonia model, *S. maltophilia* elicited a strong inflammatory response as measured by significant interleukin-8 (IL-8) and tumor necrosis factor-α (TNF-α) expression in respiratory epithelial cells and macrophages, respectively. Low rates of pneumonia and sepsis (20%) in TNF receptor-1 (TNFR1)–negative mice compared with wild-type mice (100%) suggested an important role of TNF-α signaling.[17] The most striking information drawn from the complete genome sequence of a clinical *S. maltophilia* strain (K279a) was the large number of genes conferring resistance to antimicrobials and heavy metals.[18] There were nine resistance-nodulation-division (RND)–type efflux pump genes.

Patients with CF and those with chronic granulomatous disease are predisposed to infection by Bcc bacteria. Here, colonization by *B. multivorans* or *B. cenocepacia* of the respiratory tract is associated with significantly higher morbidity and mortality[19] (Fig. 220-1), particularly after lung transplantation, increasing the mortality within the first 6 months after transplantation to up to 40%[20] and to 85% after 10 years.[21] Whether this is strictly attributable to the virulence of Bcc or rather represents the poor disease status of CF patients affected by Bcc colonization is controversial.[22,23] In principle, all Bcc species may cause infections in CF patients. *B. cenocepacia* and *B. multivorans* are by far the most frequent Bcc bacteria in this patient population, causing up to 80% of Bcc infections, whereas other Bcc species account for less than 10% of cases.

Drug resistance in Bcc is mediated by an immunodominant drug efflux pump (bcrA).[24] Bcc species express a number of different virulence factors that variably contribute to the pathogenesis of Bcc infections. By using proteomic profiling, Chung and Speert identified a number of virulence factors associated with *B. cenocepacia* survival in mice.[25] Virulence factors may be present in some but absent in other strains of a given species, enabling the respective organisms to colonize and invade lung tissue, to survive in intracellular compartments, and to induce and elicit robust inflammatory responses. This is particularly true for the epidemic E12 lineage of *B. cenocepacia*. Current knowledge about Bcc virulence determinants contributing to colonization, invasion, and intracellular survival has been summarized in a comprehensive review.[26] *B. cepacia* ET12 contains a hybrid of two insertion sequences as well as a 1.4-kilobase open reading frame, which have

been demonstrated in transmissible *B. cenocepacia* species. Transmissibility is genetically related to *esmR* and *cblA* genes, and *esmR* (or the *B. cepacia* epidemic strain marker [BCESM]) is detected only in *B. cenocepacia* strains. It has been shown that the BCESM is part of a genomic island encoding virulence and metabolism-associated genes designated *B. cenocepacia* island (cii).[27] Noteworthy is the presence of an *N*-acyl homoserine lactone (AHL) synthase gene and the corresponding regulator gene. One factor affecting the early stages of colonization is the scavenging of iron. Bcc possesses at least four iron-binding siderophores: salicylic acid, ornibactin, pyochelin, and cepabactin.[26]

Adherence in epidemic *B. cenocepacia* strains is conferred by the presence of long, flexible type II pili exhibiting cable morphology. These giant cable pili mediate attachment to respiratory epithelia.[28] Genes necessary for cable biosynthesis are encoded by the cbl operon, consisting of at least seven genes: *cblA*, the major pilin subunit; *cblB*, a proposed chaperone; *cblC*, a proposed usher protein; *cblD*, a minor pilin protein; and the regulatory genes *cblR*, *cblS*, and *cblT*. The first four genes of the cbl operon—*cblA*, *cblB*, *cblC*, and *cblD*—were shown to be sufficient for pilus assembly in *Escherichia coli*, but the regulatory genes are required for pilus biogenesis in *B. cenocepacia*.[29-31] Bcc cells lacking Cbl pili still bind to cytokeratin 13 (CK13), the 55-kDa protein expressed in CF patients preferentially in bronchiolar and respiratory epithelium,[28,29] indicating that other bacterial proteins, such as a 22-kDa protein, mediate adherence. Mutants not expressing cable pili (cblA or CblS mutants) showed reduced binding (50%). In mutants lacking the 22-kDa adhesin (adhA mutants), adhesion toward CK13 was almost completely abolished (0% to 8%). For optimal binding, both Cbl pili and the adhesin appear to be required.[32] Other fimbrial structures, such as mesh (Msh), filamentous (Fil), spine (Spn), and spike (Spk), have been identified, but their pathogenetic relevance has yet to be determined.[26,33] Nonfimbrial adhesins, a 37-kDa protein corresponding to the Bcc porin C, and an unidentified 66-kDa outer membrane protein have also been described, but detailed knowledge is still lacking.[34] Nonpiliate strains use lipid receptors expressed mainly on the basolateral surface of respiratory epithelia and alveolar type II pneumocytes.[35]

Bcc bacteria have invasive potential. They can migrate across the epithelial barrier to invade lung parenchyma and capillaries.[36,37] Invasiveness may be due to inhibition of natural pulmonary defense mechanisms such as human β-defensins.[38] Invasive clinical Bcc isolates have shown their ability to survive in macrophages and pulmonary epithelial cells, whereas environmental strains may lack this ability.[39] Adhesion by cable pili and the 22-kDa adhesin appears to be required for transmigration across the squamous epithelium because mutants lacking either adhesin, the adhA mutant in particular, were shown to be compromized in their transmigration capacity.[32] In contrast, *B. cenocepacia* expressing both pili and the 22-kDa adhesin invaded and migrated across the epithelial barrier, causing IL-8 release and epithelial damage. Bacteria were surrounded by filopodia and present in membrane-bound vesicles within the cells after 24 hours.[40] Martin and Mohr[39] compared the capacity of a clinical *B. cenocepacia* isolate and an environmental *B. multivorans* strain to invade cultured macrophages and pulmonary epithelial cells. Although both strains showed similar invasion frequencies for macrophages, the clinical strain was more invasive in epithelial cells and able to survive and replicate both in macrophages and in epithelial cells. Cable pili induce epithelial cell cytotoxicity and thus appear to play a major role in the pathogenesis of *B. cenocepacia* infection. Purified cable pili activate caspases and major cysteine proteinases involved in apoptosis.[41] Besides transcytosis and and disruption of the epithelial barrier by pilus-mediated epithelial cell death described previously, Bcc species are able to transmigrate the respiratory epithelium through paracytosis by disrupting tight junctions by dephosphorylation and dissociation of occludin from the tight junction complex.[42] It has also been shown that lipases produced by Bcc species may play a role in invasion because the lipase inhibitor Orlistat significantly decreased the invasion, affecting neither plasma membrane nor tight junction integrity.[43] Invasiveness was impaired

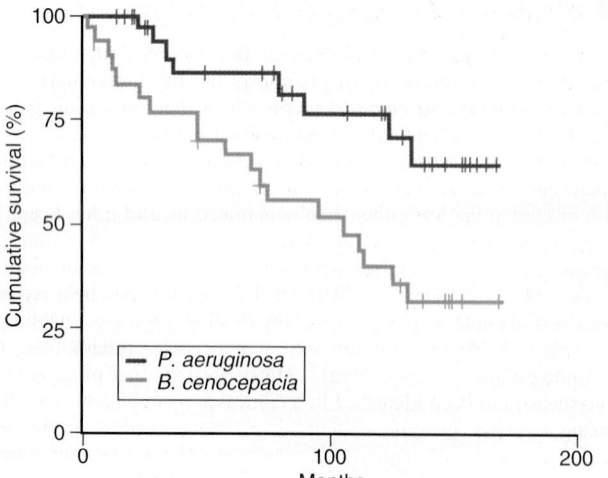

Figure 220-1 Survival of patients with cystic fibrosis infected by *Burkholderia cenocepacia* compared with *Pseudomonas aeruginosa*. *(From Jones AM, Dodd ME, Govan JR, et al. Burkholderia cenocepacia and Burkholderia multivorans: Influence on survival in cystic fibrosis. Thorax. 2004;59:948-951.)*

when two genes (i.e., *fliG*, encoding a component of the motor-switch complex, and *fliI*, encoding an ATPase required for protein translocation) were disrupted.[44] However, reduced invasion was not due to defective adherence. Invasion was inhibited by cytochalasin D, suggesting that the host-cell cytoskeleton may play a role in facilitating bacterial entry.[45] This is consistent with the observation that Bcc mutants lacking the *bscN* gene, encoding an ATP-binding protein possibly representing part of a type III secretion system, exhibited attenuated virulence in a murine model.[46] Invasion of *B. cenocepacia* can be strongly inhibited by bovine lactoferrin, an effect not influenced by its iron-binding activity.[47] This may be of clinical importance because it has been demonstrated that recombinant human lactoferrin (rhL) inhibited growth and biofilm formation in several Bcc species. Susceptibility to rifampicin was enhanced in the presence of rhl.[48] *B. cenocepacia* and some other Bcc species express two metalloproteases, ZmpA and ZmpB, that may contribute to the spread of these organisms by degrading collagen and fibronecting. They are able to inactivate major host protease inhibitors, such as α_2-macroglobulin, which may contribute to systemic dissemination and septicemia.[49] In addition, immunoglobulins, transferrin, and lactoferrin are cleaved by ZmpB, allowing *B. cenocepacia* to evade host defences.

Several mechanisms appear to enable intracellular survival. Reactive oxygen and nitrogen intermediates possess critical roles in the host defense against Bcc, as shown in p47phox$^{(-/-)}$ mice and in mice with a targeted disruption of the inducible nitric oxide synthase (*iNOS*) gene.[50] Bcc-infected macrophages primed with interferon-γ produced less nitric oxide than interferon-γ–primed, noninfected cells.[51] It could be shown that an overexpressed azurin homologue, normally involved in electron transfer during denitrification, induced apoptosis in macrophages in a caspase-dependent manner.[52] Several catalase-peroxidases of *B. cenocepacia* have been described that provide bacteria expressing these enzymes a significant advantage in resisting attack by macrophage-derived H_2O_2.[53] Similarly, superoxide dismutases like the *B. cenocepacia* periplasmic superoxide dismutase SodC protect this bacterium from exogenous O_2^-, thus contributing to intracellular survival in macrophages.[54] Pigments, such as the pyomelanin produced by some *B. cenocepacia* strains, are capable of scavenging free radicals, thus attenuating the oxidative burst.[55] Flagellum-mediated motility appears to facilitate adhesion to and penetration of epithelial barriers by Bcc.[44] Biofilm formation followed by invasion and destruction of epithelial cells has been identified as a major pattern of invasiveness in *B. cenocepacia*.[36] Strains producing abundant exopolysaccharide (EPS) persisted in a mouse model of pulmonary infection.[56,57] Eighty to 90% of clinical Bcc isolates produce the EPS cepacian. Cepacian is required for the development of thick biofilms. The initiation of biofilm formation is unaffected. No clear correlation between the ability of various strains to produce EPS and to form biofilms and persistence and virulence has been found.[58] In CF patients, pulmonary infection is characterized by an excessive accumulation of neutrophils. It has been shown that EPS from a clinical *B. cenocepacia* strain interfered with the function of neutrophils by inhibiting chemotactic migration and scavenging of ROS. This, together with the resistance of Bcc species to antibacterial peptides, a nonoxidative defense by neutrophils, explains the inability of CF patients to clear the bacteria from infected lungs.[59] Fifty-three percent of clinical *B. cenocepacia* IIIA isolates showed a nonmucoid phenotype, whereas 100% of the isolates from the *B. cenocepacia* IIIB lineage and 82.8% of the *B. multivorans* isolates were frankly mucoid.[60] Phenotypic switching, preferably mucoid-to-nonmucoid conversions, has been observed in sequential isolates from 15 patients, and it is presumed that nonmucoid isolates are associated with increased disease severity, whereas the mucoid phenotype is associated with persistence.

Bcc LPS induces the release of proinflammatory cytokines (TNF-α, IL-6, and IL-8) from blood monocytes and whole blood,[61,62] thus contributing to the severe inflammatory response observed in CF patients, who are often showing a rapidly necrotizing course. Bcc lipopolysaccharides further induce increased surface expression of CR3 on neutrophils as well as the priming of respiratory burst activity.[63]

Most *B. cenocepacia* strains, isolates of the ET12 lineage in particular, are able to induce a strong and sustained inflammatory reaction by the interaction of bacterial ligands such as LPS or flagella with toll-like receptor (TLR). It could be shown that highly purified LPS from clinical Bcc strains induced a TLR4/CD14-mediated activation of mitogen-activated protein kinase pathways and activation of NFκB.[64] LPS from different clinical isolates elicited varied immune responses. Although LPS isolated from *B. cenocepacia* strains activates cells through MyD88-dependent pathways, LPS isolated from *B. multivorans* acts through MyD88-independent pathways. This may be due to differences in the acylation patterns and may explain different clinical outcomes.[65,66] *B. cenocepacia* flagella induce a a strong TLR5-mediated NFκB activation and IL-8 secretion.[67] Interaction of LPS and flagellins with TLR4 and TLR5, respectively, does significantly contribute to pathogenesis, but other signaling events have been proposed that explain the robust inflammatory response found in epidemic *B. cenocepacia* infections. A recent report described direct binding of strain BC7 to TNFR1, activating the TNFR1 signaling pathway in a manner similar to TNF-α. This resulted in strong IL-8 production.[68] Another possibly important way of subverting the host's immune response has been described,[69] demonstrating that *B. cenocepacia*, but not *B. multivorans,* disrupted maturation and induced necrosis in human dendritic cells. Expression of virulence factors and environmental adaptation in *B. cenocepacia* are regulated by two sets of quorum sensing (QS) genes, the *cepIR* and *cciIR*, the former present in all *B. cenocepacia* strains and the latter exclusively in the epidemic strains containing the cci island.[70] CepI produces two AHL, primarily octanoyl-homoserine lactone, whereas CciI produces mainly hexanoyl-homoserine lactone. The transcriptional regulator CepR corresponds to the AHL signals by regulating respective target gene positively or negatively. CepR is also required for *cciIR* gene expression. The *cepIR* QS system regulates the expression of a variety of virulence factors, such as extracellular proteases, chitinase, ornibactin biosynthesis, biofilm maturation, and motility. QS mutants affect attachment and stability of *B. cenocepacia* biofilms.[71] Flannagan and colleagues identified a six-gene cluster encoding a two-component regulatory system and an HtrA protease required for adaptation of *B. cenocepacia* to environmental stress (e.g., exposure to osmotic or thermal stress and survival in a rat model of chronic lung infection).[72] Recently, a novel sensor kinase-response regulator, AtsR, has been described. Inactivation of the *atsR* gene resulted in overexpression of Hcp (hemolysin-coregulated protein) probably secreted by an upregulated type VI secretion system, increased biofilm production, stronger adherence to polystyrene and lung epithelial cells, and actin rearrangements in infected macrophages.[73] At present, it is unclear whether the protrusions formed in macrophages contribute to bacterial escape from macrophages or delay phagosome-lysosome fusion. Inhibition or delay of phagolysosomal fusion appears to play a crucial role in intracellular survival of *B. cenocepacia*. Here, mtgC, needed for growth of *B. cenocepacia* in magnesium-depleted medium, appears to play an important role.[74] Two alternative sigma factors, RpoE and RpoN, were shown to be crucial for regulating genes required delaying phagolysosomal fusion and phagosome maturation.[75,76]

More information will result once complete fully annotated genomes will become available. So far, more than 30 *Burkholderia* genome-sequencing projects have been initiated. The sequence of *B. cenocepacia* J2315, a strain of the ET12 lineage, has been completed at the Sanger Institute, and sequences are available for searching. The genome is very large; it totals 8 Mb in three chromosomes of 3.8, 3.2, and 0.8 Mb, respectively, and a 92.7-kb plasmid. It encodes more than 7000 genes, 10% of which have been acquired through horizontal gene transfer.[4]

Epidemiology

S. maltophilia may be acquired from diverse environmental sources, such as tap water, ready-to-eat salads, or contaminated solutions. Among CF patients, colonization with *S. maltophilia* has been reported for 10% to 15% of them[77,78] and has not been found to adversely influence patients' prognosis.[79]

Bcc organisms are distributed ubiquitously and found most commonly on plant roots, the rhizosphere, soil, and moist environments. They are of increasing importance for agriculture and bioremediation because of their antinematodal and antifungal properties as well as their capability to degrade a wide range of toxic compounds.[80,81] More than 20% of environmental Bcc strains are closely genetically related to clinical isolates,[82] and outbreaks have been reported originating from diverse sources such as contaminated faucets, nebulizers, chlorhexidine solution, alcohol-free mouthwash, multidose albuterol vials used among multiple patients, indigo-carmine dye used in enteral feeding, tap water, bottled water, cosmetics, napkins, nasal sprays, and ultrasound gels. Patients may acquire Bcc either from the environment or through patient-to-patient transmission. *B. cenocepacia* and *B. multivorans* are more predominant among CF patients than non-CF patients.[4] Some authors have detected *B. cepacia* more frequently among non-CF patients.[83] Recent progress in molecular typing methods enabled hospital epidemiologists to correctly identify outbreak strains and, hence, to identify the source and trace transmission routes. Ribotype restriction fragment length polymorphism (RFLP) profiles and pulsed-field gel electrophoresis (PFGE)-resolved RFLPs were used to identify a single dominant and highly transmissible clone in a hospital outbreak involving CF and non-CF patients. Their risk for acquisition was linked to hospitalization, and thus infection control policies must consider the transmission between non-CF and CF patients.[84] A comprehensive study evaluating multiple genomic typing systems including random amplified polymorphic DNA (RAPD) typing, PFGE, and BOX polymerase chain reaction (BOX-PCR) fingerprinting compared the results obtained by these different methods with each other as well as to data from previous studies with multilocus restriction typing (MLRT). The authors concluded that PFGE and RAPD fingerprinting were most suitable for small-scale studies (i.e., local outbreaks), whereas BOX-PCR fingerprinting appeared more appropriate for large-scale studies aimed at analyzing global epidemiology.[85] In the same study, BOX-PCR fingerprinting was considered a rapid and easy alternative to MLRT.

The availability of rapid and accurate tests for genomovar identification allowed for a comprehensive analysis of the prevalence of different Bcc species. By the age of 18 years, about 3.5% of CF patients harbor Bcc.[86] Data from the United States, Canada, and Italy show that *B. cenocepacia* and *B. multivorans* are the most prevalent genomovars among CF patients, accounting for 95% of all infections. *B. cenocepacia* are predominant, ranging from 80% to 50% (mean, 67.5%) among different CF populations studied so far. Further analysis of the different *recA* lineages revealed significant geographic differences. Whereas type IIIB strains represented 75% of all US *B. cenocepacia* isolates, type IIIA strains are more prevalent in Canada and Europe, accounting for about 70% of all genomovar III isolates.[4,87-89] The unique distribution of selected Bcc genomovars indicates the presence of epidemic strains exhibiting particular virulence and transmissibility. So far, two genetic elements have been identified that are associated with epidemic spread: *cblA*, a gene encoding a protein for cable pilus production, and *esmR*, also called BCESM, representing a 1.4-kb putative open reading frame with homology to negative transcriptional regulators. Analyzing all *B. cenocepacia* strains isolated from Canadian CF patients of different geographic origin, Speert and co-workers[89] identified four genetic lineages defined by RAPD and PFGE. Only strains from RAPD type 02, representing the ET12 clonal lineage, harbored both BCESM and *cblA*. The predominance of this RAPD type in Ontario, Canada was correlated with a significantly higher prevalence, accounting for 22% of patients in Ontario versus 5% in Quebec.

A population structure analysis of *B. cenocepacia*[90] revealed that 86.7% of all restriction types clustered into three major clonal complexes, comprising epidemic clones ET12 (RT-6 complex), PHDC (RT-46 complex), and Midwest (RT-88 complex). These clones have a wide geographic distribution and exhibit varying degrees of genetic recombination. Infection with clone ET12 has been associated with

increased mortality and the so-called cepacia syndrome, characterized by rapid, often fatal respiratory failure and septicemia.[91] PDHC is the clone responsible for almost all Bcc infections in the mid-Atlantic region of the United States.[92] A strain belonging to this clonal lineage has been isolated from organic soils in four agricultural fields that had been planted with onions for several years. This indicates that environmental strains may play a pivotal role in the epidemiology of Bcc infections and could explain the ongoing human acquisition despite infection control measures.[93] The third clone described is most prevalent in CF patients from the Midwestern region of the United States.[94] In contrast to some reports advocating the identification of the *cblA* gene as a means of influencing patient segregation and infection control strategies,[95] several authors[90,92] provided evidence that the presence of putative transmissibility factors *cblA* or *esmR* varied significantly among established epidemic clones, leading to the conclusion that infection control measures should not be based on the presence or absence of these markers. An attempt to identify other genetic elements that may be specific for epidemic Bcc strains led to the identification of a novel insertion sequence, designated *IS1363*, in clone PHDC.[96] *IS1363* was also found in most isolates of clone ET12, but not in other Bcc species except *B. ambifaria* (genomovar VII). At present, it remains unclear whether this IS element contributes to the increased capacity of both clones to infect CF patients. However, together with other IS elements, it may contribute to the genomic plasticity of Bcc species. Considering the acquisition of environmental strains by CF patients, the observation of frequent genetic recombination in *B. cenocepacia* populations may have important implications for the biotechnical use of Bcc species.[90,97]

Clinical Manifestations

STENOTROPHOMONAS MALTOPHILIA

The most frequent clinical manifestations of *S. maltophilia* infection are bloodstream infections and pneumonia.[12,98,99] *S. maltophilia* bloodstream infection results in a high fatality rate, particularly when not treated promptly with appropriate antibiotics.[100] However, most *S. maltophilia* isolates from respiratory secretions represent colonization rather than infection.[101] True *S. maltophilia* pneumonia is more likely to occur among intensive care or cancer patients and is associated with extensive use of broad-spectrum antibiotics, advanced age, mechanical ventilation, and a higher Acute Physiology and Chronic Health Evaluation II (APACHE II) score.[98] *S. maltophilia* pneumonia is among the nosocomial infections most frequently treated inappropriately[102] and is associated with a high mortality rate, particularly when associated with bacteremia or obstruction. It may be complicated by septic shock and multiple organ dysfunction syndrome. Chest radiographs may show lobar, nodular, or bronchopneumonic infiltrates, and computed tomography scans typically exhibit diffuse bilateral multifocal infiltrates and ground-glass attenuation (Fig. 220-2).[103,104] The respiratory

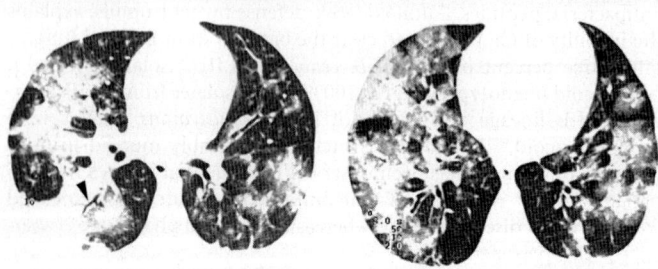

Figure 220-2 Thoracic computed tomography scan in an allogeneic hematopoietic stem cell transplant recipient with *Stenotrophomonas maltophilia* pneumonia. *(From Gasparetto EL, Bertholdo DB, Davaus T, et al. Stenotrophomonas maltophilia pneumonia after bone marrow transplantation: Case report with emphasis on the high-resolution CT findings. Br J Radiol. 2007;80:e19-e20.)*

microbial flora is often mixed, even in cases in which *S. maltophilia* is considered to be a significant pathogen. However, *S. maltophilia* may represent indirect pathogenicity through the production of at least two inducible β-lactamases, L1 and L2, hydrolyzing almost all classes of β-lactam antimicrobials and thus supporting the growth of pathogens such as *Serratia marcescens* and *Pseudomonas aeruginosa* even in the presence of imipenem or ceftazidime.[105]

S. maltophilia bacteremias are typically central venous catheter-related and may be polymicrobial.[106,107] In cancer patients, antimicrobial treatment with fluoroquinolones, trimethoprim-sulfamethoxazole, carbapenems, or cephalosporins may predispose for *S. maltophilia* bacteremia.[108,109] Single cases of other clinical manifestations to *S. maltophilia* infection, such as endocarditis on both native and prosthetic valves, endophthalmitis, sinusitis, cellulitis, meningitis, liver abscess, and myositis, have been described. Cellulitis develops around catheter insertion sites or arises hematogenously. Ecthyma gangrenosum may be a rare cutaneous complication of both Bcc and *S. maltophilia* bacteremia. In contrast, hematogenous skin lesions of *S. maltophilia* present as firm, tender, erythematous nodules. *S. maltophilia* isolated from the urinary tract often represent colonization in the presence of a Foley catheter rather than true infection. However, the urinary tract may be the focus of severe sepsis, particularly after instrumentation or surgery.

BURKHOLDERIA CEPACIA COMPLEX

Patients with CF and those with chronic granulomatous disease are predisposed to Bcc pneumonia.[4,89,110-112] Apart from chronic asymptomatic carriage, rapid and fatal clinical deterioration with necrotizing granulomatous pneumonia, called *cepacia syndrome*,[113] and bacteremia may occur (Fig. 220-3).[114]

Increased mortality has been observed in CF patients after colonization with Bcc.[19,91,115,116] CF patients colonized with *B. cepacia* genom-

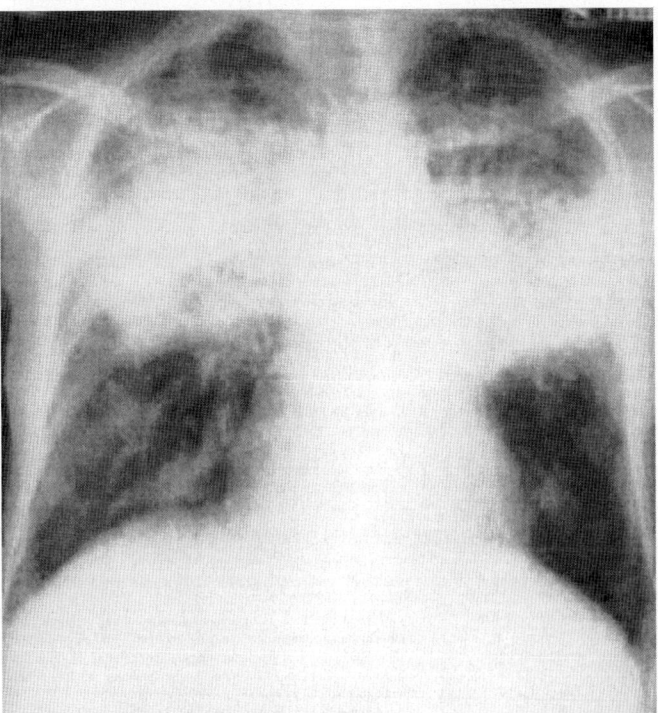

Figure 220-3 **Chest radiograph showing typical appearances of the cepacia syndrome in a patient with cystic fibrosis.** *(From Jones AM, Dodd ME, Webb AK. Burkholderia cepacia: Current clinical issues, environmental controversies and ethical dilemmas. Eur Respir J. 2001;17:295-301.)*

ovar III who are undergoing lung transplantation have been reported to carry an up to 50% risk for fatal post-transplantation complications,[20,21,117] which has led several centers to avoid lung transplantation in CF patients colonized with this organism.[118] Most CF patients colonized with Bcc, however, show little change in their clinical picture, and those who do may be effectively treated with adequate antimicrobial agents.[23]

Bcc bacteremia, most often catheter-related and polymicrobial, has been reported in cancer patients[119] and in patients undergoing hemodialysis,[120] and nosocomial pneumonia was observed in intensive care patients who were mechanically ventilated and pretreated with broad-spectrum antibiotics such as fluoroquinolones and ceftazidime.[121,122]

Bcc skin and soft tissue infection may occur in patients with burns or surgical wounds and in soldiers with prolonged foot immersion in water. Genitourinary tract infection caused by Bcc has been reported after urethral instrumentation, after transrectal prostate biopsy, or through exposure to contaminated solutions.

▮ Treatment

STENOTROPHOMONAS MALTOPHILIA

Treatment recommendations for both *S. maltophilia* and *B. cepacia* complex infections vary profoundly, and an ideal treatment standard has not been established. It is essential to distinguish between a clinically significant *S. maltophilia* infection and colonization or polymicrobial infection with other, potentially more pathogenic microorganisms involved. For treatment considerations, it should be kept in mind that prior use of fluoroquinolones, carbapenems, or third- or fourth-generation cephalosporins represents a major risk factor for the development of *S. maltophilia* bacteremia.[107,108,123]

In patients other than those with CF, who have bacteremia caused by *S. maltophilia* alone, an indwelling venous catheter is likely to be the source of infection. Removal of this foreign body hastens cure.[109] Some authors have found that the attributable mortality in non-CF patients with *S. maltophilia* or Bcc bacteremia may be similar to that observed in other bacteremias caused by gram-negative bacilli.[12,124]

Trimethoprim-sulfamethoxazole (TMP-SMZ) and ticarcillin–clavulanic acid, given alone or in combination, are agents with consistent therapeutic activity against *S. maltophilia* isolates.[106,125,126] For ticarcillin-clavulanate, high rates of in vitro resistance among *S. maltophilia* have been reported from single centers with extensive use of β-lactam antibiotics, as has been the case for TMP-SMX.[127-129] The in vitro sensitivity testing of *S. maltophilia* against antimicrobial drugs may show results contrasting to the clinical outcome in patients treated with these antibiotics.[130] This is particularly relevant for TMP-SMZ. Ceftazidime, aztreonam, moxifloxacin, or ciprofloxacin may be suitable for treatment as well, depending on susceptibility.[106,131-133] Minocycline has excellent in vitro activity; however, clinical experience with this agent is limited. Tigecycline has been reported to be a new potentially effective agent for clinical treatment of *S. maltophilia* infections but experience is limited.[134,135]

Antimicrobial therapy of *S. maltophilia* infection, pending in vitro susceptibility testing, may be initiated with a combination of TMP-SMZ and ticarcillin-clavulanate at high dosages (15 to 20 mg/kg/day of trimethoprim) for TMP-SMZ and 3.1 g every 4 hours of ticarcillin-clavulanate. Removal of foreign material or necrotic tissue is a valuable adjunct to medical therapy. In cases in which removal of an indwelling venous catheter is not suitable, systemic antimicrobial therapy in combination with antibiotic-lock treatment of the catheter has been successfully performed.[136] Some patients with a history of allergy to TMP-SMX may successfully undergo desensitization, enabling them to be treated effectively with TMP-SMX.[137] In mechanically ventilated patients with *S. maltophilia* infection of their lower respiratory tract, systemic antibiotic treatment in combination with nebulized aminoglycoside application may be considered,[106] provided that no previous application of this modality has caused the emergence of aminoglycoside-resistant *S. maltophilia*.

Multivariate analyses have shown that the presence of septic shock at onset of infection, profound neutropenia, and delay in appropriate antimicrobial therapy are significant predictors of poor outcome in patients with *S. maltophilia* bacteremia.[101,105,119,126]

BURKHOLDERIA CEPACIA COMPLEX

Antimicrobial agents that are effective against Bcc include meropenem, TMP-SMZ, chloramphenicol, and minocycline. Other potentially active single agents include the ureidopenicillins, third-generation cephalosporins, and fluoroquinolones.[138] Rates of in vitro resistance of Bcc to TMP-SMZ range from 5% in Quebec, Canada[89] and Latin America to 10% in Europe.[99] Combination antimicrobial treatment is recommended for patients with pulmonary Bcc infection.[139-141] Successful treatment with combinations of meropenem with ciprofloxacin and tobramycin has been reported, as has been for ceftazidime and tobramycin, whereas the combination of TMP-SMZ with a β-lactam may result in antagonism.[142] Additional nebulization of antimicrobial agents such as meropenem or tobramycin has been reported to be effective as well.[143] Among more recently developed antimicrobial agents, doripenem appears to have therapeutical potential against Bcc.[144]

In individual CF patients with life-threatening Bcc infection, short-term adjunctive treatment with methylprednisolone may be beneficial.[145] Future immunotherapeutic options, primarily prophylactic vaccination against Bcc[146] or nasal immunization,[147] appear to be promising, particularly in light of scarce new antimicrobial agents under development for the treatment of multidrug-resistant gram-negative bacilli.

Prevention and Control

Because both *B. cepacia* complex and *S. maltophilia* are commonly found in the environment, and patient-to-patient transmission, although repeatedly reported,[80,87,148-151] is less frequent than acquisition from other sources, strategies aiming at prevention of infections caused by these multidrug-resistant pathogens are difficult to design.[89] Accepted prophylactic measures include (1) an appropriate antibiotic policy, particularly a critical use of ciprofloxacin, cefepime, and imipenem; (2) strict hand hygiene and institution of barrier techniques for colonized or infected patients; and (3) surveillance among CF patients and identification of potential nosocomial reservoirs such as the public water system,[152] commercially available drinking water,[153] sink drains,[154] faucet aerators,[155] contaminated handwash or mouthwash solutions,[156] and medical equipment. Education of patients and health care workers is a cornerstone of such preventive measures. Isolation and segregation measures have been proved useful for prevention of transmission of Bcc between CF patients.[157] For CF patients, living with a person colonized by Bcc, contact with a Bcc-colonized patient, hospitalization, and attending a summer CF camp have been shown to be associated with an increased risk for becoming colonized or infected with these organisms.[158] Patient segregation and rigorous infection control measures should be reinforced to reduce or prevent transmission of Bcc. Patients infected with transmissible genomovar strains should not be cohorted with patients infected with *B. multivorans* or other Bcc genomovars.[157,159] However, continued efforts will be required to implement CF sputum surveillance with improved species and strain identification and to elucidate bacterial or host factors contributing to patient-to-patient transmission.[93]

A double-blind, placebo-controlled trial in adult CF patients infected with *B. cenocepacia* has not shown any benefit from nebulized taurolidine.[160] In cases in which control measures did not prevent the infection of CF patients, acquisition from natural environments should be considered.[161] The widespread use of Bcc in agriculture and bioremediation of contaminated environmental sites causes a conflict about its commercial use in light of its potentially life-threatening impact on CF patients.[113,162]

REFERENCES

1. Clark WA, Hollis DG, Weaver RE, et al. *Identification of unusual pathogenic gram negative aerobic and facultative aerobic bacteria.* Atlanta, GA: Centers for Disease Control; 1985.
2. Burdge DR, Noble MA, Campbell ME, et al. *Xanthomonas maltophilia* misidentified as *Pseudomonas cepacia* in cultures of sputum from patients with cystic fibrosis: A diagnostic pitfall with major clinical implications. *Clin Infect Dis.* 1995; 20:445-448.
3. Haussler S, Lehmann C, Breselge C, et al. Fatal outcome of lung transplantation in cystic fibrosis patients due to small-colony variants of the *Burkholderia cepacia* complex. *Eur J Clin Microbiol Infect Dis.* 2003;22:249-253.
4. Mahenthiralingam E, Baldwin A, Dowson CG. *Burkholderia cepacia* complex bacteria: Opportunistic pathogens with important natural biology. *J Appl Microbiol.* 2008;104:1539-1551.
5. Vanlaere E, Sergeant K, Dawyndt P, et al. Matrix-assisted laser desorption ionisation-time-of-flight mass spectrometry of intact cells allows rapid identification of *Burkholderia cepacia* complex. *J Microbiol Methods.* 2008;75:279-286.
6. Baldwin A, Mahenthiralingam E, Thickett KM, et al. Multilocus sequence typing scheme that provides both species and strain differentiation for the *Burkholderia cepacia* complex *J Clin Microbiol.* 2005;43:4665-4673.
7. Henry D, Campbell M, McGimpsey C, et al. Comparison of isolation media for recovery of *Burkholderia cepacia* complex from respiratory secretions of patients with cystic fibrosis. *J Microbiol.* 1999;37:1004-1007.
8. Zhou J, Garber E, Desai M, et al. Compliance of clinical microbiology laboratories in the United States with current recommendations for processing respiratory tract specimens from patients with cystic fibrosis. *J Clin Microbiol.* 2006;44: 1547-1549.
9. McMenamin JD, Zaccone TM, Coeyne T, et al. Misidentification of *B. cepacia* in US Cystic Fibrosis treatment centers. *Chest.* 2000;117:1161-1165.
10. Snyder JW, Munier GK, Johnson CL. Direct comparison of the BD Phoenix System with the MicroScan WalkAway System for identification and antimicrobial susceptibility testing of Enterobacteriaceae and nonfermenting Gram-negative organisms. *J Clin Microbiol.* 2008;46:2327-2333.
11. Zbinden A, Böttger EC, Bosshard PP, et al. Evaluation of the colorimetric VITEK 2 card for identification of Gram-negative nonfermentative rods: comparison to 16S rRNA gene sequencing. *J Clin Microbiol.* 2007;45:2270-2273.
12. Denton M, Kerr KG. Microbiological and clinical aspects of infection associated with *Stenotrophomonas maltophilia. Clin Microbiol Rev.* 1998;11:57-80.
13. Windhorst S, Frank E, Georgieva DN, et al. The major extracellular protease of the nosocomial pathogen *Stenotrophomonas maltophilia. J Biol Chem.* 2002;277:11042-11049.
14. Hagemann M, Hasse D, Berg G. Detection of a phage genome carrying a zonula occludens like toxin gene (zot) in clinical isolates of Stenotrophomonas maltophilia. *Arch Microbiol.* 2006;185:449-458.
15. Fouhy Y, Scanlon K, Schouest K, et al. Diffusible signal factor-dependent cell-cell signaling and virulence in the nosocomial pathogen Stenotrophomonas maltophilia. *J Bacteriol.* 2007;189:4964-4968.
16. Ryan RP, Fouhy Y, Garcia BF, et al. Interspecies signalling via the Stenotrophomonas maltophilia diffusible signal factor influences biofilm formation and polymyxin tolerance in Pseudomonas aeruginosa. *Mol Microbiol.* 2008;68: 75-86.
17. Waters VJ, Gómez MI, Soong G, et al. Immunostimulatory properties of the emerging pathogen Stenotrophomonas maltophilia. *Infect Immun.* 2007;75:1698-1703.
18. Crossman LC, Gould VC, Dow JM, et al. The complete genome, comparative and functional analysis of Stenotrophomonas maltophilia reveals an organism heavily shielded by drug resistance determinants. *Genome Biol.* 2008;9:R74.
19. Jones AM, Dodd ME, Govan JR, et al. *Burkholderia cenocepacia* and *Burkholderia multivorans:* influence on survival in cystic fibrosis. *Thorax.* 2004;59:948-951.
20. Aris RM, Routh JC, LiPuma JJ, et al. Lung transplantation for cystic fibrosis patients with *Burkholderia cepacia* complex: Survival linked to genomovar type. *Am J Respir Crit Care Med.* 2001;164:2102-2106.
21. de Perrot M, Chaparro C, McRae K, et al. Twenty-year experience of lung transplantation at a single center: Influence of recipient diagnosis on long-term survival. *J Thorac Cardiovasc Surg.* 2004;127:1493-1501.
22. Frangolias DD, Mahenthiralingam E, Rae S, et al. *Burkholderia cepacia* in cystic fibrosis: Variable disease course. *Am J Respir Crit Care Med.* 1999;160:1572-1577.
23. McManus TE, Moore JE, Crowe M, et al. A comparison of pulmonary exacerbations with single and multiple organisms in patients with cystic fibrosis and chronic *Burkholderia cepacia* infection. *J Infect.* 2003;46:56-59.
24. Wigfield SM, Rigg GP, Kavari M, et al. Identification of an immunodominant drug efflux pump in *Burkholderia cepacia. J Antimicrob Chemother.* 2002;49:619-624.
25. Chung JW, Speert DP. Proteomic identification and characterization of bacterial factors associated with *Burkholderia cenocepacia* survival in a murine host. *Microbiology.* 2007;153: 206-214.
26. Mohr CD, Tomich M, Herfst CA. Cellular aspects of *Burkholderia cepacia* infection. *Microbes Infect.* 2001;3:425-435.
27. Baldwin A, Sokol PA, Parkhill J, et al. The *Burkholderia cepacia* epidemic strain marker is part of a novel genomic island encoding both virulence and metabolism-associated genes in *Burkholderia cenocepacia. Infect Immun.* 2004;72:1537-1547.
28. Sajjan US, Sylvester FA, Forstner JF. Cable-piliated *Burkholderia cepacia* binds to cytokeratin 13 of epithelial cells. *Infect Immun.* 2000;68:1787-1795.
29. Sajjan US, Xie H, Lefebre MD, et al. Identification and molecular analysis of cable pilus biosynthesis genes in *Burkholderia cepacia. Microbiology.* 2003;149:961-971.
30. Tomich M, Mohr CD. Transcriptional and posttranscriptional control of cable pilus gene expression in *Burkholderia cenocepacia. J Bacteriol.* 2004;186:1009-1020.
31. Tomich M, Mohr CD. Genetic characterization of a multicomponent signal transduction system controlling the expression of cable pili in *Burkholderia cenocepacia. J Bacteriol.* 2004;186:3826-3836.
32. Urban TA, Goldberg JB, Forstner JF, et al. Cable pili and the 22-kilodalton adhesin are required for *Burkholderia cenocepacia* binding to and transmigration across the squamous epithelium. *Infect Immun.* 2005;73:5426-5437.
33. Goldstein R, Sun L, Jiang RZ, et al. Structurally variant classes of pilus appendage fibers coexpressed from *Burkholderia (Pseudomonas) cepacia. J Bacteriol.* 1995;177:1039-1052.
34. Saiman L, Cacalano G, Prince A. *Pseudomonas cepacia* adherence to respiratory epithelial cells is enhanced by *Pseudomonas aeruginosa. Infect Immun.* 1990;58:2578-2584.
35. Sylvester FA, Sajjan US, Forstner JF. *Burkholderia* (basonym *Pseudomonas*) *cepacia* binding to lipid receptors. *Infect Immun.* 1996;64:1420-1425.
36. Schwab U, Leigh M, Ribeiro C, et al. Patterns of epithelial cell invasion by different species of the *Burkholderia cepacia* complex in well-differentiated human airway epithelia. *Infect Immun.* 2002;70:4547-4555.

37. Sajjan U, Corey M, Humar A, et al. Immunolocalisation of *Burkholderia cepacia* in the lungs of cystic fibrosis patients. *J Med Microbiol.* 2001;50:535-546.
38. Baird RM, Brown H, Smith AW, et al. *Burkholderia cepacia* is resistant to the antimicrobial activity of airway epithelial cells. *Immunopharmacology.* 1999;44:267-272.
39. Martin DW, Mohr CD. Invasion and intracellular survival of *Burkholderia cepacia. Infect Immun.* 2000;8:24-29.
40. Sajjan U, Ackerley C, Forstner J. Interaction of cblA/adhesin-positive *Burkholderia cepacia* with squamous epithelium. *Cell Microbiol.* 2002;4:73-86
41. Cheung KJ, Li G, Urban TA, et al. Pilus-mediated epithelial cell death in response to infection with *Burkholderia cenocepacia. Microb Infect.* 2007;9:829-837.
42. Kim JY, Sajjan US, Krasan GP, LiPuma JJ. Disruption of tight junctions during traversal of the respiratory epithelium by *Burkholderia cenocepacia. Infect Immun.* 2005;73:7107-7112.
43. Mullen T, Markey K, Murphy P, et al. Role of lipase in *Burkholderia cepacia* complex (Bcc) invasion of lung epithelial cells. *Eur J Clin Microbiol Infect Dis.* 2007;26:869-877.
44. Tomich M, Herfst CA, Golden JW, et al. Role of flagella in host cell invasion by *Burkholderia cepacia. Infect Immun.* 2002; 70:1799-1806.
45. Burns JL, Jonas M, Chi EY, et al. Invasion of respiratory epithelial cells by *Burkholderia (Pseudomonas) cepacia. Infect Immun.* 1996;64:4054-4059.
46. Tomich M, Griffith A, Herfst CA, et al. Attenuated virulence of a *Burkholderia cepacia* type III secretion mutant in a murine model of infection. *Infect Immun.* 2003;71:1405-1415.
47. Berlutti F, Superti F, Nicoletti M. Bovine lactoferrin inhibits the efficiency of invasion of respiratory A549 cells of different iron-regulated morphological forms of *Pseudomonas aeruginosa* and *Burkholderia cenocepacia. Int J Immunopathol Pharmacol.* 2008;21:51-59.
48. Caraher EM, Gumulapurapu K, Taggart CC, et al. The effect of recombinant human lactoferrin on growth and the antibiotic susceptibility of the cystic fibrosis pathogen *Burkholderia cepacia* complex when cultured planktonically or as biofilms. *J Antimicrob Chemother.* 2007;60:546-554.
49. Kooi C, Subsin B, Chen R, et al. *Burkholderia cenocepacia* ZmpB is a broad-specificity zinc metalloprotease involved in virulence. *Infect Immun.* 2006;74:4083-4093.
50. Segal BH, Ding L, Holland SM. Phagocyte NADPH oxidase, but not inducible nitric oxide synthase, is essential for early control of *Burkholderia cepacia* and *Chromobacterium violaceum* infection in mice. *Infect Immun.* 2003;71:205-210.
51. Saini LS, Galsworthy SB, John MA, et al. Intracellular survival of *Burkholderia cepacia* complex isolates in the presence of macrophage cell activation. *Microbiology.* 1999;145:3465-3475.
52. Punj V, Sharma R, Zaborina O, et al. Energy-generating enzymes of *Burkholderia cepacia* and their interactions with macrophages. *J Bacteriol.* 2003;185:3167-3178.
53. Charalabous P, Risk JM, Jenkins R, et al. Characterization of a bifunctional catalase-peroxidase of *Burkholderia cenocepacia. FEMS Immunol Med Microbiol.* 2007;50:37-44.
54. Keith KE, Valvano MA. Characterization of SodC, a periplasmic superoxide dismutase from *Burkholderia cenocepacia. Infect Immun.* 2007;75:2451-2460.
55. Keith KE, Killip L, He P, et al. *Burkholderia cenocepacia* C5424 produces a pigment with antioxidant properties using a homogentisate intermediate. *J Bacteriol.* 2007;189:9057-9065.
56. Chung JW, Altman E, Beveridge TJ, et al. Colonial morphology of *Burkholderia cepacia* complex genomovar III: Implications in exopolysaccharide production, pilus expression, and persistence in the mouse. *Infect Immun.* 2003;71:904-909.
57. Herasimenka Y, Cescutti P, Impallomeni G, et al. Exopolysaccharides produced by clinical strains belonging to the *Burkholderia cepacia* complex. *J Cystic Fibrosis.* 2007;6:145-152.
58. Cunha MV, Sousa SA, Leitão JH, et al. Studies on the involvement of the exopolysaccharide produced by cystic fibrosis-associated isolates of the *Burkholderia cepacia* complex in biofilm formation and in persistence of respiratory infections. *J Clin Microbiol.* 2004;42:3052-3058.
59. Bylund J, Burgess LA, Cescutti P, et al. Exopolysaccharides from *Burkholderia cenocepacia* inhibit neutrophil chemotaxis and scavenge reactive oxygen species. *J Biol Chem.* 2006;5:2526-2532.
60. Zlosnik JE, Hird TJ, Fraenkel MC, et al. Differential mucoid exopolysaccharide production by members of the *Burkholderia cepacia* complex. *J Clin Microbiol.* 2008;46:1470-1473.
61. Shaw D, Poxton IR, Govan JR. Biological activity of *Burkholderia (Pseudomonas) cepacia* lipopolysaccharide. *FEMS Immunol Med Microbiol.* 1995;11:99-106.
62. Hutchison ML, Bonell EC, Poxton IR, et al. Endotoxic activity of lipopolysaccharides isolated from emergent potential cystic fibrosis pathogens. *FEMS Immunol Med Microbiol.* 2000;27: 73-77.
63. Hughes JE, Stewart J, Barclay GR, et al. Priming of neutrophil respiratory burst activity by lipopolysaccharide from *Burkholderia cepacia. Infect Immun.* 1997;65:4281-4287.
64. Bamford S, Ryley H, Jackson SK. Highly purified lipopolysaccharides from *Burkholderia cepacia* complex clinical isolates induce inflammatory cytokine responses via TLR4-mediated MAPK signalling pathways and activation of NFkappaB. *Cell Microbiol.* 2007;9:532-543.
65. De Soyza A, Silipo A, Lanzetta R, et al. Chemical and biological features of *Burkholderia cepacia* complex lipopolysaccharides. *Innate Immun.* 2008;14:127-144.
66. Ieranò T, Silipo A, Sturiale L, et al. The structure and pro-inflammatory activity of the lipopolysaccharide from *Burkholderia multivorans* and the differences between clonal strains colonizing pre- and post-transplanted lungs. *Glycobiology.* 2008;18:871-881
67. Urban TA, Griffith A, Torok AM, et al. Contribution of *Burkholderia cenocepacia* flagella to infectivity and inflammation. *Infect Immun.* 2004;72:5126-5134.
68. Sajjan US, Hershenson MB, Forstner JF, et al. *Burkholderia cenocepacia* ET12 strain activates TNFR1 signalling in cystic fibrosis airway epithelial cells. *Cell Microbiol.* 2008;10:188-201.
69. Macdonald KL, Speert DP. Differential modulation of innate immune cell functions by the *Burkholderia cepacia* complex: *Burkholderia cenocepacia* but not *Burkholderia multivorans* disrupts maturation and induces necrosis in human dendritic cells. *Cell Microbiol.* 2008;10:2138-2149.
70. Subsin B, Chambers CE, Visser MB, et al. Identification of genes regulated by the *cepIR* quorum-sensing system in *Burkholderia cenocepacia* by high-throughput screening of a random promoter library. *J Bacteriol.* 2007;189:968-979.
71. Tomlin KL, Malott RJ, Ramage G, et al. Quorum-sensing mutations affect attachment and stability of *Burkholderia cenocepacia* biofilms. *Appl Environ Microbiol.* 2005;71:5208-5218.
72. Flannagan RS, Aubert D, Kooi C, et al. *Burkholderia cenocepacia* requires a periplasmic HtrA protease for growth under thermal and osmotic stress and for survival in vivo. *Infect Immun.* 2007;75:1679-1689.
73. Aubert DF, Flannagan RS, Valvano MA. A novel sensor kinase-response regulator hybrid controls biofilm formation and type VI secretion system activity in *Burkholderia cenocepacia. Infect Immun.* 2008;76:1979-1991.
74. Maloney KE, Valvano MA. The *mgtC* gene of *Burkholderia cenocepacia* is required for growth under magnesium limitation conditions and intracellular survival in macrophages. *Infect Immun.* 2006;74:5477-5486.
75. Flannagan RS, Valvano MA. *Burkholderia cenocepacia* requires RpoE for growth under stress conditions and delay of phagolysosomal fusion in macrophages. *Microbiology.* 2008;154: 643-653.
76. Saldías MS, Lamothe J, Wu R, et al. *Burkholderia cenocepacia* requires the RpoN sigma factor for biofilm formation and intracellular trafficking within macrophages. *Infect Immun.* 2008;76:1059-1067.
77. Lambiase A, Raia V, Del Pezzo M, et al. Microbiology of airway disease in a cohort of patients with cystic fibrosis. *BMC Infect Dis.* 2006;6:4.
78. Valenza G, Tappe D, Turnwald D, et al. Prevalence and antimicrobial susceptibility of microorganisms isolated from sputa of patients with cystic fibrosis. *J Cyst Fibros.* 2008;7: 123-127.
79. Gibson RL, Burns JL, Ramsey BW. Pathophysiology and management of pulmonary infections in cystic fibrosis. *Am J Respir Crit Care Med.* 2003;168:918-951.
80. Holmes A, Govan J, Goldstein R. Agricultural use of *Burkholderia (Pseudomonas) cepacia:* a threat to human health? *Emerg Infect Dis.* 1998;4:221-227.
81. LiPuma JJ, Mahenthiralingam M. Commercial use of *Burkholderia cepacia. Emerg Infect Dis.* 1999;5:305-306.
82. Baldwin A, Mahenthiralingam E, Drevinek P, et al. Environmental *Burkholderia cepacia* complex isolates in human infections. *Emerg Infect Dis.* 2007;13:458-461.
83. Reik R, Spilker T, Lipuma JJ. Distribution of *Burkholderia cepacia* complex species among isolates recovered from persons with or without cystic fibrosis. *J Clin Microbiol.* 2005;43: 2926-2928.
84. Holmes A, Nolan R, Taylor R, et al. An epidemic of *Burkholderia cepacia* transmitted between patients with and without cystic fibrosis. *J Infect Dis.* 1999;179:1197-1205.
85. Coenye T, Spilker T, Martin A, et al. Comparative assessment of genotyping methods for epidemiologic study of *Burkholderia cepacia* genomovar III. *J Clin Microbiol.* 2002;40:3300-3307.
86. Rajan S, Saiman L. Pulmonary infections in patients with cystic fibrosis. *Semin Respir Infect.* 2002;17:47-56.
87. Agodi A, Mahenthiralingam E, Barchitta M, et al. *Burkholderia cepacia* complex infection in Italian patients with cystic fibrosis: Prevalence, epidemiology, and genomovar status. *J Clin Microbiol.* 2001;39:2891-2896.
88. LiPuma JJ, Spilker T, Gill LH, et al. Disproportionate distribution of *Burkholderia cepacia* complex species and transmissibility markers in cystic fibrosis. *Am J Respir Crit Care Med.* 2001;164:92-96.
89. Speert DP, Henry D, Vandamme P, et al. Epidemiology of *Burkholderia cepacia* complex in patients with cystic fibrosis, Canada. *Emerg Infect Dis.* 2002;8:181-187.
90. Coenye T, LiPuma JJ. Population structure analysis of *Burkholderia cepacia* genomovar III: Varying degrees of genetic recombination characterize major clonal complexes. *Microbiology.* 2003;149:77-88.
91. Ledson MJ, Gallagher MJ, Jackson M, et al. Outcome of *Burkholderia cepacia* colonisation in an adult cystic fibrosis centre. *Thorax.* 2002;57:142-145.
92. Chen JS, Witzmann KA, Spilker T, et al. Endemicity and inter-city spread of *Burkholderia cepacia* genomovar III in cystic fibrosis. *J Pediatr.* 2001;139:643-649.
93. LiPuma JJ. Preventing *Burkholderia cepacia* complex infection in cystic fibrosis: Is there a middle ground? *J Pediatr.* 2002;141:467-469.
94. Kumar A, Dietrich S, Schneider W, et al. Genetic relatedness of *Burkholderia (Pseudomonas) cepacia* isolates from five cystic fibrosis centers in Michigan. *Respir Med.* 1997;91:485-492.
95. Clode FE, Kaufmann ME, Malnick H, et al. Distribution of genes encoding putative transmissibility factors among epidemic and nonepidemic strains of *Burkholderia cepacia* from cystic fibrosis patients in the United Kingdom. *J Clin Microbiol.* 2000;38: 1763-1766.
96. Liu L, Spilker T, Coenye T, et al. Identification by subtractive hybridization of a novel insertion element specific for two widespread *Burkholderia cepacia* genomovar III strains. *J Clin Microbiol.* 2003;41:2471-2476.
97. Parke JL, Gurian-Sherman D. Diversity of the *Burkholderia cepacia* complex and implications for risk assessment of biological control strains. *Annu Rev Phytopathol.* 2001;39:225-258.
98. Gopalakrishnan R, Hawley HB, Czachor JS, et al. *Stenotrophomonas maltophilia* infection and colonization in the intensive care units of two community hospitals: A study of 143 patients. *Heart Lung.* 1999;28:134-141.
99. Gales AC, Jones RN, Forward KR, et al. Emerging importance of multidrug-resistant *Acinetobacter* species and *Stenotrophomonas maltophilia* as pathogens in seriously ill patients: Geographic patterns, epidemiological features, and trends in the SENTRY Antimicrobial Surveillance Program (1997-1999). *Clin Infect Dis.* 2001;32(Suppl 2):S104-S113.
100. Metan G, Uzun O. Impact of initial antimicrobial therapy in patients with bloodstream infections caused by *Stenotrophomonas maltophilia. Antimicrob Agents Chemother.* 2005;49: 3980-3981.
101. Pathmanathan A, Waterer GW. Significance of positive *Stenotrophomonas maltophilia* culture in acute respiratory tract infection. *Eur Respir J.* 2005;25:911-914.
102. Kollef KE, Schramm GE, Wills AR, et al. Predictors of 30-day mortality and hospital costs in patients with ventilator-associated pneumonia attributed to potentially antibiotic-resistant gram-negative bacteria. *Chest.* 2008;134:281-287.
103. Jones AM, Dodd ME, Webb AK. *Burkholderia cepacia:* Current clinical issues, environmental controversies and ethical dilemmas. *Eur Respir J.* 2001;17:295-301.
104. Gasparetto EL, Bertholdo DB, Davaus T, et al. *Stenotrophomonas maltophilia* pneumonia after bone marrow transplantation: case report with emphasis on the high-resolution CT findings. *Br J Radiol.* 2007;80:e19-20.
105. Kataoka D, Fujiwara H, Kawakami T, et al. The indirect pathogenicity of *Stenotrophomonas maltophilia. Int J Antimicrob Agents.* 2003;22:601-606.
106. Boktour M, Hanna H, Ansari S, et al. Central venous catheter and *Stenotrophomonas maltophilia* bacteremia in cancer patients. *Cancer.* 2006;106:1967-1973.
107. Safdar A, Rolston KV. *Stenotrophomonas maltophilia*: changing spectrum of a serious bacterial pathogen in patients with cancer. *Clin Infect Dis.* 2007;45:1602-1609.
108. Ansari SR, Hanna H, Hachem R, et al. Risk factors for infections with multidrug-resistant *Stenotrophomonas maltophilia* in patients with cancer. *Cancer.* 2007;109:2615-2622.
109. Meyer E, Schwab F, Gastmeier P, et al. *Stenotrophomonas maltophilia* and antibiotic use in German intensive care units: data from Project SARI (Surveillance of Antimicrobial Use and Antimicrobial Resistance in German Intensive Care Units). *J Hosp Infect.* 2006;64:238-243.
110. Taccetti G, Campana S, Marianelli L. Multiresistant non-fermentative gram-negative bacteria in cystic fibrosis patients: The results of an Italian multicenter study. Italian Group for Cystic Fibrosis Microbiology. *Eur J Epidemiol.* 1999;15:85-88.
111. Bevivino A, Dalmastri C, Tabacchioni S, et al. *Burkholderia cepacia* complex bacteria from clinical and environmental sources in Italy: Genomovar status and distribution of traits related to virulence and transmissibility. *J Clin Microbiol.* 2002; 40:846-851.
112. Winkelstein JA, Marino MC, Johnston RB Jr, et al. Chronic granulomatous disease: Report on a national registry of 368 patients. *Medicine (Baltimore).* 2000;79:155-169.
113. Belchis DA, Simpson E, Colby T. Histopathologic features of *Burkholderia cepacia* pneumonia in patients without cystic fibrosis. *Mod Pathol.* 2000;13:369-372.
114. Tablan OC, Chorba TL, Schidlow DV, et al. *Pseudomonas cepacia* colonization in patients with cystic fibrosis: Risk factors and clinical outcome. *J Pediatr.* 1985;107:382-387.
115. Beringer PM, Appleman MD. Unusual respiratory bacterial flora in cystic fibrosis: Microbiologic and clinical features. *Curr Opin Pulm Med.* 2000;6:545-550.
116. Soni R, Marks G, Henry DA, et al. Effect of *Burkholderia cepacia* infection in the clinical course of patients with cystic fibrosis: A pilot study in a Sydney clinic. *Respirology.* 2002;7:241-245.
117. De Soyza A, McDowell A, Archer L, et al. *Burkholderia cepacia* complex genomovars and pulmonary transplantation outcomes in patients with cystic fibrosis. *Lancet.* 2001;358:1780-1781.
118. LiPuma JJ. *Burkholderia cepacia* complex: A contraindication to lung transplantation in cystic fibrosis? *Transpl Infect Dis.* 2001; 3:149-160.
119. Martino R, Gomez L, Pericas R, et al. Bacteraemia caused by non-glucose-fermenting gram-negative bacilli and *Aeromonas* species in patients with haematological malignancies and solid tumours. *Eur J Clin Microbiol Infect Dis.* 2000;19:320-323.

120. Kaitwatcharachai C, Silpapojakul K, Jitsurong S, et al. An outbreak of *Burkholderia cepacia* bacteremia in hemodialysis patients: An epidemiologic and molecular study. *Am J Kidney Dis.* 2000;36:199-204.

121. Gruson D, Hilbert G, Vargas F, et al. Rotation and restricted use of antibiotics in a medical intensive care unit: Impact on the incidence of ventilator-associated pneumonia caused by antibiotic-resistant gram-negative bacteria. *Am J Respir Crit Care Med.* 2000;162:837-843.

122. Siddiqui AH, Mulligan ME, Mahenthiralingam E, et al. An episodic outbreak of genetically related *Burkholderia cepacia* among non-cystic fibrosis patients at a university hospital. *Infect Control Hosp Epidemiol.* 2001;22:419-422.

123. Hanes SD, Demirkan K, Tolley E, et al. Risk factors for late-onset nosocomial pneumonia caused by *Stenotrophomonas maltophilia* in critically ill trauma patients. *Clin Infect Dis.* 2002;35:228-235.

124. Yu WL, Wang DY, Lin CW, et al. Endemic *Burkholderia cepacia* bacteraemia: Clinical features and antimicrobial susceptibilities of isolates. *Scand J Infect Dis.* 1999;31:293-298.

125. Betriu C, Sanchez A, Palau ML, et al. Antibiotic resistance surveillance of *Stenotrophomonas maltophilia*, 1993-1999. *J Antimicrob Chemother.* 2001;48:152-154.

126. Micozzi A, Venditti M, Monaco M, et al. Bacteremia due to *Stenotrophomonas maltophilia* in patients with hematologic malignancies. *Clin Infect Dis.* 2000;31:705-711.

127. Barbier-Frebour N, Boutiba-Boubake I, Nouvello M, et al. Molecular investigation of *Stenotrophomonas maltophilia* isolates exhibiting rapid emergence of ticarcillin-clavulanate resistance. *J Hosp Infect.* 2000;45:35-41.

128. Fadda G, Spanu T, Ardito F, et al. Antimicrobial resistance among non-fermentative Gram-negative bacilli isolated from the respiratory tracts of Italian inpatients: a 3-year surveillance study by the Italian Epidemiological Survey. *Int J Antimicrob Agents.* 2004;23:254-261.

129. Tsiodras S, Pittet D, Carmeli Y, et al. Clinical implications of *Stenotrophomonas maltophilia* resistant to trimethoprim-sulfamethoxazole: A study of 69 patients at 2 university hospitals. *Scand J Infect Dis.* 2000;32:651-656.

130. Carroll KC, Cohen S, Nelson R, et al. Comparison of various in vitro susceptibility methods for testing *Stenotrophomonas maltophilia*. *Diagn Microbiol Infect Dis.* 1998;32:229-235.

131. Falagas ME, Valkimadi PE, Huang YT, et al. Therapeutic options for *Stenotrophomonas maltophilia* infections beyond co-trimoxazole: a systematic review. *J Antimicrob Chemother.* 2008;62:889-894

132. Schmitz FJ, Verhoef J, Fluit AC. Comparative activities of six different fluoroquinolones against 9,682 clinical bacterial isolates from 20 European university hospitals participating in the European SENTRY surveillance programme. The SENTRY Participants Group. *Int J Antimicrob Agents.* 1999;12:311-317.

133. Weiss K, Restieri C, De Carolis E, et al. Comparative activity of new quinolones against 326 clinical isolates of *Stenotrophomonas maltophilia*. *J Antimicrob Chemother.* 2000;45:363-365.

134. Noskin GA. Tigecycline: A new glycylcycline for treatment of serious infections. *Clin Infect Dis.* 2005;41:S303-S314.

135. Sader HS, Jones RN, Dowzicky MJ, et al. Antimicrobial activity of tigecycline tested against nosocomial bacterial pathogens from patients hospitalized in the intensive care unit. *Diagn Microbiol Infect Dis.* 2005;52:203-208.

136. Gattuso G, Tomasoni D, Ceruti R, et al. Multiresistant *Stenotrophomonas maltophilia* tunneled CVC-related sepsis, treated with systemic and lock therapy. *J Chemother.* 2004;16:494-496.

137. Yilmaz M, Celik AF, Mert A. Successfully treated nosocomial *Stenotrophomonas maltophilia* bacteremia following desensitization to trimethoprim-sulfamethoxazole. *J Infect Chemother.* 2007;13:122-123

138. Bhakta DR, Leader I, Jacobson R, et al. Antibacterial properties of investigational, new, and commonly used antibiotics against isolates of *Pseudomonas cepacia* isolates in Michigan. *Chemotherapy.* 1992;33:319-323.

139. Husain S, Singh N. *Burkholderia cepacia* infection and lung transplantation. *Semin Respir Infect.* 2002;17:284-290.

140. Blumer JL, Saiman L, Konstan MW, et al. The efficacy and safety of meropenem and tobramycin vs ceftazidime and tobramycin in the treatment of acute pulmonary exacerbations in patients with cystic fibrosis. *Chest.* 2005;128:2336-2346.

141. Zhou J, Chen Y, Tabibi S, et al. Antimicrobial susceptibility and synergy studies of *Burkholderia cepacia* complex isolated from patients with cystic fibrosis. *Antimicrob Agents Chemother.* 2007;51:1085-1088

142. Manno G, Ugolotti E, Belli ML, et al. Use of the E test to assess synergy of antibiotic combinations against isolates of *Burkholderia cepacia*-complex from patients with cystic fibrosis. *Eur J Clin Microbiol Infect Dis.* 2003;22:28-34.

143. Weidmann A, Webb AK, Dodd ME, et al. Successful treatment of cepacia syndrome with combination nebulised and intravenous antibiotic therapy. *J Cyst Fibros.* 2008;7:409-411

144. Chen Y, Garber E, Zhao Q, et al. In vitro activity of doripenem (S-4661) against multidrug-resistant gram-negative bacilli isolated from patients with cystic fibrosis. *Antimicrob Agents Chemother.* 2005;49:2510-2511.

145. Okano M, Yamada M, Ohtsu M, et al. Successful treatment with methylprednisolone pulse therapy for a life-threatening pulmonary insufficiency in a patient with chronic granulomatous disease following pulmonary invasive aspergillosis and *Burkholderia cepacia* infection. *Respiration.* 1999;66:551-554.

146. Fauré R, Shiao TC, Lagnoux D, et al. En route to a carbohydrate-based vaccine against *Burkholderia cepacia*. *Org Biomol Chem.* 2007;5:2704-2708.

147. Bertot GM, Restelli MA, Galanternik L, et al. Nasal immunization with *Burkholderia multivorans* outer membrane proteins and the mucosal adjuvant adamantylamide dipeptide confers efficient protection against experimental lung infections with *B. multivorans* and *B. cenocepacia*. *Infect Immun.* 2007;75:2740-2752

148. Agodi A, Barchitta M, Giannino V, et al. *Burkholderia cepacia* complex in cystic fibrosis and non-cystic fibrosis patients: Identification of a cluster of epidemic lineages. *J Hosp Infect.* 2002;50:188-195.

149. Heath DG, Hohneker K, Carriker C, et al. Six-year molecular analysis of *Burkholderia cepacia* complex isolates among cystic fibrosis patients at a referral center for lung transplantation. *J Clin Microbiol.* 2002;40:1188-1193.

150. Labarca JA, Leber AL, Kern VL, et al. Outbreak of *Stenotrophomonas maltophilia* bacteremia in allogenic bone marrow transplant patients: Role of severe neutropenia and mucositis. *Clin Infect Dis.* 2000;30:195-197.

151. Garcia de Viedma D, Marin M, Cercenado E, et al. Evidence of nosocomial *Stenotrophomonas maltophilia* cross-infection in a neonatology unit analyzed by three molecular typing methods. *Infect Control Hosp Epidemiol.* 1999;20:816-820.

152. Zanetti F, De Luca G, Stampi S. Recovery of *Burkholderia pseudomallei* and *B. cepacia* from drinking water. *Int J Food Microbiol.* 2000;59:67-72.

153. Mary P, Defives C, Hornez JP. Occurrence and multiple antibiotic resistance profiles of non-fermentative gram-negative microflora in five brands of non-carbonated French bottled spring water. *Microb Ecol.* 2000;39:322-329.

154. Moore JE, Thompson I, Crowe M, et al. *Burkholderia cepacia* from a sink drain. *J Hosp Infect.* 2002;50:235-237.

155. Weber DJ, Rutala WA, Blanchet CN, et al. Faucet aerators: A source of patient colonization with *Stenotrophomonas maltophilia*. *Am J Infect Control.* 1999;27:59-63.

156. Klausner JD, Zukerman C, Limaye AP, et al. Outbreak of *Stenotrophomonas maltophilia* bacteremia among patients undergoing bone marrow transplantation: Association with faulty replacement of handwashing soap. *Infect Control Hosp Epidemiol.* 1999;20:756-758.

157. Festini F, Buzzetti R, Bassi C, et al. Isolation measures for prevention of infection with respiratory pathogens in cystic fibrosis: a systematic review. *J Hosp Infect.* 2006;64:1-6.

158. Walsh NM, Casano AA, Manangan LP, et al. Risk factors for *Burkholderia cepacia* complex colonization and infection among patients with cystic fibrosis. *J Pediatr.* 2002;141:512-517.

159. Mahenthiralingam E, Vandamme P, Campbell ME, et al. Infection with *Burkholderia cepacia* complex genomovars in patients with cystic fibrosis: Virulent transmissible strains of genomovar III can replace *Burkholderia multivorans*. *Clin Infect Dis.* 2001;33:1469-1475.

160. Ledson MJ, Gallagher MJ, Robinson M, et al. A randomized double-blinded placebo-controlled crossover trial of nebulized taurolidine in adult cystic fibrosis patients infected with *Burkholderia cepacia*. *J Aerosol Med.* 2002;15:51-57.

161. LiPuma JJ, Spilker T, Coenye T, et al. An epidemic *Burkholderia cepacia* complex strain identified in soil. *Lancet.* 2002;359:2002-2003.

162. LiPuma JJ. *Burkholderia cepacia* epidemiology and pathogenesis: Implications for infection control. *Curr Opin Pulm Med.* 1998;4:337-341.

221

Burkholderia pseudomallei and *Burkholderia mallei*: Melioidosis and Glanders

BART J. CURRIE

The genus *Burkholderia* is currently composed of many species, but only three are notable pathogens for humans or animals: the former *cepacia* complex (described in Chapter 220) *pseudomallei* (the agent of melioidosis), and *mallei* (the agent of equine glanders). All three are aerobic, nonsporulating, straight or slightly curved gram-negative bacilli that were formerly placed in the genus *Pseudomonas*.

Melioidosis

Melioidosis is a disease of humans and animals; it has enormous clinical diversity, spanning asymptomatic infection, localized skin ulcers or abscesses, chronic pneumonia mimicking tuberculosis, and fulminant septic shock with abscesses in multiple internal organs. Most disease is from recent infection, but latency with reactivation is described up to 62 years after exposure. Most cases are reported from Southeast Asia and northern Australia, but melioidosis is increasingly being recognized in people infected in an endemic region who return or travel to Europe and the United States. The causative bacterium, *Burkholderia pseudomallei*, is also considered a potential biologic warfare agent.

HISTORY

In 1912, Whitmore and Krishnaswami described cases of a newly recognized septicemic disease in morphine addicts in Rangoon, Burma.[1] Fatal cases were characterized by widespread caseous consolidation of the lung and abscesses in liver, spleen, kidney, and subcutaneous tissues. The bacillus isolated from tissues was similar to that causing glanders (*Burkholderia mallei*) but was motile. Whitmore noted the clinical similarity to glanders, and Stanton and Fletcher subsequently proposed the name *melioidosis,* derived from the Greek *melis* ("distemper of asses"). Various names were used for the causative bacterium, including *Bacillus whitmori* and, for many years, *Pseudomonas pseudomallei.*[2] In 1992, seven *Pseudomonas* species were moved to a new genus, *Burkholderia.* *B. cepacia* is the type species in the genus, which includes the organisms causing melioidosis (*B. pseudomallei*) and glanders (*B. mallei*).

ETIOLOGY

B. pseudomallei is a small, gram-negative, oxidase-positive, motile, aerobic bacillus with occasional polar flagella. On staining, a bipolar "safety pin" pattern is seen. The organism is easily recovered on standard culture medium but may be misidentified as *B. cepacia, P. stutzeri,* or other *Pseudomonas* species.

The organism is present in soil and surface water in endemic regions. Humans and animals are infected by percutaneous inoculation, inhalation, or ingestion. Occasional laboratory-acquired infections are described, but person-to-person spread and zoonotic infection are very uncommon.

EPIDEMIOLOGY

After the initial account in Burma, melioidosis was documented in humans and animals in Malaysia and Singapore from 1913 and then Vietnam from 1925 and Indonesia from 1929.[3-5] Thailand has reported the largest number of cases,[6-8] with an estimated 2000 to 3000 cases of melioidosis each year.[9] Melioidosis is also common in Malaysia[10] and Singapore.[11,12] Other countries in the region where melioidosis is recognized in humans and animals include China (especially Hong Kong), Taiwan, Brunei, Vietnam, and Laos.[13-17] Melioidosis is also likely to occur in Cambodia and the Philippines.[5,9,18] Melioidosis has been increasingly recognized in India, although reports that some of the "plague" scares of 1994 may have been cases of melioidosis have been disproved.[19,20] Cases have been reported from Sri Lanka, Bangladesh, and Pakistan.[5] Despite the early documentation of melioidosis in Burma and Indonesia, recent cases had not been reported from Indonesia until after the 2004 Asian tsunami.[21] Cases of melioidosis have also been documented from Papua New Guinea, Fiji, and New Caledonia,[22] but the extent of endemicity in the Pacific islands remains to be defined.

Cases of melioidosis are increasingly being documented from outside the classic endemic region of Southeast Asia, Australasia, the Indian subcontinent, and China. These include sporadic human or animal cases or environmental isolates of *B. pseudomallei* from the Middle East, Africa, the Caribbean, and Central and South America. Although some of these reports are from incorrect species diagnosis, others are confirmed, making the endemic limitations of melioidosis very unclear.[5] Sporadic cases and occasional case clusters have recently occurred in Brazil and elsewhere in the Americas.[23] Despite recent cases from Madagascar,[24] the true extent and magnitude of the presence of *B. pseudomallei* in Africa remains entirely unknown. Global warming may well result in expansion of the endemic boundaries of melioidosis.

The two locations where melioidosis is arguably the most important single bacterial pathogen for humans are some northeast provinces in Thailand and the Top End of the Northern Territory of Australia. In northeast Thailand, 20% of community-acquired septicemic cases are caused by melioidosis, which accounts for 39% of fatal septicemias[7] and 36% of fatal community-acquired pneumonias.[25] In the Top End of the Northern Territory, melioidosis has been the most common cause of fatal community-acquired bacteremic pneumonia.[26]

In addition to endemic melioidosis, there are several documented situations where melioidosis became established in nontropical locations. In France, in the 1970s, cases of melioidosis occurred in animals in a Paris zoo, with spread to other zoos and equestrian clubs.[3] In addition to fatal animal and human cases, there was extensive soil contamination persisting for some years. *B. pseudomallei* was considered likely to have been introduced by importation of infected animals. A cluster of cases occurred over a 25-year period in southwestern Western Australia (31°S), involving animal cases and one human infection in a farmer. Ribotyping of the farm animal and human isolates and one isolate from the soil showed identical patterns.[27] This supports the suggestion of clonal introduction of *B. pseudomallei* into this temperate region, probably via an infected animal, with environmental contamination, local dissemination, and persistence over 25 years.

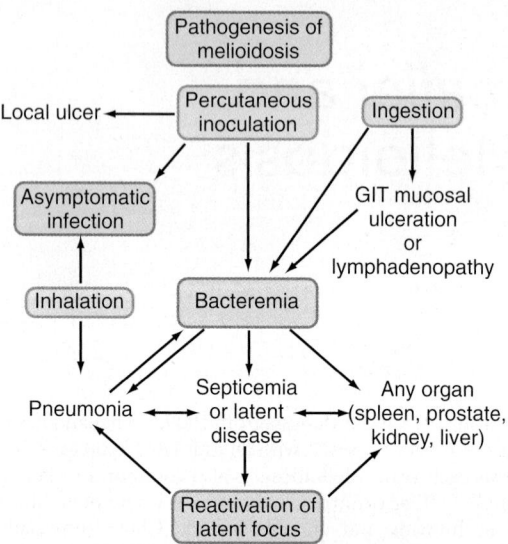

Figure 221-1 Natural history of infection with *Burkholderia pseudomallei.* GIT, gastrointestinal tract.

Melioidosis was an important cause of morbidity and mortality in foreign troops fighting in Southeast Asia. Dance has noted that at least 100 cases occurred among French forces in Indochina between 1948 and 1954.[3] By 1973, 343 cases had been reported in American troops fighting in Vietnam. Concerns of reactivation of latent infection in soldiers returning from Vietnam, with estimates from serology studies of approximately 225,000 potential cases, resulted in melioidosis being called the "Vietnamese time bomb."[28] However, although occasional cases of reactivation of *B. pseudomallei* still occur in Vietnam veterans, it is rare in comparison to the numbers exposed.

TRANSMISSION

Figure 221-1 summarizes the natural history of infection with *B. pseudomallei*. Studies from Malaysia, and more recently from Thailand[29] and Australia,[30] have found that the organism is more common in cleared, irrigated sites such as rice paddies and farms. It has been suggested that the increase in melioidosis cases in Thailand may partly be the consequence of the increased number of bacteria in such environments and partly the consequence of increased exposure to bacteria resulting from changes in behaviors, such as farming techniques.[13] In Australia, *B. pseudomallei* has been found most commonly in clay soils to a depth of 25 to 45 cm, and it has been proposed that the bacteria move to the surface with the rising water table during the wet season.[31] An alternative explanation for the variable bacterial presence found is that during times of stress, such as in prolonged dry seasons, *B. pseudomallei* may persist in soil in a viable but nonculturable state.[32] Differential gene activation may allow such environmental bacteria to respond and adapt to different environmental conditions. This possibility is also relevant to the pathogenicity, latency, and reactivation of infection with *B. pseudomallei* in humans. The role of biofilms in the persistence of *B. pseudomallei* in the environment, as well as in animal and human hosts, requires further study.[33] There is increasing interest in the intracellular survival of *B. pseudomallei*, and it has been proposed that an ecologic niche for the bacteria in the environment may be in environmental protozoa or fungi.[32]

In most endemic regions, there is a close association between melioidosis and rainfall. In northeast Thailand[34] and northern Australia,[35] 75% and 85% of cases, respectively, have occurred in the wet season. Although early animal studies showed infection with *B. pseudomallei* through oral or nasal exposure and from ingestion, more recent reviews have considered that most human cases are from percutane-ous inoculation of *B. pseudomallei* after exposure to muddy soils or surface water in endemic locations.[2,5,26] Ingestion and sexual transmission have been suggested as unusual modes of transmission of *B. pseudomallei*. Presentations of melioidosis pneumonia after presumptive inoculating skin injuries have been documented in patients with soil-contaminated burns and are also common in tropical Australia.[26] This suggests hematogenous spread to the lung rather than inhalation or spread from the upper respiratory tract. However, under certain epidemiologic conditions, the inhalation route may predominate, as suggested for soldiers exposed to dusts raised by helicopter rotor blades in Vietnam.[36] Melioidosis after near-drowning is well documented, with the probable infecting event being aspiration.[14] Intensity of rainfall is an independent predictor of melioidosis manifesting as pneumonia and of a fatal outcome,[37] suggesting that heavy monsoonal rainfall and winds may result in a shift toward inhalation as the mode of infection with *B. pseudomallei*. Several outbreaks of melioidosis in Australia have been linked to contamination of potable water with *B. pseudomallei*.[38,39] The water supplies involved were unchlorinated or the chlorination was below standard. The contamination of the water supply has been attributed to soil disturbance during excavations.

The incubation period for melioidosis is influenced by inoculating dose, mode of infection, host risk factors, and probably differential virulence of infecting *B. pseudomallei* strains. Onset of melioidosis within 24 hours has been seen in presumed aspiration after near-drowning and, in some cases, after severe weather events. In 25 cases of acute melioidosis in which a clear incubation period could be determined between the inoculating injury and the onset of symptoms, the incubation period was 1 to 21 days (mean, 9 days),[40] which is consistent with a series of nosocomial cases from Thailand, in which the incubation period was 3 to 16 days (mean, 9.5 days).[41]

PATHOGENESIS

Serology studies have shown that most infection with *B. pseudomallei* is asymptomatic.[42,43] In northeast Thailand, most of the rural population is seropositive by indirect hemagglutination (IHA),[34] with most seroconversion occurring between 6 months and 4 years of age.[43] Although melioidosis occurs in all age groups, severe clinical disease such as septicemic pneumonia is seen mostly in those with risk factors such as diabetes, renal disease, and alcoholism.

In addition to infection by inhalation, bacterial load on exposure (inoculating dose) and virulence of the infecting strain of *B. pseudomallei* are also likely to influence the severity of disease. However, it has been noted that despite the large bacterial load in severely ill patients with septicemic pulmonary melioidosis, person-to-person transmission is extremely unusual. This, together with the rarity of fulminant melioidosis in healthy people, supports the primary importance of host risk factors for development of melioidosis. Furthermore, although it is clear from laboratory studies of isolates of *B. pseudomallei* from animals, humans, and the environment that virulence differs among *B. pseudomallei* isolates,[44] the importance of this variation in virulence in determining clinical aspects of melioidosis remains uncertain. Molecular typing that shows clonality of isolates in animal and human clusters has revealed that the same outbreak strain can cause different clinical presentations, with host factors being most important in determining the severity of disease.[39] Whole-genome sequencing and subsequent molecular studies have shown that *B. pseudomallei* has two chromosomes, multiple genomic islands that are variably present in different strains and have a great propensity for horizontal gene transfer.[45] Further studies are required to unravel the global phylogeny and evolutionary history of *B. pseudomallei* and related species and to determine which genes or gene clusters may be critical for pathogenesis and disease presentation and outcome.[46]

B. pseudomallei is a facultative intracellular pathogen that can invade and replicate inside various cells, including polymorphonuclear leukocytes and macrophages and some epithelial cell lines.[47] Animal models have been unable to confirm a clinically relevant exotoxin for

B. pseudomallei.[48] However, resistance to human serum (conferred by lipopolysaccharide [LPS])[49] and the ability of *B. pseudomallei* to survive intracellularly (conferred in part by capsular polysaccharide) appear to be critical in the pathogenesis of melioidosis.[50-52] Type III secretion systems in *B. pseudomallei* have also been found to be important in cell invasion and intracellular survival.[53,54] Quorum sensing may play an important role in many aspects of virulence of *B. pseudomallei*, including cell invasion, cytotoxicity and antimicrobial resistance.[55,56] Other putative virulence factor candidates include flagella, type IV pili and other adhesins, a siderophore, and secreted proteins such as hemolysin, lipases, and proteases.[56]

Intracellular survival of *B. pseudomallei* in human and animal hosts is likely to explain the ability for latency. After internalization, *B. pseudomallei* escapes from endocytic vacuoles into the cell cytoplasm, and induction of actin polymerization at one bacterial pole leads to membrane protrusions, with cell-to-cell spread involving these actin tails.[54,56,57] Additional survival factors are the ability of *B. pseudomallei* to form antibiotic-resistant small-colony variants[58] and the ability of mucoid variants with large extracellular polysaccharide glycocalyx structures to form biofilm-encased microcolonies that are also relatively antibiotic-resistant.

There have been a number of studies showing elevated levels of various endogenous inflammatory mediators and cytokines to be associated with severity and outcomes of melioidosis. Nevertheless, whether these elevated cytokines are a cause or result of severe disease is not established. In Thailand, there was an association of severe melioidosis with tumor necrosis factor (TNF)-α gene allele 2, which is linked to higher constitutive and inducible production of TNF-α.[59] However, in a mouse model of melioidosis, neutralization of TNF-α or interleukin (IL)-12 increased susceptibility to infection in vivo, and interferon-γ (IFN-γ) was found to be important for survival, with mice treated with monoclonal anti–IFN-γ dying more quickly.[60] A role for Toll-like receptors in the innate immune response in melioidosis has been proposed.[61] There are, therefore, important host protective mechanisms against *B. pseudomallei* in cytokine responses as well as potentially detrimental ones, with the timing of cytokine release and the balance between pro- and anti-inflammatory responses likely to determine the severity of disease and outcome of infection.[56,62] The extent to which host polymorphisms in immune response contribute in comparison to differences in organism virulence, infecting dose of *B. pseudomallei*, and defined host risk factors such as diabetes remains to be clarified. Nevertheless, the predominant association with fatal melioidosis is the presence of defined patient risk factors.

Although a vigorous cell-mediated immune response may protect against disease progression,[63] there is no definitive evidence for the development of immunity from melioidosis after natural exposure to *B. pseudomallei*, and reinfection can occur with a different strain of *B. pseudomallei* after successful treatment of melioidosis.[64]

Table 221-1 summarizes the risk factors for melioidosis. The most important risk factors are diabetes, alcohol excess, and renal disease.[2,35,65] In Thailand, the adjusted odds ratios for diabetes and renal disease (chronic renal impairment or renal or ureteric calculi) in cases of melioidosis versus controls were 12.9 (95% confidence interval [CI], 5.1 to 37.2) and 2.9 (95% CI, 1.7 to 5.0), respectively.[65] Other risk factors for melioidosis include chronic lung disease (including cystic fibrosis), thalassemia (odds ratio in Thailand, 10.2; 95% CI, 3.5 to 30.8), malignancies, steroid therapy, iron overload, and tuberculosis.[65] Severe disease and fatalities are uncommon in those without risk factors who are diagnosed and treated early, with only one death in 51 patients without risk factors in one study.[35] Risk factors are less common in children than in adults.[66,67]

Evidence suggests that there may be a predisposition to melioidosis in those with diabetes, alcohol excess, or chronic renal disease, which may reflect impairment of their neutrophil and other phagocytic cell functions, such as mobilization, delivery, adherence, and ingestion.[35,68] Melioidosis has also been described in chronic granulomatous disease.[69]

TABLE 221-1	Risk Factors for Melioidosis	
Risk Factor*	**Thailand (% of cases)**	**Australia (% of cases)**
Diabetes	23-60	37
Alcohol excess	12	39
Renal disease	20-27	10
Chronic lung disease	NR	27
Thalassemia	7	Nil
No risk factors	24-36	20

*Not listed: malignancy, steroid therapy, iron overload, cardiac failure.
NR, not reported.
Thailand data from Punyagupta S. Melioidosis: Review of 686 cases and presentation of a new clinical classification. In: Punyagupta S, Sirisanthana T, Stapatayavong B, eds: *Melioidosis.* Bangkok: Bangkok Medical; 1989:217-229; Chaowagul W, White NJ, Dance DA, et al. Melioidosis: A major cause of community-acquired septicemia in northeastern Thailand. *J Infect Dis.* 1989;159:890-899; Suputtamongkol Y, Chaowagul W, Chetchotisakd P, et al. Risk factors for melioidosis and bacteremic melioidosis. *Clin Infect Dis.* 1999;29:408-413; and Limmathurotsakul D, Chaowagul W, Chierakul W, et al. Risk factors for recurrent melioidosis in northeast Thailand. *Clin Infect Dis.* 2006;43:979-986.
Australia data from Currie BJ, Fisher DA, Howard DM, et al. Endemic melioidosis in tropical northern Australia: A 10-year prospective study and review of the literature. *Clin Infect Dis.* 2000;31:981-986.

CLINICAL MANIFESTATIONS

The earliest descriptions of melioidosis documented the fulminant end of the clinical spectrum, with abscesses throughout both lungs and in many organs.[1] At the other end of the spectrum are asymptomatic infections and localized skin ulcers or abscesses without systemic illness. Howe and colleagues have classified melioidosis as acute, subacute, and chronic.[36] The Infectious Disease Association of Thailand has summarized 345 cases in these categories[2,6]:

1. Multifocal infection with septicemia (45% of cases, 87% mortality)
2. Localized infection with septicemia (12% of cases, 17% mortality)
3. Localized infection (42% of cases, 9% mortality)
4. Transient bacteremia (0.3%)

More recent bacteremia and overall mortality rates have been, respectively, 60% and 44% in Thailand,[34] 46% and 19% in Australia,[35] and 43% and 39% in Singapore.[5]

Table 221-2 summarizes the clinical presentations of patients with melioidosis in northern Australia. Pneumonia is the commonest clinical presentation of patients with melioidosis in all studies, accounting for around half of cases. Secondary pneumonia after another primary presentation occurs in around 10% of cases. Acute melioidosis pneumonia has a spectrum from fulminant septic shock (mortality up to 90%; Figs. 221-2 to 221-5) to mild undifferentiated pneumonia, which can be acute or subacute in nature, with little mortality. Septicemic patients present acutely unwell with high fevers and prostration and often little initial cough or pleuritic pain. On chest radiographs, diffuse nodular infiltrates often develop throughout both lungs and they coalesce, cavitate, and progress rapidly, consistent with the caseous necrosis and multiple metastatic abscess formation seen at autopsy. Nonsepticemic patients with pneumonia and some with septicemic pneumonia have a more predominant cough, with productive sputum and dyspnea, and their chest radiographs show discrete but progressive consolidation in one or more lobes (Fig. 221-6). In endemic regions, acute pneumonia with upper lobe consolidation warrants consideration of melioidosis, although lower lobe infiltrates are also common.

In 12% of cases in northern Australia, patients present with chronic melioidosis, defined as illness with symptoms for longer than 2 months' duration on presentation. Many of these patients have features mimicking tuberculosis, with fevers, weight loss, productive cough (sometimes with hemoptysis), and classic upper lobe infiltrates, with or without cavitation on chest radiographs (Fig. 221-7). In these patients, disease can be remitting and relapsing over many years, sometimes with an initial misdiagnosis of tuberculosis. Although acute deterioration with septicemia may occur, mortality in this group is low.

	Total		Bacteremic		Nonbacteremic	
Parameter	*No.*	*Deaths (Mortality)*	*No.*	*Deaths (Mortality)*	*No.*	*Deaths (Mortality)*
Septic Shock	111	59 (53%)	99	49 (49%)	12	13 (81%)
Pneumonia	85	44 (52%)	75	36 (48%)	10*	8 (80%)
Genitourinary	9	5 (56%)	8	4 (50%)	1†	1 (100%)
Osteomyelitis, septic arthritis	4	2 (50%)	4	2 (50%)	0	0 (0%)
No focus	13	8 (62%)	12	7 (58%)	1	1 (100%)
No Septic Shock	403	17 (4%)	181	13 (7%)	222	4 (2%)
Pneumonia	177	9 (5%)	78	8 (10%)	99	1 (1%)
Genitourinary	64	2 (3%)	39	2 (5%)	25	0 (0%)
Skin abscess(es)	64	0 (0%)	1	0 (0%)	63	0 (0%)
Soft tissue abscess(es)	14	0 (0%)	1	0 (0%)	13	0 (0%)
Neurologic	14	3 (21%)	3	0 (0%)	11	3 (47%)
Osteomyelitis, septic arthritis	12	0 (0%)	6	0 (0%)	6	0 (0%)
Other	58	3 (5%)	53	3 (6%)	5	0 (0%)
Total	514	76 (15%)	280	62 (22%)	234	14 (6%)

TABLE 221-2 Clinical Presentations and Outcomes of Melioidosis in Northern Australia

*Seven blood cultures not done, three blood cultures negative.
†Blood culture not done.
Updated from Currie BJ, Fisher DA, Howard DM, et al. Endemic melioidosis in tropical northern Australia: A 10-year prospective study and review of the literature. *Clin Infect Dis.* 2000;31:981-986.

Until recently it was thought that a colonization state did not exist for *B. pseudomallei,* with presence in sputum or throat always reflecting disease. However, it has more recently become evident that *B. pseudomallei* can both colonize airways and cause disease in patients with cystic fibrosis (CF) and bronchiectasis. The similarity to infection with *B. cepacia* complex in CF is of concern, given the association of *B. cepacia* complex with more rapid deterioration in lung function. Furthermore, likely transmission of *B. pseudomallei* between two siblings with CF has been reported.[70] Patients with CF traveling to melioidosis-endemic locations should be warned of the risk of melioidosis, which should be considered if they become sick after returning.

It is common for patients to present with skin ulcers or abscesses (Figs. 221-8 and 221-9).[71] Occasionally, they present with septic arthritis or osteomyelitis, or one of these can develop after the patient has presented with another primary diagnosis, usually pneumonia (Fig. 221-10). Also well recognized, whatever the clinical presentation, are abscesses in internal organs, especially spleen, kidney, prostate, and liver (Figs. 221-11 to 221-15). Where available, abdominopelvic computed tomography (CT) scanning is useful in all melioidosis patients to detect internal abscesses.

Three differences have been noted between Thailand and tropical Australia. First, suppurative parotitis accounts for up to 40% of melioidosis in children in Thailand[66,72] but is very rare in Australia. Second, prostatic melioidosis is well recognized but uncommon, except in Australia, where routine abdominopelvic CT scanning of all melioidosis cases has shown prostatic abscesses to be present in 18% of all male patients with melioidosis (Fig. 221-16).[35] Some were incidental in patients presenting with pneumonia or septicemia, but a primary genitourinary presentation was common with fevers, abdominal discomfort, dysuria, and sometimes diarrhea and urinary retention. Third, neurologic melioidosis accounts for around 4% of cases in northern Australia, with the distinctive clinical features being brain stem encephalitis, often with cranial nerve palsies (especially the seventh nerve), together with peripheral motor weakness, or occasionally just flaccid paraparesis alone. The CT scan is often normal, but dramatic changes are seen on magnetic resonance imaging (MRI), most notably a diffusely increased T_2-weighted signal in the midbrain, brain stem, and spinal cord (Fig. 221-17).[73] Direct bacterial invasion of the brain and spinal cord occurs with this melioidosis encephalomyelitis.[74]

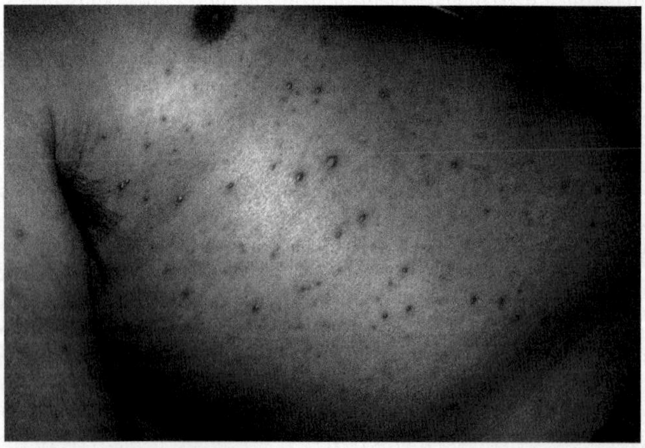

Figure 221-2 Multiple pustules in a 46-year-old diabetic man with fatal septicemic melioidosis.

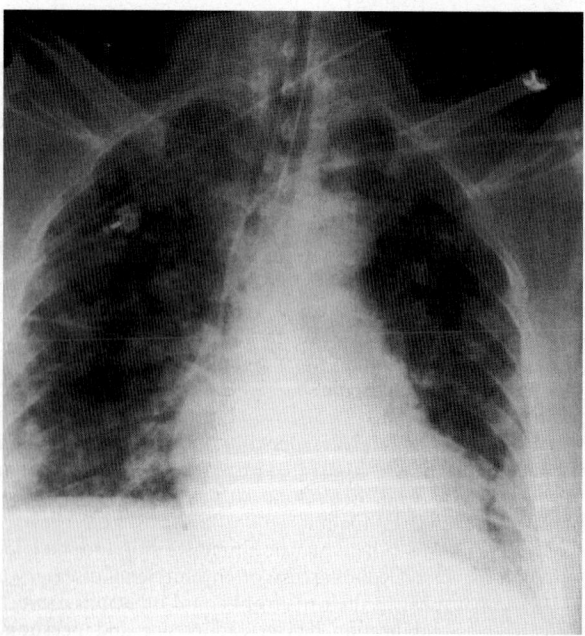

Figure 221-3 Chest radiograph of patient in Figure 221-2, showing multiple pulmonary abscesses.

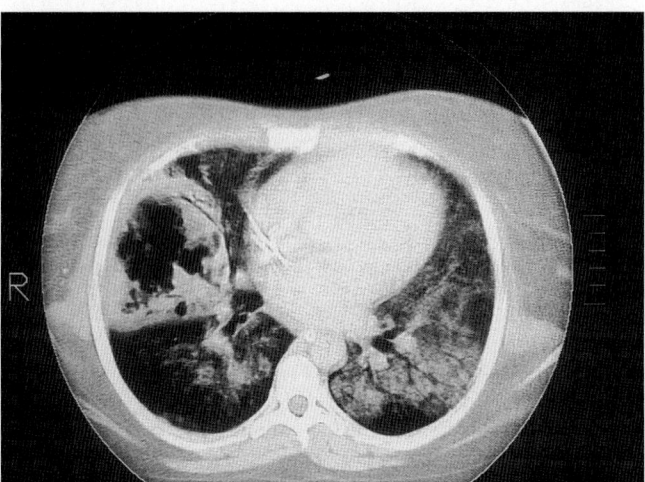

Figure 221-4 CT scan of the chest of a 26-year-old woman with fatal melioidosis, showing large pulmonary abscess.

Neurologic melioidosis is occasionally seen outside Australia, although mostly as macroscopic brain abscesses.[6,75]

Unusual foci of melioidosis infection described in case reports or case series include mycotic aneurysms, lymphadenitis resembling tuberculosis, mediastinal masses, pericardial collections, and adrenal abscesses.

It has long been recognized that *B. pseudomallei,* like tuberculosis, has the potential for reactivation from a latent focus, usually in the lung—hence the concern of the "Vietnamese time bomb" in returned soldiers. Latent periods from exposure to *B. pseudomallei* in an endemic

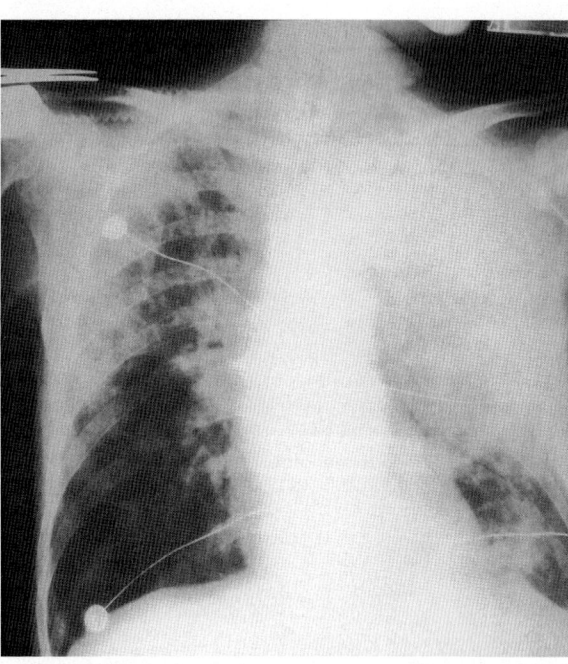

Figure 221-6 Extensive left upper lobe consolidation in 54-year-old man with fatal melioidosis pneumonia.

region to onset of melioidosis in a nonendemic region have been documented as being as long as 62 years.[76] However, cases of reactivated *B. pseudomallei* appear to be very uncommon, accounting for only 3% of cases in northern Australia. The vast majority of cases of melioidosis occur in the monsoonal wet seasons of the various endemic regions, supporting the concept that in endemic areas, most patients with melioidosis have recent infections that appear with acute illness.

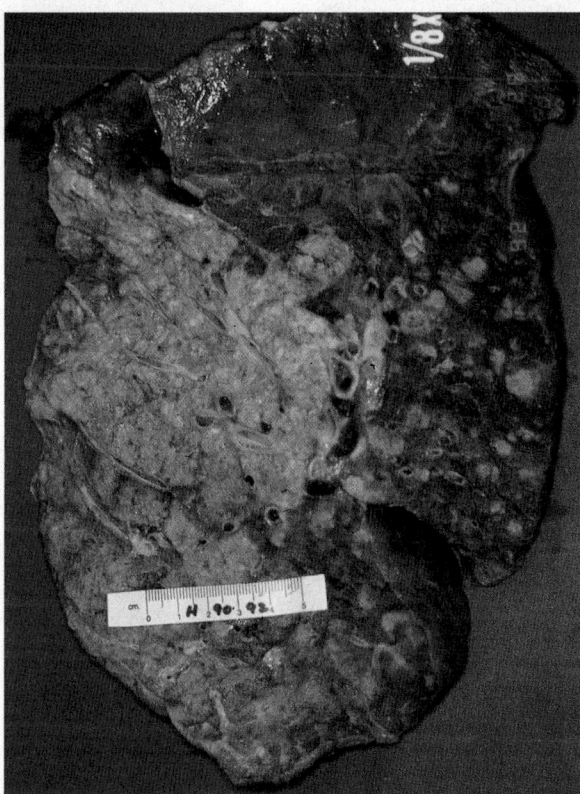

Figure 221-5 Multiple lung abscesses seen at autopsy of patient with acute melioidosis pneumonia.

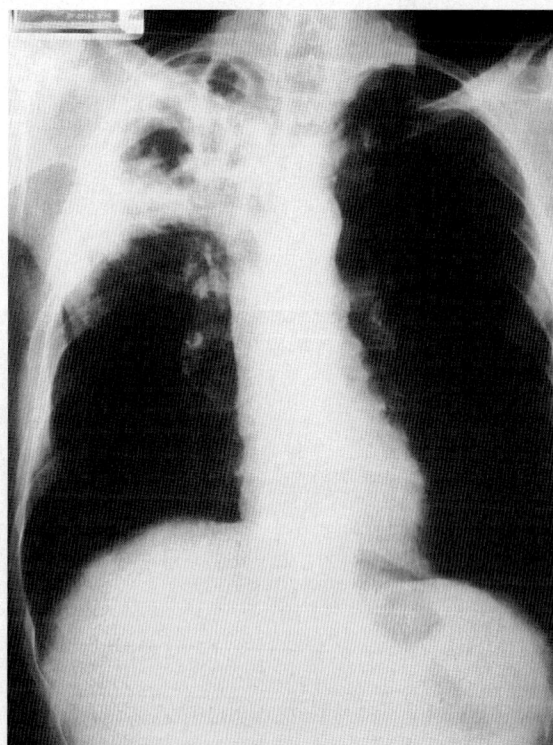

Figure 221-7 Radiograph showing right upper lobe cavitation of a 62-year-old man with nonfatal chronic melioidosis.

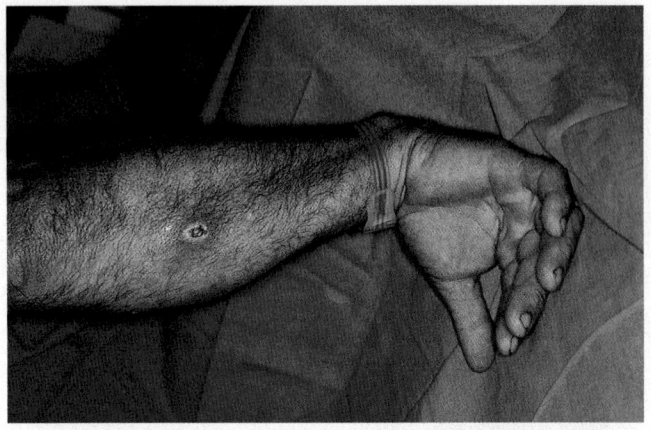

Figure 221-8 Cutaneous melioidosis seen on the right forearm of a 50-year-old man.

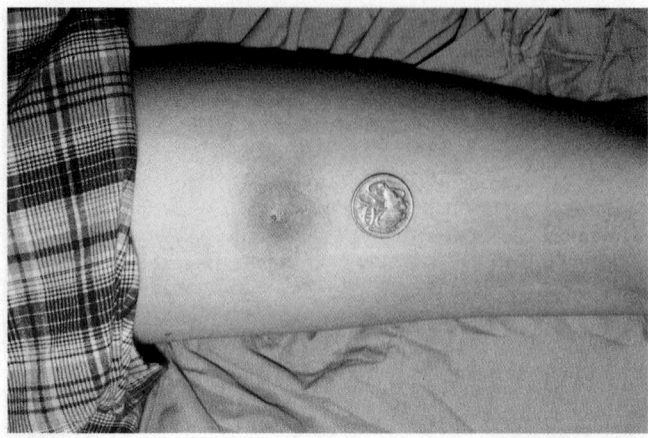

Figure 221-9 Cutaneous melioidosis of the right thigh in an 11-year-old boy.

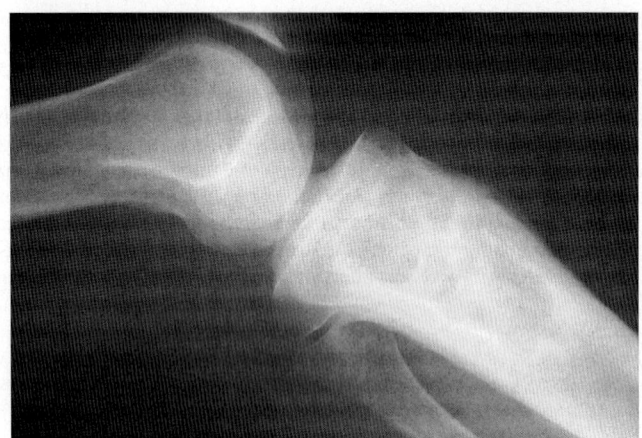

Figure 221-10 Radiograph of large lucent areas in proximal tibia of a 43-year-old man.

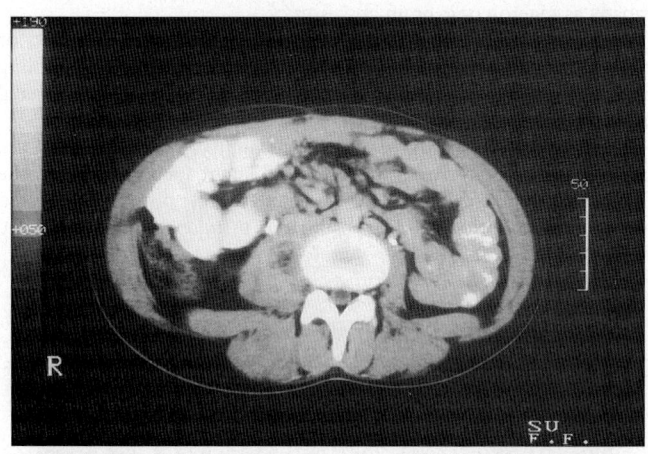

Figure 221-11 Right psoas abscess in a 17-year-old girl with melioidosis.

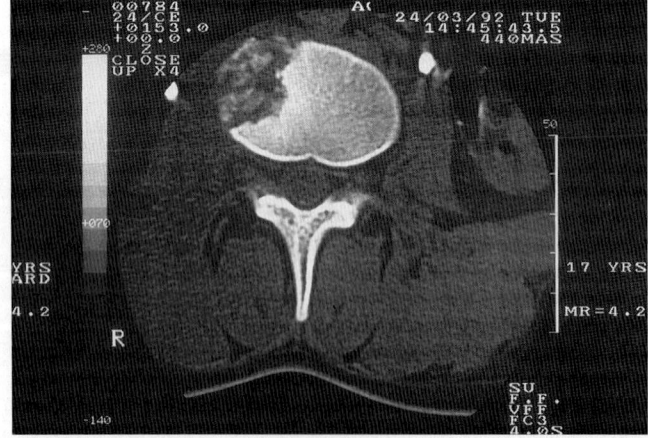

Figure 221-12 The patient in Figure 221-11 developed an L3 osteomyelitis 6 weeks later.

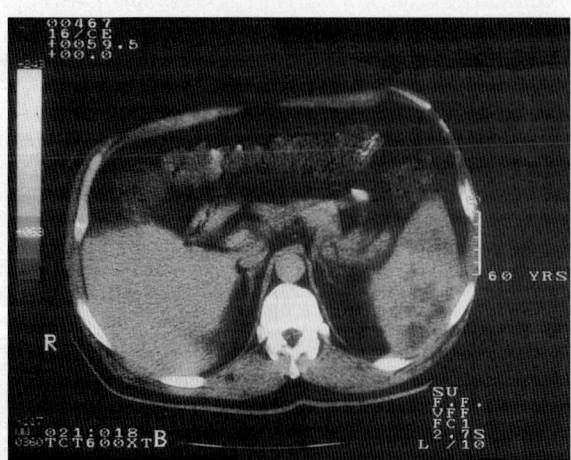

Figure 221-13 CT scan showing splenic abscesses in a 60-year-old diabetic.

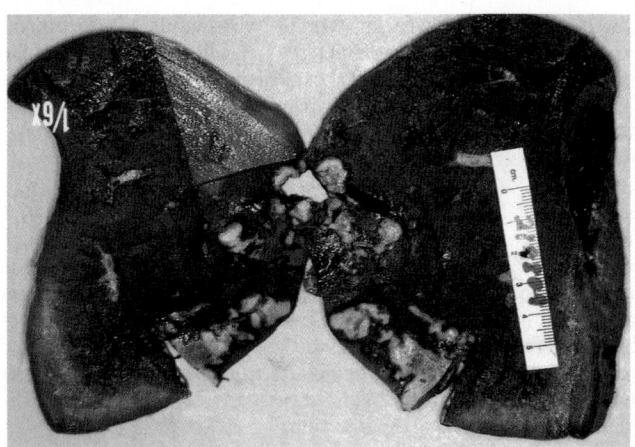

Figure 221-14   Abscesses seen at splenectomy performed on the patient in Figure 221-13.

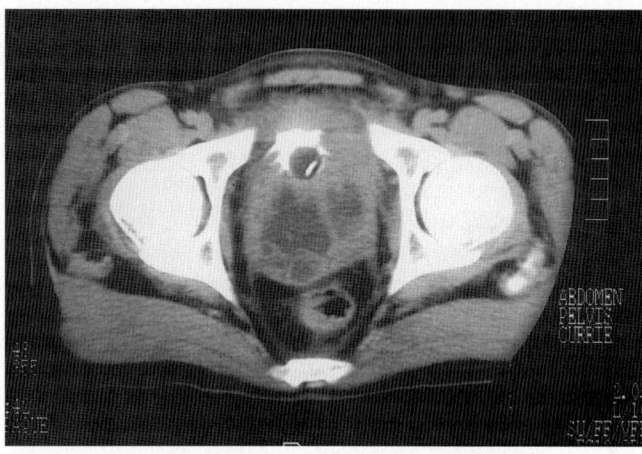

Figure 221-16   Melioidosis prostatic abscesses in a 31-year-old man who presented with fever and urinary retention.

Reactivation of melioidosis has been associated with influenza, other bacterial sepses, and development of known melioidosis risk factors such as diabetes. It remains unknown what proportion of asymptomatic seropositive people actually have latent infection with the potential for reactivation.

LABORATORY DIAGNOSIS

Definitive diagnosis of melioidosis requires a positive culture of *B. pseudomallei*. Melioidosis must be considered in febrile patients in or returning from endemic regions to enable appropriate samples to be tested. *B. pseudomallei* readily grows in commercially available blood culture media, but it is not unusual for laboratories in nonendemic locations to misidentify the bacteria as a *Pseudomonas* species, especially because some commercial identification systems are poor at identifying *B. pseudomallei*.[77] Culture from nonsterile sites increases the likelihood of diagnosis but can be problematic. The rate of successful culture is increased if sputum, throat swabs, ulcer or skin lesion swabs, and rectal swabs are placed into Ashdown's medium, a gentamicin-containing liquid transport broth that results in the selective growth of *B. pseudomallei*.[78,79] *B. pseudomallei* can be identified by combining the commercial API 20NE or 20E biochemical kit with a simple screening system involving the Gram stain, oxidase reaction, typical growth characteristics, and resistance to certain antibiotics.[80]

There are a variety of locally developed antigen and DNA detection techniques used in endemic regions for early identification of *B. pseudomallei* in culture media and patient blood or urine, but these are not yet widely available.[80-84] An indirect hemagglutination test (IHA), various enzyme-linked immunosorbent assays (ELISAs), and other serologic assays are available.[83,85,86] In endemic areas, their usefulness is limited by high rates of background antibody positivity. In acute septicemic melioidosis, IHA and ELISA are often initially negative, but repeat testing may show seroconversion. A positive IHA or ELISA in a tourist returning from a melioidosis-endemic region is useful in supporting the possibility of melioidosis, but definitive diagnosis still requires a positive culture.

TREATMENT

B. pseudomallei is characteristically resistant to penicillin, ampicillin, first- and second-generation cephalosporins, gentamicin, tobramycin, and streptomycin. Before 1989, "conventional therapy" for melioidosis consisted of a combination of chloramphenicol, sulfamethoxazole-trimethoprim, doxycycline, and sometimes kanamycin, given for 6 weeks to 6 months.[2,87] However, there were also reports of the successful use of sulfamethoxazole-trimethoprim alone and tetracycline or doxycycline alone. These conventional antibiotics are bacteriostatic rather than bactericidal, and in vitro studies have shown various combinations to be antagonistic.

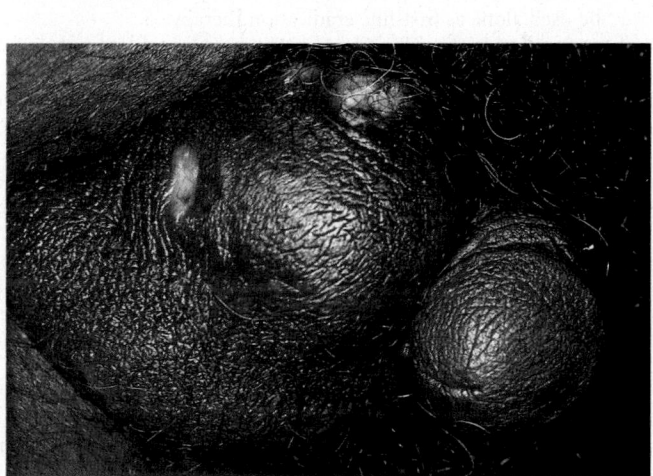

Figure 221-15   Melioidosis orchitis and scrotal ulcer in a 49-year-old man.

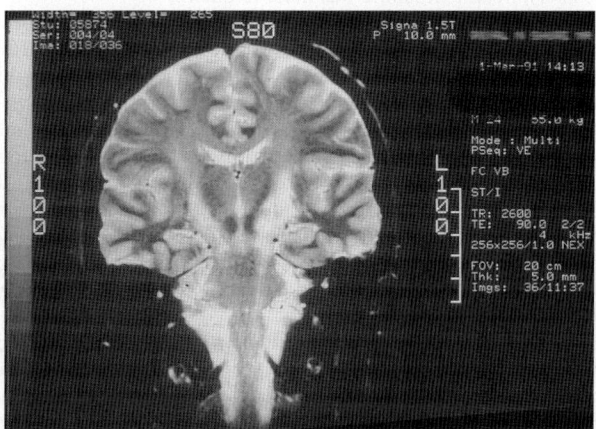

Figure 221-17   Melioidosis encephalomyelitis in a 24-year-old man. MRI shows increased T_2-weighted signal extending through brain stem and into spinal cord.

TABLE 221-3	Antibiotic Therapy for Melioidosis

Initial Intensive Therapy (minimum of 10-14 days)

Ceftazidime (50 mg/kg, up to 2 g) every 6 hr

or

Meropenem (25 mg/kg, up to 1 g) every 8 hr

or

Imipenem (25 mg/kg, up to 1 g) every 6 hr
  With or without

Any one of the three may be combined with

Sulfamethoxazole-trimethoprim (40/8 mg/kg up to 1600/320 mg) every 12 hr
  (recommended for neurologic cutaneous, bone and prostatic melioidosis)

Eradication Therapy (minimum of 3 mo)

Sulfamethoxazole-trimethoprim (40/8 mg/kg up to 1600/320 mg) every 12 hr
  With or without

Doxycycline (2.5 mg/kg up to 100 mg) every 12 hr

Subsequent studies have shown *B. pseudomallei* to be susceptible to various newer β-lactam antibiotics, especially ceftazidime, imipenem, meropenem, piperacillin, amoxicillin-clavulanate, ceftriaxone, and cefotaxime, with various degrees of bactericidal activity. Table 221-3 summarizes recommended antibiotic treatment.

Initial Intensive Therapy for Melioidosis

The most important therapeutic study for melioidosis was an open-label randomized trial in Thailand comparing ceftazidime (120 mg/kg/day) with conventional therapy, which showed that ceftazidime is associated with a 50% lower overall mortality in severe melioidosis.[87] Ceftazidime then became the drug of choice for initial intensive therapy for melioidosis. Another study from Thailand showed similar results when ceftazidime was used in combination with sulfamethoxazole-trimethoprim.[88] Whether sulfamethoxazole-trimethoprim added to ceftazidime is superior to ceftazidime alone has been studied in two randomized controlled trials in Thailand.[89] Although the addition of sulfamethoxazole-trimethoprim conferred no survival benefit, the excellent tissue penetration of sulfamethoxazole-trimethoprim is the rationale for recommending combination therapy in neurologic, cutaneous, bone and joint, and prostatic melioidosis.

After initial favorable reports of use of amoxicillin-clavulanate, another randomized comparative trial in Thailand showed that initial therapy with high-dose IV amoxicillin-clavulanate is as effective as ceftazidime in preventing deaths in severe melioidosis.[90] However, when amoxicillin-clavulanate was continued as eradication therapy (see later), treatment failure was more frequent.

The carbapenems imipenem and meropenem have the lowest minimum inhibitory concentrations against *B. pseudomallei*. Furthermore, in vitro time-kill studies to measure the rate of bacterial killing has shown the carbapenems to perform better against *B. pseudomallei* than ceftazidime.[91,92] High-dose imipenem has been shown in another comparative trial from Thailand to be at least as effective as ceftazidime for severe melioidosis, with no differences in mortality between the groups and with fewer treatment failures in those given imipenem.[93] Observational data from Australia have suggested that meropenem produces better outcomes in severe melioidosis than ceftazidime, which has led to the recommendation that meropenem be the drug of choice for melioidosis septic shock.[94]

The duration of initial intensive therapy should be 10 to 14 days, with longer treatment required for critically ill patients, or for extensive pulmonary disease, deep-seated collections or organ abscesses, osteomyelitis, septic arthritis, and neurologic melioidosis. Even with the newer regimens, the therapeutic response can be slow, with median time to defervescence up to 9 days, and longer times seen in those with deep-seated abscesses.

Ceftazidime infusions (6 g over 24 hours, adult dose) through a peripherally inserted central catheter (PICC line) using an elastomeric infusion device (Baxter, Sydney) have enabled early hospital discharge for in-home therapy.[95] The absence of any postantibiotic effect with ceftazidime gives such a continuous infusion a theoretical advantage over intermittent dosing.

Subsequent Eradication Therapy for Melioidosis

After initial intensive therapy, using ceftazidime, imipenem, or meropenem, possibly in combination with sulfamethoxazole-trimethoprim, subsequent eradication therapy is considered necessary for preventing recrudescence or later relapse of melioidosis. Both duration of eradication therapy and the best antibiotics to use remain uncertain. Molecular typing of isolates from patients with recurrent melioidosis has confirmed that most cases are true relapses from failed eradication rather than new infection.[64]

There are a number of reasons for failure of eradication therapy:

1. The most important factor responsible for most recrudescences or relapses of melioidosis is poor compliance with eradication therapy.
2. Relapses were found to be 4.7 times (95% CI, 1.6 to 14.1) more common in patients with severe disease than in those with localized melioidosis.[96] Positive blood cultures and multifocal disease were also associated with relapse.[64]
3. Use of ceftazidime in the initial intensive therapy was also associated with a halving of relapses.[96]
4. Duration of eradication therapy is also critical, with relapses after oral therapy of 8 weeks or less more likely than if eradication therapy is given for longer than 12 weeks.[64,96]
5. The choice of agents for the eradication therapy is important. Both amoxicillin-clavulanate and oral quinolones (ciprofloxacin or ofloxacin) have been found to be less effective in preventing relapse than the former conventional eradication with chloramphenicol (given usually only for the first 4 to 8 weeks), sulfamethoxazole-trimethoprim, and doxycycline.[64] Amoxicillin-clavulanate is recommended for eradication therapy in pregnancy and is an alternative to sulfamethoxazole-trimethoprim in children or those intolerant of sulfamethoxazole-trimethoprim or with a *B. pseudomallei* isolate confirmed as resistant to sulfamethoxazole-trimethoprim, with dosing guidelines recently published.[97] Quinolones should not be considered as first-line agents for melioidosis, with in vitro susceptibility testing generally showing resistance or intermediate results. A trial of eradication therapy involved a comparison of doxycycline alone versus conventional chloramphenicol (first 4 weeks only), sulfamethoxazole-trimethoprim, and doxycycline combination therapy.[98] Relapses were significantly more common in the doxycycline-alone group, resulting in a recommendation that doxycycline not be used alone as first-line eradication therapy.

A randomized trial has found no benefit in adding chloramphenicol to sulfamethoxazole-trimethoprim plus doxycycline for the eradication phase.[99] It has been suggested that sulfamethoxazole-trimethoprim is the critical component for eradication therapy, and prospective studies in Australia using sulfamethoxazole-trimethoprim alone have supported this because relapses occurred almost exclusively in noncompliant patients. Interpretation of disk diffusion sensitivity testing has been problematic for sulfamethoxazole-trimethoprim, and agar dilution methods have confirmed that most *B. pseudomallei* isolates are sensitive to sulfamethoxazole-trimethoprim. Ongoing studies will ascertain whether it is still beneficial to have combination therapy for the eradication phase of melioidosis treatment or whether sulfamethoxazole-trimethoprim without doxycycline is adequate.

Adjunctive Therapy

Surgical drainage of large abscesses is indicated, but this is usually not necessary or possible for multiple small abscesses in the spleen and liver. Parotid abscesses require careful incision and drainage. Prostatic abscesses can often be drained under ultrasound guidance using a rectal probe, with transurethral resection reserved for failures of the simpler procedure.

State-of-the-art intensive care management has resulted in decreased mortality in patients with melioidosis septic shock. The possible primary role of neutrophil function in containing *B. pseudomallei* has led to the empirical use of granulocyte colony-stimulating factor (G-CSF) in patients with strictly defined septic shock, with observational data from Australia showing a significant improvement in survival with G-CSF.[100] Nevertheless, a randomized controlled trial in Thailand has shown no survival benefit of G-CSF in that location.[101]

PREVENTION

Primary prevention involves education in endemic areas about minimizing exposure to wet season soils and surface water, especially for diabetics. Footwear and gloves while gardening are recommended in northern Australia, but preventing occupational exposure in rice farmers may be unrealistic in Southeast Asia. Cystic fibrosis patients should consider avoiding travel to high-risk areas.

Laboratory-acquired infections, person-to-person spread, and zoonotic infection are all very uncommon, but secondary prophylaxis with sulfamethoxazole-trimethoprim, doxycycline, or amoxicillin-clavulanate could be considered for exceptional circumstances, especially if the exposed person is diabetic or has other risk factors for melioidosis. Guidelines for the management of accidental laboratory exposure have recently been published.[102] Isolation of patients is recommended only for those with severe suppurative pneumonia with productive sputum.

Concerns of possible bioterrorism using the bacterium or its virulence components in genetically engineered constructs and of exposure of military personnel to *B. pseudomallei* have driven funding for recent work. Development of a melioidosis vaccine could also have substantial benefits for those living in endemic regions and for commercial livestock, although cost will be a major impediment to availability. Preliminary studies have included various conjugate, live attenuated, and heterologous vaccine candidates.[56]

Glanders

Glanders is a highly communicable disease of solipeds (horses, donkeys, and mules) that is caused by *Burkholderia mallei*. It can be transmitted to other animals and to humans.

HISTORY

Glanders was described by Hippocrates and has long been recognized as an occupational risk for horse handlers, veterinarians, equine butchers, and laboratory workers. Together with anthrax, glanders was involved in the first modern use of microbes as weapons when German agents targeted horses in the United States, Romania, Spain, Norway, and Argentina between 1915 and 1918.[103]

ETIOLOGY

B. mallei is a small, gram-negative, oxidase-positive, aerobic bacillus. Unlike *B. pseudomallei*, it is nonmotile. It is a host-adapted pathogen that, unlike *B. pseudomallei*, does not persist in the environment outside its equine host. The *Burkholderia* genome projects and multilocus sequence typing have supported the idea that *B. mallei* evolved in animals from the environmental pathogen *B. pseudomallei*.[104,105]

EPIDEMIOLOGY, TRANSMISSION, AND PATHOGENESIS

With quarantine and other control measures, glanders has been eradicated from most countries, but enzootic foci continue in the Middle East, Asia, Africa, and South America. In addition to disease in equines, glanders has occurred in cats and other carnivores eating infected horse meat. Inhalation and percutaneous inoculation also occur. Dis-

charges from the horse respiratory tract and skin are highly infectious. *B. mallei* has much greater potential for zoonotic transmission than *B. pseudomallei*, and the risk of laboratory-acquired infection also appears to be greater for *B. mallei*.[106,107] The incubation period is from as short as 1 to 2 days (e.g., with inhalation) to many months and, as occurs with melioidosis, reactivation from a latent focus after many years has been described.

There are many parallels with the pathogenesis of *B. pseudomallei*, with studies showing the *B. mallei* extracellular polysaccharide capsule to be a critical determinant of virulence.[52,108,109] There is differential susceptibility among animals and, although it is likely that diabetics are more susceptible to infection and disease progression with *B. mallei*,[107] the human host risk factors are less well defined than for melioidosis.

CLINICAL MANIFESTATIONS

Knowledge of the disease in horses is useful for understanding the potential for zoonotic transmission to humans. In acute glanders in horses, fever is accompanied by necrotic ulcers and nodules in the nasal passages that result in copious, infectious, sticky yellow discharges. Neck and mediastinal lymph nodes are enlarged, and pneumonia with nodular abscesses and dissemination to internal organs can accompany the progressive deterioration. In cutaneous glanders (known as farcy), nodular lymphatic or skin abscesses (0.5 to 2.5 cm) occur and ulcerate, discharging infectious, oily yellow pus.[110]

Human glanders, like melioidosis, can be acute or chronic, with mode of infection, inoculating dose, and host risk factors determining the clinical course. With inhaled organisms (respiratory inoculation), acute febrile illness with ulcerative necrosis of the tracheobronchial tree can occur, with mucopurulent discharge involving the nose, lips, and eyes. Lobar or bronchopneumonia, neck and mediastinal lymphadenopathy, pustular skin lesions, and septicemia with dissemination to internal organs can follow.[111] Historically, without antibiotics, death within 10 days usually occurred, but a more chronic pneumonic illness was also recognized after inhalation of *B. mallei*.[106]

After percutaneous inoculation, local skin nodules that can suppurate and regional lymphadenopathy occur, often accompanied by fever, rigors, and malaise.[107,111] Regional lymphadenopathy is much more common than with melioidosis. Lymphatic tract nodules and suppurating abscesses in the lymph nodes are common after several weeks in untreated cases. Dissemination at 1 to 4 weeks can result in infection in almost any tissue, with spleen and liver abscesses, pneumonia, lung abscesses, pleural nodules, and multiple subcutaneous and muscle abscesses all being common (Fig. 221-18). Central nervous system infection can also occur.

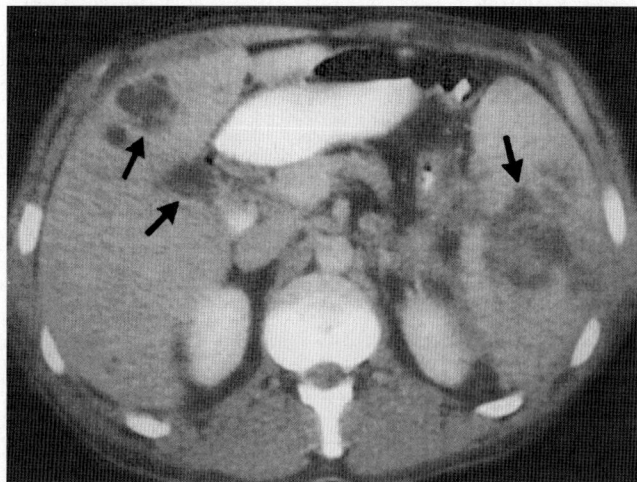

Figure 221-18 **CT scan showing abscesses (*arrows*) in liver and spleen of a patient with laboratory-acquired glanders.** (*From Srinivasan A, Kraus CN, DeShazer D, et al. Glanders in a military research microbiologist. N Engl J Med. 2001;345:256-258.*)

LABORATORY DIAGNOSIS

Definitive diagnosis of glanders requires a positive culture of *B. mallei.* Blood, exudates, and pus from abscesses should be cultured on standard media. Organisms are often very scanty in exudates and pus and are morphologically indistinguishable from those of *B. pseudomallei.* As happens with *B. pseudomallei,* some commercial identification systems may misidentify *B. mallei* as a *Pseudomonas* species, and 16S ribosomal RNA gene-sequenced analysis or a *B. mallei*–specific polymerase chain reaction assay may be required for confirmation.[107] Current serologic assays cannot distinguish *B. mallei* from *B. pseudomallei,* and the mallein skin test used extensively in animal control programs and modified for human diagnosis has poor specificity.[106]

TREATMENT

The antibiotic susceptibility profile of *B. mallei* resembles that of *B. pseudomallei,* except that gentamicin and newer macrolides (e.g., clarithromycin, azithromycin) are active against *B. mallei* but not *B. pseudomallei.*[112] Although response to treatment with older regimens was often slow, rapid improvement occurred in the recent U.S. military researcher with laboratory-acquired infection who was treated with imipenem and doxycycline.[107] This was the first reported case of glanders in the United States in more than 50 years. Recommended treatment and duration are the same as for melioidosis.

PREVENTION

Prevention depends on control of glanders in the equine species and strict precautions to prevent laboratory-acquired infection.[106,107] Unlike the case with melioidosis, isolation of all infected persons is recommended to prevent person-to-person spread. Guidelines for the management of accidental laboratory exposure have been published.[102] As with melioidosis, there is much work being done toward a vaccine to prevent disease in humans.[110]

REFERENCES

1. Whitmore A, Krishnaswami CS. An account of the discovery of a hitherto undescribed infective disease occurring among the population of Rangoon. *Indian Med Gaz.* 1912;47:262-267.
2. Leelarasamee A, Bovornkitti S. Melioidosis: Review and update. *Rev Infect Dis.* 1989;11:413-425.
3. Dance DA. Melioidosis: The tip of the iceberg? *Clin Microbiol Rev.* 1991;4:52-60.
4. White NJ. Melioidosis. *Lancet.* 2003;361:1715-1722.
5. Cheng AC, Currie BJ. Melioidosis: epidemiology, pathophysiology, and management. *Clin Microbiol Rev.* 2005;18: 383-416.
6. Punyagupta S. Melioidosis: Review of 686 cases and presentation of a new clinical classification. In: Punyagupta S, Sirisanthana T, Stapatayavong B, eds. *Melioidosis.* Bangkok: Bangkok Medical; 1989:217-229.
7. Chaowagul W, White NJ, Dance DA, et al. Melioidosis: A major cause of community-acquired septicemia in northeastern Thailand. *J Infect Dis.* 1989;159:890-899.
8. Vuddhakul V, Tharavichitkul P, Na-Ngam N, et al. Epidemiology of *Burkholderia pseudomallei* in Thailand. *Am J Trop Med Hyg.* 1999;60:458-461.
9. Leelarasamee A. Melioidosis in Southeast Asia. *Acta Trop.* 2000;74:129-132.
10. Puthucheary SD, Parasakthi N, Lee MK. Septicaemic melioidosis: A review of 50 cases from Malaysia. *Trans R Soc Trop Med Hyg.* 1992;86:683-685.
11. Yap EH, Chan YC, Goh KT, et al. Sudden unexplained death syndrome—a new manifestation in melioidosis? *Epidemiol Infect.* 1991;107:577-584.
12. Liu Y, Loh JP, Aw LT, et al. Rapid molecular typing of *Burkholderia pseudomallei,* isolated in an outbreak of melioidosis in Singapore in 2004, based on variable-number tandem repeats. *Trans R Soc Trop Med Hyg.* 2006;100:687-692.
13. Dance DA. Melioidosis as an emerging global problem. *Acta Trop.* 2000;74:115-119.
14. Lee N, Wu JL, Lee CH, et al. *Pseudomonas pseudomallei* infection from drowning: The first reported case in Taiwan. *J Clin Microbiol.* 1985;22:352-354.
15. Hsueh PR, Teng LJ, Lee LN, et al. Melioidosis: An emerging infection in Taiwan? *Emerg Infect Dis.* 2001;7:428-433.
16. Parry CM, Wuthiekanun V, Hoa NT, et al. Melioidosis in Southern Vietnam: Clinical surveillance and environmental sampling. *Clin Infect Dis.* 1999;29:1323-1326.
17. Phetsouvanh R, Phongmany S, Soukaloun D, et al. Causes of community-acquired bacteremia and patterns of antimicrobial resistance in Vientiane, Laos. *Am J Trop Med Hyg.* 2006; 75:978-985.
18. Wuthiekanun V, Pheaktra N, Putchhat H, et al. *Burkholderia pseudomallei* antibodies in children, Cambodia. *Emerg Infect Dis.* 2008;14:301-303.
19. Cherian T, Raghupathy P, John TJ. Plague in India. *Lancet.* 1995;345:258-259.
20. Dance DA, Sanders D, Pitt TL, et al. *Burkholderia pseudomallei* and Indian plague-like illness. *Lancet.* 1995;346:904-905.
21. Athan E, Allworth AM, Engler C, et al. Melioidosis in tsunami survivors. *Emerg Infect Dis.* 2005;11:1638-1639.
22. Le Hello S, Currie BJ, Godoy D, et al. Melioidosis in New Caledonia. *Emerg Infect Dis.* 2005;11:1607-1609.
23. Inglis TJ, Rolim DB, Sousa Ade Q. Melioidosis in the Americas. *Am J Trop Med Hyg.* 2006;75:947-954.
24. Borgherini GP, Poubeau F, Paganin S, et al. Melioidosis: an imported case from Madagascar. *J Travel Med.* 2006; 13:318-320.
25. Boonsawat W, Boonma P, Tangdajahiran T, et al. Community-acquired pneumonia in adults at Srinagarind Hospital. *J Med Assoc Thai.* 1990;73:345-352.
26. Currie BJ, Fisher DA, Howard DM, et al. The epidemiology of melioidosis in Australia and Papua New Guinea. *Acta Trop.* 2000;74:121-127.
27. Currie B, Smith Vaughan H, Golledge C, et al. *Pseudomonas pseudomallei* isolates collected over 25 years from a non-tropical endemic focus show clonality on the basis of ribotyping. *Epidemiol Infect.* 1994;113:307-312.
28. Clayton AJ, Lisella RS, Martin DG. Melioidosis: A serological survey in military personnel. *Mil Med.* 1973;138: 24-26.
29. Wuthiekanun V, Smith MD, Dance DA, et al. Isolation of *Pseudomonas pseudomallei* from soil in north-eastern Thailand. *Trans R Soc Trop Med Hyg.* 1995;89:41-43.
30. Kaestli M, Mayo M, Harrington G, et al. Sensitive and specific molecular detection of *Burkholderia pseudomallei,* the causative agent of melioidosis, in the soil of tropical northern Australia. *Appl Environ Microbiol.* 2007;73:6891-6897.
31. Thomas AD, Forbes Faulkner J, Parker M. Isolation of *Pseudomonas pseudomallei* from clay layers at defined depths. *Am J Epidemiol.* 1979;110:515-521.
32. Inglis TJ, Mee B, Chang B. The environmental microbiology of melioidosis. *Rev Med Microbiol.* 2001;12:13-20.
33. Vorachit M, Lam K, Jayanetra P, et al. Resistance of *Pseudomonas pseudomallei* growing as a biofilm on silastic discs to ceftazidime and co-trimoxazole. *Antimicrob Agents Chemother.* 1993; 37:2000-2002.
34. Suputtamongkol Y, Hall AJ, Dance DA, et al. The epidemiology of melioidosis in Ubon Ratchatani, northeast Thailand. *Int J Epidemiol.* 1994;23:1082-1090.
35. Currie BJ, Fisher DA, Howard DM, et al. Endemic melioidosis in tropical northern Australia: A 10-year prospective study and review of the literature. *Clin Infect Dis.* 2000;31:981-986.
36. Howe C, Sampath A, Spotnitz M. The pseudomallei group: A review. *J Infect Dis.* 1971;124:598-606.
37. Currie BJ, Jacups SP. Intensity of rainfall and severity of melioidosis, Australia. *Emerg Infect Dis.* 2003;9:1538-1542.
38. Inglis TJ, Garrow SC, Henderson M, et al. *Burkholderia pseudomallei* traced to water treatment plant in Australia. *Emerg Infect Dis.* 2000;6:56-59.
39. Currie BJ, Mayo M, Anstey NM, et al. A cluster of melioidosis cases from an endemic region is clonal and is linked to the water supply using molecular typing of *Burkholderia pseudomallei* isolates. *Am J Trop Med Hyg.* 2001;65:177-179.
40. Currie BJ, Fisher DA, Anstey NM, et al. Melioidosis: Acute and chronic disease, relapse and re-activation. *Trans R Soc Trop Med Hyg.* 2000;94:301-304.
41. Sookpranee M, Lumbiganon P, Boonma P. Nosocomial contamination of *Pseudomonas pseudomallei* in the patients at Srinagarind Hospital. In: Punyagupta S, Sirisanthana T, Stapatayavong B, eds. *Melioidosis.* Bangkok: Bangkok Medical; 1989:204-210.
42. Ashdown LR, Guard RW. The prevalence of human melioidosis in Northern Queensland. *Am J Trop Med Hyg.* 1984; 33:474-478.
43. Wuthiekanun V, Chierakul W, Langa S, et al. Development of antibodies to *Burkholderia pseudomallei* during childhood in melioidosis-endemic northeast Thailand. *Am J Trop Med Hyg.* 2006;74:1074-1075.
44. Ulett GC, Currie BJ, Clair TW, et al. *Burkholderia pseudomallei* virulence: Definition, stability and association with clonality. *Microbes Infect.* 2001;3:621-631.
45. Holden MT, Titball RW, Peacock SJ, et al. Genomic plasticity of the causative agent of melioidosis, *Burkholderia pseudomallei. Proc Natl Acad Sci U S A.* 2004;101:14240-14245.
46. Tuanyok A, Auerbach RK, Brettin TS, et al. A horizontal gene transfer event defines two distinct groups within *Burkholderia pseudomallei* that have dissimilar geographic distributions. *J Bacteriol.* 2007;189:9044-9049.
47. Egan AM, Gordon DL. *Burkholderia pseudomallei* activates complement and is ingested but not killed by polymorphonuclear leukocytes. *Infect Immun.* 1996;64:4952-4959.
48. Brett PJ, Woods DE. Pathogenesis of and immunity to melioidosis. *Acta Trop.* 2000;74:201-210.
49. DeShazer D, Brett PJ, Woods DE. The type II O-antigenic polysaccharide moiety of *Burkholderia pseudomallei* lipopolysaccharide is required for serum resistance and virulence. *Mol Microbiol.* 1998;30:1081-1100.
50. Reckseidler SL, DeShazer D, Sokol PA, et al. Detection of bacterial virulence genes by subtractive hybridization: identification of capsular polysaccharide of *Burkholderia pseudomallei* as a major virulence determinant. *Infect Immun.* 2001;69:34-44.
51. Woods DE. The use of animal infection models to study the pathogenesis of melioidosis and glanders. *Trends Microbiol.* 2002;11:483-484.
52. DeShazer D, Waag DM, Fritz DL, et al. Identification of a *Burkholderia mallei* polysaccharide gene cluster by subtractive hybridization and demonstration that the encoded capsule is an essential virulence determinant. *Microb Pathog.* 2001;30: 253-269.
53. Winstanley C, Hart CA. Presence of type III secretion genes in *Burkholderia pseudomallei* correlates with Ara⁻ phenotypes. *J Clin Microbiol.* 2000;38:883-885.
54. Stevens MP, Wood MW, Taylor LA, et al. An Inv/Mxi-Spa-like type III protein secretion system in *Burkholderia pseudomallei* modulates intracellular behaviour of the pathogen. *Mol Microbiol.* 2002;46:649-659.
55. Ulrich RL, Deshazer D, Brueggemann EE, et al. Role of quorum sensing in the pathogenicity of *Burkholderia pseudomallei. J Med Microbiol.* 2004;53:1053-1064.
56. Wiersinga WJ, van der Poll T, White NJ, et al. Melioidosis: insights into the pathogenicity of *Burkholderia pseudomallei. Nat Rev Microbiol.* 2006;4:272-282.
57. Stevens MP, Stevens JM, Jeng RL, et al. Identification of a bacterial factor required for actin-based motility of *Burkholderia pseudomallei. Mol Microbiol.* 2005;56:40-53.
58. Haussler S, Rohde M, Steinmetz I. Highly resistant *Burkholderia pseudomallei* small colony variants isolated in vitro and in experimental melioidosis. *Med Microbiol Immunol (Berl).* 1999;188:91-97.
59. Nuntayanuwat S, Dharakul T, Chaowagul W, et al. Polymorphism in the promoter region of tumor necrosis factor-alpha gene is associated with severe melioidosis. *Hum Immunol.* 1999;60:979-983.
60. Santanirand P, Harley VS, Dance DA, et al. Obligatory role of gamma interferon for host survival in a murine model of infection with *Burkholderia pseudomallei. Infect Immun.* 1999; 67:3593-3600.
61. Wiersinga WJ, Wieland CW, Dessing MC, et al. Toll-like receptor 2 impairs host defense in gram-negative sepsis caused by *Burkholderia pseudomallei* (melioidosis). *PLoS Med.* 2007;4:e248.
62. Wiersinga WJ, Dessing MC, Kager PA, et al. High-throughput mRNA profiling characterizes the expression of inflammatory molecules in sepsis caused by *Burkholderia pseudomallei. Infect Immun.* 2007;75:3074-3079.
63. Barnes JL, Warner J, Melrose W, et al. Adaptive immunity in melioidosis: a possible role for T cells in determining outcome of infection with *Burkholderia pseudomallei. Clin Immunol.* 2004;113:22-28.
64. Limmathurotsakul D, Chaowagul W, Chierakul W, et al. Risk factors for recurrent melioidosis in northeast Thailand. *Clin Infect Dis.* 2006;43:979-986.

65. Suputtamongkol Y, Chaowagul W, Chetchotisakd P, et al. Risk factors for melioidosis and bacteremic melioidosis. *Clin Infect Dis.* 1999;29:408-413.
66. Lumbiganon P, Viengnondha S. Clinical manifestations of melioidosis in children. *Pediatr Infect Dis J.* 1995;14:136-140.
67. Edmond K, Bauert P, Currie B. Paediatric melioidosis in the Northern Territory of Australia: An expanding clinical spectrum. *J Paediatr Child Health.* 2001;37:337-341.
68. Easton A, Haque A, Chu K, et al. A critical role for neutrophils in resistance to experimental infection with *Burkholderia pseudomallei. J Infect Dis.* 2007;195:99-107.
69. Tarlow MJ, Lloyd J. Melioidosis and chronic granulomatous disease. *Proc R Soc Med.* 1971;64:19-20.
70. Holland DJ, Wesley A, Drinkovic D, et al. Cystic fibrosis and *Burkholderia pseudomallei:* An emerging problem? *Clin Infect Dis.* 2002;35:e138-140.
71. Gibney KB, Cheng AC, Currie BJ. Cutaneous melioidosis in the tropical top end of Australia: a prospective study and review of the literature. *Clin Infect Dis.* 2008;47:603-609.
72. Dance DA, Davis TM, Wattanagoon Y, et al. Acute suppurative parotitis caused by *Pseudomonas pseudomallei* in children. *J Infect Dis.* 1989;159:654-660.
73. Currie BJ, Fisher DA, Howard DM, et al. Neurological melioidosis. *Acta Trop.* 2000;74:145-151.
74. Koszyca B, Currie BJ, Blumbergs PC. The neuropathology of melioidosis: two cases and a review of the literature. *Clin Neuropathol.* 2004;23:195-203.
75. Chadwick DR, Ang B, Sitoh YY, et al. Cerebral melioidosis in Singapore: A review of five cases. *Trans R Soc Trop Med Hyg.* 2002;96:72-76.
76. Ngauy V, Lemeshev Y, Sadkowski L et al. Cutaneous melioidosis in a man who was taken as a prisoner of war by the Japanese during World War II. *J Clin Microbiol.* 2005;43:970-972.
77. Lowe P, Engler C, Norton R. Comparison of automated and nonautomated systems for identification of *Burkholderia pseudomallei. J Clin Microbiol.* 2002;40:4625-4627.
78. Ashdown LR. An improved screening technique for isolation of *Pseudomonas pseudomallei* from clinical specimens. *Pathology.* 1979;11:293-297.
79. Peacock SJ, Chieng G, Cheng AC, et al. Comparison of Ashdown's medium, *Burkholderia cepacia* medium, and *Burkholderia pseudomallei* selective agar for clinical isolation of *Burkholderia pseudomallei. J Clin Microbiol.* 2005;43: 5359-5361.
80. Dance DA, Wuthiekanun V, Naigowit P, et al. Identification of *Pseudomonas pseudomallei* in clinical practice: Use of simple screening tests and API 20NE. *J Clin Pathol.* 1989;42:645-648.
81. Smith MD, Wuthiekanun V, Walsh AL, et al. Latex agglutination for rapid detection of *Pseudomonas pseudomallei* antigen in urine of patients with melioidosis. *J Clin Pathol.* 1995; 48:174-176.
82. Wuthiekanun V, Desakorn V, Wongsuvan G, et al. Rapid immunofluorescence microscopy for diagnosis of melioidosis. *Clin Diagn Lab Immunol.* 2005;12:555-556.
83. Sirisinha S, Anuntagool N, Dharakul T, et al. Recent developments in laboratory diagnosis of melioidosis. *Acta Trop.* 2000;74:235-245.
84. Meumann EM, Novak RT, Gal D, et al. Clinical evaluation of a type III secretion system real-time PCR assay for diagnosing melioidosis. *J Clin Microbiol.* 2006;44:3028-3030.
85. Cheng AC, O'Brien M, Freeman K, et al. Indirect hemagglutination assay in patients with melioidosis in northern Australia. *Am J Trop Med Hyg.* 2006;74:330-334.
86. Chantratita N, Wuthiekanun V, Thanwisai A, et al. Accuracy of enzyme-linked immunosorbent assay using crude and purified antigens for serodiagnosis of melioidosis. *Clin Vaccine Immunol.* 2007;14:110-113.
87. White NJ, Dance DA, Chaowagul W, et al. Halving of mortality of severe melioidosis by ceftazidime. *Lancet.* 1989;2:697-701.
88. Sookpranee M, Boonma P, Susaengrat W, et al. Multicenter prospective randomized trial comparing ceftazidime plus co-trimoxazole with chloramphenicol plus doxycycline and co-trimoxazole for treatment of severe melioidosis. *Antimicrob Agents Chemother.* 1992;36:158-162.
89. Chierakul W, Anunnatsiri S, Short JM, et al. Two randomized controlled trials of ceftazidime alone versus ceftazidime in combination with trimethoprim-sulfamethoxazole for the treatment of severe melioidosis. *Clin Infect Dis.* 2005;41:1105-1113.
90. Suputtamongkol Y, Rajchanuwong A, Chaowagul W, et al. Ceftazidime vs. amoxicillin/clavulanate in the treatment of severe melioidosis. *Clin Infect Dis.* 1994;19:846-853.
91. Smith MD, Wuthiekanun V, Walsh AL, et al. Susceptibility of *Pseudomonas pseudomallei* to some newer beta-lactam antibiotics and antibiotic combinations using time-kill studies. *J Antimicrob Chemother.* 1994;33:145-149.
92. Smith MD, Wuthiekanun V, Walsh AL, et al. In-vitro activity of carbapenem antibiotics against beta-lactam susceptible and resistant strains of *Burkholderia pseudomallei. J Antimicrob Chemother.* 1996;37:611-615.
93. Simpson AJ, Suputtamongkol Y, Smith MD, et al. Comparison of imipenem and ceftazidime as therapy for severe melioidosis. *Clin Infect Dis.* 1999;29:381-387.
94. Cheng AC, Fisher DA, Anstey NM, et al. Outcomes of patients with melioidosis treated with meropenem. *Antimicrob Agents Chemother.* 2004;48:1763-1765.
95. Huffam S, Jacups SP, Kittler P, et al. Out of hospital treatment of patients with melioidosis using ceftazidime in 24 h elastomeric infusors, via peripherally inserted central catheters. *Trop Med Int Health.* 2004;9:715-717.
96. Chaowagul W, Suputtamongkol Y, Dance DA, et al. Relapse in melioidosis: Incidence and risk factors. *J Infect Dis.* 1993; 168:1181-1185.
97. Cheng AC, Chierakul W, Chaowagul W, et al. Consensus guidelines for dosing of amoxicillin-clavulanate in melioidosis. *Am J Trop Med Hyg.* 2008;78:208-209.
98. Chaowagul W, Simpson AJ, Suputtamongkol Y, et al. A comparison of chloramphenicol, trimethoprim-sulfamethoxazole, and doxycycline with doxycycline alone as maintenance therapy for melioidosis. *Clin Infect Dis.* 1999;29:375-380.
99. Chaowagul W, Chierakul W, Simpson AJ, et al. Open-label randomized trial of oral trimethoprim-sulfamethoxazole, doxycycline, and chloramphenicol compared with trimethoprim-sulfamethoxazole and doxycycline for maintenance therapy of melioidosis. *Antimicrob Agents Chemother.* 2005;49:4020-4025.
100. Cheng AC, Stephens DP, Anstey NM, et al. Adjunctive granulocyte colony-stimulating factor for treatment of septic shock due to melioidosis. *Clin Infect Dis.* 2004;38:32-37.
101. Cheng AC, Limmathurotsakul D, Chierakul W, et al. A randomized controlled trial of granulocyte colony-stimulating factor for the treatment of severe sepsis due to melioidosis in Thailand. *Clin Infect Dis.* 2007;45:308-314.
102. Peacock SJ, Schweizer HP, Dance DA, et al. Management of accidental laboratory exposure to *Burkholderia pseudomallei* and *B. mallei. Emerg Infect Dis.* 2008;14:e2.
103. Wheelis M. First shots fired in biological warfare. *Nature.* 1998;395:213.
104. Godoy D, Randle G, Simpson AJ, et al. Multilocus sequence typing and evolutionary relationships among the causative agents of melioidosis and glanders, *Burkholderia pseudomallei* and *Burkholderia mallei. J Clin Microbiol.* 2003;41:2068-2079.
105. Nierman WC, DeShazer D, Kim HS, et al. Structural flexibility in the *Burkholderia mallei* genome. *Proc Natl Acad Sci U S A.* 2004;101:14246-14251.
106. Howe C, Miller WR. Human glanders: Report of six cases. *Ann Intern Med.* 1947;26:93-115.
107. Srinivasan A, Kraus CN, DeShazer D, et al. Glanders in a military research microbiologist. *N Engl J Med.* 2001; 345:256-258.
108. Fritz DL, Vogel P, Brown DR, et al. Mouse model of sublethal and lethal intraperitoneal glanders *(Burkholderia mallei). Vet Pathol.* 2000;37:626-636.
109. Burtnick MN, Brett PJ, Woods DE. Molecular and physical characterization of *Burkholderia mallei* O antigens. *J Bacteriol.* 2002;184:849-852.
110. Lopez J, Copps J, Wilhelmsen C, et al. Characterization of experimental equine glanders. *Microbes Infect.* 2003;5: 1125-1131.
111. Robins GD. A study of chronic glanders in man with report of a case: Analysis of 156 cases collected from the literature. *Stud R Victoria Hosp Montreal.* 1906;2:1-98.
112. Heine HS, England MJ, Waag DM, et al. In vitro antibiotic susceptibilities of *Burkholderia mallei* (causative agent of glanders) determined by broth microdilution and E-test. *Antimicrob Agents Chemother.* 2001;45:2119-2121.

222

Acinetobacter Species

DAVID M. ALLEN | BARRY J. HARTMAN

Bacteria that constitute the genus *Acinetobacter* were originally identified in the first decade of the 20th century. However, it was not until the advent of modern infection control that its role as a ubiquitous opportunistic pathogen was appreciated. During the past 25 years, an improved understanding of the microbiology, taxonomy, and ecology of *Acinetobacter* has emerged. Issues of continuing clinical relevance include *Acinetobacter* speciation, antimicrobial resistance, and appropriate therapy. Two recent reviews provide additional information.[1,2]

History and Microbiology

The genus *Acinetobacter* has had a colorful taxonomic history. Before the 1970s, *Acinetobacter* was frequently misidentified because of an absence of distinguishing features. Subsequent use of transformation and nutritional studies defined the genus *Acinetobacter* and placed it within the family Neisseriaceae.

Historically, rediscoveries of this ubiquitous organism led to the creation of numerous genera with resultant taxonomic chaos. Probably first described in 1908 as *Diplococcus mucosus*, *Acinetobacter* was initially identified by the absence of common characteristics—no color, nonmotile, unable to reduce nitrates, and nonfermenting.[3] The lack of distinctive characteristics was a driving force in the evolving nomenclature of the day: *Micrococcus* (small), *Mima* (mimics), *Achromobacter* (colorless), *Acinetobacter* (motionless), and *anitratus* (nitrate nonreducing). In the 1930s and 1940s, while attempting to organize *Neisseria*-like organisms morphologically, De Bord proposed a new tribe, Mimaeae, to encompass these organisms.[4] Later, Brisou and Prévot proposed the genus *Acinetobacter* to include colorless, nonmotile, saprophytic gram-negative bacilli, regardless of oxidase activity.[5] Ultimately, two of the three genera (*Mima* and *Herellea*) in the now-obsolete tribe Mimeae came to be included under the genus *Acinetobacter*. Further refinement emerged when oxidase activity was used to distinguish *Moraxella* (oxidase-positive) from *Acinetobacter* (oxidase-negative).

Although genus clarification was clearly established by 1971,[6] recent efforts are directed toward species delineation. References published before the mid-1980s recognized one species, *Acinetobacter calcoaceticus*, with two subspecies (var. *anitratus* and var. *lwoffi*) or two species,[7] *A. calcoaceticus* and *A. lwoffi*. The two subspecies and species were distinguished by the ability of *A. calcoaceticus* var. *anitratus* to produce acid from glucose and the inability of var. *lwoffi* to do so. Efforts to speciate the genus further have subsequently included bacteriocin typing, phage typing, characterization of outer membrane proteins, serotyping, phenotyping, ribotyping, transfer ribonucleic acid (tRNA) and genomic fingerprinting,[8] and DNA homology.[9] As one might anticipate, nucleic acid fingerprinting and DNA homology remain the most reliable methods for distinguishing species.

Based on DNA-DNA hybridization studies, at least 21 different *Acinetobacter* strains (genomic species, or "genospecies") have been identified (Table 222-1).[10] Despite moderate success in applying simple, reproducible phenotypic studies to speciate *Acinetobacter* without resorting to more cumbersome studies, some clusters remain; for example, phenotypically similar genospecies 1, 2, 3, and 13 make up the *A. calcoaceticus-Acinetobacter baumannii* complex. In routine clinical practice, precise species identification is not necessary and compromises in terminology (e.g., *A. calcoaceticus-A. baumannii*

complex or *A. baumannii* complex) meet clinicians' as well as microbiologists' needs. However, for epidemiologic purposes, additional investigations such as pulsed field gel electrophoresis, amplified fragment length polymorphisms (AFLP), randomly amplified polymorphic DNA–polymerase chain reaction (RAPD-PCR), or ribotyping may still be required for exact strain identification.

Acinetobacter are rod-shaped during rapid growth and coccobacillary in the stationary phase. They are generally encapsulated, nonmotile (occasionally exhibiting twitching motility), aerobic, gram-negative organisms with a tendency to retain crystal violet and therefore to be incorrectly identified as gram-positive cocci. Versatility in exploiting a variety of carbon and energy sources allows *Acinetobacter* to grow on routine laboratory media and accounts for its prevalence in nature. Colonies are 1 to 2 mm, nonpigmented, domed, and mucoid, with smooth to pitted surfaces. Frequent misidentification of *Acinetobacter* as *Neisseria* or *Moraxella* on Gram staining is readily clarified by the negative oxidase reaction of *Acinetobacter*. The inability of *Acinetobacter* spp. to reduce nitrate or to grow anaerobically distinguishes these organisms from Enterobacteriaceae. Additionally, *Acinetobacter* are indole-negative and catalase-positive. Hemolysis of red blood cells, acidification of glucose, growth at 44°C, and variability in carbon source uptake are a few of the phenotypic characteristics applied to distinguish *Acinetobacter* strains (Table 222-2).

Epidemiology

Acinetobacter differs from other members of the family Neisseriaceae by the simplicity of its growth requirements. The ability to use a variety of carbon sources via diverse metabolic pathways expands its habitat. Related genera (*Moraxella*, *Neisseria*, and *Kingella*) are parasitic in warm-blooded animals, whereas free-living *Acinetobacter* can be found on animate and inanimate objects. Almost 100% of soil and water samples yield *Acinetobacter*. *Acinetobacter* has been isolated from many sources, including pasteurized milk, frozen foods, chilled poultry, foundry and hospital air, vaporizer mist, tap water faucets, peritoneal dialysate baths, bedside urinals, washcloths, angiography catheters, ventilators, laryngoscopes, duodenoscopes, multidose medication, plasma protein fraction, hospital pillows, and soap dispensers.[11] *Acinetobacter* may survive on dry inanimate objects for months, comparable to *Staphylococcus aureus*.[12] *Acinetobacter* resistance to biocides (e.g., chlorhexidine) becomes a concern when inadvertent biocide dilution, inadequate biocide exposure time, presence of biologic debris, and/or the presence of a multidrug-resistant (MDR) *Acinetobacter* is involved.[13,14]

Acinetobacter has been grown from numerous human sources, including skin, sputum, urine, feces, and vaginal secretions. Up to 25% of healthy ambulatory adults exhibit cutaneous colonization,[15] and 7% of adults and infants have transient pharyngeal colonization.[16] It is the most common gram-negative organism persistently carried on the skin of hospital personnel,[17] and it has been found to colonize inpatient tracheostomy sites frequently.

The prevalence of *Acinetobacter* clinical isolates varies somewhat by country and by specimen site but has generally increased worldwide in the past 2 decades. Data reported to the Centers for Disease Control and Prevention (CDC) National Nosocomial Infection Surveillance (NNIS) indicated that *Acinetobacter* was the cause of 2.4% of intensive

Table 222-1	*Acinetobacter* Nomenclature

Current

Acinetobacter calcoaceticus (genomic species 1)

A. baumannii (genomic species 2)

A. haemolyticus (genomic species 4)

A. junii (genomic species 5)

A. johnsonii (genomic species 7)

A. lwoffi (genomic species 8/9)

A. radioresistens (genomic species 12)

A. baylyi

A. bouvetii

A. gerneri

A. grimontii

A. parvus

A. schindleri

A. tandoii

A. tjernbergiae

A. towneri

A. ursingii

A. venetianus

Acinetobacter spp. unnamed (≥14 other genomic species)

Before 1986

?*Diplococcus mucosus* (1908)

Micrococcus calco-aceticus (1911)

Alcaligenes haemolysis (1937)

Mima polymorpha (1939)

Moraxella lwoffi (1940)

Herellea vaginicola (1942)

Bacterium anitratum (1948)

B5W (1949)

Neisseria winogradsky (1952)

Achromobacter lwoffi (1953)

Achromobacter anitratum (1954)

Moraxella glucidolytica (1956)

Acinetobacter anitratum (1957)

Acinetobacter lwoffi (1957)

Acinetobacter polymorpha (1957)

Achromobacter citroalcaligenes (1963)

Achromobacter conjunctivae (1963)

Achromobacter hemolyticus var. *alcaligenes* (1963)

Achromobacter hemolyticus var. *glucidolytica* (1963)

Alcaligenes metalcaligenes (1963)

Acinetobacter calcoaceticus var. *anitratus* (1968)

Acinetobacter calcoaceticus var. *anitratus* (1968)

Acinetobacter calcoaceticus var. *lwoffi* (1968)

Table 222-2	Characteristics of the Family *Neisseriaceae*			
	Genus			
Characteristic	*Acinetobacter*	*Neisseria*	*Moraxella*	*Kingella*
Shape	Paired cocci to medium rods	Paired cocci	Paired cocci to short rods	Paired rods
Oxidase	−	+	+	+
Catalase	+	+	+	−
Nitrate reduction	−	+	±	+
Metabolism	Active, varied	Limited, simple	Limited, simple	Limited, simple
Acid from glucose	±	−	−	+

+, present; −, absent.

care unit (ICU) nosocomial bloodstream infections, 2.1% of surgical site infections, 1.6% of nosocomial urinary tract infections, and 6.9% (3% in 1975) of nosocomial pneumonia in sentinel U.S. hospitals in 2003.[18,19] Although constituting the largest increase in gram-negative pneumonia since 1975, *Acinetobacter* remains less frequent than *Pseudomonas*, *Klebsiella*, and *Enterobacter* in that category.

Risk factors associated with community-acquired *Acinetobacter* infection include alcoholism, cigarette smoking, chronic lung disease, diabetes mellitus, and residence in a tropical developing community.[20] Risk factors specific for nosocomial infection include length of hospital stay, surgery, wounds, previous infection (independent of previous antibiotic use),[21] fecal colonization with *Acinetobacter*,[22] treatment with broad-spectrum antibiotics, indwelling central intravenous or urinary catheters,[23] admission to a burn unit or ICU, parenteral nutrition, mechanical ventilation, and breaches in infection control protocols.[21,23]

Pathogenesis

A limited number of virulence factors reduce this bacterium to the role of an opportunist. Although growth in an acidic pH at lower temperatures may enhance its ability to invade devitalized tissue, no known cytotoxins are produced. Lipopolysaccharide is present in the cell wall, but little is known of its endotoxigenic potential in humans. Additional features that may enhance the survival of *Acinetobacter* include bacteriocin production, presence of fimbriae, presence of a capsule, and prolonged viability under dry conditions.[12,24] The capsule that surrounds most strains may inhibit phagocytosis and has been speculated to predispose those with selective complement component deficiencies to infection.[20] In summary, without disruption of normal host defense mechanisms, the role of *Acinetobacter* in human infection remains limited.

Clinical Manifestations

Acinetobacter spp. can cause suppurative infections in almost every organ system.[25] Although *Acinetobacter* is acknowledged to be an opportunist in hospitalized patients, community-acquired infections are reported. Interpreting the significance of isolates from clinical specimens is often difficult because of the wide distribution of *Acinetobacter* in nature and its ability to colonize healthy or damaged tissues. Additionally, *Acinetobacter* can be misinterpreted on Gram staining as other gram-negative organisms more commonly associated with particular clinical syndromes (e.g., in cerebrospinal fluid, *Neisseria meningitidis*; in sputum, *Haemophilus influenzae*). The *A. baumannii* complex makes up 80% of total *Acinetobacter* clinical isolates, whereas nonclinical items (e.g., food) are more likely to harbor non–*A. baumannii* species. However, repeated isolation of non–*A. baumannii* genospecies from appropriate clinical specimens should not be dismissed as contaminant.

RESPIRATORY TRACT

The respiratory system is the most common site for *Acinetobacter* infection because of its transient pharyngeal colonization of healthy persons and a high rate of tracheostomy colonization.[25]

Acinetobacter has been reported to cause community-acquired bronchiolitis and tracheobronchitis in healthy children.[26] Tracheobronchitis can also occur in compromised adults. Pulmonary toilet often eradicates the organism without the use of systemic antibiotics in these latter hosts.

Adult community-acquired *Acinetobacter* pneumonia generally occurs in patients with diminished host defenses (e.g., alcoholism, tobacco use, diabetes mellitus, renal failure, underlying pulmonary disease).[27-29] Reports from developing tropical regions document a higher local prevalence of community-acquired *Acinetobacter* pneumonia compared with temperate climates. One series from tropical northern Australia found community-acquired *Acinetobacter* pneumonia to account for 10% of all community-acquired bacteremic pneumonias and 21% of gram-negative pneumonias.[20] Mortality in various published series has been 40% to 64%.[29] The prevalence of community-acquired *Acinetobacter* pneumonia was speculated to be a consequence of the generally poor health of persons in the communities under study, frequent use of penicillins, and/or genetic predisposition.

The greatest impact of *Acinetobacter* has been as a causative agent of nosocomial pneumonia, particularly ventilator-associated cases.[19] Predisposing factors for nosocomial *Acinetobacter* pneumonia include endotracheal intubation, tracheostomy, previous antibiotic therapy, ICU residence, recent surgery, high APACHE II score, and underlying pulmonary disease. Nosocomial spread in the ICU setting has been attributed to ventilator equipment, gloves, colonized nursing, and respiratory therapy personnel among others. Recently, an ICU-based diabetic health care worker developed pneumonia, septic shock, and acute respiratory distress syndrome (ARDS) following occupational exposure to an *Acinetobacter*-infected U.S. soldier wounded in Iraq.[30] Nosocomial *Acinetobacter* pneumonias are frequently multilobar. Cavitation, pleural effusion, and bronchopleural fistula formation have been observed. Nosocomial pneumonia reports from France found the mortality rate from *Pseudomonas* and *Acinetobacter* to be higher than 70%.[31] Secondary bacteremia and septic shock are associated with a poor prognosis.[25] When attempting to determine the contribution of *Acinetobacter* to the morbidity and death of critically ill patients, it is important to note that either colonization or infection with *A. baumannii* in ICU patients has been independently associated with excess length of stay and excess mortality. Colonization of *Acinetobacter* is attributable more to the poor condition of the patient rather than the virulence of *Acinetobacter*.[21]

BACTEREMIA

True *Acinetobacter* bacteremia should be distinguished from pseudobacteremia resulting from improper blood culture technique.[15] Nosocomial *Acinetobacter* bacteremia is frequently associated with respiratory tract infections and use of IV catheters; urinary tract, wound, skin, and abdominal infections are less frequent sources.[19] Although descriptions of well-appearing patients with bacteremia have been recorded (generally in patients with indwelling catheters),[32] septic shock may be seen in up to 30% of bacteremic patients. The mortality rate from *Acinetobacter* bacteremia has been reported to be 17% to 46%.[25,33] *Acinetobacter* bacteremia with species other than *A. baumannii* tends to be less severe.

GENITOURINARY

Studies isolating *Acinetobacter* from patients with a penicillin-resistant "gonorrhea-like" urethritis led to the erroneous implication of *Acinetobacter* as a cause of this illness.[34] Despite colonization of the lower urinary tract with *Acinetobacter*, it is only rarely invasive. However, cases of cystitis and pyelonephritis have been documented in the setting of an indwelling bladder catheter or nephrolithiasis.[25]

INTRACRANIAL INFECTION

Initially described by Cowan in 1938,[3] *Acinetobacter* meningitis occurs infrequently.[35] Although it is generally identified following head trauma or neurosurgical procedures,[36] there have been reports of *Acinetobacter* meningitis occurring in healthy hosts. Meningitis can manifest abruptly or follow a more indolent course. A petechial rash has been noted in up to 30% of patients with *Acinetobacter* meningitis.[26] *Acinetobacter* may be morphologically confused with *N. meningitidis* on Gram staining of spinal fluid.

SOFT TISSUE

Acinetobacter has become a major pathogen in traumatic wounds (e.g., war wounds), postoperative incisions, and burns as a result of the organism's ability to thrive on compromised tissue and foreign bodies. As a war injury–related pathogen, an increased number of *Acinetobacter* infections were first noted during the Korean war.[37] It was the most common gram-negative bacillus to contaminate traumatic extremity injuries during the Vietnam conflict.[38] Similar findings have been reported during the Afghanistan and Iraq conflicts, except that the *Acinetobacter* strains identified are now MDR strains and readily isolated from the environment of field hospitals and ICUs.[39-42] Nosocomial *Acinetobacter* infections complicated more recent natural disasters, including the 1999 Turkish Marmara earthquake and the 2004 Southeast Asian tsunami.[43,44]

Acinetobacter can cause cellulitis in association with an indwelling venous catheter. Resolution of catheter-induced cellulitis may occur with catheter removal alone. Synergistic necrotizing fasciitis in conjunction with *Streptococcus pyogenes* has been described.[25,38,45]

MISCELLANEOUS INFECTIONS

Acinetobacter infection can occur in any body site. Reported ocular cases include conjunctivitis, endophthalmitis,[46] corneal ulceration caused by soft contact lens contamination, and corneal perforation.[47] Native and prosthetic valve endocarditis has been described.[48] Osteomyelitis, septic arthritis, and pancreatic and liver abscesses have also been reported.

▨ Antibiotic Resistance

As with other opportunistic gram-negative organisms (e.g., *Stenotrophomonas maltophilia*), increasing antibiotic resistance has hindered therapeutic management. Although there are significant differences in *Acinetobacter* antimicrobial resistance patterns according to species, country of isolation, and region,[49] the overall trend is one of increasing resistance. *Acinetobacter baumannii* isolates are frequently resistant to multiple antibiotic classes through an array of resistance mechanisms including the following: the production of antibiotic altering enzymes (e.g., cephalosporinases, carbapenemases, aminoglycoside-modifying enzymes); alterations in antibiotic targets (e.g., penicillin binding proteins, topoisomerases, DNA gyrase); limited antibiotic entry (e.g., porin mutations, limited porin production); and enhanced antibiotic egress (e.g., efflux pumps).[50,51]

Chromosomally encoded AmpC cephalosporinases are present in all *A. baumannii* isolates, but overexpression (and in vitro cephalosporin resistance) only occurs when an upstream insertion sequence (IS*Aba1*) is present. Serine oxacillinases and metallo-β-lactamases are causes of increasing carbapenem resistance existing in genetically mobile components, which facilitates resistance transmission. Relevant resistance to aminoglycosides has predominantly been via aminoglycoside-modifying enzymes; however, the recently described transposon-based *armA* gene codes for a 16S rRNA methylase that alters the target and thus creates high-level resistance to all aminoglycosides.[52] Multidrug efflux pumps can decrease quinolone, aminoglycoside, cephalosporin, carbapenem, trimethoprim, tigecycline, and tetracycline levels in the periplasmic space. The presence of additional antimicrobial resistance mechanisms working in concert with efflux pumps confounds therapeutic options. Polymyxin B and colistin resistance is thought to arise from alteration in lipopolysaccharide drug binding.[53] The presence of 45 *Acinetobacter* resistance genes was recently described by Fournier and colleagues in France as an 86-kb resistance "island"; some of the genes had not previously been reported to be associated with *Acinetobacter*.[54]

▨ Treatment

Acinetobacter may colonize the skin, pharynx, gastrointestinal tract, urethra, conjunctiva, and vagina. Interpretation of culture results must take into consideration colonization and potential environmental contamination. Isolation of *Acinetobacter* from colonized patients requires no specific therapy. Appropriate isolation precautions should be instituted on identification of *Acinetobacter* resistant to multiple antibiotic classes.

For years, β-lactams, particularly third-generation cephalosporins, extended-spectrum penicillins, penicillin–β-lactam inhibitor combinations and carbapenems, often combined with aminoglycosides in more severe infections, have been the mainstay of *Acinetobacter* therapy. However, most nosocomial *A. baumannii* are now resistant to many classes of antimicrobials. Fluoroquinolones, tigecycline, ceftazidime, trimethoprim-sulfamethoxazole, doxycycline, imipenem, meropenem, doripenem, polymyxin B, and colistin may retain activity against some nosocomial isolates.[55] Ertapenem has little intrinsic activity and should not be used. Heteroresistance to polymyxins has been reported but its clinical significance remains unclear.[56] The rapid development of significant resistance to quinolones, aminoglycosides, and carbapenems in selected areas worldwide[57] makes broad therapeutic generalizations difficult. As such, effective therapy must be individualized to reflect these differences in regional, local, and specific hospital resistance patterns.

Sulbactam has intrinsic bactericidal activity via penicillin-binding protein 2 separate from its inhibition of β-lactamases against some MDR *Acinetobacter* strains.[58] Tazobactam and clavulanic acid activities are less than that of sulbactam, and their clinical relevance is less well documented.[59] Sulbactam's efficacy is borne out by several reports documenting successful treatment of serious *Acinetobacter* infections, including meningitis and ventriculitis[36,60-62]; however, resistance to sulbactam has risen. In vitro data on more than 200 *A. baumannii* isolates have found imipenem (and meropenem) to have the lowest minimal inhibitory concentration (MIC) of available antimicrobial agents, with ampicillin-sulbactam being the most active of the remaining β-lactams.[63] Although imipenem and meropenem can be reliable agents, outbreaks of carbapenem-resistant *Acinetobacter* are of continuing concern and have been reported in the Americas, Europe, Africa, Asia, and the Middle East.[64] Imipenem or meropenem with an aminoglycoside and β-lactam–β-lactamase inhibitor with an aminoglycoside were found to be synergistic in vitro against MDR nosocomial *A. baumannii* isolates.[65] However, in vivo data assessing imipenem and amikacin synergy have been less compelling.[66] Fluoroquinolone and amikacin synergy was noted for *A. baumannii* isolates with a low quinolone minimal inhibitory MIC.[67] Species other than *A. baumannii* exhibit less overall antimicrobial resistance.

For MDR–*A. baumannii* infections combination therapy is often used and has included IV polymyxin B combined with rifampin, or imipenem or azithromycin. Polymyxins have been aerosolized for inhalational therapy of pneumonia[68,69] and injected intrathecally to treat *Acinetobacter* meningitis.[70] Imipenem combined with rifampin has been less clinically successful and associated with a high rate of rifampin resistance at the end of therapy.[71] A recent retrospective study comparing polymyxins with ampicillin-sulbactam when carbapenem resistance was present has suggested improved outcome in those who received sulbactam.[72] The clinician using β-lactams should be aware of therapeutic failures and relapses resulting from the emergence of resistance during therapy. Although experience with tigecycline is limited, use of this drug has also been associated with a gradual increase in resistance.

No strong recommendations can be made for any combination therapy. Controlled studies to evaluate the efficacy of these combinations are needed before formal recommendations can be given.

A hospital outbreak involving MDR *Acinetobacter* should prompt a review of infection control procedures involving hand washing, patient isolation,[73] ventilator care, and housekeeping. In addition, a case-control study and a review of local antimicrobial prescribing habits may be in order.[52] The use of nonabsorbable antibiotics for selective decontamination of the digestive tract has been suggested but has not gained clinical acceptance.[74]

REFERENCES

1. Maragakis LL, Perl TM. *Acinetobacter baumanii*: Epidemiology, antimicrobial resistance and treatment options. *Clin Infect Dis.* 2008;46:1254-1263.
2. Munoz-Price LS, Weinstein RA. Acinetobacter infection. *N Engl J Med.* 2008;358:1271-1281.
3. Cowan ST. Unusual infections following cerebral operations: With a description of *Diplococcus mucosus* (von Lingelsheim). *Lancet.* 1938;2:1052-1054.
4. De Bord GG. Description of Mimaeae Trib. nov. with three genera and three species and two new species of *Neisseria* from conjunctivitis and vaginitis. *Iowa State College J Sci.* 1942;16:471-480.
5. Brisou J, Prévot A-R. Etudes de systématique bactérienne: Revision des espèces réunies dans le genre Achromobacter. *Ann Inst Pasteur.* 1954;86:722-728.
6. Juni E. Interspecies transformation of *Acinetobacter*, genetic evidence for a ubiquitous genus. *J Bacteriol.* 1972;112:917-931.
7. Skerman VBD, McGowan V, Sneath PHA. Approved lists of bacterial names. *Int J Syst Bacteriol.* 1980;30:225-420.
8. Dijkshoorn L, Aucken H, Gerner-Smidt P, et al. Comparison of outbreak and nonoutbreak *Acinetobacter baumannii* strains by genotype and phenotypic methods. *J Clin Microbiol.* 1996;34:1519-1525.
9. Bouvet PJ, Grimont PAD. Taxonomy of the genus *Acinetobacter* with the recognition of *Acinetobacter baumannii* sp. nov., *Acinetobacter haemolyticus* sp. nov., *Acinetobacter johnsonii* sp. nov., and *Acinetobacter junii* sp. nov. and emended descriptions of *Acinetobacter calcoaceticus* and *Acinetobacter lwoffi*. *Int J Syst Bacteriol.* 1986;36:228-240.
10. Peleg AY, Seifert H, Paterson DL. *Acinetobacter baumannii*: Emergence of a successful pathogen. *Clin Micro Rev.* 2008;21:538-582.
11. Villegas MV, Hartstein AI. Acinetobacter outbreaks, 1977-2000. *Infect Control Hosp Epidemiol.* 2003;24:284-295.
12. Kramer A, Schwebke I, Kampf G. How long do nosocomial pathogens persist on inanimate surfaces? A systemic review. *BMC Infect Dis.* 2006;6:130-137.
13. Köljalg S, Naaber P, Mikelsaar M . Antibiotic resistance as an indicator of bacterial chlorhexidine susceptibility. *J Hosp Infect.* 2002;5:106-113.
14. Kawamura-Sato K, Wachino J, Kondo T, et al. Reduction of disinfectant bactericidal activities in clinically isolated Acineto- bacter species in the presence of organic material. *J Antimicrob Chemother.* 2008;61:568-576.
15. Al-Khoja MS, Darrell JH. The skin as the source of *Acinetobacter* and *Moraxella* species occurring in blood cultures. *J Clin Pathol.* 1979;32:497-499.
16. Baltimore RS, Duncan RL, Shapiro ED, et al. Epidemiology of pharyngeal colonization of infants with aerobic gram-negative rod bacteria. *J Clin Microbiol.* 1989;27:91-95.
17. Larson EL. Persistent carriage of gram-negative bacteria on hands. *Am J Infect Control.* 1981;9:112-119.
18. Gaynes R, Edwards JR; National Nosocomial Infections Surveillance System. Overview of nosocomial infections caused by gram-negative bacilli. *Clin Infect Dis.* 2005;41:848-854.
19. National Nosocomial Infections Surveillance System. National Nosocomial Infections Surveillance (NNIS) System Reports, data summary from January 1992 through June 2004, issued Oct 2004. *Am J Infect Control.* 2004;32:470-485.
20. Anstey NM, Currie BJ, Withnall KM. Community-acquired *Acinetobacter* pneumonia in the northern territory of Australia. *Clin Infect Dis.* 1992;14:83-91.
21. Lortholary O, Fagon J-Y, Hoi AB, et al. Nosocomial acquisition of multi-resistant *Acinetobacter baumannii*: Risk factors and prognosis. *Clin Infect Dis.* 1995;20:790-796.
22. Donskey CJ. Antibiotic regimens and intestinal colonization with antibiotic-resistant gram-negative bacilli. *Clin Infect Dis.* 2006;43(Suppl 2):S62-S69.
23. Scerpella EG, Wanger AR, Armitige L, et al. Nosocomial outbreak caused by a multiresistant clone of *Acinetobacter baumannii*: Results of the case-control and molecular epidemiologic investigations. *Infect Control Hosp Epidemiol.* 1995;16:92-97.
24. Joly-Guillou M-L. Clinical impact and pathogenicity of *Acinetobacter*. *Clin Microbiol Infect.* 2005;11:868-873.
25. Glew RH, Moellering RC Jr, Kunz LJ. Infections with *Acinetobacter calcoaceticus (Herellea vaginicola)*: Clinical and laboratory studies. *Medicine (Baltimore).* 1977;56:79-97.
26. O'Connell CJ, Hamilton R. Gram-negative rod infections: II. *Acinetobacter* infections in general hospital. *N Y State J Med.* 1981;81:750-753.
27. Goodhart GL, Abrutyn E, Watson R, et al. Community-acquired *Acinetobacter calcoaceticus* var *anitratus* pneumonia. *JAMA.* 1977;238:1516-1518.
28. Anstey NM, Currie BJ, Hassell M, et al. Community-acquired bacteremic *Acinetobacter* pneumonia in tropical Australia is caused by diverse strains of *Acinetobacter baumannii*, with carriage in the throat of at-risk groups. *J Clin Microbiol.* 2002;40:685-686.
29. Leung WS, Chu CM, Tsang KY, et al. Fulminant community-acquired *Acinetobacter baumannii* pneumonia as a distinct clinical sydrome. *Chest.* 2006;120:102-109.
30. Whitman TJ, Qasba SS, Timpone JG, et al. Occupational transmission of *Acinetobacter baumannii* from the United States servicemen wounded in Iraq to a health care worker. *Clin Infect Dis.* 2008;47:439-443.
31. Fagon J-Y, Chastre J, Domart Y, et al. Mortality due to ventilator-associated pneumonia or colonization with *Pseudomonas* or *Acinetobacter* species: Assessment by quantitative culture of samples obtained by protected specimen brush. *Clin Infect Dis.* 1996;23:538-542.
32. Robinson RG, Garrison RG, Brown BW. Evaluation of the clinical significance of the genus *Herellea*. *Ann Intern Med.* 1964;60:19-25.
33. Seifert H, Strate A, Pulverer G. Nosocomial bacteremia due to *Acinetobacter baumannii*. Clinical features, epidemiology, and predictors of mortality. *Medicine (Baltimore).* 1995;74:340-349.
34. Kozub WR, Bucolo S, Sami AW, et al. Gonorrhea-like urethritis due to *Mima polymorpha* var. *oxidans*: Patient summary and bacteriological study. *Arch Intern Med.* 1968;122:514-516.
35. Chang WN, Lu CH, Huang CR, et al. Community-acquired *Acinetobacter* meningitis in adults. *Infection.* 2000;28:395-397.
36. Allen DM, Wong SY. *Acinetobacter*: A perspective. *Singapore Med J.* 1990;31:511-514.
37. Lindberg RB, Wetzler TF, Newton A, et al. The bacterial flora of the bloodstream in the Korean battle casualty. *Ann Surg.* 1955;141:366-368.
38. Tong MJ. Septic complications of war wounds. *JAMA.* 1972;222:1044-1047.
39. Sebeny PJ, Riddle MS, Peterson K. *Acinetobacter baumannii* skin and soft tissue infections associated with war trauma. *Clin Infect Dis.* 2008;48:444-449.
40. Aronson NE, Sanders JW, Moran KA. In harm's way: Infections in deployed American military forces. *Clin Infect Dis.* 2006;43:1045-1051.

41. Scott P, Deye G, Srinivasan A, et al. An outbreak of multidrug-resistant *Acinetobacter baumanii-calcoaceticus* complex infection in the US military health care system associated with military operations in Iraq. *Clin Infect Dis.* 2007;44:1577-1584.

42. Hawley JS, Murray CK ,Griffith ME, et al. Susceptibility of *Acinetobacter* strains isolated from deployed US military personnel. *Antimicrob Agents Chemother.* 2007;51:376-378.

43. Maegele M, Gregor S, Steinhausen E, et al. The long-distance tertiary air transfer and care of tsunami victims: Injury patterns and microbiologic and psychologic aspects. *Crit Care Med.* 2005;33:1136-1140.

44. Oncul O, Keskin O, Acar HV, et al. Hospital-acquired infections following the 1999 Marmara earthquake. *J Hosp Infect.* 2002;51: 47-51.

45. Amsel MB, Horrilleno E. Synergistic necrotizing fasciitis: A case of polymicrobial infection with *Acinetobacter calcoaceticus*. *Curr Surg.* 1985;42:370-372.

46. Peyman GA, Vastine DW, Diamond JG. Vitrectomy and intra-ocular gentamicin management of *Herellea* endophthalmitis after incomplete phacoemulsification. *Am J Ophthalmol.* 1975;80: 764-765.

47. Wand M, Olive GM, Mangiaracine AB. Corneal perforation and iris prolapse due to *Mima polymorpha*. *Arch Ophthalmol.* 1975;93:239-241.

48. Gradon JD, Chapnick EK, Lutwick LI. Infective endocarditis of a native valve due to *Acinetobacter*: Case report and review. *Clin Infect Dis.* 1992;14:1145-1148.

49. Landman D, Quale JM, Mayorga D, et al. Citywide clonal outbreak of multiresistant *Acinetobacter baumannii* and *Pseudomonas aeruginosa* in Brooklyn, NY: The preantibiotic era has returned. *Arch Intern Med.* 2002;162:1515-1520.

50. Bonomo RA, Szabo D. Mechanisms of multidrug resistance in *Acinetobacter* species and *Pseudomonas aeruginosa*. *Clin Infect Dis.* 2006;43(Suppl 2):S49-S56.

51. Vila J, Martí S, Sánchez-Céspedes J. Porins, efflux pumps and multidrugresistance in *Acinetobacter baumannii*. *J Antimicrob Chemother.* 2007;59:1210-1215.

52. Doi Y, Adams JM, Yamane K, et al. Identification of 16S rRNA methylase-producing *Acinetobacter baumannii* clinical strains in North America. *Antimicrob Agents Chemother.* 2007;51: 4209-4210.

53. Peterson AA, Fesik SW, McGroarty EJ. Decreased binding of antibiotics to lipopolysaccharides from polymyxin-resistant strains of *Escherichia coli* and *Salmonella typhmurium*. *Antimicrob Agents Chemother.* 1987;31:230-237.

54. Fournier PE, Vallenet V, Berbe S, et al. Comparative genomes of multidrug resistance in *Acinetobacter baumanii*. *PLoS Genet.* 2006;2:e7.

55. Seifert H, Baginski R, Schulze A, et al. Antimicrobial susceptibility of *Acinetobacter* species. *Antimicrob Agents Chemother.* 1993; 37:750-753.

56. Li J, Rayner CR, Nation RL, et al. Heteroresistance to colistin in multidrug-resistant *Acinetobacter baumanii*. *Antimicrob Agents Chemother.* 2006;50:2946-2950.

57. Poirel L, Nordmann P. Carbapenem resistance in *Acinetobacter baumanii*: Mechanisms and epidemiology. *Clin Microbiol Infect.* 2006;12:826-836.

58. Urban C, Go E, Mariano N, et al. Effect of sulbactam on infections caused by imipenem-resistant *Acinetobacter calcoaceticus* biotype *anitratus*. *J Infect Dis.* 1993;167:448-451.

59. Amyes SGB. β-Lactam resistance and the use of inhibitor combinations. *J Med Microbiol.* 1997;46:728-731.

60. Jiménez-Mejías ME, Pachón J, Becerril B, et al. Treatment of multi-drug resistant *Acinetobacter baumannii* meningitis with ampicillin/sulbactam. *Clin Infect Dis.* 1997;24:932-935.

61. Jellison TK, Mkinnon PS, Rybak MJ. Epidemiology, resistance, and outcomes of *Acinetobacter baumannii* bacteremia treated with imipenem-cilastatin or ampicillin-sulbactam. *Pharmacotherapy.* 2001;21:142-148.

62. Wood GC, Hanes SD, Croce MA, et al. Comparison of ampicillin-sulbactam and imipenem-cilastatin for the treatment of *Acinetobacter* ventilator-associated pneumonia. *Clin Infect Dis.* 2002;34:1425-1430.

63. Visalli MA, Jacobs MR, Moore TD, et al. Activities of β-lactams against *Acinetobacter* genospecies as determined by agar dilution and e-test MIC methods. *Antimicrob Agents Chemother.* 1997; 41:767-770.

64. Tankovic J, Legrand P, De Gatines G, et al. Characterization of a hospital outbreak of imipenem-resistant *Acinetobacter baumannii* by phenotypic and genotypic typing methods. *J Clin Microbiol.* 1994;32:2677-2681.

65. Marques MB, Brookings ES, Moser SA, et al. Comparative in vitro antimicrobial susceptibilities of nosocomial isolates of *Acinetobacter baumannii* and synergistic activities of nine antimicrobial combinations. *Antimicrob Agents Chemother.* 1997; 41:881-885.

66. Bernabeu-Wittel M, Pichardo C, Garcia-Curiel A, et al. Pharmakinetic/ pharmacodynamic assessment of the *in-vivo* efficacy of imipenem alone or in combination with amikacin for the treatment of experimental multiresistant *Acinetobacter baumanii* pneumonia. *Clin Microb Infect.* 2005;11:319-325.

67. Bajaksouzian S, Visalli MA, Jacobs MR, et al. Activities of levofloxacin, ofloxacin, ciprofloxacin, alone and in combination with amikacin, against acinetobacters as determined by checkerboard and time-kill studies. *Antimicrob Agents Chemother.* 1997;41: 1073-1076.

68. Falagas ME, Kasiakou SK. Toxicity of polymyxins: A systemic review of the evidence from old and recent studies. *Crit Care.* 2006;10:R27.

69. Kwa AL, Loh C, Low JG, et al. Nebulized colistin in the treatment of pneumonia due to multidrug resistant *Acinetobacter baumanii* and *Pseudomonas aeruginosa*. *Clin Infect Dis.* 2005; 41:754-757.

70. Rahal JJ. Novel antibiotic combinations against infections with almost completely resistant *Pseudomonas aeruginosa* and *Acinetobacter* species. *Clin Infect Dis.* 2006;43(Suppl 2):S95-S99.

71. Saballs ML, Pujol M, Tubau F, et al. Rifampicin/imipenem combination in the treatment of carbapenem-resistant *Acinetobacter baumannii* infections. *J Antimicrob Chemother.* 2006;58:697-700.

72. Oliveira MS, Prado GV, Costa SF, et al. Ampicillin/sulbactam compared with polymyxins for the treatment of infections caused by carbapenem-resistant *Acinetobacter* spp. *J Antimicrob Chemother.* 2008;61:1369-1375.

73. Brooks SE, Walczak MA, Hameed R. Are we doing enough to contain *Acinetobacter* infections? *Infect Control Hosp Epidemiol.* 2000;21:304.

74. Bonten MJ. Selective digestive tract decontamination—will it prevent infection with multidrug-resistant gram-negative pathogens but still be applicable in institutions where methicillin-resistant *Staphylococcus aureus* and vancomycin-resistant enterococci are endemic? *Clin Infect Dis.* 2006;43(Suppl 2):S70-S74.

223

Salmonella Species, Including Salmonella Typhi

DAVID A. PEGUES | SAMUEL I. MILLER

Salmonellae are named for the pathologist Salmon, who first isolated *Salmonella choleraesuis* from porcine intestine.[1] *Salmonella* are effective commensals and pathogens that cause a spectrum of diseases in humans and animals, including domesticated and wild mammals, reptiles, birds, and insects. Some *Salmonella* serotypes, such as *Salmonella* Typhi, *Salmonella* Paratyphi, and *Salmonella* Sendai, are highly adapted to humans and have no other known natural hosts, whereas others, such as *Salmonella* Typhimurium, have a broad host range and can infect a wide variety of animal hosts and humans. Some *Salmonella* serotypes, such as Dublin (cattle) and Arizonae (reptiles), are mostly adapted to an animal species and only occasionally infect humans. The widespread distribution of *Salmonella* in the environment, their increasing prevalence in the global food chain, and their virulence and adaptability have an enormous medical, public health, and economic impact worldwide.

History

Before the 19th century, typhus and typhoid fever were confused. Though various clinical distinctions were proposed, none reliably distinguished these syndromes. In 1829 in Paris, P. Ch. A. Louis separated typhoid from other fevers on the basis of intestinal lymph node and spleen pathology.[2] He also described the clinical phenomena of rose spots, intestinal perforation, and hemorrhage. In the English literature, William Jenner in 1850 settled the question of whether typhus and typhoid were different diseases.[3] He distinguished typhoid based on the pathologic evidence of enlargement of the Peyer's patches and mesenteric lymph nodes. Jenner also noted that prior attacks of typhoid protected against subsequent attacks; this was not the case for typhus. In 1869, Wilson proposed the term *enteric fever* as an alternative to typhoid fever, given the anatomic site of infection.[4] Though enteric fever remains a more accurate term, the use of the term *typhoid* persists today.

In 1873 Budd demonstrated that food, water, and fomites could transmit typhoid fever.[5] Gaffkey in Germany isolated the typhoid bacillus in 1884 from the spleens of infected patients.[6] In 1896, Pfeiffer and Kalle made the first typhoid vaccine with heat-killed organisms.[7] In the same year Widal and others demonstrated that convalescent sera from typhoid patients caused the organisms to "stick together in large balls and lose their motility."[8] Widal coined the term *agglutinin* to describe this observation. The antigenic classification or serotyping of *Salmonella* used today is a result of years of study of antibody interactions with bacterial surface antigens by Kauffman and White during the 1920s to 1940s.[9] In 1948, Theodore Woodward and colleagues reported the successful treatment of Malaysian typhoid patients with chloromycetin,[10] and the modern age of antimicrobial therapy for typhoid fever began. In 1952, Zinder and Lederberg, using *S.* Typhimurium, discovered genetic transduction, the transfer of genetic information from one cell to another by a virus particle (bacteriophage P22).[11] Ames and coworkers in 1973 reported the development of the Ames test, which uses *S.* Typhimurium auxotrophic mutants to test the mutagenic activity of chemical compounds.[12] At present *Salmonella* pathogenesis is studied widely in animal and tissue culture models of mammalian infection as an important model of host-parasite interactions.

Classification and Taxonomy

Salmonella is a genus of the family of Enterobacteriaceae. Before 1983, the existence of multiple *Salmonella* species was taxonomically accepted. Currently, as a result of experiments indicating a high degree of DNA similarity, the genus *Salmonella* is separated into two species: *Salmonella enterica,* which contains six subspecies (I, II, IIIa, IIIb, IV, and VI), and *Salmonella bongori,* which was formerly subspecies V.[13] *S. enterica* subspecies I contains almost all the serotypes pathogenic for humans, except for rare human infections with subspecies IIIa and IIIb that were formerly designated by the genus *Arizonae.*

Members of the seven *Salmonella* subspecies can be serotyped into one of more than 2500 serotypes (serovars) according to antigenically diverse surface structures: somatic O antigens, the carbohydrate component of lipopolysaccharide, and flagellar (H) antigens (Table 223-1).[13] The name usually refers to the location where the *Salmonella* serotype was first isolated. According to the current *Salmonella* nomenclature system in use at the U.S. Centers for Disease Control and Prevention (CDC) and World Health Organization laboratories, the full taxonomic designation *Salmonella enterica* subspecies *enterica* serotype Typhimurium can be shortened to *Salmonella* serotype Typhimurium or *Salmonella* Typhimurium.[14] The authors have chosen to use the abbreviated form in this chapter and will omit the "serotype," for example, designating "*Salmonella* serotype Typhimurium" as "*Salmonella* Typhimurium."

The Genome

The genome sequences of 15 complete salmonellae serotypes, including two *S.* Typhi strains, two *S.* Paratyphi A strains, and one *S.* Paratyphi B strain, six nontyphoidal strains, and numerous other species-specific serotypes including Arizonae, Choleraesuis, Dublin, and Gallinarum, are available in Genbank. Twenty-five other partially completed genomes using next generation sequencing technology also are available, including 15 *S.* Typhi sequences.[15] The salmonellae genomes contain approximately 4.8 to 4.9 million base pairs with approximately 4400 to 5600 coding sequences. A characteristic phenomenon of host restriction such as that found for *S.* Typhi is gene loss. In *S.* Typhi strain CT18 there are 204 inactivated pseudogenes, which may explain its host restriction to humans, though a recent publication comparing *Salmonella* Gallinarum, which is host restricted to poultry, to *Salmonella* Enteritidis phage type 4, which infects poultry and is broad host range, found significant overlap between the defined pseudogenes in both *S.* Typhi and *S.* Gallinarum.[15,16]

Microbiology

Salmonellae are gram-negative, non-spore-forming, facultatively anaerobic bacilli that measure 2 to 3 by 0.4 to 0.6 µm in size. Like other Enterobacteriaceae, they produce acid on glucose fermentation, reduce nitrates, and do not produce cytochrome oxidase.[17] All organisms except *S.* Gallinarum-Pullorum are motile as a result of peritrichous flagella, and most do not ferment lactose. However, approximately 1% of organisms are able to ferment lactose and therefore may not be

TABLE 223-1	*Salmonella* Species, Subspecies, and Serotypes and Their Usual Habitats		
Salmonella *Species and Subspecies*		**No. of Serotypes Within Subspecies**	**Usual Habitat**
S. enterica subsp. *enterica* (I)		1504	Warm-blooded animals
S. enterica subsp. *salmae* (II)		502	Cold-blooded animals and the environment*
S. enterica subsp. *arizonae* (IIIa)		95	Cold-blooded animals and the environment*
S. enterica subsp. *diarizonae* (IIIb)		333	Cold-blooded animals and the environment*
S. enterica subsp. *houtenae* (IV)		72	Cold-blooded animals and the environment*
S. enterica subsp. *indica* (VI)		13	Cold-blooded animals and the environment*
S. bongori (V)		22	Cold-blooded animals and the environment*
Total		2541	

*Isolates of all species and subspecies have occurred in humans.
Adapted from Popoff MY, Bockemühl J, Gheesling LL. Supplement 2002 (No. 46) to the Kauffmann-White scheme. *Res Microbiol.* 2004;155:568-570.

detected if only MacConkey agar or other semiselective media are used to identify *Salmonella* based on colorimetric assay for fermentation of lactose. The differential metabolism of sugars can be used to distinguish many *Salmonella* serotypes; serotype Typhi is the only organism that does not produce gas on sugar fermentation.[17]

Freshly passed stool is preferred for the isolation of *Salmonella* and should be plated directly onto agar plates. Low-selective media, such as MacConkey agar and deoxycholate agar, and intermediate-selective media, such as Salmonella-Shigella, xylose-lysine-deoxycholate, or Hektoen agar, are widely used to screen for both *Salmonella* and *Shigella* species. Selective chromogenic media, such as CHROMagar, are more specific than other selective media, reduce the need for confirmatory testing and time to identification, and increasingly are used for the primary isolation and presumptive identification of *Salmonella* from clinical stool specimens.[18]

In addition to plating stool onto primary media, tetrathionate- and selenite-based enrichment broths are often used to facilitate the recovery of low numbers of organisms.[18] Highly *Salmonella*-selective media, such as selenite with brilliant green, should be reserved for use in stool cultures of suspected carriers and under special circumstances, such as outbreaks. Bismuth sulfite agar, which contains an indicator of hydrogen sulfite production and does not contain lactose, is preferred for the isolation of *S.* Typhi and can be used for the detection of the 1% of *Salmonella* strains (including most *Salmonella* serogroup C strains) that ferment lactose.[19] After primary isolation, possible *Salmonella* isolates can be tested in commercial identification systems or inoculated into screening media such as triple-sugar–iron and lysine-iron agar. Direct detection of *Salmonella* from stool and food specimens using polymerase chain reaction (PCR) and rapid serologic diagnosis using anti-*Salmonella* 09 IgM antibodies are under development.[20-22]

Isolates with typical biochemical profiles for *Salmonella* should be serogrouped with commercially available polyvalent antisera or sent to a reference or public health laboratory for complete serogrouping. Salmonellae are serogrouped according to their polysaccharide O (somatic) antigens, Vi (capsular) antigens, and H (flagellar) antigens according to the Kauffman-White scheme.[23] The Vi antigen is a heat-labile capsular homopolymer of *N*-acetylgalactosaminouronic acid that is used for the identification of *S.* Typhi strains and occasionally other *Salmonella* serotypes by slide agglutination.[24] In *S.* Typhi and *S.* Paratyphi C, the polysaccharide Vi antigen can inhibit O antigen agglutination because it is so abundant, and boiling is required to inactive Vi antigen and to detect O antigen. Most antigenic variability occurs in the O antigen, which is composed of chains of oligosaccharide attached to a core oligosaccharide linked covalently to lipid A.

Although serotyping of all surface antigens can be used for formal identification, most laboratories perform a few simple agglutination reactions that define specific O antigens into serogroups, designated as groups A, B, C_1, C_2, D, and E *Salmonella*. Strains in these six serogroups cause approximately 99% of *Salmonella* infections in humans and warm-blooded animals. Although this grouping is useful in epidemiologic studies and can be used to confirm genus identification, it cannot identify whether the organism is likely to cause enteric fever, because considerable cross-reactivity occurs among serogroups. For example, *S.* Enteritidis, which typically causes gastroenteritis, and *S.* Typhi, which causes enteric fever, are both group D. Similarly, another frequent cause of gastroenteritis, *S.* Typhimurium, and some *S.* Paratyphi, another cause of enteric fever, are both group B.

Subtyping methods frequently are used for epidemiologic purposes to differentiate strains of common *Salmonella* serotypes. Phenotyping methods may be useful for characterizing outbreak-associated strains and sporadic multidrug-resistant isolates, and include bacteriophage typing, plasmid profile analysis, antimicrobial susceptibility, and biotyping. More discriminative genotyping techniques, including ribotyping, pulsed-field gel electrophoresis, insertion sequences analysis, PCR-based fingerprinting, multilocus sequence typing, and genomic DNA analysis using microarrays have been used in epidemiologic studies to differentiate strains within a given serotype.

Epidemiology

SALMONELLA TYPHI AND SALMONELLA PARATYPHI

In contrast to other *Salmonella* serotypes, the etiologic agents of enteric fever—*S.* Typhi and *S.* Paratyphi serotypes A, B, and C—have no known hosts other than humans. Most commonly, foodborne or waterborne transmission occurs as a result of fecal contamination by ill or asymptomatic chronic carriers. Usually, waterborne transmission involves the ingestion of fewer microorganisms and, as a result, has a longer incubation period and lower attack rate compared with foodborne transmission. Although direct person-to-person transmission is uncommon, *S.* Typhi can be transmitted sexually, including by anal and oral sex.[25] Health care workers can acquire the disease from infected patients as a result of poor hand hygiene or handling laboratory specimens.[26]

Enteric fever continues to be a global health problem, with an estimated 21.6 million cases caused by *S.* Typhi and 5.5 million cases caused by *S.* Paratyphi A, B, or C annually and an incidence ranging from 25 to 1000 cases per 100,000 population in endemic regions.[27,28] An estimated 200,000 to 600,000 deaths occur annually, based on extrapolation from endemic regions.[27] Regions with a high incidence of typhoid fever (>100/100,000 cases/year) include south-central Asia and southeast Asia. Regions of medium incidence (10-100/100,000 cases/year) include the rest of Asia, Africa, Latin America and the Caribbean, and Oceania, except for Australia and New Zealand (Fig. 223-1).[27] The incidence of enteric fever correlates with poor sanitation and lack of access to clean drinking water. In endemic regions, typhoid fever is more common in urban than rural areas and among young children and adolescents (aged 1 to 15 years). Reported risk factors include contaminated water or ice, flooding, food and drinks purchased from street vendors, raw fruits and vegetables grown in fields fertilized with sewage, ill contacts in the household, lack of handwashing and toilets, and evidence of prior *Helicobacter pylori* infection, likely related to chronic reduced gastric acidity. Outbreaks of typhoid fever in developing countries can result in high morbidity and mortality, especially among children less than 5 years of age and when caused by antimicrobial-resistant strains.[29,30] Between 1970 and 1989, many strains of *S.* Typhi developed plasmid-mediated multidrug resistance to the common first-line antimicrobials chloramphenicol, ampicillin, and trimethoprim in many regions of the world, especially in the Indian subcontinent and south Asia.[31] Although these multidrug-resistant strains belonged to different Vi phage types, they typically contain a self-transferable 120-MDa plasmid of the H1 incompatibility

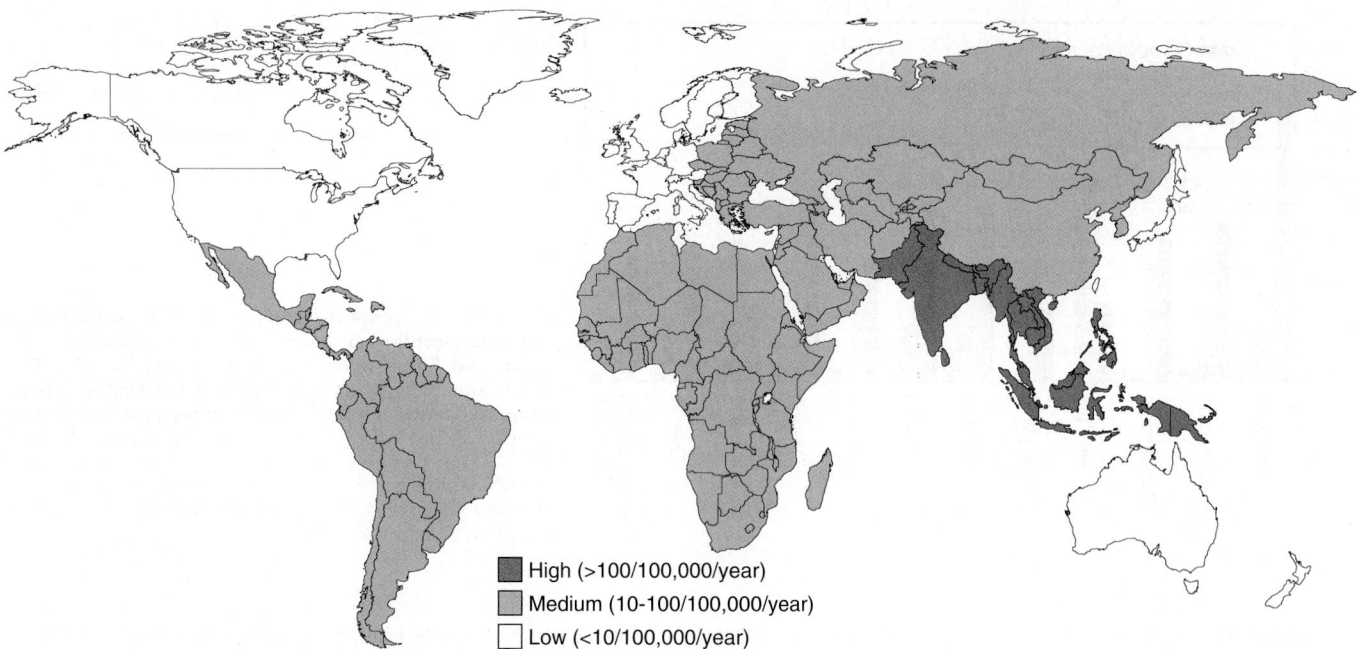

Figure 223-1 **Annual incidence of typhoid fever per 100,000 population.** *(Adapted from Crump JA, Luby SP, Mintz ED. The global burden of typhoid fever. Bull World Health Organ. 2004;82:346-353.)*

type that often also encodes resistance to streptomycin, sulfonamides, and tetracyclines.[31] In the 1990s, with the increased use fluoroquinolones for treatment of multidrug-resistant typhoid fever, chromosomal and plasmid-encoded resistance to ciprofloxacin emerged among S. Typhi and S. Paratyphi A isolates from the Indian subcontinent and south Asia.[32] In 2003, in Katmandu, Nepal, 73.3% and 94.9% of S. Typhi and S. Paratyphi A strains contained gyrA gene mutation, were resistant to nalidixic acid, and had decreased susceptibility to fluoroquinolones (ciprofloxacin minimum inhibitory concentration [MIC] 0.25-1.0 μg/mL), a phenotype associated with an increased risk of fluoroquinolone treatment failure.[33,34] Even more alarmingly, in 2005, 22% of S. Typhi strains from New Delhi, India, were resistant to ciprofloxacin and 16% were resistant to ceftriaxone.[35] Although multidrug-resistant strains remain common in many areas of Asia, in some areas antimicrobial-susceptible strains have reemerged and are genetically unrelated to the previous multidrug-resistant clones.[36]

With improvements in food handling and water/sewage treatment, enteric fever has become a rare occurrence in developed nations. In 2006, a total of 353 cases of typhoid fever were reported in the United States compared with 35,994 cases in 1920.[37] From 25% to 30% of reported cases of enteric fever in the United States are domestically acquired. Although the majority of these cases are sporadic, 7% of total cases were part of recognized outbreaks linked to contaminated food products and previously unrecognized chronic carriers.[38]

The incidence of typhoid among U.S. travelers is estimated to be 3 to 30 cases per 100,000.[38] Of 1393 cases of typhoid fever reported to the CDC between 1994 and 1999, 74% were associated with recent international travel, most commonly to India (30%), Pakistan (13%), Mexico (12%), Bangladesh (8%), the Philippines (8%), and Haiti (5%). An increased proportion of cases are associated with foreign-born U.S. residents visiting friends and relatives (~80%). Only 4% of travelers diagnosed with enteric fever gave a history of S. Typhi vaccination within the previous 5 years. Increased rates of multidrug-resistant S. Typhi and S. Paratyphi have been reported among travelers returning to the United States and United Kingdom.[39,40] In the United States, 42% of recent S. Typhi isolates and 87% of S. Paratyphi isolates were resistant to nalidixic acid and had a decreased susceptibility to ciprofloxacin (MIC ≥ 0.12 μg/mL).[39,41]

NONTYPHOIDAL SALMONELLAE

In many countries the incidence of human *Salmonella* infections has increased markedly, although good population-based surveillance data are mostly lacking. In the United States, the incidence rate of nontyphoidal *Salmonella* infection has doubled in the last two decades, with an estimated 1.4 million cases occurring annually (Fig. 223-2).[42] In 2007, the incidence rate of salmonellosis (14.9 per 100,000 population) was highest among 11 potentially foodborne diseases under active

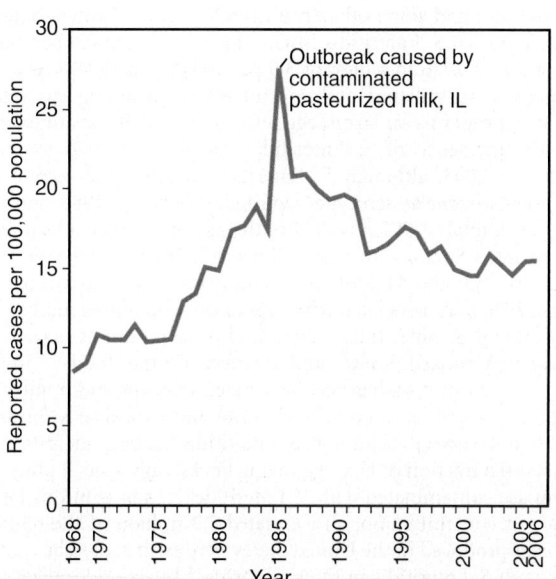

Figure 223-2 **Incidence rate per 100,000 population of nontyphoidal salmonellosis by year, United States, 1968 through 2006.** *(Adapted from McNabb SJ, Jajosky RA, Hall-Baker PA, et al. Summary of notifiable diseases—United States, 2006. MMWR Morb Mortal Wkly Rep. 2008;55:75).*

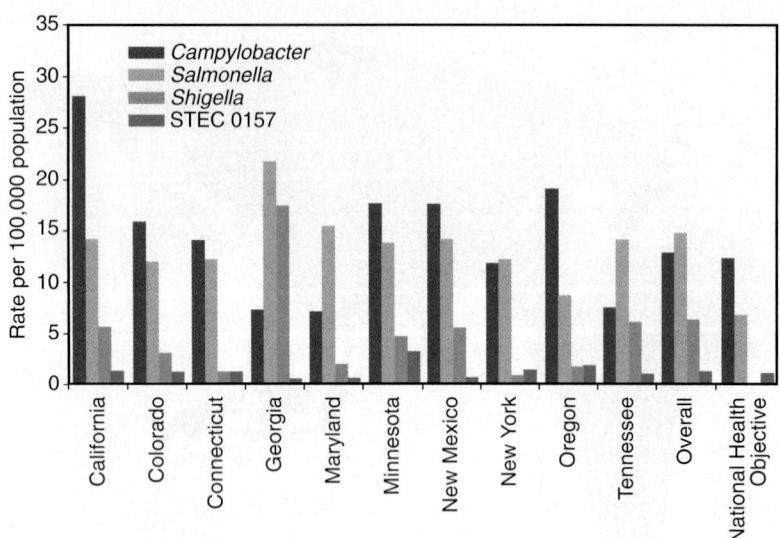

Figure 223-3 Incidence rate per 100,000 population of laboratory-confirmed *Salmonella, Campylobacter, Shigella,* and Shiga toxin producing *E. coli* O157 (STEC 1057) infections by selected sites in the United States, compared with national health objectives (Foodborne Diseases Active Surveillance Network, 2007). *(From Centers for Disease Control and Prevention (CDC). Preliminary FoodNet data on the incidence of foodborne illnesses—selected sites, United States, 2007. MMWR Morb Mortal Wkly Rep. 2008;57:366-370.)*

surveillance, ranging from 8.65 to 21.78 per 100,000 population (Fig 223-3).[43] Compared to 1996 to 1998, relative rates of *Salmonella* decreased only 8% in 2007. During this period, five *Salmonella* serotypes accounted for one-half of all human isolates reported in the United States—Typhimurium (19%), Enteritidis (14%), Newport (9%), Javiana (5%), and Heidelberg (4%).[43] The incidence of nontyphoidal *Salmonella* infection is highest during the rainy season in tropical climates and during the warmer months in temperate climates, coinciding with the peak in foodborne outbreaks.[44]

Unlike *S.* Typhi and *S.* Paratyphi, whose only reservoir is humans, nontyphoidal *Salmonella* can be acquired from multiple animal reservoirs. Transmission of *Salmonella* to humans can occur by many routes, including consumption of food animal products, especially eggs, poultry, undercooked ground meat and dairy products, fresh produce contaminated with animal waste, contact with animals or their environment, and contaminated water.[45-47] During the 1980s and 1990s, *S.* Enteritidis associated with shell eggs emerged as the predominant *Salmonella* serotype and source of foodborne disease in the United States and some other countries.[48,49] In the United States, the rate of reported *S.* Enteritidis isolates increased from 0.6 per 100,000 population in 1976 to a high of 3.9 per 100,000 in 1994.[50] As a result of intensive surveillance and control effort, including egg quality-assurance programs on farms, egg refrigeration, and consumer education, the incidence of *S.* Enteritidis infection declined to 1.7 per 100,000 in 2003, although *S.* Enteritidis remains the second most common *Salmonella* serotype reported.[50] Between 1985 and 2003, there was a total of 997 reported outbreaks of *S.* Enteritidis infection in the United States, with 33,687 illnesses, 3281 hospitalizations, and 82 deaths.[50] Of the 44% of these outbreaks with a confirmed food vehicle, 75% were associated with eggs or egg-containing ingredients.[50] Outbreaks of *S.* Enteritidis infection also have been associated with inadequately cooked poultry and a variety of other foods.[50] Sporadic *S.* Enteritidis infection has been associated with egg and poultry consumption as well as international travel and exposure to birds and reptiles in the home.[51] Although *S.* Enteritidis has been identified from a substantial fraction of U.S. egg-laying flocks, only a small proportion of eggs are contaminated with *S.* Enteritidis.[52] Even with this low frequency of contamination, an estimated 2.2 million of the 65 billion shell eggs produced in the United States were estimated to be contaminated with *S.* Enteritidis in the mid-1990s.[52] Infection localizes to the ovaries and upper oviduct tissue and is transmitted to the forming egg before shell deposition, resulting in contamination of the albumen and yolk. Although cooking eggs until all liquid yolk is solidified kills *S.* Enteritidis, the use of pasteurized egg products remains the safest alternative for institutions and the general public.

Transmission of *S.* Enteritidis from farm to farm may be facilitated by contaminated chicken manure, insects, and rodents and by ingestion of feed contaminated with mouse droppings, because *S.* Enteritidis strains cultured from the spleens of mice caught on farms have enhanced ability to contaminate eggs.[53] The loss of cross-immunity resulting from culling chickens infected with *S.* Gallinarum and *S.* Pullorum in the United States and United Kingdom also may have contributed to the emergence of *S.* Enteritidis.[54] *Salmonella* live in the intestines of most food animals, and contamination of raw poultry and meat products can occur during slaughter and processing. Retail ground poultry and meat are at high risk of contamination with *Salmonella*, including with antimicrobial resistant strains.[55] In a 2007 survey of food products, 26.3% of ground chicken, 17.9% of ground turkey, and 2.7% of ground beef specimens tested positive for *Salmonella*.[56] Although raw chicken carcasses and other meats are less commonly contaminated with *Salmonella* than is ground poultry, cross-contamination of food items from handling of raw chicken and inadequate hand hygiene are risks for sporadic salmonellosis in the home.[57] There is considerable mismatch between animal and human *Salmonella* serotypes, suggesting that the risk of transmission is not equal for all food products and serotypes.[58]

Changes in food consumption and the rapid growth of international trade in agricultural food products have facilitated the dissemination of new *Salmonella* serotypes associated with fresh fruits and vegetables. Human or animal feces may contaminate the surface of fruits and vegetables and may not be removed by washing. Recent foodborne outbreaks of salmonellosis associated with fresh produce include tomatoes (*S.* Newport), cantaloupe (multiple serotypes), unpasteurized orange juice (multiple serotypes), cilantro (*S.* Thompson), and raw seed sprouts (*S.* Muenchen and *S.* Stanley). Tomatoes can internalize *Salmonella* when imersed in water, and contamination on the tomato or melon surface can be transferred to the interior when it is cut.[59] Sprout seeds can become contaminated before sprouting, and soaking seeds with 20,000 ppm calcium hypochlorite or other disinfectant can reduce, but does not eliminate, the risk of sprout-associated illness.[60]

Manufactured food items pose an enormous potential hazard of foodborne salmonellosis in developed countries because of their centralized production and wide-scale distribution. Both pasteurized and unpasteurized milk and milk products, including powdered infant formula, have increasingly been recognized as a source of *Salmonella* infections.[61] In 1994, an estimated 224,000 cases of *S.* Enteritidis gastroenteritis developed among persons in the United States who ate a nationally distributed ice cream product. The source of the *S.* Enteritidis was most likely pasteurized ice cream premix that was contaminated during transport in tanker trailers that previously carried nonpasteurized liquid eggs.[62] In 2008 to 2009, a large multistate outbreak of *S.* Typhimurium infection was associated with peanut butter and peanut paste used in more than 180 different food products.

Salmonellosis associated with exotic pets is a resurgent public health problem, especially from exposure to reptiles, including turtles, iguanas, lizards, and snakes.[63,64] Of all *Salmonella* serotypes, 40% have been cultured predominantly from reptiles and are rarely found in other animals or humans. The recognition of pet turtle–associated salmonellosis led to the banning of shipment of small pet turtles in several countries but not to elimination of the problem.[65] Based on extrapolation from population-based surveillance, 6% of all sporadic *Salmonella* infections and 11% among persons less than 21 years old are attributable to contact with reptiles or amphibians.[64] Exposure to pet birds, pet rodents, dogs, and cats and to pet food and pet treats made from animal parts are other potential sources of human salmonellosis, including infection with multidrug-resistant strains.[66-68]

Multidrug resistance among human nontyphoidal *Salmonella* isolates is increasing in both developing and developed countries (Fig. 223-4).[41,69,70] A diversity of transferable resistance plasmids have been identified from multidrug-resistant nontyphoidal *Salmonella* strains and contribute to the conjugative transfer of resistance between enteric bacterial species.[71] Of particular concern is the worldwide emergence in the 1990s of a distinct strain of multidrug-resistant *S.* Typhimurium characterized as definitive phage type 104 (DT104) that is resistant to at least five antimicrobials—ampicillin, chloramphenicol, streptomycin, sulfonamides, and tetracyclines (R-type ACSSuT).[72] All DT104 strains contain a chromosome- and integron-encoded β-lactamase (PSE-1) that appears to have been acquired from plasmids in *Pseudomonas* species.[73] The DT104 strain has broad host reservoirs, and its widespread clonal dissemination in domestic livestock, especially among beef and dairy cattle, likely was promoted by use of antimicrobials on farms for therapeutic uses and for growth enhancement.[74,75] In the United States, the proportion of human *S.* Typhimurium R-type ACSSuT increased from 0.6% in 1979 to 34% in 1996. In 2005, resistance to at least ACSSuT was among the most common multidrug-resistant phenotypes (6.9%) among non-Typhi *Salmonella*, including 22.2% of *S.* Typhimurium and 12.6% of *S.* Newport isolates (see Fig. 223-4).[41] Acquisition of *S.* Typhimurium DT104 is associated with exposure to ill farm animals and to a variety of meat products, including raw or undercooked ground beef.[76] Although likely no more virulent than susceptible *S.* Typhimurium strains, infection with DT104 is

associated with increased risk of bloodstream infection and hospitalization, likely reflecting inadequate empirical antimicrobial therapy.[77,78]

Outbreaks and sporadic cases of nontyphoidal *Salmonella* resistant to third-generation cephalosporins increasingly have been reported.[79-81] Resistance is mediated by a transferable plasmid containing *ampC* (*bla*CMY) probably acquired by horizontal genetic transfer from *Escherichia coli* strains in food-producing animals and linked to the widespread use of the veterinary cephalosporin ceftiofur.[82] In 1998, the first reported case of ceftriaxone-resistant *Salmonella* infection acquired in the United States occurred in a child in Nebraska and was associated with exposure to cattle on his family's ranch that harbored *S.* Typhimurium with a 160-kb plasmid encoding CMY-2 AmpC β-lactamase.[79] Recent U.S. surveys found that 5.1% of *Salmonella* isolates from cattle and pigs and 1.6% of isolates from humans were ceftriaxone resistant (MIC ≥ 16 μg/mL).[41] A multidrug-resistant strain of *S.* Newport (MDR-AmpC), with decreased susceptibility to ceftriaxone (MIC > 2 μg/mL) and resistance to eight other human antimicrobials and ceftiofur, has emerged in the United States (see Fig. 223-4).[83] In 2005, MDR-AmpC was detected in 2.0% of all non-Typhi *Salmonella* and 12.6% of *S.* Newport isolates.[41] Risk factors for infection with MDR-AmpC *S.* Newport include consumption of uncooked ground beef, runny eggs or omelets, and recent exposure to an antimicrobial to which the strain is resistant.[81] Multidrug-resistant *Salmonella* strains expressing carbapenemase genes have been reported rarely.[84,85]

Nalidixic acid and fluoroquinolone-resistant *Salmonella* strains have been emerging among humans and animals, and resistance is due to chromosomal mutations of the intracellular targets DNA gyrase (gyrA or gyrB) or topoisomerase IV, to overproduction of efflux pumps, and more recently to acquisition of the plasmid-mediated quinolone resistance determinant *qnr*.[86-89] From 1996 to 2005, the proportion of non-Typhi *Salmonella* isolates in the United States that were nalidixic acid resistant (MIC ≥ 32 μg/mL) increased fivefold (from 0.4% to 2.4%), although ciprofloxacin resistance remained rare (see Fig. 223-4).[41] In comparison, in the United Kingdom, the incidence of ciprofloxacin resistance increased from 0% in 1993 to 14% in 1996 following the licensing of the enrofloxacin for veterinary use in 1993.[90] In Taiwan in 2000, a strain of ciprofloxacin-resistant (MIC ≥ 4 μg/mL) *S.* Choleraesuis caused a large outbreak of invasive infections that was linked to the use of enrofloxacin in swine feed.[69] On the basis of increased prevalence of nalidixic acid–resistant *Salmonella* and fluoroquinolone-resistant *Campylobacter* species in humans, the U.S. FDA withdrew approval of the use of fluoroquinolones in poultry in 2005.

Although health care–associated salmonellosis is infrequent, such infections have been associated with multidrug-resistant strains, sustained transmission, and substantial morbidity and mortality.[91-95] Nosocomial transmission of *Salmonella* from patients to health care workers has been associated with handling soiled linen, noncompliance with barrier precautions, and fecally incontinent residents.[96] However, the risk of transmission from health care workers to patients appears to be low if infection control measures are observed carefully.[97] In contrast, the risk of nosocomial transmission to neonates and infants from acutely or chronically infected family members appears higher.[98] Neonates are at high risk for fecal-oral transmission of *Salmonella* because of relative gastric achlorhydria and the buffering capacity of ingested breast milk and formula. High-iron infant formula may further increase the risk of infant salmonellosis compared with breast-feeding.[99] Contaminated enteral feeding and crowding also have been associated with nosocomial transmission among pediatric patients.[100] Control of outbreaks in daycare centers may be difficult because of the need for frequent diaper changing and the higher rate and longer duration of convalescent carriage seen in the preschool age group.[101]

Residents of nursing homes are at increased risk of foodborne salmonellosis and more severe morbidity and mortality because of poor infection control compliance and presence of comorbid illnesses, acid-suppressing medications, and waning immunity.[91,102,103]

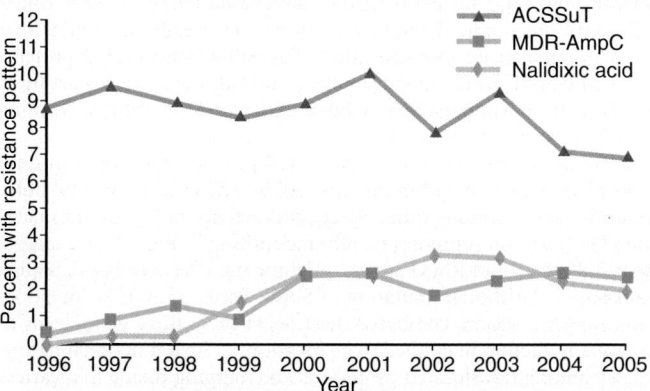

Figure 223-4 **Resistance patterns of non-Typhi *Salmonella* isolates, United States, 1996 to 2005.** ACSSuT, resistance to ampicillin, chloramphenicol, streptomycin, sulfonamides, and tetracycline; MDR-AMPC, resistance to ACSSuT + amoxicillin/clavulanic acid + ceftiofur and decreased susceptibility to ceftriaxone (MIC ≥ 2 μg/mL); Nalidixic acid, MIC ≥ 32 μg/mL. *(From Centers for Disease Control and Prevention. National Antimicrobial Resistance Monitoring System [NARMS] 2005 Annual Report. Available at: http://www.cdc.gov/narms/reports.htm.)*

Pathogenesis

Salmonella infections begin with the ingestion of bacteria in contaminated food or water. Estimates of the infectious dose vary substantially and depend on the method of determination. In studies involving administration of laboratory *Salmonella* strains to healthy human volunteers, the median dose required to produce disease was approximately 10^6 bacteria.[104] In contrast, investigations of point source outbreaks suggest that as few as 200 bacteria may produce nontyphoidal gastroenteritis in many of those exposed, and that the ingested dose is an important determinant of incubation period and disease severity.[104,105] Discrepancies in these results may stem from use of attenuated strains in the challenge experiments and from variation in disease susceptibility in the general population. Gastric acidity represents the initial barrier to *Salmonella* colonization, and conditions that increase gastric pH significantly increase susceptibility to infection. On exposure to acid in vitro, salmonellae display an adaptive acid tolerance response that probably facilitates bacterial survival in the stomach and passage to the small intestine.[106]

INTERACTIONS WITH INTESTINAL EPITHELIUM AND INDUCTION OF ENTERITIS

Salmonellae must evade host antimicrobial factors secreted into the intestinal lumen, including antimicrobial peptides, bile salts, and secretory immunoglobulin A, and traverse a protective mucous barrier before encountering intestinal epithelial cells.[107,108] Salmonellae express an array of distinct fimbriae that contribute to tight adherence to intestinal epithelial cells in culture. It is necessary to delete multiple fimbriae synthesis genes to prevent infection in animal models, suggesting that functional redundancy exists.[109] Microscopy reveals that salmonellae invade intestinal epithelial cells by a morphologically distinct process termed *bacteria-mediated endocytosis* (Fig. 223-5).[110] Shortly after bacteria adhere to the apical epithelial surface, profound cytoskeletal rearrangements occur in the host cell, disrupting the normal epithelial brush border and inducing formation of membrane ruffles that reach out and enclose adherent bacteria in large vesicles. This process resembles the membrane ruffling and macropinocytosis induced in many cell types by growth factors and is functionally distinct from receptor-mediated endocytosis, the mechanism by which

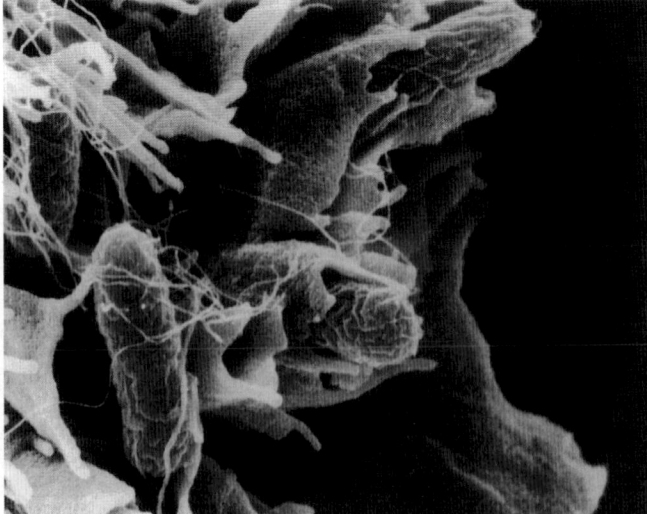

Figure 223-5 **Scanning electron micrograph showing *Salmonella* Typhimurium entering an HEp-2 cell through bacteria-mediated endocytosis.** Membrane ruffles extend from the cell surface, enclosing and internalizing adherent bacteria. *(From Ohl ME, Miller SI. Salmonella: A model for bacterial pathogenesis. Annu Rev Med. 2001;52: 259-274.)*

many other pathogens enter nonphagocytic cells. Following bacteria internalization, a fraction of the *Salmonella*-containing vesicles transcytose to the basolateral membrane, and the apical epithelial brush border reconstitutes. The epithelial cell type that serves as the principal portal for *Salmonella* invasion remains uncertain. In the mouse enteric fever model, salmonellae preferentially adhere to and enter the specialized microfold cells (M cells) that overlie lymphoid tissue within Peyer's patches.[111] In bovine and rabbit models of enteritis, however, salmonellae do not appear to interact preferentially with M cells, but instead adhere to and invade intestinal enterocytes diffusely.[112] It is possible that M cells are the principal portal of entry in the enteric fever syndrome, and that generalized invasion of enterocytes plays a greater role in the enteritis induced by nontyphoidal *Salmonella* serotypes.

Salmonellae encode a type III secretion system (T3SS) within *Salmonella* pathogenicity island 1 (the SPI-1 T3SS), which is required for bacteria-mediated endocytosis and intestinal epithelial invasion. T3SSs are complex macromolecular machines that have evolved to subvert host cell function through the translocation of virulence proteins directly from the bacterial cytoplasm into the host cell (see Chapters 1 and 3 for overview). *Salmonella* mutants lacking a functional SPI-1 T3SS do not invade epithelial cells in tissue culture and are severely attenuated in animal models of infection following oral administration.[112] In the past decade considerable attention has focused on identifying the virulence proteins translocated into epithelial cells by the SPI-1 T3SS and delineating the host cell processes these proteins target. At least five translocated proteins are essential for efficient invasion of cultured epithelial cells, though invasion in animal tissues may be more complicated and diverse.[113]

Two SPI-1 translocated proteins, SipC and SipA, promote membrane ruffling and *Salmonella* invasion through direct interactions with the actin cytoskeleton. The SipC protein inserts into the host cell plasma membrane and forms part of a protein complex that allows translocation of additional SPI-1 virulence proteins directly into the host cell cytoplasm.[114] SipC also directly nucleates actin polymerization at the site of *Salmonella* attachment and stimulates actin filament bundling.[115] The SipA protein further enhances actin polymerization through stabilization of actin filaments and reduction of the critical concentration for polymerization.[116] SipA mutants invade epithelial cells less efficiently than wild-type bacteria and induce disorganized, diffuse ruffling in host cells, in contrast to the localized ruffling induced around wild-type bacteria.

Additional SPI-1 translocated proteins contribute to *Salmonella* invasion by targeting members of the Rho family of monomeric GTP binding proteins (G proteins). Rho family members, including cdc42, rac, and rho, regulate the structure and dynamics of the actin cytoskeleton and are required for formation of the membrane ruffles that mediate *Salmonella* internalization. The SPI-1 translocated proteins SopE and SopE2 directly activate Rac1 and Cdc42 in vitro by acting as GDP/GTP exchange factors (GEFs), and induce membrane ruffling and macropinocytosis following microinjection into epithelial cells.[117] SopB is an additional SPI-1 translocated protein that targets inositol phosphate signaling within the host cell by acting as an inositol polyphosphatase.[118] Among other effects, this activity indirectly stimulates Rho GTPases and promotes membrane ruffling.[119] Recent data suggest that only Rac1 and RhoG are essential for the effects of SopE, SopE2, and SopB.[120] Although mutation of SopB, SopE, or SopE2 alone does not impact invasion, combined deletion of these three genes leads to a severe reduction in epithelial cell invasion.[119] Such functional redundancy among translocated proteins is an emerging theme in a variety of T3SSs. Overall, available data indicate that SipA and SipC act in concert with downstream cellular effectors of activated Rho GTPases to initiate and spatially direct the actin rearrangements that lead to *Salmonella* internalization.

Recent studies in mice indicate that salmonellae may also cross the intestinal epithelial border by an SPI-1–independent process involving host dendritic cells.[121,122] These cells express tight junction proteins and can intercalate between intestinal epithelial cells and access the intestinal lumen without disrupting epithelial integrity. In this manner dendritic cells may internalize bacteria in the intestinal lumen, and subsequently carry these bacteria to distant sites as they undergo their physiologic migration to lymphoid tissues. The diversity of mechanisms utilized by salmonellae to cross the intestinal barrier indicates the importance of this mechanism to its lifestyle within mammals.

In addition to invasion of intestinal epithelial cells, *Salmonella* serotypes clinically associated with gastroenteritis induce a secretory response in intestinal epithelium and initiate recruitment and transmigration of neutrophils into the intestinal lumen. The SPI-1 T3SS is also required for these responses in tissue culture and animal models of enteritis. Specifically, *Salmonella* strains unable to deliver any SPI-1 virulence proteins as a result of mutations in the secretion apparatus fail to induce fluid secretion or neutrophil accumulation in ligated bovine ileal loops, and do not cause gastroenteritis in calves.[123] In tissue culture models of enteritis, translocation of SPI-1 proteins into intestinal epithelial cells leads to synthesis and polarized secretion of inflammatory mediators and neutrophil chemoattractants, including interleukin-8 (IL-8).[124]

Several SPI-1 translocated proteins that contribute to intestinal inflammation and fluid secretion have been identified. Stimulation of Rho GTPase signaling by SopE and SopE2 also leads to activation of microtubule-associated protein kinase pathways and movement of the proinflammatory transcription factor nuclear factor–κB (NF-κB) to its site of action in the nucleus.[117] In addition to its role in invasion, the inositol polyphosphatase activity of SopB leads to accumulation of D-myo-inositol-1,4,5,6-tetrakisphosphate in epithelial cells.[125] The increased concentration of this compound ultimately leads to an increase in cellular basal chloride secretion, with associated fluid flux. The SPI-1 translocated proteins SopA and SopD also contribute to intestinal secretory and inflammatory responses in ligated ileal loops, but the molecular basis of these effects remains unclear. Many other effector proteins that are delivered by the T3SS apparatus may also effect these or similar pathways with different targets. Individual nontyphoidal salmonellae have a diverse complement of effector proteins, for instance, many strains do not have SopE2. The association of specific effector proteins could alter the pathogenicity of specific strains and their emergence in humans from animal reservoirs.[126]

Following *Salmonella* invasion, intestinal inflammation may also result from activation of the innate immune system through stimulation of proinflammatory receptors present on phagocytes and the basolateral surface of intestinal epithelia. This includes activation of Toll-like receptor 4 (Tlr4) by lipopolysaccharide and Toll-like receptor 5 (Tlr5) by bacterial flagellin.[127] The cytosolic surveillance pathway is also activated by the translocation of flagellin into the cytoplasm by the type III secretion system and its recognition by the inflammasome through the Ipaf pathway. This pathway results in the secretion of IL-1-β, an important pro-inflammatory cytokine.[128,129] Intestinal inflammation probably contributes to fluid secretion and diarrhea through disruption of the epithelial barrier and increased water flux by an exudative mechanism. In contrast to the neutrophilic inflammation and gastroenteritis induced by nontyphoidal *Salmonella* strains, S. Typhi induces monocytic inflammation in the human intestine and produces significantly less, if any, diarrhea.[130] The molecular basis of this difference in the host response remains unknown. One possibility is the presence of the Vi-polysaccharide capsule in most strains of *S.* Typhi that can prevent recognition of LPS by TLR4.[131]

Several studies demonstrate that salmonellae also utilize the SPI-1 T3SS to deliver proteins that downregulate the host inflammatory response associated with *Salmonella* invasion. The SptP protein inactivates Rho GTPase signaling by acting as a GTPase-activating protein (Rho GAP).[132] This directly opposes the activity of SopE and SopE2 and reduces membrane ruffling and proinflammatory signaling following bacterial invasion. In addition, the SspH1 and AvrA proteins inhibit NF-κB activation and related host cell cytokine synthesis.[133,134] These SPI-1 translocated proteins may promote bacterial persistence in the host by maintaining host cell integrity and allowing evasion of the host immune response. The presence of SPI-1 translocated pro-

teins with opposing molecular actions (e.g., SopE and SptP) suggests that there may be temporal ordering of protein function, with initial activity of SPI-1 proteins associated with invasion and proinflammatory signaling and subsequent activity of anti-inflammatory proteins. This dampening of the inflammatory response attributed to multiple bacterial effector proteins may contribute to the long period of relative asymptomatic colonization of the intestinal tract typical of nontyphoidal *Salmonella* infection.

INTERACTIONS WITH MACROPHAGES AND SYSTEMIC INFECTION

After crossing the epithelial barrier, salmonellae encounter and enter macrophages present in the submucosal space and Peyer's patches. Macrophage invasion may occur through bacteria-mediated macropinocytosis or through phagocytosis directed by several receptors present on the macrophage. Available data in both human infection and animal models of disease indicate that the ability of *Salmonella* to survive and replicate within macrophages is essential for dissemination within the host and induction of systemic disease. In persons with enteric fever and positive blood cultures, the majority of organisms are contained within the mononuclear fraction.[135] Furthermore, the ability of *Salmonella* mutants to replicate within macrophages in tissue culture correlates with ability to produce systemic disease in the mouse typhoid model, and microscopic examination of infected mouse liver and spleen demonstrates that the majority of organisms are located within macrophages.[136,137] Although residence within the macrophage shields the bacterium from effectors of humoral immunity, it also exposes the bacterium to the microbicidal and nutrient-poor environment of the phagosome. Within the host, salmonellae induce the expression of numerous genes that allow evasion of these antimicrobial defenses.

Once in the intracellular environment the bacteria persist within a vacuolar compartment that endures for hours to days. Salmonellae can survive within a compartment that fuses with lysosomes, and hence inhibition of phagosome fusion with lysosomes is unlikely to be a major pathogenic strategy of salmonellae. The vacuole acidifies, though its acidification may be delayed. Resistance to a variety of vacuolar bactericidal activities is essential to pathogenesis including resistance to antimicrobial peptides, nitric oxide, and oxidative killing. This is supported by experiments demonstrating that S. Typhimurium mutants sensitive to these compounds are less virulent for mice and that mice deficient in these activities are more susceptible to S. Typhimurium.[138]

Salmonella sense the acidic environment of the *Salmonella*-containing vacuole (SCV) and activate a variety of regulatory proteins required for *Salmonella* adaptation to the intracellular environment for replication within host cells. The best studied of these is the PhoP/PhoQ two-component regulatory system. The PhoP/PhoQ system senses the intracellular environment and regulates transcription of over 200 genes some of which are required for survival within macrophages. PhoQ is the sensor protein for the phagosome environment by sensing acidic pH and antimicrobial peptides to activate gene expression.[139-141] Activation of the PhoP/PhoQ and other regulons leads to widespread modifications in the protein and lipopolysaccharide components of the bacterial inner and outer membranes.[142] As many as 900 to 1000 genes are induced in response to the phagosome environment including many involved in remodeling of the cell surface to resist host cell killing mechanisms.[143] These surface modifications confer resistance to antimicrobial factors within the phagosome, including antimicrobial peptides, oxygen, and nitrogen radicals. PhoP/PhoQ-regulated lipopolysaccharide modifications include addition of aminoarabinose, ethanolamine, palmitate, and 2-hydroxymryistate to lipid A, thus altering the charge density and fluidity of the outer membrane and discouraging antimicrobial peptide insertion in the membrane.[142] Cell surface polysaccharide is also dramatically altered.[142] In addition, PhoP/PhoQ-regulated modifications in lipid A structure produce a lipopolysaccharide molecule with significantly less proinflammatory signaling activity and repress flagellin synthesis, which may facilitate bacterial survival within host tissues.[142] PhoP/PhoQ mutants of *S.* Typhi are avirulent in humans and are promising live typhoid vaccine candidates.[144] *S.* Typhi also modifies its surface through synthesis of the Vi capsule, a polysaccharide structure that confers resistance to phagocytosis by neutrophils and killing by complement, reduces recognition of lipopolysaccharide, and promotes survival within human macrophages.[145]

Salmonella have a second T3SS that is necessary for survival in the macrophage and for establishment of systemic infection.[146] Proteins delivered by both type III secretion systems are important for intracellular survival. SipA delivered by SPI1 persists on the phagosome membrane, where it promotes intracellular survival.[147] Encoded on *Salmonella* pathogenicity island 2 (SPI-2) is an additional T3SS that is adapted to be expressed by intracellular bacteria and translocates proteins across the membrane of the SCV into the macrophage cytosol. SPI-2 translocated proteins are hypothesized to alter trafficking to the SCV to promote bacterial growth such that useful nutrients are routed to the SCV. Most remarkably, salmonellae alter the phagosome to tubulate in a mechanism that requires SPI-2 translocated proteins. Such tubulation has been correlated with virulence, as SPI-2 translocated proteins implicated in this process are required for phagosome tubulation to occur. Phagosome tubulation is dynamic and rapid and appears to be dependent on the recruitment of microtubule motors, the activation of small GTPases, and membrane lipid alteration. The mechanism by which tubulation of the phagosome promotes virulence is unknown, but it could allow bacteria or their products to specifically traffic within the phagosome to different cellular localizations to promote nutrient acquisition or cell-to-cell spread. Several SPI-2 translocated proteins, including SifA, SifB, SseJ, SopD2, PipB, and PipB2, localize to the surface of the SCV. Other SPI-2 translocated proteins interact with the actin cytoskeleton surrounding the SCV and probably contribute to remodeling of vacuole-associated actin networks.[148,149] SpvB is a *Salmonella* virulence protein that is secreted into the macrophage cytoplasm, possibly by the SPI-2 T3SS, and ADP-ribosylates monomeric actin (G-actin), thus promoting disassembly of actin networks around the vacuole.[149,150] Other proteins appear to localize to the Golgi apparatus possibly to promote secretory traffic to the SCV.[138,151]

Many other bacterial factors are required for full virulence including those required for synthesis of essential nutrients and iron acquisition, and the virulence plasmids found in many nontyphoidal *Salmonella* serotypes. The virulence plasmids of *S.* Typhimurium, *S.* Dublin, *S.* Choleraesuis, and *S.* Enteritidis all contain an 8-kb region that promotes dissemination beyond the intestine in animal models and bacteremia in humans.[152] This region encodes the SpvB protein, as well as several other proteins of unknown function.

HOST RESPONSE AND IMMUNITY

The innate immune system senses invasive *Salmonella* infections using receptors that recognize conserved elements of bacterial structure. This includes recognition by plasma membrane and phagosomal membrane Toll-like receptors (Tlr) and cytoplasmic recognition receptors or the nucleotide-oligomerization domain-like receptors (Nod),[117] lipopolysaccharide by Tlr4, bacterial lipoproteins by Toll-like receptor 2 (Tlr2), and flagellin by Tlr5 flagellin by a signaling system that includes Ipaf and peptidoglycan by Nod1 and Nod2.[127] Activation of these receptors on phagocytes and epithelia leads to synthesis of cytokines that orchestrate the inflammatory response and instruct the subsequent antigen-specific immune response. Mice lacking a functional Tlr4 response are highly susceptible to *Salmonella* infection, confirming the importance of this initial response to infection.[153] Other studies indicate that caspase-1, a protease important for secretion of IL-1 and IL-18 as well as inflammatory cell death in host cells, is important for infection in mice by the oral route, indicating that recognition and activation of the cytoplasmic sensing components by Nod family members are important for control of infection in the

intestinal mucosa.[154] Studies in mice further demonstrate that the initial control of *S.* Typhimurium replication in host tissue requires recruitment and activation of macrophages. In both mice and humans, macrophage activation and efficient killing of *Salmonella* are associated with production of interferon-γ, IL-12, and tumor necrosis factor–α.[155-157] Mice with targeted disruptions in these genes are highly susceptible to infection. Rheumatoid arthritis patients treated with tumor necrosis factor antagonists have developed severe and fatal septicemias.[158] In addition, humans with mutations in the interferon-γ and IL-12 receptor genes develop severe infections with nontyphoidal *Salmonella* serotypes.[159]

Although the innate immune system is able to suppress initial *Salmonella* replication, final clearance of infection and immunity to rechallenge requires a Th1-type CD4 T-cell response and production of specific antibodies by B cells.[157] This is supported by the observation that mice lacking mature CD4 cells (H2I;AB⁻ mice) or B cells (Igh-6⁻ mice) are unable to control *Salmonella* infection.[157,160,161] The importance of cellular immunity in controlling *Salmonella* infection in humans is made apparent by the extreme susceptibility of individuals with human immunodeficiency virus (HIV) infection, lymphoproliferative diseases, or immune suppression following transplant.[162-165] A variety of other immunodeficiencies have been associated with *Salmonella* infection including common variable immunodeficiency.[166] Furthermore, vaccine studies in humans demonstrate that protection against *S.* Typhi infection correlates with development of cell-mediated immunity.[167] In accord with the importance of CD4 T cell–mediated immunity, recent population-based studies in humans have found an association between specific major histocompatibility complex class II alleles and susceptibility to typhoid fever.[168] CD8 T cells with cytolytic activity against *Salmonella*-infected host cells are also present in infected mice, but the importance of this activity in immunity remains unclear. Little is known about the antigen specificity of protective immune responses to *Salmonella* infection in humans, though antibodies against the Vi polysaccharide, lipopolysaccharide O antigen, and flagella are present in previously vaccinated or infected individuals.

Clinical Manifestations

Specific *Salmonella* serotypes most often produce characteristic clinical syndromes, including gastroenteritis, enteric fever, bacteremia and vascular infection, localized infections, and the chronic carrier state, and outcomes of infection differ substantially by serotype.[169]

GASTROENTERITIS

Infection with nontyphoidal *Salmonella* most often results in self-limited acute gastroenteritis that is indistinguishable from that caused by many other enteric bacterial pathogens. Within 6 to 48 hours after ingestion of contaminated food or water, nausea, vomiting, and diarrhea occur.[170] In most cases, stools are loose, of moderate volume, and without blood. In rare cases, stool may be watery and of large volume ("cholera-like") or of small volume associated with tenesmus ("dysentery-like"). Fever (38° to 39°C), abdominal cramping, nausea, vomiting, and chills frequently are reported. Headache, myalgias, and other systemic symptoms also may occur. Microscopic examination of stools shows neutrophils and, less frequently, red blood cells. Infrequently, *Salmonella* can cause a syndrome of pseudoappendicitis or can mimic the intestinal changes of inflammatory bowel disease.[170] Toxic megacolon is a rare but potentially life-threatening complication.[171]

Diarrhea is usually self-limited, typically lasting for 3 to 7 days.[170] Diarrhea that persists for more than 10 days should suggest another diagnosis. If fever is present, it usually resolves within 48 to 72 hours. Occasionally, patients require hospitalization because of dehydration, and death occurs infrequently. In the United States, nontyphoidal *Salmonella* infections result in an estimated rate of hospitalization of 2.2 per 1 million population and in 582 deaths per year.[172] A disproportionate number of these deaths occur among the elderly, especially those residing in long-term care facilities, and among immunocompromised patients, including persons with HIV/AIDS, lupus flares, or rheumatologic illness who are receiving anti–tumor necrosis factor antibody therapy.[46,103,158,173,174]

After resolution of gastroenteritis, the mean duration of carriage of nontyphoidal *Salmonella* in the stool is 4 to 5 weeks and varies by *Salmonella* serotype.[101] Antimicrobial therapy may increase the duration of carriage.[101] In addition, a higher proportion of neonates have prolonged carriage; in one study, 50% of neonates were still excreting *Salmonella* at 6 months.[175] However, the delayed clearance of infection in neonates does not result in permanent carriage, because almost all chronic carriers are adults.[101]

ENTERIC FEVER

Enteric fever is a severe systemic illness characterized by fever and abdominal pain that is caused by dissemination of S. Typhi and S. Paratyphi. Recent studies in Asia suggest that the incidence of enteric fever is highest in children less than 5 years of age and that young children experience similar rates of fever, signs and symptoms, and need for hospital admission compared with older people.[29] These findings contrast with earlier studies which suggested that S. Typhi infection caused a mild disease in young children.[176] Patients with immunosuppression, biliary and urinary tract abnormalities, hemoglobinopathies, malaria, schistosomiasis, bartonellosis, histoplasmosis, and *Helicobacter* co-infection are at increased risk of severe disease.[130,177-179] Although enteric fever classically is described as an acute illness with fever and abdominal tenderness, the symptoms are nonspecific and may be insidious in onset. The diagnosis of enteric fever should be considered strongly in the evaluation of any traveler who returns from tropical and subtropical areas with fever.

In the preantibiotic era, approximately 15% of patients with typhoid fever died.[180] Today the average case-fatality rate of enteric fever in the developing world is less than 1% and is 0.4% in the United States; increased mortality is associated with multidrug-resistant strains and delayed antimicrobial therapy.[37,181] The incubation period for S. Typhi averages 10 to 14 days but ranges from 5 to 21 days depending on the inoculum ingested and the health and immune status of the person. Following ingestion of the organism, persons may develop enterocolitis with diarrhea lasting several days; these symptoms usually resolve before the onset of fever. Diarrhea is more common in certain geographic areas, among patients with HIV/AIDS, and among children under 1 year of age.[176] Typically, fecal leukocytes are detected and stool protein is increased.[176] Constipation is present in 10 to 38% of patients. Although fever and abdominal pain are the classic signs of enteric fever, fever is documented on presentation in only approximately 75% of cases, and abdominal pain is reported in only 30 to 40%.[176,180] The presentation of enteric fever may be altered by comorbidities and early administration of antimicrobials. Nonspecific symptoms, such as chills, diaphoresis, dull frontal headache, anorexia, cough, weakness, sore throat, dizziness, and muscle pains, are frequent before the onset of fever.[182] Initially, fever is low grade, rises by the second week of illness to 39° to 40° C, and usually resolves by 4 weeks without antimicrobial therapy. Patients with enteric fever usually appear acutely ill, although those previously exposed to S. Typhi or S. Paratyphi or who seek early medical attention can present with a milder illness. Relative bradycardia is neither a sensitive nor a specific sign of typhoid fever, occurring in fewer than 50% of patients.[130] Approximately 30% of patients will have rose spots—a faint salmon-colored maculopapular rash on the trunk—at the end of the first week (Fig. 223-6).[130] Organisms can be cultured from punch biopsies of these lesions, and the pathology is characterized by a perivascular mononuclear cell infiltrate. The rash can be very faint in highly pigmented patients and typically resolves after 2 to 5 days. Some patients develop cervical lymphadenopathy. Crackles on auscultation are uncommon, and chest radiographs are almost always normal.[130] Frequently, abdominal examination reveals pain on deep palpation and increased peristalsis. From 20% to 50% of patients have hepatosplenomegaly. In the prean-

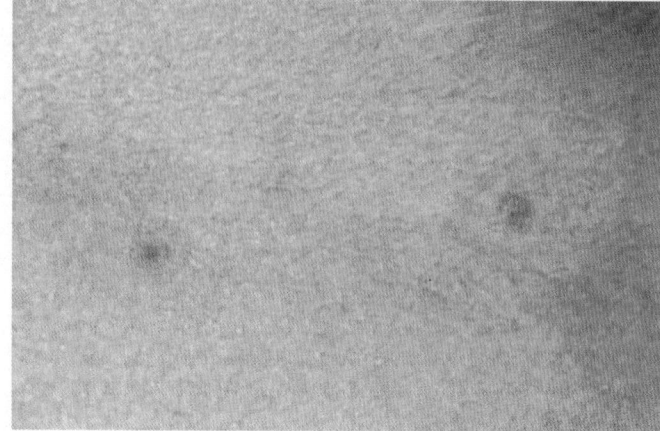

Figure 223-6 "Rose spots"—the rash of enteric fever due to *S. Typhi* or *S. Paratyphi.*

tibiotic era, two thirds of pregnancies complicated by typhoid fever resulted in fetal demise and miscarriage. Recent evidence does not suggest that enteric fever results in significant complications of pregnancy or neonatal outcomes.[183]

The development of severe disease (which occurs in ~10% to 15% of patients) depends on host factors (immunosuppression, antacid therapy, previous exposure, and vaccination), strain virulence and inoculum, and choice of antibimicrobial therapy. Gastrointestinal bleeding (10 to 20%) and intestinal perforation (1 to 3%) most commonly occur in the third and fourth weeks of illness and result from hyperplasia, ulceration, and necrosis of the ileocecal Peyer's patches at the initial site of *Salmonella* infiltration. Both complications are life threatening and require immediate fluid resuscitation and surgical interventions, with broad-spectrum antibimicrobial coverage for polymicrobial peritonitis.[130] Surgical repair may include resection and primary anastomosis, oversewing of the ulcer, and ostomy. Neurologic manifestations occur in 2% to 40% of patients, and include meningitis, Guillain-Barré syndrome, neuritis, and neuropsychiatric symptoms such as picking at bedclothes or imaginary objects, described as muttering delirium or coma vigil.[184]

Rare complications whose incidences are reduced by prompt antibiotic treatment include disseminated intravascular coagulation; hematophagocytic syndrome; pancreatitis; hepatic and splenic abscesses and granulomas; endocarditis, pericarditis, and myocarditis; orchitis; hepatitis; glomerulonephritis; pyelonephritis and hemolytic uremic syndrome; severe pneumonia; arthritis; osteomyelitis; and parotitis. Following resolution of the fever, weakness, weight loss, and debilitation may persist for months. Up to 10% of patients have a mild relapse, usually within 2 to 3 weeks of fever resolution and associated with the same strain type and susceptibility profile.

Laboratory abnormalities associated with enteric fever are nonspecific and include leukopenia, anemia, subclinical disseminated intravascular coagulopathy, and elevated creatinine kinase and liver function tests (e.g., aspartate transaminase and alanine transaminase; 300 to 500 U/dL),[185] and liver biopsies demonstrate focal Kupffer cell hyperplasia and mononuclear cell infiltration of the portal space.[186] Creatinine clearance is usually normal. Patients rarely develop proteinuria and immune complex glomerulonephritis, and irreversible loss of renal function has not been reported. Nonspecific ST- and T-wave electrocardiographic abnormalities are uncommon.

Enteric Fever Diagnosis

The definitive diagnosis of enteric fever requires the isolation of S. Typhi or S. Paratyphi from blood, bone marrow, another sterile site, rose spots, stool, or intestinal secretions. The sensitivity of blood culture is only 40% to 80%, probably because of high rates of antibimicrobial use in endemic areas and the small quantities of S. Typhi (i.e., <15 organisms/mL) typically present in the blood of patients with typhoid fever.[187]

Because almost all *S.* Typhi in blood are associated with the mononuclear cell–platelet fraction, blood clot culture, centrifugation of blood and culture of the buffy-coat fraction, or the lysis direct plating–lysis centrifugation method can substantially reduce the time to isolation of the organism and variably improve sensitivity.[188,189]

Enteric fever is the only bacterial infection of humans for which bone marrow examination is recommended routinely, but the sensitivity is variable (55% to 90%). Higher colony counts are present in the bone marrow compared with blood and, unlike blood culture, are not reduced by up to 5 days of prior antimicrobial therapy.[190] The duodenal string test is a useful noninvasive technique to sample duodenal secretions, with a sensitivity of up to 58%.[191] Children have a higher incidence of positive stool cultures compared with adults (60% vs. 27%), and stool cultures may become positive during the third week of illness in untreated patients.[192] Thus, the optimal diagnostic approach in both children and adults is to culture blood, bone marrow, and intestinal secretions (gastric and/or stool). With this approach, the diagnosis can be established in more than 90% of patients.[193]

A number of serologic tests, including the classic Widal test that is more than 100 years old, have been developed to detect *S.* Typhi antigen or antibody. The Widal test is neither sensitive (47% to 77%) nor specific (50% to 92%) and may lead to overdiagnosis of enteric fever in endemic areas. Newer commercially available kits for the rapid serologic diagnosis of enteric fever typically detect IgM antibody to lipopolysaccharide or outer membrane proteins of *S.* Typhi. These kits perform better among hospitalized patients than among those evaluated in the community setting for enteric fever.[194,195] However, in countries where resources are limited, rapid and simple tests to detect anti–*S.* Typhi antibody against lipopolysaccharide or outer membrane protein may replace the less accurate Widal test. DNA probe and PCR assays have been developed for detection of *S.* Typhi and *S.* Paratyphi in blood and are more rapid and sensitive than standard culture but are not yet commercially available and are impractical in many areas where typhoid is endemic.[196,197]

BACTEREMIA AND VASCULAR INFECTION

Up to 8% of patients with nontyphoidal *Salmonella* gastroenteritis develop bacteremia; of these, 5% to 10% develop localized infections.[198] Bacteremia and metastatic infection are more common with *S.* Choleraesuis and *S.* Dublin and among infants, the elderly, and those who are immunocompromised.[162,177,199-203] Among children, nontyphoidal *Salmonella* bacteremia usually is associated with gastroenteritis and prolonged fever, infrequently causes focal infections, and is fatal in less than 10% of cases.[200] In contrast, adults are more likely to have primary bacteremia and have a high incidence of secondary focal infections and death.[200] The mortality of nontyphoidal *Salmonella* bacteremia increases with the magnitude of bacteremia and in the presence of coma or septic shock.[204,205]

Salmonella have a propensity for infection of vascular sites, including vascular grafts, and high-grade or persistent bacteremia suggests an endovascular infection.[206] The risk of endovascular infection complicating *Salmonella* bacteremia is estimated to be 9% to 25% in persons over 50 years of age, usually involves the aorta, and most commonly results from seeding atherosclerotic plaques or aneurysms.[207-209] Mortality rates range from 14% to 60% and are lower with prompt diagnosis and combined medical and surgical therapy.[200-201] Venous septic thrombophlebitis also has been reported.[210]

SALMONELLOSIS AND HIV INFECTION

Nontyphoidal *Salmonella* are the leading cause of community-acquired bacteremia in HIV-infected persons in both developing and developed countries.[211,212] In the pre-HAART (highly active antiretroviral therapy) era, nontyphoidal *Salmonella* bacteremia occurred 20 to 100 times more commonly among those with HIV infection compared with the general population.[164,213] Among HIV-infected patients, nontyphoidal *Salmonella* bacteremia is associated with lower CD4 lymphocyte counts and a higher risk of metastatic complications, recurrent bacteremia, and mortality despite antimicrobial therapy, especially in Africa.[212,214]

Recurrent nontyphoidal *Salmonella* bacteremia is an AIDS-defining illness that apparently results from incomplete clearance of the primary infection owing to impaired cell-mediated immunity and dysregulation of proinflammatory cytokines release.[215] In the pre-HAART era, as many as 43% of patients with nontyphoidal *Salmonella* bacteremia had one or more recurrent episodes.[215] Among patients receiving HAART, the incidence of recurrent nontyphoidal *Salmonella* bacteremia has declined up to 96% compared with the pre-HAART era.[203] The risk reduction is likely due to the impact of HAART on virologic suppression and immune reconstitution, a direct bactericidal activity of some antiretrovirals on *Salmonella* species, the prophylactic use of trimethoprim-sulfamethoxazole, and the therapeutic use of ciprofloxacin.[203,216,217]

LOCALIZED INFECTIONS

Extraintestinal focal infections develop in approximately 5% to 10% of persons with *Salmonella* bacteremia, and their diagnosis and management are summarized in Table 223-2.[198]

CHRONIC CARRIER STATE

The chronic carrier state is defined as the persistence of *Salmonella* in stool or urine for periods greater than 1 year. From 0.2% to 0.6% of patients with nontyphoidal *Salmonella* infection develop chronic carriage.[218] Up to 10% of untreated patients with typhoid fever excrete *S.* Typhi in the feces for up to 3 months, and 1% to 4% develop chronic carriage.[180,207] The frequency of chronic carriage is higher in women; in persons with biliary abnormalities, gallstones, or concurrent bladder infection with *Schistosoma haematobium*; and in infants.[219,220] Chronic carriage of *S.* Typhi and *S.* Paratyphi A has been associated with an increased incidence of carcinoma of the gallbladder and of other gastrointestinal malignancies.[221] Serology for the Vi antigen may be useful in distinguishing chronic carriage from acute infection with *S.* Typhi because chronic carriers will often have a high antibody titer to this antigen.[222]

Immunization Against *S.* Typhi

Theoretically, it is possible to eliminate *Salmonella* that cause enteric fever, as the bacteria survive only in human hosts and are spread by contaminated food and water. However, given the high prevalence of the disease in developing countries that lack adequate sewage disposal and water treatment, this goal currently is unrealistic. Thus, travelers to at-risk countries should be advised to monitor their food and water intake carefully and to strongly consider vaccination.

Two typhoid vaccines currently are commercially available: (1) Ty21a, an oral, live attenuated *S.* Typhi vaccine (given on days 1, 3, 5, and 7 with a booster every 5 years); and (2) a parenteral Vi capsular polysaccharide vaccine (Vi CPS), consisting of purified Vi polysaccharide from the bacterial capsule (given as a single 0.5-mL intramuscular dose with a booster every 2 years). Ty21a vaccine is contraindicated in pregnant women, those taking antimicrobial therapy, and immunocompromised patients. The minimal age for vaccination is 6 years for Ty21a and 2 years for Vi CPS. The old parenteral whole-cell typhoid-paratyphoid A and B vaccine is no longer licensed in the United States, largely because of significant side effects.[223] In addition, an acetone-killed whole-cell vaccine is available only for use by the U.S. military. These vaccines have been most extensively evaluated in endemic populations, achieve approximately 50% to 80% efficacy depending on prior exposure, and confer protection that lasts only for several years.[224-226] Although data on typhoid vaccines in travelers are limited, some evidence suggests that efficacy may be substantially lower than that for local populations in endemic areas. Currently, there is no licensed vaccine against paratyphoid fever. Ty21a confers

TABLE 223-2	**Extraintestinal Infectious Complications of Salmonellosis**						
Site	*Incidence*	*Risk Factors*	*Manifestations*	*Complications*	*Mortality*	*Diagnosis*	*Therapy**
Endocarditis[207,254]	0.2-0.4%	Preexisting valvular heart disease	Valvular vegetation, infected mural thrombus	Valve perforation, relapse (20-25%), pericarditis	~70%	Blood culture, echocardiography	Early valve surgery + 6 wk P ceph 3, P ampicillin, or P, then PO fluoroquinolone
Arteritis[200,255,256]	Rare	Atherosclerosis, aortic aneurysm, endocarditis, prosthetic graft, myelodysplasia	Prolonged fever, pain in back, chest, or abdomen	Mycotic aneurysm, aneurysm rupture, aortoenteric fistula, vertebral osteomyelitis	14-60%	Blood culture, sonogram, MRI or CT	Early surgical intervention + 6 wk P ceph 3, P ampicillin, or P, then PO fluoroquinolone
Central nervous system[257-259]	0.1-0.9%	Infants (especially neonates)	Meningitis, ventriculitis, brain abscess, subdural empyema, encephalopathy	Seizures, mental retardation, hydrocephalus, brain infarction, relapse	~20-60%	CSF culture, CT or MRI	≥3 wk P ceph 3, P ampicillin, or a carbapenem
Pulmonary[260]	Rare	Lung malignancy, structural lung disease, sickle cell anemia	Pneumonia	Lung abscess, empyema, bronchopleural fistula	~25-60%	Respiratory culture, chest radiograph	≥2 wk P/PO abx
Bone[261,262]	<1%	Sickle cell anemia, male gender, connective tissue disease, immunosuppression	Femur, tibia, humerus, lumbar vertebrae	Relapse, chronic osteomyelitis	Very low	Bone radiograph	≥4 wk P ceph 3, P ampicillin, or P, then PO fluoroquinolone + surgery for sequestra
Joint, reactive[263-265]	0.6%	HLA-B27, antimicrobial therapy	Joints (≥3 joints) involved (especially knee, ankle, wrist, and sacroiliac)	Prolonged symptoms (mean duration, 5.5 mo)	Negligible	Joint fluid examination and culture	Nonsteroidal anti-inflammatory agent
Joint, septic[266]	0.1-0.2%	Osteoarthritis, connective tissue disease, sickle cell disease, prosthetic joint	Knee, hip, shoulder	Joint destruction, osteomyelitis	Very low	Joint fluid examination and culture	Repeated needle aspiration + ≥4 wk P/PO abx
Muscle/soft tissue[267]	Rare	Local trauma, male gender, diabetes, HIV infection	Abscess, pyomyositis	Osteomyelitis, endovascular infection, frequent relapse	~33%	Ultrasonography, aspiration	Drainage + ≥2 wk P abx
Hepatobiliary[268]	Rare	Cholelithiasis, cirrhosis, amebic abscess, echinococcal cyst, hepatocellular carcinoma	Hepatomegaly, cholecystitis, hepatic abscess	Rupture with secondary peritonitis, subphrenic abscess, spontaneous bacterial peritonitis	~10%	Ultrasonography, aspiration	Drainage + ≥2 wk P abx
Splenic[269]	Rare	Sickle cell anemia, splenic cyst, splenic hematoma	Splenomegaly	Left pleural empyema, subphrenic abscess, rupture with secondary peritonitis	<10%	Ultrasonography, aspiration	≥2 wk P abx + percutaneous drainage or splenectomy
Urinary[163,270,271]	0.6%	Urolithiasis, malignancy, renal transplant, elderly female	Cystitis, pyelonephritis	Renal abscess, interstitial nephritis, relapse	~20%	Urine culture, ultrasonography	Removal of structural abnormality + 1-2 wk P abx + ≥6 wk PO fluoroquinolone or TMP-SMX
Genital[207]	Rare	Pregnancy, renal transplant	Ovarian abscess, testicular abscess, prostatitis, epididymitis	Abscess	Very low	Ultrasonography, aspiration	Drainage of collection + 1-2 wk P abx + ≥6 wk PO fluoroquinolone or TMP-SMX
Soft tissue[272]	<1%	Local trauma, immunosuppression	Pustular dermatitis, SC abscess, wound infection	Septic thrombophlebitis, endophthalmitis	~15%	Drainage culture	≥2 wk P abx + drainage of collection

*P ceph 3, parenteral third-generation cephalosporin; P ampicillin, parenteral ampicillin; P/PO fluoroquinolone, parenteral or oral fluoroquinolone; P/PO abx, parenteral or oral antimicrobial (e.g., fluoroquinolone, ampicillin, TMP-SMX, or third-generation cephalosporin); TMP-SMX, trimethoprim-sulfamethoxazole.

CSF, cerebrospinal fluid; CT, computed tomography; HIV, human immunodeficiency virus; MRI, magnetic resonance imaging; PO, oral; SC, subcutaneous.

moderate protection (45%) against *S.* Paratyphi B infection but not against *S.* Paratyphi A.[225,227]

A meta-analysis of efficacy and toxicity vaccine trials comparing the whole-cell vaccine, Ty21a, and Vi CPS in populations in endemic areas found that, while all three vaccines have similar efficacy for the first year, the 3-year cumulative efficacy of the whole-cell vaccine (73%) exceeds that of both Ty21a (51%) and purified Vi (55%).[228] In addition, the heat-killed whole-cell vaccine maintains its efficacy for 5 years, while Ty21a and Vi CPS maintain their efficacy for 4 and 2 years, respectively. However, the whole-cell vaccine is associated with a much higher incidence of side effects than the other two vaccines: 16% of whole-cell vaccine recipients develop fever and 10% miss a day of work or school, whereas only 1% to 2% of persons receiving the alternative vaccines have any fever.

Vi CPS typhoid vaccine is poorly immunogenic in children less than 5 years of age because of T cell–independent properties.[224] The recently developed Vi-rEPA vaccine contains Vi polysaccharide bound to a nontoxic recombinant protein that is identical to *Pseudomonas aeruginosa* exotoxin A. In 2- to 4-year-olds, two injections of Vi-rEPA induced higher T cell responses and higher levels of serum antibodies to Vi than did Vi CPS in 5- to 14-year olds.[229] In a two-dose trial in 2- to 5-year-old children in Vietnam, Vi-rEPA provided 91% efficacy at 27 months and was very well tolerated.[230] At least three new live vaccines are in clinical development.

Typhoid vaccine is not required for international travel, but it is recommended for travelers to areas where there is a moderate to high risk of exposure to *S.* Typhi , especially those traveling to south Asia and other developing countries in Asia, Africa, the Caribbean, and Central and South America, who will have exposure to potentially contaminated food and drink.[226] Typhoid vaccine should be considered even for persons planning less than 2 weeks' travel to high-risk areas.[38] In addition, laboratory workers who work with *S.* Typhi and household contacts of known *S.* Typhi carriers should be vaccinated. Because vaccine protective efficacy can be overcome by high inocula that are common in foodborne exposure,[226,231] immunization is an adjunct and not a substitute for avoiding high-risk foods and beverages. Immunization is not recommended for adults residing in typhoid-endemic areas or in the management of persons potentially exposed to a common-source outbreak. In 2000, the World Health Organization recommended immunization of school-aged children in high-risk areas where antimicrobial-resistant *S.* Typhi strains are prevalent. Currently, only China and Vietnam have incorporated typhoid vaccination into routine immunization programs.[232]

Enteric fever is a notifiable disease in the United States. Individual health departments have their own guidelines for allowing food handlers or health care workers to return to work. The reporting system enables public health departments to identify potential source patients and to treat chronic carriers in order to prevent further outbreaks. In addition, since 1% to 4% of patients with *S.* Typhi infection become chronic carriers, it is important to monitor patients (especially childcare providers and food handlers) for chronic carriage and to treat this condition if indicated.

Therapy for Salmonellosis

ENTERIC (TYPHOID) FEVER

Early diagnosis and prompt administration of appropriate antimicrobial therapy prevents severe complications of enteric fever and results in case-fatality rates of less than 1%.[233] The initial choice of antimicrobial therapy depends on the susceptibility of the *S.* Typhi and *S.* Paratyphi strains in the area of residence or travel (Table 223-3). For treatment of drug-susceptible typhoid fever, fluoroquinolones are the most effective class of agents with cure rates of about 98% and rates of relapse and fecal carriage of less than 2%.[233] In a recent Cochrane review, fluoroquinolone therapy for multidrug-resistant enteric fever reduced rates of clinical failure but not microbiologic failure or relapse compared with ceftriaxone or cefixime.[234] The greatest experience is with ciprofloxacin (500 mg orally twice a day for 5 to 7 days). Ofloxacin (400 mg orally twice a day for 5 to 7 days) is similarly successful for treatment of nalidixic acid–susceptible strains. A 3-day course of oral fluoroquinolone therapy is effective for the treatment of uncomplicated, multidrug-resistant typhoid, and may be especially useful for management of typhoid epidemics.[235] However, the increased incidence of nalidixic acid–resistant *S.* Typhi in Asia, likely related to the widespread availability of these agents over the counter, is now limiting the use of fluoroquinolones for empirical therapy. Patients infected with nalidixic acid–resistant *S.* Typhi strains should be treated with ceftriaxone, azithromycin, or high-dose ciprofloxacin therapy (ciprofloxacin 750 mg twice a day) for 10 to 14 days. High-dose fluoroquinolone therapy for 7 days for treatment of nalidixic acid–resistant enteric fever has been associated with delayed resolution of fever, higher rates of treatment failure, and high rates of fecal carriage immediately post-treatment.[236]

Ceftriaxone, cefotaxime, and oral cefixime are effective agents for treatment of multidrug-resistant enteric fever, including nalidixic acid– and fluoroquinolone-resistant strains. Ceftriaxone (1 to 2 g daily in adults or 60 to 75 mg/kg daily in children) administered either intravenously or intramuscularly for 10 to 14 days or oral cefixime (200 mg twice daily in adults or 10 to 15 mg/kg twice daily in children) for 7 to 14 days resolves fever in an average of 4 days, and results in cure rates of 95%, relapse rates of 3% to 6%, and fecal carriage rates of less than 3%.[234] Oral azithromycin (1 g once a day for

TABLE 223-3	Recommended Antimicrobial Treatment for Typhoid Fever					
	Optimal Treatment			**Alternative Effective Treatment**		
Susceptibility	*Drug*	*Typical Adult Dose*	*Duration (days)*	*Drug*	*Typical Adult Dose*	*Duration (days)*
Uncomplicated Typhoid Fever						
Fully sensitive	Ciprofloxacin	500 mg PO bid	5-7*	Chloramphenicol	500 mg PO qid	14-21
	Ofloxacin	400 g PO bid	5-7	Amoxicillin	1 g PO tid	14
				TMP-SMX	160/800 mg PO bid	7
Multidrug resistance	Fluoroquinolone (e.g., ciprofloxacin)	500 mg PO bid	5-7*	Azithromycin	1 g PO daily	7
	Cefixime	200 mg PO bid	7-14			
Quinolone resistance	Azithromycin	1 g PO daily	7	Cefixime	200 mg PO bid	7-14
	Ceftriaxone	2 g IV daily	10-14			
Severe Typhoid Fever Requiring Parenteral Treatment						
Fully sensitive	Fluoroquinolone (e.g., ciprofloxacin)	400 mg IV q12h	10-14	Chloramphenicol	1.5 g IV q6h	14-21
				Ampicillin	2 g IV q6h	14
				TMP-SMX	160/800 mg IV q8-12h	14
Multidrug resistance	Fluoroquinolone (e.g., ciprofloxacin)	400 mg IV q12h	10-14	Ceftriaxone	2 g IV q12h	10-14
				Cefotaxime	2 g IV q8h	10-14
Quinolone resistance	Ceftriaxone	2 g IV q12h	10-14	Fluoroquinolone (e.g., ciprofloxacin)	400 mg IV q8h	14
	Cefotaxime	2 g IV q8h	10-14			

*Three-day course also effective.

bid, twice daily; qid, four times daily; tid, three times daily; IV, intravenously; PO, orally; TMP-SMX, trimethoprim-sulfamethoxazole.

Adapted from Bhutta ZA. Current concepts in the diagnosis and treatment of typhoid fever. *BMJ.* 2006;333:78-82; and World Health Organization (WHO) Department of Vaccines and Biologicals. Background document: The diagnosis, prevention and treatment of typhoid fever. Geneva: WHO; 2003:19-23. Available at: http://www.who.int/vaccine_research/documents/en/typhoid_diagnosis.pdf.

5 days or 1 g on day 1 followed by 500 mg orally for 6 days) results in fever clearance in 4 to 6 days with rates of relapse and convalescent stool carriage of less than 3%.[236] In a recent Cochrane review, azithromycin significantly reduced rates of treatment failure and duration of hospital stay compared with fluoroquinolones for the management of uncomplicated *S.* Typhi or *S.* Paratyphi A infection, including multidrug-resistant or nalidixic acid–resistant strains.[237] Despite efficient in vitro killing of *Salmonella*, first- and second-generation cephalosporins as well as aminoglycosides are ineffective in treating clinical infections.

Chloramphenicol (500 mg four times a day), ampicillin (1 g four times a day), amoxicillin (1 g three times a day), and trimethoprim-sulfamethoxazole (1 double-strength tablet twice a day) formerly were widely used for treatment of typhoid.[238] However, emergence of plasmid-encoded resistance first to chloramphenicol in the 1970s and then to chloramphenicol, ampicillin, and trimethoprim beginning in 1989 has limited the usefulness of these agents in many developing countries, except in Latin America and sub-Saharan Africa, where resistance remains relatively uncommon. The agents are inexpensive, widely available, and as effective as fluoroquinolones for the treatment of susceptible strains, resolving fever in 5 to 7 days.[234] However, they require 14 to 21 days of divided daily therapy, and adherence may be low. Oral chloramphenicol is not available in the United States.

Most patients with uncomplicated enteric fever can be managed at home with oral antimicrobial therapy and antipyretics. Patients with persistent vomiting, diarrhea, or abdominal distention should be hospitalized and treated with supportive therapy and a parenteral third-generation cephalosporin or fluoroquinolone, depending on the susceptibility profile. Therapy should be administered for at least 10 days, or 5 days after resolution of fever. High-dose dexamethasone (initial dose 3 mg/kg followed by eight doses of 1 mg/kg every 6 hours for 48 hours) should be considered for patients with severe typhoid fever with shock, obtundation, stupor, or coma. In a randomized, prospective, double-blind study performed in Indonesia, the administration of dexamethasone with chloramphenicol was associated with a substantially lower mortality in patients with severe typhoid fever compared with those who received chloramphenicol alone (10% vs. 55%).[239] Patients should be carefully monitored, as dexamethasone may mask signs of abdominal complications. Steroid treatment beyond 48 hours may increase the relapse rate.[240]

The 1% to 4% of patients who develop chronic carriage of *S.* Typhi can be treated for 4 to 6 weeks with an appropriate oral antimicrobial. Treatment with oral amoxicillin, trimethoprim-sulfamethoxazole, ciprofloxacin, or norfloxacin has been shown to be approximately 80% effective in eradicating chronic carriage of susceptible organisms.[241,242] Antimicrobial agents are infrequently effective in eradicating the carrier state when anatomic abnormalities, such as biliary or kidney stones, are present. In such cases, surgery combined with antimicrobial therapy is often required for eradication. Patients with urinary carriage associated with *S. haematobium* should be treated with praziquantel before eradication of *S.* Typhi is attempted. Chronic suppressive antimicrobial therapy should be considered for those patients with persistent carriage in whom no anatomic abnormality can be identified or who relapse after cholecystectomy.

NONTYPHOIDAL *SALMONELLA*

Salmonella gastroenteritis is usually a self-limited disease, and therapy primarily should be directed to the replacement of fluid and electrolyte losses. In a large meta-analysis, antimicrobial therapy for uncomplicated nontyphoidal *Salmonella* gastroenteritis, including short-course or single-dose regimens with oral fluoroquinolones, amoxicillin, or trimethoprim-sulfamethoxazole, did not significantly decrease the length of illness, including duration of fever or diarrhea, and was associated with an increased risk of relapse, positive culture after 3 weeks, and adverse drug reactions.[243] Therefore, antimicrobials should not be used routinely to treat uncomplicated nontyphoidal *Salmonella* gastroenteritis or to reduce convalescent stool excretion.

Although fewer than 5% of all patients with *Salmonella* gastroenteritis develop bacteremia, certain patients are at increased risk for invasive infection and may benefit from preemptive antimicrobial therapy. Antimicrobial therapy should be considered for neonates (probably up to 3 months of age), those older than 50 years with suspected atherosclerosis, and for persons with immunosuppression, cardiac valvular or endovascular abnormalities, or significant joint disease. Treatment should consist of an oral or intravenous antimicrobial administered for 48 to 72 hours or until the patient becomes afebrile. Immunocompromised persons, including those with AIDS, who develop *Salmonella* gastroenteritis may require 7 to 14 days of therapy, typically with a fluoroquinolone, to reduce the risk of extraintestinal spread.[244] For susceptible organisms, oral therapy with a fluoroquinolone, trimethoprim-sulfamethoxazole, or amoxicillin is adequate. Although fluoroquinolones are not recommended for administration to children younger than 10 years of age, they may have a role in treating severe nontyphoidal salmonellosis in this age group, particularly among immunocompromised patients.[245] Occasionally, antimicrobial prophylaxis has been required to control institutional outbreaks, especially in long-term care facilities or pediatric wards, where compliance with infection control measures may be difficult.[246]

BACTEREMIA

Because of the increasing prevalence of antimicrobial resistance, empirical therapy for life-threatening bacteremia or focal infection suspected to be caused by nontyphoidal *Salmonella* should include a third-generation cephalosporin and a fluoroquinolone until susceptibilities are known. High-grade bacteremia (i.e., >50% of three or more blood cultures positive) should prompt a search for endovascular abnormalities by echocardiogram or other imaging techniques, such as computerized tomography or indium-labeled white blood cell scan. Low-grade bacteremia not involving vascular structures should be treated with intravenous antimicrobial therapy for 7 to 14 days. Documented or suspected endovascular infection should be treated with intravenous ceftriaxone or ampicillin or intravenous fluoroquinolone for 6 weeks followed by oral therapy. Early surgical resection of infected aneurysms or other infected endovascular sites is recommended.[200,201] Patients with infected prosthetic vascular grafts that could not be resected have been maintained successfully on chronic suppressive oral therapy.[247]

RECURRENT *SALMONELLA* BACTEREMIA IN PERSONS WITH AIDS

In persons with AIDS and a first episode of *Salmonella* bacteremia, at least 4 to 6 weeks of therapy is recommended with a fluoroquinolone, trimethoprim-sulfamethoxazole, or ceftriaxone to attempt eradication of the organism and to decrease the risk of recurrent bacteremia.[244] Persons who relapse following 4 to 6 weeks of antimicrobial therapy should receive long-term suppressive therapy with an oral fluoroquinolone or trimethoprim-sulfamethoxazole, based on susceptibility testing.[244]

FOCAL INFECTIONS

Treatment recommendations for the management of focal *Salmonella* infections are summarized in Table 223-2. For extraintestinal nonvascular infections, antimicrobial therapy for 2-4 weeks (depending on the infection site) is usually recommended. In cases of chronic osteomyelitis, abscesses, and urinary or hepatobiliary infection associated with anatomic abnormalities, surgical resection or drainage may be required in addition to prolonged antimicrobial therapy to eradicate infection.

CARRIER STATE

Treatment of persons with asymptomatic carriage of nontyphoidal *Salmonella* is controversial. In a randomized, placebo-controlled trial conducted in Thailand among asymptomatic food workers, two 5-day regimens (norfloxacin, 400 mg twice daily, and azithromycin, 500 mg once daily) were similar to placebo in eradicating nontyphoidal *Salmonella* carriage and increased the risk of reinfection with antimicrobial-resistant *S. Schwarzengrund*.[248]

Prevention and Control

The prevention and control of salmonellosis require both an understanding of the complex cycles of transmission and ongoing surveillance to characterize trends in *Salmonella* incidence and prevalence and to identify outbreaks. Safe drinking water and effective sewage treatment can reduce the burden of enteric fever in developing countries, but substantial economic and social barriers continue to hinder progress on this front. The emergence of nalidixic acid–resistant *S.* Typhi in Asia has increasingly shifted emphasis from treatment to vaccination.[249]

In developed countries, control of foodborne salmonellosis requires identification of controllable hazards, monitoring, and verification to limit the introduction and multiplication of *Salmonella* from the farm to the table.[250] Recognition of foodborne outbreaks requires that clinicians have a high index of suspicion, order the appropriate laboratory test, and promptly report positive culture results to local public health departments. Vaccination of feed animals, further limiting the use of antimicrobials as growth promoters, and improved food safety practices should further reduce the burden of foodborne salmonellosis. Active population-based surveillance for foodborne diseases has improved estimates of disease burden,[43] and use of algorithms and rapid molecular subtyping has improved the ability to detect outbreaks of salmonellosis associated with widely distributed agricultural and manufactured foods.[251] Although most cases of *Salmonella* infection occur sporadically, large numbers of persons potentially may become infected when commercial kitchens serve *Salmonella*-contaminated foods that have not been sufficiently cooked or that have been mishandled. Commercial food service establishments can reduce the risk of foodborne *Salmonella* illness if they do not serve food containing raw or undercooked eggs, use pasteurized eggs whenever possible, and avoid cross-contamination of food items. Use of pasteurized eggs for all recipes calling for bulk-pooled eggs is recommended for all nursing homes and hospitals.[103]

The most cost-effective approach to the control of salmonellosis in food handlers is attention to good personal hygiene and maintenance of time-temperature standards for food handling. Routine screening of food handlers for carriage after gastroenteritis is commonly performed before they are allowed to return to work. However, there is little justification for this approach because few outbreaks are related to specific food handlers, prolonged carriage in food handlers after gastroenteritis is rare, and the number of organisms present is small. Therefore, it is reasonable to allow individuals to return to work after diarrhea is resolved. Two consecutive negative stool samples should be required only for food handlers whose work involves touching unwrapped foods that are consumed raw or served without further cooking. Routine surveillance of food handlers for asymptomatic stool carriage of *Salmonella* is not recommended.

To limit the risk of nosocomial transmission to patients and health care workers, patients excreting *Salmonella* should be managed with Standard Precautions, including the use of personal protective equipment, including gloves, when they perform direct patient care or handle soiled articles. Control of *Salmonella* outbreaks in long-term care facilities or neonatal care areas may be difficult because of poor compliance with isolation precautions, the increased susceptibility of these patients, and frequent transfers between health care facilities.[252,253] Although *Salmonella* infection in newborns, the elderly, or the immunocompromised can be severe, the risk of transmission of *Salmonella* from health care workers to patients appears to be very small.[97] Once the health care worker is asymptomatic and passing formed stool, the individual should be allowed to return to work if Standard Precautions are observed. However, local and state regulations should be followed because some require work exclusion for health care workers who have salmonellosis until two or more stool cultures obtained at least 24 hours apart are negative.

REFERENCES

1. Smith T. The hog-cholera group of bacteria. *US Bur Anim Ind Bull.* 1894;6:6-40.
2. Louis PCA. *Recherches anatomiques, pathologiques, et thérapeutiques sur la maladie connue sous les noms de gastroenterite, fièvre putride, adynamique, typhoide, comparée avec les maladies aigues les plus ordinaires.* Paris: J-B Ballière; 1829.
3. Jenner W. *On the Identity or Non-identity of Typhoid and Typhus Fevers.* London: C. & J. Adlard; 1850.
4. Wilson JC. *A Treatise on the Continued Fevers.* New York: Wood Pub; 1881.
5. Budd W. *Typhoid Fever: Its Nature, Mode of Spreading, and Prevention.* London: Longmans Publishing; 1873.
6. Schroeter J. In: Cohn F, ed. *Kryptogamenflora von Schlesien Bd 3.* Breslau: J. U. Kern; 1885:1-814.
7. Pfeiffer R, Kalle W. Experimentelle untersuchunger zur Frage der Schutzimpfung des Menschen geger typhus addominalis. *Dtsch Med Wocheschn.* 1896;22:735.
8. Widal F. Serodiagnostic de la fièvre typhoide. *Bull Med Hop Paris.* 1896;13:561-566.
9. Kauffman F. *The Diagnosis of Salmonella Types.* Springfield, IL: Charles C. Thomas; 1950.
10. Woodward TE, Smadel JE, Ley HL, et al. Preliminary report on the beneficial effect of chloromycetin in the treatment of typhoid fever. *Ann Intern Med.* 1948;29:131-134.
11. Zinder ND, Lederberg J. Genetic exchange in *Salmonella. J Bacteriol.* 1952;64:679-699.
12. Ames BN, Lee FD, Durston WE. An improved bacterial test system for detection and classification of mutagens and carcinogens. *Proc Natl Acad Sci U S A.* 1973;70:782-786.
13. Popoff MY, Bockemühl J, Gheesling LL. Supplement 2002 (No. 46) to the Kauffmann-White scheme. *Res Microbiol.* 2004; 155:568-570.
14. Brenner FW, Villar RG, Angulo FJ, et al. *Salmonella* nomenclature. *J Clin Microbiol.* 2000;38:2465-2467.
15. Holt KE, Parkhill J, Mazzoni CJ, et al. High-throughput sequencing provides insights into genome variation and evolution in *Salmonella* Typhi. *Nat Genet.* 2008;40:987-993.
16. Thomson NR, Clayton DJ, Windhorst D, et al. Comparative genome analysis of *Salmonella* Enteritidis PT4 and *Salmonella* Gallinarum 287/91 provides insights into evolutionary and host adaptation pathways. *Genome Res.* 2008;18:1624-1637.
17. Farmer JJ, Boatwright, KD, Janda JM. *Enterobacteriaceae: Introduction and Identification.* Washington, DC: American Society for Microbiology; 2007.
18. Perez JM, Cavalli P, Roure C, et al. Comparison of four chromogenic media and Hektoen agar for detection and presumptive identification of *Salmonella* strains in human stools. *J Clin Microbiol.* 2003;41:1130-1134.
19. Ruiz J, Nunez ML, Diaz J, et al. Comparison of five plating media for isolation of *Salmonella* species from human stools. *J Clin Microbiol.* 1996;34:686-688.
20. Pathmanathan SG, Cardona-Castro N, Sanchez-Jimenez MM, et al. Simple and rapid detection of *Salmonella* strains by direct PCR amplification of the hilA gene. *J Med Microbiol.* 2003; 52:773-776.
21. Hein I, Flekna G, Krassnig M, et al. Real-time PCR for the detection of *Salmonella* spp. in food: an alternative approach to a conventional PCR system suggested by the FOOD-PCR project. *J Microbiol Methods.* 2006;66:538-547.
22. Oracz G, Feleszko W, Golicka D, et al. Rapid diagnosis of acute *Salmonella* gastrointestinal infection. *Clin Infect Dis.* 2003; 36:112-115.
23. Nataro JP, Bopp CA, Fields PI, et al. *Escherichia, Shigella,* and *Salmonella.* In: Murray PR, Baron EJ, Jorgensens M, et al, eds. *Manual of Clinical Microbiology.* 9th ed. Washington, DC: American Society for Microbiology; 2007:467-471.
24. Daniels EM, Schneerson R, Egan WM, et al. Characterization of the *Salmonella* Paratyphi C Vi polysaccharide. *Infect Immun.* 1989;57:3159-3164.
25. Reller ME, Olsen SJ, Kressel AB, et al. Sexual transmission of typhoid fever: a multistate outbreak among men who have sex with men. *Clin Infect Dis.* 2003;37:141-144.
26. Weikel CS, Guerrant RL. Nosocomial salmonellosis. *Infection Control.* 1985;6:218-220.
27. Crump JA, Luby SP, Mintz ED. The global burden of typhoid fever. *Bull World Health Organ.* 2004;82:346-353.
28. Ochiai RL, Acosta CJ, Danovaro-Holliday MC, et al. A study of typhoid fever in five Asian countries: disease burden and implications for controls. *Bull World Health Organ.* 2008; 86:260-268.
29. Sinha A, Sazawal S, Kumar R, et al. Typhoid fever in children aged less than 5 years. *Lancet.* 1999;354:734-737.
30. Bhutta ZA, Naqvi SH, Razzaq RA, et al. Multidrug-resistant typhoid in children: presentation and clinical features. *Rev Infect Dis.* 1991;13:832-836.
31. Rowe B, Ward LR, Threlfall EJ. Multidrug-resistant *Salmonella* Typhi: a worldwide epidemic. *Clin Infect Dis.* 1997;24(Suppl 1):S106-S109.
32. Wain J, Hoa NT, Chinh NT, et al. Quinolone-resistant *Salmonella* Typhi in Viet Nam: molecular basis of resistance and clinical response to treatment. *Clin Infect Dis.* 1997;25:1404-1410.
33. Threlfall EJ, de Pinna E, Day M, et al. Alternatives to ciprofloxacin use for enteric fever, United Kingdom. *Emerg Infect Dis.* 2008;14:860-861.
34. Shirakawa T, Acharya B, Kinoshita S, et al. Decreased susceptibility to fluoroquinolones and gyrA gene mutation in the *Salmonella enterica* serovar Typhi and Paratyphi A isolated in Katmandu, Nepal, in 2003. *Diagn Microbiol Infect Dis.* 2006;54:299-303.
35. Kumar S, Rizvi M, Berry N. Rising prevalence of enteric fever due to multidrug-resistant *Salmonella*: an epidemiological study. *J Med Microbiol.* 2008;57:1247-1250.
36. Weill FX, Tran HH, Roumagnac P, et al. Clonal reconquest of antibiotic-susceptible *Salmonella enterica* serotype Typhi in Son La Province, Vietnam. *Am J Trop Med Hyg.* 2007;76: 1174-1181.
37. Mermin JH, Townes JM, Gerber M, et al. Typhoid fever in the United States, 1985-1994: changing risks of international travel and increasing antimicrobial resistance. *Arch Intern Med.* 1998;158:633-638.

38. Steinberg EB, Bishop R, Haber P, et al. Typhoid fever in travelers: who should be targeted for prevention? *Clin Infect Dis.* 2004;39:186-191.
39. Gupta SK, Medalla F, Omondi MW, et al. Laboratory-based surveillance of paratyphoid fever in the United States: travel and antimicrobial resistance. *Clin Infect Dis.* 2008;46:1656-1663.
40. Cooke FJ, Day M, Wain J, et al. Cases of typhoid fever imported into England, Scotland and Wales (2000-2003). *Trans R Soc Trop Med Hyg.* 2007;101:398-404.
41. Centers for Disease Control and Prevention. National Antimicrobial Resistance Monitoring System (NARMS) 2005 Annual Report. Available at: ⟨http://www.cdc.gov/narms/reports.htm⟩. Accessed 3/26/2009.
42. Voetsch AC, Van Gilder TJ, Angulo FJ, et al. FoodNet estimate of the burden of illness caused by nontyphoidal *Salmonella* infections in the United States. *Clin Infect Dis.* 2004;38(Suppl 3):S127-134.
43. Centers for Disease Control and Prevention (CDC). Preliminary FoodNet data on the incidence of infection with pathogens transmitted commonly through food—10 states, 2007. *MMWR Morb Mortal Wkly Rep.* 2008;57:366-370.
44. Gradel KO, Dethlefsen C, Schonheyder HC, et al. Severity of infection and seasonal variation of non-typhoid *Salmonella* occurrence in humans. *Epidemiol Infect.* 2007;135:93-99.
45. Todd EC. Epidemiology of foodborne diseases: a worldwide review. *World Health Stat Q.* 1997;50:30-50.
46. Mishu B, Koehler J, Lee LA, et al. Outbreaks of *Salmonella enteritidis* infections in the United States, 1985-1991. *J Infect Dis.* 1994;169:547-552.
47. Angulo FJ, Tippen S, Sharp DJ, et al. A community waterborne outbreak of salmonellosis and the effectiveness of a boil water order. *Am J Public Health.* 1997;87:580-584.
48. Mishu B, Griffin PM, Tauxe RV, et al. *Salmonella enteritidis* gastroenteritis transmitted by intact chicken eggs. *Ann Intern Med.* 1991;115:190-194.
49. Rodrigue DC, Tauxe RV, Rowe B. International increase in *Salmonella enteritidis*: a new pandemic? *Epidemiol Infect.* 1990;105:21-27.
50. Braden CR. *Salmonella enterica* serotype Enteritidis and eggs: a national epidemic in the United States. *Clin Infect Dis.* 2006;43:512-517.
51. Marcus R, Varma JK, Medus C, et al. Re-assessment of risk factors for sporadic *Salmonella* serotype Enteritidis infections: a case-control study in five FoodNet Sites, 2002-2003. *Epidemiol Infect.* 2007;135:84-92.
52. Ebel E, Schlosser W. Estimating the annual fraction of eggs contaminated with *Salmonella enteritidis* in the United States. *Int J Food Microbiol.* 2000;61:51-62.
53. Guard-Petter J, Henzler DJ, Rahman MM, et al. On-farm monitoring of mouse-invasive *Salmonella enterica* serovar enteritidis and a model for its association with the production of contaminated eggs. *Appl Environ Microbiol.* 1997;63:1588-1593.
54. Baumler AJ, Hargis BM, Tsolis RM. Tracing the origins of *Salmonella* outbreaks. *Science.* 2000;287:50-52.
55. White DG, Zhao S, Sudler R, et al. The isolation of antibiotic-resistant salmonella from retail ground meats. *N Engl J Med.* 2001;345:1147-1154.
56. USDA Food Safety and Inspection Service. Progress report on salmonella testing of raw meat and poultry products, 1998-2007. Available at: ⟨http://www.fsis.usda.gov/science/progress_report_salmonella_testing/index.asp⟩.
57. Parry SM, Palmer SR, Slader J, et al. Risk factors for salmonella food poisoning in the domestic kitchen—a case control study. *Epidemiol Infect.* 2002;129:277-285.
58. Sarwari AR, Magder LS, Levine P, et al. Serotype distribution of *Salmonella* isolates from food animals after slaughter differs from that of isolates found in humans. *J Infect Dis.* 2001;183:1295-1299.
59. Multistate outbreaks of *Salmonella* infections associated with raw tomatoes eaten in restaurants—United States, 2005-2006. *MMWR Morb Mortal Wkly Rep.* 2007;56:909-911.
60. Brooks JT, Rowe SY, Shillam P, et al. *Salmonella* Typhimurium infections transmitted by chlorine-pretreated clover sprout seeds. *Am J Epidemiol.* 2001;154:1020-1028.
61. Cahill SM, Wachsmuth IK, Costarrica Mde L, et al. Powdered infant formula as a source of *Salmonella* infection in infants. *Clin Infect Dis.* 2008;46:268-273.
62. Ryan CA, Nickels MK, Hargrett-Bean NT, et al. Massive outbreak of antimicrobial-resistant salmonellosis traced to pasteurized milk. *JAMA.* 1987;258:3269-3274.
63. Woodward DL, Khakhria R, Johnson WM. Human salmonellosis associated with exotic pets. *J Clin Microbiol.* 1997;35:2786-2790.
64. Mermin J, Hutwagner L, Vugia D, et al. Reptiles, amphibians, and human *Salmonella* infection: a population-based, case-control study. *Clin Infect Dis.* 2004;38(Suppl 3):S253-261.
65. Turtle-associated salmonellosis in humans—United States, 2006-2007. *MMWR Morb Mortal Wkly Rep.* 2007;56:649-652.
66. Update: recall of dry dog and cat food products associated with human *Salmonella Schwarzengrund* infections—United States, 2008. *MMWR Morb Mortal Wkly Rep.* 2008;57:1200-1202.
67. Finley R, Reid-Smith R, Weese JS. Human health implications of *Salmonella*-contaminated natural pet treats and raw pet food. *Clin Infect Dis.* 2006;42:686-691.
68. Swanson SJ, Snider C, Braden CR, et al. Multidrug-resistant *Salmonella enterica* serotype Typhimurium associated with pet rodents. *N Engl J Med.* 2007;356:21-28.
69. Chiu CH, Wu TL, Su LH, et al. The emergence in Taiwan of fluoroquinolone resistance in *Salmonella enterica* serotype choleraesuis. *N Engl J Med.* 2002;346:413-419.
70. Gordon MA, Graham SM, Walsh AL, et al. Epidemics of invasive *Salmonella enterica* serovar enteritidis and *S. enterica* serovar Typhimurium infection associated with multidrug resistance among adults and children in Malawi. *Clin Infect Dis.* 2008;46:963-969.
71. Boyd EF, Hartl DL. Recent horizontal transmission of plasmids between natural populations of *Escherichia coli* and *Salmonella enterica.* *J Bacteriol.* 1997;179:1622-1627.
72. Humphrey T. *Salmonella* Typhimurium definitive type 104: a multi-resistant *Salmonella.* *Int J Food Microbiol.* 2001;67:173-186.
73. Casin I, Breuil J, Brisabois A, et al. Multidrug-resistant human and animal *Salmonella* Typhimurium isolates in France belong predominantly to a DT104 clone with the chromosome- and integron-encoded beta-lactamase PSE-1. *J Infect Dis.* 1999;179:1173-1182.
74. Sorensen O, Van Donkersgoed J, McFall M, et al. *Salmonella* spp. shedding by alberta beef cattle and the detection of *Salmonella* spp. in ground beef. *J Food Prot.* 2002;65:484-491.
75. Beaudin BA, Brosnikoff CA, Grimsrud KM, et al. Susceptibility of human isolates of *Salmonella* Typhimurium DT 104 to antimicrobial agents used in human and veterinary medicine. *Diagn Microbiol Infect Dis.* 2002;42:17-20.
76. Dechet AM, Scallan E, Gensheimer K, et al. Outbreak of multidrug-resistant *Salmonella enterica* serotype Typhimurium Definitive Type 104 infection linked to commercial ground beef, northeastern United States, 2003-2004. *Clin Infect Dis.* 2006;42:747-752.
77. Allen CA, Fedorka-Cray PJ, Vazquez-Torres A, et al. In vitro and in vivo assessment of *Salmonella enterica* serovar Typhimurium DT104 virulence. *Infect Immun.* 2001;69:4673-4677.
78. Varma JK, Molbak K, Barrett TJ, et al. Antimicrobial-resistant nontyphoidal *Salmonella* is associated with excess bloodstream infections and hospitalizations. *J Infect Dis.* 2005;191:554-561.
79. Fey PD, Safranek TJ, Rupp ME, et al. Ceftriaxone-resistant salmonella infection acquired by a child from cattle [see comments]. *N Engl J Med.* 2000;342:1242-1249.
80. Dunne EF, Fey PD, Kludt P, et al. Emergence of domestically acquired ceftriaxone-resistant *Salmonella* infections associated with AmpC beta-lactamase. *JAMA.* 2000;284:3151-3156.
81. Varma JK, Marcus R, Stenzel SA, et al. Highly resistant *Salmonella* Newport-MDRAmpC transmitted through the domestic US food supply: a FoodNet case-control study of sporadic *Salmonella* Newport infections, 2002-2003. *J Infect Dis.* 2006;194:222-230.
82. Winokur PL, Vonstein DL, Hoffman LJ, et al. Evidence for transfer of CMY-2 AmpC beta-lactamase plasmids between *Escherichia coli* and *Salmonella* isolates from food animals and humans. *Antimicrob Agents Chemother.* 2001;45:2716-2722.
83. Gupta A, Fontana J, Crowe C, et al. Emergence of multidrug-resistant *Salmonella enterica* serotype Newport infections resistant to expanded-spectrum cephalosporins in the United States. *J Infect Dis.* 2003;188:1707-1716.
84. Armand-Lefevre L, Leflon-Guibout V, Bredin J, et al. Imipenem resistance in *Salmonella enterica* serovar Wien related to porin loss and CMY-4 beta-lactamase production. *Antimicrob Agents Chemother.* 2003;47:1165-1168.
85. Nordmann P, Poirel L, Mak JK, et al. Multidrug-resistant *Salmonella* strains expressing emerging antibiotic resistance determinants. *Clin Infect Dis.* 2008;46:324-325.
86. Heisig P. High-level fluoroquinolone resistance in a *Salmonella* Typhimurium isolate due to alterations in both gyrA and gyrB genes. *J Antimicrob Chemother.* 1993;32:367-377.
87. Giraud E, Cloeckaert A, Kerboeuf D, et al. Evidence for active efflux as the primary mechanism of resistance to ciprofloxacin in *Salmonella enterica* serovar Typhimurium. *Antimicrob Agents Chemother.* 2000;44:1223-1228.
88. Cheung TK, Chu YW, Chu MY, et al. Plasmid-mediated resistance to ciprofloxacin and cefotaxime in clinical isolates of *Salmonella enterica* serotype Enteritidis in Hong Kong. *J Antimicrob Chemother.* 2005;56:586-589.
89. Hopkins KL, Wootton L, Day MR, et al. Plasmid-mediated quinolone resistance determinant qnrS1 found in *Salmonella enterica* strains isolated in the UK. *J Antimicrob Chemother.* 2007;59:1071-1075.
90. Threlfall EJ, Frost JA, Ward LR, et al. Increasing spectrum of resistance in multiresistant *Salmonella* Typhimurium [letter]. *Lancet.* 1996;347:1053-1054.
91. Olsen SJ, DeBess EE, McGivern TE, et al. A nosocomial outbreak of fluoroquinolone-resistant salmonella infection. *N Engl J Med.* 2001;344:1572-1579.
92. Wadula J, von Gottberg A, Kilner D, et al. Nosocomial outbreak of extended-spectrum beta-lactamase-producing *Salmonella isangi* in pediatric wards. *Pediatr Infect Dis J.* 2006;25:843-844.
93. Weikel CS, Guerrant RL. Nosocomial salmonellosis [editorial]. *Infect Control.* 1985;6:218-220.
94. Nair D, Gupta N, Kabra S, et al. *Salmonella senftenberg*: a new pathogen in the burns ward. *Burns.* 1999;25:723-727.
95. Wall PG, Ryan MJ, Ward LR, et al. Outbreaks of salmonellosis in hospitals in England and Wales: 1992-1994. *J Hosp Infect.* 1996;33:181-190.
96. Wall PG, Ryan MJ. Faecal incontinence in hospitals and residential and nursing homes for elderly people [letter; comment]. *BMJ.* 1996;312:378.
97. Tauxe RV, Hassan LF, Findeisen KO, et al. Salmonellosis in nurses: lack of transmission to patients. *J Infect Dis.* 1988;157:370-373.
98. Wilson R, Feldman RA, Davis J, et al. Salmonellosis in infants: the importance of intrafamilial transmission. *Pediatrics.* 1982;69:436-438.
99. Haddock RL, Cousens SN, Guzman CC. Infant diet and salmonellosis. *Am J Public Health.* 1991;81:997-1000.
100. Bornemann R, Zerr DM, Heath J, et al. An outbreak of *Salmonella* serotype Saintpaul in a children's hospital. *Infect Control Hosp Epidemiol.* 2002;23:671-676.
101. Buchwald DS, Blaser MJ. A review of human salmonellosis. 2. Duration of excretion following infection with nontyphi *Salmonella.* *Rev Infect Dis.* 1984;6:345-356.
102. Bowen A, Newman A, Estivariz C, et al. Role of acid-suppressing medications during a sustained outbreak of *Salmonella enteritidis* infection in a long-term care facility. *Infect Control Hosp Epidemiol.* 2007;28:1202-1205.
103. Levine WC, Smart JF, Archer DL, et al. Foodborne disease outbreaks in nursing homes, 1975 through 1987. *JAMA.* 1991;266:2105-2109.
104. Blaser MJ, Neuman LS. A review of human salmonellosis: I. Infective dose. *Rev Infect Dis.* 1982;4:1096.
105. Mintz ED, Cartter ML, Hadler JL, et al. Dose-response effects in an outbreak of *Salmonella* enteritidis. *Epidemiol Infect.* 1994;112:13-23.
106. Foster JW, Hall HK. Adaptive acidification tolerance response of *Salmonella typhimurium.* *J Bacteriol.* 1990;172:771-778.
107. Michetti P, Mahan MJ, Slauch JM, et al. Monoclonal secretory immunoglobulin A protects mice against oral challenge with the invasive pathogen *Salmonella typhimurium.* *Infect Immun.* 1992;60:1786-1792.
108. Selsted ME, Miller SI, Henschen AH, et al. Enteric defensins: antibiotic peptide components of intestinal host defense. *J Cell Biol.* 1992;118:929-936.
109. van der Velden AW, Baumler AJ, Tsolis RM, et al. Multiple fimbrial adhesins are required for full virulence of *Salmonella typhimurium* in mice. *Infect Immun.* 1998;66:2803-2808.
110. Francis CL, Starnbach MN, Falkow S. Morphological and cytoskeletal changes in epithelial cells occur immediately upon interaction with *Salmonella typhimurium* grown under low-oxygen conditions. *Mol Microbiol.* 1992;6:3077-3087.
111. Jones BD, Ghori N, Falkow S. *Salmonella typhimurium* initiates murine infection by penetrating and destroying the specialized epithelial M cells of the Peyer's Patches. *J Exp Med.* 1994;180:15-23.
112. Watson PR, Paulin SM, Bland AP, et al. Characterization of intestinal invasion by *Salmonella typhimurium* and *Salmonella dublin* and effect of a mutation in the *invH* gene. *Infect Immun.* 1995;63:2743-2754.
113. Haraga A, West TE, Brittnacher MJ, et al. *Burkholderia thailandensis* as a model system for the study of the virulence-associated type III secretion system of *Burkholderia pseudomallei.* *Infect Immun.* 2008;76:5402-5411.
114. Scherer CA, Cooper E, Miller SI. The *Salmonella* type III secretion translocon protein SspC is inserted into the epithelial cell plasma membrane upon infection. *Mol Microbiol.* 2000;37:1133-1145.
115. Hayward RD, Koronakis V. Direct nucleation and bundling of actin by the SipC protein of invasive *Salmonella.* *EMBO J.* 1999;18:4926-4934.
116. Zhou D, Mooseker MS, Galan JE. Role of the *S. typhimurium* actin-binding protein SipA in bacterial internalization. *Science.* 1999;283:2092-2095.
117. Hardt W-D, Chen L-M, Schuebel KE, et al. *S. typhimurium* encodes an activator of Rho GTPases that induces membrane ruffling and nuclear responses in host cells. *Cell.* 1998;93:815-826.
118. Norris FA, Wilson MP, Wallis TS, et al. SopB, a protein required for virulence of *Salmonella dublin,* is an inositol phosphate phosphatase. *Proc Natl Acad Sci U S A.* 1998;95:14057-14059.
119. Zhou D, Chen LM, Hernandez L, et al. A *Salmonella* inositol polyphosphatase acts in conjunction with other bacterial effectors to promote host cell actin cytoskeleton rearrangements and bacterial internalization. *Mol Microbiol.* 2001;39:248-259.
120. Patel JC, Galan JE. Differential activation and function of Rho GTPases during *Salmonella*–host cell interactions. *J Cell Biol.* 2006;175:453-463.
121. Rescigno M, Urbano M, Valzasina B, et al. Dendritic cells express tight junction proteins and penetrate gut epithelial monolayers to sample bacteria. *Nat Immunol.* 2001;2:361-367.
122. Vazquez-Torres A, Jones-Carson J, Baumler AJ, et al. Extraintestinal dissemination of *Salmonella* by CD18-expressing phagocytes. *Nature.* 1999;401:804-808.
123. Watson PR, Galyov EE, Paulin SM, et al. Mutation of invH, but not stn, reduces *Salmonella*-induced enteritis in cattle. *Infect Immun.* 1998;66:1432-1438.
124. McCormick BA, Colgan SP, Delp-Archer C, et al. *Salmonella typhimurium* attachment to human intestinal epithelial monolayers: transcellular signalling to subepithelial neutrophils. *J Cell Biol.* 1993;123:895-907.
125. Eckmann L, Rudolf MT, Ptasznik A, et al. D-*myo*-Inositol 1,4,5,6-tetrakisphosphate produced in human intestinal epithelial cells in response to *Salmonella* invasion inhibits phos-

phoinositide 3-kinase signaling pathways. *Proc Natl Acad Sci U S A.* 1997;94:14456-14460.
126. Prager R, Mirold S, Tietze E, et al. Prevalence and polymorphism of genes encoding translocated effector proteins among clinical isolates of *Salmonella enterica*. *Int J Med Microbiol.* 2000;290:605-617.
127. Akira S. Mammalian Toll-like receptors. *Curr Opin Immunol.* 2003;15:5-11.
128. Miao EA, Alpuche-Aranda CM, Dors M, et al. Cytoplasmic flagellin activates caspase-1 and secretion of interleukin 1beta via Ipaf. *Nat Immunol.* 2006;7:569-575.
129. Sun YH, Rolan HG, Tsolis RM. Injection of flagellin into the host cell cytosol by *Salmonella enterica* serotype Typhimurium. *J Biol Chem.* 2007;282:33897-33901.
130. Rubin RH, Weinstein L. *Salmonellosis: Microbiologic, Pathologic, and Clinical Features.* New York: Stratton Intercontinental; 1977.
131. Wilson RP, Raffatellu M, Chessa D, et al. The Vi-capsule prevents Toll-like receptor 4 recognition of *Salmonella*. *Cell Microbiol.* 2008;10:876-890.
132. Fu Y, Galan JE. A *Salmonella* protein antagonizes Rac-1 and Cdc42 to mediate host-cell recovery after bacterial invasion. *Nature.* 1999;401:293-297.
133. Collier-Hyams LS, Zeng H, Sun J, et al. Cutting edge: *Salmonella* AvrA effector inhibits the key proinflammatory, anti-apoptotic NF-kappa B pathway. *J Immunol.* 2002;169:2846-2850.
134. Haraga A, Miller SI. A *Salmonella enterica* serovar typhimurium translocated leucine-rich repeat effector protein inhibits NF-κ-B-dependent gene expression. *Infect Immun.* 2003;71:4052-4058.
135. Rubin FA, McWhirter PD, Burr D, et al. Rapid diagnosis of typhoid fever through identification of *Salmonella* typhi within 18 hours of specimen acquisition by culture of the monomuclear cell-platelet fraction of blood. *J Clin Microbiol.* 1990;28:825-827.
136. Fields PI, Swanson RV, Haidaris CG, et al. Mutants of *Salmonella typhimurium* that cannot survive within the macrophage are avirulent. *Proc Natl Acad Sci U S A.* 1986;83:5189-5193.
137. Richter-Dahlfors A, Buchan AMJ, Finlay BB. Murine Salmonellosis studied by confocal microscopy: *Salmonella typhimurium* resides intracellularly inside macrophages and exerts a cytotoxic effect on phagocytes in vivo. *J Exp Med.* 1997;186:569-580.
138. Haraga A, Ohlson MB, Miller SI. Salmonellae interplay with host cells. *Nat Rev Microbiol.* 2008;6:53-66.
139. Bader MW, Sanowar S, Daley ME, et al. Recognition of antimicrobial peptides by a bacterial sensor kinase. *Cell.* 2005;122:461-472.
140. Prost LR, Miller SI. The Salmonellae PhoQ sensor: mechanisms of detection of phagosome signals. *Cell Microbiol.* 2008;10:576-582.
141. Prost LR, Daley ME, Bader MW, et al. The PhoQ histidine kinases of *Salmonella* and *Pseudomonas* spp. are structurally and functionally different: evidence that pH and antimicrobial peptide sensing contribute to mammalian pathogenesis. *Mol Microbiol.* 2008;69:503-519.
142. Guo L, Lim K, Gunn JS, et al. Regulation of lipid A modifications by *Salmonella* Typhimurium virulence genes *phoP-phoQ*. *Science.* 1997;276:250-253.
143. Prost LR, Sanowar S, Miller SI. *Salmonella* sensing of antimicrobial mechanisms to promote survival within macrophages. *Immunol Rev.* 2007;219:55-65.
144. Hohmann EL, Oletta CA, Killeen KP, et al. *phoP/phoQ*–deleted *Salmonella typhi* (TY800) is a safe and immunogenic single dose typhoid fever vaccine in volunteers. *J Infect Dis.* 1996;173:1408-1414.
145. Looney RJ, Steigbigel RT. Role of the Vi antigen of *Salmonella* typhi in resistance to host defense in vitro. *J Lab Clin Med.* 1986;108:506-516.
146. Shea JE, Hensel M, Gleeson C, et al. Identification of a virulence locus encoding a second type III secretion system in *Salmonella typhimurium*. *Proc Nat Acad Sci U S A.* 1996;93:2593-2597.
147. Brawn LC, Hayward RD, Koronakis V. *Salmonella* SPI1 effector SipA persists after entry and cooperates with a SPI2 effector to regulate phagosome maturation and intracellular replication. *Cell Host Microbe.* 2007;1:63-75.
148. Meresse S, Unsworth KE, Habermann A, et al. Remodelling of the actin cytoskeleton is essential for replication of intravacuolar *Salmonella*. *Cell Microbiol.* 2001;3:567-577.
149. Miao EA, Brittnacher M, Haraga A, et al. *Salmonella* effectors translocated across the vacuolar membrane interact with the actin cytoskeleton. *Mol Microbiol.* 2003;48:401-415.
150. Lesnick ML, Reiner NE, Fierer J, et al. The *Salmonella* spvB virulence gene encodes an enzyme that ADP-ribosylates actin and destabilizes the cytoskeleton of eukaryotic cells. *Mol Microbiol.* 2001;39:1464-1470.
151. Salcedo SP, Holden DW. SseG, a virulence protein that targets *Salmonella* to the Golgi network. *EMBO J.* 2003;22:5003-5014.
152. Fierer J, Krause M, Tauxe R, et al. *Salmonella typhimurium* bacteremia: association with the virulence plasmid. *J Infect Dis.* 1992;166:639-642.
153. Bernheiden M, Heinrich JM, Minigo G, et al. LBP, CD14, TLR4 and the murine innate immune response to a peritoneal *Salmonella* infection. *J Endotoxin Res.* 2001;7:447-450.
154. Lara-Tejero M, Sutterwala FS, Ogura Y, et al. Role of the caspase-1 inflammasome in *Salmonella* Typhimurium pathogenesis. *J Exp Med.* 2006;203:1407-1412.
155. Mastroeni P, Harrison JA, Robinson JH, et al. Interleukin-12 is required for control of the growth of attenuated aromatic-compound-dependent salmonellae in BALB/c mice: role of gamma interferon and macrophage activation. *Infect Immun.* 1998;66:4767-4776.
156. Everest P, Roberts M, Dougan G. Susceptibility to *Salmonella typhimurium* infection and effectiveness of vaccination in mice deficient in the tumor necrosis factor alpha p55 receptor. *Infect Immun.* 1998;66:3355-3364.
157. Hess J, Ladel C, Miko D, et al. *Salmonella typhimurium* aroA-infection in gene-targeted immunodeficient mice: major role of CD4+ TCR-alpha beta cells and IFN-gamma in bacterial clearance independent of intracellular location. *J Immunol.* 1996;156:3321-3326.
158. Netea MG, Radstake T, Joosten LA, et al. *Salmonella* septicemia in rheumatoid arthritis patients receiving anti-tumor necrosis factor therapy: association with decreased interferon-gamma production and Toll-like receptor 4 expression. *Arthritis Rheum.* 2003;48:1853-1857.
159. Jouanguy E, Doffinger R, Dupuis S, et al. IL-12 and IFN-gamma in host defense against mycobacteria and salmonella in mice and men. *Curr Opin Immunol.* 1999;11:346-351.
160. Mastroeni P, Simmons C, Fowler R, et al. Igh-6$^{-/-}$ (B-cell-deficient) mice fail to mount solid acquired resistance to oral challenge with virulent *Salmonella enterica* serovar typhimurium and show impaired Th1 T-cell responses to *Salmonella* antigens. *Infect Immun.* 2000;68:46-53.
161. Nauciel C. Role of CD4$^+$ T cells and T-independent mechanisms in acquired resistance to *Salmonella typhimurium* infection. *J Immunol.* 1990;145:1265-1269.
162. Han T, Sokal JE, Neter E. Salmonellosis in disseminated malignant diseases: a seven-year review (1959-1965). *N Engl J Med.* 1967;276:1045-1052.
163. Mussche MM, Lameire NH, Ringoir SM. *Salmonella* Typhimurium infections in renal transplant patients: report of five cases. *Nephron.* 1975;15:143-150.
164. Celum CL, Chaisson RE, Rutherford GW, et al. Incidence of salmonellosis in patients with AIDS. *J Infect Dis.* 1987;156:998-1002.
165. Angulo FJ, Swerdlow DL. Bacterial enteric infections in persons infected with human immunodeficiency virus. *Clin Infect Dis.* 1995;21(Suppl 1):S84-S93.
166. Oksenhendler E, Gerard L, Fieschi C, et al. Infections in 252 patients with common variable immunodeficiency. *Clin Infect Dis.* 2008;46:1547-1554.
167. Nencioni L, Villa L, De Magistris MT, et al. Cellular immunity against *Salmonella* typhi after live oral vaccine. *Adv Exp Med Biol.* 1987;216B:1669-1675.
168. Dunstan SJ, Stephens HA, Blackwell JM, et al. Genes of the class II and class III major histocompatibility complex are associated with typhoid fever in Vietnam. *J Infect Dis.* 2001;183:261-268.
169. Jones TF, Ingram LA, Cieslak PR, et al. Salmonellosis outcomes differ substantially by serotype. *J Infect Dis.* 2008;198:109-114.
170. Saphra I, Winter JW. Clinical manifestations of salmonellosis in man: an evaluation of 7779 human infections identified at the New York Salmonella Center. *N Engl J Med.* 1957;256:1128-1134.
171. Chaudhuri A, Bekdash BA. Toxic megacolon due to *Salmonella*: a case report and review of the literature. *Int J Colorectal Dis.* 2002;17:275-279.
172. Mead PS, Slutsker L, Dietz V, et al. Food-related illness and death in the United States. *Emerg Infect Dis.* 1999;5:607-625.
173. Lim E, Koh WH, Loh SF, et al. Non-typhoidal salmonellosis in patients with systemic lupus erythematosus: a study of fifty patients and a review of the literature. *Lupus.* 2001;10:87-92.
174. Levine WC, Buehler JW, Bean NH, et al. Epidemiology of non-typhoidal *Salmonella* bacteremia during the human immunodeficiency virus epidemic. *J Infect Dis.* 1991;164:81-87.
175. Szanton VL. Epidemic salmonellosis. *Pediatrics.* 1957;20:794-808.
176. Butler T, Islam A, Kabir I, et al. Patterns of morbidity and mortality in typhoid fever dependent on age and gender: review of 552 hospitalized patients with diarrhea. *Rev Infect Dis.* 1991;13:85-90.
177. Barrett-Connor E. Bacterial infection and sickle cell anemia: an analysis of 250 infections in 166 patients and a review of the literature. *Medicine.* 1971;50:97-112.
178. Wheat LJ, Rubin RH, Harris NL, et al. Systemic salmonellosis in patients with disseminated histoplasmosis: case for 'macrophage blockade' caused by *Histoplasma capsulatum*. *Arch Intern Med.* 1987;147:561-564.
179. Bhan MK, Bahl R, Sazawal S, et al. Association between *Helicobacter pylori* infection and increased risk of typhoid fever. *J Infect Dis.* 2002;186:1857-1860.
180. Stuart BM, Pullen RL. Typhoid: clinical analysis of three hundred and sixty cases. *Arch Intern Med.* 1946;78:629-661.
181. Bhutta ZA. Impact of age and drug resistance on mortality in typhoid fever. *Arch Dis Child.* 1996;75:214-217.
182. Roland HAK. The complications of typhoid fever. *J Trop Med Hyg.* 1961;64:143.
183. Sulaiman K, Sarwari AR. Culture-confirmed typhoid fever and pregnancy. *Int J Infect Dis.* 2007;11:337-341.
184. Verghese A. The "typhoid state" revisited. *Am J Med.* 1985;79:370-372.
185. Khan M, Coovadia YM, Connoly C, et al. The early diagnosis of typhoid fever prior to the Widal test and bacteriological culture results. *Acta Tropica.* 1998;69:165-173.
186. El-Newihi HM, Alamy ME, Reynolds TB. *Salmonella* hepatitis: analysis of 27 cases and comparison with acute viral hepatitis. *Hepatology.* 1996;24:516-519.
187. Farooqui BJ, Khurshid M, Ashfaq MK, et al. Comparative yield of *Salmonella* Typhi from blood and bone marrow cultures in patients with fever of unknown origin. *J Clin Pathol.* 1991;44:258-259.
188. Wain J, Diep TS, Ho VA, et al. Quantitation of bacteria in blood of typhoid fever patients and relationship between counts and clinical features, transmissibility, and antibiotic resistance. *J Clin Microbiol.* 1998;36:1683-1687.
189. Mantur BG, Bidari LH, Akki AS, et al. Diagnostic yield of blood clot culture in the accurate diagnosis of enteric fever and human brucellosis. *Clin Lab.* 2007;53:57-61.
190. Wain J, Pham VB, Ha V, et al. Quantitation of bacteria in bone marrow from patients with typhoid fever: relationship between counts and clinical features. *J Clin Microbiol.* 2001;39:1571-1576.
191. Benavente L, Gotuzzo E, Guerra J, et al. Diagnosis of typhoid fever using a string capsule device. *Trans R Soc Trop Med Hyg.* 1984;78:564-565.
192. Edelman R, Levine MM. Summary of an international workshop on typhoid fever. *Rev Infect Dis.* 1986;8:329-349.
193. Gilman RH, Terminel M, Levine MM, et al. Relative efficacy of blood, urine, rectal swab, bone-marrow, and rose-spot cultures for recovery of *Salmonella* Typhi in typhoid fever. *Lancet.* 1975;1:1211-1213.
194. Kawano RL, Leano SA, Agdamag DM. Comparison of serological test kits for diagnosis of typhoid fever in the Philippines. *J Clin Microbiol.* 2007;45:246-247.
195. Naheed A, Ram PK, Brooks WA, et al. Clinical value of Tubex and Typhidot rapid diagnostic tests for typhoid fever in an urban community clinic in Bangladesh. *Diagn Microbiol Infect Dis.* 2008;61:381-386.
196. Levy H, Diallo S, Tennant SM, et al. PCR method to identify *Salmonella enterica* serovars Typhi, Paratyphi A, and Paratyphi B among *Salmonella* isolates from the blood of patients with clinical enteric fever. *J Clin Microbiol.* 2008;46:1861-1866.
197. Aziah I, Ravichandran M, Ismail A. Amplification of ST50 gene using dry-reagent-based polymerase chain reaction for the detection of *Salmonella* Typhi. *Diagn Microbiol Infect Dis.* 2007;59:373-377.
198. Mandal BK, Brennand J. Bacteraemia in salmonellosis: a 15 year retrospective study from a regional infectious diseases unit. *BMJ.* 1988;297:1242-1243.
199. Wang JY, Hwang JJ, Hsu CN, et al. Bacteraemia due to ciprofloxacin-resistant *Salmonella enterica* serotype Choleraesuis in adult patients at a university hospital in Taiwan, 1996-2004. *Epidemiol Infect.* 2006;134:977-984.
200. Shimoni Z, Pitlik S, Leibovici L, et al. Nontyphoid *Salmonella* bacteremia: age-related differences in clinical presentation, bacteriology, and outcome. *Clin Infect Dis.* 1999;28:822-827.
201. Hsu RB, Tsay YG, Chen RJ, et al. Risk factors for primary bacteremia and endovascular infection in patients without acquired immunodeficiency syndrome who have nontyphoid salmonellosis. *Clin Infect Dis.* 2003;36:829-834.
202. Chen PL, Chang CM, Wu CJ, et al. Extraintestinal focal infections in adults with nontyphoid *Salmonella* bacteraemia: predisposing factors and clinical outcome. *J Intern Med.* 2007;261:91-100.
203. Hung CC, Hung MN, Hsueh PR, et al. Risk of recurrent nontyphoid *Salmonella* bacteremia in HIV-infected patients in the era of highly active antiretroviral therapy and an increasing trend of fluoroquinolone resistance. *Clin Infect Dis.* 2007;45:e60-e67.
204. Gradel KO, Dethlefsen C, Schonheyder HC, et al. Magnitude of bacteraemia is associated with increased mortality in non-typhoid salmonellosis: a one-year follow-up study. *APMIS.* 2008;116:147-153.
205. Yen YF, Lin YC, Chen TL, et al. Non-typhoidal *Salmonella* bacteremia in adults. *J Microbiol Immunol Infect.* 2007;40:227-233.
206. Parsons R, Gregory J, Palmer DL. *Salmonella* infections of the abdominal aorta. *Rev Infect Dis.* 1983;5:227-231.
207. Cohen JI, Bartlett JA, Corey GR. Extra-intestinal manifestations of *Salmonella* infections. *Medicine.* 1987;66:349-388.
208. Benenson S, Raveh D, Schlesinger Y, et al. The risk of vascular infection in adult patients with nontyphi *Salmonella* bacteremia. *Am J Med.* 2001;110:60-63.
209. Gradel KO, Schonheyder HC, Pedersen L, et al. Incidence and prognosis of non-typhoid *Salmonella* bacteraemia in Denmark: A 10-year county-based follow-up study. *Eur J Clin Microbiol Infect Dis.* 2006;25:151-158.
210. Carey J, Buchstein S, Shah S. Septic deep vein thrombosis due to *Salmonella johannesburg*. *J Infect.* 2001;42:79-80.
211. Tumbarello M, Tacconelli E, Caponera S, et al. The impact of bacteraemia on HIV infection: nine years experience in a large Italian university hospital. *J Infect.* 1995;31:123-131.
212. Arthur G, Nduba VN, Kariuki SM, et al. Trends in bloodstream infections among human immunodeficiency virus–infected adults admitted to a hospital in Nairobi, Kenya, during the last decade. *Clin Infect Dis.* 2001;33:248-256.
213. Gruenewald R, Blum S, Chan J. Relationship between human immunodeficiency virus infection and salmonellosis in 20- to

59-year-old residents of New York City. *Clin Infect Dis.* 1994;18:358-363.

214. Gordon MA, Banda HT, Gondwe M, et al. Non-typhoidal salmonella bacteraemia among HIV-infected Malawian adults: high mortality and frequent recrudescence. *AIDS.* 2002; 16:1633-1641.

215. Gordon MA, Gordon SB, Musaya L, et al. Primary macrophages from HIV-infected adults show dysregulated cytokine responses to *Salmonella*, but normal internalization and killing. *AIDS.* 2007;21:2399-2408.

216. Casado JL, Valdezate S, Calderon C, et al. Zidovudine therapy protects against *Salmonella* bacteremia recurrence in human immunodeficiency virus-infected patients. *J Infect Dis.* 1999;179:1553-1556.

217. Hung CC, Hsieh SM, Hsiao CF, et al. Risk of recurrent nontyphoid *Salmonella* bacteraemia after early discontinuation of ciprofloxacin as secondary prophylaxis in AIDS patients in the era of highly active antiretroviral therapy. *AIDS.* 2001; 15:645-647.

218. Musher DM, Rubenstein AD. Permanent carriers of nontyphosal salmonellae. *Arch Intern Med.* 1973;132:869-872.

219. Neves J, Raso P, Marinko PP. Prolonged septicemic salmonellosis intercurrent with *Schistosomiasis mansoni* infection. *J Trop Med Hyg.* 1971;74:9.

220. Balfour AE, Lewis R, Ahmed S. Convalescent excretion of *Salmonella enteritidis* in infants. *J Infect.* 1999;38:24-25.

221. Nath G, Singh H, Shukla VK. Chronic typhoid carriage and carcinoma of the gallbladder. *Eur J Cancer Prev.* 1997; 6:557-559.

222. Lanata CF, Levine MM, Ristori C, et al. Vi serology in detection of chronic *Salmonella* Typhi carriers in an endemic area. *Lancet.* 1983;2:441-443.

223. Ashcroft MT, Morrision RJ, Nicholson CC. Controlled field trial in British Guiana school children of heat-killed-phenolized and acetone-killed lyophilized typhoid vaccines. *Am J Hyg.* 1964;79:196-206.

224. Klugman KP, Gilbertson IT, Koornhof HJ, et al. Protective activity of Vi capsular polysaccharide vaccine against typhoid fever. *Lancet.* 1987;2:1165-1169.

225. Simanjuntak CH, Paleologo FP, Punjabi NH, et al. Oral immunisation against typhoid fever in Indonesia with Ty21a vaccine [see comments]. *Lancet.* 1991;338:1055-1059.

226. Arguin PM, Kozarsky PE, Reed C. *CDC Health Information for International Travel 2008.* Atlanta, GA: DHHS, Mosby Elsevier; 2008.

227. Levine MM, Ferreccio C, Black RE, et al. Ty21a live oral typhoid vaccine and prevention of paratyphoid fever caused by *Salmonella enterica* Serovar Paratyphi B. *Clin Infect Dis.* 2007;45 (Suppl 1):S24-S28.

228. Engels EA, Falagas ME, Lau J, et al. Typhoid fever vaccines: a meta-analysis of studies on efficacy and toxicity. *BMJ.* 1998;316:110-116.

229. Robbins JD, Robbins JB. Reexamination of the protective role of the capsular polysaccharide (Vi antigen) of *Salmonella* Typhi. *J Infect Dis.* 1984;150:436-449.

230. Lin FY, Ho VA, Khiem HB, et al. The efficacy of a *Salmonella* Typhi Vi conjugate vaccine in two-to-five-year-old children. *N Engl J Med.* 2001;344:1263-1269.

231. Hornick RB, Greisman SE, Woodward TE, et al. Typhoid fever: pathogenesis and immunologic control. *N Engl J Med.* 1970;283:686-691.

232. DeRoeck D, Jodar L, Clemens J. Putting typhoid vaccination on the global health agenda. *N Engl J Med.* 2007;357:1069-1071.

233. Parry CM. The treatment of multidrug-resistant and nalidixic acid-resistant typhoid fever in Viet Nam. *Trans R Soc Trop Med Hyg.* 2004;98:413-422.

234. Thaver D, Zaidi AK, Critchley JA, et al. Fluoroquinolones for treating typhoid and paratyphoid fever (enteric fever). *Cochrane Database Syst Rev.* 2008:CD004530.

235. Tran TH, Bethell DB, Nguyen TT, et al. Short course of ofloxacin for treatment of multidrug-resistant typhoid. *Clin Infect Dis.* 1995;20:917-923.

236. Parry CM, Ho VA, Phuong le T, et al. Randomized controlled comparison of ofloxacin, azithromycin, and an ofloxacin-azithromycin combination for treatment of multidrug-resistant and nalidixic acid–resistant typhoid fever. *Antimicrob Agents Chemother.* 2007;51:819-825.

237. Effa EE, Bukirwa H. Azithromycin for treating uncomplicated typhoid and paratyphoid fever (enteric fever). *Cochrane Database Syst Rev.* 2008:CD006083.

238. Herzog C. Chemotherapy of typhoid fever. *Infection.* 1976;4:166-173.

239. Hoffman SL, Punjabi NH, Kumala S, et al. Reduction of mortality in chloramphenicol-treated severe typhoid fever by high-dose dexamethasone. *N Engl J Med.* 1984;310:82-88.

240. Cooles P. Adjuvant steroids and relapse of typhoid fever. *J Trop Med Hyg.* 1986;89:229-231.

241. Freerksen E, Rosenfield M, Freerksen Rea. Treatment of chronic *Salmonella* carriers. *Chemotherapy.* 1977;23:192.

242. Ferreccio C, Morris JG Jr, Valdivieso C, et al. Efficacy of ciprofloxacin in the treatment of chronic typhoid carriers. *J Infect Dis.* 1988;157:1235.

243. Sirinavin S, Garner P. Antibiotics for treating salmonella gut infections. *Cochrane Database Syst Rev.* 2000:CD001167.

244. Benson CA, Kaplan JE, Masur H, et al. Treating opportunistic infections among HIV-infected adults and adolescents: recommendations from CDC, the National Institutes of Health, and the HIV Medicine Association/Infectious Diseases Society of America. *MMWR Recomm Rep.* 2004;53:1-112.

245. Leibovitz E, Janco J, Piglansky L, et al. Oral ciprofloxacin vs. intramuscular ceftriaxone as empiric treatment of acute invasive diarrhea in children. *Pediatr Infect Dis J.* 2000;19:1060-1067.

246. Lightfoot NF, Ahmad F, Cowden J. Management of institutional outbreaks of *Salmonella* gastroenteritis. *J Antimicrob Chemother.* 1990;26:37-46.

247. Donabedian H. Long-term suppression of *Salmonella* aortitis with an oral antibiotic. *Arch Intern Med.* 1989;149:1452-1453.

248. Sirinavin S, Thavornnunth J, Sakchainanont B, et al. Norfloxacin and azithromycin for treatment of nontyphoidal salmonella carriers. *Clin Infect Dis.* 2003;37:685-691.

249. Ochiai RL, Acosta CJ, Agtini M, et al. The use of typhoid vaccines in Asia: the DOMI experience. *Clin Infect Dis.* 2007;45(Suppl 1):S34-S38.

250. Hulebak KL, Schlosser W. Hazard analysis and critical control point (HACCP) history and conceptual overview. *Risk Anal.* 2002;22:547-552.

251. Swaminathan B, Gerner-Smidt P, Ng LK, et al. Building PulseNet International: an interconnected system of laboratory networks to facilitate timely public health recognition and response to foodborne disease outbreaks and emerging foodborne diseases. *Foodborne Pathog Dis.* 2006;3:36-50.

252. Standaert SM, Hutcheson RH, Schaffner W. Nosocomial transmission of *Salmonella* gastroenteritis to laundry workers in a nursing home. *Infect Control Hosp Epidemiol.* 1994;15:22-26.

253. Kay RS, Vandevelde AG, Fiorella PD, et al. Outbreak of healthcare-associated infection and colonization with multidrug-resistant *Salmonella enterica* serovar Senftenberg in Florida. *Infect Control Hosp Epidemiol.* 2007;28:805-811.

254. Pace F, Fanfarillo F, Giorgino F, et al. *Salmonella enteritidis* pericarditis: case report and review of the literature. *Ann Ital Med Int.* 2002;17:189-192.

255. Soravia-Dunand VA, Loo VG, Salit IE. Aortitis due to *Salmonella*: report of 10 cases and comprehensive review of the literature. *Clin Infect Dis.* 1999;29:862-868.

256. Chiu CH, Ou JT. Risk factors for endovascular infection due to nontyphoid salmonellae. *Clin Infect Dis.* 2003;36:835-836.

257. Huang LT, Ko SF, Lui CC. *Salmonella* meningitis: clinical experience of third-generation cephalosporins. *Acta Paediatr.* 1997;86:1056-1058.

258. Lee WS, Puthucheary SD, Omar A. *Salmonella* meningitis and its complications in infants. *J Paediatr Child Health.* 1999;35:379-382.

259. Karim M, Islam N. *Salmonella* meningitis: report of three cases in adults and literature review. *Infection.* 2002;30:104-108.

260. Aguado JM, Obeso G, Cabanillas JJ, et al. Pleuropulmonary infections due to nontyphoidal strains of *Salmonella*. *Arch Intern Med.* 1990;150:54-56.

261. Santos EM, Sapico FL. Vertebral osteomyelitis due to salmonellae: report of two cases and review. *Clin Infect Dis.* 1998;27:287-295.

262. Banky JP, Ostergaard L, Spelman D. Chronic relapsing salmonella osteomyelitis in an immunocompetent patient: case report and literature review. *J Infect.* 2002;44:44-47.

263. Dworkin MS, Shoemaker PC, Goldoft MJ, et al. Reactive arthritis and Reiter's syndrome following an outbreak of gastroenteritis caused by *Salmonella enteritidis.* *Clin Infect Dis.* 2001;33:1010-1014.

264. Buxton JA, Fyfe M, Berger S, et al. Reactive arthritis and other sequelae following sporadic *Salmonella* Typhimurium infection in British Columbia, Canada: a case control study. *J Rheumatol.* 2002;29:2154-2158.

265. Ekman P, Kirveskari J, Granfors K. Modification of disease outcome in *Salmonella*-infected patients by HLA-B27. *Arthritis Rheum.* 2000;43:1527-1534.

266. Chen JY, Luo SF, Wu YJ, et al. *Salmonella* septic arthritis in systemic lupus erythematosus and other systemic diseases. *Clin Rheum.* 1998;17:282-287.

267. Collazos J, Mayo J, Martínez E, et al. Muscle infections caused by *Salmonella* species: case report and review. *Clin Infect Dis.* 1999;29:673-677.

268. Lee CC, Poon SK, Chen GH. Spontaneous gas-forming liver abscess caused by *Salmonella* within hepatocellular carcinoma: a case report and review of the literature. *Dig Dis Sci.* 2002;47:586-589.

269. Torres JR, Gotuzzo E, Istúriz R, et al. Salmonellal splenic abscess in the antibiotic era: a Latin American perspective. *Clin Infect Dis.* 1994;19:871-875.

270. Ramos JM, Aguado JM, García-Corbeira P, et al. Clinical spectrum of urinary tract infections due on nontyphoidal *Salmonella* species. *Clin Infect Dis.* 1996;23:388-390.

271. Sivapalasingam S, Hoekstra RM, McQuiston JR, et al. *Salmonella* bacteriuria: an increasing entity in elderly women in the United States. *Epidemiol Infect.* 2004;132:897-902.

272. Behr MA, McDonald J. *Salmonella* neck abscess in a patient with beta-thalassemia major: case report and review. *Clin Infect Dis.* 1996;23:404-405.

224

Shigella Species (Bacillary Dysentery)

HERBERT L. DuPONT

The term *dysentery* was used by Hippocrates to indicate a condition characterized by the frequent passage of stool containing blood and mucus, accompanied by straining and painful defecation. It was not until the end of the 19th century, when the causes of amebiasis and bacillary dysentery were determined, that the two great forms of dysentery could be accurately separated. In view of the absence of liver complications, much of the dysentery in the older historical writings is considered to be of bacillary origin (shigellosis). After the causative agents of the two types of dysentery were determined, the different epidemiologic settings were described. In 1859, in Prague, Lambl and then later Osler[1] and Councilman and Lafleur[2] helped verify the pathogenicity of *Entamoeba histolytica*. In 1906, Shiga conclusively demonstrated that a bacterium was present in the stool of many patients with dysentery, and that agglutinins could be demonstrated in the serum of the infected patients.[3] At about the same time, Flexner found a similar but serologically different organism in the stools of other patients with dysentery acquired in the Philippines.[4] Rogers stated in 1913 that "epidemic dysentery in asylums, jails, or in long-occupied and unsanitary military camps during the war is almost certain to be bacillary, while sporadic cases in a warm climate are more frequently amebic."[5]

Medical writings since the beginning of recorded history have dealt with the common problems of dysentery in civilian and military populations; perhaps the greatest historical consideration is the influence that bacillary dysentery has had on military campaigns. Almost every long campaign and extended siege has produced epidemics of bacillary dysentery, particularly when sanitation and food sources could not be adequately controlled. In many battles described during the Peloponnesian War, the British campaigns in the 18th century, Napoleon's campaigns, the Crimean War, the American Civil War, the Franco-Prussian War, and the Sino-Japanese War, a heavier toll was ascribed to bacillary dysentery than to war-related injuries.[6]

Microbiology

Shigella organisms are small gram-negative rods that are members of the family Enterobacteriaceae, tribe Escherichieae, and genus *Shigella*. They are nonmotile and nonencapsulated. Both *Shigella* and enteroinvasive *Escherichia coli* evolved when transferable virulence plasmids were acquired by *E. coli*.[7]

ISOLATION TECHNIQUES

The infecting strain of *Shigella* is generally present in stool in concentrations between 10^3 and 10^9 viable cells/g of stool, depending on the stage of illness. During the postconvalescent shedding period, counts fall to 10^2 to 10^3 viable cells/g of stool. Recovery of the agent microbiologically is not usually difficult in the early stages of disease because of the higher counts present; it is more difficult during later stages of illness because of the lower counts of viable bacteria. Patients with shigellosis at the height of their illness can have negative stool cultures.[8] Careful selection of material and processing on appropriate media give a higher yield of organisms. The sooner after passage the specimen is processed, the higher is the yield. Stool that stands at room temperature for more than 24 hours has a profound drop in the number of viable cells, and recovery is less likely. A rectal swab obtained and seeded immediately at the bedside is the optimal way to perform a stool culture.

For bacteriologic identification of *Shigella*, a bit of blood or mucus is seeded onto at least two different media. Generally, stool is plated lightly onto a medium with only mild inhibiting factors for gram-negative growth, such as MacConkey's agar, xylose-lysine-deoxycholate agar, Tergitol-7, or eosin–methylene blue (EMB) agar, whereas a separate specimen is plated heavily onto a more inhibitory medium such as *Shigella-Salmonella* medium. The more plates used, the greater the recovery yield. After overnight incubation at 37°C, lactose-negative colonies are transferred to triple-sugar iron agar and lysine-iron agar slants and reincubated. Those giving a characteristic reaction—alkaline slant, acid butt, and no gas—are tested biochemically and then serologically identified with *Shigella* grouping and typing antisera.

GROUP AND TYPE IDENTIFICATION

The 47 serotypes of *Shigella* are divided into four groups, depending on serologic similarity and fermentation reactions: group A (*Shigella dysenteriae*), group B (*Shigella flexneri*), group C (*Shigella boydii*), and group D (*Shigella sonnei*). Commercial antiserum is available for determining group- and type-specific antigenicity. *S. sonnei* accounts for between 60% and 80% of the cases currently reported in the United States and other industrialized areas.

INVASIVE *ESCHERICHIA COLI*

Certain strains of *E. coli* can cause a clinical illness indistinguishable from shigellosis and should be considered as causative agents of bacillary dysentery. Almost all the *Shigella*-like *E. coli* strains have been shown to possess somatic antigens related to *Shigella* serotypes, further demonstrating the similarity of these two groups of organisms. Invasive *E. coli* (IEC) strains that cause bacillary dysentery have been shown to belong serologically to the following *E. coli* O groups: 28, 29, 112, 115, 124, 136, 143, 144, 147, 152, 164, and 167. Serotyping may ultimately prove to be useful in detecting these strains. The classic laboratory test for determining the virulence of a bacterial isolate (*Shigella* or IEC strain) was the Sereny test.[9] Keratoconjunctivitis develops after 1 to 7 days in guinea pigs (or rabbits) when an invasive bacterial strain (*E. coli* or *Shigella*) is dropped into the conjunctival sac of the animal (Fig. 224-1). This test is no longer used for diagnostic purposes.

A different form of bacillary dysentery has been shown to be caused by an O157:H7 strain of *E. coli* and other Shiga-toxin producing *E. coli* strains.[10] The source of *E. coli* O157:H7 infection has characteristically been inadequately cooked hamburgers obtained at a fast-food chain. Other non–O157:H7 serotypes of *E. coli* have also been implicated as causative agents of the syndrome (see Chapter 218).

Pathogenesis
COMMUNICABILITY AND INFECTIVITY

Bacillary dysentery is one of the most, if not *the* most, communicable of the bacterial diarrheas. Experiments in volunteers have demonstrated that shigellosis is unique among bacterial enteropathogens in that fewer than 100 viable cells can readily produce the disease in healthy adults.[11] Dose-response data obtained in volunteers for virulent strains from three species of *Shigella* are given in Table 224-1. When volunteers ingested 500 or fewer viable cells of *S. flexneri*, *S. sonnei*, or *S. dysenteriae* 1 (the Shiga bacillus), essentially the same rate

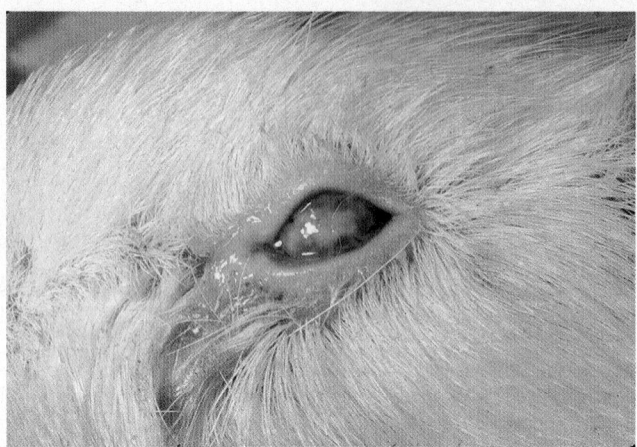

Figure 224-1   Guinea pig with keratoconjunctivitis after conjunctival inoculation of invasive *Escherichia coli*. This is a positive Sereny test result but is no longer used for diagnosis.

of clinical illness resulted, 27% to 45%.[11] This low dose of organisms probably explains how the illness can be transferred from person to person, why the secondary attack rate is so high when an index case is introduced into a family, and why recurrent bacillary dysentery is an important problem in institutionalized or crowded populations.

The reasons for this low-dose response are not completely clear. One possible explanation is that virulent shigellae can withstand the low pH of gastric juice. In a study of adult Bangladeshi men admitted to the hospital with diarrhea, normal gastric acid levels were seen in subjects with shigellosis, amebiasis, and pathogen-negative diarrhea, whereas patients with secretory diarrhea caused by *Vibrio cholerae* and enterotoxigenic *E. coli* had low gastric acid levels, offering evidence that *Shigella* did not require reduced gastric acidity to produce enteric disease.[12] In another study, *Shigella* isolates were able to survive at a pH of 2.5 for at least 2 hours, whereas *Salmonella* was not.[13] *Shigella* strains were also shown to be able to survive in acidic apple juice and tomato juice stored at 7°C and 22°C, respectively, for up to 14 days, showing its resistance to acid.[14] IEC and *Shigella* possess the same virulence determinates but IEC requires a dose 1000 times higher.[15] IEC strains have not been compared with *Shigella* to determine if relative acid susceptibility might explain the different dose response. Nonpathogenic *E. coli* appear to have similar acid susceptibility to strains of *Shigella*, suggesting that this is not the reason for the difference in dose response.[13]

MUCOSAL INVASION AND INFLAMMATION

Virulent *Shigella* and other nontoxigenic invasive *E. coli* strains produce disease after invading the intestinal mucosa.[16] Genes required for bacterial entry into epithelial cells are present on a 30-kb entry region of a 220-kb virulence plasmid.[17] *Shigella* infection is superficial, and only rarely does the organism penetrate beyond the mucosa, which explains the rarity of obtaining positive blood cultures in patients with shigellosis despite the common occurrence of hyperpyrexia and toxemia. *Shigella* and IEC invade colonic and rectal cells, including M cells of the follicle-associated epithelium, macrophages, and epithelial cells; invasion is followed by intracellular multiplication, spread of infection to adjacent cells, severe inflammation, and destruction of colonic mucosa.[18] Apoptotic destruction of macrophages in subepithelial tissue allows survival of the invading shigellae, and inflammation facilitates further bacterial entry.[19] Once the organisms are intracellular, they multiply within the cytoplasm and move from cell to cell by an actin-dependent process.

Pathogenic strains of *Shigella* and other bacterial enteropathogens have evolved a complex type III secretion mechanism that enables them to invade the intestinal mucosa.[20] Bacterial proteins (including toxins) are injected from the bacterial cytoplasm into the cytosol of host mucosal cells, where they modulate the functions of the host cells and dictate how the host and pathogen relate.[21-23] Each type III system consists of the secretion apparatus, secreted effector proteins, cytoplasmic chaperones (specialized for transporting the specific effector proteins), and specific transcriptional regulators.[24-26] The secreted proteins—there are approximately 20, including VirA, OspB to OspG, IpaA-D, and IpgD—stimulate bacterial entry into nonphagocytic cells and induce apoptosis.[23] *Shigella* strains decrease production of host antimicrobial peptides facilitating survival and colonization of the gut lining.[27]

Pathogenic strains of bacterial pathogens belonging to the type III secretion system can be detected by screening for virulence genes directly.[28] DNA probes and polymerase chain reaction techniques have been developed to detect *Shigella* and invasive *E. coli* and can be used in epidemiologic studies.

TOXIGENICITY

The Shiga bacillus (*S. dysenteriae* 1) was shown in the early 20th century to produce a neurotoxin that caused paralysis and death in mice and rabbits. Since then, it has been suspected that the toxin played an important role in the pathogenesis of clinical illness. Later, an exotoxin in the Shiga bacillus was shown to have enterotoxin activity in the ligated ileal loop model[29] and also to have cytotoxic properties when intestinal mucosa was examined.[30] Undoubtedly, invasiveness is the primary virulence characteristic of *Shigella* strains, but toxin elaboration may play a role in the evolution of the local destructive mucosal lesion once the organisms have invaded the colonic mucosa. It is possible that toxin might also help explain the watery small bowel type of diarrhea that is characteristically seen during the first or second day of illness. Shiga toxin production appears to be the important virulence property of hemorrhagic colitis and hemolytic uremic syndrome caused by *E. coli* (O157:H7).[31]

ANATOMIC LOCATION OF INFECTION

Studies in volunteers have helped establish the intestinal localization of bacteria in experimental shigellosis (H.L. DuPont and R.B. Hornick, unpublished data). Within 12 hours after subjects swallow virulent shigellae, the bacteria transiently multiply in the small bowel to concentrations of 10^7 to 10^9 viable cells/mL of luminal contents, at which time abdominal pain, cramping, and fever occur. Within a few days, the infecting strain is no longer detectable in small bowel fluid, the patient's temperature becomes lower, and pain and tenderness, generally confined to the lower abdominal quadrants, become more severe. Urgency, tenesmus, and passage of bloody mucoid stools (dysentery) often occur in the later stages of infection and correlate with a diffuse colonic localization of the bacteria. Although strains of *Shigella* appear to be resistant to acid, as discussed earlier, acid exposure may transiently inhibit the virulence properties of the organism, which may encourage transit through the small bowel to the colon, where viru-

TABLE 224-1	Response of Adult Volunteers to Experimental Challenge with Viable Virulent Strains of *Shigella*		
Shigella Species	**Inoculum (Organisms)**	**No. of Volunteers**	**No. of Cases of Clinical Shigellosis (% of total)**
S. flexneri (strain 2467T)	≤180	72	23 (32)
	≥5 × 10³	211	124 (59)
S. sonnei (53G)	500	58	26 (45)
S. dysenteriae 1*	≤200	22	6 (27)
	≥2 × 10³	22	14 (64)

*Strains A-1 and M-131.
Adapted from DuPont HL, Levine MM, Hornick RB, et al. Inoculum size in shigellosis and implications for expected mode of transmission. *J Infect Dis.* 1989;159:1126-1128.

lence characteristics are once more produced.[32] The density of intramucosal bacteria is highest at the luminal surface and extends in decreasing concentrations to reach the lamina propria and submucosa. Microabscesses form and coalesce, becoming large abscesses that slough and produce mucosal ulcerations. In shigellosis, both humoral and cellular immune mechanisms are stimulated. Cytokine levels correlate with disease severity,[33] and a number of fecal cytokines, including interleukin-8 (IL-8) and IL-1β, are higher than those seen with other enteric bacterial pathogens.[34]

Epidemiology

Hippocrates indicated that when a dry winter was followed by a rainy spring, an increase in the number of dysentery cases would follow in the summer. Generally, bacillary dysentery is a summertime illness. Shigellosis is characteristically seen in children living in crowded areas with inadequate sanitation and limited water. Because of the characteristic clinical picture of bacillary dysentery, it is one of the most accurately diagnosed and reported classes of infectious diarrhea. The greatest frequency of illness is reported in infants and younger or preschool children. Disease rates and also complications and severity parallel the degree of malnutrition. Flies may be important in the transmission of bacillary dysentery,[35,36] especially in tropical climates. Dysentery in warm countries is most prevalent when the fly population is at its highest. Bacteriologic surveys of fly populations have indicated that flies can occasionally be shown to be positive for *Shigella* bacteria.[35] The low dose required for infection at least partially explains the potential for fly transmission of shigellosis. Fly control, hand washing, and breast-feeding show protective effects against the organism.[37]

CYCLIC PATTERNS OF DISEASE

Since the description of bacteriologic isolation procedures, cyclic epidemics of bacillary dysentery have been described, each cycle lasting 20 to 50 years.[38] In Europe, during the first 25 years of the 20th century, dysentery was generally caused by *S. dysenteriae* 1 (the Shiga bacillus), and mortality was higher than subsequently seen when other serotypes became prevalent. Between 1926 and 1938, *S. flexneri* strains became more prevalent than the Shiga bacillus in the developing world, and *S. flexneri* remains the major *Shigella* type in these areas. *S. sonnei* has become the major cause of bacillary dysentery in European countries and the United States. Widespread epidemics in the developing world may be seen for the more virulent *S. dysenteriae* 1, resulting in deaths without proper antimicrobial therapy. Shiga dysentery remains a special problem in parts of Africa and in the Indian subcontinent and Bangladesh.

INCIDENCE OF SHIGELLOSIS BY GEOGRAPHY AND HOST

The annual number of *Shigella* episodes worldwide is estimated to be 165 million, of which more than 100 million occur in the developing world, with more than 1 million deaths.[39] The highest rate of *Shigella* infection (69% of cases) and the highest death rate (61% of deaths) occur in those younger than 5 years.[39] In the United Kingdom, shigellosis has been reported commonly in school-aged children where fecal contamination of lavatory seats in nursery and primary schools has been shown to result from children with diarrhea, and that infection is transmitted to the hands of the younger children.[40] Shigellosis has become an important problem in daycare centers for preschool children in the United States. Between 20,000 and 50,000 cases are reported each year in the United Kingdom and approximately 13,000 to 19,000 cases each year in the United States. The actual number of cases is clearly far greater than those reported.

In numerous published studies, a causative agent has been identified in 10% to 50% of pediatric diarrhea cases, depending on geographic location, severity of illness, and laboratory methods used.[41-43] Bacillary dysentery is primarily a disease of children 6 months to 10 years of age,

although adults often acquire the illness from their children. Bacillary dysentery does not commonly develop in children younger than 6 months. However, in industrialized countries, *Shigella* strains may rarely cause severe illness in newborns,[44] but in developing countries, where breast-feeding is more common, infants are resistant to shigellosis,[45] probably because of exclusion from contaminated food or drink, changes in the intestinal flora of breast-fed children, or the presence of specific antibody in breast milk.

MODES OF SPREAD AND RESERVOIRS IN NATURE

Many cases of bacillary dysentery in industrialized regions are a result of person-to-person transmission. Widespread epidemics have occurred in military or civilian populations and among persons on cruise ships who have ingested contaminated food or water. Water and food appear to be particularly important vectors of *Shigella* transmission in developing countries, where they may be the most important sources of infection.[46,47] Epidemics of waterborne shigellosis generally appear to be the result of wells contaminated with fecal material. Felson[48] found that dysentery strains could be recovered for up to 6 months from water samples maintained at room temperature. Wells are often located close to cesspools and outhouses in developing countries, where sanitation principles are not followed. In other areas, septic tank discharge may empty into lakes, ponds, or other bodies of water close to intake lines for camp water supplies or adjacent to bathing beaches. Chlorination of water, if appropriately maintained, will remove the threat of such infections. In the United States, foodborne[49] and waterborne[50] outbreaks of shigellosis occur occasionally.

An epidemiologic observation has been made that when water sanitation improvements are implemented in a community, the incidence of typhoid fever falls but the prevalence of bacillary dysentery remains unchanged.[48] In contrast to shigellosis, diseases caused by *Salmonella*, *Vibrio cholerae*, *Campylobacter*, and invasive *E. coli* appear to be epidemiologically associated in almost all cases with foodborne or waterborne transmission. Such a vehicle of transmission is probably necessary with the latter agents because a larger inoculum is necessary to produce illness.[51]

Hand transmission is likely to be a common means of acquiring infection. At a custodial institution, mentally retarded persons were studied for the prevalence of hand transmission of bacteria.[35] Finger and simultaneous fecal cultures were obtained from 268 institutionalized patients. A *Shigella* strain was isolated from the stool of 39 persons, and the fingers were positive in 4 (10% of those with a positive stool culture). In addition, fecal cultures were found to be negative in an additional 229 patients, whereas a *Shigella* strain was isolated from the hands and fingers of 2 of these patients with negative stool cultures. *E. coli* was recovered from the fingers of 82% of those studied, which demonstrates the common occurrence of fecal organisms on the hands of institutionalized persons. These institutionalized patients had adequate washroom and showering facilities and did not show evidence of decreased personal hygiene.

Secondary cases during outbreaks of shigellosis are common. One study demonstrated that bacillary dysentery develops in 61% of the children younger than 1 year once an index case occurs in a household.[35] The attack rate was approximately 40% for those aged 1 to 4 years and 20% for all ages once an index case was identified. Secondary attack rates are increased in homes with outhouses and are reduced in families once sanitary toilet facilities are installed. Transmission rates also correlated with poverty and overcrowding. After a bout of shigellosis without antimicrobial therapy, fecal excretion of the infecting strain generally lasts 1 to 4 weeks. Long-term *Shigella* carriage rarely occurs.[6,52] In contrast to typhoid and cholera carriers, where the gallbladder or small bowel may be a site of infection, the organisms in dysentery carriage are confined to a colonic site. In the absence of coexistent parasitic infestation of the intestine, these carriers generally respond to antimicrobial therapy. The number of organisms excreted by these persons is generally less than that seen in acute dysentery, and thus the infection in such individuals is less communicable than that in active cases.

Diagnosis

HISTORY

Bacillary dysentery should be considered in any patient with acute diarrheal illness associated with toxemia and systemic symptoms, particularly when the illness lasts longer than 48 hours, intrafamily spread occurs with an interval of 1 to 3 days between cases, fever is present, or blood or mucus is seen in stool. The occurrence of hyperpyrexia and seizures in infants and children with shigellosis has led some to the conclusion that a neurotoxin is important in the pathogenesis of clinical illness, although there is little to support this notion. In patients able to give a careful history, a descending intestinal tract infection is often described. The first symptoms may be fever and abdominal cramping, followed by voluminous watery stool during small bowel infection, followed by a decrease in fever and an increase in the number of stools passed with smaller volume ("fractional stools") as the colon becomes the site of infection. At that time, the passage of bloody mucoid stools with fecal urgency and tenesmus may develop. Abdominal pain and diarrhea occur in almost all patients with shigellosis, fever can be documented in approximately one third of cases, and mucus is seen in the stools of 50% and gross blood in 40% of cases.[8]

PHYSICAL EXAMINATION

Findings on physical examination are nonspecific and include a variable degree of systemic toxemia, fever (which may be as high as 105° F), abdominal tenderness (especially over the lower abdominal quadrants), and hyperactive bowel sounds. Rectal examination or proctoscopy is generally painful, and an abnormally friable, hyperemic rectal mucosa, increased mucus secretion, and areas of ecchymosis are generally found. Ulcerations of rectal mucosa can be seen after several days of illness. Rectal prolapse may occur with profuse stooling.

LABORATORY FINDINGS

During the acute illness, the infecting strain is present in large enough numbers that stool cultures are generally positive. In the later stages of the disease, it may be necessary first to culture material in enrichment broth before plating. Culture of colonic or rectal biopsy does not improve the efficiency of stool culture in shigellosis.[53] The key to establishing the diagnosis of shigellosis is isolation of the organism from diarrheal stool. Laboratory identification of *Shigella* was discussed earlier ("Isolation Techniques"). In research centers where the service is available, direct fluorescent antibody microscopy may be useful in detecting the organism when present in small numbers,[54] but because of the numerous serotypes potentially responsible for the infection, this procedure does not have widespread application.

The total white blood cell count demonstrates no consistent findings, although leukopenia and brisk leukocytosis are seen on occasion. A shift to the left (an increased number of band cells in comparison to segmented neutrophils) when a leukocyte differential count is performed in a patient with diarrhea suggests bacillary dysentery. The single most important laboratory test other than stool culture is direct microscopic examination of a stained fecal smear, which will show prevalent polymorphonuclear leukocytes.[55] A wet mount preparation is made by adding stool (mucus, if present) to an equal amount of methylene blue dye. The preparation is then covered with a coverslip and examined microscopically under the high dry objective. Alternatively, the specimen can be heat-fixed before staining with dilute methylene blue. The specimen can then be examined under oil after drying. This dry preparation can be stored for later review. Numerous sheets of polymorphonuclear leukocytes are normally found in shigellosis and invasive *E. coli* diarrhea (Fig. 224-2). Prevalent leukocytes indicate a diffuse colitis or proctitis. The leukocyte test, when positive,

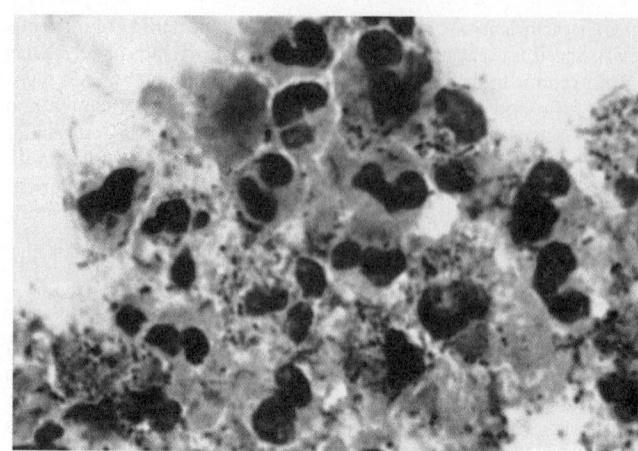

Figure 224-2   Fecal leukocytes taken from patient with diffuse colitis (methylene blue stain). This exudative response may be seen in shigellosis, salmonellosis, *Campylobacter* infection, and colitis caused by invasive or Shiga toxin–producing *Escherichia coli*.

indicates a pathologic process, not an etiologic one, and white cells are usually also seen in salmonellosis, *Campylobacter* diarrhea, and Shiga toxin–producing, invasive *E. coli* colitis, and idiopathic ulcerative colitis.

Serologic evaluation of a patient with bacillary dysentery is not generally helpful in establishing the diagnosis because humoral antibodies do not develop before recovery. Serologic procedures are helpful as an epidemiologic tool in defining the extent of an epidemic in a population known to be infected by a known *Shigella* serotype (especially the Shiga bacillus). The humoral antibody response correlates with the severity of clinical disease.[8]

Treatment and Clinical Course

In certain patients with bacillary dysentery (particularly in infants and older adults), significant dehydration may result from excessive fluid loss through diarrhea and vomiting. The fluid losses can generally be replaced by oral intake because the diarrhea associated with bacillary dysentery is not normally associated with profound fluid and electrolyte depletion. If vomiting or extreme toxemia is a prominent feature of the illness, especially in the very young or very old, IV fluid replacement may be necessary.

Antibiotics are useful in the management of shigellosis and may be lifesaving in the case of Shiga dysentery. Because the infection is normally self-limited and because antibiotic resistance commonly develops in populations after prolonged use of drugs, some think that antimicrobial therapy should be reserved for the most severely ill patients.[56] However, because the infection is generally transmitted from person to person and the infected or colonized person represents the major reservoir of infection, for public health reasons each patient with a positive stool culture or with known bacillary dysentery should be treated. The treatment of choice for shigellosis when susceptibility is unknown is a fluoroquinolone for adults. The specific drugs and dosages are indicated in Table 224-2. Trimethoprim-sulfamethoxazole had been the treatment of choice for this enteric infection, but resistance has become widespread for strains of *Shigella*.[57-59] Antibiotic resistance is a growing problem for enteric bacterial pathogens. It has occurred as a result of plasmid or transposon transmission or in an epidemic spread by chromosome-mediated mobile genetic elements (integrons) in the horizontal transfer of antibacterial resistance.[60] Although 3-day therapy is generally recommended in shigellosis, single-dose fluoroquinolones may be given for milder forms of shigellosis.[61] For children, various drugs may be used. Cephalosporins have become a common form of treatment of pediatric shigellosis.[62-64] Although not approved for use in children, short-course fluoroquino-

TABLE 224-2	Antibacterial Therapy for Patients with Shigellosis			
Adults		**Children**		
Agent	*Dosage*	*Agent*	*Dosage*	
Levofloxacin	500 mg qd × 3 days	Ceftriaxone	50 mg/kg IV once daily (maximum, 2 g/day) × 5 days	
Ciprofloxacin	500 mg bid × 3 days	Cefixime*	8 mg/kg/day as single daily dose or divided q12h × 5 days	
		Azithromycin	10 mg/kg/day in a single daily dose × 3 days	
Azithromycin	500 mg qd × 3 days	Ciprofloxacin*	25 mg/kg/day, divided q12h × 3-5 days	

*Not approved for use in children.

lones can be safely used.[65] Amdinocillin, an unlicensed drug, has been used in Bangladesh for shigellosis.[65] Azithromycin has been used successfully for treatment of multidrug-resistant *Shigella* infection in adults[66,67] and should be useful in the management of pediatric shigellosis. Nalidixic acid may be helpful in the management of pediatric shigellosis.[68] Although most of the drugs listed in Table 224-2 for treating shigellosis in adults and children are not approved for use in this disease, short-course therapy should be effective and safe.

Intestinal motility patterns may be important in recovery from infection, as well as in preventing mucosal invasion by a bacterial agent.[69] In such cases, diarrhea might be viewed as a protective mechanism, and its inhibition by motility-active drugs may not be wise. Paregoric has occasionally been shown to worsen clinical salmonellosis[69] and, in occasional patients, antidiarrheal drugs such as diphenoxylate (Lomotil) worsen bacillary dysentery and could play a role in the development of toxic dilation of the colon.[70] In dysenteric diarrhea, the antimotility drugs may be safely given if effective antimicrobial drugs are also administered.[71]

Clinical illness, if left untreated, generally lasts 1 day to 1 month, with an average of 7 days. Although mortality is unusual in shigellosis except in malnourished children and older adults, the clinical illness is more striking and more likely to lead to hospitalization than are most other forms of infectious diarrhea. Complications, which are unusual, generally consist of severe dehydration, febrile seizures, septicemia or pneumonia from coliform organisms (and, less commonly, the infecting *Shigella* strain), keratoconjunctivitis, immune complex acute glomerulonephritis, post-*Shigella* irritable bowel syndrome, and hemolytic uremic syndrome. A post-*Shigella* reactive arthritis (Reiter's syndrome) may develop in patients with HLA-B27 histocompatibility antigen and infection by group B *Shigella* (*S. flexneri*). *S. dysenteriae* 1 characteristically produces a more serious form of diarrhea, and the mortality associated with untreated disease during epidemics may be as high as 20%. Bacterial strains that produce Shiga toxin (*S. dysenteriae* 1 and *E. coli* in hemorrhagic colitis) may produce the hemolytic-uremic syndrome as a complication of illness. Now that oral rehydration therapy has reduced the incidence of most cases of dehydration-associated deaths from diarrhea, shigellosis represents the most important form of fatal enteric illness in areas of high endemicity.[72] A rare fulminating form of bacillary dysentery secondary to massive small intestine invasion by the infecting bacteria is seen in children, and death early in infection is common (the "Ikari" syndrome).

Control

ENVIRONMENTAL CONTROL

A safe water supply is important for the control of shigellosis and is probably the single most important factor in areas with substandard sanitation facilities.[73] Chlorination is another factor important in decreasing the incidence of all waterborne enteric bacterial infections. Of critical importance to the establishment of a safe water supply system are the general level of sanitation in the area and the establishment of an effective sewage disposal system. Insecticides are useful in decreasing the vector population during peak seasons, and a decrease in the incidence of shigellosis, but not salmonellosis, may be seen after their use.[36] At other times of the year, it may be helpful to attack breeding places of insects. Garbage collection and disposal of excreta and sewage may also be useful in controlling the vectors.

In many areas of the developing world, it is necessary to examine the techniques of home preparation and storage of food. Important features may be improved, such as personal and food hygienic facilities, and refrigeration may be necessary. A major prerequisite in transmission in most cases of bacillary dysentery is the degree of contact and the level of personal hygiene between patients with disease and susceptible persons. Other factors are frequent and effective hand washing, voluntary removal of persons with diarrhea from roles as food handlers, and appropriate refrigeration and proper cooking of potentially infected foods. Breast-feeding is an important means of decreasing the incidence of bacillary dysentery in developing countries and in communities with substandard hygienic practices. Also, mothers should be taught how to prepare foods to supplement breast-feeding and to ensure the safety of the diet after weaning to improve sanitation and nutrition. Finally, cases of diarrhea should be adequately diagnosed and patients isolated, and antimicrobial therapy should be instituted in cases of bacillary dysentery to decrease the reservoir of virulent strains. The degree of symptomatology, personal hygiene, and education about how enteric bacteria can be spread are important factors that may determine the rate of transmission of the agent, and these factors should influence the decision for antimicrobial therapy.

IMMUNOLOGIC CONTROL

Epidemiologic studies have indicated that a degree of homologous immunity can be demonstrated in those who have recovered from bacillary dysentery.[74-76] These observations have supported the idea that a protective vaccine might be developed. It was shown that killed parenteral vaccines fail to protect animals against experimentally produced shigellosis[77] and to protect humans against naturally occurring illness.[78] Besredka[79] suggested that the immunity against bacillary dysentery conferred by one attack of the disease was essentially the result of sensitization of the intestinal mucosa to dysentery bacilli and that the antibodies circulating in serum had a small role or none at all in protection. After more than 90 years, Besredka's concept of intestinal immunity is still held as the primary mode through which immunologic control might be feasible. However, the nature of the intestinal immune response has not been completely characterized. In natural shigellosis, IgA concentrations in stool increase, as do anti-*Shigella* secretory IgA antibodies directed to homologous lipopolysaccharide.[80] Also, lymphocytes, monocytes, and granulocytes, in the absence of complement but in the presence of antibody, may serve an anti-*Shigella* function through cell-mediated mechanisms.[81] Formal and co-workers worked with both spontaneously derived avirulent *Shigella* mutants and hybrid strains (*Shigella–E. coli*) in monkeys.[82]

The most successful outcome in the area of *Shigella* vaccine development was achieved by Mel and colleagues, who used streptomycin-dependent mutant strains of *Shigella* as orally administered immunizing agents in Yugoslavian army soldiers and in children living in areas of hyperendemicity.[83] These workers demonstrated that immunization with a live-attenuated bacterial strain given orally in multiple doses (at least four) would prevent clinical disease but not alter the carrier status, provided that gastric acidity was first decreased by sodium bicarbonate swallowed just before the vaccine. Serotype-specific protection followed vaccination and lasted for at least 6 months, and the immunizing agent remained protective when combined as a bivalent preparation. Experiments in volunteers have demonstrated that the protective immunity imparted by oral immunization approximates that after recovery from disease.[84]

In the future, immunologic control may be possible against a limited number of serotypes of shigellae when attack rates are shown to be particularly high. Further research is being directed toward developing an immunizing strain that multiplies in the intestinal tract so that fewer doses need to be administered. It may be possible to create such a strain by intergeneric hybridization.[85] Attenuated bacteria can be constructed that are better adapted to host intestinal proliferation and that combine multiple serotypes. Avirulent mutants and bioengineered strains may produce anti-*Shigella* immunity. Conjugate *Shigella* vaccines are also being evaluated. It is possible that antitoxin immunity might be important to susceptibility and that a successful immunizing agent should also include a toxoid component.

REFERENCES

1. Osler W. On the amebae coli in dysentery and in dysentery liver abscess. *Johns Hopkins Hosp Bull.* 1890;1:736.
2. Councilman WT, Lafleur HA. Amebic dysentery. *Johns Hopkins Hosp Rep.* 1891;2:395.
3. Shiga K. Observations on the epidemiology of dysentery in Japan. *Philippine J Sci.* 1906;1:485.
4. Flexner S. On the etiology of tropical dysentery. *Philadelphia Med J.* 1900;6:417.
5. Rogers L. Bacillary dysentery. In: *Dysenteries, Their Differentiation and Treatment.* London: Oxford University Press; 1913:268.
6. Davison WC. A bacteriological and clinical consideration of bacillary dysentery in adults and children. *Medicine (Baltimore).* 1922;1:389.
7. Yang J, Nie H, Chen L, et al. Revisiting the molecular evolutionary history of *Shigella* spp. *J Mol Evol.* 2007;64:71-79.
8. DuPont H, Hornick R, Dawkins A, et al. The response of man to virulent *Shigella flexneri* 2a. *J Infect Dis.* 1969;119:396-401.
9. Sereny B. Experimental *Shigella* keratoconjunctivitis: A preliminary report. *Acta Microbiol Acad Sci Hung.* 1955;2:293-296.
10. Riley LW, Remis RS, Helgerson SD, et al. Hemorrhagic colitis associated with a rare *Escherichia coli* serotype. *N Engl J Med.* 1983;308:681-685.
11. DuPont HL, Levine MM, Hornick RB, et al. Inoculum size in shigellosis and implications for expected mode of transmission. *J Infect Dis.* 1989;159:1126-1128.
12. Evans CAW, Gilman RH, Rabbani GH, et al. Gastric acid secretion and enteric infection in Bangladesh. *Trans R Soc Trop Med Hyg.* 1997;91:681-685.
13. Gorden J, Small PLC. Acid resistance in enteric bacteria. *Infect Immun.* 1993;61:364-367.
14. Bagamboula CF, Uyttendaele M, Debevere J. Acid tolerance of *Shigella sonnei* and *Shigella flexneri*. *J Appl Microbiol.* 2002;93:479-486.
15. DuPont HL, Formal SB, Hornick RB, et al. Pathogenesis of *Escherichia coli* diarrhea. *N Engl J Med.* 1971;285:1-9.
16. LaBrec E, Schneider H, Magnani T, et al. Epithelial cell penetration as an essential step in the pathogenesis of bacillary dysentery. *J Bacteriol.* 1964;88:1503-1518.
17. Sasakawa C, Kamata K, Sakai T, et al. Virulence-associated genetic regions comprising 31 kilobases of the 230-kilobase plasmid in *Shigella flexneri* 2a. *J Bacteriol.* 1988;170:2480-2484.
18. Sansonetti PJ. Rupture, invasion and inflammatory destruction of the intestinal barrier by *Shigella*, making sense of prokaryote-eukaryote cross-talk. *FEMS Microbiol Rev.* 2001;25:3-14.
19. Sansonetti PJ, Van Nhieu GT, Egile C. Rupture of the intestinal barrier and mucosal invasion by *Shigella flexneri*. *Clin Infect Dis.* 1999;28:466-475.
20. Blocker AJ, Deane JE, Veenendaal AK, et al. What's the point of the type III secretion system needle? *Proc Natl Acad Sci USA.* 2008;105:6507-6513.
21. Hueck CJ. Type III protein secretion systems in bacterial pathogens of animals and plants. *Microbiol Mol Biol Rev.* 1998;62:379-433.
22. Cheng LW, Schneewind O. Type III machines of gram-negative bacteria: Delivering the goods. *Trends Microbiol.* 2000;8:214-220.
23. Galan JE, Collmer A. Type III secretion machines: Bacterial devices for protein delivery into host cells. *Science.* 1999;284:1322-1328.
24. Tran Van Nhieu G, Bourdet-Sicard R, Dumenil G, et al. Bacterial signals and cell responses during *Shigella* entry into epithelial cells. *Cell Microbiol.* 2000;2:187-193.
25. Mavris M, Sansonetti PJ, Parsot C. Identification of the *cis*-acting site involved in activation of promoters regulated by activity of the type III secretion apparatus in *Shigella flexneri*. *J Bacteriol.* 2002;184:6751-6759.
26. Page AL, Sansonetti P, Parsot C. Spa15 of *Shigella flexneri*, a third type of chaperone in the type III secretion pathway. *Mol Microbiol.* 2002;43:1533-1542.
27. Sperandio B, Regnault B, Guo J, et al. Virulent *Shigella flexneri* subverts the host innate immune responses through manipulation of antimicrobial peptide gene expression. *J Exp Med.* 2008;205:1121-1132.
28. Stuber K, Frey J, Burnens AP, et al. Detection of type III secretion genes as a general indicator of bacterial virulence. *Mol Cell Probes.* 2003;17:25-32.
29. Keusch GT, Grady GF, Mata LJ, et al. Pathogenesis of *Shigella* diarrhea: I. Enterotoxin production by *Shigella dysenteriae* 1. *J Clin Invest.* 1972;51:1212-1218.
30. Keusch GT, Grady GF, Takeuchi A, et al. Pathogenesis of *Shigella* diarrhea: II. Enterotoxin-induced acute enteritis in the rabbit ileum. *J Infect Dis.* 1972;126:92-95.
31. O'Brien AD, Newland JW, Miller RK, et al. Shiga-like toxin-converting phages from *Escherichia coli* strains that cause hemorrhagic colitis or infantile diarrhea. *Science.* 1984;226:694-696.
32. Speelman P, Kabir I, Islam M. Distribution and spread of shigellosis: A colonic study. *J Infect Dis.* 1984;150:899-903.
33. Raqib R, Wretlind B, Anderson J, et al. Cytokine secretion in acute shigellosis is correlated to disease activity and directed more to stool than to plasma. *J Infect Dis.* 1995;171:376-384.
34. Greenberg DE, Jiang ZD, Steffen R, et al. Markers of inflammation in bacterial diarrhea among travelers, with a focus on enteroaggregative *Escherichia coli* pathogenicity. *J Infect Dis.* 2002;185:944-949.
35. Hardy A, Watt J. Studies of the acute diarrheal diseases: XVIII. Epidemiology. *Public Health Rep.* 1948;63:363-378.
36. Watt J, Lindsay D. Diarrheal disease control studies: I. Effect of fly control in a high morbidity area. *Public Health Rep.* 1948;63:1319-1333.
37. Chompook P, Todd J, Wheeler JG, et al. Risk factors for shigellosis in Thailand. *Int J Infect Dis.* 2006;10:425-433.
38. Kostrzewski J, Stypulkowska-Misiurewicz H. Changes in the epidemiology of dysentery in Poland and the situation in Europe. *Arch Immunol Ther Exp (Warsz).* 1968;16:429-451.
39. Kotloff KL, Winickoff JP, Ivanoff B, et al. Global burden of *Shigella* infections: Implications for vaccine development and implementation of control strategies. *Bull WHO.* 1999;77:651-666.
40. Cruickshank R. Diarrheal diseases in the United Kingdom. In: Pemberton J, ed. *Epidemiology Reports on Research and Teaching.* London: Oxford University Press; 1963:60.
41. Ingram V, Rights F, Khan H, et al. Diarrhea in children of West Pakistan: Occurrence of bacterial and parasitic agents. *Am J Trop Med Hyg.* 1966;15:743-750.
42. Pickering LK, Evans Jr DJ, Munoz O, et al. Prospective study of enteropathogens in children with diarrhea in Houston and Mexico. *J Pediatr.* 1978;93:282-388.
43. Nguyen T, Le Van P, Nguyen GK, et al. Etiology and epidemiology of diarrhea in children in Hanoi, Vietnam. *Int J Infect Dis.* 2006;10:298-308.
44. Haltalin K. Neonatal shigellosis: Report of 16 cases and review of the literature. *Am J Dis Child.* 1967;114:603-611.
45. Mata L, Urrutia J, Garcia B, et al. *Shigella* infection in breast-fed Guatemalan Indian neonates. *Am J Dis Child.* 1969;117:142-146.
46. Boyce JM, Hughes JM, Alim AR, et al. Patterns of *Shigella* infection in families in rural Bangladesh. *Am J Trop Med Hyg.* 1982;31:1015-1020.
47. Tjoa WS, DuPont HL, Sullivan P, et al. Location of food consumption and travelers' diarrhea. *Am J Epidemiol.* 1977;106:61-66.
48. Felson J. *Bacillary Dysentery Colitis and Enteritis.* Philadelphia: WB Saunders; 1945.
49. Donadio J, Gangarosa E. Foodborne shigellosis. *J Infect Dis.* 1969;119:666-668.
50. Lee SH, Levy DA, Craun GF, et al. Surveillance for waterborne-disease outbreaks—United States, 1999-2000. *MMWR Morb Mortal Wkly Rep.* 2002;51(SS08):1-47.
51. DuPont H, Hornick R. Clinical approach to infectious diarrheas. *Medicine (Baltimore).* 1973;52:265-270.
52. Levine MM, DuPont HL, Khodabandelou M, et al. Long-term shigella-carrier state. *N Engl J Med.* 1973;288:1169-1171.
53. Barbut F, Beaugerie L, Dalas N, et al. Comparative value of colonic biopsy and intraluminal fluid culture for diagnosis of bacterial acute colitis in immunocompetent patients. *Clin Infect Dis.* 1999;29:356-360.
54. Thomason B, Cowart G, Cherry W. Current status of immunofluorescence techniques for rapid detection of shigellae in fecal specimens. *Appl Microbiol.* 1965;13:605-613.
55. Harris J, DuPont H, Hornick R. Fecal leukocytes in diarrheal illness. *Ann Intern Med.* 1972;76:697-703.
56. Weissman J, Gangarosa E, DuPont H, et al. Changing needs in the antimicrobial therapy of shigellosis. *J Infect Dis.* 1973;127:611-613.
57. Murray BE. Resistance of *Shigella, Salmonella,* and other selected enteric pathogens to antimicrobial agents. *Rev Infect Dis.* 1986;8(Suppl):S172-S181.
58. Replogle ML, Fleming DW, Cieslak PR. Emergence of antimicrobial-resistant shigellosis in Oregon. *Clin Infect Dis.* 2000;30:515-519.
59. Flores A, Araque M, Vizcaya L. Multiresistant *Shigella* species isolated from pediatric patients with acute diarrheal disease. *Am J Med Sci.* 1998;316:379-384.
60. McIver CJ, White PA, Jones LA, et al. Epidemic strains of *Shigella sonnei* biotype g carrying integrons. *J Clin Microbiol.* 2002;40:1538-1540.
61. Bennish ML, Salam MA, Khan WA, et al. Treatment of shigellosis: III. Comparison of one- or two-dose ciprofloxacin with standard 5-day therapy: A randomized, blinded trial. *Ann Intern Med.* 1992;117:727.
62. Kabir I, Butler T, Khanam A. Comparative efficacies of single intravenous doses of ceftriaxone and ampicillin for shigellosis in a placebo-controlled trial. *Antimicrob Agents Chemother.* 1986;29:645-648.
63. Ashkenazi S, Amir J, Waisman Y, et al. A randomized, double-blind study comparing cefixime and trimethoprim-sulfamethoxazole in the treatment of childhood shigellosis. *J Pediatr.* 1993;123:817-821.
64. Varsano I, Eidlitz-Marcus T, Nussinovitch M, et al. Comparative efficacy of ceftriaxone and ampicillin for treatment of severe shigellosis in children. *J Pediatr.* 1991;118:627-632.
65. Salam MA, Dhar U, Khan WA, et al. Randomized comparison of ciprofloxacin suspension and pivmecillinam for childhood shigellosis. *Lancet.* 1998;352:522-527.
66. Khan WA, Seas C, Dhar U, et al. Treatment of shigellosis: V. Comparison of azithromycin and ciprofloxacin: A double-blind, randomized, controlled trial. *Ann Intern Med.* 1997;126:697-703.
67. Shanks GD, Smoak BL, Aleman GM, et al. Single-dose azithromycin or three-day course of ciprofloxacin as therapy for epidemic dysentery in Kenya. *Clin Infect Dis.* 1999;29:942-943.
68. Salam MA, Bennish ML. Therapy for shigellosis. I. Randomized, double-blind trial of nalidixic acid in childhood shigellosis. *J Pediatr.* 1988;113:901-907.
69. Sprinz H. Pathogenesis of intestinal infections. *Arch Pathol.* 1969;87:556-562.
70. DuPont H, Hornick R. Adverse effects of Lomotil therapy in shigellosis. *JAMA.* 1973;226:1525-1528.
71. Murphy GS, Bodhidatta L, Echeverria P, et al. Ciprofloxacin and loperamide in the treatment of bacillary dysentery. *Ann Intern Med.* 1993;118:582-586.
72. Butler T, Islam M, Azad AK, et al. Causes of death in diarrhoeal diseases after rehydration therapy: An autopsy study of 140 patients in Bangladesh. *Bull World Health Organ.* 1987;65:317-323.
73. Nyerges V, Eng N. Plan for the control of gastrointestinal diseases: Environmental sanitation, epidemiology, health education and early diagnosis and treatment. In: *Control of Gastrointestinal Diseases.* Pan-American Health Organization, Technical Discussion, Science Publication; Washington, DC: 1963;100:36.
74. Cruickshank R. Acquired immunity: Bacterial infections. In: Cruickshank R, ed. *Modern Trends in Immunology.* Washington, DC: Butterworth; 1963;102:107-129.
75. DuPont H, Gangarosa E, Reller L, et al. Shigellosis in custodial institutions. *Am J Epidemiol.* 1970;92:172-179.
76. Hardy A, Watt J. The acute diarrheal diseases. *JAMA.* 1944;124:1173-1179.
77. Formal S, Maenza R, Austin S, et al. Failure of parenteral vaccines to protect monkeys against experimental shigellosis. *Proc Soc Exp Biol Med.* 1967;125:347-349.
78. Hardy A, DeCapito T, Halbert S. Studies of acute diarrheal diseases: XIX. Immunization in shigellosis. *Public Health Rep.* 1948;63:685-688.
79. Besredka A. On the mechanism of dysenteric infection, antidysenteric vaccination per os, and the nature of antidysenteric immunity. *Ann Inst Pasteur Paris.* 1919;33:301.
80. Winsor Jr DK, Mathewson JJ, DuPont HL. Comparison of serum and fecal antibody responses of patients with naturally acquired *Shigella sonnei* infection. *J Infect Dis.* 1988;158:1108-1112.
81. Lowell GH, MacDermott RP, Summers PL, et al. Antibody-dependent cell-mediated antibacterial activity: K lymphocytes, monocytes, and granulocytes are effective against *Shigella*. *J Immunol.* 1980;125:2778-2784.
82. Formal S, Kent T, May H, et al. Protection of monkeys against experimental shigellosis with a living attenuated oral polyvalent dysentery vaccine. *J Bacteriol.* 1966;92:17-22.
83. Mel D, Arsic B, Nikolic B, et al. Studies on vaccination against bacillary dysentery: 4. Oral immunization with live monotypic and combined vaccines. *Bull World Health Organ.* 1968;39:375-380.
84. DuPont HL, Hornick RB, Snyder MJ, et al. Immunity in shigellosis: II. Protection induced by oral live vaccine or primary infection. *J Infect Dis.* 1972;125:12-16.
85. Baron LS, Kopecko DJ, Formal SB, et al. Introduction of *Shigella flexneri* 2a type and group antigen genes into oral typhoid vaccine strain *Salmonella typhi* Ty21A. *Infect Immun.* 1987;55:2797-2801.

225

Haemophilus Species (Including H. influenzae and Chancroid)

TIMOTHY F. MURPHY

Haemophilus influenzae

DESCRIPTION OF THE PATHOGEN

Haemophilus influenzae is a small, nonmotile, non–spore-forming bacterium and a pathogen of humans found principally in the upper respiratory tract, first reported by Pfeiffer in 1892. The sensational claim that it was the primary agent of epidemic influenza proved fallacious; nonetheless, it has a wide range of pathogenic potential. Its requirement for growth factors, which can be supplied by erythrocytes, accounts for the generic name *Haemophilus* (blood-loving). In microscopic appearance, it is a small $(1- \times 0.3\text{-}\mu)$ gram-negative bacterium. Stained organisms obtained from clinical specimens vary microscopically from small coccobacilli to long filaments. This variable morphologic appearance (pleomorphism) and inconsistent uptake of dyes (e.g., safranin) may result in erroneous interpretations of stained smears.

Aerobic growth of *H. influenzae* requires two supplements known as X factor and V factor, although neither refers to a single substance. X factor can be supplied by heat-stable iron-containing pigments that supply protoporphyrins. Porphyrin-based assays represent the most reliable methods for identifying *Haemophilus* species.[1] Because X factor is not required for anaerobic growth of *H. influenzae,* confusion may arise if *H. influenzae* is grown anaerobically (e.g., after stab inoculation). The heat-labile V factor, a coenzyme, may be supplied by nicotinamide adenine dinucleotide, nicotinamide adenine dinucleotide phosphate, or nicotinamide nucleoside. Although present in erythrocytes, V factor must be released from the cell to sustain optimal growth, and thus standard blood agar is an unsatisfactory medium. *H. influenzae* exhibits satellitism around colonies of hemolytic *Staphylococcus aureus* (a source of V factor), and this technique may be used to identify *H. influenzae.* Although it is not a strict requirement, some *H. influenzae* strains grow best in 5% to 10% carbon dioxide.

Strains of *H. haemolyticus* are frequently misidentified as *H. influenzae* in clinical microbiology laboratories and in published studies. The confusion results from the observation that many strains of *H. haemolyticus* are not hemolytic, and this is the sole characteristic used routinely to distinguish *H. haemolyticus* from *H. influenzae* in commercial kits and in clinical microbiology laboratories. *H. influenzae* and *H. haemolyticus* both have growth requirements for X and V factors. Analysis of 500 strains originally identified as nontypeable *H. influenzae* has revealed that 27% of nasopharyngeal isolates from children and 40% of sputum isolates from adults were in fact *H. haemolyticus.*[2] *H. haemolyticus* is a commensal and does not appear to cause disease. Strains of *H. haemolyticus* and *H. influenzae* can be distinguished from one another using a polymerase chain reaction (PCR) assay based on 16S ribosomal DNA sequences, or by differences in the superoxide dismutase C gene or outer membrane protein P6.[2-4]

Viability of *H. influenzae* is lost rapidly, so clinical specimens should be inoculated onto appropriate media without delay. A biotyping scheme devised by Kilian (based on indole production, urease, and ornithine decarboxylase activity) may be used to characterize individual isolates.[5] Biotype III includes *Haemophilus aegyptius,* the "Koch-Weeks bacillus." A clone of biotype IV strains is associated with neonatal and postpartum infections.

Colonies of *H. influenzae* are usually granular, transparent (or slightly opaque), circular, and dome-shaped. On chocolate agar, most colonies attain a size of about 0.5 to 0.8 mm during the first 24 hours of growth at 37° C, enlarging to 1.0 to 1.5 mm by 48 hours. Six serotypes, designated a to f, are based on antigenically distinct capsular polysaccharide types. Colonies of encapsulated strains are mucoid—iridescent when grown on transparent media and examined using an indirect source of light—and may attain a size of 3 to 4 mm. Capsular type b strains are important invasive pathogens in humans. Strains of *H. influenzae* that lack a polysaccharide capsule are generally referred to as nontypeable because they are nonreactive with typing antisera raised against each of the six capsules. The population structure of *H. influenzae* type b is clonal, whereas nontypeable strains demonstrate substantial genetic diversity. Most unencapsulated isolates are not capsule-deficient variants of extant capsule clones; they are genetically distinct from encapsulated strains of *H. influenzae.*

EPIDEMIOLOGY AND RESPIRATORY TRACT COLONIZATION

H. influenzae is recovered exclusively from humans; no other natural host is known. It is recovered from the upper airway and, rarely, the genital tract. Spread from one person to another occurs by airborne droplets or by direct contact with secretions.

Exposure to nontypeable *H. influenzae* begins after birth. Colonization of the respiratory tract is a dynamic process, with new strains of nontypeable *H. influenzae* being acquired and cleared from the respiratory tract frequently.[6] Varied patterns of colonization are evident in the first 2 years of life: brief colonization with one strain, prolonged colonization with one strain, and recurrent colonization with different strains.[6-9] Children who attend daycare centers are colonized at a higher rate than control children.[9,10] Nasopharyngeal colonization by *H. influenzae* in the first year of life is associated with an increased risk of recurrent otitis media compared with children who remain free of colonization.[11] The widespread administration of pneumococcal polysaccharide vaccines has caused changes in patterns of nasopharyngeal colonization. The recent increase in the proportion of cases of otitis media caused by nontypeable *H. influenzae* appears to be a result of reduction in nasopharyngeal colonization by vaccine serotypes of *S. pneumoniae,* with "replacement" of vaccine serotypes of *S. pneumoniae* by nonvaccine pneumococcal serotypes, nontypeable *H. influenzae* and *Moraxella catarrhalis.*[12,13]

Nontypeable *H. influenzae* frequently colonizes the lower respiratory tract in the setting of chronic obstructive pulmonary disease (COPD) and cystic fibrosis; multiple strains colonize the respiratory tract of these patients simultaneously.[14-17] Acquisition of new strains of nontypeable *H. influenzae* is associated with an increased risk of exacerbations of COPD.[2,18] Using selective media improves the recovery rate of *H. influenzae* from the sputum of patients with cystic fibrosis.[19]

Based on its binding to mucin and adherence to epithelial cells, *H. influenzae* has long been considered an extracellular pathogen. Several lines of evidence, however, now establish that *H. influenzae* has both an extracellular and intracellular niche in the human respiratory tract.[20-23] Therefore, *H. influenzae* is present in the airway lumen,

TABLE 225-1	Comparison of Selected Features of Nontypeable and Type b Strains of *Haemophilus influenzae*	
Feature	Nontypeable Strains	Type b Strains
Colonization rate in upper respiratory tract	30%-80%	<1% in vaccinated populations; 2%-4% in unvaccinated populations
Capsule	Unencapsulated	PRP capsule
Pathogenesis	Mucosal infections	Invasive infections
Clinical manifestations	Otitis media, exacerbations of COPD, sinusitis	Meningitis, epiglottitis, and other invasive infections in infants and children
Evolutionary history	Genetically diverse	Clonal
Vaccine	None available; under development	Highly effective PRP-conjugate vaccines

COPD, chronic obstructive pulmonary disease.

bound to mucin, adherent to respiratory cells, within the interstitium of the submucosa, and within cells of the respiratory tract. This observation has important implications for understanding the dynamics of colonization of the human respiratory tract and the human immune response to the bacterium.

Before the widespread use of conjugate vaccines, type b strains colonized the nasopharynx of children at a rate of 2% to 4%. The rate of nasopharyngeal colonization by type b strains has decreased substantially with the use of conjugate vaccines to prevent invasive infections caused by *H. influenzae* type b. Table 225-1 summarizes several features of nontypeable and type b strains.

PATHOGENESIS

Otitis Media

The first step in the pathogenesis of infection is colonization of the upper respiratory tract. *H. influenzae* expresses a variety of adhesin molecules (Table 225-2), each of which has its own specificity for host receptors.[24,25] The prevalence and distribution of adhesins varies among nontypeable strains.[25,26] In contrast to type b strains, which gain access to the bloodstream, nontypeable strains cause disease by local invasion of mucosal surfaces. The pathogenesis of otitis media involves direct extension of bacteria from the nasopharynx to the middle ear via the eustachian tube.[27] Release of lipo-oligosaccharide, lipoproteins, peptidoglycan fragments, and other antigens induces host inflammation.

Strains of nontypeable *H. influenzae* show differences in their pathogenic potential. A subset of strains that colonize the nasopharynx are capable of causing otitis media and have different sets of genes compared with strains that cause asymptomatic colonization. For example, otitis media strains are more likely to have the lipo-oligosaccharide synthesis gene *lic2B* and the histidine operon than asymptomatic colonizing strains.[28,29]

Nontypeable *H. influenzae* has also been implicated as a cause of otitis media with effusion, a term that refers to the presence of middle ear fluid in the absence of clinical signs of acute otitis media. In addition to positive cultures of some middle ear fluids, analysis by PCR reveals the presence of microbial DNA and mRNA, suggesting that *H. influenzae* is present in a viable but nonculturable form in some cases of otitis media with effusion.[30,31]

H. influenzae in the form of biofilms is present in the middle ear in animal models and in the middle ears of children with otitis media.[32,33-35] A biofilm is a community of bacteria encased in a matrix and attached to a surface. Bacteria in biofilms are more resistant to host clearance mechanisms and more resistant to antibiotics compared with planktonic bacteria.[36] Nontypeable *H. influenzae* biofilms are associated with recurrent and chronic otitis media.[35]

Exacerbations of Chronic Obstructive Pulmonary Disease

The lower respiratory tract of adults with COPD is chronically colonized by nontypeable *H. influenzae*. The course of COPD is character-

ized by intermittent exacerbations of the disease. Several lines of evidence implicate *H. influenzae* as the most common bacterial cause of exacerbations, including bronchoscopic sampling of the lower respiratory tract during exacerbations, analysis of immune responses to *H. influenzae* isolated from patients experiencing exacerbations, correlation of airway inflammation with sputum bacteriology, and molecular analysis of prospectively collected isolates.[18,37,38] Differences in pathogenic potential among strains in the setting of COPD are based on genome content.[39,40] A complex host-pathogen interaction most likely determines the outcome of the acquisition of a new strain of nontypeable *H. influenzae*; the determinants include virulence of the strain, degree of host impairment of innate immunity and pulmonary function, host inflammatory response, preexisting immunity, perception of symptoms, and other factors.[37]

Invasive Infections Caused by Haemophilus influenzae Type b

The importance of the type b capsule as a critical virulence factor in the pathogenesis of invasive disease has been well established by the use of genetic techniques and an infant rat model of bacteremia and meningitis.[41] Mutants lacking the polyribitol ribose phosphate (PRP) capsule do not cause invasive disease, whereas the isogenic parent strains are highly virulent in the infant rat model. The type b capsular polysaccharide is composed of PRP. The capsule enables the organism to invade the bloodstream following colonization of the respiratory tract (see later).

IMMUNITY

Nontypeable Haemophilus influenzae

Immunity to infection by nontypeable *H. influenzae* is complex and not completely understood. A hallmark of infections caused by nontypeable *H. influenzae* is their propensity for recurrence. The immune response to surface antigens of nontypeable strains is intimately involved in the pathogenesis of recurrent infection. Studies in animal models, in adults with COPD, and in children with otitis media have all demonstrated that the most prominent antibody response is directed at strain-specific determinants.[42-44] The clinical observation of recurrent infections in immunocompetent hosts (recurrent otitis media in children and recurrent exacerbations in COPD) suggests that strain-specific immune responses leave the host susceptible to recurrent infections by different strains of *H. influenzae*. A variety of membrane-associated surface-exposed determinants are immunogenic and potential targets of protective host immune responses. For example,

TABLE 225-2	Adhesins of *Haemophilus influenzae*	
Adhesin	Molecular Mass (kDa)	Observation
Pili (fimbriae)	20-25	*hifA-hif*E gene cluster
Type 4 pilus	~14	*pilABCD* gene cluster; mediates twitching motility
HMW1 and HMW2	120-125	Homologous with filamentous hemagglutinin of *Bordetella pertussis*
Hap	155	Homologous with IgA protease
Hsf	~240	Surface fibrils; present in type b strains; homologue of Hia
Hia	115	Hia absent from strains that express HMW1, HMW2; present in nontypeable strains
OMP P5	~35	Binds mucin; also called fimbrin; homologous with OMP A of *Escherichia coli*
OMP P2	36-42	Binds mucin
PE binding adhesin	46	Binds phosphatidyl ethanolamine
Protein E	16	Binds myeloma IgD and type 2 alveolar cells
Lipo-oligosaccharide	2.5-3.3	Adhesin for respiratory epithelial cells

outer membrane protein P2, the major porin protein, contains immunodominant strain-specific determinants on the bacterial surface. Adults with COPD make potentially protective antibodies to strain-specific determinants on P2 following infection. Patients remain susceptible to recurrent infections by other strains. Furthermore, the P2 genes of strains that colonize adults with COPD undergo point mutations in the human respiratory tract.[45,46] The mutations result in amino acid changes in the surface-exposed loops of the P2 molecule. A similar phenomenon has been observed with outer membrane protein P5.[47] These variants have a selective advantage and are able to evade the host response and cause recurrent or persistent infection.

The presence of serum bactericidal antibody is associated with protection from otitis media caused by nontypeable *H. influenzae*.[42,48] Because nontypeable *H. influenzae* causes mucosal infection, mucosal immunity likely plays a role in host defense; however, the mucosal immune response to *H. influenzae* is poorly understood. Finally, observations have suggested that cell-mediated immune responses play a role in protection against infection.[49]

Haemophilus influenzae *Type b*

Protection against invasive *H. influenzae* type b infections is mediated by antibodies to the type b capsular polysaccharide PRP. Serum anti-PRP antibodies activate complement-mediated bactericidal and opsonic activity in vitro and mediate protective immunity against systemic infections in humans. The level of maternally acquired serum antibody to PRP declines after birth and reaches a nadir at approximately 18 to 24 months of age, the peak age incidence of meningitis caused by *H. influenzae* type b in an unimmunized child. The level of antibody to PRP then gradually rises, apparently as a result of exposure to *H. influenzae* type b or cross-reacting antigens. Systemic disease is unusual after the age of 6 years, even in the absence of immunization because of, at least in part, naturally acquired antibody to PRP.

Immunization with vaccines that are composed of PRP conjugated to carrier proteins affords protection by inducing antibodies to PRP. These vaccines are now widely used and are highly effective in preventing invasive disease caused by *H. influenzae* type b in infants and children. In addition, these vaccines prevent colonization of the nasopharynx; this effect accounts for herd immunity by reducing the circulation of type b strains.

CLINICAL MANIFESTATIONS OF NONTYPEABLE *HAEMOPHILUS INFLUENZAE*

Otitis Media. Nontypeable *H. influenzae* accounts for 25% to 35% of all cases of acute otitis media. Approximately 25 million episodes of otitis media occur annually in the United States. Although such episodes occur at any age, they are most common in children aged 6 months to 5 years. The typical clinical presentation of acute otitis media in infants is fever and irritability, whereas older children also complain of ear pain. A prior viral respiratory tract infection is commonly the antecedent of an episode of otitis media. The diagnosis is made by pneumatic otoscopy. A precise causative diagnosis requires tympanocentesis, but this is not performed routinely.

Although it is not possible to determine the causative agent of otitis media in an individual child based on clinical characteristics, certain features are associated with otitis media caused by nontypeable *H. influenzae* compared with *S. pneumoniae*. Otitis media caused by nontypeable *H. influenzae* is less likely to cause fever and is less often associated with otorrhea than pneumococcal otitis media, suggesting that the former causes a less virulent form of the disease, but substantial overlap is seen.[50,51] Nevertheless, features associated with nontypeable *H. influenzae* otitis media include a history of recurrent episodes, treatment failure, concomitant conjunctivitis, previous amoxicillin treatment, bilateral otitis media, and acute otitis media within 2 weeks of completing a course of any antibiotic.[52-55] Since 2000, most infants in the United States have received the seven-valent pneumococcal conjugate vaccine. An increase in the proportion of acute otitis media caused by nontypeable *H. influenzae* in children failing initial antimi-

crobial therapy or with recurrent episodes has occurred coincident with the widespread use of this vaccine.[56,57]

Exacerbations of Chronic Obstructive Pulmonary Disease. The course of COPD is characterized by intermittent exacerbations of the disease. It is estimated that approximately half of exacerbations are caused by bacteria, and nontypeable *H. influenzae* is the most common bacterial cause.[2,18] The three cardinal signs of an exacerbation are an increase from baseline of sputum production, sputum purulence (change in sputum color), and dyspnea. Fever is generally absent or low grade and infiltrates are not present on chest radiography. A sputum Gram strain often reveals abundant gram-negative coccobacilli.

Community-Acquired Pneumonia. Nontypeable *H. influenzae* is an important cause of pneumonia in adults, particularly in older adults and those with COPD and acquired immunodeficiency syndrome.[58,59] The clinical features are indistinguishable from those of pneumonia caused by other bacteria and include fever, cough, and purulent sputum, usually of several days' duration. The chest film reveals infiltrates that may be patchy or show lobar distribution. A Gram-stained smear of the sputum shows a predominance of small gram-negative coccobacilli.

Acute Respiratory Tract Infections in Children in Developing Countries. In many countries in which adverse socioeconomic circumstances are prevalent, acute pneumonia in infants caused by nontypeable *H. influenzae* is a major cause of morbidity and mortality.[60,61] Carefully performed studies in several developing countries have established that nontypeable *H. influenzae* accounts for a significant proportion of pneumonia. The importance of acute respiratory tract infections as a major global health problem has led to the establishment of international programs (e.g., through the World Health Organization), with the aim of enhancing the recognition, appropriate management, and prevention of respiratory tract infections.

Sinusitis. Studies that have used cultures of direct sinus aspirates show that nontypeable *H. influenzae* is a common cause of acute maxillary sinusitis.[62,63] Patients experience nasal obstruction, purulent nasal discharge, headache, and facial pain. As in the case of otitis media, an invasive procedure (sinus aspiration) is required to establish a causative diagnosis.

Neonatal and Maternal Sepsis. Neonatal sepsis caused by nontypeable *H. influenzae* has been recognized with increasing frequency since the 1980s.[64] The infection is associated with 50% mortality overall and 90% mortality in premature infants. Many strains that cause neonatal sepsis are biotype IV and share several genotypic and phenotypic characteristics with one another. Indeed, studies of the genetic relationships of these potentially invasive strains and other nontypeable strains have suggested that the invasive biotype IV strains are closely related to *H. haemolyticus*.[2]

These same biotype IV strains also cause postpartum sepsis associated with endometritis. Nontypeable *H. influenzae* is a well-documented cause of tubo-ovarian abscess or chronic salpingitis. Diagnosis is established by tubal cultures at laparoscopy or cultures of peritoneal fluid by culdocentesis.

Bacteremia and Invasive Infections. Although the most common clinical manifestations of infections by nontypeable *H. influenzae* are otitis media and nonbacteremic respiratory tract infections in adults, the organism also occasionally causes bacteremia. Most invasive *H. influenzae* infections in countries in which the *H. influenzae* type b vaccines are used are caused by nontypeable strains.[65-67] Population-based studies estimate an incidence of 1.7 cases/100,000 adults of invasive disease caused by *H. influenzae* and, overall, the incidence is highest in older adults.[66,68] Most people with bacteremia have underlying conditions such as alcoholism, cardiopulmonary disease, HIV infection, or cancer. The respiratory tract is the usual source of infection when bacteremia is present. Invasive strains of nontypeable *H.*

influenzae are genetically and phenotypically diverse.[69] Bacteremic infections caused by nontypeable *H. influenzae* are associated with significant mortality.

Nontypeable *H. influenzae* is also an unusual cause of a variety of invasive infections that are documented by case reports and small series. All the invasive diseases that are commonly caused by type b *H. influenzae* are, on occasion, caused by nontypeable strains as well as types a, c, d, e, and f. These infections include adult epiglottitis, empyema, septic arthritis, cellulitis, osteomyelitis, pericarditis, cholecystitis, intra-abdominal infection, and vascular graft infection.

Conjunctivitis. Nontypeable *H. influenzae* is the most common bacterial cause of conjunctivitis in children.[70,71] In contrast to the sporadic nature of other *Haemophilus* infections, conjunctivitis can occur in outbreaks, particularly in daycare centers. Clinical features include conjunctival hyperemia and purulent discharge. Occasionally, nontypeable *H. influenzae* causes severe conjunctivitis that is characterized by copious, purulent discharge, lid edema, chemosis, and keratitis.

CLINICAL MANIFESTATIONS OF *HAEMOPHILUS INFLUENZAE* TYPE B

Meningitis. Meningitis is the most serious acute manifestation of systemic infection caused by *H. influenzae*. Antecedent symptoms of upper respiratory infection are common. Specific questioning concerning the occurrence of disease in contacts (household, daycare centers) is prudent. None of the clinical features of meningitis caused by *H. influenzae* distinguishes it from other forms of purulent meningitis. The peak age incidence varies somewhat among populations, depending in part on vaccine use, but this infection now occurs most often in those who are incompletely immunized. Adult cases are infrequent and often have a background of recent or remote head trauma, prior neurosurgery, paranasal sinusitis, otitis, or cerebrospinal fluid leak. *H. influenzae* meningitis in neonates is also rare, but such cases can resemble early-onset group B streptococcal infection. The most common signs are fever and altered central nervous system function, but the young child may have few specific signs, and nuchal rigidity is often absent. More obvious manifestations, such as seizures or coma, commonly develop as the disease progresses. Subdural effusions are a common complication. Clinical suspicion should be greatest when, after 2 or 3 days of adequate therapy, there is a tense anterior fontanelle, seizures (particularly if focal), hemiparesis, or neurologic deterioration. In older children, one looks for papilledema and altered mental status.

With appropriate management, the overall mortality rate from *H. influenzae* meningitis is less than 5%, but apparently permanent sequelae occur in many of the survivors.

Epiglottitis. Acute respiratory obstruction caused by a cellulitis of the supraglottic tissues is a potentially lethal disease with a characteristically fulminating onset. Swelling of the epiglottis and aryepiglottic folds with complete obliteration of the vallecular and piriform sinuses is typical. Usually, the patient is a child (aged 2 to 7 years), but occurrence in adults is also well known. The onset is often explosive, with initial features being sore throat, fever, and dyspnea progressing rapidly to dysphagia, pooling of oral secretions, and drooling of saliva from the mouth. The child is restless, anxious, and adopts a sitting position, with neck extended and chin protruding to reduce airway obstruction. Abrupt deterioration commonly occurs within a few hours, resulting in death in the absence of adequate treatment. The characteristic findings are seen above the larynx. The epiglottis is red and swollen and bears a striking resemblance to a bright red cherry obstructing the pharynx at the base of the tongue. The trachea appears normal. Examination of the larynx should be performed only in a setting in which an airway can be placed, because this examination, if injudiciously performed, may lead to fatal respiratory obstruction.

Pneumonia and Empyema. The true frequency of primary lung infections caused by *H. influenzae* b in children is difficult to determine

with accuracy. Typically, the patient is between 4 months and 4 years of age and becomes ill in winter or spring, presenting with a consolidative pneumonia (often with pleural involvement) that is severe enough to require hospitalization. The only clinical feature that tends to distinguish *H. influenzae* pneumonia from bacterial pneumonias caused by *S. aureus* or *Streptococcus pneumoniae* is a more insidious onset. The development of severe dyspnea, tachycardia, and evidence of cardiovascular failure suggests pericarditis, an uncommon but important complication.

Cellulitis. Cellulitis is predominantly seen in young children. The clinical features are fever and a raised, warm, tender area of distinctive reddish blue hue, most often located on one cheek or in the periorbital region. The distinctive color, its location, and age of the child should suggest the cause. The soft tissue involvement progresses rapidly over a few hours. Some of these children have, or develop, evidence of other septic foci (e.g., meningitis), because an accompanying bacteremia is extremely common.

Bacteremia without Localized Disease. Children, particularly those 6 to 36 months of age, may acquire bacteremia without evidence of local disease; *S. pneumoniae* is the most common cause of this syndrome. Typically, fever, anorexia, and lethargy prompt the visit to a physician; the examination is nondiagnostic. This condition is appreciated most often in those with a temperature higher than 102° F (39° C) and an increased peripheral neutrophil count. Children with sickle cell disease or with a previous splenectomy are particularly susceptible. Early diagnosis and therapy are critical because these patients may worsen rapidly and experience septic shock or a localized purulent focus.

Septic Arthritis. *H. influenzae* causes septic arthritis in children younger than 2 years. Typically, there is involvement of a single, large, weight-bearing joint (without osteomyelitis), displaying decreased mobility, pain on movement, and swelling. Positive cultures of blood and joint fluid are usual. However, the signs and symptoms may be more subtle; for example, septic arthritis is an important cause of prolonged fever and irritability (or prolonged antigenemia) during the treatment of other systemic *H. influenzae* diseases (e.g., meningitis).

Response to systemic antibiotics is dramatic and often curative, but long-term follow-up is important because residual joint dysfunction occurs in a significant percentage of children.

H. influenzae septic arthritis also occurs in adults. A review of 29 adults with *H. influenzae* arthritis found that 14 had multiarticular disease and 15 monoarticular disease, with 6 being in the knee only.[72] Nineteen had extra-articular infection as well, including meningitis, pneumonia, sinusitis, and cellulitis. Predisposing factors were found in 22, such as alcohol abuse, trauma, rheumatoid arthritis, systemic lupus erythematosus, diabetes mellitus, splenectomy, multiple myeloma, lymphoma, or common variable hypogammaglobulinemia.

DIAGNOSIS

Nontypeable *Haemophilus influenzae*

Because nontypeable *H. influenzae* is often present in the human upper airway in the absence of clinical disease, determining the causative pathogen in individual patients is challenging. A diagnosis of otitis media is made by pneumatic otoscopy. Culture of middle ear fluid obtained by tympanocentesis would be required to determine the microbial cause. However, because tympanocentesis is a relatively invasive procedure, empirical therapy with antibiotics is initiated based on predictions of the likely pathogens, which are known to be *Streptococcus pneumoniae*, nontypeable *H. influenzae,* and *Moraxella catarrhalis* determined by studies that have used cultures of middle ear fluid obtained by tympanocentesis. Judicious use of tympanocentesis in children with recurrent or refractory otitis media may be indicated to identify the pathogen precisely in difficult cases, but this procedure is not used routinely.[73]

The cause of exacerbations of COPD and community-acquired pneumonia in individual patients is difficult to determine. The presence of nontypeable *H. influenzae* in the sputum of patients experiencing an exacerbation of COPD or pneumonia is suggestive of the diagnosis but does not establish the organism as the pathogen because it may be present in the airways in the absence of disease. Nontypeable *H. influenzae* is the most common bacterial cause of exacerbations of COPD and causes a smaller proportion of cases of community-acquired pneumonia.

Isolating the organism from a blood culture unequivocally establishes the organism as causative. Although blood cultures are invaluable when positive, most infections caused by nontypeable *H. influenzae* are not associated bacteremia so blood cultures are relatively insensitive.

Haemophilus influenzae *Type b*

A provisional diagnosis of meningitis, epiglottitis, facial cellulitis, or septic arthritis is usually prompted by the history and clinical findings. Confirmation requires microbiologic studies. Cultures of blood, cerebrospinal fluid (CSF), and other normally sterile fluids (e.g., from joints or pleural, subdural, or pericardial spaces) are diagnostic. Even if antibiotic therapy has been started, the yield is sufficiently great to recommend that they be taken. Cultures of the inflamed epiglottis are generally positive but should be taken only when a functional airway can be guaranteed. Whenever feasible, specimens obtained for culture should also be Gram-stained; in about 70% of cases of meningitis, CSF smears reveal typical organisms. Detection of capsular antigen in serum, CSF, or concentrated urine using immunoelectrophoresis, latex agglutination, or enzyme-linked immunosorbent assay may be diagnostic and can be made in up to 90% of culture-proven cases of meningitis. Antigen is also often detected in infected pleural, pericardial, or joint fluid and can facilitate diagnosis because it persists after antibiotic therapy.

TREATMENT

Nontypeable Haemophilus influenzae

Many infections caused by nontypeable *H. influenzae*, such as otitis media and exacerbations of COPD, can be treated with oral antimicrobial agents. Overall, approximately 30% of nontypeable strains produce β-lactamase but substantial geographic variability in this rate is observed. Therefore, ampicillin and amoxicillin should be used only if the susceptibility of the infecting isolate is known. The clinician who manages patients with otitis media and exacerbations of COPD frequently chooses an antimicrobial agent empirically. In this circumstance, the antimicrobial agent should be active against *S. pneumoniae* and *M. catarrhalis* as well as *H. influenzae*.

Oral antimicrobial agents that are active against nontypeable *H. influenzae* (and also *S. pneumoniae* and *M. catarrhalis*) include amoxicillin-clavulanate, fluoroquinolones, macrolides (e.g., azithromycin, clarithromycin), and various extended-spectrum cephalosporins (e.g., cefixime, cefpodoxime, cefaclor, loracarbef, cefuroxime).

Parenteral antibiotic therapy is indicated for more serious infections caused by nontypeable *H. influenzae*. Parenteral antimicrobial agents that are active include cephalosporins (e.g., ceftriaxone, cefuroxime, ceftazidime, cefotaxime), ampicillin-sulbactam, fluoroquinolones, and azithromycin.

Those with certain immunodeficiencies, especially those with primary deficiency of antibody synthesis, have increased susceptibility to infection, especially with nontypeable *H. influenzae*. They may benefit from passive infusion of immunoglobulin preparations administered intramuscularly or intravenously. This form of immunoglobulin replacement decreases the incidence of systemic infections in these persons and the number of episodes of both upper and lower respiratory tract infections caused by nontypeable *H. influenzae*.

Haemophilus influenzae *Type b*

Without treatment, infection caused by *H. influenzae* type b can be rapidly fatal. This is particularly true of meningitis and epiglottitis. The most favored regimen is cefotaxime or ceftriaxone. For children, cefotaxime is given as 200 mg/kg/day, divided into six hourly doses. The pediatric dose of ceftriaxone is 75 to 100 mg/kg, divided into 12 hourly doses. Adult doses are ceftriaxone, 2 g every 12 hours, or cefotaxime, 2 g every 4 to 6 hours. Treatment is continued until the patient is afebrile and without clinical or laboratory signs of infection for 3 to 5 days. The usual duration of therapy is 7 to 10 days. Patients with complications such as endophthalmitis, endocarditis, pericarditis, or osteomyelitis may require 3 to 6 weeks of therapy.

Administration of corticosteroids to patients with *H. influenzae* type b meningitis reduces the incidence of neurologic sequelae (see Chapter 84 for a review of this subject). The presumed mechanism is the reduction of inflammation that results from release of bacterial cell wall fragments when bacteria are killed by antibiotics. Dexamethasone therapy (IV, 0.6 mg/kg/day in four divided doses for 4 days) should be administered to children older than 2 months.

Antibiotic therapy is only one facet of the management of the child with *H. influenzae* infection. Critical attention must also be given to supportive therapy, including maintaining oxygenation and adequate perfusion of tissues.

Chemoprophylaxis for *Haemophilus influenzae* Type b. In the absence of prior immunization, household contacts younger than 4 years with those with invasive *H. influenzae* type b infection have a substantial incidence of disease. Rifampin prophylaxis as 20 mg/kg once daily (600 mg maximum) for 4 days has eradicated the carrier state in approximately 95% of carriers and significantly reduced the incidence of secondary cases in household members. Rifampin comes in 150- and 300-mg capsules. The dose can be conveniently given to young children in applesauce.

Rifampin prophylaxis is recommended for all household members, including adults (except pregnant women) when there has been contact with an index case of *H. influenzae* type b disease by a household member who is younger than 48 months and whose immunization status with the conjugate vaccine is incomplete, or is an immunocompromised child of any age.[58] A contact is defined as a child who is a household member or who has spent 4 or more hours each day with the index case for at least 5 of the 7 days preceding the day that the index case was hospitalized. Based on efficacy of the *H. influenzae* type b vaccine, chemoprophylaxis is not recommended when all household contacts younger than 48 months have completed their immunization series. Children who were immunosuppressed at the time of vaccination may not have responded and therefore should be considered unvaccinated. If rifampin is to be effective in preventing secondary cases, it should be given within 7 days after the index patient is hospitalized. The index patient should also be given rifampin if treated with regimens other than cefotaxime or ceftriaxone. Chemoprophylaxis is usually provided just before discharge from the hospital.

Rifampin prophylaxis is indicated for all attendees and personnel at a daycare center or nursery when two or more cases of invasive *H. influenzae* type b disease have occurred within 60 days if incompletely immunized children attend the facility. The duration and dose of rifampin are the same as for household contacts. Chemoprophylaxis is not indicated for a single case at a daycare center or nursery.

Active Immunization against *Haemophilus influenzae* Type b. Conjugate vaccines for invasive *H. influenzae* type b infections in infants and children are highly effective. The vaccines induce serum antibody to the PRP capsule; this antibody is bactericidal for the organism. The protective level of serum antibody to PRP has been estimated to be approximately 0.15 μg/mL, although this estimate must be interpreted cautiously. An unexpected finding from studies that assessed the effect of vaccination on nasopharyngeal colonization was that vaccination reduces or eliminates carriage of *H. influenzae* type b strains, which has played an important role in the effectiveness of the vaccine. The widespread use of conjugate vaccines has almost eradicated invasive disease in children younger than 5 years in the

United States. These vaccines represent a dramatic success in disease prevention and health care cost savings.

Certain populations, including Native American and native Alaskan children, show a persistently elevated rate of infection, even with widespread vaccination. Furthermore, localized populations with low vaccination rates contribute to the continued circulation of *H. influenzae* type b strains, despite a national vaccination rate higher than 90%. Therefore, continued surveillance, particularly in these high-risk populations, will be important. Determination of the serotypes of disease isolates will distinguish disease that results from lack of vaccination or vaccine failure from invasive disease caused by non–type b strains. A striking reduction in the incidence of invasive infections caused by *H. influenzae* type b has been seen in countries in which conjugate vaccines have been used widely. However, the global impact has been less impressive because the vaccines are used primarily in affluent countries. Currently, it is estimated that worldwide, approximately 2% of cases of invasive *H. influenzae* type b infections are prevented by the vaccines.[74]

Two conjugate vaccines are currently licensed and available in the United States (Table 225-3). All children should be immunized with a conjugate vaccine beginning at 2 months of age. A primary series consisting of three doses at 2, 4, and 6 months of age (PRP-T) or two doses given at 2 and 4 months (PRP-OMPC), depending on the vaccine product, is recommended. After administration of the primary series, antibody titers decline, so an additional booster dose should be given between 12 and 15 months of age. Vaccines may be administered during visits when other vaccines are given. Adverse reactions are few; the most common are pain, redness, and swelling at the injection site.

There are no currently licensed vaccine for nontypeable *H. influenzae*. However, a randomized, prospective, placebo-controlled trial with a vaccine that contained protein D, a conserved surface protein, has shown partial efficacy in prevention of nontypeable *H. influenzae* otitis media.[75] Additional progress in developing vaccines to prevent infections caused by nontypeable *H. influenzae* is anticipated.

HAEMOPHILUS INFLUENZAE BIOGROUP AEGYPTIUS

H. influenzae biogroup aegyptius was formerly called *H. aegyptius*. However, recent genetic studies have established that *H. influenzae* and *H. aegyptius* are members of the same species; hence, the organism is now referred to as *H. influenzae* biogroup aegyptius.

H. influenzae biogroup aegyptius has long been known to cause conjunctivitis. In 1984, a fulminant systemic illness was described in a small Brazilian town. Following an episode of purulent conjunctivitis, children experienced high fever, vomiting, and abdominal pain. These symptoms were followed by petechiae, purpura, peripheral necrosis, and vascular collapse. Blood cultures were positive for *H. influenzae* biogroup aegyptius.[76] The mortality was 70%, but subsequent reports have described milder forms of the illness. The illness was called Brazilian purpuric fever and has now been described in several rural Brazilian towns in addition to two cases in Australia. Brazilian purpuric fever has occurred sporadically and as outbreaks. The peak age of incidence is 1 to 4 years.

H. influenzae biogroup aegyptius is remarkable in that the organism has acquired the capacity to cause a fulminant invasive disease in spite of lacking a capsule, which is often associated with invasive infections.

Strains of *H. influenzae* biogroup aegyptius are of a clonal origin. Case clone strains share several characteristics, including a unique plasmid, identical electrophoretic type in multilocus enzyme typing, typical ribosomal DNA restriction patterns, and a conserved surface epitope on outer membrane protein P1.[77,78] Case clone strains contain 16 chromosomal elements and a mobile genetic element that are unique to the clonal group.

Identifying the virulence factors that give case clone strains the ability to cause invasive disease will be important in understanding Brazilian purpuric fever. From a broader perspective, characterizing the molecular mechanisms that account for the invasive potential in an otherwise noninvasive bacterium (nontypeable *H. influenzae*) is of great interest in understanding the pathogenesis of invasive bacterial infections.

Haemophilus ducreyi

DESCRIPTION OF THE PATHOGEN

H. ducreyi is the causative agent of chancroid, an infection characterized by genital ulcer and inguinal lymphadenitis. *H. ducreyi* is a highly fastidious gram-negative coccobacillus. Its microscopic appearance and its nutritional requirement for hemin account for the classification of the bacterium in the genus *Haemophilus*. However, studies of DNA homology and chemotaxonomy have demonstrated substantial differences between *H. ducreyi* and other *Haemophilus* species. *H. ducreyi* will likely be reclassified in the future, but this issue awaits further study. The organism is a strict human pathogen and there are no known animal or environmental reservoirs.

EPIDEMIOLOGY

Chancroid is a common cause of genital ulcers in developing countries. Like other genital ulcer disease, chancroid facilitates the transmission of human immunodeficiency virus (HIV). This association between HIV and chancroid has generated increased interest in understanding the pathogenesis of *H. ducreyi* infection and in improving diagnostic tests for genital ulcer disease. In view of the limited resources in developing countries in which *H. ducreyi* infection is endemic, the true prevalence of chancroid is unknown. The development of PCR-based diagnostic assays holds promise that the epidemiology of infection will be better understood. Initial application of these tests indicates that an increasing number of patients with genital ulcer disease have multiple agents simultaneously.[79]

Several epidemiologic features of *H. ducreyi* infection are apparent. Although the bacterium is a common cause of genital ulcers in developing countries, the disease occurs primarily in sporadic outbreaks in industrialized countries. The annual number of cases reported in the United States has remained stable since 2000; there were 33 cases in 2006. Transmission is primarily heterosexual and males have outnumbered females in most studies. A high proportion of infected males report sexual contact with commercial sex workers. Chancroid has been strongly associated with illicit drug use. The transmission dynamics of the organism suggest that the disease is likely to be perpetuated in highly sexually active populations, such as commercial sex workers.[79]

TABLE 225-3	*Haemophilus influenzae* Type b Conjugate Vaccines				
Scientific Name	Brand Name (Manufacturer)	Carbohydrate	Protein Carrier	Polysaccharide-to-Protein Ratio	Recommended Dose Carbohydrate (μg)
PRP-T*	ActHIB (Sanofi Pasteur)	Native PRP	Tetanus toxoid	0.33	10
PRP-OMPC‡	PedvaxHIB (Merck)	Native PRP	OMPC†	0.05-0.10	15

*PRP-T is also marketed as TriHIBit, which contains diphtheria, tetanus, and acellular pertussis vaccines (DTaP). Because of evidence of reduced immunogenicity of the Hib component when used in combination, TriHIBit is approved only for the fourth dose of the DTaP and Hib series, not for use as the primary series at 2, 4, or 6 months of age.
†Outer membrane protein complex derived from *Neisseria meningitidis* serogroup B.
‡PRP-OMPC is also marketed as Comvax in combination with hepatitis B vaccine (Recombivax, 5 mg) for administration at 2, 4, 12, and 15 months.

PATHOGENESIS AND IMMUNE RESPONSE

Infection occurs as a result of inoculation of bacteria through breaks in the epithelium during sexual contact with an infected individual. Studies using a human model of experimental *H. ducreyi* infection have led to the identification of selected genes or gene clusters that are required for full virulence.[80,81] The bacterium colocalizes with neutrophils and macrophages but is not phagocytosed, suggesting that evasion of phagocytic killing is important in pathogenesis. Ulcers contain predominantly T cells, with low numbers of B cells. Patients who have had chancroid may have repeated infections, indicating that natural infection does not confer protective immunity; a similar phenomenon is observed in the human volunteer model as well.[82]

CLINICAL MANIFESTATIONS

The hallmark of chancroid is genital ulceration. The lesion often begins as a papule and evolves into an ulcer. Typical ulcers are painful, well circumscribed with ragged edges, and not indurated. The base of the ulcer is covered with necrotic material and bleeds easily when scraped. Little or no inflammation of the surrounding skin is present. Approximately half of patients with chancroid have inguinal lymphadenopathy. These lymph nodes sometimes become fluctuant and rupture spontaneously.

Chancroid can present in atypical ways. Multiple ulcers may coalesce to form a giant ulcer. Ulceration may resolve before the appearance of inguinal adenopathy and suppuration, resulting in presentation as suppurative inguinal adenitis in the absence of an active genital ulcer. Multiple small ulcers may resemble folliculitis. The main differential diagnostic considerations include primary syphilis (chancre), genital herpes, lymphogranuloma venereum, donovanosis, and condyloma latum of secondary syphilis. In the presence of HIV infection, the number of ulcers at initial presentation may be greater and the duration of ulceration may be longer.

DIAGNOSIS

Because a clinical diagnosis of chancroid is often inaccurate, laboratory confirmation of the diagnosis should be sought. Gram stain of a swab of the ulcer may reveal a predominance of gram-negative coccobacilli but these smears are difficult to interpret because of the presence of other bacteria. Isolation of *H. ducreyi* from a swab of the lesion or from an aspirate of suppurative lymph nodes confirms the diagnosis. Because the organism is difficult to grow, the use of selective and supplemented media is required. The most promising approach to the diagnosis of chancroid is a PCR-based assay. This sensitive and specific multiplex assay amplifies targets from *H. ducreyi*, *Treponema pallidum*, and herpes simplex virus types 1 and 2, the most common causes of genital ulcer disease.[83] When this assay becomes commercially available, it will be a useful method to establish the cause of genital ulcers.

TREATMENT

The recommendation by the Centers for Disease Control and Prevention is a single 1-g dose of azithromycin orally. Alternative regimens include ceftriaxone (250 mg IM in a single dose), ciprofloxacin (500 mg PO twice daily for 3 days), or erythromycin base (500 mg PO three times daily for 7 days). Azithromycin and ceftriaxone have the distinct advantage of single-dose treatment.

Ulcers usually improve symptomatically by 3 days and by objective evaluation by 7 days following initiation of treatment. Lack of improvement should raise several considerations, including coinfection with another pathogen (especially genital herpes or primary syphilis), coexisting HIV infection, which is associated with a delayed response to treatment of chancroid, lack of adherence to the treatment regimen and, finally, resistance of the *H. ducreyi* isolate to the antimicrobial agent prescribed. Isolates from patients who do not respond promptly to treatment should be tested for antimicrobial susceptibility.

Contacts of patients with chancroid should be identified and treated if they had sexual contact with the patient during the 10 days prior to the onset of symptoms in the patient, even in the absence of clinical symptoms in the contact.

Other *Haemophilus* Species

DESCRIPTION OF THE PATHOGEN

Haemophilus species other than *H. influenzae* and *H. ducreyi* are unusual causes of disease in humans. However, as a result of increased awareness of these bacteria as potential pathogens and as a result of improvements in isolating the bacteria in culture, it is now apparent that other *Haemophilus* species more commonly cause human infection than previously believed, particularly in the case of infective endocarditis. *Haemophilus* species are present as part of the normal bacterial flora of the human upper respiratory tract. *H. parainfluenzae* is the predominant species accounting for approximately 75% of the *Haemophilus* flora of the human upper airway.

Members of the genus *Haemophilus* are small gram-negative coccobacilli with fastidious growth requirements. The growth requirements are used to distinguish among the species. *Haemophilus* require X factor (hemin), V factor (nicotinamide adenine dinucleotide), or both for growth. These are supplied by erythrocytes but the erythrocytes must be lysed to release V factor. This growth requirement is supplied in the clinical microbiology laboratory by growing *Haemophilus* species on chocolate agar. Table 225-4 shows differential characteristics of *Haemophilus* and related species that have been documented to cause infection in humans. Species are distinguished based on their different growth requirements for X and V factor, enhancement of growth by CO_2, expression of catalase, and ability to cause hemolysis. Species designated as *A. paraphrophilus*, *H. parainfluenzae*, and *H. parahaemolyticus* require V factor but not X factor for growth, whereas *A. aphrophilus* and *H. haemolyticus* require X and V or X only.

TABLE 225-4	Differential Characteristics of *Haemophilus* and *Aggregatibacter* Species				
	Growth Factor Requirement				
Organism	X	V	CO₂ Dependence	Hemolysis	Catalase
A. aphrophilus	+	−	+	−	−
A. paraphrophilus	−	+	+	−	±
H. parainfluenzae	−	+	−	−	+
H. haemolyticus	+	+	−	±	+
H. parahaemolyticus	−	+	−	+	+
H. ducreyi	+	−	±	±	−

+, present; −, absent.

CLINICAL MANIFESTATIONS

Haemophilus species, particularly *H. parainfluenzae*, and the two species moved from *Haemophilus* to *Aggregatibacter*, *A. aphrophilus* and *A. paraphrophilus*, are now recognized increasingly as a cause of infective endocarditis, causing up to 5% of cases of endocarditis. *Haemophilus* species are included in the so-called HACEK (*Haemophilus* species, *Aggregatibacter* species [including *A. actinomycetemcomitans*, formerly *Actinobacillus actinomycetemcomitans*], *Cardiobacterium* species, *Eikenella* species, and *Kingella* species) group of bacteria, which are slow-growing bacteria known to cause endocarditis. The presence of *Haemophilus* species (and others in the HACEK group) should be suspected in patients with a strong clinical suspicion of endocarditis and negative blood cultures. Because these bacteria are slow growing, incubation of blood cultures for 2 weeks has been recommended. However, recent studies indicate that extended incubation does not increase recovery from standard automated blood cultures.[84,85] Most patients with endocarditis caused by *Haemophilus* and *Aggregatibacter* species have underlying valvular heart disease. Echocardiography, particularly transesophageal echocardiography, is useful in identifying vegetations and characterizing underlying valvular disease. The clinical course of *Haemophilus* and *Aggregatibacter* endocarditis tends to be subacute, and embolization is common.[86]

Other *Haemophilus* species are relatively rare human pathogens, presumably because of their low pathogenic potential. They have been documented as rare causes of a variety of local upper respiratory and systemic infections, including sinusitis, otitis media, conjunctivitis, dental abscess, lower respiratory tract infection, peritonitis, biliary tract infection, brain abscess, osteomyelitis, and wound infections. Most of these are documented by small series and case reports.

TREATMENT

Treatment should be guided by the antimicrobial susceptibility of the etiologic isolate. The antimicrobial susceptibility characteristics of other *Haemophilus* and related species are similar to those of *H. influenzae*, although fewer data on other *Haemophilus* species are available. Some strains produce β-lactamase and are thus resistant to ampicillin. Agents with generally good activity include trimethoprim-sulfamethoxasole, third-generation cephalosporins, fluoroquinolones, and aztreonam.

In view of the increasing incidence of β-lactamase production among strains of *Haemophilus*, the treatment of choice for *Haemophilus* species endocarditis is now third-generation cephalosporins (ceftriaxone or cefotaxime).[87] Treatment of native valve endocarditis should be given for 4 weeks and treatment for prosthetic valve endocarditis should continue for 6 weeks.

REFERENCES

1. Munson E, Pfaller M, Koontz F, et al. Comparison of porphyrin-based, growth factor-based, and biochemical-based testing methods for identification of *Haemophilus influenzae*. *Eur J Clin Microbiol Infect Dis*. 2002;21:196-203.
2. Murphy TF, Brauer AL, Sethi S, et al. *Haemophilus haemolyticus*: A human respiratory tract commensal to be distinguished from *Haemophilus influenzae*. *J Infect Dis*. 2007;195:81-89.
3. McCrea KW, Xie J, LaCross N, et al. Relationships of nontypeable *Haemophilus influenzae* strains to hemolytic and nonhemolytic *Haemophilus haemolyticus* strains. *J Clin Microbiol*. 2008; 46:406-416.
4. Fung WW, O'Dwyer CA, Sinha S, et al. Presence of copper- and zinc-containing superoxide dismutase in commensal *Haemophilus haemolyticus* isolates can be used as a marker to discriminate them from nontypeable *H. influenzae* isolates. *J Clin Microbiol*. 2006;44:4222-4226.
5. Kilian M. A taxonomic study of the genus *Haemophilus*, with the proposal of a new species. *J Gen Microbiol*. 1976;93:9-62.
6. Faden H, Duffy L, Williams A, et al. Epidemiology of nasopharyngeal colonization with nontypeable *Haemophilus influenzae* in the first 2 years of life. *J Infect Dis*. 1995;172:132-135.
7. Watson K, Carville K, Bowman J, et al. Upper respiratory tract bacterial carriage in Aboriginal and non-Aboriginal children in a semi-arid area of Western Australia. *Pediatr Infect Dis J*. 2006;25:782-790.
8. Farjo RS, Foxman B, Patel MJ, et al. Diversity and sharing of *Haemophilus influenzae* strains colonizing healthy children attending day-care centers. *Pediatr Infect Dis J*. 2004;23:41-46.
9. Barbosa-Cesnik C, Farjo RS, Patel M, et al. Predictors for *Haemophilus influenzae* colonization, antibiotic resistance and for sharing an identical isolate among children attending 16 licensed day-care centers in Michigan. *Pediatr Infect Dis J*. 2006; 25:219-223.
10. Peerbooms PG, Engelen MN, Stokman DA, et al. Nasopharyngeal carriage of potential bacterial pathogens related to day care attendance, with special reference to the molecular epidemiology of *Haemophilus influenzae*. *J Clin Microbiol*. 2002;40:2832-2836.
11. Faden H, Duffy L, Wasielewski R, et al. Relationship between nasopharyngeal colonization and the development of otitis media in children. *J Infect Dis*. 1997;175:1440-1445.
12. Leibovitz E, Jacobs MR, Dagan R. *Haemophilus influenzae*: A significant pathogen in acute otitis media. *Pediatr Infect Dis J*. 2004;23:1142-1152.
13. Revai K, McCormick DP, Patel J, et al. Effect of pneumococcal conjugate vaccine on nasopharyngeal bacterial colonization during acute otitis media. *Pediatrics*. 2006;117:1823-1829.
14. Murphy TF, Brauer AL, Schiffmacher AT, et al. Persistent colonization by *Haemophilus influenzae* in chronic obstructive pulmonary disease. *Am J Respir Crit Care Med*. 2004;170:266-272.
15. Murphy TF, Sethi S, Klingman KL, et al. Simultaneous respiratory tract colonization by multiple strains of nontypeable *Haemophilus influenzae* in chronic obstructive pulmonary disease: implications for antibiotic therapy. *J Infect Dis*. 1999;180: 404-409.
16. Moller LVM, Regelink AG, Grasselier H, et al. Multiple *Haemophilus influenzae* strains and strain variants coexist in the respiratory tract of patients with cystic fibrosis. *J Infect Dis*. 1995;172:1388-1392.
17. Starner TD, Zhang N, Kim G, et al. *Haemophilus influenzae* forms biofilms on airway epithelia: implications in cystic fibrosis. *Am J Respir Crit Care Med*. 2006;174:213-220.
18. Sethi S, Evans N, Grant BJB, et al. New strains of bacteria and exacerbations of chronic obstructive pulmonary disease. *N Engl J Med*. 2002;347:465-471.
19. Smith A, Baker M. Cefsulodin chocolate blood agar: a selective medium for the recovery of *Haemophilus influenzae* from the respiratory secretions of patients with cystic fibrosis. *J Med Microbiol*. 1997;46:883-885.
20. Bandi V, Apicella MA, Mason E, et al. Nontypeable *Haemophilus influenzae* in the lower respiratory tract of patients with chronic bronchitis. *Am J Respir Crit Care Med*. 2001;164:2114-2119.
21. Forsgren J, Samuelson A, Ahlin A, et al. *Haemophilus influenzae* resides and multiplies intracellularly in human adenoid tissue as demonstrated by in situ hybridization and bacterial viability assay. *Infect Immun*. 1994;62:673-679.
22. Swords WE, Buscher BA, Ver Steeg IK, et al. Non-typeable *Haemophilus influenzae* adhere to and invade human bronchial epithelial cells via an interaction of lipooligosaccharide with the PAF receptor. *Mol Microbiol*. 2000;37:13-27.
23. Ketterer MR, Shao JQ, Hornick DB, et al. Infection of primary human bronchial epithelial cells by *Haemophilus influenzae*: macropinocytosis as a mechanism of airway epithelial cell entry. *Infect Immun*. 1999;67:4161-4170.
24. St. Geme III JW. Molecular and cellular determinants of non-typeable *Haemophilus influenzae* adherence and invasion. *Cell Microbiol*. 2002;4:191-200.
25. St. Geme III JW, Kumar VV, Cutter D, et al. Prevalence and distribution of the *hmw* and *hia* genes and the HMW and Hia adhesins among genetically diverse strains of nontypeable *Haemophilus influenzae*. *Infect Immun*. 1998;66:364-368.
26. Krasan GP, Cutter D, Block SL, et al. Adhesin expression in matched nasopharyngeal and middle ear isolates of nontypeable *Haemophilus influenzae* from children with acute otitis media. *Infect Immun*. 1999;67:449-454.
27. Murphy TF, Bernstein JM, Dryja DD, et al. Outer membrane protein and lipooligosaccharide analysis of paired nasopharyngeal and middle ear isolates in otitis media due to nontypable *Haemophilus influenzae*: pathogenetic and epidemiological observations. *J Infect Dis*. 1987;156:723-731.
28. Pettigrew MM, Foxman B, Marrs CF, et al. Identification of the lipooligosaccharide biosynthesis gene *lic*2B as a putative virulence factor in strains of nontypeable *Haemophilus influenzae* that cause otitis media. *Infect Immun*. 2002;70:3551-3556.
29. Xie J, Juliao PC, Gilsdorf JR, et al. Identification of new genetic regions more prevalent in nontypeable *Haemophilus influenzae* otitis media strains than in throat strains. *J Clin Microbiol*. 2006; 44:4316-4325.
30. Post JC, Preston RA, Aul JJ, et al. Molecular analysis of bacterial pathogens in otitis media with effusion. *JAMA*. 1995;273: 1598-1604.
31. Hendolin PH, Paulin L, Ylikoski J. Clinically applicable multiplex PCR for four middle ear pathogens. *J Clin Microbiol*. 2000; 38:125-132.
32. Ehrlich GD, Veeh R, Wang X, et al. Mucosal biofilm formation on middle-ear mucosa in the chinchilla model of otitis media. *JAMA*. 2002;287:1710-1715.
33. Hong W, Mason K, Jurcisek J, et al. Phosphorylcholine decreases early inflammation and promotes the establishment of stable biofilm communities of nontypeable *Haemophilus influenzae* strain 86-028NP in a chinchilla model of otitis media. *Infect Immun*. 2007;75:958-965.
34. Jurcisek J, Greiner L, Watanabe H, et al. Role of sialic acid and complex carbohydrate biosynthesis in biofilm formation by non-typeable *Haemophilus influenzae* in the chinchilla middle ear. *Infect Immun*. 2005;73:3210-3218.
35. Hall-Stoodley L, Hu FZ, Gieseke A, et al. Direct detection of bacterial biofilms on the middle-ear mucosa of children with chronic otitis media. *JAMA*. 2006;296:202-211.
36. Slinger R, Chan F, Ferris W, et al. Multiple combination antibiotic susceptibility testing of nontypeable *Haemophilus influenzae* biofilms. *Diagn Microbiol Infect Dis*. 2006;56:247-253.
37. Sethi S, Murphy TF. Infection in the course and pathogenesis of chronic obstructive pulmonary disease. *N Engl J Med*. 2008; 359:2355-2365.
38. Sethi S, Wrona C, Eschberger K, et al. Inflammatory profile of new bacterial strain exacerbations of chronic obstructive pulmonary disease. *Am J Respir Crit Care Med*. 2008;177:491-497.
39. Fernaays MM, Lesse AJ, Sethi S, et al. Differential genome contents of nontypeable *Haemophilus influenzae* strains from adults with chronic obstructive pulmonary disease. *Infect Immun*. 2006;74:3366-3374.
40. Fernaays MM, Lesse AJ, Cai X, et al. Characterization of *igaB*, a second immunoglobulin A1 protease gene in nontypeable *Haemophilus influenzae*. *Infect Immun*. 2006;74:5860-5870.
41. Moxon ER, Deich RA, Connelly C. Cloning of chromosomal DNA from *Haemophilus influenzae*. *J Clin Invest*. 1984;73: 298-306.
42. Faden H, Bernstein J, Brodsky L, et al. Otitis media in children. I. The systemic immune response to nontypable *Haemophilus influenzae*. *J Infect Dis*. 1989;160:999-1004.
43. Troelstra A, Vogel L, Van Alphen L, et al. Opsonic antibodies to outer membrane protein P2 of nonencapsulated *Haemophilus influenzae* are strain specific. *Infect Immun*. 1994;62:779-784.
44. Sethi S, Wrona C, Grant BJ, et al. Strain-specific immune response to *Haemophilus influenzae* in chronic obstructive pulmonary disease. *Am J Respir Crit Care Med*. 2004; 169:448-453.
45. Duim B, Vogel L, Puijk W, et al. Fine mapping of outer membrane protein P2 antigenic sites which vary during persistent infection by *Haemophilus influenzae*. *Infect Immun*. 1996; 64:4673-4679.
46. Duim B, van Alphen L, Eijk P, et al. Antigenic drift of non-encapsulated *Haemophilus influenzae* major outer membrane protein P2 in patients with chronic bronchitis is caused by point mutations. *Mol Microbiol*. 1994;11:1181-1189.
47. Duim B, Bowler LD, Eijk PP, et al. Molecular variation in the major outer membrane protein P5 gene of nonencapsulated *Haemophilus influenzae* during chronic infections. *Infect Immun*. 1997;65:1351-1356.
48. Shurin PA, Pelton SI, Tazer IB, et al. Bactericidal antibody and susceptibility to otitis media caused by nontypeable strains of *Haemophilus influenzae*. *J Pediatr*. 1980;97:364-369.
49. Abe Y, Murphy TF, Sethi S, et al. Lymphocyte proliferative response to P6 of *Haemophilus influenzae* is associated with rela-

tive protection from exacerbations of chronic obstructive pulmonary disease. *Am J Respir Crit Care Med.* 2002;165:967-971.

50. Rodriguez WJ, Schwartz RH. *Streptococcus pneumoniae* causes otitis media with higher fever and more redness of tympanic membranes than *Haemophilus influenzae* or *Moraxella catarrhalis. Pediatr Infect Dis J.* 1999;18:942-944.

51. Leibovitz E, Satran R, Piglansky L, et al. Can acute otitis media caused by *Haemophilus influenzae* be distinguished from that caused by *Streptococcus pneumoniae? Pediatr Infect Dis J.* 2003;22:509-515.

52. Kilpi T, Herva E, Kaijalainen T, et al. Bacteriology of acute otitis media in a cohort of Finnish children followed for the first two years of life. *Pediatr Infect Dis J.* 2001;20:654-662.

53. Leibovitz E, Asher E, Piglansky L, et al. Is bilateral acute otitis media clinically different than unilateral acute otitis media? *Pediatr Infect Dis J.* 2007;26:589-592.

54. McCormick DP, Chandler SM, Chonmaitree T. Laterality of acute otitis media: Different clinical and microbiologic characteristics. *Pediatr Infect Dis J.* 2007;26:583-588.

55. Murphy TF, Faden H, Bakaletz LO, et al. Nontypeable *Haemophilus influenzae* as a pathogen in children. *Pediatr Infect Dis J.* 2009;28:43-48.

56. Casey JR, Pichichero ME. Changes in frequency and pathogens causing acute otitis media in 1995-2003. *Pediatr Infect Dis J.* 2004;23:824-828.

57. Block SL, Hedrick J, Harrison CJ, et al. Community-wide vaccination with the heptavalent pneumococcal conjugate significantly alters the microbiology of acute otitis media. *Pediatr Infect Dis J.* 2004;23:829-833.

58. Polsky B, Gold JWM, Whimbey E, et al. Bacterial pneumonia in patients with acquired immunodeficiency syndrome. *Ann Intern Med.* 1986;104:38-41.

59. Rello J, Bodi M, Mariscal D, et al. Microbiological testing and outcome of patients with severe community-acquired pneumonia. *Chest.* 2003;123:174-180.

60. Weinberg GA, Ghafoor A, Ishaq Z, et al. Clonal analysis of *Haemophilus influenzae* isolated from children from Pakistan with lower respiratory tract infections. *J Infect Dis.* 1989;160:634-643.

61. Klein JO. Role of nontypeable *Haemophilus influenzae* in pediatric respiratory tract infections. *Pediatr Infect Dis J.* 1997; 16:S5-S8.

62. Finegold SM, Flynn MJ, Rose FV, et al. Bacteriologic findings associated with chronic bacterial maxillary sinusitis in adults. *Clin Infect Dis.* 2002;35:428-433.

63. Talbot GH, Kennedy DW, Scheld WM, et al. Rigid nasal endoscopy versus sinus puncture and aspiration for microbiologic documentation of acute bacterial maxillary sinusitis. *Clin Infect Dis.* 2001;33:1668-1675.

64. Quentin R, Goudeau A, Wallace RJ, Jr., et al. Urogenital, maternal and neonatal isolates of *Haemophilus influenzae*: Identification of unusually virulent serologically non-typeable clone families and evidence for a new *Haemophilus* species. *J Gen Microbiol.* 1990;136:1203-1209.

65. Campos J, Hernando M, Roman F, et al. Analysis of invasive *Haemophilus influenzae* infections after extensive vaccination against *H. influenzae* type b. *J Clin Microbiol.* 2004;42: 524-529.

66. Dworkin MS, Park L, Borchardt SM. The changing epidemiology of invasive *Haemophilus influenzae* disease, especially in persons > or = 65 years old. *Clin Infect Dis.* 2007;44:810-816.

67. Heath PT, Booy R, Azzopardi HJ, et al. Non-type b *Haemophilus influenzae* disease: Clinical and epidemiologic characteristics in the *Haemophilus influenzae* type b vaccine era. *Pediatr Infect Dis J.* 2001;20:300-305.

68. Farley MM, Stephens DS, Brachman PS, Jr., et al. Invasive *Haemophilus influenzae* disease in adults. *Ann Intern Med.* 1992;116:806-812.

69. Erwin AL, Nelson KL, Mhlanga-Mutangadura T, et al. Characterization of genetic and phenotypic diversity of invasive nontypeable *Haemophilus influenzae. Infect Immun.* 2005;73:5853-5863.

70. Patel PB, Diaz MC, Bennett JE, et al. Clinical features of bacterial conjunctivitis in children. *Acad Emerg Med.* 2007;14:1-5.

71. Buznach N, Dagan R, Greenberg D. Clinical and bacterial characteristics of acute bacterial conjunctivitis in children in the antibiotic resistance era. *Pediatr Infect Dis J.* 2005;24:823-828.

72. Borenstein DG, Simon GL. *Hemophilus influenzae* septic arthritis in adults. A report of four cases and a review of the literature. *Medicine.* 1986;65:191-201.

73. Pelton SI. Acute otitis media in an era of increasing antimicrobial resistance and universal administration of pneumococcal conjugate vaccine. *Pediatr Infect Dis J.* 2002;21:599-604.

74. Peltola H. Worldwide *Haemophilus influenzae* type b disease at the beginning of the 21st century: global analysis of the disease burden 25 years after the use of the polysaccharide vaccine and a decade after the advent of conjugates. *Clin Microbiol Rev.* 2000;13:302-317.

75. Prymula R, Peeters P, Chrobok V, et al. Pneumococcal capsular polysaccharides conjugated to protein D for prevention of acute otitis media caused by both *Streptococcus pneumoniae* and nontypable *Haemophilus influenzae*: a randomised double-blind efficacy study. *Lancet.* 2006;367:740-748.

76. Brazilian Purpuric Fever Study Group. Brazilian purpuric fever: Epidemic purpura fulminans associated with antecedent purulent conjunctivitis. *Lancet.* 1987;2:757-761.

77. Brenner DJ, Mayer LW, Carlone GM, et al. Biochemical, genetic, and epidemiologic characterization of *Haemophilus influenzae* biogroup aegyptius (*Haemophilus aegyptius*) strains associated with Brazilian purpuric fever. *J Clin Microbiol.* 1988;26: 1524-1534.

78. Lesse AJ, Gheesling LL, Bittner WE, et al. Stable, conserved outer membrane epitope of strains of *Haemophilus influenzae* biogroup aegyptius associated with Brazilian purpuric fever. *Infect Immun.* 1992;60:1351-1357.

79. Bong CT, Bauer ME, Spinola SM. *Haemophilus ducreyi*: Clinical features, epidemiology, and prospects for disease control. *Microbes Infect.* 2002;4:1141-1148.

80. Spinola SM, Bauer ME, Munson RS, Jr. Immunopathogenesis of *Haemophilus ducreyi* infection (chancroid). *Infect Immun.* 2002;70:1667-1676.

81. Bauer ME, Fortney KR, Harrison A, et al. Identification of *Haemophilus ducreyi* genes expressed during human infection. *Microbiology.* 2008;154:1152-1160.

82. Humphreys TL, Li L, Li X, et al. Dysregulated immune profiles for skin and dendritic cells are associated with increased host susceptibility to *Haemophilus ducreyi* infection in human volunteers. *Infect Immun.* 2007;75:5686-5697.

83. Orle KA, Gates CA, Martin DH, et al. Simultaneous PCR detection of *Haemophilus ducreyi*, *Treponema pallidum*, and herpes simplex virus types 1 and 2 from genital ulcers. *J Clin Microbiol.* 1996;34:49-54.

84. Baron EJ, Scott JD, Tompkins LS. Prolonged incubation and extensive subculturing do not increase recovery of clinically significant microorganisms from standard automated blood cultures. *Clin Infect Dis.* 2005;41:1677-1680.

85. Petti CA, Bhally HS, Weinstein MP, et al. Utility of extended blood culture incubation for isolation of *Haemophilus*, *Actinobacillus*, *Cardiobacterium*, *Eikenella*, and *Kingella* organisms: a retrospective multicenter evaluation. *J Clin Microbiol.* 2006; 44:257-259.

86. Darras-Joly C, Lortholary O, Mainardi JL, et al. *Haemophilus* endocarditis: report of 42 cases in adults and review. *Haemophilus* Endocarditis Study Group. *Clin Infect Dis.* 1997;24:1087-1094.

87. Wilson WR, Karchmer AW, Dajani AS, et al. Antibiotic treatment of adults with infective endocarditis due to streptococci, enterococci, staphylococci, and HACEK microorganisms. *JAMA.* 1995;274:1706-1713.

226

Brucella Species

EDWARD J. YOUNG

Brucellosis is a disease of animals (zoonosis) that under certain circumstances can be transmitted to humans.[1] Although it occurs worldwide, brucellosis is more common in countries that do not have effective public health and animal health programs.[2,3] In the United States and other developed countries, brucellosis in domestic animals has been largely controlled or eliminated. Consequently, the incidence of human brucellosis is low, with fewer than 200 cases reported annually to the Centers for Disease Control and Prevention. As one of the first bacteria to be weaponized, *Brucella* remains a potential bioterrorism agent,[4,5] and all confirmed cases should have epidemiologic evaluation.[6]

History

Brucellosis has likely been present since man first domesticated animals; however, the early history of the disease is linked to the British military and their presence on the island of Malta.[7] It was there in 1861 that Marston first differentiated brucellosis from other clinical fevers and where 25 years later Bruce first isolated *Brucella melitensis* from victims of Malta fever.[8] From 1904 to 1907, the Mediterranean Fever Commission studied the disease on Malta, concluding that native goats were the reservoir and raw goat's milk was the vehicle of transmission from animal to human.[9] In Denmark in 1895, Bang identified *Brucella abortus* as a cause of contagious abortion in cattle, and in the United States in 1914, Traum isolated *Brucella suis* from aborted swine. However, it was not until the 1920s, from the work of Alice Evans and others, that the relatedness of these apparently disparate microorganisms was recognized and the genus was named to honor Bruce.[10] In the 1950s, *Brucella ovis* from sheep and *Brucella neotomae* from desert wood rats were added to the genus, but they have not been shown to cause disease in humans. In 1966, *Brucella canis* was isolated from kennel-bred dogs, but it is an infrequent human infection.[11] Since 1994, novel members of the genus have been isolated from a variety of marine mammals. The names *Brucella pinnipediae* and *Brucella ceteceae* have been proposed for the seal and cetacean (whales and dolphins) isolates, respectively. The role of these organisms as a source of human infection remains to be determined.[12]

The Pathogen

Brucellae are small, gram-negative, unencapsulated, nonsporulating coccobacilli. They grow aerobically, although some require supplemental CO_2 for primary isolation. All strains are catalase positive, but oxidase and urease activities and the production of H_2S are variable. The major nomen species and their biovars are differentiated based on metabolic tests, growth on media containing dyes, and lysis by specific bacteriaphages.[13]

Based on rRNA sequences, *Brucella* spp. are classified in the α-2 group of proteobacteria having a close phylogenetic relationship with *Bartonella* spp. and plant pathogens such as *Agrobacterium tumefaciens* and *Sinorhizobium meliloti*.[14] The genus is divided into six major nomen species based on natural host preferences and cultural, metabolic, and antigenic characteristics.[15] However, DNA-DNA hybridization studies have shown a remarkable degree (>90%) of homology between strains, indicating that it is a monospecific genus with subspecies corresponding to evolutionary lineages adapted to specific hosts.[16]

The *Brucella* genome contains two circular chromosomes of approximately 2.1 and 1.5 Mb except *B. suis* biovar 3, which has a single chromosome of 3.31 Mb.[16-18] The major cell wall antigen is S-LPS containing the A and M antigens first described by Wilson and Miles. The O-side chain is composed of approximately 100 residues of 4-formamide-4,6-dideoxymannose linked $\alpha_{1,2}$ in A-dominant strains, but with every fifth residue linked $\alpha_{1,3}$ in M-dominant strains.[19] Numerous outer and inner membrane, cytoplasmic, and periplasmic proteins have also been characterized, some of which appear to play a role in virulence and intracellular survival.[20,21]

Epidemiology

Brucellosis exists in animals worldwide but is especially prevalent in the Mediterranean basin, the Arabian peninsula, the Indian subcontinent, and in parts of Central Asia, Africa, Mexico, and Central and South America.[3,22] *B. melitensis* is the most frequently reported cause of human brucellosis worldwide. The usual reservoirs are goats and sheep, but in some areas, camels are of local importance. In areas where they coexist with goats or are fed sheep offal, cattle can be infected with *B. melitensis* and are a source of human disease.[23] *B. abortus* is found principally in cattle, but other bovidae such as bison, buffalo, camels, and yaks are important in some areas. *B. suis* biovars 1-3 occur in domestic and feral swine and are a cause of abattoir-associated brucellosis.[24] In Croatia, wild boars have been shown to harbor *B. suis* biovar 2,[25] and in the southern United States, approximately 20% of feral swine test positive for *B. suis* and have caused infection in hunters.[26] *B. canis* is widespread in canines in many countries but is an infrequent cause of human infection.[27]

Routes of transmission from animal to human include (1) direct contact with infected animals or their secretions through cuts or abrasions in the skin or conjunctival sac, (2) inhalation of contaminated aerosols, and (3) ingestion of unpasteurized dairy products. Consequently, brucellosis is an occupational risk for ranchers, veterinarians, abattoir workers, and laboratory personnel.[28] Meat products are rarely the source of infection because they are not usually consumed raw and the numbers of organisms in muscle tissue are low. In areas where drinking animal blood or ingesting raw liver are traditions, foodborne infection from other than dairy products is possible.[29] Person-to-person transmission of brucellosis is unusual; however, rare cases in which sexual transmission was suspected have been reported.[30] In addition, blood transfusions and bone marrow transplants[31] have been sources of brucellosis, emphasizing the need for *Brucella* antibody screening, especially in endemic areas. Although persons with HIV are at risk of a number of zoonotic agents, very few cases of brucellosis are reported.[32] Brucellosis is not uncommon in children, especially in areas where *B. melitensis* is endemic and animals and children share a common living space.[33,34] It is not unusual to find more than one case of brucellosis in a household; therefore, screening of contacts of index cases is warranted.[35]

Although once common in the United States, the eradication of bovine brucellosis has reduced the incidence of human infection to fewer than 0.5 cases per 100,000 population (Fig. 226-1). The epidemiology of brucellosis in Texas and California has changed from a disease associated with exposure to cattle to one linked to the ingestion of unpasteurized goat milk products imported from Mexico.[36] On the

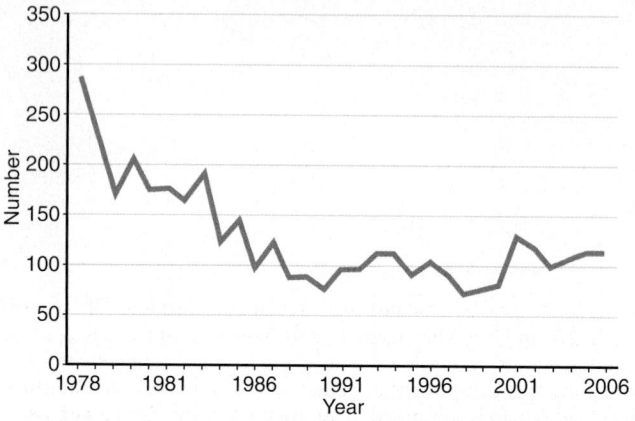

Figure 226-1 **Brucellosis.** Number of reported cases, by year—United States, 1976 to 2000. The incidence of brucellosis has remained stable in recent years, reflecting an ongoing risk of infection with *Brucella melitensis* and *Brucella abortus* acquired through exposure to unpasteurized milk products in countries with endemic brucellosis in sheep, goats, and cattle and *Brucella suis* acquired through contact with feral swine in the United States. *(From CDC. Summary of notifiable diseases—United States, 2006. MMWR Morb Mortal Wkly Rep. 2008;55:1-94.)*

border with Mexico, brucellosis is eight times more prevalent than elsewhere in the United States.[37]

Pathogenesis

Infection with any *Brucella* nomen species, including naturally rough species and attenuated *vaccine* strains, can result in serious human illness. The nutritional and immune status of the host as well as the size of the infectious inoculum and possibly the route of transmission can be determinants of disease. For example, the low pH of gastric juice appears to be more effective in preventing oral infection with *B. abortus* than *B. melitensis*,[38] and antacids have been implicated as playing a role in foodborne infections.[39]

The brucellae are facultative intracellular pathogens that can survive and multiply within phagocytic cells of the host. The mechanisms by which brucellae evade intracellular killing by professional phagocytes are not completely understood, but appear to involve inhibition of bactericidal functions, including phagolysosomal fusion, neutrophil degranulation, and the oxidative burst.[40] Brucellae within macrophages and monocytes become localized in organs of the reticuloendothelial system, such as the lymph nodes, liver, spleen, and bone marrow. Their adaptation to the intracellular milieu requires virulence genes, notably the *virB* operon, that encode a type IV secretion system.[41] This system is necessary for brucellae within membrane-bound vacuoles to obtain nutrients with which to replicate in organelles derived from the endoplasmic reticulum.[42] The eventual elimination of virulent brucellae depends on the activation of macrophages with the development of Th1-type cell–mediated immunity. The principal cytokines involved in anti-*Brucella* activity of macrophages include tumor necrosis factor-α, tumor necrosis factor-γ, interleukin-1, and interleukin-12.[43]

Host Immunity

Natural resistance to *Brucella* infection has been reported in swine, cattle, and water buffalo.[44] The *Nramp1* gene (natural resistance-associated macrophage protein 1) first recognized in mice and later renamed *Slc11a1* (solute carrier family 11 member 1) seems to play an important role in innate immunity by preventing bacterial growth in macrophages during the initial stages of infection. This gene also influences adaptive immunity through its pleiotropic effects and stabiliza-

tion of certain cytokine mRNAs.[45] The acquired immune response in brucellosis is characterized by the appearance of immunoglobulin M antibodies within the first week of infection, followed by a switch to immunoglobulin G synthesis after the second week.[46] With recovery, antibody titers decline slowly but are usually not detected after 2 to 3 years. Persistent elevation of immunoglobulin G antibodies is prognostic of chronic infection or relapse.[47,48]

Clinical Manifestations

The symptoms of brucellosis are nonspecific (e.g., fever, sweats, malaise, anorexia, headache, back pain). The onset can be insidious or acute, generally beginning within 2 to 4 weeks after inoculation. An undulant fever pattern is apparent in patients who are untreated for long periods of time, leading to the name undulant fever for brucellosis. Some patients report malodorous sweat and a peculiar taste in the mouth. Depression is common and often out of proportion to the severity of other symptoms. Compared with the plethora of somatic complaints, physical abnormalities may be few. Mild lymphadenopathy is reported in 10% to 20% and splenomegaly or hepatomegaly in 20% to 30% of cases.[49] Brucellosis is a systemic infection in which any organ or system of the body can be involved. Attempts to categorize the disease into acute, subacute, and chronic according to the length or severity of symptoms are purely arbitrary. When involvement of a specific organ predominates, the disease is often termed focal or localized; however, there is little compelling evidence that such complications necessarily represent a distinct subset of patients.

Recurrence of symptoms after therapy may or may not be associated with relapse of the disease.[50] Bacteriologic relapse generally occurs within 3 to 6 months after discontinuing therapy and is usually not caused by antibiotic resistance.[51] Chronic brucellosis is usually caused by persistent foci of infection in tissues such as bone, spleen, liver, and other organs.[52] In chronic brucellosis, symptoms can recur over long periods of time and are associated with objective signs of infection, notably fever. An important laboratory finding is the persistence of high titers of immunoglobulin G antibodies.[53] In contrast, some patients experience delayed convalescence, with persistent nonspecific symptoms, but without objective signs of illness or elevated titers of antibodies. The cause of this condition is poorly understood, but some authorities believe that it may represent preexisting psychoneurosis exacerbated by the infection.[54]

Complications

GASTROINTESTINAL TRACT

Alimentary tract symptoms such as anorexia, nausea, vomiting, pain, diarrhea, and constipation are elicited in as many as 70% of patients with brucellosis. Pathologic lesions include hyperemia of the intestinal mucosa with inflammation of Peyer's patches. Acute ileitis has been documented radiographically and histologically in patients infected with *B. melitensis*.[55]

Rare cases of acute pancreatitis have been reported.[56]

HEPATOBILIARY SYSTEM

Hepatic involvement is common in brucellosis; however, transaminase levels can be normal or only mildly elevated. The histologic findings are often subtle and can be overlooked entirely. The spectrum of hepatic pathology is quite variable depending in part on the etiologic agent. Infection with *B. abortus* is characterized by granuloma indistinguishable from sarcoidosis.[57] In contrast, infection with *B. melitensis* yields lesions ranging from small, almost insignificant aggregates of mononuclear cells surrounding foci of necrosis, to a diffuse nonspecific inflammation resembling viral hepatitis.[58] In other cases, epithelioid granulomas have been reported.[59] Infection with *B. suis* (and occasionally other brucellae) often results in hepatosplenic abscesses.[60]

Hepatitis generally resolves with antimicrobial therapy, and in the absence of other causes (e.g., hepatitis C, alcoholism), cirrhosis does not occur. In cases of suppurative abscesses, surgical intervention may be required.[61] *Brucella* spp. can also be a rare cause of acute cholecystitis and peritonitis.[62]

SKELETAL SYSTEM

Osteoarticular complications are the most common focal forms of the disease and have been reported in 10% to 80% of cases depending on the series, the ages of the patients, and the infecting *Brucella* spp.[49] The axial skeleton is the most common site with sacroiliitis occurring in younger patients[63] and spondylitis occurring in older persons, usually in the lumbar spine.[64] Vertebral osteomyelitis is a particularly serious complication, with associated paravertebral, epidural, or psoas abscesses occurring in almost one half of cases.[65] Such cases require prolonged (at least 3 months) antimicrobial therapy and may also need surgical intervention. Peripheral *Brucella* arthritis usually involves large weight-bearing joints (hips and knees); however, any joint, including sternoclavicular, can be involved.[66] Synovial fluid contains a preponderance of lymphocytes, and recovery of brucellae is improved by the use of techniques that lyse leukocytes[67] (see Chapter 17 for the lysis-centrifugation method).

Although rare, prosthetic joint infection caused by *Brucella* spp. has been reported and excisional arthroplasty may be necessary for cure.[68] Postinfectious spondyloarthritis, bursitis, and tenosynovitis have also been reported associated with brucellosis.[69]

NERVOUS SYSTEM

Depression and mental inattention are common symptoms in brucellosis; however, direct invasion of the central nervous system occurs in less than 5% of cases. Neurologic syndromes in brucellosis include meningitis, encephalitis, myelitis-radiculoneuronitis, brain abscess, epidural abscess, granuloma, and demyelinating and meningovascular syndromes. Acute or chronic meningitis is the most frequent nervous system complication.[70-72] Sensorineural hearing loss has been reported as a complication of *Brucella* meningitis.[73] Vasculitis associated with brucellosis, which may be immune mediated, can involve blood vessels throughout the body including the brain.[74,75] Analysis of cerebrospinal fluid in *Brucella* meningitis reveals a lymphocytic pleocytosis, elevated protein, and normal or low glucose concentrations. Gram stains and cultures of cerebrospinal fluid are often negative; therefore, the diagnosis depends on the presence of specific antibodies or real-time polymerase chain reaction.[76] The prognosis of treated neurobrucellosis is generally favorable; however, cases of severe neurologic sequelae have been reported.[77]

CARDIOVASCULAR SYSTEM

Endocarditis occurs in less than 2% of cases, but it accounts for the majority of brucellosis-related deaths.[78] Before effective therapy, including valve replacement surgery, *Brucella* endocarditis was nearly always fatal.[79] The aortic valve is most often involved, and both native and prosthetic valve infections, as well as infections of other vascular prostheses, have been reported.[80] Pericarditis, glomerulonephritis, and mycotic aneurysms involving the brain, aorta, and other blood vessels are secondary complications. Automated blood culture techniques and echocardiography have improved the ability to make an early diagnosis.[81]

RESPIRATORY SYSTEM

Airborne transmission of brucellosis is a problem in abattoirs and laboratories; however, respiratory manifestations are rare, even in countries where the disease is enzootic.[82,83] Respiratory involvement ranges from flulike symptoms with normal x-rays to bronchitis, pneumonia, lung nodules, abscess, miliary lesions, hilar adenopathy, and pleural effusion/empyema.[84] Rarely are brucellae identified by stain or culture of expectorated sputum.

GENITOURINARY TRACT

Although brucellae can be recovered from urine, renal complications of brucellosis are rare. Interstitial nephritis, pyelonephritis, glomerulonephritis, and immunoglobulin A nephropathy have been reported.[85] Epididymoorchitis occurs in as many as 20% of men with brucellosis. It is usually unilateral with normal urine sediment and can mimic tuberculosis or tumor.[86]

PREGNANCY

The principal manifestation of brucellosis in animals is spontaneous abortion, and erythritol in the tissues of susceptible animals is thought to enhance the growth of brucellae in the genital tract. Brucellosis can also cause abortion in humans; however, it is not clear whether it is any more common than with other bacteremic infections. Reports from areas where *B. melitensis* is endemic suggest that the incidence of abortion among pregnant women is high and that prompt therapy can be lifesaving for the fetus.[87]

HEMATOLOGIC COMPLICATIONS

Hematologic manifestations of brucellosis include anemia, leukopenia, thrombocytopenia, and clotting disorders. Such abnormalities are generally mild and resolve with therapy.[88] Granulomas are found in the bone marrow in as many as 75% of cases. Rarely, severe thrombocytopenia with cutaneous purpura and/or bleeding from mucosal sites can occur. The etiology may include hypersplenism, reactive hemophagocytosis, or immune destruction of platelets.[89]

CUTANEOUS LESIONS

Skin lesions occur in approximately 5% of patients with brucellosis. Many nonspecific, often transient lesions have been reported, including rashes, papules, ulcers, abscess, erythema nodosum, petechiae, purpura, and vasculitis.[90] Contact dermatitis was once a common finding among veterinarians exposed to infected animals.[91]

OCULAR LESIONS

A variety of ocular lesions have been reported in patients with brucellosis. Uveitis is generally a late complication, consisting variably of chronic iridocyclitis, nummular keratitis, multifocal choroiditis, and optic neuritis.[92] *Brucella* uveitis is considered a noninfectious immune reaction that responds to topical and systemic corticosteroid therapy. Rare cases of endogenous endophthalmitis have been reported in which brucellae were recovered from vitreous humor.[93]

Diagnosis

Because the symptoms of brucellosis are nonspecific, it is important to obtain a detailed history that includes occupation, avocations, travel to enzootic areas, and ingestion of high-risk foods, such as unpasteurized dairy products. The white blood cell count is often normal or low, and the erythrocyte sedimentation rate is variable. The diagnosis is made with certainty by isolation of brucellae from blood, bone marrow, or other tissue. The rate of bacterial isolation varies from 15% to more than 90%, depending on the methods used. Most laboratories now use continuous-monitoring automated blood culture systems (e.g., BACTEC or BacT/Alert) that have improved the time to isolation and have obviated the need for biphasic media techniques. Nevertheless, the handling of brucellae is a risk to laboratory personnel, and appropriate precautions should be taken.[94] Brucellae are isolated most often from blood or bone marrow; however, in selected cases, urine, cerebrospinal fluid, synovial fluid, and biopsies of the liver, lymph nodes, and other tissues can be successful. The results of rapid automated bacterial identification systems must be interpreted with caution because not all contain appropriate profiles, and brucellae have been misidentified as *Moraxella phenylpyruvica* or *Ochrobactrum anthropi.*[95] Where available, polymerase chain reaction assays using various primers have shown high sensitivity and specificity; however, standardization of methods remains a problem in comparing data between laboratories.[96-98] Interestingly, some authors have detected DNA in blood samples by polymerase chain reaction after treatment despite apparent clinical recovery.[99,100] The significance of this finding remains to be determined.

In the absence of bacteriologic confirmation, a presumptive diagnosis can be made by demonstrating high or increasing titers of specific antibodies in the serum. A variety of tests have been applied to the serologic diagnosis of brucellosis, of which the serum agglutination test is the most widely used.[53] Rose Bengal and a rapid dipstick assay are useful for screening; however, positive results should be confirmed by a serum agglutination test.[101] The *Brucella* enzyme-linked immunosorbent assay is considered to be the most sensitive and specific serologic test; however, false-positive results have been reported with some commercial products.[102] Regardless of the assay used, no single titer is *always* diagnostic; however, most cases of active infection have titers of 1:160 or higher. Most serologic assays measure antibodies directed against lipopolysaccharide, however, an enzyme-linked immunosorbent assay to detect *Brucella* cytoplasmic proteins has been reported to differentiate between active and inactive infection.[103]

■ Treatment

Antimicrobial therapy relieves symptoms, shortens the duration of illness, and decreases the incidence of complications or relapse. A variety of drugs have activity against brucellae; however, the results of in vitro susceptibility tests do not always predict clinical efficacy.[23] The intracellular localization of brucellae is believed to offer some protection against antimicrobials, and drugs with good penetration into cells are thought necessary for cure.

Tetracyclines are among the most active drugs for treating brucellosis; however, the rate of relapse with single-drug therapy is unacceptably high and combinations of drugs are generally used. A regimen of tetracycline (500 mg every 6 hours PO for 6 weeks) plus streptomycin (1 g/day IM for 2 to 3 weeks) had long been the treatment of choice. Subsequently, doxycycline was substituted for tetracycline and gentamicin for streptomycin. Currently, the combination of doxycycline (200 mg/day PO for 6 weeks) plus gentamicin (5 mg/kg/day IM for 7 days) provides excellent results.[23,104,105] The combination of doxycycline (200 mg/day PO for 6 weeks) plus rifampin (600 to 900 mg/day PO for 6 weeks) offers the advantage of an all-oral regimen, but it is not advised in cases with complications, such as spondylitis.[106,107]

Although there was initial enthusiasm for trimethoprim-sulfamethoxazole (cotrimoxazole) for the treatment of human brucellosis, some studies showed an unacceptably high relapse rate. Nevertheless, when used in combination with other drugs, such as rifampin, a quinolone, or an aminoglycoside, trimethoprim-sulfamethoxazole is useful for treating children younger than 8 years of age, in whom tetracycline is contraindicated owing to the potential for staining teeth. Both trimethoprim-sulfamethoxazole and rifampin appear to be safe drugs for treating brucellosis during pregnancy. The quinolones vary widely in activity against brucellae, but their concentration within phagocytic cells would appear to make them ideal for treating brucellosis. However, monotherapy with quinolones has been disappointing, and their use should always be in combination with other drugs.[108]

The treatment of complications, such as meningitis and endocarditis, poses special problems, and the optimal regimen of drugs remains unclear. Most authorities recommend the use of doxycycline in combination with two or more other drugs with treatment continued for several months depending on the response. Doxycycline crosses the blood-brain barrier better than generic tetracycline and has been used successfully with trimethoprim-sulfamethoxazole and rifampin for meningitis and endocarditis.[109] Some third-generation cephalosporins achieve high concentrations in cerebrospinal fluid, but susceptibility of brucellae is variable and sensitivity should be ensured. Although cases of endocarditis have occasionally been cured with antibiotics alone, many require a combined medical and surgical approach. Corticosteroids are often recommended for neurobrucellosis; however, in the absence of controlled studies, efficacy is unproven.

■ Prevention

The prevention of human brucellosis depends on the elimination of the disease in animals. Effective attenuated live bacterial vaccines exist against *B. abortus* (strain 19) and *B. melitensis* (Rev-1), but as yet none exists for *B. suis* or *B. canis*. On rare occasions, accidents with these vaccines have resulted in human infection. A stable rough mutant of *B. abortus* (RB51) has largely replaced strain 19 in the United States and seems to be less pathogenic for humans. No safe effective vaccine exists to protect humans against brucellosis, and there is controversy regarding postexposure antibiotic prophylaxis.[23,110,111]

REFERENCES

1. Pappas G, Akritidis N, Bosilkovski M, et al. Brucellosis. *N Engl J Med.* 2005;352:2325-2336.
2. Kozukeev T, Ajeilat S, Maes E, et al. Risk factors for brucellosis—Leylek and Kada districts, Batken Oblast, Kyrgyzstan, January-November, 2003. *MMWR Morb Mortal Wkly Rep.* 2006;55:31-34.
3. Pappas G, Papadimitriou P, Akritidis N, et al. The new global map of human brucellosis. *Lancet Infect Dis.* 2006;6:91-99.
4. Chang M-H, Glynn MK, Groseclose SL. Endemic, notifiable bioterrorism-related diseases, United States, 1992-1999. *Emerg Infect Dis.* 2003;9:556-564.
5. Yagupsky P, Baron EJ. Laboratory exposures to brucellae and implications for bioterrorism. *Emerg Infect Dis.* 2005;11:1180-1185.
6. CDC. Suspected brucellosis case prompts investigation of possible bioterrorism-related activity—New Hampshire and Massachusetts, 1999. *MMWR Morb Mortal Wkly Rep.* 2000;49:509-512.
7. Naudi JR. *Brucellosis: The Malta Experience, A Celebration 1905-2005.* Malta: Publishers Enterprises Group; 2005.
8. Vassallo DJ. The Corps disease: brucellosis and its historical association with the Royal Army Medical Corps. *J R Army Med Corps.* 1992;138:140-150.
9. Williams E. The Mediterranean Fever Commission: its origin and achievements. In: Young EJ, Corbel MJ, eds. *Brucellosis: Clinical and Laboratory Aspects.* Boca Raton, FL: CRC Press; 1989:11-23.
10. Spink WW. *The Nature of Brucellosis.* Minneapolis: University of Minnesota Press; 1956.
11. Wanke MM. Canine brucellosis. *Animal Reprod Sci.* 2004; 82-83:195-207.
12. Whatmore AM, Dawson CE, Groussaud P, et al. Marine mammal *Brucella* genotype associated with zoonotic infection. *Emerg Infect Dis.* 2008;14:517-518.
13. Corbel MJ. Microbiological aspects. In: Madkour MM. *Madkour's Brucellosis.* New York: Springer-Verlag; 2001:51-64.
14. Paulsen IT, Seshadri R, Nelson KE, et al. The *Brucella suis* genome reveals fundamental similarities between animal and plant pathogens and symbionts. *Proc Natl Acad Sci U S A.* 2002;99:13148-13153.
15. Cloeckaert A, Vizcaíno N. DNA polymorphism and taxonomy of *Brucella* species. In: López-Goñi I, Moriyón I, eds. *Brucella: Molecular and Cellular Biology.* Norfolk, England: Horizon Bioscience; 2004:1-24.
16. Chain PSG, Comerci DJ, Tolmasky ME, et al. Whole-genome analysis of speciation events in pathogenic brucellae. *Infect Immun.* 2005;73:8353-8361.
17. Jumas-Bilak E, Michaux-Charachon S, Bourg G, et al. Differences in chromosome number and genome rearrangements in the genus *Brucella. Mol Microbiol.* 1998;27:99-106.
18. Sanchez DO, Zandomeni RO, Cravero S, et al. Gene discovery through genomic sequencing of *Brucella abortus. Infect Immun.* 2001;69:865-868.
19. Iriarte M, González D, Delrue RM, et al. *Brucella* lipopolysaccharide: structure, biosynthesis and genetics. In: López-Goñi I, Moriyón I, eds. *Brucella: Molecular and Cellular Biology.* Norfolk, England: Horizon Bioscience; 2004:159-291.
20. Moriyon I, López-Goñi I. Structure and properties of the outer membranes of *Brucella abortus* and *Brucella melitensis. Int Microbiol.* 1997;46:101-103.
21. Guzmán-Verri C, Manterola L, Sola-Landa A, et al. The two-component system BvrR/BvrS essential for *Brucella abortus* virulence regulates the expression of outer membrane proteins with counterparts in members of the *Rhizobiaceae. Proc Natl Acad Sci U S A.* 2002;99:12375-12380.
22. Hasanjani Roushan MR, Mohrez M, Smailnejad Gangi SM, et al. Epidemiological features and clinical manifestations in 469 adult patients with brucellosis in Babol, Northern Iran. *Epidemiol Infect.* 2004;132:1109-1114.
23. Corbel MJ, ed. *Brucellosis in Humans and Animals.* Geneva: World Health Organization; 2006.
24. Trout D, Gomez TM, Bernard BP, et al. Outbreak of brucellosis at a United States pork packing plant. *J Occup Environ Med.* 1995;37:697-703.

25. Cvetnic Z, Mitak M, Ocepek M, et al. Wild boars (Sus scrofa) as reservoirs of *Brucella suis* biovar 2 in Croatia. *Acta Vet Hung.* 2003;51:465-473.

26. Starnes CT, Talwani R, Horvath JA, et al. Brucellosis in two hunt club members in South Carolina. *J S C Med Assoc.* 2004;100:113-115.

27. Wallach JC, Giambartolomei GH, Baldi PC, et al. Human infection with M-strain of *Brucella canis. Emerg Infect Dis.* 2004;10:146-148.

28. Young EJ. Human brucellosis. *Rev Infect Dis.* 1983;5:321-342.

29. Chan J, Baxter C, Wenman WM. Brucellosis in an Inuit child, probably related to caribou meat consumption. *Scand J Infect Dis.* 1989;21:337-338.

30. Mesner O, Riesenberg K, Biliar N, et al. The many faces of human-to-human transmission of brucellosis: congenital infection and outbreak of nosocomial disease related to an unrecognized clinical case. *Clin Infect Dis.* 2007;45:e135-e140.

31. Ertem M, Kürekçi AE, Aysev D, et al. Brucellosis transmitted by bone marrow transplantation. *Bone Marrow Transplant.* 2000;26:225-226.

32. Moreno S, Ariza J, Espinosa FJ, et al. Brucellosis in patients infected with the human immunodeficiency virus. *Eur J Clin Microbiol Infect Dis.* 1998;17:319-326.

33. Young EJ. *Brucella* species (brucellosis). In: Long SS, Pickering LK, Prober CG, eds. *Principles and Practice of Pediatric Infectious Diseases.* 3rd ed. Philadelphia: Elsevier; 2008:855-858.

34. Shaalan MA, Memish ZA, Mahmoud SA, et al. Brucellosis in children: clinical observations in 115 cases. *Int J Infect Dis.* 2002;6:182-186.

35. Almuneef MA, Memish ZA, Balkhy HH, et al. Importance of screening household members of acute brucellosis cases in endemic areas. *Epidemiol Infect.* 2004;132:533-540.

36. Fosgate GT, Carpenter TE, Chomel BB, et al. Time-space clustering of human brucellosis, California, 1973-1992. *Emerg Infect Dis.* 2002;8:672-678.

37. Troy SB, Rickman LS, Davis CE. Brucellosis in San Diego: epidemiology and species-related differences in acute clinical presentations. *Medicine.* 2005;84:174-187.

38. Morales-Otero P. *Studies of Brucella Infection in Puerto Rico.* San Juan: PR; 1948:46-88.

39. Steffen R. Antacids—a risk factor in traveller's brucellosis? *Scand J Infect Dis.* 1977;9:311-312.

40. Liautard J, Gross A, Köhler S. Interactions between professional phagocytes and *Brucella* spp. *Microbiol Semin.* 1996;12:197-206.

41. Boschiroli ML, Ouahrani-Battache S, Foulongne V, et al. The *Brucella suis* virB operon is induced intracellularly in macrophages. *Proc Natl Acad Sci U S A.* 2002;99:1544-1549.

42. Celli J, Salcedo SP, Gorvel J-P. *Brucella* coopts the small GTPase Sar1 for intracellular replication. *Proc Natl Acad Sci U S A.* 2005;102:1673-1678.

43. Yingst S, Hoover DL. T cell immunity to brucellosis. *Crit Rev Microbiol.* 2003;29:313-331.

44. Capparelli R, Alfano F, Amoroso MG, et al. Protective effect of the Nramp1 BB genotype against *Brucella abortus* in the water buffalo (*Bubalus bubalis*). *Infect Immun.* 2007;75:988-996.

45. Wyllie S, Seu P, Goss JA. The natural resistance-associated macrophage protein 1 Slc11a1 (formerly Nramp 1) and iron metabolism in macrophages. *Microbes Infect.* 2002;4:351-359.

46. Ariza J, Pellicer T, Pallares RN, et al. Specific antibody profile in human brucellosis. *Clin Infect Dis.* 1992;14:131-140.

47. Pellicer T, Ariza J, Foz A, et al. Specific antibodies detected during relapse of human brucellosis. *J Infect Dis.* 1988;157:918-924.

48. Gazapo E, Lahoz JG, Subiza JL, et al. Changes in IgM and IgG antibody concentrations over time: importance for diagnosis and follow-up. *J Infect Dis.* 1989;159:219-225.

49. Colmenero JD, Reguera JM, Martos F, et al. Complications associated with *Brucella melitensis* infection: a study of 530 cases. *Medicine.* 1996;75:195-211.

50. Ariza J, Corredoira J, Pallares R, et al. Characteristics of and risk factors for relapse of brucellosis in humans. *Clin Infect Dis.* 1995;20:1241-1249.

51. Ariza J, Bosch J, Gudiol F, et al. Relevance of in vitro antimicrobial susceptibility of *Brucella melitensis* to relapse rate in human brucellosis. *Antimicrob Agents Chemother.* 1986;30:958-960.

52. Spink WW. What is chronic brucellosis? *Ann Intern Med.* 1951;35:258-274.

53. Young EJ. Serologic diagnosis of human brucellosis: analysis of 214 cases by agglutination tests and review of the literature. *Rev Infect Dis.* 1991;13:359-372.

54. Cluff LE. Medical aspects of delayed convalescence. *Rev Infect Dis.* 1991;13(Suppl):138-140.

55. Petrella R, Young EJ. Acute brucella ileitis. *Am J Gastroenterol.* 1988;83:80-82.

56. Papaioannides D, Korantzopoulos P, Sinapidis D, et al. Acute pancreatitis associated with brucellosis. *JOP.* 2006;7:62-65.

57. Spink WW, Hoffbauer FW, Walker WW, et al. Histopathology of the liver in human brucellosis. *J Lab Clin Med.* 1949;34:40-58.

58. Young EJ. *Brucella melitensis* hepatitis: the absence of granulomas. *Ann Intern Med.* 1979;91:414-415.

59. Akritidis N, Tzivras M, Delladetsima I, et al. The liver in brucellosis. *Clin Gastroenterol Hepatol.* 2003;5:1109-1112.

60. Colmenero JD, Queipo-Ortuño MI, Reguera JM, et al. Chronic hepatosplenic abscesses in brucellosis: clinico-therapeutic features and molecular diagnostic approach. *Diag Microbiol Infect Dis.* 2002;42:159-167.

61. Ariza J, Pigrau C, Cañas C, et al. Current understanding and management of chronic hepatosplenic suppurative brucellosis. *Clin Infect Dis.* 2001;32:1024-1033.

62. Aziz S, Al-Anazi AR, Al-Aska AI. A review of gastrointestinal manifestations of brucellosis. *Saudi J Gastroenterol.* 2005;11:20-27.

63. Ariza J, Pujol M, Valverde J, et al. Brucellar sacroiliitis: findings in 63 episodes and current relevance. *Clin Infect Dis.* 1993;16:761-765.

64. Solera J, Lozano E, Martínez-Alfaro E, et al. Brucellar spondylitis: review of 35 cases and literature survey. *Clin Infect Dis.* 1999;29:1440-1449.

65. Colmenero JD, Ruiz-Mesa JD, Plata A, et al. Clinical findings, therapeutic approach, and outcome of brucellar vertebral osteomyelitis. *Clin Infect Dis.* 2008;46:426-433.

66. Berrocal A, Gotuzzo E, Calvo A, et al. Sternoclavicular brucellar arthritis: a report of 7 cases and a review of the literature. *J Rheumatol.* 1993;20:1184-1186.

67. Yagupsky P, Peled N. Use of the isolator 1.5 microbial tube for detection of *Brucella melitensis* in synovial fluid. *J Clin Microbiol.* 2002;40:3878.

68. Weil Y, Mattan Y, Liebergall M, et al. *Brucella* prosthetic joint infection: a report of 3 cases and a review of the literature. *Clin Infect Dis.* 2003;36:e81-e86.

69. Gotuzzo E, Alarcón GS, Bocanegra TS, et al. Articular involvement in human brucellosis: a retrospective analysis of 304 cases. *Semin Arthritis Rheum.* 1982;12:245-255.

70. Bouza E, García de la Torre M, Parras F, et al. Brucellar meningitis. *Rev Infect Dis.* 1987;9:810-822.

71. McLean DR, Russell N, Khan MY. Neurobrucellosis: clinical and therapeutic features. *Clin Infect Dis.* 1992;15:582-590.

72. Haji-Abdolbagi M, Rasooli-Nejad M, Jafari S, et al. Clinical and laboratory findings in neurobrucellosis: review of 31 cases. *Arch Iranian Med.* 2008;11:21-25.

73. Al-Sous MW, Bohlega S, Al-Kawi MZ, et al. Neurobrucellosis: clinical and neuroimaging correlation. *Am J Neuroradiol.* 2004;25:395-401.

74. Adaleti I, Albayram S, Gurses B, et al. Vasculopathic changes in the cerebral arterial system with neurobrucellosis. *Am J Neuroradiol.* 2006;27:384-386.

75. Young EJ, Tarry A, Genta RM, et al. Thrombocytopenic purpura associated with brucellosis: report of 2 cases and literature review. *Clin Infect Dis.* 2000;31:904-909.

76. Colmenero JD, Queipo-Ortuño MI, Reguera JM, et al. Real time polymerase chain reaction: a new powerful tool for the diagnosis of neurobrucellosis. *J Neurol Neurosurg Psychiatry.* 2005;76:1025-1027.

77. Seidel G, Pardo CA, Newman-Toker D, et al. Neurobrucellosis presenting as leukoencephalopathy: the role of cytotoxic T lymphocytes. *Arch Pathol Lab Med.* 2003;127:e374-e377.

78. Al-Harthi SS. The morbidity and mortality patterns of *Brucella* endocarditis. *Int J Cardiol.* 1989;25:321-324.

79. Jacobs F, Abramowicz D, Vereerstraeten P, et al. *Brucella* endocarditis: the role of combined medical and surgical treatment. *Rev Infect Dis.* 1990;12:740-744.

80. Dhand A, Ross JJ. Implantable cardioverter-defibrillator infection due to *Brucella melitensis*: case report and review of brucellosis of cardiac devices. *Clin Infect Dis.* 2007;44:e37-e39.

81. Reguera JM, Alarcón A, Miralles F, et al. *Brucella* endocarditis: clinical, diagnostic, and therapeutic approach. *Eur J Clin Microbiol Infect Dis.* 2003;22:647-650.

82. Sanford JP. *Brucella* pneumonia. *Semin Respir Infect.* 1997;12:24-27.

83. Pappas G, Bosilkovski M, Akritidis N, et al. Brucellosis and the respiratory system. *Clin Infect Dis.* 2003;37:e95-e99.

84. Theegarten D, Albrecht S, Tötsch M, et al. Brucellosis of the lung: case report and review of the literature. *Virchows Arch.* 2008;452:97-101.

85. Shoja M, Khosroshahi MT, Tubbs S, et al. Brucellosis mimicking vasculitis in a patient with renal failure and peripheral neuropathy. *Am J Med Sci.* 2008;336:285-287.

86. Navarro-Martínez A, Solera J, Corredoira J, et al. Epididymoorchitis due to *Brucella melitensis*: a retrospective study of 59 patients. *Clin Infect Dis.* 2001;33:2017-2022.

87. Khan MY, Mah MW, Memish ZA. Brucellosis in pregnant women. *Clin Infect Dis.* 2001;32:1172-1177.

88. Crosby E, Llosa L, Quesada M, et al. Hematologic changes in brucellosis. *J Infect Dis.* 1984;150:419-424.

89. Young EJ, Tarry A, Genta RM, et al. Thrombocytopenic purpura associated with brucellosis: report of 2 cases and literature review. *Clin Infect Dis.* 2000;31:904-909.

90. Ariza J, Servitje O, Pallarés R, et al. Characteristic cutaneous lesions in patients with brucellosis. *Arch Dermatol.* 1989;125:380-383.

91. Milionis H, Christou L, Elisaf M. Cutaneous manifestations in brucellosis: case report and review of the literature. *Infection.* 2000;28:124-126.

92. Rolando I, Olarte L, Vilchez G, et al. Ocular manifestations associated with brucellosis: a 26-year experience in Peru. *Clin Infect Dis.* 2008;46:1338-1345.

93. Al Faran MF. *Brucella melitensis* endogenous endophthalmitis. *Ophthalmologica.* 1990;201:19-22.

94. CDC. Laboratory-acquired brucellosis–Indiana and Minnesota, 2006. *MMWR Morb Mortal Wkly Rep.* 2008;57:39-42.

95. Elsaghir AAF, James EA. Misidentification of *Brucella melitensis* as *Ochrobactrum anthropi* by API 20NE. *J Med Microbiol.* 2003;52:441-442.

96. Morata P, Queipo-Ortuño MI, Reguera JM, et al. Development and evaluation of a PCR-enzyme-linked immunosorbent assay for diagnosis of human brucellosis. *J Clin Microbiol.* 2003;41:144-148.

97. Queipo-Ortuño MI, Colmenero JD, Baeza G, et al. Comparison between LightCycler real-time polymerase chain reaction (PCR) assay with serum and PCR-enzyme-linked immunosorbent assay with whole blood samples for the diagnosis of human brucellosis. *Clin Infect Dis.* 2005;40:260-264.

98. Mitka S, Anetakis C, Souliou E, et al. Evaluation of different PCR assays for early detection of acute and relapsing brucellosis in humans in comparison with conventional methods. *J Clin Microbiol.* 2007;45:1211-1218.

99. Navarro E, Segura JC, Castaño MJ, et al. Use of real-time quantitative polymerase chain reaction to monitor the evolution of *Brucella melitensis* DNA load during therapy and post-therapy follow-up in patients with brucellosis. *Clin Infect Dis.* 2006;42:1266-1273.

100. Vrioni G, Pappas G, Priavali E, et al. An eternal microbe: *Brucella* DNA persists for years after clinical cure. *Clin Infect Dis.* 2008;46:e131-e136.

101. Casao MA, Smits HL, Navarro E, et al. Clinical utility of a dipstick assay in patients with brucellosis: correlation with the period of evolution of the disease. *Clin Microbiol Infect.* 2003;9:301-305.

102. CDC. Public health consequences of a false-positive laboratory test result for *Brucella*: Florida, Georgia, and Michigan, 2005. *MMWR Morb Mortal Wkly Rep.* 2008;57:603-605.

103. Goldbaum FA, Velikovsky CA, Baldi PC, et al. The 18-kDa cytoplasmic protein of *Brucella* species—an antigen useful for diagnosis is a lumazine synthase. *J Med Microbiol.* 1999;48:833-839.

104. Solera J, Geijo P, Largo J, et al. A randomized, double-blind study to assess the optimal duration of doxycycline treatment for human brucellosis. *Clin Infect Dis.* 2004;39:1776-1782.

105. Roushan MRH, Mohraz M, Hajiahmadi M, et al. Efficacy of gentamicin plus doxycycline versus streptomycin plus doxycycline in the treatment of brucellosis in humans. *Clin Infect Dis.* 2006;42:1075-1080.

106. Ariza J, Bosilkovski M, Cascio A, et al. Perspectives for the treatment of brucellosis in the 21st century: the Ioannina recommendations. *PLoS Med.* 2007;4:e317.

107. Skalsky K, Yahav D, Bishara J, et al. Treatment of human brucellosis: systematic review and meta-analysis of randomized controlled trials. *Br Med J.* 2008;336:701-704.

108. Falagas ME, Bliziotis IA. Quinolones for treatment of human brucellosis: critical review of the evidence from microbiological and clinical studies. *Antimicrob Agents Chemother.* 2006;50:22-33.

109. Young EJ. An overview of human brucellosis. *Clin Infect Dis.* 1995;21:283-290.

110. Robichaud S, Libman M, Behr M, et al. Prevention of laboratory-acquired brucellosis. *Clin Infect Dis.* 2004;38:e119-e122.

111. Maley MW, Kociuba K, Chan RC. Prevention of laboratory-acquired brucellosis: significant side effects of prophylaxis. *Clin Infect Dis.* 2006;42:433-434.

227

Francisella tularensis (Tularemia)

ROBERT L. PENN

Francisella tularensis is a gram-negative pathogen primarily of animals and occasionally of humans. The disease it causes is now recognized as tularemia in most areas of the world, but it has been called rabbit fever, deer fly fever, and market men's disease in the United States; wild hare disease (yato-byo) and Ohara's disease in Japan; and water-rat trappers' disease in Russia. Tularemia continues to be responsible for significant morbidity and mortality, despite the availability of numerous antibiotics active against the organism.[1]

F. tularensis infections have become a public health issue, with increasing concerns regarding military or terrorist uses of the organism in biological warfare (see Chapter 323). Because of this, tularemia was returned to the list of reportable diseases in the United States in 2000, after being excluded in 1995, and *F. tularensis* has once again become the subject of intense investigation. With heightened surveillance has come an appreciation of the continued occurrence, often in outbreaks, of natural *F. tularensis* infections throughout the world.

History

Tularemia has been so intimately linked to investigators in the United States that it has been referred to as an "American achievement."[2] However, its history includes important contributions from many other areas of the world, including Japan and the former Soviet Union. Hare-associated illness compatible with tularemia has been known in Japan since 1818, and perhaps the earliest written description of a patient with unmistakable tularemia was provided by Homma-Soken in 1837.[3]

Credit for identifying the organism and recognizing the important clinical syndromes belongs to U.S. workers. In 1911, while evaluating possible plague outbreaks after the San Francisco earthquake, McCoy described a plague-like illness common in the California ground squirrel, and with Chapin he successfully cultured the causative agent in 1912.[4] They named it *Bacterium tularense* because this work took place in Tulare county. The first human case to have bacteriologic confirmation was an ocular infection reported in 1914 by Vail[5] and by Wherry and Lamb.[6] Although the cause was unknown at the time, tularemia was transmitted by contact with biting flies in Utah and was termed deer fly fever. Dr. Edward Francis, working for the U.S. Public Health Service, established the true cause of deer fly fever as *B. tularense* (a full decade after the organism was discovered in squirrels), proved the deer fly was the vector, and named the human disease *tularemia* to emphasize the frequent accompanying bacteremia. Francis also contributed to work that improved methods for cultivating *B. tularense* and making a serologic diagnosis, identified tick and other reservoirs for its transmission, clarified the clinical syndromes associated with tularemia, and emphasized the risk to laboratory workers and consumers from infected sources. For this lifetime of achievements, the genus in which the organism is classified was renamed *Francisella* in his honor.

In Japan, Ohara had described a rabbit-associated febrile disease, transmitted the illness to his wife by rubbing rabbit hearts over her hand, and recovered an organism from her lymph nodes; Francis later showed that this Japanese organism was identical to *B. tularense*. Tularemia was recognized in Astrakhan, Russia, in 1926, and during the subsequent decades scattered serious outbreaks occurred throughout the country. Scientists in the former Soviet Union also have intensively studied the disease and its causative organism.

Description of the Pathogen

Francisella are small, aerobic, catalase-positive, pleomorphic, gram-negative coccobacilli. They are more uniformly rod-shaped during logarithmic growth, during which they tend to exhibit bipolar staining with Gram or Giemsa methods; this staining pattern accentuates a coccoidal appearance. The cell wall of *F. tularensis* has an unusually high level of fatty acids that have a profile unique to the genus, and wild strains possess an electron-transparent lipid-rich capsule. Loss of the capsule may lead to loss of serum resistance and virulence but may not diminish viability or survival within neutrophils[7]; however, the capsule is neither toxic nor immunogenic.

Francisella spp. belong to the γ-proteobacteria and may be categorized on the basis of growth characteristics, biochemical reactions, and virulence properties (Table 227-1). The family Francisellaceae includes two species in the genus *Francisella* and four subspecies of *F. tularensis*.[8,9] Although all have been associated with human disease, only the *tularensis* and *holarctica* subspecies of *F. tularensis* are relatively common. *F. tularensis* subsp. *tularensis*, also referred to as type A, is found almost exclusively in North America and is the most virulent species. Although previously thought to be restricted to North America, *F. tularensis* subsp. *tularensis* has been isolated in Europe and its identity verified using molecular techniques.[10] *F. tularensis* subsp. *holarctica*, also referred to as type B, is found predominantly in Asia and Europe but also in North America; it is less virulent in humans and of low virulence in rabbits. The *F. tularensis* live vaccine strains (LVS) are derived from *F. tularensis* subsp. *holarctica*. *Francisella novicida* was previously classified as a separate species, but it is now known to be a subspecies of *F. tularensis*.[8,9] *F. tularensis* subsp. *novicida* is of low virulence. Strains isolated from a restricted area in central Asia have been designated *F. tularensis* subsp. *mediaasiatica*, are of low virulence, and produce acid from glycerol but not glucose.[8] Strains isolated in Japan have been designated *F. tularensis* subsp. *holarctica* biovar *japonica*, but their differentiation from other subsp. *holarctica* strains on the basis of traditional phenotypic testing was not possible.[9]

The taxonomy of *Francisella* has been complicated because biochemical reactions may be variable, weak, or delayed and also in part because of the different terms given to organisms isolated in different areas of the world. Classification of *Francisella* has been advanced by the sequencing of the whole genome from representative strains of *F. tularensis* subsp. *tularensis* (strain Schu S4), subsp. *holarctica* (including the attenuated live vaccine strain), and subsp. *novicida*, along with application of various molecular typing methods.[10-12] These have included 16S ribosomal DNA gene sequence analysis, microarray analysis of the whole genome, and multiple-locus variable-number tandem repeat analysis (MLVA).[10] Reports using these techniques have supported the currently accepted taxonomy as outlined previously and in Table 227-1, demonstrated the utility of these methods for species and subspecies typing, and identified *F. tularensis* subsp. *holarctica* biovar *japonica* as a distinct group.[12,13] When applied to a sample of isolates from North America, MLVA has been used to successfully discriminate individual strains and has identified two separate clades of *F. tularensis* subsp. *tularensis* (designated A.I and A.II).[13] Genomic sequencing and other genomic analyses have indicated that there was a common *F. tularensis* ancestor for clonal subspecies evolution, that subsp. *novicida* is the oldest, and that subspp. *tularensis* appeared before subsp. *holarctica*, which is the youngest.[14]

	F. tularensis Subspecies*			
Feature	tularensis	holarctica	novicida	F. philomiragia
Cysteine growth requirement	+	+	−	−
Growth in broth plus 6% NaCl	−	−	+†	+†
Motility	−	−	−	−
Oxidase	−	−	−	+‡
Nitrate reduction	−	−	−	−
Acid from				
Glucose	+†	+†	+†	+†
Glycerol	+	−	+	+
Gelatin hydrolysis	−	−	−	+†
Relative virulence				
Humans	High	Intermediate	Low	Low
Rabbits	High	Low	Low	NA

*The fourth F. tularensis subspecies, mediaasiatica, and the japonica biovar of F. tularensis subsp. holarctica are described in the text.
†Variable or delayed.
‡Using Kovacs test; negative using cytochrome-oxidase test.
NA, not available.
Data from Sjöstedt[9] and Lindquist and co-workers.[8]

F. tularensis requires cysteine or cystine (or another sulfhydryl source) for growth and therefore will not grow on most routine solid media or on gram-negative selective media such as MacConkey or eosin methylene blue agars. It may be recovered with the use of glucose cysteine blood agar, thioglycolate broth, chocolate agar suitable for gonococcal growth, modified Thayer-Martin medium, buffered charcoal-yeast agar, or cysteine heart agar with 9% chocolatized sheep blood.[8,9] Blood agar may support growth of some F. tularensis isolates on initial plating but not on subpassage.[15] Some strains of F. tularensis lack an overt requirement for cysteine or enriched medium for growth, and clinically significant strains of Francisella have been reported that do not show the expected fastidious growth characteristics.[9] Francisella should be suspected, however, whenever a slowly growing, small, and poorly staining gram-negative coccobacillus is isolated on chocolate agar and grows poorly or not at all on blood agar.[8] Visible colonies take 2 to 5 days to appear. Incubation at 35°C is optimal, with or without an atmosphere of increased CO_2. The recovery of F. tularensis from contaminated specimens may be facilitated by the addition of penicillin, cycloheximide, and polymyxin B to the media.[8] Virtually all F. tularensis strains are positive for β-lactamase.

Differentiation of Francisella from other bacteria can be accomplished using direct fluorescent antibody staining, slide agglutination, polymerase chain reaction (PCR), or cellular fatty acid composition analysis.[8] It is important to note that automated laboratory identification systems should not be used for the identification of Francisella because they may generate aerosols and commonly misidentify F. tularensis as Haemophilus or Actinobacillus species.[15] Whenever F. tularensis is suspected, the state public health laboratory should be notified immediately, and any local microbiological testing should be done using a biological safety cabinet and following Biosafety Level 2 procedures.[15] Isolates that cannot be excluded as F. tularensis should be sent to a reference laboratory in the Laboratory Response Network, typically the state public health laboratory. Federal regulations rigorously control transport of F. tularensis cultures and must be followed when sending an isolate to a referral laboratory for identification.

Antisera can distinguish between F. tularensis subspp. tularensis and novicida but not between subspp. tularensis and holarctica; strains within subspecies do not have antigenic differences detectable by antisera. F. tularensis produces no known exotoxins. The lipopolysaccharide (LPS) from the live vaccine strain of F. tularensis possesses at least 1000-fold less endotoxin activity than the LPS from Escherichia coli.[16]

This is in part because F. tularensis LPS has a unique structure and, unlike other gram-negative bacteria, it is not recognized by Toll-like receptor 4 (TLR4) and does not bind to LPS-binding protein.[17] However, it has been shown that human B cells produce tumor necrosis factor-α (TNF-α), interleukin-6 (IL-6), and antibody in response to purified LPS from F. tularensis.[18] The O-antigen side chains from subspp. tularensis and holarctica are identical but differ from that of subsp. novicida.[17] Mutants of F. novicida with altered LPS O-antigen side chains exhibit varying degrees of serum sensitivity and ability to grow in macrophages.[19] Pili have been visualized on the surface of F. tularensis subsp. holarctica live vaccine strain and subsp. novicida; genome sequencing has detected genes homologous to those from other bacteria that encode type IV pili in F. tularensis subspp. tularensis, holarctica, and novicida; and type IV pili assembly contributes to virulence in murine models.[20,21]

Host immune responses are directed against numerous cell wall antigens, including membrane proteins, LPS, and carbohydrates, but previously it was not possible to identify dominant antigens. Proteomic analysis using serum from donors who have had tularemia or who have been vaccinated with the live vaccine strain has identified a large number of F. tularensis protein antigens and is able to identify among them possible immunodominant antigens.[12,22] These have included many cytoplasmic and membrane proteins, as well as hypothetical proteins of unknown localization.[12,22] Further proteomic analyses will be helpful to refine future diagnostic tests for tularemia and for the construction of effective vaccines.

Phenotypic correlates of virulence have included the capsule and citrulline ureidase activity. Wild encapsulated strains of F. tularensis are resistant to the bactericidal activity of normal serum, but a capsule-deficient mutant is serum sensitive.[23] The contribution of citrulline ureidase to virulence is unclear, and there are pathogenic isolates that do not possess this activity. Plasmids that have been found in isolates of F. tularensis subspp. holarctica and novicida, and in Francisella philomiragia, have not been found in the more virulent F. tularensis subsp. tularensis and thus are not essential for virulence. Several acid phosphatases (Acp) are present in Francisella and they are important for its survival within macrophages. AcpA can inhibit the respiratory burst of neutrophils, and expression of AcpA and histidine acid phosphatase (Hap) is induced by growth within macrophages.[24] In addition, the deletion of acpA, acpB, acpC, and hap from subsp. novicida results in a mutant strain that is impaired in its ability to survive within macrophages and to escape from the phagosome.[24] A siderophore for iron acquisition is present in F. tularensis and is upregulated by growth in iron-limited conditions; this may be a virulence mechanism by enhancing Francisella intracellular growth, as it is in other intracellular pathogens.[25]

Genomic and proteomic analyses have the potential to more specifically identify virulence factors in F. tularensis.[12,22,26] F. tularensis contains a cluster of genes involved in virulence, the Francisella pathogenicity island (FPI). There are two copies of the FPI in subspp. tularensis and holarctica and one copy in subsp. novicida; although largely identical, the FPI from subsp. tularensis differs from that in subsp. holarctica and subsp. novicida.[27,28] The FPI contains 19 genes required for murine virulence and intracellular growth in macrophages, including iglABCD and pdpABCD. mglA and mglB are not located within the FPI and code for transcriptional regulators of many FPI genes as well as non-FPI genes; other FPI regulators include sspA and pmrA.[29,30] Intracellular growth, iron limitation, and exposure to H_2O_2 also regulate expression of these genes.[27,28] Disruption of many of these genes has been shown to impair the organism's ability to survive within macrophages and significantly reduces virulence in animal models. IglC, a 23-kDa protein that was originally identified because it is upregulated during Francisella growth within macrophages, is the product of the FPI gene iglC and it has been the subject of intense scrutiny. Intact mglA and iglC are required for F. tularensis growth within macrophages, virulence for mice, and also for growth within amoebae.[27] IglC is involved in F. tularensis escape from the phagosome, prevention of phagosome-lysosome fusion, and apoptosis of infected macrophages.[31,32] Many other genes can also be identified that probably play a role in *Francisella* virulence, and these are currently being explored.[26,33]

F. philomiragia was previously called *Yersinia philomiragia*. It was reclassified because it shares the unique fatty-acid profile of the *Francisella* and substantial DNA relatedness to this genus, although it has some unique biochemical features (see Table 227-1) and DNA hybridization patterns that distinguish it from *F. tularensis. F. philomiragia* is of low virulence for humans and has been isolated from muskrats and water. All strains originally tested produced β-lactamase and were most susceptible to aminoglycosides, cefoxitin, cefotaxime, fluoroquinolones, tetracycline, and chloramphenicol. However, an infection caused by *F. philomiragia* resistant to cefazolin and cefotaxime has been reported.[34]

A number of newly appreciated *Francisella*-like organisms have been identified by PCR amplification of 16S rRNA gene sequences or by culture. A survey of soil throughout Houston, Texas, using PCR amplification of DNA extracts identified multiple *Francisella*-like organisms that were distinct from known species of *F. tularensis* and *F. philomiragia*.[35] *Francisella*-like organisms have been identified as a cause of granulomatous diseases in several fish species. They have been cultured, and 16S rRNA gene sequencing has shown them to be related most closely to *F. philomiragia*. However, isolates from Atlantic cod are currently believed to be new species of *Francisella*. They have been referred to as *Francisella philomiragia* subsp. *noatunensis* subsp. nov. by Mikalsen and co-workers[36] and as *Francisella piscicida* by Ottem and associates[37]; currently, it is unclear if these represent the same or different organisms.

Several endosymbiotic bacteria of ticks have been classified within the Francisellaceae family on the basis of 16S ribosomal gene sequence data. These include *Wolbachia persica*, an endosymbiont found in Rocky Mountain wood ticks termed *Dermacentor andersoni* symbiont, and symbiont B of *Ornithodorous moubata*.[9] Similar organisms can be found in other hard and soft ticks, suggesting that they may be more widely distributed than previously observed. A *Francisella*-like organism has been found as an endosymbiont of a *Paramecium* species, and a related organism has been isolated from the waters off Hong Kong.[38,39]

Epidemiology

Tularemia is widely distributed, but it is primarily a disease of the Northern Hemisphere and is most common between 30° and 71° north latitude. It has been remarkably absent from the United Kingdom, Africa, South America, and Australia. Whipp and co-workers[40] reported the first case of tularemia from Australia in 2003, and it was caused by a subsp. *novicida*-like organism. Tularemia was very common in the United States before World War II. However, its incidence has declined steadily since the 1950s and has remained at fewer than 0.15 cases per 100,000 population since 1965.[41,42] Because of its stable and low incidence, tularemia was removed from the list of nationally reportable diseases in 1995 but was added back in 2000 in part because of the concern about its use for bioterrorism. Since 2001, the case rates have been 0.05 per 100,000 population or less.[42] Arkansas, Missouri, South Dakota, and Oklahoma reported 56% of the total U.S. cases from 1990 through 2000, with counties in Montana, Kansas, and Massachusetts also reporting high numbers of cases during this decade (Fig. 227-1).[41] In 2006, Arkansas, Kansas, Massachusetts, Missouri, and Nebraska reported 50% of the U.S. total number of tularemia cases.[42] Groups with high incidence rates include American Indians and Alaska Natives. Subtle changes have occurred in the geographic distribution of cases in the United States between 1965 and 1999.[43] The southern border of tularemia has shifted northward so that fewer cases have been reported from south-central states in recent years, and this is consistent with the predicted effects of climate change on tularemia's geographic distribution.[43] Environmental data also have been used to develop a model to predict risk of tularemia in specific geographic regions.[44] More detailed investigation using molecular typing has found that specific *F. tularensis* strains may be geographi-

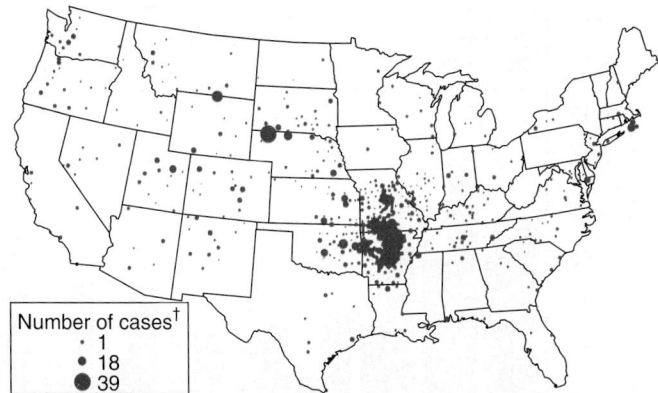

Figure 227-1 **The total number of tularemia cases reported in the lower continental United States by county of residence from 1990 through 2000.** Alaska reported 10 cases in four counties during this time. †Circle size is proportional to the number of cases, ranging from 1 to 39. *(From Centers for Disease Control and Prevention. Tularemia— United States, 1990-2000. MMWR Morbid Mortal Wkly Rep. 2002;51:181-184.)*

Number of cases†
· 1
● 18
● 39

cally limited. Farlow and associates[45] used MLVA subtyping to evaluate 83 North American isolates of *F. tularensis* subsp. *tularensis* and identified two distinct groups of organisms termed A.I and A.II. *F. tularensis* subsp. *tularensis* group A.I was found primarily in the central United States, including the states reporting the highest numbers of tularemia cases, and also in California; *F. tularensis* subsp. *tularensis* group A.II was found primarily in the western United States at higher elevations than the A.I isolates.[45] The distribution of group A.I isolates correlated with the distribution of *Amblyomma americanum* and *Dermacentor variabilis* ticks and the eastern cottontail rabbit (*Sylvilagus floridanus*); the distribution of group A.II isolates correlated with the distribution of *D. andersoni* and the deer fly *Chrysops discalis*, and also with the mountain cottontail rabbit (*Sylvilagus nuttali*). There were only a few isolates of subsp. *novicida*, but most were found in the southeastern United States.[45] In contrast, isolates of *F. tularensis* subsp. *holarctica* were widely dispersed geographically.[45] Pulse-field gel electrophoresis on 41 *F. tularensis* subp. *tularensis* U.S. isolates identified two separate patterns, with type A-east isolates corresponding to the distribution of group A.I isolates and type A-west isolates corresponding to the distribution of group A.II isolates.[46] Illness caused by type A-west isolates was relatively benign and was less severe than that caused by either type A-east isolates or subsp. *holarctica*.[46] Testing of additional U.S. isolates has identified two A1 genotypes, A1a and A1b. Genotype A1b isolates were significantly more likely to be from invasive infections and were associated with significantly higher mortality in humans than A1a and A2 isolates.[46a] Additional instances of the geographic restriction of specific *F. tularensis* strains from Eurasia have been identified as newer molecular typing methods have been more widely applied.[13,47-49] Tularemia emerged recently in new areas of Sweden for unknown reasons, and it was identified in Spain for the first time in 1996 probably from imported hares.[50,51]

Historically, in the United States tularemia incidence has been most frequent in June through August and in December. The summer peak corresponds to a greater number of tick-acquired cases, whereas the smaller peak in winter reflects an increased number of hunting-associated cases. However, only the peak in the late spring and summer was prominent in more recent years. A review of 316 available *F. tularensis* human isolates from 39 states collected between 1964 and 2004 found that 208 (66%) were subsp. *tularensis* and 108 (34%) were subsp. *holarctica*.[46] Most isolates of both subspecies occurred between May and September; a very small increase in numbers in December was noted only for subsp. *tularensis* and not for subsp. *holarctica*, and only subsp. *tularensis* was associated with lagomorph exposure.[46] Males account for the majority of cases, perhaps because of greater exposure

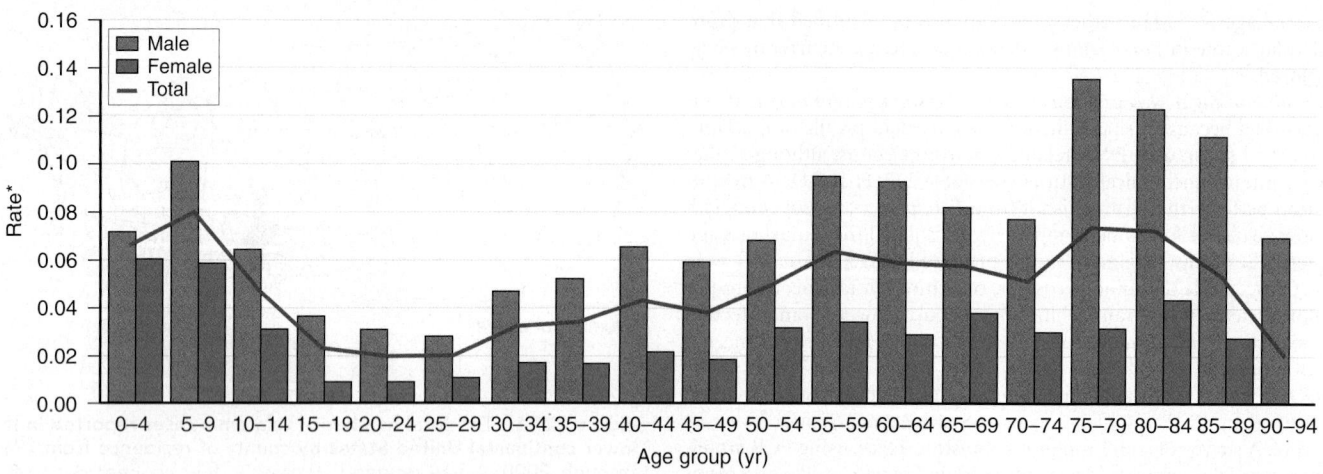

Figure 227-2   Age and gender of tularemia cases reported in the United States from 1990 through 2000. *Average annual incidence per 100,000 population. (From Centers for Disease Control and Prevention. Tularemia—United States, 1990-2000. MMWR Morbid Mortal Wkly Rep. 2002;51:181-184.)*

opportunities, and tularemia can occur in individuals of any age (Fig. 227-2). In the United States, incidence rates are highest in children age 5 to 9 years and in people 75 years or older (see Fig. 227-2).[41] Occupations that have been associated with an increased risk of tularemia are laboratory worker, farmer, landscaper, veterinarian, sheep worker, hunter or trapper, and cook or meat handler.

F. tularensis is capable of infecting hundreds of different vertebrates and invertebrates, but no more than a dozen mammalian species are important to its ecology in any geographic region. These include lagomorphs, particularly *Sylvilagus* and *Lepus* spp., and rodents such as voles, squirrels, muskrats, and beavers in North America; included in Eurasia are voles, hamsters, mice, and hares. Transmission of *F. tularensis* to humans occurs most often through the bite of an insect or contact with contaminated animal products. Other routes of transmission include aerosol droplets, contact with contaminated water or mud, and animal bites. Illness may occur in families or friends because of shared activities and exposures. Nonetheless, human-to-human spread does not occur.

Bloodfeeding arthropods and flies are the most important vectors for tularemia in the United States. Ticks predominate in the Rocky Mountain states and eastward, whereas biting flies predominate in California, Nevada, and Utah. However, an increase in human tularemia noted in Wyoming between 2001 and 2003 was linked most often to transmission by biting flies and was associated with a simultaneous outbreak of tularemia in rabbits.[52] In contrast, mosquitoes are the most frequent insect vector in Sweden and Finland, and they are also important in the former Soviet Union. At least 13 species of ticks have been found to be naturally infected with *F. tularensis*, and transovarial passage may occur. The dog tick (*D. variabilis*), wood tick (*D. andersoni*), and Lone Star tick (*A. americanum*) are commonly involved in North America. The organism may be present in tick saliva or feces and may be inoculated either directly or indirectly into the bite wound. Several outbreaks of tick-borne tularemia have involved *F. tularensis* subsp. *holarctica* (type B), although this organism is more often linked to water, rodents, and aquatic animals; tick transmission traditionally has been associated with subsp. *tularensis* (type A). Tularemia in children in endemic areas of the United States is now most often associated with tick exposure in the summer.

Animal contact is another important mode of acquiring tularemia. Skinning, dressing, and eating infected animals, including rabbits, muskrats, beavers, squirrels, and birds, have transmitted tularemia, occasionally resulting in large outbreaks in hunters. Wild animals sold as pets are also potential vectors, as occurred in 2002 when infected prairie dogs were widely commercially distributed.[53] The first outbreak in Spain was associated with processing hare carcasses and hare meat, and it was notable for a preponderance of women patients.[51] Airborne

transmission has occurred from these activities, as well as from contact with water, contaminated dust, and hay. An outbreak in 2000 of pneumonic tularemia on Martha's Vineyard was associated with mowing lawns and using a brush cutter, and since then cases of pneumonic tularemia have been regularly encountered on Martha's Vineyard each summer.[54] Serologic evidence of *F. tularensis* infection among potential animal reservoirs on Martha's Vineyard was found most frequently in raccoons (52.4%) and skunks (49.2%), although active infection in skunk and raccoon samples was not found by culture and PCR.[55] Carnivorous animals may transiently carry *F. tularensis* in the mouth or on claws after killing or feeding on infected prey, whether or not they become infected. This is thought to be the mechanism by which domestic cats occasionally transmit tularemia. *F. tularensis* may survive for prolonged periods in water, mud, and animal carcasses even if frozen; however, cooking game meats thoroughly to the proper temperatures should minimize risk from ingestion. Contaminated food and water continue to be important environmental sources of tularemia, and disruptions of infrastructure caused by wars and natural disasters may be important contributing factors.[56,57] In postwar Kosovo, an epizootic in increased rodent populations contaminated ransacked homes and food with *F. tularensis*, which led to a food- and waterborne outbreak among refugees returning to disrupted housing and sanitation.[57] The devastating effects of an earthquake in Turkey are believed to have resulted in water contamination and subsequent outbreaks of tularemia in the region.[56] It has been demonstrated that *F. tularensis* LVS strain will multiply intracellularly in *Acanthamoeba castellanii*, amoebal cysts may become infected, and coculture of the organisms enhances the growth of *F. tularensis*.[58] Such a relationship may prove relevant to natural aquatic reservoirs for tularemia.

Pathogenesis

F. tularensis is a virulent organism for susceptible species, including the accidental human host. Although the organism is reported to penetrate intact skin, most investigators believe that penetration occurs through sites of inapparent skin disruption. The infectious dose in humans depends on the portal of entry: 10 to 50 organisms when injected intradermally or when inhaled, and 10^8 organisms when ingested. That low numbers of bacteria can cause infection through the skin, mucous membranes, and airways helps to explain in part the extreme risk that *F. tularensis* poses to laboratory workers. In general, *F. tularensis* subsp. *tularensis* causes more severe disease than subspp. *holarctica* and *novicida*. The specific molecular reasons underlying these differences in virulence are unclear.

During the first 3 to 5 days after cutaneous inoculation, *F. tularensis* multiplies locally and produces a papule; ulceration occurs 2 to 4 days later. Organisms spread from the site of entry to regional lymph nodes and may disseminate via a lymphohematogenous route to involve multiple organs. Bacteremia is probably common in this early phase, although it is only occasionally detected. An elegant description of the pathogenesis is offered by Geyer and colleagues.[59] Infection with *F. tularensis* is characterized by an acute inflammatory response that involves fibrin, neutrophils, macrophages, and T lymphocytes. Neutrophils and macrophages surround earlier inflammatory cells, stimulated by the initial inoculum, that have become necrotic and degenerated. Eventually, lymphocytes, epithelioid cells, and giant cells migrate into the necrotic tissue. This extensive necrosis is noted in both lung tissue and lymph nodes. As the necrotic tissue expands, adjacent veins and arteries may thrombose. The organisms are usually present at the site of the necrotic tissue but are difficult to demonstrate on routine stains. Silver impregnation techniques (Steiner, Dieterle, and Warthin-Starry) enhance the visibility of the organisms, which are usually found in macrophages and epithelioid cells. Granulomas develop that occasionally may caseate; for this reason, specimens may be mistaken for tuberculosis. These changes can occur in any infected site and have been found at autopsy in lung, liver, spleen, lymph nodes, and bone marrow. Coalescence of necrotic foci may yield abscess formation. *F. tularensis* may remain viable in tissues for prolonged periods.

Humoral immunity, directed against carbohydrate antigens, develops between the second and third week after infection, with the almost simultaneous appearance of immunoglobulin M (IgM), IgG, and IgA agglutinating antibodies. However, antibodies alone are insufficient to protect against virulent *F. tularensis* infection.[60] Opsonizing IgG and IgM antibodies are also produced, with the most efficient opsonization involving both immune serum and complement (C3). Nonetheless, oxygen-dependent neutrophil killing of wild virulent strains is poor. Human neutrophils phagocytose opsonized *F. tularensis* live vaccine strain organisms but do not kill them, and they escape into the neutrophil cytoplasm. This is associated with disruption of neutrophil NADPH oxidase assembly, a failure of the respiratory burst, and impaired neutrophil responsiveness to other activating stimuli.[61]

F. tularensis is a facultative intracellular parasite that is capable of growing within several different cell types, including macrophages, dendritic cells, hepatocytes, alveolar epithelial cells, and endothelial cells.[62,63] However, macrophages are the primary site of its survival and replication. Entry into macrophages occurs through a unique mechanism involving engulfment by relatively capacious and asymmetrical pseudopod loops; this type of uptake is dependent on complement and complement receptors but not antibodies.[62] Mannose receptors and class A scavenger receptors may provide other pathways for *F. tularensis* uptake.[62] Inside the macrophage, virulent *F. tularensis* strains impair maturation of the endosome, thus avoiding phagosome-lysosome fusion, and quickly escape into the cytosol. Within 15 to 30 minutes after infection, phagosomes containing *F. tularensis* are transiently acidified by the vacuolar ATPase pump, and this is essential for organisms to escape into the cytoplasm.[64] Bacteria proliferate in the cytoplasm and are released upon macrophage cell death, which is induced at least in part through a pathway that involves type I interferon signaling and ASC/caspace-1.[65,66]

Complete recovery from tularemia requires cell-mediated immunity, which is demonstrable approximately 1 week earlier than antibody responses and is directed against protein antigens. This cell-mediated immunity is α/β T-cell dependent but may involve either CD4⁺ or CD8⁺ T cells. Attempts are being made to define the critical molecular determinants that induce protective immunity. Current understanding about the immunopathogenesis of tularemia has been largely derived from mice infected with *F. tularensis* subsp. *novicida* or other strains less virulent for humans, and it is not known how this relates to human tularemia caused by more virulent organisms. Furthermore, different routes of infection and infection in different mouse strains may elicit different murine immune responses.[67,68] Interferon-γ (IFN-γ) and TNF-α activate macrophages to kill *F. tularensis* through the production of nitric oxide and other reactive nitro-

gen products, although alveolar macrophages may use other mechanisms to inhibit the organism.[68]

Several mechanisms are involved in the innate response that controls infection before the development of conventional cellular immunity. Early host defense against *F. tularensis* infection involves neutrophils, dendritic cells, macrophages, TNF-α, IFN-γ, and IL-12, but these are not sufficient to resolve the infection. Neutrophils are less important in the lung than in systemic infection in mice, and neutrophils may contribute to lung damage.[69] The initial response to *F. tularensis* infection is dependent on Toll-like receptor 2 recognition, particularly in the lung.[68] In the mouse lung, virulent *F. tularensis* strains are capable of suppressing the expected early immune response.[70,71] TLR4 recognition of *F. tularensis* LPS is poor; interestingly, resistance of mice to pulmonary infection with subsp. *novicida* is enhanced by pretreatment with a TLR4 agonist.[72]

For complete resolution of systemic infection, it is necessary that α/β⁺ T cells be functional and present after the initial defenses provided by the macrophages, dendritic cells, cytokines, and neutrophils. CD4⁺ and CD8⁺ cells each contribute to survival of mice infected intradermally with the vaccine strain, but both are required to fully clear the infection.[68] The contribution of α/β⁺ T cells involves TNF-α and IFN-γ production and is dependent on IL-12 p40.[68] Impaired clearance of *F. tularensis* live vaccine strain from mice with pulmonary infection may result from increased local PGE₂ secretion and decreased numbers of IFN-γ secreting T cells.[73] Natural infection or vaccination in humans results in long-lasting memory CD4⁺ and CD8⁺ cells.[74] In mice, B cells contribute to protection against the vaccine strain that is not dependent on antibodies, but it is unknown if B cells play a similar role in human infection.[68] Immunization of mice with *F. tularensis* may protect against subsequent challenge but not prevent persistent, low-level organ infection, and the essential determinants of sterilizing immunity remain unknown.

Expansion of circulating γ/δ T cells has been documented in patients with acute tularemia. These cells respond to phosphoantigens from many different pathogens, including *F. tularensis*. The observed increase in the levels of Vγ9Vδ2 cells occurs after the first week of illness and may persist for longer than 1 year after infection.[75] However, 10 to 30 years after infection, long-lived memory cells responsive to *F. tularensis* heat shock proteins are α/β T cells and not γ/δ T cells.[74]

The organism's intracellular residence in the liver and other sites may help to protect it from these defenses and permit its early growth. *F. tularensis* is contained within granulomas in the livers of mice infected with the vaccine strain, and granuloma formation involves hepatic natural killer cells, IFN-γ production, and expression of inducible nitric oxide synthase.[76] Neutrophils and mononuclear cells accumulate at infected liver foci in mice and lyse hepatocytes harboring *F. tularensis*, thereby releasing organisms from this sequestered environment.[77]

Clinical Manifestations

The clinical consequences of *F. tularensis* infection depend on the virulence of the particular organism, the portal of entry, the extent of systemic involvement, and the immune status of the host. The result can range from asymptomatic or inconsequential illness to acute sepsis and rapid death. Patients who seek medical attention usually present with at least one of six classic forms of tularemia: ulceroglandular, glandular, oculoglandular, pharyngeal, typhoidal, and pneumonic. This somewhat artificial classification emphasizes only the predominant manifestations commonly encountered, and there is overlap in many patients.

The incubation period averages 3 to 5 days, but it ranges from 1 to 21 days. Tularemia usually starts abruptly, with the onset of fever, chills, headache, malaise, anorexia, and fatigue. Other prominent symptoms may include cough, myalgias, chest discomfort, vomiting, sore throat, abdominal pain, and diarrhea. A pulse-temperature deficit was noted in up to 42% of evaluable patients in the United States,

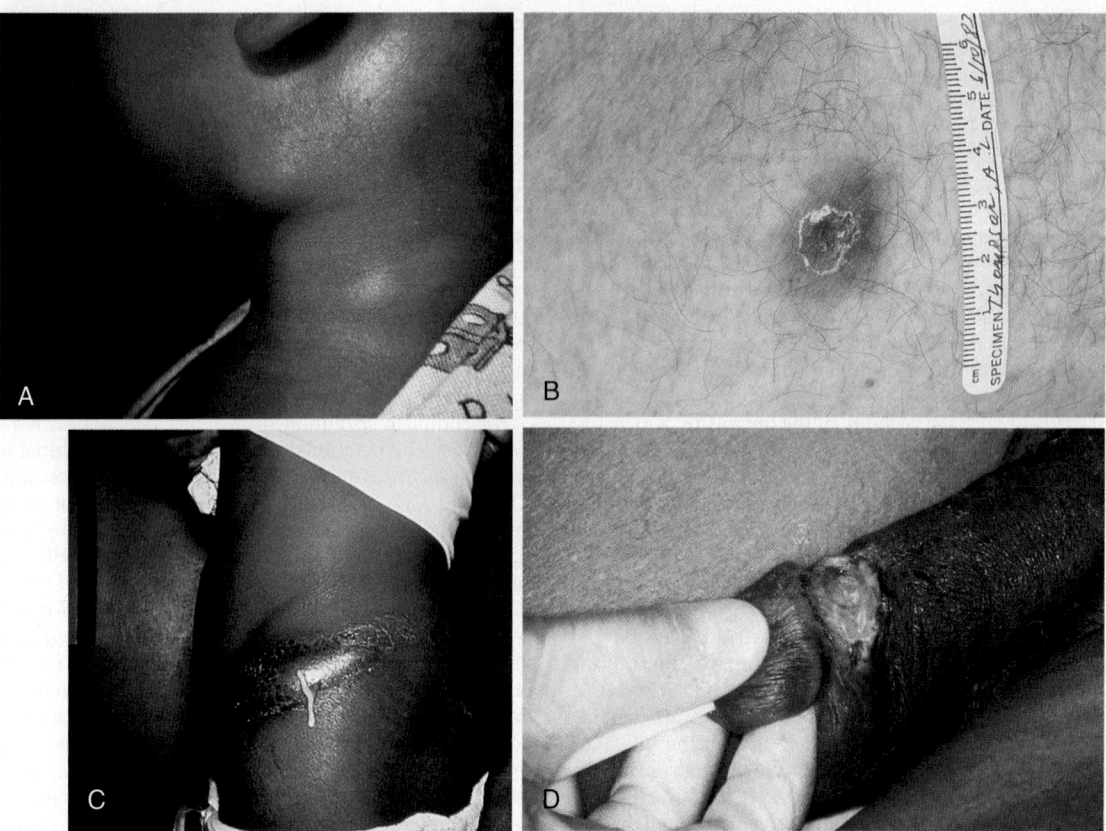

Figure 227-3 Examples of primary lesions seen in ulceroglandular tularemia. A, Large cervical and submandibular lymph nodes in a young child; an ulcer was found under the hairline on her forehead at the site of a tick bite. *(Courtesy of Dr. Joseph A. Bocchini, Louisiana State University Health Sciences Center, Shreveport, LA.)* **B,** Papule undergoing central necrosis with desquamation on the thigh of a middle-aged man. **C,** Inguinal adenopathy and suppurative mass in a young hunter who had carried a dead hare at his side. *(Courtesy of Dr. Joseph A. Bocchini, Louisiana State University Health Sciences Center, Shreveport, LA.)* **D,** Penile ulcer that was suspected of being syphilis or another sexually transmitted disease until the history of a recent tick bite was obtained by the infectious diseases consultant. *(Courtesy of Dr. John W. King, Louisiana State University Health Sciences Center, Shreveport, LA.)*

although this was found in only 5% of patients infected with subsp. *holarctica* infection in Sweden.[3,50] Fever (usually >101°F) classically lasts for several days, remits for a short interval, and then recurs along with other symptoms. Without treatment, fever lasts an average of 32 days, and chronic debility, weight loss, and adenopathy may persist for many months longer.[78] Less virulent strains cause a milder, self-limited illness that may resolve without therapy. Systemic symptoms may abate by the time medical help is sought so that the clinical picture is dominated by one or more of the six patterns listed; this may lead to confusion regarding the correct diagnosis, particularly in the 25% to 50% of patients without an evident source of infection.

Ulceroglandular tularemia has been the presentation in the majority of cases; tick bites and animal contacts are the usually recalled exposures. This is the form that is most quickly recognized as tularemia. The initial specific complaint is often of enlarged and tender localized lymphadenopathy (Fig. 227-3). The inciting skin lesion may appear before, simultaneously with, or from one to several days after the adenopathy. It starts as a red, painful papule in a region draining into the involved lymph nodes. Vesicles also may be seen, and these may be mistaken for herpes simplex or varicella infection.[79] The papule then undergoes necrosis, leaving a tender ulcer with a raised border (see Fig. 227-3). If untreated, the ulcer may take weeks to heal and leave a residual scar. Multiple lesions may occur, particularly in those with animal sources.[3] The location of the ulcer generally reflects the mode of acquisition; animal contacts tend to yield ulcers on the hands and forearms, and tick bites tend to yield ulcers on the trunk, the perineum, the lower extremities, and the head and neck. The distribution of lymphadenopathy also reflects the exposure history, as illustrated in

Figure 227-4; overall, cervical and occipital adenopathy is most common in children, and inguinal adenopathy is most common in adults. Skin changes over the involved nodes, seen in 19.1% of cases in a series from Sweden,[50] should suggest underlying suppuration. Some patients have a sporotrichoid presentation with ascending sub-

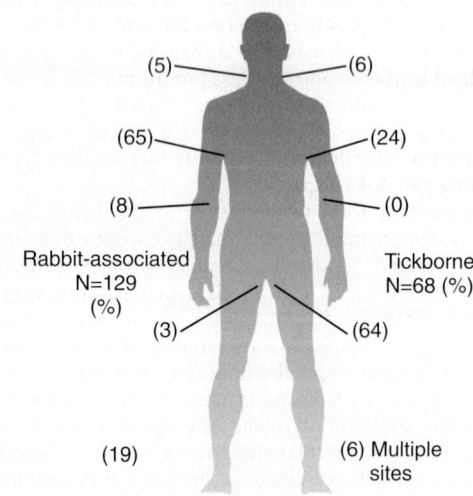

Figure 227-4 Distribution of lymphadenopathy in rabbit-associated and tick-borne tularemia.

cutaneous nodules. Lymphangitis is rare unless there is bacterial super-infection of the ulcer.

Glandular tularemia occurs when patients present with tender regional lymphadenopathy but without an evident cutaneous lesion. This form accounts for one fifth or less of cases in the United States. Glandular tularemia represents essentially the same process as ulceroglandular disease, except that a skin lesion either healed before presentation or was minimal or atypical and overlooked. Enlarged lymph nodes may persist for prolonged periods, and in some patients an exposure or prior febrile illness will be forgotten. For this reason, tularemia may not be considered in the initial differential diagnosis of some patients whose primary presentation is lymphadenopathy. In either ulceroglandular or glandular tularemia, the lymph nodes may suppurate (see Fig. 227-3). More than 20% will suppurate if left untreated or if treatment is delayed longer than 2 weeks.[2] When fluctuant, they should be needle-aspirated or surgically drained. The differential diagnosis of ulceroglandular and glandular tularemia includes pyogenic bacterial infections, cat-scratch disease, syphilis, chancroid, lymphogranuloma venereum, tuberculosis, nontuberculous mycobacterial infection, toxoplasmosis, sporotrichosis, rat-bite fever, anthrax, plague, and herpes simplex virus infection.

Oculoglandular tularemia represents only a minority of cases. In this form, organisms have gained entry through the conjunctiva, either from contaminated fingers or from contaminated splashes and aerosols. Disease may be bilateral, but this is uncommon. Early complaints may include photophobia and excessive lacrimation. Examination shows lid edema and a painful conjunctivitis, with injection, chemosis, and small, yellowish conjunctival ulcers or papules in some patients. Associated tender lymphadenopathy may occur in the preauricular, submandibular, and cervical regions. If the adenopathy is extensive and more prominent than the eye findings, then this syndrome may be mistaken for mumps.[3] Visual loss is rare, but complications include corneal ulceration, dacrocystitis, and nodal suppuration. The differential diagnosis of oculoglandular tularemia includes pyogenic bacterial infections, adenoviral infection, syphilis, cat-scratch disease, and herpes simplex virus infection.

Pharyngeal tularemia, another variant of ulceroglandular disease, is the result of primary invasion through the oropharynx. The source may be contaminated foods or water or contaminated droplets. This form, which represents a few cases overall in the United States, has been seen with increasing frequency in recent outbreaks in other countries. Children have been involved more often than adults, and several family members may be affected simultaneously. It must be distinguished from the sore throat that may accompany any of the other major clinical forms of tularemia. In pharyngeal tularemia, the patient's predominant complaint typically is of fever and severe throat pain. Exudative pharyngitis or tonsillitis is the rule, and one or more ulcers may be seen. A pharyngeal membrane has been described in some patients that is similar to a diphtheritic membrane.[78] Cervical, preparotid, and retropharyngeal adenopathy may be present, occasionally with bilateral involvement or abscess formation. When there is a delay in seeking care, the dominant manifestation may be cervical adenopathy without prominent fever or pharyngotonsillitis. The differential diagnosis includes streptococcal pharyngitis, infectious mononucleosis, adenoviral infection, and diphtheria. Tularemia should be suspected in an endemic area whenever a severe sore throat is unresponsive to penicillin therapy and routine diagnostic tests have been unrewarding.

Typhoidal tularemia refers to a febrile illness caused by *F. tularensis* that is not associated with prominent lymphadenopathy and does not fit into any of the other major forms. The typhoidal form may result from any mode of acquisition, and it is the most difficult to diagnose. Because the portal of entry is usually inapparent clinically, a history of outdoor activities with tick or animal exposure should be sought. Many patients have serious underlying chronic medical disorders and their presentation can be quite dramatic, with acute prostration and rapid death, or a protracted illness. Prominent symptoms of typhoidal tularemia may include any combination of fever with chills, headache,

myalgias, sore throat, anorexia, nausea, vomiting, diarrhea, abdominal pain, and cough. Examination may reveal dehydration, hypotension, mild pharyngitis and cervical adenopathy, meningismus, and diffuse abdominal tenderness. Hepatomegaly and splenomegaly are found uncommonly in the acute stages and become more likely the longer the duration of illness. Severe disease may be accompanied by cholestasis with jaundice. Diarrhea, a major manifestation only in typhoidal tularemia, is loose and watery but only rarely bloody. Children may have more severe intestinal involvement, including focal areas of bowel necrosis.[78] Rare gastrointestinal manifestations include cholangitis, granulomatous hepatitis, and liver abscess. Secondary pleuropulmonary involvement is common in this form, with pulmonary infiltrates or pleural effusions being found in up to 45% of typhoidal cases; it is even more frequent in laboratory-acquired infections. Additional findings in severely ill patients may include hyponatremia, elevated creatine phosphokinase, myoglobinuria, pyuria, renal failure, and positive blood cultures. The differential diagnosis of typhoidal tularemia includes typhoid fever caused by *Salmonella* spp., brucellosis, *Legionella* infection, Q fever, disseminated mycobacterial or fungal infection, rickettsioses, malaria, endocarditis, and any other cause of prolonged fever without localizing signs.

Pneumonic tularemia refers to an illness whose initial presentation is dominated by pulmonary infection. This is found in up to 20% of all tularemia cases and may occur at any age. It may result from direct inhalation of the organism or from secondary hematogenous spread to the lung. Primary pneumonic tularemia is a risk for certain occupations, including sheep shearers, farmers, landscapers, and laboratory workers. Cases also have been described as resulting from common exposure in a more casual setting.[80] Secondary pneumonia may occur early or after a delay of weeks to months in the course of tularemia.[2] Although secondary pneumonia may complicate any of the syndromes already discussed, Evans and colleagues[3] found pneumonia to be most frequent in typhoidal (83%) and ulceroglandular (31%) diseases. Scofield and associates[81] reported that patients with pneumonic involvement were more likely to be older, to recall no exposure, to present with typhoidal illness, to have positive cultures, to stay hospitalized longer, and to have a higher mortality rate. From 25% to 30% of patients have infiltrates on radiographic examination without any clinical findings of pneumonia.[3] Pneumonia from *F. tularensis* subsp. *tularensis* (type A) is a significantly more severe disease than that caused by subsp. *holarctica* (type B), but illness may be prolonged with either subspecies. Common symptoms include fever, cough, no or minimal sputum production, substernal tightness, and pleuritic chest pain. Hemoptysis may occur but is uncommon. Physical examination may be nonspecific or may reveal rales, consolidation, and a friction rub or signs of effusion. Some patients need mechanical ventilation, and adult respiratory distress syndrome may complicate the course of any form of tularemia. Routine examination of sputum does not help to suggest the diagnosis. However, a false-positive direct fluorescent antibody stain for *Legionella* on bronchoscopy specimens has been reported.[82] Infected pleural fluid is exudative, negative on Gram stain, and usually contains more than 1000 leukocytes/mm³; cells are predominantly lymphocytes, but neutrophilic effusions may occur. Pleural effusions seen with tularemia frequently mimic those seen with tuberculosis. Similar findings for both include a lymphocyte-rich exudative pleural effusion and a high adenosine deaminase concentration.[83] Granulomas may be found on pleural biopsy and may be confused with tuberculosis. Acute radiographic changes may include subsegmental or lobar infiltrates (Fig. 227-5), hilar adenopathy, pleural effusion, and apical or miliary infiltrates; less common changes include ovoid densities, cavitation, and bronchopleural fistula. However, in some patients the initial chest films are normal. Secondary pneumonias are more likely to involve the lower lobes and be bilateral, perhaps because of their hematogenous origin. Healing usually occurs without residual changes, but fibrosis and calcifications may result. Therefore, tularemia may manifest as an enigmatic community-acquired pneumonia that does not respond to routine therapies. The differential diagnosis of pneumonic tulare-

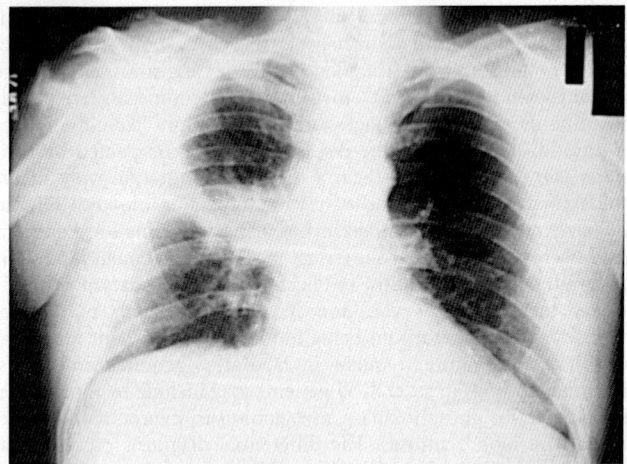

Figure 227-5   Chest radiograph of untreated tularemia pneumonia. This patient remained symptomatic for more than 3 months. The diagnosis was established serologically when poorly developed granulomas were found in a transbronchial biopsy, other causes were excluded, and the exposure history was finally obtained. *(From Penn RL, Kinasewitz GT. Factors associated with a poor outcome in tularemia. Arch Intern Med. 1987;147:265-268. Copyright 1987, American Medical Association.)*

mia includes *Mycoplasma* pneumonia, *Legionella* infection, *Chlamydophila pneumoniae* infection, Q fever, psittacosis, tuberculosis, the deep mycoses, and many other causes of atypical or chronic pneumonias.

Secondary skin rashes are an underappreciated part of tularemia and may be found in up to 43% of cases.[50,84] They usually appear within the first 2 weeks of symptoms, but in a minority of cases they are delayed. Rash is more common in women than in men. Cutaneous changes may include diffuse maculopapular and vesiculopapular eruptions, pustules, erythema nodosum, erythema multiforme, acneiform lesions, and urticaria. Sweet's syndrome has also been reported in association with tularemia.[85] Although any type of secondary rash may be part of any form of tularemia, erythema nodosum has been found to occur most commonly with pneumonic tularemia.

The clinical manifestations of infections caused by *F. tularensis* subsp. *novicida* are less well characterized than for the other subspecies but are similar to those previously described. A *novicida*-like organism was isolated from an adult with a toe abscess and regional adenopathy that complicated a cut sustained in brackish water in Australia.[40] This occurrence in the Southern Hemisphere and the molecular identification of older *F. tularensis* isolates as subsp. *novicida* after being previously classified as other subspecies suggest that infections actually caused by subsp. *novicida* may be underappreciated.[40] *F. philomiragia* infection has caused a skin vesicle, pneumonia, empyema, sepsis, peritonitis, splenic microabscesses, and meningitis. This organism predominantly infects patients with host defenses impaired by chronic granulomatous disease, near-drowning in salt water or estuaries, or myeloproliferative disorders.[86] Infections have been documented from North America and Europe, and the organism has been found in tissues, blood, cerebrospinal fluid, and other body fluids.[86]

Complications and Outcome

Suppuration of involved lymph nodes is currently the most common complication of tularemia (see Fig. 227-3), and this may occur even after specific antibiotic therapy. Nodes that suppurate after appropriate therapy are often sterile but benefit from drainage. Patients with severe disease may manifest disseminated intravascular coagulation, renal failure, rhabdomyolysis, jaundice, and hepatitis. Meningitis, encephalitis, pericarditis, peritonitis, osteomyelitis, splenic rupture, and thrombophlebitis have become very rare since antibiotic therapy has become available. Single cases of endocarditis,[87] prosthetic joint

infection with bacteremia,[88] and peritonitis[89] caused by *F. tularensis* have been reported. The cerebrospinal fluid in meningitis patients almost always shows a mononuclear cell pleocytosis, with a high protein concentration and hypoglycorrhachia.[89a] Brain abscesses may be seen as a complication of the meningitis.[90]

Tularemia may lead to months of debility in some patients, usually associated with late lymph node suppuration or persistent fatigue. Features that are associated with a worse prognosis include increasing age, serious coexisting medical conditions, symptoms lasting 1 month or longer before treatment, significant pleuropulmonary disease, typhoidal illness, renal failure, a delay in the diagnosis, and inappropriate antibiotic therapy.[1,81] Overall death rates in the antibiotic era have been 4% or less, but they were as high as 60% before the introduction of streptomycin as treatment.[91]

Diagnosis

The diagnosis of tularemia ultimately rests on clinical suspicion. Results of routine laboratory testing are nonspecific. The leukocyte count and sedimentation rate may be normal or elevated. Thrombocytopenia, hyponatremia, elevated serum transaminases, increased creatine phosphokinase, myoglobinuria, and sterile pyuria are occasionally found.[1] The organism is rarely seen on Gram-stained smears or in tissue biopsies and does not grow in routinely plated cultures. However, *F. tularensis* may be recovered from blood, pleural fluid, lymph nodes, wounds, sputum, and gastric aspirates when processed on supportive media. Because of this and its potential danger to laboratory personnel, individuals working in the area or who may come in contact with the specimens should be notified if tularemia is suspected. Isolations by blood culture have included the less virulent *holarctica* (type B) strains as well as the more virulent *tularensis* (type A) strains. Animal inoculation is rarely performed, in part because this requires Biosafety Level 3 facilities. Biosafety Level 2 is sufficient for laboratory handling of routine clinical specimens, but Biosafety Level 3 should be used to process isolates suspected of being *F. tularensis*.[8]

The rapid diagnosis of *F. tularensis* infection has become a more urgent goal as a result of its potential use as an agent of bioterrorism (see Chapter 323). Methods for rapid diagnosis that have been reported include direct fluorescent antibody staining of smears and tissues, antigen detection in urine, detection using specific monoclonal antibodies, RNA hybridization with a 16S ribosomal probe, and PCR. However, except for PCR, they have not been accepted for widespread use.

The use of PCR is appealing in that smears and cultures are usually negative, standard microbiologic isolation may be hazardous to laboratory personnel, serologic diagnosis may take several weeks to confirm, and the basic methodology is widely available. Although very sensitive in artificial media, PCR assays are less sensitive when applied to biologic specimens and false negatives may occur. A review of three reports from Sweden found that PCR using primers for the 17-kDa lipoprotein *F. tularensis* gene *tul4* was 77% sensitive and culture was 63% sensitive for the diagnosis of ulceroglandular tularemia.[91] PCR may prove useful for diagnosing tularemia in patients several weeks into their illness and in those already receiving suppressive empirical antibiotic therapy. Real-time PCR assays with multiple targets offer promise for improved sensitivity and specificity and for field use (see Chapter 323).[91]

Serologic studies are the most common way that the diagnosis of tularemia is confirmed. Antibodies to *F. tularensis* may be demonstrated by tube agglutination, microagglutination, hemagglutination, and enzyme-linked immunosorbent assay; the tube agglutination and microagglutination tests are the standard methods.[8,92] Standard serologies detect infections with *F. tularensis* subspp. *tularensis* and *holarctica* equally well, and they are usually negative with subsp. *novicida* and with *F. philomiragia*. Standard tube agglutination titers are usually negative in the first week of illness, are positive in most patients after 2 weeks, and peak after 4 or 5 weeks. The microagglutination assay is up to 100-fold more sensitive than tube agglutination. IgM and IgG antibodies appear together, and high titers of both may persist for longer than a decade after infection, limiting the value of a single positive result. A presumptive diagnosis is supported by an acute tube agglutination titer of 1:160 or more, or an acute microagglutination titer of 1:128 or more, in the face of compatible disease, but this may also reflect remote infection.[8] Definitive serologic diagnosis requires a fourfold or greater rise in titer between acute and convalescent specimens; serologies may need to be repeated at 7- to 10-day intervals before a rise is demonstrated. Antibodies may cross-react with *Brucella* spp., *Proteus* OX19, and *Yersinia* spp., but titers to *F. tularensis* are almost always higher. False-positive heterophile agglutinins also rarely occur during tularemia. Tests for cell-mediated immunity such as whole blood IFN-γ release assay in response to tularemia antigens are promising and may be positive earlier than serologies, but they are not commercially available.[92] Gene profiling of cells in whole blood samples obtained from patients with tularemia offers promise as a future rapid diagnostic tool.[93]

Therapy

The drug of first choice for the treatment of all forms of tularemia except meningitis is streptomycin, although gentamicin is an acceptable substitute. The minimum dosage of streptomycin that is effective therapy for tularemia is 7.5 to 10 mg/kg intramuscularly every 12 hours for 7 to 14 days. An alternative regimen is 15 mg/kg intramuscularly every 12 hours for the first 3 days, followed by half this dose to complete treatment. For patients who are very ill, 15 mg/kg every 12 hours may be given throughout a 7- to 10-day course. Doses greater than 2 g/day of streptomycin in adults do not increase efficacy and should not be given. The pediatric weight-based regimens for streptomycin are similar, up to a maximum of the adult dose: 30 to 40 mg/kg/day intramuscularly in two divided doses for a total of 7 days; or 40 mg/kg/day intramuscularly in two divided doses for the first 3 days, followed by 20 mg/kg/day intramuscularly in two divided doses for the next 4 days. The first few days of streptomycin rarely may induce a Jarish-Herxheimer–like reaction, with an increase in symptoms and a transient decrease of the serum agglutination titer. Gentamicin has proved to be effective therapy, including in pediatric patients. It may be given intravenously, and it may be more readily available than streptomycin. Doxycycline has a higher relapse rate compared with the aminoglycosides. Gentamicin is given intravenously at a dose of 5 mg/kg/day in divided doses for 7 to 14 days, with desired peak serum levels of at least 5.0 μg/mL. The efficacy of single daily dosing has been reported for small numbers of adult cases but has not been rigorously studied.[54,94] Nonetheless, it is efficacious and some practitioners consider once-daily gentamicin an acceptable alternative that facilitates completing treatment as an outpatient.[54] The doses of both streptomycin and gentamicin need to be adjusted for renal insufficiency. Penetration of these drugs into the cerebrospinal fluid is poor and erratic, and it may be inadequate in tularemic meningitis. Pittman and colleagues[95] reported a central nervous system shunt infection caused by *F. tularensis* that was successfully treated with intrathecal gentamicin. An additional 16 cases of tularemic meningitis have been documented. Sucessful treatment has included combinations of streptomycin with chloramphenicol or a combination of doxycycline with either streptomycin or gentamicin.[89a]

Tetracycline and chloramphenicol are bacteriostatic for *F. tularensis*, and this accounts in part for the high rate of relapse after treatment with these agents. Tetracycline should not be used in children younger than 8 years of age, during pregnancy, or during lactation. Tetracycline is most effective in adults when given as 2 g/day in divided oral doses for at least 14 days; a suggested oral regimen in children is 30 mg/kg/day, to a maximum of 2 g/day, in divided doses for the same duration. Doxycycline may also be used and provides the convenience of twice-daily dosing. In general, chloramphenicol should not be chosen to treat tularemia because of its potentially serious toxicity and the availability of more effective alternatives with less dangerous potential side effects. However, chloramphenicol, 50 to 100 mg/kg/day intravenously in divided doses, may be added to streptomycin to treat meningitis. When used in the past for other forms of tularemia, the oral dose of chloramphenicol has been 30 to 50 mg/kg/day in three or four divided doses for at least 14 days. The oral preparation is no longer available in the United States.

Drugs with well-established clinical efficacy have exhibited achievable minimal inhibitory concentrations (MICs) against *F. tularensis* on standardized in vitro susceptibility tests.[96] Other agents with relatively low MICs have included erythromycin, rifampin, cefoxitin, cefotaxime, ceftriaxone, and ceftazidime. The effectiveness of these drugs in treating tularemia is not fully established, and ceftriaxone has failed in several patients treated as outpatients.[97] Ceftriaxone exhibited poor intracellular inhibitory activity against a strain of *F. tularensis* subsp. *holarctica* grown in macrophage-like cell monolayers, whereas aminoglycosides, doxycycline, telithromycin, fluoroquinolones, and rifampin were active in this assay.[98] Although erythromycin has been used successfully in a few patients who were thought to have *Legionella* infections, resistance to erythromycin is prevalent in some areas in Europe and Russia, and in general it is considered unreliable as therapy.[82,96,99] Ikäheimo and associates[100] found that all 38 type B clinical isolates they tested were resistant to imipenem in vitro.

In vitro susceptibility studies have found that the fluoroquinolones are active against *F. tularensis* subsp. *tularensis* as well as subsp. *holarctica*.[96] Clinical experience with the fluoroquinolones as therapy for tularemia caused by *F. tularensis* subsp. *holarctica* has been favorable, even in immunocompromised hosts, and some consider ciprofloxacin and moxifloxacin to be the drugs of choice for mild to moderate subsp. *holarctica* infections.[101] Eliasson and co-workers[102] have recommended the use of gentamicin combined with a fluoroquinolone for patients with severe tularemia. However, the outcome with fluoroquinolone therapy may be suboptimal, and there is minimal experience using these agents for infections caused by the more virulent *F. tularensis* subsp. *tularensis*. Ciprofloxacin has also been effective therapy in children with tularemia. Johansson and colleagues[103] described 12 children, ranging in age from 1 to 10 years, with tularemia given ciprofloxacin 15 to 20 mg/kg daily in two divided doses. The 2 patients who completed only 3½ and 7 days of treatment relapsed, but all 12 patients were cured after completing 10 to 14 days of uninterrupted therapy. Ciprofloxacin was active in vitro against the few isolates of *F. philomiragia* tested; it was used successfully to treat a child with chronic granulomatous disease and *F. philomiragia* adenitis and lung infection, but it was part of an unsuccessful regimen in a young man with *F. philomiragia* sepsis.[86,104]

Antibodies to *F. tularensis* and serum from vaccinated people are effective passive therapies for murine infection.[60] Proteomic analysis has been used to identify target antigens for development of monoclonal antibodies that are effective in protecting mice from pulmonary intranasal challenge when given either intranasally or intraperitoneally.[105] Together, these results offer the future hope of immunotherapeutic agents for tularemia. Surgical therapies are limited to drainage of abscessed lymph nodes and chest tube drainage of empyemas.

Treatment of tularemia in the setting of a bioterrorist event is discussed in Chapter 323.

Prevention

Avoiding exposure to the organism is the best prevention of tularemia. Wild animals should not be skinned or dressed using bare hands, and bare hands should not be used to handle an animal that appears ill. Gloves, masks, and protective eye covers should be worn when performing such tasks and when disposing of dead animals brought home by household pets. Wild game should be cooked thoroughly before ingestion. Wells or other waters that are contaminated by dead animals should not be used. Treatment of community water supplies with standard chlorination protects against waterborne tularemia.[106] The most important measure to avoid tick bites in infested areas is wearing clothing that is tight at the wrists and ankles and that covers most of the body. Chemical tick repellants may also be of benefit. Frequent checks should be made for attached ticks so that they may be removed promptly; this must not be done with bare hands, and care should be taken not to crush the tick.

Hospitalized patients with tularemia do not need special isolation because person-to-person spread does not occur, and even in the preantibiotic era, secondary cases were not found. Standard universal precautions for contaminated secretions are adequate when handling drainage from wounds or eyes.

Vaccines prepared from killed *F. tularensis* are ineffective, in part because they only induce an antibody response.[107] A live vaccine based on an attenuated strain of *F. tularensis* subsp. *holarctica* (LVS), originally obtained from the former Soviet Union, has been developed in the United States. The LVS vaccine is an attenuated, live *F. tularensis* strain that occurs in two colony phenotypes, only one of which is immunogenic and has major importance for the induction of protective immunity. The nonimmunologic phenotype has a tendency to accumulate during storage, reducing the efficacy of the vaccine. In addition, the live vaccine strain of *F. tularensis* cannot provide high immune response in the presence of antimicrobial agents such as doxycycline. This vaccine does not spread from the inoculation site, induces cell-mediated and humoral immunity, is effective in preventing typhoidal disease, and reduces the severity of ulceroglandular disease but does not prevent it.[107,108] LVS vaccination was considered in the past for people who worked with *F. tularensis* and for anyone else with repeated occupational exposures. However, use of the vaccine was suspended in part because of questions about its stability, basis of attenuation, efficacy after challenge with other *Francisella* strains by varied routes of exposure, usefulness in immunocompromised patients, and the need to administer it by scarification.[107,109] A new tularemia vaccine is actively being sought using several different strategies, including developing inactivated or subunit vaccines, finding different attenuated strains with defined mutations that are immunogenic, and improving the LVS vaccine.[107] Genomic and proteomic analyses are being used to identify candidate *F. tularensis* proteins that are recognized by patients who have had tularemia for inclusion in potential subunit vaccines.[110] Immunization with native outer membrane proteins plus Freund's adjuvant given intraperitoneally protects mice against intranasal challenge with

F. tularensis subsp. *tularensis* Schu S4.[111] In humans and animal models, protection against pulmonary challenge is enhanced when the LVS vaccine is given by aerosol or intranasally. KuoLee and co-workers[112] found that oral LVS protected mice against intranasal *F. tularensis* challenge. Inactivated LVS preparations given intranasally also protect mice against intranasal *F. tularensis* challenge, and IgA is required for protection.[113,114] Together, these observations suggest that mucosal immunity, particularly mucosal IgA, may contribute to vaccine-induced protection against respiratory tularemia. Recently, an improved LVS vaccine was produced using accepted good manufacturing practices that had limited toxicity in rabbits; this vaccine induced IgG, IgM, and IgA antibodies that cross-reacted with *F. tularensis* subsp. *tularensis* strain Schu S4.[109] A phase I double-blind, placebo-controlled trial of this new LVS vaccine is under way in humans.[109] However, there are many biologic and regulatory issues that will need to be addressed before this or another vaccine is available for human use.

Antibiotic prophylaxis after potential exposures of unknown risk, such as tick bites, is not recommended. In the past, intramuscular streptomycin was given for preemptive treatment of documented exposures from laboratory accidents because streptomycin successfully aborts illness when given in the incubation period after experimental inoculation. Gentamicin should be effective for this purpose as well, but this has not been confirmed. Currently, either doxycycline or ciprofloxacin given orally for 14 days is recommended for adults with suspected or proven high-risk exposure to *F. tularensis*.[53,106] Individuals with lower-risk exposures may be observed for fever or other signs of illness without antibiotics. Observation without antibiotics is also appropriate for exposures in vaccinated individuals. No therapy is needed for someone whose only exposure is to a patient with tularemia because human-to-human transmission does not occur. Post-exposure treatment is discussed more completely in Chapter 323.

Recovery from tularemia is thought to confer protective immunity for life, although a few recurrent infections have been documented. Most recurrences have been clinically mild ulceroglandular disease, and systemic symptoms have been uncommon. Therefore, previously infected individuals are not candidates for vaccination or preemptive antibiotic therapy after a known exposure.

REFERENCES

1. Penn RL, Kinasewitz GT. Factors associated with a poor outcome in tularemia. *Arch Intern Med.* 1987;147:265-268.
2. Tärnvik A, Berglund L. Tularaemia. *Eur Respir J.* 2003;21:361-373.
3. Evans ME, Gregory DW, Schaffner W, et al. Tularemia: a 30-year experience with 88 cases. *Medicine (Baltimore).* 1985;64:251-269.
4. McCoy GW, Chapin CW. Further observations on a plaguelike disease of rodents with a preliminary note on the causative agent *Bacterium tularense. J Infect Dis.* 1912;10:61-72.
5. Vail DT. *Bacillus tularense* infection of the eye. *Ophthalmol Rec.* 1914;23:487.
6. Wherry WB, Lamb BH. Infection of man with *Bacterium tularense. J Infect Dis.* 1914;15:331-340.
7. Sandström G, Löfgren S, Tärnvik A. A capsule-deficient mutant of *Francisella tularensis* LVS exhibits enhanced sensitivity to killing by serum but diminished sensitivity to killing by polymorphonuclear leukocytes. *Infect Immun.* 1988;56:1194-1202.
8. Lindquist D, Chu MC, Probert WS. *Francisella* and *Brucella.* In: Murray PR, Baron EJ, Jorgensen JH, et al, eds. *Manual of Clinical Microbiology.* 9th ed. Washington, DC: American Society for Microbiology Press; 2007:815-834.
9. Sjöstedt AB. *Francisella.* In: Brenner DJ, Krieg NR, Staley JT, et al, eds. *Bergey's Manual of Systematic Bacteriology.* 2nd ed. vol. 2. New York: Springer-Verlag; 2005:200-210.
10. Keim P, Johansson A, Wagner DM. Molecular epidemiology, evolution, and ecology of *Francisella. Ann N Y Acad Sci.* 2007;1105:30-66.
11. Larsson P, Oyston PC, Chain P, et al. The complete genome sequence of *Francisella tularensis*, the causative agent of tularemia. *Nature Genet.* 2005;37:153-159.
12. Titball RW, Petrosino JF. *Francisella tularensis* genomics and proteomics. *Ann N Y Acad Sci.* 2007;1105:98-121.
13. Johansson A, Farlow J, Larsson P, et al. Worldwide genetic relationships among *Francisella tularensis* isolates determined by multiple-locus variable-number tandem repeat analysis. *J Bacteriol.* 2004;186:5808-5818.
14. Svensson K, Larsson P, Johansson D, et al. Evolution of subspecies of *Francisella tularensis. J Bacteriol.* 2005;187:3903-3908.
15. Centers for Disease Control and Prevention, American Society for Microbiology, Association of Public Health Laboratories. Basic Protocols for Level A Laboratories for the Presumptive Identification of *Francisella tularensis.* Available at http://www.asm.org/ASM/files/leftmarginheaderlist/downloadfilename/0000000525/tularemiaprotocol[1].pdf; Accessed August 1, 2008.
16. Ancuta P, Pedron T, Girard R, et al. Inability of the *Francisella tularensis* lipopolysaccharide to mimic or to antagonize the induction of cell activation by endotoxins. *Infect Immun.* 1996;64:2041-2046.
17. Gunn JS, Ernst RK. The structure and function of *Francisella* lipopolysaccharide. *Ann N Y Acad Sci.* 2007;1105:202-218.
18. Rahhal RM, Vanden Bush TJ, McLendon MK, et al. Differential effects of *Francisella tularensis* lipopolysaccharide on B lymphocytes. *J Leukoc Biol.* 2007;82:813-820.
19. Cowley SC, Gray CJ, Nano FE. Isolation and characterization of *Francisella novicida* mutants defective in lipopolysaccharide biosynthesis. *FEMS Microbiol Lett.* 2000;182:63-67.
20. Chakraborty S, Monfett M, Maier TM, et al. Type IV pili in *Francisella tularensis*: roles of pilF and pilT in fiber assembly, host cell adherence, and virulence. *Infect Immun.* 2008;76:2852-2861.
21. Forslund AL, Kuoppa K, Svensson K, et al. Direct repeat-mediated deletion of a type IV pilin gene results in major virulence attenuation of *Francisella tularensis. Mol Microbiol.* 2006;59:1818-1830.
22. Sundaresh S, Randall A, Unal B, et al. From protein microarrays to diagnostic antigen discovery: a study of the pathogen *Francisella tularensis. Bioinformatics.* 2007;23:i508-i518.
23. Sjöstedt A. Virulence determinants and protective antigens of *Francisella tularensis. Curr Opin Microbiol.* 2003;6:66-71.
24. Mohapatra NP, Soni S, Reilly TJ, et al. Combined deletion of four *Francisella novicida* acid phosphatases attenuates virulence and macrophage vacuolar escape. *Infect Immun.* 2008;76:3690-3699.
25. Ramakrishnan G, Meeker A, Dragulev B. fslE is necessary for siderophore-mediated iron acquisition in *Francisella tularensis* Schu S4. *J Bacteriol.* 2008;190:5353-5361.
26. Su J, Yang J, Zhao D, et al. Genome-wide identification of *Francisella tularensis* virulence determinants. *Infect Immun.* 2007;75:3089-3101.
27. Barker JR, Klose KE. Molecular and genetic basis of pathogenesis in *Francisella tularensis. Ann N Y Acad Sci.* 2007;1105:138-159.
28. Nano FE, Schmerk C. The *Francisella* pathogenicity island. *Ann N Y Acad Sci.* 2007;1105:122-137.
29. Charity JC, Costante-Hamm MM, Balon EL, et al. Twin RNA polymerase-associated proteins control virulence gene expression in *Francisella tularensis. PLoS Pathog.* 2007;3:e84.
30. Mohapatra NP, Soni S, Bell BL, et al. Identification of an orphan response regulator required for the virulence of *Francisella* spp. and transcription of pathogenicity island genes. *Infect Immun.* 2007;75:3305-3314.
31. Lai XH, Golovliov I, Sjöstedt A. Expression of IglC is necessary for intracellular growth and induction of apoptosis in murine macrophages by *Francisella tularensis. Microb Pathog.* 2004;37:225-230.
32. Santic M, Molmeret M, Klose KE, et al. The *Francisella tularensis* pathogenicity island protein IglC and its regulator MglA are essential for modulating phagosome biogenesis and subsequent bacterial escape into the cytoplasm. *Cell Microbiol.* 2005;7:969-979.
33. Weiss DS, Brotcke A, Henry T, et al. In vivo negative selection screen identifies genes required for *Francisella* virulence. *Proc Natl Acad Sci U S A.* 2007;104:6037-6042.
34. Sicherer SH, Asturias EJ, Winkelstein JA, et al. *Francisella philomiragia* sepsis in chronic granulomatous disease. *Pediatr Infect Dis J.* 1997;16:420-422.
35. Barns SM, Grow CC, Okinaka RT, et al. Detection of diverse new *Francisella*-like bacteria in environmental samples. *Appl Environ Microbiol.* 2005;71:5494-5500.
36. Mikalsen J, Olsen AB, Tengs T, et al. *Francisella philomiragia* subsp. *noatunensis* subsp. nov., isolated from farmed Atlantic

cod (*Gadus morhua* L.). *Int J Syst Evol Microbiol.* 2007;57:1960-1965.
37. Ottem KF, Nylund A, Isaksen TE, et al. Occurrence of *Francisella piscicida* in farmed and wild Atlantic cod, *Gadus morhua* L., in Norway. *J Fish Dis.* 2008;31:525-534.
38. Beier CL, Horn M, Michel R, et al. The genus *Caedibacter* comprises endosymbionts of *Paramecium* spp. related to the *Rickettsiales* (*Alphaproteobacteria*) and to *Francisella tularensis* (*Gammaproteobacteria*). *Appl Environ Microbiol.* 2002;68: 6043-6050.
39. Lau KW, Ren J, Fung MC, et al. *Fangia hongkongensis* gen. nov., sp. nov., a novel gammaproteobacterium of the order Thiotrichales isolated from coastal seawater of Hong Kong. *Int J Syst Evol Microbiol.* 2007;57:2665-2669.
40. Whipp MJ, Davis JM, Lum G, et al. Characterization of a *novicida*-like subspecies of *Francisella tularensis* isolated in Australia. *J Med Microbiol.* 2003;52:839-842.
41. Centers for Disease Control and Prevention. Tularemia—United States, 1990-2000. *MMWR Morb Mortal Wkly Rep.* 2002;51:181-184.
42. Centers for Disease Control and Prevention. Summary of notifiable diseases—United States, 2006. *MMWR Morb Mortal Wkly Rep.* 2008;55:1-92.
43. Nakazawa Y, Williams R, Peterson AT, et al. Climate change effects on plague and tularemia in the United States. *Vector Borne Zoonotic Dis.* 2007;7:529-540.
44. Eisen RJ, Mead PS, Meyer AM, et al. Ecoepidemiology of tularemia in the south central United States. *Am J Trop Med Hyg.* 2008;78:586-594.
45. Farlow J, Wagner DM, Dukerich M, et al. *Francisella tularensis* in the United States. *Emerg Infect Dis.* 2005;11:1835-1841.
46. Staples JE, Kubota KA, Chalcraft LG, et al. Epidemiologic and molecular analysis of human tularemia, United States, 1964-2004. *Emerg Infect Dis.* 2006;12:1113-1118.
46a. Kugeler KJ, Mead PS, Janusz AM, et al. Molecular epidemiology of *Francisella tularensis* in the United States. *Clin Infect Dis.* 2009;48:863-870.
47. Dempsey MP, Dobson M, Zhang C, et al. Genomic deletion marking an emerging subclone of *Francisella tularensis* subsp. *holarctica* in France and the Iberian Peninsula. *Appl Environ Microbiol.* 2007;73:7465-7470.
48. Gurcan S, Karabay O, Karadenizli A, et al. Characteristics of the Turkish isolates of *Francisella tularensis*. *Jpn J Infect Dis.* 2008;61:223-225.
49. Kantardjiev T, Ivanov I, Velinov T, et al. Tularemia outbreak, Bulgaria, 1997-2005. *Emerg Infect Dis.* 2006;12:678-680.
50. Eliasson H, Bäck E. Tularaemia in an emergent area in Sweden: an analysis of 234 cases in five years. *Scand J Infect Dis.* 2007;39:880-889.
51. Perez-Castrillon JL, Bachiller-Luque P, Martin-Luquero M, et al. Tularemia epidemic in northwestern Spain: clinical description and therapeutic response. *Clin Infect Dis.* 2001;33: 573-576.
52. Centers for Disease Control and Prevention. Tularemia transmitted by insect bites—Wyoming, 2001-2003. *MMWR Morb Mortal Wkly Rep.* 2005;54:170-173.
53. Centers for Disease Control and Prevention. Outbreak of tularemia among commercially distributed prairie dogs, 2002. *MMWR Morb Mortal Wkly Rep.* 2002;51:688, 699.
54. Matyas BT, Nieder HS, Telford SR 3rd. Pneumonic tularemia on Martha's Vineyard: clinical, epidemiologic, and ecological characteristics. *Ann N Y Acad Sci.* 2007;1105:351-377.
55. Berrada ZL, Goethert HK, Telford SR 3rd. Raccoons and skunks as sentinels for enzootic tularemia. *Emerg Infect Dis.* 2006;12:1019-1021.
56. Leblebicioglu H, Esen S, Turan D, et al. Outbreak of tularemia: a case-control study and environmental investigation in Turkey. *Int J Infect Dis.* 2008;12:265-269.
57. Reintjes R, Dedushaj I, Gjini A, et al. Tularemia outbreak investigation in Kosovo: case control and environmental studies. *Emerg Infect Dis.* 2002;8:69-73.
58. Abd H, Johansson T, Golovliov I, et al. Survival and growth of *Francisella tularensis* in *Acanthamoeba castellanii*. *Appl Environ Microbiol.* 2003;69:600-606.
59. Geyer SJ, Burkey A, Chandler FW. Tularemia. In: Connor DH, ed. *Pathology of Infectious Diseases.* Stamford, Conn.: Appleton & Lange; 1997:869-873.
60. Kirimanjeswara GS, Golden JM, Bakshi CS, et al. Prophylactic and therapeutic use of antibodies for protection against respiratory infection with *Francisella tularensis*. *J Immunol.* 2007;179:532-539.
61. McCaffrey RL, Allen LA. *Francisella tularensis* LVS evades killing by human neutrophils via inhibition of the respiratory burst and phagosome escape. *J Leukoc Biol.* 2006;80:1224-1230.
62. Clemens DL, Horwitz MA. Uptake and intracellular fate of *Francisella tularensis* in human macrophages. *Ann N Y Acad Sci.* 2007;1105:160-186.
63. Hall JD, Craven RR, Fuller JR, et al. *Francisella tularensis* replicates within alveolar type II epithelial cells in vitro and in vivo following inhalation. *Infect Immun.* 2007;75:1034-1039.
64. Santic M, Asare R, Skrobonja I, et al. Acquisition of the vacuolar ATPase proton pump and phagosome acidification are essential for escape of *Francisella tularensis* into the macrophage cytosol. *Infect Immun.* 2008;76:2671-2677.
65. Henry T, Brotcke A, Weiss DS, et al. Type I interferon signaling is required for activation of the inflammasome during *Francisella* infection. *J Exp Med.* 2007;204:987-994.
66. Mariathasan S, Weiss DS, Dixit VM, et al. Innate immunity against *Francisella tularensis* is dependent on the ASC/caspase-1 axis. *J Exp Med.* 2005;202:1043-1049.
67. Conlan JW, Zhao X, Harris G, et al. Molecular immunology of experimental primary tularemia in mice infected by respiratory or intradermal routes with type A *Francisella tularensis*. *Mol Immunol.* 2008;45:2962-2969.
68. Elkins KL, Cowley SC, Bosio CM. Innate and adaptive immunity to *Francisella*. *Ann N Y Acad Sci.* 2007;1105:284-324.
69. Malik M, Bakshi CS, McCabe K, et al. Matrix metalloproteinase 9 activity enhances host susceptibility to pulmonary infection with type A and B strains of *Francisella tularensis*. *J Immunol.* 2007;178:1013-1020.
70. Bosio CM, Bielefeldt-Ohmann H, Belisle JT. Active suppression of the pulmonary immune response by *Francisella tularensis* Schu4. *J Immunol.* 2007;178:4538-4547.
71. Mares CA, Ojeda SS, Morris EG, et al. Initial delay in the immune response to *Francisella tularensis* is followed by hypercytokinemia characteristic of severe sepsis and correlating with upregulation and release of damage-associated molecular patterns. *Infect Immun.* 2008;76:3001-3010.
72. Lembo A, Pelletier M, Iyer R, et al. Administration of a synthetic TLR4 agonist protects mice from pneumonic tularemia. *J Immunol.* 2008;180:7574-7581.
73. Woolard MD, Hensley LL, Kawula TH, et al. Respiratory *Francisella tularensis* live vaccine strain infection induces Th17 cells and prostaglandin E_2, which inhibits generation of gamma interferon-positive T cells. *Infect Immun.* 2008;76:2651-2659.
74. Ericsson M, Kroca M, Johansson T, et al. Long-lasting recall response of $CD4^+$ and $CD8^+$ $\alpha\beta$ T cells, but not $\gamma\delta$ T cells, to heat shock proteins of *Francisella tularensis*. *Scand J Infect Dis.* 2001;33:145-152.
75. Kroca M, Tärnvik A, Sjöstedt A. The proportion of circulating $\gamma\delta$ T cells increases after the first week of onset of tularaemia and remains elevated for more than a year. *Clin Exp Immunol.* 2000;120:280-284.
76. Bokhari SM, Kim KJ, Pinson DM, et al. NK cells and gamma interferon coordinate the formation and function of hepatic granulomas in mice infected with the *Francisella tularensis* live vaccine strain. *Infect Immun.* 2008;76:1379-1389.
77. Conlan JW, North RJ. Early pathogenesis of infection in the liver with the facultative intracellular bacteria *Listeria monocytogenes*, *Francisella tularensis*, and *Salmonella typhimurium* involves lysis of infected hepatocytes by leukocytes. *Infect Immun.* 1992;60: 5164-5171.
78. Dienst FT Jr. Tularemia: a perusal of three hundred thirty-nine cases. *J La State Med Soc.* 1963;115:114-124.
79. Byington CL, Bender JM, Ampofo K, et al. Tularemia with vesicular skin lesions may be mistaken for infection with herpes viruses. *Clin Infect Dis.* 2008;47:e4-e6.
80. Siret V, Barataud D, Prat M, et al. An outbreak of airborne tularaemia in France, August 2004. *Euro Surveill.* 2006;11: 58-60.
81. Scofield RH, Lopez EJ, McNabb SJ. Tularemia pneumonia in Oklahoma, 1982-1987. *J Okla State Med Assoc.* 1992;85: 165-170.
82. Roy TM, Fleming D, Anderson WH. Tularemic pneumonia mimicking Legionnaires' disease with false-positive direct fluorescent antibody stains for *Legionella*. *South Med J.* 1989;82:1429-1431.
83. Pettersson T, Nyberg P, Nordström D, et al. Similar pleural fluid findings in pleuropulmonary tularemia and tuberculous pleurisy. *Chest.* 1996;109:572-575.
84. Syrjälä H, Karvonen J, Salminen A. Skin manifestations of tularemia: a study of 88 cases in northern Finland during 16 years (1967-1983). *Acta Derm Venereol.* 1984;64:513-516.
85. Ruiz AI, Gonzalez A, Miranda A, et al. Sweet's syndrome associated with *Francisella tularensis* infection. *Int J Dermatol.* 2001;40:791-793.
86. Mailman TL, Schmidt MH. *Francisella philomiragia* adenitis and pulmonary nodules in a child with chronic granulomatous disease. *Can J Infect Dis Med Microbiol.* 2005;16:245-248.
87. Tancik CA, Dillaha JA. *Francisella tularensis* endocarditis. *Clin Infect Dis.* 2000;30:399-400.
88. Cooper CL, Van Caeseele P, Canvin J, et al. Chronic prosthetic device infection with *Francisella tularensis*. *Clin Infect Dis.* 1999;29:1589-1591.
89. Han XY, Ho LX, Safdar A. *Francisella tularensis* peritonitis in stomach cancer patient. *Emerg Infect Dis.* 2004;10:2238-2240.
89a. Hofinger DM, Cardona L, Mertz GJ, et al. Tularemic meningitis in the United States. *Arch Neurol.* 2009;66:523-527.
90. Gangat N. Cerebral abscesses complicating tularemia meningitis. *Scand J Infect Dis.* 2007;39:258-261.
91. Tärnvik A, Chu MC. New approaches to diagnosis and therapy of tularemia. *Ann N Y Acad Sci.* 2007;1105:378-404.
92. Eliasson H, Olcen P, Sjöstedt A, et al. Kinetics of the immune response associated with tularemia: comparison of an enzyme-linked immunosorbent assay, a tube agglutination test, and a novel whole-blood lymphocyte stimulation test. *Clin Vaccine Immunol.* 2008;15:1238-1243.
93. Andersson H, Hartmanova B, Bäck E, et al. Transcriptional profiling of the peripheral blood response during tularemia. *Genes Immun.* 2006;7:503-513.
94. Hassoun A, Spera R, Dunkel J. Tularemia and once-daily gentamicin. *Antimicrob Agents Chemother.* 2006;50:824.
95. Pittman T, Williams D, Friedman AD. A shunt infection caused by *Francisella tularensis*. *Pediatr Neurosurg.* 1996;24:50-51.
96. Urich SK, Petersen JM. In vitro susceptibility of isolates of *Francisella tularensis* types A and B from North America. *Antimicrob Agents Chemother.* 2008;52:2276-2278.
97. Cross JT, Jacobs RF. Tularemia: treatment failures with outpatient use of ceftriaxone. *Clin Infect Dis.* 1993;17:976-980.
98. Maurin M, Mersali NF, Raoult D. Bactericidal activities of antibiotics against intracellular *Francisella tularensis*. *Antimicrob Agents Chemother.* 2000;44:3428-3431.
99. Harrell Jr RE, Simmons HF. Pleuropulmonary tularemia: successful treatment with erythromycin. *South Med J.* 1990;83: 1363-1364.
100. Ikäheimo I, Syrjälä H, Karhukorpi J, et al. In vitro antibiotic susceptibility of *Francisella tularensis* isolated from humans and animals. *J Antimicrob Chemother.* 2000;46:287-290.
101. Meric M, Willke A, Finke EJ, et al. Evaluation of clinical, laboratory, and therapeutic features of 145 tularemia cases: the role of quinolones in oropharyngeal tularemia. *APMIS.* 2008;116: 66-73.
102. Eliasson H, Broman T, Forsman M, et al. Tularemia: current epidemiology and disease management. *Infect Dis Clin North Am.* 2006;20:289-311.
103. Johansson A, Berglund L, Gothefors L, et al. Ciprofloxacin for treatment of tularemia in children. *Pediatr Infect Dis J.* 2000; 19:449-453.
104. Friis-Møller A, Lemming LE, Valerius NH, et al. Problems in identification of *Francisella philomiragia* associated with fatal bacteremia in a patient with chronic granulomatous disease. *J Clin Microbiol.* 2004;42:1840-1842.
105. Lu Z, Roche MI, Hui JH, et al. Generation and characterization of hybridoma antibodies for immunotherapy of tularemia. *Immunol Lett.* 2007;112:92-103.
106. Dennis DT, Inglesby TV, Henderson DA, et al. Tularemia as a biological weapon: medical and public health management. *JAMA.* 2001;285:2763-2773.
107. Conlan JW, Oyston PC. Vaccines against *Francisella tularensis*. *Ann N Y Acad Sci.* 2007;1105:325-350.
108. Hepburn MJ, Purcell BK, Lawler JV, et al. Live vaccine strain *Francisella tularensis* is detectable at the inoculation site but not in blood after vaccination against tularemia. *Clin Infect Dis.* 2006;43:711-716.
109. Pasetti MF, Cuberos L, Horn TL, et al. An improved *Francisella tularensis* live vaccine strain (LVS) is well tolerated and highly immunogenic when administered to rabbits in escalating doses using various immunization routes. *Vaccine.* 2008;26:1773-1785.
110. McMurry JA, Gregory SH, Moise L, et al. Diversity of *Francisella tularensis* Schu4 antigens recognized by T lymphocytes after natural infections in humans: identification of candidate epitopes for inclusion in a rationally designed tularemia vaccine. *Vaccine.* 2007;25:3179-3191.
111. Huntley JF, Conley PG, Rasko DA, et al. Native outer membrane proteins protect mice against pulmonary challenge with virulent type A *Francisella tularensis*. *Infect Immun.* 2008;76:3664-3671.
112. KuoLee R, Harris G, Conlan JW, et al. Oral immunization of mice with the live vaccine strain (LVS) of *Francisella tularensis* protects mice against respiratory challenge with virulent type A *F. tularensis*. *Vaccine.* 2007;25:3781-3791.
113. Baron SD, Singh R, Metzger DW. Inactivated *Francisella tularensis* live vaccine strain protects against respiratory tularemia by intranasal vaccination in an immunoglobulin A-dependent fashion. *Infect Immun.* 2007;75:2152-2162.
114. Rawool DB, Bitsaktsis C, Li Y, et al. Utilization of Fc receptors as a mucosal vaccine strategy against an intracellular bacterium, *Francisella tularensis*. *J Immunol.* 2008;180:5548-5557.

228

Pasteurella Species

JOHN J. ZURLO

Pasteurella are gram-negative coccobacilli that inhabit the oral cavity and gastrointestinal tract of many animals and cause various infectious problems, including septicemia and pneumonia. In humans, infection is most often caused by dog and cat bites resulting in cellulitis, subcutaneous abscesses, and a number of other syndromes. Bacteria belonging to the genus *Pasteurella* were first isolated from birds with cholera in 1878; they were characterized 2 years later by Pasteur. In 1886, Hueppe speciated the organism, *Bacterium septicemia haemorrhagica*, as the cause of hemorrhagic septicemia in animals. The first human case of *Pasteurella* infection, a case of puerperal sepsis, was described by Brugnatelli in 1913. The isolation of *Pasteurella multocida* from an infection occurring after a cat bite was first described in 1930. Subsequently, as additional isolates were recovered and characterized, related species were grouped together, first as *Pasteurella septica*, and then by the late 1930s as the *P. multocida* group. The complete genome of *P. multocida* was sequenced in 2001, offering an opportunity to elucidate the mechanisms of pathogenicity more accurately.[1]

Description of the Pathogen

The family Pasteurellaceae includes the genera *Pasteurella*, *Haemophilus*, and *Actinobacillus*.[2] Based on the genomic sequence, it appears that *Pasteurella* and *Haemophilus* diverged approximately 270 million years ago.[1] DNA hybridization separates the *Pasteurella* species into two groups: (1) *Pasteurella sensu stricto*; and (2) *Pasteurella*-related species, with the latter more closely related to *Haemophilus* and *Actinobacillus*[2] (Table 228-1). Species of the genus *Pasteurella* are nonmotile, facultatively anaerobic, gram-negative coccobacilli measuring 1 to 2 μm in length. Organisms grow in culture on a variety of commercial media, including sheep blood and chocolate agar, but not usually on Mac-Conkey agar media. They are fastidious and can be difficult to isolate and identify from nonsterile specimens such as sputum. Most strains are catalase-, oxidase-, and indole-positive and produce acid from sucrose. The most common human isolates belong to the *P. multocida* group and appear as smooth, iridescent, blue colonies on growth media. Encapsulated isolates typically appear mucoid. Strain differences of *P. multocida* have been identified on the basis of capsular antigens that define five serogroups (A, B, D, E, F) and somatic antigens that define sixteen serotypes (1 to 16).[3] Because of their sometimes fastidious nature, specific guidelines for methodologies to accurately determine minimal inhibitory concentrations (MICs) of *Pasteurella* species have been published.[4]

Epidemiology

Based on case reports and case series of infected patients, *Pasteurella* spp., particularly *P. multocida*, appear to have a worldwide distribution. For most *Pasteurella* spp., the principal reservoir is in animals. *P. multocida* has been isolated from the upper respiratory tracts of a variety of animals, including dogs, cats and other felines, pigs, and a wide variety of domestic and wild animals. Dogs and cats have particularly high colonization rates. In most cases, carriage is asymptomatic, although both upper and lower respiratory tract infections and septicemia are well known to occur in animals.[5] Although the reservoirs of most of the non-*multocida* species (*P. canis*, *P. stomatis*, *P. dagmatis*, *P. aerogenes*, and *P. pneumotropica*) are likely animal, notable is *Pasteurella bettyae*, a cause of neonatal infection and genitourinary infection in adults, whose reservoir is not well defined.[6] Respiratory tract colonization by *P. multocida* in humans is well known to occur. In most cases, colonized patients have underlying upper or lower respiratory tract diseases including chronic sinusitis, chronic obstructive pulmonary disease (COPD), or bronchiectasis.[7-9] Most colonized patients have a history of household or domesticated animal contact.[7,10,11]

Broadly speaking, human infection with *Pasteurella* can be divided into three types: infection occurring after animal bites, usually from dogs or cats; infection occurring after other animal exposures; and infection with no known animal contact. Infection after animal bites is the most commonly reported clinical setting for the organism (see Chapter 319).[7,11,12,13-18]

Among animal bites, dog bites are most common, followed by cat bites. Approximately 15% to 20% of dog bite wounds and more than 50% of cat bite wounds become infected.[11,16] The higher incidence of infection after cat bites probably results from the fact that cat teeth are thinner and more commonly result in puncture wounds, which are known to carry a higher risk of infection. For dog bite infections, *Staphylococcus aureus* and streptococcal species are the most commonly isolated pathogens, with *Pasteurella* and other organisms next in frequency.[14,17] For cat bite infections, *Pasteurella* spp. are the most common pathogens.[17,19] Francis and associates, studying bite-related *P. multocida* infections in Oregon between 1962 and 1972, noted that 76% were the result of cat bites and the remaining 24% were from dog bites.[15] The difference in incidence of *Pasteurella* infections in dog and cat bites may reflect the higher rate of upper respiratory colonization in cats. *Pasteurella* infections also have been reported after bites from a variety of other animals, including pigs, rats, lions, opossums, and rabbits.[18] In addition to bites, *Pasteurella* infections also have been reported after dog and cat scratches and from the licking of open wounds by these animals.[12]

Pasteurella infections are well known to develop in patients exposed to animals but without a history of bites or scratches. These include skin and soft tissue infections, bone and joint infections, pneumonia, meningitis, endocarditis, and septicemia.[11,20] Persons at risk for infection from animal exposure include veterinarians, farmers, livestock handlers, pet owners, and food handlers. Although the mode of infection in most reported cases is not clear, most have been presumed to result from inadvertent direct inoculation of organisms or from upper respiratory tract colonization, with subsequent dissemination to the target organ or organs.

In a significant proportion of *Pasteurella* cases, no known animal exposure or contact can be identified. In 1970, Hubbert and associates reviewed what was then the world's literature; they identified 72 reported cases of *P. multocida* infection unrelated to bites and described 136 additional cases.[20] In 16% of the reviewed cases and 31% of their additional cases, no animal exposure or contact could be identified. Once again, the spectrum of infectious complications was wide, similar to that described for patients with nonbite animal exposures. Vertical transmission of *P. multocida* has been described rarely.[21]

Pathogenesis

Despite the fact that *Pasteurella* species have long been established as human pathogens, the precise mechanisms of pathogenicity remain uncertain. In animals, virulent *P. multocida* strains adhere to mucosal epithelial cells in the upper respiratory tract, particularly in the tonsils, and in some cases mediated by fimbriae.[22] Several virulence factors have been described in *Pasteurella* spp. Much attention has focused on

Pasteurella senso stricto	Pasteurella-*related Species*
P. multocida	*P. aerogenes*
Subspecies *multocida*	*P. bettyae*
Subspecies *septicum*	*P. caballi*
Subspecies *gallicida*	*P. pneumotropica*
P. canis	*P. trehalosi*
P. dagmatis	*Mannheimia haemolytica*
P. stomatis	
Avibacterium gallinarum	

Data from Murray PR, Baron EJ, Jorgensen JH, et al, eds. *Manual of Clinical Microbiology*, 9th ed. Washington, DC: ASM Press; 2007;621-623.

Pasteurella multocida toxin (PMT). PMT is a potent mitogen that has been shown to activate a number of intracellular signaling cascades, resulting in a multitude of deleterious effects.[23] Specifically PMT has been shown to inhibit the migratory response of dendritic cells, thereby impairing immune surveillance.[24] Along with ToxA protein, also produced by *P. multocida*, PMT is associated with progressive atrophic rhinitis in pigs.[25] In addition, most virulent *Pasteurella* strains produce polysaccharide capsules that confer many possible mechanisms of pathogenicity, including resistance to desiccation, promotion of adherence, and resistance to phagocytosis and complement-mediated killing.[26] Finally, binding of transferrin by some pathogenic *Pasteurella* strains has been demonstrated and may be a mechanism used by the bacteria to ensure an iron supply necessary for growth.[27] Indeed, based on the genomic sequence data 2.5% of the entire genome encodes for proteins involved in iron acquisition.[1]

The humoral response to *P. multocida* infection has been characterized. Antibodies to somatic and capsular antigenic determinants develop within 2 weeks after clinical infection. Capsular antibodies are more long-lasting than somatic antibodies.[28] The precise role for such antibodies in host defense in humans is not clear.

Clinical Manifestations

Most reported *Pasteurella* infections in humans are caused by *P. multocida* and involve skin and soft tissues. However, even though subspecies *septica* has been shown to cause skin and soft tissue infections almost exclusively, subspecies *multocida* also has been found to cause bacteremia and pneumonia.[29] Other species have been described much less commonly[12] (Table 228-2). Beyond skin and soft tissues, other sites of infection are uncommon and have been the subject of individual case reports or small case series.

SKIN AND SOFT TISSUE INFECTIONS

Infections of skin and soft tissues most commonly develop after a bite or scratch. Less commonly, infections develop after a dog or cat has licked an open wound. Inflammation, swelling, and tenderness develop at the site of injury, usually within 24 hours from the time of exposure.[11,13,15] Regional lymphadenopathy occurs in 30% to 40% of cases. Wound discharge, ranging from serosanguineous to frankly purulent, has been noted in 21% to 39% of cases; fever develops in approximately 20%. Anatomically, more than 50% of cases of infection from both dog and cat bites occur in the upper extremities, followed by the lower extremities, head, face, and neck; multiple sites of infection are sometimes evident.[15,18] Abscesses and tenosynovitis are the most frequent complications of *Pasteurella* soft tissue infection, with septic arthritis and osteomyelitis being less common. Bacteremia is rare. Weber and colleagues noted an overall complication rate of 39% among 23 patients studied.[11] In a large study analyzing bacterial species isolated from wounds inflicted by dog and cat bites, *P. canis* was the most common isolate from dog bites, whereas *P. multocida* subsp. *multocida* and subsp. *septicum* were the most common from cat bites.[30]

BONE AND JOINT INFECTIONS

Bone and joint infections with *Pasteurella* species have been reported uncommonly. These infections take three different forms—septic arthritis, osteomyelitis, and combined arthritis and osteomyelitis. Ewing and associates have reported 2 cases each of septic arthritis and osteomyelitis caused by *P. multocida* and reviewed the literature.[31] Among 14 cases of septic arthritis reported and reviewed, 7 (50%) involved dog or cat bites or scratches, 5 (36%) involved animal exposure without recent or known bites or scratches, and in the remaining 2 cases there were no reported animal exposures. The knee was the most common joint involved (11 cases), often in the setting of rheumatoid arthritis, osteoarthritis, or joint prosthesis. Five of the 14 patients were receiving prednisone. Osteomyelitis developed as the result of direct extension of soft tissue inflammation or by direct inoculation of the periosteum at the time of the bite. Among 13 cases of osteomyelitis reported, 9 (69%) involved animal bites or scratches, 1 (8%) involved animal exposure, and in 3 cases there was no reported exposure. In contrast with septic arthritis, most cases (69%) of osteomyelitis developed in an upper extremity bone, usually the hand or wrist. Also unlike septic arthritis, chronic medical conditions and corticosteroid therapy were not common antecedents. Finally, among 7 cases of combined septic arthritis and osteomyelitis, 6 involved bones and joints of the upper extremities, usually a phalanx and interphalangeal joint infected after a cat bite. Prosthetic joint infections caused by *P. multocida* have been reported infrequently, often in patients with rheumatoid arthritis receiving corticosteroids.[32]

CENTRAL NERVOUS SYSTEM INFECTIONS

Central nervous system infections with *P. multocida* have been reported infrequently. Meningitis is most common. There have been rare cases of focal lesions, such as brain abscess and subdural empyema.[11] Of 29 cases of meningitis reported in the English language literature through 1999, most patients had animal contact, usually licking of mucosa or nonintact skin. Bacteremia was seen in nearly two thirds of patients. Mortality was 25% overall, with decreasing mortality among later cases.[33]

SEPTICEMIA AND ENDOCARDITIS

Septicemia is another uncommon complication of *Pasteurella* infection. Two reviews of *Pasteurella* septicemia have reported that most patients have a primary source of infection (e.g., cellulitis, arthritis, meningitis, pneumonia, peritonitis) and most have had an underlying medical condition, with cirrhosis being most common, and a correspondingly high mortality. Most cases involved animal trauma or exposures.[34,35] Infective endocarditis has been reported much less frequently than septicemia. Saleh and co-workers have reported a case of "*Pasteurella gallinarum*" infectious endocarditis in an adolescent 10 years after surgery to correct a truncus arteriosus.[36] They found 17 other cases of *Pasteurella* infectious endocarditis in the medical literature caused by many different *Pasteurella* spp. In almost 50% of cases, no preexisting heart disease was evident. Also, no animal contact was evident in 11 cases. Rare cases of prosthetic valve endocarditis with *Pasteurella* species have been reported.[37]

RESPIRATORY TRACT INFECTIONS

Respiratory tract infections with *Pasteurella* spp. involve the upper respiratory tract, causing sinusitis and bronchitis, and the lower respiratory tract, causing both pneumonia and empyema. The respiratory tract is second only to skin and soft tissue in frequency of clinical isolation of *Pasteurella*. *P. multocida* subsp. *multocida* has been reported to be the most common *Pasteurella* spp. to cause respiratory tract infections.[29,38] As noted, asymptomatic *Pasteurella* colonization of the upper respiratory tract has been reported in patients with underlying respiratory tract disease, including chronic obstructive pulmonary disease

TABLE
228-2

Clinical Characteristics of 159 Strains of *Pasteurella* Species Isolated from 146 Infected Humans over a 3-Year Period

Species	N	Wound Infections or Abscesses*	Blood	Cerebrospinal Fluid	Other
P. multocida subsp. *multocida*	95	85	5	1	4[†]
P. multocida subsp. *septica*	21	20		1	
P. canis	28	28			
P. stomatis	10	10[‡]			
P. dagmatis	5	2[§]			3[¶]

*Caused by dog or cat bites, or wounds licked by dogs or cats.
[†]Includes three cases of infection from cut wounds unassociated with any known animal contact.
[‡]In eight cases of wound infection, *P. multocida* subsp. *multocida* was also recovered.
[§]In cases of wound abscesses, *P. multocida* subsp. *multocida* and *P. canis* were also recovered.
[¶]One case each of severe cellulitis, groin abscess, throat abscess.
Adapted from Holst E, Rollof J, Larsson L, et al. Characterization and distribution of *Pasteurella* species recovered from infected humans. *J Clin Microbiol.* 1992;30:2984-2987.

and bronchiectasis. Presumably for a subset of this patient group, the organism invades and causes disease. There is nothing clinically distinguishing about upper respiratory tract infections. Pneumonia usually occurs in patients with underlying lung disease and is usually lobar, with a short prodrome. Cases of multilobar and diffuse pulmonary involvement have been described.[11] *Pasteurella* empyema was the subject of a case report and review of the literature by Nelson and Hammer.[39] Most of the 14 patients were adults with a mean age of 70 years, and most had underlying pulmonary disease, either COPD or bronchiectasis. Although respiratory and constitutional complaints were the dominant presenting symptoms, fever was surprisingly uncommon. Pleural fluid was described as purulent in all patients from whom a sample was obtained.

INTRA-ABDOMINAL INFECTIONS

Of the few reported cases of *Pasteurella* intra-abdominal infections, spontaneous bacterial peritonitis and appendicitis, with or without associated peritonitis, have been the most frequent clinical syndromes. Among the reported cases of spontaneous bacterial peritonitis, almost all have had cirrhosis (usually alcoholic) and preexisting ascites.[40] Raffi and associates reported three cases of *P. multocida* appendiceal peritonitis and identified eight additional well-documented cases of appendicitis in the literature.[41] Accompanying peritonitis was variably present. It was postulated that the source of the organism was most likely from oropharyngeal colonization. Fourteen cases of peritonitis have been reported in association with peritoneal dialysis. Cats were the presumed source in all patients, and poor animal hygiene was thought to be the likely cause of infection.[42]

OTHER *PASTEURELLA* INFECTIONS

Infections of other sites with *Pasteurella* species have been reported rarely and include the genitourinary tract,[20,43] epiglottitis,[44] and endophthalmitis.[11,45] *Pasteurella* infections also have been reported in patients with a variety of immune deficiencies including bronchitis in a patient with Sweet's syndrome,[46] fatal sepsis in a patient with hairy cell leukemia,[47] cellulitis with bacteremia in a neutropenic host,[48] and malacoplakia in a patient with acquired immunodeficiency syndrome (AIDS).[49]

■ Treatment, Prevention, and Prognosis

Several decades of clinical experience with *Pasteurella* and numerous in vitro studies have indicated that penicillin is the best antimicrobial

agent for the treatment of virtually all forms of infection.[7,11,15] Penicillins with good in vitro activity include penicillin G, penicillin V, ampicillin, amoxicillin, and amoxicillin–clavulanic acid.[50] Antistaphylococcal penicillins including oxacillin, nafcillin, dicloxacillin, and cloxacillin are not as active and are not recommended for treatment of documented *Pasteurella* infections.[51] Many cephalosporins demonstrate in vitro activity against *P. multocida*. In general, activity increases with later generation cephalosporins. Goldstein and associates have reported high minimal inhibitory MICs for cephalexin, cefaclor, and cefadroxil and recommended that they not be used for treatment of documented infections.[51] The oral cephalosporins, cefuroxime and cefixime, along with parenteral agents, including ceftriaxone and cefoperazone, demonstrate excellent in vitro activity and are probably good substitutes for penicillin.[52]

Plasmid-mediated β-lactamase production has been described in *P. multocida* strains isolated from animals. At least five human cases of *Pasteurella* infection caused by β-lactamase-producing strains have been reported. All patients had pulmonary disease.[53] Among non–β-lactam antibiotics, agents with in vitro activity include tetracyclines, fluoroquinolones, macrolides, trimethoprim-sulfamethoxazole, and chloramphenicol.[50,51,54,55] A fluoroquinolone, doxycycline, or trimethoprim-sulfamethoxazole should be considered as an alternative for patients with intolerance to β-lactams. Aminoglycosides have moderate to poor activity in vitro and probably should not be used, particularly given the paucity of clinical experience. Clindamycin and erythromycin consistently demonstrate high MICs in vitro and are not recommended. The newer long-acting macrolides such as azithromycin appear to have better activity but should be used with caution because clinical experience with these agents is limited.[55]

Because animal bite wound infections are frequently polymicrobial and may include *S. aureus*, streptococcal species, and anaerobes in addition to *Pasteurella*, empirical antibiotic therapy should be directed at these organisms until or unless wound cultures define the specific bacteriology of the infection.[17] Outpatient treatment of documented, uncomplicated *Pasteurella* cellulitis can be undertaken with penicillin VK, amoxicillin, or ampicillin, with close follow-up.[11] Duration of therapy is not well defined, but 10 to 14 days is probably a reasonable time course. Patients with evidence of involvement of deeper structures (e.g., tenosynovitis, arthritis) should be hospitalized and treated parenterally, with β-lactam–β-lactamase combinations being the treatment of choice until the microbiology is defined. Drainage and débridement may be necessary for patients who have progressive infection with extensive suppuration.

Treatment of septic arthritis should consist of antimicrobial therapy along with frequent drainage of the involved joints.[31] Most patients recover fully. Similarly, the outcome for osteomyelitis appears to be good, although débridement in addition to antimicrobial therapy is often needed. The outcome of septic arthritis with osteomyelitis is not as good, with residual deformity and loss of function being common. For all bone and joint *Pasteurella* infections, antimicrobial therapy should be continued for 4 to 6 weeks.

Patients with other end-organ forms of *Pasteurella* infection do poorly overall. High mortality has been reported for most of these cases. For patients with bacteremia without endovascular infection, the mortality rate is high, probably as a result of the infection itself combined with the underlying medical problem, usually alcoholic cirrhosis. For endocarditis, among 17 reported patients, 5 died and 4 required valve replacement.[36] For patients with pneumonia, morbidity and mortality are high, almost certainly as a result of severe underlying pulmonary disease. Finally, patients with spontaneous bacterial peritonitis have an extremely high mortality rate, whereas those with appendicitis, with or without peritonitis, generally do well.[40,41]

The use of antimicrobial prophylaxis for patients presenting with animal bites shortly after the injury that are not obviously infected is controversial. Many experts recommend antibiotic treatment for crush injuries (especially when edema is obvious), hand wounds, or wounds immediately adjacent to bones or joints. Although a few small trials have been completed, none has been large enough or seen enough patients to reach significant end points to determine the efficacy of such therapy unequivocally. Amoxicillin–clavulanic acid is a commonly used agent that has activity against *S. aureus*, streptococci, anaerobes, and *Pasteurella*. The combination of cefuroxime or doxycycline, or a fluoroquinolone or trimethoprim-sulfamethoxazole, plus either metronidazole or clindamycin should be alternatives for patients with serious penicillin allergies. Courses of 3 to 5 days are usually recommended.[56]

REFERENCES

1. May BJ, Zhang Q, Li LL, et al. Complete genomic sequence of *Pasteurella multocida*, Pm70. *Proc Natl Acad Sci U S A.* 2001;98:3460-3465.
2. von Graevenitz A, Zbinden R, Mutters R. *Actinobacillus, Capnocytophaga, Eikenella, Kingella, Pasteurella*, and other fastidious or rarely encountered gram-negative rods. In: Murray PR, Baron EJ, Jorgensen JH, et al, eds. *Manual of Clinical Microbiology*, 9th ed. Washington DC: ASM Press; 2007;621-635.
3. Townsend KM, Boyce JD, Chung JY, et al. Genetic organization of *Pasteurella multocida* cap loci and development of a multiplex capsular typing system. *J Clin Microbiol.* 2001;39:924-929.
4. Jorgensen JH, Hindler JF. New consensus guidelines from the clinical and laboratory standards institute for antimicrobial susceptibility testing of infrequently isolated or fastidious bacteria. *Clin Infect Dis.* 2007;44:280-286.
5. Carter GR. Pasteurellosis: *Pasteurella multocida* and *Pasteurella hemolytica. Adv Vet Sci.* 1967;11:321-379.
6. De Leon JP, Sandfort RF, Wong JD. *Pasteurella bettyae*: Report of nine cases and evidence of an emerging neonatal pathogen. *Clin Microbiol Newsletter.* 2000;22: 190-192.
7. Jones FL, Smull CE. Infections in man due to *Pasteurella multocida. Pa Med.* 1973;76:41-44.
8. Bartley EO. *Pasteurella septica* in chronic nasal sinusitis. *Lancet.* 1960;2:581-582.
9. Cawson RA, Talbot JM. The occurrence of *Pasteurella septica* (syn. *multocida*) in bronchiectasis. *J Clin Pathol.* 1955;8: 49-51.
10. Avril JL, Donnio PY, Pouedras P. Selective medium for *Pasteurella multocida* and its use to detect oropharyngeal carriage in pig breeders. *J Clin Microbiol.* 1990;28:1438-1440.
11. Weber DJ, Wolfson JS, Swartz MN, et al. *Pasteurella multocida* infections: Report of 34 cases and review of the literature. *Medicine (Baltimore).* 1984;63:133-154.
12. Holst E, Rollof J, Larsson L, et al. Characterization and distribution of *Pasteurella* species recovered from infected humans. *J Clin Microbiol.* 1992;30:2984-2987.
13. Arons MS, Fernando L, Polayes IM. *Pasteurella multocida*: The major cause of hand infections following domestic animal bites. *J Hand Surg [Am].* 1982;7:47-52.
14. Brook I. Microbiology of human and animal bite wounds in children. *Pediatr Infect Dis J.* 1987;6:29-32.
15. Francis DP, Holmes MA, Brandon G. *Pasteurella multocida*: Infections after domestic animal bites and scratches. *JAMA.* 1975;233:42-45.
16. Dendle C, Looke D. Review article: animal bites: An update for management with a focus on infection. *Emerg Med Australasia.* 2008;20:458-467.
17. Goldstein EJC, Citron DM, Wield B, et al. Bacteriology of human and animal bite wounds. *J Clin Microbiol.* 1978;8:667-672.
18. Hubbert WT, Rosen MN. *Pasteurella multocida* infections. I. *Pasteurella multocida* infection due to animal bite. *Am J Public Health Nations Health.* 1970;60:1103-1108.
19. Westling K, Farra A, Cars B, et al. Cat bite wound infections: A prospective clinical and microbiological study at three emergency wards in Stockholm, Sweden. *J Infect.* 2006;53:403-407.
20. Hubbert WT, Rosen MN. *Pasteurella multocida* infections. II. *Pasteurella multocida* infection in man unrelated to animal bites. *Am J Public Health Nations Health.* 1970;60:1109-1117.
21. Zaramella P, Zamorani E, Freato F, et al. Neonatal meningitis due to a vertical transmission of *Pasteurella* multocida. *Pediatr Int.* 1999;41:307-310.
22. Pijoan C, Trigo F. Bacterial adhesion to mucosal surfaces with special reference to *Pasteurella multocida* isolates from atrophic rhinitis. *Can J Vet Res.* 1990;54(Suppl):S16-S21.
23. Orth JH, Lang S, Taniguchi M, et al. *Pasteurella multocida* toxin-induced activation of RhoA is mediated via two families of Gα proteins, Gαq and Gα12/13. *J Biol Chem.* 2005;280:36701-36707.
24. Blocker D, Berod L, Fluhr JW, et al. *Pasteurella multocida* toxin (PMT) activates RhoGTPases, induces actin polymerization and inhibits migration of human dendritic cells, but does not influence macropinocytosis. *Int Immunol.* 2006;18:459-464.
25. Lichtensteiger CA, Steenbergen SM, Lee RM, et al. Direct PCR analysis for toxigenic *Pasteurella multocida. J Clin Microbiol.* 1996;34:3035-3039.
26. Boyce JD, Chung JY, Adler B. *Pasteurella multocida* capsule: Composition, function and genetics. *J Biotechnol.* 2000; 83:153-160.
27. Schryvers AB, Gonzalez GC. Receptors for transferrin in pathogenic bacteria are specific for the host's protein. *Can J Microbiol.* 1990;36:145-147.
28. Choudat D, Paul G, Legoff C, et al. Specific antibody responses to *Pasteurella multocida. Scand J Infect Dis.* 1987;19:453-457.
29. Donnio PY, Lerestif-Gautier AL, Avril JL. Characterization of *Pasteurella* spp. strains isolated from human infections. *J Comp Pathol.* 2004;130:137-142.
30. Talan DA, Citron DM, Abrahamian FM, et al. Bacteriologic analysis of infected dog and cat bites. Emergency Medicine Animal Bite Infection Study Group. *N Engl J Med.* 1999;340:85-92.
31. Ewing R, Fainstein V, Musher DM, et al. Articular and skeletal infections caused by *Pasteurella multocida. South Med J.* 1980;73:1349-1352.
32. Maradona JA, Asensi V, Carton JA, et al. Prosthetic joint infection by *Pasteurella multocida. Eur J Clin Microbiol Infect Dis.* 1997;16:623-625.
33. Green BT, Ramsey KM, Nolan PE. *Pasteurella multocida* meningitis: Case report and review of the last 11 y. *Scand J Infect Dis.* 2002;34:213-217.
34. Raffi F, Barrier J, Baron D, et al. *Pasteurella multocida* bacteremia: Report of thirteen cases over twelve years and review of the literature. *Scand J Infect Dis.* 1987;19:385-393.
35. Kimura R, Hayashi Y, Takeuchi T, et al. *Pasteurella multocida* septicemia caused by close contact with a domestic cat: case report and literature review. *J Infect Chemother.* 2004;10:250-252.
36. Saleh MAF, Al-Madan MS, Erwa HH, et al. First case of human infection caused by *Pasteurella gallinarum* causing infective endocarditis in an adolescent 10 years after surgical correction for truncus arteriosus. *Pediatrics.* 1995;95:944-948.
37. Rosenbach KA, Poblete J, Larkin I. Prosthetic valve endocarditis cuased by Pasteurella dagmatis. *South Med J.* 2001;94: 1033-1035.
38. Chen HI, Hulten K, Clarridge JE 3rd. Taxonomic subgroups of *Pasteurella multocida* correlate with clinical presentation. *J Clin Microbiol.* 2002;40:3438-3441.
39. Nelson SC, Hammer GS. *Pasteurella multocida* empyema: Case report and review of the literature. *Am J Med Sci.* 1981;281:43-49.
40. Szpak CA, Woodard BH, White JO, et al. Bacterial peritonitis and bacteremia associated with *Pasteurella multocida. South Med J.* 1980;73:801-803.
41. Raffi F, David A, Mouzard A, et al. *Pasteurella multocida* appendiceal peritonitis: Report of three cases and review of the literature. *Pediatr Infect Dis.* 1986;5:695-698.
42. Antony SJ, Oglesby KA. Peritonitis associated with *Pasteurella multocida* in peritoneal dialysis patients–case report and review of the literature. *Clin Nephrol.* 2007;68:52-56.
43. Liu W, Chemaly RF, Tuohy MJ, et al. *Pasteurella multocida* urinary tract infection with molecular evidence of zoonotic transmission. *Clin Infect Dis.* 2003;36:E58-60.
44. Wine N, Lim Y, Fierer J. *Pasteurella multocida* epiglottitis. *Arch Otolaryngol Head Neck Surg.* 1997;123:759-761.
45. Dang Burgener NP, Baglivo E, Harbarth S, et al. *Pasteurella multocida* endophthalmitis: Case report and review of the literature. *Klin Monatsbl Augenheilkd.* 2005;222:231-233.
46. Boivin S, Segard M, Piette F, et al. Sweet syndrome associated with *Pasteurella multocida* bronchitis. *Arch Intern Med.* 2000;160:1869.
47. Athar MK, Karim MS, Mannam S, et al. Fatal *Pasteurella* sepsis and hairy-cell leukemia. *Am J Hematol.* 2003;72:285.
48. Gowda RV, Stout R. *Pasteurella multocida* infection in a postchemotherapy neutropenic host following cat exposure. *Clin Oncol (R Coll Radiol).* 2002;14:497-498.
49. Bastas A, Markou N, Botsi C, et al. Malakoplakia of the lung caused by *Pasteurella multocida* in a patient with AIDS. *Scand J Infect Dis.* 2002;34:536-538.
50. Goldstein EJC, Citron DM. Comparative activities of cefuroxime, amoxicillin-clavulanic acid, ciprofloxacin, enoxacin, ofloxacin against aerobic and anaerobic bacteria isolated from bite wounds. *Antimicrob Agents Chemother.* 1988;32:1143-1148.
51. Goldstein EJC, Citron DM, Richwald GA. Lack of in vitro efficacy of oral forms of certain cephalosporins, erythromycin, and oxacillin against *Pasteurella multocida. Antimicrob Agents Chemother.* 1988;32:213-225.
52. Noel GJ, Teele DW. In vitro activities of selected new and long-acting cephalosporins against *Pasteurella multocida. Antimicrob Agents Chemother.* 1986;29:344-345.
53. Lion C, Lozniewski A, Rosner V, et al. Lung abscess due to beta-lactamase-producing *Pasteurella multocida. Clin Infect Dis.* 1999;29:1345-1346.
54. Goldstein EJC, Citron DM, Merriam CV, et al. Activity of gatifloxacin compared to those of five other quinolones versus aerobic and anaerobic isolates from skin and soft tissue samples of human and animal bite wound infections. *Antimicrob Agents Chemother.* 1999;43:1475-1479.
55. Citron DM, Warren YA, Fernandez HT, et al. Broth microdilution and disk diffusion tests for susceptibility testing of *Pasteurella* species isolated from human clinical specimens. *J Clin Microbiol.* 2005;43:2485-2488.
56. Stevens DL, Bisno AL, Chambers HF, et al. Practice guidelines for the diagnosis and management of skin and soft-tissue infections. *Clin Infect Dis.* 2005;41:1373-1406.

229

Yersinia Species, Including Plague

DAVID T. DENNIS | PAUL S. MEAD

The genus *Yersinia* includes 11 species, 3 of which are important human pathogens: *Yersinia pestis, Yersinia enterocolitica,* and *Yersinia pseudotuberculosis.* The yersinioses are zoonotic infections of rodents, pigs, birds, and other domestic and wild animals; humans are considered incidental hosts that do not contribute to the natural disease cycle. *Y. pestis* causes plague and is transmitted by fleas. The most common clinical manifestation of plague is acute febrile lymphadenitis, called bubonic plague. Less common forms include septicemic, pneumonic, pharyngeal, and meningeal plague. Although life-threatening, plague can respond promptly to treatment with appropriate antimicrobials. *Y. enterocolitica* and *Y. pseudotuberculosis* typically produce an enteric infection with fever, diarrhea, and abdominal pain that can mimic acute appendicitis. Common pathologic lesions of the enteric yersinioses are acute enteritis and mesenteric lymphadenitis.

Yersinia pestis

HISTORY

Plague is a highly virulent disease credited with changing human history in ways both large and small.[1] Primarily an infection of rodents and their fleas, plague has repeatedly spread to humans, causing at least three major pandemics. The first pandemic, or Justinian Plague, originated in central Africa and affected much of the Mediterranean basin during the sixth-century Byzantine Empire. The second pandemic began in 1347 and spread rapidly throughout Europe, killing an estimated one fourth of the population. So quickly did the "Black Death" advance that some have questioned whether it was actually caused by *Y. pestis.*[2] Amplification of *Y. pestis* DNA from the dental pulp of skeletons dating from the 6th and 18th centuries,[3,4] coupled with new information on transmission mechanisms,[5] provides strong support for plague as the cause of both pandemics.

The third, or modern, pandemic began in China in the 1860s. By 1894, it had spread to Hong Kong, where Alexandre Yersin isolated the causative agent. Over the ensuing 20 years, *Y. pestis* was spread by rats on steamships to port cities on all inhabited continents, including North America. Rat-associated plague was soon brought under control in most urban areas; however, the infection spread to various species of wild rodents, becoming entrenched in rural areas of the Americas, Africa, and Asia (Fig. 229-1). In the first half of the 20th century, India was most severely affected by plague epidemics, with more than 20 million cases and 10 million deaths. In the 1960s and 1970s, war-torn Vietnam became the country most affected by plague, reporting thousands of cases annually.[6] Plague has recently resurged in the nations of sub-Saharan Africa and the adjacent island of Madagascar,[7,8] areas that now account for more than 95% of cases reported to the World Health Organization.[8]

Y. pestis was developed as an aerosol weapon during the Cold War, and its potential for misuse by terrorists is considered an important national security threat requiring special measures for medical and public health preparedness[9] (see Chapter 322). The plague bacillus is designated a category A select biologic agent whose handling is regulated by federal law.[10]

DESCRIPTION OF THE PATHOGEN

Y. pestis is a gram-negative coccobacillus that exhibits bipolar-staining with Giemsa, Wright's, or Wayson staining. A member of the Entero-

bacteriaceae,[1] it grows aerobically on most culture media, including blood agar and MacConkey agar. It also grows well in nutrient broths, such as brain-heart infusion broth. Cultures grow more slowly than most bacteria and optimally at 28°C. Small colonies are visible on MacConkey agar after 24 to 48 hours of incubation at 35°C. On triple-sugar-iron agar, *Y. pestis* produces an alkaline slant and an acid butt. It is nonmotile and non–spore forming, does not ferment lactose, and is citrate, urease, and indole negative.

Genomic studies indicate that *Y. pestis* evolved from the enteric pathogen *Y. pseudotuberculosis* as recently as 1500 to 20,000 years ago.[11] This transition from an enteric to a flea-borne pathogen was made possible by the acquisition of two unique plasmids, coupled with inactivation of genes required for survival in the mammalian gut.[12-14] The 110-kb plasmid (referred to as pMT1 or pFra) encodes a protein with phospholipase activity that is necessary for survival in the flea midgut, as well as the antiphagocytic fraction 1 (F1) envelope antigen (Table 229-1). These and other factors are differentially expressed at temperatures encountered in fleas and mammals, respectively. The 9.5-kb pPCP1 plasmid encodes a plasminogen activator protein (Pla protease) that is responsible for temperature-dependent coagulase and fibrinolysin activities. The origins of these plasmids remain uncertain; however, approximately half of the DNA sequences of the pFra plasmid are shared with a plasmid of *Salmonella* serotype *typhi.*[15] As with the other yersiniae, the plague bacillus also produces V and W antigens that confer a calcium requirement for growth at 37°C.[1] The expression of these antigens, mediated by an approximately 70-kb plasmid, is essential for virulence and plays a role in adapting the organism for intracellular survival and multiplication. Chromosome-mediated factors include a potent lipopolysaccharide endotoxin and a pigmentation factor, the hemin storage locus (*hms*), that regulates iron uptake and enables the bacteria to form blockages of the flea gut that enhance transmission.[12,13]

Three classic biovars of *Y. pestis,* Antiqua, Medievalis, and Orientalis, have been described based on the ability of isolates to ferment glycerol and convert nitrate to nitrite. It has been postulated that these phenotypes reflect strains associated with the first, second, and third pandemics, respectively. However, recent studies using a variety of molecular techniques suggest that *Y. pestis* isolates represent as many as eight genetically distinct populations that do not correlate entirely with biovar.[16] Furthermore, limited archeologic evidence suggests that all three pandemics were caused by strains of the Orientalis phenotype.[17]

EPIDEMIOLOGY

Sometimes viewed as a problem of the past, plague remains a threat in many parts of the world, especially rural Africa[8] (see Fig. 229-1). In the 15-year period from 1989 to 2003, 25 countries reported a total of 38,310 cases (average ~2500 cases per year) and 2845 deaths (7% fatality rate).[12] Madagascar, Tanzania, Democratic Republic of the Congo, Vietnam, Mozambique, Namibia, and Peru each accounted for more than 1000 cases. The potential for re-emergence of plague is underscored by the recent cases of human plague in Algeria, 50 years after the last occurrence.[18] In Madagascar, repeated outbreaks of rat-borne plague have occurred since 1990 in the port city of Mahajanga, as well as in rural areas of the central highlands.[19] In the United States, 415 cases of plague were reported from 1970 through 2007, with 59 deaths. Although wild rodent plague occurs in 17 of the contiguous western

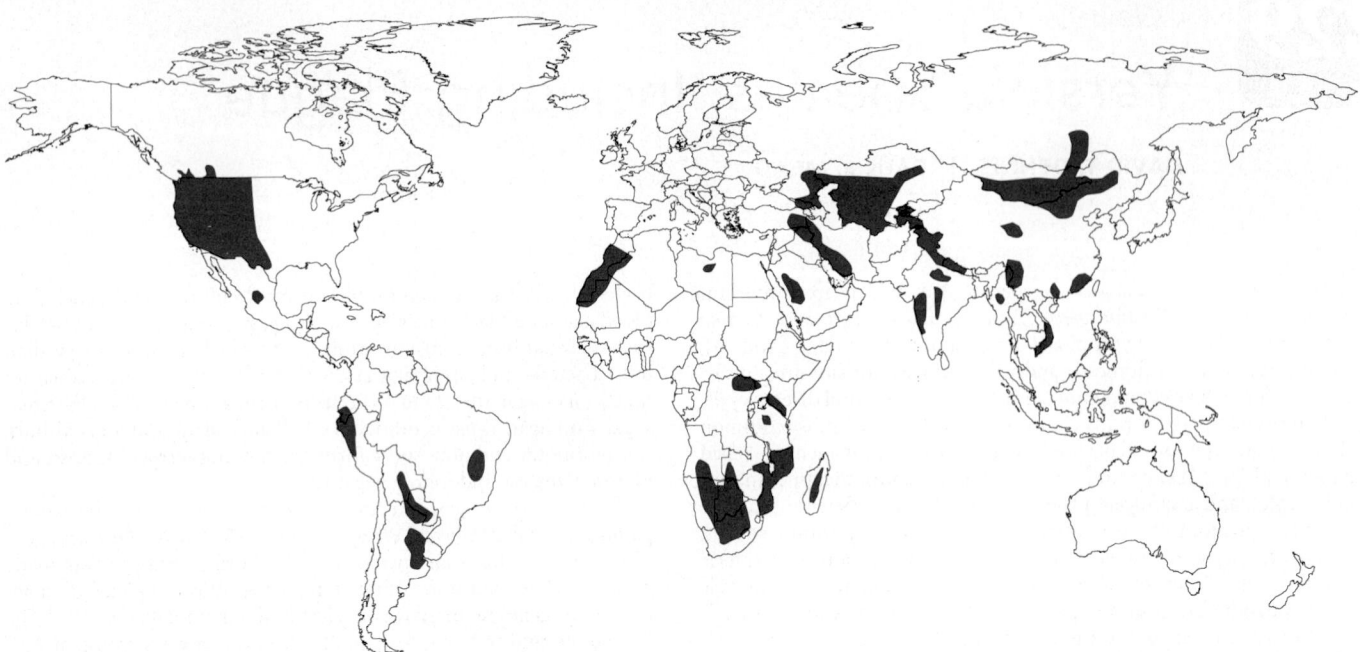

Figure 229-1 **Worldwide distribution of plague endemic areas.** *(Data compiled from the World Health Organization, Centers for Disease Control and Prevention, and other sources. From Centers for Disease Control and Prevention. Prevention of plague: recommendations of the Advisory Committee on Immunization Practices (ACIP). MMWR Recomm Rep. 1996;45:1-15.)*

TABLE 229-1	Key Virulence and Transmission Factors of *Yersinia pestis*	
Location	*Factor(s)*	*Putative Function*
pPCP1 plasmid (9.5 kb)	Plasminogen activator (Pla protease)	Protease: targeted activity at mammalian tissue barriers; adhesion: enhances invasion of mammalian cells; coagulase: promotes blockage of flea midgut
pCD1 plasmid (~70-75 kb)	*Yersinia* outer protein (Yop) virulon	Type III secretion system, inhibits phagocytosis and lymphocyte proliferation; transport of effector proteins to host cells
	V antigen	Facilitates intracellular survival; required for type III secretion system translocation pore
pMT1/pFra plasmid (~110 kb)	Fraction 1 antigen	Expressed at higher temperatures, creates capsule that interferes with phagocytosis
	Yersinia murine toxin (Ymt)	Phospholipase D activity upregulated at lower temperatures, necessary for colonization of flea midgut and blockage formation; toxic for mice and rats
Chromosome (4.6 Mb)	Hemin storage system (*hms*)	Proteins produced at lower temperatures; iron acquisition; colonization of flea proventriculus, biofilm production
	Yersiniabactin (Ybt) system	Siderophore; iron acquisition
	Yersinia Fe uptake system	ATP-binding cassette transport system; iron acquisition
	Lipopolysaccharide	Temperature-dependent remodeling of lipid A structure; prevents containment by mammalian immune response
	pH 6 fimbriae antigen (psa)	Blocks phagocytosis; pH dependent

Compiled from references 1, 12, and 14.

U.S. states extending from the Pacific Coast to the Great Plains, approximately 80% of human cases occur in New Mexico, Arizona, and Colorado, and approximately 10% in California (Fig. 229-2).[20] Since the early part of the 20th century, plague in the United States has shown clear patterns of spread from California eastward to the Great Plains states, and persons are increasingly exposed around their homes as development extends into natural settings. Plague arising in travelers (peripatetic plague) can present a diagnostic challenge and trigger concern about possible terrorist exposures.[21]

Plague is transmitted among its animal hosts through flea bites and less commonly by cannibalism or predation (Fig. 229-3). Throughout the world, the domestic rats *Rattus rattus* and *Rattus norvegicus* are considered the most dangerous reservoirs of plague, due in part to their close association with humans. The oriental rat flea *Xenopsylla cheopis* is a highly efficient vector and has long been credited as a principal source of transmission to humans. However, many other flea species can also transmit infection, and there is growing appreciation for the potential role of the human flea *Pulex irritans* as a bridging vector in regions of Africa.[22,23] Risk of spread of plague from rats to humans is positively correlated with the density of rats, the number of fleas per animal (flea index), and the *Y. pestis* infection rates in sampled rats and rat fleas.[24] In sylvatic plague foci, such as those in the western United States and the deserts, savannah, and steppes in other endemic regions, the important reservoirs are various burrowing rodents. Because humans do not contribute to the natural cycle of plague, they are considered "dead-end" hosts. Only when there are cases of pneumonic plague is the infection passed directly from person to person. Rarely, humans develop primary pneumonic plague after exposure to cats with respiratory infection.[25]

In the United States, males and females are equally affected by plague. More than half of cases occur in persons younger than 20 years of age. Although a majority of cases occur in whites, the incidence rate in endemic southwestern states is highest among Native Americans and Hispanics.[26] Within endemic areas, elevated plague risk is associated with close contact with rodents and their feline and canine predators, the presence of harborage and food sources for wild rodents in the vicinity of homes, and possibly a failure to control fleas on pet dogs

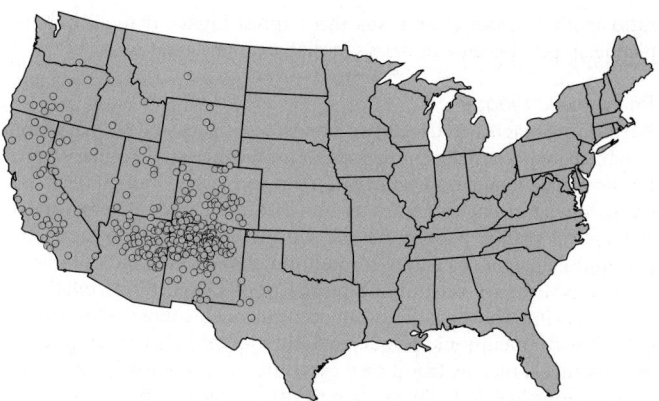

1 dot = 1 case randomly placed with county of exposure

Figure 229-2 Cases of plague in the western United States, 1970 to 2007. Each dot represents one case, with the dot placed randomly in the county of exposure. *(Map courtesy of the Centers for Disease Control and Prevention, Fort Collins, CO.)*

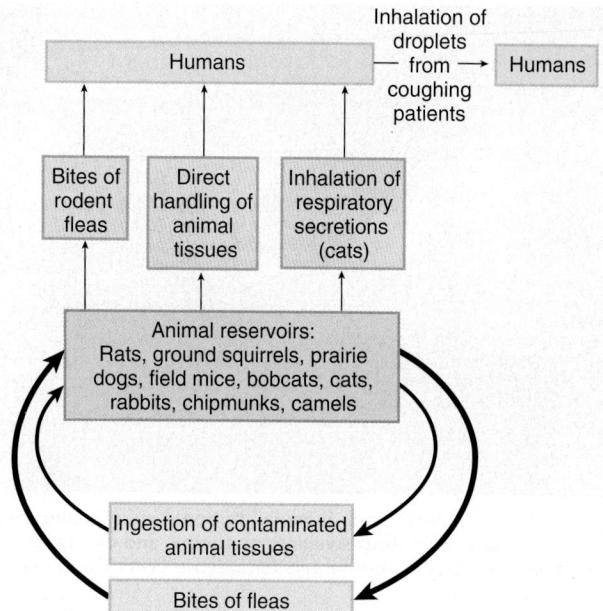

Figure 229-3 Transmission of plague. The *wide arrows* indicate common modes of transmission, the *medium arrows* indicate occasional modes of transmission, and the *thin arrow* indicates a rare kind of transmission.

and cats.[27] Sleeping with pets may increase the risk of infection.[28] Most human cases occur during May through October, when plague-bearing rodents and their fleas are most numerous and active and when people are more likely to be outdoors and exposed to natural cycles of infection.

PATHOGENESIS

Fleas become infected by feeding on a bacteremic host. In the ambient-temperature environment of the flea, transmission factors are expressed that allow the bacillus to colonize the flea midgut, replicate, and create a blockage of the flea intestine.[14] Starved of sustenance, "blocked" fleas feed aggressively, regurgitating bacteria into the bite wound at each attempt. The inoculated bacteria express very little F1 antigen, and most are likely phagocytized and killed by polymorphonuclear leukocytes. However, a few bacteria may be taken up by mononuclear cells unable to kill them.[12] Growing now at 37° C, the bacteria multiply intracellularly and begin to produce F1 envelope antigen. If lysis of the mononuclear cells occurs, the released F1-producing bacilli are relatively resistant to further phagocytosis.[1,12] The invading organisms are carried via lymphatics to the regional lymph nodes, where they initiate an intense inflammatory reaction, creating a bubo. Microscopic examination of the involved nodes reveals invasion by polymorphonuclear leukocytes, hemorrhagic necrosis with destruction of normal architecture, and dense concentrations of extracellular bacilli. Bacteremia is common and, in the absence of specific therapy, can lead to sepsis, pneumonia, and purulent, necrotic, and hemorrhagic lesions in various organs. If not treated quickly, plague sepsis and attendant endotoxemia lead to profound pathophysiologic effects, including excessive release of proinflammatory mediators, such as tumor necrosis factor-α and other kinins. The resulting systemic inflammatory response syndrome may lead to disseminated intravascular coagulation, bleeding, organ failure, and irreversible shock.[29] Affected tissues contain inflamed microvasculature occluded by fibrin thrombi, resulting in necrosis and hemorrhage. Purpuric skin lesions are the most obvious manifestations of a bleeding diathesis; they are usually found scattered across the extremities and trunk, are at first red but change to a dark purple, and, in the patients who survive, eventually slough. Blockage of vessels in acral sites, such as the tips of the fingers, toes, ears, and nose, can lead to gangrene of these parts (Fig. 229-4).[30] These startling cutaneous signs may be the origin of the term "Black Death."

CLINICAL MANIFESTATIONS

The clinical manifestations of plague vary depending in part on the route of exposure. In the United States, 80% to 85% of cases first

present as bubonic plague, approximately 15% as septicemic plague, and 1% to 3% as pneumonic or other forms of plague. The usual incubation period from exposure to illness is 2 to 7 days, but can be as short as 1 day in the setting of primary pneumonic exposure.

Bubonic Plague

Bubonic plague is characterized by the sudden onset of fever, chills, weakness, and headache, accompanied by regional lymphadenitis, usually in the groin, axilla, or neck. The swollen lymph nodes, or buboes, are so tender that the patient may avoid any motion that would provoke discomfort. For example, patients with femoral buboes often rotate the hip externally to relieve pressure on the area and walk with a limp.

The buboes of patients with plague are oval swellings that vary from 1 to 10 cm in length and elevate the overlying skin, which may be stretched, warm, and erythematous. Palpation typically elicits extreme

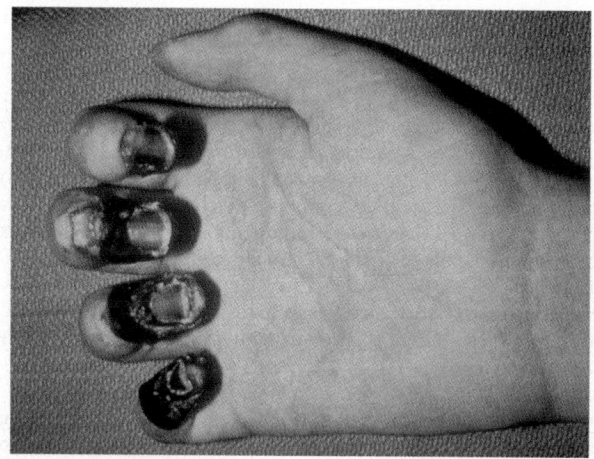

Figure 229-4 Right hand of a patient with plague displaying acral gangrene, a manifestation that may have given rise to the term "Black Death." *(Courtesy of the Centers for Disease Control and Prevention, Fort Collins, CO.)*

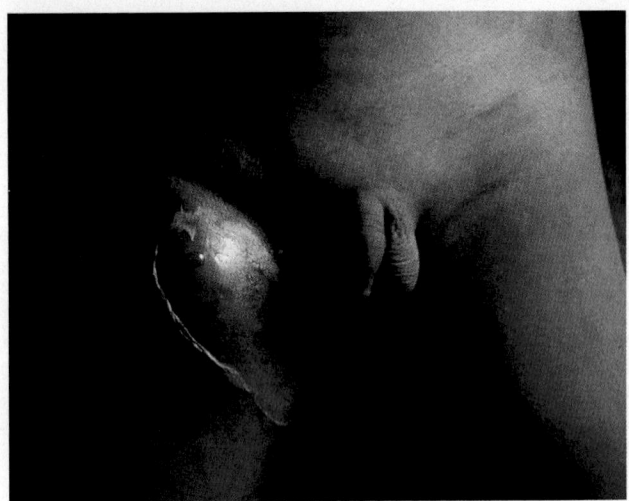

Figure 229-5 Femoral and inguinal buboes in a young male showing marked edematous swelling, erythema, and overlying desquamation. *(Courtesy of the Centers for Disease Control and Prevention, Fort Collins, CO.)*

tenderness, and the examiner feels either smooth, uniform, egg-shaped masses or an irregular cluster of several nodes with intervening and surrounding edema. The developing mass is typically firm and non-fluctuant, and the perinodal edema can be either gelatinous or pitting in nature. Although infections other than plague can produce acute lymphadenitis, plague is unique for the suddenness of onset of the fever and bubo, the intensity of inflammation in the bubo, and the absence in the majority of cases of an obvious sentinel infected skin lesion or associated ascending lymphangitis (Fig. 229-5). On careful examination, however, skin lesions are detectable in as many as one fourth of patients with bubonic plague.[29,31] Papules, vesicles, or pustules are most common and are found distal to the affected lymph nodes, presumably representing sites of the infective flea bites. Rarely, these lesions progress to extensive cellulitis or abscesses. Ulcerations may result from the breakdown of furuncles and be covered by eschars (Fig. 229-6). Examination of swabs or scrapings from skin lesions usually demonstrates collections of polymorphonuclear leukocytes and plague bacilli.

Buboes are most commonly located in the groin, with femoral nodes being more frequently affected than the inguinal nodes. The axillary and cervical regions are other commonly involved sites. The distribution of buboes is determined by the site of entry of infection. In adults, the large majority of infective flea bites occur on the lower extremities; relatively greater numbers of bites occur on the upper body in children.

Patients often do not seek care on the first days of illness. By the time of examination, they are typically prostrate and lethargic but may exhibit restlessness or agitation. Temperatures are usually elevated in the range of 38.5° C to 40.0° C. Occasionally, patients are delirious with high fever, and seizures are common in children. Pulse rates are increased to 110 to 140 beats per minute. Blood pressure is characteristically low, in the range of 100/60 mm Hg, owing to vasodilation. The liver and spleen are often palpable and tender. Without appropriate intervention, shock may ensue, and a cascading clinical course can produce death as quickly as 2 to 3 days after the onset of symptoms.

Septicemic Plague

Occasionally, bacteria proliferate in the body without producing a bubo. Patients may become ill with fever and die with sepsis but without detectable lymphadenitis. This syndrome has been termed *primary* septicemic plague to denote systemic plague without an antecedent bubo or plague pneumonia. In New Mexico, 25% of plague cases in 1980 to 1984 were of the primary septicemic form, and the case-fatality

ratio in these cases (33%) was three times higher than in bubonic plague, in part because of delays in diagnosis and treatment.[32,33]

Pneumonic Plague

Pneumonic plague occurs in two forms, secondary and primary, both of which are potentially contagious to close contacts. Secondary pneumonic plague is the more common form and arises through hematogenous spread of bacteria from a bubo or other source. Approximately 10% of all plague patients in the United States develop secondary pneumonic plague, usually as a result of delayed treatment of bubonic infections. Primary pneumonic plague results from direct inhalation of bacteria into the lungs. This can occur through contact with another patient with pneumonic plague, exposure to animals with respiratory or pharyngeal plague, laboratory exposures, or, potentially, as a result of intentional aerosol release for purposes of terrorism.

Regardless of form, pneumonic plague is a fulminant condition that progresses rapidly and is usually complicated by sepsis. Patients with plague pneumonia experience rapidly advancing tachypnea, dyspnea, hypoxia, chest pain, cough, hemoptysis, and general signs of endotoxemia. The sputum is often purulent but may be watery, frothy, and copious, and may be blood tinged or grossly hemorrhagic, at which point it may contain large numbers of plague bacilli.[34] Radiographs show patchy bronchopneumonia, cavities, or confluent consolidation,[35] and the radiologic findings may be more impressive than indicated by physical examination. Untreated pneumonic plague is almost always fatal, and mortality is very high in persons whose treatment is delayed beyond 18 to 24 hours after symptom onset. The case-fatality rate for pneumonic plague in the United States since 1950 approaches 50%.

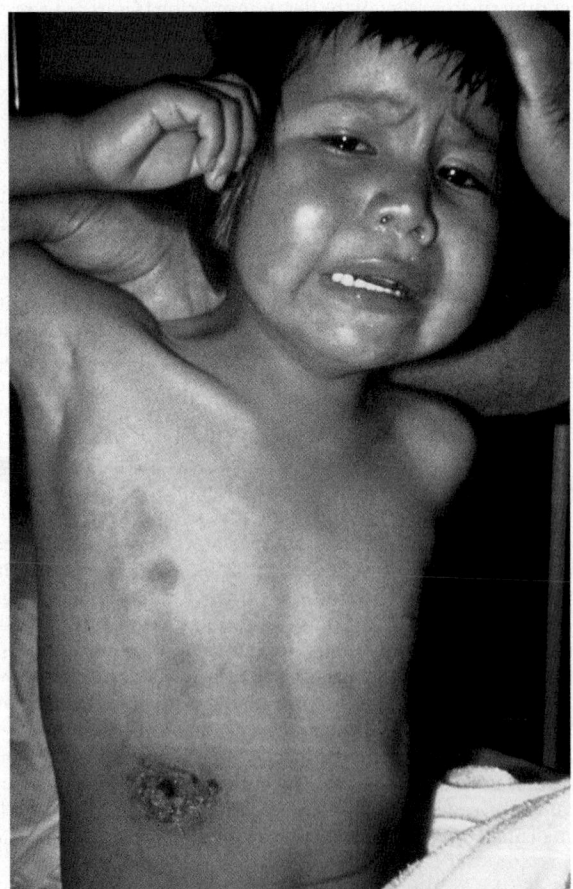

Figure 229-6 Axillary bubo with ulceration and small eschar at the site of an infective flea bite. *(Courtesy of the Centers for Disease Control and Prevention, Fort Collins, CO.)*

To prevent person-to-person transmission, patients with suspected pneumonic plague should be managed in isolation under respiratory droplet precautions.[9,36] Strict isolation under negative pressure and filtered exhausting is not necessary because infectious dispersal by fine aerosol or dried droplet nuclei does not occur. Person-to-person transmission of pneumonic plague requires close contact, typically with a patient who is in the late stages of infection and coughing copious amounts of bloody sputum.[37] The last case of person-to-person respiratory spread in the United States occurred in Los Angeles in 1924. There have been at least nine subsequent cases of primary pneumonic plague, two resulting from laboratory exposures and others from exposures to domestic cats with respiratory plague, none of which resulted in transmission to other persons.[25]

Other Syndromes

Plague meningitis is a rare complication. It may occur as a delayed manifestation of inadequately treated bubonic plague or as a manifestation of acute early disease. Plague meningitis is characterized by fever, headache, sensorial changes, meningismus, and cerebrospinal fluid pleocytosis with a predominance of polymorphonuclear leukocytes. Bacteria are frequently demonstrable with a Gram or Wayson stain of spinal fluid sediment, and endotoxin has been demonstrated in spinal fluid with the limulus test.[38]

Plague can produce pharyngitis resembling acute tonsillitis. The anterior cervical lymph nodes are usually inflamed, and *Y. pestis* may be recovered from a throat culture or by aspiration of a cervical bubo. This is a rare clinical form of plague that follows the inhalation or ingestion of plague bacilli. Asymptomatic pharyngeal colonization with *Y. pestis* has been reported in close contacts of pneumonic plague cases.

Plague manifests sometimes with prominent gastrointestinal symptoms of nausea, vomiting, diarrhea, and abdominal pain. These symptoms may precede the bubo. In septicemic plague, they may occur without a bubo and commonly result in diagnostic confusion, delays in correct treatment, and a consequent elevated mortality rate.[39]

LABORATORY FINDINGS

A distinctive feature of plague, in addition to the bubo, is a propensity for rapid multiplication of the bacillus in the blood. In the early acute stages of bubonic plague, intermittent seeding of the bloodstream is probably universal. In one series, single blood cultures obtained at the time of hospital admission were positive in 27% of cases.[31] Some patients develop high-density bacteremia, and the finding of characteristic bacilli in a stained peripheral blood smear is associated with a poor prognosis (Fig. 229-7). The peripheral blood leukocyte count is typically elevated, in the range of 10,000 to 20,000 cells/mm³, with a predominance of neutrophils. Severely ill patients tend to have the higher leukocyte counts. Occasional patients develop myelocytic leukemoid reactions with leukocyte counts as high as 100,000/mm³. Examination of the leukocytes in the peripheral blood smear typically reveals cytoplasmic vacuolations, toxic granulations, and Döhle bodies that are characteristic of acute bacterial infections. Blood eosinophils are usually diminished or absent in the acute stage of infection but return to normal or show elevated levels during convalescence. Blood platelet levels may be normal or low in the early stages of bubonic plague. Although patients with plague rarely develop a generalized bleeding tendency from profound thrombocytopenia, disseminated intravascular coagulation is common in advanced illness. Fibrinogen-fibrin degradation products in the sera are common in patients in advanced stages of illness.[29] Liver function test results, including serum aminotransferases and bilirubin, are frequently abnormal. As expected, hypotensive patients may develop impaired renal function.

DIAGNOSIS

Plague should be included in the differential diagnosis of an acute febrile illness in a patient who was recently in a plague-endemic area and at risk of exposure to infected animals or their fleas. When plague is suspected, diagnostic specimens should be obtained promptly and antimicrobial therapy initiated immediately thereafter.[40,41] Chest radiographs should be obtained to rule out pneumonia. Appropriate diagnostic specimens include blood cultures and other materials as indicated, such as bubo aspirates, sputum, tracheobronchial washes, swabs of skin lesions or pharyngeal mucosa, and cerebrospinal fluid. Bubo aspirates are especially useful and can be obtained by inserting a 20-gauge needle on a 10-mL syringe containing 2 mL of sterile saline solution into the bubo and withdrawing the plunger several times until the saline becomes blood tinged. Because the typical acute bubo does not contain liquid pus, it may be necessary to inject the saline solution into the bubo and immediately reaspirate it.

Protocols and algorithms have been developed for clinical laboratories to follow in diagnosing plague and are available online through the American Society of Microbiology (www.asm.org).[40,42] Material for culture should be inoculated onto suitable media (e.g., brain-heart infusion broth, sheep blood agar, chocolate agar, or MacConkey agar) and held for 5 to 7 days. Culture counts from blood typically range from fewer than 10 to as many as 4×10^7 colony-forming units/mL. For staining, drops of bubo aspirate, blood, or other materials should be placed onto microscopic slides and air dried. Gram stain reveals polymorphonuclear leukocytes and plump gram-negative coccobacilli ranging from 1 to 2 μm in length. With Wayson staining, *Y. pestis* appears as light blue bacilli with dark blue polar bodies, giving the organisms a closed safety-pin appearance that is characteristic of but not pathognomonic for *Y. pestis*. For more specific staining, a direct immunofluorescence test can be applied to smears of fluids or cultures.

In patients with negative cultures, plague can be confirmed by passive hemagglutination testing for antibodies to *Y. pestis* F1 antigen. A fourfold or greater change in titer between acute and convalescent serum or a single titer greater than or equal to 1:128 in an unvaccinated patient with compatible illness is considered diagnostic.[43] Although some patients will develop detectable antibodies as soon as 5 days after illness onset,[44] convalescent serum should generally be obtained at least 4 to 6 weeks later. Early specific antibiotic treatment may delay seroconversion by several weeks. Positive serologic titers diminish gradually over months to years. Enzyme-linked immunosorbent assays for detecting immunoglobulin M and G antibodies to *Y. pestis* can be used to identify antibodies in early infection and to differentiate them from antibodies developed in response to previous vaccination. Presumptive identification of *Y. pestis* can be made by polymerase chain reaction or antigen-capture enzyme-linked immunosorbent assay.[45,46] A rapid, handheld chromatographic assay designed to detect *Y. pestis* antigens in patient samples also seems promising for

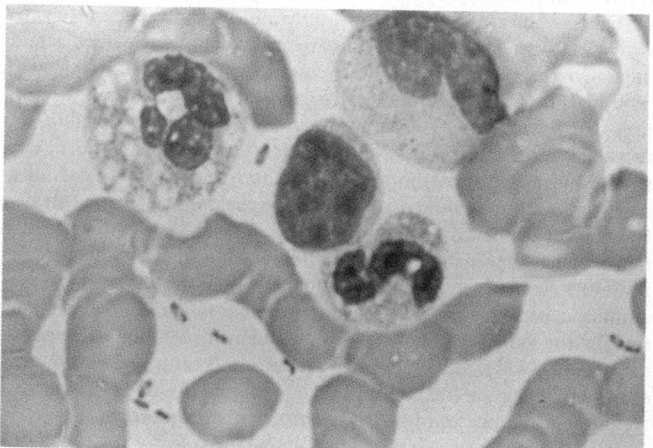

Figure 229-7 Peripheral blood smear of septicemic plague patient showing large numbers of bipolar-staining bacilli. *(Courtesy of the Centers for Disease Control and Prevention, Fort Collins, CO.)*

rapid presumptive diagnosis at the bedside, even when performed under primitive field conditions.[47]

In response to concerns regarding biologic terrorism, a national Laboratory Response Network has been established in the United States to provide upgraded, standardized diagnostic testing for *Y. pestis* and other selected agents.[10,48] This network links state and local public health laboratories with other advanced-capacity laboratories, including those at the Centers for Disease Control and Prevention. Member laboratories operate either as sentinel laboratories (level A) or as reference levels B through D, representing progressively stringent safety, containment, and technical proficiency capabilities. Sentinel laboratories include hospital and other community clinical laboratories that practice Biosafety Level 2 safety procedures and perform initial tests to presumptively identify or rule out *Y. pestis* infection, using such procedures as direct staining, bacterial culture, and biochemical screening tests. Suspicious isolates and source materials are to be forwarded to reference laboratories (federal, state, and local public health laboratories with BSL-2 and BSL-3 capabilities), which are prepared to perform advanced rapid diagnostic tests, to confirm the identification of *Y. pestis* and to characterize strain attributes. Reference laboratories are also prepared to carry out antimicrobial susceptibility studies, and some perform molecular subtyping tests, such as multiple locus variable number tandem-repeat assay, restriction fragment length polymorphism, and pulsed-field gel electrophoresis.[48]

For diagnosis in fatal cases, tissues, including samples of lymph nodes, liver, spleen, lungs, and bone marrow, should be collected at necropsy for culture, direct fluorescent antibody testing, and histologic studies, including immunohistochemical staining.

TREATMENT AND PREVENTION

Antibiotics

Without treatment, plague is fatal in more than 50% of bubonic cases and in nearly all cases of septicemic or pneumonic plague. Effective antibiotic therapy should be given immediately after obtaining diagnostic specimens. Streptomycin has been considered the drug of choice since its introduction in the 1940s, and prompt administration can reduce the mortality rate in bubonic plague to 5% or less. Streptomycin should be administered intramuscularly in two divided doses daily, in a dose for adults of 30 mg/kg body weight/day for 7 days or at least 3 days after remission of fever and other symptoms. Most patients improve rapidly and become afebrile after approximately 3 days of therapy.[29] Streptomycin is ototoxic and nephrotoxic. Although the risk of severe vestibular damage and hearing loss is considered to be small in the short courses required for treating plague, systematic measurements of these effects have not been made on plague patients, and streptomycin damage to the eighth cranial nerve, if it occurs, is permanent. Bilateral deafness and vestibular damage have been reported in children born of women given streptomycin during pregnancy for conditions other than plague. Therefore, streptomycin should be used cautiously in pregnant women, older patients, and patients with hearing difficulty. The risk of kidney damage as a result of short courses of streptomycin therapy is also small, but renal function should be monitored as a precaution. If the serum creatinine levels increase to more than 1.5 mg/dL, consideration should be given to adjusting the streptomycin dose. In mild renal impairment, the recommended dose is approximately 20 mg/kg/day, and in advanced impairment, it is 8 mg/kg every 3 days.

Where streptomycin is not available for immediate use, gentamicin has been proposed as an acceptable alternative based on in vitro susceptibility studies, animal models, and anecdotal reports of efficacy in treating humans with plague.[9,49-53] A retrospective analysis of 50 plague patients treated in New Mexico between 1985 and 1999 suggests that gentamicin, or a combination of gentamicin and doxycycline, is at least as efficacious as streptomycin.[54] All 36 gentamicin-treated patients survived without complications. In a randomized trial of 65 patients with plague in Tanzania, 94% of patients treated with gentamicin recovered.[55] Studies treating patients with other diseases indicate that

gentamicin is less ototoxic but more nephrotoxic than streptomycin. Damage to the kidneys caused by gentamicin is usually mild and reversible, so the drug is considered to be safer than streptomycin for use in pregnant women and children. As well, gentamicin is approved for use by intravenous administration, and single daily doses in adults are thought to provide more favorable blood levels and be less toxic than multiple daily doses. Because of these and other considerations, gentamicin has been recommended as an alternative in the first-line treatment of plague in the event of a bioterrorist attack[9] and is included for this reason in the national pharmaceutical emergency stockpile.

For patients with contraindications to the use of aminoglycosides, tetracycline and its congeners are satisfactory alternatives. Doxycycline is the tetracycline of choice in treating plague because of the convenience of its twice-daily dose schedule, its rapid absorption from the gut, and its superior ability to achieve peak serum concentrations. Doxycycline treatment should be initiated with a loading dose, either intravenously or orally depending on the severity of illness. In adults, a loading dose of 200 mg every 12 hours on the first day rapidly achieves a peak serum concentration of approximately 8 μg/mL[56] and is followed by a daily dose of 100 mg every 12 hours. Tetracycline is administered to adults in an initial loading dose of 2 g, followed by a usual dose of 2 g/day in four divided doses. Doxycycline or tetracycline can also be used to complete a course of treatment begun with an aminoglycoside. When used as principal treatment, a tetracycline should be given for 7 to 10 days or for at least 3 days after fever and other symptoms have subsided.

For conditions in which high tissue penetration is important, such as plague meningitis, pleuritis, or myocarditis, chloramphenicol is considered the drug of choice.[9,49] It may be used separately or in combination with an aminoglycoside. Chloramphenicol is given as a loading dose of 25 to 30 mg/kg body weight, followed by 50 to 60 mg/kg/day in four divided doses. As indicated by clinical response, the chloramphenicol dose may be reduced to a daily dose of 25 to 30 mg/kg/day to lessen the magnitude of bone marrow suppression, which is reversible. The irreversible marrow aplasia associated with chloramphenicol is so rare (estimated to occur in 1 in 40,000 patients) that its consideration should not deter its use in patients who are seriously ill with plague infection. Trimethoprim-sulfamethoxazole (cotrimoxazole) has been used successfully to treat bubonic plague, but responses may be delayed and incomplete, and it is not considered a first-line choice. Fluoroquinolones show much promise for treatment of plague based on studies conducted in vitro and in murine models[50,57-60]; however, published clinical experience is currently limited to the successful treatment of a single patient with ciprofloxacin.[49,61] Penicillins, cephalosporins, and macrolides have a suboptimal clinical effect and are not recommended for use in treating plague.

Strains of *Y. pestis* that are resistant to antimicrobials have only rarely been isolated from humans. Usually these strains have shown partial resistance to a single agent only and have not been associated with treatment failures. In 1995, two clinical isolates with plasmid-mediated drug resistance were recovered in Madagascar, one with high-level resistance to streptomycin and the second resistant to multiple drugs, including streptomycin, chloramphenicol, ampicillin, tetracycline, and sulfonamides.[49] Both patients, treated per protocol with streptomycin and trimethoprim-sulfamethoxazole, recovered. Molecular studies have identified very different plasmids in the two strains, and they are believed to have arisen independently, possibly through horizontal gene transfer in the flea midgut.[49] It is unclear whether such resistance would be expected to propagate in nature in the absence of antibiotic pressure on wild rodent populations, and to date these remain the only such natural isolates identified among thousands tested worldwide. Antimicrobial resistance is not known to have emerged during the treatment of plague in humans, and relapses after recommended courses of treatment are virtually unknown.

Supportive Therapy

Most patients are febrile and have constitutional symptoms, including nausea and vomiting. Hypotension and dehydration are common. The patient's hemodynamic status should be monitored closely and shock managed according to general principles used to combat endotoxic shock.[62] Investigational agents to counter effects of sepsis from other gram-negative bacteria, such as recombinant activated protein C,[63] have not been evaluated in plague patients. There is no evidence that corticosteroids are beneficial in treating plague.

Buboes usually recede during the first week of antibiotic treatment, but it may be several weeks before they completely resolve; occasionally, they enlarge or become fluctuant, requiring incision and drainage. The aspirate is usually sterile, but persistence of viable *Y. pestis* in buboes after apparent clinical cure has been reported. This persistence has not been associated with relapse of systemic plague.

Precautions

All suspected plague cases should be reported immediately to state health department authorities for assistance with confirmation of microbiologic diagnosis, epidemiologic investigation, and protection of the public's health. Patients with uncomplicated infections who are promptly treated present no health hazards to other persons. Those with cough or other signs of pneumonia should be placed in isolation and managed under respiratory droplet precautions for at least 48 hours after the institution of antibiotic therapy or until the sputum culture is negative. Respiratory droplet precautions include the use of fitted masks, gowns, gloves, and protective eyewear when providing direct patient care.[36,64] Cultures of clinical materials are usually negative after 24 hours of treatment. Patients without respiratory plague can be managed under standard precautions. Potentially infective clinical fluids should be handled with gloves and with care to avoid aerosolization (such as could result from dropping a specimen or by breakage of a container during centrifugation). Routine clinical specimens are managed in the laboratory under Biosafety Level 2 precautions, but manipulation of cultures should be performed in a negative pressure hood using Biosafety Level 3 procedures.

Prevention

Concern for bioterrorism has stimulated a resurgence in research on plague vaccines (see Chapter 322). For many years a formalin-killed vaccine, Plague Vaccine U.S.P., was available for use by persons who worked with *Y. pestis* in the laboratory and a few other categories of persons at high risk of exposure. It was given routinely to military personnel serving in Vietnam. However, its manufacture has been discontinued, and there is now only one source worldwide (Commonwealth Serum Laboratories Ltd., Australia). The killed vaccine does not protect against respiratory exposures, requires multiple doses over time, and has no utility in combating epidemic disease in a setting of modern sanitation and availability of prophylactic antibiotics.[65] Research is under way to develop improved plague vaccines that are likely to be protective against airborne infection and could be administered as inhalants.[66,67] At present, the most promising candidates are recombinant subunit vaccines that express F1 and V antigens of *Y. pestis* and seem to protect animals against infective aerosol exposures.[68-70] A wide variety of other approaches are also under investigation, including passive immunization with aerosolized monoclonal antibodies[71] and vaccines based on attenuated *Y. pseudotuberculosis*.[72,73]

Antibiotics can be used for chemoprophylaxis against plague in persons thought to have had an infective exposure within the previous 7 days, such as family members, care providers, and others with a close and direct contact with a patient having pneumonic plague or a laboratory worker exposed to an accident that may have created an infective aerosol.[65] Doxycycline is the prophylactic agent of first choice, given in an adult dose of 100 mg twice daily for 7 days. Postexposure prophylaxis may be an important control measure in circumstances of intentional use of *Y. pestis* in a terrorist event. Persons potentially exposed to either an aerosol release or persons with symptoms of plague pneumonia should be placed under surveillance for 7 days and be considered for prophylactic treatment. National guidelines for antimicrobial prophylaxis in the event of bioterrorism recommend doxycycline or ciprofloxacin for this purpose.[9]

Persons living in endemic areas should use personal protective measures against rodents and fleas, including living and working in rat-proofed dwellings, removing food and harborage for rodents, using repellents, and applying insecticides on their pets.[20]

Reservoir and Vector Control

The control of plague by health departments requires knowledge of the epidemiology of infected reservoir hosts, vectors, and the contact of humans with these animals in any particular area. In the United States, the Centers for Disease Control and Prevention branch in Fort Collins, Colorado, fields a team of entomologists, mammalogists, and epidemiologists to investigate cases of plague. The approach to prevent further cases is specific to each circumstance and usually consists of using insecticides around rodent runs, nests, or burrows; removing rodent harborage; and educating people on environmental sanitation, early detection and treatment of suspected plague, and avoidance of sick or dead rodents and cats. If killing of rodents is considered, flea control should be carried out before or at the time of killing to reduce the chances that infective fleas will feed on humans.

Y. Enterocolitica and Y. Pseudotuberculosis

HISTORY

The enteropathogenic yersiniae are relatively recently recognized causes of disease, and an understanding of their microbiology, epidemiology, and pathogenesis is evolving.[74] Sharing many of the virulence factors with *Y. pestis*, the enteropathogenic *Yersinia* spp. rely further on adaptive gene expressions that favor intestinal colonization, epithelial invasion, and survival in natural environments outside animal hosts. The major clinical syndromes associated with these organisms are enterocolitis, mesenteric adenitis, terminal ileitis, septicemia, and various immunoreactive conditions, especially reactive arthritis. Different disease expressions predominate in different age groups. Modes of transmission are principally fecal-oral, by hand-to-mouth transfer of organisms following handling of contaminated animals and animal carcasses, by ingestion of contaminated food or water, and rarely by transfusion of contaminated blood. Genomic studies suggest that *Y. pseudotuberculosis* is the recent progenitor of *Y. pestis*.[11]

DESCRIPTION OF THE PATHOGENS

Y. enterocolitica and *Y. pseudotuberculosis* are pleomorphic gram-negative bacilli in the family Enterobacteriaceae. They are non–lactose-fermenting, urease-positive organisms that grow at a wide range of temperatures; they are motile at 25°C but not at 37°C. Both grow on brain-heart infusion, MacConkey agar, and SS agar at room temperature and at 37°C, and in buffered saline at 4°C. Colonies are difficult to detect after incubation for 24 hours but are readily apparent at 48 hours. They can be distinguished from other enteric pathogens and from *Y. pestis* by biochemical profiles; however, rapid tests may be a cause of misidentification if not properly coded. More than 60 serotypes and 6 biotypes of *Y. enterocolitica* have been described. Most strains from patients belong to serotypes O:3, O:5.27, O:8, and O:9 and to biotypes 2, 3, and 4. There is a separate system for serotyping *Y. pseudotuberculosis*, also based on somatic antigens. Six serotypes (I through VI) and four subtypes of *Y. pseudotuberculosis* have been identified, with O group I accounting for approximately 80% of human cases.

Pathogenic strains are resistant to serum complement, penetrate human epithelial cells (HeLa cells) and guinea pig conjunctivae, are lethal to mice, and demonstrate cytotoxicity. Some of these characteristics are mediated by plasmids with weights of 41 to 82 kDa.[75-78] The 70-kb plasmid, which expresses V and W antigens, encodes for at least six proteins, called Yops, that confer various pathogenic properties, including resistance to phagocytosis by polymorphonuclear leukocytes, cytotoxicity, ability to initiate apoptosis of monocytes, suppression of tumor necrosis factor-α, and interference with platelet aggregation and complement activation.[78] The plasmid also encodes a secreted protein kinase[79] and an outer membrane protein with tyrosine phosphatase activity.[80] *Y. enterocolitica* does not produce a siderophore for iron transport and therefore grows better in the presence of other bacteria than do those that produce siderophores.[81] However, it can use host-chelated iron stores and chelating agents, such as desferrioxamine. Many strains of *Y. enterocolitica* produce a heat-stable enterotoxin that is similar to the heat-stable enterotoxin produced by *Escherichia coli*. This enterotoxin, which is produced at 22°C but not at 37°C, has not proven to be important in the pathogenesis of diarrhea associated with the yersinioses. Both *Y. enterocolitica* and *Y. pseudotuberculosis* produce a lipopolysaccharide endotoxin that has biologic properties similar to those of other gram-negative bacteria.

EPIDEMIOLOGY

Y. enterocolitica is distributed widely throughout the world and can be isolated from multiple environmental sources, including fresh water, contaminated foods, and a wide range of wild and domestic animals. It is an infrequent cause of diarrhea and abdominal pain in the United States, accounting for 15-fold fewer cases than *Shigella* in a recent survey.[82] In contrast, it is relatively common in northern Europe, and in Denmark *Y. enterocolitica* causes diarrhea more than twice as often as *Shigella*.[83] Infections have been documented in other parts of the world, including South America, Africa, and Asia, but *Y. enterocolitica* is not considered an important cause of tropical diarrhea.[84] Most isolates from Europe are serotypes O:3 and O:9, whereas most of the isolates from Canada and the United States are serotypes O:3 and O:8, respectively.

Children and adults of both sexes are susceptible, but children are affected more often than are adults. The majority of cases of the enterocolitis syndrome occur in the age group 1 to 4 years, whereas mesenteric adenitis and terminal ileitis are more common among older children and young adults. Transmission of infection occurs by ingestion of contaminated food or water and, less commonly, by direct contact with infected animals or patients (Fig. 229-8). The zoonotic reservoirs of *Y. enterocolitica* are diverse, including pigs, rodents, rabbits, sheep, cattle, horses, dogs, and cats. Transmission of infection to humans from contact with pet dogs and cats or their feces has been suggested. *Y. enterocolitica* is frequently present on the tonsils and in the alimentary tract of pigs, and transmission of infection can occur by ingestion of incompletely cooked pork and contamination of other foods by pork.[85] In Finland, butchers were shown to have been at increased risk of infection.[86] The ability of this organism to grow at 4°C means that refrigerated meats can be sources of infection. Outbreaks of foodborne disease have occurred in the United States, including outbreaks caused by contaminated milk, bean sprouts, and consumption of raw pork intestines (chitterlings) during holiday festivities.[74,87] In households where chitterlings are being prepared, infants too young to eat chitterlings may nevertheless become infected through cross-contamination of other items in the kitchen.[88] Fecal-oral transmission may account for reports of secondary infections in households; studies in children with *Y. enterocolitica* enterocolitis have shown that excretion of the organism in the stool usually persists for weeks.[89] Chronic carrier states have not been reported. The organism has been isolated from lakes, streams, and drinking water, but only a few cases have been linked to ingestion of natural water sources.

Persons with impaired immune defenses are at higher risk of septicemia and localized metastatic infections; recognized predisposing factors include diabetes, malignancy, immunosuppressive therapy, chronic liver disease, alcoholism, malnutrition, old age, and iron overload caused by hemolytic anemia, such as the thalassemias and other disorders requiring multiple transfusions.[90] The treatment of iron-overloaded patients with deferoxamine has been particularly associated with *Yersinia* sepsis because this iron chelator enhances the growth of the organism and also seems to inhibit polymorphonuclear leukocyte defenses against the infection.[91] *Y. enterocolitica* can multiply in stored blood, and banked blood has been a source of sepsis, resulting in shock and death in 50% of cases.[92]

Infection caused by *Y. pseudotuberculosis* is the most rarely recognized of the yersinioses. The organism is widespread in nature and has been recovered from various rodents, rabbits, deer, farm animals, and wild and domestic birds. Although this infection has a worldwide distribution, most cases have been reported from Europe, generally among children 5 to 14 years old. Males are affected three times as often as females, and illness occurs most frequently in the winter. The principal route of transmission is thought to be fecal-oral through contact with infected animals or contaminated food or water. In 1998, a large outbreak in Canada was linked epidemiologically to pasteurized milk, although the mechanism of contamination was never fully determined.[93] Fresh produce has been identified as the source of several recent outbreaks in Finland, including one in which over 100 schoolchildren became ill after eating raw carrots.[94,95]

PATHOGENESIS

The alimentary tract is the portal of entry in most cases. An inoculum of 10^9 organisms may be required to cause infection. After an incubation period of 4 to 7 days, infection may result in mucosal ulcerations in the terminal ileum (rarely in the ascending colon), necrotic lesions in Peyer's patches, and enlargement of mesenteric lymph nodes.[96] In severe cases, thrombosis of mesenteric blood vessels, intestinal necrosis, and hemorrhage may occur. The appendix has a normal histologic appearance or shows mild inflammation. Septicemia may lead to focal abscesses in various organs (e.g., lung, liver, meninges). A reactive polyarthritis is not uncommon[97] and has a predilection for patients with histocompatibility antigen HLA-B27, possibly as a result of a molecular mimicry between HLA-B27 antigen and *Yersinia* antigens.[74,98] Superantigenic activity has been found in cultures of *Y. enterocolitica* and could contribute to reactive arthritis.[99] The pathogenesis of yersiniosis-associated erythema nodosum is unknown.

CLINICAL MANIFESTATIONS

Enterocolitis accounts for two thirds of reported cases of symptomatic *Y. enterocolitica* infections and is characterized by fever, diarrhea, and abdominal pain lasting 1 to 3 weeks. Nausea and vomiting occur in 15% to 40% of cases. Leukocytes, blood, or mucus may be present in

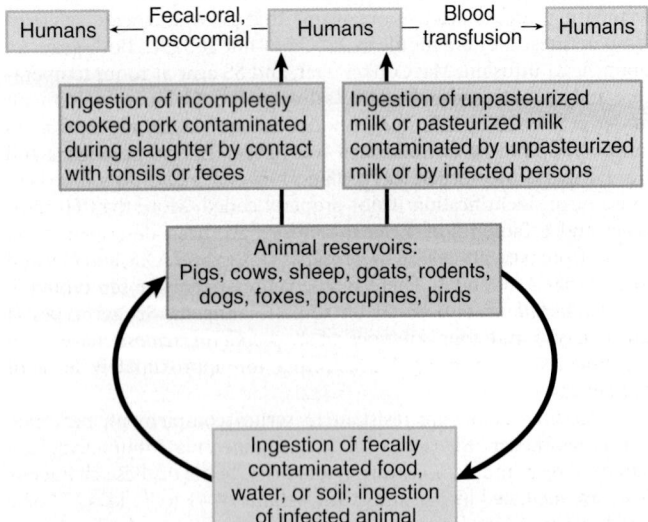

Figure 229-8 **Transmission routes of *Yersinia enterocolitica*.** *Wide arrows indicate common routes, medium arrows indicate occasional routes, and thin arrows indicate rare routes.*

the stool. In serious cases, perforation of the ileum and rectal bleeding may occur. Patients with mesenteric adenitis or terminal ileitis have fever, right lower quadrant pain and tenderness, and leukocytosis. This syndrome is most common in older children and adolescents and may be clinically indistinguishable from acute appendicitis.[100] Analysis of several common-source outbreaks in the United States disclosed that 10% of 444 patients with symptomatic undiagnosed *Y. enterocolitica* infections underwent laparotomy for suspected appendicitis.

Reactive polyarthritis occurs as a complication in approximately 15% of patients.[97] It begins a few days to a month after the onset of acute diarrhea and may involve the knees, ankles, toes, fingers, and wrists. In most cases, two to four joints become inflamed in rapid succession over a period of 2 to 14 days. Symptoms persist for more than 1 month in two thirds of cases and for more than 4 months in one third. After 12 months, most patients are asymptomatic, but a few have persistent low back pain, including sacroiliitis, which has been specifically related to the presence of HLA-B27.[98] Ankylosing spondylitis rarely occurs. Synovial fluid examination typically reveals a polymorphonuclear pleocytosis, usually with fewer than 25,000 leukocytes/mm³ of fluid. Cultures are usually negative. Reiter syndrome, with arthritis, urethritis, and conjunctivitis, has also been reported. Like arthritis, this complication is much more likely to develop in persons with the HLA-B27 antigen.[101,102]

Erythema nodosum occurs in as many as 30% of cases in Scandinavia. Skin lesions typically appear on the legs and trunk 2 to 20 days after onset of fever and abdominal pain and resolve spontaneously within a month in most cases. Women with this condition outnumber men by 2 to 1.

Exudative pharyngitis is a part of the spectrum of illness caused by *Y. enterocolitica*. In one large *Y. enterocolitica* enteritis outbreak in the United States, 8% of patients presented with acute pharyngitis and fever, without accompanying diarrhea.[103] Rare cases of pneumonia, empyema, and lung abscess have been reported.[104]

Y. enterocolitica septicemia is uncommon but severe and often fatal. It is most often reported in patients with underlying immunocompromising conditions, the elderly, and patients with iron overload. Septicemic patients may develop hepatic or splenic abscesses, peritonitis, septic arthritis, osteomyelitis, wound infections, or meningitis. Endocarditis and mycotic aneurysms caused by *Y. enterocolitica* have been reported.

The most common manifestation of *Y. pseudotuberculosis* infection in humans is mesenteric adenitis, which causes an acute appendicitis-like syndrome with fever and right lower quadrant abdominal pain.[105] Surgical exploration usually reveals a normal appendix and enlarged mesenteric lymph nodes and sometimes inflammation of the terminal ileum. The infection is usually self-limited, and computed tomography scanning of the abdomen may help avoid exploratory laparotomy. Erythema nodosum and polyarthritis have also been described in patients with *Y. pseudotuberculosis* infection. *Y. pseudotuberculosis* septicemia is infrequently reported; approximately 50% of septicemic patients have underlying chronic disease.[77] A scarlet fever–like syndrome has been described in association with certain strains of *Y. pseudotuberculosis* in far eastern Russia and Japan. This condition correlates with the ability of these strains to produce *Y. pseudotuberculosis* mitogen, a unique superantigen analogous to the superantigens implicated in staphylococcal and streptococcal toxic shock syndromes.[106] In addition, there has been long-standing speculation that *Y. pseudotuberculosis* may be implicated in the clinically similar Kawasaki disease.[107,108] In a recent review of 452 patients diagnosed with Kawasaki disease, approximately 10% had evidence of *Y. pseudotuberculosis* infection, which in turn was associated with a higher frequency of arterial lesions.[109]

DIAGNOSIS

Results of routine laboratory tests are nonspecific; leukocyte counts are usually normal or slightly elevated, with a modest shift to the left. *Yersinia* may be isolated from stool, mesenteric lymph nodes, pharyngeal exudates, peritoneal fluid, or blood and from abscesses, depending on the clinical syndrome. Recovery of organisms from otherwise sterile materials, such as blood, cerebrospinal fluid, and mesenteric lymph node tissue, is not difficult, but isolation from feces is hampered by slow growth and by overgrowth of normal fecal flora. Yield can be increased by using cold enrichment, alkali treatment, or selective CIN agar, but these methods are unnecessarily costly because usual enteric culturing methods detect most clinically significant infections.[110]

Serologic tests are useful in diagnosing *Yersinia* infections provided sera are appropriately absorbed. Agglutination tests, enzyme-linked immunosorbent assays, and immunoblotting tests are used; testing against multiple serogroups is time-consuming and costly and not usually performed for routine clinical diagnosis. *Y. enterocolitica* and *Y. pseudotuberculosis* cross-react with one another and with other organisms, such as *Brucella*, *Vibrio*, *Bartonella*, *Borrelia*, and *E. coli*. *Y. pseudotuberculosis* types II and IV cross-react with *Salmonella* groups B and D. Agglutinating antibodies appear soon after onset of illness, peak during the second week, and generally disappear within 2 to 6 months. Documentation of a fourfold or greater increase in antibodies is often not possible because the specimens collected early in the acute illness are already elevated. Polymerase chain reaction and immunohistochemical staining procedures are experimental.

Patients experiencing reactive arthritis syndromes have elevated erythrocyte sedimentation rates, but rheumatoid factor and antinuclear antibodies are usually absent. Synovial fluid from affected joints is sterile.

PREVENTION AND THERAPY

Public health measures to control *Yersinia* infection should focus on safe food handling, processing, and preparation practices, especially involving pork and pork products; limiting storage times of refrigerated but unfrozen foods before consumption; and preventing cross-contamination. Special attention should be given to protecting milk. The consumption of raw or undercooked meats, especially pork and pork products such as chitterlings, should be avoided. Hand washing and the control of environmental cross-contamination are the principal measures to reduce the spread of enteric pathogens in the home, daycare, health care, and pet care settings. The methods of slaughtering and butchering pigs can be modified to reduce contamination of meat and exposures of workers. In blood banks, donors should be asked about recent fever, abdominal pain, and diarrhea and be requested to notify the blood bank if these symptoms develop after donation.

Y. enterocolitica is usually susceptible in vitro to aminoglycosides, chloramphenicol, tetracycline, trimethoprim-sulfamethoxazole, piperacillin, ciprofloxacin, and the third-generation cephalosporins.[111] Because they produce β-lactamases, isolates are often resistant to penicillin, ampicillin, and first-generation cephalosporins. The value of antimicrobial therapy in cases of enterocolitis and mesenteric adenitis is unclear because these infections are usually self-limited. Treatment of enterocolitis with antibiotics shortens the persistence of immunoglobulin G anti-*Yersinia* antibodies to approximately 3 months. Patients with *Y. enterocolitica*–induced septicemia, which has a mortality rate of 50% despite treatment, should receive antibiotic therapy. The drug of choice has not yet been identified, but good responses have been reported with the aminoglycosides, trimethoprim-sulfamethoxazole, doxycycline, and ciprofloxacin,[103] whereas failures have occurred with cefuroxime, ceftazidime, and cefoperazone.[112]

Y. pseudotuberculosis is usually sensitive in vitro to ampicillin, tetracycline, chloramphenicol, cephalosporins, and aminoglycosides. Although antibiotic therapy is probably not warranted in most patients with mesenteric adenitis, patients with septicemia should receive ampicillin (100 to 200 mg/kg/day IV) or tetracycline, doxycycline, or a suitable aminoglycoside administered in standard doses for treating severe infections. The mortality rate in *Y. pseudotuberculosis* septicemia is 75% despite antibiotic therapy.

Patients with reactive arthritis may benefit from treatment with nonsteroidal anti-inflammatory agents, intra-articular steroid injections, and physical therapy.

Other *Yersinia* Species

Strains that were formerly considered biochemically atypical isolates of *Y. enterocolitica* have been reclassified as *Yersinia intermedia, Yer-sinia frederiksenii,* and *Yersinia kristensenii. Y. intermedia* and *Y. frederiksenii* have been recovered rarely from patients with enterocolitis and in a few instances have been reported to be associated with soft tissue infections. The pathogenic potential of these organisms remains unclear.

REFERENCES

1. Perry RD, Fetherston JD. *Yersinia pestis*—etiologic agent of plague. *Clin Microbiol Rev.* 1997;10:35-66.
2. Cohn SK. The Black Death: end of a paradigm. *Am Hist Rev.* 2002;107:703-738.
3. Drancourt M, Houhamdi L, Raoult D. *Yersinia pestis* as a telluric, human ectoparasite-borne organism. *Lancet Infect Dis.* 2006;6:234-241.
4. Wiechmann I, Grupe G. Detection of *Yersinia pestis* DNA in two early medieval skeletal finds from Aschheim (Upper Bavaria, 6th century A.D.). *Am J Phys Anthropol.* 2005;126:48-55.
5. Eisen RJ, Bearden SW, Wilder AP, et al. Early-phase transmission of *Yersinia pestis* by unblocked fleas as a mechanism explaining rapidly spreading plague epizootics. *Proc Natl Acad Sci U S A.* 2006;103:15380-15385.
6. Butler T. *Plague and Other Yersinia Infections.* New York: Plenum; 1983.
7. Chanteau S, Ratsifasoamanana L, Rasoamanana B, et al. Plague, a reemerging disease in Madagascar. *Emerg Infect Dis.* 1998;4:101-104.
8. Stenseth NC, Atshabar BB, Begon M, et al. Plague: past, present, and future. *PLoS Med.* 2008;5:e3.
9. Inglesby TV, Dennis, DT, Henderson DA, et al. Plague as a biological weapon: medical and public health management. *JAMA.* 2000;283:2281-2290.
10. Centers for Disease Control and Prevention. Biological and chemical terrorism: strategic plan for preparedness and response. Recommendations of the CDC Strategic Planning Workgroup. *MMWR Recomm Rep.* 2000;49:1-14.
11. Achtman M, Zurth K, Morelli G, et al. *Yersinia pestis,* the cause of plague, is a recently emerged clone of *Yersinia pseudotuberculosis. Proc Natl Acad Sci U S A.* 1999;24:14043-14048.
12. Zhou D, Han Y, Yang R. Molecular and physiological insights into plague transmission, virulence and etiology. *Microbes Infect.* 2006;8:273-284.
13. Parkhill J, Wren BW, Thompson NR, et al. Genome sequence of *Yersinia pestis,* the causative agent of plague. *Nature.* 2001;413:523-527.
14. Hinnebusch BJ. The evolution of flea-borne transmission in *Yersinia pestis. Curr Issues Mol Biol.* 2005;7:197-212.
15. Prentice MB, James KD, Parkhill J, et al. *Yersinia pestis* pFra shows biovar-specific differences and recent common ancestry with a *Salmonella enterica* serovar Typhi plasmid. *J Bacteriol.* 2001;183:2586-2594.
16. Achtman M, Morelli G, Zhu P, et al. Microevolution and history of the plague bacillus, *Yersinia pestis. Proc Natl Acad Sci U S A.* 2004;101:17837-17842.
17. Drancourt M, Signoli M, Dang LV, et al. *Yersinia pestis* Orientalis in remains of ancient plague patients. *Emerg Infect Dis.* 2007;13:332-333.
18. World Health Organization. Human plague in 2002 and 2003. *Wkly Epidemiol Rec.* 2004;79:301-306.
19. Boisier P, Rahalison L, Rasolomaharo M, et al. Epidemiological features of four successive annual outbreaks of bubonic plague in Mahajanga, Madagascar. *Emerg Infect Dis.* 2002;8:311-316.
20. Centers for Disease Control and Prevention. Fatal human plague—Arizona and Colorado, 1996. *MMWR Morb Mortal Wkly Rep.* 1997;46:617-620.
21. Centers for Disease Control and Prevention. Imported plague-New York City, 2002. *MMWR Morb Mortal Wkly Rep.* 2003;52:725-728.
22. Laudisoit A, Leirs H, Makundi RH, et al. Plague and the human flea, Tanzania. *Emerg Infect Dis.* 2007;13:687-693.
23. Eisen RJ, Gage KL. Adaptive strategies of *Yersinia pestis* to persist during inter-epizootic and epizootic periods. *Vet Res.* 2009;40:1.
24. Gage KL. Plague surveillance. In: *Plague Manual: Epidemiology, Distribution, Surveillance and Control.* Geneva: World Health Organization; 1999:135-166.
25. Gage KL, Dennis DT, Orloski KA, et al. Cases of cat-associated plague in the western U.S., 1977-1998. *Clin Infect Dis.* 2000;30:893-900.
26. Kaufmann AF, Boyce JM, Martone WJ. Trends in human plague in the United States. *J Infect Dis.* 1980;141:522-524.
27. Mann JM, Martone WJ, Boyce JM, et al. Endemic human plague in New Mexico: risk factors associated with infection. *J Infect Dis.* 1979;140:397-401.
28. Gould LH, Pape J, Ettestad P, et al. Dog-associated risk factors for human plague. *Zoonoses Public Health.* 2008;55:448-454.
29. Butler T. A clinical study of bubonic plague: observations on the 1970 Vietnam epidemic with emphasis on coagulation studies, skin histology and electrocardiograms. *Am J Med.* 1972;53:268-276.

30. Dennis D, Meier F. Plague. In: Horsburgh CR, Nelson AM, eds. *Pathology of Emerging Infections.* Washington, DC: ASM Press; 1997:21-47.
31. Butler T, Bell WR, Nguyen NL, et al. *Yersinia pestis* infection in Vietnam. I. Clinical and hematological aspects. *J Infect Dis.* 1974;129(Suppl):S78-S84.
32. Hull HF, Montes JM, Mann JM. Septicemic plague in New Mexico. *J Infect Dis.* 1987;155:113-118.
33. Crook LD, Tempest B. Plague: a clinical review of 27 cases. *Arch Intern Med.* 1992;152:1253-1256.
34. Wu L-T. *A Treatise on Pneumonic Plague.* Geneva: League of Nations Health Organization; 1926.
35. Alsofrom DJ, Mettler FA Jr, Mann JM. Radiographic manifestations of plague in New Mexico, 1975-1980: a review of 42 proved cases. *Radiology.* 1981;139:561-565.
36. Garner JS. Guidelines for isolation precautions in hospitals. Hospital Infection Control Practices Advisory Committee. *Infect Control Hosp Epidemiol.* 1996;17:53-80.
37. Kool JL. Risk of person-to-person transmission of pneumonic plague. *Clin Infect Dis.* 2005;40:1166-1172.
38. Butler T, Levin J, Nguyen NL, et al. *Yersinia pestis* infection in Vietnam. II. Quantitative blood cultures and detection of endotoxin in the cerebrospinal fluid of patients with meningitis. *J Infect Dis.* 1976;133:493-499.
39. Hull HF, Montes JM, Mann JM. Plague masquerading as gastrointestinal illness. *West J Med.* 1986;145:485-487.
40. Centers for Disease Control and Prevention. *Basic protocols for Level A laboratories for the presumptive identification of* Yersinia pestis (full text). 2002. Available at: <http://www.bt.cdc.gov/agent/plague/laboratory-testing.asp>. Accessed December 18, 2008.
41. Miller JM. Agents of bioterrorism: preparing for bioterrorism at the community health care level. *Infect Dis Clin North Am.* 2001;15:1127-1155.
42. American Society of Microbiology, Biological Weapons Resources Center. Detection and treatment-Sentinel (level A) laboratory. 2003. Available at: <http://www.asm.org>. Accessed December 18, 2008.
43. Chu M. Laboratory manual of plague diagnostic tests. In: *Centers of Disease Control and Prevention and World Health Organization.* 2000.
44. Butler T, Hudson BW. The serological response to *Yersinia pestis* infection. *Bull World Health Organ.* 1977;55:39-42.
45. Loiez C, Herwegh S, Wallet F, et al. Detection of *Yersinia pestis* in sputum by real-time PCR. *J Clin Microbiol.* 2003;41:4873-4875.
46. Radnedge L, Gamez-Chin S, McCready PM, et al. Identification of nucleotide sequences for the specific and rapid detection of *Yersinia pestis. Appl Environ Microbiol.* 2001;67:3759-3762.
47. Chanteau S, Rahalison L, Ralafiarisoa L, et al. Development and testing of a rapid diagnostic test for bubonic and pneumonic plague. *Lancet.* 2003;361:211-216.
48. Morse SA, Kellogg RB, Perry S. Detecting biothreat agents: the Laboratory Response Network. *ASM News.* 2003;69:433-437.
49. Galimand M, Carniel E, Courvalin P. Resistance of *Yersinia pestis* to antimicrobial agents. *Antimicrob Agents Chemother.* 2006;50:3233-3236.
50. Byrne WR, Welkos SL, Pitt ML, et al. Antibiotic treatment of experimental pneumonic plague in mice. *Antimicrob Agents Chemother.* 1998;42:675-681.
51. Wong JD, Barash JR, Sandfort RF, et al. Susceptibilities of *Yersinia pestis* strains to 12 antimicrobial agents. *Antimicrob Agents Chemother.* 2000;44:1995-1996.
52. Crook LD, Tempest B. Plague—a clinical review of 27 cases. *Arch Intern Med.* 1992;152:1253-1256.
53. Welty TK, Grabman J, Kompare E, et al. Nineteen cases of plague in Arizona: a spectrum including ecthyma gangrenosum due to plague and plague in pregnancy. *West J Med.* 1985;142:641-646.
54. Boulanger L, Ettestad P, Fogarty J, et al. Gentamicin and tetracyclines for the treatment of human plague: a review of 75 cases in New Mexico from 1985-1999. *Clin Infect Dis.* 2004;38:663-669.
55. Mwengee W, Butler T, Mgema S, et al. Treatment of plague with gentamicin or doxycycline in a randomized clinical trial in Tanzania. *Clin Infect Dis.* 2006;42:614-621.
56. Cunha BA. Doxycycline for community-acquired pneumonia. *Clin Infect Dis.* 2003;37:870.
57. Frean J, Klugman KP, Arntzen L, et al. Susceptibility of *Yersinia pestis* to novel and conventional antimicrobial agents. *J Antimicrob Chemother.* 2003;52:294-296.

58. Hernandez E, Girardet M, Ramisse F, et al. Antibiotic susceptibilities of 94 isolates of *Yersinia pestis* to 24 antimicrobial agents. *J Antimicrob Chemother.* 2003;52:1029-1031.
59. Steward J, Lever MS, Russell P, et al. Efficacy of the latest fluoroquinolones against experimental *Yersinia pestis. Int J Antimicrob Agents.* 2004;24:609-612.
60. Russell P, Eley SM, Bell DL, et al. Doxycycline or ciprofloxacin prophylaxis and therapy against experimental *Yersinia pestis* infection in mice. *J Antimicrob Chemother.* 1996;37:769-774.
61. Kuberski T, Robinson L, Schurgin A. A case of plague successfully treated with ciprofloxacin and sympathetic blockade for treatment of gangrene. *Clin Infect Dis.* 2003;36:521-523.
62. Wheeler AP, Gordon RB. Treating patients with severe sepsis. *N Engl J Med.* 1999;340:207-214.
63. Dellinger PR. Inflammation and coagulation: implications for the septic patient. *Clin Infect Dis.* 2003;36:1259-1265.
64. Siegel JD, Rhinehart E, Jackson M, et al, and the Healthcare Infection Control Practices Advisory Committee. 2007 *Guideline for Isolation Precautions: preventing Transmission of Infectious Agents in Healthcare Settings,* June 2007. Available at <http://www.cdc.gov/ncidod/dhqp/pdf/guidelines/Isolation2007.pdf>; Accessed December 18, 2008.
65. Centers for Disease Control and Prevention. Prevention of plague. Recommendations of the Advisory Committee on Immunization Practices (ACIP). *MMWR Recomm Rep.* 1996;45:1-15.
66. Titball RW, Williamson ED. Second and third generation plague vaccines. *Adv Exp Med Biol.* 2003;529:397-406.
67. Eyles JE, Williamson ED, Spiers ID, et al. Generation of protective immune responses to plague by mucosal administration of microspore coencapsulated recombinant subunits. *J Control Release.* 2000;63:191-200.
68. Morris SR. Development of a recombinant vaccine against aerosolized plague. *Vaccine.* 2007;25:3115-3117.
69. Wang D, Jia N, Li P, et al. Protection against lethal subcutaneous challenge of virulent *Y. pestis* strain 141 using an F1-V subunit vaccine. *Sci China C Life Sci.* 2007;50:600-604.
70. Williamson ED, Stagg AJ, Eley SM, et al. Kinetics of the immune response to the (F1+V) vaccine in models of bubonic and pneumonic plague. *Vaccine.* 2007;25:1142-1148.
71. Hill J, Eyles JE, Elvin SJ, et al. Administration of antibody to the lung protects mice against pneumonic plague. *Infect Immun.* 2006;74:3068-3070.
72. Taylor VL, Titball RW, Oyston PC. Oral immunization with a dam mutant of *Yersinia pseudotuberculosis* protects against plague. *Microbiology.* 2005;151:1919-1926.
73. Balada-Llasat JM, Panilaitis B, Kaplan D, et al. Oral inoculation with type III secretion mutants of *Yersinia pseudotuberculosis* provides protection from oral, intraperitoneal, or intranasal challenge with virulent *Yersinia. Vaccine.* 2007;25:1526-1533.
74. Bottone EJ. *Yersinia enterocolitica:* the charisma continues. *Clin Microbiol Rev.* 1997;10:257-276.
75. Cornelis G, Laroche Y, Balligand G, et al. *Yersinia enterocolitica,* a primary model for bacterial invasiveness. *Rev Infect Dis.* 1987;9:64-87.
76. Smego RA, Frean J, Koornhof HJ. Yersiniosis I: microbiological and clinicoepidemiological aspects of plague and non-plague *Yersinia* infections. *Eur J Clin Microbiol Infect Dis.* 1999;18:1-15.
77. Bottone EJ. *Yersinia enterocolitica:* overview and epidemiologic correlates. *Microbes Infect.* 1999;1:323.
78. Cornelis GR, Boland A, Boyd AP, et al. The virulence plasmid of *Yersinia,* an antihost genome. *Microbiol Mol Biol Rev.* 1998;62:1315-1352.
79. Gaylov EE, Hakansson S, Forsberg A, et al. A secreted protein kinase of *Yersinia pseudotuberculosis* is an indispensable virulence determinant. *Nature.* 1993;361:730-732.
80. Guan K, Dixon JE. Protein tyrosine phosphatase activity of an essential virulence determinant in *Yersinia. Science.* 1990;249:553-556.
81. Cantinieaux B, Boelaert J, Hariga C, et al: Impaired neutrophil defense against *Yersinia enterocolitica* in patients with iron overload who are undergoing dialysis. *J Lab Clin Med.* 1988;111:524-528.
82. Centers for Disease Control and Prevention. Preliminary FoodNet data on the incidence of infection with pathogens transmitted commonly through food—10 states, 2007. *MMWR Morb Mortal Wkly Rep.* 2008;57:366-370.
83. Helms M, Simonsen J, Molbak K. Foodborne bacterial infection and hospitalization: a registry-based study. *Clin Infect Dis.* 2006;42:498-506.

84. Carniel E, Butler T, Hossain S, et al. Infrequent detection of *Yersinia enterocolitica* in childhood diarrhea in Bangladesh. *Am J Trop Med Hyg.* 1986;35:370-371.

85. Tauxe RV, Vandepitte J, Wauters G, et al. *Yersinia enterocolitica* infections and pork: the missing link. *Lancet.* 1987;1:1129-1132.

86. Merilahti-Palo R, Lahesmaa R, Granfors K, et al. Risk of *Yersinia* infection among butchers. *Scand J Infect Dis.* 1991;23:55-61.

87. Lee LA, Taylor J, Carter GP, et al. *Yersinia enterocolitica* 0:3: an emerging cause of pediatric gastroenteritis in the United States. *J Infect Dis.* 1991;163:660-663.

88. Jones TF, Buckingham SC, Bopp CA, et al. From pig to pacifier: chitterling-associated yersiniosis outbreak among black infants. *Emerg Infect Dis.* 2003;9:1007-1009.

89. Abdel-Haq NM, Asmar BI, Abuhammour WM, et al. *Yersinia enterocolitica* infection in children. *Pediatr Infect Dis J.* 2000;19:945-948.

90. Adamkiewicz TV, Berkovitch M, Krishnan C, et al. Infection due to *Yersinia enterocolitica* in a series of patients with beta-thalassemia: incidence and predisposing factors. *Clin Infect Dis.* 1998;27:1362-1366.

91. Robins-Browne RM, Prpic JK. Desferrioxamine and systemic yersiniosis. *Lancet.* 1983;2:1372.

92. Centers for Disease Control and Prevention. Red blood cell transfusions contaminated with *Yersinia enterocolitica*-United States, 1991-1996, and initiation of a national study to detect bacteria-associated transfusion reactions. *MMWR Morb Mortal Wkly Rep.* 1997;46:553-555.

93. Press N, Fyfe M, Bowie W, et al. Clinical and microbiological follow-up of an outbreak of *Yersinia pseudotuberculosis* serotype Ib. *Scand J Infect Dis.* 2001;33:523-526.

94. Nuorti JP, Niskanen T, Hallanvuo S, et al. A widespread outbreak of *Yersinia pseudotuberculosis* O:3 infection from iceberg lettuce. *J Infect Dis.* 2004;189:766-774.

95. Rimhanen-Finne R, Niskanen T, Hallanvuo S, et al. *Yersinia pseudotuberculosis* causing a large outbreak associated with carrots in Finland, 2006. *Epidemiol Infect.* 2008:1-6.

96. Bradford WD, Noce PS, Gutman LT. Pathologic features of enteric infection with *Yersinia enterocolitica*. *Arch Pathol.* 1974;98:17-22.

97. Townes JM, Deodhar AA, Laine ES, et al. Reactive arthritis following culture-confirmed infections with bacterial enteric pathogens in Minnesota and Oregon: a population-based study. *Ann Rheum Dis.* 2008;67:1689-1696.

98. van der Heijden IM, Res PCM, Wilbrink B, et al. *Yersinia enterocolitica*: a cause of chronic polyarthritis. *Clin Infect Dis.* 1997;25:831-837.

99. Stuart PM, Woodward JG. *Yersinia enterocolitica* produces superantigenic activity. *J Immunol.* 1992;148:225-233.

100. Strom H, Johansson C. Appendicitis followed by reactive arthritis in an HLA B27-positive man after infection with *Yersinia enterocolitica*, diagnosed by serotype specific antibodies and antibodies to *Yersinia* outer membrane proteins. *Infection.* 1997;25:317-319.

101. Borg AA, Gray J, Dawes PT. *Yersinia*-related arthritis in the United Kingdom: a report of 12 cases and review of the literature. *Q J Med.* 1992;304:575-582.

102. Granfors K, Jalkanen S, von Essen R, et al. *Yersinia* antigens in synovial-fluid cells from patients with reactive arthritis. *N Engl J Med.* 1989;320:216-221.

103. Rose FB, Camp CJ, Antes EJ. Family outbreak of fatal *Yersinia enterocolitica* pharyngitis. *Am J Med.* 1987;82:636-637.

104. Greene JN, Herndon P, Nadler JP, et al. Case report: *Yersinia enterocolitica* necrotizing pneumonia in an immunocompromised patient. *Am J Med Sci.* 1993;305:171-173.

105. Weber J, Finlayson NB, Mark JBD. Mesenteric lymphadenitis and terminal ileitis due to *Yersinia pseudotuberculosis*. *N Engl J Med.* 1970;283:172-174.

106. Eppinger M, Rosovitz MJ, Fricke WF, et al. The complete genome sequence of *Yersinia pseudotuberculosis* IP31758, the causative agent of Far East scarlet-like fever. *PLoS Genet.* 2007;3:e142.

107. Uchiyama T, Kato H. The pathogenesis of Kawasaki disease and superantigens. *Jpn J Infect Dis.* 1999;52:141-145.

108. Vincent P, Salo E, Skurnik M, et al. Similarities of Kawasaki disease and *Yersinia pseudotuberculosis* infection epidemiology. *Pediatr Infect Dis J.* 2007;26:629-631.

109. Tahara M, Baba K, Waki K, et al. Analysis of Kawasaki disease showing elevated antibody titres of *Yersinia pseudotuberculosis*. *Acta Paediatr.* 2006;95:1661-1664.

110. Kachoris M, Ruoff KL, Welch K, et al. Routine culture of stool specimens for *Yersinia enterocolitica* is not a cost-effective procedure. *J Clin Microbiol.* 1988;26:582-583.

111. Gayraud M, Scavizzi MR, Mollaret HH, et al. Antibiotic treatment of *Yersinia enterocolitica* septicemia: a retrospective review of 43 cases. *Clin Infect Dis.* 1993;17:405-410.

112. Crowe M, Ashford K, Ispahani P. Clinical features and antibiotic treatment of septic arthritis and osteomyelitis due to *Yersinia enterocolitica*. *J Med Microbiol.* 1996;45:302-309.

230

Bordetella pertussis

VALERIE WATERS | SCOTT HALPERIN

History

The first epidemic of whooping cough was described in 1578 by DeBaillou, who wrote the following: "The lung is so irritated that, in its attempt by every effort to cast forth the cause of the trouble, it can neither admit breath nor easily give it forth again. The sick person seems to swell up, and, as if about to strangle, holds his breath clinging in the midst of his jaws. ..."[1] This vivid clinical description of whooping cough holds true to this day. In 1679, Sydenham gave this respiratory illness the name pertussis, meaning a violent cough of any type.[2] The organism that causes whooping cough was discovered in 1900 by Bordet and Gengou. They described a new gram-negative bacillus (subsequently named *Bordetella pertussis*, after Bordet) which they had found in the sputum of a 6-month-old infant with whooping cough.[3] By 1906, they had developed a culture medium to support the growth of the organism and described in detail its morphology and virulence characteristics. In 1943, Joseph Lapin, a pediatrician who worked in the whooping cough clinic at the Bronx Hospital in New York City, wrote an extensive monograph on the subject of pertussis.[1]

Description of Pathogen

Bordetella pertussis is the pathogen that causes whooping cough or pertussis.[4] It is one of 10 known *Bordetella* species, namely, *B. pertussis, B. parapertussis, B. bronchiseptica,* ovine-adapted *B. parapertussis, B. avium, B. hinzii, B. holmesii, B. trematum, B. petrii,* and *B. ansorpii. B. pertussis* and *B. parapertussis* are the most common *Bordetella* species causing respiratory illnesses in humans. Although *B. pertussis* strictly affects humans and has no known animal reservoir,[5] many of the other *Bordetella* species are recognized primarily for the diseases they cause in animals. *B. bronchiseptica* causes kennel cough in dogs and cats, and human infections occur primarily in immunocompromised patients, often after exposure to animals.[6-8] Ovine-adapted *B. parapertussis* causes respiratory tract infections in sheep.[9] *B. avium* is a pathogen of poultry[10] but has been isolated from the ear culture of a patient with chronic otitis media.[11] Similarly, *B. hinzii* also colonizes the respiratory tract of poultry and has been isolated from the sputum of cystic fibrosis patients.[12] It has been reported to cause bacteremia in immunocompromised[13,14] as well as immunocompetent patients[15] and has been described as a cause of chronic cholangitis.[16] *B. holmesii,* initially described by the Centers for Disease Control and Prevention (CDC) as nonoxidizer group 2 (NO-2),[17] is associated with bacteremia,[18] particularly in asplenic patients,[19] endocarditis,[20] and respiratory illness.[21] *B. trematum* has been isolated from patients with wounds or otitis media.[22,23] *B. petrii,* originally identified from an environmental source,[24] has been recently isolated from a patient with chronic suppurative mastoiditis[25] and from a patient with mandibular osteomyelitis.[26] Finally, in 2005, a novel species of *Bordetella, Bordetella ansorpii,* was described following the isolation of a gram-negative bacillus from the purulent exudate of an epidermal cyst.[27] 16S rRNA gene sequencing has revealed that this bacterium belongs to the *Bordetella* genus but is distinct from other *Bordetella* species. This species was subsequently isolated from an immunocompromised patient in the United Kingdom.[28]

Bordetella species are small gram-negative coccobacilli.[29] Some species are motile and, except for *B. petrii,* are strictly aerobic. All species possess catalase activity and oxidize amino acids but do not ferment carbohydrates. *Bordetella* organisms grow optimally at 35° to 37° C. *Bordetella* species are fastidious because their growth can be inhibited by components commonly found in laboratory media. In addition, their rate of growth is inversely related to their degree of fastidiousness. *B. pertussis* is the most fastidious and slowest growing of the *Bordetella* species. Its growth is inhibited by fatty acids, metal ions, sulfides, and peroxides. Isolation of *B. pertussis* requires a medium containing charcoal, blood, or starch. Traditionally, the Bordet-Gengou (BG) medium has been used and consists of a potato-starch base. Charcoal medium (Regan-Lowe [RL] medium), supplemented with glycerol, peptones, and horse or sheep blood, can also be used and may provide better isolation of *B. pertussis* than the BG medium.

Pathogenesis

B. pertussis infection and disease occur following four important steps: (1) attachment, (2) evasion of host defenses, (3) local damage, and (4) systemic manifestations.[4]

Filamentous hemagglutinin (FHA) and fimbriae (FIM) are two major adhesins and virulence determinants for *B. pertussis.* FHA is a 220-kDa surface-associated and secreted protein and FIM is a filamentous cell surface structure. They are required for tracheal colonization, are highly immunogenic, and are components of certain acellular pertussis vaccines.[4] However, there is likely redundancy in the adhesion role of *B. pertussis* proteins and it has been suggested that in the absence of FHA, virulence factors such as pertactin (PRN) may mediate attachment.[30] Pertussis toxin (PT) also acts as an adhesin[31] and has specific recognition domains for human cilia.[32]

Evasion of host defenses occurs primarily through adenylate cyclase toxin (ACT) and PT.[33] ACT is a toxin secreted by *B. pertussis* that catalyzes the conversion of adenosine triphosphate (ATP) to cyclic adenosine monophosphate (cAMP), which inhibits the migration and activation of phagocytes. It has also recently been shown to suppress T-lymphocyte activation and chemotaxis.[34] PT, one of the most important virulence factors of *B. pertussis,* also targets the innate immune system of the lung by inactivating or suppressing G protein–coupled signaling pathways. PT has two components, the A subunit and the B subunit. The B (binding) subunit binds to the cell surface to enable the A (active) subunit to ADP ribosylate G proteins, thereby altering the cell.[33] Through this mechanism of action, PT delays the recruitment of neutrophils to the respiratory tract and targets airway macrophages to promote *B. pertussis* infection.[35] The virulence factors of *B. pertussis,* such as PT, are encoded by the *Bvg* (or *vir*) gene. The Bvg operon is composed of BvgA and BvgS, members of a two-component signal transduction system that controls the genetic state or phase, of *B. pertussis.*[36] There are virulent and avirulent phases, and their expression is regulated by environmental factors.[37]

Original reports by Lapin described the local tissue damage caused by pertussis in the lung.[1] The initial pulmonary lesion is a lymphoid hyperplasia of peribronchial and tracheobronchial lymph nodes. Necrosis and desquamation of the bronchial epithelium follow, with diffuse infiltrations by macrophages (Fig. 230-1). Most of the damage to the ciliated epithelial cells is caused by tracheal cytotoxin (TCT). TCT is a disaccharide tetrapeptide derived from peptidoglycan, which triggers the production of an inducible nitric oxide (NO) synthase.[38] The synthase produces NO, which ultimately kills the tracheal epithelial cells. The induction of the NO synthase is likely caused by the cytokine interleukin-I (IL-1) generated in response to TCT.[39] Dermonecrotic toxin (DNT), a 160-kDa heat-labile secreted toxin that

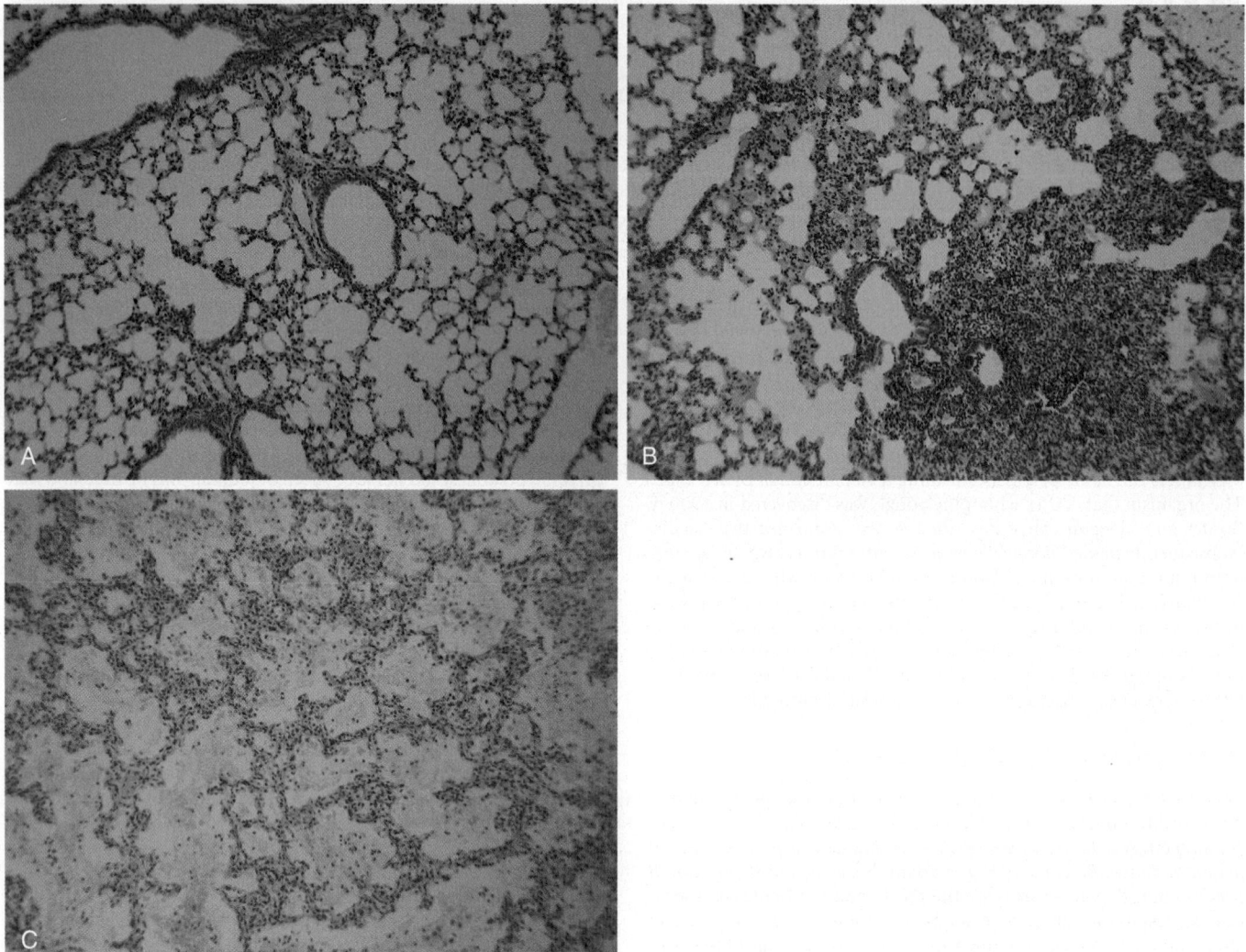

Figure 230-1 **Tissue damage caused by pertussis in the lung.** Hematoxylin and eosin (H&E) stain of lung tissue of a 21-day-old uninfected mouse **(A)**, a 21-day-old mouse infected with 5×10^8 colony-forming units of *Bordetella pertussis* **(B)**, and a 34-day-old infant who died of pertussis **(C)** showing diffuse mononuclear and neutrophilic alveolar and interstitial infiltration (all 10× objective and digital zoom).

activates intracellular Rho GTPases, may also have a role in local tissue damage.[40] DNT was first discovered by Bordet and Gengou and derives its name from the characteristic skin lesion produced when injected into test animals.

Unlike other bacterial diseases, there are few systemic manifestations of *B. pertussis* infection because it does not enter the circulation and disseminate. *B. pertussis* is relatively sensitive to killing by serum in vitro. However, in vivo, even serum-sensitive strains can efficiently infect mice.[41,42] *B. pertussis* has multiple mechanisms for avoiding antibody-mediated complement killing,[43] including the expression of BrkA, a surface-associated protein belonging to the autotransporter secretion system.[44] PT is the primary virulence determinant responsible for the systemic manifestations, of which the most prominent is leukocytosis with lymphocytosis.[33] Other systemic responses include sensitization to histamine and serotonin and sensitization of the beta-islet cells of the pancreas. This latter effect leads to hyperinsulinemia with resultant hypoglycemia, particularly in young infants.[1] Pertussis-associated encephalopathy is rarely observed[45]; some have suggested that it may be caused by the effect of pertussis toxin on the central nervous system via monocyte chemoattractant protein-1 (MCP-1) overexpression.[46] Fatal pulmonary hypertension has also been associated with pertussis in infants.[47]

In addition to the direct effects of these virulence factors in the lung, some believe that they modulate, in a more global fashion, the immune system itself.[48] Studies investigating immunomodulation by *B. pertussis* have demonstrated skewing of the host immune response toward expansion of the Th17 subset of T lymphocytes, induced by the production of cytokine IL-23.[49] The Th17 immune response may be protective against some other gram-negative bacterial respiratory pathogens,[50] but may also be associated with chronic autoimmune inflammation.[51] Some have suggested that the chronic cough seen with *B. pertussis* infection may be explained by this autoimmune phenomenon, akin to asthma.[48]

Epidemiology

Despite vaccination, pertussis disease continues to be a problem in the developing and developed world.[52] According to the World Health Organization (WHO), an estimated 50 million cases and 300,000 deaths occur every year because of *B. pertussis*[53] (Fig. 230-2). Case-fatality rates in developing countries may be as high as 3% in infants.[54] WHO recommended that a pertussis incidence of less than 1 case/100,000 population be achieved in Europe by 2000. Data from countries represented in the Global Pertussis Initiative (GPI) have indicated that this goal has not yet been achieved.[54]

Immunization coverage with DTP3 vaccines in infants, 2006

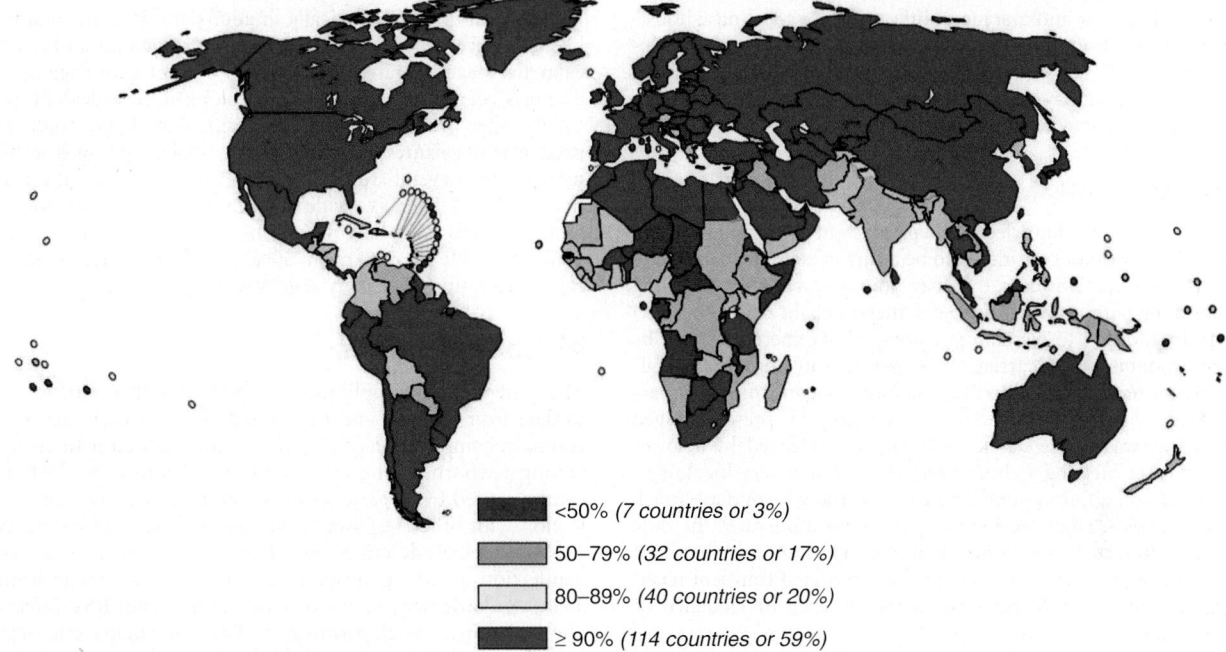

- ■ <50% *(7 countries or 3%)*
- ▨ 50–79% *(32 countries or 17%)*
- ▧ 80–89% *(40 countries or 20%)*
- ■ ≥ 90% *(114 countries or 59%)*

Figure 230-2 **Immunization coverage with DTP3 vaccines in infants, 2006.** *(From WHO/UNICEF coverage estimates 1980-2006, August 2007. ©WHO, 2007.)*

PREVACCINE ERA

In the prevaccine era, pertussis was a major childhood illness and a leading cause of death. Pertussis disease has always been cyclical, with peaks occurring every 3 to 5 years.[55] From 1940 to 1948 in the United States, pertussis was responsible for more deaths in the first year of life than measles, scarlet fever, diphtheria, poliomyelitis, and meningitis combined.[4] Unlike the current age distribution of pertussis disease, however, pertussis affected children primarily 1 to 10 years of age. From 1918-1921 in Massachusetts, for example, over 80% of pertussis cases occurred in children ages 1 to 9 years, whereas only 10% occurred in infants younger than 1 year.[56]

VACCINE ERA

With the introduction of the whole-cell pertussis vaccine in the 1940s, pertussis rates dropped dramatically. They reached a nadir in the United States in the late 1970s to early 1980s, with a reported 0.5 to 1.0 case/100,000 population between 1976 and 1982.[56] Since then, there has been a gradual increase in pertussis rates over the last 20 years, with peaks of disease continuing to occur every 3 to 5 years.[57] The age distribution of pertussis disease has changed as well, with the most cases occurring in unimmunized infants younger than 1 year. Recent data from the National Notifiable Disease Surveillance System and the Nationwide Inpatient Database in the United States have revealed that from 1993 to 2004, 86% of hospitalizations and all deaths caused by pertussis were in infants 3 months of age or younger.[58] Similarly, according to Canadian data from 1991 to 1997 from the Immunization Monitoring Program (IMPACT), almost 80% of hospitalized cases of pertussis and all deaths secondary to pertussis occurred in children 6 months of age or younger.[59]

CURRENT ISSUES FOR ADULTS AND ADOLESCENTS

In recent years, there has also been an increase in pertussis in adolescents and young adults. In the 1990s, Canada experienced a resurgence of pertussis, primarily in young adolescents.[60] This was a result of the low effectiveness of the whole-cell pertussis vaccine used between 1985

and 1998 in this country. This resulted in a "marching cohort" effect or the age of peak incidence increasing, each year, by 1 year, revealing the existence of a susceptible cohort[61] (Fig. 230-3). This was addressed with universal immunization programs to vaccinate adolescents with a more effective acellular pertussis vaccine.[60]

Despite a more effective acellular pertussis vaccine,[62] pertussis outbreaks in young adults continue to occur and have been well described worldwide.[63-67] Because adults often present with atypical pertussis and clinicians may think of whooping cough as a childhood disease, pertussis is frequently not diagnosed in older patients.[68] Adults represent a significant source of infection for infants; transmission has been reported from mothers,[69] adolescents,[70] grandparents,[71] and health care workers.[72-74] This shift in epidemiology is partly explained by

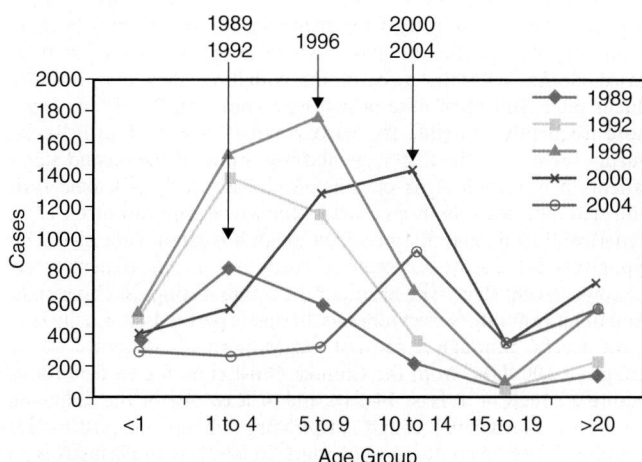

Figure 230-3 **Number of cases of pertussis reported in different age groups in Canada between 1989 and 2004.** Arrows indicate the age group in which the incidence was highest in a given year, excluding infants younger than 1 year.

waning immunity. Although, traditionally, immunity following natural pertussis infection was believed to be lifelong, there is evidence that this is not the case and that repeat infections[75] or subclinical boosting[76] likely occurs. Immunity after pertussis immunization also diminishes over time. It is estimated that immunity following acellular pertussis vaccination may begin to decline after 4 to 5 years, suggesting that a booster dose may be appropriate.[77]

THE CARRIER STATE

In the past, based on knowledge obtained from traditional culture methods, there was not considered to be a carrier state for *B. pertussis* in the nasopharynx. However, this may no longer be true, according to studies done with more sensitive polymerase chain reaction (PCR) methods. In addition to circulating among adults, there may also be transient nasopharyngeal carriage of *B. pertussis* in immunized children. A recent report[78] has described a laboratory-confirmed (primarily by PCR) outbreak of pertussis occurring in preschool-aged children. This was not a classic pertussis, as evidenced by a lower number of cases meeting a clinical case definition, a very low hospitalization rate of unimmunized infants, and a low secondary attack rate in households. High vaccine rates may have moderated the outbreak and, with respiratory co-infection in a significant proportion of cases, a positive PCR result may simply have reflected transient nasopharyngeal carriage of *B. pertussis* in the absence of evidence of seroconversion.

Clinical Presentation

There is a spectrum of disease caused by *B. pertussis* infection and its presentation will vary according to the patient's age, degree of immunity, use of antibiotics, and respiratory co-infection.[79]

YOUNG CHILDREN

Joseph Lapin wrote a detailed description of typical or classic pertussis in 1943 that remains true to this day.[1] Pertussis is classically divided into three stages: the catarrhal or prodromal stage, the paroxysmal stage, and the convalescent stage. The catarrhal stage begins after a usual incubation period of 7 to 10 days, with a range of 5 to 21 days. In the catarrhal stage, children will present with signs and symptoms of a common upper respiratory tract infection including rhinorrhea, nonpurulent conjunctivitis with excessive lacrimation, occasional cough, and low-grade fever. The catarrhal stage typically lasts 1 to 2 weeks and is followed by the paroxysmal stage. As its name suggests, the paroxysmal stage is characterized by paroxysms or fits of coughing. The child will typically have spasms of uncontrollable coughing, often 10 to 15 coughs in a row in a single expiration, the face may turn red or purple and, at the end of the paroxysm, he or she may have an inspiratory whoop. The whoop is caused by inspiring against a partially closed glottis. With the force of the coughing, they may produce mucus plugs and often have post-tussive vomiting. Paroxysms occur more frequently at night. The paroxysmal stage lasts 1 to 6 weeks. During the end of the first stage and beginning of the second stage, patients may exhibit signs of systemic disease, such as leukocytosis with lymphocytosis, both risk factors for worse clinical outcome.[80-82] Hyperinsulinemia may also occur, although it is rarely associated with hypoglycemia.[83] Lastly, as symptoms begin to wane, the patient enters the convalescent stage. The length of the cough distinguishes pertussis from other respiratory tract illnesses. In classic pertussis, it usually lasts 1 to 6 weeks, although it can last longer; pertussis is known as the "cough of 100 days" from the Chinese. Most clinical case definitions require a cough of at least 14 days and at least one of the following symptoms: paroxysmal cough, inspiratory whoop, or post-tussive vomiting.[79] The mean duration of cough in adults with pertussis is 36 to 48 days.[68] For up to 1 year following pertussis infection, it is not uncommon to have recurrences of the paroxysmal cough or inspiratory whoop with other respiratory illnesses.

INFANTS AND ADULTS

Pertussis can present atypically in adults and infants. Infants are less likely to have the characteristic inspiratory whoop and a significant catarrhal stage and are more likely to present with gagging, gasping, cyanosis, or apnea and have a prolonged convalescent phase.[82-84] Infants often present with the nonspecific sign of poor feeding and can present with seizures. In adults, paroxysmal coughing is seen in most patients and several studies have reported cough duration of longer than 21 days.[68] There is a wide range in the percentage of adult patients with pertussis who have whooping (8% to 82%) and post-tussive vomiting (17% to 65%, mean 50%). Unlike children, in adults, post-tussive vomiting is strongly suggestive of pertussis.

Complications

There are several complications associated with pertussis. According to data from Canada and the United States, pneumonia is the most common complication of pertussis in hospitalized patients, especially among newborns younger than 1 month (10% to 18%).[58,59] Pneumonia can be caused by *B. pertussis* infection itself (see Fig. 230-1) or coinfection with other respiratory pathogens. Respiratory syncytial virus (RSV) is the best described copathogen with *B. pertussis*. Rates of RSV coinfection in infants hospitalized with pertussis range from 5% to 33%.[58,84] Conversely, 8% to 16% of children with RSV infection may also be positive for *B. pertussis*.[85,86] The case-fatality rate of pertussis is highest in infants; approximately 1% of children younger than 6 months will die with pertussis infection.[59] In a case-control study done by the IMPACT surveillance network, leukocytosis and pneumonia were independent predictors of death in infants hospitalized with pertussis.[80] Encephalopathy is a rare complication of pertussis.[45] It occurs more commonly in younger nonimmunized children (in 1.4% of infants younger than 2 months)[87] but can occur in adults as well.[88] It typically presents between the second and fourth week of cough.[89] Seizures are the most common clinical manifestation, although paresis and paraplegias, ataxia, aphasia, blindness, deafness, and decerebrate posturing have also been described. Pertussis-specific antigens may cross the blood-brain barrier and directly affect the central nervous system because high cerebrospinal fluid (CSF) antibody titers to pertussis toxin and filamentous hemagglutinin have been reported in cases of pertussis encephalopathy.[45] Complications of pertussis, such as pneumonia and urinary incontinence, are surprisingly high in older patients and significantly more frequent in adults than adolescents, especially in those who smoke or who have asthma.[90] Other complications of pertussis caused by the forceful and persistent nature of the cough include subconjunctival hemorrhages, syncope, and rib fractures.

Diagnosis

The first step in the diagnosis of pertussis is to have the appropriate index of suspicion for pertussis disease. For vaccine trials, WHO defines a case of pertussis as a patient with a paroxysmal cough for 21 days or longer and one or more of the following criteria: positive culture for *B. pertussis*, significant increases in IgG and IgA antibody against FHA, agglutinogen (AGG) 2 and 3 or PT, or proven contact with a culture-confirmed case.[79] This definition favors specificity of diagnosis rather than sensitivity. According to the CDC and WHO, for pertussis surveillance, a clinical case is defined as a patient with cough for 14 days or longer and at least one of the following: paroxysmal cough, whoop, or post-tussive vomiting. This is a more sensitive definition but confirmation requires a positive laboratory finding by culture or PCR assay or a confirmed epidemiologic link.

CULTURE

Laboratory confirmation of pertussis has traditionally been made by culture methods.[29] Proper collection (including the timing of culture), transport, and storage of specimens are required to enhance the detection of *B. pertussis* by culture methods. Preferred patient specimens for the diagnosis of pertussis are nasopharyngeal (NP) aspirates and posterior NP swabs. These specimens contain the ciliated respiratory epithelial cells for which *B. pertussis* has an affinity. The advantage of NP aspirates rather than swabs is an increased culture positivity rate and added sample for any additional tests. If NP swabs are used, swab material should be calcium alginate, Dacron, or rayon, because cotton will inhibit the growth of *B. pertussis*. Specific transport media should be used for NP specimens, including 1% acid-hydrolyzed casein or Amies medium with charcoal. Specimens may be inoculated into enrichment media such as RL transport medium, which contains half-strength charcoal agar and horse blood with cephalexin to suppress normal NP flora growth. For culture testing, specimens should then be inoculated onto BG or RL medium supplemented with glycerol, peptones, and sheep (or, preferably, horse) blood. Cephalexin is added to reduce the growth of normal flora but may inhibit the growth of some strains of *B. pertussis*. After incubation in ambient air at 35° to 36°C, *B. pertussis* colonies may become visible after 3 to 4 days, although plates are typically held up to 7 days. *B. pertussis* colonies are round, domed, mercury silver–colored, and shiny and produce hemolysis on BG agar. Polyclonal or monoclonal antibodies may be used to confirm identity or *B. pertussis* can be identified by biochemical tests based on differential phenotypic characteristics.

MOLECULAR DIAGNOSIS

Culture method is the most specific way to diagnose pertussis. The sensitivity of culture for *B. pertussis*, however, varies widely depending on specimen transport and collection methods, as described earlier, as well as patient factors such as previous immunization, interval since symptom onset, antibiotic use, and age.[79] Different studies have reported culture sensitivity rates for *B. pertussis* ranging from 15% to 80%.[91-93] Many clinical microbiology laboratories now use nucleic acid detection methods such as PCR assay as a more sensitive diagnostic test for pertussis. Different PCR assays target different chromosomal regions of *B. pertussis* including the pertussis toxin (PT) promoter region, a region upstream of the porin gene, the repetitive insertion sequence IS481, the ACT gene, and a region upstream of the flagellin gene.[29] PCR methods for *B. pertussis* include the standard PCR gel assay and the reportedly more sensitive real-time assay. The main advantages of diagnosing pertussis by PCR are its aforementioned increased sensitivity and the rapidity of testing compared with culture methods. In addition, unlike culture, which is often only positive early in the course of the disease, PCR will remain positive even after 7 days of antibiotic treatment in over half of pertussis cases.[94] However, one needs to be cautious with the use of PCR testing for pertussis as well. Because PCR detects genomic material, it will detect both live and dead bacteria. As with any PCR-based method, contamination is always a concern. Although *B. pertussis* is not an environmental organism, contamination at single collection sites, with positive cultures from environmental surfaces and staff, has been described.[95] Contamination may also occur in the laboratory and may be responsible for pseudo-outbreaks of pertussis.[96] There is no standardized or U.S. Food and Drug Administration (FDA)–approved, commercially available PCR test for *B. pertussis*, and PCR assay methodologies and results may vary significantly between laboratories. Depending on where the crossing threshold is set for real-time PCR positivity, the sensitivity and specificity may also vary widely. Studies suggest that PCR may be too sensitive a test to use alone as a screening method for pertussis diagnosis in an outbreak setting[63] and, in the absence of clinical, serologic, or culture confirmation, positive results may simply reflect transient nasopharyngeal carriage.[78]

SEROLOGY

Pertussis can also be diagnosed using serologic methods.[97] The advantage of serology is that by the time the patient presents with typical symptoms of pertussis, the antibody response is usually present. In contrast, nasopharyngeal cultures are usually only positive early in the course of the disease. Most laboratories use an enzyme-linked immunosorbent assay (ELISA) to detect antibodies to *B. pertussis*. ELISAs have been developed with whole bacterial cells, PT, FHA, PRN, FIM, lipo-oligosaccharide, and adenylate cyclase toxin. Whole bacterial cell ELISAs are limited by cross-reactivity with other *Bordetella* species and other bacteria. PT is the most common antigen used for *B. pertussis* serology. PT is only produced by *B. pertussis*, making it a highly specific antigen, and it is an important protective antigen in the immune response to infection and immunization. Unfortunately, young infants may not produce an antibody response to PT. FHA has also been used as an ELISA antigen. However, the antibody response to FHA is not specific because all *Bordetella* species have FHA, and antibodies to *Haemophilus influenzae* and *Mycoplasma pneumoniae* have been shown to cross-react with FHA. In addition, the presence of FHA antibody has not been correlated with protection in human studies. PRN and FIM may also be used to detect a serologic response to *B. pertussis* but antibodies to these antigens occur less consistently than those against PT. ELISAs using lipo-oligosaccharide and adenylate cyclase have been described only in a few research laboratories. Although there are ELISAs to detect IgG, IgA, and IgM to *B. pertussis*, IgG assays are the most frequently used as a diagnostic test, are the best standardized and most widely available. IgG rises typically 2 to 3 weeks after infection or primary immunization and 1 week after booster immunization. Distinguishing between antibody responses secondary to infection and secondary to recent immunization may not be possible. Paired sera are the gold standard for serologic diagnosis and a twofold increase is considered significant evidence of seroconversion.

The difficulty with *B. pertussis* serology, however, is that one rarely obtains an acute and convalescent phase sera but rather obtains a convalescent and late convalescent phase sera, because pertussis is often recognized late in the course of the disease. In immunized individuals, the antibody response is rapid and one may not see the antibody rise in convalescent serology. Single serum antibody titers have thus been used to diagnose pertussis and typically require level 3 standard deviations (SDs) above that of healthy age-matched controls, preferably for two or more antigens. Single serum testing is particularly useful for adolescents and adults because cultures are often negative in this age group and pertussis immunizations are usually more remote. With adult and adolescent immunization campaigns, the serologic diagnosis of pertussis based on a single serum sample may become more challenging.

DIRECT FLUORESCENT ANTIBODY

Finally, direct fluorescent antibody (DFA) testing can also be used to diagnose pertussis infection. Fluorochrome-conjugated monoclonal or polyclonal antibodies recognizing a lipo-oligosaccharide epitope directly detect *B. pertussis* in nasopharyngeal secretions.[29] However, although it is a rapid and inexpensive diagnostic test, it has poor sensitivity and specificity. The sensitivity of DFA compared with culture is reported to range from 30% to 71%.[93,98] In addition, the specificity of DFA is variable because of cross-reactivity with other organisms such as *B. bronchiseptica*, *H. influenzae*, and diphtheroids.[29] DFA is not considered to be laboratory confirmation of a case of pertussis for most national surveillance systems and has been replaced in large part in clinical laboratories by the other diagnostic tests described.

▨ Treatment

ANTIMICROBIAL AGENTS

There is controversy regarding the efficacy of antibiotic therapy in the different stages of pertussis disease. The difficulty is partly caused by the fact that most studies are powered for a primary outcome of nasopharyngeal microbial eradication rather than for a clinical outcome. The classic teaching is that antibiotics improve symptoms and ablate disease when given early in the course of the disease, during the catarrhal stage, but not when given in the paroxysmal stage.[99] In an open randomized study by Bergquist and colleagues,[100] 17 patients with a positive culture for *B. pertussis* were treated with erythromycin for 10 days and compared with untreated controls. Treatment eradicated the bacterium from the nasopharynx in all but one patient and the treated group developed significantly fewer whoops than the control group. However, although patients were enrolled within the first 14 days of their illness, a significant proportion already complained of a whooping cough on their initial visit, suggesting that antibiotics may have an effect, albeit not a dramatic one, in the paroxysmal as well as the catarrhal stage of disease. The erythromycin study group from Germany[101] has also reported improvement in the frequency and severity of coughing in patients in the early paroxysmal stage of pertussis treated with erythromycin. However, a Cochrane review of 11 randomized or quasirandomized controlled trials of antibiotics for treatment of whooping cough has concluded that although antibiotics are effective in eliminating *B. pertussis*, they do not alter the subsequent clinical course of the illness.[102]

Traditionally, oral erythromycin was the antibiotic of choice to treat pertussis.[103] Erythromycin estolate is considered superior to erythromycin ethylsuccinate or erythromycin stearate because of the higher drug concentrations achieved in the serum and respiratory secretions. The CDC recommends an erythromycin dose of 40 to 50 mg/kg/day in four divided doses for children to a maximum of 2 g/day for adolescents and adults for 14 days to treat pertussis.[99] Although the CDC recommends a 14-day treatment course, 7 days of a maximum of 1g of erythromycin estolate treatment was found to be as effective for the eradication of *B. pertussis* and improved compliance in a randomized controlled clinical trial in Canada.[104] The main problem with oral erythromycin treatment for pertussis is the frequency of gastrointestinal side effects. Up to 30% of patients may experience gastrointestinal symptoms such as nausea, vomiting, or diarrhea. In addition, there is an association between oral erythromycin and hypertrophic pyloric stenosis in infants younger than 1 month and azithromycin should therefore be used in this age group.[105]

Several randomized controlled trials have assessed the role of newer macrolides in the treatment of pertussis.[106,107] A Cochrane review of these studies has determined that short-term antibiotics (azithromycin for 3 to 5 days or clarithromycin for 7 days) are as effective as long-term antibiotics (erythromycin for 10 to 14 days) in eradicating *B. pertussis* from the nasopharynx (relative risk [RR], 1.02; 95% confidence interval [CI], 0.98 to 1.05) but had fewer side effects (RR, 0.66; 95% CI, 0.52 to 0.83).[102] Trimethoprim-sulfamethoxazole for 7 days may also be effective although the efficacy data are not convincing.[108,109] Although fluoroquinolones have been shown to have in vitro activity against *B. pertussis*,[110] there is a lack of evidence of their clinical efficacy. *B. pertussis* strains are not routinely tested for antimicrobial susceptibility because there is no standardized method for antimicrobial susceptibility testing for *B. pertussis* and *B. pertussis* is often detected by molecular rather than culture methods.[103] Although erythromycin resistance, which predicts resistance to other macrolides, in *B. pertussis* strains have been identified and are likely caused by a mutation of the erythromycin-binding site in the 23S rRNA gene,[111] there is no evidence that erythromycin resistance in *B. pertussis* in increasing or spreading.[110] Continued surveillance of *B. pertussis* isolates, however, is needed.

SUPPORTIVE CARE

In addition to antibiotic therapy, supportive care is paramount for the management of pertussis, especially in infants. Intubation and mechanical ventilation may be required for infants with apnea and cyanosis.[84] Physicians should also be aware of the potential for respiratory co-infection and treat them appropriately. Adjunctive therapy such as corticosteroids, salbutamol, pertussis-specific immunoglobu-

lin, and antihistamines have been used to treat the cough of pertussis symptomatically and are the subject of a Cochrane review.[112] Only nine studies satisfied the inclusion criteria; four had insufficient data and the remaining studies were small and poorly reported. No statistically significant benefit was found for any of the interventions. Neither diphenhydramine nor salbutamol changed the frequency of coughing spells and dexamethasone did not decrease the length of hospital stay. Pertussis immunoglobulin did not affect length of hospital stay and, although it was associated with a mean reduction in the number of whoops per 24 hours, the difference was not statistically significant. An efficacy study of pertussis immune globulin for the treatment of hospitalized infants with pertussis was prematurely terminated because of expiration of the immune globulin and unavailability of additional study product.[113]

Prevention

IMMUNIZATION

Immunization is the single most effective means of preventing pertussis disease. The history of pertussis vaccination is long and began with attempts to develop a vaccine from whole *B. pertussis* organism. The difficulty lay in striking the right balance between making a vaccine with enough bacteria that it was immunogenic versus making a vaccine that was too reactogenic because of additional impurities.[4] Prior to the 1940s, the efficacy of a vaccine could only be assessed in human trials until Kendrick and associates developed the mouse potency test.[114] In the mouse potency test, the efficacy of a vaccine was determined by immunizing a mouse intraperitoneally and then infecting it intracerebrally with live *B. pertussis*. Survival was measured at 14 days and a potency unit was calculated according to WHO criteria. Using standardized potency vaccines, the British Medical Research Council performed multiple field trials during the 1940s and 1950s testing different vaccines and found a correlation between the results of the mouse potency test and degree of protection in children against pertussis disease.[115] Concurrently, the United States began routine immunization of children with whole-cell pertussis vaccines in the 1940s and observed a dramatic drop in the rates of pertussis. However, no formal prospective clinical efficacy trials were done to assess whole-cell pertussis vaccines, routinely given combined with diphtheria and tetanus toxoids (DTP vaccine). The best data available regarding their efficacy are from six vaccine trials done in four countries between 1990 and 1995 comparing acellular and whole-cell pertussis vaccines.[4] Except for the Connaught vaccine—thought to be less effective in their attempts to make it less reactogenic—the percentage efficacy of DTP against typical pertussis ranges from 89% to 96%. WHO recommends immunization with DTP and it continues to be used worldwide in many countries.[52]

WHOLE-CELL VACCINES

The problem with whole-cell pertussis vaccines is their reactogenicity. It is known that DTP vaccine causes significantly more local reactions (redness, swelling, and pain) and systemic reactions such as drowsiness, vomiting, and persistent crying than acellular pertussis vaccines and DT alone.[4] More serious adverse events such as convulsions and hypotonic and hyporesponsive episodes (HHE) are much rarer occurrences, especially after the introduction of acellular vaccines.[116] There has also been much discussion surrounding the role of pertussis vaccine in causing neurologic injury and death.[117] From the 1940s to the 1970s, there were multiple case reports and series reporting possible vaccine complications ranging from encephalopathy and coma to death.[118,119] The ensuing controversy about pertussis vaccination affected much of Europe, Japan, United States, Soviet Union, and Australia. A large case-control study, the National Childhood Encephalopathy Study (NCES), investigated the relationship between DTP immunization and neurologic injury and found the risk to be very low (1 in 111,000). In 1991, the U.S. Institute of Medicine reviewed all the literature and concluded that there was no evidence to support an association between pertussis immunization and permanent neurologic damage.[120] In addition, according to IMPACT data from 1993 to 2002 in Canada, there was no evidence of encephalopathy following more than 6.5 million doses of pertussis vaccine.[121] There was also initial concern regarding the possible association between pertussis vaccination and sudden infant death syndrome (SIDS).[122] However, several large controlled studies have failed to find a cause-and-effect relationship between pertussis immunization and SIDS.[123,124] It is likely that any possible association between pertussis immunization and infantile seizures or SIDS is a result of the fact that these conditions present coincidentally with the time at which the two- or three-dose primary series of DTP is administered.

ACELLULAR PERTUSSIS VACCINES

In response to concerns regarding reactogenicity, pertussis vaccines composed of acellular components of *B. pertussis* were developed. Sato and coworkers from Japan were the first to design an acellular pertussis vaccine containing two purified hemagglutinins (HAs): filamentous HA and leukocytosis-promoting factor HA.[125] By removing endotoxin (lipopolysaccharide [LPS]) from the preparation, they were able to produce a vaccine that was as effective as the whole-cell vaccine and caused fewer side effects. The vaccine was used for mass immunization in Japan beginning in 1981 during an epidemic of pertussis. Although efficacy data for this first acellular pertussis vaccine were limited, its use spurred the development of further prototypes. Several different versions of acellular pertussis vaccines have since been developed and include one-, two-, three-, four-, and five-component vaccines (composed of a combination of PT, FIM 2 and 3, PRN, and/or FHA). All are less reactogenic than their whole-cell counterparts because they do not contain LPS.[4] Their efficacies vary depending on the type of study done and the case definition used but range from 59% to 93% for pertussis cases defined according to the WHO criteria. Vaccines containing PT, FHA, PRN, and FIM are likely more effective against mild disease than vaccines containing PT, FHA, and/or PRN alone, suggesting that fimbriae may have a role in protection against infection and/or milder disease.[126]

VACCINATION SCHEDULES

Most North American immunization schedules recommend pertussis vaccination at 2, 4, 6, and 18 months, with a booster at 4 to 6 years. Although there are many different pertussis immunization schedules throughout the world, most will have two or three doses in the first year of life, another dose in the second year of life, and a preschool booster. Childhood immunization with pertussis containing combination vaccines has been demonstrated to be safe, immunogenic, and effective for the control of pertussis.[127] However, pertussis outbreaks continue to occur in the adult[65,74,128] and adolescent population.[67,129] Because adolescents and adults continue to be a source of pertussis transmission,[70,71] immunization of this group has recently been investigated by the Adult Pertussis Trial (APERT).[130] In this study, 2781 healthy subjects were randomized to receive either a tricomponent acellular vaccine or a hepatitis A vaccine. Vaccine protection against pertussis disease was 92% during the study follow-up period (median duration, 22 months). Several prospective randomized controlled trials have assessed the reactogenicity and immunogenicity of Tdap (Adacel) in several thousand adolescents and adults.[131-133] The Tdap vaccine elicited robust immune responses and had a similar safety profile to the Td vaccine. Follow-up data from several of these studies demonstrated that antibody titers to pertussis exceed preimmunization levels 1, 3, and 5 years later.[134] Further studies have shown that Tdap boosters can be given safely at intervals as short as 18 months after prior tetanus, diphtheria, or pertussis vaccinations in adolescents.[135] Both cellular and humoral immune responses occur after acellular pertussis immunization of

adults and adolescents, but the cell-mediated immune response may be of greater magnitude and longer duration and thus more reflective of long-term protection.[136] Both the National Advisory Committee on Immunization (NACI) and the Advisory Committee on Immunization Practices (ACIP) of the CDC have recommended routine Tdap vaccination for adolescents and to replace Td with Tdap boosters in adults.[137-139] The Canadian experience has demonstrated that an adolescent pertussis vaccine program can be implemented on a national scale,[60] is safe,[140] and can result in a further decrease in the incidence of pertussis.[141]

VACCINATION OF HEALTH CARE WORKERS

Health care workers are another potential source of pertussis transmission, particularly to patients. Multiple nosocomial pertussis outbreaks have been described,[72-74] with significant patient health consequences and costs incurred to the health care system.[142-144] Costs included direct medical center costs for treatment and prophylaxis, costs for personnel time, and indirect medical center costs for time lost from work. It is more cost-effective for health care workers to be vaccinated than to manage a nosocomial exposure of pertussis.[145] The ACIP recommends that health care workers who work in hospitals or ambulatory care settings and have direct patient contact should receive a single dose of Tdap at an interval as short as 2 years from the last dose of Td.[139] Given its cost-effectiveness, health care institutions should provide universal Tdap immunization to their health care workers.

PROTECTION OF INFANTS

Infants are most vulnerable to severe pertussis disease, so specific strategies have been examined to protect neonates from pertussis transmission.[146] A cocoon strategy of vaccinating household members may be effective in providing partial protection to unimmunized infants because parents are known to be important sources of infection in these cases. One study has shown a 70% decrease in the number of pertussis cases in infants 0 to 3 months of age in households in which a cocoon strategy had been implemented.[147] Immunizing mothers during pregnancy has also been investigated. The ACIP does not consider pregnancy a contraindication to Tdap vaccination, although it recommends that women receive Tdap before becoming pregnant or receive a dose of Tdap in the immediate postpartum period.[139] Although pertussis antibodies cross the placenta, maternal antibody levels are low and decay rapidly.[148] Administering a pertussis booster dose during pregnancy may increase neonatal antibody titers but may not help with the infant's cellular immune response to infection. Finally, neonatal pertussis vaccination has also been studied as a method of preventing pertussis. Vaccination of newborn infants with whole-cell pertussis vaccine resulted in "immune tolerance" or reduced antibody responses to *B. pertussis* antigens compared with infants who received their first pertussis vaccine at 2 months.[149,150] However, early neonatal immunization with acellular pertussis vaccine was safe, well tolerated, and accelerated the acquisition of pertussis antibodies in infants without inducing immune tolerance.[151] Future antibody responses to *H. influenzae* and hepatitis B vaccines may be dampened, however. Clinical trials are currently underway to assess the safety and efficacy of maternal and neonatal immunization against pertussis.

CHEMOPROPHYLAXIS

In addition to immunization, chemoprophylaxis may be used to prevent the transmission of *B. pertussis*. In the United States, erythromycin prophylaxis is recommended for all household contacts and other close contacts, including those in child care.[99] In Canada, chemoprophylaxis is recommended only for infant or pregnant women (third trimester) and household contacts.[152] However, erythromycin prophylaxis of pertussis contacts is not practiced uniformly throughout the world. In fact, in a Cochrane review of 2 randomized controlled trials of antibiotic treatment of contacts,[153,154] the authors concluded that chemoprophylaxis of contacts older than 6 months do not significantly improve clinical symptoms or the number of cases developing culture-positive *B. pertussis*.[102] It is important to note, however, that these randomized trials did not specifically investigate the use of erythromycin in high-risk populations, such as children younger than 6 months, who might benefit the most from any added protection. Although there are reports of successful chemoprophylaxis against pertussis, these are often the results of uncontrolled or poorly controlled studies.[155,156] It is likely in many cases that transmission occurs before pertussis is diagnosed in the index case, thus limiting the usefulness of chemoprophylaxis. If chemoprophylaxis is to be of any benefit, it needs to be given early in the course of the disease in the index case and before the occurrence of the first secondary case.[157] Chemoprophylaxis is generally not recommended if 21 days have elapsed since the onset of cough in the index case.[99]

PERTUSSIS IN SCHOOLS AND DAY CARE CENTERS

Children and staff with pertussis should be excluded from attendance until 5 days after initiation of macrolide treatment. Those untreated should be excluded for 21 days after onset of illness. Exposed children, particularly incompletely immunized children, should be observed for 21 days after the last contact.

Future Directions

Although much has been learned about pertussis since the time of Lapin, there remain several unanswered questions. How much pertussis disease is there in adults? Do adults require multiple doses of pertussis vaccine, and will this result in less cough illness? Is there a nasopharyngeal carrier state for *B. pertussis*? Is maternal immunization a safe and effective way of preventing neonatal pertussis? Future research is needed in these and other areas to further our understanding of pertussis.

REFERENCES

1. Lapin JH. *Whooping Cough.* Springfield, Ill: Charles C Thomas; 1943.
2. Sydenham T. *Opera Universa Medica.* London: Sydenham Society; 1741.
3. Bordet J, Gengou O. Le microbe de la coqueluche. *Ann Inst Pasteur.* 1906;20:731-741.
4. Mattoo S, Cherry JD. Molecular pathogenesis, epidemiology, and clinical manifestations of respiratory infections due to *Bordetella pertussis* and other Bordetella subspecies. *Clin Microbiol Rev.* 2005;18:326-382.
5. Cotter PA, Miller JF. *Bordetella.* In: Groisman EA, ed. *Principles of Bacterial Pathogenesis.* London: Academic Press; 2001:620-674.
6. Viejo G, de la Iglesia P, Otero L, et al. *Bordetella bronchiseptica* pleural infection in a patient with AIDS. *Scand J Infect Dis.* 2002;34:628-629.
7. Berkowitz DM, Bechara RI, Wolfenden LL. An unusual cause of cough and dyspnea in an immunocompromised patient. *Chest.* 2007;131:1599-1602.
8. Ner Z, Ross LA, Horn MV, et al. *Bordetella bronchiseptica* infection in pediatric lung transplant recipients. *Pediatr Transplant.* 2003;7:413-417.
9. Porter JF, Connor K, Donachie W. Isolation and characterization of *Bordetella parapertussis*-like bacteria from ovine lungs. *Microbiology.* 1994;140(Pt 2):255-261.
10. Sebaihia M, Preston A, Maskell DJ, et al. Comparison of the genome sequence of the poultry pathogen *Bordetella avium* with those of *B. bronchiseptica, B. pertussis,* and *B. parapertussis* reveals extensive diversity in surface structures associated with host interaction. *J Bacteriol.* 2006;188:6002-6015.
11. Dorittke C, Vandamme P, Hinz KH, et al. Isolation of a *Bordetella avium*-like organism from a human specimen. *Eur J Clin Microbiol Infect Dis.* 1995;14:451-454.
12. Spilker T, Liwienski AA, LiPuma JJ. Identification of Bordetella spp. in respiratory specimens from individuals with cystic fibrosis. *Clin Microbiol Infect.* 2008;14:504-506.
13. Fry NK, Duncan J, Edwards MT, et al. A UK clinical isolate of *Bordetella hinzii* from a patient with myelodysplastic syndrome. *J Med Microbiol.* 2007;56:1700-1703.
14. Cookson BT, Vandamme P, Carlson LC, et al. Bacteremia caused by a novel Bordetella species, "*B. hinzii*." *J Clin Microbiol.* 1994;32:2569-2571.
15. Kattar MM, Chavez JF, Limaye AP, et al. Application of 16S rRNA gene sequencing to identify *Bordetella hinzii* as the causative agent of fatal septicemia. *J Clin Microbiol.* 2000;38:789-794.
16. Arvand M, Feldhues R, Mieth M, et al. Chronic cholangitis caused by *Bordetella hinzii* in a liver transplant recipient. *J Clin Microbiol.* 2004;42:2335-2337.
17. Weyant RS, Hollis DG, Weaver RE, et al. *Bordetella holmesii* sp. nov., a new gram-negative species associated with septicemia. *J Clin Microbiol.* 1995;33:1-7.
18. Greig JR, Gunda SS, Kwan JTC. *Bordetella holmesii* bacteraemia in an individual on haemodialysis. *Scand J Infect Dis.* 2001; 33:716-717.
19. Shepard CW, Daneshvar MI, Kaiser RM, et al. *Bordetella holmesii* bacteremia: A newly recognized clinical entity among asplenic patients. *Clin Infect Dis.* 2004;38:799-804.
20. Tang YW, Hopkins MK, Kolbert CP, et al. *Bordetella holmesii*-like organisms associated with septicemia, endocarditis, and respiratory failure. *Clin Infect Dis.* 1998;26:389-392.
21. Dorbecker C, Licht C, Korber F, et al. Community-acquired pneumonia due to *Bordetella holmesii* in a patient with frequently relapsing nephrotic syndrome. *J Infect.* 2007;54: e203-e205.
22. Vandamme P, Heyndrickx M, Vancanneyt M, et al. *Bordetella trematum* sp. nov., isolated from wounds and ear infections in humans, and reassessment of *Alcaligenes denitrificans* Ruger and Tan 1983. *Int J Syst Bacteriol.* 1996;46:849-858.
23. Daxboeck F, Goerzer E, Apfalter P, et al. Isolation of *Bordetella trematum* from a diabetic leg ulcer. *Diabet Med.* 2004; 21:1247-1248.
24. von Wintzingerode F, Schattke A, Siddiqui RA, et al. *Bordetella petrii* sp. nov., isolated from an anaerobic bioreactor, and emended description of the genus Bordetella. *Int J Syst Evol Microbiol.* 2001;51:1257-1265.
25. Stark D, Riley LA, Harkness J, et al. *Bordetella petrii* from a clinical sample in Australia: Isolation and molecular identification. *J Med Microbiol.* 2007;56:435-437.
26. Fry NK, Duncan J, Malnick H, et al. *Bordetella petrii* clinical isolate. *Emerg Infect Dis.* 2005;11:1131-1133.
27. Ko KS, Peck KR, Oh WS, et al. New species of Bordetella, *Bordetella ansorpii* sp. nov., isolated from the purulent exudate of an epidermal cyst. *J Clin Microbiol.* 2005;43: 2516-2519.
28. Fry NK, Duncan J, Malnick H, et al. The first UK isolate of '*Bordetella ansorpii*' from an immunocompromised patient. *J Med Microbiol.* 2007;56:993-995.
29. Loeffelholz MJ, Sanden GN. *Bordetella pertussis.* In: Murray PR, Baron E, Jorgensen J, et al, eds. *Manual of Clinical Microbiology.* 9th ed, vol 1. Washington, DC: ASM Press; 2007:803-814.
30. Cherry JD. Comparative efficacy of acellular pertussis vaccines: An analysis of recent trials. *Pediatr Infect Dis J.* 1997;16: S90-S96.
31. Tuomanen E, Weiss A. Characterization of two adhesins of *Bordetella pertussis* for human ciliated respiratory-epithelial cells. *J Infect Dis.* 1985;152:118-125.
32. Saukkonen K, Burnette WN, Mar VL, et al. Pertussis toxin has eukaryotic-like carbohydrate recognition domains. *Proc Natl Acad Sci U S A.* 1992;89:118-122.
33. Pittman M. The concept of pertussis as a toxin-mediated disease. *Pediatr Infect Dis.* 1984;3:467-486.
34. Paccani SR, Dal Molin FD, Benagiano M, et al. Suppression of T lymphocyte activation and chemotaxis by the adenylate cyclase toxin of *Bordetella pertussis. Infect Immun.* 2008;76: 2822-2832.
35. Carbonetti NH, Artamonova GV, Van Rooijen N, et al. Pertussis toxin targets airway macrophages to promote *Bordetella pertussis* infection of the respiratory tract. *Infect Immun.* 2007;75: 1713-1720.
36. Stibitz S, Aaronson W, Monack D, et al. Phase variation in *Bordetella pertussis* by frameshift mutation in a gene for a novel two-component system. *Nature.* 1989;338:266-269.
37. Melton AR, Weiss AA. Environmental regulation of expression of virulence determinants in *Bordetella pertussis. J Bacteriol.* 1989;171:6206-6212.
38. Luker KE, Tyler AN, Marshall GR, et al. Tracheal cytotoxin structural requirements for respiratory epithelial damage in pertussis. *Mol Microbiol.* 1995;16:733-743.
39. Flak TA, Goldman WE. Autotoxicity of nitric oxide in airway disease. *Am J Respir Crit Care Med.* 1996;154:S202-S206.
40. Walker KE, Weiss AA. Characterization of the dermonecrotic toxin in members of the genus Bordetella. *Infect Immun.* 1994;62:3817-3828.
41. Burns VC, Pishko EJ, Preston A, et al. Role of Bordetella O antigen in respiratory tract infection. *Infect Immun.* 2003;71: 86-94.
42. Harvill ET, Cotter PA, Miller JF. Pregenomic comparative analysis between *Bordetella bronchiseptica* RB50 and *Bordetella pertussis* tohama I in murine models of respiratory tract infection. *Infect Immun.* 1999;67:6109-6118.
43. Marr N, Luu RA, Fernandez RC. *Bordetella pertussis* binds human C1 esterase inhibitor during the virulent phase, to evade complement-mediated killing. *J Infect Dis.* 2007;195:585-588.
44. Stefanelli P, Sanguinetti M, Fazio C, et al. Differential in vitro expression of the brkA gene in *Bordetella pertussis* and *Bordetella parapertussis* clinical isolates. *J Clin Microbiol.* 2006; 44:3397-3400.
45. Grant CC, McKay EJ, Simpson A, et al. Pertussis encephalopathy with high cerebrospinal fluid antibody titers to pertussis toxin and filamentous hemagglutinin. *Pediatrics.* 1998;102:986-990.
46. Huang D, Tani M, Wang J, et al. Pertussis toxin-induced reversible encephalopathy dependent on monocyte chemoattractant protein-1 overexpression in mice. *J Neurosci.* 2002;22: 10633-10642.
47. Halasa NB, Barr FE, Johnson JE, et al. Fatal pulmonary hypertension associated with pertussis in infants: does extracorporeal membrane oxygenation have a role? *Pediatrics.* 2003;112: 1274-1278.
48. Carbonetti NH. Immunomodulation in the pathogenesis of *Bordetella pertussis* infection and disease. *Curr Opin Pharmacol.* 2007;7:272-278.
49. Harrington LE, Mangan PR, Weaver CT. Expanding the effector CD4 T-cell repertoire: The Th17 lineage. *Curr Opin Immunol.* 2006;18:349-356.
50. Happel KI, Dubin PJ, Zheng M, et al. Divergent roles of IL-23 and IL-12 in host defense against *Klebsiella pneumoniae. J Exp Med.* 2005;202:761-769.
51. Langrish CL, Chen Y, Blumenschein WM, et al. IL-23 drives a pathogenic T cell population that induces autoimmune inflammation. *J Exp Med.* 2005;201:233-240.
52. World Health Organization (WHO). *Pertussis Surveillance. A Global Meeting.* Geneva: Department of Vaccines and Biologicals; 2001.
53. Plotkin S. Aims, scope and findings of the global pertussis initiative. *Pediatr Infect Dis J.* 2005;24:S5-S6.
54. Tan T, Trindade E, Skowronski D. Epidemiology of pertussis. *Pediatr Infect Dis J.* 2005;24:S10-S18.
55. Forsyth K. Pertussis, still a formidable foe. *Clin Infect Dis.* 2007;45:1487-1491.
56. Cherry JD. The epidemiology of pertussis and pertussis immunization in the United Kingdom and the United States: A comparative study. *Curr Probl Pediatr.* 1984;14:1-78.
57. Halperin SA. The control of pertussis—2007 and beyond. *N Engl J Med.* 2007;356:110-113.
58. Cortese MM, Baughman AL, Zhang R, et al. Pertussis hospitalizations among infants in the United States, 1993 to 2004. *Pediatrics.* 2008;121:484-492.
59. Halperin SA, Wang EE, Law B, et al. Epidemiological features of pertussis in hospitalized patients in Canada, 1991-1997: Report of the Immunization Monitoring Program—Active (IMPACT). *Clin Infect Dis.* 1999;28:1238-1243.
60. Halperin SA. Canadian experience with implementation of an acellular pertussis vaccine booster-dose program in adolescents: Implications for the United States. *Pediatr Infect Dis J.* 2005;24:S141-S146.
61. Ntezayabo B, De Serres G, Duval B. Pertussis resurgence in Canada largely caused by a cohort effect. *Pediatr Infect Dis J.* 2003;22:22-27.
62. Bettinger JA, Halperin SA, De Serres G, et al. The effect of changing from whole-cell to acellular pertussis vaccine on the epidemiology of hospitalized children with pertussis in Canada. *Pediatr Infect Dis J.* 2007;26:31-35.

63. Centers for Disease Control and Prevention (CDC). Outbreaks of respiratory illness mistakenly attributed to pertussis—New Hampshire, Massachusetts, and Tennessee, 2004-2006. *MMWR Morb Mortal Wkly Rep*. 2007;56:837-842.
64. Sotir MJ, Cappozzo DL, Warshauer DM, et al. Evaluation of polymerase chain reaction and culture for diagnosis of pertussis in the control of a county-wide outbreak focused among adolescents and adults. *Clin Infect Dis*. 2007;44:1216-1219.
65. Mertens PL, Borsboom GJ, Richardus JH. A pertussis outbreak associated with social isolation among elderly nuns in a convent. *Clin Infect Dis*. 2007;44:266-268.
66. Centers for Disease Control and Prevention (CDC). Pertussis outbreak in an Amish community—Kent County, Delaware, September 2004-February 2005. *MMWR Morb Mortal Wkly Rep*. 2006;55:817-821.
67. Craig AS, Wright SW, Edwards KM, et al. Outbreak of pertussis on a college campus. *Am J Med*. 2007;120:364-368.
68. von Konig CH, Halperin S, Riffelmann M, et al. Pertussis of adults and infants. *Lancet Infect Dis*. 2002;2:744-750.
69. Izurieta HS, Kenyon TA, Strebel PM, et al. factors for pertussis in young infants during an outbreak in Chicago in 1993. *Clin Infect Dis*. 1996;22:503-507.
70. Deen JL, Mink CA, Cherry JD, et al. Household contact study of *Bordetella pertussis* infections. *Clin Infect Dis*. 1995;21:1211-1219.
71. Wendelboe AM, Njamkepo E, Bourillon A, et al. Transmission of *Bordetella pertussis* to young infants. *Pediatr Infect Dis J*. 2007;26:293-299.
72. Alexander EM, Travis S, Booms C, et al. Pertussis outbreak on a neonatal unit: Identification of a healthcare worker as the likely source. *J Hosp Infect*. 2008;69:131-134.
73. Bonmarin I, Poujol I, Levy-Bruhl D. Nosocomial infections and community clusters of pertussis in France, 2000-2005. *Euro Surveill*. 2007;12:E11-E12.
74. Bassinet L, Matrat M, Njamkepo E, et al. Nosocomial pertussis outbreak among adult patients and healthcare workers. *Infect Control Hosp Epidemiol*. 2004;25:995-997.
75. Cherry JD. Epidemiological, clinical, and laboratory aspects of pertussis in adults. *Clin Infect Dis*. 1999;28(Suppl 2):S112-S117.
76. Long SS, Welkon CJ, Clark JL. Widespread silent transmission of pertussis in families: Antibody correlates of infection and symptomatology. *J Infect Dis*. 1990;161:480-486.
77. Schellekens J, von Konig CH, Gardner P. Pertussis sources of infection and routes of transmission in the vaccination era. *Pediatr Infect Dis J*. 2005;24:S19-S24.
78. Waters V, Jamieson F, Richardson SE, et al. Outbreak of atypical pertussis detected by polymerase chain reaction in immunized preschool-aged children. *Pediatr Infect Dis J*. 2009; in press.
79. Cherry JD, Grimprel E, Guiso N, et al. Defining pertussis epidemiology: Clinical, microbiologic and serologic perspectives. *Pediatr Infect Dis J*. 2005;24:S25-S34.
80. Mikelova LK, Halperin SA, Scheifele D, et al. Predictors of death in infants hospitalized with pertussis: a case-control study of 16 pertussis deaths in Canada. *J Pediatr*. 2003;143:576-581.
81. Pierce C, Klein N, Peters M. Is leukocytosis a predictor of mortality in severe pertussis infection? *Intensive Care Med*. 2000;26:1512-1514.
82. Surridge J, Segedin ER, Grant CC. Pertussis requiring intensive care. *Arch Dis Child*. 2007;92:970-975.
83. Smith C, Vyas H. Early infantile pertussis; increasingly prevalent and potentially fatal. *Eur J Pediatr*. 2000;159:898-900.
84. Crowcroft NS, Booy R, Harrison T, et al. Severe and unrecognised: Pertussis in UK infants. *Arch Dis Child*. 2003; 88:802-806.
85. Korppi M, Hiltunen J. Pertussis is common in nonvaccinated infants hospitalized for respiratory syncytial virus infection. *Pediatr Infect Dis J*. 2007;26:316-318.
86. Cosnes-Lambe C, Raymond J, Chalumeau M, et al. Pertussis and respiratory syncytial virus infections. *Eur J Pediatr*. 2008; 167:1017-1019.
87. Farizo KM, Cochi SL, Zell ER, et al. Epidemiological features of pertussis in the United States, 1980-1989. *Clin Infect Dis*. 1992;14:708-719.
88. Halperin SA, Marrie TJ. Pertussis encephalopathy in an adult: case report and review. *Rev Infect Dis*. 1991;13:1043-1047.
89. Zellweger H. Pertussis encephalopathy. *Arch Pediatr*. 1959;76:381-386.
90. De Serres G, Shadmani R, Duval B, et al. Morbidity of pertussis in adolescents and adults. *J Infect Dis*. 2000;182:174-179.
91. Dragsted DM, Dohn B, Madsen J, et al. Comparison of culture and PCR for detection of *Bordetella pertussis* and *Bordetella parapertussis* under routine laboratory conditions. *J Med Microbiol*. 2004;53:749-754.
92. Lingappa JR, Lawrence W, West-Keefe S, et al. Diagnosis of community-acquired pertussis infection: Comparison of both culture and fluorescent-antibody assays with PCR detection using electrophoresis or dot blot hybridization. *J Clin Microbiol*. 2002;40:2908-2912.
93. Loeffelholz MJ, Thompson CJ, Long KS, et al. Comparison of PCR, culture, and direct fluorescent-antibody testing for detection of *Bordetella pertussis*. *J Clin Microbiol*. 1999;37: 2872-2876.
94. Edelman K, Nikkari S, Ruuskanen O, et al. Detection of *Bordetella pertussis* by polymerase chain reaction and culture in the nasopharynx of erythromycin-treated infants with pertussis. *Pediatr Infect Dis J*. 1996;15:54-57.
95. Taranger J, Trollfors B, Lind L, et al. Environmental contamination leading to false-positive polymerase chain reaction for pertussis. *Pediatr Infect Dis J*. 1994;13:936-937.
96. Lievano FA, Reynolds MA, Waring AL, et al. Issues associated with and recommendations for using PCR to detect outbreaks of pertussis. *J Clin Microbiol*. 2002;40:2801-2805.
97. Halperin S. Serologic and molecular tools for diagnosing *Bordetella pertussis* infection. In: Detrick B, ed. *Manual of Molecular and Clinical Laboratory Immunology*, 7th ed. Washington, DC: ASM Press; 2006:540-546.
98. Halperin SA, Bortolussi R, Wort AJ. Evaluation of culture, immunofluorescence, and serology for the diagnosis of pertussis. *J Clin Microbiol*. 1989;27:752-757.
99. Pickering LK, ed. *Red Book*. 27th ed, vol 1. Elk Grove Village, Ill: American Academy of Pediatrics; 2006.
100. Bergquist SO, Bernander S, Dahnsjo H, et al. Erythromycin in the treatment of pertussis: A study of bacteriologic and clinical effects. *Pediatr Infect Dis J*. 1987;6:458-461.
101. Hoppe JE. Comparison of erythromycin estolate and erythromycin ethylsuccinate for treatment of pertussis. The Erythromycin Study Group. *Pediatr Infect Dis J*. 1992;11:189-193.
102. Altunaiji S, Kukuruzovic R, Curtis N, et al. Antibiotics for whooping cough (pertussis). Cochrane Database Syst Rev 2007 (3):CD004404.
103. von Konig CH. Use of antibiotics in the prevention and treatment of pertussis. *Pediatr Infect Dis J*. 2005;24:S66-S68.
104. Halperin SA, Bortolussi R, Langley JM, et al. Seven days of erythromycin estolate is as effective as fourteen days for the treatment of Bordetella pertussis infections. *Pediatrics*. 1997;100:65-71.
105. Maheshwai N. Are young infants treated with erythromycin at risk for developing hypertrophic pyloric stenosis? *Arch Dis Child*. 2007;92:271-273.
106. Langley JM, Halperin SA, Boucher FD, et al. Azithromycin is as effective as and better tolerated than erythromycin estolate for the treatment of pertussis. *Pediatrics*. 2004;114:e96-e101.
107. Lebel MH, Mehra S. Efficacy and safety of clarithromycin versus erythromycin for the treatment of pertussis: a prospective, randomized, single blind trial. *Pediatr Infect Dis J*. 2001;20:1149-1154.
108. Hoppe JE, Halm U, Hagedorn HJ, et al. Comparison of erythromycin ethylsuccinate and co-trimoxazole for treatment of pertussis. *Infection*. 1989;17:227-231.
109. Adcock KJ, Reddy S, Okubadejo OA, et al. Trimethoprim-sulphamethoxazole in pertussis: Comparison with tetracycline. *Arch Dis Child*. 1972;47:311-313.
110. Gordon KA, Fusco J, Biedenbach DJ, et al. Antimicrobial susceptibility testing of clinical isolates of *Bordetella pertussis* from northern California: Report from the SENTRY Antimicrobial Surveillance Program. *Antimicrob Agents Chemother*. 2001;45:3599-3600.
111. Bartkus JM, Juni BA, Ehresmann K, et al. Identification of a mutation associated with erythromycin resistance in *Bordetella pertussis*: Implications for surveillance of antimicrobial resistance. *J Clin Microbiol*. 2003;41:1167-1172.
112. Pillay V, Swingler G. Symptomatic treatment of the cough in whooping cough. Cochrane Database Syst Rev 2003(4):CD003257.
113. Halperin SA, Vaudry W, Boucher FD, et al. Is pertussis immune globulin efficacious for the treatment of hospitalized infants with pertussis? No answer yet. *Pediatr Infect Dis J*. 2007; 26:79-81.
114. Kendrick PL, Eldering G, Dixon MK, et al. Mouse protection tests in the study of pertussis vaccine: A comparative series using the intracerebral route for challenge. *Am J Publ Health Nations Health*. 1947;37:803-810.
115. VACCINATION against whooping-cough; the final report to the Whooping-Cough Immunization Committee of the Medical Research Council and to the medical officers of health for Battersea and Wandsworth, Bradford, Liverpool, and Newcastle. *BMJ*. 1959;1:994-1000.
116. Le Saux N, Barrowman NJ, Moore DL, et al. Decrease in hospital admissions for febrile seizures and reports of hypotonic-hyporesponsive episodes presenting to hospital emergency departments since switching to acellular pertussis vaccine in Canada: A report from IMPACT. *Pediatrics*. 2003;112:e348.
117. Baker JP. The pertussis vaccine controversy in Great Britain, 1974-1986. *Vaccine*. 2003;21:4003-4010.
118. Berg JM. Neurological complications of pertussis immunization. *BMJ*. 1958;2:24-27.
119. Kulenkampff M, Schwartzman JS, Wilson J. Neurological complications of pertussis inoculation. *Arch Dis Child*. 1974; 49:46-49.
120. Institute of Medicine. *Adverse Effects of Pertussis and Rubella Vaccines: A Report of the Committee to Review the Adverse Consequences of Pertussis and Rubella Vaccines*. Washington, DC: National Academy Press; 1991.
121. Moore DL, Le Saux N, Scheifele D, et al. Lack of evidence of encephalopathy related to pertussis vaccine: Active surveillance by IMPACT, Canada, 1993-2002. *Pediatr Infect Dis J*. 2004; 23:568-571.
122. Baraff LJ, Ablon WJ, Weiss RC. Possible temporal association between diphtheria-tetanus toxoid-pertussis vaccination and sudden infant death syndrome. *Pediatr Infect Dis*. 1983;2: 7-11.
123. Griffin MR, Ray WA, Livengood JR, et al. Risk of sudden infant death syndrome after immunization with the diphtheria-tetanus-pertussis vaccine. *N Engl J Med*. 1988;319:618-623.
124. Hoffman HJ, Hunter JC, Damus K, et al. Diphtheria-tetanus-pertussis immunization and sudden infant death: Results of the National Institute of Child Health and Human Development Cooperative Epidemiological Study of Sudden Infant Death Syndrome risk factors. *Pediatrics*. 1987;79:598-611.
125. Sato Y, Kimura M, Fukumi H. Development of a pertussis component vaccine in Japan. *Lancet*. 1984;1:122-126.
126. Olin P, Rasmussen F, Gustafsson L, et al. Randomised controlled trial of two-component, three-component, and five-component acellular pertussis vaccines compared with whole-cell pertussis vaccine. Ad Hoc Group for the Study of Pertussis Vaccines. *Lancet*. 1997;350:1569-1577.
127. Halperin SA. Prevention of pertussis across the age spectrum through the use of the combination vaccines PENTACEL and ADACEL. *Expert Opin Biol Ther*. 2006;6:807-821.
128. Klement E, Uliel L, Engel I, et al. An outbreak of pertussis among young Israeli soldiers. *Epidemiol Infect*. 2003;131:1049-1054.
129. Mancuso JD, Snyder A, Stigers J, et al. Pertussis outbreak in a US military community: Kaiserslautern, Germany, April-June 2005. *Clin Infect Dis*. 2007;45:1476-1478.
130. Ward JI, Cherry JD, Chang SJ, et al. Efficacy of an acellular pertussis vaccine among adolescents and adults. *N Engl J Med*. 2005;353:1555-1563.
131. Pichichero ME, Rennels MB, Edwards KM, et al. Combined tetanus, diphtheria, and 5-component pertussis vaccine for use in adolescents and adults. *JAMA*. 2005;293:3003-3011.
132. Halperin SA, Smith B, Russell M, et al. An adult formulation of a five-component acellular pertussis vaccine combined with diphtheria and tetanus toxoids is safe and immunogenic in adolescents and adults. *Vaccine*. 2000;18:1312-1319.
133. Halperin SA, Smith B, Russell M, et al. Adult formulation of a five component acellular pertussis vaccine combined with diphtheria and tetanus toxoids and inactivated poliovirus vaccine is safe and immunogenic in adolescents and adults. *Pediatr Infect Dis J*. 2000;19:276-283.
134. Barreto L, Guasparini R, Meekison W, et al. Humoral immunity 5 years after booster immunization with an adolescent and adult formulation combined tetanus, diphtheria, and 5-component acellular pertussis vaccine. *Vaccine*. 2007;25:8172-8179.
135. Halperin SA, Sweet L, Baxendale D, et al. How soon after a prior tetanus-diphtheria vaccination can one give adult formulation tetanus-diphtheria-acellular pertussis vaccine? *Pediatr Infect Dis J*. 2006;25:195-200.
136. Meyer CU, Zepp F, Decker M, et al. Cellular immunity in adolescents and adults following acellular pertussis vaccine administration. *Clin Vaccine Immunol*. 2007;14:288-292.
137. National Advisory Committee on Immunization. Prevention of pertussis in adolescents and adults. *Can Commun Dis Rep*. 2003;29:1-9.
138. Broder KR, Cortese MM, Iskander JK, et al. Preventing tetanus, diphtheria, and pertussis among adolescents: Use of tetanus toxoid, reduced diphtheria toxoid and acellular pertussis vaccines recommendations of the Advisory Committee on Immunization Practices (ACIP). *MMWR Recomm Rep*. 2006; 55:1-34.
139. Kretsinger K, Broder KR, Cortese MM, et al. Preventing tetanus, diphtheria, and pertussis among adults: Use of tetanus toxoid, reduced diphtheria toxoid and acellular pertussis vaccine recommendations of the Advisory Committee on Immunization Practices (ACIP) and recommendation of ACIP, supported by the Healthcare Infection Control Practices Advisory Committee (HICPAC), for use of Tdap among health-care personnel. *MMWR Recomm Rep*. 2006;55:1-37.
140. David ST, Hemsley MC, Pasquali PE, et al. Enhanced surveillance for adverse events following immunization: Two years of dTap catch-up among high school students in Yukon, Canada (2004, 2005). *Can J Public Health*. 2006;97:465-469.
141. Kandola K, Lea A, White W, et al. A comparison of pertussis rates in the Northwest Territories: Pre- and postacellular pertussis vaccine introduction in children and adolescents. *Can J Infect Dis Med Microbiol*. 2005;16:271-274.
142. Zivna I, Bergin D, Casavant J, et al. Impact of Bordetella pertussis exposures on a Massachusetts tertiary care medical system. *Infect Control Hosp Epidemiol*. 2007;28:708-712.
143. Calugar A, Ortega-Sanchez IR, Tiwari T, et al. Nosocomial pertussis: Costs of an outbreak and benefits of vaccinating health care workers. *Clin Infect Dis*. 2006;42:981-988.
144. Ward A, Caro J, Bassinet L, et al. Health and economic consequences of an outbreak of pertussis among healthcare workers in a hospital in France. *Infect Control Hosp Epidemiol*. 2005;26:288-292.
145. Daskalaki I, Hennessey P, Hubler R, et al. Resource consumption in the infection control management of pertussis exposure among healthcare workers in pediatrics. *Infect Control Hosp Epidemiol*. 2007;28:412-417.
146. Forsyth KD, Wirsing von Konig CH, Tan T, et al. Prevention of pertussis: Recommendations derived from the second Global Pertussis Initiative roundtable meeting. *Vaccine*. 2007;25: 2634-2642.
147. Van Rie A, Hethcote HW. Adolescent and adult pertussis vaccination: computer simulations of five new strategies. *Vaccine*. 2004;22:3154-3165.
148. Van Rie A, Wendelboe AM, Englund JA. Role of maternal pertussis antibodies in infants. *Pediatr Infect Dis J*. 2005;24: S62-S65.
149. Provenzano RW, Wetterlow LH, Sullivan CL. Immunization and antibody response in the newborn infant. I. Pertussis

inoculation within twenty-four hours of birth. *N Engl J Med.* 1965;273:959-965.

150. Barrett CD, Timm EA, Molner JG, et al. Multiple antigen for immunization against poliomyelitis, diphtheria, pertussis, and tetanus. II. Response of infants and young children to primary immunization and eighteen-month booster. *Am J Public Health Nations Health.* 1959;49:644-655.

151. Knuf M, Schmitt HJ, Wolter J, et al. Neonatal vaccination with an acellular pertussis vaccine accelerates the acquisition of pertussis antibodies in infants. *J Pediatr.* 2008;152:655-660.

152. National consensus conference on pertussis, Toronto, May 25-28, 2002. *Can Commun Dis Rep.* 2003;29(Suppl 3):1-33.

153. Halperin SA, Bortolussi R, Langley JM, et al. A randomized, placebo-controlled trial of erythromycin estolate chemoprophylaxis for household contacts of children with culture-positive *Bordetella pertussis* infection. *Pediatrics.* 1999;104:e42.

154. Prophylactic erythromycin for whooping-cough contacts. *Lancet.* 1981;1:772.

155. Sprauer MA, Cochi SL, Zell ER, et al. Prevention of secondary transmission of pertussis in households with early use of erythromycin. *Am J Dis Child.* 1992;146:177-181.

156. Granstrom G, Sterner G, Nord CE, et al. Use of erythromycin to prevent pertussis in newborns of mothers with pertussis. *J Infect Dis.* 1987;155:1210-1214.

157. De Serres G, Boulianne N, Duval B. Field effectiveness of erythromycin prophylaxis to prevent pertussis within families. *Pediatr Infect Dis J.* 1995;14:969-975.

231

Rat-Bite Fever: *Streptobacillus moniliformis* and *Spirillum minus*

RONALD G. WASHBURN

Rat-bite fever is a rare systemic febrile illness typically transmitted by the bite of a rat or other small rodent. The infection has a worldwide distribution and can be caused by either *Streptobacillus moniliformis* or *Spirillum minus*, bacteria commonly found in the oropharyngeal flora of rodents. Although the name *Spirillum minus* will be retained in this chapter, the taxonomic status of this organism is unclear and it may not be a *Spirillum*. Streptobacillary disease accounts for the vast majority of cases of rat-bite fever in the United States,[1] whereas *S. minus* infections occur mainly in Asia. Table 231-1 compares the two different forms of rat-bite fever.

Illness following rat bites has been known in India for more than 2000 years,[2] and the characteristic syndrome of rat-bite fever was recorded in the United States as early as 1839.[3] The causative gram-negative bacillus, initially named *Streptothrix muris ratti*, was recovered from an infected individual in 1916.[4] In 1925, a blood culture isolate from a laboratory worker with fever, rash, and arthritis was called *S. moniliformis,* based on its morphologic resemblance to a beaded necklace.[5] In 1926, a similar organism, *Haverhillia multiformis,* was grown from the blood of patients during an epidemic illness resembling rat-bite fever in Haverhill, Massachusetts.[6] Both *H. multiformis* and *S. muris ratti* were subsequently shown to be identical to *S. moniliformis,* the causative agent of streptobacillary rat-bite fever.[2]

Streptobacillus moniliformis

BACTERIOLOGY

S. moniliformis is a pleomorphic, nonmotile, nonsporulating, nonencapsulated gram-negative bacillus measuring 0.3 to 0.7 μm wide by 1 to 5 μm long. Filaments and beadlike chains up to 150 μm long may contain 1- to 3-μm-wide fusiform swellings.[7] The organism is microaerophilic, requiring a partial pressure of CO_2 between 8% and 10% for primary isolation. Trypticase soy agar or broth must be supplemented with 10% to 20% rabbit or horse serum, defibrinated blood, or ascites to support optimal growth. Alternatively, media may be supplemented with a papain digest of ox liver.[8] Sodium polyanethol sulfonate, a substance sometimes added to trypticase soy broth or thioglycollate broth to inhibit the antibacterial activity of human blood, impedes the growth of *S. moniliformis* in concentrations of at least 0.0125%.[8,9]

On blood agar plates, nonhemolytic cotton-like colonies, 1 to 2.5 mm in diameter, appear after approximately 3 days of incubation at 37° C. In broth media, characteristic flocculent puffballs are seen at the bottom of the broth after 2 to 10 days. Penicillin-resistant L-phase variants may form spontaneously or in the presence of penicillin both in vivo and in vitro.[10] Low muramic acid content in the cell envelope may contribute to the propensity of *S. moniliformis* to produce L forms,[11] which impart a slightly turbid appearance to broth media. Sugar fermentation is variable but often includes galactose, glucose, maltose, and salicin. Fatty acid analysis by gas-liquid chromatography is useful for the rapid identification of *S. moniliformis* isolates.[12-15] In addition, sodium dodecyl sulfate–polyacrylamide gel electrophoresis patterns of cellular proteins may be useful for epidemiologic studies of Haverhill fever.[16]

Epidemiology

In the United States, persons who are at risk for percutaneous inoculation with *S. moniliformis* include animal laboratory personnel and individuals (especially children) inhabiting crowded urban dwellings or rural areas infested with wild rats.[1,17-23] Rat-bite fever is typically transmitted by the bite or scratch of rats, mice, squirrels, or carnivores that prey on those rodents, including cats, dogs, pigs, ferrets, and weasels.[17,24] One reported case followed the bite of a gerbil.[25] The infection may also be acquired by handling rats, with no apparent breach of intact skin,[18,26] or with a portal of entry, such as varicella lesions.[27] From 50% to 100% of wild and laboratory rats harbor *S. moniliformis* in their nasopharyngeal flora,[18,28-30] and they may develop otitis media.[31] Although healthy laboratory mice are generally not colonized with streptobacilli, they do share with rats the susceptibility to epizootic infections characterized by polyarthritis, septicemia, pneumonia, otitis media, and high rates of abortion.[2,29,32-34] *S. moniliformis* has also been reported to cause pleuritis in a koala,[35] cervical abscesses and pneumonia in guinea pigs,[36] arthritis in turkeys and a monkey, and endocarditis in a macaque.[37]

Pathophysiologically, the clinical disease is probably the consequence of failed local cutaneous defenses and bacterial dissemination. The few available published pathology reports described vasculitis[38,39] and intravascular thrombi.[40]

Oral ingestion of organisms has caused several epidemics of Haverhill fever (erythema arthriticum epidemicum), an illness clinically resembling rat-bite fever. Potential sources of such outbreaks include foods such as turkey, or milk or water contaminated with rat excrement.[5,6,8,18,41-43] Presumably, once ingested, *S. moniliformis* organisms gain access to the peripheral circulation by penetrating the gastrointestinal mucosa.

Clinical Manifestations

A brief incubation period, usually less than 10 days in duration (range, 1 to 22 days), follows the bite of the rat. An abrupt onset of fever, chills, headache, vomiting, and severe migratory arthralgias and myalgias marks the beginning of clinical disease; by that time, the wound itself has usually already healed. Indeed, the diagnosis is often initially obscured by the patient's incognizance of a bite that probably occurred during sleep. Regional lymphadenopathy is minimal or absent, in contrast to *S. minus* infection. The peripheral white blood cell count may range as high as 30,000/mm^3, with a leftward shift. Up to 25% of patients have false-positive serologic test results for syphilis.

Within 2 to 4 days after the onset of fever, a nonpruritic maculopapular, morbilliform, petechial, vesicular[42] or pustular[38,44] rash erupts over the palms, soles, and extremities. Skin lesions may become purpuric[40] or confluent, and may eventually desquamate.[17] Approximately 50% of patients develop asymmetrical polyarthritis or true septic arthritis[45,46] concurrently with the rash or within a few days thereafter.[19,47-52] The knees are most commonly involved, followed by the ankles, elbows, wrists, shoulders, and hips.[41,50,51] Typically, fever subsides spontaneously after 3 to 5 days without specific antibiotic therapy, and the remaining symptoms gradually resolve within 2 weeks. However, fever may occasionally relapse in an irregular pattern for weeks or months,[10] producing a clinical picture of fever of undeter-

TABLE 231-1	Comparison of Two Different Types of Rat-Bite Fever	
	Organism	
Parameter	**Streptobacillus moniliformis**	**Spirillum minus**
Organism	Gram-negative bacillus	Gram-negative coiled rod
Geographic distribution	North America, Europe	Asia
Mode of transmission	Rat bite, ingestion	Rat bite
Clinical syndrome		
• Ulceration of initial bite wound	No	Yes
• Arthritis	Yes	No
• Regional lymphadenopathy	No	Yes
• Rash	Yes	Yes
• Relapsing fever	Yes	Yes
Diagnosis	Culture, PCR	Direct visualization, xenodiagnosis
Therapy	Penicillin G	Penicillin G

PCR, polymerase chain reaction.

mined origin, or arthritis may persist for as long as 2 years. Haverhill fever differs clinically from percutaneously acquired rat-bite fever chiefly in the heightened severity of vomiting and high incidence of pharyngitis.[8,17]

Reported complications of *S. moniliformis* infection include endocarditis,[18,41,49,53-57] myocarditis,[18,28] pericarditis,[2,53] sepsis,[58] meningitis,[56] pneumonia,[18,56] amnionitis,[59] and anemia.[2,28] Abscesses have been observed in almost all organs, including brain,[60] liver, spleen, kidney, skin,[7,61] and the female genital tract.[15] In infants and young children, diarrhea and weight loss may be prominent.[18,22,56] The mortality of untreated cases ranges as high as 13%,[56] and endocarditis in the preantibiotic era was uniformly lethal. Most of those intravascular infections involved valves previously damaged by rheumatic valvulitis or calcification.[41] A case of prosthetic valve endocarditis was recently reported.[62]

Diagnosis

In a febrile patient with rash and recent rat exposure, the diagnosis can usually be narrowed to rat-bite fever or leptospirosis. However, the physician caring for a laboratory worker may step into the trap of ascribing a seemingly benign febrile illness to viral infection. Furthermore, without a positive exposure history, the proper diagnosis may be even more elusive, and diagnoses such as meningococcemia, enteric fever, drug reaction, and viral exanthem enter into consideration. When the rash involves the palms and soles, rat-bite fever may mimic Rocky Mountain spotted fever[63] or secondary syphilis. The presence of oligoarticular or migratory polyarthritis heightens concerns about disseminated gonococcal infection, Lyme disease, brucellosis, septic arthritis, infective endocarditis, rheumatoid arthritis, and acute rheumatic fever.

Direct visualization of pleomorphic bacillary organisms in Giemsa-, Wayson-, or Gram-stained smears of blood, joint fluid, and pus may provide an early clue to the diagnosis. However, laboratory diagnosis rests ultimately on culturing *S. moniliformis* using enriched media.[64] An enzyme-linked immunosorbent assay has been developed for the detection of specific antibody against *S. moniliformis*.[65] More recently, polymerase chain reaction (PCR) techniques that amplify bacterial 16S ribosomal RNA have been used to detect *S. moniliformis* infection in rodents[66] and humans.[42,67]

Treatment and Prevention

Both agents of rat-bite fever, *S. moniliformis* and *Spirillum minus,* are susceptible to penicillin. In the past, procaine penicillin G was given

IM as 600,000 units every 12 hours for 10 to 14 days.[2,17,47] Currently, IV penicillin G appears more appropriate. The Jarisch-Herxheimer reaction may complicate initial therapy of *S. minus* infections. Oral tetracycline, 500 mg every 6 hours, is preferred for penicillin-allergic patients.[2,12] Streptomycin, 7.5 mg/kg, can be given intramuscularly every 12 hours, although potential ototoxicity makes this less desirable. Limited experience indicates that erythromycin,[68] chloramphenicol,[8,63] clindamycin,[18,28] or ceftriaxone[40,44,52] might also be effective.

Most patients respond promptly to therapy. For individuals who appear well after 5 to 7 days of parenteral therapy, the course can be completed with an additional week of oral penicillin V or ampicillin, 500 mg every 6 hours. Patients with mild disease can probably be treated orally for the entire course.

Endocarditis is so rare that optimal therapy is uncertain. Probably, 4 weeks of IV penicillin, with or without streptomycin or gentamicin,[57] is adequate. A total daily dose of 20 million units has been advocated for patients whose isolates are resistant to 0.1 µg/mL.[54]

After a rodent bite, the wound should be thoroughly cleaned and tetanus prophylaxis should be administered, if warranted by the patient's immunization history. A 3-day course of oral penicillin, 2 g/day, would seem reasonable, although the prophylactic efficacy of penicillin in this setting is unknown, and the patient should be advised to report any subsequent symptoms. Measures to limit the incidence of rat-bite fever include eradication of rats in urban areas, avoidance of nonpasteurized milk and potentially contaminated water, and the use of gloves by laboratory workers when handling rodents.

Spirillum minus

Spirillum minus causes a significant portion of cases of rat-bite fever in Asia but rarely produces infection in the United States.[69,70] In Japan, the infection is called *sodoku* (*so,* rat; *doku,* poison).

The causative organism was discovered by Carter during the 19th century.[71] In the early years of the 20th century, specimens from patients with *sodoku* were shown to contain spirochetes capable of infecting guinea pigs. Those bacteria were initially called *Spirocheta morsus muris* or *Sporozoa muris*.[72] The organism was renamed *Spirillum minus* in 1924.[73]

BACTERIOLOGY

Spirillum minus is a short, thick, gram-negative, tightly coiled spiral rod measuring 0.2 to 0.5 µm by 3 to 5 µm.[74,75] The organism has two to six regular helical turns.[75] Terminal polytrichous flagella confer darting motility, which can be demonstrated with darkfield examination. The flagella can be stained with silver impregnation methods (e.g., Fontana-Tribondeau). Despite reports to the contrary, *Spirillum minus* has not been cultured on artificial media and its name derives from its appearance alone. It may be a *Campylobacter* that causes systemic disease, such as *Campylobacter fetus* but, unlike *C. fetus,* has fastidious growth requirements. No attempt at sequence analysis of the organism in body fluids has been reported.

EPIDEMIOLOGY, PATHOGENESIS, AND PATHOLOGY

The epidemiology of *S. minus* infections is similar to that of streptobacillary rat-bite fever, with the exception that oral ingestion has not been shown to cause spirillary disease. A case occurred in a traveler returning from Vietnam to Italy.[76] The major route of transmission is through rat bites. Approximately 25% of tested rats were positive for *S. minus* in conjunctival and nasopharyngeal secretions, pulmonary lesions, and blood.[74] Human-to-human transmission has not been documented.

Relapses of spirillary rat-bite fever have been postulated to be caused by seeding of blood and distant foci during periodic reactivation of the primary bite lesion. The available recorded autopsies show granulomatous inflammation at the original site of inoculation, with epithelial necrosis and mononuclear infiltration of the dermis. Regional lymph nodes are hyperplastic. Deep tissue specimens from distant areas of skin rash contain dilated blood vessels and round cell infiltrates. Liver, spleen, renal tubules, myocardium, and meninges may be hemorrhagic, with areas of necrosis in liver and kidney.

CLINICAL MANIFESTATIONS

The initial bite wound heals promptly but then becomes painful, swollen, and purple approximately 1 to 4 weeks later; it is associated with regional lymphangitis and lymphadenitis. This local inflammatory lesion ushers in a systemic illness characterized by fever, chills, headache, and malaise. In contrast with streptobacillary rat-bite fever, arthritis and myalgias are rare in *Spirillum minus* infection. Next, the bite wound commonly progresses to chancre-like ulceration and induration with eschar formation. During the first week of fever, a blotchy violaceous or reddish-brown macular rash erupts over the extremities, face, scalp, and trunk, and then fades during subsequent afebrile intervals. Occasionally, the rash may be urticarial.[75] Leukocytosis with peripheral white blood cell counts in the range of 10,000 to 20,000/mm^3 may be observed, and up to 50% of patients have false-positive syphilis serologies.

Without specific antibiotic therapy, fevers lasting 3 to 4 days recur at regular intervals between afebrile periods of 3 to 9 days. Spontaneous cure usually occurs within 1 to 2 months, but in selected instances fevers have relapsed for years.[75]

The most serious complication of untreated spirillary rat-bite fever is endocarditis. Most of these rare intravascular infections have been observed in patients with preexisting valvular disease, but one reported case occurred on a normal aortic valve.[77] The spectrum of reported complications also includes myocarditis, pleural effusions, hepatitis, splenomegaly, meningitis, epididymitis, conjunctivitis, and anemia.[75,78] Overall mortality of untreated *S. minus* infections in the preantibiotic era was 6% to 10%.

DIAGNOSIS AND TREATMENT

Diagnosis depends on the history of rat bite, typical clinical features, and demonstration of the organisms on examination of blood, exudate, or lymph node tissue using Giemsa stain, Wright stain, or darkfield microscopy. Organisms have been recovered from mice or guinea pigs 1 to 3 weeks after intraperitoneal inoculation,[75,79] with the precaution that the animals must be prescreened to rule out the presence of preexisting spirochete infections. No specific serologic test or PCR assay is available for *S. minus* infection. Treatment is the same as for *S. moniliformis* infection.

REFERENCES

1. Anderson LC, Leary SL, Manning PJ. Rat-bite fever in animal research laboratory personnel. *Lab Anim Sci.* 1983;33:292-294.
2. Roughgarden JW. Antimicrobial therapy of rat-bite fever. *Arch Intern Med.* 1965;116:39-54.
3. Wilcox W. Violent symptoms from bite of rat. *Am J Med Sci.* 1839;26:245.
4. Blake FC. Etiology of rat-bite fever. *J Exp Med.* 1916;23:39.
5. Levaditi C, Nicolau S, Poincloux P. Sur le rôle étiologique de *Streptobacillus moniliformis* (nov spec) dans l'erythème polymorphe aigu septicemique. *C R Acad Sci.* 1925;180:1188.
6. Parker F Jr, Hudson NP. The etiology of Haverhill fever (erythema arthriticum epidemicum). *Am J Pathol.* 1926;2:357-379.
7. Torres A, Cuende E, De Pablos M, et al. Remitting seronegative symmetrical synovitis with pitting edema associated with subcutaneous *Streptobacillus moniliformis* abscess. *J Rheumatol.* 2001;28:1696-1698.
8. Shanson DC, Pratt J, Greene P. Comparison of media with and without "panmede" for the isolation of *Streptobacillus moniliformis* from blood cultures and observations on the inhibitory effect of sodium polyanethol sulphonate. *J Med Microbiol.* 1985; 19:181-186.
9. Lambe Jr DW, McPhedran AM, Mertz JA, et al. *Streptobacillus moniliformis* isolated from a case of Haverhill fever: Biochemical characterization and inhibitory effect of sodium polyanethol sulfonate. *Am J Clin Pathol.* 1973;60:854-860.
10. Dolman CE, Kerr De, Chang H, et al. Two cases of rat-bite fever due to *Streptobacillus moniliformis. Can J Public Health.* 1951;42:228-241.
11. Knipp LH, Sokatch JR. The chemical composition of the cell envelope of *Streptobacillus moniliformis. Can J Microbiol.* 1969;15:665-669.
12. Edwards R, Finch RG. Characterisation and antibiotic susceptibilities of *Streptobacillus moniliformis. J Med Microbiol.* 1986;21:39-42.
13. Rowbotham TJ. Rapid identification of *Streptobacillus moniliformis. Lancet.* 1983;2:567.
14. Rygg M, Brunn CF. Rat bite fever *(Streptobacillus moniliformis)* with septicemia in a child. *Scand J Infect Dis.* 1992;24:535-540.
15. Pins MR, Holden JM, Yang JM, et al. Isolation of presumptive *Streptobacillus moniliformis* from abscesses associated with the female genital tract. *Clin Inf Dis.* 1996;22:471-476.
16. Costas M, Owen RJ. Numerical analysis of electrophoretic protein patterns of *Streptobacillus moniliformis* strains from human, murine, and avian infections. *J Med Microbiol.* 1987;23:303-311.
17. Taber LH, Feigin RD. Spirochetal infections. *Pediatr Clin North Am.* 1979;26:410-411.
18. McHugh TP, Bartlett RL, Raymond JI. Rat bite fever: Report of a fatal case. *Ann Emerg Med.* 1985;14:1116-1118.
19. Anderson D, Marrie TJ. Septic arthritis due to *Streptobacillus moniliformis. Arthritis Rheum.* 1987;30:229-230.
20. Cole JS, Stoll RW, Bulger RJ. Rat-bite fever: Report of three cases. *Ann Intern Med.* 1969;71:979-981.
21. Collins CH. *Laboratory-Acquired Infections: History, Incidence, Causes, and Prevention.* London: Butterworths; 1983:7-13.
22. Raffin BJ, Freemark M. Streptobacillary rat-bite fever: A pediatric problem. *Pediatrics.* 1979;64:214-217.
23. Wullenweber M. *Streptobacillus moniliformis*—a zoonotic pathogen. *Lab Anim.* 1995;29:1-15.
24. Peel MM. Dog-associated bacterial infections in humans: Isolates submitted to an Australian reference laboratory, 1981-1992. *Pathology.* 1993;25:379-384.
25. Wilkins EGL, Millar JGB, Cockcroft PM, et al. Rat-bite fever in a gerbil breeder. *J Infect.* 1988;16:177-180.
26. Fordham JN, McKay-Ferguson E, Davies A, et al. Rat bite fever without the bite. *Ann Rheum Dis.* 1992;51:411-412.
27. Prager L, Frenck RW Jr. *Streptobacillus moniliformis* infection in a child with chickenpox. *Pediatr Infect Dis J.* 1994; 13:417-418.
28. Taylor AF, Stephenson TG, Giese HA, et al. Rat-bite fever in a college student—California. *MMWR Morb Mortal Wkly Rep.* 1984;33:318-320.
29. Strangeways WI. Rats as carriers of *Streptobacillus moniliformis. J Pathol.* 1933;37:45-51.
30. Koopman JP, van den Brink ME, Vennix PPCA, et al. Isolation of *Streptobacillus moniliformis* from the middle ear of rats. *Lab Anim.* 1991;25:35-39.
31. Wullenweber M, Jonas C, Kunstyr I. *Streptobacillus moniliformis* isolated from otitis media of conventionally kept laboratory rats. *J Exp Anim Sci.* 1992;35:49-57.
32. Wullenweber M, Kaspareit-Rittinghausen J, Faroug M. *Streptobacillus moniliformis* epizootic in barrier-maintained C57BL/6J mice and susceptibility to infection of different strains of mice. *Lab Anim Sci.* 1990;40:608-612.
33. Glastonbury JR, Morton JG, Matthews LM. *Streptobacillus moniliformis* infection in Swiss white mice. *J Vet Diagn Invest.* 1996;8:202-209.
34. Taylor JD, Stephens CP, Duncan RG, et al. Polyarthritis in wild mice *(Mus musculus)* caused by *Streptobacillus moniliformis. Aust Vet J.* 1994;71:143-145.
35. Russell EG, Straube EF. Streptobacillary pleuritis in a koala. *J Wild Dis.* 1979;15:391-394.
36. Kirchner BK, Lake SG, Wightman SR. Isolation of *Streptobacillus moniliformis* from a guinea pig with granulomatous pneumonia. *Lab Anim Sci.* 1992;42:519-521.
37. Valverde CR, Lowenstine LJ, Young CE, et al. Spontaneous rat bite fever in non-human primates: a review of two cases. *J Med Primatol.* 2002;31:345-349.
38. Tandon R, Lee M, Curran E, et al. A 26-year-old woman with a rash on her extremities. *Clin Infect Dis.* 2006;43:1585-1586.
39. Albedwawi S, LeBlanc C, Show A, et al. A teenager with fever, rash and arthritis. *CMAJ.* 2006;175:354.
40. Ojukwu IC, Christy C. Rat-bite fever in children: Case report and review. *Scand J Infect Dis.* 2002; 34:474-477.
41. McEvoy MB, Noah ND, Pilsworth R. Outbreak of fever caused by *Streptobacillus moniliformis. Lancet.* 1987;2:1361-1363.
42. Berger C, Altwegg M, Meyer A, et al. Broad-range polymerase chain reaction for diagnosis of rat-bite fever caused by *Streptobacillus moniliformis. Pediatr Infect Dis J.* 2001;20:1181-1182.
43. Place EH, Sutton LE. Infection with *Streptobacillus moniliformis. Arch Intern Med.* 1934;5:659.
44. Cunningham BB, Paller AS, Katz BZ. Rat bite fever in a pet lover. *J Am Acad Dermatol.* 1998;38:330-332.
45. Dendle C, Wolley IJ, Korman TM. Rat-bite fever septic arthritis: Illustrative case and literature review. *Eur J Clin Microbiol Infect Dis.* 2006;25:791-797.
46. Thong Y-H, Barkham TMS. Suppurative polyarthritis following a rat bite. *Ann Rheum Dis.* 2003;62:805-806.
47. Mandel DR. Streptobacillary fever: An unusual cause of infectious arthritis. *Clev Clin Q.* 1985;52:203-205.
48. Rumley RL, Patrone NA, White L. Rat-bite fever as a cause of septic arthritis: A diagnostic dilemma. *Ann Rheum Dis.* 1987;46: 793-795.
49. Rupp ME. *Streptobacillus moniliformis* endocarditis: Case report and review. *Clin Infect Dis.* 1992;14:769-772.
50. Azimi P. Pets can be dangerous. *Pediatr Infect Dis J.* 1990;9:670.
51. Holroyd KJ, Reiner AP, Dick JD. *Streptobacillus moniliformis* polyarthritis mimicking rheumatoid arthritis: An urban case of rat bite fever. *Am J Med.* 1988;85:711-714.
52. Hockman DE, Pence CD, Whittler RR, et al. Septic arthritis of the hip secondary to rat bite fever. *Clin Orthop.* 2000; 380:173-176.
53. Carbeck RB, Murphy JF, Britt EM. Streptobacillary rat-bite fever with massive pericardial effusion. *JAMA.* 1967;201: 703-704.
54. McCormack RC, Kaye D, Hook EW. Endocarditis due to *Streptobacillus moniliformis:* A report of two cases and review of the literature. *JAMA.* 1967;200:77-79.
55. Simon MW, Wilson D. *Streptobacillus moniliformis* endocarditis: A case report. *Clin Pediatr.* 1986;25:110-111.
56. Sens MA, Brown EW, Wilson LR, et al. Fatal *Streptobacillus moniliformis* infection in a two month old infant. *Am J Clin Pathol.* 1989;91:612-616.
57. Kondruweit M, Weyand M, Mahmoud FO, et al. Fulminant endocarditis caused by *Streptobacillus moniliformis* in a young man. *J Thor Cardiovasc Surg.* 2007;134:1579-1580.
58. Centers for Disease Control and Prevention (CDC). Fatal rat-bite fever—Florida and Washington, 2003. *MMWR Morb Mort Wkly Rep.* 2005;53:1198-1202.
59. Faro S, Walker C, Pierson RL. Amnionitis with intact amniotic membranes involving *Streptobacillus moniliformis. Obstet Gynecol.* 1980;55S:9S-11S.
60. Dijkmans BAC, Thomeer RTWM, Vielvoye GJ, et al. Brain abscess due to *Streptobacillus moniliformis* and *Actinobacterium meyerii. Infection.* 1984;12:34-36.
61. Vasseur E, Joly P, Nouvellon M, et al. Cutaneous abscess: A rare complication of *Streptobacillus moniliformis* infection. *Br J Dermatol.* 1993;129:95-96.
62. Chen P-L, Lee N-Y, Yan J-J, et al. Prosthetic valve endocarditis caused by *Streptobacillus moniliformis*: A case of rat bite fever. *J Clin Microbiol.* 2007;45:3125-3126.
63. Portnoy BL, Satterwhite TK, Dyckman JD. Rat bite fever misdiagnosed as Rocky Mountain spotted fever. *South Med J.* 1979;72:607-609.
64. Centers for Disease Control and Prevention (CDC). Rat-bite fever—New Mexico, 1996. *MMWR Morb Mortal Wkly Rep.* 1998;47:89-91.
65. Boot R, Bakker RH, Thuis H, et al. An enzyme-linked immunosorbent assay (ELISA) for monitoring rodent colonies for *Streptobacillus moniliformis* antibodies. *Lab Anim.* 1993;27:350-357.
66. Boot R, Oosterhuis A, Thuis HCW. PCR for the detection of *Streptobacillus moniliformis. Lab Anim.* 2002;36:200-208.
67. Wallet F, Savage C, Loiez C, et al. Molecular diagnosis of arthritis due to *Streptobacillus moniliformis. Diagn Microbiol Infect Dis.* 2003;47:623-624.
68. Konstantopoulos K, Skarpas P, Hitjazis F, et al. Rat-bite fever in a Greek child. *Scand J Infect Dis.* 1992;24:531-533.

69. Anderson LC, Leary SL, Manning PJ. Ratbite fever in animal research laboratory personnel. *Lab Anim Sci*. 1983;33: 292-294.

70. Cole JS, Stoll RW, Bulger RJ. Ratbite fever: Report of three cases. *Ann Intern Med*. 1969;71:979-981.

71. Hiatt JR, Hiatt N. The forgotten first career of Doctor Henry Van Dyke Carter. *J Am Coll Surg*. 1995;181:464-486.

72. Roughgarden JW. Antimicrobial therapy of ratbite fever. *Arch Intern Med*. 1965;116:39-54.

73. Robertson A. Causal organism of ratbite fever in man. *Ann Trop Med*. 1924;18:157.

74. McHugh TP, Bartlett RL, Raymond JI. Rat bite fever: Report of a fatal case. *Ann Emerg Med*. 1985;14:1116-1118.

75. Taber LH, Feigin RD. Spirochetal infections. *Pediatr Clin North Am*. 1979;26:410-411.

76. Signorini L, Colombini P, Cristini F, et al. Inappropriate footwear and rat-bite fever in an international traveler. *J Travel Med*. 2002;9(5):275.

77. McIntosh CS, Vickers PJ, Isaacs AJ. Spirillum endocarditis. *Postgrad Med J*. 1975;51:645-648.

78. Raffin BJ, Freemark M. Streptobacillary ratbite fever: A pediatric problem. *Pediatrics*. 1979;64:214-217.

79. Dow GR, Rankin RJ, Saunders BW. Ratbite fever. *N Z Med J*. 1992;105:133.

232

Legionella

PAUL H. EDELSTEIN | NICHOLAS P. CIANCIOTTO

History

Legionnaires' disease is an acute pneumonic illness caused by gram-negative bacilli of the genus *Legionella*, the most common of which is *Legionella pneumophila*. Pontiac fever is a febrile, nonpneumonic, systemic illness closely associated with, if not caused by, *Legionella* spp. Legionellosis is the term that encompasses all diseases caused by, or presumed to be caused by, the *Legionella* bacteria, including Legionnaires' disease, focal nonpulmonary infections, and Pontiac fever.

Legionnaires' disease was first recognized when it caused an epidemic of pneumonia at a Pennsylvania State American Legion convention in Philadelphia in 1976; 221 people were affected, and 34 died. Despite intensive laboratory investigation, the cause of the outbreak went undetected for many months. This mystery provoked considerable fear and widespread speculation about the cause, including claims that the disease was part of a government germ warfare experiment, a terrorist act, a hoax to cover up government incompetence, or caused by a toxin. A thorough epidemiologic investigation determined that the disease was most likely airborne, and focused primarily at one convention hotel, which closed because of adverse publicity.[1,2]

The inability to determine the cause of the outbreak confounded politicians and scientists who had thought that there were no new infectious diseases to be discovered. There was enough national and political concern to prompt two independent congressional investigations of the outbreak. About 6 months later, two investigators at the Centers for Disease Control and Prevention, Joseph McDade and Charles Shepard, announced that they had discovered the causative agent, a fastidious gram-negative bacillus.[3] Because of the historical association with the American Legion convention, this disease is now called "Legionnaires' disease" and the causative agents belong to the family Legionellaceae, with *L. pneumophila* being the agent responsible for the 1976 Philadelphia epidemic. Use of an antibody test for the disease has shown that several prior unsolved outbreaks of pneumonia had been Legionnaires' disease, including epidemics investigated in the 1950s and 1960s.[4,5] The availability of diagnostic tests uncovered a 6-year long epidemic of Legionnaires' disease among British tourists staying at one hotel in Spain.[6] An unsolved epidemic of a nonpneumonic febrile illness was also found to have been the result of exposure to *Legionella* bacteria; this illness was termed *Pontiac fever*, after Pontiac, Michigan, where this had occurred.[7,8] As with Legionnaires' disease, prior epidemics of Pontiac fever had occurred as early as 1949, without determination of a cause.[9] Bacterial culture isolates from the 1940s through the 1960s were found to be *Legionella* bacteria, although at the time they had been thought to be rickettsial agents.[10-15] Thus, both the organism and the disease had been studied decades before, but major advances in technology and epidemiology were required to classify the disease properly and determine its cause.

Even with identification of *L. pneumophila* in 1977 as the cause of Legionnaires' disease, the source of the bacterium, factors promoting its multiplication and spread, and ways to abort epidemics of Legionnaires' disease remained uncertain for several years. Epidemics of the disease, especially nosocomial ones, commonly lasted for years, even though the cause of the disease was recognized.[16-22] Eventually, it was discovered that *L. pneumophila* and other *Legionella* spp. were naturally occurring aquatic bacteria that had a propensity for growing in warm water, most particularly in cooling towers, water heaters, and potable water plumbing. These discoveries led to the end of several multiyear outbreaks of the disease, and to methods for preventing the disease.[23] It is now unusual for outbreaks of Legionnaires' disease to last more than 1 or 2 weeks because of improved diagnostic, environmental detection, and remediation methods.

Legionnaires' disease still occurs, both in sporadic and epidemic forms, sometimes involving many hundreds of victims.[24,25] The disease, although a relatively rare (1% to 5%) cause of community-acquired pneumonia, can cause severe disease and death, if treated improperly. Enough is now known about the disease so that epidemics can be aborted in days, to treat patients effectively, and to reduce the frequency of the disease by making modifications in building design and maintenance.

Causative Agents

The *Legionella* spp. are small, gram-negative bacilli with fastidious growth requirements. Proteins rather than carbohydrates are used as an energy source. The bacteria are obligate aerobes and grow at temperatures ranging from 20° to 42°C. The *Legionella* bacteria are in the taxonomic order Legionellae, which includes the families Coxiellaceae and Legionellaceae.[26] *Coxiella burnetii*, an obligate intracellular parasite and the causative agent of Q fever, is the closest relative of the *Legionellaceae*. Three different genera have been proposed for the Legionellaceae: *Legionella*, *Fluoribacter*, and *Tatlockia*; however, use of the latter two genera has never been widely accepted, and the single genus *Legionella* is almost universally used to describe all species. L-cysteine is required for the growth of all but one of the clinically important *Legionella* spp., and this amino acid is needed for the initial growth of all described *Legionella* spp. from environmental or clinical sources. Soluble iron is required for optimal growth and for initial isolation of the bacterium from clinical and environmental sources. Iron, L-cysteine, α-ketoglutarate, and charcoal-containing yeast extract agar buffered with an organic buffer (BCYEα agar) are the preferred growth media for clinical isolation. Clinically important *Legionella* spp. grow best at 35°C in humidified air on BCYEα medium, usually in 2 to 5 days after inoculation of plates. Up to 14 days of incubation may very rarely be required for the isolation of unusual *Legionella* spp.

More than 50 different *Legionella* spp. have been described, 20 of which have been reported to infect humans.[26,27] *L. pneumophila* contains at least 16 different serogroups; seven other species contain two different serogroups, with the remaining species containing only one serogroup each.[28] *L. pneumophila* serogroup 1 caused the 1976 Philadelphia outbreak and is the cause of 70% to 90% of all cases of Legionnaires' disease for which there has been a bacterial isolate.[29,30] *L. pneumophila* serogroup 1 can be further divided into multiple subtypes using various serologic, other phenotypic, and genetic methods. One particular subtype of *L. pneumophila* serogroup 1 causes 67% to 90% of cases of Legionnaires' disease caused by *L. pneumophila*, and 85% of cases caused by *L. pneumophila* serogroup 1. This subtype is distinguished by its reactivity with a particular monoclonal antibody, and is variously known as the Pontiac, Joly monclonal type 2 (MAb2), or Dresden monoclonal type 3/1 (Mab 3/1) monoclonal subtype.[31] The predominance of the Pontiac subtype has implications for diagnosis (see later).

Most clinical microbiology laboratories should be able to identify *Legionella* bacteria to the genus level by detection of their typical colony morphology and Gram stain appearance, by determination of L-cysteine growth dependence, and by excluding possible mimics using standard microbiologic identification techniques (Fig. 232-1).

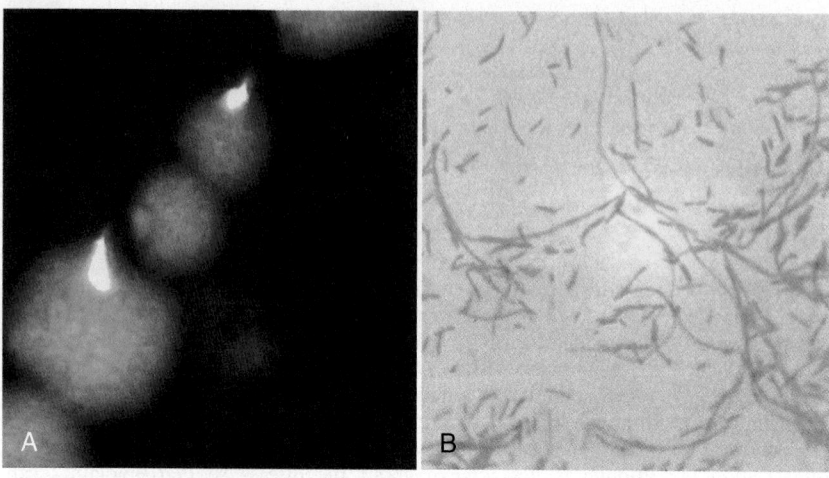

Figure 232-1   Cultures of _Legionella pneumophila._
A, Typical opal-like colony of _L. pneumophila_ grown on BCYEα agar. **B,** Gram stain of _L. pneumophila_ taken from culture plate. Basic fuchsin should be used as the counterstain, because safranin stains the bacterium poorly (**A,** 10×; **B,** 1000× magnification).

Identification of _L. pneumophila_ and _L. pneumophila_ serogroup 1, the most common clinical isolate, can be accomplished by sophisticated clinical microbiology laboratories using relatively simple serologic testing. Identification of other _L. pneumophila_ serogroups and other _Legionella_ spp. is often much more difficult, and is best left to specialized reference laboratories.[32] This is because these bacteria are relatively inert in common biochemical tests, and require sophisticated phenotypic, serologic, and molecular testing techniques. Most national reference laboratories use bacterial DNA sequencing for definitive identification.

Microbial Ecology

The _Legionella_ bacteria are found in our aqueous environment, in a large variety of habitats—from lakes, streams, and even coastal oceans—at temperatures ranging from 5° to more than 50° C.[33] Warm water (25° to 40° C) supports the highest concentration of these bacteria, and warm water is the major bacterial reservoir leading to Legionnaires' disease. Free-living amebas (e.g., _Naegleria_, _Acanthamoeba_, _Hartmannella_) in the same waters support the intracellular growth and survival of the _Legionella_ bacteria.

The interaction between amebas and _Legionella_ bacteria has been studied most comprehensively for _L. pneumophila_, which is a facultative intracellular parasite of several different amebas.[34,35] The bacterium multiplies many thousand-fold within the amebas (Fig. 232-2).

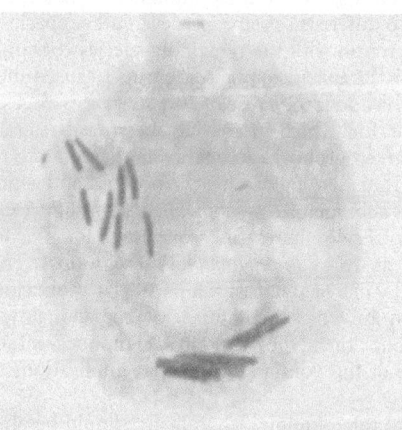

Figure 232-2   Gimenez stain of _Legionella pneumophila_ growing in an ameba (1000× magnification). Note that the bacteria are much smaller and more uniform in morphology than when the bacteria are taken from a culture plate (see Fig. 232-1B).

When faced with inimical environmental factors, such as pH changes, absence of nutrients, or temperature alteration, the _Legionella_-infected amebas encyst, guaranteeing the survival of both the host and parasite until more favorable conditions allow excystment. In both natural and man-made waters, _Legionella_-infected amebas are found in consortia of many different microorganisms, all of which exist in a biofilm.

In addition to intra-amebal survival, freely living _Legionella_ bacteria can enter a low metabolic state termed _viable but not cultivatable_, which makes them difficult to recover from the environment and probably more resistant to biocides.[36] The _Legionella_ bacteria, amebas, and other microorganisms constantly escape from the biofilm (sessile phase) because water flow and pressure fluxes into a freely moving phase (planktonic phase) and then back into the sessile phase. Environmental changes that disrupt the biofilm can result in the sudden and massive release of _Legionella_ bacteria into the surrounding water. If this water is then aerosolized or aspirated, the bacteria can cause illness in a susceptible host. Almost all cases of Legionnaires' disease result from _Legionella_ contamination of warm man-made waters, such as water heaters, air conditioning and other types of cooling towers, warm water baths, warm water plumbing systems, and recirculating water systems. One exception to this is that _L. longbeachae_ appears to be transmitted mainly through soil contact, especially potting soil used by gardeners.[37] _Legionella_ bacteria are present in very low concentrations in disinfectant-treated cold potable water, usually at levels of less than one bacterium/L; up to 50 L of this type of water may need to be sampled to detect a single _Legionella_ bacterium. However, in water distribution pipes, especially older pipes with low or no water flow, the bacterial density can be amplified by growth in biofilm. The bacteria can be further amplified in the presence of warm conditions, such as that found in many buildings or heat rejection devices. _Legionella_ bacteria concentrations in air conditioning cooling towers range from 10^2 to 10^8 colony-forming units (cfu)/L. Up to 80% of air-conditioning cooling towers tested contained the bacterium, as did 5% to 30% of home and industrial water heaters and hot water plumbing systems.[33] Contaminated water that is aerosolized serves to disseminate the bacteria into the environment. The concentration of _Legionella_ bacteria in a particular environmental site may spontaneously fluctuate over a wide range, presumably because of extrabacterial factors such as temperature, presence of biofilm disruptive forces, type and concentration of other microorganisms in the biofilm consortium, and concentrations of various organic and inorganic compounds.

Pathogenesis

Legionnaires' disease is initiated by inhalation, and probably microaspiration, of _Legionella_ bacteria into the lungs. Although _Legionella_ bacteria are ubiquitous in our environment, they rarely cause disease. A confluence of a number of factors must occur simultaneously before

Legionnaires' disease can develop. These factors include the following: presence of virulent strains in a environmental site; a means for dissemination of the bacteria, such as by aerosolization; and proper environmental conditions allowing the survival and inhalation of an infectious dose of the bacteria by a susceptible host. Strains of different virulence, at least for guinea pigs, exist for the same species, and some species and serogroups are more virulent than others.[38-41] The reasons for different virulence of strains, even within the same species, is not known with certainty, but may include aerosol stability, ability to grow in amebas, and surface hydrophobicity.

The infectious form of the bacterium is not known, but in all cases the bacteria originate from water containing the bacteria. One exception to a water-borne source is that of *L. longbeachae*, which appears to be soil-borne, although water-borne transmission may also occur.[37] Several possibilities exist for the infectious particle causing disease, including *Legionella* bacteria contained in an amebal cyst, a particle of biofilm containing *Legionella* bacteria and other microorganisms, and freely dispersed, extracellular planktonic *Legionella* bacteria. The physiologic state of the *Legionella* bacteria causing infection is unknown, but may include bacteria in stationary or logarithmic growth phases, as well as a sporelike form of the bacterium.[42] The physiologic state of *Legionella* bacteria may be important for its virulence, because virulence increases when the bacterium is grown in amebas, in the late stationary phase in vitro, or as the sporelike form.[43-45] Because aerosolization of dispersed logarithmic phase bacteria rapidly kills most bacteria within seconds to minutes, it makes sense that the infectious form of the organism would be protected by biofilm, within an amebal cyst, or as the sporelike form; all these infectious forms protect the bacteria from heat, cold, and disinfectants.

The bacterial inoculum required to cause Legionnaires' disease is unknown. Guinea pigs, which are quite susceptible to experimentally introduced *L. pneumophila* pneumonia, develop asymptomatic infection with inocula as low as 10 to 100 bacteria when delivered by aerosol, disease with about 1000 bacteria, and death after infection with 10,000 bacteria. A packet of bacteria in amebal cysts or in a biofilm fragment easily contains more than 1000 bacteria, making it possible that inhalation of a single infected amebal cyst or biofilm fragment could cause disease. Survival of extracellular *L. pneumophila* in an aerosol is dependent on relative humidity, with different relative humidity optima for each strain, meaning that the disease-causing critical concentration of bacteria in the environment may differ even for the same strain, depending on environmental conditions.[46] Recent epidemiologic evidence has suggested that relative humidity may be a key factor in disease transmission.[25,47]

Water contaminated with sufficient concentration of virulent *Legionella* bacteria can be aerosolized by water-cooled heat rejection devices such as air-conditioning cooling towers, whirlpool spas, shower heads, water misters, and some respiratory equipment. In addition, microaspiration of the contaminated water can also produce disease. Once the bacteria enter the lung, they are phagocytosed by alveolar macrophages, and perhaps also internalized by respiratory epithelial cells.[48] The *Legionella* bacteria produce virulence factors that enhance phagocytosis and then allow intracellular survival and growth (see later). After sufficient intracellular growth, the bacteria kill the macrophage, escape into the extracellular environment, and are then rephagocytosed by macrophages. The bacterial concentration in the lung increases considerably because of amplification of the bacteria in macrophages; for example, the number of *L. pneumophila* in guinea pig lungs increases by about one million–fold over a 3-day period after initial infection.

Following this intracellular multiplication, neutrophils, additional macrophages, and erythrocytes infiltrate the alveoli, and capillary leakage results in edema.[49] Chemokines and cytokines released by infected macrophages help trigger the severe inflammatory response.[50] In the A/J mouse model of Legionnaires' disease,[51] the relevant proinflammatory chemokines and cytokines include KC, MIP-2, tumor necrosis factor-α (TNF-α), interleukin-12 (IL-12), IL-18, and interferon-α (IFN-γ).[52-54] A variety of known and unknown bacterial factors prevent killing of the bacterium by neutrophils or serum complement. Systemic spread of the bacteria may be accomplished by infection of circulating monocytes. The mechanisms for systemic toxicity of the disease are unclear, but may be related to cytokine production during infection. Immune control of the infection is mediated by the cellular immune system.[55] The key role of TNF-α in the control of Legionnaires' disease has been underscored by the increased risk of the disease in people receiving TNF-α inhibitors.[56,57]

Toll-like receptors (TLRs) on macrophages and other cells form a crucial part of the innate immune response to *L. pneumophila* infection. TLR2 detects *L. pneumophila* lipopolysaccharide (unlike TLR4, which is important for the detection of enteric bacteria), TLR 5 flagellin, and TLR9 unknown ligands.[58-60] Mice lacking TLR2, 5, or 9 have accentuated disease and mortality, and humans with a TLR5 stop polymorphism are more susceptible to Legionnaires' disease; for unclear reasons, human TLR4 polymorphisms are protective.[58-61] Intracellular innate immune sensors detect bacterial flagellin via NOD-like receptors,[62] and it is the inability to sense cytosolic flagellin that makes one mouse strain genetically susceptible to *L. pneumophila* infection. Other eukaryotic cell surface receptors may be important, as demonstrated by the association of mannose-binding lectin deficiency with human susceptibility to Legionnaires' disease.[63]

The Th1 T-cell response and its associated cytokines are particularly crucial for the clearance of *Legionella* organisms.[53] IFN-γ activation renders macrophages nonpermissive for *L. pneumophila* growth.[64] This change in host permissiveness involves, among other things, a reduction in intracellular iron, a factor necessary for *L. pneumophila* replication.[65] Antibodies develop during the course of *L. pneumophila* infection, but the humoral immune response does not appear to be critical for host defense. The ability of *L. pneumophila* to grow within macrophages is central to pathogenesis.[33] Indeed, most legionellae seen in lung samples are associated with alveolar macrophages. Furthermore, the susceptibility of an animal species correlates with the ability of *L. pneumophila* to infect its macrophages, and bacterial mutants that are impaired for in vitro infection of macrophages have reduced virulence. It is widely believed that the adaptation of *L. pneumophila* to protozoan niches in nature has engendered it with the ability to infect mammalian phagocytes.[66] *L. pneumophila* enters the macrophage by conventional or coiling phagocytosis,[67-69] processes that use the host cell actin cytoskeleton.[70] Opsonization with the C3 component of complement can promote phagocytosis,[71] but entry by this pathway dampens the oxidative burst and thereby may enhance bacterial intracellular survival. However, opsonin-independent phagocytosis also appears to be important.[45] Even in the event that the oxidative burst is triggered, *L. pneumophila* strains may be resistant to hydrogen peroxide, superoxide anion, and hydroxyl radicals. After entry, legionellae reside within a nascent phagosome (Fig. 232-3) that does not fuse with endosomes or lysosomes,[72-74] thereby avoiding acidification and degradative enzymes. The phagosome soon associates with smooth vesicles, mitochondria, and rough endoplasmic reticulum.[75-77] Later in the intracellular cycle, the *L. pneumophila* phagosome fuses with acidic lysosomal compartments, but bacterial growth continues.[78] Ultimately, the *L. pneumophila* phagosome fills the host cell. On nutrient depletion (e.g., amino acid depletion), *L. pneumophila* is believed to convert to a flagellated form that is primed to seek out and infect new host cells.[43,79] Macrophage death involves an early induction of apoptosis and a late necrosis that appears to be triggered by a pore-forming activity.[80]

Processes in addition to macrophage infection likely contribute to disease caused by *L. pneumophila*. The bacterium may replicate or, at a minimum, must temporarily survive within the extracellular spaces of the alveoli.[81] The ability of *L. pneumophila* strains to resist complement and cationic peptides may be especially relevant for extracellular survival, particularly following the onset of inflammation.[82-84] The examination of infected lung tissue has suggested that *L. pneumophila* may also grow in the alveolar epithelium.[85] Based on in vitro models, the microbe grows within both alveolar types I and II cells.[86,87] The importance of extramacrophage processes is also implied by the fact

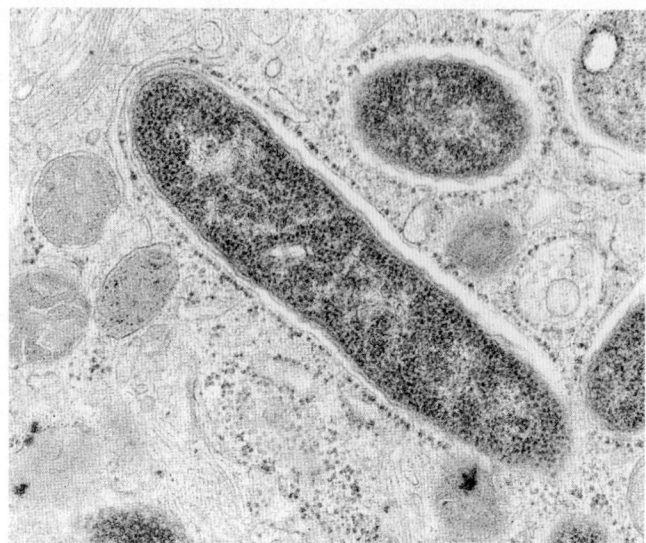

Figure 232-3 Electron micrograph of *Legionella pneumophila* growing within a phagosome of an alveolar macrophage (10,000× magnification). Note the characteristic ribosomal studding of the phagosome.

that mutants can be isolated that are not defective for macrophage infection but are impaired for virulence in animals.[88]

Neither the pathogenesis nor the cause of Pontiac fever is known with certainty. Pontiac fever is caused by inhalation of a disease-causing environmental aerosol derived from water containing microorganisms, including *Legionella* bacteria. Of patients with this disease, 30% to 85% have serum anti-*Legionella* antibody in higher concentrations than is found in the normally healthy population.[89] The prevalent assumption is that the illness is caused by inhalation of the *Legionella* bacteria. However, because the aerosols contain a vast array of other microorganisms and toxins, including endotoxin, it is unclear whether the disease is caused by inhalation of endotoxin, inhalation of a number of microorganisms, inhalation of *Legionella* bacteria alone, or a combination of all these agents.[89] Infections with non-*Legionella* bacteria can produce *Legionella* antibodies, so the presence of such antibodies does not prove that Pontiac fever is caused solely by *Legionella* infection or intoxication. Bath water fever, a clinical syndrome thought to be caused by endotoxin inhalation, is very similar to Pontiac fever, suggesting that Pontiac fever may also be caused by endotoxin inhalation.[89] Several cases of Pontiac fever have been reported to have occurred in people exposed to environmental contamination that in some others caused Legionnaires' disease; whether this is really Pontiac fever or mild Legionnaires' disease is open to question, and does not help answer the question of cause and pathogenesis.[89] Perhaps the strongest evidence implicating systemic infection with *Legionella* bacteria as the cause of Pontiac fever has been the very rare reports of positive *L. pneumophila* urinary antigen tests or positive cultures in patients with Pontiac fever.[89] The rarity of such cases and the rapid recovery without antibiotic therapy argue against systemic infection as the main cause of Pontiac fever.

LEGIONELLA PNEUMOPHILA VIRULENCE FACTORS

A variety of surface structures have been implicated in *L. pneumophila* pathogenesis. Type IV pili modestly promote bacterial attachment to macrophages and epithelial cells,[90] and flagella promote invasion independently of adherence.[91] The major outer membrane protein is a porin that also serves as a binding site for complement components and thus mediates opsonophagocytosis.[92] The Mip protein is a surface-exposed peptidyl prolyl isomerase that is required for the early stages of intracellular infection and for full virulence in animals,[93-95] whereas the heat shock protein Hsp60 has been shown to enhance epithelial

cell invasion.[96] The *rtxA* gene promotes adherence and virulence, although the structure and localization of its protein product are unclear.[97,98] *Legionella* lipopolysaccharide (LPS) contains some endotoxic activity and changes in LPS have correlated with increases in serum resistance, intracellular growth, and virulence.[99] Finally, the *rcp* gene, which appears to encode a lipid A–modifying enzyme, confers resistance to cationic peptides and promotes macrophage and lung infection.[83]

L. pneumophila secretes various proteins, degradative enzymes, and putative toxins. The release of proteins by *L. pneumophila* into the extracellular milieu or into host cells is dependent on at least two different protein secretion systems, the so-called type II and type IV protein secretion systems.[100-103] Genome sequencing also suggests the existence of types I and V secretion systems.[104] Acid phosphatases, aminopeptidases, an RNAse, a chitinase, a zinc metalloprotease, mono-, di-, and triacylglycerol lipases, a phospholipase A, a lysophospholipase A, cholesterol acyltransferase, phospholipases C, a peptidyl prolyl isomerase, and a number of novel proteins are all secreted via the *Legionella* type II system.[105-108] Mutations in the genes encoding the type II secretion system diminish infectivity for macrophages, protozoa, and animals.[107,109] The secreted zinc protease is produced during infection and promotes pathology in the guinea pig model of disease as well as intracellular infection of some ameba hosts.[105,110] Surprisingly, the type II–secreted chitinase promotes bacterial persistence in the lungs of infected mice.[106] The *Legionella* type IV secretion system known as Dot/Icm promotes intracellular infection in multiple ways.[103] First, it enhances *L. pneumophila* entry into host cells.[111,112] Second, it is essential for the ability of the *Legionella* parasite to inhibit phagosomal-endosomal-lysosomal fusions and establish its replicative niche.[73,113,114] Finally, the Dot/Icm system is important for apoptosis and bacterial egress from its spent host cell.[115,116] Mutations in *dot/icm* loci lead to loss of virulence.[88,117] Many proteins are secreted by the Dot/Icm system and in most cases these "effector" proteins translocate from the *Legionella*-containing vacuole into the host cell cytoplasm.[103,118] Some of these, including VipA, VipD, VipF, AnkX, LegC3, LegC7 (YflA), and LegC2 (YlfB), have been implicated in bacterial evasion of lysosome fusion.[119-121] Others, such as RalF, DrrA (SidM), LepB, LidA, and SidJ, play roles in the recruitment of ER-derived vesicles to the *Legionella*-containing vacuole.[122-125] Still others, including SdhA and SidF, serve to block programmed cell death and thereby permit prolonged bacterial replication.[126,127] Finally, the effectors LepA and LepB have been implicated in bacterial egress from the spent host cell.[128] *L. pneumophila* expresses various glucosyltransferases capable of inhibiting host cell protein synthesis (elongation factor 1A), and some of these are also believed to be substrates of the type IV secretion.[129,130] Although Dot/Icm is generally regarded as essential for *L. pneumophila* infection, a second type IV secretion system, known as Lvh, is under certain circumstances able to provide the requisite virulence-associated functions.[131] Interestingly, many of the type II– and type IV–secreted proteins, as well as other mediators of infection (e.g., LpnE and Lpg0971), bear a striking sequence similarity to eukaryotic proteins, suggesting that they evolved to act in a manner analogous to host cell proteins.[104,106,119,132-136]

Several infectivity factors have been localized to the *L. pneumophila* periplasm or cytoplasm. A copper-zinc superoxide dismutase resides in the periplasm, affording resistance to toxic superoxide anions, and the KatB catalase-peroxidase is needed for optimal intracellular infection.[137,138] The *Legionella* phosphoenolpyruvate phosphotransferase and HtrA protein promote intracellular growth and virulence.[139,140] *L. pneumophila* iron acquisition, important for intracellular and extracellular replication, involves, among other things, a secreted ferric iron chelator (the siderophore legiobactin), secreted pyomelanin with ferric reductase activity, and inner membrane ferrous iron transporter (FeoB).[141-144]

In addition to the identification of eukaryotic-like proteins in the *L. pneumophila* genome, another outcome of sequencing bacterial genomes is the realization that there are large segments of DNA, including plasmids and chromosomal islands, which can vary between

L. pneumophila strains.[104,145-147] It is possible that these variable regions of the genome will help explain differences in virulence that may exist between strains.

VIRULENCE FACTORS AND PATHOGENESIS OF OTHER *LEGIONELLA* SPP.

Relatively little is known about the virulence mechanisms, molecular pathogenesis, and cell biology of infections caused by *Legionella* spp. other than *L. pneumophila*. With the exception of *L. longbeachae*, infections caused by the other *Legionella* spp. are rare and found almost exclusively in severely immunocompromised patients. This implies that these other species lack critical virulence factors that allow ready intracellular multiplication. However, some strains of *L. micdadei*, *L. dumoffii*, and other species can multiply normally in guinea pig and other animal macrophages; *L. longbeachae* appears to multiply well in most cell types.[148-151] Unlike *L. pneumophila*, non–AJ strain mice are not resistant to infection with a number of other *Legionella* spp., including *L. bozemanae*, *L. dumoffii*, *L. micdadei*, and *L. longbeachae*.[152] *L. longbeachae* resides within a ribosome-studded phagosome, albeit with markers of late endosomal maturation, unlike *L. pneumophila*, which is able to block endosomal maturation at an early stage.[148,153,154] In contrast, *L. micdadei* resides in a smooth phagosome, and *L. dumoffii* grows in the cytoplasm rather than in a phagosome.[151,153,155,156] The clinical implications of these differences in pathogenesis are not clear, although it seems likely that those bacteria not multiplying in an early endosome may differ in their responses to antimicrobial administration that targets that compartment.

Epidemiology

INCUBATION PERIOD AND CONTAGIOUSNESS

The incubation period during most outbreaks of Legionnaires' disease has been reported to be between 2 to 10 days, with median values of 4 to 6 days, and some outliers of from 1 up to 28 days.[1,157] The incubation period may be slightly longer in some outbreaks. In the West Frisian Flower Show epidemic in 1999, the incubation period ranged from 2 to 19 days, with a median of 7 days; 16% of patients had an incubation period longer than 10 days. A 2-month incubation period was reported for one nosocomial case.[158] The incubation period of Pontiac fever is generally 4 hours to 3 days, with a median of 2 days, although incubation periods of up to 9 days have been reported.[7,159,160]

Person-to-person transmission of Legionnaires' disease or Pontiac fever does not occur. Apocryphal reports of Legionnaires' disease acquisition acquired from manipulation of *L. pneumophila*–infected human lung specimens exist. Disease transmission from experimentally infected animals to other animals does not occur, nor from animals to humans. Finally, laboratory transmission from bacterial cultures to humans has not been documented. The lack of contagiousness, and the apparent low infectivity of laboratory cultures for humans, support experimental studies showing that the infectiousness of the bacterium is enhanced by intra-amebal growth and by special growth conditions, and that a sporelike bacterial form, only produced under special conditions, is highly virulent.[43-45]

PATTERNS AND RATES OF DISEASE, AND MORTALITY

Legionnaires' disease occurs in sporadic and epidemic forms. About 65% to 75% of reported cases are not associated with known epidemics of the disease.[29,161] Underreporting of the disease is common because many sporadic cases are treated empirically, without diagnostic studies being performed, because of false-negative diagnostic test results, because of underreporting of diagnosed cases, and because only passive surveillance systems are in place to detect disease occurrence. Thus, only about 2800 cases of Legionnaires' disease were reported in 2006 (9.5/ million population) to the Centers for Disease Control and Prevention

(CDC). This rate is lower than that reported in France in 2007, 22.4 cases/million population, and about the same as England and Wales in 2007, 8.2/million (37% acquired abroad). In contrast, prospective studies of both sporadic community-acquired and nosocomial Legionnaires' disease have reported far more cases in the United States than would be expected based on the number of cases reported to the CDC. One prospective community-based study in Ohio of adult patients with community-acquired pneumonia requiring hospitalization found that 2.4% of these patients had Legionnaires' disease, and that the disease incidence was about 80/million population/year.[162] When extrapolated to the entire U.S. population, the authors estimated that from 8000 to 18,000 cases of Legionnaires' disease occur annually among adults requiring hospitalization for pneumonia. The incidence of Legionnaires' disease causing community-acquired pneumonia not requiring hospitalization is not known with certainty. One small regional U.S. study had estimated that the incidence of Legionnaires' disease among outpatients treated for pneumonia is 40 to 280/million population/ year.[163] Thus, somewhere between 18,000 and 88,000 U.S. cases of Legionnaires' disease are estimated to occur annually, most of which are not epidemic-related. A recent German study of community-acquired Legionnaires' disease that used sensitive diagnostic tests found that the annual rate was 180 to 360 cases/million population, which if extrapolated to the United States would mean that 56,000 to 112,000 Legionnaires' disease cases occur annually in the United States,[164] and that only about 2% to 5% of U.S. cases are currently reported to the CDC. Some geographic regions appear to have more Legionnaires' disease than others, such as western Pennsylvania and Ohio in the United States and Catalonia in Spain; whether this is because of true differences in disease incidence or better case ascertainment is uncertain. The incidence of Legionnaires' disease in the United States and elsewhere appears to be increasing, based on the numbers of cases reported to public health agencies; whether this is the result of more widespread use of the urine antigen test, better reporting and surveillance, or a true disease increase is unknown.[165] Estimates of Legionnaires' disease as a cause of community-acquired pneumonia requiring hospitalization in adults range from 0.5% to 10% of all admitted pneumonia cases; an average value is probably about 2%, even in geographic regions with excellent diagnostic capabilities.[166-170]

Legionnaires' disease of children is thought to be uncommon, representing 1% or less of causes of pneumonia in this age group, and generally occurs as a nosocomial disease of immunosuppressed children.[171] Neonates may be at relatively high risk of Legionnaires' disease because of the immaturity of their immune systems. Both nosocomially and domestically acquired cases of the disease have been reported in apparently immunologically normal newborns exposed to *Legionella*-contaminated water in incubators, or bathtubs, or during birth.

Shortly after the Philadelphia outbreak, nosocomial Legionnaires' disease outbreaks were reported in several cities throughout the United States and Europe. Because relatively little was known about the environmental ecology of *L. pneumophila*, or about optimal diagnostic methods, these outbreaks were characterized by long durations, often years in length, and high numbers of cases and fatalities. For example, the Legionnaires' disease outbreak at the Wadsworth Veterans Administration Hospital in Los Angeles resulted in more than 250 cases of disease in patients and visitors over an 8-year period.[16,23,172] A 17-year long outbreak of unrecognized nosocomial Legionnaires' disease occurred at another U.S. hospital, involving many fewer patients.[173] Nosocomial Legionnaires' disease epidemics continue to occur worldwide, albeit with durations measured in weeks rather than years.[174,175] Nosocomial pneumonia usually only affects a relatively small number of hospitalized patients, with attack rates less than 1% of patients.[16,176] During nosocomial outbreaks of Legionnaires' disease, the minority (5% to 11%) of patients with nosocomial pneumonia of all causes have been reported to have Legionnaires' disease,[16,177-179] although in some explosive outbreaks involving a single ward the attack rates may be much higher.

Community-based Legionnaires' disease epidemics continue to occur more than 25 years after the 1976 Philadelphia outbreak, some of them quite serious in terms of the number of people affected. Recent outbreaks include one in Murcia, Spain, in 2001, involving up to 700 people, with six deaths; Barrow-in-Furness, England, in 2002, more than 130 people, with six deaths; and Bovenkarspel, the Netherlands, in 1999, 188 people, 21 deaths.[180] Of note, two of these recent outbreaks involved people visiting a town center, rather than being inside a particular building. Long-distance spread of disease from industrial aerosols has been recently reported from France and Norway.[25,181]

Legionnaires' disease affecting travelers constitutes up to 50% of reported cases in some countries. In many cases, a common source outbreak has been found, but for others the cases appear to be sporadic. Multiple common source outbreaks have been uncovered in travelers by a cooperative European reporting system that collects and analyzes Legionnaires' disease cases in travelers.[182] Such a well-coordinated traveler's health monitoring and analysis system does not exist in the United States, and as a result many small epidemics of the disease are likely undetected in this country.[183]

Despite the immense publicity usually generated by epidemics of Legionnaires' disease, sporadic cases of the disease are about fourfold more common than linked cases of the disease. Some sporadic cases are undoubtedly the result of common source outbreaks involving just a few people. This is especially true of travelers who return home during the incubation period or while they are ill, but still well enough to travel. Other evidence for common source links for apparently unrelated cases has come from an observation in Glasgow showing that proximity of a residence to an air-conditioning cooling tower was a risk factor for Legionnaires' disease.[184]

Pontiac fever often causes explosive outbreaks of disease with high attack rates. Attack rates of 70% to 90% have been reported from several epidemics.[7,159,185-187]

Legionnaires' disease mortality rates are highly variable, ranging from less than 1% to as high as 80%, depending on the underlying health of the patient, promptness of specific therapy, and whether the disease is sporadic, nosocomial, or part of a large outbreak.[29,188-190] The lowest mortality rates, around 1%, have been observed in recent large outbreaks of the disease, whereas the highest mortality rates have been reported in untreated nosocomial disease in patients with severe underlying diseases.[191] The average fatality rates for sporadic disease is estimated to be about 10% to 15%. Fatality rates of nosocomial disease have declined by more than 50% in the United States over the last 20 years; a similar but less dramatic decrease in death rates of community-acquired cases has also been observed.[29] The declines in mortality rates appear to be the result of better and faster disease recognition, especially through use of the urine antigen test, and more widespread use of empirical therapy for pneumonia that includes drugs active against *L. pneumophila*.[29,191] More details on mortality rates and response to therapy is given in the treatment section of this chapter.

RISK FACTORS

Host risk factors for Legionnaires' disease are those that result in decreased local or systemic cellular immunity and those that increase the chances of exposure to an infectious aerosol or microaspiration of contaminated water. Also important in determining whether Legionnaires' disease has occurred are the relative virulence of the bacterium, its aerosol stability, probably the growth phase of the organism, and environmental factors that facilitate the spread of the bacterium from contaminated water to the host, such as wind direction, relative humidity, and aerosol formation.

Male gender, cigarette smoking, chronic heart or lung disease, diabetes, end-stage renal failure, organ transplantation, immunosuppression, some forms of cancer, and age older than 50 years have all been found to be host risk factors for Legionnaires' disease.[176,180,192,193] The approximately twofold greater risk with male gender may be caused by the higher prevalence of cigarette smoking and its complications in males. Cigarette smoking increases risk by about two- to sevenfold, probably because of the adverse effects of cigarette use on local pul-

monary defense mechanisms. Immunosuppression that decreases local or systemic cellular immunity, and particularly glucocorticoid administration, increases the risk by about two- to sixfold; cytotoxic chemotherapy was shown to be a risk factor in one study. Anti–TNF-α therapy has emerged recently as a significant risk factor for Legionnaires' disease.[56,57] Lung, but not gastrointestinal tract, cancer has been shown to be a risk factor for Legionnaires' disease.[192] Various hematologic malignancies have also been shown to be important risk factors, especially hairy cell leukemia.[177,192] Small single studies of genetic predisposition to Legionnaires' disease have shown that polymorphisms in TLR4, TLR5, and mannose-binding lectin produce minor predispositions to the disease[58,61,63]; it is unlikely that these polymorphisms account for most of the human risk for Legionnaires' disease and confirmatory studies are needed to define the risks better. Animal studies have implicated TLR2 and TLR9 as being important in host immunity but to date no human data exist on the Legionnaires' disease associated with polymorphisms in these TLRs.[59,60] Recent surgery has been an important risk factor for nosocomial disease, probably because of general anesthetic-caused defects in local lung defense or *Legionella*-contaminated water introduced into the respiratory tract in the perioperative or postoperative periods, or both factors combined.[194,195] Alcoholism has been shown to be a predisposing condition in only some studies, and has never been shown to be a risk factor in multivariate analyses.[176,177,193,196] There appear to be no predisposing host factors for Pontiac fever.

Because Legionnaires' disease cannot occur without exposure to the bacterium, activities that increase the chances of exposure to *Legionella* bacteria in water increase the risks of disease acquisition. Factors such as recent overnight travel, use of well water in the home, recent plumbing work inside the home, disruptions of water supply resulting in "brown" water at the water tap, and possibly living in a water distribution network with older plumbing or using an electric water heater all increase the risk of community-acquired Legionnaires' disease.[193,197] Other community, recreational, or travel-related activities increasing the chances of acquiring the disease include the use of, or proximity to, whirlpool spas or hot water spring spas, living in close proximity to a cooling tower, or being near decorative fountains.[180,184,198-200] Rarely reported risks are near-drowning[10,200,201] and delivery by water birth.[202]

A wide range of nosocomial exposures can result in Legionnaires' disease. Almost all involve delivery of *Legionella*-contaminated water into the respiratory tract and include the use of tap water filled or rinsed—nebulizers, humidifiers, oxygen humidifiers, ventilator tubing, and nasogastric feedings or lavages.[203-206] Consumption of *Legionella*-contaminated ice can also be a risk factor for nosocomial Legionnaires' disease.[207] These risk factors are in addition to exposure to *Legionella*-contaminated air originating from a cooling tower.[208-210] Rare cases of nosocomial *Legionella* wound infection have resulted from irrigation or bathing of wounds in *Legionella*-contaminated water.[211,212]

MODES OF TRANSMISSION

Legionnaires' disease is transmitted from the environment to people by inhalation of an infectious aerosol.[213] In an unknown fraction of cases, microaspiration of contaminated water into the lungs is the mode of transmission, rather than inhalation of an aerosol.[206,214] Finally, massive aspiration of contaminated water into the lungs during near-drownings is a very unusual but reported mode of disease transmission.[200,201]

Multiple examples of exclusive aerosol transmission of Legionnaires' disease exist, especially in epidemics having a cooling tower, water spa, water fountain, or water mister as the source of disease.[1,198,199,209,210,215-219] In these cases, proximity to the aerosol generator, duration of exposure, and presence in an area downstream of the contaminated device have all been found to be risk factors for disease acquisition. Of note, when reported, either consumption of water at the epidemic site has not occurred in most disease victims, or the drinking water of the outbreak site has been culture-negative for *L. pneumophila*.

The data supporting microaspiration of water as a major mode of transmission are less convincing, but in some specific reports the evidence is compelling. These data include examples of nosocomial disease in patients whose major risk factor was nasogastric tube irrigation with tap water and interruption of nosocomial outbreaks by substituting sterile water for tap water for drinking and nasogastric tube irrigation.[206,214,220,221] Whether microaspiration is the major transmission mode for nosocomial disease is controversial and unproven.[222] Experimental animal data are unhelpful in this regard, because both aerosol delivery and tracheal instillation produce disease.[223,224]

Rare reports of peritonitis or bowel abscesses caused by *L. pneumophila* have led to speculation that oral ingestion may be a mode of disease transmission.[225-227] In all these cases, *L. pneumophila* pneumonia or empyema occurred concurrently, making unclear which organs were the ones primarily infected. In contrast to the relative ease of producing lethal guinea pig pneumonia by the aerosol or intratracheal route, huge amounts of *L. pneumophila* delivered by oral gavage are cleared rapidly without causing severe pneumonia,[228] although another experimental study yielded somewhat different results.[229] Overall, it is very unlikely that oral ingestion of *Legionella*-contaminated water is more than a minor mode of transmission of the disease.

OUTBREAK INVESTIGATION

Prompt notification of public health authorities of any strongly suspected or confirmed case of Legionnaires' disease is critically important for detecting epidemics of the disease, and in many regions is legally required. What appears to be only a single case of the disease may be part of an epidemic, or the index case. Alert physicians have sometimes detected pneumonia clusters that led to the discovery of emerging and long-standing epidemics of Legionnaires' disease.[1,198]

In addition to reporting nosocomial Legionnaires' disease to public health authorities, the medical institution should embark on extensive investigation of even a single case of nosocomial Legionnaires' disease.[230] This is because more cases may have occurred previously, or will appear subsequently. Retrospective review of the frequency and causes of nosocomial pneumonia for a 3- to 6-month period may yield more cases, especially if combined with testing of saved lung tissues from biopsies or necropsies. Prospective laboratory testing of all patients with nosocomial pneumonia for Legionnaires' disease can also be useful in finding more cases, for a 3- to 6-month period. Hospital physicians should be notified to consider Legionnaires' disease when making diagnostic and therapeutic decisions in patients with nosocomial pneumonia until either it is clear that no more nosocomial cases have occurred, or until an ongoing nosocomial outbreak has been eradicated.

Investigation of community-acquired and nosocomial outbreaks of Legionnaires' disease requires a thorough epidemiologic investigation. This will help generate hypotheses concerning the source of the outbreak and demonstrate risk factors using controlled studies. Environmental testing without concurrent epidemiologic investigation can lead to misleading findings, even when molecular fingerprinting is used to compare clinical and environmental isolates.[231,232] It is crucially important to have only a qualified laboratory perform environmental studies because not all environmental microbiology companies are competent in the proper collection, processing, and culturing of water specimens for *Legionella* spp. bacteria. Certification is required in some countries, but not in the United States, although voluntary certification is available from the CDC.[233] If at all possible, it is crucial to obtain as many clinical isolates as possible of *Legionella* bacteria from affected patients; this affords the possibility to compare the strain identity of environmental and clinical isolates. Detailed protocols for environmental sampling are available.[233-235]

Some rough clues to an environmental source of a Legionnaires' disease epidemic can be found in the pace of the outbreak and its geographic distribution. Explosive outbreaks involving tens to hundreds of people over a several-day period are most often the result of a contaminated massive aerosol generator, usually a cooling tower, but occasionally a whirlpool spa or misting device. Potable water–associated outbreaks may produce as many cases, but generally over a much longer period of time (many weeks or months). Potable water–related outbreaks are confined to a single building or building complex if the plumbing is common among buildings. In contrast, cooling tower–related epidemics often affect building visitors and those within several hundred meters, up to 10 km from the tower.[25] Interior aerosol-generating devices, such as recreational spas and misters, cause disease only in building visitors.

ENVIRONMENTAL DECONTAMINATION FOR OUTBREAKS

All aerosol-generating sources implicated or highly suspected of being a source of epidemic Legionnaires' disease should be taken out of operation as soon as possible; this generally includes cooling towers and hot tubs. Implicated potable water sources such as plumbing systems should be shut down, if possible. Recommendations exist for emergency disinfection of such sources and may differ according to local regulations or guidelines.[230,235-237] The emergency disinfection process usually includes hyperchlorination or other oxidant applications, or heating. Long-term remediation can be complex and requires expert engineering and public health advice.

Clinical Presentation

LEGIONNAIRES' DISEASE

Legionnaires' disease causes acute consolidating pneumonia that cannot be accurately differentiated on initial presentation from pneumococcal pneumonia. Several prospective studies have shown that the two diseases have almost identical clinical and roentgenographic findings and that nonspecific laboratory test results cannot differentiate between the two diseases.[238-240] However, initial clinical findings of community-acquired and nosocomial epidemic Legionnaires' disease seemed to indicate that a distinct clinical syndrome was observed.[241] This syndrome was characterized by fever with pulse-temperature dissociation, myalgia, nonproductive cough, few pulmonary symptoms, diarrhea, confusion, hyponatremia, hypophosphatemia, and elevated liver-associated enzyme levels. Although this symptom complex does occur in Legionnaires' disease, it is not specific or frequent enough to allow differentiation of the disease from other common causes of community-acquired pneumonia. A clinical scoring system that was devised to help increase diagnostic accuracy is neither specific nor sensitive.[190,242]

A prodromal illness may occur, lasting for hours to several days, with symptoms of headache, myalgia, asthenia, and anorexia. Fever accompanies this prodrome, except in severely immunocompromised patients. Multiple rigors may occur, as well as diarrhea and abdominal pain. Cough, with or without chest pain, often develops hours to days after onset of the prodrome; the cough produces purulent sputum in only about 50% of patients with Legionnaires' disease. The initial clinical picture may be confusing because the systemic symptoms can be more impressive than those referable to the lower respiratory tract, leading some physicians to diagnose influenza, a gastrointestinal illness and, in some cases, an acute abdomen syndrome. However, careful physical examination of the chest and chest roentgenography almost always demonstrate findings of pneumonia, including focal rales and alveolar filling pulmonary infiltrates that vary from patchy infiltrates to multiple areas of consolidation.[243,244] Chest computed tomography (CT) findings include ground-glass opacities and consolidation.[245,246] Pleuritic chest pain, sometimes in concert with hemoptysis, may occur and can mislead the clinician into considering pulmonary infarction. Headache can be the most prominent feature and may be so severe as to suggest subarachnoid hemorrhage. Mental confusion is commonly reported in some series; obtundation, seizures, and focal neurologic findings may also occur less frequently.[247-249] Some patients may have negative chest x-ray films on presentation, which show focal or diffuse pulmonary infiltrates within 1 day. Cavitation of consolidated lung is seen in about 10% of immunosuppressed patients. Pleural effusion without pulmonary infiltrates may rarely be observed as the sole radiographic abnormality. Bronchoscopic findings in patients with consolidating pneumonia are often remarkable for the absence of inflammation or purulent secretions in the large airways. Abdominal examination may reveal generalized or local tenderness and, in rare cases, evidence of peritonitis. Splenomegaly is uncommon. Findings of pericarditis, myocarditis, and focal abscesses are rare. No rash is associated with this disease, except that caused by other factors such as drug therapy. Symptoms of rhinorrhea, chronic afebrile fatigue, and fever without pneumonia lasting for many weeks are not seen or are so rare as to make the diagnosis unlikely.

A number of nonspecific laboratory test abnormalities may occur in Legionnaires' disease.[55] These include hyponatremia, hypophosphatemia, increased liver-associated enzyme levelss (aspartate aminotransferase [AST], alanine aminotransferase [ALT], alkaline phosphatase), hyperbilirubinemia, leukopenia, thrombocytopenia, disseminated intravascular coagulation, leukocytosis, pyuria, and elevated creatine kinase (MM fraction) and lactate dehydrogenase (LDH) levels. A few studies have shown that patients with Legionnaires' disease are more likely to have hyponatremia than those with other causes of pneumonia, but the range of serum sodium values is too broad for this abnormality to be diagnostic in an individual patient.[250] Laboratory markers of pancreatitis are detected if this is a complication of Legionnaires' disease. Renal disease caused by Legionnaires' disease may result in the presence of urine casts and white cells, elevated serum creatinine levels, or both. Myoglobinuria is a relatively common finding, usually indicated by a positive dipstick test for blood in the absence of significant numbers of red cells in the urine. Hypoxemia occurs in proportion to the severity of the pneumonia and underlying cardiopulmonary disease.

Clinical diagnosis may be more specific if the patient's clinical course after treatment is taken into account and if epidemiologic and immunologic risk factors are considered. The chances of a patient having Legionnaires' disease are increased if an acute consolidating pneumonia fails to respond to several days of β-lactam antimicrobial therapy, or if the pneumonia is severe enough to require intensive care unit hospitalization. Important epidemiologic clues include use of a hot tub or recreational spa, travel outside the home for 1 day or more, recent pneumonia of a co-worker, fellow conference attendee or fellow traveler, and recent plumbing work done at home or at work, as indicated by air in the pipes or brown discoloration of the water. Patients with suppression of the cellular immune system are at high risk for getting Legionnaires' disease; these include those treated with glucocorticoids and with antirejection drugs after organ transplantation. Administration of very high-dose methylprednisolone or muromonab-CD3 for acute organ rejection are especially high risk factors for Legionnaires' disease. Administration of TNF-α antagonists are also a major risk factor for the disease.

The nonspecific presentation of Legionnaires' disease can make clinical diagnosis very difficult, and mandates empirical therapy for most patients with community-acquired pneumonia of uncertain cause. Diagnosis of the index or sporadic case of nosocomial Legionnaires' disease can also be difficult, especially because this disease is an uncommon cause of nosocomial pneumonia in most hospitals.

EXTRAPULMONARY INFECTIONS

Extrapulmonary infections are very rare and usually occur as metastatic complications of pneumonia in immunocompromised patients. Metastatic infection has been reported almost exclusively in immunocompromised patients or patients with fatal Legionnaires' disease who may develop abscesses and other infections of the brain, spleen, or extrathoracic lymph nodes, and skeletal and myocardial muscles.[251-255] Other reported sites of metastatic infection have been the intestines and liver, kidneys, peritoneum, pericardium, vascular shunts and grafts, bone marrow, joints, surgical wounds including prosthetic heart valves and aorta, perirectal area, and skin and subcutaneous tissues.[225,256-265] In some of these cases, the onset of symptoms of the metastatic infection precede the recognition of pneumonia by several days, and in other cases the metastatic infection presents days to weeks subsequent to onset of the pneumonia. In some cases, the metastatic infection site was the only evidence of relapse of infection. Three cases of metastatic infection have been reported in apparently previously healthy patients,[253,266,267] but otherwise immunosuppression has been reported in such patients. Metastatic infection complicating fatal Legionnaires' disease has not generally been recognized premortem. Nonmetastatic direct extension of a thoracic empyema into the soft tissues of the chest has been reported after thoracentesis.[268]

Rare cases of primary infection not preceded by Legionnaires' disease have also been reported. These appear to be the result of direct inoculation of Legionella-contaminated water into various tissues, usually in hosts with compromise of local, if not systemic, immunity. Culture-proven sites of such infections have been surgical or other wounds, prosthetic heart valves, mediastinum, and respiratory sinuses.[211,212,269-272] One unusual case of pyarthrosis in an apparently nonimmunosuppressed patient without pneumonia has been reported.[267] Some infections were introduced by bathing postoperative patients with contaminated tap water, the use of therapeutic baths, and inadvertent tap water irrigation of the mediastinum after esophageal perforation.

PONTIAC FEVER

Pontiac fever is a self-limited, short-duration febrile illness, usually diagnosed only during an outbreak of the disease.[7,89,159,160,186] The usual story is onset of symptoms 12 to 36 hours after exposure to a bacteria-contaminated aerosol, either in a workplace or some other group setting. Attack rates are high, with more than 80% to 90% of such exposed people becoming ill. The sources of contaminated aerosol have included industrial processes using sprayed water (e.g., lathes, artificial fiber plants, building humidification), recreational spas, decorative water fountains, and cooling towers. Fever, myalgia, headache, and asthenia are the dominant symptoms. Cough, dyspnea, anorexia, arthralgia, and abdominal pain occur less frequently. Most patients are not ill enough to seek medical attention, recovering without specific therapy 3 to 5 days after disease onset. There is little information about physical examination findings in the first day of illness; examination 2 to 5 days after onset may show fever and tachypnea, but little else. Pneumonia does not occur. Fatigue and nonfocal neurologic complaints have been reported to persist for up to several months in the minority of affected patients. Because the clinical findings are nonspecific, it is difficult, if not impossible, to diagnose this disease accurately in the absence of similar illnesses in co-workers or others with a common source exposure. Inquiries regarding the health of co-workers and acquaintances and a history of known water exposure may help confirm the diagnosis, but even these findings may be nonspecific and insensitive.

Laboratory Diagnosis

Specific but relatively insensitive tests are available for the diagnosis of Legionnaires' disease (Table 232-1). These include culture of lower respiratory tract secretions, tissues, and fluids, detection of L. pneumophila serogroup 1 antigenuria by immune assays, detection of L. pneumophila bacteria in lower respiratory tract secretions, tissues, and fluids by immunofluorescent microscopy, detection of L. pneumophila–specific antibodies by immunoassay, and detection of L. pneumophila DNA using molecular amplification and detection technologies.

Culture yield depends on the severity of illness, with the lowest yield (15% to 25%) for mild pneumonia and the highest yield (more than 90%) for severe pneumonia causing respiratory failure.[32,273] Prior specific antimicrobial therapy affects the yield adversely, although some patients have positive sputum cultures for days to weeks after initiation

TABLE 232-1	Specific Diagnostic Tests for Legionnaires' Disease Caused by *Legionella pneumophila****			
Test	**Specimen Types**	**Sensitivity (%)**	**Specificity (%)**	**Comments**
Culture	Sputum, other lower respiratory tract secretions; lung; pleural fluid; blood; extrapulmonary tissues, fluids	20-95	100	May be positive up to several days after treatment; requires special media and expertise
Antigenuria	Urine	60-95	>99	Highest sensitivity for *L. pneumophila* serogroup 1, Pontiac type
Immunofluorescent microscopy	Same as culture	20-50	99	Highest specificity with monoclonal antibody; requires very high level of technical expertise
Antibody	Paired serum	20-70	95-99	Highest specificity for *L. pneumophila* serogroup 1
Molecular amplification	Sputum, other lower respiratory tract secretions; urine	20-75	90-95	Not well standardized; good performance in some reference labs

*Pertains only to L. pneumophila *infections. The yield of diagnostic tests is lower for infection caused by other species, especially those tests based on immunoassay.*

of specific therapy. Expectorated sputum or, even better, endotracheal aspirates are good specimens for culture; neither bronchoscopy nor lung biopsy is required for good culture yield, assuming a good-quality sputum specimen. Sputum cultures may be positive despite the presence of epithelial cells and lack of leukocytes, making suspicion of Legionnaires' disease an exception to the usual sputum adequacy screening criteria. The major advantage of culture diagnosis is that the yield is not dependent on *L. pneumophila* serotype or on *Legionella* spp., a fault of all antibody and urine testing. Culture is also often the only test that is positive in cases of Legionnaires' disease caused by other *Legionella* species. Complete investigation of the source of an outbreak requires a clinical isolate, another reason to perform culture. Proper performance of culture requires the inoculation of multiple special selective and nonselective media, preplating decontamination of specimens, and laboratory technologists skilled in the recognition and identification of *Legionella* bacteria. Unfortunately, many clinical laboratories have neither the expertise nor the ability to perform this test properly.

Urine antigen testing has revolutionized the laboratory diagnosis of Legionnaires' disease, making it the most common laboratory test ordered for diagnosis of this disease.[29,274] This is because the test can be easily performed by those without special skills, especially the card-based immunoassay, because the test is often positive when other tests are negative and because it is highly specific. Unlike culture, urine antigen persists for days after antimicrobial therapy begins. The test is not perfect, however; it is most sensitive for the detection of the Pontiac monoclonal antibody type (MAB 2+) of *L. pneumophila* serogroup 1(up to 90%), less sensitive for other monoclonal antibody types of *L. pneumophila* serogroup 1 (60%), and very poorly sensitive (less than 5%) for other *L. pneumophila* serogroups and other species.[275-277] Because most (about 90%) cases of community-acquired Legionnaires' disease are caused by the Pontiac subtype of *L. pneumophila* serogroup 1, the average sensitivity of this test is in the range of 70% to 80%. Immunocompromised patients, patients with nosocomial Legionnaires' disease, and some Australian patients are more likely to have Legionnaires' disease caused by other serogroups and species, and hence a negative urine antigen test.[275] Yield can be increased by urine concentration.[278] Rare false-positive test results may be caused by rheumatoid-like factors, which are easy to inactivate, although most laboratories do not perform this inactivation step. A common clinical error is to order only urine antigen testing and to stop therapy for Legionnaires' disease if the urine test is negative because the urine test is not 100% sensitive and, for some patient groups, may be poorly sensitive. Positive test results are associated with more severe disease.[196] Patients with extensive bilateral Legionnaires' disease may excrete urinary antigen for weeks to months after recovery. This should not cause confusion over whether a positive test is the result of new or old pneumonia in the absence of a history of recent hospitalization for severe pneumonia.

Antibody detection is insensitive and of low specificity unless paired acute and convalescent sera are tested.[279] For optimal yield, convalescent sera should be collected at 4, 6, and 12 weeks after disease onset.

About 80% to 90% of seroconversions occur by 4 weeks, with the remaining seroconversions requiring an additional 2 to 8 weeks. Only about 75% of patients with culture-proven Legionnaires' disease will seroconvert at all, even with optimally timed and tested sera . Test specificity is affected by the type of antigen used, its fixation method, and other details of testing methodology. Few commercially available serologic tests are of optimal specificity or sensitivity because of the use of polyvalent antigen preparations and because of deviations from standardized test methodology.[280] Only seroconversion to *L. pneumophila* serogroup 1 is of high enough specificity for clinical use; measurement of antibodies to other serogroups and species is plagued by low specificity and cannot be recommended. Serologic testing is more useful for epidemiologic investigations than for clinical use in a single patient.

Detection of *L. pneumophila* in respiratory tract tissues and fluids using immunofluorescent microscopy (direct fluorescent antibody, DFA) testing is specific if a monoclonal antibody to this species is used and the test is performed by experts.[281] Use of other reagents, or testing by nonexperts, usually results in many false-positive test results. The test is insensitive, even in experienced hands, except in cases of severe pneumonia, in which the organism load is high. Many laboratories no longer perform this test because of its low yield and complexity.[282]

Molecular amplification and detection of *L. pneumophila* are available primarily as a research test, although it is increasingly available at reference and public health laboratories and one commercial assay has been approved for use in the United States. Most but not all evaluations have shown that molecular methods are about as sensitive as culture, although more recent studies have shown that molecular methods are more sensitive than culture. The addition of molecular testing increases diagnostic yield by 10% to 100% over that for urine antigen testing,[164,283] and appears to be most useful for the diagnosis of milder cases of the disease. Primers can be selected that can detect all known species and serotypes. Some studies have reported nonspecific results, but whether this is caused by the low sensitivity of culture or nonspecificity of the molecular tests is uncertain. Use of this test methodology for clinical purposes should only be undertaken for well-validated and controlled assays.[273] However, when available, these assays can increase diagnostic yield. Genetic sequencing of positive molecular products can be used in many cases for species level identification and in some cases for molecular fingerprinting.[284]

Optimal test yield requires performing more than one type of test; sputum culture and urine antigen testing are the two preferred tests. If both of these are negative and there are clinical or epidemiologic reasons for making a retrospective diagnosis weeks to months later, then antibody testing should be ordered. If a well-validated molecular assay is available, this would be another option in addition to the other tests.

The yield of all tests (but perhaps especially antibody determination) is diminished by specific therapy, requiring testing before, or within a few days, of the start of antimicrobial therapy. However, therapy should not be withheld for an inordinate time pending collection or testing of specimens, and should not be stopped based solely on a negative laboratory test result.

Treatment and Response to Therapy

Legionella bacteria are intracellular parasites of monocytic phagocytes and probably some other human cells. This means that all antimicrobial agents efficacious for Legionnaires' disease must be concentrated, and bioactive, within these cells. In addition the intracellular drugs must be distributed in the same subcellular location as the bacteria. The macrolides, quinolones, and tetracyclines all meet these criteria. In contrast, none of the β-lactams, monobactams, aminoglycosides, or phenicols are active for this disease because of their low or poorly active intracellular activity against the *Legionella* bacteria.[189]

Prospective, adequately sized clinical trials of antimicrobial therapy for Legionnaires' disease have not been performed.[189,190,285] The only comparative clinical data available are retrospective data from community-acquired or nosocomial outbreaks of the disease. Patients treated with erythromycin or tetracycline had significantly lower fatality rates than those treated with β-lactam or aminoglycoside agents; in the 1976 Philadelphia epidemic, the fatality rates for those treated with erythromycin or a tetracycline were 10% versus 20% to 40% for other drugs.[1] Similarly, in one outbreak of nosocomial disease, immunosuppressed patients treated with erythromycin had a 24% fatality rate in comparison to a 80% rate for otherwise treated patients, and erythromycin-treated nonimmunocompromised patients had a 7% fatality rate in comparison to 25% for those otherwise treated.[241] A number of small uncontrolled or underpowered prospective controlled studies of the treatment of Legionnaires' disease have been carried out. Because in most studies the expected outcome is good, with overall fatality rates of less than 10% and cure rates in excess of 80%, it is difficult to interpret the existing studies as anything but anecdotal. These studies have shown that small numbers of patients with Legionnaires' disease have responded adequately to erythromycin, tetracycline, azithromycin, dirithromycin, clarithromycin, telithromycin, pefloxacin, ciprofloxacin, gatifloxacin, grepafloxacin, sparfloxacin, trovafloxacin, and levofloxacin. One retrospective study of Legionnaires' disease with severe pneumonia has shown that patients treated with a fluoroquinolone antimicrobial agent within 8 hours of ICU admission had significantly better outcomes than those treated later, or with other drugs, including erythromycin.[286] Some more recent uncontrolled studies have shown that erythromycin and clarithromycin are inferior to levofloxacin therapy for Legionnaires' disease in terms of hospital length of stay, time to become afebrile, and complications but not mortality.[287,288] Of note, no comparison with azithromycin, the most potent anti-*Legionella* macrolide, was performed. Addition of rifampin to levofloxacin led to worse outcomes than levofloxacin alone in another uncontrolled study.[289]

In the absence of adequately sized human studies, decisions about potential antimicrobial efficacy for Legionnaires' disease must be made on the basis of experimental animal and cell culture studies. The ability of a drug to inhibit or kill intracellular *L. pneumophila* usually correlates well with its clinical effectiveness for Legionnaires' disease. Similarly, therapy studies using a guinea pig model of Legionnaires' disease correlate well with drug effectiveness for the treatment of the disease in humans. The guinea pig model is generally a severe test of drug effectiveness, giving results similar to those expected for immunosuppressed or severely ill patients. These studies have shown that β-lactam drugs, aminoglycosides, and chloramphenicol neither inhibit intracellular *L. pneumophila* nor effect cure in the guinea pig model.[189,285] In contrast, erythromycin, clarithromycin, and tetracyclines can inhibit the intracellular growth of the bacterium and cure guinea pigs with experimental Legionnaires' disease. However, these drugs are unable to kill intracellular *L. pneumophila* or clear the bacterium effectively from experimentally infected guinea pigs, despite clinical cure of the animals. Many quinolone antimicrobial agents, azithromycin, and some ketolide compounds are much more active against intracellular *L. pneumophila* than erythromycin, clarithromycin, or tetracyclines. In addition, these more active drugs have superior activity in the guinea pig model for parameters such as bacterial clearance, length of therapy and dose required for cure, and amount of residual lung inflammation. The superior intracellular and animal model activity of quinolones, azithromycin, and ketolides appears to be the result of their greater ability to kill intracellular *L. pneumophila* or have residual antibacterial activity after drug cessation and, in some cases, of their direct or indirect anti-inflammatory activities, especially azithromycin.[189,190,285,290-293]

The decision regarding which antimicrobial agent to administer for Legionnaires' disease should be guided by severity of illness, degree of immunocompromise, drug cost, drug toxicity, and drug availability (Table 232-2). Nonimmunocompromised outpatients with mild Legionnaires' disease can be treated with any of the drugs listed in the table, with drug cost, availability and toxicity being the main deciding factors. Hospitalized or immunocompromised patients with Legionnaires' disease should be treated with one of the listed quinolones or azithromycin, unless drug unavailability or cost prevents their use. Initial IV antimicrobial therapy may be required for severely ill patients. Even in these patients, oral antimicrobial therapy can be used as soon as there is clinical improvement and intestinal drug absorption is adequate. Few patients can tolerate the administration of oral eryth-

TABLE 232-2	Preferred Treatment for Legionnaires' Disease				
Clinical Condition	*First Choice*	*Dosage*[*,†,‡]		*Second Choice*	*Dosage*[*,†]
Mild pneumonia, not immunocompromised, outpatient	Erythromycin *or*	500 mg qid for 10 to 14 days			
	doxycycline *or*	200 mg load, then 100 mg bid for 10 to 14 days			
	azithromycin *or*	500 mg qd for 3 to 5 days			
	levofloxacin *or*	500 mg qd for 7 to 10 days			
	ciprofloxacin *or*	500 mg bid for 7 to 10 days			
	moxifloxacin *or*	400 mg qd for 7 to 10 days			
	clarithromycin	500 mg bid for 10 to 14 days			
Hospitalized with pneumonia or immunocompromised	Azithromycin *or*	500 mg qd for 7 to 10 days		Ciprofloxacin *or*	400 mg q8h IV or 750 mg PO bid for 14 days
				moxifloxacin	400 mg qd for 14 days
	levofloxacin	500 mg qd for 10 to 14 days		Erythromycin *plus*	750 to 1000 mg IV qid for 3 to 7 days, then 500 mg qid for a total course of 21 days
				rifampin	600 mg bid for 5 days

*Dosage adjustments have to be made for renal insufficiency for some of these drugs.
†Therapy duration may need to be considerably longer for patients with lung abscesses, empyema, endocarditis, or extrathoracic infection.
‡Oral dosing is adequate for outpatients and for those hospitalized or immunocompromised patients with mild disease and adequate absorption. Initial IV dosing is indicated for severe disease.

romycin in high doses, making the maximum oral daily dosage lower than the IV dosage. Immunocompromised patients treated with erythromycin or clarithromycin, with or without rifampin, may suffer relapse days to months after cessation of therapy, especially if the level of immunosuppression is subsequently increased. Coadministration of rifampin with drugs other than erythromycin or doxycycline may be harmful, has questionable benefit, and should not be used.[289] Whether combining azithromycin with levofloxacin is superior to either drug alone is unstudied in experimental models, although in one case azithromycin addition was thought to have been curative within 24 hours of administration in a patient thought to have failed levofloxacin therapy.[294] It is possible that the anti-inflammatory activity of azithromycin could provide some benefit in desperate situations, although initial therapy with this drug alone might carry the same benefit.

Most Legionnaires' disease patients treated with one of the recommended antimicrobial agents respond promptly to the therapy, sometimes within hours. Within 12 to 24 hours, most patients have improvement or complete clearance of myalgia, confusion, headache, abdominal pain, diarrhea, nausea, vomiting, and anorexia. Four to 7 days may be required for complete resolution of fever, but there should be a steady decrease in fever over that period, with the most improvement being seen in the first day or two. Cough, sputum production, shortness of breath, and pleuritic chest pain respond more slowly to therapy, but major improvements usually occur within the first several days. As with most types of bacterial pneumonia, convalescence may be prolonged for months and complicated by neuropsychiatric disease, including chronic fatigue.[295,296] In addition, there can be persistent (months) pulmonary physiologic abnormalities that may or may not be symptomatic.[297] It is not clear that these complications are more severe or common with Legionnaires' disease than with other common causes of pneumonia, or whether the emotional trauma of epidemic disease causes more complications. Evidence of chest consolidation on physical examination, and especially by roentgenography, may take considerably longer to resolve. It is common to observe apparent increases in the sizes of the original pulmonary infiltrates despite substantial clinical improvement over the first several days of therapy; this is not a cause for alarm as long as the patient is improving by other measures.[298] Complete clearing as seen on the chest x-ray may not occur for up to 4 months after initiation of specific antimicrobial therapy, although most patients have complete clearing after 2 months.[243,299,300] Severely immunocompromised patients, or those with severe pneumonia requiring artificial ventilation, may take longer to improve after initiation of specific therapy, or may not respond at all because of irreversible acute respiratory disease syndrome (ARDS). Even in such patients, many systemic signs of infection improve, such as fever, although the respiratory failure itself may worsen.

Failure to respond to specific therapy for Legionnaires' disease should bring into question the validity of the diagnosis, possibility of coinfection or superinfection, and possibility of extrapulmonary disease complicating the Legionnaires' disease. Up to 10% of patients with Legionnaires' disease have coinfections or superinfections with other respiratory pathogens or other pathogens, such as pneumococcus, *Haemophilus influenzae*, *Staphylococcus aureus*, enteric gram-negative bacilli, *Listeria*, *Nocardia*, *Pneumocystis*, *Aspergillus*, *Mycobacterium tuberculosis*, and *Cryptococcus* spp., and various viruses.[190,301,302] Superinfection with opportunistic pathogens is generally seen in severely immunocompromised patients and in those with nosocomial Legionnaires' disease, and coinfection with common respiratory pathogens may be seen in patients with community-acquired Legionnaires' disease. Drug fever, pancreatitis, myocarditis, hepatitis, pericarditis, metastatic infection, and pleural empyema may rarely be complications of Legionnaires' disease or its treatment, and also may be causes of prolonged fever or poor response to therapy.

Ancillary therapy of Legionnaires' disease has not been studied systematically. Excessive oxygen therapy should be avoided to prevent oxygen toxicity of the lung and progression of infection. Experiments in mice with *L. pneumophila* pneumonia have shown that hyperoxia

mediates lung damage and progression of infection, a finding that may or may not be applicable to humans.[303] Corticosteroid therapy for treatment of ARDS caused by Legionnaires' disease has been advocated by some,[190] but this therapy is of unproven benefit and could be detrimental to control of the infection.[304,305] A clinical response to administration of bactericidal quinolones is mandated before the administration of such immunosuppressive therapy, as well as continuation of the antimicrobials during and after steroid therapy. Corticosteroid therapy may be indicated for postpneumonic lung diseases such as bronchiolitis obliterans organizing pneumonia and perhaps pulmonary fibrosis.[306-308] Various unproven therapies have been used in individual cases of life-threatening Legionnaires' disease, with apparent salutary benefit, including drotrecogin-α, sivelestat, independent lung ventilation, and extracorporeal membrane oxygenation.[309-312] I (PE) am aware of several unpublished failures of the same or similar therapies.

Prevention

IMMUNIZATION AND CHEMOPROPHYLAXIS

No human vaccine for Legionnaires' disease exists, and prior infection does not necessarily prevent reinfection.[302] Experiments in guinea pigs have shown that vaccination with several different *L. pneumophila* antigens are effective in preventing death from otherwise lethal bacterial challenges.[313,314] Whether such vaccines would prove useful in humans is unknown.

Chemoprophylaxis with a macrolide antibiotic has been effective at preventing Legionnaires' disease in immunocompromised patients during nosocomial epidemics of the disease.[315,316] This is a reasonable step to take for high-risk populations prior to control of an epidemic.

ENGINEERING MODIFICATIONS AND MAINTENANCE

Proper building and plumbing design and construction can reduce the frequency and intensity of *L. pneumophila* contamination of potable water systems. These design features include properly insulating hot water pipes to prevent the warming of water in adjacent cold water pipes, eliminating blind pipe runs, eliminating stagnation, reducing or eliminating water holding tanks, eliminating the use of plumbing materials that support the growth of *L. pneumophila*, and maintaining hot water temperatures above 50°C and cold water temperatures below 20°C.[234,235,317,318] In older buildings, these modifications can be difficult and expensive. Maintaining hot water temperature above 50°C in hospitals, homes, and nursing homes can result in severe scalding burns, because third-degree burns can result after only a few seconds to minutes of immersion.[319] Installation of thermostatically controlled mixing valves is required to prevent scalding injuries. Whether any of these modifications can prevent Legionnaires' disease outbreaks has not been studied. An important part of environmental control of the disease is risk assessment, which is part of many national and international guidelines and regulations.[320,321]

Use of monochloramine, rather than chlorine, to treat public drinking water reduces the colonization of water with *Legionella* spp. and of nosocomial Legionnaires' disease.[322-324] More widespread use of this water treatment method holds promise for reducing the incidence of Legionnaires' disease.

The risk of heavy *L. pneumophila* colonization of air-conditioning cooling towers and transmission of the biocontaminated aerosol into buildings can be reduced by locating cooling towers away from and downwind of building air intakes, by installation of drift eliminators, and by proper and regular cooling tower maintenance.[234,317] Cooling tower–related outbreaks sometimes occur despite what appears to be proper design, maintenance, and operation, highlighting the technical difficulty of maintaining cooling towers completely free of the bacterium.[210,219] Determination of the effectiveness of cooling tower maintenance for preventing colonization by *L. pneumophila* is difficult without performing quantitative cultures for the bacteria.

Recreational spas must be properly constructed, regularly maintained, and closely monitored to prevent high levels of bacterial growth, which sometimes includes *Legionella* bacteria. Guidelines for such maintenance include hourly monitoring of biocide levels during use, limiting the number of users in the spa, daily hyperhalogenation, and periodic complete spa drainage and filter cleaning.[325,326] Proper construction of recreational spas includes access to interior pipes for inspection and cleaning. Preventing *Legionella* colonization of natural hot spring spas can be difficult if not impossible because elevated water temperatures and high levels of inorganic compounds can inactivate biocides.

ENVIRONMENTAL CULTURES FOR *LEGIONELLA* BACTERIA

There is little national or international consensus regarding the usefulness of routinely performing environmental cultures to help prevent Legionnaires' disease.[321] The *Legionella* bacteria that are ubiquitous in our aqueous environment almost never cause disease, so simply finding the bacteria in the environment does not mean that disease will occur. Combined with natural fluctuations and extreme heterogeneity in *Legionella* environmental concentrations, this makes it very difficult to use a specific bacterial concentration accurately as a trigger point for action. Finally, the methods used for determining *Legionella* concentrations are imprecise, although both national and international standards exist for such testing.[327,328] The low predictive value of positive cultures for disease occurrence is a major reason why many governmental and other organizations such as the CDC, United Kingdom, and American Society of Heating, Refrigerating and Air-Conditioning Engineers (ASHRAE) recommend against the routine use of environmental cultures in risk assessment. The cost and risk to the environment of remediation, without certain benefit, also add to the reluctance to perform routine environmental cultures.[230,235,329,330]

On the other hand, some governmental agencies and private organizations advocate for routine culturing for *Legionella*, arguing that knowledge of the environmental presence of the bacterium can direct monitoring for disease, and that remediation may prevent disease. Some recommend or require the use of cooling tower cultures for *Legionella* to monitor maintenance effectiveness but not directly for risk assessment.[234]

In contrast to routine culturing, many have recommended that hospital water systems supplying immunocompromised patients be cultured for *L. pneumophila*, and that remediation be carried out if positive cultures are found. Others have suggested that all hospital water supplies be checked.[234,329,331,332] Evidence from an uncontrolled retrospective study in Pittsburgh has suggested that routine cultures of the potable water distribution system of health care facilities, combined with disinfection when the culture results reach a trigger point, have dramatically reduced the frequency of nosocomial Legionnaires' disease in that city.[333] Widespread adoption of these guidelines awaits confirmatory, well-controlled prospective studies.

A reasonable approach is routinely to perform cultures of potable water supplying severely immunocompromised patients in hospitals, perhaps monthly, and to consider an annual survey in health care institutions without these patients. Negative cultures do not exclude the possibility of nosocomial Legionnaires' disease, but make it less likely. Routine environmental cultures of non–health care environments appears unwarranted, except when they are required to monitor cooling tower treatment effectiveness. Outbreak investigations will always require environmental cultures, regardless of institution type.

REFERENCES

1. Fraser DW, Tsai TR, Orenstein W, et al. Legionnaires' disease: Description of an epidemic of pneumonia. *N Engl J Med.* 1977;297:1189-1197.
2. Edelstein PH. Legionnaires' disease: History and clinical findings. In: Heuner K, Swanson MS (eds): *Legionella: Molecular Microbiology.* Norfolk, UK: Caister Academic Press; 2008: 1-18.
3. McDade JE, Shepard CC, Fraser DW, et al. Legionnaires' disease: Isolation of a bacterium and demonstration of its role in other respiratory disease. *N Engl J Med.* 1977;297:1197-1203.
4. Osterholm MT, Chin TD, Osborne DO, et al. A 1957 outbreak of Legionnaires' disease associated with a meat-packing plant. *Am J Epidemiol.* 1983;117:60-67.
5. Thacker SB, Bennett JV, Tsai TF, et al. An outbreak in 1965 of severe respiratory illness caused by the Legionnaires' disease bacterium. *J Infect Dis.* 1978;138:512-519.
6. Grist NR, Reid D, Najera R. Legionnaires' disease and the traveller. *Ann Intern Med.* 1979;90:563-564.
7. Glick TH, Gregg MB, Berman B, et al. Pontiac fever. An epidemic of unknown etiology in a health department: I. Clinical and epidemiologic aspects. *Am J Epidemiol.* 1978;107:149-160.
8. Kaufmann AF, McDade JE, Patton CM, et al. Pontiac fever: Isolation of the etiologic agent (*Legionella pneumophila*) and demonstration of its mode of transmission. *Am J Epidemiol.* 1981;114:337-347.
9. Armstrong CW, Miller GB Jr. A 1949 outbreak of Pontiac fever-like illness in steam condenser cleaners. *Arch Environ Health.* 1985;40:26-29.
10. Bozeman FM, Humphries JW, Campbell JM. A new group of rickettsia-like agents recovered from guinea pigs. *Acta Virol.* 1968;12:87-93.
11. Hébert GA, Moss CW, McDougal LK, et al. The rickettsia-like organisms TATLOCK (1943) and HEBA (1959): Bacteria phenotypically similar to but genetically distinct from *Legionella pneumophila* and the WIGA bacterium. *Ann Intern Med.* 1980;92:45-52.
12. Thomason BM, Harris PP, Hicklin MD, et al. A *Legionella*-like bacterium related to WIGA in a fatal case of pneumonia. *Ann Intern Med.* 1979;91:673-676.
13. Tatlock H. A Rickettsia-like organism recovered from guinea pigs. *Proc Soc Exp Biol Med.* 1944;57:95-99.
14. Tatlock H. Studies on a virus from a patient with Fort Bragg fever (pretibial fever). *J Clin Invest.* 1947;26:287-297.
15. Tatlock H. Clarification of the cause of Fort Bragg fever (pretibial fever)—January, 1982. *Rev Infect Dis.* 1982;4:157-158.
16. Haley CE, Cohen ML, Halter J, et al. Nosocomial Legionnaires' disease: A continuing common-source epidemic at Wadsworth Medical Center. *Ann Intern Med.* 1979;90:583-586.
17. Fisher-Hoch SP, Bartlett CL, Tobin JO, et al. Investigation and control of an outbreaks of legionnaires' disease in a district general hospital. *Lancet.* 1981;1:932-936.
18. Broome CV, Goings SAJ, Thacker SB, et al. The Vermont epidemic of Legionnaires' disease. *Ann Intern Med.* 1979;90:573-577.
19. Gerber JE, Casey CA, Martin P, et al. Legionnaires' disease in Vermont. 1972-1976. *Am J Clin Pathol.* 1981;76:816-818.
20. Klaucke DN, Vogt RL, LaRue D, et al. Legionnaires' disease: The epidemiology of two outbreaks in Burlington, Vermont, 1980. *Am J Epidemiol.* 1984;119:382-391.
21. Brown A, Yu VL, Elder EM, et al. Nosocomial outbreak of Legionnaires' disease at the Pittsburgh Veterans Administration Medical Center. *Trans Assoc Am Physicians.* 1980;93:52-59.
22. Best M, Yu VL, Stout J, et al. *Legionellaceae* in the hospital water-supply. Epidemiological link with disease and evaluation of a method for control of nosocomial legionnaires' disease and Pittsburgh pneumonia. *Lancet.* 1983;2:307-310.
23. Shands KN, Ho JL, Meyer RD, et al. Potable water as a source of Legionnaires' disease. *JAMA.* 1985;253:1412-1416.
24. Castilla J, Barricarte A, Aldaz J, et al. A large Legionnaires' disease outbreak in Pamplona, Spain: Early detection, rapid control and no case fatality. *Epidemiol Infect.* 2008;136:823-832.
25. Nygard K, Werner-Johansen O, Ronsen S, et al. An outbreak of legionnaires disease caused by long-distance spread from an industrial air scrubber in Sarpsborg, Norway. *Clin Infect Dis.* 2008;46:61-69.
26. Garrity GM, Bell JA, Lilburn T. Order VI. *Legionellales* ord. nov. In: Brenner DJ, Krieg NR, Staley JT et al, eds. *Bergey's Manual of Systematic Bacteriology.* 2nd ed. New York: Springer; 2005:210-247.
27. Kuroki H, Miyamoto H, Fukuda K, et al. *Legionella impletisoli* sp. nov. and *Legionella yabuuchiae* sp. nov., isolated from soils contaminated with industrial wastes in Japan. *System Appl Microbiol.* 2007;30:273-279.
28. Helbig JH, Benson RF, Pelaz C, et al. Identification and serotyping of atypical *Legionella pneumophila* strains isolated from human and environmental sources. *J Appl Microbiol.* 2007;102:100-105.
29. Benin AL, Benson RF, Besser RE. Trends in legionnaires disease, 1980-1998: Declining mortality and new patterns of diagnosis. *Clin Infect Dis.* 2002;35:1039-1046.
30. Yu VL, Plouffe JF, Pastoris MC, et al. Distribution of *Legionella* species and serogroups isolated by culture in patients with sporadic community-acquired legionellosis: An international collaborative survey. *J Infect Dis.* 2002;186:127-128.
31. Helbig JH, Bernander S, Castellani PM, et al. Pan-European study on culture-proven Legionnaires' disease: Distribution of *Legionella pneumophila* serogroups and monoclonal subgroups. *Euro J Clin Microbiol Infect Dis.* 2002;21:710-716.
32. Edelstein PH. Legionella. In: Murray PR, ed. *Manual of Clinical Microbiology.* 9th ed. Washington, DC: ASM Press; 2006: 835-849.
33. Fields BS, Benson RF, Besser RE. *Legionella* and Legionnaires' disease: 25 years of investigation. *Clin Microbiol Rev.* 2002;15:506-526.
34. Rowbotham TJ. Current views on the relationships between amoebae, *Legionellae* and man. *Isr J Med Sci.* 1986;22: 678-689.
35. Harb OS, Gao LY, Abu Kwaik Y. From protozoa to mammalian cells: A new paradigm in the life cycle of intracellular bacterial pathogens. *Environ Microbiol.* 2000;2:251-265.
36. Steinert M, Emody L, Amann R, et al. Resuscitation of viable but nonculturable *Legionella pneumophila* Philadelphia JR32 by *Acanthamoeba castellanii*. *Appl Environ Microbiol.* 1997;63:2047-2053.
37. O'Connor BA, Carman J, Eckert K, et al. Does using potting mix make you sick? Results from a *Legionella longbeachae* case-control study in South Australia. *Epidemiol Infect.* 2007;135:34-39.
38. Samrakandi MM, Cirillo SL, Ridenour DA, et al. Genetic and phenotypic differences between *Legionella pneumophila* strains. *J Clin Microbiol.* 2002;40:1352-1362.
39. Dennis PJ, Lee JV. Differences in aerosol survival between pathogenic and nonpathogenic strains of *Legionella pneumophila* serogroup 1. *J Appl Bacteriol.* 1988;65:135-141.
40. Bezanson G, Fernandez R, Haldane D, et al. Virulence of patient and water isolates of *Legionella pneumophila* in guinea pigs and mouse L929 cells varies with bacterial genotype. *Can J Microbiol.* 1994;40:426-431.
41. Bollin GE, Plouffe JF, Para MF, et al. Difference in virulence of environmental isolates of *Legionella pneumophila*. *J Clin Microbiol.* 1985;21:674-677.
42. Berk SG, Faulkner G, Garduno E, et al. Packaging of live *Legionella pneumophila* into pellets expelled by *Tetrahymena* spp. does not require bacterial replication and depends on a Dot/Icm-mediated survival mechanism. *Appl Environ Microbiol.* 2008;74:2187-2199.
43. Garduño RA, Garduño E, Hiltz M, et al. Intracellular growth of *Legionella pneumophila* gives rise to a differentiated form dissimilar to stationary-phase forms. *Infect Immun.* 2002;70:6273-6283.
44. Byrne B, Swanson MS. Expression of *Legionella pneumophila* virulence traits in response to growth conditions. *Infect Immun.* 1998;66:3029-3034.
45. Cirillo JD, Cirillo SL, Yan L, et al. Intracellular growth in Acanthamoeba castellanii affects monocyte entry mechanisms and

enhances virulence of Legionella pneumophila. *Infect Immun.* 1999;67:4427-4434.
46. Hambleton P, Broster MG, Dennis PJ, et al. Survival of virulent *Legionella pneumophila* in aerosols. *J Hyg (Lond).* 1983;90:451-460.
47. Fisman DN, Lim S, Wellenius GA, et al. It's not the heat, it's the humidity: Wet weather increases legionellosis risk in the greater Philadelphia metropolitan area. *J Infect Dis.* 2005;192:2066-2073.
48. Cianciotto NP. Pathogenicity of *Legionella pneumophila. Int J Med Microbiol.* 2001;291:331-343.
49. Winn WC Jr, Myerowitz RL. The pathology of the *Legionella* pneumonias. A review of 74 cases and the literature. *Hum Pathol.* 1981;12:401-422.
50. Salins S, Newton C, Widen R, et al. Differential induction of gamma interferon in *Legionella pneumophila*–infected macrophages from BALB/c and A/J mice. *Infect Immun.* 2001;69:3605-3610.
51. Brieland J, Freeman P, Kunkel R, et al. Replicative *Legionella pneumophila* lung infection in intratracheally inoculated A/J mice. A murine model of human Legionnaires' disease. *Am J Pathol.* 1994;145:1537-1546.
52. Brieland JK, Jackson C, Hurst S, et al. Immunomodulatory role of endogenous interleukin-18 in gamma interferon-mediated resolution of replicative *Legionella pneumophila* lung infection. *Infect Immun.* 2000;68:6567-6573.
53. Deng JC, Tateda K, Zeng X, et al. Transient transgenic expression of gamma interferon promotes *Legionella pneumophila* clearance in immunocompetent hosts. *Infect Immun.* 2001;69:6382-6390.
54. Tateda K, Moore TA, Newstead MW, et al. Chemokine-dependent neutrophil recruitment in a murine model of *Legionella* pneumonia: potential role of neutrophils as immunoregulatory cells. *Infect Immun.* 2001;69:2017-2024.
55. Edelstein PH, Meyer RD. Legionella. In: Weinstein RS, Graham AR, Anderson RE, et al, eds. *Advances in Pathology and Laboratory Medicine.* St. Louis: Mosby–Year Book; 1995:149-167.
56. Tubach F, Ravaud P, Salmon-Ceron D, et al. Emergence of *Legionella pneumophila* pneumonia in patients receiving tumor necrosis factor-alpha antagonists. *Clin Infect Dis.* 2006;43:e95-e100.
57. Girard LP, Gregson DB. Community-acquired lung abscess caused by *Legionella micdadei* in a myeloma patient receiving thalidomide treatment. *J Clin Microbiol.* 2007;45:3135-3137.
58. Hawn TR, Verbon A, Lettinga KD, et al. A common dominant TLR5 stop codon polymorphism abolishes flagellin signaling and is associated with susceptibility to legionnaires' disease. *J Exp Med.* 2003;198:1563-1572.
59. Akamine M, Higa F, Arakaki N, et al. Differential roles of Toll-like receptors 2 and 4 in in vitro responses of macrophages to *Legionella pneumophila. Infect Immun.* 2005;73:352-361.
60. Bhan U, Trujillo G, Lyn-Kew K, et al. Toll-like receptor 9 regulates the lung macrophage phenotype and host immunity in murine pneumonia caused by *Legionella pneumophila. Infection & Immunity.* 2008;76:2895-2904.
61. Hawn TR, Verbon A, Janer M, et al. Toll-like receptor 4 polymorphisms are associated with resistance to Legionnaires' disease. *Proc Natl Acad Sci U S A.* 2005;102:2487-2489.
62. Roy CR, Zamboni DS. Cytosolic detection of flagellin: A deadly twist. *Nat Immunol.* 2006;7:549-551.
63. Eisen DP, Stubbs J, Spilsbury D, et al. Low mannose-binding lectin complement activation function is associated with predisposition to Legionnaires' disease. *Clin Exp Immun.* 2007;149:97-102.
64. Nash TW, Libby DM, Horwitz MA. IFN-gamma–activated human alveolar macrophages inhibit the intracellular multiplication of *Legionella pneumophila. J Immunol.* 1988;140:3978-3981.
65. Byrd TF, Horwitz MA. Interferon gamma-activated human monocytes downregulate transferrin receptors and inhibit the intracellular multiplication of *Legionella pneumophila* by limiting the availability of iron. *J Clin Invest.* 1989;83:1457-1465.
66. Swanson MS, Hammer BK. *Legionella pneumophila* pathogenesis: A fateful journey from amoebae to macrophages. *Annu Rev Microbiol.* 2000;54:567-613.
67. Horwitz MA. Phagocytosis of the Legionnaires' disease bacterium (*Legionella pneumophila*) occurs by a novel mechanism: Engulfment within a pseudopod coil. *Cell.* 1984;36:27-33.
68. Rechnitzer C, Blom J. Engulfment of the Philadelphia strain of *Legionella pneumophila* within pseudopod coils in human phagocytes. Comparison with other *Legionella* strains and species. *APMIS.* 1989;97:105-114.
69. Khelef N, Shuman HA, Maxfield FR. Phagocytosis of wild-type *Legionella pneumophila* occurs through a wortmannin-insensitive pathway. *Infect Immun.* 2001;69:5157-5161.
70. Elliott JA, Winn WC Jr. Treatment of alveolar macrophages with cytochalasin D inhibits uptake and subsequent growth of *Legionella pneumophila. Infect Immun.* 1986;51:31-36.
71. Payne NR, Horwitz MA. Phagocytosis of *Legionella pneumophila* is mediated by human monocyte complement receptors. *J Exp Med.* 1987;166:1377-1389.
72. Clemens DL, Lee BY, Horwitz MA. *Mycobacterium tuberculosis* and *Legionella pneumophila* phagosomes exhibit arrested maturation despite acquisition of Rab7. *Infect Immun.* 2000;68:5154-5166.
73. Joshi AD, Sturgill-Koszycki S, Swanson MS. Evidence that Dot-dependent and -independent factors isolate the *Legionella pneumophila* phagosome from the endocytic network in mouse macrophages. *Cell Microbiol.* 2001;3:99-114.
74. Wiater LA, Dunn K, Maxfield FR, et al. Early events in phagosome establishment are required for intracellular survival of *Legionella pneumophila. Infect Immun.* 1998;66:4450-4460.
75. Kagan JC, Roy CR. *Legionella* phagosomes intercept vesicular traffic from endoplasmic reticulum exit sites. *Nat Cell Biol.* 2002;4:945-954.
76. Swanson MS, Isberg RR. Association of *Legionella pneumophila* with the macrophage endoplasmic reticulum. *Infect Immun.* 1995;63:3609-3620.
77. Tilney LG, Harb OS, Connelly PS, et al. How the parasitic bacterium *Legionella pneumophila* modifies its phagosome and transforms it into rough ER. Implications for conversion of plasma membrane to the ER membrane. *J Cell Sci.* 2001;114:24-50.
78. Sturgill-Koszycki S, Swanson MS. *Legionella pneumophila* replication vacuoles mature into acidic, endocytic organelles. *J Exp Med.* 2000;192:1261-1272.
79. Hammer BK, Tateda ES, Swanson MS. A two-component regulator induces the transmission phenotype of stationary-phase *Legionella pneumophila. Mol Microbiol.* 2002;44:107-118.
80. Abu-Zant A, Santic M, Molmeret M, et al. Incomplete activation of macrophage apoptosis during intracellular replication of *Legionella pneumophila. Infect Immun.* 2005;73:5339-5349.
81. Chandler FW, Blackmon JA, Hicklin MD, et al. Ultrastructure of the agent of Legionnaires' disease in the human lung. *Am J Clin Pathol.* 1979;71:43-50.
82. Lüneberg E, Zähringer U, Knirel YA, et al. Phase-variable expression of lipopolysaccharide contributes to the virulence of *Legionella pneumophila. J Exp Med.* 1998;188:49-60.
83. Robey M, O'Connell W, Cianciotto NP. Identification of *Legionella pneumophila rcp*, a *pagP*-like gene that confers resistance to cationic antimicrobial peptides and promotes intracellular infection. *Infect Immun.* 2001;69:4276-4286.
84. Edelstein PH, Hu B, Higa F, et al. *lvgA*, a novel *Legionella pneumophila* virulence factor. *Infect Immun.* 2003;71:2394-2403.
85. Rodgers FG. Ultrastructure of *Legionella pneumophila. J Clin Pathol.* 1979;32:1195-1202.
86. Cianciotto NP, Stamos JK, Kamp DW. Infectivity of *Legionella pneumophila mip* mutant for alveolar epithelial cells. *Curr Microbiol.* 1995;30:247-250.
87. Mody CH, Paine R, Shahrabadi MS, et al. *Legionella pneumophila* replicates within rat alveolar epithelial cells. *J Infect Dis.* 1993;167:1138-1145.
88. Edelstein PH, Edelstein MA, Higa F, et al. Discovery of virulence genes of *Legionella pneumophila* by using signature tagged mutagenesis in a guinea pig pneumonia model. *Proc Natl Acad Sci U S A.* 1999;96:8190-8195.
89. Edelstein PH. Urine antigen tests positive for Pontiac fever: Implications for diagnosis and pathogenesis. *Clin Infect Dis.* 2007;44:229-231.
90. Stone BJ, Abu Kwaik Y. Expression of multiple pili by *Legionella pneumophila*: Identification and characterization of a type IV pilin gene and its role in adherence to mammalian and protozoan cells. *Infect Immun.* 1998;66:1768-1775.
91. Dietrich C, Heuner K, Brand BC, et al. Flagellum of *Legionella pneumophila* positively affects the early phase of infection of eukaryotic host cells. *Infect Immun.* 2001;69:2116-2122.
92. Hoffman PS, Ripley M, Weeratna R. Cloning and nucleotide sequence of a gene (*ompS*) encoding the major outer membrane protein of *Legionella pneumophila. J Bacteriol.* 1992;174:914-920.
93. Cianciotto NP, Eisenstein BI, Mody CH, et al. A mutation in the *mip* gene results in an attenuation of *Legionella pneumophila* virulence. *J Infect Dis.* 1990;162:121-126.
94. Fischer G, Bang H, Ludwig B, et al. Mip protein of *Legionella pneumophila* exhibits peptidyl-prolyl-cis/trans isomerase (PPIase) activity. *Mol Microbiol.* 1992;6:1375-1383.
95. Wagner C, Khan AS, Kamphausen T, et al. Collagen binding protein Mip enables *Legionella pneumophila* to transmigrate through a barrier of NCI-H292 lung epithelial cells and extracellular matrix. *Cell Microbiol.* 2007;9:450-462.
96. Garduño RA, Garduño E, Hoffman PS. Surface-associated hsp60 chaperonin of *Legionella pneumophila* mediates invasion in a HeLa cell model. *Infect Immun.* 1998;66:4602-4610.
97. Cirillo SL, Lum J, Cirillo JD. Identification of novel loci involved in entry by *Legionella pneumophila. Microbiol.* 2000;146:1345-1359.
98. D'Auria G, Jimenez N, Peris-Bondia F, et al. Virulence factor rtx in *Legionella pneumophila*: Evidence suggesting it is a modular multifunctional protein. *BMC Genomics.* 2008;9:14.
99. Luneberg E, Mayer B, Daryab N, et al. Chromosomal insertion and excision of a 30-kb unstable genetic element is responsible for phase variation of lipopolysaccharide and other virulence determinants in *Legionella pneumophila. Mol Microbiol.* 2001;39:1259-1271.
100. Cianciotto NP. Type II secretion: A protein secretion system for all seasons. *Trends Microbiol.* 2005;13:581-588.
101. Vincent CD, Vogel JP. The *Legionella pneumophila* IcmS-LvgA protein complex is important for Dot/Icm-dependent intracellular growth. *Mol Microbiol.* 2006;61:596-613.
102. De Buck E., Anné J, Lammertyn E. The role of protein secretion systems in the virulence of the intracellular pathogen *Legionella pneumophila. Microbiology.* 2007;153:3948-3953.
103. Shin S, Roy CR. Host cell processes that influence the intracellular survival of *Legionella pneumophila. Cell Microbiol.* 2008;10:1209-1220.
104. Cazalet C, Rusniok C, Bruggemann H, et al. Evidence in the *Legionella pneumophila* genome for exploitation of host cell functions and high genome plasticity. *Nat Genet.* 2004;36:1165-1173.
105. Rossier O, Dao J, Cianciotto NP. The type II secretion system of *Legionella pneumophila* elaborates two aminopeptidases, as well as a metalloprotease that contributes to differential infection among protozoan hosts. *Appl Environ Microbiol.* 2008;74:753-761.
106. Debroy S, Dao J, Soderberg M, et al. *Legionella pneumophila* type II secretome reveals unique exoproteins and a chitinase that promotes bacterial persistence in the lung. *Proc Natl Acad Sci U S A.* 2006;103:19146-19151.
107. Soderberg MA, Cianciotto NP. A *Legionella pneumophila* peptidyl-prolyl-cis-trans isomerase present in culture supernatants is necessary for optimal growth at low temperatures. *Appl Environ Microbiol.* 2008;74:1634-1638.
108. Galka F, Wai SN, Kusch H, et al. Proteomic characterization of the whole secretome of *Legionella pneumophila* and functional analysis of outer membrane vesicles. *Infect Immun.* 2008;76:1825-1836.
109. Rossier O, Starkenburg SR, Cianciotto NP. *Legionella pneumophila* type II protein secretion promotes virulence in the A/J mouse model of Legionnaires' disease pneumonia. *Infect Immun.* 2004;72:310-321.
110. Moffat JF, Edelstein PH, Regula DP Jr, et al. Effects of an isogenic Zn-metalloprotease-deficient mutant of *Legionella pneumophila* in a guinea-pig pneumonia model. *Mol Microbiol.* 1994;12:693-705.
111. Hilbi H, Segal G, Shuman HA. Icm/dot-dependent upregulation of phagocytosis by *Legionella pneumophila. Mol Microbiol.* 2001;42:603-617.
112. Watarai M, Derre I, Kirby J, et al. *Legionella pneumophila* is internalized by a macropinocytotic uptake pathway controlled by the Dot/Icm system and the mouse Lgn1 locus. *J Exp Med.* 2001;194:1081-1096.
113. Coers J, Kagan JC, Matthews M, et al. Identification of Icm protein complexes that play distinct roles in the biogenesis of an organelle permissive for *Legionella pneumophila* intracellular growth. *Mol Microbiol.* 2000;38:719-736.
114. Dumenil G, Isberg RR. The *Legionella pneumophila* IcmR protein exhibits chaperone activity for IcmQ by preventing its participation in high-molecular-weight complexes. *Mol Microbiol.* 2001;40:1113-1127.
115. Molmeret M, Alli OA, Zink S, et al. icmT is essential for pore formation-mediated egress of *Legionella pneumophila* from mammalian and protozoan cells. *Infect Immun.* 2002;70:69-78.
116. Zink SD, Pedersen L, Cianciotto NP, et al. The Dot/Icm type IV secretion system of *Legionella pneumophila* is essential for the induction of apoptosis in human macrophages. *Infect Immun.* 2002;70:1657-1663.
117. Marra A, Blander SJ, Horwitz MA, et al. Identification of a *Legionella pneumophila* locus required for intracellular multiplication in human macrophages. *Proc Natl Acad Sci U S A.* 1992;89:9607-9611.
118. Ninio S, Roy CR. Effector proteins translocated by *Legionella pneumophila*: Strength in numbers. *Trends Microbiol.* 2007;15:372-380.
119. de Felipe KS, Glover RT, Charpentier X, et al. *Legionella* eukaryotic-like type IV substrates interfere with organelle trafficking. *PLoS Pathog.* 2008;4:e1000117.
120. Shohdy N, Efe JA, Emr SD, et al. Pathogen effector protein screening in yeast identifies *Legionella* factors that interfere with membrane trafficking. *Proc Natl Acad Sci U S A.* 2005;102:4866-4871.
121. Pan X, Luhrmann A, Satoh A, et al. Ankyrin repeat proteins comprise a diverse family of bacterial type IV effectors. *Science.* 2008;320:1651-1654.
122. Nagai H, Kagan JC, Zhu X, et al. A bacterial guanine nucleotide exchange factor activates ARF on *Legionella* phagosomes. *Science.* 2002;295:679-682.
123. Ingmundson A, Delprato A, Lambright DG, et al. *Legionella pneumophila* proteins that regulate Rab1 membrane cycling. *Nature.* 2007;450:365-369.
124. Machner MP, Isberg RR. A bifunctional bacterial protein links GDI displacement to Rab1 activation. *Science.* 2007;318:974-977.
125. Liu Y, Luo ZQ. The *Legionella pneumophila* effector SidJ is required for efficient recruitment of endoplasmic reticulum proteins to the bacterial phagosome. *Infect Immun.* 2007;75:592-603.
126. Banga S, Gao P, Shen X, et al. *Legionella pneumophila* inhibits macrophage apoptosis by targeting pro-death members of the Bcl2 protein family. *Proc Natl Acad Sci U S A.* 2007;104:5121-5126.
127. Laguna RK, Creasey EA, Li Z, et al. A *Legionella pneumophila*-translocated substrate that is required for growth within macrophages and protection from host cell death. *Proc Natl Acad Sci U S A.* 2006;103:18745-18750.
128. Chen J, de Felipe KS, Clarke M, et al. *Legionella* effectors that promote nonlytic release from protozoa. *Science.* 2004;303:1358-1361.

129. Belyi I, Popoff MR, Cianciotto NP. Purification and characterization of a UDP-glucosyltransferase produced by *Legionella pneumophila*. *Infect Immun.* 2003;71:181-186.

130. Belyi Y, Tabakova I, Stahl M, et al. Lgt: A family of cytotoxic glucosyltransferases produced by *Legionella pneumophila*. *J Bacteriol.* 2008;190:3026-3035.

131. Bandyopadhyay P, Liu S, Gabbai CB, et al. Environmental mimics and the Lvh type IVA secretion system contribute to virulence-related phenotypes of *Legionella pneumophila*. *Infect Immun.* 2007;75:723-735.

132. Aragon V, Kurtz S, Cianciotto NP. *Legionella pneumophila* major acid phosphatase and its role in intracellular infection. *Infect Immun.* 2001;69:177-185.

133. Habyarimana F, Al-Khodor S, Kalia A, et al. Role for the Ankyrin eukaryotic-like genes of *Legionella pneumophila* in parasitism of protozoan hosts and human macrophages. *Environ Microbiol.* 2008;10:1460-1474.

134. Bruggemann H, Cazalet C, Buchrieser C. Adaptation of *Legionella pneumophila* to the host environment: Role of protein secretion, effectors and eukaryotic-like proteins. *Curr Opin Microbiol.* 2006;9:86-94.

135. Sansom FM, Newton HJ, Crikis S, et al. A bacterial ecto-triphosphate diphosphohydrolase similar to human CD39 is essential for intracellular multiplication of *Legionella pneumophila*. *Cell Microbiol.* 2007;9:1922-1935.

136. Newton HJ, Sansom FM, Dao J, et al. Sel1 repeat protein LpnE is a *Legionella pneumophila* virulence determinant that influences vacuolar trafficking. *Infect Immun.* 2007;75:5575-5585.

137. Bandyopadhyay P, Steinman HM. *Legionella pneumophila* catalase-peroxidases: Cloning of the katB gene and studies of KatB function. *J Bacteriol.* 1998;180:5369-5374.

138. St John G, Steinman HM. Periplasmic copper-zinc superoxide dismutase of *Legionella pneumophila*: Role in stationary-phase survival. *J Bacteriol.* 1996;178:1578-1584.

139. Higa F, Edelstein PH. Potential virulence role of the *Legionella pneumophila* ptsP ortholog. *Infect Immun.* 2001;69:4782-4789.

140. Pedersen LL, Radulic M, Doric M, et al. HtrA homologue of *Legionella pneumophila*: An indispensable element for intracellular infection of mammalian but not protozoan cells. *Infect Immun.* 2001;69:2569-2579.

141. Allard KA, Viswanathan VK, Cianciotto NP. lbtA and lbtB are required for production of the *Legionella pneumophila* siderophore legiobactin. *J Bacteriol.* 2006;188:1351-1363.

142. Chatfield CH, Cianciotto NP. The secreted pyomelanin pigment of *Legionella pneumophila* confers ferric reductase activity. *Infect Immun.* 2007;75:4062-4070.

143. Robey M, Cianciotto NP. *Legionella pneumophila* feoAB promotes ferrous iron uptake and intracellular infection. *Infect Immun.* 2002;70:5659-5669.

144. Cianciotto NP. Iron acquisition by *Legionella pneumophila* [review]. *Biometals.* 2007;20:323-331.

145. Chien M, Morozova I, Shi S, et al. The genomic sequence of the accidental pathogen *Legionella pneumophila*. *Science.* 2004;305:1966-1968.

146. Glockner G, Albert-Weissenberger C, Weinmann E, et al. Identification and characterization of a new conjugation/type IVA secretion system (trb/tra) of *Legionella pneumophila* Corby localized on two mobile genomic islands. *Int J Med Microbiol.* 2008;298:411-428.

147. Brassinga AK, Hiltz MF, Sisson GR, et al. A 65-kilobase pathogenicity island is unique to Philadelphia-1 strains of *Legionella pneumophila*. *J Bacteriol.* 2003;185:4630-4637.

148. Asare R, Abu KY. Early trafficking and intracellular replication of *Legionella longbeachaea* (sic) within an ER-derived late endosome-like phagosome. *Cell Microbiol.* 2007;9:1571-1587.

149. Alli OA, Zink S, von Lackum NK, et al. Comparative assessment of virulence traits in *Legionella* spp. *Microbiol.* 2003;149:631-641.

150. Joshi AD, Swanson MS. Comparative analysis of *Legionella pneumophila* and *Legionella micdadei* virulence traits. *Infect Immun.* 1999;67:4134-4142.

151. Weinbaum DL, Benner RR, Dowling JN, et al. Interaction of *Legionella micdadei* with human monocytes. *Infect Immun.* 1984;46:68-73.

152. Izu K, Yoshida S, Miyamoto H, et al. Grouping of 20 reference strains of *Legionella* species by the growth ability within mouse and guinea pig macrophages. *FEMS Immunol Med Microbiol.* 1999;26:61-68.

153. Gerhardt H, Walz MJ, Faigle M, et al. Localization of *Legionella* bacteria within ribosome-studded phagosomes is not restricted to *Legionella pneumophila*. *FEMS Microbiol Letters.* 2000;192:145-152.

154. Doyle RM, Cianciotto NP, Banvi S, et al. Comparison of virulence of *Legionella longbeachae* strains in guinea pigs and U937 macrophage-like cells. *Infect Immun.* 2001;69:5335-5344.

155. Maruta K, Miyamoto H, Hamada T, et al. Entry and intracellular growth of *Legionella dumoffii* in alveolar epithelial cells. *Am J Respir Crit Care Med.* 1998;157:1967-1974.

156. Ogawa M, Takade A, Miyamoto H, et al. Morphological variety of intracellular microcolonies of *Legionella* species in Vero cells. *Microbiol Immunol.* 2001;45:557-562.

157. Hindersson P, Høiby N, Bangsborg J. Sequence analysis of the *Legionella micdadei* groELS operon. *FEMS Microbiol Lett.* 1990;61:31-38.

158. Marrie TJ, Bezanson G, Haldane DJ, et al. Colonisation of the respiratory tract with *Legionella pneumophila* for 63 days before the onset of pneumonia. *J Infect.* 1992;24:81-86.

159. Goldberg DJ, Wrench JG, Collier PW, et al. Lochgoilhead fever: Outbreak of nonpneumonic legionellosis due to *Legionella micdadei*. *Lancet.* 1989;1:316-318.

160. Lüttichau HR, Vinther C, Uldum SA, et al. An outbreak of Pontiac fever among children following use of a whirlpool. *Clin Infect Dis.* 1998;26:1374-1378.

161. Joseph CA, Harrison TG, Ilijic-Car D, et al. Legionnaires' disease in residents of England and Wales: 1998. *Commun Dis Pub Health.* 1999;2:280-284.

162. Marston BJ, Plouffe JF, File TM Jr, et al. Incidence of community-acquired pneumonia requiring hospitalization. Results of a population-based active surveillance Study in Ohio. The Community-Based Pneumonia Incidence Study Group. *Arch Intern Med.* 1997;157:1709-1718.

163. Foy HM, Broome CV, Hayes PS, et al. Legionnaires' disease in a prepaid medical-care group in Seattle 1963-75. *Lancet.* 1979;1:767-770.

164. von Baum H, Ewig S, Marre R, et al. Community-acquired *Legionella* pneumonia: New insights from the German competence network for community-acquired pneumonia. *Clin Infect Dis.* 2008;46:1356-1364.

165. Neil K, Berkelman R. Increasing incidence of legionellosis in the United States, 1990-2005: Changing epidemiologic trends. *Clin Infect Dis.* 2008;47:591-599.

166. Plouffe J, Schwartz DB, Kolokathis A, et al. Clinical efficacy of intravenous followed by oral azithromycin monotherapy in hospitalized patients with community-acquired pneumonia. *Antimicrob Agents Chemother.* 2000;44:1796-1802.

167. Plouffe JF, Herbert MT, File TM Jr, et al. Ofloxacin versus standard therapy in treatment of community-acquired pneumonia requiring hospitalization. Pneumonia Study Group. *Antimicrob Agents Chemother.* 1996;40:1175-1179.

168. File TM Jr, Segreti J, Dunbar L, et al. A multicenter, randomized study comparing the efficacy and safety of intravenous and/or oral levofloxacin versus ceftriaxone and/or cefuroxime axetil in treatment of adults with community-acquired pneumonia. *Antimicrob Agents Chemother.* 1997;41:1965-1972.

169. Trémolières F, de Kock F, Pluck N, et al. Trovafloxacin versus high-dose amoxicillin (1 g three times daily) in the treatment of community-acquired bacterial pneumonia. *Euro J Clin Microbiol Infect Dis.* 1998;17:447-453.

170. Breiman RF, Butler JC. Legionnaires' disease: Clinical, epidemiological, and public health perspectives. *Semin Resp Infect.* 1998;13:84-89.

171. Edelstein PH. Legionnaires' disease, Pontiac fever, and related illnesses. In: Feigen RD, Cherry JD, Demmler-Harrison GJ, et al, eds. *Textbook of Pediatric Infectious Diseases.* 6th ed. Philadelphia: WB Saunders; 2009.

172. Edelstein PH, Nakahama C, Tobin JO, et al. Paleoepidemiologic investigation of Legionnaires' disease at Wadsworth Veterans Administration Hospital by using three typing methods for comparison of legionellae from clinical and environmental sources. *J Clin Microbiol.* 1986;23:1121-1126.

173. Kool JL, Fiore AE, Kioski CM, et al. More than 10 years of unrecognized nosocomial transmission of legionnaires' disease among transplant patients. *Infect Control Hosp Epidemiol.* 1998;19:898-904.

174. Ozerol IH, Bayraktar M, Cizmeci Z, et al. Legionnaire's disease: A nosocomial outbreak in Turkey. *Journal of Hospital Infection.* 2006;62:50-57.

175. Gudiol C, Verdaguer R, Angeles DM, et al. Outbreak of Legionnaires' disease in immunosuppressed patients at a cancer centre: Usefulness of universal urine antigen testing and early levofloxacin therapy. *Clin Microbiol Infect.* 2007;13:1125-1128.

176. Broome CV, Fraser DW. Epidemiologic aspects of legionellosis. *Epidemiol Rev.* 1979;1:1-16.

177. Carratala J, Gudiol F, Pallares R, et al. Risk factors for nosocomial *Legionella pneumophila* pneumonia. *Am J Resp Crit Care Med.* 1994;149:625-629.

178. Marrie TJ, MacDonald S, Clarke K, et al. Nosocomial legionnaires' disease: Lessons from a four-year prospective study. *Am J Infect Control.* 1991;19:79-85.

179. Prodinger WM, Bonatti H, Allerberger F, et al. *Legionella* pneumonia in transplant recipients: a cluster of cases of eight years' duration. *J Hosp Infect.* 1994;26:191-202.

180. den Boer JW, Yzerman EP, Schellekens J, et al. A large outbreak of Legionnaires' disease at a flower show, the Netherlands, 1999. *Emerg Infect Dis.* 2002;8:37-43.

181. Nguyen TM, Ilef D, Jarraud S, et al. A community-wide outbreak of legionnaires disease linked to industrial cooling towers—how far can contaminated aerosols spread? *J Infect Dis.* 2006;193:102-111.

182. Joseph CA, Ricketts KD. From development to success: The European surveillance scheme for travel-associated Legionnaires' disease. *Eur J Public Health.* 2007;17:652-656.

183. Centers for Disease Control and Prevention (CDC): Surveillance for travel-associated legionnaires disease—United States, 2005-2006. *MMWR Morb Mortal Wkly Rep.* 2007;56:1261-1263.

184. Bhopal RS, Fallon RJ, Buist EC, et al. Proximity of the home to a cooling tower and risk of non outbreak Legionnaires' disease. *BMJ.* 1991;302:378-383.

185. Herwaldt LA, Gorman GW, McGrath T, et al. A new *Legionella* species, *Legionella feeleii* species nova, causes Pontiac fever in an automobile plant. *Ann Intern Med.* 1984;100:333-338.

186. Mangione EJ, Remis RS, Tait KA, et al. An outbreak of Pontiac fever related to whirlpool use, Michigan 1982. *JAMA.* 1985;253:535-539.

187. Friedman S, Spitalny K, Barbaree J, et al. Pontiac fever outbreak associated with a cooling tower. *Am J Public Health.* 1987;77:568-572.

188. Joseph C. New outbreak of legionnaires' disease in the United Kingdom. *BMJ.* 2002;325:347-348.

189. Edelstein PH. Antimicrobial chemotherapy for legionnaires' disease: A review. *Clin Infect Dis.* 1995;21:S265-S276.

190. Roig J, Rello J. Legionnaires' disease: A rational approach to therapy. *J Antimicrob Chemother.* 2003;51:1119-1129.

191. Sopena N, Force L, Pedro-Botet ML, et al. Sporadic and epidemic community legionellosis: Two faces of the same illness. *Eur Resp J.* 2007;29:138-142.

192. Marston BJ, Lipman HB, Breiman RF. Surveillance for Legionnaires' disease. Risk factors for morbidity and mortality. *Arch Intern Med.* 1994;154:2417-2422.

193. Straus WL, Plouffe JF, File TM Jr, et al. Risk factors for domestic acquisition of Legionnaires disease. Ohio Legionnaires Disease Group. *Arch Intern Med.* 1996;156:1685-1692.

194. Serota AI, Meyer RD, Wilson SE, et al. Legionnaires' disease in the postoperative patient. *J Surg Res.* 1981;30:417-427.

195. Korvick JA, Yu VL. Legionnaires' disease: An emerging surgical problem. *Ann Thorac Surg.* 1987;43:341-347.

196. Lettinga KD, Verbon A, Weverling GJ, et al. Legionnaires' disease at a Dutch flower show: Prognostic factors and impact of therapy. *Emerg Infect Dis.* 2002;8:1448-1454.

197. Alary M, Joly JR. Risk factors for contamination of domestic hot water systems by Legionellae. *Appl Environ Microbiol.* 1991;57:2360-2367.

198. Jernigan DB, Hofmann J, Cetron MS, et al. Outbreak of Legionnaires' disease among cruise ship passengers exposed to a contaminated whirlpool spa. *Lancet.* 1996;347:494-499.

199. Hlady WG, Mullen RC, Mintz CS, et al. Outbreak of Legionnaire's disease linked to a decorative fountain by molecular epidemiology. *Am J Epidemiol.* 1993;138:555-562.

200. Miyamoto H, Jitsurong S, Shiota R, et al. Molecular determination of infection source of a sporadic *Legionella* pneumonia case associated with a hot spring bath. *Microbiol Immunol.* 1997;41:197-202.

201. Lavocat MP, Berthier JC, Rousson A, et al. [Pulmonary legionnaires' disease in a child following drowning in fresh water.] *Presse Med.* 1987;16:780.

202. Franzin L, Scolfaro C, Cabodi D, et al. *Legionella pneumophila* pneumonia in a newborn after water birth: A new mode of transmission. *Clin Infect Dis.* 2001;33:e103-e104.

203. Arnow PM, Chou T, Weil D, et al. Nosocomial Legionnaires' disease caused by aerosolized tap water from respiratory devices. *J Infect Dis.* 1982;146:460-467.

204. Joly JR, Déry P, Gauvreau L, et al. Legionnaires' disease caused by *Legionella dumoffii* in distilled water. *Can Med Assoc J.* 1986;135:1274-1277.

205. Mastro TD, Fields BS, Breiman RF, et al. Nosocomial Legionnaires' disease and use of medication nebulizers. *J Infect Dis.* 1991;163:667-671.

206. Marrie TJ, Haldane D, MacDonald S, et al. Control of endemic nosocomial legionnaires' disease by using sterile potable water for high risk patients. *Epidemiol Infect.* 1991;107:591-605.

207. Bangsborg JM, Uldum S, Jensen JS, et al. Nosocomial legionellosis in three heart-lung transplant patients: Case reports and environmental observations. *Euro J Clin Microbiol Infect Dis.* 1995;14:99-104.

208. Brown CM, Nuorti PJ, Breiman RF, et al. A community outbreak of Legionnaires' disease linked to hospital cooling towers: An epidemiological method to calculate dose of exposure. *Int J Epidemiol.* 1999;28:353-359.

209. Fiore AE, Nuorti JP, Levine OS, et al. Epidemic Legionnaires' disease two decades later: Old sources, new diagnostic methods. *Clin Infect Dis.* 1998;26:426-433.

210. Badenoch J. *First report of the committee of inquiry into the outbreak of Legionnaires' disease in Stafford in April 1985.* London: Her Majesty's Stationery Office; 1986.

211. Lowry PW, Blankenship RJ, Gridley W, et al. A cluster of *Legionella* sternal-wound infections due to postoperative topical exposure to contaminated tap water. *N Engl J Med.* 1991;324:109-113.

212. Brabender W, Hinthorn DR, Asher M, et al. *Legionella pneumophila* wound infection. *JAMA.* 1983;250:3091-3092.

213. Fraser DW. Legionellosis: Evidence of airborne transmission. *Ann N Y Acad Sci.* 1980;353:61-66.

214. Johnson JT, Yu VL, Best MG, et al. Nosocomial legionellosis in surgical patients with head-and-neck cancer: Implications for epidemiological reservoir and mode of transmission. *Lancet.* 1985;2:298-300.

215. Addiss DG, Davis JP, LaVenture M, et al. Community-acquired Legionnaires' disease associated with a cooling tower: Evidence for longer-distance transport of *Legionella pneumophila*. *Am J Epidemiol.* 1989;130:557-568.

216. Kool JL, Warwick MC, Pruckler JM, et al. Outbreak of Legionnaires' disease at a bar after basement flooding. *Lancet.* 1998;351:1030.

217. Brown CM, Nuorti PJ, Breiman RF, et al. A community outbreak of Legionnaires' disease linked to hospital cooling towers: An epidemiological method to calculate dose of exposure. *Int J Epidemiol.* 1999;28:353-359.

218. Mahoney FJ, Hoge CW, Farley TA, et al. Communitywide outbreak of Legionnaires' disease associated with a grocery store mist machine. *J Infect Dis.* 1992;165:736-739.
219. Gabbay J. *Broadcasting House Legionnaires' disease. Report of the Westminster Action Committee convened to co-ordinate the investigation and control of the outbreak of Legionnaires' disease associated with Portland Place, London W1 in April/May 1988.* London: Department of Public Health, Parkside District Health Authority; 1988;
220. Blatt SP, Parkinson MD, Pace E, et al. Nosocomial Legionnaires' disease: aspiration as a primary mode of disease acquisition. *Am J Med.* 1993;95:16-22.
221. Dournon E, Bure A, Desplaces N, et al. Legionnaires' disease related to gastric lavage with tap water. *Lancet.* 1982;1:797-798.
222. Yu VL. Could aspiration be the major mode of transmission for *Legionella*? *Am J Med.* 1993;95:13-15.
223. Davis GS, Winn CW Jr, Gump DW, et al. Legionnaires' pneumonia in guinea pigs and rats produced by aerosol exposure. *Chest.* 1983;83:15S-16S.
224. Winn WC Jr, Davis GS, Gump DW, et al. Legionnaires' pneumonia after intratracheal inoculation of guinea pigs and rats. *Lab Invest.* 1982;47:568-578.
225. Schmidt T, Pfeiffer A, Ehret W, et al. *Legionella* infection of the colon presenting as acute attack of ulcerative colitis. *Gastroenterology.* 1989;97:751-755.
226. Dournon E, Bure A, Kemeny JL, et al. *Legionella pneumophila* peritonitis. *Lancet.* 1982;1:1363.
227. Grangeon V, Vincent L, Pacheco Y. [Digestive disorders and Legionnaires' lung disease. Accompanying signs or visceral location?] *Rev Mal Respir.* 2000;17:489-492.
228. Plouffe JF, Para MF, Fuller KA, et al. Oral ingestion of *Legionella pneumophila. J Clin Lab Immunol.* 1986;20:113-117.
229. Katz SM, Hammel JM, Matus JP, et al. A self-limited febrile illness produced in guinea pigs associated with oral administration of *Legionella pneumophila. Gastroenterology.* 1988;95:1575-1581.
230. Tablan OC, Anderson LJ, Besser R, et al. Guidelines for preventing health-care–associated pneumonia, 2003: Recommendations of CDC and the Healthcare Infection Control Practices Advisory Committee. *MMWR Recomm Rep.* 2004;53:1-36.
231. Kool JL, Buchholz U, Peterson C, et al. Strengths and limitations of molecular subtyping in a community outbreak of Legionnaires' disease. *Epidemiol Infect.* 2000;125:599-608.
232. Lawrence C, Reyrolle M, Dubrou S, et al. Single clonal origin of a high proportion of *Legionella pneumophila* serogroup 1 isolates from patients and the environment in the area of Paris, France, over a 10-year period. *J Clin Microbiol.* 1999;37:2652-2655.
233. Centers for Disease Control and Prevention. Legionellosis Resource Site (Legionnaires' Disease and Pontiac Fever). Available at <http://www.cdc.gov/legionella>.
234. Freije MR. *Legionellae Control in Health Care Facilities. A Guide for Minimizing Risk.* Indianapolis, Ind: HC Information Resources; 1996.
235. Joseph CA, Lee JV, van Wijngaarten J, et al. European Guidelines for Control and Prevention of Travel-Associated Legionnaires' Disease. 2005. Available at <http://www.ewgli.org/data/european_guidelines/european_guidelines_jan05.pdf>.
236. Sehulster L, Chinn RY, CDC, et al. Guidelines for environmental infection control in health-care facilities. Recommendations of CDC and the Healthcare Infection Control Practices Advisory Committee (HICPAC). *MMWR Recomm Rep.* 2003;52:1-42.
237. Lin YS, Stout JE, Yu VL, et al. Disinfection of water distribution systems for *Legionella. Semin Resp Infect.* 1998;13:147-159.
238. Roig J, Aguilar X, Ruiz J, et al. Comparative study of *Legionella pneumophila* and other nosocomial- acquired pneumonias. *Chest.* 1991;99:344-350.
239. Granados A, Podzamczer D, Gudiol F, et al. Pneumonia due to *Legionella pneumophila* and pneumococcal pneumonia: Similarities and differences on presentation. *Eur Respir J.* 1989;2:130-134.
240. Woodhead MA, Macfarlane JT. Comparative clinical and laboratory features of *Legionella* with pneumococcal and mycoplasma pneumonias. *Br J Dis Chest.* 1987;81:133-139.
241. Kirby BD, Snyder KM, Meyer RD, et al. Legionnaires' disease: Report of sixty-five nosocomially acquired cases and review of the literature. *Medicine (Baltimore).* 1980;59:188-205.
242. Gupta SK, Imperiale TF, Sarosi GA. Evaluation of the Winthrop-University Hospital criteria to identify *Legionella* pneumonia. *Chest.* 2001;120:1064-1071.
243. Muder RR, Yu VL, Parry MF. The radiologic manifestations of *Legionella* pneumonia. *Semin Resp Infect.* 1987;2:242-254.
244. Domingo C, Roig J, Planas F, et al. Radiographic appearance of nosocomial legionnaires' disease after erythromycin treatment. *Thorax.* 1991;46:663-666.
245. Sakai F, Tokuda H, Goto H, et al. Computed tomographic features of *Legionella pneumophila* pneumonia in 38 cases. *J Comput Assist Tomogr.* 2007;31:125-131.
246. Kim KW, Goo JM, Lee HJ, et al. Chest computed tomographic findings and clinical features of *Legionella* pneumonia. *J Comput Assist Tomogr.* 2007;31:950-955.
247. Morgan JC, Cavaliere R, Juel VC. Reversible corpus callosum lesion in legionnaires' disease. *J Neurol Neurosurg Psychiatr.* 2004;75:651-654.
248. Shelburne SA, Kielhofner MA, Tiwari PS. Cerebellar involvement in legionellosis. *South Med J.* 2004;97:61-64.
249. Johnson JD, Raff MJ, Van Arsdall JA. Neurologic manifestations of Legionnaires' disease. *Medicine (Baltimore).* 1984;63:303-310.
250. Fernandez JA, Lopez P, Orozco D, et al. Clinical study of an outbreak of Legionnaire's disease in Alcoy, Southeastern Spain. *Eur J Clin Microbiol Infect Dis.* 2002;21:729-735.
251. Watts JC, Hicklin MD, Thomason BM, et al. Fatal pneumonia caused by *Legionella pneumophila*, serogroup 3: Demonstration of the bacilli in extrathoracic organs. *Ann Intern Med.* 1980;92:186-188.
252. White HJ, Felton WW, Sun CN. Extrapulmonary histopathologic manifestations of Legionnaires' disease: Evidence for myocarditis and bacteremia. *Arch Pathol Lab Med.* 1980;104:287-289.
253. Weisenburger DD, Rappaport H, Ahluwalia MS, et al. Legionnaires' disease. *Am J Med.* 1980;69:476-482.
254. Evans CP, Winn WC Jr. Extrathoracic localization of *Legionella pneumophila* in Legionnaires' pneumonia. *Am J Clin Pathol.* 1981;76:813-815.
255. Warner CL, Fayad PB, Heffner RR Jr. *Legionella* myositis. *Neurol.* 1991;41:750-752.
256. Ferrer A, Lloveras J, Codina G, et al. [Prevention of acute tubular necrosis in immediately after a kidney transplant.] *Med Clin (Barc).* 1987;88:346-347.
257. Kalweit WH, Winn WC Jr, Rocco TA Jr, et al. Hemodialysis fistula infections caused by *Legionella pneumophila. Ann Intern Med.* 1982;96:173-175.
258. Arnow PM, Boyko EJ, Friedman EL. Perirectal abscess caused by *Legionella pneumophila* and mixed anaerobic bacteria. *Ann Intern Med.* 1983;98:184-185.
259. Ampel NM, Ruben FL, Norden CW. Cutaneous abscess caused by *Legionella micdadei* in an immunosuppressed patient. *Ann Intern Med.* 1985;102:630-632.
260. Reyes RR, Noble RC. Legionnaires' pericarditis. *J Ky Med Assoc.* 1983;81:757-758.
261. Mayock R, Skale B, Kohler RB. *Legionella pneumophila* pericarditis proved by culture of pericardial fluid. *Am J Med.* 1983;75:534-536.
262. Fogliani J, Domenget JF, Hohn B, et al. [Legionnaires' disease with digestive tract lesions. One case.] *Nouv Presse Med.* 1982;11:2699-2702.
263. Nomura S, Hatta K, Iwata T, et al. *Legionella pneumophila* isolated in pure culture from the ascites of a patient with systemic lupus erythematosus. *Am J Med.* 1989;86:833-834.
264. Guyot S, Goy JJ, Gersbach P, et al. *Legionella pneumophila* aortitis in a heart transplant recipient. *Transpl Infect Dis.* 2007;9:58-59.
265. Bemer P, Leautez S, Ninin E, et al. *Legionella pneumophila* arthritis: Use of medium specific for mycobacteria for isolation of *L. pneumophila* in culture of articular fluid specimens. *Clin Infect Dis.* 2002;35:E6-E7.
266. Monforte R, Marco F, Estruch R, et al. Multiple organ involvement by *Legionella pneumophila* in a fatal case of Legionnaires' disease. *J Infect Dis.* 1989;159:809.
267. Linscott AJ, Poulter MD, Ward K, et al. *Legionella pneumophila* serogroup 4 isolated from joint tissue. *J Clin Microbiol.* 2004;42:1365-1366.
268. Waldor MK, Wilson B, Swartz M. Cellulitis caused by *Legionella pneumophila. Clin Infect Dis.* 1993;16:51-53.
269. Tompkins LS, Roessler BJ, Redd SC, et al. *Legionella* prosthetic-valve endocarditis. *N Engl J Med.* 1988;318:530-535.
270. McCabe RE, Baldwin JC, McGregor CA, et al. Prosthetic valve endocarditis caused by *Legionella pneumophila. Ann Intern Med.* 1984;100:525-527.
271. Schlanger G, Lutwick LI, Kurzman M, et al. Sinusitis caused by *Legionella pneumophila* in a patient with the acquired immune deficiency syndrome. *Am J Med.* 1984;77:957-960.
272. Muder RR, Stout JE, Yee YC. Isolation of *Legionella pneumophila* serogroup 5 from empyema following esophageal perforation. Source of the organism and mode of transmission. *Chest.* 1992;102:1601-1603.
273. Murdoch DR. Diagnosis of *Legionella* infection. *Clin Infect Dis.* 2003;36:64-69.
274. Formica N, Yates M, Beers M, et al. The impact of diagnosis by *Legionella* urinary antigen test on the epidemiology and outcomes of Legionnaires' disease. *Epidemiol Infect.* 2001;127:275-280.
275. Helbig JH, Uldum SA, Bernander S, et al. Clinical utility of urinary antigen detection for diagnosis of community-acquired, travel-associated, and nosocomial Legionnaires' disease. *J Clin Microbiol.* 2003;41:838-840.
276. Okada C, Kura F, Wada A, et al. Cross-reactivity and sensitivity of two *Legionella* urinary antigen kits, Biotest EIA and Binax NOW, to extracted antigens from various serogroups of *L. pneumophila* and other *Legionella* species. *Microbiol Immunol.* 2002;46:51-54.
277. Edelstein PH. Urinary antigen detection for *Legionella* spp. In: Isenberg HD, ed. *Clinical Microbiology Procedures Handbook.* 2nd ed. Washington, DC: ASM Press; 2004:11.4.1-11.4.6.
278. Domínguez J, Gali N, Blanco S, et al. Assessment of a new test to detect *Legionella* urinary antigen for the diagnosis of Legionnaires' Disease. *Diagn Microbiol Infect Dis.* 2001;41:199-203.
279. Edelstein PH. Detection of antibodies to *Legionella*. In: Detrick B, Hamilton RG, Folds JD, eds. *Manual of Molecular and Clinical Laboratory Immunology.* 7th ed. Washington, DC: ASM Press; 2006:468-476.
280. Elverdal P, Jorgensen CS, Uldum SA. Comparison and evaluation of four commercial kits relative to an in-house immunofluorescence test for detection of antibodies against *Legionella pneumophila. Eur J Clin Microbiol Infect Dis.* 2008;27:149-152.
281. Edelstein PH. Detection of *Legionella* antigen by direct immunofluorescence. In: Isenberg HD, ed. *Clinical Microbiology Procedures Handbook.* 2nd ed. Washington, DC: ASM Press; 2004:11.3.1-11.3.7.
282. She RC, Billetdeaux E, Phansalkar AR, et al. Limited applicability of direct fluorescent-antibody testing for *Bordetella* sp. and *Legionella* sp. specimens for the clinical microbiology laboratory. *J Clin Microbiol.* 2007;45:2212-2214.
283. Diederen BM, Kluytmans JA, Vandenbroucke-Grauls CM, et al. Utility of real-time PCR for diagnosis of Legionnaires' disease in routine clinical practice. *J Clin Microbiol.* 2008;46:671-677.
284. Luck PC, Ecker C, Reischl U, et al. Culture-independent identification of the source of an infection by direct amplification and sequencing of *Legionella pneumophila* DNA from a clinical specimen. *J Clin Microbiol.* 2007;45:3143-3144.
285. Edelstein PH. Chemotherapy of Legionnaires' disease with macrolide or quinolone antimicrobial agents. In: Marre R, Abu Kwaik Y, Bartlett C, et al, eds. *Legionella*. Washington, DC: ASM Press; 2002:183-188.
286. Gacouin A, Le Tulzo Y, Lavoue S, et al. Severe pneumonia due to *Legionella pneumophila*: Prognostic factors, impact of delayed appropriate antimicrobial therapy. *Intens Care Med.* 2002;28:686-691.
287. Blázquez Garrido RM, Espinosa Parra FJ, Alemany Francés L, et al. Antimicrobial chemotherapy for legionnaires disease: levofloxacin versus macrolides. *Clin Infect Dis.* 2005;40:800-806.
288. Sabria M, Pedro-Botet ML, Gomez J, et al. Fluoroquinolones vs macrolides in the treatment of Legionnaires disease. *Chest.* 2005;128:1401-1405.
289. Grau S, Antonio JM, Ribes E, et al. Impact of rifampicin addition to clarithromycin in *Legionella pneumophila* pneumonia. *Int J Antimicrob Agents.* 2006;28:249-252.
290. Edelstein PH, Shinzato T, Doyle E, et al. In vitro activity of gemifloxacin (SB-265805, LB20304a) against *Legionella pneumophila* and its pharmacokinetics in guinea pigs with *L. pneumophila* pneumonia. *Antimicrob Agents Chemother.* 2001;45:2204-2209.
291. Edelstein PH, Weiss WJ, Edelstein MA. Activities of tigecycline (GAR-936) against *Legionella pneumophila* in vitro and in guinea pigs with *L. pneumophila* pneumonia. *Antimicrob Agents Chemother.* 2003;47:533-540.
292. Edelstein PH, Shinzato T, Edelstein MA. BMS-284756 (T-3811ME) a new fluoroquinolone: In vitro activity against *Legionella*, efficacy in a guinea pig model of *L. pneumophila* pneumonia and pharmacokinetics in guinea pigs. *J Antimicrob Chemother.* 2001;48:667-675.
293. Edelstein PH, Higa F, Edelstein MAC. In vitro activity of ABT-773 against *Legionella pneumophila*, its pharmacokinetics in guinea pigs, and its use to treat guinea pigs with *L. pneumophila* pneumonia. *Antimicrob Agents Chemother.* 2001;45:2685-2690.
294. Pedro-Botet ML, Garcia-Cruz A, Tural C, et al. Severe Legionnaires' disease successfully treated with levofloxacin and azithromycin. *J Chemother.* 2006;18:559-561.
295. Lettinga KD, Verbon A, Nieuwkerk PT, et al. Health-related quality of life and posttraumatic stress disorder among survivors of an outbreak of Legionnaires disease. *Clin Infect Dis.* 2002;35:11-17.
296. Metlay JP, Fine MJ, Schulz R, et al. Measuring symptomatic and functional recovery in patients with community-acquired pneumonia. *J Gen Intern Med.* 1997;12:423-430.
297. Jonkers RE, Lettinga KD, Pels Rijcken TH, et al. Abnormal radiological findings and a decreased carbon monoxide transfer factor can persist long after the acute phase of *Legionella pneumophila* pneumonia. *Clin Infect Dis.* 2004;38:605-611.
298. Tan MJ, Tan JS, Hamor RH, et al. The radiologic manifestations of Legionnaire's (sic) disease. The Ohio Community-Based Pneumonia Incidence Study Group. *Chest.* 2000;117:398-403.
299. Fairbank JT, Mamourian AC, Dietrich PA, et al. The chest radiograph in Legionnaires' disease. Further observations. *Radiology.* 1983;147:33-34.
300. Kirby BD, Peck H, Meyer RD. Radiographic features of Legionnaires' disease. *Chest.* 1979;76:562-565.
301. Marrie TJ, Haldane D, Bezanson G. Nosocomial Legionnaires' disease: Clinical and radiographic patterns. *Can J Infect Dis.* 1992;3:253-260.
302. Meyer RD, Edelstein PH, Kirby BD, et al. Legionnaires' disease: Unusual clinical and laboratory features. *Ann Intern Med.* 1980;93:240-243.
303. Tateda K, Deng JC, Moore TA, et al. Hyperoxia mediates acute lung injury and increased lethality in murine *Legionella* pneumonia: The role of apoptosis. *J Immunol.* 2003;170:4209-4216.
304. Skerrett SJ, Schmidt RA, Martin TR. Impaired clearance of aerosolized *Legionella pneumophila* in corticosteroid-treated rats: A model of Legionnaires' disease in the compromised host. *J Infect Dis.* 1989;160:261-273.
305. Amundson DE, Murray KM, Brodine S, et al. High-dose corticosteroid therapy for *Pneumocystis carinii* pneumonia in patients with acquired immunodeficiency syndrome. *South Med J.* 1989;82:711-718.
306. Shankar PS, Anderson CL, Scott JH. Legionnaires' disease with severe hypoxemia and saddleback fever. *Postgrad Med.* 1981;69:87-92.

307. Sato P, Madtes DK, Thorning D, et al. Bronchiolitis obliterans caused by *Legionella pneumophila*. *Chest.* 1985;87:840-842.

308. Hürter T, Rumpelt HJ, Ferlinz R. Fibrosing alveolitis responsive to corticosteroids following Legionnaires' disease pneumonia. *Chest.* 1992;101:281-283.

309. Ichiba S, Jenkins DR, Peek GJ, et al. Severe acute respiratory failure due to *Legionella* pneumonia treated with extracorporeal membrane oxygenation. *Clin Infect Dis.* 1999;28:686-687.

310. Narita Y, Naoki K, Horiuchi N, et al. [A case of *Legionella* pneumonia associated with acute respiratory distress syndrome (ARDS) and acute renal failure treated with methylprednisolone and sivelestat.] *Nihon Kokyuki Gakkai Zasshi.* 2007;45:413-418.

311. Bodur H, Savran Y, Koca U, et al. *Legionella* pneumonia with acute respiratory distress syndrome, myocarditis and septic shock successfully treated with drotrecogin alpha (activated). *Eur J Anaesthes.* 2006;23:808-810.

312. Fujita M, Tsuruta R, Oda Y, et al. Severe *Legionella* pneumonia successfully treated by independent lung ventilation with intrapulmonary percussive ventilation. *Respirology.* 2008;13:475-477.

313. Blander SJ, Horwitz MA. Major cytoplasmic membrane protein of *Legionella pneumophila*, a genus common antigen and member of the hsp 60 family of heat shock proteins, induces protective immunity in a guinea pig model of Legionnaires' disease. *J Clin Invest.* 1993;91:717-723.

314. Weeratna R, Stamler DA, Edelstein PH, et al. Human and guinea pig immune responses to *Legionella pneumophila* protein antigens OmpS and Hsp60. *Infect Immun.* 1994;62:3454-3462.

315. Vereerstraeten P, Stolear JC, Schoutens-Serruys E, et al. Erythromycin prophylaxis for Legionnaire's disease in immunosuppressed patients in a contaminated hospital environment. *Transplantation.* 1986;41:52-54.

316. Oren I, Zuckerman T, Avivi I, et al. Nosocomial outbreak of *Legionella pneumophila* serogroup 3 pneumonia in a new bone marrow transplant unit: Evaluation, treatment and control. *Bone Marrow Transplantation.* 2002;30:175-179.

317. Chartered Institution of Building Services Engineers: *Technical Memoranda TM13. Minimising the Risk of Legionnaires' disease*, London: Chartered Institution of Building Services Engineers; 2002.

318. *ASHRAE Guideline 12-2000. ASHRAE Standard: Minimizing the Risk of Legionellosis Associated with Building Water Systems.* Atlanta: American Society of Heating, Refrigeration, and Air-Conditioning Engineers; 2000.

319. Huyer DW, Corkum SH. Reducing the incidence of tap-water scalds: Strategies for physicians. *CMAJ.* 1997;156:841-844.

320. HSC: *Legionnaires' Disease.* London: HSE Books; 2000.

321. World Health Organization: *Legionella and the Prevention of Legionellosis.* Geneva: World Health Organization; 2007.

322. Heffelfinger JD, Kool JL, Fridkin S, et al. Risk of hospital-acquired legionnaires' disease in cities using monochloramine versus other water disinfectants. *Infect Control Hosp Epidemiol.* 2003;24:569-574.

323. Flannery B, Gelling LB, Vugia DJ, et al. Reducing *Legionella* colonization in water systems with monochloramine. *Emerg Infect Dis.* 2006;12:588-596.

324. Moore MR, Pryor M, Fields B, et al. Introduction of monochloramine into a municipal water system: Impact on colonization of buildings by *Legionella* spp. *Appl Environ Microbiol.* 2006;72:378-383.

325. Centers for Disease Control and Prevention. Suggested Health and Safety Guidelines for Public Spas and Hot Tubs, 1985. Available at <http://www.cdc.gov/healthySwimming/pdf/CDC_Public_Spa_and_Hot_Tubs_Historical_Reference.pdf>.

326. Health Protection Agency. *Management of Spa Pools: Controlling the Risks of Infection.* London: Health Protection Agency; 2006.

327. International Organization for Standardization. *Water Quality: Detection and Enumeration of Legionella, Part 1 (ISO 11731:1998).* Geneva: International Standards Organization; 1998.

328. International Organization for Standardization. *Water Quality: Detection and Eumeration of Legionella, Part 2: Direct Membrane Filtration Method for Waters with Low Bacterial Counts (ISO 11731-2:2004).* Geneva: International Standards Organization; 2004.

329. Morris JG Jr, Davis C, Perl TM, et al. Report of the Maryland Scientific Working Group to Study *Legionella* in Water Systems in Healthcare Institutions. 2000. Available at <http://www.dhmh.state.md.us/html/legionella.htm>.

330. Sehulster L, Chinn RYW. Guidelines for environmental infection control in health-care facilities. Recommendations of CDC and the Healthcare Infection Control Practices Advisory Committee. *MMWR Morb Mortal Wkly Rep.* 2003;52:1-44.

331. Tablan OC, Anderson LJ, Arden NH, et al. Guideline for prevention of nosocomial pneumonia. The Hospital Infection Control Practices Advisory Committee. *Am J Infect Control.* 1994;22:247-292.

332. Texas Department of State Health Services. Legionnaire's Disease (Legionellosis). 2002. Available at <http://www.dshs.state.tx.us/idcu/disease/legionnaires/taskforce>.

333. Squier CL, Stout JE, Krsytofiak S, et al. A proactive approach to prevention of health care-acquired Legionnaires' disease: The Allegheny County (Pittsburgh) experience. *Am J Infect Control.* 2005;33:360-367.

233

Other *Legionella* Species

ROBERT R. MUDER

Since the discovery of *Legionella pneumophila* in 1977, the family Legionellaceae has expanded to include more than 40 named species.[1] Like *L. pneumophila*, these other species are found in aquatic environments and soil. The vast majority of human infections are pneumonic, occurring after exposure to an environmental source of *Legionella*.[2] Twenty species have been documented to cause human infection based on isolation of organisms from clinical material or detection of bacterial DNA (Table 233-1). Isolates of the other species are limited to water and soil, although several have been implicated in human infection based on seroconversion in the absence of isolation.

In addition to the described species, there are other organisms that are in all probability members of the genus *Legionella*, based on analysis of 16S ribosomal RNA sequences.[3,4] These organisms, termed "*Legionella*-like amebal pathogens" (LLAPs), infect freshwater amebas and are found in aquatic environments capable of supporting the growth of *Legionella*. LLAPs grow very poorly or not at all on media supporting the growth of *Legionella*. However, there is serologic evidence implicating LLAPs as occasional causes of community-acquired pneumonia.[5]

In 1977, workers from the University of Pittsburgh and the University of Virginia visualized gram-negative, weakly acid-fast organisms from lung tissue of immunosuppressed patients with acute pneumonitis.[6,7] Almost all of the patients were receiving steroids or cytotoxic chemotherapy; renal transplant recipients were a prominent group. Although organisms could be seen on biopsy and autopsy lung specimens by various stains, they could not be grown on standard bacteriologic culture media. A *Legionella*-like organism was isolated after the clinical specimens were inoculated into guinea pigs and embryonated eggs. Sera from these patients contained high titers of antibodies against this organism, confirming its etiologic role in pneumonia.

This new organism, originally called Pittsburgh pneumonia agent, was serologically and genetically distinct from *L. pneumophila*, although it phenotypically resembled *L. pneumophila* in growth requirements and the presence of branched-chain fatty acids in the cell wall. The organism proved to be identical to organisms isolated in 1943 ("TATLOCK") and 1959 ("HEBA") from guinea pigs injected with the blood of two patients with nonpneumonic illnesses.[8,9] The first documented isolation of *Legionella bozemanii* was in 1959 from the lung tissue of a patient dying of pneumonia after immersion in fresh water.[9,10]

Description of the Pathogens

Legionella species are gram-negative aerobic bacilli that share a number of common phenotypic features, including growth on buffered charcoal yeast extract agar (BCYE), lack of growth on blood agar, catalase activity, and requirement for cysteine. Tests for urease, nitrate reduction, and fermentative activity are uniformly negative.[11] Although individual species differ in several phenotypic characteristics, such as gelatin liquification, hippurate hydrolysis, and oxidase activity, these tests are of limited utility in differentiation. When grown on yeast extract agar, *Legionella* species produce a water-soluble, extracellular compound that fluoresces yellow-green on exposure to long-wave ultraviolet light. Several species exhibit a blue-white or red autofluorescence under ultraviolet light. Most species produce β-lactamase; *Legionella micdadei*, *Legionella maceachernii*, and *Legionella feeleii* do not. Cell wall fatty acid profiles and ubiquinone content are sufficiently distinctive to permit species identification on the basis of gas-liquid chromatography.[12] Differentiation of the common species is most conveniently made in the laboratory by direct fluorescent antibody staining of the isolates. Slide agglutination can also be used for selected isolates.[2] Determination of DNA homology is the definitive method, especially for the less common strains. Other biochemical and immunologic methods for species classification of *Legionella* are described in Chapter 232.

L. micdadei is unique in that it retains the modified acid-fast stain.[6,7] *L. micdadei* can appear as weakly or partially acid-fast bacilli in clinical specimens. The acid-fast property is not usually present in organisms grown on solid media, but it may be retained in liquid culture. The modified acid-fast stain substitutes 1% sulfuric acid (a less potent decolorizing agent) for the traditional 3% hydrochloric acid. This characteristic has occasionally led to misidentification of *L. micdadei* infection as mycobacterial infection, with initiation of antituberculous agents.[7,13,14]

Like *L. pneumophila*, other *Legionella* species are pathogenic for freshwater amebas,[15,16] and a number of species are capable of vigorous intracellular growth within human macrophages.[17] All *Legionella* species tested contain the *dot/icm* loci, composed of 24 genes essential for pathogenesis, mediating uptake of *Legionella* by macrophages, evasion of lysosomal fusion, intracellular replication, and host cell lysis. However, in vitro cytopathogenicity for macrophages varies among species, with *L. pneumophila*, *L. micdadei*, and *Legionella dumoffii* being the most cytopathogenic.[17]

Epidemiology

Like *L. pneumophila*, other *Legionella* species are widely distributed in aquatic habitats and soil.[18,19] Several species associated with human disease have only been isolated from clinical specimens. In addition to *L. pneumophila*, water distribution systems may be colonized with any of a number of *Legionella* species, including *L. micdadei*, *L. bozemanii*, *L. dumoffii*, *Legionella anisa*, and *L. feeleii*.[20-25] Recovery of these species is generally less frequent and technically more demanding than is recovery of *L. pneumophila*. *L. anisa*, however, is a common inhabitant of hospital water systems; it rarely causes disease in that setting.[26] Commensal microflora and sediment known to promote proliferation of *L. pneumophila* in water distribution systems do not support the growth of *L. micdadei*.[27] Thus, the growth kinetics of *L. micdadei* may explain its infrequent presence in the water supply, such that only patients with prolonged hospitalization or immunosuppression are susceptible. Like *L. pneumophila*, other species multiply within aquatic protozoa.[15,16]

The role of non-*pneumophila Legionella* species in community-acquired pneumonia is gradually emerging. Investigators in Ohio reported seven culture-confirmed cases of community-acquired *L. bozemanii* pneumonia from a single institution during a 5-year period.[28] In a subsequent study, 14% of patients with community-acquired pneumonia showed seroconversion to *Legionella* species, including *L. bozemanii* (8%) and *L. anisa* (4%).[29] An international study of 509 cases of culture-confirmed, community-acquired *Legionella* infection[30] found that 91% were caused by *L. pneumophila*. Of the remainder, *Legionella longbeachae* (3.9%) and *L. bozemanii* (2.4%) were next in frequency, followed by *L. micdadei*, *L. feeleii*, *L. dumoffii*, *Legionella wadsworthii*, and *L. anisa*. A European study of culture-confirmed *Legionella* infection from 1995 to 2005 found that 95% of cases were caused by *L. pneumophila*; *L. micdadei*, *L. bozemanii*, and *L. longbeachae* accounted for the majority of the remainder.[31] Other

TABLE 233-1	*Legionella* Species Other Than *L. pneumophila* Causing Human Disease
L. micdadei[93,94]	*L. jordanis*[102]
L. bozemannii[10,58]	*L. gormanii*[103]
L. dumoffii[10,95]	*L. anisa*[104]
L. longbeachae[96]	*L. tusconensis*[105]
L. wadsworthii[97]	*L. sainthelensi*[106]
L. hackeliae[98]	*L. lansingensis*[107]
L. maceachernii[99]	*L. parisiensis*[108]
L. feeleii[100]	*L. oakridgensis*[109]
L. birminghamensis[61]	*L. waltersii*[110]
L. cincinnatiensis[101]	

species appear to be very rare causes of human infection; for several, only a single instance of isolation from a human has been described.

Most reported patients with non-*pneumophila Legionella* infections have been immunocompromised due to corticosteroid therapy, organ transplantation, or malignancy.[30] Patients with *L. micdadei* pneumonia are more likely to be immunosuppressed than those with *L. pneumophila* infection.[32] *Legionella* species are frequent opportunistic pathogens in patients undergoing organ transplantation.[6,14,33-36] After *L. pneumophila*, *L. micdadei*, *L. bozemanii*, and *L. dumoffii* are the most frequent causes of *Legionella* infection in transplant patients.[35]

As with *L. pneumophila*, infection with *L. longbeachae* and *L. dumoffii* has occurred in patients with hairy cell leukemia.[37,38] Human immunodeficiency virus (HIV) infection is associated with some increased risk of infection due to *L. pneumophila*; cases of *L. bozemanii*,[39] *L. feeleii*,[40] and *L. micdadei*[41] infection occurring in the setting of HIV infection have also been reported.

Most reported clusters of infection due to non-*pneumophila* species have been nosocomial and have included *L. micdadei*,[6,7,20,42-44] *L. bozemanii*,[21] and *L. dumoffii*.[45] Two outbreaks of pneumonia due to *Legionella sainthelensis* occurred in Canadian nursing homes.[46] As is typically the case with *L. pneumophila* infection, the source of these outbreaks was the facility's water system. One reported outbreak among solid-organ transplant recipients in a single center involved 12 patients during a 6-month period; the attack rate was 19%.[47] *L. micdadei* was widespread in the hospital water system, and pulsed-field gel electrophoresis of bacterial DNA showed the clinical and environmental strains to be identical. Colonization of the water system with two *Legionella* species may result in outbreaks of infection in which pneumonia may be caused by either or both species simultaneously. A simultaneous outbreak of *L. pneumophila* and *L. micdadei* infection, for example, included patients with both pathogens isolated from respiratory secretions.[47] A cluster of prosthetic valve endocarditis cases and a cluster of sternal wound infections due to *L. pneumophila* and *L. dumoffii*, singly and in combination, occurred in a single hospital.[25,48] Sternal wound infection was the result of contamination of wounds by tap water during bathing.

In contrast to *L. pneumophila*, reports of community-acquired outbreaks due to other *Legionella* species are rare. However, cases may be overlooked because cultures for *Legionella* are not obtained in most cases of community-acquired pneumonia, and the urinary antigen test only detects infection with *L. pneumophila* serogroup 1. In Australia and the United States, there have been multiple cases of community-acquired *L. longbeachae* pneumonia[49-52] associated with exposure to potting soil. Australian investigators isolated *L. longbeachae* from the soil and commercial potting mixes from many of the patient's homes. Potting mixes made in Australia contained the organism, but mixes made in Europe did not.[50] Restriction fragment length polymorphism showed that organisms isolated from the patients and soils were closely related.[51]

There are reports of outbreaks of nonpneumonic legionellosis ("Pontiac fever") associated with exposures to contaminated aerosols. One such outbreak involved 317 workers in an automobile plant in which machinery produced aerosols of water-based coolant containing *L. feeleii*.[53] A whirlpool spa contaminated with *L. micdadei* ("Lochgoilhead fever")[54] and a decorative fountain contaminated with *L. anisa*[55]

have also been implicated in outbreaks of nonpneumonic disease. An outbreak of Pontiac fever with seroconversion to both *L. pneumophila* and *L. micdadei* occurred in a group of children and adults exposed to a poorly maintained whirlpool spa.[56]

Many reported cases of pneumonia due to *Legionella* species are sporadic infections. In such cases, it has generally not been possible to identify an environmental source of the organism. The mode of transmission of the organism from the environment to humans is uncertain except in a limited number of outbreak situations cited previously. There are no reports of outbreaks of pneumonic infection due to non-*pneumophila Legionella* species associated with large aerosol-generating devices such as cooling towers. The occurrence of simultaneous infection by *L. pneumophila* and other species[25,47,48,57] suggests that these other species share common modes of transmission with *L. pneumophila*. Reports of pneumonia following immersion in fresh water[9,58,59] and aspiration[60] suggest that aspiration is a mechanism of transmission to the patient, as has been documented for *L. pneumophila*.[61] Human-to-human transmission does not occur.

Clinical Manifestations

The vast majority of human *Legionella* infections present as pneumonia. Clinically and radiographically, pneumonia caused by other *Legionella* species resembles that caused by *L. pneumophila*.[2,62] Fever is present in more than 90% of patients, exceeding 103°F (39.4°C) in half. Cough is often nonproductive or minimally productive, although most patients produce some sputum. The majority of patients complain of dyspnea. Sixty percent have some alteration in mental status, ranging from lethargy to obtundation. In immunosuppressed patients, pleuritic chest pain is a frequent complaint,[6,7] and the presentation may mimic that of pulmonary embolism. Immunosuppressed patients may have fever without any other symptoms of pneumonia despite the presence of radiographic pulmonary infiltrates.[33,63,64] Occasionally, *Legionella* infections in these patients present as incidental radiographic abnormalities in the absence of fever.[32,63,64] Documented extrapulmonic infection is rare. Four cases of prosthetic valve endocarditis due to *L. dumoffii* (including one with simultaneous *L. pneumophila* infection) occurred at a single hospital.[48] The patients presented with a chronic syndrome of persistent fever, night sweats, malaise, and weight loss without embolic phenomena. All four patients responded to prolonged therapy with erythromycin and rifampin, although three required valve replacement. There is a single case report of prosthetic valve infection due to *L. micdadei*.[65] Sternal wound infection following cardiac surgery presented as serosanguineous wound drainage in the early postoperative period.[25] Gram stain failed to demonstrate organisms, but cultures yielded *L. dumoffii* and *L. pneumophila*. Isolated cases of pericarditis due to *L. bozemanii* and *L. dumoffii* have been reported in cardiac transplant patients.[66,67]

Cutaneous infection due to *L. micdadei* has occurred following pneumonia, presumably by bacteremic seeding,[68] and in the absence of pulmonary infection.[69] Multiple recurrent soft tissue abscesses due to *L. cincinnatiensis* occurred in patient with nephrotic syndrome and monoclonal gammopathy.[70] The patient did not have pneumonia, and the route of infection was not determined. There is a single reported case of *L. longbeachae* osteomyelitis, occurring in a patient receiving corticosteroids for systemic lupus erythematosus who also had *L. longbeachae* pneumonia.[71]

Laboratory data are not distinctive. The majority of patients show a neutrophilic leukocytosis unless receiving cytotoxic agents as immunosuppressive therapy. Elevations of hepatic transaminases or alkaline phosphatase are common. Hyponatremia, reportedly more frequent in *L. pneumophila* infection than in other pneumonias, occurs in one third of cases of *L. micdadei* infection.[72]

Radiographic manifestations are similar to those of *L. pneumophila* infection.[73] In nonimmunosuppressed patients, segmental to lobar infiltrates similar to those occurring in other bacterial pneumonias are typical.[74] An expanding pulmonary nodule has been a dramatic finding in some immunosuppressed patients.[6,63,75] Cavitation of nodules or infiltrates may occur in immunosuppressed patients (Figs. 233-1 and 233-2).[42,63] The cavities often enlarge during treatment and clinical improvement, and they rarely require intervention. Small pleural effusions are common; these usually resolve without drainage, but empyema may occur.

Nonpneumonic disease due to non-*pneumophila* species closely resembles Pontiac fever, the syndrome associated with *L. pneumophila*.[53-55] Following a brief incubation period averaging 36 to 48 hours after exposure to a *Legionella*-containing aerosol, patients experience the abrupt onset of a "flulike" syndrome of fever, chills, headache, myalgias, and malaise. Attack rates may exceed 80% among those exposed. Clinical and radiologic evidence of pneumonia is absent; spontaneous recovery after 2 to 7 days is the rule. Diagnosis is made by recognition of the clinical and epidemiologic features, isolation of a *Legionella* species from an aerosol generation source, and demonstration of seroconversion to the suspected agent on the part of the patients affected. *Legionella* species are generally not detected in clinical material from these patients. There is evidence that the clinical manifestations of Pontiac fever may be the result of an immunologic reaction to high levels of endotoxin in aerosolized water containing *Legionella* rather than the result of infection.[76]

Diagnosis

Isolation of the infecting agent from clinical material (e.g., sputum or bronchoalveolar lavage fluid) on selective media is the most reliable means of diagnosis. BCYE agars with added antibiotics to suppress commensal flora are available commercially,[77] but these media often have decreased sensitivity for isolation of non-*pneumophila* strains[78]; cefamandole is especially inhibitory. *Legionella* species lacking β-lactamase, such as *L. micdadei* and *L. bozemanii*, will not grow on BCYE formulations containing cephalosporins. A more sensitive medium consists of BCYE with added vancomycin, anisomycin, and polymyxin B. The non-*pneumophila* strains are easily missed in clinical and environmental specimens if dye-containing media are not used. Colonies of *L. micdadei* and *L. maceachernii* are blue on culture media containing bromocresol purple and bromothymol blue dyes, whereas the colonies of other species are yellow-green to apple-green[2,79]; the dyes color the organism, making detection easier.

Direct fluorescent antibody (DFA) stains for the visualization of *Legionella* species in clinical specimens are commercially available for a limited number of species. The sensitivity and specificity of DFA staining for species other than *L. pneumophila* are not precisely known. A *Legionella* DNA probe can detect the presence of multiple *Legionella* species but does not differentiate among species. The DNA probe appears to have fewer false-positive reactions than does DFA staining[80]; it is no longer commercially available. The commercially available test for *Legionella* urinary antigen detects only *L. pneumophila* serogroup 1; it is not useful for other *Legionella* species. Detection of *Legionella* spp. in clinical specimens by DNA amplification is a promising technique that has been applied in a limited number of cases.[81]

Antibody seroconversion in diagnosing infection caused by non-*pneumophila* species is of uncertain specificity. Reports of infection based on seroconversion alone should be viewed with skepticism.

Treatment

There are no randomized trials of therapy for *Legionella* infection; the majority of reported clinical experiences concern infection with *L. pneumophila*. In vitro susceptibility data and more limited clinical experience indicate that response to therapies for infections caused by other species should be similar. *Legionella* species are susceptible in vitro to erythromycin, tetracycline, trimethoprim-sulfamethoxazole, rifampin, and ciprofloxacin.[82,83]

Erythromycin has been the historical drug of choice based on the observation of clinical response in the majority of patients.[2,38,84] However, there are a number of case reports of erythromycin failure in highly immunocompromised patients.[34,85-87] Failure of erythromy-

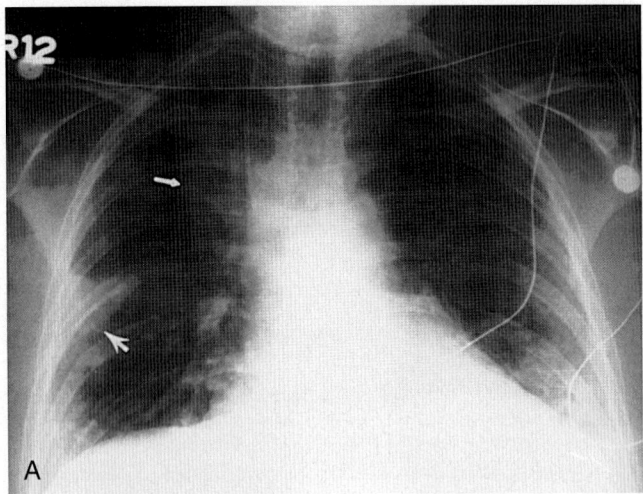
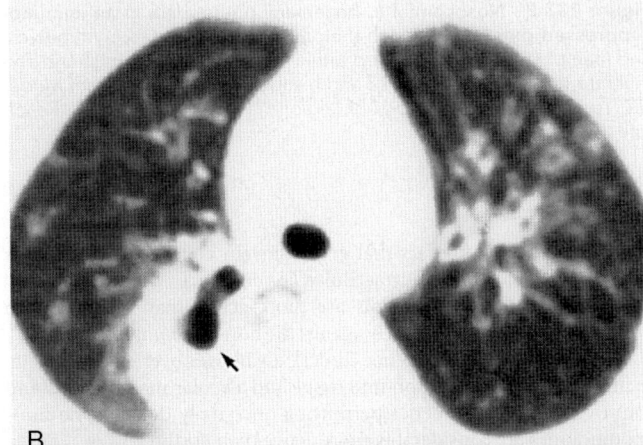
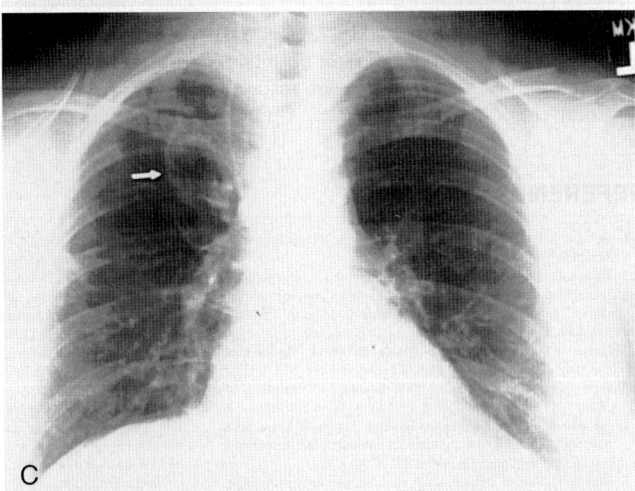

Figure 233-1 **Nosocomial *L. micdadei* in a young female receiving steroids for systemic lupus erythematosus.** On day 3, she experienced abrupt onset of fever, dyspnea, and pleuritic chest pain. **A,** Poorly marginated densities (*small arrow*) and a wedge-shaped density (*large arrow*) were seen on chest x-ray films, suggesting pulmonary embolus, although pulmonary angiography was nonconfirmatory. Direct fluorescent antibody stain and culture of sputum yielded *L. micdadei.* Cavitation in the right upper lobe was seen on day 7 and day 10. **B,** Computed tomography shows the cavity (*arrow*). **C,** A residual thin-walled cavity was still visible on day 15 (*arrow*). The patient ultimately made a full recovery. (*From Muder RR, Yu VL, Parry M. Radiology of Legionella pneumonia. Semin Respir Infect. 1987;2:242-254.*)

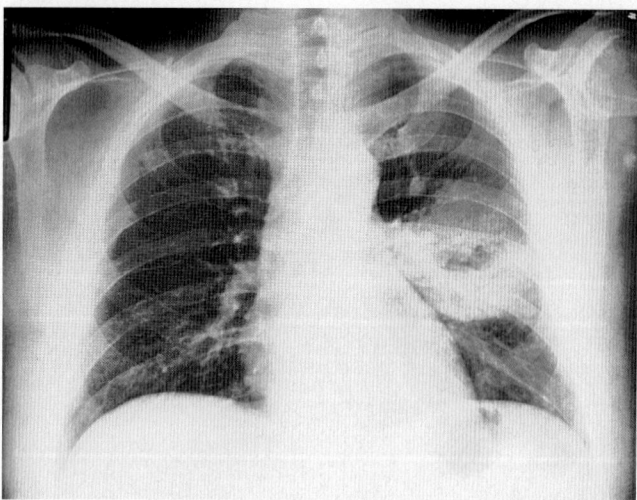

Figure 233-2 **Nosocomial *L. bozemanii* pneumonia in an immuno-suppressed patient.** Although the patient responded to erythromycin and rifampin, cavitation occurred within the left lower lobe infiltrate. The infiltrate decreased by month 3 and resolved by month 6. *(From Muder RR, Yu VL, Parry M. Radiology of Legionella pneumonia. Semin Respir Infect. 1987;2:242-254.)*

cin may be due to the fact that erythromycin is bacteriostatic rather than bactericidal against intracellular *Legionella*.

The newer macrolide agents are more active than erythromycin both in vitro and intracellularly against the non-*pneumophila* species.[88-90] They offer a number of other clinical advantages over erythromycin, including better penetration into tissue and alveolar macrophages and improved pharmacokinetics permitting once-daily dosing. The fluoroquinolones are considerably more active than erythromycin.[90] Based on these factors, the newer macrolides or quinolones are the therapy of choice for infection caused by *Legionella* species. Patients who are immunocompromised or who are hospitalized with potentially life-threatening infection should receive intravenous therapy with either azithromycin or a fluoroquinolone.[91] Quinolones are preferable when

treating transplant patients receiving cyclosporine or tacrolimus because macrolides interfere with the metabolism of these antirejection agents.

The optimal duration of therapy with these agents is uncertain. Data from clinical trials of community-acquired pneumonia suggest that in immunocompetent patients, 5 to 10 days of therapy with azithromycin or 10 to 14 days of therapy with a fluoroquinolone constitutes adequate therapy.[89] Immunocompromised patients should receive longer courses of therapy (14 to 21 days) to prevent relapse. Oral therapy may be used as initial treatment in immunocompetent patients who are not seriously ill. Patients receiving initial parenteral therapy may be switched to oral therapy once a clinical response is apparent.

Prevention

Many cases of infection due to non-*pneumophila Legionella* species are sporadic, and the source is undetermined. When identified, the source is nearly always aquatic; soil is an occasional reservoir. As with *L. pneumophila*, cases of nosocomial disease due to *L. micdadei*, *L. bozemanii*, and *L. dumoffii* have been linked to *Legionella* colonization of hospital water systems. Although the occurrence of *L. pneumophila* in a hospital water system is associated with a high risk of nosocomial legionellosis, the risk posed by the presence of other species in a facility's water system is less well-defined.

An increasing number of state and local public health departments recommend that hospitals conduct periodic surveillance of their water systems for *Legionella*. Although this surveillance is primarily directed at prevention of disease caused by *L. pneumophila*, surveillance may reveal the presence of other species. If surveillance demonstrates the presence of *L. micdadei*, *L. bozemanii*, or *L. dumoffii*, one approach would be to investigate all cases of nosocomial pneumonia occurring in highly immunocompromised patients, including transplant recipients and patients treated with high-dose corticosteroids or immunosuppressive agents, for the occurrence of *Legionella* infection. Because the urinary antigen test detects only infection due to *L. pneumophila* serogroup 1, culture of sputum or bronchoscopy specimens on selective media is required for diagnosis. Identification of cases among high-risk patients should prompt consideration of eradication of *Legionella* from the water system. Measures directed at *L. pneumophila* are effective against other *Legionella* species. Water disinfection using copper-silver ion generators has good long-term efficacy.[92]

REFERENCES

1. Benson RF, Fields BS. Classification of the genus *Legionella*. *Semin Respir Infect.* 1998;13:90-99.
2. Fang GD, Yu VL, Vickers RM. Disease due to Legionellaceae (other than *Legionella pneumophila*): historical, microbiological, clinical and epidemiological review. *Medicine.* 1989;68:116-139.
3. Birtles RJ, Rowbotham TJ, Raoult D, et al. Phylogenetic diversity of intra-amoebal legionellae as revealed by 16s rRnA gene sequence comparison. *Microbiology.* 1996;142:3525-3530.
4. Adeleke A, Pruckler J, Benson R, et al. *Legionella*-like amebal pathogens—phylogenetic status and possible role in respiratory diseases. *Emerg Infect Dis.* 1996;2:225-230.
5. Marrie TJ, Raoult D, La Scola B, et al. *Legionella*-like and other amoebal pathogens as agents of community-acquired pneumonia. *Emerg Infect Dis.* 2001;7:1026-1029.
6. Myerowitz RC, Pasculle AW, Dowling J, et al. Opportunistic lung infection due to "Pittsburgh pneumonia agent." *N Engl J Med.* 1979;301:953-958.
7. Rogers BH, Donowitz GR, Walker GK, et al. A clinicopathological study of five cases caused by an unidentified acid-fast bacterium. *N Engl J Med.* 1979;301:959-961.
8. Tatlock H. Studies on a virus from a patient with Fort Bragg fever (pretibial fever). *Clin Invest.* 1947;26:87-93.
9. Bozeman FM, Humphries JW, Campbell JM. A new group of *Rickettsia*-like agents recovered from guinea pigs. *Acta Virol.* 1968;12:87-93.
10. Brenner DJ, Steigerwalt A, Gorman GW. *Legionella bozemanii*, sp nov and *Legionella dumoffii* sp nov: classification of two additional species of *Legionella* associated with human pneumonia. *Curr Microbiol.* 1980;4:111-116.
11. Brenner DJ, Steigerwalt AG, Gorman GW, et al. Ten new species of *Legionella*. *Int J Syst Bacteriol.* 1985;35:50-59.

12. Lambert MA, Moss CW. Cellular fatty acid compositions and isoprenoid quinone contents of 23 *Legionella* species. *J Clin Microbiol.* 1989;27:465-473.
13. Hilton E, Freedman RA, Cintron F, et al. Acid-fast bacilli in sputum: a case of *Legionella micdadei* pneumonia. *J Clin Microbiol.* 1986;24:1102-1103.
14. Schwebke JR, Hackman R, Bowden R. Pneumonia due to *Legionella micdadei* in bone marrow transplant recipients. *Rev Infect Dis.* 1990;12:824-828.
15. Wadowsky RM, Wilson TM, Kapp NJ, et al. Multiselection of *Legionella* spp. in tap water containing *Hartmanella oerniformis*. *Appl Environ Microbiol.* 1991;57:1950-1955.
16. Fields BS, Barbaree JM, Sanden GN, et al. Virulence of *Legionella anisa* strain associated with Pontiac fever: an evaluation using protozoan, cell culture, and guinea pig models. *Infect Immun.* 1990;58:3139-3142.
17. Alli OAT, Zink S, von Lackum NK, et al. Comparative virulence traits in *Legionella* spp. *Microbiology.* 2003;149:631-641.
18. Tison DL, Baross JA, Seidler RJ. *Legionella* in aquatic habitats in the Mount Saint Helens blast zone. *Curr Microbiol.* 1983;9:345-348.
19. Joly JR, Boissiot M, Duchaine J, et al. Ecological distribution of Legionellaceae in the Quebec City area. *Can J Microbiol.* 1984;30:63-67.
20. Best M, Yu VL, Stout J, et al. Legionellaceae in the hospital water supply—epidemiological link with disease and evaluation of a method of control of nosocomial Legionnaires' disease and Pittsburgh pneumonia. *Lancet.* 1983;2:307-310.
21. Parry MF, Stampleman L, Hutchinson J, et al. Waterborne *Legionella bozemanii* and nosocomial pneumonia in immunosuppressed patients. *Ann Intern Med.* 1985;103:205-210.
22. Barbaree JM. Selecting a subtyping technique for use in investigations of legionellosis epidemics. In: Barbaree JM, Brieman RF,

Dufour AP, eds. *Legionella: Current Status and Emerging Perspectives.* Washington, DC: American Society for Microbiology; 1993:169-172.
23. Bornstein N, Veilly C, Marmet D, et al. Isolation of *Legionella anisa* from a hospital hot water system. *Eur J Clin Microbiol.* 1985;4:327-330.
24. Palutke WA, Crane LR, Wentworth BB, et al. *Legionella feeleii*-associated pneumonia in humans. *N Engl J Med.* 1986;86:348-351.
25. Lowry PW, Blankenship RJ, Gridley W, et al. A cluster of *Legionella* sternal wound infections due to postoperative topical exposure of contaminated tap water. *N Engl J Med.* 1991;324:109-112.
26. Stout JE, Muder RR, Mietzner S, et al. Role of environmental surveillance in determining risk for hospital-acquired legionellosis: a national surveillance study with clinical correlations. *Infect Control Hosp Epidemiol.* 2007;28:818-824.
27. Best MG, Stout J, Yu VL, et al. *Tatlockia micdadei* growth kinetics may explain its infrequent isolation from water and the low prevalence of Pittsburgh pneumonia. *Appl Environ Microbiol.* 1985;49:1521-1522.
28. McNally C, Plouffe J. *Legionella bozemanii*—an important etiological agent in community-acquired pneumonia [abstract 519]. In: Program and Abstracts of the 36th Annual Meeting of the Infectious Diseases Society of America, Denver, CO; 1998.
29. McNally C, Hackman B, Fields BS, et al. Potential importance of *Legionella* species as etiologies in community acquired pneumonia (CAP). *Diagn Microbiol Infect Dis.* 2000;38:79-82.
30. Yu VL, Plouffe JF, Castellani-Pastoris M, et al. Distribution of *Legionella* species and serogroups isolated by culture in consecutive patients with community acquired pneumonia: an

international collaborative survey. *J Infect Dis.* 2002;186: 127-128.
31. Diederen BMW. *Legionella* spp. and legionnaires' disease. *J Infect.* 2008;56:1-12.
32. Muder RR, Yu VL, Zuravleff JJ. Pneumonia due to the Pittsburgh pneumonia agent: new clinical perspective with a review of the literature. *Medicine.* 1983;62:120-128.
33. Singh N, Muder RR, Yu VL, et al. *Legionella* infection in liver transplant recipients: implications for management. *Transplantation.* 1993;56:1549-1551.
34. Harrington RD, Woolfrey AE, Bowden R, et al. Legionellosis in a bone marrow transplant center. *Clin Infect Dis.* 1996;18:361-368.
35. Ernst A, Gordon FD, Hayek J, et al. Lung abscess complication: *Legionella micdadei* pneumonia in an adult liver transplant recipient. *Transplantation.* 1998;65:130-133.
36. Chow J, Yu VL. *Legionella*: a major opportunistic pathogen in transplant recipients. *Semin Respir Infect.* 1998;13: 132-139.
37. Lang R, Miller I, Manon J, et al. *Legionella longbeachae* in a splenectomized hairy-cell leukemia patient. *Infection.* 1990; 18:31-32.
38. Fang GD, Stout JE, Yu VL, et al. Community-acquired pneumonia caused by *Legionella dumoffii* in a patient with hairy cell leukemia. *Infection.* 1990;18:383-385.
39. Harris A, Lally M, Albrecht M. *Legionella bozemanii* pneumonia in three patients with AIDS. *Clin Infect Dis.* 1998;27: 97-99.
40. Lo Presti F, Riffard S, Neyret C, et al. First isolation in Europe of *Legionella feeleii* from two cases of pneumonia. *Eur J Clin Microbiol Infect Dis.* 1998;17:64-66.
41. Johnson KM, Huseby JS. Lung abscess caused by *Legionella micdadei. Chest.* 1997;111:252-253.
42. Rudin JE, Wing EJ. A comparative study of *Legionella micdadei* and other nosocomial acquired pneumonia. *Chest.* 1984; 86:875-880.
43. Doebbeling BN, Ishak MA, Wade BH, et al. Nosocomial *Legionella micdadei* pneumonia: 10 years experience and a case-control study. *J Hosp Infect.* 1989;13:289-298.
44. Knirsch CA, Jakob K, Schoonmaker D, et al. An outbreak of *Legionella micdadei* pneumonia in transplant patients: education, molecular epidemiology, and control. *Am J Med.* 2000; 108:290-295.
45. Brooks RG, Hofflin JM, Jamieson SW, et al. Infectious complications in heart-lung transplant recipients. *Am J Med.* 1985; 79:412-422.
46. Loeb M, Simor AE, Mandell L, et al. Two nursing home outbreaks of respiratory infections with *Legionella sainthelensis. J Am Geriatric Soc.* 1999;47:547-552.
47. Muder RR, Yu VL, Vickers R, et al. Simultaneous infection with *Legionella pneumophila* and Pittsburgh pneumonia agent—clinical features and epidemiological implications. *Am J Med.* 1983;74:609-614.
48. Tompkins LS, Roessler BJ, Redd SC, et al. *Legionella* prosthetic-valve endocarditis. *N Engl J Med.* 1988;318:530-535.
49. Camerson S, Walker C, Roden D, et al. Epidemiological characteristics of *Legionella* infection in South Australia: implications for disease control. *Aust N Z Med.* 1991;21:65-70.
50. Steele TW, Moore CY, Sangster N. Distribution of *Legionella longbeachae* serogroup 1 and other legionellae in potting soil in Australia. *Appl Environ Microbiol.* 1990;56:2984-2988.
51. Lanser JA, Adams M, Doyle R, et al. Genetic relatedness of *Legionella longbeachae* isolates from human and environmental sources in Australia. *Appl Environ Microbiol.* 1990;56:2784-2790.
52. Centers for Disease Control and Prevention. Legionnaires' disease associated with potting soil—California, Oregon, and Washington, May-June 2000. *MMWR Morb Mortal Wkly Rep.* 2000;49:777-778.
53. Herwaldt LA, Gorman GW, McGrath T, et al. A new *Legionella* species, *Legionella feeleii* species nova, causes Pontiac fever in an automobile plant. *Ann Intern Med.* 1984;100:333-338.
54. Goldberg DJ, Wrench JG, Collier PW, et al. Lochgoilhead fever: outbreak of non-pneumonic legionellosis due to *Legionella micdadei. Lancet.* 1989;1:316-318.
55. Fenstersheib M, Miller M, Diggins C, et al. Outbreak of Pontiac fever due to *Legionella anisa. Lancet.* 1990;336:35-37.
56. Luttichau HR, Vinther C, Uldum SA, et al. An outbreak of Pontiac fever among children following use of a whirlpool. *Clin Infect Dis.* 1998;26:1374-1378.
57. Tompkins LS, Trout N, Wood ST, et al. Molecular epidemiology of *Legionella* species by restriction endonuclease and alloenzyme analysis. *J Clin Microbiol.* 1987;25:1875-1880.
58. Cordes LG, Gorman GW, Wilkinson HW, et al. Atypical *Legionella*-like organisms: fastidious water-associated bacteria pathogenic for man. *Lancet.* 1979;2:927-930.
59. Thompson BM, Harris PP, Hicklin MD, et al. A *Legionella*-like bacterium related to WIGA in a fatal case of pneumonia. *Ann Intern Med.* 1979;91:673-676.
60. Donegan EA, Deal MM, Melanephy MC, et al. Primary isolation of a new strain of the TATLOCK/Pittsburgh pneumonia agent (*Legionella micdadei*). *West J Med.* 1981;134:384-389.
61. Yu VL. Could aspiration be the major mode of transmission for *Legionella*? *Am J Med.* 1993;95:13-15.
62. Muder RR, Yu VL. Infection due to *Legionella* species other than *L. pneumophila. Clin Infect Dis.* 2002;35:990-998.
63. Ellis AR, Mayers DL, Martone WJ, et al. Rapid expanding pulmonary nodule caused by Pittsburgh pneumonia agent. *JAMA.* 1981;245:1558-1559.
64. Wilkinson HW, Thacker LW, Benson RF, et al. *Legionella birminghamensis* sp. nov. isolated from a cardiac transplant recipient. *J Clin Microbiol.* 1987;25:2120-2122.
65. Patel MC, Levi MH, Mahdevi P, et al. *L. micdadei* PVE successfully treated with levofloxacin/valve replacement: case report and review of the literature. *J Infect Dis.* 2005;51:e265-e268.
66. Swinburn CR, Gould FK, Corris PA, et al. Opportunist pulmonary infection with *Legionella bozemanii. Thorax.* 1989;44: 434-435.
67. Valentine HA, Hunt SA, Gibbons R, et al. Increasing pericardial effusion in cardiac transplant recipients. *Circulation.* 1989;79:603-609.
68. Ampel NM, Ruben FL, Norden CW. Cutaneous abscess caused by *Legionella micdadei* in an immunosuppressed patient. *Ann Intern Med.* 1985;102:630-632.
69. Kilborn JA, Manz LA, O'Brien M, et al. Necrotizing cellulitis caused by *Legionella micdadei. Am J Med.* 1992;92:104-106.
70. Gubler JGH, Schorr M, Gaia V, et al. Recurrent soft tissue abscess caused by *Legionella cincinnatiensis. J Clin Microbiol.* 2001;39:4568-4570.
71. McClelland MR, Vazar LT, Kagawa FT. Pneumonia and osteomyelitis due to *Legionella longbeachae* in a woman with systemic lupus erythematosus. *Clin Infect Dis.* 2004;38:e102-e106.
72. Fang GD, Yu VL, Vickers RM. Infections caused by the Pittsburgh pneumonia agent. *Semin Respir Infect.* 1987;2: 262-266.
73. Muder RR, Yu VL, Parry M. Radiology of *Legionella* pneumonia. *Semin Respir Infect.* 1987;2:242-254.
74. Muder RR, Reddy S, Yu VL, et al. Pneumonia caused by Pittsburgh pneumonia agent: radiologic manifestations. *Radiology.* 1984;150:633-637.
75. Pope TL, Armstrong P, Thompson R, et al. Pittsburgh pneumonia agent: chest film manifestations. *AJR Am J Roentgenol.* 1982;138:237-241.
76. Fields BS, Haupt T, Davis JP, et al. Pontiac fever due to *Legionella micdadei* from a whirlpool spa: possible role of bacterial endotoxin. *J Infect Dis.* 2001;15:1289-1292.
77. Vickers RM, Stout JE, Yu VL, et al. Culture methodology for the isolation of *Legionella pneumophila* and other Legionellaceae from clinical and environmental specimens. *Semin Respir Infect.* 1987;2:274-279.
78. Lee TC, Vickers RM, Yu VL, et al. Growth of 28 *Legionella* species on selective culture media: a comparative study. *J Clin Microbiol.* 1993;31:2761-2768.
79. Vickers RM, Brown A, Garrity GM. Dye-containing buffered charcoal yeast extract medium for the differentiation of members of the family Legionellaceae. *J Clin Microbiol.* 1981;13:380-382.
80. Finkelstein R, Brown P, Palutke WA, et al. Diagnostic efficacy of a DNA probe in pneumonia caused by *Legionella* species. *J Med Microbiol.* 1993;38:183-186.
81. Jaulhac B, Reinthaler FF, Pschaid A, et al. Detection of *Legionella* species in bronchoalveolar lavage fluids by DNA amplification. *J Clin Microbiol.* 1992;30:920-924.
82. Pasculle AW, Dowling JW, Weyent RS, et al. Susceptibility of Pittsburgh pneumonia agent (*Legionella micdadei*) and other newly recognized members of the genus *Legionella* to nineteen antimicrobial agents. *Antimicrob Agents Chemother.* 1981;20: 793-799.
83. Saito A, Koga H, Shigeno H, et al. The antimicrobial activity of ciprofloxacin against *Legionella* species and the treatment of experimental *Legionella* pneumonia in guinea pigs. *J Antimicrob Chemother.* 1986;18:251-260.
84. Wing EJ, Schafer FJ, Pasculle AW. Successful treatment of *Legionella micdadei* (Pittsburgh pneumonia agent) pneumonia with erythromycin. *Am J Med.* 1981;21:836-839.
85. Taylor TH, Albrecht MA. *Legionella bozemanii* cavitary pneumonia poorly responsive to erythromycin: case report and review. *Clin Infect Dis.* 1995;20:329-334.
86. Koch CA, Robyn JA, Coccia MR. Systemic lupus erythematosus: a risk factor for pneumonia caused by *Legionella micdadei*? *Arch Intern Med.* 1997;157:2670-2671.
87. Rudin JE, Evans TL, Wing EJ. Failure of erythromycin in treatment of *Legionella micdadei* pneumonia. *Am J Med.* 1984;76: 318-320.
88. Stout JE, Arnold B, Yu VL. Comparative activity of azithromycin, clarithromycin, roxithromycin, dirithromycin, quinupristin/dalfopristin, and erythromycin against *Legionella* species by broth microdilution and intracellular susceptibility testing in HL-60 cells. *J Antimicrob Chemother.* 1998;41:289-291.
89. Vergis EN, Yu VL. *Legionella* species. In: Yu VL, Merigan TC, Barriere SL, et al, eds. *Antimicrobial Therapy and Vaccines.* Baltimore: Williams & Wilkins; 1998:257-272.
90. Stout JE, Arnold B, Yu VL. Comparative activity of ciprofloxacin, ofloxacin, levofloxacin, and erythromycin against *Legionella* species by broth microdilution and intracellular susceptibility testing in HL-60 cells. *Diagn Microbiol Infect Dis.* 1998; 30:37-43.
91. Stout JE, Yu VL. Current concepts: Legionellosis. *N Engl J Med.* 1997;337:682-687.
92. Stout JE, Yu VL. Experience of the first 16 hospitals using copper-silver ionization for *Legionella* control: implications for the evaluation of other disinfection modalities. *Infect Control Hosp Epidemiol.* 2003;24:563-568.
93. Pasculle A, Myerowitz R, Rinaldo C. New bacterial agent of pneumonia isolated from renal transplant recipients. *Lancet.* 1979;2:58-61.
94. Hebert GA, Steigerwalt AG, Brenner DJ. *Legionella micdadei* species nova: classification of a third species of *Legionella* associated with human pneumonia. *Curr Microbiol.* 1980;3:257.
95. Lewallen KS, McKinney RM, Brenner DJ, et al. A newly identified bacterium phenotypically resembling, not genetically distinct from, *Legionella pneumophila*: an isolate in a case of pneumonia. *Ann Intern Med.* 1979;91:831-834.
96. McKinney RM, Porschen RK, Edelstein PH, et al. *Legionella longbeachae* species nova, another etiologic agent of human pneumonia. *Ann Intern Med.* 1981;94:739-743.
97. Edelstein PH, Brenner DJ, Moss CW, et al. *Legionella wadsworthii* species nova: a cause of human pneumonia. *Ann Intern Med.* 1982;97(6):809-813.
98. Wilkinson HW, Thacker WL, Steigerwalt AG, et al. Second serogroup of *Legionella hackeliae* isolated from a patient with pneumonia. *J Clin Microbiol.* 1985;22:488-489.
99. Wilkinson HW, Thacker WL, Brenner DJ, et al. Fatal *Legionella maceachernii* pneumonia. *J Clin Microbiol.* 1985;22:1055.
100. Thacker WL, Wilkinson HW, Plikaytis BB, et al. Second serogroup of *Legionella feeleii* strains isolated from humans. *J Clin Microbiol.* 1985;22:1-4.
101. Thacker WL, Benson RF, Staneck JL, et al. *Legionella cincinnatiensis* sp. nov. isolated from a patient with pneumonia. *J Clin Microbiol.* 1988;26:418-420.
102. Thacker WL, Wilkinson HW, Benson RF, et al. *Legionella jordanis* isolated from a patient with fatal pneumonia. *J Clin Microbiol.* 1988;28:1400-1401.
103. Griffith ME, Lindsay DS, Benson RF, et al. First isolation of *Legionella gormanii* from a patient with fatal pneumonia. *J Clin Microbiol.* 1988;26:380-381.
104. Bornstein N, Mercatello A, Marmet D, et al. Pleural infection caused by *Legionella anisa. J Clin Microbiol.* 1989;27:2100-2101.
105. Thacker WL, Benson RF, Staneck JL, et al. *Legionella tucsonesis* sp. nov. isolated from a renal transplant recipient. *J Clin Microbiol.* 1989;27:1831-1834.
106. Benson RF, Thacker WL, Fang FC, et al. *Legionella sainthelensis* serogroup 2 isolated from patients with pneumonia. *Res Microbiol.* 1990;141:453-463.
107. Thacker WL, Dyke JW, Benson RF, et al. *Legionella lansingensis* sp. nov. isolated from a patient with pneumonia and underlying chronic lymphocytic leukemia. *J Clin Microbiol.* 1992;30: 2398-2401.
108. Lo Presti F, Riffard S, Jarraud S, et al. The first clinical isolate of *Legionella parisiensis. J Clin Microbiol.* 1997;35:1706-1709.
109. Lo Presti F, Reffard S, Jarraud S, et al. Isolation of *Legionella oakridgensis* from two patients with pleural effusion living in the same geographical area. *J Clin Microbiol.* 2000;38:3128-3130.
110. Konig C, Hebestreit H, Valenza G, et al. *Legionella waltersii*—a novel cause of pneumonia? *Acta Pediatr.* 2005;55:2030-2049.

234

Capnocytophaga

J. MICHAEL JANDA | MARGOT GRAVES

Taxonomy

The genus *Capnocytophaga* consists of fermentative bacteria that morphologically appear as thin to slender gram-negative bacilli with tapered ends. The genus consists of eight named species—*C. gingivalis, C. granulosa, C. haemolytica, C. leadbetteri, C. ochracea, C. sputigena, C. canimorsus,* and *C. cynodegmi*—and one unnamed taxon (AHN8471) that can be subdivided into two major groups associated with the oral microflora of humans and animals.[1] With the exception of *C. leadbetteri* and AHN8471, all other species are recognized human pathogens. Phylogenetically, the genus *Capnocytophaga* resides in the family *Flavobacteriaceae* (rRNA superfamily V).[2]

Pathogenesis and Clinical Manifestations

There are few published data on what virulence factors are operative in *Capnocytophaga* infections. Human capnocytophaga such as *C. gingivalis* and *C. sputigena* produce a number of cell-bound or extracellular factors that may promote progression of peridontitis by enhancing the growth of bacteria in plaques and subgingival pockets or by evading host immune responses. Such factors include immunoglobulin A1 protease, phospholipase A2, aminopeptidases, and chemotaxis-guided (gliding) motility.[3,4]

C. canimorsus invades and multiplies in J774 murine macrophages with cytotoxic destruction of the monolayer, a trait that distinguishes it from *C. cynodegmi*.[4,5] Investigations by Shin and colleagues have found that multiple live and heat-killed strains of *C. canimorsus* failed to elicit immune responses from mouse and human macrophages, including cytokines, chemokines, and nitric oxide.[6] Toll-like receptors were also unable to respond to *C. canimorsus*, suggesting that in the initial stages of silent entry of the bacterium into the human host, the ability to avoid an inflammatory response may play a key role.

Human *Capnocytophaga* infections can be broken down into five major categories: (1) septicemia, (2) diseases of the central nervous system (CNS), (3) eye infections, (4) illnesses associated with pregnancy, and (5) miscellaneous complications, including infections of bone and tissue. Although most *Capnocytophaga* infections occur in persons with impaired immune function or with significant underlying disease, infections in healthy persons have been documented, but are typically less severe in nature.[7,8]

HUMAN ORAL-ASSOCIATED SPECIES

Oral *Capnocytophaga* spp. are residents of the subgingival sulcus and of supragingival plaque and have been implicated as opportunistic pathogens of gingivitis, periodontal disease, and oropharyngeal mucositis.[1,9,10] One recent study using two different molecular approaches has found *C. ochracea* and *C. granulosa* to be the two most common species associated with subgingival plaque.[11] These results closely mirror findings from a multicenter study in which *C. ochracea* predominated as the cause of *Capnocytophaga* bacteremia in cancer patients.[12]

The most common infection associated with oral capnocytophaga is septicemia, with an incidence ranging from 0.5% to 3.0%. Sepsis is most often observed in patients with underlying hematologic malignancies, including acute and chronic myelogenous leukemia, lympho-

mas, Hodgkin's disease, and multiple myeloma (Table 234-1).[12,13] Onset of sepsis typically coincides with the initiation of profound neutropenia (<500 granulocytes/mm^3) induced by chemotherapy or after hematopoietic stem cell transplantation.[8] Oral ulcerations such as severe mucositis, gingival hyperplasia, esophagitis, and peritodonitis appear to serve as portals of entry for systemic invasion. Maury and associates[13] found all 24 persons with *Capnocytophaga* bacteremia to be neutropenic; 88% of these patients had severe oral mucositis or periodontitis. Warren and Allen[14] have suggested that pediatric patients are more prone to developing *Capnocytophaga* sepsis than adults; Campbell and Edwards have reviewed the literature on this topic.[15] However, Joliet-Gougeon and co-workers[16] found that the frequency of oral carriage of capnocytophaga by children at an oncology department varies from 16% to 61% and no cases of systemic disease were detected during a 10-year period. These results suggest that whereas oral carriage of *Capnocytophaga* by children may be high, the risk of developing severe disease is relatively low.

Bloodborne disease caused by *Capnocytophaga* is typically monomicrobic (85% to 90%) in nature. When polymicrobic illnesses occur, they most often involve viridans streptococci, anaerobes, or aerobic or facultatively anaerobic rods.[8] *C. ochracea* is the species commonly implicated in sepsis, with most cases occurring in immunocompromised persons.[12,13] However, serious *C. ochraeca* sepsis and purpura fulminans have been reported in a healthy 46-year-old man 2 weeks after an uneventful dental extraction.[17] Fewer than 20 cases of *C. sputigena* or *C. gingivalis* bacteremia have been reported, and only a single case of *C. haemolytica* septicemia has been recorded. No cases of *C. granulosa* septicemia have been published.[18] The overall attributable mortality rate associated with *Capnocytophaga* bacteremia varies from 16% to 42%; later investigations have reported lower values, approaching 0%.[8,12-15]

Oral species are less frequently implicated in CNS infections than their zoonotic counterparts. Unlike septicemia, CNS illnesses most often manifest themselves in immunocompetent individuals, with the major risk factor being dental manipulations (see Table 234-1). Cases of *Capnocytophaga* subdural empyema and frontal brain abscess have been described in healthy persons who underwent tooth extraction.[19] Brain abscesses and extremely rare cases of meningitis have also been reported in pediatric patients with bloodborne dyscrasias.

Ocular infections can run the gamut from blepharoconjunctivitis to keratitis, endophthalmitis, and corneal ulceration. People prone to developing ocular disease are older than 70 years, immunosuppressed, or involved in IV or crack cocaine drug use. In one series of 10 patients with keratitis, risk factors associated with infection included corneal epithelial defects, previous ocular infections, topical steriod therapy, and intraocular surgery.[20]

Chorioamnionitis is the most common clinical presentation associated with pregnancy and *Capnocytophaga* infection. Mild to severe illnesses can develop, resulting in premature contractions, labor, or fetal death. *Capnocytophaga* species can be recovered from infected placenta, cervix, and endometrium as well as amniotic fluid. Perinatal illnessess may ensue via an ascending route of infection or through hematogenous spread.[21] Most cases of chorioamnionitis involve recent oral sex as the primary risk factor.

Other unusual monomicrobic or mixed infections involving oral capnocytophaga species include peritonitis, pyogenic arthritis, vertebral osteomyelitis, cervical and liver abscesses, pneumonia, pleural effusion and empyema, pyonephrosis, and soft tissue infections. In

TABLE 234-1	Salient Features Distinguishing Human- from Animal-Associated *Capnocytophaga*		
Characteristic		Human-associated	Animal-associated
Patient population			
Children		+	−
Adults		+	+
Underlying diseases*			
Leukemia, lymphoma		+	−
Asplenia		−	+
Ethanol abuse		−	+
Risk factors			
Neutropenia and chemotherapy		+	−
Dental manipulations		+	−
Animal bites		−	+
Laboratory tests			
Catalase		−	+
Oxidase		−	+
Arginine dihydrolase		−	+

*For invasive disease such as septicemia.

many case reports, predisposing risk factors and apparent routes of infection are not identified.

INFECTIONS ASSOCIATED WITH ZOONOTIC SPECIES

The zoonotic species *C. canimorsus* and *C. cynodegmi* are normal inhabitants of the oral cavity of dogs and cats.[22] Most life-threatening illnesses associated with these two zoonoses are attributed to *C. canimorsus* (more than 90%), which for unexplained reasons has a higher predilection for causing serious disease than *C. cynodegmi*. Extraintestinal manifestations caused by these two species (septicemia, meningitis) are more limited than observed with their human oral-associated counterparts. Zoonotic-associated infections arise via exogenous introduction of bacteria into wounds from penetrating traumas (dog bite) or by inapparent inoculation of bacilli into abraded surfaces or tissues via intimate contact with pets. Invasive diseases resulting from such exposures are associated with higher mortality rates.

Symptoms associated with *C. canimorsus* septicemia are similar to those of other gram-negative pathogens.[7,23] A prominent diagnostic feature found in 20% to 40% of cases of *C. canimorsus* septicemia is a rash that may vary from a macular or maculopapular eruption to a more severe and rapidly fatal form, such as purpura fulminans with petechial lesions, retiform purpura, or symmetrical gangrene.[24-26] The overall gross case fatality rate for *C. canimorsus* septicemia is fairly constant, 27% to 33%.[27,28]

Epidemiology

C. canimorsus sepsis occurs in males (M/F ratio, 2.8 to 3.6 : 1) older than 40 years (70% to 90%) and suffering from one or more underlying conditions (62% to 89%).[7,24,27,28] Past medical history is often significant for recent dog-bite exposure (more than 50%) or incidental contact with dogs (23% to 28%).[26-29] Persons at risk of developing bloodborne disease include dog owners, veterinarians, breeders, kennel workers, mail carriers, and hunters. On six or more occasions, cat bites or scratches have been implicated as the source of *C. canimorsus* septicemia, with one reported fatality.[30] By 1996, over 100 cases of systemic infection involving *C. canimorsus* had been published in the literature[24] and this number has more than doubled in the intervening years, with one large retrospective study reporting on 55 cases of invasive disease over a 32-year period. The authors in this latter survey[23] suggested that detection of systemic disease caused by *C. canimorsus* may be on the rise because of several factors, including more pet ownership, more opportunities for animal contact, and better laboratory methods for detecting infections.

Hicklin and colleagues[27] have found splenectomized patients are more prone to developing sepsis with disseminated intravascular coagulation (58%) than those with intact spleens (16%), and multiple case reports describing overwhelming postsplenectomy infections accompanying *C. canimorsus* sepsis have been reported. In some reviews, the incidence of those with *C. canimorsus* bacteremia and asplenia is as high as one third, but other studies suggested a value closer to 20%.[24] Other underlying conditions associated with aggressive *C. canimorsus* infections include ethanol abuse, immunosuppression, and corticosteroid therapy.[24] Job and associates[28] estimated that persons with underlying medical problems are three times more likely to contract *Capnocytophaga* disease than healthy people, although fatality rates are not appreciably different. Other complications associated with *C. canimorsus* septicemia include Waterhouse-Friderichsen syndrome, thrombotic thrombocytopenic purpura, and hemolytic uremic syndrome.[31-33] Life-threatening *C. canimorsus* illnesses can also occur in healthy people, although less frequently and typically with less severity.[34]

Meningitis is the second most common presentation and the reported mortality rate is very low (5%) in comparison to cases of septicemia without CNS involvement.[35,36] *C. canimorsus* has also been linked to endocarditis with a fatality rate approaching 33%.[37] Other miscellaneous infections have been described and include eye infections, arthritis, cellulitis, glomerulonephritis, renal failure, and pneumonia.[24,27]

Although *C. cynodegmi* is a common resident of the mouths of dogs, it rarely causes disease. Khawari and co-workers[38] have described a fatal case of *C. cynodegmi* sepsis and meningitis in a previously splenectomized 72-year-old woman who was bitten on the hand by her pet dog. She rapidly developed signs of sepsis, with facial purpura and a progressive macular rash, and succumbed to infection within 48 hours of admission. *C. cynodegmi* peritonitis has been reported in a 67-year-old man with end-stage renal disease who developed cloudy dialysate subsequent to automated peritoneal dialysis.[39] He was treated with cefuroxime, gentamicin, and metronidazole, to which he responded favorably. Although he did not own a dog, he occasionally fed his neighbor's cat.

Diagnosis and Laboratory Identification

Presumptive diagnosis of *Capnocytophaga* sepsis can be made by examination of the patient's peripheral whole blood or buffy coat using Gram or Wright-Giemsa stain.[31,40] A strong index of suspicion of the presence of *Capnocytophaga* can be made if slender, medium to long, gram-negative rods with tapered ends are observed (Fig. 234-1).

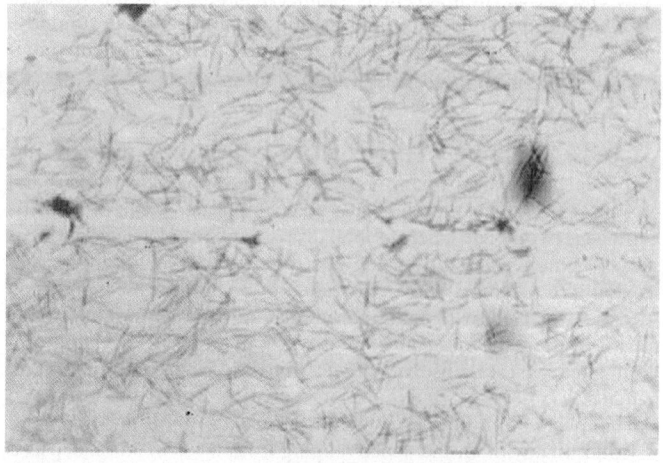

Figure 234-1 Gram stain of *Capnocytophaga* exhibiting long, slender rods. *(Courtesy of Dr. Edward J. Bottone.)*

Pers and colleagues[7] have reported seeing bacteria on initial microscopic examinations of cerebrospinal fluid (CSF), whereas another report has described slender, fusiform bacilli in conjunctival scrapings.[41] 16S rRNA gene sequencing performed directly on a clinical sample or a positive blood culture can decrease the turn-around time to diagnosis[40] and polymerase chain reaction (PCR) assay using species-specific primers can detect capnocytophaga in mixed culture in dental plaque samples.[42]

Capnocytophaga infections can be diagnosed by isolating and identifying the organism from appropriate specimens. If a clinician suspects *Capnocytophaga* septicemia, a request to the laboratory to incubate blood cultures for up to 10 days should be made to enhance recovery of this fastidious and slow-growing organism. Recovery of capnocytophagae from CSF or blood typically ranges from 3 to 7 days.[35] Some *Capnocytophaga* species appear to be sensitive to the anticoagulant SPS used in some blood culture bottles.[43] Performing a Gram stain on blood culture sediment at the first indication of growth can yield a presumptive identification, although there is a small chance that the Gram stain can be misread.[44] Sediment from terminal negative blood cultures can be either Gram-stained or subcultured for up to 5 additional days in 5% CO_2. *Capnocytophaga* spp. can also be recovered from clinical specimens, including CSF, abscess material, respiratory secretions, amniotic fluid, the urogenital tract, joint fluid, and various tissues. Prolonged incubation of these specimens may be required to recover capnocytophagae.

Capnocytophaga spp. are considered fastidious bacteria because they grow slowly on blood-enriched media and generally require an increased CO_2 atmosphere (5% to 10%). They grow on blood agar and often on chocolate agar, but not on MacConkey or Heart Infusion agars. Several authors report success isolating strains using selective media containing bacitracin, polymyxin B, vancomycin, and trimethoprim.[45] *Capnocytophaga* isolates are reported to grow on kanamycin-vancomycin laked blood (KVLB) agar medium with a reduced concentration of kanamycin (2 µg/ml)[46] and Thayer-Martin and Martin-Lewis media.[47]

Colonies may be visible at 24 hours but often require 48 to 72 hours to reach 2 to 4 mm in diameter. They are convex and smooth and can show irregular edges, indicating what is described as gliding motility. Colonies of the human oral strains can have a slight yellow pigment on initial growth, which becomes darker yellow to orange with age. Colonies are also described as having a bluish-purple hue or a metallic sheen on blood agar medium.[39] Others describe colonies as being yellowish-pinkish or bluish speckled.[46] The colonies of the zoonotic strains are not usually pigmented.

A number of methods are employed to identify these isolates to species—conventional biochemicals, protein profiles, multilocus enzyme electrophoresis, serotyping of immunoglobulin A1 proteases, DNA probes, 16S rRNA PCR restriction fragment length polymorphism analysis, and 16S rRNA gene sequencing.[11] Unfortunately, most current commercial identification kits are unable to identify this organism as to genus and species. One package insert cautions the laboratorian to consider specimen source, atmospheric preferences, Gram stain characteristics, and growth on selective agar when using their product.[48] Table 234-1 lists some biochemical tests that can help differntiate the main *Capnocytophaga* groups. A combination of some

conventional biochemical tests with 16S rRNA gene sequencing can be useful in identifying organisms as to species.[23]

Treatment

Capnocytophaga species are broadly susceptible to many antimicrobial agents. Because occasional strains produce β-lactamase, a penicillin–β-lactamase combination or a third-generation cephalosporin is the drug of first choice for parenteral therapy. Ampicillin-clavulanate, piperacillin-tazobactam, ceftriaxone, cefepime, or ceftazidime could all be useful. For oral therapy of milder infections, clindamycin, doxycycline, or a fluoroquinolone would be indicated. Carbapenems could be indicated in mixed soft tissue infections with more resistance organisms than *Capnocytophaga* species. Aminoglycosides, antistaphylococcal penicillins, colistin, and first-generation cephalosporins are not considered useful.

Because it may take at least several days before *Capnocytophaga* spp. can be presumptively recognized, clinicians should keep this organism in mind in cases if there is a history of dog or cat bite or with neutropenic patients with oral mucositis or peridontitis. This is especially true if the patient is asplenic or has a history of alcohol abuse.

Jolivet-Gougeon and colleagues[49] have reported an extensive review of the literature describing *Capnocytophaga* spp. and their susceptibility patterns. There is no standardized method of susceptibility testing for *Capnocytophaga* spp. They speculated that the differing methods used by researchers may explain the varying susceptibility results described in the literature for the same antimicrobial agents. Their review compiled a rather long list of antimicrobial agents that have variable activity against *Capnocytophaga*, including quinolones, metronidazole, vancomycin, aminoglycosides, aztreonam, penicillins, and cephalosporins. Pers and co-workers[39] have described a clindamycin-resistant *C. cynodegmi* isolate that was also resistant to gentamicin and erythromycin. Another case report described a metronidazole-resistant isolate that was successfully treated with linezolid.[50] Maury and colleagues[13] have described a high frequency of β-lactamase–producing bacteremic strains in neutropenic patients and von Graevenitz and associates[47] additionally reported that *Capnocytophaga* isolates are resistant to aminoglycosides and colistin. Despite the difficulties with obtaining susceptibility patterns for these organisms, a number of authors suggest doing antimicrobial susceptibility testing on patients' isolates if at all possible.

Prevention

Awareness and education are the most effective ways to prevent *Capnocytophaga* infections. Heightened awareness of clinicians of patient risk factors and of laboratories isolating and identifying *Capnocytophaga* organisms can reduce the time to diagnosis and result in more specific antimicrobial treatment. Rapid presumptive diagnosis may result in the patient receiving better targeted antibiotics for these organisms before a conclusive diagnosis is confirmed. High-risk factor subjects, particularly those without a spleen, can be made aware of activities that increase their risk of developing a *Capnocytophaga* infection.[51]

REFERENCES

1. Frandsen EVG, Poulsen K, Könönen E, et al. Diversity of *Capnocytophaga* species in children and description of *Capnocytophaga leadbetteri* sp. nov. and *Capnocytophaga* genospecies AHN8471. *J Syst Evol Microbiol.* 2008;58:324-336.
2. Bernardet J-F, Nakagawa Y, Holmes B. Proposed minimal standards for describing new taxa of the family *Flavobacteriaceae* and amended description of the family. *Int J Syst Evol Microbiol.* 2002;52:1049-1070.
3. Spratt DA, Greenman J, Schaffer AG. *Capnocytophaga gingivalis* aminopeptidase: A potential virulence factor. *Microbiology.* 1995;141:3087-3093.
4. Reinholdt J, Kilian M. Comparative analysis of immunoglobulin A1 protease activity among bacteria representing different genera, species, and strains. *Infect Immun.* 1997;65:4452-4459.

5. Fischer LJ, Weyant RS, White EH, et al. Intracellular multiplication and toxic destruction of cultured macrophages by *Capnocytophaga canimorsus*. *Infect Immun.* 1995;63:3484-3490.
6. Shin H, Mally M, Kuhn M, et al. Escape from immune surveillance by *Capnocytophaga canimorsus*. *J Infect Dis.* 2007;195:375-386.
7. Pers C, Gahrn-Hansen B, Frederiksen W. *Capnocytophaga canimorsus* septicemia in Denmark, 1982-1995: Review of 39 cases. *Clin Infect Dis.* 1996;23:71-75.
8. Bonatti H, Rossboth DW, Nachbaur D, et al. A series of infections due to *Capnocytophaga* spp. in immunosuppressed and immunocompetent patients. *Clin Microbiol Infect.* 2003;9:380-387.
9. Fredricks DN, Schubert MM, Myerson D. Molecular identification of invasive gingival bacterial community. *Clin Infect Dis.* 2005;41:e1-e4.

10. Ciantar M, Gilthorpe MS, Hurel SJ, et al. *Capnocytophaga* spp. in periodontitis manifesting diabetes mellitus. *J Periodontol.* 2005;76:194-203.
11. Ciantar M, Newman HN, Wilson M, et al. Molecular identification of *Capnocytophaga* spp. via 16S rRNA PCR-restriction fragment length polymorphism analysis. *J Clin Microbiol.* 2005;43:1894-1901.
12. Martino R, Rámila E, Capdevila JA, et al. Bacteremia caused by *Capnocytophaga* species in patients with neutropenia and cancer: Results of a multicenter study. *Clin Infect Dis.* 2001;33:e20-e22.
13. Maury S, Leblanc T, Rousselot P, et al. Bacteremia due to *Capnocytophaga* species in patients with neutropenia: high frequency of β-lactamase–producing strains. *Clin Infect Dis.* 1999;28:1172-1174.

14. Warren JS, Allen SD. Clinical, pathogenic, and laboratory features of *Capnocytophaga* infections. *Am J Clin Pathol.* 1986; 86:513-518.
15. Campbell JR, Edwards MS. *Capnocytophaga* species infections in children. *Pediatr Infect Dis J.* 1991;10:944-948.
16. Joliet-Gougeon A, Tamani-Shacoori Z, Desbordes L, et al. Prevalence of oropharyngeal beta-lactamase–producing *Capnocytophaga* spp. in pediatric oncology patients over a ten-year period. *BMC Infect Dis.* 2005;5:32-36.
17. Desai SS, Harrison RA, Murphy MD. *Capnocytophaga ochracea* causing severe sepsis and purpura fulminans in an immunocompetent patient. *J Infect.* 2007;54:e107-e109.
18. Gutierrez-Martin MA, Araji OA, Barquero JM, et al. Aortic valve endocarditis by *Capnocytophaga haemolytica*. *Ann Thorac Surg.* 2007;84:1008-1010.
19. Wang H-K, Chen Y-C, Teng L-J, et al. Brain abscess associated with multidrug-resistant *Capnocytophaga ochracea* infection. *J Clin Microbiol.* 2007;45:645-647.
20. Alexandrakis G, Palma LA, Miller D, et al. *Capnocytophaga* keratitis. *Ophthalmology.* 2000;107:1503-1506.
21. Howlett AA, Mailman TL, Ganapathy V. Early cystic lung disease in a premature neonate with perinatally acquired *Capnocytophaga*. *J Perinatol.* 2007;27:68-70.
22. Blanche P, Bloch E, Sicard D. *Capnocytophaga canimorsus* in the oral flora of dogs and cats. *J Infect.* 1998;36:134.
23. Janda JM, Graves MH, Lindquist D, et al. Diagnosing *Capnocytophaga canimorsus* infections. *Emerg Infect Dis.* 2006;12:340-342.
24. Lion C, Escande F, Burdin JC. *Capnocytophaga canimorsus* infections in human: Review of the literature and cases report. *Eur J Epidemiol.* 1996;12:521-533.
25. Lipsker D, Kara F. Images in clinical medicine. Retiform purpura. *N Engl J Med.* 2008;358:e1.
26. Deshmukh PM, Camp CJ, Rose FB, et al. *Capnocytophaga canimorsus* sepsis with purpura fulminans and symmetrical gangrene following a dog bite in a shelter employee. *Am J Med Sci.* 2004;327:369-372.
27. Hicklin H, Verghese A, Alvarez S. Dysgonic fermenter 2 septicemia. *Rev Infect Dis.* 1987;9:884-890.
28. Job L, Horman JT, Grigor JK et al. Dysgonic fermenter-2: A clinico-epidemiologic review. *J Emerg Med.* 1989;7:185-192.
29. Azhar SS. What really caused this woman's *Capnocytophaga canimorsus* septicemia? *Infect Med.* 2007;24:251-253.
30. McLean CR, Hargrove R, Behn E. Case study: The first fatal case of *Capnocytophaga canimorsus* sepsis caused by a cat scratch. *J R Nav Med Serv.* 2004;90:13-15.
31. Mirza I, Wolk J, Toth L, et al. Waterhouse-Friderichsen syndrome secondary to *Capnocytophaga canimorsus* septicemia and demonstration of bacteremia by peripheral blood smear. *Arch Pathol Lab Med.* 2000;124:859-863.
32. Mulder AH, Gerlag PGG, Verhoef LHM, et al. Hemolytic uremic syndrome after *Capnocytophaga canimorsus* (DF-2) septicemia. *Clin Nephrol.* 2001;55:167-170.
33. Kok RHJ, Wolfhagen MJHM, Moot BM, et al. A patient with thrombotic thrombocytopenic purpura caused by *Capnocytophaga canimorsus* septicemia. *Clin Microbiol Infect.* 1999;5:297-298.
34. Low SC-M, Greenwood JE. *Capnocytophaga canimorsus*: Infection, septicemia, recovery and reconstruction. *J Med Microbiol.* 2008;57:901-903.
35. Le Moal G, Landron C, Robert R, et al. Meningitis due to *Capnocytophaga canimorsus* after receipt of a dog bite: case report and review of the literature. *Clin Infect Dis.* 2003;36:e42-e46.
36. de Boer MGJ, Lambregts PCLA, van Dam AP, et al. Meningitis caused by *Capnocytophaga canimorsus*: when to expect the unexpected. *Clin Neurol Neurosurg.* 2007;109:393-398.
37. Sandoe JAT. *Capnocytophaga canimorsus* endocarditis. *J Med Microbiol.* 2004;53:245-248.
38. Khawari AA, Myers JW, Ferguson DA Jr, et al. Sepsis and meningitis due to *Capnocytophaga cynodegmi* after splenectomy. *Clin Infect Dis.* 2005;40:1709-1710.
39. Pers C, Tvedegaard E, Christensen JJ, et al. *Capnocytophaga cynodegmi* peritonitis in a peritoneal dialysis patient. *J Clin Microbiol.* 2007;45:3844-3846.
40. Wald K, Martinez A, Moll S. *Capnocytophaga canimorsus* infection with fulminant sepsis in an asplenic patient: diagnosis by review of peripheral blood smear. *Am J Hematol.* 2008;83:879.
41. Wasserman D, Asbell PA, Friedman AJ, et al. *Capnocytophaga ochracea* chronic blepharoconjunctivitis. *Cornea.* 1995;14:533-535.
42. Hayashi F, Okada M, Zhong X, et al. PCR detection of *Capnocytophaga* species in dental plaque samples from children aged 2 to 12 years. *Microbiol Immunol.* 2001;45:17-22.
43. Shawar R, Sepulveda J, Clarridge JF. Use of the RapID-ANA system and sodium polyanetholesulfonate disk susceptibility testing in identifying *Haemophilus ducreyi*. *J Clin Microbiol.* 1990;28:108-111.
44. Rand KH, Tillan M. Errors in interpretation of Gram stains from positive blood cultures. *Am J Clin Pathol.* 2006; 126:686-690.
45. Ciantar M, Spratt DA, Neumann HN, et al. Assessment of five culture media for the growth and isolation of *Capnocyophaga* spp. *Eur J Clin Microbiol Infect Dis.* 2001;7:158-160.
46. Jousimies-Somer H, Summanen MS, Citron DM, et al. *Wadsworth-KTL Anaerobic Bacteriology Manual*, 6th ed. Belmont, CA: Star Publishing; 2002; 98, 184.
47. von Graevenitz A, Zbinden R, Mutters R. *Actinobacillus, Capnocytophaga, Eikenella, Kingella, Pasteurella*, and other fastidious or rarely encountered gram-negative rods. In: Murray PR, Baron EJ, Jorgensen JH, et al, eds. *Manual of Clinical Microbiology.* 9th ed. Washington, DC: ASM Press; 2007;621-635.
48. Remel. RapID ANA II System, package insert, rev. December 1, 2004.
49. Jolivet-Gougeon A, Sixou J-L, Tamanai-Shacoori Z, et al. Antimicrobial treatment of *Capnocytophaga* infections. *Int J Antimicrob Agents.* 2007;29:367-373.
50. Sabbatani S, Manfredi R, Frank G, et al. *Capnocytophaga* spp. Brain abscess in an immunocompetent host: Problems with antimicrobial chemotherapy and literature review. *J Chemother.* 2004;16:497-501.
51. Brigden ML. Detection, education and management of the asplenic or hyposplenic patient. *Am Family Physician.* 2001; 63:499-506.

235

Bartonella, Including Cat-Scratch Disease

LEONARD N. SLATER | DAVID F. WELCH

Background and Classification

Members of the class Alphaproteobacteria and family Bartonellaceae, the genus *Bartonella*, are closely related to the genera *Brucella* and *Agrobacterium* on the basis of 16S ribosomal RNA (rRNA) similarity; members of the family Rickettsiaceae are more distantly related. On the basis of genetic similarity,[1,2] unification of the genera *Bartonella* and *Rochalimaea* as a single genus and the removal of the family Bartonellaceae from the order Rickettsiales were put forth in 1993.[2] The similarity of *Bartonella* to the classic pathogen *Brucella* has been further substantiated through whole genome sequencing showing that *Bartonella* contains a reduced version of the chromosomal elements of *Brucella melitensis*.[3]

The genus *Bartonella*, synonymous with *Bartonia*, was described in 1913 and referred to the erythrocyte-adherent organisms originally described by Dr. A. L. Barton in 1909.[4,5] The type species is *Bartonella bacilliformis*. Limited to the Andes mountain regions of South America, *B. bacilliformis* infection had received little attention outside its endemic zone in recent years until related bacteria, originally classified in the genus *Rochalimaea*, were found to be pathogens in acquired immunodeficiency syndrome (AIDS) and then in other circumstances.

The former genus *Rochalimaea*, previously grouped with *Bartonella* in the order Rickettsiales, had long contained only two member species, *Rochalimaea vinsonii*, the "Canadian vole agent," and *Rochalimaea quintana* (other synonyms: *Rickettsia quintana*, *Rickettsia pediculi*, *Rickettsia wolhynica*, *Rickettsia weigl*, *Burnetia* [*Rocha-limae*] *wolhynica*, and *Wolhynia quintanae*),[6,7] the agent of trench fever, a debilitating but self-limited human illness so named after it affected many military personnel in World War I.[8] Except for sporadic outbreaks, trench fever had all but disappeared from the clinical scene in recent decades. However, *R. quintana* reemerged in the 1990s as a pathogen of considerable interest[9-13] coincident with the discovery of two related species pathogenic to humans, originally named *Rochalimaea henselae* and *Rochalimaea elizabethae*.[14-17]

In 1995, a further merger of a number of species of the genus *Grahamella*, which are intraerythrocytic pathogens of rodents, birds, fish, and other animals, into the genus *Bartonella* took place.[18] Additional species and subspecies since have been identified,[19-25] and some not previously recognized as human pathogens have become newly associated with infections in humans.[26,27]

Although *Bartonella* spp. have been characterized recently as "emerging" pathogens, DNA analysis of dental pulp provides evidence that *Bartonella henselae* and *Bartonella quintana* have existed since antiquity.[28,29]

A list of validated and recently described[30-34] members of the genus *Bartonella* is provided in Table 235-1.

Epidemiology of the Common Human-Pathogenic Species

Bartonella species are primarily infectious agents of nonhuman animals. Humans are incidental hosts in most cases (even though animal hosts of *B. bacilliformis* and *B. quintana* have not yet been identified), with transmission via arthropod vectors or direct inoculation.

Presumably as a result of the limited distribution of sand fly vectors (genus *Lutzomyia* [formerly *Phlebotomus*]), natural transmission of *B. bacilliformis* infections occurs only at altitudes of 1 to 3 km in the Andes mountains. Even in the modern antibiotic era, focal outbreaks continue. *B. quintana* is globally distributed. Outbreaks of trench fever (also known as Wolhynia fever, Meuse fever, His-Werner disease, shin bone fever, shank fever, and quintan or 5-day fever) have been focal and widely separated, often associated with conditions of poor sanitation and personal hygiene, which may predispose to exposure to *Pediculus humanus*, the human body louse, *B. quintana*'s only identified vector. No nonhuman vertebrate reservoirs have been identified for *B. bacilliformis* or *B. quintana*.

B. henselae is globally endemic; serologic studies indicate that infection of domestic cats is worldwide, with the prevalence of antibodies being higher in warm, humid climates. Free-ranging and captive wild felids in California also have a substantial prevalence of antibodies reactive with *B. henselae*,[35] although infection with other *Bartonella* species could result in cross-reactive antibodies. Rates of bacteremia in cats can vary[36-39] but generally tend to be higher among feral animals in any particular locale. *B. henselae* bacteremia has been documented in healthy domestic cats that have been specifically associated with bacillary angiomatosis (BA)[37] or typical cat-scratch disease (CSD)[38,40] in their human contacts.

Transmission of *B. henselae* to humans has been linked to cats by serologic and epidemiologic studies,[41-44] its culture recovery from the lymphadenitis of CSD,[38,45] and its identification by polymerase chain reaction (PCR)-based DNA identification in further cases of CSD lymphadenitis[46-48] and conjunctival disease,[49] as well as in CSD skin test antigen.[50,51]

The major arthropod vector of *B. henselae* is the cat flea, *Ctenocephalides felis*, as evidenced by epidemiologic associations,[38,42,44] identification of *B. henselae* by culture and DNA amplification from such fleas,[36,38] and transmission of *B. henselae* among cats by such fleas under controlled experimental conditions.[52] Cat fleas appear to serve primarily as vectors for cat-to-cat transmission; their contribution to human infection is not as yet defined. Additional *Bartonella* species also have been identified in cat fleas.[53] Other types of fleas, as well as ixodid and *Dermacentor* ticks, have been found to harbor various *Bartonella* species.[54-58]

Both *Bartonella clarridgeiae* and *Bartonella koehlerae* are widespread agents of asymptomatic infection of cats,[19,20,22] capable of occasional transmission to humans and the uncommon cause of illness.[21,27] Because there has been only a single human isolate of *B. elizabethae*, little is known of its epidemiology, except that its DNA has been amplified from the blood of dogs.[59]

Clinical Manifestations of the Common Human-Pathogenic Species

OROYA FEVER AND VERRUGA PERUANA: *BARTONELLA BACILLIFORMIS*

The long-suspected link between Oroya fever and verruga peruana was confirmed tragically in 1885 by Daniel Carrión, a medical student who injected himself with blood from a verruga peruana lesion and subsequently died of "Oroya fever."[60] The eponym "Carrión's disease" has since denoted the full spectrum of *B. bacilliformis* infection.

TABLE 235-1	Bartonella Species as Currently Recognized for Potential as Human Pathogens

Common as Human Pathogens

Bartonella bacilliformis
Bartonella henselae
Bartonella quintana

Uncommon or Suspected as Human Pathogens

Bartonella alsatica
Bartonella koehlerae
Bartonella clarridgeiae
Bartonella elizabethae
Bartonella grahamii
Bartonella rochalimae
Bartonella tamiae
Bartonella vinsonii subsp. *arupensis*
Bartonella vinsonii subsp. *berkhoffii*

Not Recognized as Human Pathogens

Bartonella australis
Bartonella birtlesii
Bartonella bovis
Bartonella capreoli
Bartonella chomelii
Bartonella doshiae
Bartonella peromysci
Bartonella phoceensis
Bartonella rattimassiliensis
Bartonella schoenbuchensis
Bartonella talpae
Bartonella taylorii
Bartonella tribocorum
Bartonella vinsonii subsp. *vinsonii*

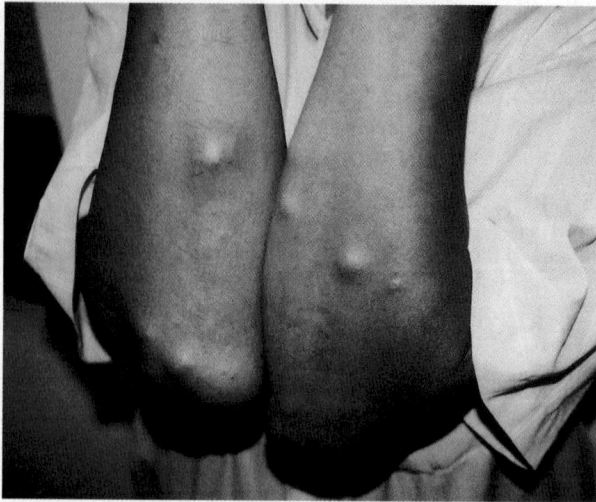

Figure 235-1 Multiple nodular subcutaneous lesions of verruga peruana in an inhabitant of the Peruvian Andes. Localization of such nodular eruptions about the flexures of the elbows and knees, as well as on the thighs and legs, is especially common. (*Courtesy of Dr. J. M. Crutcher, Oklahoma State Department of Health, Oklahoma City.*)

Oroya fever, an acute hematologic disease resulting from primary bacteremia, develops 3 to 12 weeks after inoculation.[61] In its mildest, insidiously developing form, a febrile illness can last less than a week and may go unrecognized (giving rise to subsequent cutaneous manifestations that are the first recognized clinical findings).[62-64] When illness is abrupt in onset, high fever, chills, diaphoresis, anorexia, prostration, headache, and mental status changes are associated with rapidly developing, profound anemia resulting from bacterial invasion, causing shortened life span and destruction of erythrocytes.[64-67] Intense myalgias and arthralgias, abdominal pain and emesis, jaundice, lymphadenopathy, thrombocytopenia, and complications such as seizures, delirium, meningoencephalitis, obtundation, dyspnea, hepatic/gastrointestinal dysfunction, and angina pectoris can occur during this stage,[64,68,69] most believed to be a consequence of the anemia and of microvascular thrombosis, resulting in end-organ ischemia.

Without antimicrobial therapy, fatalities are high for the severe, abrupt form of hematic illness.[68] With appropriate treatment in the modern era, mortality is reported to be less than 10%.[64] For survivors, convalescence is associated with a decline of fever and disappearance of bacteria on blood smears but also a temporarily increased susceptibility to subsequent (opportunistic) infections such as salmonellosis[64,69,70] or toxoplasmosis.[64,71,72] Asymptomatic persistent bacteremia with *B. bacilliformis* infection can occur in up to 15% of survivors of acute infection.[73] They may serve as the organism's reservoir. Whereas some modern era reports paint a picture of similar patterns of *recognized* disease,[64] others suggest that initial infection may more often be asymptomatic or mild than was previously believed.[63,74]

The eruptive phase of *B. bacilliformis* infection, "verruga peruana" lesions, usually becomes evident within weeks to months of resolution of acute infection if it was not treated with antibiotics. This late-stage manifestation is characterized by crops of skin lesions marked by an evolution of stages[64,65]: miliary, then nodular (Fig. 235-1), then mulaire (Fig. 235-2). Mulaire lesions are the most superficial and obviously blood filled of the eruptive manifestations, often bulbous, engorged with blood, and prone to ulceration and bleeding. Mucosal and internal lesions can also occur. Healing at a particular skin site, often punctuated by recurrences, usually takes place over several weeks to 3

or 4 months subsequently, and fibrosis of mulaire lesions may occur. The nodules may develop at one site while receding at another. Histology of active lesions demonstrates neovascular proliferation with occasional bacteria evident in interstitial spaces. Bacterial invasion of/replication within endothelial cells (long believed to be the cause of cytoplasmic inclusions first described by Rocha-Lima) is actually rare.[75]

BACTEREMIC ILLNESS AND ENDOCARDITIS: *BARTONELLA QUINTANA*, *BARTONELLA HENSELAE*, AND OTHER SPECIES

Acute mortality resulting from bacteremia with non-*bacilliformis* *Bartonella* species, even when persistent, is apparently uncommon. In recent years, *B. quintana* bacteremic infection outside of the context of human immunodeficiency virus (HIV) infection has been identified

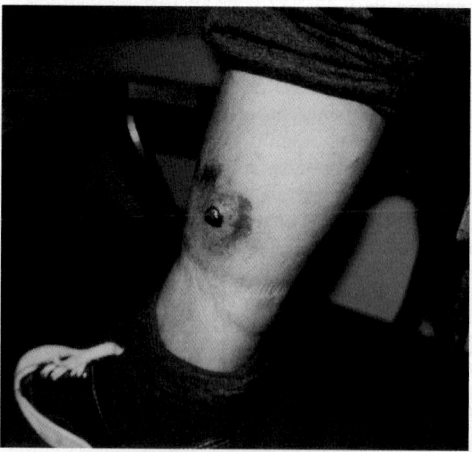

Figure 235-2 A single large mulaire lesion of verruga peruana on the leg of an inhabitant of the Peruvian Andes. Such lesions are prone to superficial ulceration, and copious bleeding may occur as a result of their vascular nature. Ecchymosis of the skin surrounding the lesion is also evident. (*Courtesy of Dr. J. M. Crutcher, Oklahoma State Department of Health, Oklahoma City.*)

sporadically and in small clusters, mainly in homeless people in North America and Europe.[76,77] "Trench fever" is characterized by a spectrum of self-limited clinical patterns.[7,8] Incubation may span 3 to 38 days before the usually sudden onset of chills and fevers. In the shortest form, a single bout of fever lasts 4 or 5 days. In the more typical periodic form, there are three to five, and sometimes up to eight, febrile paroxysms, each lasting approximately 5 days. The continuous form is manifested by 2 or 3 weeks, and up to 6 weeks, of uninterrupted fever. Afebrile infection is the least common form. Other nonspecific symptoms and signs such as headache, vertigo, retro-orbital pain, conjunctival injection, nystagmus, myalgias, arthralgias, hepatosplenomegaly, rash, leukocytosis, and albuminuria may accompany the illness.

B. quintana or *B. henselae* bacteremia in HIV-infected people is often characterized by insidious development of malaise, body aches, fatigue, weight loss, progressively higher and longer recurring fevers, and, sometimes, headache. Hepatomegaly may occur, but localizing symptoms or physical findings are often lacking. In contrast, *B. henselae* bacteremia in HIV-uninfected people more often may present with abrupt onset of fever, which may persist or become relapsing. Localizing symptoms or physical findings remain unusual.[14,16,78,79] Aseptic meningitis concurrent with bacteremia has been documented.[79,80] Both *B. henselae* and *B. quintana* bacteremia can evolve into long-term persistence if not treated appropriately.[77,79]

B. elizabethae has been isolated only once, as the cause of bacteremia and endocarditis.[17] *B. quintana* and *B. henselae* have been reported increasingly to cause endocarditis, especially of the "blood culture–negative" variety.[10,12,81-88] People with *B. quintana* endocarditis often have been alcoholic and/or homeless, whereas people with *B. henselae* endocarditis more commonly have had cat exposure. In a retrospective study of 101 patients with *Bartonella* endocarditis,[88] presentation was usually subacute but with a significant proportion (17%) of patients afebrile at the time of presentation. Embolic phenomena were reported in 44 (43%) of the patients on presentation. Fifty-eight patients (57%) had previously known valvular heart disease; irrespective of antimicrobial therapy, 76 patients required valvular surgery because of severe valvular damage. Twelve patients ultimately died; 2 were cured only after a relapse, and the remaining 87% were cured with first therapy. Despite the pediatric predominance of CSD, pediatric *B. henselae* endocarditis has been recognized only rarely.[87] Many cases have required valve resection irrespective of antimicrobial use. Diagnoses in blood culture–negative cases have been established with serology, DNA amplification from valve tissue, immunohistochemistry, or all three.

B. vinsonii, generally not considered a human pathogen, has been isolated once, as the cause of bacteremia and fever in an apparently otherwise healthy rancher from the western United States. *B. vinsonii* subsp. *berkhoffii* is now known to be a cause of bacteremia and endocarditis in dogs.[23,24] *Bartonella koehlerae* and *Bartonella alsatica* have each been associated once with endocarditis in humans.[26,27] Febrile, bacteremic illnesses have been identified once with a *B. clarridgeiae*-like isolate in a traveler returning from Peru, where she sustained numerous arthropod bites,[30] and three times with *Bartonella tamiae* in residents of Thailand who had all trapped or killed rats.[32]

BACILLARY ANGIOMATOSIS/PELIOSIS: *BARTONELLA QUINTANA* AND *BARTONELLA HENSELAE*

BA (also referred to as epithelioid angiomatosis or bacillary epithelioid angiomatosis) is a disorder of neovascular proliferation originally described involving skin and regional lymph nodes of HIV-infected people.[89-91] It has been demonstrated since to be able to involve a variety of internal organs, including liver, spleen, bone, brain, lung, bowel, and uterine cervix,[78,92-100] and to occur in other immunocompromised[78,94,101] as well as immunocompetent hosts.[102,103] *B. henselae* and *B. quintana* have been found to be a cause of BA both by direct culture[9,16,36,78,104] and by PCR amplification from tissue of specific DNA sequences.[36,42,101,103,105,106] Either species can cause cutaneous lesions,

but subcutaneous and osseous lesions are more often associated with *B. quintana* and hepatosplenic lesions only with *B. henselae*.[106]

Cutaneous BA lesions often arise in crops, but both the temporal pattern of development and the gross morphologic characteristics can vary. They can be remarkably similar to lesions of verruga peruana, but the major clinical differential diagnoses are usually Kaposi's sarcoma[107] and pyogenic granuloma. In gross appearance, BA skin lesions[108] can be subcutaneous or dermal nodules, or single or multiple dome-shaped, skin-colored or red to purple papules, or both, any of which may display ulceration, serous or bloody drainage, and crusting (Figs. 235-3 and 235-4). Lesions can range in diameter from millimeters to centimeters, number from a few to hundreds, be fixed or freely mobile, be associated with enlargement of regional lymph nodes, involve mucosal surfaces or deeper soft tissues, occur in a variety of distributions, and bleed copiously when incised. Visceral lesions can be quite dramatic as well, in both their number and their heterogeneity of gross appearance (Fig. 235-5). When cutaneous lesions are absent, diagnosis is often delayed because the features associated with visceral involvement (fever, lymphadenopathy, hepatomegaly, splenomegaly, CD4 lymphopenia, anemia, and serum alkaline phosphatase elevation) are nonspecific.[98]

BA is distinguished from other neovascular tumors histologically.[108,109] It consists of lobular proliferations of small blood vessels containing plump, cuboidal endothelial cells interspersed with mixed inflammatory cell infiltrates having neutrophil predominance (Fig. 235-6A and B). Endothelial cell atypia, mitoses, and necrosis may be present. Fibrillar- or granular-appearing amphophilic material is often present in interstitial areas when stained by hematoxylin and eosin (H&E) stain. Warthin-Starry staining or electron microscopy demonstrates these to be clusters of bacilli (see Fig. 235-6C).

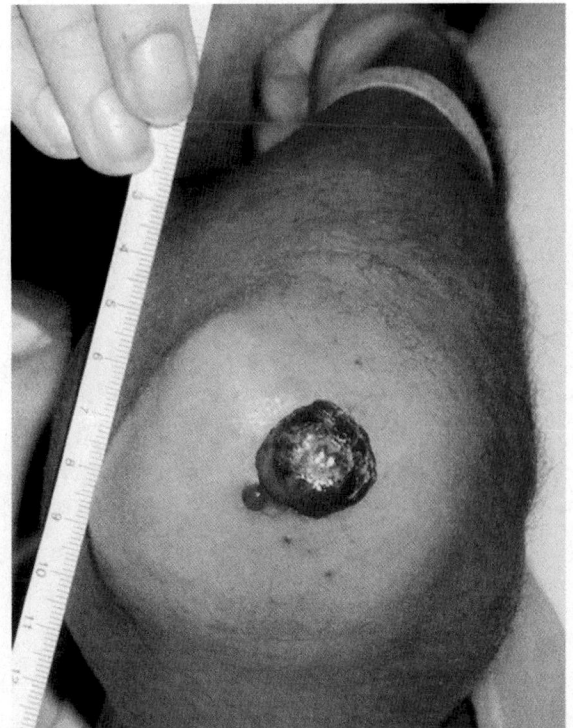

Figure 235-3 A crop of cutaneous bacillary angiomatosis lesions on the elbow of an AIDS patient. The largest lesion, resembling a mulaire lesion of verruga peruana, was of variegated purple color and had an ulcerated surface that wept serous fluid. It began a month earlier as a small cherry angioma-like lesion, much like the three adjacent smaller lesions that had all since erupted within the preceding week. All lesions involuted with doxycycline therapy.

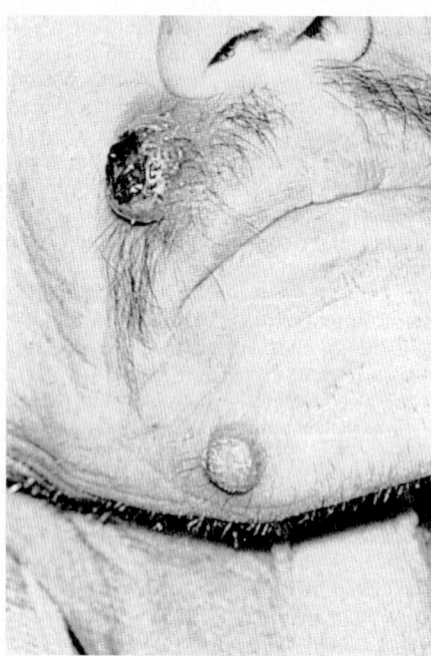

Figure 235-4 Cutaneous bacillary angiomatosis: friable, exophytic nodular lesion with serous crusting and surrounding erythema on upper lip; firm papular lesion with collarette of scale on chin. *(Courtesy of Drs. Jordan W. Tappero, Centers for Disease Control and Prevention, Atlanta, GA; and Jane E. Koehler, University of California at San Francisco.)*

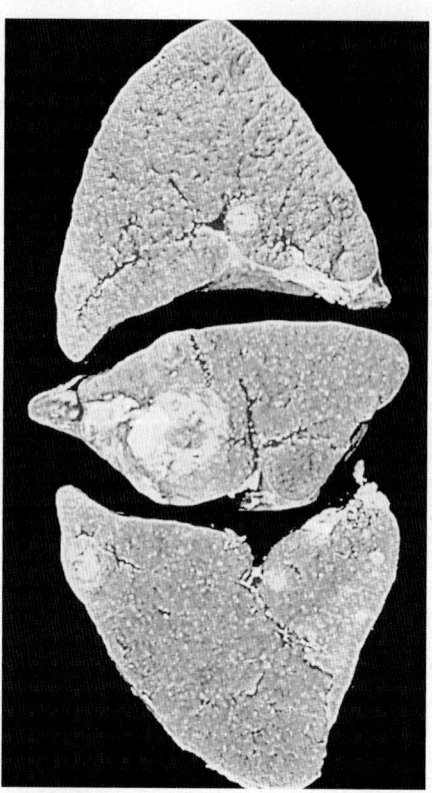

Figure 235-5 **Cut surfaces of the spleen of a pharmacologically immunosuppressed renal transplant recipient.** Numerous *B. henselae*-induced miliary-appearing nodular lesions range in size from millimeters to centimeters, some of the larger of which were necrotic, whereas others contained hemorrhage. Histologic findings included bacillary angiomatosis, bacillary peliosis, and pyogranulomatous changes. *(From Slater LN, Welch DF, Min K-W. Rochalimaea henselae causes bacillary angiomatosis and peliosis hepatis. Arch Intern Med. 1992;152:602-606.)*

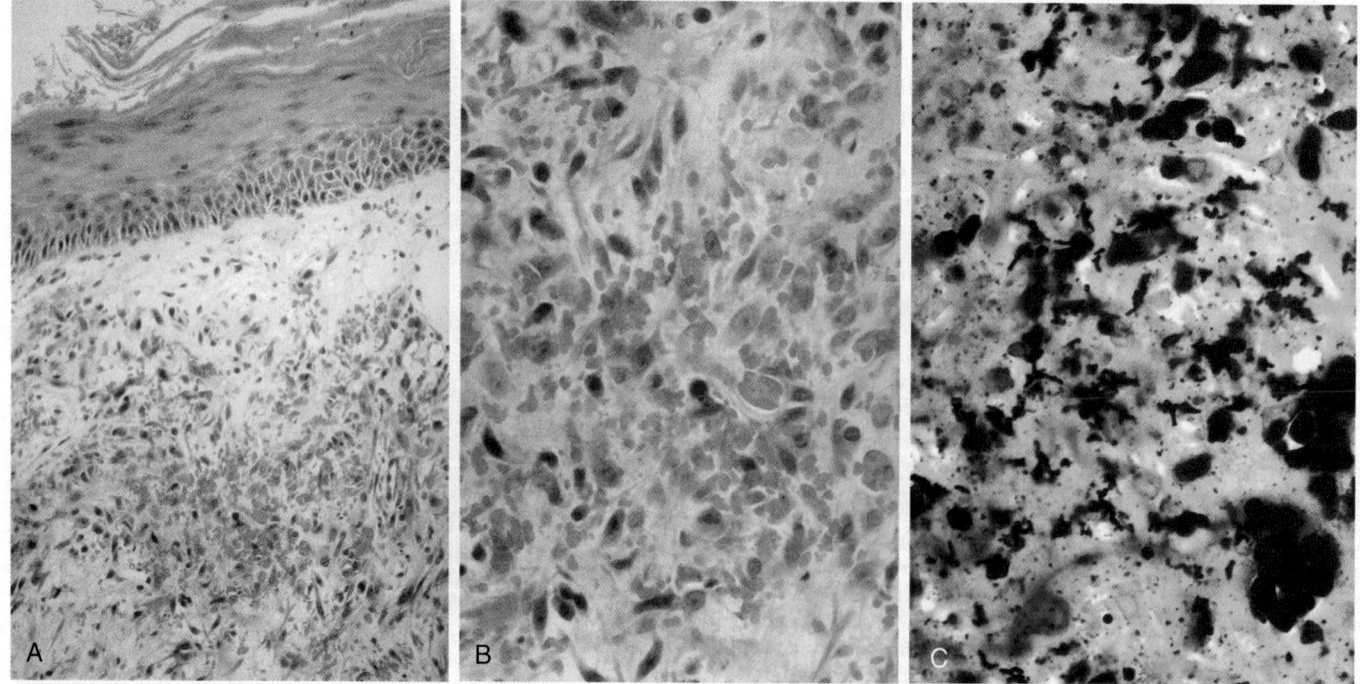

Figure 235-6 **Histology of a cutaneous lesion of bacillary angiomatosis. A,** Increased presence of erythrocytes in the dermis as a result of new capillary formation (H&E stain, original magnification ×40). **B,** Typical cuboidal endothelial cells among the increased number of erythrocytes (H&E stain, original magnification ×200). **C,** Dark-staining bacilli among the dark-staining erythrocytes (Warthin-Starry silver stain, original magnification ×1000).

Bacillary peliosis (BP), originally described involving the liver and sometimes spleen in HIV-infected people,[110] has since been identified in other immunosuppressed people and found to involve lymph nodes as well.[78,111] Involved organs contain numerous blood-filled cystic structures that can range from microscopic to several millimeters in size. H&E-stained tissue reveals partially endothelial cell–lined peliotic spaces often separated from surrounding parenchymal cells by fibromyxoid stroma containing a mixture of inflammatory cells, dilated capillaries, and clumps of granular material. Such clumps are filled with Warthin-Starry–staining bacilli.[110] Molecular epidemiologic investigation has revealed that only *B. henselae* appears to be culpable in this process.[106]

Inflammatory reactions in immunocompromised hosts caused by *B. henselae* infection without associated angiomatosis or peliosis have been reported involving liver, spleen, lymph nodes, heart, lung, and bone marrow.[112,113] They are characterized by nodular collections of lymphocytes and nonepithelioid histiocytes that may become centrally necrotic, containing aggregates of neutrophils and karyorrhexic debris suggestive of microscopic abscess formation.[112,113] These may represent a clinical-pathologic link with CSD.[114]

CAT-SCRATCH DISEASE: *BARTONELLA HENSELAE* AND *BARTONELLA CLARRIDGEIAE*

Among the *Bartonella* species, CSD has been associated nearly exclusively with *B. henselae*. Evidence indicating its cardinal role includes the serologic responses of people with CSD[41,43,44,115]; the identification of *B. henselae* in CSD lymphadenitis by culture,[45] PCR-based DNA amplification,[46-48,116-119] and immunocytochemistry[120]; detection of *B. henselae* in CSD skin test antigens by PCR[50,51]; and the recovery of *B. henselae* from the blood of healthy cats (which can be persistently bacteremic)[36,38,121] and from cat fleas.[36]

The various manifestations comprising CSD have been recognized for more than a century, but "la maladie des griffes de chat" was not defined as a syndrome until 1950.[122] CSD remained an infection in search of an agent for more than 40 years after that. Thus, most cases have been identified by clinical/pathologic criteria, supplemented by reactions to unstandardized skin test antigens in some. It is reasonable to ascribe the majority of CSD cases to *B. henselae* based on the numerous lines of evidence developed in recent years. Yet it remains likely that other agents can cause occasional "typical" CSD cases, such as has been reported with *Afipia felis*[123,124] and *B. clarridgeiae*.[21] (Non-*felis Afipia* spp. have been isolated from only skeletal or pleuropulmonary sites, or both, of one patient each and not in the setting of CSD; their roles as pathogens remain speculative.[123])

CSD is the most commonly recognized manifestation of human infection with *Bartonella*. In the United States, estimated CSD cases approach 25,000 annually.[125] Interestingly, veterinary care personnel do not have evidence of notably higher levels of infection than the general population.[126]

"Typical CSD" represents 88% to 89% of cases overall. A primary cutaneous papule or pustule develops approximately 3 to 10 days after an animal contact (most commonly a kitten or feral cat) at a site of inoculation (usually a scratch or bite) (Fig. 235-7),[127-129] and it may last for 1 to 3 weeks. Regional lymphadenopathy ipsilateral to the inoculation site (mainly head, neck, or upper extremity), which develops in 1 to 7 weeks (Figs. 235-8, 235-9, and 235-10), is the most prominent and common manifestation (>90% of typical cases) and the one that usually precipitates medical evaluation. Even at the time of such presentation, an inoculation site (scratch, bite, or primary papule or pustule) may be detected in more than two thirds of patients when actively sought. One third to 60% of patients may have low-grade fever lasting several days. One fourth of patients may report malaise or fatigue, and approximately 10% report headache or sore throat. Transient rash may occur in approximately 5% of patients. Transient mild leukocytosis, with increased neutrophils and sometimes eosinophils, and elevated erythrocyte sedimentation rate may occur.

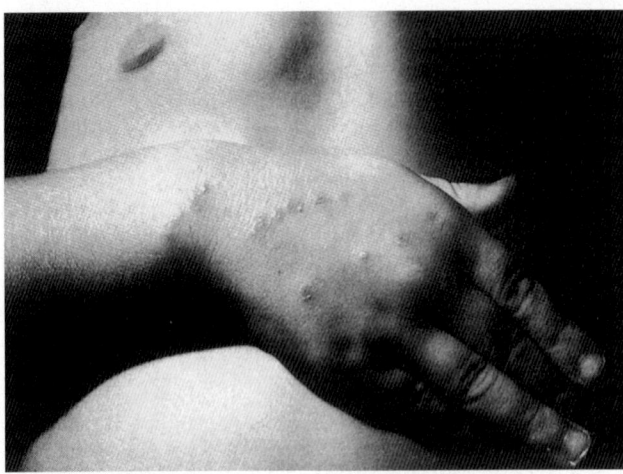

Figure 235-7 A child with typical cat-scratch disease demonstrating the original scratch injuries and the primary papule that soon thereafter developed proximal to the middle finger. *(Courtesy of Dr. V. H. San Joaquin, University of Oklahoma Health Sciences Center, Oklahoma City.)*

Nearly half of typical CSD patients have single lymph node involvement, another 20% have multiple node involvement at one site, and the remaining one third have node involvement at multiple sites. Up to one sixth of patients with typical CSD develop lymph node suppuration. Ultrasonography may assist in the assessment of lymph node size and suppuration,[38,130] and it may be used to direct needle aspiration of pus (usually done to relieve discomfort). Node enlargement usually persists for 2 to 4 months but may last considerably longer; spontaneous resolution is the rule. The histopathology of nodes includes a mixture of nonspecific inflammatory reactions including granulomata and stellate necrosis. Bacilli are best demonstrated by Dieterle, Warthin-Starry, or Steiner staining. Hypercalcemia uncommonly may complicate CSD lymphadenopathy as a result of endogenous overproduction of active vitamin D associated with granuloma formation.[131]

Previously considered to be uncommon in CSD, musculoskeletal manifestations actually occur in more than 10% of cases, as defined in an 11-year surveillance study involving 913 patients with compatible clinical presentation and confirmatory PCR and/or serologic test for

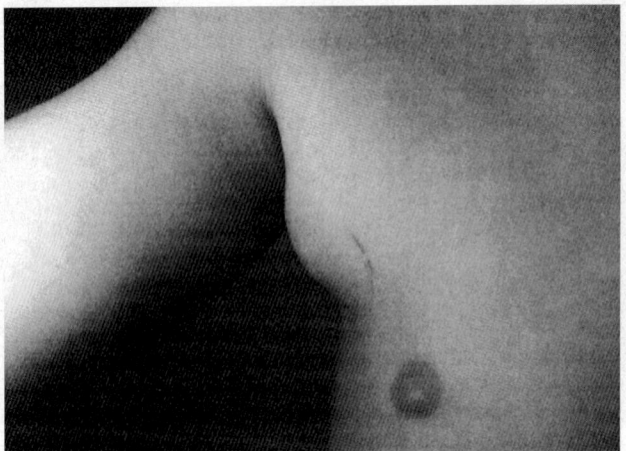

Figure 235-8 Right axillary lymphadenopathy followed the scratches and development of a primary papule in this child with typical cat-scratch disease, also illustrated in Figure 235-7. *(Courtesy of Dr. V. H. San Joaquin, University of Oklahoma Health Sciences Center, Oklahoma City.)*

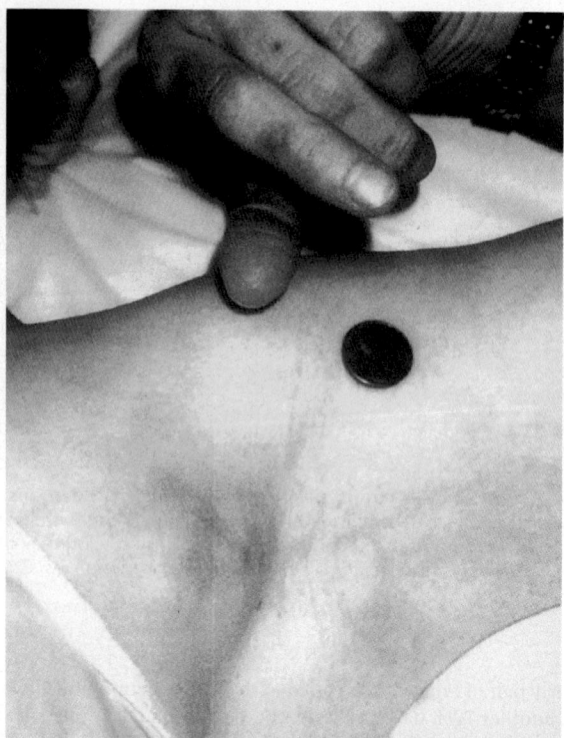

Figure 235-9 **A 45-year-old woman with left axillary CSD lymphadenitis that developed approximately 3 weeks after she sustained a cat scratch on the left index finger, on which the primary papule is still evident.** The U.S. penny was placed in the image for size comparison.

B. henselae.[132] Myalgia occurred in 5.8%, had a median duration of 4 weeks, and was often severe. Arthropathy (arthralgia or arthritis, or both) occurred in 5.5%, involving mainly the medium and large joints for a median of 5.5 weeks and characterized as moderate to severe in intensity in more than half of these patients. In a small proportion, chronic symptoms persisted for more than 1 year and could be debili-

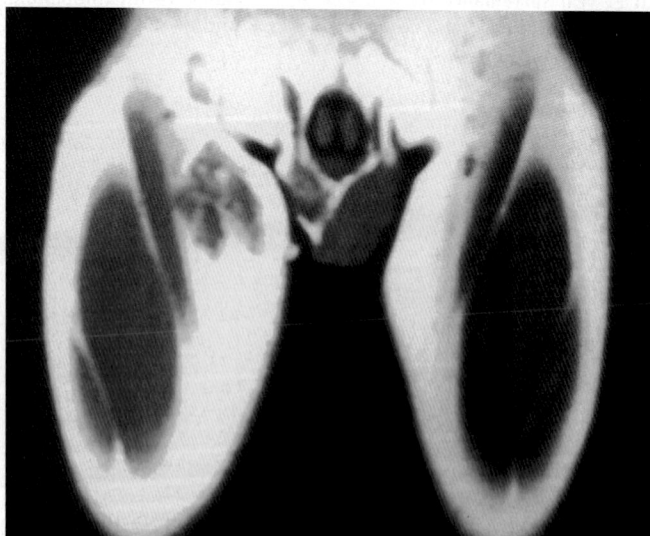

Figure 235-10 **Magnetic resonance imaging of a 25-year-old man who developed a tender, inflamed right groin mass (seen medial to the right sartorius muscle) that ultimately was proven to represent lymph node swelling of CSD lymphadenitis.** He had recently acquired previously feral kittens, which frequently scratched him on the lower extremities as he played with them.

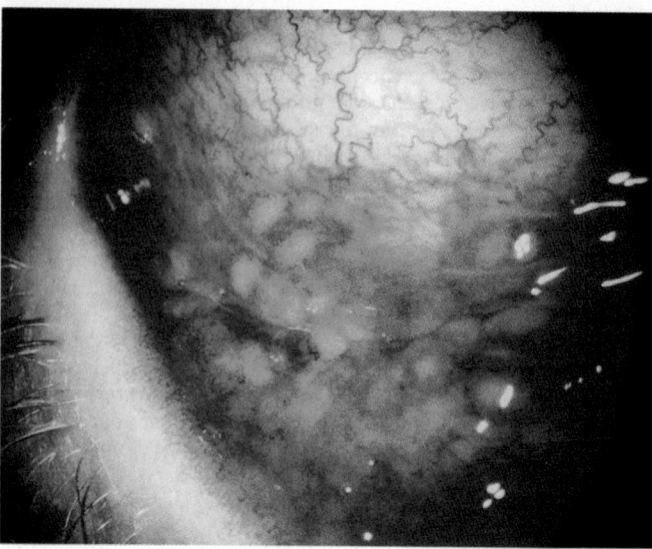

Figure 235-11 **The granulomatous conjunctivitis of Parinaud's oculoglandular syndrome is associated with ipsilateral local lymphadenopathy, usually preauricular and less commonly submandibular.**

tating. Much less commonly, tendonitis, neuralgia, and osteomyelitis were identified, all at a rate of less than 1%. Age older than 20 years increased the risk of having any of these symptoms, and female gender was also associated with increased risk of arthropathy.

Up to half of the overall 11% or 12% of CSD cases that are atypical represent Parinaud's oculoglandular syndrome, a self-limited granulomatous conjunctivitis and ipsilateral, usually preauricular, lymphadenitis (Fig. 235-11).[133,134] Various other "atypical" manifestations[135] include self-limited granulomatous hepatitis/splenitis, atypical pneumonitis,[136] osteitis,[137] and neurologic syndromes (mainly encephalopathy and neuroretinitis). A syndrome of prolonged fever of unknown origin (FUO) in children has been described as well.[138]

Because of the insidious and nonspecific nature of the fever and abdominal pain of CSD hepatitis/splenitis, diagnosis may be delayed until a history of cat exposure prompts ultrasonographic or computed tomographic abdominal imaging, which usually demonstrates multiple hypodense lesions (Fig. 235-12), and serologic testing.[114,139-141]

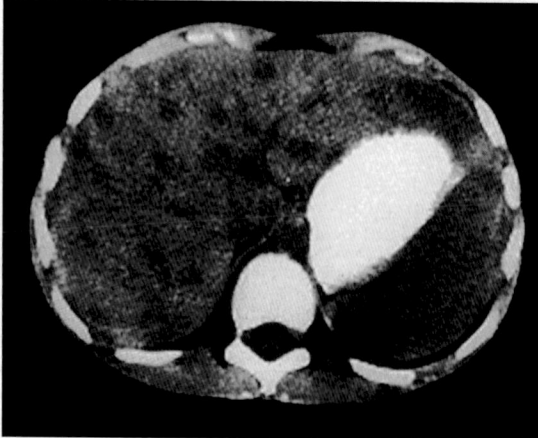

Figure 235-12 **In this computed tomographic image of a patient with hepatic involvement of cat-scratch disease, the absence of enhancement of the multiple lesions after contrast infusion is consistent with the granulomatous inflammation of this entity.** Treated empirically with various antibiotics without improvement before establishment of this diagnosis, the patient subsequently recovered fully with no further antimicrobial therapy. *(Courtesy of Dr. V. H. San Joaquin, University of Oklahoma Health Sciences Center, Oklahoma City.)*

Similarly, the nonspecific nature and rarity of many of the other atypical manifestations besides Parinaud's syndrome may result in delay in their accurate diagnosis until a history of cat exposure or suggestive findings on histopathology prompt specific evaluation directed at *B. henselae*.[127]

A dramatic if infrequent manifestation, encephalopathy, was first reported within a few years of the description and naming of CSD.[142-145] Encephalopathy probably occurs in 2% to 4% of all CSD cases recognized, although estimates range as widely as 1% to 7%.[146] Extrapolating from the estimated U.S. CSD case rate,[125] 500 to 1000 annual CSD encephalopathy cases occur in the United States. Recognition of this phenomenon may increase with the availability of serologic testing and improved blood culture techniques. It remains predominantly a clinical diagnosis, subject to laboratory confirmation by techniques described later (predominantly antibody testing). Adolescents and adults may represent a greater proportion of cases of CSD encephalopathy than they do of CSD overall.[147] Although encephalopathy usually follows the development of lymphadenopathy, it has also been reported to precede lymph node involvement or to occur in its absence. Persistent, generalized headache is a common part of the history, but fever is an inconsistent finding. Patients may become very restless, and combativeness is often described. Nearly half of patients can develop seizures that may range from focal to generalized, and from brief and self-limited to status epilepticus. Short-term anticonvulsant therapy may be required, as may be supportive therapy in the face of obtundation or coma. Concurrent acute neurologic manifestations may be present transiently (e.g., nuchal rigidity, pathologic reflexes, and pupillary dilatation). When they occur, neurologic deficits such as aphasia, cranial nerve palsy, paresis, hemiplegia, and ataxia are also usually self-limited, although time to resolution may span weeks to months to as long as 1 year. However, persistence of intellectual impairment and of seizures has been reported uncommonly.[148-150]

Laboratory studies, such as cerebrospinal fluid (CSF) analysis and culture, generally do not add specific positive diagnostic findings to the clinical picture of CSD encephalopathy but, rather, serve to exclude other processes. Elevations of CSF protein concentration and leukocytes occur in only approximately one third of patients (but do not necessarily coincide in the same patients); lymphocytes predominate. Hypoglycorrhachia is rare. CSF cultures have been consistently negative, even since the recognition of the CSD-*B. henselae* association. Studies of the brain with computed tomography and/or magnetic resonance imaging are usually normal, but a few cases of persistent structural abnormalities have been reported.[149,150] Electroencephalography during the acute phase of CSD encephalopathy commonly reveals diffuse slowing, yet another nonspecific feature that resolves with clinical recovery.

The pathogenesis of CSD encephalopathy and other central nervous system (CNS) manifestations associated with CSD remains unclear. It is unknown whether these rare complications are attributable to direct invasion of the CNS by *B. henselae* or to other mechanisms, such as vasculitis or immune response. *B. henselae* has been shown to infect feline microglial cells in vitro and to survive intracellularly for up to 4 weeks; however, no ultrastructural abnormalities were identified by electron microscopy within the infected brain cells.[151] At autopsy of a rare fatality resulting from CSD meningoencephalitis, there was marked cerebral edema with no gross evidence of acute meningitis. Microscopic examination revealed multiple granulomatous lesions as well as meningitis and encephalitis. Warthin-Starry silver stain of the brain and liver revealed pleomorphic rod-shaped bacilli consistent with *B. henselae*. Analysis of brain tissue with PCR confirmed the presence of *B. henselae* DNA.[152] Another such rare case report of the findings in a 6-year-old child who died with disseminated CSD with encephalitis demonstrated intracerebral histologic findings of perivascular lymphocytic infiltrates and microglial nodules.[153]

Apparently unrelated to CSD encephalopathy is the rare phenomenon of possible tick-transmitted coinfection of humans with *Borrelia burgdorferi* and *B. henselae*, resulting in concurrent CNS symptoms ascribed to chronic Lyme disease.[154]

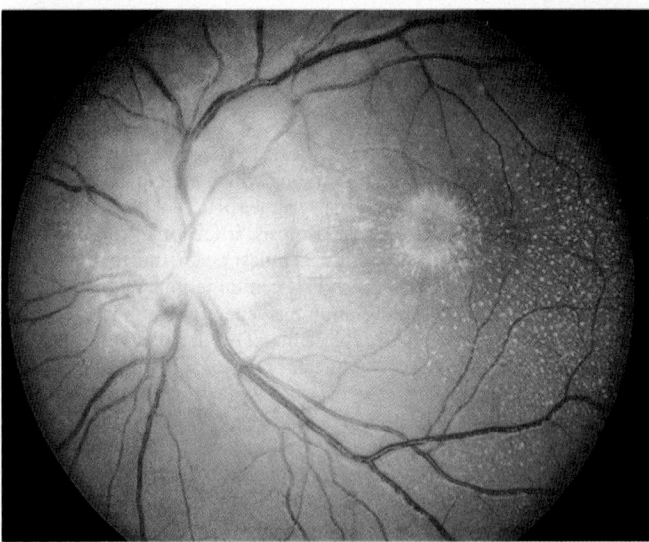

Figure 235-13 Among the most common manifestations of the neuroretinitis of cat-scratch disease, and certainly among the most striking in appearance, is papilledema associated with stellate macular exudates.

Neuroretinitis associated with CSD[80,147,155,156] has been confirmed to be related to *B. henselae*.[80,157] After its description in 1970,[155] neuroretinitis remained for years a clinical diagnosis,[51] but current culture and nonculture techniques for identification of *B. henselae* have improved diagnostic accuracy. *Bartonella grahamii* has been identified once by PCR amplification and sequence analysis in the intraocular fluid of a HIV-seronegative patient with bilateral neuroretinitis and behavioral changes; *B. elizabethae* has been implicated as the pathogen in another patient with neuroretinitis by serologic antibody studies exclusively.[158,159]

Neuroretinitis manifests as fairly sudden loss of visual acuity, usually unilaterally, sometimes preceded by an influenza-like syndrome or development of unilateral lymphadenopathy. The most striking, if not most common, retinal manifestation is papilledema associated with macular exudates in a star formation (Fig. 235-13), first associated with CSD in 1984.[156] Although this manifestation is characteristic of CSD neuroretinitis, it is not pathognomonic; other types of inflammation have also been reported. In a retrospective study of 24 CSD patients with 35 affected eyes, isolated foci of retinitis or choroiditis were the most common ocular manifestation, identified in 83% of eyes and 83% of patients. Optic disk swelling was the second most common finding (46% of eyes and 63% of patients), followed by a macular star (43% of eyes and 63% of patients) and vascular-occlusive events (14% of eyes and 21% of patients). Final visual acuity was 20/25 or better in 26 of 35 eyes (74%) and was similar in both treated and untreated patients.[160] Neuroretinitis usually has a favorable spontaneous course, and the utility of antimicrobial and/or corticosteroid therapy remains debated. Prospective follow-up of recently well-documented cases reveals that some have mild residual visual deficits.[80,161]

Historically, the diagnosis of a case of typical CSD required fulfillment of three of the four following criteria, whereas all four were necessary in an atypical case: (1) history of an animal (usually cat or dog) contact with the presence of a scratch or primary skin or eye lesion; (2) aspiration of "sterile" pus from the lymph node, or culture and other laboratory testing that excluded other etiologic possibilities; (3) a positive CSD skin test; and (4) a lymph node biopsy revealing pathology consistent with CSD. Skin test antigen, originally described by Hanger and Rose, is prepared by 56° C heating for 72 hours of saline-diluted "sterile" pus derived from CSD lymphadenitis. It has never been standardized or produced commercially. It is of historic interest because of its confirmatory role in diagnosis of CSD in the past. However, its potential for transmission of hepatitis viruses, HIV, and prions is a major contemporary concern, even if its sources are well screened. Its use in the era of other avenues of diagnosis is no longer warranted.

The differential diagnosis of typical CSD includes many causes of (unilateral) lymphadenopathy, among which are typical or atypical mycobacterial infection, tularemia, plague, brucellosis, syphilis, sporotrichosis, histoplasmosis, toxoplasmosis, infectious mononucleosis syndromes, lymphoma, and other neoplasms. In the inguinal area, tender adenopathy in the absence of a genital lesion suggests *Staphylococcus aureus*, CSD, lymphogranuloma venereum, and, in the febrile patient with a tick exposure, tularemia. The diagnosis of CSD can be easily overlooked if the clinician fails to obtain an adequate history, especially in the case of the atypical syndromes and not uncommonly in the case of adults with the typical syndrome whose clinicians are inexperienced with CSD. In elderly adults (>60 years old), manifestations tend to be less typical, further confounding the diagnosis.[162] With domestic cats representing the largest category of companion animals in the United States, the importance of an accurate history regarding animal exposure cannot be emphasized enough when evaluating a patient with findings consistent with CSD. Fortunately, in most cases, whether typical or atypical, spontaneous resolution occurs.

HIV-ASSOCIATED NEUROLOGIC SYNDROMES

B. henselae or *B. quintana*, or both, has been implicated in a small proportion of cases of HIV-associated brain lesions, meningoencephalitis, encephalopathy, and neuropsychiatric disease[80,95,163-166] that cannot be ascribed to other causes.

A case of intracerebral BA has been described.[95] *Bartonella* infection associated with neurologic manifestations complicating HIV infection has been demonstrated by serum and CSF antibodies and CSF DNA amplification,[163] although technical limitations prevented accurate species implication in these cases. A study of autopsy brain tissue reported evidence of *B. henselae* by immunofluorescence staining and by PCR amplification in three AIDS dementia patients with elevated CSF:serum indices of *B. henselae*–reactive antibody.[165] A nested case-control study has since confirmed an association between the presence of serum anti-*Bartonella* immunoglobulin M (IgM) (implying recent infection) and increased risk of development of neuropsychological decline or dementia.[166] At least 4% of new cases of HIV-associated dementia or neuropsychological decline were estimated to result from *Bartonella* infections and, therefore, to be potentially treatable with antibiotics. Additional case reports have added anecdotal evidence of the utility of antimicrobials in reversing *Bartonella*-associated neuropsychiatric abnormalities in HIV-infected people.[164]

Pathogenesis

In cats, *B. henselae* appears to be a nearly perfectly adapted parasite, capable of causing long-term and/or cyclic, high-grade bacteremia largely in the absence of illness in its usual hosts.[36,40,52,167-169] Elucidation of mechanisms of this host-parasite relationship is in its infancy. Fundamental knowledge about the pathogenic mechanisms of *Bartonella* species in humans is growing, primarily focused on interactions with erythrocytes and endothelial cells, induction of neoangiogenesis, and mechanisms of survival. Pathogenic mechanisms have been reviewed in greater detail elsewhere.[170]

The pathogenic mechanisms of *Bartonella* spp. involve complex host pathogen interactions. Using antisera from patients infected with *B. quintana*, two-dimensional immunoblotting has identified two dozen consistently recognized immunoreactive antigens from among 60 total membrane proteins identified. Among outer membrane proteins, variable outer membrane proteins (VompA and VompB), hemin-binding protein E, and peptidyl-prolyl *cis-trans*

isomerase were most frequently recognized by the sera, leading to the hypothesis that there is surface expression of these virulence factors during human infection.[171]

B. bacilliformis cells have polar flagella that confer motility and may participate in adhesion to erythrocytes.[172,173] Aggregative fimbriae may also play a role in such adhesion.[174] Erythrocyte invasion involves an extracellular deformin protein, the flagellum, and proteins encoded by the invasion-associated locus (*ialAB*).[173,175-177] Although *B. henselae* does not bind to human erythrocytes in vitro in a manner similar to *B. bacilliformis*, supernatants of in vitro growth of *B. henselae* contain a protein very similar to the deformin of *B. bacilliformis*. Also in a manner similar to *B. bacilliformis*, *B. henselae* outer membrane proteins bind with a number of erythrocyte ghost membrane proteins.[178] The 31-kDa outer membrane protein of *B. henselae* is involved in heme acquisition and may therefore be a virulence factor.[179]

After entry into erythrocytes, *B. bacilliformis* can replicate within and, occasionally, escape from the endosomal vacuoles.[180] Studies from the high-grade feline bacteremia of *B. henselae* have not resolved whether it is truly intra- or extraerythrocytic in cats.[181,182] In humans, the enhanced efficiency of recovery of these pathogens with lysis-type blood cultures suggests some degree of intracellular localization. Through the use of confocal microscopy and monoclonal antibody labeling, *B. quintana* has been shown to be able to invade human erythrocytes, both in vivo and in vitro.[183,184] From electron microscopy, there is evidence that *B. henselae* also infects human erythrocytes.[185] However, the presence of *B. henselae* within human erythrocytes has been demonstrated to be the result of invasion of CD34+ progenitor cells rather than mature erythrocytes.[186]

B. bacilliformis has been demonstrated to stimulate endothelial cell proliferation both in vitro and in vivo, likely through a sheddable stimulatory factor.[187-189] In situ hybridization of clinical specimens of verruga peruana suggests *B. bacilliformis* stimulation of endothelial production of angiopoietin-2 and epidermal production of vascular endothelial growth factor.[190] Similar in vitro proliferative effects can be induced by *B. henselae* and *B. quintana*. *B. henselae* can also induce endothelial cell migration in vitro. The proliferative effects of *B. henselae* are mediated, at least in part, by *Bartonella* adhesin A (BadA), the expression of which is required for bacterial binding to endothelial cells and fibronectin. Expression varies among strains of *B. henselae* due to unknown regulatory mechanisms.[191] In *B. quintana*, expression of the variable outer membrane proteins is required to induce the expression of vascular endothelial growth factor from human macrophage and epithelial cell lines, but Vomp expression does not increase bacterial adherence to the cells.[192] The ability of *B. henselae* and *B. quintana* to induce angiogenesis also appears to depend on their expression of a translocated protein, bepA, which is necessary and sufficient to inhibit vascular endothelial cell apoptosis by causing elevated intracellular levels of cAMP, fostering expression of cAMP-responsive genes.[193]

In the process of endothelial cell invasion by *B. bacilliformis*, the host cell appears to be an active participant through the pathogen's induction of rearrangement of the host's cytoskeleton.[194] *B. quintana* has been demonstrated to invade and multiply within endothelial cells in vitro and in vivo and form intracellular blebs in the process.[195] *B. henselae* interaction with the endothelial cell in vitro results in bacterial aggregation on the cell surface and subsequent engulfment and internalization of the bacterial aggregate by a unique structure, the invasome.[196]

Intracellular survival of *Bartonella* spp. may be facilitated by production of superoxide dismutases[197] and possibly production of stress-response-processing proteases.[198] Also, *B. henselae* and *B. quintana* produce heat shock proteins of the *groEL* genes, which share signature sequences with genes of other gram-negative bacteria known to invade eukaryotic cells.

The inflammatory response elicited by *B. henselae* in CSD appears to be mediated by the effect of the organism on dendritic cells. Introduction of *B. henselae* to dendritic cells in vitro results in rapid internalization of the bacteria by the dendritic cells, followed by their phenotypic maturation and modulation of their chemokine output. The chemokines detected are capable of influencing the development of the CSD granuloma.[199]

Laboratory Diagnosis

Presumptive diagnosis can be made by direct examination of clinical materials in the context of a *Bartonella*-associated syndrome. Definitive diagnosis of *Bartonella*-associated diseases can be achieved through modified conventional bacteriologic culture methods, coculture with endothelial cells, immunoserologic or immunocytochemical means, and/or DNA amplification. Detailed discussion of these techniques is available in other reference sources.[200,201] Approaches that are currently practical for the majority of clinical laboratories are direct examination, culture, and serology. Serologic testing is becoming a mainstay of diagnosis, particularly for that part of the clinical spectrum of diseases occupied by CSD and CNS infection. When two or more criteria are fulfilled among epidemiologic, serologic, histologic, or molecular evidence of *Bartonella*, a firm diagnosis is possible.[202]

DIRECT EXAMINATION

Giemsa-stained blood films are commonly used in endemic locales to detect *B. bacilliformis* in patients with Oroya fever. A wide morphologic range is seen in such smears, with the organisms appearing as red-violet rods or rounded forms, occurring singly or in groups and associated with erythrocytes. Bacilli are the most typical, measuring 0.25 to 0.5 by 1.0 to 3.0 μm. The cells are often curved and may show uni- or bipolar enlargement and granules. Rounded organisms measure approximately 0.75 μm in diameter, and a ringlike variety is sometimes abundant.[203] Although appearing adherent to erythrocytes by light microscopy, bacteria also have been observed within erythrocytes when viewed by electron microscopy.[204] Rarely do blood smears reveal species other than *B. bacilliformis* in patients bacteremic with *Bartonella*. The magnitude of human bacteremia associated with *B. henselae/B. quintana* does not typically afford direct observation of bacteria in blood smears; however, direct immunofluorescence may occasionally be positive.[205]

Bartonella spp. are gram-negative, are not acid fast, and stain poorly or not at all in tissue other than by silver impregnation techniques (e.g., Warthin-Starry, Steiner, and Dieterle stains). *B. henselae* and *B. quintana* are demonstrable by Warthin-Starry staining in BA/BP; *B. henselae* may be silver stained during the early stages of lymphadenopathy in CSD but typically not during the later granulomatous stage of inflammation. Species-specific direct detection of organisms in tissue by immunocytochemical labeling has also been described,[87,122,120,206] but reagents for such labeling are not widely available.

SPECIMEN COLLECTION AND HANDLING FOR CULTURE

The sources from which isolation is attempted most commonly are blood and tissue. The time interval from collection to processing should be minimized. If storage of specimens is necessary, they should be frozen. A controlled study of the effects of blood collection and handling methods has shown that blood specimens from *B. henselae*-infected cats that were collected in either ethylenediaminetetraacetic acid (EDTA) or Isolator (Wampole, Cranbury, NJ) blood-lysis tubes yielded good recovery, and that blood collected in tubes containing EDTA could be plated after 26 days at -65°C with no loss of sensitivity.[207] Whenever possible, specimens should be collected prior to antimicrobial therapy, especially with the tetracyclines and macrolides. Growth of *B. henselae* is also inhibited by concentrations of sodium polyanethol sulfonate (SPS) that are used in blood culture media.[200] The precaution of adding agents to neutralize SPS toxicity or using resin-containing media (primarily to lyse erythrocytes) should be taken if blood is cultured in commercial systems. Lytic blood culture systems (e.g., Isolator) combine the advantageous effect of neutralizing SPS toxicity by hemoglobin freed from erythrocytes with the potential release of intracellular organisms.

CULTURE

All *Bartonella* spp. can be cultured on cell-free media, unlike members of the order Rickettsiales. Recovery of *Bartonella* spp. is optimized using freshly prepared rabbit-heart infusion agar plates.[208] However, various formulations of blood or chocolate agar will support their growth, with the best results dependent on media freshness. Approaches used for recovery of other fastidious pathogens are generally suitable, except that most isolates require more than 7 days of incubation before they can be detected. Therefore, routine bacterial culture protocols rarely allow *Bartonella* spp. to be detected. Protocols designed to yield other slowly growing organisms (e.g., *Histoplasma capsulatum* or *Mycobacterium avium* complex on noninhibitory media) can also result in recovery of *Bartonella* spp. Cultures are not recommended to diagnose most cases of CSD, and in fact the sensitivity is at best only 20% compared to PCR assays.[209] Attempted isolation of *Bartonella* spp. may be useful in the settings of (1) FUO or neuroretinitis after cat exposure; (2) fever, lymphadenitis, neuroretinitis, or encephalitis of unknown origin in the immunocompromised patient; (3) endocarditis without recovery of typical pathogens; and (4) bacillary angiomatosis/peliosis.

Inoculated media should be incubated at 35° to 37°C under conditions of 5% to 10% CO_2 and greater than 40% humidity. (*B. bacilliformis* and possibly some strains of *B. clarridgeiae* spp. have a lower [25° to 30°C] optimal temperature for growth.) The medium should be as freshly prepared as possible. Plates sealed after 24 hours of incubation with plastic film or shrink wrap to preserve moisture content of the media can usually be incubated up to 30 days without notable deterioration.

Although *Bartonella* spp. usually grow best on solid or semisolid media, there are alternative approaches to use of the Isolator with direct plating, including use of broth-based blood culture systems, chemically defined fluid media,[210] or cell culture systems.[211] The sensitivity of a shell vial culture assay may be slightly better than that of agar plate techniques.[212] In the automated continuously monitored blood culture systems, *Bartonella* spp. rarely produce turbidity or convert enough oxidizable substrate for these CO_2 detection-based systems to indicate growth. However, several isolates have been detected initially using BACTEC (Becton Dickinson, Sparks, MD) and resin-containing media combined with acridine orange staining at the termination of a 7-day incubation period, with recovery subsequently achieved by subculture to solid media.[10,11,83] Of note, growth of a *B. clarridgeiae*-like blood isolate in a vacationer who returned to the United States from Peru was detected by a BACTEC system after 15 days of incubation.[30] Another CO_2 detection blood culture system, BacT/Alert (bioMérieux, Durham, NC), has been reported to yield positive growth algorithms in several cases of *B. henselae* bacteremia. Although Gram stains of the broth and routine 72-hour subcultures proved negative, acridine orange and Warthin-Starry staining demonstrated bacilli, and phase-contrast microscopy of wet mounts revealed bacilli with "rachety motility." Specific immunofluorescent labeling of organisms obtained directly from the broth or subsequently subcultured on semisolid media identified *B. henselae*.[213] Extended incubation of blood culture vials has permitted recovery of *B. quintana* in prosthetic valve endocarditis.[214]

Bartonella spp. have been isolated from liver, spleen, lymph node, and skin after homogenization either by direct plating of tissue homogenate or aspirate[16,38,45,80,85] or by cocultivation with various cell lines.[9,12] *B. henselae/B. quintana* grow in endothelial cell cultures as elongated pleomorphic organisms visible in Gimenez-stained preparations 72 hours after inoculation of the cell cultures. The cocultivation method is not practical for most microbiology laboratories, although it may result in recovering occasional isolates missed with cell-free media. In the absence of coculture, more than 1 month of incubation often has been necessary to yield evident colonies from some tissue

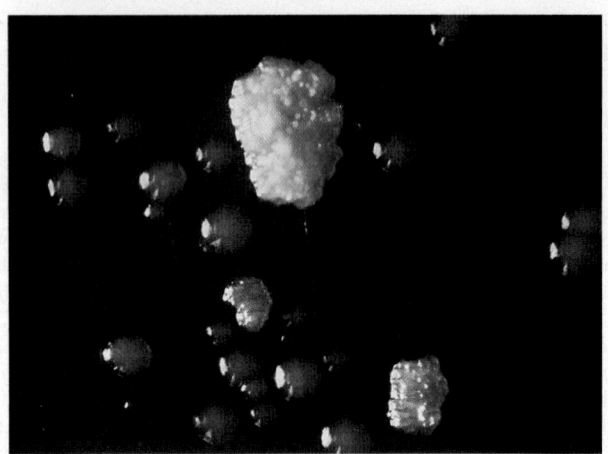

Figure 235-14   Smooth and verrucous colony types growing concurrently in a chocolate agar culture of *B. henselae* (magnification approximately ×40).

specimens.[38,45] Because selective culture techniques have not been developed, recovery of isolates from specimens such as skin may be more difficult if indigenous or contaminating flora are present.

IDENTIFICATION

Colonies of *Bartonella* spp. are of two morphologic types: (1) irregular, raised, whitish, rough, and dry in appearance (characterized as "cauliflower," "molar tooth," or "verrucous") or (2) smaller, circular, tan, and moist in appearance, tending to pit and adhere to the agar. Both are usually present in the same culture (Fig. 235-14). Colonial heterogeneity varies by species. *B. henselae* typically displays a greater proportion of rough colonies than *B. quintana*, which may even appear as uniformly smooth in primary cultures. Serial *B. henselae* subcultures tend to have increasing proportions of smooth colonies. Cultures of *B. henselae* on blood agar produce an odor similar to the caramel odor (diacetyl) of *Streptococcus milleri*. Colonies contain small, gram-negative, slightly curved rods resembling *Campylobacter*, *Helicobacter*, or *Haemophilus*. Cells, especially of *B. henselae*, are very autoadherent, demonstrable when scraping colonies from agar with a loop. Twitching motility of cells is evident in wet mounts, presumably interrelated with adherence, with both features being mediated by fine fimbriae (pili) visible in negatively stained electron microscopy. Cells of *B. bacilliformis*, *B. clarridgeiae*, and *B. rochalimae* possess polar flagella.

The features of incubation for more than 7 days before the appearance of colonies, small curved gram-negative bacilli, and negative catalase and oxidase reactions are sufficient for presumptive identification of *B. henselae* or *B. quintana*.[201,208] Additional methods to confirm the identity of isolates may be employed, or isolates may be referred to a laboratory experienced with *Bartonella* spp. for confirmatory identification. Although the reagents are not widely available, a reliable means to distinguish *B. henselae* from *B. quintana* isolates quickly is immunofluorescence with antisera monospecific for each of these two species.[208,213,215]

Commercial identification kits do not contain *Bartonella* spp. in their databases, but the MicroScan (Dade Behring, Deerfield, IL) rapid anaerobe panel distinguishes *Bartonella* spp. from species that are in its database. Using this panel with careful adjustment of inoculum size to a McFarland no. 3 standard, it is also possible to distinguish *Bartonella* species on the basis of biotype codes[200,208] (10077640 = *B. henselae*, 10073640 = *B. quintana*, and 10077240 = *B. bacilliformis*). Heavier inocula blur the distinctions. In other systems, the biochemical reactivity of *B. quintana* and *B. henselae* has been enhanced by addition of hemin to test media.[216]

Determination of the cellular fatty acid composition by gas-liquid chromatography is useful in identifying and distinguishing *Bartonella*

spp. from other genera.[14,208] The Bartonellaceae have relatively simple gas-liquid chromatography profiles consisting mainly of $C_{18:1}$, $C_{18:0}$, and $C_{16:0}$ acids. *B. elizabethae* contains a greater amount of $C_{17:0}$ than the other species. An unusual branched-chain fatty acid (11-methyloctadec-12-enoic acid) distinguishes *Afipia* spp. from *Bartonella* spp. and other organisms.[123,217]

ANTIMICROBIAL SUSCEPTIBILITY TESTING

Clinical correlation studies of susceptibility testing results with *Bartonella* spp. have not been performed to the extent necessary to ensure that meaningful data can be generated. If required, antimicrobial susceptibility testing can be performed by incorporation of antimicrobial agents into either blood or chocolate agar and testing by the agar dilution technique.[14,218] *Haemophilus* test medium with a broth microdilution technique has also been described, but the Etest (AB Biodisk, Solna, Sweden) may be the most practical means to assess susceptibility.[219-221] Testing in other types of systems has also been reported.[222-225] Because of the slow growth and fastidious nature of the organisms, some test methods may be inappropriate. Testing of isolates is problematic in any system for those strains displaying the most fastidious growth characteristics.

Generally, *B. henselae* isolates are susceptible in vitro to most antibacterial agents tested, including β-lactams, tetracyclines, macrolides, aminoglycosides, fluoroquinolones, vancomycin, rifampin, chloramphenicol, and co-trimoxazole, but are resistant to nalidixic acid. In vitro resistance to penicillin and ampicillin, tetracycline, or vancomycin has been noted. *B. quintana* is similar in its in vitro susceptibility pattern. Some investigators argue that aminoglycosides most reliably demonstrate in vitro bactericidal activity, mandating their use for therapy of bacteremia and endocarditis.[77,88,226,227]

MOLECULAR METHODS

Numerous PCR assays, some employing real-time detection technology,[228,229] have been developed for direct detection of *Bartonella* spp. in pus, skin lesions, or tissue. Sera of CSD lymphadenitis patients yield relatively low sensitivity.[230] A gene fragment specific for citrate synthase, a heat shock protein, or the *groEL* gene of *B. henselae* is demonstrable by PCR in the majority of patients with CSD.[48,117,119,229] Amplification of rRNA gene segments with universal primers followed by direct nucleotide sequence analysis of the amplification products is another approach that may generate useful results when species other than the most common ones are encountered.[101,119,231] Improved detection of *Bartonella* DNA in histologic or other material such as sera from culture-negative endocarditis has been reported using nested PCR amplification techniques.[232,233] PCR amplification has also enabled identification of *B. henselae* in CSF and brain tissue of patients with HIV-related neurologic processes in the absence of culture recovery.[163,165]

PCR-based typing techniques have proven useful for epidemiologic purposes, and some studies suggest a greater diversity of restriction fragment length polymorphism (RFLP) types in the blood of bacteremic HIV-infected people than in the CSD lesions of immunocompetent hosts.[234,235] Strain typing can be performed using PCR-based RFLP,[13,234,236] pulsed-field gel electrophoresis (PFGE), multilocus sequence typing,[237] repetitive extragenic palindromic PCR (REP-PCR),[19,238] and enterobacterial repetitive intergenic consensus PCR (ERIC-PCR) with sodium dodecyl sulfate-polyacrylamide gel electrophoresis.[39] Among these and other techniques compared to PFGE, the latter tends to be less reliable than the others in the case of *Bartonella* spp. that have been studied.[237,239]

SEROLOGIC TESTING

Using a simple sonic lysate of *B. bacilliformis* as antigen, an IgG immunoblot assay has been reported to have 70% and 94% sensitivity in people with acute and chronic infection, respectively, but with suboptimal specificity.[240] An alternative approach has been an immunofluorescence assay detecting IgG, reported to have 82% and 93% sensitivity in people with acute and chronic infection, respectively, but at the expense of substantial cross-reaction with other *Bartonella* species.[241] It can also detect IgM in patients with early acute disease. When used in the endemic region to assess patients with syndromes compatible with *B. bacilliformis* disease, the low specificity of these tests may be relatively less important than for geographically widespread *Bartonella* species. A novel serologic assay for *B. bacilliformis* has been developed using recombinant Pap 31 antigen that shows promise for use in endemic areas.[242]

Enzyme immunoassay (EIA) and radioimmunoprecipitation have been found comparably more sensitive than hemagglutination and immunofluorescence assays in older studies of human antibodies to *B. quintana*.[243] With EIA, all cases in a small series of acute primary or relapsed trench fever were found to have measurable, although often low, levels of anti-*B. quintana* antibodies.[244]

Immunofluorescence assay (IFA)[41,44,245-247] and several EIAs[43,115,208,248] have been described for *B. henselae* and *B. quintana*. To date, they have been used most commonly to demonstrate anti-*Bartonella* antibodies in people with CSD[41,43,44,115,157,245,247,248] or endocarditis[12,84-88,246] and in some cases of HIV-associated aseptic meningitis, encephalopathy, or neuropsychiatric disease.[80,163,166] Human antibody responses often have been substantially cross-reactive between *B. quintana* and *B. henselae*.[115,245] Furthermore, in some of these assays there may be serologic cross-reaction with *Chlamydia* species and *Coxiella burnetii*, other potential agents of "culture-negative endocarditis" in humans.[12,86,246,249]

IFA and EIA assays using whole bacterial cell antigens, especially if performed at only one time for a particular subject, appear to be variably and sometimes suboptimally sensitive and specific.[247,248,250] The Centers for Disease Control and Prevention's IFA that uses *B. henselae* cells fixed on slides is probably the most widely emulated, with a reported sensitivity for its detection of anti–*B. henselae* IgG of 85% to 94%. However, this method has a high rate of cross-reaction with *B. quintana* antigens from contemporary isolates. Commercially developed kits have also applied this assay to detect IgM, with similar sensitivity and specificity issues.

Alternative EIA methodology, using partially[87,208,251] or highly purified[252] or recombinant[242,253] antigen preparations, ultimately may prove more species sensitive and specific. An EIA using as antigen partially purified proteins presumed to be of outer membrane origin has been assayed with a population of CSD patients meeting stringent clinical criteria associated with proof of *B. henselae* infection on culture or PCR, or both. Anti–*B. henselae* IgG detected in 75% and IgM detected in 44% resulted in 85% combined sensitivity, comparable to that of the IFA, and specificity of more than 98%, which is much better than that of the IFA.[254]

Treatment and Prevention

Recommendations for treatment of *Bartonella* species based on best available evidence have been published.[255]

The standard therapy for acute *B. bacilliformis* infection in South America (Oroya fever) has been oral chloramphenicol in a dose of 2 g/day for 1 or 2 weeks, often co-administered with a second agent such as a β-lactam antibiotic. Oral chloramphenicol is no longer available in the United States and would not be appropriate because of adverse effects if it were available. Alternatives such as oral ciprofloxacin,[255] doxycycline, other tetracyclines, ampicillin, or trimethoprim-sulfamethoxazole can be given for a comparable duration. Parenteral therapy can be substituted if oral intake or bowel absorption is impaired. In modern-era Peru, the agent of primary choice in the treatment of eruptive phase lesions has become oral rifampin (10 mg/kg/day up to 600 mg) for 10 to 14 days, with the alternative being streptomycin (15 to 20 mg/kg/day) for 10 days.[64,255]

In vitro susceptibility of *B. henselae* and *B. quintana* does not necessarily predict in vivo response to therapy. Indeed, BA/BP can develop and organisms can be recovered in the face of therapy with co-trimoxazole, β-lactam antibiotics, and fluoroquinolone antibiotics.[106,256] In contrast, therapy with rifampin, tetracyclines, or macrolides dramatically reduces culture recovery from BA/BP lesions, and macrolide administration appears to protect against *Bartonella* infections.[106] The routine use of rifabutin, clarithromycin, and azithromycin for the prevention of *M. avium* complex infections in people with AIDS appears to have reduced the incidence of *Bartonella* infections in that population. Yet when appropriate care has not been accessed, *Bartonella* infection rates can rival those of *M. avium* complex in people with advanced HIV infection. In one area of high HIV prevalence, evidence of *B. henselae* or *B. quintana* infection was found in 18% of people evaluated for acute or persistent unexplained fever, 97% of whom were HIV-infected and had a median CD4 lymphocyte count of 35 cells/μL and no antiretroviral exposure.[257]

Ease of administration, low cost, and observed clinical effectiveness make oral erythromycin (500 mg PO four times daily) or doxycycline (100 mg PO twice daily) for 3 or 4 months the initial agents of choice to treat processes such as BA and BP.[106,255-258] As long as it is of adequate duration, such therapy appears effective for most manifestations. Exceptions may include bony or parenchymal involvement and endocarditis, for which initial parenteral therapy may be advantageous. In endocarditis, addition of intravenous gentamicin for the first 2 weeks appears beneficial and is recommended to be combined in a dose of 3 mg/kg/day with 6 weeks of doxycycline; in uncomplicated bacteremia the same regimen is applicable but with 4 weeks of doxycycline.[77,79,88,255] Hemodynamic considerations may require valve replacement irrespective of the effect of antimicrobials on bacterial proliferation. Longer durations of treatment are appropriate in the HIV-infected patient[255] or if fever or bacteremia is persistent or recurrent in the HIV-uninfected patient.[80] Relapsing disease has been seen in both immunocompromised and immunocompetent hosts, especially, but not only, if therapy is terminated prematurely. For relapses occurring after adequately long initial treatment, chronic suppressive therapy with doxycycline or erythromycin should be considered.

There have been anecdotal reports of the utility of various agents (rifampin, gentamicin, trimethoprim-sulfamethoxazole, fluoroquinolones, and azithromycin[259-263]) in the treatment of CSD. However, only azithromycin has been demonstrated to accelerate the resolution of typical CSD lymphadenopathy in a placebo-controlled, double-blind study.[130] Although the value of antibiotic therapy of CSD remains debatable in light of the usually benign outcome of most manifestations,[262] oral azithromycin (500 mg on day 1 and then 250 mg per day on days 2 through 5) should be the agent of first choice if antimicrobial administration is contemplated for treating extensive CSD lymphadenitis.[255] Utility in treatment of "atypical" manifestations of CSD remains undefined.

Although there is no definite evidence of the utility of antibiotic therapy in altering the course of neurologic manifestations of CSD, case reports of neuroretinitis associated with persistent *B. henselae* bacteremia, and of *Bartonella*-associated antibiotic-responsive neuropsychiatric manifestations in the setting of HIV infection, probably support the inclination to treat with antimicrobials. Two-agent therapy for neuroretinitis accelerates resolution in comparison to untreated historical control cases. The agents used in such cases have usually been erythromycin or doxycycline (with or without combined rifampin) or, alternatively, azithromycin, clarithromycin, or fluoroquinolones.[80,161,164] Currently, 4 to 6 weeks of oral doxycycline and rifampin therapy (100 mg and 300 mg, respectively, twice daily) is recommended.[255] Systemic corticosteroid therapy is often administered by ophthalmologists as an adjunct or alternative to antimicrobials; no definitive advantage or disadvantage to such an approach has been demonstrated.

Prevention of *B. bacilliformis* and *B. quintana* infections is probably best achieved by avoiding the locales or circumstances in which exposure to their arthropod vectors occurs. Eradication of body louse infestation should reduce risk of *B. quintana* infection.[264] In contrast, prevention of *B. henselae* (and possibly *B. clarridgeiae* and *B. koehlerae*) infection entails avoidance of interactions with cats that might result in scratches, bites, or licks and exposure to cat fleas or flea feces.[264] Feral cats, cats that are allowed outdoors, cats with fleas, and kittens (<12 months old) all have a higher chance of being *B. henselae* infected.[265] Although the role of cat fleas in the transmission of *B. henselae* to humans is inadequately defined, treatment of pet cats for such infestation may be prudent, especially if human owners or contacts are immunosuppressed. Antibiotic therapy of cats implicated in CSD transmission or otherwise demonstrated to be *B. henselae* or *B.*

clarridgeiae infected does not durably eliminate bacteremia[266-268] and is not warranted, except perhaps in the setting of immunosuppressed human contacts. In general, removal of cats from the household of immunocompetent or immunosuppressed humans is unnecessary as long as the contact precautions defined previously are maintained. Although certainly not recommended, direct contact with cat feces or urine does not appear to present a risk for human *B. henselae* infection.

REFERENCES

1. Relman DA, Lepp PW, Sadler KN, et al. Phylogenetic relationships among the agent of bacillary angiomatosis, Bartonella bacilliformis, and other alpha-proteobacteria. Mol Microbiol. 1992;6:1801-1807.
2. Brenner DJ, O'Connor SP, Winkler HH, et al. Proposals to unify the genera Bartonella and Rochalimaea, with descriptions of Bartonella quintana comb. nov., Bartonella vinsonii comb. nov., Bartonella henselae comb. nov., and Bartonella elizabethae comb. nov., and to remove the family Bartonellaceae from the order Rickettsiales. Int J Syst Bacteriol. 1993;43:777-786.
3. Alsmark CM, Frank AC, Karlberg EO, et al. The louse-borne human pathogen Bartonella quintana is a genomic derivative of the zoonotic agent Bartonella henselae. Proc Natl Acad Sci U S A. 2004;101:9716-9721.
4. Strong RP, Tyzzer EE, Brues CT, et al. Verruga peruviana, Oroya fever and uta: preliminary report of the first expedition to South America from the Department of Tropical Medicine of Harvard University. J Am Med Assoc. 1913;61:1713-1716.
5. Strong RP, Sellards AW. Oroya fever: second report. J Am Med Assoc. 1915;64:806-808.
6. Mooser H, Wyer F. Experimental infection of Macacus rhesus with Rickettsia quintana (trench fever). Proc Soc Exp Biol Med. 1953;83:699-701.
7. Liu W-T. Trench fever: a resumé of literature and a note on some obscure phases of the disease. Chinese Med J. 1984;97:179-190.
8. McNee JW, Renshaw A. "Trench fever": a relapsing fever occurring with the British forces in France. Br Med J. 1916;1:225-234.
9. Koehler JE, Quinn FD, Berger TG, et al. Isolation of Rochalimaea species from cutaneous and osseous lesions of bacillary angiomatosis. N Engl J Med. 1992;327:1625-1632.
10. Spach DH, Callis KP, Paauw DS, et al. Endocarditis caused by Rochalimaea quintana in a patient infected with human immunodeficiency virus. J Clin Microbiol. 1993;31:692-694.
11. Larson AM, Dougherty MJ, Nowowiejski DJ, et al. Detection of Bartonella (Rochalimaea) quintana by routine acridine orange staining of broth blood cultures. J Clin Microbiol. 1994;32:1492-1496.
12. Drancourt M, Mainardi JL, Brouqui P, et al. Bartonella (Rochalimaea) quintana endocarditis in three homeless men. N Engl J Med. 1995;332:419-423.
13. Spach DH, Kanter AS, Dougherty MJ, et al. Bartonella (Rochalimaea) quintana bacteremia in inner-city patients with chronic alcoholism. N Engl J Med. 1995;332:424-428.
14. Slater LN, Welch DF, Hensel D, et al. A newly recognized fastidious gram-negative pathogen as a cause of fever and bacteremia. N Engl J Med. 1990;323:1587-1593.
15. Regnery RL, Anderson BE, Clarridge III JE, et al. Characterization of a novel Rochalimaea species, R. henselae sp. nov., isolated from blood of a febrile, human immunodeficiency virus-positive patient. J Clin Microbiol. 1992;30:265-274.
16. Welch DF, Pickett DA, Slater LN, et al. Rochalimaea henselae sp. nov., a cause of septicemia, bacillary angiomatosis, and parenchymal bacillary peliosis. J Clin Microbiol. 1992;30:275-280.
17. Daly JS, Worthington MG, Brenner DJ, et al. Rochalimaea elizabethae sp. nov. isolated from a patient with endocarditis. J Clin Microbiol. 1993;31:872-881.
18. Birtles RJ, Harrison TG, Saunders NA, et al. Proposals to unify the genera Grahamella and Bartonella, with descriptions of Bartonella talpae comb. nov., Bartonella peromysci sp. nov., Bartonella taylorii sp. nov., and Bartonella doshiae sp. nov. Int J Syst Bacteriol. 1995;45:1-8.
19. Clarridge III JE, Raich TJ, Pirwani D, et al. Strategy to detect and identify Bartonella species in a routine clinical laboratory yields Bartonella henselae from human immunodeficiency virus-infected patient and unique Bartonella strain from his cat. J Clin Microbiol. 1995;33:2107-2113.
20. Heller R, Artois M, Xemar V, et al. Prevalence of Bartonella henselae and Bartonella clarridgeiae in stray cats. J Clin Microbiol. 1997;35:1327-1331.
21. Kordick DL, Hilyard EJ, Hadfield TL, et al. Bartonella clarridgeiae, a newly recognized zoonotic pathogen causing inoculation papules, fever and lymphadenopathy (cat scratch disease). J Clin Microbiol. 1997;35:1813-1818.
22. Gurfield AN, Boulouis H-J, Chomel BB, et al. Coinfection with Bartonella clarridgeiae and Bartonella henselae and with different Bartonella henselae strains in domestic cats. J Clin Microbiol. 1997;35:2120-2123.
23. Breitschwerdt EB, Kordick DL, Malarkey DE, et al. Endocarditis in a dog due to infection with a novel Bartonella subspecies. J Clin Microbiol. 1995;33:154-160.
24. Kordick DL, Swaminathan B, Greene CE, et al. Bartonella vinsonii subsp. berkhoffii subsp. nov., isolated from dogs; Bartonella vinsonii subsp. vinsonii; and emended description of Bartonella vinsonii. Int J Syst Bacteriol. 1996;46:704-709.
25. Welch DF, Carroll KC, Hofmeister EK, et al. Isolation of a new subspecies, Bartonella vinsonii subsp. arupensis, from a cattle rancher: identity with isolates found in conjunction with Borrelia burgdorferi and Babesia microti among naturally infected mice. J Clin Microbiol. 1999;37:2598-2601.
26. Raoult D, Roblot F, Rolain J-M, et al. First isolation of Bartonella alsatica from a valve of a patient with endocarditis. J Clin Microbiol. 2006;44:278-279.
27. Avidor B, Graidy M, Efrat G, et al. Bartonella koehlerae, a new cat-associated agent of culture-negative human endocarditis. J Clin Microbiol. 2004;42:3462-3468.
28. Drancourt M, Tran-Hung L, Courtin J, et al. Bartonella quintana in a 4000-year-old human tooth. J Infect Dis. 2005;191:607-611.
29. La VD, Clavel B, Lepetz S, et al. Molecular detection of Bartonella henselae DNA in the dental pulp of 800-year-old French cats. Clin Infect Dis. 2004;39:1391-1394.
30. Eremeeva ME, Gerns HL, Lydy SL, et al. Bacteremia, fever, and splenomegaly caused by a newly recognized Bartonella species. N Engl J Med. 2007;356:2381-2387.
31. Fournier PE, Taylor C, Rolain JM, et al. Bartonella australis sp. nov. from kangaroos, Australia. Emerg Infect Dis. 2007;13:1961-1962.
32. Kosoy M, Morway C, Sheff KW, et al. Bartonella tamiae sp. nov., a newly recognized pathogen isolated from three human patients from Thailand. J Clin Microbiol. 2008;46:772-775.
33. Maillard R, Riegel P, Barrat F, et al. Bartonella chomelii sp. nov., isolated from French domestic cattle (Bos taurus). Int J Syst Evol Microbiol. 2004;54:215-220.
34. Gundi VA, Davoust B, Khamis A, et al. Isolation of Bartonella rattimassiliensis sp. nov. and Bartonella phoceensis sp. nov. from European Rattus norvegicus. J Clin Microbiol. 2004;42:3816-3818.
35. Yamamoto K, Chomel B, Lowenstine L, et al. Bartonella henselae antibody prevalence in free-ranging and captive wild felids from California. J Wildlife Dis. 1998;34:56-63.
36. Koehler JE, Glaser CA, Tappero JW. Rochalimaea henselae infection: a new zoonosis with the domestic cat as reservoir. JAMA. 1994;271:531-535.
37. Chomel BB, Abbot RC, Kasten RW, et al. Bartonella henselae prevalence in domestic cats in California: risk factors and association between bacteremia and antibody titers. J Clin Microbiol. 1995;33:2445-2450.
38. Demers DM, Bass JW, Vincent JM, et al. Cat scratch disease in Hawaii: etiology and seroepidemiology. J Pediatr. 1995;127:23-26.
39. Sander A, Büler C, Pelz K, et al. Detection and identification of two Bartonella henselae variants in domestic cats in Germany. J Clin Microbiol. 1997;35:584-587.
40. Kordick DL, Wilson KH, Sexton DJ, et al. Prolonged Bartonella bacteremia in cats associated with cat-scratch disease patients. J Clin Microbiol. 1995;33:3245-3251.
41. Regnery RL, Olson JG, Perkins BA, et al. Serologic response to "Rochalimaea henselae" antigen in suspected cat-scratch disease. Lancet. 1992;339:1443-1445.
42. Tappero JW, Mohle-Boetani J, Koehler J, et al. The epidemiology of bacillary angiomatosis and bacillary peliosis. JAMA. 1993;269:770-775.
43. Barka NR, Hadfield T, Patnaik M, et al. EIA for detection of Rochalimaea henselae-reactive IgG, IgM, and IgA antibodies in patients with suspected cat scratch disease [letter]. J Infect Dis. 1993;167:1503-1504.
44. Zangwill KM, Hamilton DH, Perkins BA, et al. Cat scratch disease in Connecticut: epidemiology, risk factors, and evaluation of a new diagnostic test. N Engl J Med. 1993;329:8-13.
45. Dolan MJ, Wong MT, Regnery RL, et al. Syndrome of Rochalimaea henselae adenitis suggesting cat scratch disease. Ann Intern Med. 1993;118:331-336.
46. Waldvogel K, Regnery RL, Anderson BE, et al. Disseminated cat-scratch disease: detection of Rochalimaea henselae in affected tissue. Eur J Pediatr. 1994;153:23-27.
47. Anderson B, Sims K, Regnery R, et al. Detection of Rochalimaea henselae DNA in specimens from cat-scratch disease patients by PCR. J Clin Microbiol. 1994;32:942-948.
48. Goral S, Anderson B, Hager C, et al. Detection of Rochalimaea henselae DNA by polymerase chain reaction from suppurative nodes of children with cat-scratch disease. Pediatr Infect Dis J. 1994;13:994-997.
49. Le HH, Palay DA, Anderson B, et al. Conjunctival swab to diagnose ocular cat scratch disease. Am J Ophthalmol. 1994;118:249-250.
50. Perkins BA, Swaminathan B, Jackson LA, et al. Case 22-1992. Pathogenesis of cat scratch disease [letter]. N Engl J Med. 1992;327:1599-1600.
51. Anderson B, Kelly C, Threlkel R, et al. Detection of Rochalimaea henselae in cat-scratch disease skin test antigens. J Infect Dis. 1993;168:1034-1036.
52. Chomel BB, Kasten RW, Floyd-Hawkins K, et al. Experimental transmission of Bartonella henselae by the cat flea. J Clin Microbiol. 1996;34:1952-1956.
53. Rolain JM, Franc M, Davoust B, et al. Molecular detection of Bartonella quintana, B. koehlerae, B. henselae, B. clarridgeiae, Rickettsia felis, and Wolbachia pipientis in cat fleas, France. Emerg Infect Dis. 2003;9:338-342.
54. Chang CC, Hayashidani H, Pusterla N, et al. Investigation of Bartonella infection in ixodid ticks from California. Comp Immunol Microbiol Infect Dis. 2002;25:229-236.
55. Sanogo YO, Zeaiter Z, Caruso G, et al. Bartonella henselae in Ixodes ricinus ticks (Acari: Ixodida) removed from humans, Belluno province, Italy. Emerg Infect Dis. 2003;9:329-332.
56. Stevenson HL, Bai Y, Kosoy MY, et al. Detection of novel Bartonella strains and Yersinia pestis in prairie dogs and their fleas (Siphonaptera: Ceratophyllidae and Pulicidae) using multiplex polymerase chain reaction. J Med Entomol. 2003;40:329-337.
57. Adelson ME, Rao RV, Tilton RC, et al. Prevalence of Borrelia burgdorferi, Bartonella spp., Babesia microti, and Anaplasma phagocytophila in Ixodes scapularis ticks collected in northern New Jersey. J Clin Microbiol. 2004;42:2799-2801.
58. Billeter SA, Miller MK, Breitschwerdt EB, et al. Detection of two Bartonella tamiae-like sequences in Amblyomma americanum (Acari: Ixodidae) using 16S-23S intergenic spacer region-specific primers. J Med Entomol. 2008;45:176-179.
59. Mexas AM, Hancock SI, Breitschwerdt EB. Bartonella henselae and Bartonella elizabethae as potential canine pathogens. J Clin Microbiol. 2002;40:4670-4674.
60. Anonymous. La Verruga Peruana y Daniel A. Carrion, Estudiante de la Facultad de Medicina, Muerto el 5 de Octobre de 1885. Lima: Imprenta del Estado; 1886.
61. Ricketts WE. Carrion's disease: a study of the incubation period in thirteen cases. Am J Trop Med. 1947;27:657-659.
62. Amano Y, Rumbea J, Knobloch J, et al. Bartonellosis in Ecuador: serosurvey and current status of cutaneous verrucous disease. Am J Trop Med Hyg. 1997;57:174-179.
63. Kosek M, Lavarello R, Gilman RH, et al. Natural history of infection with Bartonella bacilliformis in a nonendemic population. J Infect Dis. 2000;182:865-872.
64. Maguina C, Garcia PJ, Gotuzzo E, et al. Bartonellosis (Carrión's disease) in the modern era. Clin Infect Dis. 2001;33:772-779.
65. Strong RP, Tyzzer EE, Brues CT, et al. Report of the First Expedition to South America, 1913. Cambridge, MA: Harvard University Press; 1915.
66. Ricketts WE. Bartonella bacilliformis anemia (Oroya fever). Blood. 1948;3:1025-1049.
67. Reynafarje C, Ramos J. The hemolytic anemia of human bartonellosis. Blood. 1961;17:562-578.
68. Ricketts WE. Clinical manifestations of Carrión's disease. Arch Intern Med. 1949;84:751-781.
69. Maguiña C, Gotuzzo E, Carcelén A, et al. Compromiso gastrointestinal bartonellosis o enfermedad de Carrión. Rev Gastroenterol Peru. 1997;17:31-43.
70. Cuadra M. Salmonellosis complication in human bartonellosis. Texas Rep Biol Med. 1956;14:97-113.
71. Pinkerton H, Weinman D. Toxoplasma infection in man. Arch Pathol. 1940;30:374-392.
72. Garcia-Caceres U, Garcia FU. Bartonellosis: an immunosuppressive disease and the life of Daniel Alcides Carrion. Am J Clin Pathol. 1991;95(Suppl 1):S56-S66.
73. Dooley JR. Bartonellosis. In: Binford CH, Connor DH, eds. Pathology of Tropical and Extraordinary Diseases. Washington, DC: Armed Forces Institute of Pathology; 1976:190-193.

74. Chamberlin J, Laughlin LW, Romero S, et al. Epidemiology of endemic *Bartonella bacilliformis*: a prospective cohort study in a Peruvian mountain valley community. *J Infect Dis*. 2002; 186:983-990.
75. Arias-Stella J, Lieberman PH, Erlandson RA, et al. Histology, immunohistochemistry, and ultrastructure of the verruga in Carrion's disease. *Am J Surg Pathol*. 1986;10:595-610.
76. Jackson LA, Spach DH. Emergence of *Bartonella quintana* infection among homeless persons. *Emerg Infect Dis*. 1996;2: 141-144.
77. Foucault C, Raoult D, Brouqui P. Randomized open trial of gentamicin and doxycycline for eradication of *Bartonella quintana* from blood in patients with chronic bacteremia. *Antimicrob Agents Chemother*. 2002;47:2204-2207.
78. Slater LN, Welch DF, Min K-W. *Rochalimaea henselae* causes bacillary angiomatosis and peliosis hepatis. *Arch Intern Med*. 1992;152:602-606.
79. Lucey D, Dolan MJ, Moss CW, et al. Relapsing illness due to *Rochalimaea henselae* in normal hosts: implication for therapy and new epidemiologic associations. *Clin Infect Dis*. 1992; 14:683-688.
80. Wong MT, Dolan MJ, Lattuada Jr CP, et al. Neuroretinitis, aseptic meningitis, and lymphadenitis associated with *Bartonella* (*Rochalimaea*) *henselae* infection in immunocompetent patients and patients infected with human immunodeficiency virus type 1. *Clin Infect Dis*. 1995;21:352-360.
81. Hadfield TL, Warren R, Kass M, et al. Endocarditis caused by *Rochalimaea henselae*. *Hum Pathol*. 1993;24:1140-1141.
82. Holmes AH, Greeough TC, Balady GJ, et al. *Bartonella henselae* endocarditis in an immunocompetent adult. *Clin Infect Dis*. 1995;21:1004-1007.
83. Spach DH, Kanter AS, Daniels NA, et al. *Bartonella* (*Rochalimaea*) species as a cause of apparent "culture-negative" endocarditis. *Clin Infect Dis*. 1995;20:1044-1047.
84. Jalava J, Kotilainen P, Nikkari S, et al. Use of polymerase chain reaction and DNA sequencing for detection of *Bartonella quintana* in the aortic valve of a patient with culture-negative infective endocarditis. *Clin Infect Dis*. 1995;21:891-896.
85. Drancourt M, Birtles R, Chaumentin G, et al. New serotype of *Bartonella henselae* in endocarditis and cat-scratch disease. *Lancet*. 1996;347:441-443.
86. Raoult D, Fournier P, Drancourt M, et al. Diagnosis of 22 new cases of *Bartonella* endocarditis. *Ann Intern Med*. 1996; 125:646-652.
87. Baorto E, Payne RM, Slater LN, et al. Culture-negative endocarditis due to *Bartonella henselae*. *J Pediatr*. 1998;132: 1052-1054.
88. Raoult D, Fournier PE, Vandenesch F, et al. Outcome and treatment of *Bartonella* endocarditis. *Arch Intern Med*. 2003;163:226-230.
89. Stoler MH, Bonfiglio TA, Steigbigel RT, et al. An atypical subcutaneous infection associated with acquired immune deficiency syndrome. *Am J Clin Pathol*. 1983;80:714-718.
90. Cockerell CJ, Webster GF, Whitlow MA, et al. Epithelioid angiomatosis: a distinct vascular disorder in patients with the acquired immunodeficiency syndrome or AIDS-related complex. *Lancet*. 1987;2:6544-6546.
91. LeBoit PE, Egbert BM, Stoler MH, et al. Epithelioid haemangioma-like vascular proliferation in AIDS: manifestation of cat scratch disease bacillus infection? *Lancet*. 1988;l:960-963.
92. Koehler JE, LeBoit PE, Egbert BM, et al. Cutaneous vascular lesions and disseminated cat-scratch disease in patients with the acquired immunodeficiency syndrome (AIDS) and AIDS-related complex. *Ann Intern Med*. 1988;109:449-455.
93. Milam MW, Balerdi MJ, Toney JF, et al. Epithelioid angiomatosis secondary to disseminated cat scratch disease involving the bone marrow and skin in a patient with acquired immune deficiency syndrome: a case report. *Am J Med*. 1990;88: 180-183.
94. Kemper CA, Lombard CM, Deresinski SC, et al. Visceral bacillary epithelioid angiomatosis: possible manifestations of disseminated cat scratch disease in the immunocompromised host: a report of two cases. *Am J Med*. 1990;89:216-222.
95. Spach DH, Panther LA, Thorning DR, et al. Intracerebral bacillary angiomatosis in a patient infected with the human immunodeficiency virus. *Ann Intern Med*. 1992;116:740-742.
96. Koehler JE, Cederberg L. Intraabdominal mass associated with gastrointestinal hemorrhage: a new manifestation of bacillary angiomatosis. *Gastroenterology*. 1995;109:2011-2014.
97. Coche E, Beigelman C, Lucidarme O, et al. Thoracic bacillary angiomatosis in a patient with AIDS. *AJR Am J Roentgenol*. 1995;165:56-58.
98. Mohle-Boetani JC, Koehler JE, Berger TG, et al. Bacillary angiomatosis and bacillary peliosis in patients infected with the human immunodeficiency virus: clinical characteristics in a case control study. *Clin Infect Dis*. 1996;22:794-800.
99. Huh YB, Rose S, Schoen RE, et al. Colonic bacillary angiomatosis. *Ann Intern Med*. 1996;124:735-737.
100. Long SR, Whitfield MJ, Eades C, et al. Bacillary angiomatosis of the cervix and vulva in a patient with AIDS. *Obstet Gynecol*. 1996;881:709-711.
101. Relman DA, Loutit JS, Schmidt TM, et al. The agent of bacillary angiomatosis: an approach to the identification of uncultured pathogens. *N Engl J Med*. 1990;323:1573-1580.
102. Cockerell CJ, Bergstresser PR, Myrie-Williams C, et al. Bacillary epithelioid angiomatosis occurring in an immunocompetent individual. *Arch Dermatol*. 1990;126:787-790.
103. Tappero JW, Koehler JE, Berger TG, et al. Bacillary angiomatosis and bacillary splenitis in immunocompetent adults. *Ann Intern Med*. 1993;118:363-365.
104. Cockerell CJ, Tierno PM, Friedman-Kien AE, et al. Clinical, histologic, microbiologic, and biochemical characterization of the causative agent of bacillary (epithelioid) angiomatosis: a rickettsial illness with features of bartonellosis. *J Invest Dermatol*. 1991;97:812-817.
105. Relman DA, Falkow S, LeBoit PE, et al. The organism causing bacillary angiomatosis, peliosis hepatis, and fever and bacteremia in immunocompromised patients [letter]. *N Engl J Med*. 1991;324:1514.
106. Koehler JE, Sanchez MA, Garrido CS, et al. Molecular epidemiology of *Bartonella* infections in patients with bacillary angiomatosis-peliosis. *N Engl J Med*. 1997;337:1876-1883.
107. Tappero JW, Koehler JE. Bacillary angiomatosis or Kaposi's sarcoma? *N Engl J Med*. 1997;337:1888.
108. Cockerell CJ, LeBoit PE. Bacillary angiomatosis: a newly characterized, pseudoneoplastic, infectious, cutaneous vascular disorder. *J Am Acad Dermatol*. 1990;22:501-512.
109. LeBoit PE, Berger TG, Egbert BM, et al. Bacillary angiomatosis: the histology and differential diagnosis of a pseudoneoplastic infection in patients with human immunodeficiency virus disease. *Am J Surg Pathol*. 1989;13:909-920.
110. Perkocha LA, Geaghan SM, Yen TSB, et al. Clinical and pathological features of bacillary peliosis hepatis in association with human immunodeficiency virus infection. *N Engl J Med*. 1990;323:1581-1586.
111. Leong SS, Cazen RA, Yu GSM, et al. Abdominal visceral peliosis associated with bacillary angiomatosis: ultrastructural evidence of endothelial cell destruction by bacilli. *Arch Pathol Lab Med*. 1992;116:866-871.
112. Slater LN, Pitha JV, Herrera L, et al. *Rochalimaea henselae* infection in AIDS causing inflammatory disease without angiomatosis or peliosis: demonstration by immunocytochemistry and corroboration by DNA amplification. *Arch Pathol Lab Med*. 1994;118:33-38.
113. Caniza MA, Granger DL, Wilson KH, et al. *Bartonella henselae*: etiology of pulmonary nodules in a patient with depressed cell-mediated immunity. *Clin Infect Dis*. 1995;20:1505-1511.
114. Liston TE, Koehler JE. Granulomatous hepatitis and necrotizing splenitis due to *Bartonella henselae* in a patient with cancer: case report and review of hepatosplenic manifestations of *Bartonella* infection. *Clin Infect Dis*. 1996;22:951-957.
115. Szelc-Kelly CM, Goral S, Perez-Perez GI, et al. Serologic responses to *Bartonella* and *Afipia* antigens in patients with cat scratch disease. *Pediatrics*. 1995;96:1137-1142.
116. Dauga C, Mira I, Grimont PAD. Identification of *Bartonella henselae* and *B. quintana* 16S rDNA sequences by branch-, genus-, and species-specific amplification. *J Med Microbiol*. 1996;45:192-199.
117. Scott MA, McCurley TL, Vnencak-Jones CL, et al. Cat scratch disease: detection of *Bartonella henselae* DNA in archival biopsies from patients with clinically, serologically and histologically defined disease. *Am J Pathol*. 1996;149:2161-2167.
118. Mouritsen CL, Litwin CM, Maiese RL, et al. Rapid polymerase chain reaction-based detection of the causative agent of cat scratch disease (*Bartonella henselae*) in formalin-fixed, paraffin-embedded samples. *Hum Pathol*. 1997;28:820-826.
119. Avidor B, Kletter Y, Abulafa S, et al. Molecular diagnosis of cat scratch disease: a two-step approach. *J Clin Microbiol*. 1997; 35:1924-1930.
120. Min K-W, Reed JA, Welch DF, et al. Morphologically variable bacilli of cat scratch disease are identified by immunocytochemical labeling with antibodies to *Rochalimaea henselae*. *Am J Clin Pathol*. 1994;101:607-610.
121. Regnery R, Martin M, Olson J. Naturally occurring "*Rochalimaea henselae*" infection in domestic cat [letter]. *Lancet*. 1992;340:557-558.
122. Debré R, Lamy M, Jammet ML, et al. La maladie des griffes de chat. *Semin Hop Paris*. 1950;26:1895-1904.
123. Brenner DJ, Hollis DG, Moss CW, et al. Proposal of *Afipia* gen. nov., with *Afipia felis* sp nov. (formerly the cat scratch disease bacillus), *Afipia clevelandensis* sp. nov. (formerly the Cleveland Clinic Foundation strain), *Afipia broomeae* sp. nov., and three unnamed genospecies. *J Clin Microbiol*. 1991;29: 2450-2460.
124. Alkan S, Morgan MB, Sandin RL, et al. Dual role for *Afipia felis* and *Rochalimaea henselae* in cat-scratch disease [letter]. *Lancet*. 1995;345:385.
125. Jackson LA, Perkins BA, Wenger JD. Cat scratch disease in the United States: an analysis of three national databases. *Am J Public Health*. 1993;83:1707-1711.
126. Noah DL, Kramer CM, Verbsky MP, et al. Survey of veterinary professionals and other veterinary conference attendees for antibodies to *Bartonella henselae* and *B. quintana*. *J Am Vet Med Assoc*. 1997;210:342-344.
127. Carithers HA. Cat-scratch disease: an overview based on a study of 1,200 patients. *Am J Dis Child*. 1985;139:1124-1133.
128. Moriarty R, Margileth A. Cat scratch disease. *Infect Dis Clin North Am*. 1987;1:575-590.
129. Margileth AM. Cat scratch disease. *Adv Pediatr Infect Dis*. 1993;8:1-21.
130. Bass JW, Freitas BD, Sisier CL, et al. Prospective randomized double-blind placebo-controlled evaluation of azithromycin for treatment of cat scratch disease. *Pediatr Infect Dis J*. 1998; 17:447-452.
131. Bosch X. Hypercalcemia due to endogenous overproduction of active vitamin D in identical twins with cat-scratch disease. *JAMA*. 1998;279:532-534.
132. Maman E, Bickels J, Ephros M, et al. Musculoskeletal manifestations of cat scratch disease. *Clin Infect Dis*. 2007;45:1535-1540.
133. Parinaud H. Conjontivite infectieuse par les animaux. *Ann Ocul*. 1889;101:252-253.
134. Cassady JV, Culbertson CS. Cat-scratch disease and Parinaud's oculoglandular syndrome. *Arch Ophthalmol*. 1953;50:68-74.
135. Margileth AM, Wear DJ, English CK. Systemic cat scratch disease: report of 23 patients with prolonged or recurrent severe bacterial infection. *J Infect Dis*. 1987;155:390-402.
136. Abbasi S, Chesney PJ. Pulmonary manifestations of cat scratch disease: a case report and review of the literature. *Pediatr Infect Dis J*. 1995;14:547-548.
137. Muszynski M, Eppes J, Riley H. Granulomatous osteolytic lesion of the skull associated with cat scratch disease. *Pediatr Infect Dis J*. 1987;6:199-201.
138. Jacobs RF, Schultze GE. *Bartonella henselae* as a cause of prolonged fever of unknown origin in children. *Clin Infect Dis*. 1998;26:80-84.
139. Lenoir AA, Storch GA, DeSchryver-Kecskemeti K, et al. Granulomatous hepatitis associated with cat scratch disease. *Lancet*. 1988;1:1132-1136.
140. Delahoussaye PM, Osborne BM. Cat-scratch disease presenting as abdominal visceral granulomas. *J Infect Dis*. 1990;161:71-78.
141. Dunn MW, Berkowitz FE, Miller JJ, et al. Hepatosplenic cat-scratch disease and abdominal pain. *Pediatr Infect Dis J*. 1997;16:269-272.
142. Stevens H. Cat-scratch fever encephalitis. *Am J Dis Child*. 1952;84:218-222.
143. Jambor J, Emura E. Benign inoculation lymphoreticulosis (cat scratch disease). *Arch Dermatol Syph*. 1953;67:439-442.
144. Thompson Jr TE, Miller KF. Cat scratch encephalitis. *Ann Intern Med*. 1953;39:146-151.
145. Weinstein L, Meade RH. Neurological manifestations of cat scratch disease. *Am J Med Sci*. 1955;229:500-505.
146. Centers for Disease Control and Prevention. Encephalitis associated with cat scratch disease—Broward and Palm Beach Counties, Florida, 1994. *MMWR Morb Mortal Wkly Rep*. 1994; 43:915-916.
147. Carithers H, Margileth A. Cat scratch disease: acute encephalopathy and other neurologic manifestations. *Am J Dis Child*. 1991;145:98-101.
148. Selby G, Walker GL. Cerebral arteritis in cat-scratch disease. *Neurology*. 1979;29:1413-1418.
149. Revol A, Vighetto A, Jouvet A, et al. Encephalitis in cat scratch disease with persistent dementia. *J Neurol Neurosurg Psychiatry*. 1992;55:133-135.
150. Hahn J, Sum J, Lee K. Unusual MRI findings after status epilepticus due to cat-scratch disease. *Pediatr Neurol*. 1994; 10:255-258.
151. Munana KR, Vitek SM, Hegarty BC, et al. Infection of fetal feline brain cells in culture with *Bartonella henselae*. *Infect Immun*. 2001;69:564-569.
152. Gerber JE, Johnson JE, Scott MA, et al. Fatal meningitis and encephalitis due to *Bartonella henselae* bacteria. *J Forensic Sci*. 2002;47:640-644.
153. Fouch B, Coventry S. A case of fatal disseminated *Bartonella henselae* infection (cat-scratch disease) with encephalitis. *Arch Pathol Lab Med*. 2007;131:1591-1594.
154. Eskow E, Rao R-VS, Mordechai E. Concurrent infection of the central nervous system by *Borrelia burgdorferi* and *Bartonella henselae*. *Arch Neurol*. 2001;58:1357-1363.
155. Sweeney VP, Drance SM. Optic neuritis and compressive neuropathy associated with cat scratch disease. *Can Med Assoc J*. 1970;103:1380-1381.
156. Dreyer RF, Hopen G, Gass DM, et al. Leber's idiopathic stellate neuroretinitis. *Arch Ophthalmol*. 1984;102:1140-1145.
157. Golnik KC, Marotto ME, Fanous MM, et al. Ophthalmic manifestations of *Rochalimaea* species. *Am J Ophthalmol*. 1994;118:145-151.
158. Kerkhoff FT, Bergmans AM, van Der Zee A, et al. Demonstration of *Bartonella grahamii* DNA in ocular fluids of a patient with neuroretinitis. *J Clin Microbiol*. 1999;37:4034-4038.
159. O'Halloran HS, Draud K, Minix M, et al. Leber's neuroretinitis in a patient with serologic evidence of *Bartonella elizabethae*. *Retina*. 1998;18:276-278.
160. Solley WA, Martin DF, Newman NJ, et al. Cat scratch disease: posterior segment manifestations. *Ophthalmology*. 1999; 106:1546-1553.
161. Reed JB, Scales JK, Wong MT, et al. *Bartonella henselae* neuroretinitis in cat scratch disease. *Ophthalmology*. 1998;105: 459-466.
162. Ben-Ami R, Ephros M, Avidor B, et al. Cat-scratch disease in elderly patients. *Clin Infect Dis*. 2005:41:969-974.
163. Schwartzman WA, Patnaik M, Barka NE, et al. *Rochalimaea* antibodies in HIV-associated neurologic disease. *Neurology*. 1994;44:1312-1316.
164. Baker J, Ruiz-Rodriguez R, Whitfield M, et al. Bacillary angiomatosis: a treatable cause of acute psychiatric symptoms in human immunodeficiency virus infection. *J Clin Psychiatry*. 1995;56:161-166.
165. Patnaik M, Schwartzman WA, Peter JB. *Bartonella henselae*: detection in brain tissue of patients with AIDS-associated neurological disease [abstract]. *J Invest Med*. 1995;43(Suppl 2): 368A.

166. Schwartzman WA, Patnaik M, Angulo FJ, et al. *Bartonella* (*Rochalimaea*) antibodies, dementia, and cat ownership in human immunodeficiency virus-infected men. *Clin Infect Dis.* 1995;21:954-959.
167. Abbot R, Chomel B, Kasten R, et al. Experimental and natural infection with *Bartonella henselae* in domestic cats. *Comp Immunol Microbiol Infect Dis.* 1997;20:41-51.
168. Guptill L, Slater L, Wu C-C, et al. Experimental infection of young specific pathogen-free cats with *Bartonella henselae. J Infect Dis.* 1997;176:206-216.
169. Kordick DL, Breitschwerdt EB. Relapsing bacteremia after blood transmission of *Bartonella henselae* to cats. *Am J Vet Res.* 1997;58:492-497.
170. Dehio C. Molecular and cellular basis of *Bartonella* pathogenesis. *Annu Rev Microbiol.* 2004;58:365-390.
171. Boonjakuakul JK, Gerns HL, Chen YT, et al. Proteomic and immunoblot analyses of *Bartonella quintana* total membrane proteins identify antigens recognized by sera from infected patients. *Infect Immun.* 2007;75:2548-2561.
172. Walker TS, Winkler HH. *Bartonella bacilliformis*: colonial types and erythrocyte adherence. *Infect Immun.* 1981;31:480-486.
173. Scherer DC, DeBuron-Conners I, Minnick MF. Characterization of *Bartonella bacilliformis* flagella and effect of antiflagellin antibodies on invasion of human erythrocytes. *Infect Immun.* 1993;61:4962-4971.
174. Minnick MF. Virulence determinants of *Bartonella bacilliformis.* In: Anderson B, Friedman H, Bendinelli M, eds. *Rickettsial Infection and Immunity.* New York: Plenum Press; 1997: 197-211.
175. Mernaugh G, Ihler GM. Deformation factor: an extracellular protein synthesized by *Bartonella bacilliformis* that deforms erythrocyte membranes. *Infect Immun.* 1992;60:937-943.
176. Xu Y-H, Lu Z-Y, Ihler GM. Purification of deformin, an extracellular protein synthesized by *Bartonella bacilliformis* which causes deformation of erythrocyte membranes. *Biochem Biophys Acta.* 1995;1234:173-183.
177. Mitchell SJ, Minnick MF. Characterization of a two-gene locus from *Bartonella bacilliformis* associated with the ability to invade human erythrocytes. *Infect Immun.* 1995;63:1552-1562.
178. Iwaki-Egawa S, Ihler GM. Comparison of the abilities of proteins from *Bartonella bacilliformis* and *Bartonella henselae* to deform red cell membranes and to bind to red cell ghost proteins. *FEMS Microbiol Lett.* 1997;157:207-217.
179. Zimmermann R, Kempf VA, Schiltz E, et al. Hemin binding, functional expression, and complementation analysis of Pap 31 from *Bartonella henselae. J Bacteriol.* 2003;185:1739-1744.
180. Benson LA, Kar S, McLaughlin G, et al. Entry of *Bartonella bacilliformis* into erythrocytes. *Infect Immun.* 1986;54:347-353.
181. Kordick DL, Breitschwerdt E. Intraerythrocytic presence of *Bartonella henselae. J Clin Microbiol.* 1995;33:1655-1656.
182. Guptill L, Wu C-C, Glickman L, et al. Extracellular *Bartonella henselae* and artifactual intraerythrocytic pseudoinclusions in experimentally infected cats. *Vet Microbiol.* 2000;76:283-290.
183. Rolain JM, Foucault C, Guieu R, et al. *Bartonella quintana* in human erythrocytes. *Lancet.* 2002;360:226-228.
184. Rolain JM, Arnoux D, Parzy D, et al. Experimental infection of human erythrocytes from alcoholic patients with *Bartonella quintana. Ann N Y Acad Sci.* 2003;990:605-611.
185. Pitassi LHU, Magalhaes RF, Barjas-Castro ML, et al. *Bartonella henselae* infects human erythrocytes. *Ultrastruct Pathol.* 2007; 31369-31372.
186. Mandle T, Einsele H, Schaller M, et al. Infection of human CD34⁺ progenitor cells with *Bartonella henselae* results in intraerythrocytic presence of *B. henselae. Blood.* 2005;106: 1215-1222.
187. Garcia FU, Wojta J, Broadley KN, et al. *Bartonella bacilliformis* stimulates endothelial cells in vitro and is angiogenic in vivo. *Am J Pathol.* 1990;136:1125-1135.
188. Garcia FU, Wojta J, Hoover RL. Interactions between live *Bartonella bacilliformis* and endothelial cells. *J Infect Dis.* 1992;165:1138-1141.
189. Conley T, Slater L, Hamilton K. *Rochalimaea* spp. stimulate endothelial cell proliferation and migration in vitro. *J Lab Clin Med.* 1994;124:521-528.
190. Cerimele F, Brown LF, Bravo F, et al. Infectious angiogenesis: *Bartonella bacilliformis* infection results in endothelial production of angiopoietin-2 and epidermal production of vascular endothelial growth factor. *Am J Pathol.* 2003;163:1321-1327.
191. Riess T, Raddatz G, Linke D, et al. Analysis of *Bartonella* adhesin A expression reveals differences between various *B. henselae* strains. *Infect Immun.* 2007;75:35-43.
192. Schulte B, Linke D, Klumpp S, et al. *Bartonella quintana* variably expressed outer membrane proteins mediate vascular endothelial growth factor secretion but not host cell adherence. *Infect Immun.* 2006;74:5003-5013.
193. Schmid MC, Scheidegger F, Dehio M, et al. A translocated bacterial protein protects vascular endothelial cells from apoptosis. *PLoS Pathog.* 2006;2:e115.
194. McGinnis-Hill E, Raji A, Valenzuela MS, et al. Adhesion to and invasion of cultured human cells by *Bartonella bacilliformis. Infect Immun.* 1992;60:4051-4058.
195. Brouqui P, Raoult D. *Bartonella quintana* invades and multiplies within endothelial cells in vitro and in vivo and forms intracellular blebs. *Res Microbiol.* 1996;147:719-731.
196. Dehio C, Meyer M, Berger J, et al. Interaction of *Bartonella henselae* with endothelial cells results in bacterial aggregation on the cell surface and the subsequent engulfment and internalisation of the bacterial aggregate by a unique structure, the invasome. *J Cell Sci.* 1997;110:2141-2154.
197. Conley TD, Wack MF, Hamilton KK, et al. Stimulation of angiogenesis and protection from oxidative damage: two potential mechanisms involved in pathogenesis by *Bartonella henselae* and other *Bartonella* species. In: Anderson B, Friedman H, Bendinelli M, eds. *Rickettsial Infection and Immunity.* New York: Plenum Press; 1997:213-232.
198. Mitchell SJ, Minnick MF. A carboxy terminal processing gene is located immediately upstream of the invasion-associated locus from *Bartonella bacilliformis. Microbiology.* 1997;143: 1221-1233.
199. Vermi W, Facchetti F, Riboldi E, et al. Role of dendritic cell-derived CXCL13 in the pathogenesis of *Bartonella henselae* B-rich granuloma. *Blood.* 2006;107:454-462.
200. Agan BK, Dolan MJ. Laboratory diagnosis of *Bartonella* infections. *Clin Lab Med.* 2002;22:937-962.
201. Chomel BB, Rolain JM. *Bartonella.* In: Murray PR, Barron EJ, Jorgensen JH, et al, eds. *Manual of Clinical Microbiology.* 9th ed. Washington, DC: American Society for Microbiology; 2007:850-861.
202. Hansmann Y, DeMartino S, Piémontet Y, et al. Diagnosis of cat scratch disease with detection of *Bartonella henselae* by PCR: a study of patients with lymph node enlargement. *J Clin Microbiol.* 2005;43:3800-3806.
203. Peters D, Wigand R. Bartonellaceae. *Bacteriol Rev.* 1955; 19:150-159.
204. Cuadra M, Takano J. The relationship of *Bartonella bacilliformis* to the red blood cell as revealed by electron microscopy. *Blood.* 1969;33:708-716.
205. Foucault C, Rolain JM, Raoult D, et al. Detection of *Bartonella quintana* by direct immunofluorescence examination of blood smears of a patient with acute trench fever. *J Clin Microbiol.* 2004;42:4904-4906.
206. Reed J, Brigati DJ, Flynn SD, et al. Immunocytochemical identification of *Rochalimaea henselae* in bacillary (epithelioid) angiomatosis, parenchymal bacillary peliosis, and persistent fever with bacteremia. *Am J Surg Pathol.* 1992;16:650-657.
207. Brenner SA, Rooney JA, Manzewitsch P, et al. Isolation of *Bartonella* (*Rochalimaea*) *henselae*: effects of methods of blood collection and handling. *J Clin Microbiol.* 1997;35:544-547.
208. Welch DF, Hensel DM, Pickett DA, et al. Bacteremia due to *Rochalimaea henselae* in a child: practical identification of isolates in the clinical laboratory. *J Clin Microbiol.* 1993;31: 2381-2386.
209. Fournier PE, Robson J, Zeaiter Z, et al. Improved culture from lymph nodes of patients with cat scratch disease and genotypic characterization of *Bartonella henselae* isolates in Australia. *J Clin Microbiol.* 2002;40:3620-3624.
210. Maggi RG, Duncan AW, Breitschwerdt EB. Novel chemically modified liquid medium that will support the growth of seven *Bartonella* species. *J Clin Microbiol.* 2005;43:2651-2655.
211. Gouriet F, Fenolla RF, Patrice J-Y, et al. Use of shell-vial cell culture assay for isolation of bacteria from clinical specimens: 13 years of experience. *J Clin Microbiol.* 2005;43: 4993-5002.
212. La Scola B, Raoult D. Culture of *Bartonella quintana* and *Bartonella henselae* from human samples: a 5-year experience (1993 to 1998). *J Clin Microbiol.* 1999;37:1899-1905.
213. Tierno PM Jr, Inglima K, Parisi MT. Detection of *Bartonella* (*Rochalimaea*) *henselae* bacteremia using BacT/Alert blood culture system. *Am J Clin Pathol.* 1995;104:530-536.
214. Sondermeijer HP, Claas EC, Orendi JM, et al. *Bartonella quintana* prosthetic valve endocarditis detected by blood culture incubation beyond 10 days. *Eur J Intern Med.* 2006; 17:441-443.
215. Slater LN, Coody DW, Woolridge LK, et al. Murine antibody responses distinguish *Rochalimaea henselae* from *Rochalimaea quintana. J Clin Microbiol.* 1992;30:1722-1727.
216. Drancourt M, Raoult D. Proposed tests for the routine identification of *Rochalimaea* species. *Eur J Clin Microbiol Infect Dis.* 1993;12:710-713.
217. Moss CW, Holzer G, Wallace PL, et al. Cellular fatty acid compositions of an unidentified organism and a bacterium associated with cat scratch disease. *J Clin Microbiol.* 1990; 28:1071-1074.
218. Myers WF, Grossman DM, Wisseman CL Jr. Antibiotic susceptibility patterns in *Rochalimaea quintana*, the agent of trench fever. *Antimicrob Agents Chemother.* 1984;25:690-693.
219. Wolfson C, Branley J, Gottlieb T. The Etest for antimicrobial susceptibility testing of *Bartonella henselae. J Antimicrob Chemother.* 1996;38:963-968.
220. Pendle S, Ginn A, Iredell J. Antimicrobial susceptibility of *Bartonella henselae* using Etest methodology. *J Antimicrob Chemother.* 2006;57:761-763.
221. Dorbecker C, Sander A, Oberle K, et al. In vitro susceptibility of *Bartonella* species to 17 antimicrobial compounds: comparison of Etest and agar dilution. *J Antimicrob Chemother.* 2006; 58:784-788.
222. Maurin M, Raoult D. Antimicrobial susceptibility of *Rochalimaea quintana, Rochalimaea vinsonii*, and the newly recognised *Rochalimaea henselae. J Antimicrob Chemother.* 1993;32: 587-594.
223. Maurin M, Gasquet S, Caroline D, et al. MICs of 28 antibiotic compounds for 14 *Bartonella* (formerly *Rochalimaea*) isolates. *Antimicrob Agents Chemother.* 1995;39:2387-2391.
224. Musso D, Drancourt M, Raoult D. Lack of bactericidal effect of antibiotics except aminoglycosides on *Bartonella* (*Rochalimaea*) *henselae. J Antimicrob Chemother.* 1995;36:101-108.
225. Ives TJ, Manzewitsch P, Regnery RL, et al. In vitro susceptibilities of *Bartonella henselae, B. quintana, B. elizabethae, Rickettsia rickettsii, R. conorii, R. akari*, and *R. prowazekii* to macrolide antibiotics as determined by immunofluorescent-antibody analysis of infected Vero cell monolayers. *Antimicrob Agent Chemother.* 1997;44:578-582.
226. Rolain JM, Maurin M, Raoult D. Bactericidal effect of antibiotics on *Bartonella* and *Brucella* spp.: clinical implications. *J Antimicrob Chemother.* 2000;46:811-814.
227. Rolain JM, Maurin M, Mallet MN, et al. Culture and antibiotic susceptibility of *Bartonella quintana* in human erythrocytes. *Antimicrob Agents Chemother.* 2003;47:614-619.
228. Ciervo A, Ciceroni L. Rapid detection and differentiation of *Bartonella* spp. by a single-run real-time PCR. *Mol Cell Probes.* 2004;18:307-312.
229. Diederen BM, Vermeulen MJ, Verbakel H, et al. Evaluation of an internally controlled real-time polymerase chain reaction assay targeting the groEL gene for the detection of *Bartonella* spp. DNA in patients with suspected cat-scratch disease. *Eur J Clin Microbiol Infect Dis.* 2007;26:629-633.
230. Vermeulen MJ, Diederen BM, Verbakel H, et al. Low sensitivity of *Bartonella henselae* PCR in serum samples of patients with cat-scratch disease lymphadenitis. *J Med Microbiol.* 2008; 57:1049-1050.
231. Ritzler M, Altwegg M. Sensitivity and specificity of a commercially available enzyme-linked immunoassay for the detection of polymerase chain reaction amplified DNA. *J Microbiol Methods.* 1996;27:233-238.
232. Margolis B, Kuzu I, Herrmann M, et al. Rapid polymerase chain reaction-based confirmation of cat scratch disease and *Bartonella henselae* infection. *Arch Pathol Lab Med.* 2003;127: 706-710.
233. Fenollar F, Sire S, Raoult D. *Bartonella vinsonii* subsp. *arupensis* as an agent of blood culture-negative endocarditis in a human. *J Clin Microbiol.* 2005;43:945-947.
234. Matar GM, Swaminathan B, Hunter SB, et al. Polymerase chain reaction-based restriction fragment length polymorphism analysis of a fragment of the ribosomal operon from *Rochalimaea* species for subtyping. *J Clin Microbiol.* 1993;31:1730-1734.
235. Bergmans AM, Schellekens JFP, van Embden JDA, et al. Predominance of two *Bartonella henselae* variants among cat-scratch disease patients in The Netherlands. *J Clin Microbiol.* 1996;34:254-260.
236. Roux V, Raoult D. Inter- and intraspecies identification of *Bartonella* (*Rochalimaea*) species. *J Clin Microbiol.* 1995;33: 1573-1576.
237. Arvand M, Viezens J. Evaluation of pulsed-field gel electrophoresis and multi-locus sequence typing for the analysis of clonal relatedness among *Bartonella henselae* isolates. *Int J Med Microbiol.* 2007;297:255-262.
238. Rodriguez-Barradas MC, Hamill RJ, Houston ED, et al. Genomic fingerprints of *Bartonella* species by repetitive element PCR for distinguishing species and isolates. *J Clin Microbiol.* 1995;33:1089-1093.
239. Foucault C, La Scola B, Lindroos H, et al. Multispacer typing technique for sequence-based typing of *Bartonella quintana. J Clin Microbiol.* 2005;43:41-48.
240. Mallqui V, Speelmon EC, Verástegui C, et al. Sonicated diagnostic immunoblot for bartonellosis. *Clin Diagn Lab Immunol.* 2000;7:1-5.
241. Chamberlin J, Laughlin L, Gordon S, et al. Serodiagnosis of *Bartonella bacilliformis* by indirect immunofluorescence assay: test development and application to a population in an area of bartonellosis endemicity. *J Clin Microbiol.* 2000;38:4269-4271.
242. Taye A, Chen H, Duncan K, et al. Production of recombinant protein Pap31 and its application for the diagnosis of *Bartonella bacilliformis* infection. *Ann N Y Acad Sci.* 2005;1063:280-285.
243. Herrmann JE, Hollingdale MR, Collins MF, et al. Enzyme immunoassay and radioimmunoprecipitation tests for the detection of antibodies to *Rochalimaea (Rickettsia) quintana* (39655). *Proc Soc Exp Biol Med.* 1977;154:285-288.
244. Hollingdale MR, Herrmann JE, Vinson JW. Enzyme immunoassay of antibody to *Rochalimaea quintana*: diagnosis of trench fever and serologic cross-reactions among other rickettsiae. *J Infect Dis.* 1978;137:578-582.
245. Dalton MJ, Robinson LE, Cooper J, et al. Use of *Bartonella* antigens for the serologic diagnosis of cat-scratch disease at a national referral center. *Arch Intern Med.* 1995;155:1670-1676.
246. La Scola B, Raoult D. Serological cross-reactions between *Bartonella quintana, Bartonella henselae*, and *Coxiella burnetii. J Clin Microbiol.* 1996;34:2270-2274.
247. Dupon M, Savin de Larclause A-M, Brouqui P, et al. Evaluation of serological response to *Bartonella henselae, Bartonella quintana*, and *Afipia felis* antigens in 64 patients with suspected cat-scratch disease. *Scand J Infect Dis.* 1996;28:361-366.
248. Bergmans AMC, Peeters MF, Schellekens JFP, et al. Pitfalls and fallacies of cat scratch disease serology: evaluation of *Bartonella henselae*-based indirect fluorescence assay and enzyme-linked immunoassay. *J Clin Microbiol.* 1997;35:1931-1937.
249. Maurin M, Eb F, Etienne J, et al. Serological cross-reactions between *Bartonella* and *Chlamydia. J Clin Microbiol.* 1997; 35:2283-2287.
250. Herremans M, Bakker J, Vermeulen MJ, et al. Evaluation of an in-house cat scratch disease IgM ELISA to detect *Bartonella*

henselae in a routine laboratory setting. *Eur J Clin Microbiol Infect Dis*. 2009;28:147-152.

251. Litwin CM, Martins TB, Hill HR. Immunologic response to *Bartonella henselae* as determined by enzyme immunoassay and Western blot analysis. *Am J Clin Pathol*. 1997;108:202-209.

252. Anderson B, Lu E, Jones D, et al. Characterization of 17-kilo-dalton antigen of *Bartonella henselae* reactive with sera from patients with cat scratch disease. *J Clin Microbiol*. 1995;33: 2358-2365.

253. Loa CC, Mordechai E, Tilton RC, et al. Production of recombinant *Bartonella henselae* 17-kDa protein for antibody-capture enzyme-linked immunosorbent assay. *Diagn Microbiol Infect Dis*. 2006;55:1-7.

254. Giladi M, Kletter Y, Avidor B, et al. Enzyme immunoassay for the diagnosis of cat-scratch disease defined by polymerase chain reaction. *Clin Infect Dis*. 2001;33:1852-1858.

255. Rolain JM, Brouqui P, Koehler JE, et al. Recommendations for treatment of human infections caused by *Bartonella* species. *Antimicrob Agents Chemother*. 2004;48:1921-1933.

256. Koehler JE, Tappero JW. Bacillary angiomatosis and bacillary peliosis in patients infected with human immunodeficiency virus. *Clin Infect Dis*. 1993;17:612-624.

257. Koehler JE, Sanchez MA, Tye S, et al. Prevalence of *Bartonella* infection among human immunodeficiency virus-infected patients with fever. *Clin Infect Dis*. 2003;37:559-566.

258. Regnery RL, Childs JE, Koehler JE. Infections associated with *Bartonella* species in persons infected with the human immunodeficiency virus. *Clin Infect Dis*. 1995;21(Suppl 1): S94-S98.

259. Bogue C, Wise JD, Gray GF, et al. Antibiotic therapy for cat-scratch disease? *JAMA*. 1989;262:813-816.

260. Holley Jr HP. Successful treatment of cat-scratch disease with ciprofloxacin. *JAMA*. 1991;265:1563-1565.

261. Collipp PJ. Cat-scratch disease: therapy with trimethoprim-sulfamethoxazole. *Am J Dis Child*. 1992;146:397-399.

262. Margileth AM. Antibiotic therapy for cat-scratch disease: clinical study of therapeutic outcome in 268 patients and a review of the literature. *Pediatr Infect Dis J*. 1992;11:474-478.

263. Chia JK, Nakata MM, Lami JL, et al. Azithromycin for the treatment of cat-scratch disease. *Clin Infect Dis*. 1998;26: 193-194.

264. Centers for Disease Control and Prevention, National Institutes of Health, and HIV Medicine Association of the Infectious Diseases Society of America. Guidelines for Prevention and Treatment of Opportunistic Infections in HIV-Infected Adults and Adolescents, pp 39-40. Available at http://www.edc.gov/mmwr/pdf/rr/rr5804.pdf. Accessed May 2009.

265. Foley JE, Chomel B, Kikuchi Y, et al. Seroprevalence of *Bartonella henselae* in cattery cats: association with cattery hygiene and flea infestation. *Vet Q*. 1998;20:1-5.

266. Greene CE, McDermott M, Jameson PH, et al. *Bartonella henselae* infection in cats: evaluation during primary infection, treatment, and rechallenge infection. *J Clin Microbiol*. 1996;34: 1682-1685.

267. Regnery RL, Rooney A, Johnson AM, et al. Experimentally induced *Bartonella henselae* infections followed by challenge exposure and antimicrobial therapy in cats. *Am J Vet Res*. 1996;57:1714-1719.

268. Kordick DL, Papich MG, Breitschwerdt EB. Efficacy of enro-floxacin or doxycycline for treatment of *Bartonella henselae* or *Bartonella clarridgeiae* infection in cats. *Antimicrob Agents Chemother*. 1997;41:2448-2455.

236

Klebsiella granulomatis (Donovanosis, Granuloma Inguinale)

RONALD C. BALLARD

Donovanosis is a chronic, progressive ulcerative disease, usually of the genital region, that is caused by an encapsulated, pleomorphic, gram-negative bacterium. The infection has previously been known by other names, including granuloma inguinale tropicum, granuloma pudenda, granuloma venereum and, most recently, granuloma inguinale. Because these names can easily be confused with that of a completely different tropical sexually transmitted disease, lymphogranuloma venereum, caused by the more invasive L-serovars of *Chlamydia trachomatis,* the term *donovanosis* has been adopted as the preferred name for the disease. The first description of donovanosis was attributed to McLeod working in India in 1881[1] and the discovery of the causative organism to Donovan in 1905.[2]

Biology of the Causative Organism

Klebsiella granulomatis, formerly known as *Calymmatobacterium granulomatis* and as *Donovania granulomatis,* is an encapsulated, pleomorphic, gram-negative bacillus measuring 1 to 2 μm by 0.5 to 0.7 μm that can be found in vacuoles in the cytoplasm of large mononuclear cells.[3] The bacteria are frequently described as having bipolar densities that give Donovan bodies the appearance of closed safety pins. The bacteria appear to multiply within these cells and are subsequently released to infect others after the rupture of mature intracytoplasmic vacuoles. Ultrastructurally, the organisms have been described as characteristically gram-negative, with a clearly defined capsule and no flagella. However, small surface projections resembling pili or fimbriae have been observed, together with electron-dense granules 35 to 45 μm in diameter in the cell periphery.[4] Formerly, it was thought that these granules provided evidence of bacteriophage infection; however, this remains contentious.[5]

Although culture of the organisms in chick embryo yolk sacs was reported in the early 1940s,[6] and subsequently in egg yolk–based media[7] and defined liquid media, no pure isolates were stored and therefore none were available for study for approximately 50 years. As a result, the organisms were poorly characterized, although a relationship with *Klebsiella* had previously been suggested because of common morphologic characteristics. Renewed efforts to isolate *Klebsiella granulomatis* from clinical material have been successful using human monocyte cultures[8] and Hep-2 cell monolayers,[9] and so progress has been made in further characterizing the causative organisms. A detailed description of the phylogeny of *C. granulomatis* based on the results of molecular studies has been published, resulting in the name *Klebsiella granulomatis* comb. nov. being formally proposed.[10,11]

Geographic Distribution and Epidemiology

Donovanosis is a relatively rare disease in the United States, with fewer than 100 cases reported annually, although in the past it was encountered more frequently in the southern states. However, it has been recognized as a cause of genital ulceration in parts of India, Papua New Guinea, the Caribbean, and South America (particularly Brazil) and has been recorded in Zambia, Zimbabwe, South Africa, Southeast Asia, and among Aboriginals and Torres Strait Islanders in Australia.[3,12]

Fortunately, the incidence of the disease has decreased significantly in recent years, either as a result of recognition of donavanosis as a public health problem with subsequent, aggressive introduction of appropriate control measures, as has occurred in Australia,[13] or as a result of unknown factors. Donovanosis has been recorded as relatively uncommon in Papua New Guinea,[14] whereas rates have decreased in Durban, South Africa,[15] parts of India,[16] and the Caribbean.[17] This situation may reflect improvements in the provision of health services and general standards of living in areas of high endemicity. Nevertheless, cases of donovanosis may still be encountered in centers remote from these endemic regions, either as a result of immigration[18] or increased vacation or business travel to these predominantly tropical areas. The disease is usually assumed to be sexually transmitted, and the possibility that it may be transmitted nonsexually remains a controversial issue. Goldberg[19] has postulated that the causative organism is a commensal of the gastrointestinal tract and that the vagina may become infected by autoinoculation. Extragenital lesions and lesions in young children all indicate alternative modes of spread; however, the age distribution of the disease in endemic areas, the frequent coexistence of other sexually transmitted diseases, and the finding that the genital area is the most frequent anatomic site of donovanosis lesions all indicate that it is primarily a sexually transmitted infection, albeit of low infectivity.

Clinical Manifestations

The primary lesion of donovanosis begins as a small painless papule or indurated nodule that manifests after an incubation period of between 8 and 80 days. The lesion soon ulcerates to form an exuberant, beefy red, granulomatous ulcer with rolled edges and with a characteristic velvet-like surface that bleeds easily on contact (Fig. 236-1). Multiple lesions may coalesce to form large ulcers, and new lesions may also form as a result of autoinoculation. Characteristically, even large ulcerative lesions are painless unless there is severe secondary infection. The disease spreads subcutaneously and may become progressively more destructive (Fig. 236-2). Spontaneous healing is accompanied by scar formation, which can also produce gross deformities (Fig. 236-3). Lymphedema, with consequent elephantiasis of the external genitalia, may occur in severe cases as a result of the blockage of the lymphatics by keloid scars. In men, the most common sites of infection are the prepuce, coronal sulcus, and penile shaft. In women, the labia and fourchette are most commonly involved, but lesions of the vaginal wall and cervix may be an uncommon cause of vaginal bleeding. Donovanosis is frequently diagnosed during pregnancy, and it has been postulated that pregnancy causes exacerbation of the disease.[20] However, the increase in diagnosis during pregnancy may just be a reflection of the asymptomatic nature of cervical infection and its detection on routine examination. Subcutaneous spread of granulomas into the inguinal region may result in the formation of groin swellings (pseudobubos), which are not a true adenitis.

Rectal lesions have been found to be associated with receptive anal intercourse among men who have sex with men (MSM),[21] whereas penile lesions are often detected among their sexual partners. Oral lesions have also been recorded in association with a history of orogenital contact.[22]

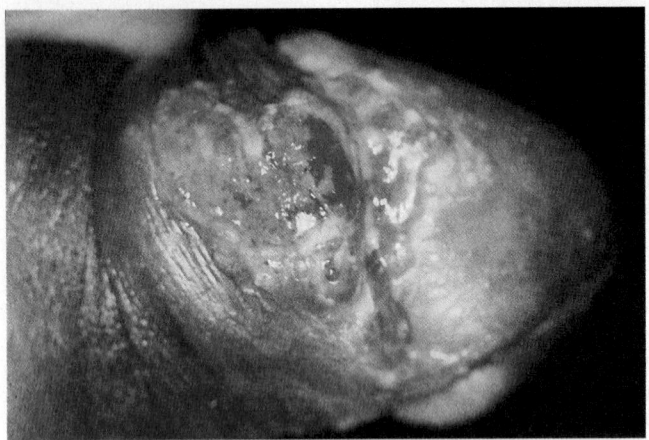

Figure 236-1   Early lesion of donovanosis.

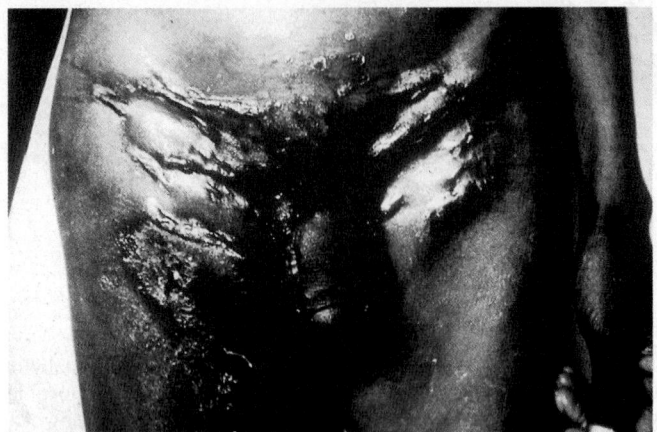

Figure 236-3   Late lesions of donovanosis showing extensive scarring and subcutaneous spread.

Systemic disease is rare, but more common in women who have primary lesions of the cervix.[23] Hematogenous spread of infection resulting in the formation of pelvic granulomas and bone and joint involvement, together with rare cases of lymphadenitis, possibly associated with lymphatic spread, have been documented.[24] Constitutional symptoms are conspicuously absent except in cases in which coinfection with other sexually transmitted diseases has been demonstrated, secondary bacterial infection is evident, or extensive spread has occurred. Donovanosis has to be distinguished from other causes of genital ulcer disease, regional lymphadenopathy, and genital elephantiasis. The lesions most likely to provide diagnostic problems on clinical grounds include cases of "pseudogranulomatous" chancroid, ulcerating genital warts, both primary and secondary syphilis, and squamous carcinoma. Multiple causative agents of genital ulceration have been noted in a single lesion.[15,25] Early reports had suggested a link between donovanosis and squamous carcinoma of the external genitalia[26]; however, this hypothesis remains unproven, and the possible coexistence of donovanosis and human papillomavirus infection, which has proven oncogenic potential, cannot be ruled out.

Diagnosis

Most cases of donovanosis are diagnosed on the basis of the characteristic clinical manifestations. However, confirmation of the diagnosis can be obtained on the basis of histologic examination of punch biopsy specimens taken from the edges of active lesions, scrapings taken from the edges of lesions, or a crush preparation made from granulation tissue obtained with a thin scalpel. In all cases, active lesions should be selected and cleansed with physiologic saline before sampling.

Although biopsy specimens are mandatory when malignancy has to be excluded, smear or crush preparations are usually adequate for the diagnosis of acute active disease of short duration. Ideally, smear preparations for microscopy should be made immediately with fresh moist tissue and should be fixed and stained with Giemsa, Leishman, or Wright stain.[3,27] Although the application of newer, rapid Giemsa techniques can provide an immediate, definitive diagnosis,[28] even in resource-poor settings, standard Giemsa and silver stains are preferred when fixed, embedded tissue specimens are prepared for histologic examination.[3] The demonstration of typical intracellular Donovan bodies in stained smears obtained from lesions (Fig. 236-4) has remained the gold standard for the diagnosis of donovanosis since they were first described by Donovan. Subsequently, Donovan bodies have also been detected in Papanicolaou-stained smears obtained from women with cervical lesions.[29,30] Earlier, isolation of *K. granulomatis* led to the development of an intradermal skin test and also a complement fixation test for the serologic diagnosis of the disease. However, these tests are no longer performed. An indirect immunofluorescence test has been devised that uses tissue sections from proven cases of donovanosis as the antigen. This test has proved both sensitive and specific[31] but is unlikely to become routine because of a lack of suitable clinical material that can be used as the antigen. The successful culture of *K. granulomatis* in monocytes[8,32] and Hep-2 cells[9] may provide an appropriate source of

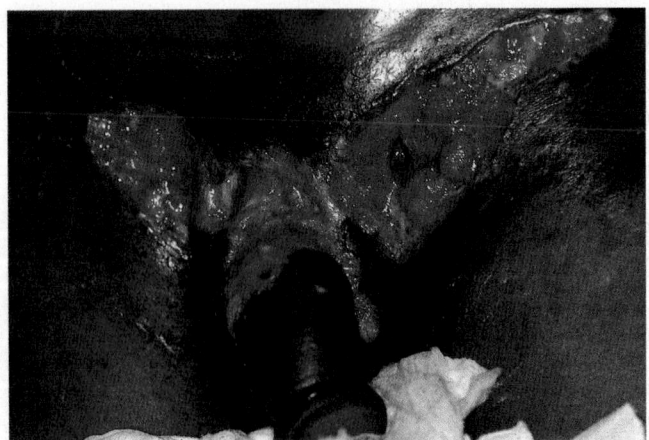

Figure 236-2   Extensive active lesions of donovanosis.

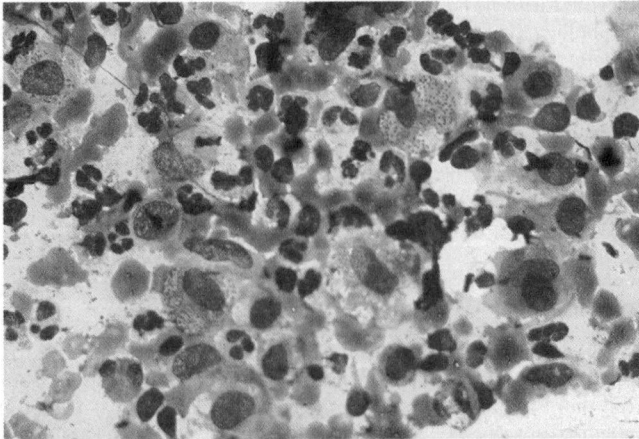

Figure 236-4   Scraping from an active lesion of donovanosis showing typical Donovan bodies in large mononuclear cells Giemsa stain (×100).

antigen for such a serologic test and offers possibilities for testing in vitro antimicrobial susceptibilities of isolates to provide a more rational basis for treatment of the disease. In particular, isolation of *K. granulomatis* in Hep-2 cell monolayers using techniques similar to those previously used for chlamydial isolation could, for the first time, provide a routine diagnostic test for donovanosis based on culture.[9]

The same Australian researchers have also demonstrated a high degree of molecular homology between *C. granulomatis* and other *Klebsiella* spp. by sequencing a region of the *pho*E (phosphatase porin) gene of *C. granulomatis* from DNA extracted from biopsy material.[33] Although there appears to be a high degree of homology between *pho*E genes of *C. granulomatis* and other *Klebsiella* spp.,[25] they were able to differentiate *C. granulomatis* from other Klebsiellae by amplifying a 700-bp region of the gene that encompasses two base changes that occur only in *C. granulomatis*. This product could subsequently be digested with the restriction endonuclease *Hae*III to yield a 167-bp fragment unique to *C. granulomatis*.[34] This molecular approach has been refined to include a colorimetric detection system.[35,36] This work represents a significant step forward in the diagnosis of the disease and may ultimately provide a viable routine alternative to culture or microscopy.

▇ Treatment

There appears to be no consensus about the ideal treatment for donovanosis because most antibiotics have been evaluated in open trials, with few data available from comparative, microbiologically controlled studies. In addition, the optimal duration of treatment for an individual case cannot be stated categorically because larger lesions appear to require longer periods of therapy.

After successful therapy, lesions begin to heal from the edges toward the center. It is my experience that treatment should be continued until complete epithelialization has taken place, which can take several weeks; otherwise, relapse may occur. Tetracycline (500 mg, four times daily by mouth) or doxycycline (100 mg twice daily by mouth) have, historically, been the treatments of choice for the disease, although many treatment failures or relapses have been recorded. Trimethoprim-sulfamethoxazole (two tablets twice daily by mouth) has also proved effective, but also with some failures.[3,12] Erythromycin (500 mg, four times daily by mouth) has also been used extensively, especially in pregnancy, with considerable success.[3,14] However, at this dosage, gastrointestinal side effects are common.

The antibiotic that exhibits the most promise in the treatment of donovanosis is azithromycin.[37] Preliminary studies have indicated that 1 g taken weekly for 4 to 6 weeks is effective.[38] It is thought that this antibiotic is particularly appropriate for the treatment of the disease because it concentrates within macrophages and is released slowly from the tissues, giving it a long tissue half-life. An added advantage of this antibiotic is that it is also active against other sexually transmitted bacteria—notably, *Haemophilus ducreyi*, *Treponema pallidum*, and *C. trachomatis*. Other antibiotics that have proved effective include the quinolones, chloramphenicol and thiamphenicol,[3] ceftriaxone,[39] and the aminoglycosides, gentamicin (1 mg/kg twice daily intramuscularly) and streptomycin (1 g twice daily intramuscularly), which have often been used to supplement tetracycline therapy in severe cases. In contrast, penicillin appears to be ineffective for treatment of the disease. Anecdotal evidence suggests that lesions may be more extensive and that prolonged periods of therapy may be required for patients with donovanosis who are coinfected with human immunodeficiency virus.

REFERENCES

1. McLeod K. Precis of operations performed in the wards of the first surgeon, Medical College O Hospital (Rio), during the year 1881. *Ind Med Gaz.* 1882;17:113.
2. Donovan C. Ulcerating granuloma of the pudenda. *Ind Med Gaz.* 1905;40:414.
3. Richens J. The diagnosis and treatment of donovanosis (granuloma inguinale). *Genitourin Med.* 1991;67:441-452.
4. Kuberski T, Papadimitriou JM, Phillips P. Ultrastructure of *Calymmatobacterium granulomatis* in lesions in granuloma inguinale. *J Infect Dis.* 1980;142:744-749.
5. Kharsany ABM, Hoosen AA, Naicker T, et al. Ultrastructure of *Calymmatobacterium granulomatis*: Comparison of culture with tissue biopsy specimens. *J Med Microbiol.* 1998;47:1069-1073.
6. Anderson K. The cultivation from granuloma inguinale of a microorganism having the characteristics of Donovan bodies in the yolk sac of chick embryos. *Science.* 1943;97:560.
7. Dulaney AD, Guo K, Packer H. Donovania granulomatis: Cultivation, antigen preparation, and immunological tests. *J Immunol.* 1948;59:335.
8. Kharsany ABM, Hoosen AA, Kiepiela P, et al. Culture of *Calymmatobacterium granulomatis* (Letter). *Clin Infect Dis.* 1996;22:391.
9. Carter J, Hutton S, Sriprakash KS, et al. Culture of the causative organism of donovanosis (*Calymmatobacterium granulomatis*) in Hep-2 cells. *J Clin Microbiol.* 1997;35:2915-2917.
10. Carter JS, Bowden FJ, Bastian I, et al. Phylogenetic evidence for reclassification of *Calymmatobacterium granulomatis* as *Klebsiella granulomatis* comb. nov. *Int J Syst Bacteriol.* 1999;49:1695-1700.
11. Kharsany ABM, Hoosen AA, Kiepiela P, et al. Phylogenetic analysis of *Calymmatobacterium granulomatis* based on 16S rRNA gene sequences. *J Med Microbiol.* 1999;48:841-847.
12. O'Farrell N. Clinico-epidemiological study of donovanosis in Durban, South Africa, *Genitourin Med.* 1993;69:108-111.
13. Bowden FJ. Donovanosis in Australia: going, going... *Sex Transm Infect.* 2005;81:365-366.
14. WHO Regional Office for the Western Pacific and National AIDS Council-National Department of Health, Papua New Guinea. Consensus Report on STI, HIV and AIDS Epidemiology, Papua New Guinea, 2000. Available at <http://www.wpro.who.int/NR/ rdonlyres/EEC64817-5D9F-4E72-9F7C-6014887E3483/0/ Consensus_Report_PNG_2000.pdf>.
15. Moodley P, Sturm PDJ, Vanmali T, et al. Association between HIV-1 infection, the etiology of genital ulcer disease, and response to syndromic management. *Sex Transm Dis.* 2003;30:241-245.
16. Kumar B, Sahoo B, Gupta S, et al. Rising incidence of genital herpes over two decades in a sexually transmitted disease clinic in North India. *J Dermatol.* 2000;29:74-78.
17. Brathwaite AR, Figueroa JP, Ward E. A comparison of prevalence rates of genital ulcers among patients attending a sexually transmitted disease clinic in Jamaica. *West Ind Med J.* 1997;46:67-71.
18. Morrone A, Toma L, Franco G, et al. Donovanosis in developed countries: Neglected or misdiagnosed disease? *Int J STD AIDS.* 2003;14: 288-289.
19. Goldberg J. Studies on granuloma inguinale. VII. Some epidemiological considerations of the disease. *Br J Vener Dis.* 1964;40:140-145.
20. O'Farrell N. Donovanosis (granuloma inguinale) in pregnancy. *Int J STD AIDS.* 1991;2:447-448.
21. Marmell M. Donovanosis of the anus in the male. An epidemiologic consideration. *Br J Vener Dis.* 1958;34:213-218.
22. Veeranna S, Raghu TY. Oral donovanosis. *Int J STD AIDS.* 2002;13:855-856.
23. Brigden MB, Guard R. Extragenital granuloma inguinale in North Queensland. *Med J Aust.* 1980;2:565-567.
24. Freinkel AL. Granuloma inguinale of cervical lymph nodes simulating tuberculosis lymphadenitis: Two case reports and review of published reports. *Genitourin Med.* 1988;64:339-343.
25. Samuel M, Aderogba K, Dutt N, et al. A hat trick of ulcerating pathogens in a single genital lesion. *Int J STD AIDS.* 2007;18:65-66.
26. Alexander LJ, Shields TL. Squamous cell carcinoma of the vulva secondary to granuloma inguinale. *Arch Dermatol Syphilol.* 1953;67:395.
27. Van Dyck E, Piot P. Laboratory techniques in the investigation of chancroid, lymphogranuloma venereum and donovanosis. *Genitourin Med.* 1992;68:130-133.
28. O'Farrell N, Hoosen A, Coetzee K, et al. A rapid stain for the diagnosis of granuloma inguinale. *Genitourin Med.* 1990;66:200201.
29. De Boer AL, de Boer F, van der Merwe JV. Cytologic identification of Donovan bodies in granuloma inguinale. *Acta Cytol.* 1984;28:126-128.
30. Leiman G, Markowitz S, Margolius KA. Cytologic detection of cervical granuloma inguinale. *Diagn Cytopathol.* 1986;2:138-143.
31. Freinkel AL, Dangor Y, Koornhof HJ, et al. A serological test for granuloma inguinale. *Genitourin Med.* 1992;68:269-272.
32. Kharsany ABM, Hoosen AA, Kiepiela P, et al. Growth and cultural characteristics of *Calymmatobacterium granulomatis*—the aetiological agent of granuloma inguinale (donovanosis). *J Med Microbiol.* 1997;46:579-585.
33. Bastian I, Bowden FJ. Amplification of *Klebsiella*-like sequences from biopsy samples from patients with donovanosis. *Clin Infect Dis.* 1996;23:1328-1330.
34. Carter JS, Bowden FJ, Sriprakash KS, et al. Diagnostic polymerase chain reaction for donovanosis. *Clin Infect Dis.* 1999;28:1168-1169.
35. Carter JS, Kemp DJ. A colorimetric detection system for *Calymmatobacterium granulomatis*. *Sex Transm Infect.* 2000;76: 134-136.
36. Mackay IM, Harnett G, Jeoffreys N, et al. Detection and discrimination of herpes simplex viruses, *Haemophilus ducreyi*, *Treponema pallidum*, and *Calymmatobacterium* (*Klebsiella*) *granulomatis* from genital ulcers. *Clin Infect Dis.* 2006;42:1431-1438.
37. Bowden FJ, Mein J, Plunkett C, et al. Pilot study of azithromycin in the treatment of genital donovanosis. *Genitourin Med.* 1996; 72:17-19.
38. Bowden FJ. Azithromycin for the treatment of donovanosis. *Sex Transm Infect.* 1998;74:78-79.
39. Merianos A, Gilles M, Chuah J. Ceftriaxone in the treatment of chronic donovanosis in central Australia. *Genitourin Med.* 1994;70:84-89.

237

Other Gram-Negative and Gram-Variable Bacilli

JAMES P. STEINBERG | EILEEN M. BURD

A large number of gram-negative aerobic bacilli have been reported to cause human infection. This chapter considers selected gram-negative organisms that have not been described in other chapters and are important in certain clinical or epidemiologic circumstances (e.g., nosocomial infection), are newly described, or are present special problems of diagnosis or therapy. Many of these organisms are saprophytic, and their clinical role is uncertain. For some of the bacteria considered here, taxonomy is in a state of flux as classifications based on phenotypic characteristics are replaced by contemporary measures of genetic relationship including 16S ribosomal RNA (rRNA) sequencing studies. Current nomenclature and previous designations are listed in Table 237-1. The gram-variable organisms *Gardnerella vaginalis* and *Mobiluncus* species are discussed at the end of the chapter.

Identification of some of these organisms is difficult; the automated systems used by many microbiology laboratories cannot identify some of these bacteria and often misidentify others. Consequently, clinical laboratories sometimes use a general description (e.g., *gram-negative nonfermenter*) rather than the genus and species name. The clinical site of infection, as shown in Table 237-2, colony morphology, and the ability of the organism to metabolize carbohydrates by fermentation provide clues that can suggest a particular organism or group of organisms. This information can help select the most effective way to provide definitive identification because for some of these organisms, special procedures for recovery, characterization, or antimicrobial susceptibility testing are required.[1,2] The decision to use alternative diagnostic methods is often based on the perceived clinical significance of the isolate, economic considerations, and available expertise. Because species identification is often not pursued, infections caused by some of these uncommon pathogens may go unrecognized. In addition, there are no published methodologic guidelines or interpretive breakpoints for susceptibility testing for most of these organisms. Consequently, reported susceptibility test results from the literature can be difficult to interpret, especially if methods and interpretive criteria are not specified. For susceptibility testing performed in clinical microbiology laboratories, reports are generally limited to the minimal inhibitory concentration (MIC) value, and an interpretation is not provided.

Glucose Fermenters

ACTINOBACILLUS AND AGGREGATIBACTER SPECIES

Actinobacillus actinomycetemcomitans, formerly the major pathogen of the genus *Actinobacillus*, is now classified in the genus *Aggregatibacter*. Other species of *Actinobacillus* that can cause human disease (*A. lignieresii, A. equuli, A. suis, A. hominis,* and *A. ureae*) are discussed at the end of this section.

Aggregatibacter actinomycetemcomitans, a cause of endocarditis, severe forms of periodontal disease, and soft tissue infection, the last of these usually in association with *Actinomyces israelii*. Based on genetic relatedness studies, this organism, *Haemophilus aphrophilus, Haemophilus paraphrophilus,* and *Haemophilus segnis* were recently transferred to the new genus *Aggretatobacter*, the name reflecting a propensity to aggregate with other bacteria.[3] *Aggretatobacter aphrophilus* and *Aggretatobacter paraphrophilus* have been combined into one species, *Aggretatobacter aphrophilus.*[3]

A. actinomycetemcomitans was first described as a human pathogen in 1912 and was initially called *Bacterium actinomycetem comitans*. Early isolates were recovered only in conjunction with *A. israelii* (hence the species designation), leading to speculation that *A. actinomycetemcomitans* was not itself capable of causing disease. *A. actinomycetemcomitans* is present in at least 30% of actinomycotic lesions.[4] After the introduction of penicillin, it was observed that *A. actinomycetemcomitans* sometimes could be recovered from persistent lesions of actinomycosis after *A. israelii* was eradicated.[5] By the early 1960s, recovery of this organism in pure culture from blood and other normally sterile body fluids was reported widely.[6] The organism also has been isolated in pure culture from patients with meningitis, brain abscess, endophthalmitis (with and without concomitant endocarditis), soft tissue infections, parotitis, septic arthritis, osteomyelitis, spinal epidural abscess, urinary tract infection, pneumonia, empyema, and pericarditis.[4,7-10] Soft tissue infections most commonly involve the cervicofacial area, although they can occur elsewhere, including chest and abdomen. There are reports of *A. actinomycetemcomitans* mimicking actinomycosis (*A. israelii* or mixed infection) and causing pneumonia with chest wall invasion.[9]

Although the organism is part of the endogenous flora of the mouth and can be recovered from about 20% of teenagers and adults, it (along with *Porphyromonas gingivalis*) is one of the major pathogens in adult and juvenile forms of periodontitis.[11] *A. actinomycetemcomitans* is present in the periodontal pockets of more than 50% of adults with refractory periodontitis and 90% of patients with localized aggressive periodontitis (formerly called *localized juvenile periodontitis*), a destructive form of periodontitis characterized by loss of the alveolar bone of the molars and incisors.[12,13] Clonal spread of the organism within families has been demonstrated using polymerase chain reaction (PCR)–based typing systems.[14] *A. actinomycetemcomitans* elaborates numerous substances that appear to contribute to periodontal disease. Some of the putative virulence factors, including a leukotoxin whose cellular receptor is a β_2-integrin, modulate the host inflammatory response.[13,15] Other candidate virulence factors contribute to tissue destruction and resorption of alveolar bone.

A. actinomycetemcomitans is one of the HACEK organisms, along with *Haemophilus parainfluenzae, Aggregatibacter (Haemophilus) aphrophilus, Aggregatibacter (Haemophilus) paraphrophilus, Cardiobacterium hominis, Eikenella corrodens,* and *Kingella kingae*, which have in common slow growth in culture, the need for incubation in an atmosphere enhanced with CO_2 for recovery in culture, and a predilection for causing endocarditis.[2] About 100 cases of endocarditis caused by *A. actinomycetemcomitans* have been reported, which is more than those caused by other HACEK organisms.[16] The onset of endocarditis is usually insidious, with a mean time to diagnosis of about 3 months. In a comprehensive review of 57 cases of *A. actinomycetemcomitans* endocarditis, 46% had periodontal disease or recent dental work, and 60% had underlying valvular disease, including 25% with prosthetic valves.[4] Fever was present in fewer than 50%; peripheral manifestations and splenomegaly each occurred in about one third. Therapy was successful in almost 80%, but significant embolization was common (39%), and 23% (13 of 57) required valve replacement. Prosthetic valve endocarditis with *A. actinomycetemcomitans* was usually recognized earlier than native valve endocarditis (42 versus 106 days), which

TABLE 237-1	Current Nomenclature and Previous Names of Gram-Negative Bacteria		
Current Designation	**Previous Names**	**Current Designation**	**Previous Names**
Glucose Fermenters		*Elizabethkingia meningoseptica*‡	*Chryseobacterium meningosepticum, Flavobacterium meningosepticum*
Actinobacillus spp.		*Methylobacterium mesophilicum* and *M. extorquens*§	*Pseudomonas mesophilica, Protomonas extorquens, Vibrio extorquens, Protaminobacter rubra,* "the pink phantom"
A. ureae	*Pasteurella ureae*		
Aeromonas spp.			
A. hydrophila		*Myroides* spp.	
A. caviae		M. odoratus	*Flavobacterium odoratum*
A. veronii biotype sobria	*A. sobria*	M. odoratimimus	
Aggregatibacter actinomycetemcomitans	*Actinobacillus actinomycetemcomitans, Bacterium actinomycetemcomitans*	*Ochrobactrum* spp.	
		O. anthropi	CDC Vd, *Achromobacter* groups A and D
Cardiobacterium spp.		O. intermedium	*Achromobacter* group C
C. hominis		*Oligella* spp.	
C. valvarum		O. ureolytica	CDC Ive
Chromobacterium violaceum		O. urethralis	*Moraxella urethralis,* CDC M4
Dysgonomonas capnocytophagoides	CDC DF-3	*Pseudomonas* spp.	
CDC EF-4		P. fluorescens	
Plesiomonas shigelloides	*Aeromonas shigelloides, Pseudomonas shigelloides*	P. putida	
		P. stutzeri	
Glucose Nonfermenters (or Weak Fermenters)		P. oryzihabitans	*Flavimonas oryzihabitans, Chromobacterium typhiflavum,* CDC Ve-2
Achromobacter spp.			
A. xylosoxidans subsp. xylosoxidans	*Alcaligenes xylosoxicans* subsp. *xylosoxidans, Achromobacter xylosoxidans, A. denitrificans*	P. luteola	*Chryseomonas luteola,* CDC group Ve-1
		Ralstonia spp.	
A. xylosoxidans subsp. denitrificans	*A. denitrificans, A. denitrificans* subsp. *denitrificans*	R. pickettii	*Pseudomonas pickettii, Burkholderia pickettii*
Alcaligenes faecalis	*A. odorans,* CDC VI	R. mannitolilytica	*R. pickettii* biovar 3/"thomasii," *Pseudomonas thomasii*
*Bergeyella zoohelcum**	*Weeksella zoohelcum,* CDC IIj	*Rhizobium radiobacter*	*Agrobacterium radiobacter, A. tumefaciens, A.* biovar 1, CDC Vd-3
Chryseobacterium spp.			
C. indologenes	*Flavobacterium indologenes*	*Roseomonas* spp.	CDC pink coccoid group I through IV
Chryseomonas luteola	*Pseudomonas luteola, Chryseomonas polytrichia,* CDC Ve-1	*Shewanella putrefaciens*	*Pseudomonas putrefaciens,* CDC Ib-1, Ib-2
Comamonas spp.		*Sphingobacterium* spp.	
C. testosteroni	*Pseudomonas testosteroni*	S. multivorum	*Flavobacterium multivorum,* CDC IIk-2
Cupriavidus spp.†		S. spiritivorum	*Flavobacterium spiritivorum,* CDC IIk-3
C. paucula	*Wautersia paucula, Ralstonia paucula,* CDC group IVc-2	*Sphingomonas paucimobilis*	*Pseudomonas paucimobilis,* CDC IIk-1
C. gilardii	*Wautersia gilardii, Ralstonia gilardii*	*Weeksella virosa*	*Flavobacterium genitale,* CDC II-f
Eikenella corrodens	*Bacteroides corrodens*		

*See *Weeksella* in text.
†See *Ralstonia* in text.
‡See *Chryseobacterium* in text.
§See *Roseomonas* in text.
CDC, Centers for Disease Control and Prevention; CSF, cerebrospinal fluid.

probably was attributable to a higher index of suspicion. This earlier diagnosis may account for the high cure rate achieved with antibiotics alone and a relative low rate of embolization reported.

Culture isolation of *A. actinomycetemcomitans* is the usual means of diagnosis, and the fastidious, slow-growing nature of the organism makes this difficult. Material obtained from soft tissue lesions should be inoculated on blood and chocolate agar because the organism grows poorly in MacConkey agar. The cultures must be incubated in an enhanced (5% to 10%) CO_2 atmosphere. By 18 to 24 hours, a few colonies (punctate, nonhemolytic) may be apparent, but the organism grows slowly, and incubation for at least 48 hours is needed. After colonies are seen, the organism continues to grow slowly, sometimes forming a star structure as part of the center of the mature colony. In broth or blood cultures, the organism often grows only in small "granules" adherent to the sides, with the medium remaining clear. In 13 patients with endocarditis, blood cultures required incubation for a mean of 5.6 days (range, 2 to 9 days) before growth was detected.[17] This finding underscores the need to hold blood culture bottles for a prolonged time if endocarditis caused by a fastidious organism is suspected. The appearance of the organism on Gram stain is coccoid to coccobacillary, similar to the appearance of *Haemophilus* species. *Actinobacillus actinomycetemcomitans* is urease negative and indole negative, reduces nitrate, and usually is oxidase negative. It is catalase positive, which helps differentiate it from *A. aphrophilus* in patients with prosthetic valve infection.[17,18]

A. actinomycetemcomitans usually is susceptible to cephalosporins (especially third-generation cephalosporins), mezlocillin, rifampin, trimethoprim-sulfamethoxazole, aminoglycosides, fluoroquinolones including ciprofloxacin and moxifloxacin, tetracycline, azithromycin, and chloramphenicol.[4,19,20] In vitro susceptibility to penicillin and ampicillin is variable, but test results do not necessarily correlate with the clinical outcome.[17] In general, treatment of actinomycosis with penicillin and surgical drainage (when necessary) is sufficient, even when mixed infection is present. Vancomycin, erythromycin, and clindamycin have little activity against *A. actinomycetemcomitans*. The organisms display variable susceptibility to metronidazole, and in vitro synergy between metronidazole and both β-lactams and ciprofloxacin has been reported.[21] Because of strain-to-strain variability, testing of clinical isolates is recommended. Unfortunately, susceptibility testing is sometimes technically difficult because of the slow growth and fastidious nature of the organism. In the past, penicillin or ampicillin combined with an aminoglycoside was the usual treatment for endo-

TABLE 237-2 Classification of Selected Gram-Negative Aerobic Bacilli by Likely Site of Infection

Organism	Most Likely Clinical Settings and Sites of Infection							
	Bloodstream	Device Associated	Intestine	Soft Tissue	Bite Wound	Urine	CSF	Nosocomial Clusters
Glucose Fermenters								
Aggregatibacter	X			X	X		X	
Aeromonas	X		X	X				
Cardiobacterium	X							
Chromobacterium	X			X				
Dysgonomonas			X					
CDC group EF-4					X			
Elizabethkingia	X							
Plesiomonas			X					
Glucose Nonfermenters (or Weak Fermenters)								
Achromobacter	X	X						X
Bergeyella					X			
Chryseobacterium	X						X	X
Comamonas								
Cupriavidus	X							X
Eikenella	X			X	X			
Methylobacterium	X	X						
Ochrobactrum	X	X						X
Oligella						X		
Pseudomonas	X	X						X
Ralstonia	X							X
Rhizobium	X	X						
Roseomonas	X	X						
Shewanella	X			X				
Sphingobacterium	X							
Sphingomonas	X	X						X
Weeksella						X		

carditis caused by this organism. Because of the potential for β-lactamase production, reports of failures with penicillin therapy, and difficulties with susceptibility testing, third-generation cephalosporins are now considered the drugs of choice. For endocarditis caused by HACEK organisms, the American Heart Association recommends ceftriaxone, 2 g daily for 4 weeks (6 weeks for prosthetic valve endocarditis).[22] Successful treatment of prosthetic valve endocarditis with oral ciprofloxacin has been reported.[23] A. actinomycetemcomitans endocarditis has developed after dental procedures despite the prophylactic use of penicillin, erythromycin, or vancomycin. Severe A. actinomycetemcomitans–associated periodontitis is usually treated with mechanical débridement in combination with oral tetracycline therapy. Tetracycline failures occur, however, and a report suggests that the combination of metronidazole and amoxicillin is effective in suppressing subgingival infection.[24]

Five species of Actinobacillus (A. lignieresii, equuli, suis, hominis, and ureae) are rare causes of human disease. The first three are commensals and opportunistic pathogens in animals,[4] whereas the latter two are commensals of the human upper respiratory tract. A. ureae was previously known as Pasteurella ureae.

A. lignieresii, A. suis, and A. equuli rarely can cause infections after bite wounds from farm animals.[25] These infections can be polymicrobial. One report has described a boar hunter who developed endocarditis caused by an Actinobacillus organism that resembled A. suis and A. hominis biochemically.[26] A recent report described 46 clinical A. hominis isolates acquired over a 22-year period, mostly from Copenhagen, Denmark.[27] Before this report, there were only a few case reports of human infections caused by this organism. Most of the isolates were from the respiratory tract; 18 of 33 respiratory isolates were reported to be pure cultures of A. hominis. The remaining respiratory cultures contained at least one other common respiratory pathogen. All the patients in this series had underlying diseases, including alcoholism, cardiovascular disease, drug addiction, chronic obstructive lung disease, and cancer. Most patients had fever and pulmonary infiltrates, and 9 of 36 patients for whom clinical information was available died, including one of the two patients with bacteremia. The identification of the A. hominis isolates was confirmed by ribotyping and DNA hybridization. In this and other reports, automated systems had difficulty identifying Actinobacillus species. Fatal A. hominis bacteremia has also been reported in two patients with severe underlying liver disease.[28] Actinobacillus ureae is a rare cause of bacteremia and meningitis. Nine of 14 cases of A. ureae meningitis were post-traumatic, and another occurred after neurosurgery.[29,30] Several patients had underlying chronic illnesses, including alcoholism and human immunodeficiency virus (HIV) infection.

Identification of Actinobacillus species is problematic. At the genus level, these organisms are biochemically similar to Pasteurella species. Species identification can be difficult without DNA hybridization studies.[31]

A. ureae meningitis has been treated successfully with penicillin and third-generation cephalosporins.[30]

AEROMONAS SPECIES

Aeromonads are ubiquitous inhabitants of fresh and brackish water. They have also been recovered from chlorinated tap water, including hospital water supplies. They occasionally cause soft tissue infections and sepsis in immunocompromised hosts and increasingly have been associated with diarrheal disease. Because of recent phylogenetic studies, Aeromonas species have been moved from the family Vibrionaceae to a new family, the Aeromonadaceae.[32,33] Taxonomy of the aeromonads is in transition. In 1984, four species of Aeromonas (hydrophila, sobria, caviae, and salmonicida) were recognized. These biochemically distinct species (phenospecies) have now been subdivided into DNA hybridization groups (genospecies), and new genospecies have been recognized. The complexity caused by the abundance of new species is compounded by attempts to reconcile genetic relatedness with the established phenospecies. For example, clinical isolates of A. sobria reside in the DNA hybridization group of A. veronii and should technically be designated A. veronii biovar sobria. There are currently 17 named species, but only 3, A. hydrophila, A. caviae, and A. veronii biovar sobria, are of major clinical importance.[34,35]

Aeromonas was first isolated more than 60 years ago, but evidence implicating this genus as a cause of gastrointestinal disease has been amassed only since the early 1980s. Reports from diverse geographic locations have associated Aeromonas species with diarrheal disease in humans; in some locales, they are recovered as commonly as Shigella or Campylobacter.[36-39] Many laboratories do not routinely culture stool for Aeromonas, so the incidence of Aeromonas-associated diarrhea may be underestimated. Evidence supporting a causative role in diarrheal disease includes (1) a higher carriage rate in symptomatic compared with asymptomatic individuals; (2) an absence of other enteric pathogens in most symptomatic patients harboring Aeromonas species; (3) identification of Aeromonas enterotoxins[40] (although the absence of an animal model has hampered efforts to directly link toxin production with disease); (4) improvement of diarrhea with antibiotics active against Aeromonas species and clinical worsening with antibiotics ineffective against the organism; and (5) evidence of a specific secretory immune response coincident with diarrheal disease.[41]

Aeromonas caviae is the predominant isolate from diarrheal stools, but in some geographic areas, A. hydrophila and A. veronii biovar sobria are frequently isolated as well.[36,38,42,43] Other Aeromonas species appear to cause asymptomatic carriage only.[34] Aeromonas-associated diarrhea usually occurs during the summer, when the concentrations of aeromonads in water are the highest. Most cases are sporadic. A recent study was unable to implicate the drinking water supply as the source of diarrheal isolates; Aeromonas isolates from diarrheal stool were genetically unrelated to those from water supplies.[44] Aeromonas is increasingly being recognized as a cause of diarrhea in travelers returning from Asia, Africa, and Latin America.[42,45,46] Daycare center outbreaks have been reported, although in one study, molecular typing did not suggest clonal spread.[47] The clinical manifestations of Aeromonas-associated diarrhea are varied. Diarrhea is usually watery and self-limited, but some persons develop fever, abdominal pain, and bloody stools. Fecal leukocytes may be present. Occasionally, diarrhea may be severe or protracted, and hospitalization may be necessary. Chronic colitis following acute Aeromonas-associated diarrhea has been reported in adults.[48] Although no controlled trials have validated antimicrobial therapy for Aeromonas-associated diarrhea, clinical improvement has occurred with antibiotics active against the organism. Hemolytic uremic syndrome associated with Aeromonas enterocolitis has been described in infants and adults.[49]

Most Aeromonas soft tissue infections are caused by A. hydrophila. Trauma followed by exposure to fresh water (and not salt water, even though aeromonad density in seawater is similar to that in fresh water[34]) usually, but not invariably, precedes infection. Cellulitis develops within 8 to 48 hours, and systemic signs are common.[50,51] Suppuration and necrosis around the wound are frequent, and surgical débridement is often necessary. Fasciitis, myonecrosis (occasionally associated with gas formation), and osteomyelitis may develop. In the setting of a rapidly progressive cellulitis after an injury related to water exposure, Aeromonas and Vibrio species infections should be considered in the differential diagnosis. Aeromonas soft tissue infections can develop after exposure to soil, in association with crush injuries, and as a complication of burns, typically when initial management of the burn included immersion in natural water sources.[51] There is one reported outbreak of A. hydrophila wound infections in participants of a mud football competition in Australia. The field was "prepared" with water from an adjacent river.[52] Aeromonas soft tissue infection is a recognized complication of the use of medicinal leeches in conjunction with reimplantation or flap surgery.[53] Aeromonas hydrophila and

other Aeromonas species are normal inhabitants of the foregut of leeches. Leeches lack the requisite proteolytic enzymes and are dependent on the symbiotic Aeromonas to digest the blood meal.[54] Aeromonas infection has developed in 7% to 20% of patients treated with leeches. Prophylactic antibiotics now have been recommended at the time of leech application.[53,54] The onset of infection after the application of medicinal leeches ranges from 1 day to more than 10 days.[55] Mild wound infection, loss of flap, myonecrosis, and sepsis may ensue.

Aeromonas bacteremia and sepsis are uncommon, but in the largest series reported to date, 143 Aeromonas bacteremias, including 104 that were monomicrobial, occurred in one institution in Taiwan over a 10-year period.[56] Aeromonas hydrophila caused 60% of the bacteremias; most of the other isolates that were identified by species were A. veronii subtype sobria and A. caviae.[57] Most patients in this series were immunocompromised, including 54% who were cirrhotic and 21% who had an underlying malignancy. Spontaneous bacterial peritonitis was common in cirrhotic patients with abdominal pain. There was a similar distribution of Aeromonas species in a study of 53 Aeromonas blood isolates collected from 27 medical centers in the United States over a 10-year period.[58] Most patients were immunocompromised, and underlying malignancy was much more common than liver disease in this series. Most patients with Aeromonas sepsis do not present with diarrhea. Interestingly, about one third of Aeromonas bacteremias are nosocomial.[57,59] In some series, the nosocomial cases were not epidemiologically linked, and endogenous gut flora was the presumed source.[59] Aeromonas has been recovered from hospital water supplies, and clusters of nosocomial Aeromonas bacteremia have been described.[60] However, in one study in which molecular typing was performed, many different genotypes were found. The mortality rate for Aeromonas sepsis is 30% to 50%.[45,57-59] Two other species, Aeromonas jandaei and Aeromonas schubertii, have rarely been isolated from the blood.[61,62] A variety of other infections caused by Aeromonas species have been reported, including intra-abdominal abscess, pancreatic abscess, hepatobiliary infection,[63] spontaneous bacterial peritonitis in patients with cirrhosis,[57] meningitis,[64] endocarditis,[65] suppurative thrombophlebitis, osteomyelitis, urinary tract infection, prostatitis, pneumonia including near-drowning–associated pneumonia,[66] empyema, lung abscess, tonsillitis, epiglottitis, keratitis, and otitis media. A. hydrophila epididymitis and bacteremia developed in a healthy man 24 hours after he had sexual intercourse with his wife in their swimming pool. Cultures obtained from the pool grew A. hydrophila.[67]

Aeromonas organisms are gram-negative, nonsporulating facultative anaerobic rods that usually are β-hemolytic on blood agar and ferment carbohydrates with acid and gas production. The organisms grow well on MacConkey agar (some strains are lactose fermenters, and some are not), but growth on thiosulfate citrate bile sucrose medium is variable. Selective techniques are often necessary for the isolation of Aeromonas species from mixed cultures. The organisms are more difficult to identify in stool cultures because enteric media may be inhibitory for some Aeromonas species. Either blood agar that contains ampicillin (10 or 30 μg/mL) or cefsulodin-irgasan-novobiocin agar can be used as a selective medium.[68] Growth of colonies on plates usually occurs within 24 hours. Aeromonas species are oxidase positive, and this test distinguishes these organisms from the oxidase-negative Enterobacteriaceae. A. hydrophila is catalase positive and motile, converts nitrate to nitrite, and is urease negative. Identification of Aeromonas to the genus level is not difficult; many automated systems (and consequently many clinical laboratories) proceed no further, reporting an Aeromonas isolate as "Aeromonas species" or "Aeromonas hydrophila complex."

The clinically relevant Aeromonas species are uniformly resistant to penicillin and ampicillin, are often resistant to cefazolin and ticarcillin, and are usually but not invariably susceptible to third-generation cephalosporins, aztreonam, and carbapenems.[69] Resistance to cefotaxime has developed on therapy.[56] Sensitivity to piperacillin and ticarcillin-clavulanate is variable. Aeromonas species produce as many as three β-lactamases, including a Bush group 2d penicillinase, a group

1 cephalosporinase, and a metallocarbapenemase.[70] Some isolates exhibit coordinated expression of these β-lactamases after both induction and selection of derepressed mutants.[71] Despite the presence of a carbapenemase, minimal inhibitory concentrations to imipenem typically remain low, although *A. jandaei* and *A. veronii* subtype *veronii* can display imipenem resistance.[72] Unlike most carbapenemases, the *Aeromonas* metallocarbapenemases have narrow substrate profiles and specifically hydrolyze carbapenems.[73] There are reports of increasing resistance to tetracycline and trimethoprim-sulfamethoxazole.[74] In one report, tigecycline was active against 200 of 201 isolates.[75] Aminoglycosides are usually active, with resistance to tobramycin being more common than resistance to gentamicin or amikacin.[69] Fluoroquinolones are highly active against *Aeromonas* species, although the existence of nalidixic acid–resistant strains containing mutations in the *gyrA* gene raise concern that fluoroquinolone resistance could easily develop.[69] *Aeromonas* species harboring a conjugative plasmid that confers multiple antibiotic resistance have been identified.[76]

CARDIOBACTERIUM SPECIES

Cardiobacterium hominis and recently described *Cardiobacterium valvarum* are the only two species in the genus *Cardiobacterium*.[77] Unlike the other HACEK organisms considered in this chapter, these organisms rarely cause disease other than endocarditis. *Cardiobacterium* species have been described as *Pasteurella*-like organisms and are part of the endogenous flora in the nose, mouth, and throat and are present occasionally on other mucous membranes as well as in the gastrointestinal tract.[78,79]

There are more than 75 reported cases of *C. hominis* infection, and all but a few have involved the heart valves. Most patients have had underlying anatomic defects (e.g., rheumatic heart disease, ventricular septal defect, congenital bicuspid valve); prosthetic cardiac valves have been involved in about 10% of reported cases.[80,81] Many patients with endocarditis have had severe periodontitis or prior dental procedures without antimicrobial prophylaxis. *Cardiobacterium hominis* endocarditis following upper gastrointestinal endoscopy has been reported.[82] A subacute presentation, with an insidious onset (mean of 2 to 5 months before diagnosis) and an absence of fever at the time of diagnosis, is common.[83] Some of the patients have splenomegaly, anemia, immune-mediated glomerulonephritis, and hematuria, consistent with a long period between infection and diagnosis. Large vegetations, and large vessel emboli, are characteristic. The mortality rate is about 10%, and valve replacement is needed in about 30% of cases.[16] Septic arthritis,[81] vertebral osteomyelitis, and mycotic aneurysms (intracranial and mesenteric) are reported complications of *C. hominis* endocarditis. Almost all clinical isolates come from blood, although meningitis associated with endocarditis has been described.[84] In one of the very rare cases of infection without endocarditis, a patient with adenocarcinoma of the kidney invading the cecum developed an abdominal abscess and bacteremia; abscess and blood cultures grew *C. hominis* and *Clostridium bifermentans*.[85] There is also a case report of *C. hominis* pacemaker lead infection without valvular involvement.[86] Because of phenotypic similarities, it is suspected that some clinical isolates identified as *C. hominis* may actually have been *C. valvarum*.[79] *C. valvarum* has been reported as a cause of insidious, afebrile endocarditis in a patient with an underlying anatomic defect and prior dental procedure without antimicrobial prophylaxis.[77] This species was first described as *Cardiobacterium* species strain B from dental plaque and has also been described among the etiologic agents in advanced lesions of children with noma.[77,87]

Cardiobacterium species are pleomorphic gram-negative rods; morphology varies considerably depending on culture conditions. They often have swelling of one or both ends and retain the crystal violet dye at the poles during the Gram stain procedure.[2] Microscopically, the organisms sometimes form rosettes, but short chains, teardrops, pairs, and clusters are also common. Supplementation of the medium with yeast extract results in a loss of the pleomorphism, and most organisms become sticklike, gram-negative rods with rounded ends.[78]

Incubation in high humidity and 3% to 5% CO_2 maximizes recovery of the organism. Both species grow better on sheep blood agar than chocolate agar and will grow on Mueller-Hinton agar or trypticase soy agar without blood but grow poorly on MacConkey agar or similar selective media. Colonies of *C. hominis* are 1 to 2 mm in diameter on sheep blood agar, usually by 48 to 72 hours after incubation at 37°C under increased CO_2. However, with some systems, incubation for 5 to 7 days before growth can be confirmed is not unusual, and cultures should be held for this period or longer if *C. hominis* is suspected.[78] *C. valvarum* is considered to be more fastidious than *C. hominis*, with tiny visible colonies, 0.2 to 0.8 mm in diameter, appearing on blood agar after 72 to 96 hours of incubation. Colonies of *C. valvarum* are nonhemolytic; however, colonies of *C. hominis* produce slight α-hemolysis after 3 to 4 days of incubation and develop a rough appearance, with a serpentine pattern of growth from the edge to adjacent colonies.[77,78] *Cardiobacterium* organisms are oxidase positive and catalase negative, and they produce indole (although positivity is weak in many strains of *C. hominis* and absent in some oral strains of *C. valvarum*). *Cardiobacterium* species may be misidentified as *Pasteurella multocida* when using the API 20NE (bioMérieux, Inc., Hazelwood, Mo) identification strip.[77] PCR amplification of 16S ribosomal DNA from heart valve tissue and arterioembolic tissue has detected *C. hominis* sequences in cases of culture-negative endocarditis.

Susceptibility tests are difficult to perform because of the organism's slow growth and unusual nutritional requirements, although a recent report suggests that the E-test appears to be a useful.[77,88] When tested, the organism is usually broadly susceptible to β-lactam drugs, fluoroquinolones, chloramphenicol, rifampin, and tetracycline.[78,88] Susceptibility to aminoglycosides, erythromycin, and clindamycin is variable. Penicillin G, with or without the addition of an aminoglycoside, has been the regimen most often employed for therapy. The first β-lactamase–producing clinical isolate was reported in 1994.[89] This isolate was also resistant to cefotaxime and piperacillin but susceptible to β-lactamase inhibitor combinations. Consequently, it is unclear whether the current recommendation to administer third-generation cephalosporins for endocarditis caused by HACEK organisms enhances coverage for *C. hominis*. The role of an aminoglycoside as part of combination therapy is unknown. Although microbiologic cure is usually achieved, complications frequently arise during the course of therapy. Systemic embolization, mycotic aneurysm, or progressive cardiac failure has necessitated replacement of the damaged valve in a number of cases.

CHROMOBACTERIUM SPECIES

Chromobacterium violaceum is a rare human pathogen but can cause life-threatening sepsis with metastatic abscesses. The organism is a common soil and water inhabitant in tropical and subtropical areas. Fewer than 200 cases have been reported worldwide, with most recent reports coming from Southeast Asia. More than 35 cases have been reported in the United States, almost all from the Southeast, primarily Florida.[90] Cases have also been reported from Australia and South America.[91,92] *C. violaceum* is the only species of this genus that causes human disease. Although not considered a normal inhabitant of the human gastrointestinal tract, *C. violaceum* was present in the feces of 3 of 65 children whose stool was cultured at the time of admission to a hospital in Atlanta.[93]

C. violaceum infection occurs in infants, children, and adults, almost always in the summer months and usually following exposure of nonintact skin to contaminated water (often stagnant) or soil. Two cases followed near-drownings. Symptoms include pain at a local site of infection, fever, nausea, vomiting, abdominal pain, and diarrhea. Local cellulitis, pustules, ulcers with necrotic base, or lymphadenitis commonly precedes evidence of systemic infection. Septic shock develops rapidly, as can pneumonia and visceral abscesses involving the liver, spleen, and lung. This presentation can be confused with septicemic melioidosis, which is more common than *C. violaceum* infection in Southeast Asia, where both diseases are endemic.[94] The mortality rate for reported cases in the United States is about 60%. Urinary tract infection, conjunctivitis, orbital cellulitis, retropharyngeal infection with prevertebral abscess, neutropenic sepsis, osteomyelitis, brain abscess,[95] meningitis, and puerperal sepsis have been reported. There are also a few case reports in the pediatric literature of *C. violaceum*–associated diarrhea.[96] A recent report from Brazil of one confirmed and two suspected cases in siblings is the first cluster of suspected *C. violaceum* infections linked to a common source.[97] *C. violaceum* infection is more common in patients with chronic granulomatous disease (CGD),[98] but cases occur in the apparently normal host. There appears to be a higher survival rate in persons with CGD compared with patients without known neutrophil dysfunction. This may reflect a selection bias because *C. violaceum* infection can be the initial manifestation of CGD, with the diagnosis of CGD being established only after recovery from the infection. Deficiency of polymorphonuclear leukocyte glucose-6-phosphate dehydrogenase and neutrophil dysfunction also were present in a 3-year-old patient who died with *C. violaceum* sepsis.[99] The pertinent virulence factors are unknown. Preliminary data from the study of only one clinical and one environmental isolate showed greater endotoxin activity and enhanced resistance to phagocytosis in the virulent strain.[100] Diagnosis is made by culture of blood, abscess fluid, or skin exudate.

C. violaceum organisms are long gram-negative bacilli; occasionally, the organisms are slightly curved and can be confused with vibrios. The organisms are facultatively anaerobic, growing readily in 18 to 24 hours on media containing tryptophan, which include common laboratory media such as sheep blood agar, chocolate agar, Mueller-Hinton agar, trypticase soy broth, and MacConkey agar. Incubation at 37°C usually is effective, although growth is enhanced if incubation occurs at 25°C. Most strains of this organism produce violacein, a pigment insoluble in water (as opposed to the water-soluble pyocyanin of *Pseudomonas* species), which imparts a violet-black color to the colonies on solid media—hence the species' name (Fig. 237-1). There are a few reports of infection caused by nonpigmented strains.[101] Violacein can induce apoptosis in tumor cell lines and is being investigated as a potential chemotherapeutic agent.[102] The color may be lost on subculture or after therapy is begun. The organisms produce hydrogen cyanide, so a faint cyanide smell may be present. The oxidase reaction is usually positive but hard to detect in pigmented strains; sometimes,

demonstration of oxidase can be enhanced by incubating the culture anaerobically, which inhibits pigment formation.[92]

C. violaceum isolates are generally susceptible to fluoroquinolones, chloramphenicol, tetracycline, trimethoprim-sulfamethoxazole, imipenem, and gentamicin.[103] The ureidopenicillins are often active, but resistance to cephalosporins is common. Although aztreonam is a natural product of some strains of *C. violaceum*,[104] most clinical isolates are susceptible to this agent. Because of the rarity of infection, the often fulminant course, and the high mortality rate, the optimal antibiotic therapy is unknown. Ciprofloxacin is the most active antibiotic in vitro, and there are recent case reports of successful treatment with fluoroquinolones, often in combination with other agents.[95] Most survivors of this infection were treated with chloramphenicol or a penicillin (carboxy or ureidopenicillin) in combination with an aminoglycoside. Relapse has occurred more than 2 weeks after the completion of therapy and apparent cure, presumably because of a residual suppurative focus.[92] Oral trimethoprim-sulfamethoxazole, doxycycline, or ciprofloxacin has been used after intravenous therapy with other antibiotics, with the oral regimen continued for several weeks to a few months to prevent relapse.

DYSGONOMONAS SPECIES

The genus *Dysgonomonas* presently contains three species, *Dysgonomonas capnocytophagoides*, *Dysgonomonas gadei*, and *Dysgonomonas mossii*, all fastidious gram-negative bacilli isolated from human sources. *D. capnocytophagoides*, formerly called DF-3, was first associated with human disease in 1988.[105,106] DF stands for *dysgonic fermenter*, indicating a fermentative organism that has difficulty growing on routine media. DF-1 and DF-2 are now *Capnocytophaga* species (see Chapter 234), but comparative 16S rRNA sequence analysis showed that DF-3 is not closely related to *Capnocytophaga*.[107]

D. capnocytophagoides has been isolated from diarrheal stools of patients with immune deficiencies, including common variable hypogammaglobulinemia, HIV infection, diabetes with chronic renal failure, and lymphoreticular and other malignancies, and from patients receiving immunosuppressive agents.[105,108-110] With the use of selective media, this organism was isolated from 11 of 690 (1.6%) stools submitted for bacterial culture at the National Cancer Institute.[108] In another prospective study of the role of *D. capnocytophagoides* in diarrheal disease, the organism was recovered from 2 of 178 specimens (1.1%) submitted for *Clostridium difficile* toxin assay and from 3 of 129 (2.3%) stool specimens from patients with HIV infection. These data suggest that the paucity of reports of recovering *D. capnocytophagoides* from stool specimens may not be attributable to its rarity (as a colonizer or pathogen) but to the inability to recover the organism on conventional media. Antibiotic therapy directed at *D. capnocytophagoides* produced a therapeutic response in some of these patients, including 4 of 11 in the first study. Some of the responders had diarrhea of several months' duration, with prompt resolution after antibiotic therapy was initiated. In other patients, the clinical significance of organism was unclear; eradication of the organism from the stool was not accompanied by resolution of diarrhea, or the diarrhea resolved without specific therapy. *D. capnocytophagoides* has also been isolated from the urine, as a cause of biliary sepsis,[111] from a polymicrobial thigh abscess in a patient with insulin-dependent diabetes,[112] and from the patients with neutropenia.[113] In one patient with acute myelocytic leukemia, a blood isolate and stool isolate of *D. capnocytophagoides* had the identical ribotype.[114] The genus *Dysgonomonas* now includes other closely related clinical isolates, including *D. gadei* and *D. mossii*, which have been isolated from the gallbladder of patients with cholecystitis.[106,115] *D. mossii* has also been recovered repeatedly from intestinal fluid in a patient with pancreatic cancer but was not associated with obvious infection.[115]

D. capnocytophagoides can be distinguished from DF-2 (*Capnocytophaga canimorsus*) by negative catalase and oxidase tests, the production of indole by most strains, and the fermentation of sucrose and xylose. It produces small gray-white colonies with a sweetish odor on

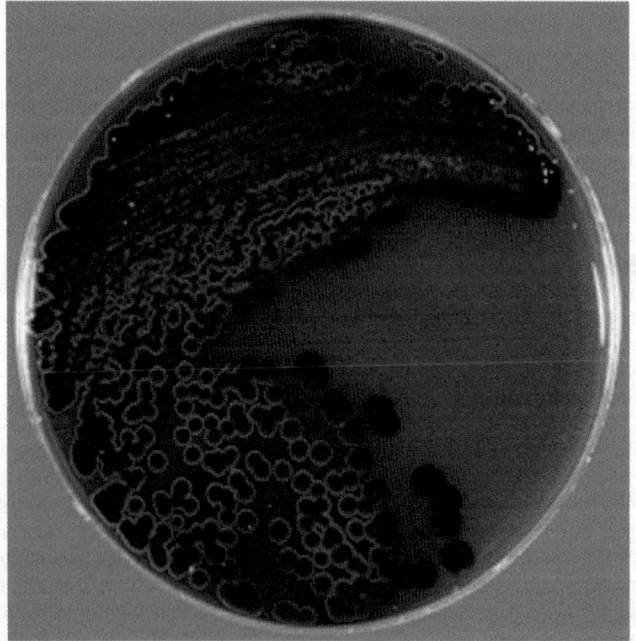

Figure 237-1 Violet-black colonies of *Chromobacterium violaceum* from production of the pigment violacein.

blood agar after 1 to 3 days of incubation. *D. capnocytophagoides* does not grow on MacConkey agar or routine enteric media. It grows on selective *Campylobacter* media when incubated at 37°C, but not 42°C, the routine incubation temperature for *Campylobacter*.[109] Selective media such as cefoperazone-vancomycin-amphotericin B blood agar inhibit normal flora and allow recovery of *D. capnocytophagoides* from stool specimens.

Despite a lack of established breakpoints, the Kirby-Bauer disk diffusion and MIC methods have been used for antimicrobial susceptibility testing.[113,115,116] *Dysgonomonas* species appear to be resistant to most β-lactam drugs, fluoroquinolones, aminoglycosides, metronidazole, vancomycin, erythromycin, and gentamicin. Many strains are susceptible to chloramphenicol, trimethoprim-sulfamethoxazole, clindamycin, and tetracycline. Tetracycline or clindamycin was used in the few reported cases of diarrheal disease that responded promptly to antibiotic administration. Despite a Kirby-Bauer zone size suggesting susceptibility, imipenem failed to clear *D. capnocytophagoides* from the bloodstream in the one reported bacteremic patient; the bacteremia resolved after therapy with trimethoprim-sulfamethoxazole was initiated.[113]

CENTERS FOR DISEASE CONTROL AND PREVENTION GROUP EF-4

EF-4 is known by its Centers for Disease Control and Prevention (CDC) letter and number designation based on growth characteristics. *EF*, or *euogenic fermenter*, refers to an organism that grows well through the fermentation of glucose. Group EF-4 bacteria are normal inhabitants of the oral cavity of dogs. Most human infections follow dog bites, although infections associated with cat bites or scratches occur as well. The organism can be isolated from bite wounds that do not demonstrate signs of inflammation, but cellulitis, abscess formation, and fever may develop. Systemic infection or infection not involving skin or skin structures is extremely rare. Endophthalmitis caused by *Pasteurella multocida* and EF-4 occurred after a cat scratch in an 8-year-old girl.[117] There is one report of bloodstream infection occurring in a patient with hepatic carcinoid who denied being bitten by a dog or cat.[118] An otherwise healthy man whose dogs often licked him in the ears developed chronic EF-4 otitis media requiring mastoidectomy.[119]

EF-4 bacteria usually appear as short rods on Gram stain, but small coccoid forms or long chains may also be present. The organisms grow well on blood-agar plates, on which colonies usually form within 24 hours, but grow poorly or not at all on MacConkey and similar agars. The colonies are small, may be slightly yellow-orange, and are smooth; some strains have a popcorn-like odor.[2] The organisms are oxidase positive and catalase-positive, and they reduce nitrate. Biovar EF-4a ferments glucose only and has arginine hydroxylase activity; biovar EF-4b does neither (and is actually a nonfermenter). Initially, EF-4 was thought to resemble the Pasteurellaceae family, but recent rRNA cistron analysis places EF-4 in the Neisseriaceae family.[120]

Penicillin G, ampicillin, tetracycline, ciprofloxacin, ofloxacin, and fluoroquinolones are all active against EF-4 at concentrations attainable with oral administration.[121] Cephalosporins, particularly first-generation agents, are less active in vitro. Chloramphenicol and aminoglycosides also have activity against EF-4.[117]

PLESIOMONAS SPECIES

Plesiomonas shigelloides, a ubiquitous freshwater inhabitant, has been implicated as a cause of acute diarrhea and, rarely, serious extraintestinal disease.[122,123] The name *Plesiomonas*, from the Greek word for "neighbor," was chosen because the organism was thought to be closely related to *Aeromonas*. It is, in fact, more closely related to *Proteus*,[124] although it is currently classified in the family Vibrionaceae. *P. shigelloides* is the only species in the genus. The organism was originally isolated in 1947 and given the name C27. It has also been named *Pseudomonas shigelloides*, *Aeromonas shigelloides*, or *Vibrio shigelloides*.

P. shigelloides is a water- and soil-associated organism that replicates at temperatures above 8°C. It is found primarily in freshwater or estuary environments within temperate and tropical climates but can exist in seawater during the warm-weather months. Asymptomatic carriage of *P. shigelloides* is very rare among healthy persons. The usual vehicles of transmission of plesiomonads to humans are water, food such as oysters, shrimp, or chicken,[112,123] and a variety of animals that may be colonized with the organism. The organism has been acquired during foreign travel.[122,125,126] *P. shigelloides* is associated with gastroenteritis, but the failure to identify an enteropathogenic mechanism, the lack of an animal model, and unsuccessful studies to induce disease in volunteers make it impossible to firmly establish a causal relationship.[127] Potential virulence factors including a β-hemolysin have been identified, but their significance is unknown.[128]

The clinical presentation of *P. shigelloides*–associated diarrhea varies from a mild self-limited illness to mucoid, bloody diarrhea with fecal leukocytes. A predominance of a secretory-type diarrhea has been reported,[123] but other series have found a high percentage with a clinical illness compatible with enteroinvasive disease featuring abdominal pain, fever, bloody diarrhea, and fecal leukocytes.[126] Most symptomatic patients have either traveled abroad or been exposed to potentially contaminated water or food. Outbreaks have been reported, particularly from Japan. The role of antibiotics for *Plesiomonas*-associated diarrhea is uncertain. Antimicrobial therapy did not shorten the duration of fever or diarrhea in Thai children with *Plesiomonas*-associated diarrhea.[129] On the other hand, in a small nonrandomized Canadian study of patients who developed *Plesiomonas*-associated diarrhea after travel abroad, 8 of 9 treated patients were asymptomatic within 2 weeks, compared with 6 of 15 controls ($P < .05$).[126]

Most descriptions of extraintestinal disease come from individual case reports. These reports include cases of osteomyelitis, septic arthritis, endophthalmitis, spontaneous bacterial peritonitis,[130] pancreatic abscess, splenic abscess, cholecystitis, cellulites, pyosalpinx,[131] and epididymo-orchitis. About 10 cases of neonatal sepsis with meningitis have been described.[132] Bacteremia is rare and usually occurs in immunocompromised hosts. In a recent case series of *Plesiomonas* bacteremia from Hong Kong, all seven patients were elderly; four had biliary tract disease, and three had underlying malignancy.[133] Bacteremia accompanying gastroenteritis has been reported in a healthy 15-year-old girl.[134]

P. shigelloides is a motile, facultatively anaerobic, gram-negative, oxidase-positive bacillus. It is readily isolated from some enteric agars such as MacConkey agar but does not grow well on thiosulfate citrate bile sucrose medium. Selective techniques may be necessary for isolation of the organism from mixed cultures, such as the use of bile peptone broth or trypticase soy broth with ampicillin.[135] The organism grows well at 35°C and produces visible colonies (nonhemolytic) within 24 hours.

P. shigelloides is usually susceptible to chloramphenicol, trimethoprim-sulfamethoxazole, quinolones, cephalosporins, and imipenem.[129,136,137] Because of β-lactamase production, most isolates are now resistant to penicillins including ureidopenicillins, although the β-lactamase inhibitor combinations appear to be active. Susceptibilities to aminoglycosides and tetracycline are variable.

Glucose Nonfermenters or Weak Fermenters

ACHROMOBACTER AND *ALCALIGENES* SPECIES

The taxonomic designations for *Achromobacter* and *Alcaligenes* species have been particularly confusing. *Achromobacter xylosoxidans* was renamed *Alcaligenes xylosoxidans* subsp. *xylosoxidans*,[138] but recent 16S rRNA sequence analysis and GC content studies support placement of this organism back in the genus *Achromobacter* (the species and subspecies designation have been maintained).[139] Other *Alcaligenes* species, *A. ruhlandii*, *A. peichaudii*, and *A. denitrificans*, have also been transferred to *Achromobacter*. Organisms formerly considered *Achromobacter* groups A, C, and D (and before that CDC groups Vd-1 and Vd-2) are now named *Ochrobactrum anthropi* and are considered separately. The *Achromobacter* species are nonfermenting gram-negative bacilli found in soil and water. They can occasionally be recovered from the respiratory tract and gastrointestinal tract, primarily in persons with health care contact. Infection results when they are introduced into wounds or colonize those with compromised host defenses. Clinically relevant species include the asaccharolytic species *A. xylosoxidans* subsp. *dentrificans, A. piechaudii*, and *Alcaligenes faecalis* (this organism remains in the genus *Alcaligenes*)[140]; the saccharolytic species *A. xylosoxidans* subsp. *xylosoxidans;* and the unnamed *Achromobacter* groups B, E, and F.[141] Although sometimes considered a contaminant, *Achromobacter* group B has been recovered from the blood of patients with clinical sepsis and endocarditis.[142-144]

A. xylosoxidans subsp. *xylosoxidans* is the most clinically important of these organisms. It probably is part of the endogenous flora of the ear and gastrointestinal tract and is a common contaminant of fluids.[145] The organism has been implicated in outbreaks of nosocomial infection associated with contaminated solutions (e.g., intravenous fluids, hemodialysis fluid, irrigation fluids, mouthwash), pressure transducers, incubators and humidifiers, and contaminated soaps and disinfectants.[146-148] Contamination of well water was the source of infection in one case of bacteremia.[149]

Clinical illness that is caused by *A. xylosoxidans* subsp. *xylosoxidans* has involved isolates from blood, peritoneal and pleural fluids, urine, respiratory secretions, and wound exudates. Bacteremia, often related to intravascular catheters, is the most commonly reported infection and is frequently polymicrobial in patients with underlying malignancies.[150-152] Biliary tract sepsis, meningitis (sometimes with lymphocytic predominance in cerebrospinal fluid), pneumonia (nosocomial and community-acquired), peritonitis (including spontaneous bacterial peritonitis and peritonitis in patients on continuous ambulatory peritoneal dialysis), urinary tract infection, conjunctivitis, osteomyelitis, prosthetic knee infection, and prosthetic valve endocarditis have been reported.[145,149-156] Patients often have an immunosuppressed state such as cancer[152,157] and HIV infection,[158] but this is not always the case, especially in nosocomial outbreaks. This organism has been recovered with increasing frequency from respiratory secretions of persons with cystic fibrosis,[159,160] and colonization has been associated with exacerbation of respiratory symptoms.[161] However, recent case-control studies have not shown more rapid deterioration in clinical or pulmonary function status among cystic fibrosis patients chronically colonized with *Achromobacter* or *Alcaligenes* species, except in a subgroup of patients with a rapid increase in specific precipitating antibodies to *A. xylosoxidans*.[159,162] Recovery in neonatal infection may result from perinatal transfer from the mother.[163]

Phylogenetically and biochemically, *Alcaligenes* and *Achromobacter* are closely related to the genus *Brucella*. Strains of *A. xylosoxidans* subsp. *xylosoxidans* grow well on blood agar and MacConkey agar plates; they produce flat, spreading and rough colonies and have peritrichous flagella, features that help distinguish them from pseudomonads. The organisms are oxidase positive and catalase positive, oxidize glucose to produce acid, and (as the species name indicates) oxidize xylose readily.[2] An isolate of *A. xylosoxidans* subsp. *xylosoxidans* can easily be mistaken for a non-*Aeruginosa* strain of *Pseudomonas* or for a strain of the *Burkholderia cepacia* complex, but the unusual susceptibility pattern suggests the correct identity.

Usually, strains of *A. xylosoxidans* subsp. *xylosoxidans* are susceptible to trimethoprim-sulfamethoxazole, ureidopenicillins, carbapenems, ceftazidime, cefoperazone, and β-lactamase inhibitor combinations.[150] Generally, they are resistant to narrow-spectrum penicillins, other cephalosporins (including cefotaxime and ceftriaxone), aztreonam, and aminoglycosides.[157,164,165] Susceptibility to the fluoroquinolones is variable.[157] High concentrations of colistin inhibit most strains.[166] Hyperproduction of β-lactamases has been implicated in resistance.[167] High rates of resistance to ciprofloxacin and aminoglycosides have been noted in strains isolated from cystic fibrosis patients.[160]

Alcaligenes faecalis can be recovered in a variety of clinical settings. Most isolates of *A. faecalis* from blood or respiratory secretions are related to the contamination of hospital equipment or fluids with the organism, with resulting human colonization or infection. The urine is the other common site of recovery, although it infrequently causes symptomatic urinary tract infection. It also has been recovered from corneal ulcers, ear discharges, wound drainage, and feces.[168,169] It is rarely recovered in pure culture from any of these sites. By contrast, *A. xylosoxidans* subsp. *denitrificans* has been recovered as a single pathogen from blood, cerebrospinal fluid, and other normally sterile body fluids as well as in mixed culture from sites usually containing normal flora. Few recent publications have addressed the pathogenic role of these organisms. *A. piechaudii* was thought to cause chronic otitis in a diabetic patient[170] and has also been recovered from blood in a patient with a hematologic malignancy and an infected Hickman catheter who had recurrent bacteremia.[171]

Identification of *Achromobacter* species is made by recovery of oxidase-positive, catalase-positive, indole-negative, and urease-negative organisms that produce flat colonies with spreading edges on blood-agar plates. Aerobic incubation is crucial for recovery in culture, and the organisms grow well at 35°C. The organisms also grow on MacConkey agar. Distinguishing the organisms and confirming identification is made difficult by their lack of reactivity in many biochemical or assimilation tests.[172] *A. faecalis* produces a distinctive sweet odor resembling that of green apples.[2]

Laboratory testing often shows *A. faecalis* strains to be susceptible to trimethoprim-sulfamethoxazole, ureidopenicillins, ticarcillin-clavulanate, carbapenems, and unlike *Achromobacter* species, most cephalosporins.[173] Results vary for aztreonam, aminoglycosides, and fluoroquinolones, whereas *A. faecalis* strains are often resistant to amoxicillin, ticarcillin, and gentamicin.[169] Extended-spectrum β-lactamase production has also been described in *A. faecalis*.[174]

CHRYSEOBACTERIUM AND ELIZABETHKINGIA SPECIES

Chryseobacterium species are inhabitants of soil and water and can be recovered from a variety of foods. They can be found in municipal water supplies despite adequate chlorination and have been recovered from the hospital environment, often in conjunction with clusters of clinical isolates. *Chryseobacterium* species are organisms of low virulence, and their presence in clinical specimens usually represents colonization and not infection. *C. indologenes* is the most frequently isolated species but is a rare cause of human disease. Intravascular catheter–related bacteremia and bacteremia associated with malignancy and neutropenia have been reported.[175] *C. meningosepticum*, however, is clinically significant in up to half of the adults and in about two thirds of the neonates from whom it is recovered.[176] Based on phylogenetic and phenotypic data, *C. meningosepticum* has recently been placed in the genus *Elizabethkingia* and is now known as *E. meningoseptica*.[177] *Chryseobacterium* species produce proteases and gelatinase, which may contribute to virulence; these are responsible for the greenish discoloration around the colonies on blood agar.

E. meningoseptica is a cause of neonatal meningitis, especially in premature infants during the first 2 weeks of life. Clusters of neonatal meningitis have been linked to many sources, including contaminated saline solution for flushing eyes, respiratory equipment, and sink drains.[176,178] Neonatal meningitis is fatal in more than half the cases, and brain abscesses and other severe sequelae are common. Most *E. meningoseptica* infections in adults are hospital acquired and occur in immunocompromised hosts. The respiratory tract is the most common site of infection, and outbreaks have been linked to contaminated ventilator tubing and aerosols.[179,180] In outbreaks, respiratory tract colonization occurs more often than infection. Bacteremia is the second most common presentation of *E. meningoseptica* infection. In one cluster of bloodstream infections related to a contaminated anesthetic, the bacteremia was transient, and systemic signs of infection resolved without specific antibiotic therapy, attesting to the low virulence of this organism in adults.[181] *E. meningoseptica* has also caused endocarditis (including prosthetic valve), cellulitis, wound infection, sepsis following extensive burns, abdominal abscess, dialysis-associated peritonitis, and endophthalmitis.[176,182] Other contaminated sources include contaminated syringes in ice chests, vials, sink drains, sink taps, tube feedings, flush solutions for arterial catheters, pressure transducers, and antiseptic solutions.[176,183,184] Infections including cellulitis, septic arthritis, community-acquired respiratory tract infection, keratitis, and bacteremia have been reported in the absence of underlying diseases.[185-189] *C. indologenes* is a rare cause of human disease. Intravascular catheter–related bacteremia and bacteremia associated with malignancy and neutropenia have been reported.[175] *Chryseobacterium* and *Elizabethkingia* species may be long, thin, slightly curved, and occasionally filamentous on Gram stain. *C. indolgenes* colonies usually form a dark-yellow pigment in culture as a result of the production of the pigment flexirubin, whereas *E. meningoseptica* colonies are smooth, large, and pale yellow (Fig. 237-2). Both organisms grow well and form colonies within 24 hours on blood or chocolate agar and grow at a much slower rate, if at all, on MacConkey agar.[190] They are not motile and produce positive catalase and oxidase reactions.

Chryseobacterium species and *E. meningoseptica* are resistant to most antibiotics, and the use of inactive drugs as empirical therapy may contribute to the poor outcome in many infections. In addition, MIC breakpoints have not been established by the Clinical and Laboratory Standards Institute (CLSI) for chryseobacteria. Results of susceptibility testing vary when different methods are used; disk diffusion methods especially are unreliable, and broth microdilution should be employed, if possible.[191] The E-test has been also suggested as a possible alternative for testing certain antibiotics.[192] *Chryseobacterium* organisms produce β-lactamases and are resistant to most β-lactam drugs, including the carbapenems and aztreonam.[191,193] Cefepime has poor activity against *E. meningoseptica,* and cefepime has only modest activity against *C. indolgenes.*[194] They are usually resistant to aminoglycosides, chloramphenicol, and erythromycin. Fluoroquinolones are usually active in vitro, and sparfloxacin, cinafloxacin, and levofloxacin are somewhat more active than ciprofloxacin.[195] In two 1997 reports, minocycline was the only agent active against all *E. meningoseptica* strains.[176,191] Doxycycline and trimethoprim-sulfamethoxazole susceptibility was variable. Rifampin is active against most strains and has been used as part of combination therapy to clear persistent infection.[196] Vancomycin, alone or in combination with other agents including rifampin, has been successful in the treatment of meningitis in infants.[197,198] In some reported cases of meningitis treated successfully with vancomycin, the MICs of vancomycin were 8 to 12 µg/mL.[199] However, two groups reported that vancomycin was inactive in vitro (MICs of 16 to more than 64 µg/mL) and called into question the

usefulness of vancomycin against *E. meningoseptica*[176,191] Thus, there is no optimal regimen for *E. meningoseptica* meningitis, and therapy should be based on properly performed susceptibility testing. Possible regimens include rifampin in combination with trimethoprim-sulfamethoxazole, vancomycin, a fluoroquinolone, or minocycline.

COMAMONAS SPECIES

Comamonas species are common environmental bacteria that occasionally cause human disease. Although these organisms are of low virulence, some of their obscurity is due to the inability of clinical laboratories to speciate them; isolates may be reported as being nonfermentative gram-negative bacilli that could not be further identified. Thus, their presence in clinical specimens may be more than appreciated.

Comamonas testosteroni, formerly *Pseudomonas testosteroni,* is the most common pathogen of the genus. This organism was isolated from 10 non-epidemiologically linked patients over a 3-year period at Parkland Memorial Hospital, where unidentified nonfermenters were sent to the state health department for speciation.[200] In five of these patients, the organism was isolated from the peritoneal cavity of patients who presented with perforated appendices; three cases occurred in intravenous drug users, one of whom had a ruptured mycotic aneurysm and *C. testosteroni* in the cerebrospinal fluid. Other reported infections include native valve endocarditis, primary bacteremia, catheter-related bacteremia, meningitis, peritonitis in a patient with alcoholic cirrhosis, and urinary tract infection. Many of these infections are polymicrobial.[201,202] *Comamonas acidovorans* has been reported to cause keratitis and other ocular infections, catheter-related bacteremia, and peritonitis in a patient receiving peritoneal dialysis.[203]

Comamonas are motile, nonpigmented, oxidase-positive, gram-negative bacilli that grow well on routine bacteriologic media. Biochemical characteristics include accumulation of β-hydroxybutyrate, acetamide hydrolysis, and reduction of nitrate to nitrite. Most currently available identification systems will identify *Comamonas* to genus level, if at all. Species are distinguished by carbon compound use patterns.

There are no guidelines for antibiotic susceptibility testing for *Comamonas* species. Aminoglycosides, fluoroquinolones, carbapenems, piperacillin-tazobactam, and ceftazidime are potentially active. *Comamonas acidovorans* is more resistant to aminoglycosides than *C. testosteroni.*

EIKENELLA SPECIES

Eikenella corrodens is a fastidious facultative anaerobic gram-negative bacillus that is part of the normal human oral flora. In 1948, Henriksen identified a gram-negative anaerobic organism that had the peculiar characteristic of creating a depression in the growth medium and referred to this organism as the *corroding bacillus.* In 1958, Eiken described and characterized a gram-negative obligate or facultative anaerobic organism for which he proposed the name *Bacteroides corrodens.* Subsequently, the strictly anaerobic organisms were renamed *Bacteroides corrodens* (and now are called *Bacteroides ureolyticus*), whereas the facultative anaerobes were reclassified in the genus *Eikenella.*[204]

E. corrodens is present as endogenous flora in the mouth and upper respiratory tract as well as on other mucous surfaces of the body. Although it is recovered most often as a component of mixed infection,[205] commonly coexisting with streptococci,[206] it has been recovered from sterile sites in pure culture.[207] Characteristic of *Eikenella* infection is an indolent course, generally taking more than 1 week from the time of injury to clinical manifestation of disease.[208] Many patients with *Eikenella* infection have underlying diseases, especially head and neck malignancies.[209,210] In recent case series and literature reviews, the head and neck were the most common sites of *Eikenella* infections in both adults and children.[207,210] Other common clinical manifestations include respiratory tract infections[205] and human bite wounds.[211] The organism

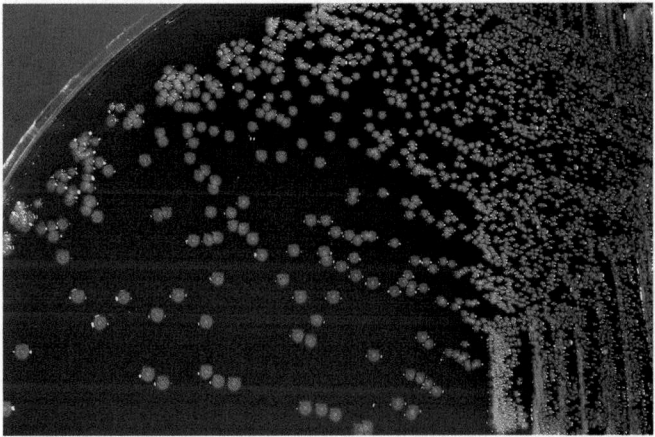

Figure 237-2 Yellow colonies of *Elizabethkingia meningosepticum* on blood agar plate.

is often present in "clenched-fist injuries," the most serious of human bite infections,[211] and infections among chronic finger or nail biters[212] and has been reported as a cause of "genital ulceration" after a human bite to the penis.[213] Because of the proximity of bone and joint spaces, these infections may lead to osteomyelitis and septic arthritis. It has also caused infection in insulin-requiring diabetic patients and drug-abusing "skin poppers" who lick their needles.[214] Severe soft tissue infection, with or without underlying osteomyelitis, may be slow to resolve.[215,216] Suppuration due to *Eikenella* infections is foul smelling, mimicking an anaerobic process. Pulmonary infections, including empyema, pneumonia, and septic emboli, in conjunction with internal jugular vein thrombosis (postanginal sepsis), can occur, typically in patients with underlying chronic illnesses or intrathoracic malignancies.[206] Gynecologic infections have been reported, including chorioamniotis resulting in preterm labor and fetal demise and infection associated with intrauterine contraceptive devices.[217,218] *Eikenella* has also been recovered in pure culture from synovial fluid, bone, cerebrospinal fluid, brain, subdural and visceral abscesses, pleuropulmonary infection, and blood.[205,206,219] *E. corrodens* is another of the so-called HACEK organisms, which, as mentioned, have in common the need for incubation in an atmosphere enhanced with CO_2 for recovery in culture and a predilection for infecting the heart valves. Endocarditis caused by *E. corrodens* typically has an indolent course, but acute presentations are reported.[204] Endocarditis usually occurs after intravenous drug use or in patients with abnormal heart valves, including prosthetic valves,[16,220] but infection on structurally normal heart valve in a patient without predisposing risk factors has been reported.[221]

E. corrodens is a gram-negative, small straight rod that at times can appear pleomorphic or coccobacillary. It grows in either aerobic or anaerobic environments. It is nonmotile and non–spore forming and does not have a capsule. Cell surface components vary from strain to strain, and these differences may relate to virulence.[222] On blood or chocolate agar, even aided by the presence of 3% to 10% CO_2, the organism grows slowly, and it often requires 2 days or more to recognize the typical pinpoint colonies. Colonies are small and grayish (older colonies may become light yellow), produce a slight greenish discoloration on the blood agar, and elaborate an odor resembling that of bleach (hypochlorite). About half produce the pitting ("corroding") of the agar that is considered characteristic. The organism grows poorly on MacConkey agar. Strains do not form acid from carbohydrates, are oxidase positive, catalase negative (a few strains are weakly catalase positive), urease negative, and indole negative and reduce nitrate to nitrite. Ampicillin, ureidopenicillins, second- and third-generation cephalosporins, and tetracyclines have been reported effective against *E. corrodens* both in vitro and in producing clinical cure.[119,223] The organism is susceptible to fluoroquinolones and azithromycin in vitro; however, it is uniformly resistant to clindamycin, erythromycin, and metronidazole and often resistant in vitro to aminoglycosides.[119,224] β-Lactamase production is uncommon at present; some of the β-lactamases produced by *Eikenella* are inhibited by clavulanate and sulbactam.[225]

FLAVOBACTERIUM AND MYROIDES SPECIES

The genus *Flavobacterium* consisted of a heterogeneous group of yellow-pigmented bacteria that did not prove to be closely related when subjected to genotypic analysis.[226] Consequently, many *Flavobacterium* species, including the clinically important species, have been reclassified to other genera and are discussed elsewhere. *Flavobacterium meningosepticum*, the most important species, is now a member of the genus *Elizabethkingia*, whereas *F. indologenes* is now in the genus *Chryseobacterium*. *Flavobacterium multivorum* and *Flavobacterium spiritivorum* now reside in the genus *Sphingobacterium*. *Flavobacterium odoratum*, an uncommon clinical isolate, has been placed in a new genus, *Myroides*, and divided into two species, *M. odoratus* and *M. odoratimimus*.[227] Although common in soil and water, *Myroides* species are rare clinical isolates and are often not considered pathogenic. However, the organism has been isolated from urine, blood, wounds,

and respiratory secretions. There are case reports of catheter-associated bacteremia and soft tissue infections, with secondary bacteremia occurring in both compromised and normal hosts.[228-230] On outbreak of catheter-related bloodstream infections was traced to ampules of water contaminated with *Myroides odoratus* and *Burkholderia cepacia*.[231]

Myroides species grow on most media, including MacConkey agar. Colonies are yellow and produce a fruity odor similar to that of *A. faecalis*. The organisms are oxidase, catalase, urease, and gelatinase positive. They reduce nitrite and do not produce indole. *Myroides* are reportedly resistant to β-lactams, including carbapenems and aminoglycosides.[229]

OCHROBACTRUM SPECIES

Organisms formerly called CDC group Vd and *Achromobacter* groups A, C, and D were renamed *Ochrobactrum anthropi* (from the Greek *ochros*, meaning "pale yellow").[138] Recent studies suggest that *Achromobacter* group C and some group A strains belong to a distinct species now designated as *O. intermedium*.[232] However, no biochemical tests currently available in clinical laboratories can separate *O. anthropi* from *O. intermedium*. *O. anthropi* is related to *Brucella* species and has been recovered from the environment and clinical sources. Published reports suggest that this organism is an emerging pathogen in immunocompromised patients and that infections caused by this organism may be increasing in frequency.[233-235]

Intravascular catheter–related bacteremia is the most common infection associated with *O. anthropi*.[233,236,237] This organism has contaminated biologic products, which have been the source of small outbreaks. Five bloodstream infections occurred in organ transplant recipients who received contaminated rabbit antithymocyte globulin.[238] Consistent with this organism's being of low virulence, bacteremia resolved in four of five immunosuppressed patients in this series without antibiotic administration. Three cases of postoperative meningitis in neurosurgical patients were traced to cadaveric pericardial patches possibly contaminated during processing.[239] *O. anthropi* has been cultured from tap water at a hematology unit in association with a small outbreak.[240] It has been reported to cause bacteremia in patients on hemodialysis and in patients with acquired immunodeficiency syndrome (AIDS),[241,242] and peritonitis in patients undergoing continuous ambulatory peritoneal dialysis.[243] *Ochrobactum* endophthalmitis has occurred following hematogenous spread and postoperatively, including a cluster of nine cases following cataract extraction with lens implantation[244] Other reported infections include infection of pacemaker leads, prosthetic valve endocarditis, pancreatic abscess, pelvic abscess complicating appendicitis, necrotizing fasciitis, and osteochondritis following a puncture wound.[234,245-247] It has also been recovered from bile, urine, wounds, stool, throat, and vagina.[248]

O. anthropi is an oxidase-positive, non–lactose-fermenting gram-negative bacillus that grows readily on MacConkey agar. The organism oxidizes glucose and xylose, but 72 hours or more of incubation may be required before this is apparent. *O. anthropi* is motile by means of peritrichous flagella, which helps to differentiate it from pseudomonads and *Chryseobacterium*. The organism is similar to *A. xylosoxidans* subsp. *xylosoxidans* in biochemical characteristics, but it can hydrolyze urea and grows poorly on cetrimide agar.[146] As previously mentioned, *O. anthropi* and *O. intermedium* are closely related to *Brucella* species, and misidentification can occur with some of the automated systems.[249]

O. anthropi is usually susceptible to trimethoprim-sulfamethoxazole and fluoroquinolones; variably susceptible to gentamicin, amikacin, netilmicin, imipenem, and tetracycline; and generally resistant to β-lactams, including most cephalosporins and penicillins, at least in part as a result of the presence of an ampC β-lactamase.[236,250] Failures with imipenem therapy have been reported.

OLIGELLA SPECIES

The genus *Oligella* was named for the small size of the bacilli on Gram stain and contains two species, *Oligella urethralis* (formerly *Moraxella urethralis* and CDC group M-4) and *Oligella ureolytica* (formerly known as CDC group IVe). *O. urethralis* is a commensal of the genitourinary tract, and most clinical isolates are from the urine, predominantly from men.[31] Although symptomatic infections are rare, bacteremia, septic arthritis mimicking gonococcal arthritis,[251] and peritonitis in two patients receiving chronic ambulatory peritoneal dialysis[252] have been described. *O. ureolytica* is also primarily found in the urine, usually from patients with long-term indwelling urinary catheters or other urinary drainage systems. These patients have a propensity to develop urinary stones that may be related to the organism's ability to hydrolyze urea and alkalinize the urine, leading to precipitation of phosphates. Bacteremia has been reported in a patient with obstructive uropathy.[253] *O. ureolytica* bacteremia has been reported in a patient with AIDS and infected decubitus ulcers.[254]

Oligella species, especially *O. urethralis*, resemble *Moraxella* and appear coccobacillary on Gram stain. Most strains will grow on blood or MacConkey agar but require extended incubation (2 to 4 days) before growth can be detected. *O. urethralis* is nonmotile, whereas most strains of *O. ureolytica* are motile by peritrichous flagella. The rapidity of the urease reaction (within 5 minutes on a Christensen urea agar slant) is a distinctive feature of *O. ureolytica*. These organisms are oxidase-positive and catalase-positive and reduce NO_3 to NO_2. Contemporary data on antimicrobial susceptibilities are sparse. Strains of *O. urethralis* are usually susceptible to β-lactam antibiotics, but β-lactamase–producing strains, as well as strains resistant to ciprofloxacin, have been reported.[252] Resistance to β-lactam antibiotics is due to acquisition of chromosomally encoded AmpC β-lactamases, either ADC-7 or ABA-1, derived from *Acinetobacter baumannii*.[255,256]

PSEUDOMONAS SPECIES

The genus *Pseudomonas* has been modified considerably and now contains the organisms previously known as *Flavimonas oryzihabitans* and *Chryseomonas luteola*.[257,258] These organisms are now included in the nonfluorescent group of pseudomonads that includes *P. stutzeri* and other rarely encountered species. The fluorescent group contains *P. fluorescens*, *P. putida*, and *P. aeruginosa*. *P. aeruginosa* is the only member of the genus that possesses significant virulence factors and is an important human pathogen; it is discussed in Chapter 219. Members of the fluorescent group produce pyoverdin, a yellow-green pigment that fluoresces under ultraviolet light. Pseudomonads are environmental organisms and have a predilection for moist environments. They can contaminate solutions such as distilled water, disinfectants, and intravenous solutions. Not surprisingly, many of the infections caused by these organisms are health care associated.

P. fluorescens is an uncommon cause of catheter-associated bacteremia[258] and pseudobacteremia due to contaminated blood collection tubes.[259] Contaminated heparin flush solution caused a large multistate outbreak of *P. fluorescens* catheter-related bacteremia; in some exposed patients with implanted ports, diagnosis was delayed for many months after exposure to the solution.[260] This organism can grow at 4° C, allowing it to proliferate in contaminated blood products and occasionally cause transfusion-related sepsis.[261] *P. fluorescens* can be misidentified by commercial laboratory systems.[258] Because isolation of this organism can reflect pseudobacteremia, proper identification is important to avoid unnecessary antimicrobial therapy. *P. putida* is also an occasional cause of nosocomial bacteremia, bacteremia in patients with cancer, pneumonia, peritonitis, urinary tract infections, and neonatal sepsis.[262-264] In an outbreak of *P. putida* catheter-related bacteremia caused by a contaminated flush solution, infection was cured without catheter removal in most patients.[264a] Isolation of this organism from clinical specimens can reflect contamination; it has also been described as a cause of a pseudo-outbreak.[265]

P. stutzeri is another uncommon clinical isolate but has been reported to cause bacteremia, nosocomial brain abscess, and meningitis in immunocompromised hosts.[266] Rare cases of community-acquired osteomyelitis, septic arthritis, and pneumonia have also been reported.[267,268] *P. stutzeri* has also been implicated as a cause of pseu-

dobacteremia and of delayed onset endophthalmitis after cataract surgery. *Pseudomonas oryzihabitans* (the species name means "inhabiting rice") is the current name for the organism that at various times has been called *Chromobacterium typhiflavum*, *Flavimonas oryzihabitans*, and CDC group Ve-2.[269] It is an infrequent cause of infection with characteristics similar to those of *P. luteola*. *P. oryzihabitans* is normally found in soil, water, and damp environments such as rice paddies. In the hospital setting, it has been recovered from sink drains and respiratory therapy equipment.[269] Central venous catheter–associated bloodstream infection is the most commonly reported infection. In an 8-year study from a major cancer center, 21 of 22 episodes of *P. oryzihabitans* bacteremia were catheter related.[270] In this series, most infections were non–hospital acquired, polymicrobial infections were common, and most bacteremias could be treated without catheter removal. In contrast, in another recent series, all *P. oryzihabitans* bacteremias were hospital acquired, and the implicated intravascular devices were removed in most cases.[271] The organism has also been associated with other foreign bodies, such as peritoneal dialysis catheters, ventriculostomy tubes, vascular grafts, prosthetic joints, and intraocular lens.[272-274] Soft tissue infections, postoperative wound infections, splenic abscesses, and meningitis have been reported.[275,276] Although most patients with *P. oryzihabitans* infection are immunocompromised, the infections are indolent and recovery is the rule.

Pseudomonas luteola is another uncommon opportunistic pathogen. It was previously known as CDC group Ve-1 and *Chryseomonas luteola*. *P. luteola* infections are often associated with foreign bodies such as central venous and peritoneal dialysis catheters. Reported infections include bacteremia, peritonitis (associated with appendicitis and colon cancer as well as catheters), osteomyelitis, endocarditis, leg ulcers, cellulitis, postoperative endophthalmitis, and meningitis.[272,275,277,278]

Pseudomonas species are aerobic, non–spore-forming, gram-negative rods. They are motile owing to the presence of one or more polar flagella. They are lactose nonfermenters and grow well on MacConkey agar. Most clinical isolates (except *P. luteola* and *P. oryzihabitans*) are oxidase positive. In addition to the negative oxidase reaction, these two species produce yellow-pigmented colonies on MacConkey agar that help distinguish them from other pseudomonads. Unlike other fluorescent pseudomonads including *P. aeruginosa*, *P. fluorescens* and *P. putida* do not reduce nitrate and oxidize xylose. *P. stutzeri* colonies are brown, dry, and wrinkled on primary isolation media.

There are limited antimicrobial susceptibility data for these pseudomonads. *P. putida* can show broad resistance to β-lactam antibiotics, and some isolates of this organism produce a metallo-β-lactamase that can readily hydrolyze carbapenems.[279] *P. oryzihabitans* is usually susceptible in vitro to ureidopenicillins, third-generation cephalosporins, aztreonam, imipenem, aminoglycosides, fluoroquinolones, and trimethoprim-sulfamethoxazole, but shows resistance to earlier-generation cephalosporins.[270,280] Clinical isolates of *P. luteola* are often resistant to first- and second-generation cephalosporins, tetracyclines, ampicillin, and trimethoprim-sulfamethoxazole but are susceptible to third-generation cephalosporins, mezlocillin, imipenem, aminoglycosides, and quinolones.[272]

RALSTONIA AND CUPRIAVIDUS SPECIES

The genus *Ralstonia* was established in 1995 and initially contained one recognized pathogen, *Ralstonia pickettii* (formerly *Pseudomonas*, then *Burkholderia*, *pickettii*).[281] Subsequently several other clinically relevant species were added to the genus, including *Ralstonia paucula* (formerly designated as CDC group IVc-2), *Ralstonia. gilardii*, and, most recently, *Ralstonia mannitolilytica* (formerly *Pseudomonas thomasii*, then *R. pickettii* biovar 3/"thomasii"). There was extensive taxonomic revision of the genus in 2004, with *R. pickettii* and similar organisms remaining in the genus *Ralstonia*, but species in the *R. eutropha* lineage, including *R. paucula* and *R. gilardii*, were transferred to the new genus *Wautersia*. 16S rRNA profiles quickly revealed that the newly named *Wautersia* organisms were synonymous with the existing genus *Cupriavidus*, which, according to nomenclature rules, has priority over the genus name *Wautersia,* and all species that had been placed in the genus *Wautersia* were transferred to the genus *Cupriavidus. Ralstonia* and *Cupriavidus* species are environmental gram-negative, nonfermentative bacilli of low virulence but can cause infection related to contaminated infusates or in immunocompromised hosts, including transplant recipients and patients with HIV infection or leukemia.[282-285]

R. pickettii can grow in saline and other fluids and has been the cause of many outbreaks related to contaminated infusates and pseudooutbreaks related to contaminated solutions used in laboratory diagnosis.[286,287] The contamination of solutions has occurred during the manufacturing process and by extrinsic manipulation. In addition to bacteremia from contaminated intravenous products, airway colonization has been caused by contaminated respiratory therapy solutions.[287] In one outbreak due to a contaminated saline solutions, only 1 of 19 patients with *R. pickettii* airway colonization received antimicrobial therapy, consistent with the low virulence of the organism.[287] Several hospital-associated outbreaks attributed to *R. mannitolilytica* have also been described.[288,289] Clinical isolates of other *Ralstonia* and *Cupriavidus* species are less common. A number of *Ralstonia* and *Cupriavidus* species have been isolated from sputum cultures of cystic fibrosis patients.[290,291] Most of the reported human infections of *C. paucula* and *C. gilardii* are intravascular catheter–related bloodstream infections, either nosocomial or community acquired.[292] Peritoneal dialysis-associated peritonitis[293] and tenosynovitis following a cat bite[294] have also been reported. Most patients have responded well to antibiotic therapy.

Ralstonia and *Cupriavidus* species grow on routine media, although growth may be slow and require more than 72 hours of incubation to visualize colonies. *Ralstonia* species have one or more polar flagella in motile species, produce acid from glucose and several other carbohydrates, and are resistant to colistin, whereas *Cupriavidus* species have peritrichous flagella, do not produce acid from glucose, and are susceptible to colistin. Extensive biochemical testing is required for identification and misidentification of these organisms by commercially available systems is common.[289] Identification may also be confused because *R. pickettii, R. mannitolilytica,* and *R. insidosa* are able to grow on selective media intended for isolation of *Burkholderia cepacia.* 16S rRNA PCR and matrix-assisted laser desorption ionization-time of flight mass spectrometry have been useful means of identification.[290,291]

There are no validated in vitro susceptibility testing methods for *Ralstonia* species or *Cupriavidus* species. *R. pickettii,* but not other *Ralstonia* or *Cupriavidus* species, produces a chromosomally encoded class D β-lactamase, OXA-22, which confers resistance or reduced susceptibility to aminopenicillins, carboxypenicillins, narrow-spectrum cephalosporins, and aztreonam.[295] An inducible chromosomal β-lactamase, OXA-60, that hydrolyzes imipenem is also widespread.[295] Isolates of *R. pickettii* have been reported to be generally susceptible to the ureidopenicillins, ciprofloxacin, and trimethoprim-sulfamethoxazole, with varied susceptibility to aminoglycosides.[296] *R. mannitolilytica* is often resistant to ampicillin, aminoglycosides, and aztreonam. *C. paucula* is reportedly susceptible to many β-lactams, along with quinolones and tetracycline, but is often resistant to aminoglycosides.[282,292]

RHIZOBIUM (FORMERLY AGROBACTERIUM) SPECIES

Based on 16S rDNA analysis, organisms previously known as *Agrobacterium* have been redesignated as *Rhizobium.*[297] These organisms are well-known plant pathogens; most contain a large tumor-inducing plasmid, and infection produces neoplastic growth in many plant species. They are present in soil and plants and have a worldwide distribution. Although most clinical isolates appear nonpathogenic, there are more than 50 reported cases of human disease caused by *Rhizobium* species, primarily *R. radiobacter.* The literature contains a few reports of disease caused by another species, *Agrobacterium tumi-*

faciens. However, *A. tumifaciens* and *R. radiobacter* differ only by the presence or absence of the tumor-inducing plasmid, and they are now combined into the new species *Rhizobium radiobacter.*[297]

More than half the reported cases of *R. radiobacter* infection are intravascular catheter–related bloodstream infections in compromised hosts, primarily patients with malignancies.[298,299] Most of these infections were not hospital acquired. However, there is a recent report of three cases of *A. tumifaciens* bacteremias occurring at a single institution in patients with tunneled intravenous catheters. Two of these cases were epidemiologically linked, and the isolates had common pulse field gel electrophoresis patterns suggesting nosocomial transmission[300] Peritonitis in patients receiving ambulatory peritoneal dialysis is the other common presentation for *R. radiobacter* infection.[301] Urinary tract infections caused by this organism have been observed in patients with nephrostomy tubes. Thus, most infections involve a device, the removal of which has been necessary in some cases to effect a cure. Other case reports include cellulitis in a patient with multiple myeloma, prosthetic valve endocarditis, bacteremias in patients with advanced AIDS, and neutropenia and bacteremic pneumonia in a patient with HIV infection.[302,303] A patient who worked in his garden the evening of cataract surgery developed *R. radiobacter* endophthalmitis 4 days later.[304] This is one of the few cases in which soil contact is mentioned. Thus, the source of the infecting organisms is for the most part unknown. Consistent with this organism's being an opportunistic pathogen of low virulence, all patients have survived. *R. radiobacter* has also caused pseudobacteremia resulting from contaminated citrated tubes used for clotting-factor studies.[305]

The organism readily grows on blood agar and MacConkey medium when incubated aerobically. Colony appearance varies for the different species. Flagellar stains show peritrichous distribution. Organisms are oxidase positive and catalase positive, and they produce gas from a variety of carbohydrates, including lactose. Rapid hydrolysis of urea and slower hydrolysis of esculin are key features that help to distinguish this organism from *Alcaligenes* species and *Pseudomonas* species, which it otherwise closely resembles.

Clinical isolates have been variably susceptible to antibiotics and display variations in susceptibility patterns within classes of antibiotics, so in vitro testing of each isolate is important. For example, most isolates are susceptible to gentamicin but resistant to tobramycin.[298] Many strains are susceptible to third-generation cephalosporins, ciprofloxacin, and trimethoprim-sulfamethoxazole. *R. radiobacter* can produce an inducible cephalosporinase as well as an aminoglycoside acetyltransferase. Monobactams are produced by some soil strains[306]; not surprisingly, clinical isolates are often resistant to aztreonam.

ROSEOMONAS SPECIES AND OTHER "PINK-PIGMENTED" GRAM-NEGATIVE BACILLI

The group of organisms previously known as CDC "pink coccoid" groups I through IV have been placed in the genus *Roseomonas* (*roseus* + *monas*, a rose-colored or pink bacterium).[31,307] Although *Roseomonas* species can be recovered from the environment, most named *Roseomonas* species, including *R. gilardii* subsp. *gilardii, R. gilardii* subsp. *rosea, R. cervicalis, R. fauriae,* and *R. mucosa,* have been isolated from clinical specimens.[308] *Roseomonas* appears to cause more clinical disease than the related pink-pigmented bacterium, *Methylobacterium.*[2,309] *Methylobacterium* species, which are so named because of their ability to facultatively use methane, were previously classified under such names as *Pseudomonas mesophilica, Protomonas extorquens, Protaminobacter rubra,* "the pink phantom," and *Vibrio extorquens.*[310] The two most clinically relevant species, *M. mesophilicum* and *M. zatmanii,* are very similar phenotypically, and some reference laboratories limit identification to the genus level only.[310]

R. gilardii is usually recovered in pure culture and, in one retrospective series, appeared to cause clinical illness more often than not.[309] Infections are often community acquired. Bloodstream infection is the most common presentation and may be related to the presence of intravascular catheters[311,312] or are secondary to processes at other sites, including intra-abdominal abscesses, respiratory tract, or urinary tract infections. These infections usually, but not invariably, occur in patients with underlying medical illnesses such as malignancies, AIDS, chronic renal disease, or diabetes. Device removal may be necessary to clear intravascular catheter-related bacteremia.[313] Peritoneal dialysis–associated peritonitis, vertebral osteomyelitis, ventriculitis, septic bursitis, soft tissue infections, and epiglottitis have also been reported.[309,314-316] Thirty-six episodes of *Roseomonas* bacteremia occurred in one referral cancer center over a 12-year period, with *R. mucosa* causing 61% of these infections.[317] Most patients had central venous catheters; line removal was necessary in six patients to clear the bloodstream infection. Most of the isolates were initially misidentified or unidentifiable; *Roseomonas* infection was confirmed by supplemental testing including 16S rRNA genotypic studies. *R. fauriae* is rarely isolated from clinical specimens but has been reported to cause peritonitis in a patient undergoing continuous ambulatory peritoneal dialysis.[318] *R. mucosa* septic arthritis has been reported in a patient with rheumatoid arthritis undergoing treatment with infliximab.

Methylobacterium has also caused intravascular catheter–related bacteremia and peritonitis in patients receiving continuous ambulatory peritoneal dialysis and soft tissue infections.[319] A pseudo-outbreak of *Methylobacterium* respiratory tract infections was traced to contaminated tap water in the bronchoscopy suite.[320]

Roseomonas species are plump gram-negative rods or coccobacilli. In contrast, *Methylobacterium* species do not stain well and can appear gram-variable and also have intracellular vacuoles. Colonies are pink pigmented and are sometimes mucoid. Both these organisms can appear weakly oxidase positive and are catalase positive and urease positive. *Roseomonas* can be distinguished from *Methylobacterium* by the inability to oxidize methanol, the inability to assimilate acetamide, and the absence of long-wave ultraviolet light absorption.[307] *Methylobacterium* has been isolated after 1 week of incubation on medium ordinarily used for the isolation of mycobacteria.[314]

Carbapenems, aminoglycosides, and tetracycline are the most active antibiotics against *Roseomonas* species.[316,317,321] They are usually resistant to penicillins and cephalosporins, with the exception of penicillin β-lactamase inhibitor combinations, which are frequently but not invariably active. *Roseomonas* species are usually susceptible to fluoroquinolones but resistant to trimethoprim-sulfamethoxazole. *Methylobacterium* grows slowly, and susceptibility testing is not always possible.[310] Many *Methylobacterium* isolates produce a β-lactamase, and the organisms are resistant to penicillins and many cephalosporins. Aminoglycosides, ciprofloxacin, and trimethoprim-sulfamethoxazole are active.

SHEWANELLA SPECIES

Shewanella putrefaciens (formerly *Pseudomonas putrefaciens, Alteromonas putrefaciens,* or CDC group Ib) is widely distributed in the environment and has infrequently been implicated as a cause of human disease. *Shewanella* can be recovered from a variety of water sources, natural gas and petroleum reserves, dairy products, meat, and fish. *S. putrefaciens* is genetically heterogeneous, and three distinct biovars have been described. Biovar 1 (CDC group Ib-1) is a major cause of spoilage of refrigerated protein-rich foods. Clinical isolates are usually biovar 2 (CDC group Ib-2), but recent data suggest that most of these isolates should be classified as the genetically distinct species *Shewanella algae* (previously *S. alga*).[322,323] However, the typing systems currently in use by most clinical microbiology laboratories identify both species as *S. putrefaciens.*[323] Thus, in all likelihood, the use of this species name will continue.

Shewanella is frequently isolated as part of a polymicrobial infection, and its pathogenic role is often unclear. Lower extremity cellulitis in association with chronic ulcers or after burns is one of the more commonly described presentations.[324] *Shewanella* bacteremia, which also is frequently polymicrobial, can accompany soft tissue infection or biliary tract disease or occur in compromised hosts, including persons with underlying liver disease or malignancy.[325,326] Compromised hosts are more likely to have accompanying signs of sepsis and have a poor outcome. A common source outbreak that led to 31 patients infected or colonized by *Shewanella* on a surgical ward was traced to a contaminated shared measuring cup.[327] In this outbreak, blood, bile, and ascitic fluid were the most common culture isolation sources. Bacteremia and respiratory distress have been described in neonates and premature infants.[325] Less commonly reported infections include peritonitis, pneumonia, empyema, purulent pericarditis, meningitis, brain abscess, osteomyelitis, otitis, urinary tract infection, endophthalmitis, keratitis, and an infected aortic aneurysm.[324,326,328] On Gram stain, *Shewanella* is a short to long rod and can be filamentous. It grows readily and produces small to medium-sized colonies that have a yellow-orange or brown to tan soluble pigment that causes greenish discoloration of the medium. Colonies may be mucoid and have a fishlike smell. *Shewanella* is oxidase-positive and is the only nonfermenter that produces hydrogen sulfide on triple sugar iron agar, a key feature that allows easy identification in the laboratory. *Shewanella algae* can be distinguished from *S. putrefaciens* by growth at 42° C, growth in 6.5% NaCl, the production of hemolysis on sheep blood agar, and the inability to produce acid from sucrose, maltose, and L-arabinose.[323] *Shewanella* is resistant to penicillin and cefazolin but susceptible to most third- and fourth-generation cephalosporins and piperacillin.[324] The organisms are also usually susceptible to aminoglycosides, chloramphenicol, erythromycin, and quinolones but less predictably susceptible to tetracycline and trimethoprim-sulfamethoxazole.[324,325,329] A report from South Africa found that most isolates were resistant to imipenem.[325] *Shewanella* may also contain a chromosomally encoded gene, *qnr3,* that confers resistance to quinolones by protecting DNA gyrase and probably also topoisomerase IV.[330] Development of resistance while on treatment has been reported with piperacillin-tazobactam and imipenem.[329]

SPHINGOBACTERIUM SPECIES

The genus *Sphingobacterium* includes organisms previously classified as *Flavobacterium* species. The organisms that were transferred to this new genus contain large amounts of sphingophospholipid compounds in their cell membranes and have other taxonomic features that distinguish them from flavobacteria.[331] Most isolates from humans are *S. multivorum* (formerly *Flavobacterium multivorum* or CDC group IIk-2) and *Sphingobacterium spiritivorum* (formerly *Flavobacterium spiritivorum* or CDC group IIk-3).

There are reported cases of *S. multivorum* causing peritonitis, septicemia in a dialysis patient, bacteremia in a patient with lymphoma as well as in a patient with diabetes, and respiratory disease in a patient with cystic fibrosis.[332-335] Most cases of *S. multivorum* infection are nosocomial, but the natural habitat of the organism is not well defined. *S. spiritivorum* has been rarely recovered from clinical specimens, primarily urine and blood.[31,336] Cellulitis presumably from soil contact with secondary bacteremia has been reported, as has hypersensitivity pneumonitis related to a water source harboring *S. spiritivorum.*[337,338]

S. multivorum and *S. spiritivorum* grow on blood agar, are oxidase and catalase positive and indole negative, and produce light-yellow colonies. They are biochemically similar to *Sphingomonas paucimobilis* (CDC group IIk-1).

Sphingobacterium species are intrinsically resistant to many commonly employed antibiotics and can grow in some antiseptics and disinfectants.[333,339] *S. multivorum* can produce an extended-spectrum β-lactamase and a metallo-β-lactamase conferring resistance to third-generation cephalosporins and carbapenems, respectively.[340] The combination of trimethoprim-sulfamethoxazole and perfloxacin produced cure in a bacteremic patient.[333] A bacteremic patient receiving hemodialysis improved clinically after receiving ampicillin and one dose of tobramycin, despite in vitro testing showing ampicillin resistance.[332]

SPHINGOMONAS SPECIES

The genus *Sphingomonas* contains at least 12 species, of which only one, *Sphingomonas paucimobilus,* is an occasional human pathogen.[341]

This organism, formerly known as *Pseudomonas paucimobilis* and CDC group IIk-1, is widely distributed in soil and water, including water sources in the hospital environment. It has been implicated in nosocomial outbreaks associated with contaminated water[342,343] and contaminated ventilator temperature probes.[344]

S. paucimobilis infections typically occur in immunocompromised persons and can be community as well as nosocomially acquired. This is an organism of low virulence, and recovery from infection is the rule, even in debilitated hosts. There are several reports of *S. paucimobilis* intravascular catheter–associated bloodstream infections, and catheter removal was necessary in some cases for cure.[345,346] Bloodstream infection has also been reported in hemodialysis patients and after infusion of contaminated autologous bone marrow.[347] Although ventilator-associated pneumonia has been described,[346] airway colonization was much more common than infection in intensive care unit outbreaks.[342,344] Peritoneal catheter–associated peritonitis, meningitis, ventriculoperitoneal shunt infection, brain abscess, soft tissue infection, wound infection, postoperative endophthalmitis, adenitis, urinary tract infection, and a variety of visceral abscesses have been reported.[346,348,349]

S. paucimobilis is strictly aerobic, weakly oxidase positive, and catalase positive. Colonies grow on blood agar but not MacConkey agar, produce a yellow pigment, and can be misidentified as *Flavobacterium* species. Despite the presence of a single polar flagellum, a low percentage of cells are actively motile, and motility can be difficult to demonstrate in the laboratory (thus the name *paucimobilis*).[350]

Susceptibility patterns reported in the literature have varied somewhat but suggest that most isolates are susceptible to trimethoprim-sulfamethoxazole, carbapenems, aminoglycosides, tetracyclines, and chloramphenicol.[345,346,350] Third-generation cephalosporins are usually active but not predictably so, and resistance to penicillins and first-generation cephalosporins is common. Although fluoroquinolones were active in some reports, resistance has been seen in others.[345,346] Patients have been noted to respond well, even when empiric treatment did not correlate with subsequent susceptibility tests.

WEEKSELLA AND *BERGEYELLA* SPECIES

The genus *Weeksella*, when proposed in 1986, contained two species, *W. zoohelcum* (CDC group IIj) and *W. virosa* (CDC group IIf), that differed from most nonfermentative gram-negative bacilli in being susceptible to penicillin. Recently, *W. zoohelcum* has been moved to the new genus *Bergeyella*.[226] *Bergeyella zoohelcum* (from the Greek "animal" + "wound") is part of the normal oral flora of dogs and other animals, and most clinical isolates come from bite wounds.[351,352] Case reports of invasive *B. zoohelcum* infections including meningitis and bacteremia are very rare; some have followed dog bites.[353,354] A 44-year-old woman developed *B. zoohelcum* bacteremia 1 day after eating a meal prepared with goat blood.[355] *W. virosa* has been isolated predominantly from the genital tract and urine of women[356,357] and is usually not a pathogen. There are case reports of dialysis-associated peritonitis and spontaneous bacterial peritonitis.[358,359] Both organisms grow well on blood agar, but most strains do not grow on MacConkey agar. They are oxidase positive, catalase positive, indole positive, and nonpigmented. In contrast to *W. virosa*, *B. zoohelcum* produces urease. *W. virosa* (from the Latin for "slimy") forms coccoid colonies that stick tenaciously to agar surfaces.[356] Both species are susceptible to β-lactam antibiotics, including penicillin, chloramphenicol, and fluoroquinolones, and are variable in susceptibility to tetracycline and trimethoprim-sulfamethoxazole. *W. virosa* is usually resistant to one or more aminoglycosides. The combination of penicillin susceptibility and aminoglycoside resistance is a clue to the identification of this organism.

CENTERS FOR DISEASE CONTROL AND PREVENTION GROUPS

The CDC's Special Bacteriology Reference Laboratory receives unusual isolates from state laboratories and other reference laboratories. Some of these isolates are unnamed and are grouped by growth characteristics. Each of these groups represents one or more species. Although many of the isolates are from sterile sites, clinical information is often limited, and the pathogenic role of these organisms is uncertain. Some of the recently described CDC groups of gram-negative rods or coccobacillary organisms include the following:

1. CDC group NO-1 (NO for nonoxidizer) consists of at least 22 strains of fastidious gram-negative bacilli isolated from human wounds, most of which were related to dog or cat bites.[31,360,361] These organisms are similar to asaccharolytic strains of *Acinetobacter* but have a negative *Acinetobacter* transformation assay, have different cellular fatty acid profiles, and, unlike most *Acinetobacter* organisms, reduce nitrate. They are susceptible to many antimicrobial agents, including β-lactams, aminoglycosides, fluoroquinolones, and tetracycline.
2. CDC Group WO-1 (WO for weak oxidizer) includes 96 oxidase-positive, motile gram-negative rods, most of which were isolated from clinical specimens.[362] One third of the clinical isolates were from blood, and 10% were from cerebrospinal fluid.[362] Signs of sepsis were present in some of the patients, but the clinical significance of this group of organisms remains unclear.
3. CDC Group WO-2 isolates now reside in the genus *Pandoraea*, which has five been named and at least three unnamed species. These organisms can colonize the airways of patients with cystic fibrosis and rarely can cause clinical disease, including bacteremia.[363-365] *Pandoraea* species are often resistant to ampicillin, extended-spectrum cephalosporins, and aminoglycosides and are variably susceptible to fluoroquinolones.[364]
4. CDC groups O-1, O-2, and O-3 are phenotypically similar; they are oxidase-positive, curved gram-negative rods that do not grow on MacConkey agar but grow on *Campylobacter*-selective media. One case of group O-1 pneumonia complicated by bronchopulmonary fistula and bacteremia has been reported.[366] One group O-3 isolate that was submitted to the CDC had been identified as a *Campylobacter* species, indicating the potential for misidentification of the O-3 group.[367] The CDC collection of group O-3 includes isolates from a variety of clinical sources, including blood, lymph nodes, joint fluid, bone, and lung. They were resistant to most β-lactam antibiotics, except imipenem; all were susceptible to aminoglycosides and trimethoprim-sulfamethoxazole but not ciprofloxacin.
5. Fifteen strains of an oxidase-positive gram-negative rod biochemically resembling *Neisseria weaveri* (CDC group M5) are currently designated *Gilardi* rod group 1 by the CDC.[368] Most of the strains were isolated from human wounds of the extremities or blood cultures.

GARDNERELLA AND *MOBILUNCUS* SPECIES

Gardnerella vaginalis is difficult to characterize in terms of its microbiologic designation and its clinical relevance. By 16S rRNA sequence analysis, it is sufficiently distinct to merit its own genus but is somewhat closely related to *Bifidobacterium* species, which are anaerobic gram-positive rods.[369] It is a facultatively anaerobic, oxidase- and catalase-negative, nonsporing, nonencapsulated, nonmotile, pleomorphic, gram-variable rod. (See the excellent review by Catlin.[370]) *G. vaginalis* has a thin cell wall, which does not retain the crystal violet-iodine complex on decolorization, accounting for the gram-variable or gram-negative appearance of the organism. However, the preponderance of evidence suggests that *G. vaginalis* has a gram-positive heritage.

The natural habitat for *G. vaginalis* is the human vagina, where it has been found in 15% to 69% of women without signs or symptoms of vaginal infection[371] and 13.5% of girls. *G. vaginalis* is almost universally present in the vagina of women with bacterial vaginosis (BV), where it is found with a mixed anaerobic flora (see Chapter 107).[372] A cytolysin has been isolated from *G. vaginalis* that may be involved in the pathogenesis of BV.[373]

The role of organisms other that *G. vaginalis* in the pathogenesis of BV remains unclear. Molecular analyses of the vaginal flora of women with BV have discovered novel species of unculturable bacteria; some of these bacterial species are highly specific for BV.[374]

Extravaginal infections caused by *G. vaginalis* are uncommon. Bacteremia is seen almost exclusively in women and is usually associated with postpartum endometritis, postpartum fever, chorioamnionitis, septic abortion, or infection after cesarean section.[375] It is a relatively infrequent (<0.5%) urinary tract isolate, and its clinical significance can be difficult to ascertain. However, it has been recovered from suprapubic bladder aspirates from pregnant women.[376] *G. vaginalis* has also been recovered from the male urogenital tract and has occasionally been associated with disease, including bacteremia and urosepsis in a previously healthy man with renal calculi.[370,376a]

Oral metronidazole, intravaginal metronidazole gel, or intravaginal clindamycin cream is the recommended treatment for BV.[377] The utility of these agents may reflect the importance of the mixed anaerobic flora in BV. Treatment of the sexual partner does not influence a woman's response to therapy or relapse rate, and the routine treatment of sexual partners is not recommended.[377] β-Lactams have been used to treat extravaginal infections caused by *G. vaginalis.* Screening and treatment of BV in pregnant women at high risk for preterm labor and before surgical abortion or hysterectomy has been recommended.[377]

Mobiluncus species are slowly growing, curved, gram-variable, motile, anaerobic bacteria predominantly found in the human vagina in association with BV. *Mobiluncus* has been isolated from the vagina of as many as 97% of women with BV[378] but in a minority of healthy controls.[379] The role of *Mobiluncus* in the pathogenesis of BV is unclear. *Mobiluncus* species, more commonly *Mobiluncus curtisii,* are associated with upper genitourinary tract infections and adverse pregnancy outcome. Extragenitourinary tract infections have included nonpuerperal breast abscesses as well as umbilical and mastectomy wounds.[380] There are five reported cases of *Mobiluncus* bacteremia, including one previously healthy woman who developed septic shock with coagulopathy, adult respiratory distress syndrome, and renal failure.[381] The only man reported to have *Mobiluncus* bacteremia had underlying ulcerative colitis.[382]*Mobiluncus* species are usually susceptible to penicillins, ampicillin, cefoxitin, clindamycin, erythromycin, imipenem, and vancomycin.[383] They can be resistant to metronidazole; the efficacy of metronidazole in the treatment of BV despite the presence of antibiotic-resistant *Mobiluncus* underscores the uncertainty of the role of this organism in the pathogenesis of the disease.

REFERENCES

1. von Graevenitz A, Zbinden R, Zmutters R. *Actinobacillus, Capnocytophaga, Eikenella, Kingella, Pasteurella,* and other fastidious or rarely encountered Gram-negative rods. In: Murray PR, Baron EJ, Jorgensen JH, et al, eds. *Manual of Clinical Microbiology.* 9th ed. Washington, DC: American Society for Microbiology Press; 2007:621-635.
2. Winn WC, Koneman EW, Allen SD, et al. *Koneman's Color Atlas and Textbook of Diagnostic Microbiology.* 6th ed. Philadelphia: JB Lippincott; 2006.
3. Nørskiv-Lauritsen N, Kilian M. Reclassification of *Actinobacillus actinomycetemcomitans, Haemophilus aphrophilus, Haemophilus paraphrophilus* and *Haemophilus segnis* as *Aggregatibacter actinomycetemcomitans* gen. nov., comb. nov., *Aggregatibacter aphrophilus* comb. nov. and *Aggregatibacter segnis* comb. nov., and emended description of *Aggregatibacter aphrophilus* to include V factor-dependent and V factor-independent isolates. *Int J Syst Evol Microbiol.* 2006;56:2135-2146.
4. Kaplan AH, Weber DJ, Oddone EZ, et al. Infection due to *Actinobacillus actinomycetemcomitans:* 15 cases and review. *Rev Infect Dis.* 1989;11:46-63.
5. Holm P. Studies on the aetiology of human actinomycosis. II. Do the "other microbes" of actinomycosis possess virulence? *Acta Pathol Microbiol Scand.* 1951;28:391-406.
6. Page MI, King EO. Infection due to *Actinobacillus actinomycetemcomitans* and *Haemophilus aphrophilus. N Engl J Med.* 1966;275:181-188.
7. Horowitz EA, Pugsley MP, Turbes PG, et al. Pericarditis caused by *Actinobacillus actinomycetemcomitans. J Infect Dis.* 1987; 155:152-153.
8. Ellner JJ, Rosenthal MS, Lerner PI, et al. Infective endocarditis caused by slow-growing, fastidious, gram-negative bacteria. *Medicine.* 1979;58:145-158.
9. Yuan A, Yang PC, Lee LN, et al. *Actinobacillus actinomycetemcomitans* pneumonia with chest wall involvement and rib destruction. *Chest.* 1992;101:1450-1452.
10. Binder MI, Chua J, Kaiser PK, et al. *Actinobacillus actinomycetemcomitans* endogenous endophthalmitis: report of two cases and review of the literature. *Scand J Infect Dis.* 2003; 35:133-136.
11. Asikainen S, Chen C, Alaluusua S, et al. Can one acquire periodontal bacteria and periodontitis from a family member? *J Am Dent Assoc.* 1997;128:1263-1271.
12. Aass AM, Preus HR, Gjermo P. Association between detection of oral *Actinobacillus actinomycetemcomitans* and radiographic bone loss in teenagers. *J Periodontol.* 1992:63:682-685.
13. Henderson B, Wilson M, Sharp L, et al. Actinobacillus actinomycetemcomitans. *J Med Microbiol.* 2002;51:1013-1020.
14. Asikainen S, Chen C, Slots J. Likelihood of transmitting *Actinobacillus actinomycetemcomitans* and *Porphyromonas gingivalis* in families with periodontitis. *Oral Microbiol Immunol.* 1996; 11:387-394.
15. Meyer DH, Fives-Taylor PM. The role of *Actinobacillus actinomycetemcomitans* in the pathogenesis of periodontal disease. *Trends Microbiol.* 1997;5:224-228.
16. Brouqui P, Raoult D. Endocarditis due to rare and fastidious bacteria. *Clin Microbiol Rev.* 2001;14:177-207.
17. Grace CJ, Levitz RE, Katz Pollak H, et al. *Actinobacillus actinomycetemcomitans* prosthetic valve endocarditis. *Rev Infect Dis.* 1988;10:922-929.
18. Wilson ME. Prosthetic valve endocarditis and paravalvular abscess caused by *Actinobacillus actinomycetemcomitans. Rev Infect Dis.* 1989;11:665-667.
19. Yogev R, Shulman D, Shulman ST, et al. In vitro activity of antibiotics alone and in combination against *Actinobacillus actinomycetemcomitans. Antimicrob Agents Chemother.* 1986;29: 179-181.
20. Muller HP, Holderrieth S, Burkhardt U, et al. In vitro antimicrobial susceptibility of oral strains of *Actinobacillus actinomycetemcomitans* to seven antibiotics. *J Clin Periodontol.* 2002; 29:736-742.
21. Pavicic MJ, van Winkelhoff AJ, de Graaff J. In vitro susceptibilities of *Actinobacillus actinomycetemcomitans* to a number of antimicrobial combinations. *Antimicrob Agents Chemother.* 1992;36:2634-2638.
22. Wilson WR, Karchmer AW, Dajani AS, et al. Antibiotic treatment of adults with infective endocarditis due to streptococci, enterococci, staphylococci, and HACEK microorganisms. *JAMA.* 1995;274:1706-1713.
23. Babinchak TJ. Oral ciprofloxacin therapy for prosthetic valve endocarditis due to *Actinobacillus actinomycetemcomitans. Clin Infect Dis.* 1995;21:1517-1518.
24. Van Winkelhoff AJ, Tijhof CJ, de Graaff J. Microbiological and clinical results of metronidazole plus amoxicillin therapy in *Actinobacillus actinomycetemcomitans*-associated periodontitis. *J Periodontol.* 1992;63:52-57.
25. Peel MM, Hornidge KA, Luppino M, et al. *Actinobacillus* spp and related bacteria in infected wounds of humans bitten by horses and sheep. *J Clin Microbiol.* 1991;29:2535-2538.
26. Arana-Domondon LC, Chen SH, Mann L, et al. Boar hunter's endocarditis. *JAMA.* 1998;279:198.
27. Friis-Moller A, Christensen JJ, Fussing V, et al. Clinical significance and taxonomy of *Actinobacillus hominis. J Clin Microbiol.* 2001;39:930-935.
28. Wust J, Gubler J, Mannheim W, et al. *Actinobacillus hominis* as a causative agent of septicemia in hepatic failure. *Eur J Clin Microbiol Infect Dis.* 1991;10:693-694.
29. Kingsland RC, Guss DA. *Actinobacillus ureae* meningitis: Case report and review of the literature. *J Emerg Med.* 1995; 13:623-627.
30. de Castro N, Pavie J, Lagrange-Xelot M, et al. Severe *Actinobacillus ureae* meningitis in an immunocompromised patient: report of one case and review of the literature. *Scand J Infect Dis.* 2007;39:1076-1079.
31. Weyant RS, Moss CW, Weaver RE, et al. *Identification of Unusual Pathogenic Gram-Negative Aerobic and Facultatively Anaerobic Bacteria.* 2nd ed. Baltimore: Williams & Wilkins; 1996.
32. Colwell RR, MacDonell MT, De Ley J. Proposal to recognize the family *Aeromonadaceae* fam nov. *Int J Syst Bacteriol.* 1986;36:473-477.
33. Abbott SL, Cheung WKW, Janda JM. The genus *Aeromonas:* Biochemical characteristics, atypical reactions, and phenotypic identification schemes. *J Clin Microbiol.* 2003;41:2348-2357.
34. Janda JM, Abbott SL. Evolving concepts regarding the genus *Aeromonas:* An expanding panorama of species, disease presentations and unanswered questions. *Clin Infect Dis.* 1998; 27:332-344.
35. Saavedra MJ, Figueras MJ, Martinez-Murcia AJ. Updated phylogeny of the genus *Aeromonas. Int J Syst Evol Microbiol.* 2006;56:2481-2487
36. Challapalli M, Tess BR, Cunningham DG, et al. *Aeromonas*-associated diarrhea in children. *Pediatr Infect Dis J.* 1988;7:693-698.
37. Gluskin I, Batash D, Shoseyov D, et al. A 15-year study of the role of *Aeromonas* spp in gastroenteritis in hospitalised children. *J Med Microbiol.* 1992;37:315-318.
38. Rautelin H, Sivonen A, Kuikka A, et al. Role of *Aeromonas* isolated from feces of Finnish patients. *Scand J Infect Dis.* 1995;27:207-210.
39. King GE, Werner SB, Kizer KW. Epidemiology of *Aeromonas* infections in California. *Clin Infect Dis.* 1992;15: 449-452.
40. Namdari H, Bottone EJ. Microbiologic and clinical evidence supporting the role of *Aeromonas caviae* as a pediatric enteric pathogen. *J Clin Microbiol.* 1990;28:837-840.
41. Jiang ZD, Nelson AC, Mathewson JJ, et al. Intestinal secretory immune response to infection with *Aeromonas* species and *Plesiomonas shigelloides* among students from the United States in Mexico. *J Infect Dis.* 1991;164:979-982.
42. Hanninen ML, Salmi S, Mattila L, et al. Association of *Aeromonas* spp with travellers' diarrhoea in Finland. *J Med Microbiol.* 1995;42:26-31.
43. Holmberg SD, Schell WL, Fanning GR, et al. *Aeromonas* intestinal infections in the United States. *Ann Intern Med.* 1986;105:683-689.
44. Borchardt MA, Semper ME, Standridge JH. *Aeromonas* isolates from human diarrheic stool and groundwater compared by pulsed-field gel electrophoresis. *Emerg Infect Dis.* 2003; 9:224-228.
45. Jones BL, Wilcox MH. *Aeromonas* infections and their treatment. *J Antimicrob Chemother.* 1995;35:453-461.
46. Vila J, Ruiz J, Gallardo F, et al. *Aeromonas* spp. and traveler's diarrhea: Clinical features and antimicrobial resistance. *Emerg Infect Dis.* 2003;9:552-555.
47. De la Morena ML, Van R, Singh K, et al. Diarrhea associated with *Aeromonas* species in children in day care centers. *J Infect Dis.* 1993;168:215-218.
48. Willoughby JM, Rahman AF, Gregory MM. Chronic colitis after *Aeromonas* infection. *Gut.* 1989;30:686-690.
49. Figueras MJ, Aldea MJ, Fernandez N, et al. *Aeromonas* hemolytic uremic syndrome. A case and a review of the literature. *Diagn Microbiol Infect Dis.* 58:231-234, 2007.
50. Gold WL, Salit IE. *Aeromonas hydrophila* infections of skin and soft tissue: Report of 11 cases and review. *Clin Infect Dis.* 1993;16:69-74.
51. Kienzle N, Muller M, Pegg S. *Aeromonas* wound infection in burns. *Burns.* 2000;26:478-482.
52. Vally H, Whittle A, Cameron S, et al. Outbreak of *Aeromonas hydrophila* wound infections associated with mud football. *Clin Infect Dis.* 2004;38:1084-1089.
53. Lineaweaver WC, Hill MK, Buncke GM, et al. *Aeromonas hydrophilia* infections following use of medicinal leeches in replantation and flap surgery. *Ann Plast Surg.* 1992;29: 238-244.
54. Mackay DR, Manders EK, Saggers GC, et al. *Aeromonas* species isolated from medicinal leeches. *Ann Plast Surg.* 1999; 42:275-279.
55. Sartor C, Limouzin-Perotti F, Legre R, et al. Nosocomial infections with *Aeromonas hydrophila* from leeches. *Clin Infect Dis.* 2002;35:E1-E5.
56. Ko WC, Lee HC, Chuang YC, et al. Clinical features and therapeutic implications of 104 episodes of monomicrobial *Aeromonas bacteraemia. J Infect.* 2000;40:267-273.
57. Ko WC, Chuang YC. *Aeromonas bacteremia:* Review of 59 episodes. *Clin Infect Dis.* 1995;20:1298-1304.

58. Janda JM, Guthertz LS, Kokka RP, et al. *Aeromonas* species in septicemia: Laboratory characteristics and clinical observations. *Clin Infect Dis.* 1994;19:77-83.
59. Dryden M, Munro R. *Aeromonas* septicemia: Relationship of species and clinical features. *Pathology.* 1989;21:111-114.
60. Cookson BD, Houang ET, Lee JV. The use of a biotyping system to investigate an unusual clustering of bacteraemias caused by *Aeromonas* species. *J Hosp Infect.* 1984;5:205-209.
61. Hickman-Brenner FW, Fanning GR, Arduino MJ, et al. *Aeromonas schubertii*, a new mannitol-negative species found in human clinical specimens. *J Clin Microbiol.* 1988;26:1561-1564.
62. Carnahan A, Fanning GR, Joseph SW. *Aeromonas jandaei* (formerly genospecies DNA group 9 *A. sobria*), a new sucrose-negative species isolated from clinical specimens. *J Clin Microbiol.* 1991;29:560-564.
63. DeFronzo RA, Murray GF, Maddrey WC. *Aeromonas* septicemia from hepatobiliary disease. *Am J Dig Dis.* 1973;18:323-331.
64. Parras F, Diaz MD, Reina J, et al. Meningitis due to *Aeromonas* species: Case report and review. *Clin Infect Dis.* 1993; 17:1058-1060.
65. Ong KR, Sordillo E, Frankel E. Unusual case of *Aeromonas hydrophila* endocarditis. *J Clin Microbiol.* 1991;29:1056-1057.
66. Ender PT, Dolan MJ, Dolan D, et al. Near-drowning-associated *Aeromonas* pneumonia. *J Emerg Med.* 1996;14:737-741.
67. Blair JE, Woo-Ming MA, McGuire PK. *Aeromonas hydrophila* bacteremia acquired from an infected swimming pool. *Clin Infect Dis.* 1999;28:1336-1337.
68. Janda JM, Abbott SL, Carnahan AM. *Aeromonas* and *Plesiomonas*. In: Murray PR, Baron EJ, Pfaller MA, et al, eds. *Manual of Clinical Microbiology*. Washington, DC: American Society for Microbiology Press; 1995:477-482.
69. Vila J, Marco F, Soler L, et al. In vitro antimicrobial susceptibility of clinical isolates of *Aeromonas caviae, Aeromonas hydrophila* and *Aeromonas veronii* biotype sobria. *J Antimicrob Chemother.* 2002;49:701-702.
70. Walsh TR, Stunt RA, Nabi JA, et al. Distribution and expression of beta-lactamase genes among *Aeromonas* spp. *J Antimicrob Chemother.* 1997;40:171-178.
71. Walsh TR, Payne DJ, MacGowan AP, et al. A clinical isolate of *Aeromonas sobria* with three chromosomally mediated inducible beta-lactamases: A cephalosporinase, a penicillinase and a third enzyme, displaying carbapenemase activity. *J Antimicrob Chemother.* 1995;35:271-279.
72. Overman TL, Janda JM. Antimicrobial susceptibility patterns of *Aeromonas jandaei, A. schubertii, A. trota,* and *A. veronii* biotype *veronii*. *J Clin Microbiol.* 1999;37:706-708.
73. Rossolini GM, Walsh T, Amicosante G. The *Aeromonas* metallo-beta-lactamases: Genetics, enzymology, and contribution to drug resistance. *Microb Drug Resist.* 1996;2:245-252.
74. Ko WC, Yu KW, Liu CY, et al. Increasing antibiotic resistance in clinical isolates of *Aeromonas* strains in Taiwan. *Antimicrob Agents Chemother.* 1996;40:1260-1262.
75. Liu CY, Huang YT, Liao CH, et al. In vitro activities of tigecycline against clinical isolates of *Aeromonas, Vibrio,* and *Salmonella* species in Taiwan. *Antimicrob Agents Chemother.* 2008;52:2677-2679.
76. Chang BJ, Bolton SM. Plasmids and resistance to antimicrobial agents in *Aeromonas sobria* and *Aeromonas hydrophila* clinical isolates. *Antimicrob Agents Chemother.* 1987;31:1281-1282.
77. Han XY, Meltzer MC, Woods JT, et al. Endocarditis with ruptured cerebral aneurysm caused by *Cardiobacterium valvarum* sp. nov. *J Clin Microbiol.* 2004;42:1590-1595.
78. Wormser GP, Bottone EJ. *Cardiobacterium hominis:* Review of microbiologic and clinical features. *Rev Infect Dis.* 1983;5: 680-691.
79 Han XY, Falsen E. Characterization of oral strains of *Cardiobacterium valvarum* and emended description of the organism. *J Clin Microbiol.* 2005;43:2370-2374.
80. Taveras JM 3rd, Campo R, Segal N, et al. Apparent culture-negative endocarditis of the prosthetic valve caused by *Cardiobacterium hominis*. *South Med J.* 1993;86:1439-1440.
81. Apisarnthanarak A, Johnson RM, Braverman AC, et al. *Cardiobacterium hominis* bioprosthetic mitral valve endocarditis presenting as septic arthritis. *Diagn Microbiol Infect Dis.* 2002; 42:79-81.
82. Pritchard TM, Foust RT, Cantely JR, et al. Prosthetic valve endocarditis due to *Cardiobacterium hominis* occurring after upper gastrointestinal endoscopy. *Am J Med.* 1991;90:516-518.
83. Robison WJ, Vitelli AS. Infectious endocarditis caused by *Cardiobacterium hominis*. *South Med J.* 1985;78:1020-1021.
84. Francioli PB, Roussianos D, Glauser MP. *Cardiobacterium hominis* endocarditis manifesting as bacterial meningitis. *Arch Intern Med.* 1983;143:1483-1484.
85. Rechtman DJ, Nadler JP. Abdominal abscess due to *Cardiobacterium hominis* and *Clostridium bifermentans*. *Rev Infect Dis.* 1991;13:418-419.
86. Nurnberger M, Treadwell T, Lin B, et al. Pacemaker lead infection and vertebral osteomyelitis presumed due to *Cardiobacterium hominis*. *Clin Infect Dis.* 1998;27:890-891.
87. Paster BJ, Falkler, WA, Enwonwu, CO, et al. Prevalent bacterial species and novel phenotypes in advanced noma lesions. *J Clin Microbiol.* 2002;40:2187-2191.
88. Kugler KC, Biedenbach DJ, Jones RN. Determination of the antimicrobial activity of 29 clinically important compounds tested against fastidious HACEK group organisms. *Diagn Microbiol Infect Dis.* 1999;34:73-76.
89. Le Quellec A, Bessis D, Perez C, et al. Endocarditis due to beta-lactamase-producing *Cardiobacterium hominis*. *Clin Infect Dis.* 1994;19:994-995.
90. Ponte R, Jenkins SG. Fatal *Chromobacterium violaceum* infections associated with exposure to stagnant waters. *Pediatr Infect Dis J.* 1992;11:583-586.
91. Huffam SE, Nowotny MJ, Currie BJ. *Chromobacterium violaceum* in tropical northern Australia. *Med J Aust.* 1998; 168:335-337.
92. de Siqueira IC, Dias J, Ruf H, et al. *Chromobacterium violaceum* in siblings, Brazil. *Emerg Infect Dis.* 2005;11:1443-1445.
93. Berkowitz FE, Metchock B. Third generation cephalosporin-resistant gram-negative bacilli in the feces of hospitalized children. *Pediatr Infect Dis J.* 1995;14:97-100.
94. Ti TY, Tan WC, Chong AP, et al. Nonfatal and fatal infections caused by *Chromobacterium violaceum*. *Clin Infect Dis.* 1993;17:505-507.
95. Moore CC, Lane JE, Stephens JL. Successful treatment of an infant with *Chromobacterium violaceum* sepsis. *Clin Infect Dis.* 2001;32:E107-E110.
96. Dromigny JA, Fall AL, Diouf S, et al. *Chromobacterium violaceum:* A case of diarrhea in Senegal. *Pediatr Infect Dis J.* 2002;21:573-574.
97. Bosch FJ, Badenhorst L, Le Roux JA, et al. Successful treatment of *Chromobacterium violaceum* sepsis in South Africa. *J Med Microbiol.* 2008;57:1293-1295.
98. Macher AM, Casale TB, Fauci AS. Chronic granulomatous disease of childhood and *Chromobacterium violaceum* infections in the Southeastern United States. *Ann Intern Med.* 1982;97:51-55.
99. Mamlok RJ, Mamlok V, Mills GC, et al. Glucose-6-phosphate dehydrogenase deficiency, neutrophil dysfunction and *Chromobacterium violaceum* sepsis. *J Pediatr.* 1987;111:852-854.
100. Miller DP, Blevins WT, Steele DB, et al. A comparative study of virulent and avirulent strains of *Chromobacterium violaceum*. *Can J Microbiol.* 1988;34:249-255.
101. Lee J, Kim JS, Nahm CH, et al. Two cases of *Chromobacterium violaceum* infection after injury in a subtropical region. *J Clin Microbiol.* 1999;37:2068-2070
102. Melo PS, Justo GZ, de Azevedo MB, et al. Violacein and its beta-cyclodextrin complexes induce apoptosis and differentiation in HL60 cells. *Toxicology.* 2003;186:217-225.
103. Aldridge KE, Valainis GT, Sanders CV. Comparison of the in vitro activity of ciprofloxacin and 24 other antimicrobial agents against clinical strains of *Chromobacterium violaceum*. *Diagn Microbiol Infect Dis.* 1988;10:31-39.
104. Duma RJ. Aztreonam, the first monobactam. *Ann Intern Med.* 1987;106:766-767.
105. Wagner DK, Wright JJ, Ansher AF, et al. Dysgonic fermenter 3-associated gastrointestinal disease in a patient with common variable hypogammaglobulinemia. *Am J Med.* 1988;84: 315-318.
106. Hofstad T, Olsen I, Eribe ER, et al. *Dysgonomonas* gen. nov. to accommodate *Dysgonomonas* gadei sp. nov., an organism isolated from a human gall bladder, and *Dysgonomonas capnocytophagoides* (formerly CDC group DF-3). *Int J Syst Evol Microbiol.* 2000;50:2189-2195.
107. Vandamme P, Vancanneyt M, van Belkum A, et al. Polyphasic analysis of strains of the genus *Capnocytophaga* and Centers for Disease Control group DF-3. *Int J Syst Bacteriol.* 1996; 46:782-791.
108. Gill VJ, Travis LB, Williams DY. Clinical and microbiological observations on CDC group DF-3, a gram-negative coccobacillus. *J Clin Microbiol.* 1991;29:1589-1592.
109. Heiner AM, DiSario JA, Carroll K, et al. Dysgonic fermenter-3: A bacterium associated with diarrhea in immunocompromised hosts. *Am J Gastroenterol.* 1992;87:1629-1630.
110. Blum RN, Berry CD, Phillips MG, et al. Clinical illnesses associated with isolation of dysgonic fermenter 3 from stool samples. *J Clin Microbiol.* 1992;30:396-400.
111. Hironaga M, Yamane K, Inaba M, et al. Characterization and antimicrobial susceptibility of *Dysgonomonas capnocytophagoides* isolated from human blood sample. *Jpn J Infect Dis.* 2008;61:212-213
112. Bangsborg JM, Frederiksen W, Bruun B. Dysgonic fermenter 3-associated abscess in a diabetic patient. *J Infect.* 1990; 20:237-240.
113. Aronson NE, Zbick CJ. Dysgonic fermenter 3 bacteremia in a neutropenic patient with acute lymphocytic leukemia. *J Clin Microbiol.* 1988;26:2213-2215.
114. Grob R, Zbinden R, Ruef C, et al. Septicemia caused by dysgonic fermenter 3 in a severely immunocompromised patient and isolation of the same microorganism from a stool specimen. *J Clin Microbiol.* 1999;37:1617-1618.
115. Matsumoto T, Kawakami Y, Oana K, et al. First isolation of *Dysgonomonas mossii* from intestinal juice of a patient with pancreatic cancer. *Arch Med Res.* 2006;37:914-916.
116. Hironaga M, Yamane K, Inaba M, et al. Characterization and antimicrobial susceptibility of *Dysgonomonas capnocytophagoides* isolated from human blood sample. *Jpn J Infect Dis.* 2008;61:212-213.
117. Vartian CV, Septimus EJ. Endophthalmitis due to *Pasteurella multocida* and CDC EF-4. *J Infect Dis.* 1989;160:733.
118. Dul MJ, Shlaes DM, Lerner PI. EF-4 bacteremia in a patient with hepatic carcinoid. *J Clin Microbiol.* 1983;18:1260-1261.
119. Roebuck JD, Morris JT. Chronic otitis media due to EF-4 bacteria. *Clin Infect Dis.* 1999;29:1343-1344.
120. Holmes B, Costas M, Wood AC. Numerical analysis of electrophoretic protein patterns of group EF-4 bacteria, predominantly from dog-bite wounds of humans. *J Appl Bacteriol.* 1990; 68:81-91.
121. Goldstein EJ, Citron DM. Comparative activities of cefuroxime, amoxicillin-clavulanic acid, ciprofloxacin, enoxacin, and ofloxacin against aerobic and anaerobic bacteria isolated from bite wounds. *Antimicrob Agents Chemother.* 1988;32:1143-1148.
122. Holmberg SD, Wachsmuth K, Hickman-Brenner FW, et al. *Plesiomonas* enteric infections in the United States. *Ann Intern Med.* 1986;105:690-694.
123. Brenden RA, Miller MA, Janda JM. Clinical disease spectrum and pathogenic factors associated with *Plesiomonas shigelloides* infections in humans. *Rev Infect Dis.* 1988;10:303-316.
124. MacDonnell MT, Colwell RR. Phylogeny of the *Vibrionaceae*, and recommendation for two new genera, *Listonella* and *Shewanella*. *Syst Appl Microbiol.* 1985;6:171-182.
125. Rautelin H, Sivonen A, Kuikka A, et al. Enteric *Plesiomonas shigelloides* infections in Finnish patients. *Scand J Infect Dis.* 1995;27:495-498.
126. Kain KC, Kelly MT. Clinical features, epidemiology, and treatment of *Plesiomonas shigelloides* diarrhea. *J Clin Microbiol.* 1989;27:998-1001.
127. Olsvik O, Wachsmuth K, Kay B, et al. Laboratory observations on *Plesiomonas shigelloides* strains isolated from children with diarrhea in Peru. *J Clin Microbiol.* 1990;28:886-889.
128. Janda JM, Abbott SL. Expression of hemolytic activity by *Plesiomonas shigelloides*. *J Clin Microbiol.* 1993;31:1206-1208.
129. Visitsunthorn N, Komolpis P. Antimicrobial therapy in *Plesiomonas shigelloides*-associated diarrhea in Thai children. *Southeast Asian J Trop Med Publ Hlth.* 1995;26:86-90.
130. Alcaniz JP, de Cuenca Moron B, Gomez Rubio M, et al. Spontaneous bacterial peritonitis due to *Plesiomonas shigelloides*. *Am J Gastroenterol.* 1995;90:1529-1530.
131. Roth T, Hentsch C, Erard P, et al. Pyosalpinx: Not always a sexual transmitted disease? Pyosalpinx caused by *Plesiomonas shigelloides* in an immunocompetent host. *Clin Microbiol Infect.* 2002;8:803-805.
132. Fujita K, Shirai M, Ishioka T, et al. Neonatal *Plesiomonas shigelloides* septicemia and meningitis: A case and review. *Acta Paediatr Jpn.* 1994;36:450-452.
133. Woo PC, Lau SK, Yuen KY. Biliary tract disease as a risk factor for *Plesiomonas shigelloides* bacteraemia: a nine-year experience in a Hong Kong hospital and review of the literature. *New Microbiol.* 2005;28:45-55.
134. Paul R, Siitonen A, Karkkainen P. *Plesiomonas shigelloides* bacteremia in a healthy girl with mild gastroenteritis. *J Clin Microbiol.* 1990;28:1445-1446.
135. Rahim Z, Kay BA. Enrichment for *Plesiomonas shigelloides* from stools. *J Clin Microbiol.* 1988;26:789-790.
136. Kain KC, Kelly MT. Antimicrobial susceptibility of *Plesiomonas shigelloides* from patients with diarrhea. *Antimicrob Agents Chemother.* 1989;33:1609-1610.
137. Stock I, Wiedemann B. Natural antimicrobial susceptibilities of *Plesiomonas shigelloides* strains. *J Antimicrob Chemother.* 2001;48:803-811.
138. Bruckner DA, Colonna P. Nomenclature for aerobic and facultative bacteria. *Clin Infect Dis.* 1993;16:598-605.
139. Yabuuchi E, Kawamura Y, Kosako Y, et al. Emendation of genus *Achromobacter* and *Achromobacter xylosoxidans* (Yabuuchi and Yano) and proposal of *Achromobacter ruhlandii* (Packer and Vishniac) comb. nov., *Achromobacter piechaudii* (Kiredjian et al.) comb. nov., and *Achromobacter xylosoxidans* subsp. *denitrificans* (Ruger and Tan) comb. nov. *Microbiol Immunol.* 1998;42:429-438.
140. Schreckenberg PC, Daneshvar MI, Weyant RS, et al. *Acinetobacter, Achromobacter, Chryseobacterium, Moraxella,* and other nonfermentative gram-negative rods. In: Murray PR, Baron EJ, Jorgensen JH, et al, eds. *Manual of Clinical Microbiology*. 8th ed. Washington, DC: American Society for Microbiology Press; 2003:749-779.
141. Holmes B, Moss CW, Daneshvar MI. Cellular fatty acid compositions of "*Achromobacter* groups B and E." *J Clin Microbiol.* 1993;31:1007-1008.
142. Jenks PJ, Shaw EJ. Recurrent septicaemia due to "*Achromobacter* group B." *J Infect.* 1997;34:143-145.
143. Holmes B, Lewis R, Trevett A. Septicaemia due to *Achromobacter* group B: A report of two cases. *Med Microbiol Lett.* 1992;1:177-184.
144. McKinley KP, Laundy TJ, Masterton RG. *Achromobacter* group B replacement valve endocarditis. *J Infect.* 1990;20:262-263.
145. Mandell WF, Garvey GJ, Neu HC. *Achromobacter xylosoxidans* bacteremia. *Rev Infect Dis.* 1987;9:1001-1005.
146. Cieslak TJ, Robb ML, Drabick CJ, et al. Catheter-associated sepsis caused by *Ochrobactrum anthropi:* Report of a case and review of related nonfermentative bacteria. *Clin Infect Dis.* 1992;14:902-907.
147. Cieslak TJ, Raszka WV. Catheter-associated sepsis due to *Alcaligenes xylosoxidans* in a child with AIDS. *Clin Infect Dis.* 1993;16:592-593.
148. Schoch PE, Cunha BA. Nosocomial *Achromobacter xylosoxidans* infections. *Infect Contr Hosp Epidemiol.* 1988;9:84-87.
149. Spear JB, Fuhrer J, Kirby BD. *Achromobacter xylosoxidans* (*Alcaligenes xylosoxidans* subsp *xylosoxidans*) bacteremia associated with a well-water source: Case report and review of the literature. *J Clin Microbiol.* 1988;26:598-599.

150. Duggan JM, Goldstein SJ, Chenoweth CE, et al. *Achromobacter xylosoxidans* bacteremia: Report of four cases and review of the literature. *Clin Infect Dis.* 1996;23:569-576.
151. Gomez-Cerezo J, Suarez I, Rios JJ, et al. *Achromobacter xylosoxidans* bacteremia: A 10-year analysis of 54 cases. *Eur J Clin Microbiol Infect Dis.* 2003;22:360-363.
152. Aisenberg G, Rolston KV, Safdar A. Bacteremia caused by *Achromobacter* and *Alcaligenes* species in 46 patients with cancer (1989-2003). *Cancer.* 2004;101:2134-2140.
153. Walsh RD, Klein NC, Cunha BA. *Achromobacter xylosoxidans* osteomyelitis. *Clin Infect Dis.* 1993;16:176-178.
154. Taylor P, Fischbein L. Prosthetic knee infection due to *Achromobacter xylosoxidans*. *J Rheumatol.* 1992;19:992-993.
155. Tang S, Cheng CC, Tse KC, et al. CAPD-associated peritonitis caused by *Alcaligenes xylosoxidans* sp. *xylosoxidans*. *Am J Nephrol.* 2001;21:502-506.
156. Castellote J, Tremosa G, Ben SL, Vazguez S. Spontaneous bacterial peritonitis due to *Alcaligenes xylosoxidans*. *Am J Gastroenterol.* 2001;96:1650-1651.
157. Legrand C, Anaissie E. Bacteremia due to *Achromobacter xylosoxidans* in patients with cancer. *Clin Infect Dis.* 1992;14:479-484.
158. Manfredi R, Nanetti A, Ferri M, et al. Bacteremia and respiratory involvement by *Alcaligenes xylosoxidans* in patients infected with the human immunodeficiency virus. *Eur J Clin Microbiol Infect Dis.* 1997;16:933-938.
159. Tan K, Conway SP, Brownlee KG, et al. *Alcaligenes* infection in cystic fibrosis. *Pediatr Pulmonol.* 2002;34:101-104.
160. Magni A, Giordano A, Mancini C, et al. Emerging cystic fibrosis pathogens: incidence and antimicrobial resistance. *New Microbiol.* 2007;30:59-62.
161. Dunne WM Jr, Maisch S. Epidemiological investigation of infections due to *Alcaligenes* species in children and patients with cystic fibrosis: Use of repetitive-element-sequence polymerase chain reaction. *Clin Infect Dis.* 1995;20:836-841.
162. Ronne-Hansen C, Pressler T, Hoiby N, et al. Chronic infection with *Achromobacter xylosoxidans* in cystic fibrosis patients; a retrospective case control study. *J Cyst Fibros.* 2006;5:245-251.
163. Hearn YR, Gander RM. *Achromobacter xylosoxidans*. An unusual neonatal pathogen. *Am J Clin Pathol.* 1991;96:211-214.
164. Mensah K, Philippon A, Richard C, et al. Susceptibility of *Alcaligenes denitrificans* subspecies *xylosoxydans* to beta-lactam antibiotics. *Eur J Clin Microbiol Infect Dis.* 1990;9:405-409.
165. Cormican MG, Jones RN. Antimicrobial activity of cefotaxime tested against infrequently isolated pathogenic species (unusual pathogens). *Diagn Microbiol Infect Dis.* 1995;22:43-48.
166. Saiman L, Chen Y, Tabibi S, et al. Identification and antimicrobial susceptibility of *Alcaligenes xylosoxidans* isolated from patients with cystic fibrosis. *J Clin Microbiol.* 2001;39:3942-3945.
167. Decre D, Arlet G, Danglot C, et al. A beta-lactamase-overproducing strain of *Alcaligenes denitrificans* subsp *xylosoxidans* isolated from a case of meningitis. *J Antimicrob Chemother.* 1992;30:769-779.
168. Tayeri T, Kelly LD. *Alcaligenes faecalis* corneal ulcer in a patient with cicatricial pemphigoid. *Am J Ophthalmol.* 1993;115:255-256.
169. Bizet J, Bizet C. Strains of *Alcaligenes faecalis* from clinical material. *J Infect.* 1997:35:167-169.
170. Peel MM, Hibberd AJ, King BM, et al. *Alcaligenes piechaudii* from chronic ear discharge. *J Clin Microbiol.* 1988;26:1580-1581.
171. Kay SE, Clark RA, White KL, Peel MM. Recurrent *Achromobacter piechaudii* bacteremia in a patient with hematological malignancy. *J Clin Microbiol.* 2001;39:808-810.
172. Pickett MJ, Greenwood JR. Identification of oxidase-positive, glucose-negative motile species of nonfermentative bacilli. *J Clin Microbiol.* 1986;23:920-923.
173. Bizet C, Tekaia F, Philippon A. In-vitro susceptibility of *Alcaligenes faecalis* compared with those of other *Alcaligenes* spp to antimicrobial agents including seven beta-lactams. *J Antimicrob Chemother.* 1993;32:907-910.
174. Pereira M, Perilli M, Mantengoli E, et al. PER-1 extended-spectrum beta-lactamase production in an *Alcaligenes faecalis* clinical isolate resistant to expanded-spectrum cephalosporins and monobactams from a hospital in Northern Italy. *Microb Drug Resist.* 2000;6:85-90.
175. Hsueh PR, Teng U, Ho SW, et al. Clinical and microbiological characteristics of *Flavobacterium indologenes* infections associated with indwelling devices. *J Clin Microbiol.* 1996;34:1908-1913.
176. Bloch KC, Nadarajah R, Jacobs R. *Chryseobacterium meningosepticum:* An emerging pathogen among immunocompromised adults. Report of 6 cases and literature review. *Medicine.* 1997;76:30-41.
177. Kim KK, Kim MK, Lim JH, et al. Transfer of *Chryseobacterium meningosepticum* and *Chryseobacterium miricola* to *Elizabethkingia* gen. nov. as *Elizabethkingia meningoseptica* and *Elizabethkingia miricola* comb. nov. *Int J Syst Evol Microbiol.* 2005;55:1287-1293.
178. Hoque SN, Graham J, Kaufmann ME, et al. *Chryseobacterium (Flavobacterium)* meningosepticum outbreak associated with colonization of water taps in a neonatal intensive care unit. *J Hosp Infect.* 2001;47:188-192.
179. Pokrywka M, Viazanko K, Medvick J, et al. A *Flavobacterium meningosepticum* outbreak among intensive care patients. *Am J Infect Control.* 1993;21:139-145.
180. Brown RB, Phillips D, Barker MJ, et al. Outbreak of nosocomial *Flavobacterium meningosepticum* respiratory infections associated with use of aerosolized polymixin B. *Am J Infect Control.* 1989;17:121-125.
181. Olsen H, Frederiksen WC, Siboni KE. Flavobacterium meningosepticum. *Lancet.* 1965;1:1294-1296.
182. Sheridan RL, Ryan CM, Pasternack MS, et al. Flavobacterial sepsis in massively burned pediatric patients. *Clin Infect Dis.* 1993;17:185-187.
183. Hoque SN, Graham J, Kaufmann ME, et al. *Chryseobacterium (Flavobacterium) meningosepticum* outbreak associated with colonization of water taps in a neonatal intensive care unit. *J Hosp Infect.* 2001;47:188-192.
184. Coyle-Gilchrist MM, Crewe P, Roberts G. *Flavobacterium meningosepticum* in the hospital environment. *J Clin Pathol.* 1976;29:824-826.
185. Bolivar R, Abramovits W. Cutaneous infection caused by *Flavobacterium meningosepticum*. *J Infect Dis.* 1989;159:150-151.
186. Sundin D, Gold BD, Berkowitz FE, et al. Community-acquired *Flavobacterium meningosepticum* meningitis, pneumonia, and septicemia in a normal infant. *Pediatr Infect Dis J.* 1991;10:73-76.
187. Ashdown LR, Previtera S. Community acquired *Flavobacterium meningosepticum* pneumonia and septicaemia. *Med J Aust.* 1992;156:69-70.
188. Bloom AH, Perry HD, Donnenfeld ED, et al. *Chryseobacterium meningosepticum* keratitis. *Am J Ophthalmol.* 2003;136:356-357.
189. Gunnarsson G, Baldursson H, Hilmarsdottir I. Septic arthritis caused by *Chryseobacterium meningosepticum* in an immunocompetent male. *Scand J Infect Dis.* 2002;34:299-300.
190. Schreckenberger PC, Daneshvar MI, Hollis DG. *Acinetobacter, Achromobacter, Chryseobacterium, Moraxella,* and other nonfermentative gram-negative rods. In: Murray PR, Baron EJ, Jorgensen JH, et al, eds. *Manual of Clinical Microbiology.* 9th ed. Washington, DC: American Society for Microbiology Press; 2007:770-802.
191. Fraser SL, Jorgensen JH. Reappraisal of the antimicrobial susceptibilities of *Chryseobacterium* and *Flavobacterium* species and methods for reliable susceptibility testing. *Antimicrob Agents Chemother.* 1997;41:2738-2741.
192. Hsueh PR, Chang JC, Teng LJ, et al. Comparison of Etest and agar dilution method for antimicrobial susceptibility testing of *Flavobacterium* isolates. *J Clin Microbiol.* 1997;35:1021-1023.
193. Marchiaro P, Ballerini V, Spalding T, et al. A convenient microbiological assay employing cell-free extracts for the rapid characterization of gram-negative carbapenemase producers. *J Antimicrob Chemother.* 2008;62:336-344.
194. Hsueh PR, Teng LJ, Yang PC, et al. Susceptibilities of *Chryseobacterium indologenes* and *Chryseobacterium meningosepticum* to cefepime and cefpirome. *J Clin Microbiol.* 1997;35:3323-3324.
195. Visalli MA, Bajaksouzian S, Jacobs MR, et al. Comparative activity of trovafloxacin, alone and in combination with other agents, against gram-negative nonfermentative rods. *Antimicrob Agents Chemother.* 1997;41:1475-1481.
196. Hirsh BE, Wong B, Kiehn TE, et al. *Flavobacterium meningosepticum* bacteremia in an adult with acute leukemia. Use of rifampin to clear persistent infection. *Diagn Microbiol Infect Dis.* 1986;4:65-69.
197. Ratner H. Flavobacterium meningosepticum. *Infect Control.* 1984;5:237-239.
198. Di Pentima MC, Mason EO Jr, Kaplan SL. In vitro antibiotic synergy against *Flavobacterium meningosepticum:* Implications for therapeutic options. *Clin Infect Dis.* 1998;26:1169-1176.
199. Hawley HB, Gump DW. Vancomycin therapy of bacterial meningitis. *Am J Dis Child.* 1973;126:261-264.
200. Barbaro DJ, Mackowiak PA, Barth SS, et al. *Pseudomonas testosteroni* infections: Eighteen recent cases and a review of the literature. *Rev Infect Dis.* 1987;9:124-129.
201. Smith MD, Gradon JD. Bacteremia due to *Comamonas* species possibly associated with exposure to tropical fish. *South Med J.* 2003;96:815-817.
202. Cooper GR, Staples ED, Iczkowski KA, et al. *Comamonas (Pseudomonas)* testosteroni endocarditis. *Cardiovasc Pathol.* 2005;14:145-149.
203. Stonecipher KG, Jensen HG, Kastl PR, et al. Ocular infections associated with *Comamonas acidovorans*. *Am J Ophthalmol.* 1991;112:46-49.
204. Patrick WD, Brown WD, Bowmer MI, et al. Infective endocarditis due to *Eikenella corrodens:* Case report and review of the literature. *Can J Infect Dis.* 1990;1:139-142.
205. Suwanagool S, Rothkopf MM, Smith SM, et al. Pathogenicity of *Eikenella corrodens* in humans. *Arch Intern Med.* 1983;143:2265-2268.
206. Joshi N, O'Bryan T, Appelbaum PC. Pleuropulmonary infections caused by *Eikenella corrodens*. *Rev Infect Dis.* 1991;13:1207-1212.
207. Paul K, Patel SS. *Eikenella corrodens* infections in children and adolescents: Case reports and review of the literature. *Clin Infect Dis.* 2001;33:54-61.
208. Brooks GF, O'Donoghue JM, Rissing JP. *Eikenella corrodens:* A recently recognized pathogen: Infections in medical-surgical patients and in association with methylphenidate abuse. *Medicine.* 1974;53:325-342.
209. Tveteras K, Kristensten S, Bach V, et al. *Eikenella corrodens:* A recently recognized pathogen in head and neck infections. *J Laryngol Otol.* 1987;101:592-594.
210. Sheng WS, Hsueh PR, Hung CC, et al. Clinical features of patients with invasive *Eikenella corrodens* infections and microbiological characteristics of the causative isolates. *Eur J Clin Microbiol Infect Dis.* 2001;20:231-236.
211. Goldstein EJC. Bite wounds and infections. *Clin Infect Dis.* 1992;14:633-640.
212. Sagerman SD, Lourie GM. *Eikenella* osteomyelitis in a chronic nail biter: A case report. *Hand Surg Am.* 1995;20:71-72.
213. Rosen T, Conrad N. Genital ulcer caused by human bite to the penis. *Sex Transm Dis.* 1999;26:527-530.
214. Swisher LA, Roberts JR, Glynn MJ. Needle licker's osteomyelitis. *Am J Emerg Med.* 1994;12:343-346.
215. Pollner JH, Khan A, Tuazon CU. Severe soft-tissue infection caused by *Eikenella corrodens*. *Clin Infect Dis.* 1992;15:740-741.
216. Raab MG, Lutz RA, Stauffer ES. *Eikenella corrodens* vertebral osteomyelitis. A case report and literature review. *Clin Orthop.* 1993:144-147.
217. Kostadinov S, Pinar H. Amniotic fluid infection syndrome and neonatal mortality caused by *Eikenella corrodens*. *Pediatr Dev Pathol.* 8:489-492, 2005
218. Drouet E, De Montclos H, Boude M, et al. *Eikenella corrodens* and intrauterine contraceptive device. *Lancet.* 1987;2:1089.
219. Stein A, Teysseire N, Capobianco C, et al. *Eikenella corrodens,* a rare cause of pancreatic abscess: Two case reports and review. *Clin Infect Dis.* 1993;17:273-275.
220. Decker MD, Graham BS, Hunter EB, et al. Endocarditis and infections of intravascular devices due to *Eikenella corrodens*. *Am J Med Sci.* 1986;292:209-212.
221. Watkin RW, Baker N, Lang S, et al. *Eikenella corrodens* infective endocarditis in a previously healthy non-drug user. *Eur J Clin Morcobiol Infect Dis.* 2002;21:890-891.
222. Chen C-K, Wilson ME. Outer membrane protein and lipopolysaccharide heterogeneity among *Eikenella corrodens* isolates. *J Infect Dis.* 1990;162:664-671.
223. Sofianou D, Kolokotronis A. Susceptibility of *Eikenella corrodens* to antimicrobial agents. *J Chemother.* 1990;2:156-158.
224. Merriam CV, Citron DM, Tyrrell KL, et al. In vitro activity of azithromycin and nine comparator agents against 296 strains of oral anaerobes and 31 strains of *Eikenella corrodens*. *Int J Antimicrob Agents.* 2006;28:244-248.
225. Goldstein EJ, Citron DM, Merriam CV, et al. In vitro activities of a new des-fluoroquinolone, BMS 284756, and seven other antimicrobial agents against 151 isolates of *Eikenella corrodens*. *Antimicrob Agents Chemother.* 2002;46:1141-1143.
226. Vandamme P, Bernardet J-F, Segers P, et al. New perspectives in the classification of the flavobacteria: Description of *Chryseobacterium* gen nov, *Bergeyella* gen nov and *Empedobacter* nom rev. *Int J Syst Bacteriol.* 1994;44:827-831.
227. Vancanneyt M, Segers P, Torck U, et al. Reclassification of *Flavobacterium odoratum* (Stutzer 1929) strains to a new genus, *Myroides,* as *Myroides odoratus* comb. Nov. and *Myroides odoratimimus* sp. nov. *Int J Syst Bacteriol.* 1996;46:926-932.
228. Hsueh PR, Wu JJ, Hsiue TR, et al. Bacteremic necrotizing fasciitis due to *Flavobacterium odoratum*. *Clin Infect Dis.* 1995;21:1337-1338.
229. Green BT, Green K, Nolan PE. *Myroides odoratus* cellulitis and bacteremia: Case report and review. *Scand J Infect Dis.* 2001;33:932-934.
230. Bachman KH, Sewell DL, Strausbaugh JL. Recurrent cellulitis and bacteremia caused by *Flavobacterium odoratum*. *J Clin Microbiol.* 1996;22:1112-1113.
231. Douce RW, Zurita J, Sanchez O, et al. Investigation of an outbreak of central venous catheter-associated bloodstream infection due to contaminated water. *Infect Control Hosp Epidemiol.* 2008;29:364-366.
232. Velasco J, Romero C, Lopez-Goni I, et al. Evolution of the relatedness of *Brucella* spp. and *Ochrobactrum anthropi* and description of *Ochrobactrum intermedium sp.* nov., a new species with a closer relationship to *Brucella* spp. *Int J Syst Bacteriol.* 1998;48:759-768.
233. Kern WV, Oethinger M, Kaufhold A, et al. *Ochrobactrum anthropi* bacteremia: Report of four cases and short review. *Infection.* 1993;21:306-310.
234. Cieslak TJ, Drabick CJ, Robb ML. Pyogenic infections due to *Ochrobactrum anthropi*. *Clin Infect Dis.* 1996;22:845-847.
235. Galanakis E, Bitsori M, Samonis G, et al. *Ochrobactrum anthropi* bacteraemia in immunocompetent children. *Scand J Infect Dis.* 2002;34:800-803.
236. Gransden WR, Eykyn SJ. Seven cases of bacteremia due to *Ochrobactrum anthropi*. *Clin Infect Dis.* 1992;15:1068-1069.
237. Stiakaki E, Galanakis E, Samonis G, et al. *Ochrobactrum anthropi* bacteremia in pediatric oncology patients. *Pediatr Infect Dis J.* 2002;21:72-74.
238. Ezzedine H, Mourad M, Van Ossel C, et al. An outbreak of *Ochrobactrum anthropi* bacteraemia in five organ transplant patients. *J Hosp Infect.* 1994;27:35-42.
239. Chang HJ, Christenson JC, Pavia AT, et al. *Ochrobactrum anthropi* meningitis in pediatric pericardial allograft transplant recipients. *J Infect Dis.* 1996;173:656-660.
240. Deliere E, Vu-Thien H, Levy V, et al. Epidemiological investigation of *Ochrobactrum anthropi* strains isolated from a haematology unit. *J Hosp Infect.* 2000;44:173-178.
241. Daxboeck F, Zitta S, Assadian O, et al. *Ochrobactrum anthropi* bloodstream infection complicating hemodialysis. *Am J Kid Dis.* 2002;40:E17.

242. Manfredi R, Nanetti A, Ferri M, et al. *Ochrobactrum anthropi* as an agent of nosocomial septicemia in the setting of AIDS. *Clin Infect Dis.* 1999;28:692-694.
243. Esteban J, Ortiz A, Rollan E, et al. Peritonitis due to *Ochrobactrum anthropi* in a patient undergoing continuous ambulatory peritoneal dialysis. *J Infect.* 2000;40:205-206.
244. Song S. Ahn JK, Lee GH, et al. An epidemic of chronic pseudophakic endophthalmitis due to *Ochrobactrum anthropi*: clinical findings and managements of nine consecutive cases. *Ocul Immunol Inflamm.* 2007;15:429-434.
245. Barson WJ, Cromer BA, Marcon MJ. Puncture wound osteochondritis of the foot caused by CDC group Vd. *J Clin Microbiol.* 1987;25:2014-2016.
246. Brivet F, Guibert M, Kiredjian M, et al. Necrotizing fasciitis, bacteremia, and multiorgan failure caused by *Ochrobactrum anthropi*. *Clin Infect Dis.* 1993;17:516-518.
247. Vaidya SA, Citron DM, Fine MB, et al. Pelvic abscess due to *Ochrobactrum anthropi* in an immunocompetent host: case report and review of the literature. *J Clin Microbiol.* 2006; 44:1184-1186.
248. Alnor D, Frimodt-Moller N, Espersen F, et al. Infections with the unusual human pathogens *Agrobacterium* species and *Ochrobactrum anthropi*. *Clin Infect Dis.* 1994;18:914-920.
249. Elsaghir AA, James EA. Misidentification of *Brucella melitensis* as *Ochrobactrum anthropi* by API 20NE. *J Med Microbiol.* 2003;52:441-442.
250. Higgins CS, Avison MB, Jamieson L, et al. Characterization, cloning and sequence analysis of the inducible *Ochrobactrum anthropi* AmpC beta-lactamase. *J Antimicrob Chemother.* 2001;47:745-754.
251. Mesnard R, Sire JM, Donnio PY, et al. Septic arthritis due to *Oligella urethralis*. *Eur J Clin Microbiol Infect Dis.* 1992; 11:195-196.
252. Riley UBG, Bignardi G, Goldberg L, et al. Quinolone resistance in *Oligella urethralis*-associated chronic ambulatory peritoneal dialysis. *J Infect.* 1996;32:155-156.
253. Rockhill RC, Lutwick LI. Group IVe-like gram-negative bacillemia in a patient with obstructive uropathy. *J Clin Microbiol.* 1978;8:108-109.
254. Manian FA. Bloodstream infection with *Oligella ureolytica, Candida krusei,* and *Bacteroides* species in a patient with AIDS. *Clin Infect Dis.* 1993;17:290-291.
255. Mammeri H, Poirel L, Mangeney N, et al. Chromosomal integration of a cephalosporinase gene from *Acinetobacter baumannii* into *Oligella urethralis* as a source of acquired resistance to beta-lactams. *Antimicrob Agents Chemother.* 2003;47: 1536-1542.
256. Hujer KM, Hamza NS, Hujer AM, et al. Identification of a new allelic variant of *Acinetobacter baumanii* cephalosporinase, ACD-7 β-lactamase: defining a unique family of class C enzymes. *Antimicrob Agents Chemother.* 2005;49:2941-2948.
257. Anzai Y, Kudo Y, Oyaizu H. The phylogeny of the genera *Chryseomonas, Flavimonas,* and *Pseudomonas* supports synonymy of these three genera. *Int J Syst Bacteriol.* 1997;47:249-251.
258. Hsueh PR, Teng LJ, Pan HJ, et al. Outbreak of *Pseudomonas fluorescens* bacteremia among oncology patients. *J Clin Microbiol.* 1998;36:2914-2917.
259. Namnyak S, Hussain S, Davalle J, et al. Contaminated lithium heparin bottles as a source of pseudobacteraemia due to *Pseudomonas fluorescens*. *J Hosp Infect.* 1999;4:23-28.
260. CDC. Update: Delayed onset *Pseudomonas fluorescens* bloodstream infections after exposure to contaminated heparin flush—Michigan and South Dakota, 2005-2006. *MMWR Morb Mortal Wkly Rep.* 2006:55:961-963.
261. Scott JF, Boulton E, Govan JRW, et al. A fatal transfusion reaction associated with blood contaminated with *Pseudomonas fluorescens*. *Vox Sang.* 1988;54:201-204.
262. Anaissie E, Fainstein V, Miller P, et al. *Pseudomonas putrida:* newly recognized pathogen in patients with cancer. *Am J Med.* 1987;82:1191-1194.
263. Yang CH, Young T, Peng MY, et al. Clinical spectrum of *Pseudomonas putida* infection. *J Formos Med Assoc.* 1996; 95:754-761.
264. Ladhani S, Bhutta ZA. Neonatal *Pseudomonas putida* infection presenting as staphylococcal scalded skin syndrome. *Eur J Clin Microbiol Infect Dis.* 1998;17:642-644.
264a. Souza Dias MB, Habert AB, Borrasca V, et al. Salvage of long-term central venous catheters during an outbreak of *Pseudomonas putida* and *Stenotrophomonas maltophilia* infections associated with contaminated heparin catheter-lock solution. *Infect Control Hosp Epidemiol.* 2008;29:125-130.
265. Romney M, Sherlock C, Stephens G, Clarke A. Pseudo-outbreak of *Pseudomonas putida* in a hospital outpatient clinic originating from a contaminated commercial anti-fog solution—Vancouver, British Columbia. *Can Commun Dis Rep.* 2000;26:183-184.
266. Yee-Guardino S, Danziger-Isakov L, Knouse M, et al. Nosocomially acquired *Pseudomonas stutzeri* brain abscess in a child: case report and review. *Infect Control Hosp Epidemiol.* 2006;27:630-632.
267. Reisler RB, Blumberg HB. Community-acquired *Pseudomonas stutzeri* vertebral osteomyelitis in a previously health patient: Case report and review. *Clin Infect Dis.* 1999;29:667-669.
268. Campos-Herrero MI, Bordes A, Rodriguez H, et al. *Pseudomonas stutzeri* community-acquired pneumonia associated with empyema: Case report and review. *Clin Infect Dis.* 1997; 25:325-326.
269. Chaudhry HJ, Schoch PE, Cunha BA. *Flavimonas oryzihabitans* (CD Group Ve-2). *Infect Control Hosp Epidemiol.* 1992; 13:485-488.
270. Lucas KG, Kiehn TE, Sobeck KA, et al. Sepsis caused by *Flavimonas oryzihabitans*. *Medicine.* 1994;73:209-214.
271. Lin RD, Hsueh PR, Chang JC, et al. *Flavimonas oryzihabitans* bacteremia: Clinical features and microbiological characteristics of isolates. *Clin Infect Dis.* 1997;24:867-873.
272. Rahav G, Simhon A, Mattan Y, et al. Infections with *Chryseomonas luteola* (CDC group Ve-1) and *Flavimonas oryzihabitans* (CDC group Ve-2). *Medicine.* 1995;74:83-88.
273. Hawkins RE, Moriarty RA, Lewis DE, et al. Serious infections involving the CDC group Ve bacteria *Chryseomonas luteola* and *Flavimonas oryzihabitans*. *Rev Infect Dis.* 1991;13:257-260.
274. Yu EN, Foster CS. Chronic postoperative endophthalmitis due to *Pseudomonas oryzihabitans*. *Am J Ophthalmol.* 2002;134: 613-614.
275. Kostman JR, Solomon F, Fekete T. Infections with *Chryseomonas luteola* (CDC group Ve-1) and *flavimonas oryzihabitans* (CDC group Ve-2) in neurosurgical patients. *Rev Infect Dis.* 1991;13:233-236.
276. Lam S, Isenberg HD, Edwards B, et al. Community-acquired soft-tissue infections caused by *Flavimonas oryzihabitans*. *Clin Infect Dis.* 1994;18:808-809.
277. Tsakris A, Hassapopoulou H, Skoura L, et al. Leg ulcer due to *Pseudomonas luteola* in a patient with sickle cell disease. *Diagn Microbiol Infect Dis.* 2002;42:141-143.
278. Rastogi S, Sperber SJ. Facial cellulitis and *Pseudomonas luteola* bacteremia in an otherwise healthy patient. *Diagn Microbiol Infect Dis.* 1998;32:303-305.
279. Docquier JD, Riccio ML, Mugnaioli C, et al. IMP-12, a new plasmid-encoded metallo-beta-lactamase from a *Pseudomonas putida* clinical isolate. *Antimicrob Agents Chemother.* 2003; 47:1522-1528.
280. Rolston KV, Ho DH, LeBlanc B, et al. In vitro activities of antimicrobial agents against clinical isolates of *Flavimonas oryzihabitans* obtained from patients with cancer. *Antimicrob Agents Chemother.* 1993;37:2504-2505.
281. Yabuuchi E, Kosako Y, Yano I, et al. Transfer of two *Burkholderia* and an *Alcaligenes* species to *Ralstonia* gen. nov.: Proposal of *Ralstonia pickettii* (Ralston, Palleroni and Doudoroff 1973) comb. nov., *Ralstonia solanacearum* (Smith 1896) comb. nov. and *Ralstonia eutropha* (Davis 1969) comb. nov. *Microbiol Immunol.* 1995;39:897-904.
282. Anderson RR, Warnick P, Schreckenberger PC. Recurrent CDC group IVc-2 bacteremia in a human with AIDS. *J Clin Microbiol.* 1997;35:780-782.
283. Thayu M, Baltimore RS, Sleight BJ, et al. CDC group IV c-2 bacteremia in a child with recurrent acute monoblastic leukemia. *Pediatr Infect Dis J.* 1999;18:397-398.
284. Vandamme P, Goris J, Coenye T, et al. Assignment of Centers for Disease Control group IVc-2 to the genus *Ralstonia* as *Ralstonia paucula* sp. nov. *Int J Syst Bacteriol.* 1999;49:663-669.
285. Osterhout GJ, Valentine JL, Dick JD. Phenotypic and genotypic characterization of clinical strains of CDC group IVc-2. *J Clin Microbiol.* 1998;36:2618-2622.
286. Maki DG, Klein BS, McCormick RD, et al. Nosocomial *Pseudomonas pickettii* bacteremias traced to narcotic tampering. A case for selective drug screening of health care personnel. *JAMA.* 1991;265:981-986.
287. Labarca JA, Trick WE, Peterson CL, et al. A multistate nosocomial outbreak of *Ralstonia pickettii* colonization associated with an intrinsically contaminated respiratory care solution. *Clin Infect Dis.* 1999;29:1281-1286.
288. Gröbner S., Heeg P, Autenrieth IB, et al. Monoclonal outbreak of catheter-related bacteraemia by *Ralstonia mannitolilytica* on two haematoncology wards. *J Infect.* 2007;55:539-544.
289. Daxboeck F, Stadler M, Assadian O, et al. Characterization of clinically isolated *Ralstonia mannitolilytica* strains using random amplification of polymorphic DNA (RAPD) typing and antimicrobial sensitivity, and comparison of the classification efficacy of phenotypic and genotypic assays. *J Med Microbiol.* 2005; 54:55-61.
290. Coenye T, Spilker T, Reik R, et al. Use of PCR analyses to define the distribution of *Ralstonia* species recovered from patients with cystic fibrosis. *J Clin Microbiol.* 2005;43:3464-3466.
291. Degand N, Carbonelle E, Dauphin B, et al. Matrix-assisted laser desorption ionization-time of flight mass spectrometry for identification of nonfermenting gram-negative bacilli isolated from cystic fibrosis patients. *J Clin Microbiol.* 2008;46:3361-3367.
292. Moissenet D, Tabone M-D, Girardet J-P, et al. Nosocomial CDC Group IVc-2 bacteremia: Epidemiological investigation by randomly amplified polymorphic DNA analysis. *J Clin Microbiol.* 1996;34:1264-1266.
293. Zapardiel J, Blum G, Caramelo C, et al. Peritonitis with CDC group IVc-2 bacteria in a patient on continuous ambulatory peritoneal dialysis. *Eur J Clin Microbiol Infect Dis.* 1991:10:509-511.
294. Musso D, Drancourt M, Bardot J, et al. Human infection due to the CDC Group IVc-2 bacterium: Case report and review. *Clin Infect Dis.* 1994;18:482-484.
295. Girlich D, Naas T, Nordmann P. OXA-60, a chromosomal, inducible, and imipenem-hydrolyzing class D β-lactamase from *Ralstonia pickettii*. *Antimicrob Agents Chemother.* 2004;48: 4217-4225.
296. Stelzmueller I, Biebl M, Wiesmayr S, et al. *Ralstonia pickettii:* Innocent bystander or a potential threat? *Clin Microbiol Infect.* 2006;12:99-101.
297. Young JM, Kuykendall LD, Martinez-Romero E, et al. A revision of *Rhizobium* Frank 1889, with an emended description of the genus, and the inclusion of all species of *Agrobacterium* Conn 1942 and *Allorhizobium undicola* de Lajudie et al. 1998 as new combinations: *Rhizobium radiobacter, R. rhizogenes, R. rubi, R. undicola* and *R. vitis*. *Int J Syst Evol Bacteriol.* 2001;51:89-103.
298. Edmond MB, Riddler SA, Baxter CM, et al. *Agrobacterium radiobacter:* A recently recognized opportunistic pathogen. *Clin Infect Dis.* 1993;16:388-391.
299. Amaya RA, Edwards MS. *Agrobacterium radiobacter* bacteremia in pediatric patients: Case report and review. *Pediatr Infect Dis J.* 2003;22:183-186.
300. Giammanco GM, Pignato S, Santangelo C, et al. Molecular typing of *Agrobacterium* species isolates from catheter-related bloodstream infections. *Infect Control Hosp Epidemiol.* 2004;25:885-887.
301. Hulse M, Johnson S, Ferrieri P. *Agrobacterium* infections in humans: Experience at one hospital and review. *Clin Infect Dis.* 1993;16:112-117.
302. Mastroianni A, Coronado O, Nanetti A, et al. *Agrobacterium radiobacter* pneumonia in a patient with HIV infection. *Eur J Clin Microbiol Infect Dis.* 1996;15:960-963.
303. Manfredi R, Nanetti A, Ferri M, et al. Emerging gram-negative pathogens in the immunocompromised host: *Agrobacterium radiobacter* septicemia during HIV disease. *New Microbiol.* 1999;22:375-382.
304. Miller JM, Novy C, Hiott M. Case of bacterial endophthalmitis caused by an *Agrobacterium radiobacter*-like organism. *J Clin Microbiol.* 1996;34:3212-3213.
305. Rogues AM, Sarlangue J, de Barbeyrac B, et al. *Agrobacterium radiobacter* as a cause of pseudobacteremia. *Infect Control Hosp Epidemiol.* 1999;20:345-347.
306. Sykes RB, Cimarusti CM, Bonner DP, et al. Monocyclic β-lactam antibiotics produced by bacteria. *Nature.* 1981; 291:489-491.
307. Rihs JD, Brenner DJ, Weaver RE, et al. *Roseomonas*, a new genus associated with bacteremia and other human infections. *J Clin Microbiol.* 1993;31:3275-3283.
308. Han XY, Pham AS, Tarrand JJ, et al. Bacteriologic characterization of 36 strains of *Roseomonas* species and proposal of *Roseomonas mucosa* sp nov and *Roseomonas gilardii* subsp *rosea* subsp nov. *Am J Clin Pathol.* 2003;120:256-264.
309. Struthers M, Wong J, Janda JM. An initial appraisal of the clinical significance of *Roseomonas* species associated with human infections. *Clin Infect Dis.* 1996;23:729-733.
310. Kaye KM, Macone A, Kazanjian PH. Catheter infection caused by *Methylobacterium* in immunocompromised hosts: Report of three cases and review of the literature. *Clin Infect Dis.* 1992;14:1010-1014.
311. Marin ME, Marco Del Pont J, Dibar E, et al. Catheter-related bacteremia caused by *Roseomonas gilardii* in an immunocompromised patient. *Int J Infect Dis.* 2001;5:170-171.
312. Lewis L, Stock F, Williams D, et al. Infections with *Roseomonas gilardii* and review of characteristics used for biochemical identification and molecular typing. *Am J Clin Pathol.* 1997; 108:210-216.
313. Richardson JD. Failure to clear a *Roseomonas* line infection with antibiotic therapy. *Clin Infect Dis.* 1997;25:155.
314. Shokar NK, Shokar GS, Islam J, et al. *Roseomonas gilardii* infection: Case report and review. *J Clin Microbiol.* 2002;40: 4789-4791.
315. Nahass RG, Wisneski R, Herman DJ, et al. Vertebral osteomyelitis due to *Roseomonas* species: Case report and review of the evaluation of vertebral osteomyelitis. *Clin Infect Dis.* 1995;21:1474-1476.
316. Nolan JS, Waites KB. Nosocomial ventriculitis due to *Roseomonas gilardii* complicating subarachnoid haemorrhage. *J Infect.* 2005;50:244-251.
317. Do I, Rolston KV, Han XV. Clinical significance of *Roseomonas* species isolated from catheter and blood samples: Analysis of 36 cases in patients with cancer. *Clin Infect Dis*, 2004;38:1579-1584.
318. Bibashi E, Sofianou D, Kontopoulou K, et al. Peritonitis due to *Roseomonas fauriae* in a patient undergoing continuous ambulatory peritoneal dialysis. *J Clin Microbiol.* 2000;38:456-457.
319. Hornei B, Luneberg E, Schmidt-Rotte H, et al. Systemic infection of an immunocompromised patient with *Methylobacterium zatmanii*. *J Clin Microbiol.* 1999;37:248-250.
320. Flournoy DJ, Petrone RL, Voth DW. A pseudo-outbreak of *Methylobacterium mesophilica* isolated from patients undergoing bronchoscopy. *Eur J Clin Microbiol Infect Dis.* 1992;11: 240-243.
321. Singal A, Malani PN, Day LJ, et al. *Roseomonas* infection associated with a left ventricular assist device. *Infect Control Hosp Epidemiol.* 2003;24:963-965.
322. Nozue H, Hayashi T, Hashimoto Y, et al. Isolation and characterization of *Shewanella alga* from human clinical specimens and emendation of the description of *S. alga*. *Int J Syst Bacteriol.* 1992;42:628-634.
323. Khashe S, Janda JM. Biochemical and pathogenic properties of *Shewanella alga* and *Shewanella putrefaciens*. *J Clin Microbiol.* 1998;36:783-787.
324. Chen YS, Liu YC, Yen MY, et al. Skin and soft-tissue manifestations of *Shewanella putrefaciens* infection. *Clin Infect Dis.* 1997;25:225-229.
325. Brink AJ, van Straten A, van Rensburg AJ. *Shewanella (Pseudomonas) putrefaciens* bacteremia. *Clin Infect Dis.* 1995;20: 1327-1332.

326. Paccalin M, Grollier G, le Moal G, et al. Rupture of a primary aortic aneurysm infected with *Shewanella alga*. *Scand J Infect Dis*. 2001;33:774-775.

327. Oh HS, Kum KA, Kim EC, et al. Outbreak of *Shewanella algae* and *Shewanella putrefaciens* infections caused by a shared measuring cup in a general surgery unit in Korea. *Infect Control Hosp Epidemiol*. 2008;29:742-748.

328. Butt AA, Figueroa J, Martin DH. Ocular infection caused by three unusual marine organisms. *Clin Infect Dis*. 1997;24:740.

329. Tan C-K, Lai C-C, Kuar W-K, et al. Purulent pericarditis with greenish pericardial effusion caused by *Shewanella algae*. *J Clin Microbiol*. 2008;46:2817-2819.

330. Lascols C, Podglagen I, Verdet C, et al. A plasmid-borne *Shewanella algae* gene, qnrA3, and its possible transfer in vivo between *Kluyvera ascorbata* and *Klebsiella pneumoniae*. *J Bacteriol*. 2008;190:5217-5223.

331. Dees SB, Moss CW, Hollis DG, et al. Chemical characterization of *Flavobacterium odoratum*, *Flavobacterium breve*, and *Flavobacterium*-like groups IIe, IIh, and IIf. *J Clin Microbiol*. 1986;23:267-273.

332. Potvliege C, Dejaegher-Bauduin C, Hansen W, et al. *Flavobacterium multivorum* septicemia in a hemodialysis patient. *J Clin Microbiol*. 1984;19:568-569.

333. Freney J, Hansen W, Ploton C, et al. Septicemia caused by *Sphingobacterium multivorum*. *J Clin Microbiol*. 1987;25:1126-1128.

334. Reina J, Borrell N, Figuerola J. *Sphingobacterium multivorum* isolated from a patient with cystic fibrosis. *Eur J Clin Microbiol Infect Dis*. 1992;11:81-82.

335. Areekul S, Vongsthongsri U, Mookto T, et al. *Sphingobacterium multivorum* septicemia: A case report. *J Med Assoc Thai*. 1996;79:395-398.

336. Holmes B, Owen RJ, Hollis DG. *Flavobacterium spiritivorum*, a new species isolated from human clinical specimens. *Int J Syst Bacteriol*. 1982;32:157-165.

337. Marinella MA. Cellulitis and sepsis due to *Sphingobacterium*. *JAMA*. 2002;288:1985.

338. Kampfer P, Engelhart S. Rolke M. et al. Extrinsic allergic alveolitis (hypersensitivity pneumonitis) caused by *Sphingobacterium spiritivorum* from the water reservoir of a steam iron. *J Clin Microbiol*. 2005;43:4908-4910.

339. Fass RJ, Barnishan J. In vitro susceptibilities of nonfermentative gram-negative bacilli other than *Pseudomonas aeruginosa* to 32 antimicrobial agents. *Rev Infect Dis*. 1980;2:841-853.

340. Blahova J, Kralikova K, Krcmery V Sr, et al. Hydrolysis of imipenem, meropenem, ceftazidime, and cefepime by multiresistant nosocomial strains of *Sphingobacterium multivorum*. *Eur J Clin Microbiol Infect Dis*. 1997;16:178-180.

341. Yabuuchi E, Yano I, Oyaizu H, et al. Proposals of *Sphingomonas paucimobilis* gen nov and comb nov, *Sphingomonas parapaucimobilis* sp nov, *Sphingomonas yanoikuyae* sp nov, *Sphingomonas adhaesiva* sp nov, *Sphingomonas capsulata* comb nov, and two genospecies of the genus *Sphingomonas*. *Microbiol Immunol*. 1990;34:99-119.

342. Crane LR, Tagle LC, Palutke WA. Outbreak of *Pseudomonas paucimobilis* in an intensive care facility. *JAMA*. 1981;246:985-987.

343. Perola O, Nousiainen T, Suomalainen S, et al. Recurrent *Sphingomonas paucimobilis*-bacteraemia associated with a multibacterial water-borne epidemic among neutropenic patients. *J Hosp Infect*. 2002;50:196-201.

344. Lemaitre D, Elaichouni A, Hundhausen M, et al. Tracheal colonization with *Sphingomonas paucimobilis* in mechanically ventilated neonates due to contaminated ventilator temperature probes. *J Hosp Infect*. 1996;32:199-206.

345. Cheong HS, Moon SY, Son JS, et al. Clinical features and treatment outcomes of infections caused by *Sphingomonas paucimobilis*. *Infect Control Hosp Epidemiol*. 2008;29:990-992.

346. Hsueh PR, Teng LJ, Yang PC, et al. Nosocomial infections caused by *Sphingomonas paucimobilis*: Clinical features and microbiological characteristics. *Clin Infect Dis*. 1998;26:676-681.

347. Lazarus HM, Magalhaes-Silverman M, Fox RM, et al. Contamination during *in vitro* procession of bone marrow for transplantation: Clinical significance. *Bone Marrow Transplant*. 1991;7:241-246.

348. Boken DJ, Romero JR, Cavalieri SJ. *Sphingomonas paucimobilis* bacteremia: Four cases and review of the literature. *Infect Dis Clin Pract*. 1988;7:286-291.

349. Reina J, Bassa A, Llompart I, et al. Infections with *Pseudomonas paucimobilis*: Report of four cases and review. *Rev Infect Dis*. 1991;13:1072-1076.

350. Holmes B, Owen RJ, Evans A, et al. *Pseudomonas paucimobilis*, a new species isolated from human clinical specimens, the hospital environment and other sources. *Int J Syst Bacteriol*. 1977;27:133-146.

351. Holmes B, Steigerwalt AG, Weaver RE, et al. *Weeksella zoohelcum* sp nov (formerly group IIj), from human clinical specimens. *Syst Appl Microbiol*. 1986;8:191-196.

352. Reina J, Borrell N. Leg abscess caused by *Weeksella zoohelcum* following a dog bite. *Clin Infect Dis*. 1992;14:1162-1163.

353. Bracis R, Seibers K, Julien RM. Meningitis caused by Group IIj following a dog bite. *West J Med*. 1979;131:438-440.

354. Montejo M, Aguirrebengoa K, Ugalde J, et al. *Bergeyella zoohelcum* bacteremia after a dog bite. *Clin Infect Dis*. 2001;33:1608-1609.

355. Beltran A, Bdiiwi S, Jani J, et al. A case of *Bergeyella zoohelcum* bacteremia after ingestion of a dish prepared with goat blood. *Clin Infect Dis*. 2006;42:891-892.

356. Holmes B, Steigerwalt AG, Weaver RE, et al. *Weeksella virosa* gen nov sp nov (formerly group IIf), found in human clinical specimens. *Syst Appl Microbiol*. 1986;8:185-190.

357. Reina J, Gil J, Alomar P. Isolation of *Weeksella virosa* (formerly CDC group IIf) from a vaginal sample. *Eur J Clin Microbiol Infect Dis*. 1989;8:569-570.

358. Faber MD, delBusto R, Cruz C, et al. Response of *Weeksella virosa* peritonitis to imipenem/cilastatin. *Adv Perit Dial*. 1991;7:133-134.

359. Boixeda D, de Luis DA, Meseguer MA, et al. A case of spontaneous peritonitis caused by *Weeksella virosa*. *Eur J Gastroenterol Hepatol*. 1998;10:897-898.

360. Hollis DG, Moss CW, Daneshvar MI, et al. Characterization of Centers for Disease Control Group NO-1, a fastidious, nonoxidative, gram-negative organism associated with dog and cat bites. *J Clin Microbiol*. 1993;31:746-748.

361. Kaiser RM, Garman RL, Bruce MG, et al. Clinical significance and epidemiology of NO-1, an unusual bacterium associated with dog and cat bites. *Emerg Infect Dis*. 2002;8:171-174.

362. Hollis DG, Weaver RE, Moss CW, et al. Chemical and cultural characterization of CDC group WO-1, a weakly oxidative gram-negative group of organisms isolated from clinical sources. *J Clin Microbiol*. 1992;30:291-295.

363. Coenye T, Liu L, Vandamme P, et al. Identification of *Pandoraea* species by 16S ribosomal DNA-based PCR assays. *J Clin Microbiol*. 2001;39:4452-4455.

364. Daneshvar MI, Hollis DG, Steigerwalt AG, et al. Assignment of CDC weak oxidizer group 2 (WO-2) to the genus *Pandoraea* and characterization of three new *Pandoraea* genomospecies. *J Clin Microbiol*. 2001;39:1819-1826.

365. Johnson LN, Han JY, Moskowitz SM, et al. *Pandoraea* bacteremia in a cystic fibrosis patient with associated systemic illness. *Pediatr Infect Dis J*. 2004;23:881-882

366. Purcell BK, Dooley DP. Centers for Disease Control and Prevention Group O1 bacterium associated pneumonia complicated by bronchopulmonary fistula and bacteremia. *Clin Infect Dis*. 1999;29:945-946.

367. Daneshvar MI, Hill B, Hollis DG, et al. CDC group O-3: Phenotypic characteristics, fatty acid composition, isoprenoid quinone content, and in vitro antimicrobic susceptibilities of an unusual gram negative bacterium isolated from clinical specimens. *J Clin Microbiol*. 1998;36:1674-1678.

368. Moss CW, Daneshvar MI, Hollis DG. Biochemical characteristics and fatty acid composition of *Gilardi* rod group 1 bacteria. *J Clin Microbiol*. 1993;31:689-691.

369. Van Esbroeck M, Vandamme P, Falsen E, et al. Polyphasic approach to the classification and identification of *Gardnerella vaginalis* and unidentified *Gardnerella vaginalis*-like coryneforms present in bacterial vaginosis. *Int J Syst Bacteriol*. 1996;46:675-682.

370. Catlin BW. *Gardnerella vaginalis*: Characteristics, clinical considerations, and controversies. *Clin Microbiol Rev*. 1992;5:213-237.

371. Aroutcheva AA, Simoes JA, Behbakht K, et al. *Gardnerella vaginalis* isolated from patients with bacterial vaginosis and from patients with healthy vaginal ecosystems. *Clin Infect Dis*. 2001;33:1022-1027.

372. Spiegel CA, Amsel R, Eschenbach D, et al. Anaerobic bacteria in nonspecific vaginitis. *N Engl J Med*. 1980;303:601-607.

373. Gelber SE, Aguilar JL, Lewis KL, et al. Functional and phylogenetic characterization of vaginolysin, the human-specific cytolysin from *Gardnerella vaginalis*. *J Bacteriol*. 2008;190:3896-3903.

374. Fredricks DN, Fiedler TL, Marrazzo. Molecular identification of bacteria associated with bacterial vaginosis. *New Engl J Med*. 2005:353:1899-1911

375. Reimer LG, Reller LB. *Gardnerella vaginalis* bacteremia: A review of thirty cases. *Obstet Gynecol*. 1984;64:170-174.

376. McFadyen IR, Eykyn SJ. Suprapubic aspiration of urine in pregnancy. *Lancet*. 1968:1:1112-1114.

376a. Lagace-Wiens PR, Ng B, Reimer A, et al. *Gardnerella vaginalis* bacteremia in a previously healthy man: case report and characterization of the isolate. *J Clin Microbiol*. 2008;46:804-806.

377. CDC. Sexually Transmitted Diseases Treatment Guidelines. *MMWR Recomm Rep*. 2006;55(RR-11).

378. Hoist E. Reservoir of four organisms associated with bacterial vaginosis suggests lack of sexual transmission. *J Clin Microbiol*. 1990;28:2035-2039.

379. Schwebke JR, Lawing LF. Prevalence of *Mobiluncus* spp among women with and without bacterial vaginosis is detected by polymerase chain reaction. *Sex Transm Dis*. 2001;28;195-199.

380. Spiegel CA. The genus *Mobiluncus*. In: Balows A, Trüper HG, Dworkin M, et al, eds. *Prokaryotes*. 2nd ed. New York: Springer-Verlag; 1992.

381. Hill DA, Seaton RA, Cameron ML, et al. Severe sepsis caused by *Mobiluncus curtisii* subsp. *ciirtisii* in a previously healthy female: case report and review. *J Infect*. 1998;37:194-196.

382. Sahuquillo-Arce JM, Ramirez-Galleymore P, Garcia J. et al. *Mobiluncus curtisii* bacteremia. *Anaerobe*. 2008;14:123-124.

383. Spiegel CA. Susceptibility of *Mobiluncus* species to 23 antimicrobial agents and 15 other compounds. *Antimicrob Agents Chemother*. 1987;31:249-252.

238

Treponema pallidum (Syphilis)

EDMUND C. TRAMONT

Syphilis is a complex systemic illness with protean clinical manifestations caused by the spirochete *Treponema pallidum*. It holds a special place in the history of Western medicine because of its earlier prevalence, the persons of historical notoriety who were (likely) infected, and its variable clinical presentations, for which it earned the epigram "the great imitator" or "the great impostor."[1-5] The first designated and recognized medical specialists were physicians treating this disease, who were called syphilologists. Special clinics were established and one of the first specialized medical journals appeared, the *American Journal of Syphilis, Gonorrhea and Venereal Disease*. Syphilis is most often transmitted by sexual contact, and, unlike most other infectious diseases, it is rarely if ever diagnosed by isolation and characterization of the causative organism. Instead, indirect methods of diagnosis are used, including the following: serologic tests (e.g., Venereal Disease Research Laboratory [VDRL] and rapid plasma reagin [RPR] tests, *Treponema pallidum* particle agglutination [TPPA], enzyme immunoassay [EIA]), darkfield microscopy, Warthin-Starry silver staining, epidemiologic data, and clinical findings. Direct immunofluorescent antibody or immunohistochemical staining and the polymerase chain reaction (PCR) assay provide more direct evidence of *T. pallidum*. Its natural course is classically divided into the following phases: (1) an incubation period lasting about 3 weeks; (2) a primary stage characterized by a nonpainful skin lesion known as a *chancre* that is usually associated with regional nonpainful lymphadenopathy, and always with early bacteremia/spirochetemia; (3) a florid secondary bacteremic or disseminated stage accompanied by generalized skin rash, mucocutaneous lesions, lymphadenopathy, and/or protean clinical findings; (4) a period of subclinical infection (early or late latent syphilis) detected only by reactive serologic tests and lasting 6 months to many years; and (5) in a small number of patients, a late or tertiary stage characterized by progressive destructive disease involving principally the ascending aorta and/or the central nervous system (CNS), including ophthalmic or auditory abnormalities, or the development of a characteristic granulomatous-like lesion known as a gumma that can involve almost any organ.

History

The historical aspects of syphilis make for fascinating reading.[5-8] Few modern clinicians are aware of the prevalence of syphilis in Western countries through the middle of the 20th century, the prominent historical figures who were infected, or the pervasiveness of this disease on medical practice. For example, syphilis was the leading cause of neurologic and cardiovascular disease among middle-aged persons at the turn of the 20th century.[2,9]

The origins of syphilis are still debated to this day and essentially come down to whether the disease was imported into the Old World (Europe) from the New World (the Caribbean and South America) by shipmates of Christopher Columbus, or was an established disease that spread throughout Europe as a consequence of urbanization. The two theories have not yet been reconciled.[7,10,11] A pandemic known as the Great Pox (as distinguished from the small pox) ravaged Europe and Asia soon after the return of Columbus from America, and also coincided with mass movements of armies and populations in Europe. It cannot be proved with certainty that *T. pallidum* was the cause of this

scourge. Nevertheless, the first clear descriptions of this illness, including the sexual mode of transmission, were recorded in the 16th century in the *Brevary of Helthe*, published in 1547:

In englyshe Morbus Gallicus (syphilis) is named the french pockes, whan that I was yonge they were named the spanyshe pockes the which be of many kyndes of the pockes, some be moyst, some be waterashe, some be drye, and some be skorvie, some be lyke skabbes, some be lyke ring wormes, some be fistuled, some be festered, some be cankarus, some be lyke wennes, some be lyke biles, some be lyke knobbles or burres, and some be ulcerous havyinge a lytle drye skabbe in the middle of the ulcerous skabbe, some hath ache in the jioyntes and no singe of the pockes and yet it may be the pockes.... The cause of these impediments or infyrmytes doth come many wayes, it maye come by lyenge in the shetes or bedde there where a pocky person hath the night before lyenin, it maye come with lyenge with a pocky person, it maye come by syttenge on a draught or sege where as a pocky person did lately syt, it may come by drynkynge oft with a pocky person, but specially it is taken when one pocky person doth synne in lechery the one with another.

Andrew Boorde

During this period, syphilis, or a disease similar to syphilis, was often accompanied by high morbidity and mortality, which attests to the extraordinarily virulent nature of the causative organism of that pestilence. It is not known whether the relatively mild nature of present-day syphilis reflects a change in the virulence of the organism, an adaptation of the human host, or the disappearance of a concomitantly occurring but unknown illness. The proponents of the New World or Columbian theory based their argument on the relatedness of endemic treponematosis in the Caribbean and South America and the purported absence of syphilitic bone lesions in pre–15th century skeletons, despite the fact that the pathologic distinction between old bone lesions attributable to leprosy, endemic treponematosis, and those of syphilis is not precise. Results of examination of medieval skeletons with modern molecular-based techniques are conflicting as to whether treponemal disease in Europe existed prior to 1492, although the exact pathogenic treponeme could not be determined because of the extreme genetic relatedness that exists among *T. pallidum* subspecies.[10,11]

One of the difficulties in sorting through older writings is that clinical distinctions between syphilis, gonorrhea, and other venereal diseases did not emerge until the late 18th century. John Hunter's unfortunate self-inoculation with urethral pus containing both *Neisseria gonorrhoeae* and *T. pallidum* only served to prolong misconceptions, because the two diseases were considered the same for some time thereafter. However, by the mid-19th century, the cause, epidemiology, and clinical manifestations of syphilis were well known.[12] Syphilis became a frequent literary subject, as evidenced by the following anonymous poem, which can be dated from the 1920s:

There was a young man from Back Bay
Who thought syphilis just went away
He believed that a chancre

Was only a canker
That healed in a week and a day.
But now he has "acne vulgaris"-
(Or whatever they call it in Paris);
On his skin it has spread
From his feet to his head,
And his friends want to know where his hair is.
There's more to his terrible plight:
His pupils won't close in the light
His heart is cavorting,
His wife is aborting,
And he squints through his gun barrel sight.
Arthralgia cuts into his slumber;
His aorta is in need of a plumber;
But now he has tabes,
And sabershinned babies,
While of gummas he has quite a number.
He's been treated in every known way,
But his spirochetes grow day by day;
He's developed paresis,
Has long talks with Jesus,
And thinks he's the Queen of the May.

The moniker "lues" came from the Latin *lues venereum,* which means disease, sickness, or pestilence, and originally was loosely applied to any venereal disease. It became a synonym for syphilis at the turn of the 20th century.

Metchnikoff successfully transferred *T. pallidum* to chimpanzees in 1903. Two years later, the organism was described in the primary lesion and adjacent lymph nodes of syphilitic patients and given the name *Spirochaeta pallida.* By 1906, Wassermann had developed the complement fixation blood test, first using an extract from the liver of a syphilitic stillborn baby; soon thereafter, however, extracts of uninfected beef livers and hearts were shown to be equally sensitive. This was the forerunner of current nontreponemal tests (see later).

With the advent of serologic testing, the prevalence of the infection was determined; between 8% and 14% of adults living in cities such as Paris, Berlin, and New York had positive serologic test results.[9] It was this high prevalence that led to the practice of screening blood donations and hospital admissions, a practice that is no longer followed, except in high-prevalence areas. During this same period, Ehrlich introduced an arsenic derivative, arsphenamine or salvarsan, as therapy. Mercury and bismuth preparations were added later but none of these disparate therapies were very efficacious. Induced-fever therapy (e.g., malaria, heat box, hot baths) was more efficacious and, in 1927, Dr. Julius Wagner von Jauregg was awarded the Nobel Prize in Medicine for describing the use of malaria injections with its subsequent fevers to treat "paralytica dementia" (neurosyphilis). These primarily palliative therapies were quickly forgotten; however, no other disease was as dramatically affected by the discovery of penicillin as syphilis.

Syphilis continues to have an impact on the practice of modern medicine. From 1932 until 1962, 431 African-American men with syphilis were prospectively followed untreated ("Tuskegee Study of Untreated Syphilis in the Negro Male") to better establish the natural history of the disease, despite the discovery of and the proven efficacy of penicillin by the late 1940s. The abuse of trust in the medical profession exemplified by this U.S. government–sponsored study led to the 1979 Belmont Report, the establishment of the National Human Investigation Board, and the requirement for the establishment of Institutional Review Boards.[13]

Etiology

The causal agent of syphilis is *T. pallidum* subsp. *pallidum,* which belongs to the order Spirochaetales, the family Spirochaetaceae, and the genus *Treponema.* Other members of the genus *Treponema* that can infect humans are *Treponema pallidum* subsp. *pertenue* (yaws),

Treponema pallidum subsp. *endemicum* (bejel, nonvenereal, or endemic syphilis) and *Treponema carateum* (pinta). The latter three are collectively known as endemic nonvenereal treponemal infections. They are all closely related morphologically, antigenically, by their ability to adhere to mammalian cells and induce antibodies detected by the routine serological tests used to diagnose syphilis, and by DNA homology, although genetic differences or signatures have emerged.[11,14,15] Hence, there arose a controversy as to whether the distinctions between these subspecies represent a biologic continuum or discrete agents.

In addition to the pathogenic spirochetes noted, a number of nonpathogenic treponemes have also been isolated from humans, particularly from the oral cavity and from the prepuce of uncircumcised men. Other organisms pathogenic for humans of the family Spirochaetaceae belong to the genera *Borrelia* and *Leptospira.*

The organisms are slender, tightly coiled, unicellular, helical cells 5 to 15 nm long and 0.09 to 0.18 nm wide. The cytoplasm is surrounded by a trilaminar membrane, peptidoglycan layer, delicate inner mucopeptide layer known as the periplast, outer lipoprotein membrane containing lipopolysaccharide, and phospholipid-rich outer membrane containing relatively few surface-exposed proteins.[16,17] This has led to the hypothesis that this microorganism acts as a "stealth" organism by minimizing the number of surface membrane–bound targets for the host's immune system to recognize until a sufficient number of spirochetes are present. The ends of the cells are tapered, and three fibrils are inserted into each end. The organism moves with a drifting, rotary, corkscrew motion and usually has a characteristic flexuose or undulating movement about its center, a distinctive feature used by experienced syphilologists to distinguish *T. pallidum* from other nonpathogenic treponemes on darkfield microscopy.

Unlike many nonpathogenic treponemes, the virulent treponemes, including *T. pallidum,* cannot be cultivated in vitro,[18,19] although limited multiplication can be obtained in tissue cultures. They have remained motile in highly enriched and specifically defined media for up to 7 days at 35°C and up to 48 hours at 37°C in a carbon dioxide–enriched environment. They can be maintained viable in liquid nitrogen, less so at −70°C, and in many mammals. Rabbits are the laboratory animals most commonly used for maintaining virulent organisms.

Because *T. pallidum* cannot be grown in vitro, it is difficult to study and determine its metabolic, physical, and pathogenic features. However, genomic sequencing has provided some insights by suggesting functional activities when its sequences are compared with those of other organisms for which the function is known.[20] The genome consists of a single circular chromosome of approximately 1,138,006 base pairs, which places it close to the lowest end of the range for bacteria. Unlike most pathogenic bacteria, its genome lacks apparent transposable elements, suggesting that the genome is extremely conserved and stable. This is the likely explanation of why *T. pallidum* has remained exquisitely sensitive to penicillin for more than 70 years and that there are few differences in DNA sequences among subspecies. Another striking feature is the relative paucity of genes involved in the biosynthesis of required nutrients or energy production. Hence, the spirochete apparently scavenges these necessary compounds from the host by transport proteins and uses only the glycolytic pathway for energy. Putative proteins that resemble hemolysins and cytotoxins have been identified but their functions have not been proven.[21]

Epidemiology

Syphilis can be acquired by sexual contact, passage through the placenta (congenital syphilis), kissing or other close contact with an active lesion, primarily a chancre or condyloma, transfusion of contaminated fresh human blood, or accidental direct inoculation.[1-3] The overwhelming majority of cases of syphilis are transmitted by sexual intercourse. A patient is most infectious early in the disease course, especially when a chancre, mucous patch, or condyloma latum is present, and gradually becomes less so over time. For all practical purposes, an immunologically intact person cannot spread syphilis by sexual contact after 4 years have elapsed since he or she acquired the illness.

Syphilis can be acquired from an infected person by kissing or touching an active lesion, which is most often present on the lips, oral cavity, breasts, or genitals. (Wet nurses occasionally spread the disease to infants, especially infants of upper class European families, for whom the employment of a wet nurse was a socially coveted status symbol.)

Congenital syphilis occurs most frequently when the fetus becomes infected in utero, although it is possible for the neonate to acquire the infection while passing through the birth canal.

Today, the acquisition of syphilis through transfused blood or blood products is now rare, at least in the developed world, because of the low incidence of disease, the requirement that all blood donors have a nonreactive nontreponemal blood test (see later) before their blood can be transfused, and because *T. pallidum* cannot survive longer than 24 to 48 hours under the current conditions of blood bank storage.

Accidental direct inoculation can occur by needlestick or during handling of infected clinical material. Syphilis of the fingers is most common in medical personnel.[22]

The number of reported new cases of syphilis in the United States has waxed and waned since the 1940s, reaching a peak incidence during World War II and, with the advent of penicillin and an aggressive public health approach, a nadir in the mid-1980s and late 1990s. The incidence rose again, dramatically, in the late 1980s and early 1990s before falling back to 1960 levels by 2000, only to rise again in specific subpopulation groups in the mid-2000s (Fig. 238-1). The highest incidence persists in the southeastern United States, from Maryland to Florida to eastern Texas and in the Southwest to southern California. Between 1986 and 1994, the rapid increase in new cases occurred strikingly among heterosexuals, as reflected by the dramatic increase of syphilis cases in women and neonates (congenital syphilis). This resurgence was linked to the exchange of sex for drugs, especially crack cocaine.[23] The smaller surge in the 2000s has been primarily in men who have sex with men (MSM). The reasons for this marked increase are likely multifold—disinhibition wrought by effective HIV treatment, the use of the Internet to meet partners, the practice of HIV serosorting, the increase in oral sex as a component of "safe sex."[24] Syphilis, nevertheless, remains a global health problem, with more than 12 million cases occurring yearly worldwide, especially in underdeveloped countries and eastern Europe, and with low-level endemicity in developed countries, with increased prevalence in specific subgroups.[24-26] Theoretically, syphilis can be eliminated by aggressive diagnostic, therapeutic, and follow-up measures.[27]

Most cases occur in the most sexually active age group (15 to 30 years of age in women, 15 to 54 years of age in men). Because contacts may be in the incubation phase and have no evidence of active disease,

aggressive contact tracing and empirical presumptive (epidemiologic treatment) of all recently exposed persons are important aspects of syphilis control. All contacts should be sought and empirically treated unless follow-up evaluations can be guaranteed.

Pathogenesis

Within hours to days after *T. pallidum* penetrates the intact mucous membrane or gains access through abraded skin, it enters the lymphatics and bloodstream and disseminates throughout the body. This is evidenced by the fact that persons who received blood transfusions from syphilitic donors in the seronegative incubation period have become infected. Almost any organ in the body can be invaded, especially the CNS.[1-3,28] The number of organisms that will establish an infection varies from patient to patient, but in rabbits an inoculum containing as few as four to eight spirochetes can result in an infection. The organism typically divides every 30 to 33 hours. Clinical lesions appear when a concentration of approximately 10^7 organisms/mg of tissue is reached. The incubation period is directly proportional to the size of the inoculum.[29,30]

In untreated cases, syphilis has traditionally been divided into the following stages: incubating, primary, secondary, early latent, late latent and late tertiary syphilis. The median incubation period is 3 weeks, but it may vary from 3 to 90 days. after which the spirochetal load expands enough to result in a chancre. This is followed in 2 to 8 weeks by immunologically mediated signs and symptoms of secondary syphilis. More than two thirds of untreated patients control their infection and do not progress to late disease. The spirochetal and host determinants of the eventual outcome are at least partially understood,[17,21,31] but it has been postulated that as in the case of many other chronic infections, the switch from a predominant Th1 (cellular) response to a Th2 (humoral) response is an important event signaling a favorable milieu for the parasite to develop into a chronic infection.[32] It has also been proposed that the paucity of proteins and lipoproteins on the outer membrane of the organism (stealth organism) contributes substantially to the organism's evasion of an effective host response,[16,17] and that antigenic variation may result in a subpopulation of spirochetes resistant to macrophage phagocytosis.[33]

The primary stage encompasses the development of the primary lesion, the chancre, which occurs at the site of inoculation. This usually painless solitary lesion does not develop in every case, or it may be so inconspicuous as to go unnoticed. Multiple chancres can occur, especially in immunocompromised persons (e.g., coinfected with HIV). Spirochetes are easily demonstrated in the lesions, especially early ones. Unless secondarily infected, chancres are conspicuously painless. They usually heal spontaneously in 2 to 8 weeks but may persist for longer periods, especially in immunocompromised hosts. (see later, HIV discussion)

The secondary or disseminated stage becomes evident 2 to 12 weeks (mean, 6 weeks) after contact. This generalized condition with parenchymal, constitutional, and mucocutaneous manifestations occurs when the greatest number of treponemes (high antigen load) is present in the body, particularly in the bloodstream. Treponemes can also be demonstrated in many other tissues, especially skin and lymph nodes. Abnormal laboratory findings and/or treponemes can be detected in the CNS, including the aqueous humor of the eye, in up to 40% of these patients.[1-3,28] The immune response of the host at this time becomes quite intense and is responsible for the more florid clinical signs and symptoms and pathologic consequences, such as an immune complex glomerulonephritis.[34]

After the secondary stage subsides, the untreated patient enters a latent period, during which the diagnosis can be made only by obtaining a positive serologic test response for syphilis. Because relapses of secondary syphilis in immunocompetent persons can occur up to 4 years after contracting syphilis, this period is divided into early latent (relapses possible) and late latent (relapses very unlikely) stages; 75% of relapses occur within the first year and are likely a consequence of waning immunity.[1-3,21] The term *late syphilis* refers both to the

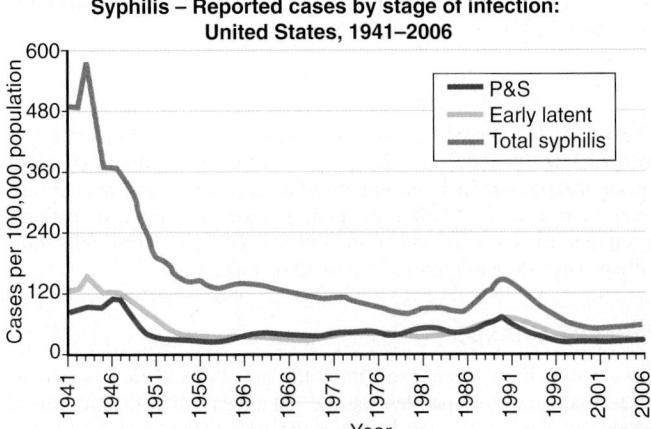

Figure 238-1 **Reported cases of syphilis, United States, 1941-2006.** *(Adapted from Centers for Disease Control and Prevention. STD Surveillance 2006: National Profile. Available at http://www.cdc.gov/std/stats06/figures/figure26.htm.)*

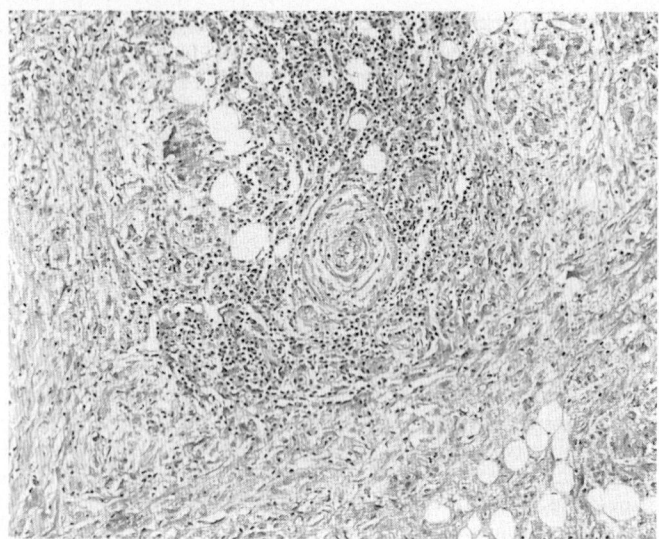

Figure 238-2 Characteristic obliterative endarteritis (hematoxylin and eosin, ×150).

clinically apparent and inapparent tertiary disease that develops in up to one third of untreated patients. Most of these lesions involve the vaso vasorum of the aorta, the small arteries of the CNS, or both; the rest consist of gummas, a unique granulomatous-like lesion with a coagulated or amorphous center and small-vessel endarteritis. The skin, liver, bones, CNS, and spleen are the most common sites in which gummas develop.

Pathologic Characteristics

Obliterative endarteritis, consisting of concentric endothelial and fibroblastic proliferative thickening, is highly suggestive of syphilis (Fig. 238-2).[2] These pathologic changes are found in all stages of syphilis. In the primary chancre, polymorphonuclear leukocytes and macrophages can often be demonstrated ingesting treponemes. Hyperkeratosis is frequently found in the skin lesions of secondary syphilis and is especially marked in condylomata. Treponemal antigens, immunoglobulin, and complement deposition in the glomeruli typical of immune complex glomerulonephritis can be demonstrated in patients who develop a nephrotic syndrome.[34] Obliterative endarteritis of the vaso vasorum and small blood vessels is the principal histopathologic finding in cardiovascular syphilis and meningovascular neurosyphilis. Appropriate staining (e.g., direct immunofluorescent antibody, immunohistochemical, or Warthin-Starry silver stain) or PCR assay can be used to demonstrate *T. pallidum*. In short, most of the pathogenesis of syphilis is the consequence of widespread microscopic vascular compromise caused by obliterative endarteritis.

Natural Course of Untreated Syphilis

The natural course of untreated syphilis was studied retrospectively in 1404 patients diagnosed clinically as having early syphilis (the Oslo study, 1891-1951).[35] There are obviously many shortcomings to this observational study, the most significant being the lack of laboratory confirmation of syphilis and the method of patient selection. (The darkfield and Wassermann tests were not available at the time the study was initiated.) However, because a similar study will never be done again, a brief review is warranted.

From 1890 to 1910, Professor Boeck of the University of Oslo, Norway, monitored patients diagnosed as having primary or secondary syphilis. Because he believed that the heavy metal–containing compounds used at that time for treatment were more harmful to the patient than the disease itself, all his patients were simply observed. Of these untreated patients, 28% developed relapsing secondary lesions

within 4 years, which led to the arbitrary designation of early latent and late latent syphilis. Twenty-eight percent eventually developed clinical complications of late syphilis; 10% developed cardiovascular syphilis, but this occurred only in patients who had acquired syphilis after 15 years of age; 6.5% developed symptomatic neurosyphilis; and 16% developed the late benign syphilis or gummas. Many of these patients had more than one "late" complication. Of those on whom autopsy was performed, 35% of the men and 22% of the women had evidence of cardiovascular involvement, especially aortitis. Syphilis was considered the primary cause of death in 15% of the men and 8% of the women. At least two thirds of these untreated patients cured themselves spontaneously.

A prospective study involving 431 African-American men with seropositive latent syphilis of 3 or more years' duration was undertaken in 1932 (the infamous Tuskegee study of 1932-1972; see earlier).This study suggested that hypertension in syphilitic black men 25 to 50 years of age was 17% more common than in black nonsyphilitic individuals. Cardiovascular complications including hypertension were more common than neurologic complications, and both were increased compared with control populations. Anatomic evidence of aortitis was found to be 25% to 35% more common in syphilitic patients on autopsy, and evidence of CNS syphilis was found in 4% of patients.[36]

A third large study, the Rosahn study, from 1917 to 1941, involving 382 autopsies of adults, revealed similar overall results.[37] Late syphilis was reported in 39% and approximately 20% were thought to have died because of these late complications. Of the late anatomic lesions at autopsy attributable to syphilis, 83% were cardiovascular, 8% were neurologic, and 9% were gummas.

These studies documented the variable waxing and waning course, the spontaneous clearing of *T. pallidum* in at least two thirds of infected persons, and an unpredictable progression of syphilis to late disease. There was an increased overall mortality in syphilitic compared with nonsyphilitic populations. The development of late complications was shown to occur about twice as often in men than in women, and a racial difference was suggested; black patients were more likely to develop cardiovascular syphilis, whereas white patients were more likely to develop neurosyphilis.

Clinical Manifestations

There was once an adage that "He who knows syphilis knows medicine." Penicillin therapy outdated this saying, but one of its legacies is the frequency of delayed and erroneous diagnoses that occur today because of the low incidence and subsequent unfamiliarity with the disease. As noted, the clinical manifestations are traditionally divided into incubating, early infectious primary and secondary stages lasting up to 4 years, often marked with periods of symptoms and signs, and latency, which progresses to a late or tertiary stage of tissue destruction in up to a third of untreated patients.

INCUBATING SYPHILIS

The median incubation period before clinical manifestations is 21 days (range, 3 to 90 days). An early spirochetemia inevitably develops during this phase, which sets the stage for secondary invasion of almost every body organ.[1,2,9] Left untreated, at least two thirds of patients spontaneously clear the infection, and the remaining third will clinically progress to late syphilis in 5 to 30 or more years.

PRIMARY SYPHILIS

The classic primary chancre begins at the site of inoculation as a single, occasionally multiple, painless papule.[38] It appears after the incubation period, quickly erodes, and becomes indurated (Figs. 238-3 and 238-4). The base is usually smooth; the borders are raised and firm and have a characteristic cartilaginous consistency. Unless secondarily infected, the ulcer has a clean appearance and no exudate; it is painless or slightly tender to the touch, a conspicuous aspect of the ulcerative

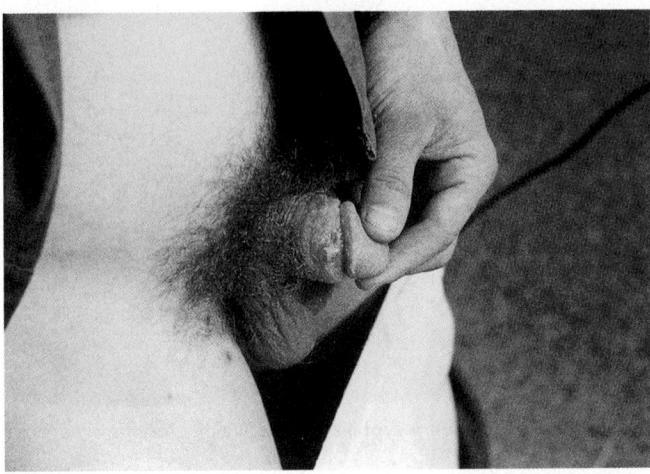

Figure 238-3 **Classic primary chancre of syphilis.** Primary syphilitic chancre of the penis.

lesion, and there is little pain or bleeding when the ulcer is scraped, such as when a specimen is obtained for a microscopic examination. Multiple chancres can occur, especially in persons who are immunosuppressed as those coinfected with HIV.[24,39] Atypical lesions occur in up to 57% of cases, and the absence of a primary skin lesion is also a possibility. The variations in presentation depend on the number of treponemes inoculated, the immune status of the patient, intercurrent antibiotic therapy, and whether the lesion becomes secondarily infected. In human volunteers with no evidence of a previous infection, a small inoculum produces only a papular lesion and a large inoculum produces an ulcerative lesion (chancre) in which treponemes can easily be identified. Persons with a history of a previous syphilitic infection may fail to develop any lesions or develop only a small darkfield-negative papule, depending on how long their natural infection went untreated.[29] Therefore, any genital lesion should raise the suspicion of syphilis, and appropriate studies to establish the diagnosis should be undertaken.

The chancre is located wherever the inoculation occurred. The external genitalia are most frequently involved. Other common sites include the cervix, mouth, perianal area, and anal canal in the female and the perianal area, anal canal, and mouth in homosexual men. A secondary infection of the primary lesion is more common with oral and anal lesions. Regional lymphadenopathy consisting of moderately enlarged, firm, nonsuppurative, painless lymph nodes or satellite buboes usually accompanies the primary lesion.

The chancre heals on its own within 3 to 6 weeks (range, 1 to 12 weeks), leaving either no trace or a thin atrophic scar. The lymphadenopathy usually persists for a longer period. The manifestations of secondary syphilis often develop while the chancre is still present,[1,2] especially in untreated HIV-infected patients.[39]

Pathologically, the chancre is characterized by an intense infiltration of plasma cells and scattered histiocytes, a concentric endothelial and fibroblastic proliferative thickening of small blood vessels and, eventually, the omnipresent and almost diagnostic obliterative endarteritis.[2] Spirochetes can be identified by silver, immunofluorescent, or other specific antibody staining methods or PCR assay (see later).

Primary syphilis must be differentiated principally from herpes virus infections, chancroid, and traumatic superinfected genital lesions. Primary genital herpes usually begins as a painful erythematous rash that develops into clusters of vesicles accompanied by regional lymphadenopathy and systemic symptoms. It runs a 10- to 14-day course in immunocompetent patients. Recurrent genital herpes is less florid and is characterized by mild to moderately painful vesicles and no lymphadenopathy. A syphilitic rash is never vesicular, except in congenital syphilis.[40] Chancroid is characterized by one or more painful, exudative, indurated ulcers associated with tender lymphadenopathy that eventually suppurate if left untreated. The ulcer has overhanging edges and bleeds easily (e.g., when scrapings are collected for a darkfield examination). Early venereal warts, granuloma inguinale, lymphogranuloma venereum, tuberculosis, atypical mycobacterial infections, tularemia, sporotrichosis, anthrax, rat bite fever, or any genital ulcer may resemble early primary syphilis.

SECONDARY SYPHILIS

The term *secondary (disseminated) syphilis* is used to describe the clinically most florid stage of the infection; it results from multiplication and wide dissemination of the spirochete and lasts until a sufficient host response develops to exert some immune control over the spirochete. It usually begins 2 to 8 weeks after the appearance of a chancre, but this period is variable. The primary chancre may still be present.[1-2,38,39,41] When the host's local immune process appears to be bringing the primary lesions under control, the spirochete disseminates widely and achieves its greatest numbers or antigenic load. Serologic tests are always positive in immunocompetent hosts and it is during this stage that the prozone phenomenon is most likely to occur (see later).

The manifestations of secondary syphilis are widespread and protean (Table 238-1). The classic and most commonly recognized lesions involve the skin. Nonpruritic macular, maculopapular, papular, or pustular lesions, and combinations and variations thereof, all occur.[1,2,41] Vesicular lesions are conspicuously absent, except in

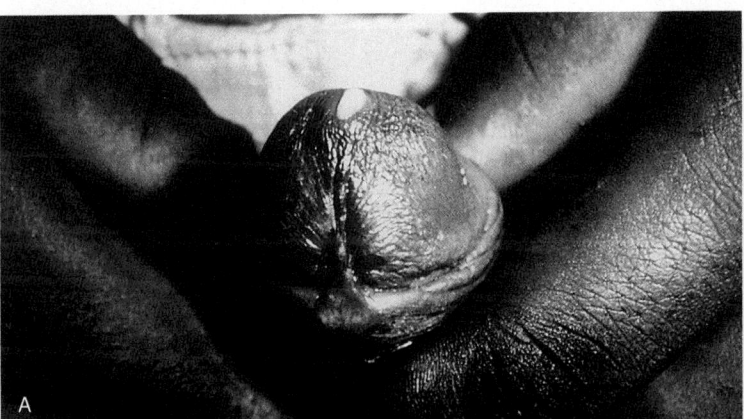
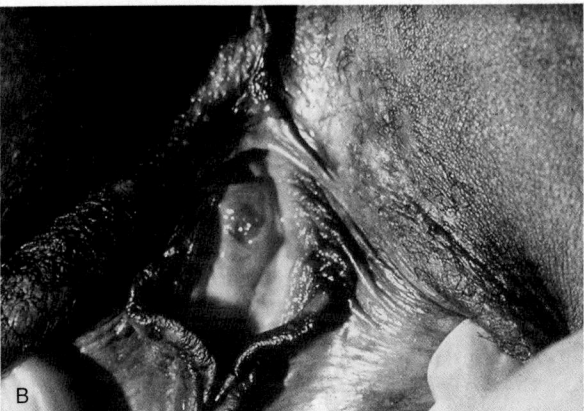

Figure 238-4 **Classic primary chancres of syphilis. A,** Primary syphilitic chancre coinfection with a pustular urethritis. **B,** Primary syphilitic chancre of the perineum.

TABLE 238-1	Clinical Manifestations of Secondary Syphilis	
Manifestation	**Percentage of Cases**	
Skin	90	
Rash*		
Macular		
Maculopapular		
Papular		
Pustular		
Condyloma latum		
Generalized lymphadenopathy		
Mouth and throat	35	
Mucous patches		
Erosions		
Ulcer (aphthous)		
Genital lesion	20	
Chancre		
Condyloma latum		
Mucous patch		
Constitutional symptoms	70	
Fever of unknown origin		
Malaise		
Pharyngitis, laryngitis		
Anorexia, weight loss		
Arthralgias		
Central nervous system	8-40	
Asymptomatic		
Symptomatic	1-2	
Headache		
Meningismus		
Meningitis		
Ocular		
Diplopia		
Impaired vision		
Otitic		
Tinnitus		
Vertigo		
Cranial nerve involvement (II-VIII)		
Renal	Unusual	
Glomerulonephritis		
Nephrotic syndrome		
Gastrointestinal	Unusual	
Hepatitis	Unusual	
Intestinal wall invasion	Unusual	
Arthritis, osteitis, and periostitis	Unusual	

*Commonly involves the palms and soles.

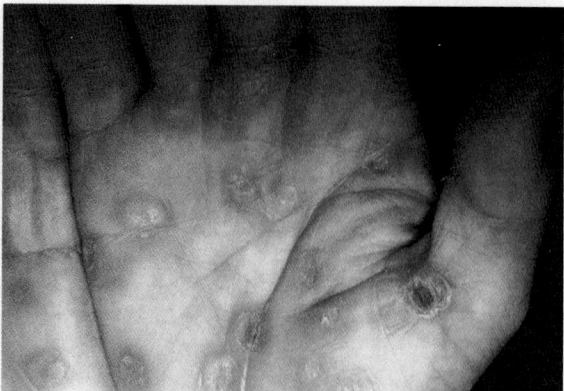

Figure 238-5 **Secondary syphilis lesions.** Palmar lesions of secondary syphilis.

painless, broad, moist, gray-white to erythematous highly infectious plaques termed *condylomata lata*. These highly infectious lesions teeming with spirochetes may also develop on mucous membranes (e.g., lips, mouth, pharynx, tonsils, vulva, vagina, glans penis, inner prepuce, cervix, anal canal). These lesions, referred to as *mucous patches*, typically manifest as a silvery gray, superficial erosion with a red periphery (Fig. 238-6). These lesions are nonpainful or minimally painful unless secondarily infected.

During relapses of secondary syphilis, the skin lesions tend to be less florid, asymmetrically distributed, and more infiltrated, suggesting a more effective host immune response. Condylomata lata, however, are common.

Constitutional symptoms are also commonly present in secondary syphilis. These manifestations include low-grade fever, malaise, pharyngitis, laryngitis, anorexia, weight loss, arthralgias, and generalized painless lymphadenopathy. Enlargement of the epitrochlear lymph nodes is a unique finding that should always suggest the diagnosis of syphilis.[1-3,41]

The CNS becomes involved in up to 40% of patients[1,2,28,42,43] as a result of seeding during the inevitable early spirochetemia. Headache and meningismus are common, increased cerebrospinal fluid (CSF) protein levels and lymphocyte counts are found in 8% to 40% of patients, and acute symptomatic aseptic meningitis occurs in 1% to 2% of patients. Importantly, spirochetes have also been isolated from the CSF of patients with no CSF abnormalities. Individual cranial nerves, especially II through VIII, can be involved.[44,45] Visual disturbances, hearing loss, tinnitus, and facial weakness are the most common manifestations. Syphilitic paraplegia (Erb's paralysis) and amyotrophic meningomyeli-

congenital syphilis. These skin lesions usually begin on the trunk and proximal extremities as bilateral, pink to red, discrete macular lesions 3 to 10 mm in diameter. Any surface area of the body can become involved. These lesions usually persist from a few days to 8 weeks and often evolve from macules into red papules (hence the term *maculopapular*); in a few patients, they finally progress to pustular lesions termed *pustular syphilids*. The degree of endarteritis and perivascular mononuclear infiltration progresses in the same manner. All the different rashes may be present at one time and may become widely distributed to involve the entire body, especially on the palms and soles, locations that strongly suggest the diagnosis (Fig. 238-5). When the hair follicles are involved (follicular syphilids), temporary patchy alopecia or thinning and a loss of eyebrows and beard may develop. Sometimes, a superficial scaling occurs (papulosquamous syphilids). In warm, moist intertriginous areas (e.g., perianal area, vulva, scrotum, inner aspects of the thighs, skin under pendulous breasts, nasolabial folds, cleft of the chin, axillary and antecubital folds, webs of the fingers and toes), the papules can enlarge, coalesce, and erode to produce

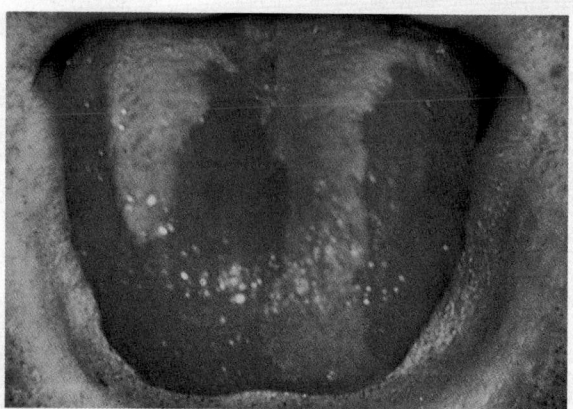

Figure 238-6 **Secondary syphilis lesion.** Mucous patch lesion of secondary syphilis.

tis characterized by the insidious onset of asymmetrical paraparesis, hyperreflexia, Babinski's sign, sphincter disturbances, spastic neurogenic bladder, and minimal back pain may occur. A waxing and waning of clinical manifestations, a classic clinical hallmark of secondary and early latent syphilis, may occur. In a significant portion of untreated patients CNS involvement (8% to 10%) will progress to late neurosyphilis. Computed tomography (CT) scanning and magnetic resonance imaging (MRI) have improved our ability to diagnose and follow patients at all stages of neurosyphilis.[46-48]

Because of the omnipresent spirochetemia, almost any organ of the body can be involved. Renal involvement may be in the form of an immune complex glomerulonephritis (subepithelial electron-dense deposits). Proteinuria is common, an acute nephrotic syndrome may develop and, rarely, hemorrhagic glomerulonephritis can occur.[34]

Syphilitic hepatitis is characterized by a disproportionately high serum alkaline phosphatase level, a normal or moderately elevated serum bilirubin concentration, and a histologic picture that includes moderate inflammation with polymorphonuclear cells and lymphocytes and some hepatocellular damage, but no cholestasis.[49] It occurs most often in conjunction with syphilitic proctitis and is seen most frequently in persons who engage in anal intercourse.

The gastrointestinal tract may also become extensively infiltrated, ulcerated, or both,[50] which can be misdiagnosed as a lymphoma or other cancers.

Anterior or panuveitis, usually mild and asymptomatic, occurs in 5% to 10% of patients with secondary syphilis, especially in HIV coinfected persons. The diagnosis is suggested whenever the uveitis is made worse by steroid treatment.[51-54]

Otosyphilis is manifested by sensorineural sudden or progressive hearing loss, tinnitus, vertigo, and dysequilibrium.[55,56]

Synovitis, osteitis, and periosteitis can also occur.[57,58] These cases are often characterized by nocturnal pain that is conspicuously increased by heat. Unusual manifestations such as bone resorption of the hands and feet (acro-osteolysis) can also occur.

The differential diagnosis of secondary syphilis is extensive. The appellation "the great imitator" or "great impostor" is appropriate.

LATENT SYPHILIS

Latent syphilis is by definition the stage of the disease during which a specific treponemal antibody test—fluorescent treponemal antibody absorption (FTA-ABS), TPPA test, *T. pallidum* hemagglutination (TPHA) or microhemagglutination for *T. pallidum* (MHA-TP), enzyme-linked immunosorbent assay (ELISA), *T. pallidum* immobilization (TPI) test, particle gel immunoassay (PaGIA)—is positive but there are no clinical manifestations of syphilis, including a normal CSF cell count and protein and glucose levels and a normal chest radiograph. However, it does not imply a lack of progression of disease, only that clinical signs and symptoms are absent. A history compatible with primary or secondary syphilis, or other sexually transmitted disease, exposure to a syphilitic person, or delivery of an infant with congenital syphilis should be sought. Early latent syphilis distinguishes the period (first 4 years) during which a clinical relapse may occur and, therefore, the patient is infectious. Ninety percent of the relapses occur in the first year, and each recurring episode is less florid. Mucocutaneous relapses are the most common.

Late latent syphilis, at least in immunocompetent patients, is associated with host resistance to reinfection and to infectious relapse.[1,2,29] However, a pregnant woman with late latent syphilis can infect her fetus in utero, and an infection can sometimes be transmitted via transfused contaminated blood.

LATE SYPHILIS

Late syphilis (tertiary syphilis) is a slowly progressive destructive inflammatory disease that can affect any organ in the body to produce clinical illness 5 to 30 or more years after the initial infection. It is generally subdivided into neurosyphilis, cardiovascular syphilis, gum-

TABLE 238-2	Indications for CSF Examination in a Syphilitic Patient
Neurologic, otologic, or ophthalmologic signs and symptoms
Late or late latent syphilis
Treatment failure (clinical recurrence or persistence of signs and symptoms, lack of nontreponemal serologic response: fourfold decrease at 24-60 mo or fourfold increase at any time).
VDRL/RPR blood titer ≥ 32

CSF, cerebrospinal fluid; RPR, rapid plasma reagin test; VDRL, Venereal Disease Research Laboratory test.

matous syphilis, and sometimes leutic osteitis (moth-eaten appearance of involved bone on radiographic studies).[1-3]

Late Neurosyphilis

The diagnosis of neurosyphilis requires an examination of the CSF (Table 238-2). Because the CNS is often invaded during the early septicemic phase, neurologic manifestations can occur during any phase or stage of the disease. Therefore, neurosyphilis is classified as acute neurosyphilis and late (chronic) neurosyphilis[1,2,42,44,45] (see Fig. 238-2). Late neurosyphilis is usually further divided into asymptomatic and symptomatic phases; the latter is further distinguished as meningovascular or parenchymatous neurosyphilis (Table 238-3). Although this classification recognizes the existence of distinctive forms of neurosyphilis that correlate with pathologic findings, there is almost always clinical overlap with combinations of meningovascular and parenchymatous features. This is not surprising, because neurosyphilis is fundamentally a chronic meningitis involving every portion of the CNS. The diagnosis of asymptomatic neurosyphilis is given to patients who have no clinical manifestation of neurologic involvement but who have one or more CSF abnormalities—pleocytosis, elevated protein concentration, decreased glucose level, or positive nontreponemal test result (e.g., VDRL/RPR), local CNS production of antibodies to *T. pallidum*, positive PCR assay, serum RPR ≥ 1:32, and suggestive CT results, which are highly suggestive of an active case of replicating spirochetes (neurosyphilis).[46-48,59-67] Asymptomatic neurosyphilis is the most common presentation of neurosyphilis.

The incidence of asymptomatic *acute* neurosyphilis in untreated patients ranges from 8% to as high as 40%, and 4% to 10% of these patients will progress to symptomatic *late* neurosyphilis. With the exception of the presentation of the highly suggestive Argyll Robertson pupil or tabes dorsalis, the symptoms and signs of neurosyphilis are nonspecific (Table 238-4), and there is evidence to suggest that

TABLE 238-3	Classification of Neurosyphilis	
Manifestation		**Percentage of Cases** (*N* = 676)
Syphilitic meningitis as a complication of secondary syphilis		8-40
Asymptomatic		7-38
Symptomatic		1-2
Asymptomatic late neurosyphilis		31
Symptomatic late neurosyphilis		69
Meningovascular		
Cerebromeningeal		6
Diffuse		
Focal		
Cerebrovascular		10
Spinal		3
Parenchymatous		
Tabetic		30
Paretic		12
Taboparetic		3
Ocular		3
Miscellaneous		2

Adapted from Merritt HH, Moore M. Acute neurosyphilitic meningitis. *Medicine (Baltimore)*. 1935;14:119.

TABLE 238-4	Clinical Manifestations of Neurosyphilis

Meningovascular
  Hemiplegia or hemiparesis
  Seizures
    Generalized
    Focal
  Aphasia

Parenchymatous
  General paresis
    Changes in personality, affect, sensorium, intellect, insight, and judgment
    Hyperactive reflexes
    Speech disturbances (slurring)
    Pupillary disturbances (Argyll Robertson pupils)
    Optic atrophy tremors (face, tongue, hands, legs)
  Tabes dorsalis
    Shooting or lightning pains into lower back or lower legs
    Ataxia
    Pupillary disturbances (Argyll Robertson pupils)
    Impotence
    Bladder disturbances
    Fecal incontinence
    Peripheral neuropathy
    Romberg sign
    Cranial nerve involvement (II-VII)

Adapted from Merritt HH, Moore M. Acute neurosyphilitic meningitis. *Medicine (Baltimore).* 1935;14:119.

symptomatic neurosyphilis may be present in as many as 4% of patients with normal CSF findings. Asymptomatic neurosyphilis is curable, a lumbar puncture is necessary to make the diagnosis of asymptomatic neurosyphilis, and asymptomatic neurosyphilis occurs in up to 40% of patients. Therefore, a lumbar puncture should be considered as part of the follow-up care for anyone who has neurologic, otologic or ophthalmologic signs and symptoms that could be attributable to syphilis, failed to have a nontreponemal serologic response (see later), had an increase in nontreponemal titer, has latent or late syphilis, or may have been treated inadequately to clear the CNS of treponemes (e.g., with benzathine penicillin; see Table 238-2).

Late symptomatic neurosyphilis is divided into two major clinical categories that have been correlated with pathologic findings: meningovascular neurosyphilis and parenchymatous neurosyphilis (see Table 238-4), but a great deal of clinical overlap occurs. (As noted, syphilitic meningitis clinically resembling aseptic meningitis may occur during early syphilis, especially during the secondary stage.) The term *meningovascular neurosyphilis* refers to the development of typical endarteritis obliterans, which affects the small blood vessels of the meninges, brain, and spinal cord and leads to multiple small areas of infarction. The term *parenchymatous neurosyphilis* refers to the actual destruction of nerve cells, principally in the cerebral cortex. The former condition represents an inflammatory process and the latter a degenerative one, but a mixture of the two pathologic processes is almost always present.

Vascular involvement (meningovascular neurosyphilis) may lead to a wide spectrum of manifestations, ranging from focal ischemia and stroke to progressive neurologic deficits, as a result of the gradual destruction of nerve tissue by small-vessel endarteritis. Hemiparesis, aphasia, and focal or generalized seizures may occur.[1-3,42,44,45]

Parenchymatous neurosyphilis[1-3,45,45a] includes general paresis (cortical involvement) and tabes dorsalis (spinal cord involvement). It is the result of widespread parenchymal damage and represents a combination of psychiatric manifestations and neurologic findings. Abnormalities correspond to the mnemonic PARESIS: **p**ersonality (emotional lability, paranoia), **a**ffect (carelessness in appearance), **r**eflexes (hyperactive); **e**ye (Argyll Robertson pupils), **s**ensorium (illusions, delusions, especially megalomania, hallucinations), **i**ntellect (decreased recent memory, judgment, insight), and **s**peech (slurred). Spinal cord damage involves principally demyelinization of the posterior column, dorsal roots, and dorsal root ganglia, which eventually results in the development of an ataxic, wide-based gait and foot slap, paresthesias, shooting or lightning pains (sudden onset, rapid radiation, and disappearance),

bladder disturbances, fecal incontinence, impotence, loss of position and vibratory sense, absent ankle and knee jerk reflexes, and loss of deep pain and temperature sensation. The Romberg sign (inability to stand with feet together and eyes closed without falling over) is classically present in patients with tabes dorsalis because of damage to the posterior columns. Trophic degenerative joint disease, known as Charcot's joints, and traumatic ulcers or sores on the lower extremities and feet resulting from the loss of sensation were prominently featured in textbooks of physical diagnosis published before the antibiotic era.

Ocular disturbances are common whenever the CNS is invaded. The Argyll Robertson pupil refers to a small irregular pupil that accommodates to near vision but does not react to light or painful stimuli. Optic atrophy occurs over a period of months to years, beginning peripherally and proceeding to the center of the nerve, producing progressive concentric constriction of the visual fields with retention of normal vision. This is referred to as gun barrel sight.

Any inflammatory manifestation of the eye can be caused by syphilitic involvement.[51-54,68] Anterior or posterior uveitis or panuveitis is the most common abnormal finding and appears to be increased in HIV coinfected persons; other ocular findings include episcleritis, vitreitis, retinitis, papillitis, interstitial keratitis, acute retinal necrosis, and retinal detachment. They may occur during any stage such as an accompanying manifestation of acute syphilitic meningitis or an isolated manifestation of secondary syphilis. Unless scarring has occurred, improvement with treatment can be dramatic.[69] The differential diagnosis of other systemic diseases includes tuberculosis, rheumatoid arthritis, sarcoidosis, toxoplasmosis, histoplasmosis, and ocular *Toxocara canis* infections.

Although any cranial nerve can be affected, those most commonly involved are the seventh and eighth cranial nerves (40%). Involvement results in the gradual development of a loss of facial expression; tremors of the lips, tongue, and facial muscles and difficulty enunciating multisyllable words (e.g., Methodist, Episcopal). The second, third, and fourth cranial nerves are the next most commonly affected (25%).

Meningovascular syphilis usually occurs 5 to 10 years after the onset of early syphilis, general paresis 15 to 20 years later, and tabes dorsalis 25 to 30 years later.

Another distinct variant of neurosyphilis is syphilitic otitis or otosyphilis.[48,55,56] The ear may be involved during any stage of the disease, including congenital syphilis. Otosyphilis is diagnosed by a combination of clinical findings, positive nontreponemal or treponemal serologic evidence of syphilis, and exclusion of other causes of sensorineural hearing loss. Symptoms include progressive and sudden unilateral or bilateral deafness, tinnitus, vertigo, and dysequilibrium. This may be the only clinically apparent symptom at presentation, and it usually presents a diagnostic dilemma, especially because the CSF parameters are often normal. In early stages, syphilitic otitis is curable[69]; if untreated, it causes irreversible damage. A positive treponemal antibody test (e.g., TPPA, TPHA, MHA-TP, EIA, FTA-ABS) is found in approximately 7% of patients with otherwise unexplained sensorineural hearing loss that is usually unilateral and in 7% of patients with cochleovestibular dysfunction (Ménière's disease), making neurosyphilis a significant cause of these disorders. Congenital otic syphilis is usually bilateral and more severe than otic involvement caused by acquired syphilis. Specialized diagnostic procedures may be required,[67] but any patient with unexplained hearing loss or vestibular disturbances who has a positive treponemal antibody test result should be treated for possible syphilitic otitis (see later).

The conditions from which neurosyphilis must be differentiated are numerous. They include any degenerative neurologic process, disorders that cause chronic inflammation (e.g., tuberculosis, fungal, parasitic, or sarcoid meningitis, tumors, subdural hematoma, Alzheimer's disease/dementia, multiple sclerosis, chronic alcoholism), and any chronic disorder that affects the vasculature of the CNS (e.g., cerebrovascular disease). The axiom that syphilis can mimic any disease is particularly apropos with regard to CNS involvement.

Given the vagaries of neurosyphilis (e.g., no routinely available single sensitive or specific test, no diagnostic clinical presentation), the clinician must use a combination of clinical and laboratory data to make the diagnosis. In modern medicine, one is loath to label a patient with a specific infectious diagnosis without specific identification of the infecting organism by culture, PCR assay, or pathologic demonstration. However, because *T. pallidum* cannot be cultured in vitro and isolation in animals is restricted to research laboratories, serologic or antibody tests alone are most often relied on to diagnose and monitor these patients. The demonstration of specific treponemal immunoglobulin G (IgG) and IgM antibody production (immunoblotting) in the CNS is helpful, and the PCR assay establishes the presence of the causative agent but not necessarily live or replicating organisms.[43,59-67,70]

The aim of treatment has been to develop a rational and safe therapeutic approach so that the patient has a reasonable expectation that the disease will be cured or will not progress to a severe neurologic disability or other late manifestation. When choosing treatment approaches, several considerations must be taken into account. First, a spirochetemia and immune response always occurs in patients with untreated syphilis. Therefore, except in patients with immune dysfunction (e.g., HIV infection), the diagnosis of neurosyphilis cannot be made without a positive serum nontreponemal antibody response (e.g., TPPA, TPHA, FTA-ABS, MHA-TP, EIA, PaGIA). Second, a positive CSF VDRL or CSF RPR test result always indicates active neurosyphilis. Third, a positive PCR test in the CSF establishes that CNS invasion has occurred but does not necessarily establish that the infection is active and the spirochetes are replicating.[70] Fourth, any CSF abnormality in the appropriate clinical setting and without an alternative explanation strongly suggests active neurosyphilis. Fifth, local CNS production of antitreponemal antibody is highly suggestive of neurosyphilis.[63] Therefore, any patient with a positive specific serum treponemal antibody test, a positive CSF VDRL/RPR, a positive CSF PCR, or evidence of local CNS antibody production with or without otherwise explained neurologic findings warrants therapy for neurosyphilis (see later).

Cardiovascular Syphilis

The underlying pathologic lesion of cardiovascular syphilis is the omnipresent endarteritis obliterans, in this case involving the vaso vasorum of the aorta. This results in a medial necrosis with destruction of elastic tissue and subsequent aortitis, with a saccular (or occasionally a fusiform) aneurysm. There is a predilection to involve the ascending aorta, which leads to weakness of the aortic valve ring and distortion of the cups and results in aortic regurgitation and coronary artery stenosis.[1-3,71] The transverse segment of the aortic arch is the next most frequently involved area; the aorta below the renal arteries is seldom involved. Symptomatic syphilitic aortitis occurs in approximately 10% of untreated cases, but the pathologic lesions can be demonstrated on postmortem examination in up to 83% of cases of untreated neurosyphilis. Asymptomatic syphilitic aortitis should be suspected whenever linear calcifications of the ascending aorta are noted on chest radiographs, a finding seldom seen in arteriosclerotic disease. Because of the inflammation-induced scarring, syphilitic aneurysms rarely dissect. Compression of surrounding mediastinal structures, such as the recurrent laryngeal nerve or other large arteries (e.g., temporal artery), may also be involved, Although once a common cause of cardiovascular disease, the success of antibiotic treatment has made cardiovascular syphilis a medical curiosity in developed countries.

Late Benign Syphilis (Gumma)

The gumma is a nonspecific, granulomatous-like lesion that occurs in late syphilis[1-3] but is rarely seen today. These indolent lesions are most commonly found in the skeletal system, skin, and mucocutaneous tissues but can develop in any organ. They may be single or multiple and vary in size from microscopic defects to large, tumor-like masses. They are of clinical importance principally as a cause of local destruction. The cutaneous manifestations range from superficial nodules to deep granulomatous lesions, which may break down to form punched-out ulcers. Involution is followed by the development of a thin, atro-

phic, noncontractile scar arranged in arciform patterns. Gummatous hepatitis may cause low-grade fever, epigastric pain and tenderness, and eventually cirrhosis (hepar lobatum). Gummas of the bone may result in fractures or joint destruction, whereas those in the upper respiratory tract can lead to perforation of the nasal system or palate. Gummas of the CNS present like any other space-occupying lesion. Trauma may predispose to involvement of a specific site. Gummas must be distinguished from other granulomatous lesions (e.g., tuberculosis, sarcoidosis, deep fungal infections) and from neoplasms. The spirochetes in these lesions are difficult to visualize on microscopic examination. A therapeutic trial of penicillin or other effective antibiotics results in a rapid and dramatic response. Gummas were the most common late complication seen in the Oslo study described earlier (approximately 15%).

CONGENITAL SYPHILIS

Infection of the fetus in utero can occur at any stage of infection in any untreated or inadequately treated mother but is most likely to occur during the spirochetemia of early syphilis. The risk of fetal infection decreases progressively thereafter. Infection of the fetus before the fourth month of gestation is unusual; therefore, early abortion is unlikely to be a result of syphilis. Adequate treatment of the mother usually but not always ensures that the fetus will not be infected. A serum VDRL/RPR higher than 1:16 and primary, secondary, and early latent syphilis in the mother during pregnancy or more than 30 days since treatment are associated with a congenitally infected neonate.[67,72-76] Depending on the severity of the infection, late abortion, stillbirth, neonatal death, neonatal disease, or latent infection may be seen.[1,2] These manifestations appear to be caused largely by dysfunction of the maternal-fetal endocrine axis, which results in decreased levels of dehydroepiandrosterone produced by the fetal adrenal glands. Of neonates with congenital syphilis, 6% to 7% will be stillborn, especially in untreated or inadequately treated mothers.

The clinical pattern is variable, but often there are no abnormal physical findings (Table 238-5).[1,2] In the perinatal period (infantile

TABLE 238-5	Clinical Signs of Congenital Syphilis	
Manifestation		**Percentage of Cases**
Early		55
Osteochondritis		
Snuffles		40
Rash		40
Anemia		30
Hepatosplenomegaly		20
Jaundice		20
Neurologic signs		20
Lymphadenopathy		5
Mucous patches		5
Late		
Frontal bosses		
Short maxillas		
Saddle nose		
Protruding mandible		
Interstitial keratitis		
Eighth nerve deafness		
High palatal arch		
Hutchinson's incisors		
Mulberry molars		
Sternoclavicular thickening (Higoumenaki's sign)		
Clutton's joints (bilateral painless swelling of knees)		
Saber shins		
Flaring scapulas		

Data from Kampmeier RH. *Essentials of Syphilogy.* 3rd ed. Philadelphia: JB Lippincott; 1943; and Stokes JH, Beerman H, Ingraham NR. *Modern Clinical Syphilogy: Diagnosis, Treatment: Case Study.* 3rd ed. Philadelphia: WB Saunders; 1945.

form), the most striking lesions affect the mucocutaneous tissues, liver, and bones. The earliest sign of congenital syphilis is usually a rhinitis (snuffles), which is soon followed by a diffuse, maculopapular, desquamative rash with extensive sloughing of the epithelium, particularly on the palms, on the soles, and about the mouth and anus. In contrast to acquired syphilis in the adult, a vesicular rash and bullae may develop. These lesions are teeming with spirochetes and have the characteristic obliterative endarteritis and perivascular mononuclear cuffing on microscopic examination that are found in other syphilitic lesions.

The liver is often heavily infected, with associated splenomegaly, anemia, thrombocytopenia, and jaundice. The generalized spirochetemia may lead to diffuse inflammatory changes of almost any organ of the body. Neonatal death is usually the result of liver failure, severe pneumonia, hypopituitarism, or pulmonary hemorrhage. Renal involvement with an immune complex glomerulonephritis may develop and usually occurs at about the fourth month of life.[34] A generalized osteochondritis and perichondritis or periostitis may affect the architecture of all bones of the skeletal system, but are most prominent in the long bones and can be easily discerned on radiographs. As in adults, CNS involvement is common, occurring in at least 22% of neonates; the CSF VDRL/RPR, cell count, and protein and glucose level determinations are of low sensitivity. Importantly, although CNS involvement is most often associated with an abnormal physical examination, conventional laboratory tests, and radiologic studies, some infants can be identified only by IgM immunoblotting of the serum or CSF or by PCR assay.[67] Neonatal congenital syphilis must be differentiated from other generalized congenital infections such as rubella, cytomegalovirus infection, and toxoplasmosis.

With a few exceptions, the untreated child who survives the first 6 to 12 months of life enters a latent period. The generalized osteochondritis, perichondritis, and periostitis may result in deformities of the nose (saddle nose) and the metaphyses of the lower extremities (anterior bowing, or saber shin). The late development of cardiovascular syphilis is rare, but interstitial keratitis is common. Photophobia, pain, circumcorneal inflammation, and superficial and deep vascularization of the cornea may occur at any time between the ages of 5 and 30 years. Asymptomatic or symptomatic neurosyphilis is also common in these patients and resembles the disease in adults. Eighth nerve deafness is particularly common. Necrotizing funisitis, an inflammatory process involving the matrix of the umbilical cord and characterized by perivascular inflammation and obliterative endarteritis, is for all practical purposes pathognomonic of congenital syphilis.[77] This disease should be suspected clinically whenever the umbilical cord is swollen and discolored red, white, and blue to resemble a barber's pole, or has a positive cord blood VDRL/RPR or PCR assay result.

Other late characteristic stigmata include recurrent arthropathy and bilateral knee effusions (Clutton's joints), centrally notched, widely spread, peg-shaped upper central incisors (Hutchinson's teeth), frontal bossing, and poorly developed maxillas.[1,2] Because at least one third of the mothers who give birth to syphilitic children have not had prenatal care and about half have had a nonreactive serologic test during the first trimester of pregnancy, serologic testing of the mother is always warranted at delivery, especially in high-risk patients. A complete evaluation of the neonate should include physical examination, routine conventional blood tests, bone radiographs, VDRL/RPR, and IgM immunoblotting on serum and CSF.[67,72-76] The best means is to combine IgM antibody determination (IgM immunoblotting) with PCR antigen detection (see later). Because giving penicillin to the neonate is almost risk-free, all neonates born to syphilitic mothers should be treated, regardless of whether the mother was treated during pregnancy.

Atypical Presentations

As noted, the clinical presentation and course of syphilis are varied, and the clinical diagnosis can sometimes elude the clinician, even under the best conditions. Because some patients may have been treated with antibiotics that are suboptimal (e.g., oral penicillin and,

in some cases, benzathine penicillin) or inadequate (e.g., macrolides, clindamycin, azithromycin), and because of the larger pool of immunocompromised HIV coinfected patients and the relative inexperience of the clinician with syphilitic patients, there is a sense that unusual patterns and atypical presentations have become more common. However, protean manifestations are the hallmark of syphilis. Older clinicians were never surprised by unusual or atypical findings, nor should clinicians today.

▣ Laboratory Diagnosis

The diagnosis of syphilis was and remains primarily indirect. Demonstration of spirochetes by a darkfield examination that does not discriminate *T. pallidum* from other spirochetes and nonspecific and specific treponemal antibody tests that yields false-positive test results are relatively common. However, direct immunostaining using antitreponemal antibodies or PCR assay establishes a more definitive diagnosis. Animal infectivity models are a research tool.

DIRECT EXAMINATION FOR SPIROCHETES

In primary, secondary, and early congenital syphilis, demonstrating the spirochete by immunostaining (e.g., direct immunofluorescent antibody [DFA] staining, immunohistochemical staining), PCR assay, or darkfield examination of mucocutaneous lesions is the quickest and most direct laboratory method of establishing the diagnosis.[1-3,78] Examination of a serous transudate from moist lesions such as a primary chancre, condyloma latum, or mucous patch is most productive because these lesions have the largest numbers of treponemes. However, *T. pallidum* can occasionally be demonstrated from dry skin lesions and from lymph nodes by saline aspiration (the saline must be free of bactericidal additives). For a darkfield examination, the surface of the suspected lesion should be cleaned with saline and gently abraded with dry gauze so as not to produce gross bleeding. The serous exudate can then be squeezed onto a glass slide, covered with a cover slip, and examined with darkfield or phase contrast microscopy. A drop of nonbactericidal saline may be added if the preparation is too thick. *T. pallidum* has a corkscrew appearance and moves in a spiraling motion, with a characteristic 90-degree undulation about its midpoint (Fig. 238-7). A lesion should be considered nonsyphilitic only after three negative examinations have been made. Specimens from mouth lesions are useless because *T. pallidum* cannot be distinguished with certainty from nonpathogenic treponemes. A scattering of a few red blood cells indicates that the specimen is adequate. Cleaning of the lesion with a topical antiseptic, soap, or bactericidal saline obscures the diagnosis because dead and nonmotile organisms are difficult to identify. However, if this is inadvertently done, direct or indirect immunofluorescent or immunohistochemical staining or PCR can be used to establish the presence of *T. pallidum*.

BIOPSY SPECIMEN

The spirochete can sometimes be demonstrated in biopsy materials. A Warthin-Starry silver stain is most commonly used, but confusion with elastic tissues can occur. Specific immunofluorescent or immunohistochemical staining of nonfrozen pathologic specimens or PCR assay is now preferred to silver staining to establish a more precise diagnosis.[79,80,80a]

SEROLOGIC TESTS

As noted, because *T. pallidum* cannot be routinely isolated and characterized and the ability to demonstrate *T. pallidum* in tissues is often not available (unlike almost all other microbial human pathogens), reliance on serologic tests has become the principal means of establishing the diagnosis. As with all serologic tests, however, sensitivity and specificity can be problematic, and these potential problems must be taken into account whenever the diagnosis is being considered. Fur-

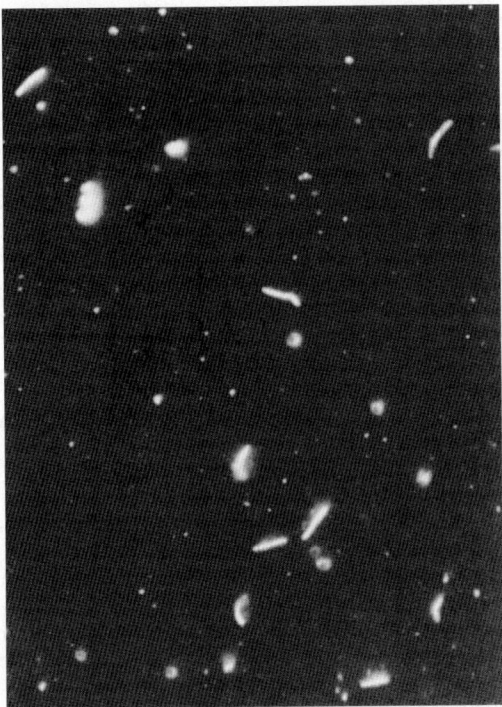

Figure 238-7 Darkfield examination. The morphologic characteristics of the spirochetes and the characteristic flexous motion about their centers can be appreciated (400×).

terminology, because it has nothing to do with the reagin IgE that is involved in allergic reactions. Syphilis reaginic antibodies are IgG and IgM antibodies directed against lipoidal antigens resulting from the interaction of host tissues with *T. pallidum* and/or from *T. pallidum* itself. The earliest cardiolipin antigens were crude extracts made from beef livers or beef hearts and false-positive reactions were common. The cardiolipin cholesterol lecithin used today is a much purer preparation and gives fewer false-positive reactions. The relationship of these tests to *T. pallidum* infection is fortuitous.

The standard nontreponemal test is the VDRL slide test, in which heated serum (56°C) is tested for its ability to flocculate or agglutinate a standardized suspension of a cardiolipin cholesterol lecithin antigen. It has distinct usefulness because it can also be used to monitor a patient's response to therapy. Most laboratories and blood banks have adapted the RPR card test modification for routine screening for syphilis and for following the response to therapy. Some use the automated reagin test (ART) or the toluidine red unheated syphilis test (TRUST). A prozone phenomenon occurs in up to 2% of infected persons, especially in secondary syphilis and pregnancy,[84] and appropriate dilutions should be performed whenever the index of suspicion is high (e.g., patients with another sexually transmitted disease, pregnant women, IV drug abusers, HIV coinfected individuals). A fourfold change in titer using the same nontreponemal test method (e.g., VDRL or RPR), is necessary to demonstrate a significant difference, and should be performed in the same laboratory and, if possible, together on the same day. Nontreponemal antibody reactivities vary during the course of untreated disease. They reach their highest prevalence and titer during the secondary and early latent stages and decline thereafter, usually to less than 1:4. Over time, at least 25% of untreated persons become VDRL- or RPR-negative and a much smaller percentage becomes serofast, almost always at a titer of less than 1:4. In fact, one of the more difficult situations to interpret is the patient with a persistently positive VDRL/RPR test result after apparently adequate therapy (chronic persistor). This may be attributable to a biologically false reaction, a persistent active infection, or reinfection, especially when the titer is higher than 1:4.[85-88] A persistently high-titer RPR or VDRL result is more common in HIV-infected persons because of the B-cell dysfunction resulting in polyclonal antibody stimulation, especially in early untreated HIV disease.

The quantitative VDRL/RPR test should become nonreactive 1 year after successful therapy in primary syphilis and 2 years after successful therapy in secondary syphilis; most patients with late syphilis will be nonreactive by the fifth year after successful therapy.[86-88a] The time required for the test to become negative correlates with the interval between contact and institution of effective therapy and with the severity of illness, especially with the type of skin lesions manifested in the secondary stage; for example, a patient with a macular rash reverts to a negative titer sooner than a patient with a papular rash. Therefore, a positive VRDL or RPR response after 1 year in a patient treated for primary syphilis or after 2 years in a patient treated for secondary syphilis suggests persistent infection, reinfection,[89] or a biologically false-positive reaction caused by another condition (e.g., untreated HIV infection, IV drug use, spirochetal infection other than syphilis, any chronic infection such as tuberculosis, any hyperimmune state such as poorly controlled lupus, or a recent vaccination[89a]).

In summary, nonspecific nontreponemal tests are inexpensive, reliable, and easy to perform. They are useful for screening sera; in areas of high prevalence (e.g., southeastern United States), they should still be used to screen hospital admissions.[90] Also, they are very useful to gauge the success of treatment but as a nonspecific test, false negatives and false positives may occur.[86]

Specific Treponemal Tests

These tests measure antibodies against specific *T. pallidum* antigens. The most common specific antitreponemal antibody tests performed today are the automated EIAs, *T. pallidum* agglutination tests (TPPA, TPHA, MHA-TP, PaGIA), and FTA-ABS, although attempts to improve the specificity continue.[82,82a,91-96] The FTA-ABS is a standard

thermore, confusion surrounds interpretation of the serologic tests for syphilis, principally because two different types of antibodies can be measured—nonspecific nontreponemal reaginic antibodies and specific antitreponemal antibodies. The test for the former is inexpensive, rapid, and convenient for screening large numbers of sera (e.g., donated blood) and monitoring the success of antibiotic treatment. Specific antibody tests establish the very high likelihood of a treponemal infection, either currently or at some time in the past (Table 238-6). To establish a diagnosis of syphilis, the two types of serologic tests were traditionally used together, although automated enzyme immunoassays, rapid dipstick (immunochromographic strip [ICS]) and particle gel immunoassay [PaGIA] syphilis antibody) tests are gaining favor as screening tests in some centers because of ease and cost.[78,81,82a,82b] It should be emphasized that as the incidence of syphilis has decreased, the quality assurance of serologic tests for syphilis has suffered, requiring diligence on the part of the clinician who suspects syphilis.[83]

Nontreponemal Reaginic Tests

Much of the confusion about these tests arises from the term *reagin*. This is the result of an unfortunate quirk in the evolution of medical

TABLE 238-6	Untreated Patients with Positive Responses to Commonly Used Serologic Tests (%)	
	Stage	
Type of Test	*Early (Primary and Secondary)*	*Late (Late Latent and Tertiary)*
Nontreponemal (reagenic) tests: VDRL, RPR, ART TRUST	70-100	60-98
Specific treponemal tests: FTA-ABS, TP-PA (TPHA, MHA-TP, EIA, PaGIA, TPI)	50-85	97-100

The nonspecific nontreponemal tests should revert to a titer < 1:4 or negative (nonreactive) when effective treatment is given except in unusual circumstances (see text). Specific treponemal tests may also revert to negative if effective treatment is given early. See text for details.

indirect immunofluorescent antibody test that uses *T. pallidum* harvested from rabbit testes as the antigen. The patient's serum is first absorbed with a nonpathogenic treponemal antigen (referred to as sorbent) to remove low-titer, natural, cross-reacting antibodies that were likely raised against saprophytic treponemes of the oral cavity or genital tract. The test has the disadvantage of being standardized at one serum dilution (1:5), requires trained technicians and, as with most immunofluorescent tests, its interpretation can be subjective, it is difficult to standardize from one laboratory to the next, and it is difficult to quantify. Hence, particle agglutination tests (TPPA, TPHA, MHA-TP) and automated EIAs and their variations (e.g., particle gel immunoassay, PaGIA) have become more widespread to measure specific treponemal antibodies. For practical purposes, these tests are all similar, but it would be advisable to consult with your referral laboratory.

Their principal use is to verify a positive nontreponemal reaginic test result. Although these tests would be relatively expensive as screening tests, some high-volume clinical laboratories have begun using automated specific treponemal tests (e.g., EIA, TPPA, TPHA, PaGIA) to screen patients.[82a,93,97] However, the clinician must consider the following caveats regarding these tests as an indication for treatment: (1) most patients with untreated syphilis will not progress to late syphilis; (2) once a specific treponemal test is positive, it remains positive for life in more than 90% of successfully treated patients, especially those who are treated late; (3) as with all serologic tests, a false-positive (or false-negative) result may occur, although all published reports reveal a high level of sensitivity and specificity for each test. Hence, a positive test should be followed with a nonspecific treponemal test (see Table 238-6). When both are positive, the probability of active disease is high but when only the specific treponemal test is positive, the diagnosis of active disease is problematic. Options include confirming with another specific treponemal test using *T. pallidum* as the antigen (TPPA, MHA-TP, FTA-ABS, PaGIA) or vice versa, or another EIA using different recombinant *T. pallidum* antigens. However, in either situation, the clinician must make a clinical judgment whether or not to treat empirically for neurosyphilis (Table 238-7)—for example, a reliable history of adequate treatment, biopsy, or PCR-proven syphilis.

The TPI test is primarily of historical interest and rarely used today, but it was the standard against which all specific treponemal tests were once compared. It determines the ability of antibody plus complement to immobilize live *T. pallidum* as visualized under a darkfield microscope (i.e., it is a bactericidal test). Because it requires maintenance of replicating *T. pallidum* in rabbits, it is expensive, time-consuming, and difficult to perform, and only a few research laboratories today have maintained the capability to perform the TPI test.

Western immunoblotting can also be used as a confirmatory test for syphilis and is particularly important for congenital syphilis.[67,73,74,94] The comparative reactivities of the most widely used tests are shown in Table 238-6. When the diagnosis of syphilis is being seriously considered in an individual patient, the TPPA, TPHA, MHA-TP, EIA, immunoblot, or FTA-ABS test should be done. Once one or more of these have become positive and the diagnosis is established, the usefulness of these tests for monitoring patients is limited, because they usually remain positive for life. In contrast, a nontreponemal antibody test (VDRL or RPR) is very helpful for monitoring the efficacy of therapy. The failure of the titer to decrease fourfold or become negative suggests a persistent infection, reinfection, or a false-positive test (see earlier).

In congenital syphilis, the combination of IgM immunoblotting (Western blot for *T. pallidum*–specific IgM), DFA for spirochetal antigen detection on nasopharyngeal and umbilical cord specimens, and/or PCR assay is the most effective laboratory means to establish the diagnosis.[67,73,74,94] The best way to monitor these infants is with serial quantitative nontreponemal tests performed over several months. As with all serial serologic determinations, the most credible results are obtained with those performed simultaneously on appropriately stored serum samples. Serum is the specimen of choice for all serologic tests; however, EDTA, sodium citrate, and heparin plasma may be used when serum cannot be obtained.

Tests for Neurosyphilis

Serologic tests for neurosyphilis have evolved over time. The CSF VDRL, the oldest test, and CSF RPR are insensitive but highly specific. A positive CSF VDRL/RPR result in the appropriate clinical setting, especially in early syphilis, establishes the diagnosis of neurosyphilis, although serum antibody contamination is possible. A negative CSF FTA unabsorbed, CSF FTA-ABS, CSF MHA-TP, CSF-TPPA, CSF-TPHA, or EIA test in essence rules out active neurosyphilis in patients with late disease but not in those with early disease.

In desperate situations, a CSF serologic diagnosis based on the production of local antitreponemal antibodies as a discriminator of CNS invasion has improved sensitivity and specificity.[59-63] The most experience has been with the intrathecal *T. pallidum* antibody (ITPA) index and the TPHA index.

The ITPA index is determined as follows:

$$ITPA\ index = (TPHA\ CSF\ IgG\ titer/total\ CSF\ IgG/TPHA) - serum\ IgG\ titer/total\ serum\ IgG$$

The total IgG measurements are in milligrams. As long as the albumin serum-to-CSF ratio is higher than 144, indicating an undamaged blood-brain barrier, then a ratio of 3.0 or higher indicates active production of local antitreponemal antibodies.

The TPHA index is determined as follows:

$$TPHA\ index = (MHA\text{-}TP\ CSF\ titer/CSF\ albumin) \times 10^3/serum\ albumin$$

The albumin measurements are in milligrams per deciliter. A TPHA index higher than 100 is indicative of local CNS antibody production.

If the patient is treated early, these indices are likely to return to normal, but if the patient is treated late (i.e., after 2 years), they are likely to remain abnormal for a prolonged period.

The PCR test for *T. pallidum* in the CSF and IgM immunoblotting are specific and sensitive.[64-67] Detection of specific oligoclonal immunoglobulins by immunofixation (enzyme-labeled antibodies) electrophoresis can also be used to detect locally produced CSF antibodies.[98] The finding of more than five mononuclear cells/mm³ of CSF in the appropriate clinical setting is also suggestive of active neurosyphilis.

In summary, the laboratory diagnosis of active neurosyphilis is dependent on the various combinations of reactive serologic tests, abnormalities in the CSF cell count and/or protein level, a reactive CSF VDRL/RPR, local CNS production of antitreponemal antibodies, or a positive PCR test.

False-Positive Serologic Test for Syphilis

The likelihood of a biologic false-positive (BFP) reaction depends on the underlying circumstances. For example, acute or transient false-positive nontreponemal reaginic test reactions may occur whenever there is a strong immunologic stimulus (e.g., acute bacterial or viral infection, vaccination, IV drug abuse, untreated HIV infection). Positive reactions persisting for months occur in the presence of continued parenteral drug abuse, with autoimmune or connective tissue diseases, especially systemic lupus erythematosus, with aging (in up to 10% of those older than 70 years), in hypergammaglobulinemic states, and in untreated or poorly controlled HIV coinfection (Table 238-8). A false-positive nontreponemal reaginic test in this setting tends to be associated with other serum factors frequently associated with autoimmune diseases, such as antinuclear, antithyroid, or antimitochondrial antibodies, rheumatoid factor, and cryoglobulins.

A false-positive nontreponemal reaginic test can usually be verified (and syphilis excluded) by obtaining a negative specific treponemal antibody test result (FTA-ABS, TPPA, TPHA, MHA-TP, EIA, PaGIA). However, at times, the same illnesses that produce a false-positive

	TABLE 238-7	Recommended Therapy for Syphilis*		

Stage	CDC Recommendation for Patients Not Allergic to Penicillin	CDC Recommendation for Patients Allergic to Penicillin	Alternative Regimens*
Early syphilis (primary, secondary, early latent), adults	Benzathine penicillin G[†] 2.4 million units IM in a single dose	Doxycycline, 100 mg PO bid for 15 days,[†] *or* Tetracycline hydrochloride, 500 mg PO qid for 15 days; *or* Desensitization to penicillin in pregnant women[†]	Amoxicillin, 500 mg plus probenecid 0.5 gm PO bid for 0-14 days *or* Procaine penicillin, 2.4 million units IM daily, plus probenecid 500 mg PO qid for 14 days *or* Ceftriaxone, 250 mg IM qd or IV for 5 days or 1g IM qd for 14 days[§] *or* Doxycycline, 100 mg PO bid for 14 days *or* Tetracycline hydrochloride, 500 mg PO qid for 15 days
Early latent syphilis	Benzathine penicillin G[†] 2.4 million units IM in a single dose	Doxycycline, 100 mg PO bid for 28 days	Amoxicillin, 500 mg, plus probenecid, 0.5 g PO bid for 0-14 days *or* Procaine penicillin, 2.4 million units IM daily, plus probenecid, 500 mg PO qid for 14 days *or* Ceftriaxone, 250 mg IM qd or IV for 5 days or 1 g IM qd for 14 days[§] *or* Doxycycline, 100 mg PO bid for 28 days
Late latent or syphilis of unknown duration, adults, or tertiary syphilis	Benzathine penicillin G[†] 2.4 million units IM given at weekly intervals × 3 (7.2 million units total)	Doxycycline, 100 mg PO bid for 28 days	Amoxicillin, 3 g PO bid with 500 mg probenecid PO bid for 10-14 days *or* Aqueous crystalline penicillin G,[†] 3.0-4.0 million units by IV infusion q4h for 10-14 days *or* Ceftriaxone, 1 g IM or IV for 14 days[§] *or* Procaine penicillin G,[†] 2.4 million units IM, plus probenecid, 0.5 g PO daily for 10 days
Neurosyphilis, adults	Aqueous crystalline penicillin G,[†] 3.0-4.0 million units by IV infusion q4h or continuous infusion for 10-14 days, *or* Procaine penicillin G,[†] 2.4 million units IM, plus probenecid, 0.5 g PO daily for 10 days Aqueous crystalline penicillin G,[†] 3.0-4.0 million units by IV infusion q4h for 10-14 days	Doxycycline, 100 mg PO bid for 28 days	Amoxicillin, 3 g PO bid, with 500 mg probenecid PO bid for 10-14 days *or* Ceftriaxone, 2 g IM or IV for 14 days[¶]
Pregnancy	Same regimen as for nonpregnant patient; only penicillin therapy reliably treats infant[‡]	Same regimen as for nonpregnant patient; only penicillin therapy reliably treats the infant[‡]	Same regimen as for nonpregnant patient; only penicillin therapy reliably treats infant[‡]
Congenital syphilis	Aqueous crystalline penicillin G, 100,000-150,000 units/kg/day, administered as 50,000 units/kg/day IV q12h for first 7 days of life and q8h for 3 days *or* Procaine penicillin G, 50,000 U/kg IM daily for minimum of 10 days	Not applicable	
Children	Benzathine penicillin G,[†] 50,000 up to 2.4 million units units/kg/day IM in single dose		

*Therapeutic regimens other than penicillin have not been well studied, especially in patients with syphilis longer than 1 year's duration; therefore, careful follow-up is mandatory.
[†]CDC recommendation; however, treatment failures with benzathine penicillin have been well documented. Patients treated with benzathine penicillin or other regimens except high-dose penicillin for ≥8 days should be reevaluated at 6-month intervals for neurosyphilis (see text); HIV-positive patients should be evaluated at 3-month intervals.
[‡]Because of the large number of well-documented treatment failures and corroborating laboratory studies, erythromycin and azithromycin are no longer recommended for the treatment of syphilis. Although *Treponema pallidum* has remained exquisitely sensitive to penicillin for more than 70 years, resistance has been engineered in the laboratory, a presage of what will likely occur someday in nature (personal communication, Stanley Falkow, Stanford University).
[§]Efficacy unknown, serologic follow-up useful. Ceftriaxone should be diluted in 1% lidocaine solution (1 g/3.6 mL) for IM injection.
[¶]Treatment failures have been reported. Chloramphenicol is theoretically beneficial treatment for neurosyphilis.
[‖]Some authorities treat syphilis with HIV infection in the same manner as syphilis without HIV infection. However, treatment failures with benzathine penicillin, ceftriaxone, procaine penicillin, and azithromycin have been reported.

TABLE 238-8	Causes of Biologic False-Positive (BFP) Serologic Test Reactions for Syphilis
Infectious Diseases	
Lyme disease*	
Leptospirosis	
Relapsing fever	
Ratbite fever (*Spirillum minus*)	
Leprosy	
Tuberculosis	
Pneumonococcal pneumonia	
Subacute bacterial endocarditis	
Chancroid	
Scarlet fever	
Rickettsial disease	
Malaria	
Trypanosomiasis	
Mycoplasma pneumonia	
Chickenpox	
Lymphogranuloma venereum	
Hepatitis (especially hepatitis C)	
Infectious mononucleosis	
Noninfectious Diseases	
Drug addiction	
Any connective tissue disease disorder	
Rheumatoid heart disease	
Blood transfusions (multiple)	
Pregnancy	
"Old age"	
Any vaccination	
Chronic liver disease (noninfectious)	

*Only specific treponemal tests, VDRL (RPR) negative. See text for details.

nontreponemal reaginic test (e.g., systemic lupus erythematosus) also result in a positive or borderline-positive FTA-ABS test reaction. Also, any specific treponemal test may be positive when the VDRL/RPR is negative, and vice versa. These false reactions can often be suggested by noting a beaded pattern of immunofluorescence on the treponemes in the FTA-ABS test, but the most definitive way to make the distinction is to carry out the functional but rarely available TPI test, PCR assay, or immunoblotting using specific *T. pallidum* antigens. Other spirochetal illnesses, such as relapsing fever (*Borrelia* spp.), the nonvenereal treponematoses (yaws, bejel, pinta), leptospirosis, or rat-bite fever *(Spirillum minus),* also yield positive nontreponemal and treponemal test results. Infection with *Borrelia burgdorferi* (Lyme disease) can result in a positive FTA-ABS test but rarely causes a positive nontreponemal reaginic reaction (VDRL or RPR).

Rarely, an infected patient, especially with an underlying immune dysfunctional state (e.g., HIV coinfection), will have a true positive nonspecific test with a false-negative specific treponemal test.

In summary, the reaginic antibody tests (RPR, VDRL, ART) are used for screening for syphilis, the specific treponemal tests (TPPA, TPHA, MHA-TP, EIA, FTA-ABS, TPI) for confirming the diagnosis, and the quantitative nontreponemal antibody tests (RPR, VDRL) for assessing the adequacy of therapy.

POLYMERASE CHAIN REACTION ASSAY

PCR tests have been developed using a variety of syphilitic DNA base pairs. They are quite specific and can be used on almost all clinical specimens, but do not distinguish live from dead organisms.[64,67,79,80] PCR tests are becoming more widely available but, when not available through a local laboratory, most local state health departments can be helpful. The specimen should be shipped immediately on ice to arrive frozen.

ISOLATION OF *TREPONEMA PALLIDUM*

Because *T. pallidum* cannot be cultivated on artificial media, inoculation of laboratory animals (primates, rabbit testes) is the only means available at present for isolating the organism.[18,19] The most experience has been with isolation in rabbits. The number of organisms that must be obtained from a human lesion to ensure a positive transfer appears to be 4 to 10 spirochetes. There has been limited success maintaining *T. pallidum* in tissue culture.

CONGENITAL SYPHILIS

The most reliable means to diagnose congenital syphilis is to test the mother at the time of birth.[67,72-77] Most infants with congenital syphilis can be identified by physical examination and radiographic and ultrasonographic studies. Delayed-onset syphilis (more than 2 days) is best diagnosed by combining tests for IgM-specific antibodies (EIA, FTA-ABS, or immunoblotting–Western blot) with antigen detection (darkfield, immunofluorescence, immunoperoxidase-labeled antibody staining; PCR). IFA staining with specifically tagged antibody is superior to darkfield examination. A calcium alginate swab is inserted into the posterior nasopharynx and rolled immediately onto slides for examination. A positive result on any test warrants a diagnosis of a treatment for congenital syphilis.

RAPID TESTS

A number of rapid (10 to 30 minutes) specific treponemal tests are now available.[81,82a] Although a few are card-based, most use a lateral flow format using recombinant antigens and are equivalent to the older specific treponemal antibody tests. They do not require instrumentation or refrigeration, which makes them particularly useful for low-resource settings. The tests can use blood, serum, or plasma depending on the manufacturer, and can use as little as a 10- to 50-µL sample. Overall, these tests are accurate but cannot distinguish between an active or inactive infection.

Treatment

Much of the controversy surrounding the treatment recommendations for syphilis stems from the primary objective that the practitioner is trying to achieve. From the public health perspective, interruption of transmission is paramount. The natural course of syphilis is helpful in that regard because infectiousness is highest when the spirochetal antigen load is highest in early infection and wanes to a nontransmissible state in 1 to 4 years (except for congenital syphilis). Also, at least two thirds of patients with untreated early syphilis do not progress to late syphilis. Hence, one to three doses of an antibiotic preparation that eliminates enough treponemes to shift the balance in favor of the host to interrupt transmission and decrease the impact of patient noncompliance to achieve that goal is an acceptable objective (e.g., benzathine penicillin). On the other hand, a clinician caring for an individual patient has a different goal—completely cure the patient of replicating treponemes, an easily achievable goal. Unfortunately, treponemes may reside in a pharmacologically difficult to reach site such as the CNS, ear, or eye, and slowly progress to a destructive clinical disease state 5 to 35 or more years after the primary infection has resolved (and the episode of syphilis often long forgotten). Obviously, the latter ensures the former, but at a practical cost-benefit ratio.

Although the efficacy of penicillin in the treatment of syphilis is well established,[30] a legacy of this old infectious disease is that there has never been a well-controlled, carefully planned, prospective study of long enough duration to determine the optimal dose or duration of therapy to ensure a cure reliably in an individual patient. Furthermore, the penicillin preparations used in earlier studies are no longer available. Therefore, the following recommendations are based on extrapolation of older data and limited clinical trial experience and must be tempered with this knowledge.[78] Hence, it should not be surprising that there are patients who have a persistent infection despite having received so-called "adequate therapy."[43,99-110]

Penicillin G, administered parenterally, is the preferred treatment for syphilis (see Table 238-7). The current Centers for Disease Control and Prevention (CDC) recommendation for the use of benzathine penicillin IM was obtained by extrapolation from the pharmacokinetics of penicillin therapy, the effect of the drug on *T. pallidum* under experimental conditions in animals, and observational clinical data, and is adequate for the great majority of patients (see Table 238-7).[78] For example, it has been shown in experimental infections that *T. pallidum* regenerates if penicillin blood levels are allowed to fall to subinhibitory levels after 18 to 24 hours.[30] Furthermore, it has been found from a variety of clinical and experimental data that a level equivalent to more than 0.03 µg/mL of penicillin is needed to ensure killing of *T. pallidum*, that maintenance of an effective blood level for at least 7 days is necessary to cure early syphilis, and that increasing the dose to more than 0.6 mg/kg over a period of 9 hours does not clear treponemes from primary chancres at an increased rate. Therefore, it can be inferred that the most effective antibiotic treatment would be one that ensures an adequate penicillin level at the site of infection over a prolonged period, 8 days or longer. The most convenient way to achieve this goal in the blood and avoid dependence on patient compliance is to treat with benzathine penicillin, despite the recognized potential inadequacies and potential failure rate of this treatment for neurosyphilis, congenital syphilis, during pregnancy, and in immunocompromised patients.[101-117] *T. pallidum* has been isolated from the CSF of patients with only a chancre and no other evidence of congenital neurosyphilis, reflecting the early spirochetemia that always occurs and the consequent propensity to invade the CNS. Therefore, to cure this readily and easily curable infection effectively, one must adequately treat treponemes in the CNS (neurosyphilis), even in patients with primary or secondary infection who have up to a 40% chance of CNS invasion. However, treponemicidal levels of benzathine penicillin are not reliably achieved in the CSF of neonates, children, or adults, and numerous treatment failures have been recorded.[43]

Nevertheless, the recommendation that benzathine penicillin be considered the treatment of choice was adopted, despite the fact that treatment failure occurs and retreatment was required in as many as 1 of 33 cases in the original study[99] and, by extrapolation, fails to cure CNS invasion between 1 in 333 to 1000 patients. On the other hand, given that at least two thirds of untreated patients cure their syphilis infection and do not progress to late syphilis, and the clinical experience of over 50 years using benzathine penicillin, the likelihood of a complete cure with relatively low doses of penicillin is increased.[30,78] Thus, treatment with benzathine penicillin, which at least provides circulating penicillin for 14 days, albeit at low levels, and does not rely on patient compliance to take an antibiotic on a daily basis, is adequate for most patients. This includes those with HIV who are coinfected and on highly active antiretroviral therapy (HAART),[24,118] especially because it decreases transmission, a major public health goal. However, when one considers the individual patient, and because of the high probability of CNS invasion, an increasing number of clinicians are uncomfortable with the risk of their patients developing late complications (5 to 35 or more years later), especially neurosyphilis, and all patients receive antibiotic therapy adequate to treat neurosyphilis.

Early incubating syphilis is likely aborted when other nonviral STDs are treated with the currently recommended regimens.

Because of the high risk of infection, presumptive or epidemiologic antibiotic treatment should be given to anyone who has been exposed to a patient with infectious syphilis within the preceding 3 months, even if she or he is seronegative, or longer if serologic tests are not immediately available or the opportunity for follow-up uncertain. All exposed persons should obviously have follow-up serologic studies to establish the diagnosis and monitor the adequacy of their response to therapy. Adequately treated non–HIV-infected and most HIV coinfected patients on HAART should have a predictable fall in their nontreponemal reaginic antibody titer.[24,86-89,118,119,119a]

All women should be serologically screened during the early stages of pregnancy and, for those at high risk, at delivery as well (e.g., drug abusers). Infected pregnant patients should receive penicillin at dosage schedules appropriate for the stage of syphilis as recommended for nonpregnant patients. If the patient has a well-documented penicillin allergy, the choice is more difficult, because the efficacy of treatment for the fetus in these cases is not well established. Hence, penicillin desensitization is recommended (see Chapter 21).[78] The patient is given gradually increasing doses of oral or IV penicillin over a period of 3 to 4 hours, until full tolerance is achieved, followed by full-dose treatment. Erythromycin and azithromycin have been effective but resistance has developed, and there have been well-documented clinical failures.[120] Pharmacologic characteristics studies in rabbit models and limited studies in humans suggest that ceftriaxone is adequate therapy.[121,122] However, conflicting clinical experience has been reported in patients who are coinfected with HIV.[123] Tetracycline, doxycycline, and chloramphenicol are *not* recommended because of potential adverse effects on the mother, fetus, or both. The mother should be monitored closely during and after the pregnancy and, if an increase in a nontreponemal reagin titer or a positive PCR test result is obtained, she and her infant must be retreated.

The risk of infection for the infant is minimal if the mother has received adequate penicillin treatment during pregnancy.[72,78] Nevertheless, the child must be examined monthly after delivery and until the nontreponemal reaginic antibody test or PCR becomes negative. Penicillin treatment should never be withheld to prove the diagnosis, and every neonate born to a syphilitic mother should be promptly treated unless adequate, serologically proven effective treatment with penicillin can be documented more than 1 month before delivery. There is no evidence that the efficacy of penicillin treatment of syphilis has diminished over 70 years,[30] probably because of the genetic fidelity of *T. pallidum*. However, there is evidence that *T. pallidum* can accept resistant plasmids, and the possibility exists that penicillin resistance may become a problem in the future.

Tetracycline, doxycycline, chloramphenicol, ceftriaxone, other cephalosporins, and azithromycin have all been shown to be effective alternative antibiotics in animal models and in small clinical trials for the treatment of early syphilis, although failures with azithromycin, erythromycin, and doxycycline have been reported. Patients who are also infected with HIV, like any other immunosuppressed group, present special problems (see later). An intact cellular immune system is an important determinant of the severity of and progression to late syphilitic disease. Therefore, most authorities believe that these patients should be treated as if they have neurosyphilis regardless of their clinical findings, especially when they are in the later stages of their HIV infection.

LATE SYPHILIS, ASYMPTOMATIC AND SYMPTOMATIC NEUROSYPHILIS

Because the CNS is invaded during the spirochetemia in up to 40% of patients and because spirochetemia occurs soon after the infection is contracted, all patients with syphilis are at risk for neurosyphilis (Fig. 238-8). A CSF examination should thus be considered. Specific indications for CSF examination include neurologic or ophthalmologic pathology, latent-stage syphilis, tertiary syphilis, clinical relapse, HIV coinfection, and serologic failure to respond to therapy with nontreponemal titers that do not fall appropriately. The finding of an elevated mononuclear cell count in the CSF, a positive reactive nontreponemal antibody test (VDRL/RPR), production of local CNS antitreponemal antibody, or positive CSF PCR test establishes the diagnosis of neurosyphilis.

Because benzathine penicillin G does not reliably produce spirocheticidal[102] levels of penicillin in the CSF, this drug cannot be relied on as a consistently curable treatment of neurosyphilis (failure rate, 1 in 333 to 1000). To ensure adequate antibiotic levels in the CNS more effectively, 12 to 24 million units of aqueous penicillin G should be given IV for 8 to 10 days; alternatives are amoxicillin (3.0 g twice daily)

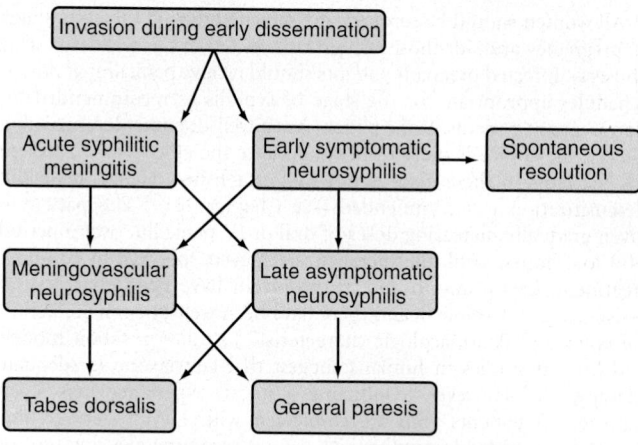

Figure 238-8   **Chronology of neurosyphilis.**

plus probenecid (0.5 to 1.0 g orally) for 14 days,[124] doxycycline (200 mg orally twice daily) for 21 days,[125] or ceftriaxone (2 g intramuscularly daily) for 14 days.[122,123] Procaine benzyl penicillin (2.4 million units intramuscularly) plus probenecid (500 mg four times daily) has been used successfully.[78] Although these regimens are recognized as adequate, some are not recommended by the CDC. Follow-up CSF examinations are not necessary unless the serum VDRL/RPR has not decreased to nonreactive in 24-month post-treatment. In these cases, the CSF should be examined every 3 to 6 months for at least 3 years unless local CNS treponemal antibodies disappear, CSF oligoclonal bands disappear, or a PCR assay turns negative. Positron emission tomography (PET), MRI, and single photon emission computed tomography (SPECT) have allowed more precise investigation of CNS invasion and have demonstrated dramatic radiographic and clinical improvement with treatment.[47,48,119a] Malignancies of the CNS have been associated with false-positive results on nontreponemal and treponemal tests, but this has almost always been associated with a negative syphilis specific serum antibody test.

OTHER TREATMENT CONSIDERATIONS

Syphilitic Otitis. Syphilitic otitis should be treated as neurosyphilis. Treatment typically includes prednisone to avert a local Jarisch-Herxheimer reaction, 30 to 60 mg every day or every other day, at least for the first 7 to 8 days,[55,78] although the benefit of steroids has not been proven. Other antibiotic treatments for neurosyphilis would be an alternative choice to parenteral penicillin.

Ocular Syphilis. Anterior and/or panuveitis is a frequent complication of acute and chronic neurosyphilis, and thus should be treated with antibiotic regimens appropriate for neurosyphilis.[78] It appears to be an increased manifestation of HIV coinfection.

HIV Coinfection. Although the presentation of syphilis is in general similar to HIV-uninfected persons, the concurrent immune dysfunction underlies the propensity for developing more severe disease and an apparent increase in treatment failures, especially in uncontrolled HIV infection.[111-117,119a,126,127] Hence, many think that coinfected persons should be treated with a course of antibiotics adequate to treat neurosyphilis.[78]

Patients with a History of Penicillin Allergy. Because penicillin G is the most reliable treatment for all stages of syphilis, desensitization of the patient should be considered.[78] This can be done orally or intravenously (see Chapter 22).

PERSISTENT INFECTION

The question of persistent infection despite adequate therapy has been a controversial subject for many years. Because untreated syphilis does not progress to late syphilis in more than two thirds of patients, coupled with the impact of a variety of antibiotics on interrupting transmission, obtaining an evidence-based outcome on the effectiveness of a treatment regimen to eliminate the development of neurosyphilis, otosyphilis, and ocular syphilis would take many years. Hence, we are left with deducing what constitutes effective therapy. Although the efficacy of treating *T. pallidum* with adequate doses of penicillin is unquestioned, in a small number of patients, spirochetes become sequestered in areas where adequate levels of penicillin can best be reliably achieved with prolonged high doses of penicillin or alternative antibiotics (e.g., the anterior chamber of the eye, CNS, and labyrinth of the inner ear; see Table 238-7). These persistent organisms can cause a clinically evident illness at some later date, as evidenced by the number of reports of unusual neurologic, optic, and otic findings for which there is little or no explanation except a positive serologic test for syphilis. *T. pallidum* can persist after inadequate treatment, particularly in the CNS, and can be isolated by inoculation of appropriate human materials into laboratory animals or by PCR assay.[43,64,67,69,79,80] The challenge facing clinicians is to identify and treat these few patients with a curable infection. Anyone with neurologic, optic, or otic abnormalities who has or has had syphilis should be considered for CSF examination and, if there are any abnormalities (see earlier) or unexplained neurologic signs or symptoms, the patient should be treated for neurosyphilis (see Table 238-7).

FOLLOW-UP AND RETREATMENT

All patients with early or congenital syphilis should have repeat quantitative nontreponemal tests at 3, 6, and 12 months (see earlier). All patients with secondary syphilis or syphilis of more than 1 year's duration should also have a repeat nontreponemal serologic test 24 months after treatment and those with late syphilis at 5 years. Examination of the CSF is also warranted in selected patients, irrespective of the serologic response (see Table 238-2). All patients with documented neurosyphilis must be monitored carefully with serologic testing and CSF examinations including MRI, PET, or SPECT until all abnormal parameters, including local CNS production of antibodies, normalize.

Retreatment should be considered whenever clinical signs and symptoms of syphilis persist or recur, there is a sustained level or increase in a nontreponemal test titer after 6 months, a positive VDRL/RPR reaction persisting beyond 12 months in primary syphilis, 24 months in secondary or latent syphilis, or 5 years in late syphilis, or there is a persistent positive PCR test result.

DEFINING THE ADEQUACY OF TREATMENT

As noted, a quantitative decrease in nontreponemal reaginic tests is reliable as a measure of the adequacy of treatment. The time required for the tests to become nonreactive depends on how long the patient was infected before curative treatment was instituted, but all patients should have a titer of less than 1:4 by year 5. Exceptions to this rule occur in those with a chronic antigenic stimulation or immune dysfunction (e.g., HIV-infected persons). Specific treponemal antibody tests can also revert to negative, especially when treatment is instituted early.

In summary, unlike almost all other pathogenic microorganisms, *T. pallidum* has remained exquisitely sensitive to penicillin. If enough penicillin G is given to reach the CNS, eye, or ear at treponemicidal levels for 8 days or longer, the patient will be cured.

JARISCH-HERXHEIMER REACTION

The Jarisch-Herxheimer (JH) reaction[128,129] is a systemic reaction resembling bacterial sepsis that usually begins 1 to 2 hours after the initial treatment of syphilis with effective antibiotics, especially penicillin. It consists of the abrupt onset of fever, chills, myalgias, headache, tachycardia, hyperventilation, vasodilation with flushing, varying degrees of obtundation, and mild hypotension. It is particularly common when secondary syphilis is treated (70% to 90%) but can occur at any stage (10% to 25%). It lasts from 12 to 24 hours and has been well correlated with the release of heat-stable protein from the spirochetes. Patients should be warned of the reaction before treatment. Varying degrees of severity occur. The reaction is self-limited but can result in acute deleterious effects. It can be prevented or treated with an anti-inflammatory agent such as aspirin every 4 hours for a period of 24 to 48 hours. Prednisone can also abort the reaction, and one dose of 60 mg PO or IV should be given as adjunctive therapy to JH patients with cardiovascular or symptomatic neurosyphilis and to pregnant patients to avoid catastrophic consequences.

IMMUNITY

Magnuson and associates[29] were able to demonstrate in human volunteers that immunity developed to reinfection. This immunity appeared not to be absolute but became more solid the longer the infection remained untreated. Humoral antibodies are only partially protective, because experimental infection in humans and rabbits can be produced when they are present. On the other hand, the granulomatous lesion (gumma), a presumed correlate of cell-mediated immunity, is produced when syphilitic reinfection is resisted. Untreated HIV-infected persons have a propensity to develop more severe disease. Similarly, malnourished patients, who also have a deficit of cellular immune function, are prone to develop more severe syphilitic disease. *T. pallidum* has evolved mechanisms to evade host immune defenses and establish a chronic infection.[16,17,21,28] Suggested reasons for this include the following: (1) a waxy, nonimmunogenic coat through which very few protein antigens protrude; (2) residence in nonimmunogenic privileged sites, such as the inner ear, eye, or CNS; (3) induction of markedly increased levels of prostaglandin E_2; and (4) a subpopulation of spirochetes that are resistant to phagocytosis presumably because of treponeme-induced macrophage downregulation.

The likelihood of development of syphilis in a susceptible person who has unprotected sexual intercourse with a patient with infectious syphilis is estimated to be about 50%. However, in controlled volunteer experiments, all volunteers without a history of serologic evidence of previous contact with *T. pallidum* developed syphilis. Obviously, the relative importance of variations in sexual and hygienic practices, immune status, inoculum size, and other factors play an important role in the transmissibility of *T. pallidum*.

Congenital syphilis appears not to confer immunity to syphilis.[130]

Syphilis in Those Coinfected with HIV

Coinfection is common.[24,131] The two diseases can affect each other in a number of ways. As with other ulcer-causing conditions, they may enhance the acquisition and transmission of each other but syphilis also upregulates CCR5 coreceptor expression[132] and causes local immune activation,[133,134] thereby further increasing the likelihood of acquisition of HIV. The natural course of syphilis may be affected, often resulting in a high antigen load, multiple chancres, and a more malignant course.[49,58,135-139] The serologic tests for syphilis may be modified, often resulting in extremely high titers and a failure to decrease in response to adequate treatment unless successfully treated with HAART.[118] In other cases, a serologic response may fail to develop.[114,140-142] Finally, with the diminished added effects of the immune system to help control the infection, high-dose or prolonged therapy may be required to effect a cure in coinfected persons.

Although patients with syphilis and HIV coinfection have shown no distinctive or unique clinical presentation or pathologic manifestations from those without concurrent HIV infection, they are at an increased risk to manifest a more protracted and malignant course, more constitutional symptoms, greater organ involvement, atypical and florid skin rashes, multiple genital ulcers, concomitant chancre during the secondary stage, and a significant predisposition to develop symptomatic neurosyphilis.,[111-113,137-140] especially uveitis. However, the failure of antibiotics to cure coinfected patients has been reported, although the actual failure rate is small. Given the known failure rate, which may be as high as 3% in non–HIV-infected persons, and the critical role that an intact cellular arm of the immune system plays in clearing the infection, this occurrence should not be surprising. Furthermore, the most conspicuous manifestations of these treatment failures are neurologic or ocular. Therefore, a more vigorous or more prolonged course of antibiotics, sufficient to cure late latent or neurosyphilis, is prudent (see Table 238-7).[78] There is also a theoretical possibility that bacteriostatic drugs such as doxycycline may be less effective because of the immune impairment.

HIV-coinfected patients are also more likely to develop aberrant serologic responses.[140-142] They may have false-positive or increasing reaginic titers despite adequate therapy, especially during the earlier phases of untreated HIV infection, when polyclonal B-cell stimulation is most prevalent. Also, they may fail to develop a response because of an overwhelming antigen load or severe immune dysfunction occurring late in the disease. Finally, as many as 11% of HIV-infected persons have a biologic false-positive serologic test result. Therefore, a high index of suspicion and extraordinary means to establish the diagnosis (e.g., special stains of biopsy specimens, PCR assay) may be required.

After treatment, aggressive serologic follow-up is recommended (at 1, 2, 3, 6, 9, 12, and 24 months). Failure of a serologic response should usually lead to retreatment, but clinical judgment must be used because HIV coinfection may lead to an aberrant response. HIV-2 infection appears not to affect the clinical course of syphilis.

In summary, HIV coinfection, especially untreated, shifts the host parasite relationship in favor of the spirochete and predisposes the patient to a more malignant course and aberrant serologic responses.

REFERENCES

1. Kampmeier RH. *Essentials of Syphilology*. 3rd ed. Philadelphia: JB Lippincott; 1943.
2. Stokes JH, Beerman H, Ingraham NR. *Modern Clinical Syphilology, Diagnosis, Treatment: Case Study*. 3rd ed. Philadelphia: WB Saunders; 1945.
3. Hook EW, Marra CM. Acquired syphilis in adults. *N Engl J Med*. 1992;326:1060-1069.
4. Tramont EC. The impact of syphilis on humankind. *Med Clin N Am*. 2004;18:101-110.
5. Tramont EC. Syphilis in adults: From Christopher Columbus to Sir Alexander Fleming to AIDS. *Clin Infect Dis*. 1995;21:1361-1371.
6. Franzen C. Syphilis in composers and musicians—Mozart, Beethoven, Paginini, Schubert, Schumann, Smetana. *Eur J Cin Microbil Infect. Dis*. 2008;27:1151-1157.
7. Waugh MA. Venereal disease in sixteenth century England. *Med Hist*. 1973;17:152-161.
8. Mays S, Crane-Kramer G, Bayliss A. Two probable cases of treponemal disease of medieval date from England. *Am J Phys Anthropol*. 2003;120:133-134.
9. Parran T. *Shadow on the Land: Syphilis*. New York: Reynal & Hitchcock; 1937.
10. Harper KB, Ocampo PS, Steiner BM, et al. On the origin of the treponematoses: A phylogenetic approach. *PLoS Negl Trop Dis*. 2008;2:e148.
11. Mulligan CJ, Norris SJ, Lukehart SA. Molecular studies in *Treponema pallidum* evolution: Toward clarity. *PLoS Negl Trop Dis*. 2008;2:e184.
12. Ricord PH. *A Treatise on Venereal Diseases*. New York: P. Gordon; 1842.
13. Fairchild AL, Bayer R. Uses and abuses of Tuskegee. *Science*. 1999;284:219-221.
14. Antal MG, Lukehart SA, Meheus AZ. The endemic treponematoses. *Microbes Infect*. 2002;4:83-94.
15. Centurion-Lara A, Moloini BJ, Godornes C, et al. Molecular differentiation of *Treponema pallidum* subspecies. *J Clin Microbiol*. 2006;44:3377-3380.
16. Blanco DR, Miller JN, Lovett MA. Surface antigens of the syphilis spirochete and their potential as virulence determinants. *Emerg Infect Dis*. 1997;3:11-20.
17. Radolf JD. Role of outer membrane architecture in immune evasion by *Treponema pallidum* and *Borelia burgdorferi*. *Trends Microbiol*. 1994;2:307-311.
18. Cox DL. Culture of *Treponema pallidum*. *Methods Enzymol*. 1994;236:390-405.
19. Lukehart SA, Marra CM. Isolation and laboratory maintenance of Treponema pallidum. *Curr Protoc Microbil*. 2007; Chapter 12:Unit 12A.1.
20. Norris SJ, Cox DL, Weinstock GM. Biology of *Treponema pallidum*: Correlation of functional activities with genome sequences. *J.Mol Microbiol Biotechnol*. 2001;3:37-62.

21. Lafond RE, Lukehart SA. Biological basis for syphilis. *Clin Microb Rev.* 2006;19:29-49.
22. Palfi Z, Ponyai K, Varkanyo V, et al. Primary syphilis of the finger. *Dermatology.* 2008:217:252-253.
23. Jones DL, Irwin K, Inciardi J, et al. The high-risk sexual practices of crack-smoking sex workers recruited from the streets of three American cities. *Sex Transm Dis.* 1998;25:187-193.
24. Zetola NM, Klausner JD. Syphilis and HIV infection: An update. *Clin Infect Dis.* 2007;44:1222-1228.
25. Buchacz,K, Klausner JD, Kerndt PR, et al. HIV incidence among men with early syphilis in Atlanta, San Francisco, and Los Angeles, 2004 to 2005. *J Acquir Immune Defic Syndr.* 2008; 47:234-240,
26. Fenton KA, Breban R, Vardavas JT, et al. Infectious syphilis in high-income settings in the 21st century. *Lancet Infect Dis*, 2008 8:244-253.
27. Rampalo AM. Can syphilis be eradicated from the world? *Curr Opin Infect Dis.* 2001;14:41-44.
28. Lukehart S, Hook EW, Baker-Zander SH, et al. Invasion of the central nervous system by *Treponema pallidum:* Implications for diagnosis and therapy. *Ann Intern Med.* 1988;109:855-862.
29. Magnuson HJ, Thomas EW, Olansky S, et al. Inoculation syphilis in human volunteers. *Medicine (Baltimore).* 1956;35:33-42.
30. Syphilotherapy, 1976. *Sex Transm Dis.* 1976;3:98.
31. Salazar JC, Karsten ROH, Radolf JD. The immune response to infection with *Treponema pallidum*, the stealth pathogen. *Microb Infect.* 2002;1133-1140.
32. Fitzgerald TJ. The Th_1/Th_2 switch in syphilitic infection: Is it detrimental? *Infect Immun.* 1992;60:3475-3479.
33. Lukehart SA, Shaffer JM, Baker Zander SA. A subpopulation of *Treponema pallidum* is resistant to phagocytosis: Possible mechanism of persistence. *J Infect Dis.* 1992;166:1449-1453.
34. O'Regan S, Fong JSC, de Chadarevian JP, et al. Treponemal antigens in congenital and acquired syphilitic nephritis. *Ann Intern Med.* 1976;85:325-327.
35. Clark EG, Danbolt N. The Oslo study of the natural course of untreated syphilis. *Med Clin North Am.* 1964;48:613-621.
36. Rockwell DH, Yobs AR, Moore MB. The Tuskeegee study of untreated syphilis: The 30th year of observation. *Arch Intern Med.* 1964;114:792.
37. Rosahn PD. Autopsy studies in syphilis. *J Vener Dis.* 1947; 649(Suppl 21).
38. Chapel TA. The variability of syphilitic chancres. *Sex Transm Dis.* 1978;5:68-72.
39. Rompalo AM, Lawlor J, Seaman P, et al. Modification of syphilitic genital ulcer manifestations by coexistent HIV infection. *Sex Transm Dis.* 2001;28:448-454.
40. Vural M, Ilikkan B, Polat E, et al. A premature newborn with vesiculobullous skin lesions. *Eur J Pediatr.* 2003;162:197-199.
41. Chapel TA. The signs and symptoms of secondary syphilis. *Sex Transm Dis.* 1980;7:161-167.
42. Merritt HH, Moore M. Acute neurosyphilitic meningitis. *Medicine (Baltimore).* 1935;14:119.
43. Tramont EC. Persistence of *Treponema pallidum* following penicillin G therapy. *JAMA.* 1976;236:2206-2209.
44. Merritt HH, Adams RD, Solomon HC. *Neurosyphilis.* New York: Oxford University Press; 1946.
45. Lauria G, Erbetta A, Pareyson D, et al. Parenchymatous neurosyphilis. *Neurol Sci.* 2001;22:281-282.
45a. Lee CH, Lin WC, Lu CH, et al. Initially unrecognized dementia in a young man with neurosyphilis. *Neurologist.* 2009;15: 95-97.
46. Lauria G, Kikuchi S, Shinpo K, et al. Subacute syphilitic meningomyelitis with characteristic spinal MRI findings. *J Neurol.* 2003;250:106-107.
47. Berbel-Garcia A, Porta-Essemann J, Martinex-Salio A, et al. Magnetic resonance image, reversible findings in a patient with general paresis. *Sex Transm Dis.* 2004;31:350-352.
48. Sonne JE, Ziefer B, Linstrom C. Manifestations of otosyphilis as visualized with computed tomography. *Otol Neurotol.* 2002;23:806-807.59.
49. Mullick CJ, Liappis AP, Benator DA, et al. Syphilitic hepatitis in HIV-infected patients: A report of 7 cases and review of the literature. *Clin Infect Dis.* 2004;39:100-105.
50. Atten MJ, Attar BM, Teopengo E, et al. Gastric syphilis: A disease with multiple manifestations. *Am J Gastroenterol.* 1994;89:2227-2229.
51. Gurvinder PT, Kaur S, Gupta R, et al. Syphilitic panuveitis and asymptomatic neurosyphilis: A marker of HIV infection. *Int J STD AIDS.* 2001;12:754-756.
52. Aldave AJ, King JA, Cunningham ET. Ocular syphilis. *Curr Opin Ophthalmol.* 2001;12:433-441.
53. Ormerod LD, Pukin JE, Sobel JD. Syphilitic posterior uveitis: Correlative findings and significance. *Clin Infect Dis.* 2001;32:1661-1673.
54. Parc CE, Chahed S. Patel SV, et al. Manifestations and treatment of ocular syphilis during an epidemic in France. *Sex Transm Dis.* 2007;34:553-33647.
55. Yimtae K, Srirompotong S, Lertsukprasert K. Otosyphilis: A review of 85 cases. *Otolaryngol Head Neck Surg.* 2007; 136:67-71.
56. Mishra S, Waimsley SL, Loufty MR, et al. Otosyphilis in HIV-co-infected individuals: A case series from Toronto Canada. *AIDS Patient Care Stds.* 2008;22:213-219.
57. Hansen K, Hvid-Jacobson H, Lindewald PS, et al. Bone lesions in early syphilis detected by bone scintigraphy. *Br J Vener Dis.* 1984;60:256-258.
58. Kastner RJ, Malone JL, Decker CF. Syphilitic osteitis in a patient with secondary syphilis and concurrent human immunodeficiency virus infection. *Clin Infect Dis.* 1994;18:250-252.
59. VanEijk RVW, Wolters EC, Tutuarima JA, et al. Effect of early and late syphilis on central nervous system: Cerebrospinal fluid changes and neurologic deficit. *Genitourin Med.* 1987; 63:77-82.
60. Lugar A, Schmidt BL, Steyer K, et al. Diagnosis of neurosyphilis by examination of the cerebrospinal fluid. *Br J Vener Dis.* 1981;57:232-237.
61. Muller F, Moskophidis M. Estimation of the local production of antibodies to *Treponema pallidum* in the central nervous system of patients with neurosyphilis. *Br J Vener Dis.* 1983; 59:80-84.
62. Prange HW, Moskophidis M, Schipper HI, et al. Relationship between neurological features and intrathecal synthesis of IgG antibodies to *Treponema pallidum* in untreated and treated human neurosyphilis. *J Neurol.* 1983;230:241-252.
63. Kotnik V, Jordan K, Stopinsek S, et al. Intrathecal antitreponemal antibody synthesis determination using INNO-LIA Syphilis Score. *Acta Dermatovenerol Alp Panonica Adriat.* 2007;16: 135-141.
64. Inagaki H, Kawai T, Miyata M, et al. Polymerase chain reaction detection of treponemal DNA in pseudolymphomatous lesions. *Hum Pathol.* 1996;27:761-765.
65. Marra CM, Maxwell CL, Smith SL, et al. Cerebrospinal fluid abnormalities in patients with syphilis: Association with clinical and laboratory features. *J Infect Dis.* 2004;189:369-376.
66. Leslie DE, Azzato F, Karapanagiotidis T, et al. Development of a real-time PCR assay to detect Treponema pallidum in clinical specimenss and assessment of assay comparison with serological testing. *J Clin Mirobiol.* 2007;45:93-96.
67. Michelow IC, Wendel GD, Norgard MV, et al. Central nervous system infection in congenital syphilis. *N Engl J Med.* 2002;346:1792-1798.
68. Da Gama RD, Cidade M. Images in clinical medicine. Interstitial keratitis as the initial expression of syphilitic reactivation. *N Engl J Med.* 2002;346:1799.
69. Balkany TJ, Dans PE. Reversible sudden deafness in early acquired syphilis. *Arch Otolaryngol.* 1978;104:60.
70. Tramont EC. Neurosyphilis in patients with human immunodeficiency virus infection. *N Engl J Med.* 1994;332:1169-1170.
71. Pugh PJ, Grech EV. Images in clinical medicine. Syphilitic aortitis. *N Engl J Med.* 2002;346:676.
72. Sheffield JS, Sanchez PJ, Morris F, et al. Congenital syphilis after maternal treatment for syphilis during pregnancy. *Am J Obstet Gynecol.* 2002;186:569-573.
73. Sanchez PJ, Wendel GD, Grimprel E, et al. Evaluation of molecular methodologies and rabbit infectivity testing for the diagnosis of congenital syphilis and neonatal central nervous system invasion by *Treponema pallidum. J Infect Dis.* 1993;167: 168-177.
74. Dorfman DH, Glaser JH. Congenital syphilis presenting in infants after the newborn period. *N Engl J Med.* 1990;323: 1299-1301.
75. Beeram MR, Chopde N, Dawood Y, et al. Lumbar puncture in the evaluation of possible congenital syphilis in neonates. *J Pediatr.* 1996;128:125-129.
76. Gust DA, Levine WC, St Louis ME, et al. Mortality associated with congenital syphilis in the United States, 1992-1998. *Pediatrics.* 2002;109:E79-E88.
77. Fojaco RM, Hensley GT, Moskowitz L. Congenital syphilis and necrotizing funisitis. *JAMA.* 1989;261:1788-1790.
78. Centers for Disease Control and Prevention, Workowski KA, Berman SM. Sexually transmitted disease treatment guidelines. *MMWR Recomm Rep.* 2006;55(RR-11):1-94.
79. Buffet M, Grange PA, Gerhardt P, et al. Diagnosis of *Treponema pallidum* in secondary syphilis by PCR and immunochemistry. *J Invest Dermatol.* 2007;127:2345-2350.
80. Bahrlof W, Springer E, Brauminger W, et al. PCR testing for Treponema pallidum in paraffin-embedded skin biopsy specimenns: Test design and impact on diagnosis. *J Clin Pathol.* 2008;61:390-395.
80a. Martin-Ezquerra G, Fernandez-Casado A, Barco D, et al. *Treponema pallidum* distribution patterns in mucocutaneous lesions of primary and secondary syphilis: An immunochemical and ultrastructural study. *Hum Pathol.* 2009;40:624-630.
81. Rydzak CE, Goldie SJ. Cost-effectiveness of rapid point-of-care prenatal syphilis screening in sub-Saharan Africa. *Sex Transm Dis.* 2008;35:775-784.
82. Marangoni A, Moroni A, Accardo S, et al. Laboratory diagnosis of syphilis with automated immunoassays. J. *Clin Lab Med.* 2009;23:1-6.
82a. Borelli S, Monn A, Meyer J, et al. Evaluation of a particle gel immunoassay as a screening test for syphilis. *Infection.* 2009;37: 26-28.
82b. Sabido M, Benzaken A, Rodrigues EJA, et al. Rapid point-of-care diagnostic test for syphilis in high-risk populations, Manaus, Brazil. *Emerg Infect Dis.* 2009;15:647-649.
83. Muller I, Brade V, Hagedron H, et al. Is serological testing a reliable tool in laboratory diagnosis of syphilis? Meta-analysis of eight external quality control surveys performed by the German Infection Serology Proficiency Testing Program. *J Clin Microbiol.* 2006;44:1335-1342.
84. Berkowitz K, Baxi L, Fox HE. False-negative syphilis screening: The prozone phenomenon, nonimmune hydrops, and diagnosis of syphilis during pregnancy. *Am J Obstet Gynecol.* 1990;163: 975-977.
85. Hutchinson CM, Rompalo AM, Reochart CA, et al. Characteristics of syphilis in patients attending Baltimore STD clinics: Multiple-risk subgroups and interactions with HIV infection. *Arch Intern Med.* 1991;151:511-516.
86. Brown ST, Akbar Z, Larsen SA, et al. Serological response to syphilis treatment. *JAMA.* 1985;253:1296-1299.
87. Fiumara NJ. Treatment of primary and secondary syphilis: Serological response. *JAMA.* 1980;243:2500-2503.
88. Fiumara NJ. Serologic responses to treatment of 128 patients with late latent syphilis. *Sex Transm Dis.* 1979;6: 243-246.
88a. Marra CM, Maxwell CL, Tantalo LC, et al. Normalization of serum rapid reagin titer predicts normalization of cerebral fluid and clinical abnormalities after treatment of neurosyphilis. *Clin Infect Dis.* 2008;47:893-899.
89. Fiumara NJ. Reinfection primary, secondary, and latent syphilis. *Sex Transm Dis.* 1980;7:111-114.
89a. Monath TP, Frey SE. Possible autoimmune reactions following smallpox vaccination: The biologic false positive test for syphilis. *Vaccine.* 2009;27:1645-1650.
90. Burton AA, Flynn JA, Neumann TM, et al. Routine serologic screening for syphilis in hospitalized patients: High prevalence of unsuspected infection in the elderly. *Sex Transm Dis.* 1994;21:133-136.
91. Sambri V, Marangoni A, Eyer C, et al. Western blotting with five *Treponema pallidum* recombinant antigens for serologic diagnosis of syphilis. *Clin Diag Lab Immunol.* 2001;8:534-539.
92. Yoshioka N, Deguchi M, Kagita M, et al. Evaluation of a chemiluminescent micparticle immunoassay for determination of Treponema pallidum antibodies. *Clin Lab.* 2007;563:597-603.
93. Martin IE, Lau A, Swatzky P, et al. Serological diagnosis of syphilis: Enzyme-linked immunosorbent assay to measure antibodies to individual recombinant Treponema pallidum antigens. *J Immunochem.* 2008;29:143-151.
94. Herrmans M, Notermans DW, Mommers M, et al. Comparison of a Treponema pallidum IgM immunoblot with a 19S fluorescent treponemal antibody absorption test for the diagnosis of congenital syphilis. *Diagn Microbiol Infect Dis.* 2007;59: 61-66.
95. Van Voorhis, WC, Barrett LK, Lukehart SA, et al. Serodiagnosis of syphilis: Antibodies to recombinant Tp0453, Tp92 and Gpd proteins are sensitive and specific indicators of infection by *Treponema pallidum. J Clin Microbol.* 2003, 41:3668-3674.
96. Manavi K, Young H, McMillan A. The sensitivity of syphilis assays in detecting different stages of early syphilis. *Int J STD AIDS.* 2006;17:768-771.
97. Borelli S, Monn A, Meyer J, et al. Evaluation of a particle gel immunoassay as a screening test for syphilis. *Infection.* 2009; 37:26-28.
98. Shen X, Tan Y. Detection of oligoclonal immunoglobulins in the cerebralspinal fluid by immunofixation electrophoresis. *Clin Chem Lab Med.* 2001;39:1209-1210.
99. Schroeter AL, Lucas JB, Price EV, et al. Treatment for early syphilis and reactivity of serologic tests. *JAMA.* 1972;221:471-476.
100. Sheffield JS, Sanchez PJ, Morris F, et al. Congential syphilis after maternal treatment for syphilis during pregnancy. *Am J Obstet Gynecol.* 2002;186:569-573.
101. Short DH, Knox JM, Glicksman J. Neurosyphilis: The search for adequate treatment. *Arch Dermatol.* 1966;93:87-91.
102. Mohr JA, Griffiths W, Jackson R, et al. Neurosyphilis and penicillin levels in cerebrospinal fluid. *JAMA.* 1976;236:2208-2210.
103. Speer ME, Taber LH, Clark DB, et al. Cerebrospinal fluid levels of benzathine penicillin G in the neonate. *J Pediatr.* 1977;91:996-997.
104. Mascola L, Pelosi R, Alexander CE. Inadequate treatment of syphilis in pregnancy. *Am J Obstet Gynecol.* 1984;150:945-947.
105. Moskovitz BL, Klimek JJ, Goldman RL, et al. Meningovascular syphilis after "appropriate" treatment of primary syphilis. *Arch Intern Med.* 1982;142:139-141.
106. Markovitz PM, Bentner KR, Maggio RP, et al. Failure of recommended treatment for secondary syphilis. *JAMA.* 1986;255: 1767-1768.
107. Goorney B, Leahy M. Relapse of early syphilis on first-line treatment. *Int J STD AIDS.* 2002;13:722-723.
108. Smith JL. *Spirochetes in Late Seronegative Syphilis, Penicillin Notwithstanding.* Springfield, Ill: Charles C Thomas; 1969.
109. Wendel GD, Sheffield JS, Hollier LM, et al. Treatment of syphilis in pregnancy and prevention of congenital syphilis. *Clin Infect Dis.* 2002;35:S200-S209.
110. Giles AJH. Tabes dorsalis progressing to general paresis after 20 years despite routine penicillin therapy. *Br J Vener Dis.* 1980;56:368.
111. Berger JR. Spinal cord syphilis associated with human immunodeficiency virus infection: A treatable myelopathy. *Am J Med.* 1992;92:101-103.
112. Flood JM, Weinstock HS, Guroy ME. Neurosyphilis during the AIDS epidemic, San Francisco, 1985-1992. *J Infect Dis.* 1998; 177:931-940.
113. Johns DR, Tierney M, Felsenstein D. Alternation in the natural history of neurosyphilis by concurrent infections with human immunodeficiency virus. *N Engl J Med.* 1987;316:1569-1572.
114. Lynn WA, Lightman S. Syphilis and HIV: A dangerous combination. *Lancet Infect Dis.* 2004;4:456-466.

115. Chen DJ. Penicillin treatment for early syphilis in the presence of HIV-1 infection: The long and short of it? *Int J STD AIDS.* 2008 19:648.
116. Fowler VG Jr, Maxwell GL, Myers SA, et al. Failure of benzathine penicillin in a case of seronegative secondary syphilis in a patient with acquired immunodeficiency syndrome: Case report and review of the literature. *Arch Dermatol.* 2001;137:1374-1376.
117. Berry CD, Hooton TM, Collier AC, et al. Neurologic relapse after benzathine penicillin therapy for secondary syphilis in a patient with HIV infection. *N Engl J Med.* 1987;316:1587-1589.
118. Ghanem KG, Moore RD, Rompalo AM, et al. Antiretroviral therapy is associated with reduced setologic failure rates for syphilis among HIV-infected patients. *Clin Inf Dis.* 2008;47: 256-265.
119. Gordon SM, Eaton ME, George R. The response of symptomatic neurosyphilis to high-dose intravenous penicillin G in patients with human immunododeficiency virus infection. *N Engl J Med.* 1994;331:1469-1473.
119a. Karp G, Schaeffer F, Jotkowitz A, et al. Syphilis and HIV co-infection. *Eur J Intern Med.* 2009;20:9-13.
120. Katz KA, Klausner JD. Azithromycin resistance in. *Curr Opin Infect Dis.* 2008;21:83-91.
121. Hook EW, Roddy RE, Handsfield HH. Ceftriaxone therapy for incubating and early syphilis. *J Infect Dis.* 1988 158:881-884.
122. Marra CM, Boutin P, McArthur JC, et al. A pilot study evaluating ceftriaxone and penicillin G as treatment agents for neurosyphilis in human immunodeficiency virus–infected individuals. *Clin Infect Dis.* 2000;30:540-544.
123. Dowell ME, Ross PG, Musler DM, et al. Response of latent syphilis or neurosyphilis to ceftriaxone therapy in persons infected with HIV. *Am J Med.* 1992;93:481-488.
124. Morrison E, Harrison S, Tramont EC. Oral amoxicillin, an alternative treatment of neurosyphilis. *Genitourin Med.* 1985;61: 359-362.
125. Yim CW, Flynn NM, Fitzgerald FT. Penetration of oral doxycycline into the cerebrospinal fluid of patients with latent or neurosyphilis. *Antimicrob Agents Chemother.* 1985;28:347-348.
126. Kastner RJ, Malone JL, Decker CF. Syphilitic osteitis in a patient with secondary syphilis and concurrent human immunodeficiency virus infection. *Clin Infect Dis.* 1994;18:250-252.
127. Manavi K, McMillan A. The outcome of treatment of early latent syphilis and syphilis of undetermined duration in HIV-infected and HIV uninfected patients. *Int J STD AIDS.* 2007;18:814-818.
128. Silberstein P, Lawrence R, Pryor D, et al. A case of neurosyphilis with florid Jarisch-Herxheimer reaction. *J Clin Neurosci.* 2002;9:689-690.
129. Klein VR, Cox SM, Mitchell MD, et al. The Jarisch-Herxheimer reaction complicating syphilotherapy in pregnancy. *Obstet Gynecol.* 1990;75:375-380.
130. Fiumara NJ. Acquired syphilis in three patients with congenital syphilis. *N Engl J Med.* 1974;290:1119-1120.
131. Buchacz K, Klausner JD, Kerndt PR, et al. HIV incidence among men diagnosed with early syphilis in Atlanta, San Francisco, and Los Angeles, 2004 to 2005. *J Acquir Immune Defic Syndr.* 2008; 47:234-240.
132. Sellati TJ, Wilkinson DA, Sheffield JS, et al. Virulent *Treponema pallidum,* lipoprotein, and synthetic lipopeptides induce CCR5 on human monocytes and enhance the susceptibility to infection of human immunodeficiency virus type 1. *J Infect Dis.* 2000;181:288-293.
133. Buchacz K, Patel P, Taylor M, et al. Syphilis increases HIV viral load and decreases CD4 cell counts in HIV-infected patients with new syphilis infections. *AIDS.* 2004;18:2075-2079.
134. Theus SA, Harrich DA, Gaynor R, et al. *Treponema pallidum,* lipoproteins, and synthetic lipoprotein analogues induce human immunodeficiency virus type 1 gene expression in monocytes via NFkB activation. *J Infect Dis.* 1998;177:941-950.
135. Hutchinson CM, Hook EW, Sheperd M, et al. Altered clinical presentation of early syphilis in patients with human immunodeficiency virus infection. *Ann Intern Med.* 1994; 121:94-99.
136. Holtom PD, Larsen RA, Leal MA. Prevalence of neurosyphilis in immunodeficiency virus infection. *J Infect Dis.* 1992; 165:1020-1025.
137. Don PC, Rubinstein R, Christie S. Malignant syphilis (lues maligna) and concurrent infection with HIV. *Int J Dermatol.* 1995;34:403-407.
138. Horowitz HW, Valsamis MP, Wicher V, et al. Brief report: Cerebral syphilitic gumma confirmed by the polymerase chain reaction in man with human immunodeficiency virus infection. *N Engl J Med.* 1994;331:1488-1491.
139. Berger JR. Spinal cord syphilis associated with human immunodeficiency virus infection: A treatable myelopathy. *Am J Med.* 1992;92:101-103.
140. Hicks CB, Benson PM, Lupton GP, et al. Seronegative secondary syphilis in a patient infected with the human immunodeficiency virus (HIV) with Kaposi sarcoma. *Ann Intern Med.* 1987; 107:492-495.
141. Tikjob G, Russel M, Petersen CS, et al. Seronegative secondary syphilis in a patient with AIDS: Identification of *Treponema pallidum* in biopsy specimen. *J Am Acad Dermatol.* 1991; 24:506-508.
142. Erbelding EJ, Vladov D, Nelson KE, et al. Syphilis serology in human immunodeficiency virus infection: Evidence for false-negative fluorescent testing. *J Infect Dis.* 1997;176:1397-1400.

Endemic Treponematoses

EDWARD W. HOOK III

Collectively, the endemic treponematoses include yaws, endemic syphilis, and pinta and are caused by *Treponema pallidum* subspecies *pertenue*, *T. pallidum* subsp. *endemicum*, and *Treponema carateum*, respectively. These relatively uncommon diseases are most often seen in developing nations and are seen in developed nations primarily as a result of immigration. The bacteria that cause the endemic treponematoses are morphologically and serologically indistinguishable from *T. pallidum* subsp. *pallidum*, the causative agent of venereal syphilis, and important parallels are found between the natural history of these diseases and syphilis. Similarly, the tools for management are adapted almost entirely from tools used as part of syphilis control efforts. Nonetheless, the endemic treponematoses differ from syphilis in terms of clinical manifestations and at the level of the genome.[1,2] Targeted for elimination in the mid 20th century, the endemic treponematoses were uncommon in the 1970s. However, more recently, rates have once again begun to increase; current estimates are that more than 2.5 million persons are affected, of whom about 460,000 represent infectious cases.[1-4]

The Organisms

Within the genus *Treponema*, four bacteria are presently recognized as human pathogens: *T. pallidum* subsp. *pallidum*, *T. pallidum* subsp. *pertenue*, *T. pallidum* subsp. *endemicum*, and *T. carateum*. Much remains to be learned about these organisms. They cannot be readily cultured in vitro, they are indistinguishable from one another morphologically and immunologically, and current understanding of their biology is based on the careful study of relatively few clinical isolates, most often in animal models.[5,6] With the sequencing of the *T. pallidum* genome,[7] however, despite more than 98% DNA homology, several genetic loci have been identified that may permit differentiation of *T. pallidum* from the treponemes that cause the endemic treponematoses.[1-3] In addition, application of evolving molecular biologic methods to the study of human treponemes promises to provide new insights into the biology of these organisms in the future.

T. pallidum and the treponemes that cause the endemic treponematoses are long, thin (8 to 13 × 0.15 μm), motile bacteria that cannot be seen with the Gram stain and are best seen in clinical specimens with darkfield microscopic examination of lesion exudate or fluorescent antibody techniques. Their regular, spiral morphology and characteristic corkscrew motility are helpful for recognition in clinical specimens. On the basis of clinical and serologic response to therapy, and studies performed in experimental animals, these treponemes are all sensitive to penicillins and the tetracyclines. Because the organisms cannot be propagated in vitro, data on minimal inhibitory and bactericidal concentrations on multiple clinical isolates are not available. Clinical and laboratory resistance to erythromycin and other macrolide antibiotics has been shown for multiple isolates of *T. pallidum* subsp. *pallidum* from North America and Western Europe,[8] and no activity is found of sulfa drugs or fluroquinolone antimicrobials against the *T. pallidum* subsp. or *T. carateum*.

Epidemiology

The endemic treponematoses are spread primarily through direct contact or, in the case of endemic syphilis, possibly as fomites (see subsequent discussion). Unlike in syphilis, however, little evidence exists of transmission via blood or blood products (although this is theoretically possible) or transplacentally in pregnant women to unborn children.

The endemic treponematoses are diseases of developing countries with varied geographic distribution, although the diseases are rare above or below the 30th parallels.[9] Yaws appears to have worldwide distribution, and endemic syphilis is most common in more arid regions of North Africa and the Arabic peninsula. Pinta has been reported only from the Caribbean islands and Central and South America. Within these regions, each of the endemic treponematoses disproportionately impacts persons living on the margins of society. Limited access to hygienic facilities has been associated with increased infection rates.

Clinical Manifestations

The endemic treponematoses can be characterized by a number of common clinical characteristics and those characteristics that distinguish them from one another.[9] Each is a chronic bacterial infection acquired through contact with infectious material. Initial lesions occur at the site of inoculation after an incubation period of 9 to 50 days (mean, 21 days). Early in the course of infection, perhaps even before primary lesions develop, the treponemes that cause these infections spread hematogenously throughout the body and, without treatment, subsequently give rise to secondary and late manifestations of infection. These diseases predictably progress from an early, localized stage to a later, more widespread stage. A minority of patients with untreated infection have development of late complications of infection. Early infection with the endemic treponematoses is characterized by the appearance of epithelial lesions at the site of inoculation. Soon after primary lesion development, regional lymphadenopathy occurs. As in the case of venereal syphilis, primary lesions of yaws and pinta resolve spontaneously without treatment and then recur over as long as 5 years, with the frequency of these recurrences declining with time. Recurrent manifestations of early endemic treponematoses are primarily dermatologic; however, on occasion, bony or cartilaginous lesions occur as well.

In a minority of untreated patients with yaws and endemic syphilis, late infection occurs. The lesions of late infections arise from hematogenously spread organisms, tend to be more destructive than the early lesions, and are most commonly manifest as either ulcerative or hyperkeratotic cutaneous lesions or bone and joint involvement.

Another distinguishing common element of the endemic treponematoses is that, unlike the situation in syphilis (*T. pallidum* subsp. *pallidum* infection), little if any evidence exists of cardiovascular involvement in late infection, neurologic sequelae of untreated infection, or transmission to children born to infected mothers who have not been treated.

YAWS

Yaws is a chronic infection caused by *T. pallidum* subsp. *pertenue* and is the most common of the endemic treponematoses. After years of relatively low levels (see discussion on Control Management), the disease apparently is once again becoming more common.[4,10,11] The disease is most common in children, with most cases in children 2 to 15 years of age. Most transmission occurs from direct (nonsexual) contact that results in the transfer of infectious exudate from lesions to uninfected individuals. Transmission is thought to be facilitated by

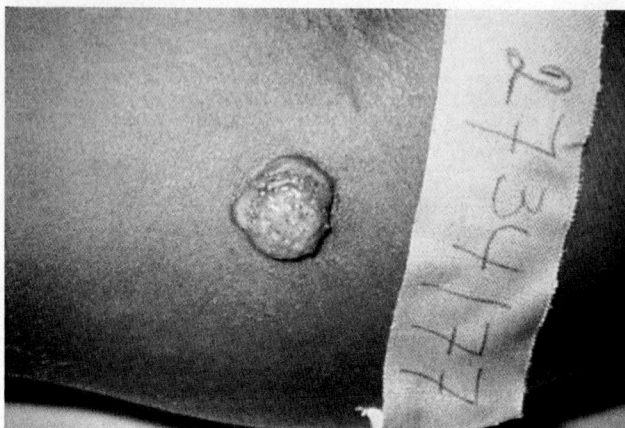

Figure 239-1 Initial papillomatous yaws lesion on upper thigh (also called primary framboesioma, mother yaw, *chancre pia nique*). Initial lesion usually commences as papule on lower extremities and slowly enlarges to form a raspberry-like lesion. (*From Perine PL, Hopkins DR, Niemel PLA, et al. Handbook of Endemic Treponematoses. Geneva: World Health Organization, 1984.*)

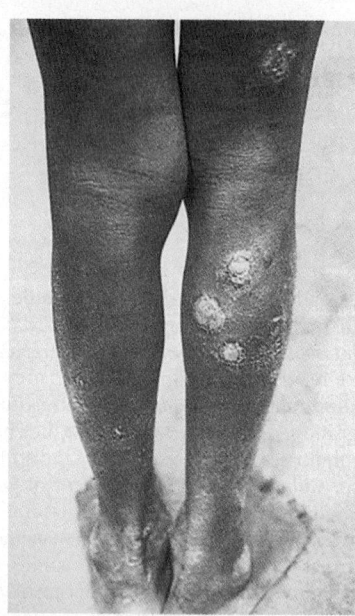

Figure 239-2 Early ulceropapillomatous yaws on the leg (also called *ulcère post-chancreux*). (*From Perine PL, Hopkins DR, Niemel PLA, et al. Handbook of Endemic Treponematoses. Geneva: World Health Organization, 1984.*)

disruption of epithelial surfaces (lacerations, insect bites, etc.) and by crowding and a relative lack of hygienic practices. These circumstances are, in general, more common in children than in adults and may help to explain why most initial infections occur in youth.

After inoculation of *T. pallidum* subsp. *pertenue* and after an incubation period of 9 to 90 days (mean, approximately 21 days), a primary papular lesion forms at the site of inoculation. Over a period of several months, the primary papule of yaws may increase in size and then heal spontaneously. Primary lesions are typically pruritic, facilitating autoinoculation; and tender regional lymphadenopathy may develop. Fever and constitutional symptoms are uncommon. At about the time the primary papule heals, secondary lesions near or distant from the initial lesion may occur. These lesions may also be papular in nature and are thought to be a consequence of both local (autoinoculation) and hematogenous spread of infection (Fig. 239-1). Secondary lesions of yaws predominately involve the skin, bone, and cartilage and, if untreated, heal without scarring (Fig. 239-2). Occasionally, secondary infection or ulceration of cutaneous lesions of yaws does occur and results in more pronounced lesions and scarring. Like the primary lesions of yaws, secondary lesions resolve spontaneously without therapy and patients enter a latent stage. The differential diagnosis of early yaws includes impetigo, scabies, molluscum contagiosum, lichen planus, and cutaneous leishmaniasis.

In a small proportion (estimated to be about 10%) of untreated patients, late lesions of yaws may occur. Late lesions are characterized by hyperkeratotic plaques and lesions, destructive bony lesions, or gummata. *Gangosa* is the term used to describe these disfiguring chronic manifestations as they destroy bone, cartilage, and soft tissue of the mouth and nose (Fig. 239-3). Bowing of the anterior tibiae (saber shins) may likewise be a late manifestation of yaws, arising from infectious periostitis.

Yaws infections may be aborted with prophylactic administration of penicillin in exposed patients. Healing is promoted with therapeutic administration of penicillin and in early cases may occur without problems. Despite appropriate therapy, serologic tests for syphilis may continue to be reactive for years.

ENDEMIC SYPHILIS (BEJEL)

Endemic syphilis is the epidemic treponematosis caused by *T. pallidum* subsp. *endemicum*.[9,11] This infection is somewhat less common than yaws and occurs primarily in dry, arid areas among nomadic and seminomadic rural populations. The disease has been most common

in North Africa, Southwest Asia, and the eastern Mediterranean region.

Endemic syphilis, like yaws, is a disease of childhood, with most cases in individuals ages 2 to 15 years. Transmission of endemic syphilis is thought to occur via direct contact and, because early lesions are often mucosal, also as fomites on shared eating or drinking utensils. The primary lesions of endemic syphilis occur as mucous patches on oral pharyngeal mucosa or as lesions at the angles of the lips (angular stomatitis). These painless lesions may resolve without therapy. Subsequently, as in other endemic treponematoses, second-

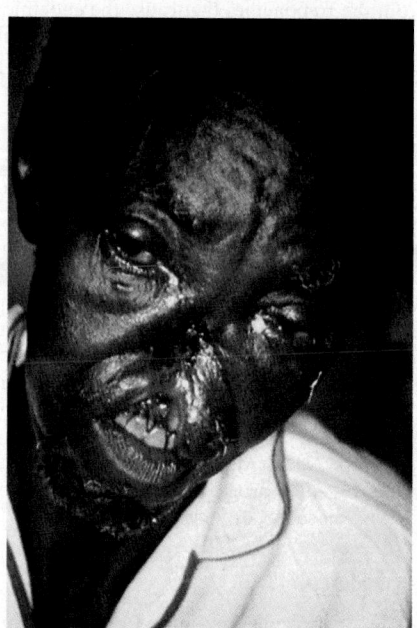

Figure 239-3 Gangosa. (*From Perine PL, Hopkins DR, Niemel PLA, et al. Handbook of Endemic Treponematoses. Geneva: World Health Organization, 1984.*)

ary lesions may become apparent. Secondary lesions of endemic syphilis may appear as rashes, mucosal lesions, or bony and cartilaginous involvement. Secondary manifestations of endemic syphilis may occur as disseminated papular rashes similar to those of secondary syphilis or as condylomata predominately in moist areas of the skin. The secondary lesions of endemic syphilis may display a wide variety of morphologies comparable with those seen in secondary syphilis.

After a period of latency, complications of endemic syphilis are relatively common. These manifestations may present as gummatous lesions or chronic ulcerative skin lesions in 25% to 50% of patients. Unlike the lesions of early endemic syphilis, late lesions tend to be destructive, chronic progressive lesions, some of which go on to cause deforming bony and cartilaginous facial lesions referred to as gangosa. In addition to the ulcerative lesions of endemic syphilis, bony involvement may occur as well and is manifested as osteoperiostitis causing disability and deformity.

PINTA

Pinta is the endemic treponematosis caused by a unique treponemal species, *T. carateum*.[9,11] Pinta, unlike yaws and endemic syphilis, which have a global distribution, is a disease limited to the New World. The disease has been described in numerous South American and Caribbean countries, including Cuba.[11-13] At the current time, the disease is quite rare; recently, however, substantial numbers of cases, including a case series of more than 200 patients, have been described in rural Brazil. The peak age prevalence for pinta is somewhat older than for yaws or endemic syphilis with individuals ages 15 to 30 years. Like other endemic treponematoses, pinta is thought to be spread through direct lesion contact. An important difference between pinta and the other endemic treponematoses is that without treatment the lesions tend to persist. The classic initial lesion of pinta is a papule or erythematous epithelial plaque. These lesions tend to occur on parts of the body that are not typically clothed, most often the leg, foot, forearm, or back of the hands. Typically, these lesions then slowly enlarge through local extension to form hyperkeratotic pigmented lesions. The lesions of pinta are accompanied by regional lymphadenopathy. In the interval of 3 to 9 months after infection, disseminated lesions may occur distal to the initial lesion and also slowly enlarge. Over time, the lesions of pinta become pigmented, initially becoming somewhat hyperpigmented and taking on a darker color described as slate blue. Late pinta is characterized further by additional pigmentary cutaneous changes; lesions may include dyschromic treponeme-containing lesions and achromic treponeme-free lesions. The depigmentation process of pinta occurs at different rates in the same lesion, giving the lesions a somewhat mottled appearance. No other disability or late complications of pinta have currently been described.

Diagnosis

The diagnosis of individual cases of the endemic treponematoses is in large part dependent on clinical recognition of appropriate clinical findings, confirmed with serologic testing with serologic tests for syphilis.[11,14] Although not widely available, visual demonstration of characteristic treponemes with darkfield microscopy of lesion exudates can provide immediate and highly specific diagnosis of the endemic treponematoses. Immunofluorescent antibody stains for treponemes are also available in some settings and likewise provide specific diagnosis of infection. In settings in which the endemic treponematoses are common, however, facilities for darkfield or immunofluorescence microscopy are rare; therefore, these methods are rarely used for diagnosis. No serologic tests have been specifically developed for diagnosis of endemic treponematoses; however, because the humoral antibody response to these diseases is indistinguishable from the response to syphilis, serologic tests for syphilis are important for confirmation of clinically suspected infections. In addition, serologic testing is useful

for estimation of population prevalence of the endemic treponematoses to guide control efforts.[9,10]

Serologic tests for syphilis (and the endemic treponematoses) are divided into nontreponemal and treponemal tests.[14] The nontreponemal tests are based on the cross reactivity of cardiolipin-cholesterol-lecithin antigens with antibodies to *T. pallidum* and are represented by tests such as the rapid plasma reagin (RPR) and venereal disease research laboratory (VDRL) tests. These tests provide quantifiable results that are useful not only for screening for infection but also for evaluation of response to therapy after treatment. In contrast, the treponemal tests are based on the reactivity of antibodies to either cloned *T. pallidum* antigens or antigens from *T. pallidum* propagated in laboratory animals. The treponemal tests are available in a variety of formats, including fluorescent treponemal antibody absorption (FTA-Abs), *T. pallidum* hemagglutination (TPHA), or a number of different commercial enzyme-linked immunosorbent assays (ELISAs). False-positive results sometimes occur with both nontreponemal and treponemal tests; however, because the tests are unrelated, use of an unrelated test to confirm an initial test result (i.e., confirmatory testing of reactive RPR or VDRL test results with a treponemal test) greatly increases the specificity of test results. Most false-positive serologic test results for syphilis are positive at a dilution of 1:4 or less. Partially on the basis of this fact, in many resource-limited settings where the prevalence of such infections is relatively high and treponemal tests are not readily available, nontreponemal test titers with a titer of greater than 1:4 are considered to represent active infection and thus to guide management decisions.

After effective treatment, most patients with active endemic treponematoses have a two-fold (four dilutions) or greater decline in serologic test result titer, although for many patients the serologic test result titers do not revert to nonreactive after successful therapy. Reinfection or relapse may be indicated with a serologic titer that rises two or more dilutions. Reversion of treponemal serologic test results to nonreactive is considerably less common than for nontreponemal tests.

Treatment

Penicillin is the preferred drug for treatment of the endemic treponematoses.[1,9,11] The drug is relatively inexpensive, available as a long-acting preparation (benzathine penicillin G) that provides treponemicidal serum levels for several weeks after administration, and highly effective. At present, the World Health Organization recommends treatment of each of the endemic treponematoses with single intramuscular doses of benzathine penicillin G, 600,000 U for children under age 10 years and 1.2 million U for persons 10 years of age or older. Treatment of all household members and close personal contacts is recommended to prevent development of infection in exposed persons. Cure rates with recommended doses of benzathine penicillin are about 97%, with treatment failure attributed to improper administration, use of out-of-date or inactive medication, or reinfection as a result of exposure to an untreated person. More recently, reports have been found of cure rates equivalent to those reported for benzathine penicillin with oral penicillin regimens[15]; however, because of potential problems related to medication adherence, benzathine penicillin remains the preferred treatment. No data suggest that any of the *T. pallidum* subspecies or *T. carateum* have clinically significant resistance to penicillin. No formal studies are found of alternative therapies for persons with penicillin allergy; however, with extrapolation from experience with venereal syphilis, tetracycline or doxycycline given for 14 days is likely to be effective.

Response to therapy may be determined through resolution of early lesions or, in persons with late infection, arrest of progression. Serologic response to therapy may also be seen as declines in nontreponemal tests for syphilis (i.e., RPR or VDRL) titers of two or more dilutions. After treatment, however, serologic test titers may not revert to seronegativity.

Public Health Management and Control Strategies

The endemic treponematoses are readily transmitted through direct contact between infected and uninfected persons. As a result, as diseases of children that do not cause systemic symptoms or limit activity, these infections not surprisingly increase in prevalence within susceptible populations. In the 1950s, the World Health Organization embarked on an ambitious global control program with use of active serologic screening and staged treatment approaches for entire communities.[1,7] In this program, communities were categorized based on seroprevalence as high prevalence (>10%), medium prevalence (5% to 10%), or low prevalence (<5%). In high-prevalence communities, the entire community was administered mass penicillin therapy; for medium-prevalence communities, all identified infected individuals, all children under 15 years, and all contacts of infected individuals were treated; and in low-prevalence settings, only individuals with active infections and their contacts were treated. In this effort, more than 450 million examinations were performed, and more than 50 million persons in 46 countries were treated. This effort was quite successful and reduced global prevalence of the endemic treponematoses by 95%; however, as the disease waned, so did resources for continuing surveillance.[4,10] Over the past two decades, infection rates have once again increased, with global prevalence of infectious cases now estimated at about 460,000 cases.[4] The potential effectiveness of community-based control efforts has been shown in India where reimplementation of the control measures reduced the number of reported cases from 3571 in 1996 to 0 in 2004; in 2006, yaws was formally declared eliminated from India.

REFERENCES

1. Antal GM, Lukehart SA, Meheus AZ. The endemic treponematoses. *Microbes Infect.* 2002;4:83-94.
2. Gray RR, Mulligan CH, Molini BJ, et al. Molecular evolution of the *tpr* C, D, I, K, G and J genes in the pathogenic genus *Treponema. Mol Biol Eval.* 2006;23:2220-2233.
3. Harper KN, Liu H, Ocampo PS, et al. The sequence of the acidic repeat protein (*arp*) gene differentiates venereal from nonvenereal *Treponema pallidum* subspecies, and the gene has evolved under strong positive subspecies in the subspecies that causes syphilis. *FEMS Immunol Med Microbiol.* 2008;53:322-332.
4. World Health Report. *Life in the 21st Century; a vision for all.* Geneva: World Health Organization; 1998.
5. Wicher K, Wicher V, Abbruscato F, et al. *Treponema pallidum* subsp. *pertenue* displays pathogenic properties different from those of *T. pallidum* subsp. *pallidum. Infect Immun.* 2000;68:3219-3225.
6. Engelkens HJ, ten Kate FJ, Judanarso J, et al. The localization of treponemes and characterization of the inflammatory infiltrate in skin biopsies from patients with primary or secondary syphilis, or early infectious yaws. *Genitourin Med.* 1993;69: 102-107.
7. Fraser CM, Norris SJ, Weinstock GM. Complete genome sequence of *Treponema pallidum*, the syphilis spirochete. *Science.* 1998;281:375-387.
8. Lukehart SA, Gordornes C, Molini BJ, et al. Macrolide resistance in *Treponema pallidum* in the United States and Ireland. *N Engl J Med.* 2004;351:154-158.
9. Perine PL, Hopkins DR, Niemel PLA, et al. *Handbook of Endemic Treponematoses.* Geneva: World Health Organization; 1984.
10. World Health Organization. Elimination of yaws in India. *Wkly Epidemiol Rec.* 2008;83:125-132.
11. Farnsworth N, Rosen T. Endemic trepanematoses: Review and update. *Clin Dermatol.* 2006;24:181-190.
12. Castro LG. Nonvenereal treponematosis [letter]. *J Am Acad Dermatol.* 1994;31:1075-1076.
13. Woltsche-Kahr I, Schmidt B, Aberer W, et al. Pinta in Austria (or Cuba?): Import of an extinct disease? *Arch Dermatol.* 1999;135: 685-688.
14. Larsen SA, Pope V, Johnson RE, et al, eds. *A Manual of Tests for Syphilis.* 9th ed. Washington: American Public Health Association; 1998.
15. Scolnik D, Aronson L, Lovinsky R, et al. Efficacy of a targeted, oral penicillin-based yaws control program among children living in rural South America. *Clin Infect Dis.* 2003;36:1232-1238.

240

Leptospira Species (Leptospirosis)

PAUL N. LEVETT | DAVID A. HAAKE

Leptospirosis is a zoonosis of global distribution, caused by infection with pathogenic spirochetes of the genus *Leptospira*. The disease is greatly underreported, particularly in tropical regions, but attempts at surveillance suggest that it may be the most common zoonosis.[1] The disease is maintained in nature by chronic renal infection of carrier animals, which excrete the organism in their urine, contaminating the environment. Human infection occurs by direct contact with infected urine or tissues or, more commonly by indirect exposure to the organisms in damp soil or water. Most human infections are probably asymptomatic; the spectrum of illness is extremely wide, ranging from undifferentiated febrile illness to severe multisystem disease with high mortality rates. The extreme variation in clinical presentation is partly responsible for the significant degree of underdiagnosis.

History

A syndrome of severe multisystem disease, presenting with profound jaundice and renal function impairment, was described by Weil in Heidelberg in 1886. Other descriptions of disease that probably represent leptospirosis were made earlier, but the cause could not be definitively ascribed to leptospiral infection.[2] Leptospires were first visualized in autopsy specimens from a patient thought to have had yellow fever,[3] but were not isolated until several years later, almost simultaneously, in Germany and Japan.[4] Diagnostic confusion between severe icteric leptospirosis and yellow fever continued, with prominent researchers such as Stokes and Noguchi dying in their attempts to discover the causative agent.[4] Several authoritative reviews have been published.[2,4-7]

Etiology

"Leptospira" derives from the Greek *leptos* (thin) and Latin *spira* (coiled). Aptly named, the leptospires are a mere 0.1 μm in diameter by 6 to 20 μm in length. The cells have pointed ends, one or both of which is usually bent into a characteristic hook (Fig. 240-1). Motility is conferred by the rotation of two axial flagella underlying the membrane sheath, which are inserted at opposite ends of the cell and extend toward the central region.[8] Because of their small diameter, leptospires are best visualized by darkfield microscopy, appearing as actively motile spirochetes (Fig. 240-2). Leptospires are readily cultured in polysorbate-albumin medium if specimens are obtained prior to initiation of antibiotic therapy.[9]

Historically, the genus *Leptospira* was classified into two species, *L. interrogans* and *L. biflexa*, comprised of pathogenic and nonpathogenic strains, respectively. Within each species, large numbers of serovars were differentiated using agglutinating antibodies. Serovar specificity is conferred by lipopolysaccharide (LPS) O antigens.[10] More than 250 serovars of pathogenic leptospires have been described; because of the large number of serovars, antigenically related serovars were grouped into serogroups for convenience in serologic testing.

Leptospires are now classified into a number of species defined by their degree of genetic relatedness, determined by DNA reassociation.[11,12] There are currently 14 named species, including pathogens (e.g., *L. interrogans*), nonpathogenic saprophytes (e.g., *L. biflexa*), and species of indeterminate pathogenicity (e.g., *L. inadai*) (Table 240-1). Some species contain both pathogenic and nonpathogenic strains. This classification is supported by 16S RNA gene sequencing (Fig. 240-3),[13] but is distinct from the former serologic classification.[5]

The system of serogroup nomenclature has no taxonomic standing, but is retained because presumptive serogroup determination by serologic testing has some epidemiologic value. However, it is doubtful whether serologic responses can be extrapolated to identification of the infecting serovar in an individual patient.[14]

The genome sequences of several *Leptospira* species and strains have been determined[15-18] and sequencing of other strains is under way. The availability of these genome sequences has already led to better understanding of leptospiral pathogenesis.

Epidemiology and Transmission

Leptospirosis is endemic throughout the world. Human infections are endemic in most regions; the peak incidence occurs in the rainy season in tropical regions and the late summer to early fall in temperate regions. Outbreaks may follow periods of excess rainfall.[19] The incidence of leptospirosis is probably grossly underestimated, because of limited diagnostic capacity in the regions where the burden of disease is greatest.[1] In the United States, the highest incidence is found in Hawaii; active surveillance in 1992 detected an annual incidence of approximately 128 cases/100,000.[20] Leptospirosis is no longer a nationally notifiable disease in the United States, although it remains notifiable in more than 20 states.

Leptospirosis is maintained in nature by chronic renal infection of carrier animals. The most important reservoirs are rodents and other small mammals, but livestock and companion animals are also significant sources of human infection. Infection of carrier animals usually occurs during infancy and, once infected, animals may excrete leptospires in their urine intermittently or continuously throughout life.

Infection occurs through direct or indirect contact with urine or tissues of infected animals. Direct contact is important in transmission to veterinarians, workers in milking sheds on dairy farms, abattoir works, butchers, hunters, and animal handlers (transmission has been reported to occur to children handling puppies and to dog handlers). Indirect contact is more common, and is responsible for disease following exposure to wet soil or water. The great majority of cases are acquired by this route in the tropics, either through occupational exposure to water, as in rice or taro farming, flooding after heavy rains, or exposure to damp soil and water during avocational activities.

Recreational exposures have become relatively more important, often in association with adventure tourism to tropical endemic areas. Several large point-source waterborne outbreaks have occurred after athletic events.[21,22] There has been an increase in leptospirosis cases in dogs in the eastern regions of North America and in the Midwest,[23] associated with a shift in the predominant serovars causing disease.[24,25] Veterinary vaccine manufacturers have responded to this problem by licensing new canine vaccines containing these emerging serovars.

Pathogenesis

Leptospires enter the body through cuts and abrasions, mucous membranes or conjunctivae, or aerosol inhalation of microscopic droplets. Swallowing contaminated lake water was the only behavioral risk factor identified in a case-control study of a large leptospirosis outbreak at the 1998 Springfield Triathlon.[21] However, the oral mucosae are probably a more important route of entry after ingestion than the intestinal tract. On entering the body, there is widespread hematogenous dissemination and penetration of tissue barriers, including

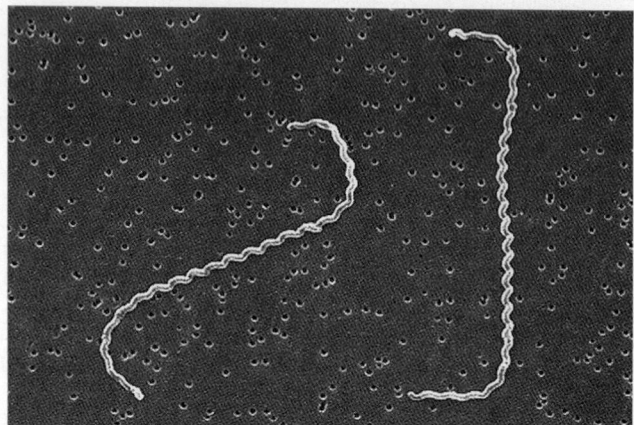

Figure 240-1 Scanning electron micrograph of cells *Leptospira interrogans* showing helical structure and curved (hooked) ends (original magnification ×60,000). *(Courtesy of Rob Weyant, Centers for Disease Control and Prevention.)*

Species	Selected Pathogenic Serovars
L. interrogans	Icterohaemorrhagiae, Copenhageni, Canicola, Pomona, Australis, Autumnalis, Pyrogenes, Bratislava, Lai
L. noguchii	Panama, Pomona
L. borgpetersenii	Ballum, Hardjo, Javanica
L. santarosai	Bataviae
L. kirschneri	Bim, Bulgarica, Grippotyphosa, Cynopteri
L. weilii	Celledoni, Sarmin
L. alexanderi	Manhao 3
Leptospira genomospecies 1	Sichuan
L. fainei	Hurtsbridge
L. meyeri	Sofia
L. inadai	Indeterminate
L. wolbachii	Nonpathogens
L. biflexa	Nonpathogens
Leptospira genomospecies 3	Nonpathogens
Leptospira genomospecies 4	Nonpathogens
Leptospira genomospecies 5	Nonpathogens
L. broomii	Indeterminate
L. licerasiae	Indeterminate

TABLE 240-1 Species of *Leptospira* and Some Pathogenic Serovars

invasion of the central nervous system and aqueous humor of the eye. Transendothelial migration of spirochetes is facilitated by a systemic vasculitis, accounting for a broad spectrum of clinical illness. Severe vascular injury can ensue, leading to pulmonary hemorrhage, ischemia of the renal cortex and tubular-epithelial cell necrosis, and destruction of the hepatic architecture, resulting in jaundice and liver cell injury, with or without necrosis.[26]

The mechanisms whereby leptospires cause disease are not clearly understood. Potential virulence factors include immune mechanisms, toxin production, adhesins, and other surface proteins. Human susceptibility to leptospirosis may be related to poor recognition of leptospiral LPS by the innate immune system.[27,28] Human toll-like receptor (TLR) 4, which responds to extremely low concentrations of gram-negative LPS (endotoxin), appears to be unable to bind leptospiral LPS,[28,29] perhaps because of the unique methylated phosphate residue of its lipid A.[30] Direct tissue damage may also be caused by production of hemolytic toxins, which may act as sphingomyelinases, phospholipases, or pore-forming proteins.[31]

Immune-mediated mechanisms have been postulated as one factor influencing the severity of symptoms.[32] Investigation of the triathlon outbreak mentioned earlier identified the human leukocyte antigen (HLA) DQ6 as an independent risk factor for leptospirosis.[33] The structural location of HLA-DQ6 polymorphisms associated with disease suggested that leptospires produce a superantigen that can cause nonspecific T-cell activation in susceptible individuals. Other

immune mechanisms, including circulating immune complexes, anti-cardiolipin antibodies, and antiplatelet antibodies, have been proposed but their significance is unproven. In horses, recurrent uveitis (moon blindness) may result from direct infection[34] or from the production of antibodies against a host epitope that is shared by common equine pathogenic serovars.[35]

A number of studies have focused on the roles of surface lipoproteins in leptospiral pathogenesis.[36] The major surface lipoprotein, LipL32, is highly conserved among pathogenic serovars.[37] LipL32 is a major target of the human immune response[38] and appears to be involved in the pathogenesis of tubulointerstitial nephritis.[39] Virulent leptospires respond to the increased osmolarity of host tissues by inducing expression of the multifunctional Lig surface proteins that mediate interactions with fibronectin, fibrinogen, and other extracellular matrix factors.[40] The Lig proteins are early antigens; IgM antibodies to their immunoglobulin-like repeats develop early in infection, offering an approach to improved detection of acute infection.[41] The endostatin-like LenA protein binds the complement regulatory protein, factor H, suggesting an important role in serum resistance.[42]

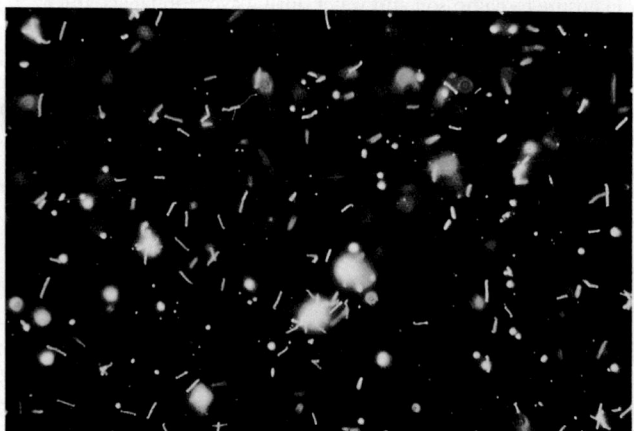

Figure 240-2 Leptospires viewed by darkfield microscopy (original magnification ×100). *(Courtesy of Mildred Galton, Public Health Image Library, Centers for Disease Control and Prevention.)*

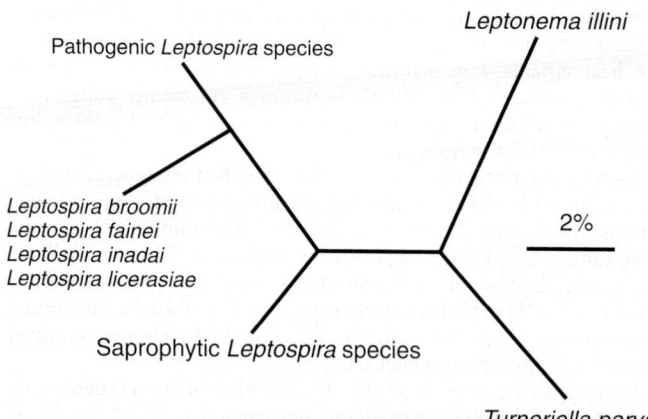

Figure 240-3 Unrooted phylogenetic tree based on 16s rRNA gene sequences of the Leptospiraceae obtained from GenBank. Species comprised of pathogenic serovars (see Table 240-1) cluster separately from nonpathogenic species. *Leptospira inadai*, *L. fainei*, *L. broomii*, and *L. licerasiae* are intermediate between pathogens and nonpathogens.

Clinical Manifestations

Leptospiral infection is associated with a very broad spectrum of severity, ranging from subclinical illness followed by seroconversion to two clinically recognizable syndromes—a self-limited systemic illness seen in approximately 90% of infections, and a severe, potentially fatal illness accompanied by any combination of renal failure, liver failure, and pneumonitis with hemorrhagic diathesis.[2,6,7] In some patients, the disease has two distinct phases, an initial septicemic stage followed by a temporary decline in fever followed by an immune phase in which the severe symptoms occur. However, in many severe cases, the distinction between these two phases is not apparent; in addition, many patients present only with the onset of the second phase of the illness.

The mean incubation period is 10 days (range, 5 to 14 days); determination of precise exposures may be difficult, leading to significant imprecision in estimated incubation times. The acute septicemic phase of illness begins abruptly with a high remittent fever (38° to 40°C) and headache, chills, rigors, and myalgias; conjunctival suffusion without purulent discharge; abdominal pain; anorexia, nausea, and vomiting; diarrhea; and cough and pharyngitis; a pretibial maculopapular cutaneous eruption occurs rarely (Table 240-2). Conjunctival suffusion (redness without exudate) and muscle tenderness, most notable in the calf and lumbar areas, are the most characteristic physical findings, but may occur in a minority of cases (see Table 240-2). Other less common signs include lymphadenopathy, splenomegaly, and hepatomegaly. The acute phase lasts from 5 to 7 days. Routine laboratory tests are nonspecific but indicative of a bacterial infection. Leptospires can be recovered from blood and cerebrospinal fluid (CSF) during the acute phase of illness, but meningeal signs are not prominent in this phase. Leptospires may also be recovered from urine, beginning about 5 to 7 days after the onset of symptoms (Fig. 240-4). Urinalysis reveals mild proteinuria and pyuria, with or without hematuria, and hyaline or granular casts. Death is rare in the acute phase of illness.

The immune phase of illness generally lasts from 4 to 30 days (see Fig. 240-4). The disappearance of leptospires from the blood and CSF coincides with the appearance of IgM antibodies.[7,52] The organisms can be detected in almost all tissues and organs, and in urine for several weeks, depending on the severity of the disease. In addition to the acute-phase symptoms described, the immune phase may be characterized by any or all of the following signs and symptoms: jaundice, renal failure, cardiac arrhythmias, pulmonary symptoms, aseptic meningitis, conjunctival suffusion with or without hemorrhage; photophobia; eye pain; muscle tenderness; adenopathy; and hepatosplenomegaly

(see Table 240-2). Abdominal pain is not uncommon and may be an indication of pancreatitis.

Aseptic meningitis, with or without symptoms, is characteristic of the immune phase of illness, occurring in up to 80% of cases. In endemic areas, a significant proportion of all aseptic meningitis cases may be caused by leptospiral infection.[53] Symptomatic patients present with an intense, bitemporal, and frontal throbbing headache, with or without delirium. A lymphocytic pleocytosis occurs, with total cell counts generally below 500/mm³. CSF protein levels are modestly elevated, between 50 and 100 mg/mL; the CSF glucose concentration is normal. Severe neurologic complications such as coma, meningoencephalitis, hemiplegia, transverse myelitis, or Guillain-Barré syndrome occur only rarely.[5]

The most distinctive form of severe illness that may develop after the acute phase of illness is Weil's disease, characterized by impaired hepatic and renal function. More severe cases may progress directly from the acute phase without the characteristic brief improvement in symptoms to a fulminant illness, with fever higher than 40°C and the rapid onset of liver failure, acute renal failure, hemorrhagic pneumonitis, cardiac arrhythmia, or circulatory collapse.[7] Mortality rates in patients developing severe disease have ranged from 5% to 40%.[2,5,6,47]

In a study of 840 hospitalized patients with severe leptospirosis (14% case-fatality rate), the risk of death was found to increase with age, especially in adults 40 years of age or older.[49,54] Altered mental status has been found to be the strongest predictor of death.[49,55] Other poor prognostic signs include acute renal failure (oliguria, hyperkalemia, serum creatinine >3.0 mg/dL), respiratory insufficiency (dyspnea, pulmonary rales, chest x-ray infiltrates), hypotension, and arrhythmias.[49] In jaundiced patients, disturbance of liver function is out of proportion to the rather mild and nonspecific pathologic findings. Conjugated serum bilirubin levels may rise to 80 mg/dL, accompanied by more modest elevations of serum transaminases, alanine aminotransferase, and aspartate aminotransferase, which rarely exceed 200 U/L.[56] This is in marked contrast to viral hepatitis. Jaundice is slow to resolve, but death caused by liver failure almost never occurs in the absence of renal failure. At autopsy, degenerative changes are seen in hepatocytes, Kupffer cells may be hypertrophied, cholestasis is evident, and erythrophagocytosis and mononuclear cell infiltrates are observed.[57] Hepatocellular necrosis is absent.

Kidney involvement is initially characterized by a unique nonoliguric hypokalemic form of renal insufficiency. Hallmarks are impaired sodium reabsorption, increased distal sodium delivery, and potassium wasting. The impairment in sodium reabsorption appears to be caused by selective loss of the ENaC sodium channel in the proximal tubular

	TABLE 240-2	**Signs and Symptoms on Admission in Patients with Leptospirosis in Large Case Series**							
Sign or Symptom (%)	*Puerto Rico, 1963*[43] (N = 208)	*China 1965*[44] (N = 168)	*Vietnam, 1973*[45] (N = 93)	*Korea, 1987*[46] (N = 150)	*Barbados, 1990*[47] (N = 88)	*Seychelles, 1998*[48] (N = 75)	*Brazil, 1999*[49] (N = 93)	*Hawaii, 2001*[50] (N = 353)	*India, 2002*[51] (N = 74)
Jaundice	49	0	1.5	16	95	27	93	39	34
Anorexia	—	46	—	80	85	—	—	82	—
Headache	91	90	98	70	76	80	75	89	92
Conjunctival suffusion	99	57	42	58	54	—	28.5	28	35
Vomiting	69	18	33	32	50	40	—	73	—
Myalgia	97	64	79	40	49	63	94	91	68
Arthralgia	—	36	—	—	—	31	—	59	12
Abdominal pain	—	26	28	40	43	41	—	51	—
Nausea	75	29	41	46	37	—	—	77	—
Dehydration	—	—	—	—	37	—	—	—	—
Cough	24	57	20	45	32	39	—	—	—
Hemoptysis	9	51	—	40	—	13	20	—	35
Hepatomegaly	69	28	15	17	27	—	—	16	—
Lymphadenopathy	24	49	21	—	21	—	—	—	15
Diarrhea	27	20	29	36	14	11	—	53	—
Rash	6	—	7	—	2	—	—	8	12

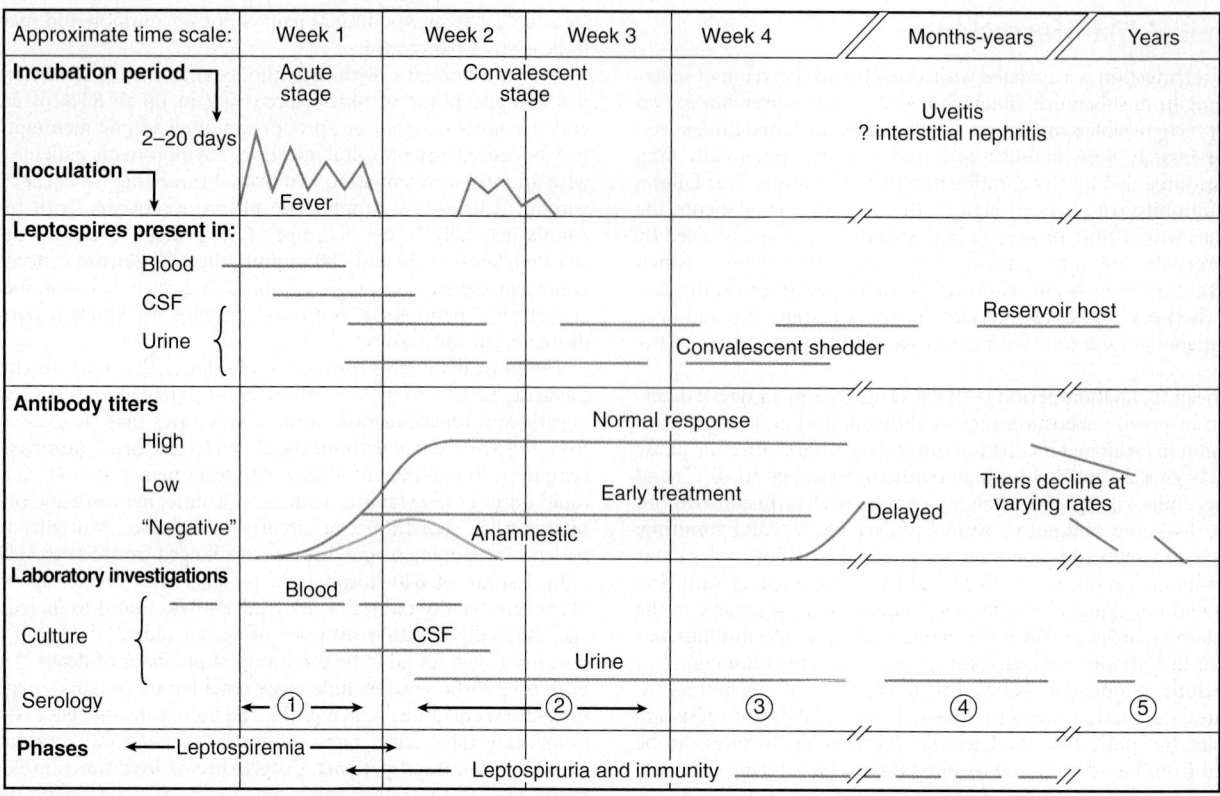

Figure 240-4 **Biphasic nature of leptospirosis and relevant investigations at different stages of disease.** Specimens 1 and 2 for serology are acute-phase specimens, 3 is a convalescent-phase sample that may facilitate detection of a delayed immune response, and 4 and 5 are follow-up samples that can provide epidemiologic information, such as the presumptive infecting serogroup. CSF, cerebrospinal fluid. (*Adapted from Levett PN. Leptospirosis. Clin Microbiol Rev. 2001;14:296-326, with permission of ASM Press.*)

epithelium. The blood urea nitrogen level is usually below 100 mg/dL, and the serum creatinine level is usually below 2 to 8 mg/dL during the acute phase of illness.[58] Thrombocytopenia occurs in the absence of disseminated intravascular coagulation and may accompany progressive renal dysfunction.[59] Renal biopsy reveals acute interstitial nephritis; immune complex glomerulonephritis may also be present.[60] If electrolyte and volume losses are not replaced, patients progress to oliguric renal failure. In fatal cases, the kidneys are swollen and yellow, with prominent cortical blood vessels.[26] Histologic findings include a diffuse, mixed tubulointerstitial inflammatory cell infiltrate of lymphocytes, plasma cells, macrophages, and polymorphonuclear leukocytes, accompanied by focal areas of tubular necrosis.[57]

Severe pulmonary hemorrhage syndrome (SPHS) can be a prominent manifestation of infection and may occur in the absence of hepatic and renal failure.[61] Frank hemoptysis can arise simultaneously with the onset of cough during the acute phase of illness.[62] However, hemorrhage is often inapparent until patients are intubated; clinicians should suspect SPHS in patients with signs of respiratory distress, whether or not they have hemoptysis. With progressive pulmonary involvement, radiographic abnormalities seen most frequently in the lower lobes evolve from small nodular densities (snowflake-like) to patchy alveolar infiltrates; confluent consolidation is uncommon but may occur.[63] The pathophysiology of SHPS is consistent with acute respiratory distress syndrome (ARDS) with diffuse lung injury, impaired gas exchange, and hemodynamic changes indicative of septic shock.[64] At autopsy, the lungs appear grossly congested and demonstrate focal areas of hemorrhage.[57] Histologically, damage to the capillary endothelium leads to congestion with foci of interstitial and intra-alveolar hemorrhage, diffuse alveolar damage, and severe air space disorganization.[65] Inflammatory infiltrates are usually absent.

Congestive heart failure occurs rarely. However, nonspecific electrocardiographic changes are common.[66] In more than 50% of patients

receiving continuous cardiac monitoring, cardiac arrhythmias may occur, including atrial fibrillation, flutter and tachycardia, and cardiac irritability, including premature ventricular contractions and ventricular tachycardia.[66] Atrial fibrillation is associated with more severe disease.[67] Cardiovascular collapse with shock can develop abruptly and, in the absence of aggressive supportive care, can be fatal. At autopsy, interstitial myocarditis with inflammatory involvement of the conduction system is seen[68]; acute coronary arteritis and aortitis are also common at postmortem examination.[69]

Laboratory Diagnosis

DIRECT DETECTION METHODS

Direct visualization of leptospires in blood or urine by darkfield microscopic examination has been used for diagnosis. However, artifacts are commonly mistaken for leptospires, and the method has both low sensitivity (40.2%) and specificity (61.5%).[70] A range of staining methods has been applied to direct detection, including immunofluorescence staining, immunoperoxidase staining, and silver staining. These methods are not widely used because of the lack of commercially available reagents and their relatively low sensitivity. Detection of leptospiral antigen in blood or urine has been attempted, but without significant success. Several polymerase chain reaction (PCR) assays have been developed for the detection of leptospires, but few have been evaluated in clinical studies,[71-73] and there have been no multicenter studies of multiple molecular diagnostic methods. The chief advantage of PCR is the prospect of confirming the diagnosis during the early acute (leptospiremic) stage of the illness, before the appearance of immunoglobulin M (IgM) antibodies, when treatment is likely to have the greatest benefit. In fulminating cases, in which death occurs before seroconversion, PCR may be of great diagnostic value.[71] Leptospiral

DNA has been amplified from serum, urine, aqueous humor, and a number of tissues obtained at autopsy.[74] For early diagnosis, serum is the optimal specimen. Urine from severely ill patients is often highly concentrated and contains significant inhibitory activity. Histologic diagnosis (Fig. 240-5) traditionally relied on silver impregnation staining,[3] but immunohistochemical staining offers greater sensitivity and specificity.[75,76]

ISOLATION AND IDENTIFICATION

Leptospires can be isolated from blood, CSF, and peritoneal dialysate fluids during the first 10 days of illness. Specimens should be collected while the patient is febrile and before antibiotic therapy is initiated. One or two drops of blood should be inoculated directly into culture medium at the bedside. Survival of leptospires in commercial blood culture media for several days has been reported.[77] Urine can be cultured after the first week of illness. Specimens should be collected aseptically into sterile containers without preservatives and must be processed within a short time of collection; best results are obtained when the delay is less than 1 hour, because leptospires do not survive well in acidic environments.[9]

Cultures are performed in albumin-polysorbate media such as EMJH (Ellinghausen-McCullough-Johnson-Harris) medium, which is available commercially. Older media contained serum.[5] Primary cultures are performed in semisolid medium, to which 5-fluorouracil is usually added as a selective agent. Cultures are incubated at 30°C for several weeks, because initial growth may be very slow.

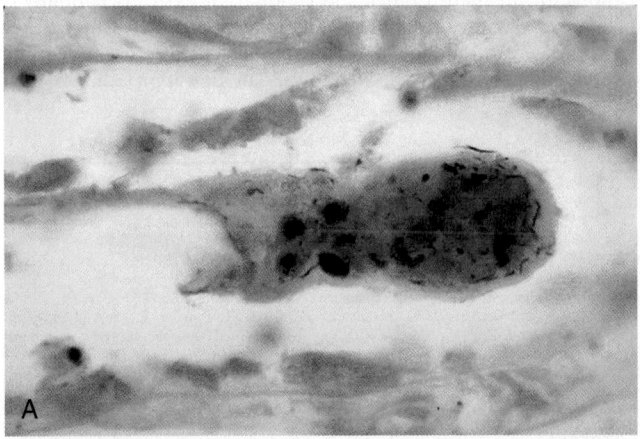

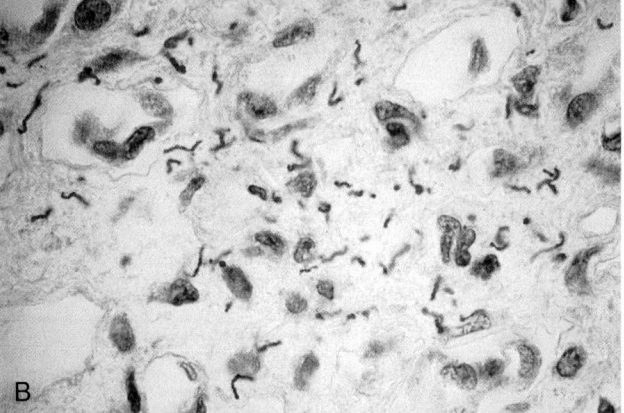

Figure 240-5 **Kidney sections stained by silver staining (A) and immunohistochemical staining (B) showing presence of multiple leptospires in tubules. (A,** *Courtesy of Dr. Martin Hicklin, Public Health Image Library, Centers for Disease Control and Prevention;* **B,** *courtesy of Juanne Layne, University of the West Indies, Barbados.)*

Isolated leptospires are identified to serovar level by traditional serologic methods or by molecular methods, such as pulsed-field gel electrophoresis.[78] These techniques are limited in availability to a few reference laboratories. Powerful molecular techniques such as multilocus sequence typing (MLST) and multiple-locus variable number tandem repeat analysis (MLVA) have been applied to the epidemiologic analysis of leptospirosis, but have yet to be widely used.[79-82]

Indirect Detection Methods

Most leptospirosis cases are diagnosed by serology. The reference standard assay is the microscopic agglutination test (MAT), in which live antigens representing different serogroups of leptospires are reacted with serum samples and then examined by darkfield microscopy for agglutination.[9] This is a complex test to maintain, perform, and interpret, and its use is restricted to a few reference laboratories.

A serologically confirmed case of leptospirosis is defined by a fourfold rise in MAT titer to one or more serovars between acute-phase and convalescent serum specimens run in parallel. A titer of at least 1:800 in the presence of compatible symptoms is strong evidence of recent or current infection.[83] Suggestive evidence for recent or current infection includes a single titer of at least 1:200 obtained after the onset of symptoms.[84] Delayed seroconversions are common, with up to 10% of patients failing to seroconvert within 30 days of the clinical onset. Cross-reactive antibodies may be associated with syphilis, relapsing fever, Lyme disease, viral hepatitis, human immunodeficiency virus (HIV) infection, legionellosis, and autoimmune diseases.[85]

The interpretation of the MAT is complicated by cross-reaction between different serogroups, especially in acute-phase samples.[5] Cross-reactivity in acute samples is attributable to IgM antibodies, which may persist for several years.[86] The MAT is a serogroup-specific assay, and should not be used to infer the identity of the infecting serovar.[14] However, knowledge of the presumptive serogroup may be of epidemiologic value in determining potential exposures to animal reservoirs.

Diagnostic application of the MAT is limited by the relatively low sensitivity when acute serum samples are tested.[87] Other agglutination assays that detect total immunoglobulins, such as the indirect hemagglutination assay, suffer from similarly low sensitivities in acute specimens, but have high case sensitivities when acute and convalescent specimens are tested.[88] IgM antibodies are detectable after about the fifth day of illness, and IgM detection assays are available in several formats.[88-91] Use of these assays as screening tests offers the potential to enhance the diagnostic capacity of many laboratories, particularly in developing countries, where most cases of leptospirosis occur.

Treatment

Antibiotic therapy should be initiated as early in the course of the disease as suspicion allows. There have been few randomized or placebo-controlled trials,[92-95] and these have produced conflicting results. Therapeutic benefits of antibiotics may be difficult to demonstrate in populations in which patients present for medical care with late and/or severe disease. Nevertheless, severe disease is usually treated with IV penicillin and mild disease with oral doxycycline (Table 240-3). Once-daily ceftriaxone has been shown to be as effective as penicillin.[96] Jarisch-Herxheimer reactions have been reported in patients treated with penicillin.[97] Patients receiving penicillin should be monitored because of the increased morbidity and mortality of such reactions.

Supportive therapy is essential for hospitalized patients. Patients with early renal disease with high-output renal dysfunction and hypokalemia should receive aggressive volume repletion and potassium supplementation to avoid severe dehydration and acute tubular necrosis. In patients who progress to oliguric renal failure, rapid initiation of hemodialysis reduces mortality and is typically required only on a short-term basis. Renal dysfunction caused by leptospirosis is typically completely reversible.[98] Patients requiring intubation for SPHS have

TABLE 240-3	Antimicrobial Agents Recommended for Treatment and Chemoprophylaxis of Leptospirosis	
Indication	Compound	Dosage
Chemoprophylaxis	Doxycycline	200 mg PO once weekly
Treatment of mild leptospirosis	Doxycycline	100 mg bid PO
	Ampicillin	500-750 mg q6h PO
	Amoxicillin	500 mg q6h PO
Treatment of moderate to severe leptospirosis	Penicillin G	1.5 MU IV q6h
	Ceftriaxone	1 g IV q24h
	Ampicillin	0.5-1 g IV q6h

decreased pulmonary compliance and should be managed as cases of ARDS. Protective ventilation strategies involving low tidal volumes (lower than 6 mL/kg) to avoid alveolar injury caused by high ventilation pressures have been shown to improve survival rates in ARDS dramatically.[99]

Prevention

Prevention of leptospirosis may be achieved by avoidance of high-risk exposures, adoption of protective measures, immunization, and use of chemoprophylaxis, in varying combinations depending on environmental circumstances and the degree of human activity.

High-risk exposures include immersion in fresh water, as in swimming, and contact with animals and their body fluids.[2] Removal of leptospires from the environment is impractical, but reducing direct contact with potentially infected animals and indirect contact with urine-contaminated soil and water remains the most effective preventive strategy available. Consistent application of rodent control measures is important in limiting the extent of contamination. Appropriate protective measures depend on the activity, but include wearing boots, goggles, overalls, and rubber gloves. In tropical environments, walking barefoot is a common risk factor.[100]

Immunization of animals with killed vaccines is widely practiced, but the immunity is short-lived and animals require periodic (usually annual) boosters.[101] Moreover, although these vaccines prevent against disease, they do not prevent infection and renal colonization; thus, they have little effect on the maintenance and transmission of the disease in the animal population in which they are applied. Current bovine and porcine vaccines used in the United States contain serovars Icterohaemorrhagiae, Canciola, Grippotyphosa, Pomona, and Hardjo, whereas canine vaccines contain all except serovar Hardjo. New vaccines for bovine use stimulate a type 1 cell-mediated immune response against serovar Hardjo[102,103] and appear to protect against renal colonization and urinary shedding.[104]

Human immunization is not widely practiced. A vaccine containing serovar Icterohaemorrhagiae is available in France for workers in high-risk occupations, and a vaccine has been developed for human use in Cuba.[105] Immunization has been more widely used in Asia to prevent large-scale epidemics in agricultural laborers.

For those who will be unavoidably exposed to leptospires in endemic environments, chemoprophylaxis is recommended (see Table 240-3). Weekly doxycycline (200 mg) has been shown to be effective in military personnel without previous exposure who underwent jungle training.[106] The use of doxycycline prophylaxis after excess rainfall in local populations in endemic areas has been studied.[107,108] Symptomatic disease was significantly reduced in one study, but serologic evidence of infection was found equally in subjects and controls.[107] Limitations of doxycycline are its photosensitivity, high frequency of gastrointestinal side effects, dietary calcium restrictions, and contraindications for pregnant women and children. In vitro susceptibility of leptospires to azithromycin[109] and its longer serum half-life suggest that this agent would be a reasonable alternative to doxycycline; however, clinical trials are needed to validate this approach.

REFERENCES

1. World Health Organization. Leptospirosis worldwide, 1999. Wkly Epidemiol Rec. 1999;74:237-242.
2. Faine S, Adler B, Bolin C, et al. Leptospira and Leptospirosis. 2nd ed. Melbourne: MedSci; 1999.
3. Stimson AM. Note on an organism found in yellow-fever tissue. Publ Health Rep. 1907;22:541.
4. Everard JD. Leptospirosis. In: Cox FEG, ed. The Wellcome Trust Illustrated History of Tropical Diseases. London: The Wellcome Trust; 1996:111-119, 416-418.
5. Levett PN. Leptospirosis. Clin Microbiol Rev. 2001;14:296-326.
6. Edwards GA, Domm BM. Human leptospirosis. Medicine. 1960;39:117-156.
7. Feigin RD, Anderson DC. Human leptospirosis. CRC Crit Rev Clin Lab Sci. 1975;5:413-467.
8. Goldstein SF, Charon NW. Motility of the spirochete Leptospira. Cell Motil Cytoskelet. 1988;9:101-110.
9. Levett PN. Leptospira. In: Murray PR, Baron EJ, Jorgensen JH, et al, eds. Manual of Clinical Microbiology. 9th ed. Washington, DC: American Society for Microbiology Press; 2007:963-970.
10. Bulach DM, Kalambaheti T, de La Peña-Moctezuma A, et al. Lipopolysaccharide biosynthesis in Leptospira. J Mol Microbiol Biotechnol. 2000;2:375-380.
11. Yasuda PH, Steigerwalt AG, Sulzer KR, et al. Deoxyribonucleic acid relatedness between serogroups and serovars in the family Leptospiraceae with proposals for seven new Leptospira species. Int J Syst Bacteriol. 1987;37:407-415.
12. Brenner DJ, Kaufmann AF, Sulzer KR, et al. Further determination of DNA relatedness between serogroups and serovars in the family Leptospiraceae with a proposal for Leptospira alexanderi sp. nov. and four new Leptospira genomospecies. Int J Syst Bacteriol. 1999;49:839-858.
13. Morey RE, Galloway RL, Bragg SL, et al. Species-specific identification of Leptospiraceae by 16S rRNA gene sequencing. Journal of Clinical Microbiology. 2006;44:3510-3516.
14. Levett PN. Usefulness of serologic analysis as a predictor of the infecting serovar in patients with severe leptospirosis. Clin Infect Dis. 2003;36:447-452.
15. Ren SX, Fu G, Jiang XG, et al. Unique physiological and pathogenic features of Leptospira interrogans revealed by whole-genome sequencing. Nature. 2003;422:888-893.
16. Nascimento AL, Ko AI, Martins EA, et al. Comparative genomics of two Leptospira interrogans serovars reveals novel insights into physiology and pathogenesis. Journal of Bacteriology. 2004;186:2164-2172.
17. Bulach DM, Zuerner RL, Wilson P, et al. Genome reduction in Leptospira borgpetersenii reflects limited transmission potential. Proc Nat Acad Sci U S A. 2006;103:14560-14565.
18. Picardeau M, Bulach DM, Bouchier C, et al. Genome sequence of the saprophyte Leptospira biflexa provides insights into the evolution of Leptospira and the pathogenesis of leptospirosis. PLoS ONE. 2008;3:e1607.
19. Trevejo RT, Rigau-Perez JG, Ashford DA, et al. Epidemic leptospirosis associated with pulmonary hemorrhage-Nicaragua, 1995. J Infect Dis. 1998;178:1457-1463.
20. Sasaki DM, Pang L, Minette HP, et al. Active surveillance and risk factors for leptospirosis in Hawaii. Am J Trop Med Hyg. 1993;48:35-43.
21. Morgan J, Bornstein SL, Karpati AM, et al. Outbreak of leptospirosis among triathlon participants and community residents in Springfield, Illinois, 1998. Clin Infect Dis. 2002; 34:1593-1599.
22. Sejvar J, Bancroft E, Winthrop K, et al. Leptospirosis in "Eco-Challenge" athletes, Malaysian Borneo, 2000. Emerg Infect Dis. 2003;9:702-707.
23. Ward MP, Glickman LT, Guptill LF. Prevalence of and risk factors for leptospirosis among dogs in the United States and Canada: 677 cases (1970-1998). J Am Vet Med Assoc. 2002;220:53-58.
24. Prescott JF, McEwen B, Taylor J, et al. Resurgence of leptospirosis in dogs in Ontario: Recent findings. Can Vet J. 2002; 43:955-961.
25. Brown CA, Roberts AW, Miller MA, et al. Leptospira interrogans serovar grippotyphosa infection in dogs. J Am Vet Med Assoc. 1996;209:1265-1267.
26. Areán VM. The pathologic anatomy and pathogenesis of fatal human leptospirosis (Weil's disease). Am J Pathol. 1962; 40:393-423.
27. de Souza L, Koury MC. Isolation and biological activities of endotoxin from Leptospira interrogans. Can J Microbiol. 1992;38:284-289.
28. Werts C, Tapping RI, Mathison JC, et al. Leptospiral endotoxin activates cells via a TLR2-dependent mechanism. Nature Immunology. 2001;2:346-352.
29. Nahori MA, Fournie-Amazouz E, Que-Gewirth NS, et al. Differential TLR recognition of leptospiral lipid A and lipopolysaccharide in murine and human cells. J Immunol. 2005;175: 6022-6031.
30. Que-Gewirth NL, Ribeiro AA, Kalb SR, et al. A methylated phosphate group and four amide-linked acyl chains in Leptospira interrogans lipid A. J Biol Chem. 2004;279:25420-25429.
31. Lee SH, Kim S, Park SC, Kim MJ. Cytotoxic activities of Leptospira interrogans hemolysin SphH as a pore-forming protein on mammalian cells. Infect Immun. 2002;70:315-322.
32. Abdulkader RC, Daher EF, Camargo ED, et al. Leptospirosis severity may be associated with the intensity of humoral immune response. Rev Inst Med Trop São Paulo. 2002;44: 79-83.
33. Lingappa J, Kuffner T, Tappero J, et al. HLA-DQ6 and ingestion of contaminated water: possible gene-environment interaction in an outbreak of leptospirosis. Genes Immun. 2004;5:197-202.
34. Faber NA, Crawford M, LeFebvre RB, et al. Detection of Leptospira spp. in the aqueous humor of horses with naturally acquired recurrent uveitis. J Clin Microbiol. 2000;38: 2731-2733.
35. Lucchesi PM, Parma AE, Arroyo GH. Serovar distribution of a DNA sequence involved in the antigenic relationship between Leptospira and equine cornea. BMC Microbiol. 2002;2:3.
36. Haake DA. Spirochaetal lipoproteins and pathogenesis. Microbiology. 2000;146:1491-1504.
37. Haake DA, Chao G, Zuerner RL, et al. The leptospiral major outer membrane protein LipL32 is a lipoprotein expressed during mammalian infection. Infect Immun. 2000;68: 2276-2285.
38. Guerreiro H, Croda J, Flannery B, et al. Leptospiral proteins recognized during the humoral immune response to leptospirosis in humans. Infect Immun. 2001;69:4958-4968.
39. Yang CW, Wu MS, Pan MJ, et al. The Leptospira outer membrane protein LipL32 induces tubulointerstitial nephritis-mediated gene expression in mouse proximal tubule cells. J Am Soc Nephrol. 2002;13:2037-2045.
40. Choy HA, Kelley MM, Chen TL, et al. Physiological osmotic induction of Leptospira interrogans adhesion: LigA and LigB bind extracellular matrix proteins and fibrinogen. Infect Immun. 2007;75:2441-2450.
41. Croda J, Ramos JG, Matsunaga J, et al. Leptospira immunoglobulin-like proteins as a serodiagnostic marker for acute leptospirosis. J Clin Microbiol. 2007;45:1528-1534.
42. Stevenson B, Choy HA, Pinne M, et al. Leptospira interrogans endostatin-like outer membrane proteins bind host fibronectin, laminin and regulators of complement. PLoS ONE. 2007;2:e1188.

43. Alexander AD, Benenson AS, Byrne RJ, et al. Leptospirosis in Puerto Rico. *Zoon Res*. 1963;2:152-227.
44. Wang C, John L, Chang T, et al. Studies on anicteric leptospirosis. I. Clinical manifestations and antibiotic therapy. *Chin Med J*. 1965;84:283-291.
45. Berman SJ, Tsai CC, Holmes KK, et al. Sporadic anicteric leptospirosis in South Vietnam. *Ann Intern Med*. 1973;79:167-173.
46. Park S-K, Lee S-H, Rhee Y-K, et al. Leptospirosis in Chonbuk province of Korea in 1987: A study of 93 patients. *Am J Trop Med Hyg*. 1989;41:345-351.
47. Edwards CN, Nicholson GD, Hassell TA, et al. Leptospirosis in Barbados: A clinical study. *W Indian Med J*. 1990;39:27-34.
48. Yersin C, Bovet P, Mérien F, et al. Human leptospirosis in the Seychelles (Indian Ocean): A population-based study. *Am J Trop Med Hyg*. 1998;59:933-940.
49. Ko AI, Galvao Reis M, Ribeiro Dourado CM, et al. Salvador Leptospirosis Study Group. Urban epidemic of severe leptospirosis in Brazil. *Lancet*. 1999;354:820-825.
50. Katz AR, Ansdell VE, Effler PV, et al. Assessment of the clinical presentation and treatment of 353 cases of laboratory-confirmed leptospirosis in Hawaii, 1974-1998. *Clin Infect Dis*. 2001;33:1834-1841.
51. Bharadwaj R, Bal AM, Joshi SA, et al. An urban outbreak of leptospirosis in Mumbai, India. *Jpn J Infect Dis*. 2002;55:194-196.
52. Turner LH. Leptospirosis I. *Trans R Soc Trop Med Hyg*. 1967;61:842-855.
53. Silva HR, Tanajura GM, Tavares-Neto J, et al. Aseptic meningitis associated with *Leptospira* in children of Salvador, Bahia. *Rev Soc Brasil Med Trop*. 2002;35:159-165.
54. Lopes AA, Costa E, Costa YA, et al. Comparative study of the in-hospital case-fatality rate of leptospirosis between pediatric and adult patients of different age groups. *Rev Inst Med Trop Sao Paulo*. 2004;46:19-24.
55. Esen S, Sunbul M, Leblebicioglu H, et al. Impact of clinical and laboratory findings on prognosis in leptospirosis. *Swiss Med Wkly*. 2004;134:347-352.
56. Edwards GA, Domm BM. Leptospirosis. II. *Med Times*. 1966;94:1086-1095.
57. Zaki SR, Spiegel RA. Leptospirosis. In: Nelson AM, Horsburgh CR, eds. *Pathology of Emerging Infections*, vol 2. Washington, DC: American Society for Microbiology Press; 1998:73-92.
58. Abdulkader RCRM, Seguro AC, Malheiro PS, et al. Peculiar electrolytic and hormonal abnormalities in acute renal failure due to leptospirosis. *Am J Trop Med Hyg*. 1996;54:1-6.
59. Edwards CN, Nicholson GD, Hassell TA, et al. Thrombocytopenia in leptospirosis: The absence of evidence for disseminated intravascular coagulation. *Am J Trop Med Hyg*. 1986;35:352-354.
60. Lai KN, Aarons I, Woodroffe AJ, et al. Renal lesions in leptospirosis. *Aust N Z J Med*. 1982;12:276-279.
61. Zaki SR, Shieh W-J; Epidemic Working Group. Leptospirosis associated with outbreak of acute febrile illness and pulmonary haemorrhage, Nicaragua, 1995. *Lancet*. 1996;347:535.
62. Yersin C, Bovet P, Mérien F, et al. Pulmonary haemorrhage as a predominant cause of death in leptospirosis in Seychelles. *Trans R Soc Trop Med Hyg*. 2000;94:71-76.
63. Im J-G, Yeon KM, Han MC, et al. Leptospirosis of the lung: Radiographic findings in 58 patients. *Am J Roentgenol*. 1989;152:955-959.
64. Marotto PC, Nascimento CM, Eluf-Neto J, et al. Acute lung injury in leptospirosis: clinical and laboratory features, outcome, and factors associated with mortality. *Clin Infect Dis*. 1999;29:1561-1563.
65. Nicodemo AC, Duarte MIS, Alves VAF, et al. Lung lesions in human leptospirosis: Microscopic, immunohistochemical, and ultrastructural features related to thrombocytopenia. *Am J Trop Med Hyg*. 1997;56:181-187.
66. Parsons M. Electrocardiographic changes in leptospirosis. *Br Med J*. 1965;2:201-203.
67. Sacramento E, Lopes AA, Costa E, et al. Electrocardiographic alterations in patients hospitalized with leptospirosis in the Brazilian city of Salvador. *Arquiv Brasil Cardiol*. 2002;78:267-270.
68. Areán VM. Leptospiral myocarditis. *Lab Invest*. 1957;6:462-471.
69. de Brito T, Morais CF, Yasuda PH, et al. Cardiovascular involvement in human and experimental leptospirosis: Pathologic findings and immunohistochemical detection of leptospiral antigen. *Ann Trop Med Parasitol*. 1987;81:207-214.
70. Vijayachari P, Sugunan AP, Umapathi T, et al. Evaluation of darkground microscopy as a rapid diagnostic procedure in leptospirosis. *Indian J Med Res*. 2001;114:54-58.
71. Brown PD, Gravekamp C, Carrington DG, et al. Evaluation of the polymerase chain reaction for early diagnosis of leptospirosis. *J Med Microbiol*. 1995;43:110-114.
72. Mérien F, Baranton G, Pérolat P. Comparison of polymerase chain reaction with microagglutination test and culture for diagnosis of leptospirosis. *J Infect Dis*. 1995;172:281-285.
73. Slack A, Symonds M, Dohnt M, et al. Evaluation of a modified Taqman assay detecting pathogenic *Leptospira* spp. against culture and *Leptospira*-specific IgM enzyme-linked immunosorbent assay in a clinical environment. *Diag Microbiol Infect Dis*. 2007;57:361-366.
74. Brown PD, Carrington DG, Gravekamp C, et al. Direct detection of leptospiral material in human postmortem samples. *Res Microbiol*. 2003;154:581-586.
75. Alves VAF, Vianna MR, Yasuda PH, et al. Detection of leptospiral antigen in the human liver and kidney using an immunoperoxidase staining procedure. *J Pathol*. 1987;151:125-131.
76. Guarner J, Shieh W-J, Morgan J, et al. Leptospirosis mimicking acute cholecystitis among athletes participating in a triathlon. *Hum Pathol*. 2001;32:750-752.
77. Palmer MF, Zochowski WJ. Survival of leptospires in commercial blood culture systems revisited. *J Clin Pathol*. 2000;53:713-714.
78. Galloway RL, Levett PN. Evaluation of a modified pulsed-field gel electrophoresis approach for the identification of *Leptospira* serovars. *Am J Trop Med Hyg*. 2008;78:628-632.
79. Ahmed N, Devi SM, Valverde Mde L, et al. Multilocus sequence typing method for identification and genotypic classification of pathogenic *Leptospira* species. *Ann Clin Microbiol Antimicrob*. 2006;5:28.
80. Salaun L, Mérien F, Gurianova S, et al. Application of multilocus variable-number tandem-repeat analysis for molecular typing of the agent of leptospirosis. *J Clin Microbiol*. 2006;44:3954-3962.
81. Slack A, Symonds M, Dohnt M, et al. An improved multiple-locus variable number of tandem repeats analysis for *Leptospira interrogans* serovar Australis: a comparison with fluorescent amplified fragment length polymorphism analysis and its use to redefine the molecular epidemiology of this serovar in Queensland, Australia. *J Med Microbiol*. 2006;55:1549-1557.
82. Thaipadungpanit J, Wuthiekanun V, Chierakul W, et al. A dominant clone of *Leptospira interrogans* associated with an outbreak of human leptospirosis in Thailand. *PLoS Negl Trop Dis*. 2007;1:e56.
83. Faine S. *Guidelines for the control of leptospirosis (offset publication No. 67)*. Geneva: World Health Organization, 1982.
84. Centers for Disease Control and Prevention. Case definitions for infectious conditions under public health surveillance. *Morbid Mortal Wkly Rep MMWR*. 1997;46(RR-10):49.
85. Bajani MD, Ashford DA, Bragg SL, et al. Evaluation of four commercially available rapid serologic tests for diagnosis of leptospirosis. *J Clin Microbiol*. 2003;41:803-809.
86. Cumberland PC, Everard COR, Wheeler JG, et al. Persistence of anti-leptospiral IgM, IgG and agglutinating antibodies in patients presenting with acute febrile illness in Barbados 1979-1989. *Eur J Epidemiol*. 2001;17:601-608.
87. Cumberland PC, Everard COR, Levett PN. Assessment of the efficacy of the IgM enzyme-linked immunosorbent assay (ELISA) and microscopic agglutination test (MAT) in the diagnosis of acute leptospirosis. *Am J Trop Med Hyg*. 1999;61:731-734.
88. Levett PN, Branch SL, Whittington CU, et al. Two methods for rapid serological diagnosis of acute leptospirosis. *Clin Diagn Lab Immunol*. 2001;8:349-351.
89. Levett PN, Branch SL. Evaluation of two enzyme-linked immunosorbent assay methods for detection of immunoglobulin M antibodies in acute leptospirosis. *Am J Trop Med Hyg*. 2002;66:745-748.
90. Smits HL, Ananyina YV, Chereshsky A, et al. International multicenter evaluation of the clinical utility of a dipstick assay for detection of *Leptospira*-specific immunoglobulin M antibodies in human serum specimens. *J Clin Microbiol*. 1999;37:2904-2909.
91. Smits HL, van Der Hoorn MA, Goris MG, et al. Simple latex agglutination assay for rapid serodiagnosis of human leptospirosis. *J Clin Microbiol*. 2000;38:1272-1275.
92. McClain JBL, Ballou WR, Harrison SM, et al. Doxycycline therapy for leptospirosis. *Ann Intern Med*. 1984;100:696-698.
93. Edwards CN, Nicholson GD, Hassell TA, et al. Penicillin therapy in icteric leptospirosis. *Am J Trop Med Hyg*. 1988;39:388-390.
94. Watt G, Padre LP, Tuazon ML, et al. Placebo-controlled trial of intravenous penicillin for severe and late leptospirosis. *Lancet*. 1988;i:433-435.
95. Costa E, Lopes AA, Sacramento E, et al. Penicillin at the late stage of leptospirosis: A randomized controlled trial. *Rev Inst Med Trop São Paulo*. 2003;45:141-145.
96. Panaphut T, Domrongkitchaiporn S, Vibhagool A, et al. Ceftriaxone compared with sodium penicillin G for treatment of severe leptospirosis. *Clin Infect Dis*. 2003;36:1507-1513.
97. Friedland JS, Warrell DA. The Jarisch-Herxheimer reaction in leptospirosis: Possible pathogenesis and review. *Rev Infect Dis*. 1991;13:207-210.
98. Andrade L, de Francesco Daher E, Seguro AC. Leptospiral nephropathy. *Semin Nephrol*. 2008;28:383-394.
99. Amato MB, Barbas CS, Medeiros DM, et al. Effect of a protective-ventilation strategy on mortality in the acute respiratory distress syndrome. *N Engl J Med*. 1998;338:347-354.
100. Douglin CP, Jordan C, Rock R, et al. Risk factors for severe leptospirosis in the parish of St. Andrew, Barbados. *Emerg Infect Dis*. 1997;3:78-80.
101. Bey RF, Johnson RC. Current status of leptospiral vaccines. *Prog Vet Microbiol Immunol*. 1986;2:175-197.
102. Naiman BM, Alt D, Bolin CA, et al. Protective killed *Leptospira borgpetersenii* vaccine induces potent Th1 immunity comprising responses by CD4 and gammadelta T lymphocytes. *Infect Immun*. 2001;69:7550-7558.
103. Brown RA, Blumerman S, Gay C, et al. Comparison of three different leptospiral vaccines for induction of a type 1 immune response to *Leptospira borgpetersenii* serovar Hardjo. *Vaccine*. 2003;21:4448-4458.
104. Bolin CA, Alt DP. Use of a monovalent leptospiral vaccine to prevent renal colonization and urinary shedding in cattle exposed to *Leptospira borgpetersenii* serovar hardjo. *Am J Vet Res*. 2001;62:995-1000.
105. Martínez R, Pérez A, Quiñones Mdel C, et al. [Eficacia y seguridad de una vacuna contra la leptospirosis humana en Cuba.] *Rev Panam Salud Publica*. 2004;15:249-255.
106. Takafuji ET, Kirkpatrick JW, Miller RN, et al. An efficacy trial of doxycycline chemoprophylaxis against leptospirosis. *N Engl J Med*. 1984;310:497-500.
107. Sehgal SC, Sugunan AP, Murhekar MV, et al. Randomized controlled trial of doxycycline prophylaxis against leptospirosis in an endemic area. *Int J Antimicrob Agents*. 2000;13:249-255.
108. Gonsalez CR, Casseb J, Monteiro FG, et al. Use of doxycycline for leptospirosis after high-risk exposure in Sao Paulo, Brazil. *Rev Inst Med Trop São Paulo*. 1998;41:59-61.
109. Hospenthal DR, Murray CK. In vitro susceptibilities of seven *Leptospira* species to traditional and newer antibiotics. *Antimicrob Agents Chemother*. 2003;47:2646-2648.

241

Borrelia Species (Relapsing Fever)

KYU Y. RHEE | WARREN D. JOHNSON, JR.

Relapsing fever is an arthropod-borne zoonosis caused by spirochetes of the genus *Borrelia*. In clinical terms, this disease is characterized by cyclical periods of fevers and nonspecific symptoms, alternating with periods of relative well-being, due to recurrent bouts of spirochetemia. *Borrelia* species associated with this disease are transmitted by two major arthropod vectors: soft ticks of the genus *Ornithodoros* and the human body louse *Pediculus humanus*. Louse-borne relapsing fever (LBRF) is associated with epidemic disease and is caused only by *Borrelia recurrentis*. Tick-borne relapsing fever (TBRF), in contrast, is associated with over 15 *Borrelia* sp. and causes endemic disease.[1-4]

Etiology

Relapsing fever *Borrelia* belongs to the family Spirochaetaceae, which also includes the genus *Treponema*.[5] Thus, these borreliae are helical, 8 to 30 μm long, 0.2 to 0.5 μm wide, have 3 to 10 loose spirals, are actively motile, and divide by transverse fission.[1,6] In structural terms, these spirochetes possess an outer slimelike layer, a cell wall, and both an outer cell wall and an inner cytoplasmic membrane, between which are anchored numerous protoplasmic filaments and flagella that wind around the cytoplasmic body.[4] While readily stained with aniline or acid dyes, strains of borreliae, however, cannot be distinguished from one another on morphologic criteria alone.

In vitro, *Borrelia* species have been cultivated in artificial media with generation times ranging from 18 hours (*Borrelia hermsii*)[7,8] to 8 to 9 hours (*B. recurrentis*).[9] Tick-borne borreliae have been reported to remain viable in their natural tick vectors for up to 12 years. Tick-mediated cultivation thus provides the optimal method for maintaining organisms.[6] While promptly killed by desiccation and ultraviolet rays, borreliae notably also survive and retain virulence when frozen at −73°C for many months.[1] Rodents (rats, hamsters, guinea pigs) injected with some strains may also develop latent brain infections.[1]

In mice, *B. hermsii* reversibly changes its major outer surface protein when it is transmitted by the tick to the mammalian host and back to the tick.[10] Tick-spirochete specificity also exists, and together, these features have been used to help identify *Borrelia* spp.[11,12]

Epidemiology and Transmission

With the exception of a few areas in the Southwest Pacific, relapsing fever occurs throughout the world.[11,12] The distribution and occurrence of TBRF (or endemic relapsing fever) is governed by the presence of enzootic cycles of the transmitting tick vector and its host. The distribution of LBRF (or epidemic relapsing fever), in contrast, is determined by socioeconomic and ecologic factors.

Louse-borne relapsing fever is caused only by *B. recurrentis* and is transmitted from person to person by the human body louse (*Pediculus humanus*).[2] Following the ingestion of infective human blood by the louse, spirochetes penetrate the midgut and multiply in the hemolymph. Tissues of the louse are not invaded by spirochetes, so disease cannot be transmitted to humans by louse saliva or excrement, or transovarially to the progeny of the louse. Epidemic relapsing fever therefore results from crushing lice, with the release of infective organisms capable of penetrating intact skin or mucous membranes.[12] Lice are infective for their lifetime (10 to 60 days), and humans are the only hosts for this organism.

Louse-borne relapsing fever usually occurs in epidemics associated with catastrophic events, such as war or famine, that result in overcrowding and dissemination of body lice. The last great epidemic occurred during World War II in North Africa and Europe and caused an estimated 50,000 deaths.[1,2] Louse-borne relapsing fever remains endemic in the highlands of Central and East Africa (Ethiopia, Sudan, Somalia, Chad) and in the South American Andes (Bolivia, Peru).[13]

Tick-borne relapsing fever is caused by at least 15 *Borrelia* spp. Each is associated with a distinct member of the transmitting argasid soft tick genus *Ornithodoros*, from which many *Borrelia* species derive their respective species names. Members of the genus *Ornithodoros* possess distinct hosts and habitats but are all obligate blood feeders at every developmental stage and orient to the presence of exhaled breath. Typically, these ticks inhabit caves, decaying wood, rodent burrows, and animal shelters. Their range of movement is limited (less than 50 yards), although rodents may carry them passively into human dwellings. Their presence often passes unnoticed because they are night feeders and lack a painful bite. In contrast to hard ticks of the genus *Ixodes*, *Ornithodoros* ticks feed quickly (5 to 20 minutes), and females return to their lair and lay clutches of eggs following each blood meal.[14] Perpetuation of *Borrelia* spirochetes is maintained via the ability of adult ticks to fast for up to 15 years while living in protected environments and, in some cases, transovarial passage to tick progeny. The specific mode of transmission appears to vary with both the species and stage of tick development. Animal reservoirs for these borreliae include rodents and small animals (chipmunks, squirrels, rabbits, rats, mice, owls, lizards).[11,12]

In TBRF, borreliae contained in the blood meal of the tick multiply rapidly and within hours invade all tissues, including salivary glands, excretory organs, and the genital system. Persistent infection of the salivary glands is thought to facilitate rapid transmission during a relatively short feeding period.[14,15] Infection of humans occurs when saliva or excrement is released by the tick while feeding.

The intrusion of humans into the ticks' environment creates the opportunity for disease transmission. The largest outbreak of tick-borne relapsing fever in the Western Hemisphere occurred in 62 campers residing in log cabins in Arizona in 1973.[16] The magnitude of this outbreak may have been related to a concurrent epizootic plague that killed many of the natural rodent hosts of the tick.[12] TBRF has been identified in regions where no cases of TBRF have been reported.

Pathophysiology

The clinical manifestations of relapsing fever mirror closely the pathophysiology of infection. During the febrile illness, borreliae multiply in the bloodstream and are often present at levels in excess of 100,000 organisms/mm^3 of blood.[2] With immune recognition, these spirochetes are cleared from the bloodstream and sequestered in internal organs, giving rise to intercurrent afebrile periods. Under immune pressure, borreliae undergo antigenic modification of their outer surface proteins and reemerge in the bloodstream both microbiologically and clinically.[17] The mechanism for this antigenic variation is mediated by both nonreciprocal *intermolecular* recombination mechanisms similar to gene conversion and *intramolecular* recombination events similar to those occurring during immunoglobulin gene rearrangements. Each of these mechanisms allows for the placement of a different surface protein (variable major protein—*vmp*) genes into a single active expression site.[18] This cyclic process of antigenic variation followed by specific antibody production is responsible for the relapsing course of this disease and can give rise to as many as 30 antigenic variants.[19] With successive relapses, borreliae revert to antigenic types similar to those present in earlier relapses. The ultimate termination of clinical disease has been attributed primarily to the development of specific borreliacidal antibody rather than to the activity of phagocytic cells.[1,20]

At autopsy, hepatitis and hepatic necrosis; miliary splenic abscesses; central nervous system lesions (hemorrhages, perivascular infiltrates, degenerative lesions); myocarditis; and hemorrhagic, gastrointestinal, and renal lesions have been described.[2,3,21]

Clinical Manifestations

Clinical manifestations of louse-borne and tick-borne relapsing fever are similar and are summarized in Table 241-1.[1-4] Variations that do occur between the two, however, are thought to be related to differences in spirochete strains, inoculating dose, host immunity, and general condition of the patients.

The incubation period of both forms of relapsing fever is often difficult to establish, because louse exposure is often long-term, and the tick bite is often unrecognized. Generally, louse-borne disease has a longer incubation period, longer febrile periods and afebrile intervals, and fewer relapses than tick-borne disease. Characteristically, both types of relapsing fever have an acute onset of high fever with rigors, severe headache, myalgias, arthralgias, and lethargy. Prodromal symptoms are rare. Initial physical findings are variable but may include altered sensorium, conjunctival suffusion, petechiae, and diffuse abdominal tenderness with hepatomegaly and splenomegaly. Less common findings include nuchal rigidity, cough, pulmonary crackles and rhonchi, lymphadenopathy, and jaundice.

During the course of illness, fever is remittent and often accompanied by tachycardia and tachypnea. Interestingly, the primary febrile episode characteristically terminates abruptly in 3 to 6 days. This crisis may be associated with fatal hypotension and shock. In addition, a truncal skin rash of 1 to 2 days' duration is common at the end of the primary febrile episode.[3] The rash can be petechial, macular, or papular.

After 7 to 10 days, fever and symptoms typically recur suddenly. The duration and the intensity of the symptoms progressively decrease with each relapse. Louse-borne relapsing fever is usually associated with a single relapse, whereas multiple relapses are the rule in tick-borne disease. During pregnancy, relapsing fever is associated with increased maternal and infant morbidity and mortality.[22-24]

Hemorrhage is common, and even more so with LBRF, but it is rarely severe (petechiae, epistaxis, hemoptysis, hematuria, hematemesis). Neurologic findings are reported in up to 30% of patients and

include coma, cranial nerve palsies, hemiplegia, meningitis, and seizures.[3,21] Rarer complications include pneumonia, bronchitis, and otitis media, as well as iritis and irdocyclitis, each of which has been reported to result in permanent impairment of vision. While rare, myocarditis with associated arrhythmias, cerebral hemorrhage, and hepatic failure are the most common causes of death. Of note, a recent report from the CDC identified several cases of the acute respiratory distress syndrome in association with TBRF cases seen in the western United States since 2001. The basis for this association, however, remains unclear.[25]

Diagnosis

The definitive diagnosis of relapsing fever is established by demonstrating the presence of borreliae in the peripheral blood of infected patients (see Table 241-1). Among febrile patients, spirochetes are found in 70% of cases when wet blood smears are examined by dark-field microscopy or in Giemsa- or Wright-stained thick and thin smears.[3,26] In contrast, organisms are rarely found during afebrile periods. Examination of acridine orange–stained smears by fluorescence microscopy or buffy coat smears can often increase the diagnostic yield of such smears.[27,28]

Agglutinating, complement-fixing, borreliacidal, and immobilizing antibodies are detectable in serum. However, these tests are not generally available and, if performed, are of limited diagnostic value owing to antigenic variation of strains and the complexity of the relapse phenomenon.[16,26] Proteus OXK agglutinin titers are elevated in relapsing fever, with the highest titers being found in patients with louse-borne disease (1:80 or greater). Antibodies to OX-19 and OX-2 are rare. Serologic tests for syphilis are positive in 5% to 10% of patients. Serologic tests for Lyme disease may also be positive.[29] Recent data suggest both louse- and tick-borne relapsing fever–associated Borreliae may be discriminated from syphilis- and Lyme disease–associated treponemes based on the presence of detectable titers against the surface protein, glycerophosphodiester phosphodiesterase (GlpQ).[30] Leukocytosis (to 25,000 cells/mm³) and an increased erythrocyte sedimentation rate (to 110 mm/hour) are common. The cerebrospinal fluid pressure is usually elevated in patients with central nervous system involvement and is associated with a pleocytosis (15 to 2200 cells/mm³) and with an elevated protein concentration (to 160 mg/100 mL).[3] The spinal fluid glucose level is normal. Spirochetes have been detected in cerebrospinal fluid by smear or by animal inoculation in up to 12% of the patients with central nervous system signs.

Early clinical diagnosis of louse-borne relapsing fever is not difficult during epidemics unless there is coexisting epidemic typhus, a disease also transmitted by the body louse. During the initial febrile episode of an isolated case of relapsing fever, the differential diagnosis can include malaria, typhoid fever, hepatitis, leptospirosis, rat-bite fever, Colorado tick fever, and dengue.[31] Epidemiologic considerations, the occurrence of relapses, and the demonstration of spirochetemia help exclude these diagnoses. In regions where Lyme disease is endemic, the diagnosis of tick-borne relapsing fever may be complicated due to similar neurologic manifestations of the diseases and cross-reactive serologic assays.[29,32]

Treatment and Prevention

Relapsing fever has been treated successfully with tetracycline, chloramphenicol, penicillin, and erythromycin.[33-36] With the possible exception of pregnant women, tetracycline, in a single oral dose (0.5 g), is the preferred therapy of louse-borne relapsing fever.[36] Erythromycin, 0.5 g in a single oral dose, is an equally effective alternative therapy.[35] Tick-borne relapsing fever is often treated with either tetracycline or erythromycin, 0.5 g every 6 hours for 5 to 10 days, because of the higher rate of treatment failures and relapses in these patients.[3,33,34] Meningitis or encephalitis should be treated with parenteral antibiotics, such as penicillin G, cefotaxime, or ceftriaxone, for 14 days

	Mean Value or Incidence	
Manifestation	Louse-Borne Disease	Tick-Borne Disease
Case-fatality rate (%)	4-40	2-5
Incubation period (days)	8 (4-18)*	7 (4-18)
Duration of first febrile attack (days)	5.5	3
Duration of afebrile interval (days)	9	7
Duration of relapses	2	2-3
Number of relapses	1-2 (1-5)*	3 (0-13)*
Maximal temperature (°F)	101-102	105
Splenomegaly (%)	77	41
Hepatomegaly (%)	66	17
Jaundice (%)	6	7
Rash (%)	8	28
Respiratory symptoms (%)	34 (cough)	16
Central nervous system involvement (%)	30	9

TABLE 241-1 Summary of Clinical Features of Relapsing Fever

*Range.

Adapted from Southern PM, Sanford JP. Relapsing fever: A clinical and microbiological review. Medicine. 1969;48:129-149.

or more.[21] The mortality of treated relapsing fever is less than 5%.[3] Untreated epidemic louse-borne disease has a mortality of up to 40%.[1,2]

Antibiotic treatment typically induces a Jarisch-Herxheimer reaction with severe rigors, leukopenia, an increase in temperature, and a decrease in blood pressure. The onset of the reaction occurs within 2 hours of initiating therapy and coincides with clearing of the spirochetemia. The reaction appears to be an exaggeration of the crisis observed in untreated patients and is most severe in louse-borne disease treated with penicillin. A significant percentage of patients with tick-borne relapsing fever, however, also develop the reaction. Recent studies suggest that the lipid component of the variable major protein possesses potent, although variable, TNFα–inducing activity.[37] Because the reaction may be life-threatening, it has been recommended that patients be kept under observation for approximately 2 hours after the initiation of treatment.[29] Release of *Borrelia* cell contents with the induction of cytokines and activation of kinins and fibrinolytic factors may have a major role in both the acute illness and the development of this reaction.[38] The Jarisch-Herxheimer reaction is associated with transient elevations of levels of plasma TNFα, interleukin-6, and interleukin-8 concentrations.[39] It is prevented by prior administration of antibodies against TNFα.[40-42] The prior administration of hydrocortisone is ineffective.[33,36]

Prevention of relapsing fever requires avoidance or elimination of the arthropod vectors. The varied habitats and the vast geographic areas populated by *Ornithodoros* ticks make their eradication impossible. However, insecticides can be used in dwellings and surrounding areas, and insect repellents applied to clothing and the skin may further decrease exposure risks. A double-blinded, placebo-controlled study of 47 patients more recently showed that following exposure to *Ornithodoros tholozoni* ticks, which harbor the causative agent of TBRF in Israel (*B. persica*), that one postexposure treatment with oral doxycycline (given 200 mg the first day and 100 mg per day for the next four days) was 100% effective among those with documented tick bites or close contacts, and no major adverse events occurred.[43] Prevention of louse-borne disease, in contrast, is best accomplished by good personal hygiene and, if necessary, delousing procedures. DDT-resistant louse strains have developed since World War II, and other insecticides may be required—for example, dimethyl dithiophosphate (malathion).[33]

REFERENCES

1. Felsenfeld O. *Borrelia: Strains, Vectors, Human and Animal Borreliosis.* St Louis: Warren H Green; 1971:180.
2. Bryceson ADM, Parry EHO, Perine PL, et al. Louse-borne relapsing fever. A clinical and laboratory study of 62 cases in Ethiopia and a reconsideration of the literature. *Q J Med.* 1970;39:129-170.
3. Southern PM Jr, Sanford JP. Relapsing fever: A clinical and microbiological review. *Medicine.* 1969;48:129-149.
4. Barbour AG, Hayes SF. Biology of *Borrelia* species. *Microbiol Rev.* 1986;50:381-400.
5. Garrity GM, ed. *Bergey's Manual of Systematic Bacteriology.* 2nd ed. New York: Springer Verlag; 2001.
6. Felsenfeld O. Borreliae, Human relapsing fever, and parasite vector host relationships. *Bacteriol Rev.* 1965;29:46.
7. Kelly RT. Cultivation and physiology of relapsing fever borreliae. In: Johnson RC, ed. *The Biology of Parasitic Spirochetes.* New York: Academic Press; 1976:87.
8. Kelly R. Cultivation of *Borrelia hermsii. Science.* 1971;173:443-444.
9. Cutler SJ, Fekade D, Hussein K, et al. Successful in-vitro cultivation of *Borrelia recurrentis. Lancet.* 1994;343:242.
10. Schwan TG, Hinnebusch BJ. Bloodstream- versus tick-associated variants of a relapsing fever bacterium. *Science.* 1998;280:1938.
11. Burgdorfer W. The enlarging spectrum of tick-borne spirochetoses: R R Parker Memorial Address. *Rev Infect Dis.* 1986;8:932-940.
12. Burgdorfer W. The epidemiology of relapsing fevers. In: Johnson RC, ed. *The Biology of Parasitic Spirochetes.* New York: Academic Press; 1976:191.
13. Felsenfeld O. The problem of relapsing fever in the Americas. *Indiana Med.* 1973;42:7.
14. Dworkin MS, Schwan TG, Anderson DE. Tick-borne relapsing fever in North America. *Med Clin NA.* 2002;86:417-433.
15. Davis GE. The endemic relapsing fevers. In: Hull TG, ed. *Diseases transmitted from Animal to Man.* Springfield, IL: Charles C Thomas; 1955:552-565.
16. Centers for Disease Control and Prevention. Relapsing fever. *Morb Mortal Wkly Rep.* 1973;22:242-246.
17. Barbour AG. Antigenic variation of a relapsing fever *Borrelia* species. *Annu Rev Microbiol.* 1990;44:155-171.
18. Barbour AG. Relapsing fevers and other *Borrelia* infections. In: Guerrant RL, Walker DH, Weller PF, eds. *Tropical Infectious Diseases.* Philadelphia: WB Saunders; 1999:535-546.
19. Schwann TG, Piesman J. Vector interactions and molecular adaptations of Lyme disease and relapsing fever spirochetes associated with transmission by ticks. *Emerg Infect Dis.* 2002;8:115-121.
20. Felsenfeld O. Immunity in relapsing fever. In: Johnson RC, ed. *The Biology of Parasitic Spirochetes.* New York: Academic Press; 1976:351-358.
21. Cadavid D, Barbour AG. Neuroborreliosis during relapsing fever: Review of the clinical manifestations, pathology, and treatment of infections in human and experimental animals. *Clin Infect Dis.* 1998;26:151.
22. Jongen VHWM, van Roosmalen J, Tiems J, et al. Tick-borne relapsing fever and pregnancy outcome in rural Tanzania. *Acta Obstet Gynecol Scand.* 1997;76:834.
23. Dupont HT, La Scola B, Williams R, et al. A focus of tick-borne relapsing fever in southern Zaire. *Clin Infect Dis.* 1997;25:139.
24. Borgnolo G, Hailu B, Ciancarelli A, et al. Louse-borne relapsing fever: A clinical and an epidemiological study of 389 patients in Asella Hospital, Ethiopia. *Trop Geogr Med.* 1993;45:66.
25. Centers for Disease Control and Prevention. Acute respiratory distress syndrome in persons with tick-borne relapsing fever—three states, 2004-2005. *MMWR Morbid Mortal Wkly Rep.* 2007;56:1073-1076.
26. Burgdorfer W. The diagnosis of relapsing fever. In: Johnson RC, ed. *The Biology of Parasitic Spirochetes.* New York: Academic Press; 1976:225.
27. Sciotto CG, Lauer BA, White WL, et al. Detection of *Borrelia* in acridine orange–stained blood smears by fluorescence microscopy. *Arch Pathol Lab Med.* 1983;107:384-386.
28. Cobey FC, Goldberg SH, Levian RA, et al. Short report: Detection of *Borrelia* (relapsing fever) in rural Ethiopia by means of the quantitative buffy coat technique. *Am J Trop Med Hyg.* 2001;65:164-165.
29. Dworkin MS, Anderson DE Jr, Schwan TG, et al. Tick-borne relapsing fever in the northwestern United States and southwestern Canada. *Clin Infect Dis.* 1998;26:122.
30. Porcella SF, Raffel SJ, Schrumpf ME, et al. Serodiagnosis of louse-borne relapsing fever with glycerophosphodiester phosphodiesterase (GlpQ) from *Borrelia recurrentis. J Clin Microbiol.* 2000;38:3561-3571.
31. Le CT. Tick-borne relapsing fever in children. *Pediatrics.* 1980;66:963-966.
32. Rawlings JA. An overview of tick-borne relapsing fever with emphasis on outbreaks in Texas. *Tex Med.* 1995;91:56.
33. Sanford JP. Relapsing fever—treatment and control. In: Johnson RC, ed. *The Biology of Parasitic Spirochetes.* New York: Academic Press; 1976:389-394.
34. Horton JM, Blaser MJ. The spectrum of relapsing fever in the Rocky Mountains. *Arch Intern Med.* 1985;145:871-875.
35. Perine PL, Teklu B. Antibiotic treatment of louseborne relapsing fever in Ethiopia: A report of 377 cases. *Am J Trop Med Hyg.* 1983;32:1096-1100.
36. Butler T. Relapsing fever: New lessons about antibiotic action. *Ann Intern Med.* 1985;102:397.
37. Vidal V, Scragg IG, Cutler SJ, et al. Variable major lipoprotein is a principal TNF-inducing factor of louse-borne relapsing fever. *Nat Med.* 1998;4:1416-1420.
38. Galloway RE, Levin J, Butler T, et al. Activation of protein mediators of inflammation and evidence for endotoxemia in *Borrelia recurrentis* infection. *Am J Med.* 1977;63:933-938.
39. Negussie Y, Remick DG, DeForge LE, et al. Detection of plasma tumor necrosis factor, interleukins 6 and 8 during the Jarisch-Herxheimer reaction of relapsing fever. *J Exp Med.* 1992;175:1207-1212.
40. Fekade D, Knox K, Hussein K, et al. Prevention of Jarisch-Herxheimer reactions by treatment with antibodies against tumor necrosis factor α. *N Engl J Med.* 1996;335:311.
41. Beutler B, Munford RS. Tumor necrosis factor and the Jarisch-Herxheimer reaction. *N Engl J Med.* 1996;335:347.
42. Coxon RE, Fekade D, Knox K, et al. The effect of antibody against TNF α on cytokine response in Jarisch-Herxheimer reactions of louse-borne relapsing fever. *Q J Med.* 1997;90:213.
43. Hasin T, Davidovitch N, Cohen R, et al. Post-exposure treatment with doxycycline for the prevention of tick-borne relapsing fever. *N Engl J Med.* 2006;355:148-155.

Borrelia burgdorferi (Lyme Disease, Lyme Borreliosis)

ALLEN C. STEERE

Lyme disease or Lyme borreliosis, which is caused by the tick-borne spirochete *Borrelia burgdorferi (sensu lato)*, occurs in temperate regions of North America, Europe, and Asia.[1] It is now the most common vector-borne disease in the United States and Europe.[2] The illness usually begins in summer (stage 1) with a characteristic expanding skin lesion, called erythema migrans (EM), which occurs at the site of the tick bite.[1,3] Within several days to weeks (stage 2), the spirochete may spread to other sites, particularly to other skin sites, the nervous system, the heart, or the joints. After months to years (stage 3), sometimes following periods of latent infection, the spirochete may cause persistent disease, most commonly affecting the joints, nervous system, or skin. Serologic testing is the most practical laboratory aid in diagnosis. All stages of the disorder are usually curable by appropriate antibiotic therapy.

Lyme disease was recognized as a separate entity in 1976 because of close geographic clustering of affected children in Lyme, Connecticut, who were thought to have juvenile rheumatoid arthritis.[4] However, parts of the illness were recognized previously in Europe and were given different names, including erythema chronicum migrans, Bannwarth's syndrome, or acrodermatitis chronica atrophicans.[3] These syndromes were linked conclusively in 1982 and 1983 with the recovery of a previously unrecognized spirochete from the tick vector[5] and from infected patients.[3] The basic outlines of the disease are similar worldwide, but there are regional variations, primarily between the illness found in America and that in Europe and Asia.[1]

Causative Organism

The agents of Lyme borreliosis belong to the eubacterial phylum of spirochetes, which are vigorously motile, corkscrew-shaped bacteria. The spirochete cell wall consists of a cytoplasmic membrane surrounded by peptidoglycan and flagella and then by a loosely associated outer membrane (Fig. 242-1).[6] Of the *Borrelia* spp., *B. burgdorferi* is the longest (20 to 30 μm) and narrowest (0.2 to 0.3 μm), and it has fewer flagella (7 to 11). The complete genome of *B. burgdorferi* has been sequenced. *B. burgdorferi* strains have a small, linear chromosome (~950 kilobases) and 17 to 21 linear and circular plasmids.[7,8]

The remarkable aspect of the *B. burgdorferi* genome is the large number of sequences for predicted and known lipoproteins,[7,8] including the plasmid-encoded outer-surface proteins (Osp) A through F. These and other differentially expressed outer-surface proteins presumably help the spirochete adapt to and survive in markedly different arthropod and mammalian environments. In addition, during the disseminated phase of the infection, another surface-exposed lipoprotein, called VlsE, undergoes extensive antigenic variation.[9] The organism has few proteins with biosynthetic activity and apparently depends on the host for much of its nutritional requirements.[7,8] The genome contains no homologues for systems that specialize in the secretion of toxins or other virulence factors. The only known virulence factors of *B. burgdorferi* are surface-exposed lipoproteins that allow the spirochete to attach to mammalian cells.

The genus *Borrelia* currently includes three pathogenic species that cause Lyme borreliosis,[10] and nine closely related species that rarely cause human infection.[11] To date, all North American strains have belonged to the first group, *B. burgdorferi (sensu stricto)*, hereafter called *B. burgdorferi*. All three groups have been found in Europe, but

most isolates there have been groups 2 (*Borrelia garinii*) and 3 (*Borrelia afzelii*) strains. Only the latter two groups have been found in Asia. These differences may well account for regional variations in the clinical picture of Lyme borreliosis. *B. burgdorferi* grows best at 33°C in a complex liquid medium called Barbour-Stoenner-Kelly medium.

Strains of *B. burgdorferi* have been subdivided according to several typing schemes, one based on sequence variation of OspC,[12] a second based on differences in the 16S-23S rRNA intergenic spacer region (RST or IGS),[13] and a third based on 8 chromosomal housekeeping genes (mutilocus typing).[14] Among *B. burgdorferi* strains in the northeastern United States, the genes encoding OspC or the IGS are in strong linkage disequilibrium, suggesting a clonal structure of strains in this geographic region.[15] From these typing systems, information is emerging concerning differential pathogenicity of strains of *B. burgdorferi*.[12,13] OspC type A (RST 1) strains seem to be the most virulent.

Vector of Transmission and Animal Hosts

The vectors of Lyme borreliosis are closely related ixodid tick species that are part of the *Ixodes ricinus* complex (also called the *Ixodes persulcatus* complex).[16] In the northeastern and midwestern United States, the deer tick, *Ixodes scapularis* (also called *Ixodes dammini*; Fig. 242-2), is the vector, and *Ixodes pacificus* is the vector in the West. In Europe, the sheep tick, *Ixodes ricinus*, and in Asia, the taiga tick, *Ixodes persulcatus*, are the primary vectors.

Ixodid ticks have larval, nymphal, and adult stages, and they require a blood meal at each stage.[11] The peak questing periods for adult *I. scapularis* are spring and fall; for nymphs, May through July; and for larvae, August and September. In the northeastern United States, from Maine to Virginia and in the north central states of Wisconsin and Minnesota, a highly efficient, horizontal cycle of *B. burgdorferi* transmission occurs among larval and nymphal *I. scapularis* ticks and certain rodents, particularly white-footed mice and chipmunks.[17] This cycle results in high rates of infection among rodents and nymphal ticks, and primarily nymphal tick bites cause many new human cases of Lyme disease during the late spring and summer months. White-tailed deer, which are not involved in the life cycle of the spirochete, are the preferred host of adult *I. scapularis*, and they seem to be critical for the survival of ticks.

The vector ecology of *B. burgdorferi* is different on the West Coast, where the frequency of Lyme disease is low. There, two intersecting cycles are necessary for the transmission of the disease,[18] one involving the dusky-footed wood rat and *Ixodes spinipalpis* (also called *Ixodes neotomae*) ticks, which do not bite humans and that maintain the cycle in nature, and the other involving wood rats and *I. pacificus* ticks, which are less often infected but do bite humans.

In the southeastern United States, immature *I. scapularis* ticks feed primarily on lizards rather than rodents, and lizards are not susceptible to *B. burgdorferi* infection. Therefore, *B. burgdorferi* infection occurs rarely in that part of the country. Instead, in the southern United States and in the mid-Atlantic states, a rash resembling erythema migrans, called southern tick-associated rash illness (STARI), has been associated with the bite of the Lone Star tick (*Amblyomma americanum*).[19] The etiology of this illness is not known, but it is not caused by B.

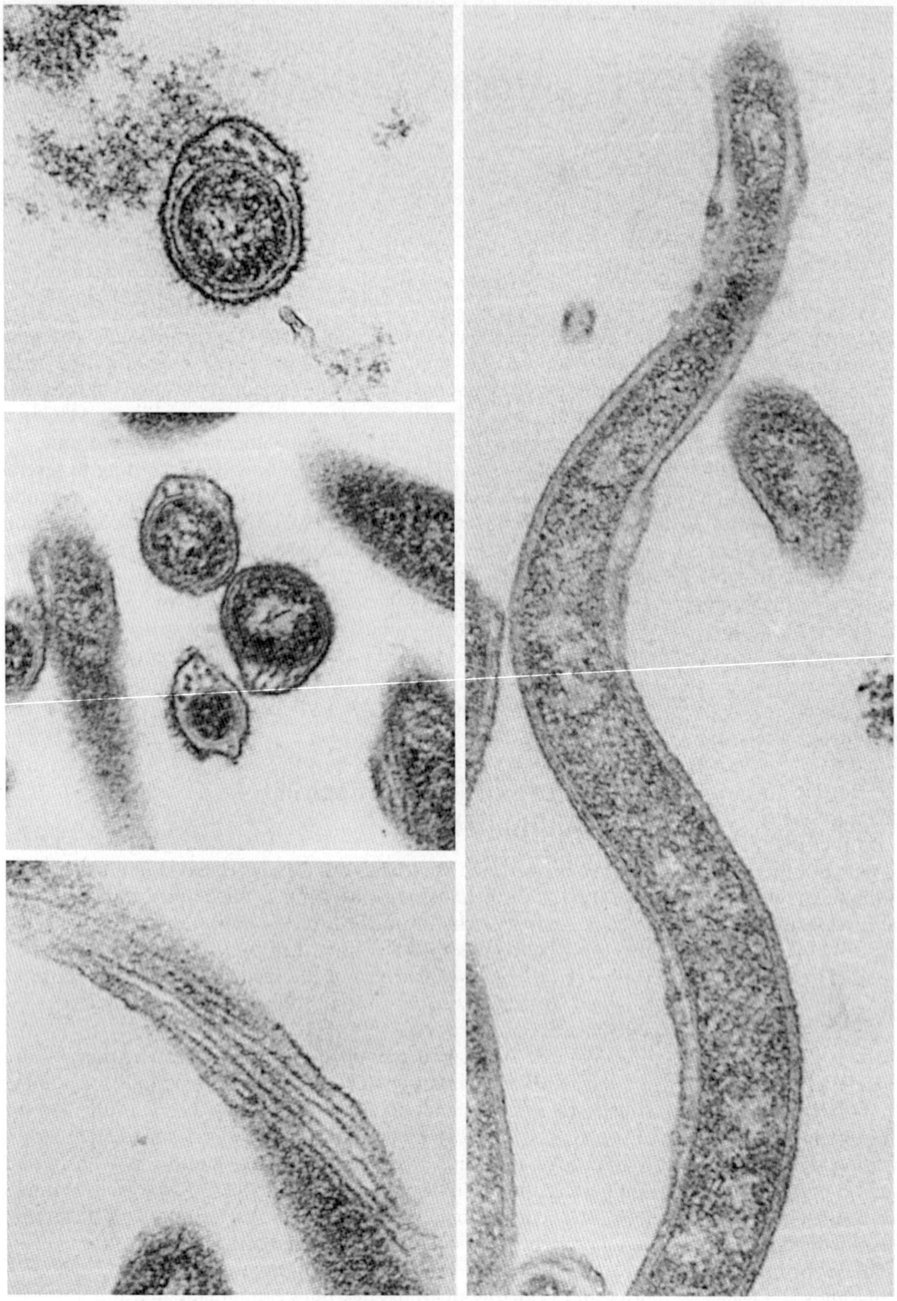

Figure 242-1 Electron micrographs of *Borrelia burgdorferi.* The spirochetes have a transverse diameter of about 0.2 mm and 7 to 11 flagella, which are shown (left panel) in cross section in the upper and middle pictures and in tangential section in the lower picture. In longitudinal section (right panel), the organism has an apparent slime layer, an outer membrane, flagellae, a cell wall, and cytoplasmic constituents; its length is 11 to 39 mm. (×40,000, except upper left [×60,000]). *(From Steere AC, Grodzicki RL, Kornblatt AN, et al. The spirochetal etiology of Lyme disease. N Engl J Med. 1983;308:733, with permission. Copyright © 1983 Massachusetts Medical Society. All rights reserved.)*

burgdorferi. STARI may be accompanied by nonspecific systemic symptoms, but it is not known to cause chronic infection.

In Europe, there is still debate about the preferred animal hosts of *I. ricinus.* These ticks feed on more than 300 animal species, including small mammals, birds, and reptiles.[20] Because the *Borrelia* species differ in their resistance to complement-mediated killing, small rodents are important reservoirs for *B. afzelii,* whereas birds are strongly associated with *B. garinii.*[21]

Epidemiology

Since surveillance was begun by the Centers for Disease Control and Prevention in 1982, the number of reported cases of Lyme disease has increased dramatically in the United States. Currently more than 20,000 cases have been noted yearly, making Lyme disease the most common vector-borne infection in the United States.[2] The disorder occurs primarily in three distinct foci: in the Northeast from Maine to

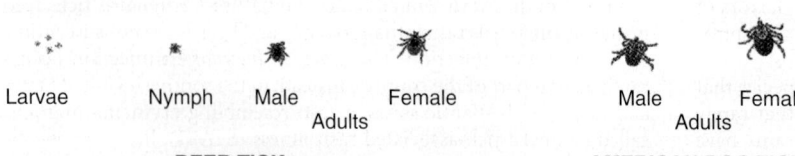

Larvae	Nymph	Male	Female		Male	Female
			Adults			Adults

DEER TICK
Ixodes scapularis

AMERICAN DOG TICK
Dermacentor variabilis

Figure 242-2 The deer tick, *Ixodes scapularis,* is the primary vector of Lyme disease in the United States. The nymph stage is most frequently implicated. For comparison, the dog tick, *Dermacentor variabilis,* is shown, but this tick does not transmit Lyme disease. Shown actual size. *(Courtesy of the Massachusetts Department of Public Health Division and the Cape Cod Cooperative Extension.)*

Virginia; in the Midwest in Wisconsin, Minnesota, and Michigan; and in the West, primarily in northern California. Lyme borreliosis also occurs in temperate regions of the Northern Hemisphere in Europe and Asia. There, the highest reported frequencies of the infection are in middle Europe, particularly in Germany, Austria, Slovenia, and Sweden.[22]

During the past 40 years, the infection in the United States has continued to spread, particularly in the Northeast. It has caused focal outbreaks in some coastal areas, and it now affects suburban locations near Boston, New York, Philadelphia, Baltimore, and Washington—the most heavily populated parts of the country.[23] Within these areas, the occurrence of Lyme disease is highly focal. In Connecticut, which has the highest reported frequency of Lyme disease in the United States, cases have been noted in all parts of the state, but most of the cases are still clustered in two counties in the southeastern part of the state, where the original epidemiologic investigation took place in the town of Lyme. In a large, two-year vaccine trial, the yearly incidence of the disease in such highly endemic areas was greater than 1 per 100 participants.[24]

Why did Lyme disease emerge in the northeastern United States during the latter part of the 20th century?[11] The infection has probably been in North America for thousands of years, but necessary ecology conditions were altered during the European colonization of North America. Woodlands were cleared for farming, and deer were hunted practically to extinction. However, during the 20th century, farmland reverted to woodland, deer proliferated, white-footed mice were plentiful, and the deer tick thrived. Soil moisture and land cover, as found near rivers and along the coast, were favorable for tick survival. Moreover, these areas became heavily populated with both humans and deer, as more rural wooded areas became wooded suburbs in which deer were without predators and hunting was prohibited. Finally, the spread of a particularly virulent spirochetal strain, *B. burgdorferi* OspC type A, may have contributed to the rise in the incidence of the infection.[25]

Pathogenesis

To maintain its complex enzootic cycle, *B. burgdorferi* must adapt to two markedly different environments: the tick and the mammalian or avian host. The spirochete survives in a dormant state in the nymphal tick midgut during the fall, winter, and spring, where it expresses primarily OspA and certain other proteins.[26] When the tick feeds during the late spring or summer, these proteins are downregulated, and another set of proteins, including OspC, is upregulated.[27,28] OspC binds mammalian plasminogen and its activators present in the blood meal, which facilitates spreading of the organism in the tick.[29] In addition, within the tick salivary gland, OspC binds a tick salivary gland protein (Salp 15), and coating of the spirochete in this tick protein is essential for initial immune evasion in the mammalian host.[30] The spirochete, which has few proteins with biosynthetic activity,[8] appears to meet its nutritional requirements by infection of a mammalian or avian host.

After injection of *B. burgdorferi* by the tick and an incubation period of 3 to 32 days, the spirochete usually first multiplies locally in the skin at the site of the tick bite. In most patients, immune cells first encounter *B. burgdorferi* at this site. Dendritic cells isolated from the dermis readily engulf *B. burgdorferi* in vitro.[31] During the initial infection, *B. burgdorferi* induces primarily pro-inflammatory responses in inflammatory cells in EM lesions,[32,33] and *B. burgdorferi*–stimulated peripheral blood mononuclear cells (PBMCs) produce primarily pro-inflammatory cytokines, particularly IFN-γ.[34] Thus, both innate and adaptive cellular elements are mobilized to fight the infection.

Within days to weeks, *B. burgdorferi* often disseminates to many sites. During this period, the spirochete has been recovered from blood and cerebrospinal fluid,[5,6,35] and it has been seen in small numbers in specimens of myocardium, retina, muscle, bone, spleen, liver, meninges, and brain.[36] To disseminate, *B. burgdorferi* binds certain host proteins and adheres to integrins, proteoglycans, or glycoproteins on host cells or tissue matrices. As in the tick, spreading though the skin and other tissue matrixes may be facilitated by the binding of plasminogen and its activators to the surface of the spirochete.[29] During dissemination, a 66-kDa spirochetal protein binds the platelet-specific integrin $\alpha_{IIb}\beta_3$, and the vitronectin receptor ($\alpha_v\beta_5$).[37] A 26-kDa glycosaminoglycan binding protein binds heparan sulfate and dermatin sulfate,[38] which are expressed on endothelial cells. A 47-kDa fibronectin-binding protein (BBK32) binds fibronectin,[39] a ubiquitous extracellular matrix protein. Finally, decorin-binding proteins A and B (DbpA and DbpB) of the spirochete bind decorin,[40] a proteoglycan on the surface of collagen, which may explain the alignment of spirochetes with collagen fibrils in the extracellular matrix in the heart, nervous system, or joints.[36]

All affected tissues show an infiltration of lymphocytes and plasma cells.[36] Some degree of vascular damage, including mild vasculitis or hypervascular occlusion, may be seen in multiple sites, suggesting that spirochetes may have been in or around blood vessels. Although *B. burgdorferi* has been identified inside cultured cells in vitro, it has not been seen in intracellular locations in histologic sections of infected tissues from patients with Lyme disease.

Despite an active immune response, *B. burgdorferi* may survive during dissemination by changing or minimizing antigenic expression of surface proteins and by inhibiting certain critical host immune responses. Two linear plasmids (lps) seem to be essential, including lp25, which encodes a nicotinamidase,[41] and lp28-1, which encodes the VlsE lipoprotein,[10] the protein that undergoes extensive antigenic variation.[42] In addition, the spirochete has a number of highly homologous, differentially expressed lipoproteins, including OspE/F paralogs, which further contribute to antigenic diversity.[43] Finally, *B. afzelii* and, to a lesser degree, *B. burgdorferi* have complement regulator-acquiring surface proteins that bind complement factor H and factor H-like protein 1.[44,45] These complement factors inactivate C3b, which protects the organism from complement-mediated killing.

Both innate and adaptive immune responses are required for optimal control of spirochetal dissemination. Membrane lipoproteins are mitogenic for B cells.[46] The specific immunoglobulin M (IgM) response is often associated with polyclonal activation of B cells, including elevated total serum IgM levels,[47] circulating immune complexes,[48] and cryoglobulins.[47] In murine *B. burgdorferi* infection, CD1d presentation of monogalactosyl diacylglycerol (MgalD, BbGL-II) to NK T cells may be important in the early innate immune response, possibly as an initial source of IFN-γ.[49] CD1d-deficient mice do not control the infection as well as their wild-type counterparts.[50]

In the human infection, the adaptive IgG response develops gradually over weeks to months to an increasing array of spirochetal proteins[51] and two borrelial glycolipids.[52] Using protein arrays that expressed approximately 1400 *B. burgdorferi* proteins, antibody responses were detected to a total of 89 proteins in a population of patients with Lyme arthritis, primarily to outer-surface lipoproteins.[53] Spirochetal killing seems to be accomplished primarily by bactericidal B cell responses,[54] which promote spirochetal killing by complement fixation and opsonization.[55] As shown in mice, the primary purpose of *B. burgdorferi*–specific CD4+ Th1 cells, which secrete mainly IFN-γ, is to prime T-cell-dependent, B-cell responses.[56] *B. burgdorferi*–specific CD8+ T cells are another important source of IFN-γ, but they do not seem to have a cytotoxic function.[57]

In the enzootic infection, *B. burgdorferi* spirochetes must survive this immune assault for only the summer months before returning to the larval ticks to begin the cycle again the next year. In contrast, infection of humans is a dead-end event for the spirochete. Within several weeks to months, innate and adaptive immune mechanisms, even without antibiotic treatment, control widely disseminated infection, and generalized systemic symptoms wane.[1] However, without antibiotic therapy, spirochetes may survive in localized niches for several more years. *B. burgdorferi*, the sole cause of the infection in the United States, may cause persistent arthritis or, in rare cases, a subtle encephalopathy or polyneuropathy accompanied by minimal, if any, systemic symptoms.[1] Patients with Lyme arthritis have very high antibody responses to many spirochetal proteins that are suggestive of hyperimmunization due to recurrent waves of spirochetal growth.[51] Even without antibiotic treatment, the number of patients who continue to have attacks of arthritis decreases by about 10% to 20% each year, and few patients have had attacks for longer than 5 years.[58] Thus, immune mechanisms seem to succeed eventually in the eradication of *B. burgdorferi* from selected niches, including the joints or nervous system.

Clinical Characteristics

As with other spirochetal infections, human Lyme borreliosis generally occurs in stages, with remissions and exacerbations and different clinical manifestations at each stage.[3] Early infection consists of stage 1 (localized EM), followed within days or weeks by stage 2 (disseminated infection). Late infection, or stage 3 (persistent infection), usually begins months to years after the disease onset, sometimes following long periods of latent infection. In an individual patient, however, the infection is highly variable, ranging from brief involvement in only one system to chronic, multisystem involvement of the skin, nerves, or joints.

EARLY INFECTION: STAGE 1 (LOCALIZED INFECTION)

In about 70% to 80% of patients, EM develops at the site of the tick bite (Fig. 242-3A and Table 242-1).[59,60] However, because of the small size of nymphal *I. scapularis,* most patients do not remember the tick bite. During the first several days, the lesion often has a homogeneous red appearance.[61] In addition, the centers of early lesions sometimes become intensely erythematous and indurated, vesicular, or necrotic. As the area of redness around the center expands, most lesions continue to have bright-red outer borders (usually flat, but occasionally raised) and partial central clearing. In some instances, migrating lesions remain an even, intense red; several red rings are found within the outside one; or the central area turns blue before it clears. Although the lesion can be located anywhere, the thigh, groin, and axilla are particularly common sites. If EM is on the head, only a linear streak might be seen to emerge from the hairline. The lesion is hot to the touch, and patients often describe it as burning or occasionally itching or painful.

In Europe, EM is often an indolent, localized infection, whereas in the United States, the lesion is associated with more intense inflammation and signs and symptoms that suggest dissemination of the spirochete.[1] In one U.S. study, spirochetes were cultured from plasma samples in 50% of patients with EM.[62] In a recent study, the EM skin lesions of *B. burgdorferi*–infected U.S. patients expanded faster, were associated with more symptoms, and had higher mRNA levels of macrophage-associated chemokines and cytokines than did EM lesions of *B. afzelii*–infected Austrian patients.[63]

EARLY INFECTION: STAGE 2 (DISSEMINATED INFECTION)

Within several days to weeks of the onset of the initial EM lesion, patients, particularly in the United States, may develop multiple annular secondary skin lesions (see Fig. 242-3B and Table 242-1),[1,60] a sign of hematogenous dissemination. Although their appearance is similar to that of the initial lesions, they are generally smaller, migrate less, and lack indurated centers; they are not associated with previous tick bites. Individual lesions sometimes appear and fade at different times, and their borders sometimes merge. During this period, some patients develop malar rash, conjunctivitis, or, rarely, diffuse urticaria. EM and secondary lesions usually fade within 3 to 4 weeks (range, 1 day to 14 months).

EM is often accompanied by malaise and fatigue, headache, fever and chills, generalized achiness, and regional lymphadenopathy.[1,60] In about 18% of patients,[59] these symptoms are the presenting picture of the infection.[64] In addition, patients sometimes have evidence of meningeal irritation with episodic attacks of excruciating headache and

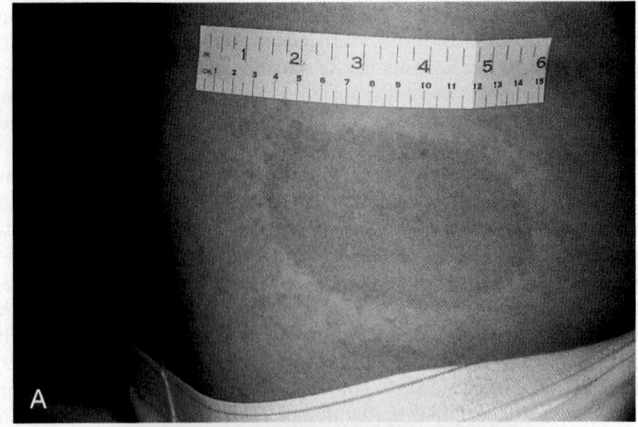

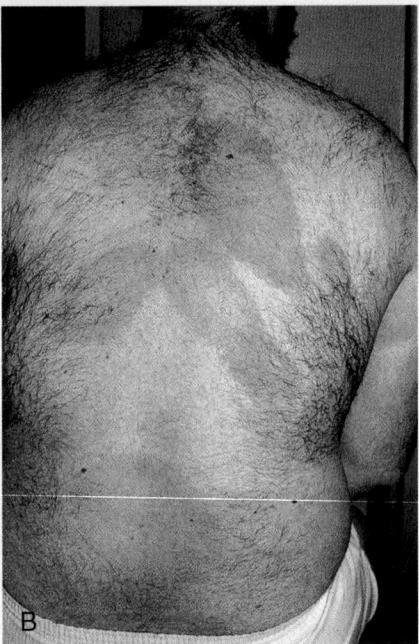

Figure 242-3 **A,** An early erythema migrans skin lesion is seen 4 days after detection. **B,** Four days after the onset of the initial skin lesion, secondary lesions have appeared, and several of their borders have merged. *(From Steere AC, Bartenhagen NH, Cratt JE, et al. The early clinical manifestations of Lyme disease. Ann Intern Med. 1983;99:76, with permission.)*

neck pain, mild encephalopathy with difficulty with mentation, migratory musculoskeletal pain, hepatitis, generalized lymphadenopathy or splenomegaly, sore throat, nonproductive cough, or testicular swelling.[60] A few patients have had microscopic hematuria, sometimes with mild proteinuria (dipstick). During the first days of illness, headache and neck stiffness are not associated with a spinal fluid pleocytosis or objective neurologic deficit. Except for fatigue and lethargy, which are often constant, the early signs and symptoms are typically intermittent and changing. For example, a patient might experience predominantly headache and a stiff neck for several days. After a few days of improvement, musculoskeletal pain might begin.

After several weeks to months, about 15% of untreated patients in the United States develop frank neurologic abnormalities, including meningitis, encephalitis, cranial neuritis (including bilateral facial palsy), motor and sensory radiculoneuritis, mononeuritis multiplex, cerebellar ataxia or myelitis—alone or in various combinations.[65] The usual pattern consists of fluctuating symptoms of meningitis with superimposed cranial (particularly facial palsy) or peripheral radicu-

TABLE 242-1	Manifestations of Lyme Disease by Stage*		
	Early Infection		**Late Infection**
System†	*Localized Stage 1*	*Disseminated Stage 2*	*Persistent Stage 3*
Skin	Erythema migrans (EM)	Secondary annular lesions Malar rash Diffuse erythema or urticaria Evanescent lesions Lymphocytoma	Acrodermatitis chronica atrophicans Localized scleroderma-like lesions
Musculoskeletal		Migratory pain in joints, tendons, bursae, muscle, bone Brief arthritis attacks Myositis‡ Osteomyelitis‡ Panniculitis‡	Prolonged arthritis attacks Chronic arthritis Peripheral enthesopathy Periostitis or joint subluxations below acrodermatitis
Neurologic		Meningitis Cranial neuritis, facial palsy Motor or sensory radiculoneuritis Subtle encephalitis Mononeuritis multiplex Pseudotumor cerebri Myelitis‡ Cerebellar ataxia‡	Chronic encephalomyelitis Spastic paraphareses Ataxic gait Subtle mental disorders Chronic axonal polyradiculopathy
Lymphatic	Regional lymphadenopathy	Regional or generalized lymphadenopathy Splenomegaly	
Heart		Atrioventricular nodal block Myopericarditis Pancarditis	
Eyes		Conjunctivitis Iritis‡ Choroiditis‡ Retinal hemorrhage or detachment‡ Panophthalmitis‡	Keratitis
Liver		Mild or recurrent hepatitis	
Respiratory		Nonexudative sore throat Nonproductive cough	
Kidney		Microscopic hematuria or proteinuria	
Genitourinary		Orchitis‡	
Constitutional systems	Minor	Severe malaise and fatigue	Fatigue

*The staging system provides a guideline for the expected timing of the different manifestations of the illness, but this may vary in an individual case.
†The systems are listed from the most to the least commonly affected.
‡Because the inclusion of these manifestations is based on one or a few cases, they should be considered possible but not proven manifestations of Lyme disease.
From Steere AC. Lyme disease. *N Engl J Med.* 1989;321:586. Copyright © 1989 Massachusetts Medical Society. All rights reserved.

loneuropathy. On examination, such patients usually have neck stiffness only on extreme flexion; Kernig's and Brudzinski's signs are not present. Facial palsy may occur alone,[66] and in rare instances, it may be the presenting manifestation of the disease. In children, the optic nerve may be affected by inflammation or increased intracranial pressure, which may lead to blindness.[1] In Europe, the most common neurologic manifestation is Bannwarth's syndrome, which consists of neuritic pain, lymphocytic pleocytosis without headache, and sometimes cranial neuritis.[1]

In patients with meningitis, cerebrospinal fluid (CSF) typically has a lymphocytic pleocytosis of about 100 cells/mm³, often with an elevated protein but a normal glucose level.[65] Specific IgG, IgM, or IgA antibody to the spirochete is produced intrathecally,[67] and *B. burgdorferi*–specific oligoclonal bands may be present. Electrophysiologic studies of affected extremities suggest primarily axonal nerve involvement.[68] Histologically, the lesions show axonal nerve injury with perivascular infiltration of lymphocytes and plasmocytes around epineural blood vessels. Stage 2 neurologic abnormalities usually last for weeks or months, but they may recur or become chronic.

Within several weeks after the onset of illness, about 5% of untreated patients develop cardiac involvement.[69] The most common abnormality is fluctuating degrees of atrioventricular block (first-degree,

Wenckebach, or complete heart block). However, some patients have evidence of more diffuse cardiac involvement, including electrocardiographic changes or a gallium scan compatible with acute myopericarditis, radionuclide evidence of mild left ventricular dysfunction, or, rarely, cardiomegaly. No patients have had heart murmurs. The duration of cardiac involvement is usually brief (3 days to 6 weeks), and the insertion of a permanent pacemaker is unnecessary.[70] One patient is known to have died of cardiac involvement of Lyme disease.[71] At autopsy, that patient had a lymphoplasmacellular infiltrate in the epicardium, myocardium, and endocardium, and a few spirochetes were seen in the myocardium. In Europe, *B. burgdorferi* has been isolated from endomyocardial biopsy samples from several patients with chronic dilated cardiomyopathy.[72] However, this complication has not been observed in the United States.[73]

During this stage, migratory musculoskeletal pain is common in joints, tendons, bursae, muscle, or bones.[1] In addition, a few patients have been described with osteomyelitis, myositis, panniculitis, or fasciitis. Conjunctivitis is the most common eye abnormality in Lyme disease, but deeper tissues in the eye may be affected as well.[1,74] There are case reports of iritis followed by panophthalmitis, choroiditis with exudative retinal detachments, or interstitial keratitis, similar to that seen in syphilis.

LATE INFECTION: STAGE 3 (PERSISTENT INFECTION)

Months after the onset of the illness, within the context of strong cellular and humoral immune responses to *B. burgdorferi*, about 60% of patients begin to experience intermittent attacks of joint swelling and pain, primarily in large joints, especially the knee, usually one or two joints at a time (see Table 242-1).[1,58] Affected knees are commonly more swollen than painful and are often hot but rarely red. Baker cysts may form and rupture early. However, both large and small joints may be affected. Attacks of arthritis generally last from a few weeks to months separated by periods of complete remission. Joint fluid white blood cell counts range from 500 to 110,000 cells/mm³, most of which, in patients with high white blood cell counts, are polymorphonuclear leukocytes. Although the total number of patients who continue to have recurrent attacks of arthritis decreases by about 10% to 20% each year, attacks of knee swelling sometimes become longer during the second or third year of illness, sometimes lasting one year or longer. However, even in untreated patients, intermittent or chronic arthritis usually resolves completely within several years.

Although most patients with either intermittent or persistent arthritis respond to oral or intravenous (IV) antibiotic treatment, a small percentage of patients have persistent joint inflammation in a knee for months or even several years after 2 months or longer of oral antibiotics or 1 month or longer of IV antibiotics, or both. This illness is defined as antibiotic-refractory Lyme arthritis.[75] Although *B. burgdorferi* DNA can often be detected in joint fluid prior to antibiotic treatment, the results of polymerase chain reaction (PCR) testing are usually negative in synovial tissue or joint fluid after antibiotic therapy,[75] suggesting that joint inflammation may continue in some patients after the near or total eradication of the spirochete from the joint with antibiotic therapy. The synovial lesion, which is similar to that seen in other forms of chronic inflammatory arthritis, shows synovial cell hyperplasia, vascular proliferation, a heavy infiltration of mononuclear cells, particularly T cells, and upregulation of adhesion molecules.[76]

Antibiotic-refractory Lyme arthritis is associated with HLA-DRB1 molecules that bind an epitope of *B. burgdorferi* OspA (OspA$_{161-175}$), particularly the HLA-DRB1*0401 and DRB1*0101 molecules,[77] and with T-cell recognition of this epitope.[78] However, as determined using tetramer reagents, the frequencies of OspA$_{161-175}$-specific T cells declined to low or undetectable levels during or soon after antibiotic therapy, months before the resolution of synovitis in patients with antibiotic-refractory arthritis, suggesting that persistent synovitis in the refractory group are not perpetuated by these cells.[79] Moreover, the antibody responses to OspA declined similarly in patients with antibiotic-responsive or antibiotic-refractory arthritis,[80] suggesting that spirochetal killing occurred in both groups.

Before and during antibiotic therapy, synovial fluid from patients with antibiotic-refractory arthritis contained exceptionally high levels of Th1 chemoattractants and cytokines, particularly CXCL9 and IFN-γ, compared with those with antibiotic-responsive arthritis.[81] Furthermore, during the postantibiotic period, when PCR results were negative and specific immune responses to *B. burgdorferi* antigens were declining, the levels of CXCL9 and IFN-γ remained high or even increased in synovial fluid and synovial tissue. A murine model was recently reported in *B. burgdorferi*–infected HLA-DR4-positive CD28-negative mice that duplicates many of the features of human antibiotic-refractory Lyme arthritis.[82] Thus, recognition of the OspA$_{161-175}$ epitope (or other unidentified epitopes) may lead to especially high levels of proinflammatory cytokines, which may not be appropriately downregulated as spirochetal killing progresses.[83] Alternately, high levels of inflammatory cytokines could lead to the breaking of tolerance to a currently unidentified self-epitope,[84] which continues to elicit synovial inflammation after spirochetal eradication.

In rare instances, along with or after episodes of Lyme arthritis, patients may develop chronic neurologic manifestations of the disorder.[1,85] In both the United States and Europe, a chronic axonal polyneuropathy may develop, manifested primarily as spinal radicular pain or distal paresthesias. Even though sensory symptoms are often localized, electrophysiologic testing frequently shows a diffuse axonal polyneuropathy affecting both proximal and distal nerve segments.[68] In Europe, *B. garinii* may cause chronic encephalomyelitis, characterized by spastic parapareses, ataxia, cognitive impairment, bladder dysfunction, and cranial neuropathy, particularly of the seventh or eighth cranial nerve, accompanied by intrathecal antibody production of IgG antibody to *B. burgdorferi*.[1]

In the United States, a mild, late neurologic syndrome has been reported, called Lyme encephalopathy, manifested primarily by subtle cognitive disturbances.[85] Although there are no inflammatory changes in CSF, intrathecal antibody production to the spirochete can often be demonstrated. Neither neuropsychological tests of memory[86] nor single photon emission computed tomography (SPECT) scanning of the brain[87] has sufficient specificity to be helpful in diagnosis. Postinfectious phenomena may also play a role in the pathogenesis of this syndrome. One unusual case of *B. burgdorferi*–induced meningoencephalitis and cerebral vasculitis has been reported that was unresponsive to antibiotics.[88] In this case, a T-cell clone recovered from the CSF responded to both spirochetal epitopes and autoantigens.

Acrodermatitis chronica atrophicans, which sometimes follows years after EM, has been observed primarily in Europe in association with *B. afzelii* infection.[89] Acrodermatitis chronica atrophicans begins with red violaceous lesions that become sclerotic or atrophic. These lesions, which may be the presenting manifestation of the disease, may last for many years, and *B. burgdorferi* has been cultured from such lesions as much as 10 years after their onset.

▨ Post–Lyme Disease Syndrome

Despite resolution of the objective manifestations of the infection with antibiotic therapy, a small percentage of patients have pain, neurocognitive, or fatigue symptoms for months or years afterwards.[90] If these symptoms last for more than 6 months, they are sometimes called post–Lyme disease syndrome or chronic Lyme disease. This syndrome is similar to or indistinguishable from chronic fatigue syndrome or fibromyalgia. Compared with active Lyme disease, these patients tend to have more generalized or disabling symptoms, which include marked fatigue, severe headache, diffuse musculoskeletal pain, multiple symmetric tender points in characteristic locations, pain and stiffness in many joints, diffuse paresthesias, difficulty with concentration, or sleep disturbance. Patients with these conditions lack evidence of joint inflammation; they have normal neurologic test results; and they usually have a greater degree of anxiety and depression. In contrast, late manifestations of Lyme disease, including arthritis, encephalopathy, or neuropathy, are usually associated with minimal systemic symptoms. There is currently no evidence that persistent subjective symptoms after recommended courses of antibiotic therapy for Lyme disease are caused by active infection.[90,91]

A counterculture has emerged that ascribes pain and fatigue syndromes to "chronic Lyme disease" when there is little or no evidence of *B. burgdorferi* infection.[90-92] In such patients, the term *chronic Lyme disease*, which is equated with chronic *B. burgdorferi* infection, is a misnomer, and the use of prolonged, potentially dangerous, and expensive antibiotic treatment for it is not warranted.

▨ Congenital Infection

In the mid-1980s, the transplacental transmission of *B. burgdorferi* was reported in two infants whose mothers had Lyme borreliosis during the first trimester of pregnancy.[1] Both infants died during the first week of life. In both, spirochetes were seen in various fetal tissues stained with the Dieterle silver stain, but cultures and serologic testing were not performed. However, in subsequent prospective studies, no cases of congenital infection have been linked to the Lyme disease spirochete.[93] Although it is still possible that *B. burgdorferi* may cause an adverse fetal outcome in humans, it has not been documented conclusively.

Coinfection

I. scapularis ticks transmit not only *B. burgdorferi*, the Lyme disease agent, but also other infectious agents, including *Babesia microti* (a red blood cell parasite) and *Anaplasma phagocytophilum* (formerly referred to as "the agent of human granulocytic ehrlichiosis"). Each of these pathogens may cause nonspecific systemic symptoms during summer, and coinfection with *B. burgdorferi* and one or both of these other tick-borne agents may lead to more severe, acute illness.[94,95] However, neither *A. phagocytophilum* nor *B. microti* is known to cause chronic infection, as with untreated *B. burgdorferi* infection.

The frequency of coinfection has been quite variable, depending on geographic location and study methodology. One problem is that anaplasmosis by itself may cause a false-positive IgM Western blot for Lyme disease. In one study of 93 patients with culture-proven EM, two patients (2%) had coinfection with *A. phagocytophilum* and two (2%) had coinfection with *B. microti*, demonstrated by PCR testing or IgG seroconversion.[94] At the other end of the spectrum, 75 of 192 patients (39%) in another study had evidence of coinfection, most commonly with Lyme disease and babesiosis.[95] In Europe and Asia, *I. ricinus* and *I. persulcatus* ticks, the vectors of *B. burgdorferi (sensu lato)*, also transmit tick-borne encephalitis virus.

Laboratory Diagnosis

Culture of *B. burgdorferi* from patient specimens in Barbour-Stoenner-Kelly (BSK) medium permits definitive diagnosis. However, positive cultures have been obtained mainly early in the illness, primarily from biopsies of EM lesions,[24] less often from plasma samples,[63] and only occasionally from CSF samples in patients with meningitis. Later in the infection, PCR testing is greatly superior to culture in the detection of *B. burgdorferi* in joint fluid.[96] *B. burgdorferi* has not been isolated from the CSF of patients with chronic neuroborreliosis, and *B. burgdorferi* DNA has been detected in CSF samples in only a small number of such patients.[97] The Lyme urine antigen test (LUAT), which has given grossly unreliable results, should not be used to support the diagnosis of Lyme disease.

Because of limited utility of microbiologic techniques, diagnosis is usually based on the recognition of a characteristic clinical picture, exposure in an endemic area, and, except in those with EM, a positive antibody response to *B. burgdorferi*.[98] For serologic testing in the United States, the Centers for Disease Control and Prevention currently recommends a two-test approach in which samples are first tested by enzyme-linked immunosorbent assay (ELISA) and those with equivocal or positive results are tested by Western blotting (Fig. 242-4).[99] These tests are usually performed with *B. burgdorferi* sonicates, most often obtained from strain B31, a RST 1 strain.

According to the CDC criteria,[99] an IgM Western blot is considered positive if two of the following three bands are present: 23, 39, and 41 kDa; however, the combination of the 23- and 41-kDa bands may still be a false-positive result. An IgG blot is considered positive if 5 of the following 10 bands are present: 18, 23, 28, 30, 39, 41, 45, 58, 66, and 93 kDa (Fig. 242-5). Approximately half of the normal population has IgG reactivity with the 41-kDa flagellar antigen of the spirochete, and this response, by itself, has no diagnostic significance. In Europe, where there is less expansion of the antibody response, no single set of criteria for immunoblot interpretation give high levels of sensitivity and specificity in all countries.[100]

Serodiagnosis is insensitive during the first several weeks of infection. During this period, approximately 30% of patients with EM in the United States have positive responses in acute phase samples, usually of the IgM isotype, but by convalescence 2 to 4 weeks later, about 65% to 75% have seroreactivity, even after antibiotic treatment.[101,102] Since these tests are usually performed with an RST 1 strain, the sensitivity of Western blotting may be somewhat lower when the patient is infected with an RST 2 or 3 strain.[103] After 4 to 8 weeks, patients with active infection have positive IgG antibody responses, regardless of the RST of the strain causing the infection. In persons with illness for longer than 4 to 8 weeks, a positive IgM test alone is likely to be a false-positive result, and thus a positive IgM response should not be used to support the diagnosis after the first two months of infection. In patients with acute neuroborreliosis, especially those with meningitis, intrathecal production of IgM, IgG, or IgA antibody

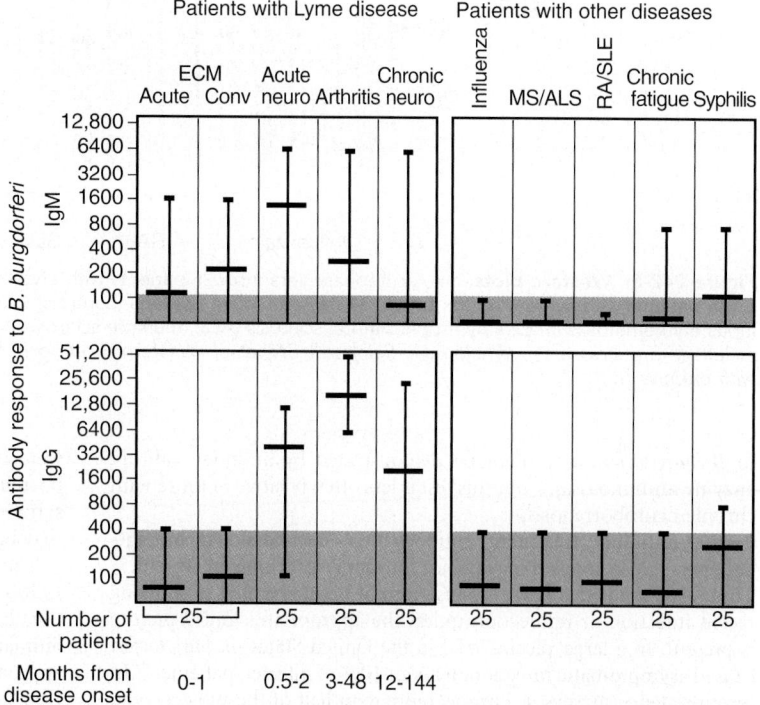

Figure 242-4 **Antibody titers to *Borrelia burgdorferi* by enzyme-linked immunosorbent assay (ELISA) in patients with various manifestations of Lyme disease and in control subjects.** Horizontal bars = mean; vertical bars = range; hatched bars = normal range. Normal range was derived from sera from 50 healthy control subjects. ALS, Amyotrophic lateral sclerosis; Con V, convalescent phase; ECM, erythema chronicum migrans; acute neuro, meningitis; chronic neuro, encephalopathy or polyneuropathy; MS, multiple sclerosis; RA, rheumatoid arthritis; SLE, systemic lupus erythematosus. *(From Dressler F, Whalen JA, Reinhardt BN, et al. Western blotting in the serodiagnosis of Lyme disease. J Infect Dis. 1993;167:392, with permission.)*

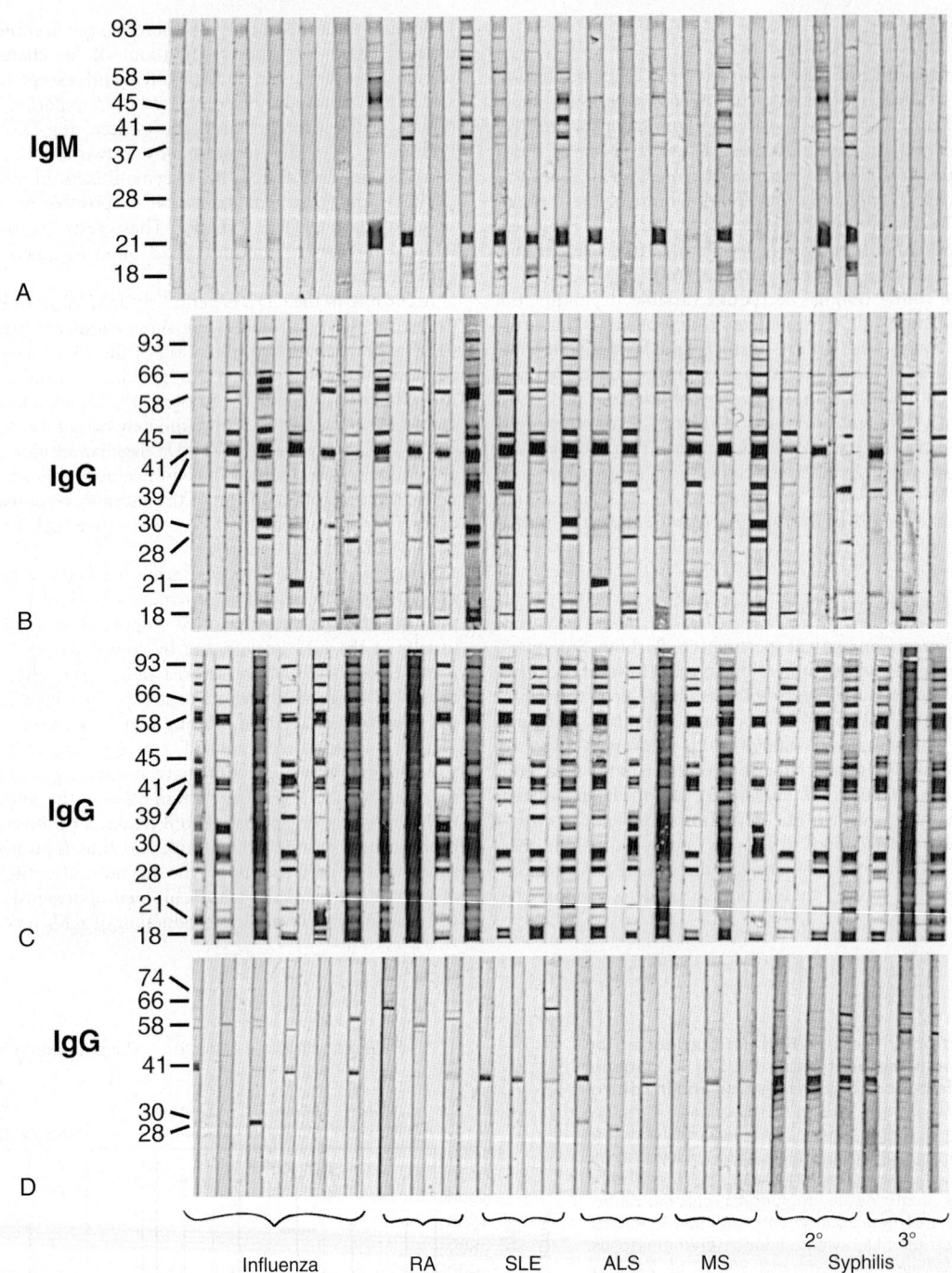

Figure 242-5 **Western blots.** If **A**, acutephase sera from 25 patients with erythema migrans; **B**, 25 patients with Lyme meningitis or facial palsy; **C**, 25 patients with Lyme arthritis; and **D**, 24 representative patients (controls) who had influenza vaccinations, rheumatoid arthritis (RA), systemic lupus erythematosus (SLE), amyotrophic lateral sclerosis (ALS), multiple sclerosis (MS), or secondary or tertiary syphilis. Molecular masses (kDa) are at left. *(From Dressler F, Whalen JA, Reinhardt BN, et al. Western Blotting in the serodiagnosis of Lyme disease. J Infect Dis. 1993;167:392, with permission.)*

to *B. burgdorferi* may often be demonstrated by antibody capture enzyme immunoassay,[67] but this test is less often positive in those with chronic neuroborreliosis.

After antibiotic treatment, antibody titers decline slowly, but IgG and even IgM responses may persist for many years after treatment.[104] Thus, even a positive IgM response cannot be interpreted as showing recent infection or reinfection unless the appropriate clinical picture is present. In a large vaccine trial in the United States, *B. burgdorferi* caused asymptomatic infection in about 10% of infected patients.[105] In seroprevalence surveys in Europe, more than half of the subjects who

were seropositive by ELISA did not remember symptoms of Lyme borreliosis.[106] If patients with past or asymptomatic infection have symptoms caused by another illness, the danger is that the symptoms may be attributed incorrectly to Lyme disease.

The most promising second-generation serologic test is an IgG ELISA that employs a 26-mer peptide of the sixth invariant region of the VlsE lipoprotein of *B. burgdorferi*, called the C6 peptide ELISA.[101,102] Similar results were obtained with this test and the standard two-test approach of sonicate IgM and IgG ELISA and Western blot. The principal advantage of the C6 peptide ELISA is the early IgG response, and therefore an IgM test is not necessary. However, the C6 ELISA is not quite as specific as sonicate Western blot. Thus, with current methods, a two-test approach that includes Western blot remains valuable for specificity and for assessing the duration of therapy. As with the sonicate tests, the response to the VlsE peptide may persist for months or years after successful antibiotic treatment; and therefore persistence of the anti-VlsE antibody response cannot be equated with spirochetal persistence in Lyme disease.[101]

Differential Diagnosis

Early in its course, a small, homogeneous EM lesion may resemble the red papule of an uninfected tick bite. If an erythema expands rapidly following a tick bite, it is more likely an allergic reaction to tick saliva than an EM lesion, which expands slowly (~1 cm/day). Patients with secondary annular EM lesions may be thought to have erythema multiforme, but Lyme disease is not associated with blistering, mucosal lesions or involvement of the palms and soles. Facial palsy caused by *B. burgdorferi* differs from that associated with herpes simplex I virus (Bell's palsy) or varicella-zoster virus (Ramsey-Hunt syndrome) by its seasonal onset (usually June through September), frequent association with EM, and positive IgM and IgG antibody responses to *B. burgdorferi*. Lyme arthritis is most like reactive arthritis in an adult or the pauciarticular form of juvenile rheumatoid arthritis in a child. Patients with Lyme arthritis usually have very high borrelia-specific IgG antibody titers by ELISA with responses to many spirochetal proteins by Western blot.

The most common mistake is to confuse chronic Lyme disease with chronic fatigue syndrome or fibromyalgia. Although subjective pain or fatigue symptoms may follow Lyme disease, the active infection usually affects one system at a time, and the patient has objective measures of involvement in that system.

Treatment

Evidence-based treatment recommendations for Lyme disease have been presented by the Infectious Diseases Society of America.[107] In brief, the various manifestations of Lyme disease can usually be treated with oral antibiotic therapy, except for patients with objective neurologic abnormalities and occasional patients with Lyme arthritis who may require intravenous therapy for successful treatment of the infection (Table 242-2). For early localized or disseminated infection, doxycycline for 14 to 21 days is recommended in persons age 8 or older, except for pregnant women. An advantage of doxycycline is its efficacy against *A. phagocytophilum*, a possible coinfecting agent. Amoxicillin, the second-choice alternative, should be used in children or pregnant women. In case of allergy, cefuroxime axetil is a third-choice alternative. Erythromycin or its cogeners, which are fourth-choice alternatives, are recommended only for patients who are unable to take doxycycline, amoxicillin, or cefuroxime axetil. Approximately 15% of patients with disseminated infection experience a Jarisch-Herxheimer–like reaction during the first 24 hours of therapy. In vitro, *B. burgdorferi* is sensitive to tetracycline, penicillin, erythromycin, and their cogeners and to third-generation cephalosporins, but it is resistant to rifampin, ciprofloxacin, and the aminoglycoside antibiotics.[107,108]

In multicenter studies of patients with EM, similar results were obtained with doxycycline, amoxicillin, and cefuroxime axetil, and more than 90% of patients had satisfactory outcomes.[109,110] Although some patients had subjective symptoms after treatment, objective evidence of persistent infection or relapse was rare, and retreatment was usually not needed. In a recent study, 10 days of doxycycline therapy was as effective as 20 days of treatment in the majority of patients with EM, and adding one 2-g dose of parenteral ceftriaxone to the beginning of a 10-day course of doxycycline did not enhance therapeutic efficacy.[111] Intravenous ceftriaxone, although effective, was not superior to oral agents in patients with EM in the absence of objective neurological involvement.[112] In contrast with second- and third-

TABLE 242-2	Treatment Regimens for Lyme Disease*
	Early Infection (Local or Disseminated)
Adults	Doxycycline, 100 mg orally two times/day for 14-21 days
	Amoxicillin, 500 mg orally three times/day for 14-21 days
	Alternatives in case of doxycycline or amoxicillin allergy:
	Cefuroxime axetil, 500 mg orally twice daily for 14-21 days
	Erythromycin, 250 mg orally four times/day for 14-21 days
Children (age 8 or younger)	Amoxicillin, 250 mg orally three times/day or 20 mg/kg/day in divided doses for 14-21 days
	Alternatives in case of penicillin allergy:
	Cefuroxime axetil, 125 mg orally twice daily for 14-21 days
	Erythromycin, 250 mg orally three times/day or 30 mg/kg/day in divided doses for 14-21 days
Arthritis (intermittent or chronic)	Doxycycline, 100 mg orally two times/day for 30-60 days
	Amoxicillin, 500 mg orally four times/day for 30-60 days
	or
	Ceftriaxone, 2 g IV once a day for 14-28 days
	Penicillin G, 20 million U IV in four divided doses daily for 14-28 days
Neurologic abnormalities (early or late)	Ceftriaxone, 2 g IV once/day for 14-28 days
	Penicillin G, 20 million U IV in four divided doses daily for 14-28 days
	Alternative in case of ceftriaxone or penicillin allergy:
	Doxycycline, 100 mg orally three times/day for 14-28 days†
Facial palsy alone	Oral regimens may be adequate
Cardiac abnormalities	
First-degree AV block (P-R interval >0.3 sec)	Oral regimens, as for early infection
High-degree AV block	Ceftriaxone, 2 g IV once/day for 14-21 days‡
	Penicillin G, 20 million U IV in four divided doses daily for 28 days‡

*Treatment failures have occurred with any of the regimens given, and a second course of therapy may be necessary.
†In the author's experience, this regimen is ineffective for the treatment of late neurologic abnormalities of Lyme disease.
‡Once the patient has stabilized, the course may be completed with oral therapy.
AV, atrioventricular.

generation cephalosporin antibiotics, first-generation cephalosporins, such as cephalexin, were ineffective.

For patients with objective neurologic abnormalities, 2- to 4-week courses of intravenous ceftriaxone are most commonly given.[85,113] Parenteral therapy with cefotaxime or penicillin G may be a satisfactory alternative. In Europe, oral doxycycline gave equivalent results to intravenous therapy in patients with acute neuroborreliosis.[114] In addition, oral doxycycline is commonly used in the United States in patients who have facial palsy alone, without more diffuse involvement of the nervous system. With antibiotic treatment, the signs and symptoms of acute neuroborreliosis usually resolve within weeks, but those of chronic neuroborreliosis improve slowly over a period of months. Objective evidence of relapse is rare after a 4-week course of therapy. In patients with high-degree atrioventricular nodal block, intravenous therapy for at least part of the course and cardiac monitoring are recommended, but insertion of a permanent pacemaker is not necessary.

Either oral or intravenous regimens are usually effective for the treatment of Lyme arthritis.[113,115] Oral therapy is easier to administer; it is associated with fewer side effects, and it is considerably less expensive. Therefore, unless the patient has concomitant neurologic involvement, the recommendation is to treat with oral doxycycline or amoxicillin for 30 days.[115] However, a small percentage of patients with Lyme arthritis require intravenous antibiotic therapy for eradication of spirochetes in the joint. Therefore, in patients who do not respond to oral antibiotics, intravenous therapy for 2 to 4 weeks is recommended. Despite treatment with either oral or intravenous antibiotic therapy, a small percentage of patients in the United States have persistent joint inflammation for months or even several years after 2 months or longer of oral antibiotics or 1 month or longer of intravenous antibiotics, termed antibiotic-refractory Lyme arthritis.[75] If patients have persistent arthritis despite this treatment and if the results of PCR testing of joint fluid are negative, such patients may be treated with anti-inflammatory agents or arthroscopic synovectomy.[75]

Following appropriately treated Lyme disease, a small percentage of patients continue to have subjective symptoms, primarily musculoskeletal pain, neurocognitive difficulties, or fatigue, in some instances, for years.[107] Among such patients, three double-blind, placebo-controlled trials failed to show a benefit from additional courses of antibiotic treatment.[116-118] In the largest of these studies, patients with post–Lyme disease syndrome received intravenous ceftriaxone for 30 days followed by oral doxycycline for 60 days or intravenous and oral placebo preparations for the same duration. However, there were no significant differences between the groups in the percentage of patients who felt that their symptoms had improved, worsened, or remained the same.[116] Such patients are best treated symptomatically rather than with prolonged courses of antibiotic therapy. Prolonged ceftriaxone therapy for unsubstantiated Lyme disease has resulted in biliary complications;[107] in one reported case, prolonged cefotaxime administration resulted in death.[107]

Although it has not been studied systematically, patients with asymptomatic infection are often given a course of oral antibiotics. Because the risk of maternal-fetal transmission seems to be very low, standard therapy for the stage and manifestation of the illness may be sufficient for pregnant patients, except that doxycycline should be avoided.[107] Reinfection may occur in patients who are treated with antibiotics early in the illness, but the author has not observed reinfection in a patient with the expanded immune response associated with Lyme arthritis.

Prevention

When possible, people should avoid tick-infested areas.[119] If not, insecticides containing DEET (N,N-diethylmetatoluamide) or permethrin effectively deter ticks, but permethrin can be applied only on clothing, and DEET can cause serious side effects when excessive amounts are applied directly to the skin.[119] Therefore, insecticides may be valuable for the occasional hike in the woods but are less helpful for people living in endemic areas who have daily tick exposures. After exposure in tick-infested areas, tick checks are important. Immature *I. scapularis* usually stay within a few inches of the ground; they often transfer to the lower extremities of the host and attach to moist parts of the body, such as the groin or axillae. In small children, they may also be found on the head and neck, which are unusual sites for tick attachment in adults. Because 24 to 72 hours of tick attachment is necessary before transmission of the spirochete occurs, removal of a tick within 24 hours of attachment is usually sufficient to prevent Lyme disease. However, if an engorged nymphal *I. scapularis* tick is found, a single, 200-mg dose of doxycycline usually prevents Lyme disease when given within 72 hours after the tick bite occurs.[107,120]

Environmental control of ticks over widespread areas is difficult.[119] Methods that may be helpful include application of acaracides, landscaping to provide desiccating barriers between tick-infested areas and lawns, and in some settings, removal or exclusion of deer. New methods of tick control, including host-targeted acaricides against rodents and deer, are being developed and may provide help in the future. A commercial Lyme disease vaccine consisting of recombinant OspA with adjuvant was marketed in 1999,[24] but it was withdrawn in 2002. Although the vaccine is not available now, the experience proved that vaccination is feasible for the prevention of Lyme disease.

REFERENCES

1. Steere AC. Lyme disease. *N Engl J Med.* 2001;345:115.
2. Dennis DT, Hayes EB. Epidemiology of Lyme Borreliosis. In: Kahl O, Gray JS, Lane RS, Stanek G, ed. *Lyme Borreliosis: Biology, Epidemiology and Control.* Oxford, England: CABI; 2002:251.
3. Steere AC. Lyme disease. *N Engl J Med.* 1989;321:586.
4. Steere AC, Malawista SE, Snydman DR, et al. Lyme arthritis: an epidemic of oligoarticular arthritis in children and adults in three Connecticut communities. *Arthritis Rheum.* 1977;20:7.
5. Burgdorfer W, Barbour AG, Hayes SF, et al. Lyme disease—a tick-borne spirochetosis? *Science.* 1982;216:1317.
6. Barbour AG, Hayes SF. Biology of *Borrelia* species. *Microbiol Rev.* 1986;50:381.
7. Fraser CM, Casjens S, Huang WM, et al. Genomic sequence of a Lyme disease spirochete, *Borrelia burgdorferi*. *Nature.* 1997;390:580.
8. Casjens S, Palmer N, Van Vugt R, et al. A bacterial genome in flux: the twelve linear and nine circular extrachromosomal DNAs in an infectious isolate of the Lyme disease spirochete *Borrelia burgdorferi*. *Mol Microbiol.* 2000;35:490.
9. Zhang JR, Hardham JM, Barbour AG, et al. Antigenic variation in Lyme disease borreliae by promiscuous recombination of VMP-like sequence cassettes. *Cell.* 1997;89:275.
10. Baranton G, Postic D, Saint-Girons I, et al. Delineation of *Borrelia burgdorferi sensu stricto*, *Borrelia garinii* sp. nov., and group VS461 associated with Lyme borreliosis. *Int J Syst Bacteriol.* 1992;42:378.
11. Steere AC, Coburn J, Glickstein L. The emergence of Lyme disease. *J Clin Invest.* 2004;113:1093.
12. Seinost G, Dykhuizen DE, Dattwyler RJ, et al. Four clones of *Borrelia burgdorferi sensu stricto* cause invasive infection in humans. *Infect Immun.* 1999;67:3518.
13. Wormser GP, Brisson D, Liveris D, et al. *Borrelia burgdorferi* genotype predicts the capacity for hematogenous dissemination during early Lyme disease. *J Infect Dis.* 2008;198:1358.
14. Margos G, Gatewood AG, Aanensen DM, et al. MLST of housekeeping genes captures geographic population structure and suggests a European origin of *Borrelia burgdorferi*. *Proc Natl Acad Sci USA.* 2008;105:8730.

15. Haninicova K, Liveris D, Sandigursky S, et al. *Borrelia burgdorferi sensu stricto* is clonal in patients with early Lyme borreliosis. *Appl Environ Microbiol* 2008;74:5008.
16. Xu G, Fang QQ, Keirans JE, et al. Molecular phylogenetic analyses indicate that the *Ixodes ricinus* complex is a paraphyletic group. *J Parasitol.* 2003;89:452.
17. LoGiudice K, Ostfeld RS, Schmidt KA, et al. The ecology of infectious disease: effects of host diversity and community composition on Lyme disease risk. *Proc Natl Acad Sci USA.* 2003;100:567.
18. Brown RN, Lane RS. Lyme disease in California: A novel enzootic transmission cycle of *Borrelia burgdorferi*. *Science.* 1992;256:1439.
19. Campbell GL, Paul WS, Schriefer ME, et al. Epidemiologic and diagnostic studies of patients with suspected early Lyme disease, Missouri, 1990-1993. *J Infect Dis.* 1995;172:470.
20. Gern L, Pierre-Francois H. Ecology of *Borrelia burgdorferi sensu lato* in Europe. In: Kahl O, Gray JS, Lane RS, Stanek G, ed. *Lyme Borreliosis: Biology, Epidemiology and Control.* Oxford, England: CABI; 2002:149.
21. Kurtenbach K, De Michelis S, Etti S, et al. Host association of *Borrelia burgdorferi sensu lato*–the key role of host complement. *Trends Microbiol.* 2002;10:74.
22. Stanek G, Satz N, Strle F, et al. Epidemiology of Lyme borreliosis. In: Weber K, Burgdorfer W, eds. *Aspects of Lyme Borreliosis.* Berlin, Germany: Springer-Verlag; 1993;358.
23. Bacon RM, Kugeler KJ, Mead PS. Surveillance for Lyme disease—United States, 1992-2006. *MMWR Surveill Summ.* 2008;57:1.
24. Steere AC, Sikand VK, Meurice F, et al. Vaccination against Lyme disease with recombinant *Borrelia burgdorferi* outer-surface lipoprotein A with adjuvant. *N Engl J Med.* 1998;339:209.
25. Qiu WG, Bruno JF, McCaig WD, et al. Wide distribution of a high-virulence *Borrelia burgdorferi* clone in Europe and North America. *Emerg Infect Dis.* 2008;14:1097.
26. Fikrig E, Narasimhan S. *Borrelia burgdorferi*–traveling incognito? *Microbes Infect.* 2006;8:1390.
27. Montgomery RR, Malawista SE, Feen KJM, et al. Direct demonstration of antigenic substitution of *Borrelia burgdorferi* ex vivo:

exploration of the paradox of the early immune response to outer surface proteins A and C in Lyme disease. *J Exp Med.* 1996;183:261.
28. Schwan TG, Piesman J. Temporal changes in outer surface proteins A and C of the Lyme disease-associated spirochete, *Borrelia burgdorferi*, during the chain of infection in ticks and mice. *J Clin Microbiol* 2000;38:382.
29. Lagal V, Portnoi D, Faure G, et al. *Borrelia burgdorferi sensu stricto* invasiveness is correlated with OspC-plasminogen affinity. *Microbes Infect.* 2006;8:645.
30. Ramamoorthi N, Narasimhan S, Pal U, et al. The Lyme disease agent exploits a tick protein to infect the mammalian host. *Nature.* 2005;436:573.
31. Filgueira L, Nestle FO, Rittig M, et al. Human dendritic cells phagocytose and process *Borrelia burgdorferi*. *J Immunol.* 1996;157:2998.
32. Muellegger RR, McHugh G, Ruthazer R, et al. Differential expression of cytokine mRNA in skin specimens from patients with erythema migrans or acrodermatitis chronica atrophicans. *J Invest Dermatol.* 2000;115:1115.
33. Salazar JC, Pope CD, Sellati TJ, et al. Coevolution of markers of innate and adaptive immunity in skin and peripheral blood of patients with erythema migrans. *J Immunol.* 2003;171:2660.
34. Glickstein L, Moore B, Bledsoe T, et al. Inflammatory cytokine production predominates in early Lyme disease in patients with erythema migrans. *Infect Immun.* 2003;71:6051.
35. Karlsson M, Hovind-Hougen K, Svenungsson B, et al. Cultivation and characterization of spirochetes from cerebrospinal fluid of patients with Lyme borreliosis. *J Clin Microbiol.* 1990;28:473.
36. Duray PH, Steere AC. Clinical pathologic correlations of Lyme disease by stage. *Ann NY Acad Sci.* 1988;539:65.
37. Coburn J, Chege W, Magoun L, et al. Characterization of a candidate *Borrelia burgdorferi* β_3-chain integrin ligand identified using a phage display library. *Mol Microbiol.* 1999;34:926.
38. Parveen N, Leong JM. Identification of a candidate glycosaminoglycan-binding adhesin of the Lyme disease spirochete *Borrelia burgdorferi*. *Mol Microbiol.* 2000;35:1220.

39. Probert WS, Johnson BJB. Identification of a 47 kDa fibronectin-binding protein expressed by *Borrelia burgdorferi* isolate B31. *Mol Microbiol.* 1998;30:1003.

40. Guo BP, Brown EL, Dorward DW, et al. Decorin-binding adhesions from *Borrelia burgdorferi*. *Mol Microbiol.* 1998;30:711.

41. Purser JE, Lawrenz MB, Caimano MJ, et al. A plasmid-encoded nicotinamidase (PncA) is essential for infectivity of *Borrelia burgdorferi* in a mammalian host. *Mol Microbiol.* 2003;48:753.

42. Bankhead T, Chaconas G. The role of VlsE antigenic variation in the Lyme disease spirochete: persistence through a mechanism that differs from other pathogens. *Mol Microbiol.* 2007;65:1547.

43. Hefty PS, Jolliff SE, Caimano MJ, et al. Changes in temporal and spatial patterns of outer surface lipoprotein expression generate population heterogeneity and antigenic diversity in the Lyme disease spirochete, *Borrelia burgdorferi*. *Infect Immun.* 2002;70:3468.

44. Kraiczy P, Hellwage J, Skerka C, et al. Complement resistance of *Borrelia burgdorferi* correlates with the expression of BbCRASP-1, a novel linear plasmid-encoded surface protein that interacts with human factor H and FHL-1 and is unrelated to Erp proteins. *J Biol Chem.* 2004;279:2421.

45. Hovis KM, Tran E, Sundy CM, et al. Selective binding of *Borrelia burgdorferi* OspE paralogs to factor H and serum proteins from diverse animals: possible expansion of the role of OspE in Lyme disease pathogenesis. *Infect Immun.* 2006;74:1967.

46. Ma Y, Weis JJ. *Borrelia burgdorferi* outer surface lipoproteins OspA and OspB possess B cell mitogenic and cytokine stimulatory properties. *Infect Immun.* 1993;61:3843.

47. Steere AC, Hardin JA, Ruddy S, et al. Lyme arthritis: correlation of serum and cryoglobulin IgM with activity, and serum IgG with remission. *Arthritis Rheum.* 1979;22:471.

48. Hardin JA, Steere AC, Malawista SE. Immune complexes and the evolution of Lyme arthritis: dissemination and localization of abnormal C1q binding activity. *N Engl J Med.* 1979;301:1358.

49. Leadbetter EA, Brigl M, Illarionov P, et al. NK T cells provide lipid antigen-specific cognate help for B cells. *Proc Natl Acad Sci USA.* 2008;105:8339.

50. Kumar H, Belperron A, Barthold SW, et al. Cutting edge: CD1d deficiency impairs murine host defense against the spirochete, *Borrelia burgdorferi*. *J Immunol.* 2000;165:4797.

51. Dressler F, Whalen JA, Reinhardt BN, et al. Western blotting in the serodiagnosis of Lyme disease. *J Infect Dis* 1993;167:392.

52. Ben-Menachem G, Kubler-Kielb J, Coxon B, et al. A newly discovered cholesteryl galactoside from *Borrelia burgdorferi*. *Proc Nat Acad Sci USA.* 2003;100:7913.

53. Barbour AG, Jasinskas A, Kayala MK, et al. A genome-wide proteome array reveals a limited set of immunogens in natural infections of humans and white-footed mice with *Borrelia burgdorferi*. *Infect Immun.* 2008;76:3374.

54. Rousselle JC, Callister SM, Schell RF, et al. Borreliacidal antibody production against outer surface protein C of *Borrelia burgdorferi*. *J Infect Dis.* 1998;178:733.

55. Montgomery RR, Lusitani D, de Boisfleury Chevance A, et al. Human phagocytic cells in the early innate immune response to *Borrelia burgdorferi*. *J Infect Dis.* 2002;185:1773.

56. Keane-Myers A, Nickell SP. T cell subset-dependent modulation of immunity to *Borrelia burgdorferi* in mice. *J Immunol.* 1995;154:1770.

57. Dong Z, Edelstein M, Glickstein LJ. CD8+ T cells are activated during the early Th1 and Th2 immune responses in the murine Lyme disease model. *Infect Immun.* 1997;65:5334.

58. Steere AC, Schoen RT, Taylor E. The clinical evolution of Lyme arthritis. *Ann Intern Med.* 1987;107:725.

59. Steere AC, Sikand VK. The presenting manifestations of Lyme disease and the outcomes of treatment (Letter). *N Engl J Med.* 2003;384:2472.

60. Steere AC, Bartenhagen NH, Craft JE, et al. The early clinical manifestations of Lyme disease. *Ann Intern Med.* 1983;99:76.

61. Smith RP, Schoen RT, Rahn DW, et al. Clinical characteristics and treatment outcomes of early Lyme disease in patients with microbiologically confirmed erythema migrans. *Ann Intern Med.* 2002;136:421.

62. Jones KL, Muellegger RR, Means TK, et al. Higher mRNA levels of chemokines and cytokines associated with macrophage activation in erythema migrans skin lesions in patients from the United States than in patients from Austria with Lyme borreliosis. *Clin Infect Dis.* 2008;46:85.

63. Wormser GP, Bittker S, Cooper D, et al. Comparison of the yields of blood cultures using serum or plasma from patients with early Lyme disease. *J Clin Microbiol.* 2000;38:1648.

64. Steere AC, Dhar A, Hernandez J, et al. Systemic symptoms without erythema migrans as the presenting picture of early Lyme disease. *Am J Med.* 2003;114:58.

65. Pachner AR, Steere AC. The triad of neurologic manifestations of Lyme disease: Meningitis, cranial neuritis, and radiculoneuritis. *Neurology.* 1985;35:47.

66. Nigrovic LE, Thompson AD, Fine AM, et al. Clinical predictors of Lyme disease among children with a peripheral facial palsy at an emergency department in a Lyme disease-endemic area. *Pediatrics.* 2008;122:1080.

67. Steere AC, Berardi VP, Weeks KE, et al. Evaluation of the intrathecal antibody response to *Borrelia burgdorferi* as a diagnostic test for Lyme neuroborreliosis. *J Infect Dis.* 1990;161:1203.

68. Logigian EL, Steere AC. Clinical and electrophysiological findings in chronic neuropathy of Lyme disease. *Neurology.* 1992;42:303.

69. Steere AC, Batsford WP, Weinberg M, et al. Lyme carditis: Cardiac abnormalities of Lyme disease. *Ann Intern Med.* 1980;93:8.

70. McAlister HF, Klementowicz PT, Andrews C, et al. Lyme carditis: An important cause of reversible heart block. *Ann Intern Med.* 1989;110:339.

71. Marcus LC, Steere AC, Duray PH, et al. Fatal pancarditis in a patient with coexistent Lyme disease and babesiosis: Demonstration of spirochetes in the heart. *Ann Intern Med.* 1985;103:374.

72. Landieri G, Salvi A, Camerini F, et al. Isolation of *Borrelia burgdorferi* from myocardium. *Lancet.* 1993;342:490.

73. Sonnesyn SW, Diehl SC, Johnson RC, et al. A prospective study of the seroprevalence of *Borrelia burgdorferi* infection in patients with severe heart failure. *Am J Cardiol.* 1995;76:97.

74. Karma A, Seppala I, Mikkila H, et al. Diagnosis and clinical characteristics of ocular Lyme borreliosis. *Am J Ophthalmol.* 1994;119:127.

75. Steere AC, Angelis SM. Therapy for Lyme arthritis; strategies for the treatment of antibiotic-refractory arthritis. *Arthritis Rheum.* 2006;54:3079.

76. Akin E, Aversa J, Steere AC. Expression of adhesion molecules in synovia in patients with treatment-resistant Lyme arthritis. *Infect Immun.* 2001;63:1774.

77. Steere AC, Klitz W, Drouin EE, et al. Antibiotic-refractory Lyme arthritis is associated with HLA-DR molecules that bind a *Borrelia burgdorferi* peptide. *J Exp Med.* 2006;203:961.

78. Gross DM, Forsthuber T, Tary-Lehman M, et al. Identification of LFA-1 as a candidate autoantigen in treatment-resistant Lyme arthritis. *Science.* 1998;281:703.

79. Kannian P, Drouin EE, Glickstein L, et al. Decline in the Frequencies of *Borrelia burgdorferi* OspA161-175-specific T cells after antibiotic therapy in HLA-DRB1*0401-positive patients with antibiotic-responsive or antibiotic-refractory Lyme arthritis. *J Immunol.* 2007;179:6336.

80. Kannian P, McHugh G, Johnson BJ, et al. Antibody responses to *Borrelia burgdorferi* in patients with antibiotic-refractory, antibiotic-responsive, or non-antibiotic-treated Lyme arthritis. *Arthritis Rheum.* 2007;56:4216.

81. Shin JJ, Glickstein LJ, Steere AC. High levels of inflammatory chemokines and cytokines in joint fluid and synovial tissue throughout the course of antibiotic-refractory Lyme arthritis. *Arthritis Rheum.* 2007;56:1325.

82. Iliopoulou BP, Alroy J, Huber BT. Persistent arthritis in *Borrelia burgdorferi*-infected HLA-DR4-positive CD28-negative mice post-antibiotic treatment. *Arthritis Rheum.* 2008;58:3892.

83. Steere AC, Glickstein L. Elucidation of Lyme arthritis. *Nat Rev Immunol.* 2004;4:143.

84. Drouin EE, Glickstein L, Kwok WW, et al. Human homologues of a *Borrelia* T cell epitope associated with antibiotic-refractory Lyme arthritis. *Mol Immunol.* 2008;45:180.

85. Logigian EL, Kaplan RF, Steere AC. Chronic neurologic manifestations of Lyme disease. *N Engl J Med.* 1990;323:1438.

86. Kaplan RF, Jones-Woodward L, Workman K, et al. Neuropsychological deficits in Lyme disease with or without other evidence of central nervous system pathology. *Appl Neuropsychol.* 1999;6:3.

87. Logigian EL, Johnson KA, Kijewski MF, et al. Reversible cerebral hypoperfusion in Lyme encephalopathy. *Neurology.* 1997;49:1661.

88. Hemmer B, Gran B, Zhao Y, et al. Identification of candidate T-cell epitopes and molecular mimics in chronic Lyme disease. *Nat Med.* 1999;5:1375.

89. Mullegger RR. Dermatological manifestations of Lyme borreliosis. *Eur J Dermatol.* 2004;14:296.

90. Feder HM Jr, Johnson BJ, O'Connell S, et al. A critical appraisal of "chronic Lyme disease". *N Engl J Med.* 2007;357:1422.

91. Sigal LH, Hassett AL. Contributions of societal and geographical environments to "chronic Lyme disease": the psychopathogenesis and aporology of a new "medically unexplained symptoms" syndrome. *Environ Health Perspect.* 2002;110:607.

92. Baker PJ. Perspectives on "chronic Lyme disease". *Am J Med.* 2008;121:562.

93. Williams CL, Stobino B, Weinstein A, et al. Maternal Lyme disease and congenital malformations: A cord blood serosurvey in endemic and control areas. *Paediatr Perinat Epidemiol.* 1995;9:320.

94. Krause, PJ, McKay K, Thompson CA, et al. Disease-specific diagnosis of coinfecting tickborne zoonoses: Babesiosis, human granulocytic ehrlichiosis, and Lyme disease. *Clin Infect Dis.* 2002;34:1184.

95. Steere AC, McHugh G, Suarez C, et al. Prospective study of co-infection in patients with erythema migrans. *Clin Infect Dis.* 2003;36:1078.

96. Nocton JJ, Dressler F, Rutledge BJ, et al. Detection of *Borrelia burgdorferi* DNA by polymerase chain reaction in synovial fluid in Lyme arthritis. *N Engl J Med.* 1994;330:229.

97. Nocton JJ, Bloom BJ, Rutledge BJ, et al. Detection of *Borrelia burgdorferi* DNA by polymerase chain reaction in cerebrospinal fluid in patients with Lyme neuroborreliosis. *J Infect Dis.* 1996;174:623.

98. Centers for Disease Control. Case definitions for public health surveillance. *Morb Mortal Wkly Rep.* 1990;39:1.

99. Centers for Disease Control. Recommendations for test performance and interpretation from the Second International Conference on serologic diagnosis of Lyme disease. *Morb Mortal Wkly Rep.* 1995;44:1.

100. Robertson J, Guy E, Andrews N, et al. A European multicenter study of immunoblotting in the serodiagnosis of Lyme borreliosis. *J Clin Microbiol.* 2000;38:2097.

101. Steere AC, McHugh G, Damle N, et al. Prospective study of serologic tests for Lyme disease. *Clin Infect Dis.* 2008;47:188.

102. Bacon RM, Biggerstaff BJ, Schriefer ME, et al. Serodiagnosis of Lyme disease by kinetic enzyme-linked immunosorbent assay using recombinant VlsE1 or peptide antigens of *Borrelia burgdorferi* compared with 2-tiered testing using whole-cell lysates. *J Infect Dis.* 2003;187:1187.

103. Wormser GP, Brisson D, Liveris D, et al. *Borrelia burgdorferi* genotype predicts the capacity for hematogenous dissemination during early Lyme disease. *J Infect Dis.* 2008;198:1358.

104. Kalish RA, McHugh G, Granquist J, et al. Persistence of immunoglobulin M and immunoglobulin G antibody responses to *Borrelia burgdorferi* 10-20 years after active Lyme disease. *Clin Infect Dis.* 2001;33:780.

105. Steere AC, Sikand VJ, Schoen RT, et al. Asymptomatic infection with *Borrelia burgdorferi*. *Clin Infect Dis.* 2003;37:528.

106. Gustafson R, Svenungsson B, Forsgren M, et al. Two-year survey of the incidence of Lyme borreliosis and tick-borne encephalitis in a high-risk population in Sweden. *Eur J Clin Microbiol Infect Dis.* 1992;11:894.

107. Wormser GP, Dattwyler RJ, Shapiro ED, et al. The clinical assessment, treatment, and prevention of Lyme disease, human granulocytic anaplasmosis, and babesiosis: clinical practice guidelines by the Infectious Diseases Society of America. *Clin Infect Dis.* 2006;43:1089.

108. Dever LL, Jorgensen JH, Barbour AG. In vitro antimicrobial susceptibility testing of *Borrelia burgdorferi*: A microdilution MIC method and timekill studies. *J Clin Microbiol.* 1992;30:2692.

109. Dattwyler RJ, Volkman DJ, Conaty SM, et al. Amoxycillin plus probenecid versus doxycycline for treatment of erythema migrans borreliosis. *Lancet.* 1990;336:1404.

110. Nadelman RB, Luger SW, Frank E, et al. Comparison of cefuroxime axetil and doxycycline in the treatment of early Lyme disease. *Ann Intern Med.* 1992;117:273.

111. Wormser GP, Ramanathan R, Nowakowski J, et al. Duration of antibiotic therapy for early Lyme disease. *Ann Intern Med.* 2003;138:697.

112. Dattwyler RJ, Luft BJ, Kunkel MJ, et al. Ceftriaxone compared with doxycycline for the treatment of acute disseminated Lyme disease. *N Engl J Med.* 1997;337:289.

113. Dattwyler RJ, Halperin JJ, Volkman DJ, et al. Treatment of late Lyme borreliosis—randomized comparison of ceftriaxone and penicillin. *Lancet.* 1988;1:1191.

114. Karlsson M, Hammers-Berggren S, Lindquist L, et al. Comparison of intravenous penicillin G and oral doxycycline for treatment of Lyme neuroborreliosis. *Neurology.* 1994;44:1203.

115. Steere AC, Levin RE, Molloy PJ, et al. Treatment of Lyme arthritis. *Arthritis Rheum.* 1994;37:878.

116. Klempner MS, Hu LT, Evans J, et al. Two controlled trials of antibiotic treatment in patients with persistent symptoms and a history of Lyme disease. *N Engl J Med.* 2001;345:85.

117. Krupp LB, Hyman LG, Grimson R, et al. Study and treatment of post Lyme disease (STOP-LD): a randomized double masked clinical trial. *Neurology.* 2003;60:1923.

118. Fallon BA, Keilp JG, Corbera KM, et al. A randomized, placebo-controlled trial of repeated IV antibiotic therapy for Lyme encephalopathy. *Neurology.* 2008;70:992.

119. Hayes EB, Piesman J. How can we prevent Lyme disease? *N Engl J Med.* 2003; 348:2424.

120. Nadelman RB, Nowakowski J, Fish D, et al. Prophylaxis with single-dose doxycycline for the prevention of Lyme disease after an *Ixodes scapularis* tick bite. *N Engl J Med.* 2001;345:79.

243

Anaerobic Infections: General Concepts

RONIT COHEN-PORADOSU | DENNIS L. KASPER

Anaerobic bacteria are a major component of the human microflora residing on mucous membranes and predominate in many infectious processes, particularly those arising from mucosal sites. These organisms generally cause disease subsequent to the breakdown of mucosal barriers and the leakage of indigenous flora into normally sterile sites. The predominance of anaerobes in certain clinical syndromes can be attributed to the large numbers of these organisms residing on mucous membranes, the elaboration of a variety of virulence factors, the ability of some anaerobic species to resist oxygenated microenvironments, synergy with other bacteria, and resistance to certain antibiotics.

Clinicians have become more aware in the last few decades of the types of infections caused by anaerobic bacteria. However, difficulty in handling specimens in which anaerobes may be important and technical difficulties in cultivating and identifying these organisms in clinical microbiology laboratories continue to lead to many cases in which the anaerobic etiology of an infectious process remains unproven. The importance of anaerobes in certain infections is further enhanced by the failure to provide appropriate antibiotic coverage for anaerobes in mixed aerobic-anaerobic infections and an increase in the number of anaerobes that have become resistant to antimicrobial agents. These various factors combine to make it crucial to understand the types of infections in which anaerobes can play a role, to use appropriate microbiologic tools to identify the organisms in clinical specimens, and to choose the most appropriate treatment, including antibiotics and surgical drainage or débridement of the infected site.

Definition of an Anaerobe

An anaerobe is an organism that requires reduced oxygen for growth, failing to grow on the surface of solid media in 10% CO_2 in air. In contrast, facultative organisms can grow in the presence or absence of air, and microaerophilic bacteria can grow in 10% CO_2 in air or under aerobic or anaerobic conditions. As opposed to several anaerobic species inhabiting human bodily surfaces, which can survive only under strict anaerobic conditions (<0.5% oxygen), anaerobes that commonly cause human infections are generally aerotolerant (i.e., they tolerate 2% to 8% oxygen) and can survive for sustained periods—but cannot replicate—in an oxygenated atmosphere. Most anaerobes do not possess catalase, but those that cause human disease often have superoxide dismutase. In general, the degree to which this enzyme is expressed dictates the aerotolerance of the organism in question.[1]

Role of Anaerobes in the Normal Flora

Several hundred species of anaerobic organisms have been identified in the human microflora. Mucosal surfaces such as the oral cavity, gastrointestinal tract, and female genital tract harbor a rich indigenous flora composed of aerobic and anaerobic bacteria. Anaerobes are dominant in these sites, accounting for 99.0% to 99.9% of the culturable flora. The microbial species and concentrations vary at different sites (Table 243-1). It is interesting that anaerobes also inhabit areas of the body that are exposed to air: skin, nose, mouth, and throat. It has been hypothesized that the ability of anaerobes to withstand oxygen at these sites is due in part to the presence of aerobes and facultative organisms that consume oxygen and reduce the oxidation-reduction potential. In addition, anaerobes are believed to reside in the portions of these sites that are relatively well protected from oxygen, such as gingival crevices.

Despite the number of anaerobic species represented in the normal flora, relatively few are involved in human infections. Infections involving anaerobes are often polymicrobial and usually result from the disruption of mucosal surfaces by surgery, trauma, tumors, or ischemia and the subsequent infiltration of resident flora. Table 243-2 shows the gram-negative and gram-positive anaerobes most commonly isolated from clinical specimens. Certain gram-negative anaerobic bacilli belonging to the genera *Bacteroides, Fusobacterium, Porphyromonas,* and *Prevotella* predominate among these isolates.[2]

Anaerobes normally abound in the oral flora, with concentrations ranging from 10^9/mL in saliva to 10^{12}/mL in gingival scrapings. The ratio of anaerobic to aerobic bacteria ranges from 1:1 on teeth to 1000:1 in the gingival crevices. The indigenous oral anaerobic flora primarily comprises *Prevotella* and *Porphyromonas* species, with *Fusobacterium* and *Bacteroides* (non–*Bacteroides fragilis* group; see below) present in lower numbers.

Low numbers of anaerobic bacteria are present in the normally acidic conditions of the stomach and upper intestine. In people with decreased gastric acidity, the microflora of the stomach resembles that of the oral cavity. The upper intestine contains relatively few organisms until the distal ileum, where the flora begins to resemble that of the colon. In the colon, there are up to 10^{12} organisms per gram of stool, with anaerobes outnumbering aerobes by approximately 1000:1 and accounting for 99.9% of the total bacterial burden. The predominant anaerobes are *Bacteroides* species (principally members of the *B. fragilis* group, including *B. fragilis, B. thetaiotaomicron, B. ovatus, B. vulgatus, B. uniformis,* and *Parabacteroides distasonis*) and *Clostridium, Peptostreptococcus,* and *Fusobacterium* species.[3]

The normal female genital tract is colonized by 10^7 to 10^9 bacteria, with an anaerobic-to-aerobic ratio of 10:1. The predominant anaerobic species are *Prevotella, Bacteroides, Fusobacterium, Clostridium,* and the anaerobic *Lactobacillus* species. *Bacteroides* species are found in the genital tract of approximately 50% of women, with *B. fragilis* making up less than 15% of this microbial population. The most common isolates from clinical specimens are *Prevotella bivia* and *P. disiens,* although *B. fragilis* is also isolated frequently from this site. The skin flora contains anaerobes as well, the predominant species being *Propionibacterium acnes* and, to a lesser extent, other species of *Propionibacterium* and *Peptostreptococcus.*

Commensal bacteria in general and commensal anaerobes in particular have been implicated as crucial mediators of several physiologic, metabolic, and immunologic functions of the mammalian host. The occupation of distinct ecologic niches within the intestinal environment that would otherwise be filled with potentially pathogenic organisms is among the most important roles that anaerobes serve as normal colonic microflora. In what is termed colonization resistance, the presence of anaerobes effectively interferes with colonization by potentially pathogenic bacterial species through the depletion of oxygen and nutrients, the production of enzymes and toxic end products,[2] and the modulation of the host's intestinal innate immune response. For example, *Bacteroides thetaiotaomicron* stimulates Paneth cells to produce RegIIIγ, a bactericidal lectin that can result in killing of gram-positive bacteria.[4] The anaerobic component of the intestinal microflora is also responsible for the production of secreted products that are helpful in human health. The production of vitamin K by anaerobes in the intestine is beneficial to the host, while the production

TABLE 243-1	Comparison of the Anaerobic Human Flora at Mucosal Surfaces			
Anatomic Site	Sampled Site	Total Bacterial Numbers (per gram/milliliter)	Anaerobe:Aerobe Ratio	
Upper airways	Nasal washings	10^3-10^4	3-5:1	
	Saliva	10^8-10^9	1:1	
	Tooth surface	10^{10}-10^{11}	1:1	
	Gingival crevices	10^{11}-10^{12}	10^3:1	
Gastrointestinal tract	Stomach	0-10^5	1:1	
	Jejunum/ileum	10^4-10^7	1:1	
	Terminal ileum and colon	10^{11}-10^{12}	10^3:1	
Female genital tract		10^7-10^9	1-10:1	

of bile by these organisms is useful in fat absorption and cholesterol regulation.[5] Carbohydrate fermentation by *Bacteroides* and other intestinal bacteria results in the production of volatile fatty acids that are reabsorbed and used by the host as an energy source.[6] Furthermore, the respective levels of the two main intestinal phyla, the Bacteroidetes and Firmicutes, have been linked to variations in the likelihood of obesity in both humans and mice.[7,8]

The anaerobic intestinal flora influences the development of an intact mucosa and of mucosa-associated lymphoid tissue. Germ-free animals exhibit reduced vascularity, digestive enzyme activity, and muscle wall thickness as well as undeveloped gut-associated lymphoid tissue. Colonization of these mice with a single species, *B. thetaiotaomicron*, affects the expression of various host genes that influence nutrient uptake, metabolism, angiogenesis, mucosal barrier function, and development of the enteric nervous system.[9] Through its symbiosis factor polysaccharide A (PSA), *B. fragilis* influences the development and function of the immune system[10] and protects mice against colitis in a model of inflammatory bowel disease.[11]

Etiology of Anaerobic Clinical Infections

It is remarkable that, despite the identification of hundreds of anaerobic species in normal flora, relatively few species seem to play a major role in infection. Infections caused by anaerobes generally occur when the organisms' commensal relationship with the host within mucosal surfaces is disrupted. Cecal contents are the source of microorganisms in the case of intra-abdominal infections following disruption of intestinal continuity and contamination of the peritoneal cavity.[12] Severe infections of the head and neck may arise from an abscessed tooth infected with commensal microflora of the mouth.

After contamination of previously sterile sites by mucosal microflora, the relatively few anaerobic bacteria that survive in the infected site are those that have resisted changes in oxidation-reduction potential and host defense mechanisms. The hallmark of infection caused by gram-negative anaerobic bacteria is abscess formation, although some sepsis syndromes have been described. Typically, abscesses form at sites of direct bacterial contamination, although distant abscesses resulting from hematogenous spread are not uncommon with the more virulent anaerobes.

Among the anaerobic gram-negative bacilli, the *B. fragilis* group is most commonly isolated from human infections. Of this group, *B.*

TABLE 243-2	Anaerobes Commonly Found in Human Infections	
Gram-negative		*Gram-positive*
Bacteroides spp.*		*Peptostreptococcus* spp.
Porphyromonas spp.		*Clostridium* spp.
Prevotella spp.		*Actinomyces* spp.
Fusobacterium spp.		

Bacteroides fragilis predominates in these infections.

fragilis is the species most often isolated from clinical cases, particularly in infections emanating from the lower intestine,[13-15] although the other members of this family are also isolated from infectious sites.[16] Other gram-negative organisms that cause human infections are *Fusobacterium, Prevotella,* and *Porphyromonas* species. The fusobacteria *F. nucleatum, F. necrophorum,* and *F. varium,* which normally reside in the oral cavity and the intestinal tract, are often isolated from sites of necrotizing pneumonia and abscesses. In the oral cavity, the pigmented anaerobes *Prevotella* and *Porphyromonas* are recognized as pathogenic species. *P. bivia* and *P. disiens* colonize the vagina and are the organisms most frequently isolated from infections arising at this site.

The major gram-positive cocci that cause disease are *Peptostreptococcus* species, while clostridia are the main pathogens among gram-positive rods. The latter organisms are commonly isolated from wounds, abscesses, and blood.

Clinical Syndromes Caused by Anaerobes

Anaerobes are remarkable in their ability to cause a variety of infections at a number of different anatomic sites. Table 243-3 summarizes the types of infections that these organisms cause. Because anaerobes colonize sites that are home to aerobes and facultative organisms as well, many infections from which anaerobes are isolated also involve these other bacteria. Figure 243-1 shows a gram-stained specimen from a site of mixed infection in a patient with Meleney's gangrene, a form of cellulitis involving *Staphylococcus aureus* and anaerobic streptococci.

ANAEROBIC INFECTIONS OF THE MOUTH, HEAD, AND NECK

Anaerobes contribute to infections associated with periodontal disease and to disseminated infections arising from the oral cavity and spread-

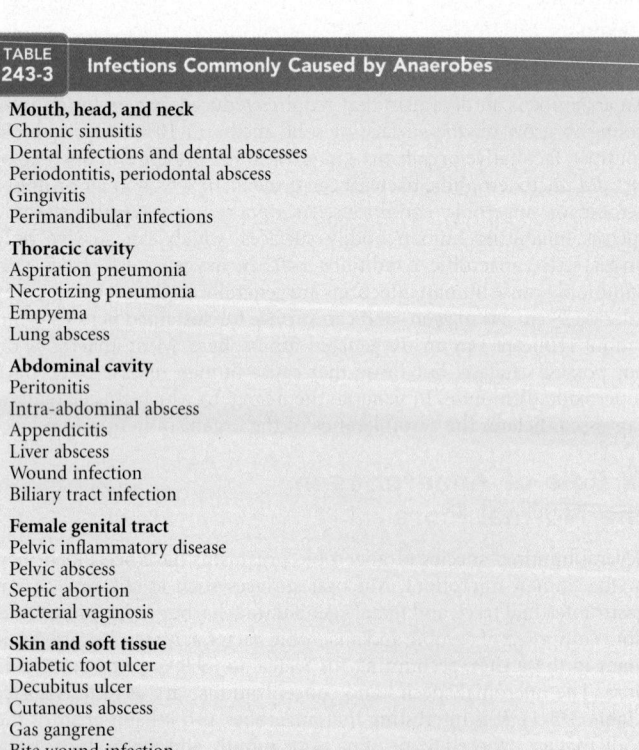

TABLE 243-3	Infections Commonly Caused by Anaerobes
Mouth, head, and neck	
Chronic sinusitis	
Dental infections and dental abscesses	
Periodontitis, periodontal abscess	
Gingivitis	
Perimandibular infections	
Thoracic cavity	
Aspiration pneumonia	
Necrotizing pneumonia	
Empyema	
Lung abscess	
Abdominal cavity	
Peritonitis	
Intra-abdominal abscess	
Appendicitis	
Liver abscess	
Wound infection	
Biliary tract infection	
Female genital tract	
Pelvic inflammatory disease	
Pelvic abscess	
Septic abortion	
Bacterial vaginosis	
Skin and soft tissue	
Diabetic foot ulcer	
Decubitus ulcer	
Cutaneous abscess	
Gas gangrene	
Bite wound infection	
Central nervous system	
Brain abscess	
Subdural empyema	
Epidural abscess	

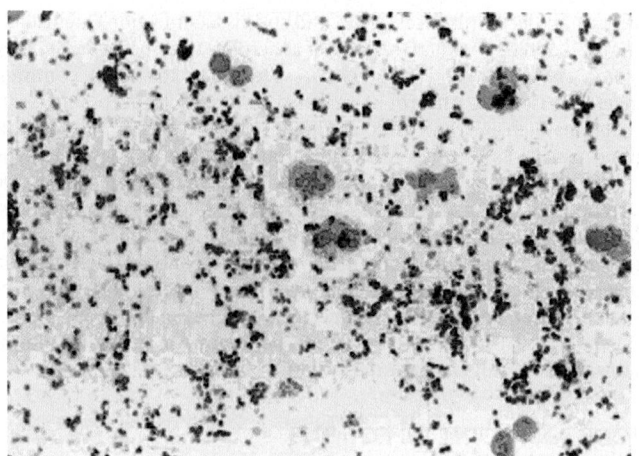

Figure 243-1 Gram-stained specimen from a patient with Meleney's gangrene. This mixed infection involving *Staphylococcus aureus* and anaerobic streptococci usually occurs around surgical wounds, stomas, and cutaneous fistulae. The infection spreads slowly and often results in skin ulceration but lacks the severe systemic toxicity observed with necrotizing fasciitis. *(Courtesy of Dr. Andrew Onderdonk.)*

ing to adjacent structures in the head and neck (see Chapter 60). The organisms isolated reflect the contiguous normal flora, among which the *Bacteroides oralis* group, pigmented *Prevotella*, *Porphyromonas asaccharolytica*, fusobacteria, peptostreptococci, and microaerophilic streptococci are dominant.

Anaerobes are involved in dental infections, including pulpitis, periapical or dental abscess, and perimandibular space infection. In the gingival crevices and gums, anaerobes are involved in gingivitis, periodontitis, and periodontal abscess. Formation of dental plaque, which is influenced by oral hygiene and other host factors, leads to the acquisition of pathogenic bacteria and the development of these infections. Infections of the periodontal area may extend into the mandible, causing osteomyelitis of the maxillary sinuses or infection of submandibular spaces.

Gingivitis may become a necrotizing ulcerative process (trench mouth, Vincent's stomatitis). This disease is usually sudden in onset and is associated with tender bleeding gums, foul breath, and a bad taste. Patients may be systemically ill with fever, cervical lymphadenopathy, and leukocytosis. The infection may spread and cause destruction of bone and soft tissue or acute necrotizing infection of the pharynx.

Perimandibular infections arise from the spread of organisms originating in the upper airways to potential spaces formed by the fascial planes of the head and neck. Two life-threatening perimandibular infections are Ludwig's angina and Lemierre syndrome. Ludwig's angina is a bilateral infection of the sublingual and submandibular spaces that results in marked local tissue swelling, tongue displacement, and potential airway compromise. Lemierre syndrome, which is now uncommon and is usually caused by *F. necrophorum*, is an infection of the posterior compartment of the lateral pharyngeal space with secondary septic thrombophlebitis of the internal jugular vein and frequent metastasis, most commonly to the lungs.

Although anaerobic bacteria play little role in acute sinusitis, they have been implicated in chronic sinusitis in both children and adults and are found in 0 to 52% of cases, depending on the specimen collection method. These infections are usually caused by a mixture of aerobic and anaerobic bacteria. The predominant anaerobic bacteria include *Peptostreptococcus*, *Fusobacterium*, and pigmented *Prevotella* species and *P. acnes*.[17] Anaerobic bacteria have been isolated in a large percentage of cases of chronic suppurative otitis media. *Bacteroides* species are found in up to 50% of cases. The role of anaerobes in acute otitis media is less clear.

Pleuropulmonary Infections

Pleuropulmonary infections are most commonly associated with the aspiration of oropharyngeal material by patients with a depressed gag reflex, impaired swallowing, or transiently impaired consciousness; these infections can also occur as a complication of periodontal disease (see Chapters 60 and 64). The anaerobes most common in pleuropulmonary infections are indigenous to the upper airways and include pigmented and nonpigmented *Prevotella*, *Peptostreptococcus*, *Bacteroides*, and *Fusobacterium* species. Four major clinical syndromes can develop: aspiration pneumonia, necrotizing pneumonia, lung abscess, and empyema. In contrast to the abrupt course of acute pneumonias (e.g., pneumococcal pneumonia), aspiration pneumonia has an indolent course. Patients usually present with chronic pulmonary symptoms and manifestations of chronic disease, including weight loss and anemia. The lobes of the lung that are affected depend most often on the position of the patient during aspiration. The sputum is not foulsmelling initially but can become malodorous with prolonged infection, and Gram stain reveals a mixed flora. Sputum samples are not reliable for culture because they contain the normal oral flora, but cultures of samples obtained by transtracheal or transthoracic aspiration, which currently are rarely used, may be of value. Protected brush or bronchoalveolar lavage samples obtained by bronchoscopy are controversial because of possible contamination and difficulty associating specific microbes with disease etiology.

Necrotizing pneumonia is characterized by the development of many small abscesses within the pulmonary parenchyma. Lung abscesses most often arise secondary to the development of periodontal disease, and, as would be expected, oral anaerobes predominate. Empyemas are a result of long-term anaerobic pulmonary infection and demonstrate foul-smelling sputum and pleuritic chest pain.

INTRA-ABDOMINAL INFECTIONS

Intra-abdominal infections—mainly peritonitis (generalized or localized) and abscesses—are usually polymicrobial and result from a breach in the continuity of the mucosal surface and spillage of the normal flora into the sterile peritoneal cavity. The cause of the breach can be appendicitis, diverticulitis, neoplasm, inflammatory bowel disease, surgery, or trauma. In infections originating from colonic sites, specimens yield, on average, four to six species, with a predominance of coliforms, anaerobes, and enterococci. The most common isolates are *Escherichia coli* and *Bacteroides* species, among which *B. fragilis* is predominant (see Chapters 71 to 76).[18] Other anaerobes commonly isolated from this type of infection include *Peptostreptococcus micros*, *Prevotella intermedia*, and *Fusobacterium* species. The involvement of clostridia can lead to severe infections. Disease originating from proximal bowel perforation reflects the flora of that site, with a predominance of aerobic and anaerobic gram-positive bacteria and *Candida*. Figure 243-2 shows the development of a pericolonic abscess in a patient with multiple diverticula. Anaerobic bacteria have been implicated in enterocolitis (typhlitis), an infection of the cecum or the entire bowel in the setting of neutropenia. *Clostridium septicum*, other clostridia, and mixed anaerobic infections have also been implicated.

B. fragilis has been associated with watery diarrhea in case-control studies of children with undiagnosed diarrheal disease.[19] Enterotoxin-producing strains are more prevalent in patients with diarrhea than in control groups. An etiologic relationship between enterotoxin-producing *B. fragilis* strains and diarrhea has been suggested.[20]

PELVIC INFECTIONS

The female genital tract is a major reservoir for anaerobes, which outnumber aerobes at this site by 10 to 1. Anaerobes are encountered in nearly all infections that are not caused by sexually transmitted agents, including pelvic abscess, septic abortion, endometritis, tuboovarian abscess, pelvic inflammatory disease, and postoperative

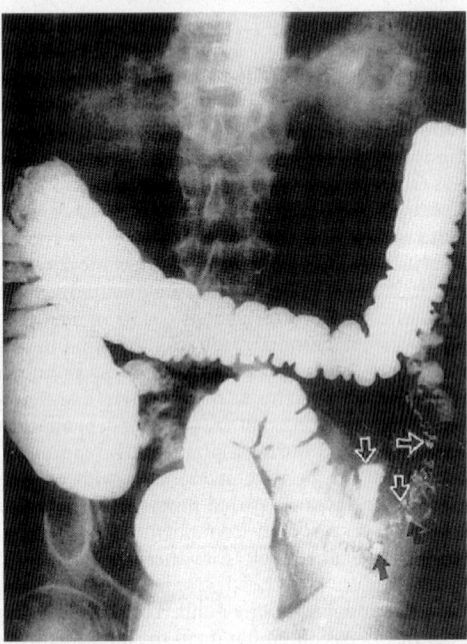

Figure 243-2 Development of a pericolonic abscess following rupture of a diverticulum. Barium enema reveals the abscesses (*arrows*). *(From Mandell G, ed.* Atlas of Infectious Diseases. *Philadelphia: Churchill Livingstone; 1995.)*

infection (see Chapter 108). The major isolates from these infections are *P. bivia, P. disiens, P. melaninogenica, B. fragilis,* peptostreptococci, and clostridia. Like intra-abdominal infections, most infections of the female genital tract are of mixed etiology, involving both anaerobes and aerobes. However, infections in which anaerobes are isolated in pure culture are more common in the pelvis than in the abdominal cavity.

Bacterial vaginosis, a disease process in which anaerobes predominate, is characterized by malodorous discharge and inflammation. Although the etiology is not clear, a change in bacterial ecology, with consequent overgrowth of certain bacterial species that replace the *Lactobacillus*-dominated normal flora, has been suggested. The anaerobic bacteria involved include *Gardnerella vaginalis* and *Prevotella, Mobiluncus,* and *Peptostreptococcus* species. A study based on 16s rRNA identification found other anaerobes that were more common in cases than in controls: *Atopobium, Leptotrichia, Megasphaera,* and *Eggerthella.*[21]

CENTRAL NERVOUS SYSTEM INFECTIONS

Central nervous system infections associated with anaerobic bacteria include brain abscess, epidural abscess, and subdural empyema. Anaerobic meningitis is rare and usually suggests a parameningeal collection or shunt infection. Either a single anaerobic species or a mixture of anaerobic and/or aerobic bacteria may be found in brain abscesses; prominent among the anaerobes are *Fusobacterium, Bacteroides,* and anaerobic or microaerophilic gram-positive cocci. Anaerobic brain abscesses may arise by hematogenous dissemination from a distant infected site or by direct extension from a site of otitis, sinusitis, or tooth infection. Figure 243-3 shows a computed tomography scan of a left parietal brain abscess.

SKIN AND SOFT TISSUE INFECTIONS

Anaerobic infections in the skin and soft tissue are most often caused by contamination with the flora from adjacent mucosal surfaces. Examples include infected sebaceous and pilonidal cysts, breast abscesses, surgical wounds, human or animal bites, diabetic foot ulcers, and decubitus ulcers. Skin and soft tissue infections are usually of mixed etiology, with a 3:2 ratio of anaerobes to aerobes. *Bacteroides, Peptostreptococcus,* and *Clostridium* species are the most common anaerobic isolates. Anaerobes can also be found in deep soft tissue infections such as necrotizing fasciitis, crepitant cellulitis, and gas gangrene, usually as part of a mixed anaerobic/aerobic etiology. This type of infection usually occurs at sites that can be contaminated from oral secretions or feces; the disease can spread rapidly and can be very destructive. Gas may be found in the infected tissues. The major pathogens in these deep infections include a combination of aerobes and anaerobes, mainly group A β-hemolytic streptococci, clostridia, peptostreptococci, and *Bacteroides* species. Fournier's gangrene is a form of cellulitis that involves the scrotum, perineum, or anterior abdominal wall and results in the extensive loss of skin.

BONE AND JOINT INFECTIONS

Infections such as osteomyelitis and septic arthritis typically arise from infected adjacent soft tissue sites. Hematogenous seeding of bones with anaerobic bacteria is uncommon. Diabetic foot ulcers and decubitus ulcers may be complicated by mixed aerobic-anaerobic osteomyelitis. *Fusobacterium* species are the most common gram-negative anaerobes isolated from infected joints; infected bone may yield a wider variety of isolates.

BACTEREMIA

Approximately 5% (range, 0.5% to 12%) of cases of bacteremia include anaerobic isolates. *B. fragilis* is the anaerobe most commonly isolated from these infections (60% to 80% of cases).[22] Anaerobic bacteremia is usually secondary to an infectious process that has emanated from an intra-abdominal source, the female genital tract, the respiratory tract, or soft tissue. Although anaerobic bacteremia accounts for only a small percentage of cases of clinically significant bacteremia, *B. fragilis* group bacteremia contributes to morbidity and mortality.[23] The rate of anaerobic bacteremia decreased from the 1970s through the early 1990s. Recent reports present conflicting data regarding rates of anaerobic bacteremia. A recent study from the Mayo Clinic compared three periods (1993-1996, 1997-2000, 2001-2004) and found a 74%

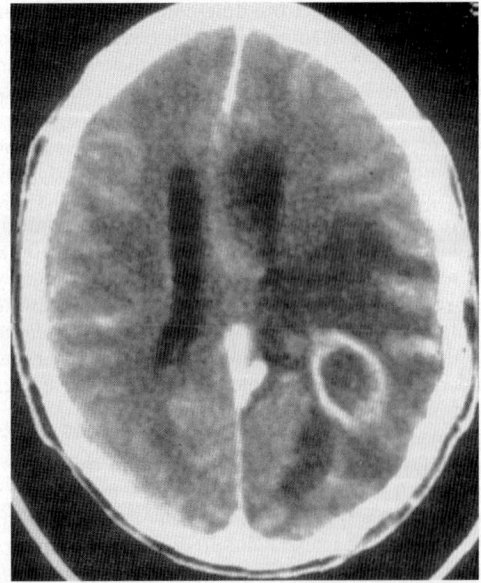

Figure 243-3 Computed tomographic image of a left parietal brain abscess. Area outlined in white demarcates the walled-off abscess. *(From Mandell G, ed.* Atlas of Infectious Diseases. *Philadelphia: Churchill Livingstone; 1995.)*

increase in anaerobic bacteremia.[24] In contrast, a report from Switzerland compared two periods (1997-2001 and 2002-2006) and found decreases in both the number of anaerobe-positive blood cultures and the proportion of all blood culture isolates that were anaerobes.[25]

Pathogenesis of Anaerobic Infections

Infections caused by anaerobes are generally a result of the breakdown of a mucosal barrier and the subsequent leakage of indigenous polymicrobial flora into previously sterile closed spaces or tissue. The introduction of many species of bacteria into otherwise sterile sites leads to a polymicrobial infection in which certain organisms predominate. The predominant gram-negative anaerobes in these infections include *B. fragilis* and *Prevotella, Fusobacterium,* and *Porphyromonas* species. Although some of these organisms are numerically dominant in the normal flora, others make up a much smaller proportion (e.g., *B. fragilis,* 0.5%); thus, their predominance among clinical isolates indicates that they possess one or more virulence factors that enhance their ability to cause disease. Typically, virulence factors associated with anaerobes confer the ability to evade host defenses, adhere to cell surfaces, produce toxins and/or enzymes, or display surface structures that contribute to pathogenic potential. Table 243-4 lists some of the virulence factors associated with anaerobic organisms commonly isolated from clinical infections.

The ability of anaerobic bacteria to act synergistically during polymicrobial infection contributes to the pathogenesis of anaerobic infections. The phenomenon of microbial synergy in these infections remains poorly characterized. It has been postulated that facultative organisms function in part to lower the oxidation-reduction potential in the microenvironment and that this change allows the propagation of obligate anaerobes. Additional studies indicate that anaerobes can produce compounds such as succinic acid and short-chain fatty acids that inhibit the ability of phagocytes to clear facultative organisms. Studies in experimental models demonstrate that facultative and obligate anaerobes synergistically potentiate abscess formation.[26]

The high frequency of abscess formation associated with *B. fragilis,* the anaerobe most commonly isolated from clinical infections,[12] led to studies of this organism's pathogenic potential in relevant animal models of disease. In an animal model of intra-abdominal sepsis, the capsular polysaccharide was identified as the major virulence factor of *B. fragilis;* this polymer plays a specific, central role in the induction

TABLE 243-4	Virulence Factors Associated with Pathogenic Anaerobes

Bacteroides fragilis
Capsular polysaccharides
Neuraminidase
Proteases
Enterotoxin
Hemagglutinin

Porphyromonas gingivalis
Proteases (gingipains)
Lipopolysaccharides
Capsule
Hemolysin

Fusobacterium necrophorum
Leukotoxin
Hemolysin
Lipopolysaccharides
Phospholipase
Proteases

Fusobacterium nucleatum
Lipopolysaccharides
Adhesins
Proteases
Leukotoxin

Prevotella spp
Lipopolysaccharides
Proteases

of abscesses.[27] A series of detailed biologic and molecular studies of this virulence factor show that *B. fragilis* produces at least eight distinct capsular polysaccharides,[28] far more than the number reported for any other encapsulated bacterium. *B. fragilis* can exhibit a wide array of distinct surface polysaccharide combinations by regulating the expression of these different capsules in an on-off manner through the reversible inversion of DNA segments containing the promoters for their expression. Structural analysis of two of these polysaccharides, PSA and PSB, revealed that each polymer consists of repeating units with positively charged free amino groups and negatively charged groups. This structural feature is rare among bacterial polysaccharides, and the ability of PSA and PSB to induce abscesses in animals depends on this zwitterionic charge motif.[29]

Mechanistic studies of the pathogenesis of intra-abdominal abscess formation by *B. fragilis* revealed a multifunctional role for its capsular polysaccharides in this process. These polymers activate host CD4 T cells and promote the release of interleukin-17 (IL-17) and chemokines.[30] In addition, the capsule induces the release of the proinflammatory cytokines tumor necrosis factor–α (TNF-α) and IL-1β from peritoneal macrophages. These cytokines potentiate the increase of cell adhesion molecules such as intracellular adhesion molecule–1 (ICAM-1) on mesothelial cell surfaces, which in turn leads to an increase in the binding of neutrophils to these cells and initiates abscess formation.[31] The capsules of *B. fragilis* also facilitate binding of the organism to mesothelial cells lining the surface of the peritoneal cavity.

B. fragilis produces other virulence factors that allow it to predominate in disease. Although the lipopolysaccharide (LPS) of *B. fragilis* possesses little biologic activity, this organism synthesizes pili, fimbriae, and hemagglutinins that aid in attachment to host cell surfaces. In addition, *Bacteroides* species produce many enzymes and toxins that contribute to pathogenicity. Enzymes such as neuraminidase, protease, glycoside hydrolases, and superoxide dismutases are all produced by *B. fragilis.* The organism produces an enterotoxin with specific effects on host cells in vitro. This toxin, termed BFT, is a metalloprotease that is cytopathic for intestinal epithelial cells and induces fluid secretion and tissue damage in ligated intestinal loops of experimental animals. Strains of *B. fragilis* associated with diarrhea in children (termed enterotoxigenic *B. fragilis,* or ETBF) produce a heat-labile 20-kDa protein toxin. The BFT specifically cleaves the extracellular domain of E-cadherin, a glycoprotein found on the surface of eukaryotic cells.[32] An association of BFT-positive *B. fragilis* with clinical episodes of diarrhea in children and adults has been suggested.[20]

A prominent etiologic agent in adult periodontitis, *Porphyromonas gingivalis,* relies on a broad range of virulence factors to cause disease. These include extracellular proteases (cysteine proteinases) that can cause attachment, degradation, or cleavage of host cell proteins and surface receptors and can modulate the host immune response; adhesins such as fimbriae and hemagglutinins; and a putative invasin (haloacid dehalogenase family phosphoserine phosphatase).[33] The capsular polysaccharide of *P. gingivalis* is a potent virulence factor that facilitates the spread of infection in mice greater than that seen with unencapsulated strains.[34] The LPS of *P. gingivalis* has strong proinflammatory activity and has been implicated in the initiation and development of periodontal disease.[35] *P. gingivalis* has been shown to invade and replicate within host cells, a mechanism that may facilitate its spread. It also evades the host immune response through modulation of innate immune function.[33]

F. necrophorum causes numerous necrotic conditions (necrobacillosis) and human oral infections. Toxins such as leukotoxin, endotoxin, and hemolysin have all been implicated as virulence factors, with leukotoxin and endotoxin playing an important role in the pathogenesis of disease. *F. nucleatum* has been isolated frequently from cases of periodontitis and contributes significantly to gingival inflammation.[36] This organism coaggregates with other oral bacteria to promote attachment to plaque; in addition, it produces several adhesins that facilitate attachment. Both *F. nucleatum* and *F. necrophorum* produce a potent LPS that is responsible for the release of numerous pro-inflammatory cytokines and other inflammatory mediators[37] that may play a pathogenic role in periodontal disease, and that presumably accounts for the severity of illness in Lemierre syndrome.

Virulence factors associated with *Prevotella* species are poorly defined. The organisms' ability to interact with other anaerobes has been reported.[38] Among their prominent virulence traits is the production of proteases and metabolic products such as volatile fatty acids and amines. This group of organisms is particularly noted for secretion of IgA proteases. The degradation of IgA produced by mucosal surfaces allows *Prevotella* to evade this first line of host defense. *P. intermedia* can invade oral epithelial cells, and antibody specific for fimbriae from this organism inhibits invasion.[39]

Diagnosis of Anaerobic Infections

Many anaerobic infections are diagnosed because the presence of anaerobes is suspected. These organisms can be difficult to culture, and their identification can be expensive or even misleading because of confusion with normal flora in some cases. Certain factors can lead the clinician to surmise that an anaerobic infection exists. Infections at particular sites, especially those proximal to mucosal surfaces with indigenous anaerobic flora, are indicative, particularly in the gastrointestinal tract, the female genital tract, or the oral cavity. Anaerobes are often associated with tissue necrosis and abscess formation. The presence of a foul odor or gas is highly suggestive as well, although the absence of these factors does not rule out anaerobic infection. A patient's failure to respond to antibiotics that are not active against anaerobes suggests anaerobic infection. Since anaerobic infections are often polymicrobial, Gram stain of exudates showing a polymicrobial flora and organisms with morphologic features of anaerobes are indicative of anaerobic infection.

When samples from suspected anaerobic infections are cultured, it is imperative that they be properly collected and transported. Samples should be collected so as to avoid contamination by indigenous flora of mucosal surfaces. The optimal specimens are normally sterile fluids (e.g., blood, pleural and peritoneal fluids, and aspirates) or biopsy samples from normally sterile sites. In general, liquids or tissues are preferable to swab specimens. Suitable commercially available anaerobic-transport media should be employed at all times. Although many anaerobes are aerotolerant, exposure to oxygen, even for the briefest period, can interfere with culture of some organisms. It is also important to remember that prior antibiotic therapy reduces cultivatability of these bacteria. Specimens should be processed as quickly as possible and handled appropriately in the clinical microbiology laboratory; they should be subjected to Gram staining, and the results should be compared with those of culture. It is not uncommon for specimens to yield no growth on culture but for numerous organisms (both gram-positive and gram-negative) to be evident on Gram staining—a result suggesting that anaerobic organisms are present. Sterile pus may indicate anaerobic infection with failed collection or identification methods. Selective and nonselective media should be used for culture in order to identify the clinically relevant anaerobes.

Treatment of Anaerobic Infections and Antibiotic Resistance

Successful therapy for anaerobic infections generally involves the administration of appropriate antimicrobial agents and/or surgical management. Because anaerobic infections can cause severe tissue damage or can result in abscess formation, débridement of necrotic tissue, drainage, restoration of airspaces, resection, and/or maintenance of blood supply is needed. Previously, surgery was uniformly required to achieve these goals. However, with the advent of computed tomography, magnetic resonance imaging, and ultrasonography, some of these procedures can be performed percutaneously.

The antibiotics used to treat anaerobic infections should be active against both aerobic and anaerobic organisms, as many of these infections are of mixed etiology. Antibiotic regimens can usually be selected empirically on the basis of the type of infection, the species of the

TABLE 243-5	Antimicrobial Agents Effective Against Medically Important Anaerobes	
Nearly Always Active	**Usually Active**
Carbapenems (imipenem, meropenem, doripenem)	Clindamycin[§] Cephamycins (cefoxitin, cefotetan)
Metronidazole*	High-dose antipseudomonal penicillins
β-Lactam/β-lactamase inhibitor combination[†]	
Chloramphenicol[‡]	

*Bactericidal against most gram-negative anaerobic strains, inactive against *Propionibacterium* spp, *Actinomyces* spp, peptostreptococci, and microaerophilic streptococci such as *S. milleri*.
[†]Such as ampicillin/sulbactam, piperacillin/tazobactam, or ticarcillin/clavulanic acid.
[‡]Despite excellent in vitro activity against all clinically important anaerobes, this drug is less desirable than other active drugs because of documented clinical failures.
[§]Resistance among the *Bacteroides fragilis* group has increased in recent years.

organisms usually present in such cases, Gram stain results, and knowledge of antimicrobial resistance patterns. Other factors influencing the selection of antibiotics include need for bactericidal activity and for penetration into compartmentalized organs (such as the brain), toxicity, and impact on the normal flora. Antibiotic susceptibility testing of anaerobic bacteria is rarely performed in clinical laboratories because of inadequate anaerobic culture techniques, difficulty in obtaining results within a useful time frame, and poor quality control of in vitro susceptibility results. It is accepted that testing is important for patients with serious or prolonged infections or in cases in which antibiotics have not had an impact. Testing is also helpful in monitoring the activity of new drugs and recording current resistance patterns among anaerobic pathogens. Nguyen and colleagues[40] showed that in vitro testing of antibiotics with activity against the *B. fragilis* group was predictive of clinical outcome in cases of anaerobic bacteremia. This report notwithstanding, antibiotic regimens still are often selected empirically with good results.

The antibiotics with the greatest activity against nearly all anaerobic bacteria include carbapenems, β-lactam/β-lactamase inhibitor combinations, metronidazole, and chloramphenicol (Table 243-5). Antibiotic resistance is increasingly reported among anaerobic bacteria[41] (Table 243-6). The medically important *Bacteroides* species are typically resistant to penicillin G (>97%). The cephamycins, cefoxitin and cefotetan, display greater activity against this group, but the prevalence of resistance has increased recently, with current figures at 8% to 14%.[42] Rates of resistance to β-lactam agents among non-*Bacteroides* anaerobes are lower but are highly variable. β-Lactamase production is a mechanism of resistance in the *B. fragilis* group, some other *Bacteroides* species, and *Prevotella, Porphyromonas,* and *Fusobacterium* species. Two distinct classes of β-lactamases have been described in B.

TABLE 243-6	Antimicrobial Agents to Which Medically Important Anaerobes Are Resistant	
Variable Resistance	**Resistance**
Penicillin*	Aminoglycosides
Cephalosporins	Trimethoprim-sulfamethoxazole
Tetracycline	Monobactams (aztreonam)
Vancomycin	
Macrolides	
Fluoroquinolones[†] (moxifloxacin, gatifloxacin)	
Tigecycline[‡]	

*Inactive against penicillinase-producing anaerobes, including most of the *Bacteroides fragilis* group.
[†]These agents exhibit weaker in vitro activity against many *Bacteroides* species other than *B. fragilis*. Resistance is increasing in the *B. fragilis* group.
[‡]Active against nearly all anaerobes, including *Bacteroides* species. Resistance has been reported.

fragilis: the active-site serine enzymes encoded by the *cepA* gene and the metallo-β-lactamases encoded by the *cfiA* gene. Any given *B. fragilis* strain contains only one of these β-lactamase-encoding genes, and taxonomic investigations have revealed that *cfiA* strains and *cepA* strains form two genotypically distinct groups. Although these groups cannot be differentiated phenotypically, *cfiA* strains exhibit a distinctive and homogeneous ribotype.

β-Lactam/β-lactamase inhibitor antibiotic combinations such as piperacillin/tazobactam and ampicillin/sulbactam are usually a good option against β-lactamase-producing anaerobes, including the *B. fragilis* group. Metronidazole is generally active against gram-negative (again including the *B. fragilis* group) and gram-positive anaerobes; resistance is rare but has been reported both in the United States and in Europe. This antibiotic is well tolerated, reaches significant levels in serum, and penetrates abscesses well. Resistance to metronidazole is more common among gram-positive anaerobes, including *P. acnes*, *Actinomyces* species, lactobacilli, and anaerobic streptococci than among gram-negative anaerobes.

Despite excellent in vitro activity against all clinically important anaerobes, chloramphenicol is less desirable than other active drugs for the treatment of anaerobic infection because of documented clinical failures. Clindamycin is active against many anaerobes. Rates of resistance to clindamycin among the *B. fragilis* group have increased in the United States from 3% in 1982 to 16% in 1996 and 26% in 2000, with rates as high as 44% in some series. Resistance to clindamycin among non-*Bacteroides* anaerobes is much less common (<10%).

Newer fluoroquinolones such as moxifloxacin have the potential to treat mixed aerobic-anaerobic infections. However, these drugs exhibit weaker in vitro activity against many *Bacteroides* species other than *B. fragilis*. A recent survey in the United States found an increase in resistance to moxifloxacin among the *B. fragilis* group.[42] Tigecycline is active against anaerobic bacteria, including most *Bacteroides* species, peptostreptococci, and *Propionibacterium*, *Prevotella*, and *Fusobacterium* species. In two phase 2 clinical trials of therapy for intra-abdominal infections, its efficacy was comparable to that of imipenem; however, resistance among *Bacteroides* and non-*Bacteroides* species has been reported.

In clinical situations, specific regimens must be tailored to the initial site of infection. Antibiotic treatment for intra-abdominal infections needs to be directed against *Bacteroides* species and the gram-negative aerobic flora of the bowel. Single agents suitable for this purpose include the carbapenems, cefoxitin, cefotetan, and β-lactam/β-lactamase inhibitor combinations. A two-drug regimen is an alternative, with one drug active against coliforms and the other against anaerobes (e.g., a third-generation cephalosporin or a quinolone with metronidazole or clindamycin). In addition, if the clinician suspects that gram-positive facultative organisms such as enterococci are involved, therapeutic regimens should include ampicillin or vancomycin.

A meta-analysis of 40 randomized or quasi-randomized controlled trials of 16 antibiotic regimens for secondary peritonitis showed equivalent clinical success for all regimens.[43] Mixed aerobic-anaerobic infections of oral origin must include drugs active against both the gram-positive aerobic and the anaerobic flora of the mouth. β-Lactamase production by anaerobic strains that are usually isolated from infections originating above the diaphragm has been reported. Suitable regimens for these infections include clindamycin, β-lactam/β-lactamase inhibitor combinations, or penicillin together with metronidazole.

The failure of antibiotic therapy against an anaerobic infection should prompt consideration of surgical drainage or débridement of the infected site. In addition, the possibility of co-infection with one or more drug-resistant aerobic organisms should be considered. In these situations, isolation of the organisms should be attempted in order to determine antibiotic susceptibility.

ACKNOWLEDGMENTS

The authors wish to acknowledge the contributions of Arthur O. Tzianabos, PhD, to this chapter in earlier editions of this book.

REFERENCES

1. Tally FP, Stewart PR, Sutter VL, et al. Oxygen tolerance of fresh clinical anaerobic bacteria. *J Clin Microbiol*. 1975;1:161-164.
2. Hentges DJ. The anaerobic microflora of the human body. *Clin Infect Dis*. 1993;16(Suppl 4):S175-S180.
3. Holdeman LV, Good IJ, Moore WE. Human fecal flora: variation in bacterial composition within individuals and a possible effect of emotional stress. *Appl Environ Microbiol*. 1976;31:359-375.
4. Cash HL, Whitham CV, Behrendt CL, et al. Symbiotic bacteria direct expression of an intestinal bactericidal lectin. *Science*. 2006;443:1126-1130.
5. Shimada K, Bricknell KS, Finegold SM. Deconjugation of bile acids by intestinal bacteria: review of literature and additional studies. *J Infect Dis*. 1969;119:73-81.
6. Hooper LV, Midtvedt T, Gordon JI. How host-microbial interactions shape the nutrient environment of the mammalian intestine. *Annu Rev Nutr*. 2002;22:283-307.
7. Ley RE, Turnbaugh PJ, Klein S, et al. Microbial ecology: human gut microbes associated with obesity. *Nature*. 2006;444:1022-1023.
8. Turnbaugh PJ, Ley RE, Mahowald MA, et al. An obesity-associated gut microbiome with increased capacity for energy harvest. *Nature*. 2006;444:1027-1031.
9. Xu J, Gordon JI. Inaugural Article: honor thy symbionts. *Proc Natl Acad Sci U S A*. 2003;100:10452-10459.
10. Mazmanian SK, Liu CH, Tzianabos AO, et al. An immunomodulatory molecule of symbiotic bacteria directs maturation of the host immune system. *Cell*. 2005;122:107-118.
11. Mazmanian SK, Round JL, Kasper DL. A microbial symbiosis factor prevents intestinal inflammatory disease. *Nature*. 2008;453:620-625.
12. Onderdonk AB, Bartlett JG, Louie T, et al. Microbial synergy in experimental intra-abdominal abscess. *Infect Immun*. 1976;13:22-26.
13. Gorbach SL, Bartlett JG. Anaerobic infections. 3. *N Engl J Med*. 1974;290:1289-1294.
14. Gorbach SL, Bartlett JG. Anaerobic infections. 2. *N Engl J Med*. 1974;290:1237-1245.
15. Gorbach SL, Bartlett JG. Anaerobic infections. 1. *N Engl J Med*. 1974;290:1177-1184.
16. Wexler HM. *Bacteroides*: the good, the bad, and the nitty-gritty. *Clin Microbiol Rev*. 2007;20:593-621.
17. Brook I. Acute and chronic bacterial sinusitis. *Infect Dis Clin North Am*. 2007;21:427-448, vii.
18. Polk BF, Kasper DL. *Bacteroides fragilis* subspecies in clinical isolates. *Ann Intern Med*. 1977;86:569-571.
19. Sears CL, Myers LL, Lazenby A, et al. Enterotoxigenic *Bacteroides fragilis*. *Clin Infect Dis*. 1995;20(Suppl 2):S142-S148.
20. Sears CL, Islam S, Saha A, et al. Association of enterotoxigenic *Bacteroides fragilis* infection with inflammatory diarrhea. *Clin Infect Dis*. 2008;47:797-803.
21. Fredricks DN, Fiedler TL, Marrazzo JM. Molecular identification of bacteria associated with bacterial vaginosis. *N Engl J Med*. 2005;353:1899-1911.
22. Aldridge KE, Ashcraft D, O'Brien M, et al. Bacteremia due to *Bacteroides fragilis* group: distribution of species, beta-lactamase production, and antimicrobial susceptibility patterns. *Antimicrob Agents Chemother*. 2003;47:148-153.
23. Redondo MC, Arbo MD, Grindlinger J, et al. Attributable mortality of bacteremia associated with the *Bacteroides fragilis* group. *Clin Infect Dis*. 1995;20:1492-1496.
24. Lassmann B, Gustafson DR, Wood CM, et al. Reemergence of anaerobic bacteremia. *Clin Infect Dis*. 2007;44:895-900.
25. Fenner L, Widmer AF, Straub C, et al. Is the incidence of anaerobic bacteremia decreasing? Analysis of 114,000 blood cultures over a ten-year period. *J Clin Microbiol*. 2008;46:2432-2434.
26. Nichols RL. Intraabdominal infections: An overview. *Rev Infect Dis*. 1985;7(Suppl 4):S709-S715.
27. Onderdonk AB, Kasper DL, Cisneros RL, et al. The capsular polysaccharide of *Bacteroides fragilis* as a virulence factor: comparison of the pathogenic potential of encapsulated and unencapsulated strains. *J Infect Dis*. 1977;136:82-89.
28. Krinos CM, Coyne MJ, Weinacht KG, et al. Extensive surface diversity of a commensal microorganism by multiple DNA inversions. *Nature*. 2001;414:555-558.
29. Tzianabos AO, Onderdonk AB, Rosner B, et al. Structural features of polysaccharides that induce intra-abdominal abscesses. *Science*. 1993;262:416-419.
30. Chung DR, Kasper DL, Panzo RJ, et al. CD4+ T cells mediate abscess formation in intra-abdominal sepsis by an IL-17-dependent mechanism. *J Immunol*. 2003;170:1958-1963.
31. Gibson FC 3rd, Onderdonk AB, Kasper DL, et al. Cellular mechanism of intraabdominal abscess formation by *Bacteroides fragilis*. *J Immunol*. 1998;160:5000-5006.
32. Chambers FG, Koshy SS, Saidi RF, et al. *Bacteroides fragilis* toxin exhibits polar activity on monolayers of human intestinal epithelial cells (T84 cells) in vitro. *Infect Immun*. 1997;65:3561-3570.
33. Yilmaz O. The chronicles of *Porphyromonas gingivalis*: the microbium, the human oral epithelium and their interplay. *Microbiology*. 2008;154:2897-2903.
34. Laine ML, van Winkelhoff AJ. Virulence of six capsular serotypes of *Porphyromonas gingivalis* in a mouse model. *Oral Microbiol Immunol*. 1998;13:322-325.
35. Ogawa T, Asai Y, Hashimoto M, et al. Cell activation by Porphyromonas gingivalis lipid A molecule through Toll-like receptor 4- and myeloid differentiation factor 88-dependent signaling pathway. *Int Immunol*. 2002;14:1325-1332.
36. Roberts GL. Fusobacterial infections: an underestimated threat. *Br J Biomed Sci*. 2000;57:156-162.
37. Sugita N, Kimura A, Matsuki Y, et al. Activation of transcription factors and IL-8 expression in neutrophils stimulated with lipopolysaccharide from *Porphyromonas gingivalis*. *Inflammation*. 1998;22:253-267.
38. Araki H, Kuriyama T, Nakagawa K, et al. The microbial synergy of *Peptostreptococcus micros* and *Prevotella intermedia* in a murine abscess model. *Oral Microbiol Immunol*. 2004;19:177-181.
39. Dorn BR, Leung KL, Progulske-Fox A. Invasion of human oral epithelial cells by *Prevotella intermedia*. *Infect Immun*. 1998;66:6054-6057.
40. Nguyen MH, Yu VL, Morris AJ, et al. Antimicrobial resistance and clinical outcome of *Bacteroides* bacteremia: findings of a multicenter prospective observational trial. *Clin Infect Dis*. 2000;30:870-876.
41. Hecht DW. Prevalence of antibiotic resistance in anaerobic bacteria: worrisome developments. *Clin Infect Dis*. 2004;39:92-97.
42. Snydman DR, Jacobus NV, McDermott LA, et al. National survey on the susceptibility of *Bacteroides fragilis* group: report and analysis of trends in the United States from 1997 to 2004. *Antimicrob Agents Chemother*. 2007;51:1649-1655.
43. Wong PF, Gilliam AD, Kumar S, et al. Antibiotic regimens for secondary peritonitis of gastrointestinal origin in adults. *Cochrane Database Syst Rev*. 2005:CD004539.

244

Clostridium tetani (Tetanus)

PAVANI REDDY | THOMAS P. BLECK

History

Tetanus was well known to the ancients; descriptions by Egyptian and Greek physicians survive to the present. They recognized the frequent relationship between injuries and the subsequent development of fatal spasms. Gowers provided the quintessential description of tetanus in 1888:

Tetanus is a disease of the nervous system characterized by persistent tonic spasm, with violent brief exacerbations. The spasm almost always commences in the muscles of the neck and jaw, causing closure of the jaws (trismus, lockjaw), and involves the muscles of the trunk more than those of the limbs. It is always acute in onset, and a very large proportion of those affected die.[1]

Nicolaier isolated a strychnine-like toxin from anaerobic soil bacteria in 1884.[2] Six years later, Behring and Kitasato described active immunization with tetanus toxoid.[3] This latter discovery should have reduced tetanus to an historical curiosity, but we still fail to fulfill this promise.

Epidemiology

The U.S. Centers for Disease Control and Prevention receive reports of about 35 to 70 domestic cases per year[4,5]; this represents underreporting of about 60%.[6] Data through 2000 are summarized in Figure 244-1. Most reported cases are in patients older than 60 years,[7] indicating that waning immunity is an important risk factor.[8] This may be a particularly serious problem in older women.[9,10] Changes in patterns of immigration may increase the number of unimmunized or inadequately immunized patients presenting for care in developed countries.[11] Injection drug abuse places patients at risk for tetanus,[12] as do other potentially unsterile practices that allow inoculation of spores.[13]

Acute injuries account for about 70% of U.S. cases, evenly divided between punctures and lacerations.[14] Other identifiable conditions are noted in 23%, leaving about 7% of cases without an apparent source. Other studies cite rates of cryptogenic tetanus as high as 23%.

In developing countries, mortality rates due to tetanus are as high as 28 per 100,000. Until recently, primary tetanus immunization programs in developing countries were ineffective. As a result, 800,000 to 1 million annual deaths were attributed to tetanus during the 1980s.[15] Two thirds of cases worldwide occurred in sub-Saharan Africa, where more than 40% of tetanus is a result of neonatal infection[15,16]; nearly one third of these infants were born to mothers of a previously afflicted child, highlighting a failure to immunize.[17]

In 1989, a worldwide commitment to the elimination of neonatal tetanus by the World Health Assembly[18,19] resulted in a decline of more than 50% in the next 10 years.[20] A resurgent effort in 1999, the Maternal and Neonatal Tetanus Elimination Program,[21] met with additional success. Current estimates suggest that worldwide neonatal tetanus now accounts for less than 200,000 deaths annually.[22] The Global Immunization Vision and Strategy, launched by the World Health Organization and the United Nations Children's Fund in 2005, continues to target tetanus as a preventable cause of neonatal death by promoting routine tetanus toxoid administration in hard-to-reach, previously underserved areas.[23]

Characteristics of *Clostridium tetani*

Clostridium tetani is an obligately anaerobic bacillus that is gram positive in fresh cultures but may have variable staining in older cultures or tissue samples.[24] The complete genome of the organism has been sequenced, and its products were recently compared with other clostridia.[25] During growth, the bacilli possess abundant flagellae and are sluggishly motile. Two toxins, tetanospasmin (commonly called *tetanus toxin*) and tetanolysin, are produced during this phase. Tetanospasmin is encoded on a plasmid that is present in all toxigenic strains.[26] Tetanolysin is of uncertain importance in the pathogenesis of tetanus. Mature organisms lose their flagella, develop a terminal spore, and begin to resemble a squash racquet (Fig. 244-2).[27] The spores are extremely stable in the environment, retaining the ability to germinate and cause disease indefinitely. They withstand exposure to ethanol, phenol, or formalin but can be rendered noninfectious by iodine, glutaraldehyde, hydrogen peroxide, or autoclaving at 121°C and 103 kPa (15 psi) for 15 minutes. Growth in culture is optimal at 37°C under strictly anaerobic conditions, but culture results are of no diagnostic value. Antibiotic sensitivity is discussed later.

Pathogenesis

The clostridial toxins that produce both tetanus and botulism are similar in structure and function despite the almost diametrically opposed clinical manifestations of the diseases. These toxins are zinc dependent matrix metalloproteinases, a category encompassing a diverse group of enzymes ranging from normal human cellular constituents necessary for cellular remodeling,[28] through determinants of neoplastic cell function,[29] to exotoxins of other microorganisms such as *Bacteroides fragilis*.[30] Tetanospasmin is synthesized as a single 151-kDa chain that is cleaved extracellularly by a bacterial protease into a 100-kDa heavy chain and a 50-kDa light chain (fragment A), which remain connected by a disulfide bridge.[31] The heavy chain can be further divided into fragments B and C by pepsin. The heavy chain appears to mediate binding to cell surface receptors and transport proteins, whereas the light chain produces the presynaptic inhibition of transmitter release that produces clinical tetanus. The nature of the receptor to which tetanospasmin binds, previously thought to be a ganglioside, remains debated.[32] The toxin enters the nervous system primarily through the presynaptic terminals of lower motor neurons, where it can produce local failure of neuromuscular transmission. It then exploits the retrograde axonal transport system and is carried to the cell bodies of these neurons in the brainstem and spinal cord, where it expresses its major pathogenic action.[33]

Once the toxin enters the central nervous system, it diffuses to the terminals of inhibitory cells, including both local glycinergic interneurons and descending γ-aminobutyric acid-ergic (GABAergic) neurons from the brainstem. The toxin degrades synaptobrevin, a protein required for docking of neurotransmitter vesicles with their release site on the presynaptic membrane.[34] By preventing transmitter release from these cells, tetanospasmin leaves the motor neurons without inhibition. This produces muscular rigidity by raising the resting firing rate of motor neurons and also generates spasms by failing to limit reflex responses to afferent stimuli. Excitatory transmitter release in the spinal cord can also be impaired, but the toxin appears to have greater affinity for the inhibitory systems. The autonomic nervous system is affected as well; this is predominantly manifested as a hyper-

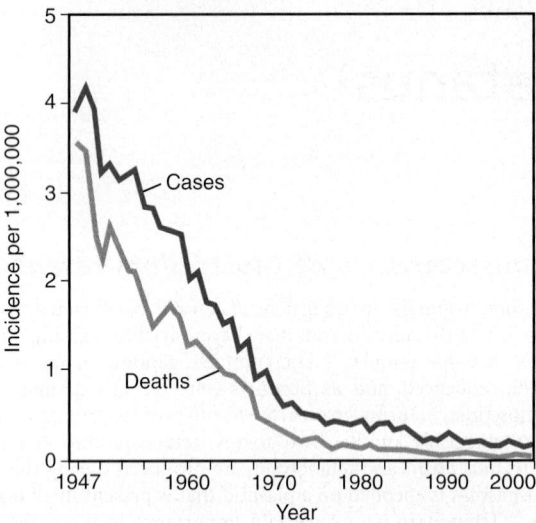

Figure 244-1 Reported cases and deaths from tetanus in the United States, 1947 to 2000. *(Data from Pascual FB, McGinley EL, Zanardi LR, et al. Tetanus surveillance—United States, 1998–2000. Centers for Disease Control and Prevention. Surveillance Summaries, June 20, 2003. MMWR Morb Mortal Wkly Rep. 2003;52:1-8.)*

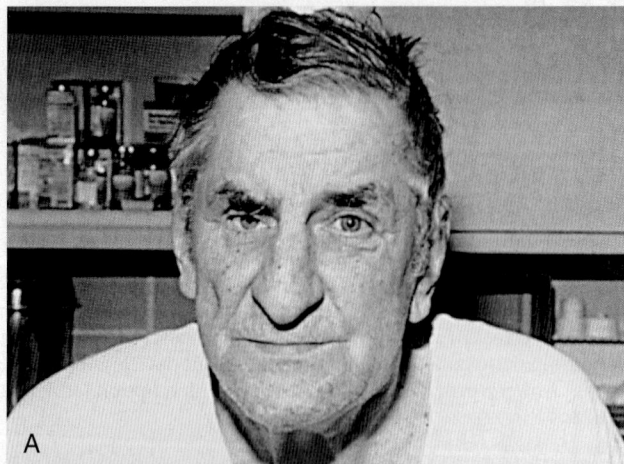

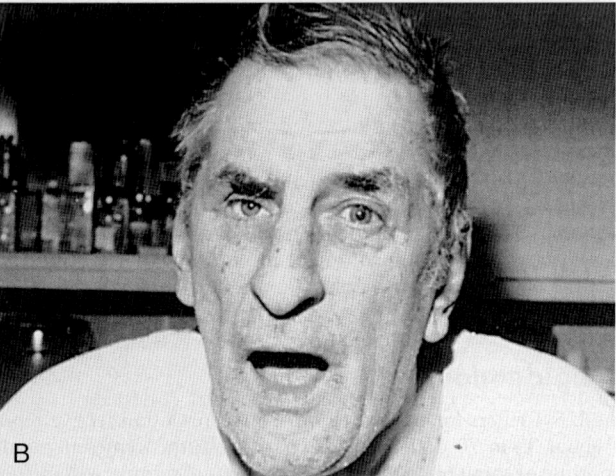

Figure 244-3 Risus sardonicus and trismus. A, Risus sardonicus. Note the straightened upper lip at rest. **B**, Trismus. The patient is opening his mouth as fully as possible. *(From Bleck TP. Tetanus. In: Scheld WM, Whitley RJ, Durack DT, eds. Infections of the Central Nervous System. New York: Raven Press; 1991:603-624.)*

sympathetic state induced by failure to inhibit adrenal release of catecholamines.

Toxin binding appears to be an irreversible event. At the neuromuscular junction, initial recovery from botulism depends on sprouting a new axon terminal; this is probably the case at other affected synapses as well. Later, the new synapses are removed when the original ones reestablish their connections.[35]

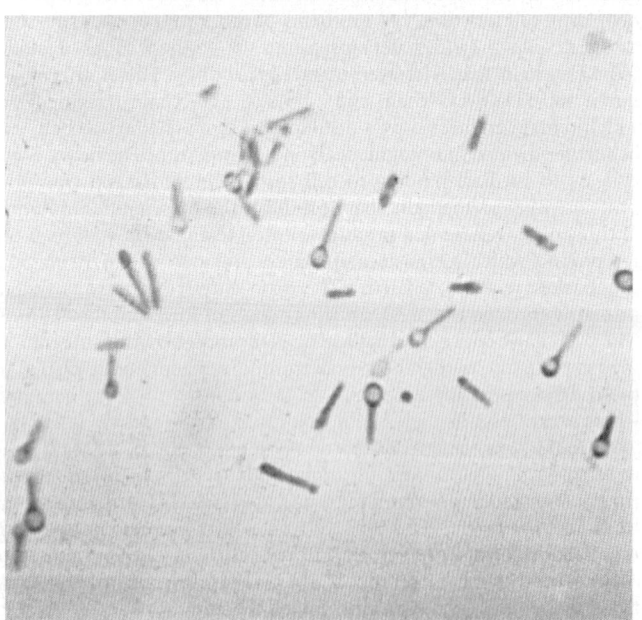

Figure 244-2 Gram stain of a culture of *Clostridium tetani*. *(From Bleck TP, Brauner JS. Tetanus. In: Scheld WM, Whitley RJ, Marra CM, eds. Infections of the Central Nervous System. 3rd ed. New York: Lippincott Williams & Wilkins; 2004:625-648. Courtesy of Paul C. Schrechenberger, Ph.D., and Alex Kuritza, Ph.D.)*

Clinical Manifestations

Tetanus is classically divided into four clinical types: *generalized, localized, cephalic,* and *neonatal.* These are valuable diagnostic and prognostic distinctions but reflect host factors and the site of inoculation rather than differences in toxin action. Terms describing the initial stages of tetanus include the *incubation period* (time from inoculation to the first symptom) and the *period of onset* (time from the first symptom to the first generalized spasm). The shorter these periods are, the worse the prognosis is.[36] Various rating scales are available.[37] Certain portals of entry (e.g., compound fractures) are associated with poorer prognoses. Tetanus may be particularly severe in narcotics addicts, for unknown reasons.[38]

Generalized tetanus is the most commonly recognized form and often begins with *risus sardonicus* (increased tone in the orbicularis oris) and *trismus* ("lockjaw"; masseter rigidity) (Fig. 244-3). Abdominal rigidity may also be present. The *generalized spasm* resembles decorticate posturing and consists of opisthotonic posturing with flexion of the arms and extension of the legs (Fig. 244-4). The patient does not lose consciousness and experiences severe pain during each spasm. The spasms are often triggered by sensory stimuli. During the spasm, the upper airway can be obstructed, or the diaphragm may participate in the general muscular contraction. Either of these compromises respiration, and even the first such spasm may be fatal. In

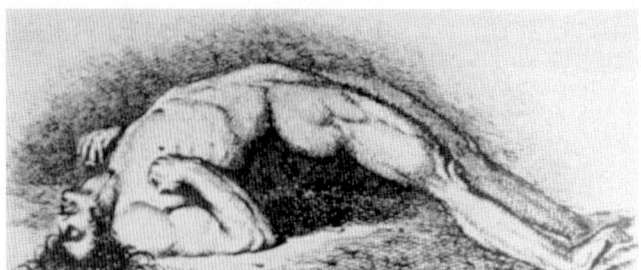

Figure 244-4 **Opisthotonus.** *(From Bell C. Essays on the Anatomy and Physiology of Expression. 2nd ed. London: J. Murray; 1824.)*

the modern era of intensive care, however, the respiratory problems are easily managed, and autonomic dysfunction, usually occurring after several days of symptoms, has emerged as the leading cause of death.[39]

The illness can progress for about 2 weeks, reflecting the time required to complete the transport of toxin, which is already intra-axonal when antitoxin treatment is given. The severity of illness may be decreased by partial immunity.[40] Recovery takes an additional month and is complete unless complications supervene. Lower motor neuron dysfunction may not be apparent until spasms remit, and recovery from this deficit in neuromuscular transmission may take additional weeks.[41] Recurrent tetanus may occur if the patient does not receive active immunization because the amount of toxin produced is inadequate to induce immunity.[42]

Localized tetanus involves rigidity of the muscles associated with the site of spore inoculation. This may be mild and persistent and often resolves spontaneously. Lower motor neuron dysfunction (weakness and diminished muscle tone) is often present in the most involved muscle. This chronic form of the disease probably reflects partial immunity to tetanospasmin.[43] Localized tetanus is more commonly a prodrome of generalized tetanus, however, which occurs when enough toxin gains access to the central nervous system.

Cephalic tetanus is a special form of localized disease affecting the cranial nerve musculature, almost always following an apparent head wound (Fig. 244-5). Although earlier reports linked cephalic tetanus to a poor prognosis, more recent studies have revealed many milder cases. A lower motor neuron lesion, frequently producing facial nerve weakness, is often apparent.[44] Extraocular muscle involvement is occasionally noted.

Neonatal tetanus (Fig. 244-6) follows infection of the umbilical stump, most commonly caused by a failure of aseptic technique if mothers are inadequately immunized.[45] Cultural practices may also contribute.[46] The condition usually presents with generalized weakness and failure to nurse; rigidity and spasms occur later. The mortality rate exceeds 90%, and developmental delays are common among survivors.[47] Poor prognostic factors include age younger than 10 days, symptoms for fewer than 5 days before presentation to hospital, and presence of risus sardonicus or fever.[48] Apnea is the leading cause of death among neonatal tetanus patients in the first week of life, and sepsis in the second week.[49] Bacterial infection of the umbilical stump leads to sepsis in almost half of infants with neonatal tetanus, which contributes to the substantial mortality despite treatment.[50]

Diagnosis

Tetanus is diagnosed by clinical observation and has a limited differential diagnosis. Laboratory testing cannot confirm or exclude the condition and is primarily useful for excluding intoxications that may mimic tetanus. Electromyographic studies are occasionally useful in questionable cases. Such testing becomes more important when no portal of entry is apparent. Antitetanus antibodies are undetectable in most tetanus patients, but many reports document the disease in

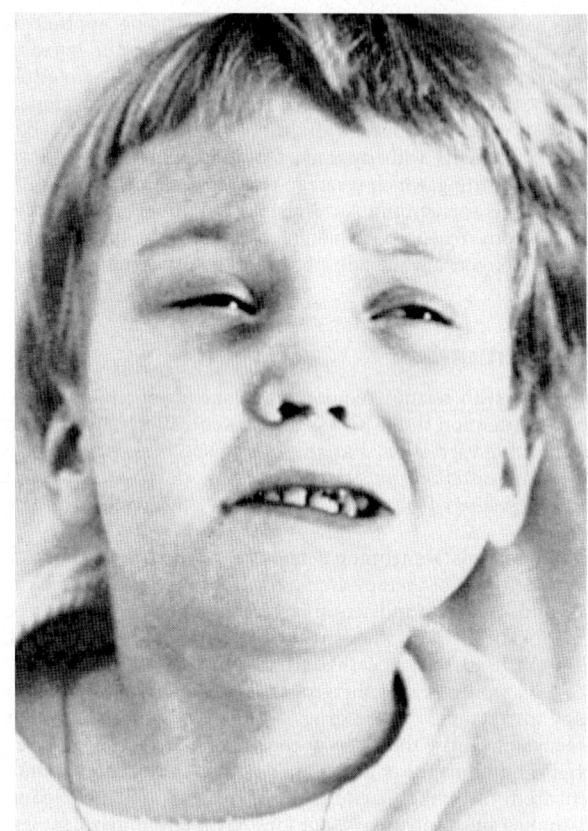

Figure 244-5 **Cephalic tetanus.** Right facial paresis is present in addition to the grimace. *(From Veronesi R, Focaccia R. The clinical picture. In: Veronesi R, ed. Tetanus: Important New Concepts. Amsterdam: Excerpta Medica; 1981:183-206.)*

patients with antibody levels above the commonly cited "protective" concentration of 0.01 IU/L.[51] Rare patients apparently develop antibodies that are not protective.[52]

Attempts to culture *C. tetani* from wounds are not useful in diagnosis because (1) even carefully performed anaerobic cultures are frequently negative; (2) a positive culture does not indicate whether the organism contains the toxin-producing plasmid; and (3) a positive culture may be present without disease in patients with adequate immunity.[53]

Strychnine poisoning, in which glycine is antagonized, is the only condition that truly mimics tetanus; toxicologic studies of serum and urine should be performed when tetanus is suspected, and tetanus

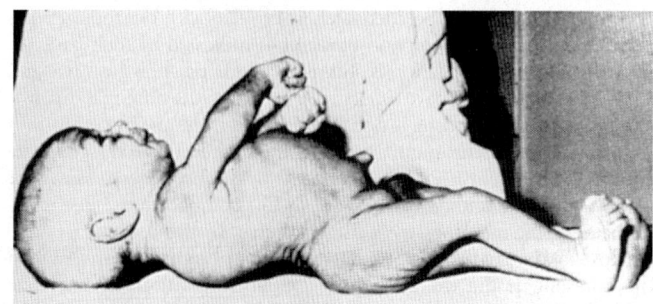

Figure 244-6 **Neonatal tetanus.** *(From Veronesi R, Focaccia R. The clinical picture. In: Veronesi R, ed. Tetanus: Important New Concepts. Amsterdam: Excerpta Medica; 1981:183-206.)*

should be considered even if strychnine poisoning appears likely. Because the initial treatments of tetanus and strychnine intoxication are similar, therapy is instituted before the assay results are available. Dystonic reactions to neuroleptic drugs or other central dopamine antagonists may be confused with the neck stiffness of tetanus, but the posture of patients with dystonic reactions almost always involves lateral head turning, which is rare in tetanus. Treatment with anticholinergic agents (benztropine or diphenhydramine) is rapidly effective against dystonic reactions. Dental infections may produce trismus and should be sought, but they do not cause the other manifestations of tetanus.

Treatment

The patient with tetanus requires simultaneous attention to several concerns. Attention to the airway and to ventilation is paramount at the time of presentation, but the other aspects of care, especially passive immunization, must be pursued as soon as the respiratory system is secure. Table 244-1 presents a suggested management protocol.

Tetanic spasms sometimes demand that the airway be secured before other lines of therapy are possible. An orotracheal tube can be passed under sedation and neuromuscular junction blockade; a feeding tube should be placed at the same time. Because the endotracheal tube may stimulate spasms, an early tracheostomy may be beneficial.[54]

Benzodiazepines have emerged as the mainstay of symptomatic therapy for tetanus.[55] These drugs are $GABA_A$ agonists and thereby indirectly antagonize the effect of the toxin. They do not restore glycinergic inhibition. The patient should be kept free of spasms and may benefit from the amnestic effects of the drugs as well. Diazepam has been studied most intensively, but lorazepam and midazolam appear equally effective. Tetanus patients have unusually high tolerance for the sedating effect of these agents and commonly remain alert at doses normally expected to produce anesthesia.[56]

The intravenous formulations of both diazepam and lorazepam contain propylene glycol. At the doses required to control generalized tetanus, this vehicle may produce lactic acidosis.[57] Nasogastric delivery of these agents is often possible, but some tetanus patients develop gastrointestinal motility disorders and do not absorb drugs well. Intravenous midazolam (5 to 15 mg/hour or more) is effective and does not contain propylene glycol, but it must be given as a continuous infusion because of its brief half-life.[58] Propofol infusion is also effective[59] but is currently very expensive, and the amount necessary to control symptoms may exceed the patient's tolerance of the lipid vehicle. When the symptoms of tetanus subside, these agents must be tapered over at least 2 weeks to prevent withdrawal symptoms. Intrathecal baclofen is also effective in controlling tetanus, but has no clear advantage over benzodiazepines. Neuroleptic agents and barbiturates, previously used for tetanus, are inferior for this indication and should not be used. Magnesium infusion may reduce the need for additional medications to control muscle spasms and cardiovascular instability, but does not appear to reduce the need for mechanical ventilation.[60]

Rare patients cannot be adequately controlled with benzodiazepines alone. Neuromuscular junction blockade is indicated in such patients, with the caveat that sedation is still required for psychological reasons. All the available drugs have side effects, including the potential for prolonged effect after the drug is discontinued. Vecuronium (by continuous infusion) and pancuronium (by intermittent injection) are adequate choices. These agents should be stopped at least once daily to assess the patient's progress and to observe for possible complications. Electroencephalographic monitoring is a useful adjunct for this purpose.[61]

Most tetanus patients still have the portal of entry apparent when they present. If the wound requires surgical attention, this may be performed after spasms are controlled. However, the course of tetanus is not affected by wound débridement.

Passive immunization with human tetanus immune globulin (HTIG) shortens the course of tetanus and may lessen its severity. A dose of 500 units appears as effective as larger doses.[62] A meta-analysis

TABLE 244-1	Suggested Management Protocol for Generalized Tetanus

I. Diagnosis and Stabilization: First Hour after Presentation

A. Assess airway and ventilation. If necessary, perform endotracheal intubation using benzodiazepine sedation and neuromuscular blockade (e.g., vecuronium, 0.1 mg/kg).

B. Obtain samples for antitoxin level, strychnine and dopamine antagonist assays, electrolytes, blood urea nitrogen, creatinine, creatine kinase, and urinary myoglobin determination.

C. Determine the portal of entry, incubation period, period of onset, and immunization history.

D. Administer benztropine (1 to 2 mg, intravenously) or diphenhydramine (50 mg, intravenously) to rule out a dystonic reaction to a dopamine-blocking agent.

E. Administer a benzodiazepine intravenously (diazepam in 5-mg increments, or lorazepam in 2-mg increments) to control spasm and decrease rigidity. Initially, employ a dose that is adequate to produce sedation and minimize reflex spasms. If this dose compromises the airway or ventilation, intubate using a short-acting neuromuscular-blocking agent. Transfer the patient to a quiet, darkened area of the intensive care unit.

II. Early Management Phase: First 24 Hours

A. Administer human tetanus immunoglobulin (HTIG), 500 units, intramuscularly; as an alternative, consider intravenous pooled immune globulin.

B. At a different site, administer adsorbed tetanus toxoid such as tetanus-diphtheria vaccine (0.5 mL) or diphtheria-pertussis-tetanus vaccine (0.5 mL), as appropriate for age, intramuscularly. Adsorbed tetanus toxoid without diphtheria toxoid is available for patients with a history of reaction to diphtheria toxoid; otherwise, the correct combination for the patient's age should be employed.

C. Begin metronidazole, 500 mg, intravenously, every 6 hr, for 7 to 10 days.

D. Perform a tracheostomy after placement of an endotracheal tube and under neuromuscular blockade if spasms produce any degree of airway compromise.

E. Débride any wounds as indicated for their management.

F. Place a soft, small-bore nasal feeding tube or a central venous hyperalimentation catheter, and begin feeding. Patients receiving total parental nutrition should also be given parenteral histamine-2 blockade or other gastric protection.

G. Administer benzodiazepines as required to control spasms and produce sedation. If adequate control is not achieved, institute long-term neuromuscular blockade (e.g., vecuronium, 6 to 8 mg/hr); continue benzodiazepines for sedation with intermittent electroencephalographic monitoring to ensure somnolence. Neuromuscular junction blockade should be discontinued daily to assess the patient's physical examination and to decrease the possibility of excessive accumulation of the blocking agent.

III. Intermediate Management Phase: The Next 2 to 3 Weeks

A. Treat sympathetic hyperactivity with labetalol (0.25 to 1.0 mg/min as needed for blood pressure control) or morphine (0.5 to 1.0 mg/kg/hr by continuous infusion). Consider epidural blockade with a local anesthetic. Avoid diuretics for blood pressure control because volume depletion will worsen autonomic instability.

B. If hypotension is present, initiate saline resuscitation. Place a pulmonary artery catheter and an arterial line, and administer fluids, dopamine, or norepinephrine as indicated.

C. Sustained bradycardia usually requires a pacemaker. Atropine or isoproterenol may be useful during pacemaker placement.

D. Begin prophylactic heparin.

E. Use a flotation bed, if possible, to prevent skin breakdown and peroneal nerve palsies. Otherwise, ensure frequent turning and employ antirotation boots.

F. Maintain benzodiazepines until neuromuscular blockade, if employed, has been terminated, and the severity of spasms has diminished substantially. Then taper the benzodiazepine dose over 14 to 21 days.

G. Begin rehabilitation planning.

IV. Convalescent Stage: 2 to 6 Weeks

A. When spasms are no longer present, begin physical therapy. Many patients require supportive psychotherapy.

B. Before discharge, administer another dose of tetanus-diphtheria vaccine or diphtheria-pertussis-tetanus vaccine.

C. Schedule a third dose of toxoid to be given 4 weeks after the second.

Adapted from Bleck TP, Brauner JS. Tetanus. In: Scheld WM, Whitley RJ, Marra CM, eds. *Infections of the Central Nervous System.* 3rd ed. New York: Lippincott Williams & Wilkins; 2004:625-648.

of the benefits of intrathecal HTIG therapy was inconclusive.[63] However, in a recent randomized trial, the administration of intrathecal HTIG with intramuscular HTIG resulted in shorter duration of spasms, shorter hospital stay, and decreased respiratory assistance demands compared with intramuscular HTIG alone.[64] Pooled intravenous immune globulin has been proposed as an alternative to HTIG,[65] although this should be approached with caution.[66] Active immunization must also be initiated.

The role of antimicrobial therapy in tetanus remains debated. The in vitro susceptibilities of *C. tetani* include metronidazole, penicillins, cephalosporins, imipenem, macrolides, and tetracycline. A study comparing oral metronidazole to intramuscular penicillin showed better survival, shorter hospitalization, and less progression of disease in the metronidazole group.[67] This may reflect a true advantage of metronidazole over penicillin, but it more likely corresponds to a negative effect of penicillin, a known GABA antagonist. Topical antibiotic application to the umbilical stump appears to reduce the risk for neonatal tetanus.[8]

Autonomic dysfunction generally reflects excessive catecholamine release and may respond to combined α- and β-adrenergic blockade with intravenous labetalol.[68] β-Blockade alone is rarely employed because the resulting unopposed α effect may produce severe hypertension. If β-blockade is chosen, the short-acting agent esmolol should be employed.[69] Other approaches to hypertension include morphine infusion,[70] magnesium sulfate infusion,[71] and epidural blockade of the renal nerves.[72] Hypotension is less common, but if present, it may require norepinephrine infusion. Myocardial dysfunction is also common[73] and may represent a further reflection of catecholamine excess.[74]

Nutritional support should be started as soon as the patient is stable. The volume of enteral feeding needed to meet the exceptionally high caloric and protein requirements of these patients may exceed the capacity of the gastrointestinal system.

The mortality rate in mild and moderate tetanus at present is about 6%; for severe tetanus, it may reach as high as 60%, even in expert centers.[75] A well-designed protocol for the critical care of tetanus patients can substantially reduce morbidity and mortality.[76] Among adults, age has little effect on mortality, with octogenarians and nonagenarians faring as well as middle-aged patients.[77] Tetanus survivors often have serious psychological problems related to the disease and its treatment that persist after recovery and may require psychotherapy.[78]

Prophylaxis

Tetanus is preventable in almost all patients, leading to its description as the "inexcusable disease."[79] Tetanus toxoid (TT), a heat-inactivated toxin, was developed in 1924.[80] The vaccine was initially used among military personnel in World War II. As a result, tetanus accounted for only 12 of nearly 3 million hospitalizations during the war; five cases were fatal.[81,82]

The Advisory Committee on Immunization Practices (ACIP) recommends a primary tetanus vaccination in combination with diphtheria and pertussis (DTaP) in the first year of life, followed by a dose at age 15 to 18 months and again at age 4 to 6 years. An adult-formulation booster (Td) should be administered at age 11 to 12 years and again 10 years later.[83] Toxoid vaccination remains the standard; DNA-based vaccination is less efficacious.[84]

In 2005, the U.S. Food and Drug Administration (FDA) approved the use of an adult formulation of tetanus, diphtheria, and acellular pertussis (Tdap) in lieu of the Td booster.[85] At this point, a single dose of Tdap should be given to adults aged 19 to 64 years if they received their last dose of Td 10 years or more ago and have never received Tdap. For adults who require tetanus toxoid–containing vaccine as part of wound management, a single dose of Tdap is preferred, if they have not received it previously and have not received Td in 5 years or more.[83] Tdap is not approved for pregnant women; pregnant women may receive Td or defer vaccination until they are able to receive Tdap in the immediate postpartum period.[86]

A dose of Tdap may also be given as soon as 2 years after the last Td dose if a booster for pertussis is desired. Settings in which a pertussis booster is indicated include the following: adults who anticipate close contact with an infant younger than 12 months, women who are considering pregnancy or who are in the immediate postpartum period, and all health care personnel.[83] Tdap is not licensed for multiple administrations; after an initial dose of Tdap, adults should receive a Td booster every 10 years (see also Chapter 320).

Serologic analysis of the U.S. population suggests that tetanus immunity wanes with age.[87,88] Although 80% of patients aged 6 to 39 years were noted to have protective antibodies to tetanus, only 28% of patients older than 70 years were seropositive.[87]

Some patients with humoral immune deficiencies may not respond adequately to toxoid injection[89]; such patients should receive passive immunization for tetanus-prone injuries regardless of the period since the last booster. About half of patients lose tetanus immunity after chemotherapy for leukemia or lymphoma.[90] Patients who have undergone bone marrow or stem cell transplantation require revaccination after the procedure[91]; two doses (given 12 and 24 months after transplantation) are probably sufficient.[92] Antibody production by the transplanted immune cells may play a minor role in subsequent host immunity.[93] Most young patients with human immunodeficiency virus (HIV) infection appear to retain antitetanus antibody production if their primary immunization series was completed before they acquired HIV[94]; however, only a minority respond adequately to booster immunization.[95] Vitamin A deficiency interferes with the response to tetanus toxoid.[96]

Neonatal tetanus may occur because of inadequate immunization of the mother. Although a full series of maternal immunizations is ideal, even one or two doses of tetanus toxoid confer substantial protection against neonatal tetanus.[97] Application of topical antimicrobial agents to the umbilical cord stump markedly decreases the incidence of neonatal tetanus when maternal immunization is insufficient.[98]

Mild reactions to tetanus toxoid (e.g., local tenderness, edema, low-grade fever) are common. More severe reactions are rare and likely are due to a hypersensitivity response to the preservative thiomersal.[99] Although there have been reports suggesting a connection between tetanus immunization and Guillain-Barré syndrome, a careful epidemiologic analysis did not confirm an association.[100]

HTIG binds directly to toxin, providing temporary immunity. Current guidelines suggest that patients with suspected tetanus or a tetanus-prone wound should receive HTIG in conjunction with vaccination if they did not complete a primary immunization series or if their immunization status is unknown.[83] Tetanus-prone wounds are characterized by devitalized tissue such as a crush injury or by a wound with potential contamination with dirt or rust.

REFERENCES

1. Gowers WR. *A Manual of Diseases of the Nervous System*. Philadelphia: Blackiston & Son; 1888.
2. Nicolaier A. Üeber infectiösen tetanus. *Dtsch Med Wochenschr*. 1884;10:842-844.
3. Behring E, Kitasato S. Üeber das zustandekommen der diphtherie-immunität und der tetanus-immunität bei thieren. *Dtsch Med Wochenschr*. 1890;16:1113-1114.
4. Pascual FB, McGinley EL, Zanardi LR, et al. Tetanus surveillance—United States, 1998–2000. Centers for Disease Control and Prevention. Surveillance Summaries, June 20, 2003. *MMWR Morb Mortal Wkly Rep*. 2003;52.
5. Centers for Disease Control. Summary of notifiable disease, 2001. *MMWR Morb Mortal Wkly Rep*. 2003;50:80.
6. Sutter RW, Cochi SL, Brink EW, et al. Assessment of vital statistics and surveillance data for monitoring tetanus mortality, United States, 1979–1984. *Am J Epidemiol*. 1990;131:132-142.
7. Gergen PJ, McQuillan GM, Kiely M, et al. A population-based serologic survey of immunity to tetanus in the United States. *N Engl J Med*. 1995;332:761-766.
8. Richardson JP, Knight AL. The prevention of tetanus in the elderly. *Arch Intern Med*. 1991;151:1712-1717.
9. Horton E, Singer C, Kozarsky P, et al. Status of immunity to tetanus, measles, mumps, rubella, and polio among U.S. travelers. *Ann Intern Med*. 1991;115:32-33.

10. Böttiger M, Gustavsson O, Svensson Å. Immunity to tetanus, diphtheria and poliomyelitis in the adult population of Sweden in 1991. *Int J Epidemiol.* 1998;27:916-925.

11. Henderson SO, Mody T, Groth DE, et al. The presentation of tetanus in an emergency department. *J Emerg Med.* 1998;16: 705-708.

12. Beeching NJ, Crowcroft NS. Tetanus in injecting drug users. *Br Med J.* 2005;330:208-209.

13. O'Malley CD, Smith N, Braun R, et al. Tetanus associated with body piercing. *Clin Infect Dis.* 1998;27:1343-1344.

14. Bleck TP. Tetanus: Dealing with the continuing clinical challenge. *J Crit Illness.* 1987;2:41-52.

15. Dietz V, Milstien JB, van Loon F, et al. Performance and potency of tetanus toxoid: implications for eliminating neonatal tetanus. *Bull World Health Organ.* 1996;74:619-628.

16. UNICEF. *Maternal and neonatal tetanus elimination by 2005: strategies for achieving and maintaining elimination.* New York: UNICEF; 2000.

17. Traverso HP, Kamil S, Rahim H, et al. A reassessment of risk factors for neonatal tetanus. *Bull World Health Organ.* 1991;69: 573-579.

18. World Health Organization. Expanded programme on immunization. The global elimination of neonatal tetanus: progress to date. *Wkly Epidemiol Rec.* 1993;68:277-282.

19. World Health Organization. *WHA 42.32 Expanded Programme on Immunization. World Health Assembly Resolutions and Decisions.* Geneva: World Health Assembly; 1989.

20. Galazka A, Birmingham M, Kurian M, et al. Tetanus. In: Murray CJL, Lopez AD, Mathers CD, eds. *The Global Epidemiology of Infectious Diseases.* Geneva: World Health Organization, 2004:151-199.

21. WHO, UNICEF, & UNFPA. *Maternal and neonatal tetanus elimination by 2005. Strategies for achieving and maintaining elimination. WHO/V&B/02.09.* Geneva: World Health Organization, United Nations Children's Fund, and United Nations Population Fund; 2000.

22. Roper MH, Vandelaer JH, Gasse FL. Maternal and neonatal tetanus. *Lancet.* 2007;370:1947-1959.

23. WHO & UNICEF. *GIVS: Global Immunization Vision and Strategy, 2006–2015.* Geneva: World Health Organization; 2005.

24. Cato EP, George WL, Finegold SM. Genus *Clostridium praemozski* 1880, 23AL. In: Smeath PHA, Mair NS, Sharpe ME, Holt JG, eds. Bergey's Manual of Systematic Bacteriology. vol. 2. Baltimore: Williams & Wilkins; 1986:1141-1200.

25. Bruggemann H, Baumer S, Fricke WF, et al. The genome sequence of *Clostridium tetani,* the causative agent of tetanus disease. *Proc Natl Acad Sci U S A.* 2003;100:1316-1321.

26. Eisel U, Jarausch W, Goretzki K, et al. Tetanus toxin: Primary structure, expression in *E. coli,* and homology with botulinum toxins. *EMBO J.* 1986;5:2495-2502.

27. Hoeniger JFM, Tauschel HD. Sequence of structural changes in cultures of *Clostridium tetani* grown on a solid medium. *J Med Microbiol.* 1974;7:425-432.

28. Geisler S, Lichtinghagen R, Boker KH, et al. Differential distribution of five members of the matrix metalloproteinase family and one inhibitor (TIMP-1) in human liver and skin. *Cell Tissue Res.* 1997;289:173-183.

29. Rooprai HK, Meter TT, Rucklidge GJ, et al. Comparative analysis of matrix metalloproteinases by immunocytochemistry, immunohistochemistry and zymography in human primary brain tumours. *Int J Oncol.* 1998;13:1153-1157.

30. Wu S, Lim KC, Huang J, et al. Bacteroides fragilis enterotoxin cleaves the zonula adherens protein, E-cadherin. *Proc Natl Acad Sci U S A.* 1998;95:14979-14984.

31. Matsuda M. The structure of tetanus toxin. In: Simpson LL, ed. *Botulinum Neurotoxin and Tetanus Toxin.* San Diego: Academic Press; 1989:69-92.

32. Middlebrook JL. Cell surface receptors for protein toxins. In: Simpson LL, ed. *Botulinum Neurotoxin and Tetanus Toxin.* San Diego: Academic Press; 1989:95-119.

33. Bleck TP, Brauner JS. Tetanus. In: Scheld WM, Whitley RJ, Durack DT, eds. *Infections of the Central Nervous System.* 2nd ed. New York: Raven Press; 1997:629-653.

34. Cornille F, Martin L, Lenoir C, et al. Cooperative exosite-dependent cleavage of synaptobrevin by tetanus toxin light chain. *J Biol Chem.* 1997;272:3459-3464.

35. Meunier FA, Schiavo G, Molgo J. Botulinum neurotoxins: From paralysis to recovery of functional neuromuscular transmission. *J Physiol Paris.* 2002;96:105-113.

36. Veronesi R, Focaccia R. The clinical picture. In: Veronesi R, ed. *Tetanus: Important New Concepts.* Amsterdam: Excerpta Medica; 1981:183-206.

37. Habermann E. Tetanus. In: Vinken PJ, Bruyn GW, eds. *Handbook of Clinical Neurology.* Amsterdam: North-Holland; 1978:491-547.

38. Cherubin CE. Clinical severity of tetanus in narcotic addicts in New York City. *Arch Intern Med.* 1968;121:156-158.

39. Edmondson RS, Flowers MWW. Intensive care in tetanus: Management, complications, and mortality in 100 patients. *Br Med J.* 1979;1401-1404.

40. Luisto M, Iivanainen M. Tetanus of immunized children. *Dev Med Child Neurol.* 1993;35:351-355.

41. Bleck TP, Calderelli DD. Vocal cord paralysis complicating tetanus. *Neurology.* 1983;33(Suppl 2):140.

42. Spenney J, Lamb RN, Cobbs CG. Recurrent tetanus. *South Med J.* 1971;64:859.

43. Risk WS, Bosch EP, Kimura J, et al. Chronic tetanus: Clinical report and histochemistry of muscle. *Muscle Nerve.* 1981;4: 363-366.

44. Mayo J, Berciano J. Cephalic tetanus presenting with Bell's palsy. *J Neurol Neurosurg Psychiatry.* 1985;48:290.

45. Schofield FD, Tucker VM, Westbrook GR. Neonatal tetanus in New Guinea: Effect of active immunization in pregnancy. *Br Med J.* 1961;2:785-789.

46. Traverso HP, Bennett JV, Kahn AJ, et al. Ghee application to the umbilical cord: A risk factor for neonatal tetanus. *Lancet.* 1989;1:486-488.

47. Anlar B, Yalaz K, Dizmen R. Long-term prognosis after neonatal tetanus. *Dev Med Child Neurol.* 1989;31:76-80.

48. Gürses N, Aydin M. Factors affecting prognosis of neonatal tetanus. *Scand J Infect Dis.* 1993;25:353-355.

49. Kurtoglu S, Caksen H, Ozturk A, et al. A review of 207 newborns with tetanus. *J Pak Med Assoc.* 1998;48:93-98.

50. Egri-Okwaji MT, Iroha EO, Kesah CN, et al. Bacteria causing septicaemia in neonates with tetanus. *West Afr J Med.* 1998;17:136-139.

51. Goulon M, Girard O, Grosbius S, et al. Les corps antitétaniques. *Nouv Presse Med.* 1972;1:3049-3050.

52. Crone NE, Reder AT. Severe tetanus in immunized patients with high anti-tetanus titers. *Neurology.* 1992;42:761-764.

53. Bleck TP. Clinical aspects of tetanus. In: Simpson LL, ed. *Botulinum Neurotoxin and Tetanus Toxin.* New York: Academic Press; 1989:379-398.

54. Mukherjee DK. Tetanus and tracheostomy. *Ann Otol.* 1977;86:67-72.

55. Vassa T, Yajnik VH, Joshi KR, et al. Comparative clinical trial of diazepam with other conventional drugs in tetanus. *Postgrad Med J.* 1874;50:755-758.

56. Bleck TP. Tetanus. *Dis Month.* 1991;37:547-603.

57. Kapoor W, Carey P, Karpf M. Induction of lactic acidosis with intravenous diazepam in a patient with tetanus. *Arch Intern Med.* 1981;141:944-945.

58. Orko R, Rosenberg PH, Himberg JJ. Intravenous infusion of midazolam, propofol and vecuronium in a patient with sever tetanus. *Acta Anaesthesiol Scand.* 1988;32:590-592.

59. Borgeat A, Dessibourg C, Rochani M, et al. Sedation by propofol in tetanus—is it a muscular relaxant? *Intensive Care Med.* 1991;17:427-429.

60. Thwaites CL, Yen LM, Loan HT, et al. Magnesium sulphate for treatment of severe tetanus: a randomised controlled trial. *Lancet.* 2006;368:1436-1443.

61. Luisto M, Seppäläinen A-M. Electroencephalography in tetanus. *Acta Neurol Scand.* 1989;80:157-161.

62. Blake PA, Feldman RA, Buchanan TM, et al. Serologic therapy of tetanus in the United States. *JAMA.* 1976;235:42-44.

63. Abrutyn E, Berlin JA. Intrathecal therapy in tetanus: A meta-analysis. *JAMA.* 1991;266:2262-2267.

64. Miranda-Filho Dde B, Ximenes RA, Barone AA, et al. Randomised controlled trial of tetanus treatment with antitetanus immunoglobulin by the intrathecal or intramuscular route. *Br Med J.* 2004;328:615.

65. Lee DC, Lederman HM. Anti-tetanus toxoid antibodies in intravenous gamma globulin: An alternative to tetanus immune globulin. *J Infect Dis.* 1992;166:642-645.

66. Bleck TP. Anti-tetanus toxoid antibodies in intravenous gamma globulin: An alternative to tetanus immune globulin. *J Infect Dis.* 1993;167:498-499.

67. Ahmadsyah I, Salim A. Treatment of tetanus: An open study to compare the efficacy of procaine penicillin and metronidazole. *Br Med J.* 1985;291:648-650.

68. Domenghetti GM, Savary S, Striker H. Hyperadrenergic syndrome in severe tetanus responsive to labetalol. *Br Med J.* 1984;288:1483-1484.

69. King WW, Cave DR. Use of esmolol to control autonomic instability of tetanus. *Am J Med.* 1991;91:425-428.

70. Rocke DA, Wasley AG, Pather M, et al. Morphine in tetanus: The management of sympathetic nervous system overactivity. *S Afr Med J.* 1986;70:666-668.

71. Lipman J, James MFM, Erskine J, et al. Autonomic dysfunction in severe tetanus: Magnesium sulfate as an adjunct to deep sedation. *Crit Care Med.* 1987;15:987-988.

72. Southorn PA, Blaise GA. Treatment of tetanus-induced autonomic dysfunction with continuous epidural blockade. *Crit Care Med.* 1986;14:251-252.

73. Udwadia FE, Sunavala JD, Jain MC, et al. Haemodynamic studies during the management of severe tetanus. *Q J Med.* 1992;83:449-460.

74. Tseuda K, Oliver PB, Richter RW. Cardiovascular manifestations of tetanus. *Anesthesiology.* 1974;40:588-592.

75. Nolla-Salas M, Garcés-Brusés J. Severity of tetanus in patients older than 80 years: comparative study with younger patients. *Clin Infect Dis.* 1993;16:591-592.

76. Brauner JS, Vieira SR, Bleck TP. Changes in severe accidental tetanus mortality in the ICU during two decades in Brazil. *Intensive Care Med.* 2002;28:930-935.

77. Jolliet P, Magnenat JL, Kobel T, et al. Aggressive intensive care treatment of very elderly patients with tetanus is justified. *Chest.* 1990;97:702-705.

78. Edwards RA, James B. Tetanus and psychiatry: Unexpected bedfellows. *Med J Aust.* 1979;1:483-484.

79. Edsall G. The inexcusable disease. *JAMA.* 1876;235:62-63.

80. McGrew RE, McGrew MP. *Encyclopedia of Medical History.* 1985;124:235-236.

81. United States Army. *The Army Immunization Program: Preventative Medicine in World War II.* Washington, DC: Government Printing Office, Medical Department, United States Army; 1955;287.

82. Glenn F. Tetanus. A preventable disease. *Ann Surg.* 1946: 1030-1040.

83. Kretsinger K, Broder KR, Cortese MM, et al, for the Centers for Disease Control and Prevention; Advisory Committee on Immunization Practices; Healthcare Infection Control Practices Advisory Committee. Preventing tetanus, diphtheria, and pertussis among adults: use of tetanus toxoid, reduced diphtheria toxoid and acellular pertussis vaccine recommendations of the Advisory Committee on Immunization Practices (ACIP) and recommendation of ACIP, supported by the Healthcare Infection Control Practices Advisory Committee (HICPAC), for use of Tdap among health-care personnel. *MMWR Recomm Rep.* 2006;15;55:1-37.

84. Saikh KU, Sesno J, Brandler P, et al. Are DNA-based vaccines useful for protection against secreted bacterial toxins? Tetanus toxin test case. *Vaccine.* 1998;16:1029-1038.

85. Pichichero ME, Rennels MB, Edwards KM, et al. Combined tetanus, diphtheria, and 5-component pertussis vaccine for use in adolescents and adults. *JAMA.* 2005;22;293:3003-3011.

86. Murphy TV, Slade BA, Broder KR, et al: Advisory Committee on Immunization Practices (ACIP) Centers for Disease Control and Prevention (CDC). Prevention of pertussis, tetanus, and diphtheria among pregnant and postpartum women and their infants recommendations of the Advisory Committee on Immunization Practices (ACIP). *MMWR Recomm Rep.* 2008;57:1-51.

87. McQuillan GM, Kruszon-Moran D, Deforest A, et al. Serologic immunity to diphtheria and tetanus in the United States. *Ann Intern Med.* 2002;136:660-666.

88. Murphy SM, Hegarty DM, Feighery CS, et al. Tetanus immunity in elderly people. *Age Ageing.* 1995;24:99-102.

89. Webster ADB, Latif AAA, Brenner MK, et al. Evaluation of test immunization in the assessment of antibody deficiency syndromes. *Br Med J.* 1984;288:1864-1866.

90. Hamarstrom V, Pauksen K, Svensson H, et al. Tetanus immunity in patients with hematological malignancies. *Support Care Cancer.* 1998;6:469-472.

91. Hammarström V, Pauksen K, Simmonsson B, et al. Tetanus immunity in autologous bone marrow and blood stem cell transplant recipients. *Bone Marrow Transplant.* 1998;22:67-71.

92. Vance E, George S, Guinan EC, et al. Comparison of multiple immunization schedules for *Haemophilus influenzae* type b-conjugate and tetanus toxoid vaccines following bone marrow transplantation. *Bone Marrow Transplant.* 1998;22:735-741.

93. Storek J, Viganego F, Dawson MA, et al. Factors affecting antibody levels after allogeneic hematopoietic cell transplantation. *Blood.* 2003;101:3319-3324.

94. Kurtzhals JAL, Kjeldsen K, Heron I, et al. Immunity against diphtheria and tetanus in human immunodeficiency virus-infected Danish men born 1950–1959. *APMIS.* 1992;100: 803-808.

95. Talesnik E, Vial PA, Labarca J, et al. Time course of antibody response to tetanus toxoid and pneumococcal capsular polysaccharides in patients infected with HIV. *J Acquir Immune Defic Syndr Hum Retrovirol.* 1998;19:471-477.

96. Semba RD, Muhilal, Scott AL, et al. Depressed immune response to tetanus in children with vitamin A deficiency. *J Nutr.* 1992;122:101-107.

97. Koenig MA, Roy NC, McElrath T, et al. Duration of protective immunity conferred by maternal tetanus toxoid immunization: Further evidence from Matlab, Bangladesh. *Am J Publ Health.* 1998;88:903-907.

98. Parashar UD, Bennett JV, Boring JR, et al. Topical antimicrobials applied to the umbilical cord stump: A new intervention against neonatal tetanus. *Int J Epidemiol.* 1998;27:904-908.

99. Jacobs RL, Lowe RS, Lanier BQ. Adverse reactions to tetanus toxoid. *JAMA.* 1982;247:40-42.

100. Tuttle J, Chen RT, Rantala H, et al. The risk of Guillain-Barre syndrome after tetanus-toxoid-containing vaccines in adults and children in the United States. *Am J Publ Health.* 1997;87: 2045-2048.

245

Clostridium botulinum (Botulism)

PAVANI REDDY | THOMAS P. BLECK

Botulism and tetanus result from intoxication with the protein neurotoxins elaborated by two related species of *Clostridium*. The toxins are very similar in structure and function, but differ dramatically in their clinical effects because they target different cells in the nervous system. Botulinum neurotoxins predominantly affect the peripheral neuromuscular junction and autonomic synapses, and primarily manifest as weakness. In contrast, although tetanus toxin can affect the same systems, its effects reflect tropism for inhibitory cells of the central nervous system (CNS) and primarily manifest as rigidity and spasm. Both conditions have potentially high fatality rates, and both are preventable through education and public health measures.

Clostridium botulinum produces most cases of botulism, with a few other clostridial strains accounting for the remainder. Botulinum toxins are designated types A through G based on antigenic differences.[1] Types A, B, E, and F produce human disease, whereas types C and D are almost exclusively confined to animals.[2] Type G toxin has not been associated with naturally acquired disease. The clinical forms of botulism include *foodborne botulism, infant botulism, wound botulism,* and *botulism of undetermined etiology.* In the past decade, botulinum A toxin has achieved prominence as a therapeutic modality in conditions that result from excessive muscle activity (e.g. torticollis) leading to rare cases of *iatrogenic botulism.* Botulinum toxin has also been developed as a weapon, which could be used to contaminate food or beverage supplies, or be aerosolized (see Chapter 326).

History of Botulism

The term *botulism* derives from the Latin word *botulus,* or sausage. Outbreaks of poisoning related to sausages and other prepared foods occurred in Europe in the 19th century. Justinus Kerner, a district health officer in southern Germany, recognized the connection between sausage and the paralytic illnesses of 230 patients in 1820, and made sausage poisoning a reportable disease.[3] At about the same time, physicians in Russia recognized a disease with similar symptoms, which they termed *fish poisoning.*[4] In 1897, van Ermengen published the first description of *C. botulinum* and showed that the organism elaborated a toxin that could induce weakness in animals.[5] This was subsequently shown to be type A toxin; type B was discovered in 1904.[6] Wound botulism was described in 1943,[7] and infant botulism in 1976.[8] The occurrence of sporadic cases without an apparent etiology, many related to gastrointestinal colonization, was first reported in 1986.[9] Type A toxin was isolated and purified in 1946.[10]

Epidemiology

Foodborne botulism is most frequently recognized in outbreaks, whereas the other forms are sporadic. Although commercially canned foods were commonly the source of toxin in the early part of this century, home-canned vegetables, fruits, and fish products are now the most common sources. In some cultures, such as among Alaskan Natives, preferred food preparation practices involving fish fermentation commonly lead to botulism.[11] In China, homemade fermented beans are the leading cause.[12] Commercial foods and restaurants are still occasional sources.[13,14] Consumption of peyote for religious reasons has resulted in botulism.[15] In the United States, 263 cases occurred due to 163 foodborne botulism events from 1990 to 2000 (17 to 43 cases per year).[16]

Infant botulism occurs with toxin types A, B, or F. In the past, infections were attributed to honey ingestion,[17] but other sources have emerged as feeding honey to infants has been discouraged.[18] In the absence of competing flora found in children and adults, *C. botulinum* colonizes the intestine of infants (ages 6 days to 12 months). Infection occurs as a consequence of absorption of toxin produced by *C. botulinum* in situ.[19] From 1992 to 2006, 2419 cases of infant botulism were identified in the United States (average, 2.1 cases per 100,000 live births).[20] Two infants without other exposures are believed to have contracted botulism through soil contamination.[21] Rare cases of infant botulism have been associated with *Clostridium baratii*[22] or *Clostridium butyricum.*[23]

Wound botulism may be caused by either type A or type B organisms. In such cases, *C. botulinum* spores contaminate the wound, leading to subsequent germination and toxin production. Almost exclusively associated with injection drug use of "black-tar" heroin, wound botulism was first reported in the United States in the 1990s. Spore contamination of heroin during preparation can lead to infection, particularly in patients who inject by "skin-popping" (i.e., drug injection into tissue rather than the vein).[24,25] More recently, black-tar heroin–related cases have also been described in Europe, including 12 cases in Germany in 2005.[26-28]

Adult botulism of unknown etiology usually involves type A toxin, but types B and F have also been implicated.[29] Affected adults become colonized with and subsequently infected by toxin-producing clostridia. Adults at risk include those with loss of bowel flora due to anatomic abnormalities, functional disorders, or antibiotic use.[30-33] Adult botulism of unknown etiology has also been attributed to types B and F[29]; in this setting, type F botulism was caused by *C. baratii.*[33]

Recently, botulinum toxin types A and B have been approved by the U.S. Food and Drug Administration (FDA) for cosmetic and therapeutic purposes (e.g., blepherospasm, strabismus, cervical dystonia). Iatrogenic botulism cases have been reported with the therapeutic[34] and unlicensed cosmetic use of botulinum toxin A.[35,36]

Rare cases of inhalational botulism have been associated with the intranasal use of contaminated cocaine.[37] Inhalation is also one of the potential routes of a bioterrorist attack with botulinum toxin (see Chapter 326). Disease due to an unusual toxin type (e.g., C, D, F, or G) or symptoms among patients with a common geographic factor may suggest an act of bioterrorism.

Characteristics of *Clostridium botulinum*

C. botulinum is a large, gram-positive, strictly anaerobic bacillus that forms a subterminal spore.[38] The species is divided into four physiologic groups. Group I organisms are proteolytic in culture and can produce toxin types A, B, and F. Group II organisms are nonproteolytic and can produce toxin types B, E, and F. Group III organisms produce toxin types C and D, and group IV produces type G. A single strain almost always produces only one toxin type. Group II organisms grow optimally between 25° and 30°C, and the other groups grow best between 30° and 37°C. Although each strain of the organism typically contains several plasmids, only type G toxin is encoded on one (e.g., *C. tetani,* in which the toxin is encoded on a plasmid).[39]

C. botulinum spores are found throughout the world in soil samples and marine sediments.[40] These spores are able to tolerate 100°C at 1 atm for several hours; because boiling renders solutions more anaerobic, it may actually favor the growth of *C. botulinum.*[41] Proper preparation of food in a pressure cooker will kill spores.

Pathogenesis

In foodborne botulism, toxin is ingested with the food in which it was produced. It is absorbed primarily in the duodenum and jejunum and passes into the bloodstream, by which it reaches peripheral cholinergic synapses (including the neuromuscular junction). In cases of wound botulism, spores are introduced into a wound, where they germinate and produce toxin. Infant botulism and probably adult botulism of unknown etiology follow ingestion of spores. Achlorhydria and antibiotic use may predispose to gastrointestinal colonization with *C. botulinum*. After inhalation, the toxin crosses through the pulmonary alveolar epithelium to gain access to the bloodstream.[42] The clinical manifestations of botulism depend on the type of toxin produced, rather than the site of its production.

Botulinum toxin is synthesized as a single polypeptide chain of low potency; the molecular weight varies from 150 to 165 kDa, depending on the toxin type. The botulinum toxins are zinc-dependent metalloproteinases,[43] as is tetanospasmin. The toxin is then nicked by a bacterial protease to produce two chains, with the light chain constituting about one third of the total mass. As with tetanospasmin, the chains remain connected by a disulfide bond. The nicked toxin type A becomes, on a molecular weight basis, the most potent toxin found in nature. In contrast to the spores, the toxin is heat labile. Different toxin types may undergo different postsynthetic processing.[44]

Once present at the synapse, the toxin prevents the release of acetylcholine (ACh). This appears to result from a three-stage process.[45] The heavy chain of the toxin mediates binding to presynaptic receptors. The nature of these receptors is uncertain; different toxin types bind to different receptors, with type B receptors outnumbering type A receptors by a factor of four.[46] The toxin enters the cell by receptor-mediated endocytosis.[47] Once inside the neuron, the toxin types differ in the mechanisms by which they inhibit ACh release.[48] The release of synaptic vesicles by an action potential is initiated by an abrupt rise in the intracellular free Ca^{2+} concentration, mediated by voltage-dependent calcium channels (Fig. 245-1).[49] This increase in free calcium triggers an interaction between synaptotagmin (in the vesicle membrane) and syntaxin (on the presynaptic cell membrane), clamping the vesicle to the presynaptic membrane. Synaptobrevin (also referred to as *vesicle-associated membrane protein*[50]) also binds to syntaxin and appears to dock the vesicle to the membrane at the proper location for fusion. There are different isoforms of synaptobrevin within neurons; a protein termed *cellubrevin* performs a similar function in non-neuronal secretory cells.[51] Synaptophysin, the third major component of this mechanism, probably forms the fusion pore that allows release of the vesicle contents into the synaptic cleft.[52]

Clostridial neurotoxins inhibit vesicle release by cleaving peptide bonds in these proteins.[53] Each toxin has a specific locus of activity. Tetanospasmin, along with botulinum neurotoxins B, D, F, and G, cleaves synaptobrevin.[54,55] Tetanospasmin and botulinum neurotoxin B appear to share the same cleavage site on synaptobrevin.[56] In contrast, botulinum toxins A[57] and E act on a 25-kDa synaptosomal-associated protein (SNAP-25),[58] and botulinum toxin C1 affects syntaxin. The toxins only affect the free proteins; once they have complexed to cause transmitter release, they are not subject to attack.[59] Synaptobrevin and synaptotagmin cleavage also occurs normally, as an effect of an endogenous protease, and these proteins are probably involved in organelle recycling.[60] The endogenous protease does not appear homologous to the clostridial toxins. However, the result is that stimulation of the presynaptic cell (e.g., the alpha motor neuron) fails to produce transmitter release, thus producing paralysis in the motor system, or autonomic dysfunction when parasympathetic nerve terminals or autonomic ganglia are involved.

Once damaged, the synapse was originally thought to be rendered useless. Because of the widespread interest in the therapeutic use of botulinum toxin, substantial research into the mechanisms of recovery is underway. The initial recovery of function in type A botulism requires sprouting of the presynaptic axon and the subsequent formation of a new synapse. Later, the original synapse recovers, and the

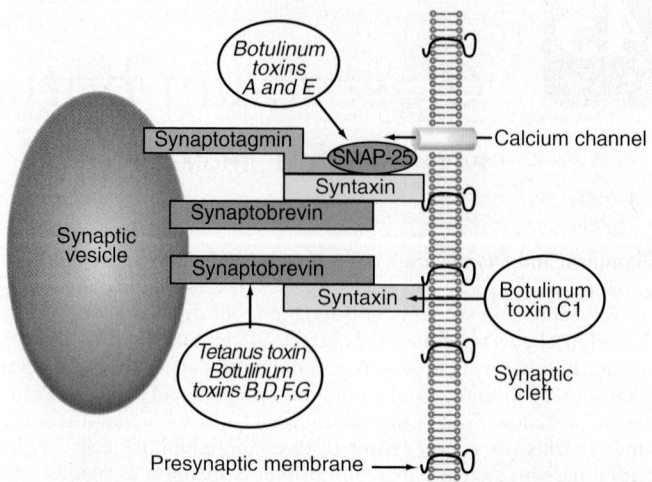

Figure 245-1 Components of the transmitter release mechanism. *(From Bleck TP, Brauner JS. Tetanus. In: Scheld WM, Whitley RJ, Durack DT, eds. Infections of the Central Nervous System. 2nd ed. New York: Raven Press; 1997:629-653.)*

newer ones are pruned away.[61] With type F botulism, recovery is substantially faster, suggesting that the original synapse regains function more rapidly.[62]

Botulinum toxin is transported within nerves in a manner analogous to tetanospasmin and can thereby gain access to the CNS. However, symptomatic CNS involvement is rare.[63]

Clinical Manifestations

The classic presentation of botulism is that of a patient who develops acute, bilateral cranial neuropathies associated with symmetrical descending weakness. The Centers for Disease Control and Prevention (CDC) suggests attention to these cardinal features: (1) fever is absent (unless a complicating infection occurs); (2) the neurologic manifestations are symmetrical; (3) the patient remains responsive; (4) the heart rate is normal or slow in the absence of hypotension; and (5) sensory deficits do not occur (except for blurred vision).[33] The first two features were important for the exclusion of poliomyelitis; rare exceptions have been noted to most of these generalizations.

Foodborne botulism usually develops between 12 and 36 hours after toxin ingestion. The patient initially complains of nausea and a dry mouth, and diarrhea may occur at this stage. Evidence of cranial nerve dysfunction most commonly starts with the eyes, reflecting parasympathetic involvement (blurred vision as a result of pupillary dilation) or involvement of cranial nerves III, IV, or VI.[64] Pupillary reactions may remain abnormal for months after motor recovery.[65] Nystagmus is occasionally noted, usually in type A disease. Lower cranial nerve dysfunction manifests as dysphagia, dysarthria, and hypoglossal weakness. Weakness then spreads to the upper extremities, the trunk, and the lower extremities. Respiratory dysfunction may result from either upper airway obstruction (the weakened glottis tending to close during attempted inspiration) or diaphragmatic weakness. Patients who need mechanical ventilation require mean periods of 58 days (type A) and 26 days (type B) for ventilatory weaning.[66] Recovery may not begin for up to 100 days.[67] Autonomic problems may include gastrointestinal dysfunction, alterations in resting heart rate, loss of responsiveness to hypotension or postural change, hypothermia, and urinary retention.[68]

Hughes summarized published reports to analyze differences in the clinical findings of intoxication with different toxin types (Table 245-1).[69] Type A is significantly more commonly associated with dysarthria, blurred vision, dyspnea, diarrhea, sore throat, dizziness, ptosis, ophthalmoplegia, facial paresis, and upper extremity weakness. Types B and E appear to produce more autonomic dysfunction. None of

TABLE 245-1	Symptoms and Signs in Patients with the Common Types of Human Botulism		
	Type A (%)	Type B (%)	Type E (%)
Neurologic Signs and Symptoms			
Dysphagia	96	97	82
Dry mouth	83	100	93
Diplopia	90	92	39
Dysarthria	100	69	50
Upper extremity weakness	86	64	NA
Lower extremity weakness	76	64	NA
Blurred vision	100	42	91
Dyspnea	91	34	88
Paresthesias	20	12	NA
Gastrointestinal Signs and Symptoms			
Constipation	73	73	52
Nausea	73	57	84
Vomiting	70	50	96
Abdominal cramps	33	46	NA
Diarrhea	35	8	39
Miscellaneous Symptoms			
Fatigue	92	69	84
Sore throat	75	39	38
Dizziness	86	30	63
Neurologic Findings			
Ptosis	96	55	46
Diminished gag reflex	81	54	NA
Ophthalmoparesis	87	46	NA
Facial paresis	84	48	NA
Tongue weakness	91	31	66
Pupils fixed or dilated	33	56	75
Nystagmus	44	4	NA
Upper extremity weakness	91	62	NA
Lower extremity weakness	82	59	NA
Ataxia	24	13	NA
DTRs diminished or absent	54	29	NA
DTRs hyperactive	12	0	NA
Initial mental status			
Alert	88	93	27
Lethargic	4	4	73
Obtunded	8	4	0

DTR, deep tendon reflex; NA, not available.
Data from references 41, 69, and 106.

these differences is diagnostic of the toxin type, however. It is important to note that the pupils are either dilated or unreactive in less than 50% of patients; although these are useful signs when present, their absence in no way diminishes the likelihood of botulism.

Patients with infant botulism present with constipation, which may be followed by feeding difficulties, hypotonia, increased drooling, and a weak cry.[70] Upper airway obstruction may be the initial sign[71] and is the major indication for intubation.[72] In severe cases, the condition progresses to include cranial neuropathies and respiratory weakness, with ventilatory failure occurring in about 50% of diagnosed patients. The condition progresses for 1 to 2 weeks and then stabilizes for another 2 to 3 weeks before recovery starts.[73] Relapses of infant botulism may occur.[74]

Infant botulism has a somewhat different pathogenesis in that it is acquired through the ingestion of spores rather than preformed toxin. The infant's intestinal flora is thought to be particularly permissive for the germination of spores, which leads to the production of toxin. The spores are acquired from environmental sources associated with areas of soil in which botulinum spore counts are high.[72]

Wound botulism lacks the prodromal gastrointestinal disorder of the foodborne form but is otherwise similar in presentation. Fever, if present, reflects wound infection rather than botulism. The wound itself may rarely appear to be healing well while neurologic manifesta-

tions are occurring. Conversely, *C. botulinum* infection may produce abscesses[75]; botulism has also been reported as a result of sinusitis with this organism after cocaine inhalation.[76] The reported incubation period varies from 4 to 14 days.

The signs and symptoms exhibited by victims of inhalational botulism are the same as those seen with ingestion. The latency between exposure and clinical disease after inhalation appears to be between 12 hours and 3 days, with maximal disease by about 5 days.[77]

Botulinum toxin has been used to treat a variety of chronic pain syndromes, achalasia, and anal fissures.[78] It has also achieved widespread notoriety for its use in cosmetic procedures. In 2004, four patients suffered from clinical symptoms of botulism after the unlicensed cosmetic use of botulinum toxin A.[35]

Diagnosis

A history appropriate to the type of botulism suspected is the most important diagnostic test. If others are already affected, the condition is easily recognized. However, because the toxin may not be evenly distributed in foodstuffs, the absence of other patients does not eliminate the diagnosis.

Botulism has a limited differential diagnosis. Myasthenia gravis and the Lambert-Eaton myasthenic syndrome (LEMS) each share some of the characteristics of botulism, but are rarely fulminant and lack autonomic features. An edrophonium test may be considered, but an improvement in strength is not pathognomonic of myasthenia gravis and has been reported in botulism.[79] Tick paralysis is excluded by a careful physical examination because the *Dermacentor* tick will still be attached. Classic acute inflammatory demyelinating polyneuropathy (AIPN; Guillain-Barré syndrome) frequently begins with sensory complaints, rapidly becomes areflexic, rarely begins with cranial nerve dysfunction, and does not alter pupillary reactivity. Patients with botulism do not become areflexic until the affected muscle group is completely paralyzed. The Miller-Fisher variant of AIPN presents with oculomotor dysfunction and may produce other cranial neuropathies but includes a prominent ataxia that is lacking in botulism. Patients with polio are febrile on presentation and have asymmetrical weakness. Magnesium intoxication may mimic botulism.[80] Rarely, botulism may be confused with diphtheria, organophosphate poisoning, or brainstem infarction.[81]

Conventional diagnosis of botulism relies on the demonstration of toxin in serum, gastric secretions, stool, or food samples. The most sensitive means of botulism toxin detection is the mouse bioassay.[82] After receiving an injection of sample, mice are followed for the development of symptoms. Toxin type may be determined by injecting infected mice with type-specific botulism antitoxin. Botulism symptoms are absent from infected mice that receive the appropriate antitoxin. Confirmation and toxin typing is obtained in almost 75% of cases.[83] The mouse bioassay is labor and resource intensive, and therefore the testing is performed in a limited number of public health laboratories. A level 2 containment facility is a minimum requirement for *C. botulinum* detection and evaluation given its potency. In addition, testing should be performed under the direction of local state or health departments or the Centers for Disease Control and Prevention (404-639-2206 or 404-639-2888) after hours.

Laboratory evaluation includes anaerobic cultures of serum, stool, and the implicated food if available. However, samples rarely yield *C. botulinum* because strict anaerobic conditions are required for growth, and competing fecal flora or nontoxigenic *C. botulinum* strains can make isolation difficult. Toxin excretion may continue up to 1 month after the onset of illness, and stool cultures may remain positive for a similar period.

Enzyme-linked immunosorbent assay has been used to detect botulinum toxin in contaminated food samples such as fish fillets, canned salmon and corned beef, pasta products, and canned vegetables.[84-87] Polymerase chain reaction may have a role as a rapid method of diagnosis, however cellular components of clinical and food samples may limit sensitivity.[88]

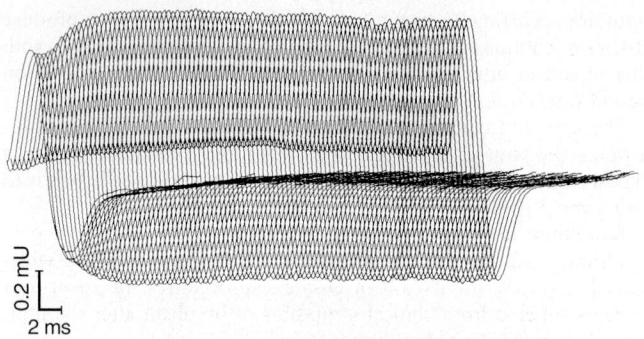

0.2 mU

2 ms

Figure 245-2 **Repetitive nerve stimulation in infant botulism.** Note the increment in response amplitude during the initial stimulations. (*Courtesy of Vern Juel, M.D., Department of Neurology and Laboratory of Electromyography, University of Virginia, Charlottesville.*)

Electrophysiologic studies reveal normal nerve conduction velocities; the amplitude of compound muscle action potentials is reduced in 85% of cases, although not all motor units may demonstrate this abnormality.[89] Repetitive nerve stimulation at high rates (20 Hz or greater, compared with the 4-Hz rate employed in the diagnosis of myasthenia gravis) may reveal a small increment in the motor response (Fig. 245-2). This test is very uncomfortable and should not be requested unless botulism or LEMS is a serious consideration. Botulism can be distinguished electrophysiologically from LEMS.[90] In infant botulism, the increments may be very dramatic. In questionable cases, single-fiber electromyography studies may be useful. There is currently some debate regarding the sensitivity of electrodiagnostic techniques in cases of infant botulism.[91] The therapeutic use of botulinum A toxin for dystonic disorders can produce electrophysiologic evidence of toxin dissemination to distant sites.[92]

If botulinum toxin is used as a biologic weapon, the diagnosis would depend on the route of exposure (see Chapter 326). Contaminated food or beverages would result in an epidemic resembling that of a natural foodborne outbreak. A deliberate release of botulinum toxin should be suspected if patients with acute flaccid paralysis and prominent bulbar palsies present in large numbers. An unusual toxin type (such as C, D, F, or G) or symptoms among patients with a common geographic location may suggest an act of bioterrorism.[77] The amount of inhaled toxin producing disease would probably not produce measurable toxin in blood or other patient samples, except perhaps for nasopharyngeal secretions.

Treatment

The importance of supportive therapy for botulism is underlined by the progressive improvement in mortality rates with advances in critical care, especially ventilatory support. The decision to intubate should be based on (1) bedside assessment of upper airway competency, and (2) changes in vital capacity (in general, an appropriately performed vital capacity measurement below 12 mL/kg frequently indicates intubation). One should not wait for the $Paco_2$ to rise or the oxygen saturation to fall before intubating the patient. In contrast to tetanus, the autonomic dysfunction of botulism is rarely life threatening, and patients who receive appropriate airway and ventilator management should recover unless complications supervene. Patients intubated with high-volume, low-pressure endotracheal tubes should not automatically undergo tracheostomy, regardless of the duration of intubation, unless required for mechanical reasons.[93] If contaminated food may still reside in the gastrointestinal tract, purgatives may be useful unless ileus has occurred. The detailed critical care management of botulism patients is beyond the scope of this text; Tacket and Rogawski have presented a useful approach.[41]

Antitoxin therapy is usually carried out with a trivalent (types A, B, and E) equine serum. Equine antitoxin is available from the CDC (510-231-7600) or state or local health departments. Its use is sup-

ported by inferential studies[94]; controlled clinical trials are lacking. Reported hypersensitivity rates vary between 9% and 20%.[95] Skin testing is performed before administering the antitoxin; a regimen for desensitization is included in the package. The standard antitoxin dose is one vial intravenously and one vial intramuscularly; although the package insert recommends repeating the dose in 4 hours in severe or progressive cases, this is not necessary.[96] A pentavalent antitoxin is available within the Department of Defense but is not available for public use. Human botulinum immune globulin (BabyBIG) was approved by the FDA in 2003 for the treatment of infant (<1 year of age) botulism. Use of BabyBIG has resulted in decreased length of intensive care unit stay, length of mechanical ventilation, and overall length of hospital stay.[97] The recommended dose is 50 mg/kg as an intravenous infusion. For suspected cases of infant botulism in any state, the California Department of Health Services, Infant Botulism Treatment and Prevention Program should be contacted (510-540-2646; http://www.infantbotulism.org). In the event of intentional dissemination of botulinum toxin, an investigational heptavalent antitoxin (ABCDEFG) may be dispensed by the Department of Defense.[77]

Patients with wound botulism should also undergo débridement, even if the wound appears to be healing well. Anaerobic cultures should be obtained at the time of surgery. The value of local instillation of antitoxin is unknown. The role of antibiotic treatment is untested, but penicillin G (10 to 20 MU daily) is frequently recommended. Metronidazole may be an effective alternative. Aminoglycosides and tetracyclines, which can impair neuron calcium entry, worsen infant botulism.[98] Lysis of *C. botulinum* in the gut by antibiotics may also increase the toxin available in infant botulism.[96] This effect has not been reported in adult cases but should be considered when gastrointestinal infection is suspected.

Agents that may improve ACh release at the neuromuscular junction have been tried in botulism without success. Guanidine has received the greatest attention.[99] Other drugs are under study.

Although the greatest improvement in muscle strength occurs in the first 3 months of recovery from botulism, patients still show improvements in strength and endurance for up to 1 year after disease onset.[77,100] With prompt attention and supportive care, the mortality rate for botulism ranges from less than 5% to 8%.[100] The mortality rate for infant botulism is less than 1%.[19]

Long-term consequences of botulism were detailed in an evaluation of 211 patients from the Republic of Georgia from 1998 to 2003. Patients interviewed at least 6 months after illness reported higher rates of fatigue, weakness, and dyspnea on exertion when compared with controls. Affected patients suffered from limitations in functional capacity and impaired psychosocial well-being.[101]

Prevention

The most important aspect of botulism prevention is proper food handling and preparation. It is impractical or undesirable to treat many foods in a manner to eliminate *C. botulinum* spores; hence, methods for the control of botulism focus on the inhibition of bacterial growth and toxin production.[96] Because the toxin is heat labile, terminal boiling or similarly intense heating of contaminated food will inactivate it. Food containers that appear to bulge may contain gas produced by *C. botulinum* and should not be opened. Other foods that appear to be spoiled should not be tasted.

In the event of an outbreak, foods suspected of being contaminated should be refrigerated until retrieval by public health personnel. Laboratory testing for botulism in the United States is only available at the CDC and several state and city public health laboratories. According to the Working Group on Civilian Biodefense, persons with potential exposure in a foodborne botulism outbreak should be monitored closely for the development of signs and symptoms; antitoxin should be administered promptly at the first signs of illness.[77]

Immunity to botulinum toxin does not develop even with severe disease, and the repeated occurrence of botulism has been reported.[102]

A pentavalent toxoid (ABCDE) vaccine is used among high-risk laboratory workers and military personnel in the United States.[103] A recombinant vaccine expressing the type A binding domain,[104] or vaccination with the carboxyl-terminal fragment,[105] promises to make vaccination less expensive and painful. Recent work suggests that inhalation of the toxin heavy chain would be immunogenic.[42]

REFERENCES

1. Hatheway CL. Bacterial sources of clostridial neurotoxins. In: Simpson LL, ed. *Botulinum Neurotoxin and Tetanus Toxin*. San Diego, CA: Academic Press; 1989:4-25.
2. Oguma K, Yokota K, Hayashi S, et al. Infant botulism due to *Clostridium botulinum* type C toxin. *Lancet*. 1990;336:1449-1450.
3. Kerner J. *Neue Beobachtungen über die in Würtemburg so haüfig vorfallen Vergiftung durch den Genuss geraüchter Würst. Tubingen, 1820. Quoted in Damon SR. Food Infections and Food Intoxications*. Baltimore: Williams & Wilkins; 1924:67.
4. Young JH. Botulism and the ripe olive scare of 1919-1920. *Bull Hist Med*. 1976;50:372-391.
5. van Ermengen E. Ueber einen neuen anaëroben Bacillus und seine Beziehungen zum Botulismus. *Z Hyg Infektionskrankh*. 1897;26:1-56.
6. Landman G. Ueber die Ursache der Darmstadter Bohnen Vergiftung. *Hyg Rundsch*. 1904;14:449-452.
7. Davis JB, Mattman LH, Wiley M. *Clostridium botulinum* in a fatal wound infection. *JAMA*. 1951;146:646-648.
8. Midura TF, Arnon SS. Infant botulism: Identification of *Clostridium botulinum* and its toxin in faeces. *Lancet*. 1976;2:934-936.
9. Chia JK, Clark JB, Ryan CA, et al. Botulism in an adult associated with food-borne intestinal infection with *Clostridium botulinum*. *N Engl J Med*. 1986;315:239-241.
10. Lamanna C, McElroy OE, Eklund HW. The purification and crystallization of *Clostridium botulinum* type A toxin. *Science*. 1946;103:613-614.
11. Shaffer N, Wainwright RB, Middaugh JP, et al. Botulism among Alaska Natives: The role of changing food preparation and consumption practices. *West J Med*. 1990;153:390-393.
12. Gao QY, Huang YF, Wu JG, et al. A review of botulism in China. *Biomed Environ Sci*. 1990;3:326-336.
13. Sheth AN, Wiersma P, Atrubin D, et al. International outbreak of severe botulism with prolonged toxemia caused by commercial carrot juice. *Clin Infect Dis*. 2008;47:1245-1251.
14. Centers for Disease Control and Prevention (CDC). Botulism associated with commercially canned chili sauce: Texas and Indiana, July 2007. *MMWR Morb Mortal Wkly Rep*. 2007;56:767-769.
15. Hashimoto H, Clyde VJ, Parko KL. Botulism from peyote. *N Engl J Med*. 1998;339:203-204.
16. Sobel J, Tucker N, Sulka A, et al. Foodborne botulism in the United States, 1990-2000. *Emerg Infect Dis*. 2004;10:1606-1611.
17. Midura TF, Snowden S, Wood RM, et al. Isolation of *Clostridium botulinum* from honey. *J Clin Microbiol*. 1979;9:282-283.
18. Spika JS, Shaffer N, Hargrett-Bean N, et al. Infant botulism in the United States: An epidemiologic study of cases occurring outside of California. *Am J Public Health*. 1983;73:1385-1388.
19. Arnon S. Infant botulism. In: Feigen RD, Cherry JD, eds. *Textbook of Pediatric Infectious Diseases*. 4th ed. Philadelphia: WB Saunders; 1998:1570-1577.
20. Koepke R, Sobel J, Arnon SS. Global occurrence of infant botulism, 1976-2006. *Pediatrics*. 2008;122:e73-82.
21. Hurst DL, Marsh WW. Early severe infantile botulism. *J Pediatr*. 1993;122:909-911.
22. Gimenez JA, Gimenez MA, DasGupta BR. Characterization of the neurotoxin isolated from a *Clostridium baratii* strain implicated in infant botulism. *Infect Immun*. 1992;60:518-522.
23. Suen JC, Hatheway CL, Steigerwalt AG, et al. Genetic confirmation of the identities of neurotoxigenic *Clostridium baratii* and *Clostridium butyricum* implicated as agents of human botulism. *J Clin Microbiol*. 1988;26:2191-2192.
24. Werner SB, Passaro DJ, McGee J, et al. Wound botulism in California, 1951-1998: a recent epidemic in heroin injectors. *Clin Infect Dis*. 2000;31:1018-1024.
25. Passaro DJ, Werner SB, McGee J, et al. Wound botulism associated with black tar heroin among injecting drug users. *JAMA*. 1998;279:859-863.
26. Kalka-Moll WM, Aurbach U, Schaumann R, et al. Wound botulism in injection drug users. *Emerg Infect Dis*. 2007;13:942-943.
27. Brett MM, Hallas G, Mpamugo O. Wound botulism in the UK and Ireland. *J Med Microbiol*. 2004;53:555-561.
28. *Update zu einer Haufung von Wundbotulismus bei injizierenden Dregenkonsumenten in Nordrhein-Westfalen Epidemiologisches Bullentin*. Berlin: Robert Koch Institut; 2005.
29. MacDonald KL, Cohen ML, Blake PA. The changing epidemiology of adult botulism in the United States. *Am J Epidemiol*. 1986;124:794-799.
30. Chia JK, Clark JB, Ryan CA, et al. Botulism in an adult associated with food-borne intestinal infection with *Clostridium botulinum*. *N Engl J Med*. 1986;315:239-241.
31. Fenicia L, Franciosa G, Pourshaban M, et al. Intestinal toxemia botulism in two young people, caused by *Clostridium butyricum* type E. *Clin Infect Dis*. 1999;29:1381-1387.
32. Griffin PM, Hatheway CL, Rosenbaum RB, et al. Endogenous antibody production to botulinum toxin in an adult with intestinal colonization botulism and underlying Crohn's disease. *J Infect Dis*. 1997;175:633-637.
33. McCroskey LM, Hatheway CL, Woodruff BA, et al. Type F botulism due to neurotoxigenic *Clostridium baratii* from an unknown source in an adult. *J Clin Microbiol*. 1991;29:2618-2620.
34. Crowner BE, Brunstrom JE, Racette BA. Iatrogenic botulism due to therapeutic botulinum toxin A injection in a pediatric patient. *Clin Neuropharmacol*. 2007;30:310-313.
35. Chertow DS, Tan ET, Maslanka SE, et al. Botulism in 4 adults following cosmetic injections with an unlicensed, highly concentrated botulinum preparation. *JAMA*. 2006;296:2476-2479.
36. Souayah N, Karim H, Kamin SS, et al. Severe botulism after focal injection of botulinum toxin. *Neurology*. 2006;67:1855-1856.
37. Roblot F, Popoff M, Carlier JP et al. Botulism in patients who inhale cocaine: the first cases in France. *Clin Infect Dis*. 2006; 43:e51-e52.
38. Cato EP, George WL, Finegold SM. Genus *Clostridium praemozski* 1880, 23AL. In: Smeath PHA, Mair NS, Sharpe ME, Holt JG, eds. Bergey's Manual of Systematic Bacteriology, vol. 2. Baltimore: Williams & Wilkins; 1986:1141-1200.
39. Eklund MW, Poysky FT, Habig WH. Bacteriophages and plasmids in *Clostridium botulinum* and Clostridium tetani and their relationship to the production of toxin. In: Simpson LL, ed. *Botulinum Neurotoxin and Tetanus Toxin*. San Diego, CA: Academic Press; 1989:25-51.
40. Hauschild AHW. Clostridium botulinum. In: Doyle MP, ed. *Foodborne Bacterial Pathogens*, New York: Marcel Dekker; 1989:112-189.
41. Tacket CO, Rogawski MA. Botulism. In: Simpson LL, ed. *Botulinum Neurotoxin and Tetanus Toxin*. San Diego, CA: Academic Press; 1989:351-378.
42. Park JB, Simpson LL. Inhalational poisoning by botulinum toxin and inhalation vaccination with its heavy-chain component. *Infect Immun*. 2003;71:1147-1154.
43. Fu FN, Lomneth RB, Cai S, et al. Role of zinc in the structure and toxic activity of botulinum neurotoxin. *Biochemistry*. 1998;37:5267-5278.
44. Critchley EMR, Mitchell JD. Human botulism. *Br J Hosp Med*. 1992;43:290-292.
45. Simpson LL. Kinetic studies on the interaction between botulinum toxin type A and the cholinergic neuromuscular junction. *J Pharmacol Exp Ther*. 1980;212:16-21.
46. Black JD, Dolly JO. Interaction of 125I-labeled botulinum neurotoxins with nerve terminals. I. Ultrastructural autoradiographic localization and quantitation of distinct membrane acceptors for types A and B on motor nerves. *J Cell Biol*. 1986;103:521-534.
47. Black JD, Dolly JO. Interaction of 125I-labeled botulinum neurotoxins with nerve terminals. II. Autoradiographic evidence for its uptake into motor nerves by receptor-mediated endocytosis. *J Cell Biol*. 1986;103:535-544.
48. Simpson LL. Peripheral actions of the botulinum toxins. In: Simpson LL, ed. *Botulinum Neurotoxin and Tetanus Toxin*. San Diego: Academic Press; 1989:153-178.
49. Bleck TP, Brauner JS. Tetanus. In: Scheld WM, Whitley RJ, Durack DT, eds. *Infections of the Central Nervous System*. 2nd ed. New York: Raven Press; 1997:629-653.
50. Trimble WS, Cowan D, Scheller RH. VAMP-1: A synaptic vesicle associated integral membrane protein. *Proc Natl Acad Sci U S A*. 1988;85:4538-4542.
51. McMahon HT, Ushkaryov YA, Edelmann L, et al. Cellubrevin is a ubiquitous tetanus-toxin substrate homologous to a putative synaptic vesicle fusion protein. *Nature*. 1993;364:346-349.
52. Buckley KM, Floor E, Kelly RB. Cloning and sequence analysis of cDNA encoding p38, a major synaptic vesicle protein. *J Cell Biol*. 1987;105:2447-2456.
53. Blasi J, Binz T, Yamasaki S, et al. Inhibition of neurotransmitter release by clostridial neurotoxins correlates with specific proteolysis of synaptosomal proteins. *J Physiol (Paris)*. 1994;88:235-241.
54. Schiavo G, Benfenati F, Poulain B, et al. Tetanus and botulinum-B neurotoxins block neurotransmitter release by proteolytic cleavage of synaptobrevin. *Nature*. 1992;359:832-835.
55. Nowakowski JL, Courtney BC, Bing QA, et al. Production of an expression system for a synaptobrevin fragment to monitor cleavage by botulinum neurotoxin B. *J Protein Chem*. 1998;17:453-462.
56. Foran P, Shone CC, Dolly JO. Differences in the protease activities of tetanus and botulinum B toxins revealed by the cleavage of vesicle-associated membrane protein and various sized fragments. *Biochemistry*. 1994;33:15365-15374.
57. Lacy DB, Tepp W, Cohen AC, et al. Crystal structure of botulinum neurotoxin type A and implications for toxicity. *Nat Struct Biol*. 1998;5:898-902.
58. Sciavo G, Santussi A, Dasgupta BR, et al. Botulinum neurotoxins serotypes A and E cleave SNAP-25 at distinct COOH-terminal peptide bonds. *FEBS Lett*. 1993;335:99-103.
59. Hayashi T, McMahon H, Yamasaki S, et al. Synaptic vesicle membrane fusion complex: Action of clostridial neurotoxins on assembly. *EMBO J*. 1994;13:5051-5061.
60. Hausinger A, Volknandt W, Zimmerman H. Calcium-dependent endogenous proteolysis of the vesicle proteins synaptobrevin and synaptotagmin. *Neuroreport*. 1995;6:637-641.
61. Meunier FA, Schiavo G, Molgo J. Botulinum neurotoxins: From paralysis to recovery of functional neuromuscular transmission. *J Physiol (Paris)*. 2002;96:1013-1015.
62. Billante CR, Zealear DL, Billante M, et al. Comparison of neuromuscular blockade and recovery with botulinum toxins A and F. *Muscle Nerve*. 2002;26:395-403.
63. Jones S, Huma Z, Haugh C, et al. Central nervous system involvement in infantile botulism. *Lancet*. 1990;335:228.
64. Terranova W, Palumbo JN, Berman JG. Ocular findings in botulism type B. *JAMA*. 1979;241:475-477.
65. Friedman DI, Fortanasce VN, Sadun AA. Tonic pupils as a result of botulism. *Am J Ophthalmol*. 1990;109:236-237.
66. Hughes JM, Blumenthal JR, Merson MH, et al. Clinical features of types A and B foodborne botulism. *Ann Intern Med*. 1981; 95:442-445.
67. Colerbatch JG, Wolff AH, Gilbert RJ, et al. Slow recovery from severe foodborne botulism. *Lancet*. 1989;2:1216-1217.
68. Vita G, Girlanda P, Puglisi RM, et al. Cardiovascular-reflex testing and single-fiber electromyography in botulism: A longitudinal study. *Arch Neurol*. 1987;44:202-206.
69. Hughes JM. Botulism. In: Scheld WM, Whitley RJ, Durack DT, ed. *Infections of the Central Nervous System*. New York: Raven Press; 1991:589-602.
70. Cornblath DR, Sladky JT, Sumner AJ. Clinical electrophysiology of infantile botulism. *Muscle Nerve*. 1983;6:448-452.
71. Oken A, Barnes S, Rock P, et al. Upper airway obstruction and infant botulism. *Anesth Analg*. 1992;75:136-138.
72. Schreiner MS, Field E, Ruddy R. Infant botulism: A review of 12 years experience at the Children's Hospital of Philadelphia. *Pediatrics*. 1991;87:159-165.
73. Angulo FJ, Getz J, Taylor JP, et al. A large outbreak of botulism: The hazardous baked potato. *J Infect Dis*. 1998;178:172-177.
74. Glauser TA, Maquire HC, Sladky JT. Relapse of infant botulism. *Ann Neurol*. 1990;28:187-189.
75. Elston HR, Wang M, Loo LK. Arm abscesses caused by *Clostridium botulinum*. *J Clin Microbiol*. 1991;29:2379-2678.
76. Kudrow DB, Henry DA, Haake DA, et al. Botulism associated with *Clostridium botulinum* sinusitis after intranasal cocaine abuse. *Ann Intern Med*. 1988;109:984-985.
77. Arnon SS, Schechter R, Inglesby TV, et al. Botulinum toxin as a biological weapon: Medical and public health management. *JAMA*. 2001;285:1059-1070.
78. Schantz EJ, Johnson EA. Botulinum toxin: The story of its development for the treatment of human disease. *Perspect Biol Med*. 1997;40:317.
79. Edell TA, Sullivan CP, Osborn KM, et al. Wound botulism associated with a positive Tensilon test. *West J Med*. 1983;139:218-219.
80. Cherington M. Botulism. *Semin Neurol*. 1990;10:27-31.
81. Dunbar EM. Botulism. *J Infect*. 1990;20:1-3.
82. Notermans S, Nagel J. Assays for botulinum and tetanus toxins. In: Simpson LL, ed. *Botulinum Neurotoxin and Tetanus Toxin*. San Diego, CA: Academic Press; 1989:319-331.
83. Dowell VR, McCroskey LM, Hatheway CL, et al. Coproexamination for botulinal toxin and *Clostridium botulinum*: A new procedure for laboratory diagnosis of botulism. *JAMA*. 1977; 238:1829-1832.
84. Roman, MG, Humber JY, Hall PA et al. Amplified immunoassay ELISA-ELCA for measuring *Clostridium botulinum* type E neurotoxin in fish fillets. *J Food Prot*. 1994;57:985-990.
85. Shone CC, Wilton-Smith P, Appleton N et al. Monoclonal antibody-based immunoassay for type A *Clostridium botulinum* toxin is comparable to the mouse bioassay. *Appl Environ Microbiol*. 1985;50:63-67.
86. Del Torre M, Stecchini ML, Peck MW. Investigation of the ability of proteolytic *Clostridium botulinum* to multiply and produce toxin in fresh Italian pasta. *J Food Prot*. 1998;61:988-993.
87. Rodriguez A, Dezfulian M. Rapid identification of *Clostridium botulinum* and botulinal toxin in food. *Folia Microbiol*. 1997;42:149-151.
88. Lindstrom M, Korleala H. Laboratory diagnosis of botulism. *Clin Microbiol Rev*. 2006;19:298-314.
89. Cherington M. Electrophysiologic methods as an aid in diagnosis of botulism: A review. *Muscle Nerve*. 1982;6:528-529.
90. Gutmann L, Pratt L. Pathophysiologic aspects of human botulism. *Arch Neurol*. 1976;33:175-179.
91. Graf W, Hays RM, Astley SJ, et al. Electrodiagnosis reliability in the diagnosis of infant botulism. *J Pediatr*. 1992;120:747-749.
92. Buchman AS, Comella CL, Stebbins GT, et al. Quantitative electromyographic analysis of changes in muscle activity following

botulinum toxin therapy for cervical dystonia. *Clin Neuropharmacol.* 1993;16:205-210.

93. Barrett DH. Endemic food-borne botulism: Clinical experience, 1973-1986. *Alaska Med.* 1991;33:101-108.

94. Tacket CO, Shandera WX, Mann JM, et al. Equine antitoxin use and other factors that predict outcome in type A foodborne botulism. *Am J Med.* 1984;76:794-798.

95. Black RE, Gunn RA. Hypersensitivity reactions associated with botulinal antitoxin. *Am J Med.* 1980;69:567-570.

96. Centers for Disease Control and Prevention. *Botulism in the United States 1899-1996: Handbook for Epidemiologists, Clinicians, and Laboratory Workers (draft).* Atlanta: Centers for Disease Control and Prevention; 1998.

97. Underwood K, Rubin S, Deakers T, et al. Infant botulism: a 30-year experience spanning the introduction of botulism immune globulin intravenous in the intensive care unit at Children's Hospital Los Angeles. *Pediatrics.* 2007;120:e1380-1385.

98. Wilson R, Morris JG, Snyder JD, et al. Clinical characteristics of infant botulism in the United States: A study of the non-California cases. *Pediatr Infect Dis.* 1982;1:148-150.

99. Kaplan JE, Davis LE, Narayan V, et al. Botulism, type A, and treatment with guanidine. *Ann Neurol.* 1979;6:69-71.

100. Wilcox PG, Morrison NJ, Pardy RL. Recovery of the ventilatory and upper airway muscles and exercise performance after type A botulism. *Chest.* 1990;98:620-626.

101. Gottlieb SL, Kretsinger K, Tarkhashvili N, et al. Long-Term Outcomes of 217 Botulism Cases in the Republic of Georgia. *Clin Infect Dis.* 2007;45:174-180.

102. Beller M, Middaugh JP. Repeated type E botulism in an Alaskan Eskimo. *N Engl J Med.* 1990;322:855.

103. Siegel LS. Human immune response to botulinum pentavalent (ABCDE) toxoid determined by a neutralization test and by an enzyme-linked immunosorbent assay. *J Clin Microbiol.* 1988;26:2351-2356.

104. Byrne MP, Smith TJ, Montgomery VA, et al. Purification, potency, and efficacy of the botulinum neurotoxin type A binding domain from Pichia pastoris as a recombinant vaccine candidate. *Infect Immun.* 1998;66:4817-4822.

105. Oshima M, Hayakari M, Middlebrook JL, et al. Immune recognition of botulinum neurotoxin type A: Regions recognized by T cells and antibodies against the protective H(C) fragment (residues 855-1296) of the toxin. *Mol Immunol.* 1997;34:1031-1040.

106. Weber JT, Hibbs RG, Darwish A, et al. A massive outbreak of type E botulism associated with traditional salted fish in Cairo. *J Infect Dis.* 1993;167:451-454.

246

Gas Gangrene and Other *Clostridium*-Associated Diseases

ANDREW B. ONDERDONK | WENDY S. GARRETT

Introduction

The genus *Clostridium* includes over 200 described species. Members of this genus participate in a variety of invasive and toxigenic processes and can cause disease that is strictly toxin mediated, such as antibiotic-associated colitis (AAC) and food-borne botulism, or they can contribute to invasive infections including bacteremia, clostridial myonecrosis (gas gangrene), and other suppurative infections resulting from the production of histotoxins and enzymes that destroy soft tissue. Historically, clostridial infections were recognized as discrete clinical syndromes well before the germ theory of disease was proposed. The clinical features of tetanus were well described by some of the earliest medical writers, such as Hippocrates, and the toxic nature of this species was noted as early as the 1870s.[1] Clostridia are often isolated as part of a mixed microflora during suppurative infections that occur as a result of fecal or soil contamination of otherwise sterile tissue. Prior to 1977, the most commonly reported clostridial infections and intoxications were those caused by *C. perfringens*. Other species, most notably *C. tetani* in nonimmunized individuals (see Chapter 243) and *C. botulinum* (see Chapter 244), also generated considerable interest due to the severity and often fatal nature of the intoxications they caused. With the discovery of the etiology of AAC first in an animal model[2] and subsequently in humans,[3] it soon became clear that in the antibiotic era, *C. difficile* was the most common clostridial species associated with human disease (CDAD). Within the hospital setting, AAC has become a significant worldwide nosocomial infection problem,[4] resulting in both toxin-mediated diarrheal disease and more fulminant presentations such as pseudomembranous enterocolitis and toxic megacolon. Recent recognition that more virulent strains of *C. difficile* occur in health care settings has provoked an increased awareness of this nosocomial infection and has prompted a demand for both rapid methods for diagnosis and more aggressive treatment of AAC.[5-7] While the well-recognized pathogenic members of the genus *Clostridium* continue to participate in a broad array of infectious processes, it is also important to note the important roles that previously obscure species, such as *C. difficile*, play in human disease.

Characteristics of *Clostridium* spp.

Members of this genus are phenotypically characterized as anaerobic, gram-positive rods that are capable of forming endospores. *Clostridium* spp. are ubiquitous in nature, found in soils and sediments throughout the world and as members of the intestinal microflora of humans and most other animals. It has been reported that over 70% of humans are colonized with clostridia at concentrations of 10^8 to 10^9 organisms per gram of feces.[8] *Clostridia* can also be isolated as part of vaginal microflora of healthy women,[9] although they tend to be transient members of the vaginal microflora, occurring in low numbers as a result of contamination by intestinal microflora rather than as part of the autochthonous community. Most members of this genus are obligate anaerobes, while strains of a few species such as *C. tertium*, *C. histolyticum*, *C. innocuum*, and *C. perfringens* are aerotolerant and can be confused with members of the genus *Bacillus* during laboratory diagnosis. Based on 16S rDNA sequence data, members of the genus *Clostridium* are part of the phylum *Firmicutes*, a diverse group of gram-positive organisms including both spore-forming and non-spore-forming genera. Based on 16S rDNA sequence analysis, the clostridia can be divided into 11 homology groups, with most of the clinically significant species belonging to homology group 1.[10] Traditional classification methods for the clostridia rely on carbohydrate fermentation profiles, detection of short-chain fatty acid end products of fermentation, Gram-stain morphology, colony morphology on agar media, and detection of specific toxins. Although many different species have been isolated from human clinical material, only a small number of species are regularly associated with human disease (Table 246-1).

Microscopically, the vegetative cells of *Clostridium* species are rod-shaped, often pleomorphic, and found as short chains, clusters, or in pairs. The cells of most species have rounded ends. This may vary with some species, which show more pointed ends (*C. ramosum*). Some species form long chains (*C. spiroforme*), which may be tightly packed to form coils. *Clostridia* usually stain gram-positively in young cultures (*C. perfringens*; Fig. 246-1A), with some species losing this staining characteristic in older cultures (*C. novyi*; see Fig. 246-1B). Species, such as *C. clostridioforme* and *C. ramosum*, rarely show the typical gram-positive appearance and present as gram-variable or gram-negative rods (see Fig. 246-1C). When spores are present, they tend to be ovoid or spherical, with the spore often distending the vegetative cell to produce a club-shaped appearance. Spores may be located centrally, subterminally, or as terminal structures, depending on the species. Spore location is used as part of the identification process. Most clostridia are motile by virtue of peritrichous flagellae, with the notable exception of the common clinical isolates, *C. perfringens* and *C. ramosum*.[10]

Clostridium spp. have diverse metabolic pathways and can be saccharolytic, proteolytic, both, or neither. *Clostridium* spp. are not known to reduce sulfate. The end products of fermentative metabolism are mixtures of short-chain fatty acids and alcohols, a characteristic that can be used for identification purposes in the clinical laboratory. Aerotolerant strains of clostridia do not form spores in the presence of oxygen, they are catalase negative, and they grow more abundantly under anaerobic conditions. Clostridia do not have a complete cytochrome system and are therefore oxidase negative.[10] Most strains are catalase and superoxide dismutase negative, although trace amounts of activity have been reported for some species. Clostridia produce a variety of biologically active proteins, including hemolysins, proteolytic enzymes, and other toxins. It is the protein toxins produced by clostridia that account for their importance in human disease. Clostridia produce a greater diversity of toxins than any other genera of bacteria.[10] These include neurotoxins, enterotoxins, collagenases, proteases, and other necrotoxins, lecithinases, lipases, DNases, and neuraminidases. The potency of some of these toxins, such as botulinum neurotoxin (BoNT) and tetanus neurotoxin (TeNT) render them among the most lethal substances yet described; less than 0.2 ng of purified toxin is fatal in mice. (See Chapters 243 and 244.)

Invasive infections caused by clostridia are invariably due to organisms that are either part of the normal intestinal and vaginal microflora or acquired by a traumatic injury that breaches the skin, which then becomes contaminated with soil, unsanitary water, or fecal material. Intoxications can occur either in response to endogenous toxin production, such as that associated with CDAD, or by ingestion of preformed toxins contaminating food, as is the case for noninfant

TABLE 246-1	Clostridial Species Commonly Associated with Human Disease					
Species	Spore Location	Lecithinase Produced	Lipase	Enterotoxins Produced	Histotoxins, Hemolysins, Proteases	Neurotoxins Produced
Tissue Infections						
C. perfringens	ST, C	+	—	Yes	Yes	No
C. ramosum	T	—	—	No	Yes	No
C. septicum	ST	—	—	No	Yes	No
C. sordellii	ST	+	—	No	Yes	No
C. bifermentans	ST	+	—	No	Yes	No
C. tertium	T	—	—	No	Yes	No
C. sphenoides	ST	—	—	No	Yes	No
C. baratii	ST	—	—	No	Yes	No
C. novyi	ST	+	+	No	Yes	No
C. histolyticum	ST	—	—	No	Yes	No
Intoxications						
C. difficile	ST	—	—	Yes	Yes	No
C. botulinum	ST, T	—	+	No	Yes	Yes
C. tetani	T	—	—	No	Yes	Yes

botulism. With the exception of environmental spread of *C. difficile* within a susceptible population, such as hospitalized patients on broad-spectrum antibiotic therapy and residents in nursing homes, clostridia rarely cause infection through person-to-person contact.

The spores of clostridia account for their persistence in hostile environments and also their exogenous acquisition by humans. In addition to their long-term survival in soil or food, clostridial spores may spread via aerosol transmission as part of naturally occurring dust clouds. *C. difficile* is of particular concern because this species may be part of the intestinal microflora of an individual or acquired through contact with individuals or contaminated surfaces and equipment within the hospital environment harboring spores. The vegetative cells of clostridia are generally susceptible to routinely used disinfectants, but spores can survive hostile environments, including heat, desiccation, and exposure to many commonly used disinfectants.[11-13] This allows pathogenic clostridia to persist in an environment, even following routine disinfection procedures. Methods for eliminating clostridial spores from some environments, such as *C. difficile* in the hospital setting, include finding methods to promote germination of the spores so the vegetative cells can be destroyed.[11,14]

Major Infections and Intoxications

CLOSTRIDIUM DIFFICILE–ASSOCIATED DISEASE (CDAD) (see Chapter 96)

Historical Perspective
Until it was identified as the primary cause of antibiotic-associated colitis in 1977, *C. difficile* was not regarded as a particularly important pathogen; however, the association of *C. difficile* with AAC has brought this organism to prominence as the most common clostridial species associated with human disease. Hall and O'Toole published the first description of *C. difficile* in 1935 and suggested that it might be involved in intestinal disease in children.[15] Interestingly, the clinical description of pseudomembranous colitis dates to the 1890s. An animal model for antibiotic-associated intestinal disease was first reported in the 1940s, with several additional observations on the induction of bowel inflammation by antibiotics in hamsters, guinea pigs, and rabbits made in the 1950s. The occurrence of pseudomembranous colitis in patients receiving broad-spectrum antibiotics before the 1970s was not uncommon. Based on laboratory analysis, it was often attributed to *Staphylococcus aureus,* one of the major nosocomial pathogens of the antibiotic era. Cultures of stool from these patients often yielded high levels of *S. aureus,* but obligately anaerobic organisms were not evaluated in these early studies. Given the common isolation of *S. aureus* from stool samples obtained from healthy indi-

viduals, these earlier observations were something of a self-fulfilling prophecy. While certain strains of *S. aureus* produce potent enterotoxins that may be responsible for some cases of AAC, there is little evidence to suggest that this species is a common cause of pseudomembranous colitis.

In 1974, investigators in St. Louis noted that about 20% of patients receiving the lincosamide antibiotic clindamycin developed diarrhea, and half of these patients had pseudomembranous colitis when examined endoscopically.[16] Publication of these observations set the stage for more detailed examination of the role of antibiotics in the occurrence of pseudomembranous colitis and led to the search for an etiologic agent. The breakthrough that ultimately led to identification of *C. difficile* as the causative agent of CDAD involved a hamster model of AAC demonstrating that vancomycin could prevent the occurrence of AAC induced by clindamycin, suggesting that a gram-positive organism was involved in the hamster disease.[17] Armed with this information and the knowledge that the disease appeared to be toxin-mediated, these same investigators isolated clostridial species from the ceca of hamsters with AAC and showed that one species, *C. difficile,* was capable of causing disease in other hamsters as pure cultures or culture filtrates in the absence of prior antibiotic exposure. The link to human disease was made when the same toxin isolated from the hamster model was found in stools of AAD patients using a combination of cytotoxicity assays and an anticlostridial antibody capable of neutralizing the cytotoxin.[18] Vancomycin remains the antibiotic of choice for treating serious CDAD in humans, and the same cytotoxicity assay used to correlate animal and human disease remains the gold standard for diagnostic assays.

Clinical Manifestations
The clinical manifestations of CDAD range from a self-limiting diarrheal disease that disappears when antibiotics are discontinued to fulminant presentations with characteristic pseudomembranes within the large intestine and progression to toxic megacolon, often with fatal complications.[19] Pseudomembranes, however, are not pathognomonic for CDAD and may also occur in AAD not caused by *C. difficile.*[20,21] Symptoms may occur while patients are receiving antibiotics, usually after 5 to 10 days of therapy, or can occur 2 to 10 weeks after antibiotic therapy has been completed.[22] All classes of antibiotics have been associated with CDAD, including the penicillins, cephalosporins, macrolides, lincosamides, and aminoglycosides. Diarrhea accompanied by fever occurs in most patients and resembles the symptoms caused by many other intestinal pathogens. In severe cases, bloody diarrhea may be present. Diarrhea is often accompanied by bloating and cramping. Leukocytosis is not uncommon. CDAD is more common in the elderly and in hospitalized patients receiving broad-spectrum antibiotic

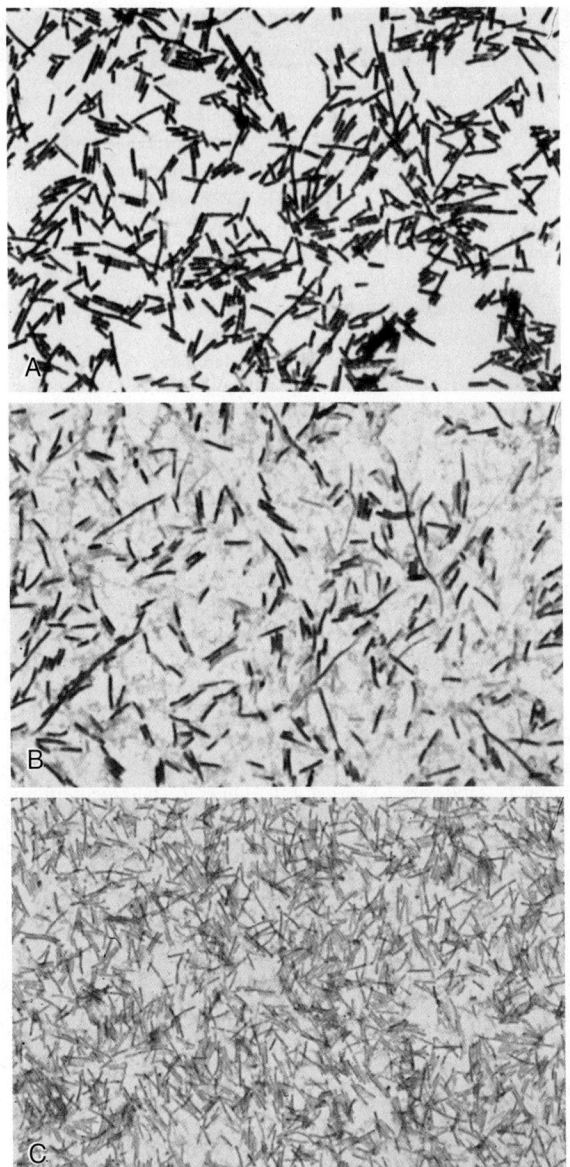

Figure 246-1 Gram stain characteristics of *Clostridium* sp.
A, *C. perfringens*. **B**, *C. novyi*. **C**, *C. ramosum*.

therapy. When surgical intervention is required for severe disease, colostomy carries a substantial risk of mortality regardless of the age of the patient.[23]

Molecular Pathogenesis

The initiating event for CDAD involves the disruption of the intestinal microbiota during treatment with antibiotics. While it is not uncommon for mild diarrhea to occur simply due to the disruption of the microbiota when broad-spectrum antibiotics are used, the presence of *C. difficile* in the intestine can lead to a more serious disease. Because *C. difficile* spores can survive even high concentrations of antibiotics, germination of spores and rapid growth of the organism may occur as antibiotic levels in the lumen of the bowel decrease below inhibitory concentrations for *C. difficile* before the recovery of the normal microbiota. The virulence of *C. difficile* is due to production of two large molecular weight toxins, TcdA and TcdB, originally described as an enterotoxin and a cytotoxin, respectively. Intestinal epithelial cells endocytose the toxins, and once internalized, the toxins irreversibly glucosylate members of the Rho family of small GTP-binding proteins. As a result, there are major alterations in the actin cytoskeleton. These changes lead to the characteristic cytotoxic effects noted in cell culture by compromising the cell's ability to internalize nutrients and carry out vesicular transport, both of which may lead to cell death. The genes for TcdA, TcdB, and an RNA polymerase sigma factor, TcdR, are carried as a pathogenicity locus. In addition, TcdC, a gene that down-regulates toxin production by interfering with TcdR, is part of this locus.[5,24-26] Hypervirulent toxin-producing strains, with a deletion in the TcdC gene, have been reported and account for the current concerns about more virulent CDAD. Deletions in the TcdC gene can contribute to unregulated toxin production resulting in much higher levels of toxin being produced. A particular outbreak-associated ribotype, O27/NAP1, is attributed with causing many cases of severe disease. Alterations in the TcdC gene have been noted in multiple ribotypes, with the O27 ribotype currently the most commonly associated with TcdC deletions.[27] In addition to the two major toxins, TcdA and TcdB, a binary ADP ribosylating toxin, CDT, a common A-B toxin motif for many clostridial species, has been reported to contribute to the occurrence of more severe CDAD.[27-30] Not all strains of *C. difficile* produce all three toxins (TcdA, TcdB, and CDT). Surveillance studies indicate that strains producing both TcdA and TcdB are most common, occurring in about 65% of strains, with TcdB (cytotoxin) produced by 97% of all strains evaluated. This likely accounts for the use of the cytotoxicity assay as a diagnostic method before the full range of toxins produced by *C. difficile* was appreciated.

Treatment and Diagnosis

Less serious presentations of CDAD have been treated with metronidazole since the late 1990s, with vancomycin reserved for treatment of serious or progressive disease (see Chapter 96).[31] Adjunct therapy using probiotics to reconstitute the normal microflora of the intestine or anion exchange resins that bind toxin have been proposed, but they appear to be of limited value and may be harmful for the patient.[31,32] The successful use of fecal bacteriotherapy has also been reported for CDAD, although it is rarely employed.[33]

Of particular concern is the recurrence of CDAD once appropriate therapy has been discontinued. This is thought to be due to the survival of the biologically inert spores during therapy and regrowth of the vegetative cells once therapy is discontinued. It has been shown in gnotobiotic mice that the concentrations of *C. difficile* can be suppressed by vancomycin but that low levels of spores survived during treatment. The concentration of *C. difficile* returned to pretreatment levels once therapy was discontinued, indicating that the spores survived antibiotic treatment and germinated when antibiotic levels declined.[34]

Laboratory diagnosis of CDAD is generally done by detection of toxin in the stool specimens of patients suspected of having disease. While culture can be performed to isolate *C. difficile*, the presence of the organism does not necessarily mean CDAD is present, because up to 4% of overtly healthy adults may carry this organism as part of their normal intestinal microflora. Initially, the cytotoxicity assay for TcdB was used to diagnose CDAD. In this assay, a monolayer cell culture is exposed to a filtrate of stool for 24 to 48 hours and examined for the characteristic cytopathic effect of TcdB. If detected, a portion of the filtrate is mixed with antibody to TcdB, and a second cell culture is used to determine if the cytopathic effect can be neutralized. While this is a very sensitive assay, the time required to make a definitive diagnosis is often 48 to 72 hours. Currently, there are a variety of enzyme immunoassays (EIA) available to provide rapid detection of both TcdA and TcdB. Assay sensitivity ranges from less than 50% to better than 93%, depending on the assay used, while assay specificity is usually greater than 90%.[35,36] Most EIA assays include detection of both TcdA and TcdB, because it is known that some strains produce one toxin but not the other. While the prevalence of CDAD varies depending on patient demographics, one large Boston teaching hospital performed over 7800 EIA assays in 2007, with over 10% yielding positive results for one or both toxins (ABO, unpublished data). PCR assays designed to detect the genes associated with toxin production are also available, although none are currently FDA approved for diagnostic use.

While *C. difficile* is responsible for many cases of antibiotic-associated diarrhea, it is not the only cause. Other clostridial species such as *C. perfringens* and *C. sordellii* are also capable of producing enterotoxins under similar circumstances that lead to diarrheal disease during antibiotic therapy.[21] Therefore, a negative assay for *C. difficile* toxins does not preclude the involvement of other clostridial species in the clinical manifestations.

When cultured on selective agar media, *C. difficile* can be readily isolated from stool samples. The colonies are generally flat, 4 to 6 mm in diameter, gray in color, with irregular margins and a ground-glass appearance. A distinctive "barnyard" odor is often detected from cultures grown on blood agar media as a result of production of *p*-cresol. Gram stain of colony growth usually shows gram-positive to gram-variable somewhat slender rods, with subterminal spores when present (Fig. 246-2). Definitive identification requires both fermentation profiles and analysis of short-chain fatty acid end products of fermentation.

It is extremely important for appropriate infection control measures to be implemented within the hospital or nursing home environment for patients diagnosed with CDAD. These measures include the rapid diagnosis of CDAD in patients on antibiotic therapy, contact precautions for patients with CDAD, appropriate therapy, and more rigorous cleaning of rooms between patient admissions.[6]

CDAD: An Emerging Public Health Crisis

The incidence of hospital-based CDAD diagnoses has skyrocketed. There was an 117% increase in the listing of CDAD on hospital discharges in the Healthcare Costs and Utilization Project Net website from 2000 to 2005.[37,38] CDAD-related death rates have steadily increased as well over the past decade. A recent study by Redelings and colleagues reported a 35% increase in mortality rates from 1999 (5.7 per million U.S. population) to 2004 (23.7 per million U.S. population).[39] Similar mortality trends have been observed in Great Britain.[40] Numerous recent studies underscore the importance of the observation that CDAD represents a major public health concern requiring increased prevention, surveillance, and reporting.

CLOSTRIDIUM PERFRINGENS AND CLOSTRIDIAL MYONECROSIS (GAS GANGRENE)

Clostridial myonecrosis, or gas gangrene, is most often caused by a traumatic injury that becomes contaminated with clostridial spores from species that cause myonecrosis, most commonly those of *C. perfringens*. Throughout history, cases of gas gangrene have increased during times of human conflict due to the numbers of traumatic injuries provoked during violent conflict. Although other clostridial species can and do cause gas gangrene, the prevalence of *C. perfringens*

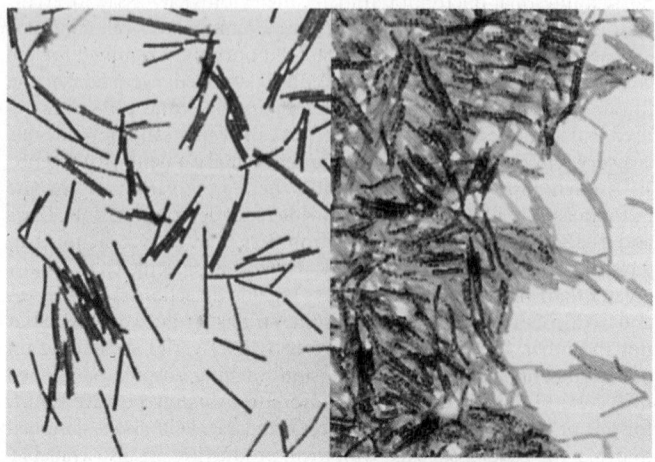

Figure 246-2 Gram stains of *C. difficile*.

TABLE 246-2	Toxins Produced by *C. perfringens*	
Toxin	*Strain types*	*Biologic Activity*
α	All strains	Lecithinase
β	B and C	Necrotoxin, necrosis of the bowel
ε	B and D	Lethal, hemorrhagic
ι	E	ADP ribosylating; lethal
cpe enterotoxin	A, C and D	Cytopathic
Neuraminidase	All strains	Hydrolyses *N*-acetylneuraminic acid
δ	B and C	Hemolysins
κ	All strains	Collagenase
λ	B, D and E	Protease
μ	All strains	Hyaluronidase
ν	All strains	DNAase

in such infections marks it as one of the major clostridial pathogens. *C. perfringens* can be isolated from soil and sediment samples from any geographic region. It is also one of the most common clostridial species isolated from the intestinal tract of humans and other animals. The ability of *C. perfringens* to cause myonecrosis is due to the production of a variety of protein toxins. Since strains of *C. perfringens* vary in their ability to produce some of the major toxins, this attribute differentiates this species into strain types (Table 246-2). Epidemiologically, *C. perfringens* type A is most common in human stool,[41] with other types more commonly associated with food poisoning and other enterotoxigenic disease (see following). Gas gangrene, while most often associated with *C. perfringens,* can be caused by other species including *C. septicum, C. sordellii, C. novyi, C. bifermentans,* and *C. histolyticum.* The common denominator for all of these species is the production of exotoxins, most often lecithinase, that devitalize tissue and promote invasive disease and myonecrosis.

Pathogenesis

All strains of *C. perfringens* produce α-toxin, a lecithinase that causes damage to cell membranes. During severe sepsis with *C. perfringens*, rapid hemolytic anemia may occur due to hemolysis caused by the α-toxin. The α-toxin is considered the major lethal toxin produced by *C. perfringens* during gas gangrene. In addition to the α-toxin, most strains produce additional hemolysins, proteases, collagenase, hyaluronidase, Dnase, and neuraminidase.

Gas gangrene is most common following traumatic injuries that result in lowered tissue oxygen tension such as crushing or penetrating injuries; the presence of foreign bodies, including soil or pieces of the object causing penetrating trauma; and mixed infections containing other organisms capable of reducing the oxygen levels at the site of infection. Studies of wounds occurring on the battlefield indicate that most are contaminated by clostridial spores, yet only a small percentage of these contaminated wounds result in clostridial myonecrosis. In the civilian population, approximately 10% of crushing wounds that occur as a result of automobile accidents have been shown to contain clostridial spores.[42] Clostridial myonecrosis may also occur following surgery, most often of the gastrointestinal or biliary tract, and following septic abortions. Contamination of lesions where vascular insufficiency is present, such as diabetic foot ulcers, the occurrence of damaged tissue associated with burns, and underlying neoplastic disease, may also contribute to the occurrence of gas gangrene.[43] Infections of the central nervous system are rare, but they do occur.[44]

Diagnosis and Treatment

Clinically, clostridial myonecrosis generally begins within 24 to 72 hours after traumatic injury or surgery. Initial symptoms may include severe pain in the absence of obvious physical findings, suggesting a deep tissue infection. When traumatic injuries penetrate the skin, redness at the site of the wound followed by a rapidly spreading brown to purple discoloration of the skin is often seen. The progression of gas gangrene is rapid, and within hours of the initial symptoms, edema and gas may be detected within the underlying tissues by physical examination, ultrasound, or radiographic evaluation. Hemorrhagic bullae may occur, along with a serosanguineous discharge and characteristic odor often described as "mousy." The odor is distinct from the putrid odor resulting from the production of volatile amines associated with gram-negative anaerobic infections. Gram stain of the discharge often reveals the typical gram-positive boxcar-shaped rods characteristic of *C. perfringens* (see Fig. 246-1A). Neutrophils are often not seen on Gram stain due to the lethal nature of α-toxin for these polymorphonuclear cells.[45] Gas gangrene leads to profound ischemia resulting from obstructed microvascular circulation caused by platelet aggregation within vessels and fibrin deposition. Unlike most soft tissue infections where the inflammatory process increases blood flow, lesions resulting from clostridial myonecrosis do not bleed readily.[46] These pro-ischemic properties are attributed to the α-toxin of *C. perfringens* and *C. septicum*, both of which have similar biologic activity. The *theta* toxin of *C. perfringens*, perfringolysin O, may also act synergistically with α-toxin to decrease microvascular perfusion. The toxins can also result in systemic hematologic derangements such as disseminated intravascular coagulation. Fever is often minimal during the early stages of disease, but progression to full-blown sepsis with its classic hypotension, renal failure, and metabolic acidosis may set in rapidly.

Rapid diagnosis of clostridial myonecrosis is critical for proper therapeutic intervention. Clinical signs such as severe pain at the site of the traumatic injury, tachycardia in the absence of fever and obvious systemic toxicity accompanied by edema, discoloration of the skin, appearance of hemorrhagic bullae, and gas detected within the tissues are typical findings. Gram stain of fluids or exudates showing the typical boxcar-shaped gram-positive rods and few polymorphonuclear cells are often the earliest laboratory findings. Spores are not seen in Gram stains of clinical specimens. Growth of *C. perfringens* on blood agar plates is rapid, with colonies often detected within 12 to 16 hours of inoculation. Colonies are yellowish to gray and opaque, 4 to 8 mm in diameter, with irregular borders and exhibit a characteristic double zone of hemolysis with an inner zone of β hemolysis surrounded by an outer zone of partial hemolysis. The lecithinase or α-toxin can be detected by growth on egg yolk agar medium, which is rich in triglycerides. An obvious white precipitation surrounding colonies is evidence of lecithinase production. Neutralization of this reaction by specific antisera—the Nagler reaction—is presumptive evidence for the identification of *C. perfringens*. Most clinical microbiology laboratories use a combination of fermentation reactions and detection of short-chain fatty acid end products for definitive identification of *Clostridium* spp. Although not widely used at present by clinical microbiology laboratories, rapid PCR methods for identification of *C. perfringens* are available.[47]

The most important part of therapy for clostridial myonecrosis is prompt surgical débridement of infected tissues. When the abdominal wall is involved, débridement of the affected muscle with generous resection margins of apparently healthy tissue is important to prevent recurrence or progression of infection. For extremities, amputation or extensive débridement is appropriate. Uterine gas gangrene most often requires hysterectomy. Early antibiotic intervention is essential for survival, and penicillin remains the most commonly employed antibiotic.[48] Although there is some concern regarding the continued susceptibility of *C. perfringens* to penicillin, most strains tested are susceptible to easily achieved levels. Other agents, including metronidazole, clindamycin, and the carbapenems, can also be used for treating clostridial myonecrosis. *C. perfringens* remains susceptible to most frontline antimicrobial agents, although resistance to antibiotics such as clindamycin has been reported.[49] The role of hyperbaric oxygen treatment as adjunctive therapy remains controversial[48,50] (see Chapter 43), as a result of the nature of the compromised tissue perfusion attributable to clostridial-driven microvascular damage. Some clinicians argue that hyperbaric oxygen treatment makes it easier to identify viable tissue, which decreases the need for more extensive surgical débridement. Other adjunctive therapy includes the use of G-CSF to stimulate hematopoietic proliferation. While some cases of clostridial myonecrosis have been successfully treated with surgical débridement and hyperbaric oxygen alone, inclusion of aggressive antibiotic therapy early in the course of treatment increases survival rates, particularly when combined with aggressive surgical débridement, and is considered the best therapeutic intervention.[48]

FOOD POISONING CAUSED BY *CLOSTRIDIUM* SP.

C. perfringens type A causes virtually all cases of clostridial food poisoning throughout the world. Contaminated food products that are not properly cooked or stored allow for the proliferation of large numbers of vegetative *C. perfringens* cells. Once consumed, the vegetative cells sporulate within the small intestine, releasing an enterotoxin that causes the characteristic symptoms. The enterotoxin appears to be a cytotoxin in that it causes demonstrable damage to mammalian cells. The enterotoxin is a small polypeptide with a molecular weight of about 35 kDa. The toxin causes fluid accumulation in the rabbit ileal loop assay, provokes vomiting with orogastric challenge in experimental animals, and produces a characteristic cytopathic effect in Vero and other cell lines.[21,51] The enterotoxin gene *cpe* can be used to detect disease-causing strains. There is some evidence that the *cpe* gene can be carried on a plasmid and spread from one *C. perfringens* strain to another. More recently, the association between some cases of presumed antibiotic-associated colitis and *C. perfringens* enterotoxin have been reported.[21]

C. perfringens food poisoning requires the ingestion of at least 10^8 viable enterotoxin-producing cells and occurs most often following the consumption of inadequately cooked and stored food. Meat and meat-containing foods are the most commonly implicated sources. Most cases occur as a common-source outbreak, usually involving commercially prepared foods and on average involve more than 20 affected individuals. Unlike *S. aureus* food poisoning and salmonellosis, home outbreaks appear to be uncommon. However, this may only reflect the fact that individual illnesses are not as likely to be identified as food poisoning when compared with group illnesses involving large numbers of people.

The incubation period for *C. perfringens* food poisoning is short, generally between 7 and 15 hours with a range of 6 to 24 hours. Symptoms include watery diarrhea, abdominal cramping, vomiting, and fever. Cases resolve spontaneously within 24 to 48 hours. When disease is suspected, culture of suspected food or stool from affected individuals is recommended, with quantitative determination of the number of *C. perfringens* present serving as a presumptive diagnostic indicator. If the isolated organisms are present at concentrations exceeding 10^6 cfu/g and the toxin gene is detected, *C. perfringens* type A is presumed to be the cause of the outbreak. Detection of the enterotoxin using a cytopathic toxin assay with neutralization can also be used as a diagnostic test. Some public health laboratories also use latex agglutination or EIA assays for detecting the enterotoxin.

Other Clostridial Infections

BACTEREMIA

Although obligate anaerobes are infrequently isolated from bacteremic patients, *Clostridia* are second only to *Bacteroides* among anaerobes isolated from blood cultures, accounting for approximately 1% of all positive cultures.[52,53] Blood culture data for a large Boston teaching hospital show that over a 5-year period, from 2003 to 2007, over 29,000 positive blood cultures were detected, with over 200 positive for obligate anaerobes. Of the positive cultures, 135 were positive for *Bacteroides fragilis* and 58 were positive for *Clostridium* spp. Of the *Clostridium* species isolated, *C. perfringens* accounted for 42 isolates, *C. septicum* for 12 isolates, and *C. difficile* for 4 isolates. Significant risk factors associated with isolation of *Clostridia* from blood include hemodialysis, intestinal malignancy, and inflammatory bowel disease.[52] Patients undergoing treatments that render them neutropenic are also at increased risk for clostridial bacteremia. *C. perfringens* followed by *C. septicum* are the most common species isolated from blood. While isolation of clostridia from blood may reflect either a transient bacteremia due to infection at another site or contamination, isolation of certain species, such as *C. septicum*, may reflect the presence of an underlying intestinal malignancy (Fig. 246-3). If not treated promptly, the toxins produced by clostridia during septicemia can result in severe disease and devastating clinical outcomes.

ABDOMINAL INFECTIONS

Infections resulting from contamination of the peritoneal cavity with intestinal contents are most often polymicrobial, and clostridia are often isolated from purulent material accompanying such infections, along with other obligate anaerobes and facultative species. Although a clear role in the infectious process has been established for organisms such as *B. fragilis* and the Enterobacteriaceae, the pathogenic significance of clostridia during these mixed infections is not clear. Gangrenous infections of the abdominal wall caused by *C. perfringens* have been well documented and usually are associated only with the presence of clostridia.

BILIARY TRACT INFECTIONS

Clostridia can be isolated from over 20% of diseased gallbladders and represents contamination of the biliary tract by normal intestinal bacteria. Biliary tract infections may either involve a single clostridial pathogen or reflect a mixed microflora. *C. perfringens* accounts for 50% of the clostridial species isolated. In some cases, gas may be present in the gallbladder lumen along with purulent material.[1] Gas gangrene of the abdominal wall is a rare complication of gallbladder surgery, resulting in contamination of the peritoneal cavity by the diseased biliary tract tissue. Demonstration of gas within the biliary tract by radiographic methods is an indication for surgical intervention and prompt antibiotic treatment directed at both obligate anaerobes including *Clostridium* and facultative enteric organisms.

FEMALE GENITAL TRACT INFECTIONS

Clostridia can be isolated from the genital tract of approximately 10% of women as part of the normal vaginal microflora. *Clostridia* are

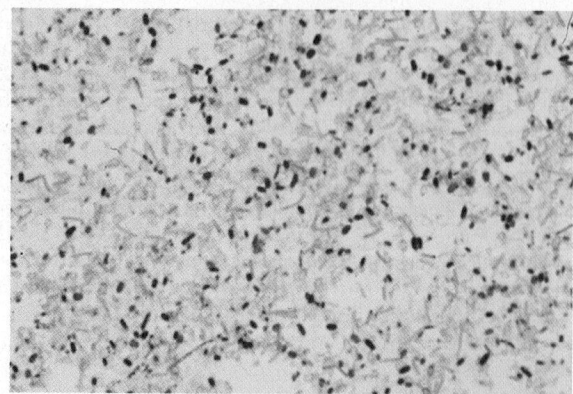

Figure 246-3 Gram stain of *C. septicum* demonstrating the gram-variable nature and the pleomorphic appearance of this species.

present in up to 20% of non-STD genital infections and may be present as part of bacterial vaginosis.[54] Although not common, postpartum and postabortion infections caused by clostridia, particularly *C. perfringens* and *C. sordellii*, can be severe.[55,56] Clostridial uterine infections start as localized chorioamnionitis as a result of infection of the fetus and placental tissues. Often a gaseous vaginal discharge is present. The infection may spread to the uterine wall and endometrial tissues, and, in the most severe cases, uterine necrosis accompanied by sepsis ensues.[1]

PLEUROPULMONARY INFECTIONS

Clostridia have been recovered from up to 10% of anaerobic pulmonary infections, with *C. perfringens* accounting for the majority of isolates.[1] Clostridia are rarely isolated as pure cultures from these specimens, suggesting that their presence as part of a mixed microflora does not necessarily reflect a causative role in the disease process. The most common sources for clostridia in such infections includes oral microflora and aspirated stomach contents. The clinical features of infections from which clostridia can be isolated are similar to those for other obligate anaerobes. On rare occasions, gas within the pleural space can be detected in association with the presence of clostridia.

REFERENCES

1. Finegold SM. *Anaerobic Bacteria in Human Disease.* New York: Academic Press; 1977:710.
2. Bartlett JG, et al. Clindamycin-associated colitis due to a toxin-producing species of Clostridium in hamsters. *J Infect Dis.* 1977;136(5):701-705.
3. Bartlett JG, et al. Role of Clostridium difficile in antibiotic-associated pseudomembranous colitis. *Gastroenterology.* 1978; 75(5):778-782.
4. Asensio A, et al. Increasing rates in Clostridium difficile infection (CDI) among hospitalised patients, Spain 1999-2007. *Euro Surveill.* 2008;13(31).
5. Kuijper EJ, et al. Update of Clostridium difficile infection due to PCR ribotype 027 in Europe, 2008. *Euro Surveill.* 2008;13(31).
6. Vonberg RP, et al. Infection control measures to limit the spread of Clostridium difficile. *Clin Microbiol Infect.* 2008;14(suppl 5):2-20.
7. Vonberg RP, et al. Costs of nosocomial Clostridium difficile-associated diarrhoea. *J Hosp Infect.* 2008;70(1):15-20.
8. Gorbach SL. Clostridum perfringens and other Clostridia. In: Gorbach SL, Bartlett JG, Blacklow NR, eds. *Infectious Diseases.* Philadelphia: W. B. Saunders Company; 1992.
9. Bartlett JG, et al. Quantitative bacteriology of the vaginal flora. *J Infect Dis.* 1977;136(2):271-277.
10. Johnson EA, Summanen P, Finegold SM. Clostridium. In: Murray PR, et al, ed. *Manual of Clinical Microbiology.* Washington D.C.: ASM Press; 2007:889-910.
11. Paredes-Sabja D, et al. Combined effects of hydrostatic pressure, temperature, and pH on the inactivation of spores of Clostridium perfringens type A and Clostridium sporogenes in buffer solutions. *J Food Sci.* 2007;72(6):M202-M206.
12. Plomp M, et al. Spore coat architecture of Clostridium novyi NT spores. *J Bacteriol.* 2007;189(17):6457-6468.

13. Roberts K, et al. Aerial dissemination of Clostridium difficile spores. *BMC Infect Dis.* 2008;8:7.
14. Paredes-Sabja D, et al. Characterization of Clostridium perfringens spores that lack SpoVA proteins and dipicolinic acid. *J Bacteriol.* 2008;190(13):4648-4659.
15. Bartlett JG. Introduction. In: Rolfe RD, Finefold SM, ed. *Clostridium difficile: Its Role in Intestinal Disease.* San Diego, CA: Academic Press, Inc.; 1988:408.
16. Tedesco FJ, Barton RW, Alpers DH. Clindamycin-associated colitis. A prospective study. *Ann Intern Med.* 1974;81(4):429-433.
17. Onderdonk A. Role of the Hamster Model of Antibiotic-Associated Colitis in Defining the Etiology of the Disease. In: Rolfe RD, Finefold SM, ed. *Clostridium difficile: Its Role in Intestinal Disease.* San Diego, CA: Academic Press, Inc; 1988:408.
18. Bartlett JG, et al. Antibiotic-associated pseudomembranous colitis due to toxin-producing Clostridia. *N Engl J Med.* 1978; 298(10):531-534.
19. Bartlett JG, Gerding DN, Clinical recognition and diagnosis of Clostridium difficile infection. *Clin Infect Dis.* 2008;46(suppl 1):S12-S18.
20. Hogenauer C, et al. Klebsiella oxytoca as a causative organism of antibiotic-associated hemorrhagic colitis. *N Engl J Med.* 2006; 355(23):2418-2426.
21. Vaishnavi C, Kaur S. Clostridium perfringens enterotoxin in antibiotic-associated diarrhea. *Indian J Pathol Microbiol.* 2008; 51(2):198-199.
22. Tedesco FJ. Pseudomembranous colitis: pathogenesis and therapy. *Med Clin North Am.* 1982;66(3):655-664.
23. Byrn JC, et al. Predictors of mortality after colectomy for fulminant Clostridium difficile colitis. *Arch Surg.* 2008;143(2):150-154; discussion 155.

24. Dupuy B, et al. Clostridium difficile toxin synthesis is negatively regulated by TcdC. *J Med Microbiol.* 2008;57(Pt 6):685-689.
25. Genth H, et al. Clostridium difficile toxins: more than mere inhibitors of Rho proteins. *Int J Biochem Cell Biol.* 2008;40(4): 592-597.
26. Matamouros S, England P, Dupuy B. Clostridium difficile toxin expression is inhibited by the novel regulator TcdC. *Mol Microbiol.* 2007;64(5):1274-1288.
27. Martin H, et al. Characterization of Clostridium difficile Strains Isolated from Patients in Ontario, Canada, from 2004 to 2006. *J Clin Microbiol.* 2008;46(9):2999-3004.
28. Barth H, Stiles BG. Binary actin-ADP-ribosylating toxins and their use as molecular Trojan horses for drug delivery into eukaryotic cells. *Curr Med Chem.* 2008;15(5):459-469.
29. Razavi B, Apisarnthanarak A, Mundy LM. Clostridium difficile: emergence of hypervirulence and fluoroquinolone resistance. *Infection.* 2007;35(5):300-307.
30. Carter GP, et al. Binary toxin production in Clostridium difficile is regulated by CdtR, a LytTR family response regulator. *J Bacteriol.* 2007;189(20):7290-7301.
31. Gerding DN, Muto CA, Owens Jr RC. Treatment of Clostridium difficile infection. *Clin Infect Dis.* 2008;46(suppl 1):S32-S42.
32. Surawicz CM. Role of probiotics in antibiotic-associated diarrhea, Clostridium difficile-associated diarrhea, and recurrent Clostridium difficile-associated diarrhea. *J Clin Gastroenterol.* 2008;42(suppl 2):S64-S70.
33. You DM, Franzos MA, Holman RP. Successful treatment of fulminant Clostridium difficile infection with fecal bacteriotherapy. *Ann Intern Med.* 2008;148(8):632-633.
34. Onderdonk AB, Cisneros RL, Bartlett JG. Clostridium difficile in gnotobiotic mice. *Infect Immun.* 1980;28(1):277-282.

35. Alcala L, et al. Comparison of Three Commercial Methods for the Rapid Detection of Clostridium difficile Toxins A and B From Fecal Specimens. *J Clin Microbiol*. 2008;46(11):2833-2835.
36. Russmann H, et al. Evaluation of three rapid assays for detection of Clostridium difficile toxin A and toxin B in stool specimens. *Eur J Clin Microbiol Infect Dis*. 2007;26(2):115-119.
37. Zilberberg MD. Clostridium difficile-related hospitalizations among US adults, 2006. *Emerg Infect Dis*. 2009;15(1):122-124.
38. Zilberberg MD, Shorr AF, Kollef MH. Increase in adult Clostridium difficile-related hospitalizations and case-fatality rate, United States, 2000-2005. *Emerg Infect Dis*. 2008;14(6):929-931.
39. Redelings MD, Sorvillo F, Mascola L. Increase in Clostridium difficile-related mortality rates, United States, 1999-2004. *Emerg Infect Dis*. 2007;13(9):1417-1419.
40. Wysowski DK. Increase in deaths related to enterocolitis due to Clostridium difficile in the United States, 1999-2002. *Public Health Rep*. 2006;121(4):361-362.
41. Carman RJ, et al. Clostridium perfringens toxin genotypes in the feces of healthy North Americans. *Anaerobe*. 2008;14(2):102-108.
42. De A, et al. Bacteriological studies of gas gangrene and related infections. *Indian J Med Microbiol*. 2003;21(3):202-204.
43. Brook I. Microbiology and management of soft tissue and muscle infections. *Int J Surg*. 2008;6(4):328-338.
44. Finsterer J, Hess B. Neuromuscular and central nervous system manifestations of Clostridium perfringens infections. *Infection*. 2007;35(6):396-405.
45. O'Brien DK, et al. The role of neutrophils and monocytic cells in controlling the initiation of Clostridium perfringens gas gangrene. *FEMS Immunol Med Microbiol*. 2007;50(1):86-93.
46. Hickey MJ, et al. Molecular and cellular basis of microvascular perfusion deficits induced by Clostridium perfringens and Clostridium septicum. *PLoS Pathog*. 2008;4(4):e1000045.
47. Loh JP, et al. The rapid identification of Clostridium perfringens as the possible aetiology of a diarrhoeal outbreak using PCR. *Epidemiol Infect*. 2008;136(8):1142-1146.
48. Smith-Slatas CL, Bourque M, Salazar JC. Clostridium septicum infections in children: a case report and review of the literature. *Pediatrics*. 2006;117(4):e796-e805.
49. Khanna N. Clindamycin-resistant Clostridium perfringens cellulitis. *J Tissue Viability*. 2008;17(3):95-97.
50. Kaide CG, Khandelwal S. Hyperbaric oxygen: applications in infectious disease. *Emerg Med Clin North Am*. 2008;26(2):571-595, xi.
51. Kobayashi S, et al. Spread of a large plasmid carrying the cpe gene and the tcp locus amongst Clostridium perfringens isolates from nosocomial outbreaks and sporadic cases of gastroenteritis in a geriatric hospital. *Epidemiol Infect*. 2008:1-6.
52. Leal J, et al. Epidemiology of Clostridium species bacteremia in Calgary, Canada, 2000-2006. *J Infect*. 2008;57(3):198-203.
53. Robert R, et al. Prognostic factors and impact of antibiotherapy in 117 cases of anaerobic bacteraemia. *Eur J Clin Microbiol Infect Dis*. 2008;27(8):671-678.
54. Brook I, Frazier EH, Thomas RL. Aerobic and anaerobic microbiologic factors and recovery of beta-lactamase producing bacteria from obstetric and gynecologic infection. *Surg Gynecol Obstet*. 1991;172(2):138-144.
55. Snow M. On alert for postpartum C. sordellii infection. *Nursing*. 2008;38(1):10.
56. McGregor JA, et al. Maternal deaths associated with Clostridium sordellii infection. *Am J Obstet Gynecol*. 1989;161(4):987-995.

247

Bacteroides, Prevotella, Porphyromonas, and Fusobacterium Species (and Other Medically Important Anaerobic Gram-Negative Bacilli)

WENDY S. GARRETT | ANDREW B. ONDERDONK

Overview

The genera *Bacteroides*, *Porphyromonas*, *Prevotella*, and *Fusobacterium* account for the majority of infections caused by anaerobic gram-negative rods. *Bilophila* and *Sutterella* also cause human infections, although they are less frequently encountered in clinical practice. These obligately anaerobic gram-negative bacteria colonize the oropharynx, distal gastrointestinal tract, and urogenital tract of humans. Several species are useful commensals, facilitating host metabolism and favorably shaping immune responses. However, many of these microbes act opportunistically, causing infections when they gain access to otherwise sterile tissues. The gram-negative anaerobic rods have a predilection for abscess formation, with the most common sites being the oropharynx, abdominal cavity, lungs, and female genital tract. These bacterial species also present clinical challenges because they are often resistant to commonly used antibiotics.

History

The turn of the 19th century was a fertile time for the discovery of gram-negative anaerobic rods (GNAR). The recognition of GNAR as important pathogens first occurred in animals in 1884 and is attributed to Loeffler. Schmorl is credited with identifying the GNAR as opportunists in humans in 1891. These discoveries stemmed from human cutaneous wound infections contracted by cross-contamination of puncture wounds in the course of experimental infection experiments with rabbits in his laboratory. Identification of the GNAR as human commensals dates back to 1898, when Halle published his discovery of *Fusobacterium* colonizing the female genital tract. At the same time, GNAR were also isolated as human pathogens from clinical specimens by Veillon and Zuber, who identified GNAR in cases of pelvic, appendiceal, and brain abscesses.[1]

The *Bacteroides* as a group were first described in the late 1890s, and for many years, the *Bacteroides* were a physiologically disparate genus of pleiomorphic obligately anaerobic gram-negative rods. Until the early 1960s, competing taxonomic systems and confusion regarding nomenclature made it difficult to determine the role of specific members of this group of organisms during infectious processes. With the advent of uniform taxonomic classification and the use of 16S rRNA phylogenetic-driven taxonomic classifications, several species were reclassified. The *Bacteroides* have been further subdivided into two additional genera—*Porphyromonas* and *Prevotella*—both of which primarily colonize the oral cavity. Identification of the genus *Fusobacterium* dates back to a similar time period.

Microbiology

BACTEROIDES

The *Bacteroides* are gram-negative, non-spore-forming, obligately anaerobic rod-shaped bacteria. There are currently over 30 recognized species of *Bacteroides*. The strictest taxonomic definition of *Bacteroides*

limits this census to under a dozen separate species. Taxonomically, the *Bacteroides* fall within the phylum Bacteroidetes. Within the Bacteroidaceae family, *Bacteroides* are distinctive in the GC-composition of their DNA, specifically 40-48 mol%. The major metabolic products of saccharolytic metabolism by this genus are acetate, succinate, and iso-valerate. The characteristic long-chain fatty acids used for identification are principally the saturated anteiso-methyl and iso-methyl branched acids. The *Bacteroides* express hexose monophosphate shunt-pentose phosphate pathway enzymes. Their sphingolipid-rich membranes also possess menaquinones, particularly MK-10 and MK-11. *Bacteroides* peptidoglycan contains meso-diaminopimelic acid.[2] Several of the *Bacteroides* express numerous capsular polysaccharides. These glycoantigens are of interest biologically for their immunomodulatory potential, particularly in the case of *B. fragilis* polysaccharide A.

The GNAR are differentiated from one another in the clinical laboratory using standard techniques: colony morphology, Gram stain, pigment production visualized in natural light and as fluorescence emission after exposure to UV light, and numerous biochemical tests. In addition to the aforementioned, short-chain fatty acid analysis by gas-liquid chromatography can also be used for species-levels *Bacteroides* discrimination. The *B. fragilis* group is of special medical importance for several reasons. It is often the predominant GNAR in polymicrobial infections, and members of this group have the potential to express beta-lactamase. *B. fragilis* group bacteremias are also associated with a high mortality rate: 27%.[3] Consequently, identifying the *B. fragilis* group by the clinical laboratory is often critical for appropriate therapeutic intervention. On blood agar, *B. fragilis* form circular, entire, white or gray, 2-3 mm colonies that are shiny and smooth. The *B. fragilis* group can be rather pleiomorphic on Gram stain, forming straight rods of varying length, as well as coccobacilli (Fig. 247-1A). When grown in liquid medium, cells develop bipolar vacuoles and show a characteristic "safety pin" appearance. A useful characteristic of the *B. fragilis* group is its bile tolerance when compared to other GNAR and, as such, its growth on *Bacteroides* Bile Esculin Agar. In addition, *B. fragilis* is highly resistant to the antibiotics, kanamycin, vancomycin, and colistin. The use of a simple disk diffusion assay for these antibiotics is often part of the identification process for GNAR (Table 247-1).

PREVOTELLA AND PORPHYROMONAS

Both *Prevotella* and *Porphyromonas* were previously considered to be part of the genus *Bacteroides*. These pigmented GNAR can be distinguished from one another metabolically as the saccharolytic *Prevotella* species and the asaccharolytic *Porphyromonas* species. There are approximately 20 *Prevotella* species that have been implicated in causing disease in humans. *Prevotella* form circular, convex, 1-2 mm, gray colonies that are shiny. On Gram stain, they form short gram-negative rods and may assume coccobacilli forms (Fig. 247-1B). *Prevotella* grow well on laked blood agar with kanamycin and vancomycin (LKV) and have variable resistance to colistin. While *Prevotella* are

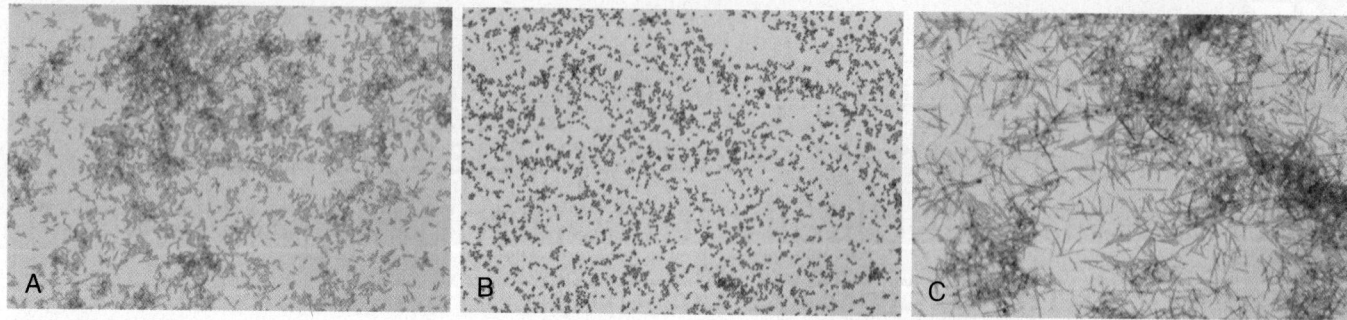

Figure 247-1 **Gram stains of selected gram negative anaerobic rods. A,** *Bacteroides fragilis.* **B,** *Prevotella intermedia.* **C,** *Fusobacterium nucleatum.*

largely regarded as pigmented GNAR, they can be unpigmented as well. Pigmented *Prevotella* form brown- or black-colored colonies after a week of growth on LKV. Before this brown or black pigment develops, *Prevotella* may fluoresce a very dark red upon exposure to a Wood's lamp (long-wave UV light). By colony morphology and Gram stain, *Porphyromonas* tend to form smaller colonies and present as shorter rods or coccobacilli on Gram stain but can be difficult to distinguish from *Prevotella*. *Porphyromonas* usually grow as pigmented colonies, initially forming gray colonies that darken to black colonies within a week after plating on laked blood agar. *Porphyromonas* do not grow on LKV media because of their sensitivity to vancomycin, but they are resistant to colistin.

FUSOBACTERIUM

Fusobacterium are obligately anaerobic filamentous gram-negative rods that are members of the phylum Fusobacter, in contrast to *Bacteroides*, *Prevotella*, and *Porphyromonas*, which are members of the Bacteroidetes. On blood agar, *Fusobacterium* form pinpoint colonies that can be circular or irregular, with some species, such as *F. nucleatum*, forming umbinate "fried egg" colonies after 3-5 days of incubation. Depending on the strain, they can be hemolytic. *Fusobacterium* species can be somewhat variable in their Gram stain and display a range of cellular morphologies from coccoid, pleiomorphic spherules (*F. necrophorum*) to rod-shaped. Rods can be short with rounded ends or long and thin with pointed ends (*F. nucleatum*), arrayed end to end (Fig. 247-1C). As a genus, they are sensitive to both kanamycin and colistin and resistant to vancomycin. *Fusobacterium* species can be distinguished by their bile sensitivity and metabolism of threonine to proprionate. Most species are indole positive and produce butyric acid during the fermentation of glucose.

COMMENSALISM

In adults, bacterial cells outnumber host cells by at least 10:1. The human microbiome is dominated by anaerobes. Gram-negative anaerobic rods colonize the mucosal surfaces of the oropharynx, gastrointestinal tract, and female urogenital tract, and *Bacteroides* and *Prevotella* are among the most abundant genera present. Mutualism and opportunism are important features of the relationship between human hosts and colonizing species of the genera *Bacteroides*, *Prevotella*, *Porphyromonas*, and *Fusobacterium*.

THE GI TRACT

The human colon is colonized by 10-100 trillion bacteria, making it the largest repository for bacteria in the body. The *Bacteroides* genus constitutes 30% of the total colonic bacteria. *Bacteroides vulgatus*, *thetaiotaomicron*, *distasonis*, *fragilis*, and *ovatus* are the most commonly encountered *Bacteroides* in the human colon.[4] There is significant variability among humans regarding the colonic colonization, with different *B. fragilis* group members as assessed by stool culture (Comstock and Onderdonk unpublished). The colonization of the gastrointestinal tract occurs during descent through the vaginal canal or postnatally for infants delivered by caesarian section. Both breast milk and exposure to environmental factors are important forces in shaping colonization. Many studies over the past several decades have been undertaken to examine this process in detail, with genomic-based technology taking central stage more recently.[5]

Symbiosis and Mutualism in Immunity and Metabolism

There has been a recent explosion of interest in clinical correlations between intestinal colonization and human health and disease. The pioneering work of Bengt Björkstén and others have examined correlations between infectious disease and atopic and allergic diseases for many decades.[6] One recent study suggests that early colonization at less than 3 weeks of age with *Bacteroides fragilis* increases the risk of asthma later in life.[7] The basic science behind these clinical observations rests in the hypothesis that certain bacterial factors may alter the balance between T-cell-based immune responses. Elegant, recent work by Mazmanian and Kasper suggests that the *Bacteroides fragilis* zwitterionic polysaccharide A (PsA) may play an essential role in maintaining immunological equilibrium in the intestine. Using both gnotobiotic mouse models and mouse models of inflammatory bowel disease, these investigators have demonstrated that PsA is a symbiosis factor that balances Th1 and Th2 T-cell subsets in the colon, in the absence of bacteria, and drives anti-inflammatory IL-10 production under proinflammatory conditions.[8,9]

The beneficial immunomodulatory effects of *Bacteroides* are not exclusive to *B. fragilis*; *B. thetaiotaomicron* also has immunomodulatory properties with the potential to dampen proinflammatory responses to commensal, intestinal bacteria. *Bacteroides thetaiotaomi-*

TABLE 247-1	Techniques and Properties to Differentiate Medically Important Gram-Negative Anaerobic Rods						
	Pencillin	*Vancomycin*	*Colistin*	*Kanamycin*	*Growth in 20% Bile*	*Pigment*	*Brick Red Fluorescence*
Bacteroides fragilis group	R	R	R	R	Y	N	N
Prevotella	S	R	V	R	N	Y	V
Porphyromonas	S	S	R	R	N	Y	V
Fusobacterium	S	R	S	S	V	N	N

N, no; R, resistant; S, sensitive; V, variable; Y, yes.

cron targets the RelA subunit of the transcription factor, NF-κB, a master regulator of proinflammatory immune responses. This process is dependent on a nuclear receptor and transcription factor called PPAR-gamma and independent of the nuclear export receptor Crm-1. However, the mechanism by which *Bacteroides thetaiotaomicron* drives this process remains to be fully understood.[10] The *Bacteroides* and other intestinal commensals also contribute to host immunity through the process of colonization resistance, the concept that the entrenched presence of commensals provides protection from invading pathogens.[11] The most central and well-understood function of *Bacteroides* resides in the mutualistic function of metabolism. The human gut at its core is a bioreactor. The saccharolytic *Bacteroides* process diverse dietary and host polysaccharides for their own metabolic needs and in doing so aids in human digestion and nutrient liberation for their human hosts. A well-nuanced understanding of the biochemistry and genomics of glycan foraging by *Bacteroides thetaiotaomicron* has emerged over the past several years.[12-15] Additionally, the work of Jeffrey Gordon and colleagues has drawn attention to the potential role of these bacteria in the human obesity epidemic.[16,17]

FEMALE UROGENITAL TRACT

The female urogenital tract and, in particular, the vagina is densely colonized by anaerobes. While the gram-positive anaerobic *Lactobacilli* are the predominant colonizers, GNAR also abound. Vaginal colonization is dynamic, with variations not only intrinsic to the female reproductive life cycle from the premenarchal through postmenopausal years but also with significant shift over a given menstrual cycle.[18-21] Pregnancy and parturition result in substantial microflora changes as well.[22]

There is also intra-individual genus-level diversity in colonization with *Bacteroides*, *Fusobacterium*, *Prevotella*, and *Porphyromonas*. In addition, there are distinct microbial community differences between the labia, urethral vestibular region, along the length of the vagina, and the cervix. Frequent isolates from the vaginal vault include *Bacteroides urealyticus* and members of the *B. fragilis* group; *Prevotella bivia*, *disiens*, *buccalis*, *melaninogenica*, and *corporis*; *Porphyromonas asaccharolytica*; and *Fusobacterium nucleatum*. Most research on the vaginal microflora and symbiotic effects has been *Lactobacillus*-centric, with the view that the GNAR may contribute to vaginal dysbiosis, negative consequences for fetal outcomes, and host mycotic and bacterial infections.[23-26]

OROPHARYNX

The oropharynx is a diverse niche for both aerobes and anaerobes. Within the mouth, the teeth, gingival crevices, saliva, and posterior pharyngeal structures provide distinctive milieus with diverse redox potentials and oxygen tensions. Gingival scrapings are particularly dense in bacteria, with estimated concentrations on the order of 10^{11-12} CFU/ml. Similar to the colonization of the lower gastrointestinal tract, colonization of the oropharynx starts at birth. Among the anaerobes, *Lactobacilli* and *Peptostreptococci* are the earliest colonizers. Fusobacterial populations emerge with the eruption of the first teeth and increase with establishment of full juvenile dentition. *Prevotella* and *Porphyromonas* colonization emerges after colonization by *Fusobacterium*. Of the GNAR, *Porphyromonas gingivalis* and *endodontalis*; *Fusobacterium nucleatum*; *Prevotella intermedia*, *melaninogenica*, *denticola*, and *loescheii*; and *Bacteroides forsythus* all commonly populate dental plaque. Poor dentition, gingivitis, and other periodontal diseases correlate with increased numbers of GNARs, as do hospitalization, residing in a long-term-care facility, and multiple medical comorbidities.

OPPORTUNISM

Commensalism should be viewed as a host-microbe relationship spanning the spectrum from mutualism through opportunism. Most, if not all, of commensal GNAR have pathogenic potential. *B. fragilis* merits especial consideration because while *B. fragilis* itself may not be the most abundant GNAR cultured from the gastrointestinal tract, it is the most common GNAR identified in clinical isolates from both blood and abscesses.[27] Multiple virulence factors underpin this observation, as well as account for the opportunism observed *by Prevotella, Porphyromonas, Fusobacterium,* and *Bilophila*. Virulence factors produced by these bacteria include capsular polysaccharides, outer-membrane proteins, lipopolysaccharide "endotoxins," attachment factors (fimbriae/pili), toxins, and numerous enzymes. Synergism is another important concept that explains the presence of GNAR in many polymicrobial infections. Several facultative anaerobes and aerobes can provide favorable environments that can promote the growth of GNAR. For example, the production of superoxide dismutase by facultative species protects obligate anaerobes that do not produce this enzyme constitutively against the highly lethal superoxide anion. Without the presence of these other microbes, the oxygen tension would not be favorable for the GNAR. In many polymicrobial infections, facultative anaerobes and aerobes function mutualistically for the GNAR, providing strong synergy for their expansion, especially for *B. fragilis*. In turn, the *B. fragilis* group with its frequent beta-lactamase activity can provide a protective environment for normally β-lactam-sensitive facultative anaerobes and aerobes.

ENDOTOXIC LPS

Endotoxic lipopolysaccharide (LPS) is a powerful mediator of systemic inflammation and a driver of septic shock. LPS can differ in its endotoxic potential. Secondary to the structure of *Bacteroides'* lipid A, the LPS does not elicit a strong host inflammatory response. This is thought to be due to the fact that these species do not contain C14-2OH fatty acid as part of the lipid A substituent. *Porphyromonas* and *Prevotella* also appear to have attenuated LPS for the same reason. Interestingly, the LPS of *Porphyromonas gingivalis* may be able to antagonize the proinflammatory effects of other LPS in mixed infections, as suggested by in vitro experiments on primary human monocytes.[28] In contrast, the LPS from *Fusobacterium* elicits a more inflammatory host response because it has a lipid A that contains C14-2OH fatty acid.[29] These observations likely stem from structural observations about Fusobacterial LPS that have demonstrated that it has a more typical LPS structure as compared to *Bacteroides*.[1,30]

CAPSULAR POLYSACCHARIDES

Bacteroides fragilis produces eight distinct polysaccharides, PS A-H, and there is complex phase variation in the expression of these polysaccharides. There is also substantial variability in these polysaccharides across *B. fragilis* strains.[31] Over the past 30 years, the work of Kasper, Onderdonk, and Comstock has led to a nuanced understanding of the role of these polysaccharides in abscess formation and immunomodulation. The capsular polysaccharide complex facilitates binding of *Bacteroides fragilis* to mesothelial cells lining the peritoneum, providing a nidus for abscess formation.[32] Abscess formation also requires both ICAM-1 and TNF-α.[33] Numerous *Prevotella* and *Porphyromonas* species, including *Prev. oralis, melaningenica*, and *Fusobacterium*, are also encapsulated and are abscessogenic.

PILI AND FIMBRIAE

In addition to capsular polysaccharide complexes promoting adherence, *Bacteroides* and *Porphyromonas* species can adhere to the epithelium via pili. There are great variations in cellular adherence of different *Bacteroides* species and strains. Pili are more frequently observed in pathogenic clinical isolates than in fecal samples from healthy subjects.[34,35] Pili have been observed specifically in *Bacteroides fragilis* and *ovatus* strains, as well as in *Porphyromonas gingivalis* and *Fusobacterium necrophorum*.

ENZYMES AND TOXINS

Numerous enzymes and toxins facilitate GNAR host mucosa invasion and immune system evasion. *Bacteroides*, *Prevotella*, *Porphyromonas*, and *Fusobacterium* can also express numerous extracellular enzymes, such as collagenase, chondroitin sulfatase, hyaluronidase, neuraminidase, DNase, phosphorylase, and proteases, that can facilitate epithelial barrier breach.[36] There are enterotoxigenic strains of *Bacteroides fragilis*, as well, that cause diarrhea in both children and adults. The toxin Btf is a 20kDa zinc-containing metalloprotease, and there are at least three isoforms. Btf is believed to cleave e-cadherin in the zonula adherens, resulting in intestinal barrier compromise. Yet another enzyme promoting GNAR pathogenic potential is superoxide dismutase, which not only reduces oxygen tension for the GNAR but provides defense against polymorphonuclear leukocyte-produced reactive oxygen species.

METABOLIC END PRODUCTS

Numerous *Bacteroides* and *Prevotella* produce significant amounts of succinate as an end product of metabolism. Several studies have suggested that succinate inhibits polymorphonuclear leukocyte (PMN) phagocytosis. In addition, a succinate-rich environment may inhibit PMN migration and perhaps drive PMN apoptosis.

HOST IMMUNE RESPONSE

Cellular and noncellular adaptive and innate immune responses play important roles in defending the host from infections from the GNAR. Neutrophils are an important first line of defense. Phagocytic and oxygen radical-generating abilities are not the neutrophil's only defense against pathogenic GNAR. Neutrophils also produce a number of antimicrobial peptides that are bactericidal for GNAR.[37] GNAR-positive abscesses are often neutrophil-rich, and neutrophils have been shown to kill *Bacteroides* and other GNAR under anaerobic conditions. Further support for the role of neutrophils in protecting the host from GNAR infections comes from studies of the prevalence of gram-negative bacteremia in neutropenic patients.[38] The complement system is another innate immune mechanism important in the clearance of these infections. Both the classical and alternative complement pathways have been shown to opsonize several *Bacteroides* and *Prevotella* species. Most discussion of dendritic cells (DC) and *Bacteroides* have not revolved around host defense but have focused on how DC-internalized glycoantigens can direct T-cell responses.[9] In mouse models, immunization with PS A has been shown to protect from *Bacteroides fragilis*–induced abscesses. The protective effects of immunization were shown to be CD4+ T-cell-dependent, despite the fact that polysaccharides are regarded as T-cell-independent antigens. Furthermore, recombinant IL-2, a potent cytokine for T-cell proliferation, was protective against *B. fragilis* abscess formation in a dose-dependent manner, further substantiating a role for T cells in host-adaptive immunity to *Bacteroides*.[39] B-cell deficiency has been shown to be a risk factor in mice for disseminated anaerobic infections, and passive immunity has been shown to be protective in mouse models.[40] However, in rat models, passive transfer has not been shown to be protective. There is little direct clinical evidence linking B- and T-lymphocyte function to host immunity to GNAR. A case study by Fisher and colleagues did report that lymphopenia was a risk factor for GNAR bacteremia in pediatric patients undergoing appendectomy.[41]

INFECTIONS

There are few initial signs and symptoms that implicate GNAR specifically on primary evaluation. The clinical signs and symptoms of GNAR infection depend on the location of the infected site. A careful history with consideration of potential sites of translocation or portal of entry may raise the suspicion for GNAR involvement—for example, bacteremia in a patient with an intra-abdominal process. Systemic infections, such as bacteremia involving GNAR, are often polymicrobial. The majority of these infections arise endogenously, from GNAR already colonizing the mucosal surfaces. Common clinical signs and symptoms associated with anaerobic infections in general include physical proximity to a mucosal site, foul-smelling purulent discharge, tissue necrosis, and palpable or imaged gas in tissues.

BACTEREMIA

The mortality of GNAR bacteremia has been reported to range from 15% to 60%, with the upper range of this mortality reflecting untreated infections.[42] In a recent retrospective, multicenter study from France, anaerobes accounted for 0.5% to 9% of all bacteremias, of which 60% were *Bacteroides* species and 22% *Clostridium* sp. These recent figures are consistent with prior data over the past several decades.[43] In the United States, the estimated prevalence of GNAR bacteremia over the past three decades has fluctuated between 0.5% and 15%. Until recently, the data suggested there was a trend toward a decreased incidence. A recent publication of a study from the Mayo Clinic reported that, at this large center, at least, cases of anaerobic bacteremia are on the rise, with 53 cases per year reported during 1993-1996; 75 cases per year during 1997-2000; and 91 cases per year during 2001-2004.[44] In 2008 in one Boston hospital, 54,448 blood cultures were performed and 5097 were positive for growth; 45 of these were positive for GNAR, and 29 of these were *B. fragilis* cases (Onderdonk AB, unpublished observation). In lieu of the lack of specific signs and symptoms of GNAR bacteremia, clinicians are highly dependent on the clinical laboratory for diagnosis. At the majority of U.S. hospitals, blood samples collected from potentially bacteremic patients are routinely collected into culture systems, allowing for evaluation of anaerobes. There should be a low clinical threshold for broad empiric coverage in critically ill patients with histories consistent with GNAR bacteremic sources.

Of all the GNAR, *Bacteroides fragilis* is most commonly isolated in bacteremias. Interestingly, there is variation in mortality rates reported among *B. fragilis* group members. Mortality rates of 24% and 31% have been associated with *B. fragilis*; 50% with *Bacteroides distasonis*; and 100% for *Bacteroides thetaiotaomicron*.[45,46] Of course, rapid susceptibility testing and administration of appropriate antibiotic therapy is essential for optimal clinical outcomes, as substantiated by a recent observational study of *Bacteroides* bacteremia that demonstrated 16% mortality with optimal therapy and 45% without.[47] Fusobacterial bacteremias represent less than 1% of all bacteremias and less than 10% of anaerobic bacteremias. Of the fusobacterial bacteremias, *F. nucleatum* and *mortiferum* are the most common.[48] Subclinical and transient bacteremia with *Prevotella* and *Fusobacterium* species have been documented following dental cleaning.[49] Clinically significant bacteremia with *Prevotella* species have been reported with both periodontal and obstetric procedures. GNAR bacteremias are not uncommon as secondary infections in the setting of other primary GNAR infections. Intra-abdominal infections are the most frequent source of these bacteremias. Frequent intra-abdominal processes associated with GNAR bacteremia include abscesses, surgical procedures, intestinal perforation, obstruction, colorectal cancer, and other malignancies. The upper and lower respiratory tract are often primary sites for fusobacterial bacteremias. The female genital tract, oropharynx, skin ulcers, and skeletal and soft tissues should be thoroughly interrogated as bacteremic sources, as they are the associated source in 5% to 25% of cases.

SKELETAL

Gram-negative anaerobes can infect both joints and bones, recently reviewed in depth by Brook.[50] Septic arthritis caused by GNAR generally results from either a hematogenous seeding of the joint space or direct extension of the bacteria via the skin. The large lower-extremity joints—hips and knees—are the most common sites, followed by the shoulders and elbows. Surgery, trauma, and multiple medical comorbidities are all risk factors. The majority of cases are associated with single species rather than a polymicrobial infection as is often seen with abscesses. In a classic review of both pediatric and adult septic arthritis cases, Finegold reported on over 1200 anaerobic joint infections and found that *Fusobacterium necrophorum* was the most common isolate recovered.[50,51] *B. fragilis* group bacteria can also cause septic arthritis, and these infections are often secondary and distant from the primary site.[52] Anaerobic osteomyelitis tends to be polymicrobial. *Bacteroides* spp. and *Fusobacterium* are most frequently cultured. Not surprisingly, *Prevotella* and *Porphyromonas* have been recovered from osteomyelitis cases involving bites. Mastoid bone infections often involve these oro-pharyngeal commensals as well. Sickle cell patients, who are at increased for osteomyelitis secondarily to sickle-related bony infarction, are the subject of several case reports of GNAR osteomyelitis involving both the axial and appendicular skeleton.[53,54] Diabetics with peripheral vascular disease are another risk group for anaerobic osteomyelitis; these infections often develop in the setting of chronic foot ulcers.[55]

SKIN AND SOFT TISSUES

GNAR are important pathogens in surgical wound infections, bites, ulcers, and infected pilonidal cysts. Following intra-abdominal or gynecological surgery, wounds can become infected with *Bacteroides* and *Prevotella* species, resulting in infections of proximal skin and soft tissues. Human, dog, and cat bites can result in GNAR skin infections. *Prevotella* is a common anaerobe that infects dog bite wounds.[56] With routine availability of anaerobic culture, anaerobes are increasingly being recovered from infected human and animal bites, especially those complicated by abscesses.[57] Pilonidal cysts and sacral decubitus ulcers can readily become contaminated by feces and subsequently infected by GNAR. Similarly, cutaneous abscesses, carbuncles, and furuncles in the perineal region can become infected with GNAR. *Bacteroides fragilis* is frequently cultured from decubitus ulcers in both the elderly and pediatric populations, as well as from foot ulcers from patients with peripheral vascular disease or diabetes.

CNS INFECTION

The most common CNS infection is meningitis. However, anaerobic meningitis is extremely rare. In Finegold's historic analysis of anaerobic infections, 298 cases of meningitis are reviewed. However, more than half are without substantiated culture data. In a more recent review by Law and Arnoff of pediatric populations, 271 cases are reviewed, of which the vast majority—over 85%—are in the setting of brain abscesses.[58] Anaerobic culture of cerebral spinal fluid is not routinely performed, and, given the rarity of these infections, there should be a compelling reason to do so. Of the GNAR reported, *Bacteroides fragilis* and *Fusobacterium necrophorum* are the most commonly isolated. In several of these cases, the upper respiratory tract or intestinal tract was the primary source that resulted in hematogenous spread in patients with medical comorbidities compromising the integrity of the blood-brain barrier. Chronic and acute otitis media has also been implicated in several of these rare cases.

Anaerobic infections of the CNS typically manifest as abscesses and are frequently polymicrobial. When abscesses develop outside of the brain parenchyma and around the dura, they are referred to as subdural empyemas or epidural abscesses, depending on the location. The location of the brain abscess correlates with the source of the infecting organism, often arising in adjacent structures—for example, frontal lobe abscess and sinus infections, and temporal lobe abscess and mastoiditis. Brain abscesses stemming from bacteremia in the absence of focal trauma can arise throughout the lobes as a focal or multifocal process. Recent neurosurgery, trauma, and the presence of ventricular shunts are risk factors for GNAR abscesses. Clearly, the site of primary infection informs not only abscess location but narrows the spectrum of causative organisms. *Bacteroides, Fusobacterium, Prevotella,* and *Porphyromonas* have all been isolated from brain abscesses.

Infections of the Aerodigestive Tract

OROPHARYNX

The GNAR are frequent culprits in infections of the tooth and peridontium. Most odontogenic infections arise in the setting of dental caries. Once opportunists have established themselves in a dental plaque, they can cause local infections or can disseminate and seed locoregional sites via extension or distant sites via hematogenous spread. Extension to and infection of the sublingual, submandibular, and perimandibular spaces can result in Ludwig's angina, a rapidly progressing infection of the floor of the mouth that can lead to death by asphyxiation without rapid surgical intervention. While *Actinomyces israelii* is the most commonly identified microorganism, among the GNAR, *Fusobacterium* has been commonly isolated. Tongue piercing, an increasingly popular trend among youths, also increases the risk of Ludwig's angina.[59,60] Locoregional spread can result in infection of the maxillary sinus, cavernous sinus, or brain parenchyma. Severe facial cellulitis, such as periorbital cellulitis, is another complication of anaerobic dental caries infection. More distal sites of dental infections involving hematogeneous spread include endocarditis, mediastinal or pleuropulmonary abscesses, or orthopedic infections.

Poor dental hygiene results in gingivitis that can lead to more severe periodontal disease. Acute necrotizing ulcerative gingivitis (ANUG) or Vincent's angina is the most severe manifestation of gingivitis. *Fusobacterium necrophorum, Prevotella melaninogenica* and *intermedia, Fusobacterum nucleatum,* and *Porphyromonas gingivalis* have all been implicated as causative agents in ANUG and odontogenic infections as well. *Bacteroides urealtyicus* and *forsythus,* but not the *B. fragilis* group, have also been identified as causative agents in oral infections.

The GNAR can result in peritonsillar abscess formation. Both *Prevotella melaninogenica* and *Fusobacterium necrophorum* are frequent GNAR isolates. One feared complication of peritonsillar abscesses that involves *Fusobacterium necrophorum* is Lemierre's syndrome—jugular vein septic thrombophlebitis. These septic emboli can seed the lungs and result in multiple systemic abscesses.

The GNAR play a role in both chronic sinusitis and acute exacerbations of chronic sinusitis but not in acute sinusitis, which in the absence of a viral etiology are caused by *Streptococcus pneumoniae, Haemophilus influenzae,* and *Moraxella catarrhalis.* The predominant anaerobes recovered in chronic sinus infections include *Prevotella* and *Porphyromonas, Fusobacterium,* and *Peptostreptococcus.*[61] Rare complications of chronic sinusitis include CNS abscesses.

EARS

Aerobes, *Streptococcus pneumoniae* and *Haemophilus influenzae,* are the predominant causative organisms in bacterial acute and chronic otitis media in the pediatric population. Anaerobes have been found in serous effusions and transmeatal biopsies from patients with chronic otitis media and acute exacerbations in the setting of chronic otitis media. Culturing serous effusions from a study of 114 otitis media patients yielded data from approximately 40% of samples; aerobes predominanted over polymicrobial anaerobic and aerobic populations, followed by single anaerobic isolates in 15%. In this study by Brook and colleagues, *Prevotella* species were the second most commonly cultured anaerobes.[62] Le Monnier and colleagues recently published a retrospective study of his institution's experience with 25 pediatric acute otitis media cases caused by *Fusobacterium necrophorum.*[63] Forty-four percent of patients had uncomplicated otitis media, 40% had acute mastoiditis, and Lemierre's syndrome was seen in four patients (16%). In a classic study of the microbiology of chronic otitis media published by Brook, the *Bacteroides fragilis* group and *Prevotella melaninogenica* were the predominant anaerobes cultured.[62]

SALIVARY GLANDS

Infection of the salivary glands, usually the parotid glands, can result from viral or bacterial pathogens. *Staphylococcus aureus* is the most frequent organism associated with acute suppurative parotitis, and mumps virus can be a cause of acute parotitis. The GNAR are the predominant anaerobes implicated in non–*Staphylococcus aureus* parotitis. *Prevotella*, *Porphyromonas*, and *Fusobacterium* spp. have all been reported.[64]

THORACIC

Anaerobic infections of the lung parenchyma and pleural space are relatively common. More specifically, these clinical infections include community-acquired and nosocomial pneumonias, lung abscesses, and pleural empyemas. Anaerobes can also result in acute mediastinitis in the setting of severe oropharyngeal infections or perforations in the upper gastrointestinal tract. Poor dentition, gingivitis, chronic obstructive pulmonary disease, cystic fibrosis, and neuromuscular diseases are all medical comorbidities that increase the risk of anaerobic pleuropulmonary infections. Smoking, alcoholism, and conditions associated with impaired consciousness, the inability to clear oral secretions (seizure disorder, dementia, severe cerebral vascular disease), or both, all increase the risk of aspiration, which is a key inciting event in these pneumonias and empyemas. Obtaining good-quality sputum samples, those not contaminated with saliva, can be a clinical challenge that confounds identification of the causative organisms in these pneumonias.

Pleuropulmonary infections linked with aspiration events are commonly polymicrobial with both aerobic and anaerobic isolates. *Streptococcus viridans* group members are commonly encountered aerobes in these infections. Regarding the GNAR, *Prevotella buccae*, *disiens*, *intermedia*, and *melaninogenica*; *Bacteroides urealyticus* and *forsythus*; and *Fusobacterium nucleatum* have all been associated with these infections.[65] A recent review of pleural infections examined the distinct microbiology of nosocomial and community-acquired infections and found that mixed streptococcal and anaerobic infectious processes had a lower associated mortality than staphylococcal, enterobacterial, or polymicrobial aerobic infections.[66] A recent study of the sputum of cystic fibrosis patients detected high levels of sputum colonization, in the absence of overt infection, particularly *Prevotella* species, and also found that *Pseudomonas aeruginosa* colonization correlated with increased anaerobic colonization.[67]

CARDIOVASCULAR

Although the GNAR are relatively uncommon causes of endocarditis and pericarditis, they are clinically important because of their antibiotic resistance and high associated mortality: 21% to 43%.[68] Of the GNAR, *Bacteroides fragilis* group bacteria are the most commons causative agent for endocarditis. However, *Fusobacterium* spp.—specifically *Fusobacterium necrophorum*—and other *Bacteroides* spp. have been cultured in endocarditis.[69] Primary sites of infectious sources include the gastrointestinal tract, head and neck, and genitourinary tract, with hematogenous spread to the cardiac valves. Anaerobic endocarditis is similar to aerobic endocarditis in terms of its valvular pattern, male predominance, and risk factors—for example, intravenous drug use. However, a prior clinical history of heart disease is not as common in GNAR endocarditis, and thromboembolic complications are more common than in aerobic endocarditis.[70] Specifically, *Bacteroides fragilis* is associated with large valvular vegetations and subsequent diffuse thrombolic phenomena. *B. fragilis* expression of heparinase and other fibrinolytic enzymes may underlie these findings.[71] In addition to the classical thromboembolic phenomena of endocarditis, temporal lobe and renal emboli as well as portal vein thrombosis have been reported.[72,73] *B. fragilis* group and *Fusobacterium* spp. are the GNARs associated with pericarditis.[74] Cardiac surgery,

trauma, gastrointestinal fistulae and perforations, and concomitant pleuropulmonary infections are all risk factors.

INTRA-ABDOMINAL

Intra-abdominal abscesses can occur after frank perforation stemming from a trauma, surgical procedure of the intestine or biliary tract, or intestinal cancer. Abscesses also form in the setting of inflammatory-infectious processes such as appendicitis, inflammatory bowel disease, diverticulitis, cholecystitis, or pancreatitis. *Bacteroides fragilis* is the prototypic anaerobe associated with intra-abdominal abscesses. *Escherichia coli* are also common isolates. The facultative anaerobe *E. coli* and *Bacteroides fragilis* can act synergistically and are often both isolated from intra-abdominal abscesses. It is the host response to the capsular polysaccharides of *Bacteroides fragilis* that results in abscess formation. Studies in mouse models using intraperitoneal injection of *B. fragilis* have provided valuable insight into how adaptive and innate immune cell subsets, as well as mesothelial cells, contribute to intra-abdominal abscess formation. It speaks to the unique biology of the *B. fragilis* that this organism that makes up less than 0.5% of the intestinal microflora is responsible for the vast majority of intra-abdominal abscesses.

PERITONITIS

Patients with end-stage renal disease on chronic peritoneal dialysis are at increased risk for peritonitis, a cause of great morbidity and mortality in these patients. A recent review by Troidle and Finkestein suggests that 80% of peritoneal samples in the setting of peritonitis are culture positive, and of these only 2.5% are associated with anaerobic organisms.[75] Peritonitis secondary to trauma, such as gunshot wounds, or perforation in the setting of intra-abdominal surgery or an intra-abdominal inflammatory process is more likely to involve the GNAR, especially the *Bacteroides fragilis* group. A recent study by Shinagawa and colleagues examined the microflora of perforation peritonitis and found that among the GNAR, *Bacteroides fragilis* was cultured most frequently in 64% of cases, followed by *Fusobacterium* spp. (40%), *Prevotella* spp./*Porphyromonas* spp. (32%), and *Bilophila wadsworthia* (28%). (*Bilophila wadsworthia* was only identified in polymicrobial infections.)[76] *Bilophila wadsworthia* is frequently (50% of reported cases) isolated in peritoneal inflammation and abscesses arising in the setting of appendiceal perforation or gangrene.[77] In neonates, peritonitis and abscesses most often occur in the setting of necrotizing enterocolitis.[78]

ENTERITIS

Enterotoxigenic *Bacteroides fragilis* (ETBF) has been implicated in enteritis, acute diarrhea in pediatric and adult populations, and as an inciting agent in inflammatory bowel disease. Diarrhea in these cases is severe, nonhemorrhagic, and accompanied by marked abdominal pain. Recent observational studies have reported on the constellation of symptoms and prevalence of ETBF in adult and pediatric populations in Bangladesh, Vietnam, and Turkey.[79-81] The prevalence of ETBF has also been investigated in cases of hospital-acquired diarrhea. Of the 152 reviewed cases, ETBF was detected in 9.2% of cases as compared to 2.3% in control cases, a statistically significant difference, $p = 0.04$.[82] The prevalence reported in healthy, asymptomatic persons ranged from 6.5% to 12.4%.[83,84] Interestingly, a recent study suggested yet another intriguing link between ETBF and human disease: In a cohort of Turkish patients, those with sporadic colorectal cancer had a higher prevalence of the bft gene by PCR than control patients—38% versus 12%.[85]

UROGENITAL TRACT

The GNAR play a central role in numerous nonsexually transmitted diseases of the urogenital tract. The bulk of these infections involve the female reproductive organs and include bacterial vaginosis, Bartholin's cyst abscess, pelvic inflammatory disease, tubo-ovarian abscess, endometritis, amniotis, and wound infections secondary to gynecologic or obstetric procedures. However, the GNAR also play a pathogenic role in acute and chronic prostatitis, prostatic and scrotal abscesses, and scrotal gangrene (Fournier's gangrene). Of these male urogenital infections, *Bacteroides fragilis*, *Prevotella*, and *Porphyromonas* spp. have been isolated, and antibiotic therapy directed at these organisms has been part of successful treatment regimens.[86] Regarding the infections afflicting female patients, bacterial vaginosis is a very common entity involving vaginal flora shifts. The vaginal microflora is usually *Lactobacillus* dominant. However, in bacterial vaginosis, there are increases in *Gardnerella vaginalis*, *Bacteroides* spp., *Prevotella* spp., *Mobiluncus* spp., and genital mycoplasmas.[26] The instigating events of bacterial vaginosis—in particular the relative importance of anaerobes versus *Gardnerella vaginalis* in disease causation—remain controversial (see Chapter 107).[87] As in other abscesses throughout the body, polymicrobial infection involving several anaerobes is often the case in tubo-ovarian and Bartholin's cyst abscesses. Bacterial vaginosis is a risk factor for preterm labor, and as such, GNAR colonization of the vagina and reproductive structures may pose a risk for adverse pregnancy outcomes.[88-90]

Treatment

While antimicrobials are the mainstay of treatment for GNAR infections, treatment regimens may also involve interventional and surgical approaches, as well as adjunctive therapies to facilitate healing and recovery. Selection of empiric antimicrobial therapy for infections involving GNAR is guided by a few general principles. Intra-abdominal infections should include coverage for both anaerobes and coliform bacteria; either two drug regimens or single agents are appropriate (specific antibiotics are discussed below). Urogenital tract infections are usually polymicrobial, involving coliforms, anaerobes, and streptococci, and broad-spectrum monotherapy or two drugs are appropriate. Similarly, skin and soft tissues infections are polymicrobial, involve both aerobes and anaerobes, and require broad coverage. CNS infections, particularly brain abscesses, should be treated with metronidazole, which has good CNS penetration, as well as a penicillin or a third-generation cephalosporin for streptococcal coverage. In addition to combating infection, there is a clear role for the prophylactic use of antibiotics in surgery (see Chapter 316). Especially in the case of colorectal surgery, prophylactic antibiotics improve patient outcomes by reducing postoperative infections. Coverage for both aerobes and anaerobes has led to a decrease in surgical wound infections by at least 75%.[91]

SURGICAL TREATMENT

Surgical treatment is a principal and essential modality for many GNAR infections. Incision and drainage is usually necessary for the treatment of abscesses. As necrosis is often a feature of infections complicated by GNAR, débridement of necrotic tissues is necessary for resolution of infections. Interventional radiologists frequently place percutaneous drains under fluoroscopic, ultrasound, or computed tomographic guidance that effectively drain abscesses. Surgical drainage in many cases ensues if relatively less invasive measures are unsuc-

cessful. Location, size, and attendant procedural risk are all prominent factors in clinical management of abscesses.

ANTIBIOTIC THERAPY

Treatment of many GNAR infections is empiric because of the polymicrobial nature of these infections and the time delays associated with anaerobic culture and susceptibility testing. Antibiotics that provide coverage across the aerobic and anaerobic spectrum should be administered when there is clinical suspicion for mixed infections. Many GNAR are resistant to a number antimicrobials as a result of extended β-lactamase resistance and metronidazole resistance, making these infections a clinical challenge (Table 247-2).

For decades, penicillin G had been the drug of choice for numerous GNAR infections. The *B. fragilis* group is penicillin-resistant, and as such, penicillin G is used for GNAR outside of the abdominopelvic cavity. Unfortunately, penicillin treatment failure has emerged secondary to β-lactamase production by certain GNAR. Penicillin resistance has been reported for *Prevotella bivia* and *disiens*, *Porphyromonas* spp., *Bacteroides splanchnicus*, and *Bilophila wadsworthia*. β-lactamase-producing strains of *Fusobacterium nucleatum*, both intra- and extra-oral, have been reported, and *Fusobacterium necrophorum* is often penicillin-resistant.[92,93] Although penicillin G is not an unreasonable choice for minor odontogenic infections, it is not recommended as empiric coverage for severe oropharyngeal or pleuropulmonary GNAR infections because of the aforementioned resistance issues.

Beta-lactam antibiotics in conjunction with beta-lactamase inhibitors—for example, ticarcillin-clavulanate or piperacillin-tazobactam—show excellent activity against *B. fragilis* group members, as well as *Prevotella*, *Porphyromonas*, *Fusobacterium*, *Bilophila*, and *Sutterella* spp. The first-generation cephalosporins are not effective against the *B. fragilis* group, *Prevotella*, and *Porphyromonas* spp., as these organisms all produce cephalosporinase.[94] Among the second-generation cepaholosporins, there is resistance among the *B. fragilis* strains to cefoxitin, and other *B. fragilis* group members are resistant to cefotetan and cefmetazole. There is variable resistance to third-generation cephalosporins, such as ceftizoxime. *Bacteroides fragilis* and *Bilophila wadsworthia* are usually resistant.

The carbapenems are a highly effective class of antibiotics for the GNAR, and several have broad-spectrum activity against both aerobic and anaerobic bacteria. Imipenem, meropenem, ertapenem, and doripenem are all FDA-approved carbapenems. Both doripenem and ertapenem provide excellent empiric coverage for complicated intra-abdominal infections.[95] However, resistance is emerging, and non-susceptibility to carbapenems has been reported for *B. fragilis*, *Fusobacterium* species, and *Prevotella* species isolates.[96] While chloramphenicol has excellent in vitro activity against GNAR, its attendant toxicities have limited its used.

Clindamycin is a highly effective antibiotic against *Prevotella* spp., *Porphyomonas*, and *Fusobacterium*. There is significant resistance among the *B. fragilis* group (5% to 35%) and *Sutterella wadsworthia* (25% to 35%).[95] Thus, while clindamycin's activity against aerobic gram-positive cocci makes it an appealing choice for the treatment of polymicrobial infections, its lack of activity against important anaerobes limits its use as a sole drug in anaerobic infections.

Tigecycline, a glycylcycline, is currently the only FDA-approved member of its class. Tigecycline has outstanding in vitro activity

TABLE 247-2	Antibiotic Sensitivities of Medically Important Gram-negative Anaerobic Rods[105]					
	Penicillin	*β-lactam*	*Clindamycin*	*Carbapenem*	*Metronidazole*	*2nd-Generation Fluoroquinolones*
Bacteroides fragilis group	R	V	V	S	S	S
Prevotella	R	V	S	S	S	S
Porphyromonas	R	V	S	S	S	S
Fusobacterium	S	V	S	S	S	S

R, resistant >30%; S, sensitive <5%; V, variable >5%.

against not only gram-positive and gram-negative anaerobes but also gram-positive aerobes.[97] Its broad spectrum makes it attractive for empiric therapy of complicated skin, soft tissues, and intra-abdominal infections.[98]

There is varying resistance among the GNAR to the quinolone antibiotics. While the GNAR are all highly susceptible to moxifloxacin, resistance rates for levofloxacin and ciprofloxacin are as high as 50%.[99]

Metronidazole has been a highly effective agent for all of the GNAR, except for *Sutterella*, for close to 50 years. Anaerobes convert this prodrug into its active form that then inhibits their nucleic acid synthesis. The rates of metronidazole resistance among the GNAR remain low—less than 1%. However, there is concern for emerging resistance. The nim resistance genes, of which six have been identified, confer resistance to metronidazole by encoding a reductase that prevents the conversion of metronidazole into its active form. A recent study of over 1500 *Bacteroides fragilis* clinical isolates from Europe detected nim gene expression in 2% of samples, raising concern for evolving resistance.[100] Use of metronidazole is limited as a single agent for many infections involving GNAR—for example, pleuropulmonary infection—because of the resistance of aerobic or microaerophilic streptococci.

REFERENCES

1. Riordan T. Human infection with *Fusobacterium necrophorum* (Necrobacillosis), with a focus on Lemierre's syndrome. *Clin Microbiol Rev.* 2007;20:622-659.
2. Tribble G. Development of a Model of Transposition for the *Bacteroides* mobilizable transposon TN4555. Volume 1999: East Carolina University, 1999.
3. Brook I. Anaerobic bacterial bacteremia: 12-year experience in two military hospitals. *J Infect Dis.* 1989;160:1071-1075.
4. Sears CL. A dynamic partnership: celebrating our gut flora. *Anaerobe.* 2005;11:247-251.
5. Palmer C, Bik EM, Digiulio DB, et al. Development of the Human Infant Intestinal Microbiota. *PLoS Biol.* 2007;5:e177.
6. Bjorksten B. Impact of gastrointestinal flora on systemic diseases. *J Pediatr Gastroenterol Nutr.* 2008;46(Suppl 1):E12-E13.
7. Vael C, Nelen V, Verhulst SL, et al. Early intestinal *Bacteroides fragilis* colonisation and development of asthma. *BMC Pulm Med.* 2008;8:19.
8. Mazmanian SK. Capsular polysaccharides of symbiotic bacteria modulate immune responses during experimental colitis. *J Pediatr Gastroenterol Nutr.* 2008;46(Suppl 1):E11-E12.
9. Mazmanian SK, Liu CH, Tzianabos AO, et al. An immunomodulatory molecule of symbiotic bacteria directs maturation of the host immune system. *Cell.* 2005;122:107-118.
10. Kelly D, Campbell JI, King TP, et al. Commensal anaerobic gut bacteria attenuate inflammation by regulating nuclear-cytoplasmic shuttling of PPAR-gamma and RelA. *Nat Immunol.* 2004;5:104-112.
11. Stecher B, Hardt WD. The role of microbiota in infectious disease. *Trends Microbiol.* 2008;16:107-114.
12. Martens EC, Chiang HC, Gordon JI. Mucosal glycan foraging enhances fitness and transmission of a saccharolytic human gut bacterial symbiont. *Cell Host Microbe.* 2008;4:447-457.
13. Lozupone CA, Hamady M, Cantarel BL, et al. The convergence of carbohydrate active gene repertoires in human gut microbes. *Proc Natl Acad Sci U S A.* 2008;105:15076-15081.
14. Koropatkin NM, Martens EC, Gordon JI, et al. Starch catabolism by a prominent human gut symbiont is directed by the recognition of amylose helices. *Structure.* 2008;16:1105-1115.
15. Coyne MJ, Chatzidaki-Livanis M, Paoletti LC, et al. Role of glycan synthesis in colonization of the mammalian gut by the bacterial symbiont *Bacteroides fragilis. Proc Natl Acad Sci U S A.* 2008;105:13099-13104.
16. Turnbaugh PJ, Hamady M, Yatsunenko T, et al. A core gut microbiome in obese and lean twins. *Nature.* 2009;457:480-484.
17. Turnbaugh PJ, Ley RE, Mahowald MA, et al. An obesity-associated gut microbiome with increased capacity for energy harvest. *Nature.* 2006;444:1027-1031.
18. Onderdonk AB, Delaney ML, Zamarchi GR, et al. Normal vaginal microflora during use of various forms of catamenial protection. *Rev Infect Dis.* 1989;11(Suppl 1):S61-S67.
19. Hammerschlag MR, Alpert S, Onderdonk AB, et al. Anaerobic microflora of the vagina in children. *Am J Obstet Gynecol.* 1978;131:853-856.
20. Bartlett JG, Moon NE, Goldstein PR, et al. Cervical and vaginal bacterial flora: ecologic niches in the female lower genital tract. *Am J Obstet Gynecol.* 1978;130:658-661.
21. Bartlett JG, Onderdonk AB, Drude E, et al. Quantitative bacteriology of the vaginal flora. *J Infect Dis.* 1977;136:271-277.
22. Ross RA, Lee ML, Delaney ML, et al. Mixed-effect models for predicting microbial interactions in the vaginal ecosystem. *J Clin Microbiol.* 1994;32:871-875.
23. Hillier SL. The complexity of microbial diversity in bacterial vaginosis. *N Engl J Med.* 2005;353:1886-1887.
24. Simhan HN, Caritis SN, Krohn MA, et al. The vaginal inflammatory milieu and the risk of early premature preterm rupture of membranes. *Am J Obstet Gynecol.* 2005;192:213-218.
25. Onderdonk AB, Lee ML, Lieberman E, et al. Quantitative microbiologic models for preterm delivery. *J Clin Microbiol.* 2003;41:1073-1079.
26. Hillier SL, Krohn MA, Rabe LK, et al. The normal vaginal flora, H_2O_2-producing lactobacilli, and bacterial vaginosis in pregnant women. *Clin Infect Dis.* 1993;16(Suppl 4):S273-S281.
27. Wexler HM. *Bacteroides*: the good, the bad, and the nitty-gritty. *Clin Microbiol Rev.* 2007;20:593-621.
28. Bostanci N, Allaker RP, Belibasakis GN, et al. *Porphyromonas gingivalis* antagonises *Campylobacter rectus* induced cytokine production by human monocytes. *Cytokine.* 2007;39:147-156.
29. Hofstad T, Skaug N, Sveen K. Stimulation of B lymphocytes by lipopolysaccharides from anaerobic bacteria. *Clin Infect Dis.* 1993;16(Suppl 4):S200-S202.
30. Hofstad T. Evaluation of the API ZYM system for identification of *Bacteroides* and *Fusobacterium* species. *Med Microbiol Immunol.* 1980;168:173-177.
31. Pantosti A, Tzianabos AO, Reinap BG, et al. *Bacteroides fragilis* strains express multiple capsular polysaccharides. *J Clin Microbiol.* 1993;31:1850-1855.
32. Gibson FC, 3rd, Onderdonk AB, Kasper DL, et al. Cellular mechanism of intraabdominal abscess formation by *Bacteroides fragilis. J Immunol.* 1998;160:5000-5006.
33. Tzianabos AO, Gibson FC 3rd, Cisneros RL, et al. Protection against experimental intraabdominal sepsis by two polysaccharide immunomodulators. *J Infect Dis.* 1998;178:200-206.
34. Guzman CA, Biavasco F, Pruzzo C. News & notes: adhesiveness of *Bacteroides fragilis* strains isolated from feces of healthy donors, abscesses, and blood. *Curr Microbiol.* 1997;34:332-334.
35. Brook I, Myhal LA, Dorsey CH. Encapsulation and pilus formation of *Bacteroides* spp. in normal flora abscesses and blood. *J Infect.* 1992;25:251-257.
36. Smith R, Paster BJ. *Prokaryotes: A Handbook on the Biology of Bacteria.* Springer; 2006.
37. Ji S, Hyun J, Park E, et al. Susceptibility of various oral bacteria to antimicrobial peptides and to phagocytosis by neutrophils. *J Periodontal Res.* 2007;42:410-419.
38. Mathur P, Chaudhry R, Kumar L, et al. A study of bacteremia in febrile neutropenic patients at a tertiary-care hospital with special reference to anaerobes. *Med Oncol.* 2002;19:267-272.
39. Tzianabos AO, Russell PR, Onderdonk AB, et al. IL-2 mediates protection against abscess formation in an experimental model of sepsis. *J Immunol.* 1999;163:893-897.
40. Hou L, Sasakj H, Stashenko P. B-Cell deficiency predisposes mice to disseminating anaerobic infections: protection by passive antibody transfer. *Infect Immun.* 2000;68:5645-5651.
41. Fisher MC, Baluarte HJ, Long SS. Bacteremia due to *Bacteroides fragilis* after elective appendectomy in renal transplant recipients. *J Infect Dis.* 1981;143:635-638.
42. Goldstein EJ. Anaerobic bacteremia. *Clin Infect Dis.* 1996;23(Suppl 1):S97-S101.
43. Zahar JR, Farhat H, Chachaty E, et al. Incidence and clinical significance of anaerobic bacteraemia in cancer patients: a 6-year retrospective study. *Clin Microbiol Infect.* 2005;11:724-729.
44. Lassmann B, Gustafson DR, Wood CM, et al. Reemergence of anaerobic bacteremia. *Clin Infect Dis.* 2007;44:895-900.
45. Brook I. The clinical importance of all members of the *Bacteroides fragilis* group. *J Antimicrob Chemother.* 1990;25:473-474.
46. Chow AW, Guze LB. Bacteroidaceae bacteremia: clinical experience with 112 patients. *Medicine (Baltimore).* 1974;53:93-126.
47. Nguyen MH, Yu VL, Morris AJ, et al. Antimicrobial resistance and clinical outcome of *Bacteroides* bacteremia: findings of a multicenter prospective observational trial. *Clin Infect Dis.* 2000;30:870-876.
48. Bourgault AM, Lamothe F, Dolce P, et al. *Fusobacterium* bacteremia: clinical experience with 40 cases. *Clin Infect Dis.* 1997;25(Suppl 2):S181-S183.
49. Bahrani-Mougeot FK, Paster BJ, Coleman S, et al. Diverse and novel oral bacterial species in blood following dental procedures. *J Clin Microbiol.* 2008;46:2129-2132.
50. Brook I. Microbiology and management of joint and bone infections due to anaerobic bacteria. *J Orthop Sci.* 2008;13:160-169.
51. Finegold SM. Therapy for infections due to anaerobic bacteria: an overview. *J Infect Dis.* 1977;135(Suppl):S25-S29.
52. Brook I. Joint and bone infections due to anaerobic bacteria in children. *Pediatr Rehabil.* 2002;5:11-19.
53. Al-Tawfiq JA. *Bacteroides fragilis* bacteremia associated with vertebral osteomyelitis in a sickle cell patient. *Intern Med.* 2008;47:2183-2185.
54. Mansingh A, Ware M. Acute haematogenous anaerobic osteomyelitis in sickle cell disease. A case report and review of the literature. *West Indian Med J.* 2003;52:53-55.
55. Lavery LA, Sariaya M, Ashry H, et al. Microbiology of osteomyelitis in diabetic foot infections. *J Foot Ankle Surg.* 1995;34:61-64.
56. Meyers B, Schoeman JP, Goddard A, et al. The bacteriology and antimicrobial susceptibility of infected and non-infected dog bite wounds: fifty cases. *Vet Microbiol.* 2008;127:360-368.
57. Brook I. Microbiology and management of human and animal bite wound infections. *Prim Care.* 2003;30:25-39, v.
58. Law DA, Aronoff SC. Anaerobic meningitis in children: case report and review of the literature. *Pediatr Infect Dis J.* 1992;11:968-971.
59. Zadik Y, Becker T, Levin L. [Intra-oral and peri-oral piercing]. *Refuat Hapeh Vehashinayim.* 2007;24:29-34, 83.
60. Perkins CS, Meisner J, Harrison JM. A complication of tongue piercing. *Br Dent J.* 1997;182:147-148.
61. Brook I. The role of anaerobic bacteria in sinusitis. *Anaerobe.* 2006;12:5-12.
62. Brook I, Finegold SM. Bacteriology of chronic otitis media. *JAMA.* 1979;241:487-488.
63. Le Monnier A, Jamet A, Carbonnelle E, et al. *Fusobacterium necrophorum* middle ear infections in children and related complications: report of 25 cases and literature review. *Pediatr Infect Dis J.* 2008;27:613-617.
64. Brook I. Current management of upper respiratory tract and head and neck infections. *Eur Arch Otorhinolaryngol.* 2008.
65. De A, Varaiya A, Mathur M. Anaerobes in pleuropulmonary infections. *Indian J Med Microbiol.* 2002;20:150-152.
66. Foster S, Maskell N. Bacteriology of complicated parapneumonic effusions. *Curr Opin Pulm Med.* 2007;13:319-323.
67. Tunney MM, Field TR, Moriarty TF, et al. Detection of anaerobic bacteria in high numbers in sputum from patients with cystic fibrosis. *Am J Respir Crit Care Med.* 2008;177:995-1001.
68. Brook I. Infective endocarditis caused by anaerobic bacteria. *Arch Cardiovasc Dis.* 2008;101:665-676.
69. Brook I. Endocarditis due to anaerobic bacteria. *Cardiology.* 2002;98:1-5.
70. Bisharat N, Goldstein L, Raz R, et al. Gram-negative anaerobic endocarditis: two case reports and review of the literature. *Eur J Clin Microbiol Infect Dis.* 2001;20:651-654.
71. Lorber B. *Bacteroides, Prevotella, Porphyromonas,* and *Fusobacterium* species (and other medically important anaerobic gram-negative bacilli). In: Mandell GL, Bennett JE, Dolin R, eds. *Mandell, Douglas, and Bennett's Principles and Practice of Infectious Diseases,* 6th ed. Philadelphia: Churchill Livingstone; 2005:2838-2846.
72. Le Goff B, Agard C, Hamidou M, et al. [Endocarditis due to *Bacteroides fragilis* revealed by portal thrombosis: a case report]. *Rev Med Interne.* 2004;25:473-475.
73. Esteban A, Wilson WR, Ruiz-Santana S, et al. Endocarditis caused by *B. fragilis. Chest.* 1983;84:104-107.
74. Brook I. Pericarditis caused by anaerobic bacteria. *Int J Antimicrob Agents.* 2008.
75. Troidle L, Finkelstein F. Treatment and outcome of CPD-associated peritonitis. *Ann Clin Microbiol Antimicrob.* 2006;5:6.
76. Shinagawa N, Tanaka K, Mikamo H, et al. [Bacteria isolated from perforation peritonitis and their antimicrobial susceptibilities]. *Jpn J Antibiot.* 2007;60:206-220.
77. Schumacher UK, Eiring P, Hacker FM. Incidence of *Bilophila wadsworthia* in appendiceal, peritoneal and fecal samples from children. *Clin Microbiol Infect.* 1997;3:134-136.
78. Brook I. Anaerobic infections in children. *Microbes Infect.* 2002;4:1271-1280.
79. Sears CL, Islam S, Saha A, et al. Association of enterotoxigenic *Bacteroides fragilis* infection with inflammatory diarrhea. *Clin Infect Dis.* 2008;47:797-803.
80. Vu Nguyen T, Le Van P, Le Huy C, et al. Diarrhea caused by enterotoxigenic *Bacteroides fragilis* in children less than 5 years of age in Hanoi, Vietnam. *Anaerobe.* 2005;11:109-114.
81. Durmaz B, Dalgalar M, Durmaz R. Prevalence of enterotoxigenic *Bacteroides fragilis* in patients with diarrhea: a controlled study. *Anaerobe.* 2005;11:318-321.

82. Cohen SH, Shetab R, Tang-Feldman YJ, et al. Prevalence of enterotoxigenic *Bacteroides fragilis* in hospital-acquired diarrhea. *Diagn Microbiol Infect Dis.* 2006;55:251-254.

83. Kato N, Liu C, Kato H, et al. Prevalence of enterotoxigenic *Bacteroides fragilis* in children with diarrhea in Japan. *J Clin Microbiol.* 1999;37:801-803.

84. Zhang G, Svenungsson B, Karnell A, et al. Prevalence of enterotoxigenic *Bacteroides fragilis* in adult patients with diarrhea and healthy controls. *Clin Infect Dis.* 1999;29:590-594.

85. Toprak NU, Yagci A, Gulluoglu BM, et al. A possible role of *Bacteroides fragilis* enterotoxin in the aetiology of colorectal cancer. *Clin Microbiol Infect.* 2006;12:782-786.

86. Brook I. Urinary tract and genito-urinary suppurative infections due to anaerobic bacteria. *Int J Urol.* 2004;11:133-141.

87. Josey WE, Schwebke JR. The polymicrobial hypothesis of bacterial vaginosis causation: a reassessment. *Int J STD AIDS.* 2008;19:152-154.

88. Onderdonk AB, Delaney ML, DuBois AM, et al. Detection of bacteria in placental tissues obtained from extremely low gestational age neonates. *Am J Obstet Gynecol.* 2008;198:110 e1-7.

89. Goyal R, Sharma P, Kaur I, et al. Bacterial vaginosis and vaginal anaerobes in preterm labour. *J Indian Med Assoc.* 2004;102:548-550, 553.

90. Urban E, Radnai M, Novak T, et al. Distribution of anaerobic bacteria among pregnant periodontitis patients who experience preterm delivery. *Anaerobe.* 2006;12:52-57.

91. Nelson RL, Glenny AM, Song F. Antimicrobial prophylaxis for colorectal surgery. Cochrane Database Syst Rev 2009:CD001181.

92. Al-Haroni M, Skaug N, Bakken V, et al. Proteomic analysis of ampicillin-resistant oral *Fusobacterium nucleatum. Oral Microbiol Immunol.* 2008;23:36-42.

93. Veldhoen ES, Wolfs TF, van Vught AJ. Two cases of fatal meningitis due to *Fusobacterium necrophorum. Pediatr Neurol.* 2007;36:261-263.

94. Tally FP, O'Keefe JP, Sullivan NM, et al. Inactivation of cephalosporins by *Bacteroides. Antimicrob Agents Chemother.* 1979;16:565-571.

95. Singer E, Calvet L, Mory F, et al. [Monitoring of antibiotic resistance of gram negative anaerobes]. *Med Mal Infect.* 2008;38:256-263.

96. Liu CY, Huang YT, Liao CH, et al. Increasing trends in antimicrobial resistance among clinically important anaerobes and *Bacteroides fragilis* isolates causing nosocomial infections: emerging resistance to carbapenems. *Antimicrob Agents Chemother.* 2008;52:3161-3168.

97. Betriu C, Culebras E, Gomez M, et al. In vitro activity of tigecycline against *Bacteroides* species. *J Antimicrob Chemother.* 2005;56:349-352.

98. Hasper D, Schefold JC, Baumgart DC. Management of severe abdominal infections. *Recent Patents Anti-Infect Drug Disc.* 2009;4:57-65.

99. Betriu C, Rodriguez-Avial I, Gomez M, et al. Changing patterns of fluoroquinolone resistance among *Bacteroides fragilis* group organisms over a 6-year period (1997-2002). *Diagn Microbiol Infect Dis.* 2005;53:221-223.

100. Lofmark S, Fang H, Hedberg M, et al. Inducible metronidazole resistance and nim genes in clinical *Bacteroides fragilis* group isolates. *Antimicrob Agents Chemother.* 2005;49:1253-1256.

248

Anaerobic Cocci

SYDNEY M. FINEGOLD | YULI SONG

Microbiology

Gram-positive anaerobic cocci are better known to most bacteriologists as peptococci or peptostreptococci. *Peptococcus* is only remotely related to other species of gram-positive anaerobic cocci and is rarely cultured from human clinical specimens. *Peptococcus niger* is now the sole remaining representative of this genus. Until recently, most clinical isolates of gram-positive anaerobic cocci were identified as species in the genus *Peptostreptococcus*, but this genus is currently being revised.[1-18] Old and new names for the most common species isolated from clinical material are given in Table 248-1. *Gemella morbillorum* is classified with streptococci and will not be discussed here. *Peptostreptococcus saccharolyticus* has been transferred to the genus *Staphylococcus* and will also not be included here.

Description of the Group

The gram-positive organisms included in this chapter are obligate, anaerobic, non–spore-forming, sometimes elongated, cocci and include the genera *Peptostreptococcus*, *Anaerococcus*, *Parvimonas*, *Finegoldia*, *Peptoniphilus*, *Peptococcus*, and *Ruminococcus*. In Gram-stained preparations of pure cultures, cells are in clumps or chains of cells varying in size from 0.3 to 2.0 mm and can be arranged in pairs, short chains, tetrads, small clusters, or irregular masses. The gram-negative cocci included here are the genera *Veillonella*, *Acidaminococcus*, *Megasphaera*, and *Anaeroglobus*. Cells vary in size from 0.3 to 2.5 mm, characteristically in pairs, but single cells, masses, or chains may also occur.

NATURAL HABITATS

Gram-positive anaerobic cocci are part of the normal flora of the mouth, upper respiratory and gastrointestinal tracts, female genitourinary system, and skin.[11] These cocci constitute 1% to 15% of the normal oral flora. Of these, *Parvimonas micra* is the predominant species in the oral flora although the presence of *Peptostreptococcus stomatis* and *Finegoldia magna* has also been reported. Many species occur in the gastrointestinal tract, with *Ruminococcus productus* being one of the most common organisms. *F. magna* and *Anaerococcus prevotii* are also common. Species of *Anaerococcus* are found in the female genitourinary tract, including *A. tetradius*, *A. lactolyticus*, *A. hydrogenalis*, *A. prevotii*, and *A. vaginalis*.[12,13] Other species found in that site include *Peptostreptococcus anaerobius*, *P. asaccharolyticus*, *F. magna*, *P. micra*, *R. productus*, and *P. niger*.[13] In the skin, *F. magna* predominates, followed by *P. asaccharolyticus* and *R. productus*. The latter may also be found in the upper respiratory tract.

Among the gram-negative anaerobic cocci, *Veillonella* and *Megasphaera* spp. are part of the normal mouth, upper respiratory tract, and gastrointestinal tract flora. *Veillonella* and *Megasphaera* are found in the vaginal flora. *Acidaminococcus* and *Megasphaera* are part of the intestinal flora and may be recovered from certain infections.

CLINICAL SIGNIFICANCE

Bacterial isolates that are predominant, virulent, and resistant to antimicrobial agents should be given the greatest attention. Bacteria present in pure culture or in large numbers are probably of major importance, as are organisms recovered in multiple cultures and isolated from normally sterile sites.

Anaerobic gram-positive cocci are opportunistic pathogens, comprising approximately 25% of all isolates from anaerobic infections.[11] They may be present in a great variety of infections involving all areas of the human body, ranging in severity from mild skin abscesses to more serious and life-threatening infections, such as brain abscess, epidural abscess, bacteremia, endocarditis, necrotizing pneumonia, and septic abortion. In a study of 114,000 blood cultures from 1997 to 2006, the overall incidence of anaerobes decreased from 12.6% to 7.0%, but the incidence of gram-positive anaerobic cocci in bacteremia increased from 5.4% to 12.0%.[14] The incidence of anaerobic cocci in pleuropulmonary infections such as lung abscess, necrotizing pneumonia, aspiration pneumonia, and empyema is about 40%. Anaerobic cocci often are isolated with other organisms in postoperative and primary wound infections, skin and soft tissue infections, including progressive bacterial synergistic gangrene, necrotizing fasciitis, and crepitant cellulitis.[15,16] Other infections in which anaerobic cocci have been recognized as significant pathogens are ocular infections, ear, nose, and throat infections, head and neck infections (including serious neck space infections), oral and dental infections, pericarditis, bone and joint infections (including prosthetic joints), infections of the female genital tract, breast abscess, intra-abdominal infections, urinary tract infections, and anorectal sepsis with and without anal fistula.[17] Although most infections involving gram-positive anaerobic cocci are polymicrobial,[18] there are many cases of their isolation in pure culture[11]; most relate to *F. magna*, but there are also reports of *P. anaerobius*, *P. asaccharolyticus*, *Peptoniphilus indolicus*, *P. micra*, *A. vaginalis*, *A. prevotii*, and *Peptoniphilus harei* in pure culture. *F. magna* is the most pathogenic and one of the most frequently isolated gram-positive anaerobic coccal species found in human clinical specimens. It has been isolated from a wide variety of infections at various body sites in pure culture. These include cases of endocarditis, meningitis, and pneumonia, some of which have been fatal.

F. magna is most commonly associated with infection of skin and soft tissue and bone and joint infections, but has also been isolated from cases of septic arthritis, prosthetic implant infections, breast abscess, diabetic foot infections, and upper respiratory tract infections, such as sinusitis and otitis media. Protein L of *F. magna* has been shown to be a B-cell superantigen.[19]

P. anaerobius is involved in polymicrobial infections, including abscess of the brain, ear, jaw, pleural cavity, pelvic, urogenital, external genitalia, abdominal regions, and nasal septum.[25] The isolation of *P. anaerobius* from endocarditis has been reported. Peptostreptococci have been associated with gingivitis and periodontitis and are found in cultures of periapical dental and peritonsillar abscesses, and in maxillary sinusitis. *P. micra* is increasingly recognized as an important oral pathogen. Although it is considered a natural commensal of the oral cavity, it may be associated with periodontal disease. It is also commonly isolated from other oral infections such as endodontic disease and peritonsillar infections, as well as from mixed infections, including brain abscess, otitis media, sinus infection, human bite wounds, pleural empyema, intra-abdominal infection, anorectal abscess, septicemia, gynecologic infection, vertebral osteomyelitis, and prosthetic joint infection. *Peptoniphilus gorbachii*, *Peptoniphilus olsenii*, and *Anaerococcus murdochii* have been seen primarily in mixed culture in soft tissue extremity infections in patients with peripheral vascular

TABLE 248-1	Changes in Classification of Gram-Positive Anaerobic Coccal Species*	
Current Classification	*Previous Classification*
Peptococcus niger	Peptococcus niger
Peptostreptococcus stomatis	Peptostreptococcus anaerobius
Peptostreptococcus anaerobius	Peptostreptococcus anaerobius
Parvimonas micra	Peptostreptococcus micros
Peptoniphilus asaccharolyticus	Peptostreptococcus asaccharolyticus
Peptoniphilus gorbachii	New species
Peptoniphilus indolicus	Peptostreptococcus indolicus
Peptoniphilus harei	Peptostreptococcus harei
Peptoniphilus ivorii	Peptostreptococcus ivorii
Peptoniphilus lacrimalis	Peptostreptococcus lacrimalis
Peptoniphilus olsenii	New species
Anaerococcus murdochii	New species
Anaerococcus prevotii	Peptostreptococcus prevotii
Anaerococcus tetradius	Peptostreptococcus tetradius
Anaerococcus octavius	Peptostreptococcus octavius
Anaerococcus hydrogenalis	Peptostreptococcus hydrogenalis
Anaerococcus lactolyticus	Peptostreptococcus lactolyticus
Anaerococcus vaginalis	Peptostreptococcus vaginalis
Finegoldia magna	Peptostreptococcus magnus
Gallicola barnesae	Peptostreptococcus barnesae
Slackia heliotrinireducens corrig	Peptostreptococcus heliotrinreducens
Atopobium parvulum	Streptococcus parvulus
Ruminococcus productus	Peptostreptococcus productus
Staphylococcus saccharolyticus	Peptostreptococcus saccharolyticus

*From human clinical specimens.

disease. *R. productus* has been found in necrotizing fasciitis, pyogenic and amebic liver abscesses, endocarditis, and epidural and orofacial abscesses.

Anaerobic gram-negative cocci are uncommonly isolated from human specimens, with *Veillonella* sp. being the most common isolate. Only rarely are *Veillonella* sp. the only etiologic agents identified in serious infections such as meningitis, osteomyelitis, prosthetic joint infection, pleuropulmonary infection, bacteremia, and endocarditis.

Clinical Specimens

COLLECTION, TRANSPORTATION, AND STORAGE

Most gram-positive anaerobic cocci isolated from human clinical material are not extremely oxygen-sensitive. Specimens suspected of harboring anaerobic cocci should be collected, transported, and stored by methods outlined in Chapter 17 and elsewhere.[20] As with other anaerobes, anaerobic cocci are prevalent in the indigenous flora of the body. Therefore, care must be taken to avoid "contamination" of clinical specimens with normal flora.

CULTURE AND ISOLATION OF ANAEROBIC COCCI

Routinely used anaerobic plate media, such as Brucella, Columbia, or Schaedler agar base supplemented with 5% sheep blood, vitamin K₁, and hemin, will support the growth of these microorganisms. However, the Centers for Disease Control and Prevention (CDC) agar base gives better recovery of gram-positive anaerobic cocci than Brucella or other agars. Tween 80 supplementation of media may improve the growth of some gram-positive anaerobic cocci. A combination of different media should be used to maximize recovery rates.

Identification

PHENOTYPIC TESTING[21]

Some gram-positive anaerobic cocci, particularly strains of *P. asaccharolyticus*, decolorize readily with Gram stain and may appear gram-negative. The cell morphology of older cultures of gram-positive anaerobic cocci can be very irregular, with many coccobacillary and rodlike forms. It is also important to distinguish gram-positive anaerobic cocci from microaerophilic organisms, such as strains of *Streptococcus* species. A simple and reliable test is to apply a 5-μg metronidazole disk to the edge of the inoculum; gram-positive anaerobic cocci show a zone of inhibition of 15 mm or larger whereas microaerophilic streptococci show no zones after incubation for 48 hours.

MOLECULAR METHODS

Several studies have used molecular techniques to identify and detect gram-positive anaerobic cocci.[23,24] DNA probes targeting the 16S rRNA gene have been used to detect *P. anaerobius* and *P. micra*. The real-time polymerase chain reaction (PCR) assay has been applied for quantitative detection of *P. micra* in clinical samples.[22] However, the methods are not standardized and substantial problems remain with molecular identification.

Treatment: Susceptibility to Antimicrobial Agents

P. anaerobius exhibits some resistance to amoxicillin, amoxicillin-clavulanate (3 of 30 strains resistant), cefoxitin (2 of 30 strains resistant), azithromycin, and moxifloxacin (1 of 30 strains resistant).[26] There was no resistance found in 31 strains of *P. stomatis*. Ednie and colleagues[27] found some resistance of *P. anaerobius* to clindamycin and ceftobiprole and of *F. magna* to clindamycin.

Penicillins are considered to be effective first-line therapy for gram-positive anaerobic cocci. Most evidence suggests that *P. asaccharolyticus*, *F. magna*, and *Parvimonas micra* are usually susceptible to penicillins, although Wren[30] has reported 16% and 8% penicillin resistance among isolates of *F. magna* and *P. micra*, respectively. Cephalosporins are usually effective and carbapenems are extremely active. Several authorities have maintained that almost all gram-positive anaerobic cocci are susceptible to metronidazole, but resistance has frequently been reported. Susceptibility to clindamycin varies widely (Table 248-2). A French multicenter study[28] has reported 28% clindamycin resistance among *Peptostreptococcus* spp. Clindamycin resistance in *F. magna* has been reported as more than 10% in one study, with 15.3% and 9% resistance in other studies.[29,30] Erythromycin and the newer macrolides clarithromycin and azithromycin have similar efficacies and are probably not active enough to be recommended. Quinolones such as ciprofloxacin have only moderate activity.[31] One report noted that only 72.4% of *F. magna* isolates are susceptible to levofloxacin. Two strains of *F. magna* have been reported to be highly resistant (minimal inhibitory concentration [MIC] > 128 μg/mL) to metronidazole, perhaps related to the *nim* gene. In studies by Brazier and associates,[32,34] taking gram-positive anaerobic cocci as a group, 7.1% of isolates were resistant to penicillin and clindamycin; these were mostly *F. magna* and *P. micra*. There was no resistance among gram-positive anaerobic cocci to piperacillin-tazobactam, cefoxitin, imipenem, or metronidazole. Others have shown that penicillin resistance is caused by changes in penicillin-binding proteins and clindamycin resistance to an RNA methylase that modifies the site of action of the drug. Linezolid and oritavancin, an investigational agent, are both very active against anaerobic gram-positive anaerobic cocci. *Veillonella* are typically resistant to penicillin.

TABLE 248-2 Antimicrobial Susceptibilities of Gram-Positive Anaerobic Cocci

Species (No. of Strains)	Pen (1)	Amp-Sul (8)*	Amp-Clav (8)*	Pip-Tazo (64)*	Cefox (32)	Imi (8)	Clinda (4)	Metro (16)	Cipro (2)	Trova (4)
Anaerococcus lactolyticus (2)	≤0.5	≤0.25	0.25		0.5	0.12	≤0.12	1		
Anaerococcus lactolyticus I (5)	≤0.5-2†	≤0.25-0.5	0.12-0.25	0.5	0.5-2	0.12-0.5	0.25-64❡	1	0.5-1	
Anaerococcus lactolyticus II (3)	≤0.5-1	≤0.25			0.5-1	0.12-0.5	≤0.12	4		
Anaerococcus murdochii (6)	≤0.5-2	≤0.25			0.5-2	0.12-1	0.25-64**	1-4		
Anaerococcus prevotii (3)	2-16	1-4	2	2	1-4	0.5-1	32-128		16	
Anaerococcus tetradius (1)	≤0.5	≤0.25			0.5	≤0.062	0.25	2		
Anaerococcus vaginalis (16)	≤0.5	0.12-0.25	0.12-0.25	0.062-0.12	≤0.12-0.25	≤0.062-0.12	0.062-0.5	0.25-4	4-8	
Finegoldia magna (12)	0.12-1	≤0.25-0.5	0.12-0.25		0.5-2	0.062-0.5	0.062-2	0.25-2	0.12-2	0.062-0.12
Peptoniphilus asaccharolyticus	≤0.5	0.12-0.25	0.12-0.25	0.062	≤0.12	≤0.062	≤0.12	0.5-4		
Peptoniphilus gorbachii	≤0.5-1	≤0.25			≤0.12-0.5	≤0.062	≤0.12-128††	0.5-4		
Peptoniphilus harei (2)	≤0.5-1	≤0.25			0.25	≤0.062	0.5	2		
Peptoniphilus olsenii (4)	≤0.5	≤0.25			≤0.12	≤0.062	≤0.12-1	0.25-1		
Peptostreptococcus anaerobius (16)	0.12-32‡	≤0.25-16¶	0.12 to 32		0.5 to 32	≤0.062-2	≤0.062-0.5	0.12-8	1	0.12
Parvimonas micra (15)	0.062-64§	0.062-0.5	0.062	0.062	0.5-1	0.062-0.12	0.062-1	0.25-1	1-16	0.062
Ruminococcus (30-60)		0.12-2	0.12-1				0.12-4	0.12-2	8-64	
Veillonella (10-20)	0.05-4	0.5-1	0.25-1			<0.06-2	0.25-0.5	0.5-4		

*Results for these three drug combinations given for amoxicillin and piperacillin.

†1 of 5 strains showed resistance.

‡3 of 16 strains showed resistance.

§2 of 15 strains showed resistance.

¶3 of 16 strains showed resistance.

❡1 of 5 strains showed resistance.

**0.25-2, 5 strains; 64, 1 strain.

††≤0.12-1, 4 strains; 64, 1 strain; 128, 1 strain.

Amp-Clav, amoxicillin-clavulanic acid; Amp-Sul, amoxicillin-sulbactam; Cefox, cefoxitin; Cipro, ciprofloxacin; Clinda, clindamycin; Imi, imipenem; Metro, metronidazole; MIC, minimum inhibitory concentration; Pen, penicillin; Pip-Tazo, piperacillin-tazobactam; Trova, trovafloxacin.

Data obtained from Wadsworth Anaerobic Bacteriology Laboratory, VA Medical Center, West Los Angeles. Strains were tested by CLSI (NCCLS) agar dilution procedures.

REFERENCES

1. Murdoch DA, Shah HN, Gharbia SE, et al. Proposal to restrict the genus *Peptostreptococcus* (Kluyver & van Niel 1936) to *Peptostreptococcus anaerobius*. *Anaerobe*. 2000;6:257-260.
2. Murdoch DA, Shah HN. Reclassification of *Peptostreptococcus magnus* (Prevot 1933, Holdeman and Moore 1972) as *Finegoldia magna* comb. nov. and *Peptostreptococcus micros* (Prevot 1933, Smith 1957) as *Micromonas micros* comb. nov. *Anaerobe*. 1999;5:555-559.
3. Tindall BJ, Euzéby JP. Proposal of *Parvimonas* gen. nov. and *Quatrionicoccus* gen. nov. as replacements for the illegitimate, prokaryotic, generic names *Micromonas* Murdoch and Shah 2000 and *Quadricoccus* Maszenan et al. 2002, respectively. *Int J Syst Evol Microbiol*. 2006;56:2711-2713.
4. Ezaki T, Kawamura Y, Li N, et al. Proposal of the genera *Anaerococcus* gen. nov., *Peptoniphilus* gen. nov. and *Gallicola* gen. nov. for members of the genus *Peptostreptococcus*. *Int J Syst Evol Microbiol*. 2001;51:1521-1528.
5. Song Y, Liu C, Finegold SM. *Peptoniphilus gorbachii* sp. nov., *Peptoniphilus olsenii* sp. nov., and *Anaerococcus murdochii* sp. nov. isolated from clinical specimens of human origin. *J Clin Microbiol*. 2007;45:1746-1752.
6. Collins MD, Wallbanks S. Comparative sequence analyses of the 16S rRNA genes of *Lactobacillus minutus*, *Lactobacillus rimae* and *Streptococcus parvulus*: Proposal for the creation of a new genus *Atopobium*. *FEMS Microbiol Lett*. 1992;95:235-240.
7. Ezaki T, Li N, Hashimoto Y, et al. 16S ribosomal DNA sequences of anaerobic cocci and proposal of *Ruminococcus hansenii* comb. nov. and *Ruminococcus productus* comb. nov. *Int J Syst Bacteriol*. 1994;44:130-136.
8. Carlier J-P, Marchandin H, Jumas-Bilak E, et al. *Anaeroglobus geminatus* gen. nov., sp. nov., a novel member of the family Veillonellaceae. *Int J Syst Evol Microbiol*. 2002;52:983-986.

9. Jumas-Bilak E, Carlier JP, Jean-Pierre H, et al. *Veillonella montpellierensis* sp. nov., a novel, anaerobic, gram-negative coccus isolated from human clinical samples. *Int J Syst Evol Microbiol*. 2004;54:1311-1316.
10. Garrity GM, Holt JG. Taxonomic outlines of the Archaea and Bacteria. In: Boone DR, Castenholz RW, eds. *Bergey's Manual of Systematic Bacteriology*, 2nd ed. New York: Springer; 2001: 155-166.
11. Murdoch DA. Gram-positive anaerobic cocci. *Clin Microbiol Rev*. 1998;11:81-120.
12. Ezaki T, Yamamoto N, Ninomiya K, et al. Transfer of *Peptococcus indolicus*, *Peptococcus asaccharolyticus*, *Peptococcus prevotii*, and *Peptococcus magnus* to the genus *Peptostreptococcus* and proposal of *Peptostreptococcus tetradius* sp. nov. *Int J Syst Bacteriol*. 1983; 33:683-698.
13. Li N, Hashimoto Y, Adnan S, et al. Three new species of the genus *Peptostreptococcus* isolated from humans: *Peptostreptococcus vaginalis* sp. nov., *Peptostreptococcus lacrimalis* sp. nov., and *Peptostreptococcus lactolyticus* sp. nov. *Int J Syst Bacteriol*. 1992;42:602-605.
14. Fenner L, Widmer AF, Straub C, et al. Is the incidence of anaerobic bacteremia decreasing? Analysis of 114,000 blood cultures over a ten-year period. *J Clin Microbiol*. 2008;46:2432-2434.
15. Bourgault A-M, Rosenblatt JE, Fitzgerald RH. *Peptococcus magnus*: A significant human pathogen. *Ann Intern Med*. 1980;93:244-248.
16. Murdoch DA, Mitchelmore IJ, Tabaqchali S. The clinical importance of gram-positive anaerobic cocci isolated at St. Bartholomew's Hospital, London, in 1987. *J Med Microbiol*. 1994;41:36-44.
17. Brook I. Intra-abdominal, retroperitoneal, and visceral abscesses in children. *Eur J Pediatr Surg*. 2004;14:265-273.

18. Finegold SM. Anaerobic infections in humans: an overview. *Anaerobe*. 1995;1:3-9.
19. Zouali M. Exploitation of host signaling pathways by B cell superantigens—potential strategies for developing targeted therapies in systemic autoimmunity. *Ann N Y Acad Sci*. 2007;1095:342-354.
20. Jousimies-Somer HR, Summanen P, Citron D, et al. *Wadsworth-KTL Anaerobic Bacteriology Manual*. 6th ed. Belmont, Calif: Star Publishing; 2002.
21. Song Y, Liu C, Finegold SM. Development of a flow chart for identification of gram-positive anaerobic cocci in the clinical laboratory. *J Clin Microbiol*. 2007;45:512-516.
22. Boutaga K, van Winkelhoff AJ, Vandenbroucke-Grauls CM, et al. Periodontal pathogens: A quantitative comparison of anaerobic culture and real-time PCR. *FEMS Immunol Med Microbiol*. 2005;45:191-199.
23. Song Y, Liu C, McTeague M, et al. 16S ribosomal DNA sequence-based analysis of clinically significant gram-positive anaerobic cocci. *J Clin Microbiol*. 2003;41:1363-1369.
24. Wildeboer-Veloo AC, Harmsen HJ, Welling GW, et al. Development of 16S rRNA-based probes for the identification of gram-positive anaerobic cocci isolated from human clinical specimens. *Clin Microbiol Infect*. 2007;13:985-992.
25. Downes J, Wade WG. *Peptostreptococcus stomatis* sp. nov., isolated from the human oral cavity. *Int J Syst Evol Microbiol*. 2006;56:751-754.
26. Könönen E, Bryk A, Niemi P, et al. Antimicrobial susceptibilities of *Peptostreptococcus anaerobius* and the newly described *Peptostreptococcus stomatis* isolated from various human sources. *Antimicrob Agents Chemother*. 2007;51:2205-2207.
27. Ednie L, Shapiro S, Appelbaum PC. Antianaerobe activity of ceftobiprole, a new broad-spectrum cephalosporin. *Diagn Microbiol Infect Dis*. 2007;58:133-136.

28. Mory F, Lozniewski A, Bland S, et al. Survey of anaerobic susceptibility patterns: A French multicentre study. *Int J Antimicrob Agents*. 1998;10:229-236.
29. Sanchez ML, Jones RN, Croco JL. Use of the E test to access macrolide-lincosamide resistance patterns among *Peptostreptococcus* species. *Antimicrob Newsletter*. 1992;8:45-49.
30. Wren MWD. Anaerobic cocci of clinical importance. *Br J Biomed Sci*. 1996;53:294-301.
31. Watt B, Brown FV. Is ciprofloxacin active against clinically important anaerobes? *J Antimicrob Chemother*. 1986;17:605-613.
32. Brazier JS, Hall V, Morris TE, et al. Antibiotic susceptibilities of gram-positive anaerobic cocci: Results of a sentinel study in England and Wales. *J Antimicrob Chemother*. 2003;52:224-228.
33. Goldstein EJ, Conrads G, Citron DM, et al. In vitro activity of gemifloxacin compared to seven other oral antimicrobial agents against aerobic and anaerobic pathogens isolated from antral sinus puncture specimens from patients with sinusitis. *Diagn Microbiol Infect Dis*. 2002;42:113-118.
34. Brazier J, Chmelar D, Dubreuil L, et al. European suveillance study on antimicrobial susceptibility of gram-positive anaerobic cocci. *Int J Antimicrob Agents*. 2008;31:316-320.

249

Anaerobic Gram-Positive Nonsporulating Bacilli

EIJA KÖNÖNEN

Anaerobic gram-positive nonsporulating bacilli belong to the commensal microbiota of the digestive tract, and some are members of the microbiota of the urogenital tract and skin. When the environment changes because of trauma, immunosuppression, or antimicrobial therapy, they can cause damage in a susceptible host and result in life-threatening infections. Most anaerobic gram-positive nonsporulating bacilli recovered from clinical specimens belong to the genera *Actinomyces*, *Propionibacterium*, *Lactobacillus*, *Atopobium*, and *Eggerthella*, and *Eubacterium*-like taxa.[1]

Taxonomy

The sequence analysis of the 16S ribosomal RNA gene has resulted in a number of changes in the taxonomy of anaerobic gram-positive nonsporulating bacilli, which are widely distributed among two gram-positive phyla, *Actinobacteria* and *Firmicutes*.[1]

Within the phylum *Actinobacteria*, the family *Actinomycetaceae* includes five genera: *Actinomyces*, *Actinobaculum*, *Arcanobacterium*, *Varibaculum*, and *Mobiluncus*. The genus *Actinomyces* is discussed in the chapter on actinomycosis (see Chapter 255). *Mobiluncus* species, *M. curtisii* and *M. mulieris*, are motile and strictly anaerobic, curved bacilli with variable Gram reactions. The genus *Propionibacterium* consists of anaerobic and aerotolerant, variable-shaped organisms of which *P. acnes* and *P. propionicum*, in particular, can be encountered in clinical material. Members of the family Bifidobacteriaceae are strictly anaerobic or occasionally microaerophilic pleomorphic rods. Human *Bifidobacterium* species and *Scardovia inopinata* and *Parascardovia denticolens*, two former *Bifidobacterium* species, reside in the intestine and mouth.[1] In addition, a closely related novel species, *Alloscardovia omnicolens*, has been isolated from various clinical specimens.[2] *Atopobium* and *Olsenella*, with variable, often coccoid, cells, have been created from the so-called anaerobic lactobacilli, currently belonging to the family *Coriobacteriaceae*. Human *Atopobium* species with clinical relevance include *A. minutum*, *A. rimae*, *A. parvulum*, and *A. vaginae*. The genus *Olsenella* includes two oral species, *O. uli* and *O. profusa*. Although most *Eubacterium* species belong to the Firmicutes, a number of former *Eubacterium* species with a high G + C content have been renamed and removed to the phylum Actinobacteria. Among those are *Eggerthella lenta*, *Collinsella aerofaciens*, and *Slackia exigua*. *E. lenta* and *C. aerofaciens* are intestinal bacteria, whereas *S. exigua* is an oral organism.[1] Two new *Eggerthella* species, *E. hongkongensis* and *E. sinensis*, and a novel genus with a motile and catalase-producing species, *Catabacter hongkongensis*, have been reported in anaerobic bacteremias.[3,4]

Within the phylum Firmicutes, the genus *Lactobacillus* constitutes a branch subdivided into groups, each named after the following species: *L. buchneri*, *L. casei*, *L. delbrueckii*, *L. plantarum*, *L. reuteri*, *L. sakei*, and *L. salivarius*. Some former *Lactobacillus* species have been reclassified and moved to other genera (e.g., *Atopobium* and *Olsenella*).[1] *Eubacterium* and *Eubacterium*-like species are widely distributed among the Firmicutes. Clinically important are *E. brachy*, *E. infirmum*, *E. minutum*, *E. nodatum*, *E. saphenum*, *E. sulci*, *Filifactor alocis*, *Mogibacterium* spp., *Pseudoramibacter alactolyticus*, *Bulleidia extructa*, and *Solobacterium moorei*. New organisms with potential clinical relevance are *Turicibacter sanguinis*, *Oribacterium sinus*, a highly motile species, and *Moryella indoligenes*.[1,5]

MEMBERS OF THE COMMENSAL MICROBIOTA

Bifidobacteria and *Collinsella* are important bacteria in the development of the gut microbiota.[6] A decrease in the levels of intestinal *Bifidobacterium* populations in older adults is seen with aging.[7] Lactobacilli form an important component of the mucosal microbiota of the gastrointestinal tract, with the most prevalent species being *L. rhamnosus*, *L. paracasei*, *L. plantarum*, and *L. salivarius*.[8] In the female genital tract and rectum, the predominant lactobacilli are *L. crispatus*, *L. gasseri*, *L. iners*, *L. jensenii*, and *L. vaginalis*.[9-12] Hydrogen peroxide production by these species, except for *L. iners*, may help control the overgrowth of bacterial vaginosis–associated organisms and protect from obstetric infections during pregnancy, such as those caused by *Mobiluncus*.[10,11] Because of their beneficial characteristics, many *Lactobacillus* strains are increasingly used as probiotics, aiming to alter the composition of the microbiota.[13]

CLINICAL ISOLATES

In infectious lesions, the organisms are often together with other anaerobic or facultative bacteria in polymicrobial consortia, typically at or close to that site; therefore, knowledge about the composition of the predominant commensal microbiota is warranted to anticipate and recognize potential organisms in clinical specimens adjacent to their natural anatomic site. Hematogenous spread of gram-positive anaerobes from the commensal microbiota and local infections along the local veins and through the general circulation expose the host to systemic infections, such as brain abscess, aortic aneurysm, and endocarditis.[14-16] The clinical significance of anaerobic bacteremia varies markedly by pathogen; if patients have an underlying condition and are not treated against anaerobes, the mortality rate can be high.[17,18] It is likely that the incidence of bacteremia caused by anaerobic gram-positive nonsporulating bacilli is underestimated because many of these organisms are slow-growing and fastidious and, if isolated, very difficult to identify by phenotypic tests.

Propionibacteria

Specimens from systemic or disseminated opportunistic infections, such as endocarditis, aortic aneurysms, central nervous system infections, osteomyelitis, osteitis, arthritis, and endodontic infections, as well as infected dog and cat bite wounds, can harbor propionibacteria.[15,19-23] Especially in cases of implantation of foreign bodies (e.g., intraocular lenses, spinal and ventriculoperitoneal shunts, prosthetic heart valves, and posterior implants for scoliosis patients) and late postoperative infections, *P. acnes* is a clinically relevant finding.[20,21,24-27] In a recent study dealing with 276 patients, the authors suggested the shoulder as having a propensity for developing *P. acnes* arthritis compared with lower limbs.[21] The predilection of *P. acnes* for prosthetic and native valves may lead to infective endocarditis, including a risk for further destruction.[24,28-31] Typically, *P. acnes* is isolated from sebaceous follicles and lesions of acne vulgaris but its connection to other conditions, such as sarcoidosis and synovitis, acne, pustulosis, hyperostosis, and osteitis (SAPHO) syndrome has been suggested.[32] Infections with involvement of *P. propionicum* include endodontic and actinomycosis-like eye infections.[33,34]

Lactobacilli

Lactobacilli are not only beneficial organisms but are among major recoveries from advanced dental caries lesions.[35] They can act as causative agents in more serious infections, especially in immunocompromised individuals with prolonged hospitalization.[16-18,36-38] In this context, the most common *Lactobacillus* species are *L. rhamnosus*, *L. casei*, *L. fermentum*, *L. gasseri*, *L. plantarum*, *L. acidophilus*, and *L. ultunensis*.[16,18,35] The presence of lactobacilli in blood specimens is of medical importance, because bacteremia and endocarditis with involvement of lactobacilli carry a relatively high mortality rate[16,18]; however, this situation may be improving.[39] A dental procedure or condition was suggested as a potential predisposing factor in 50% of cases of *Lactobacillus* endocarditis.[16] Several *Lactobacillus* species have been isolated from blood; *L. rhamnosus*, which is typically vancomycin-resistant, was the most frequent species.[16-18,40] Vancomycin-resistant lactobacilli have also been connected to dialysis-related peritonitis after extended use of glycopeptides.[37,38] Different from other *Lactobacillus* species, *L. iners* has been observed in connection to bacterial vaginosis by replacing vaginal health–associated lactobacilli, *L. crispatus*, *L. gasseri*, and *L. jensenii*.[12]

Bifidobacteria

Except for the involvement of bifidobacteria in dental caries, they are generally considered nonpathogenic. *B. adolescentis* and *B. dentium* have been occasionally isolated from other infections in immunocompromised patients.[36] In addition, *B. scardovii* has been isolated from human clinical samples, including blood, urine, and the hip.[41] Recently, the only species of a closely related genus *Alloscardovia* was named *A. omnicolens*. This refers to its presence everywhere in the human body, because it has been isolated from a number of clinical specimens, originating from blood, urine, urethra, mouth, tonsil, and abscesses of the lung and aortic valve.[2]

Atopobium and Olsenella

Both genera include several clinically relevant species. *A. vaginae* is increasingly reported to be involved in infections of the genital tract,[12,42] with high concentrations of *A. vaginae* being especially typical for bacterial vaginosis and thus a diagnostically valuable marker of this state.[12,43] *A. minutum* has been isolated from various infections of the lower part of the body, *A. parvulum* from respiratory specimens and endodontic infections, and *A. rimae* from severe odontogenic infections.[22,44,45] *Olsenella* species, especially *O. uli*, have been detected in various oral infections.[22,45] In addition, *O. uli* has been reported as one of the causative organisms in clinically significant bacteremia.[17]

Mobiluncus

Of the two *Mobiluncus* species, *M. curtisii* appears to be more virulent than *M. mulieris*. *M. curtisii* has been connected to bacterial vaginosis, in which its presence is seen as vibrio-like organisms in smears of vaginal fluid; treatment failure is the result of persistence of the organism.[46] In addition, *M. curtisii* has been occasionally isolated from endometrial smears and pus specimens of the female genital tract.[47] Some reports on extragenital infections and bacteremias with *Mobiluncus* species have been presented.[48]

Eggerthella and Related Species

Members of the genus *Eggerthella* have shown to possess particular pathogenic potential. *E. lenta* has been isolated from various clinical specimens, such as blood, abscesses, wounds, obstetric and genitourinary tract infections, and intra-abdominal infections.[36,49] All *Eggerthella* species—that is, *E. lenta*, *E. hongkongensis*, and *E. sinensis*—have been associated with bacteremias of relatively high mortality.[3,17] Also, a related species, *Catabacter hongkongensis*, was recently detected in

blood samples, with the bacteremia being mainly of gastrointestinal source.[4] An oral species, *Slackia exigua*, is frequently found in periodontal disease and severe odontogenic infections.[44,50]

Eubacterium and Other Taxa

Various *Eubacterium* (in the stricter sense) and related species (e.g., *Filifactor alocis*, *Mogibacterium timidum*, *Mogibacterium vescum*, and *Pseudoramibacter alactolyticus*), have been isolated from periodontal, endodontic, and odontogenic infectious lesions.[22,44,50] Conceivably, organisms of this group are among the anaerobic recoveries from infected human bite wounds.[51] In addition to being isolated from infections in the upper part of the body, *E. nodatum* has been found in infections of the female genital tract.[52] *E. tenue* as well as *Solobacterium moorei* have been detected in clinically significant bacteremias.[17,53,54] Taxonomic changes have hampered assessment of the role of various taxa, previously identified as *Eubacterium*, as causative infectious agents. Of the novel taxa, *Turicibacter sanguinis* has been isolated from human blood, *Oribacterium sinus* from pus of a human sinus, and *Moryella indoligenes* from abscesses below the waistline.[1,5]

Microbiologic Aspects

Most routine diagnostic laboratories identify this group of bacteria by their growth characteristics and Gram stain appearance. *Eggerthella* and *Propionibacterium* species (except *P. propionicum*) are catalase-positive, whereas other anaerobic gram-positive nonsporulating bacilli are catalase-negative. Biochemical tests are not uniformly useful. Increasingly, sequencing of the 16S rRNA gene is used for identification.

Although some species of this group can be very aerotolerant, most species are not. Proper specimen collection and transport techniques are essential for the successful recovery of these anaerobic bacteria. Avoidance of contamination by commensals of the surrounding skin, mucous membranes, and nonsterile secretions is crucial; therefore, mucosal or cutaneous swabs are not appropriate specimens, although still frequently used.[55] Transport media should be specifically designed for the survival of anaerobic bacteria. In the laboratory, specimens should be processed without delay, using appropriate culture media and prolonged incubation. As slow-growing organisms, many anaerobic gram-positive nonsporulating organisms can be easily overgrown by facultatives, leading to biased estimates of their true numbers and clinical significance in mixed cultures. Accurate identification of the isolates, especially *Eubacterium*-like organisms, to the species level, and even to the genus level, are limited if only phenotypical tests are used.[44]

Treatment

Initial diagnosis of infection and choice of antimicrobial therapy is often based on empirical information, while awaiting laboratory test results. Unfortunately, hospital laboratories seldom perform susceptibility testing for anaerobes and, if performed, very few antimicrobials are tested.[55] Table 249-1 summarizes susceptibilities of some anaerobic gram-positive bacilli to a number of antimicrobials. The most uniformly active antimicrobial agents are the penicillins and carbapenems. It is notable that species and strain-related resistance to glycopeptides is frequent in members of the genus *Lactobacillus*.[16,40] Therefore, vancomycin should not be used for the treatment of bacteremia or infections with involvement of lactobacilli without susceptibility testing. Also, cephalosporins are not consistently effective in the treatment of *Lactobacillus* bacteremia. Because metronidazole is the drug of choice in many anaerobic infections, it is also noteworthy that metronidazole-resistant strains are common among *Propionibacterium*, *Bifidobacterium*, and *Lactobacillus* and that strictly anaerobic genera, such as *Atopobium*, *Mobiluncus*, *Eggerthella*, and *Eubacterium*, harbor occasionally resistant strains.[47,56-58] Some novel drugs, such as linezolid, quinupristin-dalfopristin, moxifloxacin, and tigecycline, exhibit potential clinical activity against anaerobic gram-positive

TABLE 249-1 Susceptibilities of Some Genera of Anaerobic Gram-Positive Bacilli to Antimicrobials*

Antimicrobial Agent	Propionibacterium	Bifidobacterium	Lactobacillus	Eubacterium-like	Eggerthella lenta
Penicillin	≤0.03-0.06	≤0.03-1	≤0.03-16	≤0.03-2	≤0.03-2
Amoxicillin	<0.06-1	≤0.06-1	0.5-2	≤0.06-1	≤0.06-1
Amoxicillin-clavulanate	≤0.06-0.5	≤0.06-0.5	0.5-2	≤0.06-1	≤0.06-2
Ampicillin	≤0.03-0.25	≤0.03-32	≤0.03-8	≤0.03-8	≤0.03-16
Piperacillin-tazobactam	≤0.03-2	≤0.03-1	≤0.03-16	≤0.03-32	≤0.03-32
Cefoxitin	≤0.03-2	0.25-64	0.06->128	≤0.03-8	1-64
Imipenem	≤0.03- 0.06	≤0.03-1	≤0.03-16	≤0.03-0.5	≤0.03-2
Ertapenem	0.06-1	0.03-2[†]	0.06->16	0.06-2	ND
Meropenem	0.03-0.5	0.03->8[†]	0.03-16	0.06-4	ND
Vancomycin	0.25-2	0.25-2	0.25->256	0.25-16	0.5-4
Ramoplanin	0.06-0.25	≤0.03-2	≤0.03-0.5	≤0.03-16	0.06-256
Teicoplanin	0.12-1	≤0.06-0.5	≤0.06->64	≤0.06-0.25	0.12-1
Telavancin	0.06-0.25	ND	≤0.03->64	0.03-1	0.12-0.25
Daptomycin	0.12-8	0.25-4	0.12->32	0.06->32	1->32
Pristinamycin	≤0.03-0.12	ND	≤0.03-2	≤0.03-2	0.06-0.12
Quinupristin-dalfopristin	≤0.03-1	≤0.12-2	0.12-16	≤0.03-8	0.12-2
Linezolid	0.25-1	0.12-2	0.5-16	0.06-8	0.5-2
Ranbezolid	1-2	<0.03-1	0.03-4	<0.03	ND
Clarithromycin	≤0.03-0.12	ND	≤0.03->64	≤0.03->64	≤0.03->64
Telithromycin	≤0.03	<0.03-0.12	≤0.03->32	≤0.03->32	≤0.03-2
Garenoxacin	0.06-1	0.25-2	ND	0.12-0.5	≤0.06-2
Gatifloxacin	0.12-0.25	0.25-2	0.25-8	0.25-0.5	ND
Moxifloxacin	0.12-2	0.25-2	0.125->8	0.25-1	0.03-4
Tigecycline	≤0.06-0.5	ND	0.06-1	ND	≤0.06-1
Clindamycin	≤0.03-64	<0.03->64	≤0.03->128	≤0.03->32	≤0.03-16
Metronidazole	64->128	0.25->128	0.25->128	≤0.03->128	≤0.06->64

*Range of minimal inhibitory concentrations (MICs [mg/L]) of tested strains to indicated antimicrobial agents.[56-65]
[†]Includes eight *Bifidobacterium* strains and six *Actinomyces* strains combined together.
ND, no data available.

bacilli, as do some agents not marketed in the United States (ranbezolid, pristinamycin, garenoxacin, and gatifloxacin).[56-65]

When anaerobic gram-positive nonsporulating bacilli are involved in biofilm infections, as is the case typically with foreign bodies, antimicrobial therapy alone is ineffective, despite in vitro susceptibility of the potential causative organism to antibiotics. Partly because of biofilm formation, mechanical intervention or removal of foreign bodies is needed in the management of these infections.[20,25-27]

REFERENCES

1. Könönen E, Wade WG. *Propionibacterium, Lactobacillus, Actinomyces*, and other non-spore-forming anaerobic gram-positive rods. In: Murray PR, Baron EJ, Jorgensen J, et al, eds. *Manual of Clinical Microbiology.* 9th ed. Washington, DC: ASM Press; 2007:872-884.
2. Huys G, Vancanneyt M, D'Haene K, et al. *Alloscardovia omnicolens* gen. nov., sp. nov., from human clinical samples. *Int J Syst Evol Microbiol.* 2007;57(Pt 7):1442-1446.
3. Lau SK, Woo PC, Woo GK, et al. *Eggerthella hongkongensis* sp. nov. and *Eggerthella sinensis* sp. nov., two novel *Eggerthella* species, account for half of the cases of *Eggerthella* bacteremia. *Diagn Microbiol Infect Dis.* 2004;49:2552-2563.
4. Lau SK, McNabb A, Woo GK, et al. *Catabacter hongkongensis* gen. nov., sp. nov., isolated from blood cultures of patients from Hong Kong and Canada. *J Clin Microbiol.* 2007;45:395-401.
5. Carlier JP, K'ouas G, Han XY. *Moryella indolgenes* gen. nov., sp. nov., an anaerobic bacterium isolated from clinical specimens. *Int J Syst Evol Microbiol.* 2007;57(Pt 4):725-729.
6. Harmsen HJ, Wildeboer-Veloo AC, Grijpstra J, et al. Development of 16S rRNA-based probes for the *Coriobacterium* group and the *Atopobium* cluster and their application for enumeration of *Coriobacteriaceae* in human feces from volunteers of different age groups. *Appl Environ Microbiol.* 2000;66:4523-4527.
7. He F, Ouwehand AC, Isolauri E, et al. Differences in composition and mucosal adhesion of bifidobacteria isolated from healthy adults and healthy seniors. *Curr Microbiol.* 2001;43:351-354.
8. Ahrné S, Novaek S, Jeppsson B, et al. The normal *Lactobacillus* flora of healthy human rectal and oral mucosa. *J Appl Microbiol.* 1998;85:88-94.
9. Vasquez A, Jakobsson T, Ahrné S, et al. Vaginal *Lactobacillus* flora of healthy Swedish women. *J Clin Microbiol.* 2002; 40:2746-2749.
10. Wilks M, Wiggins R, Whiley A, et al. Identification and H₂O₂ production of vaginal lactobacilli from pregnant women at high risk of preterm birth and relation with outcome. *J Clin Microbiol.* 2004;42:713-717.
11. Antonio MA, Rabe LK, Hillier SL. Colonization of the rectum by *Lactobacillus* species and decreased risk of bacterial vaginosis. *J Infect Dis.* 2005;192:394-398.
12. De Backer E, Verhelst R, Verstraelen H, et al. Quantitative determination by real-time PCR of four vaginal *Lactobacillus* species, *Gardnerella vaginalis* and *Atopobium vaginae* indicates an inverse relationship between *L. gasseri* and *L. iners. BMC Microbiol.* 2007;7:115.
13. Reid G, Jass J, Sebulsky MT, et al. Potential uses of probiotics in clinical practice. *Clin Microbiol Rev.* 2003;16:658-672.
14. Li X, Tronstad L, Olsen I. Brain abscesses caused by oral infection. *Endod Dent Traumatol.* 1999;15:95-101.
15. Marques da Silva R, Lingaas PS, Geiran O, et al. Multiple bacteria in aortic aneurysms. *J Vasc Surg.* 2003;38:1384-1389.
16. Cannon JP, Lee TA, Bolanos JT, et al. Pathogenic relevance of *Lactobacillus*: A retrospective review of over 200 cases. *Eur J Clin Microbiol Infect Dis.* 2005;24:31-40.
17. Lau SK, Woo PC, Fung AM, et al. Anaerobic, non-sporulating, Gram-positive bacilli bacteraemia characterized by 16S rRNA gene sequencing. *J Med Microbiol.* 2004;53(Pt 12):1247-1253.
18. Salminen MK, Rautelin H, Tynkkynen S, et al. *Lactobacillus* bacteremia, clinical significance, and patient outcome, with special focus on probiotic *L. rhamnosus* GG. *Clin Infect Dis.* 2004;38:62-69.
19. Estoppey O, Rivier G, Blanc CH, et al. *Propionibacterium avidum* sacroiliitis and osteomyelitis. *Rev Rhum Engl Ed.* 1997;64:54-56.
20. Jakab E, Zbinden R, Gubler J, et al. Severe infections caused by *Propionibacterium acnes*: an underestimated pathogen in late postoperative infections. *Yale J Biol Med.* 1996;69:477-482.
21. Levy PY, Fenollar F, Stein A, et al. *Propionibacterium acnes* postoperative shoulder arthritis: an emerging clinical entity. *Clin Infect Dis.* 2008;46:1884-1886.
22. Munson MA, Pitt-Ford T, Chong B, et al. Molecular and cultural analysis of the microflora associated with endodontic infections. *J Dent Res.* 2002;81:761-766.
23. Talan DA, Citron DM, Abrahamian FM, et al. Bacteriologic analysis of infected dog and cat bites. *N Engl J Med.* 1999; 340:85-92.
24. Günthard H, Hany A, Turina M, et al. *Propionibacterium acnes* as a cause of aggressive aortic valve endocarditis and importance of tissue grinding: case report and review. *J Clin Microbiol.* 1994; 32:3043-3045.
25. Hahn F, Zbinden R, Min K. Late implant infections caused by *Propionibacterium acnes* in scoliosis surgery. *Eur Spine J.* 2005;14:783-788.
26. Lutz MF, Berthelot P, Fresard A, et al. Arthroplastic and osteosynthetic infections due to *Propionibacterium acnes*: a retrospective study of 52 cases, 1995-2002. *Eur J Clin Microbiol Infect Dis.* 2005;24:739-744.
27. Nisbet M, Briggs S, Ellis-Pegler R, et al. *Propionibacterium acnes*: An under-appreciated cause of post-neurosurgical infection. *J Antimicrob Chemother.* 2007;60:1097-1103.
28. Hinestrosa F, Djurkovic S, Bourbeau PP, et al. *Propionibacterium acnes* as a cause of prosthetic valve aortic root abscess. *J Clin Microbiol.* 2007;45:259-261.
29. van Leeuwen WJ, Kappetein AP, Bogers AJ. Acute dehiscence of a valve prosthesis 5 years after implantation. *Int J Cardiol.* 2007; 117:e79-e81.
30. Kanjanauthai S, Kanluen T. *Propionibacterium acnes*: A rare cause of late prosthetic valve endocarditis and aortic root abscess. *Int J Cardiol.* 2006;130:e66-e68.
31. Mohsen AH, Price A, Ridgway E, et al. *Propionibacterium acnes* endocarditis in a native valve complicated by intraventricular abscess: A case report and review. *Scand J Infect Dis.* 2001;33:379-380.
32. Perry AL, Lambert PA. Propionibacterium acnes. *Lett Appl Microbiol.* 2006;42:185-188.
33. Brazier JS, Hall V. *Propionibacterium propionicum* and infections of the lacrimal apparatus. *Clin Infect Dis.* 1993;17:892-893.
34. Siqueira JF Jr, Rocas IN. Polymerase chain reaction detection of *Propionibacterium propionicus* and *Actinomyces radicidentis* in

primary and persistent endodontic infections. *Oral Surg Oral Med Oral Pathol Oral Radiol Endod.* 2003;96:215-222.

35. Byun R, Nadkarni MA, Chhour K-L, et al. Quantitative analysis of diverse *Lactobacillus* species present in advanced dental caries. *J Clin Microbiol.* 2004;42:3128-3136.

36. Brook I, Frazier EH. Significant recovery of non-sporulating anaerobic rods from clinical specimens. *Clin Infect Dis.* 1993; 16:476-480.

37. Klein G, Zill E, Schindler R, et al. Peritonitis associated with vancomycin-resistant *Lactobacillus rhamnosus* in a continuous ambulatory peritoneal dialysis patient: Organism identification, antibiotic therapy, and case report. *J Clin Microbiol.* 1998;36:1781-1783.

38. Neef PA, Polenakovik H, Clarridge JE, et al. *Lactobacillus paracasei* continuous ambulatory peritoneal dialysis–related peritonitis and review of the literature. *J Clin Microbiol.* 2003;41: 2783-2784.

39. Salvana EM, Frank M. *Lactobacillus* endocarditis: Case report and review of cases reported since 1992. *J Infect.* 2006;53:e5-e10.

40. Salminen MK, Rautelin H, Tynkkynen S, et al. *Lactobacillus* bacteremia, species identification, and antimicrobial susceptibility of 85 blood isolates. *Clin Infect Dis.* 2006;42:e35-e44.

41. Hoyles L, Inganas E, Falsen E, et al. *Bifidobacterium scardovii* sp. nov., from human sources. *Int J Syst Bacteriol.* 2002;52(Pt 3): 995-999.

42. Geissdörfer W, Böhmer C, Pelz K, et al. Tuboovarian abscess caused by *Atopobium vaginae* following transvaginal oocyte recovery. *J Clin Microbiol.* 2003;41:2788-2790.

43. Menard JP, Fenollar F, Henry M, et al. Molecular quantification of *Gardnerella vaginalis* and *Atopobium vaginae* loads to predict bacterial vaginosis. *Clin Infect Dis.* 2008;47:33-43.

44. Downes J, Munson MA, Spratt DA, et al. Characterisation of *Eubacterium*-like strains isolated from oral infections. *J Med Microbiol.* 2001;50:947-951.

45. Olsen I, Johnson JL, Moore LV, et al. *Lactobacillus uli* sp. nov. and *Lactobacillus rimae* sp. nov. from the human gingival crevice and emended descriptions of *Lactobacillus minutus* and *Streptococcus parvulus*. *Int J Syst Bacteriol.* 1991;41:261-266.

46. Schwebke JR, Lawing LF. Prevalence of *Mobiluncus* spp. among women with and without bacterial vaginosis as detected by polymerase chain reaction. *Sex Transm Dis.* 2001;28:195-199.

47. Bahar H, Torun MM, Ocer F, et al. *Mobiluncus* species in gynaecological and obstetric infections: Antimicrobial resistance and prevalence in a Turkish population. *Int J Antimicrob Agents.* 2005;25:268-271.

48. Sahuquillo-Arce JM, Ramirez-Galleymore P, Garcia J, et al. *Mobiluncus curtisii* bacteremia. *Anaerobe.* 2008;14:123-124.

49. Mosca A, Summanen P, Finegold SM, et al. Cellular fatty acid composition, soluble-protein profile, and antimicrobial resistance pattern of *Eubacterium lentum*. *J Clin Microbiol.* 1998; 36:752-755.

50. Booth V, Downes J, Van den Berg J, et al. Gram-positive anaerobic bacilli in human periodontal disease. *J Periodont Res.* 2004;39:213-220.

51. Talan DA, Abrahamian FM, Moran GJ, et al; Emergency Medicine Human Bite Infection Study Group. Clinical presentation and bacteriologic analysis of infected human bites in patients presenting to emergency departments. *Clin Infect Dis.* 2003;37:1481-1489.

52. Hill GB, Ayers OM, Kohan AP. Characteristics and sites of infection of *Eubacterium nodatum*, *Eubacterium timidum*, *Eubacterium brachy*, and other asaccharolytic eubacteria. *J Clin Microbiol.* 1987;25:1540-1545.

53. Detry G, Pierard D, Vandoorslaer K, et al. Septicemia due to *Solobacterium moorei* in a patient with multiple myeloma. *Anaerobe.* 2006;12:160-162.

54. Lau SK, Teng JL, Leung KW, et al. Bacteremia caused by *Solobacterium moorei* in a patient with acute proctitis and carcinoma of the cervix. *J Clin Microbiol.* 2006;44:3031-3034.

55. Goldstein EJ, Citron DM, Goldman PJ, et al. National hospital survey of anaerobic culture and susceptibility methods: III. *Anaerobe.* 2008;14:68-72.

56. Citron DM, Merriam CV, Tyrrell KL, et al. In vitro activities of ramoplanin, teicoplanin, vancomycin, linezolid, bacitracin, and four other antimicrobials against intestinal anaerobic bacteria. *Antimicrob Agents Chemother.* 2003;47:2334-2338.

57. Hoellman DB, Kelly LM, Credito K, et al. In vitro antianaerobic activity of ertapenem (MK-0826) compared to seven other compounds. *Antimicrob Agents Chemother.* 2002;46:220-224.

58. Liebetrau A, Rodloff AC, Behra-Miellet J, et al. In vitro activities of a new des-fluoro quinolone, garenoxacin, against clinical anaerobic bacteria. *Antimicrob Agents Chemother.* 2003; 47:3667-3671.

59. Edmiston CE, Krepel CJ, Seabrook GR, et al. In vitro activities of moxifloxacin against 900 aerobic and anaerobic surgical isolates from patients with intra-abdominal and diabetic foot infections. *Antimicrob Agents Chemother.* 2004;48:1012-1016.

60. Goldstein EJ, Citron DM, Merriam CV, et al. In vitro activities of the new semisynthetic glycopeptide telavancin (TD-6424), vancomycin, daptomycin, linezolid, and four comparator agents against anaerobic gram-positive species and *Corynebacterium* spp. *Antimicrob Agents Chemother.* 2004;48:2149-2152.

61. Goldstein EJ, Citron DM, Merriam CV, et al. Comparative in vitro activities of XRP 2868, pristinamycin, quinupristin-dalfopristin, vancomycin, daptomycin, linezolid, clarithromycin, telithromycin, clindamycin, and ampicillin against anaerobic gram-positive species, actinomycetes, and lactobacilli. *Antimicrob Agents Chemother.* 2005;49:408-413.

62. Ednie LM, Rattan A, Jacobs MR, et al. Antianaerobe activity of RBX 7644 (ranbezolid), compared with those of eight other agents. *Antimicrob Agents Chemother.* 2003;47:1143-1147.

63. Goldstein EJ, Citron DM, Merriam CV, et al. Comparative in vitro susceptibilities of 396 unusual anaerobic strains to tigecycline and eight other antimicrobial agents. *Antimicrob Agents Chemother.* 2006;50:3507-3513.

64. Bradford PA, Weaver-Sands DT, Petersen PJ. In vitro activity of tigecycline against isolates from patients enrolled in phase 3 clinical trials of treatment for complicated skin and skin-structure infections and complicated intra-abdominal infections. *Clin Infect Dis.* 2005;41(Suppl 5):S315-S332.

65. Moubareck C, Gavini F, Vaugien L, et al. Antimicrobial susceptibility of bifidobacteria. *J Antimicrob Chemother.* 2005; 55:38-44.

250

Mycobacterium tuberculosis

DANIEL W. FITZGERALD | TIMOTHY R. STERLING | DAVID W. HAAS

The term *tuberculosis* describes a broad range of clinical illnesses caused by *Mycobacterium tuberculosis* (or less commonly *Mycobacterium bovis*). It is second only to human immunodeficiency virus (HIV) as a cause of death worldwide resulting from a single infectious agent. In 1993 the World Health Organization (WHO) declared tuberculosis a global public health emergency, and tuberculosis continues to be an immense global public health problem. Tuberculosis can affect virtually every organ, most importantly the lungs, and is typically associated with granuloma formation.

History

There is evidence of spinal tuberculosis in Neolithic, pre-Columbian, and early Egyptian remains. However, tuberculosis did not become a major problem until the Industrial Revolution, when crowded living conditions favored its spread. In the 17th and 18th centuries, tuberculosis caused one fourth of all adult deaths in Europe. Before antimicrobial agents became available, the cornerstone of treatment was rest in the open air in specialized sanatoria. Sanatorium regimens probably benefitted some cases diagnosed before cavitation but had little impact on cavitary disease. When it became clear that cavitation was the pivotal event in progressive pulmonary tuberculosis, most special therapies focused on cavity closure.

The modern era of tuberculosis began in 1946 with demonstration of the efficacy of streptomycin (STM). In 1952, the availability of isoniazid (INH) made tuberculosis curable in most patients, and the addition of rifampin (RMP) in 1970 allowed for even more effective combination therapy. With drug coverage it became possible to successfully resect tuberculous tissue, but with drug treatment resection was rarely necessary. Bed rest and collapse therapy added nothing to chemotherapy; treated patients rapidly became noninfectious; and specialized sanatoria ultimately disappeared. The duration of chemotherapy progressively decreased from approximately 2 years before the availability of RMP, to 9 months with INH plus RMP, and to 6 months using multidrug therapy including INH, RMP, and pyrazinamide (PZA). With INH it also became practical to treat asymptomatic people thought to harbor tubercle bacilli based on positive tuberculin tests.

In the United States, reported cases of tuberculosis had declined nearly every year since accurate statistics became available. However, in 1985 case rates began increasing, driven largely by HIV infection. Tuberculosis control programs in some large cities were not equipped to manage this emerging problem. The often-interrelated factors of illicit drug use, homelessness, and HIV infection predispose to reactivation of remote tuberculosis, to the acquisition and spread of new disease, and, because of irregular adherence to drug therapy, to the development and spread of drug-resistant strains. Epidemics involving strains that were resistant to at least INH and RMP (i.e., multidrug resistant [MDR]) emerged in these populations and spread to HIV-negative persons, including health care workers. Many outbreaks were caused by the Beijing strain, with "strain W" dominating in New York City.

Treatment programs failed because of drug resistance, patient non-adherence, and nosocomial transmission of *M. tuberculosis*. Since 1992, however, tuberculosis incidence rates in the United States have again declined and in 2007 reached the lowest in history.[1] This attests to the success that can be achieved with intensified diagnostic, treatment, and prevention efforts, and with control of HIV-induced immunocompromise by antiretroviral therapy.[2]

The global situation has, unfortunately, not been as successful. The HIV pandemic fueled increased tuberculosis case rates in resource-limited countries worldwide, especially in sub-Saharan Africa. Scant resources and fragile infrastructure, together with a high prevalence of HIV/AIDS, has driven the global burden of tuberculosis higher. As in the United States, MDR tuberculosis (MDR-TB) emerged and spread. In response, WHO worked diligently over the past decade to expand tuberculosis treatment services, including directly observed therapy, short-course (DOTS) programs. In parallel, second-line medications, including fluoroquinolones, were made increasingly available worldwide, with a functional DOTS program being a prerequisite for access to discounted drug pricing.[3]

With widespread use of second-line agents, selection for *M. tuberculosis* resistant to both first- and second-line drugs was inevitable. Extensively drug-resistant [XDR] tuberculosis (defined as resistance to at least INH, RMP, a fluoroquinolone, and an aminoglycoside) first occurred as early as 2001 in Kwazulu-Natal, South Africa,[4,5] and has since been reported in many countries on several continents. Although application of established tuberculosis public health principles, supported by ample funding, may ultimately control this dire situation,[6] the immensity of this challenge is daunting.

Microbiology

The *M. tuberculosis* complex comprises seven species in the genus *Mycobacterium*, family Mycobacteriaceae, and order Actinomycetales that are causes of human tuberculosis and zoonotic disease. The *M. tuberculosis* complex species share 99.9% sequence identity and likely evolved from a single clonal ancestor.[7] The species *M. tuberculosis* causes the vast majority of human tuberculosis. *M. bovis* causes disease in cattle and spreads to humans through animal contact and consumption of unpasteurized milk. A recent cluster investigation of six tuberculosis cases in the United Kingdom demonstrates that *M. bovis* can be transmitted from human to human.[8] *Mycobacterium africanum* and *Mycobacterium canetti* are both rare causes of tuberculosis in Africa. *Mycobacterium caprae*, another cattle pathogen, *Mycobacterium microti*, a pathogen for rodents, and *Mycobacterium pinnipedii*, a pathogen for seals, have been reported to cause zoonotic tuberculosis in humans.

Humans are the only reservoir for the species *M. tuberculosis*, although many animals are susceptible to infection.[9] Some have postulated that an ancient ancestor of *M. tuberculosis* infected hominids in East Africa 3 million years ago, and has since coevolved with its human host.[10] *M. tuberculosis* is an aerobic, non-spore-forming, non-motile bacillus with a high cell wall content of high-molecular-weight lipids. Growth is slow, the generation time being 15 to 20 hours, compared with much less than 1 hour for most common bacterial pathogens, and visible growth takes from 3 to 8 weeks on solid media. The organism tends to grow in parallel groups, producing the colony characteristic of serpentine cording. Complete genome sequences that have been reported include the H37Rv laboratory strain of *M. tuberculosis*, an XDR strain of *M. tuberculosis*, and the BCG strain of *M. bovis*.[11-13] In radical contrast to other bacteria, a very large portion of *M. tuberculosis* genes encode enzymes involved in lipogenesis and lipolysis. Comparative analyses are identifying unique *M. tuberculosis* gene products that are important for survival and may modulate the host immune response (see "Immunology").

A wide spectrum of laboratory techniques has been developed to diagnose active tuberculosis. No single test is perfect, and unfortu-

TABLE 250-1	Comparison of Assays Used in the Diagnosis of Active Tuberculosis			
Clinical Laboratory Question	*Diagnostic Assay*	*Advantages*	*Limitations*
Are mycobacteria present in a clinical specimen?	Culture on solid media (Lowenstein-Jensen egg-based or Middlebrook agar-based media)	Gold standard for isolating *Mycobacterium tuberculosis*; detects 10-100 organisms/mL; shows colony morphology, detects mixed infection, allows quantification of growth; provides organisms for speciation, strain identification, susceptibility testing	Visible growth takes 3-8 wk
	Culture in liquid broth	Sensitivity and specificity similar to solid media; automated systems decrease workload; provides organisms for speciation, strain identification, and susceptibility testing; growth detected in 7-21 days	Does not show colony morphology, detect mixed cultures, or quantify growth
	Acid-fast stain	Same-day results; simple technology; inexpensive	Less sensitive than culture, requiring 10,000 organisms/mL; cannot distinguish *M. tuberculosis* from other mycobacteria
	Nucleic acid amplification (e.g., polymerase chain reaction [PCR])	Same-day results; sensitivity intermediate between acid-fast stain and culture; identifies organisms as members of *M. tuberculosis* complex	Requires advanced laboratory techniques; cannot distinguish dead from viable organisms; culture still needed for speciation, strain identification, and susceptibility testing
Is a mycobacterium isolated from a clinical specimen a member of *M. tuberculosis* complex? (*Mycobacterium tuberculosis*, *Mycobacterium bovis*, *Mycobacterium bovis*-BCG, *Mycobacterium africanum*, *M. microti*, or *Mycobacterium canetti*)	Nucleic acid amplification	(See above)	(See above)
	Nucleic acid probes	Results available in 2 hr; sensitivity and specificity approach 100%; does not require amplification	Requires at least 10^5 organisms; most useful for pure culture, not directly on clinical specimen; cannot distinguish among members of *M. tuberculosis* complex
	BACTEC *p*-nitroacetyl-aminohydroxypropiophenone (NAP) assay	Provides preliminary identification of *M. tuberculosis*	Need for paired cultures increases cost
	High-performance liquid chromatography (HPLC)	Same-day results; sensitivity and specificity approach 100%; can distinguish *M. bovis*-BCG from other members of *M. tuberculosis* complex	Requires HPLC technology; only useful with pure culture
To which species of *M. tuberculosis* complex does a clinical isolate belong?	Colony morphology and biochemical assays (niacin test, heat sensitive catalase, nitrate reduction, PZA monodrug resistance, etc.)	Classic approach for speciation of *M. tuberculosis*	Time consuming and labor intensive
	PCR genomic analysis	May rapidly distinguish among *M. tuberculosis* complex species	Not yet commercially available for this purpose
Do different *M. tuberculosis* isolates represent the same strain?	Genotyping by restriction fragment length polymorphism (RFLP) analysis, spoligotyping, and mycobacterial interspersed repetitive unit (MIRU) analysis	The CDC offers free strain typing through the National Tuberculosis Genotyping and Surveillance Network	Sophisticated assay available only at specialized centers
Is an *M. tuberculosis* isolate drug resistant?	Agar proportion method	Quantifies the proportion of organisms resistant to a drug	Requires as long as 8 wk
	Liquid BACTEC method	Results within 5-14 days	Does not quantify proportion of resistance
	Molecular tests for chromosomal mutations associated with drug resistance	Allow same-day determination of drug resistance; most promising for rifampin resistance mutations	Need to be validated in multiple clinical settings, and not yet FDA approved

nately, some diagnostics on which clinicians still rely were developed over 100 years ago. Advantages and limitations of various methods are presented in Table 250-1.

ACID-FAST STAINING

The term *acid-fast bacilli* is practically synonymous with mycobacteria, although *Nocardia* and some other organisms are variably acid fast. In the Ziehl-Neelsen stain, a fixed smear covered with carbol-fuchsin is heated, rinsed, decolorized with acid-alcohol, and counterstained with methylene blue. The Kinyoun stain is modified to make heating unnecessary. The organisms appear as slightly bent, beaded rods 2 to 4 μm long and 0.2 to 5 μm wide. In sputum they often lie parallel, or two organisms adhere at one end to form a V. An estimated 10,000 organisms/mL of sputum are required for smear positivity, and detection of at least 10 organisms on a slide is optimal; a single organism on a slide is highly suggestive. The sensitivity of sputum acid-fast bacillus smear when compared to culture is approximately 60%.[14] Sensitivity is significantly lower with noncavitary disease and HIV infection. Sensitivity increases by approximately 10% with the collection of a second sputum sample, and 2% with a third.[15] Sputum processing with bleach and concentration before acid-fast staining also increases sensitivity.[16] Most laboratories in the United States now use a fluorochrome stain with phenolic auramine or auramine-rhodamine, a slightly modified acid-alcohol decolorization step, and potassium permanganate counterstaining. Because the mycobacteria are easily seen with a ×20 or ×40 low-magnification objective, fluorescence microscopy requires less technician time and may increase the sensitivity over conventional acid-fast bacillus smears.[17] Advances in ultrabright light-emitting diode (LED) microscopes may make the technology more robust for use in resource-poor settings.[18]

Any biologic fluid or material can be examined directly (e.g., pleural fluid, cerebrospinal fluid [CSF], urine, gastric lavage fluid), although thin fluids are best examined after sedimentation by centrifugation. Positive smears from concentrated gastric aspiration material are usually due to *M. tuberculosis* and are especially important in young children from whom sputum collection may not be possible.

CULTURE METHODS FOR *M. TUBERCULOSIS*

Culture is the gold standard for detecting mycobacteria in clinical specimens. Samples of sputum or tissue require initial decontamination to remove fast-growing nonmycobacterial organisms, and liquefaction to allow access of decontaminants to nonmycobacterial organisms and media nutrients to surviving mycobacteria. Decontamination-liquefaction is most commonly done using *N*-acetyl-L-cysteine as a mucolytic in 1% sodium hydroxide solution. Mycobacteria are relatively protected during this procedure by a fatty acid-rich cell wall. However, normally sterile tissues or fluids such as CSF or pleural fluid should not be decontaminated, as some loss of mycobacterial viability does occur. The sample is then neutralized and centrifuged, and the sediment is inoculated onto media.

Three types of media may be used for culture of mycobacteria: solid egg based (e.g., Lowenstein Jensen), solid agar based (e.g., Middlebrook 7H11), and liquid broth (e.g., Middlebrook 7H12). Media are made selective for mycobacteria by adding antibiotics. Nonselective media, on which growth is more rapid, are available. Growth is more rapid in 5% to 10% carbon dioxide. Liquid broth cultures require 1 to 3 weeks of incubation for detection of organisms, as compared to solid media, which require 3 to 8 weeks. However, solid media allow examination of colony morphology, detection of mixed cultures, and quantification of growth. Further, occasional strains of mycobacteria may only grow on solid media. For these reasons, experts suggest using liquid and solid media in conjunction, with inoculation of at least one solid medium culture.[19]

Commercial automated liquid broth systems greatly facilitate mycobacterial culture. They monitor mycobacterial growth by detection of CO_2 production or O_2 consumption through radiometric, flourometric, or colorimetric indicators. The BACTEC mycobacterial growth indicator tube (MGIT) system (Becton Dickinson Microbiology Systems, Sparks, MD), which detects growth in 1 to 3 weeks by a fluorometric method, is widely used.[20,21]

A new noncommercial liquid broth assay has been developed in which mycobacteria are cultured in liquid media on a multi-well plate and then examined microscopically for characteristic serpentine cording. The addition of antimicrobials to the media allows drug susceptibility testing to be performed simultaneously. Preliminary results show that this microscopic-observation drug-susceptibility (MODS) assay yields results in 7 to 10 days with sensitivity and specificity similar to commercially available liquid broth systems.[22] The promising, inexpensive, and rapid method for culture and drug susceptibility testing will need to be standardized before it is adopted widely.

NUCLEIC ACID AMPLIFICATION

Nucleic acid amplification assays offer another technique for the direct detection of *M. tuberculosis* in clinical specimens. There are at least two commercially available and U.S. Food and Drug Administration (FDA)-approved amplification assays: the Amplified *M. tuberculosis* Direct Test (Gen-Probe, San Diego CA), which targets ribosomal RNA, and the AMPLICOR *M. tuberculosis* Test (Roche Diagnostic Systems, Basel, Switzerland), which targets DNA. Other nucleic acid amplification tests (NAATs) available outside of the United States are

not yet FDA approved. The sensitivity of nucleic acid amplification is intermediate between acid-fast staining and culture. For smear-positive specimens, the sensitivity and specificity of nucleic acid amplification exceed 95%. For smear-negative cases, sensitivity has ranged from 40% to 77% and the specificity remains over 95%.[23]

Nucleic acid amplification complements but does not replace clinical judgment, acid-fast smear, and culture in the diagnosis of tuberculosis.[24,25] In sputum acid-fast smear-positive individuals, positive nucleic acid amplification indicates the presence of *M. tuberculosis* complex and confirms active tuberculosis. When there is a high clinical index of suspicion for pulmonary tuberculosis but with a negative acid-fast smear, a positive NAAT is highly predictive of tuberculosis and allows early initiation of therapy. NAATs perform less well when the clinical index of suspicion for tuberculosis is low, in which case the frequency of false-positive tests may approach that of true positives.[26] Case series of suspected extrapulmonary tuberculosis suggest that nucleic acid amplification of nonrespiratory specimens (e.g., pleural fluid, urine, CSF, tissue) may aid in diagnosis.[27-29] However, sensitivity is low and data are currently inadequate to provide clear usage guidelines for amplification assays in the diagnosis of extrapulmonary tuberculosis. Of note, NAATs cannot distinguish viable from dead organisms so cannot be used to monitor treatment response.

Nucleic acid amplification requires strict adherence to good laboratory practices. In one disquieting study, 20 blinded sputum samples were sent to laboratories in 18 different countries. Only 5 (16%) of 30 laboratories correctly identified the presence or absence of mycobacterial nucleic acid in all 20 samples, and 17 (57%) reported false-positive results.[30]

SPECIATION OF MYCOBACTERIA

Once mycobacteria have been identified in a clinical specimen, speciation is necessary for clinical diagnosis and epidemiologic investigation. For example, speciation may be important in immunocompromised patients at risk for nontuberculous mycobacterial infection, in localities where *M. bovis* transmission from animals to humans is possible, or in bladder cancer patients receiving bacille Calmette-Guérin (BCG) immune stimulatory therapy. Speciation generally involves two steps: first, mycobacteria are identified as members of the *M. tuberculosis* complex (*M. tuberculosis*, *M. bovis*, *M. africanum*, *M. microti*, *M. canetti*, *M. caprae*, and *M. pinnipedii*) or as mycobacteria species other than tuberculosis (MOTT). Subsequently, if necessary, mycobacteria can be speciated within the *M. tuberculosis* complex. NAATs, growth in selective antibiotic media, nucleic acid probes, and high-performance liquid chromatography are all used to place mycobacteria within the *M. tuberculosis* complex.[31] Each has advantages and limitations that are detailed in Table 250-1. Identifying individual species within the *M. tuberculosis* complex is more challenging. *M. tuberculosis* grows slowly, lacks pigment, produces niacin, reduces nitrates, has weak catalase activity that is lost by heating to 68° C at pH 7.0, does not demonstrate monodrug resistance to PZA, is resistant to thiophen-2-carboxylic acid hydrazide, and prefers aerophilic conditions. Other members of the complex show different patterns on these tests. Polymerase chain reaction (PCR)-based genomic deletion analysis, which capitalizes on available complete genome sequence for *M. tuberculosis*, can also identify species within the *M. tuberculosis* complex.[32]

GENOTYPING OF *M. TUBERCULOSIS*

Characterizing the particular strain of *M. tuberculosis* is important for epidemiologic purposes, such as tracing transmission from person to person, distinguishing exogenous reinfection from endogenous reactivation in cases of recurrent tuberculosis, and identifying laboratory cross-contamination of cultures. The Centers for Disease Control and Prevention (CDC) offers free strain typing through the National Tuberculosis Genotyping and Surveillance Network based on three standardized typing methods: restriction fragment length polymorphism (RFLP) analysis, spacer oligonucleotide typing (spoligotyping), and mycobacterial interspersed repetitive unit (MIRU) analysis.[33] In RFLP analysis, DNA cleavage fragments generated using *pvuII* are separated by electrophoresis and visualized using a probe to a repetitive DNA sequence, insertion sequence (IS) *6110*. Because numerous copies of IS*6110* are present at variable chromosomal locations in most *M. tuberculosis* isolates, identical RFLP patterns represent the same strain. Spoligotyping detects variability in the direct repeat (DR) region in *M. tuberculosis* genome. Whether the QTF-G or Elispot blood tests are more specific or sensitive than the tuberculin skin test (TST) in latent or active tuberculosis is still unclear, however, there are direct repeats of a conserved 36-base-pair sequence, separated by multiple spacer sequences. Different *M. tuberculosis* strains are distinguished by the presence or absence of 43 unique spacers. Each possible combination of spacers is designated by a unique numerical code that identifies a unique spoligotype strain. In MIRU analysis twelve different DNA sequences, each of which can be tandemly repeated in the *M. tuberculosis* genome, are analyzed. The number of tandem repeats for each of the twelve sequences (or loci) is determined by PCR to create a 12-number code. Each code corresponds to a unique MIRU strain.

DRUG SUSCEPTIBILITY TESTING

Testing of *M. tuberculosis* isolates for drug susceptibility is important to guide therapy. In the United States the agar proportion method is most commonly used. The absolute concentration method and resistance ratio method are used less commonly. The agar proportion method compares growth of appropriately diluted inocula on drug-containing media to growth on drug-free media and is reported as proportion resistant. For most drugs, resistance is significant when growth on drug-containing media exceeds 1% of control; 6% to 10% resistance or more indicates that the drug will add nothing to multiple drug therapy. Liquid broth systems, such as BACTEC, can also be used and provide results in 5 to 14 days, but they do not give the proportion of resistant organisms.[34,35]

As noted above, the MODS method shows promise as an inexpensive and rapid method for culture and drug susceptibility testing.[22]

Molecular tests to detect chromosomal mutations associated with mycobacterial drug resistance have been developed.[36-39] Most useful are tests for RMP resistance, which predicts poor treatment outcomes and is a surrogate marker for MDR-TB.[20] Assays detect mutations in the 81-bp *rpoB* gene, which encodes the β-subunit of RNA polymerase and correlates with greater than 96% of RMP resistance. Resistance to INH is more complex and is encoded by multiple genes, including the catalase peroxidase gene *katG*, the *inhA* gene involved in fatty acid biosynthesis, the *ahpC* gene, the *oxyR* gene, and the *kasA* gene.[40] Mutations associated with resistance to PZA, ethambutol (EMB), STM, and fluoroquinolones have also been identified.[41] Two line probe assays are commercially available, the INNO-LiPA Rif.TB kit (Innogenetics, Zwijndrecht, Belgium), which detects resistance to RMP on culture isolates, and the Genotype MTBDRplus assay (Hain Lifescience, Nehren, Germany), which detects resistance to INH and RMP on culture isolates and sputum samples.[42,43] The WHO recently recommended widespread use of these assays.[44] Their utility with use of large-scale implementation in many countries will need to be closely monitored.

Epidemiology

GENERAL CONSIDERATIONS

M. tuberculosis infects one third of the world's population and causes 9 million new cases of tuberculosis and approximately 2 million deaths each year.[45] Tuberculosis is second only to HIV as a cause of death worldwide resulting from a single infectious agent.[46] Immunocompromise due to HIV infection is a risk factor for tuberculosis, and 0.2 million tuberculosis deaths are in HIV-infected individuals. Drug-resistant tuberculosis is emerging globally, with approximately 0.5 million new MDR cases annually. Two factors essential for the rapid spread of *M. tuberculosis* are crowded living conditions and a popula-

tion with little native resistance. In the 19th century, tuberculosis caused more than one quarter of all adult deaths in Europe, eliminating those with the least native resistance. A downward trend had been established before the turn of the 20th century. Epidemiologists once believed the disease would eventually disappear based on the assumptions that one in twenty infections result in active cavitary disease of the lung (i.e., become contagious). Thus, each cavitary case would have to infect 20 persons to maintain case rates.[47] In Holland in the early 1900s, one infectious case produced only 13 new infections.[47] The annual decrement in mortality and morbidity from tuberculosis was approximately 5% in developed countries due to progressively higher natural residual resistance in those who survived infection and to living conditions less conducive to airborne spread. This rate of decline approximately doubled after chemotherapy became widespread. In the past decade the high incidence of tuberculosis in Africa, Asia, Eastern Europe, and South America, the HIV co-epidemic, and burgeoning MDR-TB demonstrate that predictions of the disappearance of tuberculosis were premature.

RECENT MORBIDITY AND MORTALITY TRENDS

In the United States the steady decline in tuberculosis morbidity reached a transient nadir in 1984, but from 1985 to 1992 an estimated 64,000 "excess" cases of active tuberculosis (compared to the projected decline) were reported, which peaked at 10.5 reported cases per 100,000 population.[48,49] Factors responsible for this increase included urban homelessness, intravenous drug abuse, growing neglect of tuberculosis control programs, and most notably the AIDS epidemic. After 1992, reported cases declined, reaching 4.4 cases per 100,000 population in 2007, the lowest in recorded history.[1] The tuberculosis rate in foreign-born persons was 10 times higher than in U.S.-born persons, and foreign-born persons now account for most reported cases in the United States (Fig. 250-1).[50,51] This reflects increased immigration from high-prevalence countries, especially Mexico, the Phillipines, Vietnam, India, and China which account for more than half of the foreign-born tuberculosis cases.[51] Strain genotyping suggests that tuberculosis among foreign-born persons is from reactivation of latent infection acquired before arrival in the United States. Further, the risk declines with duration of residency, also suggesting that most infections were acquired before immigration.[52] The likelihood of developing tuberculosis after immigrating varies both by country of origin and by length of time since arrival (Table 250-2).[51,53,54]

Tuberculosis has also become concentrated in certain ethnic/racial minorities and medically underserved populations often occurring in contact-based microepidemics. In 2007, rates among blacks and Hispanics were 7 to 8 times higher than in non-Hispanic whites; the rate

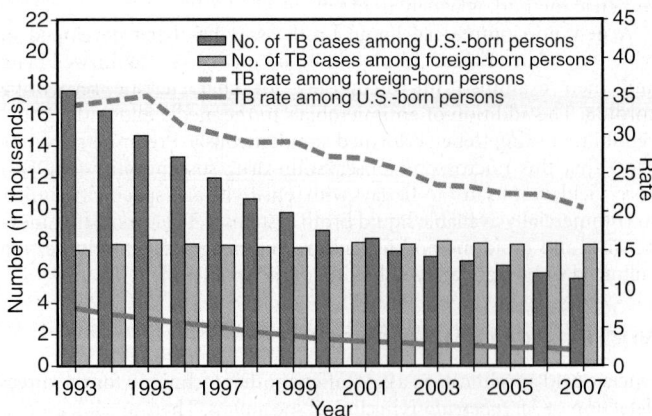

Figure 250-1 Number of reported cases of tuberculosis in the United States by country of birth, 1993-2007. Rates are per 100,000 population. Data for 2007 are provisional. (*Adapted from Centers for Disease Control and Prevention. Trends in Tuberculosis—United States, 2007. MMWR Morb Mortal Wkly Rep. 2008;57;281-285.*)

TABLE 250-2	Reported Tuberculosis Case Rates in Immigrants According to Country of Birth: Stratified by Time Since Entry into the United States	
	Crude Rate (per 100,000 Person-Years)*	
Country	*U.S. Entry ≤ 2 years*	*U.S. Entry > 2 years*
Somalia	889	179
Ethiopia and Eritrea	562	82
Vietnam	319	47
Cambodia	307	65
Philippines	283	38
Ecuador	194	31
Haiti	189	40
Honduras	177	28
Peru	159	32
Guatemala	111	21
India	106	33
China	74	26
El Salvador	73	11
Mexico	52	14
Korea	40	19
All foreign-born	75	16

*Data provided for the 15 most commonly reported countries of birth.

Adapted from Cain KP, Benoit SR, Winston CA, MacKenzie WR. Tuberculosis among foreign born persons in the United States. *JAMA* 2008;300;405-412.

TABLE 250-3	Incidence of Active Tuberculosis in Certain Groups	
Group	*Incidence per 100,000*	*Reference*
Hostel residents in Glasgow	1946	65
Hostel residents in Boston	317	66
Nursing home residents, tuberculin positive on admission	2400	67
Nursing home residents, tuberculin converters	5900	67
Diabetics, Korea	1061	68
Health care workers, South Africa	1133	69
Dialysis patients, San Francisco	5800	70
East Indian dialysis patients, London	25,000	71
AIDS patients, New York, 1986	7000	72
Haitian AIDS patients, 1984	60,000	73

in Asians was 23 times higher than in whites. A number of outbreaks have affected the urban poor, alcoholics, intravenous drug users, the homeless, migrant farm workers, and prison inmates.

The age distribution of tuberculosis reflects the degree of ongoing transmission in a given population. Disease in the elderly is generally due to reactivation of infection acquired in the remote past, whereas tuberculosis in young children indicates ongoing active transmission in the community. In this regard, 85% of childhood cases in the United States are diagnosed in racial and ethnic minorities.

Tuberculosis in the United States is most frequent in geographic regions and demographic groups where AIDS is prevalent, notably urban blacks and Hispanics between 25 and 45 years of age.[55] Persons with active tuberculosis are more frequently HIV positive than is the general population. Approximately 11% of all tuberculosis cases in the United States are HIV coinfected.[1,56] Among populations with a high prevalence of tuberculin positivity, waning immunity caused by HIV infection results in enormous tuberculosis case rates. For example, development of AIDS in Haitians, in whom tuberculin conversion in childhood is almost universal, has resulted in active tuberculosis in 60%.[57] Since 1993, the CDC AIDS surveillance case definition has included any form of active tuberculosis in an HIV-positive person.[58]

Despite a predominantly urban epidemiology, large tuberculosis outbreaks have also affected small communities.[59,60] One well-characterized outbreak began in 1988 in a coastal Maine village where tuberculosis had not been reported in the previous 3 years.[60] A ship-yard worker with cavitary tuberculosis was the source of 21 subsequent active cases and 697 new tuberculous infections. In retrospect, the source case had repeatedly sought medical attention for cough, sore throat, and hoarseness during 8 months before tuberculosis was diagnosed and treated. This report highlights the need for vigilance among all segments of the population, not just those known to have high tuberculosis case rates.

The prevalence of positive TSTs in United States Navy recruits offers insights into trends of latent tuberculosis infection over time, and risk factors for infection. From 1958 through 1969, more than 1 million U.S. Navy recruits received TSTs, and 5.2% were positive. In the 1980s and 1990s, the rate of tuberculin reactivity dropped to approximately 1.5% of new Navy recruits. The prevalence was greater in blacks (5%), Hispanics (5%), and Asian/Pacific Islanders (26%) than in whites (0.8%). Tuberculin positivity was more than 10-fold more prevalent among foreign-born recruits.[61-63] In a survey of noninstitutionalized

civilians in the United States, the prevalence of tuberculin reactivity among persons from 25 to 74 years of age decreased from 14.4% in 1972 to 5.6% in 2000.[64]

Immigrants for the most part retain the tuberculin positivity and tuberculosis rates of their country of origin (see Table 250-2).[53,54] Other groups, such as intravenous drug users, patients with end-stage renal disease or diabetes, health care workers in endemic countries, residents of institutions for the homeless, and, to a lesser degree, nursing home residents, demonstrate morbidity rates greatly in excess of the general population (Table 250-3).[65-73]

On a global scale, tuberculosis has a devastating impact in developing nations, with 12 countries accounting for 70% of all cases (Table 250-4).[45] In 1993, the WHO declared tuberculosis a global public health emergency and intensified major initiatives to address the problem. An important aspect of this strategy is supervised treatment, which may include directly observed treatment, short course (DOTS).[74] However, the challenges are daunting. Profound poverty, the HIV pandemic, civil wars, and refugee migration all impede success. Some countries have made considerable progress in recent years. In China, access to directly observed treatment (DOT) has been expanded from 31% of tuberculosis cases in 2001 to 80% in 2005.[75] Dramatic progress has also been made in India, the country with the greatest number of tuberculosis cases.[76] From 2001 to 2006, DOT coverage increased from 12% to 64%, saving hundreds of thousands of lives.[45,77] Africa, which suffers from the highest rates of HIV and tuberculosis in the world, has not seen such gains, with low case detection, low DOT coverage, and low cure rates.

Over 30 million persons worldwide are now living with HIV/AIDS.[78] The potential for continued interaction between AIDS and tuberculosis is therefore immense. In some developing countries where most

TABLE 250-4	Reported Tuberculosis Cases among Countries That Account for 70% of Reported Cases Worldwide, 2006	
Country	*Cases*	*Rate per 100,000 population*
India	1,228,827	107
China	940,889	71
South Africa	303,114	628
Indonesia	277,589	121
Pakistan	176,678	110
Philippines	147,305	171
Bangladesh	145,186	93
Russian Federation	124,689	87
Myanmar	122,472	253
Ethiopia	122,198	151
Kenya	108,342	296
Vietnam	97,363	113

Adapted from World Health Organization: Global Tuberculosis Database. Available at http://www.who.int/research/en/.

TABLE 250-5	Epidemiologic Circumstances in Which an Exposed Person Is at Increased Risk of Infection with Drug-Resistant *Mycobacterium tuberculosis**

- Exposure to a person who has known drug-resistant tuberculosis
- Exposure to a person with active tuberculosis who has had prior treatment for tuberculosis (treatment failure or relapse) and whose susceptibility test results are not known
- Exposure to persons with active tuberculosis from areas in which there is a high prevalence of drug resistance
- Exposure to persons who continue to have positive sputum smears after 2 months of combination chemotherapy
- Travel in an area of high prevalence of drug resistance

*This information is to be used in deciding whether or not to add a fourth drug (usually ethambutol [EMB]) for children with active tuberculosis, not to infer the empirical need for a second-line treatment regimen.

From Centers for Disease Control and Prevention. Treatment of tuberculosis. American Thoracic Society, CDC and Infectious Diseases Society of America. *MMWR Morb Mortal Wkly Rep.* 2003;52(RR-11):1-88.

persons harbor tubercle bacilli before adulthood, the prevalence of HIV infection becomes the only determinant of coinfection. The situation is worst in sub-Saharan Africa, where the incidence of tuberculosis has risen in parallel with the incidence of HIV. Between 1990 and 2005, the incidence of tuberculosis more than doubled from 149 to 343 per 100,000 population. In 2006, 85% of the world's HIV-positive tuberculosis cases were in Africa. It is estimated that 30% to 40% of all AIDS deaths in Africa are from tuberculosis. This dramatic increase in disease burden has overwhelmed the region's limited health care capacity. Many other regions are also being profoundly affected by the coepidemics of tuberculosis and AIDS.

DRUG-RESISTANT TUBERCULOSIS

Drug-resistant tuberculosis poses an immense challenge for tuberculosis control. Resistance to antituberculous agents can be either *primary,* that is, present before initiating therapy and due to transmission of a drug-resistant *M. tuberculosis* strain, or *secondary,* indicating emergence of resistance after having received antituberculosis therapy. Risk factors for infection with drug-resistant tuberculosis are listed in Table 250-5. Strains resistant to at least INH and RMP are defined as MDR. Strains resistant to at least INH, RMP, a fluoroquinolone, and an aminoglycoside are defined as XDR.[79]

The WHO has regularly reported global drug-resistance rates since 1994.[80-82] In the United States, the rate of primary resistance to any antituberculosis drug has remained stable at about 12%, and of MDR tuberculosis about 1%.[82] Rates of primary MDR tuberculosis vary widely among countries. Among 93 sites surveyed worldwide, an estimated 4.8% of all incident cases in 2006 were MDR,[83] an increase from 1% in 1999.[84] Some so-called hot spots of MDR tuberculosis include Estonia, Henan Province in China, Latvia, and the Russian oblasts of Ivanovo and Tomsk, in which rates exceed 5%.[81,82] Among the countries or geographical settings assessed in the most recent survey, the median prevalence of MDR tuberculosis among new cases was 1%, with a range of 0% to 14%.

Rates of secondary drug resistance are usually higher than primary drug resistance. The global median prevalence of secondary drug resistance is 18.6% (range 0% to 82%) for any drug resistance and 6.9% (range 0% to 56%) for MDR-TB.[82] Corresponding rates in the United States are 19% and 5%, respectively. Prior antituberculosis treatment is the most important risk factor for drug-resistant tuberculosis. Additional historical clues that increase the likelihood of drug resistance include infection acquired in regions where resistance is prevalent, and known contact with a drug-resistant case. One study from southern California recorded resistance in 71% of patients with tuberculosis who had been previously treated and had cavitary disease.[85] Homelessness, illicit drug use, and advanced AIDS all favor acquisition or development of drug-resistant infections.[66,86] Resistance to at least one drug was present in 33% of *M. tuberculosis* isolates during 1 month in 1991 in New York City and to both INH and RMP in a remarkable 19%.[87] Fluoroquinolone resistance was also noted. By 1994, these numbers

had declined to 24% and 13%, respectively,[88] and have continued to decline.[89]

Of immense concern is transmission of XDR tuberculosis (XDR-TB).[79] Outbreaks of XDR-TB have recently been reported in South Africa and Iran.[4,90] In South Africa, all XDR-TB cases were in HIV coinfected individuals, and 98% died. Although precise global estimates of XDR-TB prevalence are not known because many surveys do not test for resistance to second-line drugs, approximately 7% of MDR-TB isolates worldwide may be XDR-TB.[83]

MODE OF SPREAD

Almost all infections with *M. tuberculosis* are due to inhalation of droplet nuclei—infectious particles from a person with pulmonary tuberculosis aerosolized by coughing, sneezing, or talking—which dry while airborne, remain suspended for long periods, and reach the terminal air passages. A cough can produce 3000 infectious droplet nuclei, talking for 5 minutes an equal number, and sneezing many more than that.[91] Accordingly, the air in a room occupied by a person with pulmonary tuberculosis may remain infectious for approximately 30 minutes even after his or her absence. Although in theory one droplet nucleus may be sufficient to establish infection, prolonged exposure and multiple aerosol inocula are usually required. Strains may vary widely in their transmissibility,[59] but infection does not generally occur out of doors because *M. tuberculosis* is killed by ultraviolet light. Large drops of respiratory secretions and fomites are unimportant in transmission, and special housekeeping measures for dishes and bed linens are unnecessary. Other modes of transmission are rare. Infection by *M. bovis* from ingestion of contaminated milk was once commonplace. Skin inoculation of *M. tuberculosis* from contamination of an abrasion occurs in pathologists and laboratory personnel (prosector's wart), and venereal transmission has been recorded. Although the source is pulmonary in the vast majority of cases, aerosolization of organisms during irrigation of cutaneous lesions or at autopsy has caused spread to health care workers.[91,92]

RISK OF INFECTION

The most important determinants of infection of tuberculin-negative persons are closeness of contact and infectiousness of the source. Cases with positive smears are highly infectious; those positive only on culture are less so. The degree of sputum positivity and pattern of coughing are important. Compared with measles, one case of which will infect 80% of susceptible casual contacts, tuberculosis is only moderately infectious in most circumstances.

Tuberculosis morbidity in a population is determined both by the risk of infection and the risk of acquiring active disease once infected. In Holland in the 1970s, 50% of 0- to 14-year-old household contacts of smear-positive cases became tuberculin positive, but only 5% did so when the contact case was culture positive but smear negative.[47] In the United States, approximately 27% of household contacts of smear-positive cases become infected, although rates as high as 80% occur in closed environments.[93] A large epidemiologic investigation in San Francisco from 1991 to 1996 estimated that 17% of new active tuberculosis cases arose from smear-negative, culture-positive index cases.

Persons coinfected with HIV do not appear to be more infectious than HIV-negative source cases. In one large study from Democratic Republic of Congo, household contacts of HIV-positive patients with pulmonary tuberculosis were no more likely to become infected with *M. tuberculosis* than were household contacts of HIV-negative tuberculosis patients.[94] A meta-analysis of six studies involving exposed health care workers supports this finding.[95]

INFLUENCE OF CHEMOTHERAPY ON SPREAD OF INFECTION

Patients receiving appropriate chemotherapy promptly become noninfectious as cough subsides and the concentration of organisms in sputum decreases. The time required to become noninfectious depends on the patient's burden of organisms, but there is indirect evidence that this occurs within 2 weeks in patients with drug-sensitive tuberculosis.[96] Thus, case finding and treatment is the most effective method of tuberculosis control. In reaction to outbreaks of MDR-TB, the CDC in 1994 established very stringent criteria for removing patients from respiratory isolation, which now include three consecutive negative sputum smears on specimens obtained at least 8 hours apart.[97]

RISK OF PROGRESSION FROM INFECTION TO ACTIVE DISEASE

In general, approximately 3% to 4% of infected individuals acquire active tuberculosis during the first year after tuberculin conversion, and an additional 5% do so thereafter.[98] These estimates are based on heavy exposures during disease-prone periods of life. Persons infected with small inocula or during disease-resistant periods probably have a much smaller risk,[99] whereas the risk of progression in immunocompromised persons is greater. In one study of 12,876 unvaccinated adolescents, 10.4% of those who converted their tuberculin tests acquired clinical tuberculosis, 54% of these within 1 year and 78% within 2 years.[47] The three periods of life during which infection is most likely to produce disease are infancy, ages 15 to 25 years, and old age. (The effect of age on disease progression is discussed in "Influence of Age on Tuberculous Infection.")

The likelihood of active disease developing varies with the intensity and duration of exposure. Persons with intense exposures are most at risk not only for infection but also for disease.[93] The degree of tuberculin positivity has some predictive value. Malnutrition, renal failure, and immunosuppression all favor progression of infection to active disease, but by far the strongest risk factor is AIDS (see Table 250-3). Among tuberculin-positive, HIV-positive intravenous drug users in one methadone clinic population, 8% per year acquired active tuberculosis.[100] It seems likely that active tuberculosis may ultimately develop in all persons with AIDS who are tuberculin positive unless prophylactic therapy is given, another fatal complication of AIDS supervenes, or HIV-induced immunosuppression is reversed with antiretroviral therapy. During outbreaks in hospitals or hospices, as many as 40% of patients with AIDS exposed to an active case have contracted active tuberculosis, often within 2 months.[101]

INSTITUTIONAL SPREAD OF TUBERCULOSIS

Hospitals

Tuberculosis has long been a recognized risk to health care workers. However, with declining disease rates and rising confidence in chemotherapy, hospital tuberculosis control programs atrophied. Occasional microepidemics of nosocomial tuberculosis in intensive care units were reported, but generally little attention was paid to the problem. However, beginning in the 1980s, numerous explosive outbreaks of tuberculosis occurred among AIDS patients on specialized wards and hospices in the United States and Europe.[101-105] In the first reported outbreak on an HIV ward, the index patient had fever, cough, a normal chest roentgenogram, and negative acid-fast smears but a positive sputum culture for *M. tuberculosis*.[102] On the same ward, 39%of other AIDS patients acquired active tuberculosis within 60 days. Major factors contributing to these outbreaks have included (1) delays in diagnosis, especially in AIDS patients with noncavitary pulmonary disease; (2) inadequate negative-pressure ventilation in patient rooms; (3) use of aerosol-generating procedures such as bronchoscopy, sputum induction, and aerosolized pentamidine treatments; (4) rapid progression to active, infectious tuberculosis in a large percentage of AIDS patients secondarily exposed; and (5) in the case of MDR-TB, prolonged infectivity despite antituberculous chemotherapy.[106] Health care workers are also at risk. Patients with AIDS and tuberculosis may be highly infectious in the absence of cavitation and even when the chest roentgenogram is normal.[102,103]

Genotyping has confirmed the nosocomial spread of tuberculosis among AIDS patients and to HIV-negative health care workers,[101] demonstrated that AIDS patients treated for one strain of *M. tuberculosis* may be reinfected with a different strain,[107] and has confirmed cross-contamination of cultures in the laboratory.

Shelters for the Homeless

Poor nutrition, intravenous drug use, alcoholism, and crowding increase the risk for both endogenous reactivation of remote infection and acquisition of new (exogenous) infection in homeless shelter clients.[66] A review of cases between 1994 and 2003 showed that 6% of tuberculosis cases in the United States were among homeless individuals, of whom 87% were men, 34% were HIV-positive, and alcohol and drug abuse was common.[108] The extraordinary frequency of HIV infection and tuberculosis in homeless men has prompted aggressive public health measures, which include identifying active cases and administering effective therapy under supervision.

Correctional Facilities

The incidence of tuberculosis is five times higher in incarcerated persons than in the general population.[109] High-risk populations—including young black and Hispanic men, intravenous drug users, and HIV-infected persons—are overrepresented in prison populations.[110] Although most prison cases are due to reactivation of old infections, outbreaks of MDR-TB have shown that transmission of new (exogenous) infection occurs as well. Although difficult for obvious reasons, preventive and curative services in correctional facilities have been identified as high public health priorities. In addition, incarcerated persons live in close quarters that favor transmission and acquisition. Crowding may be the strongest risk factor for transmission in prisons, but this may be offset by effectively treating latent tuberculous infection.[110] Transmission in prisons and jails may also serve as a reservoir for spread to the community, especially to inner-city populations.

CONTROLLING NOSOCOMIAL SPREAD

Spread of tuberculosis in the health care setting has raised justifiable concern. Tuberculin conversion rates as high as 50% among health care workers on HIV wards were reported early in the AIDS epidemic.[103] Delays in diagnosis and initiation of therapy are critical for both outcome and infectiousness to others.[106,111] The HIV status of patients may not be known on admission, tuberculosis is often not an early consideration, an appropriate number of sputum specimens for examination (three) is often not submitted, and sputum acid-fast stains may be negative. Further, the clinical picture of extrapulmonary or disseminated tuberculosis may be confusing. Accordingly, tuberculosis must be considered in any HIV-positive patient with subacute or chronic pulmonary symptoms or symptoms compatible with extrapulmonary tuberculosis. Rapid culture methods and PCR methods may expedite diagnosis.[23,106,112]

Hospitalized HIV-positive patients with respiratory symptoms should be admitted to negative-pressure isolation rooms (so that air flows from the corridor into the room and is safely exhausted to the outside) with six air changes per hour. Procedures that stimulate coughing, such as sputum induction or bronchoscopy should be carried out in negative-pressure rooms or special booths. The use of particulate respirator masks, with appropriate training and fitting, further reduces risk and is recommended by the CDC. Ultraviolet radiation of the air—either pulled by a fan through a radiation chamber or with the ultraviolet beam directed into the uppermost parts of the room so as to avoid direct radiation of personnel—is also advised. The CDC has published extensive guidelines for control of transmission of tuberculosis in diverse health care settings.[113]

▣ Immunology

Tuberculosis is the prototype of infections that require a cellular immune response for their control (see Chapter 9).[114] Abundant antibodies are produced during infection, but play no apparent role in host defense. In the first few weeks after exposure, the host has little immune defense against infection by *M. tuberculosis*. Small inhaled inocula multiply freely in alveolar spaces or within alveolar macrophages. Entry into macrophages involves interactions with complement receptors, mannose receptors, and Fc receptors.[115] The bacteriostatic influence of alveolar macrophages on intracellular bacilli at this stage is probably minimal.

M. tuberculosis uses several strategies to survive within macrophage phagosomes while delaying or preventing effective immune responses. Mycobacterial urease helps prevent acidification of the phagosome, thus limiting the effectiveness of bactericidal enzymes. In addition, by remaining within the phagosome, the organism does not initially elicit strong CD8$^+$ cytotoxic T-cell responses via the proteosomal pathway of antigen presentation. The organism also secretes abundant superoxide dismutase, catalase, thioredoxin, and other antioxidants that detoxify reactive oxygen species generated by phagocytes. Microbial antioxidants not only provide direct protection against host-generated oxidants but also suppress early oxidant-mediated immune responses needed for efficient antigen presentation including the activation and apoptosis of macrophages.[116] This both assures the organism's continued survival within its host cell, and interferes with the development of strong adaptive T-cell responses. The recent elucidation of such pathogenic mechanisms has fostered rational strategies toward vaccine development (see "Vaccination").

Unrestrained replication proceeds for weeks, both in the initial focus and in lymphohematogenous metastatic foci. A heparin-binding hemagglutinin of *M. tuberculosis* may facilitate extrapulmonary dissemination by inducing epithelial transcytosis.[117] The development of cellular immunity ultimately supervenes. Tissue hypersensitivity is florid in comparison to other intracellular infections, perhaps fueled by the adjuvant activity of mycobacterial lipids.

All persons have a native population of lymphocytes, mostly CD4$^+$ cells bearing $\alpha\beta$ T-cell receptors, capable of recognizing mycobacterial antigens that have been processed and presented by macrophages in a major histocompatibility complex class II context. When the lymphocyte encounters antigen in this manner, it is activated and proliferates, producing a clone of similarly reactive lymphocytes. T cells, in turn, produce many distinct secretory proteins (lymphokines), which attract, retain, and activate macrophages at the site of antigen. Activated macrophages accumulate high concentrations of lytic enzymes and reactive metabolites that greatly increase their mycobactericidal competence, but if released into surrounding tissues may cause tissue necrosis. Activated macrophages also secrete regulatory molecules (e.g., tumor necrosis factor-α [TNF-α], platelet-derived growth factor, transforming growth factor-β, and fibroblast growth factor), which in concert with lymphocyte secretory proteins (e.g. interferon-γ, migration-inhibitory factor) determine the character of the pathologic and clinical response. Epithelioid cells, characteristic of the tuberculous granuloma, are highly stimulated macrophages. The Langhans giant cell consists of fused macrophages oriented around tuberculosis antigen with the multiple nuclei in a peripheral position, representing the most successful type of host tissue response. Cytotoxic CD8$^+$ T cells are also generated during infection,[118] and may directly lyse infected mononuclear phagocytes.

When the population of activated lymphocytes reaches a certain size, cutaneous delayed reactivity to tuberculin becomes manifest, generally within 3 to 9 weeks after initial infection. At the same time, enhanced macrophage microbicidal activity appears. The pathologic features of tuberculosis are the result of the degree of hypersensitivity and the local concentration of antigen. When the antigen load is small and tissue hypersensitivity is high, organization of lymphocytes, macrophages, Langhans giant cells, fibroblasts, and capillaries results in granuloma formation. Foci characterized by the resulting hard tubercles are termed *proliferative* or *productive* and constitute a successful tissue reaction with containment of infection, healing with eventual fibrosis, encapsulation, and scar formation. When both antigen load and hypersensitivity are high, epithelioid cells and giant cells are sparse

or entirely lacking; lymphocytes, macrophages, and granulocytes are present in a less organized fashion; and tissue necrosis may be present, a tissue reaction that has been called *exudative*. In the absence of necrosis, exudative lesions may heal completely, or tissue necrosis may persist. Necrosis in tuberculosis tends to be incomplete, resulting in solid or semisolid acellular material referred to as *caseous* because of its cheesy consistency. The chemical environment and oxygen tension in solid caseous material tend to inhibit microbial multiplication. However, caseous necrosis is unstable, especially in the lungs, where it tends to liquefy and discharge through the bronchial tree, producing a tuberculous cavity and providing conditions in which bacterial populations reach very high titers. Cavities may contain from 10^7 to 10^9 organisms compared with only 10^2 to 10^4 in areas of caseous necrosis.[119] Infectious material sloughed from a cavity creates new exudative foci in other parts of the lung (bronchogenic spread). A cross section of a pulmonary cavity demonstrates all these pathologic reactions, from the least to the most successful in terms of containment of infection. The central cavity, which contains myriad bacilli, is surrounded by a layer of caseous material with fewer organisms, a more peripheral layer of macrophages and lymphocytes with little organization and still fewer organisms, an area that is even more peripheral with epithelioid cells and giant cells in which the bacterial content is quite low, and, most peripherally, a bacillus-free layer of encapsulating fibrosis.

When the degree of hypersensitivity is very low, the tissue reaction may be nonspecific, consisting of a few polymorphonuclear leukocytes and mononuclear cells with huge numbers of tubercle bacilli, so-called *nonreactive tuberculosis*.[120] The immunologic spectrum from florid hypersensitivity to little or no specific tissue reaction is similar to that seen in leprosy and is recapitulated in HIV-infected persons as the CD4$^+$ T count declines.

Any immunity that follows natural infection is likely maintained by persistence of viable tubercle bacilli with *in vivo* boosting. In tuberculin-positive persons, endogenous foci may reactivate repeatedly, and active CD4$^+$ T-cell surveillance is necessary to maintain quiescence.[121] However, reactivation disease may arise from these sites of boosting. In murine models of protective immunity to tuberculosis, CD4$^+$ T cells as well as the cytokines interferon-γ and TNF-α are essential. However, activation of human monocytes with TNF-α, not interferon-γ, most effectively inhibits intracellular replication of *M. tuberculosis*. Conversely, increased production and bioactivation of transforming growth factor-β may favor bacterial survival and multiplication.[122,123] In humans, an effective response to *M. tuberculosis* tends to follow a Th1 pattern with preferential expression of interferon-γ, interleukin (IL)-2, and IL-12.

When macrophages from patients with established tuberculosis encounter *M. tuberculosis,* they produce cytokines that modulate the activity of CD4$^+$ T cells. These cells are essential for optimal macrophage bactericidal activity. Costimulatory cytokines elaborated by macrophages (IL-1, TNF-α, and IL-6) activate CD4$^+$ T cells and induce interferon-γ production. However, macrophages also produce cytokines (transforming growth factor-β and IL-10) that depress interferon-γ production, inhibit blastogenesis, and block the activity of IL-12. Mycobacterial antigens can promote the expression of inhibitory cytokines, and suppression of CD4$^+$ T-cell responses may contribute to immunosuppression, deactivation of macrophage effector function, and disease progression in tuberculosis.[121]

Various immunodominant antigens of *M. tuberculosis* have been identified, including ESAT-6 and the 30-kD (or 85B) antigen.[121] However, *M. tuberculosis* antigens necessary for protective immunity are not yet known, and there are currently no validated human surrogate markers for protective immunity.

Tuberculin Skin Test

The TST is used to determine whether an individual is infected with *M. tuberculosis*. Koch's tuberculin (old tuberculin) was an extract of a boiled culture of tubercle bacilli. In 1934, Siebert made a simple protein precipitate (purified protein derivative [PPD]) of old tuberculin, which became the preferred reagent in most areas. In 1941, a large single lot was adopted as the biologic standard (PPD-S) to which other preparations are now standardized. A 5-tuberculin unit (TU) dose of PPD is equivalent to 0.0001 mg of PPD-S protein in 0.1 mL of solution.[124]

DOSAGE

The sensitivity and specificity of the 5-TU dose were derived in populations in which the incidence of tuberculosis was accurately known. A 5-TU dose of tuberculin clearly separated groups with 100% infection, such as sanatorium patients, from groups with a very low incidence of tuberculosis, such as infants from noninfectious environments. In the former, tuberculin reactions peaked at 16 to 17 mm; in the latter 0- to 5-mm reactions were elicited.

TECHNICAL ASPECTS

Tuberculin testing is performed by intradermal injection of 5 TU of PPD in 0.1 mL of solution, usually on the volar aspect of the forearm. The injection is made with a short, beveled 26- or 27-gauge needle with the bevel facing upward (Mantoux test). Correct injection produces a raised, blanched 6 to 10 mm wheal. Deeper injections may be washed out by vascular flow, resulting in false-negative results. The loss of potency that occurs when PPD adsorbs to glass surfaces is prevented by the addition of the detergent polysorbate 80 (Tween 80). Tween-stabilized tuberculin in solution is light sensitive and must be refrigerated. The skin reaction is usually read in 48 to 72 hours. A positive test is defined by the diameter of induration, not erythema, in response to 5 TU. The diameter should be read across the forearm and can be measured by viewing the reaction tangentially against a light background. An alternative is to use a medium-point ballpoint pen to draw a line starting 1 to 2 cm away from the skin reaction and moving toward its center. The pen is lifted when resistance is felt, the procedure repeated from the opposite direction, and the distance between opposing line ends measured.

TARGETED TUBERCULIN TESTING

The American Thoracic Society and CDC guidelines on tuberculin skin testing recommend targeted tuberculin testing of persons at high risk for developing tuberculosis, and treatment of latent infection if the test is positive.[125] This includes persons at high risk for recent infection (e.g., recent immigrants, health care workers, tuberculosis contacts) and persons with clinical conditions that increase the risk for tuberculosis, regardless of age (e.g., HIV/AIDS, organ transplant). Testing of persons at lower risk is discouraged. Initial testing is also recommended for persons whose activities place them at increased risk of exposure, such as employees at medical and correctional facilities.

INTERPRETATION

Based on sensitivity and specificity of tuberculin testing, three cutoff levels have been recommended for defining positive reactions, 5 mm, 10 mm, and 15 mm (see "Treatment of Latent Tuberculous Infection").[125] The 5-mm cutoff is used for immunocompromised persons and recent contacts of patients with active tuberculosis. The 10-mm cutoff is used for other high-risk groups. The 15-mm cutoff is used for low-risk groups, although guidelines for targeted tuberculin testing suggest that low-risk persons not be tested. Ninety percent of persons with 10 mm of induration and virtually all with greater than 15 mm of induration to 5 TU are infected with *M. tuberculosis*. Induration of less than 10 mm may be cross-reactions caused by infection with other mycobacterial species or prior BCG vaccination. However, even 5- to 10-mm reactions are suspicious for tuberculous infection in geographic areas substantially free of other mycobacteria, such as the northeastern United States, and among persons with a high likelihood of tuberculosis, such as HIV-infected persons and contacts of active

cases.[126,127] Unless BCG vaccination was very recent, positive tuberculin reactions should not be attributed to BCG.[128]

BOOSTER EFFECT

Although tuberculin cannot sensitize an uninfected person, it can restimulate remote hypersensitivity that has deteriorated. This booster effect (a positive tuberculin test after a negative one) develops within several days after a first injection and may be persistent. This causes interpretative problems, because a negative test result followed by a positive test result approximately 10 weeks later may be a product of either a recent infection or a booster effect. This problem is circumvented by retesting nonreactors 1 to 3 weeks after the initial test. If the second test result is positive, this indicates boosting rather than recent tuberculin conversion.

FALSE-POSITIVE AND FALSE-NEGATIVE REACTIONS

False-positive reactions represent nontuberculous mycobacterial infection. False-negative reactions occur in at least 20% of all persons with known active tuberculosis. In one study, 25% of 200 patients with active tuberculosis were nonreactive to 5 TU, and 10% were also non-reactive to 250 TU.[129] Most false-negative test results in patients with tuberculosis are attributed to general illness and become positive 2 to 3 weeks after effective treatment is initiated. Protein malnutrition diminishes all cutaneous delayed hypersensitivity reactions. Sarcoidosis may cause false-negative tuberculin test results. Intercurrent viral infections (including HIV-1 infection with < 200 CD4$^+$ T cells/mm^3), vaccination with live-virus vaccines (measles, smallpox), reticuloendothelial disease, and corticosteroid therapy may cause false-negative tuberculin reactions. Attempts to correlate negative tuberculin tests with generalized anergy (e.g., negative skin test responses to mumps, *Candida*, and tetanus toxoid) have not been illuminating, and such "anergy testing" is therefore not recommended (see "Tuberculin Testing and HIV Infection").[130] Intraobserver reliability in reading reactivity may vary by as much as 3 mm, causing some classification uncertainty if induration is close to the cutoff value.[131] Tuberculin test results are negative during the first 3 to 9 weeks of initial infection.

VARIANT ("DELAYED") TUBERCULIN REACTIVITY

An unusual form of tuberculin response (so-called delayed reactivity) has been described among Indochinese immigrants. This involves induration of less than 10 mm at 48 to 72 hours, which increases to greater than 10 mm when the skin test is read again at 6 days.

LOSS OF TUBERCULIN REACTIVITY

Earlier in the 20th century, lifelong tuberculin positivity was maintained by frequent reexposure to tubercle bacilli or continued active disease. However, a positive tuberculin test will revert to negative unless restimulated by new aerosol inocula or persisting infection. In one tuberculin survey, 8.1% of positive reactors reverted to true negative when retested 1 year later (Table 250-6).[132] Persons with a history of a positive skin test result can be safely retested. Two negative tests a week apart (to exclude boosting) indicate true negativity.

TUBERCULIN TESTING AND HIV INFECTION

During HIV infection, tuberculin reactivity decreases as the CD4 cell count falls. One study of patients with active tuberculosis demonstrated 10 mm or greater induration in response to 5 TU in only 60% of persons with HIV infection and in 35% of those with AIDS.[133] Induration of 5 mm in persons with HIV infection is sufficient to warrant treatment of latent tuberculous infection (see "Treating Latent Tuberculous Infection in Persons with HIV Infection").[134] Testing simultaneously for cutaneous anergy with ubiquitous antigens such as mumps, tetanus toxoid, and *Candida* is not recommended. Because of

TABLE 250-6	Annual Tuberculin Conversion Rates (Positive to Negative) According to Age Groups, Victoria County, Canada, 1959-1962		
Age Groups	Positive Reactors Retested after 1 Year	Number of Reversions to Negative	Reversion Rate (%)
0-19	99	22	22.2
20-39	200	16	8.0
40-59	525	25	4.8
60 and older	377	34	9.0
Total	1201	97	8.1

From Grzybowski S, Allen EA. The challenge of tuberculosis in decline: A study based on the epidemiology of tuberculosis in Ontario, Canada. *Am Rev Respir Dis.* 1964;90: 707-720.

lack of standardization and reproducibility, and variable risk of tuberculosis among anergic persons, cutaneous anergy does not predict *M. tuberculosis* infection, and responsiveness to control antigens but not PPD does not exclude tuberculous infection (see "Treatment of Latent Tuberculous Infection"). Two studies failed to demonstrate that 6 months of INH preventive therapy administered to anergic HIV-positive persons significantly reduced tuberculosis rates.[135,136]

NEWER ASSAYS FOR LATENT *M. TUBERCULOSIS* INFECTION

The TST has limitations, including false-positive results from environmental mycobacterial exposure or BCG vaccination and operator-dependent variability in test placement and reading. Therefore, several new tests to detect latent *M. tuberculosis* infection have been developed that measure host cellular immune response to *M. tuberculosis* in whole blood samples. The Quantiferon-TB Gold (QFT-G) test (Cellestis Limited, Carnegie, Victoria, Australia) quantifies release of interferon-γ from lymphocytes in whole blood incubated overnight with three *M. tuberculosis* antigens, the early secretory antigen target-6 (ESAT-6), culture filtrate protein-10 (CFP10), and TB7.7. These three proteins are absent from BCG and from most other nontuberculous mycobacterial species. The FDA has approved the QFT-G, and the CDC has established guidelines for its use to detect latent tuberculosis.[137] According to the CDC, the QTF-G may be used in all circumstances in which TST is used and interpreted in the same way. Blood must be tested within 12 hours of collection and 5 ml are required, which may be excessive for small children.

Another assay, an enzyme-linked immunospot (ELISPOT) assay, also detects T-cell responses to *M. tuberculosis* antigens ESAT-6, CFP10, and TB7.7.[138] In an investigation of a large school outbreak of tuberculosis in the United Kingdom, the ELISPOT had 89% agreement with the TST and correlated more closely with exposure to the index case than the tuberculin test. An ELISPOT assay to detect *M. tuberculosis* infection is now commercially available, the T-SPOT.TB (Oxford Immunotec, Oxford, UK). Whether the QTF-G or ELISPOT blood tests are more specific or sensitive than the TST in latent or active tuberculosis is still unclear. Unlike TST, blood tests do not require a follow-up visit for determining results.

Pathogenesis

Airborne droplet nuclei containing tubercle bacilli reach the terminal air spaces where multiplication begins. The initial focus is usually subpleural and in the midlung zone (the lower parts of the upper lobes and the upper parts of the lower and middle lobes), where greater airflow favors deposition of bacilli. (Very rarely, nonpulmonary initial foci will involve abraded skin, the intestine, the oropharynx, or the genitalia, all associated with foci in regional lymph nodes.)

The initial pulmonary focus is typically single, although multiple foci are present in about one fourth of cases. The bacteria are ingested by alveolar macrophages, which may be able to eliminate small numbers of bacilli. However, bacterial multiplication tends to be mostly unimpeded, destroying the macrophage. Blood-borne lymphocytes and monocytes are attracted to this focus, the latter differentiating into macrophages, which ingest bacilli released from degenerating cells, and pneumonitis slowly develops. Infected macrophages are carried by lymphatics to regional (hilar, mediastinal, and sometimes supraclavicular or retroperitoneal) lymph nodes, but in the nonimmune host may spread hematogenously throughout the body. During this occult preallergic lymphohematogenous dissemination, some tissues favor retention and bacillary multiplication. These include the lymph nodes, kidneys, epiphyses of the long bones, vertebral bodies, and juxtaependymal meningeal areas adjacent to the subarachnoid space, but most importantly, the apical-posterior areas of the lungs. Before the development of hypersensitivity (tuberculin reactivity), microbial growth is uninhibited, both in the initial focus and in metastatic foci, providing a nidus for subsequent progressive disease in the lung apices and in extrapulmonary sites, either promptly or after a variable period of latency.

EVOLUTION OF THE PRIMARY INFECTION

Tuberculin positivity appears 3 to 9 weeks after infection and marks the development of cellular immunity and tissue hypersensitivity. In most instances the infection is controlled, with the only evidence of infection being a positive skin test. In a minority of cases, antigen concentration in the primary complex, consisting of the initial pulmonary focus (the Ghon focus) and the draining regional nodes, will have reached sufficient size that hypersensitivity results in necrosis and roentgenographically visible calcification, producing the Ranke complex (parenchymal and mediastinal calcific foci). Much less commonly, pulmonary apical and subapical metastatic foci contain sufficient bacilli that necrosis ensues with the onset of hypersensitivity, producing tiny calcific deposits (Simon's foci) in which viable bacilli may persist.

The onset of tuberculin hypersensitivity may be associated with erythema nodosum or phlyctenular keratoconjunctivitis (a severe unilateral inflammation of the eye), although these manifestations are unusual in the United States. The primary complex may progress. In children, large hilar or mediastinal lymph nodes may produce bronchial collapse with distal atelectasis or may erode into a bronchus and spread infection distally. Also, typically in children but also in nonwhite races with less constitutional resistance to tuberculosis, as well as those infected in advanced age[67] and AIDS patients,[139] the primary focus may become an area of advancing pneumonia, so-called progressive primary disease, which may cavitate and spread via the bronchi. Again, typically in the very young, preallergic lymphohematogenous dissemination may progress directly to hyperacute miliary tuberculosis as a result of caseous material directly reaching the blood stream, either from the primary complex or from a caseating metastatic focus in the wall of a pulmonary vein (Weigart focus). Hematogenous dissemination in the very young is often followed within weeks by tuberculous meningitis. In adolescents and young adults, the subpleural primary focus may rupture, delivering bacilli and antigen into the pleural space to produce serofibrinous pleurisy with effusion. Overwhelmingly, the most important consequence of preallergic lymphohematogenous dissemination is seeding of the apical-posterior areas of the lung, where disease may progress without interruption or after a latent period of months or years, resulting in pulmonary tuberculosis of the adult or reactivation-type tuberculosis (endogenous reinfection).

PRIMARY (CHILDHOOD) AND REINFECTION (ADULT) TUBERCULOSIS

The traditional terms *primary* or *childhood pulmonary tuberculosis* and *reinfection* or *adult pulmonary tuberculosis* followed roentgenographic observations early in the 20th century when initial (primary) infection in childhood was thought to be universal.[140] Children's roentgenograms characteristically demonstrated large mediastinal or hilar lymph nodes with inconspicuous pneumonitis in the lower or middle lung field, whereas in adolescents and adults, apical or subapical infiltrates, often with cavitation and no hilar adenopathy, were the rule. These clinical and roentgenographic differences are due to age-related immunologic factors. Although many primary infections in adolescents and adults resemble primary infection in childhood, in others in this age group, an apical-posterior, metastatic pulmonary focus progresses within weeks to "adult"-type pulmonary disease, whereas the initial focus in the lower lung field and hilar nodes involutes undetected.

Chronic Pulmonary Tuberculosis

APICAL LOCALIZATION

In adults, apical localization of pulmonary tuberculosis has often been attributed to the hyperoxic environment of the apices and the aerobic nature of the organism. A more plausible theory attributes it to deficient lymphatic flow at the lung apices, especially the posterior apices, where the pumping effect of respiratory motion is minimal. Deficient lymph traffic would favor retention of bacillary antigen and, when hypersensitivity ensues, tissue necrosis. Apical-posterior localization with a tendency to cavitation and progression is characteristic of pulmonary tuberculosis in adolescents and adults. In contrast, infection acquired by the elderly often causes nondescript lower lobe pneumonia similar to progressive primary infection of childhood.[67]

ENDOGENOUS VERSUS EXOGENOUS REINFECTION

Resistance to exogenous reinfection in otherwise healthy, previously infected individuals is generally robust, with new inocula being destroyed before substantial multiplication occurs. In countries where the level of contagion is low, most cases of active tuberculosis reflect reactivation of latent foci.[140] However, when contagion is high, exogenous reinfection may be more common.[47,141] Airflow in the apical-posterior areas of the lung is low, but when inhaled droplet nuclei reach that location, as is more likely with high levels of contagion, bacillary multiplication will be favored by the same local factors that enhance multiplication of blood-borne organisms. Support for this comes from a study from India that showed that disease in household contacts of active cases was most common in the middle-aged and elderly, who were certain to have been previously infected,[142] and from molecular epidemiology data.[66] Repeated inhalational exposures to tubercle bacilli maintain tissue hypersensitivity and cellular immunity, making superinfection more difficult; however, when the airborne inoculum is large, or in immunocompromised hosts, superinfection may occur.

INFLUENCE OF AGE ON TUBERCULOUS INFECTION

Many of the best clinical descriptions of tuberculosis come from the preantimicrobial era, when infection occurred early in life and cellular immunity was maintained by frequent exposure to tubercle bacilli. However, in industrialized countries, infection more often occurs later in life, and cellular immunity may wane in the absence of restimulation. Accordingly, clinical patterns have changed. At one time, most patients were adolescents and young adults with apical cavitary disease. In developed countries, the incidence of tuberculosis (cases per 100,000) is now greatest in older persons, in whom hypersensitivity is less marked and in whom the clinical manifestations may be different and more subtle. Hypersensitivity and cellular immunity likely become less vigorous with age (see "Epidemiology").

INFECTION IN INFANCY AND CHILDHOOD

Infection in infants often results in disease, with local progression and dissemination (miliary-meningeal disease). The younger the patient, the greater the risk of progressive disease until the age of 5 years. From age 5 until puberty is a time of relative resistance to progressive disease, although not to infection. When disease occurs, it is usually the childhood type of pulmonary tuberculosis. Involvement of lymph nodes, bones, and, less commonly, other progressive extrapulmonary foci may develop, but tuberculosis confined to the lung in this age group usually heals spontaneously. The short-term prognosis in these cases is good even if untreated, but there is a high frequency of relapse with chronic cavitary tuberculosis when the more disease-prone periods of adolescence and young adulthood arrive.[143]

INFECTION IN ADOLESCENCE AND YOUNG ADULTHOOD

Clinical disease developing after infection in adolescence or young adulthood may resemble childhood infection (lower lung field pneumonitis, hilar adenitis) but with less parenchymal and hilar calcification (Fig. 250-2). This is particularly the case in dark-skinned races and in immunocompromised patients, including those with AIDS.[140] Rarely, the roentgenographic picture may be mixed, with features of childhood disease subsiding while chronic upper lobe (adult) disease progresses. However, disease in this age group frequently first appears as chronic upper lobe tuberculosis with no clinical features of childhood disease. The tendency toward apical cavitation soon after the initial infection appears soon after puberty and is marked in young adults.[125] Because most young people in industrialized countries are tuberculin negative (Fig. 250-3), most pulmonary tuberculosis in adolescents and young adults is due to recent initial infection rather than to late progression of childhood infection.

INFECTION IN MIDADULTHOOD

Infection acquired during the middle years has a much better immediate and probably long-term prognosis than infection acquired in the teens and early 20s, presumably because of a reduced tendency to tissue necrosis.[143,144] One study demonstrated progression from infection to cavitary tuberculosis in 23% of patients infected from 15 to 19 years of age, 13% of those infected from 20 to 24 years of age, 4% of those infected from 25 to 29 years of age, and only 2% of those infected

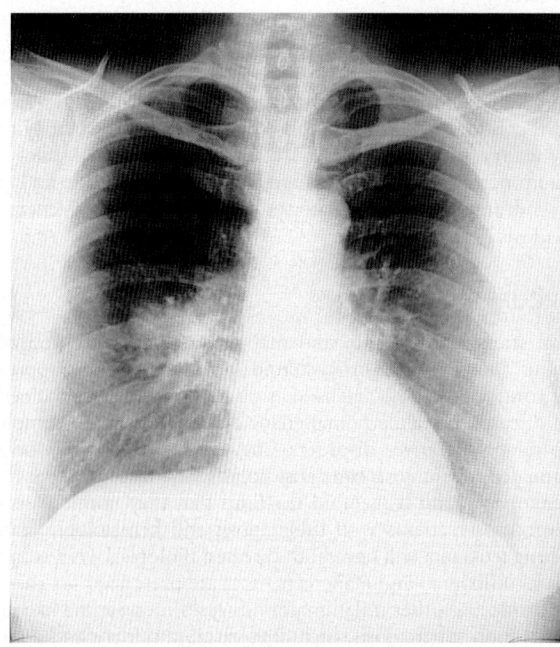

Figure 250-2 Chest roentgenogram showing marked right hilar lymphadenopathy and lower lobe opacity in a 58-year-old woman with primary tuberculosis.

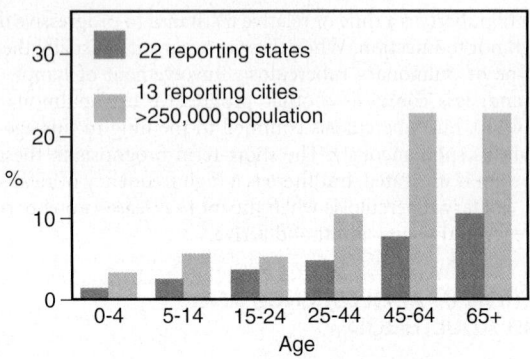

Figure 250-3 Percentage of positive tuberculin reactors by age, selected areas, United States, 1979. *(From Centers for Disease Control and Prevention [CDC], Tuberculosis Control Division. Tuberculosis in the United States, 1979. Atlanta, Ga., CDC, 1981, pp 4-31.)*

after 30 years of age. Progression occurred in 3 months in many and within 1 year in most.[145] (Elderly individuals were not included in the study.)

INFECTION IN OLD AGE

In the elderly, infection acquired years earlier can progress as age compromises immunity, producing typical apical-posterior disease. Studies of tuberculosis in nursing homes, however, have demonstrated that elderly patients are often tuberculin negative, either because they had never been infected or because remote past infection had been completely cleared, with a loss of tissue hypersensitivity. Such tuberculin-negative persons are susceptible to new infection, and if this occurs, they acquire active disease with a frequency similar to that of adolescents. This is typically a nondescript, poorly resolving pneumonitis in the lower or middle lobes or anterior segments of the upper lobes, sometimes with pleural effusion and resembling primary infection in children except for much less hilar-mediastinal lymphadenopathy.[67] Even with prompt diagnosis and treatment, tuberculosis after age 65 appears to be more frequently associated with death.

LATE HEMATOGENOUS TUBERCULOSIS

Chronic tuberculosis is probably always associated with recurrent abortive episodes of hematogenous spread. However, when aging or other factors compromise cellular immunity, such episodes may become progressively more frequent, producing the subtle and often fatal syndrome of late hematogenous or progressive generalized tuberculosis.

INTERCURRENT EVENTS

General stress, poor health, and malnutrition favor progression of infection. Therapy with corticosteroids or other immunosuppressive agents compromise host defenses, as do hematopoietic-reticuloendothelial diseases, particularly malignancies. Tuberculosis in complicating myeloproliferative disorders may cause confusion because disseminated tuberculosis can cause aplastic anemia, thrombocytopenia, leukopenia, and leukemoid reactions that may mimic leukemia. However, most patients with tuberculosis and hematologic findings suggesting leukemia will have both diseases. Biological TNF-α inhibitors (e.g., infliximab and etanercept) that are prescribed for rheumatoid arthritis and other inflammatory diseases increase the likelihood of reactivation tuberculosis, including extrapulmonary and disseminated disease.[146,147]

The postgastrectomy state, jejunal-ileal bypass surgery, and end-stage renal disease are all risk factors for progression (see "Treat-

ment of Latent Tuberculous Infection"). Viral illnesses, particularly in children, may predispose to progression of infection. Destructive local pulmonary processes such as lung abscess, carcinoma, cavitary histoplasmosis, and pulmonary resection occasionally are followed by activation of previously quiescent pulmonary foci. The development of bone and joint tuberculosis after physical injury, and late generalized hematogenous tuberculosis after major trauma both illustrate that the balance between host and infection can be altered by both systemic factors and local physical disturbance.

TUBERCULOSIS IN AIDS

The earliest descriptions of tuberculosis in AIDS emphasized the very great risk of reactivation of remote infection as a result of progressively compromised cellular immunity. Among Haitians, all of whom were likely infected with *M. tuberculosis* in childhood, AIDS was associated with development of active tuberculosis in 60%.[73] Subsequent studies of HIV-positive and tuberculin-positive methadone clinic patients in New York City showed that active tuberculosis developed in 8% yearly.[100]

As discussed in "Epidemiology," HIV-infected patients are predisposed not only to reactivation of remote infection but also to rapid progression of recently acquired infection.[101,102] It is unclear whether AIDS increases susceptibility to acquisition of new infection.

Management of tuberculosis in AIDS may be complicated by concomitant intravenous drug use and homelessness. Interestingly, long before the AIDS epidemic, illicit intravenous drug use was shown to favor an increased incidence of extrapulmonary disease.[148]

HUMAN GENETICS AND TUBERCULOSIS

Given the complex pathogenesis of *M. tuberculosis* within the human host it is certain that human genetic variants influence various aspects of infection and disease progression. Efforts to define such variants, however, have yielded inconsistent results. Tentative associations involve genes that encode HLA molecules,[149-152] IFN-γ and its receptor,[153-155] NRAMP1 (renamed SLC11A1),[156-158] TIRAP,[159-161] MCP-1,[162] TLR-4,[163] mannose-binding lectin,[164] IL12-β and its receptor,[165,166] the vitamin D receptor,[167,168] and CD14.[169] It is unclear which of these associations are valid, as many have not yet been replicated in other study populations, and functional effects of many polymorphisms are unknown.

▪ Pulmonary Tuberculosis

PRIMARY TUBERCULOSIS IN CHILDHOOD

The initial focus of pulmonary tuberculosis in children occurs most frequently in the midlung zones but may develop anywhere. At the time of tuberculin conversion, fever and lassitude and rarely erythema nodosum or phlyctenar keratoconjunctivitis may be present briefly. Clinical manifestations of the initial infection depend on the age of the patient. It is most often symptomatic in childhood because of an age-related tendency to extensive regional lymphadenitis. This may compress central bronchi, causing a brassy cough or atelectasis of a segment or lobe, or may rupture into a bronchus, seeding infection distally and causing pneumonia. In the very young, there is a tendency to progressive lymphohematogenous dissemination with miliary-meningeal disease. Uncommonly, again more in infants, local progression of the initial pneumonia results in progressive primary disease, which may spread via the bronchial tree or the blood stream. However, most infections during the relatively disease-resistant period of childhood (ages 5 to 12 years) are usually nonprogressive, with healing by involution and encapsulation.[143] Progression, if any, occurs in extrapulmonary metastatic foci or with the development of apical-posterior pulmonary tuberculosis, usually when the patient reaches puberty or young adulthood.

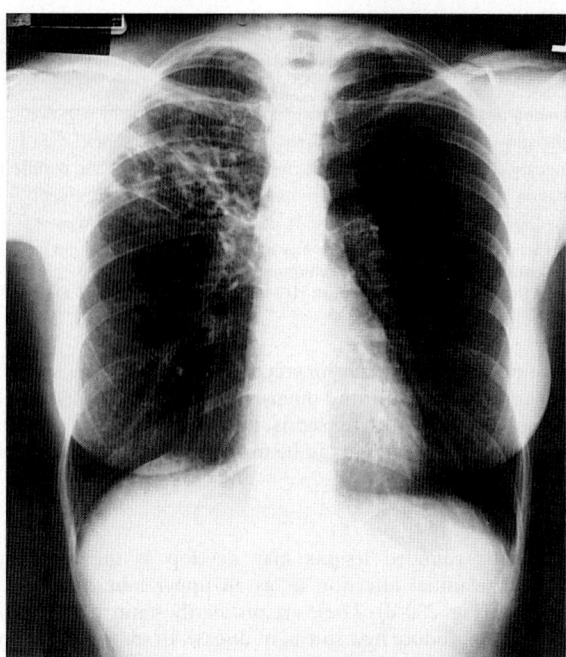

Figure 250-4 Chest roentgenogram showing a right apical infiltrate in a patient with moderately advanced postprimary tuberculosis.

POSTPRIMARY (ADULT-TYPE) PULMONARY TUBERCULOSIS

Primary infection in adolescents and adults (1) may occur without symptoms and signs, (2) may produce a typical primary complex, or (3) may result in typical chronic pulmonary tuberculosis without a demonstrable primary complex. Any pneumonic infiltrate, especially if associated with a hilar or mediastinal node, may represent primary infection. These lesions may undergo caseation, liquefaction, and bronchogenic spread just as with classic chronic pulmonary tuberculosis.

Postprimary pulmonary tuberculosis in adults is usually asymmetrical and characterized by caseation, fibrosis, and frequently cavity formation. It begins as a patch of pneumonitis in the subapical-posterior aspect of an upper lobe, usually just below the clavicle or first rib (Fig. 250-4). A less frequent location is the apex of the lower lobe, where it may be obscured by the heart and hilum on chest roentgenogram. The inflammatory response in the sensitized host produces a fibrin-rich alveolar exudate containing a mixture of inflammatory cells. Serial roentgenograms may demonstrate waxing and waning and sometimes complete regression. If the process accelerates, however, an area of caseous necrosis surrounded by epithelioid cells, granulation tissue, and eventually fibrosis develops. This may arrest by inspissation of the caseous area, fibrous encapsulation, and healing. Caseation, however, tends to liquefy and drain into the bronchial tree, spreading bacillary contents by coughing. The cavity is prevented from collapsing by the fibrous capsule and the inelasticity of the surrounding lung. For unclear reasons, the pulmonary cavity favors bacillary multiplication to enormous titers, 5 to 6 logs greater than in noncavitary lesions. The progressive nature of pulmonary tuberculosis is due to (1) the tendency of apical caseous foci to liquefy, (2) the enormous concentrations of organisms in the resulting pulmonary cavities, and (3) spread of this bacilli-rich material through the bronchial tree. Progression from minimal infiltrate to far-advanced cavitary disease can occur within a few months (Fig. 250-5).

Coughing aerosolizes infectious cavity secretions that may distribute widely throughout the lung (bronchogenic spread). New foci eventually develop that, in turn, may undergo caseation, fibrosis, and healing

or slough, resulting in new cavities. The segment or lobe containing the initial cavity is typically involved first with scattered patchy disease, but the contralateral apex is often secondarily involved with progressive disease. Bronchogenic spread may establish foci of infection in the lower lobe and anterior portions of the upper lobe, producing a polymorphous mottling on chest roentgenogram, but these are usually nonprogressive and heal with fibrosis. Although hematogenous spread from an established pulmonary focus can occur, it is usually limited by hypersensitivity-induced thrombosis.

The highly infectious secretions from a cavity always cause some degree of endobronchial inflammation and ulceration, which may be extensive. Ulcerative tuberculous laryngitis is an extension of this process, as is local disease throughout the upper airways, mouth, middle ear, and gastrointestinal tract.

Mechanisms of healing are the same whether spontaneous or under the influence of chemotherapy. Without drug therapy, solid caseous foci surrounded by contracting fibrous tissue occasionally arrest. However, viable bacilli almost always persist in such lesions, and can later reactivate. Before drug therapy, open healing of persisting cavities never occurred, and some large, thick-walled cavities in shrunken fibrotic lobes could persist for years with minimal symptoms while remaining highly infectious (chronic fibroid tuberculosis). With drug therapy, cavities may resolve or they may heal but remain open, sometimes with complete reepithelialization. The major risk of such persistent cavities is superinfection with organisms such as *Aspergillus* or nontuberculous mycobacteria.

LOWER LOBE AND ENDOBRONCHIAL TUBERCULOSIS

These terms are not appropriate for chronic pulmonary tuberculosis of the ordinary kind that happens to involve the apex of the lower lobes. In adults, *lower lung field tuberculosis* describes three different but often associated processes: (1) progressive lower lobe pneumonia

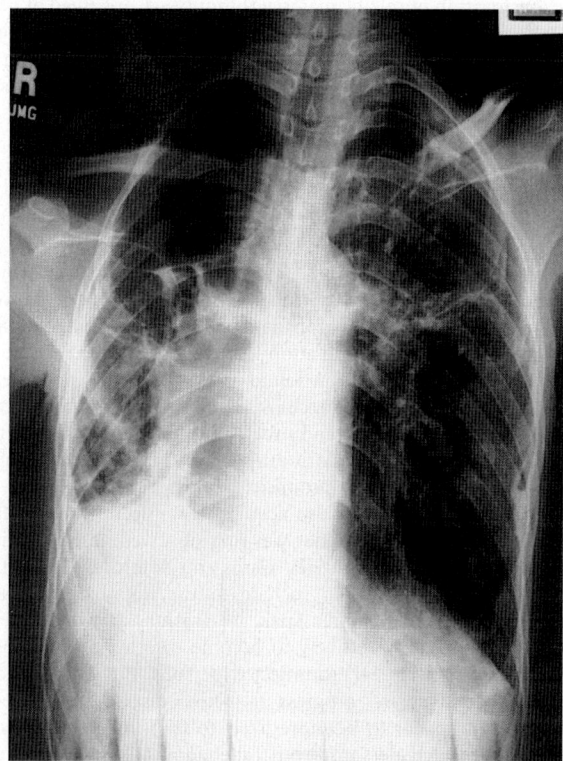

Figure 250-5 Chest roentgenogram showing far-advanced bilateral apical cavitary pulmonary tuberculosis in a 32-year-old woman from Ethiopia.

in recently infected older individuals; (2) endobronchial tuberculosis, often with parenchymal consolidation-collapse; and (3) tuberculosis complicating AIDS. These three processes differ from postprimary tuberculosis roentgenographically, and the former two have a low bacterial content.

Progressive Lower Lobe Disease in Older Persons

Tuberculosis in an older individual frequently causes a nonspecific, nonresolving pneumonitis in the lower or middle lobes or anterior segments of the upper lobes, similar to primary infection in childhood, except with less hilar and mediastinal adenopathy.[93] Tuberculosis should be considered in any slowly or nonresolving pneumonitis in an older patient.

Endobronchial Tuberculosis

In the past, superficial endobronchial lesions resulting from infectious secretions were common, sometimes spreading to the larynx and beyond or causing obstructive atelectasis with collapse. These superficial lesions responded quickly to chemotherapy. Now endobronchial disease is most frequently caused by rupture of an adjacent node into the bronchial tree, or less frequently by direct spread from parenchymal tuberculosis.[170] The chest roentgenogram typically reveals collapse-consolidation but may be normal in as many as 20% of cases. Sputum smear results are usually negative, but the bronchial wash result is frequently positive.[170]

The usual bronchoscopic findings are mucosal edema, ulceration, and narrowing, but in 30% of cases, bulky granulation tissue may resemble bronchogenic carcinoma. Endobronchial involvement is usual in lower lung field tuberculosis,[171] and endobronchial ulcers occasionally produce positive sputum smears with normal chest roentgenograms. Large parenchymal cavities may be present, at times associated with an air-fluid level resulting from intermittent obstruction and poor drainage. Bronchial perforation by tuberculous nodes with endobronchial mass formation and lower lobe consolidation has been observed in patients with AIDS.

Calcified nodes can erode into the bronchial tree and cause hemoptysis, expectoration of calcific material (lithoptysis), or spread of previously quiescent bacilli. The atelectatic pneumonitis, which may result with or without new active disease, is most frequently seen in the anterior segment of the upper lobe and medial segment of the middle lobe.

Pulmonary Tuberculosis in AIDS

Tuberculosis as first described in persons with advanced AIDS was characterized by middle or lower lung field location, absence of cavitation, a greatly increased incidence of extrapulmonary disease, and usually a negative tuberculin test result.[172,173] It resembled childhood tuberculosis except for a negative tuberculin test result and less prominent hilar and mediastinal lymphadenopathy. A later study of tuberculosis in a much less ill population in clients of tuberculosis clinics unaware of their HIV infection found a clinical picture no different from ordinary reactivation tuberculosis in HIV-negative patients, with apical, often cavitary, disease and tuberculin positivity being the rule. The clinical picture of tuberculosis during HIV infection is determined by the degree of immunocompromise (Table 250-7).[139]

HIV-positive persons may also acquire new infection from others in their environment, a risk that was first observed among patients with advanced AIDS living in HIV wards and domiciles. The clinical picture in these patients can include diffuse, rapidly progressive, noncavitary disease that is often fatal.[101,102] It is unclear whether HIV-infected persons are more likely to become infected after exposure to *M. tuberculosis* than HIV-uninfected persons, but once infected, they are more likely to progress to active disease. HIV-infected persons do not appear to be more likely to transmit *M. tuberculosis* than HIV-uninfected persons,[95] but tuberculosis disease, and therefore *M. tuberculosis* transmission, can occur even when the source case has a normal chest roentgenogram or a negative acid-fast sputum stain.[174-176]

TABLE 250-7	Clinical Manifestations of Active Tuberculosis in Early versus Late HIV Infection*	
	Early	**Late**
Tuberculin test	Usually positive	Usually negative
Adenopathy	Unusual	Common
Pulmonary distribution	Upper lobe	Lower and middle lobe
Cavitation	Often present	Typically absent
Extrapulmonary disease	10-15% of cases	50% of cases

*For practical purposes, early and late may be defined as CD4+ cell counts greater than 300 cells/mm³ and less than 200 cells/mm³, respectively.

Adapted from Murray JF. Cursed duet: HIV infection and tuberculosis. *Respiration.* 1990;57:210-220.

It is important to consider tuberculosis in HIV-positive individuals with respiratory failure in the intensive care unit. Patients may have adult respiratory distress or sepsis syndrome with multiple organ system failure. The diagnosis can be made readily by stain and culture of sputum and/or blood.

Tuberculomas

Asymptomatic rounded lesions may develop as the parenchymal residua of the initial infection or as an upper lobe caseous lesion encapsulates (Fig. 250-6). These are ordinarily static, but larger ones may cavitate to produce new spread of disease. In some persons, excessive fibrosis occurs with small caseous or granulomatous residua becoming surrounded by concentric layers of fibrous tissue, at times with central or concentric calcification resembling histoplasmomas. Most such lesions are stable and important only in being confused with cancer.

SYMPTOMS

Infection with *M. tuberculosis* is usually asymptomatic, although some persons may have a relatively brief period of symptoms.[177,178] Early pulmonary tuberculosis is asymptomatic, and may be discovered by chance on a chest roentgenogram. As the bacillary population grows, however, nonspecific constitutional symptoms such as anorexia,

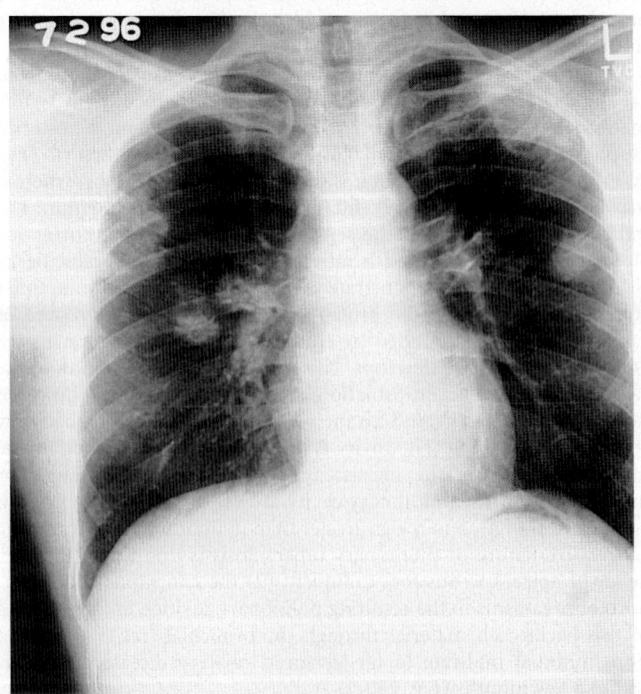

Figure 250-6 Chest roentgenogram demonstrating multiple bilateral pulmonary tuberculomas in an asymptomatic 35-year-old man from Poland.

fatigue, weight loss, chills, fever, and night sweats may ensue. A productive cough is usually present. Coughing to clear cavitary secretions is usually mild and well tolerated but may become bothersome when bronchial involvement is extensive. The mucopurulent sputum is nonspecific, and both cough and sputum may be ignored by patients with chronic bronchitis. Hemoptysis resulting from caseous sloughing or endobronchial erosion is usually minor but connotes advanced disease. Sudden massive hemoptysis resulting from erosion of a pulmonary artery by an advancing cavity (Rasmussen's aneurysm) was an occasional terminal event in the predrug era but is now seldom seen. In inactive disease, brisk hemoptysis may be due to *Aspergillus* superinfection of residual cavities (aspergilloma). Chest pain is usually due to extension of inflammation to the parietal pleura. Pleural involvement adjacent to an established cavity tends to cause visceral-parietal pleural symphysis without effusion (dry pleurisy). Serofibrinous pleurisy with effusion is often an early postprimary event but may also complicate chronic pulmonary tuberculosis. Rarely, chest pain leads to discovery of tuberculous empyema. Symptoms often pertain to site of disease, such as painful pharyngeal ulcers; indolent and nonhealing ulcers of the mouth or tongue; hoarseness and dysphagia that are due to laryngeal involvement; tuberculous otitis media; gastrointestinal symptoms that are due to enteric ulceration, perforation, or mass formation; or anal pain that is due to tuberculous perirectal abscess and fistula formation. Lower lobe tuberculosis resulting from bronchial lymph node perforation may be associated with lithoptysis (stone spitting) and characteristically produces symptoms of severe endobronchial disease with serious cough and often hemoptysis.

PHYSICAL EXAMINATION

Physical findings are not specific, in general underestimating the extent of the illness, and may be absent in spite of extensive disease. Dullness with decreased fremitus may indicate pleural thickening or fluid. Crackles may be appreciated only when the patient breathes in after a short cough (post-tussive rales) and may persist long after healing owing to permanent distortion of small airways. With large lesions, signs of consolidation with open bronchi (whispered pectoriloquy, tubular breath sounds) can be heard. Distant hollow breath sounds heard over cavities are called *amphoric*, like the sound made by blowing across the mouth of a jar (amphora).

ROENTGENOLOGIC FINDINGS

The chest roentgenogram is central to diagnosis, determination of the extent and character of disease, and evaluation of the response to therapy. Certain patterns are highly suggestive, although not diagnostic, of tuberculosis. A patchy or nodular infiltrate in the apical- or subapical-posterior areas of the upper lobes or the superior segment of a lower lobe is highly suspicious for early chronic tuberculosis, especially if bilateral or associated with cavity formation (see Fig. 250-4). Cavities may be more apparent by computed tomography (CT) or magnetic resonance imaging (MRI). Cavitation in the apical segment of the lower lobe may be obscured by the heart shadow and, in the lateral view, by the dorsal spine. Air-fluid levels are uncommon in upper lobe tuberculosis (less than 10%) but occur more frequently in lower lobe cavities. Fresh bronchogenic spread from recent spillage of infectious cavity contents appears as multiple, discrete, soft, fluffy infiltrates, or a confluent infiltrate adjacent to a cavity, or in the middle or lower lung field on the same or opposite side. These latter types of spread are seldom progressive and heal by rounding up into more discrete lesions with regular borders.

Both chronicity and histopathologic features can be estimated based on the chest roentgenogram. Granulomatous lesions tend to be small, nodular, and sharply defined, indicating few organisms and a good host response. Exudative lesions (pneumonic) tend to have soft, indistinct borders and are more unstable. Fibrotic scars have sharp margins and tend to contract. Caseation causes increased density. Healing exu-

dative lesions first become smaller and less dense and then, as scarring develops, become more sharply defined. Lower lobe tuberculosis is nonspecific roentgenographically. Other patterns include poorly resolving pneumonia, atelectasis, mass lesions, and large cavities with air-fluid levels; initial misdiagnosis is the rule. Pneumonia associated with hilar adenopathy should always suggest primary tuberculosis, regardless of the lung fields involved and patient age. Pulmonary tuberculosis can also occur in persons with a normal chest radiograph; up to 6% of HIV-seronegative and 22% of HIV-seropositive persons with pulmonary tuberculosis have a normal chest radiograph.[174,179-181]

OTHER LABORATORY FINDINGS

Normocytic, normochromic anemia, hypoalbuminemia, and hypergammaglobulinemia are characteristic of advanced disease. The white blood cell count is usually normal but may be between 10,000 and 15,000 cells/mm^3. Many HIV-negative patients with active tuberculosis have CD4$^+$ T-cell counts much lower than 500 cells/L, which return toward normal with treatment.[182] Monocytosis is seen in less than 10% of cases. Hematuria or sterile pyuria should suggest coexisting renal tuberculosis. Hyponatremia with features of inappropriate secretion of antidiuretic hormone is characteristic of tuberculous meningitis but also occurs with isolated pulmonary involvement. Hyponatremia should also suggest associated Addison's disease due to adrenal tuberculosis. Hypercalcemia is also seen during pulmonary tuberculosis, usually in the first weeks of therapy.

DIAGNOSIS

A strong presumptive diagnosis can often be made based on the roentgenographic pattern. A positive sputum smear, usual in extensive disease, provides additional evidence in support of a diagnosis. However, an intercurrent cancer or lung abscess, particularly in the apices, may erode a quiescent focus of tuberculosis and cause brief shedding of tubercle bacilli without causing active disease. The best diagnostic sputum specimen is an early morning sample. Although two sputum specimens are sufficient in some settings, three specimens are recommended because of greater sensitivity. Aspiration of gastric contents, obtained early in the morning to sample sputum swallowed during sleep, is an alternative when sputum is not produced. The specificity of gastric aspiration is diminished by the presence of nontuberculous mycobacteria, but may be higher in children than adults. Sputum induction by hypertonic saline aerosols is also an effective substitute in ambulatory patients—the yield is comparable to fiberoptic bronchoscopy.[183] Pulmonary tuberculosis in AIDS patients is often noncavitary, and therefore may have a lower bacillary burden than in HIV-seronegative persons. The high prevalence of smear-negative tuberculosis in HIV-infected persons underscores the importance of obtaining sputum culture, even in resource-poor settings.[176] Positive sputum smears are much more likely to indicate *M. tuberculosis* than *M. avium* complex, even in areas where both diseases are common.[184] NAATs, described previously, can provide a rapid distinction between the two infections in smear-positive respiratory secretions.

A negative tuberculin reaction does not exclude tuberculosis even when the dose is 250 TU; anergy can occur in the setting of active disease.[129,185] The TST is insensitive in immunocompromised persons, such as HIV-infected persons with <100 CD4$^+$ lymphocytes/mm^3.[186] Granuloma formation on histologic examination, even with acid-fast bacilli, is still only strong presumptive evidence, because similar findings may be produced by mycobacteria other than tuberculosis. Granulomas in the absence of acid-fast bacilli can be seen with other infectious diseases (e.g., histoplasmosis) and noninfectious causes (e.g., sarcoidosis, autoimmune disease). Definitive diagnosis requires culture and speciation.

Fiberoptic Bronchoscopy

Diagnostic fiberoptic bronchoscopy with transbronchial biopsy and bronchoalveolar lavage should be considered when sputum tests are inconclusive and the suspicion of tuberculosis remains high. In AIDS patients with pulmonary tuberculosis but negative smears, bronchoscopy yields a rapid diagnosis (based on smears and histologic features) in only one third of cases.[187-189] Thus, a negative acid-fast stain at bronchoscopy does not exclude tuberculosis, although such cases are certainly less contagious.

Tuberculosis Diagnosed at Autopsy

From 1985 through 1988, 5.1% of all reported tuberculosis cases in the United States were diagnosed at death.[190] Usually, the patient is old and has underlying diseases. Both nonresolving pulmonary processes and extrapulmonary tuberculosis, particularly chronic miliary and meningeal disease, are often present in such patients. The usual reason for failure to diagnose tuberculosis in such patients is failure to look for it.

TUBERCULOSIS AND CANCER

It has been estimated that 1% to 5% of tuberculosis patients also have cancer, most being male smokers. It is possible that cancer can arise in tuberculous scars, and it is certain that cancer can erode old quiescent tuberculous foci, causing active disease. However, in many patients the diseases will be anatomically remote. No one cancer cell type predominates.

When tuberculosis and cancer occur together, diagnosis of the latter is often difficult but should be kept in mind in older men with tuberculosis who smoke, and sputum cytologic studies should be performed. There are certain roentgenographic findings that suggest concomitant cancer, such as progression of one area while the remainder of the lesion is regressing, a large (>3 cm) mass lesion admixed with infiltrative disease, the presence of hilar nodes in adult chronic pulmonary tuberculosis, and postobstructive atelectasis.[191]

■ Treatment of Tuberculosis

Before effective drugs were available, 50% of patients with active pulmonary tuberculosis died within 2 years, and only 25% were cured.[47] With the advent of chemotherapy, successful treatment became a reasonable goal in all adults. In practice, failures occur because of drug resistance or an inappropriate regimen but most importantly because of nonadherence to therapy. For this reason the responsibility for adequate treatment has been shifted from the patient to the prescribing physician and to the health department, emphasizing the importance of DOT.[192]

ANTITUBERCULOUS DRUGS

Additional information on dosage and pharmacology of antituberculous drugs is provided in Chapter 39.

Isoniazid
INH is the cornerstone of therapy and should be included in all regimens unless the *M. tuberculosis* strain is INH-resistant. Occasionally, when the *M. tuberculosis* strain is resistant to low-level INH but susceptible to higher INH levels, and there is resistance to other antituberculosis drugs, INH is included in the regimen (though not considered to have full activity). The most important adverse effect of INH is hepatitis, the risk of which increases with age and underlying liver disease. Although rare, it can be fatal.[193]

Rifampin
RMP is the second major antituberculous agent. The most important complication of RMP is hepatitis, which is usually cholestatic. Although the risk of hepatitis is lower with RMP than INH,[194,195] hepatitis occurs more frequently in regimens containing both INH and RMP than in those containing INH alone.[196]

Of special concern is that RMP, by inducing hepatic P-450 cytochrome oxidases, causes many drug–drug interactions. Examples of drugs whose levels are reduced in the presence of rifampin include warfarin, hormonal contraceptives, azole antifungal agents, methadone, corticosteroids, cyclosporine, tacrolimus, non-nucleoside reverse transcriptase inhibitors and HIV-1 protease inhibitors. This can result in subtherapeutic levels of these drugs, necessitating either increases in their dosage or use of an antituberculosis drug other than RMP. The interaction between RMP and HIV-1 protease inhibitors can lead to suboptimal HIV-1 protease inhibitor levels, inadequate control of viral replication, and emergence of drug-resistant virus. In this setting, RMP may be replaced by rifabutin, which has comparable antituberculous activity but is a weaker enzyme inducer.[197]

Rifapentine
Rifapentine is a rifamycin antibiotic with a long half-life that allows once-weekly administration.[198] It may be used in HIV-seronegative persons in the continuation phase of tuberculosis treatment of noncavitary pulmonary disease that is smear negative after 2 months of treatment.[192] Rifapentine should not be used in HIV-infected persons due to the high risk of acquired rifamycin resistance.[199]

Pyrazinamide
PZA is an essential component of 6-month regimens. Early studies of PZA using high doses recorded such serious hepatotoxicity that it was largely abandoned. At currently recommended doses, PZA is associated with higher rates of hepatotoxicity and rash than other first-line drugs.[200] Recent cohort and case-control analyses found that adding PZA to INH and RMP increased the risk of hepatotoxicity appreciably.[201] In addition, severe hepatic injury and deaths have been reported among predominantly HIV-negative adults receiving short-course RMP plus PZA for latent tuberculous infection.[202] The beneficial effect of PZA is limited to the first 2 months in regimens containing both INH and RMP.[203] Side effects include hyperuricemia, mild nongouty polyarthralgias that respond to nonsteroidal anti-inflammatory agents, and gout. *M. bovis* is uniformly resistant to PZA.[204]

Ethambutol
EMB is included in initial treatment regimens until drug susceptiblity results return and resistance to the other first-line drugs has been excluded, at which time it can be discontinued. It is given at a daily dosage of 15 to 25 mg/kg. At 15 mg/kg the risk of ocular toxicity is low, but assessment of visual acuity and color discrimination should be performed at baseline and monthly while on therapy.

Streptomycin
STM, the first major antituberculous drug, was promptly replaced by INH as the cornerstone of therapy. Its activity is similar to that of EMB when either drug is given with INH, RMP, and PZA. Its use is limited by relatively high rates of resistance (particularly in high-incidence countries), parenteral administration, nephrotoxicity, and ototoxicity.

Fluoroquinolones
Although experience with these agents is not extensive, their in vitro activity and favorable clinical results suggest that some fluoroquinolones, particularly later-generation agents such as ofloxacin and moxifloxacin are effective antituberculosis drugs.[205] However, fluoroquinolones should not be used as first-line therapy but rather be reserved for patients who are intolerant of first-line drugs or who have drug-resistant tuberculosis, as part of a well-designed multidrug regimen. The potential role of fluoroquinolones as first-line antituberculosis therapy is currently under evaluation in clinical trials.

Second-Line Agents
Second-line agents are less efficacious or more toxic, or both, than first-line drugs. These include ethionamide, cycloserine, amikacin, kanamycin, capreomycin, thiacetazone, para-aminosalicylic acid (PAS), and other agents discussed in Chapter 39.

Third-Line Agents

These agents have even less activity against *M. tuberculosis* than second-line agents, and are usually given only as adjunctive therapy to persons with XDR tuberculosis. These drugs have generally not been evaluated in a systematic manner for the treatment of tuberculosis. Such drugs include amoxicillin-clavulanate, clarithromycin, clofazamine, and linezolid.

Agents under Development

There are several new drugs that are currently under investigation. These include TMC-207 (Tibotec), OPC-67683 (Otsuka), PA-0824 (Global Alliance for TB Drug Development), and SQ-109 (Sequella).[206]

SELECTING A DRUG REGIMEN

Before RMP was available, excellent results in drug-sensitive infections were obtained with INH plus either PAS or EMB given for 18 to 24 months, "reinforced" in extensive disease by STM for the first 6 to 12 weeks. Relapse rates were unacceptably high with shorter courses. However, demonstration that RMP was equal to INH in efficacy led to studies of shorter treatment regimens. In definitive studies, drug-sensitive infections responded as effectively to 9 months of INH and RMP as to 18- to 24-month regimens not containing RMP.[207,208] It was subsequently demonstrated that 6-month regimens based on an initial 2-month intensive "bactericidal phase" of INH, RMP, PZA, and either STM or EMB, followed by a "continuation phase" of INH and RMP for 4 more months, performed as well.[209,210] It was also established that "continuation phase" drugs could be administered twice or thrice weekly, facilitating DOT.[211] Next it was shown that neither STM nor EMB improved results over a three-drug regimen (INH, RMP, and PZA) during the first 2 months of intensive therapy when the isolate was fully susceptible.[209] This 6-month three-drug regimen is acceptable for drug-sensitive infections. However, given concerns about resistance, EMB should be included until susceptibility testing results are known. A 6-month continuation phase of INH and EMB is inferior to a 4-month continuation phase of INH and RMP.[212]

STANDARD REGIMENS BASED ON ISONIAZID AND RIFAMPIN

The combination of INH (5 mg/kg; maximum 300 mg), RMP (10 mg/kg; maximum 600 mg), PZA (25 mg/kg), and EMB (15 mg/kg) all given once daily by mouth should be initiated in persons suspected of having tuberculosis.[192,213] Therapy can be given daily throughout the entire course of treatment, or switched to intermittent therapy after 14 days of daily therapy. Intermittent therapy should be provided under direct observation. These four drugs should be continued for 2 months; EMB can be discontinued when susceptibility results return noting that the infecting organism is susceptible to the other 3 drugs.

At the end of 2 months, PZA and EMB can be discontinued and INH and RMP continued to complete a 6-month course. Several treatment regimens have been endorsed by the CDC, American Thoracic Society (ATS), Infectious Diseases Society of America (IDSA),[192] and WHO.[214] Several well-studied regimens are presented in Table 250-8.[192] As an alternative in persons with drug-susceptible disease, INH and RMP can be given daily during the first 2 months, followed by 7 months of either daily or twice-weekly therapy.[192,215] When given twice weekly, the RMP dose remains the same and the INH dose is increased to 15 mg/kg (900 mg maximum). In persons with a cavity on initial chest radiograph and positive sputum cultures after 2 months of therapy, tuberculosis relapse risk is high;[216] INH and RMP should be continued for an additional 3 months (9-month total course) to decrease the relapse risk.[192]

In persons with resistance to or intolerance of INH, a 6-month regimen of RMP, PZA, and EMB can be used. Results of all 6-month regimens in patients with initial resistance to RMP are poor, and such

TABLE 250-8	Drug Regimens for Culture-Positive Pulmonary Tuberculosis Caused by Drug-Susceptible Organisms				
Initial Phase			**Continuation Phase**		
Regimen	Drugs	Interval and Doses* (minimal duration)	Regimen	Drugs	Interval and Doses*† (minimal duration)	Range of Total Doses (minimal duration)
1	INH RIF PZA EMB	7 days/wk for 56 doses (8 wk) or 5 days/wk for 40 doses (8 wk)‡	1a	INH/RIF	7 days/wk for 126 doses (18 wk) or 5 days/wk for 90 doses (18 wk)‡	182-130 (26 wk)
			1b	INH/RIF	Twice weekly for 36 doses (18 wk)#	92-76 (26 wk)
			1c§	INH/RPT	Once weekly for 18 doses (18 wk)	74-58 (26 wk)
2	INH RIF PZA EMB	7 days/wk for 14 doses (2 wk), then twice weekly for 12 doses (6 wk) or 5 days/wk for 10 doses (2 wk),‡ then twice weekly for 12 doses (6 wk)	2a	INH/RIF	Twice weekly for 36 doses (18 wk)#	62-58 (26 wk)
			2b§	INH/RPT	Once weekly for 18 doses (18 wk)	44-40 (26 wk)
3	INH RIF PZA EMB	Three times weekly for 24 doses (8 wk)	3a	INH/RIF	Three times weekly for 54 doses (18 wk)	78 (26 wk)
4	INH RIF EMB	7 days/wk for 56 doses (8 wk) or 5 days/wk for 40 doses (8 wk)‡	4a	INH/RIF	7 days/wk for 217 doses (31 wk) or 5 days/wk for 155 doses (31 wk)‡	273-195 (39 wk)
			4b	INH/RIF	Twice weekly for 62 doses (31 wk)#	118-102 (39 wk)

*When DOT is used, drugs may be given 5 days/week and the necessary number of doses adjusted accordingly. Although there are no studies that compare five with seven daily doses, extensive experience indicates this would be an effective practice.

†Patients with cavitation on initial chest radiograph and positive cultures at completion of 2 months of therapy should receive a 7-month (31-week; either 217 doses [daily] or 62 doses [twice weekly]) continuation phase.

‡Five-day-a-week administration is always given by DOT.

§Options 1c and 2b should be used only in HIV-negative patients who have negative sputum smears at the time of completion of 2 months of therapy and who do not have cavitation on initial chest radiograph. For patients started on this regimen and found to have a positive culture from the 2-month specimen, treatment should be extended an extra 3 months.

#Not recommended for HIV-infected patients with CD4+ cell counts < 100 cells/mm³.

EMB, ethambutol; INH, isoniazid; PZA, pyrazinamide; RIF, rifampin; RPT, rifapentine.

Adapted from Centers for Disease Control and Prevention. Treatment of tuberculosis. American Thoracic Society, CDC and Infectious Diseases Society of America. *MMWR Morb Mortal Wkly Rep.* 2003;52(RR-11):1-88.

cases probably require 18- to 24-month courses, as was the case before RMP was available.[217]

When hepatitis (defined as transaminases > ×5 upper limit of normal regardless of symptoms or > ×3 upper limit of normal in persons with symptoms of hepatitis) occurs in patients receiving INH, RMP, and/or PZA, all drugs should be discontinued until hepatic transaminase levels normalize and symptoms resolve. Drugs may then be cautiously reintroduced in a stepwise fashion while monitoring serum transaminase levels. If persons are intolerant of INH, a regimen of RMP, PZA, and EMB can be given to complete a 6-month course. If persons are intolerant of RMP, a more prolonged (18- to 24-month) regimen based on INH and at least one companion drug (e.g., EMB and possibly a fluoroquinolone) can be continued.

DIRECTLY OBSERVED TREATMENT

Poor adherence to antituberculosis therapy over the entire course of treatment, with resultant development of drug-resistant tuberculosis and low rates of tuberculosis cure and treatment completion, has led to the recommendation to use DOT whenever feasible.[192] Importantly, DOT is cost effective, especially when considering the cost of MDR cases that are prevented.[218] Because all doses are observed, compliance is improved and the likelihood of emergence of resistance minimized. The ability of mandatory DOT to control drug resistance in a community is well established.[219,220] In some cases, recalcitrant patients must be detained for completion of therapy.

REGIMENS OF LESS THAN 6 MONTHS FOR MINIMAL DISEASE

Extent of disease can be quantified by the mycobacterial content of sputum, with smear- and culture-positive sputum representing most severe disease, smear-negative and culture-positive sputum representing intermediate disease, and smear- and culture-negative sputum representing the least amount of disease. Good results have been obtained with as little as 4 months of therapy in patients with less extensive tuberculosis.[221] A 4-month course of treatment (2 months of INH, RMP, PZA, and EMB followed by 2 months of INH and RMP) is recommended for HIV-seronegative persons with culture-negative tuberculosis.[192] In HIV-seropositive persons with culture-negative tuberculosis a 6-month regimen is recommended.

FIXED-DOSE COMBINATION TABLETS

Fixed-dose preparations containing either 150 mg of INH and 300 mg of RMP (Rifamate), or INH 50 mg, RMP 120 mg, and PZA 300 mg (Rifater) are available. These prevent the patient from omitting drugs and taking monotherapy, and therefore decrease the risk of resistance. Fixed-dose combinations are particularly useful when DOT cannot be provided.

TREATMENT OF MULTIDRUG-RESISTANT TUBERCULOSIS

Surprisingly, studies of four-drug, 6-month chemotherapy demonstrated that initial INH or STM resistance did not compromise outcome, but results were very poor (>50% lack of conversion or relapse) when initial RMP resistance was present.[217] In a recent meta-analysis, treatment failure and relapse were substantially higher in the presence of initial drug resistance.[222]

For treatment for tuberculosis that is resistant to both INH and RMP, susceptibility testing for second-line drugs should be performed and treatment individualized according to the susceptibility test results. In some settings, standardized second-line regimens are used. If a suboptimal regimen is prescribed, resistance to additional drugs may emerge and the opportunity for success may be lost. In a study from Denver, Colorado, only one half of 171 HIV-negative patients with MDR-TB ever converted sputum cultures to negative despite

prolonged administration of carefully selected regimens (not including fluoroquinolones).[223] In a follow-up study from the same institution the long-term success rate was 75%.[224] In a study from Latvia, 66% of MDR-TB patients completed therapy or were cured.[225] In contrast, two smaller studies among HIV-seronegative patients from New York City and San Francisco noted remission in virtually all evaluable HIV-negative patients treated for MDR-TB.[226,227] For tuberculosis that is INH and RMP resistant but fluoroquinolone susceptible, a fluoroquinolone should always be administered along with other drugs to which the organism is susceptible. The risk of treatment failure is increased if the *M. tuberculosis* isolate is also resistant to fluoroquinolones.[228,229] Levofloxacin may be preferred over ofloxacin, but moxifloxacin has the greatest in vitro activity against *M. tuberculosis*. Companion drugs may include aminoglycosides (STM, kanamycin, or amikacin) or capreomycin, ethionamide, and cycloserine.[226,230-232] The injectable agents are particularly important for good outcomes.

TREATMENT OF EXTENSIVELY DRUG-RESISTANT TUBERCULOSIS

Treatment of XDR-TB, which is defined as resistance to INH, RMP, any fluoroquinolone, and at least one of three injectable second-line drugs (amikacin, kanamycin, or capreomycin),[79] is difficult and is usually associated with poor outcomes. The risk of treatment failure and death has been higher than in patients with MDR-TB in some series,[233,234] but not all.[235] Treatment with at least five drugs to which the organism is susceptible is recommended.

COURSE OF TREATMENT AND DURATION OF OBSERVATION

At least three sputum samples and, if available, specimens obtained at bronchoscopy, should be submitted before beginning treatment. In patients with presumed tuberculosis, treatment should be initiated immediately; a few days of antituberculous treatment will not interfere with bacteriologic diagnosis. If cultures are negative and there are no alternative diagnoses, clinical and radiographic response to therapy after 2 months of treatment is consistent with a diagnosis of tuberculosis. Periodic chest roentgenograms are helpful, although monthly films are not necessary. Beginning 1 month after initiation of therapy, three sputum cultures should be obtained monthly to monitor conversion to negative or, if sputum cultures remain positive, to detect treatment failure and the possible emergence of drug resistance. Sputum cultures should convert to negative within 2 months. In a minority of patients, sputum smears remain positive after cultures turn negative. Sporadic positive smears for long periods presumably represent inactive bacilli released from caseous foci. When cultures remain positive after 4 months of treatment it is considered treatment failure. Causes of treatment failure include drug resistance, noncompliance with therapy, and malabsorption of antituberculosis drugs. Sensitivity testing should be performed and consideration given to adding at least two new drugs to which the organism was sensitive at the outset of treatment, at least until sensitivities are known. Addition of only one drug risks development of resistance to the added drug. Adherence to therapy should be ensured, and serum drug levels considered to assess absorption.

Patients receiving INH, RMP, and PZA should be asked about symptoms of hepatitis monthly, and hepatic transaminase levels should be checked in symptomatic persons. In persons with abnormal hepatic transaminases at baseline, such labs should be monitored regularly, particularly early in the course of therapy. Patients receiving EMB should be regularly questioned regarding visual symptoms; their visual acuity should be measured (Snellen chart) and red-green color discrimination assessed monthly. Patients receiving STM should be examined for balance and high-frequency hearing loss, and renal function monitored closely.

Relapse after adequate treatment of drug-sensitive infections is infrequent (2% to 5%). Prolonged follow-up of appropriately treated patients is not necessary except in the case of unusually extensive disease, slow bacteriologic response to treatment, suspicion of poor compliance, drug-resistant disease, or high-risk patients with intercurrent diseases. In high-incidence settings, an additional 12 months of INH after completion of a 6-month RMP-containing regimen reduces the tuberculosis recurrence rate among HIV-infected adults.[236,237] However, such a practice is often not performed due to logistical constraints.

TREATMENT ALGORITHM

A committee from the CDC, the ATS, and the IDSA has published an algorithm that embodies the principles previously discussed but also takes into account the significance of cavitation on the duration of treatment (Fig. 250-7).[192] Due to the high relapse risk among persons with pulmonary cavitation on chest radiograph and a positive sputum culture after 2 months of therapy,[216] it is recommended that treatment be extended to a total of 9 months in such patients.

RE-TREATMENT

Recurrent tuberculosis may be due to either relapse (same *M. tuberculosis* strain as the original episode) or reinfection (different *M. tuberculosis* strain). Genotyping (RFLP, MIRU, and spoligotyping) may be used to distinguish *M. tuberculosis* isolates. Clinical judgment based on experience is critical in re-treatment cases, and testing of susceptibility to first- and second-line drugs is required.[192] Some generalizations concerning re-treatment can be made:

1. In a patient with drug-susceptible tuberculosis who receives rifamycin-based DOT, relapse is likely due to a drug-susceptible organism. Such patients usually respond again to the initial regimen.

2. If compliance has been irregular, particularly if the patient has not received DOT, resistant organisms will probably be present.

3. When drug resistance is suspected, the treatment regimen should include INH, RMP, PZA, EMB, a fluoroquinolone, and an injectable agent (e.g., STM) pending susceptibility results.

4. Capreomycin or amikacin can replace STM. Kanamycin is less effective and more toxic and is used as a last resort. There is usually no cross-resistance between capreomycin and STM, amikacin or kanamycin, but amikacin and kanamycin are usually cross-resistant.

5. Tuberculosis resistant to INH and RMP (i.e., MDR-TB) should be treated with EMB, PZA, a fluoroquinolone, an injectable agent, plus probably one additional agent. The injectable agent is given for 4 to 6 months, surgery may be required, and the total treatment duration is 18 to 24 months.[232,238]

6. Tuberculosis resistant to INH, RMP, an injectable agent, and a fluoroquinolone (i.e., XDR-TB) should be treated with at least 5 drugs to which the organism is susceptible.[235] Surgical resection may be required. A prolonged course of treatment is necessary, but the optimal duration is unknown.

OTHER FORMS OF TREATMENT

Bed rest does not influence outcome when effective chemotherapy is given. Resection still has a role in the salvage of patients in whom treatment fails and who have localized, resectable disease, and extensive drug resistance.

Corticosteroids

Corticosteroids in conjunction with antituberculosis therapy improve neurological outcome and mortality in persons with tuberculous

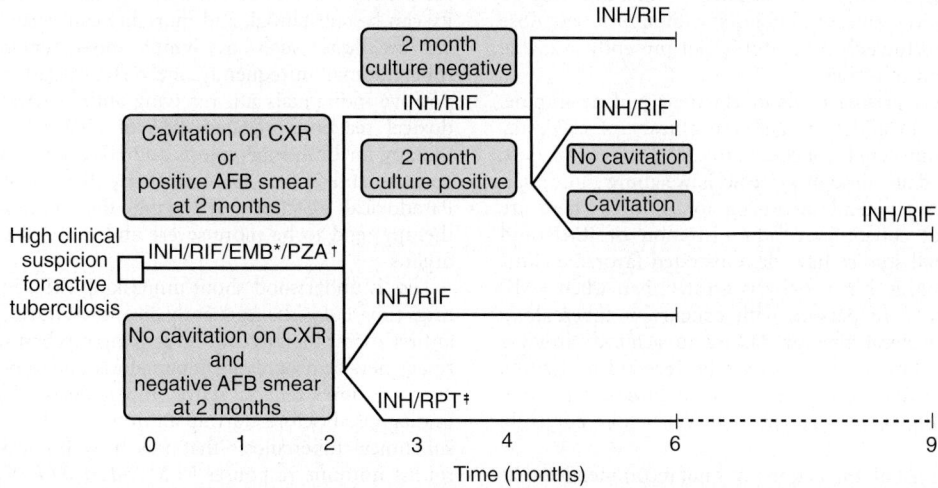

Figure 250-7 **Treatment algorithm for tuberculosis.** Patients in whom tuberculosis is proved or strongly suspected should have treatment initiated with isoniazid, rifampin, pyrazinamide, and ethambutol for the initial 2 months. A repeat smear and culture should be performed when 2 months of treatment has been completed. If cavities were seen on the initial chest radiograph or the acid-fast smear is positive at completion of 2 months of treatment, the continuation phase of treatment should consist of isoniazid and rifampin daily or twice weekly for 4 months to complete a total of 6 months of treatment. If cavitation was present on the initial chest radiograph and the culture at the time of completion of 2 months of therapy is positive, the continuation phase should be lengthened to 7 months (total of 9 months of treatment). If the patient has HIV infection and the CD4+ cell count is less than 100/mm³, the continuation phase should consist of daily or three times weekly isoniazid and rifampin. In HIV-uninfected patients having no cavitation on chest radiograph and negative acid-fast smears at completion of 2 months of treatment, the continuation phase may consist of either once-weekly isoniazid and rifapentine, or daily or twice-weekly isoniazid and rifampin, to complete a total of 6 months (*bottom*). Patients receiving isoniazid and rifapentine, and whose 2-month cultures are positive, should have treatment extended by an additional 3 months (total of 9 months). *EMB may be discontinued when results of drug susceptibility testing indicate no drug resistance. †PZA may be discontinued after it has been taken for 2 months (56 doses). ‡RPT should not be used in HIV-infected patients with tuberculosis or in patients with extrapulmonary tuberculosis. Therapy should be extended to 9 months if 2-month culture is positive. AFB, acid fast bacilli; CXR, chest radiograph; EMB, ethambutol; INH, isoniazid; PZA, pyrazinamide; RIF, rifampin; RPT, rifapentine. (*From Centers for Disease Control and Prevention [CDC]. Treatment of tuberculosis. American Thoracic Society, CDC and Infectious Diseases Society of America. MMWR Morb Mortal Wkly Rep. 2003;52[RR-11]:1-88.*)

meningitis, and improve outcome and mortality in persons with tuberculous pericarditis. Use of corticosteroids is therefore recommended in these situations. For all other clinical manifestations of tuberculosis, however, there is no long-term benefit of adjunctive corticosteroids—and therefore no therapeutic role.[239]

TREATMENT OF TUBERCULOSIS IN HIV-INFECTED PATIENTS

The treatment of HIV-related tuberculosis is complicated by major drug–drug interactions between antituberculosis and antiretroviral therapy. These interactions affect the choice of therapy (and appropriate doses) for both diseases. Invaluable websites that provide extensive advice and information regarding treatment options for HIV-related tuberculosis, including managing and avoiding drug–drug interactions, are maintained by the Department of Health and Human Services[240] and the CDC.[241] These websites are updated regularly, and should be consulted routinely because new antiretroviral agents and interactions are being discovered. Chapter 39 includes three tables from the CDC website about use of antiretrovirals together with rifampin or rifabutin.

The rifamycins interact extensively with many HIV protease inhibitors and non-nucleoside reverse transcriptase inhibitors (see Chapter 39).[242] Among the rifamycins, RMP has the most interactions, rifapentine an intermediate amount, and rifabutin the least. RMP is contraindicated for use with most HIV protease inhibitors (saquinavir, indinavir, nelfinavir, fosamprenavir, atazanavir, darunavir, tipranavir) and the non-nucleoside reverse transcript inhibitor etravirine. Miraviroc can be used with RMP if the miraviroc dose is increased to 600 mg twice daily. Raltegravir can be given with RMP with no change in dose. The RMP pharmacokinetic interaction with saquinavir–ritonavir and lopinavir–ritonavir may be overcome with increased protease inhibitor dosages.[243,244] However, several healthy volunteer studies were prematurely terminated when individuals receiving RMP promptly developed marked hepatotoxicity on adding ritonavir-boosted lopinavir,[243] saquinavir,[244] or atazanavir.[245] Rifabutin may be used in combination with protease inhibitors, with appropriate dose modification.[240,241] Unfortunately, rifabutin is not presently available in most resource-limited countries.

RMP modestly lowers plasma levels of efavirenz and nevirapine. RMP does not appear to affect the antiviral efficacy of efavirenz, and they can be administered concomitantly. The efavirenz dose can remain at 600 mg daily, though in persons weighing more than 60 kg some experts recommend increasing to 800 mg. There are greater concerns about concomitant administration of RMP and nevirapine. Several small studies have demonstrated favorable clinical and virologic responses, but toxicity is greater than when RMP is given with efavirenz.[246] In persons with concurrent tuberculosis at the start of antiretroviral therapy, failure to achieve virologic suppression was more common in persons who received nevirapine than efavirenz (both given with RMP).[247] RMP lowers maraviroc and raltegravir levels; there are no clinical data currently available.

Despite this extensive list of interactions, it is not recommended that treatment of tuberculosis be delayed or that highly active antiretroviral therapy be avoided. Because antimycobacterial drugs other than the rifamycins do not have substantial interactions, an alternative regimen with INH, STM, PZA, and EMB can be considered. However, in HIV-infected persons, regimens that are not rifamycin-based may be less effective than rifamycin-based regimens.

The CDC's Tuberculosis Trials Consortium Study 23 prescribed twice-weekly, rifabutin-based, continuation phase therapy to HIV-infected adults with active tuberculosis. Of the 169 patients enrolled, nine developed treatment failure or relapse. Of these, eight acquired rifamycin resistance.[248] Acquired rifamycin resistance is seen almost exclusively in patients with advanced AIDS who receive intermittent antituberculosis therapy. In response to this study, the CDC recommends that HIV-infected persons with fewer than 100 CD4+

T cells/mm^3 should not receive once- or twice-weekly regimens. These patients should receive daily therapy during the intensive phase, and daily or thrice-weekly doses during the continuation phase.[249]

Patients with HIV-related enteropathy may not respond to chemotherapy because of inadequate absorption of oral agents, and in rare cases pharmacokinetic monitoring may be necessary.[250]

IMMUNE RECONSTITUTION INFLAMMATORY SYNDROME

Immune reconstitution inflammatory syndrome (IRIS) results from rapid restoration of immune responses to opportunistic pathogens, most importantly *M. tuberculosis*. This has most often been described in patients receiving antiretroviral therapy. Characteristic features include initiation of virologically effective antiretroviral therapy within the previous 3 months (the period of most rapid immune recovery), clinical deterioration with exaggerated inflammation, and absence of an alternative explanation such as drug resistance, drug hypersensitivity, other infections, or lymphoma. Tuberculosis-associated IRIS comprises two main categories: (1) onset in patients who are already being treated for tuberculosis (termed *paradoxical IRIS*), and (2) onset in patients with previously unrecognized, untreated tuberculosis (termed *unmasking IRIS*). During paradoxical IRIS, patients have typically been responding to tuberculosis therapy but develop recurrent, new, or worsening manifestations such as fever, cough, lymph node enlargement, or roentgenographic abnormalities after starting antiretrovirals.[251,252] Such patients demonstrate robust peripheral blood T-cell responses to purified protein derivative, and increased pro-inflammatory cytokines.[253] Paradoxical IRIS is most likely to occur in patients with more advanced AIDS, disseminated and extrapulmonary tuberculosis, a good immunologic and virologic response to antiretrovirals, and in those who initiate antiretrovirals soon after starting antituberculous drugs.[254] Reported frequencies range from 8% to 43%.[254] Although symptoms of paradoxical IRIS are usually self-limited and last a median of 2 months,[248,255] morbidity can be substantial, and mortality can occur but is rare. Paradoxical reactions such as lymph node enlargement or cerebral tuberculomas infrequently affect HIV-negative individuals, or HIV-positive individuals not receiving antiretrovirals. In one study paradoxical reactions affected 36% of HIV-infected patients receiving therapy for both tuberculosis and HIV, but only 2% of HIV-negative patients and 7% of HIV-infected patients not on antiretrovirals.[251] Paradoxical reactions following the initiation of antiretroviral therapy tend to be more severe and more likely to involve multiple organs.

Less is understood about unmasking IRIS. In resource-limited settings tuberculosis is frequently diagnosed during the initial months of antiretroviral therapy, but underlying mechanisms vary.[256] Some represent new or progressive tuberculosis due to persistent immunodeficiency, some reflect active tuberculosis that was present but undiagnosed before starting antiretroviral therapy, and others reflect subclinical tuberculosis that was truly unmasked by restoration of robust immune responses to *M. tuberculosis*. Consensus case definitions were recently published to facilitate research into tuberculosis-associated IRIS in resource-limited settings.[254]

The optimal timing of antiretroviral therapy initiation in HIV-infected persons with tuberculosis is unclear. Factors that need to be considered include the high mortality rate in TB/HIV patients, the beneficial effects of antiretroviral therapy on survival, but also the large pill burden of treatment for both diseases, drug–drug interactions, high toxicity rates, and the risk of IRIS. To date there have been no clinical trials to asssess this issue. However, in a decision analysis pertaining to patients with less than 200 CD4+ lymphocytes/mm^3, initiation of antiretroviral therapy within 2 months of antituberculosis treatment (compared to 2 to 6 months after initiating antituberculosis therapy) was favored in almost all clinical situations.[257]

DURATION OF THERAPY

The duration of antituberculosis therapy is determined by relapse risk. Several relatively small studies noted comparable relapse rates in HIV-infected and HIV-uninfected persons after 6 months of antituberculosis therapy. Based on these data, the current recommendation is to treat for the same duration regardless of HIV status.[192] However, more recent observational studies have noted higher recurrence rates in HIV-infected than HIV-uninfected persons who receive 6 months of treatment.[258,259] A clinical trial of 6 versus 9 months of antituberculosis treatment in HIV-infected persons has not been performed. In high tuberculosis incidence settings such as Haiti, an additional 12 months of INH after completing a 6-month, RMP-containing regimen reduced the tuberculosis recurrence rate in HIV-infected adults.[236]

OTHER SPECIAL TREATMENT CIRCUMSTANCES

Childhood
Pulmonary tuberculosis in childhood should be treated with INH, RMP, and PZA for 2 months, followed by INH and RMP for 4 months. The inability to monitor visual acuity limits the use of EMB in very young children, though it can be given if the bacillary burden is high and/or drug resistance is suspected.[192]

Pregnancy
Treatment should not be deferred during pregnancy. For drug-sensitive tuberculosis, INH, RMP, and EMB is the regimen of choice. STM should not be used during pregnancy because of potential eighth nerve toxicity in the fetus. Although PZA is routinely recommended by international organizations, use has not been recommended in the United States because of inadequate teratogenicity data.[192]

Uremia and End-Stage Renal Disease
Dosages of INH and RMP need not be adjusted for renal failure but should be administered after dialysis, and pyridoxine supplementation should be routine. In patients with creatinine clearance less than 30 mL/minute and those on hemodialysis, EMB should be dosed at 15 to 25 mg/kg, and PZA 25 to 35 mg/kg, both given three times per week (after dialysis for those on hemodialysis). Biochemical monitoring of hepatotoxicity during renal failure may be complicated by abnormally low transaminase levels in uremia.

Liver Disease
The selection and dosage of antituberculous agents do not need to be modified in most patients with underlying liver disease, but hepatic transaminases and bilirubin must be followed closely. In persons intolerant of INH due to hepatotoxicity, a 6-month regimen of RMP, PZA, and EMB can be used. If PZA can be tolerated for only 2 months, RMP and EMB should be given for a total 12-month course.[192] For persons with extensive tuberculosis and severe hepatitis who should not have a prolonged treatment interruption, "bridging" regimens that include EMB, fluoroquinolone, and STM could be considered until a more standard regimen can be instituted.[192] Preexisting liver disease (e.g., hepatitis C virus infection) may complicate the detection of drug-related hepatotoxicity; accordingly, clinical and biochemical supervision should be assiduous.

Patients Receiving Immunosuppressive Drugs
Tuberculosis that develops during immunosuppressive treatment of another disease should be treated with the same regimens used to treat immunocompetent hosts. Immunosuppressive therapy need not be discontinued. Given the increased predisposition to tuberculosis among persons receiving a TNF-α inhibitor (e.g., etanercept, infliximab), discussion between all of the patient's medical providers (e.g., rheumatology, gastroenterology, pulmonology, and infectious diseases) may be helpful to determine a rational treatment strategy.

TREATMENT OF LATENT TUBERCULOUS INFECTION

Soon after INH became available, it became widely used in the United States to treat not only persons with active disease (as part of combination therapy), but also *M. tuberculosis* infection, to prevent progression to active tuberculosis. In contrast, many other countries have used a tuberculosis prevention strategy based primarily on BCG vaccination at birth rather than treatment of latent tuberculosis infection. The current strategy in the United States is to perform TST (or an interferon-γ release assay) only on persons who are at high risk of progressing to active tuberculosis, and then treat all persons with a positive test regardless of age. Criteria for TST positivity and groups for whom treatment of latent tuberculous infection is indicated are listed in Table 250-9.[125,260]

DRUG REGIMENS

Nine months of INH, up to 300 mg daily, is the preferred regimen for treating latent tuberculous infection in adults and children, regardless of HIV status.[125] Six months of INH may be more cost effective, but in a post hoc analysis of previously conducted studies, 9 to 10 months of INH provided greater protection than 6 months, thus it is the recommended duration.[261] When necessary, supervised intermittent treatment of latent tuberculous infection with INH (15 mg/kg; up to 900 mg) twice weekly, can be used. Pyridoxine supplementation, 10 to 50 mg daily, is recommended to prevent peripheral neuropathy in persons older than 65 years of age; pregnant and breastfeeding women; persons with diabetes mellitus, chronic renal failure, or alcoholism; persons undergoing treatment with anticonvulsants; and persons who are malnourished. For persons who are intolerant of INH or who are presumed to have INH-resistant infection, 4 months of RMP (10 mg/kg; 600 mg maximum) is an acceptable alternative.[125] This regimen is well tolerated,[194,195] though its effectiveness has not been studied. In a study of a 3-month regimen of RMP, tuberculosis rates were comparable to 6 months of INH, but still relatively high overall.[262] In children, a 6-month course of RMP is recommended.[260]

A 2-month regimen of daily RMP/PZA is as effective as a 12-month daily regimen of INH in HIV-infected adults.[263] Unfortunately, initial

TABLE 250-9	Criteria for Tuberculin Positivity by Risk Group	
Reaction ≥ 5 mm of Induration	**Reaction ≥ 10 mm of Induration**	**Reaction ≥ 15 mm of Induration**
HIV-positive persons	Recent immigrants (within 5 yr) from high-prevalence countries	Persons with no risk factors for tuberculosis
Recent contacts of tuberculosis case patients	Injection drug users	
Fibrotic changes on chest radiograph consistent with prior tuberculosis	Residents and employees of high-risk congregate settings (prisons and jails, nursing homes, hospitals and other health care facilities, residential facilities for patients with AIDS, and homeless shelters)	
Patients with organ transplants and other immunosuppressed patients (receiving equivalent of ≥15 mg/day of prednisone for at least 1 month)	Children less than 4 years of age, or infants, children, and adolescents exposed to adults at high risk	

Adapted from Centers for Disease Control and Prevention. Targeted tuberculin testing and treatment of latent tuberculosis infection. American Thoracic Society. *MMWR Morb Mortal Wkly Rep.* 2000;49(RR-6):1-51.

enthusiasm for this 2-month regimen waned following numerous reports of severe liver injury and death, primarily in HIV-negative individuals.[202] This regimen is no longer recommended.[264]

Optimal treatment of latent tuberculous infection when resistance to both INH and RMP (i.e., MDR-TB) is likely is not known. Regimens of PZA plus either EMB or a fluoroquinolone for 6 to 12 months have been recommended, but such regimens are poorly tolerated and their effectiveness has never been studied.[125]

RISK OF ISONIAZID HEPATOTOXICITY DURING TREATMENT OF LATENT TUBERCULOUS INFECTION

A U.S. Public Health Service survey found the incidence of probable INH-associated hepatitis increased with age: rates per 1000 persons were 0 for those younger than age 20, 3 for ages 20 to 34, 12 for ages 35 to 49, 23 for ages 50 to 64, and 8 for age older than 64.[193] The incidence in daily drinkers of alcohol was also high (26.5 to 1000). The number in the elderly was probably falsely low because of a small sample size. A much larger experience recorded hepatitis in 4.6% of patients older than 65.[265] A large European study reported a hepatitis incidence of 520 per 100,000 population; the figure was 280 per 100,000 for those younger than 35 years and 770 per 100,000 for those older than 54 years. Most hepatitis develops within the first 3 months, and the risk of death, once clinical hepatitis develops, is substantial.[193,266] Biochemical monitoring will likely prevent some deaths, because there is a subclinical phase of at least several weeks. Byrd and colleagues recorded elevated serum transaminase levels in 18.3% of patients taking INH but no deaths in a biochemically monitored population. Many patients with severe biochemical hepatitis would not have been detected by monitoring symptoms only.[267] In contrast, one public health clinic reported only 11 cases of clinical hepatotoxicity and no deaths among more than 11,000 persons receiving INH over a 7-year period.[268] Based on this and other considerations, emphasis is now placed on clinic monitoring for signs and symptoms of adverse effects, with prompt evaluation if these develop. Current recommendations advocate routine baseline and follow-up laboratory monitoring only for persons with HIV infection, pregnant and early postpartum women, and persons with chronic liver disease or who use alcohol regularly.[125]

Snider and Caras analyzed 177 cases of fatal hepatitis from various sources,[269] and estimated a case rate of 14 per 100,000 of those starting and 23 per 100,000 of those completing therapy. Sixty-nine percent were female, with clustering around pregnancy. However, many experts agree that treating latent tuberculous infection during pregnancy should not be delayed if the infection was recently acquired or in HIV-positive women.[125]

TREATMENT OF CONTACTS OF ACTIVE CASES

The U.S. Public Health Service contact study showed that treatment of latent tuberculous infection decreased the incidence of subsequent tuberculosis among contacts of active cases from 1550 to 610 cases per 100,000, a 61% reduction over 10 years.[270] In those who were tuberculin negative when first surveyed, the figures (per 100,000) were 510 without and 150 with chemoprophylaxis, a 59% reduction. Estimates of the risk to contacts in some smaller studies are much higher. One year of INH therapy is about 70% effective in preventing disease, with failures most often caused by nonadherence.[271] INH prophylaxis may also fail in drug-resistant infections. It appears unlikely that prophylactic INH monotherapy taken reliably by contacts results in subsequent INH resistance.

Treatment of latent tuberculous infection is indicated for persons found to be TST positive (5 mm of induration) after contact with an active case. In children younger than age 5 who are close contacts of an active case but have a negative TST, INH should be initiated and a TST repeated after 3 months. If the second TST is positive, a 9-month course should be completed; if it is negative, INH can be discontinued.

To address the risk to health care workers inadvertently exposed to tuberculosis, Stead reviewed 33 previously investigated hospital and nursing home outbreaks.[127] In this setting, on discovering that exposures have occurred, a list of all exposed personnel and their TST results before exposure should be assembled. Nonreactors should be retested 8 weeks after the exposure to allow time for TST conversion. However, if exposure is particularly heavy, or in HIV-positive health care workers, preventive therapy should be started even before retesting. Treatment can later be discontinued in HIV-negative persons if they remain tuberculin negative.[113]

TREATMENT OF QUIESCENT, PREVIOUSLY UNTREATED PULMONARY TUBERCULOSIS

Tuberculin-positive patients with fibrotic upper lobe lesions and patients who had active tuberculosis before drugs were available are at increased risk for developing tuberculosis.[271] Six- and 12-month regimens of INH are effective in preventing development of active disease,[271] but based on a post hoc analysis, a 9-month course of INH is advised.[192,261] The longer the lesion has been stable, the less is the risk of relapse.

TREATMENT OF INDIVIDUALS WITH RECENT INFECTION

The first 2 years after tuberculin conversion (defined as an increase in induration on tuberculin skin testing of at least 10 mm) is the period of greatest risk for development of active disease. Most authorities recommend treatment of latent tuberculous infection for any person known to have converted within 2 years, regardless of age. Reactions that require boosting to be elicited are not recent conversions and do not require treatment.

TREATING LATENT TUBERCULOUS INFECTION IN PERSONS WITH HIV INFECTION

In the era before highly active antiretroviral therapy, TST- and HIV-positive injection drug users had an annual risk of active tuberculosis of approximately 8% per year.[100] As indicated in Table 250-9, the CDC recommends that a TST of greater than 5 mm induration be considered a positive test and therefore an indication for treating latent tuberculous infection in persons with known or suspected HIV infection in whom active tuberculosis has been ruled out.[125]

Anergy testing in immunocompromised persons is unreliable, and treatment of latent tuberculosis in anergic HIV-infected persons does not decrease tuberculosis risk.[135,136] Therefore, since 1997 the CDC has recommended against routine anergy testing for HIV-positive persons at risk for tuberculosis (see "Tuberculin Testing and HIV Infection").[272]

M. TUBERCULOSIS INFECTION IN PERSONS WITH ADDITIONAL RISK FACTORS

Treatment of latent tuberculous infection is advised for persons with *M. tuberculosis* infection who are from groups with a known high incidence of tuberculosis, including immigrants from developing countries, intravenous drug users, the homeless, prisoners, and residents of long-term care facilities.[125] An argument has been made for treating latent tuberculous infection in patients after gastrectomy and jejunoileal bypass surgery for obesity. There is a greatly increased incidence of tuberculosis in patients undergoing chronic renal dialysis[70] and in renal transplant patients. Preventive therapy has been recommended for latently infected patients with silicosis, but relapse after therapy has been observed. Treatment of latent tuberculous infection has also been recommended for patients with myeloproliferative disorders and hematologic malignancies, especially when corticosteroids are given. Prolonged treatment with high doses of corticosteroids undoubtedly predisposes to activation of latent tuberculosis. Latently infected individuals who are to receive anti-TNF-α monoclonal antibodies (e.g., infliximab) should receive treatment of latent tuberculous infection.[146] Such immunosuppressive therapy may be initiated before completing INH.

Pregnant Women
Because INH treatment for latent tuberculous infection may be associated with a slightly increased risk of maternal hepatitis, added caution with respect to INH-induced hepatotoxicity is indicated.

The Nursing Home Problem
A major analysis by Stead and colleagues showed that 3.8% of men and 2.3% of women who were tuberculin positive on admission to nursing homes acquired active disease, and that this could be decreased 10-fold with treatment of latent tuberculous infection.[265] Treatment of latent tuberculous infection was clearly beneficial in patients who tuberculin converted after admission, with 11.6% of men and 7.6% of women acquiring active disease without treatment of latent tuberculous infection but only 0.2% with treatment.

VACCINATION

BCG, a live-attenuated vaccine derived from a strain of *M. bovis,* is used in young children throughout much of the world. Most evidence indicates that BCG vaccination of children results in a 60% to 80% decrease in the incidence of tuberculosis.[273] Its use is reasonable in high-prevalence situations, greater than those that now exist in the United States and most industrialized nations. It should be administered only to tuberculin-negative persons. Although BCG vaccine does not prevent infection, it usually prevents progression to clinical disease, and effectively prevents disseminated disease in young children. The risk of disseminated BCG infection after vaccination in infants born to HIV-positive mothers is small. BCG should not be given to persons known to be infected with HIV. Prior BCG vaccination does not alter guidelines for TST interpretation, particularly if at least 10 years have passed since vaccination.

The effect of BCG vaccination on tuberculin reactivity depends on the age at vaccination and interval before skin testing. In a study in Montreal, children vaccinated once with BCG before the age of 1 year had a 7.9% prevalence of positive TSTs 10 to 25 years later, comparable to those who never received BCG.[274] Prevalence of positive TSTs was 18% among those vaccinated between 1 and 5 years of age and 25.4% among those vaccinated after age 5. Although tuberculin reactivity wanes after infant BCG vaccination, later skin testing can cause a booster effect, a potential source of confusion. Interestingly, there is no relationship between tuberculin reactivity after BCG vaccination and protection against development of active tuberculosis.[128]

Intravesicular BCG, used to treat bladder cancer, is a rare cause of miliary granuloma in the liver or lung, psoas abscess, or osteomyelitis.[275-277] This mycobacteriosis responds to treatment with INH and RMP.

The development of a better vaccine for tuberculosis is a high priority.[278] Some candidates are subunit vaccines wherein immunodominant antigens are expressed by viral vectors or formulated with adjuvant. Live-attenuated vaccines have the potential advantage of inducing responses to a broader array of antigens, and the current vaccine against tuberculosis—BCG—has been modified to produce greater amounts of immunodominant antigens. An improved understanding of host pathways for presenting antigens of intracellular pathogens and mechanisms by which *M. tuberculosis* suppresses antigen presentation has fostered novel live-attenuated vaccine candidates. Promising approaches involve recombinant *M. tuberculosis* or BCG strains that have been specifically engineered to promote phagosomal permeability or induce apoptosis, or both, either by adding a phagosomal escape toxin (e.g., listeriolysin, perfringolysin)[279] or by reducing the activity and secretion of anti-apoptotic microbial enzymes.[280,281] The Stop TB Partnership regularly updates an online document describing new vaccine candidates.[282]

Extrapulmonary Tuberculosis

Extrapulmonary tuberculosis can be divided into three groups based on pathogenesis. The first comprises superficial mucosal foci resulting from the spread of infectious pulmonary secretions via the respiratory and gastrointestinal tracts. Such lesions were once almost inevitable complications of extensive cavitary pulmonary disease but are now rare. The second group comprises foci established by contiguous spread, such as from a subpleural focus into the pleural space. The third group comprises foci established by lymphohematogenous dissemination, either at the time of primary infection or, less commonly, from established chronic pulmonary or extrapulmonary foci.

AIDS AND EXTRAPULMONARY TUBERCULOSIS

Before 1985, cases of pulmonary tuberculosis in the United States decreased each year, whereas the number of extrapulmonary cases remained stable at about 4000 per year. The percentage of cases caused by extrapulmonary disease subsequently increased, largely as a result of coinfection with HIV. Unlike in non-AIDS patients, concomitant pulmonary and extrapulmonary disease is very common in AIDS patients with tuberculosis. Cases of HIV-associated pulmonary and extrapulmonary tuberculosis have declined in the United States since 1992.[48] There are certain distinguishing features of AIDS-associated extrapulmonary tuberculosis. The frequency of disseminated disease (more than one focus or progressive hematogenous disease) is high, 38% in one series,[283] and rapidly progressive forms with diffuse pulmonary infiltrates, acute respiratory failure, and disseminated intravascular coagulation have been observed. Tuberculosis pleuritis, when it occurs, is often bilateral and part of a disseminated process. Visceral lymphadenopathy, both mediastinal and abdominal, is frequent, and a contrast-enhanced CT scan showing nodes with central low attenuation suggests the diagnosis. Abscesses of the liver, pancreas, prostate, spleen, chest, abdominal wall, and other soft tissues have also been described. Extrapulmonary tuberculosis appears to predict an increased risk of developing paradoxical IRIS when antiretroviral therapy is initiated (see "Immune Reconstitution Inflammatory Syndrome").[254]

GENERAL COMMENTS ON TREATMENT OF EXTRAPULMONARY TUBERCULOSIS

Extrapulmonary foci usually respond to treatment more rapidly than does cavitary pulmonary tuberculosis due to the lower burden of organisms in the former. Therapy with four-drug regimens (INH, RMP, PZA, and EMB) for 2 months, followed by INH and RMP for 4 months, is advised in most cases caused by drug-sensitive organisms. The exceptions include bone and joint disease (6 to 9 months), and tuberculous meningitis (9 to 12 months though optimal duration unknown).[192] Adjunctive corticosteroids are recommended for persons with pericardial or central nervous system (CNS) tuberculosis.

MILIARY TUBERCULOSIS

The term *miliary tuberculosis,* first used to describe its pathologic resemblance to millet seeds, now describes any progressive disseminated hematogenous tuberculosis. Miliary tuberculosis can be roughly divided into three groups: (1) acute miliary tuberculosis associated with a brisk and histologically typical tissue reaction; (2) cryptic miliary tuberculosis, a more prolonged illness with subtle clinical findings and an attenuated histologic response; and (3) nonreactive tuberculosis characterized by huge numbers of organisms, little organized tissue response, and often a septic or typhoidal clinical picture.[120]

USUAL (ACUTE) MILIARY TUBERCULOSIS

In the prechemotherapy era, miliary tuberculosis occurred either soon after primary infection in children or young adults or as a terminal event in untreated chronic organ tuberculosis. In children, the illness

TABLE 250-10	Miliary Tuberculosis			
	Study			
	Biehl[284]	*Munt*[285]	*Maartens et al.*[286]	*Kim et al.*[287]
Number of cases	69	68	109	38%*
Mean age	51	50	—	60%*
Minority race	85%	87%	94%	79%*
Predisposing factors	15%	31%	42%	66%*
Weeks of symptoms	2-16	3-24	1-52	—
Meningitis	17%	19%	22%	—
Tuberculin positive	61%	84%	43%	28%
Miliary roentgenogram	93%	97%	—	91%*
Other foci of tuberculosis	32%	23%	—	—
Positive sputum smear	—	39%	33% (21/64)	36% (12/33)
Marrow diagnostic†	—	20%	41% (9/22)	9% (2/22)
Transbronchial biopsy diagnostic‡	—	—	76% (39/51)	62% (5/8)

*This percentage includes interstitial and diffuse alevolar patterns.
†Marrow diagnostic if caseating granuloma or acid-fast bacilli are seen.
‡Transbronchial biopsy diagnostic if any granuloma or acid-fast bacilli are seen.

is acute or subacute, with high intermittent fevers, night sweats, and occasional rigors. Pleural effusion, peritonitis, or meningitis occurs in as many as two thirds of persons. The illness in young adults is usually more chronic and initially less severe. However, miliary tuberculosis is now more frequently observed in older individuals, often with underlying illnesses or conditions that may confuse diagnosis.

Four large series in the chemotherapy era[284-287] have emphasized the frequency of miliary tuberculosis in minority racial groups, and the importance of underlying conditions such as alcoholism, cirrhosis, neoplasm, pregnancy, rheumatologic disease, and treatment with immunosuppressive agents (Table 250-10).[284-287] There is usually no prior history of tuberculosis, and the onset is often subtle. Generalized symptoms of fever, anorexia, weakness, and weight loss are nonspecific. Headache may indicate meningitis; abdominal pain may be due to peritonitis; and pleural pain may result from pleuritis. Physical findings are likewise usually nonspecific, but a careful search for cutaneous eruptions, sinus tracts, scrotal masses, and lymphadenopathy may yield a prompt biopsy diagnosis. A miliary infiltrate on chest roentgenogram is the most helpful finding and the usual reason miliary tuberculosis is suspected (Fig. 250-8). Unfortunately, many patients, particularly the elderly, succumb to miliary tuberculosis before the chest roentgenogram becomes abnormal.[288] The white blood cell count is usually normal, and anemia is the rule. Hyponatremia with the laboratory features of inappropriate secretion of antidiuretic hormone is frequent, particularly with meningitis.[285] Addison's disease should be considered as a cause of hyponatremia. Elevations of alkaline phosphatase and transaminases are common, as are hypoxemia, hypocapnia, and impairment of pulmonary diffusion capacity. Cultures of sputum, gastric contents, urine, and CSF are positive in some combination in most cases, but smears of sputum and pulmonary secretions alone are positive in fewer than one third. Immediate diagnosis often results from examination of tissue (lymph nodes, scrotal masses when present, liver biopsy, or bone marrow specimens). Mycobacterial blood cultures may also be positive. Transbronchial biopsy is an excellent way to obtain tissue and should be performed promptly when the diagnosis is suspected.[289] The finding of caseating granulomas or acid-fast bacilli is virtually diagnostic.

Rapid diagnosis is mandatory. However, treatment should be initiated immediately based on strong clinical suspicion, as mortality from miliary tuberculosis is most often due to delays in treatment. Response may be prompt or may take several weeks. Fulminant miliary tuberculosis may be associated with severe refractory hypoxemia and disseminated intravascular coagulation.

CRYPTIC MILIARY TUBERCULOSIS AND LATE GENERALIZED (CHRONIC HEMATOGENOUS) TUBERCULOSIS

Chronic organ tuberculosis is probably always associated with intermittent, nonprogressive seeding of the blood stream. In some individuals, however, especially as age or other factors compromise immunity, this becomes continuous and produces progressive hematogenous tuberculosis long after the primary infection.[290] The term *cryptic miliary tuberculosis* usually describes older patients with miliary tuberculosis in whom the diagnosis is obscure because of normal chest roentgenograms, negative tuberculin test results, and often confounding underlying illnesses to which symptoms are mistakenly attributed;[291] this term has also been applied to miliary tuberculosis diagnosed at autopsy.[288]

The foci responsible for late generalized tuberculosis are often clinically silent, for example, renal, genitourinary, osseous, or visceral lymph nodes.[290] Chronic pulmonary foci are at times involved but are rarely the only source. The clinical picture is frequently fever of unknown origin, often with a normal chest roentgenogram and a negative tuberculin test result. Fever may be absent, and in one series diagnosis was made ante mortem in only 15% of cases.[290] Late generalized tuberculosis may be associated with major hematologic abnormalities.

NONREACTIVE TUBERCULOSIS

The histologic appearance in this rare form of disseminated hematogenous tuberculosis shows nonspecific necrosis containing disintegrating neutrophils and enormous numbers of tubercle bacilli.[120] In the typical case, granulomas and epithelioid cells are lacking, although intermediate cases have areas more typical for tuberculosis. The gross pathologic findings are soft abscesses from minute to 1 cm, which always involve the liver and spleen, usually the marrow, commonly the

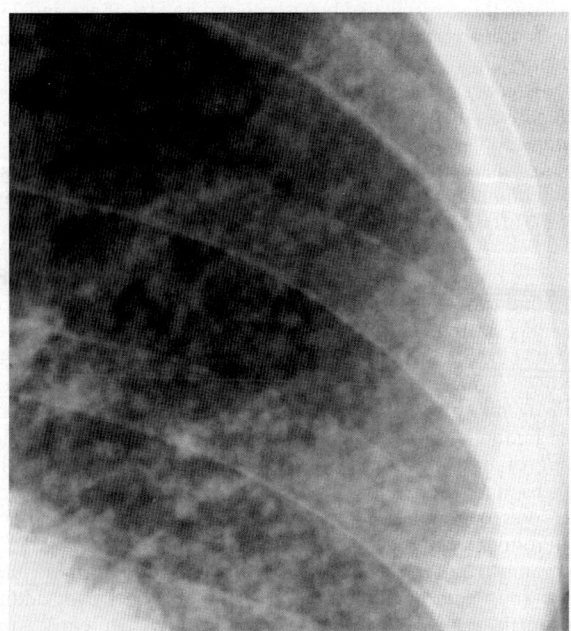

Figure 250-8 Detail of a chest roentgenogram (left midlung zone) showing countless 0.5- to 1.0-mm nodules typical of miliary tuberculosis.

lungs and kidneys, but never the meninges. The clinical picture may be overwhelming sepsis, with splenomegaly and often an inconspicuous diffuse mottling on the chest roentgenogram. Major hematologic abnormalities are common (see "Miliary Tuberculosis and Hematologic Abnormalities").

MILIARY TUBERCULOSIS AND HEMATOLOGIC ABNORMALITIES

Some patients with late generalized tuberculosis and most with nonreactive tuberculosis have serious hematologic abnormalities, including leukopenia, thrombocytopenia, anemia, leukemoid reactions, myelofibrosis, and polycythemia.[292] Leukemoid reactions may suggest acute leukemia, although most patients in whom hematogenous tuberculosis coexists with the clinical picture of leukemia have both diseases. Disseminated tuberculosis should be considered when pancytopenia is associated with fever and weight loss or as a cause of other obscure hematologic disorders.

PRIMARY HEPATIC TUBERCULOSIS

Rarely, miliary tuberculosis may mimic cholangitis with fever, liver function test abnormalities suggestive of obstructive disease, and little evidence of hepatocellular disease. Diagnosis is made by liver biopsy.

MILIARY TUBERCULOSIS IN AIDS

In AIDS patients, 10% with tuberculosis and 38% with extrapulmonary tuberculosis have miliary disease.[187,283] Major constitutional symptoms and hectic fevers are characteristic. The chest roentgenogram is abnormal in 80% and may include typical miliary mottling. Only 10% of patients are tuberculin positive.[187] The sputum smear is positive in only 25%,[283] but cultures of many materials will be positive, including blood in 50% to 60%. Biopsies during life show typical tuberculous histologic appearance but with more stainable organisms than in non-HIV miliary tuberculosis. In fatal cases, in contrast, the histologic picture is often nonreactive tuberculosis.[187]

Abscesses of various soft tissue and visceral organs have been described in patients with AIDS and tuberculosis, usually with other evidence of disseminated disease. Locations include the liver, spleen, pancreas, psoas muscle with or without spinal involvement, mediastinum, neck, chest wall, abdominal wall, and prostate.[187,283,293] Diagnosis is usually made by CT or ultrasonography and confirmed by needle or catheter aspiration. Clinical response to chemotherapy and drainage is usually good. An abscess may appear or reappear during therapy and respond to repeated aspiration.

CNS TUBERCULOSIS—TUBERCULOUS MENINGITIS

This condition is usually caused by rupture of a subependymal tubercle into the subarachnoid space rather than direct hematogenous seeding. Meningitis complicating miliary disease usually develops several weeks into the illness. In childhood, meningitis is an early postprimary event, and three fourths of these persons have a concurrently active primary complex, pleural effusion, or miliary tuberculosis. Subependymal foci may remain quiescent indefinitely before rupturing. This may follow head trauma or be associated with general depression of host immunity as a result of alcohol abuse or other factors.

Pathologic Features

Meningeal involvement is most pronounced at the base of the brain. In long-standing cases, a gelatinous mass may extend from the pons to the optic nerves, being most prominent adjacent to the optic chiasm. In more chronic cases, fibrous tissue may encase cranial nerves. Vasculitis of local arteries and veins may lead to aneurysm, thrombosis, and focal hemorrhagic infarction. Perforating vessels to the basal ganglia and pons are most often involved, producing movement dis-

orders or lacunar infarcts; involvement of branches of the middle cerebral artery may cause hemiparesis.

Clinical Findings

The usual illness begins with a prodrome of malaise, intermittent headache, and low-grade fever, followed within 2 to 3 weeks by protracted headache, vomiting, confusion, meningismus, and focal neurologic signs. The clinical spectrum is broad, ranging from chronic headache or subtle mental status changes to sudden, severe meningitis progressing to coma. Fever may be absent, and the peripheral white blood cell count is usually normal. Mild anemia is usual, and hyponatremia resulting from inappropriate antidiuretic hormone secretion is common. Evidence of concomitant extrameningeal tuberculosis is present in roughly three fourths of cases,[294] with miliary shadowing on the chest roentgenogram being most suggestive. In many cases, however, there are no clinical or historical clues to suggest tuberculosis.

The cornerstone of diagnosis is examination of the CSF. The cell count generally ranges from 0 to 1500/mm³, the protein is elevated, and the CSF glucose is characteristically low. A lymphocytic predominance is usual, although one quarter of cases have a polymorphonuclear pleocytosis, usually early in the course. Identifying bacilli often requires examination of large volumes of fluid from repeated lumbar punctures. In one study, stains of sediment revealed acid-fast bacilli in 37% of cases on initial examination, but in 90% when fluids from four large-volume lumbar punctures were examined.[294] Initial atypical findings such as neutrophilic pleocytosis, normal glucose, or even entirely normal CSF indices evolve to more typical mononuclear cell predominance with hypoglycorrhachia over time. Commercial kits for detecting *M. tuberculosis* in respiratory specimens by amplification technology (see Chapter 17) can also be used on CSF, though they are not currently approved for this purpose. Overall, the sensitivity of PCR in the CSF is low. The CSF is often culture negative for *M. tuberculosis*, but the CSF PCR has been reported to be positive in roughly 60% to 90% of CSF that eventually are culture positive.[295,296]

In patients with meningitis, CT or MRI may reveal rounded lesions presumed to be tuberculomas, basilar arachnoiditis, cerebral infarction, or hydrocephalus (Fig. 250-9).

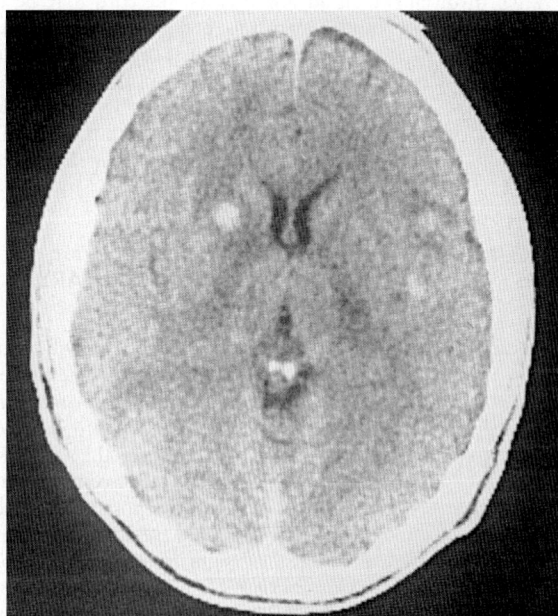

Figure 250-9 Multiple cerebral cortical densities on CT of a patient with tuberculous meningitis.

Prognosis is influenced by age, duration of symptoms, and neurologic deficits. Mortality is greatest in patients younger than age 5 (20%), older than age 50 (60%), or in whom illness has been present for more than 2 months (80%).[294] Patients without neurocognitive impairment, focal neurologic signs, or hydrocephalus at start of therapy are likely to recover, whereas approximately half of patients who are stuporous or have dense paraplegia or hemiplegia die, or recover with severe residual neurologic defects.[294] Concomitant HIV infection does not appear to alter the clinical and laboratory manifestations or the prognosis of tuberculous meningitis, except that CNS mass lesions are more likely.[297]

Treatment

In the presence of meningeal inflammation, both INH and PZA reach concentrations in the CSF equaling those in blood. RMP penetrates the blood-brain barrier less well but still adequately. In some cases PZA is given beyond the first 2 months of treatment because of its excellent CNS penetration, though its activity after 2 months of treatment is unclear. The RMP dose is sometimes increased due to its poor CNS penetration, particularly with concomitant administration of corticosteroids. Otherwise, the dosages are as for pulmonary tuberculosis.

Most authorities recommend adjunctive corticosteroids in tuberculosis meningitis, particularly stage 2 (objective neurologic findings) and stage 3 (stupor–coma) patients, beginning prednisone at 60 to 80 mg daily. This may be gradually reduced after 1 to 2 weeks and discontinued by 4 to 6 weeks, as guided by symptoms. Symptoms and CSF abnormalities may rebound transiently as steroids are tapered. Ventricular shunting may be beneficial if symptomatic hydrocephalus supervenes.[271]

TUBERCULOMAS

Intracranial tuberculomas are space-occupying lesions that may manifest with seizures. They are most frequently multiple, appearing on imaging studies as avascular masses with surrounding edema. Corticosteroids reduce edema and decrease symptoms, and chemotherapy prevents spread of infection in cases diagnosed at operation.

TUBERCULOUS SPINAL MENINGITIS

Infrequently, tuberculosis causes spinal meningitis with or without intracranial involvement. In advanced cases, the cord may be completely encased in a gelatinous exudate. An intramedullary tuberculoma or an extradural granulomatous mass can cause symptoms without meningeal involvement. Nerve root or cord compression causes pain, bladder or rectal sphincter weakness, hypesthesia, anesthesia, paresthesias in the distribution of a nerve root, or paralysis. Subarachnoid block may cause CSF protein concentrations to be extremely high, with or without cells.

TUBERCULOUS PLEURISY (SEROFIBRINOUS PLEURISY WITH EFFUSION)—EARLY POSTPRIMARY PLEURISY WITH EFFUSION

When infection occurs early in life, tuberculous pleurisy with effusion follows the primary infection within weeks or months. The pathogenesis is rupture of a large subpleural component of the primary infection and delivery of infectious, antigenic material into the pleural space, with inflammation and seeding of foci over the visceral and parietal pleura. In the past, this affected mostly adolescents and young adults, and rarely older adults. Immediate prognosis was excellent, with resolution of the effusion within several months in as many as 90% of cases. However, studies of soldiers during World War II (before chemotherapy) demonstrated that 65% relapsed with chronic organ tuberculosis within 5 years.[298] Early postprimary serofibrinous pleurisy with effusion identifies quantitatively large primary infections with a relatively poor long-term prognosis.

PLEURISY WITH EFFUSION COMPLICATING CHRONIC PULMONARY TUBERCULOSIS

In contrast to early studies,[298] an increased proportion of pleurisy with effusion since the early 1980s occurs in older individuals with chronic pulmonary tuberculosis, often with complicating illnesses such as cirrhosis or congestive heart failure to which the effusion is mistakenly attributed. In one study, one half of pleurisy cases occurred in the setting of established chronic pulmonary tuberculosis.[299]

PLEURISY WITH EFFUSION COMPLICATING MILIARY TUBERCULOSIS

Pleural effusions occur in 10% to 30% of cases of miliary tuberculosis.[284,286] These may be associated with other progressive extrapulmonary foci and involvement of other serous membranes. Cases with coexistent pleural (at times bilateral), peritoneal, and pericardial tuberculosis have been referred to as *tuberculous polyserositis*.

Clinical Features and Diagnosis of Tuberculous Pleurisy

The clinical presentation may be low grade and subtle or abrupt and severe, easily confused with acute bacterial pneumonia. Cough and pleuritic chest pain are usual, and fever may be high. The effusion is usually less than massive and almost always unilateral except when associated with miliary tuberculosis. The pleural fluid typically contains 500 to 2500 white blood cells/mm³, with more than 90% lymphocytes in two thirds of cases. However, 38% of cases in one series had predominantly neutrophils, and 15% had more than 90% neutrophils on the first tap.[300] Repeated taps demonstrate a shift to lymphocytic predominance. Mesothelial cells, characteristic of neoplastic effusions, are sparse or absent, eosinophils are rarely present, and less than 10% of effusions are serosanguineous. The pleural fluid protein usually exceeds 2.5 g/dL, glucose is usually moderately low compared with serum values but rarely less than 20 mg/dL, and the pH is almost always 7.3 or lower and may be as low as 7.0. Elevated pleural fluid adenosine deaminase levels have been suggested to be highly sensitive and specific for tuberculous pleuritis.[301] High pleural fluid adenosine deaminase levels with other conditions (e.g., neoplasia) limit its diagnostic utility in countries with a low prevalence of tuberculosis,[302] although levels with such conditions infrequently exceed the suggested cutoff for tuberculosis.[303,304] Bloody pleural fluid suggests either tuberculosis or malignancy. In the usual case of early postprimary pleurisy with effusion, the acid-fast stain of the fluid sediment is seldom positive, the culture is positive in 25% to 30%, pleural needle biopsy yields granulomas in 75%, and culture of a needle biopsy specimen may be positive even in the 25% of cases with nonspecific pleuritis on histologic examination. Cases complicating chronic pulmonary tuberculosis more often have positive pleural acid-fast smears (50%) and positive cultures (60%) but are less likely (25%) to demonstrate granulomas on pleural biopsy. Repeat pleural biopsy may be necessary to establish the diagnosis, and a small open pleural biopsy or thoracoscopy is diagnostic in virtually all cases. Smears of sputum or gastric fluid are rarely positive in early postprimary cases, and cultures are positive in 25% to 33%. In contrast, sputum smear is positive in 50% and the culture is positive in 60% of "reactivation" cases.[299] Tuberculosis is often not considered as the cause of a pleural effusion in an older person with complicating illnesses such as cirrhosis or congestive heart failure.[300] When pleural effusion complicates miliary tuberculosis, findings associated with the latter condition usually dominate the clinical picture.

Treatment of Tuberculous Pleurisy

Early postprimary pleural effusions spontaneously resolve in 2 to 4 months. Chemotherapy does not hasten resolution but prevents active disease elsewhere in the body, which will otherwise occur in 65% of cases.[298] Therapy is as described for pulmonary tuberculosis. Multiple thoracenteses are not necessary once the diagnosis is established and treatment initiated. A small minority heals with pleural fibrosis. Corticosteroid therapy hastens symptomatic improvement and fluid resorption, but no long-term benefit has been shown and therefore it is not recommended.

TUBERCULOUS EMPYEMA AND BRONCHOPLEURAL FISTULA

Tuberculous empyema occurs when a major cavity ruptures into the pleural space. This often catastrophic illness is usually associated with bronchopleural fistula formation and frank pus. Before antituberculous drugs were available, tuberculous empyema was almost always rapidly fatal. It virtually never occurs in patients being treated with chemotherapy.

TUBERCULOUS PERICARDITIS

Tuberculous pericarditis is most often caused by extension from a contiguous focus of infection, usually mediastinal or hilar nodes but also the lung, spine, or sternum. Less commonly, it occurs during miliary tuberculosis. It sometimes develops during the course of otherwise effective drug therapy. In the United States, tuberculous pericarditis is an uncommon complication of AIDS, but in two series from sub-Saharan Africa the vast majority of effusive pericarditis cases were tuberculous, and almost all patients were HIV-positive.[305,306]

Clinical Features and Diagnosis of Tuberculous Pericarditis

The onset may be abrupt, resembling acute idiopathic pericarditis, or insidious, resembling congestive heart failure. Symptoms of infection or cardiovascular compromise may be present. Individual cases may present with chronic constrictive pericarditis and may be mistaken for cirrhosis with ascites. As many as 39% also have a pleural effusion, providing a convenient source for diagnostic fluid and tissue.[307,308] Echocardiography demonstrates effusion when present and may reveal multiple loculations suggestive of tuberculosis.

Pericarditis with effusion is usually quickly diagnosed based on physical findings and radiologic examination, but establishing that it is tuberculous in nature is often difficult. The tuberculin test result may be negative and evidence of extrapericardial tuberculosis lacking. In areas of high endemicity, a presumptive diagnosis is often correctly made.[307,308] In the United States, however, many cases are initially misdiagnosed as idiopathic, uremic, or rheumatoid pericarditis.[309]

Pericardiocentesis (ideally performed in a cardiac catheterization laboratory) is indicated for hemodynamic compromise. However, because pericardiocentesis carries risk, and because 90% of acute pericarditis in the United States is idiopathic (presumed viral) and subsides spontaneously in 2 to 3 weeks, some authorities advise against early pericardiocentesis. If improvement has not occurred by that time, a subxiphoid pericardial window can be performed. This provides both fluid and tissue for diagnosis, although in some cases the biopsy demonstrates only nonspecific inflammation.[307,308] Tuberculous pericardial fluid demonstrates many of the characteristics of tuberculous pleural fluid, with acid-fast smears being rarely positive and cultures being positive in approximately 50% of cases. Bloody fluid suggests either tuberculosis or malignancy. The usefulness of adenosine deaminase determinations on pericardial fluid is not certain, but PCR for *M. tuberculosis* may be diagnostic, although sensitivity is low.

Treatment of Tuberculous Pericarditis

Antibiotic treatment is the same as for pulmonary tuberculosis. In a large study from South Africa, treatment with corticosteroids (60 mg/day for 4 weeks, 30 mg/day for 4 weeks, and 15 mg/day for 2 weeks) decreased mortality from 11% in controls to 4% in treated cases. Pericardiectomies were also less frequently necessary in patients given corticosteroids (30% in controls vs. 11% in steroid-treated patients). Adjunctive corticosteroids are therefore recommended for the treatment of tuberculous pericarditis. Surgical drainage via a subxiphoid pericardial window at the outset did not decrease either mortality or

the eventual need for pericardiectomy, although it provided diagnostic tissue and obviated the need for recurrent pericardiocenteses. However, 2% surgical mortality was associated with the procedure.[307,310]

When hemodynamic compromise persists for 6 to 8 weeks, pericardiectomy is usually indicated, and this should probably be performed earlier rather than later. Approximately two thirds of patients, however, do well without surgery.

SKELETAL TUBERCULOSIS—POTT'S DISEASE (TUBERCULOUS SPONDYLITIS)

One third of cases of skeletal tuberculosis involve the spine, as a result of past hematogenous foci, contiguous disease, or lymphatic spread from pleural disease. The earliest focus is the anterior superior or inferior angle of the vertebral body. This usually spreads to the intervertebral disk and adjacent vertebra, producing the classic roentgenographic picture of anterior wedging of two adjacent vertebral bodies with destruction of the intervening disk and the physical finding of a tender spine prominence or gibbus. The lower thoracic spine is involved most frequently, followed by the lumbar spine (Fig. 250-10).

In endemic countries, Pott's disease usually occurs in older children and young adults, but in developed countries it has become a disease of older persons.[311] Evidence of other foci of tuberculosis and systemic symptoms are often absent, early complaints may be back pain or stiffness with an initially normal roentgenogram, and diagnosis may be delayed until signs of advanced disease such as paralysis, deformity, or sinus formation develop. Bacilli are sparse, and smear and culture of pus or tissue are positive in only one half of cases. Histologic studies reveal granulomas with or without caseation in three fourths of cases.

Abscess and Sinus Formation

Paraspinal cold abscesses develop in 50% or more, in some cases appearing after treatment has been initiated, and in some cases visible only by CT or MRI. The pus, confined by tight ligamentous

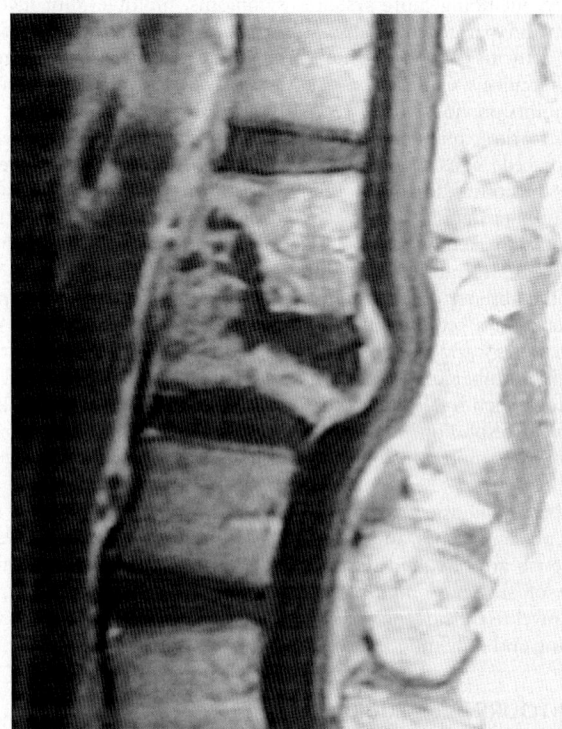

Figure 250-10 Magnetic resonance imaging study showing extensive destruction of L1 and L2 vertebral bodies and the intervening disk with posterior extension in a Pakistani man with Pott's disease.

investments, can dissect along tissue planes for long distances to present as a mass or a draining sinus in the supraclavicular space, above the posterior iliac crest in the Petit triangle, or in the groin, the buttock, or even the popliteal fossa. The abscess can spread infection to distant vertebral bodies, sometimes without affecting the intervening vertebrae. Epidural or psoas abscess can also complicate tuberculous spondylitis.

Pott's Paraplegia

In approximately half of cases, weakness or paralysis of the lower extremities is present or develops after treatment has begun, perhaps due to arachnoiditis and vasculitis.[311] Less frequently, it will be due to compression of the cord by an inflammatory mass or rarely pressure in the abscess producing ischemic changes in the subjacent cord. Inflammatory thrombosis of the anterior spinal artery can occur, and sudden cord compression may result from marked spinal instability.

Treatment

A 6- to 9-month course of therapy that contains INH and RMP is at least as effective as 18-month regimens that include INH plus PAS and ethambutol.[312,313] Adjunctive surgical debridement or resection of the involved bone plus bone grafting did not improve outcome compared to antituberculosis therapy alone. Thus, current recommendations are to treat spinal tuberculosis with a 6- to 9-month regimen that includes INH and RMP, with PZA and EMB for the first 2 months.[192] Surgical intervention may be necessary in patients who do not respond to therapy, those with cord compression with neurologic deficits, or spine instability.

PERIPHERAL OSTEOARTICULAR TUBERCULOSIS

Older reports described peripheral tuberculous arthritis as a chronic, slowly progressive monoarthritis in 90% of cases,[314] often without systemic symptoms or extraskeletal tuberculosis, and most frequently in the hip or knee. A history of trauma was common, followed weeks or months later by indolent progressive inflammation. More recent reports suggest a shift to an older population with a different clinical picture, including more systemic symptoms, multiple joint involvement, and periarticular abscess formation.[315] Tenosynovitis of the hand, arthritis of the wrist, and carpal tunnel syndrome can be caused by tuberculosis. Clinical confusion occurs when tuberculosis superinfects joints previously involved with other arthritides.

The earliest manifestation of tuberculous arthritis is pain, which may precede signs of inflammation and roentgenographic changes by weeks or months. Roentgenograms initially may show soft tissue swelling but later demonstrate osteopenia, periarticular bony destruction, periosteal thickening, and eventually destruction of cartilage and bone. Cold abscesses and draining sinuses often develop in chronic cases.

In the absence of coexistent extra-articular tuberculosis, diagnosis almost always requires biopsy. Histologic features compatible with tuberculosis warrant chemotherapy, although other chronic infections (fungi, nontuberculous mycobacteria) can cause identical clinical and histologic pictures. For early cases, prolonged chemotherapy results in complete resolution. Surgery is necessary only when serious joint instability requires fusion, and then only after chemotherapy has failed.

Tuberculous osteomyelitis can affect any bone, including the ribs, skull, phalanx, pelvis, and long bones.[316] Other causes of osteomyelitis of the rib are rare, and tuberculosis is the most common infectious cause of single or multiple osteomyelitic rib lesions. Tuberculous osteomyelitis outside the vertebral body presents as a cold abscess, with swelling and only modest erythema or pain.

GENITOURINARY TUBERCULOSIS—RENAL TUBERCULOSIS

Asymptomatic renal cortical foci may occur during all forms of tuberculosis. An autopsy study of pulmonary tuberculosis revealed unsuspected renal foci in 73% of cases, usually bilateral; 25% of miliary cases have positive urine cultures.[317] Cortical foci tend to be stable unless they penetrate to the medulla, where local factors favor accelerated infection. Most patients have evidence of concomitant extragenitourinary disease, usually pulmonary and most frequently inactive. In normal hosts, the interval between infection and active renal disease is usually years and sometimes decades. Local symptoms predominate, and advanced tissue destruction may occur long before the diagnosis is made.

The clinical features in two large series of cases are presented in Table 250-11.[318,319] Although sterile pyuria is typical of renal tuberculosis, positive cultures for routine bacterial pathogens may lead to misdiagnosis, sometimes for years. The intravenous pyelogram is usually abnormal. Early findings are nonspecific, but later changes may be more suggestive, including papillary necrosis, ureteral strictures, "pipe stem" changes, "corkscrewing," "beading," hydronephrosis, gross parenchymal cavitation, and autonephrectomy. Focal calcification is particularly suggestive. The clinical disease is usually unilateral, although microscopic changes are probably always bilateral. Culture of three morning urine specimens for mycobacteria establishes the diagnosis in 80% to 90% of cases. When a renal abnormality is present but urine cultures are negative, cytologic studies and culture of material obtained by fine-needle biopsy may be diagnostic. Ureteral cicatrization and obstruction may occur following otherwise effective chemotherapy, but surgery is rarely required.

Hypertension is not a feature of renal tuberculosis, and renal function is usually preserved. However, a rare condition called *tuberculous interstitial nephritis* may cause renal failure.[320] It is characterized by interstitial granulomas and normal-sized kidneys, usually in the presence of active extrarenal tuberculosis. Acid-fast bacilli have been seen but not cultured from renal biopsy specimens, and renal dysfunction responds to corticosteroid therapy but not antituberculous chemotherapy alone. It is unclear that tuberculous interstitial nephritis is actually caused by tuberculous infection.

MALE GENITAL TUBERCULOSIS

Eighty percent of male genital tuberculosis is associated with coexistent renal disease, and most advanced renal tuberculosis is associated with some male genital focus.[321] Spread of infection from renal foci involves the prostate, seminal vesicles, epididymis, and testis in that order. The usual clinical finding is a scrotal mass that may be tender or associated

TABLE 250-11 Clinical Features of Renal Tuberculosis in Two Series of Patients

Clinical Features	Simon et al.[318]	Christensen[319]
Number of patients	102	78
Primarily genitourinary symptoms	61%	71%
Back and flank pain	27%	10%
Dysuria, frequency	31%	34%
Constitutional symptoms	33%	14%
Abnormal urine, no symptoms	5%	20%
Abnormal urinalysis	66%	93%
Abnormal intravenous pyelogram	68%	93%
Tuberculin positive	88%	95%
Abnormal chest roentgenogram	75%	66%
Active pulmonary tuberculosis	38%	7%
Other old or active extrapulmonary disease	5%	20%
Urine culture positive		
For tuberculosis	80%	90%
For routine pathogens	45%	12%
Epididymitis, orchitis	19%	17%
Chronic prostatis	6%	6%

with a draining sinus. Stones may form with treatment of prostatic tuberculosis. Genital foci not associated with renal disease can be established by lymphohematogenous spread and usually present as a painful testicular or scrotal mass. Diagnosis may be suggested by the presence of epididymal or prostatic calcification, although the latter also occurs with nontuberculous chronic prostatitis. The diagnosis is usually established by surgery, and response to chemotherapy is excellent.

GENITOURINARY TUBERCULOSIS IN AIDS

In a study of 79 HIV-positive patients with tuberculosis, 77% had positive urine cultures, usually as an incidental finding. Only two had male genital involvement, none had symptoms of renal disease, and in only 4% was the genitourinary tract the only apparent site of tuberculosis.[283]

FEMALE GENITAL TUBERCULOSIS

Female genital tuberculosis begins with a hematogenous focus in the endosalpinx, from which it may spread to the endometrium (50%), ovaries (30%), cervix (10%), and vagina (1%).[322] In the cervix, a granulomatous ulcerating mass may resemble carcinoma. Common complaints are infertility or local symptoms consisting of menstrual disorders and abdominal pain. The clinical picture may suggest pelvic inflammatory disease that is unresponsive to therapy. Systemic symptoms are uncommon, and evidence of old tuberculosis need not be present. Pregnancies that occur in the presence of pelvic tuberculosis are often ectopic. Although cultures of menstrual blood or endometrial scrapings may be positive, the diagnosis is usually made by examination of tissue removed at operation. Response to chemotherapy is excellent, and surgery is needed only for residual large tuboovarian abscesses.

GASTROINTESTINAL TUBERCULOSIS

Before effective chemotherapy was available, 70% of patients with advanced pulmonary disease acquired gastrointestinal tuberculosis from swallowing infectious secretions, and usually developed diarrhea and abdominal pain. Although most cases at present are likely due to swallowed respiratory secretions, roentgenographic evidence of pulmonary tuberculosis is less frequent, the diagnosis being made unexpectedly by surgery or endoscopy.[323]

Any location from mouth to anus can be involved. Nonhealing ulcers of the tongue or oropharynx and nonhealing sockets after tooth extraction may be due to tuberculosis. Esophageal disease is most frequently caused by an adjacent caseous node, which leads to stricture with obstruction or tracheoesophageal fistula formation, and rarely fatal hematemesis from an aortoesophageal fistula. Stomach involvement may be ulcerative or hyperplastic and may cause gastric outlet obstruction. Isolated duodenal disease can produce symptoms of peptic ulcer or obstruction. Small bowel involvement may lead to perforation, obstruction, enteroenteric and enterocutaneous fistulas, massive hemorrhage, and severe malabsorption. Small bowel lesions are frequently multiple. The ileocecal area is the most typical site of enteric tuberculosis, producing pain, anorexia, diarrhea, obstruction, hemorrhage that may be severe, and often a palpable mass. Clinical, roentgenographic, endoscopic, and even operative findings may suggest carcinoma. A successful diagnosis is usually made by colonoscopy. In a study of 50 cases, ileocecal involvement, with or without involvement of other areas was found in 35 cases, isolated segmental colonic disease was found in 13 cases, and pancolitis was initially misdiagnosed as ulcerative colitis in 2 cases. Evidence of pulmonary tuberculosis was present in only 18 cases.[324] The response of gastrointestinal tuberculosis to chemotherapy is excellent. Once the diagnosis is established, surgery should be deferred if possible until the results of chemotherapy have been assessed.

Pancreatic tuberculosis may manifest as an abscess or as a mass involving local nodes and resembling carcinoma. The biliary tract may be obstructed by tuberculous nodes, and tuberculous ascending cholangitis has been described. Tuberculosis is a frequent cause of granulomatous hepatitis. This is usually asymptomatic but may be associated with an elevated alkaline phosphatase level that is out of proportion to bilirubin levels with normal transaminase levels. Very rarely, tuberculous granulomatous hepatitis causes jaundice without evidence of extrahepatic tuberculosis. This is called *primary tuberculosis of the liver. Focal hepatic tuberculosis* describes single or multiple tuberculous abscesses. These appear to occur most frequently in racial groups with little natural immunity to tuberculosis and in children.[325]

GASTROINTESTINAL TUBERCULOSIS IN AIDS

Bowel involvement is not a common feature of extrapulmonary tuberculosis in AIDS patients. One series reported bowel fistulas in less than 4% of such cases,[283] another reported CT evidence of gastrointestinal abnormalities in 4 of 23 cases,[326] and a third study noted positive stool cultures for *M. tuberculosis* in 4 of 10 cases.[327] Tuberculous visceral abscesses, including hepatic, splenic, and pancreatic, may occur in AIDS patients. Pain and fever are usually present. Diagnosis is often made by CT or ultrasonographically guided drainage procedures. Chemotherapy alone has not been effective in all cases.[293]

TUBERCULOUS PERITONITIS

Tuberculous peritonitis results either from spread of adjacent tuberculous disease such as an abdominal lymph node, intestinal focus, or fallopian tube, or during miliary tuberculosis. In a summary of 11 series, evidence of associated pleuropulmonary tuberculosis was present in 25% to 83% of cases and the tuberculin test was positive in 30% to 100% of cases.[328] Pleural effusion is the most frequent associated finding, but evidence of tuberculosis in other sites is often present. AIDS patients do not have an increased frequency of peritonitis.[283]

The clinical picture has been divided into *plastic* and *serous* types. The less common plastic type is characterized by tender abdominal masses and a "doughy abdomen." Serous effusions present as ascites with or without signs of peritonitis. Symptoms of fever, abdominal pain, and weight loss are common.[328] The onset may be insidious, although acute presentations resembling bacterial peritonitis also occur. In the past, diagnosis was often made at surgery for a mass or an acute abdomen. Tuberculous peritonitis often goes undiagnosed in patients with concomitant cirrhosis with ascites.[329] Of 20 patients with both conditions, the diagnosis of tuberculous peritonitis was suspected ante mortem in only 11. Tuberculous peritonitis has been reported in peritoneal dialysis patients with the clinical picture of bacterial peritonitis unresponsive to routine antibiotics.[330]

The peritoneal fluid is exudative, usually containing 500 to 2000 cells. Lymphocytes typically predominate, although in some cases neutrophils are more abundant early in the process. Acid-fast smear of peritoneal fluid is seldom positive, and culture is positive in only 25% of cases. An elevated adenosine deaminase level in ascitic fluid has been reported to have high sensitivity and specificity,[331] although among 140 patients in India the positive predictive value was only 25%.[332]

Analysis of peritoneal fluid by PCR may also be diagnostic, although sensitivity is low. In the absence of other foci of tuberculosis, peritoneal tissue must often be obtained to make the diagnosis. Histologic examination of peritoneal biopsy specimens obtained by a Cope needle were positive in 64% of cases and those obtained by peritoneoscopy in 85% in one series.[333] Fatal hemorrhages after both Cope needle biopsy and peritoneoscopy have been recorded.[328]

Treatment is the same as for pulmonary tuberculosis. There is some evidence that adjunctive corticosteroids decrease the likelihood of late intestinal obstruction,[333] but pending definitive studies, the routine use of adjunctive corticosteroids cannot be recommended.[334]

TUBERCULOUS LYMPHADENITIS (SCROFULA)— PERIPHERAL NODES

Lymphadenitis is the most frequent form of extrapulmonary tuberculosis. In HIV-negative persons, it is usually unilateral and cervical in location.[335] The most common site is along the upper border of the sternocleidomastoid muscle, where it presents as a painless, red firm mass. It is seen most frequently in young adult females of minority races, although it can affect any age or race. Children often have an ongoing primary infection, but in other age groups evidence of extranodal tuberculosis and systemic symptoms are usually absent. Lymphadenopathy outside the cervical and supraclavicular area indicates more serious tuberculosis, usually with systemic symptoms. The tuberculin test result is almost always positive. Fine-needle aspiration demonstrates cytologic evidence of granuloma, but smears or cultures are usually negative.[336] Biopsy with culture is often required for diagnosis, because nodes with a nonspecific histologic appearance have been positive for *M. tuberculosis* on culture, and material with typical histologic features may be due to other mycobacteria or fungi. Complete excision of involved nodes with no drain left in place is recommended to diminish the possibility of postoperative fistula formation. Untoward events such as node enlargement with pain, suppuration, sinus formation, and appearance of new nodes occur in 25% to 30% of cases, both during and after chemotherapy, and do not indicate failure of drug treatment. These likely represent reactions to retained tuberculous antigens rather than uncontrolled infection; they usually subside spontaneously, and short courses of corticosteroids may be beneficial when the problem persists.[337]

Conversely, in individuals with AIDS, peripheral tuberculous lymphadenitis is almost always multifocal and associated with major systemic symptoms such as fever, weight loss, and evidence of tuberculosis in the lungs (parenchyma, nodes, or pleura) or elsewhere (Fig. 250-11).[336] In one series from New York City, tuberculosis caused 57% of generalized lymphadenopathy in HIV-positive intravenous drug users.[338] In contrast to non-HIV-infected persons, material removed by fine-needle aspiration is positive on acid-fast stain in the great

majority of cases—as frequently as it is by culture. However, both cytologic and histologic findings are less specific than in HIV-negative persons.[339]

MEDIASTINAL TUBERCULOUS LYMPHADENOPATHY

Mediastinal adenopathy during primary infection is often visible roentgenologically, especially in children. In minority races, mediastinal adenopathy resulting from tuberculosis may also be seen in young adults, and cases in very old persons have been reported.[340] Associated systemic symptoms may or may not be present, causing confusion with other mediastinal masses such as histoplasmosis, lymphoma, and carcinoma. The finding of low-density areas in the nodes on CT suggests tuberculosis, but diagnosis usually requires mediastinoscopy. In HIV-infected persons with tuberculosis, in contrast, mediastinal lymphadenopathy is frequent. Multiple nodes are usually involved, coalescing into large mediastinal masses with low-density centers, peripheral contrast enhancement, and no calcification.[341,342]

FIBROSING MEDIASTINITIS

Tuberculosis can cause fibrosing mediastinitis, although less commonly than histoplasmosis. Patients present with dyspnea on exertion resulting from compression of pulmonary veins and arteries or, less commonly, superior vena cava syndrome. Hilar adenopathy or active pulmonary disease is rarely found. A perfusion lung scan helps define the extent of pulmonary vascular compression, but thoracotomy is required for diagnosis. Mediastinoscopy is either contraindicated because of superior vena cava syndrome or unsuccessful because of fibrosis.

MESENTERIC TUBERCULOUS LYMPHADENITIS

In HIV-negative persons, isolated symptomatic mesenteric lymphadenitis without bowel disease or peritonitis is rare. It may cause abdominal pain, fever, a palpable mass, or symptoms of partial small bowel obstruction. In AIDS patients with tuberculosis, abdominal lymphadenopathy is common and may be massive.[342,343] Involvement is more often intra-abdominal than retroperitoneal, and occasionally obstruction of the biliary tract, ureters, or bowel is observed. As with thoracic disease, the nodes often are low density or have low-density centers and peripheral enhancement. Other abnormalities on CT may include abscesses in the liver, spleen, pancreas, or kidney; local ileal thickening; extraluminal bowel gas indicating fistula formation; and ascites.

CUTANEOUS TUBERCULOSIS

In the past, a number of cutaneous conditions were associated with tuberculosis elsewhere in the body, although *M. tuberculosis* could not be identified in the lesions. These have been considered allergic reactions to the infection and termed *tuberculids*. They include erythema induratum of Bazin, papulonecrotic tuberculids, and others. This association has been questioned, and some have attributed tuberculids to other processes, such as sarcoidosis.[344] *M. tuberculosis* DNA has been detected in erythema induratum skin lesions by PCR.[345] Erythema nodosum has been attributed to primary tuberculosis, although organisms cannot be cultured from the lesions.

The pathogenesis of cutaneous involvement in tuberculosis is varied. Skin involvement may result from exogenous inoculation (which in the previously nonsensitized host is associated with regional lymphadenitis), spread from an adjacent focus to the overlying skin (as from lymphadenitis, osteomyelitis, or epididymitis), and hematogenous spread from a distant focus or as a part of the generalized hematogenous dissemination. This last is seen in patients with AIDS and tuberculous bacteremia.[346] The clinical picture of all cutaneous mycobacterial infections, including tuberculosis, is highly variable, and any unexplained skin lesion, especially if it has nodular or ulcer-

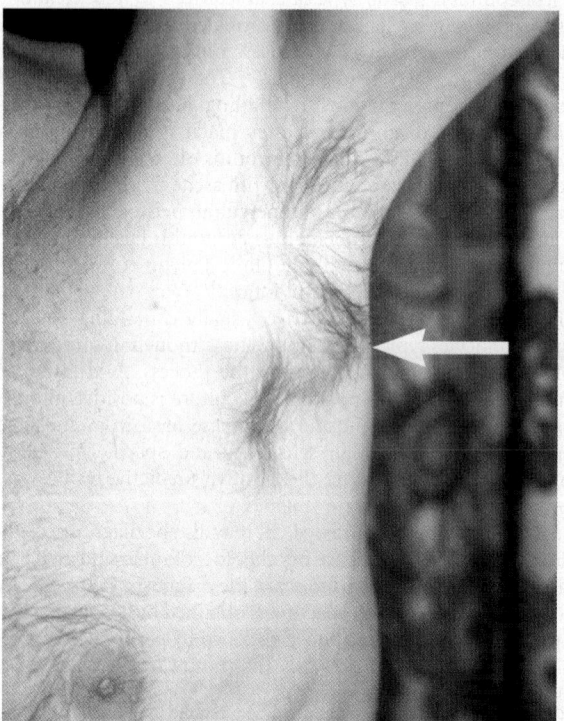

Figure 250-11 Axillary lymphadenitis caused by *Mycobacterium tuberculosis* in a patient with acquired immunodeficiency syndrome.

ative components, may be due to tuberculosis, particularly in AIDS patients.

TUBERCULOUS LARYNGITIS

In the prechemotherapy era, laryngeal tuberculosis occurred in more than a third of patients dying of pulmonary tuberculosis, often associated with painful ulcers of the epiglottis, pharynx, tonsils, and mouth, as well as middle ear involvement. Laryngeal disease was highly infectious and often caused terminal widespread bronchogenic dissemination throughout the lungs. At present, however, more than one half of laryngeal tuberculosis cases are due to hematogenous seeding. Such cases are still highly contagious. Lesions vary from erythema to ulceration and exophytic masses resembling carcinoma.[347] Symptoms include cough, wheezing, hemoptysis, dysphagia, odynophagia, and otalgia.

TUBERCULOUS OTITIS

Tuberculous otitis media is rare and frequently misdiagnosed. Half of the cases have no other evidence of present or past tuberculosis. The classic clinical picture is painless otorrhea with multiple tym-

panic perforations, exuberant granulation tissue, early severe hearing loss, and mastoid bone necrosis. The diagnosis has been missed for years by excellent otolaryngologists, even when tissue was available. Tuberculous otitis may be complicated by facial nerve paralysis. Response to drug therapy is excellent, and surgery is usually not required.[348]

MISCELLANEOUS CONDITIONS

Tuberculosis of the aorta with or without aneurysm formation can be caused by spread from contiguous diseased nodes, pericarditis, spondylitis, paravertebral abscesses, or empyema. Extensive hematogenous dissemination or aortic rupture may occur. Tuberculosis produces various ocular syndromes, including choroidal tubercles, uveitis, iritis, and episcleritis. Tuberculosis may also involve the breast, producing abscesses, sclerosing lesions resembling carcinoma, and multiple nodules. Destructive nasal lesions resembling Wegener's granulomatosis both clinically and histologically have been caused by tuberculosis.[349] Tuberculosis of the adrenal glands may cause adrenal enlargement with or without calcification, as may histoplasmosis, but granulomatous adrenal tuberculosis may cause Addison's disease without either calcification or adrenal enlargement.[350]

REFERENCES

1. Trends in tuberculosis—United States, 2007. *MMWR Morb Mortal Wkly Rep.* 2008;57:281-285.
2. Palella FJ, Delaney KM, Moorman AC, et al. Declining morbidity and mortality among patients with advanced human immunodeficiency virus infection. *N Engl J Med.* 1998;338:853-860.
3. Iseman MD. Extensively drug-resistant Mycobacterium tuberculosis: Charles Darwin would understand. *Clin Infect Dis.* 2007;45:1415-1416.
4. Gandhi NR, Moll A, Sturm AW, et al. Extensively drug-resistant tuberculosis as a cause of death in patients co-infected with tuberculosis and HIV in a rural area of South Africa. *Lancet.* 2006;368:1575-1580.
5. Pillay M, Sturm AW. Evolution of the extensively drug-resistant F15/LAM4/KZN strain of *Mycobacterium tuberculosis* in Kwa-Zulu-Natal, South Africa. *Clin Infect Dis.* 2007;45:1409-1414.
6. Dukes Hamilton C, Sterling TR, Blumberg HM, et al. Extensively drug-resistant tuberculosis: are we learning from history or repeating it? *Clin Infect Dis.* 2007;45:338-342.
7. Ernst JD, Trevejo-Nunez G, Banaiee N. Genomics and the evolution, pathogenesis, and diagnosis of tuberculosis. *J Clin Invest.* 2007;117:1738-1745.
8. Evans JT, Smith EG, Banerjee A, et al. Cluster of human tuberculosis caused by *Mycobacterium bovis*: evidence for person-to-person transmission in the UK. *Lancet.* 2007;369:1270-1276.
9. Oh P, Granich R, Scott J, et al. Human exposure following *Mycobacterium tuberculosis* infection of multiple animal species in a metropolitan zoo. *Emerg Infect Dis.* 2002;8:1290-1293.
10. Gutierrez MC, Brisse S, Brosch R, et al. Ancient origin and gene mosaicism of the progenitor of *Mycobacterium tuberculosis*. *PLoS Pathog.* 2005;1:e5.
11. Cole ST, Brosch R, Parkhill J, et al. Deciphering the biology of *Mycobacterium tuberculosis* from the complete genome sequence. *Nature.* 1998;393:537-544.
12. Broad Institute. *Mycobacterium tuberculosis* Database. Broad Institute. Available at http://www.broad.mit.edu/annotation/genome/Mycobacterium_tuberculosis_spp/MultiHome.html. Accessed November 2008.
13. Garnier T, Eiglmeier K, Camus JC, et al. The complete genome sequence of *Mycobacterium bovis*. *Proc Natl Acad Sci U S A* 2003;100:7877-7882.
14. Apers L, Mutsvangwa J, Magwenzi J, et al. A comparison of direct microscopy, the concentration method and the Mycobacteria Growth Indicator Tube for the examination of sputum for acid-fast bacilli. *Int J Tuberc Lung Dis.* 2003;7:376-381.
15. Mase SR, Ramsay A, Ng V, et al. Yield of serial sputum specimen examinations in the diagnosis of pulmonary tuberculosis: a systematic review. *Int J Tuberc Lung Dis.* 2007;11:485-495.
16. Bonnet M, Ramsay A, Githui W, et al. Bleach sedimentation: an opportunity to optimize smear microscopy for tuberculosis diagnosis in settings of high prevalence of HIV. *Clin Infect Dis.* 2008;46:1710-1716.
17. Steingart KR, Henry M, Ng V, et al. Fluorescence versus conventional sputum smear microscopy for tuberculosis: a systematic review. *Lancet Infect Dis.* 2006;6:570-581.
18. Perkins MD, Cunningham J. Facing the crisis: improving the diagnosis of tuberculosis in the HIV era. *J Infect Dis.* 2007;196(Suppl 1):S15-S27.

19. Hale YM, Pfyffer GE, Salfinger M. Laboratory diagnosis of mycobacterial infections: new tools and lessons learned. *Clin Infect Dis.* 2001;33:834-846.
20. Hanna BA, Ebrahimzadeh A, Elliott LB, et al. Multicenter evaluation of the BACTEC MGIT 960 system for recovery of mycobacteria. *J Clin Microbiol.* 1999;37:748-752.
21. Leitritz L, Schubert S, Bucherl B, et al. Evaluation of BACTEC MGIT 960 and BACTEC 460TB systems for recovery of mycobacteria from clinical specimens of a university hospital with low incidence of tuberculosis. *J Clin Microbiol.* 2001;39:3764-3767.
22. Moore DA, Evans CA, Gilman RH, et al. Microscopic-observation drug-susceptibility assay for the diagnosis of TB. *N Engl J Med.* 2006;355:1539-1550.
23. Barnes PF. Rapid diagnostic tests for tuberculosis—Progress but no gold standard. *Am J Respir Crit Care Med.* 1997; 155:1497-1498.
24. Centers for Disease Control and Prevention. Nucleic acid amplification tests for tuberculosis. *MMWR Morb Mortal Wkly Rep.* 1996;45:951.
25. Ling DI, Flores LL, Riley LW, et al. Commercial nucleic-acid amplification tests for diagnosis of pulmonary tuberculosis in respiratory specimens: meta-analysis and meta-regression. *PLoS ONE.* 2008;3:e1536.
26. Catanzaro A, Perry S, Clarridge JE, et al. The role of clinical suspicion in evaluating a new diagnostic test for active tuberculosis: results of a multicenter prospective trial. *JAMA.* 2000;283:639-645.
27. Pfyffer GE, Kissling P, Jahn EM, et al. Diagnostic performance of amplified *Mycobacterium tuberculosis* direct test with cerebrospinal fluid, other nonrespiratory, and respiratory specimens. *J Clin Microbiol.*1996;34:834-841.
28. O'Sullivan CE, Miller DR, Schneider PS, et al. Evaluation of Gen-Probe amplified *Mycobacterium tuberculosis* direct test by using respiratory and nonrespiratory specimens in a tertiary care center laboratory. *J Clin Microbiol.* 2002;40:1723-1727.
29. Piersimoni C, Scarparo C, Piccoli P, et al. Performance assessment of two commercial amplification assays for direct detection of *Mycobacterium tuberculosis* complex from respiratory and extrapulmonary specimens. *J Clin Microbiol.* 2002;40:4138-4142.
30. Noordhoek GT, vanEmbden JDA, Kolk AHJ. Reliability of nucleic acid amplification for detection of *Mycobacterium tuberculosis*: an international collaborative quality control study among 30 laboratories. *J Clin Microbiol.* 1996;34:2522-2525.
31. Diagnostic standards and classification of tuberculosis in adults and children. *Am J Respir Crit Care Med.* 2000;161:1376-1395.
32. Parsons LM, Brosch R, Cole ST, et al. Rapid and simple approach for identification of *Mycobacterium tuberculosis* complex isolates by PCR-based genomic deletion analysis. *J Clin Microbiol.* 2002;40:2339-2345.
33. National TB Controllers Association/CDC Advisory Group on Tuberculosis Genotyping. Guide to the Application of Genotyping to Tuberculosis Prevention and Control. US Department of Health and Human Services, CDC, Atlanta, Ga., 2004.
34. Tortoli E, Benedetti M, Fontanelli A, et al. Evaluation of automated BACTEC MGIT 960 system for testing susceptibility of *Mycobacterium tuberculosis* to four major antituberculous drugs:

comparison with the radiometric BACTEC 460TB method and the agar plate method of proportion. *J Clin Microbiol.* 2002; 40:607-610.
35. Bemer P, Palicova F, Rusch-Gerdes S, et al. Multicenter evaluation of fully automated BACTEC Mycobacteria Growth Indicator Tube 960 system for susceptibility testing of *Mycobacterium tuberculosis*. *J Clin Microbiol.* 2002;40:150-154.
36. Telenti A, Honore N, Bernasconi C, et al. Genotypic assessment of isoniazid and rifampin resistance in *Mycobacterium tuberculosis*: a blind study at reference laboratory level. *J Clin Microbiol.* 1997;35:719-723.
37. Williams DL, Spring L, Gillis TP, et al. Evaluation of a polymerase chain reaction–based universal heteroduplex generator assay for direct detection of rifampin susceptibility of *Mycobacterium tuberculosis* from sputum specimens. *Clin Infect Dis.* 1998;26:446-450.
38. Kim B-J, Kim S-Y, Park B-H, et al. Mutations in the rpoB gene of *Mycobacterium tuberculosis* that interfere with PCR-single-strand conformation polymorphism analysis for rifampin susceptibility testing. *J Clin Microbiol.* 1997;35:492-494.
39. Nachamkin I, Kang C, Weinstein MP. Detection of resistance to isoniazid, rifampin, and streptomycin in clinical isolates of *Mycobacterium tuberculosis* by molecular methods. *Clin Infect Dis.* 1997;24:894-900.
40. Mdluli K, Slayden RA, Zhu Y, et al. Inhibition of a *Mycobacterium tuberculosis* β-ketoacyl ACP synthetase by isoniazid. *Science.* 1998;280:1607-1616.
41. Drobniewski FA, Wilson SM. The rapid diagnosis of isoniazid and rifampicin resistance in *Mycobacterium tuberculosis*: a molecular story. *J Med Microbiol.* 1998;47:189-196.
42. Morgan MS, Kalantri S, Flores L, et al. A commercial line probe assay for the rapid detection of rifampicin resistance in *Mycobacterium tuberculosis*: a systematic review and meta-analysis. *BMC Infect Dis.* 2005;5:62.
43. Barnard M, Albert H, Coetzee G, et al. Rapid molecular screening for multidrug-resistant tuberculosis in a high-volume public health laboratory in South Africa. *Am J Respir Crit Care Med.* 2008;177:787-792.
44. World Health Organization. Molecular Line Probe Assays for Rapid Screening of Patients at Risk of Multidrug-Resistant Tuberculosis (MDR-TB). Available at <http://www.who.int/tb/features_archive/mdrtb_rapid_tests/en/index.html>; Accessed November 2008.
45. World Health Organization. Global Tuberculosis Database. Available at <http://www.who.int/research/en/>; Accessed November 2008.
46. *World Health Organization Report on the Tuberculosis Epidemic.* Geneva: World Health Organization; 1997.
47. Styblo K. Recent advances in epidemiological research in tuberculosis. *Adv Tuberc Res.* 1980;20:1-63.
48. Centers for Disease Control and Prevention. Tuberculosis morbidity—United States, 1997. *MMWR Morb Mortal Wkly Rep.* 1998;47:253-257.
49. American Thoracic Society. Control of tuberculosis in the United States. *Am Rev Respir Dis.* 1992;146:1623-1633.
50. Centers for Disease Control and Prevention. Tuberculosis morbidity among U.S.-born and foreign-born populations—United States, 2000. *MMWR Morb Mortal Wkly Rep.* 2002;51:101-104.

51. Cain KP, Haley CA, Armstrong LR, et al. Tuberculosis among foreign-born persons in the United States: achieving tuberculosis elimination. *Am J Respir Crit Care Med.* 2007;175:75-79.
52. Binkin NJ, Zuber PLF, Wells CD, et al. Overseas screening for tuberculosis in immigrants and refugees to the United States: current status. *Clin Infect Dis.* 1996; 23:1226-1232.
53. Zuber PLF, McKenna MT, Binkin NJ, et al. Long-term risk of tuberculosis among foreign-born persons in the United States. *JAMA.* 1997;278:304-307.
54. Cain KP, Benoit SR, Winston CA, et al. Tuberculosis among foreign-born persons in the United States. *JAMA.* 2008;300: 405-412.
55. Jereb JA, Kelly GD, Dooley SW, et al. Tuberculosis morbidity in the United States: final data, 1990. *MMWR Morb Mortal Wkly Rep.* 1991;40:23-27.
56. Havlir DV, Barnes PF. Tuberculosis in patients with human immunodeficiency virus infection. *N Engl J Med.* 1999; 340:367-373.
57. Barnes PF, Bloch AB, Davidson PT, et al. Tuberculosis in patients with human immunodeficiency virus infection. *N Engl J Med.* 1991;100:191-200.
58. Centers for Disease Control. 1993 Revised certification system for HIV infection and expanded surveillance case definition for AIDS among adolescents and adults. *MMWR Morb Mortal Wkly Rep.* 1992;41:1-19.
59. Valway SE, Sanchez MPC, Shinnick TK, et al. An outbreak involving extensive transmission of a virulent strain of *Mycobacterium tuberculosis. N Engl J Med.* 1998;338:633-639.
60. Mishu Allos B, Gensheimer KF, Bloch AB, et al. Management of an outbreak of tuberculosis in a small community. *Ann Intern Med.* 1996;125:114-117.
61. Cross ER, Hyams KC. Tuberculin skin testing in US Navy and Marine Corps personnel and recruits, 1980-1986. *Am J Public Health.* 1990;80:435-438.
62. Trump DH, Hyams KC, Cross ER, et al. Tuberculosis infection among young adults entering the US Navy in 1990. *Arch Intern Med.* 1993;153:211-216.
63. Smith B, Ryan MA, Gray GC, et al. Tuberculosis infection among young adults enlisting in the United States Navy. *Int J Epidemiol.* 2002;31:934-939.
64. Khan K, Wang J, Hu W, et al. Tuberculosis infection in the United States: national trends over three decades. *Am J Respir Crit Care Med.* 2008;177:455-460.
65. Patel KR. Pulmonary tuberculosis in residents of lodging houses, night shelters and common hostels in Glasgow: A 5-year prospective study. *Br J Dis Chest.* 1985;79:60-66.
66. Nardell E, McInnis B, Thomas B, et al. Exogenous reinfection with tuberculosis in a shelter for the homeless. *N Engl J Med.* 1986;315:1570-1575.
67. Stead WW, Lofgren JP, Warren E, et al. Tuberculosis as an endemic and nosocomial infection among the elderly in nursing homes. *N Engl J Med.* 1985;312:1483-1487.
68. Kim SJ, Hong YP, Lew WJ, et al. Incidence of pulmonary tuberculosis among diabetics. *Tuber Lung Dis.* 1995;76:529-533.
69. Naidoo S, Jinabhai CC. TB in health care workers in KwaZulu-Natal, South Africa. *Int J Tuberc Lung Dis.* 2006;10:676-682.
70. Andrew OT, Schoenfeld PY, Hopewell PC, et al. Tuberculosis in patients with end-stage renal disease. *Am J Med.* 1980; 68:59-65.
71. Cuss FM, Carmichael DJ, Linington A, et al. Tuberculosis in renal failure: a high incidence in patients born in the third world. *Clin Nephrol.* 1986;25:129-133.
72. Louie E, Rice LB, Holzm RS. Tuberculosis in non-Haitian patients with acquired immunodeficiency syndrome. *Chest.* 1986;90:542-545.
73. Pitchenik AE, Cole C, Russell BW, et al. Tuberculosis, atypical mycobacteriosis, and the acquired immunodeficiency syndrome among Haitian and non-Haitian patients in South Florida. *Ann Intern Med.* 1984;101:641-645.
74. World Health Organization. A World Free of TB. Available at <http://www.who.int/tb/en/>; Accessed November 2008.
75. Wang L, Liu J, Chin DP. Progress in tuberculosis control and the evolving public-health system in China. *Lancet.* 2007; 369:691-696.
76. Sharma SK, Liu JJ. Progress of DOTS in global tuberculosis control. *Lancet.* 2006;367:951-952.
77. Khatri GR, Frieden TR. Controlling tuberculosis in India. *N Engl J Med.* 2002;347:1420-1425.
78. UNAIDS. 2008 Report on the Global AIDS Epidemic. United Nations Programme on HIV/AIDS. UNAIDS, Geneva, Switzerland. Available at <http://www.unaids.org/en/>; Accessed November 2008.
79. From the Centers for Disease Control and Prevention: Morbidity and Mortality Weekly Report. Notice to readers: revised definition of extensively drug-resistant tuberculosis. *JAMA.* 2006;296:2792.
80. Pablos-Mendez A, Raviglione MC, Laszlo A, et al. Global surveillance for antituberculosis-drug resistance, 1994-1997. World Health Organization—International Union against Tuberculosis and Lung Disease Working Group on Anti-Tuberculosis Drug Resistance Surveillance. *N Engl J Med.* 1998;338: 1641-1649.
81. Espinal MA, Laszlo A, Simonsen L, et al. Global trends in resistance to antituberculosis drugs. World Health Organization—International Union against Tuberculosis and Lung Disease Working Group on Anti-Tuberculosis Drug Resistance Surveillance. *N Engl J Med.* 2001;344:1294-1303.
82. Aziz MA, Wright A, Laszlo A, et al. Epidemiology of antituberculosis drug resistance (the Global Project on Anti-tuberculosis Drug Resistance Surveillance): an updated analysis. *Lancet.* 2006;368:2142-2154.
83. World Health Organization. Anti-Tuberculosis Drug Resistance in the World. Report No. 4. Available at http://www.who.int/tb/publications/2008/drs_report4_26feb08.pdf. Accessed November 2008.
84. Espinal MA, Laszlo A, Simonsen L, et al. Global trends in resistance to antituberculosis drugs. World Health Organization—International Union against Tuberculosis and Lung Disease Working Group on Anti-Tuberculosis Drug Resistance Surveillance. *N Engl J Med.* 2001;344:1294-1303.
85. Ben-Dov I, Mason G. Drug-resistant tuberculosis in a southern California hospital: trends from 1969 to 1984. *Am Rev Respir Dis.* 1987;135:1307-1310.
86. Pablos-Mendez A, Raviglione MC, Battan R, et al. Drug resistant tuberculosis among the homeless in New York City. *NY State J Med.* 1990;90:351-355.
87. Frieden TR, Sterling T, Pablos-Mendez A, et al. The emergence of drug resistant tuberculosis in New York City. *N Engl J Med.* 1993;328:521-526.
88. Frieden TR, Fujiwara PI, Washko RM, et al. Tuberculosis in New York City—turning the tide. *N Engl J Med.* 1995;333:229-233.
89. Munsiff SS, Li J, Cook SV, et al. Trends in drug-resistant *Mycobacterium tuberculosis* in New York City, 1991-2003. *Clin Infect Dis.* 2006;42:1702-1710.
90. Masjedi MR, Farnia P, Sorooch S, et al. Extensively drug-resistant tuberculosis: 2 years of surveillance in Iran. *Clin Infect Dis.* 2006;43:841-847.
91. Frampton MW. An outbreak of tuberculosis among hospital personnel caring for a patient with a skin ulcer. *Ann Intern Med.* 1992;117:312-313.
92. Templeton GL, Illing LA, Young L, et al. The risk for transmission of *Mycobacterium tuberculosis* at the bedside and during autopsy. *Ann Intern Med.* 1995;122:922-925.
93. Stead WW. Tuberculosis among elderly persons: an outbreak in a nursing home. *Ann Intern Med.* 1981;94:606-610.
94. Klausner JD, Ryder RW, Baende E, et al. *Mycobacterium tuberculosis* in household contacts of human immunodeficiency virus type 1-seropositive patients with active pulmonary tuberculosis in Kinshasa, Zaire. *J Infect Dis.* 1993;168:106-111.
95. Cruciani M, Malena M, Bosco O, et al. The impact of human immunodeficiency virus type 1 on infectiousness of tuberculosis: a meta-analysis. *Clin Infect Dis.* 2001;33:1922-1930.
96. Cauthen GM, Dooley SW, Onorato IM, et al. Transmission of *Mycobacterium tuberculosis* from tuberculosis patients with HIV infection or AIDS. *Am J Epidemiol.* 1996;144:69-77.
97. Centers for Disease Control and Prevention. Guidelines for preventing the transmission of *Mycobacterium tuberculosis* in health-care facilities, 1994. *MMWR Morb Mortal Wkly Rep.* 1994;43:1-132.
98. Horsburgh CR Jr. Priorities for the treatment of latent tuberculosis infection in the United States. *N Engl J Med.* 2004;350:2060-2067.
99. Bates JH, Stead WW. The history of tuberculosis as a global epidemic. *Med Clin North Am.* 1993;77:1205-1217.
100. Selwyn PA, Hartel D, Lewis VA, et al. A prospective study of the risk of tuberculosis among intravenous drug users with human immunodeficiency virus infection. *N Engl J Med.* 1989; 320:545-555.
101. Daley CL, Small PM, Schecter GF. An outbreak of tuberculosis with accelerated progression among persons infected with the human immunodeficiency virus. *N Engl J Med.* 1992;36:231-235.
102. Di Perri G, Danzi MC, DeChecchi G. Nosocomial epidemic of active tuberculosis among HIV-infected patients. *Lancet.* 1989;2:1502-1504.
103. Pearson ML, Jereb JA, Frieden TR. Nosocomial transmission of multidrug-resistant *Mycobacterium tuberculosis*: a risk to patients and healthcare workers. *Ann Intern Med.* 1992;117: 191-196.
104. Fischl MA, Uttamchandani RB, Daikos GL, et al. An outbreak of tuberculosis caused by multiple-drug resistant tubercle bacilli among patients with HIV infection. *Ann Intern Med.* 1992;11:177-183.
105. Edlin BR, Tokars JI, Grieco MH, et al. An outbreak of multidrug-resistant tuberculosis among hospitalized patients with the acquired immunodeficiency syndrome. *N Engl J Med.* 1992;326:1514-1521.
106. Kramer F, Modilevsky T, Waliany AR, et al. Delayed diagnosis of tuberculosis in patients with human immunodeficiency virus infection. *Am J Med.* 1990;89:451-456.
107. Small PM, Shafer RW, Hopewell PC. Exogenous reinfection with multidrug-resistant *Mycobacterium tuberculosis* in patients with advanced HIV infection. *N Engl J Med.* 1993;328: 1137-1144.
108. Haddad MB, Wilson TW, Ijaz K, et al. Tuberculosis and homelessness in the United States, 1994-2003. *JAMA.* 2005; 293:2762-2766.
109. Prevention and control of tuberculosis in correctional and detention facilities: recommendations from CDC. Endorsed by the Advisory Council for the Elimination of Tuberculosis, the National Commission on Correctional Health Care, and the American Correctional Association. *MMWR Recomm Rep.* 2006;55:1-44.
110. Braun MM, Truman BI, Maguire B. Increasing incidence of tuberculosis in a prison inmate population: association with HIV infection. *JAMA.* 1989;261:393-397.
111. Rao VK, Iademarco EP, Fraser VJ, et al. Delays in the suspicion and treatment of tuberculosis among hospitalized patients. *Ann Intern Med.* 1999;130:404-411.
112. ATS Workshop. Rapid diagnostic tests for tuberculosis—What is the appropriate use? *Am J Respir Crit Care Med.* 1997;155:1804-1814.
113. Jensen PA, Lambert LA, Iademarco MF, et al. Guidelines for preventing the transmission of Mycobacterium tuberculosis in health-care settings, 2005. *MMWR Recomm Rep.* 2005;54: 1-141.
114. Orme IM, Andersen P, Boom WH. T cell response to *Mycobacterium tuberculosis. J Infect Dis.* 1993;167:1481-1497.
115. Aderem A, Underhill DM. Mechanisms of phagocytosis in macrophages. *Annu Rev Immunol.* 1999;17:593-623.
116. Edwards KM, Cynamon MH, Voladri RK, et al. Iron-cofactored superoxide dismutase inhibits host responses to *Mycobacterium tuberculosis. Am J Respir Crit Care Med.* 2001;164:2213-2219.
117. Pethe K, Alonso S, Biet F, et al. The heparin-binding haemagglutinin of *M. tuberculosis* is required for extrapulmonary dissemination. *Nature.* 2001;412:190-194.
118. van Soolingen D, Hoogenboezem T, de Haas PE, et al. A novel pathogenic taxon of the *Mycobacterium tuberculosis* complex, Canetti: characterization of an exceptional isolate from Africa. *Int J Syst Bacteriol.* 1997;47:1236-1245.
119. Canetti G. Present aspects of bacterial resistance in tuberculosis. *Am Rev Respir Dis.* 1965;92:687-703.
120. O'Brien JR. Nonreactive tuberculosis. *J Clin Pathol.* 1954; 7:216-225.
121. Ellner JJ. The immune response in human tuberculosis: implications for tuberculosis control. *J Infect Dis.* 1997;176:1351-1359.
122. Hirsch CS, Hussain R, Toossi Z, et al. Cross-stimulatory role for transforming growth factor β in tuberculosis: suppression of antigen driven interferon γ production. *Proc Natl Acad Sci USA.* 1996;93:3193-3198.
123. Aung H, Wu M, Johnson JL, et al. Bioactivation of latent transforming growth factor beta1 by *Mycobacterium tuberculosis* in human mononuclear phagocytes. *Scand J Immunol.* 2005; 61:558-565.
124. Snider DE Jr. The tuberculin skin test. *Am Rev Respir Dis.* 1982;125:108-118.
125. Targeted tuberculin testing and treatment of latent tuberculosis infection. American Thoracic Society. *MMWR Morb Mortal Wkly Rep.* 2000;49(RR-6):1-51.
126. Centers for Disease Control. The use of preventive therapy for tuberculous infection in the United States: recommendations of the Advisory Committee for the Elimination of Tuberculosis. *MMWR Morb Mortal Wkly Rep.* 1990;39:9-12.
127. Stead WW. Management of health care workers after inadvertent exposure to tuberculosis: a guide for the use of preventive therapy. *Ann Intern Med.* 1995;122:906-912.
128. Menzies D. What does tuberculin reactivity after bacille Calmette-Guerin vaccination tell us? *Clin Infect Dis.* 2000;31:S71-S74.
129. Nash DR, Douglass JE. Anergy in active pulmonary tuberculosis: a comparison between positive and negative reactors and an evaluation of 5 TU and 250 TU skin test doses. *Chest.* 1980;77:32-37.
130. Slovis BS, Plitman JD, Haas DW. The case against anergy testing as a routine adjunct to tuberculin skin testing. *JAMA.* 2000;283:2003-2007.
131. Pouchot J, Grasland A, Collet C, et al. Reliability of tuberculin skin test measurement. *Ann Intern Med.* 1997;126:210-214.
132. Grzybowski S, Allen EA. The challenge of tuberculosis in decline: a study based on the epidemiology of tuberculosis in Ontario, Canada. *Am Rev Respir Dis.* 1964;90:707-720.
133. Johnson MP, Coberly JS, Clermont HC, et al. Tuberculin skin test reactivity among adults infected with human immunodeficiency virus. *J Infect Dis.* 1992;166:194-198.
134. Centers for Disease Control. Purified protein derivative (PPD) tuberculin anergy and HIV infection: guidelines for anergy testing and management of anergic persons at risk of tuberculosis. *MMWR Morb Mortal Wkly Rep.* 1991;40:27-33.
135. Gordin FM, Matts J, Miller C, et al. A controlled trial of isoniazid in persons with anergy and human immunodeficiency virus infection who are at high risk for tuberculosis. *N Engl J Med.* 1997;337:315-320.
136. Whalen CC, Johnson JL, Okwera A, et al. A trial of three regimens to prevent tuberculosis in Ugandan adults infected with the human immunodeficiency virus. *N Engl J Med.* 1997;337:801-808.
137. Mazurek GH, Jereb J, Lobue P, et al. Guidelines for using the QuantiFERON®-TB Gold Test for detecting *Mycobacterium tuberculosis* infection, United States. *MMWR Recomm Rep.* 2005;54:49-55.
138. Ewer K, Deeks J, Alvarez L, et al. Comparison of T-cell–based assay with tuberculin skin test for diagnosis of *Mycobacterium tuberculosis* infection in a school tuberculosis outbreak. *Lancet.* 2003;361:1168-1173.
139. Murray JF. Cursed duet: HIV infection and tuberculosis. *Respiration.* 1990;57:210-220.
140. Stead WW. Pathogenesis of a first episode of chronic pulmonary tuberculosis in man: recrudescence of residuals of the primary infection or exogenous reinfection? *Am Rev Respir Dis.* 1967; 95:729-745.

141. Romeyn JA. Exogenous reinfection in tuberculosis. *Am Rev Respir Dis.* 1970;101:923-927.

142. Kumar RA, Saran M, Verma BL, et al. Pulmonary tuberculosis among contacts of patients with tuberculosis in an urban Indian population. *J Epidemiol Community Health.* 1984;38: 253-258.

143. Dahl RH. First appearance of pulmonary cavity after primary infection with relation to time and age. *Acta Tuberc Scand.* 1952;27:140-149.

144. Stead WW, Kerby GR, Schlueter DP, et al. The clinical spectrum of primary tuberculosis in adults: confusion with reinfection in the pathogenesis of chronic tuberculosis. *Ann Intern Med.* 1968;68:731-745.

145. Gedde-Dahl T. Tuberculous infection in the light of tuberculin matriculation. *Am J Hyg.* 1952;56:139-214.

146. Keane J, Gershon S, Wise RP, et al. Tuberculosis associated with infliximab, a tumor necrosis factor alpha-neutralizing agent. *N Engl J Med.* 2001;345:1098-1104.

147. Mohan AK, Cote TR, Block JA, et al. Tuberculosis following the use of etanercept, a tumor necrosis factor inhibitor. *Clin Infect Dis.* 2004;39:295-299.

148. Reichman LB, Felton CP, Edsall JR. Drug dependence, a possible new risk factor for tuberculosis disease. *Arch Intern Med.* 1979;139:337-339.

149. Brahmajothi V, Pitchappan RM, Kakkanaiah VM, et al. Association of pulmonary tuberculosis and HLA in South India. *Tubercle.* 1991;72:123-132.

150. Mehra NK, Rajalingam R, Mitra DK, et al. Variants of HLA-DR2/DR51 group haplotypes and susceptibility to tuberculoid leprosy and pulmonary tuberculosis in Asian Indians. *Int J Lepr Other Mycobact Dis.* 1995;63:241-248.

151. Delgado JC, Baena A, Thim S, et al. Aspartic acid homozygosity at codon 57 of HLA-DQ beta is associated with susceptibility to pulmonary tuberculosis in Cambodia. *J Immunol.* 2006; 176:1090-1097.

152. Balamurugan A, Sharma SK, Mehra NK. Human leukocyte antigen class I supertypes influence susceptibility and severity of tuberculosis. *J Infect Dis.* 2004;189:805-811.

153. Jouanguy E, Lamhamedi-Cherradi S, Lammas D, et al. A human IFNGR1 small deletion hotspot associated with dominant susceptibility to mycobacterial infection. *Nat Genet.* 1999; 21:370-378.

154. Rossouw M, Nel HJ, Cooke GS, et al. Association between tuberculosis and a polymorphic NFkappaB binding site in the interferon gamma gene. *Lancet.* 2003;361:1871-1872.

155. Cooke GS, Campbell SJ, Sillah J, et al. Polymorphism within the interferon-gamma/receptor complex is associated with pulmonary tuberculosis. *Am J Respir Crit Care Med.* 2006;174: 339-343.

156. Bellamy R, Ruwende C, Corrah T, et al. Variations in the NRAMP1 gene and susceptibility to tuberculosis in West Africans. *N Engl J Med.* 1998;338:640-644.

157. Awomoyi AA, Marchant A, Howson JM, et al. Interleukin-10, polymorphism in SLC11A1 (formerly NRAMP1), and susceptibility to tuberculosis. *J Infect Dis.* 2002;186:1808-1814.

158. Zhang W, Shao L, Weng X, et al. Variants of the natural resistance-associated macrophage protein 1 gene (NRAMP1) are associated with severe forms of pulmonary tuberculosis. *Clin Infect Dis.* 2005;40:1232-1236.

159. Hawn TR, Dunstan SJ, Thwaites GE, et al. A polymorphism in Toll-interleukin 1 receptor domain containing adaptor protein is associated with susceptibility to meningeal tuberculosis. *J Infect Dis.* 2006;194:1127-1134.

160. Khor CC, Chapman SJ, Vannberg FO, et al. A Mal functional variant is associated with protection against invasive pneumococcal disease, bacteremia, malaria and tuberculosis. *Nat Genet.* 2007;39:523-528.

161. Nejentsev S, Thye T, Szeszko JS, et al. Analysis of association of the TIRAP (MAL) S180L variant and tuberculosis in three populations. *Nat Genet.* 2008;40:261-262.

162. Flores-Villanueva PO, Ruiz-Morales JA, Song CH, et al. A functional promoter polymorphism in monocyte chemoattractant protein-1 is associated with increased susceptibility to pulmonary tuberculosis. *J Exp Med.* 2005;202:1649-1658.

163. Ferwerda B, Kibiki GS, Netea MG, et al. The toll-like receptor 4 Asp299Gly variant and tuberculosis susceptibility in HIV-infected patients in Tanzania. *AIDS.* 2007;21:1375-1377.

164. Soborg C, Madsen HO, Andersen AB, et al. Mannose-binding lectin polymorphisms in clinical tuberculosis. *J Infect Dis.* 2003;188:777-782.

165. Tso HW, Lau YL, Tam CM, et al. Associations between IL12B polymorphisms and tuberculosis in the Hong Kong Chinese population. *J Infect Dis.* 2004;190:913-919.

166. Remus N, El BJ, Fieschi C, et al. Association of IL12RB1 polymorphisms with pulmonary tuberculosis in adults in Morocco. *J Infect Dis.* 2004;190:580-587.

167. Roth DE, Soto G, Arenas F, et al. Association between vitamin D receptor gene polymorphisms and response to treatment of pulmonary tuberculosis. *J Infect Dis.* 2004;190:920-927.

168. Bornman L, Campbell SJ, Fielding K, et al. Vitamin D receptor polymorphisms and susceptibility to tuberculosis in West Africa: a case-control and family study. *J Infect Dis.* 2004;190: 1631-1641.

169. Rosas-Taraco AG, Revol A, Salinas-Carmona MC, et al. CD14 C(-159)T polymorphism is a risk factor for development of pulmonary tuberculosis. *J Infect Dis.* 2007;196:1698-1706.

170. Lee JH, Park SS, Lee DH, et al. Endobronchial tuberculosis: clinical and bronchoscopic features in 121 cases. *Chest.* 1992;102:990-994.

171. Chang S, Lee P, Perug P. Lower lung field tuberculosis. *Chest.* 1987;91:230-232.

172. Pitchenik AE, Rubinson HA. The radiographic appearance of tuberculosis in patients with the acquired immune deficiency syndrome (AIDS) and pre-AIDS. *Am Rev Respir Dis.* 1985;131:393-396.

173. Chaisson RE, Schecter GF, Theuer CP, et al. Tuberculosis in patients with the acquired immunodeficiency syndrome. Clinical features, response to therapy, and survival. *Am Rev Respir Dis.* 1987;136:570-574.

174. Perlman DC, El-Sadr WM, Nelson ET, et al. Variation of chest radiographic patterns in pulmonary tuberculosis by degree of human immunodeficiency virus–related immunosuppression. The Terry Beirn Community Programs for Clinical Research on AIDS (CPCRA). The AIDS Clinical Trials Group (ACTG). *Clin Infect Dis.* 1997 ;25:242-246.

175. Behr MA, Warren SA, Salamon H, et al. Transmission of Mycobacterium tuberculosis from patients smear-negative for acid-fast bacilli. *Lancet.* 1999;353:444-449.

176. Getahun H, Harrington M, O'Brien R, et al. Diagnosis of smear-negative pulmonary tuberculosis in people with HIV infection or AIDS in resource-constrained settings: informing urgent policy changes. *Lancet.* 2007;369:2042-2049.

177. Kline SE, Hedemark LL, Davies SF. Outbreak of tuberculosis among regular patrons of a neighborhood bar. *N Engl J Med.* 1995;333:222-227.

178. Kent DC. Tuberculosis epidemics, U.S. Navy. *Bull Int Union Tuberc.* 1968;41:79-82.

179. Greenberg SD, Frager D, Suster B, et al. Active pulmonary tuberculosis in patients with AIDS: spectrum of radiographic findings (including a normal appearance). *Radiology.* 1994;193: 115-119.

180. Marciniuk DD, McNab BD, Martin WT, et al. Detection of pulmonary tuberculosis in patients with a normal chest radiograph. *Chest.* 1999;115:445-452.

181. Pepper T, Joseph P, Mwenya C, et al. Normal chest radiography in pulmonary tuberculosis: implications for obtaining respiratory specimen cultures. *Int J Tuberc Lung Dis.* 2008; 12:397-403.

182. Jones BE, Oo MM, Taikwel EK, et al. CD4 cell counts in human immunodeficiency virus-negative patients with tuberculosis. *Clin Infect Dis.* 1997;24:988-991.

183. Conde MB, Soares SL, Mello FC, et al. Comparison of sputum induction with fiberoptic bronchoscopy in the diagnosis of tuberculosis: experience at an acquired immune deficiency syndrome reference center in Rio de Janeiro, Brazil. *Am J Respir Crit Care Med.* 2000 ;162:2238-2240.

184. Yajko DM, Nassos PS, Sanders CA, et al. High predictive value of the acid-fast smear for *Mycobacterium tuberculosis* despite the high prevalence of *Mycobacterium avium* complex in respiratory specimens. *Clin Infect Dis.* 1994;19:334-336.

185. Menzies R, Vissandjee B, Rocher I, et al. The booster effect in two-step tuberculin testing among adults in Montreal. *Ann Intern Med.* 1994;120:190-198.

186. Fisk TL, Hon HM, Lennox JL, et al. Detection of latent tuberculosis among HIV-infected patients after initiation of highly active antiretroviral therapy. *AIDS.* 2003;17: 1102-1104.

187. Salzman SH, Schindel ML, Aranda CP, et al. The role of bronchoscopy in the diagnosis of pulmonary tuberculosis in patients at risk for HIV infection. *Chest.* 1992;102:143-146.

188. Miro AM, Gibilara E, Powell S, et al. The role of fiberoptic bronchoscopy for diagnosis of pulmonary tuberculosis in patients at risk for AIDS. *Chest.* 1992;101:1211-1214.

189. Kennedy DJ, Lewis WP, Barnes PF. Yield of bronchoscopy for the diagnosis of tuberculosis in patients with human immunodeficiency virus infection. *Chest.* 1992;102:1040-1044.

190. Reider HL, Kelly GD, Bloch AB, et al. Tuberculosis diagnosed at death in the United States. *Chest.* 1991;100:678-681.

191. Mok CK, Nandi P, Ong GB. Coexistent bronchogenic carcinoma and active pulmonary tuberculosis. *J Thorac Cardiovasc Surg.* 1978;76:469-472.

192. Centers for Disease Control and Prevention. Treatment of tuberculosis. American Thoracic Society, CDC and Infectious Diseases Society of America. *MMWR Morb Mortal Wkly Rep.* 2003;52(RR-11):1-88.

193. Kopanoff DE, Snider DE Jr, Caras GJ. Isoniazid-related hepatitis: a U.S. Public Health Service cooperative surveillance study. *Am Rev Respir Dis.* 1978;117:991-1001.

194. Menzies D, Dion MJ, Rabinovitch B, et al. Treatment completion and costs of a randomized trial of rifampin for 4 months versus isoniazid for 9 months. *Am J Respir Crit Care Med.* 2004;170:445-449.

195. Page KR, Sifakis F, de Montes OR, et al. Improved adherence and less toxicity with rifampin vs isoniazid for treatment of latent tuberculosis: a retrospective study. *Arch Intern Med.* 2006;166:1863-1870.

196. Steele MA, Burk RF, Des Prez RM. Toxic hepatitis with isoniazid and rifampin: a metaanalysis. *Chest.* 1991;99:465-471.

197. Centers for Disease Control and Prevention. Clinical update: impact of HIV protease inhibitors on the treatment of HIV-infected tuberculosis patients with rifampin. *MMWR Morb Mortal Wkly Rep.* 1996;45:921-925.

198. Jarvis B, Lamb HM. Rifapentine. *Drugs.* 1998;56:607-616.

199. Vernon A, Burman W, Benator D, et al. Acquired rifamycin monoresistance in patients with HIV-related tuberculosis treated with once-weekly rifapentine and isoniazid. Tuberculosis Trials Consortium. *Lancet.* 1999;353:1843-1847.

200. Yee D, Valiquette C, Pelletier M, et al. Incidence of serious side effects from first-line antituberculosis drugs among patients treated for active tuberculosis. *Am J Respir Crit Care Med.* 2003;167:1472-1477.

201. Chang KC, Leung CC, Yew WW, et al. Hepatotoxicity of pyrazinamide: cohort and case-control analyses. *Am J Respir Crit Care Med.* 2008;177:1391-1396.

202. Ijaz K, Jereb JA, Lambert LA, et al. Severe or fatal liver injury in 50 patients in the United States taking rifampin and pyrazinamide for latent tuberculosis infection. *Clin Infect Dis.* 2006;42:346-355.

203. Zhang Y, Mitchison D. The curious characteristics of pyrazinamide: a review. *Int J Tuberc Lung Dis.* 2003;7:6-21.

204. Dankner WM, Waecker NJ, Essey MA, et al. *Mycobacterium bovis* infections in San Diego: a clinicoepidemiologic study of 73 patients and a historical review of a forgotten pathogen. *Medicine.* 1993;72:11-37.

205. Rustomjee R, Lienhardt C, Kanyok T, et al. A Phase II study of the sterilising activities of ofloxacin, gatifloxacin and moxifloxacin in pulmonary tuberculosis. *Int J Tuberc Lung Dis.* 2008;12:128-138.

206. Spigelman MK. New tuberculosis therapeutics: a growing pipeline. *J Infect Dis.* 2007;196(Suppl 1):S28-S34.

207. Perez-Stable EJ, Hopewell PC. Current tuberculosis treatment regimens: choosing the right one for your patient. *Clin Chest Med.* 1989;10:323-339.

208. Davidson PT, Le HQ. Drug treatment of tuberculosis—1992. *Drugs.* 1992;43:651-673.

209. Snider DE Jr, Zierski M, Graczyk J, et al. Short-course tuberculosis chemotherapy studies conducted in Poland during the past decade. *Eur J Respir Dis.* 1986;68:12-18.

210. British Thoracic Association. A controlled trial of six months chemotherapy in pulmonary tuberculosis. Second report: results during the 24 months after the end of chemotherapy. *Am Rev Respir Dis.* 1982;126:460-462.

211. Cohn DL, Catlin BJ, Peterson KL, et al. A 62-dose, 6-month therapy for pulmonary and extrapulmonary tuberculosis: a twice-weekly, directly observed, and cost-effective regimen. *Ann Intern Med.* 1990;112:407-415.

212. Jindani A, Nunn AJ, Enarson DA. Two 8-month regimens of chemotherapy for treatment of newly diagnosed pulmonary tuberculosis: international multicentre randomised trial. *Lancet.* 2004;364:1244-1251.

213. Hopewell PC, Pai M, Maher D, et al. International standards for tuberculosis care. *Lancet Infect Dis.* 2006;6:710-725.

214. World Health Organization. Treatment of Tuberculosis, Guidelines for National Programmes, 3rd ed., Geneva, Switzerland, 2003 (WHO/CDS/TB 2003-313).

215. Dutt AK, Moers D, Stead WW. Short-course chemotherapy for tuberculosis with mainly twice-weekly isoniazid and rifampin: community physicians' seven-year experience with mainly outpatients. *Am J Med.* 1984;77:233-242.

216. Benator D, Bhattacharya M, Bozeman L, et al. Rifapentine and isoniazid once a week versus rifampicin and isoniazid twice a week for treatment of drug-susceptible pulmonary tuberculosis in HIV-negative patients: a randomised clinical trial. *Lancet.* 2002;360:528-534.

217. Mitchison DA, Nunn AJ. Influence of initial drug resistance on the response to short-course chemotherapy of pulmonary tuberculosis. *Am Rev Respir Dis.* 1986;133:423-430.

218. Moore RD, Chaulk CP, Griffiths R, et al. Cost-effectiveness of directly observed versus self-administered therapy for tuberculosis. *Am J Respir Crit Care Med.* 1996;154:1013-1019.

219. Fujiwara PI, Cook SV, Rutherford CM, et al. A continuing survey of drug-resistant tuberculosis, New York City, April 1994. *Arch Intern Med.* 1997;157:531-536.

220. Weis SE, Slocum PC, Blais FX, et al. The effect of directly observed therapy on the rates of drug resistance and relapse in tuberculosis. *N Engl J Med.* 1994;330:1179-1184.

221. Hong Kong Chest Service Tuberculosis Research Center, Madras, British Medical Research Council. A controlled trial of 3-month, 4-month, and 6-month regimens of chemotherapy for sputum smear-negative pulmonary tuberculosis: Results at 5 years. *Am Rev Respir Dis.* 1989;139:871-876.

222. Lew W, Pai M, Oxlade O, et al. Initial drug resistance and tuberculosis treatment outcomes: systematic review and meta-analysis. *Ann Intern Med.* 2008;149:123-134.

223. Goble M, Iseman MD, Madsen LA. Treatment of 171 patients with pulmonary tuberculosis resistant to isoniazid and rifampin. *N Engl J Med.* 1993;328:527-532.

224. Chan ED, Laurel V, Strand MJ, et al. Treatment and outcome analysis of 205 patients with multidrug-resistant tuberculosis. *Am J Respir Crit Care Med.* 2004;169:1103-1109.

225. Leimane V, Riekstina V, Holtz TH, et al. Clinical outcome of individualised treatment of multidrug-resistant tuberculosis in Latvia: a retrospective cohort study. *Lancet.* 2005;365: 318-326.

226. Telzak EE, Sepkowitz K, Alpert P, et al. Multidrug-resistant tuberculosis in patients without HIV infection. *N Engl J Med.* 1995;333:907-911.

227. Burgos M, Gonzalez LC, Paz EA, et al. Treatment of multidrug-resistant tuberculosis in San Francisco: an outpatient-based approach. *Clin Infect Dis.* 2005;40:968-975.

228. Yew WW, Chan CK, Chau CH, et al. Outcomes of patients with multidrug-resistant pulmonary tuberculosis treated with ofloxacin/levofloxacin-containing regimens. *Chest*. 2000;117:744-751.
229. Yew WW, Chan CK, Leung CC, et al. Comparative roles of levofloxacin and ofloxacin in the treatment of multidrug-resistant tuberculosis: preliminary results of a retrospective study from Hong Kong. *Chest*. 2003;124:1476-1481.
230. Treatment of tuberculosis and tuberculous infection in adults and children. *Am J Respir Crit Care Med*. 1994;149:1359-1374.
231. Centers for Disease Control and Prevention. Initial therapy for tuberculosis in the era of multidrug resistance: recommendations of the Advisory Council for the Elimination of Tuberculosis. *JAMA*. 1993;270:694-698.
232. Iseman MD. Treatment of multidrug-resistant tuberculosis. *N Engl J Med*. 1993;329:784-791.
233. Kim HR, Hwang SS, Kim HJ, et al. Impact of extensive drug resistance on treatment outcomes in non-HIV-infected patients with multidrug-resistant tuberculosis. *Clin Infect Dis*. 2007;45:1290-1295.
234. Chan ED, Strand MJ, Iseman MD. Treatment outcomes in extensively resistant tuberculosis. *N Engl J Med*. 2008;359:657-659.
235. Mitnick CD, Shin SS, Seung KJ, et al. Comprehensive treatment of extensively drug-resistant tuberculosis. *N Engl J Med*. 2008;359:563-574.
236. Fitzgerald DW, Desvarieux M, Severe P, et al. Effect of post-treatment isoniazid on prevention of recurrent tuberculosis in HIV-1-infected individuals: a randomised trial. *Lancet*. 2000;356:1470-1474.
237. Churchyard GJ, Fielding K, Charalambous S, et al. Efficacy of secondary isoniazid preventive therapy among HIV-infected Southern Africans: time to change policy? *AIDS*. 2003;17:2063-2070.
238. Mukherjee JS, Rich ML, Socci AR, et al. Programmes and principles in treatment of multidrug-resistant tuberculosis. *Lancet*. 2004;363:474-481.
239. Dooley DP, Carpenter JL, Rademacher S. Adjunctive corticosteroid therapy for tuberculosis: a critical reappraisal of the literature. *Clin Infect Dis*. 1997;25:872-887.
240. The Panel on Clinical Practices for Treatment of HIV Infection. Guidelines for the Use of Antiretroviral Agents in HIV-1-Infected Adults and Adolescents. 2008. Available at http://hivatis.org. Accessed November 2008.
241. Centers for Disease Control and Prevention. *Managing Drug Interactions in the Treatment of HIV-Related Tuberculosis*. Centers for Disease Control and Prevention; 2008. Available at http://www.cdc.gov/tb/TB_HIV_Drugs/default.htm. Accessed November 2008.
242. Burman WJ, Gallicano K, Peloquin C. Therapeutic implications of drug interactions in the treatment of human immunodeficiency virus–related tuberculosis. *Clin Infect Dis*. 1999;28:419-429.
243. Nijland HM, L'homme RF, Rongen GA, et al. High incidence of adverse events in healthy volunteers receiving rifampicin and adjusted doses of lopinavir/ritonavir tablets. *AIDS*. 2008;22:931-935.
244. Grange S, Schutz M, Schmitt C, et al. Unexpected hepatotoxicity observed in a healthy volunteer study on the effects of multiple dose rifampicin on the steady-state pharmacokinetics of ritonavir-boosted saquinavir and vice versa [abstract 35]. In: Program and Abstracts of the 6th International Workshop on Clinical Pharmacology of HIV Therapy. Quebec City: 2005. Virology Education, Utrecht, The Netherlands.
245. Haas DW, Koletar SL, Laughlin L, et al. Hepatotoxicity and gastrointestinal intolerance when healthy volunteers taking rifampin add twice-daily atazanavir and ritonavir. *J Acquir Immun Defic Syndr*. 2009;50:290-293.
246. Manosuthi W, Mankatitham W, Lueangniyomkul A, et al. Standard-dose efavirenz vs. standard-dose nevirapine in antiretroviral regimens among HIV-1 and tuberculosis co-infected patients who received rifampicin. *HIV Med*. 2008;9:294-299.
247. Boulle A, Van CG, Cohen K. et al. Outcomes of nevirapine- and efavirenz-based antiretroviral therapy when coadministered with rifampicin-based antitubercular therapy. *JAMA*. 2008;300:530-539.
248. Burman W, Weis S, Vernon A, et al. Frequency, severity and duration of immune reconstitution events in HIV-related tuberculosis. *Int J Tuberc Lung Dis*. 2007;11:1282-1289.
249. Centers for Disease Control and Prevention. Acquired rifamycin resistance in persons with advanced HIV disease being treated for active tuberculosis with intermittent rifamycin-based regimens. *MMWR Morb Mortal Wkly Rep*. 2002;51:214-215.
250. Berning SE, Huitt DA, Iseman MD, Peloquin CA. Malabsorption of antituberculous medications by a patient with AIDS. *N Engl J Med*. 1992;327:1817-1818.
251. Narita M, Ashkin D, Hollender ES, Pitchenik AE. Paradoxical worsening of tuberculosis following antiretroviral therapy in patients with AIDS. *Am J Respir Crit Care Med*. 1998;158:157-161.
252. Wendel KA, Alwood KS, Gachuhi R, et al. Paradoxical worsening of tuberculosis in HIV-infected persons. *Chest*. 2001;120:193-197.
253. Bourgarit A, Carcelain G, Martinez V, et al. Explosion of tuberculin-specific Th1-responses induces immune restoration syndrome in tuberculosis and HIV co-infected patients. *AIDS*. 2006;20:F1-F7.
254. Meintjes G, Lawn SD, Scano F, et al. Tuberculosis-associated immune reconstitution inflammatory syndrome: case definitions for use in resource-limited settings. *Lancet Infect Dis*. 2008;8:516-523.
255. Olalla J, Pulido F, Rubio R, et al. Paradoxical responses in a cohort of HIV-1-infected patients with mycobacterial disease. *Int J Tuberc Lung Dis*. 2002;6:71-75.
256. Lawn SD, Wilkinson RJ, Lipman MC, et al. Immune reconstitution and "unmasking" of tuberculosis during antiretroviral therapy. *Am J Respir Crit Care Med*. 2008;177:680-685.
257. Schiffer JT, Sterling TR. Timing of antiretroviral therapy initiation in tuberculosis patients with AIDS: a decision analysis. *J AIDS*. 2007;44:229-234.
258. Nettles RE, Mazo D, Alwood K, et al. Risk factors for relapse and acquired rifamycin resistance after directly observed tuberculosis treatment: a comparison by HIV serostatus and rifamycin use. *Clin Infect Dis*. 2004;38:731-736.
259. Nahid P, Gonzalez LC, Rudoy I, et al. Treatment outcomes of patients with HIV and tuberculosis. *Am J Respir Crit Care Med*. 2007;175:1199-1206.
260. Pediatric Tuberculosis Collaborative Group. Targeted tuberculin skin testing and treatment of latent tuberculosis infection in children and adolescents. *Pediatrics*. 2004;114:1175-2101.
261. Comstock GW. How much isoniazid is needed for prevention of tuberculosis among immunocompetent adults? *Int J Tuberc Lung Dis*. 1999;3:847-850.
262. British Medical Research Council. A double-blind placebo-controlled clinical trial of three antituberculosis chemoprophylaxis regimens in patients with silicosis in Hong Kong. Hong Kong Chest Service/Tuberculosis Research Centre, Madras. *Am Rev Respir Dis*. 1992;145:36-41.
263. Gordin F, Chaisson RE, Matts JP, et al. Rifampin and pyrazinamide vs isoniazid for prevention of tuberculosis in HIV-infected persons: an international randomized trial. Terry Beirn CPCRA, the AACTG, the PAHO, and the CDC Study Group. *JAMA*. 2000;283:1445-1450.
264. Centers for Disease Control and Prevention. Update: adverse event data and revised American Thoracic Society/CDC recommendations against the use of rifampin and pyrazinamide for treatment of latent tuberculosis infection—United States, 2003. *MMWR Morb Mortal Wkly Rep*. 2003;52:735-739.
265. Stead WW, To T, Harrison RW, et al. Benefit-risk considerations in preventive treatment of tuberculosis in elderly persons. *Ann Intern Med*. 1987;107:843-845.
266. Saukkonen JJ, Cohn DL, Jasmer RM, et al. An official ATS statement: hepatotoxicity of antituberculosis therapy. *Am J Respir Crit Care Med*. 2006;174:935-952.
267. Byrd RB, Horn BR, Griggs GA, et al. Isoniazid chemoprophylaxis: association with detection and incidence of liver toxicity. *Arch Intern Med*. 1970;137:1130-1133.
268. Nolan CM, Goldberg SV, Buskin SE. Hepatotoxicity associated with isoniazid preventive therapy: a 7-year survey from a public health tuberculosis clinic. *JAMA*. 1999;281:1014-1018.
269. Snider DE Jr, Caras GJ. Isoniazid-associated hepatitis deaths: a review of available information. *Am Rev Respir Dis*. 1992;145:494-497.
270. Ferebee SH. Controlled chemoprophylaxis trials in tuberculosis: a general review. *Bibl Tuberc Med Thorac*. 1970;26:28-106.
271. International Union Against Tuberculosis. Efficacy of various durations of isoniazid preventive therapy for tuberculosis: five years of follow-up in the IUAT trial. *Bull World Health Organ*. 1982;60:555-564.
272. Centers for Disease Control and Prevention. Anergy skin testing and preventive therapy for HIV-infected persons: revised guidelines. *MMWR Morb Mortal Wkly Rep*. 1997;46:1-10.
273. Luelmo F. BCG vaccination. *Am Rev Respir Dis*. 1982;125:70-72.
274. Menzies R, Vissandjee B. Effect of bacille Calmette-Guérin vaccination on tuberculin reactivity. *Am Rev Respir Dis*. 1992;145:621-624.
275. Hakim S, Heaney JA, Heinz T, et al. Psoas abscess following intravesical bacillus Calmette-Guérin for bladder cancer: a case report. *J Urol*. 1993;150:188-189.
276. McParland C, Cotton DJ, Gowda KS, et al. Miliary *Mycobacterium bovis* induced by intravesical bacille Calmette-Guerin immunotherapy. *Am Rev Respir Dis*. 1992;146:1330-1333.
277. Lamm DL, Stogdill VD, Stogdill BJ, et al. Complications of bacillus Calmette-Guérin immunotherapy in 1278 patients with bladder cancer. *J Urol*. 1986;135:272-274.
278. Skeiky TA, Sadoff JC. Advances in tuberculosis vaccine strategies. *Nat Rev Microbiol*. 2006;4:469-476.
279. Grode L, Seiler P, Baumann S, et al. Increased vaccine efficacy against tuberculosis of recombinant *Mycobacterium bovis* bacille Calmette-Guerin mutants that secrete listeriolysin. *J Clin Invest*. 2005;115:2472-2479.
280. von Reyn CF, Vuola JM. New vaccines for the prevention of tuberculosis. *Clin Infect Dis*. 2002;35:465-474.
281. Hinchey J, Lee S, Jeon BY, et al. Enhanced priming of adaptive immunity by a proapoptotic mutant of *Mycobacterium tuberculosis*. *J Clin Invest*. 2007;117:2279-2288.
282. Stop TB Partnership. Available at http://www.stoptb.org/retooling/. Accessed November 2008.
283. Shafer RW, Kim DS, Weiss JP, et al. Extrapulmonary tuberculosis in patients with human immunodeficiency virus infection. *Medicine*. 1991;70:384-397.
284. Biehl JP. Miliary tuberculosis: a review of sixty-eight adult patients admitted to a municipal general hospital. *Am Rev Tuberc*. 1958;77:605-622.
285. Munt PW. Miliary tuberculosis in the chemotherapy era: with a clinical review in 69 American adults. *Medicine*. 1972;51:139-155.
286. Maartens G, Willcox PA, Benatar SR. Miliary tuberculosis: rapid diagnosis, hematologic abnormalities, and outcome in 109 treated adults. *Am J Med*. 1990;89:291-296.
287. Kim JH, Langston AA, Gallis HA. Miliary tuberculosis: epidemiology, clinical manifestations, diagnosis, and outcome. *Rev Infect Dis*. 1990;12:583-590.
288. Yu YL, Chow WH, Humphries MJ, et al. Cryptic miliary tuberculosis. *Q J Med*. 1986;59:421-428.
289. Willcox PA, Potgieter PD, Bateman ED, et al. Rapid diagnosis of sputum negative miliary tuberculosis using the flexible fiber-optic bronchoscope. *Thorax*. 1986;41:681-684.
290. Slavin RE, Walsh TJ, Pollock AD. Late generalized tuberculosis: a clinical pathologic analysis and comparison of 100 cases in the pre-antibiotic and antibiotic eras. *Medicine*. 1980;59:351-366.
291. Proudfoot AT, Akhar AJ, Douglas AC, et al. Miliary tuberculosis in adults. *Br Med J*. 1969;2:273-276.
292. Cameron SJ. Tuberculosis and the blood: a special relationship. *Tubercle*. 1974;55:55-72.
293. Lupatkin H, Brau N, Flomenberg P, et al. Tuberculous abscesses in patients with AIDS. *Clin Infect Dis*. 1992;14:1040-1044.
294. Kennedy DH, Fallon RJ. Tuberculous meningitis. *JAMA*. 1979;241:264-268.
295. Chedore P, Jamieson FB. Rapid molecular diagnosis of tuberculous meningitis using the Gen-Probe amplified Mycobacterium tuberculosis direct test in a large Canadian public health laboratory. *Int J Tuberc Lung Dis*. 2002;6:913-919.
296. Bonington A, Strang JI, Klapper PE, et al. Use of Roche AMPLICOR Mycobacterium PCR in early diagnosis of tuberculous meningitis. *J Clin Microbiol*. 1998;36:1251-1254.
297. Dube MP, Holtom PD, Larsen RA. Tuberculous meningitis in patients with and without human immunodeficiency virus infection. *Am J Med*. 1992;93:520-524.
298. Roper WH, Waring JJ. Primary serofibrinous pleural effusion in military personnel. *Am Rev Tuberc*. 1955;71:616-634.
299. Antoniskis D, Amin K, Barnes PF. Pleuritis as a manifestation of reactivation tuberculosis. *Am J Med*. 1990;89:447-450.
300. Epstein DM, Kline LR, Albelda SM, et al. Tuberculous pleural effusions. *Chest*. 1987;91:106-109.
301. Roth BJ. Searching for tuberculosis in the pleural space. *Chest*. 1999;116:3-5.
302. Laniado-Laborin R. Adenosine deaminase in the diagnosis of tuberculous pleural effusion: is it really an ideal test? A word of caution. *Chest*. 2005;127:417-418.
303. Lee YC, Rogers JT, Rodriguez RM, et al. Adenosine deaminase levels in nontuberculous lymphocytic pleural effusions. *Chest*. 2001;120:356-361.
304. Jimenez CD, Diaz NG, Perez-Rodriguez E, et al. Diagnostic value of adenosine deaminase in nontuberculous lymphocytic pleural effusions. *Eur Respir J*. 2003;21:220-224.
305. Taelman H, Kagame A, Batungwanayo J, et al. Pericardial effusion and HIV infection. *Lancet*. 1990;335:924.
306. Maher D, Harries AD. Tuberculous pericardial effusion: a prospective clinical study in a low-resource setting—Blantyre, Malawi. *Int J Tuberc Lung Dis*. 1997;1:358-364.
307. Strang JIG, Gibson DG, Mitchison DA, et al. Controlled clinical trial of complete open surgical drainage and of prednisolone in treatment of tuberculous pericardial effusion in Transkei. *Lancet*. 1988;2:759-763.
308. Strang JIG, Gibson DG, Nunn AJ, et al. Controlled trial of prednisolone as adjuvant in treatment of tuberculous constrictive pericarditis in Transkei. *Lancet*. 1987;23: 1418-1422.
309. Agner RC, Gallis HA. Pericarditis differential diagnostic considerations. *Arch Intern Med*. 1979;139:407-412.
310. Strang JI, Nunn AJ, Johnson DA, et al. Management of tuberculous constrictive pericarditis and tuberculous pericardial effusion in Transkei: results at 10 years follow-up. *QJM*. 2004;97:525-535.
311. Janssens JP, De Haller R. Spinal tuberculosis in a developed country: a review of 26 cases with special emphasis on abscesses and neurologic complications. *Clin Orthop*. 1990;257:67-75.
312. Five-year assessment of controlled trials of short-course chemotherapy regimens of 6, 9 or 18 months' duration for spinal tuberculosis in patients ambulatory from the start or undergoing radical surgery. Fourteenth report of the Medical Research Council Working Party on Tuberculosis of the Spine. *Int Orthop*. 1999;23:73-81.
313. Controlled trial of short-course regimens of chemotherapy in the ambulatory treatment of spinal tuberculosis. Results at three years of a study in Korea. Twelfth report of the Medical Research Council Working Party on Tuberculosis of the Spine. *J Bone Joint Surg Br*. 1993;75:240-248.
314. Davidson PT, Horowitz I. Skeletal tuberculosis: a review with patient presentations and discussion. *Am J Med*. 1970;48:77-84.
315. LiZares LF, Valcarcel A, Del Castillo JM, et al. Tuberculous arthritis with multiple joint involvement. *J Rheumatol*. 1991;18:635-636.
316. Muradali D, Gold WL, Vellend H, et al. Multifocal osteoarticular tuberculosis: report of four cases and review of management. *Clin Infect Dis*. 1993;17:204-209.

317. Bentz RR, Dimcheff DG, Nemiroff MJ, et al. The incidence of urine cultures positive for *Mycobacterium tuberculosis* in a general tuberculosis patient population. *Am Rev Respir Dis.* 1975;111:647-650.
318. Simon HB, Weinstein AJ, Pasternak MS, et al. Genitourinary tuberculosis: clinical features in a general hospital population. *Am J Med.* 1977;63:410-420.
319. Christensen WI. Genitourinary tuberculosis: Review of 102 cases. *Medicine.* 1974;53:377-390.
320. Morgan SH, Eastwood JB, Baker LRI. Tuberculous interstitial nephritis: the tip of an iceberg? *Tubercle.* 1990;71:5-6.
321. Gorse GJ, Belshe RB. Male genital tuberculosis: a review of the literature with instructive case reports. *Rev Infect Dis.* 1985;7:511-524.
322. Carter JR. Unusual presentations of genital tract tuberculosis. *Int J Gynecol Obstet.* 1990;33:171-176.
323. Jakubowski A, Elwood RK, Enarson DA. Clinical features of abdominal tuberculosis. *J Infect Dis.* 1988;158:687-692.
324. Shah S, Thomas V, Mathan M, et al. Colonoscopic study of 50 patients with colonic tuberculosis. *Gut.* 1992;33:347-351.
325. Kielhofner MA, Hamill RJ. Focal hepatic tuberculosis in a patient with acquired immunodeficiency syndrome. *South Med J.* 1991;84:401-404.
326. Hulnick DH, Megibow AJ, Naidich DP, et al. Abdominal tuberculosis: CT evaluation. *Radiology.* 1985;157:199-204.
327. Modilevsky T, Sattler FR, Barnes PF. Mycobacterial disease in patients with human immunodeficiency virus infection. *Arch Intern Med.* 1989;149:2201-2205.
328. Bastani B, Shariatzadeh MR, Dehdashti F. Tuberculous peritonitis: report of 30 cases and review of the literature. *Q J Med.* 1985;56:549-557.
329. Burack WR, Hollister RM. Tuberculous peritonitis. *Ann Intern Med.* 1960;28:510-523.
330. Cheng IKP, Chan PCK, Chan MK. Tuberculous peritonitis complicating long-term peritoneal dialysis. *Am J Nephrol.* 1989;9:155-161.
331. Fernandez-Rodriguez CM, Perez-Arguelles BS, Ledo L, et al. Ascites adenosine deaminase activity is decreased in tuberculous ascites with low protein content. *Am J Gastroenterol.* 1991;86:1500-1503.
332. Kaur A, Basha A, Ranjan M, Oommen A. Poor diagnostic value of adenosine deaminase in pleural, peritoneal & cerebrospinal fluids in tuberculosis. *Indian J Med Res.* 1992;95:270-277.
333. Singh MM, Bhargava AN, Jain KP. Tuberculous peritonitis: an evaluation of pathogenetic mechanisms, diagnostic procedures and therapeutic measures. *N Engl J Med.* 1969;281:1091-1094.
334. Haas DW. Are adjunctive corticosteroids indicated during tuberculous peritonitis? *Clin Infect Dis.* 1998;27:57-58.
335. Summers GD, McNicol MW. Tuberculosis of superficial lymph nodes. *Br J Dis Chest.* 1980;74:369-373.
336. Dandapat MC, Mishra BM, Dash SP, et al. Peripheral lymph node tuberculosis: a review of 80 cases. *Br J Surg.* 1990;77:911-912.
337. Campbell IA. The treatment of superficial tuberculous lymphadenitis. *Tubercle.* 1990;71:1-3.
338. Hewlett D Jr, Duncanson FP, Jagadha V, et al. Lymphadenopathy in an inner city population consisting principally of intravenous drug abusers with suspected acquired immunodeficiency syndrome. *Am Rev Respir Dis.* 1988;137:1275-1279.
339. Shriner KA, Mathisen GE, Goetz MB. Comparison of mycobacterial lymphadenitis among persons infected with human immunodeficiency virus and seronegative controls. *Clin Infect Dis.* 1992;15:601-605.
340. Van den Brande P, Vijgen J, Demedts M. Isolated intrathoracic tuberculous lymphadenopathy. *Eur Respir J.* 1991;4:758-760.
341. Pastores SM, Naidich DP, Arnada CP, et al. Intrathoracic adenopathy associated with pulmonary tuberculosis in patients with human immunodeficiency virus infection. *Chest.* 1993;103:1433-1437.
342. Perich J, Ayuso MC, Vilana R, et al. Disseminated lymphatic tuberculosis in acquired immunodeficiency syndrome: computed tomography findings. *Can Assoc Radiol J.* 1990;41:353-357.
343. Radin DR. Intraabdominal *Mycobacterium tuberculosis* vs *Mycobacterium avium-intracellulare* infections in patients with AIDS: distinction based on CT findings. *AJR Am J Roentgenol.* 1991;156:487-491.
344. Beyt BE Jr, Ortbals DW, Santa Cruz DJ, et al. Cutaneous mycobacteriosis: analysis of 34 cases with a new classification of the disease. *Medicine.* 1981;60:95-109.
345. Yen A, Rady PL, Cortes-Franco R, et al. Detection of *Mycobacterium tuberculosis* in erythema induratum of Bazin using polymerase chain reaction. *Arch Dermatol.* 1997;133:532-533.
346. Rohatgi PK, Palazzolo JV, Saini NB. Acute miliary tuberculosis of the skin in acquired immunodeficiency syndrome. *J Am Acad Dermatol.* 1992;26:356-359.
347. Lindell MM Jr, Jing BS, Wallace S. Laryngeal tuberculosis. *AJR Am J Roentgenol.* 1977;129:677-680.
348. Lee PY, Drysdale AJ. Tuberculous otitis media: a difficult diagnosis. *J Laryngol Otol.* 1993;107:339.
349. Harrison NK, Knight RK. Tuberculosis of the nasopharynx misdiagnosed as Wegener's granulomatosis. *Thorax.* 1986;41:219-220.
350. Kelestimur F, Ozbakir O, Saglam A. Acute adrenocortical failure due to tuberculosis. *J Endocrinol Invest.* 1993;16:281-284.

251

Mycobacterium leprae

CYBÈLE A. RENAULT | JOEL D. ERNST

Leprosy has a rich history dating to biblical times.[1] Even with the development of modern antibiotic therapy, leprosy continues to place a significant burden on individuals and society, and patients continue to be stigmatized by the diagnosis, leading some to avoid proper diagnosis and therapy. Peripheral nerve damage, the most common complication of leprosy, leads to the characteristic deformities of the disease; early detection and therapy can prevent significant morbidity and disability.

Of the chronic infectious diseases whose clinical and pathologic manifestations arise in a distinct and well-characterized spectrum, leprosy is among the best understood. At one end of the clinical spectrum, tuberculoid leprosy is characterized by a small number of skin lesions, few bacilli in lesions, and development and recruitment of T lymphocytes that contribute to control of the infection.[2,3] At the other extreme, lepromatous leprosy is characterized by a larger number of skin lesions, clinically apparent infiltration of peripheral nerves and skin lesions by a large number of bacilli, and the presence of fewer T lymphocytes in lesions whose effector mechanisms are unable to control the infection.[2,3]

The discovery of *M. leprae* has historical significance: Armauer Hansen discovered the microbe in 1873, before Koch's discovery of *M. tuberculosis*, but the inability to cultivate *M. leprae* in vitro (a problem that remains unsolved) allowed Koch to be credited with the discovery and the germ theory of disease.

Before the advent of effective antibiotics, treatment consisted of isolating patients in leprosaria, but in the past 25 years there has been a major change in both the management and understanding of leprosy. In the 1920s, the U.S. Public Health Service (USPHS) established a program for patients with leprosy that dramatically changed the manner in which this disease is managed. The United States formally adopted a multidrug treatment policy and an ambulatory care program in 1981, and under USPHS guidance the World Health Organization (WHO) adopted a similar program in 1982. Despite these advances, leprosy is still a disease that is far from being eradicated.

Epidemiology

Because detection of asymptomatic leprosy is difficult and because of the stigma associated with the diagnosis, estimates of leprosy incidence and prevalence are underestimated compared to those of other diseases. Because *M. leprae* cannot be cultured in vitro and because there is no sensitive and specific diagnostic test for the detection of individuals who are infected without clinical disease, transmission of leprosy is still poorly understood. The predominant mode of transmission is likely to be through respiratory droplets or nasal secretions, as up to 10^7 viable bacilli per day can be shed in respiratory secretions of people with multibacillary leprosy.[4] Modes of nonrespiratory transmission such as transplacental[5] or via breast milk[6] are also possible. Because *M. leprae* has been detected in skin,[7] sebaceous gland secretions, and eccrine sweat glands,[8] skin-to-skin transmission has not been excluded. Other modes of transmission such as soil, insect vectors, and exposure to infected animals (armadillos, chimpanzees, monkeys) remain speculative.

The likelihood of developing disease is determined by several variables. Age is an important factor, as clinical disease has a bimodal distribution: Adolescents aged 10-19 years of age are the most susceptible, followed by a second peak at the age of 30 years or older.[9] Gender is relevant in adult patients: In contrast to children, where there is no difference in prevalence between the sexes, adult men are twice as likely to develop the disease as adult women.[10] The risk of disease is associated with contact with infected individuals; individuals who are in contact with multibacillary patients are at highest risk of developing disease.[10]

Cases of leprosy exhibit geographic (e.g., village) and family clustering. Although clustering of leprosy in families can be due at least in part to shared environments and exposure, there is strong evidence for genetic determinants of susceptibility to leprosy.[11] Moreover, there are clearly genetic variations that influence susceptibility to the presence of infection (leprosy per se), whereas other genetic loci influence the clinical form of the disease (paucibacillary or multibacillary). Most early efforts to define the genetic determinants of susceptibility to leprosy were association studies that examined the frequency of human leukocyte antigen (HLA) types with leprosy per se or the clinical form. Although these studies demonstrated associations between HLA-DR2 (now subtyped as DRB1*1501 and DRB1*1502) and tuberculoid leprosy, they also revealed that HLA genes did not fully account for the genetic effects on susceptibility, and other genes have been identified whose variants contribute to leprosy susceptibility (Table 251-1).

A genome-wide linkage scan recently identified strong linkage between susceptibility to leprosy per se and a region on chromosome 6q25-6q26 in a Vietnamese population.[12] Subsequent analyses of that chromosomal region revealed specific single-nucleotide polymorphisms (SNPs) that formed haplotypes in the shared promoter region of the PARK2 and PACRG genes; heterozygosity and homozygosity for the susceptible haplotype were associated with very high odds ratios of 3.23 and 5.28, respectively, compared to homozygosity for the resistant haplotype; subsequent analysis in a Brazilian population confirmed the association of variation at the PARK2/PACRG locus with leprosy.[13] PARK2 is an E3 ubiquitin ligase, which indicates that regulated protein degradation in mononuclear phagocytes or Schwann cells, or both, is important for resistance to leprosy; the function of PACRG is unknown but is also thought to be related to proteasome function. In addition, high-resolution analysis of the 6p21 chromosomal region that was also linked to leprosy in Vietnamese families revealed that a hypofunctional variant (LTA+80 AA/AC) of the gene encoding the TNF-related cytokine lymphotoxin-α is associated with early-onset (i.e., before 15 years of age) leprosy, with an odds ratio of greater than 5; the same LTA+80 variant was associated with early-onset leprosy in cohorts in Brazil and India.[14]

In contrast to these findings, genetic studies have revealed a lack of association of leprosy susceptibility with the chromosomal region (5p) that contains the Th2 cytokine gene cluster.[15] Because a Th2 response is characteristic of lepromatous leprosy, this finding suggests that genetic variations in this region are not primary determinants of polarization of the immune response to *M. leprae*. Additional studies are necessary to understand more fully the genetic basis of susceptibility to leprosy and to define precisely the polymorphisms in the chromosomal regions linked to susceptibility.

GLOBAL EPIDEMIOLOGY

In 2007, WHO reported detection of 254,525 new cases of leprosy,[16] but active case finding has clearly established that there is an additional hidden caseload. In recent years, the number of incident cases has decreased by an average of almost 20% per year; this decrease can likely

TABLE 251-1	**Genetic Susceptibility in Leprosy**		
Gene or Chromosomal Region		**Clinical Form of Disease**	
	Leprosy per se	**Multibacillary**	**Paucibacillary**
HLA DRB1*1501[88]		S	
HLA DRB1*1502[89]			S
HLA DRB1*1501+1502[90]	S (Tuberculoid)		
HLA DRB1*04[91]	R		
HLA DRB1*10[91]	S		
NRAMP1 (SLC11A1) 3′ UTR[92,93]	S	S	
Vitamin D receptor nucleotide 352; homozygosity for C[94]		S	
Vitamin D receptor nucleotide 352; homozygosity for T[94]			S
TNF-α promoter (-308A)[95]		S	
TNF-α promoter (-308A)[96]	R	R	
IL-10 promoter (819TT)[96]			S
TAP2-B allele[97]			S
Toll-like Receptor 1 (TLR1) (I602S)[31]	R		
HLA/TNF haplotype segregation[98]		S	S
6q25[12]	S		
PARK2/PACRG[13]	S		
Lymphotoxin-α[14]	S		
10p13[12,99]	S		
20p12[100]	S		S

HLA, human leukocyte antigen; IL-10, interleukin-10; R, linkage or association with resistance; S, linkage or association with susceptibility; TNF, tumor necrosis factor.

be attributed to active case finding and to the widespread distribution of multidrug therapy free of cost. Of the 254,525 new cases detected in 2007, 171,552 were detected in South and East Asia, followed by 41,978 cases in the Americas and 31,037 cases in Africa.[16] The vast majority of cases in the Americas are in Brazil.

In 1982, WHO embarked on a campaign for the elimination of leprosy. The present goal of the WHO program is to reduce the prevalence of leprosy to less than 1 case per 10,000 people. The program has successfully increased the percentage of leprosy patients receiving MDT and has reduced the global prevalence of leprosy from estimates as high as 18 million to less than 2 million. At the beginning of 2008, there were only three remaining countries that reported a prevalence of more than 1 case per 10,000: Brazil, Nepal, and Timor-Leste. These three countries accounted for over one quarter of the registered cases at the beginning of 2008.[16]

UNITED STATES

The epidemiology of leprosy in the United States reflects immigration patterns, as the vast majority of cases are in Hispanic and Asian immigrants. There are currently approximately 6500 cases registered with the National Hansen's Disease Program, with 137 new cases reported in 2006. New York, California, Texas, Massachusetts, Florida, and Louisiana accounted for the largest number of cases (63%) in the 2006 surveillance report, but cases were reported from 30 states. The largest number of patients (36%) were self-identified as being of Asian or Pacific origin, followed closely (35%) by Hispanic whites and African-Americans. Almost three quarters of the patients were men, and patient age ranged from 7 to 83 years. A marked increase in cases occurred with the emigration of Southeast Asian refugees during 1978 to 1988, but this was not accompanied by an increase in cases in people born in the United States, indicating that transmission of leprosy within the United States is rare.[17] However, endemic cases have been

identified in the New York City metropolitan area, Mississippi, Louisiana, and Texas.[17-19]

Microbiology and Genome Sequence

Despite many generations of effort, *M. leprae* cannot be cultured in vitro. Consequently, knowledge of the biology of *M. leprae* has been restricted to biochemical and physiologic characterization of bacteria isolated from experimentally infected nine-banded armadillos. *M. leprae* is a straight or slightly curved rod-shaped organism, 1 to 8 μm long and 0.3 μm in diameter. It is gram positive and acid fast, although staining with carbol fuchsin can be irregular. On the basis of assays in footpads of immunodeficient mice, the doubling time of *M. leprae* has been estimated to be 11 to 13 days.[1] Like other mycobacteria, *M. leprae* possesses a highly lipid-rich cell wall, which contains diverse lipids and glycolipids, including an abundant antigenic glycolipid termed phenolic glycolipid 1 (PGL-1).

The availability of the genome sequence of *M. leprae* has provided substantial information on the biology of *M. leprae*, its relationship to other mycobacteria, potential explanations for the inability to culture it in vitro, and potential new targets for drug therapy. The genome contains approximately 3.3 million base pairs, with an average G + C content of 57.8%. It compares to the genome of *M. tuberculosis*, which contains approximately 4.4 million base pairs, with an average G + C content greater than 65%.[20] In addition to the reduction in the size of the *M. leprae* genome compared with that of *M. tuberculosis*, only 49.5% of the *M. leprae* genome is predicted to contain protein-coding genes, because of a high frequency of pseudogenes (approximately 27% of the genome) and noncoding DNA. Therefore, the functional genome of *M. leprae* appears to be less than 40% of the size of the genome of *M. tuberculosis*. Because it is generally believed that *M. leprae* and *M. tuberculosis* evolved from a common mycobacterial ancestor, *M. leprae* appears to have lost approximately 2000 genes since the divergence, which has left it dependent on highly specialized ecological niches for its survival.

Analysis of the residual functional genes of *M. leprae* in comparison with those of *M. tuberculosis* and the sequenced genomes of other bacteria has provided considerable insight into its biology. On the basis of the presence of intact operons, it appears that *M. leprae* has retained nearly all essential anabolic pathways, including synthesis of amino acids, purines, pyrimidines, nucleosides, nucleotides, and many vitamins and enzyme cofactors. In contrast, it lacks the diversity of the apparatus for lipid synthesis and modification characteristic of *M. tuberculosis*. In particular, *M. leprae* lacks methoxymycolates, probably because of the absence of the *mmaA2* and *mmaA3* genes whose products are responsible for methoxy modification of mycolic acids in *M. tuberculosis*.[21] In addition, *M. leprae* has only 6 genes encoding polyketide synthases, compared with 18 in *M. tuberculosis*. Because specific polyketides contribute to pathogenesis of *M. tuberculosis*[22] and *Mycobacterium ulcerans*,[23] the differential polyketide synthase gene content may account for some of the differences in pathogenesis of *M. leprae* compared with other virulent mycobacteria.

One of the polyketide synthases absent from the *M. leprae* genome is encoded by *mbtB*, which is essential for synthesis of salicylate-derived mycobactin siderophores in *M. tuberculosis*. An *M. tuberculosis* mutant that lacks *mbtB* is impaired in its ability to acquire iron and to grow in iron-poor media or macrophages.[22] The absence of the entire *mbt* operon from *M. leprae* implies that this species is impaired in its ability to acquire iron and must depend on other mechanisms for iron acquisition and retention, which may contribute to the narrow ecological niche occupied by *M. leprae*. A glycolipid that is important in *M. leprae* pathogenesis and that is absent from *M. tuberculosis* is phenolic glycolipid-1 (PGL-1). PGL-1 is derived from phthiocerol dimycocerosate (PDIM) by addition of O-methylated deoxy sugars, but analysis of the *M. leprae* genome sequence has not yet revealed the genes encoding the glycosyltransferases that modify PDIM to produce PGL-1.

An additional application of genome sequence data is the use of sequence variants for studies of evolution and for molecular epidemiology studies of leprosy transmission. A study using single-nucleotide polymorphisms, which are rare in the *M. leprae* genome (1 per 28,000 bp), revealed a global phylogeny of *M. leprae* that indicated that the bacteria originated in East Africa or the Near East and disseminated globally by human migration to Europe, West Africa, and the Americas.[24] In contrast, studies using variable number of tandem repeat (VNTR) typing have so far implied that their rate of variation may be excessively high for studies of human-to-human transmission, as they have revealed variable results from samples of different sites from individual patients.[25,26]

Immunology

CLINICAL AND IMMUNOLOGIC SPECTRUM OF LEPROSY

In endemic countries, clinical leprosy has long been categorized by two WHO-classified subtypes: paucibacillary, referring to five or fewer skin lesions and negative AFB skin slit smears, and multibacillary, referring to greater than five skin lesions and positive AFB skin slit smears. In resource-constrained regions where skin slit smears are not available, the advantage of the WHO classification system is that patients can be grouped on the basis of the number of skin lesions alone. The Ridley-Jopling classification system is also used to describe the subtype of disease. This system classifies patients into five types: tuberculoid (TT), borderline tuberculoid (BT), mid-borderline (BB), borderline lepromatous (BL), and lepromatous leprosy (LL), and is based on a combination of clinical manifestations (number and appearance of skin lesions, peripheral nerve thickening/impairment and systemic or mucosal involvement), the bacillary load, and histopathology.[2] Tuberculoid (TT) and lepromatous (LL) patients have *stable* cell-mediated immunity—that is, their disease manifestations do not change over time. In contrast, patients with borderline disease (BT, BB, BL) have *unstable* cell-mediated immunity, and their clinical manifestations may change over time (e.g., manifestations can "upgrade" or "downgrade" toward tuberculoid or lepromatous presentations, respectively). Some patients develop an indeterminate form of the disease that is distinct from the subtypes included within this spectrum. This form of leprosy is seen most frequently in young children, is associated with a short duration of symptoms and a lack of neurologic involvement, and can resolve without treatment.

The Ridley-Jopling classification system has been widely used, at least in part because of the clear correlation between the histologic appearance of the local immune response (abundant lymphocytes and well-formed granulomas in tuberculoid; fewer lymphocytes without well-formed granulomas in lepromatous) and the number of bacteria (few in tuberculoid; numerous in lepromatous). From these observations, a correlation between the nature of the immune response, control of bacterial growth, and clinical appearance in leprosy has provided a basis for studies of the protective cellular immune response to *M. leprae.*

MECHANISMS OF IMMUNITY

The early observation that tuberculoid leprosy is associated with large numbers of lymphocytes and low numbers of *M. leprae* in lesions supported the concept that adaptive cellular immunity contributes to control of the infection. A seminal contribution to understanding protective immunity in leprosy was the finding that tuberculoid leprosy was associated with lymphocyte expression of interleukin-2 (IL-2), lymphotoxin, and interferon-γ in lesions, whereas lepromatous leprosy was associated with expression of IL-4, IL-5, and IL-10, and not interferon-γ, in lesions.[3] This pattern of polarity of cytokine production fits the paradigm of helper T-cell type 1 (Th1) or helper T-cell type 2 (Th2) differentiation of the effector functions of T lymphocytes and has been used as the basis of further studies to understand the determinants of an effective immune response to *M. leprae.*

Given the evidence that a Th1 CD_4^+ T-cell response to *M. leprae* is associated with control of infection and a Th2 response is not, identifying the factors that determine the polarity of the immune response in leprosy has received considerable attention. Although individuals with lepromatous leprosy exhibit little, if any, Th1 immune response to *M. leprae* antigens, their CD_4^+ T lymphocytes are capable of responding to *M. tuberculosis* antigens with a Th1 (i.e., interferon-γ) response, which demonstrates that lepromatous leprosy is not the result of a global inability to generate a Th1 response.[27] This finding has focused attention on the interactions of *M. leprae* and antigen-presenting cells such as monocytes and dendritic cells because the outcome of these encounters can determine the polarity of naïve CD_4^+ T-cell differentiation (i.e., Th1 versus Th2).

As described in Chapter 9, antigen stimulation of CD_4^+ T lymphocytes is mediated by presentation of pathogen-derived peptide (bound to major histocompatibility complex class II) or glycolipid (bound to CD1a, b, c, or d) antigens on monocytes or dendritic cells for recognition by specific T-cell antigen receptors. The determinants of the polarity of differentiation of antigen-stimulated naïve T lymphocytes are imposed by antigen-presenting cells. One of the major determinants of Th1 differentiation of naïve T lymphocytes is IL-12, whose expression is approximately 10-fold higher in tuberculoid lesions than in lepromatous lesions,[28] although peripheral blood monocytes and monocyte-derived dendritic cells from patients with lepromatous leprosy and tuberculoid leprosy produce similar amounts of IL-12 in response to a triacylated lipopeptide derived from *M. leprae.*[27] Lipopeptide stimulation of antigen-presenting cell IL-12 production is mediated by Toll-like receptors 1 (TLR1) and 2 (TLR2), and expression of TLR1 and TLR2 is much higher in lesions of tuberculoid compared with lepromatous leprosy.[29] Deficient expression of TLR2 in lepromatous lesions may be secondary to the presence of IL-4, which downregulates expression of TLR2 on monocytes and monocyte-derived dendritic cells in vitro.[29]

In addition to TLR-stimulated production of IL-12, stimulation of antigen-presenting cells through CD40 by activated T cells expressing CD40L contributes to production of IL-12. Expression of CD40 and CD40L has also been found to be deficient in lepromatous compared with tuberculoid lesions.[30] The low expression of TLR1, TLR2, and CD40 in lepromatous lesions may contribute to deficient induction of IL-12, and the resulting deficiency of IL-12 in lepromatous lesions is consistent with failure to generate Th1, interferon-γ–producing CD_4^+ T cells that respond to *M. leprae* antigens. However, reports that a polymorphism in TLR1 that disrupts trafficking of TLR2 to the cell surface is associated with protection from leprosy per se[31] and from reversal reactions[32] indicates that the role of TLR2 is more complex than the in vitro studies imply.

Although understanding of the differences in the immune response in lepromatous compared with tuberculoid leprosy has advanced considerably, the essential initial determinant of the distinct responses remains to be identified. The polarity of the cellular immune response (i.e., Th1 versus Th2) is likely to be determined during the initial encounter of a naïve host with *M. leprae,* but it is not yet clear whether the essential determinant of that outcome is influenced by the route of infection, the precise phenotype of the antigen-presenting cells that present *M. leprae* antigens to naïve T cells, or other host cofactors such as infection with other pathogens. Further investigations of the determinants of T-cell differentiation are needed; in addition, studies of the contributions of other subsets of T lymphocytes, including Th17 and regulatory T cells, are likely to reveal additional insights into the immunopathogenesis of leprosy.

Pathogenesis of Nerve Damage

Peripheral sensory nerve damage is the leading cause of functional morbidity in people with leprosy and is characteristic of both paucibacillary and multibacillary disease. Peripheral nerve damage in leprosy can be mediated directly by *M. leprae*, as well as by the immune response to *M. leprae*.[33,34]

DIRECT NERVE DAMAGE BY MYCOBACTERIUM LEPRAE

M. leprae invades Schwann cells, the glial cells of the peripheral nervous system. Because Schwann cells form a functional unit with peripheral nerve axons surrounded by a basal lamina, studies have focused on the interaction of *M. leprae* with proteins of the basal lamina. These studies revealed that *M. leprae* specifically interacts with the G domain of the α_2-subunit of laminin-2, a neural-specific extracellular matrix protein.[35] This domain of laminin-2 can bind simultaneously to *M. leprae* and to the Schwann cell laminin receptor, α-dystroglycan, allowing high-affinity binding of *M. leprae* to Schwann cells by using laminin-2 as a bridging molecule.[36] Laminin-2 interacts with two distinct molecules on the surface of *M. leprae*, a 21-kDa protein and the abundant glycolipid PGL-1. The 21-kDa protein, termed *M. leprae laminin-binding protein* (ML-LBP21; also known as histone-like protein/Hlp[37]), interacts with the G4 module of the α-subunit of laminin-2, and ML-LBP21 is sufficient to mediate invasion of Schwann cells.[38] PGL-1, which is a highly abundant component of *M. leprae*, also binds to the α_2-subunit of laminin-2, through the G4 and G5 modules of the G domain.[39] PGL-1, like ML-LBP21/Hlp, is sufficient to mediate invasion of Schwann cells and interacts with laminin-2– through the unique trisaccharide of PGL-1 (3,6-di-O-methylglucose– linked α-1→4 to 2,3-di-O-methylrhamnose–linked β-1→2 to 3-O-methylrhamnose).[39,40] These studies provide considerable insight into the molecular mechanism of the direct interaction between *M. leprae* and Schwann cells of peripheral nerves and illustrate that *M. leprae* uses a neural-specific target for its apparently redundant bacterial molecules (ML-LBP21/Hlp and PGL-1) to achieve its unique tropism for peripheral nerves.

Once *M. leprae* or its PGL-1 is bound and internalized by Schwann cells, it can cause demyelination of peripheral nerves in vitro and in vivo in the absence of a cellular immune response.[33] Binding and activation of the receptor tyrosine kinase ErbB2 by one or more unidentified molecules on the surface of *M. leprae* can also lead to rapid demyelination of peripheral nerves in vitro.[41] Demyelination by *M. leprae* can promote further invasion of Schwann cells by the bacteria, as *M. leprae* preferentially invades nonmyelinated Schwann cell– axon units. *M. leprae*–mediated demyelination occurs without early cell death or toxicity, although Schwann cells and neurons can die by apoptosis later after infection.[33,42] In addition, dead *M. leprae* or PGL-1 shed from live or dying *M. leprae* can mediate peripheral nerve demyelination,[33] which may contribute to the ongoing nerve damage that can follow initiation of active chemotherapy.

In addition to PGL-1, an *M. leprae* 19-kDa lipoprotein can mediate Schwann cell apoptosis as an agonist of TLR2. TLR2 is expressed on Schwann cells in vitro and in vivo, and apoptotic Schwann cells can be found in human leprosy lesions.[42] The results of these studies clearly demonstrate that *M. leprae* is capable of direct peripheral nerve damage, even in the absence of inflammation or a cellular immune response. These mechanisms are likely to be especially responsible for peripheral nerve damage in multibacillary leprosy.

IMMUNOLOGICALLY MEDIATED PERIPHERAL NERVE DAMAGE IN LEPROSY

In addition to direct damage to peripheral nerves by *M. leprae*, there is abundant evidence that the immune response in leprosy contributes to nerve damage. This contribution is likely to account for much of the nerve damage that occurs in paucibacillary leprosy, in which the bacteria and PGL-1 are present in insufficient quantities to cause widespread nerve damage, and in reversal reactions, in which inflammation is particularly prominent.

Several distinct immunologic mechanisms probably contribute to nerve damage in leprosy.[43] Proinflammatory cytokines such as tumor

necrosis factor, IL-1β, and interferon-γ are especially prominent in lesions during reversal reactions,[44] when marked and irreversible nerve damage can occur. Because these molecules can directly and indirectly contribute to inflammatory tissue damage and can induce apoptosis of Schwann cells in vitro,[45] it is likely that these mediators play an active role in nerve damage. Reversal reactions are also characterized by an increase in the number of CD_4^+ T lymphocytes in lesions, and at least some of these CD_4^+ cells exhibit a cytotoxic phenotype and kill *M. leprae*–infected Schwann cells through antigen- and class II–dependent secretion of cytotoxic granule contents.[34] Whether similar mechanisms of nerve damage occur in chronic tuberculoid leprosy is not established, but qualitatively similar cytokines and T lymphocytes are found in tuberculoid lesions. Investigation of the potential roles of proinflammatory Th17 cells in reversal reactions and nerve damage in chronic tuberculoid leprosy are also warranted.

Clinical Manifestations

The cardinal manifestations of leprosy are hypopigmented, erythematous, or infiltrative skin lesions with or without neurologic signs or symptoms (including hypoesthesia, weakness, autonomic dysfunction, or peripheral nerve thickening); the clinical manifestations of leprosy vary significantly, depending on the subtype of disease. Patients with stable tuberculoid or borderline tuberculoid leprosy may present with skin lesions but without subjective complaints. In contrast, patients with advanced tuberculoid leprosy may present with peripheral neuropathy, which is generally asymmetric. Patients with stable lepromatous or borderline lepromatous leprosy may present with widespread infiltrative skin lesions or prominent peripheral neuropathy with secondary deformities (such as claw hand) or nonhealing painless ulcers. Reactions (described following) include reversal reactions, which present most often with increased erythema of preexisting skin lesions and progressive peripheral neuropathy, and erythema nodosum leprosum (ENL), which presents with systemic signs and painful erythematous skin nodules. The history of a patient with suspected leprosy should include whether the person has resided in an area with high prevalence and whether the person has been previously diagnosed or treated for leprosy. Certain patients may deny knowledge of a prior diagnosis or may report that skin lesions or neuropathy, or both, are acute, as they wish to avoid the stigma of a diagnosis of leprosy; this occurs even in emigrants to developed countries.

When performing the physical exam, the skin ideally should be examined in natural sunlight, as skin lesions are less likely to be noticed in artificial light. Peripheral nerves should be palpated for nerve thickness and tenderness, and both motor and sensory function (particularly for temperature and light touch) should be carefully evaluated.

Although skin lesions may involve any part of the body, they are infrequently found on the scalp, axillae, or perineum. Four typical types of skin lesions are noted: macules, plaques, diffuse infiltrated lesions, or subcutaneous nodules ("lepromas"). Patients with tuberculoid (TT) disease typically have 1-3 macules or plaques with sharp and well-defined borders. Dry, scaling lesional skin is frequent, and lesions have significant sensory loss. Borderline leprosy encompasses three subtypes: borderline tuberculoid (BT), mid-borderline (BB), or borderline lepromatous (BL); lesions in this group are often annular. Borderline tuberculoid (BT) patients typically have 5-25 macular or plaquelike skin lesions, which may have decreased sensation (although they are not fully anesthetic, as in TT patients). Mid-borderline (BB) patients have an even higher number of skin lesions, usually greater than 25. The lesions are typically papules or plaques with irregular margins and are of variable size, shape, and distribution. Borderline lepromatous (BL) patients have innumerable macules, papules, or plaques; these skin lesions may become infiltrated and nodular. The clinical manifestations of lepromatous leprosy (LL), the most severe form of the disease, are caused by a high mycobacterial load in the absence of an efficacious cell-mediated immune response. Skin lesions are characterized by the insidious onset of ill-defined macules, followed by the development of a symmetrical nonscaling infiltrative dermopathy. Skin findings are most pronounced in the cooler body areas (such as the earlobes, the central portion of the face, and the extensor surfaces of the thighs and forearms), and sensation is intact. "Leonine facies," or thickening of facial skin with accentuation of the skin creases, is a classic descriptor for this type of leprosy. Hair loss, often involving the eyelashes (ciliary madarosis) and the lateral third of the eyebrows (superciliary madarosis), is a late finding. Lepromatous patients can suffer from involvement of the eye, nasal mucosa (leading to septal perforation and to saddle nose deformity), larynx, liver, kidney, and bone—the latter leading to the characteristic bone resorption and shortening of digits that are severely disabling in these patients.

In addition to skin findings, the degree of hypoesthesia aids in clinically classifying leprosy. The degree of hypoesthesia depends on the location of the lesion, the size of the lesion, and the degree of a Th1 immune response. Tuberculoid lesions are generally hypoesthetic, although exceptions do occur—for example, small tuberculoid lesions on the highly innervated face may have intact sensation. In contrast, the skin lesions of multibacillary leprosy (borderline lepromatous and lepromatous) generally have intact sensation, although occasionally borderline lepromatous lesions may exhibit hypoesthesia. In addition to lesional hypoesthesia, peripheral neuropathies occur throughout the leprosy spectrum. Marked peripheral nerve thickening (especially in superficial nerves, such as the ulnar, median, and posterior tibial nerves) is characteristic of both borderline and lepromatous disease. In India and Nepal, a proportion (5% or higher, depending on the geographic region) of individuals with leprosy present with a pure neuritic form, which lacks skin lesions and manifests purely as asymmetrical neuropathy. Diagnosis of this form of leprosy requires nerve biopsy, and histology may reveal any of the disease subtypes.

DIFFERENTIAL DIAGNOSIS

Each of the major clinical manifestations of leprosy has a distinct differential diagnosis. Tuberculoid lesions or reactions often have an overlying fine scale, which resembles common inflammatory dermatoses such as eczema and psoriasis. The scaling appearance may be confused with pityriasis versicolor or dermatophyte infections. However, the granulomatous response in leprosy is generally more infiltrative than that seen in typical inflammatory dermatoses. In addition, there is loss of sensation in tuberculoid lesions, which is almost pathognomonic of leprosy. Hypopigmented lesions may be confused with vitiligo, although vitiligo is defined by complete loss of pigment, in contrast to the partial pigment loss seen in leprosy. At the lepromatous end of the spectrum, an infiltrative dermopathy is present, sensation is intact, and lesions lack scale. A biopsy and Fite stain distinguish leprosy from other infiltrative disorders, such as cutaneous tuberculosis, sarcoidosis, swimming pool granuloma (*Mycobacterium marinum*), granuloma annulare, granuloma multiforme, ANCA-associated (formerly Wegener's) granulomatosis, tertiary syphilis, cutaneous or post kala-azar leishmaniasis, Lyme disease, deep fungal infections, onchocerciasis, lupus profundus, or cutaneous lymphomas.

Another common presentation of leprosy is as a leprosy reaction (reversal reaction or erythema nodosum leprosum [ENL]), simulating lupus erythematosus, rheumatoid arthritis, viral exanthems, urticaria, drug eruptions, and other vascular reaction patterns such as erythema multiforme. As leprosy can itself be associated with autoimmune phenomena, including positive antinuclear antibody, rheumatoid factor, thyroid autoantibodies, and Hashimoto's thyroiditis, a biopsy and Fite stain are required to make the distinction.

The third common way for leprosy to arise is as a peripheral neuropathy. As the differential diagnosis of peripheral neuropathy is large, a high index of suspicion is required to make the diagnosis of neural leprosy. Palpation of the nerves may reveal thickened nerves, which are suggestive of leprosy, but a nerve biopsy is required to confirm the diagnosis, as other diseases (such as amyloidosis or neurofibromatosis) can also cause nerve thickening. As biopsy of peripheral nerves sacrifices function, judicious selection is required. The sural nerve is pre-

ferred, as it results in only a mild loss of sensation on the lateral aspect of the foot that can improve with time. Fite stain of the nerve usually reveals only sparse bacilli and a granulomatous tuberculoid histopathology but rarely a pure neural leprosy is multibacillary.

Diagnosis

Clinical examination, in combination with skin slit smears, is a common means of diagnosing leprosy in endemic countries. Skin slit smears play an important role in both the diagnosis and the classification of disease, as they offer a means to estimate the bacillary load. The skin slit procedure involves making a small incision through the epidermis, scraping the dermal surface of the skin (including the edge of the lesion), smearing the scrapings on a glass slide, and then using heat fixation and Ziehl-Neelsen staining (or Fite staining, if available) to detect the organism. Ideally, at least six sites should be sampled, including the skin lesions themselves, the earlobes, eyebrows, elbow, knees, and nasal mucosa. The bacillary index is based on a logarithmic scale per high-powered field (HPF), with a range from 1+ to 6+ acid-fast bacilli. For example, 1+ refers to 1-10 bacilli per HPF, and 6+ refers to more than 1000 bacilli per HPF. Although skin slit smears are poorly sensitive (especially for individuals with paucibacillary disease), their high specificity makes them clinically useful to identify the most infectious patients (i.e., patients with lepromatous disease).

When the resources are available, histopathology remains the gold standard for establishing a definitive diagnosis and for accurately classifying the subtype of disease. Skin biopsies should be taken entirely from within the active lesion; normal tissue is not helpful in the pathologic evaluation. The clinician's index of suspicion needs to be followed up by a pathologist's ability to properly perform Fite staining of tissue biopsy specimens with appropriate positive controls for the staining. The National Hansen's Program offers pathologic evaluation of biopsy specimens free of charge (http://www.hrsa.gov/hansens/clinicalcenter.htm; 1-800-642-2477).

It should be emphasized that although *M. leprae* is acid fast, it is particularly sensitive to alcohol decolorization, and the Fite or modified Fite stain is essential; Ziehl-Neelsen staining may produce false-negative results. With proper Fite staining, lepromatous leprosy reveals numerous (>1000 per HPF) acid-fast bacilli, including clumps, termed globi (Fig. 251-1). With progression toward the tuberculoid pole, the number of bacilli decreases to 100 to 1000/HPF in borderline lepromatous disease; they are frequent (10 to 100/HPF) in borderline, scattered to rare (0.1 to 10/HPF) in borderline tuberculoid, and rare or totally absent in polar tuberculoid disease. At the paucibacillary tuberculoid pole, the diagnosis of leprosy can be made in the absence of acid-fast bacilli with well-formed noncaseating granulomas and nerve involvement (Fig. 251-2).

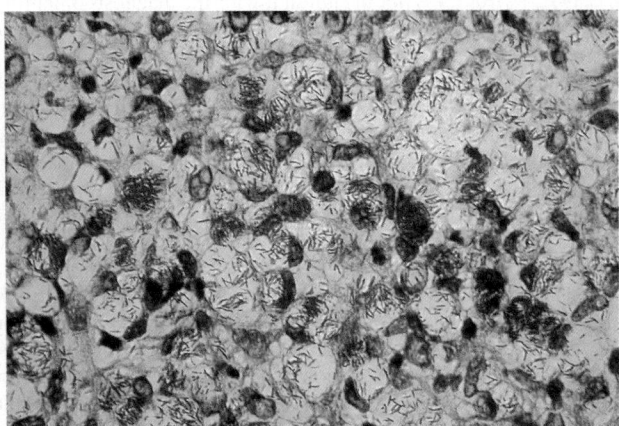

Figure 251-1 **Multibacillary, or lepromatous, leprosy shows numerous Fite-positive organisms and only rare lymphocytes.**

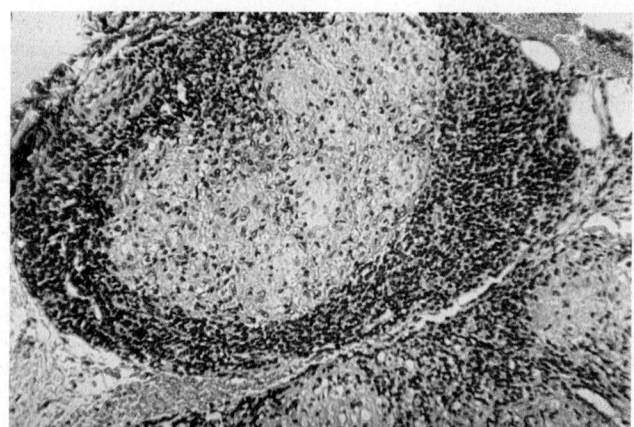

Figure 251-2 Paucibacillary, or tuberculoid, leprosy shows a "sarcoidal" granuloma with nerve involvement. Macrophages have an active secretory hyaline appearance with many lymphocytes. Fite staining may be negative or show only a few organisms.

In addition to the Fite stain, hematoxylin and eosin and immunohistochemistry are helpful in making the diagnosis and identifying the type of leprosy. In lepromatous leprosy, the macrophages (or histiocytes) are flaccid, inactive, foamy (due to accumulation of host lipids[46]) cells (termed Virchow cells) because of the lack of macrophage activation in the absence of local interferon-γ. There are also very few lymphocytes, and the lymphocytes that are present produce IL-10 or IL-4, or both, and not interferon-γ.[44] In contrast to lepromatous leprosy, in tuberculoid and borderline tuberculoid disease, macrophage stimulation by interferon-γ results in a hyaline appearance of an active secretory cell with a surrounding mantle of numerous CD4 and CD8 T lymphocytes.[47] Borderline lepromatous, borderline, and borderline tuberculoid give a picture between these two extremes. In an immunohistochemical study of lepromatous skin, an intradermal injection of interferon-γ upgraded lepromatous leprosy infiltrates toward a borderline tuberculoid picture with epidermal proliferation.[48]

Serologic assays detecting antibodies against PGL-1 have been developed in an attempt to facilitate the diagnosis of leprosy. As these assays reflect bacillary load in untreated patients, PGL-1 serology is most sensitive in individuals close to the lepromatous pole of disease (with a bacillary index of 4+ or higher) but becomes less sensitive as patients approach the tuberculoid pole (with a bacillary index less than 4+). False-positive tests may be found in nonleprosy patients, with highest rates in patients with tuberculosis and or autoimmune diseases.[49] Because of its poor ability to detect early and paucibacillary cases, PGL-1 serology is not in clinical use for the diagnosis of leprosy. Investigations are currently under way to evaluate and develop serologic tests using other *M. leprae* protein antigens.

Following the completion of *M. leprae* genomic sequencing in 2001, new diagnostic techniques have been developed, particularly using real-time or conventional polymerase chain reaction (PCR) to detect *M. leprae* DNA. Although PCR is highly sensitive in multibacillary patients, it is less sensitive in patients with paucibacillary disease.[50] Additional immunodiagnostic assays based on antigens unique to *M. leprae* as revealed by the genome sequence appear promising as new tools in diagnosis of asymptomatic as well as clinical leprosy.[51]

Similar to the intradermal tuberculin skin test (TST) for *M. tuberculosis*, a delayed-type hypersensitivity reaction, the lepromin reaction (also called the Mitsuda reaction), exists for *M. leprae*. This test involves an intradermal inoculation of heat-killed *M. leprae*, and the diameter of induration is measured, typically 4 weeks after placement. The lepromin reaction is not used in the diagnosis of leprosy but instead has been used to classify patients within the Ridley-Jopling system.

Reactions

Type 1 (reversal reactions) and type 2 (erythema nodosum leprosum) reactions can occur before, during, or following the completion of treatment, and they generally require immediate treatment in order to prevent clinical progression of neuropathy. Infectious diseases specialists in the Western world are frequently consulted for the management of these reactions; clinicians should therefore consider leprosy reactions on the differential diagnosis in patients from endemic regions who present with systemic or neurologic (or both) skin symptoms.

REVERSAL REACTIONS (LEPRA TYPE 1 REACTIONS)

Reversal reactions, a leading cause of neurologic impairment in leprosy, can occur throughout the disease spectrum with the exception of polar tuberculoid disease. These reactions are the consequence of the development of an increase in the Th1 cellular immune response and therefore represent a vigorous host response against *M. leprae* in the skin and nerves, with local production of interferon-γ and tumor necrosis factor[44] combined with the effects of cytolytic CD4+ T cells.[34]

Reversal reactions are recognized clinically by increased erythema, warmth, edema, and occasional ulceration of preexisting cutaneous plaques and nodules (Fig. 251-3), in combination with increased swelling and tenderness of peripheral nerves (especially the ulnar and the posterior tibial nerves). There may be a peripheral lymphocytosis, and skin biopsy may show an accompanying increase in lymphocytes with nerve involvement. Although focal symptoms can be severe, occasionally leading to nerve abscesses and necrosis, systemic symptoms are unusual. Type 1 reactions are most frequently seen in patients with borderline disease (BT, BB, BL), as these patients have a fluctuating (unstable) cell-mediated immune response. This type of reaction can also be seen in women postpartum, as a consequence of immune restoration following delivery.

ERYTHEMA NODOSUM LEPROSUM (LEPRA TYPE 2 REACTIONS)

Erythema nodosum leprosum (ENL) is clinically distinguished from reversal reactions by the acute development of new painful, tender, and erythematous subcutaneous nodules (Fig. 251-4). ENL is thought to result from antigen-antibody complex deposition in the skin with the subsequent activation of complement. It is associated with high levels of TNF, which may decrease with treatment.[52] The peripheral blood may show a polymorphonuclear leukocytosis with a left shift, and neutrophils infiltrate the immune complex deposits, occasionally leading to vasculitis and ulceration.

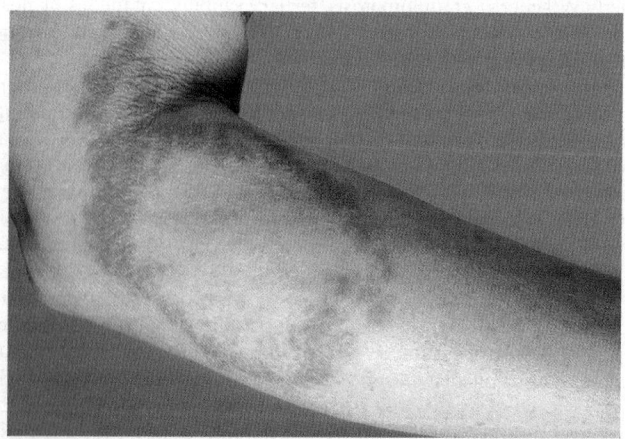

Figure 251-3 Reversal reactions are clinically recognized by erythema outlining infiltrative plaques.

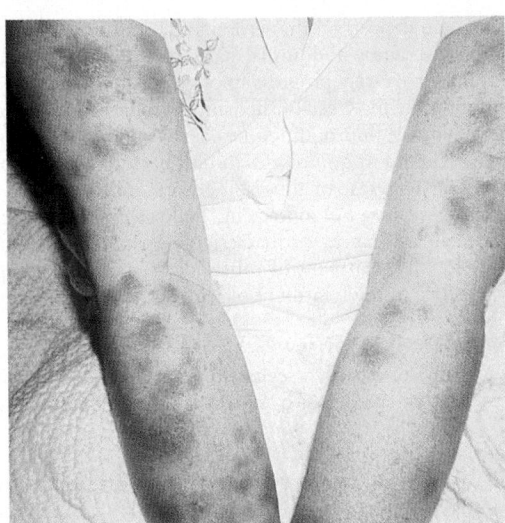

Figure 251-4 Erythema nodosum leprosum is recognized clinically by discrete subcutaneous red nodules (panniculitis).

Clinically, ENL skin lesions occur in clusters and are classically found on the extensor surfaces of the lower extremities and on the face. Although manifestations are most common in the skin, ENL can involve many organs, leading to arthralgias, frank arthritis, or dactylitis, severe neuritis, lymphadenitis, nasal involvement (rhinitis or epistaxis), eye involvement (iridocyclitis, leading to glaucoma and blindness), nephritis, orchitis (potentially leading to hypogonadism and sterility), and edema in the face or extremities. Unlike type 1 reactions, systemic symptoms are common in ENL, with patients frequently presenting with malaise and fever up to 40° C. In severe cases, ENL can be life-threatening, presenting with features similar to septic shock.

Type 2 reactions are typically seen in lepromatous (LL) and borderline lepromatous (BL) patients, as these are the two patient groups that have the highest levels of *M. leprae* antigens and antibodies. ENL typically occurs during the first 2 years after the initiation of treatment. One study found that the mean time to presentation with ENL was 3.7 months after initiation of MDT,[53] although patients may present with ENL after their course of MDT is complete. Patients with ENL may present with single acute episodes, a relapsing, remitting form comprised of multiple acute episodes, or a chronic, continuous form; one study has reported that the chronic form was most common, comprising 62.5% of cases in an Indian cohort.

LUCIO'S PHENOMENON

Lucio's phenomenon (also referred to as erythema necroticans) is an uncommon but potentially fatal form of reaction in multibacillary leprosy that is distinct from type 1 (reversal reaction) or type 2 (ENL) reactions.[54] It is a necrotizing vasculitis caused by endothelial invasion of *M. leprae* that is clinically manifest by bluish or violaceous and hemorrhagic plaques, followed by necrotic ulcerations (Fig. 251-5). These symptoms typically occur in the absence of systemic complaints or leukocytosis. This phenomenon is most commonly seen in Central America, although cases have been reported in India and Brazil.

▣ Long-Term Complications

The major chronic complications and deformities of leprosy are due to nerve damage, involving the peripheral nerve trunks, the small dermal nerves, or both. Nerve damage can be purely autonomic, leading to anhidrosis—skin drying and cracking; it can result in sensory deficits, leading to chronic, nonhealing injuries and ulcers; and it can be pure motor, resulting in muscle paralysis (especially of the small muscles of the hand and foot) due to motor trunk involvement.

Skin lesions overlying a nerve trunk distribution predict the involvement of that particular nerve, which is frequently palpable on examination. The posterior tibial nerve is the most frequently affected, followed by the ulnar, median, lateral popliteal, and facial nerves.[55] Similar to patients with diabetic neuropathy, sensory deficits in leprosy may lead to undetected trauma, ulceration, and osteomyelitis, which ultimately result in tissue damage and bone resorption. Patients should be referred to appropriate rehabilitation medicine specialists, when available, for management of chronic neuropathy and injury prevention. Facial deformity caused by facial nerve palsies and skin infiltration are amenable to reconstructive surgery.

The eye is also a site of involvement in leprosy, and all leprosy patients should be examined by an ophthalmologist. One study found that 2.8% of patients with multibacillary disease were blind, and an additional 11% of these patients had potentially blinding ocular pathology at the time of diagnosis.[56] Infection with *M. leprae* causes visual impairment via direct invasion of the skin and eye itself or through involvement of the ocular nerves. The most common causes of blindness in leprosy are lagophthalmos (an inability to close the eye, secondary to facial nerve involvement) with resulting exposure keratopathy or corneal ulceration; corneal ulceration due to trigeminal nerve involvement, resulting from decreased corneal sensation, decreased blinking and increased risk of trauma; iridocyclitis; and secondary cataracts.[57] It is important to check patients for an intact corneal reflex and, if it is absent, take appropriate precautions to avoid corneal drying, injury, and opacification. *M. leprae* can grow in the uveal tract, and frank uveitis can occur, especially in cases of ENL. It is important to be aware that ocular ENL can still be active even after ENL in the skin and joints is controlled. Ocular ENL requires topical corticosteroids. Often a low dose of thalidomide (50 to 100 mg/day) can help protect the patient from chronic active uveitis and progressive loss of sight.

The testicles are a site of predilection for multibacillary leprosy, and multibacillary patients should be screened for elevated follicle-stimulating hormone or luteinizing hormone and decreased testosterone levels. Even patients with multibacillary leprosy who have received adequate antibiotic therapy and are bacillus negative are at risk for progressive testicular dysfunction, including infertility. Hypogonadal males are also at greater risk for osteopenia and frank osteoporosis.

▣ Therapy
ANTIMICROBIAL THERAPY

Background
Before the advent of antibiotics, there was no effective treatment for leprosy, and isolation in leprosaria was the standard approach to disease control and therapy. Dapsone was the first antibiotic found to

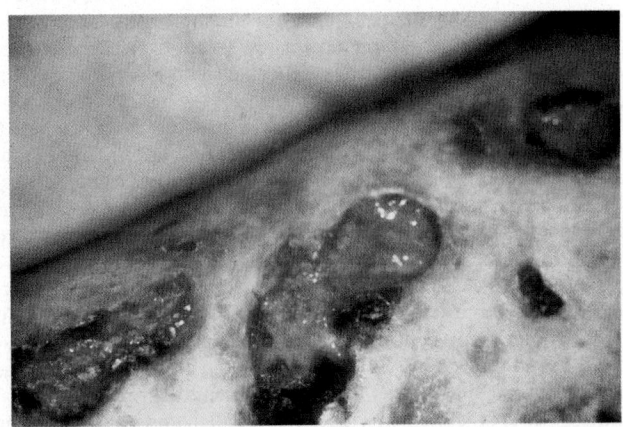

Figure 251-5 Lucio's phenomenon is recognized clinically by erosions and ulcerations secondary to underlying vasculitis.

be effective for leprosy, on the basis of trials conducted in the 1940s and 1950s. Dapsone monotherapy was the standard of care worldwide until the 1970s, when reports of treatment efficacy with rifampin and clofazimine began to appear, and when reports of *M. leprae* resistance to dapsone monotherapy (secondary to missense mutations in the *folP1* gene) emerged. In 1981 the USPHS officially adopted the policy of MDT, and WHO followed with a modified protocol shortly thereafter.

Agents to Treat Leprosy

The three established antimicrobial agents are dapsone, rifampin, and clofazimine. Minocycline is also effective[58] and has proved useful when a patient is intolerant of first-line agents. Fluoroquinolones are used in select cases (e.g., in cases when rifampin cannot be used due to potential drug interactions, or in cases of rifampin or dapsone resistance).

Dapsone, a weakly bactericidal drug that blocks folic acid synthesis, is inexpensive, well absorbed after oral administration, has a long serum half-life (28 hours), and is well tolerated by most patients. Dapsone is safe for use in pregnancy. It is routinely used at a dose of 50-100 mg/day. Glucose-6-phosphate dehydrogenase (G6PD)–deficient individuals are susceptible to dapsone-induced methemoglobinemia and hemolysis, and all patients should be screened for G6PD deficiency before starting dapsone. If a patient has mild G6PD deficiency (the African type; caused by mutations that result in instability of the enzyme), dapsone can be started at 25 mg/day, but close monitoring for anemia is necessary. In addition to methemoglobinemia and hemolytic anemia, dapsone can cause bone marrow suppression and profound neutropenia. Other rare adverse effects of dapsone include hepatitis, cholestatic jaundice, and "dapsone syndrome," which typically occurs within 6 weeks of treatment initiation and is characterized by exfoliative dermatitis, generalized lymphadenopathy, fever, and hepatosplenomegaly.[1]

Rifampin, a DNA-dependent RNA polymerase inhibitor, is the most bactericidal drug against *M. leprae*, as determined by the decrease in viability of bacteria in the mouse footpad assay. It is rapidly absorbed after oral administration and has a serum half-life of approximately 3 hours. It is routinely used at a dose of 600 mg/day for treatment of leprosy but should never be used in monotherapy, as resistance can develop with single-point mutations in its target: RNA polymerase II. Because rifampin is actively bactericidal and rapid release of components from dead bacteria can have proinflammatory effects, rifampin is contraindicated during active reversal reactions or ENL. Adverse effects of rifampin include a maculopapular skin rash, hepatotoxicity, an influenza-like syndrome (most frequent with intermittent therapy), and orange discoloration of tears, urine, saliva, and sweat. Thrombocytopenia occurs occasionally, but the platelet count rarely decreases below 10^5/L. If mild thrombocytopenia occurs, rifampin can be continued if the platelet count does not decrease below 10^5/L. Rifampin also induces cytochrome P-450 3A4, 2C8, and 2C9, and decreases serum concentrations of many drugs, including corticosteroids and oral contraceptives. Rifampin decreases serum concentrations of dapsone, but this is not clinically significant with a dapsone dose of 100 mg/day.

Clofazimine is a lipophilic dye that is bacteriostatic against *M. leprae*. Clofazimine has a very long (70-day) half-life and appears to have anti-inflammatory activity as well as direct bacteriostatic activity, although its target(s) and mechanism of action are unknown. The usual dose of clofazimine for leprosy is 50 mg/day, except when used to treat reversal reactions or ENL, when up to 200-300 mg/day may be used. Clofazimine is generally very well tolerated; its major side effect is nearly universal discoloration of the skin and conjunctiva. The skin discoloration can range from reddish tan to bluish black but is reversible within 6 to 12 months of discontinuing the drug. Clofazimine has little bone marrow toxicity or hepatotoxicity. Chronic reactional patients who are maintained with prolonged high doses of clofazimine (200-300 mg/day) need to be monitored for enteropathy, as clofazi-mine crystals can deposit on the serosal surface of the gastrointestinal tract, leading to crampy abdominal pain, mild nausea, and diarrhea. This condition may rarely progress to bowel obstruction.

In addition to the three established antimycobacterial agents for the treatment of leprosy, fluoroquinolones have been used successfully in clinical trials. The fluoroquinolones inhibit bacterial DNA replication by inhibiting DNA-gyrase or topoisomerase. Ciprofloxacin is ineffective against *M. leprae*, but ofloxacin, pefloxacin, sparfloxacin, and moxifloxacin all appear to be bactericidal. Moxifloxacin has been under study for the treatment of tuberculosis, and it also appears to be highly effective in the treatment of leprosy.[59]

Regimens to Treat Leprosy

Standard therapy for leprosy uses multiple drugs to increase the cure rate and prevent emergence of drug resistance and treatment failure.

U.S. Regimens

Paucibacillary leprosy: Dapsone 100 mg/day plus rifampin 600 mg/day for 12 months.

Multibacillary leprosy: Dapsone 100 mg/day plus rifampin 600 mg/day plus clofazimine 50 mg/day for 24 months.

World Health Organization Regimens

Single-lesion paucibacillary leprosy: Single-dose regimen with rifampin 600 mg, ofloxacin 400 mg, and minocycline 100 mg (ROM). This regimen was proposed by WHO in 1997 following the availability of results from a trial in India.[60] However, the single-dose regimen is thought to be less effective than the regimen for paucibacillary leprosy (described following)[61]; one study found that patient age 40 years or older and positive *M. leprae* PCR were risk factors for poor clinical outcome (defined as a reversal reaction, with or without neuritis) in patients treated with ROM.[62] Long-term studies are needed to assess the risk of relapse with single-dose treatment.

Paucibacillary leprosy (Intermediate, TT, or BT): Dapsone 100 mg/day, unsupervised, plus rifampin 600 mg once monthly, supervised, for 6 months.

Multibacillary leprosy (BB, BL, or LL): Dapsone 100 mg/day, plus clofazimine 50 mg/day, unsupervised, with rifampin 600 mg monthly and clofazimine 300 mg monthly, supervised. The original recommended duration of therapy was 2 years, but this recommendation was later shortened to 12 months[63]; however, some authorities recommend continuing treatment for 2 years in the setting of a high bacillary index (4+ or greater),[57] preferably until skin smears are negative. It is important to note that U.S. guidelines for the treatment of leprosy are significantly different from the WHO MDT recommendations, although they are both based on the same principle: use of multiple drugs to avoid drug resistance. Information and consultation are available through the National Hansen's Disease Program in Baton Rouge, Louisiana (http://www.hrsa.gov/hansens/clinicalcenter.htm; 1-800-642-2477). The U.S. recommendations include daily rifampin, the most bactericidal of the antibiotics against *M. leprae*, and recommend daily clofazimine only for chronically reactional patients or patients with suspected resistance. In the U.S. regimens, longer durations of therapy are recommended, but this can be individualized, and monotherapy beyond 5 or 10 years is probably not necessary when the patient is clinically bacillus negative. Because of the large initial load of bacilli in multibacillary leprosy, pockets of bacillary persistence may be detected by nerve biopsy even after "adequate" treatment.

RESPONSE TO THERAPY

Response to therapy is seen clinically as flattening and disappearance of papules, nodules, and plaques and improvement of nerve function. Quantitation of bacillary load to assess response to treatment is cumbersome and at best is semiquantitative. The number of intact Fite-positive organisms in slit smears or skin biopsies is referred to as the morphologic index and should be zero by the end of therapy. The presence of intact organisms after a patient has received chemotherapy for several months should cause concern for either noncompliance or drug resistance, although the persistence of mycobacteria on biopsy may represent non-viable *M. leprae*. In this regard, one study found that following treatment with MDT for 24 months in patients with lepromatous disease, mycobacteria noted on biopsy specimens were not viable, regardless of the initial bacillary load. In contrast, in lepromatous patients treated with MDT for 12 months, 3.3% of patients with a high bacillary index pretreatment were found to have viable organisms on biopsy.[64]

Occasionally, patients who have been adequately treated later show evidence of chronic reversal reactions and late neuropathies. Such patients, when bacillus negative, are considered not to have relapses but to have late reversal reactions, and they should be treated with low-dose clofazimine (50-100 mg, 3 times a week), with monitoring of their nerve function. If the nerves remain stable or improve, clofazimine should be continued until all signs of reaction have cleared. If the nerves show evidence of deterioration, additional therapy is warranted, including increasing the dose of clofazimine, adding a second or third antibiotic, or giving a course of corticosteroids, depending on the rate and degree of nerve deterioration.

Role of Resistance Testing

M. leprae resistance to the antimycobacterial agents has been reported and is associated with mutations in the *folP1* (dapsone), *rpoB* (rifampin), and *gyrA* (fluoroquinolone) genes. Resistance to clofazimine is uncommon. The gold-standard method for resistance testing is the labor-intensive mouse footpad susceptibility assay although DNA-based assays (e.g., PCR) have been developed and are in increasing use. Testing for resistance is currently performed only in cases of relapsed disease, although some experts also recommend intermittent testing of new cases to monitor for emerging resistance.

RELAPSES AND TREATMENT OF RELAPSES

Reported relapse rates following the recommended course of MDT are highly variable. Risk of relapse directly correlates with bacillary load; one study found that individuals with a bacillary index of 4 or greater at diagnosis or an index of 3 or greater after completion of MDT had the highest risk of relapse—up to 20%.[65] If a patient who has a history of adequate treatment later presents with new lesions that are bacillus positive, the patient should be considered as a new case and should be treated according to the recommended regimens. The more thorough U.S. regimens rather than once-monthly rifampin should be used when affordable.

TREATMENT OF REACTIONS

Treatment of Reversal Reactions

The decision on treatment of reactions should be made clinically, and antimycobacterial chemotherapy with clofazimine or dapsone, or both, should be continued throughout the course of therapy of a reactional state; rifampin should be withheld in the presence of active neuritis. In cases of borderline tuberculoid and borderline leprosy, a sudden loss of sensation requires prompt institution of corticosteroids without waiting for laboratory findings, as delay in instituting therapy can lead to permanent nerve damage and disability. In patients with subpolar lepromatous and borderline lepromatous leprosy, and in some patients with borderline and borderline tuberculoid leprosy, reversal reactions may be low grade, and management is based on clinical judgment and the patient's level of discomfort.

If the reaction is confined to the skin, as it often is in lepromatous and occasionally in borderline lepromatous leprosy, it is reasonable to allow it to smolder, as the reaction is a manifestation of a more effective cellular immune response. If there is evidence of peripheral nerve deterioration, which is common in borderline lepromatous and nearly universal in borderline and borderline tuberculoid patients with reversal reactions, it is important to institute prednisone promptly at a dosage of 40-80 mg/day. The rate of tapering needs to be individualized and in general should be 10 mg per month or less in order to avoid permanent nerve damage and residual deformity. The expected recovery of nerve function is variable and depends on the particular nerve involved; one study found neurologic improvement following steroid treatment for 3 months in 30% to 84% of patients; patients who had the shortest duration of symptoms prior to the initiation of therapy and those who had less severe symptoms at presentation had the best prognosis.[66] For chronic neuropathies with intact sensation, adding clofazimine or increasing the dose of clofazimine is an additional option. Rifampin should be withheld until the nerves become quiescent. Thalidomide, because of its ability to upregulate Th1 responses and its potential neurotoxicity, is contraindicated in pure reversal reactions. Occasionally, patients who present with ENL (see the next section) undergo a transition to mixed reactions and reversal reactions, which requires adjustment of therapy.

Treatment of Erythema Nodosum Leprosum

The treatment of choice for ENL is thalidomide. Although corticosteroids can also be used, thalidomide is preferred as a steroid-sparing agent in order to avoid complications associated with prolonged administration of the high steroid doses required to control the disease. Notably, however, corticosteroids (prednisone, 60-80 mg/day) are used to treat ENL in some thalidomide-refractory cases and in reproductive-aged women, in whom thalidomide is contraindicated.

Thalidomide is available from Celgene Corporation (www.celgene .com) and requires that patients and the prescribing physician be enrolled in the System for Thalidomide Education and Prescribing Safety (STEPS) program to avoid the well-known teratogenic effect of phocomelia. The mechanism of action of thalidomide is incompletely understood, although one of its two enantiomers suppresses the release of TNF from mononuclear cells,[67] and it is likely to have multiple relevant cellular targets in ENL.[68] To treat ENL, the clinician should initiate therapy at a dose dictated by the intensity of the signs and symptoms. If a multibacillary patient has severe ENL with large subcutaneous plaques, frank arthritis, and temperature in excess of 38.8° C, a dose of 100 mg 4 times a day is indicated. With control of the reaction, tapering at a rate of approximately 50-100 mg a week can be initiated, to a maintenance dose of 50-100 mg at night. For milder cases of ENL with low-grade fever and a few scattered subcutaneous nodules, 50-100 mg at night may be sufficient. Because the major side effect of thalidomide, other than congenital malformations and somnolence, is peripheral neuropathy, it is incumbent on the clinician to attempt periodically to taper patients off thalidomide completely. The peripheral neuropathy side effect is dose dependent with almost no neurotoxicity below 50 mg/day.[69] Because thalidomide may actually enhance Th1 immunity, it should not be used for pure reversal reactions. Occasionally, ENL is refractory to thalidomide, or the reaction is more of a reversal reaction or mixed reaction.

Management of chronic reactions, often lasting months and years, is among the most challenging problems encountered in clinical leprosy. As with chronic corticosteroid therapy for any indication, patients require monitoring for and management of hypertension, diabetes, peptic ulcers, reactivation of tuberculosis, glaucoma, and osteopenia. Bone-density evaluation and prophylactic calcium, vitamin D, and bisphosphonates are necessary, especially for postmenopausal women and hypogonadal men. Alternate-day steroids can be considered during the tapering phrase, but daily and even divided daily doses of prednisone are required for acute reactions. For chronically reactional steroid-dependent patients, there is a great need for steroid-sparing agents. Chronically reactional patients who receive corticosteroids need to be monitored for downgrading reactions, which are best diagnosed by skin biopsy, showing an increase in acid-fast bacilli. Such patients may require additional antimycobacterial chemotherapy.

SUPPORTIVE CARE AND REHABILITATION

Rehabilitation is an important component of leprosy management. The most common chronic residual deformity is that of the insensitive foot. Management is similar to that of the diabetic foot, with an emphasis on the prevention of neurotrophic ulcers. It is important that the clinician examine the plantar surface of both feet of all leprosy patients at each clinic visit. Any callosities on the distal toes, great toe, metatarsal heads, or heels are an indication of lack of proper proprioception and excessive pressure. Careful inspection and sensory examination of the feet and lower extremities followed by proper unloading of the feet are mandatory. Many plantar ulcers due to leprosy heal spontaneously if relieved from weight-bearing; however, new techniques, such as superficial flap placement, are under study. Protective footwear with molded inserts and patient education about the importance of self-examination are major tools to prevent neurotrophic ulcers.

When neurotrophic ulcers have developed, an algorithm similar to that for the diabetic foot can be used.[70] If the sedimentation rate is elevated or there is radiographic evidence of bone erosion, a bone scan or magnetic resonance imaging, or both, of the foot is indicated. Antibiotic management of chronic osteomyelitis depends on the extent of the findings and is a matter of clinical judgment and available resources. Judicious use of neurology, physical therapy, occupational therapy, and hand surgery consultation is required for individual patients. Reconstructive surgery, when available, plays a critical role in the treatment of contractures of the hands and feet: footdrop and lagophthalmos.

Prevention of Leprosy

Global leprosy eradication is difficult, if not impossible, for multiple reasons: Lepromatous patients are highly infectious, nasal swabs are positive for *M. leprae* in more than 5% of asymptomatic healthy individuals in endemic areas,[71] and *M. leprae* can persist in the environment.[72] For these reasons, the emphasis is not on eradication of *M. leprae* but on the prevention of transmission.

In the United States, the current recommendations for prevention include examination of household contacts and first- and second-degree relatives. The examination should include a complete body skin examination, accompanied by a history of neurologic symptoms (i.e., numbness, tingling, paresthesias), and examination of the peripheral nervous system including palpation of the nerves. Skin biopsy, slit smears, and nerve conduction velocities are obtained for suspected contacts. One report has recommended up to 3 years of full-dose dapsone monotherapy, but because of sporadic compliance and potential side effects, the USPHS National Hansen's Disease Program does not recommend routine dapsone prophylaxis. In some cases, contacts with suspicious skin lesions and peripheral nerve findings that fall short of a definitive diagnosis of leprosy may warrant a therapeutic trial. New strategies for prevention of leprosy depend on further understanding of the transmission of *M. leprae*, which in turn would benefit from high-resolution methods of DNA-based strain typing, such as those that have been used in tuberculosis control.

ROLE OF THE BCG VACCINE IN LEPROSY PREVENTION

Although intended to protect against tuberculosis, the BCG vaccine has been found to protect against leprosy; one study found an efficacy ranging between 32% and 86%, with decreasing benefit with age.[73] In Malawi, a single childhood BCG vaccine had a protective efficacy of 50%, and administration of a second dose conferred protection for an additional 50%.[74] Subcutaneous injection of BCG combined with killed *M. leprae* did not have an additional protective effect compared to the single BCG vaccine in the Malawi study, although this combination was found to have efficacy superior to BCG alone in a study performed in India.[75]

Leprosy in Special Patient Populations

LEPROSY AND HUMAN IMMUNODEFICIENCY VIRUS

Despite the importance of CD_4^+ T cells and the role of the cellular immune response in control of *M. leprae*, current evidence indicates that human immunodeficiency virus (HIV)–associated immunodeficiency has little effect on the course of leprosy. Although HIV is more prevalent in patients with leprosy than in healthy blood donors in some studies, this has not been a widespread finding. Unlike the well-documented increased risk of infection with *M. tuberculosis* in HIV-infected individuals, HIV is not thought to be a risk factor for acquisition of leprosy, nor is it associated with increased disease severity, rapidity of onset of disease, or a delayed response to treatment. In addition, HIV has not been found to affect the clinical form of leprosy (i.e., lepromatous disease is not more common or tuberculoid disease less common than in HIV-negative control subjects),[76-78] and HIV infection does not appear to affect the histopathologic appearance of leprosy lesions.[77] This is surprising, but despite the decreased numbers of CD_4^+ T lymphocytes in the blood of HIV-infected individuals, lymphocytes are routinely seen on skin biopsies from these patients.[79] *M. leprae* may grow too slowly to affect the clinical form of leprosy in people with HIV in developing countries, as other complications of HIV may dominate. However, as antiretroviral therapy and prophylaxis against other opportunistic infections become more common in the developing world, changes in the course and manifestations of leprosy in people with HIV are becoming apparent. Indeed, people with HIV and *M. leprae* coinfection often exhibit reversal reactions as a manifestation of immune reconstitution upon treatment with antiretroviral therapy.[80-83]

LEPROSY IN OTHER IMMUNOCOMPROMISED HOSTS

Leprosy has been reported in renal, heart, and stem cell transplant (SCT) recipients; the majority of cases have been reported in renal transplant recipients living in leprosy-endemic areas.[84] Notably, two cases diagnosed in American heart transplant recipients were in native-born individuals who presumably had indirect contact with infected armadillos through dogs.[85,86] Six cases have been reported in HLA-identical allogeneic SCT recipients.[87] One challenge in treating transplant recipients with leprosy is the potential adverse medication interactions, particularly between rifampin and cyclosporine; for this reason, treating leprosy in these patients requires the use of alternative antimycobacterial regimens. In addition, the duration of therapy in these patients is in question, as it is unclear if this group should receive a prolonged treatment course in light of their immunocompromised state.

A second population in whom leprosy has been reported are patients receiving TNF-blocking monoclonal antibodies (e.g., infliximab or adalimumab). These agents, which have been increasingly used in the treatment of autoimmune diseases, have been associated with the development or reactivation of infections typically contained by cell-mediated immunity (e.g., tuberculosis and endemic fungal infections). Two U.S.-born patients with rheumatologic diseases treated with infliximab had rapid development of borderline lepromatous lesions in the first 2 years after infliximab treatment; their disease was most likely due to reactivation of subclinical disease.[19] Both patients developed reversal reactions after infliximab was discontinued and MDT was initiated; presumably, the reactions developed when host immunity was restored following the discontinuation of the TNF antagonist. This pathophysiology may be similar to the HIV-associated immune reconstitution syndrome, when patients develop manifestations of leprosy following immune restoration while on ART.

REFERENCES

1. Hastings R, ed. *Leprosy*. 2nd ed. Edinburgh: Churchill Livingstone; 1994.
2. Ridley DS, Jopling WH. Classification of leprosy according to immunity. A five-group system. *Int J Lepr Other Mycobact Dis*. 1966;34:255-273.
3. Yamamura M, Uyemura K, Deans RJ, et al. Defining protective responses to pathogens: cytokine profiles in leprosy lesions. *Science*. 1991;254:277-279.
4. Davey TF, Rees RJ. The nasal discharge in leprosy: clinical and bacteriological aspects. *Lepr Rev*. 1974;45:121-134.
5. Melsom R, Harboe M, Duncan ME, et al. IgA and IgM antibodies against *Mycobacterium leprae* in cord sera and in patients with leprosy: an indicator of intrauterine infection in leprosy. *Scand J Immunol*. 1981;14:343-352.
6. Pedley JC. The presence of M. leprae in human milk. *Lepr Rev*. 1967;38:239-242.
7. Job CK, Jayakumar J, Kearney M, et al. Transmission of leprosy: a study of skin and nasal secretions of household contacts of leprosy patients using PCR. *Am J Trop Med Hyg*. 2008; 78:518-521.
8. Kotteeswaran G, Chacko CJ, Job CK. Skin adnexa in leprosy and their role in the dissemination of M. leprae. *Lepr India*. 1980;52:475-481.
9. Moet FJ, Pahan D, Schuring RP, et al. Physical distance, genetic relationship, age, and leprosy classification are independent risk factors for leprosy in contacts of patients with leprosy. *J Infect Dis*. 2006;193:346-353.
10. Bakker MI, Hatta M, Kwenang A, et al. Risk factors for developing leprosy–a population-based cohort study in Indonesia. *Lepr Rev*. 2006;77:48-61.
11. Alter A, Alcais A, Abel L, et al. Leprosy as a genetic model for susceptibility to common infectious diseases. *Hum Genet*. 2008;123:227-235.
12. Mira MT, Alcais A, Van Thuc N, et al. Chromosome 6q25 is linked to susceptibility to leprosy in a Vietnamese population. *Nat Genet*. 2003;33:412-415.
13. Mira MT, Alcais A, Nguyen VT, et al. Susceptibility to leprosy is associated with PARK2 and PACRG. *Nature*. 2004; 427:636-640.
14. Alcais A, Alter A, Antoni G, et al. Stepwise replication identifies a low-producing lymphotoxin-alpha allele as a major risk factor for early-onset leprosy. *Nat Genet*. 2007;39:517-522.
15. Blackwell JM. Genetics of host resistance and susceptibility to intramacrophage pathogens: a study of multicase families of tuberculosis, leprosy and leishmaniasis in north-eastern Brazil. *Int J Parasitol*. 1998;28:21-28.
16. WHO Weekly Epidemiological Record (WER). 2008;83: 293-300.
17. Mastro TD, Redd SC, Breiman RF. Imported leprosy in the United States, 1978 through 1988: an epidemic without secondary transmission. *Am J Public Health*. 1992;82:1127-1130.
18. Levis WR, Vides EA, Cabrera A. Leprosy in the eastern United States. *JAMA*. 2000;283:1004-1005.
19. Scollard DM, Joyce MP, Gillis TP. Development of leprosy and type 1 leprosy reactions after treatment with infliximab: a report of 2 cases. *Clin Infect Dis*. 2006;43:e19-22.
20. Cole ST, Eiglmeier K, Parkhill J, et al. Massive gene decay in the leprosy bacillus. *Nature*. 2001;409:1007-1011.
21. Yuan Y, Barry CE 3rd. A common mechanism for the biosynthesis of methoxy and cyclopropyl mycolic acids in *Mycobacterium tuberculosis*. *Proc Natl Acad Sci U S A*. 1996;93: 12828-12833.
22. De Voss JJ, Rutter K, Schroeder BG, et al. The salicylate-derived mycobactin siderophores of *Mycobacterium tuberculosis* are essential for growth in macrophages. *Proc Natl Acad Sci U S A*. 2000;97:1252-1257.
23. George KM, Chatterjee D, Gunawardana G, et al. Mycolactone: a polyketide toxin from *Mycobacterium ulcerans* required for virulence. *Science*. 1999;283:854-857.
24. Monot M, Honore N, Garnier T, et al. On the origin of leprosy. *Science*. 2005;308:1040-1042.
25. Monot M, Honore N, Baliere C, et al. Are variable-number tandem repeats appropriate for genotyping *Mycobacterium leprae*? *J Clin Microbiol*. 2008;46:2291-2297.
26. Young SK, Ponnighaus JM, Jain S, et al. Use of Short Tandem Repeat Sequences to Study *Mycobacterium leprae* in Leprosy Patients in Malawi and India. *PLoS Negl Trop Dis*. 2008;2:e214.
27. Kim J, Uyemura K, Van Dyke MK, et al. A role for IL-12 receptor expression and signal transduction in host defense in leprosy. *J Immunol*. 2001;167:779-786.
28. Sieling PA, Wang XH, Gately MK, et al. IL-12 regulates T helper type 1 cytokine responses in human infectious disease. *J Immunol*. 1994;153:3639-3647.
29. Krutzik SR, Ochoa MT, Sieling PA, et al. Activation and regulation of Toll-like receptors 2 and 1 in human leprosy. *Nat Med*. 2003;9:525-532.
30. Yamauchi PS, Bleharski JR, Uyemura K, et al. A role for CD40-CD40 ligand interactions in the generation of type 1 cytokine responses in human leprosy. *J Immunol*. 2000;165:1506-1512.
31. Johnson CM, Lyle EA, Omueti KO, et al. Cutting edge: A common polymorphism impairs cell surface trafficking and functional responses of TLR1 but protects against leprosy. *J Immunol*. 2007;178:7520-7524.
32. Misch EA, Macdonald M, Ranjit C, et al. Human TLR1 Deficiency Is Associated with Impaired Mycobacterial Signaling and Protection from Leprosy Reversal Reaction. *PLoS Negl Trop Dis*. 2008;2:e231.
33. Rambukkana A, Zanazzi G, Tapinos N, et al. Contact-dependent demyelination by *Mycobacterium leprae* in the absence of immune cells. *Science*. 2002;296:927-931.
34. Spierings E, de Boer T, Wieles B, et al. *Mycobacterium leprae*-specific, HLA class II-restricted killing of human Schwann cells by CD4+ Th1 cells: a novel immunopathogenic mechanism of nerve damage in leprosy. *J Immunol*. 2001; 166:5883-5888.
35. Rambukkana A, Salzer JL, Yurchenco PD, et al. Neural targeting of *Mycobacterium leprae* mediated by the G domain of the laminin-alpha2 chain. *Cell*. 1997;88:811-821.
36. Rambukkana A, Yamada H, Zanazzi G, et al. Role of alpha-dystroglycan as a Schwann cell receptor for *Mycobacterium leprae*. *Science*. 1998;282:2076-2079.
37. Soares de Lima C, Zulianello L, Marques MA, et al. Mapping the laminin-binding and adhesive domain of the cell surface-associated Hlp/LBP protein from *Mycobacterium leprae*. *Microbes Infect*. 2005;7:1097-1109.
38. Shimoji Y, Ng V, Matsumura K, et al. A 21-kDa surface protein of *Mycobacterium leprae* binds peripheral nerve laminin-2 and mediates Schwann cell invasion. *Proc Natl Acad Sci U S A*. 1999;96:9857-9862.
39. Ng V, Zanazzi G, Timpl R, et al. Role of the cell wall phenolic glycolipid-1 in the peripheral nerve predilection of *Mycobacterium leprae*. *Cell*. 2000;103:511-524.
40. Hunter SW, Fujiwara T, Brennan PJ. Structure and antigenicity of the major specific glycolipid antigen of *Mycobacterium leprae*. *J Biol Chem*. 1982;257:15072-15078.
41. Tapinos N, Ohnishi M, Rambukkana A. ErbB2 receptor tyrosine kinase signaling mediates early demyelination induced by leprosy bacilli. *Nat Med*. 2006;12:961-966.
42. Oliveira RB, Ochoa MT, Sieling PA, et al. Expression of Toll-like receptor 2 on human Schwann cells: a mechanism of nerve damage in leprosy. *Infect Immun*. 2003;71:1427-1433.
43. Wisniewski HM, Bloom BR. Primary demyelination as a non-specific consequence of a cell-mediated immune reaction. *J Exp Med*. 1975;141:346-359.
44. Yamamura M, Wang XH, Ohmen JD, et al. Cytokine patterns of immunologically mediated tissue damage. *J Immunol*. 1992;149:1470-1475.
45. Conti G, De Pol A, Scarpini E, et al. Interleukin-1 beta and interferon-gamma induce proliferation and apoptosis in cultured Schwann cells. *J Neuroimmunol*. 2002;124:29-35.
46. Cruz D, Watson AD, Miller CS, et al. Host-derived oxidized phospholipids and HDL regulate innate immunity in human leprosy. *J Clin Invest*. 2008;118:2917-2928.
47. Van Voorhis WC, Kaplan G, Sarno EN, et al. The cutaneous infiltrates of leprosy: cellular characteristics and the predominant T-cell phenotypes. *N Engl J Med*. 1982;307:1593-1597.
48. Nathan CF, Kaplan G, Levis WR, et al. Local and systemic effects of intradermal recombinant interferon-gamma in patients with lepromatous leprosy. *N Engl J Med*. 1986;315:6-15.
49. Kumar B, Sinha R, Sehgal S. High incidence of IgG antibodies to phenolic glycolipid in non-leprosy patients in India. *J Dermatol*. 1998;25:238-241.
50. Martinez AN, Britto CF, Nery JA, et al. Evaluation of real-time and conventional PCR targeting complex 85 genes for detection of *Mycobacterium leprae* DNA in skin biopsy samples from patients diagnosed with leprosy. *J Clin Microbiol*. 2006;44: 3154-3159.
51. Geluk A, van der Ploeg J, Teles RO, et al. Rational combination of peptides derived from different *Mycobacterium leprae* proteins improves sensitivity for immunodiagnosis of *M. leprae* infection. *Clin Vaccine Immunol*. 2008;15:522-533.
52. Iyer A, Hatta M, Usman R, et al. Serum levels of interferon-gamma, tumour necrosis factor-alpha, soluble interleukin-6R and soluble cell activation markers for monitoring response to treatment of leprosy reactions. *Clin Exp Immunol*. 2007; 150:210-216.
53. Pocaterra L, Jain S, Reddy R, et al. Clinical course of erythema nodosum leprosum: an 11-year cohort study in Hyderabad, India. *Am J Trop Med Hyg*. 2006;74:868-879.
54. Ang P, Tay YK, Ng SK, et al. Fatal Lucio's phenomenon in 2 patients with previously undiagnosed leprosy. *J Am Acad Dermatol*. 2003;48:958-961.
55. Croft RP, Richardus JH, Nicholls PG, et al. Nerve function impairment in leprosy: design, methodology, and intake status of a prospective cohort study of 2664 new leprosy cases in Bangladesh (The Bangladesh Acute Nerve Damage Study). *Lepr Rev*. 1999;70:140-159.
56. Courtright P, Daniel E, Sundarrao C, et al. Eye disease in multibacillary leprosy patients at the time of their leprosy diagnosis: findings from the Longitudinal Study of Ocular Leprosy (LOSOL) in India, the Philippines and Ethiopia. *Lepr Rev*. 2002;73:225-238.
57. Walker SL, Lockwood DN. Leprosy. *Clin Dermatol*. 2007; 25:165-172.
58. Gelber RH, Murray LP, Siu P, et al. Efficacy of minocycline in single dose and at 100 mg twice daily for lepromatous leprosy. *Int J Lepr Other Mycobact Dis*. 1994;62:568-573.
59. Pardillo FE, Burgos J, Fajardo TT, et al. Powerful Bactericidal Activity of Moxifloxacin in Human Leprosy. Antimicrob Agents Chemother; 2008.
60. Efficacy of single-dose multidrug therapy for the treatment of single-lesion paucibacillary leprosy. Single-lesion Multicentre Trial Group. *Indian J Lepr*. 1997;69:121-129.
61. Lockwood DN. Rifampicin/minocycline and ofloxacin (ROM) for single lesions–what is the evidence? *Lepr Rev*. 1997;68: 299-300.
62. Sousa AL, Stefani MM, Pereira GA, et al. *Mycobacterium leprae* DNA associated with type 1 reactions in single lesion paucibacillary leprosy treated with single dose rifampin, ofloxacin, and minocycline. *Am J Trop Med Hyg*. 2007;77: 829-833.
63. WHO Expert Committee on Leprosy, 7th Report. (1998): 1-43.
64. Ebenezer GJ, Daniel S, Norman G, et al. Are viable *Mycobacterium leprae* present in lepromatous patients after completion of 12 months' and 24 months' multi-drug therapy? *Indian J Lepr*. 2004;76:199-206.
65. Jamet P, Ji B. Relapse after long-term follow up of multibacillary patients treated by WHO multidrug regimen. Marchoux Chemotherapy Study Group. *Int J Lepr Other Mycobact Dis*. 1995;63:195-201.
66. van Brakel WH, Khawas IB. Nerve function impairment in leprosy: an epidemiological and clinical study—Part 2: Results of steroid treatment. *Lepr Rev*. 1996;67:104-118.
67. Walker SL, Waters MF, Lockwood DN. The role of thalidomide in the management of erythema nodosum leprosum. *Lepr Rev*. 2007;78:197-215.
68. Haslett PA, Corral LG, Albert M, et al. Thalidomide costimulates primary human T lymphocytes, preferentially inducing proliferation, cytokine production, and cytotoxic responses in the CD8+ subset. *J Exp Med*. 1998;187:1885-1892.
69. Gaspari A. Thalidomide neurotoxicity in dermatological patients: the next "STEP". *J Invest Dermatol*. 2002;119: 987-988.
70. Patout CA Jr, Birke JA, Wilbright WA, et al. A decision pathway for the staged management of foot problems in diabetes mellitus. *Arch Phys Med Rehabil*. 2001;82:1724-1728.
71. Beyene D, Aseffa A, Harboe M, et al. Nasal carriage of *Mycobacterium leprae* DNA in healthy individuals in Lega Robi village, Ethiopia. *Epidemiol Infect*. 2003;131:841-848.
72. Lavania M, Katoch K, Katoch VM, et al. Detection of viable *Mycobacterium leprae* in soil samples: Insights into possible sources of transmission of leprosy. *Infect Genet Evol*. 2008.
73. Rodrigues LC, Kerr-Pontes LR, Frietas MV, et al. Long-lasting BCG protection against leprosy. *Vaccine*. 2007;25:6842-6844.
74. Randomised controlled trial of single BCG, repeated BCG, or combined BCG and killed *Mycobacterium leprae* vaccine for prevention of leprosy and tuberculosis in Malawi. Karonga Prevention Trial Group. *Lancet*. 1996;348:17-24.
75. Gupte MD, Vallishayee RS, Anantharaman DS, et al. Comparative leprosy vaccine trial in south India. *Indian J Lepr*. 1998;70: 369-388.
76. Gebre S, Saunderson P, Messele T, et al. The effect of HIV status on the clinical picture of leprosy: a prospective study in Ethiopia. *Lepr Rev*. 2000;71:338-343.
77. Sampaio EP, Caneshi JR, Nery JA, et al. Cellular immune response to *Mycobacterium leprae* infection in human immunodeficiency virus-infected individuals. *Infect Immun*. 1995; 63:1848-1854.
78. van den Broek J, Chum HJ, Swai R, et al. Association between leprosy and HIV infection in Tanzania. *Int J Lepr Other Mycobact Dis*. 1997;65:203-210.
79. Ustianowski AP, Lawn SD, Lockwood DN. Interactions between HIV infection and leprosy: a paradox. *Lancet Infect Dis*. 2006;6:350-360.
80. Batista MD, Porro AM, Maeda SM, et al. Leprosy reversal reaction as immune reconstitution inflammatory syndrome in patients with AIDS. *Clin Infect Dis*. 2008;46: e56-e60.
81. Lawn SD, Wood C, Lockwood DN. Borderline tuberculoid leprosy: an immune reconstitution phenomenon in a human immunodeficiency virus-infected person. *Clin Infect Dis*. 2003;36: e5-6.
82. Martiniuk F, Rao SD, Rea TH, et al. Leprosy as immune reconstitution inflammatory syndrome in HIV-positive persons. *Emerg Infect Dis*. 2007;13:1438-1440.
83. Trindade MA, Valente NY, Manini MI, et al. Two patients coinfected with *Mycobacterium leprae* and human immunodeficiency virus type 1 and naive for antiretroviral therapy who exhibited type 1 leprosy reactions mimicking the immune reconstitution inflammatory syndrome. *J Clin Microbiol*. 2006;44:4616-4618.
84. Shih HC, Hung TW, Lian JD, et al. Leprosy in a renal transplant recipient: a case report and literature review. *J Dermatol*. 2005;32:661-666.
85. Launius BK, Brown PA, Cush E, et al. A case study in Hansen's disease acquired after heart transplant. *Crit Care Nurs Q*. 2004;27:87-91.
86. Modi K, Mancini M, Joyce MP. Lepromatous leprosy in a heart transplant recipient. *Am J Transplant*. 2003;3:1600-1603.

87. Pieroni F, Stracieri AB, Moraes DA, et al. Six cases of leprosy associated with allogeneic hematopoietic SCT. *Bone Marrow Transplant.* 2007;40:859-863.

88. Rani R, Fernandez-Vina MA, Zaheer SA, et al. Study of HLA class II alleles by PCR oligotyping in leprosy patients from north India. *Tissue Antigens.* 1993;42:133-137.

89. Mehra NK, Rajalingam R, Mitra DK, et al. Variants of HLA-DR2/DR51 group haplotypes and susceptibility to tuberculoid leprosy and pulmonary tuberculosis in Asian Indians. *Int J Lepr Other Mycobact Dis.* 1995;63:241-248.

90. Zerva L, Cizman B, Mehra NK, et al. Arginine at positions 13 or 70-71 in pocket 4 of HLA-DRB1 alleles is associated with susceptibility to tuberculoid leprosy. *J Exp Med.* 1996;183:829-836.

91. Vanderborght PR, Pacheco AG, Moraes ME, et al. HLA-DRB1*04 and DRB1*10 are associated with resistance and susceptibility, respectively, in Brazilian and Vietnamese leprosy patients. *Genes Immun.* 2007;8:320-324.

92. Abel L, Sanchez FO, Oberti J, et al. Susceptibility to leprosy is linked to the human NRAMP1 gene. *J Infect Dis.* 1998;177:133-145.

93. Meisner SJ, Mucklow S, Warner G, et al. Association of NRAMP1 polymorphism with leprosy type but not susceptibility to leprosy per se in west Africans. *Am J Trop Med Hyg.* 2001;65:733-735.

94. Roy S, Frodsham A, Saha B, et al. Association of vitamin D receptor genotype with leprosy type. *J Infect Dis.* 1999;179:187-191.

95. Roy S, McGuire W, Mascie-Taylor CG, et al. Tumor necrosis factor promoter polymorphism and susceptibility to lepromatous leprosy. *J Infect Dis.* 1997;176:530-532.

96. Santos AR, Suffys PN, Vanderborght PR, et al. Role of tumor necrosis factor-alpha and interleukin-10 promoter gene polymorphisms in leprosy. *J Infect Dis.* 2002;186:1687-1691.

97. Rajalingam R, Singal DP, Mehra NK. Transporter associated with antigen-processing (TAP) genes and susceptibility to tuberculoid leprosy and pulmonary tuberculosis. *Tissue Antigens.* 1997;49:168-172.

98. Mira MT, Alcais A, di Pietrantonio T, et al. Segregation of HLA/TNF region is linked to leprosy clinical spectrum in families displaying mixed leprosy subtypes. *Genes Immun.* 2003;4:67-73.

99. Siddiqui MR, Meisner S, Tosh K, et al. A major susceptibility locus for leprosy in India maps to chromosome 10p13. *Nat Genet.* 2001;27:439-441.

100. Tosh K, Meisner S, Siddiqui MR, et al. A region of chromosome 20 is linked to leprosy susceptibility in a South Indian population. *J Infect Dis.* 2002;186:1190-1193.

252

Mycobacterium avium Complex

FRED M. GORDIN | C. ROBERT HORSBURGH, JR.

Mycobacterium avium complex (MAC) comprises two closely related organisms: *M. avium* and *Mycobacterium intracellulare*. Four subspecies of *M. avium* have been described, of which *subsp. hominissuis* is the pathogen of humans. Three major disease syndromes are produced by MAC in humans: pulmonary disease, usually in adults whose systemic immunity is intact; disseminated disease, usually in patients with advanced human immunodeficiency virus (HIV) infection; and cervical lymphadenitis. Also, but rarely, MAC can cause disease in other sites, such as cutaneous disease. The frequency of MAC pulmonary and lymph node disease seems to be increasing, particularly in developed countries, but neither condition is reportable, and increases may be due to improved culture and radiographic techniques. Occurrence of disseminated MAC disease increased precipitously with the HIV pandemic but has declined subsequently with the introduction of effective antiretroviral therapy.

Epidemiology

RESERVOIR AND ROUTE OF ACQUISITION

MAC organisms are common in many environmental sites and are thought to be acquired by inhalation or ingestion. Person-to-person spread has not been observed. Environmental sites harboring MAC are diverse, including water, soil, and animals.[1,2] MAC has been found to colonize natural water sources, indoor water systems, pools, and hot tubs.[3-6] Specific sites from which patients acquire MAC are identified rarely, but exposure to recirculating hot water systems has been identified as one route of acquisition of MAC in patients with acquired immunodeficiency syndrome (AIDS).[6] Less than 15% of cases can be traced to this source, however, suggesting that other environmental reservoirs also may be important. Increased risk for disseminated MAC among patients with AIDS also has been associated with exposure to swimming pools and other water sources,[7] whereas MAC infection of the skin can occur after hot tub use.[8] Aerosols of fresh and salt water may contain MAC, and these have been proposed as vehicles leading to transmission of MAC respiratory disease.[9] The frequent occurrence of MAC in milk (even after pasteurization) and the preponderance of cases of cervical lymphadenitis in children younger than 3 years old have led some investigators to speculate that oral exposure to organisms in milk is the route of infection for this clinical presentation.[10]

PULMONARY DISEASE

MAC pulmonary disease is seen in most developed countries. In the United States[11] and in Japan,[12] there are approximately 1.3 cases per 100,000 persons, whereas in France there are 0.2 cases per 100,000 persons,[13] and in Switzerland, there are 0.9 cases per 100,000 persons.[14] An estimated 3000 cases of MAC pulmonary disease are seen annually in the United States.[11] The average age of patients with MAC pulmonary disease in the United States is 58 years, and most patients are men. Younger persons also seem to be at risk for focal MAC pulmonary disease, however.[15,16] Specific risk factors for MAC pulmonary disease have not been identified, although many reported cases have occurred in persons with a history of prior tuberculosis or heavy smoking. Chronic bronchiectasis is associated with MAC but is likely the result of the disease rather than a predisposition. MAC pulmonary disease can occur in HIV-infected persons without dissemination, although the risk of subsequent dissemination is high.[17-19] One report has identi-

fied isolates from residential bathrooms that matched isolates of patients with pulmonary disease, suggesting acquisition from this source.[20] MAC hypersensitivity pneumonitis has also been linked to exposure to pigeons and exotic birds as well as hot tubs.[21] Reports have identified MAC in the sputum of patients with cystic fibrosis, and a causal role has been proposed for this organism in the destruction of pulmonary tissue seen in cystic fibrosis patients.[22,23] MAC also may cause pulmonary disease in patients with pulmonary alveolar proteinosis.[24]

DISSEMINATED DISEASE

Disseminated MAC disease was extremely rare before 1980,[25] but then the heightened susceptibility of AIDS patients to this disease led to a marked increase in the number of cases. In 1994, an estimated 37,000 cases of disseminated MAC disease were seen in patients with AIDS, making this the most common clinical manifestation of MAC and the most common bacterial disease among patients with AIDS.[26] Since then, with the introduction of preventive antibiotic regimens and effective antiretroviral therapy, the number of patients with MAC has declined substantially.[27,28] Disseminated MAC disease also can be seen in children with primary immunodeficiency diseases, such as IFNγR1 or IL-12βR1 deficiency, and in patients with hairy cell leukemia.[29,30,31]

The greatest risk for MAC in patients with AIDS is in patients with severe depression of the CD_4^+ cell count: Disseminated MAC is seen rarely in patients with greater than 100 CD_4^+ cells/mm^3, and the median CD_4^+ cell count among patients with disseminated MAC and AIDS is 10 cells/mm^3.[32,33] The risk for MAC increases as the CD_4^+ count declines,[33] and the prior occurrence of another opportunistic condition increases the risk for MAC at any given CD_4^+ cell level.[34] Early in the HIV epidemic, similar risks for MAC in HIV-infected patients were seen when patients were compared by age, race, sex, or HIV transmission risk.[35] More recently, patients with AIDS and disseminated MAC are likely to be women and minorities, reflecting lack of preventive care and overall trends in the HIV epidemic.[27] Children with AIDS have a risk for MAC similar to that of adults.[36]

Rates of disseminated MAC disease among patients with AIDS are higher in the southern United States compared with patients in the northern United States or Canada; these differences may be due to decreased environmental exposure to MAC in the north during the winter.[37] Disseminated MAC has been reported with a frequency of 10% to 25% of AIDS patients in Europe, North America, and Australia, but the disease is less common in developing countries, particularly in Africa, where less than 1% of patients with AIDS are affected.[38,39] These differences may be due to several factors, including a smaller proportion of AIDS patients with extremely low CD_4^+ cell counts, protection from MAC by prior exposure to *Mycobacterium tuberculosis*,[40] or fewer exposures to MAC in piped water systems.

LYMPHADENITIS

An estimated 300 cases of culture-confirmed MAC lymphadenitis occur in the United States each year.[11] This number is likely to be an underestimate, however, because many cases of lymphadenitis are not cultured or fail to grow an organism. MAC cervical adenitis is largely a disease of children, with most cases occurring in children younger than age 3 years, based on reports from Europe, North America, and Australia. A recent report estimated the incidence of MAC lymphadenitis in children in the Netherlands at 51 cases per 100,000.[41] The disease shows a modest female predominance, and nearly all reported cases are in whites.[42] Before 1980, most nontuberculous lymphadenitis in the United States was due to *Mycobacterium scrofulaceum,* but in recent years, MAC has been the cause in most cases.[43] MAC lymphadenitis also is seen in HIV-infected persons, particularly as a manifestation of the immune reconstitution syndrome[44]; cervical, mediastinal, or intra-abdominal nodes may be involved.

Pathogen

CLASSIFICATION AND MICROBIOLOGY

Organism

Mycobacteria are aerobic, non-spore-forming, nonmotile bacilli. Their cell walls include mycolic acid-containing, long-chain glycolipids or glycopeptidolipids, or both, that protect these facultative intracellular parasites from lysosomal attack. The organisms grow slowly (10-21 days on solid media) and produce thin-translucent or domed-opaque colonies. Colonies are usually light tan in color, although some MAC strains produce a yellow pigment that increases with light exposure. MAC can be cultured on solid or liquid media; liquid media are more sensitive and yield results in a shorter time but do not allow quantitation of mycobacterial load.[45] Glycolipid typing has divided MAC into 28 serovars; 1-6, 8-11, and 21 are *M. avium,* and 7, 12-20, and 25 are *M. intracellulare.*[46] Pulsed-field gel electrophoresis has been able to resolve greater differences in these isolates, indicating there is considerable diversity in the strains of MAC that infect patients.[47] MAC isolates can be identified as *M. avium* or *M. intracellulare* by DNA probes or polymerase chain reaction restriction analysis.[48] In vitro susceptibility testing of MAC isolates against macrolides and azalides is clinically useful, but susceptibility testing against other antimycobacterial agents (e.g., ethambutol, rifamycins, fluoroquinolones, and aminoglycosides) has not been shown to predict clinical response and is not recommended.[45]

Virulence

MAC is relatively avirulent in the normal host. Serovars 1, 4, and 8 are uncommon in the environment, but they cause most cases of disseminated disease in AIDS patients.[46] These serovars are thought to be associated with virulence and do appear more virulent in an animal model of infection.[49] Possible relative virulence factors include adherence to intestinal epithelial cells, production of catalase, failure to acidify vesicles, and inhibition of phagosome-lysosome fusion.[50-52] Clinical isolates from patients with disseminated disease are always of the smooth-transparent colony type, rather than the domed or opaque type. Colonies that are smooth and transparent are more likely to replicate in vivo, are more likely to induce the cytokines tumor necrosis factor-α and interleukin-1, and usually have decreased susceptibility to antimycobacterial agents in vitro.[53] An isolate from a patient with MAC disease has been shown to produce increased cell lysis and increased ability to stimulate HIV replication in vitro, relative to the abilities of an animal MAC isolate.[54] MAC also seems to be able to exist symbiotically with water-borne amebas, leading to increased virulence of MAC in an animal model.[55]

Pathogenesis

MAC disease results from primary acquisition of the organism by either ingestion or inhalation. No cases of reactivation MAC disease have been reported.

Pulmonary Disease

MAC pulmonary disease develops after inhalation of MAC. The duration from inhalation to disease is unknown but presumably occurs over many months to years. More than one distinct MAC organism can be recovered from some patients,[56] suggesting that disease, superinfection, or colonization may occur concomitantly. Tissue lesions usually are localized and appear grossly as well-circumscribed nodules.

Granulomatous pleuritis, bronchitis, vasculitis, and interstitial pneumonia also have been reported.[57] The histologic features vary from poorly formed to well-formed granulomas. Giant cells are seen frequently, and in rare cases, there is central caseating necrosis and cavitation. Thoracic lymph node involvement is uncommon.

Disseminated Disease

Infection is acquired through inhalation or ingestion of MAC, followed by localized disease in the lung or gut. Dissemination ensues from either location over several months.[17] In patients with AIDS, 80% to 90% of infections are acquired by ingestion. Most disseminated disease is due to a single MAC strain, but multiple distinct isolates have been recovered from 15% of patients.[47] The organisms penetrate the gut wall, possibly through Peyer's patches, and subsequently are phagocytized by macrophages and other reticuloendothelial cells.[58,59] Histologically, epithelial cells show only mild inflammatory changes, and ulceration is uncommon. Sheets of foamy macrophages are present in the lamina propria; these massively infected cells may expand the intestinal villi, giving an appearance similar to Whipple's disease. On acid-fast staining, the cells are packed with bacilli.

The resulting thickening of the bowel wall (Fig. 252-1) can lead to intussusception, gastrointestinal hemorrhage, or obstruction, but these are rare. Mesenteric adenopathy ensues (Fig. 252-2); poorly formed granulomas, abscesses, and necrosis with neutrophilic inflammation are seen in these nodes[60,61]; the cells are filled with acid-fast bacilli. Granulomas with giant cells, epithelioid macrophages, and caseating necrosis can be seen but are less common. Subsequently, hematologic dissemination occurs.[62] Any organ can be seeded secondarily, but the most common sites are liver, spleen, and bone marrow (Fig. 252-3).[60,61] The histologic picture in these organs is similar to that in the lymph nodes. The burden of organisms in the blood is variable, ranging from 1 to greater than 10^5 colony-forming units/mL.[18,63] Higher levels of bacteremia likely represent a longer duration of dissemination and signal a poor prognosis. Untreated disseminated MAC disease leads to death by inanition. Decreased caloric intake and increased metabolic demand seem to play a role in this process.

Entry of MAC into the bloodstream leads to elevated serum levels of tumor necrosis factor-α and interleukin-6, which likely are responsible for the predominant symptoms of fever, night sweats, and cachexia.[64,65] The mechanism of the severe anemia seen in disseminated MAC disease is not well understood because bone marrow involvement can be minimal. Erythropoietin levels are variable, and clinical response to exogenous erythropoietin is unpredictable.[66]

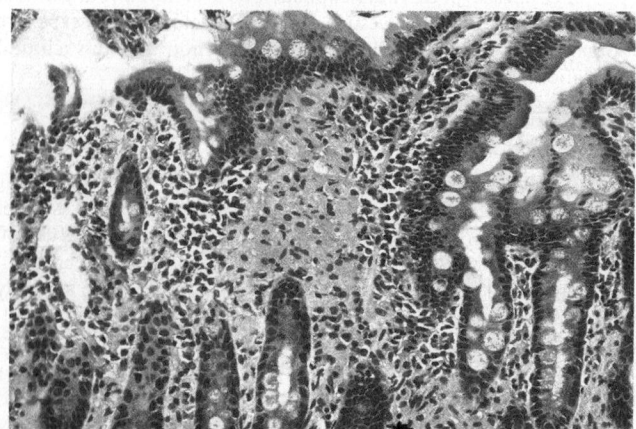

Figure 252-1 **Photomicrograph of intestinal biopsy specimen from a patient with disseminated *Mycobacterium avium* complex disease and AIDS.** Laminae propria of villi are infiltrated with histiocytes. On special stains, the histiocytes were filled with acid-fast bacilli (not evident on this hematoxylin and eosin stain).

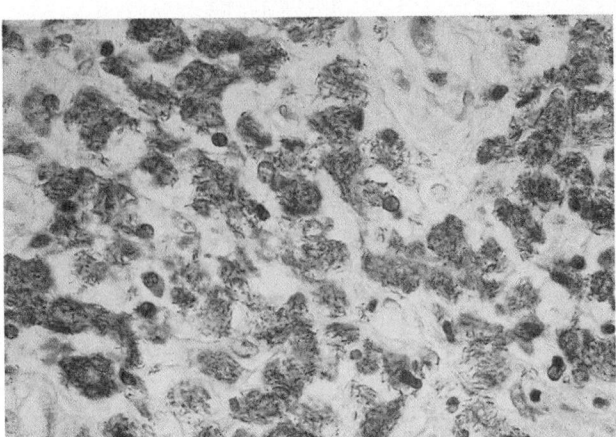

Figure 252-2 Photomicrograph of mesenteric lymph node shows histiocytes filled with acid-fast bacilli, stained in red.

A unique pathophysiologic abnormality seen with disseminated MAC disease is marked elevation of serum alkaline phosphatase, which is seen in roughly 5% of patients. Serum enzyme levels may reach 20 to 40 times the normal level, with little elevation of transaminases, bilirubin, or other parameters of hepatic function; nonetheless, fractionation shows it to be of hepatic origin. Patients have little symptomatic discomfort, and the histologic picture in the liver does not show marked abnormality, suggesting interference with enzyme metabolism rather than hepatic tissue destruction.

Lymphadenitis

MAC cervical and abdominal lymphadenitis likely is acquired through ingestion of MAC, whereas thoracic lymphadenitis presumably occurs subsequent to inhalation. Lesions reveal granulomas, usually without caseation. Ulceration and fistula formation are frequent complications, particularly when nodes have been incised or aspirated. In the immunologically normal host, acid-fast bacilli can be seen in macrophages and giant cells, but they often are single, and dissemination of disease does not occur. In HIV-infected patients without antiretroviral therapy, there is little granulomatous response, and unrestrained mycobacterial replication leads to macrophages filled with acid-fast bacilli with eventual dissemination. When antiretroviral therapy is instituted, a vigorous granulomatous response results in elimination of bacilli from the tissues.

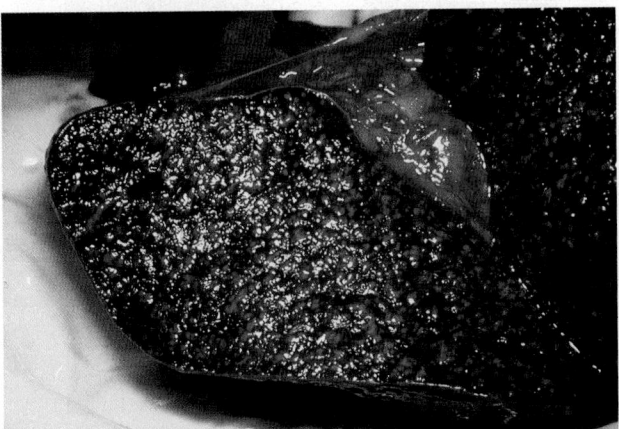

Figure 252-3 Section of spleen from a patient with disseminated *Mycobacterium avium* complex (MAC) disease and AIDS. Multiple, small, yellow-gray disseminated foci of MAC infection are seen.

HOST IMMUNITY

Pulmonary Disease

The fact that many cases of MAC pulmonary disease have occurred in persons with a history of smoking or chronic lung disease, or both, suggests that impaired pulmonary clearance mechanisms may predispose patients to MAC. No specific clearance defects have been identified, however. Patients with MAC lung disease develop antibody and delayed hypersensitivity to MAC antigens, and humoral and cell-mediated immunity remain intact.[67] The host immune response consists of granuloma formation with ingestion and intracellular killing of MAC by macrophages.

Disseminated Disease

Persons with inherited defects in the interferon (IFN)-γ signaling pathway also are exquisitely susceptible to disseminated MAC disease, confirming the importance of this cytokine in host defense against MAC. Sites of defects so far identified include the IFN-γ receptor ligand binding chain, the IFN-γ signal transducing chain, and defective IL-12-mediated modulation of IFN-γ production.[68-71] Exogenously administered IFN-γ overcomes these defects and may lead to clinical improvement.[72]

In patients with AIDS, macrophage phagocytosis of MAC is unimpaired, but intracellular killing does not occur, and organisms multiply unimpeded within macrophages. Macrophages from patients with AIDS can respond normally to cytokines,[73] although cytokine production by T cells is severely impaired in such patients, leading to failure of macrophage activation to eliminate intracellular MAC.[74] MAC-specific T cells develop during disseminated disease in AIDS patients, but these cells do not appear to be able to control the pathogen.[62] Cytotoxic CD$_4^+$ cells are important in inhibiting intracellular replication of MAC, but their function also is impaired in HIV infection.[75]

Humoral factors also may play a role in disseminated MAC disease. Antibodies against MAC are produced in response to disease in normal hosts but not in patients with AIDS.[32] Although these antibodies are not known to have a role in protection against MAC disease, they increase MAC killing in vitro.[76] Conversely, MAC growth can be stimulated by high serum levels of triglycerides and by the iron overload seen in patients with AIDS.[77]

Lymphadenitis

Patients with MAC lymphadenitis also develop antibodies and delayed hypersensitivity to MAC antigens, indicating intact humoral and cell-mediated immunity. The histologic response usually consists of non-caseating granuloma formation; few acid-fast bacilli are seen in tissue sections.

▣ Clinical Presentation

PULMONARY DISEASE

The clinical presentation of pulmonary MAC disease is nonspecific and can be confused with other mycobacterial infections and chronic pulmonary diseases. The classic presentation of pulmonary MAC is one of a subacute-to-chronic illness occurring in individuals with a prior history of underlying pulmonary pathology due to smoking, bronchiectasis, cancer, silicosis, prior tuberculosis, or other diseases.[16,78,79] Most of these individuals are middle-aged to older men, predominately white, and frequently with a history of heavy smoking and heavy alcohol consumption. The clinical picture in this population is one of a chronic disease, with the predominant symptoms being productive cough (occurring in >80% of patients), weight loss or weakness (in approximately half), and fever or night sweats (each in 10% to 20% of patients).[13,78,79] This presentation of pulmonary MAC has been reported to result in death within 2 years of diagnosis in 15% of individuals. Pulmonary MAC alone, without disseminated disease, also may occur in persons with HIV infection.[19]

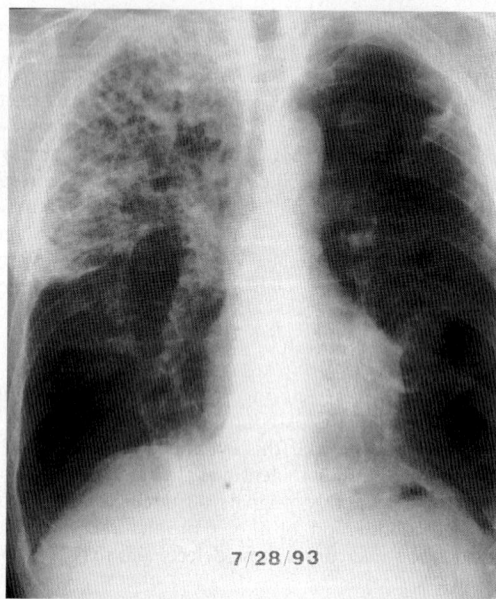

Figure 252-4 Chest radiograph of a man with cavitary *Mycobacterium avium* complex disease in the left upper lobe and infiltrative disease in the right upper lobe. *(Courtesy of James L. Cook, MD.)*

The chest radiograph in this chronic form of pulmonary MAC typically shows upper lobe fibronodular and cavitary disease, which may be associated with pleural thickening (Fig. 252-4). Rates of cavitation tend to be higher than with tuberculosis: Cavitary disease is reported in 60% to 90% of patients with MAC[78,79] compared with approximately 50% of patients with tuberculosis. The cavities in patients with MAC also are more likely to be thin-walled than in tuberculosis and may be quite large, with most in the 2- to 4-cm range.[80] MAC pulmonary disease is bilateral in almost half of patients. Pleural effusions are uncommon. Other features that may be identified on chest radiographs in patients with pulmonary MAC are pectus excavatum and scoliosis. In one report, 27% of individuals with MAC had pectus excavatum compared with 2.4% in the general population, and 52% of patients with MAC had scoliosis compared with 19% in the general population.[15] Computed tomography (CT) scans of the chest may add some useful clinical information. In a series comparing patients with pulmonary MAC with patients with pulmonary tuberculosis, nodules and consolidation were found equally in both groups; bronchiectasis was found significantly more often, however, in patients with MAC (94% versus 27%).[81] The CT finding of bronchiectasis with multiple nodular infiltrates (Fig. 252-5) is particularly suggestive of MAC pulmonary disease. Tree-in-bud opacities are seen often, but these are not specific for MAC.

Pulmonary MAC also has been recognized with increasing frequency in middle-aged to elderly women with no preexisting lung disease.[16,82,83] This syndrome, sometimes referred to as "the Lady Windermere syndrome," named for the principal character in Oscar Wilde's play. This syndrome presents with a more indolent clinical picture and with fewer chest radiograph abnormalities. Patients with this syndrome usually present with chronic cough, but other constitutional symptoms, such as weight loss and fever, are uncommon. The chest radiograph in these patients shows less lung involvement than in patients with predisposing lung disease, and changes may occur only over years of follow-up.[80,82,83] Discrete pulmonary nodules may be seen often in the middle lobe or lingular regions, although other areas of the lungs may be involved (Fig. 252-6). Cavities have been reported in only 25% of these patients. High-resolution CT (HRCT) scans can be important as a means of detecting micronodules (<5 mm) and evidence of bronchiectasis in this population (Fig. 252-7).[80,81,84]

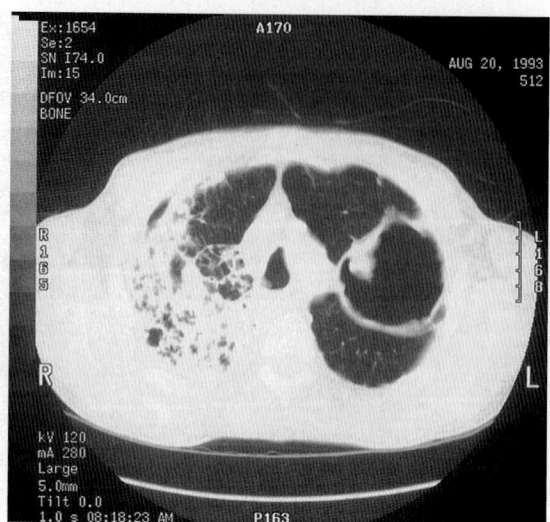

Figure 252-5 Computed tomography scan of the lung of the patient in Figure 252-4. Left upper lobe cavity is now apparent, with extensive lung destruction.

Patients with cystic fibrosis frequently are colonized with nontuberculosis mycobacteria, but the clinical importance of MAC in this population is not clear. In one multicenter prevalence study of 986 patients with cystic fibrosis, 13% had at least one of three sputum samples positive for nontuberculosis mycobacteria, most (72%) with MAC.[85] Overall, patients with cystic fibrosis and MAC had similar pulmonary function tests compared with patients without MAC.[86] Serial HRCT scans provided important information because patients with MAC and progression of HRCT abnormalities were more likely to have clinical decline than other cystic fibrosis patients with MAC. In cystic fibrosis patients, HRCT abnormalities suggestive of progressive MAC were progression of areas of cystic or cavitary disease, subsegmental or larger areas of consolidation, pulmonary nodules, and tree-in-bud opacities; these changes are not specific, however, for MAC.[86]

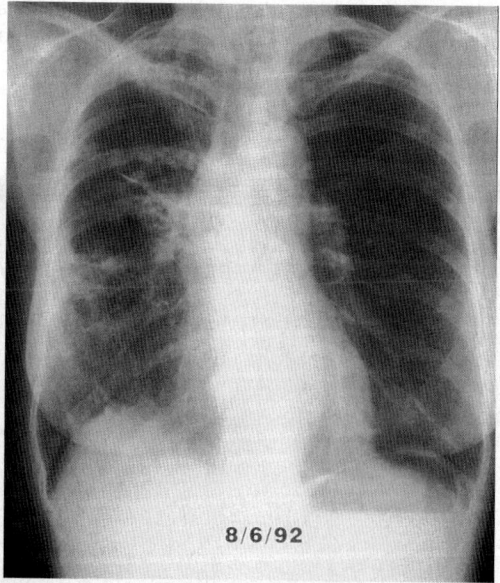

Figure 252-6 Chest radiograph of a 67-year-old woman with right-sided bronchiectasis and *Mycobacterium avium* complex pulmonary disease. Nodular densities are seen in the right middle lobe. *(Courtesy of James L. Cook, MD.)*

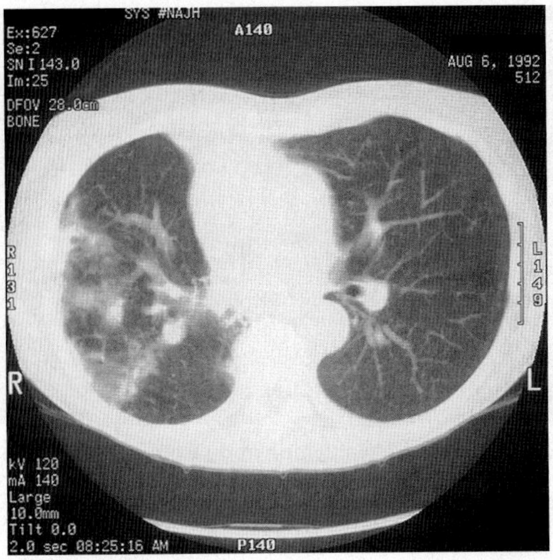

252 *Mycobacterium avium* Complex **3181**

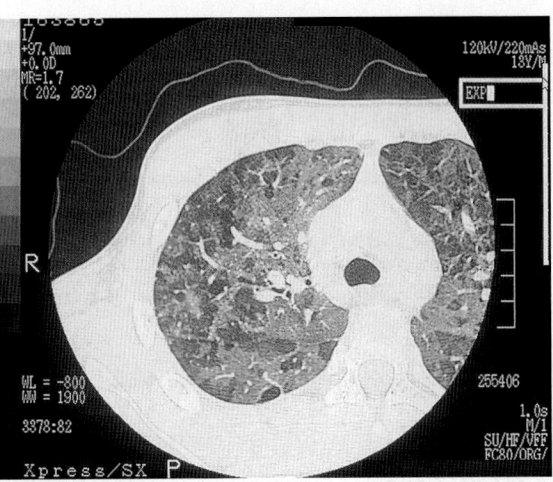

Figure 252-7 Computed tomography scan of the lung of the patient in Figure 252-6. Nodules and bronchiectasis are evident.

Figure 252-8 Computed tomography scan of a patient with hypersensitivity pneumonitis induced by *Mycobacterium avium* complex shows bilateral infiltrates that cleared rapidly with antimycobacterial agents and prednisone. *(Courtesy of James L. Cook, MD.)*

Another pattern of MAC pulmonary disease, known as "hot-tub lung disease,"[87-89] occurs in persons exposed to pools of heated water containing MAC. Patients with this condition are presumed to have inhaled aerosolized MAC, resulting in a hypersensitivity pneumonitis. These patients present with mild-to-moderate dyspnea and dry cough, with or without fever. Chest radiographs and CT scans show patterns similar to those seen in other hypersensitivity pneumonitides, with a variety of radiologic patterns, including bilateral alveolar infiltrates, centrilobular nodules, and "ground-glass" opacities (Fig. 252-8).[87-89]

DISSEMINATED DISEASE

Disseminated MAC occurs almost exclusively in persons with advanced HIV disease. In a large natural history study of patients with HIV infection, MAC bacteremia developed at a median CD$_4^+$ cell count of 13 cells/mm^3, and the median survival after diagnosis was only 134 days.[33] It is difficult to separate the clinical and laboratory features directly attributable to MAC from abnormalities attributable to advanced HIV disease. In early reports, more than 90% of persons with disseminated MAC had high fever, weight loss, night sweats, or severe anemia (hematocrit <25%).[90-92] Other features associated with MAC include abdominal pain, diarrhea, intra-abdominal lymphadenopathy, hepatosplenomegaly, and an elevated serum alkaline phosphatase level. With the advent of effective antiretroviral therapy and more widespread early detection of MAC, the clinical presentation has evolved,[27] as patients presenting in the late 1990s with MAC were less likely to have severe anemia, significant weight loss, or an elevated alkaline phosphatase than patients presenting in the early and mid-1990s. The clinical features directly attributable to the onset of disseminated MAC have been described by evaluating patients at risk, with prospective monthly blood cultures for MAC.[93] At the time blood cultures became positive, patients with MAC had more weight loss, fever, anemia, abdominal pain, or elevated alkaline phosphatase than patients who did not develop MAC. The onset of these clinical changes occurred within 2 months of the first positive blood culture for MAC.[93]

In patients with disseminated MAC, other organ-specific localizing signs and symptoms may be present as a manifestation of the involvement of these organ systems. A comprehensive autopsy series of 44 patients with AIDS and disseminated MAC showed the most common organs involved to be the spleen, lymph nodes, liver, intestines, colon, bone marrow, and, less commonly, lungs, adrenals, stomach, and central nervous system.[94] Patients may present with clinical manifestations of disease referable to any of these body systems. Patients with AIDS and disseminated MAC may have concurrent pulmonary disease,

but this is not common. Although MAC isolated from respiratory specimens may be a harbinger of disseminated MAC,[17] parenchymal lung involvement occurs in less than 10% of patients with disseminated MAC.[19] When parenchymal lung disease does occur in this population, the chest radiograph may reveal alveolar infiltrates, nodules, or cavitary disease.

Local manifestations of disseminated MAC may occur in AIDS patients with severe immune suppression who have been started on antiretroviral therapy; these patients can develop local symptoms as a result of an inflammatory reaction to MAC antigens as the cell-mediated immune response is restored. This phenomenon is called the *immune reconstitution inflammatory syndrome* (IRIS) or a "paradoxical reaction" (Figs. 252-9 through 252-11).[44,95,96] Most often, patients exhibit painful lymphadenopathy, occurring within 1 to 12 weeks of initiating antiretroviral therapy; pulmonary-thoracic disease, abdominal pain, and hepatosplenomegaly also have been reported to occur in 25% to 30% of patients.[96] Patients with immune reconstitution syndrome differ from other patients with disseminated MAC: Fever may be present, but other constitutional symptoms (e.g., weight loss and night sweats) usually are absent, and blood cultures usually do not grow MAC. Biopsy may be required to establish an accurate diagnosis and to exclude other processes.

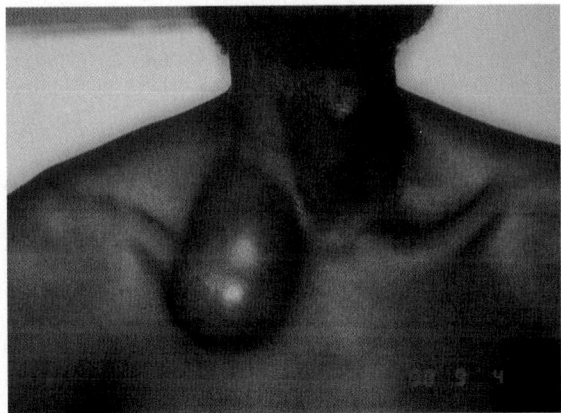

Figure 252-9 Immune reconstitution reaction in a patient with disseminated *Mycobacterium avium* complex disease and AIDS after initiation of antimycobacterial and antiretroviral therapy. This enlarged supraclavicular lymph node was not painful.

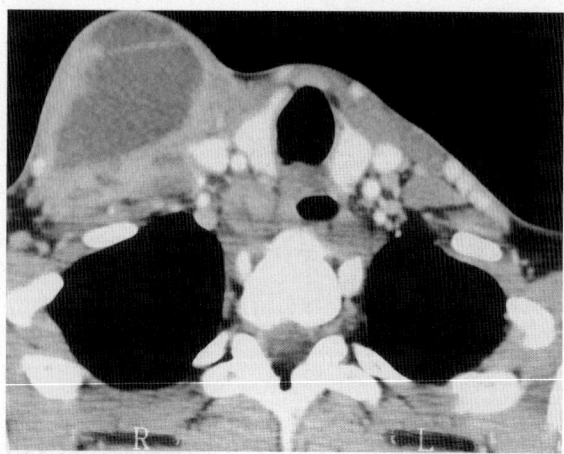

Figure 252-10 Computed tomography scan of lymph node shown in Figure 252-9. The node can be seen to be cystic. Multiple enlarged, but noncystic mediastinal lymph nodes also were present.

Disseminated infection with MAC rarely occurs in patients without AIDS. In one review of 37 patients with disseminated MAC but without AIDS, most patients either had received steroids or had an underlying hematopoietic malignancy.[25] The clinical features of disseminated MAC disease in this population were similar to the features in persons with disseminated MAC and AIDS: Fever, weight loss, and local pain occurred in 32% to 54% of patients; night sweats occurred in 14%; anemia occurred in 75%; and lymphadenopathy or hepatosplenomegaly occurred in more than 40%.

LYMPHADENITIS

Cervicofacial lymphadenitis is the most common manifestation of MAC in children, and more than 80% of patients with MAC cervical lymphadenitis are between 1 and 5 years old.[41-43,97-99] The disease also can occur in adults, but tuberculosis as a cause of lymphadenopathy is more common than MAC in patients older than 12 years.[98,99] The clinical presentation is usually painless or minimally painful unilateral enlargement of a node in the submandibular or high jugular region (Fig. 252-12).[41-43,97] Fever is uncommon. Bilateral disease occurs in less than 10% of individuals, and multiple nodes are involved in less than 20% of children. Nodes are most often firm but not fluctuant. Node size may vary from 1 to 7 cm in diameter, with the mean size in one series reported as 2.5 × 3 cm.[97,99]

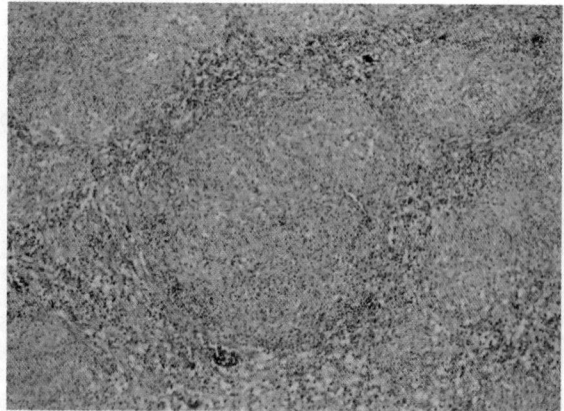

Figure 252-11 Histologic section of excised node from the patient with immune reconstitution reaction shown in Figures 252-9 and 252-10. Granulomas are seen, but no acid-fast organisms were identified. Multinucleated giant cells also were present (not shown).

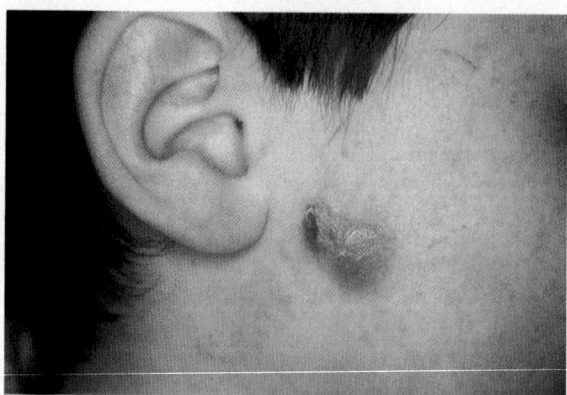

Figure 252-12 Preauricular lymph node from a 5-year-old boy with normal immunity and unilateral *Mycobacterium avium* complex lymphadenopathy.

OTHER SITES

Cutaneous disease due to MAC is uncommon and not differentiated easily from other chronic skin lesions. Lesions may be ulcers, nodules, or plaques. Cases of cutaneous MAC have been reported in immunocompetent and immunosuppressed hosts.[8,100-102] Most often, cutaneous MAC is due to direct inoculation of the skin by trauma, surgery, or injection. Local swelling, erythema, and tenderness may be present for months to years. The lesions are indolent, with little or no lymph node reaction or systemic symptoms. MAC also is a rare cause of renal disease, prostatitis, peritonitis, corneal ulceration, mastoiditis, mastitis, osteomyelitis, endocarditis, septic arthritis, and synovitis.

Diagnosis

PULMONARY DISEASE

Diagnosis of MAC pulmonary disease is difficult because of the high frequency of positive sputum cultures among persons without disease.[45] A single sputum culture that grows MAC has a low predictive value for disease. The American Thoracic Society and Infectious Diseases Society of America have developed a clinical case definition for pulmonary MAC disease: Patients must be symptomatic, have abnormalities on chest radiograph or high-resolution CT scan of the chest, and have one of the following features: (1) two positive MAC sputum cultures; or (2) a bronchial wash or lavage with a positive culture for MAC; or (3) acid-fast bacilli or granulomas, or positive MAC culture from a histopathologic specimen (if MAC is not cultured from the biopsy, MAC should be present in at least one sputum or bronchial wash sample).

Smears are neither sensitive nor specific in the diagnosis of pulmonary MAC disease because they are not commonly positive and, when positive, are less likely to be MAC than to be *M. tuberculosis* or other nontuberculous mycobacteria. Cultures usually turn positive by 21 days when performed on solid media and by 14 days when performed in broth, but the time to growth on culture depends on the inoculum size. Cultures cannot be classified definitively as negative until 6 weeks of observation have failed to yield an organism. Cultures contaminated with bacterial or fungal overgrowth before 6 weeks cannot be interpreted and should be repeated. MAC DNA can be detected directly in sputum, but no licensed tests are available; these tests also would be expected to detect colonization so that the American Thoracic Society/ Infectious Diseases Society of America diagnostic criteria for MAC pulmonary disease still must be satisfied. Patients who do not meet the diagnostic criteria should be followed closely and reevaluated because clinical disease may develop over time.

Other conditions that may mimic the infiltrative form of MAC pulmonary disease include tuberculosis and other nontuberculous mycobacterial infections, nocardiosis, histoplasmosis, blastomycosis, coccidioidomycosis, and necrotizing bacterial pneumonia. Bronchiectasis also may be caused by IgG deficiency, pulmonary ciliary disorders, cystic fibrosis, toxin exposure, or allergic bronchopulmonary aspergillosis.

MYCOBACTERIUM AVIUM COMPLEX HYPERSENSITIVITY PNEUMONITIS

Patients with hypersensitivity pneumonitis due to MAC usually give a history of exposure to aerosols from pools or hot tubs. Chest radiographs may be normal; show nodules or infiltrates; or, in the acute presentation, show total opacification of the lung fields.[4,87-89] In the acute stages, lung biopsy may show neutrophilic or lymphocytic infiltrates; later, noncaseating granulomas may be seen. Patients with hypersensitivity pneumonitis usually grow MAC from sputum, bronchoalveolar lavage, or lung biopsy specimens; this entity may be a combination of early infection and hypersensitivity. No test for serum precipitins to MAC antigens is currently available.

DISSEMINATED DISEASE

Disseminated MAC is diagnosed by recovery of MAC from blood or another usually sterile site, such as bone marrow, liver, or spleen. Although recovery from only one of these sites might indicate localized disease in that organ, such positive cultures are highly predictive of positive cultures from the other sites. MAC growth from lymph nodes may represent localized disease, whereas MAC growth from sputum, bronchial washings, gastrointestinal biopsy specimens, or stool can represent colonization or localized disease; in such cases, positive cultures from more than one organ are needed to establish a diagnosis of disseminated disease. Isolation of MAC from stool by itself does not indicate that the organism is causing disease, and treatment should not be initiated based solely on that finding. The risk of developing MAC-associated disease in severely immunocompromised patients is higher, however, if MAC is present in the stools.

Blood is the preferred specimen for culture, and greater than 90% of cases of disseminated disease are diagnosed by a positive blood culture. Blood cultures are sensitive and specific for the diagnosis of disseminated MAC disease in patients with AIDS. A single specimen yields the diagnosis in 90% to 95% of cases, and two specimens yield the diagnosis in 99% of cases.[103,104] Additional cultures should be obtained only when clinical suspicion is high. However, early in disease, bone marrow biopsy with culture may be a more sensitive diagnostic procedure.[62] Culture on liquid medium is preferable to culture on solid medium and is more rapid; growth on liquid medium often can be detected in 8 to 14 days, but cultures still must be held for 6 weeks to be negative. When growth is detected in liquid medium, hybridization with DNA or RNA probes can identify MAC definitively in a matter of hours. Blood mycobacterial burden can be quantitated using lysis-centrifugation systems with plating on solid medium, but this information has limited clinical utility.[104] When blood mycobacterial burden is high, mycobacteria may be seen on Kinyoun or auramine stain of buffy coat smears, but this method of diagnosis is neither sensitive nor specific for MAC. Direct detection of MAC in blood by polymerase chain reaction has been reported to be as sensitive and specific as culture, but this assay is not widely available.[105,106]

Disseminated MAC disease has protean manifestations, but none of its features are pathognomonic. The differential diagnosis is broad. Disseminated disease due to histoplasmosis, tuberculosis, or other nontuberculous mycobacteria is especially similar to disseminated MAC. Systemic cryptococcosis, blastomycosis, toxoplasmosis, cytomegalovirus, salmonellosis, lymphoma, and AIDS wasting syndrome also should be considered.

LYMPHADENITIS

Confirmed diagnosis of MAC lymphadenitis requires growth of MAC from the node. Excision is preferred to needle biopsy or aspirate

because fistula formation is common after needle biopsy or aspiration. In the non-HIV-infected host, cultures are likely to yield no growth when obtained more than 1 month after the appearance of adenopathy. Histologic examination that reveals noncaseating granuloma with or without acid-fast bacilli is suggestive but not diagnostic. In these cases, or when excision cannot be performed, dual skin testing that includes specific antigens for MAC is sensitive and specific, but these reagents are not licensed for use in the United States at present.[107] Skin testing with *M. tuberculosis* antigen alone (purified protein derivative-standard) has been reported to have limited sensitivity,[107,108] but in a recent report of non–tuberculous lymphadentis in children living in a low-risk setting for TB, a positive PPD skin test was a useful predictor of mycobacterial infection in the node—most cases being caused by MAC.[109]

Isolated lymphadenopathy has a large differential diagnosis. Tuberculosis and lymphoma are the most commonly encountered entities that present similarly to MAC. Mononucleosis, toxoplasmosis, syphilis, cat-scratch disease, other malignancies, and lymph nodes reactive to local bacterial infections also should be considered.

OTHER SITES

Diagnosis of MAC disease in other sites, such as skin, soft tissues, bones, and joints, is suggested by the finding of acid-fast bacilli or granulomas in tissue, but confirmation requires recovery of MAC by culture of the affected site.

Treatment

PRINCIPLES OF TREATMENT

Successful treatment of MAC is a challenge. As with therapy of other mycobacterial infections, the use of at least two active drugs is essential to prevent emergence of resistance and to achieve a long-term cure. Therapy is made difficult by the paucity of drugs that are highly active against MAC and by the frequency of adverse effects associated with the available drugs. In the premacrolide era, success rates of treatment of pulmonary MAC were 50% or less.[78,79,110] Treatment regimens included the use of multiple agents, including isoniazid, ethambutol, rifampin, streptomycin, amikacin, para-aminosalicylic acid, clofazimine, cycloserine, and ethionamide. Immediate failure rates were 25%, and eventual failure and relapse rates approached 50%. In addition, these premacrolide regimens required treatment durations of 36 months, and patients had frequent and severe adverse drug reactions—particularly with cycloserine, ethionamide, and the aminoglycosides. AIDS patients with disseminated MAC also responded poorly to non-macrolide-containing regimens.[111-113] Although the degree of bacteremia was reduced in some trials, overall failure rates and mortality remained high, and drug toxicity was substantial.

Macrolides and azalides exhibit excellent in vitro activity against MAC.[114] Using broth dilution techniques, a minimal inhibitory concentration of less than 8 μg/mL is considered susceptible to clarithromycin, and greater than 32 μg/mL is considered resistant. Greater than 99% of strains of MAC from patients not previously given a macrolide are susceptible to clarithromycin or azithromycin,[115-117] although in one series of AIDS patients newly diagnosed with disseminated MAC, 17% had baseline resistance to macrolides. This was attributed to previous macrolide exposure during MAC treatment or prophylaxis.[118] Macrolide/azalide monotherapy has been evaluated in the treatment of pulmonary MAC in non-AIDS patients. In a trial of clarithromycin monotherapy, 94% of patients showed clinical improvement, but 16% developed clarithromycin resistance.[116] In another trial, azithromycin was given as sole therapy for 4 months to patients with pulmonary MAC, resulting in clinical improvement without the development of macrolide resistance.[117] The clinical effectiveness of clarithromycin and azithromycin has been shown when employed as monotherapy for AIDS patients with disseminated MAC.[115,119,120] Treatment with these drugs resulted in a marked decrease in MAC bacteremia and concomitant reduction in clinical symptoms. When used as monotherapy, however, rates of acquired macrolide resistance are unacceptable. In the largest trial of monotherapy with clarithromycin, 46% of patients developed strains of MAC with a minimal inhibitory concentration equal to or greater than 32 μg/mL, and the development of these resistant strains was associated with recurrence of clinical symptoms.[115]

Other drugs also have been shown to have clinical activity against MAC. Rifabutin is active in vitro against MAC,[121] and in a placebo-controlled trial, rifabutin combined with ethambutol and clofazimine resulted in improvement in bacteremia in 7 of 11 AIDS patients with disseminated MAC compared with 0 of 13 patients receiving placebo with the same two other drugs.[122] Ethambutol has been shown to have activity in vitro against MAC[123] and to be effective in reducing mycobacteremia when used as monotherapy for AIDS patients with disseminated MAC.[124]

Combination therapy is essential in treating MAC to maximize the effectiveness of the macrolides and to minimize the development of macrolide resistance. Many different combination regimens have been evaluated. In pulmonary MAC in patients who have tolerated 6 or more months of macrolide therapy, sputum conversion rates have ranged from 70% to 90%.[125-127] Although there has not been a direct comparative study of azithromycin and clarithromycin in the treatment of MAC pulmonary disease, rates of culture conversion appear lower in studies of azithromycin.[128] Most patients in these macrolide studies received ethambutol, rifabutin (or rifampin), and an aminoglycoside in addition to the macrolide. The importance of the macrolide in the regimens was evident in a study of patients with pulmonary MAC who were being treated with a combination of ethambutol and rifampin without a macrolide: There was a 69% failure rate with 36% mortality.[129]

The addition of macrolides to treatment regimens for AIDS patients with disseminated MAC has shown a marked clinical benefit. Patients receiving a three-drug regimen of clarithromycin, rifabutin, and ethambutol had greater clearance of bacteremia and improved survival compared with patients receiving rifabutin, ethambutol, clofazimine, and ciprofloxacin.[130] Other trials of clarithromycin-containing regimens for the treatment of disseminated MAC have had better clinical outcomes than historical results of patients treated with nonmacrolide-containing regimens.[131,132] Azithromycin also is effective in the treatment of disseminated MAC, although fewer studies have been performed with azithromycin than with clarithromycin. In two comparison trials, patients who received azithromycin were less likely to have MAC bacteremia cleared than patients who received clarithromycin.[133,134]

Tolerability

The maximal dose of clarithromycin is 500 mg twice daily; higher doses have been associated with poorer clinical outcomes and should not be used.[115,135] Many patients, particularly elderly patients, have difficulty tolerating 500 mg twice daily of clarithromycin, largely because of gastrointestinal side effects (Table 252-1). When gastrointestinal side effects occur, doses may be reduced, either to half-dose once a day or full dose thrice weekly. A noncomparative study of treating pulmonary MAC with a thrice-weekly clarithromycin-based regimen, however, showed lower-than-expected improvement rates, particularly in patients with cavitary disease.[126] Alternatively, azithromycin may be substituted for clarithromycin because azithromycin has similar activity and provokes less gastrointestinal intolerance.[136] Patients initially intolerant of azithromycin may be able to tolerate decreased dose levels or less frequent administration. Ethambutol is well tolerated by most patients, although at higher doses, gastrointestinal intolerance or optic neuritis may occur.[137] Rifabutin is associated with gastrointestinal distress, liver function abnormalities, and neutropenia. When given at higher doses or in combination with drugs that inhibit its metabolism, rifabutin has been associated with uveitis and severe arthralgias.[138,139] For patients unable to tolerate rifabutin, rifampin may be substituted and is often better tolerated.

TABLE 252-1	Drugs Employed in the Treatment of *Mycobacterium avium* Complex Disease		
Drug	**Usual Daily Dose***	**Usual Intermittent Dose**	**Common Adverse Effects**
Clarithromycin	500 mg bid	1 g 3 times/week	GI distress, bitter taste, rash, hearing loss, drug interactions
Azithromycin	250 mg qd	500-600 mg 3 times/week	GI distress, hearing loss
Ethambutol	15 mg/kg qd	25 mg/kg 3 times/week	At high doses: optic neuritis, GI distress
Rifabutin	300 mg qd	300 mg 3 times/week	GI distress, hepatitis, neutropenia, drug interactions; at high doses: uveitis, arthralgias
Rifampin	600 mg qd	600 mg 3 times/week	GI distress, hepatitis, neutropenia, drug interactions
Amikacin	Not recommended	15 mg/kg IV 3 times/week	Vestibular and auditory abnormalities, renal toxicity
Streptomycin	Not recommended	15 mg/kg IM (maximum 3 times/week 1 g)	Vestibular and auditory abnormalities, renal toxicity

*Oral dosing unless otherwise indicated.
GI, gastrointestinal.

Aminoglycosides must be administered parenterally; streptomycin usually is given intramuscularly, and amikacin usually is given intravenously. Patients frequently become intolerant of the repeated intramuscular injections associated with long-term streptomycin treatment, so the availability of long-term intravenous access devices makes amikacin the preferable agent. Administration of aminoglycosides twice or thrice weekly is adequate for treatment of MAC, and this relative infrequency lessens inconvenience to the patient. The major toxicities of aminoglycosides are hearing loss and renal function impairment. When amikacin, kanamycin, or streptomcyin were given daily as 15 mg/kg or three times weekly as 25 mg/kg for mycobacterial infections, ototoxicity occurred in 37%, vestibular toxicity in 9%, and nephrotoxicity in 15%.[140] Aminoglycoside hearing loss is usually permanent. Audiometry should be performed at baseline and repeated monthly in all elderly patients who are beginning aminoglycoside therapy for MAC. Similarly, serum creatinine levels should be followed weekly and dosing adjusted accordingly.

Drug Interactions

Neither azithromycin nor ethambutol has clinically important drug interactions, and this is a major advantage of these agents. Clarithromycin inhibits cytochrome P-450 (CYP 3A4) and interferes with the metabolism of drugs that use this enzyme. Increased serum concentrations of theophylline, carbamazepine, omeprazole, digoxin, and terfenadine have been reported when these drugs were coadministered with clarithromycin. Serum levels of theophylline, carbamazepine, and digoxin should be monitored when taken with clarithromycin; coadministration of clarithromycin and terfenadine is contraindicated. Similarly, warfarin (Coumadin) metabolism may be affected, with potentiation of its anticoagulant effect, so prothrombin times should be monitored closely. Serum levels of clarithromycin are increased when the drug is coadministered with fluconazole or ranitidine, but these increased levels do not seem to be associated with alterations in either efficacy or toxicity.

Rifampin and rifabutin decrease clearance of other drugs by induction of the hepatic microsomal enzyme cytochrome P-450 pathway.[141,142] Many drugs potentially can be affected by rifampin/rifabutin, including clarithromycin, methadone, warfarin, estrogens, theophylline, and several classes of antiretroviral agents. When possible, serum levels of these agents should be monitored when coadministered with rifampin or rifabutin. Rifabutin has a less pronounced effect on hepatic enzyme induction than rifampin and may offer advantages in some cases. Serum levels of clarithromycin and its active metabolite, 14-OH clarithromycin, are decreased by 65% when the drug is coadministered with rifampin; when coadministered with rifabutin, the decrease is 47%.[143] Rifampin and rifabutin have substantial drug interactions with protease inhibitors and non-nucleoside reverse transcriptase inhibitors used in treating HIV infection. Rifampin is not usually recommended for use in these patients, and rifabutin doses need to be adjusted (see Chapter 39).[141] Because fluoroquinolones can affect serum levels of theophylline, dilantin, and warfarin, these agents should be monitored when coadministered with fluoroquinolones. Coadministration of fluoroquinolones with calcium-containing or magnesium-containing antacids or ferrous sulfate tablets can lead to decreased absorption and decreased serum drug levels of the fluoroquinolones.

Drug Dosing in Patients with Impaired Renal Function

Clarithromycin, ethambutol, fluoroquinolones, and aminoglycosides are excreted by the kidneys, and doses of these agents should be reduced in patients with renal insufficiency. Rifampin, rifabutin, and azithromycin are excreted largely by the liver and do not require dose reduction when given to patients with renal insufficiency.

Treatment of Macrolide-Resistant Mycobacterium avium Complex Disease

Isolates resistant in vitro to clarithromycin are uniformly cross-resistant to azithromycin, so substitution when resistant organisms are present provides no benefit.[144] Neither drug should be continued in patients with MAC disease caused by macrolide-resistant organisms. Choosing the optimal regimen for treatment of MAC disease with macrolide-resistant organisms is challenging because regimens employed before the advent of macrolides were only marginally effective. Most experts recommend a four-drug regimen comprising rifabutin, ethambutol, a fluoroquinolone, and an aminoglycoside.[45,145] For patient convenience and ease of administration, amikacin is preferable to streptomycin. Choice of the optimal fluoroquinolone is problematic because many MAC isolates are not susceptible in vitro to achievable serum levels of moxifloxacin or levofloxacin.[146] Moxifloxacin may have a better profile and is effective in animal models of MAC, but clinical experience with it is limited. Ethionamide and cycloserine may be useful but have substantial toxicities; it is advisable to consult a specialist with experience in the use of these agents. Isoniazid, pyrazinamide, and clofazimine are minimally active in vitro and do not provide clinical benefit.[129,147]

Immunomodulatory Treatment of Mycobacterium avium Complex Disease

MAC disease in patients with inherited immune defects may have a better response to antimycobacterial therapy when treatment to restore or circumvent immune defects is undertaken. When inherited defects in the IFN-γ signaling pathway are present, subcutaneously administered IFN-γ overcomes these defects and may lead to clinical improvement.[72] IFN-γ has also been shown to be of benefit as an adjunct to antibiotic treatment of patients with pulmonary MAC disease without defined immune defects.[148]

■ Specific Treatment Plans

PULMONARY MYCOBACTERIUM AVIUM COMPLEX

Drug Treatment

The decision to treat for pulmonary MAC is made difficult by the long duration of therapy required and the likelihood of substantial drug toxicity. Treatment should be initiated only for patients with active clinical symptoms, abnormal imaging studies, and positive cultures, as discussed earlier. Treatment of pulmonary MAC should include a

TABLE 252-2	Regimens for Pulmonary MAC (*Mycobacterium avium* Complex)		
Initial Therapy for Nodular/Bronchiectatic Disease	*Initial Therapy for Cavitary Disease*	*Advanced (Severe) or Previously Treated Disease*	
Clarithromycin 1000 mg TIW or azithromycin 500-600 mg TIW	Clarithromycin 500-1000 mg/d or azithromycin 250-300 mg/d	Clarithromycin 500-1000 mg/d or azithromycin 250-300 mg/d	
plus	plus	plus	
Ethambutol 25 mg/kg TIW	Ethambutol 15 mg/kg/d	Ethambutol 15 mg/kg/d	
plus	plus	plus	
Rifampin 600 mg TIW	Rifampin 600 mg/d with or without Streptomycin or amikacin§	Rifabutin 300 mg/d or rifampin 600 mg/d	
		plus	
		Streptomycin or amikacin§	

§See text for dosing recommendation. Modified from An Official ATS/IDSA Statement: Diagnosis, treatment, and prevention of nontuberculous mycobacterial diseases. *Am J Respir Crit Care Med.* 2007;175:367-416.

minimum of three drugs—usually clarithromycin, 500 mg twice daily; ethambutol, 15 mg/kg; and rifampin, 600 mg or rifabutin, 300 mg/day (Table 252-2). Most experts use rifampin in the treatment of patients with pulmonary MAC due to a lesser incidence of adverse effects. An aminoglycoside, usually amikacin or streptomycin, may be valuable for patients for the initial 2-3 months of treatment with extensive disease.[45,149] Consensus treatment guidelines suggest daily use of the oral medications, with the aminoglycoside used two to three times weekly.[45] Patients should be evaluated monthly for clinical improvement, adherence to the drug regimen, and occurrence of adverse effects. Sputum should be obtained monthly for mycobacterial smear and culture. The rate of improvement can be expected to be slow, with most patients remaining culture positive for 6-12 months.[45,125-127,150] Chest radiographs need not be repeated frequently because changes occur slowly. Patients who do not show clinical improvement and whose sputum does not clear of MAC after 6-12 months should be evaluated for adherence to the regimen. For patients who cannot tolerate the initial regimen, one option is changing from daily clarithromycin to a regimen of thrice-weekly dosing—clarithromycin, 1 g; ethambutol, 25 mg/kg; and rifabutin, 300 mg—all given on a thrice-weekly schedule, although this is not recommended for patients with extensive disease.[126] Adverse drug effects may require further dose adjustments. Another option for patients who cannot tolerate clarithromycin is to change to azithromycin, 250 mg daily, with ethambutol, 15 mg/kg, and rifampin, 600 mg, also given daily. For patients with the nodular/bronchiectatic form of pulmonary MAC, a thrice-weekly regimen may be given from the outset with either clarithromycin, 1 g, or azithromycin 500-600 mg, plus ethambutol, 25 mg/kg, and rifampin, 600 mg, each given thrice weekly.[45,128] With patients taking thrice-weekly regimens, it is essential to discuss the extreme importance of adherence to the regimen.

For patients who are not responding despite good adherence to therapy, drug resistance needs to be considered, and drug susceptibility testing for macrolides and azalides should be done. Although almost all MAC isolates from untreated patients with pulmonary disease are susceptible to macrolides and azalides, resistance can develop on treatment, leading to a poor outcome. Isolates resistant to clarithromycin also are resistant to azithromycin.[144] Drug susceptibility testing is not recommended for drugs other than the macrolides.[45]

The optimal duration of therapy is unknown, but most experts treat at least 12 months after sputum cultures have become negative. Most patients with pulmonary MAC receive a total of 18-24 months of therapy.[45] Shorter durations may be reasonable for patients with minimal disease who show a rapid clinical response to treatment. Patients should be followed every few months after therapy is discontinued because relapses can occur.

Surgery

Surgical lung resection has a limited role and is a possibility for select patients who do not respond to medical therapy. Although most surgical procedures for MAC were performed in the premacrolide era,[151] surgical resection of MAC-infected lung continues to be required occasionally despite the use of clarithromycin-containing drug regimens.[152,153] The indication for surgery is usually failure of drug treatment, with the intent of removing major areas of disease, where tissue penetration of antibiotics may be limited. Occasional patients need surgery to control complications of MAC, such as pneumothorax, bronchiectasis, or hemoptysis. Because most patients with MAC have many comorbid conditions, surgery in this population may have a high rate of complications, notably prolonged air leaks and bronchopulmonary fistulas,[151,152] although a recent report noted few negative outcomes in select patients.[153]

HYPERSENSITIVITY PNEUMONITIS

Most patients with MAC hypersensitivity pneumonitis ("hot-tub lung") have responded well to short-term interventions.[87-89] Some patients have responded simply to avoidance of the source of exposure, with no additional therapy.[89] For patients with progressive pulmonary symptoms, a short (2 months) course of prednisone with or without antimycobacterial drugs for 3-6 months has been shown to be effective.[87,89]

DISSEMINATED DISEASE

Antimycobacterial treatment should be initiated promptly for all patients with culture-confirmed evidence for disseminated MAC. Patients with clinical symptoms suggesting disseminated MAC should have blood cultured, but presumptive treatment is not recommended, as clinical suspicion is a poor predictor of disseminated MAC disease.[62] If treatment is initiated pending culture results, the clinician should discontinue treatment and evaluate for other illness if the cultures remain negative after 6 to 8 weeks. All MAC isolates from patients with AIDS should have initial susceptibility testing performed to exclude macrolide resistance, which has been reported to be as high as 17%.[118] HIV-infected patients should not be treated if they are colonized with MAC in the sputum or gastrointestinal tract but have no evidence of active infection; these patients should be followed carefully, however, because 60% may develop MAC bacteremia within 1 year.[17]

Patients with disseminated MAC should be treated with clarithromycin, 500 mg twice daily, and ethambutol, 15 mg/kg/day (Table 252-3).[145] Azithromycin may be substituted if clarithromycin cannot be tolerated, but most experts prefer clarithromycin in this setting. Some experts recommend the addition of rifabutin, 300 mg/day, but the addition of this drug is of uncertain benefit. In one trial, the addition of rifabutin did not affect bacteriologic response or survival,[132] but another trial, using a higher dose of rifabutin (450 mg/day), showed modest clinical benefit.[154] Patients with HIV infection and MAC disease have improved clinical outcomes and decreased risk of relapse if antiretroviral therapy for HIV disease is administered concurrently. This treatment is complicated by drug interactions between the rifabutin used to treat MAC disease and the protease inhibitors and nonnucleoside reverse transcriptase inhibitors (or both) used to treat HIV infection. In this situation, treatment of MAC with clarithromycin and ethambutol (alone) is preferred. If rifabutin is to be used, dose adjustment of rifabutin, protease inhibitors, or non-nucleoside reverse transcriptase inhibitors may be required (see Table 252-3).[141,142,145]

When effective antimycobacterial therapy of disseminated MAC is instituted, fevers and night sweats usually resolve within 2 to 4 weeks, and mycobacteria are cleared from the blood in 4 to 8 weeks. Severe anemia and fatigue may not resolve, however, for 2 to 6 months. Patients with a hematocrit less than 25% should receive transfusions or exogenous erythropoietin to stimulate erythrocyte production and increase the hematocrit to 28% or greater. Endogenous erythropoietin

TABLE 252-3	Regimens for Disseminated MAC (*Mycobacterium avium* Complex)	
	Preferred	*Alternative*
Treatment	Clarithromycin 500 mg bid plus	Azithromycin 500-600 mg qd plus
	Ethambutol 15 mg/kg qd with or without	Ethambutol 15 mg/kg qd with or without
	Rifabutin 300 mg qd*	Rifabutin 300 mg qd*
Prevention	Azithromycin 1200 mg every week	Clarithromycin 500 mg bid or rifabutin 300 mg qd*

*In HIV-positive patients receiving a PI or NNRTI, rifampin should be replaced by rifabutin, though the dosage depends on the antiretrovirals. The rifabutin dose should be decreased to 150 mg thrice weekly or the blood rifabutin concentration monitored in patients receiving amprenavir, atazanavir, darunavir, fosamprenavir, nelfinavir, loprinavir-ritonavir (Kaletra®), tipranavir-ritonavir, and ritonavir. Rifabutin should be increased to 450-600 mg daily or 600 mg 2-3 times weekly in patients receiving efavirenz but should not be used at all in patients taking saquinavir or delavirdine. No rifabutin dose adjustment is required for patients taking nevirapine or etravirine. There are inadequate data on use of rifabutin with maraviroc or raltegravir, but probably no rifabutin dose adjustment is required. Clairithromycin increases the rifabutin AUC by 76%, making azithromycin a better choice for combination use. Modified from recommendations of the National Institutes of Health, the Centers for Diseases Control and Prevention, and the HIV Medicine Association of the Infectious Diseases Society of America, Guidelines for Prevention and Treatment of Opportunistic Infections in HIV-Infected Adults and Adolescents. *MMWR Recomm Rep.* 2009;58:1-207.

levels do not seem to be a good predictor of success of exogenous erythropoietin,[66] and symptomatic improvement after transfusion is prompt, so transfusion often is preferable. Hematocrit should be followed monthly to assess the need for subsequent transfusion. The response of anorexia and weight loss to antimycobacterial therapy is variable, but parenteral nutritional supplementation is not indicated. Follow-up blood cultures are not necessary for patients with clinical improvement but should be done for patients who fail to improve after 4 to 8 weeks. MAC isolates from patients failing therapy should be tested for susceptibility to clarithromycin, although most isolates remain sensitive in vitro to this drug.[131,132]

Some patients beginning antiretroviral therapy experience either a local inflammatory reaction or a worsening of systemic symptoms as a manifestation of the immune reconstitution syndrome.[44,95,96] This situation is especially likely when antimycobacterial therapy and antiretroviral therapy are initiated concurrently. Common local reactions are painful lymphadenopathy, abdominal pain, or hepatosplenomegaly. Most patients with the immune reconstitution syndrome improve with no change in therapy. For patients with severe symptoms, a short course (4-8 weeks) of steroids (e.g., prednisone, 0.5 mg/kg daily, tapered as signs and symptoms permit) may relieve symptomatic discomfort.[145]

The duration of treatment depends greatly on the patient's immune status. Therapy should be continued indefinitely for patients with less than 100 CD_4^+ cells/mm^3. In several large series, AIDS patients with disseminated MAC who have had a significant elevation of CD_4^+ cell counts owing to antiretroviral therapy have had antimycobacterial therapy stopped with no apparent harm.[155,156] Based on these studies, experts suggest that it is reasonable to discontinue treatment for persons who have received MAC therapy for at least 12 months and have had equal to or greater than 100 CD_4^+ cells/mm^3 for at least 6 months.[145] Patients should continue to be followed because there have been occasional reports of patients relapsing with local or systemic MAC after discontinuation of treatment.

LYMPHADENITIS

Surgical excision is the treatment of choice for lymphadenitis due to MAC.[97-99] Complete excision of the node is recommended as a diagnostic and therapeutic intervention. For individuals for whom surgery poses a high risk, therapy with a clarithromycin-containing regimen may be successful.[43]

Prophylaxis

Patients with AIDS and CD_4^+ cell counts of less than 50 cells/mm^3 are at high risk of developing disseminated MAC disease. Disseminated MAC disease develops in approximately 20% of such patients each year.[32,33] Given the high morbidity and mortality associated with disseminated MAC, chemoprophylaxis of MAC is a crucial component of care for all patients with CD_4^+ cell counts less than 50 cells/mm^3.[145] Drugs that have been proved effective at preventing disseminated MAC in this population are clarithromycin,[157] azithromycin,[158] and rifabutin.[159] In direct comparison studies, the macrolides/azalides were more effective than rifabutin.[160,161] There is no added benefit to using combination therapy to prevent disseminated MAC because resistance rarely emerges with single-agent prophylaxis.

Before beginning antimycobacterial prophylaxis, patients with fever, weight loss, or other symptoms of disseminated MAC should have a mycobacterial blood culture performed to ensure that disseminated disease is not present. Routine screening of sputum or stools for MAC is not indicated. Azithromycin, 1200 mg once weekly, is the preferred regimen, based on ease of administration and low toxicity (see Table 252-3). Clarithromycin also is effective but must be given at a dose of 500 mg twice daily. Rifabutin, 300 mg daily, should be used only when the patient cannot tolerate azithromycin or clarithromycin. Patients receiving rifabutin monotherapy also should be screened for active tuberculosis to avoid the emergence of rifampin-resistant tuberculosis. Patients who have had a nadir CD_4^+ cell of less than 50 cells/mm^3 and who with antiretroviral therapy have achieved an increase in CD_4^+ cells to greater than 100 cells/mm^3 are no longer at increased risk for MAC. Controlled studies have shown the safety of discontinuing antimycobacterial prophylaxis for MAC in this population.[162,163] Current recommendations are to discontinue MAC prophylaxis in persons who have achieved CD_4^+ counts greater than 100 cells/mm^3 for at least 3 months.[145] Patients should be restarted on prophylaxis if their CD_4^+ cells subsequently decline to less than or equal to 50 cells/mm^3.

REFERENCES

1. Horsburgh CR Jr. Epidemiology of *Mycobacterium avium* complex. *Lung Biol Health Dis.* 1996;87:1-22.
2. Wolinsky E. Nontuberculous mycobacteria and associated diseases. *Am Rev Respir Dis.* 1979;119:107-159.
3. du Moulin GC, Stottmeier KD, Pelletier PA, et al. Concentration of *Mycobacterium avium* by hospital hot water systems. *JAMA.* 1988;260:1599-1601.
4. Marras TK, Wallace Jr RJ, Koth LL, et al. Hypersensitivity pneumonitis reaction to *Mycobacterium avium* in household water. *Chest.* 2005;127:664-671.
5. von Reyn CF, Maslow JN, Barber TW, et al. Persistent colonisation of potable water as a source of *Mycobacterium avium* infection in AIDS. *Lancet.* 1994;343:1137-1141.
6. Tobin-D'Angelo MJ, Blass MA, del Rio C, et al. Hospital water as a source of *Mycobacterium avium* complex (MAC) isolates in respiratory specimens. *J Infect Dis.* 2004;189:98-104.
7. von Reyn CF, Arbeit RD, Tosteson ANA, et al, and the International MAC Study Group. The international epidemiology of disseminated *Mycobacterium avium* complex infection in AIDS. *AIDS.* 1996;10:1025-1032.
8. Sugita Y, Ishii N, Katsuno M, et al. Familial cluster of cutaneous *Mycobacterium avium* infection resulting from use of a circulating, constantly heated bath water system. *Br J Dermatol.* 2000;142:789-793.
9. Parker BC, Ford MA, Gruft H, et al. Epidemiology of infection by nontuberculous mycobacteria: IV. Preferential aerosolization of *Mycobacterium intracellulare* from natural waters. *Am Rev Respir Dis.* 1983;128:652-656.
10. Chapman JS. The atypical mycobacteria. *Hosp Pract.* 1970;5:69-80.
11. O'Brien RJ, Geiter LJ, Snider DE. The epidemiology of nontuberculous mycobacterial diseases in the United States: Results from a national survey. *Am Rev Respir Dis.* 1987;135:1007-1014.
12. Tsukamura M, Kita N, Shimoide H, et al. Studies on the epidemiology of nontuberculous mycobacteriosis in Japan. *Am Rev Respir Dis.* 1988;137:1280-1284.
13. Maugein J, Dailloux M, Carbonnelle B, et al. Sentinel-site surveillance of *Mycobacterium avium* complex pulmonary disease. *Eur Respir J.* 2005;26:1092-1096.
14. Debrunner M, Salfinger M, Brandli O, et al. Epidemiology and clinical significance of nontuberculous mycobacteria in patients negative for human immunodeficiency virus in Switzerland. *Clin Infect Dis.* 1992;15:330-345.
15. Iseman MD, Buschman DL, Ackerson LM. Pectus excavatum and scoliosis: Thoracic abnormalities associated with pulmonary disease caused by *Mycobacterium avium* complex. *Am Rev Respir Dis.* 1991;144:914-916.
16. Reich JM, Johnson RE. *Mycobacterium avium* complex pulmonary disease: Incidence, presentation, and response to therapy in a community setting. *Am Rev Respir Dis.* 1991;143:1381-1385.
17. Chin DP, Hopewell PC, Yajko DM, et al. *Mycobacterium avium* complex in the respiratory or gastrointestinal tract and the risk of developing *Mycobacterium avium* complex bacteremia in patients with the human immunodeficiency virus. *J Infect Dis.* 1994;169:289-295.
18. Horsburgh CR, Metchock B, Gordon SM, et al. Predictors of survival in patients with AIDS and disseminated *Mycobacterium avium* complex disease. *J Infect Dis.* 1994;170:573-577.
19. Kalayjian RC, Toossi Z, Tomashefski JF Jr, et al. Pulmonary disease due to infection by *Mycobacterium avium* complex in patients with AIDS. *Clin Infect Dis.* 1995;20:1186-1194.
20. Nishiuchi Y, Maekura R, Kitada S, et al. The recovery of Mycobacterium avium-intracellulare complex (MAC) from the residential bathrooms of patients with pulmonary MAC. *Clin Infect Dis.* 2007;45:347-351.
21. Hanak V, Golbin JM, Ryu JH. Causes and presenting features in 85 consecutive patients with hypersensitivity pneumonitis. *Mayo Clinic Proc.* 2007;82:812-816.
22. Kilby JM, Gilligan PH, Yankaskas JR, et al. Nontuberculous mycobacteria in adult patients with cystic fibrosis. *Chest.* 1992;102:70-75.
23. Pinto-Powell R, Olivier KN, Marsh BJ, et al. Skin testing with *Mycobacterium avium* sensitin to identify infection with *M. avium* complex in patients with cystic fibrosis. *Clin Infect Dis..* 1996;22:560-562.
24. Witty LA, Tapson VF, Piantadosi CA. Isolation of mycobacteria in patients with pulmonary alveolar proteinosis. *Medicine.* 1994;73:103-109.
25. Horsburgh CR Jr, Mason UG, Farhi DC, et al. Disseminated infection with *Mycobacterium avium-intracellulare:* A report of 13 cases and a review of the literature. *Medicine.* 1985;64:36-48.
26. Horsburgh CR. Epidemiology of human disease caused by *Mycobacterium avium* complex. *Can J Infect Dis.* 1994;5(suppl B):5B-9B.
27. Horsburgh CR, Gettings J, Alexander LN, et al. Disseminated *Mycobacterium avium* complex disease among patients infected with human immunodeficiency virus, 1985-2000. *Clin Infect Dis.* 2001;33:1938-1943.
28. Kaplan JE, Hanson D, Dworkin MS, et al. Epidemiology of human immunodeficiency virus–associated opportunistic infections in the United States in the era of highly active antiretroviral therapy. *Clin Infect Dis.* 2000;30(suppl 1):S5-14.
29. Reichenbach J, Rosenzweig S, Doffinger R, et al. Mycobacterial diseases in primary immunodeficiencies. *Curr Opin Allergy Clin Immunol.* 2001;1:503-511.
30. Winter SM, Bernard EM, Gold JW, et al. Humoral response to disseminated infection by *Mycobacterium avium–Mycobacterium intracellulare* in acquired immunodeficiency syndrome and hairy cell leukemia. *J Infect Dis.* 1985;151:523-527.
31. Sexton P, Harrison AC. Susceptibility to nontuberculous mycobacterial lung disease. *Eur Respir Dis.* 2008; 31:1322-1333.
32. Horsburgh CR. *Mycobacterium avium* complex infection in the acquired immunodeficiency syndrome. *N Engl J Med.* 1991;324:1332-1338.
33. Nightingale SD, Byrd LT, Southern PM, et al. Incidence of *Mycobacterium avium-intracellulare* complex bacteremia in human immunodeficiency virus positive patients. *J Infect Dis.* 1992;165:1082-1085.
34. Finkelstein DM, Williams PL, Molenberghs G, et al. Patterns of opportunistic infections in patients with HIV infection. *J Acquir Immune Defic Synd.* 1996;12:38-45.
35. Horsburgh CR, Selik RM. The epidemiology of disseminated nontuberculous mycobacterial infection in the acquired immunodeficiency syndrome (AIDS). *Am Rev Respir Dis.* 1989;139:4-7.
36. Horsburgh CR, Caldwell MB, Simonds RJ. Epidemiology of disseminated nontuberculous mycobacterial infection in children with AIDS. *Pediatr Infect Dis J.* 1993;12:219-222.
37. Horsburgh CR Jr, Schoenfelder JR, Gordin FM, et al. Geographic and seasonal variation in *Mycobacterium avium* bacteremia among North American patients with AIDS. *Am J Med Sci.* 1997;313:341-345.
38. Gilks CF, Brindle RJ, Mwachari C, et al. Disseminated mycobacterium infection among HIV-infected patients in Kenya. *J Acquir Immune Defic Syndr.* 1995;8:195-198.
39. Okello DO, Sewankambo N, Goodgame R, et al. Absence of bacteremia with *Mycobacterium avium-intracellulare* in Ugandan patients with AIDS. *J Infect Dis.* 1990;162:208-210.
40. Horsburgh CR, Hanson DL, Jones JL, et al. Protection from *Mycobacterium avium* complex disease in HIV-infected persons with a history of tuberculosis. *J Infect Dis.* 1996;174:1212-1217.
41. Haverkamp MH, Arend SM, Lindeboom JA, et al. Nontuberculous mycobacterial infection in children: A 2-year prospective surveillance study in the Netherlands. *Clin Infect Dis.* 2004;39:450-456.
42. Schaad UB, Votteler TP, McCracken GH, et al. Management of atypical mycobacterial lymphadenitis in childhood: A review based on 380 cases. *J Pediatr.* 1979;95:356-360.
43. Wolinsky E. Mycobacterial lymphadenitis in children: A prospective study of 105 nontuberculous cases with long-term follow-up. *Clin Infect Dis.* 1995;20:954-963.
44. Phillips P, Kwiatkowski MB, Copland M, et al. Mycobacterial lymphadenitis associated with the initiation of combination antiretroviral therapy. *J Acquir Immune Defic Syndr Hum Retrovirol.* 1999;20:122-128.
45. An official ATS/IDSA statement: Diagnosis, treatment, and prevention of nontuberculous mycobacterial diseases. *Am J Respir Crit Care Med.* 2007;175:367-416.
46. Tsang AY, Denner JC, Brennan PJ, et al. Clinical and epidemiological importance of typing of *Mycobacterium avium* complex isolates. *J Clin Microbiol.* 1992;30:479-484.
47. Arbeit RD, Slutsky A, Barber TW, et al. Genetic diversity among strains of *Mycobacterium avium* causing monoclonal and polyclonal bacteremia in patients with AIDS. *J Infect Dis.* 1993;167:1384-1390.
48. Smole SC, McAleese F, Ngampasutadol J, et al. Clinical and epidemiological correlates of genotypes within the *Mycobacterium avium* complex defined by restriction and sequence analysis of hsp65. *J Clin Microbiol.* 2002;40:3374-3380.
49. Gangadharam PR, Perumal VK, Crawford JT, et al. Association of plasmids and virulence of *Mycobacterium avium* complex. *Am Rev Respir Dis.* 1988;137:212-214.
50. Mapother ME, Songer JC. In vitro interaction of *Mycobacterium avium* with intestinal epithelial cells. *Infect Immun.* 1984;45:67-73.
51. Pethel ML, Falkinham JO III. Plasmid-influenced changes in *Mycobacterium avium* catalase activity. *Infect Immun.* 1989;57:1714-1718.
52. Frehel C, de Chastellier C, Lang T, et al. Evidence for inhibition of fusion of lysosomal and prelysosomal compartments with phagosomes in macrophages infected with pathogenic *Mycobacterium avium. Infect Immun.* 1986;52:252-262.
53. Shiratsuchi H, Toosi Z, Mettler MA, et al. Colonial morphotype as a determinate of cytokine expression by human monocytes infected with *M avium. J Immunol.* 1993;150:2945-2954.
54. Birkness KA, Swords WE, Huang PH, et al. Observed differences in virulence-associated phenotypes between a human clinical isolate and a veterinary isolate of *Mycobacterium avium. Infect Immun.* 1999;67:4895-4901.
55. Cirillo JD, Falkow S, Tompkins LS, et al. Interaction of *Mycobacterium avium* with environmental amoebae enhances virulence. *Infect Immun.* 1997;65:3759-3767.
56. Guthertz LS, Damsker B, Bottone EJ, et al. *Mycobacterium avium* and *Mycobacterium intracellulare* infections in patients with and without AIDS. *J Infect Dis.* 1989;160:1037-1041.
57. Marchevsky A, Damsker B, Gribetz A, et al. The spectrum of pathology of non-tuberculous mycobacterial infections in open-lung biopsy specimens. *Am J Clin Pathol.* 1982;78:695-700.
58. Horsburgh CR. The pathophysiology of disseminated *M. avium* disease in AIDS. *J Infect Dis.* 1999;179(suppl 3):S461-S465.
59. Torriani FJ, Behling CA, McCutchan JA, et al. Disseminated *Mycobacterium avium* complex: Correlation between blood and tissue burden. *J Infect Dis.* 1996;173:942-949.
60. Klatt EC, Jensen DF, Meyer PR. Pathology of *Mycobacterium avium-intracellulare* infection in acquired immunodeficiency syndrome. *Hum Pathol.* 1987;709:714.

61. Wallace JM, Hannah JB. *Mycobacterium avium* complex infection in patients with the acquired immunodeficiency syndrome. *Chest.* 1988;93:926-932.
62. MacGregor RR, Hafner R, Wu JW, et al. Clinical, microbiological, and immunological characteristics in HIV-infected subjects at risk for disseminated Mycobacterium avium complex disease: an AACTG study. *AIDS Research Hum Retrovir.* 2005;21:689-695.
63. Hafner R, Inderlied CB, Peterson DM, et al. Correlation of quantitative bone marrow and blood cultures in AIDS patients with disseminated *Mycobacterium avium* complex infection. *J Infect Dis.* 1999;180:438-447.
64. Haug CJ, Aukrust P, Lien E, et al. Disseminated *Mycobacterium avium* complex infection in AIDS: Immunopathogenic significance of an activated tumor necrosis factor system and depressed serum levels of 1,25 dihydroxyvitamin D. *J Infect Dis.* 1996;173:259-262.
65. Haas DW, Lederman MM, Clough LA, et al. Proinflammatory cytokine and human immunodeficiency virus RNA levels during early *Mycobacterium avium* complex bacteremia in advanced AIDS. *J Infect Dis.* 1998;177:1746-1749.
66. Gascon P, Sathe SS, Rameshwar P. Impaired erythropoiesis in the acquired immunodeficiency syndrome with disseminated *Mycobacterium avium* complex. *Am J Med.* 1993;94:41-48.
67. Vankayalapati R, Wizel B, Samten B, et al. Cytokine profiles in immunocompetent persons infected with *Mycobacterium avium* complex. *J Infect Dis.* 2001;183:478-484 (Epub December 20, 2000).
68. Newport MJ, Huxley CM, Huston S, et al. A mutation in the interferon-gamma-receptor gene and susceptibility to mycobacterial infection. *N Engl J Med.* 1996;335:1941-1949.
69. Holland SM, Dorman SE, Kwon A, et al. Abnormal regulation of interferon-gamma, interleukin-12, and tumor necrosis factor-alpha in human interferon-gamma receptor 1 deficiency. *J Infect Dis.* 1998;178:1095-1104.
70. Dorman SE, Holland SM. Mutation in the signal-transducing chain of the interferon-gamma receptor and susceptibility to mycobacterial infection. *J Clin Invest.* 1998;101:2364-2369.
71. Frucht DM, Holland SM. Defective monocyte costimulation for IFN-gamma production in familial disseminated *Mycobacterium avium* complex infection: Abnormal IL-12 regulation. *J Immunol.* 1996;157:411-416.
72. Holland SM, Eisenstein EM, Kuhns DB, et al. Treatment of disseminated nontuberculous mycobacterial infection with interferon gamma: A preliminary report. *N Engl J Med.* 1994;330:1348-1355.
73. Johnson JL, Shiratsuchi H, Toba H, et al. Preservation of monocyte effector functions against *Mycobacterium avium-M. intracellulare* in patients with AIDS. *Infect Immun.* 1991;59:3639-3645.
74. Havlir DV, Schrier RD, Torriani FJ, et al. Effect of potent antiretroviral therapy on immune responses to *Mycobacterium avium* in human immunodeficiency virus-infected subjects. *J Infect Dis.* 2000;182:1658-1663 (Epub October 18, 2000).
75. Ravn P, Pedersen BK. *Mycobacterium avium* and purified protein derivative-specific cytotoxicity mediated by CD4+ lymphocytes from healthy HIV-seropositive and -seronegative individuals. *J Acquir Immune Defic Syndr.* 1996;2:433-441.
76. Schnittman SH, Lane C, Witebsky FG, et al. Host defense against *Mycobacterium-avium* complex. *J Clin Immunol.* 1988;8:234-243.
77. Douvas GS, May MH, Pearson JR, et al. Hypertriglyceridemic serum, very low density lipoprotein, and iron enhance *Mycobacterium avium* replication in human macrophages. *J Infect Dis.* 1994;170:1248-1255.
78. Yeager H Jr. Pulmonary disease due to *Mycobacterium intracellulare. Am Rev Respir Dis.* 1973;108:547-552.
79. Contreras MA, Cheung OT, Sanders DE, et al. Pulmonary infection with nontuberculous mycobacteria. *Am Rev Respir Dis.* 1988;137:149-152.
80. Levin DL. Radiology of pulmonary *Mycobacterium avium-intracellulare* complex. *Clin Chest Med.* 2002;23:603-612.
81. Primack SL, Logan PM, Hartman TE, et al. Pulmonary tuberculosis and *Mycobacterium avium-intracellulare:* A comparison of CT findings. *Radiology.* 1995;194:413-417.
82. Prince DS, Peterson DD, Steiner RM, et al. Infection with *Mycobacterium avium* complex in patients without predisposing conditions. *N Engl J Med.* 1989;321:863-868.
83. Reich JM, Johnson RE. *Mycobacterium avium* complex pulmonary disease presenting as an isolated lingular or middle lobe pattern. *Chest.* 1992;101:1605-1609.
84. Swenson SJ, Hartman TE, Williams DE. Computer tomographic diagnosis of *Mycobacterium avium-intracellulare* complex in patients with bronchiectasis. *Chest.* 1994;105:49-52.
85. Olivier KN, Weber DJ, Wallace RJ Jr, et al. Nontuberculous mycobacteria: I. Multicenter prevalence study in cystic fibrosis. *Am J Respir Crit Care Med.* 2003;167:828-834.
86. Olivier KN, Weber DJ, Lee J-H, et al. Nontuberculous mycobacteria: II. Nested-cohort study of impact on cystic fibrosis lung disease. *Am J Respir Crit Care Med.* 2003;167:835-840.
87. Khoor A, Leslie KO, Tazelaar HD, et al. Diffuse pulmonary disease caused by nontuberculous mycobacteria in immunocompetent people (hot tub lung). *Am J Clin Pathol.* 2001;115:755-762.
88. Mangione EJ, Huitt G, Lenaway D, et al. Nontuberculous mycobacterial disease following hot tub exposure. *Emerg Infect Dis.* 2001;7:1039-1042.
89. Hanak V, Kalra S, Aksamit TR, et al. Hot tub lung: Presenting features and clinical course of 21 patients. *Respiratory Medicine.* 2006;100:610-615.
90. Wong B, Edwards FF, Kiehn TE, et al. Continuous high-grade *Mycobacterium avium-intracellulare* bacteremia in patients with the acquired immune deficiency syndrome. *Am J Med.* 1985;78:35-40.
91. Zakowski P, Fligiel S, Berlin GW, et al. Disseminated *Mycobacterium avium-intracellulare* infection in homosexual men dying of acquired immunodeficiency. *JAMA.* 1982;248:2980-2982.
92. Greene JB, Sidhu GS, Lewin S, et al. *Mycobacterium avium-intracellulare:* A cause of disseminated life-threatening infection in homosexuals and drug abusers. *Ann Intern Med.* 1982;97:539-546.
93. Gordin FM, Cohn DL, Sullam PM, et al. Early manifestations of disseminated *Mycobacterium avium* complex disease: A prospective evaluation. *J Infect Dis.* 1997;176:126-132.
94. Torriani FJ, McCutchan JA, Bozzette SA, et al. Autopsy findings in AIDS patients with *Mycobacterium avium* complex bacteremia. *J Infect Dis.* 1994;170:1601-1605.
95. Hassell M, French MA. *Mycobacterium avium* infection and immune restoration disease after highly active antiretroviral therapy in a patient with HIV and normal CD4+ counts. *Eur J Clin Microbiol Infect Dis.* 2001;20:889-891.
96. Phillips P, Bonner S, Gataric N, et al. Nontuberculous mycobacterial immune reconstitution syndrome in HIV-infected patients: Spectrum of disease and long-term follow-up. *Clin Infect Dis.* 2005;41:1483-1497.
97. Stewart MG, Starke JR, Coker NJ. Nontuberculous mycobacterial infections of the head and neck. *Arch Otolaryngol Head Neck Surg.* 1994;120:873-876.
98. Rahal A, Abela A, Arcand PH, et al. Nontuberculous mycobacterial adenitis of the head and neck in children: Experience from a tertiary care pediatric center. *Laryngoscope.* 2002;111:1791-1796.
99. Castro DJ, Hoover L, Castro DJ, et al. Cervical mycobacterial lymphadenitis. *Arch Otolaryngol.* 1985;111:816-819.
100. Hellinger WC, Smilack JD, Greider JL Jr, et al. Localized soft-tissue infections with *Mycobacterium avium/Mycobacterium intracellulare* complex in immunocompetent patients: Granulomatous tenosynovitis of the hand and wrist. *Clin Infect Dis.* 1995;21:65-69.
101. Kayak JD, McCall CO. Sporotrichoid cutaneous *Mycobacterium avium* complex infection. *J Am Acad Dermatol.* 2002;47:S249-S250.
102. Kullavanijaya P, Sirimachan S, Surarak S. Primary cutaneous infection with *Mycobacterium avium-intracellulare* complex resembling lupus vulgaris. *Br J Dermatol.* 1997;136:264-266.
103. Stone BL, Cohn DL, Kane MS, et al. Utility of paired blood cultures and smears in diagnosis of disseminated *Mycobacterium avium* complex infections in AIDS patients. *J Clin Microbiol.* 1994;32:841-842.
104. Havlir D, Kemper CA, Deresinski SC. Reproducibility of lysis-centrifugation cultures for quantification of *Mycobacterium avium* complex bacteremia. *J Clin Microbiol.* 1993;31:1794-1798.
105. Gamboa F, Manterola JM, Lonca J, et al. Detection and identification of mycobacteria by amplification of RNA and DNA in pretreated blood and bone marrow aspirates by a simple lysis method. *J Clin Microbiol.* 1997;35:2124-2128.
106. De Francesco MA, Colombrita D, Pinsi G, et al. Detection and identification of *Mycobacterium avium* in the blood of AIDS patients by the polymerase chain reaction. *Eur J Clin Microbiol Infect Dis.* 1996;15:551-555.
107. von Reyn CF, Williams D, Horsburgh CR, et al. Dual skin testing with *Mycobacterium avium* sensitin and purified protein derivative to discriminate pulmonary disease due to *M. avium* complex from pulmonary disease due to *Mycobacterium tuberculosis. J Infect Dis.* 1998;177:730-736.
108. Daley AJ, Isaacs D. Differential avian and human tuberculin skin testing in non-tuberculous mycobacterial infection. *Arch Dis Child.* 1999;80:377-379.
109. Lindeboom JA, Kuijper EJ, Prins JM, et al. Tuberculin skin testing is useful in the screening for nontuberculous mycobacterial cervicofacial lymphadenitis in children. *Clin Infect Dis.* 2006;43(12):1547-1551.
110. Ahn CH, Ahn SS, Anderson RA, et al. A four-drug regimen for initial treatment of cavitary disease caused by *Mycobacterium avium* complex. *Am Rev Respir Dis.* 1986;134:438-441.
111. Kemper CA, Meng T-C, Nussbaum J, et al. Treatment of *Mycobacterium avium* complex bacteremia in AIDS with a four-drug oral regimen. *Ann Intern Med.* 1992;116:466-472.
112. Hoy J, Mijch A, Sandland M, et al. Quadruple-drug therapy for *Mycobacterium avium-intracellulare* bacteremia in AIDS patients. *J Infect Dis.* 1990;161:801-805.
113. Chiu J, Nussbaum J, Bozzette S, et al. Treatment of disseminated *Mycobacterium avium* complex infection in AIDS with amikacin, ethambutol, rifampin, and ciprofloxacin. *Ann Intern Med.* 1990;113:358-361.
114. Heifets L. Susceptibility testing of *Mycobacterium avium* complex isolates. *Antimicrob Agents Chemother.* 1996;40:1759-1967.
115. Chaisson RE, Benson CA, Dubé MP, et al. Clarithromycin therapy for bacteremic *Mycobacterium avium* complex disease. *Ann Intern Med.* 1994;121:905-911.
116. Wallace RJ Jr, Brown BA, Griffith DE, et al. Initial clarithromycin monotherapy for *Mycobacterium avium-intracellulare* complex lung disease. *Am J Respir Crit Care Med.* 1994;149:1335-1341.
117. Griffith DE, Brown BA, Girard WM, et al. Azithromycin activity against *Mycobacterium avium* complex lung disease in patients who were not infected with human immunodeficiency virus. *Clin Infect Dis.* 1996;23:983-989.
118. Gardner EM, Burman WJ, DeGroote MA, et al. Conventional and molecular epidemiology of macrolide resistance among new *Mycobacterium avium* complex isolates recovered from HIV-infected patients. *Clin Infect Dis.* 2005;41:1041-1044.
119. Dautzenberg B, Marc TS, Meyohas MC, et al. Clarithromycin and other antimicrobial agents in the treatment of disseminated *Mycobacterium avium* infections in patients with acquired immunodefiency syndrome. *Arch Intern Med.* 1993;153:368-372.
120. Young LS, Wiviott L, Wu M, et al. Azithromycin for treatment of *Mycobacterium avium-intracellulare* complex infection in patients with AIDS. *Lancet.* 1991;338: 1107-1109.
121. Woodley CL, Kilburn JO. In vitro susceptibility of *Mycobacterium avium* complex and *Mycobacterium tuberculosis* strains to a spiro-piperidyl rifamycin. *Am Rev Respir Dis.* 1982;126:586-587.
122. Sullam PM, Gordin FM, Wynne BA, and the Rifabutin Treatment Group. Efficacy of rifabutin in the treatment of disseminated infection due to *Mycobacterium avium* complex. *Clin Infect Dis.* 1994;19:84-86.
123. Heifets LB, Iseman M, Lindholm-Levy PJ. Combinations of rifampin or rifabutin plus ethambutol against *Mycobacterium avium* complex. *Am Rev Respir Dis.* 1988;137:711-715.
124. Kemper CA, Havlir D, Haghighat D, et al. The individual microbiologic effect of three antimycobacterial agents, clofazimine, ethambutol, and rifampin, on *Mycobacterium avium* complex bacteremia in patients with AIDS. *J Infect Dis.* 1994;170:157-164.
125. Tanaka E, Kimoto T, Tsuyuguchi K, et al. Effect of clarithromycin regimen for *Mycobacterium avium* complex pulmonary disease. *Am J Respir Crit Care Med.* 1999;160:866-872.
126. Lam PK, Griffith DE, Aksamit TR, et al. Factors related to response to intermittent treatment of *Mycobacterium avium* complex lung disease. *Am J Respir Crit Care Med.* 2006;173:1283-1289.
127. Wallace RJ Jr, Brown BA, Griffith DE, et al. Clarithromycin regimens for pulmonary *Mycobacterium avium* complex. *Am J Respir Crit Care Med.* 1996;153:1766-1772.
128. Griffith DE, Brown BA, Girard WM, et al. Azithromycin-containing regimens for treatment of *Mycobacterium avium* complex lung disease. *Clin Infect Dis.* 2001;21:1547-1553.
129. The Research Committee of the British Thoracic Society. Pulmonary disease caused by *Mycobacterium avium-intracellulare* in HIV-negative patients: Five-year follow-up of patients receiving standardised treatment. *Int J Tuberc Lung Dis.* 2002;6:628-634.
130. Shafran SD, Singer J, Zarowny DP, et al. A comparison of two regimens for the treatment of *Mycobacterium avium* complex bacteremia in AIDS: Rifabutin, ethambutol, and clarithromycin versus rifampin, ethambutol, clofazimine, and ciprofloxacin. *N Engl J Med.* 1996;335:377-383.
131. Dubé MP, Sattler FR, Torriani FJ, et al. A randomized evaluation of ethambutol for prevention of relapse and drug resistance during treatment of *Mycobacterium avium* complex bacteremia with clarithromycin-based combination therapy. *J Infect Dis.* 1997;176:1225-1232.
132. Gordin FM, Sullam PM, Shafran SD, et al. A randomized, placebo-controlled study of rifabutin added to a regimen of clarithromycin and ethambutol for treatment of disseminated infection with *Mycobacterium avium* complex. *Clin Infect Dis.* 1999;28:1080-1085.
133. Ward TT, Rimland D, Kauffman C, et al. Randomized, open-label trial of azithromycin plus ethambutol vs. clarithromycin plus ethambutol as therapy for *Mycobacterium avium* complex bacteremia in patients with human immunodeficiency virus infection. *Clin Infect Dis.* 1998;27:1278-1285.
134. Dunne M, Fessel J, Kumar P, et al. A randomized, double-blind trial comparing azithromycin and clarithromycin in the treatment of disseminated *Mycobacterium avium* infection in patients with human immunodeficiency virus. *Clin Infect Dis.* 2000;31:1245-1252.
135. Cohn DL, Fisher EJ, Peng GT, et al. A prospective randomized trial of four three-drug regimens in the treatment of disseminated *Mycobacterium avium* complex disease in AIDS patients: Excess mortality associated with high-dose clarithromycin. *Clin Infect Dis.* 1999;29:125-133.
136. Brown BA, Griffith DE, Girard W, et al. Relationship of adverse events to serum drug levels in patients receiving high-dose azithromycin for mycobacterial lung disease. *Clin Infect Dis.* 1997;24:958-964.
137. Griffith DE, Brown-Elliott BA, Shepherd S, et al. Ethambutol ocular toxicity in treatment regimens for *Mycobacterium avium* complex lung disease. *Am J Respir Crit Care Med.* 2005;172:250-253.
138. Shafran SD, Deschênes J, Miller M, et al. Uveitis and pseudojaundice during a regimen of clarithromycin, rifabutin, and ethambutol. *N Engl J Med.* 1994;330:438-439.
139. Siegal FP, Eilbott D, Burger H, et al. Dose-limiting toxicity of rifabutin in AIDS-related complex: Syndrome of arthralgias/arthritis. *AIDS.* 1990;4:433-441.

140. Peloquin CA, Berning SE, Nitta AT, et al. Aminoglycoside toxicity: daily vs thrice-weekly dosing for treatment of mycobacterial disease. *Clin Infect Dis.* 2004; 38:1538-1544.
141. CDC. Updated guidelines for the use of rifamycins for the treatment of tuberculosis among HIV-infected patients taking protease inhibitors or nonnucleoside reverse transcriptase inhibitors. http://www.cdc.gov/tb/TB_HIV_Drugs/Rifabutin/htm.
142. Panel on Antiretroviral Guidelines for Adults and Adolescents. Guidelines for the use of antiretroviral agents in HIV-1-infected adults and adolescents. Department of Health and Human Services. http://www.aidsinfo.nih.gov/ContentFiles/Adultand-AdolescentGL.pdf.
143. Wallace RJ Jr, Brown BA, Griffith DE, et al. Reduced serum levels of clarithromycin in patients treated with multidrug regimens including rifampin or rifabutin for *Mycobacterium avium-M. intracellulare* infection. *J Infect Dis.* 1995;171:747-750.
144. Heifets L, Mor N, Vanderkolk J. *Mycobacterium avium* strains resistant to clarithromycin and azithromycin. *Antimicrob Agents Chemother.* 1993;37:2364-2370.
145. Recommendations of the National Institute of Health (NIH), the Centers for Diseases Control and Prevention (CDC), and *the HIV Medicine Association of the Infectious Diseases Society of America (HIVMA/IDSA).* Guidelines for Prevention and Treatment of Opportunistic Infections in HIV-Infected Adults and Adolescents. http://AIDSinfo.nih.gov. (June 18, 2008 version).
146. Rodriguez Díaz JC, López M, Ruiz M, et al. In vitro activity of new fluoroquinolones and linezolid against non-tuberculous mycobacteria. *Int J Antimicrob Agents.* 2003;21:585-588.
147. Chaisson RE, Keiser P, Pierce M, et al. Clarithromycin and ethambutol with or without clofazimine for the treatment of bacteremic *Mycobacterium avium* complex disease in patients with HIV infection. *AIDS.* 1997;11:311-317.
148. Milanes-Virelles MT, Garcia-Garcia I, Santos-Herrera Y, et al. Adjuvant interferon gamma in patients with pulmonary atypical Mycobacteriosis: a randomized, double-blind, placebo-controlled study. *BMC Infect Dis.* 2008;8:17.
149. Kobashi Y, Matsushima T, Oka M. A double-blind randomized study of aminoglycoside infusion with combined therapy for pulmonary *Mycobacterium avium* complex disease. *Respir Med.* 2007;101:130-138.
150. Aksamit TR. *Mycobacterium avium* complex pulmonary disease in patients with pre-existing lung disease. *Clin Chest Med.* 2002;23:643-653.
151. Pomerantz M, Madsen L, Goble M, et al. Surgical management of resistant mycobacterial tuberculosis and other mycobacterial pulmonary infections. *Ann Thorac Surg.* 1991;52:1108-1112.
152. Nelson KG, Griffith DE, Brown BA, et al. Results of operations in *Mycobacterium avium-intracellulare* lung disease. *Ann Thorac Surg.* 1998;66:325-330.
153. Watanabe M, Hasegawa N, Ishizaka A, et al. Early pulmonary resection for *Mycobacterium Avium* complex lung disease treated with macrolides and quinolones. *Ann Thorac Surg.* 2006;81:2026-2030.
154. Benson CA, Williams PL, Currier JS, et al. A prospective, randomized trial examining the efficacy and safety of clarithromycin in combination with ethambutol, rifabutin, or both for the treatment of disseminated *Mycobacterium avium* complex disease in persons with acquired immunodeficiency syndrome. *Clin Infect Dis.* 2003;37:1234-1243.
155. Shafran SD, Mashinter LD, Phillips P, et al. Successful discontinuation of therapy for disseminated *Mycobacterium avium* complex infection after effective antiretroviral therapy. *Ann Intern Med.* 2002;137:734-737.
156. Aberg JA, Williams PL, Liu T, et al. A study of discontinuing maintenance therapy in human immunodeficiency virus-infected subjects with disseminated *Mycobacterium avium* complex: AIDS clinical trial group 393 study team. *J Infect Dis.* 2003;187:1046-1052.
157. Pierce M, Crampton S, Henry D, et al. A randomized trial of clarithromycin as prophylaxis against disseminated *Mycobacterium avium* complex infection in patients with advanced acquired immunodeficiency syndrome. *N Engl J Med.* 1996;335:384-391.
158. Oldfield EC, Fessel WJ, Dunne MW, et al. Once weekly azithromycin therapy for prevention of *Mycobacterium avium* complex infection in patients with AIDS: A randomized, double-blind, placebo-controlled multicenter trial. *Clin Infect Dis.* 1998;26:611-619.
159. Nightingale SD, Cameron DW, Gordin FM, et al. Two controlled trials of rifabutin prophylaxis against *Mycobacterium avium* complex infection in AIDS. *N Engl J Med.* 1993;329:828-833.
160. Benson CA, Williams PL, Cohn DL, et al. Clarithromycin or rifabutin alone or in combination for primary prophylaxis of *Mycobacterium avium* complex disease in patients with AIDS: A randomized, double-blind, placebo-controlled trial. *J Infect Dis.* 2000;181:1289-1297.
161. Havlir DV, Dubé MP, Sattler FR, et al. Prophylaxis against disseminated *Mycobacterium avium* complex with weekly azithromycin, daily rifabutin, or both. *N Engl J Med.* 1996;335:392-398.
162. El-Sadr WM, Burman WJ, Grant LB, et al. Discontinuation of prophylaxis against *Mycobacterium avium* complex disease in HIV-infected patients who have a response to antiretroviral therapy. *N Engl J Med.* 2000;342:1085-1092.
163. Currier JS, Williams PL, Koletar SL, et al. Discontinuation of *Mycobacterium avium* complex prophylaxis in patients with antiretroviral therapy–induced increases in CD4+ cell count. *Ann Intern Med.* 2000;133:493-503.

253

Infections Due to Nontuberculous Mycobacteria Other than *Mycobacterium avium-intracellulare*

BARBARA A. BROWN-ELLIOTT | RICHARD J. WALLACE, JR.

The improvement in mycobacterial culture techniques and the increasing utility of modern molecular techniques for identification of previously unidentified organisms has produced a major resurgence of interest in disease caused by the nontuberculous mycobacteria (NTM). In addition, there has been an increasing appreciation of the defects in lung structure and immune response that predispose to NTM.[1] This group of mycobacteria is composed of species other than the *Mycobacterium tuberculosis* complex, which consists of *M. tuberculosis*, *Mycobacterium africanum*, *Mycobacterium bovis*, and *Mycobacterium leprae*. Previous names for this group of organisms include "atypical mycobacteria" or "mycobacteria other than *M. tuberculosis* (MOTT)."[2] Currently there are more than 120 species of NTM, of which more than one-half are considered to be potential sources of disease. Approximately 28 of these isolates have been described in the past 5 years.[3,4] *Mycobacterium avium* complex (MAC) is described extensively in Chapter 252. Traditionally, NTM have been categorized into different groups based on characteristic colony morphology, growth rate, and pigmentation (the Runyon system of classification). This system has become less useful as we focus on more rapid molecular systems of diagnostics. However, growth rates and colony pigmentation continue to provide practical means for grouping species of mycobacteria within the laboratory and are thus still used.[2]

Rapidly Growing Mycobacteria (RGM)

This group of organisms includes nonpigmented and pigmented species that produce mature growth on media plates within 7 days. There are currently five groups or complexes of RGM based on pigmentation and genetic relatedness. Nonpigmented pathogenic species now include 12 species within the *M. fortuitum* group (*M. fortuitum*, *M. peregrinum*, *M. senegalense*,[5,6] *M. conceptionense*,[7] *M. setense*,[8] and the third biovariant complex including *M. septicum*,[9,10] *M. mageritense*,[11,12] *M. porcinum*,[13] *M. houstonense*, *M. bonickei*, *M. brisbanense*, and *M. neworleansense*[9]) and five species within the *M. chelonae/abscessus* group (*M. chelonae*, *M. abscessus*, *M. immunogenum*,[5] *M. bolletii* and *M. massiliense*).[5,14,15,16] The *M. mucogenicum* group includes three species: *M. mucogenicum* (formerly *M. chelonae*-like organism) and two newly described species, *M. aubagnense* and *M. phocaicum*.[15] A fourth group of pathogenic organisms within the RGM, is the *M. smegmatis* group.[5,17] Isolates within this group include late pigmenting or nonpigmented species. The smegmatis group is currently composed of three species: *M. smegmatis*, *M. wolinskyi*, and *M. goodii*.[17] Many of these pathogenic species grow best at 30°C, but none have special nutritional requirements. All 20 of these species, including the newly described species (*M. aubagnense*, *M. phocaicum*, *M. bolletii*, and *M. massiliense*), have been recovered from clinical specimens on multiple occasions.[5,9,15,16]

The fifth group, (early) pigmenting RGM, are difficult to identify using conventional (phenotypic) laboratory methods. The pigmented species that have been implicated in clinical disease include *M. flavescens*, *M. neoaurum*, *M. vaccae*, *M. phlei*, the thermophilic species *M. thermoresistible*, and several newly described species, including *M. canariasense*, *M. cosmeticum*, *M. monacense*, and *M. psychrotolerans*.[2,18-21]

Slowly-Growing Mycobacteria

This group includes species of mycobacteria that require more than 7 days to reach mature growth. Some species may also require nutritional supplementation of routine mycobacterial media.[2] The major clinically important established species within this group include the *M. avium* complex (*M. avium* and *M. intracellulare*, and less commonly, *M. chimaera* and *M. colombiense*), *M. kansasii*, *M. xenopi*, *M. simiae* complex (*M. simiae*, *M. lentiflavum*, and *M. triplex*), *M. szulgai*, *M. malmoense*, *M. scrofulaceum*, and the *M. terrae/M. nonchromogenicum* complex, and less commonly *M. asiaticum*.[22] In Africa and Australia, *M. ulcerans* continues to be a major pathogen. Cultivation of this species is difficult, as it requires up to several months to grow, so molecular detection and identification are currently more optimal than culture techniques.[22,23] Other organisms that require special nutritional supplements include *M. haemophilum*, which requires hemin for growth (hence its name), and *M. genavense*,[22,23] which requires mycobactin J and prolonged incubation in broth culture. Most of these slowly-growing mycobacteria grow best at 35°C to 37°C, with the exception of *M. haemophilum*, which prefers lower temperatures (28°C to 30°C), and *M. xenopi*, which grows well at 42°C.[22,24] Newly described pigmented organisms in this group include *M. nebraskense*,[28] *M. parascrofulaceum*,[24,29,30] *M. parmense*,[31] *M. saskatchewanense*,[32] *M. pseudoshottsii*,[33] and *M. seoulense*.[34] Nonpigmented newly described species include two species related to *M. avium* complex, *M. chimaera*[4,34] and *M. colombiense*,[35] and five other species, *M. florentinum*,[4,36] *M. arupense*,[4,25] *M. kumamotonense*,[26] *M. senuense*,[27] and *M. montefiorense*.[4,37]

Intermediately Growing Mycobacteria

This group of organisms includes *M. marinum* and *M. gordonae*. These organisms are pigmented and require 7 to 10 days to reach mature growth. *M. marinum* grows optimally at 28° to 30°C, whereas *M. gordonae* prefers 35° to 37°C.[22]

NTM and the Environment

Most NTM species are readily recovered from the environment. Isolates have been recovered from samples of soil, water, animals, plant material, and birds.[2,22,38] A few species that are known to cause disease, such as *M. haemophilum* and *M. ulcerans,* have rarely been recovered from the environment.[23,38] Although an association with an environmental source may be present, a direct link to the environment has not been proven except for health care–associated disease and pseudo-outbreak, and no evidence of person-to-person spread has been reported, presumably due to the lower virulence of environmental species.[2] Tap water is considered the major reservoir for most common human NTM pathogens and as such is of increasing public health interest. Species from tap water include *M. gordonae*, *M. kansasii*, *M. xenopi*, *M. simiae*, *M. avium* complex, and rapidly growing mycobacteria, especially *M. mucogenicum*.[2,5,22,39] Biofilms, which are the filmy layers at the solid and liquid interface, are recognized as a source of growth and possibly a mode of transmission for mycobacteria.[38,39] Moreover, biofilms may serve to render mycobacteria less susceptible to disinfectants and antimicrobial therapy.[40] Biofilms appear to be present in almost all collection and piping systems, so mycobacteria may often be recovered from these sites. The persistence of pathogenic NTM in water and biofilms has important implications in the epidemiology of infections related to water.

NTM and Clinical Disease

NTM produce six major clinical disease syndromes (Table 253-1), which are reviewed in the following sections.

Pulmonary Disease

Geography of Common NTM Species

Chronic pulmonary disease in a human immunodeficiency virus (HIV)–negative host is the most common localized clinical disease caused by NTM.[22] In the United States, M. avium complex (MAC), followed by M. kansasii, is the most frequently recognized pathogen.[22] In Canada, some parts of the United Kingdom, and Europe, M. xenopi ranks third, whereas M. malmoense is second after MAC in Scandinavia and northern Europe.[2,22,24] In southeast England, M. xenopi and M. kansasii (known to be present in local water supplies) are both more

TABLE 253-1 Major Clinical Syndromes Associated with Nontuberculous Mycobacterial Infection

Syndrome	Most Common Causes	Less Frequent Causes
Chronic bronchopulmonary disease (adults, patients with cystic fibrosis)	M. avium complex (M. intracellulare, and M. avium), M. kansasii, M. abscessus	M. xenopi, M. malmoense, M. szulgai, M. smegmatis, M. scrofulaceum, M. celatum, M. simiae, M. goodii, M. asiaticum, M. heckeshornense, M. branderi, M. lentiflavum, M. triplex, M. fortuitum, M. arupense, M. bolletii, M. phocaicum, M. aubagnense, M. florentinum, M. massiliense, M. nebraskense, M. saskatchewanense, M. seoulense, M. senuense
Cervical or other lymphadenitis (especially children)	M. avium complex	M. scrofulaceum, M. malmoense (northern Europe), M. abscessus, M. fortuitum, M. lentiflavum, M. tusciae, M. palustre, M. interjectum, M. elephantis, M. heidelbergense, M. parmense
Skin and soft tissue disease	M. fortuitum group, M. chelonae, M. abscessus, M. marinum, M. ulcerans (Australia, tropical countries only)	M. kansasii, M. haemophilum, M. porcinum, M. smegmatis, M. genavense, M. lacus, M. novocastrense, M. houstonense, M. goodii, M. immunogenum, M. mageritense, M. massiliense, M. arupense, M. conceptionense, M. moracense, M. montefiorense (eels), M. pseudoshottsii (fish)
Skeletal (bone, joint, tendon) infection	M. marinum, M. avium complex, M. kansasii, M. fortuitum group, M. abscessus, M. chelonae	M. haemophilum, M. scrofulaceum, M. smegmatis, M. terrae/chromogenicum complex, M. wolinskyi, M. goodii, M. arupense
Disseminated infection		
HIV-seropositive host	M. avium, M. kansasii, M. genavense, M. haemophilum, M. xenopi,	M. marinum, M. simiae, M. intracellulare, M. scrofulaceum, M. fortuitum, M. conspicuum, M. celatum, M. lentiflavum, M. triplex, M. colombiense
HIV-seronegative host	M. abscessus, M. avium, M. kansasii, M. chelonae	M. marinum, M. avium, M. kansasii, M. haemophilum, M. chimaera
Catheter-related infections	M. fortuitum, M. abscessus, M. chelonae	M. mucogenicum, M. immunogenum, M. mageritense, M. septicum, M. neoaurum

HIV, human immunodeficiency virus.

TABLE 253-2 Clinical Settings for Nontuberculous Mycobacterial Lung Disease

Radiographic Disease	Setting	Usual Pathogen* (Rare Pathogen)
Upper lobe cavitary	Male smokers, often abusing alcohol, usually early 50s	M. avium complex, M. kansasii
RML, lingular nodular bronchiectasis	Female nonsmokers, usually older than 60 years	M. avium complex, M. abscessus (M. kansasii)
Localized alveolar, cavitary disease	Prior granulomatous disease (usually tuberculosis) with bronchiectasis	M. abscessus, M. avium complex
Not established	Adolescents with cystic fibrosis	M. abscessus, M. avium complex
Reticulonodular or alveolar bilateral lower lobe disease	Achalasia, chronic vomiting secondary to GI disease, exogenous lipoid pneumonia (mineral oil aspirations, etc.)	M. fortuitum (M. abscessus, M. avium complex, M. smegmatis, M. goodii)
Reticulonodular disease	HIV-positive hosts, maybe prior bronchiectasis secondary to PCP or other cause	M. avium complex

*Too little information is available for selected pathogens such as M. xenopi, M. malmoense, M. szulgai, M. celatum, and M. asiaticum and the newly described species.
GI, Gastrointestinal; HIV, human immunodeficiency virus; PCP, Pneumocystis pneumonia; RML, right middle lobe.

common than MAC.[2,24,41] In the United States, the third most common cause of NTM pulmonary disease is M. abscessus complex, which produces 80% of pulmonary infections caused by rapidly growing mycobacteria.[22] (This study antedated recognition of M. bolletii and M. massiliense.)

NTM Species Associated Infrequently with Pulmonary Disease

Among the newly described RGM, pulmonary infection has been reported with M. bolletii,[15] M. massiliense,[16,42] M. phocaicum,[15] and M. aubagnense.[15] Other NTM that less commonly cause pulmonary disease include M. fortuitum, M. smegmatis, M. goodii,[5,16] M. szulgai,[22] M. simiae,[22] M. celatum,[22,43] M. lentiflavum,[44] M. asiaticum,[22] M. heckeshornense,[45] and, rarely, M. gordonae.[22] Recently pulmonary infections have also been attributed to newer species, including M. arupense,[26] M. chimaera,[4,46] M. florentinum,[4,36] M. kumamotonense,[26] M. nebraskense,[4,28] M. saskatchewanense,[4,32] M. senuense,[27] and M. seoulense.[34] In contrast to nodular disease caused by M. abscessus, pulmonary disease with M. goodii[5,16] usually involves lipoid pneumonia.

Pulmonary Syndromes with NTM Other than MAC

Clinical disease with M. kansasii produces upper lobe fibrocavitary disease and nodular disease similar to MAC in the same setting. M. abscessus group also produces nodular disease in the setting of bronchiectasis. Pulmonary NTM disease is rare in children, except for those with cystic fibrosis.[22]

A bilateral subacute to acute alveolar disease is well recognized in the setting of achalasia. High fevers, striking leucocytosis above 20,000, cough and mucus production, and an acute illness are common. The histopathology shows a combination of lipoid disease and acute/granulomatous infection. The usual pathogen is M. fortuitum, but M. abscessus, M. smegmatis, and M. goodii can be seen.[22]

Clinical NTM Disease

Because the signs and symptoms of NTM lung disease are often variable and nonspecific, disease with NTM is difficult to diagnose without positive respiratory cultures (Table 253-2).[47] Patients often present with chronic cough, a "throat clearing" with or without sputum production, and fatigue. Less frequently, complaints of malaise, dyspnea, fever, hemoptysis, and weight loss may also be present. Clinical studies should include microbiologic cultures for acid-fast bacilli and routine chest radiographs. High-resolution chest computed tomography is essential in patients suspected of having nodular bronchiectasis. Recovery of NTM from a single sputum sample is not proof of NTM disease, especially when the acid-fast bacillus (AFB) smear is negative and NTM are present in low numbers. The American Thoracic Society statement on the diagnosis and treatment of NTM[22] has recently revised the diagnostic criteria to determine lung disease caused by NTM (Table 253-3 and see Chapter 252).[22] For NTM disease due to organisms other than MAC, these criteria may need to be adjusted because inadequate data are available to evaluate these criteria. Expert consultation should be obtained when NTM that are infrequently encountered are recovered.[22]

Treatment of M. kansasii *Lung Disease*

Treatment of lung disease caused by *M. kansasii* has traditionally been less difficult than that for *M. avium* complex since the introduction of rifampin.[48] A regimen of daily rifampin, 600 mg, isoniazid, 300 mg, and ethambutol, 15 mg/kg, has been widely accepted in the United States and is still recommended by the American Thoracic Society (Table 253-4).[22] In HIV-positive patients receiving a PI or NNRTI, rifampin should be replaced by rifabutin, though the dosage depends on the antiretrovirals. The rifabutin dose should be decreased to 150 mg daily in patients receiving amprenavir, atazanavir, nelfinavir, and ritonavir. Rifabutin should be increased to 450 mg daily or 600 mg thrice weekly in patients receiving efavirenz but should not be used at all in patients taking saquinavir. No rifabutin dose adjustment is required for patients taking nevirapine or etravirine. There are inadequate data on use of rifabutin with maraviroc or raltegravir, but probably no rifabutin dose adjustment is required. Patients should be treated with at least 12 months of culture negativity.[22] For patients resistant or intolerant to rifampin, clarithromycin is a reasonable alternative agent.[22,49]

The usefulness of isoniazid in this regimen is controversial, with a macrolide offering a much better alternative. In the United Kingdom,

TABLE 253-3	American Thoracic Society Diagnostic Criteria for Nontuberculous Mycobacterial Lung Disease

The minimum evaluation of a patient for NTM lung disease should include:
1. Chest radiograph or, when no cavitation is present, high-resolution computed tomography (HRCT)
2. At least three sputum or respiratory samples for acid-fast bacilli (AFB) culture.
3. Exclusion of other disease such as tuberculosis (TB).

Clinical diagnosis of NTM is based on pulmonary symptoms, presence of nodules or cavities as seen on chest radiograph or an HRCT scan with multifocal bronchiectasis with multiple small nodules, and exclusion of other diagnoses.

Microbiological Diagnosis of NTM
1. At least two expectorated sputa (or at least one bronchial wash or lavage) with positive cultures for NTM or transbronchial or other lung biopsy showing the presence of granulomatous inflammation or AFB with one or more sputum or bronchial washings that are culture positive for NTM.

Data from Griffith DE, Aksamit T, Brown-Elliott BA, et al: An official ATS/IDSA statement: Diagnosis, treatment and prevention of nontuberculous mycobacterial diseases. American Thoracic Society Statement. *Am J Respir Crit Care Med.* 2007; 175:367-416.

isoniazid is omitted from the regimen. An intermittent regimen (three times weekly) using clarithromycin in place of isoniazid (the same drugs and drug concentration as for MAC) suggests that intermittent therapy for *M. kansasii* can be highly effective, but it has been reported in a limited number of patients.[49]

Untreated strains of *M. kansasii* are susceptible to low concentrations of rifampin, rifabutin, ethambutol, ethionamide, streptomycin, sulfonamides, clarithromycin, and the quinolones, although information on drugs other than rifampin or ethambutol is limited on the clinical utility of these latter three agents.[22,49] Acquired mutational resistance of rifampin to *M. kansasii* can occur, but this organism is readily treated with multidrug regimens.[22]

TABLE 253-4	Frequently Used Treatment Regimens for Common Nontuberculous Mycobacterial Pathogens other than MAC				
Species	Disease[2]	Drug	Daily Adult Doses[3]	Three Times Weekly Adult Dose	Duration
M. kansasii	Pulmonary (USA)	Isoniazid *plus*	300 mg		Culture negative at least 12 mos
		Rifampin *plus*	600 mg	600 mg	
		Ethambutol	15 mg/kg[2]	25 mg/kg	
		Clarithromycin	500 mg bid	500 mg bid	
	(UK)	Rifampin *plus*	600 mg	600 mg	9-12 mos
		Ethambutol	15 mg/kg	15 mg/kg	
	Disseminated	Same as pulmonary			
	HIV-positive	Same as pulmonary (USA) but replace rifampin with rifabutin or clarithromycin[4]	150 mg		Same as pulmonary (USA)
			500 mg bid		
M. abscessus	Pulmonary (adults)	Amikacin IV *plus*	7-10 mg/kg single dose[1]	NA	2 wk (designed to improve, not cure)
		Imipenem IV *or*	1 gm twice daily		
		Cefoxitin IV *plus*	8-12 g/d (2 or 3 doses)		2 wk
		Clarithromycin	500 mg bid		6 mos
	Cutaneous localized	Clarithromycin	500 mg bid		6 mos
	Disseminated or extensive cutaneous	Same 3 drugs as above		NA	
M. marinum	Cutaneous	Clarithromycin *or*	500 mg bid	NA	3 mos minimum for all regimens
		Minocycline *or*	100 mg bid		
		Rifampin *plus*	600 mg		
		Ethambutol	15 mg/kg		

[1]Based on age, weight, renal status (ATS).
[2]Human immunodeficiency virus (HIV)–negative host unless otherwise stated.
[3]Drugs by mouth unless otherwise stated.
[4]Patients on HIV medicines inactivated by rifampin.
MAC, *Mycobacterium avium* complex.
From: Brown-Elliott BA, Wallace RJ Jr.: Infections caused by nontuberculous mycobacteria. In: Mandell GL, Bennett JE, Dolin R, eds. *Mandell, Douglas, and Bennett's Principles and Practice of Infectious Diseases*, 6th ed. Vol 2. Philadelphia: Churchill Livingstone; 2005:2909-2916.

Treatment of M. abscessus *Complex Lung Disease*

Treatment of *M. abscessus* complex lung disease with antimicrobials alone has generally been unsuccessful.[22] Courses of therapy in adults with clarithromycin, high-dose IV cefoxitin (8-12 g/day in two to three divided doses) or imipenem (1 gm twice daily), and low-dose parenteral amikacin (peaks in 20-25 μg/mL range on once daily dosing) produce clinical improvement with limited toxicity but do not result in microbiologic cure.[22] Studies using a new IV glycylcycline antibiotic, tigecycline, are being evaluated currently. All species of RGM, including the *M. abscessus* complex, have MICs of less than 1 μg/mL to this agent.[50] This drug is now often included in multidrug therapy.

A concern for the usefulness of the macrolides for *M. smegmatis, M. fortuitum,* and the *M. abscessus* group is that they contain inducible *erm* genes (*erm* 38, *erm* 39, and *erm* 41, respectively), which induces macrolide resistance and may be responsible for treatment failure.[51-54] The microbiologic and clinical response to the macrolides for therapy of *M. abscessus* group lung disease has traditionally been poor, a response that is likely explained by the presence of the *erm* gene.[51-54]

Treatment of Other NTM

A recommended or standardized treatment for lung disease caused by other slowly growing mycobacteria such as *M. simiae, M. szulgai, M. xenopi, M. branderi,* and *M. malmoense* has not been established.[22,24] Drug combinations similar to those used with MAC, such as clarithromycin, ethambutol, rifabutin, and perhaps an aminoglycoside with 12 months of negative cultures, seem reasonable at the present time.[22,24,41]

Pseudo-outbreaks of pulmonary disease have been described, usually related to contamination of bronchoscopes or the automated endoscope washing machine.[22] *M. immunogenum* is the most common species recovered in this setting, followed by *M. abscessus* complex.[5,14] *M. immunogenum* has also been associated with hypersensitivity pneumonitis associated with occupational exposure to metalworking fluids.[14]

Lymphadenitis

Localized cervical lymphadenitis is the most common NTM disease in children, with a peak incidence between 1 and 5 years of age.[2,43,55,56] NTM-affected lymph nodes are usually in the anterior cervical chain and are unilateral and painless. The nodes may enlarge rapidly with the formation of fistulas to the skin, and prolonged drainage may occur. Occasionally, other nodes outside the head and neck, such as the mediastinal lymph nodes, may be involved.[2,55] A definitive diagnosis of NTM lymphadenitis is made by recovery of the etiologic organism from lymph node cultures. The tuberculin skin test is often weakly positive (5-10 mm), but it may be more than 10 mm.[55] Routine biopsy or incision and drainage should be avoided because these procedures often result in the formation of fistulas and chronic drainage. Fine-needle aspiration with cytology and culture has been used increasingly with apparently few associated problems.

Treatment of NTM cervical lymphadenitis is still evolving. The potential role of macrolide treatment regimens without surgery or as a supplement to surgery in complicated or recurrent disease is being considered with increasing frequency. Clarithromycin combined with ethambutol or rifabutin is the usual suggested regimen (see Table 253-4). However, the established treatment of routine NTM cervical lymphadenitis (from the premacrolide era) remains surgical excision without (antituberculous drug) chemotherapy.[22]

Since the early 1980s, 80% of cases of culture-positive NTM lymphadenitis in children in the United States have been caused by MAC.[2,22] The remainder of the cases in Australia and the United States are caused by *M. scrofulaceum,* and only about 10% of the cases have been caused by *M. tuberculosis.*[2,22,55] In parts of northern Europe, including Scandinavia and the United Kingdom, *M. malmoense* has become the second most common pathogen after MAC.[2,24,57] *M. lentiflavum* appears to be an increasing cause of cervical lymphadenitis in selected geographic areas.[44] The same is true for *M. haemophilum,* as a recent report from Israel showed that the rate of isolation of *M. haemophilum*

in cervical lymphadenitis since 1996 was 51%.[58] Rarely, other species are recovered, including rapidly growing mycobacteria,[2,5] *M. kansasii, M. interjectum, M. parmense, M. palustre, M. tusciae, M. heidelbergense, M. elephantis, M. triplex,* and *M. bohemicum.*[2-4]

Recently, a report from Thailand of 128 HIV-negative adult patients described disseminated NTM infection with bilateral lymphadenitis in 89% of the patients. The majority of infections were caused by RGM, including *M. abscessus, M. fortuitum, M. chelonae,* and *M. thermoresistibile.* The investigators noted that unlike the more common form of NTM lymphadenitis in children, all but one of 129 patients were adults whose infection spread to other organ involvement.[59]

Localized Cutaneous and Soft Tissue Infections

Although most pathogenic species of NTM have been incriminated in cutaneous NTM disease, *M. marinum, M. ulcerans,* and the rapidly growing mycobacteria most often cause localized skin infections.[5,20,22,55]

M. marinum

M. marinum causes an infection historically recognized as "swimming pool" or "fish tank" granuloma.[2,22,55,60] This common name is derived from the epidemiologic niche of the organism. Most infections occur 2 to 3 weeks after contact with contaminated water from one of these sources. The lesions are most often small violet papules on the hands and arms that may progress to shallow, crusty ulcerations and scar formation. Lesions are usually singular. However, multiple ascending lesions resembling sporotrichosis ("sporotrichoid disease") can occasionally occur.[2,22,60] Most patients are clinically healthy with a previous local hand injury that becomes infected while cleaning a fish tank, or patients may sustain scratches or puncture wounds from saltwater fish, shrimp, fins, and so forth contaminated with *M. marinum.* Swimming pools seem to be a risk only when nonchlorinated. Diagnosis is made from culture and histologic examination of biopsy material, along with a compatible history of exposure. No treatment of choice is recognized for *M. marinum* (see Table 253-3). Treatments have traditionally been a two-drug combination of rifampin plus ethambutol or monotherapy with doxycycline, minocycline, clarithromycin, or trimethoprim-sulfamethoxazole given for a minimum of 3 months. Clarithromycin has been used increasingly because of good clinical efficacy and minimal side effects, although published experience is limited.[2,22]

Rapidly Growing Mycobacteria

The rapidly growing species *M. abscessus, M. fortuitum,* and *M. chelonae* are the most common NTM involved in cases of community-acquired infections of skin and soft tissue in the USA.[2,5] The *M. fortuitum* group is responsible for 60% of localized cutaneous infections in previously healthy individuals. Unlike infections with the *M. chelonae–M. abscessus* group, the patient with *M. fortuitum* localized infection usually has no predisposing immune-suppression.[2,5] In a series of 42 patients for whom clinical history was available, the majority of infections involved some type of traumatic injury, such as metal puncture wounds from stepping on a nail (48%), motor vehicle accidents (26%), and injuries involving the foot or leg (approximately 40%).[2,5] Open lacerations or fractures were common.

In contrast, localized infections with *M. chelonae* are seen primarily in patients who are immunosuppressed, especially on long-term corticosteroids. Autoimmune diseases such as rheumatoid arthritis and systemic lupus are often predisposing factors. In a study by Wallace and colleagues, 35% of the *M. chelonae* with nonpulmonary infections were seen in localized wound infections.[5]

Disease due to *M. abscessus* is somewhat intermediate, as it causes disease in normal hosts and those with immune suppression. Examples of localized wound infection with *M. abscessus* include soft tissue infection of the cheek following an insect bite and vertebral osteomyelitis.[5]

Occasionally, localized community-acquired infections of the skin, soft tissue, or bone may involve slow-growing species, including MAC,[22] *M. kansasii*,[22] and *M. terrae/M. nonchromogenicum* complex,[22] and rarely newer species, such as *M. novocastrense*[61] and *M. lacus*.[62] Among the newly described species, *M. monacense* has been recovered from a post-traumatic wound infection in a healthy child.[20]

Health Care–Associated Infections

Sporadic cases of health care–associated skin and soft tissue disease have also been described. These cases include infections of long-term intravenous or peritoneal catheters, postinjection abscesses, surgical wound infections, such as after cardiac bypass surgery, and augmentation mammoplasty.[5,22,63,64]

A cluster of 12 cases involving *M. fortuitum* and *M. porcinum* in postaugmentation mammoplasty surgical site infections was recently described in Brazil.[63] Clustered outbreaks or pseudo-outbreaks of mycobacterial skin, soft tissue, or bone infections have been described and usually result from contaminated fluids such as ice made from tap water, irrigation or exposure to tap water, injectable medicines, and topical skin solutions/markers.[22]

The contamination of benzalkonium chloride (a quaternary ammonium commonly used as an antiseptic) with *M. abscessus* was responsible for a serious outbreak of *M. abscessus* following steroid injections and serves to emphasize the limitations of disinfectants against mycobacteria.[65] Recently there have been reports of eye disease due to RGM including post-keratoplasty and following laser-assisted in situ keratomileusis (LASIK) surgery for correction of myopia.[5,66] A cluster of *M. chelonae* keratitis was associated with hyperoptic LASIK using a contact lens mask. Thirty-one of 43 additional cases of keratitis between 2000 and 2001 were part of this outbreak, while the 12 other reported cases were sporadic.[67]

Other recent outbreaks involving nontuberculous mycobacteria have involved contamination of liposuction equipment with *M. chelonae*, with the same disease strain found in tap water used for rinsing suction tubing.[68] Most of the skin and soft tissue disease outbreaks have involved the rapidly growing species *M. fortuitum* and *M. abscessus*. However, an outbreak of four patients with alcohol-resistant mycobacterial species (two with *M. chelonae* and two with *M. nonchromogenicum*) was reported in Hong Kong after acupuncture treatments from 1999 to 2000.[69] Additionally, between 2003 and 2004, an outbreak of *M. abscessus* occurred in patients from the United States who visited the Dominican Republic for cosmetic surgery for fat removal (known as "lipotourism").[70] Although no water samples or environmental samples were available for testing in this outbreak, the reservoir for these types of outbreaks has historically been municipal or hospital water supplies.[22]

Since 2002, several outbreaks of lower-extremity folliculitis due to RGM (*M. fortuitum*, *M. abscessus*, and *M. mageritense* disease), associated with nail salons ("foot-spa disease"), have been reported.[71-75] Leg hair removal by wax stripping followed by NTM-contaminated foot baths was followed by indolent folliculitis.

Outbreaks of newly described species including *Mycobacterium cosmeticum*, *M. massiliense*, and *M. bolletii* have also been described recently from postinjection abscess following flu or cold antibiotic injections, cosmetic procedures, and following laparascopic surgeries in Korea, Brazil, Venezuela, and Ohio.[19,76,77]

Skin/Soft Tissue

Diagnosis and Treatment

Diagnosis of all types of skin and soft tissue infections is made by culture of specific NTM from drainage material or tissue biopsy. Treatment may include amikacin, cefoxitin, ciprofloxacin, moxifloxacin, clarithromycin, doxycycline, linezolid, sulfonamides, and imipenem for the *M. fortuitum* group, whereas only amikacin, cefoxitin, imipenem, and clarithromycin, or only amikacin, imipenem, tobramycin, clarithromycin, and sometimes linezolid, have activity against *M. abscessus* and *M. chelonae*, respectively.[5,22,78] Clarithromycin is gener-

ally the drug of choice for localized disease (but not for disseminated disease) caused by *M. chelonae* and *M. abscessus*.[79] However, the efficacy of macrolide treatment for *M. abscessus* (and the *M. fortuitum* group) is likely diminished by recent recognition that they carry novel *erm* genes that confer inducible resistance.[51-54] The duration of therapy is usually 4 to 6 months.

Antituberculous agents have no efficacy against any of the rapidly growing mycobacteria, other than ethambutol for *M. smegmatis*, and should not be used.[80] Monotherapy with quinolones is not recommended because of the high risk of mutational resistance of the RGM to these agents. Treatment of slowly growing species is similar to that for chronic lung disease, except that the duration of therapy may only be 6 to 12 months, depending on severity of the disease.[22]

Two unusual species causing skin and soft tissue infections in select situations are *M. ulcerans* and *M. haemophilum*. *M. ulcerans* is not endemic in the United States, but it is endemic in northern areas of Australia and tropical locations of the world, where it is commonly known as the "Buruli ulcer."[23] *M. ulcerans* is extremely slow growing, with the average incubation time around 8 to 12 weeks, and *M. haemophilum* may take up to 3 to 4 weeks to grow on primary culture.[22,24,81] Thus, newer molecular techniques for identification of these organisms have expedited diagnosis of infection with the organisms.[22] The *M. ulcerans* infection progresses from an itchy nodule, most often on the extremities, to a necrotic lesion that may result in severe limb deformity. Treatment success is common in early disease with excisional surgery, rifampin, sulfonamides, and clofazimine, but for advanced ulcerative disease, therapeutic response has generally been poor.[23] Surgical débridement and skin grafting then become the usual therapeutic measures of choice.[22,23,49] Recent studies suggest that clarithromycin is highly active in vitro.[20]

M. haemophilum causes cutaneous infections (primarily of the extremities) in immunosuppressed patients, especially in the setting of organ transplantation, long-term high-dose steroid use, or HIV.[22,81] A review cited more than 50 cases of *M. haemophilum*, with almost 80% of them involving skin and soft tissue infections.[81] *M. haemophilum* has a special growth requirement for hemin or iron and may present some diagnostic difficulties if iron- or hemin-supplemented media and lower temperatures (incubation at 28° C to 30° C) are not used.[22,81] A surprising number of specimens are acid-fast bacillus smear positive and culture negative, so a presumptive diagnosis is often based on typical caseating granulomas and a negative culture for *M. tuberculosis* in the common clinical setting. Therapy for this species usually includes clarithromycin and rifampin or rifabutin.[2,24,81] Of note, *M. montefiorense* and *M. pseudoshottsii* have been recovered from granulomatous lesions in eels and fish, respectively.[4,33,37]

Infection of Tendon Sheaths, Bones, Bursae, and Joints

Both rapidly growing and slowly growing species of NTM have been implicated in chronic granulomatous infections involving tendon sheaths, bursae, bones, and joints after direct inoculation of the pathogen through accidental trauma, surgical incisions, puncture wounds, or injections.[2,7,22,55] Most patients have no underlying immune suppression, but high risk for some pathogens such as *M. chelonae* and *M. haemophilum* is seen in patients who are immunosuppressed.[82] MAC and *M. marinum* have been described as causing tenosynovitis of the hand,[2,22,55] although the rapidly growing mycobacteria *M. kansasii* and *M. terrae* complex (especially *M. nonchromogenicum*) have also been associated with a chronic type of disease.[2,22,55] Osteomyelitis of the sternum caused by *M. fortuitum*, and *M. abscessus* has also been found in clustered outbreaks and sporadic cases after cardiac surgery.[22] Newly described species—*M. conceptionense*, *M. porcinum*, and *M. setense*—have been isolated from post-traumatic osteitis and osteomyelitis.[7,8,13,82] Additionally, *M. haemophilum* has a tendency to involve bones and joints, usually with concurrent draining skin lesions and bacteremia.[81] *M. arupense* has also been recovered from the culture of a tendon in a patient with diabetes mellitus.[83] Recently, an outbreak of 58 cases of bone and joint infections in immunocompetent patients in a French hospital involved *M. xenopi*.[41]

Management of mycobacterial rheumatologic infections often requires surgical débridement for both diagnosis and therapy, especially for the closed spaces of the hand and the wrist and for patients with infected bones such as fractured long bones or the sternum after cardiac surgery. Drug therapy for the specific pathogen is also essential.[2,22]

Disseminated Disease

HIV Disease
In the setting of advanced HIV infection, most disseminated NTM disease is due to *M. avium*. However, other NTM, including *M. kansasii*, *M. genavense*, *M. intracellulare*, *M. haemophilum*, *M. simiae*, *M. celatum*, *M. malmoense*, *M. marinum*, and rapidly growing mycobacteria, have also been recovered.[5,22,24,81,84,85] Disseminated disease among the newer species—*M. triplex*, *M. lentiflavum*, and *M. conspicuum*—has also been reported, as have multiple recoveries of the newly described species *M. colombiense*.[2-5]

Disseminated *M. kansasii* is the second most frequent cause of disseminated NTM disease in the setting of AIDS, disseminated MAC being the most common cause.[22] Pulmonary and cutaneous manifestations have occurred[22] in patients with chronic lymphocytic leukemia, after organ transplantation, and in those infected by HIV. One study reported five patients with disseminated *M. kansasii* infection, including three patients with pulmonary and extrapulmonary involvement and two patients with exclusive extrapulmonary involvement. All patients had CD_4^+ lymphocyte counts less than 200 cells/μL. The most common clinical manifestation was pulmonary disease with thin-walled cavitary lesions.[2,22] Prior to the advent of antiretroviral therapy, *M. genavense* was the second most frequently isolated species after *M. avium* in some geographic areas.

Non-HIV Disease
Disseminated disease with other NTM species has been reported and is most frequently seen with *M. chelonae*. Disseminated disease involving *M. chelonae* is primarily cutaneous and typically presents as a chronic syndrome with multiple painful, draining, red nodules, usually involving the lower extremities.[22] Almost all patients are immunosuppressed, usually from corticosteroid therapy for disease such as rheumatoid arthritis. Other types of immune suppression include autoimmune disease, leukemia, or in transplant recipients. Although the disease is presumably a consequence of hematogenous spread, a portal of entry is rarely evident, and septicemia is rare.[22]

While the majority of disseminated cutaneous disease is due to *M. chelonae*, *M. abscessus* complex has been reported in approximately 20% of the cases. Disease involving sites other than skin is rare, except in severely immunosuppressed patients. Disseminated disease with *M. abscessus* is a serious disease and can be difficult to treat.[22] Other NTM such as *M. haemophilum* produce similar clinical syndromes in similar settings with infection most often in the lower extremities in immunosuppressed patients.[22,81]

Catheter-Related Infections

Currently, catheter-related infections are the most common health care–associated NTM infections encountered.[2,5,22] Infections are seen most often with long-term central intravenous catheters, but they may also occur with peritoneal or shunt catheters. The usual pathogens are rapidly growing mycobacteria, especially *M. fortuitum*, and *M. mucogenicum* (see Table 253-1). These infections may be manifested as fever, local catheter site drainage, bacteremia, or, occasionally, lung infiltrates or granulomatous hepatitis. The usual treatment is catheter removal combined with appropriate antibiotics for 6 to 12 weeks.[2,22]

Recently an outbreak of *M. mucogenicum* and the newly described species *M. phocaicum* was reported in central venous catheters in an oncology unit of a Texas hospital.[86] Isolates of the RGM species *M. neoaurum* (pigmented) and *M. brumae* have also been incriminated in catheter-related sepsis.[87,88]

Miscellaneous Infections

Less commonly, NTM have been associated with other types of infections, including central nervous system (CNS) and ocular infections. NTM including *M. genavense*, *M. kansasii*, *M. malmoense*, and RGM, primarily *M. fortuitum*, have been identified with CNS disease.[89] The first known case of *M. abscessus* meningitis was described in 2001 in a 59-year-old woman who had no significant medical history but had sustained a knife wound to the neck months prior to her symptoms.[90]

Ocular infections have most often involved the RGM, especially the *M. abscessus/chelonae* group. The number of infections has increased to include post-keratoplasty and post-LASIK surgery. As previously discussed, infections have been associated with outbreaks and in sporadic fashion.[66,67] Treatment for patients with corneal infections due to RGM is usually complicated by the lack of available effective antimicrobials. For patients who do not respond to topical antimicrobials, surgical interventions are recommended.[91]

Laboratory Aspects

Stain and Culture
The methods used for staining and culture of *M. tuberculosis* generally work well for the NTM, although some RGM are adversely affected by harsh decontamination methods that are standard for *M. tuberculosis*.[2,22] Middlebrook 7H10 or 7H11 agar, BACTEC (Becton Dickinson, Sparks MD) broth, and the newer rapid broth systems all support growth of the commonly encountered NTM.[22] Cultures of skin and soft tissue should be plated at 28°C to 30°C, as well as 35°C, because some species such as *M. marinum*, *M. chelonae*, and *M. haemophilum* grow only at low temperatures on primary isolation. *M. genavense* (BACTEC broth for 6 to 8 weeks)[2,22] and *M. haemophilum* (iron or heme in the media and lower temperatures)[2,22,81] have special growth requirements.[2,22,81] If *M. ulcerans*, *M. genavense*, or *M. malmoense* is suspected, cultures should be held up 10 to 12 weeks before discarding. Due to the difficulty often encountered in growing *M. ulcerans* and *M. genavense* on solid media, molecular techniques may be necessary to identify these species.[2,22-24]

Identification
Identification of NTM increasingly focuses and depends on the use of rapid diagnostic systems: high-performance liquid chromatography (HPLC), which assesses the patterns of long-chain fatty acids (mycolic acids); molecular methods such as partial gene sequencing of multiple genes, including 16S r-RNA, hsp65, and rpoB[15,22,24,92]; polymerase chain reaction (PCR) restriction fragment length polymorphism analysis (PRA) of a 441-base pair fragment of the 65-kD heat shock protein gene[2,93-95]; and commercially available molecular probes. The latter probes for RNA are currently available for *M. tuberculosis* complex, *M. avium*, *M. intracellulare*, MAC, *M. gordonae*, and *M. kansasii*.[2,22] For most of the newer species, partial gene sequencing of the 16S ribosomal RNA gene, rpoB gene, or both, are important or essential for species identification.[2-5,15,22] Molecular methods, including the INNO-LiPa multiplex probe assay that targets the 16S-23S internal transcribed spacer (Innogenetics, Ghent, Belgium) and the Geno-Type assay that targets the 23S rRNA gene (Hain Lifescience, Nehren, Germany) are available in Europe and are the major methods utilized for identification of multiple species of NTM.[96,97]

Traditional biochemical testing to determine carbohydrate utilization and other standard mycobacterial tests such as arylsulfatase, nitrate reduction, and iron uptake are slow and inadequate and have largely been abandoned, especially for most newer species where molecular methods are needed to provide definitive identification.[22,24,47]

Other methods of identification include pyrosequencing, a short sequence analysis method based on detection of pyrophosphate during DNA synthesis,[98] and mass spectral identification by matrix-assisted laser desorption ionization-time-of-flight mass spectrometry (MALDI-TOF MS).[99] These methods warrant further study and to date have only been used in research or large reference labs.

Susceptibility Testing: Rapidly Growing Mycobacteria (RGM)

The three most widely accepted methods of susceptibility testing of RGM include agar disk elution, broth microdilution, and, most recently, the E-test gradient minimal inhibitory concentration.[22,80] In 2003, the CLSI (Clinical and Laboratory Standards Institute, formerly the National Committee for Clinical Laboratory Standards [NCCLS]) published a document for standardization of susceptibility testing of all mycobacteria species, including the NTM.[80] The CLSI recommended method for susceptibility testing with RGM is the broth microdilution technique.[80] The antimicrobials used are select bacterial agents because antituberculous drugs are not effective against these species. Current minimal recommendations for testing the RGM include clarithromycin (used as a class representative agent for the new macrolides), amikacin, cefoxitin, imipenem, tobramycin, doxycycline, linezolid, ciprofloxacin, and a sulfonamide.[22,80] Although newer antimicrobial agents such as moxifloxacin probably should be tested, the CLSI has not addressed breakpoints and interpretive values for these antimicrobials yet.

Susceptibility Testing: Slowly Growing NTM

The proportion method in agar, broth microdilution, E-test, and automated broth systems, including the MGIT (Becton Dickinson, Sparks, MD) and the ESP (Trek Diagnostics, Cleveland, OH), have been used for determining minimal inhibitory concentrations of the slowly growing NTM.[22,47] No single susceptibility method has been recommended by the CLSI for all slowly-growing species. For isolates of MAC, the CLSI has recommended a broth-based method with either broth microdilution or broth macrodilution by commercial systems acceptable. For susceptibility testing of the other slowly growing mycobacteria until further multicenter susceptibility studies have been performed, either broth or agar methods may be utilized as long as each laboratory validates the method for the species and antimicrobials tested and quality control and proficiency testing are in place.[22,80] Standard first-line antituberculous agents (ethambutol, rifampin, isoniazid) are commonly tested along with other agents, including clarithromycin (clarithromycin is used as the class agent for the macrolides including azithromycin), rifabutin, minocycline, streptomycin, amikacin, linezolid, quinolones (ciprofloxacin and moxifloxacin), and a sulfonamide for most species of nontuberculous slowly growing mycobacteria.[2,22,80] Susceptibility testing to pyrazinamide is not recommended because it has no efficacy against NTM. Currently, susceptibility testing is recommended for isolates of *M. kansasii* (rifampin only), MAC (clarithromycin only), and less commonly encountered slowly growing species such as *M. xenopi* (all of the aforementioned drugs).[2,22,80]

Isolates of *M. kansasii* that are resistant to rifampin should be tested against the aforementioned panel of secondary agents. Isolates that are susceptible to rifampin will also be susceptible to rifabutin and should require no additional testing.[22,80]

Isolates of *M. marinum* have a narrow range of MICs and do not require susceptibility testing unless the patient fails treatment after several months.[22,80]

Because no correlation has been shown between susceptibility results and clinical outcome for antituberculous agents, the American Thoracic Society and the CLSI recently recommended that susceptibility testing to the antituberculous agents (rifampin, rifabutin, ethambutol, streptomycin) other than clarithromycin is not indicated.[22,80] Although testing of first-line antituberculous agents does not provide useful clinical information, some experts suggest that it may be reasonable to test moxifloxacin and linezolid for patients who fail initial macrolide-based therapy. However, these agents should not be used as substitutes for the initial three-drug regimen (macrolide, rifamycin, and ethambutol), and their role in the treatment of macrolide-resistant MAC is currently uncertain.[22]

Strain Comparison

Molecular methods such as Southern hybridization with repetitive elements, random arbitrarily primed polymerase chain reaction (RAPD), and pulsed-field gel electrophoresis (PFGE) of NTM are currently used for strain comparison "DNA fingerprinting" of NTM outbreaks.[22,99] PFGE is the most widely used technique and remains the "gold standard" for definitive strain comparison of the NTM. With recent modifications to the technique to eliminate DNA degradation, strain typing by PFGE is feasible for all species of mycobacteria.[100]

REFERENCES

1. Sexton P, Harrison AC. Susceptibility to nontuberculous mycobacterial lung disease. *Eur Respir Dis.* 2008;31:1322-1333.
2. Brown-Elliott BA, Wallace Jr RJ. Infections caused by nontuberculous mycobacteria. In: Mandell, Bennett, Dolin, eds. Mandell, Douglas and Bennett's Principles and Practice of Infectious Diseases. 6th ed. Vol. 2. Elsevier Churchill Livingstone Inc.; 251: 2005:2909-2916.
3. Tortoli E. Impact of genotypic studies on mycobacterial taxonomy: the new mycobacteria of the 1990s. *Clin Microbiol Rev.* 2003;16:319-354.
4. Tortoli E. The new mycobacteria: an update. *FEMS Immunol Med Microbiol.* 2006;48:159-178.
5. Brown-Elliott BA, Wallace Jr RJ. Clinical and taxonomic status of pathogenic nonpigmented or late-pigmenting rapidly growing mycobacteria. *Clin Microbiol Rev.* 2002;15:716-746.
6. Wallace Jr RJ, Brown-Elliott BA, Brown JM, et al. Polyphasic characterization reveals that the human pathogen *Mycobacterium peregrinum* type II belongs to the bovine pathogen species *Mycobacterium senegalense. J Clin Microbiol.* 2005;43:5925-5935.
7. Adékambi T, Stein A, Carvajal J, et al. Description of *Mycobacterium conceptionense* sp. nov., a *Mycobacterium fortuitum* group organism isolated from a post-traumatic osteitis inflammation. *J Clin Microbiol.* 2006;44:1268-1273.
8. Lamy B, Marchandin H, Hamitouche K, et al. *Mycobacterium setense* sp. nov., a *Mycobacterium fortuitum* group organism isolated from a patient with soft tissue infection and osteitis. *Int J Syst Evol Microbiol.* 2008;58:486-490.
9. Schinsky MF, Morey RE, Steigerwalt AG, et al. Taxonomic variation in the *Mycobacterium fortuitum* third-biovariant complex: description of *Mycobacterium boenickei* sp. nov., *Mycobacterium houstonense* sp. nov., *Mycobacterium neworleansense* sp. nov. and *Mycobacterium brisbanense* sp. nov. and recognition of *Mycobacterium porcinum* from human clinical isolates. *Int J Syst Evol Microbiol.* 2004;54:1653-1667.
10. Schinsky MF, McNeil MM, Whitney AM, et al. *Mycobacterium septicum* sp. nov. a new rapidly growing species associated with catheter-related bacteraemia. *Int J Syst Evol Microbiol.* 2000; 50:575-581.
11. Domenech P, Jimenez MS, Menendez MC, et al. *Mycobacterium mageritense* sp. nov. *Int J Syst Bacteriol.* 1997;47:535-540.
12. Wallace Jr RJ, Brown-Elliott BA, Wilson RW, et al. Clinical and laboratory features of *Mycobacterium mageritense. J Clin Microbiol.* 2002;40:2930-2935.
13. Wallace Jr RJ, Brown-Elliott BA, Wilson RW, et al. Clinical and laboratory features of *Mycobacterium porcinum. J Clin Microbiol.* 2004;42:5689-5697.
14. Wilson RW, Steingrube VA, Böttger EC, et al. A new mycobacterial species related to *Mycobacterium abscessus: Mycobacterium immunogenum* sp. nov.—an international cooperative study on mycobacterial taxonomy. *Int J Syst Evol Microbiol.* 2001;51:1751-1764.
15. Adékambi T, Berger P, Raoult D, et al. rpoβ gene sequence-based characterization of emerging nontuberculous mycobacteria with descriptions of *Mycobacterium bolletii* sp. nov., *Mycobacterium phocaicum* sp. nov. and *Mycobacterium aubagnense* sp. nov. *Int J Syst Evol Microbiol.* 2006;56:133-143.
16. Adékambi T, Reynaud-Gaubert M, Greub G, et al. Amoebal coculture of "*Mycobacterium massiliense*" sp. nov. from the sputum of a patient with hemoptoic pneumonia. *J Clin Microbiol.* 2004;42:5493-5501.
17. Brown BA, Springer B, Steingrube VA, et al. Description of *Mycobacterium wolinskyi* and *Mycobacterium goodii*, two new rapidly growing species related to *Mycobacterium smegmatis* and associated with human wound infections: A cooperative study from the International Working Group on Mycobacterial Taxonomy. *Int J Syst Bacteriol.* 1999;49:1493-1511.
18. Jimenez MS, Campos-Herrero MI, Garcia D, et al. *Mycobacterium canariasense* sp. nov. *Int J Syst Evol Microbiol.* 2004;54:1729-1734.
19. Cooksey RC, de Waard JH, Yakrus MA, et al. *Mycobacterium cosmeticum* sp. nov., a novel rapidly growing species isolated from a cosmetic infection and from a nail salon. *Int J Syst Evol Microbiol.* 2004;54:2385-2391.
20. Reischl U, Melzl H, Kroppenstedt RM, et al. *Mycobacterium monacense* sp. nov. *Int J Syst Evol Microbiol.* 2006;56:2575-2578.
21. Trujillo ME, Velázquez E, Kroppenstedt RM, et al. *Mycobacterium psychrotolerans* sp. nov., isolated from pond water near a uranium mine. *Int J Syst Epidemiol Microbiol.* 2004;54:1459-1463.
22. Griffith DE, Aksamit T, Brown-Elliott BA, et al. An official ATS/IDSA statement: Diagnosis, treatment and prevention of nontuberculous mycobacterial diseases. American Thoracic Society Statement. *Am J Resp Crit Care Med.* 2007;175:367-416.
23. Portaels F, Traore H, De Ridder K, et al. In vitro susceptibility of *Mycobacterium ulcerans* to clarithromycin. *Antimicrob Agents Chemother.* 1998;42:2070-2073.
24. Brown-Elliott BA, Griffith DE, Wallace Jr RJ. Newly described or emerging human species of nontuberculous mycobacteria. *Infect Dis Clin N America.* 2002;16:187-220.
25. Cloud JL, Meyer JJ, Pounder JL, et al. *Mycobacterium arupense* sp. nov., a novel moderately growing nonchromogenic bacterium isolated from clinical specimens. *Int J Syst Evol Microbiol.* 2006;56:1413-1418.
26. Masaki T, Ohkusu K, Hata H, et al. *Mycobacterium kumamotonense* sp. nov. recovered from clinical specimen and the first isolation report of *Mycobacterium arupense* in Japan: Novel

slowly growing, nonchromogenic clinical isolates related to *Mycobacterium terrae* complex. *Microbiol Immunol.* 2006;50:889-897.
27. Mun H-S, Park J-H, Kim H, et al. *Mycobacterium senuense* sp. nov., a slowly growing, non-chromogenic species closely related to the *Mycobacterium terrae* complex. *Int J Syst Evol Microbiol.* 2008;58:641-646.
28. Mohamed AM, Iwen PC, Tarantolo S, et al. *Mycobacterium nebraskense* sp. nov., a novel slowly growing scotochromogenic species. *Int J Syst Evol Microbiol.* 2004;54:2057-2060.
29. Tortoli E, Chianura L, Fabbro L, et al. Infections due to the newly described species *Mycobacterium parascrofulaceum. J Clin Microbiol.* 2005;43:4286-4287.
30. Turenne CY, Cook VJ, Burdz TV, et al. *Mycobacterium parascrofulaceum* sp. nov., novel slowly growing, scotochromogenic clinical isolates related to *Mycobacterium simiae. Int J Syst Evol Microbiol.* 2004;54:1543-1551.
31. Fanti F, Tortoli E, Hall L, et al. *Mycobacterium parmense* sp. nov. *Int J Syst Evol Microbiol.* 2004;54:1123-1127.
32. Turenne CY, Thibert L, Williams K, et al. *Mycobacterium saskatchewanense* sp. nov., a novel slowly growing scotochromogenic species from human clinical isolates related to *Mycobacterium interjectum* and Accuprobe-positive for *Mycobacterium avium* complex. *Int J Syst Evol Microbiol.* 2004;54:659-667.
33. Rhodes MW, Kator H, McNabb A, et al. *Mycobacterium pseudoshottsii* sp. nov., a slowly growing chromogenic species isolated from Chesapeake Bay striped bass (*Morone saxatilis*). *Int J Syst Evol Microbiol.* 2005;55:1139-1147.
34. Mun H-S, Kim H-J, Oh E-J, et al. *Mycobacterium seoulense* sp. nov., a slowly growing scotochromogenic species. *Int J Syst Evol Microbiol.* 2007;57:594-599.
35. Murcia MI, Tortoli E, Menendez MC, et al. *Mycobacterium colombiense* sp. nov., a new member of the *Mycobacterium avium* complex and description of MAC-X as a new ITS genetic variant. *Int J Syst Evol Microbiol.* 2006;56:2049-2054.
36. Tortoli E, Rindi L, Goh KS, et al. *Mycobacterium florentinum* sp. nov., isolated from humans. *Int J Syst Evol Microbiol.* 2005;55:1101-1106.
37. Levi MH, Bartell J, Gandolfo L, et al. Characterization of *Mycobacterium montefiorense* sp. nov., a novel pathogenci mycobacterium from moray eels that is related to *Mycobacterium triplex. J Clin Microbiol.* 2003;41:2147-2152.
38. Falkinham JO III, Norton CD, LeChevallier MW. Factors influencing numbers of *Mycobacterium avium, Mycobacterium intracellulare,* and other mycobacteria in drinking water distribution systems. *App Environ Microbiol.* 2001;67:1225-1231.
39. Galassi L, Tortoli E, Burrini D, et al. Nontuberculous mycobacteria in hospital water systems: application of HPLC for identification of environmental mycobacteria. *J Water Health.* 2003;1(3):133-139.
40. Bardouniotis E, Ceri H, Olson ME. Biofilm formation and biocide susceptibility testing of *Mycobacterium fortuitum* and *Mycobacterium marinum. Curr Microbiol.* 2003;46:28-32.
41. Salliot C, Desplaces N, Boiserenoult P, et al. Arthritis due to *Mycobacterium xenopi*: a retrospective study of 7 cases in France. *Clin Infect Dis* 2006;43:987-993.
42. Simmon KE, Pounder JI, Greene JN, et al. Identification of an emerging pathogen, *Mycobacterium massiliense,* by *rpoB* sequencing of clinical isolates collected in the United States. *J Clin Microbiol.* 2007;45:1978-1980.
43. Piersimoni C, Zitti PG, Nista D, et al. *Mycobacterium celatum* pulmonary infection in the immunocompetent: Case report and review. *Emerg Infect Dis.* 2003;9:399-402.
44. Piersimoni C, Goteri G, Nista D, et al. *Mycobacterium lentiflavum* as an emerging causative agent of cervical lymphadenitis. *J Clin Microbiol.* 2004;42:3894-3897.
45. Roth A, Reischl U, Schönfeld N, et al. *Mycobacterium heckeshornense* sp. nov., a new pathogenic slowly growing *Mycobacterium* sp. causing cavitary lung disease in an immunocompetent patient. *J Clin Microbiol.* 2000;38:4102-4107.
46. Tortoli E, Rindi L, Garcia MJ, et al. Proposal to elevate the genetic variant MAC-A, included in the *Mycobacterium avium* complex, to species rank as *Mycobacterium chimaera* sp. nov. *Int J Syst Evol Microbiol.* 2004;54:1277-1285.
47. Clinical and Laboratory Standards Institute. Laboratory detection and identification of mycobacteria; approved guideline. *CLSI.* 2008; M48-A.
48. Pezzia W, Raleigh JW, Bailey MC, et al. Treatment of pulmonary disease due to *Mycobacterium kansasii*: Recent experience with rifampin. *Rev Infect Dis.* 1981;3:1035-1039.
49. Griffith DE, Brown-Elliott BA, Wallace Jr RJ. Thrice-weekly clarithromycin-containing regimen for treatment of *Mycobacterium kansasii* lung disease: Results of a preliminary study. *Clin Infect Dis.* 2003;37:1178-1182.
50. Wallace Jr RJ, Brown-Elliott BA, Crist CJ, et al. Comparison of the in vitro activity of the glycylcycline tigecycline (formerly GAR-936) with those of tetracycline, minocycline, and doxycycline against isolates of nontuberculous mycobacteria. *Antimicrob Agents Chemother.* 2002;46:3164-3167.
51. Nash KA. Intrinsic macrolide resistance in *Mycobacterium smegmatis* is conferred by a novel *erm* gene, *erm*(38). *Antimicrob Agents Chemother.* 2003;47:3053-3060.
52. Nash KA, Andini N, Zhang Y, et al. Intrinsic macrolide resistance in rapidly growing mycobacteria. *Antimicrob Agents Chemother.* 2006;50:3476-3478.
53. Nash KA, Zhang Y, Brown-Elliott BA, et al. Molecular basis of intrinsic macrolide resistance in clinical isolates of *Mycobacterium fortuitum. J Antimicrob Chemother.* 2005;55:170-177.
54. Nash KA. A novel gene, *erm*(41), confers inducible macrolide resistance to clinical isolates of *Mycobacterium abscessus*, but is absent from *Mycobacterium chelonae. Antimicrob Agents Chemother.* 2009;53:1367-1376.
55. Wolinsky E. Mycobacterial lymphadenitis in children: A prospective study of 105 nontuberculous cases with long-term follow-up. *Clin Infect Dis.* 1995;20:954-963.
56. Cabria F, Torres M-V, García-Cía J-I, et al. Cervical lymphadenitis caused by *Mycobacterium lentiflavum. Ped Infect Dis J.* 2002;21:574-575.
57. Zaugg M, Salfinger M, Opravil M, et al. Extrapulmonary and disseminated infections due to *Mycobacterium malmoense*: Case report and review. *Clin Infect Dis.* 1993;16:540-549.
58. Cohen YH, Amir J, Ashkenazi S, et al. *Mycobacterium haemophilum* and lymphadenitis in immunocompetent children, *Israel Emerg Infect Dis.* 2008;14:1437-1439.
59. Chetchotisakd P, Kiertiburanakul S, Mootsikapun P, et al. Disseminated nontuberculous mycobacterial infection in patients who are not infected with HIV in Thailand. *Clin Infect Dis.* 2007;45:421-427.
60. Aubry A, Chosidow O, Caumes E, et al. Sixty-three cases of *Mycobacterium marinum* isolates. *Arch Intern Med.* 2002;162:1746-1752.
61. Shojaei H, Goodfellow M, Magee JG, et al. *Mycobacterium novocastrense* sp. nov., a rapidly growing photochromogenic mycobacterium. *Int J Syst Bacteriol.* 1997;47:1205-1207.
62. Turenne C, Chedore P, Wolfe J, et al. *Mycobacterium lacus* sp. nov., a new slow-growing non-chromogenic clinical isolate. *Int J Syst Evol Microbiol.* 2002;52:2135-2140.
63. Sampaio JL, Chimara E, Ferrazoli L, et al. Application of four molecular typing methods for analysis of *Mycobacterium fortuitum* group strains causing post-mammaplasty infections. *Clin Microbiol Infect.* 2006;12:142-149.
64. Wallace Jr RJ, Musser JM, Hull SI, et al. Diversity and sources of rapidly growing mycobacteria associated with infections following cardiac surgery. *J Infect Dis.* 1989;159:708-716.
65. Tiwari TSP, Ray B, Jost Jr KC, et al. Forty years of disinfectant failure: Outbreak of postinjection *Mycobacterium abscessus* infection caused by contamination of benzalkonium chloride. *Clin Infect Dis.* 2003;36:954-962.
66. Sampaio JLM, Junior DN, de Freitas D, et al. An outbreak of keratitis caused by *Mycobacterium immunogenum. J Clin Microbiol.* 2006;44:3201-3207.
67. Winthrop KL, Steinberg EB, Holmes G, et al. Epidemic and sporadic cases of nontuberculous mycobacterial keratitis associated with laser in situ keratomileusis. *Am J Ophthalmol.* 2003;135:223-224.
68. Meyers H, Brown-Elliott BA, Moore D, et al. An outbreak of *Mycobacterium chelonae* infection following liposuction. *Clin Infect Dis.* 2002;34:1500-1507.
69. Woo PCY, Leung K-W, Wong SSY, et al. Relatively alcohol-resistant mycobacteria are emerging pathogens in patients receiving acupuncture treatment. *J Clin Microbiol.* 2002;40:1219-1224.
70. Furuya EY, Paez A, Srinivasan A, et al. Outbreak of *Mycobacterium abscessus* wound infections among "Lipotourists" from the United States who underwent abdominoplasty in the Dominican Republic. *Clin Infect Dis.* 2008;46:1181-1188.
71. Gira AK, Reisenauer AH, Hammock L, et al. Furunculosis due to *Mycobacterium mageritense* associated with footbaths at a nail salon. *J Clin Microbiol.* 2004;42:1813-1817.
72. Sniezak PJ, Graham BS, Busch HB, et al. Rapidly growing mycobacterium infections following pedicures. *Arch Dermatol.* 2003;139:629-634.
73. Winthrop KL, Abrams M, Yakrus M, et al. An outbreak of mycobacterial furunculosis associated with footbaths at a nail salon. *N Engl J Med.* 2002;346:1366-1371.
74. Winthrop KL, Albridge K, South D, et al. The clinical management and outcome of nail salon-acquired *Mycobacterium fortuitum* skin infection. *Clin Infect Dis.* 2004;38:38-44.
75. Vugia DJ, Jang Y, Zizek C, et al. Mycobacteria in nail salon whirlpool footbaths, *California Emerg Infect Dis.* 2005;11:616-618.
76. Kim H-Y, Yun Y-J, Park CG, et al. Outbreak of *Mycobacterium massiliense* infection associated with intramuscular injections. *J Clin Microbiol.* 2007;45:3127-3130.
77. Viana-Niero C, Lima KVB, Lopes ML, et al. Molecular characterization of *Mycobacterium massiliense* and *Mycobacterium bolletii* in isolates collected from outbreaks of infections after laparoscopic surgeries and cosmetic procedures. *J Clin Microbiol.* 2008;46:850-855.
78. Wallace RJ Jr, Brown-Elliott BA, Ward SC, et al. Activities of linezolid against rapidly growing mycobacteria. *Antimicrob Agents Chemother.* 2001;45:764-767.
79. Vemulapalli RK, Cantey JR, Steed LL, et al. Emergence of resistance to clarithromycin during treatment of disseminated cutaneous *Mycobacterium chelonae* infection: Case report and literature report. *J Infect.* 2001;43:163-168.
80. Woods GL, Brown-Elliott BA, Desmond EP, et al. *Susceptibility testing of mycobacteria, nocardiae, and other aerobic actinomycetes; Approved Standard.* NCCLS, 2003; M24-A.
81. Saubolle MA, Kiehn TE, White MH, et al. *Mycobacterium haemophilum*: Microbiology and expanding clinical and geographic spectra of disease in humans. *Clin Microbiol Rev.* 1996;9:435-447.
82. Toro A, Adekambi T, Cheynet F, et al. *Mycobacterium setense* infection in humans. Letter to the Editor. *Emerg Infect Dis.* 2008;14:1330-1332.
83. Tsai T-F, Lai C-C, Tsai I-C, et al. Tenosynovitis caused by *Mycobacterium arupense* in a patient with diabetes mellitus. *Clin Infect Dis.* 2008;47:861-863.
84. Shafran SD, Singer J, Zarowny DP, et al. A comparison of two regimens for the treatment of *Mycobacterium avium* complex bacteremia in AIDS: Rifabutin, ethambutol, and clarithromycin versus rifampin, ethambutol, clofazimine, and ciprofloxacin. *N Engl J Med.* 1996;335:377-383.
85. Bonomo RA, Briggs JM, Gross W, et al. *Mycobacterium celatum* infection in a patient with AIDS. *Clin Infect Dis.* 1998;26:243-245.
86. Cooksey RC, Jhung MA, Yakrus MA, et al. Multiphasic approach reveals genetic diversity of environmental and patient isolates of *Mycobacterium mucogenicum* and *Mycobacterium phocaicum* associated with an outbreak of bacteremias at a Texas Hospital. *App Environ Microbiol.* 2008;74:2480-2487.
87. Lee SA, Raad II, Adachi JA, et al. Catheter-related bloodstream infection caused by *Mycobacterium brumae. J Clin Microbiol.* 2004;42:5429-5431.
88. Simmon KE, Low YY, Brown-Elliott BA, et al. Phylogenetic analysis of *Mycobacterium aurum* and *Mycobacterium neoaurum* with re-description of *M. aurum* culture collection strains. *Int J Syst Evol Microbiol.* 2009;59:1371-1375.
89. Wallace Jr RJ. Infections due to nontuberculous mycobacteria. In: Scheld WM, Whitley RJ, Marra CM, eds. Infections of the Central Nervous System. 3rd ed. Vol 26. 2004:461-478.
90. Maniu CV, Hellinger WC, Chu S-Y, et al. Failure treatment of chronic *Mycobacterium abscessus* meningitis despite adequate clarithromycin levels in cerebrospinal fluid. *Clin Infect Dis.* 2001;33:745-748.
91. Garg P, Bansal AK, Sharma S, et al. Bilateral infectious keratitis after laser in situ keratomileusis. *Ophthalmology.* 2001;108:121-125.
92. Stout JE, Hopkins GW, McDonald JR, et al. Association between 16S-23S internal transcribed spacer sequence groups of *Mycobacterium avium* complex and pulmonary disease. *J Clin Microbiol.* 2008;46:2790-2793.
93. Patel JB, Leonard DGB, Pan X, et al. Sequence-based identification of *Mycobacterium* species using the MicroSeq 500 16S rDNA bacterial identification system. *J Clin Microbiol.* 2000;38:246-251.
94. Steingrube VA, Gibson JL, Brown BA, et al. PCR amplification and restriction endonuclease analysis of a 65-kilodalton heat shock protein gene sequence for taxonomic separation of rapidly growing mycobacteria. *J Clin Microbiol.* 1995;33:149-153.
95. Telenti A, Marchesi F, Balz M, et al. Rapid identification of mycobacteria to the species level by polymerase chain reaction and restriction enzyme analysis. *J Clin Microbiol.* 1993;31:175-178.
96. Russo C, Tortoli E, Menichella D. Evaluation of the new GenoType mycobacterium assay for identification of mycobacterial disease. *J Clin Microbiol.* 2006;44:334-339.
97. Wagner D, Young LS. Nontuberculous mycobacterial infections: a clinical review. *Infection.* 2004;32:257-270.
98. Tuohy MJ, Hall GS, Sholtis M, et al. Pyrosequencing as a tool for the identification of common isolates of *Mycobacterium* sp. *Diagn Microbiol Infect Dis.* 2005;51:245-250.
99. Pignone ML, Greth KM, Cooper J, et al. Identification of mycobacteria by matrix-assisted laser desorption ionization-time-of-flight mass spectrometry. *J Clin Microbiol.* 2006;44:1963-1970.
100. Zhang Y, Yakrus MA, Graviss EA, et al. Pulsed-field gel electrophoresis study of *Mycobacterium abscessus* isolates previously affected by DNA degradation. *J Clin Microbiol.* 2004;42:5582-5587.

254

Nocardia Species

TANIA C. SORRELL | DAVID H. MITCHELL | JONATHAN R. IREDELL | SHARON C-A. CHEN

*N*ocardia is a genus of aerobic actinomycetes responsible for localized or disseminated infections in animals and humans. The genus is named after Edmond Nocard, who in 1888 described the isolation of an aerobic actinomycete from cattle with bovine farcy. The first human case of nocardiosis was reported by Eppinger in 1890. Cases of human disease have increased substantially in the past two decades, in association with an increasing population of immunocompromised hosts and improved methods for detection and identification of *Nocardia* species in the clinical laboratory.

Classification

The aerobic actinomycetes are a large and diverse group of gram-positive bacteria[1] that appear on microscopy as branching, filamentous cells. Members of the group are often only distantly related phylogenetically. A subgroup, the "aerobic nocardiform actinomycetes," is the most important cause of human infection and includes the genera *Mycobacteria, Corynebacteria, Nocardia, Rhodococcus, Gordona,* and *Tsukamurella.* All members of the group have cell walls containing mesodiaminopimelic acid, arabinose, galactose (type IV cell wall[1]), and mycolic acids of various chain lengths. The latter are responsible for varying degrees of acid fastness on appropriate staining. In addition, *Nocardia* species are characterized by an ability to form aerial hyphae and to grow in media containing lysozyme and by an inability to grow at 50°C.[1]

Traditional laboratory methods for identification of *Nocardia* species,[1,2] which are based on simple biochemical reactions and hydrolysis tests, and by cell wall mycolic acid analysis, are limited in their ability to differentiate these organisms, especially between phylogenetically closely related species.[1,2] To overcome these difficulties, various molecular tools have been developed to facilitate accurate species determination.

The application of molecular methods, such as sequence analysis of the *Nocardia* 16S ribosomal (rRNA) gene,[3,4] has greatly expanded the spectrum of pathogenic *Nocardia* species and has led to significant taxonomic changes and species reassignment within the genus. This is particularly evident among isolates belonging to the "*Nocardia asteroides* complex."[2] More than 80 *Nocardia* species have now been described (NCBI taxonomy for *Nocardia*: http://www.ncbi.nlm.nih.gov/Taxonomy/) of which at least 33 have been implicated in human disease.[2,3] The main pathogenic taxonomic groups include members of the former *N. asteroides* complex (e.g., *N. asteroides* sensu stricto, *Nocardia nova,* and *Nocardia transvalensis* complexes), *Nocardia otitidiscaviarum, Nocardia farcinica,* and *Nocardia brasiliensis,*[2] but an increasing number of novel species have also been described. Those reported to cause human infection include two that were formerly part of the *N. asteroides* complex, *Nocardia abscessus,*[5] *Nocardia cyriacigeorgica,*[6] *Nocardia paucivarans,*[7] *Nocardia africana,*[8] *Nocardia veterana,*[9] and most recently, *Nocardia wallacei* and *Nocardia blacklockiae.*[10] The genomes of some *Nocardia* species (including *N. farcinica* and *N. nova*) have been published.

Ecology and Epidemiology

Nocardia species are ubiquitous environmental saprophytes, occurring in soil, organic matter, and water.[1,2] Human infection usually arises from direct inoculation of the skin or soft tissues or by inhalation. Mycetoma due to *N. brasiliensis* is the most common nocardial infection reported from tropical regions of the southern United States, Central and South America, and Australia. Worldwide, respiratory and disseminated infections are most often due to members of the previously broadly defined *N. asteroides* complex.[1,2,11] In a contemporary study of nocardiosis in organ transplant recipients, *N. nova* and *N. farcinica* were more common than *N. asteroides.*[12]

Nocardia species are well-recognized causes of infection in animals, with bovine mastitis being the most common.[2] There are no reports of animal-to-human transmission. Clusters of invasive nocardiosis acquired by patients in oncology and transplantation units, presumed to be associated with inhalation of contaminated dust, have been described.[2] Concurrent transmission by the hands of staff or contaminated fomites appeared likely in one of these outbreaks.[2] Hospital construction work may have been a risk factor in separate clusters of postsurgical wound infections due to *Nocardia* species.[2,13] Pulsed-field gel electrophoresis[13] and random amplification of polymorphic DNA (RAPD) fingerprinting[14] have been successfully used for confirming clusters and defining common sources.

Pathology and Pathogenesis

Sections of tissues infected with *Nocardia* species usually demonstrate an acute pyogenic inflammatory reaction. Branching, beaded, filamentous bacteria, similar to those seen in smears taken from cultures, may be demonstrated within the abscesses on Gram staining (Fig. 254-1). "Sulfur granules" (bacterial macrocolonies) similar to those seen in actinomycosis, may be found in nocardial mycetomas. *Nocardia* species usually stain acid fast in tissue sections if a method such as that of Fite-Faraco is used, whereas *Actinomyces* species do not.[1]

The interaction between the host and parasitizing nocardia has been comprehensively reviewed.[15] Disease manifestations of nocardiosis are determined principally by the portal of entry, tissue tropism, growth rates in vivo, ability to survive phagocyte attack, the nature of the host immune reaction, and the characteristics of the infecting strain. Protective immune responses to *Nocardia* species are primarily T-cell mediated, and nocardiosis is more problematic in patients with impaired cell-mediated immunity, eliciting little in the way of an effective humoral response.[15]

In murine models of infection, virulent nocardia are cleared from the blood within a few hours of intravenous inoculation and localize in a number of organs (lung, brain, kidneys, liver, spleen). The outcome of infection is largely determined by the ability of a given strain to resist the initial neutrophil leukocyte response and subsequent attack by activated macrophages.[15] Early neutrophil mobilization, although often insufficient to abort infection, appears to retard the process until lymphocyte-mediated cytotoxicity and activated macrophages effect a definitive response.[15,16] Healing is associated with strong sustained rises in interferon-γ (IFN-γ) in animal models and IFN-γ may have a therapeutic role in humans with chronic granulomatous disease.[17]

Specific Virulence Determinants

The nocardial envelope is structurally similar to that of other actinomycetes. Fifteen to 25% of the cell wall mass in rapidly growing organisms, and nearly twice that in stationary phase, is composed of peptidoglycan.[18,19] Differences in cell wall ultrastructure and chemical composition are evident during logarithmic and stationary phases of growth. Intrastrain differences in toxicity to host cells as well as virulence in animal models[15,19] may also result from differences in the

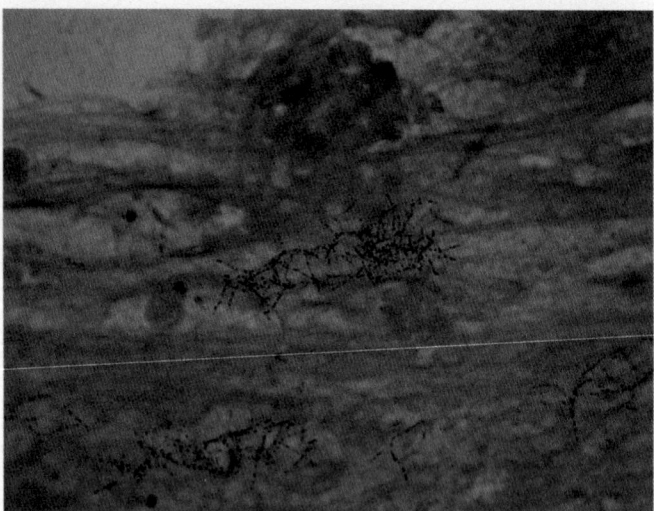

Figure 254-1   Pulmonary nocardiosis. Photomicrograph of direct Gram-stained smear from a patent with pulmonary nocardiosis, showing typical branching rods.

expression of virulence factors and hence specific cell tropisms. Mycolic acid polymers such as trehalose-6,6′-dimycolate ("cord factor") are members of a group of biologically active cell wall glycolipids found in many actinomycetes, including *Nocardia* species,[18] and are associated with virulence.[20,21] They are toxic in vitro and in animal models,[20,22] insert themselves into phospholipid bilayers in vitro and contribute to inhibition of phagosome-lysosome fusion and acidification in macrophages.[21]

Nocardia species contain no cell wall lipopolysaccharide, exopolysaccharide capsule, or surface fimbriae. However, strain-dependent specific adhesins and invasion properties influence the outcome of infection in animal models.[23,24] Virulent strains of *N. asteroides* are relatively resistant to neutrophil-mediated killing,[25] and organisms in the logarithmic growth phase are more toxic to macrophages.[18] They inhibit phagosome-lysosome fusion more successfully in vitro,[26] giving rise to L-forms, which can be isolated from within macrophages many days later.[27,28] Cell wall–deficient forms (L-forms) of *Nocardia* species have been isolated from serious human and animal infections[29,30] and may explain occasional late relapse of nocardial infections. Nonspecific interactions with neutrophils may contribute to the indolence of nocardiosis in the context of reduced cell-mediated immunity.[11] Patients with specific defects in the phagocyte oxidative burst (e.g., chronic granulomatous disease)[11,17] may be more vulnerable to this infection. The ability to use macrophage lysosomal acid phosphatase as a sole carbon source may be significant in vivo,[31] but inhibition of macrophage phagosome acidification and resistance to the oxidative burst of neutrophils and macrophages are probably more important. Highly pathogenic *Mycobacterium tuberculosis* and *N. asteroides* secrete superoxide dismutase (SOD) into growth media, whereas nonpathogenic mycobacteria and *Nocardia* species do not.[32,33] Antibodies to surface-presented SOD halved the survival of a virulent strain of *N. asteroides* (but not a less virulent strain) in the presence of activated neutrophils in vitro, with added catalase having a protective effect for the less virulent strain.[33] Specific toxins, including hemolysins and proteases, have been identified but are not thought to be widespread or important virulence factors.[15,34,35]

Ciliated epithelia appear relatively resistant to invasion by *Nocardia* species. However, a range of susceptible lung- and airway-associated cell types has been observed in rat models of infection.[24] Seeding of the central nervous system (CNS) may follow hematogenous spread from any focus, and tropism for cerebral tissue is evident experimentally. Neuroinvasiveness and macrophage penetration vary significantly between strains. Electron microscopic studies of infected macrophage and astrocytoma-derived or -related cell lines suggest that the penetration competence of invasive *N. asteroides* is localized to the bacterial apex.[34] Specific lectins have been shown to determine site specificity in the murine brain,[34] intrinsic differences in expression of which may contribute to variations in host susceptibility.[36]

Clinical Epidemiology

Members of the broadly defined *N. asteroides* complex are responsible for about 80% of noncutaneous invasive disease, and for most systemic and CNS disease.[15] *N. farcinica* is an important[37] and generally more antibiotic-resistant member of this complex. There is evidence from mouse models that it may be more virulent than other *Nocardia* species.[38] *N. brasiliensis* is the most oft-reported cause of cutaneous and lymphocutaneous disease, particularly in tropical areas. *N. pseudobrasiliensis*, a new species recently separated from *N. brasiliensis*, appears to be associated with systemic, including CNS, infections.[39] Noncutaneous disease is the most frequent presentation of nocardiosis caused by the less common pathogens, *N. transvalensis*[40] and *N. otidiscavarium*,[15] although both may cause severe cutaneous infection.[41] Superficial nocardiosis following implantation is not necessarily associated with compromised cell-mediated immunity but may progress to disseminated disease in that setting.[41]

Immunocompromise is a well-established risk factor for nocardiosis. *Nocardia* species may therefore be considered as opportunistic pathogens, which cause serious and disseminated disease in settings such as organ transplantation and lymphoreticular neoplasia, with the relative risk for progressive disease reflecting the level of immunosuppression. A compilation of more than a thousand randomly selected cases from the literature showed that more than 60% of all reported nocardiosis cases are associated with preexisting immune compromise, ranging from alcoholism and diabetes to organ transplantation and AIDS.[20] In a contemporary study of nocardiosis in recipients of solid organ transplants, significant risk factors included receipt of high-dose corticosteroids or cytomegalovirus disease within the preceding 6 months and high serum levels of calcineurin inhibitors within the preceding 30 days.[12] Preexisting immunocompromise was present in more than one third of *N. farcinica* infections in another study.[37] Persons with chronic pulmonary disorders, notably, pulmonary alveolar proteinosis, and almost any condition requiring long-term corticosteroid use, are also at risk. Although cases of nocardiosis have been described in patients with AIDS, the overall incidence is low and not fully explained by the use of sulfonamide prophylaxis against *Pneumocystis jirovecii* pneumonia.[42]

Clinical Manifestations

SUPERFICIAL INFECTION AND MYCETOMA

Ubiquitous in soil, all the nocardia can establish superficial infection after relatively trivial inoculation injuries (Fig. 254-2), which may vary from insect and animal bites to puncture wounds and contaminated abrasions. *N. brasiliensis* is the most common cause of progressive cutaneous and lymphocutaneous (sporotrichoid) disease, whereas *N. asteroides* more commonly causes self-limited infection.[11,15] Because the initial response to *Nocardia* is pyogenic, self-limited skin lesions may initially be disregarded or treated as staphylococcal in origin. Severe and invasive systemic disease is almost certainly overrepresented in the literature, and the extent to which mycetoma is relatively underreported and nocardial infection underdiagnosed overall is unknown. Mycetoma is a chronically progressive, destructive disease, occurring days to months after inoculation, and is typically located distally on the limbs. Eumycetoma (of fungal etiology) and actinomycetoma (due to actinomycetes) are equally prominent in the literature, the epidemiology varying with geographic location[43] (see Chapter 262). Overall, *Streptomyces* and *Actinomadura* species appear to be of equal or greater importance than *Nocardia* species among causative agents of actinomycetoma. Suppurative granulomas, progressive

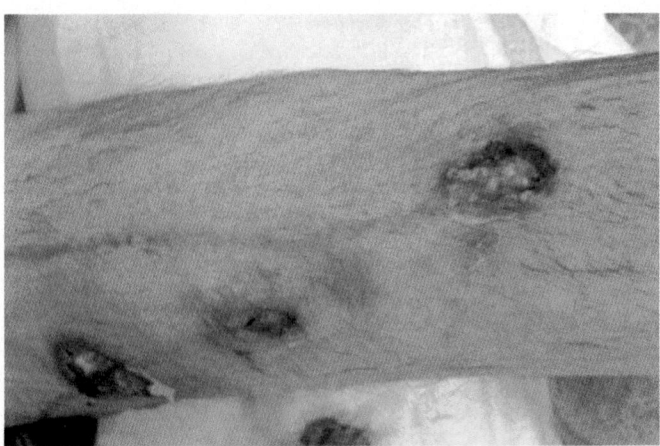

Figure 254-2 Skin lesions. Nocardial skin lesions due to direct inoculation in an immunosuppressed landscape gardener.

fibrosis and necrosis, sinus formation with destruction of adjacent structures, and macroscopically visible infective granules are regular features of nocardial mycetoma.[43] Inoculation injury occasionally results in infection of the cornea.

PULMONARY MANIFESTATIONS

Pulmonary disease is the predominant clinical presentation, occurring in more than 40% of reported cases.[12,15] Almost 90% of these are caused by members of the *N. asteroides* complex, broadly defined. Pulmonary nocardiosis is usually suppurative in nature, but granulomatous or mixed responses may occur. Clinical manifestations of established infection include endobronchial inflammatory masses, pneumonia, lung abscess, and cavitary disease with contiguous extension to surface and deep structures, including effusion and empyema. Radiologic manifestations include irregular nodules (usually cavitating when large), reticulonodular or diffuse pneumonic infiltrates, and pleural effusions (Fig. 254-3). The "halo sign," considered characteristic of aspergillosis in neutropenic patients, has been described. Progressive fibrotic disease may develop following inadequate therapy, and diagnosis is often difficult. Pulmonary nocardiosis may be a fatal complication of advanced HIV infection and often presents as alveolar infiltrates that progress during therapy rather than as cavitary disease.[44-46] It occurs most commonly in severely immunocompromised patients (CD4 < 200/mm³)[47] in whom nonspecific radiologic appearances oblige a search for a definitive diagnosis. Nocardiosis should always be considered in the differential diagnosis of indolent pulmonary disease, particularly in the setting of cellular immune compromise, along with other actinomycetes (e.g., mycobacteria, *Actinomyces* species) and Eumycetes (e.g., *Cryptococcus neoformans*, *Aspergillus* species). Clues to a nocardial etiology include spread to contiguous structures, especially with soft tissue swellings or external fistulas, and to the CNS. Secondary cerebral localization and clinically silent destructive infection are sufficiently common that cerebral imaging, preferably magnetic resonance imaging (MRI), should be performed in all cases of pulmonary and disseminated nocardiosis. Invasive diagnostic procedures should be considered early in the immune compromised host because disease may follow a rapidly progressive course in patients with severe immunodeficiency, and coincident pathology with similar clinical characteristics (e.g., aspergillosis, tuberculosis, malignancy) is well documented.[48]

DISSEMINATED DISEASE

CNS involvement was recognized in more than 44% of cases of all systemic nocardiosis in one large survey.[20] Up to one fourth of reported nocardial disease other than mycetoma involves the CNS, with nearly half of these cases exclusively involving the CNS.[11,49,50] Insidious presentations are often mistaken for neoplasia because of the paucity of clinical and laboratory signs of bacterial inflammation, and silent invasion and persistence make diagnosis and management more difficult.[11,15] Clinical manifestations of CNS nocardiosis usually result from local effects of granulomas or abscesses in the brain, and less commonly, the spinal cord or meninges (Fig. 254-4). Disease frequently progresses over months to years and causes a broad range of neurologic deficits, including chronic behavioral and psychiatric disturbance, which reflect localization in the cerebral cortices, basal ganglia, and midbrain. Tissue diagnosis of a cerebral mass in the setting of proven pulmonary nocardiosis is not always necessary.[11] However, cerebral biopsy should be considered early in the immunocompromised patient because of the higher incidence of serious coexisting pathology and a more aggressive course than that traditionally ascribed to cerebral nocardiosis.

Disseminated infection is characterized by widespread abscess formation. The most commonly reported sites include the CNS and eyes (particularly the retina), skin and subcutaneous tissues, kidneys, joints, bone, and heart (Fig. 254-5).

COLONIZATION

Occasional instances of transient colonization of sputum and skin by *Nocardia* species have been reported and appear to indicate aerosol contamination or soil-derived contamination. Colonization of the sputum is typically found in patients with underlying pulmonary pathology who are not receiving steroid therapy and requires no specific therapy. Significant isolates of *Nocardia* should be visible on Gram stain, produce a pure or predominant growth in culture, and be isolated repeatedly from clinical specimens.[51] However, the extent to which spontaneously resolving or subclinical pulmonary infection occurs in the population is ill defined, and at least one leading authority warns against dismissing positive sputum cultures as harmless.[15]

Laboratory Diagnosis

The microbiology laboratory should always be informed when nocardiosis is suspected because the diagnosis may be missed by routine laboratory methods. Respiratory secretions, skin biopsy specimens, or aspirates from deep collections are the most common specimens from which *Nocardia* species are isolated. Direct smears from such specimens typically show gram-positive, beaded, fine right-angled branching filaments (<1 µm diameter) that are usually acid fast; filaments may fragment to form rods and coccoid forms of varying sizes. Standard blood culture media support the growth of *Nocardia* organisms, but prolonged incubation (up to 2 weeks) and blind subcultures may be required for their detection.[1] Bacteremia, as demonstrated by positive blood cultures, is rare in patients with nocardiosis,[2] yet has been described in cases of central venous catheter infection due to *Nocardia* species.[2] *Nocardia* species will grow on most nonselective media used routinely for culture of bacteria, fungi, and mycobacteria. However, in specimens containing mixed flora (e.g., respiratory secretions), nocardial colonies are easily obscured by those of more rapidly growing bacteria, and the yield is increased by use of selective media, such as Thayer-Martin agar with antibiotics[52] or Paraffin agar.[53] Buffered charcoal-yeast extract (BCYE) medium, which is commonly used for selective growth of *Legionella* species, may also be used for isolation of *Nocardia* species from respiratory specimens.[54] Decontamination methods used for mycobacterial culture are too harsh for *Nocardia* species and may substantially reduce the numbers of viable organisms present in the specimen.[55]

Growth of *Nocardia* species may take 48 hours to several weeks, but typical colonies are usually seen after 3 to 5 days. *Nocardia* species appear as either buff or pigmented, waxy cerebriform colonies (Fig. 254-6) or have a dry, chalky-white appearance if aerial hyphae are produced.[1] They have a characteristic earthy odor. Most isolates are acid fast by a method such as the modified Kinyoun technique, but

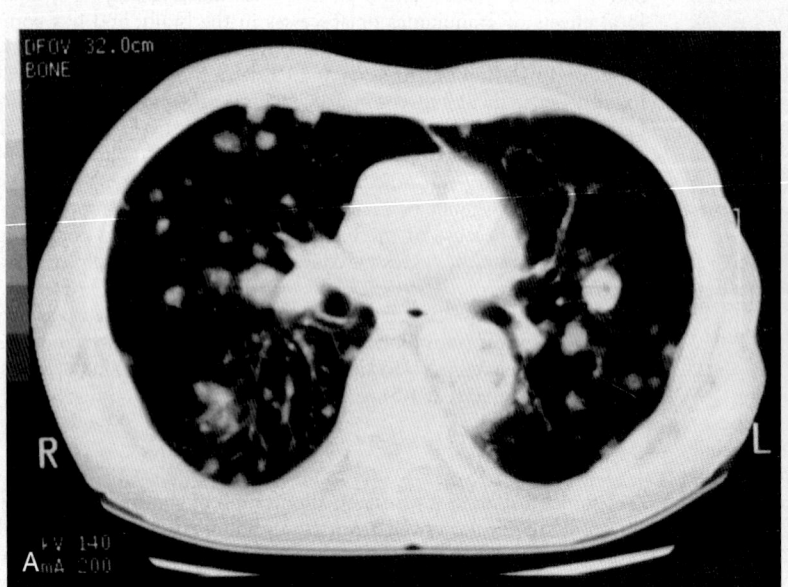
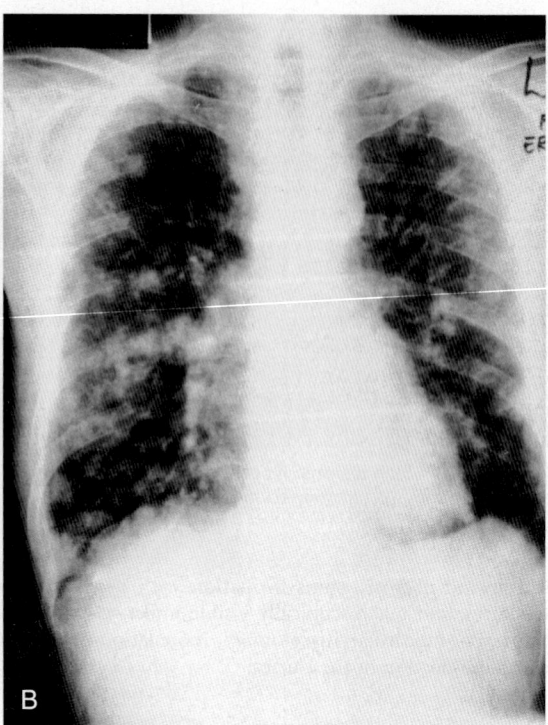

Figure 254-3 Pulmonary nodules. Multiple pulmonary nodules, demonstrated by computed tomography (**A**) and chest radiograph (**B**), in an immunosuppressed patient with disseminated nocardiosis.

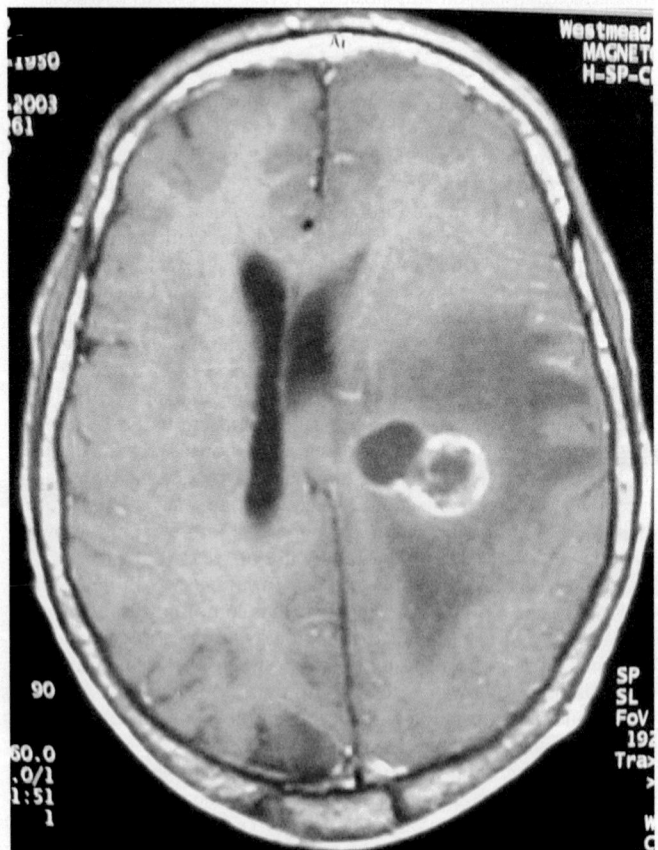

Figure 254-4 Brain abscess. Magnetic resonance image showing *Nocardia* brain abscess.

this characteristic may vary with strain and culture media used. Of note, smears from cultures often show greater fragmentation of filaments than direct smears from clinical specimens and require careful differentiation from other actinomycetes.

Accurate species identification is important because this enables predictions regarding antimicrobial susceptibility in many cases. Presumptive *Nocardia* isolates can be assigned to traditional groupings based on the hydrolysis of casein, tyrosine, xanthine, hypoxanthine, and testosterone and by sugar use tests.[1,2] These methods allow characterization of many clinically relevant *Nocardia* species but are relatively expensive, slow, and limited by their inability to differentiate members of, for example, the *N. asteroides* complex and *N. nova*

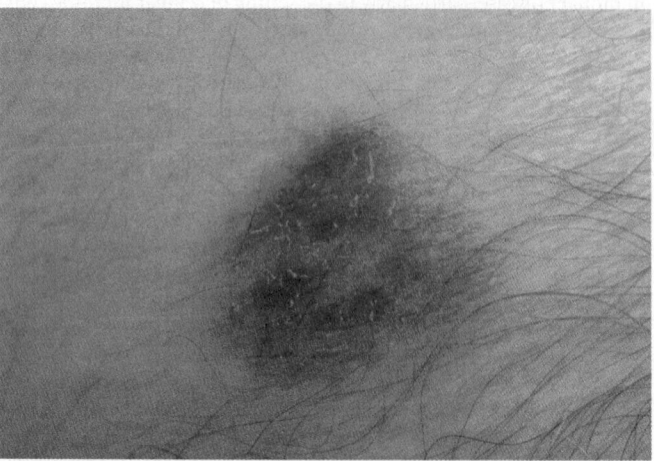

Figure 254-5 Skin lesion. Skin lesion from disseminated *Nocardia farcinica* infection.

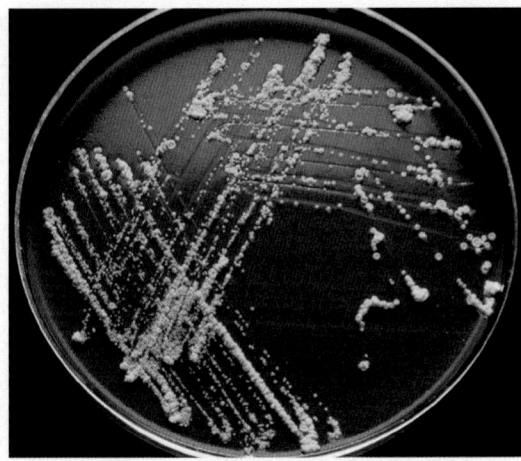

Figure 254-6 Culture. Typical colonies of *Nocardia* species growing on selective media.

complex, or to identify newly described species.[1,2] A number of commercial identification systems, such as the API 20C,[56] may allow more rapid identification and differentiation of *Nocardia* species but suffer from the same limitations of traditional phenotypic tests.

MOLECULAR IDENTIFICATION OF *NOCARDIA* SPECIES

The availability of molecular techniques has enabled not only rapid, accurate species identification of *Nocardia* but also the recognition and characterization of numerous new species. Approaches that have been developed include ribotyping, polymerase chain reaction (PCR), restriction fragment length polymorphism (RFLP) analyses, and DNA sequencing.[2] Most analyses have exploited genetic variation within the *Nocardia* 16S rRNA gene region or the heat shock protein 65 (*hsp65*) gene.

Ribotyping has been used for identification of a limited number of *Nocardia* species[57,58] and to differentiate between *N. asteroides* sensu stricto[57] and *N. farcinica*. Its widespread application is limited by the need for multiple probes to identify different species. PCR-RFLP analysis generates species-specific RFLP patterns that result from the presence or absence of restriction endonuclease recognition sites within variable regions of a specific gene. Both the *Nocardia* 16S rRNA gene and the *hsp65* gene (441 bp) have been targeted for this purpose.[59-61] In general, results obtained by *hsp65*- and 16S rRNA-based RFLP assays showed good, but variable, agreement for species identification, and the more unusual *Nocardia* isolates were not identified by either method.[61] Another limitation was the observation of variable or ambiguous RFLP profiles within species owing to base changes within a restriction endonuclease recognition site or the presence of sequence variation in multiple copies of the gene of interest, such as that noted for the 16S rRNA gene of *N. nova*.[2,62] If PCR-RFLP is used to identify *Nocardia* organisms, analyses of two different genetic loci is recommended to maximize accuracy of identification.

DNA sequencing is currently the best tool for species identification of *Nocardia* because it is rapid and identifies most *Nocardia* isolates reliably. Sequencing of the first 500 to 606 base pairs (bp) of the 5′ end of the 16S rRNA gene is the currently recommended method.[2-4] There is consensus that this region contains sufficient sequence variability for species identification,[4,61] even though analysis of longer gene fragments (e.g., 999 bp) may give more precise identifications.[4] Using this method, *N. abscessus* was found to represent 5.8% and *N. cyriacigeorgica*, 15% of a recent collection of 86 clinical isolates in Belgium.[63]

Species identification of *Nocardia* by 16S rRNA sequence analysis; however, does have limitations. Accuracy of identification is dependent on the quality of the gene repositories used for sequence comparisons, and public databases are known to contain inaccuracies or incorrect sequence entries.[64] Partial sequencing of a single gene may not distinguish between closely related species, and species identification from a database containing a single strain or small number of strains (which are potentially nonrepresentative) must also be interpreted with caution. Errors may also arise because multiple but different 16S rRNA genes are present in certain *Nocardia* species such as *N. nova*.[51,62] Finally, there is a lack of consensus on the criterion for species identification. Indeed, isolates from distinct species have been reported to have as much as 99.8% sequence similarity.[3] In such cases, DNA-hybridization studies are required to determine whether the isolates belong to the same species. Superior results from partial sequence analysis of other genes, including *hsp65* and *secA1*, have been reported, but the sequences are not available in public databases, and the findings require substantiation.[59,64,65]

Management

Clinical experience has shown that successful therapy requires the use of antimicrobial drugs and, in some cases, appropriate surgical drainage or débridement. Optimal antimicrobial regimens have not been established by controlled clinical trials. Thus, initial selection of a therapeutic regimen should take into account the site and severity of infection, the host immune status, potential drug interactions or toxicity, and the species of *Nocardia*.

Antimicrobial susceptibility testing is a useful guide to therapy in many settings (Table 254-1), but results should be interpreted with caution, given the paucity of studies correlating in vitro susceptibility data with clinical outcome. Nevertheless, with the exception of nocardial brain abscesses,[66] therapy based on in vitro susceptibility results is often effective. The Clinical Laboratory Standards Institute (CLSI; formerly National Committee for Clinical Laboratory Standards) has recently approved a broth microdilution method for antimicrobial testing of the aerobic actinomycetes.[67] Other methods include the E-test (AB Biodisk Solna, Sweden) and the BACTEC radiometric methods, which have been shown to correlate well with broth microdilution[68] and are simpler to use in the routine clinical laboratory. At present, it is recommended that isolates be sent to a specialized reference laboratory for susceptibility testing or confirmation of susceptibility. Testing is especially indicated when patients present with deep-seated or disseminated infection, fail to respond to initial therapy or relapse after therapy, and when alternatives to sulfonamides are being considered. Testing is also indicated when relatively resistant *Nocardia* species, such as *N. farcinica*, or one of the newly described species, such as *N. abscessus*, has been identified. Susceptibility profiles of *Nocardia* species are summarized in Table 254-1.

Sulfonamides, which have been the mainstay of therapy since their introduction in the 1940s, have substantially improved outcomes. However, the mortality rate with sulfonamide monotherapy is as high as 50%,[69-71] particularly in severely ill patients, those with cerebral involvement or disseminated nocardiosis, and immunosuppressed patients. In these groups, empirical combination therapy is generally commenced pending susceptibility test results. Amikacin combined with imipenem (or meropenem) is a suitable regimen for empiric therapy. Three-drug regimens consisting of a sulfonamide, amikacin, and either a carbapenem or third-generation cephalosporin have also been used for high-risk patients,[11,12] although there is no evidence of increased efficacy.

Among the sulfonamides, sulfadiazine and sulfisoxazole were the antimicrobial agents of choice for many years. Sulfadiazine may cause oliguria, azotemia, and crystalluria in patients with a low fluid intake and can be prevented by alkalinizing the urine. Sulfisoxazole is less likely to cause oliguria. Trisulfapyrimidine combinations should be as effective and less toxic.[11] In adults with normal renal function, dose schedules of 6 to 12 g/day in four to six oral doses after a loading dose of 4 g should lead to a therapeutic serum level of 100 to 150 mg/L 2 hours after a dose.[11] Although doses of 3 to 6 g/day are effective in most cases of pulmonary and systemic disease,[50] higher doses have

TABLE 254-1	Antimicrobial Susceptibility of Selected *Nocardia* Species (% Isolates Susceptible)					
Antimicrobial*	**N. asteroides**	**N. farcinica**	**N. nova**	**N. brasiliensis**	**N. transvalensis**	**N. otitidiscaviarum**
Sulfamethoxazole	96-99	89-100	89-97	99-100	90	V
Trimethoprim-sulfamethoxazole	100	100	NR	100	88	V
Ampicillin	40-93	0-5	100	14	10	NR
Amoxicillin-clavulanate	53-67	47-71	3-6	65-97	30	R
Ceftriaxone	94-100	0-73	100	88-100	50	NR
Imipenem	77-98	64-100	100	20-30	90	R
Amikacin	100	100	100	100	†82	S
Doxycycline	48-88	0-14	19-94	NR	NR	NR
Minocycline	78-94	12-96	89-100	75-90	54	S
Ciprofloxacin	38-98	68-100	0	12-30	60	R
Moxifloxacin	50	NR	NR	NR	NR	NR
Erythromycin	23-93	0-3	100	40	50	NR
Clarithromycin	42	5	NR	NR	NR	NR
Linezolid	100	100	100	100	100	100

*Based on a small number of isolates. Amikacin resistance has been considered a characteristic of the *N. transvalensis* complex.
R, resistant; V, variable susceptibility; S, sensitive; NR, not reported.

been favored in immunosuppressed patients with AIDS[46] and in patients after cardiac transplantation.[72]

Trimethoprim-sulfamethoxazole (TMP-SMX) is the formulation currently preferred by most clinicians, despite the absence of conclusive clinical data supporting increased efficacy of the combination compared with sulfadiazine and sulfisoxazole, and increased myelotoxicity. TMP-SMX (available in the fixed ratio of 1:5) has potential advantages over the older sulfonamide drugs in that in vitro synergistic activity between the two drug components has been demonstrated against a majority of *Nocardia* isolates.[69,70] Optimal ratios of TMP to SMX for demonstration of synergy vary between 1:10 to 1:5 or less in different studies.[70,73] The usual ratio of these drugs in serum and cerebrospinal fluid (CSF) is 1:20.[74] Relative drug levels in tissues and pus, including cerebral nocardial abscesses, approximate 1:7 or less.[69,75]

In adults with normal renal function and localized disease, the recommended dose of TMP-SMX is 5 to 10 mg/kg TMP and 25 to 50 mg/kg SMX in two to four divided doses, depending on the extent of disease.[69] In patients with primary cutaneous infection, including sporotrichoid nocardiosis, 5 mg/kg/day of TMP component is sufficient, in combination with appropriate surgical débridement.[69] Higher initial doses (15 mg/kg TMP and 75 mg/kg SMX) intravenously or by mouth are frequently used in patients with cerebral abscesses; severe, extensive, or disseminated infection; or AIDS.[47,70] Doses can generally be reduced and therapy changed from intravenous to oral after 3 to 6 weeks, depending on clinical response. Cure of cerebral nocardiosis has been noted with lower doses of TMP-SMX (about 10 mg/kg/day of the TMP component)[76,77] or less.[78] Immunocompromised patients do not necessarily need higher doses of TMP-SMX, for example, 5 mg/kg/day (TMP component) in two doses has been successful in the treatment of pulmonary infection in renal transplant recipients.[79] However, in these patients, two or more drugs, which may include sulfonamides, are frequently prescribed.[70,71] It has been recommended that a serum sulfonamide level performed 2 hours after an oral dose at steady state is useful to confirm that gastrointestinal absorption is adequate and that recommended therapeutic levels of sulfonamide (100 to 150 mg/L) have been achieved.[80] In practice, measurement of serum drug levels should be considered when absorption from the gastrointestinal tract is uncertain, patients requiring high doses of TMP-SMX and who are at risk for dose-related toxicity (e.g., renal and bone marrow failure) and in cases of poor therapeutic response.

Clinical decisions to initiate sulfonamides depend in part on the causative *Nocardia* species. Sulfonamides are the treatment of choice for infections due to *N. brasiliensis*,[69,81] members of the former *N. asteroides* complex,[2] and *N. transvalensis*.[11,40] These drugs are less active in vitro against *N. otitidiscaviarum* (see Table 254-1) but have been

reported to be curative in cases of localized cutaneous infection.[82] Other *Nocardia* species displaying inconsistent susceptibility to sulfonamides include *N. farcinica*. Alternative antimicrobial agents therefore should be considered in infections caused by these species (see Table 254-1) or in those failing sulfonamide therapy or those intolerant of sulfonamide-containing regimens because of hypersensitivity, gastrointestinal toxicity, or myelotoxicity. Sulfonamide intolerance occurs in up to 55% of patients with AIDS.[83] Desensitization is an option for continuation of TMP-SMX in the presence of hypersensitivity reactions. Although desensitization has been used successfully in patients with AIDS,[84] severe reactions have been reported in other settings.[74] Renal transplantation is associated with an increased risk for sulfonamide-induced myelotoxicity in patients receiving azathiaprine[85] and of nephrotoxicity in patients receiving cyclosporine or tacrolimus.

The choice of alternative therapeutic drugs has necessarily been based on in vitro susceptibility data and efficacy in animal models, especially short-term murine models of cerebral and pulmonary nocardiosis.[86,87] Assessment of these regimens in human nocardiosis is complicated by the relative paucity of (albeit increasing) clinical experience, the fact that multiple antimicrobial drugs have often been employed either in combination or sequentially,[12,88] and the variable, chronic course of nocardiosis.

Most clinical experience has been obtained with amikacin and imipenem, which appear to be the most active agents in vitro and in animal models.[11,88] In vitro, amikacin exhibits excellent activity against all species of *Nocardia*, with the exception of *N. transvalensis* (see Table 254-1). Imipenem is also highly active *in vitro* except against *N. brasiliensis*, although more than 10% of isolates of *N. farcinica*, *N. transvalensis*, and in one study, *N. asteroides* sensu strictu were resistant (see Table 254-1). Of note, minimal inhibitory concentrations of imipenem may be high for certain newly described species, for instance, *N. abscessus*.[2] Synergy between TMP-SMX and amikacin has been demonstrated in vitro; with imipenem, the effect is predominantly additive.[89] In the short-term, murine models of cerebral and pulmonary nocardiosis, imipenem and amikacin were significantly more effective than TMP-SMX,[86,87] but the apparent inferior efficacy of TMP-SMX may be model dependent.[90]

Amikacin has been used successfully, usually in combination with other agents, including sulfonamides, in patients with nocardiosis involving several different body sites, and in immunocompromised patients.[88,91] Although amikacin is potentially nephrotoxic and ototoxic, once-daily dose regimens make it a amenable to use in-home intravenous therapy programs. In one study, cure was effected in seven of eight patients given amikacin in combination with agents demonstrating synergy *in vitro*.[92] An initial parenteral regimen of imipenem and amikacin (10 to 15 mg/kg/day in two divided doses) has been recommended as primary therapy in pulmonary nocardiosis[93] and in the very ill patient,[11] although there are no data from clinical trials that support this approach. Meropenem is an attractive alternative to imipenem in patients with cerebral nocardiosis because it has a similar pharmacokinetic profile, has good CSF penetration, and is associated with a lower incidence of seizures. It has good in vitro activity against most *Nocardia* species,[94,95] although one study found that meropenem was less active than imipenem against *N. farcinica* and *N. nova*.[2] The few published reports of the use of meropenem in nocardiosis have been in the setting of combination therapy with other antinocardial agents and have resulted in varying efficacy.[96,97] Of note, the carbapenem ertapenem appears to be inactive against *Nocardia* species.[98]

Despite its broad-spectrum activity against *Nocardia* species, the use amikacin is problematic in many risk groups because of underlying poor renal function. Third-generation cephalosporins have the advantages of excellent CSF penetration and low toxicity. Those with long serum half-lives are suitable for use in ambulatory intravenous therapy programs. In several case reports, the efficacy of ceftriaxone-containing regimens in the treatment of nocardiosis has been documented.[88] Ceftriaxone, cefotaxime (see Table 254-1), and cefuroxime[11] exhibit significant in vitro activity against *Nocardia* species, with the exceptions of *N. farcinica*, *N. transvalensis,* and *N. ototidiscaviarum*. Synergy between cefotaxime and imipenem has been noted against susceptible strains of *Nocardia* in vitro, although not in a murine model of cerebral nocardiosis.[99] Cefuroxime and amikacin also exhibit synergistic activity in vitro.[92]

The most frequently used oral alternatives to sulfonamides include minocycline, despite its poor therapeutic index, and amoxicillin-clavulate. Minocycline (100 to 200 mg twice daily), has been effective when used alone, in combination with other drugs, as sequential therapy or in patients who are allergic to sulfonamides.[47,100-106] Amoxicillin-clavulanate has also been effective in individual patients when used as sequential therapy or in combination with other agents[47,106,107] and may be especially useful in treatment of cutaneous infections due to *N. brasiliensis*, a consistent β-lactamase producer.[108] However, mutation in the β-lactamase gene of *N. brasiliensis* has resulted in relapse during therapy with amoxicillin-clavulanate.[109] In continental Europe, amoxicillin-clavulanate or imipenem combined with amikacin has been recommended, especially for infections due to *N. farcinica*.[71] The use of amoxicillin-clavulanate should be guided by in vitro sensitivity data because susceptibility is variable and species dependent (see Table 254-1), demonstration of β-lactamase production is not necessarily predictive of resistance to β-lactam drugs, and although species such as *N. nova* can test as susceptible to ampicillin, in other tests they appear to be resistant to amoxicillin-clavulanic acid.[110]

Linezolid is an oral alternative with good in vitro activity against all clinically important species of *Nocardia*.[2] Its bioavailability is close to 100%, CSF penetration is good, and efficacy has been demonstrated predominantly in a few patients unable to tolerate TMP-SMX.[84,111,112] Long-term therapy carries a risk for significant toxicity requiring discontinuation of therapy. This includes hematologic toxicity, lactic acidosis, retrobulbar optic neuritis, and peripheral neuropathy.[111]

In vitro susceptibility results should also be used to guide the choice of alternative agents for which few clinical data are available such as the macrolides, fluoroquinolones, and possibly tigecycline. Information regarding the in vitro activity of the fluoroquinolones is limited. Many isolates of the former *N. asteroides* complex, *N. brasiliensis,* and *N. otitidiscaviarum* are resistant to ciprofloxacin.[113] In a more recent study, the newer fluoroquinolones gatifloxacin and moxifloxacin demonstrated greater activity than ciprofloxacin against a number of *Nocardia* species with a trend toward greater susceptibility in *N. farcinica*.[114] Thus far, clinical experience with patients treated with moxifloxacin has been mainly in infections due to *N. farcinica* as salvage therapy or in combination with other agents or surgical débridement. Results have been mixed with both successful and poor outcomes reported.[115,116] In vitro and clinical data with regard to the use of macrolides to treat nocardiosis are similarly few. Oral clarithromycin has

been used in a small number of patients who were allergic to or intolerant of sulfonamides.[117,118] There are in vitro data for the intravenous drug tigecycline, which appears to be active against the many *Nocardia* species, including imipenem- and TMP-SMX-resistant isolates.[119]

SURGICAL MANAGEMENT

The place of surgery in the management of nocardiosis depends on the site and extent of infection. In extraneural disease, indications for aspiration, drainage, or excision of abscesses are similar to those for other chronic bacterial infections. Therapeutic aspiration is generally inadequate in patients with thick-walled multiloculated abscesses, which contain little free-flowing pus, including patients with mycetomas.[120] In patients with brain abscesses, surgery should be performed when abscesses are accessible and relatively large, the patient's condition deteriorates or lesions progress within 2 weeks of therapy, or there is no reduction in abscess size within 1 month.[121] Decompression of lesions can be accomplished by stereotactic aspiration, although cure in many cases is effected only after craniotomy and total excision.[121] Small abscesses can be cured by prolonged antimicrobial therapy. Because abscesses may progress in the face of appropriate therapy, all patients must be monitored frequently with cranial computed tomography or other imaging modalities.

DURATION OF THERAPY AND PROGNOSIS

Clinical improvement is generally evident within 3 to 5 days[90] or, at the most, 7 to 10 days after the initiation of appropriate therapy.[80] Parenteral therapy can usually be safely changed to an oral regimen after 3 to 6 weeks, depending on clinical response. Initial high doses of TMP-SMX can also be reduced at this time. Patients with extensive nocardiosis, necrotic foci not amenable to surgery, or those who respond slowly may benefit from prolongation of parenteral and subsequently oral therapy.[11] Lack of response to initial therapy may be due to primary drug resistance, inadequate penetration of drug into sites of infection (dependent on dose, bioavailability of oral drugs, abscess location and pathology, and patient compliance), the presence of a sequestered abscess requiring surgical drainage, and in an immunocompromised host, overwhelming nocardial infection or a coexisting or secondary opportunistic infection.

Patients receiving immunosuppressive medications should generally continue to receive these medications during treatment of nocardiosis in order to contain the underlying disease or to prevent transplant rejection. However, reduction or cessation of immunosuppressive drugs may be required if the *Nocardia* infection is uncontrolled and progressive despite therapeutic serum levels of antimicrobial drugs.

Recommendations on the duration of therapy are necessarily empirical and based primarily on reports of relapse after sulfonamide therapy of different durations.[46,69,70,76,81,122] There are rare case reports of cure of extrapulmonary abscesses after short-course parenteral therapy (7 to 8 weeks) with amikacin and surgical drainage,[37,123] or amikacin plus ceftriaxone, as in a case of cerebral nocardiosis.[124] One- to 3-month courses of therapy are curative in patients with primary cutaneous infection, including sporotrichoid nocardiosis and superficial ulcers.[50,69] Prolonged therapy is required in patients with mycetoma.[120] Nonimmunosuppressed patients with pulmonary or systemic nocardiosis (excluding CNS involvement) should be treated for at least 6 months, and those with CNS involvement, for 12 months. These patients should be monitored for at least 1 year after completion of therapy to detect late relapses.[76,122] In HIV-negative, immunosuppressed patients, isolated pulmonary disease should be treated for at least 6 months and disseminated disease for 6 to 12 months, depending on the underlying state of immunosuppression and response to therapy. Therapy should be continued for 12 months or longer if there are intercurrent increases in immunosuppression, for example, due to episodes of graft rejection. For patients who must be maintained on steroid or cytotoxic therapy, prolonged low-dose maintenance therapy may be required. The most suitable maintenance regimen has not been defined, but daily low-dose therapy seems appropriate because TMP-SMX administered two or three times weekly did not prevent the development of nocardiosis after bone marrow transplantation[91,125] or solid organ transplantation.[12] In patients with AIDS, early institution of a prolonged primary course of antinocardial therapy is essential because treatment of patients with late presentations or those whose nocardial infection has relapsed has usually been unsuccessful.[46] In this group, low-dose maintenance therapy may be required for life. There are no data on whether such therapy can be discontinued in patients with responding well to HAART (highly active antiretroviral therapy).

PROPHYLAXIS

Primary prophylaxis against nocardial infection is not generally necessary for patients who are immunosuppressed after transplantation, because of the low incidence of nocardiosis, especially since the introduction of cyclosporine.[106] The daily use of TMP-SMX as prophylaxis against alternative infections may prevent some cases of nocardiosis, as has been observed after renal transplantation,[126] although the overall impact of such therapy is dependent on the dose regimen used for prophylaxis[12] and is reduced by the late occurrence of cases of nocardiosis after transplantation.[106] TMP-SMX prophylaxis has not been of proven benefit in the prevention of nocardiosis in patients with AIDS, possibly because the overall incidence based on autopsy series is low.[127] It is notable, however, that cases of nocardiosis in AIDS patients were usually found in those who had not been receiving sulfonamide prophylaxis against other pathogens.[47]

CLINICAL OUTCOMES

The clinical outcome of therapy for nocardiosis is dependent on the site and extent of disease and underlying host factors. Cure rates of almost 100% are found in patients with skin or soft tissue involvement, compared with 90% in pleuropulmonary disease, 63% in disseminated infection, and 50% in brain abscess.[70] Mortality in patients with brain abscesses diagnosed antemortem approximates 31% but is higher (41%) in patients with multiple abscesses and in immunocompromised patients (55%).[121] In an early, large series of patients with nocardiosis, mortality was increased significantly in patients with Cushing disease and those receiving corticosteroids or antineoplastic drugs, but was not related to the severity of the underlying disease.[128] Although immunosuppressive therapy increases the risk for pulmonary and disseminated nocardiosis in recipients of organ transplants, it is not clear to what extent maintenance of immunosuppressive therapy during treatment of nocardiosis interferes with outcome. In fact most patients can be cured with appropriate antimicrobial therapy even if immunosuppressive drugs are continued, provided the diagnosis is made early and appropriate full-dose therapy is continued for an adequate period of time.[72,106,125] On the other hand, delay in diagnosis and early cessation of therapy are poor prognostic factors, which in patients with AIDS have been associated with failure of subsequent therapy.[46]

In summary, the choice and dose of antimicrobial drugs and the duration of therapy depend on the sites and extent of infection, underlying host factors, the species of *Nocardia,* and the clinical response to initial management. Therapy with TMP-SMX remains the mainstay of treatment for patients with nocardiosis. The use of additional or alternative drugs in severely ill patients, for example, amikacin, a carbapenem, or ceftriaxone, may improve prognosis, especially in the immunocompromised. Alternative regimens are required in patients unable to tolerate, or who fail therapy with, sulfonamides, and often in those with infections due to relatively resistant species. Linezolid, the new quinolones, and macrolides that are effective orally offer promise for the future.

REFERENCES

1. Conville PS, Witebsky FG. *Nocardia, Rhodococcus, Gordonia, Actinomadura, Streptomyces,* and other aerobic actinomycetes. In: Murray PR, Baron EJ, Jorgensen JH, et al, eds. *Manual of Clinical Microbiology.* 9th ed. Washington: ASM Press; 2007.
2. Brown-Elliott B, Brown JM, Conville P, et al. Clinical and laboratory features of the *Nocardia* spp. Based on current molecular taxonomy. *Clin Microbiol Rev.* 2006;19:259-282.
3. Roth A, Andrees S, Kroppenstedt RM, et al. Phylogeny of the genus nocardia based on reassessed 16SrRNA gene sequences reveals underspeciation and division of strains classified as *Nocardia* asteroids into three established species and two unnamed taxons. *J Clin Microbiol.* 2003;41:851-856.
4. Cloud J, Conville P, Croft A, et al. Evaluation of partial 16SS DNA sequencing for identification of nocardia species by using the Micro Seq 500 system with an expanded database. *J Clin Microbiol.* 2004;42:578-584.
5. Yassin AF, Raney F, Mendrock U, et al. *Nocardia abscessus* sp. nov. *Int J Syst Evol Microbiol.* 2000.50:1487-1493.
6. Yassin AF, Rainey FA, Steiner U. *Nocardia cyriacigeorgici* sp. nov. *Int J Syst Evol Microbiol.* 2001;51:1419-1423.
7. Eisenblatter M, Disko U, Stoltenburg-Didinger G, et al. Isolation of *Nocardia paucivorans* from the cerebrospinal fluid of a patient with relapse of cerebral nocardiosis. *J Clin Microbiol.* 2002;40:3532-3534.
8. Hamid ME, Mohamed MF, Saeed NS, et al. *Nocardia africana* sp. nov., a new pathogen isolated from patients with pulmonary infections. *J Clin Microbiol.* 2001;625-630.
9. Gurtler V, Smith R, Mayall B, et al. *Nocardia veterana* sp. nov., isolated from human bronchial lavage. *Int J Syst Evol Microbiol.* 2001;51:933-936.
10. Conville PS, Brown JM, Steigerwalt AG, et al. *Nocardia wallacei* sp. nov. and *Nocardia blacklockiae* sp. nov., human pathogens and members of the "*Nocardia transvalensis* Complex". *J Clin Microbiol.* 2008;46:1178-1184.
11. Lerner PI. Nocardiosis. *Clin Infect Dis.* 1996;22:891-905.
12. Peleg AY, Hussain S, Qureshi ZA, et al. Risk factors, clinical characteristics, and outcome of *Nocardia* infection in organ transplant recipients: a matched case-control study. *Clin Infect Dis.* 2007;44:1307-1314.
13. Blumel J, Blumel E, Yassin AF, et al. Typing of *Nocardia farcinica* by pulsed-field electrophoresis reveals an endemic strain as source of hospital infections. *J Clin Microbiol.* 1998;36:118-122.
14. Provost F, Laurent F, Camacho Uzcategui LR, et al. Molecular study of persistence of *Nocardia asteroides* and *Nocardia otitidiscaviarum* strains in patients with long-term nocardiosis. *J Clin Microbiol.* 1997;35:1157-1160.
15. Beaman L, Beaman BL. *Nocardia* species: host-parasite relationships. *Clin Microbiol Rev.* 1994;7:213-264.
16. Deem RL, Doughty FA, Beaman BL. Immunologically specific direct T lymphocyte mediated killing of *Nocardia asteroides. J Immunol.* 1983;130:2401-2406.
17. Dorman SE, Guide SV, Conville PS, et al. *Nocardia* infection in chronic granulomatous disease. *Clin Infect Dis.* 2002;35:390-394.
18. Beaman BL. Structural and biochemical alterations of *Nocardia asteroides* cell walls during its growth cycle. *J Bacteriol.* 1975;123:1235-1253.
19. Beaman BL, Moring SE. Relationship among cell wall composition, stage of growth, and virulence of *Nocardia asteroides* GUH-2. *Infect Immun.* 1988;56:557-563.
20. Tamplin ML, McClung NM. Quantitative studies of the relationship between trehalose lipids and virulence of *Nocardia asteroides* isolates. In: Ortiz-Ortiz L, Bojalil LF, Yakeloff V, eds. *Biological, biochemical and biomedical aspects of actinomycetes.* Orlando, Fla: Academic Press, Inc; 1984:251-258.
21. Spargo BJ, Crowe LM, Ioneda T, et al. Cord factor (α,α-trehalose 6,6′-dimycolate) inhibits fusion between phospholipid vesicles. *Proc Natl Acad Sci U S A.* 1991;88:737-740.
22. Silva CL, Tinciani I, Brandao-Filho SL, et al. Mouse cachexia induced by trehalose dimycolate from *Nocardia asteroides. J Gen Microbiol.* 1988;134:1629-1633.
23. Beaman BL. The cell wall as a determinant of pathogenicity in *Nocardia*: the role of L-forms in pathogenesis. In: Ortiz-Ortiz L, Bojalil LF, Yakeloff V, eds. *Biological, biochemical and biomedical aspects of actinomycetes.* Orlando, Fla: Academic Press, Inc; 1984:89-105.
24. Beaman BL. Differential binding of *Nocardia asteroides* in the murine lung and brain suggest multiple ligands on the nocardial surface. *Infect Immun.* 1996;64(11):4859-4862.
25. Filice GA, Beaman BL, Krick JA, et al. Effects of human neutrophils and monocytes on *Nocardia asteroides*: failure of killing despite occurrence of the oxidative metabolic burst. *J Infect Dis.* 1980;142:432-438.
26. Davis-Scibienski C, Beaman BL. Interaction of *Nocardia asteroides* with rabbit alveolar macrophages: association of virulence, viability, ultrastructural damage, and phagosome- lysosome fusion. *Infect Immun.* 1980;28:610-619.
27. Bourgeois L. Beaman BL. In vitro sphaeroplast and L-form induction within the pathogenic nocardiae. *J Bacteriol.* 1976;127:584-594.
28. Beaman BL, Smathers M. Interaction of *Nocardia asteroides* with cultured rabbit alveolar macrophages. *Infect Immun.* 1976;13:1126-1131.
29. Beaman BL, Scates SM. Role of L-forms of *Nocardia caviae* in the development of chronic mycetomas in normal and immunodeficient murine models. *Infect Immun.* 1981;33:893-907.
30. Buchanan AM, Beaman BL, Pedersen NC, et al. *Nocardia asteroides* recovery from a dog with steroid- and antibiotic-unresponsive idiopathic polyarthritis. *J Clin Microbiol.* 1983;18:702-708.
31. Black CM, Beaman BL, Donovan RM, et al. Intracellular acid phosphatase content and the ability of different macrophage populations to kill *Nocardia asteroides. Infect Immun.* 1985;47:375-383.
32. Kusunose E, Ichihara K, Noda Y, et al. Superoxide dismutase from *mycobacterium tuberculosis. J Biochem.* 1976;80:1343-1352.
33. Beaman L, Beaman BL. Monoclonal antibodies demonstrate that superoxide dismutase contributes to protection of *Nocardia asteroides* within the intact host. *Infect Immun.* 1990;58:3122-3128.
34. Beaman BL, Ogata SA. Ultrastructural analysis of attachment to and penetration of capillaries in the murine pons, mid-brain, thalamus, *and hypothalamus by* Nocardia asteroides. *Infect Immun.* 1993;61:955-965.
35. Licon-Trillo A, Angeles Castro-Corona M, Salinas-Carmona MC. Immunogenicity and biophysical properties of a *Nocardia brasiliensis* protease involved in pathogenesis of mycetoma. *FEMS Immunol Med Microbiol.* 2003;37:37-44.
36. Kuipers S, Aerts PC, van Dijk H. Differential microorganism-induced mannose-binding lectin activation. *FEMS Immunol Med Microbiol.* 2003;36:33-39.
37. Schiff TA, McNeil MM, Brown JM. Cutaneous *Nocardia farcinica* infection in an immunocompromised patient: case report and review. *Clin Infect Dis.* 1993;16:756-760.
38. Desmond EP, Flores M. Mouse pathogenicity studies of *Nocardia asteroides* complex species and clinical correlation with human isolates. *FEMS Microbiol Lett.* 1993;110:281-284.

39. Ruimy R, Riegel P, Carlotti A, et al. Nocardia pseudobrasiliensis sp. nov., a new species of *Nocardia* which groups bacterial strains previously identified as *Nocardia brasiliensis* and associated with invasive diseases. *Int J Syst Bacteriol.* 1996;46:259-264.
40. McNeil MM, Brown JM, Georghiou PR, et al. Infections due to *Nocardia transvalensis*: clinical spectrum and antimicrobial therapy. *Clin Infect Dis.* 1992;15:453-463.
41. Forbes GM, Harvey FAH, Philpott-Howard J, et al. Nocardiosis in liver transplantation: variation in presentation, diagnosis and therapy *J Infect.* 1990;20:11-19.
42. Kim J, Minamoto GY, Grieco MH. Nocardial infection as a complication of AIDS: report of six cases and review. *Rev Infect Dis.* 1991;13:624-629.
43. Mahgoub ES. Agents of mycetoma. In: Mandell GL, Bennett JE, Dolin R. *Mandell, Douglas and Bennett's principles and practice of infectious diseases.* 4th ed. vol. 2. NY: Churchill Livingstone; 1995:2327-2330.
44. Kramer MR, Uttamchandani RB. The radiographic appearance of pulmonary nocardiosis associated with AIDS. *Chest.* 1990;98:382-385.
45. Lucas SB, Hounnou A, Peacock C, et al. Nocardiosis in HIV-positive patients: an autopsy study in West Africa. *Tuber Lung Dis.* 1994;75:301-307.
46. Uttamchandani RB, Daikos GL, Reyes RR, et al. Nocardiosis in 30 patients with advanced Human Immunodeficiency Virus infection: clinical features and outcome. *Clin Infect Dis.* 1994;18:348-353
47. Javaly K, Horowitz HW, Wormser GP. Nocardiosis in patients with human immunodeficiency virus infection: report of two cases and review of the literature. *Medicine.* 1992;71:128-138.
48. Farina C, Boiron P, Goglio A, et al. Human nocardiosis in northern Italy from 1982 to 1992. Northern Italy Collaborative Group on Nocardiosis. *Scand J Infect Dis.* 1995;27:23-27.
49. Boiron P, Provost F, Chevrier G, et al. Review of nocardial infections in France 1987 to 1990. *Eur J Clin Microbiol Infect Dis.* 1992;11:709-714.
50. Georghiou PR, Blacklock ZM. Infection with *Nocardia* species in Queensland: a review of 102 clinical isolates. *Med J Aust.* 1992;156:692-697.
51. Conville PS, Witebsky FG. Analysis of multiple differing copies of the 16S rRNA gene in five clinical isolates and three type strains of *Nocardia* species and implications for species assignment. *J Clin Microbiol.* 2007;45:1146-1151.
52. Ashdown LR. An improved screening technique for isolation of *Nocardia* species from sputum specimens. *Pathology.* 1990;22:157-161.
53. Shawar RM, Moore DG, La Rocco MT. Cultivation of *Nocardia* spp. on chemically defined media for selective recovery of isolates from clinical specimens. *J Clin Microbiol.* 1990;28:508-512.
54. Vickers RM, Rihs JD, Yu VL. Clinical demonstration of isolation of *Nocardia asteroides* on buffered charcoal-yeast-extract media. *J Clin Microbiol.* 1992;30:227-228.
55. Murray PR, Heeren RA, Niles AC. Effect of decontamination procedures on recovery of *Nocardia* spp. *J Clin Microbiol.* 1987;25:2010-2011.
56. Kiska DL, Hicks K, Pettit DJ. Identification of medically relevant *Nocardia* species with an abbreviated battery of tests. *J Clin Microbiol.* 2002;40:1346-1351.
57. McNeil MM, Ray S, Kozarsky PE, et al. *Nocardia farcinica* pneumonia in a previously healthy woman: species characterisation with use of digoxigenin-labelled cDNA probe. *Clin Infect Dis.* 1997;25:933-934.
58. Chapman G, Beaman BL, Loeffler A, et al. In situ hybridization for detection of nocardial 16S rRNA: reactivity within intracellular inclusions in experimentally infected cynomolgus monkeys—and in Lewy body-containing human brain specimens. *Exp Neurol.* 2003;184:715-725.
59. Steingrube VA, Brown BA, Gibson JL, et al. DNA amplification and restriction endonuclease analysis for differentiation of 12 species and taxa of *Nocardia*, including recognition of four new taxa within the *Nocardia asteroides* complex. *J Clin Microbiol.* 1995;33:3096-3101.
60. Steingrube VA, Wilson RW, Brown BA, et al. Rapid identification of clinically significant species and taxa of aerobic actinomycetes, including *Actinomadura, Gordona, Nocardia, Rhodococcus, Streptomyces*, and *Tsukamurella* isolates, by DNA amplification and restriction endonuclease analysis. *J Clin Microbiol.* 1997;35:817-822.
61. Conville PS, Fischer SH, Cartwright CP, et al. Identification of *Nocardia* species by restriction endonuclease analysis of an amplified portion of the 16S rRNA gene. *J Clin Microbiol.* 2000;38:158-164.
62. Conville PS, Witebsky FG. Multiple copies of the 16S rRNA gene in *Nocardia nova* isolates and implications for sequence-based identification procedures. *J Clin Microbiol.* 2005;43:2881-2885.
63. Wauters G, Avasani V, Charlier J, et al. Distribution of *Nocardia* species in clinical samples and their routine rapid identification in the laboratory. *J Clin Microbiol.* 2005;43:2624-2628.
64. Patel JB, Wallace RJ, Brown-Elliot BA, et al. Sequence-based identification of aerobic actinomycetes. *J Clin Microbiol.* 2004;42:2530-2540.
65. Conville PS, Zelazny AM, Witebsky FG. Analysis of secA1 gene sequences for identification of *Nocardia* species. *J Clin Microbiol.* 2006;44:2760-2766.
66. Corti ME, Villafane-Fioti MF. Nocardiosis: a review. *Int J Infect Dis.* 2003;7:243-250.
67. Clinical and Laboratory Standards Institute/NCCLS. *Susceptibility testing of mycobacteria, nocardiae, and other aerobic actinomycetes; approved standard.* CLSI/NCCLS Document M24-A. 2003.
68. Ambaye A, Kohner PC, Wollan PC, et al. Comparison of agar dilution, broth microdilution, disk diffusion, E-test and BACTEC radiometric methods for antimicrobial susceptibility testing of clinical isolates of the *Nocardia asteroides* complex. *J Clin Microbiol.* 1997;35:847-852.
69. Wallace RJ Jr, Septimus EJ, Williams TW Jr, et al. Use of trimethoprim-sulfamethoxazole for treatment of infections due to *Nocardia. Rev Infect Dis.* 1982;4:315-325.
70. Smego RA Jr, Moeller MB, Gallis HA. Trimethoprim-sulfamethoxazole therapy for *Nocardia* infections. *Arch Intern Med.* 1983;143:711-718.
71. Beaman BL, Boiron P, Beaman L, et al. *Nocardia* and nocardiosis. *J Med Vet Mycol.* 1992;30(Suppl 1):317-331.
72. Simpson GL, Stinson EB, Egger MJ, et al. Nocardial infections in the immunocompromised host: a detailed study in a defined population. *Rev Infect Dis.* 1981;3:492-507.
73. Bennett JE, Jennings AE. Factors influencing susceptibility of *Nocardia* species to trimethoprim-sulfamethoxazole. *Antimicrob Agents Chemother.* 1978;13:624-627.
74. Moylett EH, Pacheco SE, Brown-Elliott BA, et al. Clinical experience with linezolid for the treatment of *Nocardia* infection. *Clin Infect Dis.* 2003;36:313-318.
75. Maderazo EG, Quintiliani R. Treatment of nocardial infection with trimethoprim and sulfamethoxazole. *Am J Med.* 1974;57:671-675.
76. Byrne E, Brophy BP, Perrett LV. *Nocardia* cerebral abscess: new concepts in diagnosis management, and prognosis. *J Neurol Neurosurg Psychiat.* 1979;42:1038-1045.
77. Smith PW, Steinkraus GE, Henricks BW, et al. CNS nocardiosis. Response to sulfamethoxazole-trimethoprim. *Arch Neurol.* 1980;37:729-730.
78. Maderazo EG, Quintiliani R. Treatment of nocardial infection with trimethoprim and sulfamethoxazole. *Am J Med.* 1974;57:671-675.
79. Wilson JP, Turner HR, Kirchner KA, et al. Nocardial infections in renal transplant recipients. *Medicine (Baltimore).* 1989;68:38-57.
80. McNeil MM, Brown JM, Hutwagner LC, et al. Evaluation of therapy for *Nocardia asteroides* complex infections. *Infect Dis Clin Pract.* 1995;4:287-292.
81. Smego RA Jr, Gallis HA. The clinical spectrum of *Nocardia brasiliensis* infection in the United States. *Rev Infect Dis.* 1984;6:164-180.
82. Clark NM, Braun DK, Pasternak A, et al. Primary cutaneous *Nocardia otitidiscaviarum* infection: case report and review. *Clin Infect Dis.* 1995;20:1266-1270.
83. Gordin FM, Simon GL, Wofsy CB. Adverse reactions to trimethoprim-sulfamethoxazole in patients with the acquired immunodeficiency syndrome. *Ann Intern Med.* 1984;100:495-499.
84. Maclean S, Iwamoto GK, Richerson HB, et al. Trimethoprim-sulfamethoxazole desensitization in the acquired immunodeficiency syndrome. *Ann Intern Med.* 1987;106:335.
85. Bradley PP, Warden GD, Maxwell JG, et al. Neutropenia and thrombocytopenia in renal allograft recipients treated with trimethoprim-sulfamethoxazole. *Ann Intern Med.* 1980;93:560-562.
86. Gombert ME, Aulicino TM, duBouchet L, et al. Therapy of experimental cerebral nocardiosis with imipenem, amikacin, trimethoprim-sulfamethoxazole, and minocycline. *Antimicrob Agents Chemother.* 1986;30:270-273.
87. Gombert M, Berkowitz L, Aulicino T, et al. Therapy of pulmonary nocardiosis in immunocompromised mice. *Antimicrob Agents Chemother.* 1990;34:1766-1768.
88. Threlkeld SC, Hooper DC. Update on management of patients with *Nocardia* infection. *Curr Clin Top Infect Dis.* 1997;17:1-23.
89. Gombert ME, Aulicino TM. Synergism of imipenem and amikacin in combination with other antibiotics against *Nocardia asteroides. Antimicrob Agents Chemother.* 1983;24:810-811.
90. Filice GA, Simpson GL. Management of *Nocardia* infections. *Curr Clin Topics Infect Dis.* 1984;5:49-64.
91. Choucino C, Goodman SA, Greer JP, et al. Nocardial infections in bone marrow transplant recipients. *Clin Infect Dis.* 1996;23:1012-1019.
92. Goldstein FW, Hautefort B, Acar JF. Amikacin containing regimens for treatment of nocardiosis in immunocompromised patients. *Eur J Clin Microbiol Infect Dis.* 1987;6:198-200.
93. Menendez R, Cordero PJ, Santos M, et al. Pulmonary infection with *Nocardia* species: a report of 10 cases and review. *Eur Resp J.* 1997;10:1542-1546.
94. Yazawa K, Mikami Y. Ohashi S, et al. In-vitro activity of new carbapenem antibiotics: comparative studies with meropenem, L-627 and imipenem against pathogenic *Nocardia* spp. *J Antimicrob Chemother.* 1992;29:169-172.
95. Wiseman LR, Wagstaff AJ, Brogden RN, et al. Meropenem. A review of its antibacterial activity, pharmacokinetic properties and clinical efficacy. *Drugs.* 1995;50:73-101.
96. Velasco N, Farrington K, Greenwood R, et al. Atypical presentation of systematic nocardiosis and successful treatment with meropenem. *Nephrol Dial Transplant.* 1996;11:709-710.
97. Hartmann A, Halvorsen CE, Jenssen T, et al. Intracerebral abscess caused by *Nocardia otitidiscaviarum* in a renal transplant patient: Cured by evacuation plus antibiotic therapy. *Nephron.* 2000;86:79-83.
98. Cercenado E, Marin M, Sanchez-Martinez M, et al. In vitro activities of tigecycline and eight other antimicrobials against different *Nocardia* species identified by molecular methods. *Antimicrob Agents Chemother.* 2007;51:1102-1104.
99. Gombert ME, duBouchet, Aulicino TM, et al. Antimicrobial synergism in the therapy of experimental cerebral nocardiosis. *J Antimicrob Chemother.* 1989;23:39-43.
100. Bach MC, Monaco AP, Finland M. Pulmonary nocardiosis. Therapy with minocycline and with erythromycin plus ampicillin. *JAMA.* 1973;224:1378-1380.
101. Wren MV, Savage AM, Alford RD. Apparent cure of intracranial *Nocardia asteroides* infection by minocycline. *Arch Intern Med.* 1979;139:249-250.
102. Curry WA. Human nocardiosis: a clinical review with selected case reports. *Arch Intern Med.* 1980;140:818-826.
103. Norden CW, Ruben FL, Selker R. Nonsurgical treatment of cerebral nocardiosis. *Arch Neurol.* 1983;40:594-595.
104. Hall WA, Martinez AJ, Dummer JS, et al. Nocardial brain abscess: diagnostic and therapeutic use of stereotactic aspiration. *Surg Neurol.* 1987;28:114-118.
105. Bross JE, Gordon G. Nocardial meningitis: case reports and review. *Rev Infect Dis.* 1991;13:160-165.
106. Arduino RC, Johnson PC, Miranda AG. Nocardiosis in renal transplant recipients undergoing immunosuppression with cyclosporine. *Clin Infect Dis.* 1993;16:505-512.
107. Wortman PD. Treatment of a *Nocardia brasiliensis* mycetoma with sulfamethoxazole and trimethoprim, amikacin and amoxicillin and clavulanate. *Arch Dermatol.* 1993;129:564-567.
108. Wallace RJ, Nash DR, Johnson WK, et al. β-lactam resistance in *Nocardia brasiliensis* is mediated by β-lactamase and reversed in the presence of clavulanic acid. *J Infect Dis.* 1987;156:959-966.
109. Steingrube VA, Wallace RJ Jr, Brown BA, et al. Acquired resistance of *Nocardia brasiliensis* to clavulanic acid related to a change in beta-lactamase following therapy with amoxicillin-clavulanic acid. *Antimicrob Agents Chemother.* 1991;35:254-258.
110. Wallace RJ, Brown BA, Tsukamura M, et al: Clinical and laboratory features of *Nocardia nova. J Clin Microbiol.* 1991;29:2407-2411.
111. Jodlowski TZ, Melnychuk I, Conry J. Linezolid for the treatment of *Nocardia* spp. infections. *Ann Pharmacother.* 2007;41:1694-1699.
112. Rivero A, Garcia-Lazaro M, Perez-Camacho I, et al. Successful long-term treatment with linezolid for disseminated infection with multiresistant *Nocardia farcinica. Infection.* 2008;36:389-391.
113. Khardori N, Shawar R, Gupta R, et al. In vitro antimicrobial susceptibilities of *Nocardia* species. *Antimicrob Agents Chemother.* 1993;37:882-884.
114. Hansen G, Swanzy S, Gupta R, et al. In vitro activity of fluoroquinolones against clinical isolates of *Nocardia* identified by partial 16S rRNA sequencing. *Eur J Clin Microbiol Infect Dis.* 2008;27:115-120.
115. Fihman V, Bercot B, Mateo J, et al. First successful treatment of *Nocardia farcinica* brain abscess with moxifloxacin. *J Infect.* 2006;52:e99-102.
116. Dahan K, El Kabbag D, Venditto M, et al. Intracranial *Nocardia* recurrence during fluorinated quinolones therapy. *Transpl Infect Dis.* 2006;8:161-165.
117. Naik S, Mateo-Bibeau R, Shinnar M, et al. Successful treatment of *Nocardia nova* bacteremia and multilobar pneumonia with clarithromycin in a heart transplant patient. *Transplant Proc.* 2007;39:1720-1722.
118. Kashima M, Kano R, Mikami Y, et al. A successfully treated case of mycetoma due to *Nocardia veterana. Br J Dermatol.* 2005;152:1349-1352.
119. Cercenado E, Marin M, Sanchez-Martinez M, et al. In vitro activities of tigecycline and eight other antimicrobials against different *Nocardia* species identified by molecular methods. *Antimicrob Agents Chemother.* 2007;51:1102-1104.
120. Lopes CF. Trimethoprim-sulfamethoxazole in the treatment of actinomycotic mycetoma by *Nocardia brasiliensis. Folha Medica.* 1996;73:89-92.
121. Mamelak AN, Obana WG, Flaherty JF, et al. Nocardial brain abscess: treatment and factors influencing outcome. *Neurosurgery.* 1994;35:622-631.
122. Geiseler PJ, Andersen BR. Results of therapy in systemic nocardiosis. *Am J Med Sci.* 1979;278:188-194.
123. Meier B, Metzger U, Müller F, et al. Successful treatment of a pancreatic *Nocardia asteroides* abscess with amikacin and surgical drainage. *J Clin Microbiol.* 1986;29:150-151.
124. Garlando F, Bodmer T, Lee C, et al. Successful treatment of disseminated nocardiosis complicated by cerebral abscess with ceftriaxone and amikacin: case report. *Clin Infect Dis.* 1992;15:1039-1040.
125. van Burik JA, Hackman RC, Nadeem SQ, et al. Nocardiosis after bone marrow transplantation: a retrospective study. *Clin Infect Dis.* 1997;24:1154-1160.
126. Peterson PK, Ferguson R, Fryd DS, et al. *Infectious diseases* in hospitalized renal transplant recipients: a prospective study of a complex and evolving problem. *Medicine.* 1982;61:360-372.
127. Niedt GW, Schinella RA. Acquired immunodeficiency syndrome. *Arch Path Lab Med.* 1985;109:727-734.
128. Presant CA, Wiernik PH, Serpick AA. Factors affecting survival in nocardiosis. *Am Rev Resp Dis.* 1973;108:1444-1448.

255 Agents of Actinomycosis

THOMAS A. RUSSO

Actinomycosis is an indolent, slowly progressive infection caused by anaerobic or microaerophilic bacteria, primarily from the genus *Actinomyces*, which normally colonize the mouth, colon, and vagina. Disruption of mucosa may lead to infection of virtually any site. When the organisms invade tissue, they form tiny but visible clumps, called grains or "sulfur granules," named for their yellow color. In this chapter, the terms *grain* and *sulfur granule* are used interchangeably. Lesions of actinomycosis are purulent foci surrounded by dense fibrosis. Clinical presentations are myriad. Once common in the preantibiotic era, today the incidence of actinomycosis is diminished and, as a result, so is its timely recognition.[1] At the time actinomycosis was much more common, it was called "the most misdiagnosed disease," and stated that "no disease is so often missed by experienced clinicians."[2] Needless to say, actinomycosis still remains as a diagnostic challenge today despite technological advances.[3] Three clinical presentations that should prompt consideration of this unique infection include (1) the combination of chronicity, progression across tissue boundaries, and masslike features, which mimics malignancy (with which it is often confused); (2) the development of a sinus tract, which may spontaneously resolve and recur; and (3) a refractory or relapsing infection after a short course of therapy, because cure of established actinomycosis requires prolonged treatment. An awareness of the full spectrum of disease manifestations prompting clinical suspicion will expedite diagnosis and treatment and minimize unnecessary surgical interventions and morbidity and mortality that all too often occur with actinomycosis.

Etiologic Agents

Actinomycosis is most commonly caused by the gram-positive higher bacterium *Actinomyces israelii*.[4] Additional species that are established but less common causes of actinomycosis include *A. naeslundii*,[5] *A. viscosus*,[6] *A. odontolyticus*,[7] *A. meyeri*,[8] and *A. gerencseriae* (formerly *A. israelii* serotype II). Although *Propionibacterium propionicum* (formerly *Arachnia propionica*) has been described to cause actinomycosis,[4] recent reports primarily describe this pathogen as causing lacrimal canaliculitis.[9,10]

Until recently, classification of *Actinomyces* spp. was based on differences in phenotypic testing (see "Diagnosis"). However, advances in microbiologic taxonomy, using genotypic methods such as comparative 16S ribosomal RNA (rRNA) gene sequencing have demonstrated that certain "classic" *Actinomyces* species were misclassified within the genera.[10] These methods have also led to the identification of several new *Actinomyces* species from both human and animal specimens and the reclassification of some actinomycetes as *Arcanobacterium*, *Actinobaculum* or Cellulomonas.[10-12] Although their role in causing human disease has not always been optimally established, an increasing body of data supports that *A. europaeus*,[10,11,13,14] *A. neuii*,[14-18] *A. radingae*,[10,11,14,19,20] *A. graevenitzii*, *A. turicensis*,[10,11,14,19-22] *A. georgiae*,[23] *Arcanobacterium* (*Actinomyces*) *pyogenes*,[24] *Arcanobacterium* (*Actinomyces*) *bernardiae*,[25,26] *A. funkei*,[14,27,28] *A. lingnae*,[14] *A. houstonensis*,[14] and *A. cardiffensis*[29] are capable of causing a variety of human infections, including the syndrome of actinomycosis.[29] Although *Eubacterium* species have been reported to cause pelvic disease in association with intrauterine contraceptive devices (IUCDs) and "lumpy jaw,"[30] additional reports would be desirable to confirm the species of this genus as agents of actinomycosis.

Despite some conflicting reports, the bulk of evidence supports the concept that most if not all actinomycotic infections are polymicrobial in nature.[1,4] Although monomicrobial infections undoubtedly occur, inadequate bacteriologic evaluation or diagnoses made on clinical or pathologic grounds will result in a failure to identify concomitant bacterial species. *Aggregatibacter* (*Actinobacillus*) *actinomycetemcomitans*, *Eikenella corrodens*, *Fusobacterium*, *Bacteroides*, *Capnocytophaga*, *Staphylococcus*, *Streptococcus*, and Enterobacteriaceae have been commonly isolated in various combinations, depending on the site of the infection. The contribution of these additional isolates to the pathogenesis of actinomycosis is difficult to assess; however, it seems reasonable to consider them as being potential copathogens when designing therapeutic regimens.

Epidemiology

The agents of actinomycosis have been clearly established as members of the endogenous flora of mucous membranes. The frequency of oral cavity colonization with *Actinomyces* is nearly 100% by 2 years of age.[31] It is also often cultured from the gastrointestinal tract, bronchi, and female genital tract. It has never been cultured from nature, and there are no documented cases of person-to-person transmission.[32] Although the normal habitats for the more recently identified *Actinomyces* spp. have not been optimally defined, data to date suggest that these species are also members of the endogenous oral, gastrointestinal, and genital flora.[14]

Actinomycosis has no geographic boundaries. Infection may occur in individuals of all ages. The peak incidence of actinomycosis is reported to be in the mid-decades, with cases in individuals younger than 10 and older than 60 years being less frequent.[4,33] Nearly all series have reported males to be infected more frequently than females, at an approximately 3:1 ratio.[1,4,33,34] Plausible, but unproven explanations for this discordance include poorer dental hygiene and increased oral trauma in males.[33]

Studies on the occurrence of actinomycosis estimated a yearly incidence of 1:100,000 in the Netherlands and Germany in the 1960s, and 1:300,000 in the Cleveland area during the 1970s, making this disease uncommon but not rare.[33] Its frequency is undoubtedly diminished since the preantibiotic era, when this disease was not only common but more malignant in nature. Improved dental hygiene and early antimicrobial treatment of infections prior to the development of a characteristic actinomycotic syndrome are likely contributing factors. However, individuals or populations that do not have access to dental and/or medical care, prolonged use of an IUCD (see "Pelvic Disease"), and bisphosphonate use (see "Oral-Cervicofacial Disease") are likely at higher risk. Furthermore, many unrecognized cases probably occur, especially oral-cervicofacial disease, that are successfully treated empirically.

Pathogenesis and Pathology

A pivotal step in the pathogenesis of actinomycosis is disruption of the mucosal barrier. Oral and cervicofacial disease is frequently associated with dental procedures, trauma, oral surgery, head and neck radiotherapy, or oncologic surgical procedures.[35] Likewise, pulmonary infections often arise in the setting of aspiration, and abdominal infection is usually preceded by conditions that result in loss of mucosal integrity, such as gastrointestinal surgery, diverticulitis, appendicitis, or foreign bodies (e.g., fish bones).[1,33] Recognition of factors that enable bacterial entry into deep tissues, however, may be absent.[34] The lack of such a history should not prevent consideration of this disease when the clinical circumstance is appropriate.

Other bacterial species concomitantly present have been designated "companion microbes." They may serve as copathogens by aiding in the inhibition of host defenses or by reducing oxygen tension. The difficulty in establishing an animal model of infection with *Actinomyces* alone and enhancement of infection by coinoculation of *E. corrodens* support the concept that additional organisms are important for the initiation of infection.[36] Further, coaggregation of *Actinomyces* and *Streptococcus* spp. occurs and results in increased resistance to phagocytosis and killing.[37]

An acute inflammatory phase manifested by a painful, cellulitic reaction is occasionally observed with oral-cervicofacial disease or with soft tissue infection elsewhere in the body. The chronic phase of this disease is more often seen.[34] Classic disease is characterized as a densely fibrotic lesion that undergoes slow, contiguous spread and ignores tissue planes. However, no studies have addressed the bacterial factor(s) responsible for the unique pathogenesis of this disease. Lesions usually appear as either single or multiple indurated swellings. As the lesion matures, it becomes soft and fluctuant and suppurates centrally. The fibrous walls of the mass have been characteristically described as "wooden" and, in the absence of suppuration, have been frequently confused with neoplasms. This extensive fibrosis, which is one of the hallmarks of this disease, may be minimal, especially in pulmonary and central nervous system lesions. Given time, sinus tracts will often extend from the abscess to either the skin or adjacent organs or bone, depending on the location of the lesion. Sinus tracts can spontaneously close and then reform. Overlying skin may assume a red to bluish hue. Hematogenous dissemination can occur from these local sites and occasionally be fulminant, although in the antibiotic era this clinical syndrome has become rare.

Microscopically, lesions have an outer zone of granulation, consisting of collagen fibers and fibroblasts. There is a central purulent loculation that contains neutrophils that surround the sulfur granules present. Granules are conglomerations of organisms and are virtually diagnostic of this disease. Bacterial biofilms may contribute to granule formation.[38] One to six may be present per loculation, and they range from microscopic to macroscopic in size (see "Diagnosis"). As many as 50 loculations may be present per lesion, and these loculations are separated by granulation tissue or foamy macrophages and may undergo coalescence. Lymphocytes and plasma cells are usually present, and eosinophils are seen in 15% of abscesses. Multinucleated giant cells are occasionally seen, primarily in pulmonary lesions, but they have also been described in disease elsewhere.[34] Suppuration is a constant feature of active disease but may not be present in all areas of the lesion.

The association of pelvic actinomycosis with IUCDs suggests that at least this foreign body contributes to pathogenesis. Associations with actinomycosis and foreign material elsewhere are less strong. Several reports describe periapical actinomycosis associated with root canal fillings, mandibular osteomyelitis associated with wire used in the treatment of a fracture, and infection of the tongue in the presence of a foreign body. *Actinomyces* infecting prosthetic joints, through presumed hematogenous spread, is rare but reported.[39] Whether aspirated or ingested foreign bodies contribute to pathogenesis via mucosal disruption, or facilitate the growth and survival of *Actinomyces,* or both, is unclear.

Cases of actinomycosis have been described in the setting of steroid use,[40] infliximab treatment,[41,42] bisphosphonate treatment,[43] acute leukemia during chemotherapy,[44] lung and renal transplantation,[45] and human immunodeficiency virus infection.[46] Ulcerative mucosal lesions (herpes simplex virus, cytomegalovirus, chemotherapy) and abnormalities in host defenses likely facilitated the development of actinomycosis in some HIV-associated cases; however, it remains unclear which arm(s) of the host defense are critical in preventing or controlling this infection and the degree to which the incidence of infection is increased in these settings.

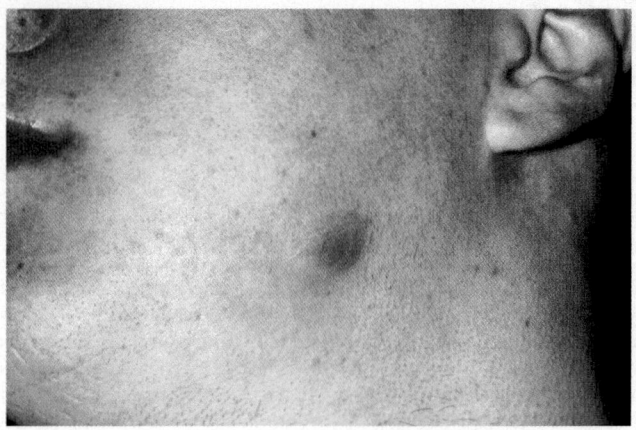

Figure 255-1 **Submandibular actinomycotic abscess.**

Clinical Manifestations

ORAL-CERVICOFACIAL DISEASE

Actinomycosis most commonly occurs and is best recognized in this location, with a mean of 55% of cases.[33] Oral-cervicofacial disease probably accounts for even a greater majority because it is underrepresented in autopsy and referral center series.

Oral-cervicofacial disease can present as a soft tissue swelling, an abscess, a mass lesion,[33,47] or occasionally an ulcerative lesion.[48] The diagnosis of actinomycosis should not only be considered in the classic setting of a painless mass at the angle of the jaw (Fig. 255-1) but should be included in the differential diagnosis of any lesion in the head and neck region. When lesions appear solid, neoplasm is the usual diagnostic consideration. Soft tissue infections of the head and neck may also present as chronic, recurring abscesses. This common scenario of temporary improvement with a short course of empirical antibiotic therapy, followed by relapse, should always arouse suspicion for actinomycosis, regardless of the location. As the disease spreads to adjacent structures, there is little regard for normal tissue planes. Lymphatic spread and associated lymphadenopathy are uncommon. Computed tomography (CT) or magnetic resonance images usually reveal an infiltrative, well- or ill-defined mass with inflammatory changes.[49] Extension to any contiguous structure may occur, including the carotid artery, orbital cavity, cranium, cervical spine, trachea, or thorax.[50-52] Pain, fever, and leukocytosis are variably present.[33]

Periapical and endodontic infection caused by *Actinomyces* probably occurs far more frequently than is recognized.[53] Appropriate dental intervention and antibiotic therapy usually result in cure before more extensive disease develops.

The most common location for diagnosed actinomycosis is the perimandibular region. Periapical infection or trauma is often, but not always, the inciting event. The classic lesion located at the angle of the jaw is the most frequent location (submandibular), but the cheek, submental space, retromandibular space, and temporomandibular joint may be affected.[54,55] As noted, a hallmark of this disease is the potential for unrestricted contiguous extension. Spread to the skin may result in sinus tract(s) formation, and these can spontaneously close and open elsewhere. The overlying skin often develops a bluish or purplish red hue. Involvement of the muscles of mastication frequently occurs, resulting in trismus.[1] Associated mandibular periostitis or osteomyelitis may also be present but is surprisingly infrequent.[56] A lytic lesion, rarefaction with sclerosis, or sclerosis alone may be seen, and this latter pattern may be confused with tumor.[57] Maxillary disease, including osteomyelitis, occurs less frequently.[58] Associated soft tissue lesions and maxillary sinus or cutaneous fistulas, or both, can occur. Maxillary and ethmoid sinusitis may present as isolated disease or can be concomitant with infection of the maxilla.[59,60]

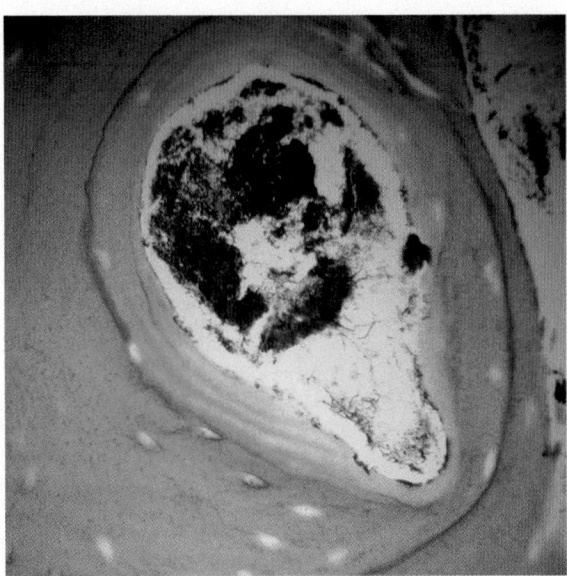

Figure 255-2 Maxillary osteomyelitis due to *A. viscosus* in a patient with multiple myeloma who was treated with biphosphonates and underwent several dental procedures. Pictured is a sulfur granule within necrotic maxilla.

The hard palate may also be involved, with presentation as a mass lesion.[1]

Two clinical settings have been recently recognized for contributing to an increased incidence of actinomycotic infection of the mandible and maxilla.[43] The first is infected osteoradionecrosis, a complication of radiation therapy used in the treatment of head and neck cancer. The second has been termed bisphosphate-associated osteonecrosis (Fig. 255-2). Bisphosphonates are increasingly used to reduce bone disease; particularly due to multiple myeloma and for the prevention of osteoporosis. Although our understanding of the pathogenesis of these syndromes is evolving. It appears that the first insult is radiation therapy and/or bisphosphonates altering the local host defenses followed by disruption of the mucosa, usually from dental procedures, thereby enabling Actinomyces to access and infect the gingival and bone.[61]

Isolated masses or ulcerative lesions can also occur in the tongue,[62] vallecula,[63] nasal cavity,[64] nasopharynx,[65] soft tissues of the head and neck,[33,66] salivary glands,[67] patent thyroglossal duct,[68] thyroid,[69] branchial cleft cyst, and hypopharynx, larynx, or both.[70] It is unclear whether Actinomyces causes tonsillitis. Although Actinomyces is frequently isolated and sulfur granules are occasionally identified in the setting of recurrent tonsillitis or tonsillar hypertrophy, the absence of a pathologic tissue reaction and lack of correlation between the isolation of Actinomyces and recurrent tonsillitis and tonsillar hypertrophy support Actinomyces as a colonizer, making a causal role in disease unlikley.[71,72]

Actinomycosis is also an uncommon but important cause of otitis media; untreated cases may result in fatal extension into the mastoid and then the central nervous system. It is characterized by numerous episodes of otitis media that transiently respond to conventional short-course therapy and resistance to myringotomy. Diagnosis can be made by the pathologic and microbiologic examination of infected material from the affected middle ear that may appear to be a cholesteatoma.[73] Infection of the external ear and temporal bone may occur from the spread of facial disease.

Actinomyces, and more commonly *P. propionicum,* can cause lacrimal canaliculitis.[74] *Actinomyces* has also caused postoperative endophthalmitis after intraocular lens implant[75] and keratitis after LASIK.[76] Rarely, secondary extension into the orbit from infected maxillary or ethmoid sinuses can occur.

THORACIC DISEASE

Thoracic involvement comprises approximately 15% of cases of actinomycosis.[77] Aspiration of organisms from the oropharynx is the usual source of infection. Direct extension may occur from disease in either the head and neck or abdominal cavity; however, such secondary spread has become increasingly uncommon since the advent of efficacious antimicrobial therapy.

The most common clinical presentation is an indolent, slowly progressive process that involves some combination of the pulmonary parenchyma and pleural space. Chest pain, fever, weight loss, and, less commonly, hemoptysis are prominent symptoms, and a cough, when present, is variably productive.[77] There are no specific radiographic manifestations, and any lobe may be involved. The usual appearance is either a mass lesion or pneumonia with or without pleural involvement (Fig. 255-3).[78] Pleural thickening, effusion, or empyema is present in greater than 50% of cases of thoracic actinomycosis (Fig. 255-3B). Rarely, actinomycosis may present as an isolated effusion. The spontaneous drainage of an empyema through the chest wall should raise suspicion for this disease.[79] Cavitary disease may develop and is more readily detected by CT scans, because multiple small cavities are more common than large ones.[80] Hilar adenopathy may be present. Pulmonary disease that extends across fissures or pleura (Fig. 255-3C), involves the mediastinum, or has contiguous bony disease should suggest actinomycosis and is also more readily appreciated by CT.[78] Extension to the chest wall with the development of a soft tissue mass, a draining sinus, or both, is a telltale sign when present (Fig. 255-3A). In the absence of this classic scenario, however, thoracic actinomycosis is almost never suspected. It is mistaken for either malignant disease, with the diagnosis made by the pathologist postresection, or for an empyema or pneumonia secondary to more usual causes. Tuberculosis, nocardiosis, histoplasmosis, blastomycosis, cryptococcosis, mixed anaerobic infection, bronchogenic carcinoma, lymphoma, mesothelioma, and pulmonary infarction are among the entities confused with pulmonary actinomycosis.

Other less common manifestations of thoracic actinomycosis include multiple pulmonary nodules, miliary disease, and endobronchial lesions, which may be associated with aspirated foreign bodies.[87,88] Primary breast disease either presents as a persistent or recurring abscess(es) or mimics malignancy,[20] and infection of a mammary prosthesis has also been described.[89]

Endocarditis, Pericarditis, and Mediastinal Disease

Mediastinal actinomycosis is an uncommon event. The structures within the anterior or posterior mediastinum and the heart can be involved alone or in combination, resulting in a diverse array of clinical presentations. Infection usually results from contiguous spread from the thorax but can arise from perforation of the esophagus, chest trauma, or extension of head and neck or abdominal disease.[81] Involvement of cardiac structures represents the majority of mediastinal infections reported. Pericarditis is most common and may be initially asymptomatic or hemodynamically insignificant, but if allowed to progress, cardiac tamponade and constrictive or adhesive pericarditis will develop.[82] Less frequently, myocardial or endocardial infection occurs, either via extension from the pericardium[83] or by initial hematogenous seeding of the endocardium.[18] Anterior mediastinal involvement may present as an isolated mass or rarely superior vena cava syndrome.[84] Concomitant anterior chest wall infection is common, but associated sternal disease is rare. Posterior mediastinal involvement may result in paraspinous muscle and soft tissue disease, esophageal fistula or encasement, or vertebral body infection, or both. Because of the slow progression of the disease, both vertebral body destruction and new bone formation occur, resulting in a mottled, saw-toothed or honeycombed appearance of bone on x-ray. The transverse processes, and with disease progression the pedicles and spinous processes, are similarly involved as the bodies, in contrast to their usual sparing with

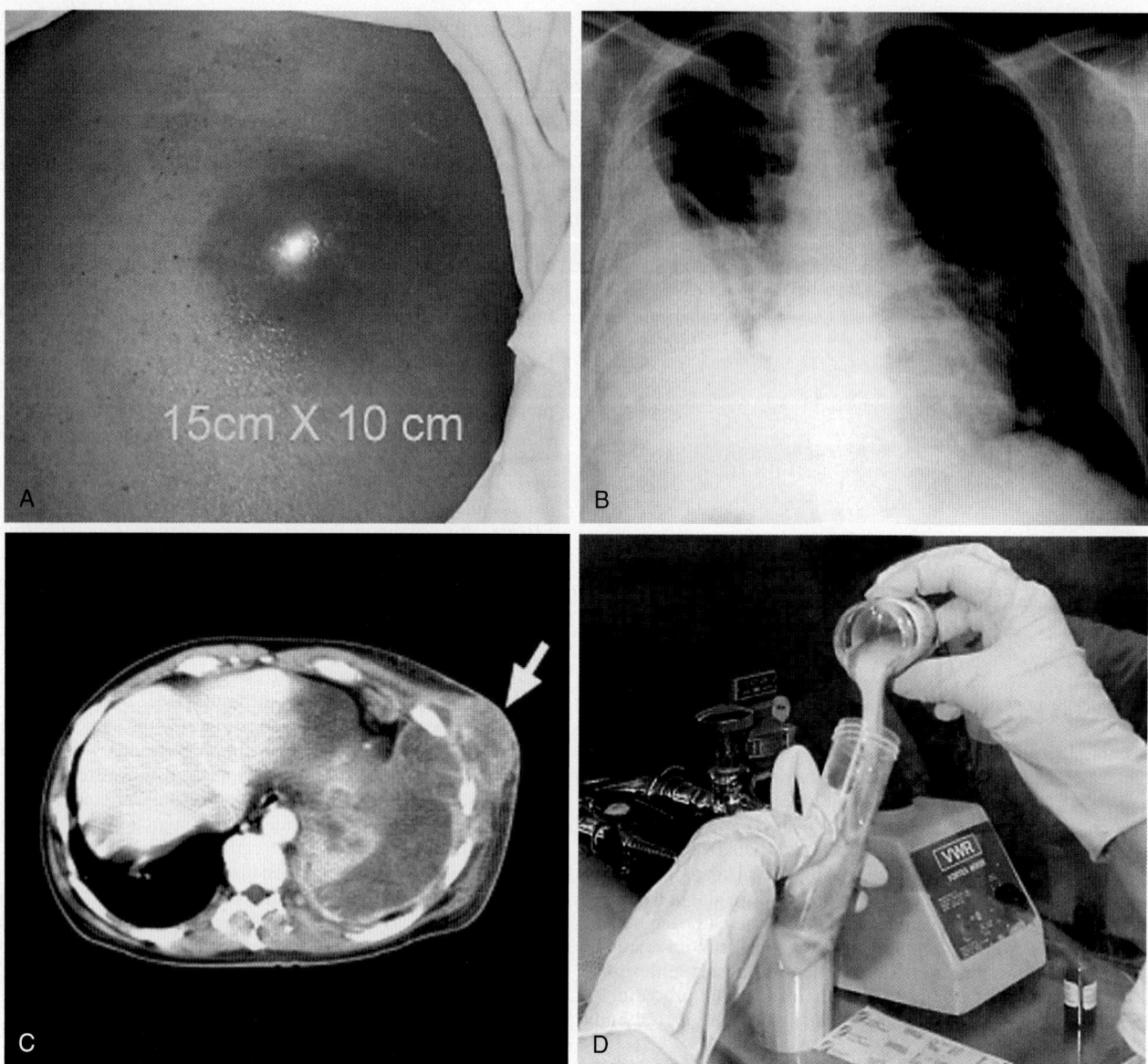

Figure 255-3   A, Chest wall mass. **B** and **C,** Chest x-ray and computed tomography demonstrating the pulmonary infiltrate, pleural effusion, and pleural and chest wall extension (*arrow*). **D,** Purulent pleural fluid obtained from aspiration. (*Courtesy of Dr. C.-B. Hsiao.*)

tuberculosis. The corresponding posterior ends of ribs are usually involved, and a typical wavy periostitis may be present, but, unlike tuberculosis, vertebral body collapse and disk space narrowing are not usually seen. Extension to the epidural space with spinal cord compression may occur.[85] Primary esophageal disease with and wihtout HIV infection has also been described.[86]

ABDOMINAL DISEASE

The proportion of reported cases involving the abdomen averages 20%.[33] Any disease or event that allows the agents of actinomycosis to breach the gastrointestinal mucosa has the potential to be complicated by this infection. The majority of abdominal infections are due to this mechanism, although the inciting conditions are not always apparent. However, it is important to note that ascension from the female genital tract of IUCD-associated actinomycosis has become an increasingly recognized source of abdominal disease[90] Hematogenous dissemination, extension from the thorax, and spillage of gallstones during laparoscopic cholecystectomy[91] are other portals of entry. As a consequence of the flow of peritoneal fluid, direct extension of primary disease, or

both, virtually any abdominal organ, region, or space can be involved either alone or in combination regardless of the initial site of infection. Abdominal actinomycosis is perhaps the greatest diagnostic challenge. This infection is rarely considered prior to the clinical laboratory or pathologist establishing the diagnosis. Months to years usually pass from the time of the inciting event to clinical recognition of this indolent disease.[34] Associated symptoms are generally nonspecific, with fever, weight loss, change in bowel habits, abdominal pain, or a sensation of a mass being most common. Abdominal actinomycosis usually presents either as an abscess or as a firm to hard mass lesion that is often fixed to the underlying tissue and mistaken for tumor.[92] Sinus tracts with drainage from either the abdominal wall or perianal region may develop (Fig. 255-4). CT findings usually demonstrate a mass lesion with focal areas of decreased attenuation or a thick-walled cystic mass, both of which frequently enhance with contrast. Lesions often appear invasive, suggesting a tumor, but associated lymphadenopathy is uncommon.[93,94] With colonic involvement, mucosal nodules with associated inflammation may be observed.[95]

Appendicitis, especially with perforation, is the most common predisposing event and is associated with 65% of the cases of actinomy-

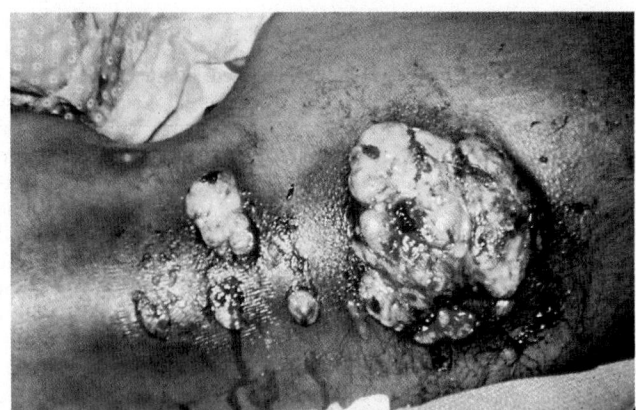

Figure 255-4 Multiple draining sinuses of the right flank secondary to intra-abdominal actinomycosis associated with appendicitis.

cosis originating in the abdomen. As a result, the right iliac fossa is the most frequent primary site of abdominal disease and right-sided abdominal infection is more common than left. It is also one of the potential inciting events for tuboovarian infection. Diverticulitis or foreign body perforation of the transverse or sigmoid colon tends to be associated with left-sided disease and accounts for 7.3% of cases, a surprisingly low percentage considering the incidence of diverticulitis. The loss of gastric mucosal integrity from peptic ulcer disease or gastrectomy may result in abdominal infection and is associated with 4.4% of cases. Isolated gastric disease, including a case after gastric bypass, has also been described.[96] Additional associations with abdominal infection include antecedent bowel surgery, typhoid fever, amebic dysentery, chicken or fish bones, trauma, and hemorrhagic pancreatitis. Interestingly, actinomycosis rarely develops as a consequence of Crohn's disease or ulcerative colitis.

Perirectal or perianal disease may result from extension of pelvic infection or, less commonly, abdominal disease. Primary disease occurs with either local mucosal damage or infection of anal crypts. The most common presentation is single or multiple perianal abscesses, sinus or fistula tract formation, or both. Infiltrating masses may develop in the buttock, posterior thigh, scrotum, or inguinal region.[97] Recurrent disease over months to years or wounds that fail to heal after drainage or fistulotomy are clues that should suggest actinomycosis,

particularly in the absence of documented inflammatory bowel disease. Strictures of the rectum can also occur and cause an alteration of bowel habits, mimicking primary bowel or metastatic prostatic or pelvic tumors.[98] This presentation is most often due to extension of pelvic disease.

Hepatic infection was present in 5% of all cases of actinomycosis.[34] Spread to the liver occurs via extension from a contiguous abdominal focus or hematogenously from more distant but established abdominal or extraabdominal foci. A case associated with a pancreatic stent has also been described.[99] Hepatic involvement is common in disseminated actinomycosis. The entity of primary or isolated disease is presumably hematogenous seeding from cryptic foci. Single or multiple abscesses or lesions suggesting neoplasia are the usual presentation (Fig. 255-5).[100] Generally, a more indolent course is observed compared to the more usual causes of pyogenic hepatic abscesses, but "companion organisms" may contribute to a more acute presentation.[101] Symptoms and laboratory findings often point to the right upper quadrant, but liver functions tests may be normal. The presently available imaging modalities and percutaneous diagnostic techniques have allowed for an increasing number of cases to be diagnosed without surgery. Uncommon presentations or sequelae of hepatic actinomycosis include cholangitis, portal vein occlusion/thrombosis, cholestasis, and extension into the thorax.[102,103] Splenic infection is less common.[104]

All levels of the urogenital tract can be infected by the agents of actinomycosis. Renal involvement can occur as either a result of hematogenous dissemination from a cryptic or defined focus, or via direct extension within the pelvis, peritoneum, or thorax. The disease usually manifests as pyelonephritis, renal carbuncle, perinephric abscess, or tumor. Tuberculosis, neoplasm, or more usual bacterial agents are usually considered as the causative agents.[105,106] Hematuria and pyuria are often present, and *Actinomyces* can be successfully detected in the urine if appropriate stains and anaerobic cultures are performed. Renal arteriography usually demonstrates a normal or diminished pattern of vascularization. Extension from pelvic disease or rectal disease may result in ureteric obstruction, infiltration, compression or encasement of the bladder, a pubic mass, or vesicocolic, ileovesical, vesicouterine, or vesicocutaneous fistulas and hydronephrosis and renal failure.[107,108] Prostatic, testicular, primary vesical, penile pilonidal sinus, and urachal involvement are described.[109-111]

Actinomycosis of the gallbladder presenting as cholecystitis or suspected neoplasm can occur but is exceedingly rare,[112] as is pancreatic involvement. "Primary" actinomycosis of the omentum, abdominal

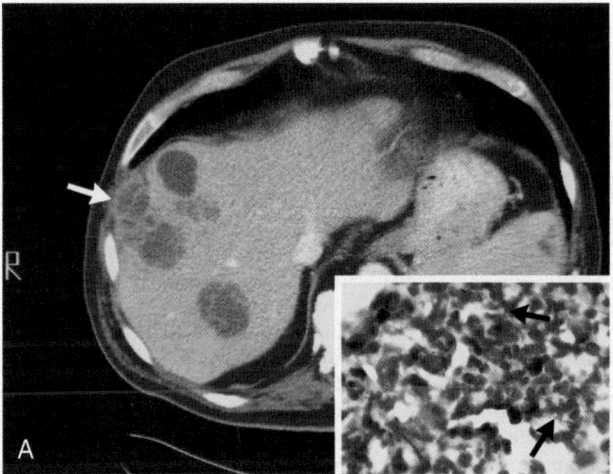
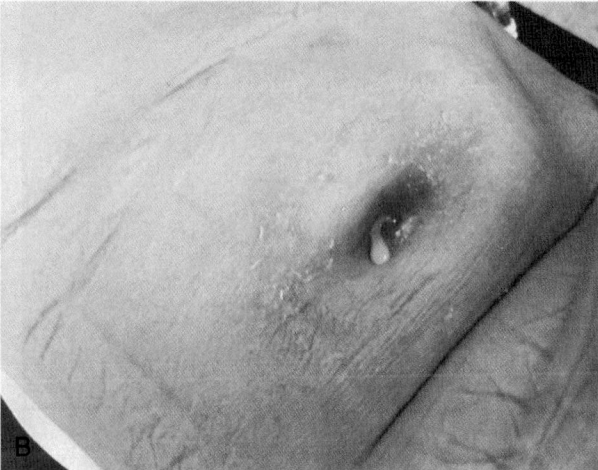

Figure 255-5 **Hepatic-splenic actinomycosis. A,** Computed tomogram showing multiple hepatic abscesses and a small splenic lesion due to *A. israelii* (inset: Gram stain of abscess fluid demonstrating beaded filamentous gram-positive rods). Arrow demonstrates extension outside of the liver. **B,** Subsequent formation of a sinus tract. *(Reprinted with permission from Saad M: Actinomyces hepatic abscess with cutaneous fistula. N Engl J Med. 353:e16,2005. Copyright 2005 Massachusetts Medical Society. All rights reserved.)*

wall, and retroperitoneum has been reported, but the majority of these cases are likely due to secondary spread from a cryptic or obscured abdominal source.[113] Isolated peritonitis associated with peritoneal dialysis has also been reported.

PELVIC DISEASE

Actinomycotic involvement of the pelvis may occur as a consequence of an intra-abdominal inciting event, such as appendicitis or rectal disease. However, the most common portal of entry is ascension from the uterus in association with the presence of any type of IUCD, which has become a widely recognized risk factor for pelvic infection.[10,114] Pelvic infection has also been described without and with other pelvic foreign bodies, including pessaries, an endocervical contraceptive device, a retained hairpin used for an abortion, mesh used with intravaginal slingplasty, and a retained intrauterine fetal bone.[115,116] On average, an IUCD is in place for 8 years in pelvic actinomycosis–associated cases. Disease rarely develops when an IUCD has been in place for less than 1 year, and risk of infection likely increases with time.[114] Pelvic actinomycosis has presented months after the removal of the IUCD; therefore, a history of prior use is important when this disease is a diagnostic consideration. Although the precise risk of IUCD-associated actinomycosis has not been quantitated, it would appear to be small.

Presentation is typically indolent, with fever, weight loss, abdominal pain, and abnormal vaginal bleeding or discharge being common symptoms. The earliest form of pelvic actinomycosis associated with an IUCD may be an endometritis. A pelvic mass or uni- or bilateral tuboovarian abscesses represents the next stage of disease progression (Fig. 255-6). Unfortunately diagnosis is often delayed. A "frozen pelvis" mimicking malignancy or endometriosis is commonly present by the time of recognition; however, CT and magnetic resonance imaging may suggest actinomycosis.[117] Disease frequently involves the ureters, bladder, or both, resulting in hydroureter and hydronephrosis.[118] Rectal involvement is also common. Extension to the abdominal wall may lead to sinus tract development, and entrapment of small or large bowel may cause fistula or bowel obstruction.[119] Rarely, the presentation of acute peritonitis, disseminated peritoneal lesions, pelvic bone involvement, extension to the thorax, or hematogenous dissemination may occur.[114,120,121]

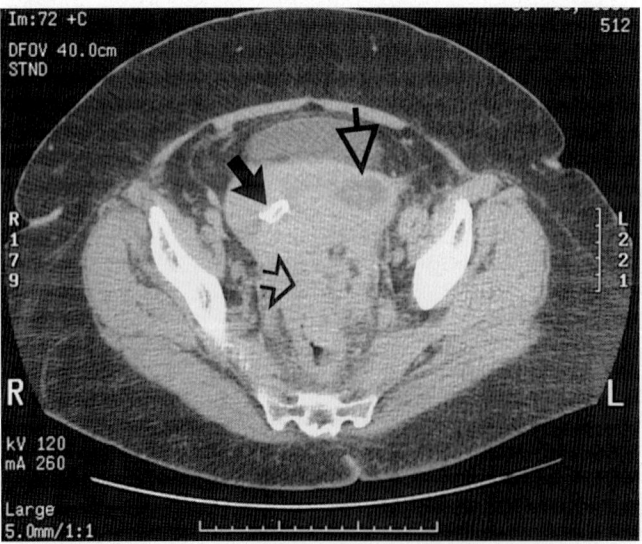

Figure 255-6 IUCD-associated pelvic actinomycosis. An IUCD encased by endometrial fibrosis (*solid arrowhead*), paraendometrial fibrosis (*open arrow*), and an area of suppuration (*open arrowhead*) can be appreciated.

One of the management issues that has received considerable attention is the presence of *Actinomyces*-like organisms (ALOs) on Papanicolaou-stained cervical specimens, which occurs on average in 7% of women using an IUCD.[122] Unfortunately this finding alone has a low postive predictive value for diagnosing pelvic infection. The detection of ALOs in the absence of symptoms warrants patient education and close follow-up but not removal of the IUCD, unless an equally suitable means of contraception can be agreed upon.[122-124] Considering the overall women-years of IUCD use and the limited number of reported cases of pelvic actinomycosis, the risk appears to be small, but the consequences of infection are significant. Therefore, in the absence of more quantitative data, it would appear prudent to remove IUCDs if symptoms of pain, abnormal bleeding, or discharge cannot be attributed to other pathogens, regardless of whether *Actinomyces* or ALOs are detected. A 14-day course of a penicillin or tetracycline should be given for treatment of possible early pelvic actinomycosis.

CENTRAL NERVOUS SYSTEM DISEASE

Actinomycosis of the central nervous system is rare. The source may be hematogenous, or it may develop through extension of oral-cervicofacial disease. In a recent review, the mean duration of symptoms prior to diagnosis was 2.1 months, longer than with most causes of central nervous system infections.[125] Brain abscess is the most common presentation. Headache and focal neurologic findings are the most common clinical features. Fever is variably present. Single or multiple abscesses may be present. The most frequent CT/MRI appearance is a ring-enhancing lesion(s) with a thick wall that may be irregular or nodular. Multiloculation, edema, and contiguous areas of low attenuation may be present. These findings are also consistent with brain abscess and tumor.[126] Less commonly, solid nodular or mass lesions termed *actinomycetomas* or *actinomycotic granuloma* occur. MR perfusion and spectroscopy findings have also been described.[127] A chronic meningitis may develop as a consequence of spread from a parameningeal focus, most commonly the middle ear or paranasal sinuses. Presentation may be acute, particularly with rupture of an abscess into the subarachnoid space, or chronic, with the cerebrospinal fluid having a normal or low glucose level, elevated protein, lymphocytic pleocytosis, and negative culture. Diagnosis can be made by microscopic examination or rarely by culture of cerebrospinal fluid. Extension of disease from foci of cranial osteomyelitis, sinus, or middle ear disease can result in cranial epidural or subdural infection, or both.[128] Spinal epidural disease may occur from direct extension of abdominal, thoracic, or cervical disease, is usually associated with a contiguous osteomyelitis, and may result in spinal cord compression.[129] Cavernous sinus syndrome, spinal intrathecal, and ventriculoperitoneal shunt infection have also been reported.[17,130-132]

MUSCULOSKELETAL DISEASE

Actinomycotic infection of the bone is usually a result of an adjacent soft tissue infection but may also be associated with trauma (e.g., fracture of the mandible), osteoradionecrosis and bisphosphonates (limited to mandibular and maxillary bones[43]; see "Oral-Cervicofacial Diseasae"), or hematogenous spread. In the preantibiotic era, the unchecked spread of thoracic and abdominal disease resulted in vertebral infection being the most common site for osseous actinomycosis (see "Thoracic Disease"). Less commonly, hematogenous vertebral osteomyelitis may originate from an occult source and clinically resemble skeletal tuberculosis. Presently, the facial bones, particularly the mandible and maxilla associated with and without osteoradionecrosis and bisphosphonate therapy, are the most frequent site of involvement.[43] Actinomycosis of the skull, ribs, clavicle, sternum, scapula, or pelvis may also occur from extension of oral-facial, thoracic, or abdominal disease. The clinical and radiographic features of infection in these locations have been discussed earlier.

Infection of the extremities, although uncommon, often poses diagnostic difficulties. Blunt or penetrating trauma of the affected area or injections are inciting events.[133,134] Some cases are a result of hematogenous dissemination from apparent or cryptic foci.[8,135,136] Skin, subcutaneous tissue, muscle, and bone may be involved alone or in various combinations. Cutaneous sinus tracts or abscesses are present in the majority of cases, as is bony involvement in the form of periostitis or acute or chronic osteomyelitis. Presentation is usually indolent. Although actinomycotic infections of the lower extremities have been described as *mycetomas,* this term is best reserved for the group of infections designated as actinomycetoma.

Actinomycotic infections of hip and knee prostheses have been described in several reports.[137] Early presentations suggest that *Actinomyces* may be introduced perioperatively, whereas late presentations suggest hematogenous seeding from a cryptic distant site. Actinomycotic arthritis of the knee has developed in association with trauma or injection of hyaluronate,[138] or as a consequence of hematogenous seeding. Actinomycosis is rarely a result of closed fist injury.

DISSEMINATED DISEASE

Although uncommon, all of the agents of actinomycosis are capable of hematogenous dissemination resulting in multiorgan involvement. *Actinomyces meyeri* appears to have the greatest capability of causing this syndrome. Disease in any location may serve as the source for spread. The lungs and liver are the most commonly affected organs, and the presentation of multiple nodules mimics disseminated malignancy. The kidneys, brain, spleen, skin, soft tissues of the extremities, and, less commonly, the heart valves may also be infected in various combinations. The clinical presentation may be surprisingly indolent when the extent of disease is appreciated.[8,135,139]

Diagnosis

The diagnosis of actinomycosis, particularly when it mimics malignancy, is rarely considered. All too often the first mention of actinomycosis is from the pathologist after extensive surgery has been performed. An increasing body of evidence suggests that medical therapy alone is usually sufficient for cure, including extensive invasive disease. Therefore, the challenge for the clinician is to consider the possibility of actinomycosis so that this unique infection can be diagnosed in the least invasive fashion and unnecessary surgery can be avoided.[140] Clinical or radiographic presentations that suggest actinomycosis have been discussed previously. Of note, actinomycotic disease has demonstrated hypermetabolism on positive emission tomography scanning.[141] Fine-needle aspiration or biopsy and CT- or ultrasound-guided aspirations or biopsies are being successfully used to obtain clinical material for diagnosis.[125,142,143] However, actinomycosis should not be excluded if the characteristic pathologic findings are not present. When only small quanties of tissue are available, sulfur granules are easily missed and only fibrosis with or without inflammation may be identified. Multiple sections may increase diagnostic sensitivity. Transbronchial biopsies have been less successful in providing diagnostic material for thoracic actinomycosis. Surgery may be required for diagnostic purposes. Even when this diagnosis is considered, suitable sampling and handling of clinical specimens is necessary for confirmation. A combination of appropriate microbiologic, molecular, and pathologic studies will maximize the chances of success. The most important step for optimal microbiologic yield is the avoidance of any antimicrobial therapy prior to obtaining the specimen. The agents of actinomycosis are exceedingly sensitive to a wide variety of agents, and even a single dose can interfere with their isolation.

The bacteriologic identification of one of the agents of actinomycosis from a sterile site will confirm the diagnosis. However, the microbiologic identification of the agents of actinomycosis occurs in only a minority of cases.[34] Although 16S rRNA gene amplification and sequencing will increase the sensitivity of diagnosis, the clinical utilization of this approach is just beginning to be explored.[144,145] Because these organisms are normal inhabitants of the oral cavity and female genital tract, the identification of organisms alone, in the absence of sulfur granules or an appropriate clinical syndrome, from sputum, bronchial washings, and cervicovaginal secretions is of little significance.

Although most strains of *Actinomyces* are microaerophilic or facultative (except *A. meyeri*), strict anaerobic processing and anaerobic growth should be utilized for primary isolation. The laboratory should receive specimens expeditiously or in anaerobic transport media. Tissue, pus, or sulfur granules are ideal, and swabs should be avoided. The microbiology laboratory should be alerted prior to receiving any specimen that may harbor the agents of actinomycosis. A Gram stain of the specimen is usually more sensitive than culture, especially if the patient has received prior antibiotics. If granules are identified, they should be washed and crushed between two slides for examination (Fig. 255-7A). The agents of actinomycosis are non-spore-forming rods. Except for *A. meyeri*, which is small and nonbranching, their usual appearance is that of branching, filamentous rods. Growth usually appears within 5 to 7 days, but primary isolation may take up to 2 to 4 weeks. Although specialized media are not required, the use of semiselective media may increase isolation rates of *Actinomyces,* particularly when more rapidly growing organisms are also present. (146) *A. israelii* characteristically forms a "molar tooth" colony on agar and grows as clumps within broth. *A. odontolyticus* colonies usually appear as rust-brown or red colored. *Actinomyces* are indole negative. Traditional identification is based on these features in combination with tests for urease, catalase, gelatin hydrolysis, and fermentation of cellobiose, trehalose, and arabinose. However, classification of *Actinomyces* based on phenotypic tests may result in misidentification.[10] Sequencing or restriction analysis of amplified 16S ribosomal DNA can assist in resolving ambiguities in identification of the non-spore-forming, gram-positive rods,[10,53,147] but its use on clinical specimens has not been broadly applied as of yet.

The single most helpful diagnostic maneuver for actinomycosis is to demonstrate grains (sulfur granules) in pus (see Fig. 255-7A) or histologic section of a surgical specimen (Fig. 255-7B, C). Grains represent a conglomeration of microorganisms that forms only in vivo. Hematoxylin-eosin staining of tissue suffices to demonstrate the grain, but a special stain (e.g., Gram, silver) is needed to show that the grain is composed of branching bacteria and not fungi (eumycetoma), cocci, or bacilli (botryomycosis). If branching bacteria are seen on staining of the grain and the infection did not originate in subcutaneous tissue (a characteristic of mycetoma) or tonsillar tissue (see "Oral-Cervicofacial Disease"), then the diagnosis of actinomycosis is established. Grains may be either micro- or macroscopic and are usually yellow (hence their name) but may be white, pinkish gray, gray, or brown. Grains may be identified grossly from draining sinus tracts, other purulent material, or sputum, but they may easily escape notice unless sought after. When pus is poured down the side of a glass tube, grains will adhere and are identified more readily. A magnifying glass may aid in their identification. In tissue sections, grains are most commonly found within microabscesses. Although they may be abundant, they are usually scanty. Only a single granule was identified from 26% of specimens in one series.[34] Because grains are surrounded by neutrophils, several histologic sections containing purulent foci need to be examined to find a grain. Microscopically, grains are round, oval, or horseshoe shaped. Although bacilli within the grain are rarely visible with the hematoxylin-eosin stain, tissue Gram stains, Gomori methenamine silver, and Giemsa stains will demonstrate gram-positive, filamentous, branching bacteria at its periphery (see Fig. 255-7). On hematoxylin-eosin stain the grains may be eosinophilic or variably surrounded by a radiating fringe of eosinophilic clubs. This eosinophilic, proteinaceous coating around organisms in tissue has been called the Splendore-Hoeppli phenomena. It represents an ill-defined host response, but may be accounted for, in part, by eosinophil granule major basic protein. This coating is not specific for actinomycosis and can also be seen in schistosomiasis, sporotrichosis, subcutaneous zygomycosis, botryomycosis, mycetoma, and other indolent infections. A combination of the clinical scenario and stains of the grain can be used to distinguish actinomycotic sulfur granules from others.

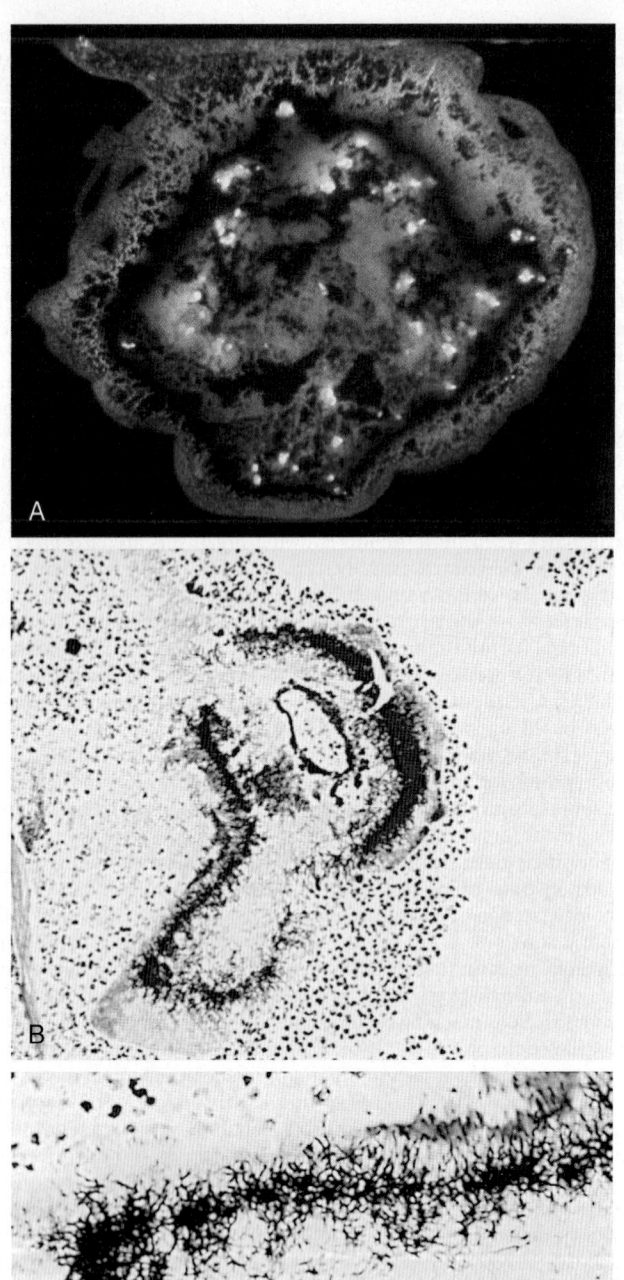

Figure 255-7 A, Macroscopic actinomycotic sulfur granules demonstrated by placing pus between two slides. **B,** Microscopic actinomycotic sulfur granule surrounded by inflammatory cells (Brown-Brenn stain, x250). **C,** Increased magnification (x1000) demonstrates the delicate, branched filaments of Actinomyces.

Clinically, nocardiosis may closely resemble actinomycosis but does not form grains in visceral lesions.[148] When *Nocardia* is the causative agent of mycetoma, granules are formed. On Gram stain, the branching gram-positive bacilli are indistinguishable from *Actinomyces,* but they may be stained by a Fite-modified acid-fast stain, whereas *Actinomyces* is not. The granules formed by the fungal agents of mycetoma show branching hyphae on periodic acid–Schiff or Gomori methenamine silver stain. Botryomycosis is a chronic bacterial soft tissue and rarely visceral infection that produces loose clumps of bacteria that resemble grains. Etiologic agents include *Staphylococcus, Streptococcus, Escherichia, Pseudomonas,* and *Proteus,* which are easily distinguished from the agents of actinomycosis by the presence of cocci or nonbranching bacilli.[149] Specimens obtained from mucus-producing locations, such as the endocervix, the bronchus, or ventricular colloid cysts, may possess pseudoactinomycotic radiate granules. If hematoxylin-eosin stain alone is used, they may mimic actinomycotic granules, as a central region is bordered by the Splendore-Hoeppli phenomena. However, special stains will reveal the absence of microorganisms.[150]

Treatment

The discovery and use of penicillin in the treatment of actinomycosis has dramatically altered the course of this disease. Two principles of therapy, based on the clinical experience of the last 60 years, have evolved. It is necessary to treat this disease both with high doses and for a prolonged period of time. Although therapy needs to be individualized, 18 to 24 million units of penicillin intravenously for 2 to 6 weeks, followed by oral therapy with penicillin or amoxicillin for 6 to 12 months, is a reasonable guideline for serious infections and bulky disease. If the duration of therapy is extended beyond the resolution of measurable disease, then relapses, one of the clinical hallmarks of this infection, will be minimized. CT and MRI studies are generally the most objective modalities to accomplish this goal. MRI scans are often more sensitive than CT scans for detecting residual infection and should be employed if possible, particularly in areas where the consequences of relapse are particularly significant (e.g., CNS).[153]

Cases with less extensive involvement, particularly in the oral-cervicofacial region, may be cured with a shorted duration of therapy.[151,152] Further, in some cases of low bulk, oral-cervico-facial disease therapy can be initiated with an oral agent. For penicillin-allergic patients, tetracycline has been used most extensively with success. Erythromycin, doxycycline, and clindamycin are other suitable alternatives. In the pregnant penicillin-sensitive patient, erythromycin is a safe alternative. Little clinical information is available on the newer antimicrobial agents except for anecdotal successes with imipenem,[154,155] and ceftriaxone[156] (Table 255-1). Limited in vitro data demonstrate that vancomycin, quinupristin-dalfopristin, linezolid, and moxifloxacin are active against *Actinomyces* spp.[157-161] In vitro data also suggest that oxacillin, dicloxacillin, cephalexin, metronidazole, and aminoglycosides should be avoided. Although in vitro data is limited and no clinical correlation exists, some variation in in vitro susceptibility exists between species.[157]

For home parenteral therapy, the ease of once-a-day dosing makes ceftriaxone appealing in certain circumstances; however, a greater body of literature supporting its efficacy would be desirable. The availability of portable infusion pumps for home therapy allows for both the appropriate dosing and practical administration of IV penicillin. For infections in critical sites (e.g., CNS) this approach remains the safest until more information is available on other agents. The pharmacokinetic properties, availability of oral and parenteral formulations, and potential efficacy of azithromycin and ertapenem also makes these agent appealing. Unfortunately little in vitro and no clinical data exist on their use to treat actinomycosis.

It is unclear whether other bacteria frequently coisolated with the etiologic agents of actinomycosis require treatment, but many of them are pathogens in their own right. Designing a therapeutic regimen that includes coverage for these organisms during the initial treatment course is reasonable. If microbiology is not available, it is important

TABLE 255-1	Appropriate and Inappropriate Antibiotic Therapy for Actinomycosis*

Group 1: Extensive Successful Clinical Experience[†]
‡Penicillin (3-4 million units IV q4h or amoxicillin 500 mg PO q6h)
Erythromycin (500-1000 mg IV q6h or 500 mg PO q6h)
Tetracycline (500 mg PO q6h)
Doxycycline (100 mg IV q12h or 100 mg PO q12h)
Minocycline (100 mg IV q12h or 100 mg PO q12h)
Clindamycin (900 mg IV q8h or 300-450 mg PO q6h)

Group 2: Anecdotal Successful Clinical Experience
‡Ceftriaxone
Ceftizoxime
Imipenem-cilastatin
Piperacillin-tazobactam

Group 3: Agents That Should Be Avoided
Metronidazole
Aminoglycosides
Oxacillin
Dicloxacillin
Cephalexin

Group 4: Agents Predicted to Be Efficacious Based on In Vitro Activity
Moxifloxacin
Vancomycin
Linezolid
Quinupristin-dalfopristin
‡Ertapenem
‡Azithromycin

*Additional coverage for concomitant "companion" bacteria may be required.
†Controlled evaluations have not been performed. Dose and duration require individualization, depending on the host site and extent of infection. As a general rule, a maximum antimicrobial dose for 2 to 6 weeks of parenteral therapy followed by oral therapy for a total duration of 6 to 12 months is required for serious infections and bulky disease, whereas a shorter duration may suffice for less extensive diseases, particularly in the oral-cervicofacial region. Monitoring therapeutic effect with computed tomography or magnetic resonance images is advisable when appropriate.
‡Agents to consider for home parenteral therapy (see text for details).

to consider the site of infection when designing empiric coverage. For example, *Aggregatibacter (Actinobacillus) actinomycetemcomitans*, *Eikenella corrodens*, *Fusobacterium*, and *Capnocytophaga* are more likely to be coisolates in head and neck infection, whereas the Enterobacteriaceae and Bacteroides are more commonly coisolated in abdominal infection.

In the preantibiotic era surgical removal of infected tissue was the only beneficial treatment. Despite the advent of efficacious antimicrobial therapy, combined medical and surgical therapy is still advocated in some reports. However, an increasing body of literature now sup-

ports the approach of initially attempting a cure with medical therapy alone.[125,162-164] Successes have been reported in cases of extensive disease, which initially appeared to be incurable using antibiotics alone. CT and magnetic resonance imaging should be used to monitor the response to therapy.[94,165] In most cases surgery can either be avoided altogether or require a less extensive procedure. This approach is particular important when the possibility of sparing critical organs is involved, such as the bladder or reproductive organs in women of childbearing age. In a patient with disease in a critical location (e.g., epidural space, selected central nervous system disease) or in whom suitable medical therapy fails, surgical intervention may be appropriate. In the setting of actinomycosis presenting as a well-defined abscess, percutaneous drainage in combination with medical therapy is a reasonable approach.

It is unclear which host defense components are most critical in affording protection against actinomycosis and whether certain hosts are more susceptible to infection. Actinomycosis has been described in association with HIV-infection, steroid use, and lymphoproliferative tumors. Whether these infections were due to disease-associated disruptions of mucosa (e.g., CMV infection with HIV infection), host defense abnormalities, immunosuppressive therapy, or some combination of these is unclear. From a treatment perspective, it is reasonable to initially use the same approach as that for noncompromised hosts. Aggressive treatment direct against HIV (e.g., HAART) and minimizing immunosuppressive therapy are also desirable if possible. There is no data on the use of immunomodulatory therapy (e.g., interferonγ or immunoglobulins).

Usually actinomycosis responds well to medical therapy. However, refractory or perceived refractory disease has been described in HIV-infected individuals as well as apparently normal hosts. In this setting basic principles of infectious disease apply. Exclude infection elsewhere (e.g., intravenous catheter-acquired bacteremia, *C. difficile* colitis) or noninfectious causes, or both (e.g., drug fever, unrelated disease) as being responsible. Confirm that high dose parenteral therapy is being utilized for initial treatment. Identify and drain significant purulent collections associated with the actinomycotic infection. Consider the possibility that untreated coisolates ("companion organisms") may be responsible. Although penicillin-resistant strains or evolution of resistance during therapy has not yet been clearly documented in vivo, this possibility should be considered when other more likely scenarios are excluded. Finally, surgery should be considered when infection is refractory to medical therapy, although as stated previously, this usually can be avoided, at least initially.

REFERENCES

1. Weese WC, Smith IM. A study of 57 cases of Actinomycosis over a 36-year period. *Arch Intern Med.* 1975;135:1562-1568.
2. Cope Z. Visceral actinomycosis. *Br Med J.* 1949:1311-1316.
3. Acevedo F, Baudrand R, Letelier LM, et al. Actinomycosis: a great pretender. Case reports of unusual presentations and a review of the literature. *Int J Infect Dis.* 2008;12(4):358-362. Epub 2008 Mar 4.
4. Pulverer G, Schutt-Gerowitt H, Schaal KP. Human cervicofacial actinomycoses: microbiological data for 1997 cases. *Clin Infect Dis.* 2003;37(4):490-497. Epub 2003 Jul 30.
5. Bonnez WLG, Mohanraj NA. Actinomycosis naeslundii as an agent of pelvic actinomycosis in the presence of an intra-uterine device. *J Clin Microbiol.* 1985;21:273-275.
6. Eng RH, Corrado ML, Cleri D, et al. Infections caused by Actinomyces viscosus. *Am J Clin Pathol.* 1981;75:113-116.
7. Cone LA, Leung MM, Hirschberg J. Actinomyces odontolyticus bacteremia. *Emerg Infect Dis.* 2003;9(12):1629-1632.
8. Apothéloz C, Regamey C. Disseminated infection due to Actinomyces meyeri: Case report and review. *Clin Infect Dis.* 1996;22:621-625.
9. Brazier JS, Hall V. Propionibacterium propionicum and infections of the lacrimal apparatus. *Clin Infect Dis.* 1993;17:892-893.
10. Hall V, Talbot P, Stubbs S, et al. Identification of clinical isolates of Actinomyces species by amplified 16S ribosomal DNA restriction analysis. *J Clin Microbiol.* 2001;39:3555-3562.
11. Sabbe L, Van De Merwe D, Schouls L, et al. Clinical spectrum of infections due to the newly described Actinomyces species A. turicensis, A. radingae, and A. europaeus. *J Clin Microbiol.* 1999;37(1):8-13.

12. Collins MD, Pascual C. Reclassification of Actinomyces humiferus (Gledhill and Casida) as Cellulomonas humilata nom. corrig., comb. nov. *Int J Syst Evol Microbiol.* 2000;50(Pt 2):661-663.
13. Funke G, Alvarez N, Pascual C, et al. Actinomyces europaeus sp. nov., isolated from human clinical specimens. *Int J Syst Bacteriol.* 1997;47:687-692.
14. Clarridge JE 3rd, Zhang Q. Genotypic diversity of clinical Actinomyces species: phenotype, source, and disease correlation among genospecies. *J Clin Microbiol.* 2002;40(9):3442-3448.
15. Funke G, von Graevenitz A. Infections due to Actinomyces neuii (Former "CDC Coryneform Group 1" bacteria). *Infection.* 1995;23:73-75.
16. Perez-Santonja JJ, Campos-Mollo E, Fuentes-Campos E, et al. Actinomyces neuii subspecies anitratus chronic endophthalmitis after cataract surgery. *Eur J Ophthalmol.* 2007;17(3):445-447.
17. Watkins RR, Anthony K, Schroder S, et al. Ventriculoperitoneal shunt infection caused by Actinomyces neuii subsp. neuii. *J Clin Microbiol.* 2008;46(5):1888-1889. Epub 2008 Mar 26.
18. Cohen E, Bishara J, Medalion B, et al. Infective endocarditis due to Actinomyces neuii. *Scand J Infect Dis.* 2007;39(2):180-183.
19. Wust J, Stubbs S, Weiss N, et al. Assignment of Actinomyces pyogenes-like (CDC coryneform group E) bacteria to the genus Actinomyces as Actinomyces radingae sp. nov. and Actinomyces turicensis sp. nov. *Lett Appl Microbiol.* 1995;20:76-81.
20. Attar KH, Waghorn D, Lyons M, et al. Rare species of actinomyces as causative pathogens in breast abscess. *Breast J.* 2007;13(5):501-505.

21. Tietz A, Aldridge KE, Figueroa JE. Disseminated coinfection with Actinomyces graevenitzii and Mycobacterium tuberculosis: case report and review of the literature. *J Clin Microbiol.* 2005;43(6):3017-3022.
22. Riegert-Johnson DL, Sandhu N, Rajkumar SV, et al. Thrombotic thrombocytopenic purpura associated with a hepatic abscess due to Actinomyces turicensis. *Clin Infect Dis.* 2002;35(5):636-637.
23. Jitmuang A. Primary actinomycotic endocarditis: a case report and literature review. *J Med Assoc Thai.* 2008;91(6):931-936.
24. Plamondon M, Martinez G, Raynal L, et al. A fatal case of Arcanobacterium pyogenes endocarditis in a man with no identified animal contact: case report and review of the literature. *Eur J Clin Microbiol Infect Dis.* 2007;26(9):663-666.
25. Funke G, Ramos C, Fernandez-Garayzabal J, et al. Description of human-derived Centers for Disease Control coryneform group 2 bacteria as Actinomyces bernardiae sp. nov. *Int J Syst Bacteriol.* 1995;45:57-60.
26. Ieven M, Verhoeven J, Gentens P, et al. Severe infection due to Actinomyces bernardiae: Case report. *Clin Infect Dis.* 1996;22:157-158.
27. Lawson P, Nikolaitchouk N, Falsen E, et al. Actinomyces funkei sp. nov., isolated from human clinical specimens. *Int J Syst Evol Microbiol.* 2001;51:853-855.
28. Westling K, Lidman C, Thalme A. Tricuspid valve endocarditis caused by a new species of actinomyces: Actinomyces funkei. *Scand J Infect Dis.* 2002;34(3):206-207.
29. Hall V, Collins MD, Hutson R, et al. Actinomyces cardiffensis sp. nov. from human clinical sources. *J Clin Microbiol.* 2002;40(9):3427-3431.

30. Hill GB. *Eubacterium nodatum* mimics *Actinomyces* in intrauterine device-associated infections and other settings within the female genital tract. *Obstet Gynecol*. 1992;79:534-538.
31. Sarkonen N, Kononen E, Summanen P, et al. Oral colonization with *Actinomyces* species in infants by two years of age. *J Dent Res*. 2000;79(3):864-867.
32. Smego RA Jr, Foglia G. Actinomycosis. *Clin Infect Dis*. 1998;26(6):1255-1261; quiz 62-63.
33. Bennhoff D. Actinomycosis: Diagnostic and therapeutic considerations and a review of 32 cases. *Laryngoscope*. 1984;94:1198-1217.
34. Brown J. Human actinomycosis. A study of 181 subects. *Hum Pathol*. 1973;4:319-330.
35. Zitsch RP 3rd, Bothwell M. Actinomycosis: a potential complication of head and neck surgery. *Am J Otolaryngol*. 1999;20(4):260-262.
36. Jordon H, Kelly D, Heeley J. Enhancement of experimental actinomycosis in mice by *Eikenella corrodens*. *Infect Immun*. 1984;46:367-371.
37. Ochiai K, Kurita-Ochiai T, Kamino Y, et al. Effect of co-aggregation on the pathogenicity of oral bacteria. *J Med Microbiol*. 1993;39:183-190.
38. Nair PN, Brundin M, Sundqvist G, et al. Building biofilms in vital host tissues: a survival strategy of Actinomyces radicidentis. *Oral Surg Oral Med Oral Pathol Oral Radiol Endod*. 2008;[Epub ahead of print].
39. Cohen O, Keiser J, Pollner J, et al. Prosthetic joint infection with *Actinomyces viscosus*. *Infect Dis Clin Pract*. 1993;2:349-351.
40. Gaffney R, Walsh M. Cervicofacial actinomycosis: an unusual cause of submandibular swelling. *J Laryngol Otol*. 1993;107:1169-1170.
41. Cohen RD, Bowie WR, Enns R, et al. Pulmonary actinomycosis complicating infliximab therapy for Crohn's disease. *Thorax*. 2007;62(11):1013-1014.
42. Marie I, Lahaxe L, Levesque H, et al. Pulmonary actinomycosis in a patient with diffuse systemic sclerosis treated with infliximab. *QJM*. 2008;101(5):419-421. Epub 2008 Mar 10.
43. Hansen T, Kunkel M, Springer E, et al. Actinomycosis of the jaws–histopathological study of 45 patients shows significant involvement in bisphosphonate-associated osteonecrosis and infected osteoradionecrosis. *Virchows Arch*. 2007;451(6):1009-1017. Epub 2007 Oct 20.
44. Chen CY, Chen YC, Tang JL, et al. Splenic actinomycotic abscess in a patient with acute myeloid leukemia. *Ann Hematol*. 2002;81(9):532-534.
45. Leach TD, Sadek SA, Mason JC. An unusual abdominal mass in a renal transplant recipient. *Transpl Infect Dis*. 2002;4(4):218-222.
46. Chaudhry SI, Greenspan JS. Actinomycosis in HIV infection: a review of a rare complication. *Int J STD AIDS*. 2000;11(6):349-355.
47. Sa'do B, Yoshiura K, Yuasa K, et al. Multimodality imaging of cervicofacial actinomycosis. *Oral Surg Oral Med Oral Pathol*. 1993;76:772-782.
48. Alamillos-Granados FJ, Dean-Ferrer A, Garcia-Lopez A, et al. Actinomycotic ulcer of the oral mucosa: an unusual presentation of oral actinomycosis. *Br J Oral Maxillofac Surg*. 2000;38(2):121-123.
49. Park JK, Lee HK, Ha HK, et al. Cervicofacial actinomycosis: CT and MR imaging findings in seven patients. *AJNR Am J Neuroradiol*. 2003;24(3):331-335.
50. Freidman HDEPA, Emko P. Postoperative carotid artery rupture caused by actinomyces infection. *Otolaryngol Head Neck Surg*. 1996;114:145-147.
51. Smego R. Actinomycosis of the central nervous system. *Rev Infect Dis*. 1987;9:855-865.
52. Nithyanandam S, D'Souza O, Rao SS, et al. Rhinoorbitocerebral actinomycosis. *Ophthal Plast Reconstr Surg*. 2001;17(2):134-136.
53. Xia T, Baumgartner JC. Occurrence of Actinomyces in infections of endodontic origin. *J Endod*. 2003;29(9):549-552.
54. Samuels R, Martin M. A clinical and microbiologic study of actinomycetes in oral and cervicofacial lesions. *Brit J Oral Maxillofac Surg*. 1988;26:458-463.
55. Richtsmeier W, Johns ME. Actinomycosis of the head and neck. *CRC Crit Rev Clin Lab Sci*. 1979;11:175-202.
56. Bartkowski SB, Zapala J, Heczko P, et al. Actinomycotic osteomyelitis of the mandible: review of 15 cases. *J Craniomaxillofac Surg*. 1998;26(1):63-67.
57. Ohlms L, Jones D, Schreibstein J, et al. Sclerosing osteomyelitis of the mandible. *Otolaryngol Head Neck Surg*. 1993;109:1070-1073.
58. Liu C, Chang K, Ou C. Actinomycosis in a patient treated for maxillary osteoradionecrosis. *J Oral Maxillofac Surg*. 1998;56:251-253.
59. Damante JH, Sant'Ana E, Soares CT, et al. Chronic sinusitis unresponsive to medical therapy: a case of maxillary sinus actinomycosis focusing on computed tomography findings. *Dentomaxillofac Radiol*. 2006;35(3):213-216.
60. Woo HJ, Bae CH, Song SY, et al. Actinomycosis of the paranasal sinus. *Otolaryngol Head Neck Surg*. 2008;139(3):460-462.
61. Dodson TB, Raje NS, Caruso PA, et al. Case records of the Massachusetts General Hospital. Case 9-2008. A 65-year-old woman with a nonhealing ulcer of the jaw. *N Engl J Med*. 2008;358(12):1283-1291.
62. Habibi A, Salehinejad J, Saghafi S, et al. Actinomycosis of the tongue. *Arch Iran Med*. 2008;11(5):566-568.
63. Thomas R, Kameswaran M, Ahmed S, et al. Actinomycosis of the vallecula: report of a case and review of the literature. *J Laryngol Otol*. 1995;109:154-156.
64. Ozcan C, Talas D, Gorur K, et al. Actinomycosis of the middle turbinate: an unusual cause of nasal obstruction. *Eur Arch Otorhinolaryngol*. 2005;262(5):412-415. Epub 2004 Nov 12.
65. Chiang CW, Chang YL, Lou PJ. Actinomycosis imitating nasopharyngeal carcinoma. *Ann Otol Rhinol Laryngol*. 2000;109(6):605-607.
66. Pant R, Marshall TL, Crosher RF. Facial actinomycosis mimicking a desmoid tumour: case report. *Br J Oral Maxillofac Surg*. 2008;46(5):391-393. Epub 2007 Oct 17.
67. Appiah S, Tickke M. Actinomycosis-an unusual presentation. *Brit J Oral Maxillo Surg*. 1995;33:248-249.
68. Cobb R, Ross H. Actinomycosis in a persistent thyroglossal duct. *Br J Surg*. 1986;73:751.
69. Karatoprak N, Atay Z, Erol N, et al. Actinomycotic suppurative thyroiditis in a child. *J Trop Pediatr*. 2005;51(6):383-385. Epub 2005 Jun 9.
70. Hagan M, Klotz S, Bartholomew W, et al. Actinomycosis of the trachea with acute tracheal obstruction. *Clin Infect Dis*. 1996;22:1126-1127.
71. Toh ST, Yuen HW, Goh YH. Actinomycetes colonization of tonsils: a comparative study between patients with and without recurrent tonsillitis. *J Laryngol Otol*. 2007;121(8):775-778. Epub 2006 Oct 11.
72. van Lierop AC, Prescott CA, Sinclair-Smith CC. An investigation of the significance of Actinomycosis in tonsil disease. *Int J Pediatr Otorhinolaryngol*. 2007;71(12):1883-1888. Epub 2007 Oct 4.
73. Mehta D, Statham M, Choo D, et al. Actinomycosis of the temporal bone with labyrinthine and facial nerve involvement. Pediatric salivary gland lesions. *Laryngoscope*. 2007;117(11):1999-2001.
74. Briscoe D, Edelstein E, Zacharopoulos I, et al. Actinomyces canaliculitis: diagnosis of a masquerading disease. *Graefes Arch Clin Exp Ophthalmol*. 2004;242(8):682-686. Epub 2004 Jun 22.
75. Garelick JM, Khodabakhsh AJ, Josephberg RG. Acute postoperative endophthalmitis caused by *Actinomyces neuii*. *Am J Ophthalmol*. 2002;133(1):145-147.
76. Karimian F, Feizi S, Nazari R, et al. Delayed-onset Actinomyces keratitis after laser in situ keratomileusis. *Cornea*. 2008;27(7):843-846.
77. Mabeza GF, Macfarlane J. Pulmonary actinomycosis. *Eur Respir J*. 2003;21(3):545-551.
78. Cheon JE, Im JG, Kim MY, et al. Thoracic actinomycosis: CT findings. *Radiology*. 1998;209(1):229-233.
79. Pérez-Castrillon J, Gonzalez-Castaneda C, del Campo-Matias F, et al. Empyema necessitatis due to *Actinomyces odontolyticus*. *Chest* 1996;1144.
80. Kim TS, Han J, Koh WJ, et al. Thoracic actinomycosis: CT features with histopathologic correlation. *AJR Am J Roentgenol*. 2006;186(1):225-231.
81. Esposti D, Lippolis A, Cipolla M, et al. An uncommon cause of pericardial actinomycosis. *Ital Heart J*. 2000;1(9):632-635.
82. Fife T, SM. F, Grennan T. Pericardial actinomycosis: Case report and review. *Rev Infect Dis*. 1991;13:120-126.
83. Peters GL, Davies RA, Veinot JP, et al. Cardiac actinomycosis: an unusual cause of an intracardiac mass. *J Am Soc Echocardiogr*. 2006;19(12):1530.e7-1530.e11.
84. Morgan D, Nath H, Sanders C, et al. Mediastinal actinomycosis. *Amer J Roentgol*. 1990;155:735-737.
85. Honda H, Bankowski MJ, Kajioka EH, et al. Thoracic vertebral actinomycosis: Actinomyces israelii and Fusobacterium nucleatum. *J Clin Microbiol*. 2008;46(6):2009-2014. Epub 8 Mar 12.
86. Abdalla J, Myers J, Moorman J. Actinomycotic infection of the oesophagus. *J Infect*. 2005;51(2):E39-43.
87. Kim YS, Suh JH, Kwak SM, et al. Foreign body-induced actinomycosis mimicking bronchogenic carcinoma. *Korean J Intern Med*. 2002;17(3):207-210.
88. Ho JC, Ooi GC, Lam WK, et al. Endobronchial actinomycosis associated with a foreign body. *Respirology*. 2000;5(3):293-296.
89. Brunner S, Graf S, Riegel P, et al. Catalase-negative *Actinomyces neuii* subsp. neuii isolated from an infected mammary prosthesis. *Int J Med Microbiol*. 2000;290(3):285-287.
90. Lee IJ, Ha HK, Park CM, et al. Abdominopelvic actinomycosis involving the gastrointestinal tract: CT features. *Radiology*. 2001;220(1):76-80.
91. Vyas JM, Kasmar A, Chang HR, et al. Abdominal abscesses due to actinomycosis after laparoscopic cholecystectomy: case reports and review. *Clin Infect Dis*. 2007;44(2):e1-4. Epub 2006 Dec 6.
92. Meyer P, Nwariaku O, McClelland RN, et al. Rare presentation of actinomycosis as an abdominal mass: report of a case. *Dis Colon Rectum*. 2000;43(6):872-875.
93. Ha H, Lee H, Kim H, et al. Abdominal actinomycosis: CT findings in 10 patients. *Am J Roent*. 1993;161:791-794.
94. Ko S, Ng S, Lee T, et al. Retroperitoneal actinomycosis with intraperitoneal spread. Stellate pattern on CT. *Clin Imaging*. 1996;20:133-136.
95. Kim JC, Ahn BY, Kim HC, et al. Efficiency of combined colonoscopy and computed tomography for diagnosis of colonic actinomycosis: a retrospective evaluation of eight consecutive patients. *Int J Colorectal Dis*. 2000;15(4):236-242.
96. Oksuz M, Sandikci S, Culhaci A, et al. Primary gastric actinomycosis: A case report. *Turk J Gastroenterol*. 2007;18(1):44-46.
97. Bauer P, Sultan S, Atienza P. Perianal actinomycosis: diagnostic and management considerations: a review of six cases. *Gastroenterol Clin Biol*. 2006;30(1):29-32.
98. Dayan K, Neufeld D, Zissin R, et al. Actinomycosis of the large bowel: unusual presentations and their surgical treatment. *Eur J Surg*. 1996;162:657-660.
99. Harsch IA, Benninger J, Niedobitek G, et al. Abdominal actinomycosis: complication of endoscopic stenting in chronic pancreatitis? *Endoscopy*. 2001;33(12):1065-1069.
100. Sharma M, Briski LE, Khatib R. Hepatic actinomycosis: an overview of salient features and outcome of therapy. *Scand J Infect Dis*. 2002;34(5):386-391.
101. Miyamoto M, Fang F. Pyogenic liver abscess involving *Actinomyces*: Case report and review. *Clin Infect Dis*. 1993;16:303-309.
102. Islam T, Athar MN, Athar MK, et al. Hepatic actinomycosis with infiltration of the diaphragm and right lung: a case report. *Can Respir J*. 2005;12(6):336-337.
103. Ubeda B, Vilana R, Bianchi L, et al. Primary hepatic actinomycosis: association with portal vein thrombosis. *Am J Roent*. 1995;164:231-232.
104. Jabr FI, Skeik N. Splenic abscess caused by actinomycosis. *Intern Med*. 2007;46(23):1943-1944. Epub 2007 Dec 3.
105. Yenarkarn P, Thoeni RF, Hanks D. Case 117: actinomycosis of left kidney with sinus tracts. *Radiology*. 2007;244(1):309-313.
106. Horino T, Yamamoto M, Morita M, et al. Renal actinomycosis mimicking renal tumor: case report. *South Med J*. 2004;97(3):316-318.
107. Ord J, Mishra V, Hudd C, et al. Ureteric obstruction caused by pelvic actinomycosis. *Scand J Urol Nephrol*. 2002;36(1):87-88.
108. de Feiter PW, Soeters PB. Gastrointestinal actinomycosis: an unusual presentation with obstructive uropathy: report of a case and review of the literature. *Dis Colon Rectum*. 2001;44(10):1521-1525.
109. Lin CY, Jwo SC, Lin CC. Primary testicular actinomycosis mimicking metastatic tumor. *Int J Urol*. 2005;12(5):519-521.
110. Al-Kadhi S, Venkiteswaran KP, Al-Ansari A, et al. Primary vesical actinomycosis: a case report and literature review. *Int J Urol*. 2007;14(10):969-971.
111. Yeung Y, Cheung MC, Chan GS, et al. Primary actinomycosis mimicking urachal carcinoma. *Urology*. 2001;58(3):462.
112. Lee YH, Kim SH, Cho MY, et al. Actinomycosis of the gallbladder mimicking carcinoma: a case report with US and CT findings. *Korean J Radiol*. 2007;8(2):169-172.
113. Filipovic B, Milinic N, Nikolic G, et al. Primary actinomycosis of the anterior abdominal wall: case report and review of the literature. *J Gastroenterol Hepatol*. 2005;20(4):517-520.
114. Fiorino A. Intrauterine contraceptive device-associated actinomycotic abscess and *Actinomyces* detection on cervical smear. *Obstet Gynecol*. 1996;87:142-149.
115. Eleuterio Junior J, Giraldo PC, Cavalcante DI, et al. Actinomyces-like organisms from a vaginal granuloma following intravaginal slingplasty with polypropylene mesh. *Int J Gynaecol Obstet*. 2008;102(2):172-173. Epub 2008 Apr 18.
116. White T, Felix JC. Pelvic actinomycosis with retained intrauterine fetal bone: a case report. *J Reprod Med*. 2007;52(3):220-222.
117. Kim SH, Kim SH, Yang DM, et al. Unusual causes of tubo-ovarian abscess: CT and MR imaging findings. *Radiographics*. 2004;24(6):1575-1589.
118. Zbar AP, Karayiannakis AJ, Chiappa AC. Obstructive uropathy and pelvic actinomycosis. *Dis Colon Rectum*. 2002;45(12):1708; author reply -9.
119. Valko P, Busolini E, Donati N, et al. Severe large bowel obstruction secondary to infection with Actinomyces israelii. *Scand J Infect Dis*. 2006;38(3):231-234.
120. Devendra K, Chen CM. Pelvic actinomycosis masquerading as an acute abdomen from a small bowel perforation. *Singapore Med J*. 2008;49(2):158-159.
121. Lawson E. Systemic actinomycosis mimicking pelvic malignancy with pulmonary metastases. *Can Respir J*. 2005;12(3):153-154.
122. Westhoff C. IUDs and colonization or infection with Actinomyces. *Contraception*. 2007;75(6 Suppl):S48-50. Epub 2007 Mar 23.
123. Penney G, Brechin S, de Souza A, et al. FFPRHC Guidance (January 2004). The copper intrauterine device as long-term contraception. *J Fam Plann Reprod Health Care*. 2004;30(1):29-41; quiz 2.
124. Kalaichelvan V, Maw AA, Singh K. Actinomyces in cervical smears of women using the intrauterine device in Singapore. *Contraception*. 2006;73(4):352-355. Epub 2005 Nov 2.
125. Pauker S, Kopelman R. A rewarding pursuit of certainty. *New Engl J Med*. 1993;329:1103-1107.
126. Sharma B, Banerjee A, Sobti M, et al. Actinomycotic brain abscess. *Clin Neurol Neurosurg*. 1990;92:373-376.
127. Wang S, Wolf RL, Woo JH, et al. Actinomycotic brain infection: registered diffusion, perfusion MR imaging and MR spectroscopy. *Neuroradiology*. 2006;48(5):346-350. Epub 2006 Apr 14.
128. Soto-Hernandez JL, Morales VA, Lara Giron JC, et al. Cranial epidural empyema with osteomyelitis caused by *Actinomyces*, CT, and MRI appearance. *Clin Imaging*. 1999;23(4):209-214.
129. Oruckaptan HH, Senmevsim O, Soylemezoglu F, et al. Cervical actinomycosis causing spinal cord compression and multisegmental root failure: case report and review of the literature. *Neurosurgery*. 1998;43(4):937-940.

130. David C, Brasme L, Peruzzi P, et al. Intramedullary abscess of the spinal cord in a patient with a right-to-left shunt: case report. *Clin Infect Dis.* 1997;24:89-90.

131. Ohta S, Nishizawa S, Namba H, et al. Bilateral cavernous sinus actinomycosis resulting in painful ophthalmoplegia. Case report. *J Neurosurg.* 2002;96(3):600-602.

132. Ushikoshi S, Koyanagi I, Hida K, et al. Spinal intrathecal actinomycosis: a case report. *Surg Neurol.* 1998;50(3):221-225.

133. Vandevelde A, Jenkins S, Hardy P. Sclerosing osteomyelitis and *Actinomyces naeslundii* of surrounding tissues. *Clin infect Dis.* 1995;20:1037-1039.

134. Metgud SC. Primary cutaneous actinomycosis: a rare soft tissue infection. *Indian J Med Microbiol.* 2008;26(2):184-186.

135. Liaudet L, Erard P, Kaeser P. Cutaneous and muscular abscesses secondary to *Actinomyces meyeri* pneumonia. *Clin infect Dis.* 1996;22:185-186.

136. Johnston J. Case 29-1993. *New Engl J Med.* 1993;329:264-269.

137. Zaman R, Abbas M, Burd E. Late prosthetic hip joint infection with Actinomyces israelii in an intravenous drug user: case report and literature review. *J Clin Microbiol.* 2002;40(11):4391-4392.

138. Lequerre T, Nouvellon M, Kraznowska K, et al. Septic arthritis due to *Actinomyces naeslundii:* report of a case. *Joint Bone Spine.* 2002;69(5):499-501.

139. Colmegna I, Rodriguez-Barradas M, Rauch R, et al. Disseminated *Actinomyces meyeri* infection resembling lung cancer with brain metastases. *Am J Med Sci.* 2003;326(3):152-155.

140. Lee YC, Min D, Holcomb K, et al. Computed tomography guided core needle biopsy diagnosis of pelvic actinomycosis. *Gynecol Oncol.* 2000;79(2):318-323.

141. Ho L, Seto J, Jadvar H. Actinomycosis mimicking anastomotic recurrent esophageal cancer on PET-CT. *Clin Nucl Med.* 2006;31(10):646-647.

142. Bakhtawar I, Schaefer RF, Salian N. Utility of Wang needle aspiration in the diagnosis of actinomycosis. *Chest.* 2001;119(6):1966-1968.

143. Hyldgaard-Jensen J, Sandstrom HR, Pedersen JF. Ultrasound diagnosis and guided biopsy in renal actinomycosis. *Br J Radiol.* 1999;72(857):510-512.

144. Siqueira JF, Rocas IN, Moraes SR, et al. Direct amplification of rRNA gene sequences for identification of selected oral pathogens in root canal infections. *Int Endod J.* 2002;35(4):345-351.

145. Lecouvet F, Irenge L, Vandercam B, et al. The etiologic diagnosis of infectious discitis is improved by amplification-based DNA analysis. *Arthritis Rheum.* 2004;50(9):2985-2994.

146. Lewis R, McKenzie D, Bagg J, et al. Experience with a novel selective medium for isolation of *Actinomyces* spp. from medical and dental specimens. *J Clin Microbiol.* 1995;33:1613-1616.

147. Hall V, O'Neill GL, Magee JT, et al. Development of amplified 16S ribosomal DNA restriction analysis for identification of *Actinomyces* species and comparison with pyrolysis-mass spectrometry and conventional biochemical tests. *J Clin Microbiol.* 1999;37(7):2255-2261.

148. Robboy S, Vickery A. Tinctorial and morphologic properties distinguishing actinomycosis and nocardiosis. *New Engl J Med.* 1970;282:593-595.

149. Bersoff-Matcha SJ, Roper CC, Liapis H, et al. Primary pulmonary botryomycosis: case report and review. *Clin Infect Dis.* 1998;26(3):620-624.

150. Pritt B, Mount SL, Cooper K, et al. Pseudoactinomycotic radiate granules of the gynaecological tract: review of a diagnostic pitfall. *J Clin Pathol.* 2006;59(1):17-20.

151. Sudhakar SS, Ross JJ. Short-term treatment of actinomycosis: two cases and a review. *Clin Infect Dis.* 2004;38(3):444-447. Epub 2004 Jan 13.

152. Choi J, Koh WJ, Kim TS, et al. Optimal duration of IV and oral antibiotics in the treatment of thoracic actinomycosis. *Chest.* 2005;128(4):2211-2217.

153. Tambay R, Cote J, Bourgault AM, et al. An unusual case of hepatic abscess. *Can J Gastroenterol.* 2001;15(9):615-617.

154. Garduno E, Rebollo M, Asencio MA, et al. Splenic abscesses caused by *Actinomyces meyeri* in a patient with autoimmune hepatitis. *Diagn Microbiol Infect Dis.* 2000;37(3):213-214.

155. Yew WW, Wong PC, Lee J, et al. Report of eight cases of pulmonary actinomycosis and their treatment with imipenem-cilastatin. *Monaldi Arch Chest Dis.* 1999;54(2):126-129.

156. Skoutelis A, Petrochilos J, Bassaris H. Successful treatment of thoracic actinomycosis with ceftriaxone. *Clin Infect Dis.* 1994;19:161-162.

157. Smith AJ, Hall V, Thakker B, et al. Antimicrobial susceptibility testing of Actinomyces species with 12 antimicrobial agents. *J Antimicrob Chemother.* 2005;56(2):407-409. Epub 2005 Jun 21.

158. LeCorn DW, Vertucci FJ, Rojas MF, et al. In vitro activity of amoxicillin, clindamycin, doxycycline, metronidazole, and moxifloxacin against oral Actinomyces. *J Endod.* 2007;33(5):557-560. Epub 2007 Mar 26.

159. Citron DM, Merriam CV, Tyrrell KL, et al. In vitro activities of ramoplanin, teicoplanin, vancomycin, linezolid, bacitracin, and four other antimicrobials against intestinal anaerobic bacteria. *Antimicrob Agents Chemother.* 2003;47(7):2334-2338.

160. Goldstein EJ, Citron DM, Merriam CV, et al. In vitro activities of daptomycin, vancomycin, quinupristin- dalfopristin, linezolid, and five other antimicrobials against 307 gram-positive anaerobic and 31 Corynebacterium clinical isolates. *Antimicrob Agents Chemother.* 2003;47(1):337-341.

161. Goldstein EJ, Citron DM, Merriam CV, et al. Activities of telithromycin (HMR 3647, RU 66647) compared to those of erythromycin, azithromycin, clarithromycin, roxithromycin, and other antimicrobial agents against unusual anaerobes. *Antimicrob Agents Chemother.* 1999;43(11):2801-2805.

162. Khalaff H, Srigley J, Klotz L. Recognition of renal actinomycosis: nephrectomy can be avoided. Report of a case. *Can J Surg.* 1995;38:77-79.

163. Nozawa H, Yamada Y, Muto Y, et al. Pelvic actinomycosis presenting with a large abscess and bowel stenosis with marked response to conservative treatment: a case report. *J Med Case Reports.* 2007;1:141.

164. Wang PT, Su SC, Hung FY, et al. Huge pelvic mass, cutaneous and vaginal fistulas, and bilateral hydronephrosis: a rare presentation of actinomycosis with a good response to conservative treatment and with long-term sequelae of renal atrophy and hydronephrosis. *Taiwan J Obstet Gynecol.* 2008;47(2):206-211.

165. Hawnaur JM, Reynolds K, McGettigan C. Magnetic resonance imaging of actinomycosis presenting as pelvic malignancy. *Br J Radiol.* 1999;72(862):1006-1011.

256

Introduction to Mycoses

JOHN E. BENNETT*

The advent of the human immunodeficiency virus epidemic and the ever-increasing use of immunosuppressive drugs has dramatically increased the incidence of deep mycoses and substantially broadened the range of fungi causing potentially lethal disease. Fortunately, the number of effective antifungal drugs has also increased. Together, these changes have made it essential for physicians to increase their awareness and understanding of medically important fungi. A number of useful texts on medical mycology are available.[1-5]

Fungal Taxonomy

Mycoses are most often named for the organisms that cause them. Changes in names of organisms have often confounded searches of the medical literature, confused clinicians, and complicated teaching young physicians. Despite these disadvantages, discovery of new relationships among seemingly divergent groups of organisms can lead to improved understanding of pathogenesis or epidemiology. Taxonomy, which is the science of classifying organisms, is drawing increasing reliance on genomic structure. As an example, a second species, called *Coccidioides posadasii*, has been distinguished within *Coccidioides immitis* using nucleotide sequences. These two species cannot be distinguished by clinical features or any of the usual laboratory tests, such as biochemical tests or appearance, but the species appear to have a different geographic distribution (Chapter 266). *Candida dubliniensis* was distinguished within *Candida albicans* based originally on molecular tests, although phenotypic differences have now been found. Subtle clinical differences between the two species are emerging, such as the higher frequency of *C. dubliniensis* in mucosal as contrasted with deep isolates (Chapter 257). As distasteful as it may be to clinicians, changes in fungal names will certainly continue. Names of diseases are most likely to be retained when they describe a clinical entity caused by more than one species (see later for an example).

A recent change in high-level taxonomy has affected the clinical use of the word zygomycosis. To understand how the word zygomycosis originated and why it is being disestablished, a brief look at the history of the description of the clinical entity mucormycosis is presented.

The first case of mucormycosis was described in 1885 by Paltauf in Germany, who described it as a case of "mucorina."[6] From the drawing in this paper, the isolate may have been a *Rhizopus* species but insufficient details were provided to identify the agent. The clinical course of rhinocerebral mucormycosis was reported in 1943, in an article using that disease name.[7] This name, mucormycosis, was retained subsequently in several hundred publications. However, Chester Emmons, the eminent mycologist, suggested the term *phycomycosis* to describe infections which had broad aseptate hyphae in common.[8] The term originated from the name of the class, Phycomycete, which at the time included agents of mucormycosis and those responsible for entomophthoramycosis, uncommon subcutaneous and paranasal sinus infections seen in the tropics. The name phycomycosis fell into disuse when the class Phycomycetes was removed and replaced by two different classes, Zygomycetes and Chytridiomycetes. The agents of both mucormycosis and entomophthoramycosis were placed in the class Zygomycetes, leading to use of the term *zygomycosis* to replace phycomycosis as a term to encompass both infections. The more specific term, *mucormycosis,* continued to be used, often leading to confusion.

Because of a recent change in high-level taxonomy, the class name Zygomycetes has been replaced by Glomeromycetes.[9] Although future research could create even further changes in taxonomy, there seems little doubt that Zygomycetes will disappear as a class name. In this new classification, all the agents of mucormycosis have been placed under the subphylum Mucormycotina and the agents of entomophthoramycosis are now in the subphylum Entomophthoramycotina. If one wished to retain a name for both infections, it would be glomeromycosis, a confusing term without precedent. Fortunately for the disease name mucormycosis, most agents are not only in the subphylum Mucormycotina, preserving the word, "mucor," but are in the order Mucorales. The single exception is the rare pathogen, *Mortierella,* which is in the order Mortierellales.

With the disappearance of the term *Zygomycetes,* it is consequently time to retire zygomycosis and return to using the word mucormycosis. The name describes a well-recognized clinical entity and is firmly embedded in 50 years of medical literature.

Common Features of Pathogenic Fungi

Some specialized terms used in this chapter are listed in Table 256-1. It is important for all infectious disease specialists to understand the distinction between yeasts and molds. Even at the first recognition in a diagnostic laboratory that a fungus has been found in a smear or culture, the laboratory can distinguish between a yeast and a mold. Yeastlike fungi are typically round or oval, generally form smooth flat colonies, and reproduce by budding. Biochemical tests are important for identification. Molds are composed of tubular structures called hyphae and grow by branching and longitudinal extension. Mold colonies typically appear fuzzy. Not all pathogenic fungi can be categorized neatly by their appearance in tissue as yeasts or molds, however. *Coccidioides* species, *Rhinosporidium seeberi,* and *Pneumocystis jirovecii* are round in tissue but do not bud. Instead, the cytoplasm divides up to form numerous internal spores that on rupture of the "mother" cell, are released to form new spherical structures. Some fungi can grow either yeastlike or as a mold. In candidiasis and tinea versicolor, the fungus is often seen in both tubular and rounded forms. The so-called dimorphic fungi grow in the host as yeastlike forms but grow at room temperature in vitro as molds. These fungi include the agents of histoplasmosis, blastomycosis, sporotrichosis, coccidioidomycosis, paracoccidioidomycosis, and chromoblastomycosis.

Almost all fungi reproduce by forming spores through mitosis, a process in which the chromosome number remains the same. A fungal colony with only this asexual spore formation or with no spore formation is said to be an anamorph, or in the imperfect (asexual) state. Several decades ago, most fungi pathogenic for humans were found only in the imperfect state. Many have subsequently been induced to form sexual spores and have been given names. Fungi growing spores that have the specialized appearance known for sexual spores are said to be teleomorphs, or in the perfect state. The name given to a fungus in the perfect state shows its similarity to other fungi in their perfect state. Although the fungus may have two names, the diagnostic laboratory uses the single name that is oldest and best established.

---

*The chapter was written by Dr. Bennett in his personal capacity. The views expressed herein do not necessarily represent the views of the NIH, DHHS, or the United States.

TABLE 256-1	Lexicon of Mycology Terms for the Clinician

Aleurioconidia/aleuriospore—spore growing at the end of a specialized hypha. The spore is released by breakage of the hypha adjacent to the spore.

Anamorph—a fungus forming only asexual spores.

Arthrospore—a spore formed by a hypha breaking at a septum.

Asexual spores—spores formed by mitosis, a form of cell division that creates an exact copy of the original cell.

Basidiomycete—one of the four major classes of fungi; includes mushrooms and *Cryptococcus neoformans*.

Basidiospore—a sexual spore that arises on a specialized structure, usually club-shaped, in a basidiomycete (e.g., *Cryptococcus neoformans* forms basidiospores in its sexual state, called *Filobasidiella neoformans*).

Blastospore—an asexual spore formed by budding (e.g., *Cryptococcus neoformans*, *Candida* species).

Conidiophore—specialized hyphae that bear a conidium (spore) on the end.

Conidium (plural, conidia)—an asexual spore usually produced at the tip or side of a hypha.

Dimorphic—capable of producing both hyphae and yeast (e.g., the agents of coccidioidomycosis, blastomycosis, histoplasmosis, sporotrichosis, and chromoblastomycosis).

Diploid—having two sets of chromosomes.

Endemic fungi—fungi having a limited geographic distribution (e.g., blastomycosis, histoplasmosis and coccidioidomycosis).

Endospore—spore formed within a larger cell, such as a *Coccidioides* spherule.

Entomophthoramycosis—infections caused by molds of the order Entomophthorales, including species of *Conidiobolus* and *Basidiobolus*.

Germ tube—a hypha emerging from a yeastlike structure, characteristic of *Candida albicans* cells placed on specialized culture medium.

Haploid—having a single set of chromosomes.

Heterothallic—a fungus that can only mate between different colonies of an opposite mating type.

Homothallic—a fungus in which mating can take place within the same colony (e.g., *Pseudallescheria boydii*).

Hyaline—colorless, transparent.

Hyalohyphomycosis—infection caused by molds with light-colored colonies. This term includes most of the pathogenic molds and is so broad it has not proven useful.

Hypha (plural, hyphae)—the tubular element that forms the body of a fungus.

Imperfect state—fungus producing only asexual spores.

Meiosis—process in a dividing cell that allows re-assorting of chromosomes and reduces the number of chromosomes by half, from diploid to haploid.

Mitosis—process in a dividing cell that produces two genetically identical copies of the original cell.

Morphology—appearance of the fungus.

Mold—filamentous fungus. A colony on agar generally appears fuzzy, rather than smooth.

Mucormycosis—infection by molds of the subphylum Mucormycotina.

Mycelium (plural mycelia)—the mass of hyphae making up a fungal colony.

Perfect state—fungus capable of producing sexual spores.

Phaeohyphomycosis—infection caused by molds with dark-colored colonies caused by pigmentation in the hyphae. Individual hyphae may not have enough pigment to be dark-colored under the microscope. A colony can be dark-colored because of the spores, such as *Sporothrix schenckii*, and may not be an agent of phaeohyphomycosis.

Phenotype—genetically determined properties that help distinguish an organism from otherwise similar organisms (e.g., requirement for exogenous uracil is a useful phenotype in some yeast mutants).

Pseudohyphae—a string of budding cells (e.g., those formed by most *Candida* species).

Sexual spores—spores formed by meiosis, a form of division in which the number of chromosomes is reduced by half.

Spherule—large round cell of *Coccidioides* species that forms spores inside.

Sporangium—a sacklike structure with asexual spores (sporangiospores) inside. Spores are released when the sack breaks.

Spp.—abbreviation for species (plural).

Teleomorph—a fungus forming sexual spores.

Thallus—the vegetative body of a fungus, such as a fungal colony.

Yeast—technically, a fungi of the family Saccharomycetaceae, including *Saccharomyces cerevisiae* (baker's yeast). The terms *yeast form* or *yeastlike* are generally used to denote fungi that reproduce by budding.

Sexual spores arise as a result of nuclear fusion followed by meiosis, a process that reduces the chromosome number by half. If the two nuclei are from the same colony (thallus), the fungus is said to be homothallic. If the nuclei are from different colonies that fuse their cytoplasm when grown adjacent to one another, the fungus is said to be heterothallic. Such fungi only join with colonies having a different, compatible mating type. Heterothallic fungi include the agents of histoplasmosis, blastoplasmosis, and cryptococcosis, as well as some fungi causing ringworm and mucormycosis.

Spores of fungi pathogenic for humans are nonmotile and spread by wind, water, and contact. Fungal cells have rigid walls of glucans and often chitin. All fungal cell walls are stained by Gomori methenamine silver. The periodic acid–Schiff reagent will stain the polysaccharide in the cell wall. All fungi, including *P. jirovecii*, stain with calcofluor, which appears brilliant white under the fluorescent microscope. This stain has replaced the wet mount or KOH stain in many diagnostic laboratories because fungi are easier to see. Gram stain is not usually helpful because most fungi, except *Candida*, remain unstained. India ink smear of cerebrospinal fluid allows visualization of a polysaccharide capsule around the cell wall and is characteristic of only one genus pathogenic for humans, the genus *Cryptococcus*. An India ink smear from a colony on a culture plate is less helpful because the capsule may be too thin to be seen. Inside the fungal cell wall is the sterol-containing cytoplasmic membrane, which is the site affected by azoles, allylamines, and the polyene macrolide antibiotics amphotericin B and nystatin. Some fungi can produce mycotoxins under specialized conditions, including species of *Stachybotrys* and *Aspergillus*, but these toxins are not known to contribute to pathogenesis of mycoses. Gliotoxin in *Aspergillus* may prove to be an exception.

Diagnosis of Mycoses

The optimal method of diagnosis is culture. Because Chapter 17 is rich in details about laboratory identification of fungal cultures, only a few generalities about these techniques are given here. Most yeasts are identified by a series of biochemical tests, although morphology (appearance of the colony and of cells on microscopic examination) also plays a role. Molds are identified almost exclusively by their morphology, particularly how they sporulate on agar. A nonsporulating mold may be termed *mycelia sterila* by the laboratory, meaning it cannot be identified. Use of molecular identification tests in reference laboratories can circumvent the need for identification based on sporulation.

Fungi can often be identified in tissue, even in the absence of culture, by taking into account the clinical findings, body site, inflammatory response, and fungal appearance (Fig. 256-1; Table 256-2). Culture diagnosis is potentially more accurate than diagnosis by histologic features, but many smaller laboratories encounter difficulties in isolating and identifying fungi. The histologic features of a biopsy specimen can be more rapidly diagnostic than culture when mycoses are caused by slow-growing fungi. Biopsy slides are more readily mailed to consultants than cultures, which may arrive nonviable or contaminated. Finally, biopsy may provide proof that the fungus is invading tissue and is not just a contaminant or saprophyte growing on debris in a lung cavity or skin ulcer. Ideally, both histologic examination and culture should be done together. As yet, detection of fungal DNA by polymerase chain reaction has not proved useful for detecting or identifying fungi in tissue. In contrast, luminescent DNA probes for hybridization to fungal RNA are commercially available and valuable for identifying colonies of *Histoplasma capsulatum*, *Coccidioides* spp., *Blastomyces dermatitidis*, and *Cryptococcus neoformans*. Identification of fungi in tissue by immunohistochemistry and molecular methods remains experimental.

Serologic Diagnosis

Despite a rich history of serologic studies of mycoses, the only mycosis for which serodiagnosis has an established role is coccidioidomycosis (Chapter 266). Even with this infection, lack of standardization of tests among laboratories and among methods has made it difficult for the clinician to interpret the results. The situation is even worse for histoplasmosis and blastomycosis, for which the most promising test in the literature, complement fixation, has been considered too labor

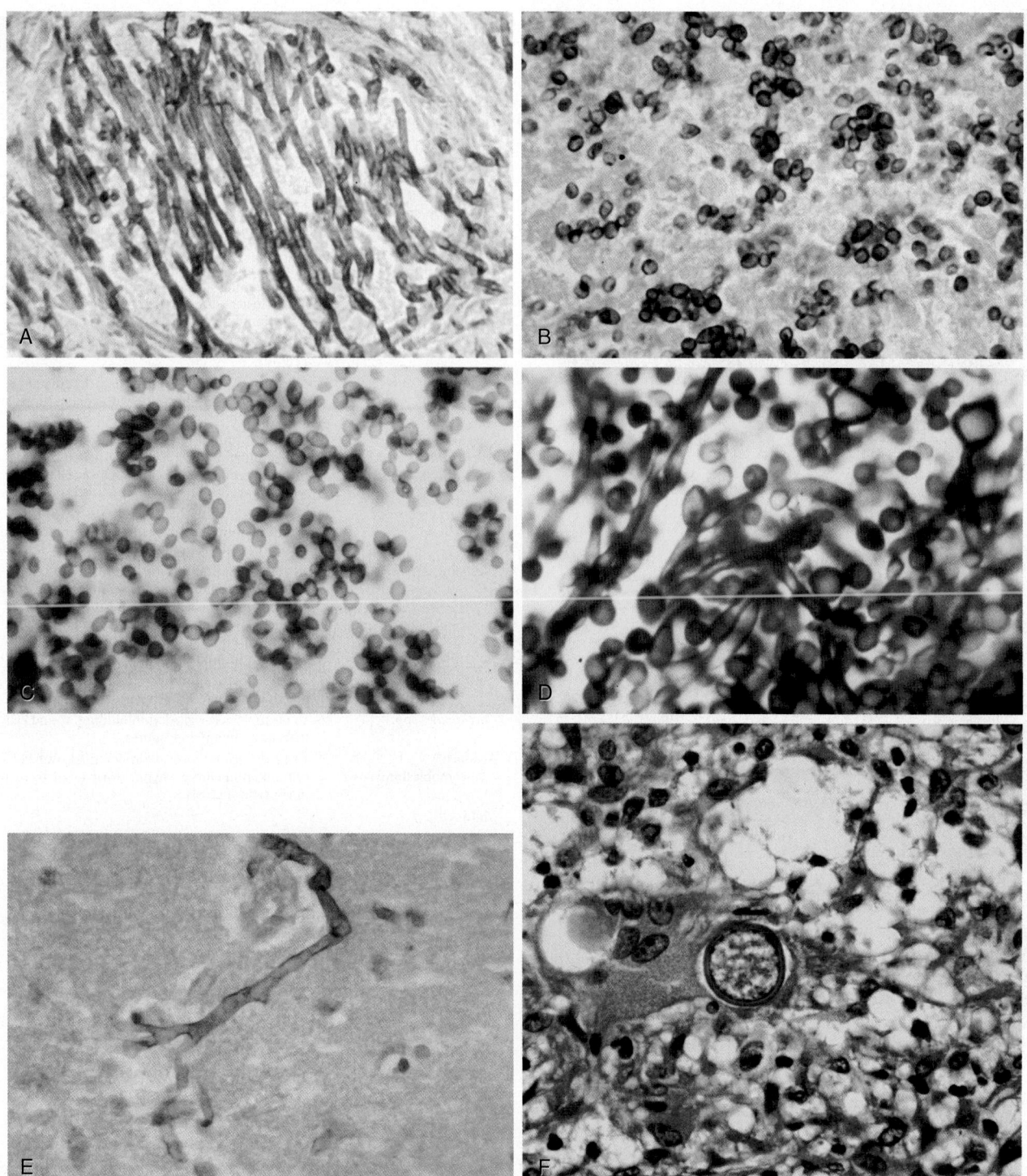

Figure 256-1 **Appearance of fungi in tissue. A,** *Aspergillus* sp., periodic acid–Schiff (PAS) stain. **B,** *Histoplasma capsulatum*, Gomori methenamine silver (GMS) stain. **C,** *Candida glabrata* yeast cells, PAS stain. **D,** *Candida albicans,* GMS stain. **E,** *Rhizomucor* sp., GMS stain. **F,** *Coccidioides* sp., hematoxylin and eosin (H&E) stain. Appearance of fungi in tissue.

Continues

intensive and replaced in commercial laboratories by tests of unknown significance. Serodiagnosis for any mycosis should be used with great caution and with knowledge of the technique and laboratory performing the test.

Diagnosis by antigen detection has proved very useful in disseminated histoplasmosis and cryptococcosis. Severe cases of aspergillosis, coccidioidomycosis, and blastomycosis may also be amenable to diagnosis by antigen detection. Tests are commercially available for

detecting β-glucan, a cell component, in patient serum. Refer to the relevant chapters for further discussion of these tests.

Epidemiology

With rare exception, mycoses are not transmissible from patient to patient. Gown, glove, or mask isolation of hospitalized patients with mycoses is not indicated. Ringworm of the scalp in children is

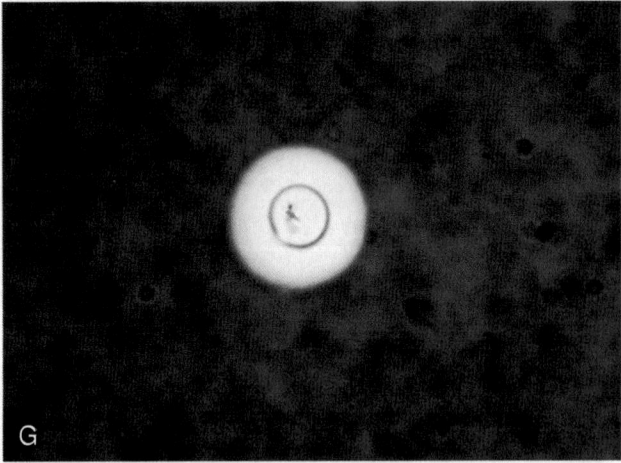
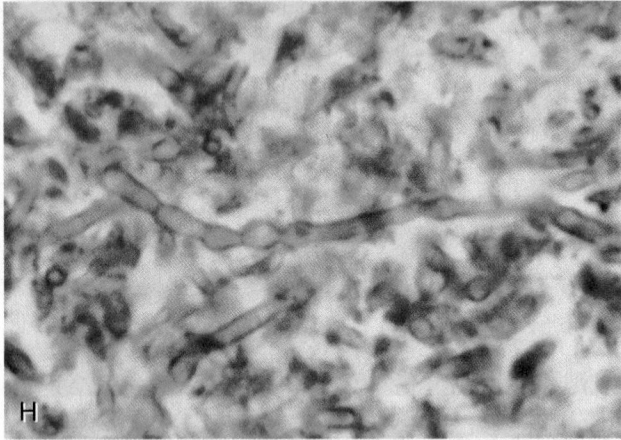
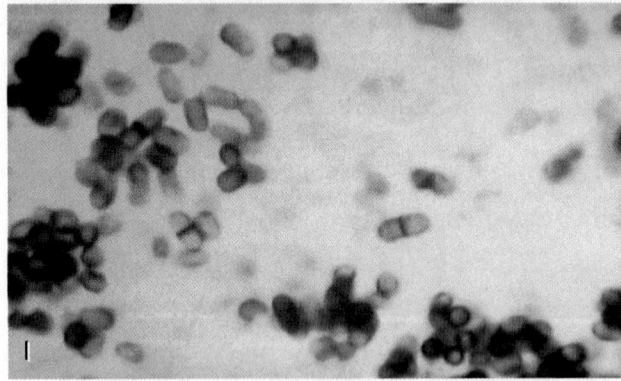

Figure 256-1, cont'd **G,** *Cryptococcus neoformans,* India ink smear of cerebrospinal fluid. **H,** *Cladophialophora bantiana,* H&E stain. **I,** *Penicillium marneffei,* GMS stain.

TABLE 256-2	Typical Appearance of Fungi in Tissue
Fungi	*Description*
Yeastlike Fungi	
Histoplasma capsulatum	2-3 × 3-4-μm oval, budding uninucleate cells; often intracellular; granulomatous inflammation. Caseous necrosis can occur. Cells in African histoplasmosis (var. *duboisii*) are 6-15 μm in diameter.
Penicillium marneffei	2-3 × 2-6-μm oblong yeasts, some with central cross septum; often intracellular except in areas of necrosis.
Pneumocystis jirovecii	3.5- to 7-μm cysts resemble *H. capsulatum* on methenamine silver stain or calcofluor but do not bud. Clusters of cysts occur in alveoli surrounded by eosinophilic amorphous material.
Candida glabrata	2.5-3 × 4-5-μm oval budding cells; pyogenic necrosis.
Candida albicans	3 × 5-μm oval, budding cells usually by tubular structures (pseudohyphae), with constrictions at septae and branching only at septations.
Cryptococcus neoformans	4- to 6-μm round uninucleate cell with large surrounding capsule; narrow pore between mother and daughter cell; daughter cell detached while small. Stains red with mucicarmine.
Sporothrix schenckii	1-3 × 3-10-μm cigar-shaped cell or 2- to 10-μm round budding cell; pyogenic and granulomatous inflammation.
Blastomyces dermatitidis	8- to 15-μm round multinucleate cell with large pore between mother and daughter cell; daughter cell remains attached until almost the size of mother cell; pyogenic and granulomatous inflammation.
Paracoccidioides brasiliensis	2- to 30-μm multiple, budding, round cells with tiny pore between mother and daughter cell; daughter cell released when small.
Coccidioides spp.	5- to 60-μm thick-walled, nonbudding, round cells that may contain endospores.
Agents of chromoblastomycosis	4- to 12-μm round or oval, brown, thick-walled cells, often in clumps; hyphal forms may be seen in superficial crusts.
Molds	
Aspergillus spp.	2- to 5-μm-wide hyphae, frequently septate, even diameter, Y-shaped branching; propensity for vascular invasion; necrosis.
Agents of mucormycosis	4- to 15-μm-wide hyphae, rarely septate, uneven diameter, often branch at broad angles; propensity for vascular invasion; necrosis.

transmissible to other children, so caps and combs should not be shared by infected children and playmates. Airborne transmission of *P. jirovecii* has been postulated, but isolation of these patients is not routine. Bandages or casts that become contaminated with draining pus from patients with coccidioidomycosis require care to ensure that the fungus does not remain on the fomite for several days because at room temperature, the fungus will grow as the infectious, spore-bearing mold form.

The diagnostic laboratory should be alerted when specimens from patients suspected of having coccidioidomycosis or histoplasmosis are sent for culture. Once these cultures grow in the mold form, they can be hazardous to laboratory personnel.

REFERENCES

1. Anaissie EJ, McGinnis MR, Pfaller MA, eds. *Clinical Mycology.* New York: Churchill Livingstone; 2003.
2. Connor D. *Pathology of Infectious Diseases.* Stamford, CT: Appleton & Lange; 1997.
3. Dismukes WE, Pappas PG, Sobelk JD. *Clinical Mycology.* New York: Oxford University Press; 2003.
4. Hospenthal DR, Rinaldi MG, eds. *Diagnosis and Treatment of Human Mycoses.* Totowa, NJ: Humana Press; 2008.
5. Kwon-Chung KJ, Bennett JE. *Medical Mycology.* Philadelphia: Lea & Febiger; 1992.
6. Paltauf A. Mycosis mucorina: Ein Beitrag zur Kenntnis der menschlichen Fadenpilzerkrankungen. *Virchows Arch Pathol Anat.* 1885;102:543-564.
7. Gregory JE, Golden A, Haymaker W. Mucormycosis of the central nervous system: Report of three cases. *Bull Johns Hopkins Hosp.* 1943;73:409-419.
8. Emmons CW, Binford CH, Utz JP. *Medical Mycology.* Philadelphia: Lea & Febiger; 1963.
9. Hibbett DS, Binder M, Bischoff JF, et al. A higher-level phylogenetic classification of the fungi. *Mycol Res.* 2007;111:509-547.

257

Candida Species

JOHN E. EDWARDS, JR.

Written descriptions of oral lesions that were probably thrush date to the time of Hippocrates and Galen. Langenbeck, in 1839, found fungi in oral lesions of a patient.[1] By 1841, Berg established the fungal cause of thrush by inoculating healthy babies with aphthous "membrane material." In 1843, Robin attached to the organism the name *Oidium albicans*. There have been more than 100 synonyms for *Candida albicans*; the two that have persisted are *Monilia albicans*, originated by Zopf in 1890, and *C. albicans*, used by Berkhout in 1923.[2]

In 1861, Zenker described the first well-documented case of deep-seated *Candida*. The first case of *Candida*-induced endocarditis was described in 1940.[3] The most interesting period in the history of *Candida* infections began in the 1940s, when the widespread use of antibiotics was introduced. Since then, previously undocumented manifestations of *Candida* infections have occurred, and the incidence of practically all forms of *Candida* infections has risen abruptly. *Candida* spp. have been the fourth most common organisms recovered from blood of hospitalized patients in the United States during recent decades.[4] Between 2000 to 2005, the incidence of candidemia-related hospitalizations per 100,000 population has risen by 52%.[5] The burden of this illness in terms of morbidity, mortality, and expense is considerable.[6] Estimates describe expenditures adding to hospital costs of approximately $1 billion for the management of candidemia in the United States.[7] Excellent comprehensive reviews detailing the emergence of *Candida* as a common pathogen are available.[8-11] These emerging infections have included not only bloodstream infection but also arthritis, osteomyelitis, endophthalmitis, myocarditis, pericarditis, pacemaker endocarditis, ventricular assist device infection, meningitis, peritonitis, myositis, pancreatitis, and others that are elaborated upon in detail in their respective sections of this chapter. The increasing incidence of human immunodeficiency virus–1 infection, the use of therapeutic modalities for advanced life support, and certain surgical procedures, such as organ transplantation and the implantation of prosthetic devices, have continued to be important in the expanding incidence of *Candida* infections.

Two interesting trends are developing with the extensive, rapidly evolving literature on *Candida* infections. First, as developing countries have introduced advanced medical care, including primarily more complex surgical procedures and more comprehensive cancer treatments, their increasing reports of the epidemiology and predisposing factors for *Candida* infections have recapitulated those that have been noted during the past two decades from countries with advanced medical care. Second, there has been a steady and significant increase in reports on the incidence and manifestations of *Candida* infections caused by non-*albicans* species.[12]

Pathogen

Candida organisms are yeasts—that is, fungi—that exist predominantly in a unicellular form. They are small (4-6 μm), thin-walled, ovoid cells (blastospores) that reproduce by budding. They grow well in vented routine blood culture bottles and on agar plates and do not require special fungal media for cultivation. Several automated blood culture methods offer more rapid detection of *Candida*. Yeast forms, pseudohyphae, and hyphae may be found in microscopic examination of clinical specimens; identification of the hyphae and pseudohyphae is facilitated with 10% potassium hydroxide, which clears the epithelial cells, and with fluorescent microscopic examination of calcofluor white–stained smears. The organism also stains gram-positive.

Candida organisms form smooth, creamy white, glistening colonies that may resemble staphylococcal colonies. A rapid, presumptive identification of *C. albicans* can be made by placing the organism in serum and observing germ tube formation—small projections from the cell surface that appear within 90 minutes. However, both false-negative and false-positive germ tube formation may occur. The remainder of the identification and speciation procedures are based primarily on physiologic parameters rather than on morphologic characteristics. Metabolic tests include carbohydrate assimilation and fermentation reactions, nitrate utilization, and urease production. Chlamydospore formation is also used to identify *C. albicans*. Because of variation in species pathogenicity, speciation is desirable. There are more than 150 species of *Candida*, but only a small percentage are regarded as frequent pathogens for humans. They are *C. albicans*, *C. guilliermondii*, *C. krusei*, *C. parapsilosis*, *C. tropicalis*, *C. pseudotropicalis*, *C. lusitaniae*, *C. dubliniensis*, and *C. glabrata* (formerly classified as *Torulopsis glabrata*). *C. dubliniensis* is a relatively newly described species that was formerly included within *C. albicans*.[13] *C. dubliniensis* forms germ tubes and chlamydospores and is identified as *C. albicans* by the most common methods. However, it will not grow at 45°C, is darker green when initially isolated on CHROMagar candida, and hybridizes poorly to the Ca3 probe. Because it is not yet clear how the clinical features may differ from those of *C. albicans*, if at all, the two are considered synonymous in this chapter. Infections by other species are being reported with increasing frequency, such as the azole-resistant species *Candida inconspicua*.[14] The API Yeast 20C strip is a commercial kit that gives accurate identification of most *Candida* spp. in 2 to 5 days. Rapid methods have been developed for speciation, such as fluorescent in situ hybridization (FISH), but they are not widely used at present (see Chapter 17).[15,16]

Epidemiology and Ecology

C. albicans organisms have been recovered from soil, animals, hospital environments, inanimate objects, and food. Nonalbicans species may live in animal or nonanimal environments, as well. Only rarely are *Candida* spp. laboratory contaminants. That principle has not been generally appreciated, and interpretation of positive cultures as laboratory or skin contaminants has led to important errors in patient management.

The organisms are normal commensals of humans and are commonly found on skin, throughout the entire gastrointestinal (GI) tract, in expectorated sputum, in the female genital tract, and in the urine of patients with indwelling Foley catheters. There is a relatively high incidence of carriage on the skin of health care workers. Although the vast majority of *Candida* infections are of endogenous origin, human-to-human transmission is possible. Examples are thrush of the newborn, which may be acquired from the maternal vagina, and balanitis in the uncircumcised man, which may be acquired through contact with a partner having *Candida* vaginitis. There is also important, emerging evidence that *Candida* infection can be acquired from the hospital environment. Molecular biology tools are improving considerably the understanding of *Candida* epidemiology.[17,18,19,20] Important studies in recent years suggest that Candida has many of the genetic components necessary for mating and suggest that mating may actually occur in vivo.[21,22,23] If *Candida* can be forced to mate in vitro and undergo meiosis, by exploitation of these genetic components, a significant breakthrough will occur in elucidating pathogenetic factors of *Candida* through molecular genetics.

Pathogenesis and Pathologic Findings

Normal defense mechanisms against *Candida* have been reviewed extensively recently.[24,25,26] Only highlights of this complex topic can be discussed herein, and the reader is referred to the cited references for more details of this evolving field.

The defense mechanism of intact integument is of importance in maintaining resistance to cutaneous candidiasis. Any process causing skin maceration leaves the involved site susceptible to *Candida* invasion, even in healthy individuals. In recent years the importance of the dendritic cell for maintaining skin and mucosal integrity and as an immune effector cell has been recognized.[24,27] The role of Toll receptors and the cathelicidins has also recently been reviewed.[28,29] The defense mechanisms of the mucosa have also been extensively reviewed and the importance of innate immunity, rather than adoptive adaptive immunity, has been emphasized.[30,31] Once the organism invades the dermis or enters the bloodstream, polymorphonuclear leukocytes play a role in defense because they have the capacity to damage pseudohyphae and to phagocytize and to kill blastospores. In addition to neutrophils, monocytes and eosinophils also ingest and kill *Candida,* as do dendritic cells.[32,33] Other cells, such as endothelial cells[34] and epithelial cells, may also ingest the organisms in vivo but do not have a direct killing effect. Platelets may also have anti-*Candida* activity.[35] A platelet-derived factor stimulates germ tube production, and *Candida* cell wall fractions agglutinate platelets.[36] Serum and plasma alone, even though they contain antibodies and complement components, are incapable of killing *Candida.*

Neutrophils and monocytes lacking myeloperoxidase or the capacity to generate hydrogen peroxide and superoxide anion fail to kill *C. albicans* effectively. This observation and additional related studies suggest that the myeloperoxidase, hydrogen peroxide, or superoxide anion system, or all of these, are a major mechanism responsible for intracellular killing of *C. albicans.* In addition, studies have identified a ferrous ion–hydrogen peroxide–iodide system that is operative in intracellular killing.[37] A further intracellular killing mechanism for phagocytes involves chymotrypsin-like cationic proteins.[38] These proteins probably act by increasing candidal membrane permeability. The role of macrophages and sessile reticuloendothelial cells has also been investigated.[39] Rabbit and mouse alveolar and peritoneal and human lung macrophages have *Candida*-killing capacities.

Of interest is a study of Taschdjian and colleagues that showed, by immunofluorescent techniques, organisms within tissue macrophages and sessile reticuloendothelial cells throughout the body in patients with disseminated candidiasis. This observation suggests a defense role for these tissue macrophages. A large number of other components are directly involved with or interactive, or both, in the mediation of phagocytosis and in some instances, the regulation of function of lymphocytes by phagocytes; they included mannose receptors, complement receptors, Fc receptors, proinflammatory cytokines, proinflammatory chemokines, INF-γ, TNF-α, IL-4, IL-10, vitronectin, IL-12, IL-17, IL-8, IL-18, and TGF-β, Toll-like receptors, T reg cells, γδ T cell, NK cells, MBL, dectin-1, MyD88, indoleamine, and 2,3 dioxygenase, just to name a few. The reader is directed to the comprehensive reviews of these additional inflammatory and immune components.[24,25]

The role of lymphocytes in defense against *Candida* and the regulation of *Candida*-induced cell-mediated immunity, within the context of the Th1/Th2 paradigm, are exceptionally complex subjects and are in a state of evolution.[40] They can be only superficially addressed herein. The importance of the defensive role of the lymphocyte can be gleaned from clinical observations: Patients with chronic mucocutaneous candidiasis are afflicted with *Candida* infection as a result of dysfunction of their lymphocyte system,[41] and patients with acquired immunodeficiency syndrome (AIDS) are highly susceptible to mucocutaneous candidiasis. However, it should be noted that there is experimental evidence for congenitally athymic (nude) mice having more resistance to *Candida* challenge than controls with normal T lymphocytes.[42]

T helper cells are pivotal for the regulation of phagocytosis. When *Candida* is recognized by both dendritic cells and polymorphonuclear leukocytes, both cell types produce IL-12, which activates Th1 cells. The activated Th1 cells then secrete INF-γ and IL-2, both of which stimulate phagocytic cells. Downregulation of phagocytosis occurs through the stimulation of Th2 cells by IL-4, primarily secreted by the resident dendritic cells. These Th2 cells secrete IL-4 and IL-10, which inhibit phagocytosis.

The role of B lymphocytes and antibody has been investigated for years. Several lines of evidence point to an important role for antibodies in defense against candidiasis. The rate of ingestion of *C. albicans* by neutrophils is increased by both heat-labile and heat-stable serum opsonins. Immunoglobulin G (IgG) and other serum constituents effectively opsonize *C. albicans.*

Evidence exists for the presence of both protective and nonprotective antibodies. Evidence for protective antibody is based in part from experimental data showing that sera from patients who recovered from disseminated candidiasis protect mice when passively transferred. Additionally, preclinical data and clinical trials have shown some benefit with an antibody to break down products of a heat shock protein from *Candida.*[43-45] Polyclonal sera and IgM monoclonal antibodies to an adhesin of *Candida* confer protection in mice.[46]

Other humoral factors are likely operative in defense against *Candida* infections. Serum iron-binding proteins have been shown to inhibit the growth of *Candida,* presumably by binding iron, which is a *Candida* growth factor. Finally, there are humoral substances that induce *C. albicans* to form pseudohyphae and to clump the organisms in vitro[47] and numerous other humoral substances that have inhibitory effects on *Candida* growth.

Complement is necessary for optimal opsonization of *Candida* blastospores[48] in vitro, and animals deficient in alternate pathway activation are more susceptible to *Candida* challenge.[49] Furthermore, C3b has been found to bind to *Candida* blastospores.[50] Also, evidence for an important role of complement is the finding of complement components deposited in the basement membrane of cutaneous lesions in patients with chronic mucocutaneous candidiasis. Both the classic and the alternate pathways are activated by *Candida.* The weight of the evidence suggests that the alternate pathway is the most important. *Candida* cells, particularly pseudohyphae, have surface molecules that resemble human complement receptors CR2 and CR3.[51,52]

The capabilities of *Candida* to adhere to vaginal, gastrointestinal, and oral epithelial cells, fibronectin, platelet fibrin clots, acrylic, endothelium, lymphocytes, and plastics have all been demonstrated. The molecular genetics of adherence have been reviewed comprehensively and are beyond the scope of this discussion.[53]

For this human commensal organism to become a pathogen, interruption of normal defense mechanisms is necessary. The factors responsible for this immunocompromise fall into two categories: naturally occurring and iatrogenic. Included in the first category is diabetes mellitus, which predisposes to cutaneous but not disseminated candidiasis.

The most important predisposing factors to *Candida* infection, and especially to disseminated candidiasis, are iatrogenic. The introduction of newer therapeutic modalities for advanced life support into clinical medicine has been primarily responsible for the dramatic change in incidence of this disease. Of these factors, probably the most important have been the introduction of antibiotics and the widespread use of indwelling intravenous catheters. Antibiotics suppress normal bacterial flora and allow *Candida* organisms to proliferate, especially in the GI tract. Sulfonamides decrease neutrophil *Candida* intracellular killing,[54] and tetracycline, doxycycline, and aminoglycosides have been shown to decrease neutrophil phagocytosis.

Factors that may provide a route for *Candida* to enter from the environment into the vascular system of susceptible patients include the use of heroin, hyperalimentation fluids, polyethylene catheters, and pressure-monitoring devices. The implantation of prosthetic materials, especially cardiac valves, ventricular assist devices, and the artificial heart, is also associated with an increased incidence of *Candida* infection. Clinical situations associated with general immune suppression may be further complicated by the use of antibiotics, hyperalimentation fluid, and the other therapeutic modalities mentioned earlier, usually in the setting of multiple abdominal surgeries, renal transplantation, neoplastic diseases, the use of steroids, and severe burns.

Two observations support the hypothesis that the GI tract is a likely source for entrance of *Candida* into the bloodstream. Krause and associates reported drinking a suspension containing a massive amount of *Candida*.[55] Despite no recognizable GI disease, the investigator became candidemic and candiduric. Stone and coworkers have shown that yeasts can cross the GI tract of animals.[56] One would expect patients who have had abdominal surgery and therapy with multiple antibiotics to be at double risk for dissemination from the GI source by having both overgrowth of *Candida* in the GI tract and interruptions of the normal GI-tract mucosal integrity. GI-tract surgery is now a well-recognized predisposing factor to disseminated candidiasis. It is possible that loss of integrity of the GI tract due to either the disease or the cytotoxic chemotherapy creates a portal by which *Candida* passes from the GI-tract lumen into the bloodstream. Alternatively, the growing body of literature regarding *Candida* as a cause of septic thrombophlebitis suggests that in many cases the skin site of vascular catheter entry, rather than the GI tract, is the most likely portal of entry.

When the organism invades visceral tissue, microabscesses are formed, generally with normal parenchyma between the microabscesses. In tissue, both yeast forms and hyphal forms are present. Whether the formation of filamentous forms of *Candida* is a factor associated with virulence is one of the major unresolved controversies within the field. The initial cellular reaction is granulocytic. Histiocytes, giant cells, and epithelioid cells appear early, and the reaction may take the form of a granulomatous response. Although organisms may be seen on hematoxylin-eosin stains, optimal staining is accomplished with period acid–Schiff or methenamine silver. In the severely immunocompromised patient, the inflammatory reaction may be minimal or almost nonexistent, leaving the abscess composed only of *Candida* and necrotic tissue.

In superficial candidiasis, the histopathologic change is a chronic dermatitis with the yeast confined to the stratum corneum. However, *Candida* granuloma (see "Clinical Manifestations") is characterized by invasion into both the epidermis and the dermis, as well as by marked hyperkeratosis and acanthosis.

The factors associated with the organism rather than the host being responsible for virulence are under extensive investigation. An incomplete list includes the germ tube, proteases, phospholipases, adherence capabilities, hydrophobicity, morphologic switching, the presence of human-like integrins, and resistance to platelet-derived microbicidal peptides. A detailed review of the interesting topic of virulence factors is beyond the scope of this discussion, but the reader is referred to the recent compendium of discussions on the topic.[53] Most notable in recent years has been the evolving studies on the role of biofilm as a pathogenesis factor for *Candida*.[57-60]

Clinical Manifestations

As the frequency of diseases due to *Candida* has increased, a relatively large number of manifestations, which were previously either not recognized or extremely infrequent, have become well documented. The discussion of these clinical manifestations is facilitated by their subdivision into mucocutaneous and deep organ involvement.

MUCOUS MEMBRANE INFECTIONS

Thrush

Oral *Candida* infections are common and have been reviewed extensively recently.[61,62,63] The term *thrush* is applied to a specific form of oral candidiasis characterized by creamy white, curdlike patches on the tongue (Fig. 257-1) and on other oral mucosal surfaces; the patches

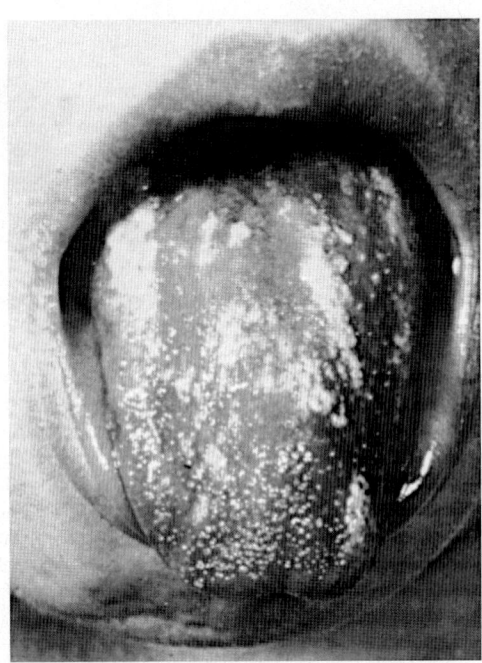

Figure 257-1 **Typical oral thrush with curdlike white patches over the tongue.** (*Courtesy of Dr. Arnold Gurevitch.*)

are removable by scraping and leave a raw, bleeding, and painful surface. The patches are actually a pseudomembrane consisting of *Candida*, desquamated epithelial cells, leukocytes, bacteria, keratin, necrotic tissue, and food debris.[64] The diagnosis can be made by the clinical appearance of the lesion and by scraping, using either a potassium hydroxide smear, Calcofluor white, or Gram stain to show masses of hyphae, pseudohyphae, and yeast forms. Simple culturing does not solidify the diagnosis because *Candida* grows easily from normal mouths. In addition to the classic lesions, which have been described by Lehner,[64] other manifestations include (1) acute atrophic candidiasis, a nonspecific atrophy of the tongue that is thought to be a sequela of acute pseudomembranous candidiasis; (2) chronic atrophic candidiasis or "denture sore mouth," which is a chronic inflammatory reaction and epithelial thinning under the dental plates; (3) angular cheilitis, an inflammatory reaction at the corners of the mouth (not due exclusively to *Candida*)[65]; and (4) *Candida* leukoplakia, which are firm, white plaques affecting the cheek, lips, and tongue that have a protracted course (and, in rare instances, may be precancerous). Since the introduction of inhaled steroids for the treatment of asthma, especially in children, oral thrush has been reported extensively in patients treated with these agents.[66] Incidence has ranged from 0% to 77%. Thrush developing in patients who use inhaled steroids usually resolves spontaneously without a change in the dosage of the agent or is successfully managed with topical nystatin suspension or clotrimazole troches. Other patients with a high incidence of thrush are cancer patients and those with AIDS. Patients with thrush for no obvious reason should be evaluated for AIDS. Because of the introduction of potent antiretroviral therapy, the incidence of thrush has declined in patients with AIDS.

Candida *Esophagitis*

Although there have been a small number of reports of *Candida* esophagitis occurring in patients with no known underlying illness, it is more commonly associated with treatment of malignancy of the hematopoietic or lymphatic systems (Fig. 257-2) and in AIDS patients.[67] Additionally, omeprazole has been implicated as a risk factor. The expression of a gene family within the organism has been shown when it invades the esophagus, suggesting the role of these genes in the pathogenesis of esophagitis.[68] Esophageal disease was believed to occur by direct

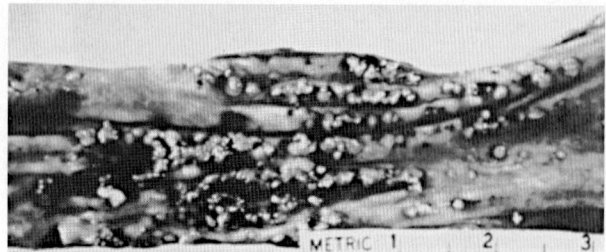

Figure 257-2 Severe *Candida* esophagitis at autopsy.

spread from oral disease (thrush), but reviews have shown that *Candida* esophagitis may occur frequently without thrush. The most common symptoms of *Candida* esophagitis include painful swallowing, a feeling of obstruction on swallowing, and substernal chest pain. Nausea and vomiting may also occur. The diagnosis is made definitively by biopsy during endoscopy (Fig. 257-3). However, the appropriate clinical settings, associated with the endoscopic appearance of white patches resembling thrush that show masses of hyphae and pseudohyphae on brushing, are enough evidence to initiate therapy without a histopathologic demonstration of the organisms invading the mucosa.

It is important to recognize that *Candida* esophagitis can occur simultaneously with herpes simplex virus or cytomegalovirus infection in severely immunocompromised patients. Radiographic examination may be helpful in making a clinical diagnosis; irregularity of the esophageal mucosa as a result of ulcerations may be seen, as well as shoulder defects, diverticulae, fistulas, and dilatation of the esophagus from denervation. Endoscopy is the preferred procedure for definitive diagnosis, however. The pseudomembrane which forms may become so extensive that it causes intraluminal protrusions and partial esophageal obstruction. Perforation of the esophagus due to esophageal candidiasis is very rare. Generally, if perforation occurs, it is in the lower two thirds of the esophagus. Some patients have had extensive esophageal disease and been almost asymptomatic, probably as a result of dener-

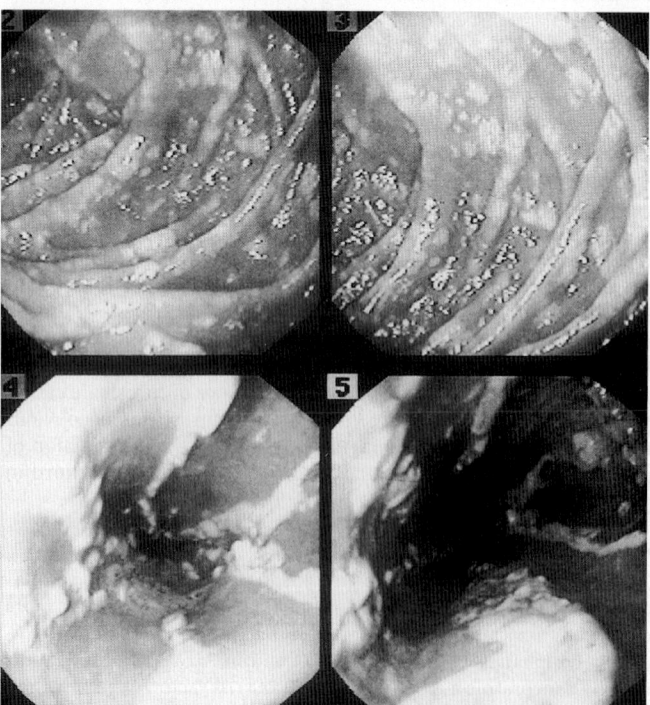

Figure 257-3 Numerous *Candida* plaques seen in the duodenum (upper panels) and esophagus (lower panels).

vation of the esophagus from the disease. Other complications include bleeding and, presumably, dissemination (see Chapter 82).

Nonesophageal Gastrointestinal Candidiasis

The most common clinical setting for GI-tract candidiasis is in patients with neoplastic disease. The esophagus is the most common site, followed by the stomach. The most frequent lesions are single or multiple ulcerations containing *Candida* deep in the ulcer beds. In addition, but with lesser frequency, chronic gastric ulcer, gastric perforation, and malignant gastric ulcer with concomitant *Candida* infection are seen. Small bowel and large bowel infection occur also. Ulceration is the most common lesion. Pseudomembrane formation and ulceration in association with tumor occurs also. As in other mucous membrane *Candida* infections, white plaques may be seen on endoscopy of the duodenum, and there may be thickening of mucosal folds in the duodenum and jejunum. Equal in frequency to the involvement of the small bowel is involvement of the large bowel, which again may be characterized by ulceration, superficial erosions, pseudomembrane formation, penetrating ulcers, and perforation. Gastric candidiasis has two forms: diffuse mucosal involvement (rare) and focal invasion of benign gastric ulcers. Comprehensive reviews of defensive mechanisms of mucosal and gastrointestinal candidiasis exist.[69,70] The importance of neutropenia facilitating hematogenous dissemination from the intestine has been demonstrated in the experimental murine model.[71]

Candida *Vaginitis*

This common infection is most frequently seen in a setting of diabetes mellitus, antibiotic therapy, and pregnancy (see Chapter 107). In addition, the use of birth control pills may be a predisposing factor, although this association is controversial. However, estimates are that 75% of women have an episode of candidal vaginitis during their lifetime; many have no recognizable underlying predisposing factor. *Candida* has assumed the role of the most common cause of vaginitis with higher frequency rates than those of *Trichomonas* or bacterial vaginosis. The widespread use of antibiotic therapy may be the most important factor responsible for the emergence of *Candida*-induced vaginitis. Reviews of the current trends in the epidemiology and pathogenesis of vaginal candidiasis are now available.[31,72,73] In these reviews the rising incidence of non-albicans *Candida* species is emphasized.

Although *Candida*-induced vaginitis may be accompanied by a thick, curdlike discharge, scanty discharge may instead characterize the infection. Edema and intense pruritus of the vulva are almost always present. The discharge consists of epithelial cells and masses of hyphae and pseudohyphae; a polymorphonuclear leukocyte response is not a component of the inflammatory reaction. The vagina and labia are usually erythematous, and extension onto skin of the perineum can occur (Fig. 257-4). In addition, endometritis due to *Candida* has been reported, and the urethra may become secondarily infected.

Vaginal candidiasis is not clearly more common or more refractory to treatment in patients with AIDS. The causes of recurrent vulvovaginal candidiasis, a particularly difficult and complex problem, may be related to deficiencies in both systemic cell-mediated immunity and local mucosal immunity.[74,75-78]

CUTANEOUS CANDIDIASIS SYNDROMES

Generalized Cutaneous Candidiasis

This condition is an unusual form of cutaneous candidiasis and is characterized by widespread eruptions over the trunk, thorax, and extremities, with increased severity in the genitocrural folds, anal region, axillae, hands, and feet (Fig. 257-5). The process begins as individual lesions that spread into large confluent areas. It occurs in both adults and children.[79,80]

Erosio Interdigitalis Blastomycetica

This term applies to *Candida* infection occurring between the fingers or toes (Fig. 257-6). It has a red base, may extend onto the sides of the digits, is painful, and is predisposed to by maceration.[81,82]

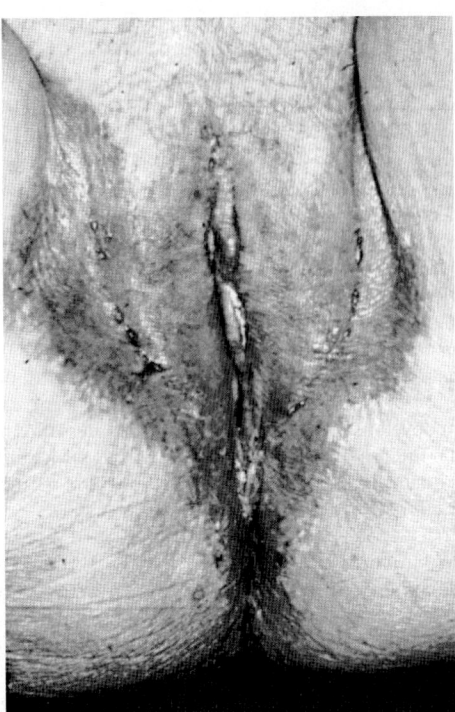

Figure 257-4 Extension of *Candida* vaginitis onto the perineum. *(Courtesy of Dr. Victor Newcomer.)*

Candida *Folliculitis*

Infection at the hair follicles with *Candida* can occur (Fig. 257-7).[83] Rarely, the condition may become extensive. It must be distinguished from folliculitis caused by the dermatophytes and tinea versicolor. This folliculitis has been described in immunocompromised hosts and

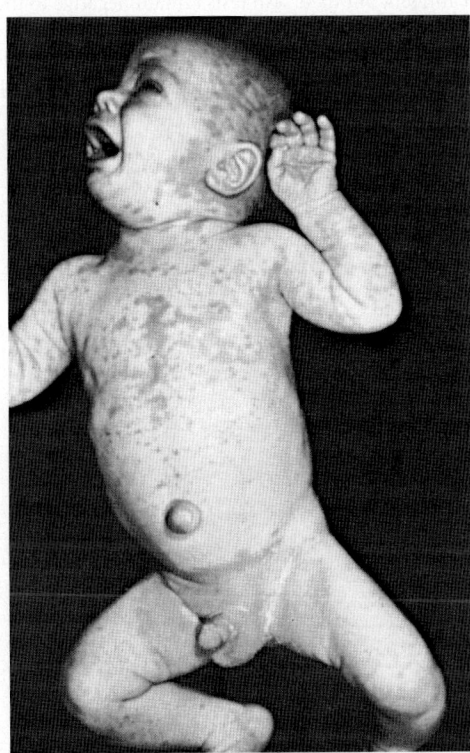

Figure 257-5 Generalized candidiasis. *(Courtesy of Dr. Victor Newcomer.)*

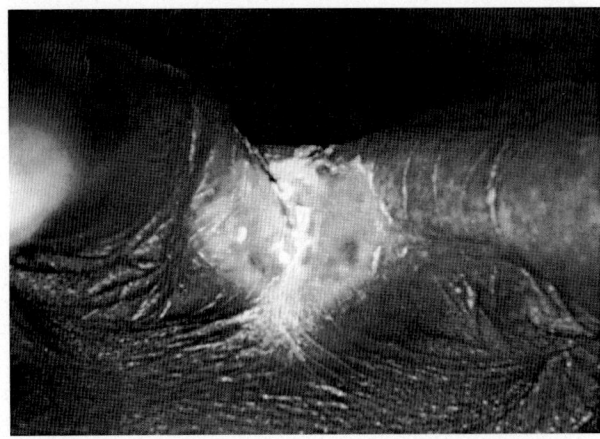

Figure 257-6 Erosio interdigitalis blastomycetica. *(Courtesy of Dr. Arnold Gurevitch.)*

intravenous drug abusers. As expected, its incidence is increased in obesity.[84]

Candida *Balanitis*

This process begins as vesicles on the penis that develop into patches resembling thrush and are accompanied by severe itching and burning. It may spread to the thighs, gluteal folds, buttocks, and scrotum. It can be acquired through sexual intercourse with a partner having vaginal candidiasis.[85] *Candida* is one of the more common causes of balanitis.[86]

Cutaneous Lesions of Disseminated Candidiasis

Four distinct types of lesions associated with disseminated candidiasis have been described. The macronodular lesions (Fig. 257-8) are 0.5 to 1 cm in diameter, pink to red, and may either be single or occur widely distributed over the entire body.[87,88] The most accurate method of making a specific diagnosis is by punch biopsy and demonstration of organisms on histologic section. Most patients with these lesions are

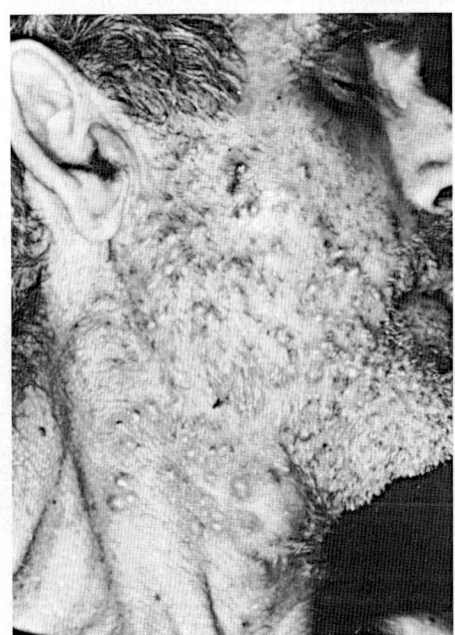

Figure 257-7 Severe *Candida* folliculitis in beard distribution. *(Courtesy of Dr. Victor Newcomer.)*

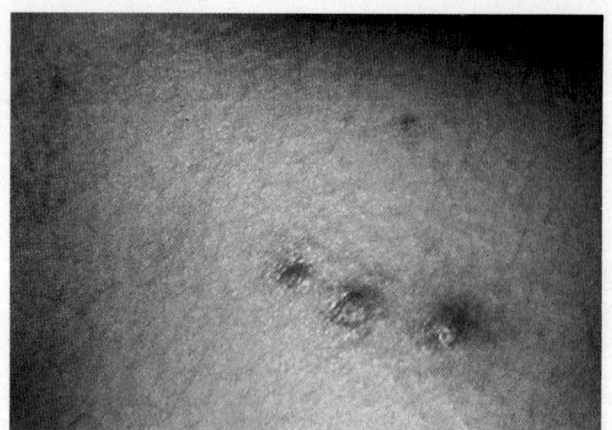

Figure 257-8 Macronodular lesions of disseminated candidiasis. *(Courtesy of Dr. Richard Meyer.)*

neutropenic, and all have disseminated candidiasis, not local inoculation. Additionally, lesions resembling ecthyma gangrenosum,[89,90] purpura fulminans,[91] and leukocytoclastic vasculitis[92] have been described. Chronic lesions of pyoderma gangrenosa may become superinfected with *Candida* and delay their definitive diagnosis.

Intertrigo
This common skin condition affects any site in which skin surfaces are in close proximity and provide a warm, moist environment. It begins as vesicopustules, which enlarge and rupture, causing maceration and fissuring. The area of involvement has a scalloped border with a white rim consisting of necrotic epidermis, which surrounds an erythematous, macerated base. Frequently, satellite lesions are found that may coalesce and extend the affected area. A variant form of cutaneous candidiasis in the intertriginous region has a miliary appearance resembling miliaria rubra with erythematous macules or vesicopustules.

Paronychia and Onychomycosis
Candida is one of the most common causes of paronychia. Species other than albicans may be causative.[93] Many skin bacteria, as well as *Candida*, can usually be recovered by culture of the infected area. The appearance of the reaction is that of a relatively well-localized area of inflammation that becomes warm, glistening, and tense and may extend extensively under the nail (Fig. 257-9). Unless the disease process is stopped, secondary thickening, ridging, and discoloration occur, and nail loss may result.

Candida paronychia occurs in association with frequent immersion of the hands in water. People who may contract paronychia include dishwashers, laundry workers, and parents of young children. There is also a higher incidence of paronychia among diabetic patients than in the nondiabetic population. Specific diagnosis is made by Gram stain or potassium hydroxide preparation and culture showing predominantly *Candida* organisms. In addition to paronychia, *Candida* may cause infection in the nail itself and is a cause of onychomycosis.[94]

Diaper Rash
Candida is a common cause of diaper rash in infants.[95] The condition generally starts in the perianal area and spreads over the perineum in the region of diaper contact (Fig. 257-10). The process is facilitated by maceration caused by wet diapers. The probable origin is the GI tract. Diagnosis is made by scraping the area and demonstrating the organisms on potassium hydroxide preparation.

In the case of perianal candidiasis, although numerous organisms and combinations of organisms have been associated with pruritus ani either alone or in combination, *Candida* is a frequent cause.[96] The perianal skin develops marked erythema and progresses to maceration (Fig. 257-11). Intense pruritus results. Complications include involvement of the anal canal and extensive spread over the perineum.

Chronic Mucocutaneous Candidiasis
The term *chronic mucocutaneous candidiasis* (CMC) is used to describe a heterogeneous group of *Candida* infections of the skin, mucous membranes, hair, and nails that have a protracted and persistent course despite what is usually adequate therapy. The subject has been reviewed comprehensively.[41] *Candida* esophagitis can occur and, over the years, cause esophageal stenosis. The major problem, however, is disfiguring lesions of the face, scalp, and hands. Alopecia in areas of infection is common and may be permanent. These infections have been associated with definable, relatively specific, immunologic abnormalities, which may be responsible for their persistent nature.

The major immune defect associated with CMC is failure of T-cell lymphocytes (thymus derived) to respond to stimulation with *Candida* antigen in vitro by either lymphocyte transformation or the synthesis of cytokines. An in vivo manifestation of this abnormality is reflected in the cutaneous anergy found in approximately one half of the patients. Various combinations of the T-cell function abnormalities exist. Some patients' lymphocytes transform in vitro when stimulated by *Candida* antigen, but their skin tests remain negative to the antigen. Certain patients with positive transformations do not synthesize macrophage inhibition factor; virtually all patients with negative transformations lack macrophage inhibition factor production. Despite these

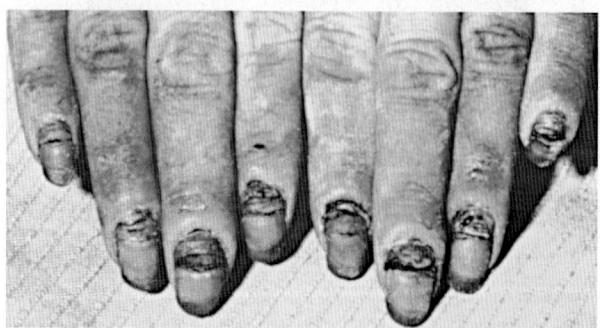

Figure 257-9 *Candida* paronychia and onychomycosis. *(Courtesy of Dr. Victor Newcomer.)*

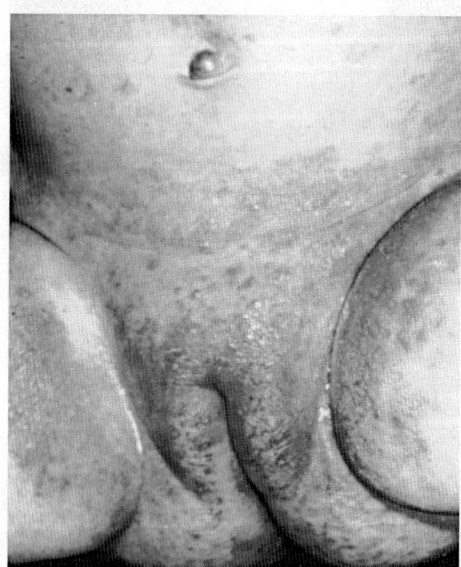

Figure 257-10 Severe *Candida* diaper rash. *(Courtesy of Dr. Victor Newcomer.)*

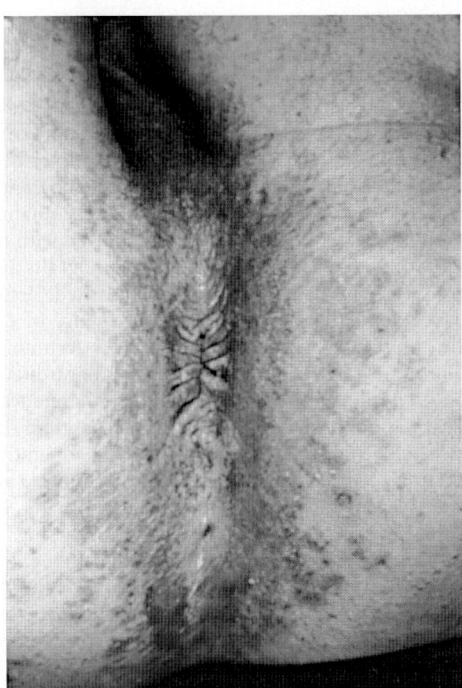

Figure 257-11 Perianal candidiasis. (*Courtesy of Dr. Victor Newcomer.*)

abnormalities of T-cell function (T-cell numbers, lymphocyte proliferative responses to nonspecific mitogens such as phytohemagglutinins and allogeneic cells), B-cell lymphocyte numbers and serum immunoglobulins are usually normal. However, a group of patients with selective immunoglobulin deficiency has been described.[97] Some patients have other immune abnormalities, such as cutaneous anergy to such antigens as streptokinase-streptodornase, mumps virus, and tetanus toxoid; defective lymphocyte transformations to nonspecific mitogens (e.g., phytohemagglutinin); defective monocyte chemotaxis; a lack of anti-*Candida* antibody in salivary IgAs; plasma inhibitors to *Candida*-stimulated lymphocyte transformations; suppressor lymphocytes; and various degrees of thymic aplasia. Not all patients have these identifiable immune abnormalities.

Most forms of CMC begin in infancy or within the first 2 decades; rarely, the onset may be after the age of 30 years. The first manifestation is usually oral thrush followed by nail infections and then skin involvement. There is a considerable spectrum of severity, ranging from chronic involvement of an isolated nail to a severely disfiguring form (*Candida* granuloma) (Fig. 257-12). An additional facet of CMC is the association of several endocrine disorders in approximately one half of the patients.[98,99] This entity is called the autoimmune polyendocrine syndrome type 1 (APS-1) and is associated with mutations in the AIRE gene.[99a] Endocrinopathy tends to follow, not precede, CMC, often after an interval of several years. The most common endocrinopathies are hypoparathyroidism and Addison's disease. Hypothyroidism and diabetes mellitus occur also. Autoimmune antibodies to adrenal, thyroid, and gastric tissues are present in approximately one half of the cases. Additionally, antibodies to interferon have been reported also.[100] Thymoma, chronic dermatophytosis, and dental dysplasia have also been associated with CMC. Associations have also been made with vitiligo, polyglandular autoimmune disease, and autoantibodies to melanin-producing cells.

Although most patients with CMC survive for a prolonged period with their disease, patients may succumb if the cutaneous condition and immunodeficiencies are severe enough. Disseminated candidiasis has been a rare complication of this disease; the most common cause of death is bacterial sepsis. The topic of *Candida* skin infection in general has been reviewed extensively.[101]

DEEP ORGAN INVOLVEMENT

Central Nervous System Candidiasis

Candida infects both parenchymal brain tissue and the meninges, usually as a complication of hematogenously disseminated candidiasis. Approximately 50% of patients with *Candida* meningitis have had disseminated disease in other organs. When infection occurs in brain parenchyma, it generally forms multiple microabscesses and small macroabscesses scattered throughout the tissue. Rarely, larger abscesses have occurred and may be visualized by MRI.

Virtually all patients with *Candida* meningitis have had cerebrospinal fluid pleocytosis. Fifty percent have had a lymphocyte pleocytosis, with an average count of 600 cells/mm³. Sixty percent have had hypoglycorrhachia and elevated protein levels; organisms have been present on wet mount or Gram stain in approximately 40%. *C. albicans* has been the responsible pathogen in 90% of cases. Occasional cases due to *C. tropicalis* are being reported. In a small series of cases, the CSF mannan has been positive, suggesting its possible usefulness as a diagnostic tool.[102]

The clinical manifestations of central nervous system involvement with diffuse microabscesses may be variable. If the patient is comatose or noncommunicative, detection of abnormalities may be exceptionally difficult. When meningitis is present, the signs of meningeal irritation (headache, stiff neck, irritability), typical of any meningeal infection, are frequently present. In the newborn, particularly the very low birth weight neonate, diagnosis is often difficult and delayed, leading to permanent neurologic sequelae. Lumbar puncture should be considered when the blood culture of such infants contains *Candida*.

In addition to occurring as a complication of disseminated candidiasis, *Candida* meningitis may result from infection of a ventricular shunt or may be introduced by lumbar puncture, trauma, or neurosurgery. The signs and symptoms are nonspecific, with typically an indolent onset. Untreated, the mortality rate is very high; it is reduced substantially with antifungal therapy. Hydrocephalus is a reasonably frequently occurring complication of the infection. An increase in the

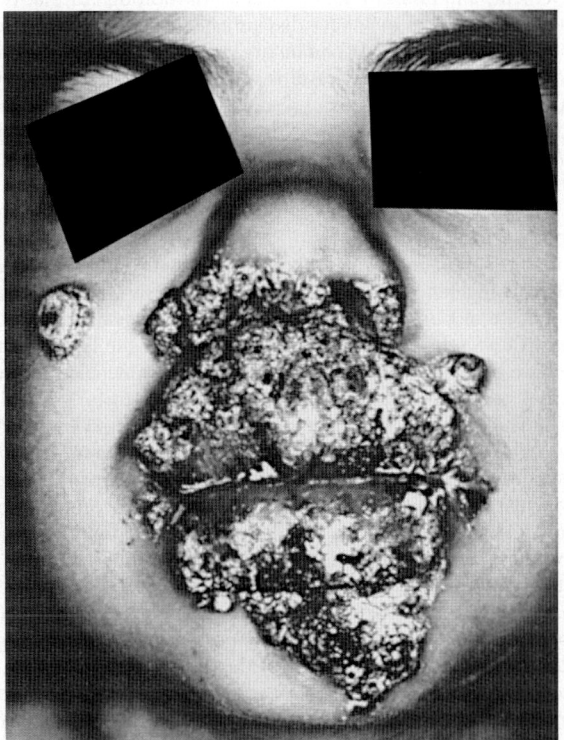

Figure 257-12 *Candida* granuloma. (*Courtesy of Dr. Victor Newcomer.*)

number of cases of *Candida* meningitis reported in neonates is occurring. AIDS is considered a predisposing factor for *Candida* meningitis.

Respiratory Tract Candidiasis

In general, *Candida* pneumonia occurs in two forms: either local or diffuse bronchopneumonia originating from endobronchial inoculation of the lung, a very rare event, or as a hematogenously seeded, finely nodular, diffuse infiltrate, which in its early stages may be difficult to distinguish from congestive heart failure or *Pneumocystis* pneumonia. Other forms of *Candida* pneumonia are very rare; those that have been described are necrotizing pneumonia, *Candida* pulmonary mycetoma, and transient infiltrates due to *Candida*. Radiographic and computed tomographic findings are nonspecific, and definitive diagnosis depends on biopsy-proven fungal invasion of pulmonary tissue. Because of a relatively high prevalence of yeasts colonizing the respiratory tract, especially in ill patients, a diagnosis of *Candida* pneumonia cannot be made on radiographic findings and recovery of yeasts from sputum or endotracheal tube aspirate.[103,104] *Candida* has also caused bronchial infection, laryngitis, epiglottitis, and infection of laryngeal prostheses. The entity of "fungal empyema thoracis" has been described as an emerging clinical entity.[105] Infection with *Candida* alone or in association with bacteria has been frequent within the population of patients with this entity. The crude mortality has been very high, and aggressive management has been advocated.

Cardiac Candidiasis

In addition to causing endocarditis, *Candida* infects both the pericardium and the myocardium. *Candida* myocarditis occurs as diffuse microabscesses scattered throughout the myocardium with normal intervening myocardial tissue. The relatively high incidence of myocarditis has been stressed by Franklin and coworkers, who found that 62% of their 50 patients with disseminated candidiasis had myocardial involvement.[106] Other retrospective autopsy studies have shown a range from 8.4% to 93%. *Candida* myocarditis has also occurred in AIDS patients. Autopsy series of disseminated candidiasis reveal a surprisingly high incidence of myocarditis (without associated valvular involvement) and point to the importance of thorough cardiac evaluation in patients who may have disseminated candidiasis. Of interest has been the emergence of *Candida* organisms as a cause of pericarditis. A review of purulent pericarditis spanning the years 1960 to 1974 revealed that *Candida* organisms were either the single cause or combined with *Aspergillus* in 15% of the 26 cases.[107] The association of *Candida* pericarditis with either cardiac surgery or burns has been emphasized.

Candida *Endocarditis*

This manifestation of *Candida* was once a distinctly rare phenomenon, but its true incidence has increased simultaneously with the generalized increase in *Candida* infections. Of all the forms of fungal endocarditis, *Candida* is by far the most common. In the last 4 decades, there have been well over 214 reported cases. In a detailed review of 319 cases of fungal endocarditis, *Candida* accounted for 67% of the cases.[108] The entity of *Candida* endocarditis has been reviewed extensively.[109,110] Additional cases have been reported in children.[111] *Candida* endocarditis occurs in association with six clinical factors: (1) underlying valvular heart disease, (2) heroin addiction, (3) cancer chemotherapy, (4) implantation of prosthetic valves, (5) prolonged use of intravenous catheters (endocarditis, right atrial fungal masses, and infection of atrial myxomas have all been described), and (6) preexisting bacterial endocarditis, on which it is superimposed. Of these associations, by far the most frequent is the postoperative cardiac surgery, accounting for approximately 50% of the cases. Of interest is the frequency of species other than *C. albicans* that have caused endocarditis; a minimum of 41% of the cases have been due to organisms of other species, some of which have been very rarely recovered species. Newer species continue to be reported.[112] In heroin addicts, *C. parapsilosis* has been the most common causative organism.[113] Of interest is that

heroin abuse has diminished in percentage of underlying predisposing conditions relative to iatrogenic causes.

The pathogenic mechanisms for fungal endocarditis are not fully understood, but patients who undergo cardiac surgery are at risk for candidemia by being exposed to multiple antibiotics, prolonged intravenous fluid administration, and intravenous plastic catheters. Both the damaged endocardium and prosthetic material apparently serve as foci for the localization of *Candida* organisms. Also, contamination of suture material has been implicated in cases reported with concentration along the suture line. Contamination of homografts and heterografts before insertion has also been documented. Experimental evidence for a role in the pathogenesis of adherence of *Candida* to platelet fibrin complexes or fibronectin, or both, is accumulating.[114,115] The most common valves involved in *Candida* endocarditis have been the aortic and the mitral. In postoperative *Candida* endocarditis, the type of surgery has not been as important as the length of the postoperative course and complications during the postoperative period. *Candida* infection has been seen in simple valvulotomies and in prosthetic material placement, heterografts, and homografts. Pacemaker endocarditis has also been described. The physical findings and usual symptoms of *Candida* endocarditis are not significantly different from those of bacterial endocarditis, with the exception of the occurrence of large emboli to major vessels. Osler's nodes, Janeway lesions, splinter hemorrhages, hepatosplenomegaly, hematuria, proteinuria, pyuria, and casts all can occur. In addition, although the lesions of hematogenous *Candida* endophthalmitis have been described much more frequently in the setting of disseminated candidiasis without endocarditis, they may also be seen with endocarditis.

The complications of *Candida* endocarditis are very similar to those of bacterial endocarditis and include valve perforation, myocarditis, congestive heart failure, mycotic aneurysms, and major emboli. Although most cases of postoperative *Candida* endocarditis occur in the first 2 postoperative months, some have occurred later, and some patients who have been treated have had recurrent active disease after 2 years[116] and perhaps as long as 8 years. Therefore, in following patients treated for postoperative endocarditis, careful follow-up must be extended over a prolonged period.

Most patients with *Candida* endocarditis have positive blood cultures. Seelig and associates, in their 1974 analysis of 91 published cases of *Candida* endocarditis following cardiac surgery, noted that only 24 patients (26%) had negative blood cultures.[117] Modern blood culture methods likely provide better sensitivity. Echocardiography is becoming progressively more helpful, and large vegetations may be detected with this technique. False-negative results are common, especially in cases of mural endocarditis without valvular involvement. Transesophageal echocardiography has improved the sensitivity, particularly in the mitral valve. Serologic tests for *Candida* antibodies are associated with a high incidence of false negatives and false positives and are not clinically useful in the diagnosis of *Candida* endocarditis.

The therapy for *Candida* endocarditis is discussed in detail in the section on therapy. Before the introduction of surgical procedures for the management of *Candida*-induced endocarditis, the mortality rate from this disease was approximately 90%. With combined surgical and medical therapy, this high mortality rate has dropped to approximately 45%. Because of the introduction of newer antifungals, there has been a greater propensity for chronic suppression in selected patients. *Candida* endocarditis has been seen in association with bacterial endocarditis. *Candida* is a superinfection introduced by prolonged intravenous catheterization for antibiotic treatment.

Urinary Tract Candidiasis

This topic has been reviewed comprehensively.[118-121] Urethral candidiasis can occur in both men and women. In men, it usually results from sexual contact with women with *Candida* vaginitis. In women, it is generally thought to be acquired from extension of *Candida* vaginitis. *Candida* prostatic infection has also been reported.[122,123] A history of previous antibiotic use has been frequent in most patients.

The presence of *Candida* in the urine is common and usually does not indicate renal tract infection. Antibiotics and Foley catheters have been associated with the acquisition of candiduria.[121] Visualization (cystoscopy) or biopsy proof of either fungus balls or tissue invasion is requisite for linking candiduria to infection. Although the use of colony counting in urine has been attempted to separate colonization from infection, it is not useful. However, finding *Candida* in urine casts may be helpful in diagnosing renal tissue invasion of the upper renal tract. Most patients with iatrogenic candiduria have spontaneous resolution; however, long-term persistence or a bladder fungus ball may be a complication, particularly in patients with diabetes mellitus, urinary stones, or obstruction. Hematogenous dissemination from the urinary tract may occur, usually with instrumention.[124]

Candida cystitis is most commonly a complication of an indwelling Foley catheter. In the absence of bladder instrumentation, *Candida* cystitis has been associated most often with diabetes mellitus. Symptoms may be absent or may be essentially identical to those of bacterial cystitis. The cystoscopic appearance of the condition is that of a chronic nonspecific cystitis. A typical thrush membrane has been observed; it resembles deposits of coagulated milk and bleeds on removal. The condition may be so severe that perforation occurs.

Candida infection of the upper urinary tract has been classified into two distinct forms: primary—that is, presumably from an ascending route—and secondary, from hematogenous spread. Papillary necrosis, calyceal invasion, fungus ball formation, and perinephric abscess can result from ascending infection, particularly in the presence of urinary tract obstruction, renal stones, or diabetes mellitus. Percutaneous nephrostomy can introduce *Candida* into the renal pelvis. The hematogenous form of the disease is by far the most common. The pathologic changes are those of multiple microabscesses, especially in the cortical areas. Emphysematous pyelonephritis may occur.[125] A case of cystitis emphysematosa has been reported also.[126] Pneumaturia has occurred as well.[127] The kidney is one of the organs most frequently involved in disseminated disease.

Candida *Arthritis, Osteomyelitis, Costochondritis, and Myositis*

These manifestations of *Candida* infections were once extremely rare, but their true incidence has increased appreciably.[128,129] Sites of localization for hematogenous *Candida*–caused osteomyelitis include the spine (vertebrae and intervertebral disks; Fig. 257-13), wrist, femur, cervical spine, and costochondral junctions of the ribs, scapula, and proximal humerus. Prosthetic joints may also be infected.[130] Blood cultures have usually been negative, and diagnosis has been made by percutaneous needle aspiration of the involved area. In children, the long bones are generally affected, whereas in adults the axial skeleton predominates. Spinal involvement may be accompanied by disk infection. Bone infection may require surgery. Osteomyelitis may be a late complication of candidemia. Radiographic examination findings are nonspecific. Osteomyelitis as a result of contiguous spread from the skin has also been documented, and there is one reported case of extension of thrush of the mouth into the mandibular bone.

Candida arthritis occurs most frequently as a complication of disseminated candidiasis. It can also occur from trauma, surgery, and intra-articular injections of steroids, and as a complication of heroin injection, rheumatoid arthritis, and AIDS. The topic of fungal arthritis in general has been reviewed.[131] In *Candida* arthritis occurring unassociated with disseminated candidiasis, non-*albicans* species have been the most common. Although the majority of cases of *Candida* arthritis have been acute, chronic *Candida* arthritis has been reported, especially in leukemic patients. Generally, *Candida* arthritis has begun as a suppurative synovitis, and a high percentage of cases have extended to form osteomyelitis. *Candida* costochondritis can occur from hematogenous seeding or as a complication of median sternotomy wound infection.

Candida infection of muscle has been described. The majority of patients have been neutropenic, had hematogenously disseminated candidiasis, and had pain in the involved muscle. The organisms may

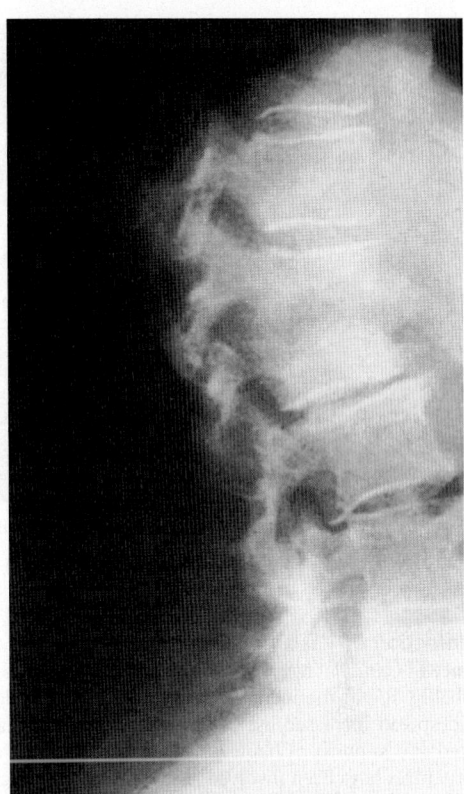

Figure 257-13 *Candida* **spinal osteomyelitis.** Note the involvement of the intervertebral disk and adjacent vertebrae. *(Reprinted from Edwards JE Jr, Turkel SB, Elden HA, et al. Hematogenous candida osteomyelitis. Am J Med. 1975;59:89-94, with permission from Excerpta Medica Inc.)*

be seen on biopsy of the involved muscle. Cases have also been reported in drug addicts. Generally, the muscle involvement is diffuse. However, a discrete muscle abscess may occur.

Candida *Infection of Peritoneum, Liver, Spleen, and Gallbladder*

Candida infection of the peritoneum is a complication of peritoneal dialysis, GI surgery, and perforation of an abdominal viscus.[132-133,134] Prior antibiotic administration has been an important predisposing factor. For reasons not completely understood, the peritoneal process usually remains localized to the abdomen; the incidence of dissemination is approximately 25% in patients acquiring the disease from GI-tract perforation. In patients with peritonitis caused by chronic ambulatory peritoneal dialysis, dissemination is distinctly uncommon. Low-birth-weight neonates disseminate more frequently from intra-abdominal sites, such as complications of surgical correction of intestinal or renal congenital abnormalities. Other GI organs infected with *Candida* that have been reported include the gallbladder,[135] liver and spleen, spleen alone, and pancreas. Hepatosplenic candidiasis has emerged as an important clinical problem in immunocompromised hosts and is particularly difficult to treat successfully. Most of these infections have occurred in severely immunocompromised patients and become manifest during their recovery from neutropenia. When the liver and spleen are involved, there is frequently involvement of other organs also, such as the kidney. Computed tomography, ultrasonography, or magnetic resonance imaging may visualize liver, kidney, or spleen abscesses (Fig. 257-14). Laparoscopic techniques have been used successfully for diagnosis. The incidence of this entity has diminished in recent years, probably as a function of the increased use of prophylaxis strategies. Fungus balls may form in the gallbladder and bile ducts.

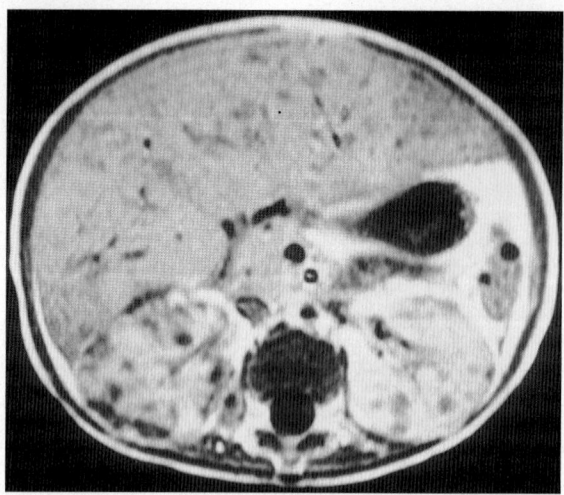

Figure 257-14 *Candida* abscesses in the liver, kidney, and spleen on magnetic resonance imaging.

Candida *Infection of Vasculature*

The incidence of *Candida* intravascular infection has increased significantly, probably due to the increased number of susceptible patients and the widespread increased use of indwelling intravascular devices for advanced life support (Chapter 79). Both peripheral and deep vascular structures have been involved, as well as both the venous and the arterial sides of the circulation and implanted prosthetic vascular materials. Although the exact pathogenesis is not known, presumably the damaged endothelium becomes susceptible to *Candida* invasion. *Candida* adherence to catheters may also play a role. Complications have included superior cava obstruction, mural endocarditis of the right atrium, tricuspid endocarditis, and pulmonary venous thrombosis. Of importance is that in patients with peripheral septic thrombophlebitis, there may be minimal symptoms and the extent of the disease may be greater than is apparent on initial clinical assessment. These patients require aggressive surgical exploration to determine the extent of the disease process. Culture of the blood and involved veins is frequently positive.

Ocular Candidiasis

Candida can infect the eye by either hematogenous spread or direct inoculation, especially during eye surgery. *Candida* can infect virtually any eye structure, including conjunctiva, cornea, lens, ciliary body, vitreous humor, and the entire uveal tract. Once endophthalmitis occurs, therapy is difficult, and the incidence of permanent intraocular damage is high (Chapters 112 and 113).

Through the 1970s there was increased reporting of hematogenous *Candida* endophthalmitis and an actual increase in incidence of this complication of candidemia.[136-141] Previous estimates of the incidence of the lesions in candidemic patients ranged as high as 28%.[142] Recent studies report a lower incidence.[137-143] An increased use of empiric and prophylactic antifungals may be an explanation for this possible decrease in incidence. A high association of retinopathy of prematurity with candidemia in very low birth weight neonates has been described.[144] Case reports include *Candida* endophthalmitis as a complication of tatooing, childbirth, abortion, therapy for HIV infection, and intravenous administration of contaminated dextrose infusion solution for minor ailments in a rural setting.

The lesions are important because they can cause permanent blindness, and they may indicate underlying disseminated candidiasis. Chorioretinal lesions are single or multiple, white, round, and initially sharply defined. As a lesion progresses over several days, the overlying vitreous humor becomes hazy, making the lesion margins indistinct. Eventually, *Candida* and neutrophils form white, cotton ball–like abscesses in a densely clouded vitreous. (Fig. 257-15). Use of the indirect ophthalmoscope facilitates visualization of their three-dimensional characteristics. Neutropenia inhibits the formation of ocular lesions in the experimental rabbit model[145] and may be associated with a lack of formation of easily seen lesions in some neutropenic patients. Diagnosis can be made by the characteristic fundoscopic picture, plus, in half the cases, an episode of known candidemia. Aspiration of the anterior chamber is rarely diagnostic. However, elective pars plana vitrectomy may be helpful both diagnostically and therapeutically in patients with vitreous abscesses.[137] Centrifuged sediment of vitrectomy fluid should be examined by smear and culture. Diagnosis may be facilitated with *Candida* specific polymerase chain reaction (PCR) of vitrectomy fluid or vitreous aspirate. Symptoms include visual blurring, floating scotomas, and, with extension to the anterior chamber, bulbar pain. Importantly, many patients in intensive care units are too ill to complain of symptoms. Although *C. albicans* has been the most frequent species causing endophthalmitis, other species have been reported with increasing frequency.

Syndrome of Disseminated Candidiasis and Candidemia

The problems of management of candidemia and detection of underlying disseminated candidiasis present major enigmas for clinicians dealing with patients who are predisposed to the disseminated form of this disease. The problem is compounded by the absence of positive blood cultures in many patients with disseminated disease. The interpretation of the significance of recovery of increased numbers of *Candida* from sites such as sputum, urine, feces, and skin is difficult because the organisms can frequently be recovered from these sites without causing infection.

The clinical setting associated with disseminated candidiasis has been previously described. As expected, the populations of patients most commonly affected are those with neoplastic disease, patients who have had complicated postoperative courses, burn patients, patients who have received organ transplants, and low-birth-weight neonates. In the neoplastic group, the most common association has been with the acute leukemic population. In the postoperative group, the patients who have had organ transplantations, heart surgery, or GI-tract surgery are at greatest risk.

When *Candida* disseminates, multiple organs are usually involved, with the kidney, brain, myocardium, and eye the most common. In cancer patients receiving extensive immunosuppressive therapy, recognition of liver and spleen involvement increased substantially, but the incidence of this complication has been in a downward trajectory. Other organs less frequently infected include the lungs, GI tract, skin, and endocrine glands. The hallmarks of the pathologic changes are

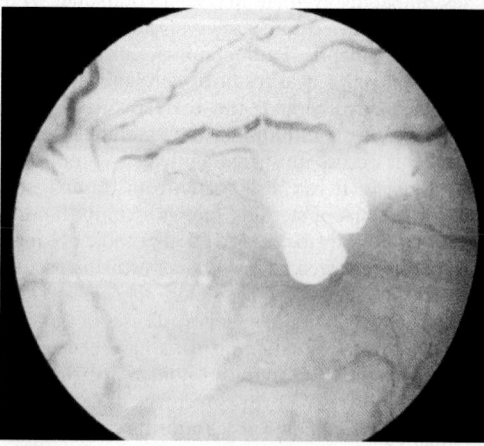

Figure 257-15 **Advanced hematogenous *Candida* endophthalmitis.** (From Fishman LS, Griffin JR, Sapico FL, et al. Hematogenous Candida endophthalmitis—a complication of candidemia. N Engl J Med. 1972;286:675. Copyright © 1972 Massachusetts Medical Society. All rights reserved.)

diffuse microabscesses with a combined acute suppurative and granulomatous reaction and small macroabscesses. Macroabscesses more than a centimeter in diameter may also form, especially in the liver and spleen.

The rate of premortem diagnosis of disseminated candidiasis has been very low; only approximately 15% to 40% of cases have been diagnosed early enough for appropriate therapy. As an aid to earlier diagnosis, considerable attention has been focused on the detection of serum antibodies to *Candida* and the detection of *Candida* antigen. Despite the appearance of a very large number of publications on the serologic diagnosis of disseminated candidiasis, spanning at least three decades, controversies remain regarding the value of various serodiagnostic procedures.[146] Problems with the older diagnostic tests have been reviewed in detail.[147,148,149,150] Currently, there is no validated serodiagnostic test that is widely used. Data are accumulating with the β-glucan assay on serum, but the place of the test in clinical management remains uncertain.[149]

The premortem diagnosis of disseminated candidiasis, therefore, remains a clinical diagnosis. Definitive diagnosis is made by histopathologic demonstration of the organism invading tissues. Of greatest importance in facilitating the diagnosis is awareness of, and persistent evaluation for, the variety of manifestations of disseminated candidiasis that serve as diagnostic clues. Candidemia is detected in about 24 hours with automated blood cultures and once detected, should prompt repeat blood culture, intravenous catheter change, and administration of an antifungal.[151-155] Some retrospective studies have correlated rapid institution of antifungal therapy with improved outcome in candidemia. The logical extension of this conclusion would be empirical therapy in patients at high risk of having candidemia. Selection of patients for empirical therapy remains incompletely defined, as discussed following.

Miscellaneous *Candida* Infections

Candida infections that have been described but are beyond the scope of this discussion include ear infections, nasal ulcers, lymphadenitis (in patients with leukemia), laryngeal infection, diarrhea, and the "drunken disease" syndrome described in Japan (thought to be due to *Candida* fermentation of carbohydrate in the GI tract). Also, *Candida* infections of numerous types have been reported with increasing frequency in antenates, neonates, and older children. Additionally, the emergence of *C. glabrata* and *C. krusei*, and *C. tropicalis* should be noted. The isolation of unusual *Candida* species continues to increase in frequency. A partial list is represented in the following descriptions.[156-158]

Treatment and Prophylaxis

GENERAL COMMENTS

Treatment strategies for nearly all forms of *Candida* infections have been reviewed in comprehensive detail for both neutropenic and nonneutropenic patients.[104] This review has been formulated into guidelines recently published under the auspices of the Infectious Diseases Society of America (IDSA). The discussion contained within this chapter will rely heavily on both other, current reviews and on the newer IDSA guideline document.[104] Significant advances for the treatment of *Candida* infections made in recent years include the introduction of the echinocandins and the development of advanced generation azoles. Of note, the intravenous preparation of itraconazole is no longer available.[159] The treatment options included herein will be limited to those agents currently approved by regulatory agencies.

Granulocyte transfusions have been given for *Candida* infection, but they are not used on a wide-scale basis, and their efficacy has not been clearly established from the limited experience to date. Experimental evidence in mice with a transfused myeloid cell line has shown beneficial results, but human trials have not been done.[161,162] Granulocytic colony–stimulating factor and other cytokines or immunomodulators

are discussed in Chapters 42 and 310 and have had limited application to the treatment of deeply invasive candidiasis.[163,164]

Antifungal Sensitivity Testing is being used increasingly for directing management of *Candida* infections, especially in refractory cases.[165,166] In general, once the species of *Candida* is defined, it is possible to predict with relatively high accuracy the minimum inhibitory concentration (MIC). The need for routine sensitivity testing on all isolates has not developed to this point.

Prophylaxis of *Candida* infection has been highly controversial. However, prospective controlled trials have shown successful results in allogeneic bone marrow transplant recipients.[167,168] Fluconazole, posaconazole, or micafungin are recommended.[104] Current guidelines recommend prophylaxis for solid organ transplant recipients, including high-risk liver, pancreas, and small bowel recipients. Fluconazole prophylaxis is recommended as postoperative prophylaxis for surgical intensive care units where there is a high incidence of disseminated candidiasis. Current recommendations are now for giving prophylaxis to patients with cytotoxic chemotherapy-induced neutropenia for the duration of the neutropenia. Fluconazole, posaconazole, caspofungin, or itraconazole may be used (Chapter 308). It should be noted that fluconazole prophylaxis does not provide protection against molds.

Empiric therapy is recommended for suspected invasive candidiasis in non-neutropenic patients. Fluconazole is the primary recommendation, but the choice really depends on the hospital epidemiology with reference to the frequency of recovery of non-*albicans* species. If non-*albicans* species are frequent or if the patient has already been treated with fluconazole (or both), with or without severe illness, an echinocandin is recommended. Either a lipid formulation of amphotericin B or conventional amphotericin B (LFAMB or AMB) are alternatives. For patients at high risk of mold infections (Chapter 308), LFAMB, voriconazole, or an echinocandin are all possibilities. Voriconazole should not be used in patients who have already received prophylaxis with fluconazole.

SYSTEMIC DRUGS FOR CANDIDIASIS

Refer to Chapter 40 for more information.

Polyenes

Amphotericin B generally remains the cornerstone of therapy for disseminated and deep organ *Candida* infection, especially those infections that may be rapidly fatal or refractory to azoles or to echinocandins. In the overall longitudinal experience of treatment of *Candida* infections, most of the experience has been with amphotericin B deoxycholate (AMB-D). However, three lipid formulations of amphotericin B (LFAMB) have been approved by regulatory agencies and are used extensively now. While evidence does not exist that the LFAMBs are more efficacious for the management of candidal infections, their use has become very popular, due mainly to their lower level of renal toxicity.

Triazoles

The triazoles currently available for the treatment of *Candida* infections include fluconazole, itraconazole, voriconazole, and posaconazole. All of the triazoles have diminished activity against *C. glabrata* and *C. krusei*. Of these, fluconazole remains the primary choice, and the majority of experience has been with it. It has excellent oral absorption, which is not affected by food consumption. It is considered the standard of therapy for oropharyngeal candidiasis and esophageal and vaginal infection.[104] It also has the high penetration into the cerebral spinal fluid and ocular fluids and highest level of renal excretion. The aggressiveness for treating patients with candidemia was changed dramatically when fluconazole was found to have equal efficacy to AMB in non-neutropenic patients.[169,170] The considerably less toxicity associated with fluconazole compared to AMB and the lack of reliable diagnostic criteria for establishing the presence or absence of disseminated candidiasis in candidemic patients, made the risk-to-benefit ratio of treating highly in favor of treatment rather than watchful waiting. The use of the other triazoles for *Candida* infections is applied mainly to situations where they may have a specific advantage regarding the susceptibility of an isolate, when fluconazole has failed, or when it is desirable to cover mold infections in addition to treating *Candida*. Posaconazole does not have a primary indication for *Candida* infections and is currently not available in an intravenous form.

Echinocandins

Three echinocandins are now approved by regulatory agencies for treatment of *Candida* infections. They are caspofungin, micafungin and anidulafungin. These drugs have the advantage of low minimal inhibitory concentrations (MIC) for a broader spectrum of species of *Candida*, including *C. glabrata* and *C. krusei*. However, *C. parapsilosis* has higher MICs. The clinical significance of these higher MICs is not clear at this time. They have the disadvantage of not being available in an oral preparation.

The enchinocandins have had a very favorable toxicity profile. They have highly comparable pharmacodynamics. In patients with moderate to severe hepatic dysfunction a dose reduction is recommended for caspofungin but not for the others. In general, the three echinocandins are considered to have equal efficacy. Many clinicians prefer to use these drugs as first line therapy for patients with candidemia, until the species of *Candida* is identified, especially if their recovery of *C. glabrata* is at high rates in their institutions. The expense of these agents is relatively high.

Flucytosine

This agent is virtually never used alone for management of *Candida* infections. It is used in combination with AMB or LFAMB for *Candida* endocarditis, meningitis, hepatosplenic candidiasis, and occasionally progressive endophthalmitis. However, there are no controlled studies demonstrating an advantage with the combination therapy. It has broad-spectrum activity against the *Candida* species, except *C. krusei*.

CANDIDEMIA IN NON-NEUTROPENIC PATIENTS

The decision to administer treatment for candidemia has been discussed previously in this chapter, and the consensus that all candidemic patients should be treated with antifungals was described. For non-neutropenic patients, fluconazole or an echinocandin is recommended. If a patient has already been on fluconazole prior to the onset of the candidemia, an echinocandin is preferred. The echinocandin is also preferred for patients with moderately severe or severe illness, or if the patient is hospitalized in an institution where there is a high incidence of *C. glabrata*, or both. Fluconazole is recommended for those patients who are less seriously ill and have not been on fluconazole previously. For patients with *C. parapsilosis* and mild to moderate illness, fluconazole is recommended. Although voriconazole is effective for candidemia, it is recommended primarily as step-down oral therapy for candidemia due to *C. krusei* or cases due to voriconazole susceptible *C. glabrata*. Although controversial, removal or at least changing of intravenous lines is recommended. For patients who are clinically unstable and on a downhill trajectory, LFAMB or AMB are recommended.

CANDIDEMIA IN NEUTROPENIC PATIENTS

For most neutropenic patients, an echinocandin, LFAMB, or AMB is recommended for initial therapy. For patients who are less ill, and in whom no fluconazole prophylaxis has been given, fluconazole is an alternative. For *C. glabrata* infections, an echinocandin is preferred, but LFAMB or AMB are less desirable alternatives. However, if the patient has already been on an azole and is doing well clinically with negative follow-up cultures, the azole could be continued. For patients with *C. parapsilosis*, fluconazole, LFAMB, or AMB are alternatives. Similar to the recommendations regarding fluconazole for *C. glabrata*, if the patient has been receiving an echinocandin, is doing well clini-

cally, and follow-up cultures are negative, they could be continued on the echinocandin. For infection with *C. krusei*, an echinocandin, LFAMB, AMB, or voriconazole is preferred. Continuation of treatment for two weeks beyond the documentation of the clearance of *Candida* from the blood and the resolution of signs and symptoms of infection referable to *Candida* and resolution of the neutropenia is recommended. If possible, intravenous lines should be removed or changed.

CANDIDA INFECTIONS OF THE CARDIOVASCULAR SYSTEM

The mortality rate is lowest with combined medical and surgical therapy, compared with either medical or surgical treatment alone. Once the diagnosis of *Candida*-caused endocarditis is made, the procedure of choice is to initiate LFAMB, with or without flucytosine. Although AMB is an alternative, due to the length of postoperative therapy, a LFAMB is preferred to reduce nephrotoxicity. Valve replacement should be performed as soon as possible. The desirability of waiting for an effect of antifungal therapy before surgery is unknown and currently it is recommended to perform surgery as soon as it is logistically feasible. After surgery, antifungal therapy should be given for at least 6 to 10 weeks because of the significant incidence of relapse. At the time of removal of the valve and surrounding vegetations, the area can be washed with an amphotericin-B–containing solution (the current IDSA guidelines do not address topical application of antifungals during surgery).[171] If there is a perivalvular abscess, or other evidence of residual *Candida*, extended suppressive therapy beyond the 6 to 10 weeks should be administered. Some patients with *Candida* endocarditis have had relapses years after surgery. Patients with *Candida* endocarditis should be monitored carefully for a minimum of 2 years postoperatively. Fluconazole is commonly used as long-term suppressive therapy. Occasional cases of successful, nonsurgical therapy are reported in both adults and children.[172,173]

For prosthetic valve endocarditis, the recommendations are the same as for native valve disease. Suppressive therapy should be lifelong if it is not feasible to remove the valve. Most patients break through suppressive therapy, usually with a fatal outcome. For other forms of cardiovascular infection, such as pericarditis or myocarditis, in general, prolonged administration of LFAMB is recommended, with modifications of the therapeutic strategy made depending on the susceptibility of the isolate to fluconazole, voriconazole, or the echinocandins. For suppurative thrombophlebitis, incision and drainage of infected vein and removal of the catheter should be done in combination with the administration of the antifungal. For pacemaker and defibrillator infections, removal of the device with administration of antifungals for similar durations used for endocarditis is recommended. If only the generator or pocket is infected, four weeks of therapy following removal of the device is recommended, whereas if the wire is infected, at least 6 weeks of therapy is recommended following the wire removal. For ventricular assist devices that cannot be removed, treatment is the same as for endocarditis.

CENTRAL NERVOUS SYSTEM *CANDIDA* INFECTION

Based on analysis of current literature, combined LFAMB or AMB and 5-fluorocytosine (5-FC) therapy, without intrathecal instillation, is the most rational treatment for both meningitis and diffuse parenchymal infection. This recommendation is based entirely on observational studies. There is experimental evidence that liposomal AMB may have a higher brain concentration.[174] The clinical significance of this evidence remains to be established, but most experts use liposomal AMB in documented central nervous system infection (personal observation). In exceptionally severe cases, intrathecal antifungals should be considered. Removal and replacement of infected ventricular devices by a two-step process is recommended (Chapter 85). Indications for surgery of *Candida*-caused brain abscesses remain unclear.

CANDIDA PERITONITIS, GALLBLADDER INFECTION, AND INTRA-ABDOMINAL ABSCESSES

Candida peritonitis due to peritoneal dialysis of adults, if there is no evidence of spread to other organs, may respond to instillation of local amphotericin B at a concentration of 2 to 4 µg/ml in dialysate fluid.[175] However, many patients experience pain with this treatment. Local inflammation from amphotericin may decrease the dialysis surface area by causing adhesions. Successful treatment with fluconazole has been reported.[176,177] Removal of the catheter is almost always necessary.[177,178] However, there are few reports of successful treatment without catheter removal.[179,180] The topic of fungal peritonitis has been reviewed recently without change in the basic therapeutic strategies outlined here.[181]

Candida coming from an abdominal drain placed at the time of GI surgery should not ordinarily prompt antifungal therapy.[152] The topic of when to begin therapy in patients with an abdominal drain that grows *Candida* on culture and the controversy regarding therapy has been discussed and reviewed in detail recently.[132] In general, there has been a lowering in the threshold for treating such patients, but the impact of treatment on their clinical outcome remains to be fully defined. Discovery of *Candida* in ascites from an undrained abdomen usually means that therapy is required. Hematogenous dissemination from the peritoneum can occur. Fluconazole prophylaxis has been successful in preventing the development of *Candida* peritonitis in a population of high-risk surgical patients with interruption of the integrity of the gastrointestinal tract.[182] *Candida* has been a cause of peritonitis in association with peritoneal dialysis, and there is substantial experience of treating it without removal of the dialysis catheter.[183]

Historically, the failure rate for the cure of hepatosplenic candidiasis has been high with both amphotericin B alone and in combination with 5-FC. Currently, LFAMB or AMB is recommended for patients who are moderately ill or have refractory disease. While fluconazole alone has been recommended for patients who are stable, an attractive alternative is to initiate therapy with either a LFAMB or AMB for two weeks followed by long-term oral fluconazole. Reports of cures with liposomal amphotericin, caspofungin, and LFAMB have appeared and are promising.[184-186] In some instances, splenectomy may be necessary for large or refractory abscesses. Recently the use of adjuvant corticosteroid therapy has been addressed in a large study, and favorable results were obtained in refractory cases.[187]

Candida-caused cholecystitis may respond to intravenous amphotericin B or fluconazole.[188] In candidiasis of the gallbladder or biliary tract, drainage may be necessary[189] in addition to antifungal therapy. *Candida* may complicate necrotizing pancreatitis and has been an increasing cause of pancreatitis. This entity should be treated with either LFAMB or AMB until the patient is stable. The role of follow-up or primary therapy with the newer agents is not clear at present (author's opinion). *Candida* pancreatic abscess has been successfully drained with computed tomography–guided percutaneous aspiration in addition to systemic antifungal therapy.

URINARY CANDIDIASIS

Postcatheterization asymptomatic candiduria usually resolves without specific antifungal therapy. Current recommendations are to not treat it unless the patient is symptomatic or in a high-risk group for dissemination. These groups include symptomatic patients, neutropenic patients, renal transplant patients, low-birth-weight infants, and patients who are undergoing urinary tract manipulations. Local amphotericin (a solution of 50 mg of amphotericin B in 1 liter of sterile water infused at 40 ml/hour through a Foley catheter) was used extensively in the past but has become unpopular due to the efficacy of oral fluconazole (200-400 mg/d for 7-14 days). However, it may be useful still for patients with resistant *Candida*, especially *C. glabrata*. For fluconazole-resistant isolates, LFAMB or AMB with or without flucytosine or voriconazole are alternatives.[104] Treatment should be continued until cultures are negative and the patient is asymptomatic. Selected patients may require irrigation with amphotericin B through nephrostomy tubes placed directly in the collecting systems. If fungus balls form in the urinary tract, they require surgical removal. For kidney involvement, intravenous LFAMB or AMB is indicated. However, oral fluconazole may be an alternative in patients with mild to moderate infection. The drug is excreted in high concentration in the urine. 5-FC is another alternative, but less popular, especially in patients with renal insufficiency, and resistance may develop. Any stents, catheters, or other prosthetic materials in the urinary tract should be removed in order to prevent recurrence.

Eradication of candiduria in patients who require a persistent indwelling Foley catheter is particularly problematic. A placebo-controlled trial found that fluconazole at 200mg/d for 14 days resulted in eradication of the candiduria, but there was a high rate of recurrence, suggesting the futility of antifungal therapy.[190] A large observational study has also verified the futility of antifungal therapy.[191] Alternatively, it is possible that the urinary tract may be a source for hematogenous dissemination, and the presence of candiduria may indicate hematogenous seeding to the kidney and widespread disseminated candidiasis. The selection of patients requiring persistent indwelling Foley catheters and the approach to their therapy must be individualized according to their clinical setting. As long as the Foley catheter remains in place, the goal of eradicating the candiduria may be impossible to attain. More data is necessary to determine the role of the newer of the azoles under development and of caspofungin.

MUCOCUTANEOUS CANDIDIASIS

Oral thrush should be treated with topical agents whenever possible. The least expensive is nystatin. The usual adult dose is 4-6 ml of 100,000 units/ml four times daily. Clotrimazole 10-mg troches given five times per day is an attractive alternative. Clotrimazole is approximately equally as effective as nystatin but is not bitter like nystatin. For more severe or refractory disease, oral fluconazole at 100-200 mg daily is recommended. For cases that are refractory to fluconazole, itraconazole solution or posaconazole suspension are alternatives. In patients with AIDS, chronic suppressive therapy may be necessary with fluconazole. Intermittent suppression is associated with higher success rates and a lower level of development of resistance. Therapy for denture sore mouth is the same as that for thrush, with the addition of meticulous cleaning of the dentures and correction of ill-fitting plates. Angular cheilitis, which is frequently associated with denture sore mouth, should be treated with either topical clotrimazole or miconazole cream.

The diagnosis of *Candida* esophagitis can be made presumptively on the basis of the presence of oral pharyngeal thrush and symptoms of esophagitis in patients with AIDS or cancer, and a trial with systemic antifungals is considered appropriate prior to endoscopic confirmation of the diagnosis. Topical therapy with clotrimazole troches, amphotericin B suspension, or nystatin suspension usually fails. Treatment with fluconazole or itraconazole capsules is recommended. Ketoconazole has lost popularity. Fluconazole is considered superior to itraconazole capsules, but itraconazole solution is considered comparable to fluconazole.

For refractory esophagitis, itraconazole solution is considered the first-choice strategy. Posaconazole suspension and voriconazole are alternatives. If necessary, intravenous therapy with LFAMB, AMB, or the echinocandins may be used. In refractory esophageal infections, low-dose (10-20 mg/day) intravenous amphotericin B has been successful.[192] Long-term suppressive therapy may be necessary in patients with AIDS.[193]

Candida intertrigo is most successfully managed by decreasing the moisture of the involved area and by the application of amphotericin B lotion or nystatin cream several times a day or topical miconazole or clotrimazole. Management of *Candida* diaper rash has been successful with nystatin powder or cream in combination with a corticosteroid, such as Mycolog-II cream. Amphotericin cream or lotion may also be used. The same agents used for diaper rash are generally successful for pruritus ani.

Uncomplicated *Candida* vaginitis responds to short courses of topical or oral therapy in the vast majority of patients. The following regimens used from 1 to 7 days are considered comparable: clotrimazole (over the counter); butoconazole (over the counter); miconazole (over the counter); tioconazole (over the counter); terconazole; oral azoles (ketoconazole, 400 mg twice daily for 5 days [not approved in the United States]); itraconazole, 200 mg twice daily for 1 day or 200 mg a day for 3 days (not approved in the United States); and fluconazole, 150 mg once orally.[194] Other regimens include nystatin, 100,000 units daily for 2 weeks, and boric acid, 600 mg in a gelatin capsule once daily (vaginal) for 14 days.[195] Recurrent *Candida* vaginitis requires eradication of causal factors as much as possible. Then treatment for 2 weeks with topical or oral azoles should be used, followed by 6 months of fluconazole, of which 150 mg orally per week is recommended. This topic has been reviewed comprehensively.[73]

Candida-caused paronychia is best managed by preventing immersion of the hands in water as much as possible and applying clotrimazole or miconazole cream twice daily. Drainage is also important.

CHRONIC MUCOCUTANEOUS CANDIDIASIS

Topical therapy to skin and mucous membranes achieves only slight improvement in this disease. Intravenous amphotericin B therapy has been effective, but nearly all patients relapse. Oral 5-FC has not been effective. The most important advance in the therapy of this disease is systemically administered azoles: ketoconazole, fluconazole, or itraconazole.[41] Fluconazole is recommended as the primary therapy.[104]

Numerous reports illustrate successful treatment. Therapy for months or years may be necessary. Development of resistance with long-term therapy is a potential problem. Those patients should be treated similarly to AIDS patients with chronic fluconazole refractory *Candida* infections.

OCULAR CANDIDIASIS

The distinction between the treatment of chorioretinitis and endophthalmitis due to *Candida* is critical and well described in Chapter 112. Whereas chorioretinitis usually responds to systemic therapy alone, endophthalmitis may require intravitreal therapy in addition to systemic therapy, particularly in the presence of a vitreous abscess.[196-197] Often, pars plana vitrectomy provides vitreal fluid for confirmation of diagnosis, offers a means of administering intravitreal therapy, and removes fungal masses from the vitreous.

MISCELLANEOUS *CANDIDA*-CAUSED INFECTIONS

The topic of *Candida* laryngeal infection has been reviewed.[198,199] Most patients have been managed with intravenous amphotericin B. Fluconazole may be appropriate as follow-up therapy. The medical treatment of *Candida* epididymo-orchitis occasionally suffices, but most patients have required drainage or orchiectomy.[200] Most cases of *Candida* pneumonia have been treated with amphotericin B. There is a paucity of information on treatment of this entity. Most patients who have isolates of *Candida* from the respiratory tract do not need specific treatment.[104,201] However, in patients who have had lung transplantation, there is a concern for infection of the transplanted lung and infection at the sites of surgical manipulations.[201]

REFERENCES

1. Langenbeck B. Auffingung von Pilzen aus der Schleimhaut der Speiseröhre einer Typhus-Leiche. *Neue Not Geb Natur Heilk (Froriep).* 1839;12:145-147.
2. Rippon JW. Candidiasis and the pathogenic yeasts. In: *Medical Mycology, The Pathogenic Fungi and the Pathogenic Actinomycetes.* Philadelphia: WB Saunders; 1988:532-581.
3. Joachim H, Polayes S. Subacute endocarditis and systemic mycosis (monilia). *JAMA.* 1940;115:205-208.
4. Pappas PG. Invasive candidiasis. *Infect Dis Clin North Am.* 2006;20:485-506.
5. Zilberberg MD, Shorr AF, Kollef MH. Secular Trends in Candidemia-Related Hospitalization in the United States, 2000-2005. *Infect Control Hosp Epidemiol.* 2008.
6. Morgan J, Meltzer MI, Plikaytis BD, et al. Excess mortality, hospital stay, and cost due to candidemia: a case-control study using data from population-based candidemia surveillance. *Infect Control Hosp Epidemiol.* 2005;26:540-547.
7. Miller LG, Hajjeh RA, Edwards JE Jr. Estimating the cost of nosocomial candidemia in the United States. *Clin Infect Dis.* 2001;32:1110.
8. Wisplinghoff H, Bischoff T, Tallent SM, et al. Nosocomial bloodstream infections in US hospitals: analysis of 24,179 cases from a prospective nationwide surveillance study. *Clin Infect Dis.* 2004;39:309-317.
9. Davis SL, Vazquez JA, McKinnon PS. Epidemiology, risk factors, and outcomes of *Candida albicans* versus non-albicans candidemia in nonneutropenic patients. *Ann Pharmacother.* 2007;41:568-573.
10. Tortorano AM, Kibbler C, Peman J, et al. Candidaemia in Europe: epidemiology and resistance. *Int J Antimicrob Agents.* 2006;27:359-366.
11. Bassetti M, Righi E, Tumbarello M, et al. *Candida* infections in the intensive care unit: epidemiology, risk factors and therapeutic strategies. *Expert Rev Anti Infect Ther.* 2006;4:875-885.
12. Sobel JD. The Emergence of Non-albicans *Candida* Species as Causes of Invasive Candidiasis and Candidemia. *Curr Infect Dis Rep.* 2006;8:427-433.
13. Hannula J, Saarela M, Dogan B, et al. Comparison of virulence factors of oral *Candida dubliniensis* and *Candida albicans* isolates in healthy people and patients with chronic candidosis. *Oral Microbiol Immunol.* 2000;15:238-244.
14. Pfaller MA, Diekema DJ, Messer SA, et al. In vitro activities of voriconazole, posaconazole, and four licensed systemic antifungal agents against *Candida* species infrequently isolated from blood. *J Clin Microbiol.* 2003;41:78-83.
15. Zhou X, Kong F, Sorrell TC, et al. Practical method for detection and identification of *Candida, Aspergillus,* and *Scedosporium* spp. by use of rolling-circle amplification. *J Clin Microbiol.* 2008;46:2423-2427.

16. Alexander BD, Ashley ED, Reller LB, et al. Cost savings with implementation of PNA FISH testing for identification of *Candida albicans* in blood cultures. *Diagn Microbiol Infect Dis.* 2006;54:277-282.
17. Odds FC, Jacobsen MD. Multilocus sequence typing of pathogenic *Candida* species. *Eukaryot Cell.* 2008;7:1075-1084.
18. Marol S, Yucesoy M. Molecular epidemiology of *Candida* species isolated from clinical specimens of intensive care unit patients. *Mycoses.* 2008;51:40-49.
19. Garland JS, Alex CP, Sevallius JM, et al. Cohort study of the pathogenesis and molecular epidemiology of catheter-related bloodstream infection in neonates with peripherally inserted central venous catheters. *Infect Control Hosp Epidemiol.* 2008;29:243-249.
20. Asmundsdottir LR, Erlendsdottir H, Haraldsson G, et al. Molecular epidemiology of candidemia: evidence of clusters of smoldering nosocomial infections. *Clin Infect Dis.* 2008;47:e17-e24.
21. Ibrahim AS, Magee BB, Sheppard DC, et al. Effects of ploidy and mating type on virulence of *Candida albicans. Infect Immun.* 2005;73:7366-7374.
22. Magee BB, Magee PT. Induction of mating in *Candida albicans* by construction of MTLa and MTLalpha strains. *Science.* 2000;289:310-313.
23. Hull CM, Raisner RM, Johnson AD. Evidence for mating of the "asexual" yeast *Candida albicans* in a mammalian host. *Science.* 2000;289:307-310.
24. Romani L. Innate and Acquired Cellular Immunity to Fungi. In: Heitman J, Filler SG, Edwards JE Jr, Mitchell AP, eds. *Molecular Principles of Fungal Pathogenesis.* Washington, D.C.: American Society for Microbiology; 2006:471-486.
25. Fernandes L, Bocca AL, Ribeiro AM, et al. In: *Pathogenic Fungi: Insights in Molecular Biology.* Horizon Scientific Press; Caister Academic Press; 2008.
26. Blanco JL, Garcia ME. Immune response to fungal infections. *Vet Immunol Immunopathol.* 2008;125:47-70.
27. Vonk AG, Netea MG, van der Meer JW, et al. Host defence against disseminated *Candida albicans* infection and implications for antifungal immunotherapy. *Expert Opin Biol Ther.* 2006;6:891-903.
28. Kang SS, Kauls LS, Gaspari AA. Toll-like receptors: applications to dermatologic disease. *J Am Acad Dermatol.* 2006;54:951-983; quiz 83-86.
29. Lopez-Garcia B, Lee PH, Yamasaki K, et al. Anti-fungal activity of cathelicidins and their potential role in *Candida albicans* skin infection. *J Invest Dermatol.* 2005;125:108-115.
30. Vilanova M, Correia A. Host defense mechanisms in invasive candidiasis originating in the GI tract. *Expert Rev Anti Infect Ther.* 2008;6:441-445.

31. Fidel PL Jr. History and update on host defense against vaginal candidiasis. *Am J Reprod Immunol.* 2007;57:2-12.
32. Romani L, Montagnoli C, Bozza S, et al. The exploitation of distinct recognition receptors in dendritic cells determines the full range of host immune relationships with *Candida albicans. Int Immunol.* 2004;16:149-161.
33. Gank KD, Yeaman MR, Kojima S, et al. SSD1 is integral to host defense peptide resistance in *Candida albicans. Eukaryot Cell.* 2008;7:1318-1327.
34. Barker KS, Park H, Phan QT, et al. Transcriptome profile of the vascular endothelial cell response to *Candida albicans. J Infect Dis.* 2008;198:193-202.
35. Yeaman MR, Cheng D, Desai B, et al. Susceptibility to thrombin-induced platelet microbicidal protein is associated with increased fluconazole efficacy against experimental endocarditis due to *Candida albicans. Antimicrob Agents Chemother.* 2004;48:3051-3056.
36. Robert R, Senet JM, Mahaza C, et al. Molecular basis of the interactions between *Candida albicans,* fibrinogen, and platelets. *J Mycol Med.* 1992;2:19-25.
37. Levitz SM, Diamond RD. Killing of aspergillus fumigatus spores and *Candida albicans* yeast phase by the iron-hydrogen peroxide-iodide cytotoxic system: Comparison with the myeloperoxidase-hydrogen peroxide-halide system. *Infection and Immunity.* 1984;43:1100-1102.
38. Ganz T, Selsted ME, Szklark D, et al. Natural peptide antibiotics of human neutrophils. *Journal of Clinical Investigation.* 1985;76:1427-1435.
39. Roilides E, Lyman CA, Sein T, et al. Antifungal activity of splenic, liver and pulmonary macrophages against *Candida albicans* and effects of macrophage colony-stimulating factor. *Medical Mycology.* 2000;38:161-168.
40. Spellberg B, Edwards JE. The Pathophysiology and Treatment of *Candida* Sepsis. *Curr Infect Dis Rep.* 2002;4:387-399.
41. Kirkpatrick CH. Chronic mucocutaneous candidiasis. *Pediatr Infect Dis J.* 2001;20:197-206.
42. Lee KW, Balish E. Systemic candidiasis in germ free, flora-defined and conventional mice. *J Reticuloendothel Soc.* 1981;29:71-77.
43. Hodgetts S, Nooney L, Al-Akeel R, et al. Efungumab and caspofungin: pre-clinical data supporting synergy. *J Antimicrob Chemother.* 2008;61:1132-1139.
44. Pachl J, Svoboda P, Jacobs F, et al. A randomized, blinded, multicenter trial of lipid-associated amphotericin B alone versus in combination with an antibody-based inhibitor of heat shock protein 90 in patients with invasive candidiasis. *Clin Infect Dis.* 2006;42:1404-1413.

45. Matthews RC, Burnie JP. Human recombinant antibody to HSP90: a natural partner in combination therapy. *Curr Mol Med*. 2005;5:403-411.
46. Cutler JE, Granger BL, Han Y. Immunoprotection against candidiasis, Chapter 17. In: Calderone RA, ed. *Candida and Candidiasis*. Washington, D.C.: American Society for Microbiology; 2002:243-256.
47. Louria DB, Smith JK, Brayton RG, et al. Anti-*Candida* factors in serum and their inhibitors: I. Clinical and laboratory observations. *Journal of Infectious Diseases*. 1972;125:102-114.
48. Ashman RB, Papadimitriou JM, Fulurija A, et al. Role of complement C5 and T lymphocytes in pathogenesis of disseminated and mucosal candidiasis in susceptible DBA/2 mice. *Microb Pathog*. 2003;34:103-113.
49. Gelfand JA, Hurley DL, Fauci AS, et al. Role of complement in host defense against experimental disseminated candidiasis. *Journal of Infectious Diseases*. 1978;139:9.
50. Kozel TR, Brown RR, Pformmer GS. Activation and binding of C3 by *Candida albicans*. *Infection and Immunity*. 1987;55: 1890-1894.
51. Hostetter MK. Adhesins and ligands involved in the interaction of *Candida* spp. with epithelial and endothelial surfaces. *Clin Microbiol Rev*. 1994;7:29-42.
52. Edwards JE Jr, Gaither TA, O'Shea JJ, et al. Expression of specific binding sites on *Candida* with functional and antigenic characteristics of human complement receptors. *Journal of Immunology*. 1986;137:3577-3583.
53. Heitman J, Filler SG, Edwards JE Jr, et al., eds. *Molecular Principles of Fungal Pathogenesis*. Washington, D.C.: American Society for Microbiology Press; 2006.
54. Lehrer RI. Inhibition by sulfonamides of the Candidacidal activity of human neutrophils. *Journal of Clinical Investigation*. 1971;50:2498-2505.
55. Krause W, Matheis H, Wulf K. Fungemia and funguria after oral administration of *Candida albicans*. *Lancet*. 1969;1:598-599.
56. Stone HH, Kolb LD, Currie CA, et al. *Candida* sepsis: Pathogenesis and principles of treatment. *Ann Surg*. 1974:697-711.
57. Nobile CJ, Schneider HA, Nett JE, et al. Complementary adhesin function in *C. albicans* biofilm formation. *Curr Biol*. 2008;18: 1017-1024.
58. Dominic RM, Shenoy S, Baliga S. *Candida* biofilms in medical devices: Evolving trends. *Kathmandu Univ Med J (KUMJ)*. 2007;5:431-436.
59. Viale P, Stefani S. Vascular catheter-associated infections: a microbiological and therapeutic update. *J Chemother*. 2006; 18:235-249.
60. Kumar CP, Menon T. Biofilm production by clinical isolates of *Candida* species. *Med Mycol*. 2006;44:99-101.
61. Davies AN, Brailsford SR, Beighton D, et al. Oral candidosis in community-based patients with advanced cancer. *J Pain Symptom Manage*. 2008;35:508-514.
62. Villar CC, Kashleva H, Nobile CJ, et al. Mucosal tissue invasion by *Candida albicans* is associated with E-cadherin degradation, mediated by transcription factor Rim101p and protease Sap5p. *Infect Immun*. 2007;75:2126-2135.
63. Shen YZ, Qi TK, Ma JX, et al. Invasive fungal infections among inpatients with acquired immune deficiency syndrome at a Chinese university hospital. *Mycoses*. 2007;50:475-480.
64. Lehner T. Classification and clinico-pathological features of *Candida* infections in the mouth. In: Winner HI, Hurley R, eds. *Symposium on Candida Infections*. Edinburgh: Churchill Livingstone; 1966:119-137.
65. Terai H, Shimahara M. Cheilitis as a variation of *Candida*-associated lesions. *Oral Dis*. 2006;12:349-352.
66. Vigneswaran N, Anderson GB. Oral and maxillofacial pathology case of the month. Oral candidiasis associated with inhaled corticosteroid use. *Tex Dent J*. 2006;123(618):22-23.
67. Mimidis K, Papadopoulos V, Margaritis V, et al. Predisposing factors and clinical symptoms in HIV-negative patients with *Candida* oesophagitis: are they always present? *Int J Clin Pract*. 2005;59:210-213.
68. Staib P, Kretschmar M, Nichterlein T, et al. Differential activation of a *Candida albicans* virulence gene family during infection. *Proc Natl Acad Sci U S A*. 2000;97:6102-6107.
69. Vazquez JA, Sobel JD. Mucosal candidiasis. *Infect Dis Clin North Am*. 2002;16:793-820, v.
70. Naglik JR, Fidel PL Jr, Odds FC. Animal models of mucosal *Candida* infection. *FEMS Microbiol Lett*. 2008;283:129-139.
71. Koh AY, Kohler JR, Coggshall KT, et al. Mucosal damage and neutropenia are required for *Candida albicans* dissemination. *PLoS Pathog*. 2008;4:e35.
72. Cassone A, De Bernardis F, Santoni G. Anticandidal immunity and vaginitis: novel opportunities for immune intervention. *Infect Immun*. 2007;75:4675-4686.
73. Sobel JD. Vulvovaginal candidosis. *Lancet*. 2007;369:1961-1971.
74. Fidel PL Jr. The protective immune response against vaginal candidiasis: lessons learned from clinical studies and animal models. *Int Rev Immunol*. 2002;21:515-548.
75. Ringdahl EN. Recurrent vulvovaginal candidiasis. *Mo Med*. 2006;103:165-168.
76. Meyer H, Goettlicher S, Mendling W. Stress as a cause of chronic recurrent vulvovaginal candidosis and the effectiveness of the conventional antimycotic therapy. *Mycoses*. 2006;49:202-209.
77. Ventolini G, Baggish MS. Post-menopausal recurrent vaginal candidiasis: effect of hysterectomy on response to treatment, type of colonization and recurrence rates post-treatment. *Maturitas*. 2005;51:294-298.
78. Farage MA, Stadler A. Risk factors for recurrent vulvovaginal candidiasis. *Am J Obstet Gynecol*. 2005;192:981-982; author reply 2-3.
79. Aldana-Valenzuela C, Morales-Marquec M, Castellanos-Martinez J, et al. Congenital candidiasis: a rare and unpredictable disease. *J Perinatol*. 2005;25:680-682.
80. Adler A, Litmanovitz I, Regev R, et al. Breakthrough *Candida* Infection in a preterm infant with congenital cutaneous *Candida albicans* infection. *Am J Perinatol*. 2005;22:169-172.
81. Domonkos AN, Arnold HL Jr, Odom RB. Disease due to fungi. In: Domonkos AN, Arnold HL Jr, Odom RB, eds. *Andrews' Diseases of the Skin Clinical Dermatology*. Philadelphia: WB Saunders; 1982:341-403.
82. Adams SP. Dermacase. Erosio interdigitalis blastomycetica. *Can Fam Physician*. 2002;48:271, 7.
83. Kapdagli H, Ozturk G, Dereli T, et al. *Candida* folliculitis mimicking tinea barbae. *Int J Dermatol*. 1997;36:295-297.
84. Scheinfeld NS. Obesity and dermatology. *Clin Dermatol*. 2004;22:303-309.
85. Edwards S. Balanitis and balanoposthitis: a review [see comments]. *Genitourin Med*. 1996;72:155-159.
86. Mayser P. Mycotic infections of the penis. *Andrologia*. 1999;31(Suppl 1):13-16.
87. Darcis JM, Etienne M, Demonty J. *Candida albicans* Septicemia in Heroin Addicts. *American Journal of Dermatopathology*. 1986;8:501-504.
88. Bodey GP, Luna M. Skin lesions associated with disseminated candidiasis. *JAMA*. 1974;229:1466-1468.
89. Agarwal S, Sharma M, Mehndirata V. Solitary ecthyma gangrenosum (EG)-like lesion consequent to *Candida albicans* in a neonate. *Indian J Pediatr*. 2007;74:582-584.
90. Leslie KS, McCann BG, Levell NJ. Candidal ecthyma gangrenosum in a patient with malnutrition. *Br J Dermatol*. 2005;153: 847-848.
91. Silverman RA, Rhodes AR, Dennehy PH. Disseminated intravascular coagulation and purpura fulminans in a patient with *Candida* sepsis. Biopsy of purpura fulminans as an aid to diagnosis of systemic *Candida* infections. *American Journal of Medicine*. 1986;80:679-684.
92. Glaich AS, Krathen RA, Smith MJ, et al. Disseminated candidiasis mimicking leukocytoclastic vasculitis. *J Am Acad Dermatol*. 2005;53:544-546.
93. Dorko E, Jautova J, Pilipcinec E, et al. Occurrence of *Candida* strains in cases of paronychia. *Folia Microbiol (Praha)*. 2004;49:591-595.
94. Hay RJ. Antifungal therapy of yeast infections. *J Am Acad Dermatol*. 1994;31:S6-S9.
95. Concannon P, Gisoldi E, Phillips S, et al. Diaper dermatitis: a therapeutic dilemma. Results of a double-blind placebo controlled trial of miconazole nitrate 0.25%. *Pediatr Dermatol*. 2001;18:149-155.
96. Kranke B, Trummer M, Brabek E, et al. Etiologic and causative factors in perianal dermatitis: results of a prospective study in 126 patients. *Wien Klin Wochenschr*. 2006;118:90-94.
97. Kalfa VC, Roberts RL, Stiehm ER. The syndrome of chronic mucocutaneous candidiasis with selective antibody deficiency. *Ann Allergy Asthma Immunol*. 2003;90:259-264.
98. Perniola R, Congedo M, Rizzo A, et al. Innate and adaptive immunity in patients with autoimmune polyendocrinopathy-candidiasis-ectodermal dystrophy. *Mycoses*. 2008;51:228-235.
99. Perheentupa J. Autoimmune polyendocrinopathy-candidiasis-ectodermal dystrophy. *J Clin Endocrinol Metab*. 2006;91: 2843-2850.
99a. Michels AW, Eisenbarth GS. Autoimmune polyendocrine syndrome type 1 (APS-1) as a model for understanding autoimmune polyendocrine syndrome type 2 (APS-2). *J Intern Med*. 2009;265:530-540.
100. Meager A, Visvalingam K, Peterson P, et al. Anti-interferon autoantibodies in autoimmune polyendocrinopathy syndrome type 1. *PLoS Med*. 2006;3:e289.
101. Chapman SW, Daniel CR. Cutaneous manifestations of fungal infection. *Infect Dis Clin North Am*. 1994;8:879-910.
102. Verduyn Lunel FM, Voss A, Kuijper EJ, et al. Detection of the *Candida* antigen mannan in cerebrospinal fluid specimens from patients suspected of having *Candida* meningitis. *J Clin Microbiol*. 2004;42:867-870.
103. Wood GC, Mueller EW, Croce MA, et al. *Candida* sp. isolated from bronchoalveolar lavage: clinical significance in critically ill trauma patients. *Intensive Care Med*. 2006;32:599-603.
104. Pappas PG, Kauffman CA, Andes D, et al. Clinical practice guidelines for the management of candidiasis: 2009 update by the Infectious Diseases Society of America. *Clin Infect Dis*. 2009;48:503-535.
105. Ko SC, Chen KY, Hsueh PR, et al. Fungal empyema thoracis: an emerging clinical entity. *Chest*. 2000;117:1672-1678.
106. Franklin WG, Simon AB, Sodeman TM. *Candida* myocarditis without valvulitis. *Am J Cardiol*. 1976;38:924-928.
107. Rubin RH, Moellering RC. Clinical microbiologic and therapeutic aspects of purulent pericarditis. *American Journal of Medicine*. 1975;59:68-78.
108. Reyes MP, Lerner AM. Endocarditis caused by *Candida* species. In: Bodeg GP, Fainstein V, eds. *Candidiasis*. New York: Raven Press; 1985:203-209.
109. Varghese GM, Sobel JD. Fungal endocarditis. *Curr Infect Dis Rep*. 2008;10:275-279.
110. Baddley JW, Benjamin DK Jr, Patel M, et al. *Candida* infective endocarditis. *Eur J Clin Microbiol Infect Dis*. 2008;27:519-529.
111. Hauser M, Hess J, Belohradsky BH. Treatment of *Candida albicans* endocarditis: case report and a review. *Infection*. 2003;31:125-127.
112. Carr MJ, Clarke S, O'Connell F, et al. First reported case of endocarditis caused by *Candida* dubliniensis. *J Clin Microbiol*. 2005;43:3023-3026.
113. Odds FC. *Candida* endocarditis, myocarditis, and other cardiovascular *Candida* infections. In: *Candida and Candidosis A review and bibliography*. London: Bailliere Tindall; 1988: 175-180.
114. Yeaman MR, Soldan SS, Ghannoum MA, et al. Resistance to platelet microbicidal protein results in increased severity of experimental *Candida albicans* endocarditis. *Infection and Immunity*. 1996;64:1379-1384.
115. Calderone RA, Scheld WM. Role of fibronectin in the pathogenesis of candidal infections. *Reviews of Infectious Diseases*. 1987;9: S400-S403.
116. Galgiani JN, Stevens DA. Fungal endocarditis: need for guidelines in evaluating therapy. *J Thorac Cardiovasc Surg*. 1977; 73:293-296.
117. Seelig MS, Speth CP, Kozinn PJ, et al. Patterns of *Candida* endocarditis following cardiac surgery. *Importance of early diagnosis and therapy (an analysis of 91 cases)*. 1974;27:125-160.
118. Toya SP, Schraufnagel DE, Tzelepis GE. Candiduria in intensive care units: association with heavy colonization and candidaemia. *J Hosp Infect*. 2007;66:201-206.
119. Paul N, Mathai E, Abraham OC, et al. Factors associated with candiduria and related mortality. *J Infect*. 2007;55: 450-455.
120. Binelli CA, Moretti ML, Assis RS, et al. Investigation of the possible association between nosocomial candiduria and candidaemia. *Clin Microbiol Infect*. 2006;12:538-543.
121. Kauffman CA. Candiduria. *Clin Infect Dis*. 2005;41(Suppl 6):S371-S376.
122. Wise GJ, Shteynshlyuger A. How to diagnose and treat fungal infections in chronic prostatitis. *Curr Urol Rep*. 2006;7: 320-328.
123. Mahlknecht A, Pecorari V, Richter A. Sepsis due to asymptomatic *Candida* prostatitis. *Arch Ital Urol Androl*. 2005;77: 155-156.
124. Toshikuni N, Ujike K, Yanagawa T, et al. *Candida albicans* endophthalmitis after extracorporeal shock wave lithotripsy in a patient with liver cirrhosis. *Intern Med*. 2006;45:1327-1332.
125. Kamaliah MD, Bhajan MA, Dzarr GA. Emphysematous pyelonephritis caused by *Candida* infection. *Southeast Asian J Trop Med Public Health*. 2005;36:725-727.
126. Singh CR, Lytle WF. Cystitis emphysematosa caused by *Candida* tropicalis. *J Urol*. 1983;130:1171-1173.
127. Sultana SR, McNeill SA, Phillips G, et al. Candidal urinary tract infection as a cause of pneumaturia. *J R Coll Surg Edinb*. 1998;43: 198-199.
128. Shaikh Z, Shaikh S, Pujol F, et al. *Candida tropicalis* osteomyelitis: case report and review of literature. *Am J Med*. 2005; 118:795-798.
129. Arias F, Mata-Essayag S, Landaeta ME, et al. *Candida albicans* osteomyelitis: case report and literature review. *Int J Infect Dis*. 2004;8:307-314.
130. Lerch K, Kalteis T, Schubert T, et al. Prosthetic joint infections with osteomyelitis due to *Candida albicans*. *Mycoses*. 2003; 46:462-466.
131. Hansen BL, Andersen K. Fungal arthritis. *A review*. 1995; 24:248-250.
132. Blot SI, Vandewoude KH, De Waele JJ. *Candida* peritonitis. *Curr Opin Crit Care*. 2007;13:195-199.
133. Rex JH. *Candida* in the peritoneum: passenger or pathogen? *Crit Care Med*. 2006;34:902-903.
134. Montravers P, Dupont H, Gauzit R, et al. *Candida* as a risk factor for mortality in peritonitis. *Crit Care Med*. 2006;34: 646-652.
135. Domagk D, Fegeler W, Conrad B, et al. Biliary tract candidiasis: diagnostic and therapeutic approaches in a case series. *Am J Gastroenterol*. 2006;101:2530-2536.
136. Edwards JE Jr. Ocular manifestations of *Candida* septicemia: review of seventy-six cases of hematogenous *Candida* endophthalmitis. *Medicine*. 1974;53:47.
137. Shah CP, McKey J, Spirn MJ, et al. Ocular candidiasis: a review. *Br J Ophthalmol*. 2008;92:466-468.
138. Ness T, Pelz K, Hansen LL. Endogenous endophthalmitis: microorganisms, disposition and prognosis. *Acta Ophthalmol Scand*. 2007;85:852-856.
139. Mehta S, Jiandani P, Desai M. Ocular lesions in disseminated candidiasis. *J Assoc Physicians India*. 2007;55:483-485.
140. Khan FA, Slain D, Khakoo RA. *Candida* endophthalmitis: focus on current and future antifungal treatment options. *Pharmacotherapy*. 2007;27:1711-1721.
141. Gregori NZ, Flynn HW Jr, Miller D, et al. Clinical features, management strategies, and visual acuity outcomes of *Candida* endophthalmitis following cataract surgery. *Ophthalmic Surg Lasers Imaging*. 2007;38:378-385.
142. Brooks RG. Prospective study of *Candida* endophthalmitis in hospitalized patients with candidemia. *Archives of Internal Medicine*. 1989;149:2226-2228.

143. Fisher RG, Gary Karlowicz M, Lall-Trail J. Very low prevalence of endophthalmitis in very low birth weight infants who survive candidemia. *J Perinatol.* 2005;25:408-411.

144. Noyola DE, Bohra L, Paysse EA, et al. Association of candidemia and retinopathy of prematurity in very low birth weight infants. *Ophthalmology.* 2002;109:80-84.

145. Henderson DK, Hockey LB, Vukalcic LJ, et al. Effect of immunosuppression on the development of experimental hematogenous *Candida* endophthalmitis. *Infection and Immunity.* 1980;27:628-631.

146. Ponton J, Moragues MD, Guillermo Q. Non-culture-based diagnosis. Chapter 27. In: Calderone RA, ed. *Candida and Candidiasis.* Washington, D.C.: American Society for Microbiology; 2002:395-425.

147. Edwards JE Jr. Invasive *Candida* Infections. *N Engl J Med.* 1991;324:1060-1062.

148. Mitsutake K, Miyazaki T, Tashiro T, et al. Enolase antigen, mannan antigen, Cand-Tec antigen, and beta-glucan in patients with candidemia. *Journal of Clinical Microbiology.* 1996;34: 1918-1921.

149. Senn L, Robinson JO, Schmidt S, et al. 1,3-Beta-D-glucan antigenemia for early diagnosis of invasive fungal infections in neutropenic patients with acute leukemia. *Clin Infect Dis.* 2008;46:878-885.

150. Krick JA, Remington JS. Opportunistic invasive fungal infections in patients with leukemia and lymphoma. *Clin Haematol.* 1976;5:249-310.

151. Young RC, Bennett JE, Geelhoed GW, et al. Fungemia with compromised host resistance. A study of 70 cases. *Annals of Internal Medicine.* 1974;80:605-612.

152. Edwards JE Jr, Bodey GP, Bowden RA, et al. International Conference for the Development of a Consensus on the Management and Prevention of Severe Candidal Infections [see comments]. *Clinical Infectious Diseases.* 1997;25: 43-59.

153. Hockey LJ, Fujita NK, Gibson TR, et al. Detection of fungemia obscured by concomitant bacteremia: in vitro and in vivo studies. *Journal of Clinical Microbiology.* 1982;16:1080-1085.

154. Wey SB, Mori M, Pfaller MA, et al. Hospital-acquired candidemia. The attributable mortality and excess length of stay. *Arch Intern Med.* 1988;148:2642-2645.

155. Rex JH. Editorial response: catheters and candidemia. *Clinical Infectious Diseases.* 1996;22:467-470.

156. Yong PV, Chong PP, Lau LY, et al. Molecular identification of *Candida* orthopsilosis isolated from blood culture. *Mycopathologia.* 2008;165:81-87.

157. Vervaeke S, Vandamme K, Boone E, et al. A case of *Candida* lambica fungemia misidentified as *Candida* krusei in an intravenous drug abuser. *Med Mycol.* 2008:1-4.

158. Samonis G, Kofteridis DP, Saloustros E, et al. *Candida albicans* versus non-*albicans* bloodstream infection in patients in a tertiary hospital: an analysis of microbiological data. *Scand J Infect Dis.* 2008;40:414-419.

159. Zonios DI, Bennett JE. Update on azole antifungals. *Semin Respir Crit Care Med.* 2008;29:198-210.

160. Safdar A, Hanna HA, Boktour M, et al. Impact of high-dose granulocyte transfusions in patients with cancer with candidemia: retrospective case-control analysis of 491 episodes of *Candida* species bloodstream infections. *Cancer.* 2004;101: 2859-2865.

161. Spellberg BJ, Collins M, Avanesian V, et al. Optimization of a myeloid cell transfusion strategy for infected neutropenic hosts. *J Leukoc Biol.* 2007;81:632-641.

162. Spellberg BJ, Collins M, French SW, et al. A phagocytic cell line markedly improves survival of infected neutropenic mice. *J Leukoc Biol.* 2005.

163. Kullberg BJ. Trends in immunotherapy of fungal infections. *Eur J Clin Microbiol Infect Dis.* 1997;16:51-55.

164. Grigull L, Beilken A, Schmid H, et al. Secondary prophylaxis of invasive fungal infections with combination antifungal therapy and G-CSF-mobilized granulocyte transfusions in three children with hematological malignancies. *Support Care Cancer.* 2006;14:783-786.

165. Pfaller MA, Diekema DJ, Ostrosky-Zeichner L, et al. Correlation of MIC with outcome for *Candida* species tested against caspofungin, anidulafungin, and micafungin: analysis and proposal for interpretive MIC breakpoints. *J Clin Microbiol.* 2008;46: 2620-2629.

166. Pfaller MA, Boyken LB, Hollis RJ, et al. Validation of 24-Hour Fluconazole MIC Readings Versus the CLSI 48-Hour Broth Microdilution Reference Method: Results from a Global *Candida* Antifungal Surveillance Program. *J Clin Microbiol.* 2008.

167. Slavin MA, Osborne B, Adams R, et al. Efficacy and safety of fluconazole prophylaxis for fungal infections after marrow transplantation—a prospective, randomized, double-blind study. *J Infect Dis.* 1995;171:1545-1552.

168. Goodman JL, Winston DJ, Greenfield RA, et al. A controlled trial of fluconazole to prevent fungal infections in patients undergoing bone marrow transplantation. *N Engl J Med.* 1992;326:845-851.

169. Rex JH, Bennett JE, Sugar AM, et al. A randomized trial comparing fluconazole with amphotericin B for the treatment of candidemia in patients without neutropenia. *N Engl J Med.* 1994;331:1325-1330.

170. Rex JH, Pappas PG, Karchmer AW, et al. A randomized and blinded multicenter trial of high-dose fluconazole plus placebo versus fluconazole plus amphotericin B as therapy for candidemia and its consequences in nonneutropenic subjects. *Clin Infect Dis.* 2003;36:1221-1228.

171. Turnier E, Kay JH, Bernstein S, et al. Surgical treatment of *Candida* endocarditis. *Chest.* 1975;67:262-268.

172. Stripeli F, Tsolia M, Trapali C, et al. Successful medical treatment of Candida endocarditis with liposomal amphotericin B without surgical intervention. *Eur J Pediatr.* 2008;167: 469-470.

173. Williams J, Lye DC. Cure of *Candida* glabrata native tricuspid valve endocarditis by continuous infusion of conventional amphotericin B in a patient with nephrotic syndrome. *Int J Antimicrob Agents.* 2007;30:192-193.

174. Groll AH, Giri N, Petraitis V, et al. Comparative efficacy and distribution of lipid formulations of amphotericin B in experimental *Candida albicans* infection of the central nervous system. *Journal of Infectious Diseases.* 2000;182:274-282.

175. Bayer AS, Blumenkrantz MJ, Montgomerie JZ, et al. *Candida* peritonitis. Report of 22 cases and review of the English literature. *American Journal of Medicine.* 1976;61:832-840.

176. Amici G, Grandesso S, Mottola A, et al. Fungal peritonitis in peritoneal dialysis: critical review of six cases. *Adv Perit Dial.* 1994;10:169-173.

177. Montenegro J, Aguirre R, Gonzalez O, et al. Fluconazole treatment of *Candida* peritonitis with delayed removal of the peritoneal dialysis catheter. *Clin Nephrol.* 1995;44:60-63.

178. Chan TM, Chan CY, Cheng SW, et al. Treatment of fungal peritonitis complicating continuous ambulatory peritoneal dialysis with oral fluconazole: a series of 21 patients [see comments]. *Nephrol Dial Transplant.* 1994;9:539-542.

179. Rodriguez-Perez JC. Fungal peritonitis in CAPD—which treatment is best? *Contrib Nephrol.* 1987;57:114-121.

180. Struijk DG, Krediet RT, Boeschoten EW, et al. Antifungal treatment of *Candida* peritonitis in continuous ambulatory peritoneal dialysis patients. *Am J Kidney Dis.* 1987;9:66-70.

181. Salvaggio MR, Pappas PG. Current Concepts in the Management of Fungal Peritonitis. *Curr Infect Dis Rep.* 2003;5: 120-124.

182. Eggimann P, Francioli P, Bille J, et al. Fluconazole prophylaxis prevents intraabdominal candidiasis in high-risk surgical patients. *Crit Care Med.* 1999;27:1066-1072.

183. Wong PN, Lo KY, Tong GM, et al. Treatment of fungal peritonitis with a combination of intravenous amphotericin B and oral flucytosine, and delayed catheter replacement in continuous ambulatory peritoneal dialysis. *Perit Dial Int.* 2008;28:155-162.

184. Arda B, Soyer N, Sipahi OR, et al. Possible hepatosplenic candidiasis treated with liposomal amphotericin B and caspofungin combination. *J Infect.* 2006;52:387-388.

185. Altintas A, Ayyildiz O, Isikdogan A, et al. Successful initial treatment with caspofungin alone for hepatosplenic candidiasis in a patient with acute myeloblastic leukemia. *Saudi Med J.* 2006;27:1423-1424.

186. Elouennass M, Doghmi K, Fagot T, et al. Hepatosplenic and kidneys candidasis complicating an acute myeloblastic leukemia. A case treated with voriconazole and caspofungin. *Ann Biol Clin (Paris).* 2005;63:423-427.

187. Legrand F, Lecuit M, Dupont B, et al. Adjuvant corticosteroid therapy for chronic disseminated candidiasis. *Clin Infect Dis.* 2008;46:696-702.

188. Bozzette SA, Gordon RL, Yen A, et al. Biliary concentrations of fluconazole in a patient with candidal cholecystitis: case report. *Clinical Infectious Diseases.* 1992;15:701-703.

189. Diebel LN, Raafat AM, Dulchavsky SA, et al. Gallbladder and biliary tract candidiasis. *Surgery.* 1996;120:760-764.

190. Sobel JD, Kauffman CA, McKinsey D, et al. Candiduria: a randomized, double-blind study of treatment with fluconazole and placebo. The National Institute of Allergy and Infectious Diseases (NIAID) Mycoses Study Group. *Clinical Infectious Diseases.* 2000;30:19-24.

191. Kauffman CA, Vazquez JA, Sobel JD, et al. Prospective multicenter surveillance study of funguria in hospitalized patients. The National Institute for Allergy and Infectious Diseases (NIAID) Mycoses Study Group. *Clinical Infectious Diseases.* 2000;30:14-18.

192. Medoff G. Controversial areas in antifungal chemotherapy: Short-course and combination therapy with amphotericin B. *Reviews of Infectious Diseases.* 1987;9:403-407.

193. Agresti MG, de Bernardis F, Mondello F, et al. Clinical and mycological evaluation of fluconazole in the secondary prophylaxis of esophageal candidiasis in AIDS patients. An open, multicenter study. *European Journal of Epidemiology.* 1994;10: 17-22.

194. Reef SE, Levine WC, McNeil MM, et al. Treatment options for vulvovaginal candidiasis, 1993. *Clinical Infectious Diseases.* 1995;20(Suppl 1):S80-S90.

195. Sobel JD. Vaginitis. *N Engl J Med.* 1997;337:1896-1903.

196. Christmas NJ, Smiddy WE. Vitrectomy and systemic fluconazole for treatment of endogenous fungal endophthalmitis. *Ophthalmic SurgLasers.* 1996;27:1012-1018.

197. Darling K, Singh J, Wilks D. Successful treatment of *Candida* glabrata endophthalmitis with amphotericin B lipid complex (ABLC). *Journal of Infection.* 2000;40:92-94.

198. De Pasquale K, Sataloff RT. *Candida* of the larynx. *Ear Nose Throat J.* 2003;82:419.

199. Wang JN, Liu CC, Huang TZ, et al. Laryngeal candidiasis in children. *Scand J Infect Dis.* 1997;29:427-429.

200. Jenkin GA, Choo M, Hosking P, et al. Candidal epididymo-orchitis: case report and review. *Clinical Infectious Diseases.* 1998;26:942-945.

201. Sole A, Salavert M. Fungal infections after lung transplantation. *Transplant Rev (Orlando).* 2008;22:89-104.

258

Aspergillus Species

THOMAS F. PATTERSON

Invasive aspergillosis is a major cause of morbidity and mortality in immunosuppressed patients. This infection is caused by *Aspergillus*, a hyaline mold that is the etiologic agent responsible not only for invasive aspergillosis but also a variety of noninvasive or semi-invasive conditions. These syndromes range from colonization with the organism, such as fungus ball due to aspergillus (also known as aspergilloma); allergic responses to *Aspergillus*, including allergic bronchopulmonary aspergillosis (ABPA); and semi-invasive or invasive infections, which span a spectrum from chronic necrotizing pneumonia to invasive pulmonary aspergillosis and other syndromes of tissue invasion.

In recent years *Aspergillus* and aspergillosis have been a major focus of clinical mycology because the number of patients with this disease has risen dramatically and because of the difficulty in diagnosing and treating invasive infection.[1] The increased number of *Aspergillus* infections has occurred because more patients are at risk for this opportunistic pathogen and because preventing the diseases it causes is difficult. Patients with established invasive aspergillosis have poor outcomes even with recent advances in therapy.[2-5] Successful therapy depends not only on an early diagnosis—which is often difficult to establish—but, even more important, on reversal of underlying host immune defects, such as neutropenia or high doses of immunosuppressive therapy.[1] Non–culture-based tests and radiologic approaches can be used to establish an early diagnosis of infection and may result in improved outcomes of infection.[6-8] Even when therapy is begun promptly, efficacy of many treatment regimens, including amphotericin B deoxycholate, is poor, particularly in patients with disseminated or central nervous system disease.[1,3] New diagnostic approaches have been introduced and antifungal agents have been developed for this disease, including the newer azoles, lipid formulations of amphotericin B, and an additional drug class—the echinocandins.[1] In this chapter, clinical mycology, epidemiology, pathogenesis, clinical presentation, diagnosis, treatment, and prevention of aspergillosis are described.

Mycology

The genus *Aspergillus* was first recognized in 1729 by Micheli, in Florence, who noted the resemblance between the sporulating head of an *Aspergillus* species and an aspergillum used to sprinkle holy water.[9] In 1856, Virchow published the first complete microscopic descriptions of the organism.[10] *Aspergillus flavus* was formally named by Link in 1809.[11] Thom and Church first classified the genus in 1926 with 69 *Aspergillus* species in 11 groups. The term "group" is now more correctly referred to as "section," but this reporting is not commonplace in clinical mycology laboratories.[12] Because phenotypic methods and DNA internal transcribed spacer sequencing only identify isolates within a section and not individual species, it has been recommended that for clinical reporting individual species should be reported as members of a "species complex."[13] With the recent use of molecular techniques to characterize pathogenic fungi, aspergilli have now increased dramatically to include more than 250 species in 7 subgenera and in multiple sections.[13,14]

Most species of *Aspergillus* reproduce asexually, but a teleomorph (or sexual form) has been identified for some species, including pathogenic species such as *Aspergillus nidulans* (teleomorph, *Emericella nidulans*), *Aspergillus amstelodami* (*Eurotium amstelodami*), and recently the most common pathogen, *A. fumigatus* (*Neosartorya fumigata*) and others.[15-17] Even though the correct taxonomic nomenclature would rename these organisms using the sexual form, generally the generic name *Aspergillus* has been retained to simplify nomenclature regardless of their teleomorphs, rather than separating the organisms into unfamiliar species based on discovery of a sexual state.[18] As with other pathogenic fungi, the taxonomy of *Aspergillus* has undergone extensive reclassification with utilization of molecular studies, such as sequencing of ribosomal genes, β-tubulin, or calmodulin, which has allowed more natural subgroupings of ascomycetous fungi.[19]

The genus *Aspergillus* is an anamorphic member (asexual form) of the family Trichocomaceae. The teleomorphs of *Aspergillus* species are classified in seven genera in the order Eurotiales in the phylum Ascomycota.[14] *Aspergillus* is distinct but is closely related to the genus *Penicillium*.[15] Identification of the genus and of common pathogenic species is usually not difficult, but species level identification of less common members can be laborious and misidentification of atypical or "cryptic" members of sections—such as poorly sporulating forms—is common.[20]

The most common species causing invasive infection is *Aspergillus fumigatus*, the most common pathogen in the section *Fumigati*, which historically has made up a vast majority of invasive isolates; *A. flavus*; *Aspergillus terreus*; and, less commonly for invasive infection, *Aspergillus niger*.[3] Recent studies have shown emergence of less common species, including *A. terreus* and unusual less pathogenic species as the etiologic agents of invasive infection (Table 258-1).[21] With more prolonged and profound immunosuppression, the list of rare species causing invasive infection continues to increase, including *A. alliaceus* (teleomorph *Petromyces alliaceus*), *A. avenaceus*, *A. caesiellus*, *A. candidus*, *A. carneus*, *A. chevalieri* (teleomorph *Eurotium chevalieri*), *A. clavatus*, *A. calidoustus*, *A. flavipes*, *A. fumigataffinis*, *A. glaucus*, *A. granulosus*, *A. lentulus*, *A. novofumigatus*, *A. nidulans* (*Emericella nidulans*), *A. ochraceus*, *Aspergillus oryzae*, *A. puniceus*, *A. pseudodeflectus*, *A. restrictus*, *A. sydowii*, *E. quadrilineatus*, *A. tamarii*, *A. versicolor*, *A. vitus* (teleomorph *Eurotium amstelodami*), *A. wentii*, *Neosartorya pseudofischeri*, and many others, although the authenticity of at least some of these has been questioned.[12,14,22-24]

Pathogenic *Aspergillus* species are easily cultured from pathologic samples and grow rapidly (within 24-72 hours) at a broad range of temperatures on a variety of media. Blood cultures are still uncommonly positive and often reflect contamination rather than invasive disease.[25] A distinguishing characteristic of pathogenic *Aspergillus* species is their ability to grow at 37°C. In addition, strains of *A. fumigatus* are able to grow at temperatures of 50°C, a feature that, in addition to morphology, can also be used to identify this species.[23] Most species initially appear as small, fluffy white colonies on culture plates within 48 hours. Presumptive identification of an *Aspergillus* species is usually readily accomplished by appearance of the fungus on gross and microscopic inspection of the colony growing on medium, which provides typical sporulation.

Microscopic features and colony morphology for the most common clinical isolates, *A. fumigatus*, *A. flavus*, *A. terreus*, and *A. niger*, are described in Table 258-1 and shown in Figures 258-1 to 258-4. Species identification of *Aspergillus* has become important because differences in antifungal drug susceptibility and likely pathogenicity may be identified.

Aspergillus fumigatus is the most pathogenic species and is the most common species in invasive infection, constituting more than 90% of the isolates in some series, although recently a lower prevalence has been described.[3] Colonies of *A. fumigatus* are typically gray-green with a wooly to cottony texture (see Fig. 258-1A).[23] Like other species of *Aspergillus*, hyphae are hyaline (lightly pigmented), have septa, and are

TABLE 258-1	Characteristics of *Aspergillus* Species Associated with Invasive Infection			
Aspergillus Species	*Frequency Isolated in Clinical Infection (%)*[3]	*Colony Characteristics*[23]	*Microscopic Features*[23]	*Clinical Significance*
A. fumigatus (Fig. 258-1A and B)	66	Smoky gray green; may have pale yellow or lavender reverse; grows at 50°C	Columnar; uniseriate; smooth to finely roughened conidia 2-3.5 μm	Most common invasive species; most pathogenic
A. flavus (Fig. 258-2A and B)	14	Olive to lime green	Radiate to loosely columnar; uniseriate or biseriate; rough conidiophore; conidia 3-6 μm	Sinusitis; skin infection; produces aflatoxin
A. terreus (Fig. 258-3A to C)	5	Beige to cinnamon buff	Columnar; biseriate; globose; small 2-2.5 μm conidia; globose accessory conidia along hyphae	Increasingly detected; resistant to amphotericin B; more susceptible to newer azoles
A. niger. (Fig. 258-4A and B)	5	Initially white, rapidly turning black with yellow reverse	Radiate; biseriate; globose, black, very rough conidia 4-5 μm	Uncommon in invasive infections; superficial agent of otic disease; colonization

Data from Patterson TF, Kirkpatrick WR, White M, et al. Invasive aspergillosis. Disease spectrum, treatment practices, and outcomes. I3 Aspergillus Study Group. *Medicine* (*Baltimore*). 2000;79:250-260; Sutton DA, Fothergill AW, Rinaldi MD, eds. *Guide to Clinically Significant Fungi.* 1st ed. Baltimore: Williams & Wilkins; 1998.

usually branched at acute (typically 45 degrees) angles. The conidial head is columnar with conidiophores that are smooth walled and uncolored, or darkened in the upper portion near the vesicle. This species is uniseriate (a term describing phialides that are attached directly to the vesicle), with closely compacted phialides borne only on the upper portion of the vesicle (see Fig. 258-1A). Conidia are smooth to finely roughened and are 2 to 3.5 μm in diameter. The fruiting head (the conidiophore and conidia) is not commonly seen in clinical speci-

mens, although it may be detected in sites exposed to air, such as wounds or lung cavities.[23] Like other *Aspergillus* spp., it is widespread in nature—found in soil, on decaying vegetation, in the air, and, more recently, in water supplies.[26,27]

Other "cryptic" members of the section *Fumigati* have been described that are human pathogens, including *A. lentulus, A. fumigataffinis, A. novofumigatus,* and others. These species are frequently poorly sporulating and fail to grow at 50°C.[20,24] Importantly, some of

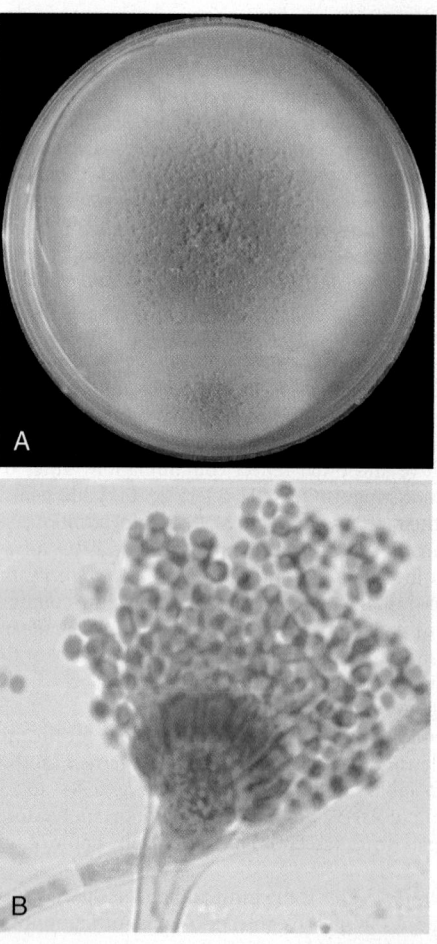

Figure 258-1 *Aspergillus fumigatus.* **A,** Gray-green colony morphology on potato flakes agar. **B,** Uniseriate conidiophore with columnar conidia (all photomicrograph magnifications ×420). (*Courtesy of Dr. Deanna Sutton.*)

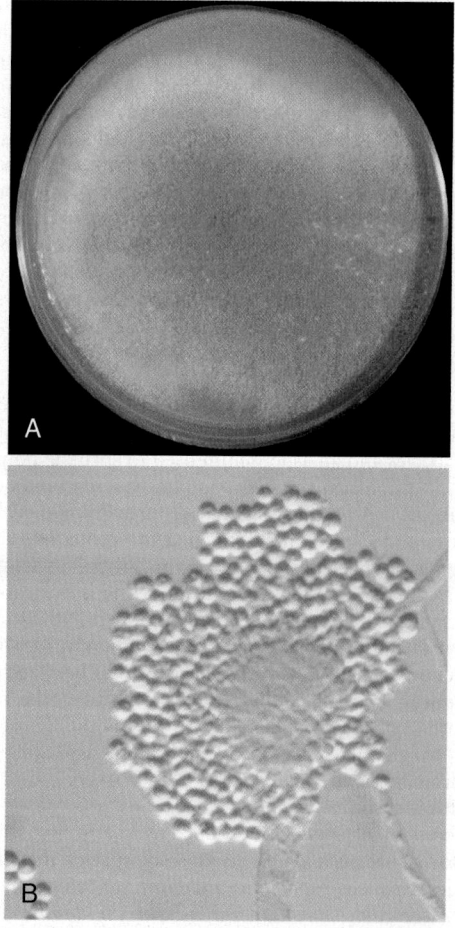

Figure 258-2 *Aspergillus flavus.* **A,** Olive–lime green colony on potato flakes agar. **B,** Radiate, biseriate conidia. (*Courtesy of Dr. Deanna Sutton.*)

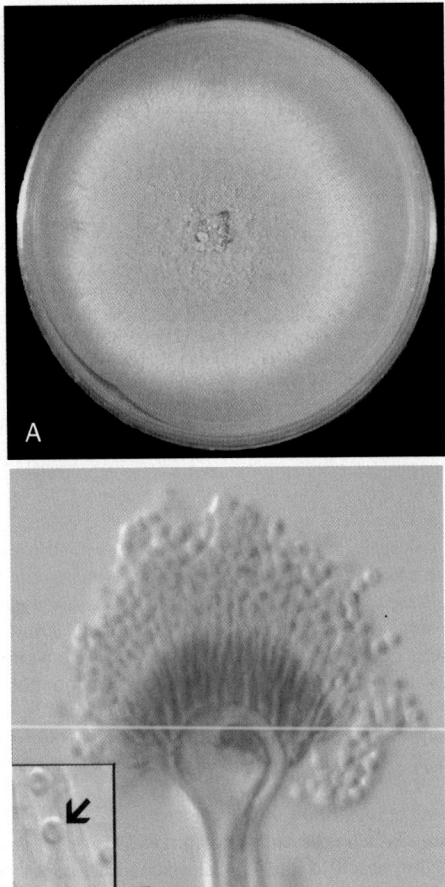

Figure 258-3 *Aspergillus terreus.* **A,** Buff-cinnamon colony on potato flakes agar. **B,** Columnar, biseriate smooth conidia. **C,** Globose, sessile accessory conidia along hyphae. *(Courtesy of Dr. Deanna Sutton.)*

these species, like *A. lentulus*, exhibit decreased antifungal susceptibility and can be associated with a poor clinical outcome.[28] When these species are only identified phenotypically, they should be referred to as members of the *Aspergillus fumigatus* species complex.

Aspergillus flavus is a common isolate in sinusitis as well as in skin and invasive infections. This species, which produces an aflatoxin, is found in soil and decaying vegetation.[29] Colonies are olive to lime green and grow at a rapid rate (see Fig. 258-2A). Some isolates are uniseriate, but it is typically biseriate. In biseriate species, sterile cells known as metulae are attached to the vesicle, and these in turn, support the phialides. This species also has noticeably rough conidiophores and smooth conidia 3 to 6 μm (see Fig. 258-2B).[23] If characterized by morphology alone, *A. flavus* and other species in the section *Flavi* should be referred to as members of the *Aspergillus flavus* species complex.

Aspergillus terreus is a common soil-related isolate that has been increasingly reported in invasive infection in immunocompromised hosts.[21] *A. terreus* conidia are small (2.0-2.5 μm), and the colony color and fruiting structures are characteristic for this species (see Fig. 258-3A and B). Colonies range in color from buff to beige to cinnamon (see Fig. 258-3A).[23] Conidiophores are smooth-walled and hyaline, and the conidial heads are biseriate and columnar (see Fig. 258-3B). A distinguishing feature of this species is the presence of globose accessory conidia that are produced on hyphae (see Fig. 258-3C). These accessory conidia can be detected in histopathologic samples, which may be used to establish presumptive identification of the species.[30] Identification of this species has become increasingly important because of its resistance to many antifungals, including amphotericin

B, although improved susceptibility and better outcomes with newer azoles have been reported.[31,32] Molecular characterization has shown *A. terreus* is also a species complex.

Aspergillus niger (see Fig. 258-4A and B) is found in soil, on plants, and even in food and condiments (such as pepper). Colonies are initially white but quickly become black with the production of the pigmented fruiting structures (see Fig. 258-4A). It grows rapidly with a pale yellow reverse. Conidial heads are biseriate and cover the entire vesicle. Conidia are brown to black and are very rough (4-5 μm) (see Fig. 258-4B), although the hyphae are hyaline.[23] The species may produce oxalate crystals in clinical specimens.[33] The role of *A. niger* in invasive infection is less well established, with its decreased pathogenicity perhaps due in part to the fact that its larger conidia do not readily reach deep into lung tissues. However, it is a common colonizing isolate and can cause superficial infection, such as otitis externa.[25,34] This species complex also contains several related species.

Other species of *Aspergillus* are less common in invasive infection, but are increasingly reported in invasive infection, perhaps reflecting a heightened awareness of their significance.[3,25] *Aspergillus nidulans*, for example, has been reported as a cause of infection in patients with chronic granulomatous disease and is a species that may be resistant to amphotericin B.[35] *Aspergillus calidoustus* is a species in the section *Ustus*, which grows at 37°C (formerly called *A. ustus*, a species that fails to grow at 37°C) and exhibits high minimum inhibitory concentrations (MICs) to several classes of antifungal agents.[36,37] Thus, even these previously "nonpathogenic" *Aspergillus* species must be considered potentially clinically significant in an appropriate clinical setting and host.[12]

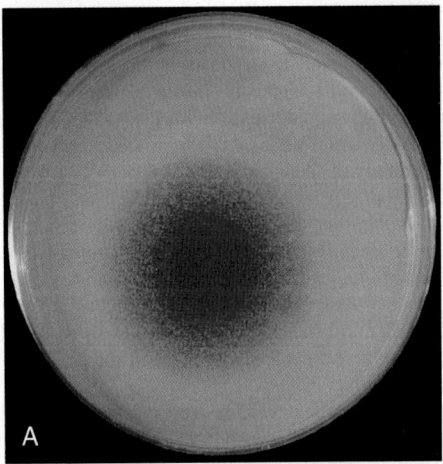
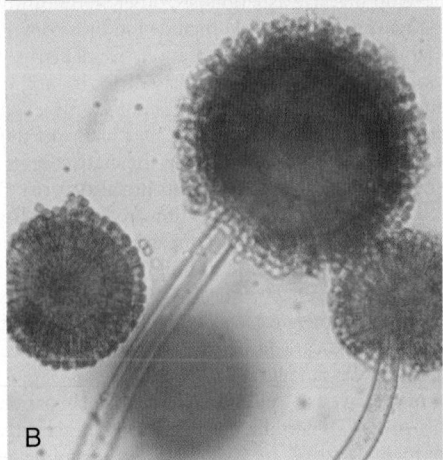

Figure 258-4 *Aspergillus niger.* **A,** Black colony on potato flakes agar. **B,** Large, radiate, biseriate and uniseriate conidia. *(Courtesy of Dr. Deanna Sutton.)*

Epidemiology

Aspergillus is ubiquitous worldwide. The organism is found in soil, water, food, and air, and is particularly common in decaying vegetation.[14] The inoculum for establishing infection is not known, but it is apparent that hosts with normal pulmonary host defenses very rarely develop disease despite routine exposure to the organism with normal daily living—through airborne conidia, through foodstuffs like pepper, and so on. In contrast, patients with altered host immunity, particularly those with reduced pulmonary host defenses (e.g., those who use corticosteroids) that inhibit the activity of pulmonary macrophages or those who are neutropenic, have increased susceptibility to the organism.[38]

Patients with prolonged and profound neutropenia (<100 neutrophils/μL) are at high risk for invasive aspergillosis, but changing treatment patterns in chemotherapy and transplantation, along with the use of growth factors, have limited the numbers of persistently neutropenic patients.[39] It is important to recognize that even among high-risk patients with hematological malignancy there is substantial heterogeneity of risk. In patients with acute myelogenous leukemia, the incidence of invasive aspergillosis has been reported to range from as low as 2% to rates as high as 25% to 28% or more, with mean incidence in recent series of 4% to 7%.[40-42] Other patients at high risk for invasive aspergillosis include patients undergoing organ and bone marrow transplantation and those receiving corticosteroids or other newer immunosuppressive therapies, including the tumor necrosis factor-α (TNF-α) antagonists such as infliximab and others.[43]

In patients undergoing hematopoietic stem cell or marrow transplantation, a recent increase in the incidence of invasive aspergillosis has been reported, and the epidemiology of infection has changed (Table 258-2).[44] In patients undergoing hematopoietic stem cell transplantation, the major periods of risk are bimodal, with peak incidence occurring at an early time after transplantation (<40 days) but also very late, more than 100 days after transplantation.[39,45] One of the factors in the changing epidemiology in this patient population is the use of nonmyeloablative transplantation procedures, which has shifted the major risk factor in these patients from neutropenia to that of the use of high doses of corticosteroids for the treatment of acute or chronic graft-versus-host disease.[39] In fact, only 31% of the hematopoietic stem cell transplant recipients with invasive aspergillosis reported by Wald and colleagues were neutropenic. Acute or chronic graft-versus-host disease may occur an extended time after marrow or stem cell transplantation, which dramatically increases the risk for *Aspergillus* infection and prolongs the period for which these patients are at risk.[39,45]

Although patients undergoing marrow or stem cell transplants and those receiving cytotoxic chemotherapy still constitute a majority of those who develop invasive aspergillosis, other significantly immunosuppressed patients are also at risk. Included in those other groups are patients undergoing organ transplantation, particularly lung transplantation (see Table 258-2).[46] The increased risk in lung transplantation is because the transplanted organ is constantly exposed to the environment, ciliary clearance is reduced, and many of these patients are colonized with *Aspergillus* in either the native or transplanted lung.[47] Other immunosuppressed patients are also at risk for invasive aspergillosis, although the rates of infection are lower in these patients, including patients with pulmonary diseases, acquired immunodeficiency syndrome (AIDS), chronic granulomatous disease and other hereditary immunodeficiency syndromes, patients who use steroids, and others.[3,38] For example, invasive aspergillosis can occur in critically ill patients in intensive care units independent of other risk factors suggesting additional risk factors for this disease.[48]

Outbreaks of invasive aspergillosis have occurred in patients exposed to aerosols of *Aspergillus* conidia in association with construction and other environmental risks.[49] In severely immunosuppressed patients, aspergillosis may occur from other exposures as well, including aerosols of contaminated water, which has recently been described.[27,50] Aspergillosis may also occur as endogenous reactivation from prior

| TABLE 258-2 | Incidence and Mortality of Invasive Aspergillosis in Transplantation |

Type of Transplant	Incidence (%)		Mortality (%)
	Range	*Mean*	
Allogeneic stem cell	2.3-11	7	76
Autologous stem cell	0.5-4	2	54
Lung	2.4-6	6	68
Liver	1-8	2	87
Heart	0.3-6	5.2	78
Kidney	0.1-4	0.7	77

Data from: Singh N, Paterson DL. Aspergillus infections in transplant recipients. *Clin Microbiol Rev.* 2005;18:44-69; Barnes PD, Marr KA. Aspergillosis: spectrum of disease, diagnosis, and treatment. *Infect Dis Clin North Am.* 2006;20:545-61; Marr KA, Carter RA, Boeckh M, Martin P, Corey L. Invasive aspergillosis in allogeneic stem cell transplant recipients: changes in epidemiology and risk factors. *Blood.* 2002;100:4358-66; Morgan J, Wannemuehler KA, Marr KA, et al. Incidence of invasive aspergillosis following hematopoietic stem cell and solid organ transplantation: interim results of a prospective multicenter surveillance program. *Med Mycol.* 2005;43:Suppl 1:S49-58.

infection or colonization, so even when it occurs in a hospital setting, it may not be possible to prevent all cases by reducing environmental exposures.[51] It should also be noted that with the prolonged period of risk—more than 100 days after transplantation in some patients—these infections become very difficult to prevent with protective environments as much of their health care will occur in a non–hospital-based setting.[51]

Pathogenicity and Host Defenses

The usual route of infection for invasive aspergillosis is through inhalation of *Aspergillus* conidia into the lungs. Although less common, invasive infection may also follow local tissue invasion such as through surgical wounds or contaminated intravenous catheters or armboards, leading to cutaneous infection.[52]

In the absence of effective host defenses following pulmonary exposure, the inhaled small resting condida enlarge and germinate, resulting in transformation into hyphae with subsequent vascular invasion and eventual disseminated infection. The incubation period for conidial germination in pulmonary tissue is variable, estimated to range from 2 days to months and may even vary by species.[30] The growth rate at 37°C may be one determinant of the rate of disease progression and possible pathogenicity of the organism. Hydrocortisone significantly increases the growth rates of *Aspergillus*, further enhancing the role of corticosteroids as a risk factor for invasive disease.[53] The process of hyphal growth and tissue invasion results in a hallmark feature of invasive aspergillosis: vascular invasion (Fig. 258-5) and pulmonary infarction (Fig. 258-6), which are classic features of invasive pulmonary aspergillosis due to the angioinvasive nature of the organism.

Although infection in apparently normal hosts can occur, invasive aspergillosis is uncommon in immunocompetent hosts.[3] Normal pulmonary defense mechanisms are usually able to contain the organism in a host with intact pulmomary defenses. The first line of defense against *Aspergillus* is ciliary clearance of the organism from the airways and limited access to the alveoli due to conidial size. This feature is one reason for the increased pathogenicity of *A. fumigatus* as compared with other species of *Aspergillus*.[54] After conidia reach the alveoli, the major line of defense becomes the pulmonary macrophage, which is capable of ingesting and killing *Aspergillus* conidia.[55] After the cells germinate, polymorphonuclear leukocytes act to extracellularly kill both swollen conidia and hyphae.[56] Efficacy of host defenses against the organism may be enhanced by opsonization of conidia with complement or other molecules such as mannose-binding protein and surfactant proteins.[57] *A. fumigatus* produces a complement inhibitor, which may increase its pathogenicity.[58] Antibodies against *Aspergillus* are common because of the ubiquitous nature of the organism, although they are not protective nor are they useful in the diagnosis

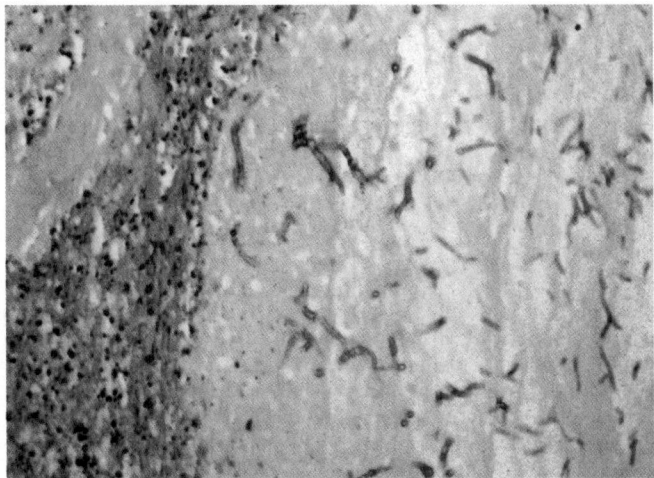

Figure 258-5 Lung tissue section showing narrow, acutely branching septated hyphae on hematoxylin-eosin stain showing vascular invasion (original magnification ×420).

of infection in high-risk patients owing to the lack of consistent seroconversion following exposure or infection.[59]

Many *Aspergillus* species produce toxins including aflatoxins, ochratoxin A, fumagillin, and gliotoxin—the last of which may reduce macrophage and neutrophil function, although the role of these toxins as major virulence factors is not established.[60] *Aspergillus* species possess other potential virulence factors including production of proteases, phospholipases, and metabolites although strains deficient in those genes are still capable of producing experimental infection.[61]

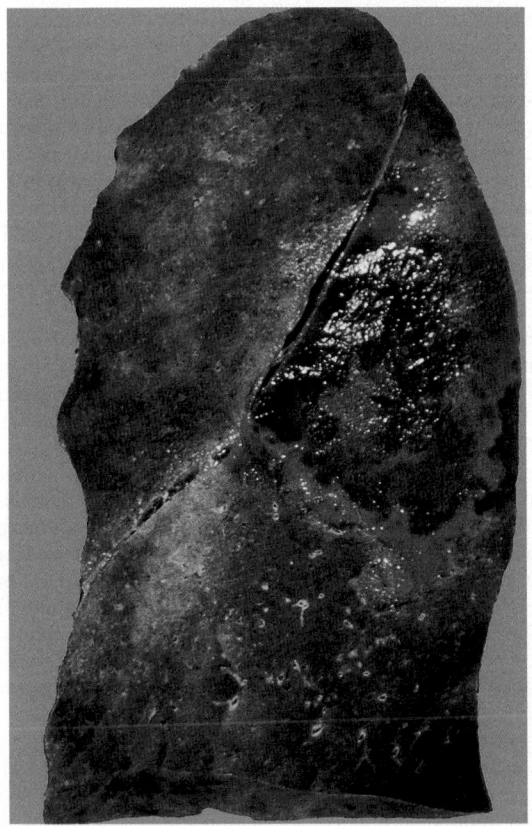

Figure 258-6 Infarcted lung tissue due to *Aspergillus* angioinvasion on gross lung specimen.

T-helper (Th) cytokines have vital roles in innate and adaptive defense against *Aspergillus*. Studies in experimental aspergillosis have shown that a Th1 response is associated with a favorable response.[62] Pathogen recognition receptors including Toll-like receptors (TLRs) and dectin-1 also mediate defense against *A. fumigatus*.[63,64] Recognition of *Aspergillus* motifs by TLR2 and dectin-1 results in activation of intracellular pathways leading to pro-inflammatory cytokine production.[65,66] These events are needed for an effective initial antifungal defense and bridge the gap between the innate and acquired immunity.[67] Polymorphisms in host genes mediating innate immune defenses influence susceptibility to invasive aspergillosis. TLR4 haplotypes and polymorphisms in plasminogen gene alleles have both been shown to be associated with increased risk of invasive aspergillosis in hematopoietic stem cell transplant patients.[68,69]

In contrast to the deficient host responses that lead to invasive *Aspergillus* infections, the pathogenesis of ABPA and allergic fungal sinusitis relates to aberrant inflammatory host responses to the organism.[70] The immune response to *Aspergillus* antigens in ABPA as in both asthmatic patients and those with cystic fibrosis is a Th2 response.[54] ABPA begins with an allergic inflammatory response that follows after *Aspergillus* conidia are inhaled into the bronchi, where they germinate and form hyphae.[70] These mycelial cells release allergens that are processed by antigen-presenting cells bearing HLA-DR2 or HLA-DR5 and presented to T cells within the bronchoalveolar lymphoid tissue. The T-cell response to these allergens favors a Th2 response, with release of cytokines IL-4, IL-5, and IL-13.[54] The inflammatory response in the bronchial submucosa leads to excessive mucin production, extravasation of eosinophils into the bronchial mucin, intermittent bronchial obstruction with atelectasis, and, over time, to bronchiectasis in some patients. Allergic fungal sinusitis is also characterized by submucosal inflammation and eosinophil-rich mucin in the sinus cavity.

Aspergilloma, called *fungus ball of the lung*, is a mass of hyphae in a preexisting cavity. *Aspergillus* causes a brisk IgG antibody response to the organism even though invasion of the cavity wall is rarely observed. Increased risk for chronic forms of pulmonary aspergillosis have been linked to subtle immune defects including polymorphisms in mannose-binding protein or alterations in surfactant D.[71]

Clinical Presentation

The spectrum of clinical syndromes associated with aspergillosis is diverse, ranging from allergic responses to the organism, asymptomatic colonization, superficial infection, and acute or subacute invasive disease. Generally, the clinical presentation reflects the underlying immune defects and risk factors associated with each patient group, with greater immune suppression correlating with increased risk for invasive disease.

ALLERGIC MANIFESTATIONS OF DISEASE

Allergic Bronchopulmonary Aspergillosis

ABPA is a long-term allergic response to *Aspergillus* that is characterized by transient pulmonary infiltrates due to atelectasis. Central bronchiectasis occurs in some patients after several years of disease.[70] The incidence of ABPA is estimated to range from 1% to 2% in patients with persistent asthma and in approximately 7% (with a range from 2% to 15%) of patients with cystic fibrosis.[54,70] Specific criteria are used to establish the diagnosis of ABPA because no single finding except for central bronchiectasis in a patient with asthma is diagnostic for the condition. These classic criteria include (1) asthma, (2) central bronchiectasis on chest computed tomography, (3) immediate cutaneous reactivity to *Aspergillus* species (or *A. fumigatus*), (4) total serum IgE concentration greater than 417 IU/mL (1000 ng/mL), (5) elevated serum IgE and/or IgG antibody to *A. fumigatus*, (6) fleeting infiltrates on chest radiograph, (7) serum precipitating antibodies to *A. fumigatus*, and (8) peripheral blood eosinophilia.[70] It has been suggested that the first five are the minimal essential criteria for ABPA in patients with asthma, with the presence of precipitating antibodies further supporting the diagnosis and total IgE levels correlating with exacerbation of disease.[70] Other clinical features may be present that can be used to support the diagnosis including positive sputum cultures for *Aspergillus* or smears with hyphae consistent with *Aspergillus,* brown mucus plugs with degenerated eosinophils (Charcot-Leyden crystals) in sputa, and chest radiographic findings suggesting bronchial inflammation.[72] These latter chest radiographic findings include the "ring sign," indicating bronchial thickening without mucus plugs, and "parallel lines" or "tram tracks" suggesting bronchiectasis, which contrasts to tapering seen in the normal bronchus.[73]

The diagnosis of ABPA in cystic fibrosis may be particularly difficult because many of the diagnostic criteria overlap with common manifestations of cystic fibrosis (Table 258-3).[54] In these patients eosinophilia is not a useful diagnostic tool because the patients may have elevated peripheral blood eosinophils from other causes.

ABPA typically progresses through a series of remissions and exacerbations but can eventually lead to pulmonary fibrosis, which is associated with a poor long-term prognosis.[72] Management of ABPA is directed at reducing acute asthmatic symptoms and avoiding end-stage fibrosis. Corticosteroid therapy is commonly used for treating exacer-

bations, although few randomized trials have been conducted for their use.[74] Guidelines suggest that worsening diagnostic or clinical parameters may warrant a trial of corticosteroid therapy.[1] The role for antifungal therapy was evaluated with a randomized double-blind, placebo-controlled trial that showed itraconazole at 200 mg per day for 16 weeks significantly reduced daily corticosteroid use, reduced levels of IgE, and improved exercise tolerance and pulmonary function.[75]

Other Allergic Manifestations

Aspergillus is an occasional cause of allergic fungal sinusitis, although most cases in the United States are due to dark-walled molds. This entity occurs in patients with a history of chronic allergic rhinitis, often with hyperplastic nasal mucosa forming nasal polyps. A mass of inspissated mucus forms in sinus cavity with *Aspergillus* hyphae and Charcot-Leyden crystals. The sinus mucosa is hyperplastic but not invaded.[76] Management is directed at aerating the sinus and ensuring that tissue invasion is not present. The benefit of treating with either intranasal steroids or systemic antifungal agents has not been shown.[1]

SAPROPHYTIC COLONIZATION AND SUPERFICIAL ASPERGILLOSIS

Fungus Balls Due to Aspergillus

A pulmonary fungus ball due to *Aspergillus*—or *aspergilloma*—is a solid mass of hyphae growing in a previously existing pulmonary cavity. Typically *Aspergillus* fungus balls of the lung develop in preexisting cavities in the pulmonary apex of patients with chronic lung disease such as bullous emphysema, sarcoidosis, tuberculosis, histoplasmosis, congenital cyst, bacterial lung abscess, or, very rarely, in a pulmonary bleb from *Pneumocystis* pneumonia in patients with AIDS.[77] On chest radiograph, a pulmonary aspergilloma appears as a solid round mass in a cavity. The detection of *Aspergillus* in sputum cultures or detection of high titers of *Aspergillus* antibodies are further evidence that the radiographic findings are consistent with a diagnosis of fungus ball due to *Aspergillus* so that a biopsy is not usually necessary except to diagnose the underlying lung disease.[78]

In many patients the fungus ball due to *Aspergillus* remains asymptomatic, but in a significant number of patients, hemoptysis occurs and can be fatal.[78] Surgical resection is considered the definitive therapy but the dense pleural adhesions adjacent the fungus ball and the poor pulmonary reserve of most patients make surgery hazardous. Contamination of the pleural space with *Aspergillus* and the common complication of bronchopleural fistula in the postoperative period can lead to chronic *Aspergillus* empyema. Dense adhesions make pleural drainage difficult, often requiring pleural stripping, further compromising lung function.[78]

Aspergillus can also be associated with fungus balls of the sinuses without tissue invasion. The maxillary sinus is the most common site for a sinus aspergilloma to occur.[79] Clinical presentation is similar to that for any chronic sinusitis. Computed tomography of the sinus can be used to confirm the fungus ball, along with cultures of *Aspergillus*, usually *A. flavus* or *A. fumigatus*. Management is usually directed at surgical removal and a generous maxillary antrostomy for sinus drainage, along with confirmation that invasive disease has not occurred.

Denning and colleagues have described three distinct syndromes of chronic pulmonary aspergillosis to better characterize those patients who develop chronic pulmonary disease related to *Aspergillus*.[80] These conditions include (1) chronic cavitary pulmonary aspergillosis, characterized by the formation and expansion of multiple cavities, which may contain fungus balls; (2) chronic fibrosing aspergillosis, which, as its name suggests, involves extensive fibrosis; and (3) chronic necrotizing, or subacute, aspergillosis, in which slowly progressive infection occurs, usually in a single thin-walled cavity with demonstration of hyphae invading tissue. In all of these conditions, the diagnosis is suggested by radiologic and clinical features and the role of therapy remains speculative, although it appears that long-term antifungal therapy may be beneficial in a subset of patients.[1,80]

TABLE 258-3	Criteria for Diagnosis and Management of Allergic Bronchopulmonary Aspergillosis (ABPA) in Patients with Cystic Fibrosis	

Diagnostic Criteria	*Comment*
Clinical deterioration (increased cough, wheezing, exercise intolerance, exercise-induced asthma, increased sputum, decrease in pulmonary function)	Clinical signs not attributed to another etiology
Immediate cutaneous reactivity to *Aspergillus* or presence of IgE to *A. fumigatus*	Pinprick skin test wheal of greater than 3 mm with surrounding erythema while not receiving antihistamines
Total serum IgE concentration greater than 500 IU/mL (>1200 ng/mL)	If ABPA is suspected and level is 200-500 repeat in 1-3 months; if taking steroids, repeat after discontinuation
One of the following: (1) precipitins (or IgG) to *A. fumigatus* or (2) new or recent abnormalities on computed tomography (bronchiectasis) or chest radiograph (mucus plugging/infiltrates)	Failure of infiltrates or abnormalities to clear after antibiotic therapy and standard physiotherapy

Recommendations for Screening for ABPA

Maintain clinical suspicion for diagnosis	Especially in patients older than 6 years
Determine total serum IgE annually	If total IgE is greater than 500 IU/mL, consider skin test or measure IgE to *Aspergillus*
If total IgE 200-500 IU/mL, repeat if clinical suspicion is high	Consider retesting with disease exacerbation and perform other diagnostic tests

Therapy for Exacerbations of ABPA

Corticosteroids: 0.5-2 mg/kg/day oral prednisone equivalent (maximum 60 mg/day) for 1-2 weeks, tapered over 2-3 months	Recommended for disease exacerbation in all patients except those with steroid toxicity
Antifungal therapy (itraconazole—or other azole with *Aspergillus* activity—voriconazole, posaconazole)	Slow steroid response or toxicity; itraconazole 5 mg/kg/day up to 400 mg/kg/day—levels necessary (other azoles may be effective but not studied); monitor liver function tests; duration 3-6 months
Adjunctive therapy: inhaled corticosteroids; bronchodilators; environmental manipulation	No evidence for efficacy in ABPA but may be useful in asthma; reasonable to search for source of extensive mold exposure

Data from Stevens DA, Moss RB, Kurup VP, et al. Allergic bronchopulmonary aspergillosis in cystic fibrosis—State of the art: Cystic Fibrosis Foundation Consensus Conference. *Clin Infect Dis.* 2003;37(Suppl 3):S225-S264.

Other Superficial or Colonizing Syndromes of Aspergillosis

Otomycosis is a condition of superficial colonization typically due to *A. niger*.[1] The clinical features include findings similar to other causes of external otitis, with the external auditory canal potentially revealing mold growing on cerumen and desquamated epithelial debris. *A. fumigatus* looks greenish, and *A. niger* forms a black tuft. Treatment is to focus on the underlying chronic otitis externa rather than the fungus. In immunocompromised patients, invasive otitis externa can occur and resembles that due to *Pseudomonas aeruginosa* clinically.[34]

Onychomycosis due to *Aspergillus* is another superficial condition that, although rare, can become chronic and respond poorly to antifungal agents.[81] Antifungal agents in the setting of nail infection may have a spectrum of activity limited to yeasts; thus, a nail culture can be useful in patients with nonresponsive disease to establish a specific fungal etiology so that appropriate therapy can be initiated.

Aspergillus is an occasional etiology of keratitis, particularly following trauma or corneal surgery (see Chapter 111).[82] The diagnosis can be established with smears demonstrating hyphae, which may be indistinguishable from other molds like *Fusarium* that also cause keratitis, but culture results are usually positive to confirm the diagnosis. Therapy consists of topical antifungal agents, usually amphotericin B or natamycin (pimaricin) drops administered hourly, although studies demonstrating efficacy of either agent—but particularly the latter—are limited. Surgical intervention may be required for deep lesions or those nonresponsive to medical therapy.[1] Azoles with *Aspergillus* activity, including itraconazole, voriconazole, and posaconazole, have been used (in addition to topical therapy) systemically for this infection, but their role is not well studied. Some of these agents, particularly voriconazole, have been also been administered topically with successful outcomes.[1,83,84] Amphotericin B has been injected intracamerally when corneal penetration has occurred.[85]

INVASIVE SYNDROMES CAUSED BY *ASPERGILLUS*

Invasive aspergillosis most frequently begins in the lung following inhalation of *Aspergillus* conidia. Invasion of hyphae into the pulmonary vasculature is common, occurring in as many as a third of patients with invasive pulmonary aspergillosis. Disseminated disease occurs either by hematogenous spread to distant sites or by contiguous extension from the lung. Hematogenous dissemination to the central nervous system or other organs, including the thyroid, liver, spleen, kidney, bone, heart, and skin, is common in patients with severe immunosuppression such as those undergoing allogeneic hematopoietic stem cell or marrow transplants and heralds an ominously poor prognosis.[3]

Invasive Pulmonary Aspergillosis

The most common manifestation of invasive aspergillosis is invasive pulmonary aspergillosis (IPA). Invasive pulmonary aspergillosis rarely manifests before 10 to 12 days of profound neutropenia, which until recently has been the major risk factor for developing infection.[86] In recent series, even with an approximate doubling of disease incidence compared with historical rates of infection, less than a third of patients undergoing marrow or hematopoietic stem cell transplantation were neutropenic at the time of diagnosis of IPA, emphasizing the shifting epidemiology to other forms of immunosuppression, such as the use of high doses of corticosteroids for treating graft-versus-host disease.[39,45] The incubation period for developing IPA after inhalation of conidia is not known, but a significant number of patients have manifestations of IPA on admission or within the first 2 weeks of hospital admission, suggesting that community-acquired exposure is common.[51,87]

Symptoms of IPA include progressive dry cough, dyspnea, pleuritic chest pain, fever despite coverage with broad-spectrum antibiotics, and pulmonary infiltrates. These symptoms may be reduced in patients who are unable to mount an inflammatory response owing to profound neutropenia. In addition, although fever is common, it may be absent in those receiving high doses of corticosteroids. Other clinical

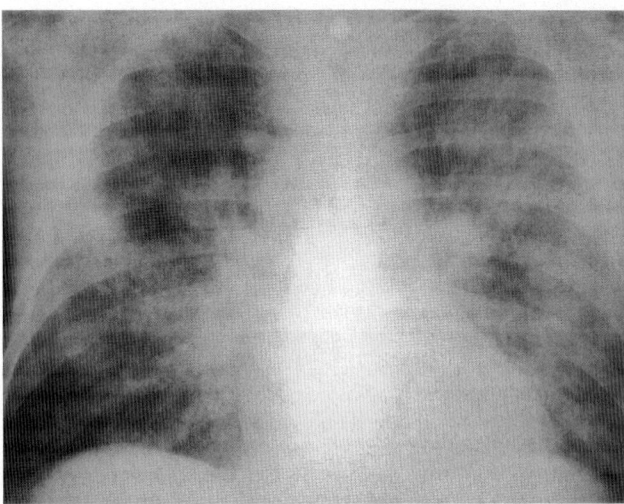

Figure 258-7 **Chest radiograph showing diffuse pulmonary infiltrates of invasive pulmonary aspergillosis.**

features of IPA include hemoptysis, pleural effusion, and pneumothorax. However, all the physical findings are nonspecific and may lag significantly behind the disease process. Clinical characteristics may resemble a pulmonary embolism with pleuritic chest pain, hemoptysis, and dyspnea, which reflect the angioinvasive nature of the organism. Laboratory studies are also nonspecific but may include elevation in bilirubin and lactate dehydrogenase, coagulation abnormalities, and elevation in C-reactive protein. Life-threatening hypoxia may occur in patients with extensive or progressive infection.

In extensive infection, multiple diffuse nodular pulmonary infiltrates are readily seen on chest radiographs or chest computed tomography (Fig. 258-7). While these are not diagnostic, diffuse nodular lesions are associated with a poor prognosis.[7,88] Other pulmonary radiographic findings of IPA include the classic pleural-based, wedge-shaped densities or cavitary lesions, although the former are not commonly detected and the latter are present late in the course of infection.[6,7] Pleural effusions are more common than previously considered, but whether they are a specific manifestation of IPA is not established.[7] The presence of a "halo" of low attenuation surrounding a nodular lesion on computed tomography is an early finding in invasive aspergillosis (Fig. 258-8A).[6,7] Later in the course of infection these nodular lesions may cavitate (usually in temporal association with recovery of neutrophils), forming an "air-crescent" sign (see Fig. 258-8B). These radiographic features are characteristic of IPA, but similar findings can also occur with other angioinvasive organisms, including *Mucorales, Fusarium,* and *Scedosporium,* as well as bacterial pathogens.

Tracheobronchitis

Aspergillus in the airways can range in significance from colonization, which is common in lung transplantation, to ulcerative tracheobronchitis.[47] The syndrome of *Aspergillus* tracheobronchitis typically occurs in patients undergoing lung transplantation and in patients with AIDS and is characterized by extensive pseudomembranous or ulcerative lesions due to *Aspergillus*.[47,89] In patients undergoing lung transplantation, the infection often occurs at the suture line of the lung transplant and can lead to dehiscence of the anastomotic site. Symptoms of tracheobronchitis are nonspecific and include dyspnea with associated pulmonary function abnormalities, cough, chest pain, fever, or hemoptysis. Symptoms may be mild and can be confused with other causes including rejection. In more severe disease, unilateral wheeze or stridor may develop because of local obstruction. Results of plain radiographs may be normal so that clinical suspicion is needed to establish the diagnosis, which is accomplished by bronchoscopy with biopsy to document tissue invasion. A prolonged course of a systemic antifungal agent therapy is usually required for treatment, although

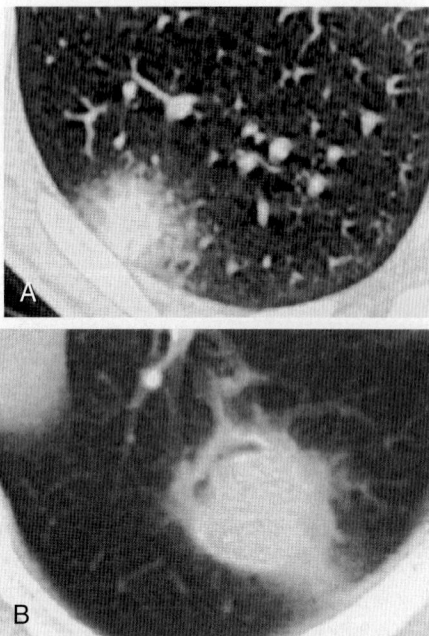

Figure 258-8 **Computed tomography of chest. A,** "Halo" sign of low attenuation surrounding a nodular lung lesion detected in early pulmonary aspergillosis. **B,** "Air-crescent" sign in a nodular lung lesion found in late disease. *(Radiographs courtesy of Dr. Reginald Greene.)*

aerosols of liposomal formulations of amphotericin B have been used for localized disease.[1]

Sinusitis
Aspergillus infection of the sinuses and nasal cavities in immunocompromised patients manifests as acute invasive rhinosinusitis often in association with invasive pulmonary aspergillosis.[76] The clinical manifestations are not specific to *Aspergillus* and include fever, cough, epistaxis, sinus discharge, and headaches. Clinical signs are also nondiagnostic but findings of an ulcerative nasal lesion with an eschar or nonsensitive area may be a clue to a fungal diagnosis.[90] Presence of epistaxis or unexplained fever in a high-risk patient may be enough to warrant endoscopy and biopsy of any nasal mucosal lesion. In patients with progressive infection, the disease spreads to contiguous paranasal sinuses, palate, orbit, or brain. The mortality in invasive cases is high, ranging from 20% in patients with leukemia in remission to up to 100% in patients with relapsed leukemia or those undergoing bone marrow transplantation.[1] Plain radiographs are not diagnostic and do not distinguish fungal etiologies from other causes of sinusitis. Sinus computed tomography (CT) scans are useful for establishing extent of infection and determining local tissue invasion (Fig. 258-9). Routine surveillance cultures of the nose have been advocated, but these lack specificity and sensitivity. Cultures from sinus aspirates are useful to demonstrate the presence of *Aspergillus,* but a biopsy with tissue invasion is needed for the diagnosis.[91] Therapy for these infections is often difficult and requires long-term administration of antifungal medications.[1] The role of surgery is controversial. Efficacy of antifungal prophylaxis has not been demonstrated, but attempts at reduction of environmental exposures in high-risk patients may be beneficial.[92]

Disseminated Infection
Progressive invasive pulmonary aspergillosis often results in disseminated invasive aspergillosis, a complication associated with an extremely high mortality.[2] In patients with severe and ongoing immunosuppression, such as patients with persistent granulocytopenia, extensive graft-versus-host disease, and progressive underlying malignancy, disseminated infection can occur. In this widespread infection,

mortality rates approach 90%, with favorable responses to antifungal therapy seen in less than 20%.[2,3]

OTHER INVASIVE SYNDROMES

Cerebral Aspergillosis
Cerebral aspergillosis is associated with the highest mortality of invasive aspergillosis syndromes, with mortality rates of more than 90% reported in most historical series.[3,93] The incidence of cerebral aspergillosis is difficult to determine because the diagnosis is often unsuspected and difficult to confirm, but it has been estimated to occur in 10% to 20% of all cases of invasive aspergillosis, usually in patients with persistent immunosuppression and disseminated disease.[3,94] In a recent series of patients undergoing allogeneic stem cell transplant, the incidence of proven or suspected cerebral aspergillosis was only 3%, but all suspected cases were fatal.[95] In one series of patients undergoing allogeneic transplantation, *Aspergillus* was found in 58% of biopsied cerebral mass lesions.[96] In transplantation the diagnosis may occur an extended time after transplant (>100 days) and is nearly always associated with extensive immunosuppression, such as therapy for graft-versus-host disease.[95] Concomitant pulmonary infection is usually but not always present.[96] Isolated cerebral aspergillosis can occur in immunocompetent patients or in the setting of injection drug use, in which case it may be associated with a slightly better prognosis provided the diagnosis is made and surgical drainage or removal is performed.[94] *Aspergillus* meningitis is rare. The clinical presentation of cerebral aspergillosis is nonspecific and is characterized by focal neurologic signs, alteration in mental status, and headaches.[97] On CT of the brain the appearance is nonspecific and is similar to that of other infectious causes of brain abscess with ring enhancement of the abscess along with surrounding edema (Fig. 258-10) and may be hemorrhagic.[98] Magnetic resonance imaging (MRI) scans may reveal additional lesions, but the findings are still nonspecific. Confirmation of the diagnosis requires biopsy, but in the setting of documented disseminated disease, the diagnosis is often presumed. However, in patients

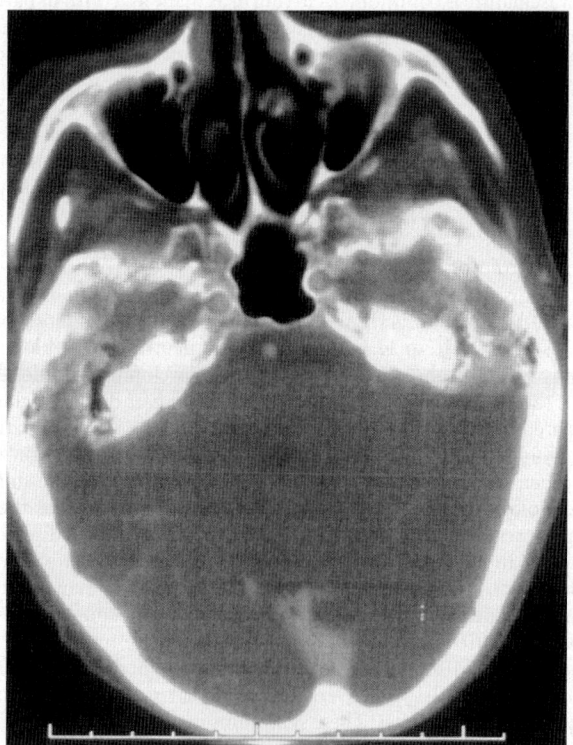

Figure 258-9 **Computed tomography of sinuses showing sinus wall thickening.**

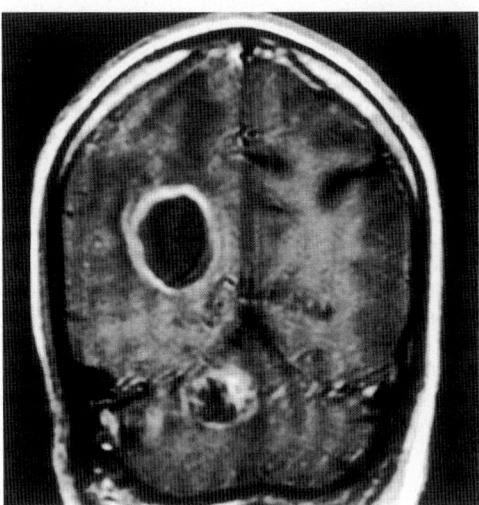

Figure 258-10 Brain abscess of invasive aspergillosis with ring enhancement and extensive edema.

without a clear diagnosis, biopsy is recommended because the differential diagnosis is extensive, including other fungi and an extensive array of opportunistic diseases. Until recently, the outcome of this infection has been almost universally fatal, although in recent trials voriconazole has been associated with favorable responses in approximately 30% of patients.[93,94]

Bone Aspergillosis

Aspergillus osteomyelitis is an uncommon finding of invasive aspergillosis. Vertebral osteomyelitis can result from local extension of an *Aspergillus* empyema. *Aspergillus* osteomyelitis can also be seen as a complication of disseminated infection or as a primary infection in certain risk groups such as chronic granulomatous disease or in intravenous drug use. Vertebral osteomyelitis is the most common site for hematogenous spread to bone, usually involving the lumbar region.[99] The lesions can be seen on plain radiographs (Fig. 258-11) as well as on a CT or an MRI scan, which can be useful to stage the infection and to guide needle biopsy of the lesion. Favorable responses in *Asper-*

gillus osteomyelitis of the spine exceeded 60% in one review, although the need for long-term therapy and surgical intervention in medically nonresponsive patients is noted.[100] Infection of an intervertebral disk is a rare complication of hematogenous spread or surgery on the disk.

Cutaneous Infection

Skin involvement by *Aspergillus* can either represent disseminated hematogenous infection or local inoculation of infection that may arise around an intravenous catheter insertion site or the surrounding areas covered by adhesive dressings.[52] Whereas most lesions occur in patients with neutropenia or in other immunocompromised patients, *Aspergillus* can also invade patients with burns or surgical wounds. Clinically, the lesion is an area of rapidly increasing erythema with a necrotic, often ulcerated, center (Fig. 258-12). The lesions resemble pyoderma gangrenosum. Pathologically, invasion of blood vessels and cutaneous ulceration occurs. Cutaneous disease can also be a manifestation of widespread disseminated disease, and in that setting a skin biopsy can be a relatively easy method to obtain tissue to establish the diagnosis of invasive aspergillosis.

Other Sites

Invasive aspergillosis has also been reported in anecdotal cases to cause infection in virtually all body sites, including the heart, kidney, esophagus, intestine, and others.[1] *Aspergillus* endocarditis can occur in either native or prosthetic heart valves.[101] Diagnosis is difficult because blood cultures usually remain negative even with extensive disease.[102] Even with surgical intervention, long-term survival is limited although favorable outcomes with newer agents, particularly voriconazole, have been reported.[103] *Aspergillus* pericarditis is also associated with disseminated infection but can occur because of local extension of invasive pulmonary aspergillosis and can be complicated with cardiac tamponade. Some of these uncommon syndromes appear more common in certain epidemiologic settings. Renal infection occurs in patients with AIDS or with a history of injection drug use.[1]

▦ Diagnosis and Susceptibility Testing

A proven diagnosis of invasive aspergillosis requires a tissue biopsy showing invasion with hyphae and a positive culture for *Aspergillus*.[91] The diagnosis can also be established with positive cultures from a normally sterile site such as a needle biopsy or cerebrospinal fluid (CSF), although blood cultures are rarely positive.[104] Tissue biopsies may not be possible in some immunosuppressed patients because of potential risks, although *Aspergillus* hyphae are easily seen with

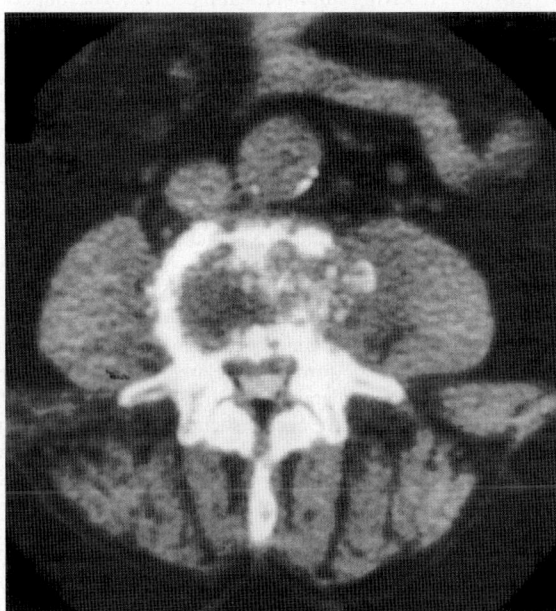

Figure 258-11 Radiograph of spine showing bone destruction associated with spinal aspergillosis.

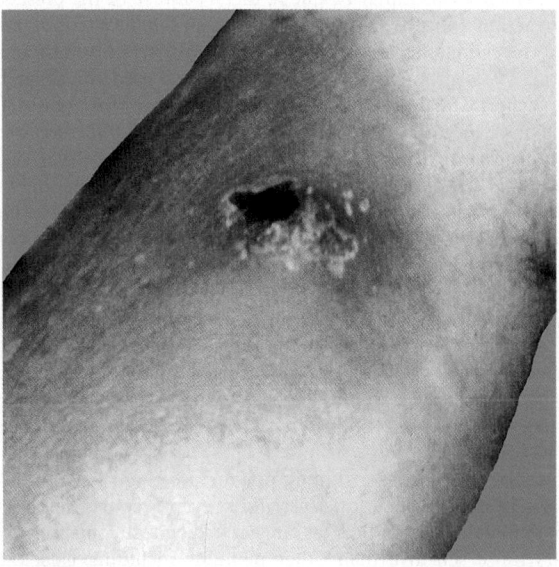

Figure 258-12 Necrotic skin lesion of cutaneous aspergillosis.

common fungal stains such as Gomori methenamine silver (GMS) or periodic acid–Schiff (PAS). *Aspergillus* hyphae are hyaline, septate, acute-angle branched, and 3 to 6 μm in width.[23] Although these features usually distinguish *Aspergillus* from agents of mucormycosis, they are not distinguishable from a number of other opportunistic molds, including *Fusarium, Scedosporium (Pseudallescheria),* and others so that a positive culture is needed to confirm the diagnosis.[23]

Cultures for *Aspergillus* in respiratory samples in high-risk patients, particularly if obtained via bronchial alveolar lavage, can support the diagnosis of probable invasive aspergillosis.[91] In current definitions of invasive mycoses, a positive respiratory culture with a clinical illness compatible with the diagnosis and new pulmonary infiltrates in an immunosuppressed patient is defined as a probable case of invasive pulmonary aspergillosis for the purposes of clinical trials.[91] *Aspergillus* is also cultured from patients in whom no clinical illness is apparent so that positive cultures in patients with a low risk for invasive aspergillosis should be interpreted with caution.[25]

Radiographic findings can also be used in the diagnosis and management of invasive pulmonary aspergillosis. Plain chest radiographs are of limited diagnostic utility because they are insensitive and findings are nonspecific.[7] However, as previously discussed chest CT can be very useful for establishing a diagnosis because the presence of a "halo" of low attenuation surrounding a nodular lesion is an early finding in invasive pulmonary aspergillosis and has been used as a marker for initiating early antifungal therapy.[4,7,105] Notably, the volume of lesions may increase over the first 7 days of infection, even when therapy is successful, so that early radiologic progression should be interpreted cautiously.[6] The CT findings of IPA have been validated in high-risk, neutropenic, and bone marrow transplant recipients, but in other patients, including solid organ transplant recipients, the CT findings are not as useful. Nonculture methods have been used to establish a rapid diagnosis of invasive aspergillosis.[106] Antibody detection is of limited utility because immunosuppressed hosts fail to mount an antibody response even with invasive infection.[59] Detection of galactomannan by EIA has contributed substantially to the diagnosis of invasive aspergillosis.[107] This assay has been validated in animal models and in clinical studies in a variety of hosts. Studies have suggested a sensitivity as high as 89% and a specificity of 92% in high-risk HSCT patients.[108] Other studies have found the assay to be less sensitive (40-50%), reflecting the impact of prior antifungal therapy in reducing the level of circulating galactomannan, a limited number of samples per patient, extent of infection, and other variables.[107-109] This has resulted in recommendations for a lower cutoff for a positive test result, especially in high-risk patients with greater probability of infection.[108,110] False-positive results have been reported, including in some neonates, which may be due to dietary intake or the presence of cross-reacting antigens with bacteria such as *Bifidobacterium,* and in patients receiving therapy with piperacillin/tazobactam and other antibiotics.[107,111,112] Although the method has been used for other body fluids such as CSF and in bronchial alveolar lavage (BAL) fluid, these samples have been less extensively evaluated compared with serum.[107,113] Results from BAL fluid testing demonstrate sensitivity that may be greater than that seen in serum testing.[114] Despite its potential value, several questions of the EIA remain, including the value of routine surveillance testing, frequency of testing, role of false-positive results, importance of prior antifungal therapy, and correlation with clinical outcome.

Other potential markers also include nonspecific fungal marker β-glucan using a variation of the limulus assay to detect endotoxin. This assay is approved for clinical diagnosis of invasive fungal infection and is included in the lastest EORTC/MSG diagnostic criteria, although few cases of invasive aspergillosis have been included in studies evaluating its utility.[115,116]

Molecular diagnostics including polymerase chain reaction (PCR) have also been developed for *Aspergillus*. Several reports demonstrate the potential for using PCR as an early diagnostic marker, which appears more sensitive than other methods including galactomannan.[117-120] These assays are not standardized and remain investiga-

tional, although this approach is very promising for improving the diagnosis of invasive aspergillosis.[121]

Susceptibility testing for molds including *Aspergillus* has been standardized, but correlation with clinical responses has not been established.[122,123] Antifungal resistance to itraconazole has been reported, which correlated with lack of efficacy in an animal model, suggesting the potential utility of susceptibility testing.[124] Multiple triazole-resistant *Aspergillus* species have been reported, including spread of a single resistance mechanism.[125,126] In that report, all cases were observed since 1999 and the prevalence of resistant *A. fumigatus* ranged from 1.7% to 6%. The authors speculated that resistance in *A. fumigatus* could be related to the widespread use of agricultural triazole fungicides.[126] Other species, such as *Aspergillus terreus,* may be resistant to amphotericin B and susceptible to the newer azoles, so testing of those species may be warranted,[127] although the indications for susceptibility testing of *Aspergillus* at the present time are unclear.

▓ Therapy

Historical efficacy of antifungal therapy in invasive aspergillosis has been extremely poor, with favorable responses in less than 40% of patients, and overall mortality rates are almost 60%.[2,3] Response to antifungal therapy depends on several factors, including the immune status of the host and the extent of infection at time of diagnosis. In severely immunosuppressed patients, such as those undergoing allogeneic bone marrow transplantation, and in patients with widely disseminated infection, extremely poor outcomes have been reported, with mortality rates in the highest-risk groups greater than 90%.[1,3]

PRIMARY ANTIFUNGAL THERAPY

Voriconazole

Voriconazole is a potent, broad-spectrum triazole that has become the recommended primary therapy for most patients with invasive aspergillosis.[1] The drug can be given either orally or intravenously and at the same dosage (Chapter 40). Voriconazole has potent fungicidal activity against various *Aspergillus* species, including *A. terreus*.[123] The recommendation for voriconazole for primary therapy is based on a randomized trial that compared voriconazole with amphotericin B deoxycholate, with each agent followed by other licensed antifungal therapy if needed for intolerance or progression of disease.[4] In this trial, voriconazole was successful in 52% of patients as compared with only 31% in those receiving amphotericin B deoxycholate. Superiority of voriconazole was demonstrated in patients at high risk for mortality, including those undergoing bone marrow transplantation and in those with extrapulmonary disease, including central nervous system involvement, as had previously been seen in open-labeled studies.[94,128] A survival benefit of voriconazole was also shown as compared with amphotericin B.[4] The efficacy of voriconazole is further demonstrated in adult and pediatric patients receiving voriconazole for treatment of invasive aspergillosis in patients who were refractory to or intolerant of conventional antifungal therapy.[31,129] Finally, voriconazole has also demonstrated efficacy in very difficult to treat clinical conditions, with responses of approximately 34% in central nervous system infection and in 52% of patients with osteomyelitis.[94,100]

Although voriconazole is generally adequately tolerated and exhibits a favorable pharmacokinetic profile, there are a number of issues to consider, including drug intolerance and drug interactions, especially those with immunosuppressive agents such as cyclosporine, tacrolimus, and sirolimus, the latter of which is contraindicated for use with voriconazole. The most common adverse event has been a transient and reversible visual disturbance that has been reported in approximately 30% of patients receiving the drug.[4] This effect is dose related and described as an altered or increased light perception that is temporary and not associated with pathologic sequelae. Other adverse events have been less common, including liver abnormalities in 10% to 15%, skin rash in 6%, nausea and vomiting in 2%, and anorexia in 1%.

Amphotericin B Deoxycholate

The other antifungal therapy licensed for primary therapy of invasive aspergillosis is amphotericin B deoxycholate. For more than four decades, amphotericin B deoxycholate has been the gold standard therapy for critically ill patients with invasive aspergillosis.[1] Several recent studies have consistently documented the limited efficacy and substantial toxicity of amphotericin B deoxycholate in high-risk patients.[4,130,131] The overall response rates of amphotericin B deoxycholate are less than 25%, with responses of only 10% to 15% in more severely immunosuppressed patients.[3,4] Wingard and colleagues have recently documented the increased morbidity and mortality associated with standard amphotericin B therapy in patients receiving bone marrow transplantation and those receiving concomitant nephrotoxic agents.[131] Similar findings were documented by Bates and colleagues, who found that renal toxicity occurred in approximately 30% of patients receiving amphotericin B deoxycholate and that this toxicity was associated with a sixfold increase in mortality as well as a dramatic increase in hospital costs.[130] These unacceptably high mortality rates and significant toxicity have highlighted the need for new therapeutic approaches to this disease; thus, for most patients with invasive aspergillosis, primary therapy with amphotericin B can no longer be recommended.[1] New antifungal therapies with activity against Aspergillus have been developed, including lipid forms of amphotericin B, the newer azoles (voriconazole, posaconazole, isavuconazole, and ravuconazole), and an additional class of antifungal therapy, the echinocandins (caspofungin, micafungin, and anidulafungin) (Table 258-4), all of which offer new options for therapy for this disease.[132,133]

OTHER ANTIFUNGAL AGENTS

Lipid Amphotericin Formulations

The lipid formulations of amphotericin B offer the advantage of less toxicity and allow higher doses of therapy.[134] Lipid formulations of amphotericin are approved for use as salvage therapy of invasive aspergillosis. The efficacy and role of lipid formulations of amphotericin B in the treatment of invasive aspergillosis remain debatable, in part, because few randomized trials have been conducted for patients with this disease.[134,135] A recent clinical trial compared the utility of high initial doses of liposomal amphotericin B (10 mg/kg/day versus 3 mg/kg/day for 2 weeks) followed by standard antifungal regimens. In this trial, similar efficacy of 50% and 46% in the 2 groups, respectively.[134] These results suggest that standard doses of liposomal amphotericin are adequate as primary therapy in some patients.[1] Another study evaluated amphotericin B colloidal dispersion for primary therapy for invasive aspergillosis, which showed similar efficacy with reduced renal toxicity of the lipid formulation but with serious pulmonary toxicities.[136] Meta-analysis of studies using lipid formulations of amphotericin B show reduced nephrotoxicity and favorable results as salvage therapy with these agents for invasive aspergillosis.[137]

Other Triazoles

Another approach to the therapy of aspergillosis has been with the triazole antifungals. Among these compounds, itraconazole is approved for use as salvage therapy of aspergillosis, but its utility has been limited because of unfavorable pharmacokinetic and tolerability profile. Although an intravenous formulation obviated bioavailability concerns, that formulation is no longer clinically available. For these reasons, itraconazole is more frequently used in less immunosuppressed patients who are able to take oral therapy and for use as sequential oral therapy and for those patients with saprophytic or allergic conditions.[3]

In addition to voriconazole, other extended-spectrum triazoles, include posaconazole, isavuconazole, and ravuconazole, have activity in vitro against Aspergillus.[138] Posaconazole is available in only an oral formulation. Posaconazole is approved for prophylaxis of invasive fungal infection including aspergillosis and has been shown to have activity in salvage therapy as well.[41,139,140] Isavuconazole, which is available both orally and intravenously, has in vitro and in vivo activity against Aspergillus and is currently in clinical development.[141]

TABLE 258-4	Antifungal Agents for Invasive Aspergillosis				
Agent	Class	Route of Administration	Dose		Comments
Primary Therapy					
Voriconazole	Azole	IV/oral	6 mg/kg (IV) q12h × 2 doses, followed by 4 mg/kg (IV) q12h or 200 mg (PO) q12h. Some experts advise oral dosing as 4 mg/kg (PO) q12h.		Recommended for primary therapy in most patients due to randomized trial demonstrating improved survival as compared with amphotericin B deoxycholate[1,4,128]; caution for use in patients with potential liver toxicity and for drug interactions
Other Agents					
Amphotericin B	Polyene	IV	1-1.5 mg/kg/day		Previous gold standard; significant toxicity in higher doses; limited efficacy in high-risk patients[130,131]
Liposomal amphotericin B	Polyene	IV	3-5 mg/kg/day		Well tolerated; minimal infusion reactions or nephrotoxicity; initial doses of 10 mg/kg/day more toxic and not more effective[134]
Amphotericin B lipid complex	Polyene	IV	5 mg/kg/day		Indicated for patients intolerant or refractory to standard therapy; case-controlled data suggest better efficacy than amphotericin B deoxycholate[172]
Amphotericin B colloidal dispersion	Polyene	IV	3-6 mg/kg/day		More infusion-related toxicity than other lipid formulations; efficacy similar to amphotericin B in primary treatment[136]
Itraconazole	Azole	Oral	200 mg bid (PO)		Oral solution improved bioavailability; intravenous formulation not currently available[3]
Posaconazole	Azole	Oral	Investigational for Aspergillus treatment: 400 mg (PO) bid; prophylaxis 200 mg (PO) tid		Oral formulation; efficacy in salvage therapy and prophylaxis[41,139,140]
Ravuconazole	Polyene	Oral	Investigational		In vitro and animal model studies; early clinical development; long half-life; intravenous formulation under study[142]
Caspofungin	Echinocandin	IV	50-70 mg/day		Approved for refractory infection and intolerance to standard therapy; well tolerated; possible interaction with cyclosporine.[146] Preclinical and anecdotal data showing improved efficacy in combination with azoles[143,150]
Micafungin	Echinocandin	IV	Investigational for Aspergillus treatment [U.S.] (50-100 mg/day)		Efficacy for prevention and salvage treatment of aspergillosis[147,173]
Anidulafungin	Echinocandin	IV	Investigational for Aspergillus (100 mg/day)		In clinical development for Aspergillus[174]

Ravuconazole has been evaluated in early-phase clinical trials and has also shown activity in animal models of invasive aspergillosis.[142]

Echinocandins

The echinocandins are an additional class of antifungals with *Aspergillus* activity.[143,144] These agents, which are administered intravenously, target glucan synthase, which is needed for production of β-1,3-glucan in fungal cells walls.[145] These effects are not fungicidal but significantly alter the growing fungal cell wall. Included in these agents are caspofungin, micafungin, and anidulafungin. Caspofungin is approved for treating patients refractory to or intolerant of standard therapies for invasive aspergillosis but is not recommended for primary therapy.[146] In one prophylaxis study, micafungin reduced the number of *Aspergillus* infections as compared with standard prophylaxis with fluconazole and has activity in salvage therapy of the disease.[147] Anidulafungin is another echinocandin with *Aspergillus* activity and appears to have favorable toxicity profile similar to those of the other echinocandins.

Combination Antifungal Therapy

The availability of several antifungal drugs and drug classes against *Aspergillus* has increased interest in combination antifungal therapy for this infection.[1,148-150] None of these combinations has been evaluated in clinical trials. At present, no convincing evidence is available for use of combination therapy. Previous studies showed in vivo (in murine aspergillosis) and in vitro antagonism between amphotericin B and ketoconazole, an early imidazole with limited *Aspergillus* activity.[151] This antagonism occurred with pretreatment of *Aspergillus* with the azole, reducing the cell wall ergosterol and eliminating the site of action of amphotericin B. Although other studies with newer azoles have not consistently shown this effect, some experimental studies have shown antagonism with combination therapy.[152,153]

Combinations of other drug classes have been attempted in the past, including amphotericin B and rifampin, flucytosine, and others (such as terbinafine).[154] Unfortunately, preclinical and in vitro studies have had limited utility in guiding clinical combination therapy. Problems with rifampin combinations include increased metabolism of the azoles, which makes that combination not generally recommended. Similarly, flucytosine has limited activity against *Aspergillus* and can cause pancytopenia that worsens immunosuppression. Recent animal model studies have demonstrated the potential for echinocandins with the new azoles (especially voriconazole) or with polyene therapy in reducing tissue burden and in sterilizing tissues.[143,155] A randomized comparison of liposomal amphotericin B 3 mg/kg plus caspofungin versus liposomal amphotericin 10 mg/kg was stopped before adequate patient accrual occurred.[156] A retrospective comparison of voriconazole plus caspofugin for salvage therapy in 16 patients found better results than prior use of voriconazole alone in 31 patients for salvage therapy.[150] This comparison did not address the use of combination drugs for initial therapy and compared drugs used in different time periods. A later retrospective analysis from the same institution showed no effect on outcome of voriconazole plus caspofungin as initial therapy and found that improved outcomes were observed over time irrespective of treatment modality.[157] A randomized clinical trial is currently in progress, comparing voriconazole to the combination of voriconazole plus anidulafungin.[143,150,155] The Infectious Diseases Society of America (IDSA) guidelines considered combination therapy to be experimental, while the Australian and German guidelines considered the data inadequate to recommend combination therapy.[1,158,159]

Adjuvant Therapy

Adjuvant therapies including surgical resection or use of granulocyte transfusions and growth factors in invasive aspergillosis can augment antifungal therapy, although their utility has not been established in randomized trials. Surgical resection of isolated pulmonary nodules before additional immunosuppressive therapies has been shown to improve outcome of infection,[88,160] although favorable outcomes with voriconazole suggest that in some patients surgical resection may not be necessary.[1] Surgical resection should also be considered in patients with severe hemoptysis or lesions near the hilar vessels or pericardium.[1]

Other adjuvant therapies include granulocyte and granulocyte-macrophage colony-stimulating factors, interferon-γ, and granulocyte transfusions, especially granulocyte colony-stimulating factor mobilized cells.[161] All these approaches have all been shown in anecdotal reports to improve outcomes but are not generally recommended for routine use.[1]

Approach to Therapy

Guidelines for treating invasive aspergillosis have been published by the IDSA.[1] Unfortunately, few randomized controlled trials exist in this area for evidence-based approaches to therapy. A prompt diagnosis and effective initial therapy are both critical in improving the outcome of this infection.[162] Radiography and use of galactomannan EIA may facilitate an early detection of aspergillosis in high-risk patients.[8,163] Most patients should receive primary therapy with voriconazole, which has been shown to be superior to amphotericin B, the other antifungal approved for primary therapy for this infection.[4] In patients who are intolerant of voriconazole, have a contraindication to the drug, or have progressive infection, alternative agents include lipid forms of amphotericin B, the echinocandins, or another triazole.[134,139,146,147] Primary use of combination therapy is not recommended at the present time because of the lack of prospective clinical trial data, but the addition of another agent or a switch to another antifungal class in a salvage setting may be considered due to the poor outcomes of a single agent in progressive infection.[1] Sequential therapy with oral azoles after initial intravenous therapy may be a useful option.[3] Although the optimal duration of antifungal therapy is not known, improvement in underlying host defenses is crucial to successful therapy.

Prevention and Prophylaxis

Prevention of invasive aspergillosis in high-risk patients is difficult. Nosocomial outbreaks of aspergillosis have been linked to construction, contaminated ventilation systems, and possibly to contaminated water.[50,164,165] For high-risk patients, such as those undergoing hematopoietic stem cell transplantation, the use of high-efficiency particulate air (HEPA) filters, frequent air exchanges, and positive pressure ventilation has been recommended to limit exposures in the hospital setting.[49,166] Infection control measures such as construction barriers will limit exposure to aerosols.[87] In addition, attention to routine maintenance and cleaning of showers and water systems may further reduce risk.[167] Some patients will still develop infection with these precautions, and an increasing number of immunosuppressed patients receive care outside of the hospital setting so that community-acquired infection is common.[51]

Efficacy of antifungal prophylaxis has been limited until recently because of the toxicity of amphotericin B and the limited activity of other oral agents against *Aspergillus*. Agents evaluated in this setting include low-dose amphotericin B, low doses of lipid formulations of amphotericin B, and nasal and aerosolized forms of amphotericin B—none of which has demonstrated conclusively to be beneficial in a large randomized clinical trial. Recent studies of aerosolized formulations of lipid amphotericin B demonstrate its safety and potential efficacy in lung transplant recipients at high risk for invasive aspergillosis.[168] Itraconazole has been suggested to have benefit against prevention of molds, but its poor tolerance in high-risk patients has also limited its use.[169,170] In a single, long-term randomized, double-blind, placebo-controlled study of fungal prophylaxis in patients with chronic granulomatous disease, itraconazole appeared to reduce the incidence of serious fungal infections, including those due to *Aspergillus*.[171]

Two recent randomized trials have established the safety and efficacy of posaconazole in high-risk patients. Posaconazole was compared to fluconazole in a randomized, double-blind trial in patients undergoing HSCT with graft-versus-host disease. In that trial, posaconazole significantly reduced the number of breakthrough fungal infections including invasive aspergillosis.[140] In the companion trial, posaconazole was compared to standard of care (either fluconazole or itraconazole) for patients with acute myelogenous leukemia or myelodysplastic syndrome.[134] In that trial, prophylaxis with posaconazole reduced breakthrough fungal infections and significantly prolonged survival. Although posaconazole was generally well tolerated, more serious adverse drug events occurred with posaconazole therapy so that a risk-benefit analysis should be considered when recommending posaconazole prophylaxis.[40] From the results of these trials, guidelines recommend the use of posaconazole prophylaxis in patients with acute myelogenous leukemia or with graft-versus-host disease who are are high risk for invasive aspergillosis.[1]

REFERENCES

1. Walsh TJ, Anaissie EJ, Denning DW, et al. Treatment of aspergillosis: clinical practice guidelines of the Infectious Diseases Society of America. *Clin Infect Dis*. 2008;46:327-360.
2. Lin SJ, Schranz J, Teutsch SM. Aspergillosis case—Fatality rate: Systematic review of the literature. *Clin Infect Dis*. 2001;32:358-366.
3. Patterson TF, Kirkpatrick WR, White M, et al. Invasive aspergillosis. Disease spectrum, treatment practices, and outcomes. I3 *Aspergillus* Study Group. *Medicine (Baltimore)*. 2000;79:250-260.
4. Herbrecht R, Denning DW, Patterson TF, et al. Voriconazole versus amphotericin B for primary therapy of invasive aspergillosis. *N Engl J Med*. 2002;347:408-415.
5. Neofytos D, Horn D, Anaissie E, et al. Epidemiology and outcome of invasive fungal infection in adult hematopoietic stem cell transplant recipients: analysis of Multicenter Prospective Antifungal Therapy (PATH) Alliance registry. *Clin Infect Dis*. 2009;48:265-273.
6. Caillot D, Couaillier JF, Bernard A, et al. Increasing volume and changing characteristics of invasive pulmonary aspergillosis on sequential thoracic computed tomography scans in patients with neutropenia. *J Clin Oncol*. 2001;19:253-259.
7. Greene RE, Schlamm HT, Oestmann JW, et al. Imaging findings in acute invasive pulmonary aspergillosis: clinical significance of the halo sign. *Clin Infect Dis*. 2007;44:373-379.
8. Maertens J, Theunissen K, Verhoef G, et al. Galactomannan and computed tomography-based preemptive antifungal therapy in neutropenic patients at high risk for invasive fungal infection: a prospective feasibility study. *Clin Infect Dis*. 2005;41:1242-1250.
9. Mackenzie DW. Aspergillus in man. In: *Proceedings of the Second International Symposium on Topics in Mycology*. Antwerp, Belgium: University of Antwerp; 1987.
10. Kwon-Chung KJ. Aspergillus: Diagnosis and description of the genus. In: *Proceedings of the Second International Symposium on Topics in Mycology*. Antwerp, Belgium: University of Antwerp; 1987.
11. Link H. Observations in ordines plantarum naturales. *Gesellschaft Naturforschender Freunde zu Berlin, Magazin*. 1809;3:1.
12. Sutton DA. Rare and emerging agents of hyalohyphomycosis. *Curr Fungal Infect Reports*. 2008;2:134-142.
13. Balajee SA, Houbraken J, Verweij PE, et al. *Aspergillus* species identification in the clinical setting. *Stud Mycol*. 2007;59:39-46.
14. Summerbell R. Ascomycetes. *Aspergillus, Fusarium, Sporothrix, Piedraia*, and Their Relatives. In: Howard DH, ed. *Pathogenic fungi in humans and animals*. 2nd ed. New York: Marcel Dekker; 2003:237-498.
15. Klich M, Pitt J. *A laboratory guide to common Aspergillus species and their teleomorphs*. North Ryde, New South Wales, Australia: Commonwealth Scientific and Industrial Research Organization; 1988.
16. Iwen PC, Rupp ME, Langnas AN, et al. Invasive pulmonary aspergillosis due to *Aspergillus terreus*: 12- year experience and review of the literature. *Clin Infect Dis*. 1998;26:1092-1097.
17. O'Gorman CM, Fuller HT, Dyer PS. Discovery of a sexual cycle in the opportunistic fungal pathogen *Aspergillus fumigatus*. *Nature*. 2008.
18. Pitt JI, Samson RA. Nomenclatural considerations in naming species of *Aspergillus* and its teleomorphs. *Stud Mycol*. 2007;59:67-70.
19. Geiser DM, Klich MA, Frisvad JC, et al. The current status of species recognition and identification in *Aspergillus*. *Stud Mycol*. 2007;59:1-10.
20. Balajee SA, Nickle D, Varga J, et al. Molecular studies reveal frequent misidentification of *Aspergillus fumigatus* by morphotyping. *Eukaryot Cell*. 2006;5:1705-1712.
21. Steinbach WJ, Benjamin DK Jr, Kontoyiannis DP, et al. Infections due to *Aspergillus terreus*: a multicenter retrospective analysis of 83 cases. *Clin Infect Dis*. 2004;39:192-198.
22. Pitt J. The current role of *Aspergillus* and *Penicillium* in human and animal health. *J Med Vet Mycol*. 1994;1:17-21.
23. Sutton DA, Fothergill AW, Rinaldi MG, eds. *Guide to Clinically Significant Fungi*. 1st ed. Baltimore: Williams & Wilkins; 1998:471.
24. Balajee SA, Gribskov JL, Hanley E, et al. *Aspergillus lentulus* sp. nov., a New Sibling Species of A. fumigatus. *Eukaryot Cell*. 2005;4:625-632.
25. Perfect JR, Cox GM, Lee JY, et al. The impact of culture isolation of *Aspergillus* species: A hospital-based survey of aspergillosis. *Clin Infect Dis*. 2001;33:1824-1833.
26. Anaissie EJ, Stratton SL, Dignani MC, et al. Pathogenic *Aspergillus* species recovered from a hospital water system: A 3-year prospective study. *Clin Infect Dis*. 2002;34:780-789.
27. Warris A, Voss A, Abrahamsen TG, et al. Contamination of hospital water with *Aspergillus fumigatus* and other molds. *Clin Infect Dis*. 2002;34:1159-1160.
28. Balajee SA, Imhof A, Gribskov JL, et al. Determination of antifungal drug susceptibilities of *Aspergillus* species by a fluorescence-based microplate assay. *J Antimicrob Chemother*. 2005;55:102-105.
29. Denning DW. Aflatoxin and human disease. A review. *Adverse Drug React Acute Poison Rev*. 1987;4:175-209.
30. Walsh TJ, Petraitis V, Petraitiene R, et al. Experimental pulmonary aspergillosis due to *Aspergillus terreus*: pathogenesis and treatment of an emerging fungal pathogen resistant to amphotericin B. *J Infect Dis*. 2003;188:305-319.
31. Perfect JR, Marr KA, Walsh TJ, et al. Voriconazole treatment for less-common, emerging, or refractory fungal infections. *Clin Infect Dis*. 2003;36:1122-1131.
32. Sutton DA, Sanche SE, Revankar SG, et al. In vitro amphotericin B resistance in clinical isolates of *Aspergillus terreus*, with a head-to-head comparison to voriconazole. *J Clin Microbiol*. 1999;37:2343-2345.
33. Geyer SJ, Surampudi RK. Photo quiz—Birefringent crystals in a pulmonary specimen. *Clin Infect Dis*. 2002;34:481,551-552.
34. Bellini C, Antonini P, Ermanni S, et al. Malignant otitis externa due to *Aspergillus niger*. *Scand J Infect Dis*. 2003;35:284-288.
35. Kontoyiannis DP, Lewis RE, May GS, et al. *Aspergillus nidulans* is frequently resistant to amphotericin B. *Mycoses*. 2002;45:406-407.
36. Houbraken J, Due M, Varga J, et al. Polyphasic taxonomy of *Aspergillus* section Usti. *Stud Mycol*. 2007;59:107-128.
37. Varga J, Houbraken J, Van Der Lee HA, et al. *Aspergillus calidoustus* sp. nov., causative agent of human infections previously assigned to *Aspergillus ustus*. *Eukaryot Cell*. 2008;7:630-638.
38. Barnes PD, Marr KA. Aspergillosis: spectrum of disease, diagnosis, and treatment. *Infect Dis Clin North Am*. 2006;20:545-561.
39. Wald A, Leisenring W, van Burik J-A, et al. Epidemiology of *Aspergillus* infections in a large cohort of patients undergoing bone marrow transplantation. *J Infect Dis*. 1997;175:1459-1466.
40. De Pauw BE, Donnelly JP. Prophylaxis and aspergillosis—has the principle been proven? *N Engl J Med*. 2007;356:409-411.
41. Cornely OA, Maertens J, Winston DJ, et al. Posaconazole vs. fluconazole or itraconazole prophylaxis in patients with neutropenia. *N Engl J Med*. 2007;356:348-359.
42. Pagano L, Fianchi L, Leone G. Fungal pneumonia due to molds in patients with hematological malignancies. *J Chemother*. 2006;18:339-352.
43. Warris A, Bjorneklett A, Gaustad P. Invasive pulmonary aspergillosis associated with infliximab therapy. *N Engl J Med*. 2001;344:1099-1100.
44. Marr KA, Carter RA, Crippa F, et al. Epidemiology and outcome of mould infections in hematopoietic stem cell transplant recipients. *Clin Infect Dis*. 2002;34:909-917.
45. Marr KA, Carter RA, Boeckh M, et al. Invasive aspergillosis in allogeneic stem cell transplant recipients: changes in epidemiology and risk factors. *Blood*. 2002;100:4358-4366.
46. Gavalda J, Len O, San Juan R, et al. Risk factors for invasive aspergillosis in solid-organ transplant recipients: a case-control study. *Clin Infect Dis*. 2005;41:52-59.
47. Singh N, Paterson DL. *Aspergillus* infections in transplant recipients. *Clin Microbiol Rev*. 2005;18:44-69.
48. Vandewoude KH, Blot SI, Depuydt P, et al. Clinical relevance of *Aspergillus* isolation from respiratory tract samples in critically ill patients. *Crit Care*. 2006;10:R31.
49. Haiduven D. Nosocomial aspergillosis and building construction. *Med Mycol*. 2008:1-7.
50. Anaissie EJ, Costa SF. Nosocomial aspergillosis is waterborne. *Clin Infect Dis*. 2001;33:1546-1548.
51. Patterson JE, Zidouh A, Miniter P, et al. Hospital epidemiologic surveillance for invasive aspergillosis: patient demographics and the utility of antigen detection. *Infect Control Hosp Epidemiol*. 1997;18:104-108.
52. Walsh TJ. Primary cutaneous aspergillosis—An emerging infection among immunocompromised patients. *Clin Infect Dis*. 1998;27:453-457.
53. Ng T, Robson G, Denning DW. Hydrocortisone-enchanced growth of *Aspergillus* spp: implications for pathogenesis. *Microbiology*. 1994;140:2475-2480.
54. Stevens DA, Moss RB, Kurup VP, et al. Allergic bronchopulmonary aspergillosis in cystic fibrosis—state of the art: Cystic Fibrosis Foundation Consensus Conference. *Clin Infect Dis*. 2003;37(Suppl 3):S225-S264.
55. Schaffner A, Douglas H, Braude A. Selective protection against conidia by mononuclear and against mycelia by polymorphonuclear phagocytes in resistance to *Aspergillus*. Observations on these two lines of defense in vivo and in vitro with human and mouse phagocytes. *J Clin Invest*. 1982;69:617-631.
56. Levitz SM, Selsted ME, Ganz T, et al. In vitro killing of spores and hyphae of *Aspergillus fumigatus* and *Rhizopus oryzae* by rabbit neutrophil cationic peptides and bronchoalveolar macrophages. *J Infec Dis*. 1986;154:483-489.
57. Crosdale DJ, Poulton KV, Ollier WE, et al. Mannose-binding lectin gene polymorphisms as a susceptibility factor for chronic necrotizing pulmonary aspergillosis. *J Infect Dis*. 2001;184:653-656.
58. Washburn RG, Hammer CH, Bennett JE. Inhibition of complement by culture supernatants of *Aspergillus fumigatus*. *J Infect Dis*. 1986;154:944-951.
59. Young RC, Bennett JE. Invasive aspergillosis. Absence of detectable antibody response. *Am Rev Resp Dis*. 1971;104:710-716.
60. Latge JP. The pathobiology of *Aspergillus fumigatus*. *Trends Microbiol*. 2001;9:382-389.
61. Cramer RA Jr, Gamcsik MP, Brooking RM, et al. Disruption of a nonribosomal peptide synthetase in *Aspergillus fumigatus* eliminates gliotoxin production. *Eukaryot Cell*. 2006;5:972-980.
62. Cenci E, Perito S, Enssle KH, et al. Th1 and Th2 cytokines in mice with invasive aspergillosis. *Infect Immun*. 1997;65:564-570.
63. Steele C, Rapaka RR, Metz A, et al. The beta-glucan receptor dectin-1 recognizes specific morphologies of *Aspergillus fumigatus*. *PLoS Pathog*. 2005;1:e42.
64. Gersuk GM, Underhill DM, Zhu L, et al. Dectin-1 and TLRs permit macrophages to distinguish between different *Aspergillus fumigatus* cellular states. *J Immunol*. 2006;176:3717-3724.
65. Meier A, Kirschning CJ, Nikolaus T, et al. Toll-like receptor (TLR) 2 and TLR4 are essential for *Aspergillus*-induced activation of murine macrophages. *Cell Microbiol*. 2003;5:561-570.
66. Marr KA, Balajee SA, Hawn TR, et al. Differential role of MyD88 in macrophage-mediated responses to opportunistic fungal pathogens. *Infect Immun*. 2003;71:5280-5286.
67. Mambula SS, Sau K, Henneke P, et al. Toll-like receptor (TLR) signaling in response to *Aspergillus fumigatus*. *J Biol Chem*. 2002;277:39320-39326.
68. Bochud PY, Chien JW, Marr KA, et al. Toll-like receptor 4 polymorphisms and aspergillosis in stem-cell transplantation. *N Engl J Med*. 2008;359:1766-1777.
69. Zaas AK, Liao G, Chien JW, et al. Plasminogen alleles influence susceptibility to invasive aspergillosis. *PLoS Genet*. 2008;4:e1000101.
70. Greenberger PA. Allergic bronchopulmonary aspergillosis. *J Allergy Clin Immunol*. 2002;110:685-692.
71. Vaid M, Kaur S, Sambatakou H, et al. Distinct alleles of mannose-binding lectin (MBL) and surfactant proteins A (SP-A) in patients with chronic cavitary pulmonary aspergillosis and allergic bronchopulmonary aspergillosis. *Clin Chem Lab Med*. 2007;45:183-186.
72. Patterson R, Greenberger PA, Radin RC, et al. Allergic bronchopulmonary aspergillosis: Staging as an aid to management. *Ann Intern Med*. 1982;96:286-291.
73. Malo JL, Hawkins R, Pepys J. Studies in chronic allergic bronchopulmonary aspergillosis. 1. Clinical and physiological findings. *Thorax*. 1977;32:254-261.
74. Wark PA, Gibson PG and Wilson AJ. Azoles for allergic bronchopulmonary aspergillosis associated with asthma. Cochrane Database Syst Rev 2003:CD001108.
75. Stevens DA, Schwartz HJ, Lee JY, et al. A randomized trial of itraconazole in allergic bronchopulmonary aspergillosis. *N Engl J Med*. 2000;342:756-762.
76. DeShazo RD, Chapin K, Swain RE. Fungal sinusitis. *N Engl J Med*. 1997;337:254-259.
77. Mylonakis E, Barlam TF, Flanigan T, et al. Pulmonary aspergillosis and invasive disease in AIDS—Review of 342 cases. *Chest*. 1998;114:251-262.
78. Kauffman CA. Quandary about treatment of aspergillomas persists. *Lancet*. 1996;347:1640.
79. Ferguson BJ. Fungus balls of the paranasal sinuses. *Otolaryngol Clin N Amer*. 2000;33:389-398.
80. Denning DW, Riniotis K, Dobrashian R, et al. Chronic cavitary and fibrosing pulmonary and pleural aspergillosis: case series, proposed nomenclature change, and review. *Clin Infect Dis*. 2003;37(Suppl 3):S265-S280.
81. Torres-Rodriguez JM, Madrenys-Brunet N, Siddat M, et al. *Aspergillus versicolor* as cause of onychomycosis: report of 12

cases and susceptibility testing to antifungal drugs. *J Eur Acad Dermatol Venereol*. 1998;11:25-31.
82. Kuo IC, Margolis TP, Cevallos V, et al. *Aspergillus fumigatus* keratitis after laser in situ keratomileusis. *Cornea*. 2001;20:342-344.
83. Bunya VY, Hammersmith KM, Rapuano CJ, et al. Topical and oral voriconazole in the treatment of fungal keratitis. *Am J Ophthalmol*. 2007;143:151-153.
84. Jurkunas UV, Langston DP, Colby K. Use of voriconazole in the treatment of fungal keratitis. *Int Ophthalmol Clin*. 2007;47:47-59.
85. Kaushik S, Ram J, Brar GS, et al. Intracameral amphotericin B: initial experience in severe keratomycosis. *Cornea*. 2001;20:715-719.
86. Gerson SL, Talbot GH, Hurwitz S, et al. Prolonged granulocytopenia: the major risk factor for invasive pulmonary aspergillosis in patients with acute leukemia. *Ann Intern Med*. 1984;100:345-351.
87. Patterson JE, Peters J, Calhoon JH, et al. Investigation and control of aspergillosis and other filamentous fungal infections in solid organ transplant recipients. *Transpl Infect Dis*. 2000;2:22-28.
88. Yeghen T, Kibbler CC, Prentice HG, et al. Management of invasive pulmonary aspergillosis in hematology patients: A review of 87 consecutive cases at a single institution. *Clin Infect Dis*. 2000;31:859-868.
89. Patterson TF, Graybill JR. Mycoses caused by molds. In: Dolin R, Masur H, Saag MS, eds. *AIDS Therapy*. 3rd ed. Philadelphia: Churchill Livingstone; 2008:815-828.
90. de Carpentier J, Ramamurthy M, Taylor P, et al. An algorithmic approach to *Aspergillus* sinusitis. *J Laryngol Otol*. 1994;108:314-318.
91. De Pauw B, Walsh TJ, Donnelly JP, et al. Revised definitions of invasive fungal disease from the European Organization for Research and Treatment of Cancer/Invasive Fungal Infections Cooperative Group and the National Institute of Allergy and Infectious Diseases Mycoses Study Group (EORTC/MSG) Consensus Group. *Clin Infect Dis*. 2008;46:1813-1821.
92. Malani PN, Kauffman CA. Prevention and prophylaxis of invasive fungal sinusitis in the immunocompromised patient. *Otolaryngol Clin North Am*. 2000;33:301-312,VIII.
93. Schwartz S, Ruhnke M, Ribaud P, et al. Poor efficacy of amphotericin B-based therapy in CNS aspergillosis. *Mycoses*. 2007;50:196-200.
94. Schwartz S, Ruhnke M, Ribaud P, et al. Improved outcome in central nervous system aspergillosis, using voriconazole treatment. *Blood*. 2005;106:2641-2645.
95. Jantunen E, Volin L, Salonen O, et al. Central nervous system aspergillosis in allogeneic stem cell transplant recipients. *Bone Marrow Transplant*. 2003;31:191-196.
96. Hagensee ME, Bauwens JE, Kjos B, et al. Brain abscess following marrow transplantation: experience at the Fred Hutchinson Cancer Research Center, 1984-1992. *Clin Infect Dis*. 1994;19:402-408.
97. Walsh TJ, Hier DB, Caplan LR. Aspergillosis of the central nervous system: Clinicopathological analysis of 17 patients. *Ann Neurol*. 1985;18:574-582.
98. Ashdown B, Tien R, Felsberg G. Aspergillosis of the brain and paranasal sinuses in immunocompromised patients: CT and MR imaging findings. *AJR Am J Roentgenol*. 1994;162:155-159.
99. Vinas PC, King PK, Diaz FG. Spinal *Aspergillus* osteomyelitis. *Clin Infect Dis*. 1999;28:1223-1229.
100. Mouas H, Lutsar I, Dupont B, et al. Voriconazole for invasive bone aspergillosis: a worldwide experience of 20 cases. *Clin Infect Dis*. 2005;40:1141-1147.
101. Gumbo T, Taege AJ, Mawhorter S, et al. *Aspergillus* valve endocarditis in patients without prior cardiac surgery. *Medicine*. 2000;79:261-268.
102. Petrosillo N, Pellicelli AM, Cicalini S, et al. Endocarditis caused by *Aspergillus* species in injection drug users. *Clin Infect Dis*. 2001;33:E97-E99.
103. Reis LJ, Barton TD, Pochettino A, et al. Successful treatment of *Aspergillus* prosthetic valve endocarditis with oral voriconazole. *Clin Infect Dis*. 2005;41:752-753.
104. Kontoyiannis DP, Sumoza D, Tarrand J, et al. Significance of aspergillemia in patients with cancer: A 10-year study. *Clin Infect Dis*. 2000;31:188-189.
105. Caillot D, Casasnovas O, Bernard A, et al. Improved management of invasive pulmonary aspergillosis in neutropenic patients using early thoracic computed tomographic scan and surgery. *J Clin Oncol*. 1997;15:139-147.
106. Mennink-Kersten MA, Verweij PE. Non-culture-based diagnostics for opportunistic fungi. *Infect Dis Clin North Am*. 2006;20:711-727.
107. Mennink-Kersten MA, Donnelly JP, Verweij PE. Detection of circulating galactomannan for the diagnosis and management of invasive aspergillosis. *Lancet Infect Dis*. 2004;4:349-357.
108. Marr KA, Balajee SA, McLaughlin L, et al. Detection of galactomannan antigenemia by enzyme immunoassay for the diagnosis of invasive aspergillosis: variables that affect performance. *J Infect Dis*. 2004;190:641-649.
109. Herbrecht R, Letscher-Bru V, Oprea C, et al. *Aspergillus* galactomannan detection in the diagnosis of invasive aspergillosis in cancer patients. *J Clin Oncol*. 2002;20:1898-1906.
110. Maertens J, Theunissen K, Verbeken E, et al. Prospective clinical evaluation of lower cut-offs for galactomannan detection in adult neutropenic cancer patients and haematological stem cell transplant recipients. *Br J Haematol*. 2004;126:852-860.
111. Sulahian A, Touratier S, Leblanc T, et al. False positive *Aspergillus* antigenemia related to concomitant administration of tazocillin (abstract M-2062a). In: *Abstracts of the 43rd Interscience Conference on Antimicrobial Agents and Chemotherapy,* Chicago, IL, September, 14-17. Washington, D.C.: American Society for Microbiology; 2003.
112. Viscoli C, Machetti M, Cappellano P, et al. False-positive galactomannan platelia *Aspergillus* test results for patients receiving piperacillin-tazobactam. *Clin Infect Dis*. 2004;38:913-916.
113. Viscoli C, Machetti M, Gazzola P, et al. *Aspergillus* galactomannan antigen in the cerebrospinal fluid of bone marrow transplant recipients with probable cerebral aspergillosis. *J Clin Microbiol*. 2002;40:1496-1499.
114. Musher B, Fredricks D, Leisenring W, et al. *Aspergillus* galactomannan enzyme immunoassay and quantitative PCR for diagnosis of invasive aspergillosis with bronchoalveolar lavage fluid. *J Clin Microbiol*. 2004;42:5517-5522.
115. Ostrosky-Zeichner L, Alexander BD, Kett DH, et al. Multicenter clinical evaluation of the (1->3) beta-D-glucan assay as an aid to diagnosis of fungal infections in humans. *Clin Infect Dis*. 2005;41:654-659.
116. Obayashi T, Negishi K, Suzuki T, et al. Reappraisal of the serum (1->3)-beta-D-glucan assay for the diagnosis of invasive fungal infections–a study based on autopsy cases from 6 years. *Clin Infect Dis*. 2008;46:1864-1870.
117. Hebart H, Loffler J, Meisner C, et al. Early detection of *Aspergillus* infection after allogeneic stem cell transplantation by polymerase chain reaction screening. *J Infect Dis*. 2000;181:1713-1719.
118. Loeffler J, Hebart H, Cox P, et al. Nucleic acid sequence-based amplification of *Aspergillus* RNA in blood samples. *J Clin Microbiol*. 2001;39:1626-1629.
119. White PL, Linton CJ, Perry MD, et al. The evolution and evaluation of a whole blood polymerase chain reaction assay for the detection of invasive aspergillosis in hematology patients in a routine clinical setting. *Clin Infect Dis*. 2006;42:479-486.
120. Costa C, Costa JM, Desterke C, et al. Real-time PCR coupled with automated DNA extraction and detection of galactomannan antigen in serum by enzyme-linked immunosorbent assay for diagnosis of invasive aspergillosis. *J Clin Microbiol*. 2002;40:2224-2227.
121. Donnelly JP. Polymerase chain reaction for diagnosing invasive aspergillosis: Getting closer but still a ways to go. *Clin Infect Dis*. 2006;42:487-489.
122. Espinel-Ingroff A, Fothergill A, Peter J, et al. Testing conditions for determination of minimum fungicidal concentrations of new and established antifungal agents for *Aspergillus* spp.: NCCLS collaborative study. *J Clin Microbiol*. 2002;40:3204-3208.
123. Espinel-Ingroff A, Johnson E, Hockey H, et al. Activities of voriconazole, itraconazole and amphotericin B in vitro against 590 moulds from 323 patients in the voriconazole Phase III clinical studies. *J Antimicrob Chemother*. 2008;61:616-620.
124. Mosquera J, Denning DW. Azole cross-resistance in *Aspergillus fumigatus*. *Antimicrob Agents Chemother*. 2002;46:556-557.
125. Verweij PE, Mellado E, Melchers WJ. Multiple-triazole-resistant aspergillosis. *N Engl J Med*. 2007;356:1481-1483.
126. Snelders E, van der Lee HA, Kuijpers J, et al. Emergence of azole resistance in *Aspergillus fumigatus* and spread of a single resistance mechanism. *PLoS Med*. 2008;5:e219.
127. Steinbach WJ, Perfect JR, Schell WA, et al. In vitro analyses, animal models, and 60 clinical cases of invasive *Aspergillus terreus* infection. *Antimicrob Agents Chemother*. 2004;48:3217-3225.
128. Denning DW, Ribaud P, Milpied N, et al. Efficacy and safety of voriconazole in the treatment of acute invasive aspergillosis. *Clin Infect Dis*. 2002;34:563-571.
129. Walsh TJ, Lutsar I, Driscoll T, et al. Voriconazole in the treatment of aspergillosis, scedosporiosis and other invasive fungal infections in children. *Pediat Inf Dis J*. 2002;21:240-248.
130. Bates DW, Su L, Yu DT, et al. Mortality and costs of acute renal failure associated with amphotericin B therapy. *Clin Infect Dis*. 2001;32:686-693.
131. Wingard JR, Kubilis P, Lee L, et al. Clinical significance of nephrotoxicity in patients treated with amphotericin B for suspected or proven aspergillosis. *Clin Infect Dis*. 1999;29:1402-1407.
132. Patterson TF. Advances and challenges in management of invasive mycoses. *Lancet*. 2005;366:1013-1025.
133. Steinbach WJ, Stevens DA. Review of newer antifungal and immunomodulatory strategies for invasive aspergillosis. *Clin Infect Dis*. 2003;37(Suppl 3):S157-S187.
134. Cornely OA, Maertens J, Bresnik M, et al. Liposomal amphotericin B as initial therapy for invasive mold infection: a randomized trial comparing a high-loading dose regimen with standard dosing (AmBiLoad trial). *Clin Infect Dis*. 2007;44:1289-1297.
135. Rex JH, Walsh TJ, Nettleman M, et al. Need for alternative trial designs and evaluation strategies for therapeutic studies of invasive mycoses. *Clin Infect Dis*. 2001;33:95-106.
136. Bowden R, Chandrasekar P, White MH, et al. A double-blind, randomized, controlled trial of amphotericin B colloidal dispersion versus amphotericin B for treatment of invasive aspergillosis in immunocompromised patients. *Clin Infect Dis*. 2002;35:359-366.
137. Barrett JP, Vardulaki KA, Conlon C, et al. A systematic review of the antifungal effectiveness and tolerability of amphotericin B formulations. *Clin Ther*. 2003;25:1295-1320.
138. Dodds Ashley ES, Alexander BD. Posaconazole. *Drugs Today (Barc)*. 2005;41:393-400.
139. Walsh TJ, Raad I, Patterson TF, et al. Treatment of invasive aspergillosis with posaconazole in patients who are refractory to or intolerant of conventional therapy: an externally controlled trial. *Clin Infect Dis*. 2007;44:2-12.
140. Ullmann AJ, Lipton JH, Vesole DH, et al. Posaconazole or fluconazole for prophylaxis in severe graft-versus-host disease. *N Engl J Med*. 2007;356:335-347.
141. Warn PA, Sharp A, Denning DW. In vitro activity of a new triazole BAL4815, the active component of BAL8557 (the water-soluble prodrug), against *Aspergillus* spp. *J Antimicrob Chemother*. 2006;57:135-138.
142. Kirkpatrick WR, Perea S, Coco BJ, et al. Efficacy of ravuconazole (BMS-207147) in a guinea pig model of disseminated aspergillosis. *J Antimicrob Chemother*. 2002;49:353-357.
143. Kirkpatrick WR, Perea S, Coco BJ, et al. Efficacy of caspofungin alone and in combination with voriconazole in a Guinea pig model of invasive aspergillosis. *Antimicrob Agents Chemother*. 2002;46:2564-2568.
144. Petraitis V, Petraitiene R, Groll AH, et al. Comparative antifungal activities and plasma pharmacokinetics of micafungin (FK463) against disseminated candidiasis and invasive pulmonary aspergillosis in persistently neutropenic rabbits. *Antimicrob Agents Chemother*. 2002;46:1857-1869.
145. Bowman JC, Hicks PS, Kurtz MB, et al. The antifungal echinocandin caspofungin acetate kills growing cells of *Aspergillus fumigatus* in vitro. *Antimicrob Agents Chemother*. 2002;46:3001-3012.
146. Maertens J, Raad I, Petrikkos G, et al. Efficacy and safety of caspofungin for treatment of invasive aspergillosis in patients refractory to or intolerant of conventional antifungal therapy. *Clin Infect Dis*. 2004;39:1563-1571.
147. Denning DW, Marr KA, Lau WM, et al. Micafungin (FK463), alone or in combination with other systemic antifungal agents, for the treatment of acute invasive aspergillosis. *J Infect*. 2006;53:337-349.
148. Aliff TB, Maslak PG, Jurcic JG, et al. Refractory *Aspergillus* pneumonia in patients with acute leukemia: successful therapy with combination caspofungin and liposomal amphotericin. *Cancer*. 2003;97:1025-1032.
149. Kontoyiannis DP, Hachem R, Lewis RE, et al. Efficacy and toxicity of caspofungin in combination with liposomal amphotericin B as primary or salvage treatment of invasive aspergillosis in patients with hematologic malignancies. *Cancer*. 2003;98:292-299.
150. Marr KA, Boeckh M, Carter RA, et al. Combination antifungal therapy for invasive aspergillosis. *Clin Infect Dis*. 2004;39:797-802.
151. Schaffner A, Frick PG. The effect of ketoconazole on amphotericin B in a model of disseminated aspergillosis. *J Infect Dis*. 1985;151:902-910.
152. Meletiadis J, Petraitis V, Petraitiene R, et al. Triazole-polyene antagonism in experimental invasive pulmonary aspergillosis: in vitro and in vivo correlation. *J Infect Dis*. 2006;194:1008-1018.
153. Meletiadis J, Stergiopoulou T, O'Shaughnessy EM, et al. Concentration-dependent synergy and antagonism within a triple antifungal drug combination against *Aspergillus* species: analysis by a new response surface model. *Antimicrob Agents Chemother*. 2007;51:2053-2064.
154. Steinbach WJ, Stevens DA, Denning DW. Combination and sequential antifungal therapy for invasive aspergillosis: review of published in vitro and in vivo interactions and 6281 clinical cases from 1966 to 2001. *Clin Infect Dis*. 2003;37(Suppl 3):S188-S224.
155. Petraitis V, Petraitiene R, Sarafandi AA, et al. Combination therapy in treatment of experimental pulmonary aspergillosis: synergistic interaction between an antifungal triazole and an echinocandin. *J Infect Dis*. 2003;187:1834-1843.
156. Caillot D, Thiébaut A, Herbrecht R, et al. Liposomal amphotericin B in combination with caspofugin for invasive aspergillosis in patients with hematologic malignancies: a randomized pilot study (Combistrat trial). *Cancer*. 2007;110:2740-2746.
157. Upton A, Kirby KA, Carpenter P, et al. Invasive aspergillosis following hemtopoietic cell transplantation: outcomes and prognostic factors associated with mortality. *Clin Infect Dis*. 2007;44:431-440.
158. Thursky KA, Playford EG, Seymor JF, et al. Recommendations for treatment of established fungal infections. *Intern Med J*. 2008;38:496-520.
159. Cornely OA, Einsele H, Enzensberger R, et al. Treatment of invasive fungal infections in cancer patients—recommendations of the Infectious Diseases Working Party (AGIHO) of the German Society of Hematology and Oncology (DGHO). *Ann Hematol*. 2009;88:97-110.
160. Caillot D, Mannone L, Cuisenier B, et al. Role of early diagnosis and aggressive surgery in the management of invasive pulmonary aspergillosis in neutropenic patients. *Clin Microbiol Infect*. 2001;7:54-61.
161. Schiffer CA. Granulocyte transfusion therapy 2006: The comeback kid? *Med Mycol*. 2006;44(Suppl):383-386.
162. Patterson TF, Boucher HW, Herbrecht R, et al. Strategy of following voriconazole versus amphotericin B therapy with other licensed antifungal therapy for primary treatment of invasive

aspergillosis: impact of other therapies on outcome. *Clin Infect Dis.* 2005;41:1448-1452.

163. Herbrecht R. Improving the outcome of invasive aspergillosis: new diagnostic tools and new therapeutic strategies. *Ann Hematol.* 2002;81(Suppl 2):S52-S53.

164. Sherertz RJ, Belani A, Kramer BS, et al. Impact of air filtration on nosocomial *Aspergillus* infections: unique risk of bone marrow transplant recipients. *Am J Med.* 1987;83:709-718.

165. Walsh TJ, Dixon DM. Nosocomial aspergillosis: environmental microbiology, hospital epidemiology, diagnosis and treatment. *Eur J Epidemiol.* 1989;5:131-142.

166. Warris A, Klaassen CH, Meis JF, et al. Molecular epidemiology of *Aspergillus fumigatus* isolates recovered from water, air, and patients shows two clusters of genetically distinct strains. *J Clin Microbiol.* 2003;41:4101-4106.

167. Anaissie EJ, Owens S, Dignani MC, et al. Cleaning bathrooms: A novel approach to reducing patient exposure to aerosolized *Aspergillus* spp. *Blood.* 2001;98:207A.

168. Palmer SM, Drew RH, Whitehouse JD, et al. Safety of aerosolized amphotericin B lipid complex in lung transplant recipients. *Transplantation.* 2001;72:545-548.

169. Marr KA, Crippa F, Leisenring W, et al. Itraconazole versus fluconazole for prevention of fungal infections in patients receiving allogeneic stem cell transplants. *Blood.* 2004;103:1527-1533.

170. Winston DJ, Maziarz RT, Chandrasekar PH, et al. Intravenous and oral itraconazole versus intravenous and oral fluconazole for long-term antifungal prophylaxis in allogeneic hematopoietic stem-cell transplant recipients. A multicenter, randomized trial. *Ann Intern Med.* 2003;138:705-713.

171. Gallin JI, Alling DW, Malech HL, et al. Itraconazole to prevent fungal infections in chronic granulomatous disease. *N Engl J Med.* 2003;348:2416-2422.

172. Walsh TJ, Hiemenz JW, Seibel NL, et al. Amphotericin B lipid complex for invasive fungal infections: Analysis of safety and efficacy in 556 cases. *Clin Infect Dis.* 1998;26:1383-1396.

173. van Burik JA, Ratanatharathorn V, Stepan DE, et al. Micafungin versus fluconazole for prophylaxis against invasive fungal infections during neutropenia in patients undergoing hematopoietic stem cell transplantation. *Clin Infect Dis.* 2004;39:1407-1416.

174. Groll AH, Mickiene D, Petraitiene R, et al. Pharmacokinetic and pharmacodynamic modeling of anidulafungin (LY303366): Reappraisal of its efficacy in neutropenic animal models of opportunistic mycoses using optimal plasma sampling. *Antimicrob Agents Chemother.* 2001;45:2845-2855.

259

Agents of Mucormycosis and Entomophthoramycosis

DIMITRIOS P. KONTOYIANNIS | RUSSELL E. LEWIS

For reasons discussed in Chapter 256, Introduction to Mycoses, disappearance of the class Zygomycetes has made the term *zygomycosis* inappropriate. The term zygomycosis encompassed both mucormycosis and entamophthoramycosis. These two infections are so different that no new name has been proposed or is needed to include both. Most of this chapter discusses mucormycosis, a group of filamentous fungi in the subphylum Mucormycotina capable of causing severe, frequently life-threatening infections in humans, especially in the immunocompromised hosts. The first description of human mucormycosis is credited to Platauf, who in 1885 described a disseminated infection in a cancer patient caused by angioinvasive hyphae with a ribbon-like appearance in tissue that he termed *Mycosis mucorina*.[1] Subsequent descriptions of the infection in the following decades relied on tissue morphology and, as often is the case today, were infrequently confirmed by culture. Hence, the findings of poorly septated, angioinvasive hyphae in tissue, assumed to be *Mucor* species, have become synonymous with the clinical term *mucormycosis* or simply *mucor infection*. This terminology is further justified by the fact that all but the rare *Mortierella* species are within the order Mucorales.[2] However, the number of species causing human mucormycosis has expanded considerably in the past two decades with improvements in culture-based morphologic identification and the application of more precise molecular diagnostics for fungal identification (Table 259-1).[2] In fact, members of the genus *Rhizopus*, not *Mucor*, are now recognized as the predominant cause of human infections.[3]

Etiology

Agents of mucormycosis are ubiquitous fungi in the environment that are commonly found in decaying organic substrates, including bread, fruits, vegetable matter, soil, compost piles, and animal excreta.[2] These fungi characteristically produce large, ribbon-like hyphae that are irregular in diameter with only occasional septae—hence the characterization of these organisms as aseptate fungi.[4] Identification can be confirmed by observing the characteristic, saclike fruiting structures (sporangia), which produce internally spherical yellow or brown spores (sporangiospores) (Fig. 259-1).[2,5] Spores range from 3 to 11 μm in diameter are easily aerosolized and dispersed and cause infections in humans when inhaled or introduced through a cutaneous or percutaneous route.[2,6,7]

Although several species of the order Mucorales have been reported to predominate as causes of human mucormycosis, culture recovery of these fungi from infected tissue is suboptimal and may skew the current understanding of the etiologic spectrum of mucormycosis. The widening application of molecular diagnostic techniques (i.e., in situ hybridization) in culture-negative cases is likely to provide new insights into the prevalence and etiology of this infection. In review of more than 900 reported cases of mucormycosis, *Rhizopus* species (47%) were the most common causes of culture-confirmed mucormycosis, followed by *Mucor* species (18%), *Cunninghamella bertholletiae* (7%), *Apophysomyces elegans* (5%), *Absidia* species (5%), *Saksenaea* species (5%), and *Rhizomucor pusillus* (4%), with other species representing less than 3% of cultured confirmed cases.[3,8] Although *Actinomucor elegans* was first isolated in 1898, the species has rarely been reported to cause mucormycosis.[9]

Seasonal variations may affect the incidence of mucormycosis, with most infections occurring late August to November.[8] Likewise, major weather events have also been associated with infections due to less frequently isolated species, such as *Syncephalastrum racemosum* from respiratory samples following Hurricane Katrina,[10] or post-tsunami wound infections due to *Apophysomyces elegans*.[11]

Epidemiology

The primary mode of acquisition of mucormycosis is inhalation of spores from environmental sources.[2] Acquisition through the cutaneous or percutaneous route also occurs with traumatic disruption of skin barriers, burns, or direct injection or catheters.[6] Gastrointestinal mucormycosis, although less common, has been reported in immunosuppressed patients with repeated ingestion of spores during periods of severe malnutrition, ingestion of non-nutritional substances (pica), fermented porridges and alcoholic drinks prepared from corn, or herbal or homeopathic products contaminated with spores.[12,13]

Agents of mucormycosis are unique among filamentous fungi in their ability to infect a broader, more heterogeneous population of human hosts compared with other opportunistic molds. Although most cases of mucormycosis are community acquired, nosocomial acquisition or pseudonosocomial outbreaks have been linked to contaminated bandages and bandage tape,[14-16] needles,[17,18] or tongue depressors used to construct splints for intravenous and arterial cannulation sites in preterm infants.[19,20] The most common underlying risk factors for invasive mucormycosis include poorly controlled diabetes mellitus (both type 1 and type 2), metabolic acidosis, high-dose glucocorticoid therapy, penetrating trauma or burns, persistent neutropenia, and chelation therapy with deferoxamine in patients on dialysis or chronically transfusion dependent.[2,3,6] Less commonly, mucormycosis is a cause of infection in the setting of renal failure, diarrhea, and malnutrition in low-birth-weight infants and in HIV patients.[3] Patients who develop mucormycosis in the absence of underlying disease or immunosuppression at the time of infection often have a history of penetrating trauma, burns, surgery, or illicit intravenous drug use before the infection.[3] For example, a recent case series of mucormycosis at a nononcology, tertiary care center found that traumatic wounds or surgical sites were the most common infections sites (31%), followed by rhinocerebral (25%) and disseminated (12.5%) infections.[21]

Because mucormycosis is not a reportable disease, the true incidence of infection is not known. A population-based survey in the United States estimated an annual incidence of 1.7 cases per million people, which translates to about 500 cases per year.[3,22] This figure probably underestimates the true incidence of mucormycosis because of the difficulties associated with antemortem diagnosis of this infection. In autopsy series, the prevalence of mucormycosis has ranged from 1 to 5 cases per 10,000 autopsies, making the infection 10- to 50-fold less common than infections with *Candida* or *Aspergillus* species.[23] Historically, most published mucormycosis cases have been reported in diabetic patients or patients with no clear underlying immunosuppression.[3]

A significant increase in the rates of mucormycosis has been observed among patient groups classically at risk for other opportu-

TABLE 259-1	Taxonomic Organization of the Most Common Agents of Mucormycosis and Entomophthoramycosis	
Mucormycosis		*Entomophthoramycosis*
Rhizopus arrhizus (Rhizopus oryzae)		*Conidiobolus coronatus*
Rhizopus microsporus		*Conidiobolus incongruus*
Rhizomucor pusillus		*Basidiobolus ranarum*
Rhizopus stolonifer		
Cunninghamella bertholletiae		
Apophysomyces elegans		
Saksenaea vasiformis		
Absidia corymbifera		
Mucor circinelloides		
Syncephalastrum racemosum		
Actinomucor elegans		
Cokeromyces recurvatus		
Mortierella wolfii		

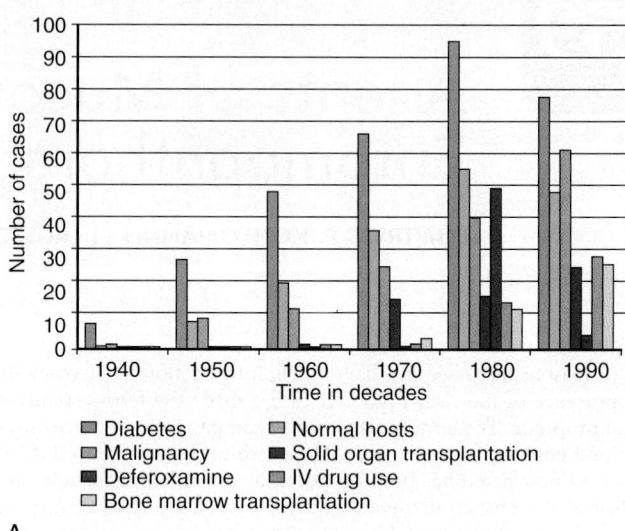

A

nistic mold infections, such as patients with hematologic malignancy, recipients of hematopoietic stem cell transplantation, and patients undergoing solid organ transplantation (Fig. 259-2). Data from the Centers for Disease Control and Prevention (CDC) Transplant Associated Infection Surveillance Network (TRANSNET) acquired from prospective surveys of 25 U.S. transplantation centers from 2001 to 2006 noted 1-year cumulative incidence rates for mucormycosis of 3.8 per 1000 in stem cell transplantations and 0.6 per 1000 organ transplantations,[24] accounting for 7% and 2%, respectively, of fungal infections diagnosed in these populations. Notably, the overall incidence of mucormycosis during the period of active surveillance at transplantation centers increased from 1.7 per 1000 in 2001 to more than 6.2 per 1000 in 2004, with *Rhizopus* species as the predominant pathogens.[24] Of concern, a growing proportion of mucormycosis cases since 2002 have presented as breakthrough infection on antifungal prophylaxis or treatment effective against aspergillosis, but not mucormycosis (i.e., voriconazole, echinocandins).[25-29] Case series in high-risk leukemia and allogeneic hematopoietic stem cell transplant (HSCT) patients suggest that mucormycosis should be considered in these populations whenever fungal sinusitis develops on *Aspergillus*-active antifungal prophylaxis (i.e., voriconazole), especially in patients with prolonged immunosuppression and underlying diabetes or malnutrition (albumin <3 g/dL).[25] Breakthrough mucormycosis in cancer patients receiving voriconazole prophylaxis has been associated with an overall mortality rate of 73%.[24,25]

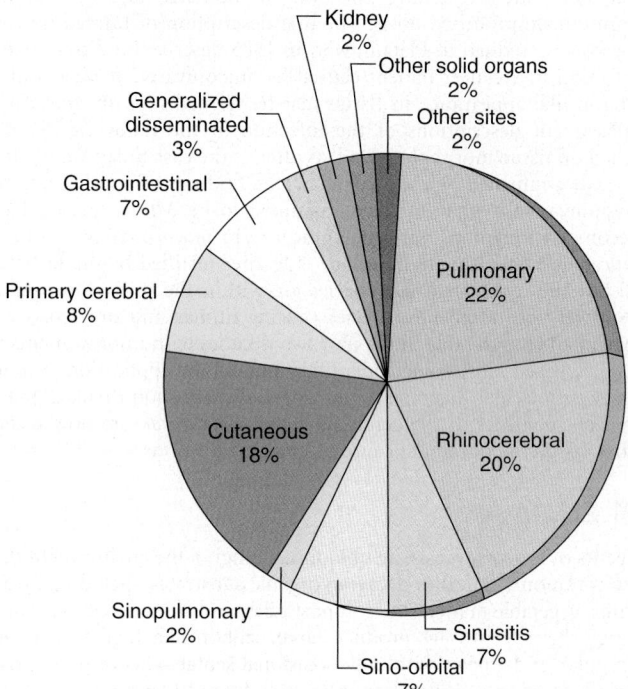

B

Figure 259-2 Mucormycosis incidence. Incidence of mucormycosis over six decades by host population (**A**) and site of infection (**B**). *(Adapted from Roden MM, Zaoutis TE, Buchanan WL, et al. Epidemiology and outcome of zygomycosis: A review of 929 reported cases. Clin Infect Dis. 2005;41:634-653.)*

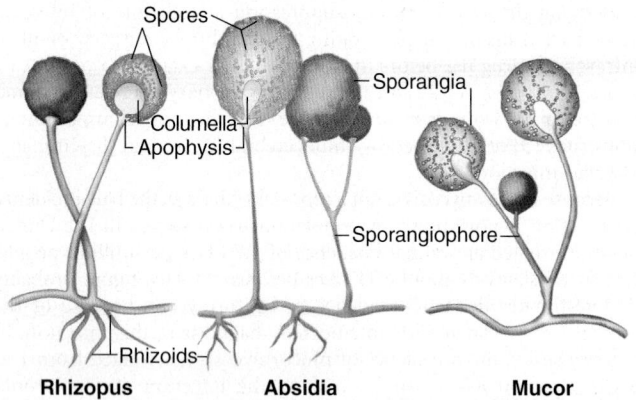

Figure 259-1 Mucormycosis agents. Illustration of the major differentiating morphologic features of three of the most common agents of mucormycosis isolated from patients. Note the presence and location of the rhizoids and columella, and the shape of the sporangia. The infectious spores reside within the sporangia. *(Illustration by Lori Messenger.)*

Pathogenesis and Immunology

Healthy humans have a strong innate immune response to mucormycosis. To establish infection, spores must overcome killing by mononuclear and polymorphonuclear phagocytes to germinate into hyphal forms—the angioinvasive form of infection. (Fig. 259-3).[6] Most spores are sufficiently small to avoid upper host airway defenses and reach the distal alveolar spaces. Larger spores (>10 μm) may lodge in the nasal turbinates predisposing patients to isolated sinusitis.[2] Inhalation of a high spore inoculum, which can occur with excavation, construction, or work in contaminated air ducts, can lead to a slowly progressing pulmonary mucormycosis even in immunocompetent hosts.[30-32] In

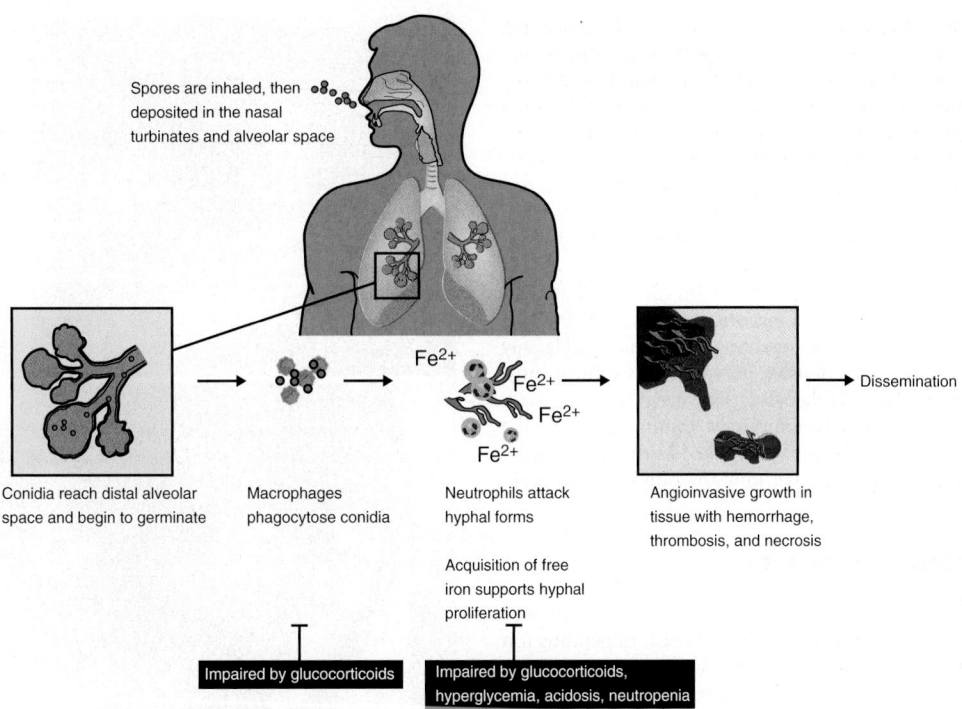

Spores are inhaled, then deposited in the nasal turbinates and alveolar space

Fe^{2+}

Fe^{2+}

Fe^{2+}

Fe^{2+}

Dissemination

Conidia reach distal alveolar space and begin to germinate

Macrophages phagocytose conidia

Neutrophils attack hyphal forms

Angioinvasive growth in tissue with hemorrhage, thrombosis, and necrosis

Acquisition of free iron supports hyphal proliferation

Impaired by glucocorticoids

Impaired by glucocorticoids, hyperglycemia, acidosis, neutropenia

Figure 259-3 Pathogenesis of invasive mucormycosis.

the case of primary cutaneous mucormycosis, subcutaneous inoculation of spores is the most common event leading to infection in normal hosts. Cutaneous mucormycosis have been described with even minor trauma, including insect bites and tattooing.[33,34]

Both mononuclear and polymorphonuclear phagocytes prevent germination of Mucorales spores and kill the hyphal forms of the fungus.[2,6,35-38] Defects in phagocytic activity due to deficiency in cell number (i.e., neutropenia) or function (i.e., associated with glucocorticoids, hyperglycemia, or acidosis) allow unimpeded growth of the hyphal form.[36,38,39] Glucocorticoids are known to impair the migration, ingestion, and phagolysosome fusion of bronchoalveolar macrophages essential for clearing spores from the alveoli.[40] Neutrophils collected from patients with severe hyperglycemia and diabetic ketoacidosis, burn stress pseudodiabetes, or glucocorticoid-treated graft-versus-host disease typically have impaired chemotaxis and diminished oxidative and nonoxidative fungicidal mechanisms against Mucorales spores and hyphae.[41]

Prolonged neutropenia is the sole identifying risk factor in about 15% of all reported cases of mucormycosis.[3] Like aspergillosis, mucormycosis is increasingly reported as a late infection in hematopoietic stem cell transplant recipients after recovery from neutropenia (stem cell engraftment).[8] Mucormycosis is increasingly encountered in the setting of multiple, overlapping, and cumulative mechanisms of immunosuppression.[24] A typical example would be a leukemic patient with graft-versus-host disease after allogeneic stem cell transplantation, who is receiving high-dose glucocorticoid therapy with either cyclosporine, tacrolimus, mycophenolate, or tumor necrosis factor-α (TNF-α) inhibitors and has steroid-associated diabetes and chronic malnutrition.[28,42,43] Not surprisingly, the prognosis of mucormycosis is especially poor in these populations.[42]

Patients with hemochromatosis may be predisposed to mucormycosis, a fact that might illustrate the relatively unique requirement of this fungus to acquire iron in tissue or bloodstream for invasive growth.[6] Fungi can acquire iron from the host using low-molecular-weight iron chelators (siderophores) or high-affinity iron permeases such as ferrirhizoferrin.[44] Of the two mechanisms, it is believed that iron permeases play a more critical role for adaptive survival of the

fungus in the human host.[45] Iron overload in organs such as the liver has also been reported to enhance fungal virulence.[46]

Patients with diabetic ketoacidosis are particularly susceptible to developing rhinocerebral forms of mucormycosis, perhaps because of diminished capacity of transferrin to bind and sequester free iron at a pH of more than 7.4. The growth of *Rhizopus oryzae* is markedly different in sera collected from patients with diabetic acidosis compared with healthy controls.[47,48] Artis and colleagues found that normal human serum is not capable of supporting the growth of *R. oryzae* even with the addition of free iron. However, under acidic conditions (pH < 7.4), the addition of exogenous iron markedly enhances the growth of *R. oryzae* hyphae. Similarly, sera collected from patients with ketoacidosis supports exuberant growth of *R. oryzae* without exogenous iron, provided the pH was maintained at less than 7.4, suggesting that acidosis disrupts the ability of transferrin to bind and sequester free iron.[47,48]

Historically, patients with severe hemochromatosis or aluminum toxicity received treatment with the metal chelator deferoxamine. Paradoxically, deferoxamine therapy is associated with an increased risk for fulminant mucormycosis.[3] Subsequent experimental models of mucormycosis demonstrated that *R. oryzae* can use deferoxamine as a xenosiderophore to form the ferrioxamine complex, which will make iron available for use previously unavailable to the fungus.[49-51] Specifically, *Rhizopus* can bind deferoxamine complexes and strip away free iron through a reductive process that allows intracellular uptake of free iron through the enzyme iron permease.[52] Interestingly, uptake of radiolabeled-iron in the presence of deferoxamine is 8- to 40-fold lower in *Candida* and *Aspergillus* compared with *R. oryzae*, suggesting this mechanism is a relatively unique pathogenic trait of this fungus. This observation has been confirmed in invertebrate and vertebrate animal models in which administration of deferoxamine worsens survival of guinea pigs infected with *R. oryzae*,[53] but not *Candida albicans*.[49,51]

Unlike deferoxamine, newer iron chelator agents such as deferiprone and deferasirox have not been associated with increased risk for mucormycosis because of their limited capacity to act as xenosidophores for *Rhizopus* species. Indeed, both deferiprone and deferasirox have shown protective effects in fly,[53] murine,[53,54] and guinea pig models of mucormycosis,[49] with several case reports suggesting a possible benefit of adjunctive deferasirox therapy in human mucormycosis.[55,56] Interestingly, the iron-starvation effects of these newer chelators have been shown to produce direct fungicidal activity against a variety of *Mucorales* species in vitro.[54] Additionally, treatment with deferasirox appears to restore proinflammatory responses in iron-overloaded tissues heavily infected with *R. oryzae*.[54] The utility of adjunctive iron chelation therapy in combination with systemic antifungal therapy for refractory mucormycosis is under investigation.

Mucorales have an exceptional capacity to invade blood vessels, resulting in necrosis of vessel walls and mycotic thrombi.[4] Thrombosis of vessels leads to infarction and hematogenous dissemination. Heavily infected tissue typically reveals extensive necrosis with diffuse infiltration of polymorphonuclear leukocytes. However, in areas with ischemic necrosis, inflammation is sometimes minimal despite the presence of numerous hyphae.[4] In the otherwise healthy host, a pyogenic or pyogranulomatous response without angioinvasion is usual.

Clinical Manifestations of Mucormycosis

The clinical presentation of mucormycosis is broad, depending on the underlying immune status and comorbidities of the host (Table 259-2). Mucormycosis in the impaired host presents as a fulminant angioinvasive infection that frequently disseminates with fatal consequences.[2,6] Although some overlap exists, mucormycosis cases are grouped according to the clinical presentation and anatomic predilection into one of six syndromes: (1) rhinocerebral infections and (2) pulmonary, (3) cutaneous, (4) gastrointestinal, (5) disseminated, and (6) unusual presentations of zygomycosis.

RHINOCEREBRAL INFECTIONS

Rhinosinusitis, rhino-orbital, and rhinocerebral infections are classic manifestations of human mucormycosis. Infection is initially localized to the nasal turbinates and paranasal sinuses following inhalation of spores but can rapidly progress to the orbit (sino-orbital) or brain (rhinocerebral), particularly in patients with diabetic ketoacidosis or profound neutropenia.[21] Patterns of progression for the infection demonstrate some host specificity (see Table 259-2). The rhino-orbital form occurs more frequently in patients with poorly controlled diabetes, whereas patients with underlying leukemia or lymphoma are more likely to present with sinopulmonary infections (Fig. 259-4). Indeed, rhino-orbital mucormycosis may be the first manifestation of undiagnosed diabetes mellitus.[57]

Initial symptoms of sinus invasion by mucormycosis are indistinguishable from other more common causes of sinusitis. Sinus pain, congestion, headache, mouth or facial pain, otologic symptoms, and hyposmia and anosmia are common. A concomitant nonproductive cough often reflects lung involvement. Involved tissues become red,

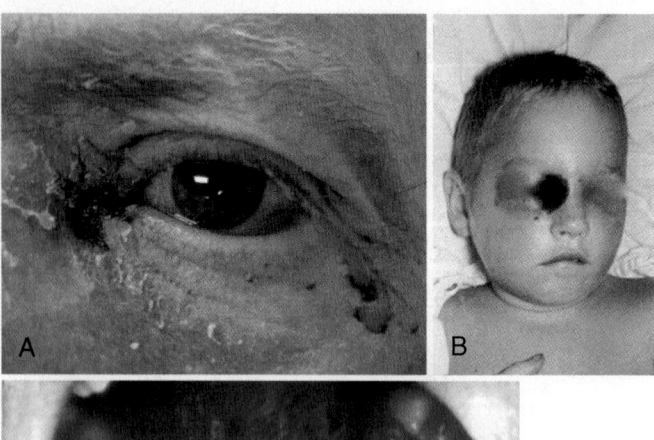
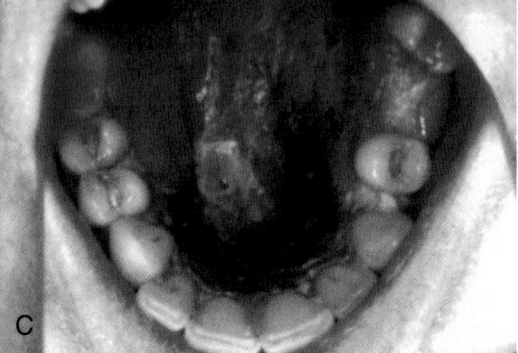

Figure 259-4 **Sino-orbital involvement of mucormycosis. A,** Orbital involvement in cancer patient. Note the periorbital ecchymosis and sanguineous discharge from the eye. **B,** Orbital involvement with ecchymosis and necrosis of the right turbinate. **C,** Necrotic eschar on the hard palate of a cancer patient with rhinocerebral mucormycosis. *(Courtesy of Drs. Gerald Bodey, the University of Texas M. D. Anderson Cancer Center, and George Viola, Baylor College of Medicine, Houston.)*

TABLE 259-2	Patterns of Mucormycosis by Host Population	
Predisposing Condition	*Predominant Sites of Infection*
Diabetes mellitus	Rhinocerebral, sino-orbital, cutaneous
Malignancy	Pulmonary, sinus, cutaneous, sino-orbital
Hematopoietic stem cell transplantation	Pulmonary, disseminated, rhinocerebral
Solid organ transplantation	Sinus, cutaneous, pulmonary, rhinocerebral, disseminated
Intravenous drug use	Cerebral, endocarditis, cutaneous, disseminated
Malnutrition	Gastrointestinal, disseminated
Deferoxamine therapy	Disseminated, pulmonary, rhinocerebral, cerebral, cutaneous, gastrointestinal
Trauma	Cutaneous, ocular

then violaceous, and finally black with thrombosis and tissue necrosis. Necrotic eschars of the nasal cavity and turbinates, facial lesions, and exophytic or necrotic lesions of the hard palate are signs of rapidly progressing infection.[58] The absence of lesions or necrotic eschars does not rule out the possibility of rhinocerebral infection, because necrotic nasal or palate lesions may be seen in only 50% of patients within 3 days of the onset of infection.[58]

Extension of sinus disease is primarily into contiguous structures. Maxillary sinus infection extends into the hard palate, nasal cavity, and ethmoid sinus. Sphenoid disease invades the cavernous sinus, contiguous temporal lobe, and the internal carotid artery in the siphon.[59] Septic emboli from the carotid artery into the frontal and parietal lobes can occur. Ethmoid sinus disease may invade the face or frontal lobe but easily crosses the lamina papyracea into the orbit.[59] The frontal sinus is an uncommon primary site. Invasion of the orbit is typically unilateral (see Fig. 259-4). Periorbital edema, proptosis, chemosis, and preseptal and orbital cellulitis are early signs of orbital extension. Pain and blurring or loss of vision often indicate invasion of the globe or optic nerve. Infraorbital facial numbness follows invasion of the infraorbital nerve within the orbit. Patients with extensive rhino-orbital or rhinocerebral disease may present with trigeminal and facial cranial nerve palsy following cavernous sinus invasion.[60] A bloody nasal discharge may be the only sign that the infection has invaded through the nasal turbinates and into the brain.[61] Intracranial complications include epidural and subdural abscesses, cavernous, and less commonly saggital sinus thrombosis.[62-64] Frank meningitis in patients with mucormycosis is less common.[8]

Radiographic imaging is often suggestive of severe sinusitis but lacks the specificity to diagnose rhinocerebral manifestations of mucormycosis. Patients with fungal or surgical disruption of the dura mater may present with superimposed bacterial meningitis, or bacterial sinusitis

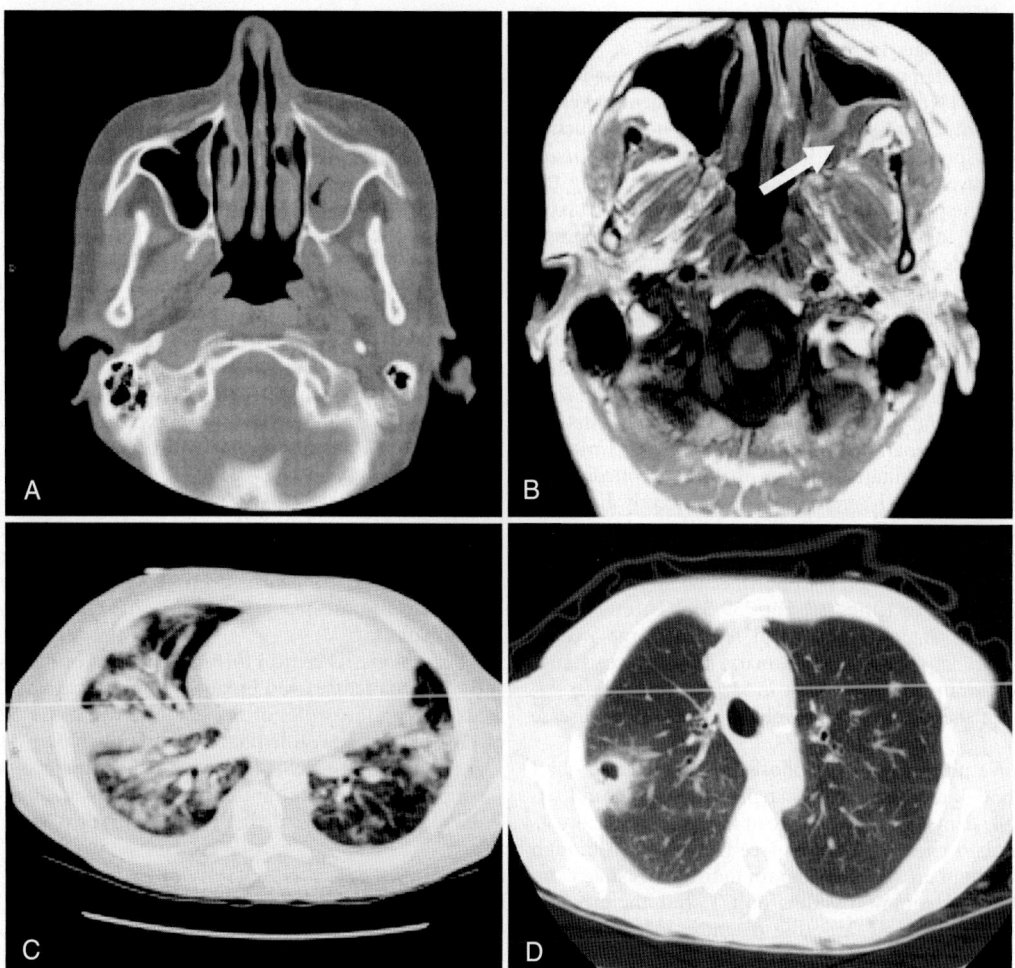

Figure 259-5 Radiographic findings in sinopulmonary mucormycosis. A, Left maxillary sinus air-fluid level is evident in this computed tomography (CT) scan that is indistinguishable from bacterial sinusitis. **B,** Magnetic resonance image reveals T2 signal hyperintensity in the left pterygoid musculature (*arrow*) in conjunction with a left maxillary sinus air-fluid level. **C,** Multiple heterogeneous nodular and consolidative lesions with a large pulmonary vessel infarct (wedge) and modest pleural effusions are shown in a cancer patient with pulmonary mucormycosis. **D,** Contrast-enhanced CT scan demonstrates the reverse halo sign in a patient with acute myelogenous leukemia and pulmonary mucormycosis. A solid ring surrounds a central area of ground-glass opacities. *(Courtesy of Dr. Edith Marom, University of Texas M. D. Anderson Cancer Center, Houston.)*

may complicate postoperative management.[65] Computed tomography (CT) of the sinuses typically reveals mucosal thickening, air-fluid levels, and bony erosion (Fig. 259-5).[66,67] Highly immunosuppressed patients often present with pansinusitis that is highly suggestive of an aggressive fungal infection.[25] Orbital thickening may also be detected on CT scans but can be detected earlier by magnetic resonance imaging (MRI).[67] CT and MRI scans of the orbits may be unremarkable during the initial stages of the infection, highlighting the importance of serial radiographic imaging for monitoring disease progression.[67] The frequency of radiographic imaging is patient dependent but may be required every 2 to 3 days in patients with suspected progression. Therefore, rhinoscopy or nasal endoscopy is critical for confirming tissue ischemia and the extent of disease.[65] Extraorbital muscle thickening is often the first sign on CT or MRI of orbital involvement and should prompt empirical antifungal therapy until surgical exploration or biopsy of the sinus and orbits can be performed, which should be done as soon as possible.[66] Every effort should be made to establish an early definitive diagnosis of mucormycosis by biopsy and culture of necrotic lesions and rapid histologic assessment of frozen sections.[68] Impression smears from the biopsy or surgical margin may also reveal hyphae consistent with Zygomycetes.

PULMONARY INFECTIONS

Pulmonary mucormycosis is most commonly encountered in patients with prolonged neutropenia, recipients of solid organ or hematopoietic stem cell transplantation, and patients receiving deferoxamine therapy.[3,22] The infection frequently occurs concomitantly with sinus infection.[22] However, the clinical manifestations of the infection are indistinguishable from more common molds such as invasive pulmonary aspergillosis (IPA). Therefore, timely diagnosis is a critical factor in the outcome on the infection because first-line antifungals typically used for aspergillosis such as voriconazole lack activity against Zygomycetes.[25] A recent case series of 61 leukemia and transplant patients with evidence of fungal pneumonia found that 84% of patients who were eventually documented to have pulmonary mucormycosis were receiving ineffective antifungal therapy at the time of their diagnosis.[69] Similarly, an analysis of 70 hematologic malignancy patients with pulmonary mucormycosis demonstrated that a delay in the administration of appropriate antifungal therapy (typically an amphotericin B formulation) as little as 6 days was associated with a doubling of 4-week (35.1% vs. 66.6%; $P = .006$) and 12-week (48.6% vs. 82.9%; $P = .029$) crude mortality rates.[70]

Clinical symptoms of pulmonary mucormycosis are subtle and nonspecific even at late stages in the infection, especially in patients receiving therapies that temper immune responses (i.e., high-dose glucocorticoid therapy, TNF-α blockers).[71] Patients frequently present with refractory fever on broad-spectrum antibiotics, nonproductive cough, progressive dyspnea, and pleuritic chest pain.[22,71] Pulmonary mucormycosis can traverse tissue planes in the lung, including the bronchi, diaphragm, chest wall, and pleura.[71] A pleural friction rub on auscultation is present in some patients. Hyphal invasion of blood vessels results in necrosis of the surrounding parenchyma, ultimately leading to cavitation or potentially fatal hemoptysis.[72-74] In patients with hematologic malignancies, clues for distinguishing pulmonary mucormycosis from invasive pulmonary aspergillosis may include the presence of severe sinusitis, prophylaxis with antifungals that possess activity against aspergillosis, but not mucormycosis (i.e., voriconazole and the echinocandins), and possibly the repeated absence of detectable *Aspergillus* galactomannan antigen in the serum.[25,71] Unfortunately, it is common in debilitated patients to have a concomitant polymicrobial pneumonia, which can further confound early diagnosis of pulmonary mucormycosis.[71,72]

The radiographic presentation of pulmonary mucormycosis is broad, including focal consolidation with nonspecific infiltrates, cavitary lesions, or even diffuse opacities (see Fig. 259-5).[71] Thrombosis of pulmonary vessels with angioinvasion often leads to large wedge-shaped infarcts.[71] Earlier studies of pulmonary mucormycosis suggested a predilection for upper lobar disease in 55% to 84% of cases.[75,76] However, any part of the lung may be involved, and bilateral disease is common.[71]

Similar to invasive pulmonary aspergillosis, high-resolution chest CT is the best method of determining the extent of pulmonary mucormycosis and typically demonstrates evidence of the infection before its appearance on standard chest radiographs (see Fig. 259-5). Although nodular opacities without an air bronchogram indistinguishable from aspergillosis are the most common finding on CT scan, the presence of multiple nodules (≥10) may favor the diagnosis of pulmonary mucormycosis.[71] Halo and air crescent signs are encountered less frequently in leukemic patients with pulmonary mucormycosis compared with pulmonary aspergillosis.[66,70] However, centrally located lesions demonstrating the air-crescent sign are often associated with an increased risk for pulmonary artery erosion and massive hemoptysis.[70] One case series suggested that a reverse halo sign, a focal round area of ground-glass attenuation surrounded by a ring consolidation, may be a more common early radiographic finding in patients with invasive pulmonary mucormycosis compared with aspergillosis (see Fig. 259-5).[77]

Pulmonary mucormycosis rapidly spreads to the contralateral lung and distal organs if not promptly treated. Although patients with pulmonary mucormycosis usually die from disseminated disease before respiratory failure occurs, dissemination is rarely detected antemortem.[22] The overall mortality rate of pulmonary mucormycosis ranges from 50% to 70% but increases to 95% with extrathoracic dissemination.[3,25]

In more immunocompetent hosts, pulmonary mucormycosis may present with more atypical, slowly progressing forms.[2] Mycotic pulmonary artery aneurysms and pseudoaneurysms, bronchial obstruction, and even asymptomatic solitary nodules have been described without clear underlying immune dysfunction. Patients with diabetes mellitus have a predilection for developing endobronchial lesions that present with a less fulminant course than pulmonary mucormycosis in the neutropenic or transplant population.[75] Occasionally, endobronchial lesions may lead to obstruction of the major airways or erosion of major pulmonary blood vessels and fatal hemoptysis.

Like *Aspergillus* species, Mucorales in rare instances can form mycetomas in preexisting lung cavities or cause slowly necrotizing pneumonia and hypersensitivity syndromes.[78] *Rhizopus* species have also been implicated in an allergic alveolitis described in farm workers as well as Scandinavian sawmill workers (wood-trimmer's disease).[79,80]

SKIN AND SOFT TISSUE INFECTIONS

Cutaneous mucormycosis is typically the result of direct spore inoculation or exposure of skin already compromised by burns or extensive trauma. Necrotizing soft tissue infections with cutaneous mucormycosis have been reported in victims of cataclysmic events such as volcanic eruptions or the tsunami tragedy of Southeast Asia.[11,81] Mucorales-contaminated bandages and needles have also been implicated in outbreaks of soft tissue infections in hospitalized patients.[14-16]

Cutaneous mucormycosis typically starts as erythema and induration of the skin at a puncture site and progresses to necrosis with a black eschar (Fig. 259-6). Cutaneous infections can quickly extend into the deep fascia and muscle layers. Necrotizing fasciitis has been reported in patients with progressive cutaneous mucormycosis and is associated with an extremely poor prognosis.[82-87] Neutropenic patients, in particular, are susceptible to lymphatic and blood vessel invasion, infarction, and necrosis with eventual dissemination. Unlike many other molds (*Aspergillus*, *Fusarium*, *Scedosporium* phaeohyphomycetes), the skin appears to be a much less common site of secondary involvement in disseminated mucormycosis.[3] Atypical dermatologic manifestations have also been reported in leukemic patients and solid organ transplant recipients that mimic erythema nodosum, panniculitis.[88,89]

Skin biopsy is critical for diagnosis as necrotic skin lesions in neutropenic patients have a broad differential diagnosis. Biopsy specimens taken from the center of the lesion down to the subcutaneous fat are most likely to reveal hyphae invading the blood vessels of the dermis and subcutis. Excision and wide débridement of cutaneous lesions, coupled with systemic antifungal therapy and, on occasion, hyperbaric oxygen therapy, can further reduce mortality rates.

GASTROINTESTINAL MUCORMYCOSIS

Primary gastrointestinal mucormycosis is a rare infection, with protean manifestations occurring primarily in malnourished patients and premature infants where it can present as necrotizing enterocolitis.[2] The infection often starts in the stomach with ulceration but can involve any compartment of the gastrointestinal tract.[90] Patients may present with peritonitis after the fungus has invaded through the gastric mucosa and bowel wall.[91] Liver abscesses have also been described after ingestion of herbal products contaminated with *Mucor indicus*.[92] In neutropenic patients, seeding of the gastrointestinal tract is probably more common than previously thought because only 25% of infections are identified antemortem.[8] Patients may present with subtle findings of fever, enterocolitis, or hematochezia that can progress to colonic ischemia with necrosis and perforation of the gut. Masslike appendiceal or ileal lesions have also been described.[91] Unfortunately, gastrointestinal mucormycosis is often diagnosed late because the nonspecific presentation and a high degree of suspicion is required for early diagnosis by endoscopic biopsy.[91]

DISSEMINATED MUCORMYCOSIS

Disseminated mucormycosis is rarely apparent before death.[93] The symptoms vary depending on the site of dissemination and degree of vascular invasion and affected organs. The patient groups classically at risk for this infection are patients receiving treatment with deferoxamine for iron overload, persistently neutropenic patients with active leukemia, and allogeneic stem cell transplant recipients with graft-versus-host disease receiving high-dose glucocorticoid therapy or perhaps TNF-α inhibitors.[3,42] Pneumonia is common in patients with disseminated mucormycosis and is assumed to be the primary source in most patients even when not detectable radiologically.[3,93] Because blood cultures are nearly always negative and recovery of the fungus from the respiratory tract is suboptimal, biopsy of the suspected sites is critical for diagnosis of the infection. Hematologically compromised patients and diabetic patients with disseminated mucormycosis have

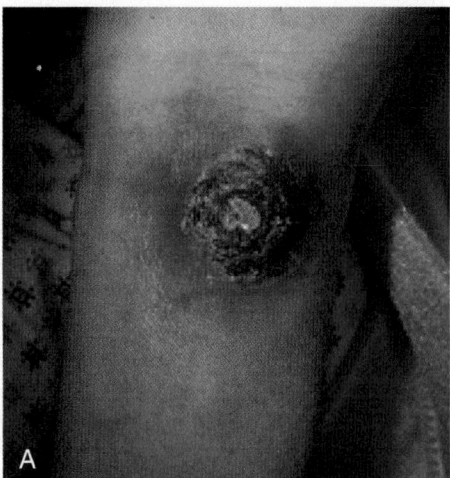

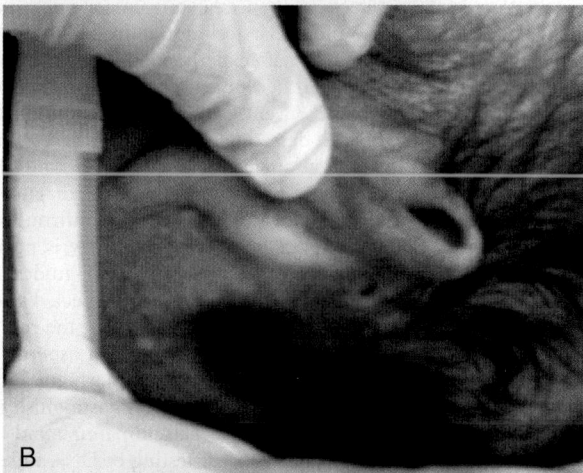

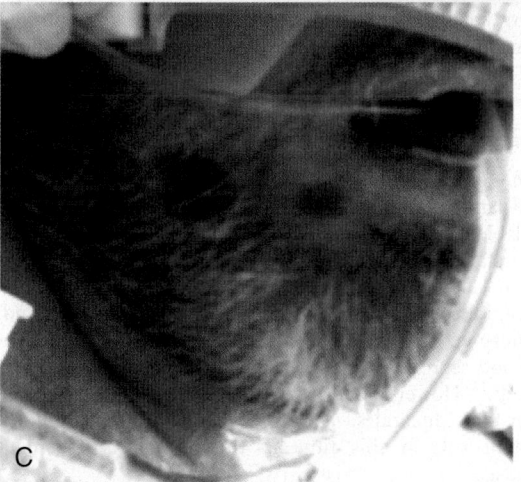

Figure 259-6 Cutaneous presentation of mucormycosis. A, Chronic, nonhealing ulcer with necrosis following traumatic inoculation. Cutaneous ecthyma gangrenosum lesions on the neck (**B**) and face (**C**) of a neutropenic patient with disseminated mucormycosis. *(Courtesy of Drs. Gerald Bodey and Saud Ahmed, the University of Texas M. D. Anderson Cancer Center, Houston.)*

presented with acute myocardial infarction or bowel ischemia after arterial occlusion by fungal thrombi.[94-97]

LESS COMMON PRESENTATIONS OF MUCORMYCOSIS

Although rare, peritonitis has been described in patients undergoing continuous ambulatory peritoneal dialysis.[98-100] The infection tends to have a slowly progressive course, although the attributable mortality rate in patients who received delayed or inappropriate therapy can exceed 60%.[98] In peritoneal dialysis catheter-related mucormycosis, prompt removal of the catheter and several weeks of systemic antifungal therapy are essential.

Isolated reports of mucormycosis of the trachea,[101] mediastinum,[102,103] bone,[104] heart,[105,106] and kidney[107] have been described. Other manifestations such as otitis externa,[108] corneal infection, and superior vena cava syndrome[109] have also been reported. Intravenous drug abusers are particularly vulnerable to central nervous system manifestations of mucormycosis, often presenting as a brain abscess involving the basal ganglia in conjunction with infective endocarditis.[110,111]

Diagnosis

The signs and symptoms of mucormycosis are nonspecific, emphasizing the importance of a high index of suspicion in susceptible patient populations. Because of the ubiquitous nature of the fungus in the environment, positive cultures may occasionally reflect culture contamination rather than true infection. However, discovery of fungal elements in a specimen from an immunocompromised host is an important diagnostic clue that should be confirmed whenever possible with histopathologic documentation of fungal invasion.[112] Not surprisingly, the site of infection has a major impact on the likelihood of histopathologic confirmation. The ease of accessibility of the skin or sinuses allows for more definite diagnosis of infections at these sites. Tissue swabs and cultures of sputum, sinus secretions, nasal mucosa, and bronchial alveolar lavage fluid are usually nondiagnostic but may be an important indication of disease in immunocompromised patients.[7] Blood cultures rarely grow Mucorales despite the angioinvasive nature of these pathogens.

In tissue, Mucorales hyphae can often be distinguished from other more common opportunistic molds such as *Aspergillus* and *Fusarium* by their broad (3 to 25 μm diameter), empty, thin-walled, mostly aseptate hyphae.[4] Frequently, these hyphae have focal bulbous dilation and nondichomatous irregular branching at occasional right angles (Fig. 259-7). Tissue sections may show a variety of mixed hyphal forms that include folded, twisted, or compressed hyphae that may be mistaken for septae or, when transected, large empty spherules of *Coccidioides immitis*. Reproductive hyphal structures containing spores (sporangia) are rarely observed in deep tissue, even in well-aerated sites of infection. Mistaken histologic identification is not rare and can lead to inappropriate therapy.

A variety of stains, including hematoxylin and eosin, Grocott-Gomori methenamine silver, and periodic acid–Schiff stains, will reveal characteristic hyphal elements in tissue. Perineural invasion is found in 90% of tissues that contain nerves.[113] The inflammatory process can range from neutrophilic, granulomatous, or pyogranulomatous to minimal inflammation with hemorrhage depending on the degree, chronicity, and type of underlying immune deficit.[4] Fungal hyphae can also be examined directly with a potassium hydroxide preparation of the tissue specimen or bronchial alveolar lavage fluid. Treatment with fluorescent stains such as Calcofluor white, Blankofluor, or Uvitex may enhance detection of hyphal elements during microscopic examination and improve the discrimination between septate and aseptate molds in biopsy specimens.[69,114]

Identification of Mucorales to the genus and species level requires cultivation of the fungus in culture to examine reproductive fruiting structures of the fungus.[2] Most species grow rapidly on fungal media

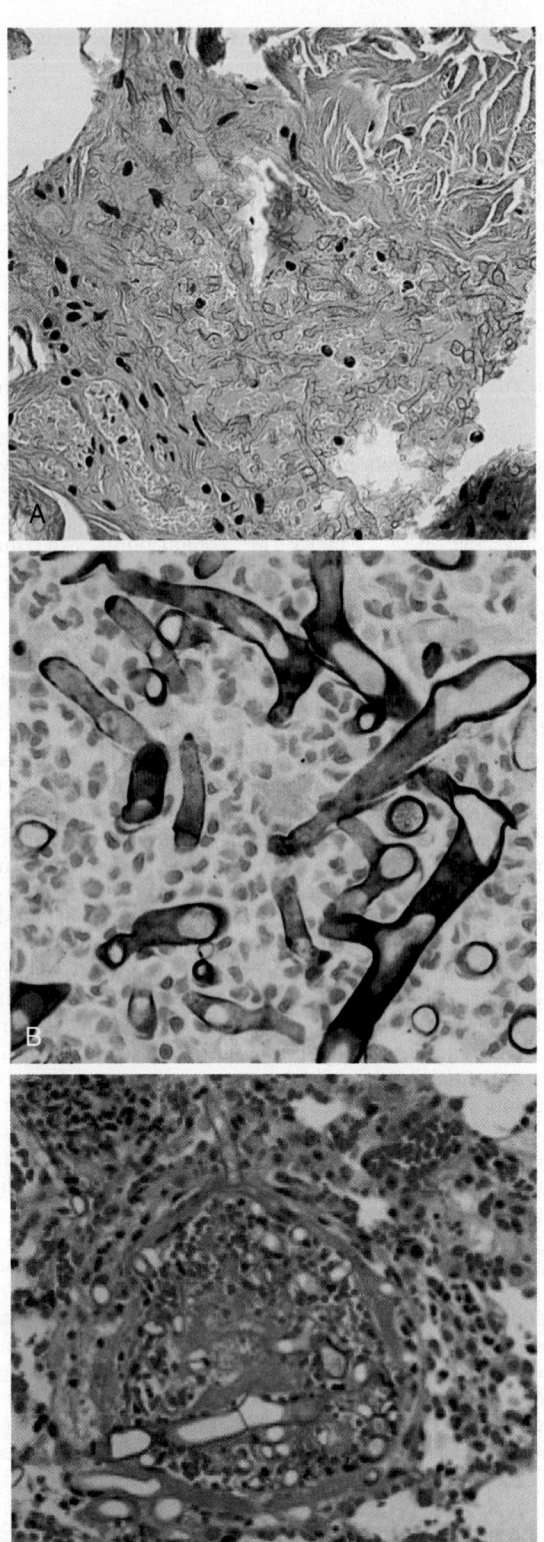

Figure 259-7 Histopathologic features of invasive mucormycosis.
A, Hematoxylin and eosin (H&E) stain of tissue taken from the inferior turbinate of a patient with sinus mucormycosis demonstrating necrosis and presence of fungal elements. **B,** Gomori methenamine silver stain of broad fungal hyphae in the lung of patient with pulmonary mucormycosis. **C,** H&E stain demonstrating invasion of a vessel wall by *Rhizopus* and pyogenic response in pulmonary mucormycosis.

such as Sabouraud dextrose agar incubated at 25° to 30°C. The level of development of the rhizoids, the shape of the sporangium, and the location of the sporangiospores are the morphologic features used to identify different genera of Mucorales (see Fig. 259-1). Nucleic acid sequencing of polymerase chain reaction (PCR) products is being used increasingly to identify cultures without typical morphologic features. Recent applications of PCR-based identification have suggested that up to 20% of species may be misidentified at the species level by morphology alone.[25] Unfortunately, culture recovery of the agents of mucormycosis from tissue is inherently poor owing to the friability of the nonseptated hyphae, making them more susceptible to damage during tissue manipulation.[2] Recovery from tissue can be improved by mincing (not homogenizing) tissue and using culture techniques that simulate in vivo growth, including incubation at 35° to 37°C in semi-anaerobic conditions.[115,116]

The importance of early differentiation of mucormycosis from other mold infections has generated considerable interest in the development of non–culture-dependent or non–histopathology-dependent diagnostic tests such as detection of specific antigens or nucleic acid by PCR. Unfortunately, few molecular techniques are in use for the diagnosis of mucormycosis and remain experimental. Antigen tests for *Aspergillus* (galactomannan) and other fungal species (β-D-glucan) are not useful for mucormycosis. Several studies have attempted to improve early diagnosis through detecting nucleic acid in serum using PCR assays or in situ hybridization techniques.[117-121] To date, these techniques have shown the greatest utility as adjunctive diagnostics, for molecular typing in epidemiologic studies, or for confirming the presumptive genus of the pathogen when histopathology is positive but cultures are negative.[119] In a prospective study of CT-guided percutaneous lung biopsy samples from patients with suspected fungal pneumonia, Lass-Florl and colleagues demonstrated that the rapidity of diagnosis and differentiation of mucormycosis from aspergillosis could be improved using a three-step analysis approach for biopsy specimens: (1) Calcofluor white staining to rapidly distinguish septated versus aseptate hyphae, (2) *Aspergillus* galactomannan and PCR testing for rapid identification, and (3) PCR testing of DNA in select biopsy specimens in which aseptate hyphae were observed or *Aspergillus* markers were negative.[69] These promising results will require further confirmation in a wider range of patients before PCR becomes a standard of care adjunctive diagnostic test for mucormycosis.

ANTIFUNGAL SUSCEPTIBILITY

Data on the antifungal susceptibility of the agents of mucormycosis are limited, and minimal inhibitory concentration (MIC) testing is rarely available outside of mycology reference or research laboratories. Although a standardized method has been proposed for filamentous fungi,[122] MIC end points from broth-based microdilution methods from this rapidly growing fungus are sometimes inconsistent and difficult to interpret. Agar-based methods such as the E-test have shown relatively good reproducibility and agreement with broth microdilution methods.[123] However, interpretive MIC breakpoints have not been defined for the Mucorales. Therefore, MIC testing does not have an important role at this time in the routine management of mucormycosis.

Mucorales are inherently resistant to many antifungal drugs used to treat systemic mycoses including ketoconazole, fluconazole, voriconazole, flucytosine (5-FC), and the echinocandins.[124-128] The lack of voriconazole activity in mucormycosis is clearly reflected in numerous case reports and case series of breakthrough cases of mucormycosis in patients receiving this triazole.[25-29] Mucorales have variable susceptibility to itraconazole and the squalene-epoxidase inhibitor terbinafine.[129,130] Amphotericin B is active against most agents of mucormycosis with MIC_{50} to MIC_{90} ranging from 0.25 to 1 μg/mL, although many species display tolerance to the fungicidal effects of amphotericin B in vitro.[124,131] Posaconazole, a newer triazole approved for the prevention of invasive fungal infections in patients with graft-versus-host disease or high-risk leukemia, has been shown to have activity against several agents of mucormycosis, with MIC_{90} ranging from 0.25 μg/mL for *Saksenaea vasiformis* to 8 μg/mL for *Rhizopus* species.[124] In general, *Rhizopus* and *Cunninghamella* species are less susceptible to itraconazole, posaconazole, terbinafine, and amphotericin B compared with *Absidia* and *Mucor* species.[7]

Synergy is occasionally observed when combinations of antifungal agents are tested in vitro against *Rhizopus* and *Absidia* species.[132] Combinations of amphotericin B plus rifampin, amphotericin B plus terbinafine, and terbinafine plus voriconazole may be synergistic, although the activity of these combinations has yet to be proved in vivo.[132] Although echinocandins are generally not considered active against Mucorales, high concentrations of caspofungin have been shown to inhibit 1,3-β-D-glucan synthase in *R. oryzae*[127] and increases exposure of immunogenic epitopes on the fungal cell wall that may enhance immune system recognition and hyphal damage.[133] Combinations of either caspofungin or micafungin with a liposomal amphotericin B were shown in some experiments, but not in others, to improve animal survival over lipid amphotericin B alone in nonneutropenic murine models of *R. oryzae* bloodstream infection.[127,134] One case series suggested a benefit for combined echinocandin-liposomal amphotericin B use in rhino-orbital cerebral and pulmonary mucormycosis in diabetic patients.[135] However, these regimens have not been investigated in randomized, prospective studies.

Treatment

Successful treatment of mucormycosis relies on timely diagnosis, reversal of underlying predisposing factors, early surgical débridement of infected tissue, and rapid initiation of effective, high-dose systemic antifungal therapy. Early diagnosis, in particular, is critical to the outcome of mucormycosis because small focal lesions can be surgically resected before the lesions progress to involve critical structures or distal organs. Patients often have an indolent clinical presentation until extensive invasion or dissemination of the infection.[68,93] Delays in the administration of systemic antifungal therapy increase the probability of patient death due to disseminated infection.[70]

Patients with suspected rhinocerebral mucormycosis should undergo a thorough examination, including CT of the paranasal sinuses and endoscopic examination of nasal turbinates with biopsy of any suspicious lesions or necrotic eschars. Patient outcome can be improved if initial treatment decisions are based on frozen tissue samples from biopsy rather than waiting for tissues to be fixed and stained for histology.[136] Rapid correction of underlying conditions, such as control of hyperglycemia and reversal of ketoacidosis and rapid tapering of glucocorticoid therapy, is critical to outcome.[6] If deferoxamine were still to be used, discontinuation of the drug would be logical but has not seemed to affect the dismal outcome in these cases. In rare cases, correction of diabetic ketoacidosis was sufficient to allow recovery from cavitary pulmonary mucormycosis without antifungal treatment.[3] In neutropenic patients, granulocyte transfusions may be beneficial as a temporary approach until granulocyte recovery.[137]

ANTIFUNGAL TREATMENT

No prospective studies of the primary treatment of mucormycosis have been performed, owing to the rarity and heterogeneous nature of this mycosis. Most evidence concerning the activity of existing antifungals has come from small case series, anecdotal case reports, and animal models of infection. Because both surgical and medical interventions are simultaneously or sequentially performed, it is difficult to ascertain the relative efficacy of drug therapy alone. The bulk of clinical data surrounding the treatment of mucormycosis has been with the use of conventional amphotericin B–deoxycholate, administered at the maximal tolerated doses of 1.0 to 1.5 mg/kg/day.[138] Unfortunately, high doses of amphotericin B are usually not tolerated for more than several days before renal function deteriorates, especially in patients with preexisting renal dysfunction (e.g., diabetic patients, those taking concomitant nephrotoxic agents, and transplant recipients).[139] Conse-

quently, lipid formulations of amphotericin B are safer than amphotericin B–deoxycholate for long-term administration and, in our opinion, are the preferred first-line treatment for severe mucormycosis.[70,139] Of the lipid formulations available in the United States, liposomal amphotericin B (L-AMB) and amphotericin B lipid complex (ABLC) have been reported useful in mucormycosis. Insufficient information is available about amphotericin B colloidal dispersion (ABCD). Although no comparative studies have been performed, outcomes with the use of the two lipid amphotericin B formulations are similar to those historically reported for conventional amphotericin B–deoxycholate, albeit with lower rates of nephrotoxicity.[138]

In one of the few published case series, 24 patients with mucormycosis and diabetes as the predominant underlying risk factor were treated with ABLC after failure or intolerance of the conventional amphotericin B–deoxycholate formulation.[139,140] The overall response rate (improvement or cure of infection) was 71% (17 of 24 patients), with few reported toxic effects, even in patients with preexisting renal dysfunction.[139] Several case reports have reported the successful treatment of mucormycosis with the liposomal formulation of amphotericin B, sometimes administered at high doses (i.e., 10 mg/kg/day) for prolonged treatment courses.[141-143] The necessity of administering high doses of lipid formulations of AMB may be questionable given the biopharmaceutical properties of free (bioactive) amphotericin (high protein binding and limited water solubility),[144] and the results of the AmBiLoad trial, which demonstrated no benefit and enhanced renal toxic effects of an initial 2-week 10 mg/kg/day versus 3 mg/kg/day regimen of L-AMB for possible or probable aspergillosis.[145] Nevertheless, the dose-response curve for L-AMB is somewhat broader for *R. oryzae* than for *A. fumigatus* in animal models of pulmonary mucormycosis, suggesting possible benefit for up-front dosage escalation strategies.[146] Clearly, the most important variable affecting efficacy of antifungal therapy is timely initiation of therapy. Any delay in the institution of systemic antifungals is associated with higher mortality.[70]

Aerosolized administration of amphotericin B, used in conjunction with concomitant systemic therapy, has been reported in several cases of patients with pulmonary mucormycosis, although the contribution of the aerosolized drug was inevaluable. Abscess drainage and direct instillation of amphotericin B were reported in several patients with cavitary pulmonary mucormycosis.[127] One case report described the successful treatment of a cancer patient with pulmonary mucormycosis using systemic therapy and ABLC aerosolized with a Respiguard II nebulizer.[147] Topical therapy with amphotericin B or other polyene macrolide antifungals (natamycin) has also been reported in primary cutaneous and corneal mucormycosis.[68,148]

Successful treatment of mucormycosis with combinations of amphotericin B, terbinafine, and rifampicin has also been described in single case reports.[149,150] A combination ABLC and caspofungin treatment regimen was associated with improved therapeutic success (100% vs. 45%; *P* = .02) in 41 patients with biopsy-proven rhino-orbital cerebral mucormycosis.[135] Interestingly, the greatest benefit was observed in patients with cerebral involvement (success rate 100% vs. 25%; *P* = .01), despite the limited penetration of echinocandins into the central nervous system. Further studies are required to compare this combination regimen to amphotericin B monotherapy for rhino-orbital cerebral mucormycosis.

Most azoles, including fluconazole and voriconazole, have no meaningful activity in mucormycosis. However, posaconazole, an orally available broad-spectrum triazole (800 mg/day administered in divided doses) appears to have clinically useful activity against several species of Mucorales.[151] In an open-label study evaluating posaconazole as salvage therapy, the overall success rate of posaconazole (800 mg/day) was 70% in 24 patients, and it was well tolerated with only minimal gastrointestinal side effects.[152,153] Similarly, a retrospective survey of posaconazole-based salvage therapy in 91 patients with refractory mucormycosis indicated an overall success rate of 61%, including 65% in patients with pulmonary mucormycosis.[136] Among patients who were not categorized as treatment successes, 21% had evidence of stable disease after 12 weeks of treatment.[136] At present, the U.S. Food and Drug Administration (FDA) has not approved posaconazole for primary or salvage therapy of mucormycosis, indicating the need for further studies.

Treatment with oral posaconazole has some important limitations because absorption of the oral suspension may be suboptimal in patients with mucositis[154] or severe diarrhea,[155,156] during cimetidine therapy,[157,158] or in patients with poor dietary intake.[157] Absorption of the drug is maximized when posaconazole is administered with a high-fat food (e.g., ice cream) in divided doses (4 times daily).[159-161] Because absorption of posaconazole is limited above 800 mg/day, dosage escalation above this daily dose will not improve concentrations in the bloodstream. Steady-state plasma concentrations of posaconazole are not reached until after about 1 week of therapy.[159,160] Therefore, it is our opinion that patients with mucormycosis should initially receive several days of a lipid amphotericin B formulation when the patient is started on posaconazole therapy. Plasma drug level monitoring may be necessary in some patients to document adequate posaconazole absorption, especially when dietary intake is poor or the patient is switched to oral posaconazole monotherapy for a documented infection.

Because mucormycosis is a relatively rare infection, primary prophylaxis is generally not recommended. Secondary prophylaxis is often desired in patients requiring further immunosuppression after treatment for mucormycosis. Posaconazole appears to be a favorable option for patients who require continuous, long-term antifungal therapy because they remain at high risk for relapsing infection.[152] Alternatively, we have successfully used intermittent infusions (i.e., 1 to 2 times weekly) of liposomal amphotericin B (5 to 10 mg/kg/day) or, in select patients, intermittent granulocyte transfusions to support patients with a prior history of disseminated mucormycosis undergoing reinduction chemotherapy.

The duration of treatment required for mucormycosis is highly individualized to the patient. Near normalization of radiographic imaging, negative biopsy specimens, and cultures from the affected site and recovery from immunosuppression are indicators that a patient is a candidate for stopping antifungal therapy.

SURGICAL MANAGEMENT

In rhinosinusitis, surgical débridement of infected tissue is a crucial component of therapy and should be urgently performed to limit the aggressive spread of infection to contiguous structures. Repeated removal of necrotic tissue or radical surgical resection (e.g., exenteration of the orbit) with subsequent reconstructive surgeries may be required for life-saving control of the infection.[76] However, rhinosinus mucormycosis has been treated successfully in select patients without radical resection, particularly when multimodality treatment options are used with careful follow-up.[162] Extension to the brain usually portends a fatal outcome. Decisions regarding the extent of surgical débridement are highly individualized to the patient. Intraoperative frozen sections can help determine the extent of involved tissue and tissue margins. Conditions such as low platelet counts and other bleeding problems must be corrected with sufficient transfusions before surgical intervention. Unfortunately, bleeding risks may limit surgical options in some patients with profound thrombocytopenia.

In patients with pulmonary mucormycosis, surgical treatment in conjunction with systemic antifungal therapy has been shown to significantly improve survival compared with antifungal therapy alone.[76,163] One large case series reported a mortality rate of 55% in patients who received systemic antifungal therapy alone compared with 27% in patients who received antifungal therapy plus surgical intervention.[72] Although the reported outcomes may reflect a selection bias in offering surgery to less severely ill patients with unifocal disease, removal of infected or devitalized tissue early when the infection is localized provides the greatest benefit. Lobectomy is often adequate in most patients, but pneumonectomy may be necessary for proximal or extensive involvement. Repeated surgeries are also necessary in some

cases. The benefit of pulmonary resection is unknown in patients with multifocal or disseminated mucormycosis.

ADJUNCTIVE THERAPIES

Several adjunctive measures have been explored for improving tissue viability, impeding fungal proliferation, and improving host immunity. Hyperbaric oxygen therapy was reported to be a beneficial adjunct to standard surgical and antifungal therapy for mucormycosis, particularly for diabetic patients with rhinocerebral disease.[164-167] Although this is not one of the approved uses of hyperbaric oxygen (see Chapter 43), the increased oxygen pressure achieved with hyperbaric oxygen may improve neutrophil activity and the putative oxidative killing effects of polyene antifungals.[168] High oxygen concentrations have also been reported to inhibit growth of Mucorales in vitro and to improve the rate of wound healing by increasing the release of tissue growth factors.[169] Lack of vigorous clinical evidence supporting the benefit of hyperbaric oxygen therapy, however, limits its recommendation for routine clinical use for this expensive and logistically difficult intervention for mucormycosis.

Multiple immune-augmentation strategies have been proposed for mucormycosis, including administration of cytokines that enhance phagocytic activity such as granulocyte colony-stimulating factor, granulocyte-macrophage colony-stimulating factor, or interferon-γ alone or in combination with granulocyte transfusions. Various combinations of these approaches have been reported with some favorable outcomes in case reports.[168,170] However, many of these immune-augmentation strategies carry some risk for enhancing inflammatory lung injury[171]; therefore, the relative benefits of such adjunctive strategies must be balanced for the risk for increased harm to the patient. The central role of iron acquisition in the pathogenesis of mucormycosis suggests that iron chelators without xenosiderophore activity in Mucorales (deferiprone and deferasirox) could be effective adjunctive antifungal therapies. Available case reports have suggested that the administration of deferasirox with antifungals may be more effective in patients with diabetic ketoacidosis compared with neutropenic patients.[55,56] Moreover, the bioavailability of oral deferasirox in patients with impaired absorption due to mucositis, graft-versus-host disease of the gut, or severe diarrhea is unknown. A pilot multicenter prospective trial examining the feasibility of this adjunctive treatment approach is underway.

PROGNOSIS

The site of infection and underlying host factors are the key prognostic determinants of mucormycosis outcome. Active hematologic malignancy, allogeneic hematopoietic stem cell transplantation, and disseminated infection are associated with poor outcome. In a series of 391 patients with hematologic malignancies with invasive fungal infections, Pagano and colleagues found that mucormycosis has significantly poorer outcome than aspergillosis.[172] In our experience, most patients who develop mucormycosis die within 12 weeks of diagnosis.[3,25,70,93] Correction of underlying immune impairment (e.g., rapid tapering of glucocorticoids), combined with aggressive multimodality treatment approaches, offer the best chance for patient survival.

Entomophthoramycosis

Infections caused by fungi in the subphylum Entomophthoramycotina, called entomophthoramycosis, include both conidiobolomycosis and basidiobolomycosis. These are rare infections of the paranasal sinus and subcutaneous tissues principally encountered in the tropics. In contrast to mucormycosis, entomophthoramycosis is usually a chronic, nonangioinvasive infection in relatively immunocompetent individuals. Although rare, case clusters of invasive disease have been reported in both immunocompromised and immunocompetent patients.[173,174] Conidiobolomycosis affects primarily the head and face, whereas basidiobolomycosis is often localized to the subcutaneous tissues of the trunk and arms. Both fungi are common inhabitants of the soil throughout the world, including the United States. However, most cases of conidiobolomycosis are found in tropical Africa, South America, Central America, and Asia.[175] Similarly, reports of basidiobolomycosis are primarily concentrated in tropical areas of Africa and Southeast Asia and in the tropical and subtropical regions of Asia, Australia, and South America.[176] Entomophthoramycosis also demonstrate some age specificity: conidiobolomycosis is uncommon in children, but 88% of basidiobolomycosis cases occur in patients younger than 20 years.[177]

CONIDIOBOLOMYCOSIS

Subcutaneous rhinofacial conidiobolomycosis is the most common manifestation of infection caused by *Conidiobolus coronatus*. Symptoms typically begin with nasal discharge, epistaxis, unilateral nasal obstruction, sinus tenderness, and extensive and persistent facial swelling that may result in disfiguration. The infection slowly progresses with granulomatous inflammation in the subcutaneous tissue without bone involvement or ulceration of the skin.[178] Systemic symptoms are rare, but disseminated conidiobolomycosis has been observed.[173] Infections with *Conidiobolus incongruus* are extremely rare but often more aggressive.[7]

BASIDIOBOLOMYCOSIS

Infections caused by *Basidiobolus ranarum* often begin as a nodular subcutaneous lesion on the trunk, arms, or buttocks. The mode of transmission for *B. ranarum* is assumed to be through minor trauma and insect bites. Fungal spores are found in the bristles of mites and are probably carried by other insects.[179] *Basidiobolus ranarum* has been theorized to be present on "toilet leaves" used for skin cleaning after a bowel movement, resulting in direct inoculation of the perineum.[180,181] The predominance of lesions in the buttocks, thighs, and perineum would appear to support this theory. The subcutaneous lesions elicited by *B. ranarum* are typically firm, but not painful, with edema around the involved sites. Deeper invasion of muscle underlying the subcutaneous tissue has been reported.[176] Several cases have been reported of otherwise healthy children with gastrointestinal tract basidiobolomycosis, most often in the colon, that may present as obstruction or mimic the presentation of Crohn's disease.[180,181] Clinical features of gastrointestinal basidiobolomycosis include abdominal pain, nausea, vomiting, diarrhea, or abdominal mass.[182] Most cases are slowly progressive locally or may spread unless appropriate therapy is administered. Chronic fibrotic-appearing lesions, including angioinvasive disease reminiscent of mucormycosis seen in diabetic and immunocompromised patients, have also been described.[174]

DIAGNOSIS

In areas where entomophthoramycosis is common, the diagnosis is often suspected from the clinical appearance of the patient and characteristic lesions or swelling.[171,172] Definitive diagnosis requires biopsy of the involved site, with characteristic findings of broad, sparsely septated hyphae surrounded by eosinophilic granular material (Splendore-Hoeppli phenomenon).[180,183] Tissue eosinophilia and granulomatous inflammation are usual. Peripheral eosinophilia may also be present, but cultures from the infected site are often negative.

DIFFERENTIAL DIAGNOSIS

Pythiosis is usually a disease of horses, cattle, dogs, and cats but is a rare cause of subcutaneous disease in human that can resemble entomophthoramycosis or can cause gastrointestinal or disseminated infection resembling mucormycosis. Although the histologic appearance of the hyphae is similar, the appearance of motile zoospores on water culture of the causative organism, *Pythium insidiosum*, can distinguish the entities.[184]

THERAPY AND PREVENTION

No standard treatment regimens have been proposed for entomophthoramycosis. *Conidiobolus* species are generally more resistant to systemic antifungals than *Basidiobolus* species.[185] Agents used to treat entomophthoramycosis include potassium iodide, trimethoprim-sulfamethoxazole, ketoconazole, itraconazole, and amphotericin B with varying success and clinical outcome.[175,176,186-189] Few clinical data are available for newer triazoles such as voriconazole, posaconazole, or the echinocandins. Surgical removal of nodules and reconstructive surgery for grossly swollen or disfigured tissues, combined with medical therapy, often provides the best chance for complete recovery. Disseminated disease should be treated as aggressively as mucormycosis.[188]

REFERENCES

1. Platauf AP. Mycosis mucorina. *Virchows Arch*. 1885;102:543-564.
2. Ribes JA, Vanover-Sams CL, Baker DJ. Zygomycetes in human disease. *Clin Microbiol Rev*. 2000;13:236-301.
3. Roden MM, Zaoutis TE, Buchanan WL, et al. Epidemiology and outcome of zygomycosis: a review of 929 reported cases. *Clin Infect Dis*. 2005;41:634-653.
4. Chandler F, Kaplan W, Awjello L. *A colour atlas and textbook of the histopathology of mycotic diseases*. London: Wolfe Medical Publishing, LTD.; 1980.
5. Larone DH. *Medically Important Fungi: A Guide to Identification*. 3rd ed. Washington, DC: ASM Press; 1995.
6. Spellberg B, Edwards J Jr, Ibrahim A. Novel perspectives on mucormycosis: pathophysiology, presentation, and management. *Clin Microbiol Rev*. 2005;18:556-569.
7. Chayakulkeeree M, Ghannoum MA, Perfect JR. Zygomycosis: the re-emerging fungal infection. *Eur J Clin Microbiol Infect Dis*. 2006;25:215-229.
8. Kontoyiannis DP, Lewis RE. Invasive zygomycosis: update on pathogenesis, clinical manifestations, and management. *Infect Dis Clin North Am*. 2006;20:581-607.
9. Khan ZU, Ahmad S, Mokaddas E, et al. *Actinomucor elegans* var. *kuwaitiensis* isolated from the wound of a diabetic patient. *Antonie van Leeuwenhoek*. 2008;94:343-352.
10. Kuruckulararante C, Garcia-Diaz J, Reed D, et al. Beyond *Rhizopus* and *Mucor*: Hurricane Katrina Stirs Up Syndephalastrum in New Orleans. In: Focus on Fungal Infections 16. Las Vegas, Nevada; 2006.
11. Andresen D, Donaldson A, Choo L, et al. Multifocal cutaneous mucormycosis complicating polymicrobial wound infections in a tsunami survivor from Sri Lanka. *Lancet*. 2005;365:876-878.
12. Lawson HH, Schmaman A. Gastric phycomycosis. *Br J Surg*. 1974;61:743-746.

13. Neame P, Rayner D. Mucormycosis: a report on twenty-two cases. *Arch Pathol*. 1960;70:143-150.
14. Gartenberg G, Bottone EJ, Keusch GT, et al. Hospital-acquired mucormycosis (*Rhizopus rhizopodiformis*) of skin and subcutaneous tissue: epidemiology, mycology and treatment. *N Engl J Med*. 1978;299:1115-1118.
15. Mead JH, Lupton GP, Dillavou CL, et al. Cutaneous *Rhizopus* infection. Occurrence as a postoperative complication associated with an elasticized adhesive dressing. *JAMA*. 1979;242:272-274.
16. Paparello SF, Parry RL, MacGillivray DC, et al. Hospital-acquired wound mucormycosis. *J Infect Dis*. 1992;14:390-392.
17. Chakrabarti A, Kumar P, Padhye AA, et al. Primary cutaneous zygomycosis due to Saksenaea vasiformis and Apophysomyces elegans. *Clin Infect Dis*. 1997;24:580-583.
18. Jain JK, Markowitz A, Khilanani PV, et al. Localized mucormycosis following intramuscular corticosteroid. Case report and review of the literature. *Am J Med Sci*. 1978;275:209-216.
19. Verweij PE, Voss A, Donnelly JP, et al. Wooden sticks as the source of a pseudoepidemic of infection with *Rhizopus microsporus* var. rhizopodiformis among immunocompromised patients. *J Clin Microbiol*. 1997;35:2422-2423.
20. Paydas S, Yavuz S, Disel U, et al. Mucormycosis of the tongue in a patient with acute lymphoblastic leukemia: a possible relation with use of a tongue depressor. *Am J Med*. 2003;114:618-620.
21. Sims CR, Ostrosky-Zeichner L. Contemporary treatment and outcomes of zygomycosis in a non-oncologic tertiary care center. *Arch Med Res*. 2007;38:90-93.
22. Kontoyiannis DP, Wessel VC, Bodey GP, et al. Zygomycosis in the 1990s in a tertiary-care cancer center. *Clin Infect Dis*. 2000;30:851-856.

23. Rees JR, Pinner RW, Hajjeh RA, et al. The epidemiological features of invasive mycotic infections in the San Francisco Bay Area, 1992-1993: Results of population-based laboratory active surveillance. *Clin Infect Dis*. 1998;27:1138-1147.
24. Park BJ, Pappas P, Marr K, et al. Recent epidemiology and zygomycosis among organ transplant and stem cell transplant recipients: Results from the TRANSNET surveillance network. In: Microbiology ASM, ed. *47th Interscience Conference on Antimicrobial Agents and Chemotherapy*. Chicago: ASM Press; 2007.
25. Kontoyiannis DP, Lionakis MS, Lewis RE, et al. Zygomycosis in a tertiary-care cancer center in the era of Aspergillus-active antifungal therapy: a case-control observational study of 27 recent cases. *J Infect Dis*. 2005;191:1350-1360.
26. Imhof A, Balajee SA, Fredricks DN, et al. Breakthrough fungal infections in stem cell transplant recipients receiving voriconazole. *Clin Infect Dis*. 2004;39:743-746.
27. Siwek GT, Dodgson KJ, de Magalhaes-Silverman M, et al. Invasive zygomycosis in hematopoietic stem cell transplant recipients receiving voriconazole prophylaxis. *Clin Infect Dis*. 2004;39:584-587.
28. Marty FM, Cosimi LA, Baden LR. Breakthrough zygomycosis after voriconazole treatment in recipients of hematopoietic stem-cell transplants. *N Engl J Med*. 2004;350:950-952.
29. Trifilio S, Singhal S, Williams S, et al. Breakthrough fungal infections after allogeneic hematopoietic stem cell transplantation in patients on prophylactic voriconazole. *Bone Marrow Transplant*. 2007;40:451-456.
30. England AC, 3rd, Weinstein M, Ellner JJ, et al. Two cases of rhinocerebral zygomycosis (mucormycosis) with common epidemiologic and environmental features. *Am Rev Respir Dis*. 1981;124:497-498.

31. Lueg EA, Ballagh RH, Forte V. Analysis of the recent cluster of invasive fungal sinusitis at the Toronto Hospital for Sick Children. *J Otolaryngol*. 1996;25:366-370.
32. Munckhof W, Jones R, Tosolini FA, et al. Cure of *Rhizopus* sinusitis in a liver transplant recipient with liposomal amphotericin B. *Clin Infect Dis*. 1993;16:183.
33. Prevoo RL, Starink TM, de Haan P. Primary cutaneous mucormycosis in a healthy young girl. Report of a case caused by Mucor hiemalis Wehmer. *J Am Acad Dermatol*. 1991;24:882-885.
34. Park S, Wong M, Marras SAE, et al. Rapid identification of *Candida dubliniensis* using a species-specific molecular beacon. *J Clin Microbiol*. 2000;38:2829-2836.
35. Ibrahim AS, Spellberg B, Avanessian V, et al. Rhizopus oryzae adheres to, is phagocytosed by, and damages endothelial cells in vitro. *Infect Immun*. 2005;73:778-783.
36. Waldorf AR, Diamond RD. Neutrophil chemotactic responses induced by fresh and swollen *Rhizopus oryzae* spores and *Aspergillus fumigatus* conidia. *Infect Immun*. 1985;48:458-463.
37. Waldorf AR, Levitz SM, Diamond RD. In vivo bronchoalveolar macrophage defense against *Rhizopus oryzae* and *Aspergillus fumigatus*. *J Infect Dis*. 1984;150:752-760.
38. Waldorf AR, Ruderman N, Diamond RD. Specific susceptibility to mucormycosis in murine diabetes and bronchoalveolar macrophage defense against Rhizopus. *J Clin Invest*. 1984;74:150-160.
39. Waldorf AR, Ruderman N, Diamond RD. Specific susceptibility to mucomycosis in murine diabetes and bronchoalveolar macrophage defense against *Rhizopus*. *J Clin Invest*. 1984;74:150-160.
40. Lionakis MS, Kontoyiannis DP. Glucocorticoids and invasive fungal infections. *Lancet*. 2003;362:1828-1838.
41. Chinn RY, Diamond RD. Generation of chemotactic factors by Rhizopus oryzae in the presence and absence of serum: relationship to hyphal damage mediated by human neutrophils and effects of hyperglycemia and ketoacidosis. *Infect Immun*. 1982;38:1123-1129.
42. Marty FM, Lee SJ, Fahey MM, et al. Infliximab use in patients with severe graft-versus-host disease and other emerging risk factors of non-*Candida* invasive fungal infections in allogeneic hematopoietic stem cell transplant recipients: a cohort study. *Blood*. 2003;102:2768-2776.
43. Stelzmueller I, Lass-Floerl C, Geltner C, et al. Zygomycosis and other rare filamentous fungal infections in solid organ transplant recipients. *Transpl Int*. 2008;21:534-546.
44. Griffiths E, Williams P. Iron uptake of pathogenic bacteria, fungi and protozoa. In: Bullen JJ, Griffiths E, eds. *Iron and infection: Molecular, physiological, and clinical aspects*. 2nd ed. London: Wiley and Sons; 1999:87-213.
45. Howard DH. Acquisition, transport, and storage of iron by pathogenic fungi. *Clin Microbiol Rev*. 1999;12:394-404, CP2.
46. Alexander J, Limaye AP, Ko CW, et al. Association of hepatic iron overload with invasive fungal infection in liver transplant recipients. *Liver Transpl*. 2006;12:1799-1804.
47. Artis WM, Patrusky E, Rastinejad F, et al. Fungistatic mechanism of human transferrin for Rhizopus oryzae and Trichophyton mentagrophytes: alternative to simple iron deprivation. *Infect Immun*. 1983;41:1269-1278.
48. Artis WM, Fountain JA, Delcher HK, et al. A mechanism of susceptibility to mucormycosis in diabetic ketoacidosis: transferrin and iron availability. *Diabetes*. 1982;31:1109-1114.
49. Boelaert JR, Van Cutsem J, de Locht M, et al. Deferoxamine augments growth and pathogenicity of Rhizopus, while hydroxypyridinone chelators have no effect. *Kidney Int*. 1994;45:667-671.
50. Boelaert JR, de Locht M, Schneider YJ. The effect of deferoxamine on different Zygomycetes. *J Infect Dis*. 1994;169:231-232.
51. Boelaert JR, de Locht M, Van Cutsem J, et al. Mucormycosis during deferoxamine therapy is a siderophore-mediated infection. In vitro and in vivo animal studies. *J Clin Invest*. 1993;91:1979-1986.
52. de Locht M, Boelaert JR, Schneider YJ. Iron uptake from ferrioxamine and from ferrirhizoferrin by germinating spores of Rhizopus microsporus. *Biochem Pharmacol*. 1994;47:1843-1850.
53. Chamilos G, Lewis RE, Hu J, et al. Drosophila melanogaster as a model host to dissect the immunopathogenesis of zygomycosis. *Proc Natl Acad Sci U S A*. 2008;105:9367-9372.
54. Ibrahim AS, Gebermariam T, Fu Y, et al. The iron chelator deferasirox protects mice from mucormycosis through iron starvation. *J Clin Invest*. 2007;117:2649-2657.
55. Soummer A, Mathonnet A, Scatton O, et al. Failure of deferasirox, an iron chelator agent, combined with antifungals in a case of severe zygomycosis. *Antimicrob Agents Chemother*. 2008;52:1585-1586.
56. Reed C, Ibrahim A, Edwards JE Jr, et al. Deferasirox, an iron-chelating agent, as salvage therapy for rhinocerebral mucormycosis. *Antimicrob Agents Chemother*. 2006;50:3968-3969.
57. Bhansali A, Bhadada S, Sharma A, et al. Presentation and outcome of rhino-orbital-cerebral mucormycosis in patients with diabetes. *Postgrad Med J*. 2004;80:670-674.
58. Yohai RA, Bullock JD, Aziz AA, et al. Survival factors in rhino-orbital-cerebral mucormycosis. *Surv Ophthalmol*. 1994;39:3-22.
59. Ochiai H, Iseda T, Miyahara S, et al. Rhinocerebral mucormycosis–case report. *Neurol Med Chir (Tokyo)*. 1993;33:373-376.
60. Frater JL, Hall GS, Procop GW. Histologic features of zygomycosis: emphasis on perineural invasion and fungal morphology. *Arch Pathol Lab Med*. 2001;125:375-378.
61. Ferguson BJ. Mucormycosis of the nose and paranasal sinuses. *Otolaryngol Clin N Am*. 2000;33:349-365.
62. Tsai TC, Hou CC, Chou MS, et al. Rhinosino-orbital mucormycosis causing cavernous sinus thrombosis and internal carotid artery occlusion: radiological findings in a patient with treatment failure. *Kaohsiung J Med Sci*. 1999;15:556-561.
63. Sehgal A, Raghavendran M, Kumar D, et al. Rhinocerebral mucormycosis causing basilar artery aneurysm with concomitant fungal colonic perforation in renal allograft recipient: a case report. *Transplantation*. 2004;78:949-950.
64. Delbrouck C, Jacobs F, Fernandez Aguilar S, et al. Carotid artery occlusion due to fulminant rhinocerebral mucormycosis. *Acta Otorhinolaryngol Belg*. 2004;58:135-140.
65. Howells RC, Ramadan HH. Usefulness of computed tomography and magnetic resonance in fulminant invasive fungal rhinosinusitis. *Am J Rhinol*. 2001;15:255-261.
66. Fatterpekar G, Mukherji S, Arbealez A, et al. Fungal diseases of the paranasal sinuses. *Semin Ultrasound CT MR*. 1999;20:391-401.
67. Greenberg MR, Lippman SM, Grinnell VS, et al. Computed tomographic findings in orbital Mucor. *West J Med*. 1985;143:102-103.
68. Greenberg RN, Scott LJ, Vaughn HH, et al. Zygomycosis (mucormycosis): emerging clinical importance and new treatments. *Curr Opin Infect Dis*. 2004;17:517-525.
69. Lass-Florl C, Resch G, Nachbaur D, et al. The value of computed tomography-guided percutaneous lung biopsy for diagnosis of invasive fungal infection in immunocompromised patients. *Clin Infect Dis*. 2007;45:e101-e104.
70. Chamilos G, Lewis RE, Kontoyiannis DP. Delaying amphotericin B-based front-line therapy significantly increases mortality in hematologic malignancy patients with zygomycosis. *Clin Infect Dis* 2008;47(4):503-509.
71. Chamilos G, Marom EM, Lewis RE, et al. Predictors of pulmonary zygomycosis versus invasive pulmonary aspergillosis in patients with cancer. *Clin Infect Dis*. 2005;41:60-66.
72. Lee FY, Mossad SB, Adal KA. Pulmonary mucormycosis: the last 30 years. *Arch Intern Med*. 1999;159:1301-1309.
73. Gupta KL, Khullar DK, Behera D, et al. Pulmonary mucormycosis presenting as fatal massive haemoptysis in a renal transplant recipient. *Nephrol Dial Transplant*. 1998;13:3258-3260.
74. Funada H, Matsuda T. Pulmonary mucormycosis in a hematology ward. *Intern Med*. 1996;35:540-544.
75. McAdams HP, Rosado de Christenson M, Strollo DC, et al. Pulmonary mucormycosis: radiologic findings in 32 cases. *AJR Am J Roentgenol*. 1997;168:1541-1548.
76. Tedder M, Spratt JA, Anstadt MP, et al. Pulmonary mucormycosis: results of medical and surgical therapy. *Ann Thorac Surg*. 1994;57:1044-1050.
77. Wahba H, Truong MT, Lei X, et al. Reversed halo sign in invasive pulmonary fungal infections. *Clin Infect Dis*. 2008;46:1733-1737.
78. Alonso A, Rodriguez SR, Rodriguez SM, et al. Interstitial pneumonitis induced in guinea pigs by the antigens of *Rhizopus nigricans*. *J Investig Allergol Clin Immunol*. 1997;7:103-109.
79. O'Connell MA, Pluss JL, Schkade P, et al. *Rhizopus*-induced hypersensitivity pneumonitis in a tractor driver. *J Allergy Clin Immunol*. 1995;95:779-780.
80. Hedenstierna G, Alexandersson R, Belin L, et al. Lung function and *Rhizopus* antibodies in wood trimmers. A cross-sectional and longitudinal study. *Int Arch Occup Environ Health*. 1986;58:167-177.
81. Patino JF, Castro D, Valencia A, et al. Necrotizing soft tissue lesions after a volcanic cataclysm. *World J Surg*. 1991;15:240-247.
82. De Decker K, Van Poucke S, Wojciechowski M, et al. Successful use of posaconazole in a pediatric case of fungal necrotizing fasciitis. *Pediatr Crit Care Med*. 2006;7:482-485.
83. Devi SC, Kanungo R, Barreto E, et al. Favorable outcome of amphotericin B treatment of zygomycotic necrotizing fascitis caused by Apophysomyces elegans. *Int J Dermatol*. 2008;47:407-409.
84. Jain D, Kumar Y, Vasishta RK, et al. Zygomycotic necrotizing fasciitis in immunocompetent patients: a series of 18 cases. *Mod Pathol*. 2006;19:1221-1226.
85. Kordy FN, Al-Mohsen IZ, Hashem F, et al. Successful treatment of a child with posttraumatic necrotizing fasciitis caused by *Apophysomyces elegans*: case report and review of literature. *Pediatr Infect Dis J*. 2004;23:877-879.
86. Lakshmi V, Rani TS, Sharma S, et al. Zygomycotic necrotizing fasciitis caused by *Apophysomyces elegans*. *J Clin Microbiol*. 1993;31:1368-1369.
87. Thami GP, Kaur S, Bawa AS, et al. Post-surgical zygomycotic necrotizing subcutaneous infection caused by *Absidia corymbifera*. *Clin Exp Dermatol*. 2003;28:251-253.
88. Nouri-Majalan N, Moghimi M. Skin mucormycosis presenting as an erythema-nodosum-like rash in a renal transplant recipient: a case report. *J Med Case Reports*. 2008;2:112.
89. Vernon SE, Dave SP. Cutaneous zygomycosis associated with urate panniculitis. *Am J Dermatopathol*. 2006;28:327-330.
90. Bittencourt AL, Ayala MA, Ramos EA. A new form of abdominal zygomycosis different from mucormycosis: report of two cases and review of the literature. *Am J Trop Med Hyg*. 1979;28:564-569.
91. Park YS, Lee JD, Kim TH, et al. Gastric mucormycosis. *Gastrointest Endosc*. 2002;56:904-905.
92. Oliver MR, Van Voorhis WC, Boeckh M, et al. Hepatic mucormycosis in a bone marrow transplant recipient who ingested naturopathic medicine. *Clin Infect Dis*. 1996;22:521-524.
93. Kontoyiannis DP, Wessel VC, Bodey GP, et al. Zygomycosis in the 1990s in a tertiary-care cancer center. *Clin Infect Dis*. 2000;30:851-856.
94. Joshita S, Kitano K, Nagaya T, et al. Zygomycosis presenting as acute myocardial infarction during hematological malignancies. *Intern Med*. 2008;47:839-842.
95. Naumann R, Kerkmann ML, Schuler U, et al. *Cunninghamella bertholletiae* infection mimicking myocardial infarction. *Clin Infect Dis*. 1999;29:1580-1581.
96. Benbow EW, McMahon RF. Myocardial infarction caused by cardiac disease in disseminated zygomycosis. *J Clin Pathol*. 1987;40:70-74.
97. Tuder RM. Myocardial infarct in disseminated mucormycosis: case report with special emphasis on the pathogenic mechanisms. *Mycopathologia*. 1985;89:81-88.
98. Polo JR, Luno J, Menarguez C, et al. Peritoneal mucormycosis in a patient receiving continuous ambulatory peritoneal dialysis. *Am J Kidney Dis*. 1989;13:237-239.
99. Branton MH, Johnson SC, Brooke JD, et al. Peritonitis due to *Rhizopus* in a patient undergoing continuous ambulatory peritoneal dialysis. *Rev Infect Dis*. 1991;13:19-21.
100. Nakamura M, Weil WB Jr, Kaufman DB. Fatal fungal peritonitis in an adolescent on continuous ambulatory peritoneal dialysis: association with deferoxamine. *Pediatr Nephrol*. 1989;3:80-82.
101. Schwartz JR, Nagle MG, Elkins RC, et al. Mucormycosis of the trachea: an unusual cause of acute upper airway obstruction. *Chest*. 1982;81:653-654.
102. Connor BA, Anderson RJ, Smith JW. Mucor mediastinitis. *Chest*. 1979;75:525-526.
103. Marwaha RK, Banerjee AK, Thapa BR, et al. Mediastinal zygomycosis. *Postgrad Med J*. 1985;61:733-735.
104. Echols RM, Selinger DS, Hallowell C, et al. *Rhizopus* osteomyelitis. A case report and review. *Am J Med*. 1979;66:141-145.
105. Mishra B, Mandal A, Kumar N. Mycotic prosthetic-valve endocarditis. *J Hosp Infect*. 1992;20:122-125.
106. Roy TM, Anderson KC, Farrow JR. Cardiac mucormycosis complicating diabetes mellitus. *J Diabetes Complications*. 1990;4:132-135.
107. Lussier N, Laverdiere M, Weiss K, et al. Primary renal mucormycosis. *Urology*. 1998;52:900-903.
108. Tierney MR, Baker AS. Infections of the head and neck in diabetes mellitus. *Infect Dis Clin North Am*. 1995;9:195-216.
109. Bosken CH, Szporn AH, Kleinerman J. Superior vena cava syndrome due to mucormycosis in a patient with lymphoma. *Mt Sinai J Med*. 1987;54:508-511.
110. Sanchez-Recalde A, Merino JL, Dominguez F, et al. Successful treatment of prosthetic aortic valve mucormycosis. *Chest*. 1999;116:1818-1820.
111. Zhang R, Zhang JW, Szerlip HM. Endocarditis and hemorrhagic stroke caused by *Cunninghamella bertholletiae* infection after kidney transplantation. *Am J Kidney Dis*. 2002;40:842-846.
112. Glazer M, Nusair S, Breuer R, et al. The role of BAL in the diagnosis of pulmonary mucormycosis. *Chest*. 2000;117:279-282.
113. Frater JL, Hall GS, Procop GW. Histologic features of zygomycosis: Emphasis on perineural invasion and fungal morphology. *Arch Pathol Lab Med*. 2001;125:375-378.
114. Ruchel R, Schaffrinski M, Seshan KR, et al. Vital staining of fungal elements in deep-seated mycotic lesions during experimental murine mycoses using the parenterally applied optical brightener Blankophor. *Med Mycol*. 2000;38:231-237.
115. Kontoyiannis DP, Chamilos G, Hassan SA, et al. Increased culture recovery of Zygomycetes under physiologic temperature conditions. *Am J Clin Pathol*. 2007;127:208-212.
116. Tarrand JJ, Lichterfeld M, Warraich I, et al. Diagnosis of invasive septate mold infections: A correlation of microbiological culture and histologic or cytologic examination. *Am J Clin Pathol*. 2003;119:854-858.
117. Kobayashi M, Togitani K, Machida H, et al. Molecular polymerase chain reaction diagnosis of pulmonary mucormycosis caused by *Cunninghamella bertholletiae*. *Respirology*. 2004;9:397-401.
118. Rickerts V, Loeffler J, Bohme A, et al. Diagnosis of disseminated zygomycosis using a polymerase chain reaction assay. *Eur J Clin Microbiol Infect Dis*. 2001;20:744-745.
119. Rickerts V, Mousset S, Lambrecht E, et al. Comparison of histopathological analysis, culture, and polymerase chain reaction assays to detect invasive mold infections from biopsy specimens. *Clin Infect Dis*. 2007;44:1078-1083.
120. Bialek R, Konrad F, Kern J, et al. PCR based identification and discrimination of agents of mucormycosis and aspergillosis in paraffin wax embedded tissue. *J Clin Pathol*. 2005;58:1180-1184.
121. Tveteras K, Kristensen S, Dommerby H. Septic cavernous and lateral sinus thrombosis: modern diagnostic and therapeutic principles. *J Laryngol Otol*. 1988;102:877-882.
122. National Committee for Clinical Laboratory Standards. *Reference method for broth dilution antifungal susceptibility testing of filamentous fungi; Approved standard NCCLS document M38-A*. Wayne, Pa: National Committee for Clinical Laboratory Standards; 2002.

123. Espinel-Ingroff A. Comparison of the E-test with the NCCLS M38-P method for antifungal susceptibility testing of common and emerging pathogenic filamentous fungi. *Journal of Clinical Microbiology*. 2001;39:1360-1367.

124. Sun QN, Fothergill AW, McCarthy DI, et al. In vitro activities of posaconazole, itraconazole, voriconazole, amphotericin B, and fluconazole against 37 clinical isolates of Zygomycetes. *Antimicrob Agents Chemother*. 2002;46:1581-1582.

125. Dannaoui E, Meis JF, Loebenberg D, et al. Activity of posaconazole in treatment of experimental disseminated zygomycosis. *Antimicrob Agents Chemother*. 2003;47:3647-3650.

126. Dannaoui E, Meletiadis J, Mouton JW, et al. In vitro susceptibilities of Zygomycetes to conventional and new antifungals. *J Antimicrob Chemother*. 2003;51(1):45-52.

127. Ibrahim AS, Bowman JC, Avanessian V, et al. Caspofungin inhibits *Rhizopus oryzae* 1,3-beta-D-glucan synthase, lowers burden in brain measured by quantitative PCR, and improves survival at a low but not a high dose during murine disseminated zygomycosis. *Antimicrob Agents Chemother*. 2005;49:721-727.

128. Espinel-Ingroff A. In vitro antifungal activities of anidulafungin and micafungin, licensed agents and the investigational triazole posaconazole as determined by NCCLS methods for 12,052 fungal isolates: review of the literature. *Rev Iberoam Micol*. 2003;20:121-136.

129. Antachopoulos C, Meletiadis J, Roilides E, et al. Rapid susceptibility testing of medically important Zygomycetes by XTT assay. *J Clin Microbiol*. 2006;44:553-560.

130. Dannaoui E, Meletiadis J, Mouton JW, et al. In vitro susceptibilities of Zygomycetes to conventional and new antifungals. *J Antimicrob Chemother*. 2003;51:45-52.

131. Espinel-Ingroff A. In vitro fungicidal activities of voriconazole, itraconazole, and amphotericin B against opportunistic moniliaceous and dematiaceous fungi. *J Clin Microbiol*. 2001;39:954-958.

132. Dannaoui E, Afeltra J, Meis JF, et al. In vitro susceptibilities of Zygomycetes to combinations of antimicrobial agents. *Antimicrob Agents Chemother*. 2002;46:2708-2711.

133. Lamaris GA, Lewis RE, Chamilos G, et al. Caspofungin-Mediated β-Glucan Unmasking and Enhancement of Human Polymorphonuclear Neutrophil Activity Against Aspergillus and Non-Aspergillus Molds. *J Infect Dis*. 2008;198:186-192.

134. Ibrahim AS, Gebremariam T, Fu Y, et al. Combination echinocandin-polyene treatment of murine mucormycosis. *Antimicrob Agents Chemother*. 2008;52:1556-1558.

135. Reed C, Bryant R, Ibrahim AS, et al. Combination Polyene-Caspofungin Treatment of Rhino-Orbital-Cerebral Mucormycosis. *Clin Infect Dis*. 2008;47:364-371.

136. van Burik JA, Hare RS, Solomon HF, et al. Posaconazole is effective as salvage therapy in zygomycosis: a retrospective summary of 91 cases. *Clin Infect Dis*. 2006;42:e61-e65.

137. Grigull L, Beilken A, Schmid H, et al. Secondary prophylaxis of invasive fungal infections with combination antifungal therapy and G-CSF-mobilized granulocyte transfusions in three children with hematological malignancies. *Support Care Cancer*. 2006;14:783-786.

138. Gleissner B, Schilling A, Anagnostopolous I, et al. Improved outcome of zygomycosis in patients with hematological diseases? *Leuk Lymphoma*. 2004;45:1351-1360.

139. Perfect JR. Treatment of non-*Aspergillus* moulds in immunocompromised patients, with amphotericin B lipid complex. *Clin Infect Dis*. 2005;40(Suppl 6):S401-S408.

140. Walsh TJ, Hiemenz JW, Seibel NL, et al. Amphotericin B lipid complex for invasive fungal infections: Analysis of safety and efficacy in 556 cases. *Clin Infect Dis*. 1998;26:1383-1396.

141. Walsh TJ, Goodman JL, Pappas P, et al. Safety, tolerance, and pharmacokinetics of high-dose liposomal amphotericin B (AmBisome) in patients infected with *Aspergillus* species and other filamentous fungi: Maximum tolerated dose study. *Antimicrob Agents Chemother*. 2001;45:3487-3496.

142. Garbino J, Adam A. Use of high-dose liposomal amphotericin B: efficacy and tolerance. *Acta Biomed*. 2006;77(Suppl 4):19-22.

143. Revankar SG, Hasan MS, Smith JW. Cure of disseminated zygomycosis with cerebral involvement using high dose liposomal amphotericin B and surgery. *Med Mycol*. 2007;45:183-185.

144. Lewis RE, Wiederhold NP. The solubility ceiling: A rationale for continuous infusion amphotericin B therapy? *Clin Infect Dis*. 2003;37:871-872.

145. Cornely OA, Maertens J, Bresnik M, et al. Liposomal amphotericin B as initial therapy for invasive mold infection: a randomized trial comparing a high-loading dose regimen with standard dosing (AmBiLoad trial). *Clin Infect Dis*. 2007;44:1289-1297.

146. Dannaoui E, Mouton JW, Meis J, et al. Efficacy of antifungal therapy in a nonneutropenic murine model of zygomycosis. *Antimicrob Agents Chemother*. 2002;46:1953-1959.

147. Safdar A, O'Brien S, Kouri IF. Efficacy and feasibility of aerosolized amphotericin B lipid complex therapy in caspofungin breakthrough pulmonary zygomycosis. *Bone Marrow Transplant*. 2004;34:467-468.

148. Buchta V, Kalous P, Otcenasek M, et al. Primary cutaneous Absidia corymbifera infection in a premature newborn. *Infection*. 2003;31:57-59.

149. Francis P, Walsh TJ. Approaches to management of fungal infections in cancer patients. *Oncology*. 1992;6:133-144.

150. Ng TT, Campbell CK, Rothera M, et al. Successful treatment of sinusitis caused by *Cunninghamella bertholletiae*. *Clin Infect Dis*. 1994;19:313-316.

151. Almyroudis NG, Sutton DA, Fothergill AW, et al. In vitro susceptibilities of 217 clinical isolates of Zygomycetes to conventional and new antifungal agents. *Antimicrob Agents Chemother*. 2007;51:2587-2590.

152. Raad II, Graybill JR, Bustamante AB, et al. Safety of long-term oral posaconazole use in the treatment of refractory invasive fungal infections. *Clin Infect Dis*. 2006;42:1726-1734.

153. Greenberg RN, Mullane K, van Burik JA, et al. Posaconazole as salvage therapy for zygomycosis. *Antimicrob Agents Chemother*. 2006;50:126-133.

154. Gubbins PO, Krishna G, Sansone-Parsons A, et al. Pharmacokinetics and safety of oral posaconazole in neutropenic stem cell transplant recipients. *Antimicrob Agents Chemother*. 2006;50:1993-1999.

155. Krishna G, Martinho M, Chandrasekar P, et al. Pharmacokinetics of oral posaconazole in allogeneic hematopoietic stem cell transplant recipients with graft-versus-host disease. *Pharmacotherapy*. 2007;27:1627-1636.

156. Walsh TJ, Raad I, Patterson TF, et al. Treatment of invasive aspergillosis with posaconazole in patients who are refractory to or intolerant of conventional therapy: an externally controlled trial. *Clin Infect Dis*. 2007;44:2-12.

157. Schering. NDA 22-003. Noxafil (posaconazole) oral suspension, 2006.

158. Jain R, Pottinger P. The effect of gastric Acid on the absorption of posaconazole. *Clin Infect Dis*. 2008;46:1627; author reply, 8.

159. Courtney R, Radwanski E, Lim J, et al. Pharmacokinetics of posaconazole coadministered with antacid in fasting or nonfasting healthy men. *Antimicrob Agents Chemother*. 2004;48:804-808.

160. Courtney R, Pai S, Laughlin M, et al. Pharmacokinetics, safety, and tolerability of oral posaconazole administered in single and multiple doses in healthy adults. *Antimicrob Agents Chemother*. 2003;47:2788-2795.

161. Ezzet F, Wexler D, Courtney R, et al. Oral bioavailability of posaconazole in fasted healthy subjects: comparison between three regimens and basis for clinical dosage recommendations. *Clin Pharmacokinet*. 2005;44:211-220.

162. Hamilton JF, Bartkowski HB, Rock JP. Management of CNS mucormycosis in the pediatric patient. *Pediatr Neurosurg*. 2003;38:212-215.

163. Raj P, Vella EJ, Bickerton RC. Successful treatment of rhinocerebral mucormycosis by a combination of aggressive surgical debridement and the use of systemic liposomal amphotericin B and local therapy with nebulized amphotericin—a case report. *J Laryngol Otol*. 1998;112:367-370.

164. Bitterman H. Hyperbaric oxygen for invasive fungal infections. *Isr Med Assoc J*. 2007;9:387-388.

165. John BV, Chamilos G, Kontoyiannis DP. Hyperbaric oxygen as an adjunctive treatment for zygomycosis. *Clin Microbiol Infect*. 2005;11:515-517.

166. Ferguson BJ, Mitchell TG, Moon R, et al. Adjunctive hyperbaric oxygen for treatment of rhinocerebral mucormycosis. *Rev Infect Dis*. 1988;10:551-559.

167. Bentur Y, Shupak A, Ramon Y, et al. Hyperbaric oxygen therapy for cutaneous/soft-tissue zygomycosis complicating diabetes mellitus. *Plast Reconstr Surg*. 1998;102:822-824.

168. Gil-Lamaignere C, Simitsopoulou M, Roilides E, et al. Interferon-gamma and granulocyte-macrophage colony-stimulating factor augment the activity of polymorphonuclear leukocytes against medically important Zygomycetes. *J Infect Dis*. 2005;191:1180-1187.

169. Barratt DM, Van Meter K, Asmar P, et al. Hyperbaric oxygen as an adjunct in zygomycosis: Randomized controlled trial in a murine model. *Antimicrob Agents Chemother*. 2001;45:3601-3602.

170. Abzug MJ, Walsh TJ. Interferon-gamma and colony-stimulating factors as adjuvant therapy for refractory fungal infections in children. *Pediatr Infect Dis J*. 2004;23:769-773.

171. Hubel K, Dale DC, Engert A, et al. Current status of granulocyte (neutrophil) transfusion therapy for infectious diseases. *J Infect Dis*. 2001;183:321-328.

172. Pagano L, Girmenia C, Mele L, et al. Infections caused by filamentous fungi in patients with hematologic malignancies. A report of 391 cases by GIMEMA Infection Program. *Haematologica*. 2001;86:862-870.

173. Walker SD, Clark RV, King CT, et al. Fatal disseminated *Conidiobolus coronatus* infection in a renal transplant patient. *Am J Clin Pathol*. 1992;98:559-564.

174. Bigliazzi C, Poletti V, Dell'Amore D, et al. Disseminated basidiobolomycosis in an immunocompetent woman. *J Clin Microbiol*. 2004;42:1367-1369.

175. Gugnani HC. Entomophthoromycosis due to *Conidiobolus*. *Eur J Epidemiol*. 1992;8:391-396.

176. Gugnani HC. A review of zygomycosis due to *Basidiobolus ranarum*. *Eur J Epidemiol*. 1999;15:923-929.

177. Mugerwa JW. Subcutaneous phycomycosis in Uganda. *Br J Dermatol*. 1976;94:539-544.

178. Martinson FD. Clinical, epidemiological and therapeutic aspects of entomophthoromycosis. *Ann Soc Belg Med Trop*. 1972;52:329-342.

179. Ibrahim A, Edwards J Jr, Filler SG. Zygomycoses. In: Dismukes WE, Pappas P, Sobekl JD, eds. *Clinical Mycology*. New York: Oxford University Press; 2003:241-251.

180. Khan ZU, Khoursheed M, Makar R, et al. Basidiobolus ranarum as an etiologic agent of gastrointestinal mucormycosis. *J Clin Microbiol*. 2001;39:2360-2363.

181. Khan ZU, Prakash B, Kapoor MM, et al. Basidiobolomycosis of the rectum masquerading as Crohn's disease: case report and review. *Clin Infect Dis*. 1998;26:521-523.

182. Lyon GM, Smilack JD, Komatsu KK, et al. Gastrointestinal basidiobolomycosis in Arizona: clinical and epidemiological characteristics and review of the literature. *Clin Infect Dis*. 2001;32:1448-1455.

183. Yousef OM, Smilack JD, Kerr DM, et al. Gastrointestinal basidiobolomycosis. Morphologic findings in a cluster of six cases. *Am J Clin Pathol*. 1999;112:610-616.

184. Bosco, DMG, Bagagli E, Araújo JP et al. Human pythiosis, Brazil. *Emerg Infect Dis*. 2005;11:715-718.

185. Guarro J, Aguilar C, Pujol I. In-vitro antifungal susceptibilities of *Basidiobolus* and *Conidiobolus* spp. strains. *J Antimicrob Chemother*. 1999;44:557-560.

186. Dworzack DL, Pollock AS, Hodges GR, et al. Mucormycosis of the maxillary sinus and palate caused by *Basidiobolus haptosporus*. *Arch Intern Med*. 1978;138:1274-1276.

187. Pasha TM, Leighton JA, Smilack JD, et al. Basidiobolomycosis: an unusual fungal infection mimicking inflammatory bowel disease. *Gastroenterology*. 1997;112:250-254.

188. Taylor GD, Sekhon AS, Tyrrell DL, et al. Rhinofacial mucormycosis caused by *Conidiobolus coronatus*: a case report including in vitro sensitivity to antimycotic agents. *Am J Trop Med Hyg*. 1987;36:398-401.

189. Foss NT, Rocha MR, Lima VT, et al. Entomophthoramycosis: therapeutic success by using amphotericin B and terbinafine. *Dermatology*. 1996;193:258-260.

260

Sporothrix schenckii

JOHN H. REX | PABLO C. OKHUYSEN

Sporotrichosis usually begins when the causative agent, *Sporothrix schenckii*, is inoculated into a site of a minor skin injury and produces an ulcerated, verrucous, or erythematous nodule, sometimes associated with local lymphatic spread. On rare occasions, the fungus is inhaled and causes a granulomatous pneumonitis that often cavitates, producing a clinical pattern very similar to tuberculosis. The fungus may also disseminate hematogenously and cause isolated osteoarticular, central nervous system, or ocular lesions in the normal host or widespread multifocal disease in the immunosuppressed host.

Mycology

S. schenckii is a dimorphic fungus that exists in a hyphal form in vitro at temperatures lower than 37°C. Colonies are initially white, but gradually become brown to black because of the production of pigmented conidia. In vivo, or at 37°C on rich media such as brain-heart infusion, the organism converts to an oval- or cigar-shaped budding yeast. Along with the characteristic morphology of the sporulating mold, identification is based on demonstration of this conversion to a yeast form. *S. schenckii* var. *luriei* has been rarely isolated from humans and differs by producing a variety of unusual shapes in vivo.[1] Further subdivision of the species *S. schenckii* into several closely related species has been proposed.[2]

Epidemiology

Sporotrichosis has been reported from locations around the globe, but most case reports come from the tropical and subtropical regions of the Americas.[3] Regions of hyperendemicity are known.[4] *S. schenckii* is most often isolated from soil, plants, or plant products such as straw, wood, sphagnum moss, and thorny plants, although the fungus is not a plant pathogen. Scratches on exposed skin of florists, rose gardeners, horticulturalists, farmers, miners, and armadillo hunters have increased risk of infection.[3,5,6] As most cases appear to be to the result of occupational or avocational exposure to these materials, typically in the form of gardening or farming, patients with suggestive syndromes should be asked about these activities. Cases of animal-to-human transmission involving squirrels, horses, dogs, cats, pigs, mules, insects, and birds have been described,[7,8] including multiple human cases in parallel with epidemic feline sporotrichosis.[9] Finally, sporotrichosis was apparently transmitted from the infected cheek of a mother to her infant.[10]

Clinical Syndromes

Infections caused by *S. schenckii* can be divided into several syndromes. The lymphocutaneous forms are the most common.

LYMPHOCUTANEOUS SPOROTRICHOSIS

Cutaneous disease arises at sites of minor trauma and inoculation of the fungus into the skin. The initial lesion is most often on a distal extremity, but almost any site may be involved, including such central locations as the nose and ocular adnexa.[6,11,12] This preference for cooler parts of the body corresponds to the known intolerance of some strains of *S. schenckii* to growth at 37°C.[13] Initial lesions are papulonodular, often erythematous, and range in size from a few millimeters to 2 to 4 cm. The lesions may be smooth or verrucous, and they often ulcerate

and develop raised erythematous borders.[11] Secondary lesions may develop proximally along lymphatic channels; these secondary lesions evolve in the same fashion as the primary lesion (Fig. 260-1). Secondary lesions do not usually involve a lymph node, although lymphadenopathy may develop. The lesions are typically painless, even after they ulcerate. The fixed, or plaque, form of sporotrichosis differs by not demonstrating any tendency to spread locally. Although spontaneous resolution of fixed sporotrichosis has been described,[11] the lesions of sporotrichosis usually wax and wane over months to years. The patient will not have systemic symptoms and laboratory examinations will be normal.

The indolent progression and physical examination features that suggest lymphocutaneous and fixed sporotrichosis are also produced by a number of other organisms (Table 260-1). Cultures of the drainage from skin lesions are occasionally helpful, but culture of biopsy material is preferred and is diagnostic when positive. Microscopic examination will reveal pyogranulomas in the mid and upper dermis, but examination of multiple sections may be required to demonstrate the organism.[14]

EXTRACUTANEOUS SPOROTRICHOSIS

Osteoarticular involvement is the most common form of extracutaneous sporotrichosis.[15] Involvement is of the major joints of the extremities (wrist [Fig. 260-2], elbow, ankle, and knee [Fig. 260-3]); the hip, shoulder, and spine are not involved.[16] Most patients present with involvement of a single joint without previously having had sporotrichosis at any another site. The joint is swollen and painful on motion, an effusion is present, and a sinus tract may develop. The overlying skin may or may not be erythematous. Systemic symptoms are minimal and, other than elevation of the erythrocyte sedimentation rate, laboratory examinations are unrevealing. Untreated, other joints may become involved. Tenosynovitis associated with carpal tunnel syndrome or nerve entrapment has been reported.[17] The radiologic changes of osteomyelitis develop slowly and include loss of articular cartilage, periosteal reaction, and periarticular osteopenia and cystic changes. Failure to consider the diagnosis has resulted in an average 25-month delay before diagnosis.[18] Repeated culture of fluid from joint aspiration, as well as culture and microscopic examination of tissue from synovial biopsies, are often required to make the diagnosis. Differential considerations include pigmented villonodular synovitis, tuberculosis, gout, osteoarthritis, and rheumatoid arthritis.

Pulmonary sporotrichosis is well described.[19] The typical patient is a 30- to 60-year-old man. Approximately one third of the patients are alcoholic, one third have another concomitant medical illness such as pulmonary tuberculosis, diabetes mellitus, sarcoidosis, or steroid use, and one third are apparently normal. Patients are occasionally asymptomatic, but will usually have a productive cough, low-grade fever, or weight loss. Other than elevation of the erythrocyte sedimentation rate, laboratory abnormalities are minimal. The chest x-ray reveals unilateral or bilateral cavitary lesions, usually with an associated parenchymal infiltrate (Fig. 260-4). Pleural effusions and hilar lymphadenopathy are occasionally noted. Gram stain or cytologic examination of sputum or bronchial washings will sometimes reveal elongated budding yeast,[20] and sputum culture will usually yield the organism. With some patients, however, repeated cultures and long-term follow-up are necessary to make the diagnosis.[21] Untreated, the cavities of pulmonary sporotrichosis gradually enlarge and produce progressive pulmonary

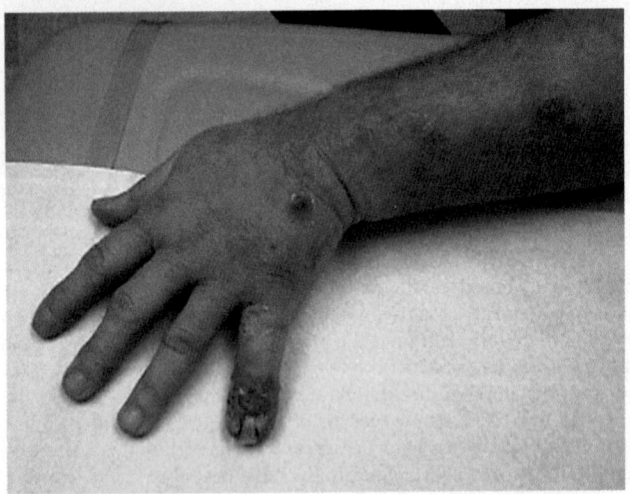

Figure 260-1 **Sporotrichosis of the fifth finger in a gardener.** Three nodular lesions are visible on the hand and arm.

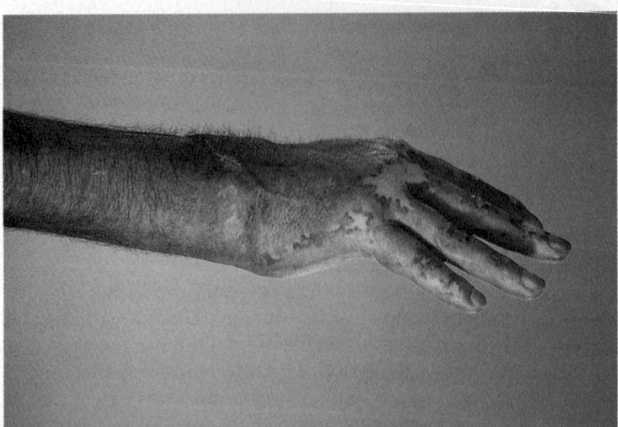

Figure 260-2 **Sporotrichosis of the bones of the wrist.**

dysfunction. A single case of spontaneous resolution of noncavitary infection has been reported.[22] The differential diagnosis includes mycobacterial infections (caused by both *M. tuberculosis* and atypical mycobacteria), histoplasmosis, and coccidioidomycosis.

Meningitis caused by *S. schenckii* has been described in a small number of patients. The patients present with an indolent meningitis. Cerebrospinal fluid (CSF) analysis demonstrates a lymphocytic pleocytosis, an elevated protein level, and hypoglycorrhachia. Culture of the CSF may be negative, and repeated cultures of large volumes of CSF or serologic studies may be required to make the diagnosis.[23] The differential diagnosis is broad and includes tuberculosis, cryptococcosis, coccidioidomycosis, and histoplasmosis.

Infections of a variety of other sites have been reported but are uncommon. Involvement of the ocular adnexa, sometimes with spread to the eye, has been described.[12] Endophthalmitis may even occur without prior trauma or other evidence of sporotrichosis.[24] Cases of isolated involvement of the sinuses, kidney, testes, and epididymis have also been reported.[15,25]

MULTIFOCAL EXTRACUTANEOUS SPOROTRICHOSIS

In otherwise normal patients with extracutaneous sporotrichosis, the lesions are generally restricted to a single site and are only locally progressive. Occasionally, a patient with osteoarticular sporotrichosis will have involvement of several joints, but the presentation is otherwise identical to that of patients with involvement of only a single joint. A much smaller group of patients, on the other hand, present with weight loss, variable low-grade fever, and often have several widely

TABLE 260-1	Differential Diagnosis of Sporotrichoid Lesions

Lesions Resembling Lymphocutaneous Sporotrichosis
(papulonodular lesions with or without central ulceration and with one or more nodules in the proximal skin along paths of presumed lymphatic spread)
  Nocardiosis caused by *N. brasiliensis*
  Cutaneous leishmaniasis
  Mycobacterial infection caused by
    M. tuberculosis (tuberculosis cutis verrucosa)
    M. marinum
    M. chelonae
    M. kansasii
    M. fortuitum
    M. leprae

Lesions Resembling Plaque Sporotrichosis
(chronic, indurated hyperkeratotic plaques)
  Infections: as for lymphocutaneous disease and also
    Blastomycosis
    Paracoccidioidomycosis
    Chromoblastomycosis
    Lobomycosis
  Neoplasms
    Squamous carcinoma
    Basal cell carcinoma
    Mycosis fungoides
  Other
    Psoriasis
    Lupus vulgaris
    Pyoderma gangrenosum

Adapted from Kostman JR, DiNubile MJ. Nodular lymphangitis: A distinctive but often unrecognized syndrome. *Ann Intern Med.* 1993;118:883-888; and Smego RA Jr, Castiglia M, Asperilla MO. Lymphocutaneous syndrome—a review of non-sporothrix causes. *Medicine.* 1999;78:38-63.

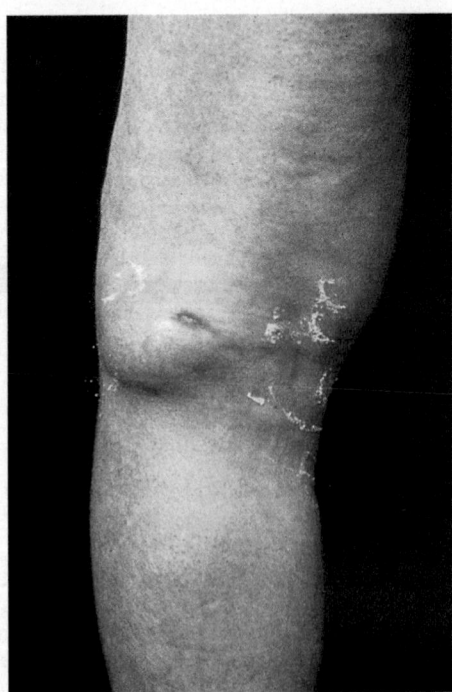

Figure 260-3 **Sporotrichosis of the knee, with formation of a Baker's cyst.** (*From Kwon-Chung KJ, Bennett JE, eds.* Medical Mycology. *Philadelphia: Lea & Febiger; 1992:712.*)

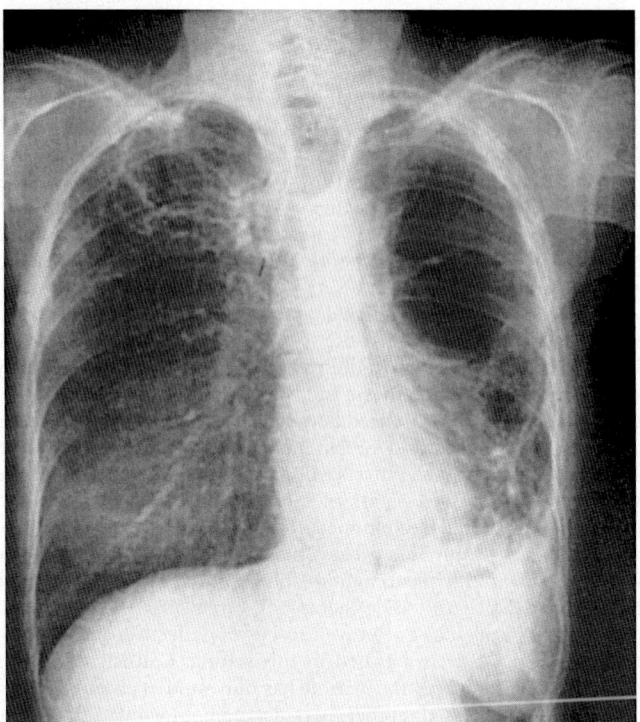

Figure 260-4 Chest roentgenogram demonstrating extensive bilateral cavitation caused by sporotrichosis.

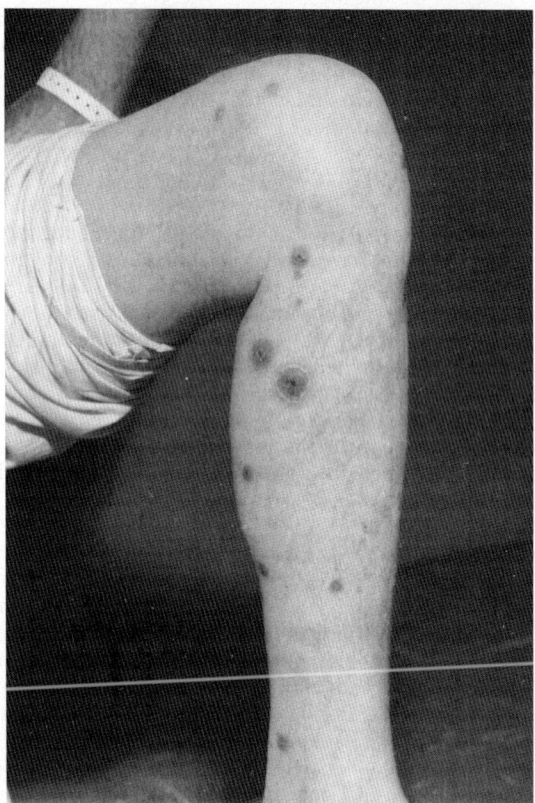

Figure 260-5 Hematogenously disseminated skin lesions scattered over the skin of a previously normal male farmer who also had joint lesions.

scattered cutaneous lesions without necessarily showing a single primary distal extremity lesion with the pattern of lymphangitic spread (Fig. 260-5). Mild anemia, leukocytosis, and elevation of the erythrocyte sedimentation rate may be present. Osteolytic bone lesions and arthritis are common and spread to the palate, eyes, and central nervous system may develop.[15,26] Noncavitary lung lesions may also be seen. Untreated infection is ultimately fatal. Patients with this form of sporotrichosis almost always have some form of immunosuppression, commonly hematologic malignancy, or HIV infection (see later). Cultures of skin lesions and joints are usually positive, whereas blood and bone marrow cultures are occasionally positive. Immunosuppressed patients who present with what appears to be simple cutaneous sporotrichosis should be carefully examined for other sites of infection and a technetium pyrophosphate bone scan should be obtained.

Clinical Manifestations of Sporotrichosis in the HIV-Infected Patient

Infection with the human immunodeficiency virus predisposes to invasive, atypical, or disseminated manifestations of sporotrichosis. When CD^4 counts are relatively well preserved, localized infection may follow direct cutaneous inoculation in a pattern analogous to that in immunocompetent patients.[27] However, widespread lymphocutaneous sporotrichosis or multifocal extracutaneous disease may be seen in patients with more advanced HIV infection. In a review of AIDS patients with disseminated sporotrichosis,[28] almost all had less than 100 CD4+ T cells/μL. Multiple ulcerative skin lesions are usually present. Sporotrichosis may also present as multifocal tenosynovitis and arthritis with or without overt cutaneous disease or systemic dissemination. Thus, it may resemble disseminated gonococcal infection or the seronegative spondyloarthropathies, such as acute reactive arthritis (Reiter's syndrome) or psoriatic arthritis (Fig. 260-6), which are seen with a higher frequency in the setting of AIDS.[29] Widespread visceral dissemination also occurs, as evidenced by reports of meningitis with parenchymal brain lesions,[30] lung abscess, liver, and spleen

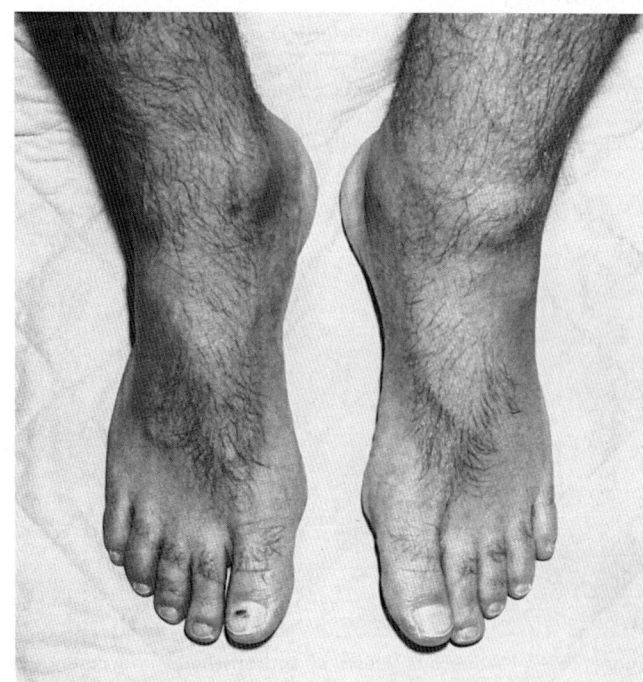

Figure 260-6 **Extensive multifocal sporotrichosis with tenosynovitis of the toes, arthritis of the ankles, and associated lymphedema in a patient with advanced AIDS.** This patient also had tenosynovitis of the wrists and hands, along with arthritis of the wrists and knees.

involvement,[31] endophthalmitis,[32] and fungemia with spread to the esophagus, colon, testes, bone marrow, and lymph nodes.[32] Sinusitis with invasion of the contiguous bone and soft tissues has also been described,[33] and emphasizes the potential for the respiratory tract as the initial focus of infection in HIV-infected patients.

Diagnosis

Diagnosis is best made by culture of the affected site, although repeated attempts at culture may have to be made. A positive culture from any site is ordinarily diagnostic of infection; however, a case of saprophytic involvement of the respiratory tract has been described.[34] A positive blood culture strongly suggests the multifocal form of sporotrichosis seen in immunocompromised hosts, although the lysis-centrifugation system may be more sensitive in detecting fungemia in non-immuno-compromised patients.[35] Serologic techniques have been described and may be useful in such obscure forms of sporotrichosis as meningitis, but are confounded by the presence of antibody in individuals without evidence of sporotrichosis.[36] No standard method of serologic testing is available.

Examination of biopsy specimens reveals a pyogranulomatous response and is diagnostic if characteristic 1- to 3-μm × 3- to 10-μm cigar-shaped yeast forms are seen. Unfortunately, the yeast may be difficult to detect unless multiple sections are examined,[14] although lesions from immunocompromised hosts may contain numerous yeasts (Fig. 260-7). In addition, *S. schenckii* often assumes a more rounded tissue form, making the biopsy suggestive but not diagnostic. The organisms may be surrounded by a stellate, periodic acid Schiff (PAS)–positive, eosinophilic material known as an asteroid body. In the brain or eye, a capsule has sometimes been demonstrable around the yeastlike cells.

As with other immunosuppressed patients, individuals with advanced AIDS may have a high fungal load that results in positive smears and cultures.[20] Skin biopsy may reveal fungal elements with a limited inflammatory response, and this should prompt the clinician to initiate a search for a systemic immunodeficiency.[37]

Therapy

Treatment guidelines for sporotrichosis have been proposed.[38] Because of its convenience and consistent efficacy,[39] itraconazole at 200 mg/day has become the therapy of choice for cutaneous sporotrichosis.[38] Therapy with itraconazole is given for 2 to 4 weeks beyond complete resolution of all lesions and usually requires 3 to 6 months to effect a

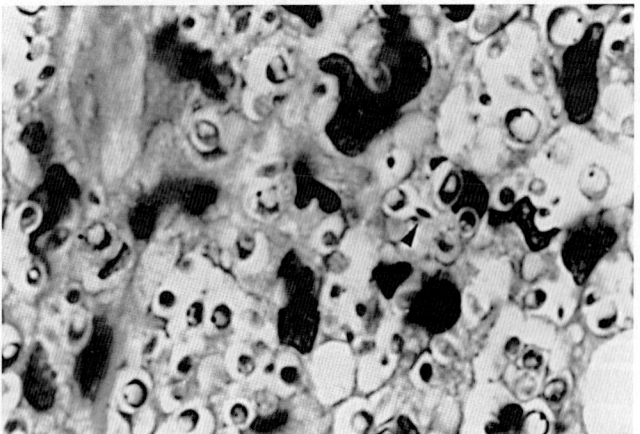

Figure 260-7 Numerous yeasts of sporotrichosis in a cutaneous lesion from an immunosuppressed patient. In the normal host, organisms are usually difficult to locate. Although a single cigar-shaped form is present (*arrowhead*), most of the yeasts have a rounded form that is consistent with, but not diagnostic of, sporotrichosis. (*Courtesy of Dr. Ronald Rapini, Houston.*)

clinical cure. Relapse has been observed on occasion after cessation of therapy. Should relapse develop, a higher dose of itraconazole (200 mg twice daily), terbinafine (see later), or iodide (see later) may be tried. Limited data suggest that terbinafine at 1000 mg/day may have efficacy similar to that of itraconazole for lymphocutaneous sporotrichosis,[40] but direct comparative data do not exist. Further, the maximum U.S. Food and Drug Administration (FDA)-approved terbinafine regimen is 250 mg daily for 12 weeks; the safety of extended therapy with 1000-mg dose has not yet been extensively validated. Iodides are an effective and inexpensive but poorly tolerated therapy for cutaneous sporotrichosis. Iodide therapy is prescribed as a saturated solution of potassium iodide (SSKI), with therapy begun at 5 to 10 drops taken orally three times daily. The dose is gradually advanced to 25 to 40 drops three times daily for children or 40 to 50 drops three times daily for adults. SSKI has a bitter taste and is made more palatable by taking it in milk, juice, or a carbonated beverage. Side effects include nausea, anorexia, diarrhea, parotid or lacrimal gland enlargement, and an acneiform rash. These side effects will remit with reduction of the dose of SSKI or temporary cessation of therapy. For both terbinafine and iodide, therapy should be continued until 2 to 4 weeks after the cutaneous lesions have resolved, a process that usually takes 3 to 6 months. Some patients are allergic to iodides and, in others, cutaneous disease may respond slowly to iodide therapy or, rarely, may fail to respond at all. Ketoconazole has not proven to be very effective, and ampho-tericin B is too toxic to be used in this setting. Consistent with its limited in vitro activity,[41] fluconazole has only modest clinical activity and should only be used if other therapies are not tolerated.[38,42] Of the newer azoles, posaconazole appears more active in vitro than voricon-azole, but no clinical data are available.[43] Because of the temperature sensitivity of this organism, heat is a useful adjunct therapy and on occasion has been curative.[44] Given the toxicity of both the azoles and iodides in pregnant women (skeletal bone deformities and goiter, respectively),[45] use of heat may be especially valuable during pregnancy.[38,46]

Therapy of extracutaneous sporotrichosis is often difficult. Itracon-azole, 200 mg PO twice daily for at least a year, is probably the drug of choice for osteoarticular sporotrichosis, although response is slow and may be incomplete. Treatment with IV amphotericin B is also effective (a lipid-associated preparation is recommended because of the improved safety profile of these formulations).[38] Ketoconazole (400 to 800 mg/day) and fluconazole (200 to 400 mg/day) appear less efficacious.[42,47] No clinical data are available for the newer azoles (vori-conazole and posaconazole) and the echinocandins do not appear consistently active.[43,48,49] Intra-articular amphotericin B is sometimes given, although its role has not been clearly defined. Surgical débride-ment is often used, but its usefulness is also uncertain. SSKI has rarely been reported to be effective, but usually is not.

If diagnosed before the development of cavities, pulmonary sporo-trichosis may be treated with SSKI or amphotericin B.[19] Cure of cavi-tary disease typically requires pulmonary resection plus a perioperative course of itraconazole or amphotericin B.[38] Treatment failure is often associated with incomplete resection. The limited available data for ketoconazole, fluconazole, or itraconazole in this setting include both successes and failures with each,[19,39] and they are not generally recommended.[38]

S. schenckii meningitis does not consistently respond to amphoteri-cin B, and the addition of 5-fluorocytosine may be warranted. Limited data suggest that itraconazole might be useful as suppressive or step-down therapy.[38] The number of reported cases of involvement of other specific sites is too limited to permit generalization. Extracutaneous sporotrichosis in the immunocompromised host usually responds, at least partially, to amphotericin B or itraconazole, although relapse is common.

THERAPY OF PATIENTS WITH AIDS

Therapy of sporotrichosis in AIDS should be tailored to the presenting syndrome. Itraconazole appears to be the drug of choice, and individuals with limited cutaneous disease can be treated with 200 mg twice daily. Amphotericin B should be used as initial therapy of disseminated disease, with lipid-associated formulations preferred over amphotericin B deoxycholate.[38] Based on the observation of frequent relapse and dissemination, chronic suppressive therapy with itraconazole appears warranted following initial control of infection. Although unsupported by direct data, it is appears reasonable to discontinue therapy in individuals who have been treated for itraconazole for a least 1 year and whose CD4+ cell counts have been at 200 cells/µL for at least 1 year.[38]

Both anecdotal and published experience suggest that multifocal extracutaneous disease in HIV-infected patients may respond poorly, if at all, to current therapies.[50,51] Therapy should be initiated with amphotericin B, followed by lifetime suppression with itraconazole. Progression may occur despite amphotericin therapy. Because disseminated disease has been reported to develop despite ongoing fluconazole being given for other indications,[52] fluconazole is not a first-line choice. As has been demonstrated for other opportunistic pathogens, the use of potent new combination antiretroviral therapies may also assist in clearing the infection.[53]

ITRACONAZOLE BLOOD LEVEL MONITORING

When itraconazole is used for noncutaneous infection or in HIV-infected subjects, confirmation of adequate blood levels is recommended. Drug levels may also be altered because of drug interactions that interfere with drug metabolism. In HIV in particular, levels may be reduced by achlorhydria, malabsorption, or diarrhea caused by other opportunistic pathogens. Plasma levels should be determined at steady state, generally after 2 weeks of therapy. Because of itraconazole's long half-life, specimens for testing may be obtained without specific regard for the timing of drug administration. Although strong data showing the correlation between itraconazole levels and response to sporotrichosis are not available, data from other settings (most notably aspergillosis) suggest that levels of the parent (unmetabolized) itraconazole molecule of 500 ng/mL by high-performance liquid chromatography would likely be adequate to produce a clinical response. This target plasma level for the parent molecule is similar to the 1000-ng/mL target for the parent and its bioactive metabolite that was suggested in recent guidelines.[38] The increased bioavailability of the newer itraconazole cyclodextrin suspension is helpful in achieving such blood levels.

Prognosis

Cutaneous sporotrichosis responds well to therapy and has an excellent prognosis. Osteoarticular sporotrichosis may require prolonged therapy but is not life-threatening. Other forms of extracutaneous sporotrichosis can be difficult to treat and may have substantial morbidity and mortality.

REFERENCES

1. Ajello L, Kaplan W. A new variant of *Sporothrix schenckii*. Mykosen. 1969;12:633-644.
2. Marimon R, Cano J, Gene J, et al. *Sporothrix brasiliensis, S. globosa*, and *S. mexicana*, three new *Sporothrix* species of clinical interest. J Clin Microbiol. 2007;45:3198-3206.
3. Travassos LR, Lloyd KO. *Sporothrix schenckii* and related species of *Ceratocystis*. Microbiol Rev. 1980;44:683-721.
4. Pappas PG, Tellez I, Deep AE, et al. Sporotrichosis in Peru: Description of an area of hyperendemicity. Clin Infect Dis. 2000;30:65-70.
5. Feeney KT, Arthur IH, Whittle AJ, et al. Outbreak of sporotrichosis, Western Australia. Emerg Infect Dis. 2007;13:1228-1231.
6. da Rosa ACM, Scroferneker ML, Vettorato R, et al. Epidemiology of sporotrichosis: A study of 304 cases in Brazil. J Am Acad Dermatol. 2005;52:451-459.
7. Saravanakumar PS, Eslami P, Zar FA. Lymphocutaneous sporotrichosis associated with a squirrel bite: Case report and review. Clin Infect Dis. 1996;23:647-648.
8. Reed KD, Moore FM, Geiger GE, et al. Zoonotic transmission of sporotrichosis—case report and review. Clin Infect Dis. 1993;16:384-387.
9. Schubach A, Schubach TMP, Barros MBD, et al. Cat-transmitted sporotrichosis, Rio de Janeiro, Brazil. Emerg Infect Dis. 2005;11:1952-1954.
10. Smith LM. Sporotrichosis: report of four clinically atypical cases. South Med J. 1945;38:505-515.
11. Bargman HB. Sporotrichosis of the nose with spontaneous cure. Can Med Assoc J. 1981;124:1027.
12. Gordon D. Ocular sporotrichosis. Arch Ophthalmol. 1947;37:56-72.
13. Kwon-Chung KJ. Comparison of isolates of *Sporothrix schenckii* obtained from fixed cutaneous lesions with isolates from other types of lesions. J Infect Dis. 1979;139:424-431.
14. Bullpitt P, Weedon D. Sporotrichosis: A review of 39 cases. Pathology. 1978;10:249-256.
15. Wilson DE, Mann JJ, Bennett JE, et al. Clinical features of extracutaneous sporotrichosis. Medicine. 1967;46:265-279.
16. Janes PC, Mann RJ. Extracutaneous sporotrichosis. J Hand Surg. 1987;12A:441-445.
17. Stratton CW, Lichtenstein KA, Lowenstein SR, et al. Granulomatous tenosynovitis and carpal tunnel syndrome caused by *Sporothrix schenckii*. Am J Med. 1981;71:161-164.
18. Crout JE, Brewer NS, Tompkins RB. Sporotrichosis arthritis: Clinical features in seven patients. Ann Intern Med. 1977;86:294-297.
19. Pluss JL, Opal SM. Pulmonary sporotrichosis: Review of treatment and outcome. Medicine. 1986;65:143-153.
20. Gori S, Lupetti A, Moscato G, et al. Pulmonary sporotrichosis with hyphae in a human immunodeficiency virus-infected patient. A case report. Acta Cytologica. 1997;41:519-521.
21. Khan FA, Guarneri JJ, Sierra MF. Primary pulmonary sporotrichosis complicated by perirectal abscess. Am Rev Respir Dis. 1975;112:119-123.
22. Pueringer RJ, Iber C, Deike MA, et al. Spontaneous remission of extensive pulmonary sporotrichosis. Ann Intern Med. 1986;104:366-367.
23. Scott EN, Kaufman L, Brown AC, et al. Serologic studies in the diagnosis and management of meningitis due to *Sporothrix schenckii*. N Engl J Med. 1987;317:935-940.
24. Font RL, Jakobiec FA. Granulomatous necrotizing retinochoroiditis caused by *Sporotrichum schenckii*. Arch Ophthalmol. 1976;94:1513-1519.
25. Friedman SJ, Doyle JA. Extracutaneous sporotrichosis. Int J Dermatol. 1983;22:171-173.
26. Lynch PJ, Voorhees JJ, Harrell ER. Systemic sporotrichosis. Ann Intern Med. 1970;73:23-30.
27. Keiser P, Whittle D. Sporotrichosis in human immunodeficiency virus-infected patients: Report of a case. Rev Infect Dis. 1991;13:1027-1028.
28. Al-Tawfiq JA, Wools KK. Disseminated sporotrichosis and *Sporothrix schenckii* fungemia as the initial presentation of human immunodeficiency virus infection. Clin Infect Dis. 1998;26:1403-1406.
29. Oscherwitz SL, Rinaldi MG. Disseminated sporotrichosis in a patient infected with human immunodeficiency virus. Clin Infect Dis. 1992;15:568-569.
30. Silva-Vergara ML, Maneira FRZ, de Oliveira RM, et al. Multifocal sporotrichosis with meningeal involvement in a patient with AIDS. Med Mycol. 2005;43:187-190.
31. Lipstein-Kresch E, Isenberg HD, Singer C, et al. Disseminated *Sporothrix schenckii* infection with arthritis in a patient with acquired immunodeficiency syndrome. J Rheumatol. 1985;12:805-808.
32. Heller HM, Fuhrer J. Disseminated sporotrichosis in patients with AIDS: Case report and review of the literature. AIDS. 1991;5:1243-1246.
33. Morgan M, Reves R. Invasive sinusitis due to *Sporothrix schenckii* in a patient with AIDS. Clin Infect Dis. 1996;23:1319-1320.
34. Lowenstein M, Markowitz SM, Nottebart HC, et al. Existence of *Sporothrix schenckii* as a pulmonary saprophyte. Chest. 1978;73:419-421.
35. Kosinski RM, Axelrod P, Rex JH, et al. *Sporothrix schenckii* fungemia without disseminated sporotrichosis. J Clin Microbiol. 1992;30:501-503.
36. Scott EN, Muchmore HG. Immunoblot analysis of antibody responses to *Sporothrix schenckii*. J Clin Microbiol. 1989;27:300-304.
37. Fitzpatrick JE, Eubanks S. Acquired immunodeficiency syndrome presenting as disseminated cutaneous sporotrichosis. Int J Dermatol. 1988;27:406-407.
38. Kauffman CA, Bustamante B, Chapman SW, et al. Clinical practice guidelines for the management of sporotrichosis: 2007 update by the infectious diseases society of America. Clin Infect Dis. 2007;45:1255-1265.
39. Sharkey-Mathis PK, Kauffman CA, Graybill JR, et al. Treatment of sporotrichosis with itraconazole. NIAID Mycoses Study Group. Am J Med. 1993;95:279-285.
40. Chapman SW, Pappas P, Kauffmann C, et al. Comparative evaluation of the efficacy and safety of two doses of terbinafine (500 and 1000 mg day(-1)) in the treatment of cutaneous or lymphocutaneous sporotrichosis. Mycoses. 2004;47:62-68.
41. Espinel-Ingroff A, Boyle K, Sheehan DJ. In vitro antifungal activities of voriconazole and reference agents as determined by NCCLS methods: Review of the literature. Mycopathologia. 2001;150:101-115.
42. Kauffman CA, Pappas PG, McKinsey DS, et al. National Institute of Allergy and Infectious Diseases Mycoses Study Group. Treatment of lymphocutaneous and visceral sporotrichosis with fluconazole. Clin Infect Dis. 1996;22:46-50.
43. Marimon R, Serena C, Gen J, et al. In vitro antifungal susceptibilities of five species of *Sporothrix*. Antimicrob Agents Chemother. 2008;52:732-734.
44. Galiana J, Conti-Díaz IA. Healing effects of heat and a rubefacient on nine cases of sporotrichosis. Sabouraudia. 1963;3:64-71.
45. Sobel JD. Use of antifungal drugs in pregnancy: A focus on safety. Drug Safety. 2000;1:77-85.
46. Vanderveen EE, Messenger AL, Voorhees JJ. Sporotrichosis in pregnancy. Cutis. 1982;30:761-763.
47. Calhoun DL, Washkin H, White MP, et al. Treatment of systemic sporotrichosis with ketoconazole. Rev Infect Dis. 1991;13:47-51.
48. Espinel-Ingroff A. Comparison of in vitro activities of the new triazole SCH56592 and the echinocandins MK-0991 (L-743,872) and LY303366 against opportunistic filamentous and dimorphic fungi and yeasts. J Clin Microbiol. 1998;36:2950-2956.
49. Nakai T, Uno J, Ikeda F, et al. In vitro antifungal activity of micafungin (FK463) against dimorphic fungi: Comparison of yeast-like and mycelial forms. Antimicrob Agents Chemother. 2003;47:1376-1381.
50. Kauffman CA. Old and new therapies for sporotrichosis. Clin Infect Dis. 1995;21:981-985.
51. Donabedian H, O'Donnell E, Olszewski C, et al. Disseminated cutaneous and meningeal sporotrichosis in an AIDS patient. Diagn Microbiol Infect Dis. 1994;18:111-115.
52. Goldani LZ, Aquino VR, Dargel AA. Disseminated cutaneous sporotrichosis in an AIDS patient receiving maintenance therapy with fluconazole for previous cryptococcal meningitis. Clin Infect Dis. 1999;28:1337-1338.
53. Carr A, Marriott D, Field A, et al. Treatment of HIV-1-associated microsporidiosis and cryptosporidiosis with combination antiretroviral therapy. Lancet. 1998;351:256-261.

261

Agents of Chromoblastomycosis

DUANE R. HOSPENTHAL*

Chromoblastomycosis (chromomycosis) is a chronic localized fungal infection of the skin and subcutaneous tissue that produces raised scaly lesions, usually of the lower extremities. The lesions of chromoblastomycosis are frequently warty or cauliflower-like in appearance, with pathognomonic muriform cells (also called "copper penny" or sclerotic bodies) found on histologic examination. This disease of tropical and subtropical distribution is produced by inoculation of the infecting fungi in association with minor trauma. Alexandrino Pedroso, for whom the major etiologic agent is named, first noted the disease in 1911, although the first publication to describe what was likely chromoblastomycosis appeared in 1914, authored by Max Rudolph.[1] The first reports to include identification of the fungal cause of this disease were published 1 year later by Medlar and Lane, who described a patient with disease acquired not in the tropics, but in New England.

Etiologic Agents

Infection is caused by one of several dark-walled (dematiaceous) fungi found in the soil, and in association with cacti, thorny plants, and other live or decaying vegetation. *Fonsecaea pedrosoi* is the most common cause of chromoblastomycosis, although disease caused by *Cladophialophora (Cladosporium) carrionii*, *Phialophora verrucosa*, and *Rhinocladiella aquaspersa* also occurs. In the largest reports from Brazil,[2] Mexico,[3] Sri Lanka,[4] and Japan,[5] *F. pedrosoi* has been responsible for 86% to 96% of all infections. *Fonsecaea compacta* is currently believed to be a variant of *F. pedrosoi* and not a distinct species. Recent molecular evaluation of *F. pedrosoi* has resulted in the division of chromoblastomycosis isolates into *F. pedrosoi* and *Fonsecaea monophora*.[6] Rare or isolated reports of disease caused by *Botryomyces caespitosus*, *Chaetomium funicola*, *Cladophialophora arxii*, *Cladophialophora boppii*, *Exophiala (Wangiella) dermatitidis*, *Exophiala jeanselmei*, *Exophiala spinifera*, *Phaeosclera dermatioides*, and *Rhytidhysteron* spp. have been published.[1,7-9]

Epidemiology

Chromoblastomycosis has been described to occur throughout the world, although most cases arise in tropical and subtropical regions, especially those with high annual rainfall. Large numbers of cases have been described from Madagascar, Brazil, Mexico, Venezuela, and Costa Rica. Disease is more prevalent in males (4:1 ratio), ages 40 to 69,[2] in association with outdoor activities such as farming and woodcutting, and in the absence of footwear use. In Madagascar, a unique epidemiology has been described in what is probably the largest focus of endemic disease.[10] Madagascar has two distinct foci of infection, with disease secondary to *F. pedrosoi* occurring in the humid, rainy, northern evergreen forest region and disease secondary to *C. carrionii* found in the arid southern desert region. In a study of 1343 cases of disease over 40 years in that country, the prevalence of 1 case/1920 inhabitants in the southern desert region has been described, with an incredible 1 in 910 prevalence in a single district of that region.

Pathology and Pathogenesis

The traumatic inoculation of the agents of chromoblastomycosis results in a mixed chronic suppurative and granulomatous host response.[11] The epidermis typically becomes thickened in a process called pseudoepitheliomatous hyperplasia, a histologic morphology that may be misidentified as malignancy by more inexperienced microscopists. Foci of polymorphonuclear cells and microabscesses are seen in both the epidermis and dermis. In the dermis, granulomas that include multinucleated giant cells and epithelioid cells are present, along with varying amounts of fibrosis. Fibrosis is increased in older lesions and can extend into the subcutaneous tissue, although disease rarely extends deep into the subcutaneous tissue. The hallmark of chromoblastomycosis, the muriform cells—also called sclerotic, copper penny, or Medlar bodies—may be found intracellularly in macrophages or extracellularly in abscesses. These are darkly pigmented (brown-golden), thick-walled, rounded cells, 4 to 12 μm in diameter, with cross walls in one or two planes (Fig. 261-1). Hyphae may also occasionally be seen, usually in the epidermis. The host response to these structures results in a process termed *transepithelial elimination*, in which fungi and damaged tissue are expelled through the epidermis, a process similar to that seen in calcinosis cutis.[12] The immunologic response of the host in this mycosis is still not well understood. Disease appears to be associated with an ineffective immune response to the organism, with chronic inflammation produced in response to persistence of the fungi in tissue. The cell-mediated immune response appears to play a central role. High interleukin-10 (IL-10) levels, low interferon-γ levels, and inefficient T-cell proliferation have been noted in patients with severe disease, with the opposite seen in those with milder chromoblastomycosis.[13] Antibody responses have shown association with disease chronicity and extent but do not appear to provide any degree of protection in this infection.[14]

Clinical Manifestations

Weeks to months following inoculation of the causative organisms through minor trauma, subjects typically develop a small scaly papule on the lower extremity at the site of the trauma (Figs. 261-2 to 261-4). This lesion slowly develops into a superficial nodule, commonly with an irregular friable surface. Frequently, these nodules later spread out to become purplish, irregular, raised plaques. In descriptions by Carrion,[15] lesions of chromoblastomycosis were categorized into five types: (1) early nodular lesions, described as soft and pink-violaceous in color, with smooth, verrucous, or scaly surfaces; (2) tumorous lesions, large, papillomatous, often lobulated masses with crusting, sometimes described as cauliflower-like; (3) verrucous lesions with prominent hyperkeratosis; (4) plaque lesions; and (5) cicatricial lesions. Most lesions have black dots associated with their outer surface that are composed of fungi and necrotic debris, the products of transepithelial elimination. Although not typically painful, lesions may be associated with pruritus, are easily traumatized, and bleed readily. Ulceration is generally limited to those lesions with bacterial superinfection. Large lesions may become hyperkeratotic, and limb distortion, including elephantiasis, can occur as a result of blockage of normal lymphatic drainage.

Although lesions have been described to occur chiefly on the lower extremities (80% to 85%) in most regions of the world,[2,16] an exception to this pattern is reported from Japan. Evaluation of 290 lesions from

---

*The views expressed are those of the author and do not reflect the official policy or position of the Department of the Army, the Department of Defense, or the U.S. Government.

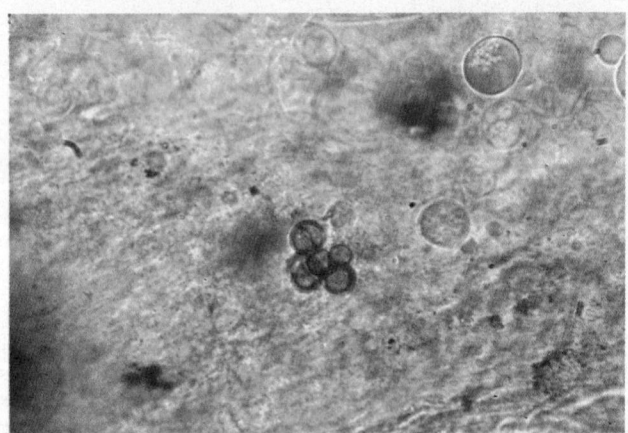

Figure 261-1 Sclerotic bodies of chromoblastomycosis. *(From Beneke ES, Rogers AL. Medical Mycology and Human Mycoses. Belmont, Calif: Star Publishing; 1996.)*

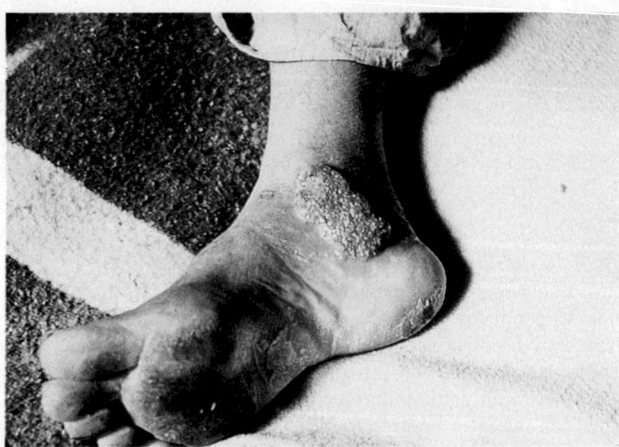

Figure 261-2 Chromoblastomycosis of the foot. *(From Beneke ES, Rogers AL. Medical Mycology and Human Mycoses. Belmont, Calif: Star Publishing; 1996.)*

that country found that chromoblastomycosis occurs most commonly on the upper extremities of male subjects and on the face or neck of females.[5]

Persistence of the lesions of chromoblastomycosis for 30 years has been reported, and delays in diagnosis of 1 to 3 years are not unusual. Although most lesions remain localized without spread to deeper structures, localized dissemination may occur via autoinoculation or via the lymphatics. Hematogenous spread has only rarely been described, but does include reports of dissemination to the central nervous system.[5] The occurrence of secondary bacterial infection has been reported to affect as many as 63% of persons with chromoblastomycosis.[3] Although apparently rare, at least eight cases of malignancy associated with chromoblastomycosis lesions have been reported in the literature.[17,18] Seven of these have been squamous cell carcinomas and one was a melanoma; all occurred after 10 or more years of disease.

The differential diagnosis of chromoblastomycosis includes psoriasis, other mycoses (e.g., blastomycosis, coccidioidomycosis, lobomycosis, mycetoma, paracoccidioidomycosis, cutaneous phaeohyphomycosis, sporotrichosis, tinea), cutaneous tuberculosis, leprosy, leishmaniasis, protothecosis, keratoacanthoma, squamous cell carcinoma, and sarcoidosis.

Diagnosis

Chromoblastomycosis should be suspected in persons with chronic scaly or friable lesions of the extremities, especially in rural tropical climates. Microscopic examination of skin scrapings can provide a rapid diagnosis of chromoblastomycosis because the characteristic muriform cells can be seen in potassium hydroxide preparations, especially those containing black dots (see Fig. 261-1). These unique structures may also be readily observed with standard staining of skin punch biopsy specimens with hematoxylin and eosin (Fig. 261-5). Although not absolutely necessary, culture should be performed to identify the specific cause of infection. Standard mycologic media (Sabouraud glucose agar), with and without cycloheximide, should be used and cultures incubated for at least 4 weeks. In culture, the fungal agents of chromoblastomycosis appear as dark molds. Under standard culture conditions, these fungi may be identified by the microscopic appearance of hyphae and reproductive structures. The muriform structures seen in tissue have been produced in vitro using low pH and the addition of propranolol, but this is not necessary for clinical diagnosis.[19] Exoantigen testing has been developed to aid in the diagnosis, although this is not commonly used.[20] Serologic and skin tests have

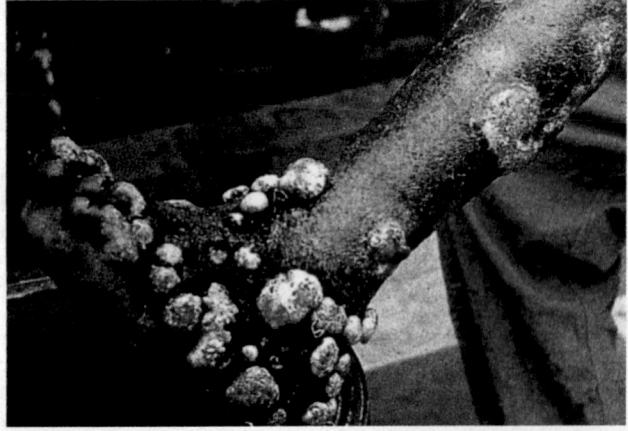

Figure 261-3 Chromoblastomycosis with multiple verrucous nodules. *(From McGinnis MR, Chandler FW. Chromoblastomycosis. In: Connor DH, Chandler FW, Schwartz DA, et al, eds. Pathology of Infectious Diseases. Norwalk, Conn: Appleton & Lange; 1997.)*

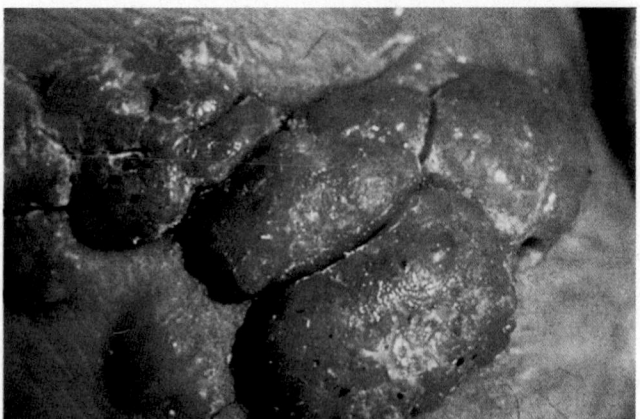

Figure 261-4 Chromoblastomycosis of the lower leg with lobulated, confluent nodules with focal ulcerations. *(From McGinnis MR, Chandler FW. Chromoblastomycosis. In: Connor DH, Chandler FW, Schwartz DA, et al, eds. Pathology of Infectious Diseases. Norwalk, Conn: Appleton & Lange; 1997.)*

with this azole antifungal agent, but the numbers of cures were small (3 of 10 patients treated for 12 to 24 months).[24] Treatment of chromoblastomycosis caused by *C. carrionii* with itraconazole has met with much greater success than treatment of that caused by other agents. One study reported cure in 2 of 5 patients with disease secondary to *F. pedrosoi* and 8 of 9 patients with *C. carrionii*, all given 100 to 400 mg of the drug daily for 4 to 8 months.[25] Queiroz-Telles and colleagues have reported the cure of 42% of patients (8 of 19) treated with 200 to 400 mg of itraconazole for a median of 7 months.[26] Another group described the therapy of 10 patients with disease secondary to *F. pedrosoi*, 4 of whom had failed prior therapy with ketoconazole.[27] All patients received 200 to 400 mg of itraconazole daily, and 8 also received monthly cryotherapy with liquid nitrogen. Nine patients were cured with 3 to 12 months of therapy; 2 of these responded with sustained cures after only 3 months of itraconazole at the lower dose of 200 mg daily. The remaining patient had marked improvement without cure. Recurrence was noted in a single patient who had been cured with a 6-month course of itraconazole (400 mg daily) and cryotherapy. Decreased in vitro susceptibility to itraconazole has been reported in one study of sequential clinical isolates of *F. pedrosoi*, potentially accounting for treatment failures.[28] Bonifaz and associates described good success with smaller lesions treated with itraconazole or cryosurgery, and in larger lesions treated with itraconazole followed by cryosurgery.[29] In that study, which included 4 patients in each group and dosing of itraconazole at 100 mg three times daily for 5 to 14 months, 8 of 12 patients (67%) were cured and the remaining 4 showed improvement. In addition to daily therapy, success with itraconazole given as pulse therapy, 400 mg daily for 7 days/month for 6 to 12 months, has also been reported.[30]

The allylamine antifungal agent terbinafine has produced excellent results in the treatment of chromoblastomycosis. In the largest study to date, terbinafine, 500 mg daily, was given to 35 patients for up to 12 months.[31] In that study, 16 patients had failed thiabendazole in the past and almost half had lesions of longer than 10 years' duration. Improvement defined as lack of bacterial superinfection and resolution of edema was seen after 2 to 4 months of therapy and, after 12 months, 86% obtained mycologic cures (72% with clinical cures).[16] Patients with *C. carrionii* infections were noted to respond more quickly than those with *F. pedrosoi* infection in that study. Unexpectedly, partial reversal of fibrosis of the lesions of chromoblastomycosis has also been reported to occur with terbinafine therapy. This reversal has been suggested to be independent of mycologic cure of infection in those receiving terbinafine.[32,33] Terbinafine used in alternate-week or combination therapy with itraconazole to treat 4 patients with resistant infections successfully has also been reported.[34]

The newer broad-spectrum azole antifungals may potentially be useful in this disease. In vitro testing has shown that the minimum inhibitory concentrations of voriconazole for *F. pedrosoi* and *F. compacta* is lower than those seen with itraconazole.[35] *F. pedrosoi* has also been shown to be susceptible to the echinocandin caspofungin in one small in vitro study.[36] Posaconazole (800 mg/day in divided doses for 6 to 2 months) has been used to successfully treat a small number of patients (five of six) with disease refractory to itraconazole and terbinafine.[37]

No vaccinations exist to prevent chromoblastomycosis. Proper protective clothing, especially footwear, and early treatment of the lesions are the only available preventive measures against this disease.

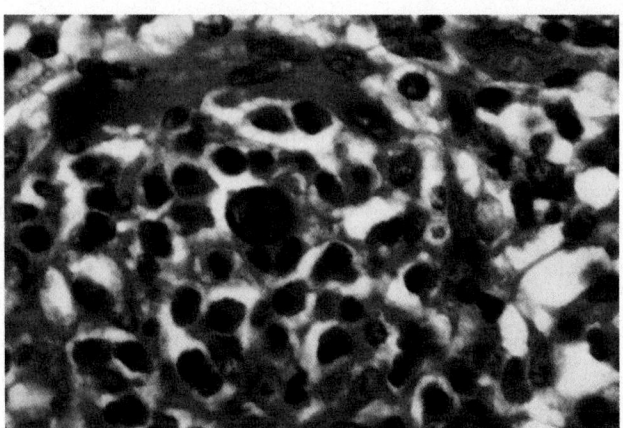

Figure 261-5 **Dermal abscess with quadrate cluster of organisms in a mixture of neutrophils, macrophages, eosinophils, and a giant cell (hematoxylin and eosin).** *(From McGinnis MR, Chandler FW. Chromoblastomycosis. In: Connor DH, Chandler FW, Schwartz DA, et al, eds. Pathology of Infectious Diseases. Norwalk, Conn: Appleton & Lange; 1997.)*

also been developed, but their use in this rare disease is limited to specialized centers in more endemic regions of the world.

Treatment

Although spontaneous resolution has been reported,[21] this is only a rare occurrence, and most chromoblastomycosis is a chronic indolent infection. When caused by its most common agent, *F. pedrosoi*, it is difficult to eradicate, even with prolonged therapy. Multiple modalities have been used to treat patients with chromoblastomycosis, including surgery, local (physical) treatments, and antifungal agents. Unfortunately, no single reproducibly successful treatment strategy has been identified. Surgical removal of small lesions appears to be effective, as does local application of liquid nitrogen, topical heat, and photocoagulation. Local curettage or electrocautery has been reported sometimes to result in disease spread and is to be discouraged. Heat therapy (42° to 46°C) with pocket warmers and other devices providing prolonged daily warmth directly to the lesions has been described as effective with 2 to 12 months of treatment.[22] Cryotherapy with liquid nitrogen sprays or applied with soaked cotton swabs or balls has been successful in the cure of small early lesions, and may be used effectively in combination with antifungal medications on larger lesions. Use of topical ajoene (a garlic extract) and 5-fluorouracil has been reported to be effective against disease secondary to *C. carrionii*.[23]

Currently, the best therapy appears to be itraconazole or terbinafine, perhaps with adjunctive cryotherapy with liquid nitrogen or other local treatments. Other antifungal agents, including amphotericin B (IV or intralesional), 5-fluorocytosine, ketoconazole, and fluconazole, have been used with poor to mixed success, alone or in combination.

Itraconazole has been reported to be effective in many patients in uncontrolled, nonrandomized studies. Early study with lower doses (100 to 200 mg daily) of itraconazole documented high response rates

REFERENCES

1. Kwon-Chung KJ, Bennett JE. *Medical Mycology*. Philadelphia: Lea & Febiger, 1992.
2. Minotto R, Bernardi CD, Mallmann LF, et al. Chromoblastomycosis: A review of 100 cases in the state of Rio Grande do Sul, Brazil. *J Am Acad Dermatol*. 2001;44:585-592.
3. Bonifaz A, Carrasco-Gerard E, Saul A. Chromoblastomycosis: Clinical and mycologic experience of 51 cases. *Mycoses*. 2001;44:1-7.
4. Attapattu MC. Chromoblastomycosis—a clinical and mycological study of 71 cases from Sri Lanka. *Mycopathologia*. 1997;137:145-151.
5. Fukushiro R. Chromomycosis in Japan. *Int J Dermatol*. 1983;22:221-229.
6. de Hoog GS, Attili-Angelis D, Vicente VA, et al. Molecular ecology and pathogenic potential of *Fonsecaea* species. *Med Mycol*. 2004;42:405-416.
7. Barba-Gomez JF, Mayorga J, McGinnis MR, et al. Chromoblastomycosis caused by *Exophiala spinifera*. *J Am Acad Dermatol*. 1992;26:367-370.
8. Chowdhary A, Guarro J, Randhawa HS, et al. A rare case of chromoblastomycosis in a renal transplant recipient caused by a non-sporulating species of *Rhytidhysteron*. *Med Mycol*. 2008;46:163-166.
9. Piepenbring M, Mendez OAC, Espinoza AAE, et al. Chromoblastomycosis casued by *Chaetomium funicola*: A case report from Western Panama. *Br J Dermatol*. 2007;157:1025-1029.
10. Esterre P, Andriantsimahavandy A, Ramarcel ER, et al. Forty years of chromoblastomycosis in Madagascar: A review. *Am J Trop Med Hyg*. 1996;55:45-47.
11. Uribe F, Zuluaga AI, Leon W, et al. Histopathology of chromoblastomycosis. *Mycopathologia*. 1989;105:1-6.
12. Batres E, Wolf JE Jr, Rudolph AH, et al. Transepithelial elimination of cutaneous chromomycosis. *Arch Dermatol*. 1978;114:1231-1232.

13. Gimenes VMF, Sousa MG, et al. Cytokine and lymphocyte proliferation in patients with different clinical forms of chromoblastomycosis. *Microbes Infect.* 2005;7:708-713.

14. Esterre P, Jahevitra M, Andriantsimahavandy A. Humoral immune response in chromoblastomycosis during and after therapy. *Clin Diagn Lab Immunol.* 2000;7:497-500.

15. Carrion AL. Chromoblastomycosis. *Ann N Y Acad Sci.* 1950;50:1255-1282.

16. Silva JP, de Souza W, Rozental S. Chromoblastomycosis: A retrospective study of 325 cases in Amazonic Region (Brazil). *Mycopathologia.* 1999;143:171-175.

17. Paul C, Dupont B, Pialoux G, et al. Chromoblastomycosis with malignant transformation and cutaneous-synovial secondary localization: The potential therapeutic role of itraconazole. *J Med Vet Mycol.* 1991;29:313-316.

18. Gon A, Minelli L. Melanoma in a long-standing lesion of chromoblastomycosis. *Int J Dermatol.* 2006;45:1331-1333.

19. da Silva JP, Alviano DS, Alviano CS, et al. Comparison of *Fonsecaea pedrosoi* sclerotic cells obtained in vivo and in vitro: Ultrastructure and antigenicity. *FEMS Immunol Med Microbiol.* 2002;33:63-69.

20. Espinel-Ingroff A, Shadomy S, Dixon D, et al. Exoantigen test for *Cladosporium bantianum, Fonsecaea pedrosoi,* and *Phialophora verrucosa. J Clin Microbiol.* 1986;23:305-310.

21. Nishimoto K, Yoshimura S, Honma K. Chromomycosis spontaneously healed. *Int J Dermatol.* 1984;23:408-410.

22. Tagami H, Ginoza M, Imaizumi S, et al. Successful treatment of chromoblastomycosis with topical heat therapy. *J Am Acad Dermatol.* 1984;10:615-619.

23. Perez-Blanco M, Valles RH, Zeppenfeldt GF, et al. Ajoene and 5-fluorouracil in the topical treatment of *Cladophialophora carrionii* chromoblastomycosis in humans: A comparative open study. *Med Mycol.* 2003;41:517-520.

24. Restrepo A, Gonzalez A, Gomez I, et al. Treatment of chromoblastomycosis with itraconazole. *Ann N Y Acad Sci.* 1988;544:504-516.

25. Borelli D. A clinical trial of itraconazole in the treatment of deep mycoses and leishmaniasis. *Rev Infect Dis.* 1987;9(Suppl 1):S57-S63.

26. Queiroz-Telles F, Purim KS, Fillus JN, et al. Itraconazole in the treatment of chromoblastomycosis due to *Fonsecaea pedrosoi. Int J Dermatol.* 1992;31:805-812.

27. Kullavanijaya P, Rojanavanich V. Successful treatment of chromoblastomycosis due to *Fonsecaea pedrosoi* by the combination of itraconazole and cryotherapy. *Int J Dermatol.* 1995;34:804-807.

28. Andrade TS, Castro LGM, Nunes RS, et al. Susceptibility of sequential *Fonsecaea pedrosoi* isolates from chromoblastomycosis patients to antifungal agents. *Mycoses.* 2004;47:216-221.

29. Bonifaz A, Martinez-Soto E, Carrasco-Gerard E, et al. Treatment of chromoblastomycosis with itraconazole, cryosurgery, and a combination of both. *Int J Dermatol.* 1997;36:542-547.

30. Ungpakorn R, Reangchainam S. Pulse itraconazole 400 mg daily in the treatment of chromoblastomycosis. *Clin Exp Dermatol.* 2006;31:245-247.

31. Esterre P, Inzan CK, Ratsioharana M, et al. A multicentre trial of terbinafine in patients with chromoblastomycosis. Effect on clinical and biologic criteria. *J Dermatol Treat.* 1998;9(Suppl 1):S29-S34.

32. Esterre P, Risteli L, Ricard-Blum S. Immunohistochemical study of type I collagen turnover and of matrix metalloproteinases in chromoblastomycosis before and after treatment by terbinafine. *Pathol Res Pract.* 1998;194:847-853.

33. Ricard-Blum S, Hartmann DJ, Esterre P. Monitoring of extracellular matrix metabolism and cross-linking in tissue, serum and urine of patients with chromoblastomycosis, a chronic skin fibrosis. *Eur J Clin Invest.* 1998;28:748-754.

34. Gupta AK, Taborda PR, Sanzovo AD. Alternate week and combination itraconazole and terbinafine therapy for chromoblastomycosis caused by *Fonsecaea pedrosoi* in Brazil. *Med Mycol.* 2002;40:529-534.

35. Radford SA, Johnson EM, Warnock DW. *In vitro* studies of activity of voriconazole (UK-109,496), a new triazole antifungal agent, against emerging and less common mold pathogens. *Antimicrob Agents Chemother.* 1997;41:841-843.

36. Del Poeta M, Schell WA, Perfect JR. *In vitro* antifungal activity of pneumocandin L-743,872 against a variety of clinically important molds. *Antimicrob Agents Chemother.* 1997;41:1835-1836.

37. Negroni R, Tobon A, Bustamante B, et al. Posaconazole treatment of refractory eumycetoma and chromoblastomycosis. *Rev Inst Med Trop S Paulo.* 2005;47:339-346.

262

Agents of Mycetoma

DUANE R. HOSPENTHAL*

Mycetoma is a chronic progressive granulomatous infection of the skin and subcutaneous tissue most often affecting the lower extremities, typically a single foot. Disease is unique from other cutaneous or subcutaneous diseases in its triad of localized swelling, underlying sinus tracts, and production of grains or granules (comprised of aggregations of the causative organism) within the sinus tracts. These infections may be caused by fungi and termed *eumycotic mycetoma* or *eumycetoma*, or by filamentous higher bacteria, termed *actinomycotic mycetoma* or *actinomycetoma*. The term *mycetoma* can also be found in the literature incorrectly referring to a fungus ball found in a pre-existing cavity in the lung or within a paranasal sinus, most often caused by *Aspergillus* spp. Grain formation by infecting organisms is restricted to the diseases mycetoma, actinomycosis (see Chapter 255), and botryomycosis. Actinomycosis is a disease produced by the anaerobic and microaerophilic higher bacteria that normally colonize the mouth and gastrointestinal and urogenital tracts. The portal of entry in actinomycosis is from those colonized sites, whereas in mycetoma the portal is the skin and subcutaneous tissue into which the organism was inoculated by minor trauma. Botryomycosis is a chronic bacterial infection of soft tissues in which the causative organism, often *Staphylococcus aureus*, is found in loose clusters among the pus. In a rare form of ringworm called *dermatophyte mycetoma*, there are also loosely compacted clusters of hyphae in subcutaneous pus. In contrast, mycetoma grains are dense clusters of organisms.

Etiologic Agents

The agents of mycetoma are fungi and aerobic filamentous bacteria that have been found on plants and in the soil.[1] The predominance of bacterial versus fungal causes of mycetoma varies amoung geographic location. Eumycotic (true fungal) disease is caused by a variety of fungal organisms. These can be divided into those that form dark grains and those that form pale or white grains (Table 262-1). Color distinctions are made by observing unstained specimens. Among the fungi causing dark-grained mycetoma, the most common are *Madurella mycetomatis, Leptosphaeria senegalensis,* and *Madurella grisea.* Other agents include *Corynespora cassicola, Curvularia geniculata, Curvularia lunata, Exophiala jeanselmei, Exophiala oligosperma, Leptosphaeria tompkinsii, Phialophora verrucosa, Plenodomas avramii, Pseudochaetosphaeronema larense, Rhinocladiella atrovirens, Pyrenochaeta mackinnonii,* and *Pyrenochaeta romeroi. Pseudallescheria boydii* (anamorph *Scedosporium apiospermum*) is the most common cause of pale-colored grains. Other fungi in that category include *Acremonium (Fusarium) falciforme, Acremonium kiliensis, Acremonium recifei, Aspergillus flavus, Aspergillus hollandicus, Aspergillus (Emericella) nidulans, Cylindrocarpon cyanescens, Cylindrocarpon destructans, Fusarium solani, Fusarium moniliforme (verticillioides), Neotestudina rosatii, Phaeoacremonium* species, and *Polycytella hominis.*[2-5] Actinomycetoma is caused by members of the order Actinomycetales, most commonly *Nocardia brasiliensis, Actinomadura madurae, Streptomyces somaliensis,* and *Actinomadura pelletieri.* Cases have been reported tha were caused by *Actinomadura latina, Nocardia asteroides, Nocardia caviae, Nocardia farcinica, Nocardia otitidiscaviarum, Nocardia mexicana, Nocardia*

transvalensis, Nocardia veterana, Nocardiopsis dassonvillei, and *Streptomyces sudanensis.*[2,6-8] Actinomycetoma grains are typically white or pale yellow, except those caused by *Actinomadura pelletieri,* which are red to pink.

Epidemiology

The oldest description of this disease appears to date back to the ancient Indian Sanskrit text *Atharva Veda,* in which reference is made to *pada valmikam,* translated to mean "anthill foot."[2] More modern descriptions from Madras, India, in the 19th century led to this disease initially being called "madura foot," or *maduromycosis,* a term still used by some today to describe eumycotic mycetoma. Mycetoma is most commonly found in tropical and subtropical climates, with the highest incidence being reported from endemic areas in the Indian subcontinent, the Middle East, Africa, and Central and South America. One of the largest current group of cases is in Sudan. Only scattered reports describe cases originating in the United States, Europe, and Japan. Disease occurs around five times more frequently in males, commonly in the 20- to 40-year-old age range. Disease is more common in agricultural workers and outdoor laborers, but is not exclusively seen in rural areas. Disease occurs sporadically throughout most areas of the world, and some postulate that the increased numbers in tropical regions may also be in part the result of decreased use of protective clothing, chiefly shoes, in the warmer, poorer endemic regions.

The causative agents of mycetoma vary from region to region and with climate. Worldwide, *M. mycetomatis* is the most common cause of this affliction, but *A. madurae, M. mycetomatis,* and *S. somaliensis* are more commonly reported from drier regions, whereas *P. boydii, Nocardia* species, and *A. pelletieri* are more common in those areas with higher annual rainfall. In India, *Nocardia* species and *M. grisea* are the most common causes of mycetoma; in the Middle East, *M. mycetomatis* and *S. somaliensis;* in West Africa, *L. senegalensis;* and in East Africa, *M. mycetomatis* and *S. somaliensis.* In Central and South America, *M. grisea* and *Nocardia* species are the common causes of mycetoma, and in the United States, *P. boydii* (*S. apiospermum*) is the most commonly recovered causative agent.[9]

Pathology and Pathogenesis

Infection follows inoculation of organisms, frequently through thorn punctures, wood splinters, or preexisting abrasions or trauma. After inoculation, these normally nonpathogenic organisms grow and survive through the production of grains (also called granules or sclerotia), structures composed of masses of mycelial fungi or bacterial filaments and a matrix component. The matrix material has been shown to be host-derived with some pathogens. In eumycetoma, hyphal elements often have thickened cell walls toward the periphery of grains, potentially conferring protection against the host immune system.[10] Grains are seen in histopathology within abscesses containing polymorphonuclear cells. Complement-dependent chemotaxis of polymorphonuclear leukocytes has been shown to be induced by both fungal (*M. mycetomatis* and *P. boydii*) and actinomycotic (*S. somaliensis*) antigens in vitro.[11] Cells of the innate immune system attempt to engulf and inactivate these organisms, but in disease ultimately fail to accomplish this goal. Abscesses containing grains are seen in association with granulomatous inflammation and fibrosis. Three types of

---

*The views expressed are those of the author and do not reflect the official policy or position of the Department of the Army, the Department of Defense, or the U.S. Government.

TABLE 262-1	Typical Morphologic Features of Mycetoma Grains	
Grain Color	*Causative Agent*
Eumycetoma (Eumycotic Mycetoma)*	
Black grains	*Madurella* spp., *Leptosphaeria* spp., *Curvularia* spp., *Exophiala* spp., *Phaeoacremonium* spp., *Phialophora verrucosa*, *Pyrenochaeta mackinnonii*, *P. romeroi*
Pale grains (white to yellow)	*Pseudallescheria boydii* (*Scedosporium apiospermum*), *Acremonium* spp., *Aspergillus* spp., *Fusarium* spp., *Neotestudina rosatii*
Actinomycetoma (Actinomycotic Mycetoma)†	
Pale grains (white to yellow)	*Actinomadurae madurae*, *Nocardia* spp.
Yellow to brown grains	*Streptomyces* spp.
Red to pink grains	*Actinomadurae pelletieri*

*2- to 5-μm diameter hyphae are observed within grain.
†0.5- to 1-μm diameter filaments are observed within grain.

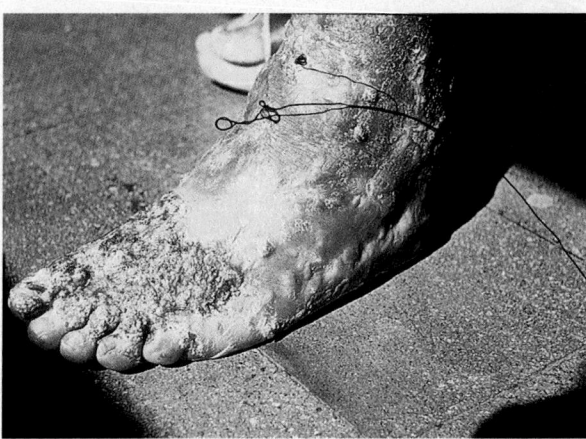

Figure 262-1 Mycetoma of the foot. (*From Beneke ES, Rogers AL. Medical Mycology and Human Mycoses. Belmont, Calif: Star Publishing; 1996.*)

immune responses have been described in response to the grains of mycetoma.[12] The type I response is seen as neutrophils degranulate and adhere to the grain surface, leading to gradual disintegration of the grain. Type II response is characterized by the disappearance of neutrophils and arrival of macrophages to clear grains and neutrophil debris. Type III response is marked by the formation of epithelioid granuloma. This host response does not appear to be able to control infection, but likely accounts for the partial spontaneous healing that is seen in the disease.

It is not clear whether persons who develop mycetoma have predisposing immune deficits. Disease does not appear to be more common in immunocompromised hosts, and early studies of immune function in persons with mycetoma have not clearly documented a common deficit.[13,14] Recent work examining genes responsible for innate immune functions has identified polymorphisms that appear to predispose people to this infection, which may be linked with neutrophil function.[15] It has been suggested that the greater frequency of disease in men is not completely explained by increased frequency of exposure to soil and plant material. Progesterone has been shown in vitro to inhibit the growth of *M. mycetomatis*, *P. romeroi*, and *N. brasiliensis*.[16,17] In the study of *N. brasiliensis*, estradiol limited disease produced in animals.[16]

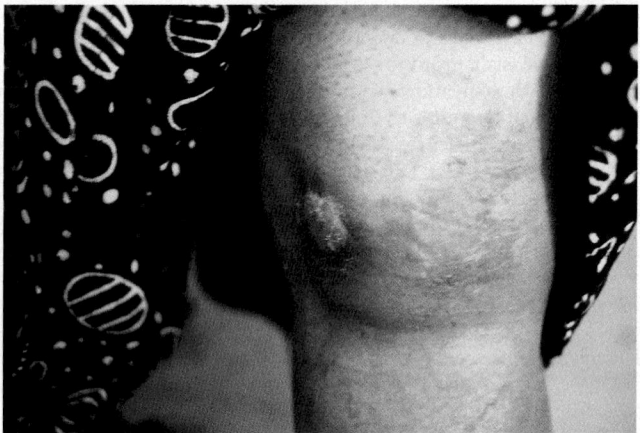

Figure 262-2 Mycetoma of the leg (seen from back of knee). (*Courtesy of Dr. Glenn W. Wortmann.*)

Clinical Manifestations

More than 75% of persons with mycetoma have a lesion of a lower extremity, most commonly in the foot (70%) (Figs. 262-1 and 262-2). Next in frequency is disease of the hand (15%), followed by the upper extremities and other areas of the body that may be exposed by carrying firewood or thorny brush, including the upper back and adjacent neck, top of the head, and, rarely, the face (Fig. 262-3). Lesions in more than one anatomic site are extraordinarily rare. Disease begins in most cases as a single, small, painless subcutaneous nodule. This nodule slowly increases in size, becomes fixed to the underlying tissue, and ultimately develops sinus tracts beneath the lesion. These tracts open to the surface and drain purulent material with grains. Grains are several millimeters in diameter and may be seen by close inspection of a gauze bandage covering the sinus tract. Progression to draining sinus tracts can take weeks, months, and even years, occurring more rapidly in actinomycetoma. In a study of patients in India, the average time to presentation with disease from history of probable inciting trauma was 3 years for *N. brasiliensis*, 7 years for *A. madurae*, and 9 years for *M. grisea*.[18]

Disease can affect the skin, subcutaneous tissue, and eventually contiguous bone, spreading along fascial planes. Overlying skin appears smooth and shiny, and is commonly fixed to the underlying tissue. Skin may be hypo- or hyperpigmented, with signs of both old healed and active sinuses, displaying the cycle of spontaneous healing of older sinuses tracts and simultaneous spread of infection to new areas typical

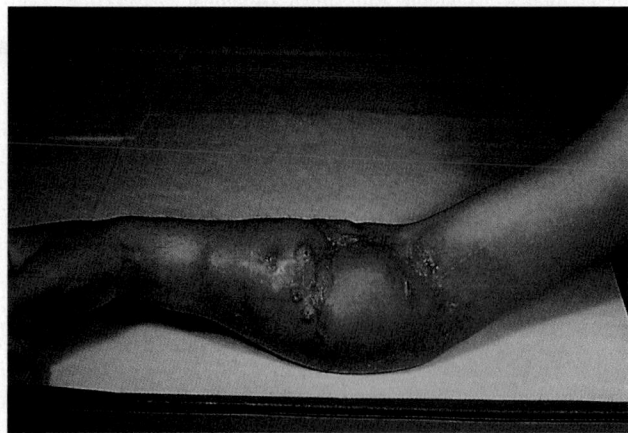

Figure 262-3 Mycetoma of the arm caused by *Madurella mycetomatis*. (*From Chandler FW, Ajello L. Mycetoma. In: Connor DH, Chandler FW, Schwartz DA, et al, eds. Pathology of Infectious Diseases. Norwalk, Conn: Appleton & Lange; 1997:1035-1044.*)

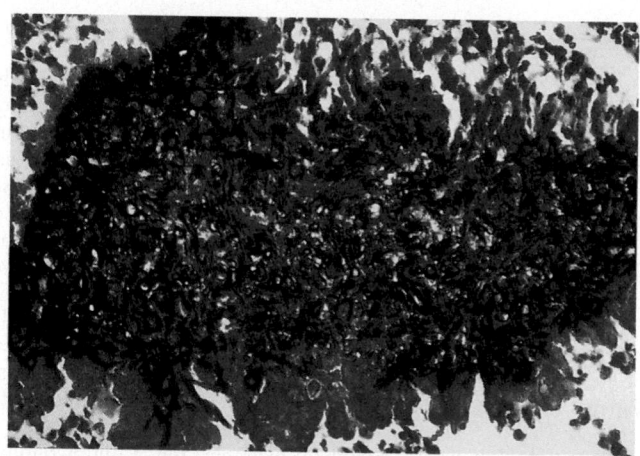

Figure 262-4 **Eumycetoma grain of *Acremonium falciforme*.** (Gomori methenamine-silver and hematoxylin and eosin stain.) *(From Chandler FW, Ajello L. Mycetoma. In: Connor DH, Chandler FW, Schwartz DA, et al, eds. Pathology of Infectious Diseases. Norwalk, Conn: Appleton & Lange; 1997:1035-1044.)*

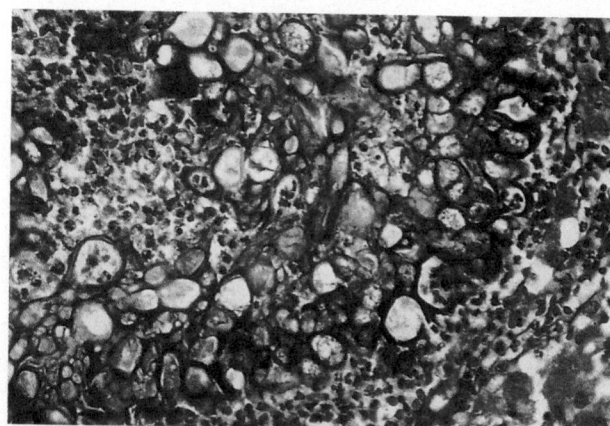

Figure 262-6 **Eumycetoma grain of *Curvularia geniculata*.** (Hematoxylin and eosin stain.) *(From Chandler FW, Ajello L. Mycetoma. In: Connor DH, Chandler FW, Schwartz DA, et al, eds. Pathology of Infectious Diseases. Norwalk, Conn: Appleton & Lange; 1997:1035-1044.)*

of this disease. Swelling is often firm and nontender, and the overlying skin is not erythematous. Muscle, tendons, and nerves are generally spared direct infection, but extensive local damage may lead to muscle wasting, bone destruction, and limb deformities. Lymphatic spread is rare, although it may follow surgical manipulation. Hematogenous spread has not been documented. This disease and its effects are generally localized, and thus no signs or symptoms of systemic illness are usually seen in mycetoma unless secondary bacterial infection occurs. When left untreated, disease continues to progress, and bacterial superinfection can lead to increased morbidity from local abscess formation, cellulitis, bacterial osteomyelitis, and, rarely, septic death.

Differential diagnosis includes botryomycosis, chronic bacterial osteomyelitis, tuberculous osteomyelitis, chromoblastomycosis, phaeohyphomycosis, and soft tissue or bone tumor.

Diagnosis

A diagnosis of mycetoma can be made by the classic triad of painless soft tissue swelling, draining sinus tracts, and extrusion of grains. Diagnosis of the causative organism can be made by microscopic

observation and culture of a grain. Deep biopsy with histopathology and culture is usually not necessary, although obtaining a deep tissue biopsy avoids the bacterial contamination of surface cultures. Grains may not be seen in any one histopathologic section because they are scattered along the tracts. When a grain is present in the section, its large size and surrounding cluster of neutrophils make it difficult to miss, even without fungal or bacterial stains (Figs. 262-4 to 262-9). Organisms are usually not seen outside the grain. An alternate strategy is the aspiration of grains directly from an unopened sinus tract for microscopic observation and culture. Evaluation of spontaneously extruded grains may not allow diagnosis, because these grains may be composed of dead organisms and are frequently associated with contaminating bacteria that grow more rapidly than the mycetomatous agent.

The grains (or granules or sclerotia) of mycetoma are usually 0.2 to 5 mm in diameter and thus may be observed grossly, without magnification. Microscopic evaluation of crushed grains prepared with potassium hydroxide or stained with Gram stain is useful in differentiating fungal from bacterial causes. On inspection, actinomycetes are recognized by the production of 0.5- to 1-μm-wide filaments and fungi

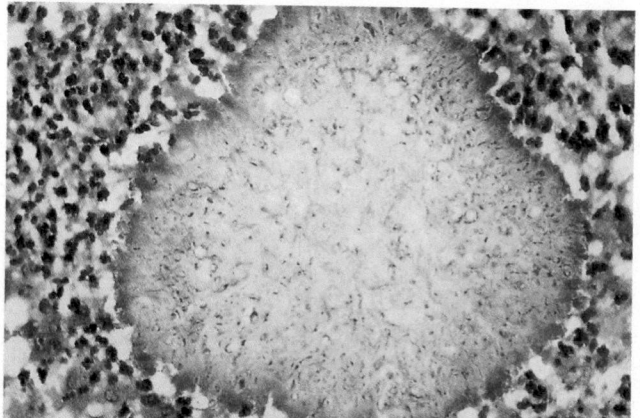

Figure 262-5 **Eumycetoma grain of *Pseudallescheria boydii*.** (Hematoxylin and eosin stain.) *(From Chandler FW, Ajello L. Mycetoma. In: Connor DH, Chandler FW, Schwartz DA, et al, eds. Pathology of Infectious Diseases. Norwalk, Conn: Appleton & Lange; 1997:1035-1044.)*

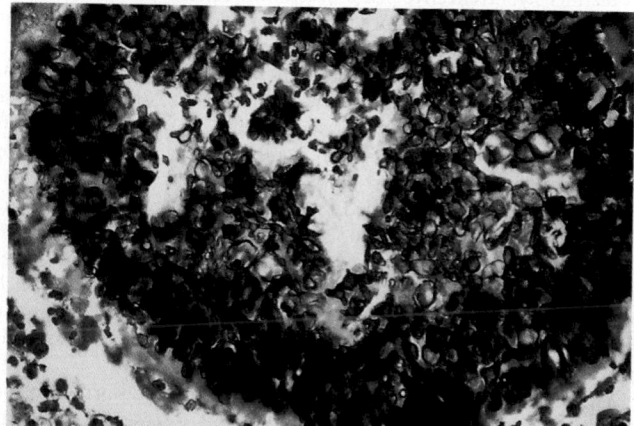

Figure 262-7 **Eumycetoma grain of *Neotestudina rosatii*.** (Gomori methenamine-silver and hematoxylin and eosin stain.) *(From Chandler FW, Ajello L. Mycetoma. In: Connor DH, Chandler FW, Schwartz DA, et al, eds. Pathology of Infectious Diseases. Norwalk, Conn: Appleton & Lange; 1997:1035-1044.)*

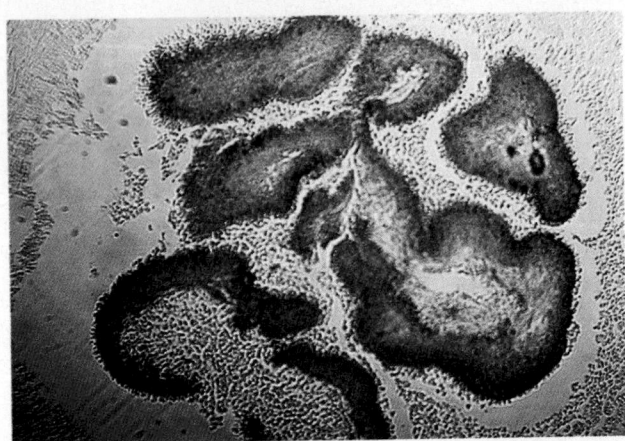

Figure 262-8 **Actinomycetoma grain** (Gridley stain.) (From Beneke ES, Rogers AL. Medical Mycology and Human Mycoses. Belmont, Calif: Star Publishing; 1996.)

by 2- to 5-µm-wide hyphae. Many reports and reviews have detailed the use of grain color, size, and consistency to diagnose the specific cause of mycetoma, but recovery of the causative agents in culture is more accurate and of greater clinical usefulness when resources are available.

Culture of grains recovered from aspirated material or biopsy specimens can be used to diagnose the specific cause of mycetoma. If extruded grains are used, most experts suggest rinsing these in 70% alcohol, or with antibiotic-containing saline solutions, to decrease bacterial contamination. Specimens should be cultured on mycologic and mycobacteriologic media and held for at least 4 weeks.

The role of radiology in the management of mycetoma is that of adjunctive assessment of disease extent, involvement of bone, and perhaps long-term follow-up of disease regression or progression. Radiographic studies can help define the extent of disease and aid in the differentiation of mycetoma from other disease. Standard radiographic studies can reveal bony involvement such as periosteal erosion secondary to invasion, osteoporosis, and changes consistent with osteomyelitis, including lytic lesions. Ultrasonography has been used successfully in the differentiation of mycetoma from osteomyelitis or tumor. In a study of 100 patients with foot swelling who underwent ultrasonography prior to surgical excision, these lesions were found to have distinct characteristics that distinguished them from other diseases.[19] Eumycetoma were found to produce single or multiple thick-walled cavities, without acoustic enhancement, with grains represented as distinct hyperreflective echoes. Actinomycetoma produced similar results except grains produced fine echoes that were found at the bottom of the cavities. Magnetic resonance imaging (MRI) and computed tomography (CT) have also been evaluated in the management of mycetoma. Both modalities provide accurate assessment of disease extent when compared with surgical findings, especially in the soft tissues.[20] When compared directly, CT appears to be more sensitive for detecting early changes consistent with bone involvement. A dot-in-circle sign has been described as a potentially specific diagnostic finding seen with MRI.[21] The dots are tiny hypointense foci (believed to be grains) within spherical, high-intensity lesions (the circle) surrounded by low-intensity matrix on T2-weighted imaging, which represent granulomas scattered in areas of fibrosis. T1-weighted, fat-saturated, postgadolinium images may also produce this appearance.

The use of serology has been advocated by some authorities in the diagnosis and long-term management of this disease. Of the tests described, counterimmunoelectrophoresis has been the most commonly used. Lack of standardization or widespread availability limit the use of these tests to centers that see a large volume of such patients. In the United States, the infrequency of the diagnosis and the diverse number of pathogens renders serology of no practical use.

Treatment

Treatment of this disease has proven to be difficult, and typically includes antimicrobial agents and surgery. Short of amputation, surgery alone is rarely successful in the treatment of mycetoma, but removal of smaller lesions or debulking of larger ones does play an important role, especially in the management of fungal disease. Because chemotherapy varies for actinomycetoma and eumycetoma, at a minimum the clinician must differentiate whether a mycetoma is caused by actinomycetes or fungi. Ideally, recovery of the causative organism can allow identification of species, and perhaps even susceptibility testing, to guide therapy. Treatment regimens are currently based on expert opinion as no randomized controlled trials have been performed. Duration of therapy is also not defined, and most patients receive 3 to 24 months of therapy to obtain an adequate response.

The most commonly described regimens for actinomycetoma include streptomycin plus either trimethoprim-sulfamethoxazole (TMP-SMX) or dapsone. In this regimen, streptomycin (14 mg/kg/day IM) is given for the first month (and sometimes three times weekly thereafter for several months) in addition to a long course of TMP-SMX, usually one double-strength tablet (160 mg trimethoprim and 800 mg sulfamethoxazole) twice daily, or dapsone (1.5 mg/kg/day twice daily). Alternate regimens include TMP-SMX plus dapsone[6] and amikacin plus TMP-SMX. The patient should be tested for glucose-6-phosphate dehydrogenase (G6PD) deficiency before dapsone use. Cycled dosing of amikacin (15 mg/kg/day, divided into two daily doses for 3 weeks) in addition to TMP-SMX for 5 weeks has also been described.[22] Most patients improved with only one or two cycles of this therapy. Gentamicin (80 mg IV) plus TMP-SMX (two double-strength tablets) given twice daily for 4 weeks followed by continuation of TMP-SMX plus doxycycline (100 mg twice daily) has more recently been reported.[23] Response to TMP-SMX alone has also been reported.[24] Other regimens that have been used include streptomycin with either sulfadoxine-pyrimethamine or rifampin, a combination of penicillin, gentamicin, and TMP-SMX followed by TMP-SMX and amoxicillin[25] and regimens that include amoxicillin-clavulanate,[26] fusidic acid, clindamycin, or imipenem-cilastatin.

Antifungal therapy of eumycetoma most commonly includes the use of azole antifungals, because amphotericin B has not been effective in producing long-term cures. Itraconazole (400 mg/day) or ketoconazole (200 to 400 mg/day) are considered first-line azole agents in the treatment of this disease. Early study using ketoconazole, 200 mg twice daily, noted marked improvement or cure in 72% of a group of 50 patients with mycetoma secondary to M. mycetomatis receiving 9 to 36 months of therapy.[6] Itraconazole at a dosage of 100 mg twice daily in

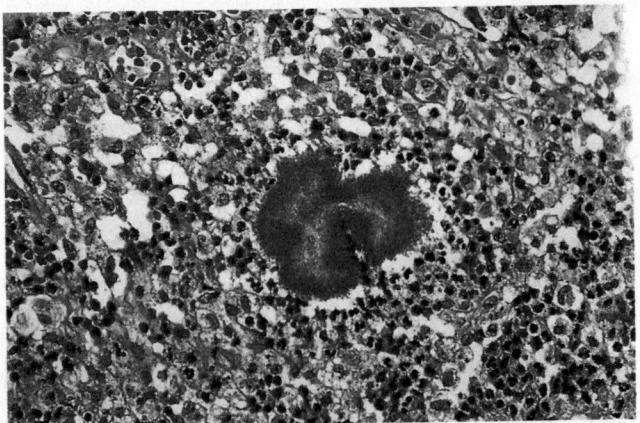

Figure 262-9 **Nocardia brasiliensis grain** (Hematoxylin and eosin stain.) (From Chandler FW, Ajello L. Mycetoma. In: Connor DH, Chandler FW, Schwartz DA, et al, eds. Pathology of Infectious Diseases. Norwalk, Conn: Appleton & Lange; 1997:1035-1044.)

the same population produced marked improvement in 42% of subjects, but no cures.[22] Multiple case reports and case series have reported mixed success with the use of itraconazole in a range of doses.[6,27,28] Fluconazole has proven to be even less effective for the treatment of mycetoma. *P. boydii* (*S. apiospermum*) is not responsive to ketoconazole therapy and is often resistant to itraconazole in vitro and in clinical therapy. In vitro, both of the newer azoles, posaconazole and voriconazole, have good activity against many of the causative agents of eumycetoma. Case reports of successful therapy with voriconazole have been published,[29-31] as has a small case series of successful therapy of previously azole refractory disease that responded to posaconazole.[32] Successful therapy with terbinafine, an allylamine antifungal, has also

been reported. Improvement or cure was seen in 16 of 20 patients who completed 24 to 48 weeks of terbinafine therapy (500 mg twice daily).[33]

Prevention

No preventive vaccine is available against any of the causative agents of mycetoma. Disease prevention is best accomplished by reduction of the incidence of the traumatic inoculation of the causative organisms. Wearing of shoes and clothing to protect against splinters and thorn pricks should be stressed. Debilitating disease can be prevented by early identification and treatment of lesions, usually with minor surgery and chemotherapy.

REFERENCES

1. Ahmed A, Adelmann D, Fahal A, et al. Environmental occurrence of *Madurella mycetomatis*, the major agent of human eumycetoma in Sudan. *J Clin Microbiol*. 2002;40:1031-1036.
2. Kwon-Chung KJ, Bennett JE. Mycetoma. In: *Medical Mycology*. Philadelphia: Lea & Febiger; 1992:560-593.
3. Smith MD, McGinnis MR. Subcutaneous fungal infections (chromoblastomycosis, mycetoma, and lobomycosis). In: Hospenthal DR, Rinaldi MG, eds. *Diagnosis and Treatment of Human Mycoses*. Totowa, NJ: Humana Press; 2008:383-392.
4. Desnos-Ollivier M, Bretagne S, Dromer F, et al. Molecular identification of black-grain mycetoma agents. *J Clin Microbiol*. 2006;44:3517-3523.
5. Hemashettar BM, Siddaramappa B, Munjunathaswamy BS, et al. *Phaeoacremonium krajdenii*, a cause of white grain eumycetoma. *J Clin Microbiol*. 2006;44:4619-4622.
6. Welsh O, Salinas MC, Rodriguez MA. Treatment of eumycetoma and actinomycetoma. *Curr Top Med Mycol*. 1995;6:47-71.
7. Quintana ET, Wierzbicka K, Mackiewicz P, et al. *Streptomyces sudanensis* sp. nov., a new pathogen isolated from patients with actinomycetoma. *Antonie van Leeuwenhoek*. 2008;93:305-313.
8. Rodriquez-Nava V, Couble A, Molinard C, et al. *Nocardia mexicana* sp. nov., a new pathogen isolated from human mycetomas. *J Clin Microbiol*. 2004;42:4530-4535.
9. Green WO, Adams TE. Mycetoma in the United States: A review and report of seven additional cases. *Am J Clin Pathol*. 1964;42:75-91.
10. Wethered DB, Markey MA, Hay RJ, et al. Ultrastructural and immunogenic changes in the formation of mycetoma grains. *J Med Vet Mycol*. 1986;25:39-46.
11. Yousif MA, Hay RJ. Leucocyte chemotaxis to mycetoma agents—the effect of the antifungal drugs griseofulvin and ketoconazole. *Trans R Soc Trop Med Hyg*. 1987;81:319-321.
12. Fahal AH, el Toum EA, el Hassan AM, et al. The host tissue reaction to Madurella mycetomatis: New classification. *J Med Vet Mycol*. 1995;33:15-17.
13. Bendl BJ, Mackey D, Al-Saati F, et al. Mycetoma in Saudi Arabia. *J Trop Med Hyg*. 1987;90:51-59.
14. Mahgoub ES, Gumaa SA, El Hassan AM. Immunological status of mycetoma patients. *Bull Soc Pathol Exot Filiales*. 1977; 70:48-54.
15. van de Sande WWJ, Fahal A, Verbrugh H, et al. Polymorphisms in genes involved in innate immunity predispose toward mycetoma susceptibility. *J Immunol*. 2007;179:3065-3074.
16. Hernández-Hernández F, López-Martínez R, Méndez-Tovar LJ, et al. *Nocardia brasiliensis*: In vitro and in vivo growth in response to steroid sex hormones. *Mycopathologia*. 1995;132:79-85.
17. Méndez-Tovar LJ, de Biève C, López-Martínez R. Effets des hormones sexuelles humaines sur le dévelopment in vitro des agents d'eumycétomes. *J Mycol Méd*. 1991;1:141-143.
18. Maiti PK, Ray A, Bandyopadhyay S. Epidemiological aspects of mycetoma from a retrospective study of 264 cases in West Bengal. *Trop Med Int Health*. 2002;7:788-792.
19. Fahal AH, Sheik HE, Homeida MM, et al. Ultrasonographic imaging of mycetoma. *Br J Surg*. 1997;84:1120-1122.
20. Sharif HS, Clark DC, Aabed MY, et al. Mycetoma: Comparison of MR imaging with CT. *Radiology*. 1991;178:865-870.
21. Sarris I, Berendt AR, Athanasous N, et al. MRI of mycetoma of the foot: Two cases demonstrating the dot-in-circle sign. *Skeletal Radiol*. 2003;32:179-183..
22. Hay RJ, Mahgoub ES, Leon G, et al. Mycetoma. *J Med Vet Mycol*. 1992;30(Suppl 1):41-49.
23. Raman M, Bhat R, Garg T, et al. A modified two-step treatment for actinomycetoma. *J Dermatol Venereol Leprol*. 2007; 73:235-239.
24. Khatri ML, Al-Halali HM, Fouad Khalid M, et al. Mycetoma in Yemen: Clinicoepidemiologic and histopathologic study. *Int J Dermatol*. 2002;41:586-593.
25. Ramam M, Garg T, D'Souza P, et al. A two-step schedule for the treatment of actinomycotic mycetomas. *Acta Derm Venereol*. 2000;80:378-380.
26. Wortman PD. Treatment of a *Nocardia brasiliensis* mycetoma with sulfamethoxazole and trimethoprim, amikacin, and amoxicillin and clavulanate. *Arch Dermatol*. 1993;129:564-567.
27. Resnik BI, Burdick AE. Improvement of eumycetoma with itraconazole. *J Am Acad Dermatol*. 1995;33:917-919.
28. Smith EL, Kutbi S. Improvement of eumycetoma with itraconazole. *J Am Acad Dermatol*. 1997;36:279-280.
29. Lacroix C, de Kerviler E, Morel P, et al. *Madurella mycetomatis* mycetoma treated successfully with oral voriconazole. *Br J Dermatol*. 2005;152:1062-1094.
30. Loulergue P, Hot A, Dannaoui E, et al. Short report. Successful treatment of black-grain mycetoma with voriconazole. *Am J Trop Med Hyg*. 2006;75:1106-1107.
31. Porte L, Khatibi S, El Hajj L, et al. *Scedosporium apiospermum* mycetoma with bone involvement successfully treated with voriconazole. *Trans R Soc Trop Med Hyg*. 2006;100:891-894.
32. Negroni R, Tobon A, Bustamante B, et al. Posaconazole treatment of refractory eumycetoma and chromoblastomycosis. *Rev Inst Med Trop S Paulo*. 2005;47:339-346.
33. N'Diaye B, Dieng MT, Perez A, et al. Clinical efficacy and safety of oral terbinafine in fungal mycetoma. *Int J Dermatol*. 2006;45:154-157.

263

Cryptococcus neoformans

JOHN R. PERFECT

Cryptococcus neoformans is an encapsulated heterobasidiomycetous fungus that has progressed from being a rare human pathogen, with just over 300 cases of cryptococcosis reported in the literature before 1955, to being a common worldwide opportunistic pathogen, as immunocompromised human populations have dramatically increased over the past 2 decades. Cryptococcosis crosses the entire spectrum of patient populations, from the apparently immunocompetent host without an underlying disease to those severely immunocompromised from infection with the human immunodeficiency virus (HIV), an organ transplantation, or a malignancy.[1] Furthermore, it has a wide range of clinical presentations, which can vary from asymptomatic colonization of the respiratory airways to dissemination of infection into any part of the human body. *C. neoformans* enters the host primarily through the lungs but has a special predilection for invading the central nervous system (CNS) of the susceptible host. Pulmonary infections are common and may have multiple clinical presentations and management issues. On the other hand, cryptococcal meningoencephalitis represents the primary life-threatening infection for this fungal pathogen and has required the most clinical attention.

History

The first identification of *Cryptococcus* from an environmental source was made by Sanfelice in 1894, from peach juice in Italy.[2] Within a year, Busse and Buschke[3] independently reported the first human case of cryptococcosis in a young woman who developed a chronic ulcer over the skin above her tibia, with yeasts identified in the tissue and later at autopsy; this yeast was also found to have spread to multiple organs in her body. By 1914, Versé described a human case of cryptococcal meningitis, and in 1916 Stoddard and Cutler gave a complete description of the CNS pathology for this infection, including in their report that the yeast forms had surrounding areas of clearing within the tissue.[4,5] This finding was the first description of the signature structure for this yeast, the polysaccharide capsule. During the early years of clinical cryptococcosis, there were several names, including *Saccharomyces neoformans*, *Cryptococcus hominis*, and *Torula histolytica*. In 1935, Benham attempted to categorize these poorly defined yeasts based on morphology, fermentation, and serologic studies.[6] She named one yeast *C. hominis* and its disease, cryptococcosis. The name was later changed to *C. neoformans* based on temporal priority, because Sanfelice had first used the species name of *neoformans*. However, despite Benham's proposal, it took another 25 years before cryptococcosis became the primary nomenclature for this infection rather than torulosis. In 1976, Kwon-Chung discovered and characterized the sexual stage of *Cryptococcus* and the teleomorphs were named *Filobasidiella neoformans* and *Filobasidiella bacillospora*.[7] It was proposed in 2002 that there be two varieties (*Cryptococcus neoformans* var. *neoformans* [serotype D] and *Cryptococcus neoformans* var. *grubii* [serotype A] and another species, *Cryptococcus gattii* [serotypes B and C]).[8] In 2005, the genome sequence of *C. neoformans* was released and several more strains have been sequenced for comparisons as we enter the genome age for fungal pathogens.[9]

Mycology

LIFE CYCLE AND GENETICS

The life cycle of *C. neoformans* involves two distinct forms, asexual and sexual. The asexual stage exists as encapsulated yeast cells that reproduce by simple, narrow-based budding. The haploid (occasionally diploid in nature), unicellular yeasts are the primary forms recovered from environmental sources and human infections. The asexual forms represent the primary structures seen in tissue and recovered from cultures during clinical disease. However, this fungus has a more complex life cycle, with a bipolar mating system that can be observed under certain in vitro conditions and even on plants.[10] For example, yeasts exist in one of two mating types, "alpha" or "a." When two strains of opposite mating types are physically placed together on specific, nutrient-poor media such as V8 juice agar, the cells undergo conjugation, producing filaments with true clamp connections. Basidia form at the ends of these filaments and within these basidia, meiosis occurs and chains of basidiospores are produced. The 1- to 2-μ basidiospores, with their size and shape, have been hypothesized to be the infectious propagules. They may deposit in the lung, where the spores rapidly convert to the yeast form. However, the sexual stage at present remains a laboratory observation, and the sexual structures such as basidiospores have yet to be identified in nature, but recombination does appear to be occurring in nature. Studies continue to make progress in understanding the molecular signaling networks that control the sexual cycle, and in some cases genes in these mating pathways have been linked to both morphogenesis and virulence of the yeast.[11]

In the 1980s, an interesting epidemiologic observation was made and confirmed by others that more than 95% of environmental and clinical *C. neoformans* isolates appear to contain only the alpha mating locus.[12] The reason for this genetic bias remains unclear, but two factors may be important. First, it has been discovered that under certain environmental conditions, *C. neoformans* undergoes haploid fruiting.[13] Haploid fruiting occurs when haploid yeast strains under specific conditions produce hyphae and basidiospores without mating and exchange of genetic information through meiosis. It is possible that this fruiting with sporulation allows wider dissemination of the fungus in the environment and thus more exposure, leading to clinical disease. Second, it has now been shown that sexual reproduction can occur between partners with the same mating type,[14] which allows recombination and improved fitness of progeny. The alpha mating–type strains are much more likely to produce haploid fruiting structures or perform same sex matings. An alternative explanation for the alpha mating locus bias is that the approximately 100-kb locus or its adjacent genomic areas contain virulence genes that make the strains more fit in the environment (or in the host). Initial studies with congenic strains of *C. neoformans* var. *neoformans* differing primarily in mating-type locus did suggest that the alpha mating strain was more virulent in mice.[15] On the other hand, the alpha and "a" mating-type loci have been identified in *C. neoformans* var. *grubii*, and experiments with two congenic strains in this variety differing only in the mating locus appear to be identical in virulence.[16] It is still uncertain how much the mating loci contribute to the virulence of this yeast, and the alpha mating–type bias is not yet precisely explained. Clearly, however, as witnessed in the Vancouver Island *C. gattii* outbreak, recombination in nature between strains can play an important part in the evolution of pathologic fitness for strains.[17]

TAXONOMY

The genus *Cryptococcus* comprises 19 species, loosely characterized as a variety of encapsulated yeasts. There continue to be occasional reports of human infections with several of these non-*neoformans* species, such as *Cryptococcus albidus* and *Cryptococcus laurentii*.[18,19]

However, such clinical reports are uncommon, and the infection is occasionally poorly documented. Therefore, any human infection with a cryptococcal species other than *C. neoformans* or *C. gattii* needs rigorous histopathology and cultural proof of infection.

For several decades, *C. neoformans* strains had been grouped into two varieties that included five serotypes based on capsule structure. *C. neoformans* var. *neoformans* and *C. neoformans* var. *grubii* included strains with serotypes D, A, and AD, and *C. gattii* contained strains with serotypes B and C. The serotype classification (A to D) describes antigenic differences in the structure of the polysaccharide capsule; these differences can be detected by antibodies from rabbit sera[20] or by specific monoclonal antibodies.[21,22]

The stable taxonomic classification of these varieties and serotypes has been updated through new genomic analyses, and several changes have been proposed. With the use of specific DNA typing methods and other physiologic factors, it has been proposed that the serotype A strains be classified into a separate variety, *C. neoformans* var. *grubii*.[23] Serotype D isolates are to remain as *C. neoformans* var. *neoformans*. The varietal status of serotype AD strains has not been proposed. It has also become clear that many of the serotype AD strains represent stable diploid strains, possibly occurring as incomplete genetic crosses between varieties *C. neoformans* and *C. grubii*. However, genetic mapping of A and D strains suggests that these varieties biologically diverged from each other more than 18 million years ago.[24] Thus, there are proposals to abolish the varietal system and replace it with three separate species that contain a grouping of several genotypes in each species. A strong argument has been proposed to change *C. neoformans* var. *gattii* (serotypes B and C) to a separate species named *Cryptococcus gattii*, and that convention will be followed here. As rapid advances in the understanding of genetic diversity are made among these fungi in the genome era, taxonomic relationships and nomenclature will remain in some flux. However, at present, for clinicians the standard serotype classification used for a half-century and the split into two varieties, *C. neoformans* and *C. gattii*, still remain useful nomenclature for describing the clinical strain differences in epidemiology, pathogenesis, and clinical features. In this chapter, the term "var. *grubii*" will be appended to the designation of serotype A because most isolates continue to be identified by serotype, not by genotype.

The anamorph (yeast or asexual stage) dominates clinical discussion of this encapsulated yeast. On the other hand, the teleomorph, with its more complex structure and genome sequences, place this fungus in the basidiomycete family, and its teleomorph genus name is *Filobasidiella*. Thus, the teleomorph of serotypes A and D strains is called *Filobasidiella neoformans*; the teleomorph of serotype B and C strains is designated *Filobasidiella bacillospora*.

Epidemiologic and clinical studies have frequently used a colored growth medium (see later) to distinguish serotype A, D, and AD isolates, from serotype B and C isolates. When referring to the results of such studies, the term "var. *neoformans*" should be understood to include what some authorities also call var. *grubii*.

IDENTIFICATION

On most routine laboratory agar media, colonies of *C. neoformans* appear within 48 to 72 hours after plating a specimen. Some selective media containing cycloheximide inhibit the growth of this yeast and thus should not be used. For blood cultures, the lysis-centrifugation method works very well for isolating *Cryptococcus*, but is no longer necessary because automated blood culture methods have been improved, and cryptococcemia is commonly detected in severely immunosuppressed patients.[25] In some populations of the world with high rates of HIV infection, cryptococcemia has become a common finding in patients during the workup of fever with blood cultures. However, it rarely produces symptoms of hypotension or shock during cryptococcemia.

On agar plates, the yeast colony grows as a white to cream–colored opaque colony several millimeters in diameter. The colonies typically become mucoid with prolonged incubation, reflecting polysaccharide

capsule formation. Colonies occasionally develop sectors that differ in pigmentation or exhibit morphologic changes (e.g., smooth or wrinkled). *C. neoformans* has been shown to possess the ability to produce a morphologic switching phenotype, which explains this variety of colony shapes in some strains.[26,27] The optimal environmental growth temperature for most *C. neoformans* strains is between 30° and 35°C, with a maximum tolerated temperature for most strains at 40°C. Serotype A strains tend to tolerate higher temperatures better than serotype D and serotype B/C strains.[28] *C. neoformans* and *C. gattii* strains generally grow well at 37°C, with generation times of 3 to 6 hours; this is a primary virulence phenotype that separates them from other cryptococcal species that generally do not tolerate mammalian body temperatures and are rarely human pathogens.

In the clinical laboratory, *C. neoformans* can be readily differentiated from other yeasts on the basis of its morphology and biochemical tests. The specific identification can be confirmed by a battery of biochemical tests available commercially in kits.[29,30] However, there are three direct tests that predict that a yeast may be *C. neoformans*. First, placing the yeast into an India ink preparation may reveal encapsulation of the yeast. The capsule is generally better seen in direct clinical specimens from the host and may not be as apparent in wet mounts made from in vitro cultures. This finding occurs because capsule production is induced by certain environmental cues, such as elevated carbon dioxide concentrations, serum, or limited iron conditions. The host environment provides an ideal condition for capsule production.

Second, a rapid urease test is positive in most *Cryptococcus* species. *Cryptococcus* spp., unlike *Candida* spp., possess urease, an enzyme that hydrolyzes urea to ammonia and increases the ambient pH. A positive urease test can be detected within minutes.[31] Several nonpathogenic yeasts produce abundant urease and *Trichosporon* species may be weakly urease positive.

Third, *C. neoformans* is one of the few yeast species that possess prominent laccase activity,[32] an enzyme that allows the conversion of diphenolic compounds into melanin. Detection of this unique biologic characteristic is possible with media containing niger seed (birdseed), caffeic acid, or dopamine. Yeast colonies that turn brown to black on these special agars are identified as melanin-positive. In a clinical specimen, such a yeast colony might well be *C. neoformans*. Other cryptococcal species also possess laccase. However, these selective agar assays are particularly helpful when attempting to identify pigmented cryptococcal colonies from environmental samples contaminated by other fungi and bacteria.

Histopathologically, *C. neoformans* has several characteristic features. In most clinical cases, *C. neoformans* in tissue exhibits a prominent capsule. Microscopically, most clinical isolates appear as spherical, narrow-based, budding, encapsulated yeast cells in both tissue and culture. Short hyphal or pseudohyphal structures may exist in vivo or under certain stress conditions in vitro, but these structures are rarely observed unless certain in vitro nutrient conditions for mating or haploid fruiting are met. The yeast cells vary in size from 5 to 10 μ in diameter, and exhibit single or multiple buds. Because the buds are readily detached from their parental cells, most yeast cells in tissue and culture lack buds. Finally, the size of the capsule under direct observation varies with the individual strain and its immediate environment.

There are three methods for identifying the four serotypes. First, antibodies had been commercially available to distinguish differences in the capsular structures, although at present there is no commercial source. Second, there are known differences between the biochemistry pathways of the serotypes. Most serotype B and C isolates assimilate glycine as a sole carbon source, whereas serotype A and D isolates generally do not. An agar containing L-canavanine, glycine, and bromothymol blue (CGB) uses a color change to separate serotypes A and D from B and C. Third, analysis of DNA base composition is extremely accurate. Comparison of sequenced genomes of these serotypes shows an approximately 6% to 8% overall difference in nucleotides between serotype A and D strains and an even greater difference between these strains and serotype B and C strains. It is clear from a variety of molecular methods, including random amplified polymorphic DNA (RAPD), karyotypes, polymerase chain reaction (PCR) fingerprinting, multilocus sequencing typing (MLST), and direct sequencing of strains, can be used to identify an isolate readily as belonging to a certain serotype or clade. Furthermore, strains can even be classified into certain genotypes by PCR fingerprint patterns. There are presently eight distinct genotypes for *C. neoformans*—VN1 to VN4 for serotype A, and VG1 to VG4 for serotypes B and C—and within these eight genotypes there are subgroup genotypes identified by MLST that possess epidemiologic relevance.[33] Serotype D isolates have proven difficult to cluster into distinct genotypes.

Ecology

C. neoformans is a saprobe in nature.[34] It was first described in fruits, but after years of investigation it is clear that it has an environmental niche or habitat associated with certain trees and rotting wood. A second consistent finding is that *C. neoformans* has frequently been isolated from soil contaminated by guano from birds.[35,36]

C. NEOFORMANS SEROTYPES A, D, AND AD (VAR. NEOFORMANS AND VAR. GRUBII)

In the 1950s, Emmons first isolated *C. neoformans* from soil and from the droppings and nests of pigeons.[35,36] Since the original reports, the fungus has been found in soil samples from around the world. However, the soils most enriched in *C. neoformans* are those that are frequented by birds, especially pigeons, turkeys, and chickens. Guano from other birds, such as canaries and parrots, has also yielded the yeast. Despite this consistent ecologic observation, the precise link between the yeast's natural habitat and birds has still not been definitively ascertained. Occasionally, birds develop disease that involves *C. neoformans*, but this is relatively unusual. The resistance of birds to disease may result from their very high body temperature, which is not conducive to growth of *C. neoformans*. However, the yeast may transiently colonize the gastrointestinal tract of the birds. The most likely environmental niche for these serotypes remains rotting vegetation or wood of certain trees. The birds may simply represent vectors, spreading the fungus from vegetations into the soils and dusts of human traffic.

C. GATTII SEROTYPES B AND C (VAR. GATTII)

Unlike *C. neoformans*, *C. gattii* has never been cultured from bird guano. Furthermore, there appears to be a certain geographic limitation to the occurrence of infections with this variety. With this knowledge base, investigators were able to culture *C. gattii* from vegetation around and associated with the river red gum trees (*Eucalyptus camaldulensis*) and forest red gum trees (*Eucalyptus tereticornis*) in Australia.[37] Because these trees were exported to other areas of the world where *C. gattii* is also observed, it was reasoned that *Eucalyptus* species might be a vector for infection. It was suggested that the yeasts or basidiospores might be released in relationship to the flowering of these trees, but this has not been proven. However, despite the association of these trees with *C. gattii*, an ongoing outbreak of cryptococcosis on Vancouver Island, British Columbia, has suggested that other trees such as firs, maples, and oaks may also be an ecologic niche for specific strains of *C. gattii*.[38]

Another ecologic factor that may be important to the human pathogenicity of this fungus is its association with other organisms. For example, it has been found in soil associated with a variety of bacteria, amebas, mites, worms, and sow bugs. The stress of this biotic area, with its abundant predatory scavengers, may have selected for a yeast species that can survive such harsh conditions. In fact, work has shown that *C. neoformans* can survive in amebas, which in some respects may provide an environment similar to that in a human macrophage.[39] Furthermore, nonpathogenic cryptococci can act as food for the nematode *Caenorhabditis elegans*, but *C. neoformans* can actually kill the

worm and several invertebrate models (worms, grubs and ameba) have been used in pathogenesis and treatment experiments.[40,41].

Epidemiology

C. neoformans is not generally considered to be a routine constituent of the human microbial biota. Although there are clinical reports of its being isolated from nonsterile sites on patients with no signs or symptoms of cryptococcosis,[42] and although it can be detected as a commensal in dogs, endobronchial colonization is more frequently observed in humans with underlying chronic pulmonary disease. When *C. neoformans* is isolated from nonsterile clinical specimens, the clinician must examine the patient for evidence of disease or analyze risk factors for the development of disease before planning further management strategies. Several methods have been used to study the existence of prior infection with *C. neoformans* without evidence for disease. Research has shown that patients with cryptococcosis have delayed hypersensitivity to cryptococcal antigens,[43] and the prevalence of positive skin test reactions in pigeon fanciers and laboratory workers engaged in research activities with this yeast have been reported to be high.[44] Unfortunately, there is no established skin test for routine clinical use in patients with cryptococcosis, and this reduces the ability to assess the magnitude of infection. However, most adults possess antibody to *C. neoformans* antigens; in New York City, most children acquire antibodies to cryptococcal antigens before the age of 10 years.[45,46] These observations suggest that there are frequent asymptomatic infections. Recent studies examining serologic evidence of cryptococcal exposure in children have emphasized that in some respects there are certain areas of high exposure and other geographical sites of much lower exposure.[47] Although exposure to this yeast is limited in certain areas of the world, infections have been reported on all continents.

The vast majority of patients with symptomatic disseminated cryptococcosis have an identified underlying immunocompromised condition (Table 263-1). The most common underlying conditions worldwide include the acquired immunodeficiency syndrome (AIDS), prolonged treatment with corticosteroids, organ transplantation, advanced malignancy, diabetes, and sarcoidosis. Cryptococcosis may identify an underlying idiopathic CD4 lymphocytopenia[48] or may be associated with the use of immune-modifying monoclonal antibodies such as alemtuzumab, infliximab, etanercept, or adalimumab.[49,50] Finally, it has been estimated that approximately 20% of patients who have cryptococcosis without HIV infection have no apparent underlying disease or risk factor.[51]

The best estimates for rates of cryptococcosis in the United States in the pre-AIDS era predicted an overall incidence of 0.8 case/million persons/year. In 1992, during the peak of the AIDS epidemic in the United States, the rate reached almost five cases of cryptococco-

TABLE 263-1	Conditions Known or Possibly Associated with Predisposition to *Cryptococcus neoformans* Infections
HIV infection	Systemic lupus erythematosus*
Lymphoproliferative disorders	HIV-negative CD4+ T-cell lymphocytopenia
Sarcoidosis	Diabetes mellitus†
Corticosteroid therapy	Organ transplantation*
Hyper-IgM syndrome	Peritoneal dialysis
Hyper-IgE syndrome	Cirrhosis
Monoclonal antibodies (e.g., infliximab intercept, adalimumab, alemtuzumab)	

*Immunosuppressive therapy may account for the predisposition.
†Diabetes mellitus has historically been considered a risk factor for cryptococcal infection. However, diabetes is a common disease, and it is unclear whether this condition is truly a specific risk factor for cryptococcosis.
From Casadevall A, Perfect JR. *Cryptococcus neoformans*. Washington DC: ASM Press; 1998:410.

sis/100,000 persons/year in several large cities. In the mid-1990s, before highly active antiretroviral therapy (HAART) but with widespread use of fluconazole for oral candidiasis, the rate was reduced, and it stabilized in the cities at approximately one case/100,000/ year.[52,53] With the widespread use of HAART in developed countries by the beginning of the 21st century, the incidence of cryptococcosis has declined and appears to have reached a stable number of new infections.[54] In the AIDS population in developed countries, it now represents an infection that identifies a disadvantaged patient or an untreated and undiagnosed HIV infection. Thus, cryptococcosis in patients with AIDS identifies this group as having less access to medical care.[55]

In less well-developed countries with major epidemics of HIV, such as sub-Saharan Africa, cryptococcosis appears to reach very high prevalences. Although the data are not precise, some reports have indicated that 15% to 45% of those with advanced HIV infection succumb to cryptococcosis.[56,57] In a more recent population-based surveillance study for cryptococcosis in an antiretroviral-naïve South Africa population, the overall incidence rate in HIV-infected patients was 95 cases/100,000 and those with AIDS had a rate of 14 cases/1000.[58] In many African medical centers, cryptococcosis represents the most common cause of culture-proven meningitis, even surpassing *Neisseria meningitidis* and *Streptococcus pneumoniae* meningitis.[59] In fact, the risk of cryptococcosis appears higher for African-born individuals even when they move to industrialized nations.[60] Increasing cases of cryptococcosis have consistently followed the pattern of HIV infections and, in countries such as Thailand, blood cultures containing this yeast have become common, but with the availability of HAART, this may change.[61]

The varieties of *C. neoformans* identified as causing disease differ by geographic location and by whether the patient has a concomitant HIV infection. Prior to the AIDS epidemic, Kwon-Chung and Bennett found that at least 80% of clinical isolates worldwide were *C. neoformans* serotype A (var. *grubii*).[62] *C. neoformans* serotype B was almost exclusively found in tropical and subtropical areas, such as southern California, Hawaii, Brazil, Australia, Southeast Asia, and central Africa. Serotype C was rare in all localities but seemed to follow the same geographic distribution as serotype B. *C. neoformans* serotype D (var. *neoformans*) was predominantly isolated from Europe, especially Denmark, Germany, Italy, France, and Switzerland, and some strains of this variety were found in the United States.[62-64] In AIDS patients, the vast majority of isolates are serotype A (var. *grubii*), although serotype D has constituted a significant percentage of isolates in several areas of France. A small measurable portion of cases with AIDS have been reported to be caused by *C. gattii*. The numbers of *C. gattii* infections were very small, even in areas where this variety was commonly observed to cause disease in the pre-AIDS era, but clinical presentations and outcomes were similar to *C. neoformans* infections in this risk group.[65]

Cryptococcosis has a measurable rate of infection in two other major risk groups, cancer patients and recipients of solid organ transplants. Since the 1950s, it has been known that patients with lymphoproliferative disorders and certain hematologic malignancies, such as chronic lymphocytic leukemia, were at higher risk than the general population for cryptococcosis.[65-69] A retrospective analysis of case reports from a single large cancer center from 1989 to 1999 reported that the incidence of cryptococcosis was 18 cases/100,000 admissions, and the incidence may increase with further use of cell-mediated immune inhibitors such as alemtuzumab and fludarabine for the management of certain malignancies.[70] Because of their profound and prolonged immunosuppression, organ transplant recipients also became a target for this infection. In one study, cryptococcosis occurred in 2.8% of all solid organ transplant recipients.[71] Kidney and liver transplant recipients appeared to have the highest risk for cryptococcosis.[72,73] However, in bone marrow transplant recipients, who have a very high incidence of fungal infections, cryptococcosis is not common. In rare circumstances, the transplanted organ (e.g., cornea, kidney,

lung) has been shown to carry the cryptococcal infection into a susceptible recipient.[73-75]

Sarcoidosis, with or without corticosteroid therapy, predisposes to cryptococcosis. The lung, skin, bone, and central nervous system lesions of the two diseases overlap clinically and by histopathology. Despite uncertain pathophysiology, diabetes as an underlying disease is frequently mentioned in those without HIV or transplant recipient risk factors.

Before the AIDS epidemic, there was a small but consistently higher rate of cryptococcosis in males than in females. Cryptococcosis can occur before puberty, but even in children with several known risk factors, the incidence is uncommon. Interestingly, there have been several reports of cryptococcosis in children with a hyper-IgM syndrome.[76,77] In adults, idiopathic CD4$^+$ T-cell lymphocytopenia may be identified by the development of disseminated cryptococcosis and, paradoxically, this underlying condition with cryptococcosis actually may have a good prognosis for treatment outcome.[48,78] With much less precision, it has been suggested that smoking and outdoor activities may increase the risk of cryptococcosis.[52,79]

There is general agreement that most cryptococcal infections are acquired primarily by inhalation of infectious propagules, and there are occasional cases of direct traumatic inoculation through contaminated environmental projectiles or laboratory or clinical accidents, such as needlesticks.[80,81] However, neither the environmental source of infection nor the infectious form of *C. neoformans* has been precisely established in most cases of cryptococcosis. It is hypothesized that either dehydrated, poorly encapsulated yeast cells or basidiospores (<5 μ) are needed as infectious propagules for alveolar deposition in the lungs. Studies at sites with contaminated soils or trees have found that the air contains the correct size of propagule for airway infection.[82-84] Molecular typing methods have confirmed that clinical isolates can be indistinguishable from environmental isolates.[85-87] Although associations between infection and environmental exposure have been reported for many of the classic dimorphic fungi, this association is rare for *C. neoformans*. However, the outbreak of *C. gattii* infections on Vancouver Island and in the Pacific Northwest has linked humans and animals molecularly to common environmental exposures.[38] There has been no consistent seasonal association for the occurrence of cryptococcosis. Although one study did observe more cases in the fall and winter,[88] another study found no seasonal association. These confusing observations likely reflect the host reactivation pathophysiology of this disease in many cases.

Human-to-human transmission of cryptococcosis has not been reported, except in cases of contaminated transplant tissue.[73-75] Many species of animals, including dogs and cats, can develop cryptococcosis,[89-91] but there is little evidence of zoonotic transmission between them and humans. However, in one case, *C. neoformans* isolated from the cage of a pet cockatoo was molecularly linked with the strain that caused infection in a transplant recipient who was exposed to the cage.[92] Also, several cryptococcal cases have been linked to intense bird exposures.[93]

Pathogenicity

The encapsulated yeast *C. neoformans* has been studied extensively for more than 50 years. In the past decade, genetic and molecular biologic research, in concert with well-established and robust animal models, has rapidly increased our understanding of its pathobiology. Progress in cryptococcal molecular biology has led to the use of karyotypes, repetitive elements, transposons and sequencing to identify yeast strains through a variety of analytic techniques, including restriction fragment length polymorphism (RFLP), RAPD, PCR fingerprints, and MLST. Recently, the entire genomes of several strains of *C. neoformans* and *C. gattii* have been sequenced. Several transformation systems are available for introducing DNA into this yeast, and site-specific gene disruptions and replacements are now routine. Dozens of specific null mutants in a variety of pathways or for specific enzymes have been made to examine their impact on the virulence composite of the yeast in robust animal models.[94] Furthermore, differential display PCR, cDNA subtraction techniques, serial analysis of gene expression (SAGE), and microarray analysis have been used to document and understand *C. neoformans* transcription profiles.[39,95,96] Proteomic and metabolomic approaches can also be used to study pathophysiology.

All these molecular tools have been used to determine the components and mechanisms that make this yeast such an efficient and deadly pathogen. The following sections describe its most prominent virulence phenotypes.

CAPSULE

The most distinctive feature of *C. neoformans* is a polysaccharide capsule containing an unbranched chain of α-1,3-linked mannose units substituted with xylosyl and β-glucuronyl groups. The serotype specificity appears to be determined by structural differences in the glucuronoxylomannan (GXM) related to the number of xylose residues and the degree of *O*-acetylation of hydroxyl groups. The capsular polysaccharide has a high negative cell surface charge and is attached to the cell wall by α-1,3-glucan residues. However, it is easily released into the immediate growth media or tissue. Capsular thickness, which varies among isolates, is regulated by several environmental cues, including both ambient P_{CO_2}, serum, and low iron concentrations, which increase capsular size in many strains. These environmental signals appear to augment the yeast's ability to produce disease and may help explain why the capsule may be small in in vitro cultures but is much larger when observed in the host. Mutant cryptococci that are made to be hypocapsular or acapsular are dramatically less virulent than the parental strains in animal models.[97] However, infections caused by capsule-free or poorly encapsulated strains have been rarely observed in a mammalian host.

The impact of the capsular polysaccharide on host immunity can be profound at many pathophysiologic levels. For example, it has been shown to produce the following effects on the host[98]:

1. It acts as an antiphagocytosis barrier.
2. It depletes complement.
3. It produces antibody unresponsiveness.
4. It dysregulates cytokine secretion.
5. It interferes with antigen presentation.
6. It produces brain edema.
7. It creates selectin and tumor necrosis factor receptor loss.
8. It allows a highly negative charge around yeast cells.
9. It extrudes itself into the intracellular environment with the potential for local toxicity on cellular organelles.
10. It enhances HIV replication.

The attached capsule with its ability to shed the structural GXM component has multiple mechanisms to abrogate a successful host immune challenge and confers resistance to oxidative stress, which may improve its intracellular survival.[99] When the GXM is shed into the host environment, it affects host immunity, but fortunately its detection in host fluids permits a successful diagnostic test.

The biochemistry of this imposing structure remains poorly understood but new insights continue to occur for this structure.[100] On the other hand, multiple genes related to capsule synthesis have been identified. Through creation of specific null mutants, it has been shown that any disturbance in efficient capsular synthesis (e.g., reduced formation, secretion, or elimination of the structure) attenuates the ability of the mutated yeast to produce disease.[97] Furthermore, there have been new insights into the many molecular signaling pathways that control expression of the capsule. For example, one critical pathway necessary for efficient capsular production uses a G protein that signals through a cyclic adenosine monophosphate (cAMP)–mediated pathway. Downregulation of this pathway with a concomitant reduction in capsule size produces an attenuated virulence phenotype, but if a mutation in the pathway upregulates capsule production, the mutant yeast becomes hypervirulent.[101]

MELANIN

The production of melanin is observed in many fungi, including some pathogenic species.[32] *C. neoformans* possesses laccase, an enzyme that catalyzes the conversion of diphenolic compounds such as L-DOPA, norepinephrine, epinephrine, and other related aromatic compounds to quinones, which rapidly autopolymerize to form melanin that is bound to the inner aspect of the yeast's cytoplasmic membrane. The production of this pigment can help identify the yeast in the laboratory, but it is also a major virulence factor for the yeast. A gene encoding for this laccase has been identified and a site-directed mutant has been created. This laccase-negative or albino mutant has been attenuated for virulence in animal models.[102]

One proposed mechanism whereby melanin may protect the yeast is through its ability to act as an antioxidant, and it has been shown that yeast cells without the ability to form melanin are more susceptible to oxidative stress. Other mechanisms whereby melanin protects the yeast from host damage involve the following:

1. Cell wall support or integrity
2. Alteration in cell wall charge
3. Interference with T-cell response
4. Abrogation of antibody-mediated phagocytosis
5. Protection from temperature changes and antifungal agents

It remains unclear whether the catecholamine-rich CNS, with its excellent substrates for melanin formation, provides some tissue tropism or rich environment that enhances this yeast's ability to produce disease. However, it has clearly been shown that melanin is formed in yeast cells within the brain.[103,104]

HIGH-TEMPERATURE GROWTH

A basic trait of all pathogenic fungi is their ability to grow well at mammalian body temperature. For example, *C. neoformans* and *C. gattii* are the only cryptococcal species to grow at 37° C, and when mutants are made that cannot grow well at this temperature, they are avirulent, even when they can make capsules and produce melanin. There appears to be some evolutionary drift in high-temperature growth in that isolates of *C. gattii* and serotype D (var. *neoformans*) generally appear to be more sensitive to growth inhibition and killing at high temperatures than serotype A (var. *grubii*), and the less heat-tolerant isolates quickly lose viability at temperatures of 40° C and above.[28]

There has been progress in understanding the genetic controls for high-temperature growth in *C. neoformans*. First, two signaling pathways (calcineurin and RAS) have been associated with the yeast's ability to grow at mammalian body temperatures, and these are linked to its virulence composite.[105,106] It is also clear that a vacuolar ATPase activity[107] and the stress sugar (trehalose) are important for high-temperature growth of this yeast. *C. neoformans* has evolved a series of molecular pathways and mechanisms to withstand host temperatures, and this is a major reason why it is a pathogen.[108]

OTHER PATHOGENICITY FACTORS

Detailed research has focused on the three classic virulence factors of *C. neoformans* (capsule, melanin, and growth at 37° C), but this complex pathogen has many other tools to produce disease. First, individual clinical or environmental strains vary in their ability to produce disease in animal models, despite possessing all known virulence factors. Strains can also rapidly change their virulence potential by passage through animals. Although many strains are clonal, there have been recombination events in nature to produce A/D hybrids and progeny that are more fit or virulent than the parental strains.[17]

Second, a series of genetic loci have been associated with the virulence composite.[1] Phospholipase activity has been linked to virulence by a gene knockout of the phospholipase B gene (PLB1). Null mutants of PLB1 are hypovirulent[109] and may have an impact on the immunologic response of the host to infection.[2] *C. neoformans* makes large amounts of urease and, if the gene for this is disrupted, infection with the mutant is attenuated in mice but not in rabbits.[3,110] A vacuolar ATPase gene is an example of a locus that appears to have an impact on several virulence phenotypes, and the absence of the encoding gene attenuates virulence of the strain.[6,107] There are multiple examples in *C. neoformans* in which a gene or pathway controls multiple virulence phenotypes. In addition to melanin as an antioxidant, several other genes such as those for superoxide dismutase, alternative oxidase, and flavohemoglobin are associated with oxidative or nitrosative stress and have been linked to the virulence composite of this yeast.

It is clear that mechanisms for stress responses are important for the yeast to establish a robust infection, but there is also some redundancy in these systems, because the yeast can still survive in the host without these protective features.[7] The alpha mating locus has been linked to the virulence of *C. neoformans* serotype D (var. *neoformans*) strains by the demonstration that the alpha mating strain is more virulent than its congenic "a" mating pair.[9] These results suggest that the mating locus, which is larger than 100 kb, may contain some virulence genes. On the other hand, studies have found that congenic *C. neoformans* serotype A (var. *grubii*) strains had no apparent difference in virulence between alpha and "a" strains in several animal models.[111] It has also been shown with several other genetic loci that virulence genes in one variety are not used by another variety or species, and vice versa. Thus, some evolutionary drift may explain the variability and complexity of the entire virulence composite of *C. neoformans* strains.

Host Responses

Because serologic and skin hypersensitivity studies frequently identify cryptococcal infections and yet the incidence of cryptococcosis is low, it has been concluded that host immunity in humans is generally effective after initial exposure to this yeast.[112,113] In fact, the vast majority of cryptococcal infections are diagnosed in patients with a compromised cell-mediated immunity. Furthermore, there is general agreement among clinicians that a strong cellular immune response producing granulomatous inflammation is essential for containment of infection.[113-116] Because granuloma formation is a result of a helper T-cell 1 (Th1)–polarized response, cytokines such as tumor necrosis factor, interferon-γ, and interleukin (IL)-2 are required.[117,118] Proinflammatory cytokines, such as IL-12, IL-18, and chemokines, such as monocyte chemotactic protein (MCP)-1 and macrophage inflammatory protein (MIP)-1α, are critically important for recruitment of inflammatory cells to the site of infection.[119,120]

Several immune cell populations, such as natural killer cells, and certain types of lymphocytes have been shown to possess direct anticryptococcal effects. Human lymphocytes (CD4, CD8) inhibit the growth of *C. neoformans* by direct contact.[121] A primary effector cell against *C. neoformans* is the macrophage, which produces anticryptococcal activity when it is activated.[122] Other professional phagocytes, such as monocyte-derived macrophages, microglial cells, and polymorphonuclear neutrophils, may kill or at least significantly inhibit *C. neoformans*. It has been shown that a major factor in the infectivity of *C. neoformans* is its ability to survive inside cells, and it has been shown that this yeast can actually be extruded from professional phagocytes to infect other cells or contain vacuoles with virulence proteins.[123-125]

It is not only the state of cellular activation or the type of host cell, but also the number of cells at the site of infection that appear to provide an effective host immune response. It is clear from natural history studies in patients with AIDS that the risk of infection dramatically increases as total CD4 lymphocyte counts drop below 50 to 100 cells/μL of blood.[126] In these patients, the paucity of inflammatory cells at the site of infection, such as the subarachnoid space, is impressive. Animal studies have further confirmed the importance of cell-mediated immunity by showing that T-cell–depleted mice are dramatically more susceptible to infection.

A series of innate factors, such as the anticryptococcal activity of saliva and serum, may discourage active infection or disease with *C.*

neoformans. Although surfactant A, dectin-1, and Toll receptors appear to have little influence on cryptococcosis,[127-129] there are other innate factors such as surfactant D, which appear to have an impact on infection. Phagocytosis of *C. neoformans* is optimally performed in the presence of complement or antibody. The intracellular fate of yeasts depends on cytokines such as interferon-γ or granulocyte-macrophage colony-stimulating factor (GM-CSF) to improve intracellular inhibition or killing of the yeasts by host oxidative or nonoxidative mechanisms. Human genome and immunogenetic studies in the future should reveal whether patients who have cryptococcosis, despite having an apparently normal immune system and no risk factors, might have subtle defects in innate or acquired immunity to this yeast. For example, it has already been shown that long-term survivors of cryptococcal meningitis have measurable persistent specific cell-mediated defects against *C. neoformans*. Recently, it was shown that there is an association of common functional genetic polymorphisms in low-affinity Fc gamma receptors with cases of cryptococcosis.[130,131]

It appears that *C. neoformans* has extracellular and intracellular components or stages of infection. The results of histologic examination of tissues and fluids range from virtual absence of an inflammatory reaction to intense granulomatous inflammation with caseous necrosis. The immune reaction appears to be primarily a function of the host status, but the yeast can participate in the inflammatory response, because switch variants in a single strain can produce vastly different histologic responses.[26] The immune response may be influenced by not only the shedding of polysaccharide into tissue but also other yeast factors such as mannitol,[132] melanin,[133] and prostaglandins,[134] which may have profound direct effects on immunomodulation of these infections.

There is substantial evidence that the humoral immunity arm can contribute to an effective immune response.[135-139] Several groups have shown that monoclonal antibody strategies directed against the polysaccharide capsule can reduce the burden of yeasts and improve survival in animal models. In fact, a polysaccharide–tetanus toxoid conjugate vaccine was shown to elicit high titers of antibody to the capsule and subsequently to protect against an IV inoculation of cryptococci in mice. These antibodies provide for (1) efficient phagocytosis, (2) enhanced natural killer cell function, and (3) improvement in clearing capsular polysaccharide. Antibodies to other structural components such as melanin[140] and glucosylceramide in the cell wall[141] have also been able to improve the host's ability to fight infection. Sophisticated serologic studies of the host have suggested that there are qualitative and quantitative differences in the individual types of immunoglobulins that may predispose to disseminated cryptococcal disease.[142] Finally, a pilot study in humans has been performed to determine the safety and dynamics of a murine monoclonal antibody for treatment of cryptococcosis.[143]

Pathogenesis

The pathogenesis of cryptococcosis is determined by three broad factors: (1) the status of the host defenses; (2) the virulence of the strain of *C. neoformans*; and (3) the size of the inoculum. The relative importance of each factor as a determinant of clinical disease remains uncertain, but it is clear that the complexities of these interactions together produce the ultimate presentation.

A reasonable scenario for the pathophysiology of cryptococcosis is that the susceptible host comes into contact with cryptococci from the environment through inhalation of infectious propagules. In the alveoli, the yeasts contact the alveolar macrophages, which recruit other inflammatory cells through cytokines or chemokines, and a proper Th1 response and granulomatous inflammation is elicited. The infection can then take one of three pathways:

1. In an immunosuppressed host, the yeast continues to proliferate and disseminate, causing clinical disease.
2. The effective immune response completely eliminates the yeast from the host.

3. The yeasts produce a small lung–lymph node complex and remain dormant in tissues but are not dead.

The third scenario may be a common occurrence. Baker and colleagues, in elegant postmortem studies of asymptomatic individuals, showed the existence of pulmonary foci and hilar nodes containing yeasts in individuals with no antecedent complaints.[144,145] The yeasts remain dormant and the host is clinically asymptomatic until loss of local immunity occurs through, for example, corticosteroid use or progression of an HIV infection. Then, the yeasts begin to replicate in the pulmonary lymph node complex and eventually disseminate into organs outside the lung. This pathophysiology is similar to the scenario proposed for reactivation of tuberculosis and histoplasmosis. Studies in France have given epidemiologic support for this concept of reactivation. In African ex-patriots who lived in Europe for many years prior to their development of cryptococcosis, the infecting strain possessed a genotype consistent with strains from an African origin.[146]

Clinical Manifestations

The two common sites for infection with this encapsulated yeast, the lung and CNS,[147] were emphasized in a review of cryptococcosis in HIV-negative patients. In this cohort, 109 (36%) were diagnosed with only pulmonary involvement and 157 (51%) presented with initial evidence of CNS disease.[51] Three other sites of infection (skin, prostate, eye) have clinical features worthy of mention. However, it should be noted that *C. neoformans* has been found to infect any organ of the human body (Table 263-2) and, in the severely immunosuppressed patient, cryptococcosis may present with involvement of multiple body sites.

Cryptococcosis demonstrates a few differences, depending on whether the patient has or does not have an underlying HIV infection.[88,148-151] HIV-infected patients present with more CNS and extrapulmonary infections, higher rates of positive India ink examinations, higher polysaccharide antigen titers, more frequent positive blood cultures, and fewer cerebrospinal fluid (CSF) inflammatory cells. These clinical distinctions are primarily a function of the severity of immunosuppression and the resulting high burden of yeast. They most likely do not reflect a specific interaction between HIV and *C. neoformans* growth.

LUNG

The respiratory tract is the most common portal of entry for this yeast, and symptoms there range from asymptomatic colonization of the airway[152] to life-threatening pneumonia with evidence of an acute respiratory distress syndrome.[153-155] In at least a third of normal hosts, the infection is asymptomatic on presentation and is detected by an abnormal chest radiograph. On the other hand, patients can present with acute symptoms of fever, chest pain, cough, weight loss, and sputum production.[156] Common and unusual pulmonary presentations are listed in Table 263-2. Cryptococcosis occasionally occurs with another pathogen; coinfections of the lung have been reported with tuberculosis, nocardiosis, and echinococcosis.[157-159] Also, *C. neoformans* may be isolated from the sputum repeatedly over months and years in patients with prior chronic lung disease but no immunosuppression, no evidence of active pulmonary parenchymal disease, negative serum cryptococcal antigen, and negative fungal cultures from urine and CSF. These patients are considered to have chronic endobronchial colonization. A pulmonary nodule in such a patient may be considered to be cryptococcal in origin but may represent a malignancy.

In normal hosts, chest radiographs commonly show well-defined, noncalcified single (Fig. 263-1) or multiple nodules. An initial presentation may be that of a radiographic lesion (or more than one) that is worrisome for a lung malignancy but then is proven by lung biopsy to be a cryptococcal infection. Other radiographic characteristics include indistinct masslike infiltrates, hilar lymphadenopathy, lobar infiltrates (Fig. 263-2), pleural effusions, and lung cavitation.[160] When infection

TABLE 263-2 Clinical Manifestations of Cryptococcosis

Central nervous system
  Acute, subacute, chronic meningitis
  Cryptococcomas of brain (abscesses)
  Spinal cord granuloma
  Chronic dementia (from hydrocephalus)
Lung
  Nodules (single or multiple)
  Lobar infiltrates
  Interstitial infiltrates
  Cavities
  Endobronchial masses
  Endobronchial colonization
  Acute respiratory distress syndrome
  Mediastinal adenopathy
  Hilar adenopathy
  Pneumothorax
  Pleural effusions/empyema
  Miliary pattern
Skin
  Papules and maculopapules
  Subcutaneous abscess
  Vesicles
  Plaques
  Cellulitis
  Purpura
  Acne
  Draining sinuses
  Ulcers
  Bullae
  Herpetiformis-like
  Molluscum contagiosum-like
Eye
  Papilledema
  Extraocular muscle paresis
  Keratitis
  Chorioretinitis
  Endophthalmitis
  Optic nerve atrophy
Genitourinary tract
  Prostatitis
  Renal cortical abscess
  Positive urine culture from occult source
  Genital lesions
Bone and joints
  Osteolytic lesion (single or multiple sites)
  Arthritis (acute/chronic)
Muscle
  Myositis
Heart, blood vessels
  Cryptococcemia
  Endocarditis (native and prosthetic)
  Mycotic aneurysm
  Myocarditis
  Pericarditis
  Infected vascular graft
Gastrointestinal tract
  Esophageal nodule
  Nodular or ulcerated lesions in stomach or intestines (may resemble Crohn's)
  Hepatitis
  Peritonitis
  Pancreatic mass
Breast
  Breast abscess
  Lymph nodes
  Lymphadenopathy
Thyroid
  Thyroiditis
  Thyroid mass
Adrenal gland
  Adrenal insufficiency
  Adrenal mass
Head and neck
  Gingivitis
  Sinusitis
  Salivary gland enlargement

From Casadevall A, Perfect JR. *Cryptococcus neoformans.* Washington DC: ASM Press; 1998:409.

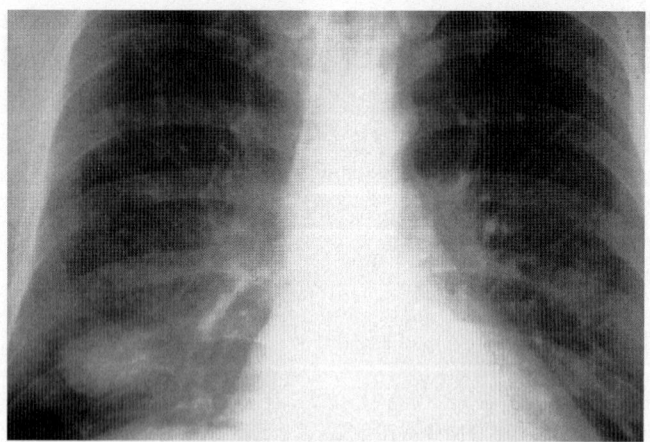

Figure 263-1 Cryptococcal nodule. This was a previously healthy, asymptomatic patient with a right lung nodule.

is limited to the lung, the test for serum cryptococcal antigen is generally negative. If there is pulmonary cryptococcosis with a positive test for serum cryptococcal antigen, it is prudent to examine for an extrapulmonary source of infection, although workups may still be negative for another infection site (e.g., blood, skin, CSF). When *C. neoformans* has been isolated from the lung in patients at high risk for dissemination, a lumbar puncture should be considered to rule out CNS infection, even in the absence of symptoms. Early asymptomatic spread to the CNS may be manifested only by a positive CSF fungal culture, with otherwise normal CSF and a negative antigen test. The number of cryptococci may be so low that several milliliters of CSF must be cultured for a positive culture to be obtained. Because positive CSF cultures are infrequent, some clinicians advocate treating previously normal patients with lung disease who are asymptomatic and have no apparent underlying disease with long-term fluconazole and omitting the lumbar puncture.[161,162]

In the severely immunosuppressed host with AIDS or who is receiving high-dose corticosteroids, cryptococcal pneumonia can progress more rapidly (over days instead of weeks).[153,155] Unlike immunocompetent hosts, most immunosuppressed individuals have constitutional symptoms such as fever, malaise, chest pain, shortness of breath, and weight loss. In these patients, pneumonia can progress to features of acute respiratory compromise, even without evidence of CNS involvement. However, because of the ability of the yeast to disseminate outside the primary lung focus to the CNS, these very high-risk patients frequently present with a meningeal rather than a pulmonary

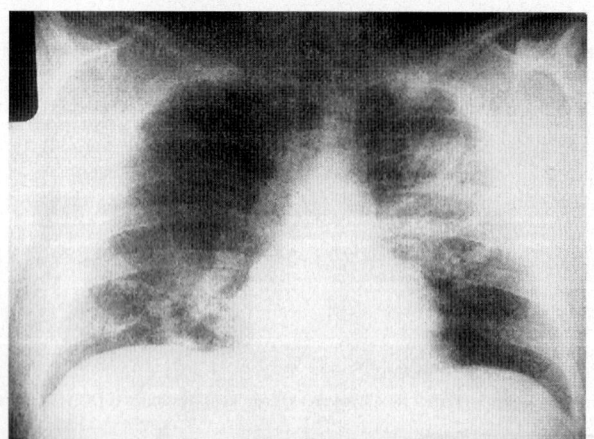

Figure 263-2 Cryptococcal pneumonia. This was a previously healthy patient with fever, cough, shortness of breath, and left lobar infiltrate.

syndrome. In AIDS patients, cryptococcal pneumonia may not be symptomatic, and over 90% may present with concomitant CNS infection at the initial diagnosis. Chest radiographs in these immunocompromised hosts are similar in their range of presentations to those of immunocompetent hosts. However, alveolar and interstitial infiltrates are particularly common and thus might be confused with *Pneumocystis* infection. Because the severely immunosuppressed patient with pulmonary cryptococcosis and AIDS generally has a CD4 count substantially below 100 cells/μL, it is always prudent to consider the possibility of coinfection with other opportunists such as typical and atypical mycobacterium, cytomegalovirus, *Nocardia*, and *Pneumocystis*.

CENTRAL NERVOUS SYSTEM

Most patients with cryptococcosis of the CNS present with signs and symptoms of subacute meningitis or meningoencephalitis, such as headache, fever, cranial nerve palsies, lethargy, coma, or memory loss over several weeks (see Table 263-2).[147] Symptoms may not be typical, and patients may present with acute (several days) symptoms of severe headaches, with intermittent headaches, or even with no headache but with altered mental status.

HIV-infected patients with cryptococcal meningitis exhibit few differences at presentation from those without HIV. However, several clinical aspects may be more prominent in patients with AIDS.[51] First, the burden of yeast is generally higher, and this may be reflected in higher polysaccharide antigen titers, slower conversion of CSF to sterilization during treatment, and a tendency toward a higher incidence of increased intracranial pressure. Second, there is a greater likelihood of finding the yeast in extracranial locations during the initial workup. Third, the possibility is greater that a second CNS event may occur, such as infection with *Toxoplasma gondii* or development of a lymphoma.

Fourth, the use of HAART in AIDS patients has created a new immune reconstitution syndrome in cryptococcal infections.[163] It appears in two forms, unmasking and paradoxical. In the unmasking form, after starting HAART, some patients develop acute symptoms of cryptococcal meningitis or pain and swelling in peripheral, hilar, or mediastinal lymph nodes. In the paradoxical form, new symptoms may also occur during otherwise successful treatment of cryptococcal meningitis in the first few weeks or months after HAART is introduced. It appears to correlate with a significant drop in HIV load, but there may be only a modest rise in the number of CD4 cells.[164] It is hypothesized that as immunity improves with HAART, silent or latent cryptococcal infections are made clinically apparent as inflammation is mobilized to interact with the yeasts or polysaccharide antigen. During treatment for cryptococcal meningitis, this immune reconstitution syndrome may be marked by increasing headaches, new neurologic signs, appearance of more inflammatory cells in the CSF, and possibly increased intracranial pressure.[165] Distinction between immune reconstitution and progressive infection can be difficult, but cultures from the CSF and lymph node aspirates are generally negative in immune reconstitution syndromes, even though cryptococci may be present on a smear.

There are limited data that relate the severity of the meningitis to the particular infecting strain and, in most cases, the host defense responses determine the clinical manifestations. However, some clinical presentations may depend on the particular infecting strain. For example, in areas of the world that have infections with both *C. neoformans* serotypes A, D, and AD (var. *neoformans* or *grubii*) and *C. gattii*, cerebral cryptococcomas (Fig. 263-3) and hydrocephalus with or without large pulmonary mass lesions in immunocompetent hosts were found more commonly with the *C. gattii* infections.[166-168] Although patients infected with this variety have higher survival rates, a subgroup of patients with *C. gattii* infections have brain parenchymal lesions by scan, complications of hydrocephalus and increased intracranial pressure, cranial neuropathies, and a poor response to therapy. These observations suggest that some strains may have a greater pro-

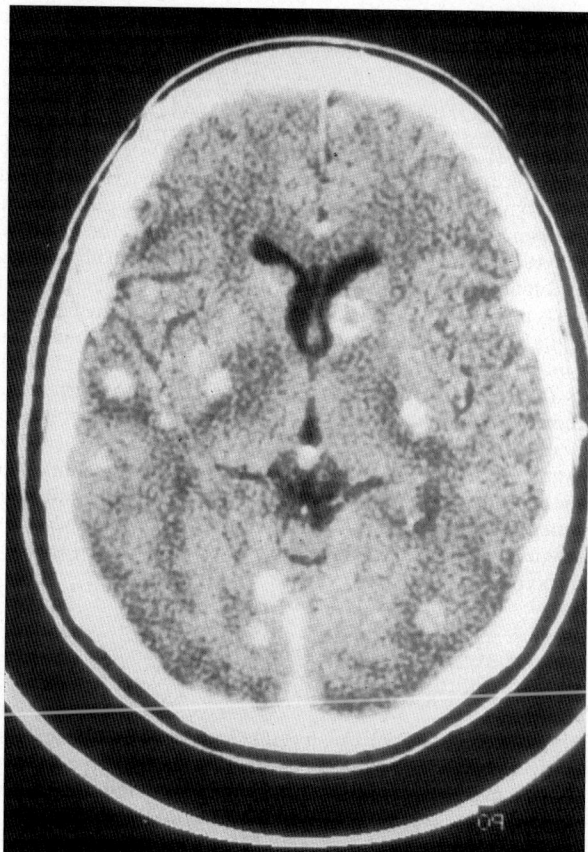

Figure 263-3   Multiple cryptococcomas. This CT scan is of a previously healthy patient.

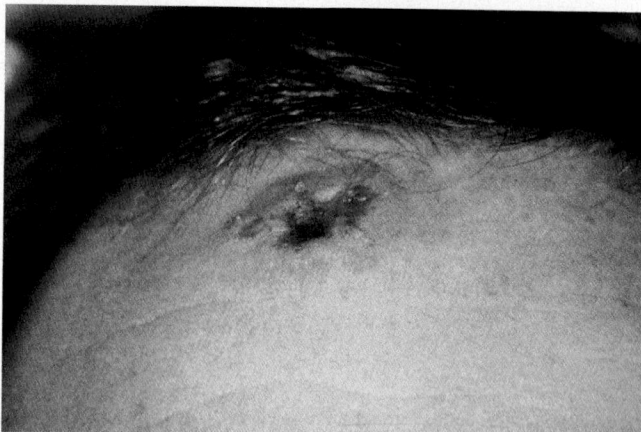

Figure 263-4   Forehead ulcer. This is in an HIV-infected host with *Cryptococcus neoformans* seen in histopathology.

pensity for invading the brain parenchyma than for producing a primary presentation of meningitis. Another example of the strain affecting disease production is from the Vancouver outbreak, wherein it was found that a recombinant strain was created in nature that was more virulent in animal models than the parental strain and had taken over most of the environmental and clinical isolates in this outbreak.[17]

SKIN

C. neoformans can produce almost any type of skin lesion (see Table 263-2). A common lesion is a papule or maculopapule, with a soft or ulcerated center (Fig. 263-4). A draining sinus usually originates in an underlying bone lesion or occasionally a subcutaneous abscess. Some lesions are easily mistaken for molluscum contagiosum, acne vulgaris, squamous carcinoma, or basal cell carcinoma. After pulmonary and CNS sites of infection, the skin is the third most common organ for appearance of infection. Skin manifestations can be extraordinarily varied.[169-172] In severely immunosuppressed patients, skin infections may present as a cellulitis (Fig. 263-5) or an abscess that mimics a bacterial skin infection in both appearance and rapidity of onset.[173,174] Because of the variety of skin manifestations, a correct diagnosis requires a biopsy with proper histopathology and culture. This is extremely important in the immunocompromised host.

In most cases, the skin lesions represent a sentinel finding for disseminated cryptococcal infection. In fact, severely immunosuppressed patients can present with both cutaneous cryptococcosis and another pathogenic fungus in the skin as a manifestation of disseminated fungal disease.[175] However, there is strong evidence that rare cases of skin cryptococcosis represent primary cutaneous cryptococcosis from direct inoculation or exposure rather than being a marker of dissemi-

nated disease. In a large retrospective review of patients with cutaneous findings, a series of immunocompetent patients had (1) solitary skin lesion(s) on unclothed areas of the skin, (2) a history of skin injury, participation in outdoor activities, or exposure to bird droppings, (3) isolation of *C. neoformans*, and (4) no evidence of disseminated disease.[176] There have been reports of direct inoculation of yeast into skin by laboratory or clinical accidents and defined episodes of trauma.[80,81] In these cases, there has been no evidence for dissemination of infection from this body site of infection.

Involvement of skin may be influenced by several factors. First, some strains of *C. neoformans* have been described as being dermotropic in animal models. Second, an observation made in a cohort of recipients of solid organ transplants has suggested that patients receiving tacrolimus appeared to develop a higher ratio of skin and soft tissue infections to CNS infections when compared with previous immunosuppressive regimens.[72] Because tacrolimus has anticryptococcal activity at temperatures of 37° to 39°C[177] but loses its anticryptococcal activity at environmental temperatures, the skin involvement might result from the lower temperatures at this body site.

PROSTATE

Like *Blastomyces* and *Mycobacterium tuberculosis*, *C. neoformans* can invade the prostate gland, although in most cases of cryptococcal infection this involvement is asymptomatic.[178] In fact, asymptomatic or silent prostate infection may first be identified during urologic surgery and may spread into the bloodstream during surgery.[179] For *C. neofor-*

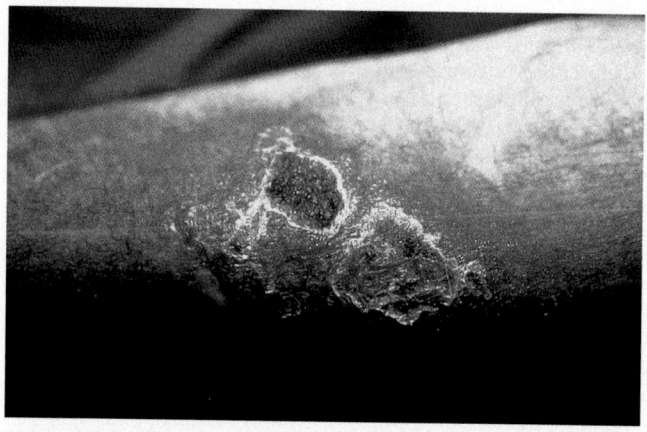

Figure 263-5   Cellulitis of the arm caused by *Cryptococcus neoformans.* This patient was severely immunosuppressed.

mans, this gland was considered an important site for sanctuary of this yeast from antifungal treatment in HIV-infected patients prior to HAART.[180,181] Frequently, in follow-up of patients with AIDS and cryptococcal meningitis after initial antifungal therapy, cultures of urine (with or without prostatic massage) or seminal fluid were positive for the yeast. In many patients, the location of relapse after therapy remains uncertain, but the prostate is clearly a site that requires prolonged therapy to clear infection in the severely immunosuppressed patients. In addition to the prostate, penile[182] and vulvar[183] lesions with *C. neoformans* have been reported, but there has been no evidence for conjugal spread of this yeast, and isolated cyptococcuria is a marker for disseminated disease.

EYE

In the early reviews of cryptococcal meningitis, ocular signs and symptoms were reported in 45% of cases.[184] The most common manifestations are ocular palsies and papilledema. Small white retinal exudates, without overlying vitritis, are probably the next most common finding. In this era of severely immunosuppressed patients, several new features of ocular involvement have arisen. First, cryptococcal eye infections can occur simultaneously with infections with other pathogens, such as HIV and cytomegalovirus.[185] Second, the presence of extensive retinal lesions, particularly with vitritis, frequently leads to blindness and only occasionally is it successfully managed.[186,187] Third, there are reports of catastrophic loss of vision without evidence for endophthalmitis.[188,189]

In these cases of blindness, which may occur while receiving therapy, two pathogenic processes have been identified. First, there is a visual loss secondary to an optic neuritis produced by infiltration of the optic nerve with yeasts and, as for endophthalmitis, there are few options for successful management. Second, other patients present with visual loss in one or both eyes during antifungal therapy. In these patients, symptoms are probably related to the development of cerebral edema and unrelieved high intracranial pressure. The probable pathogenesis is compression of the ophthalmic artery within the optic sheath. Treatment is decrease of CSF pressure by repeated lumbar punctures, CSF shunting, or perhaps slitting the optic sheath within the posterior orbit. Once blindness has occurred, return of visual acuity is rare. A central scotoma or optic atrophy may be the only sequela of cured ocular cryptococcosis.

OTHER BODY SITES

C. neoformans can produce infection in most areas of the body (see Table 263-2), and several require further discussion. Cryptococcemia occurs during severe immunosuppression and when there is a high burden of yeast in the body and is a common finding in advanced AIDS. Cryptococcemia rarely produces vascular instability, and only a few cases of endocarditis have been described.

Bone lesions prior to the AIDS epidemic were reported in up to 5% of disseminated cases.[190] Bone lesions are typically one or more well-circumscribed osteolytic lesions in almost any bone and may have a contiguous soft tissue abscess ("cold abscess"). Bone lesions of sarcoidosis resemble cryptococcal lesions on x-ray films but are more often on the hands or feet, and have no contiguous soft tissue abscess.[191] In AIDS patients, the yeast may be found in bone marrow biopsies cultured for other reasons.

Cryptococcal peritonitis can present in two distinct patient groups—those receiving chronic ambulatory peritoneal dialysis and those with underlying liver disease and cirrhosis.[192,193]

Rare body sites for cryptococcosis (less than a dozen reported cases) include the genital and urinary tracts (renal cortical abscess, positive urine culture from an occult site), muscle (myositis), heart (native and prosthetic valve endocarditis), mycotic aortitis or aneurysm, myocarditis, pericarditis, vascular foreign body, thyroid (thyroiditis, mass), adrenal gland (adrenal insufficiency), head and neck (gingivitis, sinusitis, salivary gland enlargement), gastrointestinal nodules or ulcers, hepatitis, breast (inflammatory mass), and lymph node (lymphadenopathy).

IMMUNE RECONSTITUTION INFLAMMATORY SYNDROME IN ORGAN TRANSPLANT RECIPIENTS

Immune reconstitution inflammatory syndrome (IRIS) causing increased symptoms of cryptococcosis has been described earlier as a complication of HAART therapy of HIV infection. More recently, it has been realized that IRIS also occurs as a complication of solid organ transplantation[194] and perhaps even in normal hosts whose immune status has improved.[195,196] IRIS in solid organ transplant recipients can be manifest as new radiographic signs and new or worsening symptoms, including fever and signs of increased intracranial pressure. IRIS occurs in patients whose potent antirejection regimens have been reduced after initiation of antifungal therapy. It occurs at a mean of 6 weeks after starting antifungal therapy and may be associated with organ graft loss. IRIS in cryptococcosis needs to be identified and, because there are no specific tests for it, the diagnosis relies on clinical guidelines and judgment.[197] It is important to recognize because its management is different than that for relapse or persistence of cryptococcosis.

Laboratory Diagnosis

MICROSCOPIC EXAMINATION

The simple procedure of mixing together India ink and biologic fluids to identify the 5- to 10-μ-diameter encapsulated yeasts remains a rapid and effective method for diagnosing cryptococcal meningitis (Fig. 263-6). Approximately 50% of non-AIDS patients with cryptococcal meningitis and over 80% of patients with AIDS have a positive India ink examination of the CSF. Experience is required to distinguish an encapsulated yeast from a lymphocyte with surrounding proteinaceous debris. India ink smears of urine, sputum, and bronchoalveolar lavage specimens are almost impossible to interpret. With calcofluor white and a fluorescent microscope, yeasts can be detected in a specimen when numbers are reduced. With routine histopathologic stains such as hematoxylin and eosin, the yeasts are surrounded by empty spaces, which reflect the capsule. The polysaccharide capsule can be identified with stains such as mucicarmine and Alcian blue (Fig. 263-7), and its ability to produce melanin allows it to be stained with the Fontana-Masson stain. Gomori's methenamine silver (GMS) fungal stain identifies the narrow-based budding yeast in tissue (Fig. 263-8), and a Gram stain usually reveals a poorly stained gram-positive yeast. Both biopsies and cytologies (Fig. 263-9) can be extremely helpful in the diagnosis of cryptococcosis.

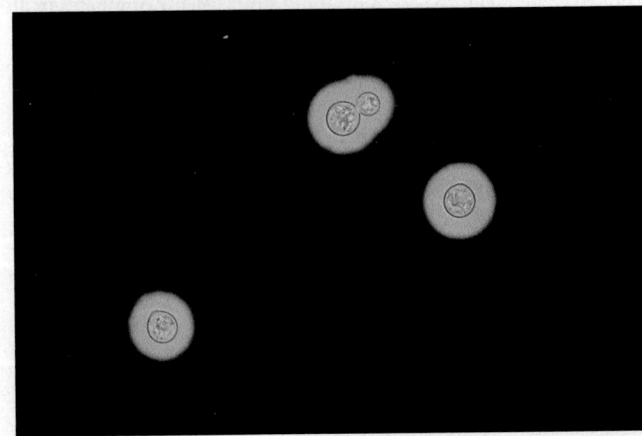

Figure 263-6 **India ink preparations from cerebrospinal fluid of patient with meningitis.** Note the encapsulated yeasts.

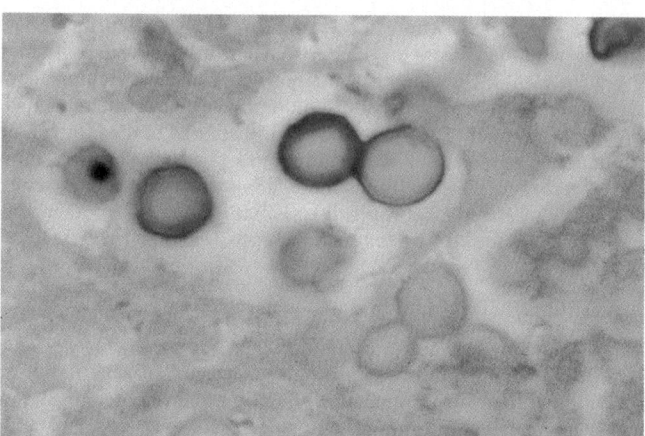

Figure 263-7 **Alcian blue stain of lung tissue from patient with cryptococcal pneumonia.** Note the blue staining of the polysaccharide capsules.

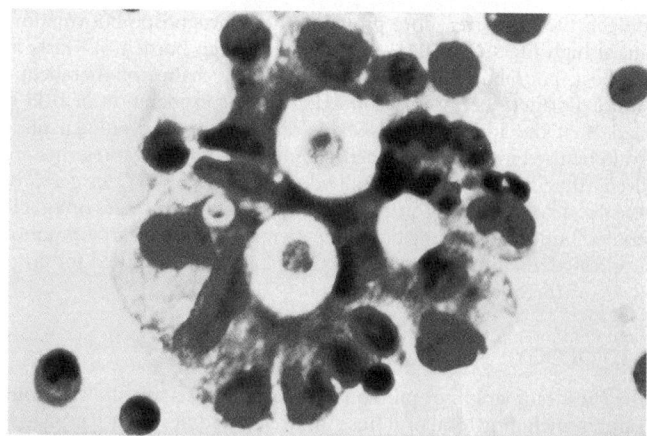

Figure 263-9 **Cytospin CSF preparation of host with cryptococcal meningitis.** This shows an encapsulated yeast surrounded by a mixed inflammatory reaction.

CULTURES

Cryptococcus neoformans can grow on most bacterial and fungal media. Both automated and lysis centrifugation methods are effective in detecting cryptococcemia, and the finding of positive blood cultures has been more common during the AIDS epidemic. Most *C. neoformans* isolates from untreated patients can be detected in culture 3 to 7 days after the specimen is collected and placed into or on culture media.

Isolates can be identified by biochemical reactions[29,30] or DNA-based methods.[198,199] Other methods to presumptively identify the yeast are to perform a rapid urease test or to inoculate the yeast onto Staib's birdseed,[200] DOPA, or caffeic acid media (in which colonies will produce melanin and turn brown to black). However, some other yeasts produce urease, and the highly mucoid colonies of some strains of *C. neoformans* may not produce enough melanin to be clearly positive.

The identification of the varieties for *C. neoformans* and *C. gattii* can be made by several methods: (1) a color reaction on concanavalin-glycine-thymol agar, which distinguishes serotypes A, D, and AD from B and C[201]; (2) an antibody kit for serotyping (not commercially available at present)[202]; and (3) fingerprinting with DNA-based methods, which can further separate strains into eight genotypes.[203-205]

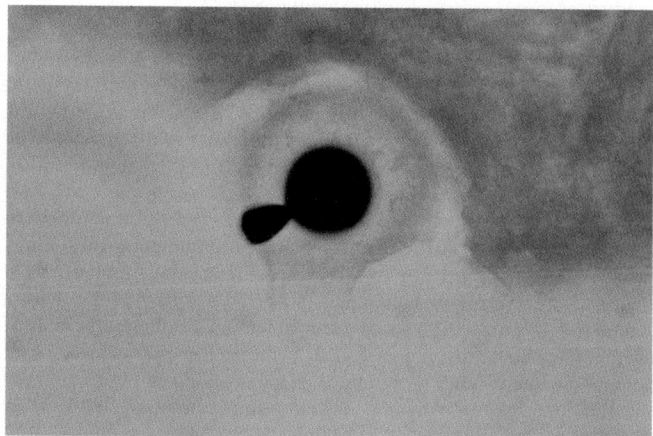

Figure 263-8 **Narrow-based yeast with a faint capsule.** (Gomori's methenamine silver stain.)

SEROLOGY

The serologic tests for detection of cryptococcal polysaccharide antigen in serum and CSF are extremely accurate for the diagnosis of invasive disease.[206] Both latex agglutination and enzyme immunoassay tests are more than 90% sensitive and specific.[207] With the proper treatment of specimens (boiling and pronase, 2-mercaptoethanol treatment), false-positive test results are not common when CSF titers are 1:4 or higher.[208] False-positive latex agglutination test results are usually negative by enzyme immunoassay, and vice versa. An occasional false-positive test result is observed when there is a cross-reactive antigen in the specimen, which may occur with microorganisms such as *Trichosporon asahii* (*beigelii*)[209] or other infections.[210] The false-negative test results may be present in early asymptomatic meningitis and in chronic indolent meningitis. The clinical experience with, and preciseness of, this test has been studied in sera and in CSF, and it is not recommended for detecting polysaccharide antigen in the urine and bronchoalveolar lavage fluid, despite some reports to the contrary.[211]

There are a number of clinical issues related to the use of cryptococcal polysaccharide antigen. Serum cryptococcal polysaccharide antigen tests have been used successfully to screen very high-risk febrile AIDS patients, particularly those with headache, in areas in which the incidence of cryptococcal meningitis is high,[212] but these tests may be less useful in areas in which the prevalence of infection is low.[213] In patients with cryptococcal infection of the lung who have a positive serum polysaccharide antigen test result, there is heightened concern that the infection has become extrapulmonary. It is also unlikely that this high-molecular-weight molecule can cross the blood-CSF barrier, and thus its presence in CSF probably confirms the presence of the yeast in this compartment. In fact, there are occasional cases of meningitis in which CSF antigen is detected early in infection before there is a high enough colony count for the routine laboratory to detect a positive culture, particularly with small volumes of CSF. There are also isolated cases of serum cryptococcal polysaccharidemia in asymptomatic HIV-infected patients with negative fungal cultures from CSF and urine. Management of these asymptomatic antigenemia cases can be confusing, but in these high-risk patients it is wise to start empirical antifungal therapy because many of them will eventually develop cryptococcosis.[214,215] If available, it is advisable to confirm a positive latex agglutination with an enzyme immunoassay, and vice versa, before beginning prolonged therapy with fluconazole.

Despite its excellence as a diagnostic test, the polysaccharide antigen is not sufficiently accurate to use in making treatment decisions. Serial polysaccharide antigen titers are imprecise and should not be used to develop treatment guidelines.[216] The cryptococcal polysaccharide antigen titer, however, does provide general prognostic information. Initial high titers (≥1 : 1024) demonstrate a high burden of yeasts in the host, poor host immunity, and a greater chance of therapeutic failure. Furthermore, it is encouraging when consideration of IRIS is made that the antigen titer is stable or dropping, and antigen titers could be used in follow-up when maintenance antifungal regimens are discontinued in HIV-infected individuals. Antibodies to *C. neoformans* may be detected during infection and are helpful for epidemiologic studies, but because many of these patients with disease are immunosuppressed, the titers are inconsistent and not generally used for diagnostic or treatment decisions.

RADIOLOGY

The chest radiograph of pulmonary cryptococcosis can show various features, including local or diffuse infiltrates, nodules, hilar lymphadenopathy, cavitation, and pleural effusion(s).[217-221] In AIDS patients, the diffuse interstitial infiltrates may be confused with coexistent *Pneumocystis* infection.[222,223]

Computed tomography (CT) and magnetic resonance imaging (MRI) of the brain are frequently used in the management of cryptococcal meningoencephalitis.[224-228] Approximately 50% of CT scans are normal in CNS infection. However, CT can reveal hydrocephalus, gyral enhancement, or single or multiple nodules that may or may not be enhancing. Cryptococcomas may be single or multiple and, in some populations (e.g., those with *C. gattii* infection), they can occur in up to 25% of non-AIDS and apparently immunocompetent patients. In patients with AIDS, the CT scan differs only in that approximately one third of patients demonstrate cortical atrophy from the underlying HIV infection. MRI scans are more sensitive than CT scans for detecting abnormalities in cryptococcal meningoencephalitis. MRI findings can include numerous clustered foci that are hyperintense on T2-weighted images and nonenhancing on postcontrast T1-weighted images in the basal ganglia or midbrain. Rarely, there may also be multiple miliary enhancing parenchymal and leptomeningeal nodules.

There are several points to emphasize with regard to CNS radiology. First, there is no pathognomonic scan, and patients with cryptococcal meningitis may simply present with evidence of idiopathic hydrocephalus.[229] Second, in AIDS patients, CNS parenchymal lesions may represent lymphoma or a second infection, such as toxoplasmosis or nocardiosis. Third, follow-up scans may actually show worsening of lesions, with enlargement, new lesions, or persistence of cryptococcomas or more leptomeningeal enhancement. This finding is not necessarily a sign of treatment failure. It simply represents enhancement by inflammation as microscopic yeast foci are being eliminated. Especially with the use of HAART and the potential for immune reconstitution, these radiographs need to be judged carefully in the context of the patient's cultures and clinical signs and symptoms before deciding that the radiograph signifies treatment failure. Lesions on MRI scans may not decrease in size for months or years, despite resolution of disease.[230]

🔲 Treatment

The management of cryptococcosis has been the subject of a series of evidence-based studies. Guidelines have been established for therapy and are in revision,[231] and the general recommendations should be helpful to clinicians, but there remain many unanswered questions. It is clear that cryptococcal meningitis is uniformly fatal without antifungal treatment. However, prior to the availability of antifungals, there were several reports of patients who survived for years before succumbing to infection. Today, in contrast, with the severe immunosuppression of HIV infection, and if adequate treatments are not available, a very high percentage of untreated patients die within the first 2 weeks of hospitalization.[232] The rapidity of the progression is likely to depend on host factors. Conversely, it has been shown that some individuals have asymptomatic endobronchial colonization with no detectable pulmonary lesions on CT scan, negative serum cryptococcal

antigen, and negative fungal cultures from CSF and urine. These patients without disease may not need antifungal treatment. In a review of non-AIDS patients with positive pulmonary cultures for *C. neoformans*, approximately 20% did not receive treatment.[51] Previously healthy patients with cryptococcosis confined to the lung healed spontaneously. However, because pulmonary cryptococcosis in immunosuppressed patients or those who will become immunosuppressed can progress or become chronic disease in the lung, and in others disseminates later to the CNS, all such patients should be treated.

IN VITRO DRUG ANALYSIS

Methods for in vitro susceptibility testing of *Cryptococcus neoformans* have been modified and standardized.[233] Most initial isolates have a low minimal inhibitory concentration (MIC) to amphotericin B, flucytosine, and azoles but a high MIC to caspofungin. By in vitro susceptibility testing, isolates have been detected that are resistant to flucytosine, azoles, and polyenes. There appears to be some correlation between MIC and clinical resistance.[234-236] However, by molecular typing methods, most of the refractory cases represent relapse isolates rather than reinfection,[237] and they possess an MIC similar to that of the primary isolates.[238] However, in one case, it was suggested by molecular techniques that reinfection occurred with a novel strain.[239] When the MIC of an isolate rises while the patient is being treated, or when the MIC is initially 16 μg/mL or higher for fluconazole or 128 μg/mL or higher for flucytosine, failure of treatment might possibly be related directly to drug resistance.[240] In fact, in HIV-associated cryptococcal meningoencephalitis in Africa. where fluconazole is used to treat mucocutaneous candidiasis and as primary therapy for cryptococcal disease, culture-positive relapses were associated with isolates that had reduced susceptibility to fluconazole (MIC ≥64 μg /mL).[241] *C. neoformans* strains have been isolated that possess known drug resistance mechanisms.

STRATEGIES

Cryptococcal Meningitis

Amphotericin B remains the cornerstone of therapy for cryptococcal meningitis and, from early studies when it was used alone[242] to its use in combinations, it has performed reasonably well for this infection, with successes in the non-AIDS era of between 60% and 75%.[243,244] With polyene therapy, two issues have been noted. First, studies have suggested that higher daily doses of amphotericin B might be more effective in sterilization of the CSF.[245] A standard induction dose for amphotericin B deoxycholate has now been established at 0.7 mg/kg/day. Second, liposomal amphotericin B (AmBisome) and amphotericin B lipid complex (ABLC) at 3 to 6 mg/kg/day have had treatment success similar to that of amphotericin B deoxycholate, with reduced toxicity.[246-250] In patients with or at risk for renal dysfunction, the lipid product of amphotericin B is frequently used.

Flucytosine has been used alone in treatment of cryptococcal meningitis,[251] but frequent development of direct drug resistance on monotherapy means that it cannot be recommended as a single agent for treatment of this infection. It is primarily used in combination therapy with amphotericin B[243,244,252-255]; dosages in patients with normal renal function are typically 100 mg/kg/day but will need to be adjusted in those with renal dysfunction. Drug levels should be monitored to keep 2-hour postdose levels under 100 μg/mL[256] or careful following complete blood counts to reduce the development of bone marrow depression in those with risk for this toxicity, such as patients with renal dysfunction or receiving high doses of polyenes. One report has concluded that adding flucytosine to amphotericin B reduces the rates of relapse compared with amphotericin B monotherapy,[257] and another retrospective report has shown reduced rates of failure in severe cryptococcal meningitis with the combination compared with other regimens.[258]

Azoles have been used effectively in the management of cryptococcal meningitis. Fluconazole has been used extensively in cryptococcal meningitis because of its excellent CSF pharmacokinetics and long-term oral safety.[259-263] Clinical trials have shown that it penetrates well into CSF and is excellent for use in the suppressive phase of cryptococcal meningitis management.[264,265] However, it tends to be fungistatic and is probably best used in the stage of infection in which there is a low burden of yeasts in the CSF; thus, it is not recommended for the primary induction phase of therapy for meningitis.

Itraconazole, despite its poor CSF penetration and inconsistent oral bioavailability, has been successfully used in the treatment of cryptococcal meningitis,[266,267] but has been shown to be inferior to fluconazole for the suppressive phase of treatment.[257] Its place in therapy for cryptococcal meningitis is probably as an alternative to first-line therapy with fluconazole, and it can be used in the clearance and suppressive phases of meningitis management if drug levels are monitored, but it is not recommended for primary induction phase therapy. Other azoles have been studied for treatment of cryptococcosis, but miconazole and ketoconazole are no longer used. The new triazoles, voriconazole and posaconazole, have been studied in a small number of refractory cases of cryptococcosis with moderate success,[268,269] but it is not clear what advantage they possess over fluconazole.

The new antifungal class of β-glucan synthase inhibitors, such as caspofungin, micafungin, and anidulafungin, does not possess reliable anticryptococcal activity. These agents are not likely to be used for cryptococcal infections.

Combination therapy for the management of cryptococcal meningitis has been extremely well studied. The combination of amphotericin B and flucytosine has become standard therapy for meningitis, and in patients without AIDS it reliably sterilizes CSF after 2 weeks of therapy. In fact, it clears CSF yeast counts significantly faster than amphotericin B alone, amphotericin B plus fluconazole, or all three agents together.[270] Flucytosine and fluconazole have been studied in animals and in open clinical trials, with some benefit, but combination therapy needs further study.[271] Finally, three-drug regimens have occasionally been reported with a polyene, an azole, and flucytosine, but the added benefit of a three-drug regimen has not been proven.

A standard algorithm for the management of cryptococcal meningitis in patients with HIV is a three-stage regimen.[253] Induction phase treatment is initiated with amphotericin B, 0.7 mg/kg/day, plus flucytosine, 100 mg/kg/day, for at least 2 weeks. Patients who have responded clinically may be switched to fluconazole, 400 to 800 mg/day for 8 to 10 weeks, as a consolidation phase. Finally, a suppressive phase is begun with fluconazole, 200 mg once daily. The use of suppressive or maintenance phase therapy for cryptococcal meningitis became a concept during the pre-HAART AIDS epidemic, when 50% to 60% of patients relapsed after therapy was stopped. With the use of fluconazole daily, suppression was better than that obtained with intermittent amphotericin B or itraconazole, and there was a reduction in the relapse rate to less than 5%.[264,265] Data from several studies have shown that administration of HAART, with its ability to produce immune reconstitution (rising CD4 counts and lower HIV loads), allows antifungal therapy to be stopped after 1 to 2 years in patients with a CD4 count above 100/μL for at least 3 months, nondetectable viral load, and negative serum cryptococcal antigen.[272,273]

Patients without AIDS can be given either a 4-week induction phase regimen of amphotericin B, with or without initial flucytosine or, more commonly, the above regimen for AIDS patients. If induction therapy included only a polyene, this phase should be extended at least another 2 weeks. If this is a transplant recipient with known renal toxicity issues, a lipid polyene substitution is favored. Patients then receive a consolidation phase of fluconazole, 400 to 800 mg for 8 weeks, and finally placed on suppressive doses of fluconazole, 200 mg/day. Criteria for stopping therapy are not well defined but include resolution of symptoms, at least two negative CSF cultures from several milliliters of CSF, and a normal CSF glucose level. A negative CSF or serum cryptococcal antigen, or a normal CSF, does not appear to be required to discontinue therapy. Patients with continuing immunosuppression may benefit from prolonged fluconazole therapy after these criteria are met because relapse rates are substantial. Because there was a 15% to

25% relapse rate, primarily in the first year after stopping therapy, before the AIDS epidemic, most patients will receive 6 to 12 months of suppressive fluconazole therapy.

The site of infection may modify the treatment recommendation.[231] Any presentation of disseminated cryptococcosis should probably follow the recommendations for cryptococcal meningitis. On the other hand, cryptococcosis confined to the lung in previously healthy persons responds well to fluconazole, 200 to 400 mg/day for 3 to 6 months.[51,260,261] Patients who are nonimmunosuppressed, with endobronchial colonization but without radiologic evidence of pulmonary parenchymal disease, do not require antifungal treatment. However, if the patient is symptomatic, immunocompromised, or at risk for immunosuppression, treatment should be started. CNS cryptococcomas tend to be treated for longer periods with fluconazole, but they rarely need surgical removal.[274] MRI scans of the brain may not show a decrease in lesion size for many months. Edema around a lesion, if present, decreases more rapidly.[230]

Identifying a relapse or persistence can be difficult in patients with cryptococcal infections. The two clearest signs of relapse after at least 4 weeks of an established antifungal regimen that suggest a change in management are development of new clinical signs and symptoms and repeat positive cultures. The persistence of a positive India ink examination or changing versus fixed polysaccharide antigen titers are not precise indications of relapse. An immune reconstitution syndrome in cryptococcosis has been described.[164] It is marked by a rapid return of an inflammatory response that may produce new symptoms such as fever, headaches with or without increasing intracranial pressure, and increased number of host cells in the CSF. This syndrome may occur from several weeks to months to a year after beginning HAART or after immunosuppressive dose reduction in transplant recipients. It is still not certain when it is best to initiate HAART during the treatment of cryptococcal meningitis to prevent this syndrome but recommendations range from 2 to 10 weeks after the initiation of antifungal therapy. It is important to recognize that this syndrome is not an indication of direct antifungal failure and might be improved with corticosteroid therapy in seriously ill patients with CNS disease.

A critical management issue in cryptococcal meningitis is the role of increased intracranial pressure.[275,276] Patients with severe infection often present with CSF opening pressures in excess of 250 mm of CSF and rapidly progressing signs of cerebral edema. Symptoms include confusion, somnolence, severe headache, emesis, cranial nerve palsies, and fading vision. The pathophysiology for this elevated subarachnoid pressure, even as antifungal treatment is started, remains uncertain, but cerebral edema is obvious at autopsy, with uncal grooving, midbrain compression, and herniation of the cerebellar tonsils. Control of increased intracranial pressures with external drainage, such as by repeated lumbar punctures with large-bore needles and ventricular or lumbar drains, may be necessary during the early treatment phase.[277] Persistent, symptomatic, high CSF pressures may warrant placement of a permanent CSF shunt. In a retrospective review, corticosteroid treatment without IRIS was not found to be generally useful,[275] but cases need to be examined on an individual basis. Unfortunately, despite intervention, blindness, permanent dementia, or death may result.

It is vital to distinguish cerebral edema from hydrocephalus. The latter is diagnosed by the presence of dilated cerebral ventricles and dementia, with or without gait ataxia or urinary incontinence. CSF pressure may or may not be elevated. A loculated temporal horn of the lateral cerebral ventricle may present as a space-filling mass and cause transfalciform herniation. Symptoms of hydrocephalus need to be identified in the follow-up period and can occur months after the initial diagnosis. A shunt for hydrocephalus can be placed successfully during effective therapy for cryptococcal meningitis.[229,278] There is nothing to suggest that shunt placement after institution of antifungal therapy presents a foreign body that impairs cure, but it needs to be placed after the start of appropriate antifungal regimen.

Every attempt to improve the immunity of the patient with cryptococcosis should be made. For example, a goal is to reduce the daily dose of prednisone to 20 mg/day or less during therapy. Adjunctive cytokine therapies, such as with granulocyte colony-stimulating factor (G-CSF), GM-CSF, and interferon-γ, have in vitro support, and phase 2 human studies with interferon-γ as adjunctive therapy encountered no serious toxicity.[279] However, clinical trials of immunomodulation for management of cryptococcosis await further definitive studies and must be aware of the potential for causing IRIS. At present, they should probably be used as adjunctive therapies for refractory cases. A single dose trial of a murine monoclonal antibody to cryptococcal capsular antigen was inconclusive.[143] Finally, HAART has a major influence on improving immunity and has made a significant impact on a patient's long-term prognosis for cryptococcal meningitis.[280] HAART should be instituted and monitored in all HIV-infected patients during treatment for cryptococcal meningitis. It is essential to gain control of the HIV infection for long-term success.

Prognosis

The most important prognostic factor for success in the treatment of cryptococcosis remains the ability to control the patient's underlying disease. It has been shown that cancer victims have shorter survival than patients with AIDS because of the inability to control their underlying neoplasm.[281] In another major group of patients with cryptococcosis, those who received solid organ transplants, the results are conflicting. Some studies have shown an outcome similar to that of patients without an underlying disease,[51] but another study reported a death rate of 42%.[71]

Several studies have examined the prognostic features of cryptococcal meningitis.[243,252,282,283] A summary of the different populations, treatment modalities, and end point evaluations has suggested that there are two major prognostic findings: (1) burden of yeasts at presentation; and (2) level of the patient's sensorium at presentation. For example, a poor prognosis is indicated by a strongly positive India ink examination, a high polysaccharide antigen titer (1 : 1024), and a poor inflammatory response in the CSF (less than 20 cells/μL). In one cohort, cryptococcosis was more severe in males, HIV-seropositive patients, and those with serotype A infection.[283] Patients who present with a lucid sensorium have a better prognosis than those who are stuporous or in a coma, and abnormal brain imaging at baseline is associated with reduced survival. The prognosis is also influenced by the ability to manage the underlying disease and to detect and treat elevated intracranial pressure. For example, very poor prognostic underlying conditions are severe liver disease and cryptococcosis or a hematologic malignancy. Identification of these high-risk patients so that failure and relapse can be predicted may allow the clinician to design a specific antifungal regimen for this refractory subset. In most cases in developed countries, the immediate mortality rate (at 6 to 12 months) of cryptococcal meningitis unfortunately still remains at 10% to 25%[284] and, in undeveloped countries with limited resources, the mortality rate at 6 months reaches 100%.[232]

Prevention

There are four potential methods for preventing infection in high-risk patients. First, in the pre-HAART era, fluconazole prophylaxis in patients with AIDS and CD4 counts under 100 cells/μL has been shown to be effective in reducing the incidence of cryptococcosis.[285-287] However, both the use of HAART and concern about drug resistance with its widespread use have reduced enthusiasm for this approach. Second, active immunization with a vaccine in high-risk patients has been considered. A cryptococcal GXM–tetanus toxoid conjugate vaccine was developed that protected mice,[288] and several new potential protective antigens have been identified. However, human trials have not yet been conducted, and the use of a vaccine in nonimmunosuppressed populations with potential risk factors for disease are hard to define. Third, the use of protective serotherapy with specific monoclonal antibodies[289,290] could be attempted in high-risk patients, but protection would require repeated injections. Finally, high-risk patients can attempt to avoid high-risk environments, such as sites where high numbers of yeasts might be aerosolized from bird droppings.

REFERENCES

1. Perfect JR, Casadevall A. Cryptococcosis. *Infect Dis Clin North Am.* 2002;16:837-874.
2. Sanfelice F. [Contributo alla morfologia e biologia dei blastomiceti che si sviluppano nei succhi di alcuni frutti.] *Ann d'Igiene.* 1894;4:463-495.
3. Buschke A. [Ueber eine durch coccidien hervorgerufene krankheit des menschen.] *Dtsch Med Wochenschr.* 1895;21:14.
4. Versé M. [Über einen Fall von generalisierter Blastomykose beim Menschen.] *Ver Dtsch Path Ges.* 1914;17:275-278.
5. Stoddard JL, Cutler EC. Torula infections in man. *Rockefeller Inst Med Res.* 1916;Monograph 6:1-98.
6. Benham RW. Cryptococcosis and blastomycosis. *Ann N Y Acad Sci.* 1950;50:1299-1314.
7. Kwon-Chung KJ. Morphogenesis of *Filobasidiella neoformans,* the sexual state of *Cryptococcus neoformans. Mycologia.* 1976;68:821-833.
8. Kwon-Chung KJ, Boekhout T, Fell JW, et al. Proposal to conserve the name *Cryptococcus gattii* against *C. hondurianus* and *C. bacillisporus* (*Basidiomycota, Hymenomycetes, Tremellomycetidae*). *Taxon.* 2002;51:804-806.
9. van Duin D, Casadevall A, Nosanchuk JD. Melanization of *Cryptococcus neoformans* and *Histoplasma capsulatum* reduces their susceptibilities to amphotericin B and caspofungin. *Antimicrob Agents Chemother.* 2002;46:3394-3400.
10. Xue C, Tada Y, Dong X, et al. The human fungal pathogen *Cryptococcus* can complete its sexual cycle during a pathogenic association with plants. *Cell Host Microbe.* 2007;14;1:263-273.
11. Hull C, Heitman J. Genetics of *Cryptococcus neoformans. Ann Rev Genet.* 2002;36:557-615.
12. Kwon-Chung KJ, Bennett JE. Distribution of "alpha" and "a" mating types of *Cryptococcus neoformans* among natural and clinical isolates. *Am J Med.* 1978;108:337-340.
13. Wickes BL, Mayorga ME, Edman U, et al. Dimorphism and haploid fruiting in *Cryptococcus neoformans:* Association with the alpha-mating type. *Proc Natl Acad Sci U S A.* 1996;93:7327-7331.
14. Lin X, Hull CM, Heitman J. Sexual reproduction between partners of the same mating type in *Cryptococcus neoformans. Nature.* 2005;434:1017-1021.
15. Kwon-Chung KJ, Edman JC, Wickes BL. Genetic association of mating types and virulence in *Cryptococcus neoformans. Infect Immun.* 1992;60:602-605.
16. Nielsen K, Cox GM, Wang P, et al. Sexual cycle of *Cryptococcus neoformans* variety *grubii* and virulence of congenic a and alpha isolates. *Infect Immun.* 2003;71:4831-4841.
17. Fraser JA, Giles SS, Wenink EC, et al. Same-sex mating and the origin of the Vancouver Island Cryptococcus gattii outbreak. *Nature.* 2005;437:1360-1364.
18. Luna J, Lusins J. Cryptococcus albidus meningitis. *South Med J.* 1973;66:1230.
19. Kromery V, Kunova A, Mardiak J. Nosocomial *Cryptococcus laurentii* fungemia in a bone marrow transplant patient after prophylaxis with ketoconazole successfully treated with oral fluconazole. *Infection.* 1997;25:130.
20. Ikeda R, Shinoda T, Fukuzawa Y, et al. Antigenic characterization of *Cryptococcus neoformans* serotypes and its application to serotyping of clinical isolates. *J Clin Microbiol.* 1982;36:22-29.
21. Dromer F, Gueho E, Ronin O, et al. Serotyping of *Cryptococcus neoformans* by using a monoclonal antibody specific for capsular polysaccharide. *J Clin Microbiol.* 1993;31:359-363.
22. Cleare W, Casadevall A. The different binding patterns of two IgM monoclonal antibodies to *Cryptococcus neoformans* serotype A and D strains correlates with serotype classification and differences in functional assays. *Clin Diagn Lab Immunol.* 1998;5:125-129.
23. Franzot SP, Salkin IF, Casadevall A. *Cryptococcus neoformans* var. *grubii:* Separate variety status for *Cryptococcus neoformans* serotype A isolates. *J Clin Microbiol.* 1999;37:838-840.
24. Xu J, Vilgalys R, Mitchell TG. Multiple gene genealogies reveal recent dispersion and hybridization in the human fungus, *Cryptococcus neoformans. Mol Ecol.* 2002;9:1471-1481.
25. Perfect JR, Durack DT, Gallis HA. Cryptococcemia. *Medicine.* 1983;62:98-109.
26. Goldman DL, Fries BC, Franzot SP, et al. Phenotypic switching in the human pathogenic fungus, *Cryptococcus neoformans,* is associated with changes in virulence and pulmonary inflammatory response in rodents. *Proc Natl Acad Sci U S A.* 1998;95:14967-14972.
27. Fries BC, Goldman DL, Casadevall A. Phenotypic switching in *Cryptococcus neoformans. Microbiol Infect Dis.* 2002;4:1345-1353.
28. Martinez LR, Garcia-Rivera J, Casadevall A. *Cryptococcus neoformans* var. *neoformans* (serotype D) strains are more susceptible to heat than *C. neoformans* var. *grubii* (serotype A strains). *J Clin Microbiol.* 2001;39:3365-3367.
29. el-Zaatari M, Pasarell L, McGinnis MR, et al. Evaluation of the updated Vitek yeast identification data base. *J Clin Microbiol.* 1990;28:1938-1941.
30. St. Germain G, Beauchesne D. Evaluation of the microscan rapid yeast identification panel. *J Clin Microbiol.* 1991;29:2296-2299.
31. Zimmer BL, Roberts GD. Rapid selective urease test for presumptive identification of *Cryptococcus neoformans. J Clin Microbiol.* 1979;10:380-381.
32. Langfelder K, Streibel M, John B, et al. Biosynthesis of fungal melanins and their importance for human pathogenic fungi. *Fungal Genet Biol.* 2003;38:143-158.
33. Meyer W, Castaneda A, Jackson S, et al. Molecular typing of Ibero American *Cryptococcus neoformans* isolates. *Emerg Infect Dis.* 2003;9:189-195.
34. Levitz SM. The ecology of *Cryptococcus neoformans* and the epidemiology of cryptococcosis. *Rev Infect Dis.* 1991;13:1163-1169.
35. Emmons CW. Isolation of *Cryptococcus neoformans* from soil. *J Bacteriol.* 1951;62:685-690.
36. Emmons CW. Saprophytic sources of *Cryptococcus neoformans* associated with the pigeon. *Am J Hyg.* 1955;62:227-232.
37. Ellis DH, Pfeiffer TJ. Ecology, life cycle, and infectious propagule of *Cryptococcus neoformans. Lancet.* 1990;336:923-925.
38. Stephen C, Lester S, Black W, et al. Multispecies outbreak cryptococcosis on southern Vancouver Island, British Columbia. *Can J Vet Res.* 2002;43:792-794.
39. Steenbergen JN, Shuman HA, Casadevall A. *Cryptococcus neoformans* interactions with amoebae suggest an explanation for its virulence and intracellular pathogenic strategy in macrophages. *Proc Natl Acad Sci.* 2001;98:15245-15250.
40. Mylonakis E, Casadevall A, Ausubel FM. Exploiting amoeboid and non-vertebrate animal model systems to study the virulence of human pathogenic fungi. *PLoS Pathog.* 2007;3:e101.
41. Mylonakis E, Ausubel FM, Perfect JR, et al. Killing of Caenorhabditis elegans by *Cryptococcus neoformans* as a model of yeast pathogenesis. *Proc Natl Acad Sci U S A.* 2002;99:15675-15680.
42. Howard DH. The commensalism of *Cryptococcus neoformans. Sabouraudia.* 1973;11:171-174.

43. Schimpff SC, Bennett JE. Abnormalities in cell-mediated immunity in patients with *Cryptococcus neoformans* infection. *J Allergy Clin Immunol.* 1975;55:430-441.
44. Newberry WM Jr, Walter JE, Chandler JW Jr, et al. Epidemiologic study of *Cryptococcus neoformans. Ann Intern Med.* 1967;67:724-732.
45. Chen L-C, Goldman DL, Doering TL. Antibody response to *Cryptococcus neoformans* proteins in rodents and humans. *Infect Immun.* 1999;67:2218-2224.
46. Goldman DL, Khine H, Abadi J. Serologic evidence for *Cryptococcus* infection in early childhood. *Pediatrics.* 2001;107:66.
47. Davis J, Zheng WY, Glatman-Freedman A, et al. Serologic evidence for regional differences in pediatric cryptococcal infection. *Pediatr Infect Dis J.* 2007;26:549-551.
48. Zonios DI, Falloon J, Huang CY, et al. Cryptococcosis and idiopathic CD4 lymphocytopenia. *Medicine (Baltimore).* 2007;86:78-92.
49. Nath DS, Kandaswamy R, Gruessner R, et al. Fungal infections in transplant recipients receiving alemtuzumab. *Transplant Proc.* 2005;37:934-936.
50. Tsiodras S, Samonis G, Boumpas DT, et al. Fungal infections complicating tumor necrosis factor alpha blockade therapy. *Mayo Clin Proc.* 2008;83:181-194.
51. Pappas PG, Perfect JR, Cloud GA, et al. Cryptococcosis in HIV-negative patients in the era of effective azole therapy. *Clin Infect Dis.* 2001;33:690-699.
52. Hajjman A, Conn LA, Stephens DS. Cryptococcosis: Population-based multistate active surveillance and risk factors in human immunodeficiency virus-infected persons. Cryptococcal Active Surveillance Group. *J Infect Dis.* 1999;179:449-454.
53. McNeil JI, Kan VL. Decline in the incidence of cryptococcosis among HIV-related patients. *J Acquir Immune Defic Syndr Hum Retrovirol.* 1995;9:206-208.
54. van Elden LJ, Walenkamp AM, Lipovsky MM. Declining number of patients with cryptococcosis in the Netherlands in the era of highly active antiretroviral therapy. *AIDS.* 2000;14:2787-2788.
55. Mirza S, Phelan M, Rimland D, et al. The changing epidemiology of cryptococcosis: An update from population-based active surveillance in 2 large metropolitan areas, 1992-2000. *Clin Infect Dis.* 2002;36:789-794.
56. Clumeck N, Sonnet J, Taelman H, et al. Acquired immunodeficiency syndrome in African patients. *N Engl J Med.* 1984;310:492-497.
57. Van de Perre P, Lepage P, Kestelyn P. Acquired immunodeficiency syndrome in Rwanda. *Lancet.* 1984;2:62-65.
58. McCarthy KM, Morgan J, Wannemuehler KA, et al. Population-based surveillance for cryptococcosis in an antiretroviral-naive South African province with a high HIV seroprevalence. *AIDS.* 2006;20:2199-2206.
59. Hakim JG, Gangaidzo IT, Heyderman RS. Impact of HIV infection on meningitis in Harare, Zimbabwe: A prospective study of 406 predominantly adult patients. *AIDS.* 2000;14:1401-1407.
60. Dore GJ, Li Y, McDonald A, et al. Spectrum of AIDS-defining illnesses in Australia, 1992 to 1998: Influence of country/region of birth. *J Acquir Immune Defic Syndr.* 2000;26:283-290.
61. Archibald LK, McDonald LC, Rheanpumikankit S. Fever and human immunodeficiency virus infection as sentinels for emerging mycobacterial and fungal bloodstream infections in hospitalized patients >15 years old, Bangkok. *J Infect Dis.* 1999;180:87-92.
62. Kwon-Chung KJ, Bennett JE. Epidemiologic differences between the two varieties of *Cryptococcus neoformans. Am J Epidemiol.* 1984;120:123-140.
63. Bennett JE, Kwon-Chung KJ, Howard DH. Epidemiology differences among serotypes of *Cryptococcus neoformans. Am J Epidemiol.* 1977;105:582-586.
64. Steenbergen JN, Casadevall A. Prevalence of *Cryptococcus neoformans* var *neoformans* (serotype D) and *Cryptococcus neoformans* var. *grubii* (serotype A) isolates in New York City. *J Clin Microbiol.* 2000;38:1974-1976.
65. Morgan J, McCarthy KM, Gould S, et al. *Cryptococcus gattii* infection: Characteristics and epidemiology of cases identified in a South African province with high HIV seroprevalence, 2002-2004. *Clin Infect Dis.* 2006;43:1077-1080.
66. Collins VP, Gellhorn A, Trimble JR. The coincidence of cryptococcosis and disease of the reticulo-endothelial and lymphatic systems. *Cancer.* 1995;4:883-889.
67. Zimmerman LE, Rappaport H. Occurrence of cryptococcosis in patients with malignant disease of reticuloendothelial system. *Am J Clin Pathol.* 1954;24:1050.
68. Kaplan MH, Rosen PP, Armstrong D. Cryptococcus in a cancer hospital: Clinical and pathological correlates in forty-six patients. *Cancer.* 1977;39:2265-2274.
69. Hutter RVP, Collins HS. The occurrence of opportunistic fungus infections in a cancer hospital. *Lab Invest.* 1962;11:1035-1045.
70. Kontoyiannis DP, Peitsch WK, Reddy BT. Cryptococcosis in patients with cancer. *Clin Infect Dis.* 2001;32:145-150.
71. Husain A, Wagener MM, Singh N. *Cryptococcus neoformans* infection in organ transplant recipients: Variables influencing clinical characteristics and outcome. *Emerg Infect Dis.* 2001;7:375-381.
72. Singh N, Gayowski T, Wagener MM, et al. Clinical spectrum of invasive cryptococcosis in liver transplant recipients receiving tacrolimus. *Clin Transpl.* 1997;11:66-70.
73. Beyt BE, Waltman SR. Cryptococcal endophthalmitis after corneal transplantation. *N Engl J Med.* 1978;298:825-826.
74. Kanj SS, Welty-Wolf K, Madden J, et al. Fungal infections in lung and heart-lung transplant recipients, report of 9 cases and review of the literature. *Medicine.* 1996;75:142-156.
75. Ooi BS, Chen BT, Lim CH, et al. Survival of a patient transplanted with a kidney infected with *Cryptococcus neoformans. Transplantation.* 1971;11:428-429.
76. Iseki M, Anzo M, Yamashita N, et al. Hyper-IgM immunodeficiency with disseminated cryptococcosis. *Acta Paediatr.* 1994;83:780-782.
77. Tabone MD, Leverger G, Landman J, et al. Disseminated lymphonodular cryptococcosis in a child with x-linked hyper-IgM immunodeficiency. *Pediatr Infect Dis J.* 1994;13:77-79.
78. Dev D, Basran GS, Slater D. Consider HIV negative immunodeficiency in cryptococcosis. *BMJ.* 1994;308:1436.
79. Olson PE, Earhart KC, Rossetti RJ. Smoking and risk of cryptococcosis in patients with AIDS. *JAMA.* 1997;277:629.
80. Casadevall AJ, Mukherjee J, Ruong R, et al. Management of *Cryptococcus neoformans* contaminated needle injuries. *Clin Infect Dis.* 1994;19:951-953.
81. Glaser JB, Garden A. Inoculation of cryptococcosis without transmission of the acquired immunodeficiency syndrome. *N Engl J Med.* 1985;313:264.
82. Powell KE, Dahl BA, Weeks RJ, et al. Airborne *Cryptococcus neoformans*: Particles from pigeon excreta compatible with alveolar deposition. *J Infect Dis.* 1972;126:412-415.
83. Wiest PM, Flanigan T, Salata RA, et al. Serious infectious complications of corticosteroid therapy for COPD. *Chest.* 1989;95:1180-1183.
84. Ruiz A, Bulmer GS. Particle size of airborne *Cryptococcus neoformans* in a tower. *Appl Environ Microbiol.* 1980;41:1225-1229.
85. Sorrell TC, Chen S, Ruma P, et al. Concordance of clinical and environmental isolates of *Cryptococcus neoformans* var. *gattii* by random amplification of polymorphic DNA analysis and PCR fingerprinting. *J Clin Microbiol.* 1996;34:1253-1260.
86. Currie BP, Freundlich LF, Casadevall A. Restriction fragment length polymorphism analysis of *Cryptococcus neoformans* isolates from environmental (pigeon excreta) and clinical sources in New York City. *J Clin Microbiol.* 1994;32:1188-1192.
87. Yamamoto Y, Kohno S, Koga H, et al. Random amplified polymorphic DNA analysis of clinically and environmentally isolated *Cryptococcus neoformans* in Nagasaki. *J Clin Microbiol.* 1995;33:3328-3332.
88. Sorvillo F, Beall G, Turner PA. Incidence and factors associated with extrapulmonary cryptococcosis among persons with HIV infection in Los Angeles County. *AIDS.* 1997;11:673-679.
89. Faggi E, Gargani G, Pizzirani C, et al. Cryptococcosis in domestic mammals. *Mycoses.* 1993;36:165-170.
90. Malik R, Dill-Mackey E, Martin P, et al. Cryptococcosis in dogs: A retrospective study of 20 consecutive cases. *J Med Vet Mycol.* 1995;33:291-297.
91. Malik R, Wigney DI, Muir DB, et al. Cryptococcosis in cats: Clinical and mycological assessment of 29 cases and evaluation of treatment using orally administered fluconazole. *J Med Vet Mycol.* 1992;30:133-144.
92. Nosanchuk JD, Shoham S, Fries BC, et al. Evidence for zoonotic transmission of *Cryptococcus neoformans* from a pet cockatoo to an immunocompromised patient. *Ann Intern Med.* 2000;132:205-208.
93. Fessel WJ. Cryptococcal meningitis after unusual exposures to birds. *N Engl J Med.* 1993;328:1354-1355.
94. Perfect JR. *Cryptococcus neoformans*: A sugar-coated killer with designer genes. *FEMS Immunol Med Microbiol.* 2005;45:395-404.
95. Del Poeta M, Toffaletti DL, Rude TH, et al. *Cryptococcus neoformans* differential gene expression detected *in vitro* and *in vivo* with green fluorescent protein. *Infect Immun.* 1999;67:1812-1820.
96. Chow ED, Liu OW, O'Brien S, et al. Exploration of whole-genome responses of the human AIDS-associated yeast pathogen Cryptococcus neoformans var grubii: nitric oxide stress and body temperature. *Curr Genet.* 2007;52:137-148.
97. Chang YC, Kwon-Chung KJ. Complementation of a capsule-deficiency mutation of *Cryptococcus neoformans* restores its virulence. *Mol Cell Biol.* 1994;14:4912-4919.
98. Casadevall A, Perfect JR. *Cryptococcus neoformans.* Washington: ASM Press; 1998:409.
99. Zaragoza O, Chrisman CJ, Castelli MV, et al. Capsule enlargement in *Cryptococcus neoformans* confers resistance to oxidative stress suggesting a mechanism for intracellular survival. *Cell Microbiol.* 2008;10:2043-2057.
100. Klutts JS, Doering TL. Cryptococcal xylosyltransferase 1 (Cxt1p) from Cryptococcus neoformans plays a direct role in the synthesis of capsule polysaccharides. *J Biol Chem.* 2008 May 23;283(21):14327-14334.
101. Alspaugh JA, Perfect JR, Heitman J. *Cryptococcus neoformans* mating and virulence are regulated by the G-protein gamma subunit GPA1 and cAMP. *Genes Dev.* 1997;11:3206-3217.
102. Salas SD, Bennett JE, Kwon-Chung KJ, et al. Effect of the laccase gene, CNLAC1, on virulence of *Cryptococcus neoformans. J Exp Med.* 1996;184:377-386.
103. Nosanchuk JD, Rosas AL, Lee SC. Melanisation of *Cryptococcus neoformans* in human brain tissue. *Lancet.* 2000;355:2049-2050.
104. Rosas AL, Nosanchuk JD, Feldmesser M. Synthesis of polymerized melanin by *Cryptococcus neoformans* in infected rodents. *Infect Immun.* 2000;68:2845-2853.
105. Odom A, Muir S, Lim E, et al. Calcineurin is required for virulence of *Cryptococcus neoformans. EMBO J.* 1997;16:2576-2589.
106. Alspaugh JA, Cavallo LM, Perfect JR, et al. *RAS1* regulates filamentation, mating, and growth at high temperature of *Cryptococcus neoformans. Mol Microbiol.* 2000;36:352-365.
107. Erickson T, Liu L, Gueylkian A, et al. Multiple virulence factors of *Cryptococcus neoformans* are dependent on VPH1. *Mol Microbiol.* 2001;42:1121-1131.
108. Perfect JR. *Cryptococcus neoformans:* The yeast that likes it hot. *FEMS Yeast Res.* 2006;6:463-468.
109. Cox GM, McDade HC, Chen SC, et al. Extracellular phospholipase activity is a virulence factor for *Cryptococcus neoformans. Mol Microbiol.* 2001;39:166-175.
110. Cox GM, Mukherjee J, Cole GT, et al. Urease as a virulence factor in experimental cryptococcosis. *Infect Immun.* 2000;68:443-448.
111. Del Poeta M, Cruz MC, Cardenas ME, et al. Synergistic antifungal activities of bafilomycin A(1), fluconazole, and the pneumocandin MK-0991/caspofungin acetate (L-743,873) with calcineurin inhibitors FK506 and L-685,818 against *Cryptococcus neoformans. Antimicrob Agents Chemother.* 2000;44:739-746.
112. Murphy JW. Cryptococcal immunity and immunostimulation. *Adv Exp Med Biol.* 1992;319:225-230.
113. Levitz SM. Overview of host defenses in fungal infections. *Clin Infect Dis.* 1992;14:S37-S42.
114. Schwartz DA. Characterization of the biological activity of *Cryptococcus* infections in surgical pathology. *Ann Clin Lab Sci.* 1988;18:388-397.
115. Lipscomb MF. Lung defenses against opportunistic infections. *Chest.* 1989;96:1393-1399.
116. Lee SC, Dickson DW, Casadevall A. Pathology of cryptococcal meningoencephalitis: Analysis of 27 patients with pathogenetic implications. *Hum Pathol.* 1996;27:839-847.
117. Aguirre K, Havell EA, Gibson GW, et al. Role of tumor necrosis factor and gamma interferon in acquired resistance to *Cryptococcus neoformans* in the central nervous system of mice. *Infect Immun.* 1995;63:1725-1731.
118. Kawakami K, Tohyama M, Teruya K. Contribution of interferon-gamma in protecting mice during pulmonary and disseminated infection with *Cryptococcus neoformans. FEMS Immunol Med Microbiol.* 1996;13:133-140.
119. Huffnagle GB, Strieter RM, McNeil LK. Macrophage inflammatory protein-1 alpha (MIP-alpha) is required for the efferent phase of pulmonary cell-mediated immunity to a *Cryptococcus neoformans* infection. *J Immunol.* 1997;159:318-327.
120. Huffnagle GB, Traynor TR, McDonald RA. Leukocyte recruitment during pulmonary *Cryptococcus neoformans* infection. *Immunopharmacology.* 2000;48:231-236.
121. Hill JO. CD4+ T cells cause multinucleated giant cells to form around *Cryptococcus neoformans* and confine the yeast within the primary site of infection in the respiratory tract. *J Exp Med.* 1992;175:1685-1695.
122. Levitz SM. Macrophage-*Cryptococcus* interactions. In: Zwilling BS, Eisenstein TK, eds. *Macrophage-Pathogen Interactions.* New York: Marcel Dekker; 1994:533-543.
123. Alvarez M, Casadevall A. Cell-to-cell spread and massive vacuole formation after Cryptococcus neoformans infection of murine macrophages. *BMC Immunol.* 2007;8:16.
124. Feldmesser M, Kress Y, Novikoff P, et al. *Cryptococcus neoformans* is a facultative intracellular pathogen in murine pulmonary infection. *Infect Immun.* 2000;68:4225-4237.
125. Feldmesser M, Tucker SC, Casadevall A. Intracellular parasitism of macrophages by *Cryptococcus neoformans. Trends Microbiol.* 2001;9:273-278.
126. Crowe SM, Carlin JB, Stewart KI, et al. Predictive value of CD4 lymphocyte numbers for the development of opportunistic infections and malignancies in HIV-infected persons. *J Acquir Immune Defic Syndr.* 1991;4:770-776.
127. Giles SS, Zaas AK, Reidy MF, et al. Cryptococcus neoformans is resistant to surfactant protein A mediated host defense mechanisms. *PLoS ONE.* 2007;2:e1370.
128. Nakamura K, Kinjo T, Saijo S, et al. Dectin-1 is not required for the host defense to Cryptococcus neoformans. *Microbiol Immunol.* 2007;51:1115-1119.
129. Nakamura K, Miyagi K, Koguchi Y, et al. Limited contribution of Toll-like receptor 2 and 4 to the host response to a fungal infectious pathogen, Cryptococcus neoformans. *FEMS Immunol Med Microbiol* 2006;47:148-154.
130. Meletiadis J, Walsh TJ, Choi EH, et al. Study of common functional genetic polymorphisms of FCGR2A, 3A and 3B genes and the risk for cryptococcosis in HIV-uninfected patients. *Med Mycol.* 2007;45:513-518.
131. Henderson DK, Bennett JE, Huber MA. Long-lasting specific immunologic unresponsiveness associated with cryptococcal meningitis. *J Clin Invest.* 1982;69:1185-1190.
132. Wong B, Perfect JR, Beggs S, et al. Production of the hexitol D-mannitol by *Cryptococcus neoformans* in vitro and in rabbits with experimental meningitis. *Infect Immun.* 1990;58:1664-1670.
133. Williamson PR. Biochemical and molecular characterization of the diphenol oxidase of *Cryptococcus neoformans*: Identification as a laccase. *J Bacteriol.* 1994;176:656-664.

134. Noverr MC, Phare SM, Toews GB, et al. Pathogenic yeasts *Cryptococcus neoformans* and *Candida albicans* produce immunomodulatory prostaglandins. *Infect Immun.* 2001;69:2957-2963.
135. Vecchiarelli A, Casadevall A. Antibody-mediated effects against *Cryptococcus neoformans*: Evidence for interdependency and collaboration between humoral and cellular immunity. *Res Immunol.* 1998;149:321-333.
136. Mukherjee J, Sharff MD, Casadevall A. Protective murine monoclonal antibodies to *Cryptococcus neoformans*. *Infect Immun.* 1992;60:4534-4541.
137. Sanford JE, Lupan DM, Schlageter AM, et al. Passive immunization against *Cryptococcus neoformans* with an isotype-switch family of monoclonal antibodies reactive with cryptococcal polysaccharide. *Infect Immun.* 1990;58:1919-1923.
138. Dromer F, Charreire J, Contrepois A, et al. Protection of mice against experimental cryptococcosis by anti-*Cryptococcus neoformans* monoclonal antibody. *Infect Immun.* 1987;55:749-752.
139. Casadevall A. Antibody immunity and invasive fungal infections. *Infect Immun.* 1995;63:4211-4218.
140. Rosas AL, Nosanchuk JD, Casadevall A. Passive immunization with melanin-binding monoclonal antibodies prolongs survival in mice with lethal *Cryptococcus neoformans* infection. *Infect Immun.* 2001;69:3410-3412.
141. Rodrigues ML, Travassos LR, Miranda KR. Human antibodies against a purified glucosylceramide from *Cryptococcus neoformans* inhibit cell budding and fungal growth. *Infect Immun.* 2000;68:7049-7060.
142. Fleuridor R, Lyles RH, Pirofski L. Quantitative and qualitative differences in the serum antibody profiles of human immunodeficiency virus-infected persons with and without *Cryptococcus neoformans* meningitis. *J Infect Dis.* 1999;180:1526-1535.
143. Larsen RA, Pappas PG, Perfect J, et al. Phase I evaluation of the safety and pharmacokinetics of murine-derived anticryptococcal antibody 18B7 in subjects with treated cryptococcal meningitis. *Antimicrob Agents Chemother.* 2005;49:952-958.
144. Baker RD. The primary pulmonary lymph node complex of cryptococcosis. *Am J Clin Pathol.* 1976;65:83-92.
145. Salyer WR, Salyer DC, Baker RD. Primary complex of *Cryptococcus* and pulmonary lymph nodes. *J Infect Dis.* 1974;130:74-77.
146. Garcia-Hermoso D, Janbon G, Dromer F. Epidemiological evidence for dormant *Cryptococcus neoformans* infection. *J Clin Microbiol.* 1999;37:3204-3209.
147. Perfect JR. Cryptococcosis. *Infect Dis Clin North Am.* 1989;3:77-102.
148. Kovacs JA, Kovacs AA, Polis M, et al. Cryptococcosis in the acquired immunodeficiency syndrome. *Ann Intern Med.* 1985;103:533-538.
149. Zuger A, Louie E, Holzman RS, et al. Cryptococcal disease in patients with acquired immunodeficiency syndrome: Diagnostic features and outcome of treatment. *Ann Intern Med.* 1986;104:234-240.
150. Chuck SL, Sande MA. Infections with *Cryptococcus neoformans* in the acquired immunodeficiency syndrome. *N Engl J Med.* 1989;321:794-799.
151. Clark RA, Greer D, Atkinson W, et al. Spectrum of *Cryptococcus neoformans* infection in 68 patients infected with acquired immunodeficiency virus. *Rev Infect Dis.* 1990;12:768-777.
152. Duperval R, Hermans PE, Brewer NS, et al. Cryptococcosis, with emphasis on the significance of isolation of *Cryptococcus neoformans* from the respiratory tract. *Chest.* 1977;72:13-19.
153. Henson DJ, Hill AR. Cryptococcal pneumonia: A fulminant presentation. *Am J Med.* 1984;228:221.
154. Kent TH, Layton JM. Massive pulmonary cryptococcosis. *Am J Clin Pathol.* 1962;38:596-604.
155. Murray RJ, Becker P, Furth P, et al. Recovery from cryptococcemia and the adult respiratory distress syndrome in the acquired immunodeficiency syndrome. *Chest.* 1988;93:1304-1307.
156. Warr W, Bates JH, Stone A. The spectrum of pulmonary cryptococcosis. *Ann Intern Med.* 1968;69:1109-1116.
157. Kahn FW, England DM, Jones JM. Solitary pulmonary nodule due to *Cryptococcus neoformans* and *Mycobacterium tuberculosis*. *Am J Med.* 1985;78:677-681.
158. Riley E, Cahan WG. Pulmonary cryptococcosis followed by pulmonary tuberculosis: A case report. *Am Rev Respir Dis.* 1972;106:594-599.
159. Dalgleish AG. Concurrent hydatid disease and cryptococcosis in a 16-year-old girl. *Med J Aust.* 1981;2:144-145.
160. Feigin DS. Pulmonary cryptococcosis: Radiologic-pathologic correlates of its three forms. *AJR Am J Roentgenol.* 1983;141:1263-1272.
161. Aberg JA, Mundy LM, Powderly WG. Pulmonary cryptococcosis in patients without HIV infection. *Chest.* 1999;115:734-740.
162. Baddley JW, Perfect JR, Oster RA, et al. Pulmonary cryptococcosis in patients without HIV infection: Factors associated with disseminated disease. *Eur J Clin Microbiol Infect Dis.* 2008;27:937-943.
163. Woods ML, MacGinley R, Eisen DP, et al. HIV combination therapy: Partial immune restitution unmasking latent cryptococcal infection. *AIDS.* 1998;12:1491-1494.
164. Jenny-Avital ER, Abadi M. Immune reconstitution cryptococcosis after initiation of successful highly active antiretroviral therapy. *Infect Immun.* 2002;35:128-133.
165. Cinti SK, Armstrong WS, Kaufman CA. Recurrence of increased intracranial pressure with antiretroviral therapy in an AIDS patient with cryptococcal meningitis. *Mycoses.* 2003;44:497-501.
166. Mitchell DH, Sorrell TC, Allworth AM, et al. Cryptococcal disease of the CNS in immunocompetent hosts: Influence of cryptococcal variety on clinical manifestations and outcome. *Clin Infect Dis.* 1995;20:611-616.
167. Speed B, Dunt D. Clinical and host differences between infections with the two varieties of *Cryptococcus neoformans*. *Clin Infect Dis.* 1995;21:28-34.
168. Chen S, Sorrell T, Nimmo G, et al. Epidemiology and host and variety-dependent characteristics of infection due to *Cryptococcus neoformans* in Australia and New Zealand. *Clin Infect Dis.* 2000;31:499-508.
169. Borton LK, Wintroub BU. Disseminated cryptococcosis presenting as herpetiform lesions in a homosexual man with acquired immunodeficiency syndrome. *J Am Acad Dermatol.* 1984;10:387-390.
170. Schupbach CW, Wheeler CE, Briggaman RA. Cutaneous manifestations of disseminated cryptococcosis. *Arch Dermatol.* 1976;112:1734-1744.
171. Concus AP, Helfand RF, Imber MJ, et al. Cutaneous cryptococcosis mimicking *Molluscum contagiosum* in a patient with AIDS. *J Infect Dis.* 1988;158:897-898.
172. Pema K, Diaz J, Guerra LG, et al. Disseminated cutaneous cryptococcosis: Comparison of clinical manifestations in the pre-AIDS and AIDS eras. *Arch Intern Med.* 1994;154:1032-1034.
173. Gauder JP. Cryptococcal cellulitis. *JAMA.* 1977;237:672-673.
174. Mayers DL, Martone WJ, Mandell GL. Cutaneous cryptococcosis mimicking gram-positive cellulitis in a renal transplant patient. *South Med J.* 1981;74:1032-1033.
175. Pierard GE, Pierard-Franchimont C, Estrada JA, et al. Cutaneous mixed infections in AIDS. *Am J Dermatopathol.* 1990;12:63-66.
176. Neuville S, Dromer F, Morin O, et al. Primary cryptococcosis: A distinct clinical entity. *Clin Infect Dis.* 2003;36:347.
177. Odom A, Del Poeta M, Perfect J, et al. The immunosuppressant FK506 and its non-immunosuppressive analog L-685,818 are toxic to *Cryptococcus neoformans* by inhibition of a common target protein. *Antimicrob Agents Chemother.* 1997;41:156-161.
178. Braman RT. Cryptococcosis (torulopsis) of prostate. *Urology.* 1981;17:284-286.
179. Plunkett JM, Turner BI, Tallent MB. Cryptococcal septicemia associated with urologic instrumentation in a renal allograft recipient. *J Urol.* 1981;125:241-242.
180. Larsen RA, Bozzette S, McCutchan A, et al. Persistent *Cryptococcus neoformans* infection of the prostate after successful treatment of meningitis. *Ann Intern Med.* 1989;111:125-128.
181. Staib F, Seibold M, L'age M, et al. *Cryptococcus neoformans* in the seminal fluid of an AIDS patient: A contribution to the clinical course of cryptococcosis. *Mycoses.* 1989;32:171-180.
182. Perfect JR, Seaworth B. Penile cryptococcosis with a review of mycotic infections of the penis. *Urology.* 1985;25:528-531.
183. Blocher KS, Weeks JA, Noble RC. Cutaneous cryptococcal infection presenting as vulvar lesion. *Genitourin Med.* 1987;63:341-343.
184. Okun E, Butler WT. Ophthalmologic complications of cryptococcal meningitis. *Arch Ophthalmol.* 1964;71:52-57.
185. Doft BH, Curtin VT. Combined ocular infection with cytomegalovirus and cryptococcosis. *Arch Ophthalmol.* 1982;100:1800-1803.
186. Crump JR, Elner SG, Elner VM, et al. Cryptococcal endophthalmitis: Case report and review. *Clin Infect Dis.* 1992;14:1069-1073.
187. Denning DW, Armstrong RW, Fishman M, et al. Endophthalmitis in a patient with disseminated cryptococcosis and AIDS who was treated with itraconazole. *Rev Infect Dis.* 1991;13:1126-1130.
188. Johnston SR, Corbett EL, Foster O, et al. Raised intracranial pressure and visual complications in AIDs patients with cryptococcal meningitis. *J Infect.* 1992;24:185-189.
189. Rex JH, Larsen RA, Dismukes WE, et al. Catastrophic visceral loss due to *Cryptococcus neoformans* meningitis. *Medicine.* 1993;72:207-224.
190. Behrman RE, Masci JR, Nicholas P. Cryptococcal skeletal infections: Case report and review. *Rev Infect Dis.* 1990;12:181-190.
191. Ross JJ, Katz JD. Cryptococcal meningitis and sarcoidosis. *J Infect Dis.* 2002;34:937-939.
192. Yinnon AM, Solages A, Treanor JJ. Cryptococcal peritonitis: report of a case developing during continuous ambulatory peritoneal dialysis and review of the literature. *Clin Infect Dis.* 1993;17:736-741.
193. Sungkanuparph S, Vibhagool A, Pracharktam R. Spontaneous cryptococcal peritonitis in cirrhotic patients. *J Postgrad Med.* 2002;48:201-202.
194. Singh N, Lortholary O, Alexander BD, et al. An immune reconstitution syndrome-like illness associated with Cryptococcus neoformans infection in organ transplant recipients. *Clin Infect Dis.* 2005;40:1756-1761.
195. Singh N, Perfect JR. Immune reconstitution syndrome and exacerbation of infections after pregnancy. *Clin Infect Dis.* 2007;45:1192-1199.
196. Ecevit IZ, Clancy CJ, Schmalfuss IM, et al. The poor prognosis of central nervous system cryptococcosis among nonimmunosuppressed patients: A call for better disease recognition and evaluation of adjuncts to antifungal therapy. *Clin Infect Dis.* 2006;42:1443-1447.
197. Singh N, Perfect JR. Immune reconstitution syndrome associated with opportunistic mycoses. *Lancet Infect Dis.* 2007;7:395-401.
198. Huffnagle KE, Gander RM. Evaluation of Gen-probe's *Histoplasma capsulatum* and *Cryptococcus neoformans* ACCU probes. *J Clin Microbiol.* 1993;31:419-421.
199. Mitchell TG, Freedman EZ, White TJ, et al. Unique oligonucleotide primers in PCR for identification of *Cryptococcus neoformans*. *J Clin Microbiol.* 1994;32:253-255.
200. Staib F. *Cryptococcus neoformans* und *Guizotia abyssinica* (syn. *G. oleifera*) Farbreaktion fur *C. neoformans*. *Zbl Hyg.* 1962;148:466-475.
201. Kwon-Chung KJ, Polacheck I, Bennett JE. Improved diagnostic medium for separation of *Cryptococcus neoformans* var. *neoformans* (serotypes A and D) and *Cryptococcus neoformans* var *gattii* (serotypes B and C). *Ann Intern Med.* 1985;103:533-538.
202. Ikeda R, Shinoda R, Fukazawa Y, et al. Antigenic characterization of *Cryptococcus neoformans* serotypes and its application of serotyping of clinical isolates. *J Clin Microbiol.* 1982;16:22-29.
203. Crampin AC, Matthews RC, Hall D, et al. PCR fingerprinting *Cryptococcus neoformans* by random amplification of polymorphic DNA. *J Med Vet Mycol.* 1993;31:463-465.
204. Spitzer ED, Spitzer SG. Use of a dispersed repetitive DNA element to distinguish clinical isolates of *Cryptococcus neoformans*. *J Clin Microbiol.* 1992;30:1094-1097.
205. Varma A, Kwon-Chung KJ. DNA probe for strain typing of *Cryptococcus neoformans*. *J Clin Microbiol.* 1992;30:2960-2967.
206. Goodman JS, Kaufman L, Loening MG. Diagnosis of cryptococcal meningitis: Detection of cryptococcal antigen. *N Engl J Med.* 1971;285:434-436.
207. Kauffman CA, Bergman AG, Severance PJ, et al. Detection of cryptococcal antigen. Comparison of two latex agglutination tests. *Am J Clin Pathol.* 1981;75:106-109.
208. Snow RM, Dismukes WE. Cryptococcal meningitis: Diagnostic value of cryptococcal antigen in cerebrospinal fluid. *Arch Intern Med.* 1975;135:1155-1157.
209. McManus EJ, Jones JM. Detection of a *Trichosporon beigelii* antigen cross-reactive with *Cryptococcus neoformans* capsular polysaccharides in serum from a patient with disseminated trichosporon infection. *J Clin Microbiol.* 1985;21:681-685.
210. Chanock SJ, Toltzis P, Wilson C. Cross-reactivity between *Stomatococcus mucilaginosus* and latex agglutination for cryptococcal antigen. *Lancet.* 1993;342:1119-1120.
211. Baughman RP, Rhodes JC, Dohn MN, et al. Detection of cryptococcal antigen in bronchoalveolar lavage fluid: A prospective study of diagnostic utility. *Am Rev Respir Dis.* 1992;145:1226-1229.
212. Desmet P, Kayembe KD, DeVroey C. The value of cryptococcal serum antigen screening among HIV-positive AIDS patients in Kinshasa, Zaire. *AIDS.* 1989;3:77-78.
213. Hoffman S, Stenderup J, Mathiesen LR. Low yield of screening for cryptococcal antigen by latex agglutination assay on serum and cerebrospinal fluid from Danish patients with AIDS or ARC. *Scand J Infect Dis.* 1991;23:697-702.
214. Feldmesser M, Harris C, Reichberg S, et al. Serum cryptococcal antigen in patients with AIDS. *Clin Infect Dis.* 1996;23:827-830.
215. Manfredi R, Moroni A, Mazzoni A, et al. Isolated detection of cryptococcal polysaccharide antigen in cerebrospinal fluid samples from patients with AIDS. *Clin Infect Dis.* 1996;23:849-850.
216. Powderly WG, Cloud GA, Dismukes WE, et al. Measurement of cryptococcal antigen in serum and cerebrospinal fluid: Value in the management of AIDS-associated cryptococcal meningitis. *Clin Infect Dis.* 1994;18:789-792.
217. Hunt KK Jr, Enquist RW, Bowen TE. Multiple pulmonary nodules with central cavitation. *Chest.* 1976;69:529-530.
218. Khoury MB, Godwin JD, Ravin CE, et al. Thoracic cryptococcosis: Immunologic competence and radiologic appearance. *AJR Am J Roentgenol.* 1984;141:893-896.
219. McAllister CK, Davis CE Jr, Ognibene AJ, et al. Cryptococcal pleuro-pulmonary disease: Infection of the pleural fluid in the absence of disseminated cryptococcosis—case report. *Milit Med.* 1984;149:684-686.
220. Young EJ, Hirsh DD, Fainstein V, et al. Pleural effusions due to *Cryptococcus neoformans*: A review of the literature and report of two cases with cryptococcal antigen determinations. *Am Rev Respir Dis.* 1980;121:743-746.
221. Zlupko GM, Fochler FJ, Goldschmidt ZH. Pulmonary cryptococcosis presenting with multiple pulmonary nodules. *Chest.* 1980;77:575.
222. Clark RA, Greer DL, Valainis GT, et al. *Cryptococcus neoformans* pulmonary infection in HIV-1–infected patients. *J Acquir Immune Defic Syndr.* 1990;3:480-485.
223. Miller WT, Edelman JM. Cryptococcal pulmonary infection in patients with AIDS: Radiographic appearance. *Radiology.* 1990;175:725-728.
224. Cornell SH, Jacoby CG. The varied computed tomographic appearance of intracranial cryptococcosis. *Radiology.* 1982;143:703-707.
225. Tan CT, Kuan BB. *Cryptococcus* meningitis, clinical–CT scan considerations. *Neuroradiology.* 1987;29:43-46.
226. Long JA, Herdt JR, DiChiro G, et al. Cerebral mass lesions in torulosis demonstrated by computed tomography. *J Comput Assist Tomogr.* 1980;4:766-769.
227. Poprich MJ, Arthur RH, Helmer E. CT of intracranial cryptococcosis. *AJR Am J Roentgenol.* 1990;154:603-606.

228. Wehn SM, Heinz R, Burger PC. Dilated Virchow-Robin spaces in cryptococcal meningitis associated with AIDS: CT and MR findings. *J Comput Assist Tomogr*. 1989;13:756-762.
229. Ingram CW, Haywood HB, Morris VM, et al. Cryptococcal ventricular peritoneal shunt infection: Clinical and epidemiological evaluation of two closely associated cases. *Infect Immun*. 1993;14:719-722.
230. Hospenthal D, Bennett JE. Persistence of cryptococcomas on neuroimaging. *Clin Infect Dis*. 2000;31:1303-1306.
231. Saag MS, Graybill JR, Larsen RA, et al. Practice guidelines for the management of cryptococcal disease. Infectious Disease Society of America. *Clin Infect Dis*. 2000;30:710-718.
232. Mwaba P, Mwansa J, Chintu C, et al. Clinical presentation, natural history and cumulative death rates of 230 adults with primary cryptococcal meningitis in Zambian AIDS patients treated under local conditions. *Postgrad Med*. 2001;77:769-773.
233. Ghannoun MA, Ibrahim AS, Fu Y, et al. Susceptibility testing of *Cryptococcus neoformans*: A microdilution technique. *J Clin Microbiol*. 1992;30:2881-2886.
234. Valez JD, Allendoerfer R, Luther M, et al. Correlation of *in vitro* azole susceptibility with in vivo response in a murine model of cryptococcal meningitis. *J Infect Dis*. 1993;168:508-510.
235. Aller AI, Martin-Manzuelos E, Lozano F, et al. Correlation of fluconazole MICs with clinical outcome in cryptococcal infection. *Antimicrob Agents Chemother*. 2000;44:1544-1548.
236. Witt MD, Lewis RJ, Larsen RA, et al. Identification of patients with acute AIDS-associated cryptococcal meningitis who can be effectively treated with fluconazole: The role of antifungal susceptibility testing. *Clin Infect Dis*. 1996;22:322-328.
237. Spitzer ED, Spitzer SG, Freundlich LF, et al. Persistence of initial infection in recurrent *Cryptococcus neoformans* meningitis. *Lancet*. 1993;341:595-596.
238. Casadevall A, Spitzer ED, Webb D, et al. Susceptibilities of serial *Cryptococcus neoformans* isolates from patients with recurrent cryptococcal meningitis to amphotericin B and fluconazole. *Antimicrob Agents Chemother*. 1993;37:1383-1386.
239. Haynes KA, Sullivan DJ, Coleman DC, et al. Involvement of multiple *Cryptococcus neoformans* strains in a single episode of cryptococcosis and reinfection with novel strains in recurrent infection demonstrated by random amplification of polymorphic DNA and DNA fingerprinting. *J Clin Microbiol*. 1995; 33:99-102.
240. Perfect JR, Cox GM. Drug resistance in *Cryptococcus neoformans*. *Drug Resist Updat*. 1999;2:259-269.
241. Bicanic T, Harrison T, Niepieklo A, et al. Symptomatic relapse of HIV-associated cryptococcal meningitis after initial fluconazole monotherapy: The role of fluconazole resistance and immune reconstitution. *Clin Infect Dis*. 2006;43:1069-1073.
242. Sarosi GA, Parker JD, Doto IL, et al. Amphotericin B in cryptococcal meningitis: Long-term results of treatment. *Ann Intern Med*. 1969;71:1079-1087.
243. Bennett JE, Dismukes W, Duma RJ, et al. A comparison of amphotericin B alone and combined with flucytosine in the treatment of cryptococcal meningitis. *N Engl J Med*. 1979;301:126-131.
244. Utz JP, Garrigues IL, Sande MA, et al. Therapy of cryptococcosis with a combination of flucytosine and amphotericin B. *J Infect Dis*. 1975;132:368-373.
245. deLalla F, Pellizzer G, Vaglia A. Amphotericin B as primary therapy for cryptococcosis in patients with AIDS: Reliability of relatively high doses administered over a relatively short period. *Clin Infect Dis*. 1995;20:263-266.
246. Leenders AC, Reiss P, Portegies P, et al. Liposomal amphotericin B (AmBisome) compared with amphotericin B both followed by oral fluconazole in the treatment of AIDS-associated cryptococcal meningitis. *AIDS*. 1997;11:1463-1471.
247. Sharkey PK, Graybill JR, Johnson ES, et al. Amphotericin B lipid complex compared with amphotericin B in the treatment of cryptococcal meningitis in patients with AIDS. *Clin Infect Dis*. 1996;22:315-321.
248. Baddour LM, Perfect JR, Ostrosky-Zeichner L. Successful use of amphotericin B lipid complex in the treatment of cryptococcosis. *Clin Infect Dis*. 2005;40(Suppl 6):S409-S413.
249. Coker RJ, Viviani M, Gazzard BG, et al. Treatment of cryptococcosis with liposomal amphotericin B (AmBisome) in 23 patients with AIDS. *AIDS*. 1993;7:829-835.
250. Tansuphaswadikul S, Nantawat W, Phonrat B, et al. Comparison of one-week with two-week regimens of amphotericin B both followed by fluconazole in the treatment of cryptococcal meningitis among AIDS patients. *J Med Assoc Thai*. 2006;89:1677-1685.
251. Utz JP, Shadomy S, McGehee RF. Flucytosine. *N Engl J Med*. 1972;286:777-778.
252. Dismukes WE, Cloud G, Gallis HA, et al. Treatment of cryptococcal meningitis with combination amphotericin B and flucytosine for four as compared with six weeks. *N Engl J Med*. 1987;317:334-341.
253. van der Horst C, Saag MS, Cloud GA, et al. Treatment of cryptococcal meningitis associated with the acquired immunodeficiency syndrome. *N Engl J Med*. 1997;337:15-21.
254. DeGans J, Portegies P, Tiessens G. Itraconazole compared with amphotericin B plus flucytosine in AIDS patients with cryptococcal meningitis. *AIDS*. 1992;6:185-190.
255. Larsen RA, Leal MAE, Chan LS. Fluconazole compared with amphotericin B plus flucytosine for cryptococcal meningitis in AIDS. *Ann Intern Med*. 1990;113:183-187.
256. Stamm AM, Diasio RB, Dismukes WE, et al. Toxicity of amphotericin B plus flucytosine in 194 patients with cryptococcal meningitis. *Am J Med*. 1987;83:236-242.
257. Saag MS, Cloud GA, Graybill JR, et al. A comparison of itraconazole versus fluconazole as maintenance therapy for AIDS-associated cryptococcal meningitis. *Clin Infect Dis*. 1999; 28:291-296.
258. Dromer F, Bernede-Bauduin C, Guillemot D, et al. Major role for amphotericin B-flucytosine combination in severe cryptococcosis. *PLoS ONE*. 2008;3:e2870.
259. Stern JJ, Hartman BJ, Sharkey P, et al. Oral fluconazole therapy for patients with the acquired immunodeficiency syndrome and cryptococcosis: Experience with 22 patients. *Am J Med*. 1988;85:477-480.
260. Dromer F, Mathoulin S, Dupont B, et al. Comparison of the efficacy of amphotericin B and fluconazole in the treatment of cryptococcosis in human immunodeficiency virus-negative patients: Retrospective analysis of 83 cases. *Clin Infect Dis*. 1996;22(Suppl 2):S154-S160.
261. Yamaguchi H, Ikemoto H, Watanabe K, et al. Fluconazole monotherapy for cryptococcosis in non-AIDS patients. *Eur J Clin Microbiol Infect Dis*. 1996;15:787-792.
262. Saag MS, Powderly WG, Cloud GA, et al. Comparison of amphotericin B with fluconazole in the treatment of acute AIDS-associated cryptococcal meningitis. *N Engl J Med*. 1992;326:83-89.
263. Berry AJ, Rinaldi MG, Graybill JR. Use of high-dose fluconazole as salvage therapy for cryptococcal meningitis in patients with AIDS. *Antimicrob Agents Chemother*. 1992;36:690-692.
264. Bozette SA, Larsen RA, Chiu J, et al. A placebo-controlled trial of maintenance therapy with fluconazole after treatment of cryptococcal meningitis in the acquired immunodeficiency syndrome. *N Engl J Med*. 1991;324:580-584.
265. Powderly WG, Saag MS, Cloud GA, et al. A controlled trial of fluconazole or amphotericin B to prevent relapse of cryptococcal meningitis in patients with the acquired immunodeficiency syndrome. *N Engl J Med*. 1992;326:793-798.
266. Denning DW, Tucker RM, Hanson LH, et al. Itraconazole therapy for cryptococcal meningitis and cryptococcosis. *Arch Intern Med*. 1989;149:2301-2308.
267. Viviani MA, Tortorano AM, Langer M, et al. Experience with itraconazole in cryptococcosis and aspergillosis. *J Infect*. 1989;18:151-165.
268. Perfect JR, Marr KA, Walsh TJ, et al. Voriconazole treatment for less common, emerging or refractory fungal infections. *Clin Infect Dis*. 2003;36:1122-1131.
269. Pitisuttithum P, Negroni R, Graybill JR, et al. Activity of posaconazole in the treatment of central nervous system fungal infections. *J Antimicrob Chemother*. 2005;56:745-755.
270. Brouwer AE, Rajanuwong A, Chierakul W, et al. Combination antifungal therapies for HIV-associated crytpococcal meningitis: Feasibility and power of quantitative CSF cultures to determine fungicidal activity. *Lancet*. 2004;363:1764-1767.
271. Larsen RA, Bozzette SA, Jones BE, et al. Fluconazole combined with flucytosine for treatment of cryptococcal meningitis in patients with AIDS. *Clin Infect Dis*. 1994;19:741-745.
272. Martinez E, Garcia-Viejo MA, Marcos MA. Discontinuation of secondary prophylaxis for cryptococcal meningitis in HIV-infected patients responding to highly active antiretroviral therapy. *AIDS*. 2000;14:2615-2617.
273. Vibhagool A, Sungkanuparph S, Mootsikapun P, et al. Discontinuation of secondary prophylaxis for cryptococcal meningitis in human immunodeficiency virus–infected patients treated with highly active antiretroviral therapy: A prospective, multicenter randomized study. *Clin Infect Dis*. 2003;36:1329-1331.
274. Fujita NK, Reynard M, Sapico FL, et al. Cryptococcal intracerebral mass lesions. *Ann Intern Med*. 1981;94:382-388.
275. Graybill JR, Sobel J, Saag M, et al. Diagnosis and management of increased intracranial pressure in patients with AIDS and cryptococcal meningitis. *Clin Infect Dis*. 2000;30:47-54.
276. Denning DW, Armstrong RW, Lewis BH, et al. Elevated cerebrospinal fluid pressures in patients with cryptococcal meningitis and acquired immunodeficiency syndrome. *Am J Med*. 1991;91:267-272.
277. Van Gemert HM, Vermeulen M. Treatment of impaired consciousness with lumbar punctures in a patient with cryptococcal meningitis and AIDS. *Clin Neurol Neurosurg*. 1991;93:257-258.
278. Yadav YR, Perfect JR, Friedman A. Successful treatment of cryptococcal ventriculo-atrial shunt infection with systemic therapy alone. *Neurosurgery*. 1988;23:317-322.
279. Pappas PG, Bustamante B, Ticona E, et al. Recombinant interferon-gamma 1b as adjunctive therapy for AIDS-related acute cryptococcal meningitis. *J Infect Dis*. 2004;189:2185-2191.
280. Jongwutiwes U, Kiertiburanakul S, Sungkanuparph S. Impact of antiretroviral therapy on the relapse of cryptococcosis and survival of HIV-infected patients with cryptococcal infection. *Curr HIV Res*. 2007;5:355-360.
281. White M, Cirrincione C, Blevins A, et al. Cryptococcal meningitis with AIDS and patients with neoplastic disease. *J Infect Dis*. 1992;165:960-966.
282. Diamond RD, Bennett JE. Prognostic factors in cryptococcal meningitis: A study of 111 cases. *Ann Intern Med*. 1974;80: 176-181.
283. Dromer F, Mathoulin-Pelissier S, Launay O, et al. Determinants of disease presentation and outcome during cryptococcosis: the CryptoA/D study. *PLoS Med*. 2007;4:e21.
284. Chayakulkeeree M, Perfect JR. Cryptococcosis. *Infect Dis Clin North Am*. 2006;20:507-544.
285. Nightingale SD, Cal SX, Peterson DM, et al. Primary prophylaxis with fluconazole against systemic fungal infections in HIV-positive patients. *AIDS*. 1992;6:191-194.
286. Powderly WG, Finkelstein DM, Feinberg J, et al. A randomized trial comparing fluconazole with clotrimazole troches for the prevention of fungal infections in patients with advanced human immunodeficiency virus infection. *N Engl J Med*. 1995;332:700-705.
287. Chetchotisakd P, Sungkanuparph S, Thinkhamrop B, et al. A multicentre, randomized, double-blind, placebo-controlled trial of primary cryptococcal meningitis prophylaxis in HIV-infected patients with severe immune deficiency. *HIV Med*. 2004;5: 140-143.
288. Devi SJ, Scheerson R, Egan W, et al. *Cryptococcus neoformans* serotype A glucuronoxylomannan protein conjugate vaccines: Synthesis, characterization, and immunogenicity. *Infect Immun*. 1991;59:3700-3707.
289. Mukherjee J, Pirofski LA, Scharff MD, et al. Antibody-mediated protection in mice with lethal intracerebral *Cryptococcus neoformans* infection. *Proc Natl Acad Sci U S A*. 1993;90:3636-3640.
290. Mukherjee J, Zuckier LS, Scharff MD, et al. Therapeutic efficacy of monoclonal antibodies to *Cryptococcus neoformans* glucuronoxylomannan alone and in combination with amphotericin B. *Antimicrob Agents Chemother*. 1994;38:580-587.

264

Histoplasma capsulatum

GEORGE S. DEEPE, JR.

Histoplasma capsulatum is one of the more common causes of infection in the U.S. Midwest and Southeast. Histoplasmosis, acquired by inhalation of mycelial fragments and microconidia, is most often self-limiting but can cause potentially lethal infection in patients with preexisting conditions. It remains a frequent cause of opportunistic infection in patients whose immune system is impaired by pharmaceutical agents or by the human immunodeficiency virus (HIV). This accelerating trend is unlikely to abate because the reservoir of *H. capsulatum* (soil) will never disappear.

History

The discovery of *H. capsulatum* was made in December 1905, when Samuel Darling, a pathologist stationed in Panama, examined visceral tissues and bone marrow from a young man from Martinique whose death was originally attributed to miliary tuberculosis.[1] Peering through his microscope, Darling was struck by the presence of many small bodies, most of which were intracellular. Having been influenced by reports from Leishman and Donovan, he mistakenly thought that this organism was a protozoan. Because it lacked a kinetoplast, Darling assumed that it was a different *Leishmania* species. He termed this new species *Histoplasma capsulatum* because it seemingly exhibited a capsule. It was not until 1912, after reviewing tissue specimens, that da Rocha-Lima suggested that the organism resembled a yeast rather than a protozoan.[2] A little more than 20 years later, the organism was finally isolated on artificial medium and observed to grow as a mold at room temperature and as a yeast at 37° C.[3]

For many years, the presence of pulmonary calcifications had become synonymous with healed tuberculosis by physicians. Amos Christie, a pediatrician at Vanderbilt University, dispelled that dictum.[4,5] The presence of cutaneous reactivity to a skin test reagent, prepared from the mycelial phase of the organism, in an infant with disseminated histoplasmosis prompted large-scale testing during the 1930s. This endeavor unearthed the surprising finding that histoplasmosis was highly prevalent in the Ohio and Mississippi river valleys.[5] Moreover, many cases of presumed tuberculosis that were based on the presence of calcified nodules on chest roentgenograms were determined to be histoplasmosis instead.[6] Eventually, many individuals residing in tuberculosis sanatoriums in the midwestern and southeastern United States were recognized to have been mistakenly admitted. They suffered from histoplasmosis, not tuberculosis. Some of these individuals contracted tuberculosis while housed in open wards with patients who had active pulmonary tuberculosis.

Ecology and Epidemiology

Cases of histoplasmosis have been reported from every continent except Antarctica. *H. capsulatum* is a soil-based fungus that has been isolated from many regions of the world and is most often associated with river valleys; the most highly endemic region is the Ohio and Mississippi river valleys (Fig. 264-1).[6] The conditions that favor the growth of this fungus in soil are a mean temperature of 22° to 29° C, an annual precipitation of 35 to 50 inches, and a relative humidity of 67% to 87%. These conditions are typically found in the temperate zone between latitudes 45 degrees north to 30 degrees south.[7] The organism is typically found within 20 cm of the surface, and it prefers soil that is acidic, has a high nitrogen content, and is moist. In areas where avians roost, the fungus is found most often where the guano is decaying and mixed with soil.[8] In such areas, infectious particles can exceed 10^5/g of soil. Fresh guano is less likely to contain any infectious particles. There is a strong association between the presence of bird and bat guano and the presence of *H. capsulatum*. In fact, the first isolation of the organism from an environmental source was from an area adjacent to a chicken house. Birds are not infected by the fungus, and attempts to isolate *H. capsulatum* from their cloaca have been unsuccessful. Bats, on the other hand, carry the fungus in their gastrointestinal tracts and shed it.[9]

Disruption of the soil by excavation or construction is one of the most common means of releasing infectious elements that are inhaled and eventually settle into the lungs. Those involved in recreational or work activities that expose them to disrupted soil are at highest risk for infection. Persons at risk include spelunkers who roam caves where bats reside and those who are engaged in agriculture, outdoor construction, or rehabilitation of buildings that have been inhabited by birds or bats. Human-to-human transmission via the pulmonary route has not been reported.

Although skin test reactivity to histoplasmin is equally distributed among men and women, disease develops in males more frequently than in females by a 4 : 1 ratio.[10] The disease incidence may be skewed because of the association of chronic pulmonary histoplasmosis with smoking, which for many years was a male-dominated activity. Unlike coccidioidomycosis, there are no known differences in susceptibility or resistance to infection among racial or ethnic groups.

H. capsulatum contains between four and seven chromosomes.[11] Differences in numbers of chromosomes are evident among strains. Originally, the organism could be distinguished by two chemotypes, but the advent of molecular biology has improved methods to distinguish strains of *H. capsulatum*. Eight clades of this fungus have been identified using molecular analysis[12]—two North American, two Latin American, and one each of Australian, Indonesian, Eurasian, and African clades. The spread of this fungus appears to have originated from Latin America between 3 and 13 million years ago. Interestingly, many of the isolates recovered from acquired immunodeficiency syndrome (AIDS) patients in St. Louis were found to be in clade 1, and these isolates are much less virulent in mice.[13] Genetic differences can be associated with varied clinical manifestations. *H. capsulatum* from specific regions of South America often produce skin lesions, whereas isolates from North America do not. The findings suggest that *H. capsulatum* is highly diverse at the genetic level, perhaps based on the fact that the fungus undergoes sexual recombination in nature, thus allowing for exchange of genetic material.

Mycology

H. capsulatum is classified as a member of the family of Ascomycetes and has a heterothallic form designated *Ajellomyces capsulatum* (see Chapter 256). Mating types (+) and (−) have been described and, when combined onto sporulating medium, they produce fruiting bodies containing asci. Isolates from patients carry the (−) mating type two to seven times more frequently than the (+) type, although the ratio of mating types in soil is 1 : 1.[14]

The organism has two forms, the mycelial phase and the yeast phase. The former is present at ambient temperature and the latter at 37° C or higher. The saprobic or mycelial phase can be divided into two colony types, brown (B) and albino (A). The A type grows more rapidly in culture and loses the capability to produce spores after

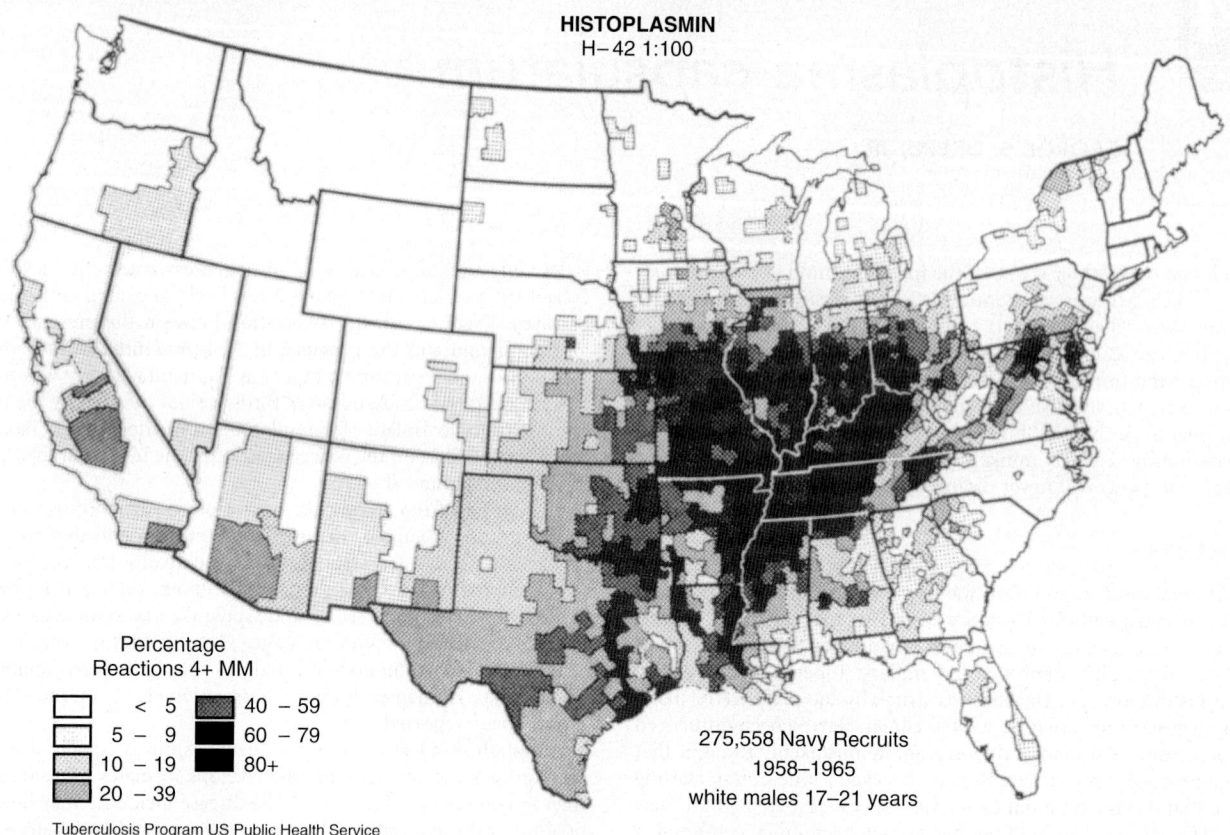

Figure 264-1 Histoplasmin reactivity in the continental United States among naval recruits. *(From Edwards LB, Acquaviva FA, Livesay VT, et al. An atlas of sensitivity to tuberculin, PPD-B, and histoplasmin in the United States. Am Rev Respir Dis. 1969;99[Part 2]:1-111, with permission.)*

prolonged subculturing. The B type generates a brown pigment. Yeast cells from the B type are more virulent in mice than those from the A type.

The basic elements of the nutritional needs of the organism are poorly defined because of the lack of a standardized medium. The organism requires vitamins, thiamine, biotin, and iron. Sulfhydryl groups in the form of cysteine or cystine are necessary for growth and maintenance of the yeast phase. The mycelial and yeast phases differ in their requirements for calcium. Chelation of this element from medium inhibits the growth of the mycelial but not the yeast phase. The transition from the mycelial to the yeast phase is associated with upregulation in the transcription of a putative calcium-binding protein messenger RNA (mRNA) and synthesis of the protein. Although this protein binds calcium, its influence on the acquisition of calcium remains unclear.[15]

Microscopic evaluation of the mycelial phase reveals two types of conidia. Macroconidia are large ovoid bodies that span 8 to 15 μm in diameter. The surface is decorated with slender protrusions that are referred to as tuberculate. Microconidia are small, smooth oval bodies with a diameter ranging from 2 to 5 μm (Fig. 264-2). These forms are believed to be the infective phase because their size is small enough to lodge in the terminal bronchioles and alveoli.

The transition from the saprobic to the yeast phase is a critical step in infectivity of the fungus. On exposure to 37°C, the organism undergoes genetic, biochemical, and physical alterations that result in the production of yeast cells that are uninucleate. These forms are small, typically 2 to 5 μm in diameter, and reproduce by multipolar budding (Fig. 264-3). The stimulus for the transition is heat, and the shift in temperature may be sensed by a change in the fluidity of the yeast membrane. Analysis of the conversion using microarrays has revealed

numerous alterations in gene expression. The shift was associated with induction of genes contributing to conidiation, cell polarity, and melanin.[16] Using insertional mutagenesis, a transcription factor termed *Ryp1* has been found to be essential for growth of yeast cells at 37°C.[17] Thus, the complexity of the shift from mycelium to yeast is just beginning to be delineated.

Three biochemical stages have been identified during the conversion following exposure to 37°C. Stage 1 is characterized by an uncoupling of oxidation-phosphorylation and a decrease in RNA and protein syn-

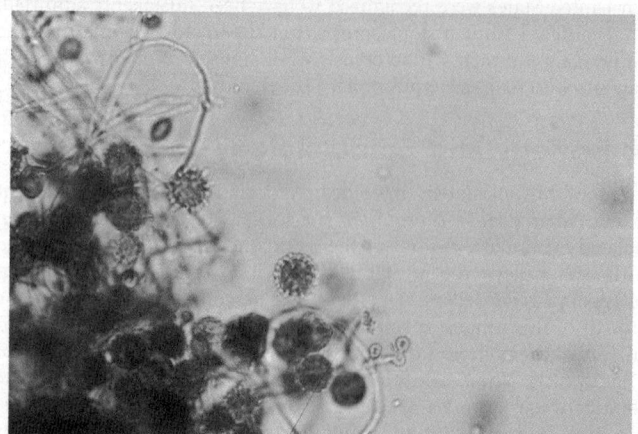

Figure 264-2 Mycelial phase of *Histoplasma capsulatum*. Both macroconidia and microconidia are evident.

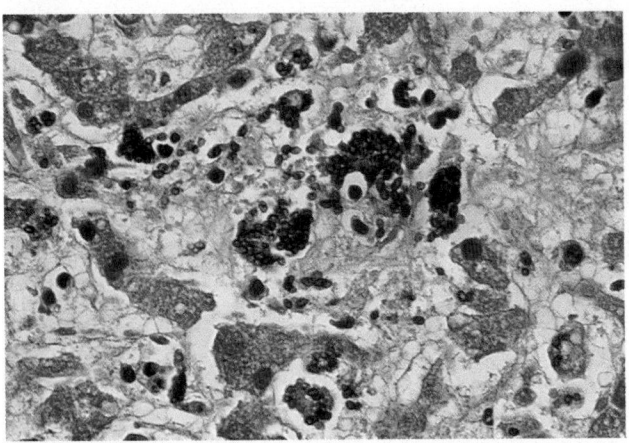

Figure 264-3 Yeast cells of *Histoplasma capsulatum* a section of liver. (Gomori methenamine silver, ×1000).

thesis. In stage 2, no respiration is detectable, and in stage 3 there is a resumption of respiration. Chitin and α- and β-glucan content differ between the two phases.

Within tissues, yeast cells may possess a morphology that differs from the usual ovoid shape. Misshapen or large yeasts have been observed in tissues and epithelial cells. These allomorphs may contain less α-1,3-glucan and appear to be less virulent in mice than oval-shaped yeasts.

Pathogenesis

The study of the pathogenesis of this fungus has been hampered by the lack of suitable tools to alter gene expression within the fungus. Technologic advances have led to several developments including a transformation system to delete genes, silencing RNA, and insertional mutagenesis using *Agrobacterium tumifaciens*. These tools create the foundation for examining the influence of genes or gene regulators on the pathobiology of *H. capsulatum*.[18,19]

The transition from the mycelial to the yeast phase is the most critical determinant in the establishment of infection.[20] This contention is supported by several findings. First, it is rare to find mycelial particles in tissues of humans or mammals with established infection. Rather, yeast cells are commonly detected. Second, exposure of *H. capsulatum* mycelia to *p*-chloromercuriphenylsulfonic acid (PCMS), a sulfhydryl inhibitor, irreversibly blocks the conversion to yeasts but does not alter growth of yeasts or mycelia. PCMS-treated mycelia fail to infect animals.

In addition to calcium, iron is another vital element required for survival of *H. capsulatum*. The organism can acquire iron from the intracellular environment by three means: release of iron scavenging siderophores, production of a ferric reductase, and modulating pH to remove iron from transferrin. α-1,3-Glucan has been found to be a key virulence factor in the pathogenesis of *H. capsulatum*.[18] Synthesis of this carbohydrate, which is regulated by an amylase, and glucan appears to bind dectin-1 and thereby suppress generation of important proinflammatory cytokines.

After conidia settle into the alveoli, they bind to the CD11-CD18 family of integrins and are engulfed by neutrophils and macrophages.[21] It is likely that the conversion of mycelia to the yeast phase transpires, at least partially if not entirely, intracellularly. The duration of the phase transition ranges from hours to days. Following transformation of the conidia into yeasts in the lungs, yeasts migrate, presumably intracellularly, to local draining lymph nodes and subsequently to distant organs rich in mononuclear phagocytes (e.g., liver and spleen). The yeasts grow readily within resting macrophages. Activation of cellular immunity is necessary for restricting growth, and in primary infection this arm of immunity matures by 2 weeks.

In experimental pulmonary infection, neutrophils constitute one of the prominent cell populations that emigrate early into infected foci of lungs.[22] These cells are capable of inhibiting the growth of yeast cells. Constituents from the azurophilic granules express fungistatic activity, and defensins also inhibit the growth of yeast cells.[23] Elimination of murine neutrophils enhances considerably the susceptibility of mice to sublethal inocula with yeast cells.[24] Neutrophils mount a respiratory burst in response to the fungus, but the oxygen intermediates are trapped intracellularly. Despite the burst, there is little evidence that toxic oxygen intermediates contribute to the anti-*Histoplasma* activity of these phagocytes.

Macrophages and dendritic cells are the principal effector cells in host resistance to this fungus.[21,25] The fate of yeast cells in each of these cell populations differs. Yeast proliferate within resting mononuclear phagocytes, but this form is killed by dendritic cells. As noted, macrophages engulf yeast via CD11-CD18 receptors, whereas dendritic cells use the fibronectin receptor. Engagement of two disparate receptors may explain in part the different fates within these cell populations.

In murine macrophages, a high percentage of yeast cells are located within phagolysosomes. Binding to the CD11-CD18 receptors and subsequent entry into human macrophages are mediated by heat shock protein 60 expressed on the surface of yeast.[26] The fungus must contend with the adverse contents (e.g., acid proteinases) of this intensely hostile environment. A mechanism whereby yeasts survive is by alkalinization of the phagolysosome.[27] Yeast cells raise the pH of the phagocytic compartment to 6.0 to 6.5. One reason for maintaining the pH within a narrow range is that yeast cells require iron to grow and, if the pH exceeds 6.5, they cannot acquire iron from the host.[21]

Nitric oxide produced by activated murine macrophages is a major mediator of anti-*Histoplasma* activity. The ability of this nitrogen intermediate to oxidize iron may explain its potent fungicidal activity.[28] However, its influence in human infection remains unknown because human macrophages infected with *H. capsulatum* have not been reported to produce nitric oxide.

The interaction between human macrophages and yeast differs substantially from that found with murine macrophages. The former cell population mounts a vigorous respiratory burst in response to unopsonized yeasts,[21] whereas murine cells do not unless yeasts are opsonized with antibody and are therefore engulfed through Fc receptors. Another contrast is that yeast cells do not predominantly reside in phagolysosomes of plastic-bound human macrophages, but rather reside in endosomes. However, if human macrophages that are adherent to collagen gels are exposed to yeast cells, massive phagolysosomal fusion develops. This process is correlated with a pronounced inhibition of growth of *H. capsulatum* yeasts.

Macrophages from HIV-infected individuals manifest defective activity in their interaction with *H. capsulatum*. These cells bind fewer yeasts than cells from uninfected individuals, and a direct correlation exists between the CD4+ T-cell count and the capacity of macrophages to bind yeast cells. On entry into cells, yeasts grow more rapidly within macrophages from HIV-infected individuals or in macrophages that have been infected in vitro with a macrophage-tropic strain of HIV. The envelope glycoprotein 120 from the virus is responsible for the inhibition of binding yeasts to macrophages,[21] but not the altered growth characteristics of the yeasts in phagocytes.

Within the elements of the acquired immune response, T cells are pivotal in clearance of the fungus. Experimental studies indicate that neither B cells nor antibodies influence host resistance, although the data are limited. CD4+ cells are extremely important in controlling primary infection in mice.[24] The central role of CD4+ cells in this species is supported by the finding that in HIV-infected individuals, most cases of histoplasmosis develop when the CD4+ cell count is lower than 200/μL.[29] Mice deficient in CD8+ cells are impaired in their ability to reduce the fungal burden, but they can eventually eliminate the fungus. Similarly, β2-microglobulin knockout mice that lack CD8+ T cells and major histocompatibility complex I antigens are more susceptible to infection than controls, but they are able to sterilize tissues.[24] In contrast, in secondary infection, the absence of CD4+ or CD8+ cells diminishes the efficiency of yeast elimination, but mice survive. The loss of protective immunity only develops when both subsets are eliminated.

The primary contribution of T cells to host defense is the release of cytokines that eventually activate mononuclear phagocytes. Blockade of endogenous interferon-γ or mice congenitally deficient in this lymphokine are exceptionally susceptible to infection.[24] Other cytokines in mice that are necessary for host clearance are interleukin-12 and tumor necrosis factor-α. Blockade of endogenous production of either of these leads to the death of mice. The effect of interleukin-12 is mediated through the induction of interferon-γ.[24] Interestingly, interleukin-12 is important in primary infection but not in reexposure histoplasmosis.[24] Tumor necrosis factor-α and interferon-γ are both necessary for controlling primary infection and the former is required for secondary infection.[24]

In vitro, recombinant interferon-γ activates murine peritoneal macrophages to inhibit the growth of yeast cells. Macrophages from other tissue sources are either nonresponsive to this stimulus or require costimulation with lipopolysaccharide.[21] The anti-*Histoplasma* action of interferon-γ is mediated by limiting iron acquisition, and this effect can be reversed by exposure to additional iron.[28] Human macrophages, on the other hand, do not respond to human recombinant interferon-γ to inhibit yeast cell growth.[21] The cytokines that activate these cells are macrophage colony-stimulating factor, granulocyte-macrophage colony-stimulating factor, and interleukin-3,[21] but the mechanism whereby these cytokines induce fungistatic activity has not been established.

Although the infection is limited by cell-mediated immunity, tissues are not sterilized. Infected individuals contain yeasts, some of which remain viable for many years. The dormant organisms pose little risk unless the individual becomes immunosuppressed as a result of potent immunosuppressive agents used to combat various clinical conditions or immunosuppressive viruses such as HIV. The metabolic state of *H. capsulatum* in tissues is unknown. It is likely that some of the yeasts remain viable, because individuals who have moved from endemic to nonendemic areas many years ago may have reactivated infection. The cascade of immunologic events that leads to activation of this form of the infection remains largely unknown; however, reports of patients developing disseminated histoplasmosis after treatment with monoclonal antibody to tumor necrosis factor-α may implicate this cytokine in reactivation.[30] A murine model of reactivation histoplasmosis has been developed that should facilitate studies of the organism and the host in this form of infection. In mice, CD4+, CD8+, and a Thy-1.2, CD4−, CD8− cell must be eliminated to achieve progressive infection. B cells also appear to be important in the severity of reactivation disease.

The hallmark of the tissue response to this fungus is the development of caseating or noncaseating granulomas in which calcium may be deposited (Fig. 264-4). The granuloma consists of an admixture of mononuclear phagocytes and lymphocytes, principally T cells. The putative function of the granuloma is to contain fungal growth. Although interferon-γ and tumor necrosis factor-α are important in the generation of granulomas formed in response to other microbes, neutralization of these two cytokines does not prevent their formation in response to *H. capsulatum*. The organization of the *Histoplasma* granuloma has been characterized in mouse livers and lungs. CD4+ and CD8+ cells are present in the granulomas of mice. T-cell composition is polyclonal and these cells are the source of interferon-γ and interleukin-17. Macrophages are the principal source of tumor necrosis factor-α.[31]

Organized granulomatous inflammation is typically observed in self-limited disease. Conversely, in progressive disseminated histoplasmosis, the more common histopathologic appearance of tissue is a massive influx of macrophages with scattered lymphocytes. Well-circumscribed granulomas are infrequently present, and the lack of an organized inflammatory response is indicative of a perturbed cellular immune response. Occasionally, the inflammatory response in mediastinal lymph nodes is exaggerated, resulting in excessive granuloma

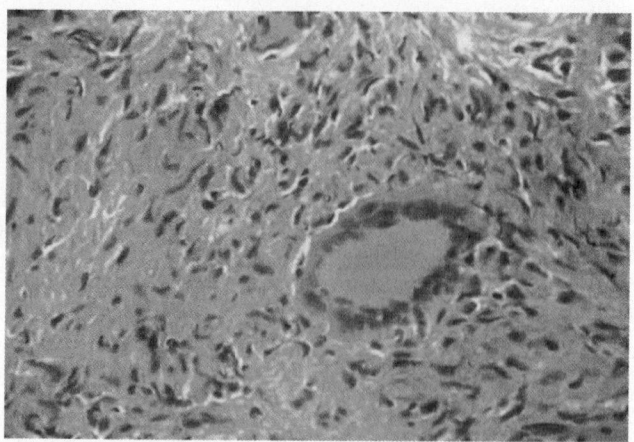

Figure 264-4 Granuloma in the lung of a patient with histoplasmosis.

formation followed by fibrosis. The progressive scarring may affect the patency of the airways and major blood vessels.[32]

In experimental infection, either cutaneous or in vitro delayed-type hypersensitivity responses to *H. capsulatum* antigens are detected approximately 2 weeks after exposure.[24] In humans, delayed-type hypersensitivity responses are manifest within 3 to 6 weeks after exposure.[33] These values are simply approximations because the precise time at which individuals are exposed in endemic areas is exceptionally difficult to determine. Reexposure to *H. capsulatum* in previously sensitized individuals is characterized by a more rapid tissue response. This finding is not surprising because *H. capsulatum* induces a memory response in which the immune system reacts in a much shorter time frame.

Infection with *H. capsulatum* produces a broad array of clinical and pathologic manifestations that must be recognized to diagnose and treat individuals afflicted with this fungus correctly. A summary of the clinicopathologic manifestations is depicted in Table 264-1.

Pulmonary Histoplasmosis

ACUTE INFECTIONS

These can be either be a primary infection or a reinfection.

Acute Primary Infection

The vast majority of primary infections (more than 90%) go unrecognized medically. Usually, they are asymptomatic or result in mild influenza-like illness for which individuals do not seek medical attention. However, there is a small proportion of patients who become overtly ill. The major determinant for the development of symptoms is likely to be the inoculum size, although differences in strain virulence cannot be excluded.[34,35] Other contributing factors include age and underlying diseases. Thus, older adults, those younger than 2 years of age, and individuals whose immune systems are compromised are more likely to develop progressive disseminated disease symptoms.

In those who become ill, the typical incubation time is 7 to 21 days, and most individuals manifest symptoms by day 14.[34-36] Fever that may reach 42° C, headache, nonproductive cough, chills, and chest pain are the most common symptoms noted. The latter is described usually as a substernal discomfort, although in an outbreak in children, it was more often located in the anterior chest.[36] Pleuritic chest pain is uncommon. The chest pain is believed to be caused by enlargement of the mediastinal or hilar lymph nodes, or both. Malaise, weakness, fatigue, and myalgia are observed in a distinctly smaller percentage of patients. Most symptoms resolve within 10 days, but can persist for several weeks if there is an exposure to a heavy inoculum. Acute pulmonary infection can be accompanied by a number of rheumatologic

TABLE 264-1	**Spectrum of *Histoplasma capsulatum*–Induced Disease**		
Manifestations	*Acute Pulmonary Disease*	*Acute Cavitary Pulmonary Disease*	*Disseminated Disease*
Clinical	Often asymptomatic	Fever, productive cough, chest pain	Fever, weight loss, hepatosplenomegaly, hematologic disturbances*
Immunologic			
Positive skin test	>90%	70%-90%	30%-55%
Lymphocyte transformation	+++†	+ to +++	±
Antibody to *Histoplasma capsulatum*‡	25%-85%§	75%-95%	70%-90%
Antigenuria	20%§	40%	60%-90%
Pathologic			
Positive culture from lungs	<25%	5%-70%	50%-70%
Histology	Caseating and noncaseating granulomas, few yeasts, giant cells	Noncaseating granulomas, interstitial fibrosis, necrosis, yeasts, cavities, few to moderate yeasts	Diffuse macrophage proliferation, abundant few giant cells

*Hematologic disturbances include anemia, leukopenia, and thrombocytopenia.
†+, Indicates a proliferative response to antigen or mitogen that is 3- to 5-fold higher than background; ++, five- to tenfold higher than background; +++, more than tenfold higher.
‡Complement fixation titer of greater than or equal to 1:8.
§Higher incidence in those with symptomatic infection.
From Deepe GS Jr, Bullock WE. Histoplasmosis: A granulomatous inflammatory response. In: Gallin JI, Goldstein IM, Synderman R, eds. *Inflammation: Basic Principles and Clinical Correlates.* 2nd ed. New York: Raven Press; 1992:943, with permission.

manifestations. Arthralgias, erythema nodosum, and erythema multiforme are present in approximately 6% of patients, most of whom are women.[37] In some, these manifestations of histoplasmosis may be the presenting complaint. Frank arthritis is distinctly uncommon.

Physical findings in acute pulmonary histoplasmosis are minimal. Crackles may be detected on auscultation of the lungs and, rarely, hepatosplenomegaly. The common roentgenographic features are characterized by a patchy pneumonitis that eventually calcifies and hilar lymphadenopathy (Fig. 264-5). If a heavy exposure has transpired, numerous patches of pneumonitis that calcify may develop, and these produce the so-called buckshot appearance on the chest roentgenogram.[34] Pleural effusions are distinctly uncommon. The white blood cell count is usually within the normal range, but approximately 30% of patients will have leukocytosis or leukopenia during the course of this infection. Another laboratory abnormality is a transient increase in the serum alkaline phosphatase level. Pulmonary function studies, performed in only a few patients, have demonstrated reversible restrictive defects, impaired diffusing capacity of lung for carbon monoxide (DL_{CO}), and obstructive defects.[38]

At least 6% of patients who acquire histoplasmosis suffer from acute pericarditis.[39] This figure may underestimate the true incidence because only those most seriously affected seek medical attention. Precordial chest pain and fever are frequent. A high proportion of patients report a respiratory illness approximately 6 weeks before the onset of the pericarditis. A pericardial friction rub is auscultated in more than 75% of patients with pericarditis, and pulsus paradoxus is also present in more than 75%. An enlarged cardiac silhouette is usually seen on chest roentgenogram. Electrocardiographic abnormalities indicative of pericarditis—for example, ST segment elevation—are often observed. Only a small percentage of individuals develop cardiac tamponade. The likely cause of the pericarditis is not direct invasion of the organism, because it is rarely found in tissue specimens or in pericardial fluid, but rather the granulomatous inflammatory response that is mounted in mediastinal lymph nodes adjacent to the pericardium.

Acute pulmonary histoplasmosis must be distinguished from influenza and from other forms of community-acquired pneumonia.[40] This task is difficult unless a thorough exposure history is obtained. Of greater concern, however, are patients who present with mediastinal lymphadenopathy. This finding is often considered to be caused by a hematologic malignancy rather than histoplasmosis. In such cases, patients may undergo unnecessary surgical procedures in an attempt to establish a diagnosis. Sarcoidosis also should be considered and distinguishing between histoplasmosis and sarcoidosis can be difficult at best. Both may have similar histopathologic features, and serum angiotensin-converting enzyme levels are elevated in each disease.[41] Thus, in all patients who present with mediastinal or hilar lymphadenopathy, it is critically important that histoplasmosis be considered in the differential diagnosis in patients who reside or have recently been in an endemic region.

A Ghon complex and pulmonary calcifications are common in healed pulmonary histoplasmosis. Another characteristic feature of resolved primary infection is the presence of splenic or liver calcifica-

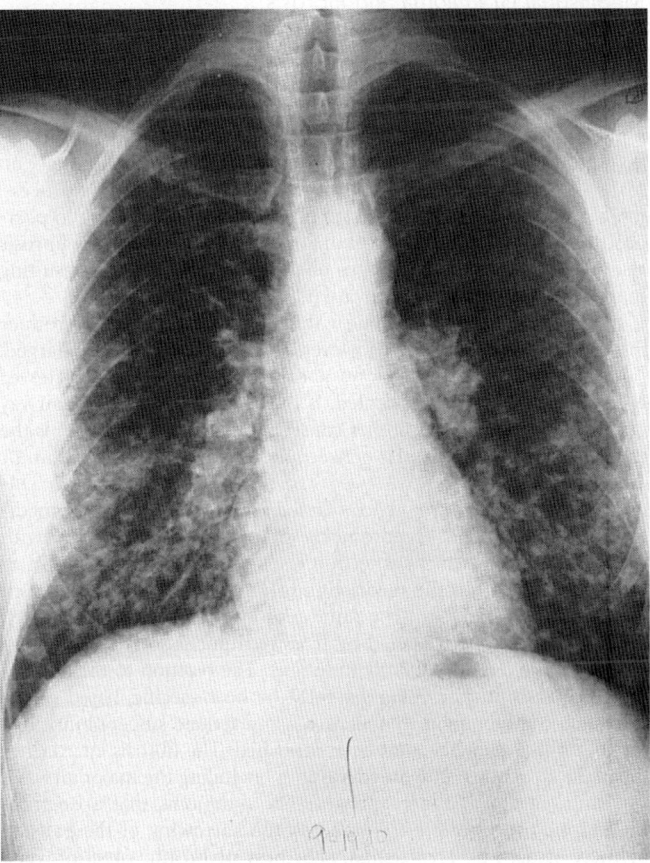

Figure 264-5 **Chest roentgenogram of patient with acute pulmonary histoplasmosis.**

tions. In fact, the presence of these on a routine roentgenogram should be considered evidence of resolved histoplasmosis if the patient has been in an endemic area. Although splenic and liver calcifications also are noted in healed tuberculosis, the most likely cause of these findings remains histoplasmosis because the incidence of tuberculosis in the United States is much lower than that of histoplasmosis.

Acute Reinfection

It is not uncommon for those who reside in endemic areas to be exposed more than once to *H. capsulatum*. Those who are reexposed to a large inoculum in heavily endemic areas present with a milder influenza-like illness. The onset can begin within 3 days, which is shorter than in primary infection. The characteristic chest roentgenogram is one of numerous small nodules that are diffusely scattered throughout both lung fields. This feature has been referred to as miliary granulomatosis. Hilar or mediastinal lymphadenopathy is absent. The duration of illness often is briefer than in primary infection.[34,35,42]

COMPLICATIONS OF PRIMARY HISTOPLASMOSIS

Histoplasmoma

A very infrequent complication of primary histoplasmosis is the development of a mass lesion that resembles a fibroma.[43] When it arises, it is found most often in the lung. Instead of resolving, a nidus of infection gradually enlarges over years to form a concentric mass. Presumably, the growth is caused by persistent antigenic stimulus from the yeasts. It is composed of active inflammation at the periphery and fibrous tissue within the inner sphere and eventually the central portion calcifies. Roentgenographically, the histoplasmoma may have a central core of calcium or rings of calcium, and these findings are useful in distinguishing it from a neoplastic growth.

Mediastinal Granuloma and Fibrosis

Another complication of primary infection is a massive enlargement of the mediastinal lymph nodes that is caused by the granulomatous inflammation mounted in response to the fungus.[34] The diameter of these nodes can reach 8 to 10 cm. The nodes are caseous and contain a fibrotic shell that may be up to 5 mm thick. Often, this process is asymptomatic. Occasionally, however, the nodes may impinge on major airways and impair gas exchange. During the healing process, the fibrotic tissue can cause retraction of the airways, leading to postobstructive pneumonias, hypoxemia, and bronchiectasis. The fibrosis also may constrict the esophagus or the superior vena cava, resulting in dysphagia, superior vena cava syndrome, or both.[43,44]

Calcific deposits that originate within the lungs occasionally produce lithoptysis. More common, however, is the penetration of enlarged, calcified nodes into the airways and the generation of particles of calcium that can be expectorated. If the calcific mass is large, airway obstruction may ensue. Another consequence of enlarged nodes is the creation of sinuses or fistulas between the airways and pericardium or esophagus.[43]

A rare but dire consequence of mediastinal involvement is mediastinal fibrosis.[45] This syndrome is similar to that observed with tuberculosis, in which the infection leads to a massive deposition of fibrotic tissue within the mediastinum (Fig. 264-6). The mechanism underlying this exuberant immune response is unknown. However, it appears not to be triggered by massive numbers of yeast, because they are observed infrequently in lesions. The reaction to the antigen or antigens from *H. capsulatum* must be host-specific, based on its infrequent development. If there exist any genetic susceptibility loci for this entity, they have not been identified. The fibrosis encroaches on all the structures of the mediastinum, including the major airways, superior vena cava, and esophagus. The symptoms that arise from the fibrotic process are attributable to the narrowing of the patency of these structures. Hypoxemia, shortness of breath, superior vena cava syndrome, and dysphagia may ensue as the fibrotic process progresses.

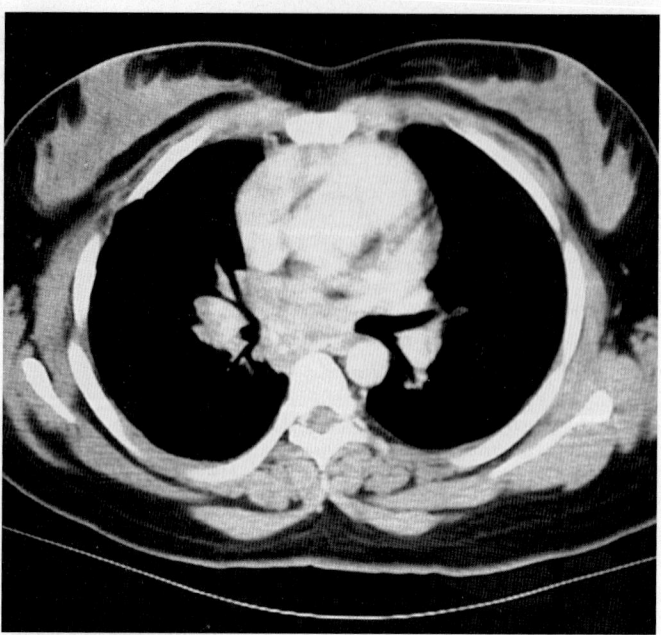

Figure 264-6 CT scan of the mediastinum in a patient with mediastinal fibrosis.

Chronic Pulmonary Histoplasmosis

Cavitary pulmonary histoplasmosis and chronic pulmonary histoplasmosis have been considered for many years to be synonymous terms. However, one review called for reconsideration. Although the precise incidence was not known because of the sporadic nature of the disease, approximately 8% of individuals developed fibrocavitary disease following two large epidemics in Indianapolis.[46] Cavitary lesions were found in the upper lobes in more than 90% of cases (Fig. 264-7). Men older than 50 years with preexisting chronic lung disease, usually emphysema, were reported to constitute the highest proportion of patients, and it was quite unusual in those younger than age 40 (less than 5% of all cases).[46,47] However, a recent review has called this association into question. Among a group of patients with pulmonary

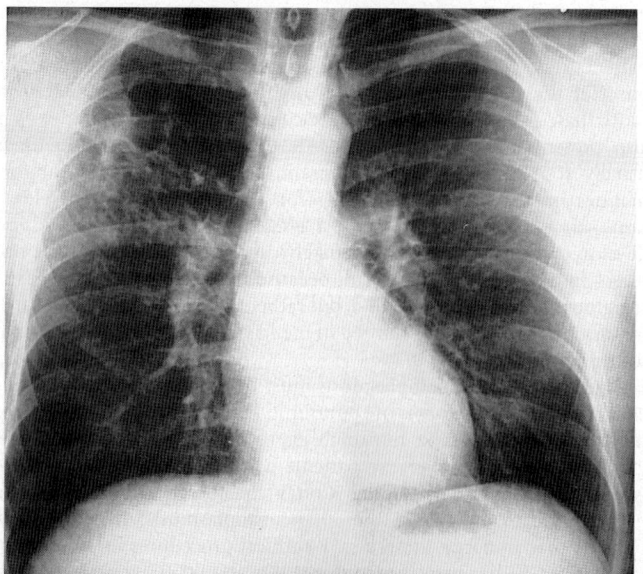

Figure 264-7 Chest roentgenogram of a patient with cavitary histoplasmosis.

symptoms that extended for at least 6 weeks, nearly 50% were women and 20% had chronic obstructive pulmonary disease (COPD). Cavities were detected in less than 40%.[48] The causes for the changing face of this illness are not clearly defined, but the decrease in tobacco use is certainly a contributing factor. It also suggests that there are at least two forms of chronically active lung disease, cavitary and noncavitary.

In the classic form of cavitary disease, the most frequent symptoms are low-grade fever, productive cough, dyspnea, and weight loss of insidious onset. Night sweats, chest pain, hemoptysis, and malaise are less common. Hemoptysis is rare. Completely asymptomatic intervals with radiologic stability are interspersed with periods of recurrent symptoms and radiologic progression. Both an early and a late stage have been described. The major difference between the two forms is the symptomatology. In the early stage, the illness, characterized by chest pain, productive cough, fever, and weakness, begins abruptly and persists for several weeks before medical attention is sought. In the late stage, the proportion of patients experiencing productive cough and hemoptysis is much higher, whereas chest pain and fever are much less frequent. Bronchogenic transmission from one segment of the lung to another may occur during cough or aspiration.[47]

Roentgenographically, patchy infiltrates appear and develop areas of dense consolidation that progress to cavitation. Over months or years, extensive fibrosis, retraction, and areas of compensatory emphysema appear unless effective treatment is given. The most common location is the upper lobes. Almost all patients have a history of heavy cigarette use or exhibit evidence of emphysema coexisting with COPD, and therefore the cavities must be distinguished from preexisting bullae. Thin-walled or thick-walled cavities may form in response to *H. capsulatum*. Enlarged hilar or mediastinal lymph nodes are notably absent, and distinctive laboratory features are not present. Leukocytosis and elevated alkaline phosphatase levels are detected in about one third of symptomatic patients, and anemia is present in half.[46,47]

The earliest lesion on histopathology is an interstitial pneumonitis. The inflammatory infiltrate is composed primarily of lymphocytes and macrophages and is often found adjacent to bullae. The alveolar walls are thickened, and the peribronchial lymphatics contain a similar type of inflammatory infiltrate. Subsequently, necrosis develops, and it resembles that caused by infarction. Vascular compromise, as denoted by subintimal thickening and vessel obliteration, is present in inflamed regions. Proteinaceous exudate can be found in bullae and yeasts are present in the necrotic lining of a cavity or in small encapsulated necrotic lesions. Areas of infarction are slowly replaced by scarring of the involved parenchyma. The healing phase is characterized by fibrosis and retraction, some leaving central areas of caseous necrosis surrounded by epithelioid cells, lymphocytes, and giant cells. Neighboring bullae may enlarge from compensatory emphysema. Following healing, recurrence of cavitary lesions will develop in approximately 20% of patients, but the prognosis of recurrence is no different from that of the initial infection.[47]

Spontaneous resolution of thin-walled and thick-walled cavities ranges from 10% to 60%, and thin-walled cavities have a higher healing rate. Despite shrinking and fibrosis of individual lesions, new lesions continue to appear and radiologic progression occurs in an estimated 79%. In individuals with COPD, cavitary histoplasmosis can exacerbate the existing pulmonary dysfunction, and the destructive nature of the inflammation irreversibly compromises pulmonary function. Death caused by cavitary histoplasmosis is distinctly unusual but is attributable to respiratory failure, cor pulmonale, or secondary bacterial pneumonia.

The association between the presence of COPD and chronic cavitary histoplasmosis suggests that the anatomic defect present in these lungs predisposes patients to this clinical form of infection and promotes the formation of cavities. This intriguing postulate has been proposed and is most likely correct, although no experimental data exist to support it.[47] The difficulty in testing this hypothesis is that a suitable animal model has not been developed. In addition, it does not explain the development of cavities in other patients. At present, *H. capsulatum* is not known to elaborate any elastinolytic or proteolytic enzymes that digest collagen.

The most common symptoms of those with the redefined chronic pulmonary histoplasmosis who did not necessarily have cavitary lesions are cough, weight loss, and fever and chills. Radiographic changes commonly include nodules, infiltrates, and lymphadenopathy. Less common are fibrosis, thickened pleura, and volume loss. Arthralgias, dyspnea, fatigue, and chest pain are observed in less than 50% of patients. The most striking difference is that in those without cavities, positive cultures are highly unusual. Most patients in this series were treated with antifungal therapy and 70% of those resolved infection. Of the remaining patients who received therapy, 10% manifested a protracted illness, 15% suffered a recurrence, and 5% did not resolve infection. Among the group that did not receive antifungal therapy (13 of 46), 2 manifested progressive infection and 1 did not clear the infiltrate.[48]

Progressive Disseminated Histoplasmosis

Although all primary infections can be considered disseminated because yeast cells migrate from the lungs to organs rich in mononuclear phagocytes, the term *progressive disseminated histoplasmosis* (PDH) refers to the relentless growth of the organism in multiple organ systems. Because *H. capsulatum* is not a reportable disease, only estimates of incidence or prevalence are available. The estimated incidence is 1/2000 cases of histoplasmosis. Following the two Indianapolis epidemics, 8% of clinically recognized cases of histoplasmosis were PDH.[49] The major risk factors in those two epidemics for this manifestation of histoplasmosis were age older than 54 years and immunosuppression. In patients with AIDS, the incidence may approach 25%. The outcome of infection with *H. capsulatum* was poor among HIV-infected individuals, including the presence of a chronic medical condition and a history of herpes simplex virus infection. Conversely, the use of antiretrovirals and triazoles was associated with a decreased risk. In an analysis of 1074 renal allograft recipients, 0.4% developed clinically recognized PDH over a 25-year span.[50] This value is moderately different from the one reported during the Indianapolis epidemic, in which 2.1% of renal allograft recipients exhibited PDH.[51] Another risk factor for acquiring PDH is the use of tumor necrosis factor-α antagonists.[30]

The exposure leading to PDH is inapparent, without an antecedent episode of acute pulmonary histoplasmosis. PDH can develop by reexposure to a large inoculum of the fungus or by reactivation of dormant endogenous foci. Many cases are believed to arise from endogenous reactivation because some cases develop in those who remotely resided in an endemic area. Reactivation of latent infection can develop from transplanted organs.[52] In one such case, kidney transplantation from one donor was associated with infection in recipients who were not residents of an endemic area. These types of cases are difficult to discern in endemic areas. Most cases of PDH are now observed in immunosuppressed individuals.[49,53] However, there still exist cases in previously normal individuals, often at the extremes of age, who were not known to exhibit preexisting immunologic dysfunction. The perturbations that cause a breach in the integrity of the immune system and therefore lead to reactivation of quiescent infected foci have not been delineated.

Although infection with *H. capsulatum* produces a broad range of disease, PDH also can be categorized by clinical and pathologic manifestations. There is an acute form associated with a fulminant course. Histopathologically, massive macrophage infiltration and scattered lymphocytes are apparent. Tissue macrophages are engorged with yeast cells, and tests of cellular immunity often reveal poor to absent responses. At the other extreme is the chronic form, characterized by an indolent course and the presence of well-circumscribed granulomas in involved tissues. In tissues, few yeasts are seen, and delayed-type hypersensitivity responses are intact in a high proportion of individuals.

ACUTE PROGRESSIVE DISSEMINATED HISTOPLASMOSIS

In the era before aggressive immunosuppressive or cytotoxic therapy, this entity was principally seen in infants—hence its moniker, the infantile form. To date, however, it is most often observed in those who are severely immunosuppressed, especially those with AIDS and hematologic malignancies such as Hodgkin's and non-Hodgkin's lymphoma. In infants and young children, it is believed that this form of histoplasmosis is a progression of a primary exposure or reinfection because pulmonary symptoms dominate the early phases of illness. The onset is usually abrupt, extending over just a few days. Fever and malaise are the two most common manifestations, followed by weight loss, cough, and diarrhea. Physical findings include hepatosplenomegaly in almost all patients, lymphadenopathy, especially of the cervical chain, in about 30%, and crackles. Jaundice is observed in a minority, and oropharyngeal ulcers develop in less than 20%.[53]

Hematologic disturbances are frequent. Anemia is present in more than 90% of cases, of whom most have a hematocrit lower than 20%. Leukopenia and thrombocytopenia are observed in more than 80% of children. Serum levels of the liver enzymes alanine aminotransferase and alkaline phosphatase are elevated in a high proportion. Chest roentgenograms most often reveal a patchy pneumonitis with mediastinal and hilar node enlargement. This finding supports the contention that acute PDH in children represents an extension of an exogenous exposure. Untreated, the mortality is 100% and, before the introduction of effective antifungal agents, most children died within 5 to 6 weeks after onset of symptoms. Terminal events include disseminated intravascular coagulation, gastrointestinal hemorrhage, probably resulting from severe thrombocytopenia, and secondary bacterial sepsis associated with profound granulocytopenia.

In HIV-infected individuals, the risk factors for the development of histoplasmosis are a CD4+ cell count lower than 200 cells/mL, history of exposure to chicken coops, and a known positive serology for complement-fixing antibodies before illness.[54] Most AIDS patients who develop PDH have had at least one opportunistic infection. Although PDH may develop in approximately 25% of AIDS patients residing in an endemic area, there is no comparable information in the era of highly active antiretroviral therapy, although anecdotal reports suggest a decline in the incidence of cases. On seeking medical attention, almost all patients manifest evidence of disseminated disease. Fever and weight loss are found in more than 90% of those with AIDS and PDH. The most common physical findings include rales, hepatosplenomegaly, and lymphadenopathy. Mucosal ulcers are distinctly uncommon, but as many as 10% of patients will exhibit cutaneous lesions.[55] The common cutaneous findings are a maculopapular eruption, petechiae, or ecchymosis. The maculopapular rash does not display any unique pattern of distribution. The finding of skin lesions is much more common in those infected with the South American strains of *H. capsulatum*. In a small study, up to 66% of South American AIDS patients with disseminated histoplasmosis manifested skin lesions. The most common appearance is a papular eruption with crusting. Less frequent are nodular or purely pustular lesions. Histopathology of skin lesions reveals necrosis circumscribing the superficial dermal vessels. There is perivascular cuffing with lymphocytes and neutrophils, but the number of cells is very few. Yeasts are present both intra- and extracellularly. In addition to the skin findings, a number of other unusual manifestations have been reported, including colonic masses, perianal ulcers, chorioretinitis, meningitis, and encephalitis. It is estimated from results of one series that up to 20% of patients with PDH will have central nervous system involvement.[56] The more aggressive forms include encephalitis, acute meningitis, and encephalopathy in acute PDH. Histoplasmoma of the central nervous system and chronic meningitis are manifestations of a more indolent form of PDH.

Anemia, thrombocytopenia, and leukopenia are common laboratory features of PDH in the immunosuppressed population. In AIDS patients, the alteration in the peripheral blood counts may be attributable in part to the disease or to the drugs that they are receiving. Ele-

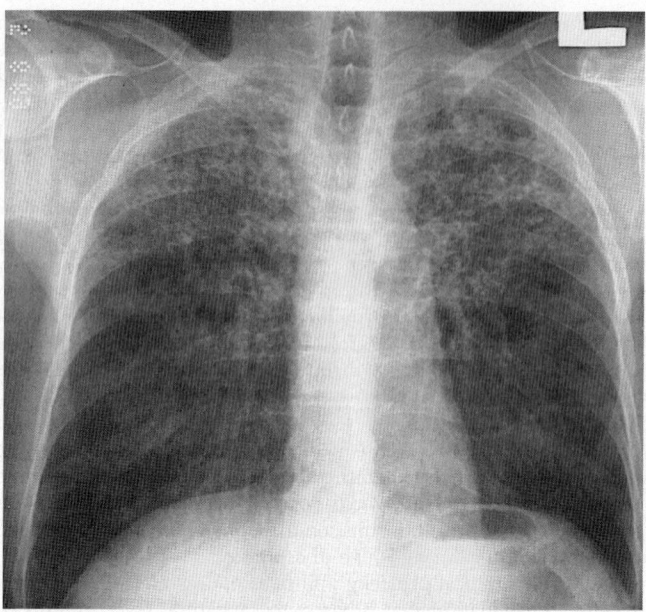

Figure 264-8 Diffuse infiltrates in patients with progressive disseminated histoplasmosis and acquired immunodeficiency syndrome.

vated serum levels of hepatic enzymes are frequently detected. Again, concomitant drugs may obscure the laboratory abnormalities caused strictly by *H. capsulatum*. Chest roentgenograms typically demonstrate widely scattered nodular opacities or a diffuse reticular pattern (Fig. 264-8). However, a substantial percentage (30%) may present with a normal roentgenogram.[57]

The fatality rate of acute PDH in the immunocompromised patient is 100% if untreated. With therapy, survival rates of the acute episode exceed 80%. Infrequently, patients exhibit a sepsis-like syndrome characterized by disseminated intravascular coagulation, encephalopathy, acute respiratory distress syndrome, vascular collapse, and, subsequently, multiorgan failure. In some patients, bone marrow biopsy has demonstrated the presence of histiocytes phagocytosing erythrocytes. This form of PDH has been termed the *reactive hemophagocytic syndrome* and, despite aggressive management and therapy, the outcome is usually catastrophic.

SUBACUTE PROGRESSIVE DISSEMINATED HISTOPLASMOSIS

Subacute PDH is distinguished from the acute form primarily by the more prolonged nature of the symptoms before the patient seeks medical attention. Fever and weight loss are common at some time during the course of infection, but fever is a presenting complaint in only about 50%. Physical findings include hepatosplenomegaly and oropharyngeal ulcers. In contrast to the ulcers observed in acute PDH, these are deeper and more likely to be confused with malignancy. Laboratory abnormalities are much less striking than in acute PDH. Although anemia and leukopenia are noted in up to 40%, the percentage of patients with severe depression of the hematocrit or leukocyte count is low. Thrombocytopenia is evident in about 20%, and is usually mild. Rarely is the platelet count lower than 20,000/μL.[53]

One of the notable features of subacute PDH is the presence of focal lesions in various organ systems, including the gastrointestinal tract, endovascular structures, central nervous system, and adrenal glands.[53,58] Aside from the liver and spleen, the gastrointestinal tract is one of the most common organs affected in subacute PDH. Yeast cells can be found in the bowel mucosa in up to 70% of autopsy cases. Macroscopic ulcerations of the small and large bowel are present in about 40%, and perforation from a penetrating ulcer has been reported. The terminal ileum and cecum are the sites most frequently involved. Symptoms referable to the bowel are not frequent but if present, diarrhea and crampy abdominal pain are typical complaints. Intestinal obstruction of the ileum also has been reported.

Endocarditis and infection of other vascular structures may be a manifestation of subacute PDH.[59] The aortic and mitral valves are affected more commonly than right-sided valves, and the aortic valve is the single most common valve involved. In about 50% of cases, there is prior evidence of valvular disease, such as a bicuspid aortic valve. Echocardiography shows that the lesions tend to be extensive, and large-vessel embolization can be the presenting symptom. Clumps of yeasts embedded in a fibrin mesh is the characteristic histopathologic feature. Occasionally, allomorphs that are as large as 20 μ in diameter have been observed. In addition, hyphal forms of *H. capsulatum* have been detected in endocarditis. If untreated, death usually ensues. Other endovascular manifestations include prosthetic valve endocarditis, infection of abdominal aortic aneurysms, and prosthetic grafts. Previous reports have indicated that blood cultures are rarely positive. However, those reports preceded improved methods for isolating *H. capsulatum* from blood.

Central nervous system infection involves all age groups and causes a number of manifestations, including chronic meningitis, mass lesion, and cerebritis. Among these, chronic meningitis is the most frequent.[56] Symptoms of central nervous system histoplasmosis may antedate medical attention for several weeks, and they include headache, altered sensorium, and cranial nerve deficits. Seizures, ataxia, meningismus, and other focal deficits constitute much of the remaining symptomatology. It must be emphasized that only half of patients may complain of symptoms localized to the central nervous system. Associated physical findings consist of hepatosplenomegaly in about one third, lymphadenopathy, and mucocutaneous lesions.

In cases of meningitis, pleocytosis of the cerebrospinal fluid is present in all patients. Cell counts usually range from 10 to 100/μL with a preponderance of lymphocytes. Hypoglycorrhachia and elevated protein levels are detected in 80%. Histopathology of the brain parenchyma and meninges characteristically reveals granulomatous inflammation. A perivenous granulomatosis in which parasitized macrophages are observed beneath the intima of parenchymal and meningeal veins is commonly seen. The basilar meninges are the most severely affected area of the central nervous system. Hydrocephalus may contribute to the symptomatology.

An intracerebral granulomatous mass, or histoplasmoma, causes a mass effect and may initially be mistaken for a malignancy or abscess by computed tomography (CT) because it exhibits ring enhancement with the administration of contrast. Dense fibrotic tissue surrounds a caseous center in which yeasts are detected. Histoplasmomas may be associated with meningitis, but often are independently present. Cerebrospinal fluid pleocytosis is common but hypoglycorrhachia is not.

Although symptoms arising from involvement of adrenal glands is not frequent, autopsy series indicate that yeasts invade this organ system in approximately 80% of cases.[60] Macrophages containing yeasts are found scattered throughout the parenchyma of the adrenal gland. There is no particular predilection for either the cortex or the medulla. The severity of infection ranges from focal areas containing parasitized macrophages to diffuse involvement of the adrenal parenchyma. The former is most commonly detected. Tissue necrosis is seen, but usually involves only a small portion of the gland. Grossly, the adrenal glands are enlarged. This postmortem discovery has been supported by findings on CT in which a high percentage of patients with subacute PDH display enlarged adrenals. Overt Addison's disease is uncommon, occurring in less than 10%. There is little information concerning the incidence of an impaired pituitary-adrenal axis.

CHRONIC PROGRESSIVE DISSEMINATED HISTOPLASMOSIS

Chronic PDH can be distinguished from subacute PDH by the prolonged chronicity of symptoms that are often very mild. This form is

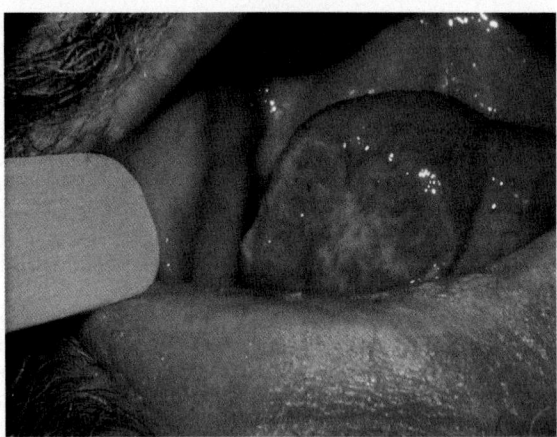

Figure 264-9 Tongue ulcer in a patient with chronic disseminated histoplasmosis.

seen almost exclusively in previously normal adults. Malaise and lethargy stand out as the most frequent complaints. Fever is much less frequent (less than 30%) and is often low grade. The most common physical finding (50%) is an oropharyngeal ulcer that is well circumscribed, indurated, and usually deep and painless (Fig. 264-9).[53] The tongue, buccal mucosa, larynx, gums, and lip are the most affected structures. Occasionally the lesion is on the labia or glans penis. These lesions are often confused with squamous carcinoma oral malignancy. Hence, it is incumbent for the clinician to consider the diagnosis of histoplasmosis; otherwise, tissue will be sent only for histology. Histopathologically, the center of the lesion contains macrophages with many yeasts, but the number of such macrophages decreases in the periphery of the lesion. Unlike the histologic reaction in other viscera, the response in the mucosa is an admixture of acute and chronic inflammation. Thus, plasma cells, lymphocytes, eosinophils, and granulocytes are found infiltrating the ulcer, and fibrosis is a characteristic feature. Areas of intact mucosa may show hyperplasia that can be confused with squamous carcinoma on superficial biopsy. Well-circumscribed granulomas are typically found, usually at the periphery.

Other symptoms include hepatosplenomegaly in about one third of patients. Chronic meningitis or chronic granulomatous hepatitis may be the only manifestation of infection. Unlike subacute PDH, there is a notable absence of disease involvement of other organ systems, including central nervous system, heart, and adrenals. Bone infection, Addison's disease, and endocarditis all have been described, but these entities are uncommon. Hematologic abnormalities are distinctly uncommon and often not significant. This illness may persist for years, with periods of spontaneous improvement in symptoms, without being recognized. On occasion, there may be an abrupt worsening caused by involvement of a particular organ such as the central nervous system, adrenals, or heart.[53] Usually, however, the illness remains undiagnosed until symptoms arising from a single organ are observed. Without appropriate therapy, infection progresses to death.

Ocular Histoplasmosis

Two different syndromes of ocular involvement are described. The less common is a uveitis or panophthalmitis in association with active progressive disseminated histoplasmosis. Granulomas are present in the uvea, and yeasts are recovered from lesions. Much more frequent is the presumed ocular histoplasmosis syndrome (POHS), which consists of a posterior uveitis or choroiditis in individuals who manifest skin test positivity to histoplasmin and intrathoracic calcifications.[61] However, it must be stressed that a skin test and the presence of intrathoracic calcifications do not prove cause and effect.

Typically, there are peripheral atrophic scars and a lack of vitreous or anterior segment inflammation. The scars or "histospots" are located posterior to the equator of the eye. They range in size from 0.2

to 0.7 disk diameters, and can vary in number from 1 to 70 in a single eye. Involvement of both eyes is uncommon (less than 10%). Most individuals are between 20 and 50 years of age when this syndrome is diagnosed, and the prevalence may be as high as 10% in endemic regions. The major destructive consequence of this lesion is macular hemorrhage, which develops 10 to 20 years after the appearance of scars. Neovascularization and scarring can lead to loss of vision in up to 60% of patients.[59] Because neovascularization can exert such devastating effects, efforts have been made to understand its cause. It has been shown that the integrin $\alpha_v\beta_3$ is expressed on blood vessels from patients with POHS.

The histopathology of POHS reveals a lymphocytic infiltration in the scarred areas. Yeasts are rarely observed in the eye or elsewhere. A model for this syndrome has been developed in primates to define the cellular immunopathology. Chronic lesions contain a preponderance of B and CD4+ cells. As in affected human eyes, yeasts are not found in the lesions. Within the choroidal lesions, there is an increase in the percentage of CD4+ cells and macrophages. There is no definitive proof that *H. capsulatum* causes the scars that are observed in humans, although the primate model establishes that this fungus can produce choroidal scars. The pathogenesis appears to be an exuberant cellular immune reaction to inert fungal antigens, thus somewhat resembling the tissue response in mediastinal fibrosis. Corticosteroid treatment of POHS does not activate latent histoplasmosis.

African Histoplasmosis

In Africa, the classic *H. capsulatum* var. *capsulatum* coexists with *H. capsulatum* var. *duboisii*. The yeast form of the latter is typically much larger, with a diameter up to 15 μm, and has a thicker wall. The mycelial form of both is indistinguishable. The pathogenesis of this fungus is presumed to be inhalation from the soil, although a primary pulmonary infection has not been demonstrated. Cutaneous inoculation is certainly an alternative mode of acquisition of the infection. Spontaneous disease has been reported in baboons and *Cynocephalus* monkeys. Most cases have been reported from Uganda, Nigeria, Zaire, and Senegal.

The clinical picture associated with infection by *H. capsulatum* var. *duboisii* is distinctly different from that caused by *H. capsulatum* var. *capsulatum*.[62] Skin and skeleton are the most frequent organs affected by this pathogen. In the skin, the usual findings are ulcers, nodules, or psoriatic-like lesions that may spontaneously resolve. Involvement of the subcutaneous tissue may present with tender nodules ("cold" abscesses) in which the typical manifestations of inflammation are absent. Osteolytic bone lesions are fairly common and are noted in up to 50% of cases. The skull and ribs are the most frequent bones affected, followed by vertebrae. The organism produces granulomatous inflammation within the bone. This type of inflammation can lead to sinus formation and cystic bone lesions. In a high proportion of patients, multiple bones may be infected. Even in the presence of overt skin or bone lesions, chest roentgenograms are often free of evidence of previous exposure to *H. capsulatum*. Draining lymph nodes also may become inflamed.

A progressive disseminated disease has been recognized. Patients are febrile, with hematologic abnormalities. There is multiorgan involvement, including liver, spleen, kidney, and lung, and miliary lesions are observed in the lungs. The histopathology resembles that induced by *Blastomyces dermatitidis* or *Coccidioides immitis*—that is, a pyogranulomatous reaction in which there is a combination of granulomas and suppuration. One likely reason for this pathologic reaction is the large size of *H. capsulatum* var. *duboisii*, which prevents avid ingestion by macrophages. Thus, neutrophils may ingress to assist in the clearance of the fungus.

Reports of African histoplasmosis in HIV-infected individuals are emerging. A variety of manifestations in individual patients has been observed. Disseminated infection with fever, cutaneous infection, and bone infection have been recognized.[63] The outcome has been favorable only in a minority of patients.

Diagnosis

Histoplasmosis only can be definitively established by isolation from body fluids or tissues. The typical medium that is used to recover the fungus from sterile fluids includes brain heart infusion agar, with the addition of antibiotics and cycloheximide when culturing nonsterile fluids such as sputum. Cultures are incubated at 30°C for up to 6 weeks. Often, growth is noted within 3 weeks, and more than 90% of cultures exhibit fungus within 7 days. Previously, confirmation that the fungus was *H. capsulatum* required exoantigen testing or conversion of the mycelial form to the yeast form, but this step is no longer necessary. All mycelial isolates are confirmed using a DNA probe that recognizes ribosomal RNA.

The incidence of positive cultures varies considerably and often is correlated with the number of specimens collected, the source of the specimen, and the burden of infection. Recovery of *H. capsulatum* from sputa of patients with acute pulmonary histoplasmosis ranges from 10% to 15%, whereas in cavitary histoplasmosis, cultures are positive in up to 60% of patients.[64] The yield of positive cultures increases with the number of specimens collected. Three or more specimens are more likely to display growth of *H. capsulatum*. In AIDS patients with pulmonary manifestations, up to 90% of cultures from the lungs obtained from bronchoscopic samples will grow *H. capsulatum*. Bone marrow and blood cultures are positive in up to 50%.[64] Yields for blood cultures are considerably higher if the lysis centrifugation technique is used. The organism can be frequently isolated from oropharyngeal ulcers in patients with chronic PDH. In endocarditis, valve cultures are positive in a high percentage but blood cultures often are negative. However, much of the evidence concerning blood cultures used the biphasic medium, which may not be as sensitive as lysis centrifugation. In meningitis, the organism is recovered from the cerebrospinal fluid (CSF) in 25% to 65% of patients,[56] and the yield is improved if a large volume (20 mL or more) is removed, because *H. capsulatum* invades the basilar meninges. The organism is unlikely to be isolated from pericardial or pleural fluid, but more likely from their respective serosal tissues. Similarly, *H. capsulatum* rarely is isolated from mediastinal tissues in patients with mediastinal fibrosis.

ANTIGEN DETECTION AND POLYMERASE CHAIN REACTION ANALYSIS

The antigen assay, which detects polysaccharide antigen in serum or urine by enzyme-linked immunosorbent assay (ELISA), is the mainstay of diagnosis, especially in those with PDH. Several laboratories now offer the test. Antigen is detected in up to 90% of patients with acute PDH, 40% with cavitary disease, and 20% with acute pulmonary histoplasmosis.[64] The test also is very useful for monitoring relapses of acute PDH, especially in immunosuppressed patients. An increase of the arbitrary value of 2 units is significantly associated with relapse of infection. Antigen detection is much more sensitive than serology for identifying relapsing cases, and it has been applied successfully to CSF in patients with meningitis. The test was positive in 12 of 14 cases. Thus, it has a high degree of sensitivity and specificity. Cross-reactivity in the urine test has been found for patients infected with *B. dermatitidis*, *Coccidioides immitis*, *Paracoccidioides brasiliensis*, or *Penicillium marneffei*, but with improvements in the test, cross-reactions are becoming less frequent.

Several reports of the usefulness of the polymerase chain reaction have been published and, although not in clinical use yet, they show promise. The future prospects for this test are unknown.

SEROLOGY

Since the late 1940s, serology has been a vital instrument in the diagnosis of infection with *H. capsulatum*. Complement-fixing (CF) antibodies and precipitin bands have been the most common tests used in the clinical laboratory. The greatest usefulness has been in the retrospective diagnosis of acute histoplasmosis, using a fourfold or greater rise in CF titer between acute and convalescent serum. This has been particularly helpful in outbreaks that are recognized in time to collect acute sera but the antibody titer rise occurs too late to be of value in patient management. For chronic pulmonary or progressive disseminated histoplasmosis, fourfold rises are not observed and antibody tests have insufficient sensitivity and specificity to be of clinical value. For CF antibodies, a titer of 1:8 to yeast or mycelial antigen is considered positive, and a titer of 1:32 indicates the need to pursue a possible diagnosis of histoplasmosis. Titers that fall between these two values neither exclude nor suggest the diagnosis. On occasion, a result is returned that states that the test is anticomplementary. This result signifies that the serum contained a substance or substances that interfered with the CF test. Repeat of the test with a new serum specimen frequently yields a result.

Low levels of CF antibodies are detected in approximately 10% of healthy individuals who reside in an endemic region. A low percentage of individuals with acute pulmonary histoplasmosis will develop CF antibodies within the first 3 weeks of infection, but by 6 weeks, at least 75% of patients manifest a positive CF antibody titer or a fourfold rise. Over the course of months, the antibody titer will decline, although it may remain serofast for years, especially in those with cavitary pulmonary disease or with chronic PDH. The false-positive rate is estimated to be 15% and is most commonly observed in those with coccidioidomycosis or with blastomycosis.[65] The reason for the cross-reactivity is the presence of a carbohydrate antigen common to the three fungi.

Another test is the detection of H and M bands during the illness. On the agar gel precipitin test, these bands are identified by lines of identity with bands formed by control sera known to have precipitating antibody to H or M antigens. These two precipitin bands were originally identified using immunodiffusion as specific to sera from patients with histoplasmosis. The H and M antigens are glycoproteins released by mycelial and yeast phase cultures. The H antigen has been cloned and sequenced, and it demonstrates homology to β-glucosidases. It is infrequently detected (less than 10%) in the sera of patients but, when present, signifies active infection. The M antigen also has been cloned and sequenced, and it has a high degree of homology to catalase. Unlike the H antigen, it is detected in up to 80% of individuals following exposure to the fungus. However, it is present in patients who have recovered from infection or who have active disease. Therefore, it is not useful in discriminating remote from current infection. A major limitation of the serologic tests is that even in the presence of active infection, they are negative in up to 50% of immunosuppressed patients, especially those with AIDS. One explanation for the poor anti-*Histoplasma* antibody response is that the immunosuppressive agents or HIV induce dysfunctional B cells and/or CD4+ T cells, thus rendering serologic assays almost useless.

HISTOCHEMICAL IDENTIFICATION

Stains for the presence of *H. capsulatum* can be extremely useful for rapid identification of the fungus in various tissues or body fluids. The yeast is visualized poorly by hematoxylin-eosin stain, but is more apparent using the periodic acid–Schiff (PAS) stain. The most useful stain is either the Gomori methenamine (GMS) or Grocott silver stain. The organism can be detected in peripheral blood smears stained with Wright-Giemsa in up to 40% of cases of acute PDH (Fig. 264-10). This percentage is much lower if the reader of the blood smear is scrutinizing the slide only to determine a differential. Examination of the peripheral blood smear can be useful if the clinician suspects PDH as a cause of a patient's illness. The yeast must be discriminated from *Pneumocystis jirovecii* in the lung. This organism is larger, nonbudding, and usually extracellular. Moreover, it is exceedingly rare to find *P. jirovecii* outside the lung or in an area of caseous necrosis. Although *Leishmania* spp. and *Toxoplasma gondii* may on occasion be confused morphologically with *H. capsulatum*, neither stains with silver.

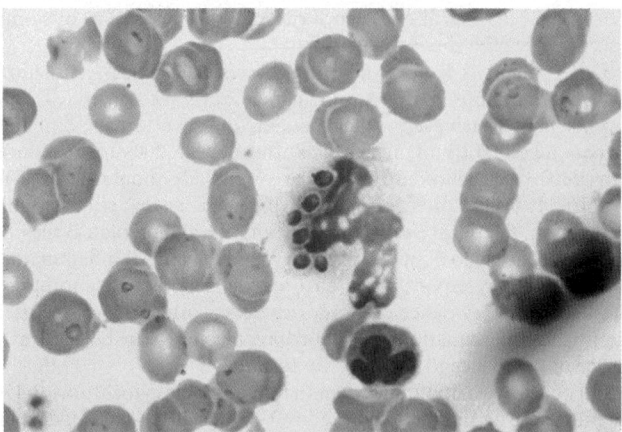

Figure 264-10 **Circulating neutrophil with intracellular yeast cells.** (Wright-Giemsa stain, ×400.)

SKIN TEST

The histoplasmin skin test has been used for several decades to determine who has been exposed to *H. capsulatum*. The skin test reagent is the supernatant from the mycelial growth and has been standardized by the World Health Organization. This reagent has been exceptionally useful as an epidemiologic tool but has practically no value as a diagnostic tool because it only indicates past exposure. The skin test antigen is no longer available commercially.

MISCELLANEOUS LABORATORY TESTS

One retrospective study has suggested that patients with AIDS who are admitted to the hospital with pulmonary infiltrates and fever higher than 38°C and serum lactate dehydrogenase (LDH) levels higher than 600 IU/mL are highly likely to have disseminated histoplasmosis.[66] Other studies have suggested that elevated serum ferritin levels are strongly suggestive of histoplasmosis.[67]

◼ Treatment

The increasing incidence of fungal infections has prompted the development and testing of a number of new antifungal agents, some of which are available commercially. The introduction of azoles has moved the treatment of histoplasmosis from an inpatient to outpatient setting. Several azoles and polyenes are now available for the treatment of this fungal disease. Updated practice guidelines for the treatment of various forms of histoplasmosis have been published.[68]

ACUTE PULMONARY HISTOPLASMOSIS

The vast majority of cases of acute pulmonary histoplasmosis do not require therapeutic intervention. Bed rest and antipyretics suffice for these individuals. Treatment should be instituted for those who have not improved after 1 month of illness or who exhibit hypoxemia. In those who have not spontaneously resolved their illness after 1 month, oral itraconazole, 200 mg three times daily for 3 days, followed by 200 mg once or twice daily for 6 to 12 weeks will be sufficient. Fluconazole is not as active as itraconazole and should be avoided. If the patient cannot ingest an oral medication or tolerate an azole, liposomal amphotericin B is the preferred agent. A dosage of 3 to 5 mg/kg IV can be given every day until the symptoms subside, often within 2 weeks. The dosage for the lipid complex formulations of amphotericin B (ABLC) is 5 mg/kg. Daily administration is useful for those who have large catheters for venous access. The deoxycholate formulation can be used at 0.7 to 1 mg/kg daily if there is a low risk of serious nephrotoxicity. No comparative trials of amphotericin B and azoles have been performed, but clinical experience suggests that resolution of symptoms is faster with the former.

If the patient is hypoxemic and requires mechanical ventilation, liposomal amphotericin B, 3 to 5 mg/kg/day, is recommended until improvement is achieved. When patients improve to the point that they can ingest food and medications, itraconazole, 200 mg three times daily for 3 days, followed by once or twice daily should be used to complete 12 weeks of therapy. If the patient is at low risk for renal dysfunction, the deoxycholate preparation of amphotericin B may be substituted at a dose of 0.7 to 1.0 mg/kg/day. The inflammatory response may be responsible in part for the respiratory compromise. Although ample evidence does not exist, corticosteroids may be used to mitigate inflammation. IV methylprednisolone can be used at a dosage of 0.5 to 1 mg/kg/day for up to 14 days.

Itraconazole is a lipophilic agent that inhibits the cytochrome P-450 system (see drug interactions listed in Chapter 40). The cyclodextrin oral liquid formulation of itraconazole increases absorption by 50% and makes administration to young children much easier.

MEDIASTINAL GRANULOMA, MEDIASTINAL FIBROSIS, AND HISTOPLASMOMA

Hilar and mediastinal lymphadenopathy from acute pulmonary histoplasmosis usually is asymptomatic but can cause a brassy cough or compress the middle lobe bronchus, leading to temporary atelectasis. Although no therapy is usually necessary, persistent symptoms could be treated with itraconazole, 200 mg three times daily for 3 days, followed by 200 mg once or twice daily for 6 to 12 weeks. Rarely, large caseous mediastinal nodes will compress the esophagus or erode into both the esophagus and bronchus, causing a bronchoesophageal fistula. Surgical resection of the nodes may be indicated, although the nodes may be densely adherent to the pulmonary veins and other surrounding structures. Corticosteroids may be used if the enlarged nodes cause significant compression of surrounding structures. Prednisone at a dose not to exceed 80 mg may be tried, with a rapid taper over 1 to 2 weeks.

Mediastinal fibrosis is an exceptionally difficult clinical problem for which there is no consensus on optimal management. Surgery, corticosteroids, and antifungal agents have been used in the treatment of this condition, with minimal success. Surgery to remove the fibrosis area and placement of intravascular stents can alleviate the life-threatening situation, but the fibrosis often progresses. Moreover, the surgery may jeopardize essential venous collaterals, such as the hemiazygos or azygos veins. Addition of azoles after surgery has been proposed, but the usefulness of this approach is debatable.[68]

A histoplasmoma of the lung, which is a fibrocaseous nodule resulting from healed acute pulmonary histoplasmosis, does not require any therapy. Surgical resection or biopsy may be needed to exclude malignancy in a solitary pulmonary nodule if no central calcification is evident. Serology is of no value in proving the nodule is a histoplasmoma.

CAVITARY PULMONARY HISTOPLASMOSIS

Although some patients with fibrocavitary disease will eventually stabilize their disease without treatment, the inability to predict which patients will eventually progress has led to the recommendation that all patients should be treated, even those who are currently asymptomatic. Treatment does not improve pulmonary function already lost and, in fact, healing may lead to some further loss of function because of fibrosis. Discontinuing cigarette smoking is an important adjunct in preventing further loss of pulmonary capacity. Many patients with only thin-walled cavities spontaneously resolve infection without therapeutic intervention. Such patients, if untreated, should be followed by serial chest roentgenography every 2 to 3 months. Those who have thick-walled cavities, progressive pulmonary infiltrates, or persistent cavities associated with declining respiratory function should be treated. Oral itraconazole, 200 mg three times daily for 3 days, followed

by once or twice daily, should be given for 12 to 24 months.[68] This regimen will arrest progression in 75% to 85% of patients. Relapse may be difficult to detect radiologically in patients with extensive prior lung damage. Sputum culture is the best means for detecting relapse, although *Aspergillus* and other rapidly growing molds may overgrow the culture plate. Fluconazole is not recommended. Itraconazole levels should be determined after 2 weeks of therapy to determine if adequate levels have been achieved. A trough blood level of 2 μg/mL by bioassay or the sum of native itraconazole and its hydroxymetabolite by high-performance liquid chromatography (HPLC) has been proposed (see Chapter 40). If there is progression of infection while on azoles or the patient has relapsed following azole therapy, amphotericin B is preferable. The total dose is 30 to 35 mg/kg, and can be given as 0.7 mg/kg/day or approximately 50 mg daily.[68] If renal dysfunction is a consideration, a lipid formulation may be used at 3 to 5 mg/kg/day.

The relapse rates for cavitary pulmonary histoplasmosis are as high as 20%, with the highest relapse rates seen in patients with thick-walled cavities. If there is a failure of antifungal therapy, surgical resection may be indicated if the patient has sufficient pulmonary reserve.

ACUTE PROGRESSIVE DISSEMINATED HISTOPLASMOSIS

Prompt institution of amphotericin B therapy is necessary for treatment of patients with acute, life-threatening PDH. Patients should be begun on liposomal amphotericin B at a dosage of 3 mg/kg/day. If the lipid complex (ABLC) is used, the dose should be 5 mg/kg/day. Within 1 to 2 weeks, most patients are symptomatically improved, and laboratory abnormalities begin to return to baseline values. If deoxycholate amphotericin B is used, the starting dose should be 25 mg followed by a rapid escalation to 1 mg/kg. Once the patient has become afebrile and clinically stable, amphotericin B can be administered at a lower dose of 0.4 to 0.5 mg/kg daily. Patients who demonstrate resolution of symptoms while on amphotericin B may be switched to itraconazole 200 mg three times daily for 3 days, followed by 200 mg twice daily for a total duration of 12 months. In acute PDH that is not associated with hemodynamic instability or severe illness, itraconazole may be used initially. Therapy should begin with 200 mg three times daily for 3 days, followed by 200 mg twice daily for at least 12 months. Itraconazole interacts with many antiretrovirals, including elevating serum concentrations of several protease inhibitors.

In patients with AIDS, lifelong suppressive therapy with itraconazole 200 mg daily is recommended for most patients. Although there are no reliable data to make this decision, it may be reasonable to discontinue maintenance therapy in patients receiving highly active antiretroviral therapy, and who have a CD4 count higher than 150 cells/μL for 6 months, a nondetectable viral load, at least 12 months of antifungal therapy, and a negative test for *Histoplasma* antigen in urine. If the patient relapses while receiving azole maintenance therapy, amphotericin B should be given.[68] Following treatment of the relapse, the patient should receive amphotericin B as maintenance therapy with 0.7 to 1 mg/kg once or twice weekly. A self-limiting immune reconstitution syndrome has been recognized occasionally in HIV patients being treated for PDH and who have had an effective response to highly active antiretroviral therapy. The syndrome presents as fever, with or without an elevated alkaline phosphatase level. Management is supportive.

Relapse of PDH is common in other persistently immunosuppressed patients and may be difficult to detect until far advanced. Indefinite suppressive therapy with itraconazole may be a useful option.

SUBACUTE AND CHRONIC PROGRESSIVE DISSEMINATED HISTOPLASMOSIS

Because many of these cases develop in patients whose immune system is intact, itraconazole 200 mg three times daily followed by 200 mg twice daily is highly efficacious. The success rate in these individuals approaches 90%. If the patient requires hospitalization, fails to improve on azole therapy, is immunosuppressed, or demonstrates intolerance to azoles, lipid-based preparations of amphotericin B, 3 to 5 mg/kg/day, should be given. When the infection is controlled by this drug, it is possible to switch them to itraconazole to complete a total of 12 months of therapy.

MENINGITIS

Patients with meningitis should be given liposomal amphotericin B, 3 to 5 mg/kg/day for 4 to 6 weeks, followed by itraconazole, 200 mg two or three times daily for at least 1 year. Blood levels of itraconazole should be determined. Cerebrospinal fluid should have a normal glucose level and no detectable cerebrospinal fluid *Histoplasma* antigen at the end of therapy. Repeat lumbar punctures should be performed approximately every week for the first 6 weeks and every 2 weeks thereafter to assess therapy. Although a high percentage of patients may respond initially to therapy, they frequently relapse. Overall cure rates are no better than 50%, and immunocompetent patients respond much better to treatment than immunosuppressed persons.

ENDOCARDITIS

As with bacterial causes of endocarditis, a microbicidal agent should be used. Therefore, liposomal amphotericin B, 3 to 5 mg/kg/day, should be given. If using another lipid formulation, 5 mg/kg should be administered. Alternatively, if there is a low risk of nephrotoxicity, deoxycholate amphotericin B, 0.7 to 1 mg/kg, may be used. Administration of an antifungal agent alone is not sufficient and must be used in combination with surgical removal of the affected valve(s). One issue is how long to treat after the valve has been removed. If there are other foci of active histoplasmosis, then treatment guidelines for progressive disseminated histoplasmosis should be used. However, if the valve was the only site involved, treatment with a lipid formulation or the deoxycholate preparation for 2 weeks following surgical extraction may be sufficient. If the patient cannot undergo surgery, an amphotericin B preparation in the highest tolerated dose, should be given daily.[68]

PERICARDITIS

Pericarditis following acute pulmonary histoplasmosis does not require antifungal therapy. Most patients can be treated symptomatically with nonsteroidal anti-inflammatory drugs (NSAIDs) for 2 to 12 weeks.[68] If patients fail to respond to these agents, or if the patient manifests hemodynamic instability, corticosteroids are indicated for 1 to 2 weeks followed by nonsteroidal agents. One must be cautious because if there are active lesions of histoplasmosis, the infection may become more aggressive during corticosteroid therapy. Itraconazole, 200 mg three times daily for 3 days, followed by 200 mg once or twice daily for 6 to 12 weeks, should be included if corticosteroids are necessary. The rationale for the antifungal is to prevent reactivation, although there is little information regarding the frequency with which this occurs in short-term usage of corticosteroids. Cardiac tamponade associated with *H. capsulatum* pericarditis is uncommon, but when it occurs, it must be treated as a medical emergency with pericardiocentesis. Despite the severity of illness, antifungal therapy is not indicated. Unlike tuberculous pericarditis, constrictive pericarditis rarely develops, but patients should be monitored for several years after the acute attack. In the uncommon situation in which the pericardium is infected as a manifestation of PDH, antifungal therapy with amphotericin B or azoles is indicated, depending on the severity of illness.

ARTHROPATHIES

NSAIDs should be continued until resolution of symptoms. If corticosteroids are used to alleviate symptoms, itraconazole should be used concomitantly, as noted earlier.

PRESUMED OCULAR HISTOPLASMOSIS

This condition does not require antifungal therapy. Laser therapy is used to prevent additional neovascularization within the choroid, but lesions that abut the fovea cannot be subjected to this treatment.[61] Photodynamic therapy for this region of the eye appears promising, as does the implementation of intravitreous antiangiogenic agents. The role of retrobulbar local injection of corticosteroids is unclear.

OTHER CONSIDERATIONS

Histoplasmosis in pregnancy should be treated with amphotericin B, preferably a lipid formulation, but the deoxycholate preparation can be used if nephrotoxicity is of low concern. The dose of liposomal preparation should be 3 to 5 mg/kg/day for 4 to 6 weeks, and that of the deoxycholate formulation 0.7 to 1.0 mg/kg/day. If using another lipid formulation of amphotericin B, 5 mg/kg is the preferred dosage.

No clear guidelines exist for patients receiving tumor necrosis factor-α antagonists. Those from the endemic area pose the highest risk for reactivation or reinfection. If a patient develops histoplasmosis while on therapy, the biologic agent should be stopped and therapy for disseminated histoplasmosis completed. Once treatment has concluded and the patient requires the antagonist, it may be prudent to administer itraconazole prophylaxis when the antagonist is instituted. Prophylaxis should be continued while tumor necrosis factor-α is being administered.

Prevention

PROPHYLAXIS OF IMMUNOCOMPROMISED PERSONS

For immunosuppressed patients who have a high risk of acquiring histoplasmosis from the environment because of their work or their residence, itraconazole, 200 mg/day, is useful. Such patients would include those with AIDS whose CD4 cell count is less than 150/μL or those who require potent immunosuppressive therapy. In the former group, prophylaxis with itraconazole reduced the incidence of infection by more than twofold. Another indication for prophylaxis in immunosuppressed patients would be for those residing in areas that have a high incidence of infection, as defined by at least 10 cases/100 patient-years.[69]

OTHER CONSIDERATIONS

Educational efforts must be ongoing to alert those who work in areas in which a substantial risk of infection exists. Dust control and the use of N95 masks should be considered. For example, construction workers who are restoring buildings that have served as homes for starlings and bats must be warned about the possibility of exposure and steps taken to remove the guano safely. Spraying 3% formalin on guano deposits will kill the fungus within several days, and the material can then be removed. However, formaldehyde decontamination is rarely used because the vapor is toxic, it can seep into groundwater (thus posing an environmental hazard), and it does not penetrate dried guano uniformly.

There is a continuing resurgent effort to develop a vaccine preventive against *H. capsulatum* pathogenic fungi because of their escalating incidence. Among those in which animal studies have defined a vaccine is *H. capsulatum*. Vaccine candidates containing heat shock protein 60 and H antigen from *H. capsulatum* have been demonstrated to confer protection to mice given a pulmonary challenge. A region of heat shock protein 60 that spans amino acids 174 to 445 appears to contain the protective activity of the entire protein. In mice, a monoclonal antibody to the cell surface has been shown to augment the efficacy of antifungal therapy.[70]

REFERENCES

1. Darling ST. A protozoal general infection producing pseudotubercles in the lungs and focal necrosis in the liver, spleen, and lymph nodes. *JAMA.* 1906;46:1283-1285.
2. da Rocha-Lima H. Histoplasmose und epizootische Lymphangitis. *Arch Schiffs Tropenhyg.* 1912;16:79.
3. DeMonbreun WA. The cultivation and cultural characteristics of Darling's *Histoplasma capsulatum. Am J Trop Med Hyg.* 1934;14: 93-125.
4. Christie A. Histoplasmosis and pulmonary calcification. *Ann N Y Acad Sci.* 1950;50:1283-1298.
5. Furcolow ML, Schubert J, Tosh FE, et al. Serologic evidence of histoplasmosis in sanitariums in the U.S. *JAMA.* 1962;180:109-114.
6. Ajello L. Distribution of *Histoplasma capsulatum* in the United States. In: Ajello L, Chick W, Furculow MF, eds. *Histoplasmosis.* Springfield, Ill: Charles C Thomas; 1971:103-122.
7. Zeidberg LD, Ajello L, Webster RH. Physical and chemical factors in relation to *Histoplasma capsulatum* in soil. *Science.* 1955; 122:33-34.
8. Emmons CW. Isolation of *Histoplasma capsulatum* from soil. *Public Health Rep.* 1949;64:892-896.
9. DiSalvo AF, Ajello L, Palmer JW, et al. Isolation of *Histoplasma capsulatum* from Arizona bats. *Am J Epidemiol.* 1969;89:606-614.
10. Schwarz J. Immunity. In: Schwarz J, ed. *Histoplasmosis.* New York: Praeger; 1981:147-176.
11. Steele PE, Carle GF, Kobayashi GS, et al. Electrophoretic analysis of *Histoplasma capsulatum* chromosomal DNA. *Mol Cell Biol.* 1989;9:983-987.
12. Kasuga T, White TJ, Koenig G, et al. Phylogeography of the fungal pathogen *Histoplasma capsulatum. Mol Ecol.* 2003;12:3383-3401.
13. Spitzer ED, Keath EJ, Travis SJ, et al. Temperature-sensitive variants of *Histoplasma capsulatum* isolated from patients with acquired immunodeficiency syndrome. *J Infect Dis.* 1990; 162:258-261.
14. Kwon-Chung KJ, Weeks RJ, Larsh HW. Studies on *Emonsiella capsulata* (*Histoplasma capsulatum*). II. Distribution of the two mating types in 13 endemic states of the United States. *Am J Epidemiol.* 1974;99:44-49.
15. Batanghari JW, Deepe GS Jr, Di Cera E, et al. Histoplasma acquisition of calcium and expression of CBP1 during intracellular parasitism. *Mol Microbiol.* 1998;27:531-539.
16. Hwang L, Hocking-Murray D, Bahrami AK, et al. Identifying phase-specific genes in the fungal pathogen *Histoplasma capsulatum* using a genomic shotgun microarray. *Mol Biol Cell.* 2003; 14:2314-2326.
17. Nguyen V, Sil A. Temperature-induced switch to the pathogenic yeast form of *Histoplasma capsulatum* requires Ryp1, a conserved transcriptional regulator. *Proc Natl Acad Sci U S A.* 2008;105: 4880-4885.
18. Rappleye CA, Goldman WE. Defining virulence genes in the dimorphic fungi. *Annu Rev Microbiol.* 2006;60:281-303.
19. Woods JP. *Histoplasma capsulatum* molecular genetics, pathogenesis, and responsiveness to its environment. *Fungal Genet Biol.* 2002;35:81-97.
20. Medoff G, Sacco M, Maresca B, et al. Irreversible block of the mycelial to yeast phase transition of *Histoplasma capsulatum. Science.* 1986;231:476-479.
21. Newman SL. Macrophages in host defense against *Histoplasma capsulatum. Trends Microbiol.* 1999;7:67-71.
22. Baughman RP, Kim CK, Vinegar A, et al. The pathogenesis of experimental pulmonary histoplasmosis. Correlative studies of histopathology, bronchoalveolar lavage, and respiratory function. *Am Rev Respir Dis.* 1986;134:771-776.
23. Newman SL, Gootee L, Gabay J. Human neutrophil-mediated fungistasis against *Histoplasma capsulatum.* Localization of fungistatic activity to the azurophil granules. *J Clin Invest.* 1993;92:624-631.
24. Deepe GS Jr, Seder RA. Molecular and cellular determinants of immunity to *Histoplasma capsulatum. Res Immunol.* 1998;149: 397-406.

25. Gildea L, Morris RE, Newman SL. *Histoplasma capsulatum* yeasts are phagocytosed via very late antigen-5, killed, and processed for antigen presentation by human dendritic cells. *J Immunol.* 2001;166:1049-1056.
26. Long KH, Gomez FJ, Morris RE, et al. Identification of heat shock protein 60 as the ligand on *Histoplasma capsulatum* that mediates binding to the CD18 receptors on human macrophages. *J Immunol.* 2003;170:487-494.
27. Eissenberg LG, Goldman WE, Schlesinger PH. *Histoplasma capsulatum* modulates the acidification of phagolysosomes. *J Exp Med.* 1993;177:1605-1611.
28. Lane TE, Wu-Hsieh BA, Howard DH. Iron limitation and the gamma interferon-mediated antihistoplasma state of murine macrophages. *Infect Immun.* 1991;59:2274-2278.
29. Wheat LJ, Connolly-Stringfield PA, Baker RL, et al. Disseminated histoplasmosis in the acquired immune deficiency syndrome: Clinical findings, diagnosis and treatment, and review of the literature. *Medicine (Baltimore).* 1990;69:361-374.
30. Lee JH, Slifman NR, Gershon SK, et al. Life-threatening histoplasmosis complicating immunotherapy with tumor necrosis factor α antagonists infliximab and etanercept. *Arthritis Rheum.* 2002;46:2565-2570.
31. Heninger E, Hogan LH, Karman J, et al. Characterization of the *Histoplasma capsulatum*-induced granuloma. *J Immunol.* 2006; 177;3303-3313.
32. Vanek J, Schwarz J. The gamut of histoplasmosis. *Am J Med.* 1971;50:89-104.
33. Loosli CG, Grayston JT, Alexander ER, et al. Epidemiological studies of pulmonary histoplasmosis in a farm family. *Am J Hyg.* 1952;55:392-401.
34. Goodwin RA Jr, Loyd JE, Des Prez RM. Histoplasmosis in normal hosts. *Medicine (Baltimore).* 1981;60:231-266.
35. Goodwin RA Jr, Des Prez RM. Histoplasmosis. *Am Rev Respir Dis.* 1978;117:929-956.
36. Storch G, Burford JG, George RB, et al. Acute histoplasmosis: Description of an outbreak in northern Louisiana. *Chest.* 1980; 77:38-42.
37. Rosenthal J, Brandt KD, Wheat LJ, et al. Rheumatologic manifestations of histoplasmosis in the recent Indianapolis epidemic. *Arthritis Rheum.* 1983;26:1065-1070.
38. Ploy-Song-Sang YY, Loudon RG, Beach BC, et al. Pulmonary function studies in acute pulmonary histoplasmosis. *South Med J.* 1979;72:568-572.
39. Wheat LJ, Stein L, Corya BC, et al. Pericarditis as a manifestation of histoplasmosis during two large urban outbreaks. *Medicine (Baltimore).* 1983;62:110-119.
40. Wheat LJ, Slama TG, Eitzen HE, et al. A large urban outbreak of histoplasmosis: Clinical features. *Ann Intern Med.* 1981;94: 331-337.
41. Davies SF, Rohrbach MS, Thelen V, et al. Elevated serum angiotensin-converting enzyme (SACE) activity in acute pulmonary histoplasmosis. *Chest.* 1984;85:307-310.
42. Powell KE, Hammerman KJ, Dahl BA, et al. Acute reinfection pulmonary histoplasmosis. A report of six cases. *Am Rev Respir Dis.* 1973;107:374-378.
43. Goodwin RA, Snell JD. The enlarging histoplasmoma. Concept of a tumor-like phenomenon encompassing the tuberculoma and coccidioidoma. *Am Rev Respir Dis.* 1969;100:1-12.
44. Schwarz J, Schaen MD, Picardi JL. Complications of the arrested primary histoplasmic focus. *JAMA.* 1976;236:1157-1161.
45. Loyd JE, Tillman BF, Atkinson JB, et al. Mediastinal fibrosis complicating histoplasmosis. *Medicine.* 1988;67:295-310.
46. Wheat LJ, Wass J, Norton J, et al. Cavitary histoplasmosis occurring during two large urban outbreaks: Analysis of clinical, epidemiologic, roentgenographic, and laboratory features. *Medicine (Baltimore).* 1984;63:201-209.
47. Goodwin RA, Owens FT, Snell JD, et al. Chronic pulmonary histoplasmosis. *Medicine (Baltimore).* 1976;55:413-452.
48. Kennedy CC, Limper AH. Redefining the clinical spectrum of chronic pulmonary histoplasmosis. A retrospective case series of 46 patients. *Medicine.* 2007;86:252-258.

49. Wheat LJ, Slama TG, Norton JA, et al. Risk factors for disseminated or fatal histoplasmosis. *Ann Intern Med.* 1982;96:159-163.
50. Peddi VR, Hariharan S, First MR. Disseminated histoplasmosis in renal allograft recipients. *Clin Transplant.* 1996;10:160-165.
51. Wheat LJ, Smith EJ, Sathapatayavongs B, et al. Histoplasmosis in renal allograft recipients: Two large urban outbreaks. *Arch Intern Med.* 1983;143:703-707.
52. Limaye AP, Connolly PA, Sagar M, et al. Transmission of *Histoplasma capsulatum* by organ transplantation. *N Engl J Med.* 2000;343:11163-11166.
53. Goodwin RA Jr, Shapiro JL, Thurman GH, et al. Disseminated histoplasmosis: Clinical and pathological correlations. *Medicine (Baltimore).* 1980;59:1-31.
54. McKinsey DS, Spiegel RA, Hutwagner L, et al. Prospective study of histoplasmosis in patients infected with human immunodeficiency virus: Incidence, risk factors, and pathophysiology. *Clin Infect Dis.* 1997;24:1195-1203.
55. Eidbo J, Sanchez RL, Tschen JA, et al. Cutaneous manifestations of histoplasmosis in the acquired immune deficiency syndrome. *Am J Surg Pathol.* 1993;17:110-116.
56. Wheat LJ, Batteiger BE, Sathapatayavongs B. Histoplasma capsulatum infections of the central nervous system: A clinical review. *Medicine (Baltimore).* 1990;69:244-260.
57. Conces DJ, Stockberger, SM, Tarver RD, et al. Disseminated histoplasmosis in AIDS: Findings on chest radiographs. *AJR.* 1993;160:15-19.
58. Sturim HS, Kouchoukos NT, Ahluvin RC. Gastrointestinal manifestations of disseminated histoplasmosis. *Am J Surg.* 1965; 110:435-440.
59. Blair TP, Waugh RA, Pollack M, et al. *Histoplasma capsulatum* endocarditis. *Am Heart J.* 1980;99:783-788.
60. Wilson DA, Muchmore HG, Tisdal RG, et al. Histoplasmosis of the adrenal glands studied by CT. *Radiology.* 1984;150: 779-783.
61. Ciulla TA, Piper HC, Xiao M, et al. Presumed ocular histoplasmosis syndrome: Update on epidemiology, pathogenesis, and photodynamic, antiangiogenic, and surgical therapies. *Curr Opin Ophthalmol.* 2001;12:442-449.
62. Cockshott WP, Lucas AO. Histoplasma dubosii. *Q J Med.* 1964;33:223-238.
63. Manfredi R, Mazzoni A, Nanetti A, et al. *Histoplasma capsulati* and *duboisii* in Europe: The impact of the HIV pandemic, travel, and immigration. *Eur J Epidemiol.* 1994;10:675-681.
64. Kauffman CA. Histoplasmosis: A clinical and laboratory update. *Clin Micro Rev* 2007;20:115-132.
65. Terry PB, Rosenow EC, Roberts GD. False-positive complement fixation serology in histoplasmosis. A retrospective study. *JAMA.* 1978;239:2453-2456.
66. Corcoran GR, Al-Abdely H, Glanders CD. Markedly elevated serum lactate dehydrogenase levels are a clue to the diagnosis of disseminated histoplasmosis in patients with AIDS. *Clin Infect Dis.* 1997;24:942-944.
67. Kirn DH, Fredericks D, McCutchan JA, et al. Serum ferritin levels correlate with disease activity in patients with AIDS and disseminated histoplasmosis. *Clin Infect Dis.* 1995;21:1048-1049.
68. Wheat LJ, Freifeld AG, Kleiman MB, et al. Clinical practice guidelines for the management of patients with histoplasmosis: 2007 update by the Infectious Diseases Society of America. *Clin Infect Dis.* 2007;45:807-825.
69. Kaplan JE, Benson C, Holmes KH, et al. Guidelines for prevention and treatment of opportunistic infections in HIV-infected adults and adolescents: recommendations from CDC, the National Institutes of Health, and the HIV Medicine Association of the Infectious Diseases Society of America. *MMWR Recomm Rep.* 2009;58(RR-4):1-207.
70. Nosanchuk JD, Steenbergen JN, Shi L, et al. Antibodies to a cell surface histone-like protein protect against *Histoplasma capsulatum. J Clin Invest.* 2003;112:1164-1175.

265

Blastomyces dermatitidis

STANLEY W. CHAPMAN | DONNA C. SULLIVAN

Blastomyces dermatitidis is the dimorphic fungus that causes the systemic pyogranulomatous disease blastomycosis. Initial infection is through the lungs and is often subclinical. Hematogenous dissemination may occur, culminating in a disease with protean manifestations. Clinical disease most often involves the lungs, skin, bones, and genitourinary system.

History

Blastomycosis was first reported in 1894 by T. C. Gilchrist,[1] who initially postulated that the disease was caused by a protozoan. In collaboration with Stokes, Gilchrist subsequently isolated the organism, established that the disease was caused by a fungus, and, finally, infected a dog with the newly isolated fungus.[2-4] Although blastomycosis was originally believed to involve only the skin, a number of cases of systemic disease were soon reported. Analysis of these early cases[5,6] led to the concept that two forms of the disease existed—cutaneous and systemic—and that they represented different portals of entry (skin and lung, respectively). This concept was not disproved until the work of Schwartz and Baum.[7] Through careful clinical and pathologic studies, they established definitively that the lung was the primary route of infection and that skin disease or other organ involvement was secondary to dissemination.

The Organism

B. dermatitidis is the imperfect (asexual) stage of *Ajellomyces dermatitidis*. The imperfect stage exhibits dimorphism, growing as a mycelial form at room temperature and as a yeast form at 37° C.[8,9] The mycelial form grows as a white mold that slowly turns light brown. On primary isolation, colonies appear in 1 to 3 weeks. The branching hyphae are usually 2 to 3 μm in diameter. Arising at right angles to the hyphae are conidiophores that produce single terminal conidia that vary from 2 to 10 μm in diameter and are round or oval in shape. The conidia are thought to be infectious for humans when the mycelia are disturbed. Conversion of the mycelial form to the yeast form at 37° C is necessary for positive identification. The physiologic events associated with this phase shift are similar to those associated with *Histoplasma capsulatum* and include heat-related stress, followed by uncoupling of oxidative phosphorylation.[10,11] Yeastlike colonies are wrinkled and cream or tan in color. The yeast cells (Fig. 265-1) may vary in diameter from 5 to 30 μm but are usually 8 to 15 μm, with a thick cell wall that is highly refractile. The yeast cells are multinucleate, containing 8 to 12 nuclei, and reproduce by single buds with a broad base between parent and bud. The daughter cell is often nearly as large as the mother cell before detachment. The same yeast cell in vitro characteristics are also noted in tissue or secretions and are used to distinguish *B. dermatitidis* from other fungi.

Two serotypes of *B. dermatitidis* have been identified by exoantigen analysis of yeast organisms.[12] Initial studies indicate that the A antigen–deficient serotypes are restricted to Africa.[13] The sexual form, *A. dermatitidis*, is heterothallic and requires opposite mating types (+ and −) for fertile cultures.[14,15] Both mating types are pathogenic, and infection occurs with equal frequency with each mating type.[16] Both types are occasionally isolated from a single patient.

Studies employing genomic restriction fragment length polymorphism analysis among isolates of *B. dermatitidis* obtained from diverse geographic regions in North America and Africa reveal a high degree of genetic similarity among isolates.[17,18] Three major groups, however, could be identified by a polymerase chain reaction (PCR)–based typing system. Strains could be further differentiated by a PCR fingerprinting method employing different primers. The use of this typing system could prove invaluable as a tool for studying the epidemiology of endemic blastomycosis as well as epidemic or case cluster situations.

Epidemiology

A complete understanding of the incidence and epidemiology of blastomycosis has been hindered by the lack of a sensitive, specific skin test reagent and the difficulty in establishing the ecologic niche of *B. dermatitidis* in nature. Our knowledge of blastomycosis is based on the collected reports of sporadic cases in humans and dogs[19-25] as well as the studies of 14 epidemics or clusters of disease.[26-39] On the basis of these data, the endemic area in North America (Fig. 265-2) includes the southeastern and south central states, especially those bordering the Mississippi and Ohio River basins; the midwestern states and Canadian provinces that border the Great Lakes; and a small area in New York and Canada along the St. Lawrence River. Maximal entropy modeling of exposure sites from human and canine cases of blastomycosis in Wisconsin predict areas of highest occurrence in proximity to waterways especially, with ecologic conditions suitable for *B. dermatitidis* present in both urban and rural environments.[40] Several studies in these endemic regions have documented hyperendemic areas with unusually high rates of blastomycosis.[24,36] Outside North America, well-documented autochthonous cases have been reported most frequently in Africa.[41] Occasional cases have also been reported in Central America, South America, India, and the Middle East.[42,43] Although most cases are reported in Mississippi, Arkansas, Kentucky, Tennessee, and Wisconsin, blastomycosis has been reported in nonendemic areas including a cluster of human and canine cases in North Carolina,[44] Colorado,[45] and Nebraska.[46]

Initial analysis of sporadic cases indicated that middle-aged men with outdoor occupations that exposed them to soil were at greatest risk for blastomycosis.[21,22,45,46] These findings, however, may reflect only the demographics of the rural states from which most of the cases were reported. In contrast, review of the 16 case clusters reported to date[22,26-40] indicates that there is no sex, age, race, occupational, or seasonal predilection for blastomycosis. In eight of the outbreaks, recreational activities in wooded areas along waterways were the major risk identified. Exposure to dust clouds associated with construction projects or crop harvesting was the only potential risk for infection identified in four of the outbreaks. Thus, exposure to soil, whether at work or at play, appears to be the common link in reports of sporadic disease and outbreaks. One report, however, concludes that many cases of blastomycosis result from exposure in the home, especially in the attic or basement. In this same article, repeat cases occurred in different families in four homes, and most cases were separated by 1 year or more. This indicates that *B. dermatitidis* may be relatively persistent at certain properties.[47]

Attempts to isolate the organism in nature have been difficult and the results inconsistent. Denton and co-workers[48-50] reported multiple isolations of *B. dermatitidis* from soil and rotting wood during environmental surveys between 1958 and 1963. Yeast-phase organisms were purportedly recovered from pigeon manure after a single case of blastomycosis, but this report lacks crucial details.[51] Isolation from soil samples from an earthen floor was also reported after a single case of

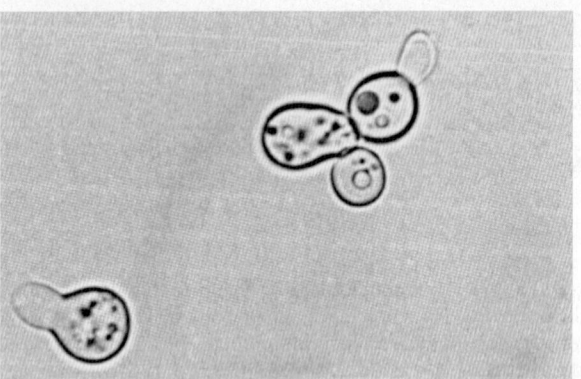

Figure 265-1 Yeast cells of *Blastomyces dermatitidis* in wet smear (× 1000).

disease in Canada.[52] The environmental isolations of *B. dermatitidis* by Klein and co-workers[32,33] in association with two outbreaks of disease represented an important breakthrough in defining the ecologic niche of the organism. In both instances, the organism was isolated from soil containing decayed vegetation or from decomposed wood. Humidity probably played an important role in promoting the growth of the organism because of the proximity to water and recent rainfall in both outbreaks. These studies, together with other in vitro work,[53,54] indicate that *B. dermatitidis* exists in nature in warm, moist soil of wooded areas that is also rich in organic debris, such as decaying vegetation. The conditions that support the growth of *B. dermatitidis* in these microfoci probably exist for only short periods of time. Thus, when a sporadic case or outbreak of blastomycosis is recognized, environmental isolation is often impossible because the appropriate local and environmental conditions may no longer exist at the site of exposure. Alternatively, a more complete understanding of the ecology of *B. dermatitidis* may also result from a more sensitive culture technique for the organism. The recently reported isolation of *B. dermatitidis* from environmental sources by Baumgardner and Paretsky using a two-step procedure may be useful in such studies.[54,55]

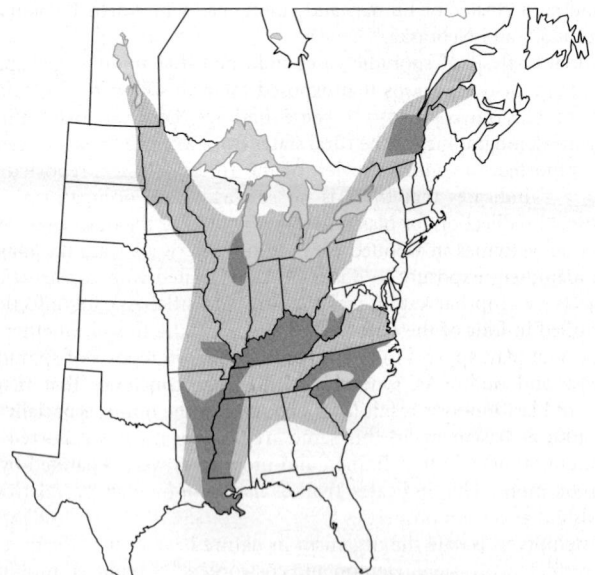

Figure 265-2 **Incidence and prevalence of blastomycosis in North America.** *Brown areas* indicate the known endemic region; *green areas* are those with the highest incidence. *(From Rippon JW. Medical Mycology: The Pathogenic Fungi and Pathogenic Actinomycetes. 3rd ed. Philadelphia: WB Saunders; 1988:474.)*

Pathogenesis and Pathology

The studies of Schwartz and Baum[7] were the first to establish that the usual portal of entry for blastomycosis in humans is the lungs. Thus, disease at other body sites is the result of dissemination from a primary pulmonary infection, even if the infection is clinically undetected. Primary cutaneous blastomycosis has occurred after accidental inoculation in the laboratory, at autopsy,[56] and after dog bites.[57] Person-to-person transmission of disease by yeast-phase organisms has not been documented, except for a rare vaginal infection acquired from a man with genitourinary blastomycosis[58] and two instances of perinatal transmission.[59,60]

Pulmonary infection occurs by inhalation of the conidia, which convert to the yeast phase in the lung. The typical inflammatory response consists of clusters of neutrophils and noncaseating granulomas with epithelioid and giant cells. This response is similar to that seen with coccidioidomycosis and sporotrichosis. Although this histopathologic picture is duplicated to a variable degree in extrapulmonary sites, the response in cutaneous disease is unique in that prominent pseudoepitheliomatous hyperplasia is present with microabscess formation that clinically and histologically may mimic a variety of cutaneous diseases, including giant keratoacanthoma and squamous cell carcinoma of the skin.[61] The same pseudoepitheliomatous response may also be seen when mucosal surfaces of the mouth, oropharynx, or larynx are involved.[62,63] The gross and histopathologic appearance of laryngeal disease is similar to that of well-differentiated squamous cell carcinoma and is not infrequently misdiagnosed as such.

Immunity

Our understanding of the immunologic defenses against *B. dermatitidis* is incomplete owing to the lack of appropriate antigens. Advances in characterizing specific yeast antigens have facilitated our study of both humoral and cellular immunity. Specific antibody against *B. dermatitidis* does not appear to confer resistance to or hasten recovery from disease. The major acquired host defense against *B. dermatitidis* is cellular immunity, mediated by antigen-specific T lymphocytes and lymphokine-activated macrophages.

NATURAL IMMUNITY AND VIRULENCE

Investigations of point-source outbreaks indicate that infection rates are high but that symptomatic disease occurs in less than half of infected individuals.[32,33] Studies using antigen-specific lymphocyte proliferation as a marker of remote infection suggest that subclinical cases of sporadic blastomycosis also occur, probably more commonly than symptomatic cases.[64] This high frequency of asymptomatic infection supports the concept that healthy people are fairly resistant to infection by *B. dermatitidis*. The presence of natural resistance may, in part, explain why blastomycosis is infrequently reported as an opportunistic infection in the immunocompromised host. When conidia are inhaled into the lungs, natural resistance is probably mediated by neutrophils, monocytes, and alveolar macrophages, which can phagocytize and kill the conidia of *Blastomyces*.

Striking differences in the susceptibilities of immature and mature mice to infection with *Blastomyces* have been linked to differences in nonspecific immunity, specifically effector cell function.[65] These studies indicate enhanced susceptibility resulting from depressed capacity of polymorphonuclear leukocytes harvested from immature mice to kill *B. dermatitidis*. Peripheral blood neutrophils from mature animals killed *B. dermatitidis* in greater numbers than those neutrophils from immature animals (41% vs. 10%). Peritoneal inflammatory cells, enriched for neutrophils, showed a similar pattern (70% for peritoneal cells from mature animals vs. 25% for immature).[65] Sugar and Picard [66] have also shown that alveolar macrophages inhibit transformation of conidia to the pathogenic yeast form. Once converted in tissue, the yeast forms are relatively resistant to phagocytosis and killing. This conidia-to-yeast conversion most likely results in a survival advantage for the organism when inhaled into the lungs and contributes to the pathogenicity of *B. dermatitidis*. The conidia-to-yeast conversion is a common virulence factor shared by the dimorphic fungi *B. dermatitidis*, *Histoplasma capsulatum*, *Coccidioides* species, *Paracoccidioides brasiliensis*, *Sporothrix schenckii*, and *Penicillium marneffei*. Nemecek and co-workers[67] have identified a dimorphism regulating gene, *DRK1*, encoding a histidine kinase, which is responsible for sensing changes in the environment, including temperature shifts, and the activation of the virulence gene for WI-1 (recently renamed BAD1).

Although the thick cell wall of the yeast form has been postulated to be antiphagocytic, specific structural and chemical components of the cell wall have been associated with virulence. Early studies by DiSalvo and Denton[68] reported a higher concentration of lipid in the yeast cells of virulent strains of *B. dermatitidis* than in less virulent strains. Conversely, Cox and Best[69] noted more phospholipid in a single virulent strain than in a less virulent strain. These two studies were limited by the genetic disparity in the strains employed. The elegant work of Klein and associates[70-72] has defined other important virulence factors associated with the yeast form of *B. dermatitidis*. These investigators identified the novel 120-kDa glycoprotein antigen, BAD-1 (WI-1), on the cell wall surface of the yeast form that serves as the major immunodominant epitope for both humoral and cellular immunity. The BAD-1 also functions as an adhesin that binds to host cell receptors, including CR3 and CD14 of human macrophages.[73] This adhesin activity is mediated by a 24–amino acid tandem repeat that shares 90% homology with the *Yersinia* adhesin invasin.[74] Binding to extracellular matrix may also be mediated by a cysteine-rich domain at the carboxyl-terminal end of BAD-1 that is similar to epidermal growth factor.[74] Using three genetically related strains, Klein and colleagues[75] have shown that alterations in the quantity of BAD-1 expressed on the cell surface, the amount of BAD-1 shed, and the modification of shed BAD-1 are different in two hypovirulent strains compared with the parental (virulent) strain. Using the same strains, Hogan and Klein[76] have also shown that the quantity and distribution of cell wall α-1,3-glucan are different in the hypovirulent and virulent strains. Collectively, these experiments indicate that the adhesin BAD-1 is a major virulence factor of *B. dermatitidis* but that other cell wall components, such as α-1,3-glucan, may modulate the BAD-1–mediated interactions between the yeast and host cell and thereby also modulate virulence.[73,77]

In addition to its role as an antigen and adhesin, both surface-bound and soluble forms of BAD-1 protein have been shown in a murine model to interfere with innate immune responses by blocking production of tumor necrosis factor-α (TNF-α) by both macrophages and neutrophils through both transforming growth factor-β1 (TGF-β1)–dependent and –independent mechanisms.[78,79] Using null mutants, these same investigators were able to show that increasing TNF-α by adenovirus-mediated gene therapy improved outcome as determined by decreased tissue burden in the lungs. Therefore, BAD-1 interferes with the immune response by blocking the induction rather than binding or inactivation of TNF-α. Finally, the BAD-1 antigen inhibits complement activation by *Blastomyces* yeast cells. In contrast, β-glucan supports complement activation.[80] These studies, analogous to the results noted for the adhesin property, indicate that surface glucan and BAD-1 have distinct regulatory roles with regard to complement activation.

POLYMORPHONUCLEAR LEUKOCYTES

The histopathologic response previously noted implicates both a neutrophil response and a cellular immune response. The polymorphonuclear leukocyte reaction is probably initiated by the release of chemotactic factors from the organism.[81] Human neutrophils efficiently phagocytize and kill the conidia of *B. dermatitidis*. Phagocytosis of conidia is optimal when complement and divalent cations are present, and killing is predominantly by oxidative mechanisms.[82,83]

Conversely, phagocytosis and killing of yeast forms are inefficient; this is probably an important factor in disease progression.

Wüthrich and colleagues[84] employed BAD-1 null mutants and wild-type *B. dermatitidis* in a murine model and found a shift toward type 1 from type 2 cytokines in the cellular profile of the inflammatory response after pulmonary infection with Δbad-1 mutants. These findings revealed that, in addition to interference of the innate phagocytic response through TNF-α, infection with wild-type yeast was associated with less interleukin-12 (IL-12) and interferon-γ (IFN-γ), and more IL-10, and an influx of inflammatory cells rich in neutrophils and poor in CD3+ T cells, compared with infection with the BAD-1 null strain.[85] The importance of IL-12 in resistance to blastomycosis has been demonstrated in the context of vaccine-induced memory, where it was found to be required for induction of protective memory responses but not their maintenance.[86] Indeed, IL-12 treatment of susceptible mice induced resistance as measured by survival and decreased yeast in the lungs, less morbidity, increased macrophage responsiveness to IFN-γ for killing, upregulation of IFN-γ, and downregulation of IL-10.[87]

Despite activating the neutrophil NADPH oxidase system, yeast forms do not efficiently stimulate the production of myeloperoxidase-dependent microbicidal products.[88] The fungicidal activity of neutrophils can be enhanced by either lymphokine-rich supernatants from immunologically stimulated T lymphocytes or IFN-γ, providing a link between cellular immunity and neutrophil function.[89,90]

CELLULAR IMMUNITY

Delayed hypersensitivity can be induced in mice by subcutaneous injections of live or killed *B. dermatitidis*. Decreased susceptibility to infection parallels the development of the cellular immune response,[91,92] and resistance to infection in mice has been transferred by T lymphocytes.[93] Macrophages harvested from mice with experimental blastomycosis have also been reported to inhibit the replication of *B. dermatitidis*, and both in vivo and in vitro IFN-γ treatments have been shown to enhance killing of *B. dermatitidis* by murine alveolar macrophages.[94,95] Interestingly, therapeutic concentrations of hydrocortisone and cyclosporine do not inhibit macrophage activation by IFN-γ.[96]

The study of cellular immunity in humans has been hindered by the lack of a sensitive, specific antigen for both in vitro studies and skin testing. The development of specific cellular immunity, as monitored by antigen-induced lymphocyte proliferation, has been documented in patients with blastomycosis using whole yeast-phase organisms; an alkali-soluble, water-soluble yeast extract; and BAD-1.[71,97,98] Chang and colleagues investigated peripheral blood mononuclear cell responses from patients with blastomycosis to segments of the WI-1 antigen recognized by T cells.[99] These studies defined a 25–amino acid segment in the amino terminus of the peptide recognized by T-cell clones and the human leukocyte antigen molecules that displayed these epitopes to T cells. BAD-1 administration produced both antibody- and cell-mediated immunity in a murine model of pulmonary blastomycosis.[100] Furthermore, use of IL-12 as an adjuvant for WI-1 significantly augmented delayed-type hypersensitivity and enhanced resistance to experimental *B. dermatitidis* infection, although the level of resistance was modest.[101]

The attenuated strain of *B. dermatitidis* with a mutated *WI-1/BAD-1* gene has been shown to be an effective live vaccine in a murine model of lethal pulmonary infection.[102] The attenuated vaccine, cell wall–membrane extract, and a yeast cytosol extract of the vaccine strain induce polarized and protective immune responses in mice. These delayed-type hypersensitivity and polarized type I cytokine responses are linked to resistance and are dependent on the presence of thymus-derived CD4+ or CD8+ lymphocytes, depending on the immune competency of the host.[84,86,103,104] In immune-competent mice, CD4+ T cells are dependent on the production of IFN-γ, TNF-α, and granulocyte-macrophage colony-stimulating factor.[103] In immunosuppressed hosts deficient for CD4+ cells, CD8+ cells compensate and mediate protective immunity.[104] Immunization of mice with cell wall–membrane and yeast cytosol extract further indicates a bias in the T-cell receptor repertoire of Vβ1 for protective T-cell clones and Vβ8.1/8.2 for non-protective and disease-enhancing clones.[105]

Macrophages from patients recovering from blastomycosis have also been shown to have enhanced inhibition of intracellular growth of *B. dermatitidis* compared with control macrophages.[106] Finally, supernatants of antigen-stimulated human lymphocytes have been shown to enhance phagocytosis and intracellular inhibition of the growth of *B. dermatitidis* by both alveolar and monocyte-derived macrophages.[106]

Despite these advances, however, an antigen for skin testing is not yet available. Blastomycin, a culture filtrate of mycelial-phase organisms, lacks both specificity and sensitivity. In the Veterans Administration Cooperative Study, only 40% of patients with blastomycosis had a positive skin test to blastomycin.[19] Further clarification of cellular immunity in human cases of blastomycosis awaits more definitive characterization of the fungal antigens.

HUMORAL IMMUNITY

Yeast antigens have been used to evaluate humoral immunity in a variety of serologic tests of different sensitivities and specificities. The complement fixation test has not proved useful because it lacks both sensitivity and specificity. At most, 50% of patients with blastomycosis have a positive complement fixation reaction to *B. dermatitidis* antigens.[13] Cross-reactivity with *H. capsulatum* and, to a lesser degree, *Coccidioides* species has also been a problem.

The immunodiffusion test, which detects precipitin antibodies to the A and B antigens located in the cell wall of the yeast, is more specific for blastomycosis. Using the modifications suggested by Kaufman and associates, the presence of antibody to the A antigen has been noted in as many as 70% to 80% of patients with blastomycosis.[107,108] However, patients with localized disease and those with symptoms of less than 50 days' duration are less likely to have a positive antibody response.[109,110] Furthermore, detectable antibody is present only a short time after cure of disease. These findings emphasize the limitations of immunodiffusion serology for both clinical and epidemiologic studies. Using the A antigen in an enzyme immunoassay has improved sensitivity, but false-positive reactions, especially in patients with histoplasmosis and other fungal infections, are more common.[110-112] Studies by Klein and Jones[113] indicate that the cross-reactive determinants reside in the carbohydrate component of the A antigen. Commercial kits for both the immunodiffusion assay and enzyme immunoassay are available.

As noted previously, Klein and Jones[70] identified the novel 120-kDa surface protein of *B. dermatitidis* yeasts designated as BAD-1. These investigators purified and characterized BAD-1 and compared it immunologically with the commercially available A antigen.[113] The results of this study indicate that the tandem repeat of BAD-1 is the major antibody recognition site of both BAD-1 and A antigen. When used in a radioimmunoassay, antibody to BAD-1 was detected in 85% of patients with blastomycosis and in only 3% of patients with other fungal infections.[70] In a second study from the same laboratory, similar sensitivity (83%) was noted for the detection of anti–BAD-1 antibodies by radioimmunoassay.[114] All patients with proven blastomycosis whose serum was obtained within 60 days of onset of symptoms or diagnosis had at least one serum sample positive for anti–BAD-1. Furthermore, anti–BAD-1 antibody titers fell as the infection resolved, and antibody titers in most patients were undetectable after 8 months from the onset of symptoms. Enhanced diagnostic sensitivity did not result from modification of the radioimmunoassay to detect immunoglobulin M antibody. Comparison of antibody detection of BAD-1 antigen by radioimmunoassay or A antigen by agar gel diffusion in dogs revealed a BAD-1 sensitivity of 92% compared with 41% for antigen A; both tests had 100% specificity in this study.[115] Further studies, including the development of a nonradiometric test, will be necessary to clarify the role of the BAD-1 antigen in the serodiagnosis of blastomycosis.

Clinical Manifestations

Our knowledge of the clinical manifestations of blastomycosis is derived from careful studies of symptomatic, sporadic cases and the few case clusters reported.[116] It must be emphasized that blastomycosis is a systemic disease with a wide variety of pulmonary and extrapulmonary manifestations. Pulmonary disease may be acute or chronic and mimics infection with pyogenic bacteria, tuberculosis, infection with other fungi, and malignancy. Cutaneous disease, the most common extrapulmonary manifestation, appears similar to disease seen with bromoderma, pyoderma gangrenosum, Majocchi granuloma, leishmaniasis, *Mycobacterium marinum* infection, mycosis fungoides, giant keratoacanthoma, and squamous cell carcinoma.

B. dermatitidis infection may involve almost every organ of the body (Table 265-1), resulting in the diversity of clinical manifestations. Skin, bone, and genitourinary sites of infection are the most common and are most likely to be clinically manifest. Extrapulmonary disease is seen most commonly during the chronic form of illness, in which about

TABLE 265-1	**Organ Involvement in Blastomycosis from Clinical and Autopsy Findings in Seven Studies**							

Organ System Involved	Cherniss & Waisbren [40]	Abernathy [35]	VA Cooperative Study [198]	Witorsch & Utz [63]	Lockwood et al. [63]	Duttera & Osterhout [63]	Busey et al. [84]	Total[†]
Lungs	28 (70)[‡]	27 (77)	118 (60)	28 (70)	59 (80)	33 (52)	76 (90)	369/534 (69)
Skin	30 (75)	28 (80)	118 (60)	29 (73)	33 (45)	36 (57)	32 (38)	306/534 (57)
Bone	19 (48)	12 (34)	46 (23)	11 (28)	10 (14)	12 (19)	6 (7)	116/534 (22)
Genitourinary system	11 (28)	5 (14)	32 (16)	13 (33)	13 (18)	6 (10)	12 (14)	92/534 (17)
Reticuloendothelial system (liver, spleen, lymph nodes)	5 (13)	13 (37)	25 (13)	7 (18)	NS[†]	3 (5)	3 (4)	56/460 (12)
Central nervous system	4 (10)	1 (3)	9 (5)	1 (3)	5 (7)	4 (6)	4 (5)	29/534 (5)
Mucous membranes	3 (8)	2 (6)	11 (6)	10 (25)	NS	NS	NS	26/273 (10)
Subcutaneous	25 (63)	NS	NS	15 (38)	NS	NS	NS	40/80 (30)
Other[§]	5 (13)	9 (26)	18 (9)	5 (13)	NS	7 (11)	2 (2)	46/460 (10)

*Number of cases given in square brackets.
†Total number based on studies where stated; NS, not stated.
‡Number of cases followed by percentage in parentheses.
§Other: thyroid, 10; gastrointestinal, 8; adrenal, 7; pleura, 6; joints, 5; heart, 2; peritoneum, 1; eye, 1; psoas, 1; retropharynx, 1.

Data from the following studies: Cherniss EI, Waisbren BA. North American blastomycosis: A clinical study of 40 cases. *Ann Intern Med.* 1956;44:105-123; Abernathy RS. Clinical manifestations of pulmonary blastomycosis. *Ann Intern Med.* 1959;51:707-727; Witorsch P, Utz JP. North American blastomycosis: A study of 40 patients. *Medicine (Baltimore).* 1968;47:169-200; Lockwood WR, Allison F, Batson BE, et al. The treatment of North American blastomycosis: Ten years experience. *Am Rev Respir Dis.* 1969; 100:314-320; Duttera MJ, Osterhout S. North American blastomycosis: A survey of 63 cases. *South Med J.* 1969; 62:295-301; Busey JF. The Veterans Administrative Cooperative Group: Blastomycosis: III. A comparative study of 2-hydroxystilbamidine and amphotericin B therapy. *Am Rev Respir Dis.* 1972; 105:812-818.

TABLE 265-2	**Clinical Experience with Blastomycosis***			

Involvement	Arkansas [44][117]	Wisconsin [73][118]	Mississippi [326][119]	Total [443]
Single-organ disease	30 (69)†	62 (85)	270 (83)	362 (82)
Lung	26 (50)	56 (77)	245 (75)	327 (74)
Skin	2 (5)	3 (4)	16 (5)	21 (5)
Other	2 (5)	3 (4)	9 (3)	14 (3)
Multiorgan disease	14 (31)	11 (15)	56 (17)	81 (18)

*Number of cases given in square brackets.
†Number of cases followed by percentage in parentheses.
 Data from the following studies: Arkansas: Bradsher RW, Rice DC, Abernathy RS: Ketoconazole therapy for endemic blastomycosis. *Ann Intern Med.* 1985;103:872-879; Wisconsin: Baumgardner DJ, Buggy BP, Mattson BJ, et al. Epidemiology of blastomycosis in a region of high endemicity in north central Wisconsin. *Clin Infect Dis.* 1992;15:629-635; Mississippi: Chapman SW, Lin AC, Hendricks KA, et al. Endemic blastomycosis in Mississippi: Epidemiological and clinical studies. *Semin Respir Infect.* 1997;12:219-228.

two thirds of patients have been reported with multiple organ involvement. Many of the reports noting this high frequency of extrapulmonary dissemination, however, were autopsy based or appeared before the availability of effective treatments. In contrast to these earlier studies, later clinical experience in Arkansas,[117] Wisconsin,[118] and Mississippi,[119] three states in which blastomycosis is endemic, has indicated a lower frequency of extrapulmonary disease (Table 265-2). About three fourths of the patients reported in these studies had isolated pulmonary disease. Similar results were recently reported by Crampton and associates for cases of blastomycosis diagnosed in Manitoba hospitals.[25] Specifically, isolated pulmonary involvement was reported in 70% of 143 patients with blastomycosis. Extrapulmonary disease is usually seen in conjunction with active pulmonary infection. In some patients, however, especially those with skin involvement, extrapulmonary lesions may be present without clinically overt pulmonary infection.

Although a variety of clinical schemata may be used in discussing blastomycosis, that proposed by Sarosi and Davies[120] appears most comprehensive. A modification of this schema is presented in Figure 265-3. The occurrence of reactivation blastomycosis is a controversial issue, with only a few cases being suggestive.[121] Cases attributed to extrapulmonary reactivation may represent the late clinical manifestations of chronic, subclinical disease that remains active after pulmo-

nary healing. The factors determining the clinical course after acute infection are not well defined but probably involve a complex interaction of pulmonary anatomy, host defenses, and microbial factors.

ACUTE PNEUMONIA

Acute pulmonary infection is often unrecognized unless related to group exposure. Analysis of point-source outbreaks indicates that only about half of infected individuals develop symptomatic disease and that the median incubation period is 30 to 45 days.[24,30-33] Symptoms are nonspecific and tend to mimic those of influenza or bacterial infection with abrupt onset of myalgias, arthralgias, chills, and fever. Pleuritic pain may be prominent but is usually transient. Cough is initially nonproductive but in many cases becomes productive of purulent sputum. The radiologic findings in the acute stage of disease, whether symptomatic or asymptomatic, are also nonspecific but are usually those of lobar or segmental consolidation (Fig. 265-4).[122,123] Pleural effusion is uncommon and, if present, is found only in small amounts. Hilar adenopathy is also uncommon.

Spontaneous resolution of symptomatic acute pneumonia has been recognized in a few sporadic cases, in case clusters, and after accidental laboratory infection.[124-126] The frequency of this has not been established. In these cases, symptoms have usually resolved in less than 4 weeks, but radiologic abnormalities have taken longer to clear.

CHRONIC OR RECURRENT INFECTION

Most patients in whom blastomycosis is diagnosed have an indolent onset and progressive disease. The clinical manifestations are diverse, including pulmonary disease, extrapulmonary disease, or both. For clarity, these are discussed separately.

Pulmonary Manifestations

The clinical manifestations of pulmonary disease are those of chronic pneumonia, including productive cough, hemoptysis, weight loss, and pleuritic chest pain. Fever, if present, tends to be low grade. The radiologic findings in these patients are variable. Lobar or segmental alveolar infiltrates, with or without cavitation, are most frequently reported (Fig. 265-5).[122,123] The specific lobar distribution of infiltrates is not clinically helpful, although upper lobe infiltrates are reported more commonly. Mass lesions that mimic bronchogenic carcinoma occur

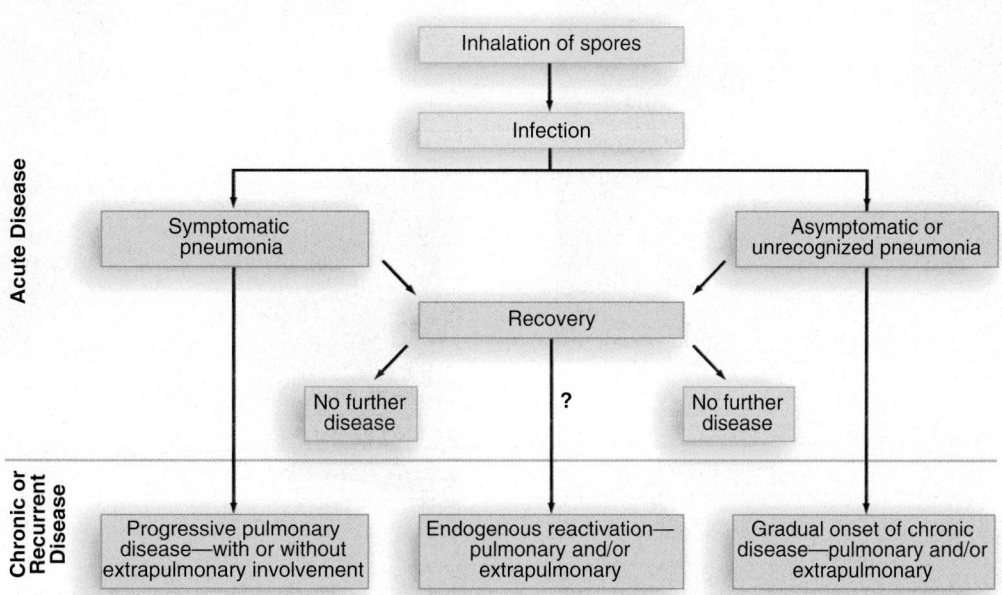

Figure 265-3 Clinical classification of blastomycosis. *(Adapted from Sarosi GA, Davies SF. Blastomycosis. Am Rev Respir Dis. 1979; 120:911-938.)*

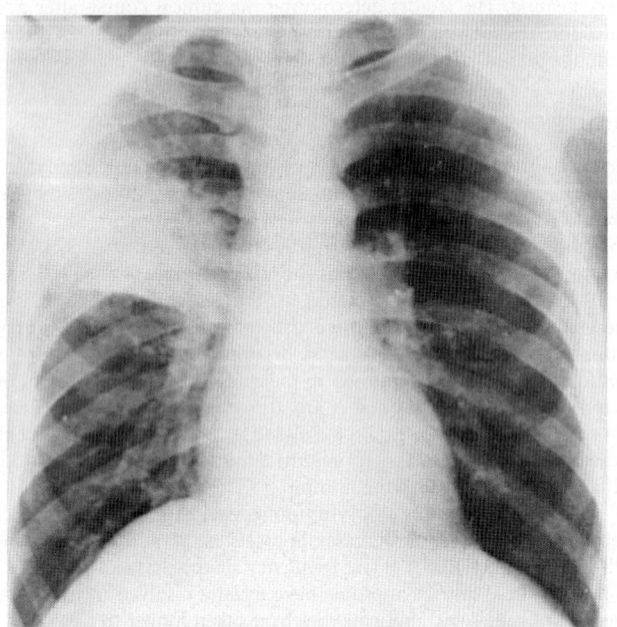

Figure 265-4 **A confluent infiltrate with a segmental distribution in a patient with blastomycosis.**

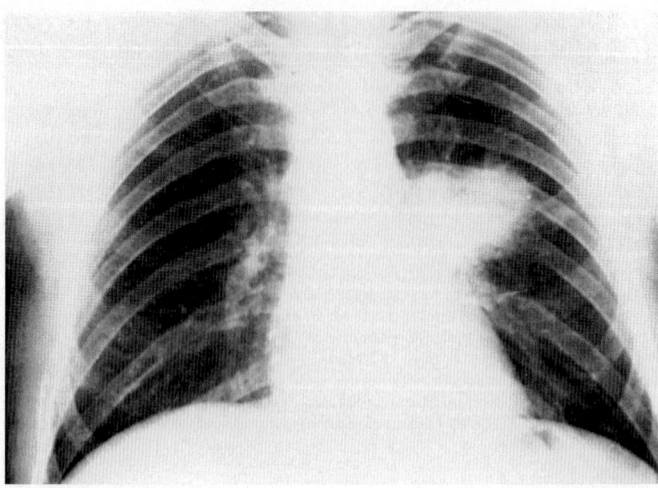

Figure 265-6 **Perihilar mass lesion in a patient with blastomycosis.** This radiographic appearance mimics that of carcinoma of the lung. To rule out a coexisting malignancy, patients with this radiographic picture should have bronchoscopy even if wet preparations of sputum reveal the organism.

almost as frequently as do alveolar infiltrates (Fig. 265-6).[127] Other radiographic features include intermediate-size nodules, solitary cavities, and fibronodular infiltrates, often with cavities (Fig. 265-7). Hilar adenopathy is variably reported. Postinfectious calcification of lymph nodes or pulmonary parenchyma is rare. An occasional patient has acute deterioration associated with miliary disease resulting from hematogenous spread[128] (Fig. 265-8) or diffuse pneumonitis from presumed endobronchial spread.[129] When either of these radiographic findings is accompanied by respiratory failure, the mortality rate usually exceeds 50%.[129] Although pleural thickening and small pleural effusions may occur, large pleural effusions are uncommon.[130]

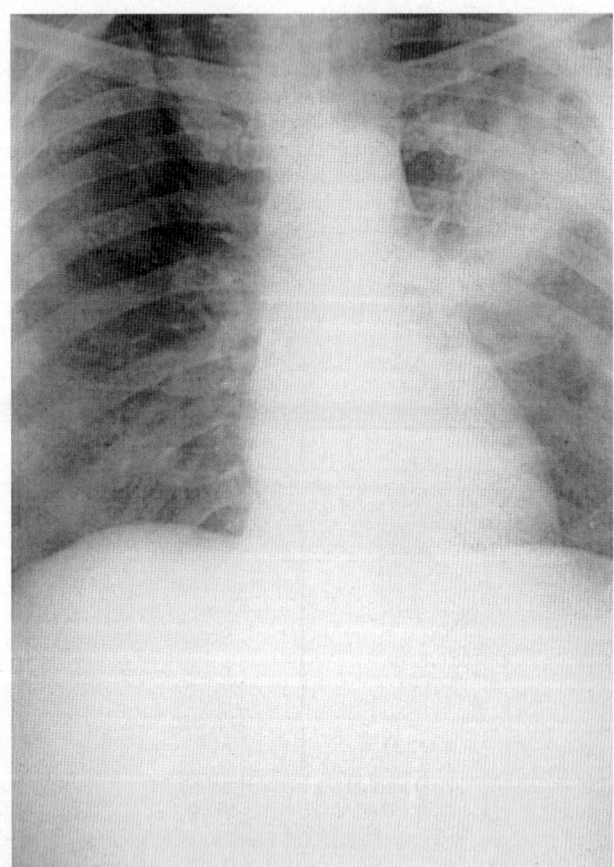

Figure 265-5 **Multinodular densities with consolidation of the left upper lobe in a patient with blastomycosis.**

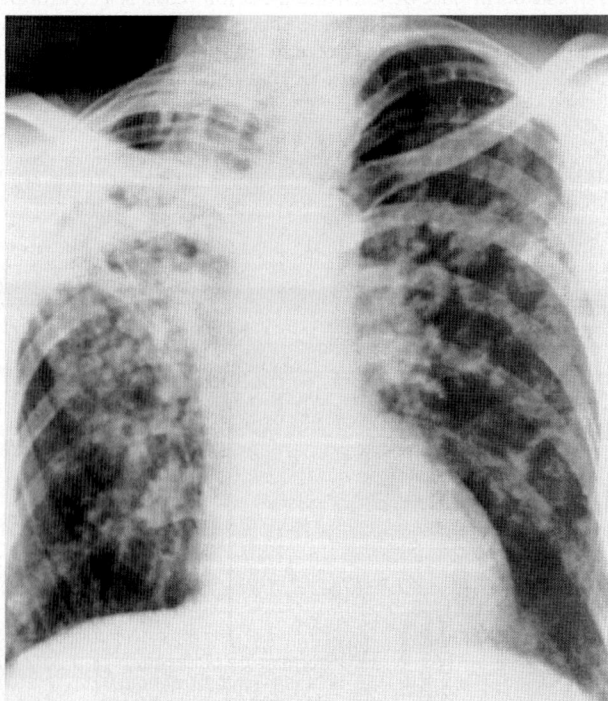

Figure 265-7 **Bilateral fibronodular infiltrates with cavitation and volume loss in the right upper lobe.** This radiographic appearance cannot be distinguished from that of tuberculosis or other granulomatous diseases.

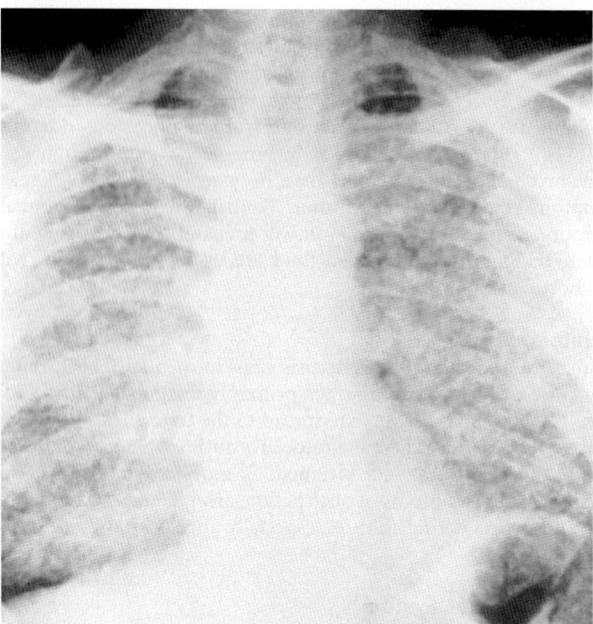

Figure 265-8 **Miliary blastomycosis in a patient with respiratory failure.** *(Courtesy of Dr. Guy Campbell, Jackson, MS.)*

Skin

Skin disease is the most common extrapulmonary manifestation of blastomycosis, being reported in 40% to 80% of cases (see Tables 265-1 and 265-2). Although extrapulmonary disease is usually seen in conjunction with active pulmonary disease, skin involvement may occur alone.[45,131-133] In some patients with skin disease, asymptomatic pulmonary disease is found. In our experience, skin disease occurs in about one third of patients with blastomycosis but is a marker for multiorgan infection, being present in three fourths of patients with disease in two or more organs.[119]

Two types of skin lesions may be seen. The first are the more characteristic verrucous lesions that usually appear on exposed body areas. These often begin as small papulopustular lesions (Fig. 265-9) and slowly spread to form crusted, heaped-up lesions that can vary in color from gray to a violaceous hue (Fig. 265-10). These lesions are often mistaken for squamous cell carcinoma. Older lesions may show central clearing with scar formation and depigmentation. Microabscess formation tends to occur at the periphery of such lesions, and removal of the eschar peripherally reveals purulent material in which the yeast forms are usually visible on wet preparation.

The second type of lesion is described as ulcerative (Fig. 265-11); the initial pustule spreads as a superficial ulcer or slightly raised lesion, with a bed of red friable granulation tissue that bleeds easily. Skin lesions of both types may be seen in the same patient. Lesions may also occur on the mucosa of the nose, mouth, and larynx. With skin lesions associated with a pulmonary pathogenesis, there is little or no regional lymph node involvement or lymphadenitis, in contrast to that seen with inoculation blastomycosis.[56,57]

Subcutaneous Nodules

Although subcutaneous nodules are often discussed as a skin manifestation, the clinical syndrome seen in patients with subcutaneous nodules is different from that associated with other skin lesions. Subcutaneous nodules are cold abscesses that are usually seen in conjunction with pulmonary and other extrapulmonary disease. The patient often appears acutely ill, systemic manifestations may be prominent, and rapid deterioration may result unless therapy is initiated promptly. Lesions sometimes drain spontaneously. Drainage or aspirated pus has abundant numbers of organisms that are readily visible on microscopic examination.

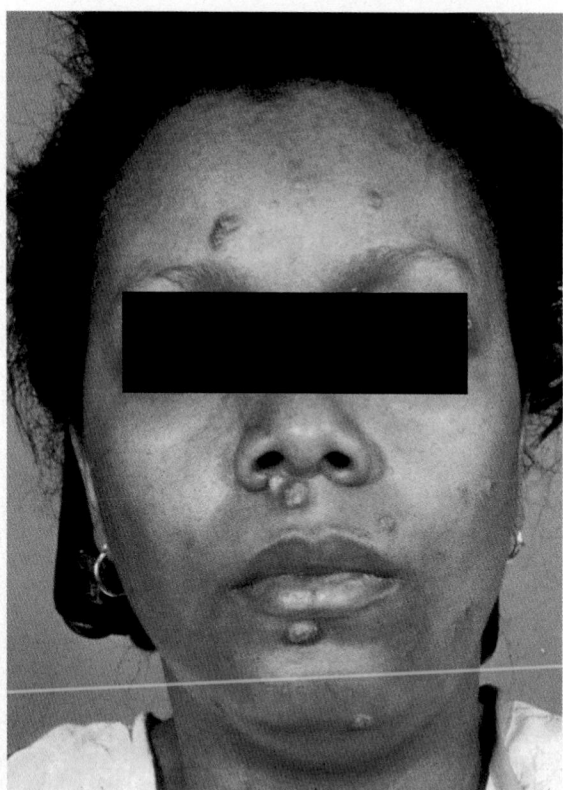

Figure 265-9 **Multiple papulopustular lesions in a patient with blastomycosis.**

Bone and Joint

After skin disease, skeletal blastomycosis is next in frequency (see Table 265-2). A recent retrospective study of 45 patients hospitalized with blastomycosis of bones or joints revealed 41 cases of osteomyelitis and 12 cases of septic arthritis, including 8 patients in whom both bone and joint were infected.[134] Cutaneous disease was present in 33 patients (73%), pulmonary disease in 29 (64%). Although almost any bone can be infected, the long bones, vertebrae, and ribs are most commonly involved.[135] A well-circumscribed osteolytic lesion is typical (Fig. 265-12). Patients with bone lesions rarely present with bone pain but instead present with contiguous soft tissue abscesses or chronic drain-

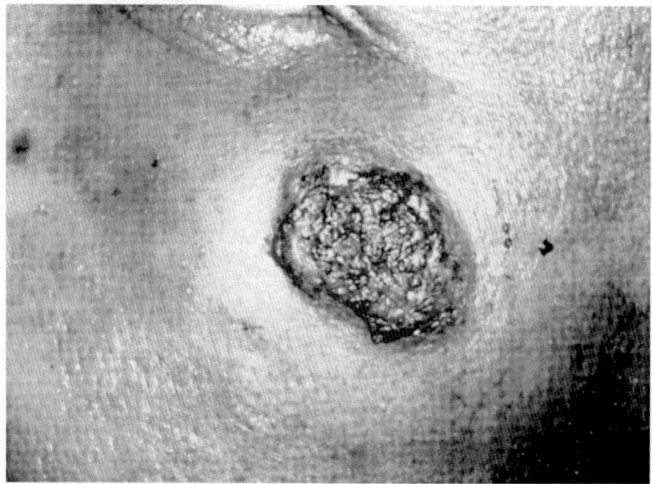

Figure 265-10 **Typical verrucous skin lesion of blastomycosis on the cheek.** Note the circumscribed edges.

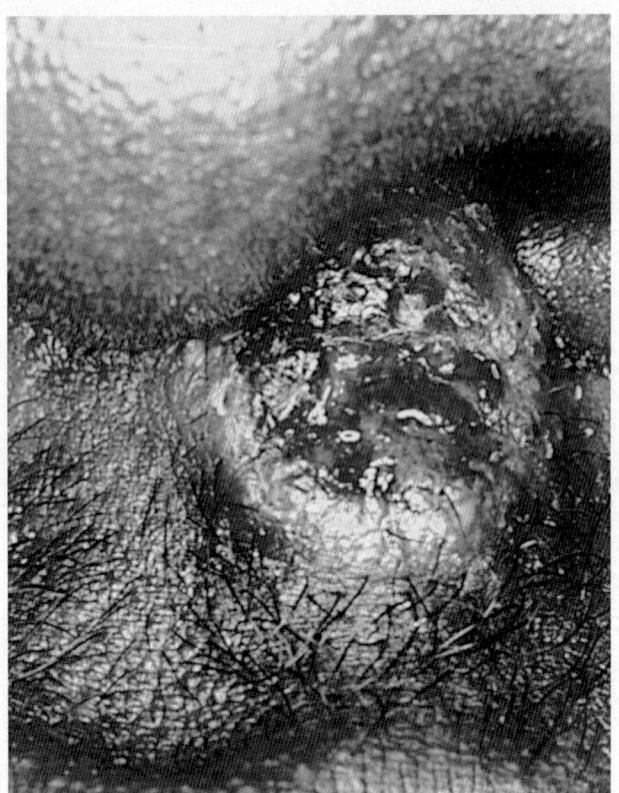

Figure 265-11 Ulcerative skin lesion of blastomycosis. These lesions bleed easily.

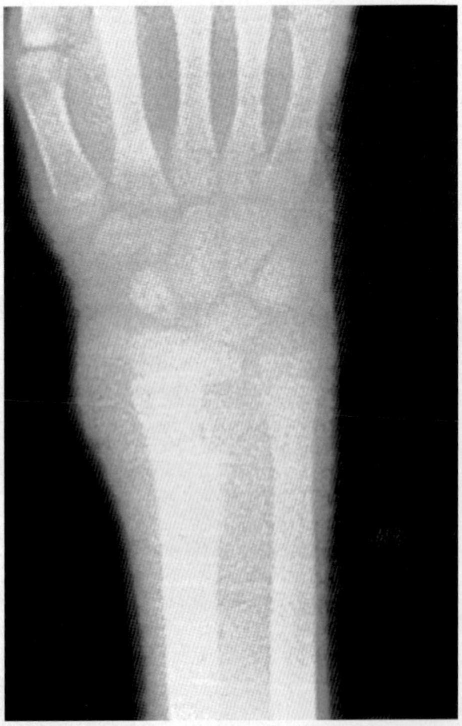

ing sinuses. Vertebral disease mimics tuberculosis, with anterior involvement of the vertebral body, destruction of the interspace, and development of large paraspinous abscesses.[136]

Arthritis associated with blastomycosis, although well described, is rare and usually occurs by extension from a contiguous osteomyelitis.[135,137-139] The arthritis is usually monoarticular, although several cases involving multiple joints have been reported.[132,138,139] Signs and symptoms may be acute or chronic. Synovial fluid is usually purulent, with organisms readily visible on wet preparation.[140] Fungal cultures and KOH staining of synovial fluid are useful in diagnosis, with a diagnostic yield of 82%.[141]

Genitourinary Tract

From 10% to 30% of blastomycosis cases in men have been reported to involve the genitourinary tract, primarily the prostate and epididymis.[142] Epididymal disease may spread to the testes. The variable incidence reported may reflect the respective authors' tenacity in pursuing the diagnosis. Prostatic involvement is most common and usually manifests with symptoms of obstruction, an enlarged and tender prostate, and pyuria. Urine cultures, especially after prostatic massage, are often positive.

Central Nervous System

In the normal host, disease involving the central nervous system (CNS) is uncommon, being reported in less than 5% of cases. Ten cases of recurrent CNS blastomycosis have been reported.[143-146] In patients with AIDS, however, CNS complications of blastomycosis are common. A review noted that 40% of AIDS patients with blastomycosis had CNS disease, usually associated with dissemination to multiple organs.[147] When present, it manifests as either an abscess or meningitis.[148-150] Abscesses present as mass lesions and may be intracranial (Fig. 265-13) or, occasionally, spinal in location. Surgical management of mass lesions may be necessary to establish the diagnosis and to prevent progressive neurologic deterioration.[151] Meningitis is usually a late and fulminant complication of widely disseminated blastomycosis.

Figure 265-12 Osteolytic lesion affecting the ulnar aspect of the distal left radius and extending to the epiphysis. Note the extensive soft tissue swelling. This child had a recent history of chronic pneumonia. (Courtesy of Dr. Blair Batson, Jackson, MS.)

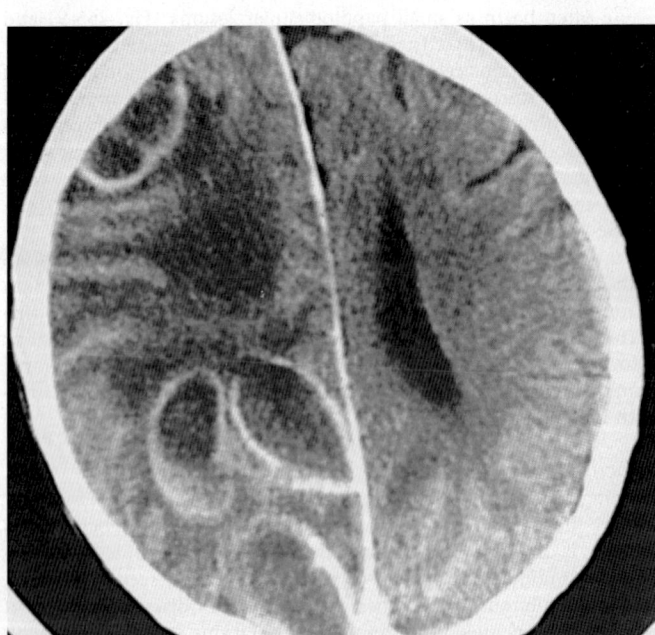

Figure 265-13 Multiple ring-enhancing lesions affecting the right frontal and parietal lobes. There is extensive surrounding edema with effacement of the sulci and right ventricle. This patient simultaneously had pulmonary blastomycosis.

Other Sites

Blastomycosis may infrequently affect the liver, spleen, gastrointestinal tract, thyroid, pericardium, adrenal glands, and other sites (see Tables 265-1 and 265-2). Reports of such cases largely represent findings at autopsy in patients with widely disseminated disease. Of note, gastrointestinal disease below the esophagus and overt adrenal insufficiency are rare.

SPECIAL CIRCUMSTANCES

Blastomycosis in Children

Although blastomycosis in children is considered rare by some authors, most recent reports have estimated that children constitute 3% to 10% of all those affected by blastomycosis.[152] Children commonly have pulmonary disease that can be associated with a variety of symptoms, and radiographic appearances can be misdiagnosed as bacterial pneumonia, tuberculosis, sarcoidosis, or malignant neoplasm.[153] Children may present with acute or chronic disseminated disease associated with cutaneous lesions,[131,154,155] osteomyelitis or septic arthritis,[132,156] or CNS involvement.[145] Skin lesions can be nodular, verrucous, or ulcerative, often with minimal inflammation. In a large common-source outbreak of disease involving 46 children, the attack rate for infection was about 50%. Of the infected patients, about half were symptomatic.[32] Pediatric patients manifest the full clinical spectrum of disease as outlined for adults.[153,157,158] However, clinical reviews from Arkansas and Toronto noted greater difficulty in establishing the diagnosis and a poorer response to oral azole treatment in children with blastomycosis.[137,156]

Blastomycosis in Pregnancy

Despite the depressed cellular immunity associated with pregnancy, blastomycosis has been reported only infrequently in pregnant women.[159-162] Disseminated disease is common, and a case of adult respiratory distress syndrome in a woman who developed blastomycosis in the third trimester of pregnancy is noteworthy.[163] In the 21 cases of blastomycosis during pregnancy, 15 patients were treated with amphotericin B, 13 were cured, 2 were lost to follow-up.[159-161] Perinatal blastomycosis has been reported in two infants born to mothers with untreated blastomycosis.[59,60] Both infants died as a result of overwhelming pulmonary disease. Infection of the infant may result from aspiration into the lungs of vaginal secretions colonized with *B. dermatitidis*, an ascending vaginal infection associated with partially ruptured membranes, or transplacental intrauterine infection.[60] Although a presumptive case of intrauterine transmission has been reported,[59] the placenta in this case was never examined. It is therefore not possible to state with certainty that the child acquired blastomycosis by intrauterine transmission. In a case reported by MacDonald and Alguire,[163] however, *B. dermatitidis* was demonstrated on both the maternal and fetal sides of the placenta. Regardless of the pathogenesis of infection, perinatal transmission remains a definite possibility, and all pregnant women with blastomycosis should be treated without delay. Amphotericin B has been used successfully for blastomycosis and other fungal infections during pregnancy, with no documented adverse outcome for the pregnancy or fetus.[160-162]

Blastomycosis in the Compromised Host

Although invasive fungal diseases are common in the immunosuppressed host, only a few reports have indicated that *B. dermatitidis* can act as an opportunistic pathogen.[147,164-166] As suggested previously, this may be related to natural host defenses that are active against the inhaled conidia.

Blastomycosis has been reported as a late infectious complication in AIDS patients.[147] Most patients have had previous AIDS-defining illnesses, and their CD4$^+$ counts are usually less than 200 cells/mm^3. Disease, whether pulmonary or disseminated, is more aggressive and more often rapidly fatal than disease in the healthy host. Pulmonary disease is more likely to present with diffuse interstitial infiltrates or a miliary pattern on the chest radiograph. Central nervous system disease is especially common, being noted to occur in 40% of patients.[147]

Blastomycosis has also been reported in other immunocompromised hosts, including transplant recipients, patients receiving glucocorticosteroid therapy, and patients receiving cytotoxic chemotherapy for hematologic malignancies or solid tumors.[164-166] A large series of patients reported by Pappas and colleagues[166] has helped to clarify the clinical spectrum of blastomycosis in the immunocompromised host. Blastomycosis in these patients was more often disseminated, more aggressive, and associated with higher mortality than in the immunocompetent host. Diffuse pulmonary infiltrates, pleural effusions, and respiratory failure were common. Multiple visceral organ dissemination and CNS disease occurred frequently but not as often as in AIDS patients.

Mortality rates of 30% to 40% have been reported for immunocompromised patients with blastomycosis. In addition, most deaths attributed to blastomycosis occur within the first few weeks of disease. Thus, early aggressive therapy with amphotericin B is indicated. Frequent relapses have been noted in AIDS patients and those with continued immunosuppressive therapy. Chronic suppressive therapy with an oral azole should therefore be strongly considered for individuals who respond to a primary course of amphotericin.[167]

Blastomycosis in Solid Organ Transplant Recipients

Blastomycosis is rare in solid organ transplant recipients, with a cumulative incidence of 0.14% (11 of 8104) reported in a retrospective case series.[168] A presumptive case of primary cutaneous blastomycosis has been reported in an immunosuppressed child following bilateral lung transplantation.[131] The mechanism by which infection develops in individual patients could not be determined. It was suggested that onset soon after transplantation was due to reactivation of old disease or concurrent asymptomatic infection, or donor transmission associated with intense immunosuppression. Because this study was done in an endemic area, primary infection could not be excluded.

Diagnosis

No clinical syndrome is characteristic of blastomycosis. Definitive diagnosis requires the growth of the organism from clinical specimens. A presumptive diagnosis may be made by visualization of the characteristic yeast in pus, sputum, other secretions, or histopathologic sections. In the appropriate clinical setting, visualization of the fungus can prompt the initiation of antimicrobial therapy.

DIRECT EXAMINATION OF SECRETIONS

Sputum or pus is easily examined by wet preparation. A drop of the specimen is placed on a microscope slide, covered with a coverslip, and examined under the high-dry objective. In a retrospective study of patients with a confirmed diagnosis of blastomycosis, Martynowicz and Prakash[169] reported that KOH smears were underused and were performed on only 30% of all microbiologic specimens collected. Wet preparations had a relatively low diagnostic yield (e.g., 36% for a single specimen and 46% for multiple specimens). Despite these low diagnostic results, the simplicity and low cost of the procedure, as well as its potential for rapid diagnosis, warrant a wet preparation on all specimens collected. Although 10% potassium hydroxide has been recommended to aid in finding the organism, it is usually not necessary because the large, characteristic yeast cell is easily seen despite cellular debris. Sometimes it is also useful to digest sputum with trypsin and smear the centrifuged sediment. Body fluids such as urine, pleural fluid, and cerebrospinal fluid (CSF) should be centrifuged and the sediment evaluated in the same way. Calcofluor white stain requires use of a fluorescence microscope but is easy, rapid, and particularly useful when organisms are sparse.

Cytology has been shown to be particularly useful in diagnosis, permitting identification of the etiologic agent in 56% of all cases and 72% of pulmonary cases of blastomycosis in a retrospective study at the University of Mississippi Medical Center.[170] When visualized, the yeast cells are easily differentiated from others on the basis of their size, refractile cell wall, and single, broad-based buds (see Fig. 265-1). Occasionally, the endospores of *C. immitis* may resemble single yeast cells, but the presence of budding can be used to distinguish *B. dermatitidis*. *Paracoccidioides brasiliensis*, rarely seen in the United States, is distinguished by the presence of multiple, narrow-based buds. *B. dermatitidis* may sometimes be as small as *Cryptococcus neoformans*, although the capsule and narrow-based bud of the latter aid in differentiation.

Bronchoscopy is useful for diagnosis, especially in patients who are not producing sputum or in whom the radiograph indicates the possibility of malignancy.[169] Bronchial washings, lavage fluid, and post-bronchoscopy sputum samples should be sent for cytology as well as smear and culture because the organism is often visualized on Papanicolaou preparations.[171]

HISTOPATHOLOGIC EXAMINATION

The presence of pyogranulomas should alert one to the possibility of blastomycosis. Yeast forms can be difficult to visualize with routine hematoxylin and eosin stains, and special stains should be used to enhance visualization. The Gomori methenamine silver stain is best used for screening tissue for the presence of fungal elements (Fig. 265-14). The Gomori methenamine silver counterstain does not allow evaluation of the inflammatory response in the tissue. The periodic acid–Schiff stain, which colors the cell wall pink or red, has a counterstain that does allow evaluation of cell morphology and tissue response. Mayer mucicarmine stains the cell wall of *B. dermatitidis* faintly or not at all, which may be useful in differentiating it from *C. neoformans* when necessary. A variety of fluorescent microscopic techniques and reagents have also been used to facilitate the histopathologic review of specimens.[172-174] Although these are occasionally helpful when fungal elements in a specimen are atypical or sparse, in our experience their routine use is not warranted because a presumptive diagnosis of *B. dermatitidis* can usually be made by review of Gomori methenamine silver– or periodic acid–Schiff–stained tissue sections.

CULTURE

Culture of *B. dermatitidis* from environmental sources remains difficult, although Baumgardner and Paretsky have recently reported successful isolation using a two-step procedure.[54,55] In patients with pulmonary blastomycosis, sputum culture has a high positive yield (e.g., 75% per single sample, 86% per patient). Specimens obtained for culture by bronchoscopy yielded a positive diagnosis in 92% of patients. Any material obtained should be placed on Sabouraud agar or, preferably, more enriched agar (e.g., Sabhi, brain-heart infusion, Gorman medium). Because initial growth is more dependable at 30° C, this temperature is recommended. Specimens contaminated with bacteria should also be cultured on medium containing an antibacterial antibiotic such as chloramphenicol. Cycloheximide can be incorporated in the medium to inhibit other fungal contaminants. This selective medium should never be used at 37° C, however, because the yeast phase of *B. dermatitidis* and some opportunistic fungi are sensitive to cycloheximide, and growth may be inhibited. The mycelial form of *B. dermatitidis* is not diagnostic, and conversion to the yeast form is required for confirmation. Early identification of mycelial cultures is possible, however, with commercially available chemiluminescent DNA probes that recognize unique RNA sequences of *Blastomyces*.[175]

SEROLOGIC METHODS

Owing to the tremendous problems associated with cross-reactivity noted for the endemic mycoses, serology is not thought to be useful for the diagnosis of blastomycosis.[176] Immunodiffusion assays that measure antibody to *Blastomyces dermatitidis* A antigen are relatively specific, and their sensitivity is 28% to 64%.[109,110] Complement fixation tests fare even worse, with sensitivities of 9% to 43% and less specificity.[109,110] Enzyme immunoassays employing A antigen demonstrated greater sensitivity, but their specificity is below that of either complement fixation or immunodiffusion.[109-112] Although the BAD-1 recombinant protein in a radioimmunoassay has shown high sensitivity and specificity,[114] it has not been adapted for clinical testing. Recently, yeast-phase lysates from multiple sources of *B. dermatitidis* have been prepared and employed to develop enzyme-linked immunoassays for immunoglobulin M (IgM) and IgG antibody detection in an effort to improve immunodiagnostic testing for blastomycosis.[177,178] These tests have not been extensively tested with human specimens.

In summary, complement fixation, immunodiffusion, and enzyme-linked immunosorbent assay serologic tests are available to aid in the diagnosis of blastomycosis. Unfortunately, sensitivity and specificity vary with the test employed. Because false-positive and false-negative results occur commonly, a negative antibody titer, regardless of which test is used, should never be used to rule out disease. Nor should a positive titer alone be an indication for therapy; it should instead stimulate the clinician to look carefully for the disease.

NUCLEIC ACID DETECTION

Molecular identification of *B. dermatitidis* in culture has been accomplished by a variety of techniques,[179] including chemiluminescent DNA probe hybridization (Accuprobe, Gen Probe, San Diego, CA),[180] PCR assays for ribosomal genes,[181,182] the ITS region,[181] repetitive sequences,[182] and species- or genus-specific genes.[183,184] The commercially available chemiluminescent DNA probe was shown to have a sensitivity of 87.4% and a specificity of 100% when 74 target and 219 nontarget fungi were tested.[185] In situ hybridization employing a pair of oligonucleotides complementary to the 18S and 28S rDNA has a reported sensitivity of 95% and a specificity of 100% in tissue sections.[186,187] To date, molecular techniques are used primarily to supplement traditional methods of diagnosing endemic mycoses. Their major contributions may be in identification of specific pathogens in tissue samples without the possibility of culture owing to formaldehyde fixation or from difficult-to-culture environmental samples.[185] PCR techniques, although promising, are labor intensive, are not generally available, and have not yet been examined in large prospective studies.

ANTIGEN DETECTION

The detection of fungal antigens in serum and urine has proved useful in the diagnosis and treatment of patients with invasive mycoses.[176] An antigen detection assay for blastomycosis is available for clinical use.[186] The sensitivity for this immunoassay is 89% in

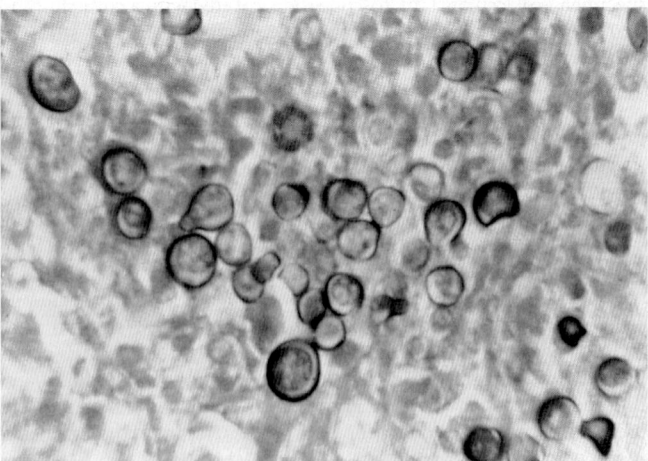

Figure 265-14 Gomori methenamine silver stain of a laryngeal biopsy specimen in a patient with suspected carcinoma of the larynx. *(Courtesy of James Gorman, Jackson, MS.)*

disseminated blastomycosis and 93% overall. Sensitivity is higher in urine than in serum, but antigen has also been detected with high sensitivity (about 80%) in other body fluids, including CSF in patients with CNS disease and bronchoalveolar lavage from patients with pulmonary involvement. Specificity was modest, 79.3% overall, owing to cross-reactive antigens present in specimens obtained from patients with histoplasmosis, paracoccidioidomycosis, and penicilliosis.[187] Cross-reactivity was less than 5% for patients with aspergillosis or cryptococcosis and less than 2% in healthy adults.[176] Antigen levels decline with successful treatment and increase with recurrence of illness. Urine antigen detection has been shown to be useful for follow-up during therapy of blastomycosis in pediatric patients and pregnancy.[161,188] *Blastomyces* antigen clearances during therapy are similar to those reported for the histoplasmosis antigen, with clearance correlating well with successful therapy and clinical improvement.[188,189] Failure to clear *Blastomyces* antigenuria is indicative of treatment failure.[161,188] Usefulness in diagnosis is limited by the ease of diagnosis using conventional methods and modest specificity once blastomycosis is considered.

CELLULAR IMMUNITY TESTING

No reagent is available for skin testing of patients with suspected blastomycosis. Lymphocyte transformation to yeast-phase organisms, the BAD-1 surface protein, and alkali-soluble, water-soluble antigens have been used as indicators of cell-mediated immunity in patients with blastomycosis.[71,93,98] In an outbreak, 81% of definite and probable cases of blastomycosis had positive lymphocyte transformation tests with the alkali-soluble, water-soluble antigen.[32] This test does not appear to be useful early in the acute disease because positive tests are not obtained in the first 2 weeks of disease. Furthermore, because this immunity appears to be long lived, a positive test does not necessarily indicate recent infection.[98] Finally, there are only limited data on the specificity of this test. Lymphocyte transformation assays are therefore not yet clinically useful and should be considered investigational tests.

Treatment

CHEMOTHERAPY

Before the availability of chemotherapy for treatment of blastomycosis, the disease as reported had a progressive course with eventual extrapulmonary disease and a mortality rate exceeding 60%. Even though isolated cutaneous disease had a better prognosis, skin lesions were progressive, and spontaneous recovery was uncommon. Thus, after the introduction of effective antifungal therapy, it was accepted that all patients with blastomycosis should be treated. This concept was questioned after the description of self-limited pulmonary blastomycosis.[125] The decision to withhold therapy for patients with acute pulmonary blastomycosis is difficult and remains a controversial issue. Although it is true that in some patients, blastomycotic pneumonia may resolve without therapy, there is no way to determine which patients will present later with extrapulmonary disease, often with serious sequelae.[190] Furthermore, some patients while under observation may suffer acute exacerbation with miliary disease or endobronchial spread, both associated with high mortality.[128,129] For these reasons, it is the policy at our medical center that all patients with active disease be treated. If a culture-based diagnosis is made after spontaneous recovery from blastomycotic pneumonia, patients are carefully evaluated for the presence of extrapulmonary disease before a decision is made to withhold treatment. If treatment is withheld, patients must be followed carefully for many years for evidence of reactivation or progressive disease.

Amphotericin B was previously considered the treatment of choice for all clinical forms of blastomycosis.[191,192] However, ketoconazole, itraconazole, and fluconazole are now considered effective alternatives for immunocompetent patients with mild to moderate disease (Table 265-3).[192] Azoles should not be used in patients with life-threatening

TABLE 265-3	Treatment Guidelines for Blastomycosis[193]	
Type of Disease	**Primary Therapy**	**Alternate Therapy**
Pulmonary		
Mild to moderate	Itraconazole, 200-400 mg/kg/day	Fluconazole, 400-800 mg/day, or Ketoconazole, 400-800 mg/day
Serious	Lipid AmB, 3-5 mg/kg/day, or Deoxycholate AmB, 0.7-1 mg/kg/day, for 1-2 wk*	Itraconazole, 200-400 mg/day (once patient is stabilized)
Disseminated		
Mild to Moderate		
Non CNS disease	Itraconazole, 200-400 mg/kg/day	Ketoconazole, 400-800 mg/day or Fluconazole, 400-800 mg/day
Serious		
CNS	Lipid AmB, 3-5 mg/kg/day, or Deoxycholate AmB, 0.7-1 mg/kg/day, for 1-2 wk*	Fluconazole, 800 mg/day (if intolerant to full course of amphotericin B)
Non-CNS	Lipid AmB, 3-5 mg/kg/day, or Deoxycholate AmB, 0.7-1 mg/kg/day, for 1-2 wk*	Itraconazole, 200-400 mg/day (once patient is stabilized)

*Followed by azole therapy.

disease or with central nervous system blastomycosis. Hydroxystilbamidine, the first effective drug available for the treatment of blastomycosis, is no longer available.

Ketoconazole

Ketoconazole is now infrequently used because of its adverse effects and variable absorption, but several useful studies have been done on blastomycosis and were the first indication that azoles were effective agents. In a prospective, randomized multicenter trial of patients treated with ketoconazole for at least 6 months, the cure rates were 100% in patients treated with 800 mg/day and 79% in those treated with 400 mg/day.[193] Toxicity was greater with the higher dose. A second study noted a cure rate of 81% in 43 patients who completed at least 1 month of therapy with 400 mg/day.[117] A retrospective study documented a cure rate of 82% for patients treated with ketoconazole at a daily dose of 400 mg or greater.[119] Therapy should be continued for at least 6 months.[192,194,195] Relapse of blastomycosis is more common after ketoconazole than after amphotericin B (10% to 14% vs. 4% or less with amphotericin B). Rates of 10% to 14% have been reported after ketoconazole therapy.[117,119,192]

Itraconazole

Itraconazole has excellent in vitro and in vivo activity against *B. dermatitidis* and has replaced ketoconazole as the first-line agent for the treatment of non–life-threatening, non-CNS blastomycosis.[196] In a prospective phase II clinical trial, itraconazole at doses ranging from 200 to 400 mg/day was effective in 90% of patients.[197] For compliant patients with at least 2 months of therapy, a successful outcome was noted in 95%. Although the study design did not allow comparison of the relative efficacy of the different doses, most patients received 200 mg/day, and no further improvement in outcome was noted in patients receiving higher doses. Itraconazole was well tolerated, and only one patient had to discontinue therapy because of drug toxicity. When compared with ketoconazole in a similar study design,[193] itraconazole appeared to be better tolerated. Bradsher[198] noted similar success in 42 patients treated with itraconazole at a daily dose of

200 mg. Thus, the recommended initial dose of itraconazole is 200 mg/day, which should effect a cure in most patients with blastomycosis. For patients whose disease persists or progresses, the dose should be increased in increments of 100 mg daily to a maximal daily dose of 400 mg. The optimal duration of therapy has not been determined, but it is recommended that treatment be continued for 6 months. Itraconazole is now the drug of choice for patients with indolent blastomycosis. The greater rapidity of the clinical response to amphotericin B has made itraconazole less desirable in severely ill patients.

Attention must be paid to the pharmacology of itraconazole, particularly the numerous drug interactions[199-202] (see Chapter 40).

Fluconazole

Fluconazole, a triazole that is available in both oral and intravenous preparations, has been used to treat only a small cohort of patients with blastomycosis. It is our opinion that, compared with ketoconazole and itraconazole, fluconazole has a limited role in the treatment of blastomycosis. The results of a pilot study employing lower-dose fluconazole were disappointing, with a successful outcome noted in only 65% of the 23 patients treated with daily doses of 200 and 400 mg.[203] A study employing higher doses of fluconazole (400 to 800 mg daily) showed enhanced efficacy.[204] A successful outcome was noted in 87% of the 39 patients treated for a mean of 8.9 months. Adverse events were usually mild. Cessation of therapy owing to an adverse event was necessary in only 1 of 39 patients; a second patient required a dosage reduction. In both patients, however, treatment was successful. These results indicate that fluconazole is similar in efficacy to ketoconazole at equivalent doses but has less serious toxicity. However, fluconazole is not as efficacious as itraconazole for the treatment of patients with mild to moderate blastomycosis. Because fluconazole has excellent penetration into the central nervous system, it may have some role in the treatment of blastomycotic meningitis and cerebral abscesses, although clinical experience in treating these conditions is limited to only a few cases.

Newer Azoles

Voriconazole, a newly released triazole, and posaconazole have shown excellent in vitro and in vivo activity against isolates of *B. dermatitidis*. Voriconazole has been used successfully to treat refractory blastomycosis and for treatment of immunosuppressed patients.[168,205] Owing to its ability to achieve adequate concentrations in the brain and CSF,[206] voriconazole has been used to treat patients with CNS blastomycosis.[145,146,179,207] Posaconazole has not been reported for the treatment of blastomycosis. These agents presently do not appear to offer any advantage for blastomycosis but may prove to offer an option in the treatment of patients failing or intolerant to amphotericin B and not tolerating itraconazole.

Amphotericin

Three lipid formulations of amphotericin B (amphotericin B lipid complex [ABLC], amphotericin B cholesteryl sulfate [ABCD], and liposomal amphotericin B [AmBisome]) are marketed in the United States. Because of lesser toxicity, ABLC and AmBisome have largely replaced conventional amphotericin B for treatment of blastomycosis in the United States despite their higher cost.[196] An amphotericin B formulation remains the drug of choice for patients who are severely immunocompromised; for patients with life-threatening disease, CNS disease, or progression of disease during treatment with an azole; and for those who are unable to tolerate an azole because of toxicity.[165,192,196] Although the exact dose and optimal duration of therapy are uncertain, most experts recommend ABLC or AmBisome, 3 to 5 mg/kg per day, or amphotericin B deoxycholate, 0.7 to 1 mg/kg per day, for 1 to 2 weeks or until improvement is noted. Although effective, amphotericin B is not currently used as sole therapy for blastomycosis.[196] Current guidelines recommend step-down therapy to an azole after an initial therapeutic response to amphotericin B. Patients who are immunocompetent and do not have CNS disease may be switched to step-down therapy of oral itraconazole, 200 mg 3 times per day for 3 days, and then 200 mg twice per day for a total of 6 to 12 months.[196] Relapse rates of most patients treated with amphotericin B are less than 5%. Relapse is more common in immunocompromised patients, especially those with AIDS.[196] Some authorities recommend lifelong suppressive therapy with itraconazole.[196] These patients still require close follow-up.

Echinocandins

The echinocandins (e.g., caspofungin, anidulafungin, and mycafungin) show only variable activity against *B. dermatitidis*. Presently, there are no clinical data to support the use of echinocandins for the therapy of blastomycosis.

SURGERY

Apart from diagnosis, surgery has little role in the treatment of blastomycosis.[196] In conjunction with antifungal therapy, surgery appears indicated for the drainage of large abscesses, for the rare patient with large accumulations of empyema fluid or bronchopleural fistula, and for the débridement of devitalized bone tissue in patients with osteomyelitis who are responding poorly to therapy. Unless patients have repeated relapses in the lung or remain culture positive with appropriate therapy, the surgical resection of large or residual lung cavities is not indicated. Furthermore, we have seen patients who developed acute, life-threatening disease after surgical resection of lung tissue for diagnostic purposes when blastomycosis was left untreated. Therefore, it is our policy to treat any patient whose resected lung tissue contains *B. dermatitidis*.

REFERENCES

1. Gilchrist TC. Protozoan dermatitis. *J Cutan Gen Dis.* 1894;12:496-499.
2. Gilchrist TC. A case of blastomycetic dermatitis in man. *Johns Hopkins Hosp Rep.* 1896;1:269-283.
3. Gilchrist TC, Stokes WR. The presence of an oidium in the tissues of a case of pseudo-lupus vulgaris. *Johns Hopkins Hosp Rep.* 1896;7:129-133.
4. Gilchrist TC, Stokes WR. Case of pseudo-lupus vulgaris caused by *Blastomyces. J Exp Med.* 1898;3:53-78.
5. Martin DS, Smith DT. Blastomycosis I: A review of the literature. *Am Rev Tuberc.* 1939;39:275-304.
6. Martin DS, Smith DT. Blastomycosis II: A report of thirteen new cases. *Am Rev Tuberc.* 1939;39:488-515.
7. Schwartz J, Baum GL. Blastomycosis. *Am J Clin Pathol.* 1951;21:999-1029.
8. Kwon-Chung KJ, Bennett JE. *Medical Mycology.* Philadelphia: Lea & Febiger; 1992:248.
9. Bradsher RW. *Blastomycosis.* In: Dismukes WE, Pappas PG, Sobel JD, ed. *Clinical Mycology.* New York: Oxford University Press; 2003:299-310.
10. Medoff G, Painter A, Kobayashi GS. Mycelial-to-yeast phase transitions of the dimorphic fungi *Blastomyces dermatitidis* and *Paracoccidioides brasiliensis. J Bacteriol.* 1987;169:4055-4060.
11. Maresca B, Kobayashi GS. Dimorphism in *Histoplasma capsulatum* and *Blastomyces dermatitidis. Contrib Microbiol.* 2000;5:201-216.
12. Kaufman L, Standard PG, Weeks RJ, et al. Detection of two *Blastomyces dermatitidis* serotypes by exoantigen analysis. *J Clin Microbiol.* 1983;18:110-114.
13. Turner S, Kaufman L. Immunodiagnosis of blastomycosis. *Semin Respir Infect.* 1986;1:22-28.
14. McDonough ES, Lewis AL. *Blastomyces dermatitidis*: Production of the sexual state. *Science.* 1967;156:528-529.
15. McDonough ES, Lewis AL. The ascigerous state of *Blastomyces dermatitidis. Mycologia.* 1968;60:76-83.
16. McDonough ES, McNamara WJ, Chan DM, et al. Geographic distribution of "+" and "–" isolates of *Blastomyces (Ajellomyces) dermatitidis* in North America. *Am J Epidemiol.* 1973;98:63-67.
17. Yates-Ciilata KE, Sander DM, Keith EJ. Genetic diversity in clinical isolates of the dimorphic fungus *Blastomyces dermatitidis* detected by PCR based random amplified polymorphic DNA assay. *J Clin Microbiol.* 1995;33:2171-2175.
18. McCullough MJ, DiSalvo AF, Clemons KV, et al. Molecular epidemiology of *Blastomyces dermatitidis. Clin Infect Dis.* 2003;328-335.
19. Blastomycosis Cooperative Study of the Veterans Administration. Blastomycosis I: A review of 198 collected cases in Veterans Administration hospitals. *Am Rev Respir Dis.* 1964;89:659-672.
20. Menges RW, Doto IL, Weeks RJ. Epidemiologic studies of blastomycosis in Arkansas. *Arch Environ Health.* 1969;18:956-971.
21. Furcolow ML, Chick EW, Busey JF, et al. Prevalence and incidence studies of human and canine blastomycosis. I: Cases in the United States, 1885–1968. *Am Rev Respir Dis.* 1970;102:60-67.
22. Furcolow ML, Busey JF, Menges RW, et al. Prevalence and incidence studies of human and canine blastomycosis. II: Yearly incidence studies in three selected states, 1960–1967. *Am J Epidemiol.* 1970;92:121-131.
23. Sekshon AS, Borgurus MS, Sims HV. Blastomycosis: Report of three cases from Alberta with a review of Canadian cases. *Mycopathologia.* 1979;1:53-63.
24. Klein BS, Vergeront JM, Davis JP. Epidemiologic aspects of blastomycosis, the enigmatic systemic mycosis. *Semin Respir Infect.* 1986;1:29-39.
25. Crampton TL, Light RB, Berg GM, et al. Epidemiology and clinical spectrum of blastomycoses diagnosed at Manitoba hospitals. *Clin Infect Dis.* 2002;34:1310-1316.

26. Smith Jr JD, Harris JS, Conant NF, et al. An epidemic of North American blastomycosis. *JAMA*. 1955;158:641-646.
27. Tosh FE, Hammerman KJ, Weeks RJ, et al. A common source epidemic of North American blastomycosis. *Am Rev Respir Dis*. 1974;109:525-529.
28. Centers for Disease Control. Blastomycosis: North Carolina. *MMWR Morb Mortal Wkly Rep*. 1976;25:205-206.
29. Kitchen MS, Reiber CD, Eastin GB. An urban epidemic of North American blastomycosis. *Am Rev Respir Dis*. 1977;115:1063-1066.
30. Cockerill III FR, Roberts GD, Rosenblatt JE, et al. Epidemic of pulmonary blastomycosis (Nanekagan fever) in Wisconsin canoeists. *Chest*. 1984;86:688-692.
31. Armstrong CW, Jenkins SR, Kaufman L, et al. Common source outbreak of blastomycosis in hunters and their dogs. *J Infect Dis*. 1987;155:568-570.
32. Klein BS, Vergeront JM, Weeks RJ, et al. Isolation of *Blastomyces dermatitidis* in soil associated with a large outbreak of blastomycosis in Wisconsin. *N Engl J Med*. 1986;314:529-534.
33. Klein BS, Vergeront JM, DiSalvo AF, et al. Two outbreaks of blastomycosis along rivers in Wisconsin: Isolation of *Blastomyces dermatitidis* from riverbank soil and evidence of its transmission along waterways. *Am Rev Respir Dis*. 1987;136:1333-1338.
34. Baumgardner DJ, Burdick JS. An outbreak of human and canine blastomycosis. *Rev Infect Dis*. 1991;13:898-905.
35. Frye MD, Seifer FD. An outbreak of blastomycosis in eastern Tennessee. *Mycopathologia*. 1991;116:15-21.
36. Proctor ME, Klein BS, Jones JM, et al. Cluster of pulmonary blastomycosis in a rural community: Evidence for multiple high-risk environmental foci following a sustained period of diminished precipitation. *Mycopathologia*. 2002;153:113-120.
37. Dworkin MS, Kuckro AN, Proia L, et al. The epidemiology of Blastomycosis in Illinois and factors associated with death. *Clin Infect Dis*. 2005;41:e107-111.
38. Moris SK, Brophy J, Richardson SE, et al. Blastomycosis in Ontario, 1994-2003. *Emerg Infect Dis*. 2006;12:274-279.
39. Bumgardner DJ, Knavel EM, Steber D, et al. Geographic distribution of human blastomycosis cases in Milwaukee, Wisconsin, USA: Association with urban watersheds. *Mycopathologia*. 2006;161:275-282.
40. Reed KD, Meece JK, Archer JR, et al. Ecologic niche modeling of *Blastomyces dermatitidis* in Wisconsin. *PLoS ONE*. 2008;3:e2034.
41. Baily GG, Robertson VJ, Neill P, et al. Blastomycosis in Africa: Clinical features, diagnosis and treatment. *Rev Infect Dis*. 1991;13:1005-1008.
42. DiSalvo AF. The ecology of Blastomyces dermatitidis. In: Al-Doory Y, DiSalvo AF, eds. *Blastomycosis*. New York: Plenum. Publishing Corp; 1992:43-69.
43. Chander B, Deb P, Sarkar C, et al. Cerebral blastomycosis: A case report. *Indian J Pathol Microbiol*. 2007;50:821-824.
44. MacDonald PD, Langley RL, Gerkin SR, et al. Human and canine pulmonary blastomycosis, North Carolina, 2001-2002. *Emerg Infect Dis*. 2006;12:1242-1244.
45. De Groote MA, Bjerke R, Smith H, et al. Expanding epidemiology of blastomycosis: Clinical features and investigation of 2 cases in Colorado. 2000;30:582-584.
46. Veliganda SR, Hinrichs SH, Rupp ME, et al. Delayed diagnosis of osseous blastomycosis in two patients following environmental exposure in nonendemic areas. *Am J Clin Pathol*. 2002;118:536-541.
47. Baumgardner DJ, Paretsky DP. Blastomycosis: More evidence for exposure near one's domicile. *WMJ*. 2001;100:4-5.
48. Denton JF, McDonough ES, Ajello L, et al. Isolation of *Blastomyces dermatitidis* from soil. *Science*. 1961;133:1126-1127.
49. Denton JF, DiSalvo AF. Isolation of *Blastomyces dermatitidis* from natural sites in Augusta, Georgia. *Am J Trop Med Hyg*. 1964;13:716-722.
50. Denton JF, DiSalvo AF. Additional isolations of *Blastomyces dermatitidis* from natural sites. *Am J Trop Med Hyg*. 1979;28:697-700.
51. Sarosi GA, Serstock DA. Isolation of *Blastomyces dermatitidis* from pigeon manure. *Am Rev Respir Dis*. 1976;114:1179-1183.
52. Bakerspigel A, Kane J, Schaus D. Isolation of Blastomyces dermatitidis from an earthen floor in southwestern Ontario, Canada. *J Clin Microbiol*. 1986;24:890-891.
53. Dixon DM, Shadomy HJ, Shadomy S. In vitro growth and sporulation of *Blastomyces dermatitidis* on woody plant material. *Mycologia*. 1977;69:1193-1195.
54. Baumgardner DJ, Laundre B. Studies on the molecular ecology of *Blastomyces dermatitidis*. *Mycopathologia*. 2001;152:51-58.
55. Baumgardner DJ, Paretsky DP. The in vitro isolation of *Blastomyces dermatitidis* from a woodpile in north central Wisconsin, USA. *Med Mycol*. 1999;37:163-168.
56. Larson DM, Eckman MR, Alber RL, et al. Primary cutaneous (inoculation) blastomycosis: An occupational hazard to pathologists. *Am J Clin Pathol*. 1983;79:253-255.
57. Gnann Jr JW, Bressler GS, Bodet CA, et al. Human blastomycosis after a dog bite. *Ann Intern Med*. 1983;98:48-49.
58. Craig MW, Davey WN, Green RA. Conjugal blastomycosis. *Am Rev Respir Dis*. 1970;102:86-90.
59. Watts EA, Gard Jr PD, Tuthill SW. First reported case of intrauterine transmission of blastomycosis. *Pediatr Infect Dis*. 1983;2:308-310.
60. Maxson S, Miller SF, Tryka AF, et al. Perinatal blastomycosis: A review. *Pediatr Infect Dis*. 1992;11:760-763.
61. Daniel WP, Danaar SC, Perry HD. Blastomycosis-like pyoderma. *Arch Dermatol*. 1979;115:170-173.
62. Reder PA, Neel III HB. Blastomycosis in otolaryngology: Review of a large series. *Laryngoscope*. 1993;103:53-58.
63. Ebeo CT, Olove K, Byrd Jr RP, et al. Blastomycosis of the vocal folds with life threatening upper airway obstruction: A case report. *Ear Nose Throat J*. 2002;81:852-855.
64. Vaaler AK, Bradsher RW, Davies SF. Evidence of subclinical blastomycosis in forestry workers in northern Minnesota and northern Wisconsin. *Am J Med*. 1990;89:470-476.
65. Ganer A, Brummer E, Stevens DA. Correlation of susceptibility of immature mice to fungal infection (blastomycosis) and effector cell function. *Infect Immun*. 2000;68:6833-6839.
66. Sugar AM, Picard M. Macrophage- and oxidant-mediated inhibition of the ability of live *Blastomyces dermatitidis* conidia to transform to the pathogenic yeast phase: Implications for the pathogenesis of dimorphic fungal infections. *J Infect Dis*. 1991;163:371-375.
67. Nemecek JC, Wüthrich M, Klein BS. Global Control of Dimorphism and Virulence in Fungi. *Science*. 2006;312:583-588.
68. DiSalvo AF, Denton JF. Lipid content of four strains of *Blastomyces dermatitidis* of different mouse virulence. *J Bacteriol*. 1963;85:927-931.
69. Cox RA, Best GK. Cell wall composition of two strains of *Blastomyces dermatitidis* exhibiting differences in virulence for mice. *Infect Immun*. 1972;5:449-453.
70. Klein BS, Jones JM. Isolation, purification, and radiolabeling of a novel 120-kD surface protein on *Blastomyces dermatitidis* yeasts to detect antibody in infected patients. *J Clin Invest*. 1990;85:152-161.
71. Klein BS, Sondel PM, Jones JM. WI-1, a novel 120-kilodalton surface protein on *Blastomyces dermatitidis* yeast cells, is a target antigen of cell-mediated immunity in human blastomycosis. *Infect Immun*. 1992;60:4291-4300.
72. Klein BS, Hogan LH, Jones JM. Immunologic recognition of a 25-amino acid repeat arrayed in tandem on a major antigen of *Blastomyces dermatitidis*. *J Clin Invest*. 1993;92:330-337.
73. Klein BS, Newman SL. Role of cell-surface molecules of *Blastomyces dermatitidis* in host-pathogen interactions. *Trends Microbiol*. 1996;4:246-251.
74. Hogan LH, Josvai S, Klein BS. Genomic cloning, characterization and functional analysis of the major surface adhesin WI-1 on *Blastomyces dermatitidis* yeasts. *J Biol Chem*. 1995;270:30725-30732.
75. Klein BS, Chaturvedi S, Hogan LH, et al. Altered expression of surface protein WI-1 in genetically related strains of *Blastomyces dermatitidis* that differ in virulence regulates recognition of yeasts by human macrophages. *Infect Immun*. 1994;62:3536-3542.
76. Hogan LH, Klein BS. Altered expression of surface α-1,3-glucan in genetically related strains of *Blastomyces dermatitidis* that differ in virulence. *Infect Immun*. 1994;62:3543-3546.
77. Brandhorst T, Klein B. Cell wall biogenesis of *Blastomyces dermatitidis*: Evidence for a novel mechanism of self service localization of a virulence-associated adhesin by an extracellular release and reassociation with cell wall chitin. *J Biol Chem*. 2000;275:7925-7934.
78. Finkel-Jimenez B, Wuthichm M, Brandhorst T, et al. WI-1 adhesin blocks phagocytic TNF-α production, imparting pathogenicity in *Blastomyces dermatitidis*. *J Immun*. 2001;166:2665-2673.
79. Finkel-Jimenez B, Wuthichm M, Klein BS. BAD1, an essential virulence factor of *Blastomyces dermatitidis*, suppresses host TNF-α production through TGF-β-dependent and independent mechanisms. *J Immun*. 2002;168:5746-5755.
80. Ahang MX, Brandhorst TT, Kozel TR, et al. Role of glucan and surface protein BAD1 in complement activation of *Blastomyces dermatitidis* yeast. *Infect Immun*. 2001;69:7559-7564.
81. Thurmond LM, Mitchell TG. *Blastomyces dermatitidis* chemotactic factor: Kinetics of production and biological characterization evaluated by a modified chemotaxis assay. *Infect Immun*. 1984;46:87-93.
82. Drutz DJ, Frey CL. Intracellular and extracellular defenses against *Blastomyces dermatitidis* conidia and yeasts. *J Lab Clin Med*. 1985;105:737-750.
83. Schaffner A, Davis CE, Schaffner T, et al. In vitro susceptibility of fungi to killing by neutrophil granulocytes discriminates between primary pathogenicity and opportunism. *J Clin Invest*. 1986;78:511-524.
84. Wüthrich M, Fisette PL, Filutowicz HI, et al. Differential requirements of T cell subsets for CD40 costimulation in immunity to *Blastomyces dermatitidis*. *J Immun*. 2006;176:5538-5547.
85. Wüthrich M, Finkel-Jimenez B, Brandhorst TT, et al. Analysis of non adhesive pathogenic mechanisms of BAD1 on *Blastomyces dermatitidis*. *Med Mycol*. 2006;44:41-49.
86. Wüthrich M, Warner T, Klein BS. IL-12 is required for induction but not maintenance of protective, memory responses to *Blastomyces dermatitidis*: Implications for vaccine development in immune deficient hosts. *J Immun*. 2005;175:5288-5297.
87. Brummer E, Vinoda V, Stevens DA. IL-12 induction of resistance to pulmonary blastomycosis. *Cytokine*. 2006;35:221-228.
88. Brummer E, Kurita N, Yoshida K, et al. A basis for resistance of *Blastomyces dermatitidis* killing by human neutrophils: Inefficient generation of myeloperoxidase system products. *J Med Vet Mycol*. 1992;30:233-243.
89. Brummer E, Stevens DA. Activation of murine polymorphonuclear neutrophils for fungicidal activity with supernatants from antigen-stimulated immune spleen cell cultures. *Infect Immun*. 1984;45:447-452.
90. Morrison CJ, Brummer E, Isenberg RA, et al. Activation of murine polymorphonuclear neutrophils for fungicidal activity by recombinant gamma interferon. *J Leukoc Biol*. 1987;41:434-440.
91. Cozad GC, Chang C. T-cell mediated immunoprotection in blastomycosis. *Infect Immun*. 1980;78:393-403.
92. Morozumi PA, Brummer E, Stevens DA. Protection against pulmonary blastomycosis. *Infect Immun*. 1982;37:670-678.
93. Brummer E, Morozumi PA, Vo PT, et al. Protection against pulmonary blastomycosis: Adaptive transfer with T lymphocytes, but not serum, from resistant mice. *Cell Immunol*. 1982;73:349-359.
94. Brummer E, Morozumi A, Philpott DE, et al. Virulence of fungi: Correlation of virulence of *Blastomyces dermatitidis* in vivo with escape from macrophage inhibition of replication in vitro. *Infect Immun*. 1981;32:864-871.
95. Brummer E, Hanson LH, Restrepo A, et al. In vivo and in vitro activation of pulmonary macrophages by IFN-γ for enhanced killing of *Paracoccidioides brasiliensis* or *Blastomyces dermatitidis*. *J Immunol*. 1988;140:2786-2789.
96. Brummer E, Hanson LH, Stevens DA. Kinetics and requirements for activation of macrophages for fungicidal activity: Effect of protein synthesis inhibitors and immunosuppressants on activation and fungicidal mechanisms. *Cell Immunol*. 1991;132:236-245.
97. Bradsher RW. Live *Blastomyces dermatitidis* yeast-induced responses of immune and non-immune human mononuclear cells. *Mycopathologia*. 1984;87:159-166.
98. Klein PS, Bradsher RW, Vergeront JM, et al. Development of long-term specific cellular immunity after acute *Blastomyces dermatitidis* infection: Assessments following a large point-source outbreak in Wisconsin. *J Infect Dis*. 1990;161:97-101.
99. Chang WL, Audet RG, Aizenstein BD, et al. T cell epitopes and human leukocyte antigen restriction elements in an immunodominant antigen of *Blastomyces dermatitidis*. *Infect Immun*. 2000;68:502-510.
100. Wüthrich M, Chang WL, Klein BS. Immunogenicity and protective efficacy of the WI-1 adhesin of *Blastomyces dermatitidis*. *Infect Immun*. 1998;66:5443-5449.
101. Wüthrich M, Finkel-Jimenez BE, Klein BS. Interleukin 12 as an adjuvant to WI-1 adhesin immunization augments delayed-type hypersensitivity, shifts the subclass distribution of immunoglobulin G antibodies, and enhances protective immunity to *Blastomyces dermatitidis*. *Infect Immun*. 2000;68:7172-7174.
102. Wüthrich M, Filutowicz HI, Klein BS. Mutation of the WI-1 gene yields an attenuated *Blastomyces dermatitidis* strain that induces host resistance. *J Clin Invest*. 2000;106:1381-1389.
103. Wüthrich M, Filutowicz HI, Warner T, et al. Requisite elements in vaccine immunity to *Blastomyces dermatitidis*: Plasticity uncovers vaccine potential in immune-deficient hosts. *J Immunol*. 2002;169:6969-6976.
104. Wüthrich M, Filutowicz HI, Warner T, et al. Vaccine immunity to pathogenic fungi overcomes the requirement for CD4 help in exogenous antigen presentation to CD8+ T cells: Implication for vaccine development in immune-deficient hosts. *J Exp Med*. 2003;197:1405-1416.
105. Wüthrich M, Filutowicz HI, Allen HL, et al. Vβ1+ Jβ1.1/Vα2+Jα49+ CD4+ T cells medicate resistance against infection with *Blastomyces dermatitidis*. *Infect Immun*. 2007;75:193-200.
106. Bradsher RW, Balk RA, Jacobs RF. Growth inhibition of *Blastomyces dermatitidis* in alveolar and peripheral macrophages from patients with blastomycosis. *Am Rev Respir Dis*. 1987;135:412-417.
107. Kaufman L, McLaughlin DW, Clark MJ, et al. Specific immunodiffusion test for blastomycosis. *Appl Microbiol*. 1973;26:244-247.
108. Williams JE, Murphy R, Standard PG, et al. Serologic response in blastomycosis: Diagnostic value of double immunodiffusion assay. *Am Rev Respir Dis*. 1981;123:209-212.
109. Klein BS, Kuritsky WAC, Kaufman L, et al. Comparison of enzyme immunoassay, immunodiffusion and complement fixation in detecting antibody in human serum to the A antigen in *B. dermatitidis*. *Am Rev Respir Dis*. 1986;133:144-148.
110. Klein BS, Vergeront JM, Kaufman L, et al. Serological test for blastomycosis: Assessments during a large point-source outbreak in Wisconsin. *J Infect Dis*. 1987;155:262-268.
111. Bradsher RW, Pappas PG. Detection of specific antibodies in human blastomycosis by enzyme immunoassay. *South Med J*. 1995;88:1256-1259.
112. Sekhorn AS, Kaufman L, Kobayashi AS, et al. The value of the Premier enzyme immunoassay for diagnosing *Blastomyces dermatitidis* infections. *J Med Vet Mycol*. 1995;33:123-125.
113. Klein BS, Jones JM. Purification and characterization of the major WI-1 from *Blastomyces dermatitidis* yeast and immunological comparison with A antigen. *Infect Immun*. 1994;62:3890-3900.
114. Soufleris AJ, Klein BS, Courtney BT, et al. Utility of anti-WI-1 serological testing in the diagnosis of blastomycosis in Wisconsin residents. *Clin Infect Dis*. 1994;19:87-92.
115. Klein BS, Squires RA, Lloyd JK, et al. Canine antibody response to *Blastomyces dermatitidis* WI-1 antigen. *Am J Vet Res*. 2000;61:554-558.

116. Bradsher RW, Chapman SW, Pappas PG. Blastomycosis. *Infect Dis Clin North Am.* 2003;17:21-40.
117. Bradsher RW, Rice DC, Abernathy RS. Ketoconazole therapy for endemic blastomycosis. *Ann Intern Med.* 1985;103:872-879.
118. Baumgardner DJ, Buggy BP, Mattson BJ, et al. Epidemiology of blastomycosis in a region of high endemicity in north central Wisconsin. *Clin Infect Dis.* 1992;15:629-635.
119. Chapman SW, Lin AC, Hendricks KA, et al. Endemic blastomycosis in Mississippi: Epidemiological and clinical studies. *Semin Respir Infect.* 1997;12:219-228.
120. Sarosi GA, Davies SF. Blastomycosis. *Am Rev Respir Dis.* 1979;120:911-938.
121. Ehni W. Endogenous reactivation in blastomycosis. *Am J Med.* 1989;86:831-832.
122. Sheflin JR, Campbell JA, Thompson GP. Pulmonary blastomycosis: Findings on chest radiographs in 63 patients. *AJR Am J Roentgenol.* 1990;154:1177-1180.
123. Brown LR, Sweasen SJ, VanScoy RE, et al. Roentgenologic features of pulmonary blastomycosis. *Mayo Clin Proc.* 1991;66:29-38.
124. Sarosi GA, Davies SF, Phillips JR. Self-limited blastomycosis: A report of 39 cases. *Semin Respir Infect.* 1986;1:40-44.
125. Sarosi GA, Hammerman KJ, Tosh FE, et al. Clinical features of acute pulmonary blastomycosis. *N Engl J Med.* 1974;290:540-543.
126. Baum GL, Lerner PI. Primary pulmonary blastomycosis: A laboratory acquired infection. *Ann Intern Med.* 1970;73:263-265.
127. Poe RH, Vassallo CL, Plessinger VA, et al. Pulmonary blastomycosis versus carcinoma: A challenging differential. *Am J Med Sci.* 1972;263:145-155.
128. Stelling CB, Woodring JH, Rehm SR, et al. Miliary pulmonary blastomycosis. *Radiology.* 1984;150:7-13.
129. Meyer KC, McManus EJ, Maki DG. Overwhelming pulmonary blastomycosis associated with the adult respiratory distress syndrome. *N Engl J Med.* 1993;329:1231-1236.
130. Kinasewitz GT, Penn RL, George RB. The spectrum and significance of pleural disease in blastomycosis. *Chest.* 1984;86:580-584.
131. Zampogna JC, Hoy MJ, Ramos-Caro FA. Primary cutaneous North American blastomycosis in an immunosuppressed child. *Pediatr Dermatol.* 2003;20:128-130.
132. Head AJ, Meyers LK, Thompson JD, et al. Disseminated blastomycosis presenting as oligoarticular septic arthritis in a 12 year old girl. *Arthritis Rheum.* 2005;53:138-141.
133. Mercurio MG, Elewski BE. Cutaneous blastomycosis. *Cutis.* 1992;50:422-424.
134. Oppenheimer M, Embil JM, Black B, et al. Blastomycosis of bones and Joints. *South Med J.* 2007;100:570.
135. MacDonald PB, Black GB, MacKenzie R. Orthopaedic manifestations of blastomycosis. *J Bone Joint Surg Am.* 1990;72:860-864.
136. Guler N, Palanduz A, Ones U, et al. Progressive vertebral blastomycosis mimicking tuberculosis. *Pediatr Infect Dis J.* 1995;14:816-818.
137. Schutze GE, Hickerson SL, Fortin EM, et al. Blastomycosis in children. *Clin Infect Dis.* 1996;22:496-502.
138. Abril A, Campbell MD, Cotton VR Jr, et al. Polyarticular blastomycotic arthritis. *J Rheumatol.* 1998;25:1019-1021.
139. Robert ME, Kauffman CA. Blastomycosis presenting as polyarticular septic arthritis. *J Rheumatol.* 1988;15:1438-1442.
140. Bayer AS, Scott VJ, Guze LB. Fungal arthritis IV. Blastomycotic arthritis. *Semin Arthritis Rheum.* 1979;9:145-151.
141. George AL Jr, Hayes JT, Grahm BS. Blastomycosis presenting as monoarticular arthritis: The role of synovial fluid cytology. *Arthritis Rheum.* 1985;28:516.
142. Eikenberg HA, Amin M, Lich RJ. Blastomycosis of the genitourinary tract. *J Urol.* 1975;113:650-652.
143. Chowfin A, Tight R, Mitchell S. Recurrent blastomycosis of the central nervous system: Case report and review. *Clin Infect Dis.* 2000;30:969-971.
144. Bakleh M, Aksamit AJ, Tleyjeh IM, et al. Successful treatment of cerebral blastomycosis with voriconazole. *Clin Infect Dis.* 2005;40:e69-e71.
145. Panicker J, Walsh T, Kamani N. Recurrent central nervous system blastomycosis in an immunocompetent child treated successfully with sequential liposomal amphotericin B and voriconazole. *Pediatr Infect Dis J.* 2006;25:377-381.
146. Borgia SM, Fuller JD, Sarabia A, et al. Cerebral blastomycosis: A case series incorporating voriconazole in the treatment regimen. *Med Mycol.* 2006;44:659-664.
147. Pappas PG, Pottage JC, Powderly WG, et al. Blastomycosis in patients with acquired immunodeficiency syndrome. *Ann Intern Med.* 1992;116:847-853.
148. Gonyea EF. The spectrum of primary blastomycotic meningitis: A review of central nervous system blastomycosis. *Ann Neurol.* 1978;3:26-39.
149. Kravitz GR, Davies SF, Eckman MR, et al. Chronic blastomycotic meningitis. *Am J Med.* 1981;71:501-505.
150. Roos KL, Bryan JP, Maggio WW, et al. Intracranial blastomycoma. *Medicine (Baltimore).* 1987;66:224-235.
151. Ward BA, Parent AD, Raila F. Indications for the surgical management of central nervous system blastomycosis. *Surg Neurol.* 1995;43:379-388.
152. Varkey B. Blastomycosis in children. *Semin Respir Infect.* 1997;12:235.
153. Alkrinawi S, Reed MH, Pasterkamp H. Pulmonary blastomycosis in children: Findings on chest radiographs. *AJR Am J Roentgenol.* 1995;165:651-654.
154. Walsh CM, Morris SK, Brophy JC, et al. Disseminated blastomycosis in an infant. *Pediatr Infect Dis J.* 2006;25:656-659.
155. Garvey K, Hinshaw M, Vanness E. Chronic disseminated cutaneous blastomycosis in an 11 year old, with a brief review of the literature. *Pediatr Dermatol.* 2006;23:541-545.
156. Bernstein S, Brunner HI, Summerbell R, et al. Blastomycosis acquired by three children in Toronto. *Can J Infect Dis.* 2002;13:259-263.
157. Laskey WK, Sarosi GA. Blastomycosis in children. *Pediatrics.* 1980;65:111-114.
158. Steele RW, Abernathy RS. Systemic blastomycosis in children. *Pediatr Infect Dis.* 1983;2:304-307.
159. Lemos LB, Soofi M, Amir E. Blastomycosis and Pregnancy. *Ann Diagn Pathol.* 2002;6:211-215.
160. Pipitone MA, Gloster HM. A case of blastomycosis in pregnancy. *J Am Acad Dermatol.* 2005;53:740-741.
161. Tarr M, Marcinak J, Mogkolrattanothai K, et al. *Blastomyces* antigen detection for monitoring progress of blastomycosis in a pregnant adolescent. *Infect Dis Obstet Gynecol.* 2007;2007:89059.
162. Ismail MA, Lerner SA. Disseminated blastomycosis in a pregnant woman: Review of amphotericin B usage in pregnancy. *Am Rev Respir Dis.* 1982;126:350-353.
163. MacDonald D, Alguire PC. Adult respiratory distress syndrome due to blastomycosis during pregnancy. *Chest.* 1990;98:1527-1528.
164. Recht AD, Davies SF, Eckman MR. Blastomycosis in immunosuppressed patients. *Am Rev Respir Dis.* 1982;125:359-362.
165. Serody JS, Mill MR, Detterbeck FC, et al. Blastomycosis in transplant recipients: Report of a case and review. *Clin Infect Dis.* 1993;16:54-58.
166. Pappas PG, Threlkeld MG, Bedsole GD, et al. Blastomycosis in immunocompromised patients. *Medicine (Baltimore).* 1993;72:311-325.
167. Wheat J. Endemic mycoses in AIDS: A clinical review. *Clin Microbiol Rev.* 1995;8:146-159.
168. Gauthier GM, Safdar N, Klein BS, et al. Blastomycosis in solid organ transplant recipients. *Transpl Infect Diseases.* 2007;9:310-317.
169. Martynowicz MA, Prakash UBS. Pulmonary blastomycosis: An appraisal of diagnostic techniques. *Chest.* 2002;121:768-773.
170. Lemos LB, Guo M, Baliga M. Blastomycosis: Organ involvement and etiologic diagnosis. A review of 123 patients from Mississippi. *Ann Diagn Pathol.* 2000;4:391-406.
171. Lemos LB, Baliga M, Taylor BD, et al. Bronchoalveolar lavage for diagnosis of fungal disease: Five years experience in a southern United States rural area with many blastomycosis cases. *Acta Cytol.* 1995;39:1101-1111.
172. Graham AR. Fungal autofluorescence with ultraviolet illumination. *Am J Clin Pathol.* 1983;79:231-234.
173. Monheit JG, Cowman DF, Moore DG. Rapid detection of fungi in tissues using calcofluor white and fluorescence microscopy. *Arch Pathol Lab Med.* 1984;108:616-618.
174. Kaplan W, Kaufman L. Specific fluorescent antiglobulins for the detection and identification of *Blastomyces dermatitidis* yeast phase cells. *Mycopathologia.* 1963;19:173-180.
175. Stockman L, Clark MA, Hunt JM, et al. Evaluation of commercially available acridine ester-labeled chemiluminescent DNA probes for culture identification of *Blastomyces dermatitidis, Coccidioides immitis, Cryptococcus neoformans* and *Histoplasma capsulatum. J Clin Microbiol.* 1993;31:845-850.
176. Wheat LJ. Antigen detection, serology, and molecular diagnosis of invasive mycoses in the immunocompromised host. *Transpl Infect Dis.* 2006;8:128-139.
177. Abuodeh RO, Chester EM, Scalarone BM. Comparative serological evaluation of 10 *Blastomyces dermatitidis* yeast phase lysate antigens from different sources. *Mycoses.* 2004;47:143-149.
178. Sestero CM, Scalarone BM. Detection of IgG and IgM in sera from canines with blastomycosis using eight *Blastomyces dermatitidis* yeast phase antigens. *Mycopathologia.* 2006;162:33-37.
179. Bakleh M, Aksamit AJ, Tleyjeh IM, et al. Successful Treatment of Cerebral Blastomycosis with Voriconazole. *Clin Infect Dis.* 2005;40:e69-e71.
180. Stockman L, Clark KA, Humt JM, et al. Evaluation of commercially available acridinium ester-labeled chemiluminescent DNA probes for culture identification of *Blastomyces dermatitidis, Coccidioides immitis, Cryptococcus neoformans,* and *Histoplasma capsulatum. J Clin Microbiol.* 1993;31:845-850.
181. Sandhu GS, Kline BC, Stockman L, et al. Molecular probes for diagnosis of fungal infections. *J Clin Microbiol.* 1995;33:2913-2919.
182. Bialek R, Cirera AC, Herrmann T, et al. Nested PCR assay for detection of *Blastomyces dermatitidis* DNA in paraffin-embedded canine tissue. *J Clin Microbiol.* 2003;41:205-208.
183. Hayden RT, Qian X, Roberts GD, et al. In situ hybridization for the identification of yeastlike organisms in tissue section. *Diagn Mol Pathol.* 2001;10:15-23.
184. Abbott JJ, Hamacher KL, Ahmed I. In situ hybridization in cutaneous deep fungal infections: A valuable diagnostic adjunct to fungal morphology and tissue cultures. *J Cutan Pathol.* 2006;33:426.
185. Burgess JW, Schawan WR, Volk TJ. PCR-based detection of DNA from the human pathogen *Blastomyces dermatitidis* from natural soil samples. *Med Mycol.* 2006;44:741-748.
186. Durkin M, Witt J, LeMonte A, et al. Antigen assay with the potential to aid in diagnosis of blastomycosis. *J Clin Microbiol.* 2004;42:4873-4875.
187 Wheat J, Wheat H, Connolly P, et al. Cross-reactivity in *Histoplasma capsulatum* variety *capsulatum* antigen assays of urine samples from patients with endemic mycoses. *Clin Infect Dis.* 1997;24:1169-1171.
188. Mongkolrattanothai K, Peev M, Wheat LJ, et al. Urine antigen detection of blastomycosis in pediatric patients. *Pediatr Infect Dis J.* 2006;25:1076-1078.
189. Wheat LJ. Current diagnosis of histoplasmosis. *Trends Microbiol.* 2003;11:488-494.
190. Lagging LM, Breland CM, Kennedy DJ, et al. Delayed treatment of pulmonary blastomycosis causing vertebral osteomyelitis, paraspinal abscess and spinal cord compression. *Scand J Infect Dis.* 1994;26:111-115.
191. Sarosi GA. Management of fungal disease. *Am Rev Respir Dis.* 1983;127:250-253.
192. Chapman SW, Bradsher Jr RW, Campbell Jr GD, et al. Practice guidelines for the management of patients with blastomycosis. *Clin Infect Dis.* 2000;30:679-683.
193. National Institute of Allergy and Infectious Diseases Study Group. Treatment of blastomycosis and histoplasmosis with ketoconazole: Results of a prospective randomized trial. *Ann Intern Med.* 1985;103:861-872.
194. Sagg MS, Dismukes WE. Treatment of histoplasmosis and blastomycosis. *Chest.* 1988;93:848-851.
195. Johnson P, Sarosi G. Current therapy of major fungal diseases of the lung. *Infect Dis Clin North Am.* 1991;5:635-645.
196. Chapman SW, Dismuckes WE, Proia LA, et al. Clinical practice guidelines for the management of blastomycosis: 2008 Update by the Infectious Disease Society of America. *Clin Infect Dis.* 2008;46: 1801-1812.
197. Dismukes WE, Bradsher RW, Cloud GC, et al. Itraconazole therapy for blastomycosis and histoplasmosis. *Am J Med.* 1992;93:489-497.
198. Bradsher RW. Histoplasmosis and blastomycosis. *Clin Infect Dis.* 1996;22:5102-5111.
199. Tucker RM, Denning DW, Hanson LH, et al. Interactions of azoles with rifampin, phenytoin, and carbamazepine: In vitro and clinical observations. *Clin Infect Dis.* 1992;14:165.
200. Daneshmend TK, Warnock DW. Clinical pharmacokinetics of ketoconazole. *Clin Pharmacokinet.* 1988;14:13-34.
201. Cleary JD, Taylor JW, Chapman SW. Itraconazole in antifungal therapy. *Ann Pharmacother.* 1992;26:502-509.
202. Wise GJ, Goldberg PE, Kozinin PJ. Do the imidazoles have a role in the management of genitourinary fungal infections? *J Urol.* 1985;133:61-64.
203. Pappas PG, Bradsher RW, Chapman SW, et al. Treatment of blastomycosis with fluconazole: A pilot study. *Clin Infect Dis.* 1995;20:267-271.
204. Pappas PG, Bradsher RW, Kaufman CA, et al. Treatment of blastomycosis with higher dose fluconazole. *Clin Infect Dis.* 1997;25:200-205.
205. Freifeld A, Proia LA, Andes D, et al. Voriconazole use for endemic fungal infections (abstract 572). In: *Program and Abstracts of the 44th Annual Meeting of the Infectious Diseases Society of America (Toronto, Canada).* Alexandria, VA: Infectious Diseases Society of America; 2006:157.
206. Lutsar I, Roffey S, Troke P. Voriconazole concentrations in the cerebrospinal fluid and brain tissue of guinea pigs and immunocompromised patients. *Clin Infect Dis.* 2003;37:728-732.
207. Lentnek AL, Lentnek IA. Successful management of *Blastomyces dermatitidis* meningitis. *Infect Med.* 2006;23:39-41.

266

Coccidioides Species

JOHN N. GALGIANI

Although the systemic fungal infection, now known as coccidioidomycosis, has been recognized for more than a century,[1] it has more recently become more prevalent throughout the nonendemic and the endemic regions of the world.[2] A medical intern is credited with first identifying in 1892 a patient who had widespread disease.[3] Organisms seen microscopically were mistakenly thought to be parasites, and only several years later was the true mycotic etiology determined and the agent given the name *Coccidioides immitis*.[4] For three decades, coccidioidomycosis was thought to be a rare and nearly always fatal infection. In 1929, an accidental laboratory exposure of a medical student at Stanford University resulted in only a transient respiratory infection. His unexpected survival stimulated a reassessment of the natural history of coccidioidal infections, which soon led to the recognition that a common respiratory condition in the San Joaquin Valley of California (valley fever) was the more usual result of infection.[5] This conclusion was corroborated with the development by Smith and colleagues[6] of a specific skin test and serologic assays for coccidioidomycosis. With these tools, the clinical spectrum was well described by the mid-1950s (an excellent monograph published by Fiese[7] remains a valuable contemporary reference on the disease).

The reemergence of coccidioidomycosis can be attributed to changes in demography and in contemporary medicine. First, the populations at risk of exposure are greatly expanded. Regions in which *Coccidioides* spp. are endemic, which previously were sparsely populated, now encompass major metropolitan centers, such as Phoenix, Arizona. With this growth has come greatly increased tourism and commerce-related movement of people into and out of endemic areas. As a result, increased numbers of people are acquiring coccidioidal infections.[8] Second, a major segment of the population has emerged with compromised cellular immunity because of either underlying diseases or immunosuppressive therapies to control other diseases.[9-22] These patients are unusually susceptible to serious coccidioidal infections, and as a result, the severity of coccidioidal infections as a public health problem has increased. Third, advances in prevention and treatment of fungal infections offer new opportunities for management. These trends have made coccidioidomycosis more relevant to physicians everywhere.[23] Finally, the emergence of *Coccidioides* spp. as potential agents of bioterrorism was identified by the Centers for Disease Control and Prevention (CDC) in 1997. Since then, awareness of this possibility has become even greater with the increased incidence of terrorism as an international tactic and because of technical advances in genetic transformation, which adds to the potential to use *Coccidioides* spp. as a biologic weapon.[24-26]

Mycology

Coccidioides spp. are dimorphic fungi that exist as either a mycelium or a unique structure known as a spherule.[27] Both forms of growth are asexual, and it is not possible to classify *Coccidioides* spp. in relation to other fungi by classic taxonomy. By molecular analysis, however, *Coccidioides* spp. appear related most to other ascomycetes, most closely to the medically important organisms *Blastomyces dermatitidis* and *Histoplasma capsulatum*.[28] Although a sexual phase has not been found, population genetic studies suggest that one does exist.[29,30] Two genetically distinct populations have been identified among the etiologic agents of coccidioidomycosis. The occurrence of two populations was correlated with separate endemic regions where patients resided. This finding prompted classification of the previously known single

species, *C. immitis*, into two species: *C. immitis* and *Coccidioides posadasii*. Most of the *C. immitis* isolates have been obtained from California, whereas *C. posadasii* isolates have been obtained from patients in other states and from countries other than the United States.[31] DNA sequence analysis of *C. posadasii* strains enabled investigators to deduce the approximate geographic origin of infection.[32] The two species have shown few phenotypic differences; the clinical manifestations resulting from infection with either species appear the same, and in vitro susceptibility to antifungals is similar.[33,34] Molecular identification methods for differentiation of *C. immitis* from *C. posadasii* have been described[34] but are not yet routinely employed. Thus, references in the literature to *C. immitis* may actually be referring to either species. Isolates for which the species has not been determined are best designated as simply *Coccidioides* spp., which is the convention followed in this chapter.

MYCELIAL (SAPROBIC) GROWTH

On routine microbiologic nutrient agar media and presumably in the soil, *Coccidioides* spp. grow as mycelia by apical extension, and true septa form along its course. Maturation within 1 week of growth results in alternating mycelial cells' undergoing a process of autolysis and thinning of the cell walls. The remaining cells (arthroconidia), which become barrel-shaped and approximately 5 µm in length, develop a hydrophobic outer layer and become capable of remaining viable for long periods. Because the attachments of arthroconidia to adjacent cell remnants are fragile, they are prone to separation by physical disruption or mild air turbulence. As a result, arthroconidia become airborne in a form capable of deposition in the lungs if inhaled.

SPHERULE (PARASITIC) GROWTH

In the lungs, arthroconidia remodel into spherical cells, shedding their hydrophobic outer wall.[35,36] During this phase, nuclear division and cell multiplication occur and septa extend from the internal surface of the wall to transect the growing spherule into scores of subcompartments, each containing viable daughter cells or endospores. In tissue, spherules can become 75 µm in diameter (Fig. 266-1). Spherules grown in vitro demonstrate nuclear division throughout maturation, although their size is smaller and the number of endospores is fewer.[37] As a spherule matures, its outer wall thins and eventually ruptures. Early in the course of experimental infections, this rupture occurs in approximately 4 days, and with the release of endospores, the number of viable fungal units is amplified by approximately 100-fold, each of which may continue to propagate in tissue or to revert to mycelial growth if removed from the site of an infection.

Epidemiology

GEOGRAPHIC RANGE

Coccidioides spp. are endemic to the soils of only certain regions of the Western Hemisphere, nearly all of which are within the north and south 40-degree latitudes. Well-described transport of arthroconidia, either in soil on fomites[38,39] or as the result of unusually severe dust storms,[40] has produced infections in persons without endemic exposure, but this generally has not led to the establishment of new areas

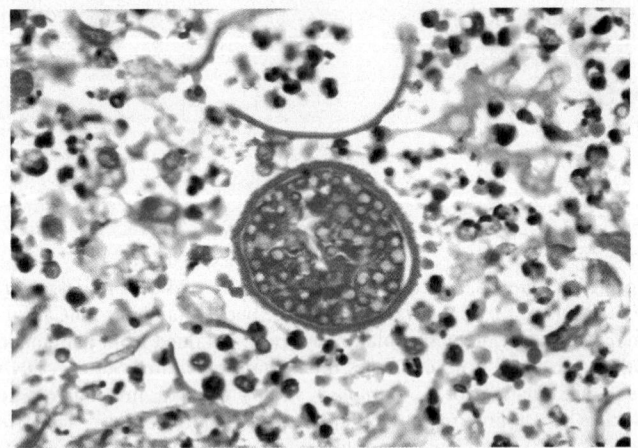

Figure 266-1 **Photomicrograph of a spherule in a tissue.** Hematoxylin and eosin staining. *(Courtesy of Richard Sobonya, MD, University of Arizona.)*

of endemicity. Regions of the United States in which *Coccidioides* spp. are endemic are shown in Figure 266-2. Noncontiguous foci of endemicity also exist such as that studied at Dinosaur National Monument, Utah.[41] These regions generally have the characteristics of the "lower Sonoran life zone," which include an arid climate, yearly rainfall of 5 to 20 inches, hot summers, winters with little freezing weather, and alkaline soil. Other areas where *Coccidioides* spp. have been identified include Mexico (adjacent to the U.S. border; western portions of Sonora, Nayarit, Jalisco, and Michoacan; central regions, including Coahulia, Durango, and San Luis Potosi), Central America (Guatemala, Honduras, Nicaragua), and South America (Argentina, Paraguay, Venezuela, Colombia, Brazil).[42] An archeologic investigation has provided evidence that *Coccidioides* spp. infected bison 8500 years ago in Nebraska, far beyond the current endemic regions.[43] This raises the possibility that climatic change could potentially affect the geographic distribution of *Coccidioides* spp.

Within the endemic regions, the likelihood of finding *Coccidioides* spp. in soil samples varies considerably among different locations[30,44] and different seasons. The fungus is recovered most easily toward the

end of winter rains.[45] This is opposite to the seasonal relationship for acquisition of new infections, which in California and Arizona occur most frequently during the summer months, after the soil has become dry. In Arizona, there is a second peak of new clinical infections from October until the winter rains, which corresponds to a similar dry period after the late summer rains in that region.[46] Colonies of *Coccidioides* spp. seem not to be distributed uniformly within the endemic region and may be quite sparse.[44]

RATES OF COCCIDIOIDAL INFECTION

Prevalence surveys in the 1950s of skin test reactivity to coccidioidal antigens in school-aged children of California's central valley suggested that the annual risk of infection was approximately 15%.[47] Smith and colleagues[48] showed that in 25% to 50% of military personnel in the San Joaquin Valley, skin test results converted to positive during a single year. More contemporary estimates from the same areas in California and from Tucson, Arizona, indicate that the risk has declined to approximately 3% per year.[47,49] Because of these lower rates and because of the large influx of new residents to the endemic regions from nonendemic locales (in 2005, estimated to total >7 million persons for southern Arizona and southern central California), the proportion of persons within the endemic region with prior infection is approximately 30%. The expected number of infections is on the order of 150,000 annually.

The numbers of infections reported to state departments of public health differ significantly from year to year. Some variation has been associated with total winter rainfall; more cases occur in the summers after wetter winters.[50] On occasion, epidemics also have been associated with disruption of infected soil, by human intent, such as with excavation[51]; after natural events, such as severe dust storms or earthquakes[52]; or during military maneuvers.[53] Some fluctuations in rates of infections are not explained, however. Such is the case for an exceptionally large epidemic in California's Central Valley in the period 1992 to 1995, in which the incidence of infection at times was more than 10 times that normally reported.[54] Since the second half of the 1990s, the incidence has also increased in Arizona (Fig. 266-3).[8,55]

Pathogenesis and Control

Nearly all infections are the result of inhaling arthroconidia. Cutaneous inoculations have been reported, producing lymphatic extension to regional lymph nodes and resolving without treatment. These occurrences are exceedingly rare, however.[56]

A single arthroconidium may be sufficient to produce a naturally acquired respiratory infection. This is the case for experimental infections in mice,[57] and air sampling within coccidioidal endemic regions

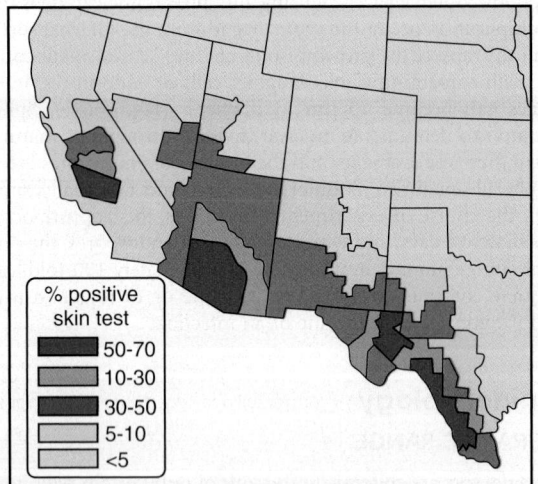

Figure 266-2 **Map of the U.S. regions endemic for coccidioidomycosis, as evidenced by a survey of skin test reactivity to coccidioidin.** *(From Edwards PQ, Palmer CD. Prevalence of sensitivity to coccidioidin, with special reference to specific and nonspecific reactions to coccidioidin and to histoplasmin. Dis Chest. 1957;31:35-60.)*

% positive skin test
- 50-70
- 10-30
- 30-50
- 5-10
- <5

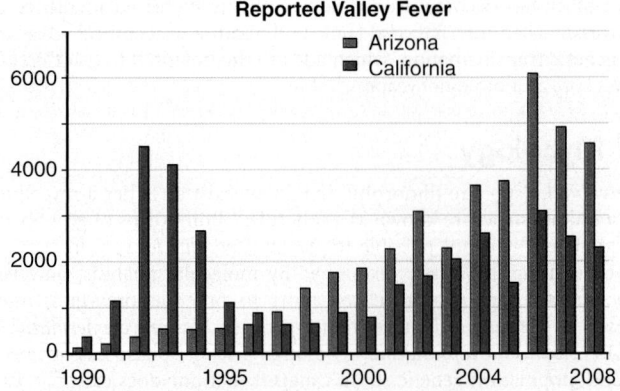

Figure 266-3 **Annually reported numbers of patients with coccidioidomycosis in Arizona and California.** *(Compiled from statistics reported by the Centers for Disease Control and Prevention and by state departments of health.)*

suggests that the ambient density of arthroconidia in the air is very low.[58,59] The size of the arthroconidium would allow its deposition within the terminal bronchiole but probably not as deeply as the alveolar space. As an arthroconidium transforms into a spherule, inflammation ensues, forming a local pulmonary lesion. Extracts of *Coccidioides* spp. have been shown to react with complement, releasing mediators of chemotaxis for neutrophils.[60] In some infections, *Coccidioides* spp. leave the lungs to establish disseminated lesions in other parts of the body. In this sequence of events, fungal elements must move from the distal bronchiole into the lung parenchyma, gain entry into the vascular space, and leave the vascular space to create extrapulmonary sites of infection. It is possible that endospores within macrophages travel through lymphatic vessels to the bloodstream, as has been described for dissemination of tuberculosis and histoplasmosis. This possibility also is compatible with the common finding of infected hilar, peritracheal, supraclavicular, and cervical lymph nodes in patients with extrapulmonary coccidioidal infections.[61]

HISTOPATHOLOGY

Microscopic examination of tissue infected with *Coccidioides* spp. shows elements of acute and chronic inflammation. Acute inflammation, including neutrophils and eosinophils, is associated with active infections and rupturing spherules.[61,62] Granulomatous lesions that include lymphocytes, histiocytes, and multinucleated giant cells are associated with chronic or arrested infections and with mature unruptured spherules.[63] In patients with widespread infections, it is common to find both inflammatory responses represented concurrently at different anatomic sites.

HOST DEFENSES

Control of coccidioidomycosis depends on T lymphocytes. This conclusion is supported by studies of experimentally produced infections in mice[64-68] and by the increased severity of naturally acquired infections in T cell–deficient patients.[10-12,15-19] Peripheral mononuclear blood cells from patients with disseminated coccidioidomycosis have virtually no interferon-γ response to coccidioidal antigens.[69] This is in contrast to the brisk stimulation of similar leukocyte preparations from patients in whom coccidioidal infections are competently controlled and who have delayed-type dermal hypersensitivity to coccidioidal skin-testing antigens.[70-72] These findings are consistent with an absent type 1 helper T cell (Th1)–type response described in some experimental animals[73,74] and human infectious diseases in which cellular immunity plays a role. In humans, however, despite the observed depression of interferon-γ levels, interleukin-4 and interleukin-10 levels were not reciprocally elevated,[70] which would be indicative of a type 2 helper T cell (Th2) response.

In addition to T cell–mediated control of infection, innate cellular responses may contribute to host defense. Inhibition of growth of *Coccidioides* spp. can be shown in vitro by human neutrophils and mononuclear cells from persons with or without prior coccidioidal infection as judged by skin test reactivity to coccidioidal antigens.[75] Although neutrophils do not seem to be fungicidal against *Coccidioides* spp., mononuclear cells or natural killer cells have been shown to reduce fungal viability.[76,77] These innate cellular inhibitory effects are most evident against arthroconidia or endospores and are lost as spherules increase in size and mature.[78] These in vitro observations can be extrapolated to indicate that innate defenses may serve primarily to slow fungal proliferation after infection, transforming what otherwise might be a more fulminant infection to a more subacute or chronic process.

Coccidioidal infections engender a variety of humoral responses to several different antigens in patients, and, as discussed subsequently, several are diagnostically useful. *Coccidioides*-infected B cell–deficient mice are not as protected by vaccination as are normal mice.[79] However, a specific defensive roll for immunoglobulins has thus far not been defined.

▣ Clinical Manifestations

At least half to two thirds of all infections caused by *Coccidioides* spp. are either inapparent or sufficiently mild not to prompt medical evaluation.[48] Of those that do become medically significant, a large majority result in a respiratory illness that is indistinguishable without specific testing from community-acquired pneumonia caused by other entities.[80] In an observational study in southern Arizona, coccidioidomycosis was estimated to be responsible for approximately one third of all cases of community-acquired pneumonia in that endemic area.[81] Nonetheless, misunderstandings of the manifestations of coccidioidomycosis or the perceived unimportance of diagnosis of early infections has led to gross disparities between the numbers of expected and reported coccidioidal infections.[82] For example, the number of coccidioidal infections reported to Arizona's Department of Health Services (see Fig. 266-3) represent only a small fraction of the expected 30,000 new illnesses. Underdiagnosis may be even more likely for patients with coccidioidomycosis evaluated outside the endemic region.[51,83] Most coccidioidal infections, whether detected or not, follow a self-limited course; only a few produce residual sequelae or chronic progressive infections. Although complications typically are manifested within weeks or up to 2 years after the original infection, the severity of the initial respiratory infection is frequently not correlated with the likelihood of complications. In this context, the identification of even mild primary infections takes on added significance and clinical relevance.

EARLY RESPIRATORY INFECTION

The first symptoms of the primary infection usually appear 7 to 21 days after exposure. Most infections seem to develop as a result of exposure to small numbers of arthroconidia; however, when exposure is unusually intense, symptoms are more likely to appear early. In an epidemic of coccidioidomycosis that occurred in the San Joaquin Valley of California between 1991 and 1994,[84] the findings in 536 patients with new infections included cough (73%), chest pain (44%), shortness of breath (32%), fever (76%), and fatigue (39%). These findings are typical of earlier reports. Although the infection often is subacute in development, patients occasionally report abrupt onset of symptoms, especially that of pleurisy. Weight loss also is a common sign, and headache has been noted in 21% of patients in the absence of meningeal infection.[46] Skin manifestations develop as part of the primary illness. Most frequent and easily missed is a nonpruritic fine papular rash that occurs early and transiently during the illness. More striking are erythema nodosum and erythema multiforme, which occur predominantly in women. Migratory arthralgias also are common complaints, and the triad of fever, erythema nodosum, and arthralgias (especially of the knees and ankles) has been termed *desert rheumatism*. Routine laboratory findings are usually normal except for an increase in the erythrocyte sedimentation rate. Peripheral blood eosinophilia may be present, occasionally accounting for two thirds of the circulating leukocytes. Chest radiograph results are abnormal in more than half of patients. Common findings include unilateral infiltrates, hilar adenopathy, and pleural effusions. Persistent hilar or peritracheal adenopathy is associated with extrathoracic spread of infection. Lung cavities are present initially in approximately 8% of infections recognized in adults but are less frequent in children.

Uncommonly, coccidioidal pneumonia manifests as a diffuse process leading to respiratory failure, either because of high-inoculum exposure[85,86] or because of fungi in the bloodstream that seed the lung in many sites (Fig. 266-4).[16] The manifestation is often fulminant, mimicking that of septic shock or a bacterial infection, and despite treatment, the rate of mortality is high. Approximately one third of human immunodeficiency virus (HIV)–infected patients exhibit this radiographic appearance. Although fungemia associated with diffuse pulmonary infiltrates may occur in immunologically intact patients,[87] it is nearly always attributable to a recognizable cellular immunodefi-

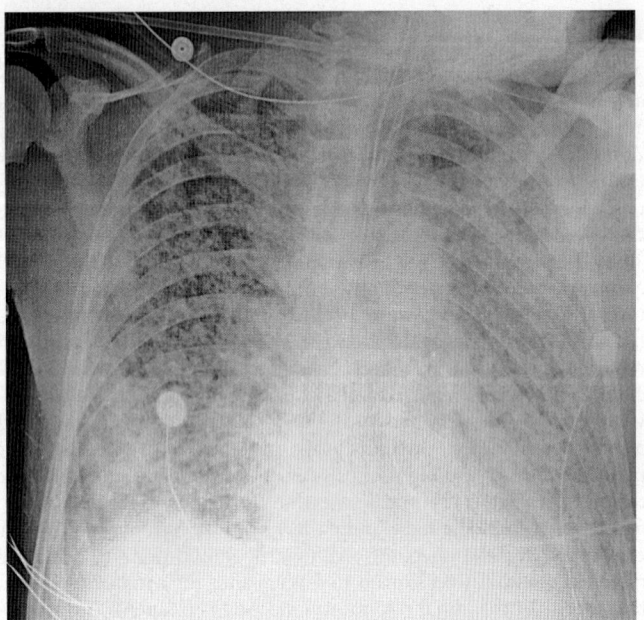

Figure 266-4 Diffuse reticulonodular infiltrates due to *Coccidioides immitis* in a patient with human immunodeficiency virus infection.

ciency state. In HIV-infected patients, the CD4$^+$ counts are typically less than 100 cells/mm^3, and the viral load is probably high.

Although some of the presenting symptoms are statistically more likely to occur with coccidioidal infections than with respiratory illness of other causes, the overlap of clinical syndromes is substantial.[80,81] For most patients, specific testing is necessary to secure a definite diagnosis of coccidioidomycosis.

Most coccidioidal respiratory infections resolve without complications, taking several weeks to many months to do so. When resolution of the self-limited illness is protracted, the symptom of fatigue, disproportionate to other evidence of infection, is frequently the last to resolve and may be a source of considerable distress. A few patients

with infections develop various pulmonary sequelae, and even fewer patients manifest disseminated infection outside the lungs. Despite their relative infrequency, these complications pose significant difficulties in diagnosis and management (discussed later).

PULMONARY NODULES AND CAVITIES

Approximately 4% of pulmonary infections result in a nodule, ranging up to 5 cm in diameter. A nodule typically causes no symptoms but may be indistinguishable from a neoplasm without histologic examination.[88] On occasion, nodules liquefy and drain into a bronchus to form a cavity (Fig. 266-5).

Pulmonary cavities may be present initially or in the later stages of the primary infection. They usually are peripheral and solitary, and with time, most develop a distinctive thin wall.[89] Cavities may not cause any symptoms, and half close within 2 years. Others are associated with local symptoms of pleuritic pain, cough, or hemoptysis (Figs. 266-6 and 266-7). Mycetoma may develop within cavities, either from mycelia of *Coccidioides* spp.[90] or with other species of fungi (Fig. 266-8). Another infrequent but well-recognized complication is rupture of a peripheral coccidioidal cavity into the pleural space and its manifestation as a pneumothorax. Ruptures commonly occur in athletic young men and are not associated with underlying immunodeficiency. Because the fungal walls of *Coccidioides* spp. are inflammatory, ruptured coccidioidal cavities often produce fluid in the pleural space, and the presence of an air-fluid level within the pleural space is a clue that the process is not a spontaneous pneumothorax or a ruptured pulmonary bleb (Fig. 266-9). If the cavity is diagnosed early, surgical resection of the cavity and closure of the pulmonary leak is the preferred treatment.[91]

CHRONIC FIBROCAVITARY PNEUMONIA

In contrast to thin-walled coccidioidal cavities, a chronic fibrotic pneumonic process that develops in some patients is characterized by pulmonary infiltrates and pulmonary cavitation.[92] This form of infection is not common among patients with T-cell deficiencies but seems to be associated with diabetes or preexisting pulmonary fibrosis related to smoking or other causes.[93] Involvement of more than one lobe is more common, and these lesions may cause systemic symptoms, such as night sweats and weight loss, and local symptoms.

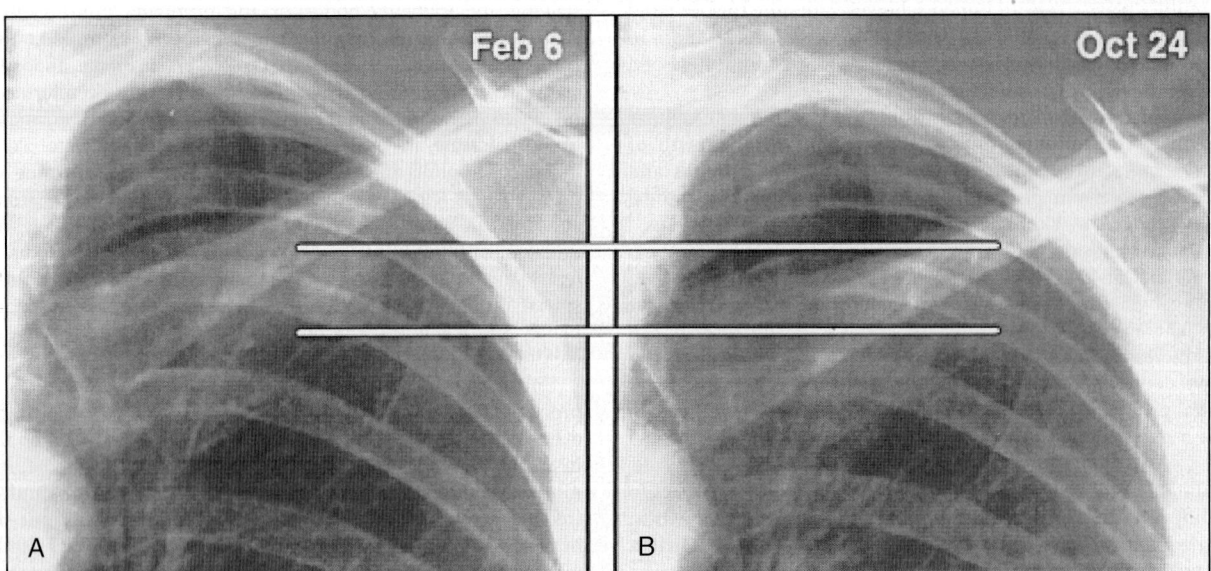

Figure 266-5 Cavitation of a coccidiodal nodule. **A,** A 1.8-cm nodule can be seen. **B,** Eight months later, this lesion has become a thin-walled cavity.

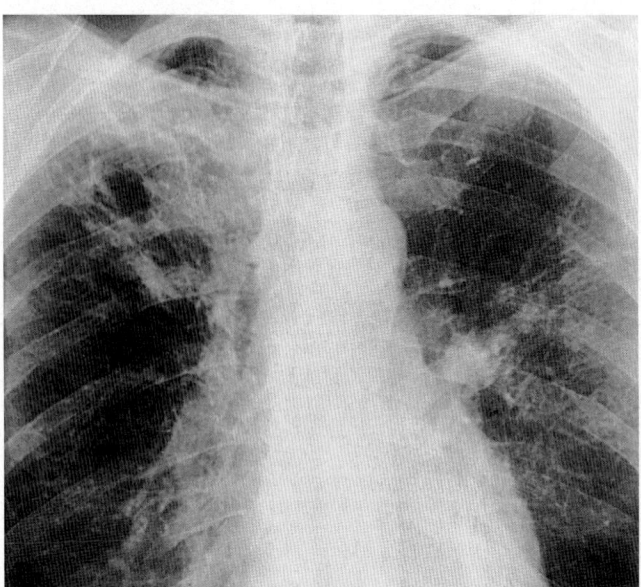

Figure 266-6 Pulmonary cavity in the right upper lobe with surrounding fibrosis.

EXTRAPULMONARY DISSEMINATION

C. immitis spreads beyond the lungs in approximately 0.5% of all infections in the general population. Several factors dramatically increase the risk of dissemination, however: immunodeficiency conditions, such as the later stages of HIV infection and Hodgkin's lymphoma, and therapies that suppress immune function, such as therapy to prevent solid organ rejection, high-dose corticosteroid therapy (equivalent to long-term prednisone doses >20 mg/day), and therapeutic inhibitors of tumor necrosis factor.[9-11,16-20,22,23] In two thirds of renal transplant recipients who developed coccidioidal infection, the infection progressed to dissemination.[11,12] With transplantation, the risk is heightened mostly by either newly acquired disease or reactivation of prior infection. Transmission by the engrafted organ has been

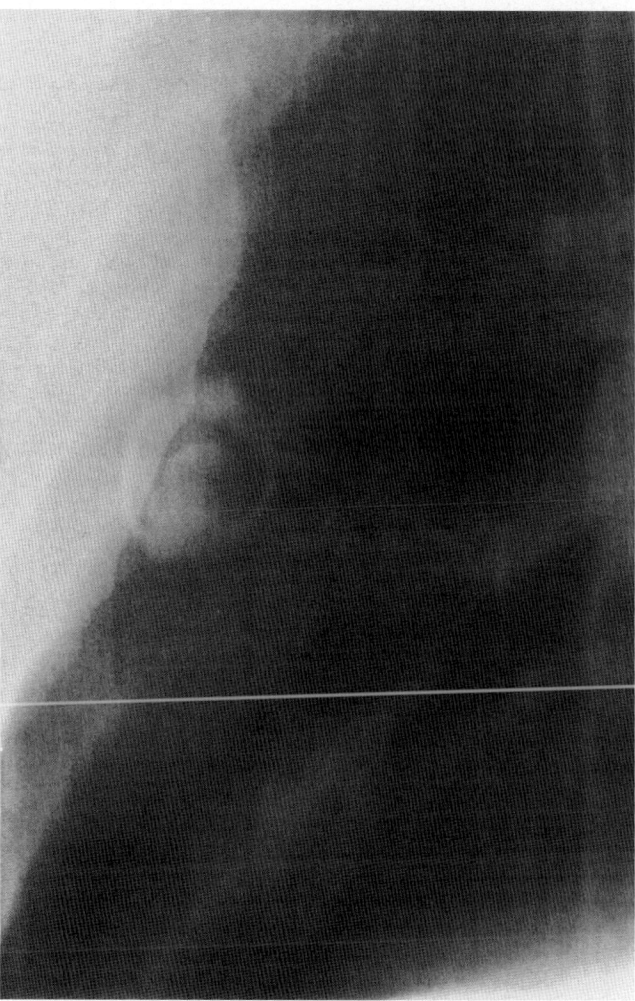

Figure 266-8 Mycetoma in the right lung of a coccidioidal cavity. Bronchoscopy specimens yielded *Coccidioides immitis* in culture. *(From Winn RE, Johnson R, Galgiani JN, et al. Cavitary coccidioidomycosis with fungus ball formation. Chest. 1994;105:412-416.)*

reported but is rare.[13,14] Dissemination is more likely to develop in men than in women.[44] Dissemination also is more likely, however, if infection is diagnosed first during pregnancy, especially during the third trimester or in the immediate postpartum period.[94,95] The risk of dissemination also appears to be increased among persons of African or Filipino ancestry, although the exact magnitude of the risk is controversial.[96]

Extrapulmonary dissemination is not associated often with pulmonary complications. Many patients with disseminated coccidioidal infection have entirely normal chest radiographs. The most common site of dissemination is the skin. The range of lesions includes superficial maculopapular lesions, keratotic and verrucose ulcers, and subcutaneous fluctuant abscesses. There is a predilection for lesions at the nasolabial fold (Fig. 266-10). Although most extrapulmonary dissemination is the result of hematogenous spread, supraclavicular and cervical lymphadenopathy also is a frequent manifestation and probably represents lymphatic drainage from the primary pulmonary infection.

Joints and bones also are common sites of dissemination. Joint infections differ from the self-limited joint complaints of desert rheumatism in that infections typically are asymmetrically distributed and are associated with a prominent synovitis and effusion. Although any joint can become infected, the knee is involved most frequently; other

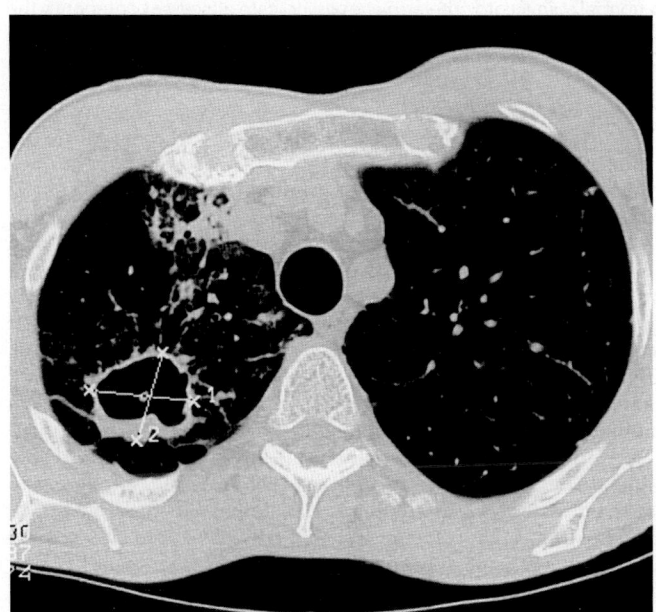

Figure 266-7 Computed tomographic scan of the cavity shown in Figure 266-4.

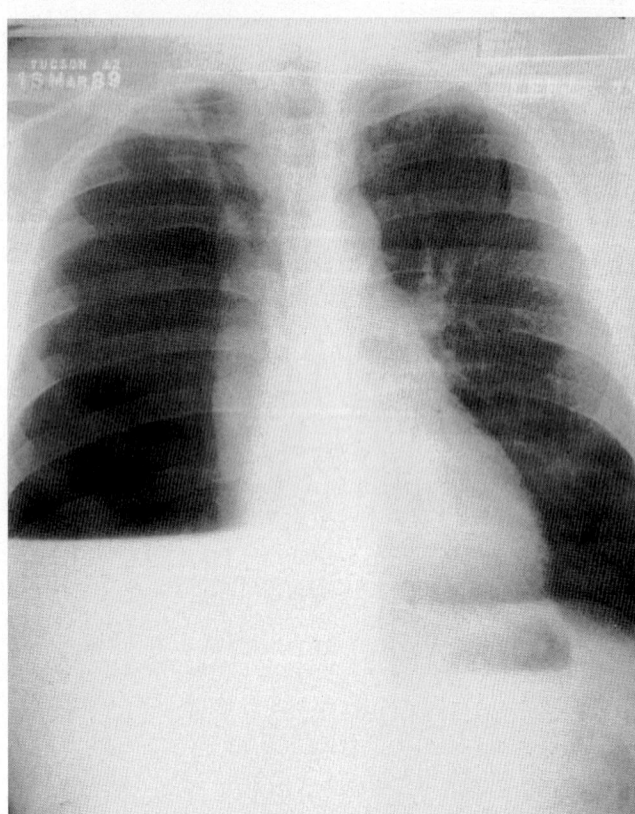

Figure 266-9 **Pyopneumothorax resulting from a ruptured coccidi-oidal cavity.** *(From Snyder LS, Galgiani JN. Coccidioidomycosis: the initial pulmonary infection and beyond. Semin Respir Crit Care Med. 1997;18:235-247.)*

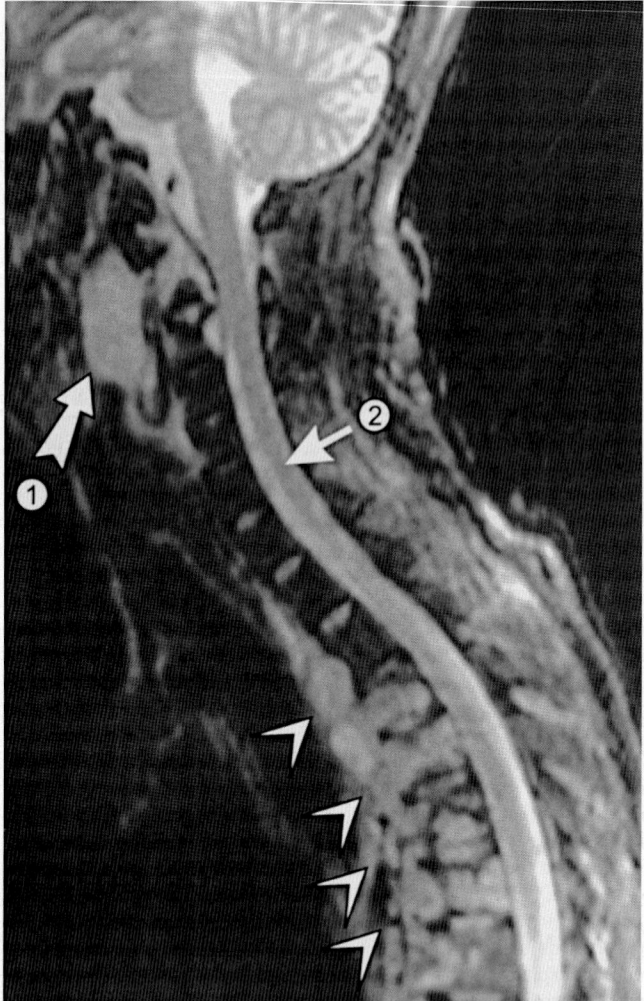

Figure 266-11 **Sagittal magnetic resonance imaging shows an anterior paraspinous abscess extending from the base of the skull to the midthoracic vertebrae.** *Arrow 1* points to an abscess that origi-nated in a cervical vertebra and dissected anteriorly. *Arrow 2* identifies a normal spinal cord. The *arrowheads* indicate abscesses anterior to the thoracic vertebrae. Multiple surgical procedures were necessary to control this infection.

common locations include the joints of the hands and wrists, the feet and ankles, and the pelvis.[97-99] Infection may be limited to the synovium or may erode to involve the underlying bone. Alternatively, bones may be involved first with secondary extension into the joint.[100] Although long bones may be affected, vertebral infection is much more common. Involvement of multiple vertebrae is typical. These may coalesce to produce anterior or posterior paraspinous soft tissue abscesses or an epidural abscess (Fig. 266-11). Magnetic

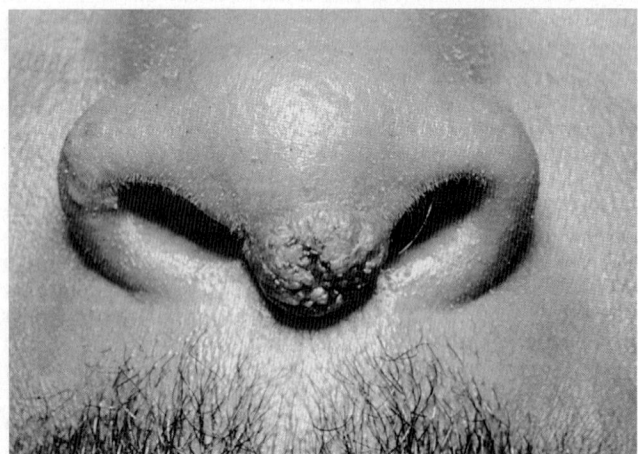

Figure 266-10 **Ulcerative lesion of disseminated coccidioidal infec-tion.** *(From Galgiani JN. Coccidioidomycosis. West J Med. 1993;159: 153-171.)*

resonance imaging (MRI) is often helpful in defining the exact loca-tion of these lesions.[101]

Coccidioidal meningitis is the most serious form of disseminated infection. Untreated, it is nearly always fatal within 2 years of diagno-sis.[102,103] Like most other complications of coccidioidomycosis, menin-gitis usually develops relatively soon after the initial infection. In one study, of 22 patients who developed meningitis after a large dust storm, CNS symptoms developed on average after 5.4 weeks of illness.[104] Similarly, a review of cases from the Department of Veterans Affairs and military records showed that of 25 patients who developed men-ingitis, 20 did so within 6 months of their first symptoms of infec-tion.[103] Common presenting symptoms are headache, vomiting, and altered mental status. In addition to CSF findings of an elevated white blood cell count, elevated protein levels, and a depressed glucose level, CSF eosinophils are occasionally prominent.[105] The main areas of involvement are the basilar meninges. Hydrocephalus is a common complication, especially in children.[106] Attention has been drawn to vasculitis and focal intracerebral coccidioidal abscesses as less frequent complications.[107-109]

Diagnosis

The manifestations of most early coccidioidal infections overlap substantially with those of other respiratory infections.[80] Specific laboratory testing usually is necessary to establish a diagnosis of coccidioidomycosis. In regions where *Coccidioides* spp. are endemic, this testing is commonplace. In most of the rest of the United States, the possibility of coccidioidomycosis is unlikely to be considered, unless a geographic exposure is identified. Obtaining a detailed travel history is a crucial first step in diagnosis. Because the incubation period usually is 1 to 3 weeks, endemic exposure within this period should raise the possibility of coccidioidomycosis to account for a respiratory condition of new onset. Exposure need not be extensive. Infections have occurred in patients whose only exposure occurred while changing airplanes at the Phoenix airport or during a single drive across California's Central Valley. Complications of the initial infection, such as chronic pneumonia or extrathoracic dissemination, may take longer to become apparent but nearly always emerge within 2 years after exposure. One exception to this rule is the detection of a pulmonary nodule or a solitary pulmonary cavity, which may persist without symptoms for many years after the original infection. Another special case is the setting of waning immunity, such as after the development of acquired immunodeficiency syndrome or with immunosuppressive therapy associated with solid organ transplantation. In such circumstances, exposure to *Coccidioides* spp. in the distant past may be sufficient to account for the current clinical illness.[110]

When the possibility of coccidioidomycosis has been raised, diagnosis may be established in two ways: (1) identifying spherules in, or recovering *C. immitis* from, a clinical specimen or (2) detecting specific anticoccidioidal antibodies in serum, cerebrospinal fluid, or other body fluid.

DIRECT EXAMINATION AND CULTURE

Isolating *Coccidioides* organisms from a patient is definitive evidence of a coccidioidal infection, and this diagnostic approach is used most frequently for patients with complicated pulmonary or disseminated syndromes. Sputum or other clinical specimens can be collected at no risk to personnel because the infection is not transmitted from the primary specimen. Direct microscopic examination of secretions can be performed immediately or after the addition of potassium hydroxide. Calcofluor staining of the cell wall in a wet mount also may help to distinguish spherules from leukocytes. *Coccidioides* spp. cannot be detected on Gram stains. Spherules also can be detected by cytology stains (e.g., in bronchoscopy specimens)[111]; by hematoxylin and eosin stains; and by other specialized procedures, such as silver or periodic acid–Schiff staining. Hematoxylin and eosin staining of spherules produces a distinctive autofluorescence that may help to identify a few organisms in tissues.[112] Using species-specific probes, researchers found that in situ hybridization was not as sensitive as silver staining but was more specific.[113] Although culture results are more sensitive, identification of spherules by direct examination is more rapid and may speed diagnosis. Direct detection of *Coccidioides* in sputum by polymerase chain reaction (PCR) has been reported but is not yet generally available.[114]

Coccidioides spp. grow well on most mycologic or bacteriologic media after 5 or 7 days of incubation. Aerobic conditions are required. When growth occurs, it is typically as a white (nonpigmented) mold. There are many exceptions to this general appearance, however, and the morphologic appearance is not reliable in determining whether the fungus is *Coccidioides* spp.[115] When growth is evident on culture medium, care should be taken not to open the culture container except in an appropriate biocontainment cabinet. Cultures at this stage are highly infectious, and infections have occurred in laboratory personnel when cultures have not been handled properly.[116]

The mycelial form of growth is not specific for *Coccidioides* spp., and further testing is required for species identification. The two most common ways for microbiologists to test this are to detect a specific coccidioidal antigen (exoantigen) in an extract of the fungus and to detect a specific ribosomal RNA sequence using a commercially available DNA probe (Gen-Probe, San Diego, CA).[117-119] At present, molecular methods (28B) to differentiate between *C. immitis* and *C. posadasii* are not commercially available. When the fungal isolate is identified as *Coccidioides* spp., it is subject to strict federal security regulations developed for all select agents of bioterrorism as listed by the CDC. Laboratories that are not registered with the CDC are liable for severe criminal penalties if isolates are not transferred to a registered laboratory or destroyed within 7 days after identification. In place of maintaining these capabilities, many clinical laboratories refer the culture to a reference laboratory where identification is completed.

SEROLOGIC TESTING

Serologic testing is the most frequent means of diagnosing primary coccidioidal infections because the patients may not be able to produce a sputum specimen, and fungal cultures often are not practical in an ambulatory setting. It also may be indispensable in establishing the cause of chronic meningitis because cultures of cerebrospinal fluid are commonly negative in coccidioidal meningitis. Of the variety of tests available, most are highly specific for an active infection.[120] Minimally reactive test results often are diagnostically important and should not be dismissed as insignificant. A negative serologic test result never excludes the presence of a coccidioidal infection, however. Performing one or more repeated serologic tests over the course of 2 months increases the sensitivity of serologic diagnosis, especially for recently acquired infections.

TUBE PRECIPITIN ANTIBODIES

Tube precipitin antibodies of this type originally were detected by the presence of a precipitin button that formed at the bottom of a test tube after overnight incubation of the patient's serum mixed with coccidioidal antigen.[121] Because immunoglobulin M (IgM) is most avid at forming immune precipitins, and because these reactions were detected early after the onset of infection, this test sometimes is referred to as the *IgM test*. The antigen responsible for this reaction is a polysaccharide from the fungal cell wall. At some time within the first 3 weeks of symptoms, tube precipitin antibodies are detected in 90% of patients; this prevalence declines to less than 5% more than 7 months after the onset of a self-limited illness.

COMPLEMENT-FIXING ANTIBODIES

When the patient's serum is mixed with coccidioidal antigen, an immune complex forms that consumes complement.[6] This event is detected by the subsequent addition of antibody-coated red blood cells, which normally lyse in the presence of complement but remain intact if the complement is depleted. Because immunoglobulin G (IgG) is the immunoglobulin class usually involved in these immune complexes, this test sometimes is referred to as the *IgG test*. Although this test originally was developed through the use of various complex extracts of *C. immitis*, it now is known that the antigen involved in this reaction is a chitinase.[122-125] In early coccidioidal infections, complement-fixing antibodies are detected later and for longer periods than are tube precipitin antibodies. Complement-fixing antibodies can be detected in other body fluids, and their detection in cerebrospinal fluid is an especially important aid to the diagnosis of coccidioidal meningitis. Complement-fixing antibody concentration is expressed as a titer, such as 1:4 or 1:64, indicating the greatest dilution of serum at which complement consumption still is detected. Traditionally, a titer of 1:16 or greater has been associated frequently with extrathoracic dissemination. Because of technical factors, however, end point results for the same serum samples may vary considerably on testing by different laboratories. More useful are serial determinations of complement-fixing antibody concentrations performed by the same laboratory. In general, higher titers reflect more extensive coccidioidal infection, increasing complement-fixing antibody concentrations are associated with worsening disease, and decreasing titers are useful in monitoring response to therapy.

IMMUNODIFFUSION TESTS

Antibodies that were detected by the original tube precipitin or complement-fixing tests can be detected by alternative procedures known as the *immunodiffusion tube precipitin* and *immunodiffusion complement-fixing* tests. Although these tests are conducted similarly, different antigens are used to measure different types of antibodies. As with the original tests, the immunodiffusion tube precipitin test result is reported by some laboratories as the IgM test result, and the immunodiffusion complement-fixing result is reported as the IgG test result. Both tests have been found to be at least as sensitive as their original counterparts.[126,127] Immunodiffusion tests are more amenable to being manufactured and distributed in commercially prepared kits, which allow them to be performed in laboratories not fully dedicated to a mycology specialty.

ENZYME-LINKED IMMUNOASSAYS

An enzyme immunoassay for coccidioidal antibodies is available commercially (Meridian Diagnostics, Cincinnati, OH). The test kit allows the specific detection of IgM or IgG antibodies. These results are not interchangeable, however, with the complement fixation or immunodiffusion test results. Positive results with this commercial kit are highly sensitive for coccidioidal infection. On occasion, false-positive results are noted, especially with the IgM enzyme immunoassay. At present, enzyme immunoassay results should ordinarily be confirmed with immunodiffusion tube precipitin, immunodiffusion complement-fixing, or complement-fixing test results. When the more established tests fail to corroborate the enzyme immunoassay, the diagnosis is less firmly established.[128-130]

LATEX TESTS

Latex tests for coccidioidal antibodies also are available commercially. They are attractive to clinical laboratories because they are easy to use, and results are obtained rapidly. There are significant numbers of false-positive reactions, however, and the latex test is not as reliable as the other tests described in this section.[120]

SKIN TESTING

Dermal delayed-type hypersensitivity to coccidioidal antigens is highly specific for coccidioidal infection.[131] Because skin test results remain positive after infection in most people for life, however, a result may not be related to the current illness. In addition, some of the most serious infections may be associated with selective anergy, and the skin test may not reveal reactivity. As useful as skin test results are for epidemiologic studies, the tests have important limitations as screening procedures for recent infection. For patients in whom coccidioidomycosis has been diagnosed by other means, skin testing may have prognostic significance.[132] At present, coccidioidal skin testing reagents are not available commercially.

OTHER APPROACHES TO DIAGNOSIS

Antigenemia may occur either with early or chronic coccidioidal infections and could be the basis of a diagnostic test.[133-136] A commercial test is available for detecting coccidioidal antigens.[137] In addition, the commercially available antigen test for histoplasmosis can be positive in severe cases of coccidioidomycosis. PCR has been used to detect *C. immitis*–specific nucleic acid sequences in patient specimens[114,138] but is currently not available commercially.

Management

GENERAL APPROACHES

The three components of managing coccidioidal infections are (1) assessment of the need for intervention, (2) selection of antifungal agents for patients who would benefit from treatment, and (3) choice of surgical procedures for débridement and reconstruction of destructive lesions. A revised practice guideline has been published[23] and is available online from the Infectious Diseases Society of America (http://www.IDSociety.org).

In patients with newly diagnosed coccidioidal infections, it is crucial to assess the extent of disease at present and the factors that increase the risk of future complications. The current extent of disease usually can be assessed with a careful review of systems, physical examination, and chest radiographs. When new focal complaints of discomfort or swelling are identified, these should be evaluated further with appropriate imaging or, if necessary, biopsy. Pain referable to bones might be assessed with a radionuclide bone scan[139,140] or an MRI. An effusion that develops in a joint could be aspirated for cell count and culture; a progressively severe headache may necessitate MRI and lumbar puncture to evaluate the possibility of meningitis; and a nonhealing skin lesion may necessitate biopsy.

In the general population, pulmonary or extrapulmonary complications are uncommon. There is a special risk of disseminated infection, however, with conditions that prominently suppress T-cell immunity. The best recognized of these are HIV infection, immunosuppression to prevent rejection of a transplanted solid organ, and treatment with high doses of corticosteroids. A growing population at risk consists of patients with rheumatologic conditions or ulcerative colitis treated with anti–tumor necrosis factor.[141] Pregnancy, especially during the third trimester or the immediate peripartum period, also seems to predispose patients to a high risk of widespread dissemination.[142] Patients with any of these risk factors nearly always should be treated with antifungal therapy even if there is no evidence of extrapulmonary spread. Patients with diabetes mellitus are not prone to extrapulmonary dissemination. They are more likely to develop pulmonary cavitation or chronic pneumonia, however, and may be more likely to require treatment.[93]

Available antifungal agents include amphotericin B and the azole antifungal agents. Their pharmacology is described in detail in Chapter 40. In coccidioidomycosis, selecting between amphotericin B and azole antifungals is based primarily on the degree of respiratory compromise in pulmonary infections or rate of progression of disseminated infections. Amphotericin B is perceived to have a more rapid onset of action; therefore, despite its well-known toxic effects, it is the preferred initial therapy for patients who have developed serious respiratory compromise or who are deteriorating rapidly. There is no evidence that a lipid formulation of amphotericin B improves on the efficacy of amphotericin B suspended with deoxycholate. Azole antifungals often are selected for patients with chronic processes because possible differences in rate of response to azole antifungals would be outweighed by their ease of administration and lack of toxicity. Ketoconazole is the only orally available azole antifungal approved by the U.S. Food and Drug Administration for the treatment of coccidioidomycosis but is no longer the preferred drug for this disease. Several clinical trials have indicated that fluconazole and itraconazole are efficacious.[143-150] No studies have demonstrated general superiority of one azole antifungal over another. In a comparison of fluconazole (400 mg once a day) and itraconazole (200 mg twice daily), the primary analysis showed that the two drugs were within 20% of each other in producing responses.[151] In a secondary analysis of skeletal lesions, response was obtained in twice as many subjects treated with itraconazole as those treated with fluconazole. The newer azoles, voriconazole and posaconazole, have also been used to treat coccidioidomycosis. In one study, 17 of 20 patients treated with 400 mg per day of posaconazole improved.[152] However, of 9 patients in whom treatment was discontinued, 3 suffered relapse. In another study of 15 patients in whom previous treatments had failed, 11 treated with 800 mg per day of posaconazole improved.[153] For voriconazole, there is less published literature, but case reports suggest that it may also be effective.[154,155]

Because the manifestations, locations, and severity of progressive forms of coccidioidomycosis vary among patients, the need for surgery is determined by the nature of specific lesions on a case-by-case basis. In some patients, especially in whom skeletal involvement is extensive, débridement and drainage of infected sites may be essential to achieving control of the infection. Even if therapy is effective in arresting fungal proliferation, fungal debris already present may continue to produce tissue destruction until it is surgically removed. Patients with persistent fever and malaise may benefit from drainage of large collections of pus. Also, surgery may be needed to stabilize bones that are structurally unsound or when the spinal cord is at risk of compression. Advances in imaging with computed tomography or MRI have aided greatly in the evaluation of specific lesions.[99,101,156,157] Repeated use of these modalities often helps to identify lesions that are progressing despite the current management strategy and patients who may benefit from additional surgical intervention or other changes in management.

EARLY UNCOMPLICATED INFECTIONS

For patients with neither risk factors nor evidence of extrapulmonary spread, treatment is of unproven benefit. To date, no placebo-controlled trials concerning this self-limited form of infection have determined whether treatment hastens the resolution of symptoms or prevents the risk of complications. Experts familiar with coccidioidomycosis have widely varying recommendations for management of specific patients in this category. Although some physicians recommend treatment for all patients, others recommend treating only patients with more severe manifestations. Even with selective therapy, its benefit is uncertain.[157a] Evidence that often is considered to indicate more severe infection includes loss of more than 10% of body weight, intense night sweats for more than 3 weeks, infiltrates involving more than half of one lung or portions of both lungs, prominent or persistent hilar or peritracheal adenopathy, anticoccidioidal complement–fixing antibody titer greater than 1 : 16, failure to develop dermal hypersensitivity to coccidioidal antigens, inability to work, or symptoms that persist for more than 2 months.[140] Because persons of African or Filipino descent seem to have some increased risk of dissemination, this factor sometimes also weighs in the decision for treatment. If treatment is recommended, commonly prescribed therapies include currently available oral azole antifungal agents, such as ketoconazole, fluconazole, or itraconazole, for courses ranging from 3 to 6 months.

DIFFUSE PNEUMONIA

Diffuse bilateral infiltrates represent either hematogenous infection of the lungs or multiple foci of infection resulting from exposure to a high inoculum of arthroconidia. In either case, even early infections are regarded as serious and warranting therapy. Initial therapy in such cases is usually with amphotericin B, at least for the first several weeks and until the illness seems to be improving. Concomitant use of a brief course of corticosteroids in this situation is controversial but advocated by some authorities.[149] After this time, therapy often is switched to an antifungal azole agent for at least 1 year. Fungemia resulting in diffuse pulmonary infiltrates is often the consequence of severe immunodeficiency, and in affected patients, treatment may need to be continued indefinitely to prevent relapse.

PULMONARY CAVITY

Cavitation as a sequela of coccidioidal pneumonia is often asymptomatic and may not necessitate treatment. With the passage of time, some cavities disappear. Cavities that do not close spontaneously over 1 to several years are sometimes resected to prevent future complications, especially if the cavity shows progressive enlargement or is immediately adjacent to the pleura. This potential benefit must be weighed against the risks of the surgical procedure, which vary according to the general health of the patient and the skill of the surgeon.

Pulmonary cavities occasionally produce symptoms, such as local pain, superinfection, or hemoptysis. When this occurs, treatment usually is instituted with oral antifungal azole therapy. This therapy often is accompanied by a diminution of symptoms, but recurrences are frequent if therapy is stopped. For these patients, resection is a reasonable alternative to long-term suppressive medical therapy. Extrapulmonary dissemination from a solitary pulmonary cavity is very uncommon.

CHRONIC FIBROCAVITARY PNEUMONIA

Persistent coccidioidal pneumonia is ordinarily treated with oral azole antifungal agents. Responses to these agents are approximately 55% to 60% as judged by improved symptoms and radiographic appearance. Treatment options for patients who do not respond include surgical resection of infection localized to a single lobe; switching to an alternative antifungal azole; for fluconazole, raising the dosage; or instituting amphotericin B therapy.

EXTRAPULMONARY DISSEMINATION

For most patients with nonmeningeal dissemination, initial therapy is with an oral antifungal azole. Exceptional patients with rapidly progressive infection or infection in critical locations, such as vertebrae, may respond faster to initial therapy with amphotericin B, but this has not been proved. As discussed previously, surgical débridement or drainage of selected lesions may be an important component of controlling infection. As in chronic coccidioidal pneumonia, treatment is continued for at least 1 year and for 6 months past the point at which all evidence of further improvement has ceased. Even so, relapses occur in approximately one third of patients when therapy is stopped, and some patients may require suppressive therapy indefinitely.

In the management of coccidioidal meningitis, most patients now are treated initially with fluconazole. This is a major departure from therapy with intrathecal amphotericin B, which until the early 1990s was still standard treatment.[158] Although there have been no comparative trials of intrathecal amphotericin B and fluconazole, the response rate of approximately 70% with fluconazole at 400 mg/day is probably at least as good as that achieved with intrathecal amphotericin B, and use of fluconazole avoids most of the toxicity associated with amphotericin B. Higher doses of fluconazole have produced responses in some patients who did not respond initially to 400 mg/day. Similar results have been obtained in patients treated with itraconazole, although there is less clinical experience with this drug than with fluconazole.

Patients who do not respond to oral azole therapy may benefit from intrathecal amphotericin B.[159] Routes of administration include repeated percutaneous intracisternal injection, injection into Ommaya reservoirs that drain to either the cistern or a ventricle, lumbar puncture with medication in a hyperbaric glucose solution, and lateral cervical injection. The technique, frequency, and dosage of intrathecal amphotericin B vary widely among practitioners.

In addition to antifungal therapy to control the meningeal inflammation, interventions are required for two other manifestations. Hydrocephalus is a common complication of coccidioidal meningitis. Hydrocephalus ordinarily does not respond to antifungal therapy, and a shunting procedure is required. Ventriculoperitoneal shunts become a conduit for *Coccidioides* spp. from the cerebrospinal space to the peritoneum, but this usually does not result in clinically apparent abdominal complications. Although infection affects predominantly the basilar meninges, intracerebral abscesses occasionally develop.[108] These lesions may necessitate drainage or resection, in addition to systemic antifungal drug therapy. Ventricular cerebrospinal fluid is unreliable for assessing therapy because WBC, protein, and glucose measurements are less abnormal during infection than is found in lumbar cerebrospinal fluid.[160]

NEW THERAPIES

Because the fungal wall of *Coccidioides* organisms contains β-1,3-glucan and chitin,[35] antifungals that interfere with synthesis of these polysaccharides potentially could be therapeutic for coccidioidomycosis. Caspofungin (Cancidas) has been effective in treatment of experimental coccidioidal infections.[161,162] However, clinical experience is limited.[163]

Nikkomycin Z, a chitin synthase inhibitor discovered in the 1970s, was subsequently shown to be very effective as a therapy against experimental murine coccidioidal infection.[164,165] Clinical trials were initiated in the 1990s but were soon interrupted because the sponsoring pharmaceutical company went out of business.[166] In 2005, the inactive project was transferred to the University of Arizona, which has reactivated the clinical studies and is currently conducting multidose safety trials.[166a]

Prevention

Developing a vaccine as a means of preventing coccidioidomycosis has been an attractive goal for many years. This strategy might be useful because immunity develops in most persons who are infected naturally.[167] A formalin-killed, whole-cell spherule vaccine was found to be exceptionally protective against lethal intranasal infections in mice.[56,168-176] The whole-cell vaccine also induced a great deal of local inflammation at the injection site, however, and thus the dose in humans is limited to 1.84 mg.[177] For an average human, this is approximately ⅟₁₀₀₀ of the vaccine dose (milligrams per kilogram) required for protection in mice. When this dose of formalin-killed spherule vaccine was used in a human field trial, vaccination failed to result in significantly fewer symptomatic cases of coccidioidal pneumonia than were detected in placebo recipients.[178] One plausible explanation for the failure is that the inflammatory reactions to the whole-cell vaccine prevented use of a sufficient dose of the antigens responsible for protection. If this is the case, use of a purified or recombinant antigen might circumvent this limitation.

Several antigens have been expressed as recombinant proteins and, when used with Th1-based adjuvants, have evoked protection against experimental coccidioidal infections in mice.[179] Current efforts are focusing on developing a formulation suitable for moving this discovery phase into clinical testing.

REFERENCES

1. Hirschmann JV. The early history of coccidioidomycosis: 1892-1945. *Clin Infect Dis.* 2007;44:1202-1207.
2. Galgiani JN. Coccidioidomycosis: a regional disease of national importance: rethinking approaches for control. *Ann Intern Med.* 1999;130:293-300.
3. Posada A. Un nuevo case de micosis fungoidea con psorospermias. *Annales del Circulo Medico Argentino.* 1892;15:585-597.
4. Ophuls W, Moffitt HC. A new pathogenic mould (formerly described as a protozoon: *Coccidioides immitis*): Preliminary report. *Phila Med J.* 1900;5:1471-1472.
5. Gifford MA. San Joaquin fever. *Kern County Dept Public Health Annu Rep.* 1936:22-23.
6. Smith CE, Saito MT, Simons SA. Pattern of 39,500 serologic tests in coccidioidomycosis. *JAMA.* 1956;160:546-552.
7. Fiese MJ. *Coccidioidomycosis.* Springfield, IL: Charles C Thomas; 1958.
8. Sunenshine RH, Anderson S, Erhart L, et al. Public Health Surveillance for coccidioidomycosis in Arizona. *Ann N Y Acad Sci.* 2007;1111:96-102.
9. Riley DK, Galgiani JN, O'Donnell MR, et al. Coccidioidomycosis in bone marrow transplant recipients. *Transplantation.* 1994;56:1531-1533.
10. Hall KA, Copeland JG, Zukoski CF, et al. Markers of coccidioidomycosis before cardiac or renal transplantation and the risk of recurrent infection. *Transplantation.* 1993;55:1422-1424.
11. Blair JE, Logan JL. Coccidioidomycosis in solid organ transplantation. *Clin Infect Dis.* 2001;33:1536-1544.
12. Logan JL, Blair JE, Galgiani JN. Coccidioidomycosis complicating solid organ transplantation. *Semin Respir Infect.* 2001;16:251-256.
13. Wright P, Pappagianis D, Taylor J, et al. Transmission of *Coccidioides immitis* from donor organs: a description of two fatal cases of disseminated coccidioidomycosis. *Clin Infect Dis.* 2001;33:1194.
14. Tripathy U, Yung GL, Kriett JM, et al. Donor transfer of pulmonary coccidioidomycosis in lung transplantation. *Ann Thorac Surg.* 2002;73:306-308.
15. Ampel NM, Dols CL, Galgiani JN. Coccidioidomycosis during human immunodeficiency virus infection: results of a prospective study in coccidioidal endemic area. *Am J Med.* 1993;94:235-240.
16. Rempe S, Sachdev MS, Bhakta R, et al. Coccidioides immitis fungemia: clinical features and survival in 33 adult patients. *Heart Lung.* 2007;36:64-71.
17. Deresinski SC, Stevens DA. Coccidioidomycosis in compromised hosts: experience at Stanford University Hospital. *Medicine (Baltimore).* 1974;54:377-395.
18. Rutala PJ, Smith JW. Coccidioidomycosis in potentially compromised hosts: the effect of immunosuppressive therapy in dissemination. *Am J Med Sci.* 1978;275:283-295.
19. Woods CW, McRill C, Plikaytis BD, et al. Coccidioidomycosis in human immunodeficiency virus–infected persons in Arizona, 1994-1997: incidence, risk factors, and prevention. *J Infect Dis.* 2000;181:1428-1434.
20. Ampel NM. Coccidioidomycosis among persons with human immunodeficiency virus infection in the era of highly active antiretroviral therapy (HAART). *Semin Respir Infect.* 2001;16:257-262.
21. Logan JL, Blair JE, Galgiani JN. Coccidioidomycosis complicating solid organ transplantation. *Semin Respir Infect.* 2001;16:251-256.
22. Ramzan NN, Shapiro MS, Robinson E, et al. Use of infliximab leading to extensive pulmonary coccidioidomycosis. *Am J Gastroenterol.* 2002;97:S157.
23. Galgiani JN, Ampel NM, Blair JE, et al. Coccidioidomycosis. *Clin Infect Dis.* 2005;41:1217-1223.
24. Dixon DM. *Coccidioides immitis* as a select agent of bioterrorism. *J Appl Microbiol.* 2001;91:602-605.
25. Warnock DW. *Coccidioides* species as potential agents of bioterrorism. *Future Microbiol.* 2007;2:277-283.
26. Abuodeh RO, Orbach MJ, Mandel MA, et al. Genetic transformation of *Coccidioides immitis* facilitated by *Agrobacterium tumefaciens. J Infect Dis.* 2000;181:2106-2110.
27. Sun SH, Sekhon SS, Huppert M. Electron microscopic studies of saprobic and parasitic forms of *Coccidioides immitis. Sabouraudia.* 1979;17:265-273.
28. Bowman BH, Taylor JW, Brownlee AG, et al. Molecular evolution of the fungi: relationship of the Basidiomycetes, Ascomycetes, and Chytridiomycetes. *Mol Biol Evol.* 1992;9:285-296.
29. Burt A, Carter DA, Koenig GL, et al. Molecular markers reveal cryptic sex in the human pathogen *Coccidioides immitis. Proc Natl Acad Sci U S A.* 1996;93:770-773.
30. Mandel MA, Barker BM, Kroken S, et al. Genomic and population analyses of the mating type loci in *Coccidioides* species reveal evidence for sexual reproduction and gene acquisition. *Eukaryot Cell.* 2007;6:1189-1199.
31. Fisher MC, Koenig GL, White TJ, et al. Molecular and phenotypic description of *Coccidioides posadasii* sp nov., previously recognized as the non-California population of *Coccidioides immitis. Mycologia.* 2002;94:73-84.
32. Fisher MC, Rannala B, Chaturvedi V, et al. Disease surveillance in recombining pathogens: multilocus genotypes identify sources of human *Coccidioides* infections. *Proc Natl Acad Sci U S A.* 2002;99:9067-9071.
33. Ramani R, Chaturvedi V. Antifungal susceptibility profiles of *Coccidioides immitis* and *Coccidioides posadasii* from endemic and non-endemic areas. *Mycopathologia.* 2007;163:315-319.
34. Tintelnot K, De Hoog GS, Antweiler E, et al. Taxonomic and diagnostic markers for identification of *Coccidioides immitis* and *Coccidioides posadasii. Med Mycol.* 2007;45:385-393.
35. Hector RF, Pappagianis D. Enzymatic degradation of the walls of spherules of *Coccidioides immitis. Exp Mycol.* 1982;6:136-152.
36. Huppert M, Sun SH, Harrison JL. Morphogenesis throughout saprobic and parasitic cycles of *Coccidioides immitis. Mycopathologia.* 1982;78:107-122.
37. Li L, Schmelz M, Kellner EM, et al. Nuclear labeling of *Coccidioides posadasii* with green fluorescent protein. *Ann N Y Acad Sci.* 2007;1111:198-207.
38. Ogiso A, Ito M, Koyama M, et al. Pulmonary coccidioidomycosis in Japan: case report and review. *Clin Infect Dis.* 1997;25:1260-1261.
39. Stagliano D, Epstein J, Hickey P. Fomite-transmitted coccidioidomycosis in an immunocompromised child. *Pediatr Infect Dis J.* 2007;26:454-456.
40. Pappagianis D, Einstein H. Tempest from Tehachapi takes toll or *Coccidioides* conveyed aloft and afar. *West J Med.* 1978;129:527-530.
41. Perera P, Stone S. Coccidioidomycosis in workers at an archeologic site—Dinosaur National Monument, Utah, June-July 2001. *Ann Emerg Med.* 2002;39:566-569.
42. Eulalio KD, de Macedo RL, Cavalcanti MA, et al. *Coccidioides immitis* isolated from armadillos (*Dasypus novemcinctus*) in the state of Piaui, northeast Brazil. *Mycopathologia.* 2001;149:57-61.
43. Morrow W. Holocene coccidioidomycosis: valley fever in early Holocene bison (*Bison antiquus*). *Mycologia.* 2006;98:669-677.
44. Greene DR, Koenig G, Fisher MC, et al. Soil isolation and molecular identification of *Coccidioides immitis. Mycologia.* 2000;92:406-410.
45. Pappagianis D. Epidemiology of coccidioidomycosis. *Curr Top Med Mycol.* 1988;2:199-238.
46. Kerrick SS, Lundergan LL, Galgiani JN. Coccidioidomycosis at a university health service. *Am Rev Respir Dis.* 1985;131:100-102.
47. Larwood TR. Coccidioidin skin testing in Kern County, California: decrease in infection rate over 58 years. *Clin Infect Dis.* 2000;30:612-613.
48. Smith CE, Beard RR, Whiting EG, et al. Varieties of coccidioidal infection in relation to the epidemiology and control of the disease. *Am J Public Health.* 1946;36:1394-1402.
49. Dodge RR, Lebowitz MD, Barbee RA, et al. Estimates of *C. immitis* infection by skin test reactivity in an endemic community. *Am J Public Health.* 1985;75:863-865.
50. Comrie AC. Climate factors influencing coccidioidomycosis seasonality and outbreaks. *Environ Health Perspect.* 2005;113:688-692.
51. Cairns L, Blythe D, Kao A, et al. Outbreak of coccidioidomycosis in Washington State residents returning from Mexico. *Clin Infect Dis.* 2000;30:61-64.
52. Jibson RW. A public health issue related to collateral seismic hazards: the valley fever outbreak triggered by the 1994 Northridge, California, earthquake. *Surveys in Geophysics.* 2002;23:511-528.
53. Crum N, Lamb C, Utz G, et al. Coccidioidomycosis outbreak among United States Navy SEALs training in a *Coccidioides immitis*–endemic area—Coalinga, California. *J Infect Dis.* 2002;186:865-868.
54. Centers for Disease Control and Prevention. Coccidioidomycosis—United States, 1991-1992. *MMWR Morb Mortal Wkly Rep.* 1993;42:21-24.
55. Leake JA, Mosley DG, England B, et al. Risk factors for acute symptomatic coccidioidomycosis among elderly persons in Arizona, 1996-1997. *J Infect Dis.* 2000;181:1435-1440.
56. Chang A, Tung RC, McGillis TS, et al. Primary cutaneous coccidioidomycosis. *J Am Acad Dermatol.* 2003;49:944-949.
57. Shubitz L, Peng T, Perrill R, et al. Protection of mice against *Coccidioides immitis* intranasal infection by vaccination with recombinant antigen 2/PRA. *Infect Immun.* 2002;70:3287-3289.
58. Hoggan MD, Ransom JP, Pappagianis D, et al. Isolation of *Coccidioides immitis* from the air [Abstract]. *Stanford Med Bull.* 1956;14:190.
59. Ajello L, Maddy K, Crecelius G, et al. Recovery of *Coccidioides immitis* from the air. *Sabouraudia.* 1965;4:92-95.
60. Galgiani JN, Isenberg RA, Stevens DA. Chemotaxigenic activity of extracts from the mycelial and spherule phases of *Coccidioides immitis* for human polymorphonuclear leukocytes. *Infect Immun.* 1978;21:862-865.
61. Huntington RW Jr, Waldmann WJ, Sargent JA, et al. Pathologic and clinical observations on 142 cases of fatal coccidioidomyco-

sis with necropsy. In: Ajello L, ed. *Coccidioidomycosis*. Tucson: University of Arizona Press; 1967:221-225.

62. Echols RM, Palmer DL, Long GW. Tissue eosinophilia in human coccidioidomycosis. *Rev Infect Dis*. 1982;4:656-664.
63. Li L, Dial SM, Schmelz M, et al. Cellular immune suppressor activity resides in lymphocyte cell clusters adjacent to granulomata in human coccidioidomycosis. *Infect Immun*. 2005;73: 3923-3928.
64. Beaman L, Pappagianis D, Benjamini E. Mechanisms of resistance to infection with *Coccidioides immitis* in mice. *Infect Immun*. 1979;23:681-685.
65. Beaman L, Benjamini E, Pappagianis D. Role of lymphocytes in macrophage-induced killing of *Coccidioides immitis* in vitro. *Infect Immun*. 1981;34:347-353.
66. Beaman L, Benjamini E, Pappagianis D. Activation of macrophages by lymphokines: enhancement of phagosome-lysosome fusion and killing of *Coccidioides immitis*. *Infect Immun*. 1983;39:1201-1207.
67. Beaman L. Fungicidal activation of murine macrophages by recombinant gamma interferon. *Infect Immun*. 1987;55: 2951-2955.
68. Beaman L. Effects of recombinant gamma interferon and tumor necrosis factor on in vitro interactions of human mononuclear phagocytes with *Coccidioides immitis*. *Infect Immun*. 1991;59: 4227-4229.
69. Ampel NM, Christian L. In vitro modulation of proliferation and cytokine production by human peripheral blood mononuclear cells from subjects with various forms of coccidioidomycosis. *Infect Immun*. 1997;65:4483-4487.
70. Corry DB, Ampel NM, Christian L, et al. Cytokine production by peripheral blood mononuclear cells in human coccidioidomycosis. *J Infect Dis*. 1996;174:440-443.
71. Ampel NM, Nelson DK, Li L, et al. The mannose receptor mediates the cellular immune response in human coccidioidomycosis. *Infect Immun*. 2005;73:2554-2555.
72. Dionne SO, Podany AB, Ruiz YW, et al. Spherules derived from *Coccidioides posadasii* promote human dendritic cell maturation and activation. *Infect Immun*. 2006;74:2415-2422.
73. Appelberg R, Castro AG, Pedrosa J, et al. Role of gamma interferon and tumor necrosis factor alpha during T-cell–independent and –dependent phases of *Mycobacterium avium* infection. *Infect Immun*. 1994;62:3962-3971.
74. Reiner SL, Locksley RM. The regulation of immunity to *Leishmania major*. *Annu Rev Immunol*. 1995;13:151-177.
75. Galgiani JN, Payne CM, Jones JF. Human polymorphonuclear-leukocyte inhibition of incorporation of chitin precursors into mycelia of *Coccidioides immitis*. *J Infect Dis*. 1984;149: 404-412.
76. Ampel NM, Bejarano GC, Galgiani JN. Killing of *Coccidioides immitis* by human peripheral blood mononuclear cells. *Infect Immun*. 1992;60:4200-4204.
77. Petkus AF, Baum LL. Natural killer cell inhibition of young spherules and endospores of *Coccidioides immitis*. *J Immunol*. 1987;139:3107-3111.
78. Frey CL, Drutz DJ. Influence of fungal surface components on the interaction of *Coccidioides immitis* with polymorphonuclear neutrophils. *J Infect Dis*. 1986;153:933-943.
79. Magee DM, Friedberg RL, Woitaske MD, et al. Role of B cells in vaccine-induced immunity against coccidioidomycosis. *Infect Immun*. 2005;73:7011-7013.
80. Yozwiak ML, Lundergan LL, Kerrick SS, et al. Symptoms and routine laboratory abnormalities associated with coccidioidomycosis. *West J Med*. 1988;149:419-421.
81. Valdivia L, Nix D, Wright M, et al. Coccidioidomycosis as a common cause of community-acquired pneumonia. *Emerg Infect Dis*. 2006;12:958-962.
82. Chang DC, Anderson S, Wannemuehler K, et al. Testing for coccidioidomycosis among patients with community-acquired pneumonia. *Emerg Infect Dis*. 2008;14:1053-1059.
83. Standaert SM, Schaffner W, Galgiani JN, et al. Coccidioidomycosis among visitors to a *Coccidioides immitis*–endemic area: an outbreak in a military reserve unit. *J Infect Dis*. 1995;171: 1672-1675.
84. Johnson RH, Caldwell JW, Welch G, et al. The great coccidioidomycosis epidemic: clinical features. In: Einstein HE, Catanzaro A, eds. *Coccidioidomycosis*. Proceedings of the Fifth International Conference. Washington, DC: National Foundation for Infectious Diseases; 1996:77-87.
85. Lopez AM, Williams PL, Ampel NM. Acute pulmonary coccidioidomycosis mimicking bacterial pneumonia and septic shock: a report of two cases. *Am J Med*. 1993;95:236-239.
86. Arsura EL, Bellinghausen PL, Kilgore WB, et al. Septic shock in coccidioidomycosis. *Crit Care Med*. 1998;26:62-65.
87. Arsura EL, Kilgore WB. Miliary coccidioidomycosis in the immunocompetent. *Chest*. 2000;117:404-409.
88. Chitkara YK. Evaluation of cultures of percutaneous core needle biopsy specimens in the diagnosis of pulmonary nodules. *Am J Clin Pathol*. 1997;107:224-228.
89. Smith CE, Beard RR, Saito MT. Pathogenesis of coccidioidomycosis with special reference to pulmonary cavitation. *Ann Intern Med*. 1948;29:623-655.
90. Winn RE, Johnson R, Galgiani JN, et al. Cavitary coccidioidomycosis with fungus ball formation: diagnosis by fiberoptic bronchoscopy with coexistence of hyphae and spherules. *Chest*. 1994;105:412-416.
91. Cunningham RT, Einstein H. Coccidioidal pulmonary cavities with rupture. *J Thorac Cardiovasc Surg*. 1982;84:172-177.
92. Sarosi GA, Parker JD, Doto IL, et al. Chronic pulmonary coccidioidomycosis. *N Engl J Med*. 1970;283:325-329.
93. Santelli AC, Blair JE, Roust LR. Coccidioidomycosis in patients with diabetes mellitus. *Am J Med*. 2006;119:964-969.
94. Walker MP, Brody CZ, Resnik R. Reactivation of coccidioidomycosis in pregnancy. *Obstet Gynecol*. 1992;79:815-817.
95. Peterson CM, Schuppert K, Kelly PC, et al. Coccidioidomycosis and pregnancy. *Obstet Gynecol Surv*. 1993;48:149-156.
96. Louie L, Ng S, Hajjeh R, et al. Influence of host genetics on the severity of coccidioidomycosis. *Emerg Infect Dis*. 1999;5: 672-680.
97. Bisla RS, Taber TH Jr. Coccidioidomycosis of bone and joints. *Clin Orthop*. 1976;121:196-204.
98. Bried JH, Galgiani JN. *Coccidioides immitis* infections in bones and joints. *Clin Orthop*. 1986;211:235-243.
99. Lund PJ, Chan KM, Unger EC, et al. Magnetic resonance imaging in coccidioidal arthritis. *Skeletal Radiol*. 1996;25: 661-665.
100. Dalinka MK, Dinnenberg S, Greendyke WH, et al. Roentgenographic features of osseous coccidioidomycosis and differential diagnosis. *J Bone Joint Surg Am*. 1971;53:1157-1164.
101. Erly WK, Carmody RF, Seeger JF, et al. Magnetic resonance imaging of coccidioidal spondylitis. *Int J Neuroradiol*. 1997;3: 385-392.
102. Einstein HE, Holeman CW Jr, Sandidge LL, et al. Coccidioidal meningitis: the use of amphotericin B in treatment. *Calif Med*. 1961;94:339-343.
103. Vincent T, Galgiani JN, Huppert M, et al. The natural history of coccidioidal meningitis: VA–Armed Forces Cooperative Studies, 1955-1958. *Clin Infect Dis*. 1993;16:247-254.
104. Pappagianis D. Coccidioidomycosis. In: Balows A, Hausler WJ Jr, Lennette EH, eds. *Laboratory Diagnosis of Infectious Diseases*. Berlin: Springer-Verlag; 1988:600-623.
105. Ismail Y, Arsura EL. Eosinophilic meningitis associated with coccidioidomycosis. *West J Med*. 1993;158:300-301.
106. Harrison HR, Galgiani JN, Reynolds AF Jr, et al. Amphotericin B and imidazole therapy for coccidioidal meningitis in children. *Pediatr Infect Dis*. 1983;2:216-221.
107. Mischel PS, Vinters HV. Coccidioidomycosis of the central nervous system: neuropathological and vasculopathic manifestations and clinical correlates. *Clin Infect Dis*. 1995;20:400-405.
108. BaZuelos AF, Williams PL, Johnson RH, et al. Central nervous system abscesses due to *Coccidioides* species. *Clin Infect Dis*. 1996;22:240-250.
109. Williams PL. Vasculitic complications associated with coccidioidal meningitis. *Semin Respir Infect*. 2001;16:270-279.
110. Hernandez JL, Echevarria S, Garcia-Valtuille A, et al. Atypical coccidioidomycosis in an AIDS patient successfully treated with fluconazole. *Eur J Clin Microbiol Infect Dis*. 1997;16: 592-594.
111. Sarosi GA, Lawrence JP, Smith DK, et al. Rapid diagnostic evaluation of bronchial washings in patients with suspected coccidioidomycosis. *Semin Respir Infect*. 2001;16:238-241.
112. Graham AR. Fungal autofluorescence with ultraviolet illumination. *Am J Clin Pathol*. 1983;79:231-234.
113. Hayden RT, Qian X, Roberts GD, et al. In situ hybridization for the identification of yeastlike organisms in tissue section. *Diag Mol Pathol*. 2001;10:15-23.
114. Cordeiro RD, Brilhante RSN, Rocha MFG, et al. Rapid diagnosis of coccidioidomycosis by nested PCR assay of sputum. *Clin Microbiol Infect*. 2007;13:449-451.
115. Huppert M, Sun SH, Bailey JW. Natural variability in *Coccidioides immitis*. In: Ajello L, ed. *Coccidioidomycosis. The Second Symposium on Coccidioidomycosis*. Tucson: University of Arizona Press; 1965:323-328.
116. Pappagianis D. Coccidioidomycosis (San Joaquin or valley fever). In: DiSalvo A, ed. *Occupational Mycoses*. Philadelphia: Lea & Febiger; 1983:13-28.
117. Huppert M, Sun SH, Rice EH. Specificity of exoantigens for identifying cultures of *Coccidioides immitis*. *J Clin Microbiol*. 1978;8:346-348.
118. Padhye AA, Smith G, Standard PG, et al. Comparative evaluation of chemiluminescent DNA probe assays and exoantigen tests for rapid identification of *Blastomyces dermatitidis* and *Coccidioides immitis*. *J Clin Microbiol*. 1994;32:867-870.
119. Sandhu GS, Kline BC, Stockman L, et al. Molecular probes for diagnosis of fungal infections. *J Clin Microbiol*. 1995;33: 2913-2919.
120. Pappagianis D, Zimmer BL. Serology of coccidioidomycosis. *Clin Microbiol Rev*. 1990;3:247-268.
121. Smith CE, Whiting EG, Baker EE, et al. The use of coccidioidin. *Am Rev Tuberc Pulm Dis*. 1948;57:330-360.
122. Johnson SM, Pappagianis D. The coccidioidal complement fixation and immunodiffusion-complement fixation antigen is a chitinase. *Infect Immun*. 1992;60:2588-2592.
123. Pishko EJ, Kirkland TN, Cole GT. Isolation and characterization of two chitinase-encoding genes (*cts1, cts2*) from the fungus *Coccidioides immitis*. *Gene*. 1995;167:173-177.
124. Yang CM, Zhu YF, Magee DM, et al. Molecular cloning and characterization of the *Coccidioides immitis* complement fixation chitinase antigen. *Infect Immun*. 1996;64:1992-1997.
125. Zimmermann CR, Johnson SM, Martens GW, et al. Cloning and expression of the complement fixation antigen-chitinase of *Coccidioides immitis*. *Infect Immun*. 1996;64:4967-4975.
126. Huppert M, Bailey JW. The use of immunodiffusion tests in coccidioidomycosis: II. An immunodiffusion test as a substitute for the tube precipitin test. *Am J Clin Pathol*. 1965;44:369.
127. Wieden MA, Galgiani JN, Pappagianis D. Comparison of immunodiffusion techniques with standard complement fixation assay for quantitation of coccidioidal antibodies. *J Clin Microbiol*. 1983;18:529-534.
128. Kaufman L, Sekhon AS, Moledina N, et al. Comparative evaluation of commercial Premier EIA and microimmunodiffusion and complement fixation tests for *Coccidioides immitis* antibodies. *J Clin Microbiol*. 1995;33:618-619.
129. Wieden MA, Lundergan LL, Blum J, et al. Detection of coccidioidal antibodies by 33-kDa spherule antigen, *Coccidioides* EIA, and standard serologic tests in sera from patients evaluated for coccidioidomycosis. *J Infect Dis*. 1996;173:1273-1277.
130. Zartarian M, Peterson EM, De la Maza LM. Detection of antibodies to *Coccidioides immitis* by enzyme immunoassay. *Am J Clin Pathol*. 1997;107:148-153.
131. Drutz DJ, Catanzaro A. Coccidioidomycosis: part I. *Am Rev Respir Dis*. 1978;117:559-585.
132. Oldfield EC, Bone WD, Martain CR, et al. Prediction of relapse after treatment of coccidioidomycosis. *Clin Infect Dis*. 1997;25:1205-1210.
133. Yoshinoya S, Cox RA, Pope RM. Circulating immune complexes in coccidioidomycosis: detection and characterization. *J Clin Invest*. 1980;66:655-663.
134. Weiner MH. Antigenemia detected in human coccidioidomycosis. *J Clin Microbiol*. 1983;18:136-142.
135. Galgiani JN, Dugger KO, Ito JI, et al. Antigenemia in primary coccidioidomycosis. *Am J Trop Med Hyg*. 1984;33:645-649.
136. Galgiani JN, Grace GM, Lundergan LL. New serologic tests for early detection of coccidioidomycosis. *J Infect Dis*. 1991;163: 671-674.
137. Durkin M, Connolly P, Kuberski T, et al. Diagnosis of coccidioidomycosis with use of the Coccidioides antigen enzyme immunoassay. *Clin Inf Dis*. 2008;47:e69-e73.
138. Clark KA, McAllister D. Direct detection of *Coccidioides immitis* in clinical specimens using target amplification. In: Einstein HE, Catanzaro A, eds. *Coccidioidomycosis*. Proceedings of the Fifth International Conference. Washington, DC: National Foundation for Infectious Diseases; 1996:129-136.
139. Stadalnik RC, Goldstein E, Hoeprich PD, et al. Diagnostic value of gallium and bone scans in evaluation of extrapulmonary coccidioidal lesions. *Am Rev Respir Dis*. 1980;121:673-676.
140. Boddicker JH, Fong D, Walsh TE, et al. Bone and gallium scanning in the evaluation of disseminated coccidioidomycosis. *Am Rev Respir Dis*. 1980;122:279-287.
141. Bergstrom L, Yocum DE, Ampel NM, et al. Increased risk of coccidioidomycosis in patients treated with tumor necrosis factor alpha antagonists. *Arthritis Rheum*. 2004;50:1959-1966.
142. Hooper JE, Lu Q, Pepkowitz SH. Disseminated coccidioidomycosis in pregnancy. *Arch Pathol Lab Med*. 2007;131:652-655.
143. Galgiani JN, Stevens DA, Graybill JR, et al. Ketoconazole therapy of progressive coccidioidomycosis: comparison of 400- and 800-mg doses and observations at higher doses. *Am J Med*. 1988;84:603-610.
144. Tucker RM, Denning DW, Dupont B, et al. Itraconazole therapy for chronic coccidioidal meningitis. *Ann Intern Med*. 1990;112: 108-112.
145. Galgiani JN, Catanzaro A, Cloud GA, et al. Fluconazole therapy for coccidioidal meningitis. *Ann Intern Med*. 1993;119:28-35.
146. Stevens DA. Itraconazole and fluconazole for treatment of coccidioidomycosis. *Clin Infect Dis*. 1994;18:470.
147. Catanzaro A, Galgiani JN, Levine BE, et al. Fluconazole in the treatment of chronic pulmonary and nonmeningeal disseminated coccidioidomycosis. *Am J Med*. 1995;98:249-256.
148. Holley K, Muldoon M, Tasker S. *Coccidioides immitis* osteomyelitis: a case series review. *Orthopedics*. 2002;25:827-831.
149. Shibli M, Ghassibi J, Hajal R, et al. Adjunctive corticosteroids therapy in acute respiratory distress syndrome owing to disseminated coccidioidomycosis. *Crit Care Med*. 2002;30: 1896-1898.
150. Perez JA Jr, Johnson RH, Caldwell JW, et al. Fluconazole therapy in coccidioidal meningitis maintained with intrathecal amphotericin B. *Arch Intern Med*. 1995;155:1665-1668.
151. Galgiani JN, Catanzaro A, Cloud GA, et al. Comparison of oral fluconazole and itraconazole for progressive, nonmeningeal coccidioidomycosis: a randomized, double-blind trial. Mycoses Study Group. *Ann Intern Med*. 2000;133:676-686.
152. Catanzaro A, Cloud GA, Stevens DA, et al. Safety, tolerance, and efficacy of posaconazole therapy in patients with nonmeningeal disseminated or chronic pulmonary coccidioidomycosis. *Clin Infect Dis*. 2007;45:562-568.
153. Stevens DA, Rendon A, Gaona-Flores V, et al. Posaconazole therapy for chronic refractory coccidioidomycosis. *Chest*. 2007;132:952-958.
154. Prabhu RM, Bonnell M, Currier BL, et al. Successful treatment of disseminated nonmeningeal coccidioidomycosis with voriconazole. *Clin Infect Dis*. 2004;39:e74-e77.
155. Proia LA, Tenorio AR. Successful use of voriconazole for treatment of *Coccidioides* meningitis. *Antimicrob Agents Chemother*. 2004;48:2341.
156. Garvin GJ, Peterfy CG. Soft tissue coccidioidomycosis on MRI. *J Comput Assist Tomogr*. 1995;19:612-614.
157. Erly WK, Bellon RJ, Seeger JF, et al. MR imaging of acute coccidioidal meningitis. *AJNR Am J Neuroradiol*. 1999;20: 509-514.

157a. Ampel NM, Giblin A, Mourani JP, Galgiani JN. Factors and outcomes associated with the decision to treat primary pulmonary coccidioidomycosis. *Clin Infect Dis*. 2009;48:172-178.

158. Labadie EL, Hamilton RH. Survival improvement in coccidioidal meningitis by high-dose intrathecal amphotericin B. *Arch Intern Med*. 1986;146:2013-2018.

159. Stevens DA, Shatsky SA. Intrathecal amphotericin in the management of coccidioidal meningitis. *Semin Respir Infect*. 2001; 16:263-269.

160. Goldstein E, Winship MJ, Pappagianis D. Ventricular fluid and the management of coccidioidal meningitis. *Ann Intern Med*. 1972;77:243-246.

161. Gonzalez GM, Tijerina R, Najvar LK, et al. Correlation between antifungal susceptibilities of *Coccidioides immitis* in vitro and antifungal treatment with caspofungin in a mouse model. *Antimicrob Agents Chemother*. 2001;45:1854-1859.

162. Gonzalez GM, Gonzalez G, Najvar LK, et al. Therapeutic efficacy of caspofungin alone and in combination with amphotericin B deoxycholate for coccidioidomycosis in a mouse model. *J Antimicrob Chemother*. 2007;60:1341-1346.

163. Antony S. Use of the echinocandins (caspofungin) in the treatment of disseminated coccidioidomycosis in a renal transplant recipient. *Clin Infect Dis*. 2004;39:879-880.

164. Hector RF, Zimmer BL, Pappagianis D. Evaluation of nikkomycins X and Z in murine models of coccidioidomycosis, histoplasmosis, and blastomycosis. *Antimicrob Agents Chemother*. 1990;34:587-593.

165. Fiedler HP, Schuz T, Decker H. An overview of nikkomycins: history, biochemistry, and applications. In: Rippon JW, Fromtling RA, eds. *Cutaneous Antifungal Agents: Selected Compounds in Clinical Practice and Development*. New York: Marcel Dekker, 1993:325-352.

166. Galgiani JN. Coccidioidomycosis: changing perceptions and creating opportunities for its control. *Ann N Y Acad Sci*. 2007;1111:1-18.

166a. Nix DE, Swezey RR, Hector R, Galgiani JN. Pharmacokinetics of nikkomycin Z after single rising oral doses. *Antimicrob Agents Chemother*. 2009;53:2517-2521.

167. Barnato AE, Sanders GD, Owens DK. Cost-effectiveness of a potential vaccine for *Coccidioides immitis*. *Emerg Infect Dis*. 2001;7:797-806.

168. Levine HB, Cobb JM, Smith CE. Immunity to coccidioidomycosis induced in mice by purified spherule, arthrospore, and mycelial vaccines. *Trans N Y Acad Sci*. 1960;22:436-447.

169. Levine HB, Cobb JM, Smith CE. Immunogenicity of spherule-endospore vaccines of *Coccidioides immitis* for mice. *J Immunol*. 1961;87:218-227.

170. Levine HB, Miller RL, Smith CE. Influence of vaccination on respiratory coccidioidal disease in cynomolgus monkeys. *J Immunol*. 1962;89:242-251.

171. Kong Y-C, Levine HB, Smith CE. Immunogenic properties of nondisrupted and disrupted spherules of *Coccidioides immitis* in mice. *Sabouraudia*. 1963;2:131-142.

172. Levine HB, Kong Y-C, Smith CE. Immunization of mice to *Coccidioides immitis*: dose, regimen and spherulation stage of killed spherule vaccines. *J Immunol*. 1965;94:132-142.

173. Levine HB. Purification of the spherule-endospore phase of *Coccidioides immitis*. *Sabouraudia*. 1961;1:112-115.

174. Kong Y-C, Savage DC, Levine HB. Enhancement of immune responses in mice by a booster injection of *Coccidioides* spherules. *J Immunol*. 1966;95:1048-1056.

175. Huppert M, Levine HB, Sun SH, et al. Resistance of vaccinated mice to typical and atypical strains of *Coccidioides immitis*. *J Bacteriol*. 1967;94:924-927.

176. Pappagianis D. Histopathologic response of mice to killed vaccines of *Coccidioides immitis*. *J Invest Dermatol*. 1967;49:71-77.

177. Williams PL, Sable DL, Sorgen D, et al. Immunologic responsiveness and safety associated with the *Coccidioides immitis* spherule vaccine in volunteers of white, black and Filipino ancestry. *Am J Epidemiol*. 1984;119:591-602.

178. Pappagianis D. Valley Fever Vaccine Study Group: evaluation of the protective efficacy of the killed *Coccidioides immitis* spherule vaccine in humans. *Am Rev Respir Dis*. 1993;148:656-660.

179. Galgiani JN. Vaccines to prevent systemic mycoses: holy grails meet translational realities. *J Infect Dis*. 2008;197:938-940.

267

Dermatophytosis and Other Superficial Mycoses

RODERICK J. HAY

The superficial fungal infections include some of the most common infectious conditions, such as ringworm, tinea corporis, and pityriasis versicolor, as well as rare disorders such as tinea nigra. Their prevalence varies in different parts of the world, but in many tropical countries, they are the most common causes of skin disease. Dermatophyte infections and other superficial mycoses are described in this chapter. Superficial candidiasis is discussed in Chapter 257.

Dermatophytosis

The dermatophytes are molds that can invade the stratum corneum of the skin or other keratinized tissues derived from epidermis, such as hair and nails. They may cause infections (dermatophytoses) at most skin sites, although the feet, groin, scalp, and nails are most commonly affected.[1] The dermatophytes are among the earliest microorganisms that were found to cause infections in humans. *Trichophyton schoenleinii*, the cause of the scalp infection favus, was isolated from a patient and the culture shown to reproduce the typical lesions after inoculation onto human skin as early as 1841. Dermatophyte infections had been described many years before this, although the identity of the cause had not been recognized. The ancient Greek physicians knew about ringworm, and there are descriptions of the manifestations of dermatophytosis in more unlikely sources, such as the records of the early Dutch explorers of the 16th century who reported a strange disease of the skin, subsequently known as *tinea imbricata*, caused by *Trichophyton concentricum*, in the islanders of the western Pacific.

THE DERMATOPHYTES

There are three genera of pathogenic dermatophyte fungi: *Trichophyton*, *Microsporum*, and *Epidermophyton*. The last genus is represented by only a single species, *Epidermophyton floccosum*. These keratinophilic organisms probably arose as saprophytic soil fungi, and some dermatophytes, which have been isolated only from soil, have not been shown to cause disease in either animals or humans. Most of the 39 dermatophyte species, however, are parasitic and can cause disease in either humans or animals, often being adapted to a single or narrow range of host species. The dermatophytes are referred to as *zoophilic*, *anthropophilic*, or *geophilic*, depending on whether their primary source is an animal, human, or soil, respectively.

The taxonomy of these fungi is complicated by the fact that most clinical isolates are imperfect fungi (organisms that do not produce sexual structures in culture). However, sexual forms of many of these species are known and have been assigned to one genus, *Arthroderma*, which corresponds to the imperfect genera *Trichophyton* and *Microsporum*. The classification of these fungi is difficult, and their exact taxonomic status remains a subject of debate, although the wider use of molecular tools to determine species has enabled a scientifically based classification to evolve.[2]

The relationships among different dermatophytes are not simply a subject for intellectual dispute. To understand the spread of infections, for instance, it is important to attempt to differentiate strains of the same species. There have been significant advances both in the molecular taxonomy of these organisms and in the development of schemes for strain differentiation through the use of molecular tools.[3] These advances have not altered the conventional classification based on morphology; rather, they have enhanced the understanding of key issues in pathogenesis, such as spread of infection in populations and relapse after apparently successful treatment. Attempts have also been made to classify the dermatophytes according to their protein composition[4] and production of antibiotics or enzymes such as urease. Both antibiotics and enzymes may play a role in determining pathogenicity. Proteinases produced by dermatophytes are inducible by, for instance, amino acids.[5] *Trichophyton rubrum* secretes a number of enzymes with different protein affinities, including keratin, the largest of which is a 200-kDa glycosylated metalloprotease, and the genes encoding subtilisin proteinases in *Microsporum canis* (Sub1, Sub2, and so forth) have been identified.[6] The significance of the production of antibiotics by dermatophytes is uncertain. The main groups detected have been the penicillins and fusidates, and these are produced by dermatophytes not only under laboratory culture conditions but also after growth on epidermal sheets in vitro.

EPIDEMIOLOGY

The factors affecting the distribution and transmission of dermatophytosis are largely dependent on the source of the infection[7]: animal, soil, or human.

Zoophilic Dermatophyte Infections

The main zoophilic dermatophyte fungi are listed in Table 267-1. Each organism is primarily an animal pathogen that sometimes causes human infection. In each case, there is usually a range of host specificities, from organisms such as *Microsporum nanum*, whose natural host is the pig and which does not infect other animals, to *Trichophyton mentagrophytes*, which affects a range of different rodent species, or, rarely, cats, dogs, and horses.

The host preferences of *T. mentagrophytes*, coupled with small clinical and cultural differences, have led many mycologists to subdivide this group. Under this classification, *T. mentagrophytes quinckeanum* (*Trichophyton quinckeanum*) is used to describe the fungus that causes the clinical pattern of favus in mice, an infection associated with the formation of epithelial crusts. However, the organisms are difficult to distinguish genetically. In most temperate countries, *Trichophyton verrucosum*, the cause of cattle ringworm, and *M. canis*, a dermatophyte that causes infections in cats or dogs, are the most common zoophilic dermatophytes that cause human infections.

Of all the zoophilic dermatophytes, *M. canis* is probably the most prevalent throughout the world, both in temperate regions and some tropical regions.[7] On occasion, the distribution of zoophilic dermatophytes may appear to be difficult to explain, but usually it reflects the distribution of the animal host. For instance, *Trichophyton erinacei* (part of the *T. mentagrophytes* complex) is confined mainly to Europe and New Zealand. It is carried by hedgehogs, which were introduced into New Zealand in the 19th century from England. *Microsporum persicolor* is a rare cause of human infections in Europe, where it has been isolated from the bank vole, whose distribution is similarly restricted. *Trichophyton simii* is associated with monkeys in India and the Far East, and infections in humans are observed only in these areas.[8]

TABLE 267-1	Classification of the Main Dermatophytic (*Trichophyton*, *Microsporum*, and *Epidermophyton*) Organisms		
		Zoophilic	
Anthropophilic	**Geophilic**	*Organism*	*Sources*
Trichophyton concentricum	*Trichophyton ajelloi*	*Trichophyton erinacei**	Hedgehogs
Trichophyton gourvilii	*Trichophyton terrestre*	*Trichophyton equinum*	Horses
Trichophyton mentagrophytes interdigitale*	*Microsporum fulvum*	*Trichophyton mentagrophytes mentagrophytes**	Rodents
Trichophyton megnini	*Microsporum gypseum*	*Trichophyton quinckeanum**	Mice
Trichophyton rubrum		*Trichophyton simii*	Monkeys
Trichophyton schoenleinii		*Trichophyton verrucosum*	Cattle
Trichophyton soudanense		*Microsporum canis*	Cats, dogs
Trichophyton tonsurans		*Microsporum gallinae*	Chickens
Trichophyton violaceum		*Microsporum nanum*	Pigs
Trichophyton yaoundei		*Microsporum persicolor*	Bank voles
Microsporum audouinii			
Microsporum ferrugineum			
Epidermophyton floccosum			

*These organisms are part of the "mentagrophytes" complex and may be classified as a single species.

Geophilic Dermatophyte Infections

Dermatophytes originating from soil, such as *Microsporum gypseum*, are infrequent causes of human disease, although they may be seen more commonly in certain parts of the tropics such as the western Pacific and Central America. In other areas, they usually cause sporadic infections, although on occasion they are responsible for outbreaks of disease among humans in appropriately exposed occupational groups, such as gardeners or farmworkers.[8]

Anthropophilic Dermatophyte Infections

Dermatophytes that are natural pathogens of humans are the most common cause of human dermatophytosis. They include organisms that mainly cause infections of glabrous skin of the feet or hands, as well as a range of pathogens whose invasion may involve penetration of the hair shaft. The most common of these organisms in most parts of the world is *T. rubrum*, which causes tinea pedis or tinea cruris in temperate climates and, particularly in the tropics, tinea corporis. Cases of infection that are caused by *T. rubrum* were once rare in the Western Hemisphere, but the infection has spread rapidly since the 1960s. This dermatophyte can cause noninflammatory chronic infections of the feet, among other sites, that are easily transmitted; this is probably an important factor that has determined its spread.[7] The large population movements during World War II are also thought to have contributed to the spread of the disease. Despite this, a variant with distinct morphologic appearances may be isolated from patients with tinea corporis,[9] particularly in the tropics, which suggests that although endemic disease caused by this species has been present for a considerable time, the key adaptation leading to spread was the appearance of strains capable of causing indolent and noninflammatory infections of peripheral skin sites.

The organisms that infect glabrous skin spread largely through contact with infected desquamated skin scales. Classically, this occurs in bathing areas or shower rooms where large numbers of individuals share common facilities: for instance, in military camps or factories.[10]

Workers in industries such as mines or nuclear fuels may have a high frequency of foot infection, mainly due to *T. rubrum*, although *Trichophyton interdigitale* (part of the *T. mentagrophytes* complex) may also be isolated.[11] Changing rooms used by the police and armed forces, schools, and public swimming pools are also sites for infection. In contrast, transmission within the home as a reflection of conjugal or familial cases is not common, although it has been suggested that some patients show immunologic and genetic susceptibility.[12] *E. floccosum* may also cause foot infections, although it is particularly associated with tinea cruris either as a sporadic disease or in institutions such as prisons or military barracks. These infections are not geographically restricted, even though there are variations in different countries. In many tropical areas, particularly the Far East, *T. mentagrophytes* is less commonly a cause of interdigital foot disease, and patients are infected by the zoophilic variety of this species on sites other than the feet.[13]

Tinea imbricata (a variant of tinea corporis), caused by the anthropophilic dermatophyte *T. concentricum*, has an unusual distribution confined to remote parts of the humid tropics.[14] The main endemic areas are the western Pacific islands, Malaysia, Assam, and parts of the Amazon basin in Brazil. Infants may be affected shortly after birth, and spontaneous recovery is unusual. Large numbers of viable organisms can be cultured from the houses of infected families. Visitors to endemic areas are rarely infected. Cases have also been described in Chiapas, southern Mexico, where the severity of the disease appears to fluctuate with the season.

The distribution of some of the other anthropophilic dermatophytes that cause tinea capitis in children, as well as other clinical forms of disease such as tinea corporis or onychomycosis, may be more restricted. The reasons for this are not entirely clear, except that because these infections are prevalent in children, who form a relatively stable population with little opportunity for travel, the spread of the disease within the continent may be limited to certain localities. Whatever the reason, these scalp infections are often found in defined endemic areas (Table 267-2). The situation is best illustrated by the distribution of *Trichophyton* spp. that cause tinea capitis in West Africa, where the endemic areas for *Trichophyton soudanense*, *Trichophyton yaoundei*, and *Trichophyton gourvilii* are distinct, although there is some overlap.[15] The predominant cause of scalp infection is *Trichophyton tonsurans* in the United Kingdom, United States, and Mexico and *Trichophyton violaceum* in India, East Africa, and the Middle East. The situation does not always remain stable, and the slow increase in numbers of *T. tonsurans* in the United States was followed by spread to the United Kingdom and some parts of Europe, Latin America, and Africa.[7] In addition, other anthropophilic *Trichophyton* infections such as *T. violaceum* and *T. soudanense* are seen in immigrants in Europe and elsewhere. Endemic anthropophilic scalp infections that are caused by *Microsporum* spp. are less common. For instance, *Microsporum ferrugineum* is found occasionally in the Far East or central Europe. *Microsporum rivalieri* is seen

TABLE 267-2	Distribution of *Trichophyton* and *Microsporum* Species Causing Tinea Capitis
Dermatophyte	*Distribution*
Trichophyton gourvilii	Central Africa
Trichophyton tonsurans	North America and Central America (Europe: some inner cities)
Trichophyton soudanense	West and central Africa
Trichophyton schoenleinii	North Africa (United States, Middle East, South Africa, South America [sporadic])
Trichophyton verrucosum	Europe
Trichophyton violaceum	Indian subcontinent, Middle East, North Africa
Trichophyton yaoundei	Central Africa
Microsporum audouinii	Central America, West Africa (Europe: uncommon)
Microsporum canis	Worldwide but uncommon in India and Far East
Microsporum ferrugineum	Central Africa, Far East

in Africa, Democratic Republic of Congo, and Angola. The most widely distributed of this genus is *Microsporum audouinii*. Once common throughout Europe, it almost disappeared but has been reintroduced by immigration from regions that remained endemic, such as West Africa, and it is still a major cause of tinea capitis in Africa. *M. canis* is a major but sporadic cause of zoophilic tinea capitis in many countries.

Favus—the infection caused by *T. schoenleinii*—has characteristic clinical features. It was once common in Europe but has now largely disappeared from many areas, although pockets of infection still exist in parts of sub-Saharan Africa. One of the features of this disease is the development of crusts, or scutula, on the scalp. Hairs are invaded, but shedding is delayed because they are not structurally damaged until late in the course of the infection. Although tinea capitis is normally a disease of children, occasionally women have favus.

Dermatophytes causing scalp disease may be carried on the skin surface without invading the skin or hair. A small proportion of carriers develop infections within 6 months, in others the fungus disappears, and the rest remain carriers.[16] It is likely, however, that some carriers are simply patients with limited but undetected infections.

Age Incidence. Tinea capitis is mainly a disease of childhood, and cases rarely occur after puberty. But this infection may occur in adults and may also be associated with scarring alopecia. The reason for the preponderance of the disease in children is thought to be the presence of medium-chain–length fatty acids (C_8 to C_{12}) in sebum that inhibit the growth of dermatophytes in postpubertal individuals. In contrast, tinea pedis is usually seen in adolescents or young adults.[17] Foot infections occasionally occur in young children, but in this age group, the nails may be invaded without concomitant skin infection.

PATHOGENESIS

Transfer of infecting organisms from soil, animals, or humans is accomplished by means of arthrospores, which are vegetative cells with thickened cell walls formed by dermatophyte hyphae in vitro and in vivo. These structures are probably shed by the primary host with skin scales or hair. It has been shown that dermatophyte arthrospores can survive for considerable periods outside the host: in some cases, for more than 15 months. Direct contact between the infected individual and another individual is not necessary for the development of dermatophytosis in the latter. The process of transfer itself is little understood, but invasion of the skin appears to follow adherence of fungal cells to keratinocytes in vitro, a process that is maximal after about 2 or 3 hours. Keratinocytes from different sites do not appear to differ in their binding capacity for arthrospores. Subsequent germination leads to invasion.[18]

Susceptibility to infection is not universal. Studies of mice experimentally infected with *T. quinckeanum* have shown considerable interstrain variation in susceptibility to dermatophytosis.[19] In humans it has been suggested that susceptibility to tinea imbricata is mediated through an autosomal recessive gene; the evidence was based on population studies among tribes of Papua New Guinea.[20] Similar studies of the more common infections have not been carried out, although the existence of family cases of dermatophytosis has led to the assumption that this is proof of underlying genetic susceptibility. The factors determining individual susceptibility to dermatophytosis are not understood, but variations in the composition of inhibitory fatty acids in sebum (described earlier) offer one explanation. Other skin surface factors thought to be important in determining the outcome of infection include the local carbon dioxide tension and the presence of surface moisture, as well as unsaturated transferrin. After invasion, dermatophytes secrete proteinases such as zinc-containing metalloproteinases, which aid penetration.[21] In experimentally infected mice and guinea pigs, the inflammatory response to dermatophytosis is maximal after 9 to 16 days, and after this stage there is resolution of the infection. The main efferent limb of immunologic resistance is the T lymphocyte. Studies of mice with *T. quinckeanum*

infections have shown that resistance can be transferred to sublethally irradiated mice with T cells bearing the phenotype of helper-inducer T cells (Thy-1).[19] Suppressor lymphocyte activity can be detected in cells from the draining lymph nodes at the peak of infection. Immunity cannot be transferred with antibody to uninfected animals. Although it is difficult to extrapolate these data to infected humans, there is evidence that the kinetics of the immune response in humans is similar. For instance, the development of delayed-type hypersensitivity in children with naturally acquired scalp ringworm caused by *T. tonsurans* is correlated with recovery. Experimentally infected humans develop both delayed-type skin reactions to trichophytin and T-lymphocyte blastogenic responses at the time of recovery.[22] Patients with chronic *T. rubrum* or *T. concentricum* infections appear to have defective T-lymphocyte–mediated responses and patients with persistent dermatophyte infections elicit a cytokine profile suggestive of a helper T cell type 2 (Th2) response.[23] These observations suggest that appropriate T-lymphocyte activation is crucial for recovery in dermatophytosis.

The afferent limb of the immune response is provided by epidermal Langerhans cells, which have been shown to act as antigen-presenting cells in mixed cultures with human lymphocytes. The mechanisms by which T lymphocytes affect recovery are less well understood. Phagocytes—mainly neutrophils and, to a lesser extent, macrophages—can kill dermatophytes both intracellularly and extracellularly, mainly through oxidative pathways.[19] Dermatophyte antigens have been shown to be chemotactic to human leukocytes and may activate the alternative pathway of complement activation. However, except in inflammatory ringworm, neutrophils are not commonly seen as part of the inflammatory infiltrate in dermatophytosis, and other mechanisms of fungal clearance must be involved. It has been shown that increased epidermal turnover occurs during infection. Although this also occurs in heterologous skin grafted onto T-cell–deficient (*nu/nu*) mice, which suggests that an intrinsic response is involved, it is maximal at the time of development of the maximal immune responses.[24] It is possible that elimination of dermatophytes is also accomplished by increased shedding of the stratum corneum and that the immune system amplifies an endogenous epidermal response to infection.

Different dermatophyte species vary in their ability to elicit an immune response; some organisms, such as *T. rubrum*, cause chronic or relapsing infections, and others, including *T. verrucosum*, lead to long-term resistance to reinfection. Some dermatophytes produce glycopeptides, which are capable of reversibly inhibiting T-lymphocyte blastogenesis in vitro.[5] This may account for in vivo modulation of immunity.

CLINICAL FEATURES

The archetypal lesion of dermatophytosis is an annular scaling patch with a raised margin that exhibits a variable degree of inflammation; the center is usually less inflamed than the edge. The word *tinea* is used to refer to dermatophyte infections, and it is usually followed by the Latin description of the appropriate site. Hence, tinea pedis is an infection of the feet, and tinea capitis is an infection of the scalp. The term *tinea incognito* is used to describe infections that do not have any of the usual characteristic features of dermatophytosis, often because of inappropriate application of corticosteroid creams. Disease associated with immunosuppression, including infection with the human immunodeficiency virus (HIV) and acquired immunodeficiency syndrome (AIDS), affects the clinical expression of dermatophytosis; the result is often diminished scaling but prominent folliculitis and the formation of pustules.

The clinical appearances of the infection vary with the site, the fungal species involved, and the host's immune response. Zoophilic fungi often cause inflammatory lesions, and in some cases, large pustular lesions (kerions) may develop. In contrast, lesions caused by anthropophilic dermatophytes often exhibit little inflammation and may become chronic (see "Pathogenesis" section).

Tinea Pedis

Tinea pedis is usually caused by infection with either *T. rubrum* or *T. interdigitale* (part of the *T. mentagrophytes* complex) or, less commonly, with *E. floccosum.* The infection usually starts in the lateral interdigital spaces of the foot or on the undersurface of the lateral aspects of the toes. The main symptom is itching, although the severity is variable. The skin usually cracks and may become severely macerated. In some cases, often when *T. mentagrophytes* is the causative organism, bullae are formed, and itching is severe. The infection may also spread onto the dorsum of the feet, usually on the lateral side of the foot. Involvement of the sole is common in *T. rubrum* infections, and part of or the entire sole becomes erythematous and covered with dry scales. This is most noticeable along the lateral borders of the sole, where the appearance is often characterized as *moccasin* or *dry-type* infection. Blisters may also be formed in small clusters on the sole. The course of infection is variable. In noninflammatory forms, the interdigital scaling is often chronic or intermittent, whereas if blisters are formed, the infection usually resolves but may recur several months later. The main complications of tinea pedis are bacterial cellulitis and fungal invasion of the toenails (onychomycosis) or the skin of the dorsum of the foot and leg.

Tinea pedis usually occurs in young adults or teenagers. It is particularly common in institutions or places where common bathing facilities are used. The clinical manifestations of infection are altered in patients with T-lymphocyte abnormalities, in whom there is often extensive spread of the lesions onto the dorsal surface of the foot.

Scaling between the toes is often referred to as *athlete's foot,* but similar clinical signs may be produced by a variety of organisms. Erythrasma that is due to *Corynebacterium minutissimum* may manifest with scaling and, in particular, maceration of the toe webs. Gram-negative bacteria such as *Pseudomonas* and *Proteus* spp. may contribute to interdigital disease in patients with closely apposed web spaces or whose work involves immersion in water. These organisms may replace the original dermatophytes in this site, an infection known as *dermatophytosis complex.*[25] *Staphylococcus aureus* may cause secondary infections of the foot, but this characteristically starts on the dorsum of the foot over the first two digits. The mold fungi *Scytalidium dimidiatum* (formerly known as *Hendersonula toruloidea*) and *Scytalidium hyalinum* may cause interdigital scaling, nail disease, and sole involvement that is indistinguishable from dry-type infections caused by dermatophytes. Cracking between the toes is conducive to cellulitis in predisposed patients such as those with chronic lymphedema.

Tinea Cruris

The most common dermatophytes associated with groin infections are *T. rubrum* and *E. floccosum.* This infection is also called *jock itch.* The infection starts with scaling and irritation in the groin. The rash usually involves the anterior aspect of the thighs, less commonly the scrotum. The leading edge extending onto the thighs is prominent and may contain follicular papules and pustules. The infection may also spread to the anal cleft. Although tinea cruris is mainly a disease of young men, it may affect women, particularly in the tropics, where the infection may spread in a band around the waist area.

As with tinea pedis, there may be clustering of cases of tinea cruris in institutionalized groups, such as those in military camps. The toe webs are also often infected in patients with tinea cruris.

Erythrasma of the groin may also cause a localized rash with itching. However, here the leading edge is less prominent than in tinea cruris, and the rash is covered with fine wrinkles. Erythrasma fluoresces pink under Wood's light. Candidiasis of the groin may also mimic tinea cruris, but an important clue to the presence of *Candida* is the appearance of small satellite pustules beyond the free margin of the rash. Flexural psoriasis causes a vivid red and uniformly scaling rash in the groin, and there is usually at least one other site with typical psoriatic plaques.

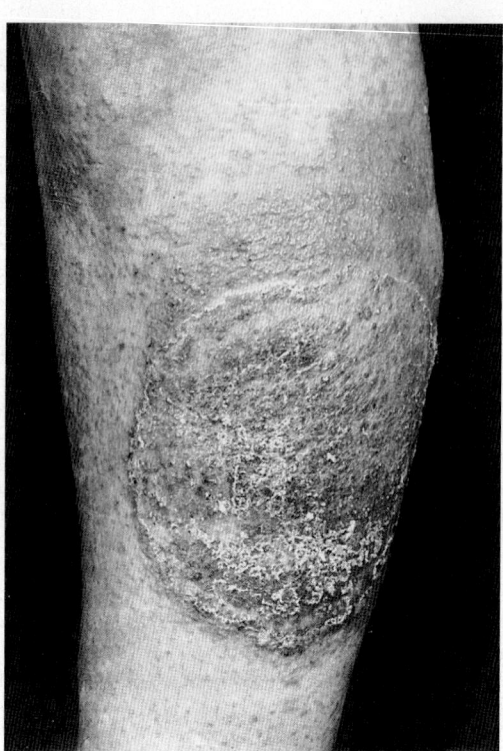

Figure 267-1 Inflammatory tinea corporis caused by *Trichophyton erinacei* (part of the *T. mentagrophytes* complex).

Tinea Corporis

Tinea corporis is one of the most commonly misdiagnosed skin diseases. Cases of this infection are not common in temperate climates, although it is seen more frequently in the tropics. This form of dermatophytosis has various clinical manifestations. Most lesions have a prominent edge that may contain pustules or follicular papules, and the center of the lesion is often less inflamed and scaly (Fig. 267-1). Sites commonly involved are the trunk and legs. Itching is variable, and lesions may be single or multiple. In general, infections caused by anthropophilic dermatophytes such as *T. rubrum* are less inflammatory and less clearly demarcated, and in some patients it is necessary to search for the margin carefully to delineate the rash. Lesions are usually hyperpigmented in pigmented skins. In contrast, zoophilic infections such as those caused by *M. canis* and *T. verrucosum* are more inflammatory, and lesions may become elevated and contain pustules. Infections caused by *M. gypseum* are also usually inflammatory and may have a brick-red appearance.

These clinical patterns vary with the site of infection. *T. rubrum* infections on the lower parts of the legs may lead to the formation of single or multiple deep nodules that may mimic erythema nodosum.[26] The overlying skin is dry, red, and scaly, which is a useful clue to the correct diagnosis. This form of infection, *nodular folliculitis,* follows follicular penetration of the hair follicles of the lower portions of the legs by the fungus. It occurs mainly in women. In patients with defective T-lymphocyte function, scaling is often minimal, and the rash of tinea corporis consists of grouped papules or pustules without significant erythema.

Tinea corporis can occur at any age, although in temperate countries, it is most often seen in children and is associated with zoophilic infections.

A number of different conditions should be considered in the differential diagnosis of tinea corporis, including eczema, psoriasis, and annular erythema. The important points to look for are the annular scaling margin of lesions and follicular prominence, which are features of dermatophytosis. However, it may be necessary to take scrapings for laboratory culture when there is doubt.

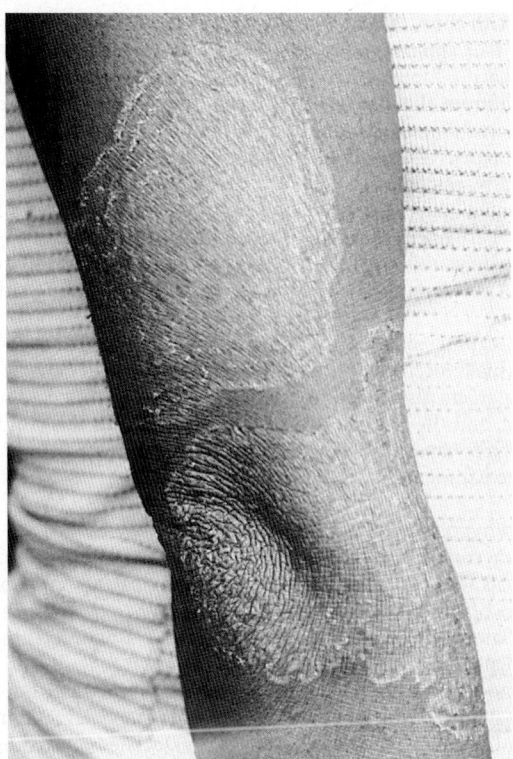

Figure 267-2 Early lesions of tinea imbricata, showing the first signs of concentric rings.

Tinea Imbricata

Tinea imbricata is a variant of tinea corporis that is caused by *T. concentricum*. The geographic distribution of the disease is shown in Table 267-2. Patients may be infected at any age, although infants and young children are most frequently affected. The main characteristic of the rash is the formation of concentric rings of scales (Fig. 267-2) over large parts of the body that amalgamate to form waves of scaling.[14] Other clinical varieties of tinea imbricata include the diffuse scaling variety, in which large flakes of skin are prominent. The disease gets its name *imbricata* (Latin for "tiled") from this clinical pattern. Other patients may have itchy lichenified lesions on the forearms. The face may be affected, as well as the sides of the fingers, but the feet, scalp, axillae, and groin are usually spared. Tinea imbricata is seldom mistaken for other diseases, and the inhabitants of endemic areas easily recognize the appearance of the infection and have specific names for it. In Papua New Guinea, it is called *sipoma* or *grille*.

Tinea Manuum

The term *tinea manuum* is used for dermatophyte infections involving the hand. In some patients, the dorsum of the hand may be affected, but most commonly the disease occurs on the palmar surface. A characteristic of dry-type infections at this site is involvement of only one palm, although in some patients, both may be affected. The clinical features are identical to those seen with dry-type infections of the sole. The usual cause is *T. rubrum*, and the feet are often involved, in addition to the hands.

Dermatophytosis affecting the palm may be confused with eczema, but the unilateral distribution of the infection and the common accompanying findings of onychomycosis and tinea pedis are helpful clues. Patients with palmoplantar keratoderma (tylosis) are particularly susceptible to superinfection of the palms and soles with dermatophytes.[27] This complication may be difficult to identify, but the skin may blister, and the hand usually itches. In such patients, fungi other than *T. rubrum* may be implicated.

Tinea Faciei

Dermatophyte infections of the face are usually caused by the same organisms associated with tinea corporis. Infections with *T. rubrum* at this site are often particularly difficult to recognize (tinea incognito). The facial skin becomes itchy and red, but the margin of the rash may be difficult to discern (Fig. 267-3). Some patients report that the facial rash is exacerbated by sun exposure. In other instances, lesions are more readily noticeable and affect the ears. Tinea faciei has been reported more frequently in patients with AIDS.

Tinea barbae (infection of the neck and beard area) may be pustular and inflamed because it is often caused by zoophilic organisms such as *T. verrucosum*. It is more localized than sycosis barbae, which is caused by *S. aureus;* this difference is helpful in distinguishing the two conditions.

Tinea Capitis

Scalp ringworm, or tinea capitis, is a disease of childhood. Its prevalence varies considerably in different parts of the world. The disease is widespread in some urban areas in the United States, Africa, and Europe. Tinea capitis is also common in parts of India. In northern Europe the disease is sporadic. The main reasons for these differences in the prevalence of infection in different localities are the nature of the infecting organisms and the availability of control measures. Endemic infections affecting large numbers of children are associated with anthropophilic organisms; sporadic disease is associated with zoophilic fungi. Tinea capitis is usually classified by the pattern of hair shaft invasion. Dermatophyte infections in which arthrospores are formed on the outside of the hair shaft are known as *ectothrix* infections; those in which the spores develop within the hair itself are known as *endothrix* infections. In *T. schoenleinii* infections, the fungi invade the hair medulla but then regress and leave tunnels containing air within the hair shaft (the "favic" pattern). Although it is identified

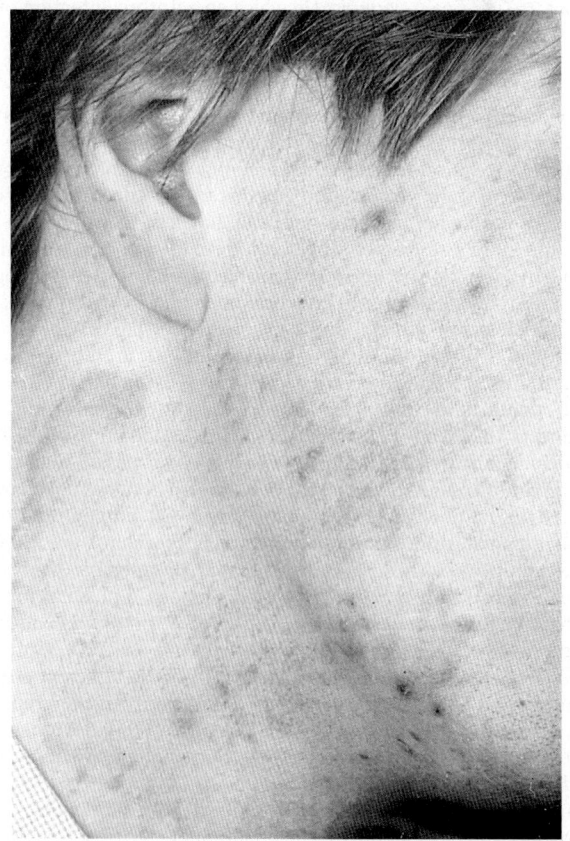

Figure 267-3 Tinea faciei caused by *Trichophyton rubrum*.

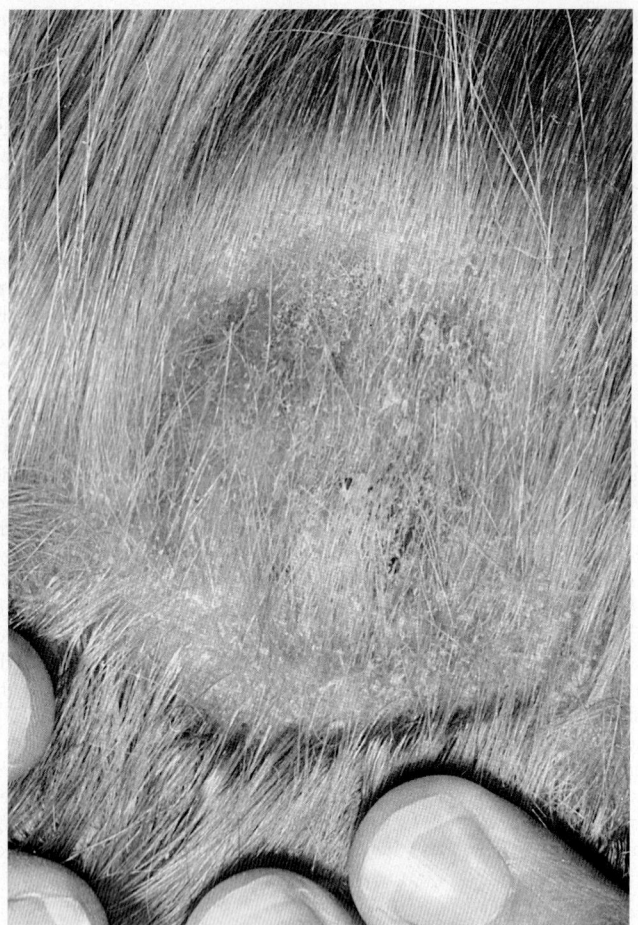

Figure 267-4 Scalp ringworm in which an ectothrix infection of the hair is caused by *Microsporum canis.*

as a childhood disease, adults exposed to *T. tonsurans* infections and patients with AIDS may develop tinea capitis.

The main clinical feature of dermatophyte scalp infections are the appearance of scaling of the scalp skin that is associated with a variable degree of erythema, inflammation, and alopecia. In some cases, the infection closely resembles seborrheic dermatitis or dandruff of the scalp. The infection is often accompanied by itching. A pathognomonic feature is hair loss. In ectothrix infections, hairs often break a few millimeters or more above the skin surface (Fig. 267-4). Broken or infected hairs are also slightly swollen and have a dull appearance. In endothrix infections, parasitized hairs break at the skin level. In some endothrix infections, scattered stumps can be seen within areas of hair loss (black-dot ringworm). In such cases, inflammation may be minimal. A further element in tinea capitis is the variable amount of inflammation, but in some cases, the whole area becomes pustular and covered with a thick scale or exudative crust. Often one of these elements dominates the clinical pattern. For instance, in some children there is little overt hair loss; the whole infection resembles seborrheic dermatitis. Likewise, in some ectothrix infections, a pustular form of dermatophytosis (kerion) develops. This is less common in endothrix infections. In most kerions, the pustules are not a sign of secondary bacterial infection,[28] although this may occur under adherent crusts.

Tinea capitis is uncommon in adults, although it has been reported with a variety of fungi such as *T. tonsurans* or *T. violaceum.* It has been associated with scarring alopecia of unknown etiology (pseudopelade) in adults.

In favus the same processes occur, but an important clinical characteristic is the formation of an inflammatory crust, or scutulum, composed of neutrophils and serous exudate around individual hair shafts. With time, these amalgamate over the surface of the scalp, so that the hair appears to be matted together with a thick crust that is said to have a mousy odor. In many patients, the signs are indistinguishable from those seen with other forms of scalp ringworm. Two other characteristics of favus are late shedding of hairs and a tendency to develop scarring alopecia. The infection may persist into adulthood, particularly in women.

Untreated scalp ringworm usually remits spontaneously after puberty. Permanent hair loss is uncommon unless the response has been severely inflammatory or the patient has favus. A surprising degree of recovery of hair growth occurs, even in children with severe kerions.

Tinea capitis must be distinguished from seborrheic dermatitis, which usually occurs in older children and does not cause hair loss. Alopecia areata also causes circumscribed areas of hair loss but does not scale, and the "exclamation mark" hairs seen in this condition—broken hairs tapering from the fractured end toward the skin surface—are pathognomonic.

Onychomycosis Caused by Dermatophytes
Onychomycosis, or fungal infection of the nails, usually occurs in individuals with infections of adjacent toe or palmar skin, except in rare cases of childhood nail infection in which nail plate invasion may develop without skin involvement. There are several different patterns of nail plate invasion.[29]

The most common clinical pattern of onychomycosis is distal and subungual onychomycosis, in which the nail plate is invaded from the distal and lateral borders. There is usually associated thickening of the nail, which becomes white, yellow, or brown. The brown discoloration is more common in the rare instances of *T. mentagrophytes* nail disease. In onychomycosis caused by endothrix scalp fungi such as *T. soudanense,* the thickening may be minimal, and the nail surface is pitted with small fissures.[30] The most common cause of onychomycosis is *T. rubrum,* which often accompanies long-standing disease, and the infection involves the entire nail plate.

Superficial white onychomycosis occurs when the nail plate is invaded from the top surface, which is eventually covered with white crumbly plaques. Other fungi, such as *Fusarium* spp., more commonly cause this pattern of nail invasion, but this may be followed by deeper penetration. However, in its pure form, superficial white onychomycosis can occur with *T. mentagrophytes,* and it may accompany distal and subungual onychomycosis in some *T. rubrum* infections. It may also accompany proximal subungual onychomycosis (described later).

In rare cases, invasion appears to originate from the proximal nail plate. This is usually a feature of relapse of treated nails, but rapidly spreading proximal nail plate invasion has also been described in patients with AIDS.[31] Patterns of infection differ with striate or continuous areas of infection. They may be caused by dermatophytes as well as nondermatophyte fungi such as *Fusarium* spp.

Onychomycosis can occur at any age, although it is more common with increasing age. Men and women are affected in equal numbers.

This infection must be distinguished from onychomycosis caused by *Candida,* in which there is little nail plate thickening but toenail infection is rare. *Scytalidium* infections may also lead to nail plate invasion. These are difficult to distinguish from infections caused by dermatophytes, but the nail plate is often not grossly thickened and may be severely undermined, and invasion affects predominantly the lateral border of the plate in the early stages of disease. Psoriasis of the nail also causes onycholysis, but the nail plate is typically covered with fine pits.

Deep Dermatophyte Infections
On rare occasions, patients known to be immunocompromised or otherwise healthy individuals develop dermatophyte infections in which the fungi invade subcutaneous tissues via the lymphatic vessels, usually causing clusters of granulomas, lymphedema (Fig. 267-5), and draining sinuses.[32] Sometimes aggregates of fungal hyphae resembling

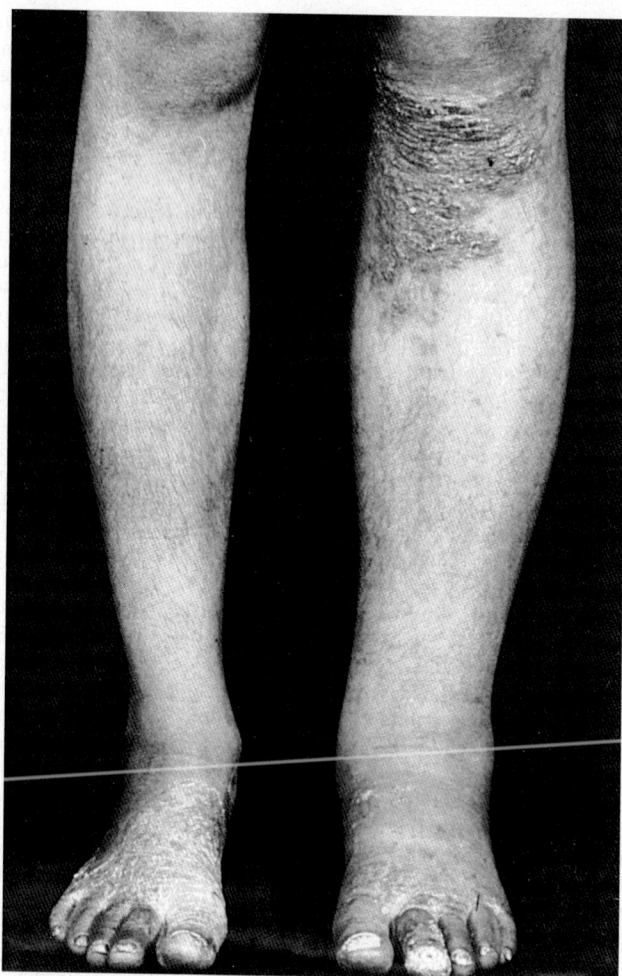

Figure 267-5 Deep dermatophytosis in which *Trichophyton rubrum* infection is causing unilateral lymphedema after invasion of the lymphatic vessels.

granuloma. It is usually sterile, although sometimes fragments of mycelium can be seen in histologic sections, and it resolves slowly with time.

LABORATORY DIAGNOSIS

In some cases it is possible to screen patients with scalp infections by using a filtered ultraviolet light source (Wood's light). Infections caused by *Microsporum* spp. fluoresce green. However, *Trichophyton* infections do not fluoresce, apart from favus, in which the hairs appear yellowish. Fluorescent hairs are infected, and apart from its use as a screening procedure, Wood's light examination may be helpful as a method of selecting hairs for microscopy and culture.

The laboratory diagnosis of dermatophytosis depends on the examination and culture of scrapings or clippings from lesions. It is important to sample the edge of skin lesions and infected nails. In the case of infected hairs, it is best to select broken stubs, which can be removed with forceps without undue trauma. Material should be allowed to soften in 10% to 20% potassium hydroxide before being examined under the microscope. Nails often take up to 2 hours to soften, although the process can be hastened by gentle warming. Fungal hyphae can be seen as chains of arthrospores in cleared scales or clippings. The fluorescent whitener calcofluor may also be used to stain fungi, but preparations have to be viewed with fluorescence microscopy; however, it may enhance the yield of positive samples.

Dermatophytes infecting hair have characteristic appearances that are helpful in recognition. Some form arthrospores on the outside of the hair shaft (ectothrix infections). The small spores can be seen by focusing the microscope on the edge of the epilated hair shaft. With most of the pathogenic *Microsporum* spp. that cause tinea capitis, small arthrospores are clustered around the outside of hair. By contrast, few *Trichophyton* spp. form ectothrix spores, but those that do, such as *T. verrucosum*, produce large arthrospores. The majority of *Trichophyton* spp. causing scalp ringworm form arthrospores within the hair shaft (endothrix infection). With some practice, it is possible to make a preliminary identification of the likely genus of invading fungus from the findings of the microscopic study of infected hair. *T. schoenleinii* invades hair, but hyphae regress and leave airspaces within the hair shaft.

Skin scrapings or nail clippings may also be cultured. Primary isolation is carried out at room temperature, usually on Sabouraud's agar containing antibiotics (penicillin-streptomycin or chloramphenicol) and cycloheximide (Acti-Dione), an antifungal agent that suppresses the growth of environmental contaminant fungi. In the case of nail disease, it is important to use media without cycloheximide because certain fungi, such as *Scytalidium*, that may infect nails are sensitive to the latter. Most dermatophytes can be identified within 2 weeks, although *T. verrucosum* grows best at 37° C and may have formed into only small and granular colonies at this stage. Identification depends on the gross colonial and microscopic morphologic features. In some cases, other tests involving nutritional requirements and hair penetration in vitro are necessary to confirm the identification. Molecular diagnosis of dermatophytosis is still in its beginning stages, although it has been used for this purpose.

In general, the identification of dermatophytes in skin material is simple and worth the effort necessary to obtain samples. It is particularly helpful in scalp infections, in which it is important to identify the likely source of infection.

TREATMENT

The usual approach to the management of dermatophyte infections is to treat with topical therapy if possible, but most nail and all hair infections and widespread dermatophytosis are best treated with oral drugs (Table 267-3).[33]

The main topical agents used for dermatophytosis are compounds with specific antifungal activity. The keratolytic agents such as Whit-

those found in eumycetomas may be observed in histologic sections. These dermatophyte "pseudomycetoma" grains may be surrounded by neutrophil abscesses, but the fungal hyphae are often engulfed by giant cells in tissue sections. Deep dermatophyte infections may extend further to involve draining lymph nodes or other sites, including the liver and brain, and they may be fatal.

Dermatophyte "Id" Reactions

The immune mechanisms in dermatophytosis may lead to the appearance of secondary rashes called *id reactions*. The most common of these is a type of acute vesicular eczema or pompholyx that occurs on the hands and feet in patients with inflammatory ringworm of the feet, mainly caused by *T. mentagrophytes*. These events are thought to be linked if the original dermatophyte infection becomes inflamed before the appearance of the secondary rash, if the latter is maximal on the affected foot, and if the patient has a strong delayed-type hypersensitivity reaction to intradermal trichophytin. The histologic pattern of this id reaction is that of eczema. A second form of id reaction, seen in patients with inflammatory tinea capitis or tinea corporis and usually caused by zoophilic organisms, consists of small follicular papules, some of which appear necrotic. This is a form of cutaneous vasculitis that usually subsides spontaneously. Both reactions may be triggered by antifungal therapy. Other less common types of id reactions include annular erythema and erythema nodosum.

Patients with follicular invasion by dermatophytes may develop a residual granuloma in the late stages of the disease called Majocchi's

TABLE 267-3 Treatment of Dermatophytosis

Dermatophytosis, Clinical Disease Pattern	Treatment
Tinea pedis	
• Interdigital	*Topical cream/ointment:* terbinafine, imidazoles (miconazole, econazole, clotrimazole, etc.), undecenoic acid, tolnaftate
• "Dry type"	*Oral:* terbinafine, 250 mg/day for 2-4 weeks; itraconazole, 400 mg/day for 1 week per month (repeated if necessary); fluconazole 200 mg weekly for 4-8 weeks
Tinea corporis	*Topical cream/ointment:* terbinafine, imidazoles (e.g., miconazole, econazole, clotrimazole)
• Small, well-defined lesions	*Oral:* terbinafine, 250 mg/day for 2 weeks; itraconazole, 200 mg/day for 1 week; fluconazole, 250 mg weekly for 2-4 weeks
• Larger lesions	Griseofulvin, 10-20 mg/kg/day for minimum 6 weeks
Tinea capitis	Terbinafine
	• <20 kg: 62.5 mg/day
	• 20-40 kg: 125 mg/day
	• >40 kg: 250 mg/day
	Itraconazole, 4-6 mg/kg pulsed dose weekly
Onychomycosis	Fluconazole, 3-8 mg/kg pulsed dose weekly
• Fingernails	Terbinafine, 250 mg daily for 6 weeks
	Itraconazole, 400 mg/day for 1 week each month, repeated for 2-3 months
	Fluconazole, 200 mg weekly for 8-16 weeks
• Toenails	Terbinafine, 250 mg daily for 12 weeks
	Itraconazole, 400 mg/day for 1 week each month, repeated for 2-4 months
	Fluconazole, 200 mg weekly for 12-24 weeks

field's ointment (salicylic and benzoic acid compound) are sometimes used. In the past, therapy relied on the use of substances, including dyes with weak antifungal activity, such as brilliant green and Castellani paint (magenta and resorcinol). Currently, a large group of specific antifungals may be used in treatment of dermatophytosis, although the use of some of these is largely confined to the treatment of tinea pedis. These drugs include chlorphenesin, undecylenate, and tolnaftate, which are available in cream or, in some cases, powder form. In few comparative studies have their relative merits been examined. Nonetheless, they are effective in uncomplicated cases. The most frequently used medications are the azole antifungals, which include miconazole, clotrimazole, econazole, tioconazole, ketoconazole, oxiconazole, bifonazole, isoconazole, and fenticonazole.[34] These are active against all the common skin fungi, and many can be taken once daily. Other potent antifungals used in the treatment of dermatophytosis are ciclopirox olamine, terbinafine, butenafine, and naftifine. It is difficult to choose between the different groups of these agents on the basis of well-constructed comparative studies.

In general, topical therapy for tinea pedis has to be continued for at least 2 and possibly 4 weeks. Topical terbinafine can be used to clear lesions of tinea pedis in 1 to 7 days and is also available as a single-dose film-forming solution applied to the soles of the feet. Tinea cruris usually responds within 2 or 3 weeks of the outset of treatment. Some of the azole agents can be used only once daily. Topical treatments for scalp and nail infections are generally ineffective, although cures of nail disease have been claimed for topically applied azoles. Three other preparations are of potential value in the management of nail disease. The first, a topically applied nail solution containing 28% tioconazole, has been found to produce mycologic and clinical remission on its own or in conjunction with oral griseofulvin. The second preparation is a combination of 40% urea and bifonazole. Urea is a potent hydrating agent and softens nails after application under occlusion. The 40% urea paste may be used to remove residual areas of infection after oral

therapy for onychomycosis.[35] This combination may also prove useful in addition to oral therapy for nail disease. Third, solutions with penetration enhancers, such as ciclopirox olamine and amorolfine used as a nail lacquer, are effective in a proportion of early cases of dermatophyte and *Candida* nail infection; these can also be applied once or twice weekly or as combination therapy with oral drugs in severe infections.[36]

The main oral antifungals used for dermatophytosis are terbinafine, itraconazole, and fluconazole. Griseofulvin is an alternative treatment but is still the treatment of choice for most cases of tinea capitis. Terbinafine is given in dosages of 250 mg daily for 2 weeks for tinea cruris or corporis, 6 weeks for fingernail infections, and 12 weeks for toenail infections. It produces rapid and long-lasting remissions for dry-type dermatophytosis and other skin infections. Itraconazole can be given continuously in dosages of 200 mg daily and is curative for tinea cruris or corporis after 1 week. Fluconazole can also be used as a treatment for dermatophytosis, but current regimens entail 150 to 300 mg weekly for infections of the skin. All three drugs are well tolerated and involve a low risk of hepatic injury (less than 1 per 70,000); in rare instances, terbinafine causes disturbance or loss of taste. All show evidence of efficacy; there is more information on terbinafine and itraconazole.[37,38]

Griseofulvin is given in dosages of 10 to 20 mg/kg daily in either tablet or syrup form and is still used in the treatment for tinea capitis. Adverse effects include headache, nausea, and abdominal discomfort. Less common reactions are urticaria, diarrhea, and photosensitivity. Griseofulvin may precipitate acute intermittent porphyria and systemic lupus erythematosus in predisposed subjects. Newer triazoles such as posaconazole, voriconazole, pramiconazole, and albaconazole are still under assessment in dermatophytosis. Oral therapy is used for scalp ringworm and nail infections. Scalp infections take 6 to 12 weeks to respond to griseofulvin. It is often useful to use a topical azole cream or shampoo in addition and, if crusts are present, to remove these with saline soaks. For the treatment of large numbers of infected children, intermittent therapy with up to 1 g of griseofulvin has been suggested; treatment may be repeated after 6 weeks. A substantial percentage of those infections may respond to single-dose therapy. Itraconazole and terbinafine are also effective in treating scalp disease, and pediatric formulations are in development.[39] Terbinafine is very effective against *Trichophyton* scalp infections but less active against *Microsporum*, for which a double dosage is advised; treatment is for 4 weeks. It is important to attempt to identify the organism causing scalp infection because, if the infection is of human origin, it can spread to other contacts, and it may be necessary to screen classmates or members of the families of children with anthropophilic infections. Zoophilic infections do not usually spread from child to child, although several family members exposed to the same source of infection may develop scalp disease.

Onychomycosis caused by dermatophytes can be treated with oral therapy. Terbinafine and itraconazole have replaced griseofulvin for this indication. For instance, in 70% to 80% of patients, terbinafine produces cure in 6 weeks for fingernails and 12 weeks for toenails.[40] Itraconazole is also effective against toenail infections at a dose of 200 mg daily for 3 months. However, for nail infections, it is usually administered as a "pulsed" treatment given for 1 week of each month at a dosage of 400 mg daily, the week's course being repeated once more for fingernail infections (two pulses) and twice or three times for toenail disease (three or four pulses).[41] Reported remission rates are above 60%. Intermittent regimens with fluconazole (300 and 450 mg weekly) are used in the treatment of onychomycosis.[42] There have been no large comparative studies of fluconazole versus the other two treatments for nail disease. However, one large double-blind study was conducted in which terbinafine, given continuously at 250 mg daily for 12 or 16 weeks, was compared with pulsed itraconazole, at 200 mg twice a day for 1 week each month repeated three or four times, in toenail onychomycosis. The results revealed significantly better responses for both terbinafine groups in both mycologic and clinical remission rates.[43]

Scytalidium Infections

Infections caused by the pigmented fungus *S. dimidiatum* closely resemble dry-type dermatophytosis caused by *T. rubrum. S. dimidiatum* (proposed to be reclassified as *Neoscytalidium dimidiatum*) was originally described as a pathogen in plants, but it appears to be a genuine cause of human infection. A similar type of infection has been ascribed to a nonpigmented mold, *S. hyalinum.* In both cases, the affected patients came from the tropics.

The precise mechanisms of infection with either organism are unknown. *S. hyalinum* has never been isolated from the environment, and although *S. dimidiatum* is a pathogen of certain plants such as fruit trees, patients do not usually give a specific history of exposure. It has been found that healthy individuals in some tropical areas carry these organisms on the feet but do not have overt disease, which suggests that asymptomatic carriage may, under the appropriate conditions, be followed by infection. Infections have been described in immigrants from tropical areas to the United Kingdom, Canada, and France. They have also been identified in the southern United States, Trinidad, Colombia, Ecuador, and India, and it is likely that it is more widespread. On occasion, it may be seen in patients who have paid short visits to the tropics.

CLINICAL FEATURES

The clinical signs of skin infection with both *Scytalidium* species are identical to those associated with dry-type *T. rubrum* infections.[44] There is scaling of the lateral interdigital spaces, over the soles, and on one or both palms. Itching is usually minimal. Onychomycosis may also develop. Often there is early invasion of the lateral border of the nail without significant thickening of the nail plate (Fig. 267-6), but eventually the whole nail plate may be undermined, and onycholysis may lead to shedding of the complete nail. Hyperpigmented streaks may occur in the nails, although these are not pathognomonic for these infections and can be seen with other forms of inflammatory nail dystrophy. Deep infections such as sporotrichoid *Scytalidium* infections and a brain abscess have rarely been reported, mainly in immunocompromised patients.[45]

DIAGNOSIS

Scrapings or nail clippings examined after treatment with potassium hydroxide contain sinuous fungal hyphae. Close inspection reveals that the structure is different from that normally seen with dermatophyte hyphae, but accurate discrimination requires experience. Both organisms grow on Sabouraud's agar but are inhibited if cycloheximide (Acti-Dione) is incorporated in the medium.

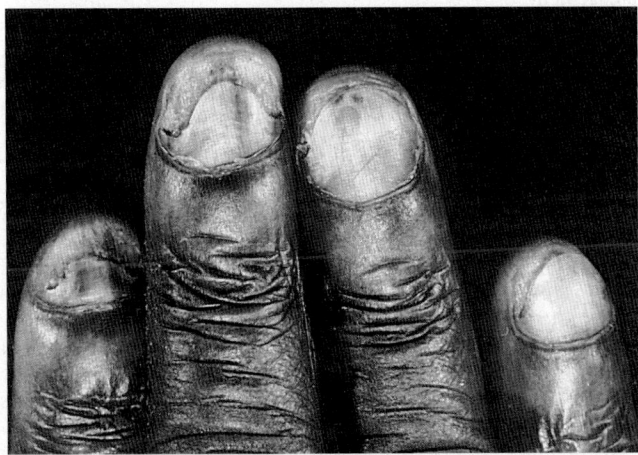

Figure 267-6 Onychomycosis caused by *Scytalidium dimidiatum.*

TREATMENT

There is no satisfactory therapy for either infection. Whitfield's ointment (6% benzoic acid and 3% salicylic acid) may be used to treat *Scytalidium* infections of the sole or the palm. However, none of the specific antifungal drugs currently available produces consistent results.

Other Forms of Onychomycosis

A number of other fungi may cause onychomycosis. The most common of these is *Scopulariopsis brevicaulis,* which usually causes infection of the great toenails. Some patients with this form of infection have previously abnormal toenails (e.g., onychogryphosis). *Scopulariopsis* infections of the nails have a typical cinnamon color that is caused by the presence of fungal spores seen on direct microscopic views of the nail. The fungus is easy to isolate in culture. Treatment may be difficult, but chemical nail removal with 40% urea may be useful.

Superficial white onychomycosis may be caused by *Acremonium* or *Fusarium* species. These infections are similar to those caused by *T. mentagrophytes,* and the identity of the causative organisms should be confirmed by culture.

On occasion, other fungi are isolated from nail material. In many cases, they appear to be colonizing the undersurface of dystrophic nail plate. On rare occasions, however, they may contribute to the nail disease by invasion. This is best established by repeated attempts at culture, and if the organism is isolated on numerous occasions and if hyphae are present in the nail, it is likely that the organism is involved in the nail disease. Examples of infections caused by a range of different organisms, such as *Aspergillus, Fusarium,* and *Acremonium* spp., have been recorded. *Fusarium* is now known to cause a range of fungal nail infections from superficial white onychomycosis to paronychia and proximal subungual disease; in severely neutropenic patients, nail infection may be followed by systemic dissemination of the fungus. Oral therapy is seldom effective against these infections,[46] and nail removal with 40% urea is probably the best alternative treatment.

Pityriasis Versicolor

Pityriasis versicolor, or tinea versicolor, is a superficial infection caused by *Malassezia* species, which are lipophilic yeasts that are normal commensals on the skin surface.[47] The infection is confined to the trunk or proximal aspects of the limbs. It does not cause hair and nail plate invasions.

ORGANISMS

The normal skin is colonized in late childhood and adult life by lipophilic yeasts. Morphologically, these are either oval (most common on the scalp) or round (mainly on the trunk), and they were previously called *Pityrosporum ovale* and *Pityrosporum orbiculare,* respectively. These organisms have now been reclassified as members of the genus *Malassezia,* among which there are seven pathogenic species: *Malassezia furfur, Malassezia pachydermatis* (not associated with human skin infections), *Malassezia sympodialis, Malassezia globosa, Malassezia restricta, Malassezia obtusa,* and *Malassezia slooffiae.*[47] Round yeasts, usually *M. globosa,* are seen in lesions of pityriasis versicolor accompanied by short, stubby hyphae; *M. furfur* may produce filaments as well but is less common.

PATHOGENESIS

The infection is associated with transformation of yeast-phase organisms into hyphal forms, although occasional patients with pityriasis versicolor have only oval yeasts. The stimulus for this phase change is unknown. Infections are more common in the tropics and may appear after sun exposure, which may therefore be a trigger factor. Patients with Cushing's syndrome may also develop this infection, but diseases related to T-lymphocyte suppression are not necessarily associated with pityriasis versicolor.[48]

A carboxylic acid called *azelaic acid,* thought to be produced by the organism in the stratum corneum, is believed to lead to the depigmentation seen in lesions.[49] *Malassezia* yeasts grow in the presence of medium-chain fatty acids.

Different species of *Malassezia* obviously play a role in the development of disease, although it is not known why, for instance, *M. globosa* in particular should be associated with pityriasis versicolor.

CLINICAL FEATURES

Pityriasis versicolor is usually seen on the trunk or proximal portions of the limbs, although more extensive infections involving the face and waist area occur in the tropics. Lesions may be hypopigmented or hyperpigmented macules that amalgamate to cover the affected area with scaling plaques. The lesions are usually not itchy. In some patients, lesions may remit spontaneously. Rare clinical variants include some infections that result in anetoderma, or localized skin atrophy.

The diagnosis can be confirmed by direct microscopic study of lesions, on which the characteristic round yeast forms and short hyphae can be seen. The scrapings can be viewed after clearing with potassium hydroxide but are seen more clearly after staining with a mixture of Parker ink and potassium hydroxide. Lesions fluoresce yellow-green under Wood's light, although this may not be seen on all affected areas. *Malassezia* yeasts are difficult to culture unless oil is added to the medium. An overlay of Tween 80 encourages growth.

TREATMENT

The most appropriate therapy for pityriasis versicolor is a topical azole or terbinafine cream; cheaper alternatives, now less often used, are 2% selenium sulfide lotion or 20% sodium thiosulfate applied daily for 10 to 14 days. These alternative preparations may be irritative. In some cases, intermittent applications of 50% propylene glycol in water prevent a relapse.[50] In severe cases, itraconazole produces remissions. The effective dosage of itraconazole is 200 mg daily for 5 days. Ketoconazole, in dosages of 200 mg daily for 5 to 10 days or a single 400-mg dose, may be used.

Patients usually have to be warned that the pigmentary changes may return to normal only after many months, even when the infection has been successfully treated.

◼ Other *Malassezia* Infections

Two other skin conditions are associated with *Malassezia* yeasts: *Malassezia* folliculitis and seborrheic dermatitis. In addition, this fungus has caused catheter-acquired sepsis (see Chapter 269).

MALASSEZIA FOLLICULITIS

There are three main forms of this condition. The first is a folliculitis on the back or upper part of the chest that consists of scattered follicular papules or pustules. These are itchy and often appear after sun exposure. In the second form, which is seen in patients with seborrheic dermatitis, there are numerous small follicular papules over the upper and lower portions of the back and chest. Erythema and greasy perifollicular scales are often seen in these patients. In the third form, multiple pustules are seen on the trunk and face in patients with HIV infection. This type is similar to the second form, and affected patients usually have severe seborrheic dermatitis.

Scrapings or biopsy specimens from lesions show numerous yeasts occluding the mouths of follicles. Treatment with topical azole antifungals may be effective, but oral therapy with itraconazole is often necessary.

SEBORRHEIC DERMATITIS

In the early part of the 20th century, seborrheic dermatitis and dandruff of the scalp were thought to be caused by *Malassezia* yeasts because numerous organisms were present in skin scales. This view was subsequently superseded by the belief that the yeasts were secondary to a hyperproliferative state. However, evidence suggests that *Malassezia* is implicated in the pathogenesis of the condition.[51]

In most cases, seborrheic dermatitis responds to oral ketoconazole or topical azole antifungals. Improvement is associated with disappearance of the organisms, and relapse is associated with recolonization. Furthermore, the clinical appearances can be mimicked in animals with the application of both live and killed organisms to the skin. Some patients with seborrheic dermatitis have high titers of antibody to *Malassezia* species.

It is unlikely that invasion of the epidermis is responsible for the appearance of seborrheic dermatitis, but an indirect disease mechanism such as sensitization or toxic damage is possible.

Seborrheic dermatitis can appear in any individual, although it is said to be particularly common in patients with neurologic disease, such as parkinsonism. In patients with AIDS, the onset of seborrheic dermatitis may be sudden and the rash more extensive than in other individuals.[52] The histology of seborrheic dermatitis is similar in all groups. Acanthosis and hyperkeratosis with elongation of dermal papillae are seen. An infiltrate of polymorphs in the epidermis above the dermal papillae is also often seen. HIV-positive patients tend to have more plasma cells in the infiltrate. These changes are similar to those seen in some forms of psoriasis.

Clinical Features

The classic features of seborrheic dermatitis make up a range of different clinical appearances. These include erythema and scaling of the central part of the anterior aspect of the chest and the upper part of the back that are accompanied by a variable degree of itching. On the face, there is erythema with greasy scales in the eyebrows, around the alae nasi, behind the ears, and in the external ears. Scaling may also appear in the presternal areas of the chest and on the back. Scaling on the scalp is accompanied by the appearance of pustules in some patients. The clinical appearances are typical, and fungal scrapings are unnecessary.

Other forms of skin disease, including severe erythroderma in infants and an intertriginous rash in adults, have also been called "seborrheic dermatitis," but these lesions do not appear to be related to the variety discussed here.

Treatment

The main therapy involves the use of topical azole creams and weak topical corticosteroids such as 1% hydrocortisone. Relapse is common, but repeated treatment when necessary is the simplest approach to management.

Malassezia is also associated with a form of atopic dermatitis affecting the face in young adults. It is believed that sensitization may play a role in exacerbating the inflammatory responses in eczematous skin.[53]

◼ Tinea Nigra

Tinea nigra is a superficial form of phaeohyphomycosis caused by *Phaeoannellomyces werneckii* (also called *Hortaea werneckii* and *Exophiala werneckii*). The infection is confined to the stratum corneum of the palms or soles and occurs mainly in the tropics or subtropics in children or young adults.

The typical lesion of tinea nigra is a superficial scaling macule that is brown or black on the palms or soles. The pigmentation is irregularly distributed over larger lesions. Spread of the infection to other sites is rare, and lesions remain asymptomatic.

The main differential diagnosis is a superficial form of melanoma or a pigmented nevus. The pigmented hyphae can be seen by direct microscopic study of skin scrapings treated with potassium hydroxide. The organism can also be cultured from scrapings.

The best therapy is treatment with a topical azole or a keratolytic agent such as Whitfield's ointment or 5% to 10% salicylic acid ointment.

White Piedra

White piedra is an uncommon infection caused by yeasts of the genus *Trichosporon*, namely, *Trichosporon ovoides* (scalp hair), *Trichosporon inkin* (pubic hair), and *Trichosporon asahii* (rare in piedra). The infection occurs in both the tropics and temperate zones. It is a superficial infection of the hair shafts of the scalp, body, or pubic hair. *Trichosporon* species may also cause a systemic infection in neutropenic patients (see Chapter 269).

The organisms may be carried on the skin or around the anus. In some patients, the infection appears to be sexually transmitted. White piedra is asymptomatic and manifests with small yellow concretions on the hair shafts.[54] The pathogenesis of this infection is still unclear, but it is likely to result from synergy between the fungi and coryneform bacteria.[55] The lesions are circumscribed and appear as small nodules, unlike the more diffuse coating of axillary or pubic hair seen in trichomycosis axillaris, which is caused by the presence of bacteria on the hair.

The diagnosis may be confirmed by examining an epilated hair mounted in potassium hydroxide. Each nodule contains fungal hyphae, and the organisms can be cultured from infected hairs without difficulty.

Treatment is difficult. Nodules may be removed simply by shaving. Otherwise, coating the hairs with an azole such as econazole or treating the patient with oral ketoconazole may cure the infection. Relapse is common after therapy.

Black Piedra

Black piedra is another infection of the hair shafts that is caused by a black yeast, *Piedraia hortae*. The disease is rare and confined mainly to parts of the humid tropics. The infection manifests with small black nodules on the hairs of the scalp and less commonly elsewhere. These have to be distinguished from pediculosis, but itching is usually absent in black piedra. With direct microscopy, these nodules can be shown to be composed of hyphal elements and small ascospores of the causative agent within a dark cement-containing stroma. Treating hairs with a topical salicylic acid, 2% formaldehyde, or an azole cream is usually sufficient, although relapse is common.

REFERENCES

1. Midgley M, Clayton YM, Hay RJ. *Medical Mycology*. London: Gower; 1997.
2. Gräser Y, De Hoog S, Summerbell RC. Dermatophytes: recognizing species of clonal fungi. *Med Mycol*. 2006;44:199-209.
3. Tsuboi R, Okeke CN, Inoue A, et al. Identification and viability assessment of dermatophyte infecting nail based on quantitative PCR of dermatophyte actin (ACT) mRNA. *Nippon Ishinkin Gakkai Zasshi*. 2002;43:91-93.
4. Giddey K, Favre B, Quadroni M, et al. Closely related dermatophyte species produce different patterns of secreted proteins. *FEMS Microbiol Lett*. 2007;267:95-101.
5. Baeza LC, Favre B, Borges CL, et al. cDNA representational difference analysis used in the identification of genes expressed by *Trichophyton rubrum* during contact with keratin. *Microbes Infect*. 2007;9:1415-1421.
6. Mignon B, Tabart J, Baldo A, et al. Immunization and dermatophytes. *Curr Opin Infect Dis*. 2008;21:134-140.
7. Ghannoum M, Isham N, Hajjeh R, et al. Tinea capitis in Cleveland: survey of elementary school students. *J Am Acad Dermatol*. 2003;48:189-193.
8. Weitzman I, Summerbell RC. The dermatophytes. *Clin Microbiol Rev*. 1995;8:240-259.
9. Seyfarth F, Ziemer M, Gräser Y, et al. Widespread tinea corporis caused by *Trichophyton rubrum* with non-typical cultural characteristics—diagnosis via PCR. *Mycoses*. 2007;50(Suppl 2):26-30.
10. Gentles JC, Evans EGV. Foot infections in swimming baths. *BMJ*. 1973;3:260-262.
11. Hope YM, Clayton YM, Hay RJ, et al. Foot infection in coal miners: a review (western Africa). *Br J Dermatol*. 1985;112:405-413.
12. Gazit R, Hershko K, Ingbar A, et al. Immunological assessment of familial tinea corporis. *J Eur Acad Dermatol Venereol*. 2008;22:871-874.
13. Blank H, Taplin D, Zaias N. Cutaneous *Trichophyton mentagrophytes* infections in Vietnam. *Arch Dermatol*. 1969;99:135-144.
14. Hay RJ. Tinea imbricata. *Curr Top Med Mycol*. 1987;2:55-72.
15. Ménan EI, Zongo-Bonou O, Rouet F, et al. Tinea capitis in schoolchildren from Ivory Coast (western Africa). A 1998-1999 cross-sectional study. *Int J Dermatol*. 2002;41:204-207.
16. Ive FA. The carrier state of tinea capitis in Nigeria. *Br J Dermatol*. 1966;22:219-221.
17. Blank F, Mann SJ, Peak PA. Distribution of dermatophytosis according to age, ethnic group and sex. *Sabouraudia*. 1974;12:352-361.
18. Zurita J, Hay RJ. The adherence of dermatophyte microconidia and arthroconidia to human keratinocytes in vitro. *J Invest Dermatol*. 1987;89:529-534.
19. Hay RJ. Fungal infections. In: Bos JD, ed. *Skin Immune System (SIS)*. Boca Raton, FL: CRC Press; 2006:598-607.
20. Serjeantson S, Lawrence G. Autosomal recessive inheritance of susceptibility to tinea imbricata. *Lancet*. 1977;1:13-15.

21. Brouta F, Descamps F, Monod M, et al. Secreted metalloprotease gene family of *Microsporum canis*. *Infect Immun*. 2002;70:5676-5683.
22. Jones HE, Reinhardt JH, Rinaldi MG. Acquired immunity to dermatophytosis. *Arch Dermatol*. 1974;109:840-848.
23. Shiraki Y, Ishibashi Y, Hiruma M, et al. Cytokine secretion profiles of human keratinocytes during *Trichophyton tonsurans* and *Arthroderma benhamiae* infections. *J Med Microbiol*. 2006;55:1175-1185.
24. Green F, Lee KW, Balish E. Chronic *T. mentagrophytes* dermatophytosis of guinea pig skin grafts on nude mice. *J Invest Dermatol*. 1982;79:125-131.
25. Leyden JJ, Kligman AM. Interdigital athletes foot, the interaction of dermatophytes and residual bacteria. *Arch Dermatol*. 1978;114:1466-1472.
26. Das S, Saha R, Bhattacharya SN. Disseminated nodular granulomatous perifolliculitis. *Indian J Med Microbiol*. 2007;25:288-290.
27. Elmros T, Liden S. Hereditary palmo-plantar keratoderma: incidence of dermatophyte infections and the results of topical treatment with retinoic acid. *Acta Derm Venereol*. 1983;63:254-257.
28. Martin ES, Elewski BE. Tinea capitis in adult women masquerading as bacterial pyoderma. *J Am Acad Dermatol*. 2003;49(2 Suppl.):S177-S179.
29. Baran R, Hay RJ, Tosti A, et al. A new classification of onychomycosis. *Br J Dermatol*. 1998;139:567-571.
30. Kalter DC, Hay RJ. Onychomycosis due to *Trichophyton soudanense*. *Clin Exp Dermatol*. 1988;13:221-227.
31. Weismann K, Knudsen EA, Pedersen C. White nails in AIDS/ARC due to *Trichophyton rubrum* infection. *Clin Exp Dermatol*. 1988;13:24-27.
32. Allen DE, Snyderman R, Meadows L, et al. Generalized *Microsporum audouinii* infection and depressed cellular immunity associated with a missing plasma factor required for lymphocyte blastogenesis. *Am J Med*. 1977;63:991-1000.
33. Gupta AK, Ryder JE, Chow M, et al. Dermatophytosis: the management of fungal infections. *Skinmed*. 2005;4:305-310.
34. Fernandez-Obregon AC, Rohrback J, Reichel MA, et al. Current use of anti-infectives in dermatology. *Expert Rev Anti Infect Ther*. 2005;3:557-591.
35. Hay RJ, Roberts D, Richardson M, et al. The evaluation of bifonazole 1% and 40% urea paste in the management of onychomycosis. *Clin Exp Dermatol*. 1988;13:164-167.
36. Baran R, Sigurgeirsson B, de Berker D, et al. A multicentre, randomized, controlled study of the efficacy, safety and cost-effectiveness of a combination therapy with amorolfine nail lacquer and oral terbinafine compared with oral terbinafine alone for the treatment of onychomycosis with matrix involvement. *Br J Dermatol*. 2007;157:149-157.
37. Roberts DT, Taylor WD, Boyle J. British Association of Dermatologists: guidelines for treatment of onychomycosis. *Br J Dermatol*. 2003;148:402-410.

38. Bell-Syer SE, Hart R, Crawford F, et al. Oral treatments for fungal infections of the skin of the foot. *Cochrane Database Syst Rev*. 2002(2):CD003584.
39. Elewski B. Cutaneous mycoses in children. *Br J Dermatol*. 1996;134(Suppl. 46):7-11.
40. Drake LA, Shear NH, Arlette JP, et al. Oral terbinafine in the treatment of toe nail onychomycosis: North American multicenter trial. *J Am Acad Dermatol*. 1997;37:740-745.
41. Odom RB, Aly R, Scher RK, et al. A multicenter, placebo-controlled, double-blind study of intermittent therapy with itraconazole for the treatment of onychomycosis of the finger nail. *J Am Acad Dermatol*. 1997;36:231-235.
42. Scher RK, Breneman D, Rich P, et al. Once-weekly fluconazole (150, 300 or 450 mg) in the treatment of distal subungual onychomycosis of the toenail. *J Am Acad Dermatol*. 1998;38:S77-S86.
43. Evans EG, Sigurgeirsson B. Double blind, randomised study of continuous terbinafine compared with intermittent itraconazole in treatment of toenail onychomycosis. The LION study group. *BMJ*. 1999;318:1031-1035.
44. Hay RJ, Moore MK. The clinical features of superficial infections caused by *Hendersonula toruloidea* and *Scytalidium hyalinum*. *Br J Dermatol*. 1984;110:677-684.
45. Mani RS, Chickabasaviah YT, Nagarathna S, et al. Cerebral phaeohyphomycosis caused by *Scytalidium dimidiatum*: a case report from India. *Med Mycol*. 2008;46:705-711.
46. Gupta AK, Gregurek-Novak T, Konnikov N, et al. Itraconazole and terbinafine treatment of some nondermatophyte molds causing onychomycosis of the toes and a review of the literature. *J Cutan Med Surg*. 2001;5:206-210.
47. Crespo Erchiga V, Delgado Florencio V. *Malassezia* species in skin diseases. *Curr Opin Infect Dis*. 2002;15:133-142.
48. Ashbee HR, Evans EG. Immunology of diseases associated with *Malassezia* species. *Clin Microbiol Rev*. 2002;15:21-57.
49. Nazzaro-Porro M, Passi S. Identification of tyrosinase inhibitors in cultures of *Pityrosporum*. *J Invest Dermatol*. 1978;71:205-208.
50. Faergemann J, Fredriksson T. Propylene glycol in the treatment of pityriasis versicolor. *Acta Derm Venereol*. 1980;60:92-93.
51. Shuster S. The aetiology of dandruff and the mode of action of therapeutic agents. *Br J Dermatol*. 1984;111:235-242.
52. Garman ME, Tyring SK. The cutaneous manifestations of HIV infection. *Dermatol Clin*. 2002;20:193-214.
53. Johansson C, Eshaghi H, Linder MT, et al. Positive atopy patch test reaction to *Malassezia furfur* in atopic dermatitis correlates with a T helper 2–like peripheral blood mononuclear cells response. *J Invest Dermatol*. 2002;118:1044-1051.
54. Kalter DCA, Tschen JA, Cernoch PL, et al. Genital white piedra: epidemiology, microbiology and therapy. *J Am Acad Dermatol*. 1986;14:982-993.
55. Youker SR, Andreozzi RJ, Appelbaum PC, et al. White piedra: further evidence of a synergistic infection. *J Am Acad Dermatol*. 2003;49:746-749.

268

Paracoccidioides brasiliensis

ANGELA RESTREPO | ANGELA MARÍA TOBÓN

Paracoccidioidomycosis is a chronic, systemic, and progressive disease that usually afflicts men engaged in agriculture. Although the lungs are the site of primary infection, medical consultation is usually sought because of disseminated lesions, mainly in the mucous membranes, skin, system, and adrenals.

Description of the Pathogen

The causative agent is a thermally dimorphic fungus, *Paracoccidioides brasiliensis,* recently classified in the phylum Ascomycota, order Onygenales, family Onygenaceae (sensu lato), despite the fact that the teleomorph has not been discovered.[1,2] Recent rRNA analyses have further divided the Onygenaceae into several clades, one of which, the Ajellomycetacea, encompasses *P. brasiliensis.* Multilocus genealogies have revealed that this fungus is actually composed of three distinct phylogenetic species (S1, PS2, PS3), which are confined to particular endemic regions.[3]

Microscopically, in cultures at 37°C, as well as in tissues and exudates, the fungus appears as an oval to round yeast cell that is variable in size (4 to 40 μm) and surrounded by a translucent double-contoured cell wall; intracytoplasmic lipid globules are characteristic and prominent. It reproduces by multiple budding; typically, numerous blastoconidia, usually small (4 to 6 μm), surround the mother cell, to which they are connected by short cytoplasmic bridges mimicking a "pilot wheel." This cell is a hallmark of *P. brasiliensis* (Figs. 268-1 and 268-2). Colonies produced at 37°C grow in approximately 10 days and are soft, cream-colored, and wrinkled.[4-6] The fungus develops as a slow-growing mold (20 to 30 days) at lower temperatures, below 26°C and including 4°C if in liquid substrates. In solid media, colonies are white and demonstrate short tufts of white aerial mycelia, but then they become cotton-like and adhere strongly to the agar. The area beneath is often brownish because of the production of melanin-like substances.[7] Microscopically, only chlamydoconidias and thin septate hyphae are observed when the mold is grown in regular mycologic media. Media with reduced carbohydrate content may give rise to arthroconidia and other types of microconidia, propagules considered to be the infectious particles in nature. Conidia have a single nucleus whereas yeasts and mycelia are multinucleated.[8] These propagules are small (4 to 5 μm) and, when given to mice intranasally, convert into yeast cells in approximately 72 hours, giving rise to progressive disease as well as pulmonary fibrosis. Thus, *P. brasiliensis* undergoes a complex transformation in vivo and also in vitro at 36° to 37°C; there is a transformation from a mycelial saprobic form growing at environmental temperatures to a virulent yeast form occurring at the mammalian host's temperature.[9-11] Morphologic transition is an important virulence trait. Together with the fungal capacity for adherence, production of proteolytic enzymes and melanin, and other traits, this prepares the fungus for its interaction with the accidental human host. Genomic studies are permitting a more refined characterization of those genes involved in host adaptation and survival.

Ecology and Epidemiology

The most notable ecologic characteristic of paracoccidioidomycosis is, perhaps, its restricted geographic distribution. It has been reported only in Latin America from Mexico (23 degrees N) to Argentina (34 degrees S); however, some countries within these latitudes are not affected (e.g., some Caribbean islands and Chile). Furthermore, the disorder does not afflict persons living in every region of the affected areas. Endemic centers are located in regions with relatively well-defined ecologic characteristics—in the tropical and subtropical forests, where temperatures are mild and humidity is relatively high and constant throughout the year.[5,6,12]

Brazil constitutes the heart of the endemic area and is followed at a distance by Colombia, Venezuela, Ecuador, Argentina, and other Latin American countries.[4,6,13] The annual incidence rate in Brazil varies from 10 to 30/million inhabitants; the mean mortality rate is 1.4/million.[14] In Colombia, the incidence is much lower and fluctuates (between 0.5 and 2.2/million) from year to year.[12] In a 21-year period, 1950 fatal cases of this mycosis were reported in São Paulo State, Brazil (92 patients/year), with the mycosis being the direct cause of death in 60% of cases.[15] Despite the fact that approximately 60 nonautochthonous cases have now been reported in North America, Europe, and Asia, every patient had previously resided in a recognized endemic country.[16-18]

Molecular tools have shown that fungal isolates obtained from various endemic countries are restricted geographically, which indicates that they occupy specialized endemic niches in nature.[19] Restricted geographic distribution indicates an equally limited habitat for *P. brasiliensis,* one that has proved elusive. The fungus has been isolated from nonhuman sources only sporadically, six times from soil and once each from a commercial chow and from penguin feces.[20] Naturally acquired animal infection has been repeatedly demonstrated in armadillos (*Dasypus novemcinctus*), a mammal distributed in areas that coincide closely to the distribution of the mycosis.[12,21] Disease in dogs and other mammals has also been reported. Despite the clue offered by such isolations, attempts to locate the precise microniche of the fungus have failed. Outbreaks have not been reported and consequently valuable information pointing toward the fungus niche is unavailable. Skin test surveys have revealed a significant prevalence of delayed hypersensitivity reactions to paracoccidioidin (close to 70%) among farm workers.[4,6,13] An ecologic analysis centered on the conditions prevailing in endemic countries has revealed that coffee- and tobacco-growing regions, as well as high humidity and heavy annual precipitation, correlate significantly with the presence of the mycosis. This has been confirmed in children and the indigenous population of the Brazilian Amazon basin, and in both occasions the unusual number of paracoccidioidomycosis cases revealed that changes in the traditional economic system and agricultural practices in the corresponding regions had resulted in increased contact with the fungus.[22,23] Paracoccidioidomycosis is not contagious from person to person. The imprecise knowledge on *P. brasiliensis* habitat has hindered determination of the route of infection. Nonetheless, clinical and pathophysiologic observations plus experimental animal studies have ruled out traumatic implantation and indicated inhalation as the infectious route.[2,24]

The age and gender distribution of clinical cases is peculiar. The mycosis is rare in children and teenagers, and most patients are 30 years of age or older.[4,23,25-28] Men are more commonly afflicted than women, at a mean ratio of 15:1. This is in contrast to the rate of infection as determined by a paracoccidioidin skin test, which is similar for both genders. Of interest is the fact that when the disease occurs in prepubertal patients, this gender difference does not exist.[5,6,13] It has been suggested that the marked gender difference seen in adults could be explained by the inhibitory action of estrogens on the conidia or mycelium transition to yeast cells. Male mice infected with *P. brasiliensis* conidia were shown to develop a progressively disseminated

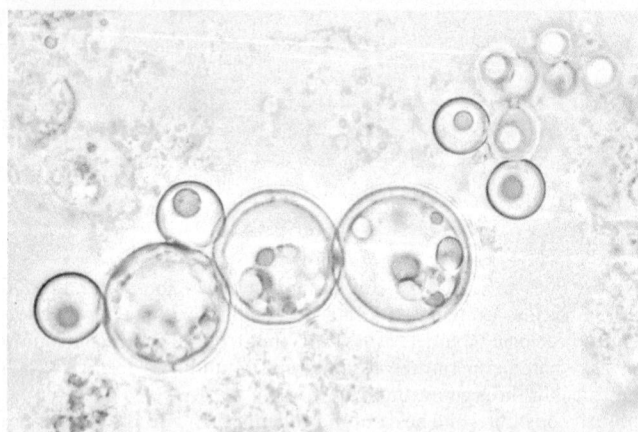

Figure 268-1 *Paracoccidioides brasiliensis.* Multiple budding and variation in cell size are apparent (potassium hydroxide preparation from pus, × 1000).

disease, whereas female mice could arrest the conidia to yeast transition, and promptly controlled the infection. The occupational distribution reveals a predilection for persons who work (or had worked) in agriculture-related occupations. The disease is characterized by long periods of latency, as demonstrated by the nonautochthonous cases reported outside the endemic area. Some of these patients developed overt paracoccidioidomycosis 30 or more years after leaving the endemic regions.[16-18] There are indications suggesting that a certain number of the yeasts present in residual lung tissues adapt to the reduced oxygen tension in walled-off residual lesions, where they remain dormant.[29]

Pathogenesis and Clinical Manifestations

Paracoccidioidomycosis encompasses a subclinical infection resulting from the initial contact with the fungus and an overt disease manifested later. The infection is evidenced by a reactive skin test, presence of anti-GP43 antibodies in healthy blood donors, and especially by the demonstration of *P. brasiliensis* in residual lesions.[4,5,13,30,31] The overt disease has two main clinical presentations, a chronic adult form previously categorized as unifocal or multifocal according to the extent of organ involvement, and the juvenile form, which is an acute or subacute more severe disease.[26,29] The latter is characterized by marked involvement of the reticuloendothelial system and occurs in less than 15% of cases; it is thought to represent progression after a rather recent exposure.[24-28] The hallmarks of the chronic adult type of disease are significant lung involvement and extrapulmonary lesions. This is the predominant form occurring in approximately 90% of cases, and represents endogenous reactivation years after initial contact with the fungus.[6,7,32] This classification does not agree with the results of gallium 67 scans, which have revealed multiorganic involvement in almost all the adult cases; in patients with the juvenile form, however, extralymphatic involvement is not infrequent.[33] A residual form represented by fibrotic scarring of previously active lesions is also recognized.[34,35] A recent cluster analysis done in patients with concomitant lung and mucosal and/or skin lesions has strongly supported the existence of two different sets. The first one included patients with mucosal damage, odynophagia, and/or dysphagia, plus alveolointerstitial infiltrates, and the second consisted of patients exhibiting dermal lesions, dyspnea, and lung fibrosis. The former would represent the early stages while the latter would correspond to the chronic host-fungus interactions.[36]

P. brasiliensis infection may become dormant and be reactivated later on under conditions that have not been clearly defined but that

may be related to immunosuppression or debilitating disease, as well as to associated conditions common to most rural patients, such as chronic alcoholism, malnutrition, and smoking.[4,6,13,27,28,32]

The host's immune defenses directly influence the clinical presentation and severity of the mycosis.[37-39] The first line of defense is represented by polymorphonuclear leukocytes, alveolar macrophages, dendritic cells, natural killer (NK) cells, complement, peptides, proinflammatory cytokines, and chemokines, all of which hinder fungal multiplication but are unable to destroy the invading microorganism.[13,40] This chain of events results in an effective innate immunity that controls fungal adaptation and growth, resulting in preferential activation of Th1 CD4$^+$ cells.[41] Once in the lungs, *P. brasiliensis* propagules interact with lung cells, as well as with the extracellular matrix proteins (ECMp). Adhesins expressed on the *P. brasiliensis* cell surface act to bring molecules for the recognition of ECMp, facilitating fungal adherence. Humoral immunity is intact. In patients with the juvenile form, specific antibodies of the IgA, IgG, and IgE subclasses are markedly increased.[42,43] Patients with the multifocal adult-type disease also have elevated antibody titers, but patients with the unifocal adult form have significantly lower antibody production than other patient groups. Additionally, patients with the juvenile form show eosinophilia and increased levels of transforming growth factor-β (TGF-β), a switching factor for IgA.

Cell-mediated immunity is crucial to defense; it is usually depressed at the peak of the infection but is restored with successful treatment. The dichotomy between humoral and cellular immune responses suggests a helper T-cell 2 (Th2) pattern of immune response.[13,39] Thus, juvenile patients and those with the adult multifocal disease exhibit nonreactive paracoccidioidin skin tests, detectable anti–*P. brasiliensis* antibodies, depressed lymphoproliferative responses to the specific gp43 antigen, and cytokine patterns corresponding to the Th2 type immunity—for example, low interferon (IFN)-γ secretion, high levels of interleukin (IL)-4, -5, and -10, plus defective synthesis of IL-12.[13,39] Addition of IL-12 to patients' macrophages and neutralization of IL-10 increase IFN-γ levels, which suggests the possibility of introducing immune modulation to restore patients' defenses. In patients with the unifocal adult disease, intermediate immune responses are observed (e.g., their specific lymphoproliferative response is higher than in the juvenile patients). Thus, patient profiles are compatible with the presence of low and high resistance to fungal invasion. In contrast to patients, infected individuals (i.e., skin test–reactive) living in the endemic area who have no clinical manifestations of the disease exhibit an opposite, normal Th1 immune profile. Cytokine and chemokine expression kinetics appear to distinguish *P. brasiliensis* infection from overt disease because *P. brasiliensis*–infected individuals demonstrate

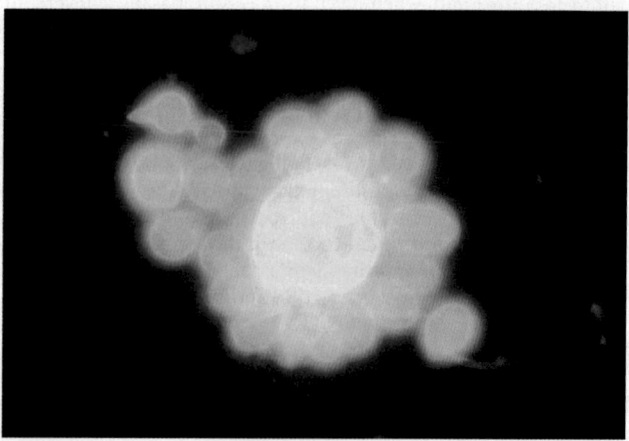

Figure 268-2 *Paracoccidioides brasiliensis* from a 37° C culture. Multiple buds surrounding the mother cell can be observed (calcofluor, × 1000).

expression of various mRNAs for specific cytokines or chemokines, all of which differ in quantity and timing of expression according to the disease form.[42]

Macrophages represent the major cellular defense against *P. brasiliensis*. When activated by IFN-γ, they ingest and kill both conidia and yeast cells through expression of inducible nitric oxide synthase (iNOS).[44,45] Nitric oxide, however, may play a dual role (resistance and susceptibility), depending on the degree of expression.[46]

Compact granulomas are considered to be the most evolved and effective biologic defense weapon against *P. brasiliensis*.[4,13,39,40] Granuloma formation involves the activity of T lymphocytes (helper and cytotoxic subsets), activated effector cells (mainly macrophages but also neutrophils), and several cytokines, especially IFN-γ and IL-12. Th2 cytokines (IL-4, IL-10, TGF-α or -β) are associated with increased host susceptibility, probably because they interfere with correct macrophage function.

Paracoccidioidomycosis is a polymorphic progressive disease, often severe, although self-limited cases have been occasionally reported.[4,5,13,31] The genetic background commanding susceptibility or resistance toward overt disease is still unknown, although it has been suggested that class II allele DRB1*11 is associated with the less severe, chronic, unifocal form of the mycosis, suggesting that it may confer resistance against *P. brasiliensis* dissemination.[47]

The lungs are the site of the primary infection, but the patient's symptoms may not reflect this.[5,6,13,28,32,33,36] In juvenile patients, the disorder is subacute and severe, and carries a bad prognosis. It is manifested by marked involvement of the reticuloendothelial system, with hypertrophy of various lymph node chains and liver and spleen enlargement; respiratory complaints are minimal.[4-7,24,27] In the adult form of the disease, the course is chronic but, contingent on specific therapy, recovery usually ensues. However, residual fibrotic sequelae, present in 38% of patients at diagnosis and in over 50% of patients after treatment, hinder complete restoration of their health.[26,35] Lesions occur mainly (over 90%) in the lungs but are frequently accompanied by secondary lesions in the mucous membranes, reticuloendothelial system, skin, adrenals, and other organs. Usually, more than one lesion is present at the time of the initial consultation.[25,28] In both clinical forms, the mycosis is also manifested by constitutional symptoms such as weakness, fever, general malaise, and weight loss.

Characteristics of the Lesions

LUNGS

In paracoccidioidomycosis, the primary lung infection tends to remain silent but progresses over time so that at diagnosis, patients frequently present with a dry cough, although at times expectoration and even hemoptysis is noticed. Usually, there is some degree of dyspnea. Auscultation reveals minimal abnormalities in comparison with radiologic findings, with a clear dissociation between the clinical manifestations and the damage observed in all image studies.[4,6,13,26,28,32] Pulmonary function studies show abnormal ventilation-perfusion and alveolar-interstitial destruction. However, findings are difficult to interpret because of the high frequency of smoking in patients with the mycosis. This combination results in an obstructive pattern involving the small airways, usually accompanied by an increase in the dead space and in the alveolar-arterial oxygen gradient.

At diagnosis, and in patients with active disease, chest x-ray images reveal mostly interstitial infiltrates (64%), followed by mixed lesions with linear and nodular infiltrates and alveolar patterns, occasionally confluent, located preferentially in the central and lower fields, and frequently bilateral and symmetrical (Fig. 268-3).[6,13,29,33] High-resolution computed tomography (HRCT) may demonstrate abnormal findings in a larger number of patients with chronic pulmonary disease (over 93%). The most common patterns are interlobular septal thickening (88%), peribronchovascular interstitial thickening (78%), centrilobular opacities (63%), intralobular lines (59%), ground-glass opacities (34%), cavities (17%), and air-space consolidation (12%)[48]

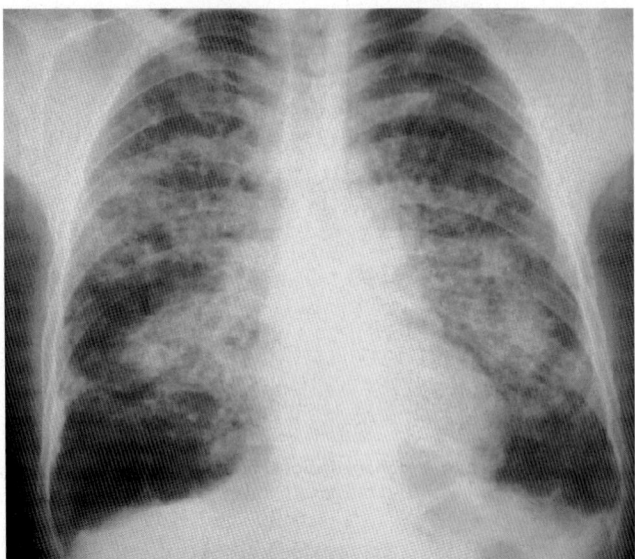

Figure 268-3   Chest x-ray in paracoccidioidomycosis. Bilateral alveolointerstitial infiltrates are seen that involve the central and lower fields, sparing the apices.

(Fig. 268-4). Gallium 67 scans revealed that pulmonary lesions were present in all juvenile and chronic adult form patients studied, thus confirming that the lungs are the preferred target of entry. At diagnosis, one third of patients who have had long-lasting disease present with serious pulmonary sequelae such as bilateral fibrosis (32%), bullae (27%), and emphysematous areas; additionally, indirect signs of pulmonary hypertension and enlargement of the right ventricle (cor pulmonale in approximately 24%) are observed.[32,36] After treatment, these residual lesions tended to increase with time. A Brazilian study examined 1059 deaths caused by the mycosis and found that mortality could be attributed to pulmonary fibrosis, chronic lower airway diseases, and pneumonic processes, thus signaling the importance of lung lesions in paracoccidioidomycosis.[15]

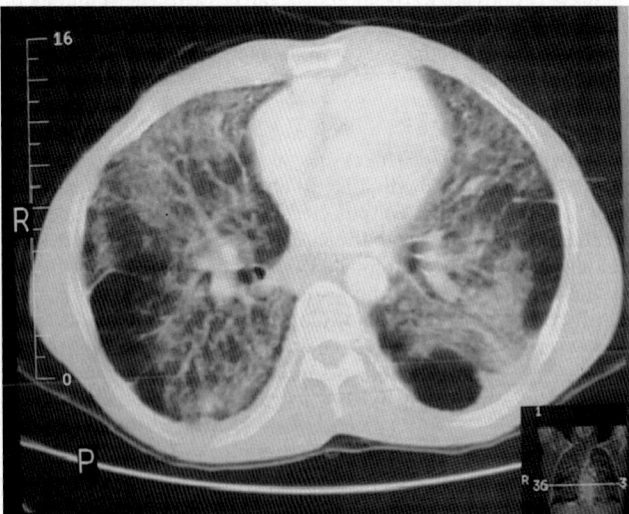

Figure 268-4   Chest high-resolution CT scan in paracoccidioidomycosis. Bilateral interlobular septa, peribronchovascular interstitial thickening, air space consolidation, areas of residual emphysema, and architectural distortion are present.

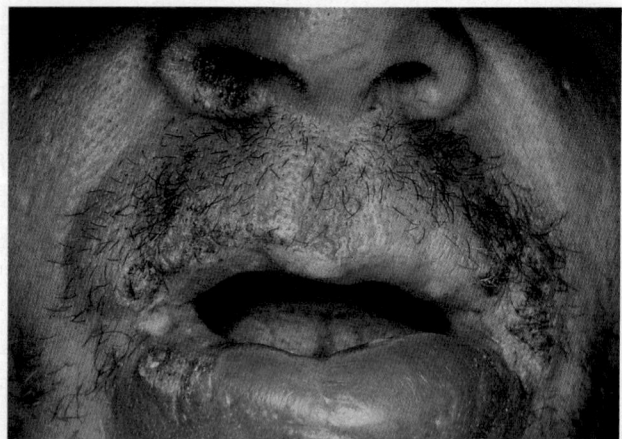

Figure 268-5 Extrapulmonary lesions of paracoccidioidomycosis. Note edema, ulceration, and crusting.

MUCOSA

Infiltrated, ulcerated, and painful lesions with ragged borders are observed regularly and occur in the cephalic segment (47.6%), as well as in the trunk (14.9%), upper limbs (14.9%), lower limbs (21.7%), and genital region (0.7%). When in the mouth, lips, gingiva, tongue, palate, larynx, and pharynx, they cause great discomfort. Dysphagia, odynophagia, and dysphonia are common; diarrhea and emaciation, although not very common, are important in patients with intestinal involvement. All these lesions have a granulomatous appearance and a mulberry-like aspect, and may produce edema of the affected area. On healing, they produce scarring and diminished sensation (Fig. 268-5).[4,6,7,13,48,49] The larynx is the third most commonly involved organ. Endoscopic studies have shown that 80% of patients with laryngeal lesions had two or more laryngeal structures involved, with vocal fold alterations in all patients, leading to dysphonia in 66.7% of them.

SKIN

Cutaneous lesions are present in approximately 25% of cases; they are variable in form and aspect and tend to appear around the natural orifices and in the lower limbs. Most commonly, they involve the head and neck. Lesions are warty, ulcerated, and crusted. They infiltrate the subcutaneous tissues and are granulomatous on biopsy. Often, lung, skin, and mucosal lesions coexist in the same patient.[4,6,7,13,26,49-51]

Lymph Nodes

Although all lymph node chains may be involved, there is a preference for cervical, axillary, mediastinal, and mesenteric nodes, although other nodes are also regularly affected. Patients with the juvenile form and at least half of those with the chronic multifocal form present with clinically detectable hypertrophied lymph nodes. Lymphatic hypertrophy can cause disease by compressing contiguous structures, such as bronchi.[4,6,7,13,25,26,28,32,36] Reticuloendothelial lesions are most easily detected by gallium 67 scans.[33] Draining fistulas may form. In adult patients with mucosal or skin lesions, enlargement of the draining lymph nodes is frequently noted.[48,49]

ADRENALS

The frequency of adrenal involvement in paracoccidioidomycosis depends on the criteria used to determine abnormalities. In necropsy reports, adrenal gland invasion is as high as 85%.[32] According to adrenocorticotropic hormone (ACTH) stimulation tests, decreased adrenal reserve is present in approximately 44% of patients. Such involvement

is lower (14%) when the early morning serum cortisol level is measured. Approximately 7% of patients exhibit an overt addisonian crisis. Image studies reveal hypertrophied glands with damage to the cortical and medullary regions. Calcifications are rare (Fig. 268-6). Proper patient surveillance allows early detection of hypoadrenalism, prompting adequate replacement therapy.[6,8,13,28,31] A significant inverse correlation between plasma levels of dehydroepiandrosterone sulfate and IL-6 has been found, indicating that this interaction may be of significance in this disease.[50]

OTHER LESIONS

Lesions in other organs and systems are occasionally noted, such as nodular lesions in the spleen and liver, masses in the central nervous system (CNS), ulcers in the gastrointestinal tract, and granulomatous lesions in the male genitourinary tract, vascular system, bone, and bone marrow. Clinical presentations vary according to the organ damaged.[4,25,26,50-54] Gallium scanning, CT, and magnetic resonance imaging (MRI) have revealed unexpected but common lesions in all organs and systems, reflecting the disseminated nature of this mycosis.[13,34,35]

Differential Diagnosis

Paracoccidioidomycosis should be suspected in men who work or had worked in agriculture in the recognized endemic areas and who present lung lesions (either active or residual) and/or mucocutaneous lesions.[13,29,32,33,36] The most important differential diagnosis is tuberculosis, a disease that may coexist with the mycosis in 15% of patients.[55] Other diseases to be considered are cancer and neoplastic disorders (including lymphoma), histoplasmosis, leishmaniasis, leprosy, and syphilis.[4,48,54,56] Only the laboratory is capable of establishing the correct diagnosis.[6,8] It should be noted that paracoccidioidomycosis is not a frequent opportunistic disorder, although it behaves as such in AIDS patients. These patients suffer severe and disseminated disease that runs a rapid course and involves preferentially the reticuloendothelial system and skin. In Brazil, its prevalence is low (1.7%) but it carries a high mortality. Paracoccidioidomycosis occurs in patients with CD4 T-cells counts below 50 cells/mL. Mortality rates are high and late relapses are common.[57,58] The mycosis has been occasionally reported in other immunosuppressed patients.

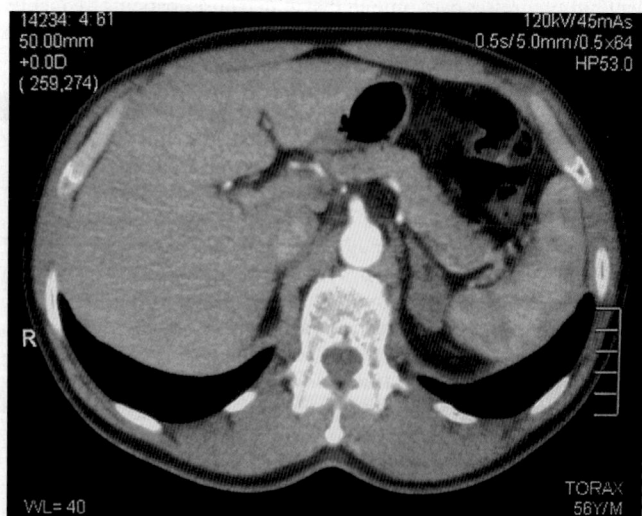

Figure 268-6 CT scan of adrenal glands in paracoccidioidomycosis. There is hypertrophy with deformity of the left gland and hypodense parenchyma.

Treatment

Paracoccidioidomycosis is the only endemic mycosis amenable to treatment with sulfa drugs. Amphotericin B and various imidazole derivatives are also effective. Because patients are usually malnourished, treatment directed merely at suppressing the multiplication of the causative agent may not be successful. Appropriate supportive therapeutic measures (e.g., improved diet, rest, correction of anemia) are essential.[4,13,59-61]

SULFONAMIDES

Either sulfadiazine or the long-acting compounds (sulfamethoxypyridazine, sulfadimethoxine, sulfamethoxazole) can be used. With sulfadiazine, the maximum therapeutic dosage is 4 g/day for adults and 60 to 100 mg/kg/day for children in divided doses. This treatment must be continued without interruption for several months until clinical and mycologic responses become apparent; then the dosage can be reduced to half. The long-acting compounds require a 1-to-2-g/day dose for adults and half that dose for children during the first 2 to 3 weeks of treatment; after clinical improvement, 500 mg/day suffices. Sulfonamide treatment should be continued for 3 to 5 years to avoid relapses, which occur in 20% to 25% of cases.[4,13,59,60] The daily use of a combination of sulfamethoxazole (400 mg) and trimethoprim (80 mg) given in one tablet two or three times daily for 12 to 24 months is preferred by some. Young children can be treated with an oral solution, 8 to 10 mg/kg of trimethoprim combined with 40 to 50 mg/kg of sulfamethoxazole in two divided doses.[28,61]

AMPHOTERICIN B

In paracoccidioidomycosis, amphotericin B is administered according to recommendations given for other systemic mycoses. Cumulative total dosages vary from 1000 to 2000 mg. Amphotericin B is not fungicidal in vivo, and all patients thus treated should also receive maintenance sulfonamide or azole therapy. Amphotericin B should be reserved for severe cases and for those patients unresponsive to other therapies.[4,13,59-61] There has been little experience with the lipid formulations of amphotericin B, largely based on cost and limited availability.

Treatment with sulfonamides and/or amphotericin B is not always successful, and the mortality rate is rather high (17% to 25%). Improvement is obtained in 65% to 70% of cases, and the remainder relapse or fail to improve.[4,13,59-61]

IMIDAZOLE COMPOUNDS

Ketoconazole treatment has resulted in major improvement (over 84%), with a 10% relapse rate after 5 years.[5,6,13,32,59,61] Ketoconazole should be given at a dosage of 200 to 400 mg/day for a minimum of 6 months and for as long as 12 to 18 months, depending on the patient's response and the results of mycologic tests. Long-lasting ketoconazole therapy mandates regular check-ups for hepatic dysfunction and gonadal alterations. At present, however, itraconazole is considered to be superior to ketoconazole, is based on its shorter treatment period (mean, 6 months), lower daily dose (100 or 200 mg once daily), lack of major interference with endocrine metabolism, little or no liver toxicity, and lower relapse rate (3% to 5%).[4] When properly controlled, patients with the severe juvenile form—including AIDS patients—and those with CNS disease respond to itraconazole. Failures, however, are occasionally encountered. Fluconazole is not recommended, because there is a need to administer high doses (up to 600 mg/day) for long periods, and also because relapses are too common. As yet unpublished clinical studies with posaconazole, a new triazole, have revealed that this compound is effective and well tolerated. Voriconazole, given orally for 6 months, has shown a complete or partial global response in 88.6% of patients in a Brazilian pilot study, but did not prove superior to itraconazole.[62] Immuno-

therapy with a peptide vaccine as an adjuvant to antifungal therapy is now being investigated and the experimental results appear promising.[63]

Laboratory Diagnosis

Diagnostic tests are oriented toward the visualization of the causative fungus in clinical samples and/or its isolation in culture. Detection of antibodies against certain fungal antigens or determining the presence of such antigens in the patient's body fluids constitute indirect diagnostic criteria.[4,6,13,64-66] *P. brasiliensis* visualization and isolation are not difficult to attain. However, prompt diagnosis is hindered by the lack of awareness on the part of many physicians.

DIRECT EXAMINATION

In specimens such as sputum, exudates, and pus, a simple wet mount suffices to reveal *P. brasiliensis* in 93% of patients. If results are negative, repeat samples should be collected and sputum should be digested and concentrated. The relatively large size of the fungal cells, their translucent walls, and their multiple budding make diagnosis simple.[4,6,13] Occasionally, however, single buds and small yeast cells may be confused with other fungi, requiring more extensive observations.[5] Direct fungal DNA detection in exudates and tissue samples by polymerase chain reaction (PCR) assay has been reported to be helpful, although the corresponding techniques are still in the experimental stage.[67,68]

HISTOLOGIC STUDIES

Biopsy is very often diagnostic. Gomori methenamine silver stain is recommended. If the typical multiple budding cells are not abundant, distinction from other fungi (e.g., *Blastomyces dermatitidis*, *Histoplasma capsulatum*, *Cryptococcus neoformans*) is necessary. Frequently, infected tissues reveal a mixed inflammatory reaction characterized by the presence of granulomas centered on yeast cells, some of which have been phagocytized. The granuloma is further characterized by the presence of neutrophils, mononuclear cells, epithelioid cells, and multinucleated giant cells, all arranged concentrically around the yeast cells (Fig. 268-7). This type of response is also present in mucocutaneous lesions and in ruptured lymph nodes. Skin lesions reveal pseudoepitheliomatous hyperplasia and intraepithelial microabscesses. In the juvenile form, tissue reactions are diffuse and phagocytosis is sparse. Lymph nodes have hyperplastic germinal centers and increased numbers of plasmocytes.[4,13,32,40]

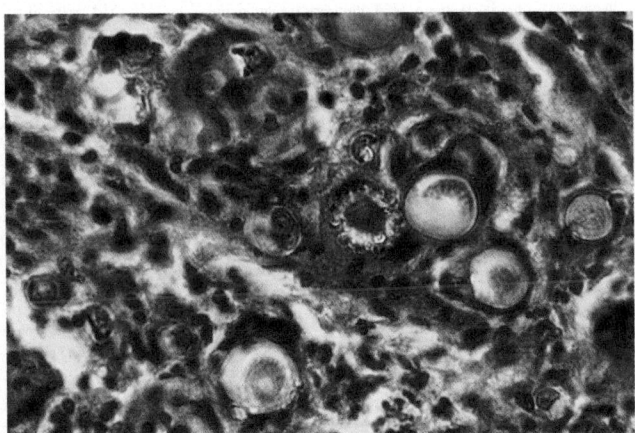

Figure 268-7 Paracoccidioidomycosis histology. Yeast cells in tissue demonstrate multiple budding and mononuclear infiltration (hematoxylin and eosin, × 400).

CULTURES

Isolation of *P. brasiliensis* in culture evidences active disease, but the test is positive in only 85% of cases and requires 20 to 30 days for growth to occur. Various culture media such as Mycosel agar (BBL) and Sabouraud agar, plus antibiotics and the mold inhibitor compound cycloheximide, can be used and incubated, preferably at room temperature (20° to 25° C). Colonies obtained require temperature-mediated transformation to the yeast form for confirmation. Incubation at 37° C carries the risk of contamination, especially in specimens rich in normal flora, such as respiratory secretions. Primary isolation often requires multiple samples (e.g., sputum) and a variety of culture media.[4,5,13]

SEROLOGIC TESTS

Serology for antibody detection is useful not only for diagnosis but also for follow-up studies. Antibodies of the immunoglobulin classes IgG, IgM, and IgE are regularly detected.[13,30,66] The easiest antibody detection method, the agar gel immunodiffusion test, demonstrates circulating antibodies in over 90% of cases. The test is highly specific, and the presence of a precipitin band practically makes the diagnosis.[4-6] However, the diagnosis cannot be based solely on this, because these antibodies can be detected years after apparently successful therapy. Another useful test, albeit a cumbersome one, is the complement fixa-tion test. Its quantitative nature allows a more precise evaluation of the patient's response to treatment. In this test, and in contrast to the immunodiffusion test, cross-reactions with *Histoplasma capsulatum* antigens are important. Other tests, such as immunofluorescence, counterimmunoelectrophoresis, the dot blot test, enzyme-linked immunosorbent assay, and immunoblotting, are also used. Improvements in serodiagnosis include the detection of antibodies against chemically characterized and/or recombinant *P. brasiliensis* antigens, notably gp43, pb27, and the 87-kilodalton HS protein. A combination of the latter two has resulted in increased sensitivity (92%) and specificity (88%).[69-71]

Antigen detection may be preferred for early diagnosis in immunocompromised individuals or when antibody detection appears inconclusive; over 60% of the active patients react in this type of test.[13,66,71] Monitoring circulating antigens is also important as a criterion of cure.[72] Parallel testing for antibody levels in the same patients has revealed that titers are rather unpredictable.

SKIN TESTS

Paracoccidioidin skin testing is not reliable for diagnosis, because many active cases (35% to 50%) are nonreactive at the time of diagnosis. Cross-reactions with histoplasmin are to be expected, although the use of the purified antigen gp43 appears to be more specific.[4,5,13]

REFERENCES

1. San-Blas G, Nino-Vega G, Iturriaga T. Paracoccidioides brasiliensis and paracccidioidomycosis: Molecular approaches to morphogenesis, diagnosis, epidemiology, taxonomy and genetics. *Med Mycol.* 2002;40:225-242.
2. Travassos LR, Goldman G, Taborda CP, et al. Insights in Paracoccidioides brasiliensis Pathogenicity. In: Kavanagh K, ed. *New Insights in Medical Mycology.* Dordrecht, The Netherlands: Springer; 2007:241-266.
3. Matute DR, McEwen JG, Puccia R, et al. Cryptic speciation and recombination in the fungus *Paracoccidioides brasiliensis* as revealed by gene genealogies. *Molec Biol Evol.* 2006;23:65-73.
4. Lacaz CS, Porto E, Martins JEC, et al. Paracoccidioidomicose. In: Lacaz CS, Porto, Martins JEC, et al, eds. *Tratado de Micologia Médica Lacaz.* 9th ed. Sao Paulo, Brazil: Sarvier; 2002: 639-729.
5. Restrepo A. Paracoccidioidomycosis. In: Dismukes WE, Pappas PG, Sobel JK, eds. *Clinical Mycology.* New York: Oxford University Press; 2003:328-345.
6. Restrepo A, Tobón AM, Agudelo CA. Paracoccidioidomycosis. In: Hospenthal DR, Rinaldi MG, eds. *Diagnosis and Treatment of Human Mycoses.* Totowa, NJ: Humana Press; 2008:331-342.
7. Taborda CP, da Silva MB, Nosanchuk JD, et al. Melanin as a virulence factor of *Paracoccidioides brasiliensis* and other dimorphic pathogenic fungi. *Mycopathologia.* 2008;165:331-340.
8. Almeida AJ, Matute DR, Carmona JA, et al. Genome size and ploidy of *Paracoccidioides brasiliensis* reveal a haploid DNA content: Flow cytometry and GP43 sequence analysis. *Fungal Gen Biol.* 2007;44:25-31.
9. Tavares AH, Silva SS, Dantas A, et al. Virulence insights from *Paracoccidiodes brasiliensis* transcriptome. *Genet Mol Res.* 2005;4:372-389.
10. Bastos KP, Bailao AM, Borges CL, et al. The transcriptome analysis of early morphogenesis in *Paracoccidioides brasiliensis* mycelium reveals novel and induced genes potentially associated to the dimorphic process. *BMC Microbiology.* 2007;7:1-14.
11. Silva SS, Paes HC, Soares CMA, et al. Insights into the pathobiology of *Paracoccidioides brasiliensis* from transcriptome analysis—advances and perspectives. *Mycopathologia.* 2008;165:249-258.
12. Restrepo A, McEwen JG, Castañada E. The habitat of *Paracoccidioides brasiliensis*: How far from solving the riddle? *Med Mycol.* 2001;39:232-241.
13. Restrepo A, Benard G, Castro C, et al. Pulmonary paracoccidioidomycosis. *Semin Resp Crit Care Med.* 2008;29:182-197.
14. Coutinho ZF, Silva D, Lazera M, et al. Paracoccidioidomycosis mortality in Brazil (1980-1995). *Cad Saude Publica.* 2002;18:1441-1454.
15. Santo AH. Tendência da mortalidade relacionada à paracoccidioidomicose, Estado de São Paulo, Brasil, 1985 a 2005: Estudo usando causas múltiplas de morte. *Rev Panam Salud Publica.* 2008;23:313-324.
16. Van Damme PA, Bierenbroodspot F, Telgtt DS, et al. A case of imported paracoccidioidomycosis: An awkward infection in the Netherlands. *Med Mycol.* 2006;44:13-18.
17. Poisson M, Heitzmann A, Mille C, et al. *Paracoccidioides brasiliensis* in a brain abscess: First French case. *J Mycol Med.* 2007; 17:114-118.
18. Mayayo E, Gómez-Aracil V, Fernández-Torres B, et al. Report of an imported cutaneous disseminated case of paracoccidioidomycosis. *Rev Iberoam Micol.* 2007;24:44-46.
19. Niño-Vega GA, Calgano AM, San Blas G, et al. RFLP analysis reveals marked geographical isolation between strains of *Paracoccidioides brasiliensis. Med Mycol.* 2000;38:437-441.
20. Franco M, Bagagli E, Scapolio S, et al. A critical analysis of isolations of *Paracoccidioides brasiliensis* from soil. *Med Mycol.* 2000; 38:185-191.
21. Bagagli E, Theodoro RC, Bosco SMG, et al. *Paracoccidioides brasiliensis*: Phylogenetic and ecological aspects. *Mycopathologia.* 2008;165:197-207.
22. Coimbra CEA, Wanke B, Santos RV, et al. Paracoccidioidin and histoplasmin sensitivity in the Tupí-Mondé Amerindian populations from the Brazilian Amazonia. *Ann Trop Med Parasitol.* 1994;88:197-207.
23. Rios-Gonçalves AJ, Londero AT, Terra GMF, et al. Paracoccidioidomycosis in children in the State of Rio de Janeiro (Brazil). Geographic distribution and the study of a "reservarea." *Rev Inst Med Trop São Paulo.* 1998;40:11-13.
24. Benard G, Kavakama J, Mendes-Giannini MJS, et al. Contribution to the natural history of paracoccidioidomycosis: Identification of the primary pulmonary infection in the acute severe form of the disease. A case report. *Clin Infect Dis.* 2005;40: e1-e14.
25. Campos MVS, Penna GO, De Castro CN, et al. Paracoccidioidomycosis at Brasilia's University hospital. *Rev Soc Brasileira Med Trop.* 2008;41:169-172.
26. Blotta MH, Mamoni RL, Oliveira SJ, et al. Endemic regions of paracoccidioidomycosis in Brazil: A clinical and epidemiologic study of 584 cases in the southeast region. *Am J Trop Med Hyg.* 1999;61:390-394.
27. Pereira RM, Bucaretchi F, Barison EM, et al. Paracoccidioidomycosis in children: Clinical presentation, follow-up and outcome. *Rev Inst Med Trop São Paulo.* 2004;46:127-131.
28. Paniagoa AM, Aguiar JI, Aguiar ES, et al. Paracoccidioidomicose: A clinical and epidemiological study of 422 cases observed in Mato Grosso do Soul. *Rev Soc Bras Med Trop.* 2003;36: 455-459.
29. Restrepo A. Morphological aspects of *Paracoccidioides brasiliensis* in lymph nodes: Implications for the prolonged latency of paracoccidioidomycosis? *Med Mycol.* 2000;38:317-322.
30. Botteon FA, Camargo ZP, Benard G, et al. *Paracoccidioides brasiliensis*: Reactive antibodies in Brazilian blood donors. *Med Mycol.* 2002;40:387-391.
31. Angulo-Ortega A, Pollak L. Paracoccidioidomycosis. In: Baker RD, ed. *The Pathologic Anatomy of the Mycoses.* New York: Springer-Verlag; 1971:507-576.
32. Tobón AM, Agudelo CA, Osorio ML, et al. Residual pulmonary abnormalities in adult patients with chronic paracoccidioidomycosis: Prolonged observations after itraconazole therapy. *Clin Infect Dis.* 2003;37:898-904.
33. Yamaga LY, Benard G, Hironaka FH, et al. The role of gallium-67 scan in defining the extent of disease in an endemic deep mycosis, paracoccidioidomycosis: A predominantly multifocal disease. *Eur J Nucl Med Mol Imaging.* 2003;30:888-894.
34. Trad HS, Trad CS, Elias Jr, et al. Radiological review of 173 consecutive cases of paracoccidioidomycosis. *Radiol Brasileira.* 2006;39:175-179.
35. Souza A, Gasparetto EL, Davaus T, et al. High-resolution CT findings of 77 patients with untreated pulmonary paracoccidioidomycosis. *Am J Radiol.* 2006;187:1248-1252.
36. Restrepo A, Tobón AM, Agudelo CA, et al. Co-existence of integumentary lesions and lung X-ray abnormalities in patients with paracoccidioidomycosis. *Am J Trop Med Hyg.* 2008;79: 159-163.
37. Camargo ZP, Franco MF. Current knowledge on pathogenesis and immunodiagnosis of paracoccidioidomycosis. *Rev Iberoam Micol.* 2000;17:41-48.
38. Calich VL, Costa TA, Felonato M, et al. Innate immunity to *Paracoccidioides brasiliensis* infection. *Mycopathologia.* 2008;165: 223-234.
39. Benard G. An overview of the immunopathology of human paracoccidioidomycosis. *Mycopathologia.* 2008;165:209-221.
40. Mendes-Giannini MJ, Monteiro da Silva JL, de Fátima da Silva J, et al. Interactions of *Paracoccidioides brasiliensis* with host cells: Recent advances. *Mycopathologia.* 2008;165:237-248.
41. Kashino SS, Fazioli RA, Cafalli-Favati C, et al. Resistance to *Paracoccidioides brasiliensis* infection is linked to a preferential Th1 immune response, whereas susceptibility is associated with absence of IFN-gamma production. *J Interferon Cytokine Res.* 2000;20:89-97.
42. Mamoni RL, Nouer SA, Oliveira SJ, et al. Enhanced production of specific IgG4, IgE, IgA and TGF-beta in sera from patients with the juvenile form of paracoccidioidomycosis. *Med Mycol.* 2002;40:153-159.
43. Mamoni RL, Blotta MH. Kinetics of cytokines and chemokines gene expression distinguishes *Paracoccidioides brasiliensis* infection from disease. *Cytokine.* 2005;32:20-29.
44. Calvi SA, Peracoli MT, Mendes RP, et al. Effect of cytokines on the in vitro fungicidal activity of monocytes from paracoccidioidomycosis patients. *Microbes Infect.* 2003;5:107-113.
45. Gónzalez A, Aristizabal BH, Caro E, et al. Production of nitric oxide and TNF-β and expression of INOS and NF κβ in peritoneal macrophages activated with interferon gamma. *Ann Rev Biomed Sci.* 2002;4:133-139.
46. Nascimento FR, Calich VL, Rodriguez D, et al. Dual role for nitric oxide in paracoccidioidomycosis: Essential for resistance, but overproduction associated with susceptibility. *J Immunol.* 2002; 168:4593-4600.
47. Sadahiro A, Roque AC, Shikanai YMA. Generic human leukocyte antigen class II (DRB1 and QB1) alleles in patients with paracoccidioidomycosis. *Med Mycol.* 2007;45:35-40.
48. Marques SA, Cortez DB, Lastória JC, et al. Paracoccidioidomycosis: Frequency, morphology, and pathogenesis of tegumentary lesions. *An bras Dermatol.* 2007;82:411-417.
49. Weber SAT, Brasolotto A, Rodrigues J, et al. Dysphonia and laryngeal sequelae in paracoccidioidomycosis: A morphological and phoniatric study. *Med Mycol.* 2006;44:219-225.
50. Leal AM, Magalhaes PK, Martínez R, et al. Adrenocortical hormones and interleukin patterns in paracoccidioidomycosis. *J Infect Dis.* 2003;187:124-127.

51. de Almeida SM, Queiros-Telles F, Teive HAG, et al. Central nervous system paracoccidioidomycosis: Clinical features and laboratory findings. *J Infect.* 2004;48:193-198.
52. Fagundes-Pereyra WJ, Cardoso Carvalho GT, Góes ADM, et al. Central nervous system paracoccidioidomycosis: Analysis of 13 cases. *Arq Neuro-Psiquiatr.* 2006;64:269-276.
53. Severo LC, Kauer CL, Oliveira FD, et al. Paracoccidioidomycosis of the male genital tract: Report of eleven cases and review of the Brazilian literature. *Rev Inst Med Trop Sao Paulo.* 2000;42:38-40.
54. Resende LSR, Mendes RP, Bacchi MM, et al. Infiltrative myelopathy by paracoccidioidomycosis: A review and report of nine cases with emphasis on bone marrow morphology. *Histopathology.* 2006;48:377-386.
55. Quagliato R, Grangeia TAG, Carvalho, RA, et al. Association between paracoccidioidomycosis and tuberculosis: reality and misdiagnosis. *J Bras Pneumol.* 2007;33:295-300.
56. Shikanai-Yasuda MA, Conceicão YMT, Kono A, et al. Neoplasia and paracoccidioidomycosis. *Mycopathologia.* 2008;165:303-311.
57. Paniago AM, de Freitas AC, Aguiar ES, et al. Paracoccidioidomycosis in patients with human immunodeficiency virus: Review of 12 cases observed in an endemic region in Brazil. *J Infect.* 2005;51:248-252.
58. Castro G, Martinez R. Disseminated paracoccidioidomycosis coinfection with HIV. *N Engl J Med.* 2006;355:2677

59. Visbal G, San Blas G, Murgich J, et al. *Paracoccidioides brasiliensis,* paracoccidioidomycosis, and antifungal antibiotics. *Curr Drug Targets Infect Disord.* 2005;5:211-226.
60. Shikanai-Yasuda MA. Pharmacological management of paracoccidioidomycosis. *Expert Opin Pharmacother.* 2005;6:385-397.
61. Shikanai-Yasuda MA, Telles Filho FDQ, Mendes RP, et al. Guidelines in paracoccidioidomycosis. *Rev Soc Brasileira Med Trop.* 2006;39:297-310.
62. Queiroz-Telles F, Luciano GZ, Haran TS, et al. An open label comparative pilot study of oral voriconazole and itraconazole for long-term treatment of Paracoccidioidomycosis. *Clin Infect Dis.* 2007;45:1462-1469.
63. Travassos LR, Taborda CP, Colombo AL. Treatment options for paracoccidioidomycosis and new strategies investigated. *Expert Rev anti-infective Ther.* 2008;6:251-262.
64. Camargo ZP. Serology of paracoccidioidomycosis. *Mycopathologia.* 2008;165:289-302.
65. Ricci G, Guerreiro Da Silva IDC, et al. Detection of *Paracoccidioides brasiliensis* by PCR in biopsies from patients with paracoccidioidomycosis: Correlation with the histopathological pattern. *Pathologica.* 2007;99:41-45.
66. Charbel CE, Levi JE, Martins JE. Evaluation of polymerase chain-reaction for the detection of *Paracoccidioides brasiliensis* DNA on serum samples from patients with paracoccidioidomycosis. *Mem Inst Oswaldo Cruz.* 2006;101:219-221.

67. Panunto-Castelo A, Freitas da-Silva G, Bragheto IC, et al. *Paracoccidioides brasiliensis* exoantigens: Recognition by IgG from patients with different clinical forms of paracoccidioidomycosis. *Microbes Infect.* 2003;5:1205-1211.
68. Diez S, Gómez BL, Restrepo A, et al. Combined use of *Paracoccidioides brasiliensis* recombinant 27 kDa and purified 87 kDa antigens in an ELISA test for the serodiagnosis of paracoccidioidomycosis. *J Clin Microbiol.* 2003;341:1536-1552.
69. Reis BS, Bozzi A, Prado FL, et al. Membrane and extracellular antigens of *Paracoccidioides brasiliensis* (Mexo): Identification of a 28-kDa protein suitable for immunodiagnosis of paracoccidioidomycosis. *J Immunol Med.* 2005;307:118-126.
70. Gómez BL, Figueroa JI, Hamilton AJ, et al. Antigenemia in patients with paracoccidioidomycosis: Detection of the 87-kilodalton determinant during and after antifungal therapy. *J Clin Microbiol.* 1998;36:3309-3316.
71. Marques da Silva SH, Mattos-Grosso D, Lopes JD, et al. Detection of *Paracoccidioides brasiliensis* gp70 circulating antigen and follow-up of patients undergoing antimycotic therapy. *J Clin Microbiol.* 2004;42:4480-4486.

Uncommon Fungi and *Prototheca*

269

DUANE R. HOSPENTHAL*

Pseudallescheria Boydii

In humans, infection with *Pseudallescheria boydii* (anamorph [asexual state] *Scedosporium apiospermum*) can produce two distinct rare diseases: mycetoma and pseudallescheriasis (scedosporiosis). Mycetoma is a chronic subcutaneous infection characterized by the production of grains (see Chapter 262), whereas pseudallescheriasis includes all other infections caused by *P. boydii*. The most common sites of pseudallescheriasis are lung, bone, joints, and the central nervous system (CNS).[1] Sinusitis, keratitis, endophthalmitis, skin and soft tissue infections, prostatitis, and endocarditis have also been described. The fungus is found in soil and fresh water, especially stagnant or polluted water, throughout the world. Disease is acquired after inhalation of this organism into the lungs or paranasal sinuses or after traumatic inoculation through the skin. There are at least 14 reported cases of *Pseudallescheria*-related pneumonia after near-drowning in contaminated water. Although colonization is more common than infection with this organism, an invasive pulmonary disease similar to invasive pulmonary aspergillosis occurs, usually in immunocompromised patients. Local trauma is the most common cause of eye, soft tissue, and osteoarticular infections in previously healthy persons. CNS infection is seen in both immunocompromised and healthy individuals.[2] Infections in immunocompetent patients usually have subacute to chronic courses, whereas those in immunocompromised patients are frequently acute and severe.

P. boydii can colonize bronchiectatic lungs, including those of patients with cystic fibrosis, or intermittently obstructed paranasal sinuses. Masses of *P. boydii* hyphae (fungus balls) have been found in lung cavities.[3] *P. boydii* has also been reported as a cause of allergic bronchopulmonary disease (similar to allergic bronchopulmonary aspergillosis),[4] pleural space infection, lung abscess, pneumonia (including aspiration pneumonia), and invasive sinusitis.[5] As with invasive pulmonary aspergillosis, invasive pulmonary pseudallescheriasis most commonly occurs in patients with prolonged neutropenia, those receiving prolonged high-dose corticosteroid therapy, or those who have undergone allogeneic bone marrow transplantation.[6] Invasive pulmonary disease with associated dissemination appears common[7] and has also occurred in patients with acquired immunodeficiency syndrome (AIDS) and after solid-organ transplantation.[8] Pulmonary disease in severely immunocompromised patients usually manifests with fever, cough, pleuritic pain, and often hemoptysis. Chest films show areas of nodularity, alveolar infiltrate, or, most commonly, consolidation.[9] Later, cavitation may be noted. Disseminated disease that manifests with only painful cutaneous nodules or endophthalmitis has also been described in immunocompromised patients.[10,11] Invasive pulmonary disease with extension to the vertebrae has been described in a patient without apparent immunocompromise.[12]

Localized disease—including infections of the eye, bone, cutaneous tissue, subcutaneous tissue (Fig. 269-1), and osteoarticular tissue—may be seen both with and without immunocompromise. Infection is commonly initiated through traumatic implantation of the fungus from soil or water. Surgery, intravenous drug injection, and repeated corticosteroid injections have less frequently been associated with localized infections.[13] Osteoarticular infection in immunocompetent patients often manifests as a painful, swollen joint with overlying erythema after penetrating injury. In occasional patients, weeks to even years may pass between antecedent trauma and the development of septic arthritis.[14,15]

Brain abscesses may result from a known or unsuspected lung lesion in immunocompromised patients, including those with AIDS.[2,16] CNS infection appears to be disproportionately prevalent among patients with pseudallescheriasis, in comparison with many other mycoses. For example, of 23 solid-organ transplant recipients with pseudallescheriasis, 11 (48%) had CNS involvement.[8] Cerebral abscesses are usually multiple; in the immunocompetent hosts, they are often reported in association with near-drownings in polluted water, such as ponds, pig troughs, and roadside ditches.[2] CNS infection from contiguous spread of sinusitis[17] and after penetrating trauma[18] has also been described. Indolent, severe neutrophilic meningitis has been reported occasionally, usually in patients with intravenous drug abuse or human immunodeficiency virus (HIV) infection. Cerebrospinal fluid culture and smear have yielded negative results; the diagnosis was made at autopsy. The first described human case of pseudallescheriasis was meningitis that was probably iatrogenic after lumbar puncture for the administration of anesthesia.[19]

Isolation of *P. boydii* from normally sterile sites is diagnostic. Only rarely is *P. boydii* cultured from blood.[1] Growth of the organism from sputum, bronchoalveolar lavage, draining wounds, or paranasal sinus aspirates is less convincing evidence of infection, unless it is accompanied by hyphae on smear or biopsy. Histologically, *P. boydii* resembles *Aspergillus* spp., with dichotomously branching septate hyphae seen in tissue. In neutropenic patients, blood vessel invasion and thrombosis are usual. The fungus grows well in standard mycologic media. After a few days, the mold colony takes on a tan color and has sporulating structures that are quite different from those of *Aspergillus*. Cultures that produce asexual conidia but do not produce the sexual reproductive structure, the cleistothecia, after 2 to 3 weeks are designated by the anamorph name *S. apiospermum*. No clinically useful serologic or other rapid identification tests are currently available.

Effective therapy of pseudallescheriasis remains elusive. In vitro and clinical resistance to amphotericin B, as well as breakthrough infections, have been reported repeatedly. Surgical débridement has been an important adjunct in treatment of pseudallescheriasis of soft tissue, bone, joint, and pleural and paranasal sinuses, although it is not curative by itself. Intra-articular instillation of amphotericin B may have contributed to success of treatment in a few patients. The rate of mortality with brain abscess has traditionally been noted to exceed 75%.[2] In the past, intravenous miconazole and surgery had been associated with most successful outcomes in CNS infection.[18] Successes have been reported with ketoconazole and itraconazole, mostly in patients with localized infection, and in conjunction with débridement.[14,20,21] Combination therapy with liposomal amphotericin B and itraconazole has been used successfully in at least one case of disseminated infection.[22] The new broad-spectrum azole antifungals (including voriconazole, posaconazole, ravuconazole, and albaconazole) and the echinocandin caspofungin have been shown to have activity against *P. boydii* in vitro.[23-28] Clinical response to voriconazole therapy has been reported in growing numbers of patients,[29-31] and response to posaconazole was achieved in a single reported case of brain abscess.[32] Voriconazole is

*The views expressed are those of the author and do not reflect the official policy or position of the Department of the Army, the Department of Defense, or the U.S. government.

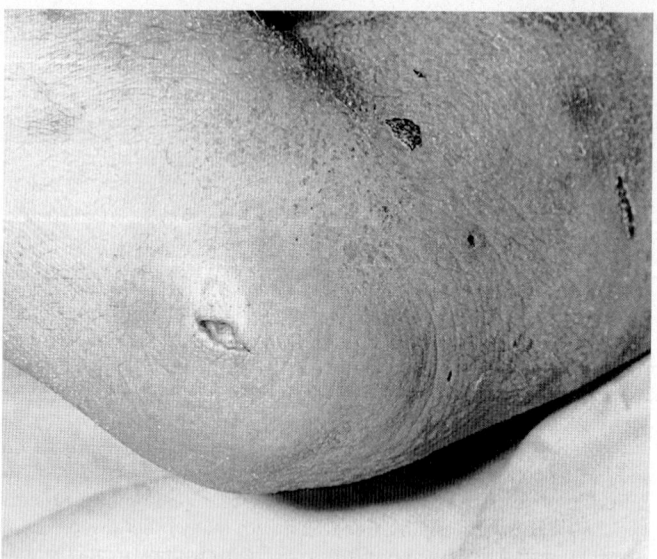

Figure 269-1 *Pseudallescheria boydii* olecranon bursitis in a corticosteroid-treated patient who fell on his elbow in the garden. Photograph shows the incision site over the subcutaneous abscess, which began in the bursa.

approved by the U.S. Food and Drug Administration (FDA) for patients with pseudallescheriasis refractory to other approved antifungal agents and for patients who cannot tolerate those agents. This indication was based on success reported in 15 of 24 patients treated with this agent (including 6 of 10 with CNS infection). Because of poor response to the only approved agent, amphotericin B, most experts believe that voriconazole is the drug of choice in the treatment of pseudallescheriasis.

Scedosporium prolificans

Scedosporium prolificans (formerly known as *S. inflatum*), a fungus found in soil, was first described in 1984 as an agent of human disease.[33] Since that time, several dozen cases have been reported from Spain,[34] as have others from Australia, Canada, France, Germany, the Netherlands, and the United States, in both immunocompromised and immunocompetent patients.[35] Patients with intact immunity most frequently have focal infections (usually osteoarticular), whereas immunocompromised persons more frequently have disseminated disease. In one review, 29 of 30 patients with disseminated *S. prolificans* infections were immunosuppressed.[35]

In immunocompetent patients, infection is usually localized and associated with trauma, including surgery.[36,37] These cases have included infections of bone and joints (Fig. 269-2), onychomycosis, and endophthalmitis. Immunocompromised patients, commonly those undergoing cytoreductive chemotherapy or bone marrow transplantation, present with fungemia and fever with neutropenia.[6,7,38,39] Skin lesions, myalgia, endophthalmitis, and pulmonary infiltrates have been described in this setting.[11,40] Skin lesions have been described as a papular rash, later becoming necrotic. Disseminated disease without neutropenia was described in patients who have undergone lung and kidney transplantation.[41] Fatal localized CNS infection was reported in a child with acute leukemia who had received six intrathecal chemotherapeutic injections.[42] *S. prolificans* has also been recovered from the external ear and sputum of patients without apparent disease.[34,36,37] Sputum colonization has been observed in patients with AIDS and cystic fibrosis and in those who have undergone liver or lung transplantation.[37,43,44]

Diagnosis is most commonly established by the recovery of the organism from culture of infected sites, including skin biopsy samples.

Disseminated disease in immunocompromised patients is usually diagnosed through blood culture.[39] Identification of *S. prolificans* is based chiefly on the morphologic characteristics of the asexual structures produced by the mold in culture.[45]

No antifungal therapy currently available is effective in treating these infections. *S. prolificans* appears to be intrinsically resistant to most antifungals. Successful therapy of joint infections has, however, been reported with the use of surgical débridement with or without intra-articular amphotericin B.[36] Disseminated infection is usually resistant to antifungal agents and carries a high mortality rate.[38] Survival was reported in one patient with disseminated disease and neutropenia who received granulocyte colony-stimulating factor (G-CSF) and amphotericin B, followed by itraconazole.[39] In one animal model, liposomal amphotericin B with the addition of G-CSF improved survival.[46] Of the currently available antifungal agents, voriconazole appears most promising in vitro, with better activity than amphotericin B, itraconazole, or posaconazole.[23,26,27] Unfortunately, current dosing regimens of voriconazole are not associated with serum concentrations at which the drug appears to be effective in vitro. One report described a 44% response rate (16 of 36 patients) with voriconazole.[29] The investigational azole, albaconazole (UR-9825), appears more active than voriconazole in vitro and has shown potential in one animal model.[23,47] Because of the in vitro and in vivo resistance of *S. prolificans* to currently available agents, the effect of combining agents has been examined. In laboratory studies, synergy has been shown through the use of combinations of amphotericin B with pentamidine[48] and of terbinafine with voriconazole, itraconazole, or miconazole.[49,50] Clinical support for this in vitro synergy is limited, although anecdotal experiences have been reported with voriconazole and terbinafine.[51,52]

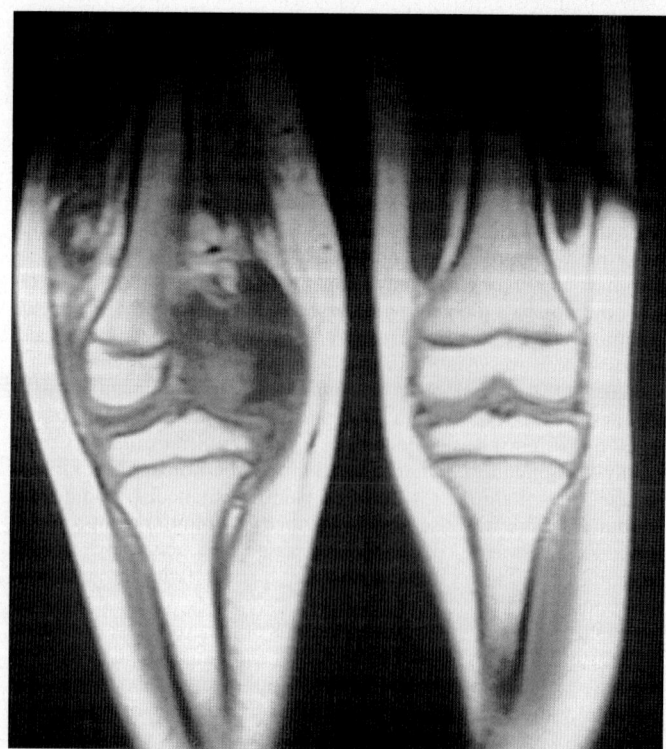

Figure 269-2 *Scedosporium prolificans* septic arthritis of the knee in an otherwise healthy 12-year-old boy. This condition developed in association with a splinter obtained during a playground fall. T_2-weighted magnetic resonance imaging depicts osteomyelitis of the medial condyle.

TABLE 269-1	Cutaneous and Subcutaneous Infections Caused by Dark-Walled Fungi		
Disease	*Lesions*	*Pathologic Features*	*Organisms**
Chromoblastomycosis	Scaly, friable, often verrucous nodules, commonly pruritic	Muriform cells (golden brown cells with cross walls in more than one plane)	*Fonsecaea pedrosoi* *Cladophialophora carrionii* *Phialophora verrucosa* *Rhinocladiella aquaspersa*
Mycetoma (eumycetoma, eumycotic mycetoma)	Nodular with draining sinuses, areas of healing	Grains composed of septate hyphae	*Madurella mycetomatis* *Leptosphaeria senegalensis* *Madurella grisea*
Subcutaneous phaeohyphomycosis	Painless, subcutaneous nodules	Septate hyphae (pseudohyphae or yeasts may also be apparent)	*Bipolaris* spp. *Exophiala* spp. *Exserohilum* spp. *Phaeoacremonium* spp. *Phialophora* spp. *Wangiella* spp.

*The most common causes are listed. See individual chapters for more complete listings (Chapter 261, Chromoblastomycosis; Chapter 262, Mycetoma).

Dark-Walled Fungi and Agents of Phaeohyphomycosis

Phaeohyphomycosis is a loosely defined term used to group infections caused by molds (and a few yeasts) that produce dark cell walls. Also described as *dematiaceous*, these are a diverse group of fungi found in the soil and air and growing on plants and in organic debris. The number of genera and species of fungi causing phaeohyphomycosis is quite large.[53,54] Frequent changes in species names have compounded the difficulty in comparing similar cases from the literature. Chromoblastomycosis (see Chapter 261) and mycetoma (see Chapter 262) are distinct infections that include dark-walled fungi as etiologic agents that are generally not included in this loose classification (Table 269-1). *P. boydii* and *Scedosporium prolificans* produce dark structures in culture, and some authorities currently consider *S. prolificans* infection one of the phaeohyphomycoses.[35] The syndromes most commonly produced by the dark-walled fungi include cutaneous and subcutaneous disease (other than chromomycosis or mycetoma), brain abscesses, and sinusitis. Fungemia[55] and disseminated disease[35] are more commonly being described in immunocompromised individuals. Meningitis, pneumonia, prosthetic valve endocarditis, contamination of saline-filled breast implants, infections in peritoneal dialysis and central venous catheters, osteomyelitis, and septic arthritis have also been reported. For most clinical purposes, it is preferable to describe disease by the type of infection and species name, such as "*Cladophialophora bantiana* brain abscess" and to reserve the term *phaeohyphomycosis* for cases in which no culture data exist or in which recovered fungi have not yet been identified.

Subcutaneous phaeohyphomycosis typically begins as a single red nodule, usually on the extremities. In an immunocompetent person, an indolent, painless expansion in the skin and subcutaneous tissue occurs, sometimes with cyst formation (Fig. 269-3). More rapid local progression and, in rare cases, extension to the brain can occur in immunosuppressed patients. A history of minor trauma is often present, or a splinter is found in the resected lesion. The fungi causing subcutaneous phaeohyphomycosis are extraordinarily diverse, but species of *Bipolaris, Exophiala, Exserohilum, Phialophora,* and *Wangiella* are particularly common.

Brain abscess is one of the best-described syndromes produced by the dark-walled fungi.[53,56,57] Disease manifests with headache of indolent onset, low-grade or no fever, and development of focal neurologic signs. There is rarely a history of exposure to dust or mold, no obvious pulmonary portal, and no evidence of dissemination outside the CNS. Affected male patients have outnumbered female patients 3:1, the median age of diagnosis is 38 years, and most patients have been immunocompetent.[57-59] Abscesses may be single or multiple and, on computed tomography or magnetic resonance imaging, are well localized within the cerebral cortex (Fig. 269-4).[60] Purulent meningitis, with or without brain abscess, may also be observed (Fig. 269-5).[61] Hematoxylin and eosin (H&E) staining reveals abscesses to have purulent centers with surrounding granulomatous reaction, and organisms appear as septate hyphae with golden brown cell walls. As in other forms of infections with the dark-walled fungi, hyphae are commonly irregular in diameter, and yeastlike cells are seen with some species. The species most commonly causing these infections is *C. bantiana* (previously named *Xylohypha bantiana, Cladosporium bantianum,* and

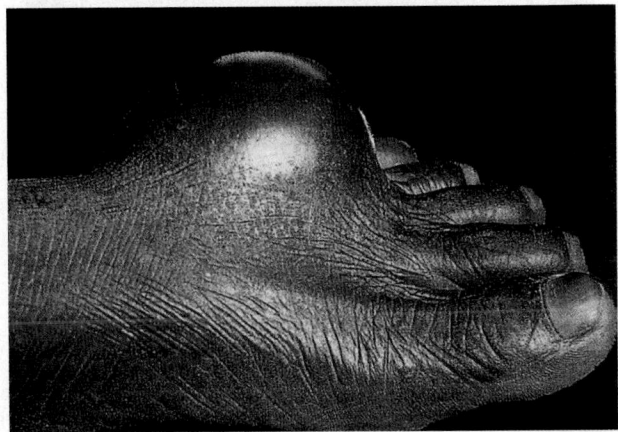

Figure 269-3 **Phaeohyphomycosis manifesting as a cyst.** *(From Chandler FW, Watts JC. Phaeohyphomycosis. In: Connor DH, Chandler FW, Schwartz DA, et al, eds. Pathology of Infectious Diseases. Norwalk, CT: Appleton & Lange; 1997.)*

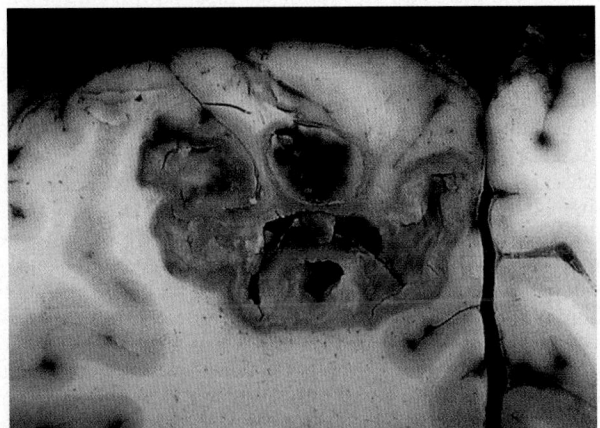

Figure 269-4 **Phaeohyphomycosis of the brain caused by *Cladophialophora* sp.** *(From Chandler FW, Watts JC. Phaeohyphomycosis. In: Connor DH, Chandler FW, Schwartz DA, et al, eds. Pathology of Infectious Diseases. Norwalk, CT: Appleton & Lange; 1997.)*

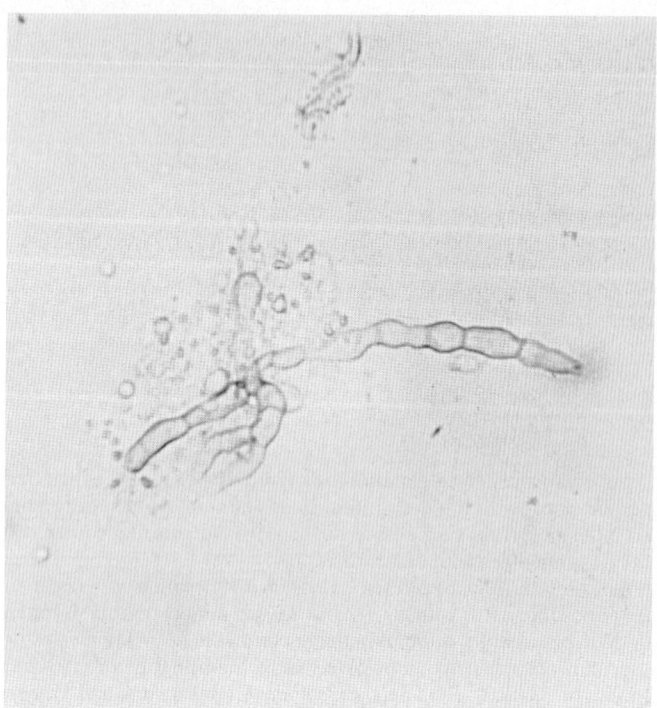

Figure 269-5   Weakly pigmented, segmented hyphae of *Clado-phialophora bantiana* in the wet mount of pus from the base of the brain.

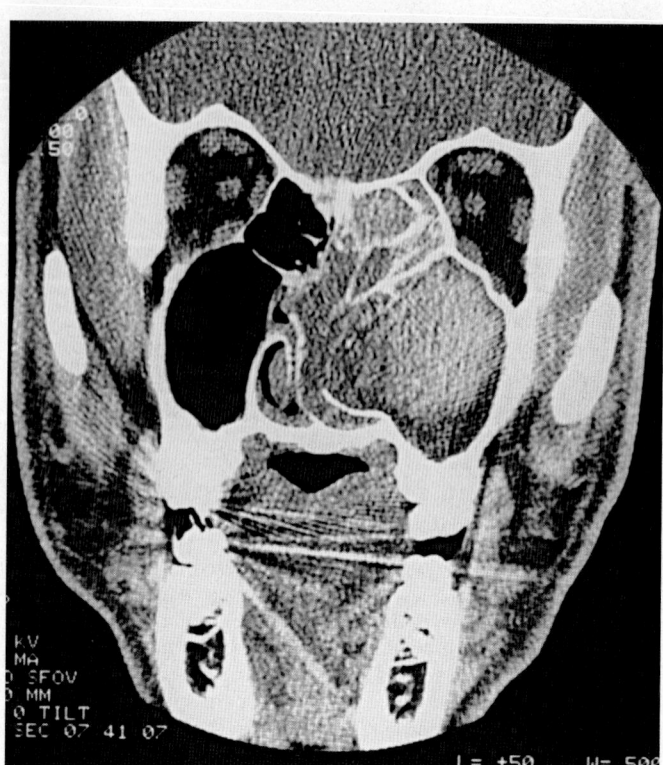

Figure 269-6   Computed tomographic scan showing outward-bulging mass in the maxillary and ethmoid sinuses of a patient with allergic fungal sinusitis.

Cladosporium trichoides), but disease is also caused by *Ramichloridium mackenziei, Ochroconis gallopavum* (formerly known as *Dactylaria constricta* var. *gallopava*), *Wangiella dermatitidis, Bipolaris spicifera, Bipolaris hawaiiensis, Chaetomium* species, and, even more rarely, other phaeohyphomycetes.[57,59,62] *R. mackenziei* infections are reported chiefly from the Middle East and India,[63,64] and *W. dermatitidis* cases predominate in the Far East. *Fonsecaea monophora* (formerly classified with *Fonsecaea pedrosoi*) has been recognized as an etiologic agent of CNS phaehyphomycosis.[65]

Allergic fungal sinusitis may be caused by a wide variety of fungi, although the dark-walled fungi (usually *Bipolaris, Exserohilum, Curvularia,* or *Alternaria* spp.) and *Aspergillus* spp. are the most common causes.[66] By definition, disease is allergic and confined to the lumen of the paranasal sinuses. Patients present with an indolent onset of sinus pain or painless proptosis. A history of seasonal or allergic rhinitis is common, and there may be a history of nasal polyps. On computed tomography or magnetic resonance imaging, one or more paranasal sinuses appear full of fluid, with outward pressure on the thinner bony sinus walls, such as the lamina papyracea, medial maxillary wall, or midline sphenoidal septum. Maxillary and ethmoid sinuses are usually involved, but sphenoid and frontal sinuses may be diseased (Fig. 269-6). Surgical débridement of the paranasal sinus removes dark, inspissated mucus; histopathologic examination reveals that this mucus has eosinophils with Charcot-Leyden crystals (degenerated eosinophils) and scattered septate hyphae.[67] The walls of the hyphae may not appear as dark as those seen in brain abscess. Irregular diameter and bulbous swellings may help distinguish these hyphae from *Aspergillus,* but culture is essential for diagnosis. The most serious sequela of allergic fungal sinusitis is brain invasion, which, when it occurs, usually does so in immunocompromised hosts (Fig. 269-7). Extension from the ethmoid or frontal sinus into the frontal lobe of the brain can be clinically silent. Erosion into the clivus, pterygoid space, or middle fossa occurs but is rare. Sudden blindness can result from compression of the optic nerve posterior to the orbital fissure. Compression of the orbit by lateral bulging of the lamina papyracea does not decrease visual acuity but does cause proptosis.

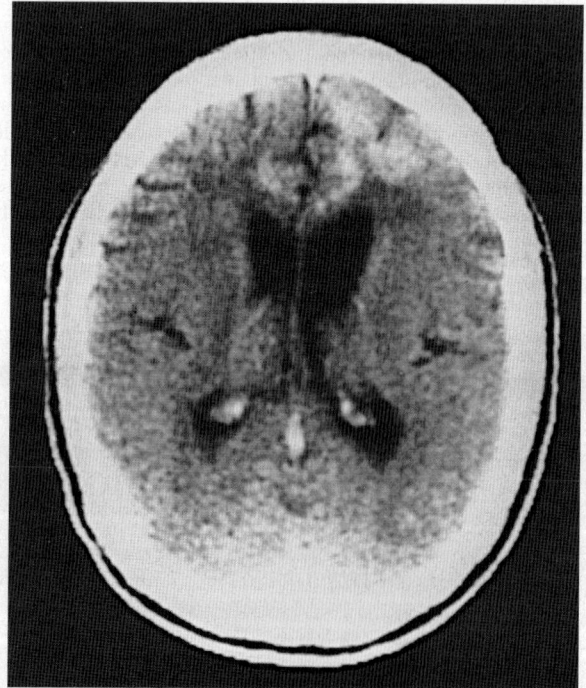

Figure 269-7   T$_2$-weighted magnetic resonance image depicting extension into the frontal lobe of a patient with *Bipolaris hawaiiensis* sinusitis.

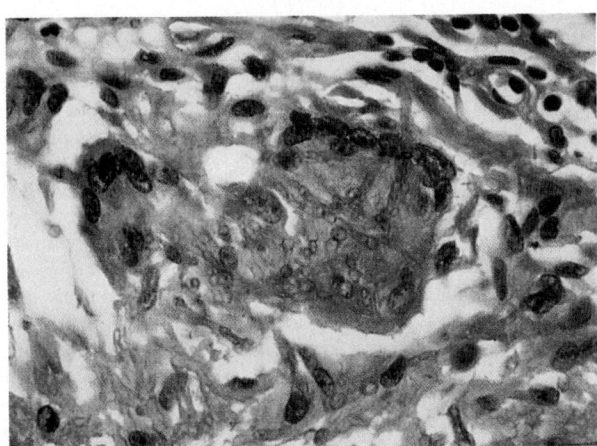

Figure 269-8 Cutaneous phaeohyphomycosis caused by *Exophiala jeanselmei.* Note the brown hyphae. (Hematoxylin and eosin stain.) *(From Chandler FW, Watts JC. Phaeohyphomycosis. In: Connor DH, Chandler FW, Schwartz DA, et al, eds.* Pathology of Infectious Diseases. *Norwalk, CT: Appleton & Lange; 1997.)*

Diagnosis of these infections requires observation of the fungi invading tissue or recovery of the fungi in culture from an otherwise sterile site. Lack of tissue invasion is necessary for the diagnosis of allergic fungal sinusitis by definition. In disease outside the CNS, these organisms may not always appear dark-walled on standard histopathologic stains. Cell wall melanin may be visible as a brownish-yellow color on H&E stain (Fig. 269-8). If melanin is not evident on fresh preparations of H&E stain, it can be stained by the Fontana-Masson method, which better enables diagnosis, especially if culture results are negative or if culture is not performed.[68] Fontana-Masson stain is, however, not 100% specific for the dark-walled fungi because the cell walls of some *Aspergillus* and other fungi with hyaline hyphae have been shown to stain dark with this method.[69]

Surgical débridement is essential to the cure of most of the infections caused by the dark-walled fungi. Good surgical curettage often suffices in treating allergic sinusitis if the cranial cavity has not been invaded. Amphotericin B is probably the drug of choice for life-threatening infection, including CNS infection. Itraconazole has been used frequently with success in infections that are not life-threatening.[70,71] To help prevent further recurrence in patients who have recurrent allergic fungal sinusitis, long-term itraconazole therapy may be used after repeated surgical drainage. In vitro, in response to most of these fungi, voriconazole commonly produces minimum inhibitory concentrations that are similar to or lower than those seen with itraconazole, which makes this new drug a potentially useful therapeutic agent.[28] Posaconazole and caspofungin have also been shown to have in vitro activity against many of these fungi.[24,25] Posaconazole has been reported to produce a good clinical response in single cases of CNS and disseminated infection caused by *R. mackenziei* and *Exophiala spinifera,* respectively.[72,73] Response of a skin and soft tissue infection to terbinafine, after poor response to amphotericin B and itraconazole, has also been reported.[74]

Fusarium Species

Species in the genus *Fusarium* are common in soil and organic debris and are frequently the cause of disease in plants. Disease in humans is rare, usually occurring after traumatic inoculation in the healthy host. Inhalation or minor trauma can lead to fusariosis in immunocompromised patients. *Fusarium,* usually *Fusarium solani,* is one of the more common causes of fungal keratitis.[75] *Fusarium* can also cause onychomycosis,[76] endophthalmitis, and skin and musculoskeletal infections (including mycetoma).[77,78] Since the early 1970s, pneumonia, fungemia, and disseminated infection with *Fusarium* have become increasingly common problems in persons with hematologic malignancy and other immunocompromising disorders (including AIDS).

Rare cases of dissemination have been described in the clinical setting of severe burns,[79] trauma,[80] and heat stroke.[81] Most commonly, however, fusariosis occurs in patients with acute leukemia (70% to 80% of cases)[82,83] and prolonged neutropenia (more than 90% of cases).[82,84] In one review of 43 patients, the median duration of neutropenia was more than 3 weeks.[82] Fusariosis is also increasingly reported in patients undergoing bone marrow transplantation.[85] The portal of entry in most of these cases of disseminated infection is not known. Inhalation, ingestion, and entry through skin trauma have been suggested. Sinusitis has preceded dissemination in a few reports. Hematogenous spread has been attributed to indwelling intravascular catheters.[86,87] Onychomycosis has been postulated to be a source of this infection in some patients.[82,88] More recently, water has been suggested as a source of these infections; the fungus was found in one hospital water supply system and in several water sources at a dialysis center.[89,90]

Infection commonly manifests with fever and myalgia unresponsive to broad-spectrum antibacterial antibiotics during periods of profound neutropenia. Disseminated fusariosis has been recognized in patients who have been receiving empiric or prophylactic antifungal therapy.[83,85,91] Skin lesions occur in 60% to 80% of infections, usually appearing as multiple papules or deep-set, painful nodules (Fig. 269-9). They may initially be flat (macular) with a central pallor, but later they become raised, erythematous, and necrotic (Fig. 269-10).[77,82,84] Lesions are most common on the extremities but have been reported on the trunk and face as well. In profoundly neutropenic patients, this infection can progress rapidly to death, in a manner similar to that in invasive aspergillosis. Skin lesions, denoting dissemination, can occur within a day of the onset of fever. In patients whose neutrophil level starts returning to normal, the infection can progress slowly over weeks until death or can become controlled and eventually cured.

Recovery of the fungus from the blood and biopsy of suspect skin lesions are the two most common and effective ways to diagnose this infection. In contrast to aspergillosis, in which blood culture results are nearly always negative, fusariosis is accompanied by positive blood culture results about 50% of the time (48 of 98 patients in one review[82]). Although nonspecific for *Fusarium* spp., a finding of septate hyphal elements in a skin biopsy specimen should aid in making rapid therapeutic decisions. *Fusarium* organisms can usually be recovered in culture of skin biopsy tissue and seen in histopathologic studies. The hyphae resemble *Aspergillus* organisms. *Fusarium* organisms have a predilection for small blood vessels, which results in angioinvasion and

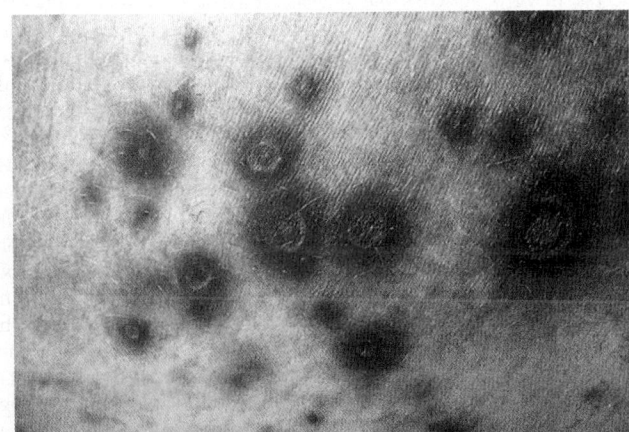

Figure 269-9 Cutaneous lesions of disseminated infection caused by *Fusarium moniliforme. (From Beneke ES, Rogers AL.* Medical Mycology and Human Mycoses. *Belmont, CA: Star Publishing Company; 1996.)*

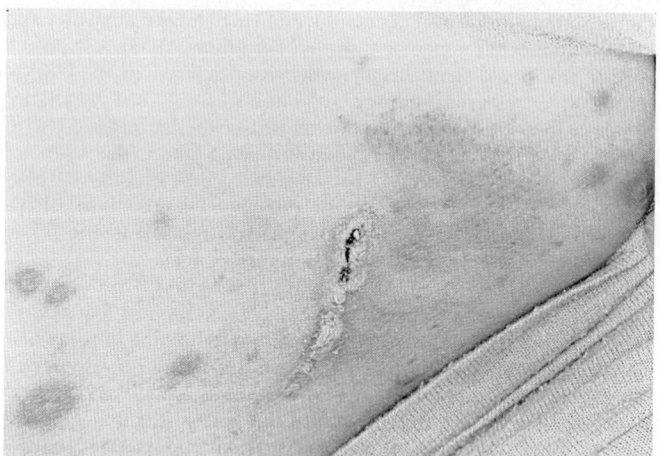

Figure 269-10 Multiple necrotic skin lesions in a neutropenic patient with hematogenously disseminated fusariosis.

associated thrombosis, although not as prominently as with *Aspergillus*. The septate hyphae of *Fusarium* spp. are difficult to visualize with routine H&E staining but are easily identified when tissue is prepared with Gomori methenamine-silver or periodic acid–Schiff stains. In culture, the characteristic feature of *Fusarium* is the production of sickle (banana)–shaped multiseptate macroconidia.[92] *F. solani* is the species most commonly recovered (when speciated), followed by *Fusarium oxysporum* and *Fusarium moniliforme* (also known as *Fusarium verticilloides*).[78,82,84]

The optimal treatment for disseminated fusariosis has not been established. Overall mortality in this infection has been reported to range from 50% to 80%.[78,85] Survival is almost always associated with the recovery from neutropenia, although corticosteroid use also impairs response to therapy.[82,84,93] In an analysis of responders versus nonresponders in one study of 43 patients, investigators noted associations with malignancy in remission (100% vs. 10%), adequate neutrophil counts (100% vs. 0%), and lack of significant (grade II or greater) graft-versus-host disease (0% vs. 66%).[82] Removal of indwelling venous catheters has been associated with improvement and thus should be considered in all cases of fungemia.[87] Amphotericin B has been included in the regimens of most successfully treated patients, and many authorities thus still consider high-dose (1.0 to 1.5 mg/kg/day) amphotericin B the drug of choice. Treatment with lipid-based amphotericin B formulations,[82,94] caspofungin,[95] and combinations of other approved antifungal agents has been reported,[96] with mixed success. In vitro, voriconazole and posaconazole have been shown to be of potential value.[24,25,27,28,97] Susceptibility varies among *Fusarium* species, however; *F. solani* is routinely less susceptible to both of these agents.[97] In vitro synergy has been shown between voriconazole and terbinafine,[98] and amphotericin B minimum inhibitory concentrations are decreased when this drug is combined with azithromycin.[99] Animal models have shown liposomal amphotericin B,[100] posaconazole,[101] and voriconazole[102] to be potentially useful in this difficult-to-treat mycosis. On the basis of successful therapy in 9 (43%) of 21 patients who received voriconazole, the FDA approved this agent for second-line use in fusariosis. Unfortunately, at least one case of breakthrough infection in a patient receiving voriconazole has been reported.[103] Successful therapy in 10 of 21 (48%) patients with posaconazole has also been reported.[104] The addition of colony-stimulating factors (G-CSF or granulocyte-macrophage colony-stimulating factor) or granulocyte transfusions to specific antifungal therapy has also been reported,[77,82,84,105] but the benefit of these adjunctive therapies is also not proven. With the current lack of clarity on how to best approach these infections, the author suggests starting patients with life-threatening infections on both a broad spectrum azole and amphotericin B.

Other Opportunistic Molds

In immunocompromised hosts, virtually any of the normally nonpathogenic fungi may cause disease. In addition to more common infections caused by *Aspergillus* and *Fusarium* spp., other rare light-colored (hyaline) molds, including species of *Paecilomyces*,[106] *Acremonium*,[107] *Trichoderma*,[108] and *Scopulariopsis*,[109] have been described as causing clinical disease more frequently than do other rare fungi. Some authorities have grouped disease caused by molds with light-colored cell walls into a group, termed the *hyalohyphomycoses*. As with the dark-walled fungi, description of these infections by the causative organisms is preferable, to minimize confusion. *Paecilomyces* has been reported to cause keratitis, endophthalmitis, and cutaneous and subcutaneous infections, as well as catheter-related fungemia, sinusitis, and disseminated infection. Like *Fusarium*, both *Paecilomyces* and *Acremonium* organisms have been reported to form reproductive structures in vivo in a process called *adventitious sporulation*.[110] This is believed to account for the much higher frequency of recovery in blood culture observed in infections involving these three genera. Also like *Fusarium*, both are typically associated with poor response to amphotericin B and the older azoles, although resistance varies among species. *Paecilomyces varioti* is susceptible to amphotericin B, and infections have been treated successfully with this agent. *Paecilomyces lilacinus* responds poorly to amphotericin B and, in vitro, is resistant to this agent, to caspofungin, and to the older azoles.[111] In vitro testing has shown multiple strains of these fungi to be more susceptible to voriconazole, ravuconazole, and posaconazole, but clinical treatment results are limited to case reports and small case series.[28,106]

Trichosporon Species

The genus *Trichosporon* is characterized by the production of septate hyphae, arthroconidia, yeasts, and pseudohyphae and by yeastlike growth on culture media. As a result of revisions in taxonomy, most of the agents of deeply invasive human *Trichosporon* infections are considered the species *Trichosporon asahii* or, less commonly, *Trichosporon mucoides*.[112-115] According to this schema, *Trichosporon asteroides* and *Trichosporon cutaneum* cause superficial infections of humans. White piedra of the scalp is caused by *Trichosporon ovoides*, and similar disease of the pubic hair is caused by *Trichosporon inkin* (see Chapter 267). *Trichosporon* can be found in soil and water, on plants, and colonizing human stool, skin, or urine.[116] More than 100 patients with deep trichosporonosis have been described; approximately 60% have been severely neutropenic, usually with acute leukemia.[115,117,118] A few have had organ transplantation, HIV infection, burns, chronic ambulatory peritoneal dialysis, or catheter-acquired fungemia.[119] Seven patients had prosthetic valve infections.[116]

Trichosporonosis is an acute, febrile, often fatal infection with dissemination to multiple deep organs and is associated with a mortality rate as high as 64%. Pneumonia is not a consistent or early feature, and thus the portal of entry is often not apparent. Renal involvement is common in disseminated disease and is associated with hematuria and funguria. Multiple red papular skin lesions may occur early on and assist diagnosis.[120,121] On biopsy, *Trichosporon* is seen as a mixture of true hyphae, pseudohyphae, budding yeasts, and arthroconidia, and it is easily mistaken for candidiasis (which does not produce arthroconidia). *Trichosporon* grows readily on most culture media, but blood cultures tend to yield positive results late in the course. In the past, therapy with amphotericin B was recommended, but poor response and failures with this drug have occurred. Minimum inhibitory concentrations of the echinocandins for these fungi are very high, and multiple incidences of breakthrough infections in patients receiving echinocandins have been reported.[122] These fungi are usually susceptible in vitro to fluconazole, itraconazole, and the new broad-spectrum azoles[123]; thus, therapy should include use of one of these azole antifungals.

Malassezia furfur

Malassezia furfur, a lipophilic yeast, commonly colonizes normal human skin and is the cause of a superficial mycosis, pityriasis (tinea) versicolor (see Chapter 267). The fungus can also cause catheter-related sepsis, almost always in patients who are receiving parenteral lipids through a central venous catheter.[124] Most reported patients have been neonates with extended stays in intensive care units, although a few have been adults with malignancy or immunosuppression.[125] Fever has been the most common finding, but bradycardia, apnea, thrombocytopenia, and catheter blockage have been observed in some infants. In the autopsy study of one case, the yeast was observed in lipid-containing areas of pulmonary vascular endothelium. *M. furfur* is rarely detected by conventional culture techniques because the yeast requires fatty acids for growth. Organisms are better recovered with culture of blood drawn back through the catheter through the use of the lysis-centrifugation technique and lipid-enriched agar.[124] The fungus adheres to the lumen of the catheter and has not been eradicated by discontinuing lipid infusions or administering miconazole or amphotericin B through the catheter.[126] Catheter removal and discontinuing parenteral lipids have been curative. In vitro, *M. furfur* appears to be susceptible to both amphotericin B and azole antifungals, including itraconazole and voriconazole.[127,128] Results of cultures or smears of peripheral blood are occasionally positive.[129] The yeast is identified on smear by its size and shape and the distinctive collarette between mother and daughter cells. Lipid requirement for growth also aids identification. It is likely that some cases attributed to *M. furfur* were caused by other lipid-requiring species in the *M. furfur* complex, which includes *Malassezia sympodialis, Malassezia globosa, Malassezia obtusa, Malassezia restricta,* and *Malassezia slooffiae*.[130] *Malassezia pachydermatis* has the same appearance and has caused similar infections, including an outbreak in a neonatal intensive care unit,[131] but does not require lipids for growth.

Other Uncommon Yeasts

Blastoschizomyces capitatus (formerly known as *Trichosporon capitatum* or *Geotrichum capitatum*) has reportedly caused severe infection in more than 75 patients, most of whom also had acute leukemia.[132,133] Blood culture findings are usually positive, and skin lesions similar to those seen in leukemic patients with disseminated candidiasis have been observed. *B. capitatus* may colonize the skin, respiratory tract, and gastrointestinal tract. Intravenous catheters are a possible portal of entry.[134] Intravenous amphotericin B with or without flucytosine[134] and voriconazole or high-dose fluconazole with amphotericin B[133] have been advocated for treatment of these infections. High-dose fluconazole was shown in an animal model to be more efficacious than amphotericin B, flucytosine, or voriconazole monotherapy.[135] Catheter removal was associated with improved outcome in the largest and most recent report.[133]

Other noncandidal yeasts may also rarely cause infection in humans.[136] These include *Pichia (Hansenula) anomala,*[137,138] the black yeast *Exophiala (Wangiella) jeanselmei,*[55] *Rhodotorula* spp.,[139] and *Saccharomyces cerevisiae*.[140] Infection is usually seen in immunocompromised individuals, most commonly as catheter-associated fungemia. Localized outbreaks secondary to *E. jeanselmei* and *P. anomala* have been described.[55,138]

Penicillium marneffei

Penicillium marneffei is a thermally dimorphic fungus that causes life-threatening disseminated infection (penicilliosis marneffei) in a geographically distinct area of the world. The expansion of the AIDS epidemic in Southeast Asia has led to a marked rise in the incidence of disseminated infection with *P. marneffei*. Before the first reports of HIV-related infection in 1988, fewer than 30 cases had been described since the first human infection in 1959.[141,142] Between 1984 and 2004, more than 6000 *P. marneffei* infections were diagnosed in Thailand.[143]

In the mid-1990s, this was the third most common opportunistic infection seen in HIV-infected individuals in northern Thailand.[144] Infection with *P. marneffei* has a limited geographic distribution, affecting persons residing in or those who have visited Southeast Asia or southern China. Endogenous cases have been reported from Myanmar (Burma), Hong Kong, Indonesia, Laos, Malaysia, Singapore, Taiwan, Thailand, Vietnam, and the Guangxi province of China.[145-147] Although most commonly seen in young adults infected with HIV, the disease has been reported in children[148,149] and adults, both with and without detectable immunocompromise.[145,146] *P. marneffei* has been isolated from the organs of apparently healthy bamboo rats (*Rhizomys pruinosis, Rhizomys sinensis, Rhizomys sumatrensis,* and *Cannomys badius*)[150,151] and the soil around their burrows.[152] The role of these rats in human infection is unknown. A case-control study of the disease in 80 persons with AIDS revealed an association with recent history of occupational or other exposure to soil.[153] In that study, no association between infection and exposure to bamboo rats was found. According to one report, infection occurs more commonly during the rainy season in northern Thailand.[154] It is likely that this infection is acquired by inhalation of conidia from an environmental source such as the soil.

Patients typically present with a chronic illness averaging 4 weeks in duration associated with low-grade fever, weight loss, and one or more skin lesions.[144] The most common clinical characteristics are fever, malaise, anemia, leukocytosis, weight loss, and, in 60% to 70% of patients, skin lesions.[144,146] Fungemia, generalized lymphadenopathy, and cough are reported in about half of patients. Subcutaneous and mucosal lesions, diarrhea, colonic lesions, hepatomegaly with or without splenomegaly, hemoptysis, osteoarticular lesions, and pericarditis have also been described.[145,155,156] Skin lesions commonly occur on the face, upper trunk, and extremities. They may occur as papules, pustules, nodules, ulcers, or abscesses. In HIV-infected individuals, lesions commonly become umbilicated and resemble those of molluscum contagiosum. Pharyngeal and palatal lesions are also more commonly seen in HIV-infected patients.[156] Lung lesions can appear as reticulonodular, nodular, or diffuse alveolar infiltrates, but on occasion they are cavitary and cause hemoptysis.[157] Autopsy studies have revealed involvement of lymph nodes, liver, spleen, lung, kidney, skin, bone, bone marrow, adrenal, tonsil, bowel, and meninges.[145,158]

Consideration of the diagnosis of *P. marneffei* infection should be made in persons who have resided in or visited an endemic area. Laboratory exposure to the organism was causally linked to disseminated infection in one immunocompromised individual.[159] The duration of incubation is not currently known, and reactivation disease may be possible. In one report, a severely immunocompromised individual acquired disseminated infection more than 10 years after visiting an endemic area.[160] Diagnosis is based on identification of the organism on smear, histopathologic studies, or culture. Diagnosis has been made most frequently from smears of skin lesions and biopsy samples of lymph node and bone marrow.[144] The organism has also been noted on peripheral blood smear in at least one report.[161] Isolation of *P. marneffei* from culture of bone marrow, blood, lymph node, skin lesions, bronchoalveolar lavage, or sputum can be diagnostic. Microscopic examination of clinical materials reveals yeast forms (2×2 to 3×6.5 μm) both within phagocytes and extracellularly.[145] The intracellular forms are smaller, resembling *Histoplasma capsulatum*, whereas the extracellular forms are larger and often have a transverse septum (asexual fission or schizogony) (Fig. 269-11). The extracellular forms may also appear as "sausage forms," consisting of three cells (8 to 13 μm in length) divided by two transverse septa or, rarely, as short hyphae. Three types of histopathologic reactions have been noted in association with *P. marneffei* infection: granulomatous, suppurative, and necrotizing inflammation.[158] Granulomatous or suppurative changes are most commonly seen in patients with normal immunity. The necrotizing reaction is more commonly seen in immunocompromised patients and is characterized by focal necrosis with surrounding histiocytes and extracellular fungi. Culture at 30°C produces a mold with sporulating structures typical of *Penicillium* organisms. Identification is aided by the formation of a soluble red pigment that diffuses

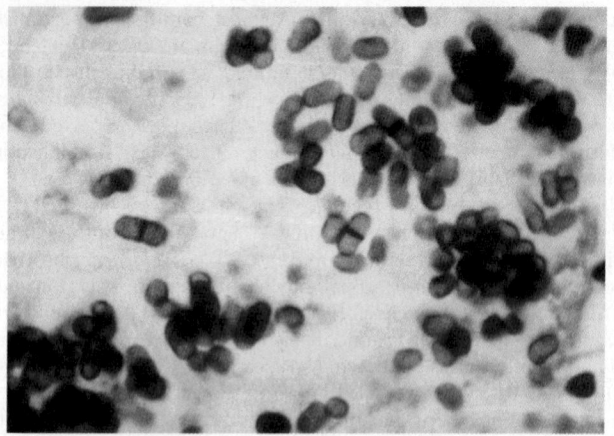

Figure 269-11 *Penicillium marneffei* **in a splenic abscess.** Note the transverse septa. (Gomori methenamine-silver stain.) *(From McGinnis MR, Chandler FW. Penicilliosis marneffei. In: Connor DH, Chandler FW, Schwartz DA, et al, eds. Pathology of Infectious Diseases. Norwalk, CT: Appleton & Lange; 1997.)*

into the agar. The mold form can be converted to a yeast form by incubation at 37° C; such dimorphism is not found in other known members of the genus *Penicillium*.[162] Because disease normally appears to result from inhalation of conidia, it seems reasonable to use Biosafety Level II precautions when working with the mold form. Diagnosis by specific immunologic techniques, including serum antibody and antigen tests, is still in the experimental stage.[163,164] The currently available galactomannan test for *Aspergillus* may assist in the diagnosis; two thirds of patients with *P. marneffei* infection had positive test results in one study.[165]

Successful treatment of disseminated infection has been reported with amphotericin B with or without the addition of flucytosine.[145] Therapy with itraconazole has also been successful, as has voriconazole in smaller series.[166] Although no randomized comparative studies have been performed, the failure rates in a study of 86 HIV-infected patients were as follows: 8 of 35 patients (22.9%) taking amphotericin B; 3 of

12 (25%) taking itraconazole; and 7 of 11 (63.6%) taking fluconazole.[167] Excellent response (97.3%) was achieved with a regimen of intravenous amphotericin B for 2 weeks (0.6 mg/kg/day) followed by oral itraconazole for 10 weeks (200 mg twice daily) in 74 HIV-infected patients.[168] This regimen allowed shortened hospital stays while producing a clearing of fungemia that was more rapid than that produced by itraconazole alone. Itraconazole has been shown to prevent relapse of this disease in patients with HIV infection.[169] Secondary prophylaxis in HIV-infected patients with itraconazole (200 mg once daily) has been suggested to prevent relapse.[144] As with secondary prophylaxis in other fungal diseases, it appears safe to stop this therapy after response to antiretroviral therapy (CD4+ cell count of 100 cells/μL or greater for at least 6 months).[170]

Lacazia loboi

Lobomycosis (Lobo's disease, keloidal blastomycosis) is a chronic skin infection most commonly afflicting the indigenous people of the Amazon regions of Colombia and Brazil. The etiologic agent of lobomycosis has never been isolated in culture, but it has been shown to be closely related to *Paracoccidioides brasiliensis* by 18S ribosomal DNA (rDNA) sequencing.[171] This fungus has been known by many genus names; most recently, *Lacazia loboi* has been proposed to replace *Loboa loboi* and other previous designations.[172] More than 100 cases have been reported from countries in Central and South America. The disease has not been acquired in the United States, except perhaps a form that was reported in dolphins.[53] The fungus remains confined to the skin, progressing slowly over decades. Probably because of this slow progression, rare cases outside of the endemic area have been reported, often many years after potential exposure.[173] Lesions are typically nodules or keloidal plaques that are red, hard, and shiny, in association with fibrosis and a granulomatous reaction on histologic examination (Figs. 269-12 and 269-13). The diagnosis is made by finding the typical globose to lemon-shaped cells (about 9 μm in diameter), either singly or in short chains (Fig. 269-14). Surgical excision is the only useful therapy.

Rhinosporidium seeberi

Rhinosporidiosis is a chronic, usually painless localized infection of the mucous membranes.[53] Formerly believed to be a fungus, the causative agent *Rhinosporidium seeberi* has also never been cultured. With 18S rDNA sequencing, this organism has been shown to be a protistan parasite.[174,175] Rhinosporidiosis occurs worldwide; the greatest numbers of cases are found in southern India and Sri Lanka.[176] Disease affects the nose and nasopharynx most commonly, the ocular structures less

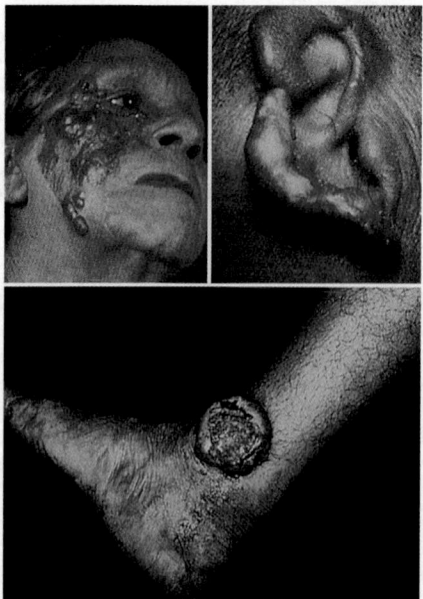

Figure 269-12 **Lobomycosis.** *(From Nikolaidis G, Rosen T. Lobomycosis. In: Connor DH, Chandler FW, Schwartz DA, et al, eds. Pathology of Infectious Diseases. Norwalk, CT: Appleton & Lange; 1997.)*

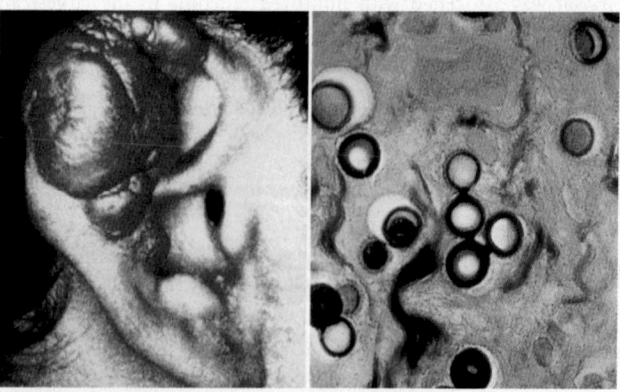

Figure 269-13 **Lobomycosis of the ear (*left*) with associated histologic findings (*right*).** (Gomori methenamine-silver stain.) *(From Herr RA, Herr E, Tarcha PR, et al. Phylogenetic analysis of Lacazia loboi places this previously uncharacterized pathogen with the dimorphic Onygenales. J Clin Microbiol. 2001;39:309-314.)*

269 Uncommon Fungi and *Protheca***

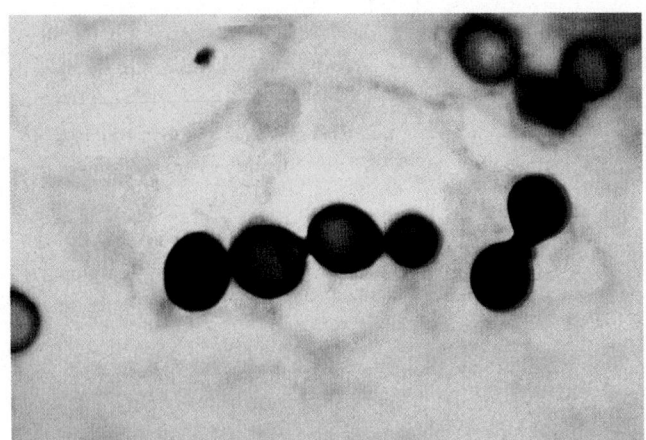

Figure 269-14 Histologic appearance of *Lacazia loboi*, the agent of lobomycosis. (Gomori methenamine-silver stain.) *(From Nikolaidis G, Rosen T. Lobomycosis. In: Connor DH, Chandler FW, Schwartz DA, et al, eds. Pathology of Infectious Diseases. Norwalk, CT: Appleton & Lange; 1997.)*

commonly, and the skin more rarely. Disseminated disease is quite rare. Lasser and Smith[177] reviewed 28 U.S. cases, finding 19 that affected the nose and 9 the conjunctiva, with 24 occurring in men and 4 in women. Lesions increase in size over months to years to form friable pedunculated masses, typically in the nose, upper airway, or conjunctiva.[178] Nasal lesions manifest as nasal obstruction or epistaxis.[179] One or more pedunculated or verrucous skin lesions, with or without nasal or conjunctival lesions, are occasionally observed.[180,181] In rare cases, polyps occur in the vagina, urethra, or penis. *R. seeberi* forms round, thick-walled cysts (sporangium) in the submucosa, varying in diameter from 10 to 200 μm, often visible through the mucosa as white dots. Mature cysts become filled with numerous spores (endospores), which on release become new cysts (Fig. 269-15). Treatment of choice is surgery.[178]

◾ *Protheca* Species

Protheca are unicellular algae that lack chlorophyll and reproduce by endosporulation. Although not fungi, these organisms are described in this chapter because they are often preliminarily misidentified in

tissue and culture as a yeast. These organisms are found in a wide range of environmental sites, including tree slime, sewage, fresh and marine water, soil, and foodstuffs. They may colonize human skin, the respiratory tract, and the gastrointestinal tract.[182] A little more than 100 cases of human infection have been reported,[53,183] almost all in adults and from widely scattered geographic areas. *Protheca wickerhamii* is the most common cause of infection in humans; infection secondary to *Protheca zofii* has also been reported.

The most common manifestation of protothecosis is a single lesion of the skin or subcutaneous tissue. The typical manifestation is a painless, slowly progressive, well-circumscribed plaque or papulonodular lesion that may become eczematoid or ulcerated. Soft tissue lesions favor the olecranon bursa, sites of minor trauma or corticosteroid injection,[184] and surgical wounds exposed to soil or water, such as that of a hand tendon repair. Lesions typically enlarge gradually over weeks to months. Skin lesions in HIV-infected patients have not differed from those seen in other patients.[185,186] Disseminated and deep-seated infections, such as peritonitis, meningitis, and endocarditis, have also been reported in rare cases.[183,187]

Protothecosis is best diagnosed through biopsy for histologic study and culture. The inflammatory response consists of both microabscesses and granulomas with multinucleate giant cells. *Protheca* cells usually range from 3 to 30 μm in diameter, are well visualized with Gomori methenamine-silver or periodic acid–Schiff stain, and often contain two to eight tightly packed endospores in each cell or sporangium (Fig. 269-16). White opaque colonies appear in a few days on standard mycologic media. Identification is made by gross and microscopic appearance plus biochemical testing (the algae is identified by most commercially available yeast identification systems).

Protothecosis has little, if any, tendency toward self-healing. There have been few cases of disseminated disease in the setting of solid organ or stem cell transplantation; all resulted in mortality.[187] Both surgical excision of lesions and intravenous amphotericin B have been used successfully.[185] *Protheca* spp. are resistant to flucytosine, but prolonged therapy with ketoconazole, itraconazole, or fluconazole has been reported to benefit some patients with skin lesions.[184,188,189] Short-course itraconazole (200 mg daily for 2 months) has been used successfully.[190]

◾ Summary

Key features of the uncommon fungi in this chapter are listed in Table 269-2.

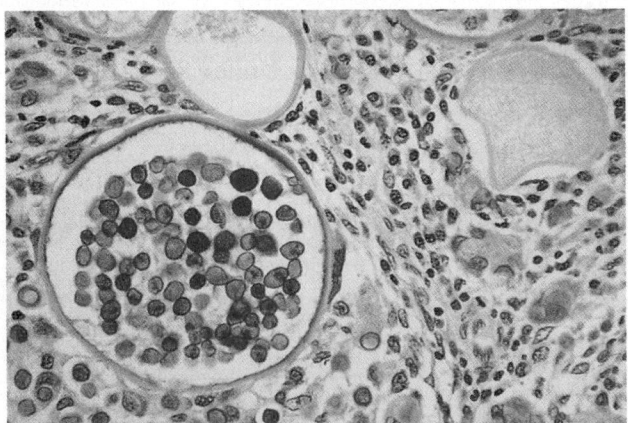

Figure 269-15 Mature sporangium of *Rhinosporidium seeberi*. (Mayer's mucicarmine stain.) *(From Watts JC, Chandler FW. Rhinosporidiosis. In: Connor DH, Chandler FW, Schwartz DA, et al, eds. Pathology of Infectious Diseases. Norwalk, CT: Appleton & Lange; 1997, with permission of the McGraw-Hill Companies.)*

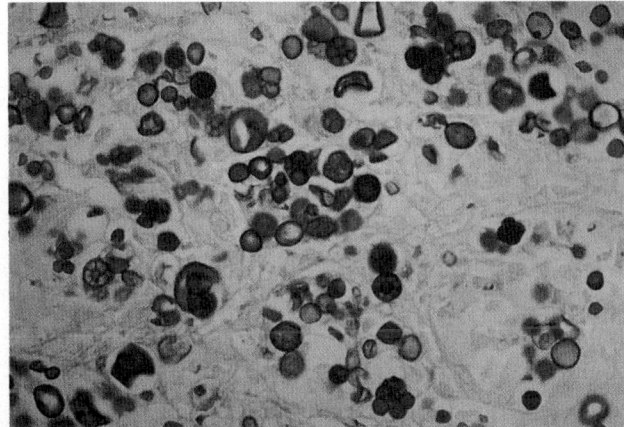

Figure 269-16 *Protheca wickerhamii* in an olecranon bursa biopsy sample. (Gridley stain.) *(From Ramsay E, Chandler FW, Connor DH. Protothecosis. In: Connor DH, Chandler FW, Schwartz DA, et al, eds. Pathology of Infectious Diseases. Norwalk, CT: Appleton & Lange; 1997.)*

TABLE 269-2	Key Features of the Uncommon Fungi, *Rhinosporidium* Species, and *Prototheca* Species					

Organism(s)	Risks Factors/Risk Groups	Geographic Epidemiologic Range	Ecologic Niche	Clinical Manifestations	Tissue Forms	Treatment
Pseudallescheria boydii (*Scedosporium apiospermum*)	Trauma, immunocompromise	Worldwide	Soil, fresh water, respiratory tract colonization	Pneumonia; osteoarticular, CNS, or disseminated infection; mycetoma	Septate hyphae	Voriconazole
Scedosporium prolificans	Severe immunocompromise, trauma	Worldwide	Soil, respiratory tract colonization	Disseminated infection, osteoarticular infection	Septate hyphae	Unknown (consider voriconazole or high-dose L-AMB)
Dark-walled fungi (including *Alternaria, Bipolaris, Cladophialophora, Curvularia, Exophiala, Exserohilum,* and *Wangiella* spp.)	Trauma, allergic rhinitis, immunocompromise	Worldwide	Soil, decaying organic matter, air, plants	Localized subcutaneous lesions, brain abscess, allergic sinusitis; disseminated infections (rare)	Septate hyphae; yeast or pseudohyphae (rarely)	High-dose D-AMB, L-AMB, itraconazole, or voriconazole
Fusarium spp.	Severe immunocompromise	Worldwide	Soil, plants	Disseminated infection, fungemia	Septate hyphae	Voriconazole +/− high-dose D-AMB or L-AMB
Trichosporon spp.	Immunocompromise, central venous catheters	Worldwide	Skin and gastrointestinal flora	Fungemia	Yeast, hyphae, arthroconidia, pseudohyphae	Fluconazole +/− high-dose D-AMB or L-AMB
Penicillium marneffei	AIDS	Southeastern Asia, southern China	Unknown	Disseminated infection	Yeasts or "sausage forms"	D-AMB +/− 5-FC or itraconazole or voriconazole
Lacazia loboi	Rural outdoor labor, minor trauma	Central and South America	Unknown	Localized cutaneous/ subcutaneous infection	Chains of large yeasts	Surgery
Rhinosporidium seeberi	Rural outdoor labor	India, Sri Lanka; very rare worldwide	Unknown	Localized mucous membrane polypoidal lesions	Spores in large (10 to 200 µm) cysts (sporangia)	Surgery
Prototheca spp.	Trauma	Worldwide	Water, soil, foodstuffs	Localized subcutaneous lesions	2-8 Endospores in sporangia	Surgery or itraconazole

AIDS, acquired immunodeficiency syndrome; CNS, central nervous system; high-dose D-AMB, deoxycholate amphotericin B (1.0 to 1.5 mg/kg/day); 5-FC, 5-fluorocytosine (should only be used when monitoring of levels is available locally); L-AMB, lipid preparations of amphotericin B (AmBisome, Abelcet, Amphotec).

REFERENCES

1. Guarro J, Kantarcioglu AS, Horre R, et al. *Scedosporium apiospermum*: changing clinical spectrum of a therapy-refractory opportunist. *Med Mycol.* 2006;44:295-327.
2. Kantarcioglu AS, Guarro J, de Hoog GS. Central nervous system infections by members of the *Pseudallescheria boydii* species complex in healthy and immunocompromised hosts: epidemiology, clinical characteristics and outcome. *Mycoses.* 2008;51:275-290.
3. Arnett JC, Hatch HB. Pulmonary allescheriasis: report of a case and review of the literature. *Arch Intern Med.* 1975;135:1250-1253.
4. Miller MA, Greenberger PA, Amerian R, et al. Allergic bronchopulmonary mycosis caused by *Pseudallescheria boydii. Am Rev Respir Dis.* 1993;148:810-812.
5. Bates DD, Mims JW. Invasive fungal sinusitis caused by *Pseudallescheria boydii:* case report and literature review. *Ear Nose Throat J.* 2006;85:729-737.
6. Husain S, Munoz P, Forrest G, et al. Infections due to *Scedosporium apiospermum* and *Scedosporium prolificans* in transplant recipients: clinical characteristics and impact of antifungal agent therapy on outcome. *Clin Infect Dis.* 2005;40:89-99.
7. Lamris GA, Chamilos G, Lewis RE, et al. *Scedosporium* infection in a tertiary care cancer center: a review of 25 cases from 1989-2006. *Clin Infect Dis.* 2006;43:1580-1584.
8. Castiglioni B, Dutton DA, Rinaldi MG, et al. *Pseudallescheria boydii* (anamorph *Scedosporium apiospermum*): Infection in solid organ transplant recipients in a tertiary medical center and review of the literature. *Medicine.* 2002;81:333-348.
9. Nomdedeu J, Brunet S, Martino R, et al. Successful treatment of pneumonia due to *Scedosporium apiospermum* with itraconazole: case report. *Clin Infect Dis.* 1993;16:731-733.
10. Bernstein EF, Schuster MG, Stieritz DD, et al. Disseminated cutaneous *Pseudallescheria boydii. Br J Dermatol.* 1995;132:456-460.
11. Larocco A, Barron JB. Endogenous *Scedosporium apiospermum* endophthalmitis. *Retina.* 2005;25:1090-1093.
12. Hung CC, Chang SC, Yang PC, et al. Invasive pulmonary pseudallescheriasis with direct invasion of the thoracic spine in an immunocompetent patient. *Eur J Clin Microbiol Infect Dis.* 1994;13:749-751.
13. Halpern AA, Nagel DA, Schurman DJ. *Allescheria boydii* osteomyelitis following multiple steroid injections and surgery. *Clin Orthop.* 1977;126:232-234.

14. Lavy D, Morin O, Venet G, et al. *Pseudallescheria boydii* knee arthritis in a young immunocompetent adult two years after a compound patellar fracture. *Joint Bone Spine.* 2001;68:517-520.
15. Tirado-Miranda R, Solera-Santos J, Brasero JC, et al. Septic arthritis due to *Scedosporium apiospermum*: case report and review. *J Infect.* 2001;43:210-212.
16. Montero A, Cohen JE, Fernandez MA, et al. Cerebral pseudallescheriasis due to *Pseudallescheria boydii* as the first manifestation of AIDS. *Clin Infect Dis.* 1998;26:1476-1477.
17. Bryan CS, DiSalvo AF, Kaufman L, et al. *Petriellidium boydii* infection of the sphenoid sinus. *Am J Clin Pathol.* 1980;74:846-851.
18. Dworzack DL, Clark RB, Borkowski WJ, et al. *Pseudallescheria boydii* brain abscess: association with near-drowning and efficacy of high-dose, prolonged miconazole therapy in patients with multiple abscesses. *Medicine.* 1989;68:218-224.
19. Benham RW, Georg LK. *Allescheria boydii*, causative agent in a case of meningitis. *J Invest Dermatol.* 1948;10:99-110.
20. Galgiani JN, Stevens DA, Graybill JR, et al. *Pseudallescheria boydii* infections treated with ketoconazole: clinical evaluations of seven patients and in vitro susceptibility results. *Chest.* 1984;82:219-224.
21. Piper JP, Golden J, Brown D, et al. Successful treatment of *Scedosporium apiospermum* suppurative arthritis with itraconazole. *Pediatr Infect Dis J.* 1990;9:674-675.
22. Barbaric D, Shaw PJ. *Scedosporium* infection in immunocompromised patients: successful use of liposomal amphotericin B and itraconazole. *Med Pediatr Oncol.* 2001;37:122-125.
23. Carrillo AJ, Guarro J. In vitro activities of four novel triazoles against *Scedosporium* spp. *Antimicrob Agents Chemother.* 2001;45:2151-2153.
24. Del Poeta M, Schell WA, Perfect JR. In vitro antifungal activity of pneumocandin L-743,872 against a variety of clinically important molds. *Antimicrob Agents Chemother.* 1997;41:1835-1836.
25. Espinel-Ingroff A. Comparison of in vitro activities of the new triazole SCH56592 and the echinocandins MK-0991 (L-743,872) and LY303366 against opportunistic filamentous and dimorphic fungi and yeasts. *J Clin Microbiol.* 1998;36:2950-2956.
26. Meletiadis J, Meis JF, Mouton JW, et al. In vitro activities of new and conventional antifungal agents against clinical *Scedosporium* isolates. *Antimicrob Agents Chemother.* 2002;46:62-68.

27. Pfaller MA, Marco F, Messer SA, et al. In vitro activity of two echinocandin derivatives, LY303366 and MK-0991 (L-743,792), against clinical isolates of *Aspergillus, Fusarium, Rhizopus,* and other filamentous fungi. *Diagn Microbiol Infect Dis.* 1998;30:251-255.
28. Radford SA, Johnson EM, Warnock DW. In vitro studies of activity of voriconazole (UK-109,496), a new triazole antifungal agent, against emerging and less-common mold pathogens. *Antimicrob Agents Chemother.* 1997;41:841-843.
29. Troke P, Aguirrebengoa K, Arteaga C, et al. Treatment of scedosporiosi with voriconazole: clinical experience with 107 patients. *Antimicrob Agents Chemother.* 2008;52:1743-1750.
30. Nesky MA, McDougal EC, Peacock JE Jr. *Pseudallescheria boydii* brain abscess successfully treated with voriconazole and surgical drainage: case report and literature review of central nervous system pseudallescheriasis. *Clin Infect Dis.* 2000;31:673-677.
31. Poza G, Montoya J, Redondo C, et al. Meningitis caused by *Pseudallescheria boydii* treated with voriconazole. *Clin Infect Dis.* 2000;30:981-982.
32. Mellinghoff IK, Winston DJ, Mukwaya G, et al. Treatment of *Scedosporium apiospermum* brain abscesses with posaconazole. *Clin Infect Dis.* 2002;34:1648-1650.
33. Malloch D, Salkin IF. A new species of *Scedosporium* associated with osteomyelitis in humans. *Mycotaxon.* 1984;21:247-255.
34. Idigoras P, Perez-Trallero E, Pineiro L, et al. Disseminated infection and colonization by *Scedosporium prolificans*: a review of 18 cases, 1990-1999. *Clin Infect Dis.* 2001;32:e158-e165.
35. Revankar SG, Patterson JE, Sutton DA, et al. Disseminated phaeohyphomycosis: review of an emerging mycosis. *Clin Infect Dis.* 2002;34:467-476.
36. Wilson CM, O'Rourke EJ, McGinnis MR, et al. *Scedosporium inflatum*: clinical spectrum of a newly recognized pathogen. *J Infect Dis.* 1990;161:102-107.
37. Wood GM, McCormack JG, Muir DB, et al. Clinical features of human infection with *Scedosporium inflatum. Clin Infect Dis.* 1992;14:1027-1033.
38. Alvarez M, Ponga BL, Rayon C, et al. Nosocomial outbreak caused by *Scedosporium prolificans (inflatum)*: four fatal cases in leukemia patients. *J Clin Microbiol.* 1995;33:3290-3295.
39. Bouza E, Munoz P, Vega L, et al. Clinical resolution of *Scedosporium prolificans* fungemia associated with reversal of neutropenia following administration of granulocyte colony-stimulating factor. *Clin Infect Dis.* 1996;23:192-193.

40. Farag SS, Firkin FC, Andrew JH, et al. Fatal disseminated *Scedosporium inflatum* infection in a neutropenic immunocompromised patient. *J Infect.* 1992;25:201-204.

41. Rabodonirina M, Paulus S, Thevenet F, et al. Disseminated *Scedosporium prolificans* (*S. inflatum*) infection after single-lung transplantation. *Clin Infect Dis.* 1994;19:138-142.

42. Madrigal V, Alonso J, Bureo E, et al. Fatal meningoencephalitis caused by *Scedosporium inflatum* (*Scedosporium prolificans*) in a child with lymphoblastic leukemia. *Eur J Clin Microbiol Infect Dis.* 1995;14:601-603.

43. del Palacio A, Garau M, Amor E, et al. Case reports. Transient colonization with *Scedosporium prolificans*: report of four cases in Madrid. *Mycoses.* 2001;44:321-325.

44. Hopwood V, Evans EGV, Matthews J, et al. *Scedosporium prolificans*, a multi-resistant fungus, from a UK AIDS patient. *J Infect.* 1995;30:153-155.

45. Salkin IF, McGinnis MR, Dykstra MJ, et al. *Scedosporium inflatum*, an emerging pathogen. *J Clin Microbiol.* 1988;26:498-503.

46. Ortoneda M, Capilla J, Pujol I, et al. Liposomal amphotericin B and granulocyte colony-stimulating factor therapy in a murine model of invasive infection by *Scedosporium prolificans*. *J Antimicrob Chemother.* 2002;49:525-529.

47. Capilla J, Yustes C, Mayayo E, et al. Efficacy of albaconazole (UR-9825) in treatment of disseminated *Scedosporium prolificans* infection in rabbits. *Antimicrob Agents Chemother.* 2003;47:1948-1951.

48. Afeltra J, Dannaoui E, Meis JF, et al. In vitro synergistic interaction between amphotericin B and pentamidine against *Scedosporium prolificans*. *Antimicrob Agents Chemother.* 2002;46:3323-3326.

49. Meletiadis J, Mouton JW, Meis JF, et al. In vitro drug interaction modeling of combinations of azoles with terbinafine against clinical *Scedosporium prolificans* isolates. *Antimicrob Agents Chemother.* 2003;47:106-117.

50. Meletiadis J, Mouton JW, Rodriguez-Tudela JL, et al. In vitro interaction of terbinafine with itraconazole against clinical isolates of *Scedosporium prolificans*. *Antimicrob Agents Chemother.* 2000;44:470-472.

51. Tong SYC, Peleg AY, Yoong J, et al. Breakthrough *Scedosporium prolificans* infection while receiving voriconazole prophylaxis in an allogeneic stem cell transplant recipient. *Transpl Infect Dis.* 2007;9:241-243.

52. Howden BP, Slavin MA, Schwarer AP, et al. Successful control of disseminated *Scedosporium prolificans* infection with a combination of voriconazole and terbinafine. *Eur J Clin Microbiol Infect Dis.* 2003;22:111-113.

53. Kwon-Chung KJ, Bennett JE. *Medical Mycology*. Philadelphia: Lea & Febiger; 1992.

54. Rinaldi MG. Phaeohyphomycosis. *Dermatol Clin.* 1996;14:147-153.

55. Nucci M, Akiti T, Barreiros G, et al. Nosocomial fungemia due to *Exophiala jeanselmei* var. *jeanselmei* and a *Rhinocladiella* species: newly described causes of bloodstream infection. *J Clin Microbiol.* 2001;39:514-518.

56. Rossman SNB, Cernoch PL, Davis JR. Dematiaceous fungi are an increasing cause of human disease. *Clin Infect Dis.* 1996;22:73-80.

57. Revankar SG, Sutton DA, Rinaldi MG. Primary central nervous system phaeohyphomycosis: a review of 101 cases. *Clin Infect Dis.* 2004;38:206-216.

58. Aldape KD, Fox HS, Roberts JP, et al. *Cladosporium trichoides* cerebral phaeohyphomycosis in a liver transplant recipient. *Am J Clin Pathol.* 1991;95:499-502.

59. Filizzola MJ, Martinez F, Rauf SJ. Phaeohyphomycosis of the central nervous system in immunocompetent hosts: report of a case and review of the literature. *Int J Infect Dis.* 2003;7:282-286.

60. Buxi TBS, Prakash K, Vohra R, et al. Imaging in phaeohyphomycosis of the brain. Case report. *Neuroradiology.* 1996;38:139-141.

61. Walz R, Bianchin M, Chaves ML, et al. Cerebral phaeohyphomycosis caused by *Cladophialophora bantiana* in a Brazilian drug abuser. *J Med Vet Mycol.* 1997;35:427-431.

62. Barron MA, Sutton DA, Veve R, et al. Invasive mycotic infections caused by *Chaetomium perlucidum*, a new agent of cerebral phaeohyphomycosis. *J Clin Microbiol.* 2003;41:5302-5307.

63. Kanj SS, Amr SS, Roberts GD. *Ramichloridium mackenziei* brain abscess: report of two cases and review of the literature. *Med Mycol.* 2001;39:97-102.

64. Sutton DA, Slifkin M, Yakulis R, et al. U.S. case report of cerebral phaeohyphomycosis caused by *Ramichloridium obovoideum* (*R. mackenziei*): criteria for identification, therapy, and review of other known dematiaceous neurotropic taxa. *J Clin Microbiol.* 1998;36:708-715.

65. Surash S, Tyagi A, de Hoog GS, et al. Cerebral phaeohyphomycosis caused by *Fonsecaea monophora*. *Med Mycol.* 2005;43:465-472.

66. deShazo RD, Chapin K, Swain RE. Fungal sinusitis. *N Engl J Med.* 1997;337:254-259.

67. Washburn RG, Kennedy DW, Begley MG, et al. Chronic fungal sinusitis in apparently normal hosts. *Medicine.* 1988;67:231-247.

68. Oliveira Ramos AM, Oliveira Sales A, Andrade MC, et al. A simple method for detecting subcutaneous phaeohyphomycosis with light colored fungi. *Am J Surg Pathol.* 1995;19:109-114.

69. Kimura M, McGinnis MR. Fontana-Masson–stained tissue from culture-proven mycoses. *Arch Pathol Lab Med.* 1998;122:1107-1111.

70. Sharkey PK, Graybill JR, Rinaldi MG, et al. Itraconazole treatment of phaeohyphomycosis. *J Am Acad Dermatol.* 1990;23:577-586.

71. Whittle DI, Kominos S. Use of itraconazole for treating subcutaneous phaeohyphomycosis caused by *Exophiala jeanselmei*. *Clin Infect Dis.* 1995;21:1068.

72. Al-Abdely HM, Alkunaizi AM, Al-Tawfiq JA, et al. Successful therapy of cerebral phaeohyphomycosis due to *Ramichloridium mackenziei* with the new triazol posaconazole. *Med Mycol.* 2005;43:91-95.

73. Negroni R, Helou SH, Petri N, et al. Case study: Posaconazole treatment of disseminated phaeohyphomycosis due to *Exophiala spinifera*. *Clin Infect Dis.* 2004;38:e15-e20.

74. Agger WA, Andes D, Burgess JW. *Exophiala jeanselmei* infection in a heart transplant recipient successfully treated with oral terbinafine. *Clin Infect Dis.* 2004;38:e112-e115.

75. Chang DC, Grant GB, O'Donnell K, et al. Multistate outbreak of *Fusarium* keratitis associated with use of a contact lens solution. *JAMA.* 2006;296:953-963.

76. Guilhermetti E, Takahachi G, Shinobu CS, et al. *Fusarium* spp. as agents of onychomycosis in immunocompetent hosts. *Int J Dermatol.* 2007;46:822-826.

77. Nucci M, Anaissie E. Cutaneous infection by *Fusarium* species in healthy and immunocompromised hosts: implications for diagnosis and management. *Clin Infect Dis.* 2002;35:909-920.

78. Nucci M, Anaissie E. *Fusarium* infections in immunocompromised patients. *Clin Microbiol Rev.* 2007;20:695-704.

79. Wheeler MS, McGinnis MR, Schell WA, et al. *Fusarium* infection in burned patients. *Am J Clin Pathol.* 1981;75:304-311.

80. Testerman GM, Steagald MK, Colquitt LA, et al. Disseminated *Fusarium* infection in a multiple trauma patient. *South Med J.* 2008;101:320-323.

81. Strum AW, Grave W, Kwee WS. Disseminated *Fusarium oxysporum* infection in a patient with heat stroke. *Lancet.* 1989;1:968.

82. Boutati EI, Anaissie EJ. *Fusarium*, a significant emerging pathogen in patients with hematologic malignancy: ten years' experience at a cancer center and implications for management. *Blood.* 1997;90:999-1008.

83. Krcméry V, Jesenska Z, Spanik S, et al. Fungaemia due to *Fusarium* spp. in cancer patients. *J Hosp Infect.* 1997;36:223-228.

84. Martino P, Gastaldi R, Raccah R, et al. Clinical patterns of *Fusarium* infections in immunocompromised patients. *J Infect.* 1994;28(suppl. 1):7-15.

85. Nucci M, Marr KA, Queiroz-Telles F, et al. *Fusarium* infection in hematopoietic stem cell transplant recipients. *Clin Infect Dis.* 2004;38:1237-1242.

86. Ammari LK, Puck JM, McGowan KL. Catheter-related *Fusarium solani* fungemia and pulmonary infection in a patient with leukemia in remission. *Clin Infect Dis.* 1993;16:148-150.

87. Raad I, Hachem R. Treatment of central venous catheter–related fungemia due to *Fusarium oxysporum*. *Clin Infect Dis.* 1995;20:709-711.

88. Girmenia C, Arcese W, Micozzi A, et al. Onychomycosis as a possible origin of disseminated *Fusarium solani* infection in a patient with severe aplastic anemia. *Clin Infect Dis.* 1992;14:1167.

89. Anaissie EJ, Kuchar RT, Rex JH, et al. Fusariosis associated with pathogenic *Fusarium* species colonization of a hospital water system: a new paradigm for the epidemiology of opportunistic mold infections. *Clin Infect Dis.* 2001;33:1871-1878.

90. Pires-Goncalves RH, Sartori FG, Montanari LB, et al. Occurrence of fungi in water used at a haemodialysis centre. *Lett Appl Microbiol.* 2008;46:542-547.

91. Krcméry V, Spanik S, Kunova A, et al. Breakthrough fungemia appearing during empiric therapy with amphotericin B. *Chemotherapy.* 1997;43:367-370.

92. Nelson PE, Dignani MC, Anaissie EJ. Taxonomy, biology, and clinical aspects of *Fusarium* species. *Clin Microbiol Rev.* 1994;7:479-504.

93. Nucci M, Anaissie EJ, Queiroz-Telles F, et al. Outcome predictors of 84 patients with haematologic malignancies and *Fusarium* infection. *Cancer.* 2003;98:315-319.

94. Wolff MA, Ramphal R. Use of amphotericin B lipid complex for treatment of disseminated cutaneous *Fusarium* infection in a neutropenic patient. *Clin Infect Dis.* 1995;20:1568-1569.

95. Apostolidis J, Bouzani M, Platsouka E, et al. Resolution of fungemia due to *Fusarium* species in a patient with acute leukemia treated with caspofungin. *Clin Infect Dis.* 2003;36:1349-1350.

96. Neuburger S, Massenkeil G, Seibold M, et al. Successful salvage treatment of disseminated cutaneous fusariosis with liposomal amphotericin B and terbinafine after allogeneic stem cell transplantation. *Transpl Infect Dis.* 2008;10:290-293.

97. Paphitou NI, Ostrosky-Zeichner L, Paetznick VL, et al. In vitro activities of investigational triazoles against *Fusarium* species: effects of inoculum size and incubation time on broth microdilution susceptibility test results. *Antimicrob Agents Chemother.* 2002;46:3298-3300.

98. Cordoba S, Rodero L, Vivot W, et al. In vitro interactions of antifungal agents against clinical isolates of *Fusarium* spp. *Int J Antimicrob Agents.* 2008;31:171-174.

99. Clancy CJ, Nguyen MH. The combination of amphotericin B and azithromycin as a potential new therapeutic approach to fusariosis. *J Antimicrob Chemother.* 1998;41:127-130.

100. Ortoneda M, Capilla J, Pastor FJ, et al. Efficacy of liposomal amphotericin B in treatment of systemic murine fusariosis. *Antimicrob Agents Chemother.* 2002;46:2273-2275.

101. Lozano-Chiu M, Arikan S, Paetznick VL, et al. Treatment of murine fusariosis with SCH 56592. *Antimicrob Agents Chemother.* 1999;43:589-591.

102. Graybill JR, Najvar LK, Gonzalez GM, et al. Improving the mouse model for studying the efficacy of voriconazole. *J Antimicrob Chemother.* 2003;51:1373-1376.

103. Cudillo L, Girmenia C, Santilli S, et al. Breakthrough fusariosis in a patient with acute lymphoblastic leukemia receiving voriconazole prophylaxis. *Clin Infect Dis.* 2005;40:1212-1213.

104. Raad II, Hachem RY, Herbrecht R, et al. Posaconazole as salvage treatment for invasive fusariosis in patients with underlying hematologic malignancy and other conditions. *Clin Infect Dis.* 2006;42:1398-1403.

105. Spielberger RT, Falleroni MJ, Coene AJ, et al. Concomitant amphotericin B therapy, granulocyte transfusions, and GM-CSF administration for disseminated infection with *Fusarium* in a granulocytopenic patient. *Clin Infect Dis.* 1993;16:528-530.

106. Pastor FJ, Guarro J. Clinical manifestations, treatment and outcome of *Paecilomyces lilacinus* infections. *Clin Microbiol Infect.* 2006;12:948-960.

107. Guarro J, Gams W, Pujol I, et al. *Acremonium* species: new emerging fungal opportunists—in vitro antifungal susceptibilities and review. *Clin Infect Dis.* 1997;25:1222-1229.

108. Chouaki T, Lavarde V, Lachaud L, et al. Invasive infections due to *Trichoderma* species: report of 2 cases, findings of in vitro susceptibility testing, and review of the literature. *Clin Infect Dis.* 2002;35:1360-1367.

109. Steinbach WJ, Schell WA, Miller JL, et al. Fatal *Scopulariopsis brevicaulis* infection in a paediatric stem-cell transplant patient treated with voriconazole and caspofungin and a review of *Scopulariopsis* infections in immunocompromised patients. *J Infect.* 2004;48:112-116.

110. Liu K, Howell DN, Perfect JR, et al. Morphologic criteria for the preliminary identification of *Fusarium*, *Paecilomyces*, and *Acremonium* species by histopathology. *Am J Clin Pathol.* 1998;109:45-54.

111. Castelli MV, Alastruey-Izquierdo A, Cuesta I, et al. Susceptibility testing and molecular classification of *Paecilomyces* spp. *Antimicrob Agents Chemother.* 2008;52:2926-2928.

112. Gueho E, Improvisi L, de Hoog GS, et al. *Trichosporon* in humans, a practical account. *Mycoses.* 1994;37:3-10.

113. Sugita T, Nishikawa A, Shinoda T. Identification of *Trichosporon asahii* by PCR based on sequences of the internal transcribed spacer regions. *J Clin Microbiol.* 1998;36:2742-2744.

114. Sugita T, Nishikawa A, Shinoda T, et al. Taxonomic position of deep-seated, mucosa associated, and superficial isolates of *Trichosporon cutaneum* from trichosporonosis patients. *J Clin Microbiol.* 1995;33:1368-1370.

115. Itoh T, Hosokawa H, Kohdera U, et al. Disseminated infection with *Trichosporon asahii*. *Mycoses.* 1996;39:195-199.

116. Haupt HM, Merz WG, Beschorner WE, et al. Colonization and infection with *Trichosporon* species in the immunosuppressed host. *J Infect Dis.* 1983;147:199-203.

117. Hung CC, Chang SC, Chen YC, et al. *Trichosporon beigelii* fungemia in patients with acute leukemia: report of three cases. *J Formos Med Assoc.* 1995;94:127-131.

118. Hajjeh RA, Blumberg HM. Bloodstream infection due to *Trichosporon beigelii* in a burn patient: case report and review of therapy. *Clin Infect Dis.* 1995;20:913-916.

119. Mirza SH. Disseminated *Trichosporon beigelii* infection causing skin lesions in a renal transplant patient. *J Infect.* 1993;27:67-70.

120. Nahass GT, Rosenberg SP, Leonardi CL, et al. Disseminated infection with *Trichosporon beigelii*. *Arch Dermatol.* 1993;129:1020-1023.

121. Walsh TJ, Newman KR, Moody M, et al. Trichosporonosis in patients with neoplastic disease. *Medicine.* 1986;65:268-279.

122. Matsue K, Uryu H, Koseki M, et al. Breakthrough trichosporonosis in patients with hematologic malignancies receiving micafungin. *Clin Infect Dis.* 2006;42:753-757.

123. Paphitou NI, Ostrosky-Zeichner L, Paetznick VL, et al. In vitro antifungal susceptibilities of *Trichosporon* species. *Antimicrob Agents Chemother.* 2002;46:1144-1146.

124. Dankner WM, Spector SA, Fierer J, et al. *Malassezia* fungemia in neonates and adults: complication of hyperalimentation. *Rev Infect Dis.* 1987;9:743-753.

125. Barber GR, Brown AE, Kiehn TE, et al. Catheter-related *Malassezia furfur* fungemia in immunocompromised patients. *Am J Med.* 1993;95:365-370.

126. Powell DA, Marcon MJ. Failure to eradicate *Malassezia furfur* Broviac catheter infection with antifungal therapy. *Pediatr Infect Dis J.* 1987;6:579-588.

127. Gupta AK, Kohli Y, Li A, et al. In vitro susceptibility of the seven *Malassezia* species to ketoconazole, voriconazole, itraconazole and terbinafine. *Br J Dermatol.* 2000;142:758-765.

128. Marcon MJ, Durrell DE, Powell DA, et al. In vitro activity of systemic antifungal agents against *Malassezia furfur*. *Antimicrob Agents Chemother.* 1987;31:951-953.

129. Brooks R, Brown L. Systemic infections with *Malassezia furfur* in an adult receiving long-term hyperalimentation therapy. *J Infect Dis.* 1987;156:410-411.

130. Boekhout T, Kamp M, Geuho E. Molecular typing of *Malassezia* species with PFGE and *RAPD*. *Mol Mycol.* 1998;36:365-372.

131. Chang HJ, Miller HL, Watkins N, et al. An epidemic of *Malassezia pachydermatis* in an intensive care nursery associated with colonization of health care workers' pet dogs. *N Engl J Med*. 1998;338:706-711.

132. Perez-Sanchez I, Anguita J, Martin-Rabadan P, et al. *Blastoschizomyces capitatus* infection in acute leukemia patients. *Leuk Lymphoma*. 2000;39:209-212.

133. Martino R, Salavert M, Parody R, et al. *Blastoschizomyces capitatus* infection in patients with leukemia: report of 26 cases. *Clin Infect Dis*. 2004;38:335-341.

134. Sanz MA, Lopez FA, Martinez ML, et al. Disseminated *Blastoschizomyces capitatus* infection in acute myeloblastic leukemia. *Support Care Cancer*. 1996;4:291-293.

135. Serena C, Marine M, Marimon, R, et al. Effect of antifungal treatment in a murine model of blastoschizomycosis. *Int J Antimicrob Agents*. 2007;29:79-83.

136. Hazen KC. New and emerging yeast pathogens. *Clin Microbiol Rev*. 1995;8:462-478.

137. da Matta VLR, Melhem MC, Colombo AL, et al. Antifungal drug susceptibility profile of *Pichia anomala* isolates from patients presenting with nosocomial fungemia. *Antimicrob Agents Chemother*. 2007;51:1573-1576.

138. Thuler LC, Faivichenco S, Velasco E, et al. Fungaemia caused by *Hansenula anomala*—an outbreak in a cancer hospital. *Mycoses*. 1997;40:193-196.

139. Zaas AK, Boyce M, Schell W, et al. Risk of fungemia due to *Rhodotorula* and antifungal susceptibility testing of *Rhodotorula* isolates. *J Clin Microbiol*. 2003;41:5233-5235.

140. Munoz P, Bouza E, Cuenca-Estrella M, et al. *Saccharomyces cerevisiae* fungemia: an emerging infectious disease. *Clin Infect Dis*. 2005;40:1625-1634.

141. DiSalvo AF, Fickling AM, Ajello L. Infection caused by *Penicillium marneffei*: description of first natural infection in man. *Am J Clin Pathol*. 1973;59:259-263.

142. Segretain G. *Penicillium marneffei* n. sp., agent d'une mycose du système réticulo-endothélial. *Mycopathol Mycol Appl*. 1959; 11:327-353.

143. Vanittanakom N, Cooper CR, Fisher MC, et al. *Penicillium marneffei* infection and recent advances in the epidemiology and molecular biology aspects. *Clin Microbiol Rev*. 2006;19:95-110.

144. Supparatpinyo K, Khamwan C, Baosoung V, et al. Disseminated *Penicillium marneffei* infections in Southeast Asia. *Lancet*. 1994;344:110-113.

145. Drouhet E. Penicilliosis due to *Penicillium marneffei*: a new emerging systemic mycosis in AIDS patients traveling or living in Southeast Asia: review of 44 cases reported in HIV infected patients during the last 5 years compared to 44 cases of non AIDS patients reported over 20 years. *J Mycol Med*. 1993;4:195-224.

146. Duong TA. Infection due to *Penicillium marneffei*, an emerging pathogen: review of 155 reported cases. *Clin Infect Dis*. 1996;23: 125-130.

147. Hung C, Hsueh P, Chen M, et al. Invasive infection caused by *Penicillium marneffei*: an emerging pathogen in Taiwan. *Clin Infect Dis*. 1998;26:202-203.

148. Kwan EYW, Lau YL, Yuen KY, et al. *Penicillium marneffei* infection in a non–HIV infected child. *J Paediatr Child Health*. 1997; 33:267-271.

149. Sirisanthana V, Sirisanthana T. *Penicillium marneffei* infection in children infected with human immunodeficiency virus. *Pediatr Infect Dis J*. 1993;12:1021-1025.

150. Ajello L, Padhye AA, Sukroongreung S, et al. Occurrence of *Penicillium marneffei* infections among wild bamboo rats in Thailand. *Mycopathologia*. 1995;131:1-8.

151. Cooper CR. From bamboo rats to humans: the odyssey of *Penicillium marneffei*. *ASM News*. 1998;64:390-396.

152. Chariyalertsak S, Vanittanakom P, Nelson KE, et al. *Rhizomys sumatrensis* and *Cannomys badius*, new natural animal hosts of *Penicillium marneffei*. *J Med Vet Mycol*. 1996;34:105-110.

153. Chariyalertsak S, Sirisanthana T, Supparatpinyo K, et al. Case-control study of the risk factors for *Penicillium marneffei* infection in human immunodeficiency virus–infected patients in northern Thailand. *Clin Infect Dis*. 1997;24:1080-1086.

154. Chariyalertsak S, Sirisanthana T, Supparatpinyo K, et al. Seasonal variation of disseminated *Penicillium marneffei* infections in northern Thailand: a clue to the reservoir? *J Infect Dis*. 1996; 173:1490-1493.

155. Ko CI, Hung CC, Chen MY, et al. Endoscopic diagnosis of intestinal penicilliosis marneffei: report of three cases and review of the literature. *Gastrointest Endosc*. 1999;50:111-114.

156. Wortmann PD. Infection with *Penicillium marneffei*. *Int J Dermatol*. 1996;35:393-399.

157. Cheng NC, Won WW, Fung CP, et al. Unusual pulmonary manifestations of disseminated *Penicillium marneffei* infection in three AIDS patients. *Med Mycol*. 1998;36:429-432.

158. Deng Z, Ribas JL, Gibson DW, et al. Infections caused by *Penicillium marneffei* in China and southeast Asia: review of eighteen published cases and report of four more Chinese cases. *Rev Infect Dis*. 1988;10:640-652.

159. Hilmarsdottir I, Coutellier A, Elbaz J, et al. A French case of laboratory-acquired disseminated *Penicillium marneffei* infection in a patient with AIDS. *Clin Infect Dis*. 1994;19:357-358.

160. Jones PD, See J. *Penicillium marneffei* infection in patients infected with human immunodeficiency virus: late presentation in an area of nonendemicity. *Clin Infect Dis*. 1992;15:744.

161. Supparatpinyo K, Sirisanthana T. Disseminated *Penicillium marneffei* infection diagnosed on examination of a peripheral blood smear of a patient with human immunodeficiency virus infection. *Clin Infect Dis*. 1994;18:246-247.

162. Cooper CR, McGinnis MR. Pathology of *Penicillium marneffei*: an emerging acquired immunodeficiency syndrome–related pathogen. *Arch Pathol Lab Med*. 1997;121:798-804.

163. Chaiyaroj SC, Chawengkirttikul R, Sirisinha S, et al. Antigen detection assay for identification of *Penicillium marneffei* infection. *J Clin Microbiol*. 2003;41:432-434.

164. Desakorn V, Simpson AJH, Wuthiekanun V, et al. Development and evaluation of rapid urinary antigen detection tests for diagnosis of *Penicillium marneffei*. *J Clin Microbiol*. 2002;40:3179-3183.

165. Huang Y, Hung C, Liao C, et al. Detection of circulating galactomannan in serum samples for diagnosis of *Penicillium marneffei* infection and cryptococcosis among patients infected with human immunodeficiency virus. *J Clin Microbiol*. 2007;45: 2858-2862.

166. Supparatpinyo K, Schlamm HT. Voriconazole as therapy for systemic *Penicillium marneffei* infections in AIDS patients. *Am J Trop Med Hyg*. 2007;77:350-353.

167. Supparatpinyo K, Nelson KE, Merz WG, et al. Response to antifungal therapy by human immunodeficiency virus–infected patients with disseminated *Penicillium marneffei* infections and in vitro susceptibilities of isolates from clinical specimens. *Antimicrob Agents Chemother*. 1993;37:2407-2411.

168. Sirisanthana T, Supparatpinyo K, Perriens J, et al. Amphotericin B and itraconazole for treatment of disseminated *Penicillium marneffei* infection in human immunodeficiency virus–infected patients. *Clin Infect Dis*. 1998;26:1107-1110.

169. Supparatpinyo K, Perriens J, Nelson KE, et al. A controlled trial of itraconazole to prevent relapse of *Penicillium marneffei* infec-

tion in patients infected with the human immunodeficiency virus. *N Engl J Med*. 1998;339:1739-1743.

170. Chaiwarith R, Charoenyos N, Sirisanthana T, et al. Discontinuation of secondary prophylaxis against penicilliosis marneffei in AIDS patients after HAART. *AIDS*. 2007;21:365-379.

171. Herr RA, Tarcha EJ, Taborda PR, et al. Phylogenetic analysis of *Lacazia loboi* places this previously uncharacterized pathogen with the dimorphic Onygenales. *J Clin Microbiol*. 2001;39: 309-314.

172. Taborda PR, Taborda VA, McGinnis MR. *Lacazia loboi* gen. nov., comb. nov., the etiologic agent of lobomycosis. *J Clin Microbiol*. 1999;37:2031-2033.

173. Elsayed S, Kuhn SM, Barber D, et al. Human case of lobomycosis. *Emerg Infect Dis*. 2004;10:715-718.

174. Fredricks DN, Jolley JA, Lepp PW, et al. *Rhinosporidium seeberi*: a human pathogen from a novel group of aquatic protistan parasites. *Emerg Infect Dis*. 2000;6:273-282.

175. Herr RA, Ajello L, Taylor JW, et al. Phylogenetic analysis of *Rhinosporidium seeberi*'s 18S small-subunit ribosomal DNA groups this pathogen among members of the protoctistan *Mesomycetozoa* clade. *J Clin Microbiol*. 1999;37:2750-2754.

176. Sudarshan V, Goel NK, Gahine R, et al. Rhinosporidiosis in Raipur, Chhattisgarh: a report of 462 cases. *Indian J Pathol Microbiol*. 2007;50:718-721.

177. Lasser A, Smith HW. Rhinosporidiosis. *Arch Otolaryngol*. 1976; 102:308-310.

178. Reidy JJ, Sudesh S, Klafter AB, et al. Infection of the conjunctiva by *Rhinosporidium seeberi*. *Surv Ophthalmol*. 1997;41:409-413.

179. Snidvongs ML, Supanakorn S, Supiyaphun P. Severe epistaxis from rhinosporidiosis: a case report. *J Med Assoc Thai*. 1998;81: 555-558.

180. Thappa DM, Venkatesan S, Sirka CS, et al. Disseminated cutaneous rhinosporidiosis. *J Dermatol*. 1998;25:527-532.

181. Ghorpade A, Ramanan C. Verrucoid cutaneous rhinosporidiosis. *J Eur Acad Dermatol Venereol*. 1998;10:269-270.

182. Lass-Florl C, Mayr A. Human protothecosis. *Clin Microbiol Rev*. 2007;20:230-242.

183. Krcméry V Jr. Systemic chlorellosis, an emerging infection in humans caused by algae. *Int J Antimicrob Agents*. 2000;15: 235-237.

184. Kim ST, Suh KS, Chae YS, et al. Successful treatment with fluconazole of prototheosis at the site of an intralesional corticosteroid injection. *Br J Dermatol*. 1996;135:803-806.

185. Carey WP, Kaykova Y, Bandres JC, et al. Cutaneous prototheosis in a patient with AIDS and severe functional defect: successful therapy with amphotericin B. *Clin Infect Dis*. 1997;25:1265-1266.

186. Polk P, Sanders DY. Cutaneous prototheosis in association with the acquired immunodeficiency syndrome. *South Med J*. 1997;90:831-832.

187. Narita M, Muder RR, Cacciarelli TV, et al. Prototheosis after liver transplantation. *Liver Transpl*. 2008;14:1211-1215.

188. Matsumoto Y, Shibata M, Adachi A, et al. Two cases of prototheosis in Nagoya, Japan. *Australas J Dermatol*. 1996;37(suppl 1):S42-S43.

189. Tang WY, Lo KK, Lam WY, et al. Cutaneous prototheosis: report of a case in Hong Kong. *Br J Dermatol*. 1995;133: 479-482.

190. Okuyama Y, Hamaguchi T, Teramoto T, et al. A human case of prototheosis successfully treated with itraconazole. *Nippon Ishinkin Gakkai Zasshi*. 2001;42:143-147.

270

Pneumocystis Species

PETER D. WALZER | A. GEORGE SMULIAN*

*P*neumocystis was discovered in 1909 by Chagas, who mistakenly interpreted the organism as a trypanosome. Several years later, the Delanöes identified *Pneumocystis* as a separate genus and species and named the organism in honor of Dr. Carini, another early worker. *Pneumocystis* first came to medical attention when it was implicated as the cause of interstitial plasma cell pneumonia, a disorder of institutionalized and debilitated infants in central and Eastern Europe after World War II. In the 1960s, *Pneumocystis* became widely appreciated as an important cause of pneumonia in immunocompromised hosts; however, with the development of safe and effective antimicrobial drugs, interest in the organism waned. The dramatic rise in the incidence of *Pneumocystis carinii* pneumonia (PCP; now renamed *Pneumocystis jirovecii* pneumonia) associated with human immunodeficiency virus (HIV) infection in the 1980s rekindled interest in *Pneumocystis* as a major medical and public health problem. During the 1990s, advances in the treatment of HIV reduced the frequency of *Pneumocystis* pneumonia and other complications. Nevertheless, *Pneumocystis* remains a leading cause of opportunistic infection, morbidity, and mortality in these patients.[1,2] Interest in the organism has also been spurred by the more recent identification of *Pneumocystis* in individuals with chronic obstructive pulmonary disease (COPD).[3]

The Pathogen

Pneumocystis describes a genus of closely related unicellular fungi of low virulence found in the lungs of humans and a variety of mammals. The taxonomic status of the genus was resolved in the late 1980s, when analysis of the rRNA gene in the 1980s suggested that the organism is more closely related to fungi than to protozoa.[4,5] This conclusion has been confirmed at every molecular locus analyzed.[6,7] Phylogenetic studies suggest that the organism is most closely related to the ascomycetes as a deep basal branch among the archiascomycetes; however, *Pneumocystis* is unusual among fungi in that the organism lacks ergosterol in its plasma membranes and is insensitive to available antifungal drugs that target ergosterol biosynthesis.

Species within the genus demonstrate genotypic and phenotypic differences manifested by antigenic differences, ultrastructural morphologic differences, and host specificity.[4,5] Genetic studies have demonstrated differences between *Pneumocystis* species at a karyotypic level, in the organization and structure of gene families within specific genomes, and at a sequence level within individual genes. Not only are there genetic differences in *Pneumocystis* among different animal hosts, but there are also species and/or strain differences in organisms from the same host. Ultrastructural morphologic differences are evident only at the level of electron microscopy, whereas other phenotypic differences between species require specialized reagents to determine antigenic characterization or multilocus enzyme electrophoresis.

Experimental models have demonstrated that *Pneumocystis* taken from a given host species appear unable to proliferate in other host species. Associated with a better understanding of the host specificity and genetic differences among members of the genus *Pneumocystis,* a need has arisen to define individual species within the genus. In recognition that the organisms described by the Delanöes were isolated from infected rats, a formal taxonomic description of rat-derived species was made, retaining the name of *P. carinii.*[8,9] *Pneumocystis* isolated from humans was formally described as *P. jirovecii* in recogni-

tion of Otto Jirovec, whose group first identified *Pneumocystis* as a human pathogen and the causative agent of interstitial plasma cell pneumonia. Subsequently, the Latin was corrected to *jirovecii.* A second species identified in rats has been named *P. wakefieldiae,* whereas *P. murina* and *P. oryctolagi* have been identified in mice and rabbits, respectively.[9]

Despite the strenuous efforts by many investigators, the lack of a reliable *Pneumocystis* in vitro cultivation system remains an intractable problem. Limited (up to 10-fold) replication of rat-derived organisms has been achieved in different cell lines and in axenic media.[10] A continuous culture system for rat- and human-derived *Pneumocystis* has been described, but has proven difficult to reproduce and maintain. Short-term culture has been used to study *Pneumocystis* metabolism and susceptibility to antimicrobial drugs, but standardization and reproducibility among laboratories have not yet been achieved.

Studies of the life cycle of *Pneumocystis* have been based mainly on light and electron microscopic analysis of forms seen in infected lungs or in short-term culture (Fig. 270-1).[5] Three developmental stages of the organism are commonly seen in conjunction with additional intermediate forms. The trophozoite or trophic form is small (1 to 4 μm), pleomorphic, and commonly exists in clusters; this stage can be identified on Giemsa stain by its reddish nucleus and blue cytoplasm. In the asexual phase of the life cycle, the trophic forms multiply by binary fission, although trophic binary fission is rarely visualized or documented. In the sexual phase, the haploid trophic forms are postulated to conjugate to form a diploid zygote that becomes a 4- to 6-μm precyst or sporocyte; this form is difficult to distinguish from the other developmental stages at the light microscopic level. The precyst undergoes meiosis followed by mitosis, leading to the formation of the cyst or spore case, which contains eight haploid intracystic bodies or spores. The expression of meiosis-specific genes, such as the functionally conserved meiotic control kinase, Ran1, and the meiotic activator, Mei2, have been confirmed in the lungs of infected mammalian hosts, suggesting sexual replication occurs in the lungs of infected mammalian hosts.[11] The 5- to 8-μm cyst has a thick cell wall that stains well with stains such as methenamine silver or toluidine blue O. The intracystic bodies are formed by compartmentalization of nuclei and cytoplasmic organelles, exhibit different shapes, and appear to be released through a rent in the cell wall. Studies using echinocandin inhibitors of β-1,3-glucan synthase suggest that the cystic form is an integral part of the life cycle.[12]

Biochemical and metabolic studies of *Pneumocystis* have been limited by the problems of culturing the organism.[13,14] The surface of *Pneumocystis* is rich in glucose and mannose, *N*-acetylglucosamine, and galactose *N*-acetylgalactosamine residues. The cell walls of cysts and trophic forms contain a number of immunogenic glycoproteins that may be part of a large complex[15] (Fig. 270-2). β-1,3-Glucans are a major component of the cell wall, whereas little or no chitin has been detected. Lipids have received considerable attention because of their relationship with antifungal therapy. Cholesterol is the dominant sterol present in *Pneumocystis.*[14] Instead of ergosterol, the organism synthesizes distinct Δ^7,C-24 alkylated sterols. Coenzyme Q10 (CoQ10) is the major ubiquinone homologue synthesized by the organism; CoQ10 homologues, such as 8-aminoquinolones and hydroxynaphthoquinones, have shown good activity against the organism. A variety of enzymes and metabolic pathways have been characterized as potential therapeutic targets.

Several major groups of *Pneumocystis* antigens have been identified. The most widely studied is a 95- to 140-kDa moiety, termed the *major surface glycoprotein* (MSG) or gpA, is highly immunogenic, exhibits

---

*All material in this chapter is in the public domain, with the exception of any borrowed figures or tables.

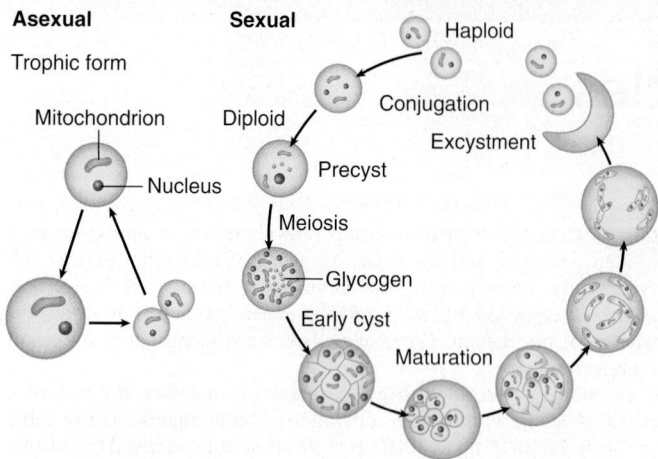

Figure 270-1 Proposed *Pneumocystis* life cycle involving asexual and sexual stages. *(Adapted from Cushion M. Pneumocystis carinii. In: Collier A, Sussman M, eds. Topley and Wilson's Microbiology and Microbial Infections, vol 4. New York: Oxford University Press; 1998:645-683, with permission.)*

shared and species-specific antigenic determinants, and contains protective B- and T-cell epitopes.[16-21] Immunization with MSG also elicits a protective response in some, but not all, animal models.[22] MSG actually represents a family of proteins encoded by multiple genes that are arranged in clusters at the ends of chromosomes. Transcription of MSG genes occurs at a single expression site, termed the *upstream conserved sequence* (UCS), which is thought to result in only one MSG isoform being expressed on the surface of *Pneumocystis* at a time.[16,23,24] Changing the MSG gene at the UCS, by recombination and gene conversion, changes the surface MSG resulting in antigenic variation.

The ability of MSG to undergo antigenic variation may be an important mechanism whereby *Pneumocystis* evades the host immune response.[16] The other important function of MSG is to facilitate interaction with host cells by adherence to the extracellular matrix proteins fibronectin, vitronectin, possibly laminin, the surfactant proteins A and D, and the mannose receptor.[25-30] MSG is composed of up to 10% N-linked carbohydrates, particularly mannose, which participate in the binding to these proteins.

A second family of surface antigens was identified during studies characterizing MSG. A subtilisin-like serine protease encoded by the *PRT1*, also known as the *KEX* multigene family, was localized to the surface of rat-derived *Pneumocystis*.[31-33] In *P. murina* and *P. jirovecii*,

only a single KEX gene has been identified.[34,35] In other fungi, these proteases are involved in the processing of preproteins as they make their way to the cell surface, and may play a role in antigenic variation in *Pneumocystis*.

The third major antigen complex is a glycoprotein that migrates as a broad band of 45 to 55 and 35 to 45 kDa in rat and human *Pneumocystis*, respectively. The gene encoding a rat *Pneumocystis* 45- to 55-kDa antigen (p55) has been cloned and sequenced; the 3′ end of the molecule stimulates a host immune response.[36,37] Immunization with recombinant p55 antigen afforded partial protection to subsequent infection.[38] Gene variation has also been demonstrated in the p55 gene, with up to five variants identified within the *Pneumocystis* genome.[39] The predicted amino acid sequence of p55 shows a repeated motif rich in glutamic acid residues that, in other microbes—for example, *Plasmodia*—has been suggested as a mechanism to divert the host immune response.[40] The 35- to 45-kDa band of human *Pneumocystis* is frequently found in respiratory tract specimens and is also recognized by serum antibodies.

Epidemiology

When first recognized, *Pneumocystis* pneumonia was known primarily as a disease affecting malnourished and premature infants. Infants are probably the natural host for the disease, becoming colonized in the first few months of life as maternal antibodies wane. This is supported by studies that report finding the organism itself or *Pneumocystis* DNA to be present in clinical or autopsy samples from infants.[41] Similar observations have been made in animal models; in rabbits, for example, the young serve as the primary dispersal host for the agent. Seroepidemiologic surveys have demonstrated that most healthy children are exposed to *Pneumocystis* by an early age.[40,42] The clinical picture of primary infection is unclear. Long presumed to be asymptomatic, evidence of *Pneumocystis* colonization has been demonstrated in respiratory secretions in 16% to 32% of children presenting with acute respiratory illnesses by sensitive molecular techniques, and serologic responses to *Pneumocystis* have been demonstrated in infants with upper respiratory tract infections.[42,43] Additional children were identified with evidence of seroconversion in the absence of a history of any respiratory symptoms. Serologic studies have shown that *Pneumocystis* has a worldwide distribution, but that the prevalence of antibodies to specific antigens varies among different geographic regions.[44,45] The frequency of *Pneumocystis* pneumonia in HIV patients in tropical and developing countries has generally been thought to be much lower than that in industrialized nations; however, studies have suggested that this may reflect rather a failure to diagnose the infection because of limited access to sophisticated medical care in third world coun-

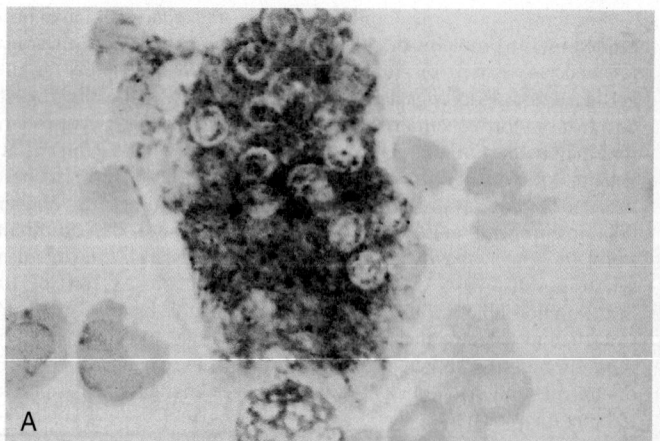
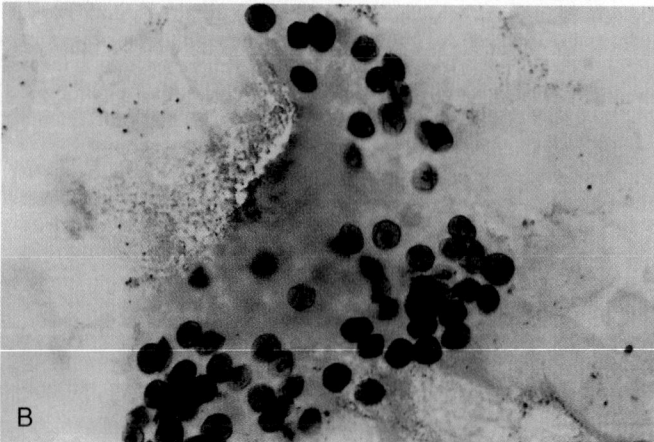

Figure 270-2. ***Pneumocystis* organisms. A,** Cluster of *Pneumocystis* trophic forms and cysts (Diff-Quik, × 1000). **B,** Cluster of *Pneumocystis* cysts (methenamine silver stain, × 1250).

tries.[46-48] Under these conditions, *Pneumocystis* infection is often seen in conjunction with more virulent infections, such as tuberculosis. The demographic features of patients with PCP generally reflect those of the underlying disease. *Pneumocystis* pneumonia has also been recognized with increased frequency in Africa in HIV-infected infants. Studies report that *Pneumocystis* organisms can be detected in up to 80% of infants with known or suspected HIV infection presenting with severe pneumonia. Attempts to compare the frequency of *Pneumocystis* pneumonia among different racial and ethnic groups have been complicated by social and cultural factors.[49] There have been conflicting reports about the seasonal occurrence of PCP.

Animal model studies have shown that *Pneumocystis* is communicable and that the principal mode of transmission is the airborne route, although the infective form of the organism is unknown.[4,5] There is debate about how long the organism resides in the host once *Pneumocystis* infection is acquired. One school of thought believes that the organism becomes part of the host's resident microbial flora and remains quiescent for long periods of time; as immune defenses become compromised, the organism causes disease by reactivation of latent infection. This view is supported by the presence of the same genetic strain of *Pneumocystis* in animal colonies for several years, the high host specificity of *Pneumocystis,* which implies coevolution of the organism and host, and the capability of MSG for antigenic variation. The other view is that *Pneumocystis* infection is transient, but that people are frequently exposed to sources of the organism throughout their lives. One line of support for this hypothesis comes from the limited duration of carriage in recent animal model studies. Healthy adult mice inoculated with *Pneumocystis* clear the infection from the lungs within a short period of time; the process takes slightly longer in neonates. Immunocompromised animals clear *Pneumocystis* from the lungs after normal immune function is restored.

Molecular epidemiologic approaches have shed new light on the natural history and epidemiology of *Pneumocystis* infection.[4,5] Although a number of molecular targets have been examined, most information has been obtained from the internal transcribed spacer (ITS) regions of the nuclear rRNA gene, the large subunit mitochondrial rRNA gene, and the dihydropteroate synthase (DHPS) gene sequence. Studies show that *Pneumocystis* isolates from HIV patients are similar to those from non-HIV patients, and that patients may harbor more than one strain of the organism. Three lines of evidence support the view that active transmission of *Pneumocystis* occurs in humans. AIDS patients with recurrent episodes of PCP were found to have *Pneumocystis* genotypes that differed from those seen in previous episodes.[50] A second study examined geographic variation of *Pneumocystis* genotypes from PCP patients in different U.S. cities.[51] This study found that genotypes at the time of an episode of *Pneumocystis* pneumonia reflected the patient's place of diagnosis and not his or her place of birth, suggesting recently acquired infections rather than reactivated latent infection. A third study noted that 53% of AIDS-defining PCP patients presented with mutant DHPS genotypes.[52] Because these patients had not been receiving prophylactic sulfa, the mutant genotypes could not have resulted from selection but rather as a result of acquisition of a mutant *Pneumocystis* strain. These data strongly suggest that *Pneumocystis* is transmitted directly from person to person, and that active acquisition rather than latency and reactivation results in most PCP episodes in adults.

The source of exposure for infants, as well as adults, is probably other individuals with active PCP or transient subclinical colonization. With the advent of AIDS, HIV-infected individuals provide an additional source of exposure. In the pre-HIV era, the prevalence of latent *Pneumocystis* infection in immunocompromised patients autopsy varied from 0% to 8%; the frequency of PCP at some institutions was related to the type or intensity of immunosuppressive therapy.[38] Other evidence supporting this concept comes from the occurrence of outbreaks or clusters of *Pneumocystis* pneumonia at orphanages and hospitals and in immunocompromised patients who had prolonged contact with each other. Geographic clustering of PCP has been reported in two U.S. cities.[39,40]

Prevalence surveys using the polymerase chain reaction (PCR) assay have detected *P. jirovecii* colonization commonly in HIV patients, other immunocompromised hosts, and patients with COPD and other chronic diseases, occasionally in pregnant females, and uncommonly in healthy people.[3] Other risk factors for colonization include CD4 count, smoking, geography, lung cancer, older age, and corticosteroid treatment. The duration of colonization varies but may persist for a few months. Colonization in HIV patients does not necessarily lead to PCP.[53]

Pathology and Pathogenesis

Once *Pneumocystis* is inhaled, it escapes the defenses of the upper respiratory tract and is deposited in alveoli. The trophic form preferentially attaches to the alveolar type I cell, and is thought to initiate infection by this act.[54] Ultrastructural analysis has shown that the adherence is characterized by close apposition of the cell surfaces, without fusion of the membranes or changes in the intramembranous particles. Although the type I cell does not replicate, in vitro studies using different cell lives have enhanced our understanding about the interaction of the organism and the host. In one report, *Pneumocystis* attachment increased as cultured alveolar type II cells differentiated into a type I cell-like phenotype.[55] Other studies have shown that the adherence occurs via extracellular matrix glycoproteins, as mentioned earlier, but involves different ligands for the specific glycoproteins.

The attachment for *Pneumocystis* to lung epithelial cells requires an intact cytoskeleton and results in changes in both the organism and host. One effect is to enhance *Pneumocystis* proliferation.[4,56] *Pneumocystis* maintains an extracellular existence within alveoli, and probably obtains essential nutrients from the alveolar fluid or living cells.[54] Knowledge of how the organism responds to its alveolar microenvironment might lead to an in vitro culture system.

The adherence of *Pneumocystis* suppresses the growth of lung epithelial cells through cyclin-dependent kinase regulatory pathways.[57] Other reports have shown that the organism alters lung guanosine triphosphate (GTP)–binding regulatory proteins and induces expression of the intracellular adhesion molecule 1 (ICAM-1) and fibrinogen.[58] These properties may influence both the lung damage and host inflammatory and reparative responses in *Pneumocystis* pneumonia.

Recent studies have begun to uncover the consequences of *Pneumocystis* attachment and the colonization that may result. Colonization in mice, macaques infected with the similar immunodeficiency virus, and HIV patients elicits an inflammatory response similar to that found with COPD.[3,59-62] There is an influx of CD8 cells, neutrophils, and macrophages, along with an increase in local and systemic proinflammatory cytokines. These changes are worsened by smoking accompanied by a decline in lung function.

Host defenses against *Pneumocystis* include innate immunity and adaptive or acquired immunity. The innate immune system, which is the first level of defense, is comprised of alveolar macrophages, surfactant protein (SP)–A, SP-D, and other factors. Because alveolar macrophages have early and late actions in the infection, they are discussed later in this chapter. SP-A is a pulmonary collectin that functions in host defense (e.g., as a nonimmune opsonin) and as an immune modulator. Immunosuppressed SP-A knockout mice develop higher infection levels of *Pneumocystis* and an increased host inflammatory response compared with wild-type mice.[63-65] The role of SP-D in host defenses is less clear, but it appears to modulate the inflammatory response.[66,67]

There is accumulating evidence that B cells are important contributors to the acquired immune response to *Pneumocystis*. *Pneumocystis* pneumonia has been reported in patients and mice with B-cell defects.[40] A positive therapeutic effect has been found with the passive administration of hyperimmune serum or monoclonal antibodies to MSG and other antigens in experimental models of PCP.[18,19,68] Immunization with live *Pneumocystis* or DNA vaccines before or after CD4 cell depletion protects mice from organism challenge, and appears to be medicated by antibodies via Th1- or Th2-type responses.[69-71] B cells not only function as the source of antibodies but also as antigen-presenting cells and help in the development of memory CD4 cells.[72] Antibodies contribute to host defenses against *Pneumocystis* by acting as opsonins.[40]

Analysis of the role of antibodies in humans has been difficult because of the high prevalence of serum antibodies in the population and the lack of information about which antigen epitopes are protective. HIV induces abnormalities in B-cell number and function, which results in impaired antibody responses to vaccines or microbial antigens.[73] Recombinant MSG antigen fragments have shown promise as serologic reagents. HIV patients who recovered from PCP have higher antibody levels to MSG than patients who never had the disease.[45] The best antibody responses were found in HIV patients with a first episode of PCP or a CD4 count of 50 cells/mm^3 or higher.[74] Although local bronchoalveolar lavage fluid (BALF) antibodies have received only limited attention, there is evidence of decreased antibody responses in HIV patients.[75,76]

Impaired cellular immunity has long been considered to be an important predisposing factor in the development of PCP.[54] Naturally occurring outbreaks of *Pneumocystis* pneumonia have occurred in immunodeficient animals, particularly colonies of severe combined immunodeficiency disease (SCID) mice and athymic nude mice and rats.[77,78] The central role of CD4 cells in host defenses against this organism has been shown by cell depletion and reconstitution experiments and by knockout mice.[22,79,80] Other contributors to these defenses include T-cell costimulatory molecules such as CD28 and CD2, the CD40 to CD40L pathway, which facilitates the interaction of T cells with B cells, and CD8 cells, which function as cytotoxic cells or by secreting cytokines.[81-88] PCP can be induced in normal rodents by the administration of corticosteroids, and these models have been used for more than 3 decades.[54] Protein malnutrition and an immature immune system also impair host defenses against *Pneumocystis*, although the defect in neonatal mice is related more to factors in the lung milieu than to T cells.[89,90] The clearest evidence of the role of defective cell-mediated immunity in the development of PCP in humans comes from persons infected with HIV. The risk of developing *Pneumocystis* pneumonia in adult HIV patients increases greatly when circulating CD4 cells fall below 200/mm^3.[91] Because CD4 counts are much higher in young children than in adults, different criteria must be used. The presence of other clinical complications of HIV—for example, fever and oral candidiasis—increases the risk of PCP independent of the CD4 count. Cases of PCP associated with low CD4 counts have been encountered in cancer patients receiving cytotoxic drugs, in adults with idiopathic CD4 lymphopenia, and in otherwise healthy individuals with subtle T-cell defects.[92,93] The issue of evaluating CD4 counts as a risk factor for *Pneumocystis* pneumonia in immunosuppressed patients has also been raised.[94,95] A few studies have found a correlation between the number of CD4 cells in peripheral blood or bronchoalveolar lavage fluid, with a poor prognosis.[96]

The interaction of HIV and *Pneumocystis* with CD4 and other T cells in humans is of considerable potential interest, but has received only limited attention. One report has suggested that HIV depletes *Pneumocystis*-specific T-cell clones horizontally—that is, by lowering the number of memory cells in the progeny without affecting the number of clones.[97] On the other hand, *Pneumocystis* infection enhances HIV replication in the lung, and may possibly accentuate the depletion of CD4 cells.[98] HIV patients who have recovered from PCP have higher proliferative and Th2-like cytokine (interleukin-4 [IL-4]) responses to native MSG than HIV patients who never had the disease.[99]

The occurrence of PCP in other patient populations with impaired cellular immunity has included premature debilitated infants, children with primary immunodeficiency diseases, particularly SCID (which involves both T- and B-cell defects) and the hyper-IgM syndrome (which involves disruption of the CD40-CD40L pathway),[85] and patients receiving immunosuppressive drugs for the treatment of a variety of conditions.[54] The principal immunocompromised hosts at risk for PCP include patients with hematologic malignancies and solid tumors (e.g., brain tumors), solid organ and bone marrow transplant recipients, and collagen vascular disorders (e.g., Wegener's granulomatosis).[92,100-102] The number of these individuals has grown over the years with better survival and the more widespread use of cytotoxic and immunosuppressive therapies. Corticosteroids, used alone or in combination with other agents, remain the most common immunosuppressive drugs implicated in the development of PCP. The relationship of corticosteroids to *Pneumocystis* has been emphasized by the occurrence of PCP in patients with Cushing's syndrome and children receiving corticosteroids for diseases such as asthma not known to predispose to opportunistic infections.[103,104] Cases of *Pneumocystis* pneumonia in patients on chemotherapy regimens without corticosteroids have also been well documented.[74] Protein malnutrition is an important risk factor for the development of *Pneumocystis* pneumonia, both by itself and as a complication of the patient's underlying disease or its chemotherapy. Lymphopenia and lung factors (e.g., radiation and fibrosis) have been suggested as additional predisposing factors in non-HIV patients.[54]

Alveolar macrophages are the first line of defense against *Pneumocystis* and the principal effector cell in clearing the organism from the lung.[105] However, activated macrophages, in the absence of CD4 cells, are unable to control *P. jirovecii* infection.[106] Also needed for *Pneumocystis* clearance is the urokinase-type plasminogen activator, which aids the recruitment of inflammatory cells.[107] An enolase produced by *Pneumocystis* can activate plasminogen, and thus may impair the host plasminogen activator.[108] Recognition and adherence of *Pneumocystis* to macrophages occur by multiple pathways involving MSG and β-glucan in the organism, extracellular matrix and surfactant proteins, and mannose, Dectin-1, and Fc receptors.[25,26,28-30,109] Toll-like receptor (TLR) 2 and TLR4 help regulate host cytokine responses.[110,111] Macrophages ingest, degrade, and kill *Pneumocystis*, releasing cytokines such as tumor necrosis factor-α (TNF-α), eicosanoids, nitric acid, and reactive oxidants.[112-114] Macrophages also undergo apoptosis, which is mediated by polyamines.[115]

Alveolar macrophage function is impaired in HIV patients as well as in cancer and transplant patients receiving immunosuppressive drugs. HIV downregulates mannose receptor expression, which results in decreased binding and uptake of *Pneumocystis*.[116,117] HIV also changes the macrophage cytokine response.[118] *Pneumocystis* itself impairs phagocytosis by promoting shedding of the mannose receptor.[119]

Exposure to *Pneumocystis* or its antigens stimulates production of a multitude of cytokines, and chemokines. Two proinflammatory cytokines, TNF-α and IL-1, have been shown to be important in host defenses against the organism, particularly in the early stages of the infections.[120,121] TNF helps recruit lymphocytes and monocytes, which contribute to *Pneumocystis* clearance, and chemokines (e.g., IL-8) from alveolar epithelial cells as part of the inflammatory response.[4] IL-6, another proinflammatory cytokine, has been produced in response to *Pneumocystis*, but its contributions to host resistance to the organism are unclear.[122] IFN-γ and granulocyte macrophage-stimulating factor (GM-CSF) are important contributors to host defense by macrophage activation or in cooperation with TNF-α.[123,124] The role of IFN-γ is particularly complex, and the results obtained can vary, depending on the experimental design. Recent studies have shown that IL-12 and IL-23 also contribute to host defenses to *Pneumocystis*.[125,126] IL-10 has also been shown to modulate the host inflammatory response, but no role in the host defense against *Pneumocystis* has been found for IL-4 or granulocyte colony-stimulating factor (G-CSF).[127,128]

The pathologic changes that occur during the development of PCP in animal models and in humans are similar.[54] As the host defenses become compromised, *Pneumocystis* organisms begin to proliferate and gradually fill alveolar lumens. In the corticosteroid-treated rat model, the organism number increases from 10^5/lung or fewer to 10^9 to 10^{10}/lung after 8 to 10 weeks of corticosteroid administration. The principal histologic finding is the formation of a foamy, eosinophilic alveolar exudate (Fig. 270-3); as the PCP increases in severity, there may also be hyaline membrane formation, along with interstitial fibrosis and edema. The host inflammatory response is usually inconspicu-

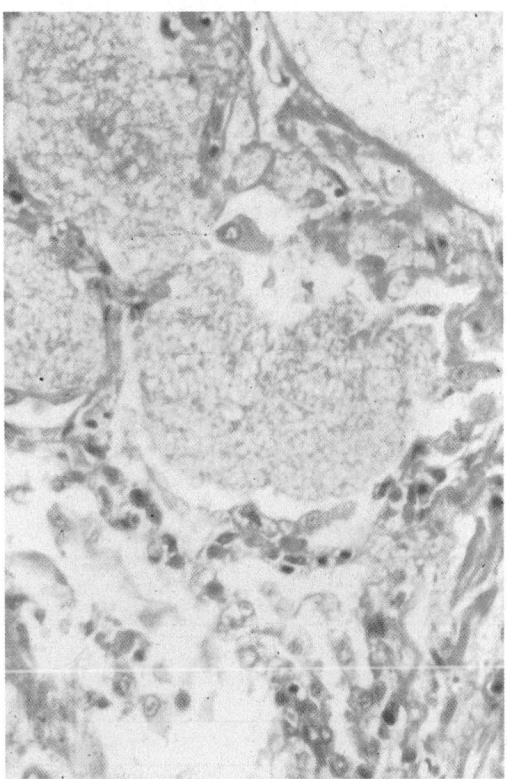

Figure 270-3. Histologic findings in pneumocystosis. *Pneumocystis* pneumonia illustrating frothy eosinophilic honeycombed material filling the alveolar space (H&E stain, × 400).

ous and is characterized by type II cell proliferation (a typical reparative response) and scanty mononuclear cell infiltrate. SCID mice exhibit cytokine production only late in the course of PCP, when elevated levels of TNF-α and IL-1 are found in the lungs.[129] Several studies have shown that rats with corticosteroid-induced PCP, as well as HIV and non-HIV patients with the disease, have elevated levels of proinflammatory cytokines in their respiratory tract but not in the peripheral blood.[130-132] Some patients exhibit atypical findings, such as lack of the alveolar exudate or the development of cavitary lesions, granulomas, or microcalcifications.[133] On electron microscopy, there is increased alveolar-capillary permeability followed by evidence of damage to the type I cell.[54,134]

Physiologic changes include hypoxemia with an increased alveolar-arterial (PAo_2-Pao_2) oxygen gradient and respiratory alkalosis, impaired diffusing capacity, suggesting alveolar-capillary block, and alterations in lung compliance, total lung capacity, and vital capacity.[135,136] The resulting picture suggests diffuse lung damage similar to that seen in the adult respiratory distress syndrome (ARDS).

The pathophysiologic changes described are caused not only by the effects of *Pneumocystis* on the type I cell, but also by alterations in the surfactant system and host inflammatory response. There is a fall in surfactant phospholipids (mainly phosphatidylcholine) that is caused by inhibition of phospholipid secretion mediated by MSG and other organism contituents.[137-140] Changes in the surfactant proteins include a decline in SP-B and SP-C and rise in SP-A and SP-D levels.[141,142] Fractionation of the surfactant has shown that most of the increased SP-A and SP-D levels are localized mainly in the small aggregate compartment.[143] There is now a considerable body of evidence showing that the immune inflammatory response to *Pneumocystis* can have harmful and helpful effects on the host lung. These effects are complex and depend to some degree on the experimental model being used. Immune reconstitution and cell depletion studies using SCID mice have shown that the clearance of PCP is associated with a hyperinflammatory response composed of increased proinflammatory cytokines

and chemokines and reduced oxygenation and compliance.[79,144-147] These effects not only involve the complex interaction of CD4 cells and CD8 cells,[148] but also subsets of CD4 cells (CD25+, CD25−) and CD8 cells (TC1, TC2), which have effector or immunomodulatory functions.[82,149-153] In contrast to humans, neutrophils are a marker of inflammation and lung damage in these animals, but do not cause lung damage.[154] The administration of a large number of splenocytes or CD4 cells sensitized to MSG in rats with corticosteroid-induced *Pneumocystis* pneumonia results in clinical illness and a cytokine cascade, along with a reduction in organism burden.[155] The presence of steroids has no apparent effect on these events. The contribution of the host inflammatory response to lung damage in HIV patients with PCP has been suggested by studies that have correlated increased numbers of neutrophils and levels of IL-8 in bronchoalveolar lavage fluid with more severe pneumonia and worse prognosis.[156,157] IL-8 functions as a potent chemoattractant, interaction with *P. jirovecii* is mediated by MSG, and its interaction with alveolar macrophages requires the coexpression of the mannose receptor and TLR2.[158-160] Alterations in eicosanoids, TNF-α, IL-1, other cytokines, and inflammatory mediators have also been noted in these and other studies; however, the pathogenic significance of these changes is unclear. HIV patients with *Pneumocystis* pneumonia also frequently experience a worsening of respiratory function soon after receiving antimicrobial drugs. Corticosteroids, if given promptly, can ameliorate or prevent this outcome and improve survival.[161] It is thought that the beneficial effects of corticosteroids are attributable to their anti-inflammatory properties or their effects on surfactant components[2]; however, studies examining these issues have produced inconsistent results.[162-165]

Clinical Manifestations

Interstitial plasma cell pneumonia, so named because of the distinctive lung infiltrate, has occurred classically in debilitated infants 6 weeks to 4 months of age who are housed in orphanages or foundling homes under crowded conditions.[54] The disease begins insidiously with symptoms such as poor feeding and progresses gradually to overt respiratory distress and cyanosis. Cases sometimes occurred in explosive outbreaks, giving rise to the term *epidemic form* of *Pneumocystis* pneumonia. Interstitial plasma cell pneumonia has largely disappeared from industrialized countries but still exists in parts of the world (and in their refugees) where poor socioeconomic conditions abound. PCP is being recognized with increasing frequency in HIV-infected children in Africa.[166]

The major presenting symptoms of PCP in the compromised host are shortness of breath, fever, and a nonproductive cough.[54,167] Occasionally sputum is produced and, rarely, hemoptysis; chest pain may also occur. Patients receiving immunosuppressive drugs frequently develop these clinical manifestations after the corticosteroid dose has been tapered, and are typically sick for about 1 to 2 weeks before seeking medical attention. *Pneumocystis* pneumonia in HIV patients usually is a subtler disease, with symptoms lasting from weeks to months; the organism burden is higher but lung damage is less severe.[168,169] Studies have also compared the clinical features of PCP in adult HIV patients by age and underlying risk group.[170,171] In both AIDS and non-AIDS patients, however, the clinical picture is variable; for example, lung allograft recipients who develop PCP frequently are asymptomatic at the time of diagnosis.

On physical examination, tachypnea and tachycardia are found in acutely ill patients. Children may demonstrate cyanosis, flaring of the nasal alae, and intercostal retractions in severe disease. Lung auscultation is usually not helpful, although rales can be heard in about one third of adults with the disease.

The chest radiograph classically exhibits bilateral diffuse infiltrates extending from the perihilar region (Fig. 270-4). Atypical manifestations have ranged from normal films to unilateral infiltrates, nodules, cavities, pneumatoceles, lymphadenopathy, and effusions.[54,167] Patients receiving prophylactic aerosol pentamidine have an increased incidence of apical infiltrates and pneumothoraces.[172] Techniques such as

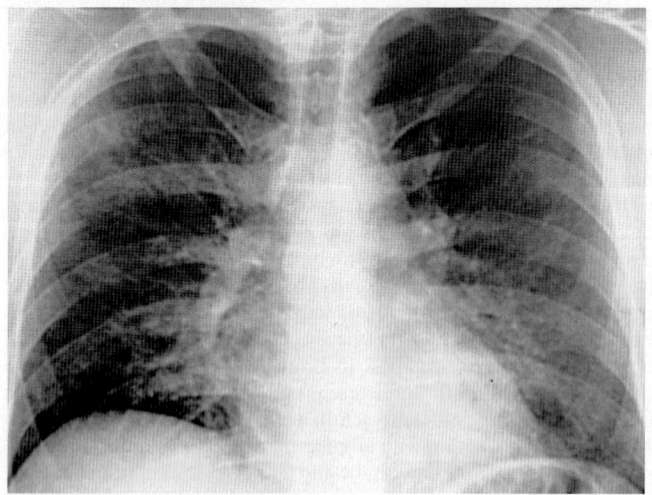

Figure 270-4   Chest radiograph. Shown are bilateral infiltrates of *Pneumocystis* pneumonia.

ultrasound and computed tomography (CT) scans have been helpful in studying mass lesions and extrapulmonary infection. High-resolution CT (HRCT) is important in the evaluation of patients with normal or equivocal chest radiographs.[167] Nuclear medicine procedures have demonstrated increased lung uptake on scans using gallium-67 citrate, indium 111, human IgG, and technetium 99–labeled monoclonal antibody to *Pneumocystis* MSG.[173,174]

Impaired oxygenation is the most frequent laboratory abnormality found in PCP; analysis of the magnitude of hypoxemia or the alveolar-oxygen gradient has been used to evaluate disease severity and monitor progression.[161] Serum lactic dehydrogenase (LDH) levels, which appear to reflect lung injury, rise frequently in *Pneumocystis* pneumonia and decline with successful therapy. However, the usefulness of serum LDH has been limited because there is much overlap among different patient groups and elevations can be produced by other diseases.[175]

OTHER CLINICAL MANIFESTATIONS

The spread of *P. jirovecii* beyond the lungs occurs mainly in patients with advanced HIV infection who are taking no prophylaxis or only aerosolized pentamidine. The actual incidence of extrapulmonary pneumocystosis is unclear because the diagnosis is made by histologic examination of sites where there are clinical manifestations or at autopsy.[176] The main sites of involvement are lymph nodes, spleen, liver, bone marrow, gastrointestinal tract, eyes, thyroid, adrenal glands, and kidneys. The clinical manifestations, which may occur with or without lung involvement, vary from incidental findings at autopsy to a rapidly progressive multisystem disease. Among the focal manifestations of extrapulmonary pneumocystosis are a rapidly enlarging thyroid mass, pancytopenia from bone marrow necrosis, retinal cotton wool spots, and numerous hypodense lesions in the spleen on CT scan. Biopsy or fine-needle aspiration shows areas of necrosis filled with foamy material. Gomori methenamine silver or fluorescent monoclonal antibody stain reveals numerous organisms.

Another clinical problem of interest is the immune reconstitution inflammatory syndrome (IRIS). IRIS is a condition in which an HIV patient's immune system begins to recover with a rise in CD4 cells days to months after starting antiretroviral therapy, and is manifested as worsening of a known condition or a new condition.[177-179] IRIS occurs in up to 25% of HIV patients undergoing antiretroviral therapy. The inciting agent can be a viable subclinical pathogen or a residual antigen from that pathogen. This distinction is important because antimicrobial drugs are administered for infection, whereas anti-inflammatory agents are needed for inflammation. In the case of *P. jirovecii*, clinical

manifestations include shortness of breath, cough, and pulmonary infiltrates of varying severity.[180]

Diagnosis

PCP should be considered in any immunocompromised patient who develops respiratory symptomatology, fever, and an abnormal chest radiograph. Because these clinical manifestations may be produced by a long list of infectious and noninfectious agents, diagnosis of *Pneumocystis* pneumonia must be made by histopathologic demonstration of the organism. With extrapulmonary pneumocystosis, the diagnosis may be suspected by the presence of the typical eosinophilic honeycombed material at the affected site.

One approach to the management of patients with suspected *Pneumocystis* pneumonia is presented in Figure 270-5. Patients with a compatible clinical picture and chest radiograph demonstrating a reticular or granular infiltrate should undergo a diagnostic procedure to collect

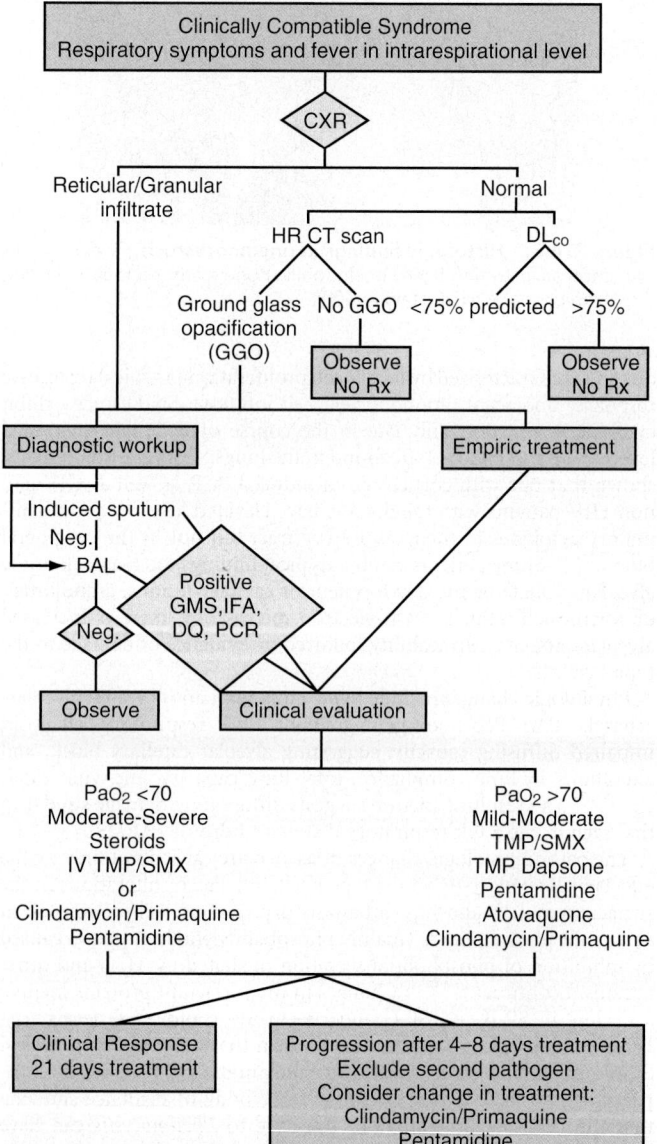

Figure 270-5   Algorithm for the diagnostic evaluation and management of patients with suspected *Pneumocystis* pneumonia. BAL, bronchoalveolar lavage; DL_co, single breath diffusing capacity for carbon monoxide; GGO, ground-glass opacities; HRCT, high-resolution CT.

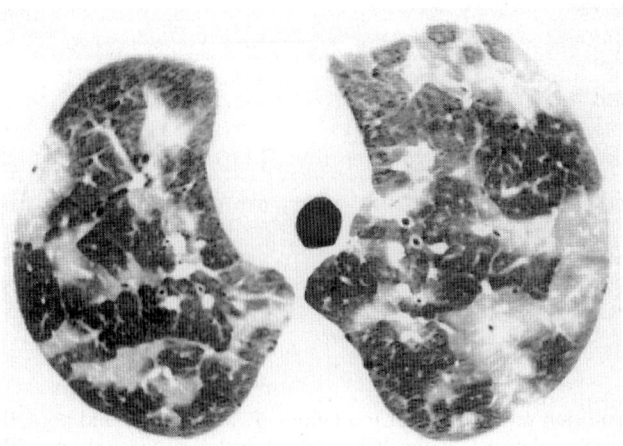

Figure 270-6 **HRCT scan of HIV patient with *Pneumocystis* pneumonia.** This patient had a normal chest radiograph. The HRCT scan demonstrates the characteristic ground-glass opacities. *(Courtesy of L. Huang.)*

respiratory secretions to detect the organism. In patients with a normal chest radiograph, additional testing should be performed to assess the probability of early *Pneumocystis* infection. Either HRCT scanning of the chest or pulmonary function testing can be used to identify patients unlikely to have *Pneumocystis* pneumonia and who may be observed without specific anti-*Pneumocystis* treatment. A prospective study has found that a normal, unchanged, or equivocal chest radiograph and a chest HRCT scan without ground-glass opacities rule out PCP.[181] Similarly, studies have shown that a normal or unchanged chest radiograph and a single breath diffusing capacity for carbon monoxide (DL_{CO}) of more than 75% of predicted almost rules out the diagnosis of *Pneumocystis* pneumonia[182] (Fig. 270-6). A DL_{CO} of less than 75% of predicted is, however, of low specificity and patients with ground-glass opacities on HRCT or a DL_{CO} of less than 75% of predicted should undergo a diagnostic workup to detect the organism.

A variety of stains have been used to identify *Pneumocystis* in respiratory tract secretions; in the hands of experienced microscopists, all are highly efficient in detecting the organism.[54,183,184] Stains such as methenamine silver or one of its simpler variants (e.g., toluidine blue O, cresyl violet), which selectively stain the wall of *Pneumocystis* cysts, have been popular among pathologists because they can be used on imprint smears or tissue sections and are easy to interpret. Reagents such as Wright-Giemsa or one of its more rapid variants (e.g., Diff-Quik) stain all *Pneumocystis* developmental stages as well as host cells. Calcofluor white is a chemifluorescent agent that binds to B-linked polymers of *Pneumocystis* and other fungi. The Papanicolaou stain, which is used by cytopathologists, is a very sensitive method to detect the foamy eosinophilic material surrounding *Pneumocystis*, although individual organisms do not stain well. Laboratories may use a rapid staining technique to screen for *Pneumocystis*, which is then followed by a more time-consuming procedure for definitive identification.

Immunofluorescence has been the most widely used immunologic technique for *Pneumocystis* diagnosis.[183,185] Commercial kits using monoclonal antibodies have been shown to be somewhat more sensitive than histologic stains in detecting *Pneumocystis*; however, this has to be balanced against the need for specialized facilities and increased cost. Immunohistochemistry has been used to detect *Pneumocystis* organisms in tissue sections. Soluble *Pneumocystis* antigens have been found in patients with PCP by immunoblotting.[186] The development of DNA amplification by PCR has introduced a new level of sensitivity in *Pneumocystis* detection. In recent years, PCR has proven to be a highly efficient method of detecting *Pneumocystis* in a variety of respiratory specimens; when performed under carefully controlled conditions, specificity has been reasonable.[187-189] The presence of a positive PCR product in a specimen that cannot be confirmed by other methods

of detection presents a diagnostic dilemma. Such a situation might result from the recent administration of anti-*Pneumocystis* drugs or may represent subclinical infection or colonization. Reverse transcriptase (RT)–PCR has been used to differentiate RNA from viable organisms from DNA and may be of use in following the response to therapy. PCR has been modified so it can be used in the clinical microbiology laboratories; if commercial kits become approved, PCR could gain acceptance as one of the standard techniques available for the diagnosis of PCP. PCR also offers promise in allowing the use of specimens obtained using noninvasive approaches, such as oropharyngeal washes to be used to establish the diagnosis. In contrast to respiratory specimens, the results of PCR in detecting *Pneumocystis* in serum have been inconsistent.

The collection of specimens that accurately reflect the disease process in the lungs is an essential component of the diagnostic evaluation of patients with suspected PCP. The collection procedures used in adults can usually be performed in children, although infants present special problems.[190] In general, the more invasive the procedure, the better the diagnostic yield. These procedures usually have a higher diagnostic yield in AIDS patients than in other immunocompromised hosts because of the higher organism burden. Although *Pneumocystis* organisms are rarely found in expectorated sputum, the organisms can be frequently detected in sputum that has been induced by inhalation of a saline mist. Induced sputum has emerged as a simple noninvasive technique that can be used to screen for the presence of *Pneumocystis*. The diagnostic yield from induced sputum ranges from less than 50% to 90% at different medical centers, depending on the level of interest and expertise in performing the procedure.[175,184] Success in the use of induced sputum requires a serious institutional commitment in terms of specially dedicated and trained personnel, and care in the processing of specimens. Several studies comparing PCR assay from oropharyngeal wash or gargle specimens with standard microscopy from induced sputum or bronchoalveolar lavage (BAL) specimens have reported promising results, but differentiation between infection and colonization still requires additional studies prior to recommendation as a standard clinical approach.[53,191,192]

Fiberoptic bronchoscopy is the most commonly performed invasive procedure, and results in the diagnosis of PCP in more than 90% of cases.[54,184] BAL specimens are usually obtained instead of washings and brushings because they have greater sensitivity and low morbidity. The diagnostic yield of BAL specimens can be increased if multiple lobes are sampled or the procedure is directed toward the sites of greatest involvement[193]; BAL specimens also provide information that cannot be obtained from induced sputum about *Pneumocystis* organism burden, the presence of other infectious agents, and the host inflammatory response.[194] Transbronchial biopsy may provide information not obtainable from BAL specimens, but is associated with a higher rate of complications (e.g., pneumothorax and bleeding).

Open lung biopsy, which requires the use of operating room facilities and general anesthesia, long served as the standard reference procedure for the diagnosis of *Pneumocystis* because it provided the greatest amount of tissue.[54] Open lung biopsy can be helpful when bronchoscopy is nondiagnostic, in evaluating another infection or condition complicating PCP, and in diagnosing Kaposi's sarcoma of the lung. Open lung biopsy is performed less frequently than in the past and minithoracotomy or thoracoscopically performed biopsies are more commonly performed.

Most serologic studies are not specific for *Pneumocystis*. Serum LDH levels are frequently elevated in *Pneumocystis* pneumonia and decline with successful therapy; however, the usefulness of serum LDH has been limited because there is much overlap among different patient groups and elevations can be produced by other diseases.[175] Other laboratory tests studied in PCP include hemoglobin, leukocyte and lymphocyte counts, and serum albumin, angiotensin-converting enzyme, thyroxine, triiodothyronine, and carcinoembryonic antigen levels.[167,183] Unfortunately, the specificity of all of these tests for *Pneumocystis* is low. The measurement of plasma S-adenosylmethionine concentrations has been proposed as a sensitive test for *Pneumocystis* pneumonia.[195,196] In laboratory animal studies, it has been shown to be depleted in *Pneumocystis*-infected animals. A more recent study demonstrated significantly lower AdoMet concentration in 28 HIV-AIDS patients with PCP compared with those in 28 control HIV-AIDS patients with bacterial or mycobacterial pneumonia. In addition, serial S-adenosylmethionine levels appeared to parallel the clinical course of disease. These results will need to be confirmed in additional controlled clinical trials. Similarly, β-D-glucan, a component of many fungal cell walls, has been detected in patients with PCP, but the usefulness of this assay as an indirect indicator of *P. jirovecii* infection needs additional investigation.[197]

Since the onset of the HIV pandemic, PCP has placed a strain on health care facilities. As managed care with its singular focus on controlling costs has come to dominate health care, *Pneumocystis* pneumonia has served as a model for studies examining the allocation of resources devoted to the care of HIV patients.[198,199] One way to reduce costs has been to replace invasive diagnostic procedures with algorithms and simple diagnostic techniques that are predictive of PCP.[167,182,184,191] The major problem with this approach is that none of the tests can reliably distinguish *Pneumocystis* infection from multiple other causes of pulmonary infiltrates in HIV patients. Another way to lower costs has been to use empirical therapy.[200] This approach may be appropriate in tropical or developing countries; historically, however, at hospitals in the United States, patients treated empirically for PCP had higher mortality than patients in whom a specific diagnosis was made by bronchoscopy, although more recent studies have suggested that this may be a cost-effective approach.[201,202] Financial considerations were cited as a major contributing factor in the decision not to perform bronchoscopy. Empirical therapy may also impair later attempts to establish a specific causative diagnosis.[203]

Course and Prognosis

The natural history of untreated PCP in HIV patients and other immunocompromised hosts is characterized by progressive respiratory insufficiency, leading to death. Prognosis is related to the degree of hypoxemia at the time of presentation; an arterial oxygen pressure of 70 mm Hg while breathing room air has been established to separate the milder from the more serious forms of disease.[161] When this is expressed as the alveolar-arterial oxygen gradient, *Pneumocystis* pneumonia has been classified as mild (less than 35 mm Hg), moderate (35 to 45 mm Hg), and severe (higher than 45 mm Hg). Other prognostic indicators in HIV patients include extensive infiltrates on chest radiograph, interstitial fibrosis and edema on biopsy, increased neutrophils and IL-8 levels in BALF, elevated LDH levels and reduced albumin levels in serum, age over 60 years, CD4 counts in BALF and blood, and general markers of disease severity.[136,156,157,167,175,183,204] Concurrent pulmonary infection with other microorganisms can complicate management of all patients, and the presence of cytomegalovirus in the respiratory tract of HIV patients may be an independent predictor of poor prognosis.[205] Other prognostic host factors in non-HIV patients include severity of the underlying disease and prior lung damage.

The introduction of highly active antiretroviral therapy (HAART) in about 1996 extended the lives of HIV-infected patients and reduced the frequency of PCP and other opportunistic infections. It is less clear whether the survival from PCP has improved over this time and, if improvement did occur, whether it was the result of HAART. A recent study has examined the mortality predictors present at the time of hospitalization in 494 patients with 54 episodes of PCP at a single institution from 1985 to 2006.[204] Six independent risk factors ranging from low oxygenation to a previous episode of PCP were identified (Table 270-1). None of the patients had received HAART. The overall case fatality rate was 13.5%, and did not change significantly over time.

A second study at this medical center was reported on HIV patients with PCP admitted to the intensive care unit (ICU).[206] Mortality dropped from 71% in the pre-HAART era to 34% in the HAART era. Because none of the patients received HAART, the better survival was thought to be caused by improved ICU care. A third study at this

TABLE 270-1	Mortality Risk Factors in 494 HIV Patients with 547 Episodes of Proven *Pneumocystis* Pneumonia		
Risk Factor	**Adjusted Odds Ratio (95% CI)***	**P**
Older age	1.57 (1.11-2.23)	.011
Subsequent episode of *Pneumocystis* pneumonia	2.27 (1.14-4.52)	.019
Low hemoglobin level	0.70 (0.60-0.83)	.001
Low Pao$_2$ on room air	0.70 (0.60-0.81)	.001
Medical comorbidity	3.93 (1.77-8.72)	.001
Pulmonary Kaposi's sarcoma	6.95 (2.26-21.37)	.001

*CI, confidence interval.

institution revealed similar mortality rates among HIV and non-HIV patients admitted to the ICU, and no better survival among HIV patients receiving HAART.[207]

Optimal management of PCP depends on prompt diagnosis and institution of therapy. Early in the HIV epidemic, survival of *Pneumocystis* patients was better at hospitals with greater familiarity with the disease; however, improvement in management has occurred throughout the medical community. In contrast to HIV patients, the mortality of PCP in several large series of non-HIV patients is 30% to 50%, a figure that has not changed appreciably in 2 decades.[100,101,169,208,209] The lack of improvement in the survival in non-HIV patients probably reflects a lack of recognition and delays in diagnosis.

Patients who recover from PCP are at risk for developing recurrent episodes of the disease as long as the immunosuppressive conditions persist.[54] HIV patients are much more likely to develop recurrence than non-HIV patients. Studies have shown that recurrent episodes occurring within 6 months of the first episode are more likely to be relapses, whereas episodes occurring at more than 6 months are more likely to represent a new episode of infection.[210] Earlier studies found that the prognosis of recurrent episodes of PCP is similar to that of initial episodes, although more recent analyses have shown a worse outcome with subsequent episodes.[204,211]

Another complication plaguing patients who recover from *Pneumocystis* pneumonia is pneumothorax.[136,167,212] Risk factors include a previous episode of PCP, the use of aerosol pentamidine, and cigarette smoking. Pneumatoceles, pneumomediastinum, and subcutaneous emphysema also occur. Management is difficult and should be individualized; measures have included chest tube, surgical or chemical pleurodesis, and thoracostomy with stapling. The previous use of corticosteroids may increase risk of morbidity.[212]

Treatment

Trimethoprim-sulfamethoxazole (TMP-SMX) is the drug of choice for all forms of pneumocystosis.[213] This agent, which acts by inhibiting folic acid synthesis, has been used for 2 decades against *Pneumocystis* with a high degree of success.[214-217] Among the attractive features of TMP-SMX are its availability in oral and parenteral forms, well-known pharmacokinetics, antibacterial properties, and cost. TMP-SMX is administered orally or intravenously in a dosage of 15 to 20 mg/kg/day (TMP) and 75 to 100 mg/kg/day (SMX) in three or four divided doses. The parenteral preparation should be used in patients who are seriously ill or have gastrointestinal disturbances. As with all anti-*Pneumocystis* drugs, treatment should be continued for 21 days in HIV patients and 14 days in non-HIV patients. The reason for the longer duration in HIV patients is thought to be the fact that these individuals have a higher organism burden and respond more slowly.

TMP-SMX is well tolerated by non-HIV patients, with gastrointestinal symptoms and skin rashes being the most common complaints. By contrast, HIV patients experience a high frequency (up to 80% or more) of adverse reactions, which usually begin during the second week of TMP-SMX therapy and may result in discontinuation of the drug in up to 50% of these individuals.[213,218] The side effects include skin rash, fever, cytopenias, nausea and vomiting, hepatitis, pancreatitis, nephritis, hyperkalemia, metabolic acidosis, central nervous system manifestations, and an anaphylactoid reaction. Most of these reactions appear to be caused by the sulfonamide component, but the mechanisms are not well understood. Among the possible contributing factors are elevated serum drug levels, the formation of hydroxylamine metabolites, glutathione deficiency, hypersensitivity, and high CD4 counts.[218-220] Hyperkalemia has been attributed to trimethoprim, which acts like a potassium-sparing diuretic.[221]

Some investigators have recommended adjusting the dosage of TMP-SMX to achieve serum concentrations of 5 to 8 µg/mL TMP and 100 to 150 µg/mL SMX to achieve maximum efficacy and minimum toxicity[216,218]; however, others have not found this approach to be beneficial or practical.[222] N-Acetylcysteine and folinic acid have not helped prevent side effects from TMP-SMX, and folinic acid may actually be harmful. Skin reactions to TMP-SMX range from mild to life-threatening—for example, toxic epidermal necrolysis, Stevens-Johnson syndrome, and anaphylaxis. In some cases, the skin rash and manifestations such as fever may resolve spontaneously or respond to conservative measures, whereas in other cases they may require discontinuation of the drug. Corticosteroids may also be helpful.[223] Desensitization regimens have been successful in patients who have experienced non–life-threatening reactions to TMP-SMX, but should be undertaken with caution.[224] Several alternative regimens have been developed for the treatment of mild to moderate PCP.[213] Although these studies have been performed mainly in HIV patients, the results should be applicable to non-HIV patients with PCP. TMP administered at a dose of 15 to 20 mg/kg/day orally combined with dapsone 100 mg/day orally has been shown to be as effective as TMP-SMX and less toxic.[225] The major adverse reactions to dapsone are methemoglobinemia, rash, fever, nausea, and vomiting; hemolysis can occur in patients who have glucose-6-phosphate dehydrogenase (G6PD) deficiency. Dapsone can be administered to patients intolerant of sulfonamides, but must be approached with caution because there are few reliable guidelines to predict who might experience a serious reaction. The serum levels of dapsone and TMP are higher when these drugs are used together than when used alone and suggest bidirectional interference with clearance.[226] Controlled studies have shown that the combination of clindamycin and primaquine exhibits comparable efficacy and toxicity to TMP-SMX and TMP and dapsone in the therapy of PCP.[225,227] The mechanism of action of clindamycin and primaquine against *Pneumocystis* is not known. The usual doses are clindamycin (600 mg every 6 hours intravenously or 300 to 450 mg every 6 hours orally) and primaquine (15 to 30 mg base/day orally). Treatment may also be initiated with intravenous clindamycin and then switched to oral administration. Adverse effects include skin rash, fever, neutropenia, gastrointestinal complaints, and methemoglobinemia.[213] Primaquine also causes hemolysis in patients with G6PD deficiency.

Atovaquone is a hydroxynaphthoquinone that was originally developed as an antimalarial agent. Atovaquone acts on the mitochondrial electron transport chain of plasmodia and, based on mutations found in *Pneumocystis* isolates from patients failing atovaquone prophylaxis, drug targets are similar in *Pneumocystis*. One study compared atovaquone with TMP-SMX and another with pentamidine isethionate for the treatment of mild to moderate PCP in HIV patients.[228,229] Atovaquone was less effective than TMP-SMX and about as effective as pentamidine; however, atovaquone was better tolerated in both studies. Adverse reactions to atovaquone include skin rash, fever, gastrointestinal symptoms, and abnormal liver function tests. An oral suspension, administered at a dose of 750 mg/5 mL twice daily with food, results in better absorption than earlier preparations.[230]

There appears to be an emerging consensus that the combination of clindamycin and primaquine is the preferred alternative regimen to TMP-SMX for moderate to severe PCP. A recent systematic review that also included new data from the authors' patient populations supported a previous meta-analysis that clindamycin and primaquine are superior to pentamidine as "salvage" treatment of PCP (i.e.,

patients who failed PCP).[231,232] A higher dose of clindamycin (600 to 900 mg every 6 to 8 hours) has usually been used.[233,234]

Other drugs that have been used are pentamidine isethionate and trimetrexate.[213] Pentamidine is an old drug that was first used to treat African trypanosomiasis; pentamidine appears to exert its antimicrobial activity by binding to DNA, but its precise mode of action against *Pneumocystis* is unknown. A number of reports have shown that pentamidine is about as effective as TMP-SMX in the therapy of PCP in HIV and non-HIV patients.[214-217] Pentamidine is usually administered as a single daily dosage of 4 mg/kg, although a dosage of 3 mg/kg has been used in some studies. The IV route is preferred over the IM route of administration; pentamidine is diluted in 50 to 250 mL of a 5% dextrose solution and infused over a period of at least 1 hour. Pentamidine administered by aerosol has also been used in the treatment of *Pneumocystis* pneumonia; however, because this form of administration is less effective than oral drugs, it is not recommended.

Pharmacokinetic studies have shown that pentamidine follows a three-compartment model with rapid passage to tissues, secondary distribution, and long (about 12 days) elimination half-life. Only a small amount of the drug is cleared by the kidney.[218,235] Pentamidine is a toxic drug; adverse reactions occur in 80% or more of HIV and non-HIV patients, and are severe enough to necessitate discontinuation of the drug in about half of cases. Side effects include hypotension, cardiac arrhythmias (e.g., torsades de pointes), azotemia, pancreatitis, dysglycemias, hyperkalemia, hypomagnesemia, hypocalcemia, neutropenia, hepatic disturbances, bronchospasm, and problems at intramuscular injection sites. Hypoglycemia, which is caused by damage of pancreatic β cells with insulin release, occurs early in therapy, and may later be followed by diabetes mellitus. The frequency of hypoglycemia and azotemia has been correlated with high serum pentamidine levels, total drug dose, and duration of treatment.[236,237] The mechanism of hyperkalemia caused by pentamidine is similar to that caused by TMP.[238]

Trimetrexate, a lipid-soluble derivative of methotrexate, is a highly potent inhibitor of *Pneumocystis* dihydrofolate reductase (DHFR). Trimetrexate is no longer commercially available. A controlled study has shown that trimetrexate is less effective but better tolerated than TMP-SMX in the therapy of PCP in hospitalized patients.[239] Other studies have shown that trimetrexate may have been valuable as salvage therapy in patients who failed or could not tolerate TMP-SMX.[213]

The response to anti-*Pneumocystis* drugs generally mirrors other clinical features of the infection. Non-HIV patients, who become ill rather quickly, usually show a clinical response by 4 days of treatment; if there is no response by 4 to 8 days, it is wise to consider switching to another drug. HIV patients typically respond more slowly and take longer to clear *Pneumocystis* from their lungs. It is prudent to wait for at least 8 days before declaring a treatment failure. As noted, clindamycin and primaquine are the preferred drugs for those patients who fail TMP-SMX; conversely, TMP-SMX is the preferred regimen for patients failing other regimens.[231] Adding anti-*Pneumocystis* drugs to the regimen is no more effective than substituting one agent for another, and may increase the risk of adverse reactions.

HIV patients frequently experience worsening of their blood oxygenation during the first few days of therapy; such a clinical deterioration can be particularly dangerous if the initial hypoxemia is marked. Several studies have shown that the administration of corticosteroids during the first 72 hours of treatment can lessen the decline in oxygenation and improve survival. These studies led to a recommendation by an expert panel that steroids be added to the treatment of all patients with moderate to severe PCP—that is, an arterial oxygen pressure less than 70 mm Hg or an alveolar-arterial oxygen gradient higher than 35 mm Hg in the following dosage regimen for adults: prednisone, 40 mg orally twice daily, days 1 to 5; 40 mg once daily, days 6 to 10; and 20 mg once daily, days 11 to 20.[161] The use of corticosteroids became widely adopted by the medical community. A subsequent report showed that steroids do not improve the outcome of PCP other than reducing the frequency of hypersensitivity reactions to TMP-SMX.[240] However, a meta-analysis and a more recent systematic review of the literature has supported the use of corticosteroids both in reducing mortality and the need for mechanical ventilation.[232,241,242]

Corticosteroids used in the manner described have generally been well tolerated.[161] The principal side effects are oral candidiasis, mucocutaneous herpes simplex, and metabolic changes, such as hyperglycemia. Concerns have been raised about increased frequency of cytomegaloviral, other fungal, and mycobacterial infections but so far have not materialized. Nevertheless, the lack of efficacy of steroids in some studies,[240,242] along with the risk of other opportunistic infections and other possible complications (e.g., increased morbidity of pneumothorax associated with the use of corticosteroids) emphasize the need for careful patient selection and follow-up.

Recommendations about the use of adjunctive corticosteroids in other *Pneumocystis* patient populations are difficult to formulate because of the limited available information. The studies that have been performed so far have suggested that corticosteroids may speed clinical improvement, but conflicting results have been obtained about whether survival is enhanced. The problem with non-HIV patients is that most of these individuals have been on corticosteroids shortly before or at the time they developed PCP. Rapid withdrawal of steroids may have serious adverse consequences, and thus it seems prudent either to maintain the current dose or return to the previous steroid dose when instituting anti-*Pneumocystis* therapy. The steroid dose can then be slowly tapered. The place of corticosteroids in non-HIV patients who have received immunosuppressive drugs other than steroids is unknown.

Future clinical advances in the treatment of PCP might come from several current lines of investigation. Although the development of a continuous culture system remains elusive, it might be possible to use molecular techniques to identify markers of virulence or antimicrobial resistance. Sequence variation in dihydropteroate synthetase, the target enzyme of sulfonamides, in human *Pneumocystis* has been identified.[243] These mutations, at positions associated with sulfonamide resistance in other organisms, have been associated with failure in prophylaxis but no clear association with treatment failure or altered outcome has been demonstrated. A systematic review in 2004 showed that patients receiving sulfa drugs for PCP prophylaxis had a significantly higher risk of developing these mutations, but concluded that there was not enough evidence that the mutations adversely affected disease outcome.[244] Since then, two of three studies found a trend toward more severe disease and worse outcome associated with these mutations.[245-247] Mutations have also been described in the gene encoding cytochrome B and have been associated with failure of atovaquone prophylaxis.[248] New drugs with improved efficacy, less toxicity, and different mechanism of action are needed. Animal models, which are the principal test system, have identified several new types of drugs (e.g., echinocandins, 8-aminoquinolines, diamidines); however, clinical trials have been held up because of market considerations. A more promising approach has been to investigate drugs that are already licensed for other agents for activity against *Pneumocystis*. Echinocandins, which inhibit the synthesis of β-1-3 glucans, are now widely used in the treatment of *Aspergillus* and *Candida* infections. Caspofungin, the prototype of these agents, has been active against *Pneumocystis* in animal models. There are case reports of success and failure of caspofungin in the treatment of PCP in humans,[249-252] but no clinical trials have yet been conducted. Manipulation of the host immune or inflammatory response could improve defenses against *Pneumocystis* while lessening their deleterious effects on the host. These studies might lead to the development of drugs with greater specificity than corticosteroids. Finally, there is increasing evidence that the physiologic changes that accompany the development of *Pneumocystis* pneumonia and result in lung injury cannot be reversed by antimicrobial therapy alone; however, they can be improved by the administration of surfactant.[253,254] Clinical trials of surfactants or other agents that improve lung physiology are needed.

Prevention

Controlled studies demonstrating the safety and efficacy of daily or intermittent TMP-SMX in preventing PCP in pediatric cancer patients have stimulated considerable interest in developing prophylactic regimens for HIV patients and other immunocompromised hosts.[1] Prophylaxis can be considered primary (directed at the first bout of *Pneumocystis* pneumonia) or secondary (directed at recurrent episodes). The decision about whether to institute chemoprophylaxis depends on such factors as the incidence of PCP in the target population as well as drug effectiveness, safety, ease of administration, and cost. Because none of the available anti-*Pneumocystis* drugs used in humans has proven to be lethal for *Pneumocystis*, they should be continued for as long as the immunosuppressive conditions exist.

Guidelines for the prevention and treatment of opportunistic infections in HIV-infected adults and adolescents have recently been updated by an expert panel from the National Institutes of Health, Centers for Disease Control and Prevention (CDC), and HIV Medicine Association of the Infectious Diseases Society of America (IDSA).[255] Chemoprophylaxis is indicated for all adults with CD4 counts less than 200/mm^3 or a history of oropharyngeal candidiasis. Persons with a CD4 cell percentage lower than 14% or a history of an AIDS-defining illness, but do not otherwise qualify, should be considered for prophylaxis. Chemoprophylaxis is also indicated for children born to HIV-infected mothers, beginning at 4 to 6 weeks of age. Medication should be continued until the child's HIV status is determined. If the child is infected with HIV, prophylaxis should be continued throughout the first year of life. The subsequent need for chemoprophylaxis is determined by age-specific CD4 counts.

Three drug regimens are currently recommended for *Pneumocystis* prophylaxis. The doses used here are for adults and adolescents; the U.S. Public Health Service (USPHS)–IDSA Guidelines should be consulted for doses in children. TMP-SMX, the drug of choice, is administered at a dosage of one double-strength tablet (160 mg TMP to 800 mg SMX) daily. One single-strength tablet (80 mg TMP to 400 mg SMX) daily is very effective and one double-strength tablet three times weekly is also acceptable. TMP-SMX protects not only against *Pneumocystis* but also against *Toxoplasma gondii* and bacterial infections. Adverse reactions to TMP-SMX occur in up to 50% or more of patients and require discontinuation of the drug in up to 30% to 40% of cases. The frequency of side effects is somewhat lower with the use of single-strength tablets or three times weekly administration. Guidelines for desensitization or rechallenge with TMP-SMX for prophylaxis are similar to those for use of TMP-SMX in treatment.

Recommended drug regimens for HIV patients who cannot tolerate TMP-SMX include dapsone, aerosolized pentamidine, and atovaquone. Dapsone may be administered at a dosage of 100 mg/day alone or 50 mg/day combined with 50 mg of pyrimethamine (a DHFR inhibitor) weekly and 25 mg of leucovorin weekly. Additional dosage schedules have also been used. Overall, the dapsone regimens have shown efficacy and toxicity similar to those of the TMP-SMX regimens. Dapsone and pyrimethamine protect against *T. gondii* but not against bacterial infections. Atovaquone suspension, 1500 mg/day day, has been shown to have similar efficacy to dapsone in patients intolerant of TMP-SMX. Pentamidine is administered at a dose of 300 mg in a Respirgard nebulizer once monthly. Aerosolized pentamidine is less effective, better tolerated, and much more expensive than TMP-SMX or dapsone. The major side effects are cough and bronchospasm, which can be controlled by a β-agonist. Aerosolized pentamidine requires a negative pressure room with adequate ventilation, and should not be performed in patients with tuberculosis.

A number of other drug regimens have been considered as possible *Pneumocystis* prophylactic agents, but there is insufficient supportive information to recommend their use. Examples include pyrimethamine combined with sulfonamides (e.g., sulfadoxine-pyrimethamine [Fansidar], clindamycin), pentamidine administered as an aerosol using other nebulizers or administered intravenously, and clindamycin plus primaquine. Prophylactic regimens for *Mycobacterium avium* complex that contain azithromycin or clarithromycin lower the incidence of PCP. Mycophenolate mofetil, an immunosuppressive agent, has demonstrated anti-*Pneumocystis* activity in experimental models.

Several studies have documented the safety of discontinuing primary and secondary *Pneumocystis* pneumonia prophylaxis in patients responding to active antiretroviral therapy. It is safe to discontinue primary and secondary prophylaxis in patients who have responded to antiretroviral therapy with a CD4 cell increase to more than 200 cells/mm³ that is sustained for longer than 3 months. However, patients who developed a prior episode of *Pneumocystis* pneumonia with CD4 cell levels higher than 200 cells/mm³ should remain on secondary prophylaxis for life.

The widespread use of *Pneumocystis* chemoprophylaxis has had a major impact on the care of HIV patients.[256] Not only has this practice reduced the incidence of PCP, but it has also improved survival and quality of life while decreasing resource use and cost. Despite this success, studies performed before the introduction of the protease inhibitors have shown that breakthrough cases of *Pneumocystis* pneumonia occur in about 20% of patients.[257] The most important predictor of failure was very low CD4 counts (less than 50 to 100/mm³).[257,258] These breakthrough infections may also have atypical manifestations, particularly in patients taking aerosol pentamidine.[259] Examples include upper lobe disease, pneumothorax, extrapulmonary pneumocystosis, and fever of unknown origin.

Recent reviews have examined the efficacy of PCP prophylaxis among non-HIV immunocompromised patients. In the randomized and quasirandomized studies examined, the event rate of *Pneumocystis* pneumonia was 7.5%. Patients receiving TMP-SMX experienced a 91% reduction in the occurrence of PCP compared with controls, for a need to treat 15 patients to prevent one episode.[260,261] Based on the trials analyzed, chemoprophylaxis should be considered in patients with autologous bone marrow and solid organ transplantation or hematologic malignancies. Prophylaxis may also be considered in the following cases: (1) primary immune deficiency diseases; (2) severe protein malnutrition; (3) persistent CD4 counts of less than 200/mm³; and (4) cytotoxic or immunosuppressive therapy for the treatment of cancers of all types, collagen vascular diseases, and other disorders. If a corticosteroid is the sole drug, a reasonable guide for the need for *Pneumocystis* prophylaxis is the equivalent of 20 mg of prednisone for longer than 1 month. Some exclude diseases (e.g., asthma) that are usually not associated with *Pneumocystis* from this recommendation; however, in light of case reports of PCP in children with asthma, these guidelines may become blurred.

TMP-SMX is the chemoprophylactic agent of choice and should be used in the same doses as are used in HIV patients. Although there is limited clinical experience with dapsone plus pyrimethamine and aerosol pentamidine, there is no reason to doubt the effectiveness of these agents in non-HIV patients.

Another method of preventing PCP is to boost the host immune response. This could be done by improving general immune function or focusing on organism-specific immunity. In the latter case, MSG is one potential candidate, but other antigens might also be explored. Immunization of immunocompromised patients at an early stage of their disease—for example, HIV patients with a higher than 500 cells/mm³ CD4 count or newly diagnosed cancer patients—might prevent, delay, or lessen the severity of PCP. Boosting the host immune response might also lessen the need for or lower the dosage of antimicrobial drugs. Alternate approaches involve administration of specific antibodies or immune modulators.

A third method of preventing PCP is by preventing exposure. The communicability of *Pneumocystis* has been shown in experimental animals.[5] However, infection control guidelines for health care facilities have not recommended isolating *Pneumocystis* patients because person-to-person transmission has seldom been convincingly demonstrated, and the disease was thought to occur by reactivation of latent infection. This outlook seems to be changing because of the continued occurrence of outbreaks or cluster of PCP, the development of sensitive techniques to detect *Pneumocystis* DNA in asymptomatic individuals and the air, and the ability to distinguish among *Pneumocystis* isolates, particularly in patients with recurrent episodes of PCP. The practice of isolating *Pneumocystis* patients from direct contact with other immunocompromised hosts is recommended by the for CDC Hospital Infection Control Practice Advisory Committee.[262] Little is also known about the behavior of the organism in the environment, although a study has suggested that *Pneumocystis* is susceptible to common antiseptic agents.[263] Despite these limitations, recent advances in technology offer promise of providing valuable insight into the epidemiologic features of this interesting and enigmatic organism.

REFERENCES

1. Barry SM, Johnson MA. *Pneumocystis carinii* pneumonia: A review of current issues in diagnosis and management. *HIV Med.* 2001;2:123-132.
2. Thomas CF Jr, Limper AH. *Pneumocystis* pneumonia. *N Engl J Med.* 2004;350:2487-2498.
3. Morris A, Wei K, Afshar K, et al. Epidemiology and clinical significance of *Pneumocystis* colonization. *J Infect Dis.* 2008;197:10-17.
4. Thomas CF Jr, Limper AH. Current insights into the biology and pathogenesis of *Pneumocystis* pneumonia. *Nat Rev Microbiol.* 2007;5:298-308.
5. Cushion M. *Pneumocystis* pneumonia. In: Merz WG, Hay RJ, eds. *Topley and Wilson's Microbiology and Microbial Infections.* 10th ed. London: Hodder and Arnold; 2005:763-806.
6. Cushion MT, Smulian AG, Slaven BE, et al. Transcriptome of *Pneumocystis carinii* during fulminate infection: Carbohydrate metabolism and the concept of a compatible parasite. *PLoS ONE.* 2007;2:e423.
7. Keely SP, Fischer JM, Stringer JR. Evolution and speciation of *Pneumocystis. J Eukaryot Microbiol* 2003;50(Suppl):624-626.
8. Stringer JR, Beard CB, Miller RF, et al. A new name (*Pneumocystis jiroveci*) for *Pneumocystis* from humans. *Emerg Infect Dis.* 2002;8:891-896.
9. Redhead SA, Cushion MT, Frenkel JK, et al. *Pneumocystis* and *Trypanosoma cruzi*: Nomenclature and typifications. *J Eukaryot Microbiol.* 2006;53:2-11.
10. Sloand E, Laughon B, Armstrong M, et al. The challenge of *Pneumocystis carinii* culture. *J Eukaryot Microbiol.* 1993;40:188-195.
11. Burgess JW, Kottom TJ, Limper AH. *Pneumocystis carinii* exhibits a conserved meiotic control pathway. *Infect Immun.* 2008;76:417-425.
12. Schmatz DM, Powles M, McFadden DC, et al. Treatment and prevention of *Pneumocystis carinii* pneumonia and further elucidation of the *P. carinii* life cycle with 1,3-beta-glucan synthesis inhibitor L-671,329. *J Protozool.* 1991;38:151S-153S.
13. Kaneshiro ES. *Pneumocystis carinii* pneumonia: The status of *Pneumocystis* biochemistry. *Int J Parasitol.* 1998;28:65-84.
14. Kaneshiro ES. Sterol metabolism in the opportunistic pathogen *Pneumocystis*: Advances and new insights. *Lipids.* 2004;39:753-761.
15. De Stefano JA, Myers JD, Du Pont D, et al. Cell wall antigens of *Pneumocystis carinii* trophozoites and cysts: Purification and carbohydrate analysis of these glycoproteins. *J Eukaryot Microbiol.* 1998;45:334-343.
16. Stringer JR. Antigenic variation in pneumocystis. *J Eukaryot Microbiol.* 2007;54:8-13.
17. Linke MJ, Sunkin SM, Andrews RP, et al. Expression, structure, and location of epitopes of the major surface glycoprotein of *Pneumocystis carinii* f. sp. carinii. *Clin Diagn Lab Immunol.* 1998;5:50-57.
18. Gigliotti F, Hughes WT. Passive immunoprophylaxis with specific monoclonal antibody confers partial protection against *Pneumocystis carinii* pneumonitis in animal models. *J Clin Invest.* 1988;81:1666-1668.
19. Gigliotti F, Haidaris CG, Wright TW, et al. Passive intranasal monoclonal antibody prophylaxis against murine *Pneumocystis carinii* pneumonia. *Infect Immun.* 2002;70:1069-1074.
20. Theus SA, Smulian AG, Sullivan DW, et al. Cytokine responses to the native and recombinant forms of the major surface glycoprotein of *Pneumocystis carinii. Clin Exp Immunol.* 1997;109:255-260.
21. Theus SA, Walzer PD. Adoptive transfer of specific lymphocyte populations sensitized to the major surface glycoprotein of *Pneumocystis carinii* decreases organism burden while increasing survival rate in the rat. *J Eukaryot Microbiol.* 1997;44:23S-24S.
22. Theus SA, Smulian AG, Steele P, et al. Immunization with the major surface glycoprotein of *Pneumocystis carinii* elicits a protective response. *Vaccine.* 1998;16:1149-1157.
23. Keely SP, Linke MJ, Cushion MT, et al. *Pneumocystis murina* MSG gene family and the structure of the locus associated with its transcription. *Fungal Genet Biol.* 2007;44:905-919.
24. Kutty G, Ma L, Kovacs JA. Characterization of the expression site of the major surface glycoprotein of human-derived *Pneumocystis carinii. Mol Microbiol.* 2001;42:183-193.
25. Pottratz ST, Paulsrud J, Smith JS, et al. *Pneumocystis carinii* attachment to cultured lung cells by pneumocystis gp 120, a fibronectin binding protein. *J Clin Invest.* 1991;88:403-407.
26. Ezekowitz RA, Williams DJ, Koziel H, et al. Uptake of *Pneumocystis carinii* mediated by the macrophage mannose receptor. *Nature.* 1991;351:155-158.
27. Kottom TJ, Kennedy CC, Limper AH. *Pneumocystis* PCINT1, a molecule with integrin-like features that mediates organism adhesion to fibronectin. *Mol Microbiol.* 2008;67:747-761.
28. Limper AH, Standing JE, Hoffman OA, et al. Vitronectin binds to *Pneumocystis carinii* and mediates organism attachment to cultured lung epithelial cells. *Infect Immun.* 1993;61:4302-4309.
29. McCormack FX, Festa AL, Andrews RP, et al. The carbohydrate recognition domain of surfactant protein A mediates binding to the major surface glycoprotein of *Pneumocystis carinii. Biochemistry.* 1997;36:8092-8099.
30. O'Riordan DM, Standing JE, Kwon KY, et al. Surfactant protein D interacts with *Pneumocystis carinii* and mediates organism adherence to alveolar macrophages. *J Clin Invest.* 1995;95:2699-2710.
31. Lugli EB, Bampton ET, Ferguson DJ, et al. Cell surface protease PRT1 identified in the fungal pathogen *Pneumocystis carinii. Mol Microbiol.* 1999;31:1723-1733.
32. Ambrose HE, Keely SP, Aliouat EM, et al. Expression and complexity of the PRT1 multigene family of *Pneumocystis carinii. Microbiology.* 2004;150:293-300.
33. Schaffzin JK, Sunkin SM, Stringer JR. A new family of *Pneumocystis carinii* genes related to those encoding the major surface glycoprotein. *Curr Genet.* 1999;35:134-143.
34. Kutty G, Kovacs JA. A single-copy gene encodes Kex1, a serine endoprotease of *Pneumocystis jiroveci. Infect Immun.* 2003;71:571-574.

35. Lee LH, Gigliotti F, Wright TW, et al. Molecular characterization of KEX1, a kexin-like protease in mouse *Pneumocystis carinii*. *Gene*. 2000;242:141-150.
36. Smulian AG, Stringer JR, Linke MJ, et al. Isolation and characterization of a recombinant antigen of *Pneumocystis carinii*. *Infect Immun*. 1992;60:907-915.
37. Theus SA, Sullivan DW, Walzer PD, et al. Cellular responses to a 55-kilodalton recombinant *Pneumocystis carinii* antigen. *Infect Immun*. 1994;62:3479-3484.
38. Smulian AG, Sullivan DW, Theus SA. Immunization with recombinant *Pneumocystis carinii* p55 antigen provides partial protection against infection: Characterization of epitope recognition associated with immunization. *Microbes Infect*. 2000; 2:127-136.
39. Ma L, Kutty G, Jia Q, Kovacs JA. Characterization of variants of the gene encoding the p55 antigen in *Pneumocystis* from rats and mice. *J Med Microbiol*. 2003;52:955-960.
40. Walzer PD. Immunologic features of *Pneumocystis carinii* infection in humans. *Clin Diagn Lab Immunol*. 1999;6:149-155.
41. Morgan DJ, Vargas SL, Reyes-Mugica M, et al. Identification of *Pneumocystis carinii* in the lungs of infants dying of sudden infant death syndrome. *Pediatr Infect Dis J*. 2001;20:306-309.
42. Vargas SL, Hughes WT, Santolaya ME, et al. Search for primary infection by *Pneumocystis carinii* in a cohort of normal, healthy infants. *Clin Infect Dis*. 2001;32:855-861.
43. Larsen HH, von Linstow ML, Lundgren B, et al. Primary *Pneumocystis* infection in infants hospitalized with acute respiratory tract infection. *Emerg Infect Dis*. 2007;13:66-72.
44. Smulian AG, Keely SP, Sunkin SM, et al. Genetic and antigenic variation in *Pneumocystis carinii* organisms: Tools for examining the epidemiology and pathogenesis of infection. *J Lab Clin Med*. 1997;130:461-468.
45. Daly KR, Koch J, Levin L, et al. Enzyme-linked immunosorbent assay and serologic responses to *Pneumocystis jiroveci*. *Emerg Infect Dis*. 2004;10:848-854.
46. Russian DA, Kovacs JA. *Pneumocystis carinii* in Africa: An emerging pathogen? *Lancet*. 1995;346:1242-1243.
47. van Oosterhout JJ, Laufer MK, Perez MA, et al. Pneumocystis pneumonia in HIV-positive adults, Malawi. *Emerg Infect Dis*. 2007;13:325-328.
48. Fisk DT, Meshnick S, Kazanjian PH. *Pneumocystis carinii* pneumonia in patients in the developing world who have acquired immunodeficiency syndrome. *Clin Infect Dis*. 2003;36:70-78.
49. Hu DJ, Fleming PL, Castro KG, et al. How important is race/ethnicity as an indicator of risk for specific AIDS-defining conditions? *J Acquir Immune Defic Syndr Hum Retrovirol*. 1995; 10:374-380.
50. Keely SP, Baughman RP, Smulian AG, et al.. Source of *Pneumocystis carinii* in recurrent episodes of pneumonia in AIDS patients. *AIDS*. 1996;10:881-888.
51. Beard CB, Carter JL, Keely SP, et al. Genetic variation in *Pneumocystis carinii* isolates from different geographic regions: Implications for transmission. *Emerg Infect Dis*. 2000;6: 265-272.
52. Huang L, Beard CB, Creasman J, et al. Sulfa or sulfone prophylaxis and geographic region predict mutations in the *Pneumocystis carinii* dihydropteroate synthase gene. *J Infect Dis*. 2000; 182:1192-1198.
53. Davis JL, Welsh DA, Beard CB, et al. *Pneumocystis* colonisation is common among hospitalised HIV infected patients with non-*Pneumocystis* pneumonia. *Thorax*. 2008;63:329-334.
54. Walzer PD, Kim CK, Cushion MT. Pneumocystis carinii. In: Walzer PD, Genta RM, ed. *Parasitic Infection in the Compromised Host*. New York: Marcel Dekker; 1989:83-178.
55. Pottratz ST, Weir AL. Attachment of *Pneumocystis carinii* to primary cultures of rat alveolar epithelial cells. *Exp Cell Res*. 1995;221:357-362.
56. Kottom TJ, Kohler JR, Thomas CF Jr, et al. Lung epithelial cells and extracellular matrix components induce expression of *Pneumocystis carinii* STE20, a gene complementing the mating and pseudohyphal growth defects of STE20 mutant yeast. *Infect Immun*. 2003;71:6463-6471.
57. Limper AH, Edens M, Anders RA, et al. *Pneumocystis carinii* inhibits cyclin-dependent kinase activity in lung epithelial cells. *J Clin Invest*. 1998;101:1148-1155.
58. Yu ML, Limper AH. *Pneumocystis carinii* induces ICAM-1 expression in lung epithelial cells through a TNF-alpha-mediated mechanism. *Am J Physiol*. 1997;273:L1103-L1111.
59. Christensen PJ, Preston AM, Ling T, et al. *Pneumocystis murina* infection and cigarette smoke exposure interact to cause increased organism burden, development of airspace enlargement, and pulmonary inflammation in mice. *Infect Immun*. 2008;76:3481-3490.
60. Norris KA, Morris A, Patil S, et al. *Pneumocystis* colonization, airway inflammation, and pulmonary function decline in acquired immunodeficiency syndrome. *Immunol Res*. 2006;36: 175-187.
61. Morris A, Sciurba FC, Lebedeva IP, et al. Association of chronic obstructive pulmonary disease severity and *Pneumocystis* colonization. *Am J Respir Crit Care Med*. 2004;170:408-413.
62. Calderon EJ, Rivero L, Respaldiza N, et al. Systemic inflammation in patients with chronic obstructive pulmonary disease who are colonized with *Pneumocystis jiroveci*. *Clin Infect Dis*. 2007;45:e17-e19.
63. Linke MJ, Harris CE, Korfhagen TR, et al. Immunosuppressed surfactant protein A-deficient mice have increased susceptibility to *Pneumocystis carinii* infection. *J Infect Dis*. 2001;183:943-952.
64. Linke M, Ashbaugh A, Koch J, et al. Surfactant protein A limits *Pneumocystis murina* infection in immunosuppressed C3H/HeN mice and modulates host response during infection. *Microbes Infect*. 2005;7:748-759.
65. Atochina EN, Beck JM, Preston AM, et al. Enhanced lung injury and delayed clearance of *Pneumocystis carinii* in surfactant protein A-deficient mice: Attenuation of cytokine responses and reactive oxygen-nitrogen species. *Infect Immun*. 2004;72:6002-6011.
66. Vuk-Pavlovic Z, Mo EK, Icenhour CR, et al. Surfactant protein D enhances *Pneumocystis* infection in immune-suppressed mice. *Am J Physiol Lung Cell Mol Physiol*. 2006;290:L442-L449.
67. Atochina EN, Gow AJ, Beck JM, et al. Delayed clearance of *Pneumocystis carinii* infection, increased inflammation, and altered nitric oxide metabolism in lungs of surfactant protein-D knockout mice. *J Infect Dis*. 2004;189:1528-1539.
68. Bartlett MS, Angus WC, Shaw MM, et al. Antibody to *Pneumocystis carinii* protects rats and mice from developing pneumonia. *Clin Diagn Lab Immunol*. 1998;5:74-77.
69. Harmsen AG, Chen W, Gigliotti F. Active immunity to *Pneumocystis carinii* reinfection in T-cell–depleted mice. *Infect Immun*. 1995;63:2391-2395.
70. Garvy BA, Wiley JA, Gigliotti F, et al. Protection against *Pneumocystis carinii* pneumonia by antibodies generated from either T helper 1 or T helper 2 responses. *Infect Immun*. 1997;65: 5052-5056.
71. Zheng M, Ramsay AJ, Robichaux MB, et al. CD4+ T cell-independent DNA vaccination against opportunistic infections. *J Clin Invest*. 2005;115:3536-3544.
72. Lund FE, Hollifield M, Schuer K, et al. B cells are required for generation of protective effector and memory CD4 cells in response to *Pneumocystis* lung infection. *J Immunol*. 2006; 176:6147-6154.
73. Moir S, Fauci AS. Pathogenic mechanisms of B-lymphocyte dysfunction in HIV disease. *J Allergy Clin Immunol*. 2008;122: 12-19.
74. Daly KR, Huang L, Morris A, et al. Antibody response to *Pneumocystis jirovecii* major surface glycoprotein. *Emerg Infect Dis*. 2006;12:1231-1237.
75. Laursen AL, Jensen BN, Andersen PL. Local antibodies against *Pneumocystis carinii* in bronchoalveolar lavage fluid. *Eur Respir J*. 1994;7:679-685.
76. Jalil A, Moja P, Lambert C, et al. Decreased production of local immunoglobulin A to *Pneumocystis carinii* in bronchoalveolar lavage fluid from human immunodeficiency virus-positive patients. *Infect Immun*. 2000;68:1054-1060.
77. Walzer PD, Kim CK, Linke MJ, et al. Outbreaks of *Pneumocystis carinii* pneumonia in colonies of immunodeficient mice. *Infect Immun*. 1989;57:62-70.
78. Furuta T, Fujita M, Machii K, et al. Fatal spontaneous pneumocystosis in nude rats. *Lab Anim Sci*. 1993;43:551-556.
79. Harmsen AG, Stankiewicz M. Requirement for CD4+ cells in resistance to *Pneumocystis carinii* pneumonia in mice. *J Exp Med*. 1990;172:937-945.
80. Shellito J, Suzara VV, Blumenfeld W, et al. A new model of *Pneumocystis carinii* infection in mice selectively depleted of helper T lymphocytes. *J Clin Invest*. 1990;85:1686-1693.
81. Beck JM, Blackmon MB, Rose CM, et al. T cell costimulatory molecule function determines susceptibility to infection with *Pneumocystis carinii* in mice. *J Immunol*. 2003;171:1969-1977.
82. McAllister F, Steele C, Zheng M, et al. In vitro effector activity of *Pneumocystis murina*–specific T-cytotoxic-1 CD8+ T cells: Role of granulocyte-macrophage colony-stimulating factor. *Infect Immun*. 2005;73:7450-7457.
83. Theus SA, Andrews RP, Steele P, et al. Adoptive transfer of lymphocytes sensitized to the major surface glycoprotein of *Pneumocystis carinii* confers protection in the rat. *J Clin Invest*. 1995;95:2587-2593.
84. Wiley JA, Harmsen AG. CD40 ligand is required for resolution of *Pneumocystis carinii* pneumonia in mice. *J Immunol*. 1995;155:3525-3529.
85. Levy J, Espanol-Boren T, Thomas C, et al. Clinical spectrum of X-linked hyper-IgM syndrome. *J Pediatr*. 1997;131:47-54.
86. Beck JM, Newbury RL, Palmer BE, et al. Role of CD8+ lymphocytes in host defense against *Pneumocystis carinii* in mice. *J Lab Clin Med*. 1996;128:477-487.
87. Kolls JK, Habetz S, Shean MK, et al. IFN-gamma and CD8+ T cells restore host defenses against *Pneumocystis carinii* in mice depleted of CD4+ T cells. *J Immunol*. 1999;162:2890-2894.
88. Steele C, Zheng M, Young E, et al. Increased host resistance against *Pneumocystis carinii* pneumonia in gamma delta T-cell-deficient mice: Protective role of gamma interferon and CD8(+) T cells. *Infect Immun*. 2002;70:5208-5215.
89. Qureshi MH, Garvy BA. Neonatal T cells in an adult lung environment are competent to resolve *Pneumocystis carinii* pneumonia. *J Immunol*. 2001;166:5704-5711.
90. Garvy BA, Qureshi MH. Delayed inflammatory response to *Pneumocystis carinii* infection in neonatal mice is due to an inadequate lung environment. *J Immunol*. 2000;165:6480-6486.
91. Phair J, Munoz A, Detels R, et al. The risk of *Pneumocystis carinii* pneumonia among men infected with human immunodeficiency virus type 1. Multicenter AIDS Cohort Study Group. *N Engl J Med*. 1990;322:161-165.
92. Kulke MH, Vance EA. *Pneumocystis carinii* pneumonia in patients receiving chemotherapy for breast cancer. *Clin Infect Dis*. 1997;25:215-218.
93. Smith DK, Neal JJ, Holmberg SD. Unexplained opportunistic infections and CD4+ T-lymphocytopenia without HIV infection. An investigation of cases in the United States. The Centers for Disease Control Idiopathic CD4+ T-lymphocytopenia Task Force. *N Engl J Med*. 1993;328:373-379.
94. Festic E, Gajic O, Limper AH, Aksamit TR. Acute respiratory failure due to *Pneumocystis* pneumonia in patients without human immunodeficiency virus infection: outcome and associated features. *Chest*. 2005;128:573-579.
95. Mansharamani NG, Balachandran D, Vernovsky I, et al. Peripheral blood CD4 + T-lymphocyte counts during *Pneumocystis carinii* pneumonia in immunocompromised patients without HIV infection. *Chest*. 2000;118:712-720.
96. Agostini C, Adami F, Poulter LW, et al. Role of bronchoalveolar lavage in predicting survival of patients with human immunodeficiency virus infection. *Am J Respir Crit Care Med*. 1997;156: 1501-1507.
97. Li Pira G, Fenoglio D, Bottone L, et al. Preservation of clonal heterogeneity of the *Pneumocystis carinii*–specific CD4 T cell repertoire in HIV infected, asymptomatic individuals. *Clin Exp Immunol*. 2002;128:155-162.
98. Koziel H, Kim S, Reardon C, et al. Enhanced in vivo human immunodeficiency virus-1 replication in the lungs of human immunodeficiency virus-infected persons with *Pneumocystis carinii* pneumonia. *Am J Respir Crit Care Med*. 1999;160: 2048-2055.
99. Theus SA, Sawhney N, Smulian AG, et al. Proliferative and cytokine responses of human T lymphocytes isolated from human immunodeficiency virus-infected patients to the major surface glycoprotein of *Pneumocystis carinii*. *J Infect Dis*. 1998;177:238-241.
100. Sepkowitz KA. Opportunistic infections in patients with and patients without acquired immunodeficiency syndrome. *Clin Infect Dis*. 2002;34:1098-1107.
101. Yale SH, Limper AH. *Pneumocystis carinii* pneumonia in patients without acquired immunodeficiency syndrome: Associated illness and prior corticosteroid therapy. *Mayo Clin Proc*. 1996;71:5-13.
102. Godeau B, Coutant-Perronne V, Le Thi Huong D, et al. *Pneumocystis carinii* pneumonia in the course of connective tissue disease: report of 34 cases. *J Rheumatol*. 1994;21:246-251.
103. Graham BS, Tucker WS Jr. Opportunistic infections in endogenous Cushing's syndrome. *Ann Intern Med*. 1984;101: 334-338.
104. Abernathy-Carver KJ, Fan LL, Boguniewicz M, et al. *Legionella* and *Pneumocystis* pneumonias in asthmatic children on high doses of systemic steroids. *Pediatr Pulmonol*. 1994;18:135-138.
105. Limper AH, Hoyte JS, Standing JE. The role of alveolar macrophages in *Pneumocystis carinii* degradation and clearance from the lung. *J Clin Invest*. 1997;99:2110-2117.
106. Hanano R, Reifenberg K, Kaufmann SH. Activated pulmonary macrophages are insufficient for resistance against *Pneumocystis carinii*. *Infect Immun*. 1998;66:305-314.
107. Beck JM, Preston AM, Gyetko MR. Urokinase-type plasminogen activator in inflammatory cell recruitment and host defense against *Pneumocystis carinii* in mice. *Infect Immun*. 1999; 67:879-884.
108. Fox D, Smulian AG. Plasminogen-binding activity of enolase in the opportunistic pathogen *Pneumocystis carinii*. *Med Mycol*. 2001;39:495-507.
109. Steele C, Marrero L, Swain S, et al. Alveolar macrophage-mediated killing of *Pneumocystis carinii* f. sp. muris involves molecular recognition by the Dectin-1 beta-glucan receptor. *J Exp Med*. 2003;198:1677-1688.
110. Zhang C, Wang SH, Liao CP, et al. Toll-like receptor 2 knockout reduces lung inflammation during *Pneumocystis* pneumonia but has no effect on phagocytosis of *Pneumocystis* organisms by alveolar macrophages. *J Eukaryot Microbiol* 2006;53(Suppl 1):S132-S133.
111. Ding K, Shibui A, Wang Y, et al. Impaired recognition by Toll-like receptor 4 is responsible for exacerbated murine *Pneumocystis* pneumonia. *Microbes Infect*. 2005;7:195-203.
112. Laursen AL, Moller B, Rungby J, et al. *Pneumocystis carinii*-induced activation of the respiratory burst in human monocytes and macrophages. *Clin Exp Immunol*. 1994;98:196-202.
113. Vassallo R, Kottom TJ, Standing JE, et al. Vitronectin and fibronectin function as glucan-binding proteins augmenting macrophage responses to *Pneumocystis carinii*. *Am J Respir Cell Mol Biol*. 2001;25:203-211.
114. Vassallo R, Standing JE, Limper AH. Isolated *Pneumocystis carinii* cell wall glucan provokes lower respiratory tract inflammatory responses. *J Immunol*. 2000;164:3755-3763.
115. Lasbury ME, Merali S, Durant PJ, et al. Polyamine-mediated apoptosis of alveolar macrophages during *Pneumocystis* pneumonia. *J Biol Chem*. 2007;282:11009-11020.
116. Kandil O, Fishman JA, Koziel H, et al. Human immunodeficiency virus type 1 infection of human macrophages modulates the cytokine response to *Pneumocystis carinii*. *Infect Immun*. 1994;62:644-6450.
117. Koziel H, Eichbaum Q, Kruskal BA, et al. Reduced binding and phagocytosis of *Pneumocystis carinii* by alveolar macrophages from persons infected with HIV-1 correlates with mannose receptor downregulation. *J Clin Invest*. 1998;102: 1332-1344.
118. Fraser IP, Takahashi K, Koziel H, et al. *Pneumocystis carinii* enhances soluble mannose receptor production by macrophages. *Microbes Infect*. 2000;2:1305-1310.

119. Stehle SE, Rogers RA, Harmsen AG, et al. A soluble mannose receptor immunoadhesin enhances phagocytosis of *Pneumocystis carinii* by human polymorphonuclear leukocytes in vitro. *Scand J Immunol.* 2000;52:131-137.
120. Limper AH. Tumor necrosis factor alpha-mediated host defense against *Pneumocystis carinii. Am J Respir Cell Mol Biol.* 1997; 16:110-111.
121. Chen W, Havell EA, Moldawer LL, et al. Interleukin 1: An important mediator of host resistance against *Pneumocystis carinii. J Exp Med.* 1992;176:713-718.
122. Chen W, Havell EA, Gigliotti F, et al. Interleukin-6 production in a murine model of *Pneumocystis carinii* pneumonia: Relation to resistance and inflammatory response. *Infect Immun.* 1993; 61:97-102.
123. Beck JM, Liggitt HD, Brunette EN, et al. Reduction in intensity of *Pneumocystis carinii* pneumonia in mice by aerosol administration of gamma interferon. *Infect Immun.* 1991;59: 3859-3862.
124. Paine R 3rd, Preston AM, Wilcoxen S, et al. Granulocyte-macrophage colony-stimulating factor in the innate immune response to *Pneumocystis carinii* pneumonia in mice. *J Immunol.* 2000;164:2602-2609.
125. Ruan S, McKinley L, Zheng M, et al. Interleukin-12 and host defense against murine *Pneumocystis* pneumonia. *Infect Immun.* 2008;76:2130-2137.
126. Rudner XL, Happel KI, Young EA, et al. Interleukin-23 (IL-23)–IL-17 cytokine axis in murine *Pneumocystis carinii* infection. *Infect Immun.* 2007;75:3055-3061.
127. Qureshi MH, Harmsen AG, Garvy BA. IL-10 modulates host responses and lung damage induced by *Pneumocystis carinii* infection. *J Immunol.* 2003;170:1002-1009.
128. Ieki R, Furuta T, Asano S, et al. Effect of recombinant human granulocyte colony-stimulating factor on *Pneumocystis carinii* infection in nude mice. *Jpn J Exp Med.* 1989;59:51-58.
129. Wright TW, Johnston CJ, Harmsen AG, et al. Analysis of cytokine mRNA profiles in the lungs of *Pneumocystis carinii*–infected mice. *Am J Respir Cell Mol Biol.* 1997;17:491-500.
130. Perenboom RM, Sauerwein RW, Beckers P, et al. Cytokine profiles in bronchoalveolar lavage fluid and blood in HIV-seropositive patients with *Pneumocystis carinii* pneumonia. *Eur J Clin Invest.* 1997;27:333-339.
131. Perenboom RM, Beckers P, Van Der Meer JW, et al. Pro-inflammatory cytokines in lung and blood during steroid-induced *Pneumocystis carinii* pneumonia in rats. *J Leukoc Biol.* 1996;60:710-715.
132. Perenboom RM, van Schijndel AC, Beckers P, et al. Cytokine profiles in bronchoalveolar lavage fluid and blood in HIV-seronegative patients with *Pneumocystis carinii* pneumonia. *Eur J Clin Invest.* 1996;26:159-166.
133. Travis WD, Pittaluga S, Lipschik GY, et al. Atypical pathologic manifestations of *Pneumocystis carinii* pneumonia in the acquired immune deficiency syndrome. Review of 123 lung biopsies from 76 patients with emphasis on cysts, vascular invasion, vasculitis, and granulomas. *Am J Surg Pathol.* 1990; 14:615-625.
134. Benfield TL, Prento P, Junge J, et al. Alveolar damage in AIDS-related *Pneumocystis carinii* pneumonia. *Chest.* 1997;111: 1193-1199.
135. D'Angelo E, Calderini E, Robatto FM, et al. Lung and chest wall mechanics in patients with acquired immunodeficiency syndrome and severe *Pneumocystis carinii* pneumonia. *Eur Respir J.* 1997;10:2343-2350.
136. Stansell JD, Hopewell, PC. *Pneumocystis carinii* pneumonia: Risk factors, clinical presentation and natural history. In: Sattler FR, Walzer PD, eds. *Pneumocystis carinii.* London: Bailliere Tindall; 1995:449-459.
137. Wang Z, Foye A, Chang Y, et al. Inhibition of surfactant activity by *Pneumocystis carinii* organisms and components in vitro. *Am J Physiol Lung Cell Mol Physiol.* 2005;288:L1124-L1131.
138. Su TH, Natarajan V, Kachel DL, et al. Functional impairment of bronchoalveolar lavage phospholipids in early *Pneumocystis carinii* pneumonia in rats. *J Lab Clin Med.* 1996;127:263-271.
139. Hoffman AG, Lawrence MG, Ognibene FP, et al. Reduction of pulmonary surfactant in patients with human immunodeficiency virus infection and *Pneumocystis carinii* pneumonia. *Chest.* 1992;102:1730-1736.
140. Lipschik GY, Treml JF, Moore SD, et al. *Pneumocystis carinii* glycoprotein A inhibits surfactant phospholipid secretion by rat alveolar type II cells. *J Infect Dis.* 1998;177:182-187.
141. Sternberg RI, Whitsett JA, Hull WM, et al. *Pneumocystis carinii* alters surfactant protein A concentrations in bronchoalveolar lavage fluid. *J Lab Clin Med.* 1995;125:462-469.
142. Beers MF, Atochina EN, Preston AM, et al. Inhibition of lung surfactant protein B expression during *Pneumocystis carinii* pneumonia in mice. *J Lab Clin Med.* 1999;133:423-433.
143. Atochina EN, Beck JM, Scanlon ST, et al. *Pneumocystis carinii* pneumonia alters expression and distribution of lung collectins SP-A and SP-D. *J Lab Clin Med.* 2001;137:429-439.
144. Roths JB, Sidman CL. Both immunity and hyperresponsiveness to *Pneumocystis carinii* result from transfer of CD4+ but not CD8+ T cells into severe combined immunodeficiency mice. *J Clin Invest.* 1992;90:673-678.
145. Wright TW, Gigliotti F, Finkelstein JN, et al. Immune-mediated inflammation directly impairs pulmonary function, contributing to the pathogenesis of *Pneumocystis carinii* pneumonia. *J Clin Invest.* 1999;104:1307-1317.
146. Wright TW, Johnston CJ, Harmsen AG, et al. Chemokine gene expression during *Pneumocystis carinii*–driven pulmonary inflammation. *Infect Immun.* 1999;67:3452-3460.
147. Wright TW, Notter RH, Wang Z, et al. Pulmonary inflammation disrupts surfactant function during *Pneumocystis carinii* pneumonia. *Infect Immun.* 2001;69:758-764.
148. Bhagwat SP, Gigliotti F, Xu H, et al. Contribution of T cell subsets to the pathophysiology of *Pneumocystis*-related immunorestitution disease. *Am J Physiol Lung Cell Mol Physiol.* 2006;291:L1256-L1266.
149. Hori S, Carvalho TL, Demengeot J. CD25+ CD4+ regulatory T cells suppress CD4+ T cell-mediated pulmonary hyperinflammation driven by *Pneumocystis carinii* in immunodeficient mice. *Eur J Immunol.* 2002;32:1282-1291.
150. Gigliotti F, Crow EL, Bhagwat SP, et al. Sensitized CD8+ T cells fail to control organism burden but accelerate the onset of lung injury during *Pneumocystis carinii* pneumonia. *Infect Immun.* 2006;74:6310-6316.
151. Meissner NN, Lund FE, Han S, et al. CD8 T cell–mediated lung damage in response to the extracellular pathogen *Pneumocystis* is dependent on MHC class I expression by radiation-resistant lung cells. *J Immunol.* 2005;175:8271-8279.
152. McKinley L, Logar AJ, McAllister F, et al. Regulatory T cells dampen pulmonary inflammation and lung injury in an animal model of *Pneumocystis* pneumonia. *J Immunol.* 2006;177: 6215-6226.
153. Swain SD, Meissner NN, Harmsen AG. CD8 T cells modulate CD4 T-cell and eosinophil-mediated pulmonary pathology in *Pneumocystis* pneumonia in B-cell–deficient mice. *Am J Pathol.* 2006;168:466-475.
154. Swain SD, Wright TW, Degel PM, et al. Neither neutrophils nor reactive oxygen species contribute to tissue damage during *Pneumocystis* pneumonia in mice. *Infect Immun.* 2004;72: 5722-5732.
155. Thullen TD, Ashbaugh AD, Daly KR, et al. Sensitized splenocytes result in deleterious cytokine cascade and hyperinflammatory response in rats with *Pneumocystis* pneumonia despite the presence of corticosteroids. *Infect Immun.* 2004;72: 757-765.
156. Mason GR, Hashimoto CH, Dickman PS, et al. Prognostic implications of bronchoalveolar lavage neutrophilia in patients with *Pneumocystis carinii* pneumonia and AIDS. *Am Rev Respir Dis.* 1989;139:1336-1342.
157. Benfield TL, Vestbo J, Junge J, et al. Prognostic value of interleukin-8 in AIDS-associated *Pneumocystis carinii* pneumonia. *Am J Respir Crit Care Med.* 1995;151:1058-1062.
158. Tachado SD, Zhang J, Zhu J, et al. *Pneumocystis*-mediated IL-8 release by macrophages requires coexpression of mannose receptors and TLR2. *J Leukoc Biol.* 2007;81:205-211.
159. Benfield TL, Kharazmi A, Larsen CG, et al. Neutrophil chemotactic activity in bronchoalveolar lavage fluid of patients with AIDS-associated *Pneumocystis carinii* pneumonia. *Scand J Infect Dis.* 1997;29:367-371.
160. Benfield TL, Lundgren B, Levine SJ, et al. The major surface glycoprotein of *Pneumocystis carinii* induces release and gene expression of interleukin-8 and tumor necrosis factor alpha in monocytes. *Infect Immun.* 1997;65:4790-4794.
161. The National Institutes of Health-University of California Expert Panel for Corticosteroids as Adjunctive Therapy for *Pneumocystis* Pneumonia. Consensus statement on the use of corticosteroids as adjunctive therapy for *Pneumocystis* pneumonia in the acquired immunodeficiency syndrome. *N Engl J Med.* 1990;323:1500-1504.
162. Benfield TL, van Steenwijk R, Nielsen TL, et al. Interleukin-8 and eicosanoid production in the lung during moderate to severe *Pneumocystis carinii* pneumonia in AIDS: A role of interleukin-8 in the pathogenesis of P. carinii pneumonia. *Respir Med.* 1995;89:285-290.
163. Huang ZB, Eden E. Effect of corticosteroids on IL1 beta and TNF alpha release by alveolar macrophages from patients with AIDS and *Pneumocystis carinii* pneumonia. *Chest.* 1993;104: 751-755.
164. Benfield TL, Schattenkerk JK, Hofmann B, et al. Differential effect on serum neopterin and serum beta 2-microglobulin is induced by treatment in *Pneumocystis carinii* pneumonia. *J Infect Dis.* 1994;169:1170-1173.
165. Dichter JR, Lundgren JD, Nielsen TL, et al. *Pneumocystis carinii* pneumonia in HIV-infected patients: Effect of steroid therapy on surfactant level. *Respir Med.* 1999;93:373-378.
166. Zar HJ. Pneumonia in HIV-infected and HIV-uninfected children in developing countries: epidemiology, clinical features, and management. *Curr Opin Pulm Med.* 2004;10: 176-182.
167. Huang L. Clinical Pesentation and Diagnosis of *Pneumocystis* pneumonia in HIV-infected Patients. In: Walzer PD, Cushion MT, ed. Pneumocystis pneumonia. New York: Marcell Dekker; 2005:349-406.
168. Haverkos HW. Assessment of therapy for *Pneumocystis carinii* pneumonia. PCP Therapy Project Group. *Am J Med.* 1984;76: 501-508.
169. Kovacs JA, Hiemenz JW, Macher AM, et al. *Pneumocystis carinii* pneumonia: A comparison between patients with the acquired immunodeficiency syndrome and patients with other immunodeficiencies. *Ann Intern Med.* 1984;100:663-671.
170. Chen HX, Ryan PA, Ferguson RP, et al. Characteristics of acquired immunodeficiency syndrome in older adults. *J Am Geriatr Soc.* 1998;46:153-156.
171. Laing R, Brettle R, Leen C, Hulks G. Features and outcome of *Pneumocystis carinii* pneumonia according to risk category for HIV infection. *Scand J Infect Dis.* 1997;29:57-61.
172. Fahy JV, Chin DP, Schnapp LM, et al. Effect of aerosolized pentamidine prophylaxis on the clinical severity and diagnosis of *Pneumocystis carinii* pneumonia. *Am Rev Respir Dis.* 1992;146:844-848.
173. Tumeh SS, Belville JS, Pugatch R, et al. Ga-67 scintigraphy and computed tomography in the diagnosis of *Pneumocystis carinii* pneumonia in patients with AIDS. A prospective comparison. *Clin Nucl Med.* 1992;17:387-394.
174. Goldenberg DM, Sharkey RM, Udem S, et al. Immunoscintigraphy of *Pneumocystis carinii* pneumonia in AIDS patients. *J Nucl Med.* 1994;35:1028-1034.
175. Benson CA, Spear J, Hines D, et al. Combined APACHE II score and serum lactate dehydrogenase as predictors of in-hospital mortality caused by first episode *Pneumocystis carinii* pneumonia in patients with acquired immunodeficiency syndrome. *Am Rev Respir Dis.* 1991;144:319-323.
176. Ng VL, Yajko DM, Hadley WK. Extrapulmonary pneumocystosis. *Clin Microbiol Rev.* 1997;10:401-418.
177. Murdoch DM, Venter WD, Van Rie A, et al. Immune reconstitution inflammatory syndrome (IRIS): Review of common infectious manifestations and treatment options. *AIDS Res Ther.* 2007;4:9.
178. Ratnam I, Chiu C, Kandala NB, et al. Incidence and risk factors for immune reconstitution inflammatory syndrome in an ethnically diverse HIV type 1-infected cohort. *Clin Infect Dis.* 2006; 42:418-427.
179. Hirsch HH, Kaufmann G, Sendi P, et al. Immune reconstitution in HIV-infected patients. *Clin Infect Dis.* 2004;38:1159-1166.
180. Takahashi T, Nakamura T, Iwamoto A. Reconstitution of immune responses to *Pneumocystis carinii* pneumonia in patients with HIV infection who receive highly active antiretroviral therapy. *Res Commun Mol Pathol Pharmacol.* 2002;112: 59-67.
181. Gruden JF, Huang L, Turner J, et al. High-resolution CT in the evaluation of clinically suspected *Pneumocystis carinii* pneumonia in AIDS patients with normal, equivocal, or nonspecific radiographic findings. *AJR Am J Roentgenol.* 1997;169:967-975.
182. Huang L, Stansell J, Osmond D, et al. Performance of an algorithm to detect *Pneumocystis carinii* pneumonia in symptomatic HIV-infected persons. Pulmonary Complications of HIV Infection Study Group. *Chest.* 1999;115:1025-1032.
183. Montaner JS, Zala C. The role of the laboratory in the diagnosis and management of AIDS-related *Pneumocystis carinii* pneumonia. In: Sattler FR, Walzer PD, eds. *Pneumocystis carinii.* London: Bailliere Tindall; 1995:471-485.
184. Kroe DM, Kirsch CM, Jensen WA. Diagnostic strategies for *Pneumocystis carinii* pneumonia. *Semin Respir Infect.* 1997;12: 70-78.
185. Aslanzadeh J, Stelmach PS. Detection of *Pneumocystis carinii* with direct fluorescence antibody and calcofluor white stain. *Infection.* 1996;24:248-250.
186. Smulian AG, Linke MJ, Cushion MT, et al. Analysis of *Pneumocystis carinii* organism burden, viability and antigens in bronchoalveolar lavage fluid in AIDS patients with pneumocystosis: Correlation with disease severity. *AIDS.* 1994;8:1555-1562.
187. Huggett JF, Taylor MS, Kocjan G, et al. Development and evaluation of a real-time PCR assay for detection of *Pneumocystis jirovecii* DNA in bronchoalveolar lavage fluid of HIV-infected patients. *Thorax.* 2008;63:154-159.
188. Robberts FJ, Liebowitz LD, Chalkley LJ. Polymerase chain reaction detection of *Pneumocystis jiroveci*: Evaluation of 9 assays. *Diagn Microbiol Infect Dis.* 2007;58:385-392.
189. Alvarez-Martinez MJ, Miro JM, Valls ME, et al. Sensitivity and specificity of nested and real-time PCR for the detection of *Pneumocystis jiroveci* in clinical specimens. *Diagn Microbiol Infect Dis.* 2006;56:153-160.
190. Birriel JA Jr, Adams JA, Saldana MA, et al. Role of flexible bronchoscopy and bronchoalveolar lavage in the diagnosis of pediatric acquired immunodeficiency syndrome–related pulmonary disease. *Pediatrics.* 1991;87:897-899.
191. Helweg-Larsen J. *Pneumocystis jiroveci.* Applied molecular microbiology, epidemiology and diagnosis. *Dan Med Bull.* 2004;51:251-273.
192. Miller RF, Huang L. A need for standardized definitions for clinical studies of *Pneumocystis. J Eukaryot Microbiol.* 2006;53 (Suppl 1):S87-S88.
193. Cadranel J, Gillet-Juvin K, Antoine M, et al. Site-directed bronchoalveolar lavage and transbronchial biopsy in HIV-infected patients with pneumonia. *Am J Respir Crit Care Med.* 1995; 152:1103-1106.
194. Huang L, Hecht FM, Stansell JD, et al. Suspected *Pneumocystis carinii* pneumonia with a negative induced sputum examination. Is early bronchoscopy useful? *Am J Respir Crit Care Med.* 1995;151:1866-1871.
195. Skelly M, Hoffman J, Fabbri M, et al. *S*-Adenosylmethionine concentrations in diagnosis of *Pneumocystis carinii* pneumonia. *Lancet.* 2003;361:1267-1268.
196. Skelly MJ, Holzman RS, Merali S. *S*-Adenosylmethionine levels in the diagnosis of *Pneumocystis carinii* pneumonia in patients with HIV infection. *Clin Infect Dis.* 2008;46:467-471.
197. Kawagishi N, Miyagi S, Satoh K, et al. Usefulness of beta-D-glucan in diagnosing *Pneumocystis carinii* pneumonia and monitoring its treatment in a living-donor liver-transplant recipient. *J Hepatobiliary Pancreat Surg.* 2007;14:308-311.

198. Bennett CL, Curtis JR, Achenbach C, et al. U.S. hospital care for HIV-infected persons and the role of public, private, and Veterans Administration hospitals. *J Acquir Immune Defic Syndr Hum Retrovirol.* 1996;13:416-421.
199. Curtis JR, Ullman M, Collier AC, et al. Variations in medical care for HIV-related *Pneumocystis carinii* pneumonia: A comparison of process and outcome at two hospitals. *Chest.* 1997; 112:398-405.
200. Masur H, Shelhamer J. Empiric outpatient management of HIV-related pneumonia: Economical or unwise? *Ann Intern Med.* 1996;124:451-453.
201. Glassroth J. Empiric diagnosis of *Pneumocystis carinii* pneumonia. Questions of accuracy and equity. *Am J Respir Crit Care Med.* 1995;152:1433-1434.
202. Parada JP, Deloria-Knoll M, Chmiel JS, et al. Relationship between health insurance and medical care for patients hospitalized with human immunodeficiency virus–related *Pneumocystis carinii* pneumonia, 1995-1997: Medicaid, bronchoscopy, and survival. *Clin Infect Dis.* 2003;37:1549-1555.
203. Gracia JD, Miravitlles M, Mayordomo C, et al. Empiric treatments impair the diagnostic yield of BAL in HIV-positive patients. *Chest.* 1997;111:1180-1186.
204. Walzer PD, Evans HE, Copas AJ, et al. Early predictors of mortality from *Pneumocystis jirovecii* pneumonia in HIV-infected patients: 1985-2006. *Clin Infect Dis.* 2008;46:625-633.
205. Benfield TL, Helweg-Larsen J, Bang D, et al. Prognostic markers of short-term mortality in AIDS-associated *Pneumocystis carinii* pneumonia. *Chest.* 2001;119:844-851.
206. Miller RF, Allen E, Copas A, et al. Improved survival for HIV infected patients with severe *Pneumocystis jirovecii* pneumonia is independent of highly active antiretroviral therapy. *Thorax.* 2006;61:716-721.
207. Dickson SJ, Batson S, Copas AJ, et al. Survival of HIV-infected patients in the intensive care unit in the era of highly active antiretroviral therapy. *Thorax.* 2007;62:964-968.
208. Haverkos HW, Drotman DP. The epidemiology of the acquired immunodeficiency syndrome. *Diagn Immunol.* 1984;2:67-72.
209. Mansharamani NG, Garland R, Delaney D, et al. Management and outcome patterns for adult *Pneumocystis carinii* pneumonia, 1985 to 1995: Comparison of HIV-associated cases to other immunocompromised states. *Chest.* 2000;118:704-711.
210. Keely SP, Stringer JR, Baughman RP, et al. Genetic variation among *Pneumocystis carinii* hominis isolates in recurrent pneumocystosis. *J Infect Dis.* 1995;172:595-598.
211. Dohn MN, Baughman RP, Vigdorth EM, et al. Equal survival rates for first, second, and third episodes of *Pneumocystis carinii* pneumonia in patients with acquired immunodeficiency syndrome. *Arch Intern Med.* 1992;152:2465-2470.
212. Metersky ML, Colt HG, Olson LK, et al. AIDS-related spontaneous pneumothorax. Risk factors and treatment. *Chest.* 1995;108:946-951.
213. Larsen HH, Masur H, Kovacs JA. Current regimens for treatment and prophylaxis of *Pneumocystis jirovecii* pneumonia. In: Walzer PD, Cushion MT, eds. Pneumocystis pneumonia. New York: Marcel Dekker; 2005:505-538.
214. Hughes WT, Feldman S, Chaudhary SC, et al. Comparison of pentamidine isethionate and trimethoprim-sulfamethoxazole in the treatment of *Pneumocystis carinii* pneumonia. *J Pediatr.* 1978;92:285-291.
215. Wharton JM, Coleman DL, Wofsy CB, et al. Trimethoprim-sulfamethoxazole or pentamidine for *Pneumocystis carinii* pneumonia in the acquired immunodeficiency syndrome. A prospective randomized trial. *Ann Intern Med.* 1986;105:37-44.
216. Sattler FR, Cowan R, Nielsen DM, et al. Trimethoprim-sulfamethoxazole compared with pentamidine for treatment of *Pneumocystis carinii* pneumonia in the acquired immunodeficiency syndrome. A prospective, noncrossover study. *Ann Intern Med.* 1988;109:280-287.
217. Klein NC, Duncanson FP, Lenox TH, et al. Trimethoprim-sulfamethoxazole versus pentamidine for *Pneumocystis carinii* pneumonia in AIDS patients: Results of a large prospective randomized treatment trial. *AIDS.* 1992;6:301-305.
218. Stein DS, Stevens RC. Treatment-associated toxicities: Incidence and mechanisms. In: Sattler FR, Walzer PD, eds. *Pneumocystis carinii.* London: Bailliere Tindall; 1995:505-530.
219. Carr A, Swanson C, Penny R, et al. Clinical and laboratory markers of hypersensitivity to trimethoprim-sulfamethoxazole in patients with *Pneumocystis carinii* pneumonia and AIDS. *J Infect Dis.* 1993;167:180-185.
220. Veenstra J, Veugelers PJ, Keet IP, et al. Rapid disease progression in human immunodeficiency virus type 1-infected individuals with adverse reactions to trimethoprim-sulfamethoxazole prophylaxis. *Clin Infect Dis.* 1997;24:936-941.

221. Velazquez H, Perazella MA, Wright FS, et al. Renal mechanism of trimethoprim-induced hyperkalemia. *Ann Intern Med.* 1993; 119:296-301.
222. Joos B, Blaser J, Opravil M, et al. Monitoring of co-trimoxazole concentrations in serum during treatment of *Pneumocystis carinii* pneumonia. *Antimicrob Agents Chemother.* 1995;39: 2661-2666.
223. Caumes E, Roudier C, Rogeaux O, et al. Effect of corticosteroids on the incidence of adverse cutaneous reactions to trimethoprim-sulfamethoxazole during treatment of AIDS-associated *Pneumocystis carinii* pneumonia. *Clin Infect Dis.* 1994; 18:319-323.
224. Leoung GS, Stanford JF, Giordano MF, et al. Trimethoprim-sulfamethoxazole (TMP-SMZ) dose escalation versus direct rechallenge for *Pneumocystis carinii* pneumonia prophylaxis in human immunodeficiency virus–infected patients with previous adverse reaction to TMP-SMZ. *J Infect Dis.* 2001;184:992-997.
225. Safrin S, Finkelstein DM, Feinberg J, et al. Comparison of three regimens for treatment of mild to moderate *Pneumocystis carinii* pneumonia in patients with AIDS. A double-blind, randomized, trial of oral trimethoprim-sulfamethoxazole, dapsone-trimethoprim, and clindamycin-primaquine. ACTG 108 Study Group. *Ann Intern Med.* 1996;124:792-802.
226. Lee BL, Medina I, Benowitz NL, et al. Dapsone, trimethoprim, and sulfamethoxazole plasma levels during treatment of *Pneumocystis* pneumonia in patients with the acquired immunodeficiency syndrome (AIDS). Evidence of drug interactions. *Ann Intern Med.* 1989;110:606-611.
227. Toma E, Fournier S, Dumont M, et al. Clindamycin/primaquine versus trimethoprim-sulfamethoxazole as primary therapy for *Pneumocystis carinii* pneumonia in AIDS:a randomized, double-blind pilot trial. *Clin Infect Dis.* 1993;17:178-184.
228. Hughes W, Leoung G, Kramer F, et al. Comparison of atovaquone (566C80) with trimethoprim-sulfamethoxazole to treat *Pneumocystis carinii* pneumonia in patients with AIDS. *N Engl J Med.* 1993;328:1521-1527.
229. Dohn MN, Weinberg WG, Torres RA, et al. Oral atovaquone compared with intravenous pentamidine for *Pneumocystis carinii* pneumonia in patients with AIDS. Atovaquone Study Group. *Ann Intern Med.* 1994;121:174-180.
230. Rosenberg DM, McCarthy W, Slavinsky J, et al. Atovaquone suspension for treatment of *Pneumocystis carinii* pneumonia in HIV-infected patients. *AIDS.* 2001;15:211-214.
231. Benfield T, Atzori C, Miller RF, et al. Second-line salvage treatment of AIDS-associated *Pneumocystis jirovecii* pneumonia: a case series and systematic review. *J Acquir Immune Defic Syndr.* 2008;48:63-67.
232. Smego RA Jr, Nagar S, Maloba B, et al. A meta-analysis of salvage therapy for *Pneumocystis carinii* pneumonia. *Arch Intern Med.* 2001;161:1529-1533.
233. Black JR, Feinberg J, Murphy RL, et al. Clindamycin and primaquine therapy for mild-to-moderate episodes of *Pneumocystis carinii* pneumonia in patients with AIDS: AIDS Clinical Trials Group 044. *Clin Infect Dis.* 1994;18:905-913.
234. Noskin GA, Murphy RL, Black JR, et al. Salvage therapy with clindamycin/primaquine for *Pneumocystis carinii* pneumonia. *Clin Infect Dis.* 1992;14:183-188.
235. Sattler FR, Jelliffe RW. Pharmacokinetic and pharmacodynamic considerations for drug dosing in the treatment of *Pneumocystis carinii* pneumonia. In: Walzer PD, ed. *Pneumocystis carinii* Pneumonia. New York: Marcel Dekker; 1994:467-486.
236. Comtois R, Pouliot J, Vinet B, et al. Higher pentamidine levels in AIDS patients with hypoglycemia and azotemia during treatment of *Pneumocystis carinii* pneumonia. *Am Rev Respir Dis.* 1992;146:740-744.
237. Lidman C, Bronner U, Gustafsson LL, et al. Plasma pentamidine concentrations vary between individuals with *Pneumocystis carinii* pneumonia and the drug is actively secreted by the kidney. *J Antimicrob Chemother.* 1994;33:803-810.
238. Kleyman TR, Roberts C, Ling BN. A mechanism for pentamidine-induced hyperkalemia: Inhibition of distal nephron sodium transport. *Ann Intern Med.* 1995;122:103-106.
239. Sattler FR, Frame P, Davis R, et al. Trimetrexate with leucovorin versus trimethoprim-sulfamethoxazole for moderate to severe episodes of *Pneumocystis carinii* pneumonia in patients with AIDS: A prospective, controlled multicenter investigation of the AIDS Clinical Trials Group Protocol 029/031. *J Infect Dis.* 1994;170:165-172.
240. Walmsley S, Levinton C, Brunton J, et al. A multicenter randomized double-blind placebo-controlled trial of adjunctive corticosteroids in the treatment of *Pneumocystis carinii* pneumonia complicating the acquired immune deficiency syndrome. *J Acquir Immune Defic Syndr Hum Retrovirol.* 1995;8:348-357.

241. Briel M, Bucher HC, Boscacci R, Furrer H. Adjunctive corticosteroids for *Pneumocystis jiroveci* pneumonia in patients with HIV-infection. Cochrane Database Syst Rev 2006;(3):CD006150.
242. Bozzette SA, Morton SC. Reconsidering the use of adjunctive corticosteroids in *Pneumocystis* pneumonia? *J Acquir Immune Defic Syndr Hum Retrovirol.* 1995;8:345-347.
243. Kazanjian P, Armstrong W, Hossler PA, et al. *Pneumocystis carinii* mutations are associated with duration of sulfa or sulfone prophylaxis exposure in AIDS patients. *J Infect Dis.* 2000; 182:551-557.
244. Stein CR, Poole C, Kazanjian P, et al. Sulfa use, dihydropteroate synthase mutations, and *Pneumocystis jirovecii* pneumonia. *Emerg Infect Dis.* 2004;10:1760-1765.
245. Crothers K, Beard CB, Turner J, et al. Severity and outcome of HIV-associated *Pneumocystis* pneumonia containing *Pneumocystis jirovecii* dihydropteroate synthase gene mutations. *AIDS.* 2005;19:801-805.
246. Valerio A, Tronconi E, Mazza F, et al. Genotyping of *Pneumocystis jiroveci* pneumonia in Italian AIDS patients. Clinical outcome is influenced by dihydropteroate synthase and not by internal transcribed spacer genotype. *J Acquir Immune Defic Syndr.* 2007;45:521-528.
247. Alvarez-Martinez MJ, Moreno A, Miró JM, et al. *Pneumocystis jirovecii* pneumonia in Spanish HIV-infected patients in the combined antiretroviral therapy era: Prevalence of dihydropteroate synthase mutations and prognostic factors of mortality. *Diagn Microbiol Infect Dis.* 2008 ;62:34-43.
248. Kazanjian P, Armstrong W, Hossler PA, et al. *Pneumocystis carinii* cytochrome b mutations are associated with atovaquone exposure in patients with AIDS. *J Infect Dis.* 2001;183: 819-822.
249. Utili R, Durante-Mangoni E, Basilico C, et al. Efficacy of caspofungin addition to trimethoprim-sulfamethoxazole treatment for severe pneumocystis pneumonia in solid organ transplant recipients. *Transplantation.* 2007;84:685-688.
250. Kamboj M, Weinstock D, Sepkowitz KA. Progression of *Pneumocystis jiroveci* pneumonia in patients receiving echinocandin therapy. *Clin Infect Dis.* 2006;43:e92-e94.
251. Waters L, Nelson M. The use of caspofungin in HIV-infected individuals. *Expert Opin Invest Drugs.* 2007;16:899-908.
252. Hof H, Schnulle P. *Pneumocystis jiroveci* pneumonia in a patient with Wegener's granulomatosis treated efficiently with caspofungin. *Mycoses.* 2008;51(Suppl 1):65-67.
253. Hughes WT, Sillos EM, LaFon S, et al. Effects of aerosolized synthetic surfactant, atovaquone, and the combination of these on murine *Pneumocystis carinii* pneumonia. *J Infect Dis.* 1998;177:1046-1056.
254. Creery WD, Hashmi A, Hutchison JS, et al. Surfactant therapy improves pulmonary function in infants with *Pneumocystis carinii* pneumonia and acquired immunodeficiency syndrome. *Pediatr Pulmonol.* 1997;24:370-373.
255. Centers for Disease Control and Prevention (CDC). Guidelines for the prevention and treatment of opportunistic infections in HIV-infected adults and adolescents. *MMWR Morb Mortal Wkly Rep.* 2009;58(RR04):1-198.
256. Freedberg KA, Scharfstein JA, Seage GR 3rd, et al. The cost-effectiveness of preventing AIDS-related opportunistic infections. *JAMA.* 1998;279:130-136.
257. Saah AJ, Hoover DR, Peng Y, et al. Predictors for failure of *Pneumocystis carinii* pneumonia prophylaxis. Multicenter AIDS Cohort Study. *JAMA.* 1995;273:1197-11202.
258. Bozzette SA, Finkelstein DM, Spector SA, et al. A randomized trial of three antipneumocystis agents in patients with advanced human immunodeficiency virus infection. NIAID AIDS Clinical Trials Group. *N Engl J Med.* 1995;332:693-699.
259. Sepkowitz KA. Effect of prophylaxis on the clinical manifestations of AIDS-related opportunistic infections. *Clin Infect Dis.* 1998;26:806-810.
260. Green H, Paul M, Vidal L, et al. Prophylaxis of *Pneumocystis* pneumonia in immunocompromised non-HIV-infected patients: Systematic review and meta-analysis of randomized controlled trials. *Mayo Clin Proc.* 2007;82:1052-1059.
261. Green H, Paul M, Vidal L, Leibovici L. Prophylaxis for Pneumocystis pneumonia (PCP) in non-HIV immunocompromised patients. Cochrane Database Syst Rev 2007;(3):CD005590.
262. Siegel JD, Rhinehart E, Jackson M, et al; Health Care Infection Control Practices Advisory Committee. Guideline for isolation precautions: Preventing transmission of infectious agents in healthcare settings. *Am J Infect Control.* 2007;35(Suppl 2): S65-S164.
263. Kuramochi T, Hioki K, Ito M. *Pneumocystis carinii* cysts are susceptible to inactivation by chemical disinfectants. *Exp Anim.* 1997;46:241-245.

271

Microsporidiosis

LOUIS M. WEISS

The Microsporidia are a group of obligate eukaryotic intracellular parasites that were recognized about 150 years ago with the description of *Nosema bombycis*, a parasite of silkworms that causes the disease pébrine in these economically important insects. The class or order Microsporidia was elevated to the phylum Microspora by Sprague in 1977.[1] In 1998, Sprague and Becnel suggested that the term *Microsporidia* instead be used for the phylum name.[2] Microsporidia is a proper name and should be capitalized.

Microsporidia have historically been considered "primitive" protozoa, although molecular phylogenetic analysis has led to the recognition that these organisms are not primitive but degenerate, and that they are related to the fungi and not to other protozoa. Such molecular phylogeny has also led to the recognition that the traditional phylogeny of these organisms based on structural observations may not reflect the true relationships among the various microsporidian species and genera.

The Microsporidia infect almost all animal phyla, including other protists. They are important agricultural parasites in insects, fish, laboratory rodents, rabbits, fur-bearing animals, and primates, and they have been described in dogs and birds kept as household pets.[3,4] Some species of Microsporidia have been used as pesticides for the biologic control of destructive species of grasshoppers and locusts.[5] In their hosts, most Microsporidia infect the digestive tract, but infections of the reproductive, respiratory, muscle, excretory, and nervous systems have been documented.[6] Microsporidia were recognized in mammalian tissue samples more than 75 years ago[7] and were first suspected as being a cause of human disease in 1959,[8] when they were found in a child with encephalitis. These organisms are most likely zoonotic or water-borne infections, or both. In the immunosuppressed host (e.g., those treated with immunosuppressive drugs or infected with human immunodeficiency virus [HIV], particularly at advanced stages of the disease), Microsporidia can produce a wide range of clinical diseases. Reports of diarrheal syndromes associated with microsporidiosis and HIV infection were first reported in 1985,[9] and the number of articles describing human disease increased rapidly after 1990. In addition to gastrointestinal tract involvement, it has been recognized that Microsporidia can infect almost any organ system and patients with encephalitis, ocular infection, sinusitis, myositis, and disseminated infection are well described in the literature. These organisms have also been reported in immunocompetent individuals.

The phylum Microsporidia (Microspora) contains more than 1000 species distributed into over 150 genera, of which the following have been demonstrated in human disease (Table 271-1)[3,10]: *Nosema* (*N. corneum* renamed *Vittaforma corneae*[11]; *N. algerae* reclassified initially as *Brachiola algerae*[12] and now as *Anncaliia algerae*[13]), *Pleistophora*, *Encephalitozoon*, *Enterocytozoon*,[9] *Septata*[14] (reclassified as *Encephalitozoon*[15]), *Trachipleistophora*,[16,17] *Brachiola*,[12] *Anncaliia*[13] and *Microsporidium*.[3] *Encephalitozoon hellem* (*E. hellem*) has been associated with superficial keratoconjunctivitis, sinusitis, respiratory disease, prostatic abscesses, and disseminated infection.[3,6,18] *Encephalitozoon cuniculi* (*E. cuniculi*) has been associated with hepatitis, encephalitis, and disseminated disease.[19-21] *Encephalitozoon* (*Septata*) *intestinalis* is associated with diarrhea, disseminated infection, and superficial keratoconjunctivitis.[14,22,23] *Nosema*, *Vittaforma*, and *Microsporidium* have been associated with stromal keratitis associated with trauma in immunocompetent hosts.[18,24] *Pleistophora*, *Anncaliia*, and *Trachipleistophora* have been associated with myositis.[16,25-27] *Trachipleistophora* has been associated with encephalitis, keratitis and disseminated disease.[17,28] *Enterocyto-*

zoon bieneusi (*E. bieneusi*), originally described in humans,[9] is associated with malabsorption, diarrhea, and cholangitis.[29,30]

General Characteristics

The Microsporidia are eukaryotes containing a nucleus with a nuclear envelope, an intracytoplasmic membrane system, chromosome separation on mitotic spindles, and vesicular Golgi.[31] In addition, a mitochondrial remnant organelle was reported in the microsporidian *Trachipleistophora hominis*.[32] Microsporidia are ubiquitous in the environment and infect almost all animal phyla (invertebrate and vertebrate hosts).[3,6,10] Microsporidia form characteristic unicellular spores (Fig. 271-1) that are environmentally resistant. The spore size and shape vary depending on the species. Whereas microsporidian spores can be as large as 12 μm, the microsporidia infecting humans have spores that range from 1.0 to 3.0 μm × 1.5 to 4.0 μm in size and are usually ovoid. The structure of the spore is characteristic of the phylum.[33] The spore coat consists of an electron-dense, proteinaceous exospore, an electronlucent endospore composed of chitin and protein, and an inner membrane or plasmalemma.[34] Proteins making up the spore coat have adhesion domains that may facilitate the binding of microsporidian spores to either the cell surface or mucus of the gastrointestinal tract prior to germination.[35] A defining characteristic of all microsporidia is an extrusion apparatus that consists of a polar tube attached to the inside of the anterior end of the spore by an anchoring disk and, depending on the species, forms 4 to approximately 30 coils around the sporoplasm in the spore. Proteomic and genetic studies have defined some of the proteins of the polar tube and spore wall[36] as well as the presence of *O*-mannosylation on these proteins.[37,38] During germination, the polar tube rapidly everts, forming a hollow tube that brings the sporoplasm into intimate contact with the host cell (Fig. 271-2). The polar tube provides a bridge to deliver the sporoplasm to the host cell. The mechanism whereby the polar tube interacts with the host cell membrane is not known, but it may require the participation of host cell proteins such as actin.[39] It is possible that the sporoplasm interacts with the host cell membrane as it emerges from the polar tube. If a spore is phagocytosed by a host cell, germination occurs, and the polar tube can pierce the phagocytic vacuole, delivering the sporoplasm into the host cell cytoplasm. The overall process of germination and formation of the polar tube delivers the sporoplasm to the host cell, functioning essentially like a hypodermic needle.[40,41]

Conditions that promote germination vary widely among species, presumably reflecting the organisms' adaptation to their host and external environment[42,43] (reviewed by Keohane and Weiss[44]). Conditions that promote spore discharge include pH shifts, dehydration followed by rehydration, various cations and anions, mucin or polyanions, hydrogen peroxide, ultraviolet irradiation, and the calcium ionophore A23187. Inhibitors of spore discharge include magnesium chloride, ammonium chloride, low salt concentrations, sodium fluoride, ultraviolet light, temperatures higher than 40°C, calcium channel antagonists, calmodulin inhibitors, cytochalasin D, demecolcine, and itraconazole. Regardless of the stimuli required for activation, most Microsporidia appear to exhibit the same response to the stimuli, an increase in intrasporal osmotic pressure. This results in an influx of water into the spore accompanied by swelling of the polaroplasts and posterior vacuole prior to spore discharge. In *A.* (*N.*) *algerae*, it has been proposed that activation brings trehalose in contact with the

TABLE 271-1	Microsporidia Identified as Pathogenic to Humans	
Genus and Species	*Reported Infections*	*Animal Hosts*‡
Encephalitozoon		
E. cuniculi*	Hepatitis, peritonitis, encephalitis,† urethritis, prostatitis, nephritis, sinusitis, keratoconjunctivitis, cystitis, diarrhea,† cellulitis, disseminated infection	Mammals (rabbits, rodents, carnivores, primates)
E. hellem*	Keratoconjunctivitis, sinusitis, pneumonitis, nephritis, prostatitis, urethritis, cystitis, diarrhea, disseminated infection	Psittacine birds (parrots, lovebirds, parakeets), birds (ostrich, hummingbirds, finches)
E. intestinalis*	Diarrhea,† intestinal perforation, cholangitis, nephritis, keratoconjunctivitis	Mammals (donkeys, dogs, pigs, cows, goats, primates)
Enterocytozoon bieneusi	Diarrhea,† wasting syndrome, cholangitis, rhinitis, bronchitis	Mammals (pigs, primates, cows, dogs, cats), birds (chickens)
Trachipleistophora		
T. hominis*	Myositis, keratoconjunctivitis, sinusitis	None
T. anthropopthera	Encephalitis, disseminated infection, keratitis	None
Pleistophora		
P. ronneafiei	Myositis	None
Pleistophora sp.	Myositis†	Fish
Annicaliia		
A. vesicularum	Myositis	None
A. algerae*	Keratoconjunctivitis, myositis, skin infection	Mosquitoes
A. connori	Disseminated infection	None
Nosema		
N. ocularum	Keratoconjunctivitis†	None
Vittaforma corneae*	Keratoconjunctivitis,† urinary tract infection	None
Microsporidium		
M. africanus	Corneal ulcer†	None
M. ceylonesis	Corneal ulcer†	None

*Organism can be grown in tissue culture.
†Cases reported in immunocompetent hosts.
‡Animals in which organism has been found other than humans.
§Previously called *Brachiola* and *Nosema*.[12,13]

enzyme trehalase, causing an increase in osmotic pressure.[45,46] The polar tube discharges from the anterior pole of the spore in an explosive reaction, occurring within less than 2 seconds, and it is thought to form a hollow tube by a process of eversion, similar to everting the finger of a glove.[40]

Microsporidia display a number of characteristics that are unusual for eukaryotic organisms. They have prokaryotic-size ribosomes[47] that do not have a 5.8S ribosome subunit but do have sequences homologous to the 5.8S region in the 23S subunit.[48] The small subunit rRNA of several Microsporidia have been sequenced and found to be significantly shorter than both eukaryotic and prokaryotic small-subunit rRNA.[49,50] These rRNA genes are in a subtelomeric location on each chromosome of *E. cuniculi*[51,52] and lack the paromomycin binding site seen in protozoa and animals.[53] The karyotype of several members of the phylum Microspora has been determined by pulsed-field electrophoresis. The genome size of the microsporidia varies from 2.3 to 19.5 Mb.[54] The genomic size of the Encephalitizoonidae is less than 3.0 Mb, making them among the smallest eukaryotic nuclear genomes so far identified. There are almost no introns in the compact genome of *E. cuniculi*, the gene density is high, and proteins are shorter than the corresponding genes in *Saccharomyces cerevisiae*. There appears to be a high degree of gene conservation among the Microsporidia.[55]

Genome data on the Microsporidia are available at the BioHealthBase Bioinformatics Resource Center (http://www.biohealthbase.org). Chromosomal analysis of *E. cuniculi* suggests that it is diploid.[56] The karyotypes of a few members of the phylum Microspora have been determined by pulsed-field electrophoresis. Small subunit rRNA (16S rRNA) diverges greatly from the small subunit rRNA sequences of other eukaryotes, and microsporidian rRNA genes are significantly shorter than those of eukaryotes and prokaryotes.[57] Sequence data of rRNA from the microsporidia have been used to develop diagnostic polymerase chain reaction (PCR) primers and to study phylogenetic relationships[58,59] (reviewed by Weiss and Vossbrinck[50]).

Use of cloned rRNA genes for the development of a microsporidian molecular phylogeny provides additional evidence for the assignment of a microsporidian to specific genera and gives us the ability to distinguish morphologically similar Microsporidia at the species level. Analysis of the rRNA genes of a variety of Microsporidia highlights the polyphyletic nature of the Microsporidia and brings into doubt the use of any single character for developing higher taxonomic groupings. For example, *E. hellem* and *E. cuniculi* are indistinguishable at the ultrastructural level, and *E. intestinalis* has a distinct extracellular matrix surrounding the sporoblasts and spores. Based on rDNA analysis, *E. intestinalis* and *E. cuniculi* are more similar to each other than to *E. hellem*.[60]

Molecular relationships are also useful for identifying environmental reservoirs for microsporidia that infect humans. *E. cuniculi* isolates

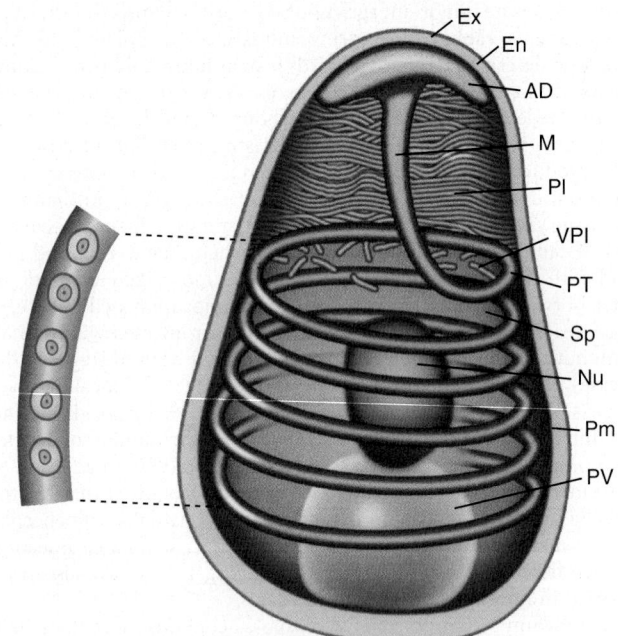

Figure 271-1 Structure of a microsporidian spore. Depending on the species, the size of the spore can vary from 1 to 10 μm and the number of polar tubule coils can vary from a few to 30 or more. Extrusion apparatus consists of the polar tube (PT), vesiculotubular polaroplast (VPl), lamellar polaroplast (Pl), anchoring disk (AD) and manubrium (M). This organelle is characteristic of the Microsporidia. The insert demonstrates a cross section of the polar tube coils (five coils in this spore), demonstrating the various concentric layers of different electron density and electon-dense core present in such cross sections. The nucleus (Nu) may be single (such as in *Encephalitozoon* spp.) or a pair of abutted nuclei known as a diplokaryon (such as in *Nosema* spp.). The endospore (En) is an inner, thicker, electron-lucent region. The exospore (Ex) is an outer electron-dense region. The plasma membrane (Pm) separates the spore coat from the sporoplasm (Sp), which contains ribosomes in a coiled helical array. The posterior vacuole (PV) is a membrane-bound structure. (*Adapted with permission from Wittner M, Weiss LM, eds. The Microsporidia and Microsporidiosis. Washington, DC: ASM Press; 1999:199.*)

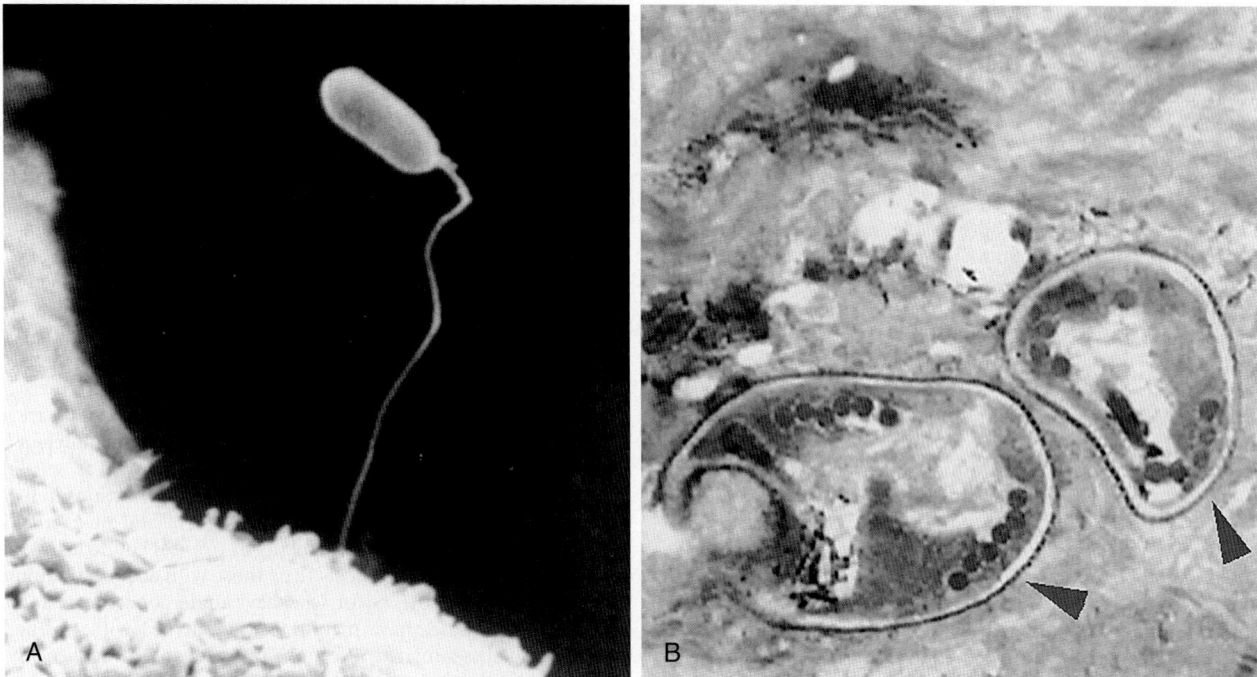

Figure 271-2 **Microsporidian polar tube. A,** Scanning electron micrograph of a tissue culture demonstrating *Encephalitozoon intestinalis* invading a Vero cell in vitro. **B,** Transmission electron micrograph of conjunctival scraping demonstrating Microsporidia (*Encephalitozoon hellem*). Arrowheads identify thick-walled spores with single nuclei and five or six coils of polar tubes. (**A** *from Kock NP. Diagnosis of Human Pathogenic Microsporidia. Dissertation, Berhard Nocht Institute for Tropical Medicine, Hamburg, Germany. With permission of N.P. Kock, C. Schmetz, and J. Schottelius.*)

from various animal species have been identified and separated based on the number of tetranucleotide repeats (5′-GTTT3′) in the intergenic spacer region of their rRNA genes.[61] Differences have also been found in the intergenic spacer region of rRNA genes of *E. bieneusi* and have been used to identify isolates associated with particular animals or environments.[62] Currently, all the different isolates that have been identified within an animal species are considered to be the same microsporidian species; however, it is possible that there may be more than one species of *Enterocytozoon* in its mammalian and avian hosts.

Phylogeny of the Microsporidia

Microsporidia are currently classified based on their ultrastructural features, including the size and morphology of the spores, number of coils of the polar tube, developmental life cycle, and host-parasite relationship (see Fig. 271-2). Tuzet and colleagues,[63] Sprague,[1] Larsson,[64] Issi,[65] Weiser,[66] and Sprague and associates[10] have provided overviews of the history, ultrastructural and structural characteristics, and life cycle differences among taxa of Microsporidia. Microsporidia can be divided into three main groups:

1. The "primitive" (Metchnikovellidae) hyperparasites of gregarines in annelids may be distinguished from the other Microsporidia by the presence of a rudimentary polar filament and a spore without a polaroplast.
2. The Chytridopsidae, Hesseidsae, and Burkeidae may be seen as "intermediates," having a short polar filament and minimal development of the polaroplast and endospore.
3. The "higher" Microsporidia have a well-developed polar filament, polaroplast, and posterior vacuole.

Differences among modern classifications of Microsporidia focus on the characteristics used to divide the third group, the higher Microsporidia, into subgroups. Molecular analysis of rRNA genes has begun to alter this classification system.[50,67] Antigenic differences between Microsporidia demonstrable by sodium dodecylsulfate polyacyramide

gel electrophoresis and immunoblot analysis have been used as adjunctive evidence when determining phylogenetic relationships among the Microsporidia infecting humans.[15,68]

The general features of the life cycle are as follows:

1. Spores are ingested or inhaled and then germinate, resulting in extension of the polar tube, which injects the sporoplasm into the host cell.
2. Merogony follows, during which the injected sporoplasm develops into meronts (the proliferative stage), which multiply, depending on the species, by binary fission or multiple fission, forming multinucleate plasmodial forms.
3. The next step is sporogony, during which meront cell membranes thicken to form sporonts.

After subsequent division, the sporonts give rise to sporoblasts, which go on to form mature spores without additional multiplication. Once a host cell becomes distended with mature spores, the cell ruptures, releasing mature spores into the environment and thereby completing the life cycle. The combination of multiplication during merogony and sporogony results in a large number of spores being produced from a single infection and illustrates the enormous reproductive potential of these organisms.

Molecular phylogenetic data indicate that the Microsporidia are related to fungi and are not primitive eukaryotes.[69-71] As early as 1994, based on β-tubulin sequence analysis, it was suggested that the Microsporidia were not ancient eukaryotes but were related to the fungi.[72] Keeling and Doolittle reported similar results for α-tubulin from three species of Microsporidia (*E. hellem, Nosema locustae, Spraguea lophii*) and for β-tubulin from *Encephalitozoon hellem*.[73] Analysis of the heat shock protein gene (*hsp70*) for *Nosema locustae, Vairimorpha necatrix, E. cuniculi, Nosema locustae,* and *E. hellem* provided confirmatory evidence of this relationship.[74-77] Comparative analysis of the largest subunit of the RNA polymerase II (*RPB1*) gene produced a phylogeny similar to the result obtained from an analysis of *hsp70* or the β-tubulin gene. Additional evidence for the relationship of Microsporidia to the fungi includes the following:

1. The *E. cuniculi* genes for thymidylate synthase and dihydrofolate reductase are separate genes.[78]
2. The small subunit rRNA gene of microsporidia lacks a paromomycin binding site, similar to the fungi.[79]
3. The EF-1α sequence of the microsporidian *Glugea plecoglossi* has an insertion that is found only in fungi and animals, not in protozoa.[79,80]
4. Microsporidia display similarities to the fungi during mitosis (e.g., closed mitosis and spindle pole bodies[81]) and meiosis.[82]
5. Microsporidia have chitin in their spore wall and store trehalose, as do fungi.
6. Analyses of glutamyl-tRNA synthetase, seryl-tRNA synthetase, vacuolar ATPase, TATA box binding protein, transcription initiation factor IIB, subunit A of vacuolar ATPase, and guanosine triphosphate (GTP)-binding protein and transcription factor IIB sequences[83,84] support a relationship between the Microsporidia and fungi.
7. Analysis of the *E. cuniculi* genome demonstrates that many of the *E. cuniculi* proteins are most similar to fungal homologues.[84]
8. The presence in *E. cuniculi* of the principal enzymes for the synthesis and degradation of trehalose confirm that this disaccharide could be the major sugar reserve in Microsporidia, as is seen in many fungi.

Analysis of glycosylation pathways has suggested that O-mannosylation (e.g., O-linked glycosylation with mannose), as seen in fungi, also occurs in Microsporidia. Evidence suggests that such O-mannosylation does indeed occur on the major polar tube protein PTP1.[37] Keeling,[85] in an analysis of β-tubulin data that included additional species of Microsporidia and more fungal phyla, suggested that the Microsporidia were a sister group to the Zygomycota.

Epidemiology

Microsporidian spores are commonly found in surface water, and human pathogenic Microsporidia have been found in municipal water supplies, tertiary sewage effluent, and ground water.[86-89] It is likely that many of the Microsporidia are water-borne pathogens. Water contact has been found to be an independent risk factor for microsporidiosis in some studies[90,91] but not in others.[92,93] *E. cuniculi* spores remain viable for 6 days when in water and 4 weeks when dry at 22°C, and *Nosema bombycis* spores may remain viable for 10 years in distilled water.[94] Spores may be killed, however, by exposure for 30 minutes to 70% ethanol, 1% formaldehyde, or 2% Lysol or by autoclaving at 120°C for 10 minutes.[95] Most microsporidian infections are transmitted by oral ingestion of spores, with the site of initial infection being the gastrointestinal tract. Viable infective spores of Microsporidia are present in a number of body fluids (e.g., stool, urine, respiratory secretions) during infection, suggesting that person-to-person transmission can occur and that ocular infection may be transmitted by external autoinoculation caused by contaminated fingers.[96] It has been possible to transmit *E. cuniculi* via rectal infection in rabbits, suggesting the possibility of sexual transmission.[97] *E. hellem* has been demonstrated in the respiratory mucosa as well as in the prostate and urogenital tract of patients, raising the possibility of respiratory and sexual transmission in humans.[98,99] Person-to-person transmission is supported by concurrent infections in cohabiting homosexual men.[100] Although congenital transmission of *E. cuniculi* has been demonstrated in rabbits, mice, dogs, horses, alpaca, foxes, and squirrel monkeys, no such congenital transmission has been demonstrated in humans.[101]

Many of the Microsporidia probably cause zoonotic infections in humans (see Table 271-1).[102] Microsporidia of the genus *Encephalitozoon* are widely distributed parasites of mammals and birds, and the onset of microsporidiosis has been associated with exposure to livestock, fowl, and pets.[103] *E. hellem* infections have been described in lovebirds and budgerigars (parakeets),[4] and one case of *E. hellem* infection has been reported in a patient who had two pet lovebirds.[104] Up to 30% of dogs in animal shelters may excrete microsporidia in their stools. Microsporidia of the genus *Encephalitozoon* were found in the stools of many animals in an epidemiologic survey in Mexico.[90] *Enterocytozoon bieneusi* appears to be widely distributed and has been reported in many mammals including pigs,[105] dogs,[106] chickens,[107] pigeons,[108] falcons, and simian immunodeficiency virus (SIV)–infected rhesus monkeys.[109] There is a documented case of transmission of *E. bieneusi* between a child and guinea pigs.[110] Enterocytozoonidae such as *Nucleospora* (previously *Enterocytozoon*) *salmonis* are pathogens found in fish. *Nosema* and *Vittaforma* infections are believed to be caused by traumatic inoculation of environmental spores of insect pathogens into the cornea.[11,24,111]

Although initially regarded as rare, Microsporidia are now believed to be common enteric pathogens that cause self-limited or asymptomatic infections in normal hosts.[103,112] Cases of microsporidiosis have been identified from all continents except Antarctica.[100,113-119] Surveys of pathogens seen in stool samples in Africa, Asia, South America, and Central America have demonstrated that Microsporidia are often found during careful stool examinations. In immunocompetent hosts, most reported cases of microsporidiosis manifested as self-limited diarrhea. They have included cases of *E. bieneusi* infections in travelers to and residents of tropical countries[87,115,120-127] and of *E. intestinalis* infections in travelers to and residents of tropical countries.[128] In contrast, in immunodeficient hosts (e.g., those with acquired immunodeficiency syndrome [AIDS] or who have undergone transplantation), most reported cases have manifested as diarrhea with wasting syndrome and disseminated infection. Infections with *E. bieneusi* have been reported in patients who have undergone liver or heart-lung transplantation, and *Encephalitozoon* sp. infections have been reported in patients who have undergone kidney, pancreas, liver, or bone marrow transplantation.[129-136] A case of chronic bilateral keratoconjunctivitis caused by *Encephalitozoon* sp. has been reported in a patient taking prednisone (20 mg/day).[137]

Reported prevalence rates in the 25 studies conducted on patients with HIV infection before the widespread use of highly active antiretroviral therapy (HAART; 1989-1998) varied between 2% and 70%, depending on the symptoms of the population studied and the diagnostic techniques used.[6,100,103,113,119,138-143] These studies suggest that asymptomatic carriage can occur in immunocompromised patients. Coinfection with different Microsporidia or other enteric pathogens can occur. There was no overall trend in these prevalence studies with regard to country of origin or other demographic characteristics. When combined, these studies identified 375 *E. bieneusi* infections among 2400 patients with chronic diarrhea, for a prevalence of 15% in this population. It is clear that since the institution of HAART and its associated immune reconstitution, the prevalence of diarrhea among AIDS patients has decreased, as has the incidence of microsporidiosis. Based on these studies, Microsporidia appear to demonstrate strength of association, coherence, and reproducibility with respect to being causative for a diarrheal syndrome. Further evidence of the association of Microsporidia with diarrhea is provided by the usefulness of albendazole in the treatment of microsporidian infection. Therapy with albendazole results in cure of the diarrhea associated with elimination of *Encephalitozoon intestinalis* from the stool of infected patients.[144] Treatment with fumagillin has a similar effect in patients with *E. bieneusi* infection.[145,146]

Serosurveys in humans have demonstrated a high prevalence of antibodies to *E. cuniculi* and *E. hellem,* suggesting that asymptomatic infection may be common.[116,147] Serologic cross-reactivity among microsporidia has been demonstrated by both immunofluorescence[148] and immunoblot testing.[149] Singh and co-workers found positive titers in 6 of 69 healthy adults in England, 38 of 89 Nigerians with tuberculosis, 13 of 70 Malaysians with filariasis, and 33 of 92 Ghanaians with malaria.[150] In another study, 14 of 115 travelers returning from the tropics and 0 of 48 nontravelers were seropositive.[151] In a study of HIV-positive men, 10 of 30 were seropositive, and all had traveled to the tropics.[152] Antibodies to *E. intestinalis* were found in 5% of pregnant French women and 8% of Dutch blood donors.[153] In HIV-positive Czech patients, 5.3% were seropositive to *E. cuniculi* and 1.3% to *E. hellem.*[154] In Slovakia, 5.1% of slaughterhouse workers were seropositive to *Encephalitozoon* spp.[155] In a survey of blood donors in the United States, 5% of donors had antibodies to *E. hellem* PTP1 antigen (LM Weiss, unpublished observations). Overall, these studies suggest that exposure to Microsporidia is common and that asymptomatic infection may be more common than originally suspected.

Immunology

Infection with *E. cuniculi* in many mammals results in chronic infection with persistently high antibody titers and ongoing inflammation (e.g., persistent encephalitis in rabbits and chronic renal disease and congenital transmission in foxes). In immunocompetent murine models of *E. cuniculi* infection, ascites develops and then clears; however, if corticosteroids are administered, the mice redevelop ascites, consistent with latent persistence of Microsporidia in these animals.[156] In mice with severe combined immunodeficiency (SCID) or athymic mice, infection with *E. cuniculi* results in death, with visceral dissemination of the organism and persistent ascites.[157] Adoptive transfer of sensitized syngeneic T-enriched spleen cells protects athymic or SCID mice against lethal *E. cuniculi* infection.[158,159] Transfer of naive lymphocytes or hyperimmune serum failed to protect or prolong the survival of these mice. Cytokine-activated murine peritoneal macrophages can inhibit the replication of *E. cuniculi* in vitro.[160] This inhibition is probably mediated by nitric oxide; studies have demonstrated that inhibition of nitric oxide synthesis inhibits such killing.[161] Mice deficient in inducible nitric oxide synthase had no change in susceptibility to *E. cuniculi* infection[162]; therefore, nitric oxide is not the major mechanism for controlling this organism.

Humoral immunity is not sufficient for protection against *E. cuniculi* infection, because adoptive transfer of immune B lymphocytes into athymic BALB/c (nu/nu) or SCID mice or passive transfer of hyperimmune serum into athymic mice does not protect these animals from death after infection. Nonetheless, during *E. cuniculi* infection, there is a strong antibody response to many components of this organism, and many of these antibodies are cross-reactive with other microsporidia. Maternal antibodies protect newborn rabbits from infection with *E. cuniculi* during the first 2 weeks of life.[163] The in vitro infectivity of microsporidia is reduced by treatment with immune serum and complement,[158] monoclonal antibody (mAb 3B6) to the spore coat,[164] or polyclonal antibodies to polar tube protein-1 (PTP1) (LM Weiss, unpublished data). IgM antibodies against PTP1 in normal human serum may play a role in preventing infection with *E. cuniculi*.[165] Overall, it is probable that antibodies play a role in limiting infection in the host, although they are clearly not sufficient to prevent mortality or to cure infection.

Interferon gamma-γ (IFN-γ) and interleukin-12 (IL-12) are important for protective immunity against a number of intracellular viral, bacterial, and parasitic infections.[166] Based on in vitro observations, it has been suggested that IFN-γ plays an important role in the protective immunity against *E. cuniculi* infection. Both natural killer (NK) cells and γδ T cells, which are increased at early stages of infection, are likely important sources of IFN-γ production. Studies with *E. intestinalis* and *E. cuniculi* have demonstrated that IFN-γ knockout mice cannot clear infection.[167] Treatment of *E. cuniculi*–infected mice with neutralizing antibody to IFN-γ or IL-12 results in increased mortality.[162] The importance of IL-12 is illustrated by the fact that lethal infection with *E. cuniculi* also occurs in p40 knockout mice, which are unable to produce IL-12.[168] IFN-γ production by dendritic cells has been demonstrated to be important for priming the gut intraepithelial lymphocyte response following oral infection with *E. cuniculi*.[169]

The role of individual T-cell subtypes during *E. cuniculi* infection has been evaluated in murine models.[168] Phenotypic analysis of the spleen cells from infected animals has revealed an increase in the CD8+ T-cell population starting at day 10 after infection, with no significant increase in CD4+ T cells. Mice deficient in CD8+ cells succumb to the parasitic challenge. In contrast, there was no change in mortality for mice deficient in CD4+ cells. The protective effect of CD8+ T cells is mediated by their ability to produce cytokines and to reduce the para-

site load by killing the infected targets in the host tissue.[170] The major killing mechanism exhibited by CD8+ T cells is via the perforin pathway, and mice lacking the perforin gene die when infected with *E. cuniculi*. These observations suggest that the cytotoxic T-cell response is a key factor in the immune response to *E. cuniculi*–infected mice. In most cases, CD8+ T cells are primed via IL-2–producing CD4+ T cells, although a normal in vivo CD8+ T cell response in the absence of CD4+ T cells has been described with many viral infections and appears also to occur with *E. cuniculi* infection. A normal antigen-specific CD8+ T-cell response to *E. cuniculi* infection has been found to occur in CD4 knockout mice.

There are scant data to confirm the immune response to Microsporidia in humans. It is clear that a strong humoral response occurs during infection and that it includes antibodies that react with the spore wall and polar tube. The immunosuppressive states associated with microsporidiosis (e.g., AIDS and transplantation) are those that inhibit cell-mediated immunity. Microsporidiosis is usually seen in HIV-infected patients when there is a profound defect in cell-mediated immunity (e.g., a CD4+ cell count lower than 100/mm³); spontaneous cure of microsporidiosis can be induced by immune reconstitution with HAART.[171-173] Overall, these data are consistent with observations on the immunology of the mouse model of microsporidiosis and suggest that restoration of cell-mediated immunity and possibly administration of IFN-γ or IL-12 are useful adjuncts for treating microsporidiosis.

Pathology and Pathogenesis
GASTROINTESTINAL TRACT INFECTIONS

Infection of the epithelium of the gastrointestinal tract (small intestine and biliary epithelium) is the most frequent presentation of microsporidiosis (Fig. 271-3). More than 90% of these infections are caused by *E. bieneusi*, with the remainder mostly caused by *E. intestinalis*.[30,33,100,103] Because most of these infections are acquired by ingesting spores, it is likely that other species of microsporidia also cause asymptomatic gastrointestinal infections. Granulomatous hepatitis caused by *E. cuniculi* is commonly seen in mammals infected with this organism, and granulomatous hepatitis caused by *Encephalitozoon* has been reported in patients with HIV infection.[174] Hepatitis with infection of the biliary system (including the portal triad and gallbladder epithelium) caused by *E. bieneusi* has been seen in SIV-infected *Macaca mulatta* (rhesus macaques).[175] Chronic gallbladder infection with *E. bieneusi* is seen in pigs. *E. bieneusi* and *E. intestinalis* infections of the biliary tract can result in sclerosing cholangitis in AIDS patients.[176,177] These observations suggest that the biliary epithelium may be a reservoir for relapse of *E. bieneusi* and perhaps other Microsporidia.

E. bieneusi infection does not produce active enteritis or ulceration, although the infection results in variable degrees of villous blunting and crypt hyperplasia. There is a gradient in parasite burden along the small intestine, with the distal duodenum and proximal jejunum having higher burdens than the proximal duodenum.[176] The organism can be found in the ileum but is rarely found in the colon. On endoscopy, scalloping of the valvulae conniventes and villous fusion may be evident.[178] The organism is located on the apical surface of the enterocytes of the small intestine and epithelial cells of the biliary tract and pancreas. Spores are rarely found on the basal surface or in the lamina propria.[179,180] This organism rarely disseminates, unlike the Encephalitizoonidae, which are commonly found in the lamina propria and disseminate to visceral organs. Infection may be associated with increased intraepithelial lymphocytes and epithelial disarray. At the villous tips, teardrop-shaped cells can be seen during the process of sloughing, which is characteristic of infection with *E. bieneusi*. Spores are smaller (1.0 × 1.5 μm) than those of *Encephalitozoon* spp. (1.2 × 2.2 μm) and more difficult to find in tissue sections (see Fig. 271-3). Infection is associated with malabsorption because of decreased mucosal surface area and functional immaturity of the villous epithelial cells.

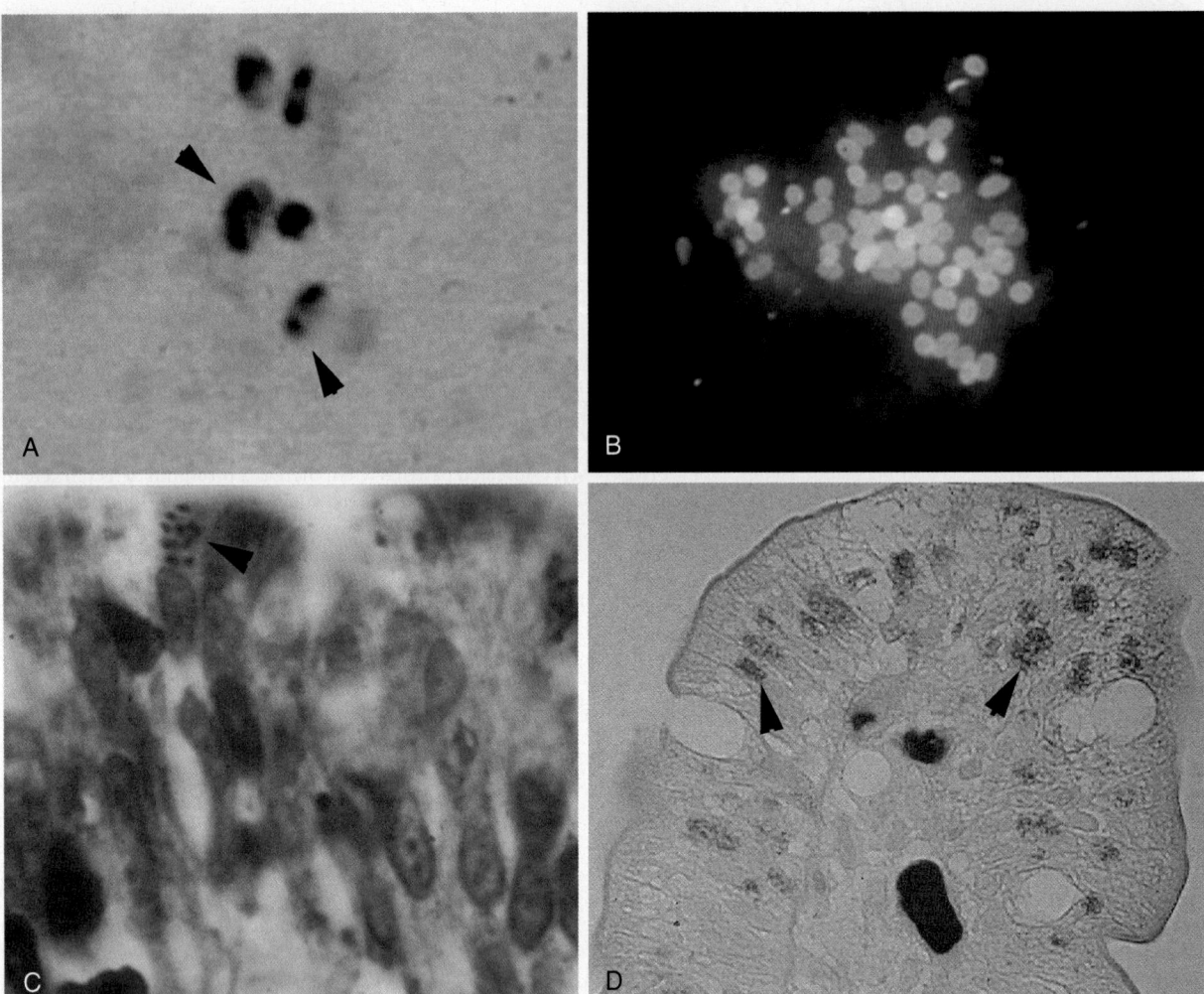

Figure 271-3 **Demonstration of microsporidia in stool, urine, and tissue samples. A,** Chromotrope 2R stain (modified trichrome stain) of a stool sample from a patient with microsporidian enteritis due to *Enterocytozoon bieneusi. Arrowheads* point to microsporidian spores. Using chromotrope 2R-based stains spores appear as 1- to 3-μm ovoid light pink structures with a belt-like stripe girding them diagonally and equatorially. **B,** Calcofluor white stain (a chemofluorescent optical brightening agent that stains chitin) demonstrating fluorescent *Encephalitozoon hellem* spores in the urine of a patient with disseminated infection. **C,** Giemsa stain of a small intestinal biopsy from a patient with electron microscopy proven *Enterocytozoon bieneusi* enteritis. The *arrowhead* points to a collection of microsporidian spores at the apical end of an enterocyte. Spores are not found on the basal side or in the lamina propria with this organism. **D,** Chromotrope 2R tissue stain of a small intestinal biopsy from a patient with electron microscopy-proven *Encephalitozoon intestinalis* infection. *Arrowheads* point to microsporidian spores. Note that spores are found in the apical and basal sides of the enterocytes as well as in the lamina propria. This is consistent with the ability of this microsporidian to disseminate. (**B** *courtesy of E. Didier, Tulane Regional Primate Research Center, Covington, LA;* **D** *courtesy of D. Kotler, St. Lukes-Roosevelt Hospital Center and J. M. Orenstein, George Washington University School of Medicine, Washington DC.*)

This parasite displays a unique intracellular developmental life cycle. A characteristic feature of the organism is the presence of electronlucent inclusions with a lamellar structure. These inclusions are closely associated with the nuclear envelope, the endoplasmic reticulum, or both. The earliest intraepithelial stages of the parasite are rounded proliferative cells limited by a typical unit membrane in direct contact with the host cell cytoplasm. Nuclear division is not immediately followed by cytokinesis in these cells, resulting in the production of multinucleate proliferative plasmodia. After the production of multiple nuclei, the parasites form electron-dense disklike structures that cluster in stacks of three to six, eventually forming the coiled portion of the polar tube. When these multinucleated sporagonial plasmodia divide by invagination of the plasmalemma, multiple spores are formed. In mature spores, the polar tubule has five to seven coils that appear in two rows when seen in cross section by transmission electron microscopy.

E. intestinalis is invasive, and spores are commonly found in the apical and basal sides of infected intestinal enterocytes as well as in cells in the lamina propria, including fibroblasts, endothelial cells, and macrophages[181] (see Fig. 271-3). This pattern of infection is also seen with other *Encephalitozoon* spp. and probably reflects the ability of these infections to disseminate to visceral organs following ingestion. Dissemination can result in necrosis of areas of the bowel, with a presentation resembling that of an acute abdomen.[19,182] Histopathology can demonstrate areas of necrosis and mucosal erosion. In pathology sections, the septated parasitophorous vacuole can be seen surrounding the developing spores. *E. intestinalis* spores are easier to detect than *E. bieneusi* spores because of their larger size, strong birefringence, and bluish color on hematoxylin and eosin staining. In addition, spores of *E. intestinalis* are more numerous in tissue. Sporogony is tetrasporous, and tubular appendages originate from the sporont surface and terminate in an enlarged bulblike structure. Unlike infections with other Encephalitizoonidae, *E. intestinalis*–infected cells have a unique parasite-secreted fibrillar network surrounding the developing organisms so the parasitophorous vacuole appears septate. Mature spores in cross section have a single row of four to seven coils of polar tubules.

Encephalitozoon cuniculi has been described in a case of peritonitis.[183] At autopsy, a mass of omentum was found that displayed focal necrosis, nongranulomatous inflammation, and microsporidian spores. *E. hellem* and *E. cuniculi* have similar developmental life cycles.[31] The genus is characterized by the presence of a phagosome-like parasitophorous vacuole. Nuclei of all stages are unpaired. Meronts divide repeatedly by binary fission. Sporonts divide into two sporoblasts that mature into spores. No tubular appendages or fibrillar networks are produced, as is seen with *E. intestinalis*. In cross section, the mature spore has five to seven coils in single rows.

GENITOURINARY TRACT INFECTION

Encephalitozoon spp. infect the genitourinary system in most mammals. Contamination of the environment by spores passed in urine is believed to be the mechanism of transmission of these organisms between successive hosts, which appears to be the case in human infections,[112,144,179,184] in whom infection discovered in any organ (e.g., eye, gastrointestinal tract, liver, central nervous system) is often associated with the shedding of spores in the urine. In HIV-infected patients with keratitis, there is usually asymptomatic infection of the urinary tract and bronchial tree. Granulomatous interstitial nephritis composed of plasma cells and lymphocytes is the most frequent pathologic finding. It is associated with tubular necrosis, with the lumen of the tubules containing amorphous granular material. Occasionally, microabscesses and granulomas form around necrotic tubules. Spores are located in the necrotic tubes and sloughing tubular epithelial cells. Organisms may also be found in the interstitium. Glomerular involvement is rarely seen. This pattern of interstitial nephritis has been seen in AIDS patients as well as in those with renal transplants complicated by microsporidiosis.[131,135,185,186] An identical pattern has been described in rabbits with *E. cuniculi* infection.

As spores and infected tubular cells are shed into the bladder, they can infect other epithelial cells of the urogenital tract. Microsporidia have been reported to cause necrotizing ureteritis and cystitis.[179] Inflammatory cystitis has been seen during cystoscopy. The organism can disseminate from the urogenital epithelial cells and can be found in macrophages, muscle, and supporting fibroblasts of the associated mucosa. Genital tract infection with *Encephalitozoon* has been reported to occur in association with urinary shedding of spores and has included prostatitis with abscess formation.[98] The frequency of microsporidian prostatitis is not known, nor is it known if sexual transmission occurs. A case of urinary tract infection and chronic prostatitis caused by *Vittaforma corneae* has also been reported in a patient with AIDS.[111]

CENTRAL NERVOUS SYSTEM INFECTION

Granulomatous encephalitis is the classic presentation of *Encephalitozoon cuniculi* infection in many mammals, such as rabbits. This infection has been recognized in a few patients with HIV infection, in whom it "mimicked" toxoplasmic encephalitis.[21] At autopsy, central nervous system (CNS) involvement was documented in a case of disseminated *E. cuniculi* (type III or dog strain) involving almost all organs.[187] Spores were present in the cerebral parenchyma, perivascular spaces, and macrophages but were not seen in oligodendrocytes, neurons, astrocytes, or meningeal cells. A second case of *E. cuniculi* encephalitis was caused by the type II or rabbit strain. There have also been two case reports of encephalitis caused by *Trachipleistophora anthropopthera*.[17,28] Both these patients had multiple ring-enhancing lesions on computed tomography (CT) scans suggestive of CNS toxoplasmosis. On pathologic examination, the 2.0×2.8 μm birefringent spores were located in the gray matter, and there was extensive necrosis. The disease also involved the heart, kidney, pancreas, thyroid, parathyroid, liver, bone marrow, lymph nodes, and spleen in addition to the brain. The most heavily infected cells were epithelial cells, cardiac myocytes, and astrocytes.

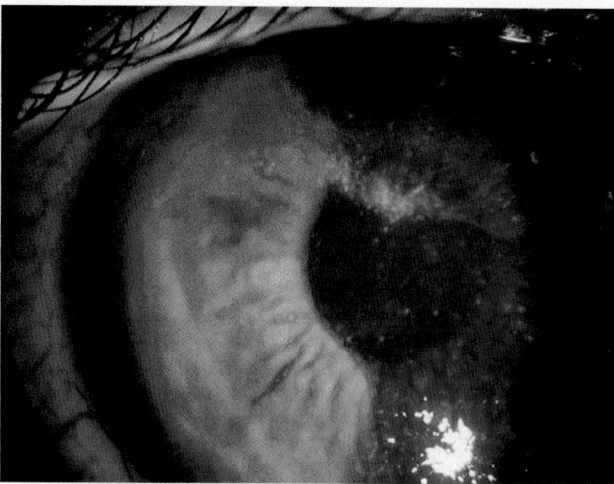

Figure 271-4 **Ocular examination of a patient with keratoconjunctivitis caused by *Encephalitozoon hellem*.** Slit-lamp examination findings in a patient with punctuate keratoconjunctivitis. A conjunctival scraping from this patient demonstrated spores consistent with *E. hellem* (see Fig. 271-2B). Sequencing of the small-subunit rRNA gene obtained by the polymerase chain reaction from this conjunctival biopsy confirmed that the infection was caused by *E. hellem*.

OCULAR INFECTION

Infection with *E. cuniculi*, *E. hellem*, or *E. intestinalis* can result in punctate keratopathy and conjunctivitis characterized by multiple punctate corneal ulcers (e.g., superficial epithelial keratitis; Fig. 271-4). Microsporidian spores are present in corneal and conjunctival epithelium, which can be obtained by scraping or biopsying the lesions. The organisms do not invade the corneal stroma but remain limited to the epithelium. Inflammatory cells are rarely present. *Trachipleistophora anthropopthera* can also cause keratitis.[188] Ocular disease may be the presenting manifestation when there is disseminated infection with any of the *Encephalitozoon* spp.[68,96,104,174,189] These infections most often occur in the setting of HIV or other immune dysfunction, although there are case reports of superficial epithelial keratitis caused by *Encephalitozoon* spp. in immunocompetent patients. Most of these immunocompetent cases have occurred in contact lens wearers. *V. corneae*, *Microsporidium africanum*, *Microsporidium ceylonensis,* and *Nosema ocularum* have also been reported to cause infection in immunocompetent patients.[190] Infections with these species of microsporidia have usually involved deeper levels of the corneal stroma and have often been associated with trauma. Biopsies have demonstrated necrosis and acute inflammatory cells with some giant cells in several cases. Clinically, these patients have a corneal stromal keratitis and occasionally uveitis.

MUSCULOSKELETAL INFECTION

Myositis with inflammation caused by several Microsporidia has been described in humans. The organisms in these case reports have included *Pleistophora ronneafiei*, *Pleistophora* sp., *Trachipleistophora hominis*, *Anncaliia vesicularum*, and *A. algerae*.[12,16,26,27,191]

The prevalence or incidence of microsporidian myositis in human is not known. Biopsies from the cases of *Pleistophora* spp. infection have demonstrated atrophic and degenerating muscle fibers infiltrated with focal clusters of large microsporidian spores that were up to 3.4 μm in length. There was a mixed inflammatory response consisting of plasma cells, lymphocytes, eosinophils, and histiocytes that was mild in the two cases occurring in AIDS patients but severe in the case involving an HIV-seronegative person.[26,192,193] The *T. hominis* infection that occurred in a patient with AIDS was associated with degeneration, atrophy, scarring, and intense inflammation.[16] The *A. vesicularum* infection occurred in an AIDS patient and was associated with cytolysis around the spores in the muscle fibers, but no cellular immune response was seen.[12] The *A. algerae* infection occurred in a patient with rheumatoid arthritis treated with steroids and monoclonal antibody to tumor necrosis factor-α (TNF-α).[191] There was a minimal cellular response to the numerous spores present in the muscle fibers.

SINUS AND RESPIRATORY INFECTION

Respiratory tract involvement is often seen with disseminated infections caused by the Encephalitozoonidae.[194] The pathologic features are nonspecific and may include rhinitis, sinusitis, and nasal polyposis in any combination.[195-201] A tongue ulcer containing *E. cuniculi* spores was reported in a patient with disseminated infection with this organism.[202] In a study of patients presenting with keratitis caused by *E. hellem*, spores of this organism were present in many of these patients' sputum samples in the absence of respiratory symptoms.[203] *E. hellem* infection of the entire length of the respiratory tract including the terminal bronchioles, associated with erosive tracheitis, bronchitis, and bronchiolitis, has been described in an autopsy report. Spores were seen in the epithelial cells, neutrophils in the bronchiolar wall, cells lining the alveoli, and extracellularly in the alveolar spaces. Case reports have confirmed that *E. cuniculi*, *E. hellem*, and *E. intestinalis* can cause bronchiolitis with or without pneumonia. Sinus biopsies in AIDS patients with chronic sinusitis and microsporidiosis have demonstrated spores in epithelium and supporting structures.[204] The inflammatory response has been variable, with lymphocytes, neutrophils, macrophages, and occasional granuloma formation. Respiratory tract infection caused by *E. bieneusi* has been reported twice, with spores found in stool, bronchoalveolar lavage fluid, and transbronchial biopsy specimens.[205,206] A case of rhinosinusitis caused by *E. bieneusi* has also been reported.[207] It has been suggested that these cases reflect contamination and colonization of the respiratory tract as a result of vomiting rather than dissemination of this organism from the gastrointestinal tract.

SKIN

Microsporidia infections of the skin have been described. In a child with leukemia, the infection was caused by *A. algerae*, with spores infecting the cellular elements of the dermis.[208] In a second case, an *Encephalitozoon* sp. was reported to be the cause of nodular skin lesions.[209,210]

▪ Clinical Manifestations

The clinical manifestations of microsporidiosis are shown in Table 271-1.

MICROSPORIDIAN INFECTION IN NON-AIDS PATIENTS

Levaditi and colleagues suggested that Microsporidia were associated with human disease as early as 1923,[211] but the first definitive proof of human infection was not reported for another 50 years. In 1973, a 4-month-old athymic male infant died with severe diarrhea and malabsorption. At autopsy, the microsporidian *Anncaliia (Nosema) conorii* was discovered in the lungs, stomach, small and large bowel, kidneys, adrenal glands, myocardium, liver, and diaphragm.[212]

In all patients (those with or without HIV infection), the most common symptomatic microsporidian infection is probably diarrhea.[90,100,114,115,120,123,128-130,213] *E. bieneusi* has been identified as a cause of self-limited diarrhea in immunocompetent hosts, including travelers[112,125-128,214,215] and, in epidemiologic studies, *E. bieneusi* has been identified in 1% to 10% of African children with diarrhea[113,216,217] and in patients undergoing liver and bone marrow transplantation.[129-136,185,186,218,219] Clinical manifestations have included watery, nonbloody diarrhea, nausea, diffuse abdominal pain, and fever. Diar-

rhea tends to be self-limited in immunocompetent patients but is persistent in patients with immunosuppression as a result of transplantation. *E. intestinalis* was found in 7.8% of the stools of patients in a survey regarding the causes of diarrhea in Mexico[90] and has been described in travelers with chronic diarrhea.

Ocular infections with ulcer or deep cornea stroma infection associated with eye pain have also been reported in immunocompetent patients. In 1973 and 1981, two cases of corneal microsporidiosis caused by *Microsporidium africanus* in Botswana[220] and *Microsporidium ceylonensis* in Sri Lanka were described (*Microsporidium* is used at the generic level for Microsporidia of unknown phylogenetic placement).[221] Additional cases of microsporidian keratitis have been identified in immunocompetent hosts.[3,190] One of these organisms was classified as *N. ocularum*,[222] and the other, which was successfully propagated in vitro, was named *N. corneum*[24] (now *V. corneae*[11]). *A. algerae* infection of the cornea has also been reported.[208] Among these immunologically normal patients with corneal infections the outcomes included enucleation, unsuccessful penetrating keratoplasty, successful treatment with a corneal transplant,[189] and therapy with topical agents until keratoplasty.[223]

Cerebral infections caused by *E. cuniculi* are commonly described in many animals but have been reported only rarely in immunocompetent humans. *Encephalitozoon* infection was demonstrated in a 3-year-old boy with seizures and hepatomegaly by positive immunoglobulin G (IgG) and IgM indirect immunofluorescence assays (using *E. cuniculi* as the antigen).[147] Recurrent fever infection with *Encephalitozoon* sp. was also reported in a 9-year-old Japanese boy with headache, vomiting, and spastic convulsions.[8]

Pleistophora sp. was identified in the skeletal muscle of an HIV-negative patient as well as HIV-positive patients with myositis associated with normal creatine phosphokinase (CPK) levels.[26,27,192,193] *A. algerae* infection of the skin has been seen in a patient with leukemia[208] and in another patient with myositis who had significant elevations in CPK and muscle pain; the latter patient had rheumatoid arthritis treated with steroids and antibody to TNF-α.[191]

MICROSPORIDIAN INFECTION IN AIDS PATIENTS

Microsporidia were recognized as opportunistic pathogens causing diarrhea and wasting in AIDS patients in 1985.[9] Since then, although most reported cases still involved diarrhea, the spectrum of diseases caused by these organisms has expanded to include keratoconjunctivitis, disseminated disease, hepatitis, myositis, sinusitis, kidney and urogenital infection, ascites, and cholangitis, as well as no symptoms at all.[3,6,30]

Enterocytozoonidae

Gastrointestinal infection is most common with *E. bieneusi*, and the presentation classically involves chronic diarrhea (which can last years[224]), anorexia, weight loss, and bloating without associated fever. It is most frequently seen in AIDS patients with CD4+ counts lower than 50 cells/mL. Frequent (3 to 10) bowel movements occur daily, consisting of loose to watery stool that does not contain blood or fecal leukocytes.[6,33,225,226] There is no fever when infection is limited to the intestinal mucosa. Diarrhea is often associated with malabsorption and is worsened by food ingestion. Malabsorption can result in weight loss and a wasting syndrome. The mortality of patients with advanced HIV disease and chronic diarrhea with wasting has been reported to be in excess of 50%.[177] Other intestinal pathogens may occur simultaneously or sequentially with the presence of this or other Microsporidia.[227]

Although originally thought to invade only enterocytes, it has been demonstrated that *E. bieneusi* can also invade cholangioepithelium.[177] When present in the cholangioepithelium, this organism has been associated with sclerosing cholangitis, AIDS cholangiopathy, and cholecystitis.[228] Presentations include abdominal pain, nausea, vomiting, and fever; jaundice is rarely seen. Fever is most likely the result of concomitant bacterial biliary infection, which produces the typical clinical manifestations of cholangitis. Imaging studies, including abdominal ultrasonography, CT, endoscopic ultrasonography, and endoscopic retrograde cholangiopancreatography (ERCP), usually demonstrate dilated biliary ducts, irregularities of the bile duct wall, and gallbladder abnormalities such as thickening, distention, or the presence of sludge. Papillary stenosis has also been seen. Bilirubin is normal, although most patients have elevated liver function tests (e.g., alkaline phosphatase, γ-glutamyltransferase, aspartate aminotransferase, alanine aminotransferase). Interestingly, an *E. bieneusi*–like organism has been identified a causative factor for cholangitis and hepatitis in SIV-infected rhesus monkeys.[109]

Systemic dissemination is rare with *E. bieneusi*. One case report described this organism in nasal mucosa, which probably resulted from direct inoculation of spores from gastrointestinal secretions.[229] There are two case reports of respiratory tract involvement with *E. bieneusi* associated with chronic diarrhea, persistent cough, dyspnea, wheezing, and chest radiographs showing interstitial infiltrates.[205,224] Spores of *E. bieneusi* were detected in these cases in stool, bronchoalveolar lavage fluid, and transbronchial biopsy specimens. *E. bieneusi* has been found to be a cause of proliferative serositis (peritonitis) in macaques (*Macaca mulatta*).

Encephalitizoonidae

Encephalitizoonidae are widely distributed among animals.[230] Three members of the family Encephalitizoonidae have been associated with disease in humans—*E. cuniculi*, *E. hellem*, and *E. intestinalis* (previously known as *Septata intestinalis*). It appears that these Microsporidia have the capacity to disseminate widely in their hosts, and their involvement in most organs has now been documented.[3,19,30,33] The ability of these organisms to disseminate correlates with their ability to grow in many cell types in vivo and in vitro. These organisms have been associated with gastroenteritis, keratitis, sinusitis, bronchiolitis, nephritis, cystitis-ureteritis, urethritis, prostatitis, hepatitis, fulminant hepatic failure, peritonitis, cerebritis, and disseminated infection.[19-21,179,183,187,231] An *Encephalitozoon* sp. has also been reported in a case of nodular skin lesions.[209,210]

The major syndrome associated with microsporidiosis is diarrhea and wasting. This is usually caused by *E. bieneusi* (more than 90% of cases in the United States) and occasionally *E. intestinalis* (although in Europe this organism may be a more frequent cause of diarrhea[232]). *E. intestinalis* also can cause cholangitis,[14,233] keratoconjunctivitis, osteomyelitis of the mandible,[234] upper respiratory infections, renal failure, keratoconjunctivitis, and disseminated infection in AIDS patients.[144,176,235] Elimination of this parasite by treatment with albendazole correlates with the resolution of symptoms.[236]

E. cuniculi has been associated with hepatitis,[174] peritonitis,[183] hepatic failure,[20] disseminated disease with fever,[187] renal insufficiency, and intractable cough.[237] Granulomatous encephalitis caused by *E. cuniculi* was first described in rabbits in 1922, and cases of encephalitis and seizures caused by *E. cuniculi* have been reported in AIDS patients.[21,187] These infections have been reported to respond to albendazole.[19,237]

E. hellem has been reported to cause disseminated disease associated with renal failure, nephritis, pneumonia, bronchitis, and keratoconjunctivitis.[203,238,239] Punctate keratoconjunctivitis is the most commonly recognized clinical manifestation of infection with this organism. Most of the reports of ocular infection caused by Encephalitizoonidae in the literature have been attributed to *E. hellem*, including three cases originally classified as *E. cuniculi*.[18,240] The remaining cases were caused by *Encephalitozoon* sp. or *E. intestinalis*.[187] Patients present with bilateral coarse punctate epithelial keratopathy and conjunctival inflammation resulting in redness, foreign body sensation, photophobia, excessive tearing, blurred vision, and changes in visual acuity. Ocular microsporidian infection in HIV-1-infected patients has been restricted to the superficial epithelium of the cornea and conjunctiva (i.e., superficial keratoconjunctivitis), and it rarely progresses to corneal ulceration (see Fig. 271-4). Physical examination reveals conjunctival hyperemia and superficial punctate keratopathy, without deep corneal ulcers or retinal involvement. Slit-lamp examination usually demonstrates punctate epithelial opacities, granular epithelial cells with irregular

fluorescein uptake, conjunctival injection, superficial corneal infiltrates, and a noninflamed anterior chamber. Infection may be bilateral or unilateral. It is often associated with disseminated disease.[202,241,242] Examination of the urine in patients with keratoconjunctivitis often reveals microsporidian spores.[99] This organism is also recognized as an important cause of infection of the nasal epithelium, which in turn causes sinusitis in AIDS patients.[204]

Other Microsporidia

Trachipleistophora hominis is a pansporoblastic microsporidian that has been described in several patients with disseminated disease in the setting of AIDS.[16] It has been reported to cause myositis, sinusitis, and keratoconjunctivitis. *Trachipleistophora anthropopthera* infection presents as encephalitis, myositis, and keratoconjunctivitis.[17,28,188] Several of these patients responded clinically to albendazole. *Anncaliia (Brachiola) vesicularum* caused myositis in an HIV-1-infected patient that responded to a regimen of albendazole and itraconozole.[12] Cases of myositis caused by *Pleistophora* sp. and *Pleistophora ronneafiei* have also been reported in patients with AIDS.[26,27,192,243] The myositis presentation of these microsporidia has included myalgias, weakness, elevated serum CPK and aldolase levels, and abnormal electromyograms consistent with inflammatory myopathy. A case of urinary tract infection, prostatitis, and *V. corneae* infection has been reported in an AIDS patient.[111]

Diagnosis

Examination of stool specimens by light microscopy has become the standard method for diagnosing gastrointestinal microsporidiosis (see Fig. 271-3). Because renal involvement with shedding of spores in the urine is common in all the species of Microsporidia that disseminate, urine specimens should be obtained whenever the diagnosis of microsporidiosis is considered. This has therapeutic implications because the Microsporidia that disseminate (e.g., *Encephalitozoon* spp.) are usually sensitive to albendazole, whereas those that do not disseminate (e.g., *E. bieneusi*) are resistant. Definitive identification of the Microsporidia causing an infection can be done using ultrastructural examination (e.g., electron microscopy) or molecular techniques (e.g., species-specific polymerase chain reaction [PCR] assay). If stool examination is negative in the setting of chronic diarrhea (longer than 2 months' duration), endoscopy should be performed. A summary of the available diagnostic tests and their usefulness in patients with suspected microsporidiosis is presented in Table 271-2.

Demonstration of Microsporidia by light microscopy is accomplished with staining methods that produce differential contrast between the spores of the Microsporidia and the cells and debris in clinical samples in which Microsporidia are found. Adequate magnification using a 60× to 100× objective is required for visualization, because the spores are 1 to 3 μm in size. Chromotrope 2R,[244] calcofluor white (fluorescent brightener 28),[245] and Uvitex 2B[246] are useful selective stains for Microsporidia in stool specimens and other body fluids. The chromotrope 2R-based method of Weber and associates[244] is a modification of a standard trichrome stain using a 10-fold higher chromotrope 2R concentration and a longer staining time. The Weber method, modified by Ryan and co-workers[247] (which uses aniline blue in place of fast green) and by Kokoskin and colleagues[248] (which uses a higher temperature), are preferred by some laboratories. With a chromotrope 2R–based stain, the spores appear as 1- to 3-μm ovoid, light pink structures with a beltlike stripe girding them diagonally and equatorially against a green (Weber chromotrope stain) or blue (Ryan modification) background (see Fig. 271-3A). A rapid (11-minute) stain, the Gram-chromotrope stain, combines chromotrope 2R staining with a Gram staining step and results in violet-staining spores.[249] Microsporidian spores can also be visualized by ultraviolet (UV) microscopy using chemifluorescent optical brightening agents such as Calcofluor white M2R (fluorescent brightener 28; Fungi-Fluor) or Uvitex 2B (Fungiqual A; Medical Diagnostics, Kandern, Germany), which stain chitin in the spore wall (endospore layer) (see Fig. 271-3B).

TABLE 271-2	Diagnostic Tests for Microsporidiosis	
Test	*Specimens*	*Usefulness*
Chromotrope or chemofluorescent stain	Urine	This is often positive in cases of disseminated microsporidiosis (e.g., *Encephalitozoon* spp.). It should be done in all suspected microsporidia cases.
	Stool	At least three stools should be examined. The combination of chromotrope and chemofluorescence stains provides the highest sensitivity and specificity. Monoclonal antibodies for immunofluorescent antigen (IFA) detection are also useful.
	Conjunctival scrapings	This is useful for the diagnosis of keratoconjunctivitis. Urine should also be examined in suspected cases to screen for disseminated microsporidiosis.
	Nasal scrapings	This can be useful for the diagnosis of Microsporidian sinusitis. Because most Microsporidia associated with sinusitis are present in the kidneys, examination of urine should be routine for suspected sinusitis cases. If these tests are negative, biopsy of the nasal mucosa may be useful for diagnosis.
Endoscopy	Touch preparations	Touch preparations are useful for rapid diagnosis (within 24 hours).
	Biliary fluid	Examination is useful for diagnosis of microsporidian cholangitis.
	Biopsy (small intestine)	Biopsy should be considered for all patients with chronic diarrhea longer than 2 months' duration and negative stool and urine examinations. In this group, endoscopy has yielded a diagnosis of microsporidia in up to 30% of patients. Tissue can be examined with chromotrope 2R, tissue Gram, or silver stain. If Microsporidia are demonstrated to invade the lamina propria, urine examination should be repeated because *Encephalitozoon* spp. are the most likely causative agents. In this setting, albendazole has high treatment efficacy.
Polymerase chain reaction (PCR)	Urine, stool, or tissue	Available from reference laboratories (e.g., CDC). PCR allows species identification.
Electron microscopy	Tissue	It provides species identification; it is crucial for identifying new species or for the characterization of Microsporidia in unusual or new locations.
Serology	Serum	Not useful for diagnosis but may be useful for epidemiologic surveys.

Such stains also stain fungi and other fecal elements; however, microsporidian spores can be distinguished from yeast as they have a uniformly oval shape and are nonbudding.

In a study that examined 50 electron microscopy-proven Microsporidia-positive stool specimens, both the chromotrope 2R and chemifluorescent brightening stains identified 100% of specimens if at least fifty 100× objective fields were examined.[250] With Uvitex 2B, all the 186 stool samples examined from 19 patients with biopsy-proven *E. bieneusi* infection were positive, whereas none of the 55 stool samples from 16 biopsy-negative patients were positive.[246] In another study evaluating Uvitex 2B staining, Microsporidia were identified in all the samples known to be chromotrope 2R stain-positive as well as in seven additional samples that were chromotrope-negative on initial examination.[251] On reexamination, however, these seven stool samples were found also to be positive with the chromotrope 2R stain. All patients with positive duodenal biopsies had positive stool examinations according to the chromotrope or chemifluorescent methods. The limit of detecting Microsporidia by these techniques appears to be 50,000 organisms/mL. Overall, the sensitivity of the chemifluorescent brightener-based stains is slightly higher than chromotrope-based stains (especially when low numbers of spores are present in a sample); however, the specificity of the chemifluorescent stains is lower (90% vs. 100% in one study). Neither the chromotrope nor the chemifluorescent stain provides information on the species of Microsporidia being identified. Although it has been reported that microsporidian spores in food can give a false-positive result, and despite the fact that Microsporidia are common in the environment, it does not appear to be a common problem when using stool specimens for diagnosing these infections.

Microsporidia in body fluids other than stool (e.g., urine, cerebrospinal fluid, bile, duodenal aspirates, bronchoalveolar lavage fluid, and sputum) have been visualized using chemifluorescent optical brightening agents or Chromotrope 2R, Giemsa, Brown-Hopps Gram, acid-fast, or Warthin-Starry silver stain.[33,252,253] Generally, it is easier to identify microsporidian spores in body fluids other than in stool because of the absence of bacteria and debris, which can be confused with microsporidian spores. Because microsporidian infections usually involve mucosa or epithelium, cytologic preparations are especially useful for diagnosis.[33] Specimens that have been useful for diagnosing microsporidian infections include intestinal and biliary epithelium, epithelium of the cornea and conjunctivae, epithelium of the sinonasal

and tracheobronchial regions, renal tubular epithelium, and urothelium. Diagnosis has also been accomplished by examining touch preparations of biopsy material. Microscopic examination of corneal tissue in patients with microsporidian keratitis, obtained by gently rubbing the conjunctiva and cornea with a tissue swab, usually reveals multiple, gram-positive, oval organisms in epithelial cells.

Histologically, microsporidian spores are easily discernible with a modified tissue chromotrope 2R or tissue Gram stain (Brown-Hopp or Brown-Brenn) in sections prepared from tissue fixed using routine procedures, Most microsporidian spores are gram-positive in tissue sections. With experience, Microsporidia can also be seen on hematoxylin and eosin-stained sections. Other stains that may be useful include periodic acid–Schiff, Giemsa, and Steiner silver stains. Some Microsporidia are also acid-fast stain-positive. Fresh tissue can also be examined by phase contrast microscopy; because of their thick wall, unstained spores are refractile, appearing green, and such spores can be birefringent. If possible, biopsy or autopsy material should also be placed in electron microscopy fixative when microsporidiosis is suspected, because the definitive diagnosis of species requires ultrastructural information. It is possible, however, to use formalin-fixed tissue for ultrastructural analysis. Molecular methods can also be used on formalin-fixed tissue, although unfixed tissue or tissue fixed in ethanol yields the best results with PCR techniques.

Polyclonal serum prepared to other Microsporidia (*E. cuniculi*) has been reported to react with *E. bieneusi*.[149,254] Monoclonal antibodies to *E. hellem*,[255] *E. intestinalis*,[256] and *E. bieneusi*[257-260] have been described. These methods have been used to detect Microsporidia in tissue sections using immunofluorescence techniques. Several of these antibodies have been demonstrated to be useful for the examination of stool specimens and have demonstrated good sensitivity and specificity. Detection kits for microsporidia in stool and environmental samples using antibodies to Encephalitozoonidae and *Enterocytozoon bieneusi* are now commercially available (Waterborne, New Orleans).

V. corneae,[24] *E. cuniculi*, *E. hellem*,[68] *T. hominis*,[16] *T. anthropopthera*,[188] and *E. intestinalis*[23] have been cultivated in tissue culture systems in vitro (for a review, see Visvesvara[261]). *E. bieneusi* has not been cultivated continuously in vitro, although limited in vitro cultivation of *E. bieneusi* has been reported (Dr. S. Tzipori, personal communication, 2006).[262] Adenovirus can mimic the cytopathologic effect of Microsporidia.[263] Experimental infection of SIV-infected rhesus monkeys with *E. bieneusi* from human tissue has been demonstrated[264] and serial propagation has been described in immunocompromised rodents.[265] The isolation of Microsporidia from clinical specimens is not a routine procedure and is available in only a few specialized research laboratories.

Serologic tests for diagnosing microsporidiosis have been developed and used for epidemiologic studies. Such serologic tests have, for the most part, not been proven useful for diagnosing microsporidiosis. In a study of 12 AIDS patients with *E. bieneusi*, 2 AIDS patients with *E. intestinalis*, and 2 immunocompetent patients with *V. corneae*, enzyme-linked immunosorbent assay (ELISA) titers for *E. hellem, E. cuniculi*, or *V. corneae* were not useful for diagnosis.[266] False-negative titers were present in 7 of the patients with microsporidiosis, and half of the control patients (without clinical microsporidiosis) had positive serology to Microsporidia. This is consistent with other AIDS-associated infections in which serology has not proven useful.

A number of molecular diagnostic tests have been developed for pathogenic Microsporidia. Weiss and Vossbrinck[54] have reviewed the PCR assays for microsporidiosis. Homology cloning of the rRNA genes of many of the Microsporidia pathogenic in humans has been accomplished using PCR techniques, and over a hundred Microsporidia species are now in the GenBank database. It has been possible to design PCR primers to these small-subunit rRNA genes to identify Microsporidia at the species level in clinical samples without the need for ultrastructural examination. Two main approaches have been used for constructing PCR primers for Microsporidia, the use of universal pan-Microsporidia primers and of species-specific primer pairs. These PCR techniques have been applied to biopsy specimens, urine, cultures and, more recently, stool specimens, and should greatly facilitate diagnostic and epidemiologic studies.[59,190,267-269] Currently, these molecular tests are available in reference laboratories such as the Centers for Disease Control and Prevention.

Treatment

Treatment for microsporidiosis is outlined in Table 271-3.

GASTROINTESTINAL AND SYSTEMIC DISEASE

Microsporidian infection often occurs in immunocompromised hosts, particularly in those with HIV infection and CD4+ cell counts lower than 50/mL. Clinical studies have demonstrated that improved immune function can result in the clinical response of patients with gastrointestinal microsporidiosis, with elimination of the organism and normalization of the intestinal architecture.[172,173,270-272] Relapse has been reported in patients who developed failure of their antiretroviral therapy associated with a decline in immune function and falling CD4+ counts. Overall, these observations suggest that part of the primary treatment of microsporidiosis in the setting of AIDS is the institution of effective HAART. There have been no reports of immune reconstitution syndromes with HAART and microsporidiosis.

Although several species of Microsporidia that infect humans can be grown in vitro (but not without a host cell monolayer), the most common human pathogenic microsporidian, *E. bieneusi*, has yet to be grown continuously in vitro. This has limited in vitro testing of antimicrosporidial agents to those active against *Encephalitozoon* spp. and *V. corneae*.[11,273,274] Several agents have also been evaluated in animal models of microsporidiosis, but until recently no practical animal model had been developed for in vivo studies of *E. bieneusi*.[265] Costa and Weiss[275] have reviewed drugs used against microsporidiosis in humans and animals.

Among the compounds tested in vitro and in vivo for treatment of microsporidiosis, fumagillin and albendazole have demonstrated the most consistent activity and have been demonstrated to have clinical efficacy in human infections with various Microsporidia.[145,146,196,198,235,276-283] Albendazole binds to β-tubulin and is active against all the Encephalitozoonidae *(E. hellem, E. cuniculi, E. intestinalis)* in vitro at concentrations lower than 0.1 mg/mL; it is also active in animal models of microsporidiosis.[276] Data on *Encephalitozoon* β-tubulin genes have demonstrated an amino acid sequence associated with sensitivity to benzimidazoles,[284] whereas the sequences of *Enterocytozoon*[285] and *Vittaforma*[286] demonstrate amino acids associated with

TABLE 271-3	Current Treatment Options for Microsporidiosis	
Organism	*Drug*	*Dosage and Duration*[†]
All microsporidian infections	HAART with immune restoration (an increase of CD4+ count to >100 cells/μL) is associated with resolution of symptoms of enteric microsporidiosis. All patients should be offered HAART as part of the initial management of microsporidial infection. Severe dehydration, malnutrition, and wasting should be managed by fluid support and nutritional supplement. Antimotility agents can be used for diarrhea control if required.	
Enterocytozoon bieneusi	No effective commercial treatment. Fumagillin (oral) has been effective in a clinical trial. *Alternatives:* Albendazole* resulted in clinical improvement in up to 50% of patients in some studies, but was not effective in other studies. Nitazoxanide, 1000 mg bid with food for 60 days, has been used, but is less effective in patients with low CD4 counts.	20 mg tid (e.g., 60 mg/day)
Encephalitozoonidae infection (e.g., systemic, sinusitis, encephalitis, hepatitis)		
E. cuniculi	Albendazole	400 mg bid[†]
E. hellem	Albendazole	400 mg bid
E. intestinalis	Albendazole	400 mg bid
Encephalitozoonidae keratoconjunctivitis	Fumagillin solution[‡] (70 μg/mL) Patients may also need albendazole* if systemic infection is present.	2 drops every 2 hours for 4 days then 2 drops 4 times a day[§]
Trachipleistophora hominis	Albendazole	400 mg bid
Annicaliia (formerly *Brachiola*) *vesicularum*	Albendazole	400 mg bid
	±Itraconazole	400 mg qd

HAART, highly active antiretroviral therapy.

*Albendazole, 400 mg bid.

[†]The duration of treatment for microsporidiosis has not been established. Relapse of infection has occurred on stopping treatment. Patients should be maintained on treatment for at least 4 weeks, and most patients should continue on treatment until their CD4 count is higher than 200 cells/μL for at least 6 months following the initiation of HAART.

[‡]Fumidil B (fumagillin bicylohexylammonium; Mid-Continent Agrimarketing, Overland Park, KS, USA) is used at 3 mg/mL in saline (final concentration of fumagillin, 70 μg/mL).

[§]Eye drops should be continued indefinitely; relapse is common on stopping treatment.

Adapted from Costa S, Weiss LM. Drug treatment of microsporidiosis. Drug Resistance Updates 2000;3:1-16.

albendazole resistance. This is consistent with the observed clinical responses to albendazole in these Microsporidia.

Albendazole is 70% protein-bound. It is distributed to blood, bile, and cerebrospinal fluid and eliminated by the kidneys. Peak serum levels 2 hours after an oral dose are 0.20 to 0.94 μg/mL. Drug absorption is increased if albendazole is taken with food containing relatively high concentrations of fat. After oral administration, the hepatic metabolism converts albendazole to albendazole sulfoxide, which is detectable in the systemic circulation. Albendazole is not carcinogenic or mutagenic, although in rats and rabbits at dosages of 30 mg/kg it is embryotoxic and teratogenic. Albendazole is therefore not recommended for use in pregnant women. Side effects are rare, although the following have been reported: hypersensitivity (rash, pruritus, fever), neutropenia (reversible), CNS effects (dizziness, headache), gastrointestinal disturbances (abdominal pain, diarrhea, nausea, vomiting), hair loss (reversible), and elevated hepatic enzyme levels (reversible). There is a report of pseudomembranous colitis following albendazole treatment.

There are few placebo-controlled comparative treatment trials of microsporidiosis caused by Encephalitozoon spp., but there are numerous case reports demonstrating the efficacy of 2 to 4 weeks of albendazole 400 mg twice daily for these infections. In a double-blind, placebo-controlled trial of eight patients with AIDS and diarrhea caused by E. intestinalis, treatment with albendazole (400 mg twice daily for 3 weeks) resulted in resolution of the diarrhea and elimination of the organism in all eight patients, similar to that seen in several case reports.[144,184,198,235,236,287,288] In case reports of chronic sinusitis, respiratory infection, and disseminated infection caused by E. hellem, treatment with 400 mg of albendazole twice daily resulted in resolution of symptoms and clearance of the organism.[289,290] Clinical improvement was demonstrated with albendazole treatment in a patient with disseminated E. cuniculi infection involving the CNS, conjunctiva, sinuses, kidneys, and lungs.[21] It has also been reported to be effective in cases of urethritis,[282] renal failure,[281] and disseminated infection.[237] In addition to its efficacy in Encephalitozoon spp., disseminated infections with other Microsporidia have also been reported to respond to albendazole treatment. In patients with disseminated infection accompanied by myositis due to T. hominis and in a patient with myositis caused by A. vesicularum, albendazole (400 mg twice daily) resulted in clinical improvement.[12,16]

In contrast to its success in treating patients with the species of Microsporidia that disseminate, albendazole has displayed only limited efficacy against E. bieneusi infection. In two studies examining 66 patients with diarrhea caused by E. bieneusi during the pre-HAART era, symptoms were alleviated in about 50% of patients treated with albendazole, but the presence of E. bieneusi persisted during treatment in all patients and there was no improvement in any patient's D-xylose absorption test.[280,283,291] The symptoms rapidly recurred on discontinuation of albendazole therapy in the patients who had reported symptom alleviation with it. Most other studies have found that albendazole has no efficacy against E. bieneusi infection.[292]

Despite a few case reports indicating that metronidazole was effective for E. bieneusi intestinal infection, most studies have demonstrated that this drug is not effective against this infection.[184,279,293] In vitro studies have also demonstrated that metronidazole has no activity against Microsporidia (e.g., E. cuniculi).[273] Other medications used without success to treat gastrointestinal microsporidiosis are azithromycin, paromomycin (Microsporidia lack the rRNA binding site for this drug), and quinacrine. Atovaquone has been anecdotally reported to have limited efficacy in patients with microsporidiosis,[279,294] although it has no in vitro activity.[273] Transient clinical remission has been reported with furazolidone or nitazoxanide (1000 mg twice daily) treatment.[180,295] Sparfloxacin and chloroquine have demonstrated in vitro activity against Microsporidia but have not been used clinically. Prophylaxis with trimethoprim-sulfamethoxazole is not effective for preventing microsporidiosis, and this drug has no in vitro or in vivo activity against these organisms.[296] Thalidomide and octreotide have both been reported to decrease diarrhea in about 50% of patients with

microsporidiosis, which is probably secondary to the effect of these agents on the physiology of enterocytes.[297] Examination of the biopsies of patients treated with thalidomide (100 mg daily for 1 month) demonstrated persistence of the parasite and no change in parasite load.

Fumagillin was isolated from Aspergillus fumigatus in 1949 and, because of its efficacy against Entamoeba histolytica in vitro, it was used during the 1950s to treat amebiasis. Fumagillin is used commercially to treat honeybees infected with the microsporidian Nosema apis and has been used to treat infections by microsporidia and myxosporeans in various types of fish.[298,299] Fumagillin and its semisynthetic analogue TNP-470 have been found to have activity in vitro and in vivo against Microsporidia pathogenic for humans, including E. cuniculi, E. hellem, E. intestinalis, V. corneae, and E. bieneusi.[145,146,276,277,279,300,301] A dose escalation trial of fumagillin performed on AIDS patients infected with E. bieneusi used dosages of 10 mg/day for 14 days, 20 mg/day for 14 days, 40 mg/day for 14 days, and 60 mg/day for 14 days. Altogether, 21 of 29 patients exhibited transient clearing of parasites from their stool; all these patients were in the first three dosage groups. In the 60-mg/day group, 8 of 11 patients did not have spores in their stools at week 6 and remained free of spores in stool specimens for a mean of 11 months. Duodenal biopsies on the same eight patients did not demonstrate Microsporidia by light or electron microscopy. A subsequent randomized trial based evaluating 12 patients (with either AIDS or transplants) confirmed that 60 mg/day (given as 20 mg three times daily) effectively treated E. bieneusi intestinal infection.[145] Treatment was associated with resolution of diarrhea, clearance of spores, improvement of Karnofsky scores, and improvement in D-xylose absorption tests. The main limiting toxicity of this treatment was thrombocytopenia, which was reversible on stopping fumagillin treatment.

Fumagillin, ovalicin, and their analogues (e.g., TNP-470) bind in a selective, covalent fashion to the metalloprotease methionine aminopeptidase type 2 (MetAP2). Methionine aminopeptidase activity is essential for eukaryotic cell survival, because removal of the terminal methionine of a protein is often essential for its function and posttranslational modification. Homology PCR assay has been used to demonstrate the presence of MetAP2 genes in several microsporidia.[302] The crystal structure of E. cuniculi MetAP2 has recently been determined (MMDB ID: 63862; PDB ID: 3CMK). Data from the E. cuniculi genome project[84] indicates that E. cuniculi does not have a methionine aminopeptidase type 1 gene (MetAP1), unlike mammalian cells, which have both MetAP1 and MetAP2; therefore, MetAP2 is an essential enzyme in microsporidia.

OCULAR DISEASE

Solutions of the soluble salt fumagillin bicylohexylammonium (Fumidil B; Mid-Continent Agrimarketing, Overland Park, KS) applied topically have been demonstrated to be nontoxic to the cornea. Treatment of ocular microsporidiosis can be accomplished using a 3-mg/mL solution of Fumidil B in saline (fumagillin, 70 μg/mL);[277,278,303-305] the treatment should be continued indefinitely, because recurrence has been reported on stopping these drops. Although clearance of Microsporidia from the eye can be demonstrated, the organism is still often present systemically and can be demonstrated in the urine or in nasal smears. In such cases, the use of albendazole as a systemic agent is reasonable and effective. Topical treatment with thiabendazole (0.4% suspension), a related benzimidazole, was ineffective in one case of keratitis caused by E. hellem. Two patients with Encephalitozoon-like organisms were reported to respond to imidazole (fluconazole and itraconazole) administration.[306] Yee and associates described complete improvement with oral itraconazole (200 mg twice daily) in a patient with E. hellem infection over a 6-week period after debulking the cornea.[104] However, Diesenhouse and co-workers observed no improvement in a patient with E. hellem treated with itraconazole, 100 mg three times daily.[277] In vitro data have not confirmed antimicrosporidial activity for imidazole compounds. Sulfa drugs have had variable results in vitro and in vivo and are not recommended for treatment. Polymyxin B, propamidine isethionate 0.1% (Brolene), gramicidin, neomycin sulfate, and tetracycline appear to have limited efficacy for the treatment of microsporidian infection and should not be used except to treat secondary bacterial infections. Keratoplasty appears to provide temporary improvement in some cases, and debulking by corneal scraping may be useful in cases not responding to medical treatment. Steroids may be useful for decreasing the associated inflammatory response but have no direct action on Microsporidia.

Prevention

There are limited data on effective preventive strategies for microsporidiosis. Currently, no prophylactic agents have been identified for these organisms. Patients have developed microsporidiosis while on trimethoprim-sulfamethoxazole prophylaxis,[296] and microsporidiosis has occurred in patients receiving dapsone, pyrimethamine, itraconazole, azithromycin, and atovaquone.[171] No studies have evaluated albendazole for prophylaxis but given its relative lack of efficacy for E. bieneusi infections, it is unlikely to be effective in preventing most cases of intestinal microsporidiosis. The most effective prophylaxis is the restoration of immune function in immunocompromised hosts. Several studies in AIDS patients have demonstrated that HAART can produce remission of intestinal microsporidiosis.[172,173,270-272] Moreover, the declining incidence of microsporidiosis and other opportunistic infections during the HAART era suggests that it also prevents symptomatic infection.

Microsporidian spores can survive and remain infective in the environment for prolonged periods. Experiments with E. cuniculi have demonstrated that they can survive for years in the environment with the correct humidity and temperature.[94] In the typical hospital environment, E. cuniculi spores can survive and remain infectious for at least 1 month. Spores can be rendered noninfectious by a 30-minute exposure to most common disinfectants, so the procedures used to clean most hospital rooms should be sufficient to limit infection. Spores are also killed by the methods commonly used for sterilization.

Although the epidemiology of the Microsporidia that infect humans has not been fully elucidated, it is likely they are food- or water-borne pathogens, and the usual sanitary measures that prevent contamination of food and water with animal urine and feces should decrease the chance for infection. Hand washing and general hygienic habits probably reduce the chance of contamination of the conjunctiva and cornea with microsporidian spores. It is not known whether person-to-person respiratory transmission occurs. Given the presence of microsporidian spores in respiratory secretions in cases of disseminated microsporidiosis, it may be useful to consider preventing contact of these patients with other immunosuppressed patients until the infection has been treated. Existing guidelines for the prevention of opportunistic infections that address food, water, and animal contact may be useful for preventing microsporidiosis. The presence of these organisms in genitourinary secretions raises the possibility of sexual transmission of these infections. It is reasonable to screen close contacts of patients with index cases of microsporidiosis for the presence of these organisms. Their importance and prevalence in our water supplies is an open question, but severely immunocompromised patients may wish to consider using bottled or filtered water in some settings.

REFERENCES

1. Sprague V. Systematics of the microsporidia. In: Bulla LA, Cheng TC, eds. *Comparative Pathobiology*. Vol 2. New York: Plenum Press; 1977:1-510.
2. Sprague VV, Becnel JJ. Note on the name-author-date combination for the taxon Microsporidies Balbiani, 1882, when ranked as a phylum. *J Invertebr Pathol*. 1998;71:91-94.
3. Wittner M, Weiss LM. *The Microsporidia and Microsporidiosis*. Washington DC: ASM Press; 1999.
4. Black SS, Steinohrt LA, Bertucci DC, et al. Encephalitozoon hellem in budgerigars (Melopsittacus undulatus). *Vet Pathol*. 1997;34:189-198.
5. American Mosquito Control Association. *Biological Control of Mosquitoes. AMCA Bulletin No. 6.* Fresno, Calif: American Mosquito Control Association; 1985:218.
6. Weber R, Bryan RT, Schwartz DA, et al. Human microsporidial infections. *Clin Microbiol Rev*. 1994;7:426-461.
7. Levaditi C, Nicolau S, Schoen R. L'agent etiologique de l'enchalite epizootique du lapin (Encephalitozoon cuniculi). *C R Soc Biol*. 1923;89:984-986.
8. Matsubayashi H, Koide T, Mikata T, et al. A case of Encephalitozoon-like body infection in man. *Arch Pathol Lab Med*. 1959;67:181-185.
9. Desportes I, Le Charpentier Y, Galian A, et al. Occurrence of a new microsporidan: Enterocytozoon bieneusi n. g., n. sp., in the enterocytes of a human patient with AIDS. *J Protozool*. 1985;32:250-254.
10. Sprague V, Becnel JJ, Hazard EI. Taxonomy of phylum microspora. *Crit Rev Microbiol*. 1992;18:285-395.
11. Silveira H, Canning EU. Vittaforma corneae n. comb. for the human microsporidium Nosema corneum Shadduck, Meccoli, Davis & Font, 1990, based on its ultrastructure in the liver of experimentally infected athymic mice. *J Eukaryot Microbiol*. 1995;42:158-165.
12. Cali A, Takvorian PM, Lewin S, et al. Brachiola vesicularum, n. g., n. sp., a new microsporidium associated with AIDS and myositis. *J Eukaryot Microbiol*. 1998;45:240-251.
13. Franzen C, Nassonova ES, Scholmerich J, et al. Transfer of the genus Brachiola (microsporidia) to the genus Anncaliia based on ultrastructural and molecular data. *J Eukaryot Microbiol*. 2006;53:26-35.
14. Cali A, Kotler DP, Orenstein JM. Septata intestinalis N. G., N. Sp., an intestinal microsporidian associated with chronic diarrhea and dissemination in AIDS patients. *J Eukaryot Microbiol*. 1993;40:101-112.
15. Hartskeerl RA, Van Gool T, Schuitema AR, et al. Genetic and immunological characterization of the microsporidian Septata intestinalis Cali, Kotler and Orenstein, 1993: reclassification to Encephalitozoon intestinalis. *Parasitology*. 1995;110(Pt 3):277-285.
16. Field AS, Marriott DJ, Milliken ST, et al. Myositis associated with a newly described microsporidian, Trachipleistophora hominis, in a patient with AIDS. *J Clin Microbiol*. 1996;34:2803-2811.
17. Yachnis AT, Berg J, Martinez-Salazar A, et al. Disseminated microsporidiosis especially infecting the brain, heart, and kidneys: Report of a newly recognized pansporoblastic species in two symptomatic AIDS patients. *Am J Clin Pathol*. 1996;106:535-543.
18. Rastrelli P, Didier E, Yee R. Microsporidial keratitis. *Ophthalmol Clin North Am*. 1994;7:614-635.
19. Orenstein JM, Gaetz HP, Yachnis AT, et al. Disseminated microsporidiosis in AIDS: Are any organs spared? *AIDS*. 1997;11:385-386.
20. Sheth SG, Bates C, Federman M, et al. Fulminant hepatic failure caused by microsporidial infection in a patient with AIDS. *AIDS*. 1997;11:553-554.
21. Weber R, Deplazes P, Flepp M, et al. Cerebral microsporidiosis due to Encephalitozoon cuniculi in a patient with human immunodeficiency virus infection. *N Engl J Med*. 1997;336:474-478.
22. Sheikh RA, Prindiville TP, Yenamandra S, et al. Microsporidial AIDS cholangiopathy due to Encephalitozoon intestinalis: Case report and review. *Am J Gastroenterol*. 2000;95:2364-2371.
23. Visvesvara GS, da Silva AJ, Croppo GP, et al. In vitro culture and serologic and molecular identification of Septata intestinalis isolated from urine of a patient with AIDS. *J Clin Microbiol*. 1995;33:930-936.
24. Shadduck JA, Meccoli RA, Davis R, et al. Isolation of a microsporidian from a human patient. *J Infect Dis*. 1990;162:773-776.
25. Cali A, Takvorian PM, Lewin S, et al. Identification of a new Nosema-like microsporidian associated with myositis in an AIDS patient. *J Eukaryot Microbiol*. 1996;43:108S.
26. Chupp GL, Alroy J, Adelman LS, et al. Myositis due to Pleistophora (Microsporidia) in a patient with AIDS. *Clin Infect Dis*. 1993;16:15-21.
27. Cali A, Takvorian PM. Ultrastructure and development of Pleistophora ronneafiei n. sp., a microsporidium (Protista) in the skeletal muscle of an immune-compromised individual. *J Eukaryot Microbiol*. 2003;50:77-85.
28. Vavra J, Yachnis AT, Shadduck JA, et al. Microsporidia of the genus Trachipleistophora—causative agents of human microsporidiosis: Description of Trachipleistophora anthropophthera n. sp. (Protozoa: Microsporidia). *J Eukaryot Microbiol*. 1998;45:273-283.
29. Pol S, Romana CA, Richard S, et al. Microsporidia infection in patients with the human immunodeficiency virus and unexplained cholangitis. *N Engl J Med*. 1993;328:95-99.
30. Franzen C, Muller A. Microsporidiosis: Human diseases and diagnosis. *Microbes Infect*. 2001;3:389-400.
31. Desportes-Livage I. Biology of microsporidia. *Contrib Microbiol*. 2000;6:140-165.
32. Williams BA, Hirt RP, Lucocq JM, et al. A mitochondrial remnant in the microsporidian Trachipleistophora hominis. *Nature*. 2002;418:865-869.
33. Weber R, Deplazes P, Schwartz D. Diagnosis and clinical aspects of human microsporidiosis. *Contrib Microbiol*. 2000;6:166-192.
34. Vavra J. Structure of the microsporidia. In: Bulla LA Jr, Cheng TC, eds. Comparative Pathobiology. vol 1. New York: Plenum Press; 1976:1-85.
35. Southern TR, Jolly CE, Lester ME, et al. EnP1, a microsporidian spore wall protein that enables spores to adhere to and infect host cells in vitro. *Eukaryot Cell*. 2007;6:1354-1362
36. Xu Y, Weiss LM. The microsporidian polar tube: A highly specialised invasion organelle. *Int J Parasitol*. 2005;35:941-953.
37. Xu Y, Takvorian PM, Cali A, et al. Glycosylation of the major polar tube protein of Encephalitozoon hellem, a microsporidian parasite that infects humans. *Infect Immun*. 2004;72:6341-6350.
38. Xu Y, Takvorian P, Cali A, et al. Identification of a new spore wall protein from Encephalitozoon cuniculi. *Infect Immun*. 2006;74:239-247
39. Foucault C, Drancourt M. Actin mediates Encephalitozoon intestinalis entry into the human enterocyte-like cell line, Caco-2. *Microb Pathog*. 2000;28:51-58.
40. Lom J. On the structure of the extruded microsporidian polar filament. *Z Parasitenkd*. 1972;38:200-213.
41. Weidner E. Ultrastructural study of microsporidian invasion into cells. *Z Parasitenkd*. 1972;40:227-242.
42. Undeen AH, Frixione E. The role of osmotic pressure in the germination of Nosema algerae spores. *J Protozool*. 1990;37:561-567.
43. Lom J, Vavra J. The mode of sporoplasm extrusion in microsporidian spores. *Acta Protozool*. 1963;1:81-89.
44. Keohane E, Weiss LM. The structure, function, and composition of the microsporidian polar tube. In: Wittner M, Weiss LM, eds. *The Microsporidia and Microsporidiosis*. Washington DC: ASM Press; 1999:196-224.
45. Undeen AH, Solter LF. Sugar acquisition during the development of microsporidian (Microspora: Sosematidae) spores. *J Invertebr Pathol*. 1997;70:106-112.
46. Undeen AH, Vander Meer RK. Microsporidian intrasporal sugars and their role in germination. *J Invertebr Pathol*. 1999;73:294-302.
47. Curgy JJ, Vavra J, Vivares C. Presence of ribosomal RNAs with prokaryotic properties in Microsporidia, eukaryotic organisms. *Biol Cell*. 1980;38:49-52.
48. Vossbrinck CR, Woese CR. Eukaryotic ribosomes that lack a 5.8S RNA. *Nature*. 1986;320:287-288.
49. Vossbrinck CR, Maddox JV, Friedman S, et al. Ribosomal RNA sequence suggests microsporidia are extremely ancient eukaryotes. *Nature*. 1987;326:411-414.
50. Weiss LM, Vossbrinck CR. Microsporidiosis: Molecular and diagnostic aspects. *Adv Parasitol*. 1998;40:351-395.

51. Vivares CP, Metenier G. Towards the minimal eukaryotic parasitic genome. *Curr Opin Microbiol.* 2000;3:463-467.
52. Brugere JF, Cornillot E, Metenier G, et al. Encephalitozoon cuniculi (Microspora) genome: Physical map and evidence for telomere-associated rDNA units on all chromosomes. *Nucleic Acids Res.* 2000;28:2026-2033.
53. Katiyar SK, Visvesvara GS, Edlind TD. Comparisons of ribosomal RNA sequences from amitochondrial protozoa: Implications for processing, mRNA binding and paromomycin susceptibility. *Gene.* 1995;152:27-33.
54. Weiss LM, Vossbrinck CR. Molecular biology, molecular phylogeny, and molecular diagnostic approaches to the microsporidia. In: Wittner M, Weiss LM, eds. *The Microsporidia and Microsporidiosis.* Washington, DC: ASM Press; 1999:129-171.
55. Corradi N, Akiyoshi DE, Morrison HG, et al. Patterns of genome evolution among the microsporidian parasites Encephalitozoon cuniculi, Antonospora locustae and Enterocytozoon bieneusi. *PLoS ONE.* 2007;2:e1277.
56. Brugere JF, Cornillot E, Metenier G, et al. Occurrence of subtelomeric rearrangements in the genome of the microsporidian parasite Encephalitozoon cuniculi, as revealed by a new fingerprinting procedure based on two-dimensional pulsed field gel electrophoresis. *Electrophoresis.* 2000;21:2576-2581.
57. Vossbrinck CF, Maddox JV, Friedman S, et al. Ribosomal RNA sequence suggests microsporidia are extremely ancient eukaryotes. *Nature.* 1987;326:411-414.
58. Baker MD, Vossbrinck CR, Maddox JV, et al. Phylogenetic relationships among Vairimorpha and Nosema species (Microspora) based on ribosomal RNA sequence data. *J Invertebr Pathol.* 1994;64:100-106.
59. Franzen C, Muller A. Molecular techniques for detection, species differentiation, and phylogenetic analysis of microsporidia. *Clin Microbiol Rev.* 1999;12:243-285.
60. Baker MD, Vossbrinck CR, Didier ES, et al. Small subunit ribosomal DNA phylogeny of various microsporidia with emphasis on AIDS related forms. *J Eukaryot Microbiol.* 1995;42:564-570.
61. Didier ES, Vossbrinck CR, Baker MD, et al. Identification and characterization of three Encephalitozoon cuniculi strains. *Parasitology.* 1995;111(Pt 4):411-421.
62. Rinder H, Thomschke A, Dengjel B, et al. Close genotypic relationship between Enterocytozoon bieneusi from humans and pigs and first detection in cattle. *J Parasitol.* 2000;86:185-188.
63. Tuzet O, Maurand J, Fize JA, et al. Proposition d'un nouveau cadre systematique pour les genres de Microsporidies. *C R Acad Sci (Paris).* 1971;272:1268-1271.
64. Larsson JIR. Identification of microsporidian genera: A guide with comments on the taxonomy. *Arch Protistenkd.* 1988;136:1-37.
65. Issi IV. Microsporidia as a phylum of parasitic protozoa [in Russian]. *Protozoology.* 1986;10:6-135.
66. Weiser J. A proposal of the basis for microsporidian taxonomy. *Proc Int Congr Protozool.* 1977;5:267.
67. Baker MD. *Phylogenetic Relationships of Five Microsporidian Genera Based on Ribosomal RNA Sequence Data.* Urbana-Champaign: University of Illinois; 1987.
68. Didier ES, Didier PJ, Friedberg DN, et al. Isolation and characterization of a new human microsporidian, Encephalitozoon hellem (n. sp.) from three AIDS patients with keratoconjunctivitis. *J Infect Dis.* 1991;163:617-621.
69. Keeling PJ, McFadden GI. Origins of microsporidia. *Trends Microbiol.* 1998;6:19-23.
70. Weiss LM, Edlind TD, Vossbrinck CR, et al. Microsporidian molecular phylogeny: The fungal connection. *J Eukaryot Microbiol.* 1999;46:17S-18S.
71. Hirt RP, Logsdon JM Jr, Healy B, et al. Microsporidia are related to fungi: Evidence from the largest subunit of RNA polymerase II and other proteins. *Proc Natl Acad Sci U S A.* 1999;96:580-585.
72. Edlind T, Katiyar S, Visvesvara G, et al. Evolutionary origins of microsporidia and basis for benzimidazole sensitivity: An update. *J Eukaryot Microbiol.* 1996;43:109S.
73. Keeling PJ, Doolittle WF. Alpha-tubulin from early-diverging eukaryotic lineages and the evolution of the tubulin family. *Mol Biol Evol.* 1996;13:1297-1305.
74. Arisue N, Sanchez LB, Weiss LM, et al. Mitochondrial-type hsp70 genes of the amitochondriate protists, Giardia intestinalis, Entamoeba histolytica and two microsporidians. *Parasitol Int.* 2002;51:9-16.
75. Germot A, Philippe H, Le GH. Evidence for loss of mitochondria in microsporidia from a mitochondrial-type hsp70 in Nosema locustae. *Mol Biochem Parasitol.* 1997;87:159-168.
76. Hirt RP, Healy B, Vossbrinck CR, et al. A mitochondrial Hsp70 orthologue in Vairimorpha necatrix: Molecular evidence that microsporidia once contained mitochondria. *Curr Biol.* 1997;7:995-998.
77. Peyretaillade E, Broussolle V, Peyret P, et al. Microsporidia, amitochondrial protists, possess a 70-kDa heat shock protein gene of mitochondrial evolutionary origin. *Mol Biol Evol.* 1998;15:683-689.
78. Vivares C, Biderre C, Duffieux F, et al. Chromosomal localization of five genes in Encephalitozoon cuniculi (Microsporidia). *J Eukaryot Microbiol.* 1996;43:97S.
79. Edlind T. Phylogenetics of protozoan tubulin with reference to the amitochondriate eukaryotes. In: Coombs GH, Vickerman K, Sleigh MA, Warren A, eds. *Evolutionary Relationships Among Protozoa.* London: Chapman & Hall; 1998:91-108.
80. Kamaishi T, Hashimoto T, Nakamura Y, et al. Protein phylogeny of translation elongation factor EF-1 alpha suggests microsporidians are extremely ancient eukaryotes. *J Mol Evol.* 1996;42:257-263.
81. Desportes I. Ultratrastructure de Stempellia mutabilis leger et Hess, microsporidie parasite de l'ephemere Ephemera vulgatta. *L Protistologica.* 1976;12:121-150.
82. Flegel TW, Pasharawipas T. A proposal for typical eukaryotic meiosis in microsporidians. *Can J Microbiol.* 1995;41:1-11.
83. Fast NM, Logsdon JM Jr, Doolittle WF. Phylogenetic analysis of the TATA box binding protein (TBP) gene from Nosema locustae: Evidence for a microsporidia-fungi relationship and spliceosomal intron loss. *Mol Biol Evol.* 1999;16:1415-1419.
84. Katinka MD, Duprat S, Cornillot E, et al. Genome sequence and gene compaction of the eukaryote parasite Encephalitozoon cuniculi. *Nature.* 2001;414:450-453.
85. Keeling PJ. Congruent evidence from alpha-tubulin and beta-tubulin gene phylogenies for a zygomycete origin of microsporidia. *Fungal Genet Biol.* 2003;38:298-309.
86. Avery SW, Undeen AH. The isolation of microsporidia and other pathogens from concentrated ditch water. *J Am Mosq Control Assoc.* 1987;3:54-58.
87. Cotte L, Rabodonirina M, Chapuis F, et al. Waterborne outbreak of intestinal microsporidiosis in persons with and without human immunodeficiency virus infection. *J Infect Dis.* 1999;180:2003-2008.
88. Sparfel JM, Sarfati C, Liguory O, et al. Detection of microsporidia and identification of Enterocytozoon bieneusi in surface water by filtration followed by specific PCR. *J Eukaryot Microbiol.* 1997;44:78S.
89. Dowd SE, Gerba CP, Pepper IL. Confirmation of the human-pathogenic microsporidia Enterocytozoon bieneusi, Encephalitozoon intestinalis, and Vittaforma corneae in water. *Appl Environ Microbiol.* 1998;64:3332-3335.
90. Enriquez FJ, Taren D, Cruz-Lopez A, et al. Prevalence of intestinal encephalitozoonosis in Mexico. *Clin Infect Dis.* 1998;26:1227-1229.
91. Hutin YJ, Sombardier MN, Liguory O, et al. Risk factors for intestinal microsporidiosis in patients with human immunodeficiency virus infection: A case-control study. *J Infect Dis.* 1998;178:904-907.
92. Conteas CN, Berlin OG, Lariviere MJ, et al. Examination of the prevalence and seasonal variation of intestinal microsporidiosis in the stools of persons with chronic diarrhea and human immunodeficiency virus infection. *Am J Trop Med Hyg.* 1998;58:559-561.
93. Wuhib T, Silva TMJ, Newman RD, et al. Cryptosporidial and microsporidial infections in human immunodeficiency virus-infected patients in northeastern Brazil. *J Infect Dis.* 1994;170:494-497.
94. Waller T. Sensitivity of Encephalitozoon cuniculi to various temperatures, disinfectants and drugs. *Lab Anim.* 1979;13:227-230.
95. Li X, Fayer R. Infectiviety of microsporidian spores exposed to temperature extremes and chemical disinfectants. *J Eukaryot Microbiol.* 2006;53(suppl 1):S77-S79.
96. Schwartz DA, Visvesvara GS, Diesenhouse MC, et al. Pathologic features and immunofluorescent antibody demonstration of ocular microsporidiosis (Encephalitozoon hellem) in seven patients with acquired immunodeficiency syndrome. *Am J Ophthalmol.* 1993;115:285-292.
97. Fuentealba IC, Mahoney NT, Shadduck JA, et al. Hepatic lesions in rabbits infected with Encephalitozoon cuniculi administered per rectum. *Vet Pathol.* 1992;29:536-540.
98. Schwartz DA, Visvesvara G, Weber R, et al. Male genital tract microsporidiosis and AIDS: Prostatic abscess due to Encephalitozoon hellem. *J Eukaryot Microbiol.* 1994;41:61S.
99. Schwartz DA, Bryan RT, Hewanlowe KO, et al. Disseminated microsporidiosis and AIDS; pathologic evidence for respiratory transmission of Encephalitozoon infection. In: Proceedings of the International Conference on AIDS, July 19-24, 1992, v. 8.
100. Bryan RT, Schwartz DA. Epidemiology of microsporidiosis. In: Wittner M, Weisss LM, eds. *The Microsporidia and Microsporidiosis.* Washington DC: ASM Press; 1999:502-516.
101. Hunt RD, King NW, Foster HL. Encephalitozoonosis: evidence for vertical transmission. *J Infect Dis.* 1972;126:212-214.
102. Matthis A, Weber R, Deplazes P. Zoonotic potential of the microsporidia. *Clin Microbiol Rev.* 2005;18:423-445.
103. Deplazes P, Mathis A, Weber R. Epidemiology and zoonotic aspects of microsporidia of mammals and birds. *Contrib Microbiol.* 2000;6:236-260.
104. Yee RW, Tio FO, Martinez JA, et al. Resolution of microsporidial epithelial keratopathy in a patient with AIDS. *Ophthalmology.* 1991;98:196-201.
105. Deplazes P, Mathis A, Muller C, et al. Molecular epidemiology of Encephalitozoon cuniculi and first detection of Enterocytozoon bieneusi in faecal samples of pigs. *J Eukaryot Microbiol.* 1996;43:93S.
106. Del Aguila C, Izquierdo F, Navajas R, et al. Enterocytozoon bieneusi in animals: Rabbits and dogs as new hosts. *J Eukaryot Microbiol.* 1999;46:8S-9S.
107. Reetz J, Rinder H, Thomschke A, et al. First detection of the microsporidium Enterocytozoon bieneusi in non-mammalian hosts (chickens). *Int J Parasitol.* 2002;32:785-787.
108. Graczyk TK, Sunderland D, Rule AM, et al. Urban feral pigeons (Columba livia) as a source for air- and waterborne contamination with Enterocytozoon bieneusi spores. *Appl Environ Microbiol.* 2007;73:4357-4358.
109. Mansfield KG, Carville A, Shvetz D, et al. Identification of an Enterocytozoon bieneusi-like microsporidian parasite in simian-immunodeficiency-virus-inoculated macaques with hepatobiliary disease. *Am J Pathol.* 1997;150:1395-1405.
110. Deplazes P, Mathis A, van Saanen M, et al. Dual microsporidial infection due to Vittaforma corneae and Encephalitozoon hellem in a patient with AIDS. *Clin Infect Dis.* 1998;27:1521-1524.
111. Weber R, Bryan RT. Microsporidial infections in immunodeficient and immunocompetent patients. *Clin Infect Dis.* 1994;19:517-521.
112. Cama VA, Pearson J, Cabrera L, et al. Transmission of *Enterocytozoon bieneusi* betweeen a child and guinea pigs. *J Clin Microbiol.* 2007;45:2708-2710.
113. Drobniewski F, Kelly P, Carew A, et al. Human microsporidiosis in African AIDS patients with chronic diarrhea. *J Infect Dis.* 1995;171:515-516.
114. Aoun K, Bouratbine A, Datry A, et al. Presence of intestinal microsporidia in Tunisia: a case report. *Bull Soc Pathol Exot.* 1997;90:176.
115. Hautvast JL, Tolboom JJ, Derks TJ, et al. Asymptomatic intestinal microsporidiosis in a human immunodeficiency virus-seronegative, immunocompetent Zambian child. *Pediatr Infect Dis J.* 1997;16:415-416.
116. Van Gool T, Luderhoff E, Nathoo KJ, et al. High prevalence of Enterocytozoon bieneusi infections among HIV-positive individuals with persistent diarrhoea in Harare, Zimbabwe. *Trans R Soc Trop Med Hyg.* 1995;89:478-480.
117. Morakote N, Siriprasert P, Piangjai S, et al. Microsporidium and Cyclospora in human stools in Chiang Mai, Thailand. *Southeast Asian J Trop Med Public Health.* 1995;26:799-800.
118. Brazil P, Sodre FC, Cuzzi-Maya T, et al. Intestinal microsporidiosis in HIV-positive patients with chronic unexplained diarrhea in Rio de Janeiro, Brazil: Diagnosis, clinical presentation and follow-up. *Rev Inst Med Trop Sao Paulo.* 1996;38:97-102.
119. Weitz JC, Botehlo R, Bryan R. Microsporidiosis in patients with chronic diarrhea and AIDS, in HIV asymptomatic patients and in patients with acute diarrhea. *Rev Med Chil.* 1995;123:849-856.
120. Cegielski JP, Ortega YR, McKee S, et al. Cryptosporidium, Enterocytozoon, and Cyclospora infections in pediatric and adult patients with diarrhea in Tanzania. *Clin Infect Dis.* 1999;28:314-321.
121. Maiga I, Doumbo O, Dembele M, et al. Human intestinal microsporidiosis in Bamako (Mali): the presence of Enterocytozoon bieneusi in HIV seropositive patients. *Sante.* 1997;7:257-262.
122. Wanke CA, DeGirolami P, Federman M. Enterocytozoon bieneusi infection and diarrheal disease in patients who were not infected with human immunodeficiency virus: Case report and review. *Clin Infect Dis.* 1996;23:816-818.
123. Gainzarain JC, Canut A, Lozano M, et al. Detection of Enterocytozoon bieneusi in two human immunodeficiency virus-negative patients with chronic diarrhea by polymerase chain reaction in duodenal biopsy specimens and review. *Clin Infect Dis.* 1998;27:394-398.
124. Albrecht H, Sobottka I. Enterocytozoon bieneusi infection in patients who are not infected with human immunodeficiency virus. *Clin Infect Dis.* 1997;25:344.
125. Sandfort J, Hannemann A, Gelderblom H, et al. Enterocytozoon bieneusi infection in an immunocompetent patient who had acute diarrhea and who was not infected with the human immunodeficiency virus. *Clin Infect Dis.* 1994;19:514-516.
126. Sobottka I, Albrecht H, Schottelius J, et al. Self-limited traveller's diarrhea due to a dual infection with Enterocytozoon bieneusi and Cryptosporidium parvum in an immunocompetent HIV-negative child. *Eur J Clin Microbiol Infect Dis.* 1995;14:919-920.
127. Wichro E, Hoetzl D, Krause R, et al. Microsporidosis in travel-associated chronic diarrhea in immune-competent patients. *Am J Trop Med Hyg.* 2005;73:285-287.
128. Raynaud L, Delbac F, Broussolle V, et al. Identification of Encephalitozoon intestinalis in travelers with chronic diarrhea by specific PCR amplification. *J Clin Microbiol.* 1998;36:37-40.
129. Rabodonirina M, Bertocchi M, Desportes-Livage I, et al. Enterocytozoon bieneusi as a cause of chronic diarrhea in a heart-lung transplant recipient who was seronegative for human immunodeficiency virus. *Clin Infect Dis.* 1996;23:114-117.
130. Sax PE, Rich JD, Pieciak WS, et al. Intestinal microsporidiosis occurring in a liver transplant recipient. *Transplantation.* 1995;60:617-618.
131. Gumbo T, Hobbs RE, Carlyn C, et al. Microsporidia infection in transplant patients. *Transplantation.* 1999;67:482-484.
132. Kelkar R, Sastry PS, Kulkarni SS, et al. Pulmonary microsporidial infection in a patient with CML undergoing allogeneic marrow transplant. *Bone Marrow Transplant.* 1997;19:179-182.
133. Mahmood MN, Keohane ME, Burd EM. Pathologic quiz case: A 45-year-old renal transplant recipient with persistent fever. *Arch Pathol Lab Med.* 2003;127:224-226.
134. Metge S, Van Nhieu JT, Dahmane D, et al. A case of Enterocytozoon bieneusi infection in an HIV-negative renal transplant recipient. *Eur J Clin Microbiol Infect Dis.* 2000;19:221-223.

135. Mohindra AR, Lee MW, Visvesvara G, et al. Disseminated microsporidiosis in a renal transplant recipient. *Transpl Infect Dis.* 2002;4:102-107.
136. Sing A, Tybus K, Heesemann J, et al. Molecular diagnosis of an Enterocytozoon bieneusi human genotype C infection in a moderately immunosuppressed human immunodeficiency virus seronegative liver-transplant recipient with severe chronic diarrhea. *J Clin Microbiol.* 2001;39:2371-2372.
137. Silverstein BE, Cunningham ETJ, Margolis TP, et al. Microsporidial keratoconjunctivitis in a patient without human immunodeficiency virus infection. *Am J Ophthalmol.* 1997;124:395-396.
138. Weiss LM. And now microsporidiosis. *Ann Intern Med.* 1995;123:954-956.
139. Van Gool T, Dankert J. Human microsporidiosis: Clinical, diagnostic and therapeutic aspects of an increasing infection. *Clin Microbiol Infect.* 1995;1:75-85.
140. Bryan RT, Cali A, Owen RL, et al. Microsporidia: Opportunistic pathogens in patients with AIDS. In: Sun T, ed. Progress in Clinical Parasitology. vol 2. New York: Field & Wood; 1991:1-26.
141. Coyle CM, Wittner M, Kotler DP, et al. Prevalence of microsporidiosis due to Enterocytozoon bieneusi and Encephalitozoon (Septata) intestinalis among patients with AIDS-related diarrhea: Determination by polymerase chain reaction to the microsporidian small-subunit rRNA gene. *Clin Infect Dis.* 1996;23:1002-1006.
142. Voglino MC, Donelli G, Rossi P, et al. Intestinal microsporidiosis in Italian individuals with AIDS. *Ital J Gastroenterol.* 1996;28:381-386.
143. Kyaw T, Curry A, Edwards-Jones V, et al. The prevalence of Enterocytozoon bieneusi in acquired immunodeficiency syndrome (AIDS) patients from the northwest of England: 1992-1995. *Br J Biomed Sci.* 1997;54:186-191.
144. Molina JM, Oksenhendler E, Beauvais B, et al. Disseminated microsporidiosis due to Septata intestinalis in patients with AIDS: Clinical features and response to albendazole therapy. *J Infect Dis.* 1995;171:245-249.
145. Molina JM, Tourneur M, Sarfati C, et al. Fumagillin treatment of intestinal microsporidiosis. *N Engl J Med.* 2002;346:1963-1969.
146. Molina JM, Goguel J, Sarfati C, et al. Trial of oral fumagillin for the treatment of intestinal microsporidiosis in patients with HIV infection; ANRS 054 Study Group: Agence Nationale de Recherche sur le SIDA. *AIDS.* 2000;14:1341-1348.
147. Bergquist NR, Stintzing G, Smedman L, et al. Diagnosis of encephalitozoonosis in man by serological tests. *BMJ.* 1984;288:902.
148. Aldras AM, Orenstein JM, Kotler DP, et al. Detection of microsporidia by indirect immunofluorescence antibody test using polyclonal and monoclonal antibodies. *J Clin Microbiol.* 1994;32:608-612.
149. Weiss LM, Cali A, Levee E, et al. Diagnosis of Encephalitozoon cuniculi infection by Western blot and the use of cross-reactive antigens for the possible detection of microsporidiosis in humans. *Am J Trop Med Hyg.* 1992;47:456-462.
150. Singh M, Kane GJ, Mackinlay L, et al. Detection of antibodies to Nosema cuniculi (Protozoa: Microscoporidia) in human and animal sera by the indirect fluorescent antibody technique. *Southeast Asian J Trop Med Public Health.* 1982;13:110-113.
151. WHO parasitic diseases surveillance: Antibody to Encephalitozoon cuniculi in man. *Wkly Epidemiol Rec.* 1983;58:30.
152. Bergquist R, Morfeldt-Mansson L, Pehrson PO, et al. Antibody against Encephalitozoon cuniculi in Swedish homosexual men. *Scand J Infect Dis.* 1984;16:389-391.
153. Van Gool T, Vetter JC, Weinmayr B, et al. High seroprevalence of Encephalitozoon species in immunocompetent subjects. *J Infect Dis.* 1997;175:1020-1024.
154. Pospisilova Z, Ditrich O, Stankova M, et al. Parasitic opportunistic infections in Czech HIV-infected patients: A prospective study. *Cent Eur J Public Health.* 1997;5:208-213.
155. Cislakova L, Prokopcakova H, Stef'kovic M, et al. Encephalitozoon cuniculi—clinical and epidemiologic significance: results of a preliminary serologic study in humans. *Epidemiol Mikrobiol Immunol.* 1997;46:30-33.
156. Didier ES, Varner PW, Didier PJ, et al. Experimental microsporidiosis in immunocompetent and immunodeficient mice and monkeys. *Folia Parasitol.* 1994;41:1-11.
157. Koudela B, Vitovec J, Kucerova Z, et al. The severe combined immunodeficient mouse as a model for Encephalitozoon cuniculi microsporidiosis. *Folia Parasitol (Praha).* 1993;40:279-286.
158. Schmidt EC, Shadduck JA. Mechanisms of resistance to the intracellular protozoan Encephalitozoon cuniculi in mice. *J Immunol.* 1984;133:2712-2719.
159. Hermanek J, Koudela B, Kucerova Z, et al. Prophylactic and therapeutic immune reconstitution of SCID mice infected with Encephalitozoon cuniculi. *Folia Parasitol (Praha).* 1993;40:287-291.
160. Didier ES, Shadduck JA. IFN-gamma and LPS induce murine macrophages to kill Encephalitozoon cuniculi in vitro. *J Eukaryot Microbiol.* 1994;41:34S.
161. Didier ES. Reactive nitrogen intermediates implicated in the inhibition of Encephalitozoon cuniculi (phylum Microspora) replication in murine peritoneal macrophages. *Parasite Immunol.* 1995;17:405-412.
162. Khan IA, Moretto M. Role of gamma interferon in cellular immune response against murine Encephalitozoon cuniculi infection. *Infect Immun.* 1999;67:1887-1893.
163. Bywater JE, Kellett BS. Humoral immune response to natural infection with Encephalitozoon cuniculi in rabbits. *Lab Anim.* 1979;13:293-297.
164. Enriquez FJ, Ditrich O, Palting JD, et al. Simple diagnosis of Encephalitozoon sp. microsporidial infections by using a panspecific antiexospore monoclonal antibody. *J Clin Microbiol.* 1997;35:724-729.
165. Furuya K, Omura M, Kudo S, et al. Recognition profiles of microsporidian Encephalitozoon cuniculi polar tube protein 1 with human immunoglobulin M antibodies. *Parasite Immunol.* 2008;30:13-21.
166. Shtrichman R, Samuel CE. The role of gamma interferon in antimicrobial immunity. *Curr Opin Microbiol.* 2001;4:251-259.
167. Achbarou A, Ombrouck C, Gneragbe T, et al. Experimental model for human intestinal microsporidiosis in interferon gamma receptor knockout mice infected by Encephalitozoon intestinalis. *Parasite Immunol.* 1996;18:387-392.
168. Khan IA, Schwartzman JD, Kasper LH, et al. CD8+ CTLs are essential for protective immunity against Encephalitozoon cuniculi infection. *J Immunol.* 1999;162:6086-6091.
169. Moretto MM, Weiss LM, Combe CL, et al. INF gamma-producing dendritic cells are important for priming of the gut intraepithelial lymphocyte response against intracellular parasitic infection. *J Immunol.* 2007;179:2485-2492.
170. Wong P, Pamer EG. CD8 T cell responses to infectious pathogens. *Annu Rev Immunol.* 2003;21:29-70.
171. Conteas CN, Berlin OG, Speck CE, et al. Modification of the clinical course of intestinal microsporidiosis in acquired immunodeficiency syndrome patients by immune status and anti-human immunodeficiency virus therapy. *Am J Trop Med Hyg.* 1998;58:555-558.
172. Goguel J, Katlama C, Sarfati C, et al. Remission of AIDS-associated intestinal microsporidiosis with highly active antiretroviral therapy. *AIDS.* 1997;11:1658-1659.
173. Foudraine NA, Weverling GJ, van Gool T, et al. Improvement of chronic diarrhoea in patients with advanced HIV-1 infection during potent antiretroviral therapy. *AIDS.* 1998;12:35-41.
174. Terada S, Reddy KR, Jeffers LJ, et al. Microsporidan hepatitis in the acquired immunodeficiency syndrome. *Ann Intern Med.* 1987;107:61-62.
175. Schwartz DA, Anderson DC, Klumpp SA, et al. Ultrastructure of atypical (teratoid) sporogonial stages of Enterocytozoon bieneusi (Microsporidia) in naturally infected rhesus monkeys (Macaca mulatta). *Arch Pathol Lab Med.* 1998;122:423-429.
176. Orenstein JM, Tenner M, Kotler DP. Localization of infection by the microsporidian Enterocytozoon bieneusi in the gastrointestinal tract of AIDS patients with diarrhea. *AIDS.* 1992;6:195-197.
177. Pol S, Romana CA, Richard S, et al. Microsporidia infection in patients with the human immunodeficiency virus and unexplained cholangitis. *N Engl J Med.* 1993;328:95-99.
178. Orenstein JM. Diagnostic pathology of microsporidiosis. *Ultrastruct Pathol.* 2003;27:141-149.
179. Schwartz DA, Sobottka I, Leitch GJ, et al. Pathology of microsporidiosis: Emerging parasitic infections in patients with acquired immunodeficiency syndrome. *Arch Pathol Lab Med.* 1996;120:173-188.
180. Schwartz DA, Abou-Elella A, Wilcox CM, et al. The presence of Enterocytozoon bieneusi spores in the lamina propria of small bowel biopsies with no evidence of disseminated microsporidiosis. Enteric Opportunistic Infections Working Group. *Arch Pathol Lab Med.* 1995;119:424-428.
181. Orenstein JM, Dieterich DT, Kotler DP. Systemic dissemination by a newly recognized intestinal microsporidia species in AIDS. *AIDS.* 1992;6:1143-1150.
182. Soule JB, Halverson AL, Becker RB, et al. A patient with acquired immunodeficiency syndrome and untreated Encephalitozoon (Septata) intestinalis microsporidiosis leading to small bowel perforation: response to albendazole. *Arch Pathol Lab Med.* 1997;121:880-887.
183. Zender HO, Arrigoni E, Eckert J, et al. A case of Encephalitozoon cuniculi peritonitis in a patient with AIDS. *Am J Clin Pathol.* 1989;92:352-356.
184. Gunnarsson G, Hurlbut D, DeGirolami PC, et al. Multiorgan microsporidiosis: Report of five cases and review. *Clin Infect Dis.* 1995;21:37-44.
185. Guerard A, Rabodonirina M, Cotte L, et al. Intestinal microsporidiosis occurring in two renal transplant recipients treated with mycophenolate mofetil. *Transplantation.* 1999;68:699-707.
186. Latib MA, Pascoe MD, Duffield MS, et al. Microsporidiosis in the graft of a renal transplant recipient. *Transpl Int.* 2001;14:274-277.
187. Mertens RB, Didier ES, Fishbein MC, et al. Encephalitozoon cuniculi microsporidiosis: Infection of the brain, heart, kidneys, trachea, adrenal glands, and urinary bladder in a patient with AIDS. *Mod Pathol.* 1997;10:68-77.
188. Pariyakanok L, Jongwutiwes S. Keratitis caused by Trachipleistophora anthropopthera. *J Infect.* 2005;51:325-328.
189. Cali A, Meisler DM, Rutherford I, et al. Corneal microsporidiosis in a patient with AIDS. *Am J Trop Med Hyg.* 1991;44:463-468.
190. Joseph J, Sharma S, Murthy SI, et al. Microsporidial keratitis in India: 16S rRAN gene-based PCR assay for diagnsois and species identification of microsporidia in clnical samples. *Invest Ophthalmol Vis Sci.* 2006;47:4468-4473.
191. Coyle CM, Weiss LM, Rhodes LV III, et al. Fatal myositis due to the microsporidian *Brachiola algerae,* a mosquito pathogen. *N Engl J Med.* 2004;351:42-47.
192. Grau A, Valls ME, Williams JE, et al. Myositis caused by Pleistophora in a patient with AIDS. *Med Clin (Barc).* 1996;107:779-781.
193. Ledford DK, Overman MD, Gonzalvo A, et al. Microsporidiosis myositis in a patient with the acquired immunodeficiency syndrome. *Ann Intern Med.* 1985;102:628-630.
194. Schwartz DA, Visvesvara GS, Leitch GJ, et al. Pathology of symptomatic microsporidial (Encephalitozoon hellem) bronchiolitis in the acquired immunodeficiency syndrome: A new respiratory pathogen diagnosed from lung biopsy, bronchoalveolar lavage, sputum, and tissue culture. *Hum Pathol.* 1993;24:937-943.
195. Didier ES, Rogers LB, Orenstein JM, et al. Characterization of Encephalitozoon (Septata) intestinalis isolates cultured from nasal mucosa and bronchoalveolar lavage fluids of two AIDS patients. *J Eukaryot Microbiol.* 1996;43:34-43.
196. Dunand VA, Hammer SM, Rossi R, et al. Parasitic sinusitis and otitis in patients infected with human immunodeficiency virus: report of five cases and review. *Clin Infect Dis.* 1997;25:267-272.
197. Franzen C, Muller A, Salzberger B, et al. Chronic rhinosinusitis in patients with AIDS: Potential role of microsporidia. *AIDS.* 1996;10:687-688.
198. Gritz DC, Holsclaw DS, Neger RE, et al. Ocular and sinus microsporidial infection cured with systemic albendazole. *Am J Ophthalmol.* 1997;124:241-243.
199. Josephson GD, Sarlin J, Reidy J, et al. Microsporidial rhinosinusitis: Is this the next pathogen to infect the sinuses of the immunocompromised host? *Otolaryngol Head Neck Surg.* 1996;114:137-139.
200. Moss RB, Beaudet LM, Wenig BM, et al. Microsporidium-associated sinusitis. *Ear Nose Throat J.* 1997;76:95-101.
201. Pedro-de-Lelis FJ, Sabater-Marco V, Herrera-Ballester A. Necrotizing maxillary sinus mucormycosis related to candidiasis and microsporidiosis in an AIDS patient. *AIDS.* 1995;9:1386-1388.
202. Degroote MA, Visvesvara G, Wilson ML, et al. Polymerase chain reaction and culture confirmation of disseminated Encephalitozoon cuniculi in a patient with AIDS: Successful therapy with albendazole. *J Infect Dis.* 1995;171:1375-1378.
203. Schwartz DA, Bryan RT, Hewanlowe KO, et al. Disseminated microsporidiosis (Encephalitozoon hellem) and acquired immunodeficiency syndrome: Autopsy evidence for respiratory acquisition. *Arch Pathol Lab Med.* 1992;116:660-668.
204. Franzen C, Mueller A, Salzberger B, et al. Chronic rhinosinusitis in patients with AIDS: potential role of microsporidia. *AIDS.* 1996;10:687-688.
205. Del Aguila C, Lopez-Velez R, Fenoy S, et al. Identification of Enterocytozoon bieneusi spores in respiratory samples from an AIDS patient with a 2-year history of intestinal microsporidiosis. *J Clin Microbiol.* 1997;35:1862-1866.
206. Weber R, Kuster H, Keller R, et al. Pulmonary and intestinal microsporidiosis in a patient with the acquired immunodeficiency syndrome. *Am Rev Respir Dis.* 1992;146:1603-1605.
207. Hartskeerl RA, Schuitema AR, van Gool T, et al. Genetic evidence for the occurrence of extra-intestinal Enterocytozoon bieneusi infections. *Nucleic Acids Res.* 1993;21:4150.
208. Visvesvara GS, Belloso M, Moura H, et al. Isolation of Nosema algerae from the cornea of an immunocompetent patient. *J Eukaryot Microbiol.* 1999;46:10S.
209. Kester KE, Visvesara GS, McEvoy P. Organism responsible for nodular cutaneous microsporidiosis in a patient with AIDS. *Ann Intern Med.* 2000;133:925.
210. Kester KE, Turiansky GW, McEvoy PL. Nodular cutaneous microsporidiosis in a patient with AIDS and successful treatment with long-term oral clindamycin therapy. *Ann Intern Med.* 1998;128:911-914.
211. Levaditi C, Nicolau S, Schoen R. Nouvelles donnees sur L'Encephalitozoon cuniculi. *C R Soc Biol.* 1923;89:1157-1162.
212. Margileth AM, Strano AJ, Chandra R, et al. Disseminated nosematosis in an immunologically compromised infant. *Arch Pathol.* 1973;95:145-150.
213. Desportes-Livage I, Doumbo O, Pichard E, et al. Microsporidiosis in HIV-seronegative patients in Mali. *Trans R Soc Trop Med Hyg.* 1998;92:423-424.
214. Lopez-Velez R, Turrientes MC, Garron C, et al. Microsporidiosis in travelers with diarrhea from the tropics. *J Travel Med.* 1999;6:223-227.
215. Muller A, Bialek R, Kamper A, et al. Detection of microsporidia in travelers with diarrhea. *J Clin Microbiol.* 2001;39:1630-1632.
216. Orenstein JM, Chiang J, Steinberg W, et al. Intestinal microsporidiosis as a cause of diarrhea in human immunodeficiency virus-infected patients: A report of 20 cases. *Hum Pathol.* 1990;21:475-481.
217. Tumwine JK, Kekitiinwa A, Nabukeera N, et al. Enterocytozoon bieneusi among children with diarrhea attending Mulago Hospital in Uganda. *Am J Trop Med Hyg.* 2002;67:299-303.
218. Goetz M, Eichenlaub S, Pape GR, et al. Chronic diarrhea as a result of intestinal microsporidiosis in a liver transplant recipient. *Transplantation.* 2001;71:334-337.

219. Kelkar R, Sastry PS, Kulkarni SS, et al. Pulmonary microsporidial infection in a patient with CML undergoing allogeneic marrow transplant. *Bone Marrow Transplant.* 1997;19:179-182.
220. Pinnolis M, Egbert PR, Font RL, et al. Nosematosis of the cornea: Case report, including electron microscopic studies. *Arch Ophthalmol.* 1981;99:1044-1047.
221. Ashton N, Wirasinha PA. Encephalitozoonosis (nosematosis) of the cornea. *Br J Ophthalmol.* 1973;57:669-674.
222. Cali A, Meisler DM, Lowder CY, et al. Corneal microsporidioses: Characterization and identification. *J Protozool.* 1991;38:215S-217S.
223. Davis RM, Font RL, Keisler MS, et al. Corneal microsporidiosis: A case report including ultrastructural observations. *Ophthalmology.* 1990;97:953-957.
224. Weber R, Muller A, Spycher MA, et al. Intestinal Enterocytozoon bieneusi microsporidiosis in an HIV-infected patient: Diagnosis by ileo-colonoscopic biopsies and long-term follow up. *Clin Invest.* 1992;70:1019-1023.
225. Rijpstra AC, Canning EU, Van Ketel RJ, et al. Use of light microscopy to diagnose small-intestinal microsporidiosis in patients with AIDS. *J Infect Dis.* 1988;157:827-831.
226. Molina JM, Sarfati C, Beauvais B, et al. Intestinal microsporidiosis in human immunodeficiency virus-infected patients with chronic unexplained diarrhea: Prevalence and clinical and biologic features. *J Infect Dis.* 1993;167:217-221.
227. Hewan-Lowe K, Furlong B, Sims M, et al. Coinfection with Giardia lamblia and Enterocytozoon bieneusi in a patient with acquired immunodeficiency syndrome and chronic diarrhea. *Arch Pathol Lab Med.* 1997;121:417-422.
228. Beaugerie L, Teilhac MF, Deluol AM, et al. Cholangiopathy associated with microsporidia infection of the common bile duct mucosa in a patient with HIV infection. *Ann Intern Med.* 1992;117:401-402.
229. Hartskeerl RA, van Gool T, Schuitema ARJ, et al. Genetic and immunological characterization of the microsporidian Septata intestinalis Cali, Kotler and Orenstein, 1993: Reclassification to Encephalitozoon intestinalis. *Parasitology.* 1995;110:277-285.
230. Didier ES, Didier PJ, Snowden KF, et al. Microsporidiosis in mammals. *Microbes Infect.* 2000;2:709-720.
231. Schwartz DA, Visvesvara GS, Leitch GJ, et al. Pathology of symptomatic microsporidial (Encephalitozoon hellem) bronchiolitis in the acquired immunodeficiency syndrome: A new respiratory pathogen diagnosed from lung biopsy, bronchoalveolar lavage, sputum, and tissue culture. *Hum Pathol.* 1993;24:937-943.
232. Van Gool T, Canning EU, Gilis H, et al. Septata intestinalis frequently isolated from stool of AIDS patients with a new cultivation method. *Parasitology.* 1994;109:281-289.
233. Willson R, Harrington R, Stewart B, et al. Human immunodeficiency virus 1-associated necrotizing cholangitis caused by infection with Septata intestinalis. *Gastroenterology.* 1995;108:247-251.
234. Belcher JW Jr, Guttenberg SA, Schmookler BM. Microsporidiosis of the mandible in a patient with acquired immunodeficiency syndrome. *J Oral Maxillofac Surg.* 1997;55:424-426.
235. Dore GJ, Marriott DJ, Hing MC, et al. Disseminated microsporidiosis due to Septata intestinalis in nine patients infected with the human immunodeficiency virus: Response to therapy with albendazole. *Clin Infect Dis.* 1995;21:70-76.
236. Weber R, Sauer B, Spycher MA, et al. Detection of Septata intestinalis in stool specimens and coprodiagnostic monitoring of successful treatment with albendazole. *Clin Infect Dis.* 1994;19:342-345.
237. De Groote MA, Visvesvara G, Wilson ML, et al. Polymerase chain reaction and culture confirmation of disseminated Encephalitozoon cuniculi in a patient with AIDS: Successful therapy with albendazole. *J Infect Dis.* 1995;171:1375-1378.
238. Weber R, Kuster H, Visvesvara GS, et al. Disseminated microsporidiosis due to Encephalitozoon hellem: Pulmonary colonization, microhematuria, and mild conjunctivitis in a patient with AIDS. *Clin Infect Dis.* 1993;17:415-419.
239. Visvesvara GS, Leitch GJ, da Silva AJ, et al. Polyclonal and monoclonal antibody and PCR-amplified small-subunit rRNA identification of a microsporidian, Encephalitozoon hellem, isolated from an AIDS patient with disseminated infection. *J Clin Microbiol.* 1994;32:2760-2768.
240. Lowder CY, Meisler DM, McMahon JT, et al. Microsporidia infection of the cornea in a man seropositive for human immunodeficiency virus. *Am J Ophthalmol.* 1990;109:242-244.
241. Lacey CJN, Clarke AMT, Fraser P, et al. Chronic microsporidian infection of the nasal mucosae, sinuses and conjunctivae in HIV disease. *Genitourin Med.* 1992;68:179-181.
242. Franzen C, Schwartz DA, Visvesvara GS, et al. Immunologically confirmed disseminated, asymptomatic Encephalitozoon cuniculi infection of the gastrointestinal tract in a patient with AIDS. *Clin Infect Dis.* 1995;21:1480-1484.
243. Macher AR, Neafie R, Angritt P, et al. Microsporidia myositis and the acquired immunodeficency syndrome (AIDS): A four-year followup. *Ann Intern Med.* 1988;109:343-344.
244. Weber R, Bryan RT, Owen RL, et al. Improved light-microscopal detection of microsporidia spores in stool and duodenal aspirates. *N Engl J Med.* 1992;326:161-166.
245. Vavra J, Dahbiova R, Hollister WS, et al. Staining of microsporidian spores by optical brighteners with remarks on the use of brighteners for the diagnosis of AIDS-associated human microsporidiosis. *Folia Parasitol (Praha).* 1993;40:267-272.
246. Van Gool T, Snijders F, Reiss P, et al. Diagnosis of intestinal and disseminated microsporidial infections in patients with HIV by a new rapid fluorescence technique. *J Clin Pathol.* 1993;46:694-699.
247. Ryan NJ, Sutherland G, Coughlan K, et al. A new trichrome-blue stain for detection of microsporidial species in urine, stool, and nasopharyngeal specimens. *J Clin Microbiol.* 1993;31:3264-3269.
248. Kokoskin E, Gyorkos TW, Camus A, et al. Modified technique for efficient detection of microsporidia. *J Clin Microbiol.* 1994;32:1074-1075.
249. Moura H, Schwartz DA, Bornay-Llinares F, et al. A new and improved "quick-hot Gram-chromotrope" technique that differentially stains microsporidian spores in clinical samples, including paraffin-embedded tissue sections. *Arch Pathol Lab Med.* 1997;121:888-893.
250. Didier ES, Orenstein JM, Aldras A, et al. Comparison of three staining methods for detecting microsporidia in fluids. *J Clin Microbiol.* 1995;33:3138-3145.
251. DeGirolami PC, Ezratty CR, Desai G, et al. Diagnosis of intestinal microsporidiosis by examination of stool and duodenal aspirate with Weber's modified trichrome and Uvitex 2B strains. *J Clin Microbiol.* 1995;33:805-810.
252. Field AS, Marriott DJ, Hing MC. The Warthin-Starry stain in the diagnosis of small intestinal microsporidiosis in HIV-infected patients. *Folia Parasitol (Praha).* 1993;40:261-266.
253. Field AS. Light microscopic and electron microscopic diagnosis of gastrointestinal opportunistic infections in HIV-positive patients. *Pathology.* 2002;34:21-35.
254. Zierdt CH, Gill VJ, Zierdt WS. Detection of microsporidian spores in clinical samples by indirect fluorescent-antibody assay using whole-cell antisera to Encephalitozoon cuniculi and Encephalitozoon hellem. *J Clin Microbiol.* 1993;31:3071-3074.
255. Croppo GP, Visvesvara GS, Leitch GJ, et al. Identification of the microsporidian Encephalitozoon hellem using immunoglobulin G monoclonal antibodies. *Arch Pathol Lab Med.* 1998;122:182-186.
256. Beckers PJ, Derks GJ, Gool T, et al. Encephalitozoon intestinalis-specific monoclonal antibodies for laboratory diagnosis of microsporidiosis. *J Clin Microbiol.* 1996;34:282-285.
257. Accoceberry I, Thellier M, Desportes-Livage I, et al. Production of monoclonal antibodies directed against the microsporidium Enterocytozoon bieneusi. *J Clin Microbiol.* 1999;37:4107-4112.
258. Zhang Q, Singh I, Sheroan A, et al. Producution and characterization of monoclonal antibodies against Enterocytozoon bieneusi purified from rhesus macaques. *Infect Immun.* 1994;73:5166-5172.
259. Sheoran AS, Feng X, Singh I, et al. Monoclonal antibodies against Enterocytozoon bieneusi of human origin. *Clin Diagn Lab Immunol.* 2005;12:1109-1113.
260. Signh I, Sheroran AS, Zhang Q, et al. Sensitivity and specificity of a monoclonal antibody-based fluorescence assay for detecting Enterocytozoon bieneusi spores in feces of simian immunodeficny virus-infected macaques. *Clin Diagn Lab Immunol.* 2005;12:1141-1144.
261. Visvesvara GS. In vitro cultivation of microsporidia of clinical importance. *Clin Microbiol Rev.* 2002;15:401-413.
262. Visvesvara GS, Leitch GJ, Pieniazek NJ, et al. Short-term in vitro culture and molecular analysis of the microsporidian, Enterocytozoon bieneusi. *J Eukaryot Microbiol.* 1995;42:506-510.
263. Visvesvara GS, Leitch GJ, Wallace S, et al. Adenovirus masquerading as microsporidia. *J Parasitol.* 1996;82:316-319.
264. Tzipori S, Carville A, Widmer G, et al. Transmission and establishment of a persistent infection of Enterocytozoon bieneusi, derived from a human with AIDS, in simian immunodeficiency virus-infected rhesus monkeys. *J Infect Dis.* 1997;175:1016-1020.
265. Feng X, Akiyoshi DE, Sheroran A, et al. Serial propagation of the microsporidian Enterocytozoon bieneusi of human origin in immunocompromised rodents. *Infect Immun.* 2006;74:4424-4429.
266. Didier ES. Immunology of microsporidiosis. *Contrib Microbiol.* 2000;6:193-208.
267. Katzwinkel-Wladarsch S, Deplazes P, Weber R, et al. Comparison of polymerase chain reaction with light microscopy for detection of microsporida in clinical specimens. *Eur J Clin Microbiol Infect Dis.* 1997;16:7-10.
268. Fedorko DP, Nelson NA, Cartwright CP. Identification of microsporidia in stool specimens by using PCR and restriction endonucleases. *J Clin Microbiol.* 1995;33:1739-1741.
269. Ombrouck C, Ciceron L, Biligui S, et al. Specific PCR assay for direct detection of intestinal microsporidia Enterocytozoon bieneusi and Encephalitozoon intestinalis in fecal specimens from human immunodeficiency virus-infected patients. *J Clin Microbiol.* 1997;35:652-655.
270. Maggi P, Larocca AM, Quarto M, et al. Effect of antiretroviral therapy on cryptosporidiosis and microsporidiosis in patients infected with human immunodeficiency virus type 1. *Eur J Clin Microbiol Infect Dis.* 2000;19:213-217.
271. Martins SA, Muccioli C, Belfort R Jr, et al. Resolution of microsporidial keratoconjunctivitis in an AIDS patient treated with highly active antiretroviral therapy. *Am J Ophthalmol.* 2001;131:378-379.
272. Miao YM, Awad-El-Kariem FM, Franzen C, et al. Eradication of cryptosporidia and microsporidia following successful antiretroviral therapy. *J Acquir Immune Defic Syndr.* 2000;25:124-129.
273. Beauvais B, Sarfati C, Challier S, et al. In vitro model to assess effect of antimicrobial agents on Encephalitozoon cuniculi. *Antimicrob Agents Chemother.* 1994;38:2440-2448.
274. Franssen FF, Lumeij JT, van Knapen F. Susceptibility of Encephalitozoon cuniculi to several drugs in vitro. *Antimicrob Agents Chemother.* 1995;39:1265-1268.
275. Costa SF, Weiss LM. Drug treatment of microsporidiosis. *Drug Resist Update.* 2000;3:384-399.
276. Didier ES. Effects of albendazole, fumagillin, and TNP-470 on microsporidial replication in vitro. *Antimicrob Agents Chemother.* 1997;41:1541-1546.
277. Diesenhouse MC, Wilson LA, Corrent GF, et al. Treatment of microsporidial keratoconjunctivitis with topical fumagillin. *Am J Ophthalmol.* 1993;115:293-298.
278. Garvey MJ, Ambrose PG, Ulmer JL. Topical fumagillin in the treatment of microsporidial keratoconjunctivitis in AIDS. *Ann Pharmacother.* 1995;29:872-874.
279. Molina JM, Goguel J, Sarfati C, et al. Potential efficacy of fumagillin in intestinal microsporidiosis due to Enterocytozoon bieneusi in patients with HIV infection: Results of a drug screening study. The French Microsporidiosis Study Group. *AIDS.* 1997;11:1603-1610.
280. Blanshard C, Peacock C, Ellis D, et al. Treatment of intestinal microsporidiosis with albendazole. In: *Proceedings of the VII International Conference on AIDS: Science Challenging AIDS*, vol 1. *Clinical Science and Trials.* Florence, Italy, July 16-21, 1991.
281. Aarons EJ, Woodrow D, Hollister WS, et al. Reversible renal failure caused by a microsporidian infection. *AIDS.* 1994;8:1119-1121.
282. Corcoran GD, Isaacson JR, Daniels C, et al. Urethritis associated with disseminated microsporidiosis: Clinical response to albendazole. *Clin Infect Dis.* 1996;22:592-593.
283. Dieterich DT, Lew EA, Kotler DP, et al. Treatment with albendazole for intestinal disease due to Enterocytozoon bieneusi in patients with AIDS. *J Infect Dis.* 1994;169:178-183.
284. Li J, Katiyar SK, Hamelin A, et al. Tubulin genes from AIDS-associated microsporidia and implications for phylogeny and benzimidazole sensitivity. *Mol Biochem Parasitol.* 1996;78:289-295.
285. Akiyoshi DE, Weiss LM, Feng X, et al. Analysis of the beta-tubulin genes from Enterocytozoon bieneusi isolates form a human and rhesus macaque. *J Eukaryot Microbiol.* 2007;54:38-41.
286. Franzen C, Salzberger B. Analysis of the beta-tubulin gene from Vittaforma corneae suggests bensimidazole resistance. *Antimicrobial Agents Chemother.* 2008;52:790-793.
287. Molina JM, Chastang C, Goguel J, et al. Albendazole for treatment and prophylaxis of microsporidiosis due to Encephalitozoon intestinalis in patients with AIDS: A randomized double-blind controlled trial. *J Infect Dis.* 1998;177:1373-1377.
288. Sobottka I, Albrecht H, Schafer H, et al. Disseminated Encephalitozoon (Septata) intestinalis infection in a patient with AIDS: Novel diagnostic approaches and autopsy-confirmed parasitological cure following treatment with albendazole. *J Clin Microbiol.* 1995;33:2948-2952.
289. Lecuit M, Oksenhendler E, Sarfati C. Use of albendazole for disseminated microsporidian infection in a patient with AIDS. *J Infect Dis.* 1994;19:332-333.
290. Visvesvara GS, Leitch GJ, Dasilva AJ, et al. Polyclonal and monoclonal antibody and PCR-amplified small-subunit rRNA identification of a microsporidian, Encephalitozoon hellem, isolated from an AIDS patient with disseminated infection. *J Clin Microbiol.* 1994;32:2760-2768.
291. Blanshard C, Ellis DS, Tovey DG, et al. Treatment of intestinal microsporidiosis with albendazole in patients with AIDS. *AIDS.* 1992;6:311-313.
292. Leder K, Ryan N, Spelman D, et al. Microsporidial disease in HIV-infected patients: a report of 42 patients and review of the literature. *Scand J Infect Dis.* 1998;30:331-338.
293. Eeftinck Schattenkerk JK, van Gool T, van Ketel RJ, et al. Clinical significance of small-intestinal microsporidiosis in HIV-1-infected individuals. *Lancet.* 1991;337:895-898.
294. Anwar-Bruni DM, Hogan SE, Schwartz DA, et al. Atovaquone is effective treatment for the symptoms of gastrointestinal microsporidiosis in HIV-1-infected patients. *AIDS.* 1996;10:619-623.
295. Bicart-Sée A, Massip P, Linas MD, et al. Successful treatment with nitazoxanide of Enterocytozoon bieneusi microsporidiosis in a patient with AIDS. *Antimicrob Agents Chemother.* 2000;44:167-168.
296. Albrecht H, Sobottka I, Stellbrink HJ, et al. Does the choice of Pneumocystis carinii prophylaxis influence the prevalence of Enterocytozoon bieneusi microsporidiosis in AIDS patients? *AIDS.* 1995;9:302-303.
297. Sharpstone D, Rowbottom A, Francis N, et al. Thalidomide: A novel therapy for microsporidiosis. *Gastroenterology.* 1997;112:1823-1829.
298. Kano T, Fukui H. Studies on Pleistophora infection in eel, Anguilla japonica. I. Experimental induction of microsporidiosis and fumagillin efficacy. *Fish Pathol.* 1982;16:193-200.

299. Higgins MJ, Kent ML, Moran JD, et al. Efficacy of the fumagillin analog TNP-470 for Nucleospora salmonis and Loma salmonae infections in chinook salmon Oncorhynchus tshawytscha. *Dis Aquat Organ*. 1998;34:45-49.

300. Coyle C, Kent M, Tanowitz HB, et al. TNP-470 is an effective antimicrosporidial agent. *J Infect Dis*. 1998;177:515-518.

301. Didier PJ, Phillips JN, Kuebler DJ, et al. Antimicrosporidial activities of fumagillin, TNP-470, ovalicin, and ovalicin derivatives in vitro and in vivo. *Antimicrob Agents Chemother*. 2006;50:2146-2155.

302. Weiss LM, Costa SF, Zhang H. Microsporidian methionine aminopeptidase type 2. *J Eukaryot Microbiol*. 2001;48(suppl): 88S-90S.

303. Rosberger DF, Serdarevic ON, Erlandson RA, et al. Successful treatment of microsporidial keratoconjunctivitis with topical fumagillin in a patient with AIDS. *Cornea*. 1993;12:261-265.

304. Wilkins JH, Joshi N, Margolis TP, et al. Microsporidial keratoconjunctivitis treated successfully with a short course of fumagillin. *Eye*. 1994;8(Pt 6):703-704.

305. Lowder CY, McMahon JT, Meisler DM, et al. Microsporidial keratoconjunctivitis caused by Septata intestinalis in a patient with acquired immunodeficiency syndrome. *Am J Ophthalmol*. 1996;121:715-717.

306. Orenstein JM, Seedor J, Friedberg DN, et al. Microsporidian keratoconjunctivitis in patients with AIDS. *MMWR Morb Mortal Wkly Rep*. 1990;39:188-189.

272

Introduction to Protozoal Diseases

JONATHAN I. RAVDIN | WILLIAM A. PETRI, JR

The protozoans known to infect humans are a diverse group, as indicated by phylogeny (Table 272-1), epidemiology (Table 272-2), clinical manifestations (Table 272-3), preferred diagnostic studies (Table 272-4), and chemotherapeutic agents effective in eradicating or arresting infection (see Chapter 44).[1,2] The phylum Protozoa is composed of morphologically simple eukaryotic organisms. Protozoa may be divided, for convenience, into four distinct groups based on method of locomotion: mastigophora (flagella), sarcodina (pseudopodia), apicomplexa (microtubule complex, commonly referred to as sporozoa), and ciliophora (ciliates) (see Table 272-1). Protozoans such as *Plasmodium* spp., *Entamoeba histolytica*, *Trypanosoma* spp., and *Leishmania* spp. are major worldwide pathogens and are among the leading causes of morbidity and mortality in areas of Africa, Asia, and Central and South America. *Giardia lamblia* and *Cryptosporidium* are frequent causes of diarrhea in developing areas and established industrialized countries. *Toxoplasma gondii*, *Cryptosporidium* spp., *Cyclospora*, *Trypanosoma cruzi*, and *Leishmania* spp. all have been noted to cause severe diseases in patients with acquired immunodeficiency syndrome.

Dramatic advancements in the last several years include the first vaccine for a parasite shown to be effective in humans, the RTS,S circumsporozoite-based vaccine for malaria, radical changes in parasite diagnostic techniques as micoscopy is replaced with more accurate and sensitive techniques (e.g., antigen detection and the polymerase chain reaction [PCR] assay), and improved understanding of pathogenesis as host, parasite, and environmental factors influencing disease are unraveled.

Advances even in taxonomy of the protozoan parasites have been profound. A fifth species of malaria, *Plasmodium knowlesi*, is now known to infect humans, as well as a third member of the *Entamoeba histolytica-dispar* complex, *E. moshkovskii*.[3,4] Cryptosporidia that infect humans are now recognized to include not only *Cryptosporidium parvum* but also *C. hominis* and additional zoonotic species.[5] Within

---

TABLE 272-1 Classification of Protozoans that Infect Humans

Phylum 1. Sarcomastigophora (flagella, pseudopodia)
  Subphylum I. Mastiglophora (flagella)
    Class 2. Zoomastigophorea
      Order 2. Kinetoplastida
        Suborder 2. Trypanosomatina
          Leishmania, Trypanosoma
      Order 5. Diplomonadida
        Suborder 2. Diplomonadina
          Giardia
      Order 7. Trichomonadida
        Dientamoeba, Trichomonas
  Subphylum III. Sarcodina (pseudopodia)
    Super class 1. Rhizopoda
      Class 1. Lobosea
        Subclass 1. Gymnamoebia
          Order 1. Amoebida
            Suborder 1. Tubulina
              Entamoeba
            Suborder 5. Acanthopodina
              Acanthamoeba
          Order 2. Schizopyrenida
            Naegleria
Phylum III. Apicomplexa (apical microtubule complex)
  Class 2. Sporozoea
    Subclass 2. Coccidia
      Order 1. Piroplasmida
        Babesia
      Order 3. Eucoccidia
        Suborder 2. Eimeriina
          Cryptosporidium, Isospora, Sarcocystis, Toxoplasma
        Suborder 3. Haemosporina
          Plasmodium
        Suborder 3. Piroplasmia
Phylum VII. Ciliophora (ciliated)
  Class I. Kinetofragminophorea
    Subclass 2. Vestibuliferia
      Order 1. Trichostomatida
        Suborder 1. Trichostomatina
          Balantidium

Data from Committee on Systematics and Evolution of the Society of Protozoologists. A newly revised classification of the protozoa. *J Protozool*. 1980;27:37-58.

TABLE 272-2 Geographic Distribution and Mechanism of Transmission of Protozoal Infections

Organism	Geographic Distribution	Means of Transmission
Acanthamoeba spp.	Undefined	Water
Babesia spp.	North America, Europe	Tick-borne, blood transfusions
Balantidium coli.	Worldwide	Zoonosis (pigs), water,* fecal-oral
Blastocystis hominis	Unknown	Fecal-oral, water
Cryptosporidium spp.	Worldwide	Water, fecal-oral, zoonosis
Entamoeba histolytica	Worldwide	Water, fecal-oral, foodborne
Giardia lamblia	Worldwide	Water, fecal-oral, foodborne
Isospora spp.	Worldwide	Fecal-oral, suspected zoonosis
Leishmania spp.[†]		Sand fly
L. donovani	India, Pakistan, East Africa, China	
L. tropica	Middle East, Central Asia	
L. major	Middle East, India, Pakistan	
L. aethiopica	Ethiopia, Kenya	
L. mexicana	Central America, Texas	
L. amazonensis	South America	
L. chagasi	Latin America	
L. viannia braziliensis	Latin America	
Naegleria spp.	Worldwide	Fresh water, intranasal exposure
Plasmodium spp.	Africa, Asia, South and Central America, Oceania	Female anopheline mosquitoes, inoculation of infected blood
Sarcocystis spp.	Unknown	Foodborne (meat)
Toxoplasma gondii	Worldwide	Zoonosis (cats), foodborne (meat), blood or organ transplant, congenital
Trichomonas vaginalis	Worldwide	Venereal, during birth (?); nonvenereal, sexually transmitted
Trypanosoma spp.		
T. cruzi	South and Central America	Reduviid bugs
T. brucei gambiense	West Africa	Tsetse fly
T. brucei rhodesiense	East Africa	Tsetse fly

*Ingestion of water contaminated with fecal material.
[†]Other *Leishmania* spp. also infect humans but are less common.

TABLE 272-3	Clinical Syndromes Caused by Protozoan Infection
Organism (Disease)	*Major Clinical Syndrome*
Acanthamoeba spp.	Keratitis, granulomatous amebic encephalitis
Babesia spp. (babesiosis)	Fever, malaise, hepatosplenomegaly, and hemolytic anemia, especially in the asplenic
Balantidium coli (balantidiosis)	Colitis
Blastocystis hominis (blastocystis)	Diarrhea
Cryptosporidium spp. (crytosporidiosis)	Self-limiting noninflammatory diarrhea; chronic severe diarrhea and cholangitis in AIDS patients
Dientamoeba fragilis	Diarrhea
Entamoeba histolytica (amebiasis)	Diarrhea, colitis, liver abscess
Giardia lamblia (giardiasis)	Noninflammatory diarrhea with malabsorption
Isospora spp. (isosporiasis)	Diarrhea
Leishmania spp. (cutaneous and visceral leishmaniasis)	Cutaneous or mucosal ulceration; visceral disease with fever, hepatosplenomegaly
Leptomyxida	Granulomatous amebic encephalitis
Naegleria spp.	Meningoencephalitis
Plasmodium spp. (malaria)	Paroxysmal fever, chills, headache, hepatosplenomegaly
Sarcocystis spp.	Myositis, fever
Toxoplasma gondii (toxoplasmosis)	Fever, malaise, lymphadenopathy; chorioretinitis; congenital abnormalities; in immunocompromised host, encephalitis, myocarditis, pneumonitis
Trichomas vaginalis (trichomoniasis)	Vaginitis, urethritis
Trypanosoma spp. (African sleeping sickness and Chagas' disease)	Fever, lymphadenopathy, meningoencephalitis, myocarditis; megaesophagus and megacolon, congestive cardiopathy

AIDS, acquired immunodeficiency syndrome.

TABLE 272-4	Diagnostic Tests for Protozoal Diseases
Disease	*Preferred Diagnostic Tests*
Amebiasis	
Intestinal	Stool antigen or PCR, serologic tests, colonoscopy
Liver	Ultrasound examination, serologic tests, PCR on liver abscess aspiration
Amebic keratitis	Corneal scraping for microscopy and culture
Babesiosis	Thin and thick blood smears, PCR
Cryptosporidiosis	Stool antigen or PCR or acid-fast and auramine-rhodamine staining of fecal samples
Giardiasis	Stool antigen or PCR
Granulomatous amebic encephalitis	Brain biopsy
Leishmaniasis	
Cutaneous and mucocutaneous	PCR, antigen detection, biopsy, touch preparation, culture, serologic tests
Visceral	PCR, antigen detection, bone marrow or splenic aspiration, touch preparation, culture, serologic tests, lymph node biopsy
Malaria	Wright or Giemsa stain of thin and thick blood smear, antigen detection or PCR
Primary amebic meningitis	Cerebrospinal fluid examination, culture for amebae
Toxoplasmosis	Serologic tests, PCR, Wright-Giemsa stain of tissue, antigen detection
Trichomoniasis	Microscopy, culture, PCR or antigen detection in genital secretions
Trypanosomiasis	
Chagas' disease	Fresh blood or stained smear, PCR, xenodiagnosis; serologic tests for chronic disease
African sleeping sickness	Blood smear, PCR, serologic tests

PCR, polymerase chain reaction.

species, differentiation of genotypes is proving to be important for organisms such as *Giardia*, *Blastocystis*, and *Toxoplasma*, where it is becoming clear that genotypes differ in their pathogenicity for humans.[5-7]

The key to the recognition of protozoal infection is a knowledge of epidemiologic risk factors such as the parasites' geographic distribution (see Table 272-2) and the most common modes of clinical presentation (see Table 272-3). The clinical diagnosis of protozoal infection presenting outside normal areas of high prevalence is usually dependent on physicians considering this possibility in their differential diagnosis. Given present levels of travel, changing immigration patterns, and the immunosuppressive effects of infection with human immunodeficiency virus, all clinicians need to have a heightened awareness of diseases caused by the protozoans. Diagnosis and therapy often require a specialized expertise with the use of tests (see Table 272-4) or drugs with which most physicians lack experience. Infectious disease consultants will frequently be called on to diagnose and manage protozoal infection; this requires the maintenance of an updated, in-depth database as provided by the chapters in this section.

REFERENCES

1. Dacks JB, Walker G, Field MC. Implications of the new eukaryotic systematics for parasitologists. *Parasitol Int.* 2008;57:97-104.
2. Morrison DA. Phylogenetic analyses of parasites in the new millennium. *Adv Parasitol.* 2006;63:1-124.
3. Pain A, Böhme U, Berry AE, et al. The genome of the simian and human malaria parasite Plasmodium knowlesi. *Nature.* 2008;455:799-803.
4. Ali IKM, Hossain MB, Roy S, et al. Entamoeba moshkovskii infections in children, Bangladesh. *Emerg Infect Dis.* 2003;9:580-584.
5. Haque R, Mondal D, Karim MA, et al. Prospective case-control study of the association between common enteric protozoan parasites and diarrhea in Bangladesh. *Clin Infect Dis.* 2009;48:1191-1197.
6. Tan KS. New insights on classification, identification, and clinical relevance of Blastocystis spp. *Clin Microbiol Rev.* 2008;21:639-665.
7. Dardé ML. Toxoplasma gondii, "new" genotypes and virulence. *Parasite.* 2008;15:366-371.

273

Entamoeba Species, Including Amebiasis

WILLIAM A. PETRI, JR. | **RASHIDUL HAQUE**

*E*ntamoeba histolytica is an invasive enteric protozoan parasite that is the cause of amebiasis.[1] *Entamoeba dispar* and *Entamoeba moshkovskii* are nonpathogenic parasites that are identical morphologically to *E. histolytica*.[2-6] *E. histolytica*, *E. dispar*, and *E. moshkovskii* therefore cannot be distinguished by a stool ova and parasite (O&P) test, which has been the traditional diagnostic method. Because *E. dispar* and *E. moshkovskii* are often as prevalent as *E. histolytica*, it is important clinically to use *E. histolytica*–specific diagnostic tests (stool antigen detection or polymerase chain reaction [PCR]).[7-10]

Entamoeba spp. are taxonomically within the subphylum Sarcodina, class Lobosea, and family Entamoebidae.[11] At least seven additional species of amebae (*Entamoeba coli*, *Entamoeba hartmanni*, *Entamoeba polecki*, *Entamoeba chattoni*, *Dientamoeba fragilis*, *Iodamoeba butschlii*, and *Endolimax nana*) infect the human intestine.[11-19] However, these are generally accepted as commensal organisms, although *E. polecki*, *Dientamoeba fragilis*, and *I. butschlii* have occasionally been implicated as causes of diarrhea.[14-16]

Hippocrates (460-377 BC) wrote that "Dysentery, if it commence with black bile, is mortal," and the Old Testament and Huang Ti's *Classic in Internal Medicine* (140-87 BC) also made reference to dysentery. In 1828, James Annesley may have made the first association of dysentery to liver abscess when he wrote in *Prevalent Diseases of India* that "… hepatic disease seems to be induced by the disorder of the bowels, more particularly when this disorder is of a subacute or chronic kind." Approximately three decades later, in 1855, Vilém Lambl described amebae in the stool of a child who had diarrhea.[20] In 1875, Fedor Lösch described ameba in the stool of a young farmer with chronic dysentery that resulted in death. He described the amebae as "round, pear shaped or irregular form and which are in a state of almost continuous motion." Autopsy studies revealed ulcerations of the colon, and Robert Koch's postulates were met when the patient's stool inoculated orally and rectally into a dog caused dysentery with amebic ulcers.[21] Stephen Kartulis is credited with first demonstrating amebae in liver and brain abscess in the 1880s.[22,23]

The first North American case of amebiasis was reported in 1890 by Sir William Osler: "Dr. B., age 29, resident in Panama for nearly six years, where he had had several attacks of dysentery, or more correctly speaking a chronic dysentery, came north in May, 1889…." Subsequently in 1890 the patient developed tenderness and hepatosplenomegaly, and amebae were observed in the stool and abscess fluid: "The general character of the amoeba [found in the stool] correspond in every particular with those found in the liver."[22] A year later, Osler's colleagues William Councilman and Henri Lafleur proceeded through a classic investigation of 14 cases of amebic dysentery to distinguish amebiasis from bacterial dysentery, and they coined the terms *amebic dysentery* and *amebic liver abscess*.[23]

Ipecac bark was used in the treatment of dysentery for centuries in Peru. Piso introduced ipecac bark to Europe in 1658. Helvetius used ipecac to successfully treat the dysentery of King Louis XIV, and subsequently sold it as a secret remedy to the French government. Not until 1858 was the use of large doses of ipecac for the treatment of dysentery promoted by the surgeon E. S. Docker in Mauritius. He demonstrated that ipecac (60 grains two to three times a day) decreased mortality from as much as 18% to only 2%. However, large doses of ipecac by mouth were complicated by severe nausea and vomiting and necessitated the co-administration of opium, chloral hydrate, or tannic acid. An alternative therapy was discovered by Leonard Rogers in India, who found that emetine, the principal alkaloid in ipecac, killed amebae in the mucus of stools from patients with dysentery at dilu-

tions as high as 1/100,000. In 1912 he reported successfully treating three patients in Calcutta, who had been unable to tolerate oral ipecac, by injection of emetine.[24]

The life cycle of *E. histolytica* was described by Dobell.[25] The cyst form of *E. histolytica* was implicated as the infective form of the parasite by Walker and Sellards[26] in Philippines in 1913, and the parasite's life cycle was outlined by Dobell in 1925. Brumpt[27] proposed that *E. histolytica* and *E. dispar* were identical morphologically, but only *E. histolytica* was pathogenic for humans. Axenic culture of *E. histolytica* (free of any associated microorganisms) was accomplished by Diamond[28] at the National Institutes of Health in 1961. In 1978, Sargeaunt and colleagues[2] wrote that *Entamoeba histolytica* and *E. dispar* species could be differentiated using zymodeme analysis, and in 1989, Tannich and associates[3] demonstrated that their DNA genomes were distinct.

Organism

SPECIES OF *ENTAMOEBA*

Many *Entamoeba* species infect humans, but only *E. histolytica* is a cause of amebiasis.[1,4-6] Of greatest significance are the three prevalent and morphologically identical amebae *E. histolytica*, *E. dispar*, and *E. moshkovskii*. All three species are in the quadrinucleated cyst clade of *Entamoeba*. The *E. histolytica* and *E. dispar* genomes share 90% identity in genic regions, and *E. moshkovskii* is also closely genetically related.[29] In most industrialized countries, *E. dispar* is 10 times more common than *E. histolytica*,[1,30-34] and *E. histolytica* and *E. dispar* can be equally prevalent even in a developing country.[18] The presence of ingested erythrocytes was the sole morphologic characteristic of some usefulness in identifying *E. histolytica*, but in one study, this characteristic was present in only 68% of cases of *E. histolytica* but also in 16% of cases of *E. dispar*.[18] *E. moshkovskii* is also prevalent and geographically widely distributed.[5,6,29,35-37] In preschool children from an urban slum, *E. moshkovskii* was present in 21%, *E. histolytica* in 16%, and *E. dispar* in 36%.[6,30] In another study in Tanzania, among approximately 100 human immunodeficiency virus (HIV)–infected individuals with diarrhea, *E. histolytica* was present in 4%, *E. moshkovskii* in 13%, and *E. dispar* in 5%.[36] In Sydney, Australia, 50% of cases of *Entamoeba* identified by stool O&P examination were *E. moshkovskii*.[37]

E. hartmanii is also in the quadrinucleated cyst clade, but it is smaller than *E. histolytica*, having trophozoites of 3 to 12 μm in diameter and cysts of 10 μm in diameter, whereas *E. histolytica* trophozoites are 12 to 60 μm in diameter, and cysts are 10 to 20 μm in diameter. *E. coli* cysts have up to eight nuclei, with trophozoites of size similar to those of *E. histolytica*. *Entamoeba gingivalis* does not form a cyst and is not an inhabitant of the intestine; instead it is observed in the mouth in gingival scrapings. Human infection with the uninucleated cyst amebae *E. polecki*, *E. chattoni*, and *Entamoeba suis* is generally rare. *E. polecki* and *E. suis* infections are linked to contact with pigs, and *E. chattoni* infection to monkeys.[38-40] Other nonpathogenic amebae include *I. butschlii*, which has characteristic glycogen vacuoles in the cysts; *E. nana*, which has a characteristic nuclear structure that lacks peripheral chromatin; and *D. fragilis*, which is more closely related to the flagellates than to the ameba with binucleate trophozoites.[12,13]

GENOTYPES OF *ENTAMOEBA HISTOLYTICA*

In addition to the genetic differences between the three morphologically identical amebae *E. histolytica*, *E. dispar*, and *E. moshkovskii*,[4,5,11] genetically distinct strains or genotypes also exist within *E. histolytica*. Genotypes have been distinguished by the use of isoenzymes, polymorphisms in protein-coding DNA, and most powerfully by polymorphisms in short tandem repeat loci linked to transfer RNA genes (reviewed by Ali and colleagues[30]). Important findings from genotyping include the following: *E. histolytica* contains many genotypes[41-47]; patients may be infected with more than one genotype at a time[47]; and certain genotypes are associated with diarrhea, others with colonization, and others with amebic liver abscess formation.[46,47] In contrast to this high level of diversity in repetitive noncoding DNA, individual protein-encoding genes such as the galactose and *N*-acetyl-D-galactosamine (Gal/GalNAc) lectin are conserved between genotypes.[45] An additional nuance to genotypes is that in a study of patients with amebic liver abscess, comparison of the amebae in the intestine and liver demonstrated in every case that each patient had different genotypes in the two locations. This surprising result suggested that there is a genetic bottleneck between the intestine and liver, and only a subset of intestinal isolates are capable of causing extraintestinal disease.[47]

LIFE CYCLE

The life cycle of *E. histolytica* begins with an infectious quadrinucleated cyst and continues with an invasive uninucleated trophozoite. The cyst is ingested from fecally contaminated food or water or through oral-anal sexual practices and, in the intestine, excysts to eight trophozoites (Fig. 273-1). The environmental stability of the cyst and relative resistance to chlorine has resulted in water-borne outbreaks caused by contamination of municipal water supplies.[48] In most laboratory-based studies of the cyst, the reptilian parasite *E. invadens* has been used because *E. histolytica* does not encyst in culture. Studies of the process of encystation in *E. invadens* have demonstrated the role of quorum sensing through a surface Gal/GalNAc lectin to initiate encystation[49] after an initial environmental signal such as osmotic shock, low glucose level, or interaction with colonic mucins. Later steps in formation of the cyst require signaling through β-adrenergic receptors and autophagy.[50,51] The cyst wall of *E. invadens* contains a chitin-binding lectin.[52] Transcriptional networks associated with encystation were identified in cultures of clinical isolates of *E. histolytica* that contain encysting organisms.[53] A total of 672 cyst-specific transcripts were identified, including chitin synthetase, some of the transmembrane kinases, and cysteine proteinases, as well as genes involved in transcription, such as chromodomain proteins, and an *myb*-like protein, EhMyb.[53]

METABOLISM

No tricarboxylic acid cycle or oxidative phosphorylation exists for *E. histolytica*.[54] Many metabolic enzymes appear to have been acquired through lateral gene transfer from bacteria.[55] Functional mitochondria, or any other compartmentalized energy generation system, are lacking, although there is a remnant of the mitochondria called the *mitosome*.[56] Glycolysis is the major pathway for adenosine triphosphate (ATP) generation and occurs in the cytosol.[57] Catabolism of amino acids is a second energy source.[58] Pyruvate ferredoxin oxidoreductase is essential in both glycolysis and amino acid catabolism and also serves to activate metronidazole through its reduction of ferredoxin, which suggests that metronidazole resistance would probably not develop.[54] Energy stores are predominantly in glycogen that occurs in cytoplasmic granules.[54]

Pathways for the biosynthesis of amino acids, with the exception of serine and cysteine, are lacking.[59,60] Cysteine is of special importance because it is the major thiol. Synthetic enzymes for cholesterol fatty acid and phospholipids also have been identified. In contrast, de novo purine synthesis is lacking.[61] More than 100 transporters have been identified in the genome, but their characterization is incomplete at this time.[54]

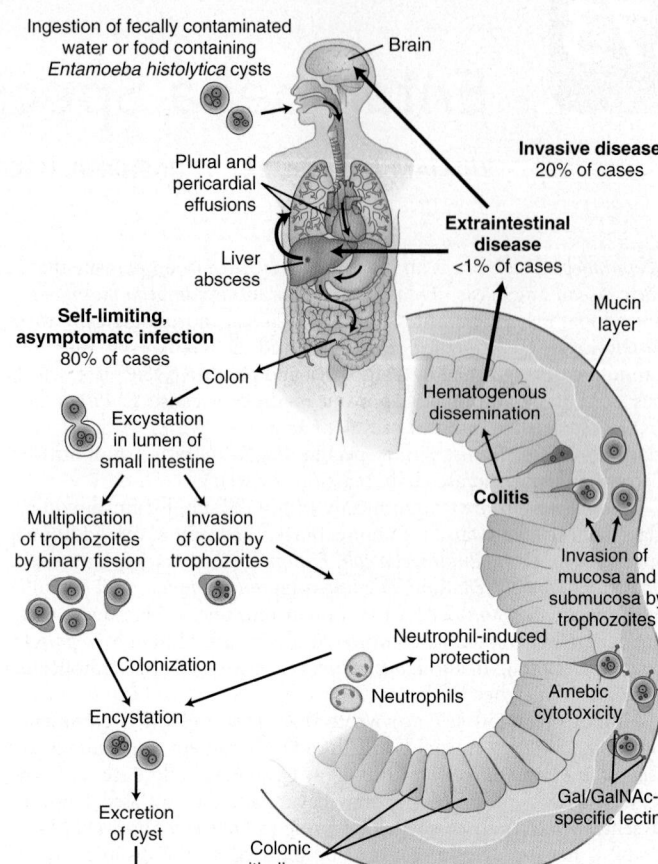

Figure 273-1 **Life cycle of *Entamoeba histolytica*.** Infection is normally initiated by the ingestion of fecally contaminated water or food containing *E. histolytica* cysts. The infective cyst form of the parasite survives passage through the stomach and small intestine. Excystation occurs in the bowel lumen, where motile and potentially invasive trophozoites are formed. In most infections, the trophozoites aggregate in the intestinal mucin layer and form new cysts, which results in a self-limited and asymptomatic infection. In some cases, however, adherence to and lysis of the colonic epithelium, mediated by the galactose and *N*-acetyl-D-galactosamine (Gal/GalNAc)–specific lectin, initiates invasion of the colon by trophozoites. Neutrophils responding to the invasion contribute to cellular protection at the site of invasion. Once the intestinal epithelium is invaded, extraintestinal spread to the peritoneum, liver, and other sites may follow. Factors controlling invasion, as opposed to encystation, probably include parasite "quorum sensing" signaled by the Gal/GalNAc-specific lectin, interactions of amebae with the bacterial flora of the intestine, and innate and acquired immune responses of the host. *(From Haque R, Huston CD, Hughes M, Houpt E, et al. Current concepts: amebiasis. N Engl J Med. 2003;348:1565-1573.)*

CELL BIOLOGY

Vesicular trafficking is of paramount importance to the parasite, inasmuch as endocytosis and phagocytosis serve as mechanisms of nutritional uptake. Exocytosis of the cysteine proteinases and ameba pores implicated in virulence and cyst wall components are also important functions of vesicular trafficking, in addition to the more typical roles in transport to and from the endoplasmic reticulum to the Golgi complex and cell surfaces. This complexity of function is reflected in the presence of 91 *Rab* genes (in comparison with 11 in *Saccharomyces cerevisiae*) involved in vesicle fusion.[62-64] N-linked glycosylation of proteins is unusual in that $Man_5GlcNAc_2$ is the most abundant N-linked glycan, whereas in other eukaryotes this would typically be processed by the addition of branching sugars.[65]

Transmembrane kinases are present and extraordinarily diverse (Fig. 273-2).[66-69] These kinases number more than 100 and are part of

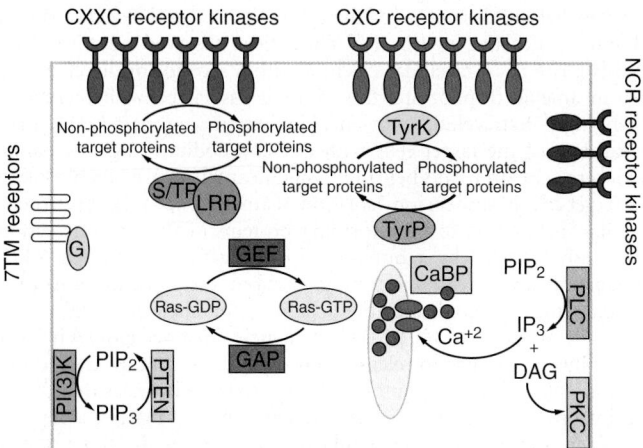

Figure 273-2 **Predicted signal transduction mechanisms of** ***Entamoeba histolytica,*** **based on analysis of the genome sequence data.** *E. histolytica* possesses three types of receptor serine/threonine kinases: one group has CXXC repeats in the extracellular domain; a second has CXC repeats; and a third has non–cysteine rich (NCR) repeats. *E. histolytica* has cytosolic tyrosine kinases (TyrK), but not receptor tyrosine kinases. Some serine/threonine phosphatases (S/TP) have an attached leucine-rich repeat (LRR) domain. CaBP, calcium-binding protein; DAG, diacylglycerol; G, G protein; GAP, guanosine triphosphatase (GTPase)–activating protein; GEF, guanine nucleotide exchange factor; IP_3, inositol-1,4,5-trisphosphate; PI(3)K, phosphatidylinositol-3-OH kinase; PIP_2, phosphatidylinositol-4,5-bisphosphate; PIP_3, phosphatidylinositol-3,4,5-trisphosphate; PKC, protein kinase C; PLC, phospholipase C; PTEN, phosphatase and tensin homologue; Ras-GDP, Ras protein–guanosine diphosphate; Ras-GTP, Ras protein–guanosine triphosphate; TyrP, tyrosine phosphatase; 7TM receptors, seven-transmembrane receptors. *(From Loftus B, Anderson I, Davies R, et al. The genome of the protist parasite* Entamoeba histolytica. *Nature. 2005;433:865-868.)*

the family of Gal/GalNAc lectin–related proteins that share the extracellular CXXC and CXC motifs of the lectin intermediate (igl) subunit. The kinase activity (ser/thr vs. tyr) of the transmembrane kinases, their substrates, ligands and biologic functions are all yet to be determined. The immediate downstream effectors of the transmembrane kinases are also yet to be identified, although more than 100 protein phosphatases are known to be present in the genome.[69] An unusual feature of these phosphatases is the presence of leucine-rich repeat domains implicated in protein-protein interactions. There are numerous seven-transmembrane G-coupled receptors and trimeric G proteins. A G protein–regulated adenylyl cyclase that functions downstream of an adrenergic ligand receptor has been biochemically identified. Cytosolic proteins involved in signal transduction include Ras, rac, rab, rho, and arf and their exchange factors: EF-hand calcium-binding proteins, phosphatidylinositol-3-OH kinase, and protein kinase C (PKC) and mitogen-activated protein (MAP) kinases.[69] It seems likely that this complex signaling system is required for the adaptation of the parasite to its host.

Some of the unique aspects of the cytoskeleton include the lack of dependence on microtubules for motility, which is instead mediated by actin-myosin motors, and the lack of intermediate filament proteins such as keratins, desmin, and vimentin. Polymerization of actin into polymers of F-actin leads to microfilament assembly, which, through the myosin family of molecular motors, provides vesicular transport and motility by means of pseudopods.[69,70]

GENOME STRUCTURE

The genome sequence is from the HM-1:IMSS strain originally isolated from the rectal biopsy sample of a Mexican man with amebic dysentery.[69] Because of a high content of repetitive DNA, the genome

has not been completely assembled but instead exists in approximately 1800 fragments, with the average of 12 sequencing reads per fragment. The incomplete nature of the genome ensures that some genes will be missing and that some misassembly will occur. The *E. histolytica* genome is estimated to be 14 chromosomes, 8000 genes, and 24 million base pairs of DNA, a size that is approximately comparable with those of *Plasmodium* and *Trypanosoma* spp. The average gene length of 389 amino acids, however, is approximately half that of *Plasmodium.*[54,69] Approximately 50% of the genome is noncoding DNA, including 20% of the genome that is dedicated to ribosomal RNA genes that are encoded in extrachromosomal circles, and another 10% that encodes transfer RNA genes organized in repetitive linear arrays (probably at chromosome ends). Additional repetitive DNA in the genome includes long interspersed repeated sequence (LINE) and short interspersed repeated sequence (SINE) transposable elements.[69]

The DNA content of *Entamoeba* appears to vary under different growth conditions. The nuclear DNA content of *E. histolytica* was shown to be 10-fold higher in axenic (bacteria-free) than xenic culture. In addition, 40-fold increases in DNA content were observed as trophozoites emerged from *E. invadens* cysts. The most plausible explanation for these observations is that the ploidy of *E. histolytica* varies through a growth-dependent process of DNA replication without nuclear division.[71]

Control of messenger RNA (mRNA) expression in *E. histolytica* shares similarities with later branching eukaryotes: The parasite transcribes mRNA monocistronically by using RNA polymerase II under the control of upstream regulatory elements.[72] Thirty percent of genes are predicted to contain introns, and the pre-mRNA splicing machinery includes conserved U2, U4, and U5 small nuclear RNAs.[73] Most of the protein subunits of RNA polymerase II are also conserved, but not all general transcription factors are identified yet. Other differences from yeast and metazoans include the presence of a third core promoter regulatory element for RNA polymerase II,[74] altered histone code,[75,76] and unique aspects of mRNA silencing through small RNAs.[53,77]

Pathogenesis

The pathogenesis of amebiasis centers on the unique tissue-destructive properties for which the organism was named *histolytica*. The process of host cell destruction has been experimentally separated into three steps: adherence, contact-dependent cytolysis, and phagocytosis of the host cell corpse (Fig. 273-3).[78-80]

ADHERENCE

The initial contact of parasite to host is mediated by the parasite's Gal/GalNAc lectin, which binds to carbohydrate determinants on the

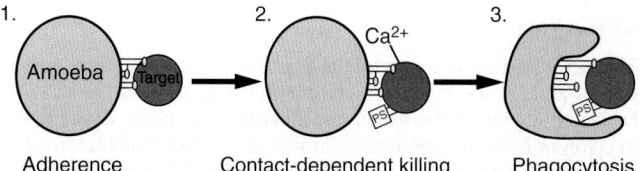

Figure 273-3 **Pathogenesis of amebiasis.** Adherence to host cells is mediated by the *N*-acetyl-D-galactosamine (Gal/GalNAc) lectin of the parasite. Contact-dependent killing (cytolysis) requires the lectin, amebic vacuole acidification, an intact cytoskeleton, and the amebapore. Death of the host cell involves rapid increases in host cytosolic Ca^{2+}, calpain activation, and caspase 3–induced apoptosis. Cell death leads to exposure of phosphatidylserine (PS) on the outer leaflet of the plasma membrane. Phagocytosis follows death of the target cell and involves both the Gal/GalNAc lectin and an amebic receptor for PS. Transmembrane kinase 96 (TMK96) has been identified as part of the initial amebic phagosome and is postulated to regulate one step in the sequential processes of adherence, killing, and ingestion of host cells.

host.[79-83] Adherence to human colonic mucin glycoproteins,[84] human neutrophils and erythrocytes,[85] certain bacteria,[86] and a variety of cell culture lines[87,88] is inhibited by up to 90% by Gal or GalNAc.[84] Blockade of lectin activity with Gal or GalNAc prevents contact-dependent cytolysis,[79] and glycosylation-deficient mutant cell lines lacking terminal Gal/GalNAc residues on N- and O-linked sugars are nearly totally resistant to amebic adherence and cytolytic activity.[88]

The colonic mucin layer of the large intestine is the first receptor encountered by the trophozoite lectin. Binding of the lectin to colonic mucins inhibits Gal/GalNAc and is of very high affinity (dissociation constant of 8.2×10^{-11} M^{-1}).[84] The mucin layer may protect the host from the parasite's contact-dependent cytolysis by binding to and neutralizing the lectin, while at the same time serving as a site of attachment for the parasite to colonize the large bowel. Interaction of trophozoites with colonic mucins appears to be a dynamic process, whereby trophozoites both induce the secretion of colonic mucins and degrade them.[89]

The Gal/GalNAc lectin is composed of a 260-kDa heterodimer of disulfide-linked heavy (170-kDa) and light (35- to 31-kDa) subunits that is noncovalently associated with an intermediate subunit of 150 kDa.[80-83] The 170-kDa subunit contains a carboxyl-terminal cytoplasmic and transmembrane domain adjacent to a cysteine-rich extracellular domain.[90,91] Five distinct genes (termed *hgl1* to *hgl5*) encoding the lectin's heavy subunit have been identified, sequenced, and shown to be expressed in trophozoites.[92] The sequence of the *hgl* genes is nearly completely conserved in isolates of *E. histolytica* from different continents, an important consideration for vaccine design.[45] The carbohydrate recognition domain is located within the cysteine-rich domain of the heavy subunit.[93] The lectin localizes to lipid rafts in the plasma membrane.[94] The lectin can be specifically released from the cell surface through the action of an amebic rhomboid protease, which probably explains earlier observations of both membrane-bound and soluble forms of the lectin.[80,81,95]

The Gal/GalNAc lectin appears to have other biologic functions in addition to adherence. Interference with lectin activity blocks chemotaxis in response to tumor necrosis factor-α (TNF-α).[96] The function of the light subunits may include lateral mobility of the Gal/GalNAc lectin, as evidenced by defects in capping of the lectin in ameba silenced for one of the genes that encodes the light subunits (*lgl* genes).[97] In an animal model, disruption of lectin function by expression of a dominant negative mutant blocked the ability of the parasite to cause liver abscess.[98,99] The lectin may serve as an organizing site for cytoplasmic proteins, with cytoplasmic proteins of the amebae that bind directly or indirectly to the lectin, including a thiol-specific antioxidant, spectrin, actin, myosin, talin, calreticulin, and cysteine proteinase 2.[100-102] The lectin has a role in evasion of serum lytic activity by inhibiting the formation of the complement membrane attack complex through blockade of C5b-9 assembly.[103] As mentioned previously, the lectin also appears to play an initiating role in cyst production.[49]

CYTOLYSIS

The lectin participates in cytolysis after mediating adherence. Apposition of amebic and target cell plasma membranes, as can be achieved by centrifugation of target cells and amebae into a pellet, does not lead to cytolysis if the amebic lectin is inhibited with Gal/GalNAc[78] or if the target cell lacks Gal and GalNAc on its surface.[86-88] This is consistent with the fact that lectin not only mediates adherence but also participates in the cytolytic event. In one study, anti–lectin monoclonal antibody directed against epitope 1 of the lectin heavy subunit blocked cytotoxicity but not adherence, which implicates the lectin directly in the cytotoxic event.[104] Killing occurs after the lectin engages GalNAc on O-linked target cell surface oligosaccharides: lectin-mediated capping of the O-linked structures (sialic acid-Gal-[sialic acid]–GalNAc) could be deduced to mediate killing.

Killing of host cells is not caused by an isolated toxin, inasmuch as parasite extracts have no cytotoxic activity. Cytolysis does require an intact parasite cytoskeleton, as demonstrated by inhibition of Rho,[105]

by cytochalasin disruption of the cytoskeleton,[79] and by expression of dominant-negative myosin II.[106] The earliest observed event in a dying cell is a rise in intracellular calcium within seconds of direct contact by an amebic trophozoite; this event is associated with membrane blebbing.[107] Extracellular ethylenediaminetetraacetic acid (EDTA) and treatment of the target cells with the slow sodium-calcium channel blockers verapamil and bepridil[108] significantly reduce amebic killing of target cells in suspension. Isolation of amebic pore-forming proteins similar in function to pore-forming proteins of the immune system has been reported by a number of investigators. A purified 5-kDa amebapore and a synthetic peptide based on the sequence of its third amphipathic α-helix has cytolytic activity for nucleated cells at high concentrations (10 to 100 μM).[109,110] Silencing of amebapore A blocked the ability of amebae to release monolayer tissue culture cells from a plastic well, although apoptosis was not specifically measured.[111] The optimal pH of amebapore is 5.3, and amebapore is inactive at a pH of 7, which may be of some significance in view of the inhibition of cytotoxicity with weak base treatment of amebae.[112] Interestingly, no DNA degradation was observed in cells lysed in vitro by the purified amebapore, which is suggestive of a different mechanism of cell killing by the purified amebapore than by the intact parasite.[113]

Cells killed by the parasite undergo nuclear chromatin condensation, membrane blebbing, and internucleosomal DNA fragmentation.[113] There is evidence of a nonclassical mechanism of apoptotic killing by *E. histolytica*. Overexpression of the Bcl-2 protein that inhibits apoptosis caused by a variety of cellular stresses (e.g., serum starvation and ultraviolet radiation) did not prevent murine cell DNA fragmentation after exposure to *E. histolytica*.[113] Furthermore, *E. histolytica* caused hepatocyte apoptosis in mice deficient in the Fas/Fas ligand and TNF receptor 1 signaling pathways.[114] Caspase 8–deficient cells, resistant to killing by Fas ligand, were readily killed by *E. histolytica*. Caspase 8–deficient cells treated with a caspase 9 inhibitor (Ac-LEHD-fmk) (at a level sufficient to inhibit apoptosis through etoposide) were readily killed as well. Together, these data suggest that *E. histolytica* initiates host cell apoptosis by directly activating the host cell's distal apoptotic machinery. Caspase 3 was activated within minutes of *E. histolytica* adherence, and the caspase 3 inhibitor Ac-DEVD-CHO at 100 μmol (sufficient to block killing through actinomycin D) blocked *E. histolytica* killing, as measured both by DNA fragmentation and by Cr51 release; this outcome indicates that both apoptotic death phenotype and necrosis were necessary.[115] In conclusion, amebic killing of the host is a result of parasite activation of apoptosis in the host cell, at the level of caspase 3 activation.

PHAGOCYTOSIS

In multicellular organisms, phagocytosis is the final step in the apoptotic pathway and serves to limit inflammation by preventing spillage of toxic intracellular contents of dead cells. Amebic ingestion of killed cells could similarly limit the host inflammatory response and enable *E. histolytica* to establish a persistent infection. Ingestion of erythrocytes and nucleated host cells occurred only after they were first killed by the amebae.[68,116,117] This indicated that changes in the surface of the host cell that occur upon apoptosis led to its engulfment. Phosphatidylserine was exposed on the surface of erythrocytes killed by *E. histolytica*, and phospho-L-serine, as well as phospho-D-serine, inhibited *E. histolytica* ingestion of erythrocytes. Inhibition of endocytosis by galactose and phosphatidylserine was additive, consistent with the Gal/GalNAc lectin and an as yet unidentified phosphatidylserine receptor acting as co-receptors for ingestion. The recognition and ingestion of the apoptotic corpse involves multiple ligands and receptors, in addition to the Gal/GalNAc lectin and the currently unidentified phosphatidylserine receptor; the roles of the serine-rich *E. histolytica* protein and collectins have been demonstrated.[118,119] Understanding the molecular mechanisms of engulfment of the corpse of the host promises to reveal much about pathogenesis, inasmuch as amebae that are defective in phagocytosis are also defective in virulence.[68,120]

ROLE OF BACTERIA

The effect of the gut bacteria on the biologic properties of *E. histolytica* may be profound. As mentioned previously, the genome content of *Entamoeba* is lower when the parasite is grown in the presence of bacteria.[54] In addition, amebae cultured with bacteria are better able to destroy monolayers of tissue culture cells and resist oxidative stress.[121-125]

CYSTEINE PROTEINASES

E. histolytica encodes at least 44 genes that are cysteine proteinases, some of which are membrane bound and others predicted to be soluble.[54] These activities are implicated in a number of potentially important activities, include degradation of colonic mucin glycoproteins,[126] digestion of hemoglobin and villin,[127,128] inactivation of interleukin-18,[129] and digestion of extracellular matrix.[130]

NOVEL RECEPTORS

Antisense-RNA knockdown of expression of a lysine- and glutamate-rich protein named KERP decreased virulence in an animal model of amebic liver abscess.[131] A serine-, threonine-, and isoleucine-rich protein that participates in adhesion and cytotoxicity has also been identified.[132]

Immune Response and Immunity

INNATE IMMUNITY

Neutrophils

Neutrophils are the earliest innate cellular immune response (occurring within 1 to 2 days) for both intestinal and hepatic amebiasis. They occur as a dominant infiltration of polymorphonuclear leukocytes surrounding trophozoites. Lymphocytes, macrophages, and epithelioid cells are recruited to these sites by day 3, in association with the formation of granulomas, which contribute to the confinement of invading trophozoites.[133-137] Neutrophils may be recruited by the chemotactic activity of an amebic membrane-bound peptide and chemokines secreted by epithelial cells exposed to *E. histolytica*.[138-141] As the consequence of interaction with trophozoites, neutrophils become activated and release reactive oxygen species and antimicrobial peptides. Many in vitro studies have reported neutrophil amebicidal activity after stimulation by interferon-γ (IFN-γ), TNF-α, lipopolysaccharide, or amebic antigens.[142,143] In accordance with a protective role for neutrophils, depletion of neutrophils with anti–Gr-1 neutralizing antibodies resulted in exacerbated amebic hepatic and intestinal disease.[144-146] It is worth noting that the GR-1 antibodies also deplete other granulocytes such as eosinophils, which are also observed as part of the innate immune response.[147] However, neutrophils can also be lysed by virulent ameba.[147-148] This can occur through disruption of the oxidase activities of the reduced form of nicotinamide adenine dinucleotide phosphate (NADPH)[149,150]; through protection of the amebae from oxidative damage by amebic peroxiredoxin, a 29-kDa surface protein conferring resistance to host reactive oxygen defenses[100,151,152]; or by inducing neutrophil apoptosis.[150] Neutrophil destruction in turn could result in tissue damage through the release of cytotoxic oxidase and lytic peptidases.[147]

Macrophages

Macrophages acquire amebicidal activity after in vitro stimulation with IFN-γ, TNF-α, or colony-stimulating factor-1 (Fig. 273-4).[153-155] The Gal/GalNAc lectin of *E. histolytica* upregulates Toll-like receptor (TLR)–2 expression in macrophages, resulting in activation of nuclear factor kappa B (NF-κB) and production of proinflammatory cytokine.[156] Macrophages lacking TLR-2 and TLR-4 showed impaired response to *E. histolytica* lipopeptidophosphoglycan (LPPG), which suggests that pattern recognition is essential in the macrophage

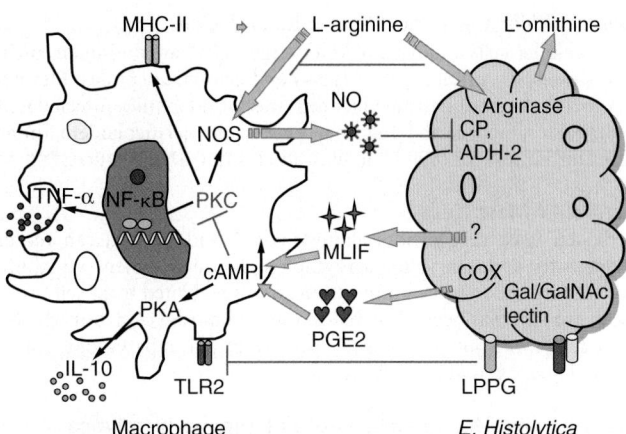

Figure 273-4 Modulation of macrophage functions by *Enteramoeba histolytica*. The killing of *E. histolytica* trophozoites by macrophages is mainly mediated by nitric oxide, derived from L-arginine by nitric oxide synthase (NOS). Nitric oxide (NO) could inhibit amebic cysteine proteinases (CP) and alcohol dehydrogenase 2 (ADH-2), the critical enzymes conferring virulence of *E. histolytica*. The arginase activity was detected in *E. histolytica*, which putatively converts L-arginine into L-ornithine, in turn limiting NO production by macrophage NOS. Prostaglandin E2 (PGE2) is an immunoregulatory molecule produced by cyclooxygenase (COX) in ameba or ameba-exposed macrophages. By activating the cyclic adenosine monophosphate (cAMP)–protein kinase A (PKA) pathway, PGE2 suppresses macrophage effector functions by inhibiting protein kinase C (PKC)–mediated expression of major histocompatibility complex class II (MHC-II) and production of tumor necrosis factor-α (TNF-α), while favoring production of interleukin-10 (IL-10). Monocyte locomotion inhibitory factor (MLIF) produced by ameba may suppress macrophage functions in a manner similar to that of PGE2. Amebic lipopeptidophosphoglycan (LPPG) might downregulate Toll-like receptor 2 (TLR-2) expression on macrophages and thus control the effector mechanisms triggered through TLR-2 signaling. Gal/GalNAc, *N*-acetyl-D-galactosamine; LPPG, lipopeptidophosphoglycan. *(From Guo X, Houpt E, Petri WA Jr. Crosstalk at the initial encounter: interplay between host defense and ameba survival strategies. Curr Opin Immunol. 2007;19:376-384.)*

response.[157] Inducible nitric oxide synthase (iNOS)–deficient mice were more susceptible to amoebic liver abscess and to *E. histolytica*-induced hepatocytic apoptosis,[29] which suggests that nitric oxide plays a critical role in host defense against amebiasis.

Despite the sensitivity of *E. histolytica* to nitric oxide–mediated cytotoxicity,[157,158] impaired macrophage function has been observed in human and experimental amebiasis, which suggests that amebae have developed strategies to modulate macrophage responses (see Fig. 273-4). Macrophage exposure to *E. histolytica* trophozoites or amebic components suppresses the respiratory burst and nitric oxide production.[159,160] A decrease in TNF-α secretion and IFN-γ–induced expression of major histocompatibility complex class II (MHC-II) has also been observed.[161,162] Macrophage suppression may depend at least partially on prostaglandin E2 (PGE2), an immunoregulator produced by *E. histolytica*, or on macrophages exposed to amebic proteins.[163,164] PGE2 elevates cyclic adenosine monophosphate (cAMP) levels in macrophages, triggering the protein kinase A (PKA) pathway, which in turn inhibits the expression of MHC-Ia molecules, the release of helper T cell type 1 (Th1) cytokines, NADPH-mediated oxidative burst, and nitric oxide synthesis through the PKC pathway (see Fig. 273-4). In addition, an immunosuppressor synthesized by ameba, monocyte locomotion inhibitory factor (MLIF), also contributes to the modulation of host immune responses. MLIF is a soluble pentapeptide with anti-inflammatory properties.[164,165]

Natural Killer Cells and Natural Killer T Cells

Natural killer cells and natural killer target cells have an innate role in host defense by production of IFN-γ and cytolytic peptides. Elevated cytotoxic activity of natural killer cells was found in mice infected with pathogenic amebae, and this may explain gender-dependent differences in the control of amebic liver abscess in C57BL/6 mice.[166,167]

Activated Mast Cells

Activated mast cells produce interleukin-6 and TNF-α, can recruit phagocytes, and can influence lymphocytic development and functions. Increased mast cell infiltration and upregulated mast cell protease expression has been observed in infected mouse ceca, but whether mast cells contribute to parasite clearance or play a pathologic role in tissue damage remains unanswered.[168]

Complement-Mediated Lysis of Entamoeba histolytica

After trophozoites penetrate the epithelial layer, the alternative complement pathway is initiated at least in part through cleavage of C3 and C5 by the amebic cysteine proteinase.[169,170] C3a and C5a act to chemoattract neutrophils to the site of infection. The Gal/GalNAc lectin heavy subunit of E. histolytica inhibits the assembly of C8 and C9 into the C5b-9 membrane attack complex, thereby preventing complement-mediated lysis of the parasite.[103]

Intestinal Epithelial Cells

Intestinal epithelial cells serve as the effectors of the mucosal immune system. Coculture of epithelial cell lines with E. histolytica trophozoites resulted in increased production of TNF-α, interleukin-1α, interleukin-6, interleukin-8, growth-regulated peptide α, and granulocyte-macrophage colony-stimulating factor by the epithelial cells.[171-173] In the murine model of intestinal amebiasis, innate resistance is conferred by nonhemopoietic cells, which suggests that the epithelial response is critical.[174] Of note is that hemopoietic interleukin-10 is required for intestinal epithelial resistance to amebiasis.[174]

ACQUIRED IMMUNITY

Mucosal Immunoglobulin A Response

A mucosal immunoglobulin A (IgA) response directed at the carbohydrate recognition domain of the parasite Gal/GalNAc lectin is linked to protection from both infection and disease (Fig. 273-5).[33,175] In contrast to mucosal IgA, serum immunoglobulin G (IgG) levels have not been correlated with protection. The lectin-specific IgG level was higher in amebic liver abscess and patients with intestinal amebiasis than in asymptomatic controls,[176] and in another study, the frequency of new E. histolytica infections was increased in children with serum IgG antibodies to the lectin.[177] These findings suggested that systemic antilectin antibody response might not provide direct protection from amebiasis.

Cell-Mediated Response

Cell-mediated production of IFN-γ would be expected to provide protection from amebiasis through its ability to activate neutrophils and macrophages to kill the parasite. In a prospective study of a cohort of preschool children in Dhaka, Bangladesh, amebic antigen stimulated IFN-γ production by peripheral blood mononuclear cells was associated with protection from future diarrhea caused by E. histolytica (Fig. 273-6).[178] An experimental amebic colitis model suggested that CD4+ T cells that produced helper T cell type 2 (Th2) cytokines mediated pathogenesis[168]; therefore, the pattern of CD4+ T-cell response may be critical. During amebic infection, T cells appear to be hyporesponsive to mitogen- or antigen-stimulated proliferation.[179] The amebic molecules conferring this suppression remain to be determined, but perhaps include MLIF activity.[164,165] The shift from Th1 to Th2 during amebic infection might result in a retarded T-cell response directed to amebic antigen. Because amebas have mitogenic effects on lymphocytes, nonspecific polyclonal activation may also disrupt antigen-specific antiamebic immunity mediated by Th1 cells.

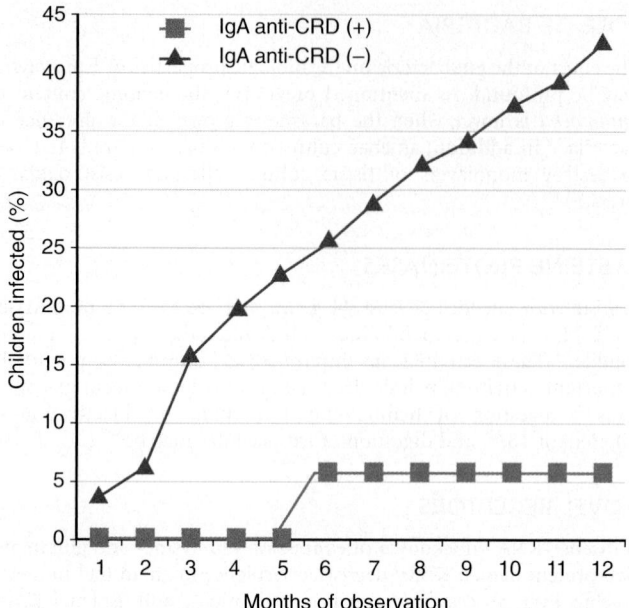

Figure 273-5 Immunoglobulin A (IgA) anti–carbohydrate recognition domain (CRD) is associated with immunity to Entamoeba histolytica infection. Children with fecal IgA antibodies against the N-acetyl-D-galactosamine (Gal/GalNAc) lectin CRD (IgA anti-CRD+; n = 81) had a lower incidence of new intestinal E. histolytica infection than did children who lacked this response (IgA anti-CRD−; n = 149). The two groups were statistically significantly different (P ≤ 0.04) at every time point. The average duration of protection was 437 days (95% confidence interval, 346 to 528 days). (From Haque R, Mondal D, Duggal P, et al. Entamoeba histolytica infection in children and protection from subsequent amebiasis. Infect Immun. 2006;74:904-909.)

Epidemiology

The prevalence of E. histolytica infection remains unknown because most of the existing data were collected in methods through which investigators could not distinguish the pathogen E. histolytica from the nonpathogenic E. dispar and E. moshkovskii.[1,180] Fortunately, most of the 500 million people worldwide previously believed to be infected with E. histolytica actually carry E. dispar or E. moshkovskii, which together are about 10 times more common.[180] Most individuals infected with E. histolytica also remain asymptomatic.[33] The best current estimate is that E. histolytica infection results in 34 to 50 million symptomatic cases worldwide each year and as many as 100,000 deaths. The bulk of the morbidity and mortality from amebiasis occurs in Central and South America, Africa, and the Indian subcontinent.[180] Local prevalence rates in these regions can be astounding. A carefully conducted national serologic survey in Mexico demonstrated antibody to E. histolytica in 8.4% of the population.[181] In the urban slums of Fortaleza, Brazil, 25% of the population tested carried antibody to E. histolytica, and the prevalence in children 6 to 14 years of age was 40%.[182] In Dhaka, Bangladesh, where diarrheal diseases are the leading cause of childhood death, the annual incidence of infection in a cohort of preschool children was 40%.[33] The annual incidence of amebic liver abscess was reported to be 21 cases per 100,000 inhabitants in Hue City, Vietnam.[183] Country-specific prevalence data for amebiasis have been reviewed.[30]

In the United States, amebiasis is the third most common parasitic infection, after giardiasis and cryptosporidiosis (1.2 cases per 100,000 U.S. population). Travelers to and immigrants from endemic regions and institutionalized individuals are at increased risk of acquiring amebiasis.[184] In returning travelers, diarrhea is the predominant reason

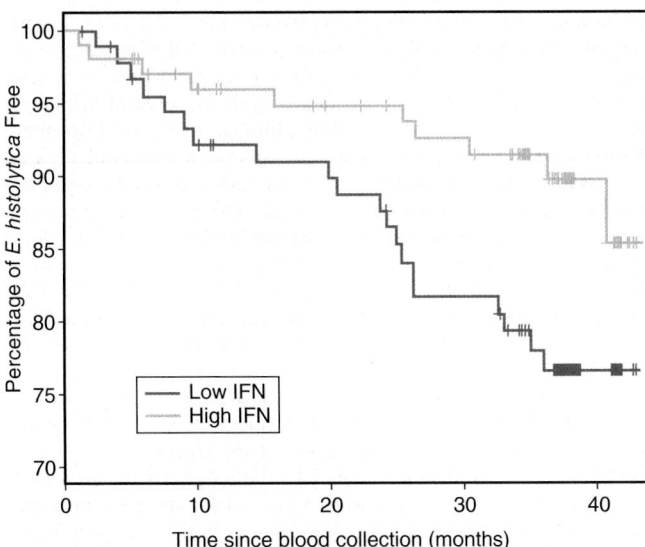

Figure 273-6 High levels of interferon (IFN)–γ are predictive of increased survival free of *Entamoeba histolytica* diarrhea. Peripheral blood mononuclear cells were stimulated with soluble amebic extract, and children were grouped by IFN-γ production in response to stimulation with soluble amebic antigen. Children were then monitored for 44 months, and the incidence of *E. histolytica* diarrhea was measured. The *upper line* and *lower line* indicate percentages of children with and without IFN-γ response, respectively, above the median for all children (580 pg/mL). The two lines are significantly different: Logrank test *P* = 0.03; *n* = 92 for low IFN-γ; and *n* =103 for high IFN-γ. (*From Haque R, Mondal D, Shu J, et al. Correlation of interferon-gamma production by peripheral blood mononuclear cells with childhood malnutrition and susceptibility to amebiasis. Am J Trop Med Hyg. 2007;76:340-344.*)

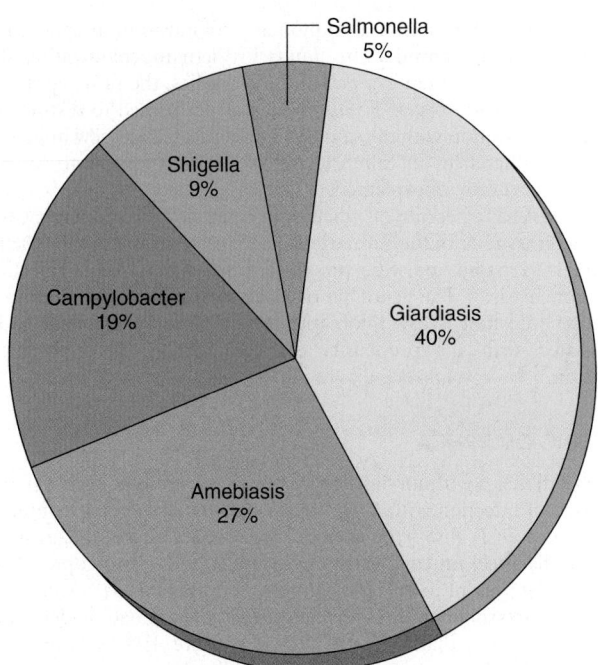

Figure 273-7 Amebiasis is the second most common cause of diarrhea in returning travelers, according to the GeoSentinel Surveillance Network of 30 travel or tropical-medicine clinics on six continents. (*Data from Freedman DO, Weld LH, Kozarsky PE, et al. Spectrum of disease and relation to place of exposure among ill returned travelers. N Engl J Med. 2006;354:119-130.*)

for a patient to visit a physician, and amebiasis is the second most common cause of diarrhea in returning travelers (Fig. 273-7).[184] Previously reported high rates of *E. histolytica* infection in homosexual men in the United States actually reflect a high prevalence of *E. dispar* infection in this population.[1] In contrast, in Asia, amebiasis is more frequently a presenting symptom of HIV infection and acquired immunodeficiency disease (AIDS); through the sexual practices of men who have sex with men, the risks of acquiring both HIV and amebiasis are similar.[185,186] The typical patient presenting with an amebic liver abscess in the United States is a 20- to 40-year-old Hispanic male immigrant. Several groups are at increased risk of severe amebiasis, including very young or old persons, malnourished persons, pregnant women, and patients receiving corticosteroids. The National Institute of Allergy and Infectious Diseases also considers *Entamoeba histolytica* a Biodefense category B pathogen because of its low infectious dose (<100 organisms), chlorine resistance, and environmental stability. All these properties make it a threat to food and water supplies, as the municipal water outbreak of amebic liver abscess in Tblisi, Republic of Georgia, demonstrated (Fig. 273-8).[187]

Clinical Manifestations

ASYMPTOMATIC INTRALUMINAL AMEBIASIS

The most common type of amebic infection is an asymptomatic cyst-passing carrier state. All *E. moshkovskii* and *E. dispar* infections and as many as 80% of *E. histolytica* infections are asymptomatic. Asymptomatically infected individuals represent a risk to the community because they are a source of new infections. Asymptomatic infection with *E. histolytica* also carries a small but definite risk to the carrier for the subsequent development of invasive amebiasis. In a study in Ban-

gladesh of children 2 to 5 years old who were colonized with *E. histolytica*, there was a small risk of developing invasive amebiasis with *E. histolytica* colonization: 2 of 17 colonized children developed dysentery during a 1-year follow-up period.[188] A subsequent study in Bangladesh revealed that 4% (25) of 651 asymptomatically infected children went on to develop amebic diarrhea or dysentery.[189] A study in South Africa revealed that of individuals colonized with *E. histolytica*, 10% developed invasive disease within 1 year.[190]

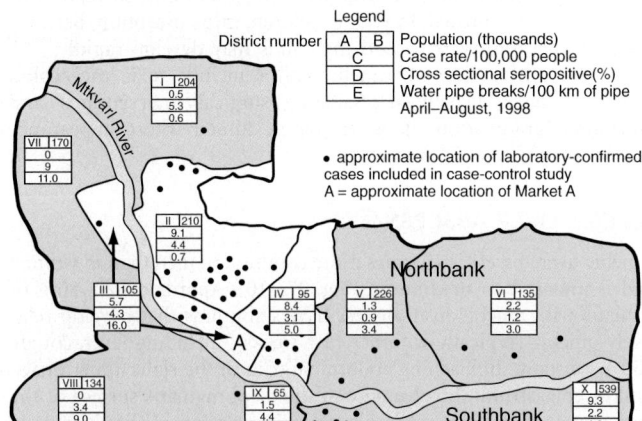

Figure 273-8 Location of cases of amebic liver abscess in Tblisi, Republic of Georgia. Cases were mapped by area of residence during the 1998 outbreak. Interruptions in water supply, decreases in water pressure, and increased water consumption were all significantly associated with infection. (*From Barwick R, Uzicanin A, Lareau S, et al. Outbreak of amebiasis in Tbilisi, Republic of Georgia, 1998. Am J Trop Med Hyg. 2002;67:623-631.*)

The median duration of asymptomatic colonization in children in Bangladesh was 2 months[33]; in adults in Vietnam, colonization was observed for more than 1 year.[32] In both studies, the same approach to DNA fingerprinting of *E. histolytica* was performed to distinguish continued infection with the same isolate from a second new infection; thus, the differences in duration of colonization appear to be real although currently unexplained.

The host has a bearing on whether infection is asymptomatic: Children heterozygous for the human leukocyte antigen class II DQB1*0601/DRB1*1501 haplotype were protected from symptomatic infection with amebiasis.[191] The genotype of *E. histolytica* also may determine whether infection is asymptomatic; certain genotypes appear to be associated with the propensity for colonization, as opposed to invasion.[47,48]

AMEBIC DIARRHEA

Amebic diarrhea without dysentery is the most common disease manifestation of infection with *E. histolytica*. Amebic diarrhea is defined as diarrhea in an *E. histolytica*-infected individual (for the diagnosis of amebic diarrhea, mucus need not be visible and microscopic blood need not be present in the stool). In one community-based study of a cohort of preschool children in Bangladesh, the annual incidences of amebic infection, diarrhea, and dysentery were 45%, 9%, and 3% respectively.[33] In a case-control study of diarrhea severe enough to prompt a patient to go to the hospital, approximately 2% of all such cases were caused by *E. histolytica*. This was true for all age groups. The mean duration of amebic diarrhea was 3 days.[33]

AMEBIC DYSENTERY OR COLITIS

Amebic dysentery, or amebic colitis, is defined as diarrhea with mucus or visible or microscopic blood in a patient with *E. histolytica* infection (Fig. 273-9). Approximately 15% to 33% of cases of *E. histolytica* diarrhea are accompanied by amebic dysentery.[33,192] Of patients with either condition, 70% have a gradual onset of symptoms over the 3 or 4 weeks after infection; increasingly severe diarrhea is the primary complaint, accompanied by general abdominal tenderness. On occasion, the onset may be acute or may be delayed for several months after infestation. This is different from bacterial causes of dysentery, in which patients usually have symptoms for only 1 to 2 days. The diarrhea is associated with abdominal pain and may be of such severity that an acute abdomen is suspected.[193,194] Surprisingly, fever is present in only the minority of patients with amebic colitis.[193] Abdominal distention or dehydration are unusual. In young children, intussusception, perforation, and peritonitis or necrotizing colitis may develop rapidly.[193-195] Unusual manifestations of amebic colitis include toxic megacolon (0.5% of cases, usually necessitating surgical intervention) and ameboma (granulation tissue in colonic lumen whose appearance mimics that of colonic cancer).

AMEBIC LIVER ABSCESS

Amebic liver abscess is 10 times more common in men than in women and is uncommon in children (Fig. 273-10). Approximately 80% of patients with amebic liver abscess have symptoms that develop relatively quickly (typically within 2 to 4 weeks), including fever, cough, and a constant, dull, aching abdominal pain in the right upper quadrant or epigastrium. Involvement of the diaphragmatic surface of the liver may lead to right-sided pleural pain or referred shoulder pain. Associated gastrointestinal symptoms, which occur in 10% to 35% of patients, include nausea, vomiting, abdominal cramping, abdominal distention, diarrhea, and constipation. Hepatomegaly with point tenderness over the liver, below the ribs, or in the intercostal spaces is a typical finding.[196,197]

The typical patient with an amebic liver abscess in the United States is an immigrant, usually a Hispanic man, 20 to 40 years old, who has fever, right upper quadrant pain, leukocytosis, abnormal serum levels of transaminases and alkaline phosphatase, and a defect on hepatic imaging study. Approximately 90% of patients with liver abscess are male. The abscess is usually single and is in the right lobe of the liver in 80% of cases.[195-200] Most frequently, patients present with liver abscess but without concurrent colitis, although a history of dysentery within the previous year is often present. Amebae are infrequently seen in the stool at the time of diagnosis of liver abscess. Liver abscess can manifest acutely (with fever and right upper abdominal tenderness and pain) or subacutely (with prominent weight loss and less frequent fever and abdominal pain). The peripheral white blood cell count is elevated, as is the alkaline phosphatase level, in many patients. Early evaluation of the hepatobiliary system with ultrasonography or computed tomography is essential for demonstrating the abscess in the liver.

The differential diagnosis of the lesion in the liver includes pyogenic abscess (less likely if the gallbladder and ducts appear normal), hepatoma and echinococcal cyst. Aspiration of the abscess is occasionally necessary in order to diagnose amebiasis (although amebas are visualized in the pus in only the minority of cases; if the abscess is pyogenic, the responsible bacteria is seen or cultured, or both). If a space-filling defect in the liver is observed, the differential diagnosis includes (1) amebiasis (most common in men with a history of travel or residence in a developing country; (2) pyogenic or bacterial abscess (suspected in women, patients with cholecystitis, elderly patients, individuals with diabetes, and patients with jaundice); (3) echinococcal abscess (an incidental finding, inasmuch as echinococcal abscess should not cause pain or fever); and (4) cancer. Most patients with amebic liver abscess have detectable circulating antigen in serum, as well as serum antiamebic antibodies.

In children, abdominal pain is reported infrequently with amebic liver abscess.[195,198,199] More commonly, high fever, abdominal distention, irritability, and tachypnea are noted. Some of these children are admitted to the hospital with a fever of unknown origin. Hepatomegaly occurs frequently, but elicitation of hepatic tenderness is not well documented. In one report, four of five children younger than 5 years of age died with amebic liver abscesses because the diagnosis was not suspected. Unusual extraintestinal manifestations of amebiasis include direct extension of the liver abscess to pleura or pericardium, and brain abscess. Death usually results from rupture of the liver abscess into the peritoneum, thorax, or pericardium but may follow extensive hepatic damage and liver failure.[195,198-200]

METASTATIC AMEBIASIS

Extra-abdominal amebiasis presumably follows direct extension from liver abscesses rather than direct dissemination from the intestine.[1,197,201] Thoracic amebiasis is the most common type of extra-abdominal amebiasis and occurs in about 10% of patients with amebic liver abscess.[195,197] Symptoms depend on the type of involvement. Empyema, bronchohepatic fistulas, or extension of a pleuropulmonary abscess into the pericardium may occur. Pericardial involvement is the next most common form of extraintestinal amebiasis and may result from rupture of a liver abscess in the left lobe of the liver into the pericardium or through extension of the right-sided pleural amebiasis.[195,201-203] It is estimated to occur in 3% of patients with hepatic abscesses. It manifests as acute pericarditis with tamponade and, on occasion, as pneumopericardium.[202,203] Amebic liver abscess in the left lobe also may rupture directly into the left side of the chest. Cerebral amebic abscesses were found in 0.66% to 4.7% of patients with amebic liver abscess.[204] In 18 patients with proven cerebral amebiasis, initial neurologic examination yielded normal findings in 13, and only 1 later developed seizures. Other foci of infection are rare, but amebic rectovesical fistula formation and involvement of pharynx, heart, aorta, and scapula have been reported. Cutaneous extension after the adherence of perforated, inflamed bowel to the skin is an extremely painful but rare complication.[205,206] This situation also may arise after invasion of the skin by trophozoites emerging from the rectum.

Figure 273-9 **Endoscopic and pathological features of intestinal amebiasis.** **A,** Colonoscopic appearance of intestinal amebiasis. **B,** Colonic ulcers averaging 1 to 2 mm in diameter, on gross pathological examination. **C,** Cross-section of a flask-shaped colonic ulcer (hematoxylin and eosin stain; magnification, ×20). **D,** Inflammatory response to intestinal invasion by *Entamoeba histolytica* (hematoxylin and eosin stain; magnification, ×100). *Arrows* indicate *E. histolytica* trophozoites. **E** and **F,** *E. histolytica* cysts in a saline preparation (magnification, ×1000). **G,** Iodine-stained cyst from stool (magnification, ×1000). **H,** *E. histolytica* trophozoite with an ingested erythrocyte, in a saline preparation from stool (magnification, ×1000). **I,** Trophozoite from stool stained with trichrome (magnification, ×1000). (Panels B, C, and D are from the slide collection of the late Dr. Harrison Juniper.) *(From Haque R, Huston CD, Hughes M, et al. Current concepts: amebiasis. N Engl J Med. 2003;348:1565-1573.)*

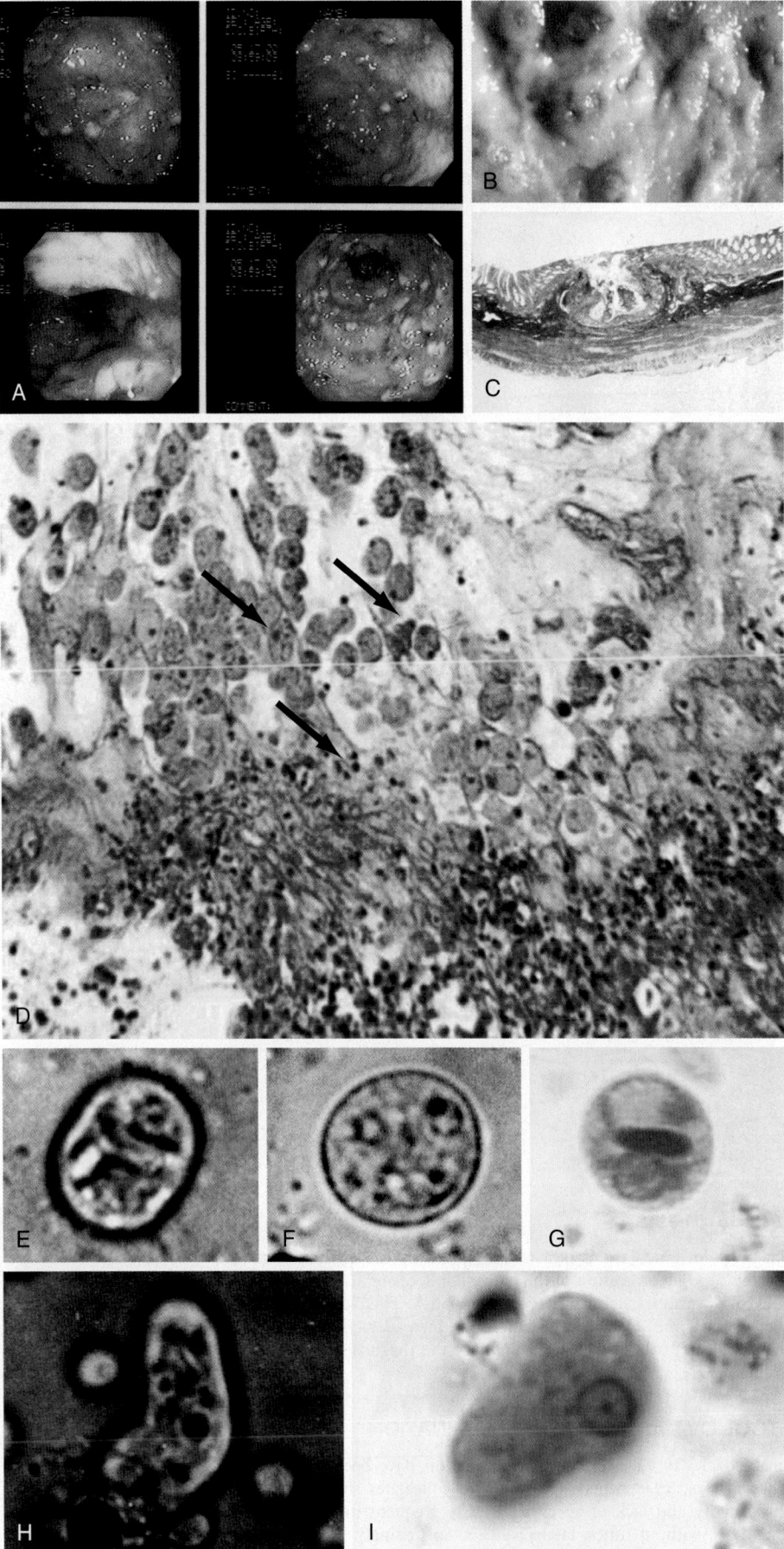

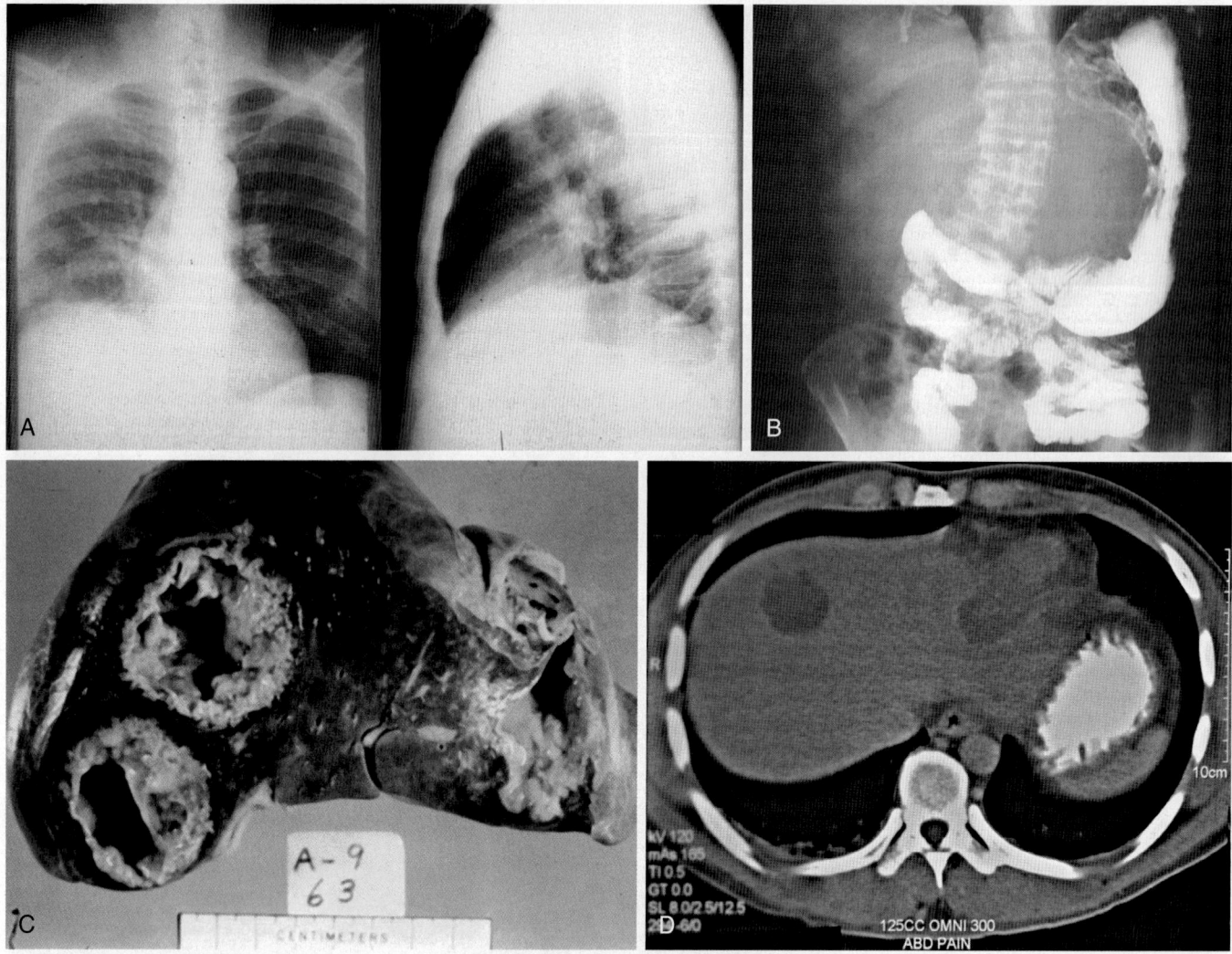

Figure 273-10   **Radiographic and pathologic features of extraintestinal amebiasis. A,** Left posteroanterior and right lateral chest radiographs in a patient with amebic liver abscess. The findings include elevated right hemidiaphragm and evidence of atelectasis. **B,** Luminal narrowing (*arrow*) revealed by a barium-enema examination in a patient with ameboma. **C,** Two abscesses in the right lobe and one abscess in the left lobe of a patient with amebic liver abscess. **D,** One abscess in the right lobe and one abscess in the left lobe in a patient with amebic liver abscess, shown on abdominal computed tomography. *(From Haque R, Huston CD, Hughes M, et al. Current concepts: amebiasis.* N Engl J Med. *2003;348:1565-1573.)*

Diagnosis

Diagnosis of amebiasis is best accomplished by the combination of serology and identification of the parasite in feces or at extraintestinal sites of invasion (such as liver abscess pus). This section reviews the use of the O&P examination, antigen detection, serologic study, culture, colonoscopy, and PCR for the diagnosis of amebiasis (Table 273-1).

STOOL OVA AND PARASITE EXAMINATION

Inadequacies of the stool O&P examination have been appreciated since at least 1978, when Krogstad and colleagues showed that its insensitivity and lack of specificity led to frequent misdiagnosis of amebiasis, with, at times, fatal results.[207] Surprisingly, 30 years later,

TABLE 273-1	Sensitivity of Tests for Diagnosis of Amebiasis		
*Test**		*Colitis*	*Liver Abscess*
Microscopy: stool		25%-60%	10%-40%
Stool antigen detection		80%	≈40%
Serum antigen detection		65%	>95%
Microscopy: abscess fluid		N/A	≤20%
Real-time PCR		>95%	>95%
Serologic testing (indirect hemagglutination)			
• Acute		70%	70%-80%
• Convalescent		>90%	>90%

Adapted from Haque R, Huston CD, Hughes M, et al. Current concepts: amebiasis. *N Engl J Med.* 2003;348:1565-1573.
N/A, not applicable; PCR, polymerase chain reaction.
*Diagnostic test sensitivity reported is for before the initiation of therapy.

the stool O&P examination remained the most common test ordered by United States physicians when intestinal amebiasis was suspected.[208] In one survey of 2800 physicians from five U.S. states, 97% of respondents believed that a routine O&P examination tested for *Entamoeba histolytica*.[208] The glaring problems with stool O&P examination were highlighted in a prospective study of 112 patients presenting at three Canadian centers with amebiasis symptoms (at least three loose bowel movements per day, abdominal pain, bloody stool, or weight loss) or risk factors (travel to or immigration from the tropics in the previous 2 years; men who have sex with men) or both. The specificity of stool O&P examination in community laboratories was an astoundingly low 10%.[209] The problems with stool O&P examination were magnified by the fact that only 5% (3) of the 65 positive results for *E. histolytica–E. dispar* complex were in fact *E. histolytica*.[209] This is because it is not possible with a stool O&P examination to distinguish morphologically the three closely related and common amebae: pathogenic *E. histolytica* and commensal *E. dispar* and *E. moshkovskii*.

In most industrialized countries, *E. dispar* is 10 times more common than *E. histolytica*,[1,30,209] and even in a developing country, *E. histolytica* and *E. dispar* can be equally prevalent.[18] The presence of ingested erythrocytes was the sole morphologic characteristic that was of some use in identifying *E. histolytica*; however, in one study, it was present in only 68% of cases of *E. histolytica* but also present in 16% of cases of *E. dispar*.[18] A third species of *Entamoeba* that is morphologically identical to *E. histolytica* is *E. moshkovskii*.[5,6,35-37] In a study of preschool children from an urban slum, *E. moshkovskii* was present in 21%, *E. histolytica* in 16%, and *E. dispar* in 36%[6]; in another study from Tanzania of approximately 100 HIV-infected individuals with diarrhea, *E. moshkovskii* was present in 13%, *E. histolytica* in 4%, and *E. dispar* in 5%.[36] In Sydney, Australia, 50% of *Entamoeba* organisms identified by stool O&P examination were *E. moshkovskii*.[37]

Anecdotal experience confirms continued difficulties in misdiagnosis in the United States.[195,210] We conclude that the stool O&P examination suffers from insensitivity and the inability to distinguish *E. histolytica* from *E. dispar* and *E. moshkovskii*.

CULTURE

Culture of *E. histolytica* from stool samples is available in only a few research laboratories worldwide.[211] Culture is, in general, more sensitive than stool O&P examination but significantly less sensitive than antigen detection or PCR.[7] It is also not specific for *E. histolytica*, and thus an *E. histolytica*-specific antigen detection or PCR test must be used on the cultured material.

COLONOSCOPY AND BIOPSY

Colonoscopy and biopsy can be helpful in the diagnosis of intestinal amebiasis.[212-214] Amebas can be difficult to visualize in the biopsy samples, and periodic acid–Schiff stains or, ideally, immunoperoxidase with anti–*E. histolytica* antibodies, can help to identify the parasites (see Fig. 273-9).[215] A limitation of colonoscopy is that it is an invasive procedure and not widely available in developing nations.

POLYMERASE CHAIN REACTION TESTING FOR AMEBIASIS

Real-time PCR is superior in sensitivity to stool antigen detection (see next section)[216] but unfortunately is still a technically complex means for the diagnosis of amebiasis. There are several real-time PCR assay formats for *E. histolytica*[9,216-218] (reviewed by Qvarnstrom and colleagues[219] and Fotedar and associates[220]). These tests are more sensitive than conventional PCR. Real-time PCR is also a sensitive test for detection of *E. histolytica* in liver abscess pus.[221] In one study, real-time PCR yielded positive results in 20 of 23 liver abscess pus specimens; the 3 specimens with negative findings had been collected from patients who had already received antiamebic therapy (8 days for one patient and 30 days for two patients).[216]

ANTIGEN TESTING FOR AMEBIASIS

The only fecal antigen test that distinguishes *E. histolytica* from *E. dispar* and *E. moshkovskii* is the TechLab *E. histolytica* II enzyme-linked immunosorbent assay (ELISA). This microwell ELISA, which detects the Gal/GalNAc adherence lectin of *E. histolytica*, is more sensitive than stool O&P examination or culture, and it is rapid (<2 hours).[7] A limitation is the need for fresh or frozen stool samples for the analysis by antigen detection. Other antigen detection tests are the RIDASCREEN *Entamoeba* (R-Biopharm, Germany) and the Triage Micro Parasite Panel (Biosite Diagnostics Inc., San Diego, California).[222] Neither of these tests can distinguish *E. histolytica* from *E. dispar*, and so they would at best serve as screening tools, with additional specific testing for *E. histolytica* required for all positive results. The TechLab *E. HISTOLYTICA* II, an ELISA, was also found to be more sensitive than the RIDASCREEN assay.[223] The Triage Panel has the advantage of coupling the testing of *E. histolytica–E. dispar* with that of *Giardia lamblia* and *Cryptosporidium parvum*, covering the three most common parasites that cause diarrhea in the United States; its disadvantage is that it requires a tedious multistep process of fecal processing and filtration. The TechLab *E. histolytica* stool antigen detection test has proved sensitive and specific in studies from Bangladesh,[7] Canada,[34] The Netherlands,[224] the United Kingdom,[225] and India.[226] In a single study, researchers observed a discrepancy between results of PCR and antigen detection,[227] and it is not clear if this discrepancy was attributable to false-positive PCR results, which is a recognized issue with some PCR formats for *E. histolytica*.[219]

Antigen detection is also useful in the diagnosis of amebic liver abscess. In one study, the TechLab *E. histolytica* II assay detected Gal/GalNAc lectin in the sera of 96% (22) of 23 patients with amebic liver abscess before they underwent treatment with the antiamebic drug metronidazole.[7] For liver abscess pus, it was 41% to 74% sensitive[7,216] for detection of the parasite. Furthermore, for stool specimens collected at the time of diagnosis of amebic liver abscess (and before metronidazole treatment), it detected the parasite in 43% (3 of 7).[7]

We conclude that the TechLab *E. histolytica* II ELISA antigen detection test has sensitivity and specificity superior to those of stool O&P examination, and its sensitivity inferior but its specificity comparable with those of PCR, but it is technically simpler to perform.

SEROLOGIC TESTS FOR AMEBIASIS

Serologic tests are a cornerstone of the diagnosis of amebic liver abscess and are an important adjunct in the diagnosis of intestinal amebiasis. However, it is important to realize that false-negative results may be obtained early in the course of intestinal amebiasis and amebic liver abscess.[7,193,196,228] The serologic tests are therefore best used in conjunction with antigen detection or PCR for *E. histolytica*.

In general, different assays for amebic antibodies behave similarly.[229,230] In one study, the RIDASCREEN kit (R-Biopharm AG, Darmstadt, Germany) enzyme immunoassay for serum antibody was reported to have sensitivity of 97%.[231] Microtiter ELISA (LMD Laboratories Inc., Carlsbad, California), ImmunoTab (Institut Virion, Wurzburg, Germany) and indirect hemagglutinin assay (Behring Diagnostics, Marburg, Germany) were compared in one study of amebic liver abscess patients from Kuwait.[230] All three tests had equal sensitivities of 98% to 99%. The ImmunoTab and Microtiter ELISA specificities were 95%, less than the 99.8% calculated specificity of the indirect hemagglutinin assay. The lower sensitivity was attributed to the high (5%) background titer of *E. histolytica* infection in individuals from endemic countries. The specificity of antibody tests for amebiasis is limited by the 5% to 10% baseline seropositivity of populations from endemic countries.

Serologic tests for *E. histolytica* intestinal infection are generally less sensitive than those for amebic liver abscess.[7,31,232] In a study in Egypt, IgG antibodies to the Gal/GalNAc lectin were found in the sera of 89% of patients with amebic colitis,[233] and in a small study from the Netherlands, 86% (six) of seven patients with intestinal amebiasis

TABLE 273-2	Drug Therapy for Treatment of Amebiasis	
Drug	*Adult Dosage*	*Side Effects*
Amebic Liver Abscess*		
Metronidazole[†]	750 mg po tid × 10 days	Primarily GI side effects: anorexia, nausea, vomiting, diarrhea, abdominal discomfort, or unpleasant metallic taste Disulfiram-like intolerance reaction to alcoholic beverages Neurotoxicity, including seizures, peripheral neuropathy, dizziness, confusion, irritability
or		
Tinidazole[‡]	2 g po once daily × 5 days	Primarily GI side effects and disulfiram-like intolerance reaction to alcoholic beverages for metronidazole or secnidazole
Followed by a luminal agent		
Paromomycin	30 mg/kg/day po in three divided doses per day × 5-10 days	Primarily GI side effects: diarrhea, GI upset
or		
Diloxanide furoate	500 mg po tid × 10 days	Primarily GI side effects: flatulence, nausea, vomiting Pruritus, urticaria
Amebic Colitis[§]		
Metronidazole	750 mg po tid × 5-10 days	Same as for amebic liver abscess
Plus a luminal agent (same as for amebic liver abscess)		
Asymptomatic Intestinal Colonization		
Treatment with luminal agent as for amebic liver abscess		

*Amebic liver abscess may necessitate antiparasitic treatment plus percutaneous or surgical drainage. Nitazoxanide may be effective therapy as well, but clinical experience is limited.
[†]Drug of choice for treatment of amebic liver abscess.
[‡]Not available in the United States.
[§]Amebic colitis may necessitate antiparasitic treatment plus surgical treatment.
GI, gastrointestinal.
Adapted from Haque R, Huston CD, Hughes M, et al. Current concepts: amebiasis. *N Engl J Med.* 2003;348:1565-1573.

were seropositive. Serologic study can be particularly helpful when *E. histolytica*–specific stool diagnostic techniques (antigen detection or PCR) are not available, because infection with *E. histolytica,* and not *E. dispar* or *E. moshkvskii,* results in seroconversion.[1,228] In conclusion, serologic study is an important part of the diagnosis of intestinal and extraintestinal amebiasis. A limitation of current tests is the lack of a point-of-care test for single use at the patient's bedside.

Treatment

Therapy for invasive infection differs from therapy for noninvasive infection (Table 273-2). Noninvasive infections may be treated with paromomycin. Nitroimidazoles, particularly metronidazole, are the mainstay of therapy for invasive amebiasis[234] (see Table 273-2). Nitroimidazoles with longer half-lives (namely, tinidazole, secnidazole, and ornidazole) are better tolerated and allow shorter periods of treatment but none except tinidazole is available in the United States. Approximately 90% of patients with mild to moderate amebic dysentery have a response to nitroimidazole therapy. In the rare case of fulminant amebic colitis, it is prudent to add broad-spectrum antibiotics to treat intestinal bacteria that may spill into the peritoneum; surgical intervention is occasionally required for acute abdomen, gastrointestinal bleeding, or toxic megacolon. Parasites persist in the intestine in as many as 40% to 60% of patients who receive nitroimidazole. Therefore, nitroimidazole treatment should be followed with paromomycin or the second-line agent diloxanide furoate to cure luminal infection. Metronidazole and paromomycin should not be given at the same time because diarrhea, a common side effect of paromomycin, may make it difficult to assess the patient's response to therapy.[235-237]

Therapeutic aspiration of an amebic liver abscess is occasionally required as an adjunct to antiparasitic therapy. Drainage of the abscess should be considered in patients who have no clinical response to drug therapy within 5 to 7 days or those with a high risk of abscess rupture, as defined by a cavity with a diameter of more than 5 cm or by the presence of lesions in the left lobe.[238] Bacterial coinfection of amebic

liver abscess has occasionally been observed (both before and as a complication of drainage), and it is reasonable to add antibiotics, drainage, or both to the treatment regimen in the absence of a prompt response to nitroimidazole therapy. Imaging-guided percutaneous treatment (needle aspiration or catheter drainage) has replaced surgical intervention as the procedure of choice for reducing the size of an abscess.[238]

Prevention

Prevention of fecal contamination of food and water has dramatically reduced transmission of amebiasis in industrialized nations. Transmission can be further reduced by the use of safe sexual practices in men who have sex with men and by proper maintenance of municipal water supplies to prevent access of chlorine-resistant amebic cysts to the treated water supply. In developing nations, however, more than 1 billion people still have no access to safe food and water.[239]

An effective vaccine is a desirable and feasible goal. The high incidence of amebiasis in community-based studies suggests that an effective vaccine would improve child health in developing countries. Because humans naturally acquire partial immunity against intestinal infection, an effective acquired immune response should be achieved. Aiding vaccine design is the demonstration that several recombinant antigens, including the Gal/GalNAc-specific lectin, provide protection in animal models of amebiasis and that human immunity is linked to intestinal IgA against the lectin.[240-245] The clonal-population structure of *E. histolytica* and, specifically, the high degree of sequence conservation of the Gal/GalNAc-specific lectin suggest that a vaccine could be broadly protective. Finally, the absence of epidemiologically significant animal reservoirs suggests that herd immunity could interrupt fecal-oral transmission in humans. The challenges will be to design vaccines capable of eliciting durable mucosal immunity, to understand the correlates of acquired immunity, and, most important, to enlist the continued support of industrialized nations to combat diarrheal diseases of children in developing countries.

REFERENCES

1. Haque R, Huston CD, Hughes M, et al. Current concepts: amebiasis. *New Engl J Med*. 2003;348:1565-1573.
2. Sargeaunt PG, Williams JE, Grene JD. The differentiation of invasive and non-invasive *Entamoeba histolytica* by isoenzyme electrophoresis. *Trans R Soc Trop Med Hyg*. 1978;72:519-521.
3. Tannich E, Horstmann RD, Knobloch J, et al. Genomic DNA differences between pathogenic and nonpathogenic *Entamoeba histolytica*. *Proc Natl Acad Sci U S A*. 1989;86:5118-5122.
4. Diamond LS, Clark CG. A redescription of *Entamoeba histolytica* Schaudinn, 1903 (Emended Walker, 1911) separating it from *Entamoeba dispar* Brumpt, 1925. *J Eukaryot Microbiol*. 1993;40: 340-344.
5. Haque R, Ali IKM, Clark CG, et al. A case report of *Entamoeba moshkovskii* infection in a Bangladeshi child. *Parasitol Int*. 1998;47:201-202.
6. Ali IKM, Hossain MB, Roy S, et al. *Entamoeba moshkovskii* infections in children, Bangladesh *Emerg Infect Dis*. 2003;9:580-584.
7. Haque H, Mollah NU, Ali IKM, et al. Diagnosis of amebic liver abscess and intestinal infection with the TechLab *Entamoeba histolytica* II antigen detection and antibody tests. *J Clin Microbiol*. 2000;38:3235-3239.
8. Blessmann J, Buss H, Nu PA, et al. Real-time PCR for detection and differentiation of *Entamoeba histolytica* and *Entamoeba dispar* in fecal samples. *J Clin Microbiol*. 2002;40:4413-4417.
9. Haque R, Roy S, Siddique A, et al. Multiplex real-time PCR assay for detection of *Entamoeba histolytica*, *Giardia lamblia* and *Cryptosporidium* spp. *Am J Trop Med Hyg*. 2007;76:713-717.
10. Tanyuksel M, Petri WA Jr. Laboratory diagnosis of amebiasis. *Clin Microbiol Rev*. 2003;16:713-729.
11. Silberman JD, Clark CG, Diamond LS, et al. Phylogeny of the genera *Entamoeba* and *Endolimax* as deduced from small-subunit ribosomal RNA sequences. *Mol Biol Evol*. 1999;16: 1740-1751.
12. Markell EK, John DT, Krotoski WA. *Lumen-Dwelling Protozoa*. 8th ed. Philadelphia: WB Saunders, 1999.
13. John DT, Petri WA Jr. *Markell and Voge's Medical Parasitology*. 9th ed. Philadelphia: Elsevier; 2006.
14. Chacin-Bonilla L. *Entamoeba polecki:* human infections in Venezuela. *Trans R Soc Trop Med Hyg*. 1992;86:634.
15. Graczyk TK, Shiff CK, Tamang L, et al. The association of *Blastocystis hominis* and *Endolimax nana* with diarrheal stools in Zambian school-age children. *Parasitol Res*. 2005;98:38-43.
16. Wahlgren M. *Entamoeba coli* as cause of diarrhoea? *Lancet*. 1991;337:675.
17. González-Ruiz A, Haque R, Aguirre A, et al. Value of microscopy in the diagnosis of dysentery associated with invasive *Entamoeba histolytica*. *J Clin Pathol*. 1994;47:236-239.
18. Haque R, Neville LM, Hahn P, et al. Rapid diagnosis of *Entamoeba* infection using the *Entamoeba* and *Entamoeba histolytica* stool antigen detection kits. *J Clin Microbiology*. 1995;33:2558-2561.
19. Verweij JJ, Polderman AM, Clark CG. Genetic variation among human isolates of uninucleated cyst-producing *Entamoeba* species. *J Clin Microbiol*. 2001;39:1644-1646.
20. Stilwell GG. Amebiasis: its early history. *Gastroenterology*. 1955;28:606.
21. Lösch F. Massenhafte Entwicklung von Amoben in Dickdarm. *Virchows Arch A*. 1975;65:196-211.
22. Kartulis S. Zur aetiologie der leberabscesse. *Centralbl Bakt*. 1887;2:745-748.
23. Councilman WT, Lafleur HA. Amoebic dysentery. *Johns Hopkins Hosp Rep*. 1891;2:395-548.
24. Rogers L. The rapid cure of amoebic dysentery and hepatitis by hypodermic injection of solle salts of emetine. *BMJ*. 1912;1:1424.
25. Dobell C. *The Amoebae Living in Man*. London: John Bale, Sons & Danielson; 1919.
26. Walker EL, Sellards AW. Experimental entamoebic dysentery. *Philippine J Sci B Trop Med*. 1913;8:253.
27. Brumpt E. Étude sommaire de l' "*Entamoeba dispar*" n. sp. Amibe à kystes quadrinuclees, parasite de l'homme. *Bull Acad Med Paris*. 1925;94:943-952.
28. Diamond LS. Axenic cultivation of *Entamoeba histolytica*. *Science*. 1961;134:336.
29. Tawari B, Ali IKM, Scott C, et al. Patterns of evolution in the unique tRNA gene arrays of the genus *Entamoeba*. *Mol Biol Evol*. 2008;25:187-198.
30. Ali IK, Clark CG, Petri WA Jr. Molecular epidemiology of amebiasis. *Infect Genet Evol*. 2008;8:698-707.
31. Gathiram V, Jackson TF. A longitudinal study of asymptomatic carriers of pathogenic zymodemes of *Entamoeba histolytica*. *S Afr Med J*. 1987;72:669-672.
32. Blessmann J, Ali IKM, Nu PA, et al. Longitudinal study of intestinal *Entamoeba histolytica* infections in asymptomatic adult carriers. *J Clin Microbiol*. 2003;41:4745-4750.
33. Haque R, Mondal D, Duggal P, et al. *Entamoeba histolytica* infection in children and protection from subsequent amebiasis. *Infect Immun*. 2006;74:904-909.
34. Pillai DR, Keystone JS, Sheppard DC, et al. *Entamoeba histolytica* and *Entamoeba dispar:* epidemiology and comparison of diagnostic methods in a setting of nonendemicity. *Clin Infect Dis*. 1999;29:1315-1318.
35. Parija SC, Khairnar K. *Entamoeba moshkovskii* and *Entamoeba dispar* associated infections in Pondicherry, India. *J Health Popul Nutr*. 2005;23:292-295.
36. Beck DL, Dogan N, Maro V, et al. High prevalence of *Entamoeba moshkovskii* in a Tanzanian HIV population. *Acta Tropica*. 2008;107(1):48-49.
37. Fotedar R, Stark D, Marriott D, et al. *Entamoeba moshkovskii* infections in Sydney, Australia. *Eur J Clin Microbiol Infect Dis*. 2008;27:133-137.
38. Desowitz RS, Barnish G. *Entamoeba polecki* and other intestinal protozoa in Papua New Guinea Highland children. *Ann Trop Med Parasitol*. 1986;80:399-402.
39. Sargeaunt PG, Patrick S, O'Keeffe D. Human infections of *Entamoeba chattoni* masquerade as *Entamoeba histolytica*. Trans *R Soc Trop Med Hyg*. 1992;86:633-634.
40. Verweij JJ, Polderman AM, Clark CG. Genetic variation among human isolates of uninucleated cyst-producing *Entamoeba* species. *J Clin Microbiol*. 2001;39:1644-1646.
41. Clark CG, Diamond LS. *Entamoeba histolytica:* a method for isolate identification. *Exp Parasitol*. 1993;77:450-455.
42. Ayeh-Kumi PF, Ali IKM, Lockhart LA, et al. *Entamoeba histolytica:* genetic diversity of clinical isolates from Bangladesh as demonstrated by polymorphisms in the serine-rich gene. *Exp Parasitol*. 2001;99:80-88.
43. Simonishvili S, Tsanava S, Sanadze K, et al. *Entamoeba histolytica:* the serine-rich gene polymorphism-based genetic variability of clinical isolates from Georgia. *Exp Parasitol*. 2005;110: 313-317.
44. Samie A, Obi CL, Bessong PO, et al. *Entamoeba histolytica:* genetic diversity of African strains based on the polymorphism of the serine-rich protein gene. *Exp Parasitol*. 2008;118: 354-361.
45. Beck DL, Tanyuksel M, Mackey A, et al. Sequence conservation of the Gal/GalNAc lectin from clinical isolates. *Exp Parasitol*. 2002;101:157-163.
46. Ali IKM, Mondal U, Roy S, et al. Evidence for a link between parasite genotype and outcome of infection with *Entamoeba histolytica*. *J Clin Microbiol*. 2007;45:285-289.
47. Ali IKM, Solaymani-Mohammadi S, Akhter J, et al. Tissue invasion by *Entamoeba histolytica:* evidence of genetic selection and/or DNA reorganization events in organ tropism. *PLoS Negl Trop Dis*. 2008;2:e219. [Erratum published 2008;2(6).]
48. Barwick R, Uzicanin A, Lareau S, et al. Outbreak of amebiasis in Tbilisi, Republic of Georgia, 1998. *Am J Trop Med Hyg*. 2002;67:623-631.
49. Turner NA, Eichinger D. *Entamoeba* invadens: the requirement for galactose ligands during encystment. *Exp Parasitol*. 2007;116: 467-474.
50. Coppi A, Merali S, Eichinger D. The enteric parasite *Entamoeba* uses an autocrine catecholamine system during differentiation into the infectious cyst stage. *J Biol Chem*. 2002;277:8083-8090.
51. Picazarri K, Nakada-Tsukui K, Nozaki T. Autophagy during proliferation and encystation in the protozoan parasite *Entamoeba* invadens. *Infect Immun*. 2008;76(1):278-288.
52. Frisardi M, Ghosh SK, Field J, et al. The most abundant glycoprotein of amebic cyst walls (Jacob) is a lectin with five Cys-rich, chitin-binding domains. *Infect Immun*. 2000;68: 4217-4224.
53. Ehrenkaufer GM, Haque R, Hackney JA, et al. Identification of developmentally regulated genes in *Entamoeba histolytica*: insights into mechanisms of stage conversion in a protozoan parasite. *Cell Microbiol*. 2007;9:1426-1444.
54. Clark CG, Alsmark UC, Tazreiter M, et al. Structure and content of the *Entamoeba histolytica* genome. *Adv Parasitol*. 2007;65: 51-190.
55. Nixon JE, Wang A, Field J, et al. Evidence for lateral transfer of genes encoding ferredoxins, nitroreductases, NADH oxidase, and alcohol dehydrogenase 3 from anaerobic prokaryotes to *Giardia lamblia* and *Entamoeba histolytica*. *Eukaryot Cell*. 2002;1:181-190.
56. Leon-Avila G, Tovar J. Mitosomes of *Entamoeba histolytica* are abundant mitochondrion-related remnant organelles that lack a detectable organellar genome. *Microbiology*. 2004;150: 1245-1250.
57. Saavedra E, Encalada R, Pineda E, et al. Glycolysis in *Entamoeba histolytica*. Biochemical characterization of recombinant glycolytic enzymes and flux control analysis. *FEBS J*. 2005;272: 1767-1783.
58. Anderson IJ, Loftus BJ. *Entamoeba histolytica:* observations on metabolism based on the genome sequence. *Exp Parasitol*. 2005;110:173-177.
59. Ali V, Hashimoto T, Shigeta Y, et al. Molecular and biochemical characterization of D-phosphoglycerate dehydrogenase from *Entamoeba histolytica*. A unique enteric protozoan parasite that possesses both phosphorylated and nonphosphorylated serine metabolic pathways. *Eur J Biochem*. 2004;271:2670-2681.
60. Nozaki T, Asai T, Sanchez LB, et al. Characterization of the gene encoding serine acetyltransferase, a regulated enzyme of cysteine biosynthesis from the protist parasites *Entamoeba histolytica* and *Entamoeba dispar*. Regulation and possible function of the cysteine biosynthetic pathway in *Entamoeba*. *J Biol Chem*. 1999;274:32445-32452.
61. Reeves RE. Metabolism of *Entamoeba histolytica* Schaudinn, 1903. *Adv Parasitol*. 1984;23:105-142.
62. Temesvari LA, Harris EN, Stanley Jr SL, et al. Early and late endosomal compartments of *Entamoeba histolytica* are enriched in cysteine proteases, acid phosphatase and several *Ras*-related Rab GTPases. *Mol Biochem Parasitol*. 1999;103:225-241.
63. Saito-Nakano Y, Yasuda T, Nakada-Tsukui K, et al. Rab5-associated vacuoles play a unique role in phagocytosis of the enteric protozoan parasite *Entamoeba histolytica*. *J Biol Chem*. 2004;279:49497-49507.
64. Saito-Nakano Y, Loftus BJ, Hall N, et al. The diversity of Rab GTPases in *Entamoeba histolytica*. *Exp Parasitol*. 2005; 110:244-252.
65. Samuelson J, Banerjee S, Magnelli P, et al. The diversity of dolichol-linked precursors to Asn-linked glycans likely results from secondary loss of sets of glycosyltransferases. *Proc Natl Acad Sci U S A*. 2005;102:1548-1553.
66. Beck DL, Boettner DR, Dragulev B, et al. Identification and gene expression analysis of a large family of transmembrane kinases related to the Gal/GalNAc lectin in *Entamoeba histolytica*. *Eukaryot Cell*. 2005;4:722-732.
67. Mehra A, Frederick J, Petri WA Jr, et al. Expression and function of a family of transmembrane kinases from the protozoan parasite *Entamoeba histolytica*. *Infect Immun*. 2006;74:5341-5351.
68. Boettner DR, Huston CD, Linford AS, et al. *Entamoeba histolytica* phagocytosis of human erythrocytes involves PATMK, a novel protein found in the amebic phagosome. *PloS Pathog*. 2008;4(1):e8.
69. Loftus B, Anderson I, Davies R, et al. The genome of the protist parasite *Entamoeba histolytica*. *Nature*. 2005;433:865-868.
70. Voigt H, Olivo JC, Sansonetti P, et al. Myosin IB from *Entamoeba histolytica* is involved in phagocytosis of human erythrocytes. *J Cell Sci*. 1999;112(Pt 8):1191-1201.
71. Mukherjee C, Clark CG, Lohia A. *Entamoeba* shows reversible variation in ploidy under different growth conditions and between life cycle phases. *PLoS Negl Trop Dis*. 2008;2(8):e281.
72. Purdy JE, Pho LT, Mann BJ, et al. Upstream regulatory elements controlling expression of the *Entamoeba histolytica* lectin. *Mol Biochem Parasitol*. 1996;78:91-103.
73. Davis CA, Brown MP, Singh U. Functional characterization of spliceosomal introns and identification of U2, U4, and U5 snRNAs in the deep-branching eukaryote *Entamoeba histolytica*. *Eukaryot Cell*. 2007;6:940-948.
74. Singh U, Rogers JB, Mann BJ, et al. Transcription initiation is controlled by three core promoter elements in the protozoan parasite *Entamoeba histolytica*. *Proc Natl Acad Sci U S A*. 1997;94:8812-8817.
75. Abhyankar MM, Hochreiter AE, Hershey J, et al. Characterization of an *Entamoeba histolytica* high-mobility-group box protein induced during intestinal infection. *Eukaryot Cell*. 2008;7:1565-1572.
76. Ramakrishnan G, Gilchrist CA, Musa H, et al. Histone acetyltransferases and deacetylase in *Entamoeba histolytica*. *Mol Biochem Parasitol*. 2004;138:205-216.
77. Linford AS, Moreno H, Good KR, et al. Short hairpin RNA-mediated knockdown of protein expression in *Entamoeba histolytica*. *BMC Microbiol*. 2009;9:38.
78. Ravdin JI, Croft BY, Guerrant RL. Cytopathogenic mechanisms of *Entamoeba histolytica*. *J Exp Med*. 1980;152:377-390.
79. Ravdin JI, Guerrant RL. Role of adherence in cytopathogenic mechanisms of *Entamoeba histolytica*. Study with mammalian tissue culture cells and human erythrocytes. *J Clin Invest*. 1981;68:1305-1313.
80. Petri WA Jr, Mann BJ, Haque R. The bittersweet interface of parasite and host: lectin-carbohydrate interactions during human invasion by the parasite *Entamoeba histolytica*. *Annu Rev Microbiol*. 2002;56:39-64.
81. Petri WA Jr, Smith RD, Schlesinger PH, et al. Isolation of the galactose binding adherence lectin of *Entamoeba histolytica*. *J Clin Invest*. 1987;80:1238-1244.
82. Petri WA Jr, Chapman MD, Snodgrass T, et al. Subunit structure of the galactose and *N*-acetyl-D-galactosamine-inhibitable adherence lectin of *Entamoeba histolytica*. *J Biol Chem*. 1989;264:3007-3012.
83. Cheng X-J, Hughes MA, Huston CD, et al. The 150 kDa Gal/GalNAc lectin co-receptor of *Entamoeba histolytica* is a member of a gene family containing multiple CXXC sequence motifs. *Infect Immun*. 2001;69:5892-5898.
84. Chadee K, Petri WA Jr, Innes DJ, et al. Rat and human colonic mucins bind to and inhibit the adherence lectin of *Entamoeba histolytica*. *J Clin Invest*. 1987;80:l245-l254.
85. Guerrant RL, Brush J, Ravdin JI, et al. Interaction between *Entamoeba histolytica* and human polymorphonuclear neutrophils. *J Infect Dis*. 1981;143:83-93.
86. Bracha R, Mirelman D. Adherence and ingestion of *Escherichia coli* serotype 055 by trophozoites of *Entamoeba histolytica*. *Infect Immun*. 1983;40:882-887.
87. Li E, Becker A, Stanley SL. Chinese hamster ovary cells deficient in *N*-acetyl-glucosaminyltransferase I activity are resistant to *Entamoeba histolytica*–mediated cytotoxicity. *Infect Immun*. 1989;57:8-12.
88. Ravdin JI, Stanley P, Murphy CF, et al. Characterization of cell surface carbohydrate receptors for *Entamoeba histolytica* adherence lectin. *Infect Immun*. 1989;57:2179-2186.
89. Lidell ME, Moncada DM, Chadee K, et al. *Entamoeba histolytica* cysteine proteases cleave the MUC2 mucin in its C-terminal domain and dissolve the protective colonic mucus gel. *Proc Natl Acad Sci U S A*. 2006;103:9298-9303.

90. Tannich E, Ebert F, Horstmann RD. Primary structure of the 170-kDa surface lectin of pathogenic *Entamoeba histolytica*. *Proc Natl Acad Sci U S A*. 1991;88:1849-1853.
91. Mann BJ, Torian BE, Vedvick TS, et al: Sequence of the cysteine-rich heavy subunit of the galactose lectin of *Entamoeba histolytica*. *Proc Natl Acad Sci U S A*. 1991;88:3248-3252.
92. Ramakrishnan G, Ragland BD, Purdy JE, et al. Physical mapping and expression of gene families encoding the *N*-acetyl D-galactosamine adherence lectin of *Entamoeba histolytica*. *Mol Microbiol*. 1996;19(1):91-100.
93. Dodson JM, Lenkowski PW Jr, Eubanks AC, et al. Role of the *Entamoeba histolytica* adhesin carbohydrate recognition domain in infection and immunity. *J Infect Dis*. 1999;179:460-466.
94. Mittal K, Welter BH, Temesvari LA. *Entamoeba histolytica:* lipid rafts are involved in adhesion of trophozoites to host extracellular matrix components. *Exp Parasitol*. 2008;120:127-134.
95. Baxt LA, Baker RP, Singh U, et al. An *Entamoeba histolytica* rhomboid protease with atypical specificity cleaves a surface lectin involved in phagocytosis and immune evasion. *Genes Dev*. 2008;22:1636-1646.
96. Blazquez S, Guigon G, Weber C, et al. Chemotaxis of *Entamoeba histolytica* towards the pro-inflammatory cytokine TNF is based on PI3K signalling, cytoskeleton reorganization and the galactose/*N*-acetylgalactosamine lectin activity. *Cell Microbiol*. 2008;10:1676-1686.
97. Bracha R, Nuchamowitz Y, Wender N, et al. Transcriptional gene silencing reveals two distinct groups of *Entamoeba histolytica* Gal/GalNAc-lectin light subunits. *Eukaryot Cell*. 2007;6:1758-1765.
98. Vines RR, Ramakrishnan G, Rogers J, et al. Regulation of adherence and virulence by the *Entamoeba histolytica* lectin cytoplasmic domain, which contains a β2 integrin motif. *Mol Biol Cell*. 1998;9:2069-2079.
99. Blazquez S, Rigothier MC, Huerre M, et al. Initiation of inflammation and cell death during liver abscess formation by *Entamoeba histolytica* depends on activity of the galactose/*N*-acetyl-D-galactosamine lectin. *Int J Parasitol*. 2007;37:425-433.
100. Hughes MA, Lee CW, Holm CF, et al. Identification of *Entamoeba histolytica* thiol-specific antioxidant as a GalNAc lectin–associated protein. *Mol Biochem Parasitol*. 2003;127:113-120.
101. Okada M, Huston CD, Mann BJ, et al. Proteomic analysis of phagocytosis in the enteric protozoan parasite *Entamoeba histolytica*. *Eukaryot Cell*. 2005;4:827-831.
102. McCoy JJ, Mann BJ. Proteomic analysis of Gal/GalNAc lectin–associated proteins in *Entamoeba histolytica*. *Exp Parasitol*. 2005;110:220-225.
103. Braga LL, Ninomiya H, McCoy JJ, et al. Inhibition of the complement membrane attack complex by the galactose-specific adhesin of *Entamoeba histolytica*. *J Clin Invest*. 1992;90:1131-1137.
104. Saffer LD, Petri WA Jr. Role of the galactose lectin of *Entamoeba histolytica* in adherence-dependent killing of mammalian cells. *Infect Immun*. 1991;59:4681-4683.
105. Godbold GD, Mann BJ. Cell killing by the human parasite *Entamoeba histolytica* is inhibited by the Rho-inactivating C3 exoenzyme. *Mol Biochem Parasitol*. 2000;108:147-151.
106. Arhets P, Olivo JC, Gounon P, et al. Virulence and functions of myosin II are inhibited by overexpression of light meromyosin in *Entamoeba histolytica*. *Mol Biol Cell*. 1998;6:1537-1547.
107. Ravdin JI, Moreau F, Sullivan JA, et al. Relationship of free intracellular calcium to the cytolytic activity of *Entamoeba histolytica*. *Infect Immmun*. 1988;56:1505-1512.
108. Ravdin JI, Sperelakis N, Guerrant RL. Effect of ion channel inhibitors on the cytopthogenicity of *Entamoeba histolytica*. *J Infect Dis*. 1982;146:335-340.
109. Leippe M, Ebel S, Schoenberger OL, et al. Pore-forming protein of pathogenic *Entamoeba histolytica*. *Proc Natl Acad Sci U S A*. 1991;88:7659-7663.
110. Leippe M, Tannich E, Nickel R, et al. Primary and secondary structure of the pore-forming peptide of pathogenic *Entamoeba histolytica*. *EMBO J*. 1992;11:3501-3506.
111. Bracha R, Nuchamowitz Y, Mirelman D. Transcriptional silencing of an amoebapore gene in *Entamoeba histolytica:* molecular analysis and effect on pathogenicity. *Eukaryot Cell*. 2003;2:295-305.
112. Ravdin JI, Schlesinger PH, Murphy CF, et al. Acid intracellular vesicles and the cytolysis of mammalian target cells by *Entamoeba histolytica* trophozoites. *J Protozool*. 1986;33:478-486.
113. Ragland BD, Ashley LS, Vaux DL, et al. *Entamoeba histolytica:* target cells killed by trophozoites undergo apoptosis which is not blocked by *bcl*-2. *Exp Parasitol*. 1994;79:460-467.
114. Seydel KB, Stanley SL Jr. *Entamoeba histolytica* induces host cell death in amebic liver abscess by a non-*Fas*-dependent, non–tumor necrosis factor α–dependent pathway of apoptosis. *Infect Immun*. 1998;66:2980-2983.
115. Huston CD, Houpt ER, Mann BJ, et al. Caspase 3 dependent killing of human cells by the parasite *Entamoeba histolytica*. *Cell Microbiol*. 2000;2:617-625.
116. Boettner DR, Huston CD, Sullivan JA, et al. *Entamoeba histolytica* and *Entamoeba dispar* utilize externalized phosphatidylserine for recognition and phagocytosis of erythrocytes. *Infect Immun*. 2005;73:3422-3430.
117. Huston CD, Boettner DR, Miller-Sims V, et al. Apoptotic killing and phagocytosis of host cells by the parasite *Entamoeba histolytica*. *Infect Immun*. 2003;71:964-972.
118. Teixeira JE, Heron BT, Huston CD. C1q- and collectin-dependent phagocytosis of apoptotic host cells by the intestinal protozoan *Entamoeba histolytica*. *J Infect Dis*. 2008;198:1062-1070.
119. Teixeira JE, Huston CD. Participation of the serine-rich *Entamoeba histolytica* protein in amebic phagocytosis of apoptotic host cells. *Infect Immun*. 2008;76:959-966.
120. Orozco E, Rodriquez MA, Murphy CF, et al. *Entamoeba histolytica:* Cytopathogenicity and lectin activity of avirulent mutants. *Exp Parasitol*. 1987;63:157-165.
121. Bracha R, Mirelman D. Virulence of *Entamoeba histolytica* trophozoites. Effects of bacteria, microaerobic conditions, and metronidazole. *J Exp Med*. 1984;160:353-368.
122. Bos HJ, Hage AJ. Virulence of bacteria-associated, *Crithidia*-associated, and axenic *Entamoeba histolytica:* experimental hamster liver infections with strains from patients and carriers. *Z Parasitenkd*. 1975;47(2):79-89.
123. Wittner M, Rosenbaum RM. Role of bacteria in modifying virulence of *Entamoeba* Histolytica. Studies of amebae from axenic cultures. *Am J Trop Med Hyg*. 1970;19:755-761.
124. Anaya-Velázquez F, Padilla-Vaca F. Effect of intestinal bacteria on the virulence of *Entamoeba histolytica*. *Arch Med Res*. 1992;23:183-185.
125. Galván-Moroyoqui JM, Domínguez-Robles MDC, Franco E, et al. The interplay between *Entamoeba* and enteropathogenic bacteria modulates epithelial cell damage. *PLoS Negl Trop Dis*. 2008;2(7):e266.
126. Moncada D, Keller K, Ankri S, et al. Antisense inhibition of *Entamoeba histolytica* cysteine proteases inhibits colonic mucus degradation. *Gastroenterology*. 2006;130:721-730.
127. Mora-Galindo J, Anaya-Velazquez F, Ramirez-Romo S, et al. *Entamoeba histolytica:* correlation of assessment methods to measure erythrocyte digestion, and effect of cysteine proteinases inhibitors in HM-1:IMSS and HK-9:NIH strains. *Exp Parasitol*. 2004;108:89-100.
128. Lauwaet T, Oliveira MJ, Callewaert B, et al. Proteolysis of enteric cell villin by *Entamoeba histolytica* cysteine proteinases. *J Biol Chem*. 2003;278:22650-22656.
129. Que X, Kim SH, Sajid M, et al. A surface amebic cysteine proteinase inactivates interleukin-18. *Infect Immun*. 2003;71:1274-1280.
130. Que X, Reed SL. Cysteine proteinases and the pathogenesis of amebiasis. *Clin Microbiol Rev*. 2000;13:196-206.
131. Santi-Rocca J, Weber C, Guigon G, et al. The lysine- and glutamic acid–rich protein KERP1 plays a role in *Entamoeba histolytica* liver abscess pathogenesis. *Cell Microbiol*. 2008;10:202-217.
132. MacFarlane RC, Singh U. Identification of an *Entamoeba histolytica* serine-, threonine-, and isoleucine-rich protein with roles in adhesion and cytotoxicity. *Eukaryot Cell*. 2007;6:2139-2146.
133. Guo X, Houpt E, Petri WA Jr. Crosstalk at the initial encounter: interplay between host defense and ameba survival strategies. *Curr Opin Immunol*. 2007;19:376-384.
134. Chadee K, Meerovitch E. The pathogenesis of experimentally induced amebic liver abscess in the gerbil (*Meriones unguiculatus*). *Am J Pathol*. 1984;117:71-80.
135. Tsutsumi V, Mena-Lopez R, Anaya-Velazquez F, et al. Cellular bases of experimental amebic liver abscess formation, *Am J Pathol*. 1984;117:81-91.
136. Martinez-Palomo A, Tsutsumi V, Anaya-Velazquez F, et al. Ultrastructure of experimental intestinal invasive amebiasis, *Am J Trop Med Hyg*. 1989;41:273-279.
137. Jarillo-Luna RA, Campos-Rodriguez R, Tsutsumi V. *Entamoeba histolytica:* immunohistochemical study of hepatic amoebiasis in mouse. Neutrophils and nitric oxide as possible factors of resistance. *Exp Parasitol*. 2002;101:40-56.
138. Chadee K, Moreau F, Meerovitch E. *Entamoeba histolytica:* chemoattractant activity for gerbil neutrophils in vivo and in vitro. *Exp Parasitol*. 1987;64:12-23.
139. Salata RA, Ahmed P, Ravdin JI. Chemoattractant activity of *Entamoeba histolytica* for human polymorphonuclear neutrophils. *J Parasitol*. 1989;75:644-646.
140. Yu Y, Chadee K. *Entamoeba histolytica* stimulates interleukin 8 from human colonic epithelial cells without parasite-enterocyte contact. *Gastroenterology*. 1997;112:1536-1547.
141. Sengelov H. Complement receptors in neutrophils. *Annu Rev Immunol*. 1995;15:107-131.
142. Denis M, Chadee K. Human neutrophils activated by interferon-γ and tumor necrosis factor-α kill *Entamoeba histolytica* trophozoites in vitro. *J Leukoc Biol*. 1989;46:270-274.
143. Guerrant RL, Brush J, Ravdin JI, et al. Interaction between *Entamoeba histolytica* and human polymorphonuclear neutrophils. *J Infect Dis*. 1981;143:83-93.
144. Seydel KB, Zhang T, Stanley SL Jr. Neutrophils play a critical role in early resistance to amebic liver abscesses in SCID mice. *Infect Immun*. 1997;65:3951-3953.
145. Velazquez C, Shibayama-Salas M, Aguirre-Garcia J, et al. Role of neutrophils in innate resistance to *Entamoeba histolytica* liver infection in mice. *Parasite Immunol*. 1998;20:255-262.
146. Asgharpour A, Gilchrist C, Baba D, et al. Resistance to intestinal *Entamoeba histolytica* infection is conferred by innate immunity and Gr-1^{+} cells. *Infect Immun*. 2005;73:4522-4529.
147. Salata RA, Ravdin JI. The interaction of human neutrophils and *Entamoeba histolytica* increases cytopathogenicity for liver cell monolayers. *J Infect Dis*. 1986;154:19-26.
148. Arbo A, Hoefsloot M, Ramirez A, et al. *Entamoeba histolytica* inhibits the respiratory burst of polymorphonuclear leukocytes. *Arch Invest Med (Mex)*. 1990;21:57-61.
149. Bruchhaus I, Richter S, Tannich E. Recombinant expression and biochemical characterization of an NADPH:flavin oxidoreductase from *Entamoeba histolytica*. *Biochem J*. 1998;330:1217-1221.
150. Sim S, Yong TS, Park SJ, et al. NADPH oxidase–derived reactive oxygen species–mediated activation of ERK1/2 is required for apoptosis of human neutrophils induced by *Entamoeba histolytica*. *J Immunol*. 2005;174:4279-4288.
151. Bruchhaus I, Richter S, Tannich E. Removal of hydrogen peroxide by the 29 kDa protein of *Entamoeba histolytica*. *Biochem J*. 1997;326:785-789.
152. Choi MH, Sajed D, Poole L, et al. An unusual surface peroxiredoxin protects invasive *Entamoeba histolytica* from oxidant attack. *Mol Biochem Parasitol*. 2005;143:80-89.
153. Salata RA, Martinez-Palomo A, Murray HW, et al. Patients treated for amebic liver abscess develop cell mediated immune responses effective in vitro against *Entamoeba histolytica*. *J Immunol*. 1986;136:2633-2639.
154. Lin JY, Seguin R, Keller K, et al. Tumor necrosis factor α augments nitric oxide–dependent macrophage cytotoxicity against *Entamoeba histolytica* by enhanced expression of the nitric oxide synthase gene. *Infect Immun*. 1994;62:1534-1541.
155. Ghadirian E, Denis M. *Entamoeba histolytica* extract and interferon-γ activation of macrophage-mediated amoebicidal function. *Immunobiology*. 1992;185:1-10.
156. Maldonado-Bernal C, Kirschning CJ, Rosenstein Y, et al. The innate immune response to *Entamoeba histolytica* lipopeptidophosphoglycan is mediated by Toll-like receptors 2 and 4. *Parasite Immunol*. 2005;27:127-137.
157. Seydel KB, Smith SJ, Stanley SL Jr. Innate immunity to amebic liver abscess is dependent on gamma interferon and nitric oxide in a murine model of disease. *Infect Immun*. 2000;68:400-402.
158. Wang W, Keller K, Chadee K. *Entamoeba histolytica* modulates the nitric oxide synthase gene and nitric oxide production by macrophages for cytotoxicity against amoebae and tumour cells. *Immunology*. 1994;83:601-610.
159. Lin JY, Keller K, Chadee K. *E. histolytica* proteins modulate the respiratory burst potential by murine macrophages. *Immunology*. 1993;78:291-297.
160. Elnekave K, Siman-Tov R, Ankri S. Consumption of L-arginine mediated by *Entamoeba histolytica* L-arginase (EhArg) inhibits amoebicidal activity and nitric oxide production by activated macrophages. *Parasite Immunol*. 2003;25:597-608.
161. Séguin R, Keller K, Chadee K. *Entamoeba histolytica* stimulates the unstable transcription of *c-fos* and tumor necrosis factor-α messenger RNA by protein kinase C signal transduction in macrophages. *Immunology*. 1995;86:49-57.
162. Wang W, Chadee K. *Entamoeba histolytica* suppresses gamma interferon–induced macrophage class II major histocompatibility complex Ia molecule and I-A beta mRNA expression by a prostaglandin E_2-dependent mechanism. *Infect Immun*. 1995;63:1089-1094.
163. Dey I, Keller K, Belley A, et al. Identification and characterization of a cyclooxygenase-like enzyme from *Entamoeba histolytica*. *Proc Natl Acad Sci U S A*. 2003;100:13561-13566.
164. Rico G, Leandro E, Rojas S, et al. The monocyte locomotion inhibitory factor produced by *Entamoeba histolytica* inhibits induced nitric oxide production in human leukocytes. *Parasitol Res*. 2003;90:264-267.
165. Rojas-Dotor S, Rico G, Perez J, et al. Cytokine expression in CD4(+) cells exposed to the monocyte locomotion inhibitory factor produced by *Entamoeba histolytica*. *Parasitol Res*. 2006;98:493-495.
166. Lotter H, Jacobs T, Gaworski I, et al. Sexual dimorphism in the control of amebic liver abscess in a mouse model of disease. *Infect Immun*. 2006;74:118-124.
167. Kim KH, Shin CO, Im K. Natural killer cell activity in mice infected with free-living amoeba with reference to their pathogenicity. *Korean J Parasitol*. 1993;31:239-248.
168. Houpt ER, Glembocki DG, Obrig TG, et al. The mouse model of amebic colitis reveals mouse strain susceptibility to infection and exacerbation of disease by CD4^{+} T cells. *J Immunol*. 2002;169:4496-4503.
169. Reed SL, Gigli I. Lysis of complement-sensitive *Entamoeba histolytica* by activated terminal complement components. *J Clin Invest*. 1990;86:1815-1822.
170. Reed SL, Ember JA, Herdman DS, et al. The extracellular neutral cysteine proteinase of *Entamoeba histolytica* degrades anaphylatoxins C3a and C5a. *J Immunol*. 1995;155:266-274.
171. Seydel KB, Li E, Zhang Z, et al. Epithelial cell–initiated inflammation plays a crucial role in early tissue damage in amebic infection of human intestine. *Gastroenterology*. 1998;115:1446-1453.
172. Eckmann L, Reed SL, Smith JR, et al. *Entamoeba histolytica* trophozoites induce an inflammatory cytokine response by cultured human cells through the paracrine action of cytolytically released interleukin-1 alpha. *J Clin Invest*. 1995;96:1269-1279.
173. Kammanadiminti SJ, Chadee K. Suppression of NF-κB Activation by *Entamoeba histolytica* in intestinal epithelial cells is mediated by heat shock protein 27. *J Biol Chem*. 2006;281:26112-26120.
174. Hamano S, Asgharpour A, Stroup SE, et al. Resistance of C57BL/6 mice to amoebiasis is mediated by nonhemopoietic cells but requires hemopoietic IL-10 production. *J Immunol*. 2006;177:1208-1213.

175. Haque R, Ali IKM, Sack RB, et al. Amebiasis and mucosal IgA antibody against the *Entamoeba histolytica* adherence lectin in Bangladeshi children. *J Infect Dis.* 2001;183:1787-1793.
176. Kaur U, Sharma AK, Sharma M, et al. Distribution of *Entamoeba histolytica* Gal/GalNAc lectin–specific antibody response in an endemic area. *Scand J Immunol.* 2004;60:524-528.
177. Haque R, Duggal P, Ali IKM, et al. Innate and acquired resistance to amebiasis in Bangladeshi children. *J Infect Dis.* 2002;186:547-552.
178. Haque R, Mondal D, Shu J, et al. Correlation of interferon-gamma production by peripheral blood mononuclear cells with childhood malnutrition and susceptibility to amebiasis. *Am J Trop Med Hyg.* 2007;76:340-344.
179. Talamás-Rohana P, Schlie-Guzmán MA, Hernández-Ramírez VI, et al. T-cell suppression and selective in vivo activation of Th2 subpopulation by *Entamoeba histolytica* 220-kilodalton lectin. *Infect Immun.* 1995;63:3953-3958.
180. World Health Organization. Amebiasis. *Wkly Epidemiol Rec.* 1997;72:97-100.
181. Caballero-Salcedo A, Viveros-Rogel M, Salvatierra B, et al. Seroepidemiology of amebiasis in Mexico. *Am J Trop Med Hyg.* 1994;50:412-419.
182. Braga LL, Mendonca Y, Paiva CA, et al. Seropositivity for and intestinal colonization with *Entamoeba histolytica* and *Entamoeba dispar* in individuals in northeastern Brazil. *J Clin Microbiol.* 1998;36:3044-3045.
183. Blessmann J, Van Linh P, Nu PA, et al. Epidemiology of amebiasis in a region of high incidence of amebic liver abscess in central Vietnam. *Am J Trop Med Hyg.* 2002;66:578-583.
184. Freedman DO, Weld LH, Kozarsky PE, et al. Spectrum of disease and relation to place of exposure among ill returned travelers. *N Engl J Med.* 2006;354:119-130.
185. Hsu MS, Hsieh SM, Chen MY, et al. Association between amebic liver abscess and human immunodeficiency virus infection in Taiwanese subjects. *BMC Infect Dis.* 2008;8:48.
186. Hung CC, Deng HY, Hsiao WH, et al. Invasive amebiasis as an emerging parasitic disease in patients with human immunodeficiency virus type 1 infection in Taiwan. *Arch Intern Med.* 2005;165:409-415.
187. Barwick R, Uzicanin A, Lareau S, et al. Outbreak of amebiasis in Tbilisi, Republic of Georgia, 1998. *Am J Trop Med Hyg.* 2002;67:623-631.
188. Haque R, Ali IKM, Petri WA Jr. Prevalence and immune response to *Entamoeba histolytica* in preschool children in an urban slum of Dhaka, Bangladesh. *Am J Trop Med Hyg.* 1999;60:1031-1034.
189. Haque, R, Mondal D, Kirkpatrick BD, et al. Epidemiologic and clinical characteristics of acute diarrhea with emphasis on *E. histolytica* infections in preschool children in urban slum of Dhaka, Bangladesh. *Am J Trop Med Hyg.* 2003;69:398-405.
190. Gathiram V, Jackson TF. A longitudinal study of asymptomatic carriers of pathogenic zymodemes of *Entamoeba histolytica*. *South Afr Med J.* 1987;72:669-672.
191. Duggal P, Haque R, Roy S, et al. Influence of human leukocyte antigen class II alleles on susceptibility to *Entamoeba histolytica* infection in Bangladeshi children. *J Infect Dis.* 2004;189:520-526.
192. Haque R, Mondal D, Karim A, et al. Association of common enteric protozoan parasites with severe diarrhea in Bangladesh: a prospective case-control study. *Clin Infect Dis.* 2009;48:1191-1197.
193. Adams EB, MacLeod IN. Invasive amebiasis. I. Amebic dysentery and its complications. *Medicine.* 1977;56:315-323.
194. Balikian JP, Bitar JG, Rishani KK, et al. Fulminant necrotizing amebic colitis in children. *Am J Proctol.* 1977;28:69-73.
195. Rao S, Solaymani-Mohammadi S, Petri WA Jr, et al. Hepatic amebiasis: a reminder of the complications. *Curr Opin Pediatr.* 2009;21(1):145-149.
196. Katzenstein D, Rickerson V, Braude A, et al. New concepts of amebic liver abscess derived from hepatic imaging, serodiagnosis, and hepatic enzymes in 67 consecutive cases in San Diego. *Medicine (Baltimore).* 1982;61:237-246.
197. Adams EB, MacLeod IN. Invasive amebiasis. II. Amebic liver abscess and its complications. *Medicine.* 1977;56:325-334.
198. Haffar A, Boland J, Edwards MS. Amebic liver abscess in children. *Pediatr Infect Dis.* 1982;1:322-327.
199. Merritt RJ, Coughlin E, Thomas DW, et al. Spectrum of amebiasis in children. *Am J Dis Child.* 1982;136:785-789.
200. Ramachandran S, Goonatillake HD, Induruwa PAC. Syndromes in amoebic liver abscess. *Br J Surg.* 1976;63:220-225.
201. Brandt H, Tamayo RP. Pathology of human amebiasis. *Hum Pathol.* 1970;1:351-385.
202. Freeman AL, Bhoola KD. Pneumopericardium complicating amoebic liver abscess: a case report. *S Afr Med J.* 1976;50:551-553.
203. Ganesan TK, Kandaswamy S. Amebic pericarditis. *Chest.* 1975;67:112-113.
204. Solaymani-Mohammadi S, Lam M, Zunt JR, et al. *Entamoeba histolytica* encephalitis diagnosed by polymerase chain reaction of cerebrospinal fluid. *Trans R Soc Trop Med Hyg.* 2007;101:311-313.
205. Magana ML, Fernandez-Diez J, Magana M. Cutaneous amebiasis in pediatrics. *Arch Dermatol.* 2008;144:1369-1372.
206. Al-Daraji WI, Ilyas M, Robson A. Primary cutaneous amebiasis with a fatal outcome. *Am J Dermatopathol.* 2008;30:398-400.
207. Krogstad DJ, Spencer HC Jr, Healy GR, et al. Amebiasis: epidemiologic studies in the United States, 1971-1974. *Ann Intern Med.* 1978;88:89-97.
208. Hennessy TW, Marcus R, Deneen V, et al. Emerging Infections Program FoodNet Working Group. Survey of physician diagnostic practices for patients with acute diarrhea: clinical and public health implications. *Clin Infect Dis.* 2004;38(Suppl. 3):S203-S211.
209. Pillai DR, Keystone JS, Sheppard DC, et al. *Entamoeba histolytica* and *Entamoeba dispar:* epidemiology and comparison of diagnostic methods in a setting of nonendemicity. *Clin Infect Dis.* 1999;29:1315-1318.
210. Solaymani-Mohammadi S, Coyle CM, Factor SM, et al. Amebic colitis in an antigenically and serologically negative patient: usefulness of a small-subunit ribosomal RNA (SSU-rRNA) gene-based PCR in diagnosis. *Diagn Microbiol Infect Dis.* 2008;62:333-335.
211. Clark CG, Diamond LS. Methods for cultivation of luminal parasitic protists of clinical importance. *Clin Microbiol Rev.* 2002;15:329-341.
212. Simsek H, Elsurer R, Sokmensuer C, et al. Ameboma mimicking carcinoma of the cecum: case report. *Gastrointest Endosc.* 2004;59:453-454.
213. Okamoto M, Kawabe T, Ohata K, et al. Amebic colitis in asymptomatic subjects with positive fecal occult blood test results: clinical features different from symptomatic cases. *Am J Trop Med Hyg.* 2005;73:934-935.
214. Hardin RE, Ferzli GS, Zenilman ME, et al. Invasive amebiasis and ameboma formation presenting as a rectal mass: an uncommon case of malignant masquerade at a western medical center. *World J Gastroenterol.* 2007;13:5659-5661.
215. McCarthy JS, Peacock D, Trown KP, et al. Endemic invasive amoebiasis in northern Australia. *Med J Australia.* 2002;177:570.
216. Roy S, Kabir M, Mondal D, et al. Real-time PCR assay for the diagnosis of *Entamoeba histolytica* infection. *J Clin Microbiol.* 2005;43:2168-2172.
217. Blessmann J, Buss H, Nu PA, et al. Real-time PCR for detection and differentiation of *Entamoeba histolytica* and *Entamoeba dispar* in fecal samples. *J Clin Microbiol.* 2002;40:4413-4417.
218. Verweij JJ, Blange RA, Templeton K, et al. Simultaneous detection of *Entamoeba histolytica, Giardia lamblia,* and *Cryptosporidium parvum* in fecal samples by using multiplex real-time PCR. *J Clin Microbiol.* 2004;42:1220-1223.
219. Qvarnstrom Y, James C, Xayavong M, et al. Comparison of real-time PCR protocols for differential laboratory diagnosis of amebiasis. *J Clin Microbiol.* 2005;43:5491-5497.
220. Fotedar R, Stark D, Beebe N, et al. Laboratory diagnostic techniques for *Entamoeba* species. *Clin Microbiol Rev.* 2007;20:511-532.
221. Calderaro AC, Gorrini S, Bommezzadri G, et al. *Entamoeba histolytica* and *Entamoeba dispar:* comparison of two PCR assays for diagnosis in a non-endemic setting. *Trans R Soc Trop Med Hyg.* 2006;100:450-457.
222. Sharp SE, Suarez CA, Duran Y, et al. Evaluation of the Triage Micro Parasite Panel for detection of *Giardia lamblia, Entamoeba histolytica/Entamoeba dispar,* and *Cryptosporidium parvum* in patient stool specimens. *J Clin Microbiol.* 2001;39:332-334.
223. Buss SN, Kabir M, Petri WA Jr, et al. Comparison of two immunoassays for detection of *Entamoeba histolytica*. *J Clin Microbiol.* 2008;46:2778-2779.
224. Visser LG, Verweij JJ, Van Esbroeck M, et al. Diagnostic methods for differentiation of *Entamoeba histolytica* and *Entamoeba dispar* in carriers: performance and clinical implications in a non-endemic setting. *J Med Microbiol.* 2006;296:397-403.
225. Furrows SJ, Moody AH, Chiodini PL. Comparison of PCR and antigen detection methods for diagnosis of *Entamoeba histolytica* infection. *J Clin Pathol.* 2004;57:1264-1266.
226. Sharma AK, Chibbar S, Bansal G, et al. Evaluation of newer diagnostic methods for the detection and differentiation of *Entamoeba histolytica* in an endemic area. *Trans R Soc Trop Med Hyg.* 2003;97:396-397.
227. Stark D, van Hal S, Fotedar R, et al. Comparison of stool antigen detection kits to PCR for diagnosis of amebiasis. *J Clin Microbiol.* 2008;46:1678-1681.
228. Stanley SL Jr, Jackson TF, Foster L, et al. Longitudinal study of the antibody response to recombinant *Entamoeba histolytica* antigens in patients with amebic liver abscess. *Am J Trop Med Hyg.* 1998;58:414-416.
229. Krupp IM. Comparison of counterimmunoelectrophoresis with other serologic tests in the diagnosis of amebiasis. *Am J Trop Med Hyg.* 1974;23:27-30.
230. Hira PR, Iqbal J, Al-Ali F, et al. Invasive amebiasis: challenges in diagnosis in a non-endemic country (Kuwait). *Am J Trop Med Hyg.* 2001;65:341-345.
231. Knappik M, Borner U, Jelinek T. Sensitivity and specificity of a new commercial enzyme-linked immunoassay kit for detecting *Entamoeba histolytica* IgG antibodies in serum samples. *Eur J Clin Microbiol Infect Dis.* 2005;24:701-703.
232. Ravdin JI, Jackson TF, Petri WA Jr. Association of serum anti-adherence lectin antibodies with invasive amebiasis and asymptomatic *Entamoeba histolytica* infection. *J Infect Dis.* 1990;162:768-772.
233. Abd-Alla MD, El-Hawey AM, Ravdin JI. Use of an enzyme-linked immunosorbent assay to detect anti-adherence protein antibodies in sera of patients with invasive amebiasis in Cairo, Egypt. *Am J Trop Med Hyg.* 1992;47:800-804.
234. Powell SJ, MacLeod I, Wilmot AL, et al. Metronidazole in amoebic dysentery and amoebic liver abscess. *Lancet.* 1966;2:1329-1331.
235. Blessmann J, Tannich E. Treatment of asymptomatic intestinal *Entamoeba histolytica* infection. *N Engl J Med.* 2002;347:1384.
236. McAuley JB, Herwaldt BL, Stokes SL, et al. Diloxanide furoate for treating asymptomatic *Entamoeba histolytica* cyst passers: 14 years' experience in the United States. *Clin Infect Dis.* 1992;15:464-468.
237. McAuley JB, Juranek DD. Paromomycin in the treatment of mild-to-moderate intestinal amebiasis. *Clin Infect Dis.* 1992;15:551-552.
238. van Sonnenberg E, Mueller PR, Schiffman HR, et al. Intrahepatic amebic abscesses: indications for and results of percutaneous catheter drainage. *Radiology.* 1985;156:631-635.
239. Water and sanitation: the neglected health MDG. *Lancet.* 2006;368:1212.
240. Houpt E, Barroso L, Lockhart L, et al. Prevention of intestinal amebiasis by vaccination with the *Entamoeba histolytica* Gal/GalNAc lectin. *Vaccine.* 2004;22:612-617.
241. Ivory CP, Chadee K. Intranasal immunization with Gal-inhibitable lectin plus an adjuvant of CpG oligodeoxynucleotides protects against *Entamoeba histolytica* challenge. *Infect Immun.* 2007;75:4917-4922.
242. Gaucher D, Chadee K. Prospect for an *Entamoeba histolytica* Gal-lectin–based vaccine. *Parasite Immunol.* 2003;25(2):55-58.
243. Abd Alla MD, White GL, Rogers TB, et al. Adherence-inhibitory intestinal immunoglobulin α antibody response in baboons elicited by use of a synthetic intranasal lectin-based amebiasis subunit vaccine. *Infect Immun.* 2007;75:3812-3822.
244. Stanley SL Jr. Vaccines for amoebiasis: barriers and opportunities. *Parasitology.* 2006;133(Suppl):S81-S86.
245. Lotter H, Russmann H, Heesemann J, et al. Attenuated recombinant *Yersinia* as live oral vaccine carrier to protect against amoebiasis. *Int J Med Microbiol.* 2008;298(1-2):79-86.

Free-Living Amebas

ANITA A. KOSHY | **BRIAN G. BLACKBURN** | **UPINDER SINGH**

Overview

The free-living amebas are aerobic, eukaryotic protists that comprise several genera. Infection of humans with free-living amebas is an infrequent but often fatal occurrence in both normal and immunocompromised individuals. Central nervous system (CNS) invasion by *Naegleria fowleri*, *Acanthamoeba* spp., and *Balamuthia mandrillaris* has been reported in hundreds of patients worldwide, with thousands of *Acanthamoeba* keratitis cases described.[1-4] A single report of human infection with *Sappinia* increases to four the number of genera of known pathogenic free-living ameba in humans, and raises the possibility of the identification of additional organisms as human pathogens in the future.[5] Distinct from other pathogenic protozoa by nature of their free-living existence, these organisms have no known insect vectors, no human carrier states of epidemiologic importance, and little relationship between poor sanitation and their transmission. Four distinct clinical syndromes are caused by the free-living amebas that infect humans: (1) primary amebic meningoencephalitis (PAM); (2) granulomatous amebic encephalitis (GAE); (3) disseminated granulomatous amebic disease (e.g., skin, pulmonary, and sinus infection); and (4) amebic keratitis (AK).

PAM is caused by *Naegleria fowleri* and occurs most commonly in healthy children and young adults with recent recreational freshwater exposure. *Naegleria* gain access to the CNS by direct invasion through the nasal mucosa and the cribriform plate and cause a rapidly fatal meningoencephalitis. GAE, caused by *Acanthamoeba* spp., *B. mandrillaris*, and *Sappinia*, is a subacute infection that likely spreads hematogenously from pulmonary or skin lesions to the CNS. The resultant focal neurological deficits progress over days to months to a diffuse meningoencephalitis and death. Disseminated granulomatous amebic disease involving the skin, lungs, or sinuses but without CNS infection with *Acanthamoeba* and *Balamuthia* have also been reported.[6,7] *Acanthamoeba* spp. also cause a subacute to chronic keratitis that is most often associated with contact lens use or corneal trauma, with rare reports of cases occurring after radial keratotomy.[4]

Organisms

NAEGLERIA

N. fowleri was named after Malcolm Fowler of Adelaide Children's Hospital of Australia, who (with R.F. Carter) described the initial cases of PAM.[8] Of the approximately 30 species in the genus, *N. fowleri* is the only known pathogen of humans, although other species cause disease in mice (e.g., *Naegleria australiensis* and *N. italica*).[9] *Naegleria* spp. have three life cycle stages: trophozoites, flagellates, and cysts (Fig. 274-1). The trophozoites are the reproductive stage of the parasite and cause invasive human disease. Trophozoites feed predominantly on bacteria, are 10 to 25 μm in diameter, have pseudopodia, and a clear nucleus with a prominent dense central nucleolus (Fig. 274-2). The granular cytoplasm can contain ingested red blood cells and leukocytes along with cytoplasmic organelles. On transfer to distilled water or a non-nutrient medium, trophozoites can transform rapidly to a transitory flagellate form, which does not divide or feed; the flagellate form can spontaneously revert to the trophozoite. When trophozoites encyst, they produce a cyst (~9 μm diameter with a central nucleus and a single-layered wall containing an average of two pores), which is resistant to environmental stresses. *N. fowleri* is thermophilic, with trophozoites growing well at temperatures as high as 45° C.[9] Organisms

can be cultivated from clinical specimens and grow well in vitro. Like *Acanthamoeba* and *Balamuthia*, *N. fowleri* can be grown in a cell-free axenic medium as well as in a chemically defined medium.

ACANTHAMOEBA

Acanthamoeba species recognized as pathogenic for humans include *A. castellanii*, *A. polyphaga*, *A. culbertsoni*, *A. palestinensis*, *A. astronyxis*, *A. hatchetti*, *A. healyi*, *A. rhysodes*, *A. divionesis*, and *A. griffini*.[1] Previously, *Acanthamoeba* were grouped by morphology and cyst size into 3 groups (I, II, and III). Given the availability of newer molecular mechanisms of determining genomic sequence, a movement to genotype *Acanthamoeba* spp. and group them by genetic similarity is underway.[1,10] Generally the genotyping is consistent with the morphologic grouping. Thus far, 15 genotypes (T1-15) have been described, with genotype T4 (correlating to *A. castellanii* complex) being the most commonly identified in the environment and in human disease.[1,10] The life cycle of *Acanthamoeba* consists of trophozoite and cyst stages (see Fig. 274-1). Trophozoites are 15-50 μm in diameter, contain a single nucleus with a prominent central nucleolus, and have distinctive slender, spinelike projections of the plasma membrane (Fig. 274-3). The cysts have a double-layered wall, are less than 18-30 μm in diameter, and like *Naegleria*, may contain pores in the cyst wall (Fig. 274-4). Trophozoites are the active form of *Acanthamoeba*, feeding on bacteria and environmental debris, whereas the cyst is the inactive but environmentally resistant stage. *Acanthamoeba* spp. can be easily cultivated in the laboratory; this is best accomplished by the use of tryptic soy agar with rabbit or horse blood, buffered charcoal yeast extract agar, and non-nutrient agar overlaid with live organisms such as *E. coli*, or *Enterobacter aerogenes*.[1,11] Like *N. fowleri*, most *Acanthamoeba* spp. can be grown in a cell-free axenic medium as well as in a chemically defined medium.[1]

BALAMUTHIA

B. mandrillaris, formerly referred to as leptomyxid ameba, is the only known species of this genus and was originally isolated from the brain of a mandrill baboon in 1986.[2,12] The life cycle consists of the trophozoite and cyst stages (see Fig. 274-1). *B. mandrillaris* trophozoites have a mean diameter of 30 μm (range 12-60 μm) and are uninucleate (Fig. 274-5). Cysts have a mean diameter of 15 μm (range 12-30 μm) with a wavy and irregular outer wall that is composed of three layers (Fig. 274-6).[1] On hematoxylin and eosin (H&E)–stained specimens, the organism cannot be reliably differentiated from *Acanthamoeba*. Laboratory growth of *Balamuthia* is more difficult than for *Acanthamoeba* or *Naegleria*, as it does not grow on bacteria-coated agar plates and has a long doubling time. Until recently, these factors and a lack of knowledge about its food source in nature have hampered isolation of environmental samples. However, the recent development of a cell-free growth medium and axenization should make the clinical and environmental isolation of this organism much easier. In addition, *Balamuthia* can be grown in the laboratory using mammalian cell cultures, and in vitro, *Balamuthia* can feed on small amebas.[2]

SAPPINIA

Sappinia, another free-living ameba, are a more recently recognized human pathogen.[5] *Sappinia* trophozoites are 40-80 μm in size, with a single large cytoplasmic vacuole and two nuclei (Fig. 274-7). The

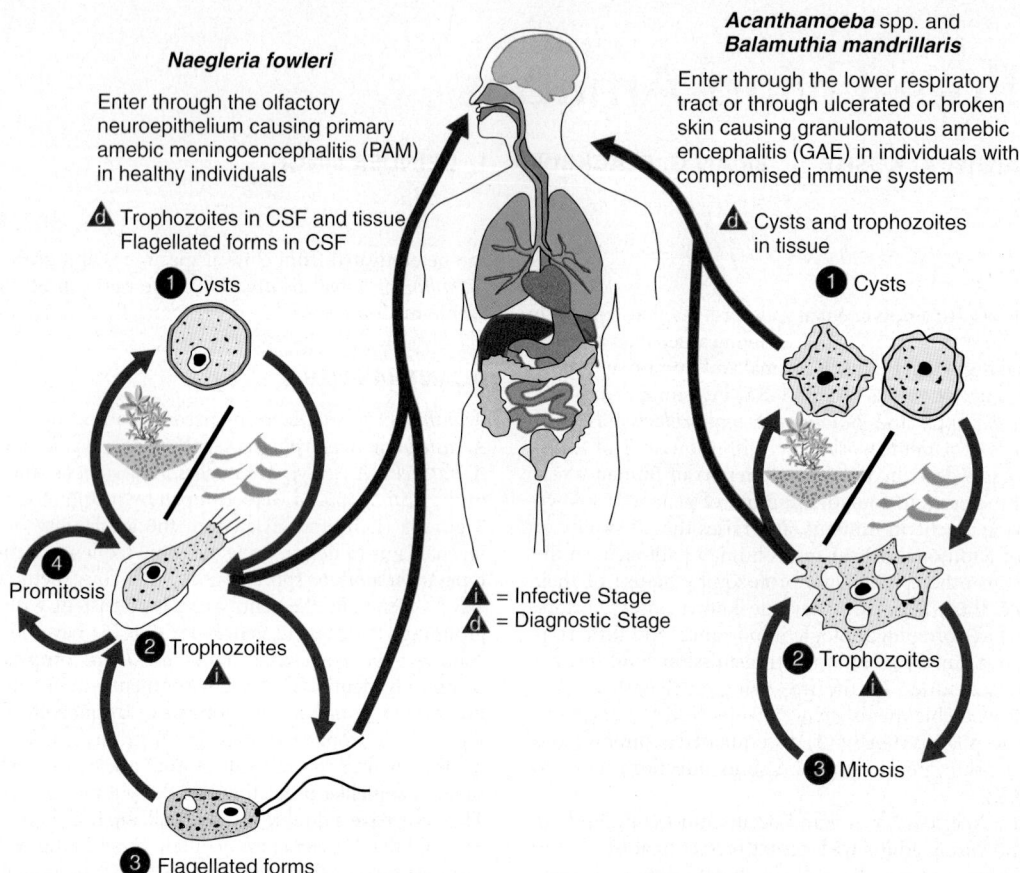

Figure 274-1 Life cycles of *Naegleria fowleri*, *Acanthamoeba* spp., and *Balamuthia*, showing stages as well as proposed portals of entry. *(Courtesy Division of Parasitic Diseases/Centers for Disease Control and Prevention, with permission.)*

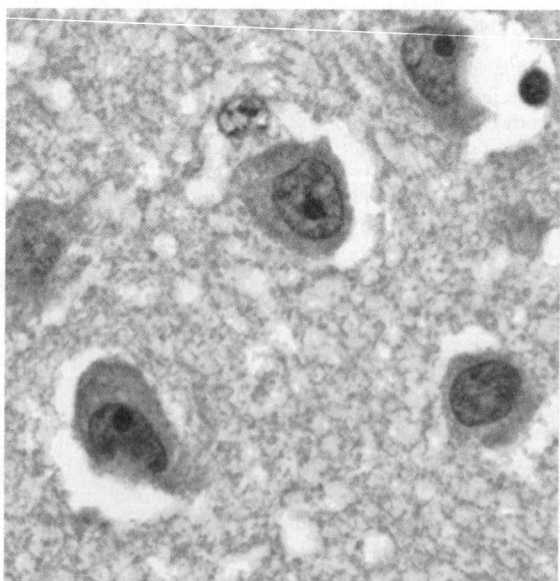

Figure 274-2 Trophozoites of *Naegleria fowleri* in brain tissue stained with hematoxylin and eosin. Note the clear nucleus with a prominent dense central nucleolus. *(Courtesy Division of Parasitic Diseases/Centers for Disease Control and Prevention, with permission.)*

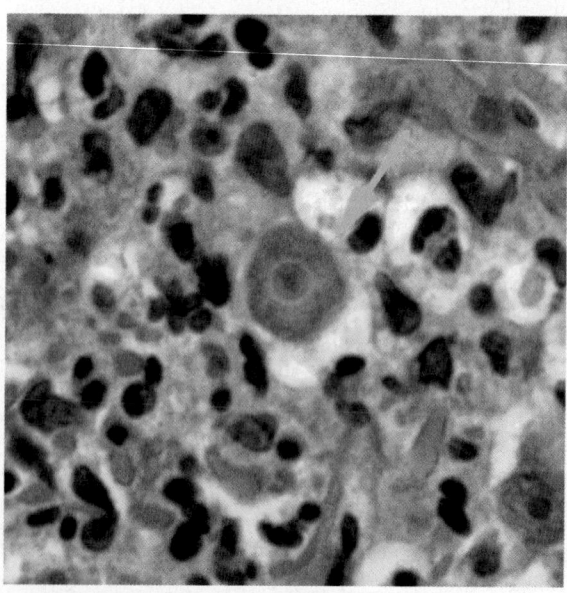

Figure 274-3 *Acanthamoeba* **trophozoite (*green arrow*) in tissue stained with hematoxylin and eosin.** Note the single nucleus with prominent central nucleolus. *(Courtesy Division of Parasitic Diseases/Centers for Disease Control and Prevention, with permission.)*

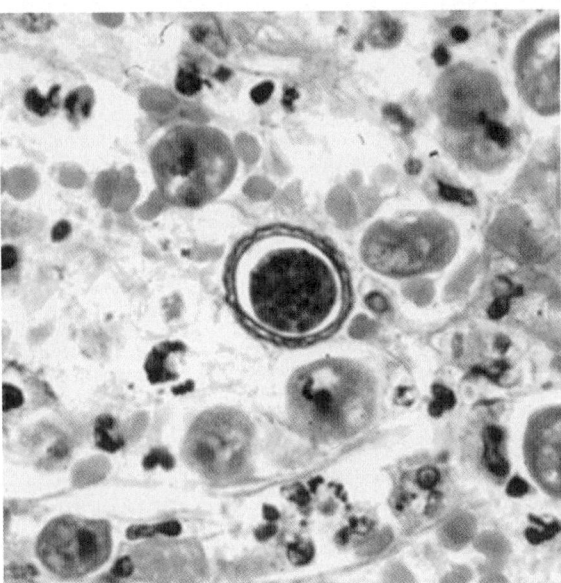

Figure 274-4 *Acanthamoeba* **cyst in brain tissue stained with hematoxylin and eosin.** Note the double wall of the cyst. *(Courtesy Division of Parasitic Diseases/Centers for Disease Control and Prevention, with permission.)*

double nucleus with a central flattening is a distinctive characteristic of this species and indicative of the sexual reproduction of these parasites, another unusual feature among free-living ameba.[13] Microbiological and clinical characteristics of the free-living amebas known to cause human disease are highlighted in Table 274-1.

EPIDEMIOLOGY

NAEGLERIA

N. fowleri has been found worldwide in soil, river, and lake water samples.[14] Importantly, *N. fowleri* is not found in seawater. Pathogenic

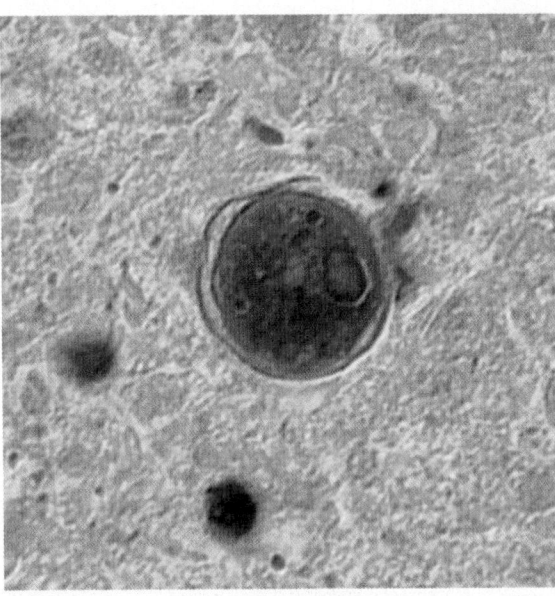

Figure 274-6 *Balamuthia* **cyst in brain tissue stained with hematoxylin and eosin.** By light microscopy only two walls can be distinguished. Specific immunostaining reliably distinguishes *Balamuthia* cysts from those of *Acanthamoeba* spp. *(From the Division of Parasitic Diseases/Centers for Disease Control and Prevention and the University of Kentucky Hospital, Lexington, Kentucky, with permission.)*

N. fowleri are thermophilic and proliferate at temperatures up to 45°C.[9] The presence of *N. fowleri* in fresh water is directly related to water temperature,[15] and *N. fowleri* has been frequently isolated from thermally polluted waters in temperate climates, including as far north in the United States as Connecticut.[16] In semitropical locations such as Florida, it is not uncommon to isolate at least one *N. fowleri* organism per 25 mL of water.[15] As water temperatures drop in winter, *Naegleria* is typically isolated from lake-bottom sediments; *Naegleria*

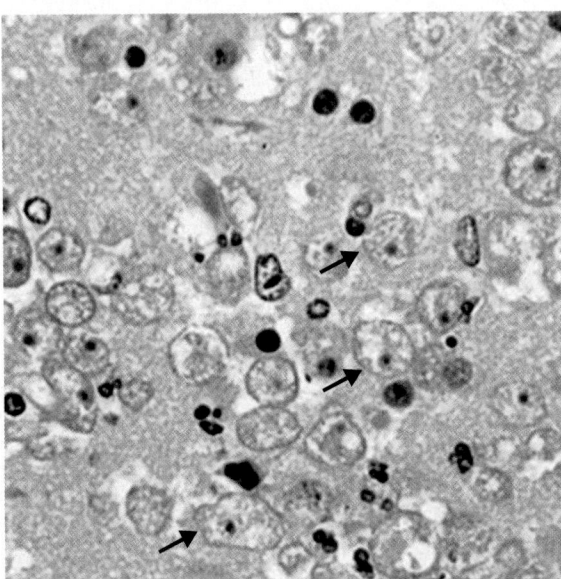

Figure 274-5 *Balamuthia* **trophozoites (*black arrows*) in brain tissue stained with hematoxylin and eosin.** Trophozoites are uninucleate and cannot be reliably distinguished from *Acanthamoeba* spp. trophozoites without specific immunostaining. *(Courtesy Division of Parasitic Diseases/Centers for Disease Control and Prevention, with permission.)*

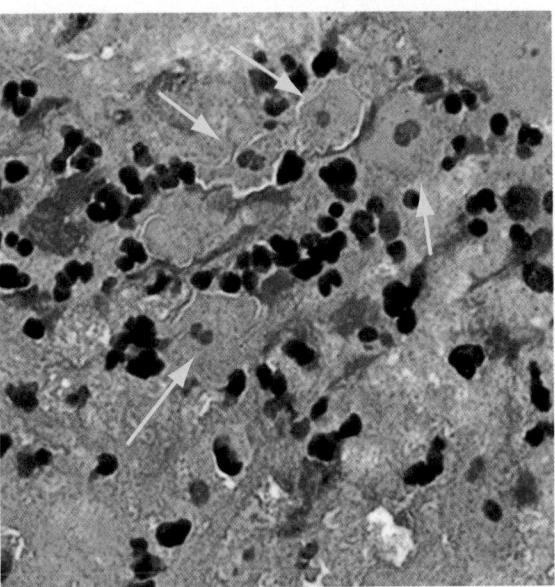

Figure 274-7 **Trophozoites of** *Sappinia* **(*yellow arrows*) in brain tissue stained with hematoxylin and eosin.** Note the distinctive double nucleus that defines this species. *(Courtesy Division of Parasitic Diseases/Centers for Disease Control and Prevention, with permission.)*

TABLE 274-1	Microbiologics and Clinical Characteristics of the Free-Living Amebas Known to Cause Human Disease				
	Naegleria fowleri	*Acanthamoeba* spp. (non-keratitis disease)	*Acanthamoeba* spp. (keratitis)	*Balamuthia mandrillaris*	*Sappinia**
Disease	Primary amebic meningoencephalitis (PAM)	Granulomatous amebic encephalitis (GAE); cutaneous lesions; sinus infections	Amebic keratitis	GAE; cutaneous lesions; sinus infections	Amebic encephalitis (granuloma not seen)
Epidemiology	Most human cases associated with exposure to recreational warm fresh water	Can acquire from soil, water, air	Corneal trauma; poor contact lens hygiene; association with certain commercial lens solutions	Can acquire from soil, water, air	Can acquire from soil, water, air
Groups at risk	Healthy children and young adults, usually male	Immunocompromised individuals	Contact lens wearers (>80% of cases)	Immunocompromised individuals; healthy children and elderly; Hispanic Americans	Single patient was immunocompetent
Signs and symptoms at presentation	Headache, neck stiffness, seizures, coma	Headache, neck stiffness, behavioral changes, coma; sinus disease; skin ulcers	Intense pain, photophobia, tearing; dendriform epitheliopathy (early); stromal ring	Headache, neck stiffness, seizures, hydrocephalus; sinus infection; skin nodules	Headache, vomiting, photophobia; preceding sinus infection
Clinical course	Prodrome of few days; fulminant disease; without treatment, death occurs within 1-2 weeks	Prodrome of weeks to months; subacute course; acute stage fatal in weeks	Prodrome of days; subacute to chronic keratitis	Prodrome of weeks to months; subacute course; acute stage fatal in weeks	Patient recovered following treatment
Laboratory diagnosis	CSF wet mount positive for ameba; CSF with polymorphonuclear pleocytosis; no cysts seen in brain tissue; PCR from CSF	Ameba rarely seen in CSF wet mount; cysts seen in brain tissue—test by IFA, IIF, or PCR for definitive identification	Corneal scraping or biopsy to find trophozoites or cysts; confocal microscopy	Ameba rarely isolated from CSF, but CSF can have highly elevated protein; cysts seen in brain tissue—test by IFA, IIF, and PCR	Binucleate ameba seen in brain tissue—test by PCR
Distinct morphologic features	Vesicular nucleus; limacine movement of ameba; flagellate stage; cysts with pores flush at surface	Vesicular nucleus; fingerlike pseudopodia projecting from surface; cyst wall with two layers and with pores		Vesicular nucleus with single or multiple nucleoli; ameboid and "spiderlike" movements in culture; cyst wall with 3 layers	Two abutting nuclei in ameba and cyst stage
In vitro cultivation	Axenic, bacterized, and defined media; tissue culture cells; optimal growth at ≥37°C	Axenic, bacterized, and defined media; tissue culture cells; optimal growth at 37°C (CNS isolates) or optimal growth at 30°C (corneal isolates)		Axenic medium; tissue culture cells; optimal growth at 37°C (bacterized medium not useful)	Bacterized cultures
CT/MRI of head	Non-specific	Space–occupying or ring-enhancing lesion	Not applicable	Space–occupying or ring-enhancing lesion	Space–occupying lesion, slight ring enhancement
Antimicrobial therapy	Intrathecal and intravenous amphotericin B, miconazole, rifampin	Pentamidine, azole compounds, flucytosine, sulfadiazine, miltefosine, amikacin IV & IT	PHMB, chlorhexidine, propamidine, hexamidine	Pentamidine, azithromycin, fluconazole, sulfadiazine, flucytosine	Azithromycin, pentamidine, itraconazole, flucytosine

*Based on a single case report.

IFA, immunofluorescent antibody staining; IIF, indirect immunofluorescent staining; PCR, polymerase chain reaction; PHMB, polyhexamethylene biguanide; IV, intravenous; IT, intrathecal.

Adapted from Visvesvara GS, Moura H, Schuster FL. Pathogenic and opportunistic free-living amoebae: *Acanthamoeba* spp, *Balamuthia mandrillaris*, *Naegleria fowleri*, and *Sappinia diploidea*. *FEMS Immunol Med Microbiol*. 2007;50:1-26.

cysts are stable for up to 8 months at 4°C.[17] Although there have probably been billions of exposures of people to *Naegleria*-contaminated fresh water, very few develop PAM.[15] The factors that protect most individuals from invasive *Naegleria* infection are not understood. In the southern United States, the presence of serum-agglutinating activity for *N. fowleri* in many young adults, but not infants, indicates that subclinical infection or exposure to *Naegleria* is common.[18] PAM has been reported in the central and southern United States, southern Australia, New Zealand, Europe, Africa, Asia, and Latin America.[19] While the true incidence of this entity is unknown, hundreds of cases of PAM have been reported worldwide. Most patients have a history of recreational freshwater exposure, although one case of PAM in an arid region of Nigeria may have been caused by inhalation of *Naegleria* cysts.[20] In the United States, 121 cases of PAM were reported from 1937 to 2007, with annual case numbers ranging from 0 to 8 per year. The median age of patients was 12 years, 78% were male, and only one patient survived. Eighty-five percent of cases occurred in the summer months, and all were in southern-tier states.[21] New reports of PAM continue to appear in the literature, and the current incidence is undoubtedly higher.[22] Clusters of cases of PAM with common environmental exposures have occurred, including 16 deaths over a three-year period that were retrospectively traced to a swimming pool in

Czechoslovakia with a low chlorine concentration.[23] A recent outbreak in Arizona highlights an additional potentially disturbing means of spread for *Naegleria*.[24] Two previously healthy children from the same neighborhood died of PAM due to *N. fowleri* within one day of each other. Neither child had any contact with recreational water during the incubation period except at private homes, nor did the two families associate with each other. Drinking water for the respective families came from the same untreated community well water system, and polymerase chain reaction (PCR) testing revealed *N. fowleri* in the water system.[25] These children were presumed to be infected during bathing; these cases were the first association of a drinking water system with *N. fowleri* infection in the United States.[24] A subsequent study demonstrated *N. fowleri*, detected by PCR, in 16% of 185 wells sampled in Arizona, indicating that transmission in this manner does pose a potential risk.[26]

ACANTHAMOEBA

Acanthamoeba spp. have been isolated from soil, water, and air in diverse geographic locations.[19,27] In contrast to *Naegleria*, *Acanthamoeba* growth is inhibited by temperatures above 35°C to 39°C. Many people are likely exposed to *Acanthamoeba* spp., as evidenced by the organism being cultured from pharyngeal swabs of healthy individuals.[1] In addition, serologic surveys have detected serum antibodies directed against *Acanthamoeba* in 50% to 100% of some cohorts of healthy people. Persons of Hispanic descent may be less likely to develop antibodies to *Acanthamoeba*, especially *A. polyphaga*, than whites; the clinical significance of this finding is currently unclear.[28,29] Although exposure of the general population to *Acanthamoeba* appears to be common, GAE caused by *Acanthamoeba* spp. occurs predominantly in debilitated or immunosuppressed individuals.[1,30] Underlying conditions reported in patients with GAE have included AIDS,[30] liver disease, diabetes mellitus, organ transplantation, steroid therapy, chemotherapy, and exposure to rituximab.[1,31,32] Recently, a number of cases of GAE with *Acanthamoeba* spp. in children with no clear immunosuppression, other than malnourishment, have been described.[33] Disseminated *Acanthamoeba* infection without overt CNS manifestations has been increasingly described, most commonly in AIDS patients but also in transplant patients and those with long-term steroid use.[27,31,34,35] Most commonly these patients have cutaneous manifestations, although involvement of the liver, lungs, and bones has been reported.[7,34]

AK occurs predominantly in healthy people who wear contact lenses or have had corneal trauma. An estimated 5000 cases have been reported in the United States, although some estimate the incidence to range as high as 1 per 10,000 contact lens wearers per year.[1,3] Of the reported cases, more than 80% were likely related to contact lens use.[1,36,37] Prior to 2005, poor contact lens hygiene—such as improperly cleaning the lens, swimming or showering with the lenses, or rinsing the lens case with tap water—was commonly associated with this disease, although it has also occurred in persons who reported none of these behaviors.[3,4] In the United States, from 2005 to 2007, an outbreak involving at least 138 patients was associated with a specific commercial contact lens multipurpose solution.[37] Though no specific contamination was found in this particular solution, and many of the affected did exhibit poor contact lens hygiene, this outbreak highlighted the fact that commercially available disinfectant solutions are not required to be effective against *Acanthamoeba* spp. to obtain FDA approval.[37,38]

BALAMUTHIA

Though *B. mandrillaris* infects animals and humans worldwide, it has only rarely been isolated from the soil and water, presumptively because it does not grow on bacterized agar plates.[2,39] The first human cases of infection with this organism were reported in 1990.[12] The isolation of *Balamuthia* from potting soil in the home of a fatally infected 3-year-old child that matched the clinical isolate from the patient confirmed the free-living and pathogenic status of *B. mandrillaris*.[40] Worldwide, there have been over 150 cases of human disease reported to date, with an extremely high mortality rate.[2,41] Approximately 55 of these have been from the United States, with only 4 survivors.[41] *Balamuthia* infections occur in both immunocompetent and immunocompromised people. In a recent review of serum from 500 patients with encephalitis in California, 10 (2%) had serologic evidence of *Balamuthia* infection; all later had more definitive testing (mostly by indirect immunofluorescence or PCR of brain tissue) that confirmed CNS infection with *Balamuthia*.[41] In this cohort of 10 patients, the median age was 16 years, 9 were male, and 9 died. Five patients had preexisting medical conditions (including diabetes, splenectomy, nephrotic syndrome, and possible lymphoma), 5 patients had a known recent exposure to soil, and 8 were of Hispanic ancestry. In the United States, individuals of Hispanic origin appear to be overrepresented among *Balamuthia* cases.[41,42] Whether this is as a result of common environmental exposures or a genetic predisposition is curretly unknown.

SAPPINIA

The only human case with *Sappinia* was reported in 2001 and involved a previously healthy 38-year-old man who developed chronic meningoencephalitis.[5] First isolated in 1908 and not previously known to be pathogenic to humans,[43] this ameba is found worldwide in soil and animal feces.[1] Recently, PCR was used to re-classify the organism from this patient, which was originally identified as *S. diploidea*, but based on PCR analysis, the organism more closely resembles *S. pedata* rather than *S. diploidea*.[43b]

Pathogenesis and Pathologic Findings

NAEGLERIA

PAM produces a diffuse meningoencephalitis, which affects the cortical gray matter most severely. Animal models[44,45] and autopsy studies[14,19] indicate that CNS invasion by *N. fowleri* occurs after nasal inoculation with amebas by disruption of the olfactory mucosa. The amebas penetrate the respiratory epithelium,[16] as well as the submucosal nervous plexus and the cribriform plate and gain access to the CNS. In the CNS, cortical hemorrhage and edema are seen, and the olfactory bulbs are hemorrhagic and necrotic. *Naegleria* trophozoites are found in the olfactory nerves and the adventitia and perivascular spaces of small to midsize arteries and arterioles,[1] and can be identified in wet mounts of cerebrospinal fluid (CSF) in patients with acute meningoencephalitis.[19,46] No cysts are seen in the brain.[1] Additionally, in a series of 16 autopsies of patients with PAM, myocarditis was present in 7, though no congestive heart failure or arrhythmias were noted. The inflammatory infiltrate was predominantly neutrophilic, and no amebas were seen in the myocardium.[47] The tissue necrosis elicited by *Naegleria* is likely mediated in part by secreted cysteine proteases and direct phagocytosis by feeding cups found on the trophozoites.[48] The protein Nfa1 mediates contact between *N. fowleri* pseudopods and target cells, and appears to be an important virulence factor for this organism.[49,50] Other potential virulence determinants including nitric oxide production, pore-forming proteins, low-molecular mass thiol compounds, and calcium-mediated complement resistance.

ACANTHAMOEBA

The histologic appearance of GAE from *Acanthamoeba* spp. is of parenchymal necrosis and granulomas, though granulomatous tissue reaction may not be present in immunocompromised individuals.[1] When the leptomeninges are involved, two patterns are seen: infiltrates containing equal numbers of polymorphonuclear cells, lymphocytes, and macrophages, or infiltrates that are predominantly of lymphocytes and macrophages.[51] Moderate to severe cerebral edema occurs, and thus bilateral uncal or cerebellar tonsillar herniations can occur. Necrotizing granulomatous lesions containing perivascular trophozoites and cysts are most frequently located in the cerebellum, midbrain, and brainstem. Multinucleated giant cells are occasionally present within the granulomas.[19] The perivascular location of amebic trophozoites and cysts suggests a hematogenous dissemination of *Acanthamoeba* to the CNS; this is also supported by identification of *Acanthamoeba* in the skin, lung, adrenals, and lymph nodes. Amebic skin lesions,[1] sinusitis,[6] and pneumonitis[52] may be sites of primary human infection that lead to hematogenous dissemination.[19]

The histologic appearance of AK is similar to that of *Acanthamoeba* infections of other organs. Both amebic cysts and trophozoites are found within the cornea. There is an acute or mixed inflammatory infiltrate that may contain epithelial and giant cells. However, amebas have also been found in tissue in the absence of an inflammatory infiltrate. Corneal neovascularization occurs to a variable extent.[53,54] Involvement of the posterior chamber of the eye is a rare complication of AK. Sterile inflammation of the posterior segment occurs without isolation or visualization of amebic cysts or trophozoites.[53] The corneal ringlike infiltrate caused by *Acanthamoeba* appears to be caused by the neutrophil chemoattractant effect of antigen-antibody complexes in the cornea.[53,54]

Significant progress has been made toward understanding the molecular basis of pathogenesis in *Acanthamoeba* infections, especially keratitis. Keratitis begins with trophozoites using a mannose binding protein to adhere to mannose glycoproteins on the corneal epithelium. These mannose glycoproteins are often upregulated after corneal trauma and with contact lens use. After adherence, *Acanthamoeba* mediates corneal cell death by a variety of mechanisms, including phagocytosis, induction of apoptosis, and direct cytolysis.[55,56] In addition to mediating adherence, the mannose glycoproteins stimulate the release of cytopathic factors from the parasites. *Acanthamoeba* also evades the immune response by degrading human IgA antibodies with secreted proteases, switching from trophozoites to cysts, and infecting the cornea, a site that lacks resident antigen-presenting cells, thus avoiding a delayed-type hypersensitivity response or a serum IgG response.[55,56] An interesting development in the cellular understanding of *Acanthamoeba* pathogenesis is that various bacteria including *Legionella* spp., *Chlamydia* spp., *Pseudomonas aeruginosa,* and *Burkholderia* spp. can survive intracellularly within the ameba.[57] This endosymbiosis has two potential sequelae: first, it may render the intracellular bacteria more pathogenic for the human host, and second, in coinfections, the *Acanthamoeba* may shield the intracellular bacteria from the immune response as well as antibiotics, thus leading to more fulminant infections with these bacterial species.[57,58]

BALAMUTHIA AND SAPPINIA

B. mandrillaris causes a subacute or chronic meningoencephalitis clinically similar to that caused by *Acanthamoeba* spp. However, the histopathological changes in *Balamuthia* GAE are much broader than what is observed in *Acanthamoeba* GAE. In balamuthiasis, the histopathology of lesions in the brain parenchyma or the meninges can range from an acute or neutrophilic immune response to a primarily chronic or granulomatous response.[51] Cysts and trophozoites of *B. mandrillaris* are seen in a perivascular pattern and are associated with angiitis and hemorrhagic necrosis of the underlying meninges and brain tissue. The angiotropic location as well as the fact that organisms have been isolated from other tissues (skin,[31] adrenals,[2] and kidneys[2]) suggests that it may be spread hematogenously. An animal model of encephalitis with *B. mandrillaris* has been developed[59] and may be useful in studying the disease pathogenesis. Both immunocompetent and immunocompromised mice are susceptible to intranasal and oral challenge with *B. mandrillaris*; the most likely portal of entry for human disease remains to be determined.[59,60]

The pathogenic potential of *Sappinia* for causing human disease is not known. Whether the case reported to date is the first of many to follow or an isolated occurrence remains to be determined.

Clinical Manifestations

A comparison of the clinical manifestations of disease by *Naegleria, Acanthamoeba, Balamuthia,* and *Sappinia* is listed in Table 274-1.

NAEGLERIA

PAM usually occurs in otherwise healthy children and young adults who have had recreational exposure to warm fresh water.[21] The onset of symptoms usually occurs two to five days after exposure, but apparent incubation periods of up to two weeks have been reported. Very early in the illness and consistent with the involvement of the olfactory nerves, the patient may notice changes in taste or smell followed by an abrupt onset of fever, anorexia, nausea, and vomiting. On initial presentation, headache and meningismus are noted in 86% to 100% of patients, and mental status changes in 66%. Patients rapidly progress to coma and death within one week after the onset of illness, usually without developing focal neurologic signs.[19] Spinal cord involvement has been reported, and one AIDS patient with *Naegleria* CNS infection has been reported.[61,62]

ACANTHAMOEBA

In contrast to PAM, GAE with *Acanthamoeba* spp. is an illness of immunocompromised and debilitated individuals, has an insidious onset, and presents with focal neurologic deficits.[1,30] Signs and symp-

toms in a series of 15 patients with GAE included mental status abnormalities (86%); seizures (66%); fever, headache, and hemiparesis (53%); meningismus (40%); visual disturbances (26%); and ataxia (20%).[63] The duration of illness from presentation until death was 7-120 days (mean 39 days). The incubation period of GAE is difficult to determine given the ubiquitous environmental presence of these organisms, but *Acanthamoeba* skin ulcers and lesions have often been present for months before the onset of CNS disease.[19,31,64] The skin lesions can be ulcerative, nodular, or subcutaneous abscesses and on biopsy demonstrate amebic granulomas.[31,64] Other clinical syndromes that have been described with *Acanthamoeba* infection include pneumonitis,[52] adrenalitis,[52] leukocytoclastic vasculitis,[65] osteomyelitis,[34] sinusitis,[6,64] and infection of a peptic ulcer.[66]

AK is generally a unilateral, sight-threatening infection that leads to corneal ulceration, blindness, and enucleation if not treated promptly. It is frequently misdiagnosed as herpetic, bacterial, or fungal keratitis, resulting in a delay to definitive treatment. The symptoms begin with a foreign-body sensation in the affected eye followed by severe pain out of proportion to the extent of tissue involvement, photophobia, tearing, blepharospasm, conjunctivitis, and blurred vision. Periods of temporary remission are common, which lead to further delays in diagnosis because they are interpreted as responses to antibacterial or antiviral therapy. Signs of AK include dendritiform epitheliopathy, a characteristic corneal ring infiltrate (Fig. 274-8), radial perineuritis, hypopyon, and anterior scleritis.[4] The dendriform epithelial pattern has been described as an early sign of AK before stromal involvement. Recognition of this manifestation and high clinical suspicion are important, as early treatment effects more rapid cure.[4]

BALAMUTHIA AND SAPPINIA

Balamuthia can cause disease in both immunocompetent and immunocompromised hosts.[2] Subacute or chronic granulomatous meningoencephalitis is the most common clinical presentation, resulting in death from one week to several months after the onset of neurologic symptoms. Important signs and symptoms include fever, headache, nausea, vomiting, seizure, and focal neurologic signs. Patients with balamuthiasis often have other concurrent illnesses, such as diabetes, renal failure, alcoholism, and IV drug use.[2]

Balamuthiasis also sometimes manifests with skin lesions; one report suggests these are particularly common in Peruvian patients.[67] These lesions are usually solitary, nodular, and often appear on the central face, although other locations such as the lower face, abdomen, and extremities have been reported.[67] As a rule, *Balamuthia* skin lesions precede CNS involvement, although in one Peruvian patient, a skin biopsy showed *B. mandrillaris* cysts, but the patient spontaneously recovered without treatment or CNS involvement.[1,67]

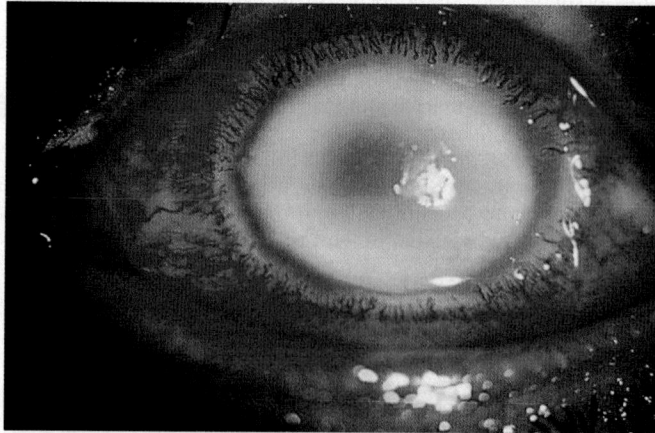

Figure 274-8 ***Acanthamoeba* keratitis with the characteristic ring infiltrate.** *(Reproduced with permission from J Comm Eye Health. 1999; 12(30): 21, Figure 1.)*

Only one case of human infection with *Sappinia* has been reported, so it is unclear whether the clinical manifestations seen in this patient will be reproduced in future infections. This patient was a previously healthy man who had an antecedent sinusitis and subsequently presented with a single temporal lobe mass that contained *Sappinia* organisms. The patient was treated with multiple drugs and survived. What implications this has regarding the virulence of *Sappinia* in comparison to the other free-living ameba remains to be determined.[5]

Laboratory Diagnosis

NAEGLERIA

PAM should be included in the differential diagnosis of children and young adults with meningoencephalitis or suspected bacterial meningitis with recent exposure to fresh water. The peripheral white cell count is usually elevated, with a predominance of neutrophils. Neuroradiologic imaging ranges from unremarkable to showing diffuse contrast enhancement of the gray matter, cisternal exudates and obliteration, and infarction.[19,68,69] The CSF pressure can be elevated, and the CSF is hemorrhagic, especially late in the course of the disease. CSF cell counts may be low early in disease but later range from 400-26,000 white blood cells/μL, with neutrophils predominating. The CSF glucose level is low to normal, and protein level is elevated. In patients with purulent CSF indices but a negative Gram stain, it is very important to examine a wet mount of CSF for amebic trophozoites. *Naegleria* trophozoites are generally destroyed by the fixation procedure for Gram stain and missed if not looked for on a wet mount. Motile trophozoites in the CSF have been seen in 14 of 16 reported patients with PAM in which a wet mount of CSF was made.[1]

Serologic diagnosis of PAM has limited utility in the clinical setting because most PAM patients die soon after infection, which leaves insufficient time to mount a detectable immune response. Nevertheless, a specific antibody response to *N. fowleri* was detected in a Californian patient who recovered from this disease. In addition, sera collected from several individuals with a history of extensive swimming in freshwater lakes in both the southeastern United States and California had detectable antibodies to *N. fowleri*. Whether these antibodies have protective activity is not clear. More recent diagnostic tools for *Naegleria* infections include molecular methods such as monoclonal antibodies and PCR for detecting organisms in the CSF, isoenzyme profile analysis from clinically isolated, cultured organisms, and DNA probes.[1] A nested PCR test has recently been developed that appears to be highly sensitive and that may make a rapid clinical diagnosis more achievable.[70]

ACANTHAMOEBA

In the past, GAE due to *Acanthamoeba* frequently was diagnosed only at autopsy. Brain biopsy is the most reliable diagnostic approach because *Acanthamoeba* spp. have only rarely been isolated from the CSF or seen on wet mount.[33,71] Exposure to *Acanthamoeba* results in detectable serum antibodies, but whether protective immunity results is unknown. Serologic studies are generally not useful for diagnosis. Previous studies have shown that antibodies to *Acanthamoeba* exist both in sera of persons without symptoms of disease as well as in patients who developed GAE or skin infections or both.[28,29]

Neuroimaging generally shows multiple space occupying lesions in the brain, with or without enhancement.[1,19,72] The differential diagnosis in these patients is extensive and includes toxoplasmosis, primary CNS lymphoma, tuberculosis, neurocysticercosis, nocardiosis, aspergillosis, bacterial brain abscess, and GAE secondary to *Balamuthia*. Radiographically, these entities cannot be differentiated reliably, and tissue stained with *Acanthamoeba*-specific antibodies is required for definitive diagnosis. Given the mass lesions, lumbar puncture may be contraindicated because of the risk of herniation. When performed, CSF results have been nondiagnostic, with intermediate elevations in the white blood cell count, elevated protein, and decreased glucose

levels.[1,19] As some GAE cases with wet mounts positive for *Acanthamoeba* have been reported, CSF wet mount is recommended if lumbar puncture is performed.

Acanthamoeba skin infections are often present in patients with GAE. Thus, skin nodules or ulcers should be biopsied and examined for *Acanthamoeba* in patients at risk of having GAE. *Acanthamoeba* have been successfully cultured from brain and cutaneous biopsy specimens. PCR of brain tissue has also demonstrated *Acanthamoeba* spp., including on formaldehyde-fixed or paraffin-embedded tissue.[32,72]

The successful treatment of AK depends on early diagnosis and treatment. Diagnosis rests on a high clinical suspicion and demonstrating *Acanthamoeba* in corneal scrapings or biopsy specimens by histopathologic examination, culture, or molecular mechanisms such as PCR or DNA probes.[3,4,73] Initial corneal scrapings, Gram stains, and cultures may be misleading because many AK cases are associated with coinfection with *Staphylococcus epidermidis*, *Staphylococcus aureus*, β-hemolytic streptococcus, or *Propionibacterium*. Culture of contact lenses and contact lens saline solution has also yielded *Acanthamoeba*.[3,4] Corneal scrapings should be examined under wet mount for motile trophozoites. Spray fixatives may best preserve the morphology of the trophozoites before air drying occurs.[74] The cysts and trophozoites can be visualized with a number of different stains, including H&E, Wright, Giemsa, periodic acid–Schiff, calcofluor white, and acridine orange.[3,4] Recently, confocal microscopy, which can be done in vivo, has been used to visualize cysts and diagnose AK.[3]

BALAMUTHIA AND SAPPINIA

Like *Acanthamoeba*, *Balamuthia* GAE is often diagnosed at autopsy, and several of the reported cases of *B. mandrillaris* had initially been ascribed to *Acanthamoeba* because of the difficulty in distinguishing the two morphologically. Given the lack of laboratory or clinical findings specific for *Balamuthia* GAE, tissue stained with *Balamuthia* specific antibodies is required for definitive diagnosis.[2] In brain biopsy specimens of patients with *B. mandrillaris* infection, both the cysts and trophozoites of the organism have been identified. Isolation of *B. mandrillaris* from CSF has only been reported once; nevertheless, in patients for whom GAE is suspected, wet mount of the CSF should be done if lumbar puncture is performed.[75] The CSF findings resemble those of *Acanthamoeba* infections and include a mononuclear pleocytosis (10-500 cells), moderate hypoglycorrhachia, and an elevated protein level, although these levels can exceed 1000 mg/dL.[2] Neuroimaging yields the same findings as in *Acanthamoeba* GAE.[2] A recent report suggests that serologic diagnosis may be possible, but this method of diagnosis has not been confirmed with prospective studies.[41,76] PCR for *Balamuthia* is a developing means of diagnosis.[41,77]

Real-time PCR, based on the 18s rRNA, was recently developed as a means to identify *Sappinia* infection.[43b] The diagnosis of *Sappinia* infection combines PCR testing with identification of trophozoites with the characteristic features (see Fig. 274-7); negative tests for *Naegleria*, *Acanthamoeba*, and *Balamuthia* species; and a clinical course consistent with acute encephalitis.[5]

A multiplex real-time PCR assay that can simultaneously detect *N. fowleri*, *Acanthamoeba* spp., and *Balamuthia* has recently been developed. This assay targets the 18S rRNA gene and appears to be both specific and sensitive.[78] The real-time PCR for *Sappinia* has been added to this triplex assay.[43] Thus, this PCR-based assay would identify any of these organisms in patients suspected of having CNS disease due to a free-living ameba.[43b,78]

Treatment

NAEGLERIA

Optimum treatment for PAM has not been well defined, and few patients have survived this disease process.[1,79] Treatment options are reviewed in the text that follows.

Clinical Evidence

Amphotericin products appear to form a cornerstone of therapy for PAM due to *Naegleria*. Many of the patients who have survived well-documented PAM received high-dose systemic and intrathecal amphotericin B.[1,79] Additional drugs used in patients who have recovered from PAM include systemic and intrathecal miconazole, fluconazole, rifampin, and sulfisoxazole.[1,79]

Animal Models and In Vitro Assays

A recent report demonstrated that azithromycin has activity against *N. fowleri* in a mouse model of primary amebic encephalitis.[80] The authors report that azithromycin had less activity against *N. fowleri* in vitro but nonetheless protected 100% of mice challenged in a PAM model; other macrolides appear to be less effective. Another report describes the synergistic activity of azithromycin plus amphotericin, both in vitro and in a mouse model.[81] Artemesinin derivatives were investigated in an animal model, but these agents were all inferior to amphotericin B.[82] Passive immunotherapy in animal models has been attempted, and intrathecal administration of anti-*Naegleria* immune serum or monoclonal antibody prolonged the survival of rabbits inoculated intracisternally with *N. fowleri*.[83] In vitro studies suggest that that both miltefosine and voriconazole may have good activity against *N. fowleri*.[84] Phenothiazines (chlorpromazine and trifluoperazine) have also demonstrated inhibitory effects on *N. fowleri* in vitro.[79]

Recommendations

Patients with suspected PAM should receive high-dose intravenous amphotericin products as part of their empirical anti-infective regimen; intrathecal amphotericin may have an additional role in confirmed or highly suspect cases. In the absence of clinical trials to guide therapeutic decisions for this rapidly fatal infection, combination antimicrobial therapy seems warranted given that most survivors received multiple drugs. The possible addition of azoles, rifampin, or other antimicrobials should also be considered. The role of newer drugs (e.g., azithromycin, miltefosine, voriconazole) as part of combination regimens in the treatment of PAM remains to be determined.

ACANTHAMOEBA GAE AND DISSEMINATED DISEASE

Data are limited regarding the treatment of *Acanthamoeba* GAE. Most cases were diagnosed postmortem, and premortem diagnosis has generally preceded death by only a few days, making evaluation of therapy difficult.

Clinical Evidence

Among the cases of successfully treated patients with GAE and disseminated *Acanthamoeba* disease, all except two were given a combination of antimicrobials. These combination regimens included trimethoprim-sulfamethoxazole (TMP/SMX), flucytosine, and sulfadiazine[79]; penicillin G and chloramphenicol[79]; sulfadiazine, pyrimethamine, and fluconazole[79]; pentamidine, levofloxacin, amphotericin B, flucytosine, rifampin, and itraconazole[79]; pentamidine, flucytosine, itraconazole, topical chlorhexidine, and ketoconazole[79]; intravenous pentamidine and oral itraconazole[31]; fluconazole, sulfadiazine, and surgical debulking[31]; ketoconazole, rifampin, and TMP/SMX[33]; TMP/SMX, rifampin, and surgical debulking[85]; and oral and topical miltefosine with intrathecal and systemic amikacin.[86] The two successfully treated cases in which only a single antimicrobial was used received sulfamethazine or TMP/SMX.[79,87] In one patient with disseminated *Acanthamoeba* and AIDS, the initiation of HAART was felt to be a critical component of the patient's survival, in addition to treatment with itraconazole, flucytosine, rifampin, and topical chlorhexidine.[64]

Animal Models and In Vitro Assays

In mice, *Acanthamoeba* infections can be treated with sulfadiazine, rifampin, and flucytosine; however, this requires treatment either before or within 24 hours of infection, an unlikely clinical scenario.[27] In general, the diamidine derivatives (including pentamidine) have the greatest activity against *Acanthamoeba*. Other drugs with in vitro activity include ketoconazole, miconazole, paromomycin, polymyxin, sulfadiazine, TMP/SMX, azithromycin, neomycin, flucytosine, and, to a lesser extent, amphotericin B.[27,53] Recent in vitro data suggest that both miltefosine and voriconazole may have good activity against *Acanthamoeba* spp.[84]

Recommendations

The mainstay of successful treatment appears to be early diagnosis and multidrug therapy. Based on the experience gained from successfully treated patients, combination regimens might include pentamidine, an azole, a sulfonamide, and possibly flucytosine. However, given the wide range of anecdotally successful regimens previously listed, it is difficult to determine the most efficacious empirical or definitive regimen. As it is now possible to test clinical isolates in vitro for drug susceptibilities, this testing offers one way of guiding definitive therapy.[86,88]

ACANTHAMOEBA KERATITIS

Treatment of AK has been notably more successful than that of GAE or PAM, with medical success rates ranging from 75% to 84%.[4,37] Successful treatment requires early diagnosis and aggressive medical management, though surgical débridement and corneal transplantation are sometimes necessary. Recognition of the dendriform pattern on the corneal epithelium, the earliest recognized sign of AK, should be followed immediately with institution of antiamebic medical therapy.[3,4] In vitro susceptibility testing for *Acanthamoeba* spp. is available and may prove useful to guide medical therapy; however, there are reports of a poor correlation between in vitro drug susceptibilities and in vivo response of patients with AK.[89]

The topical cationic antispectic agents chlorhexidine (0.02%) and polyhexamethylene biguanide (PHMB, 0.02%) are effective against both the trophozoites and the cysts and have become the mainstay of therapy for AK.[3,4] Using chlorhexidine or PHMB with a diamidine-propamidine (Brolene) or hexamidine (Desmodine) is common, but neither of the latter medications is available in the United States. Hexamidine monotherapy has been used in France.[4] Other agents that have been used in conjunction with chlohexidine or PHMB include oral ketoconazole, itraconazole, voriconazole, and topical imidazoles (1%).[4] Miltefosine has excellent activity against trophozoites and is partially active against cysts,[84] but its use in combination with the cationic antiseptics is still investigational.[4] Propamidine isethionate has caused a reversible epithelial keratopathy after prolonged treatment that can be confused with recurrent AK.[90]

The use of corticosteroids in AK is controversial. Crystalline keratopathy caused by viridans streptococci has occurred after topical corticosteroid therapy of AK in two patients.[91] In animals models and in vitro studies, steroid treatment made the disease worse. However, recent studies revealed no increased risk of treatment failure in patients treated with adjuvant steroids and improved graft survival in patients who did not have inflammation at the time of graft placement.[4,92]

Recommendations

Topical chlorhexidine or PHMB with or without adjuvant diamidine or other agent should be applied every hour for the first several days. Treatment is then tapered based on the clinical response. Medical therapy may fail or require adjunctive surgical therapy.[3,4] Neomycin should not be used as it is ineffective against cysts, has limited clinical efficacy data, and can cause hypersensitivity.[4,89]

BALAMUTHIA

Therapy for *B. mandrillaris* infections is not well defined. Systemic infections are associated with a high mortality rate.

Clinical Evidence

In the United States, four survivors have been reported. Three of the surviving patients were treated with flucytosine, pentamidine, fluconazole, sulfadiazine, and a macrolide (azithromycin or clarithromycin); the fourth patient's treatment regimen is unknown.[41] These patients had timely diagnoses, highlighting the importance of a high index of suspicion and appropriate diagnostic measures in treating this infection. In Peru, three patients with balamuthiasis have survived. Of these, one patient (with no CNS involvement) received no treatment, but the other two received prolonged therapy with albendazole and itraconazole. Surgical débridement was performed in one of these patients with cutaneous disease.[1,41]

In Vitro Assays

Pentamidine, azithromycin, and clarithromycin appear to have some activity, although clarithromycin[93,94] appears amebastatic. In the same study, fluconazole and ketoconazole were poor inhibitors of *Balamuthia* growth, amphotericin B was marginal, and TMP/SMX had minimal effect.[93] Recent in vitro data suggest that that miltefosine may inhibit *Balamuthia*, but voriconazole had virtually no effect on this organism.[84]

Recommendations

The mainstay of successful regimens is multidrug therapy as evidenced from the preceding, but given the various combinations used, it is difficult to determine the most effective regimen. Early diagnosis and drug therapy appear to be essential, as dissemination of *Balamuthia* to the CNS carries an extremely poor prognosis.

SAPPINIA

The single patient with a *Sappinia* infection was treated with azithromycin, pentamidine, itraconazole, and flucytosine, and survived.[5]

Prevention

Given the ubiquitous nature of *Acanthamoeba* and *B. mandrillaris*, primary prevention efforts will likely prove difficult. PAM occurs so rarely that active surveillance for *N. fowleri* in public swimming areas is probably not justified as a public health measure. However, a single source of infection, such as a popular swimming area, can cause an outbreak of PAM. Thus, because of the occurrence of clusters of patients with PAM with common environmental exposures,[8,23] health officials should consider closing implicated lakes, rivers, or streams to swimming. A domestic water supply has recently been implicated as the source of *N. fowleri* in Arizona,[24] and new water treatment measures are being developed to eliminate free-living ameba.[95] *N. fowleri* is susceptible to chlorine and can be controlled in swimming pools by adequate chlorination.

AK associated with contact lens use is generally preventable. Contact lenses should not be worn while swimming or showering, new contact lens cleaning solution should be used every night, homemade saline solutions should be avoided, contact lens cases should be allowed to air dry each day, and orthokeratology should be avoided. Some authors advocate either daily disposable lens, disposing of the contact lens case after three months of use, or microwaving the lens case for three minutes on high power. Finally, commercially available contact lens disinfectant solutions that are specifically effective against *Acanthamoeba* are needed.[3,4,37,38]

Resources

In the United States, two reference laboratories currently perform diagnostic testing for free-living amebas: one at the Centers for Disease Control and Prevention (testing for all free-living amebas) and the other at the California Department of Public Health (testing for *Balamuthia* only). Contact information for testing, as well as for advice about cases includes Govinda S. Visvesvara, Ph.D (Division of Parasitic Diseases [DPD], CDC, Atlanta, GA) at phone: 770-488-4417 and e-mail: *gsv1@cdc.gov*. Alternate contact at DPD/CDC: phone: 770-488-7775 (business hours); 770-488-7100 (after hours emergencies); e-mail: *parasites@cdc.gov*. California Department of Public Health contact: Carol Glaser, Chief, Viral & Rickettsial Disease Laboratory, California Department of Public Health, phone: 510-307-8613.

REFERENCES

1. Visvesvara GS, Moura H, Schuster FL. Pathogenic and opportunistic free-living amoebae: *Acanthamoeba* spp, *Balamuthia mandrillaris*, *Naegleria fowleri*, and *Sappinia diploidea*. *FEMS Immunol Med Microbiol*. 2007;50:1-26.
2. Matin A, Siddiqui R, Jayasekera S, et al. Increasing importance of *Balamuthia mandrillaris*. *Clin Micro Rev*. 2008;21:435-448.
3. Hammersmith KM. Diagnosis and management of *Acanthamoeba* keratitis. *Curr Opin Ophthalmol*. 2006;17:327-331.
4. Chong EM, Dana MR. *Acanthamoeba* keratitis. *Int Ophthal Clin*. 2007;47:33-46.
5. Gelman BB, Rauf SJ, Nader R, et al. Amoebic encephalitis due to *Sappinia diploidea*. *JAMA*. 2001;285:2450-2451.
6. Dunand VA, Hammer SM, Rossi R, et al. Parasitic sinusitis and otitis in patients infected with human immunodeficiency virus: Report of five cases and review. *Clin Infect Dis*. 1997;25:267-272.
7. Selby DM, Chandra RS, Rakusan TA, et al. Amebic osteomyelitis in a child with acquired immunodeficiency syndrome: A case report. *Pediatr Pathol Lab Med*. 1998;18:89-95.
8. Fowler M, Carter RF. Acute pyogenic meningitis probably due to *Acanthamoeba* sp: A preliminary report. *Br Med J*. 1965;5464:740-742.
9. Schuster FL. Cultivation of pathogenic and opportunistic free-living amebas. *Clin Microbiol Rev*. 2002;15:342-354.
10. Booton GC, Visvesvara GS, Byers TJ, et al. Identification and distribution of *Acanthamoeba* species genotypes associated with nonkeratitis infections. *J Clin Micro*. 43:1689-1693.
11. Gordon SM, Steinberg JP, DuPuis MH, et al. Culture and isolation of *Acanthamoeba* species and leptomyxid amebas from patients with amebic meningoencephalitis, including two patients with AIDS. *Clin Infect Dis*. 1992;15:1024-1030.
12. Visvesvara GS, Martinez AJ, Schuster FL, et al. Leptomyxid ameba, a new agent of amebic meningoencephalitis in humans and animals. *J Clin Microbiol*. 1990;28:2750-2756.
13. Goodfellow L, Belcher J, Page F. A light and electron microscopical study of *Sappinia diploidea*, a sexual amoeba. *Protistologica*. 1974;Xfas:207-216.

14. John DT. Primary amebic meningoencephalitis and the biology of *Naegleria fowleri*. *Annu Rev Microbiol*. 1982;36:101-123.
15. Wellings FM, Amuso PT, Chang SL, et al. Isolation and identification of pathogenic *Naegleria* from Florida lakes. *Appl Environ Microbiol*. 1977;34:661-667.
16. Rojas-Hernández S, Jarillo-Luna A, Rodríguez-Monroy M, et al. Immunohistochemical Characterization of the Initial Stages of *Naegleria Fowleri* Meningoencephalitis in Mice. *Parasitol Res*. 2004;94:31-36.
17. Warhurst DC, Carman JA, Mann PG. Survival of *Naegleria fowleri* cysts at 4 degrees C for eight months with retention of virulence. *Trans R Soc Trop Med Hyg*. 1980;74:832.
18. Marciano-Cabral F, Cline ML, Bradley SG. Specificity of antibodies from human sera for *Naegleria* species. *J Clin Microbiol*. 1987;25:692-697.
19. Martinez AJ. *Free-Living Amebas: Natural History, Prevention, Diagnosis, Pathology and Treatment of Disease*. Boca Raton, FL: CRC Press; 1985.
20. Lawande RV, John I, Dobbs RH, et al. A case of primary amebic meningoencephalitis in Zaria, Nigeria. *Am J Clin Pathol*. 1979;71:591-594.
21. Centers for Disease Control and Prevention. Primary Amebic Meningoencephalitis—Arizona, Florida, and Texas, 2007. *MMWR*. 2008;57:573-577.
22. Okuda DT, Coons S. *Naegleria fowleri* meningoencephalitis. *Neurology*. 2003;61:E1.
23. Schuster FL, Visvesvara GS. Free-living amoebae as opportunistic and non-opportunistic pathogens of humans and animals. *Int J Parasitol*. 2004;34:1001-1027.
24. Blackburn BG, Craun GF, Yoder JS, et al. Surveillance For Waterborne-Disease Outbreaks Associated With Drinking Water-United States, 2001-2002. *MMWR*. 2004;53(SS-8):23-46.
25. Marciano-Cabral F, MacLean R, Mensah A, et al. Identification of *Naegleria fowleri* in domestic water sources by nested PCR. *Appl Environ Microbiol*. 2003;69:5864-5869.
26. Blair B, Sarkar P, Bright KR, et al. *Naegleria fowleri* in well water. *Emerg Infect Dis*. 2008;14:1499-1501.

27. Marciano-Cabral F, Cabral G. *Acanthamoeba* sp as agents of disease in humans. *Clin Microbiol Rev*. 2003;16:273-307.
28. Cerva L. *Acanthamoeba culbertsoni* and *Naegleria fowleri*: Occurrence of antibodies in man. *J Hyg Epidemiol Microbiol Immunol*. 1989;33:99-103.
29. Chappell CJ, Wright JA, Coletta M, et al. Standardized method of measuring *Acanthamoeba* antibodies in sera from healthy human subjects. *Clin Diag Lab Immunol*. 2001;8(4):724-730.
30. Sison JP, Kemper CA, Loveless M, et al. Disseminated *Acanthamoeba* infection in patients with AIDS: Case reports and review. *Clin Infect Dis*. 1995;20:1207-1216.
31. Walia R, Montoya JG, Visvesvara GS, et al. A case of successful treatment of cutaneous *Acanthamoeba* infection in a lung transplant recipient. *Transpl Infect Dis*. 2006;9:51-54.
32. Meersseman W, Lagrou K, Sciot R, et al. Rapidly fatal *Acanthamoeba* encephalitis and treatment of cryoglobulinemia. *Emerg Infect Dis*. 2007;13:469-471.
33. Singhal T, Bajpai A, Kalra V, et al. Successful treatment of *Acanthamoeba* meningitis with combinations oral antibiotics. *Pediatric Infect Dis*. 2001;20:623-627.
34. Steinberg JP, Galindo RL, Kraus ES, et al. Disseminated acanthamebiasis in a renal transplant recipient with osteomyelitis and cutaneous lesions: Case report and literature review. *Clin Infect Dis*. 2002;35:e43-49.
35. Slater CA, Sickel JZ, Visvesvara GS, et al. Brief report: Successful treatment of disseminated *Acanthamoeba* infection in an immunocompromised patient. *N Engl J Med*. 1994;331:85-87.
36. Stehr-Green JK, Bailey TM, Brandt FH, et al. *Acanthamoeba* keratitis in soft contact lens wearers. A case-control study. *JAMA*. 1987;258:57-60.
37. Centers for Disease Control and Prevention. *Acanthamoeba* keratitis—multiple states, 2005-2007. *MMWR*. 2007;56:532-534.
38. Patel A, Hammersmith K. Contact lens-related microbial keratitis: recent outbreaks. *Curr Opin Ophthalmal*. 2008;19:302-306.
39. John DT, Howard MJ. Seasonal distribution of pathogenic free-living amebae in Oklahoma waters. *Parasitol Res*. 1995;81:193-201.

40. Schuster FL, Dunnebacke TH, Booton GC, et al. Environmental isolation of *Balamuthia mandrillaris* associated with a case of amebic encephalitis. *J Clin Microbiol.* 2003;41:3175-3180.

41. Centers for Disease Control and Prevention. Balamuthia amebic encephalitis—California, 1999-2007. *MMWR.* 2008;57:768-771.

42. Schuster FL, Glaser C, Honarmand S, et al. *Balamuthia* amebic encephalitis risk, Hispanic Americans. *Emerg Infect Dis.* 2004;10:1510-1512.

43. Hartmann M, Nagler K. Copulation bei Ameoba diploidea mit Selbstsamdigbleiben der Gametenkerne wahrend des ganzen lebenscyclus. *Sitz-Ber der Ges naturf Freunde Berlin.* 1908;5:112-125.

43b. Qvarnstrom Y, da Silva AJ, Schuster FL, et al. Molecular confirmation of *Sappinia pedata* as a causative agent of amoebic encephalitis. *Clin Infect Dis.* 2009;199:1139-1142.

44. Martinez J, Duma RJ, Nelson EC, et al. Experimental *Naegleria* meningoencephalitis in mice. Penetration of the olfactory mucosal epithelium by *Naegleria* and pathologic changes produced: A light and electron microscope study. *Lab Invest.* 1973;29:121-133.

45. Jaroli KL, McCosh JK, Howard MJ. The role of blood vessels and lungs in the dissemination of *Naegleria fowleri* following intranasal inoculation in mice. *Folia Parasitol (Praha).* 2002;49:183-188.

46. Loschiavo F, Ventura-Spagnolo T, Sessa E, et al. Acute primary meningoencephalitis from entamoeba *Naegleria fowleri.* Report of a clinical case with a favourable outcome. *Acta Neurol (Napoli).* 1993;15:333-340.

47. Markowitz SM, Martinez AJ, Duma RJ, et al. Myocarditis associated with primary amebic (*Naegleria*) meningoencephalitis. *Am J Clin Pathol.* 1974;62:619-628.

48. Aldape K, Huizinga H, Bouvier J, et al. *Naegleria fowleri:* Characterization of a secreted histolytic cysteine protease. *Exp Parasitol.* 1994;78:230-241.

49. Jeong SR, Lee SC, Song KJ, et al. Expression of the nfa1 gene cloned from pathogenic *Naegleria fowleri* in nonpathogenic *N. gruberi* enhances cytotoxicity against CHO target cells in vitro. *Infect Immun.* 2005;73(Jul(7)):4098-4105.

50. Lee YJ, Kim JH, Jeong SR, et al. Production of Nfa1-specific monoclonal antibodies that influences the in vitro cytotoxicity of *Naegleria fowleri* trophozoites on microglial cells. *Parasitol Res.* 2007;101:1191-1196.

51. Guarner J, Bartlett J, Shieh W-J, et al. Histopathologic spectrum and immunohistochemical diagnosis of amebic meningoencephalitis. *Modern Path.* 2007;20:1230-1237.

52. Anderlini P, Przepiorka D, Luna M, et al. *Acanthamoeba* meningoencephalitis after bone marrow transplantation. *Bone Marrow Transplant.* 1994;14:459-461.

53. Auran JD, Starr MB, Jakobiec FA. *Acanthamoeba* keratitis. A review of the literature. *Cornea.* 1987;6:2-26.

54. Baum J. In: Case records of the Massachusetts General Hospital Case 10-1985. *N Engl J Med.* 1985;312:634-641.

55. Clarke DW, Niederkorn JY. The pathophysiology of *Acanthamoeba* keratitis. *Trends Parasitol.* 2006;22(4):175-180.

56. Clarke DW, Niederkorn JY. The immunobiology of *Acanthamoeba* keratitis. *Microbes and Infection.* 2006;8(5):1400-1405.

57. Horn M, Wagner M. Bacterial endosymbionts of free-living amoebae. *J Eukaryot Microbiol.* 2004;51:509-514.

58. Hammer BK, Swanson MS. *Legionella pneumophila* pathogenesis: a fateful journey from amoeba to macrophages. *Ann Rev Micro.* 2000;54:567-613.

59. Janitschke K, Martinez AJ, Visvesvara GS, et al. Animal model *Balamuthia mandrillaris* CNS infection: contrast and comparison in immunodeficient and immunocompetent mice: A murine model of "granulomatous" amebic encephalitis. *J Neuropathol Exp Neurol.* 1996;55:815-821.

60. Kiderlen AF, Laube U, Radam E, et al. Oral infection of immunocompetent and immunodeficient mice with *Balamuthia mandrillaris* amebae. *Parasitol Res.* 2007;100:775-782.

61. Viriyavejakul P, Rochanawutanon M, Sirinavin S. *Naegleria* meningomyeloencephalitis. *Southeast Asian J Trop Med Public Hlth.* 1997;28:237-240.

62. De Jonckheere JF, Brown S. Primary amebic meningoencephalitis in a patient with AIDS—Unusual protozoological findings. *Clin Infect Dis.* 1997;25:943-944.

63. Martinez AJ. Is *Acanthamoeba* encephalitis an opportunistic infection? *Neurology.* 1980;30:567-574.

64. Carter W, Gompf S, Toney J, et al. Disseminated *Acanthamoeba* sinusitis in a patient with AIDS: a possible role for early antiretroviral therapy. *AIDS Reader.* 2004;14:41-49.

65. Helton J, Loveless M, White CR Jr. Cutaneous *Acanthamoeba* infection associated with leukocytoclastic vasculitis in an AIDS patient. *Am J Dermatopathol.* 1993;15:146-149.

66. Thamprasert K, Khunamornpong S, Morakote N. *Acanthamoeba* infection of peptic ulcer. *Ann Trop Med Parasitol.* 1993;87:403-405.

67. Bravo F, Sanchez MR. New and re-emerging cutaneous infectious diseases in Latin America an other geographic areas. *Derm Clin.* 2003;21:655-668.

68. Kidney DD, Kim SH. CNS infections with free-living amebas: neuroimaging findings. *Am J Roentgenol.* 1998;17:809-812.

69. Singh P, Kochhar R, Vashita RK, et al. Amebic meningoencephalitis: spectrum of imaging findings. *Am J Neuroradiol.* 2006;27:1217-1221.

70. Reveiller FL, Cabanes PA, Marciano-Cabral F. Development of a nested PCR assay to detect the pathogenic free-living amoeba *Naegleria fowleri. Parasitol Res.* 2002;88:443-450.

71. Petry F, Torzewski M, Bohl J, et al. Early diagnosis of *Acanthamoeba* infection during routine cytological examination of cerebrospinal fluid. *J Clin Micro.* 2006;44:1903-1904.

72. Shirwadkar CG, Samant R, Sankhe M, et al. *Acanthamoeba* encephalitis in patient with systemic lupus, India. *Emerg Infect Dis.* 2006;12:984-986.

73. Lai S, Asgari M, Henney HR Jr. Non-radioactive DNA probe and polymerase chain reaction procedures for the specific detection of *Acanthamoeba. Mol Cell Probes.* 1994;8:81-89.

74. Wright P, Warhurst D, Jones BR. *Acanthamoeba* keratitis successfully treated medically. *Br J Ophthalmol.* 1985;69:778-782.

75. Jayasekera S, Sissons J, Tucker J, et al. Postmortem culture of *Balamuthia mandrillaris* from the brain and cerebrospinal fluid of a case of granulomatous amoebic meningoencephalitis, using human brain microvascular epithelial cells. *J Med Microbiol.* 2004;53:1007-1012.

76. Schuster FL, Yagi S, Wilkins PP, et al. *Balamuthia mandrillaris,* agent of amebic encephalitis: detection of serum antibodies and antigenic similarity of isolates by enzyme immunoassay. *J Eukaryot Micro.* 2008;55:313-320.

77. Yagi S, Booton GC, Visvesvara GS, et al. Detection of *Balamuthia* mitochondrial 16S rRNA gene DNA in clinical specimen by PCR. *J Clin Microbiol.* 2005;43:3192-3197.

78. Qvarnstrom Y, Visvesvara GS, Sriram R, et al. Multiplex Real-time PCR assay for simultaneous detection of *Acanthamoeba* spp, *Balamuthia mandrillaris,* and *Naegleria fowleri. J Clin Microbiol.* 2006;44(10):3589-3595.

79. Schuster FL, Visvesvara GS. Opportunistic amoebae: challenges in prophylaxis and treatment. *Drug Resist Updates.* 2004;7:41-51.

80. Goswick SM, Brenner GM. Activities of azithromycin and amphotericin B against *Naegleria fowleri* in vitro and in a mouse model of primary amebic meningoencephalitis. *Antimicrob Agents Chemother.* 2003;47:524-528.

81. Soltow SM, Brenner GM. Synergistic activities of azithromycin and amphotericin B against *Naegleria fowleri* in vitro and in a mouse model of primary amebic meningoencephalitis. *Antimicrob Agents Chemother.* 2007;51:23-27.

82. Gupta S, Ghosh PK, Dutta GP, et al. In vivo study of artemisinin and its derivatives against primary amebic meningoencephalitis caused by *Naegleria fowleri. J Parasitol.* 1995;81:1012-1013.

83. Lallinger GJ, Reiner SL, Cooke DW, et al. Efficacy of immune therapy in early experimental *Naegleria fowleri* meningitis. *Infect Immun.* 1987;55:1289-1293.

84. Schuster FL, Guglielmo BJ, Visvesvara GS. In-vitro activity of miltefosine and voriconazole on clinical isolates of free living amebas: *Balamuthia, Acanthamoeba* spp., and *Naegleria fowleri. J Eukaryot Microbiol.* 2006;53:121-126.

85. Fung KT, Dhillon AP, McLaughlin JE, et al. Cure of *Acanthamoeba* cerebral abscess in a liver transplant patient. *Liver Transplantation.* 2008;14:308-312.

86. Walochnik J, Aichelburg A, Assadian O, et al. Granulomatous amebic encephalitis caused by *Acanthamoeba* of genotype T2 in human immunodeficiency virus-negative patient. *J Clin Microbiol.* 2008;46:338-340.

87. Sharma PP, Gupta P, Murali MV, et al. Primary amebic meningoencephalitis caused by *Acanthamoeba* successfully treated with cotrimoxazole. *Indian Pediatr.* 1993;30:1219-1222.

88. McBride J, Ingram PR, Henriquez FL, et al. Development of colorimetric microtiter plate assay for assessment of antimicrobials against *Acanthamoeba. J Clin Microbiol.* 2005;43:629-634

89. Perez-Santonja JJ, Kilvington S, Hughes R, et al. Persistently culture positive *Acanthamoeba* keratitis: In vitro resistance and in vitro sensitivity. *Ophthalmology.* 2003;110:1593-1600

90. Johns KJ, Head WS, O'Day DM. Corneal toxicity of propamidine. *Arch Ophthalmol.* 1988;106:68-69.

91. Davis RM, Schroeder RP, Rowsey JJ, et al. *Acanthamoeba* keratitis and infectious crystalline keratopathy. *Arch Ophthalmol.* 1987;105:1524-1527.

92. Park DH, Palay DA, Daya SM, et al. The role of topical corticosteroids in the management of *Acanthamoeba* keratitis. *Cornea.* 1997;16:277-283.

93. Schuster FL, Visvesvara GS. Axenic growth and drug sensitivity studies of *Balamuthia mandrillaris,* an agent of amebic meningoencephalitis in humans and other animals. *J Clin Microbiol.* 1996;34:385-388.

94. Schuster FL, Visvesvara GS. Efficacy of novel antimicrobials against clinical isolates of opportunistic amebas. *J Eukaryot Microbiol.* 1998;45:612-618.

95. Vernhes MC, Benichou A, Pernin P, et al. Elimination of free-living amoebae in fresh water with pulsed electric fields. *Water Res.* 2002;36:3429-3438.

275

Plasmodium Species (Malaria)

RICK M. FAIRHURST* | THOMAS E. WELLEMS

The Malaria Problem

Malaria is an overwhelming problem in tropical developing countries, accounting for an estimated 250 to 500 million febrile illnesses and up to a million deaths annually.[1-4] It is estimated that up to 40% of the world's population is at risk for acquiring malaria. In sub-Saharan Africa, most severe cases and deaths occur in children younger than 5 years old and in pregnant women.

The introduction of chloroquine and dichlorodiphenyltrichloroethane (DDT) at the end of World War II brought dramatic new power to malaria control efforts. With postwar economic recovery and a renewed spirit of international cooperation, optimism ran high that these new tools might be used to eliminate malaria, and in 1955 the World Health Organization launched its campaign to eradicate the disease. This goal proved overly optimistic, and the centrally organized DDT-spraying programs at the core of the campaign were discontinued in 1967. The campaign nevertheless brought regional successes that coincided with other factors to reduce malaria incidence rates in many areas of the world (e.g., in Asia)[5] (Fig. 275-1A).

A stark exception to this general progress is sub-Saharan Africa, where malaria remains deeply entrenched. Even the most committed spraying and eradication programs in endemic areas of this region could not defeat malaria's efficient transmission by the Anopheles gambiae mosquito.[6] The wide availability and use of chloroquine did, however, boost the health of young African children who suffer most from Plasmodium falciparum, the species responsible for the deadliest form of malaria. As chloroquine became increasingly available in the 1950s to 1970s, death rates from malaria in Africa began to drop, approaching half the level of the prechloroquine years.[7] Unfortunately, the massive use of chloroquine (hundreds of tons sufficient for hundreds of millions of treatments annually) in the 1980s[8] selected for chloroquine-resistant P. falciparum strains that entered and spread across Africa. In the 1980s and 1990s, malaria resurged and death rates increased. The impact of chloroquine resistance was especially evident in young children, who do not have the partially protective antimalarial immunity that usually develops after repeated episodes of the illness (Fig. 275-1B).[9,10] Unfortunately, the safety and low cost of chloroquine were unmatched by other, more expensive drugs that have been largely unaffordable in developing countries.[11] In the absence of an effective vaccine, successful treatment of malaria in Africa depends on new drugs becoming affordable and readily available.

Plasmodium and Its Life Cycle

Plasmodium parasites belong to the Apicomplexa group of protozoa, which includes other pathogens such as Babesia, Toxoplasma, and Cryptosporidium species. Apicomplexa are distinguished morphologically by the presence of a specialized complex of apical organelles (micronemes, rhoptries, and dense granules) involved in host cell invasion (see Fig. 275-4A).[12] Four Plasmodium species are classified as human malaria parasites: P. falciparum, P. vivax, P. ovale, and P. malariae. Some malaria parasites of other primates (e.g., P. knowlesi, P. cynomolgi, and P. simium) can also infect humans under natural conditions.[13] Indeed, with the recently appreciated extent of human infections from P. knowlesi, a natural pathogen of macaque monkeys,

this parasite has been proposed to be a "fifth human malaria parasite" responsible for significant morbidity and mortality in Malaysia.[14,15]

In 1880, Alphonse Laveran first observed malaria parasites in a human blood sample, including the exflagellation of microgametes that usually emerge in the mosquito.[16] It was eventually established that parasites in the bloodstream reproduce asexually in the haploid state (Fig. 275-2). During erythrocytic development, some parasites undergo a poorly understood switch to sexual forms: male and female gametocytes. These are the forms that are taken up by and infect anopheline mosquitoes, as proven by Ronald Ross and Battista Grassi in the 1890s.[17,18] Gametocytes emerge from erythrocytes in the mosquito midgut as male and female gametes that cross-fertilize to form diploid zygotes, which in turn differentiate into ookinetes that burrow across the midgut wall. Each ookinete develops into an oocyst containing up to 1000 sporozoites that emerge and are then carried by the insect hemolymph to invade the salivary glands. These processes in the mosquito require an extrinsic incubation period of about 1 to 2 weeks.

Mosquitoes inject sporozoites into humans when they bite. Shortt and Garnham demonstrated in 1948 that sporozoites must first invade and replicate in hepatocytes before they can differentiate into merozoites capable of entering the intraerythrocytic cycle.[19] The injected sporozoites typically take several hours to travel through dermal tissues and migrate across host cell barriers before they enter blood and lymphatic systems and are carried to the liver.[20] A molecular motor installed between the sporozoite plasma membrane and a double inner-membrane complex powers motility in this journey, while sporozoite surface proteins that are linked to this motor provide traction for gliding and crossing cellular barriers in tissue transit and invasion.[21,22]

Invasion of sporozoites into hepatocytes takes place by a coordinated series of steps including host cell contact, signaling events with discharge of calcium, release of ligands and processing molecules from micronemes and other organelles of the sporozoite apical complex, and active entry of the sporozoite into an induced parasitophorous vacuole in the cytoplasm of the hepatocyte. The host tetraspanin molecule CD81 is important for sporozoite entry into hepatocytes.[23,24] Two recent studies have shown the class B type I scavenger receptor SR B1, a known co-receptor with CD81 for invasion of hepatocytes by hepatitis C virus (HCV), also promote efficient Plasmodium infection of hepatocytes.[25,26] A likely role for SR B1 is the organization of CD81 into tetraspanin-enriched microdomains that are preferred membrane areas for sporozoite entry.[25] Since SR-B1 is vital in providing cholesterol to the hepatocyte by HDL-cholesteryl ester uptake, its exploitation by Plasmodium and HCV represents the evolutionary selection of a dependable invasion pathway by these pathogens. SR B1's role in HDL-cholesteryl ester uptake and activation of the liver fatty-acid carrier L-FABP also supports the transformation and growth requirements of the parasite inside the hepatocyte. Individual infected hepatocytes support the development of 10,000 to 30,000 merozoites, a process that is not associated with symptoms. All P. falciparum and P. malariae parasites complete their liver stage development in about 1 to 2 weeks.[27] P. vivax and P. ovale liver stages also can develop promptly or can remain latent as hypnozoites in the liver for months to years before emerging to produce relapses of malaria (see Fig. 275-2).

Once a merozoite breaks out by protease activity from its host hepatocyte (or from its host erythrocyte in the bloodstream cycle),[28] it engages loosely with a noninfected erythrocyte and then reorients so that its apical end faces the surface.[29] The merozoite then drives itself into the erythrocyte through a ring-shaped, electron-dense junction that moves from the front to back end of the merozoite by the power

*All material in this chapter is in the public domain, with the exception of any borrowed figures or tables.

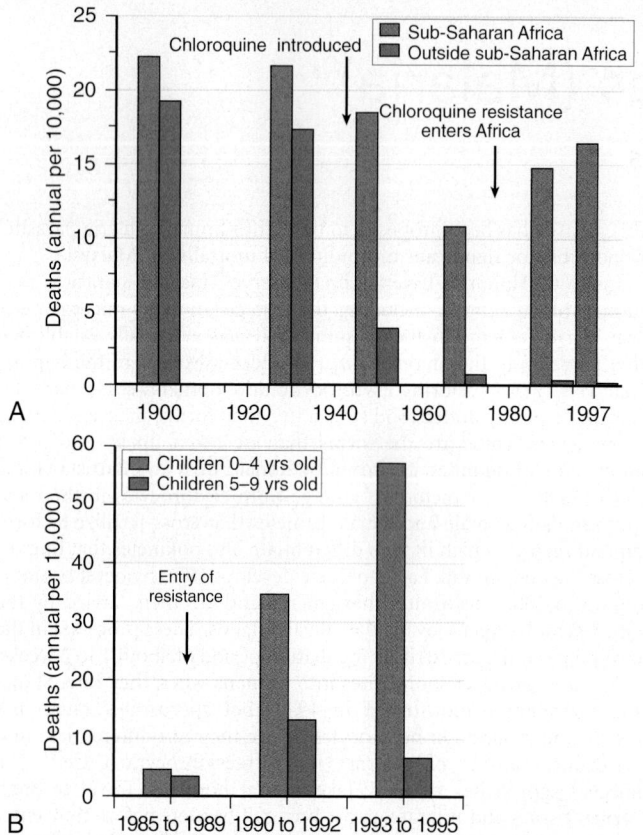

Figure 275-1 **Malaria death rates after the introduction of chloroquine and subsequent evolution of chloroquine-resistant *P. falciparum*. A,** Malaria death rates in the 20th century. Dramatic reductions in mortality have been achieved outside sub-Saharan Africa. Mortality rates declined after the introduction of chloroquine but rose again after the spread of chloroquine resistance across the continent. **B,** Rise in mortality among children in the village of Mlomp, Senegal. Increased death rates were observed after chloroquine resistance entered the village, chiefly among children younger than 5 years old, the most susceptible age group in highly endemic areas. (*A, Adapted from Carter R, Mendis KN. Evolutionary and historical aspects of the burden of malaria. Clin Microbiol Rev. 2002;15:564-594. B, Adapted from Trape JF, Pison G, Preziosi MP, et al. Impact of chloroquine resistance on malaria mortality. C R Acad Sci III. 1998;321:689-697.*)

of an actin-myosin motor.[29] An envelope of invaginated membrane surrounds the merozoite as it enters, forming the parasitophorous vacuole once invasion is complete.[30] These steps of invasion are supported by cellular signaling events, energy-dependent migration, and discharge of contents from the rhoptries, micronemes, dense granules and perhaps other compartments of the apical complex.[31] In *P. falciparum* infection, this invasion process can be supported by multiple different interactions between parasite molecules and erythrocyte surface molecules, including glycophorins.[32,33] Successful invasion of *P. vivax*, by contrast, depends on an interaction with erythrocyte Duffy antigen. Within erythrocytes, merozoites develop from ring forms into trophozoites and then into schizonts over 48 hours (*P. falciparum, P. vivax, P. ovale*) or 72 hours (*P. malariae*). After breaking down their host cell membrane by enzymatic digestion, 24 to 32 merozoites exit into the bloodstream, each of which is capable of infecting a new erythrocyte. Cycles of invasion and growth in erythrocytes produce a parasite biomass that enlarges exponentially, causing fever and leading to pathological processes such as erythrocyte loss (anemia) and sequestration of infected erythrocytes in microvascular beds (cerebral malaria).

Pathophysiology

THE MALARIA PAROXYSM AND GENERAL CONSIDERATIONS

Malaria presents as an acute febrile illness that is often but not always characterized by the classic malaria paroxysm: chills and rigors, followed by fever spikes up to 40°C (104°F), and then profuse sweating that can ultimately give way to extreme fatigue and sleep. Paroxysms last several hours, can occur with a regular periodicity coinciding with the synchronous rupture of blood schizonts, may alternate with relatively asymptomatic periods, and are associated with high levels of tumor necrosis factor-α (TNF-α).[34] Paroxysms can occur in tertian 48-hour or quartan 72-hour cycles, or in other more complicated patterns.[35] TNF-α may originate from monocytes stimulated by glycosyl phosphatidylinositol moieties or other substances released on schizont rupture.[36,37]

Malaria can be acutely malignant and painful, or more indolent and asymptomatic. It increases the morbidity and mortality associated with other diseases by stressing host systems and producing effects such as dehydration, anemia, and some degree of immune suppression. Malaria is tremendously debilitating and impedes economic development through its adverse effects on fertility, population growth, saving and investment, worker productivity, absenteeism, premature mortality, and medical costs.[38,39] A single episode of malaria has been estimated to result in a loss of 5 to 20 working days, and an agricultural family afflicted by malaria may be up to 60% less productive than a family without malaria.[40]

PLASMODIUM FALCIPARUM

P. falciparum malaria can be much more acute and severe than malaria caused by other *Plasmodium* species (Fig. 275-3). Although *P. vivax* can cause serious and fatal illness,[41,42] by far the largest fraction of deaths directly attributable to malaria are caused by severe complications of *P. falciparum* infection, including cerebral malaria, severe anemia, respiratory failure, renal failure, and severe malaria of pregnancy.[43,44] Important contributory factors include metabolic acidosis, hypoglycemia, and superimposed bacterial infections. Fatal *P. falciparum* infections are often associated with the failure of multiple organ systems.

An important feature of the pathogenesis of *P. falciparum* is the ability of its mature trophozoite and schizont forms to sequester in the deep venous microvasculature. This sequestration is promoted by a number of processes: the adherence of infected erythrocytes to endothelial cells[45,46] (Fig. 275-4F and G), rosetting—the binding of infected erythrocytes to noninfected erythrocytes[47,48] (Fig. 275-4H), reduced red cell deformability[49,50] (Fig. 275-4C and D), and platelet-mediated clumping of infected erythrocytes.[51,52] In malaria of pregnancy, erythrocytes accumulate within the proteoglycan matrix of placental intervillous spaces. *P. falciparum*–infected erythrocytes can thus accumulate throughout the body, including the heart,[53] lung, liver,[54] brain,[55-57] kidney,[58] dermis, bone marrow,[59] and placenta.[60] Noninfected erythrocytes, monocytes and macrophages, platelets, and depositions of thrombin are often found in association with these infected erythrocytes.[55,57,58,61]

By sequestration, *P. falciparum* may avoid filtration and destruction by the spleen and thus multiply to high densities.[62] The survival and propagation of parasites may be aided when they sequester in the low oxygen gas environment of postcapillary venules. Attachment points to endothelium have been shown by electron microscopy to be dense protrusions, termed knobs, on the surface of infected erythrocytes (Fig. 275-4D and E), where antigenically variable cytoadherence proteins (PfEMP-1; see later) are anchored. Attachment at knobs (Fig. 275-4F) supports cytoadherence in vitro and sequestration in vivo (Fig. 275-4G).[63,64] Under flow conditions, cytoadherence events are reminiscent of leukocyte adhesion, involving distinct phases of tethering, rolling, and stable adhesion.[65]

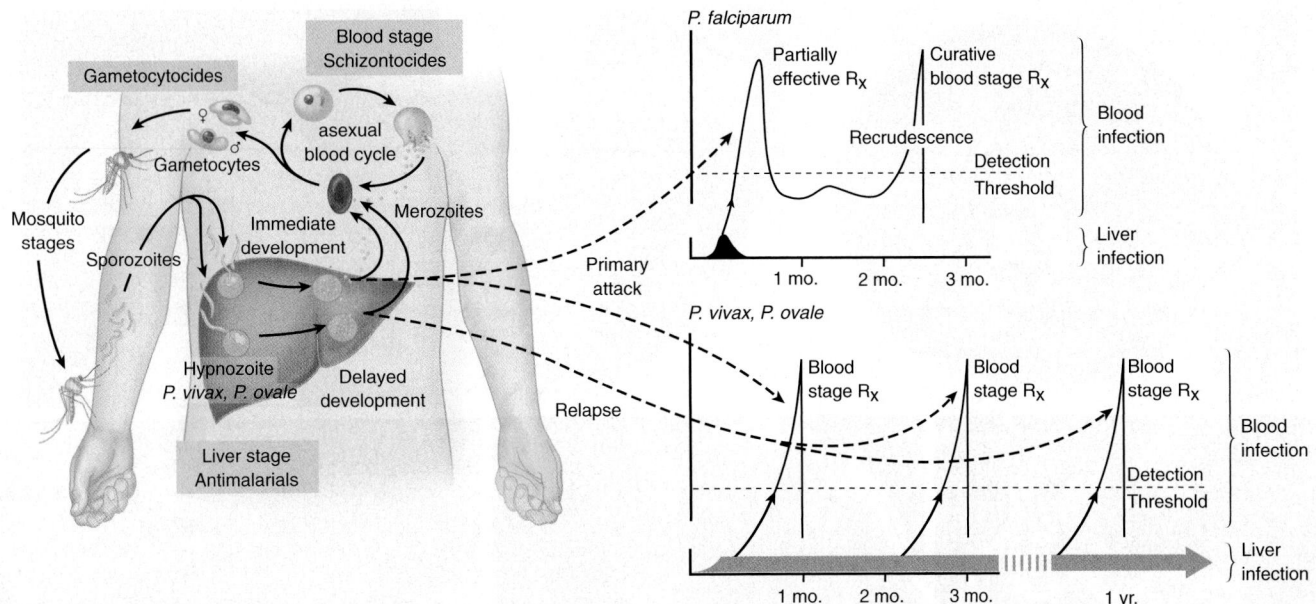

Figure 275-2 **The *Plasmodium* life cycle and disease patterns of recrudescence and relapse.** Anopheline mosquitoes transmit malaria by injecting sporozoites into the human host. The sporozoites then invade hepatocytes, in which they develop into schizonts. Each infected hepatocyte ruptures to liberate 10,000 to 30,000 merozoites that invade circulating erythrocytes. Growth and development of the parasites in red cells result in subsequent waves of merozoite invasion. This asexual blood cycle repeats every 48 (*P. falciparum, P. vivax, P. ovale*) or 72 (*P. malariae*) hours, leading to amplification of parasite density; paroxysms of chills, fevers, and sweats; and other manifestations of disease. Malaria symptoms are typically experienced 2 to 4 weeks after the mosquito bite. If the parasites are not cleared (e.g., patient receives partially effective therapy), recrudescence of parasitemia and malaria symptoms can occur. Eradicating parasites with an effective drug regimen cures malaria. Some *P. vivax* and *P. ovale* parasites can postpone their development in the liver, persisting as latent forms called hypnozoites. Hypnozoites are not eradicated by standard therapy (e.g., chloroquine) directed against blood stages. Resumption of hypnozoite development months to years after initial infection can lead to malaria relapse that requires an additional round of drug therapy to treat recurrent symptoms and eradicate blood stages. Treating hypnozoites with primaquine can prevent relapses of malaria.

P. falciparum erythrocyte membrane protein-1 (PfEMP-1) is central to malaria pathogenesis.[66] PfEMP-1 is a family of major antigenically variant proteins encoded by a multicopy gene family termed *var*.[67] Approximately 60 different *var* genes are present in the haploid genome of each parasite, encoding variants of PfEMP-1 with unique antigenic and cytoadherence properties.[68,69] A single PfEMP-1 variant is thought to be predominantly expressed on the surface of an individual infected erythrocyte,[70] while others are silenced.[71] Switches in expression between individual members of the *var* gene family occur at an estimated rate of 2% to 18% per cell per generation[72,73] and produce the antigenic variation in *P. falciparum* populations during the course of an infection. PfEMP-1 proteins exposed on knobs have

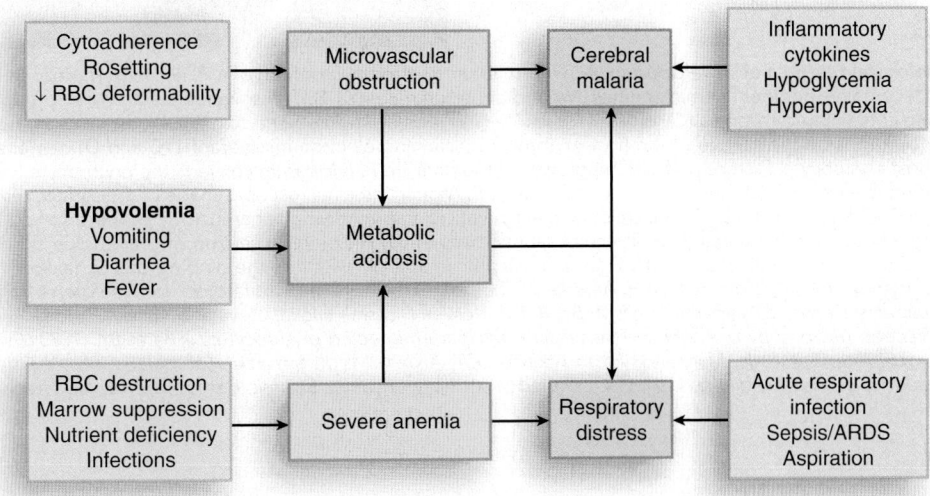

Figure 275-3 **Pathogenesis of severe *P. falciparum* malaria.** Deaths from severe falciparum malaria are commonly attributable to the effects of severe anemia, cerebral malaria, and respiratory distress in young children. This schematic illustrates how multiple pathogenic events such as cytoadherence, destruction of noninfected erythrocytes, and production of inflammatory cytokines combine to produce the microvascular sequestration and metabolic acidosis that are central to the development of severe disease.

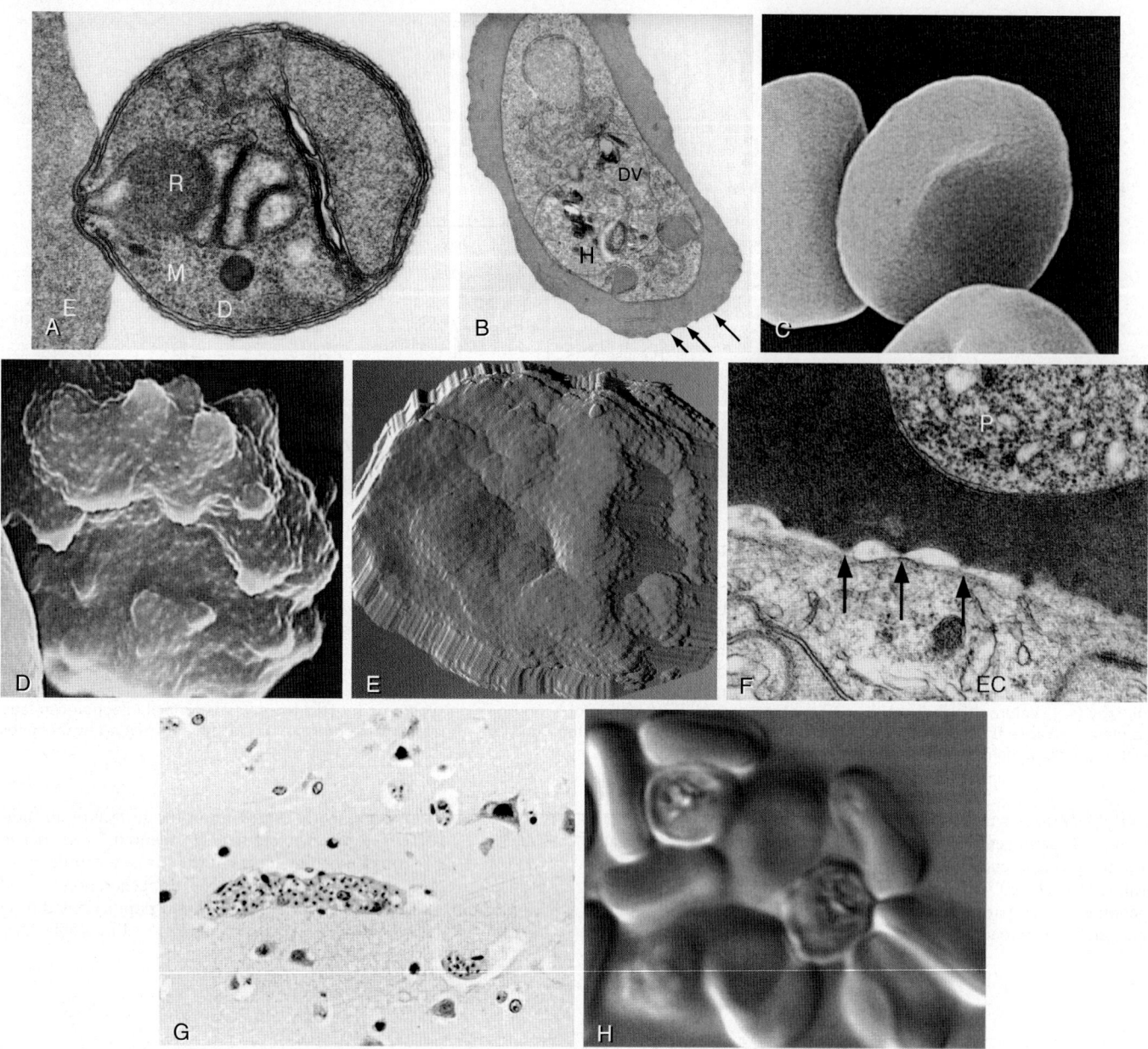

Figure 275-4 Morphological features of *P. falciparum*. A, Transmission electron micrograph of a *P. knowlesi* merozoite invading an erythrocyte E via its apical end, which contains rhoptries (R), micronemes (M), and dense granules (D). **B,** Transmission electron micrograph of an intraerythrocytic *P. falciparum* trophozoite containing cytosomes (C), digestive vacuole (DV), and crystalline hemazoin (H). *Arrows* identify numerous small electron-dense protrusions termed knobs on the surface of the host erythrocyte. Scanning electron micrographs (**C** and **D**) demonstrate the effects of the malaria parasite on its host erythrocyte. Distension from the growth of the parasite *P. falciparum* converts the erythrocyte from a deformable bicon-cave disk C to a nondeformable cell D displaying knobs over its surface. **E,** Atomic force microscopic image of the surface of a *P. falciparum*–infected erythrocyte showing numerous knob structures. **F,** Transmission electron micrograph showing adherence via knobs (*arrows*) between a *P. falciparum*–infected erythrocyte and a host endothelial cell (EC) of a cerebral microvessel. **G,** Histological section of brain tissue showing pigmented mature *P. falciparum* parasites sequestered in microvessels. **H,** Light microscopic image of rosetting, the binding of a *P. falciparum*–infected erythrocyte to multiple noninfected erythrocytes. (**A,** *From Fujioka H, Aikawa M. The malaria parasite and its life cycle. In: Wahlgren M, Perlmann P, eds.* Malaria: Molecular and Clinical Aspects. *Harwood Academic; 1999:19-55.* **B,** *Courtesy of Hisashi Fujioka, Cleveland, Ohio.* **C** *and* **D,** *From Aikawa M, Rabbege JR, Udeinya IJ, et al. Electron microscopy of knobs in Plasmodium falciparum-infected erythrocytes.* J Parasitol. *1983;69:435-437.* **E,** *Courtesy of James Dvorak and Takayuki Arie, Bethesda, Maryland. [From Atkinson CT, Aikawa M. Ultrastructure of malaria-infected erythrocytes.* Blood Cells. *1990;16:351-368.]* **G,** *Courtesy of Hisashi Fujioka, Cleveland, Ohio.* **H,** *Courtesy of James Dvorak, Bethesda, Maryland [reprinted with permission].*)

binding domains that adhere to host molecules, including CD36, intercellular adhesion molecule-1 (ICAM-1), thrombospondin, platelet-endothelial cell adhesion molecule (PECAM/CD31),[65,74-76] and chondroitin sulfate A.[77,78] Broods of parasites infecting a human host may express several variants in their subpopulations.

There is some evidence that *P. falciparum* strains may be associated with pathological developments of different severity because of the particular variants of PfEMP-1 expressed as well as the distribution of host receptors.[45,79-82] CD36 is an important cytoadherence receptor expressed on microvascular endothelium as well as on monocytes and platelets and is thought to mediate the sequestration of parasites as well as immune response to infection.[83] CD36, however, may have a more limited role in the brain, where ICAM-1 is believed to be a principal cytoadherence receptor. This concept is supported by evidence of ICAM-1 upregulation in autopsy brain specimens and studies that have correlated cerebral malaria with the ability of parasite field isolates to bind ICAM-1.[84-87] Recently, parasitized erythrocytes were also found to bind the globular head of C1q receptor on brain microvascular endothelial cells.[88] Parasitized erythrocytes that bind chondroitin sulfate A (CSA) expressed by syncytiotrophoblasts usually do not bind CD36,[89] which accounts for their selective sequestration in placental tissue and role in malaria of pregnancy.

PfEMP-1 is also an important parasite ligand in rosetting,[90] as it can adhere to complement receptor 1 (CR1)[91] and blood group A antigen[92] on host erythrocytes. A human CR1 polymorphism that reduces *P. falciparum* rosetting was found in one study to protect against severe malaria[93]; data from other studies of rosetting and disease severity have in some cases shown an association[94-98] and in others have not.[99,100] Forms of PfEMP-1 that bind to surface glycoprotein CD36 on platelets are also thought to have an important role in the platelet-mediated clumping of infected erythrocytes.[51]

High parasite densities,[101] increased parasite multiplication rates,[102] and evidence of high parasite biomass (e.g., intraleukocytic pigment, mature trophozoites, and schizonts) on peripheral blood smear, are associated with increased severity of malaria and death.[103,104] *P. falciparum* can infect erythrocytes of all ages,[105] which aids in producing heavy parasite burdens; *P. vivax* is selective for reticulocytes[106,107] and does not achieve high densities.

CEREBRAL MALARIA

The classic histopathological finding of fatal cerebral malaria is the intense sequestration of parasitized erythrocytes in the cerebral microvasculature (see Fig. 275-4G), often accompanied by ring hemorrhages, perivascular leukocyte infiltrates, thrombin deposition, activated platelets,[56,108-112] and immunohistochemical evidence for endothelial cell activation.[55,86,113] In one autopsy series of patients who died from cerebral malaria, 94% of brain microvessels contained adherent parasitized erythrocytes versus 13% of controls who died from noncerebral malaria.[114] In another study, 7 of 31 (24%) African children who received a clinical diagnosis of cerebral malaria were found at autopsy to have nonmalarial causes of coma, underscoring the possibility that other illnesses may mimic the cerebral malaria presentation in areas where incidental parasitemia is common.[110]

Sequestration of parasitized erythrocytes stimulates the local production of inflammatory cytokines and mediators such as TNF-α, elevated levels of which may correlate with disease severity.[115-117] These cytokines also upregulate adhesion molecules such as ICAM-1 in the cerebral microvasculature,[118,119] which may lead to further sequestration of infected and noninfected erythrocytes, leukocytes, and activated platelets.[108] Impaired nitric oxide bioavailability may also contribute to endothelial dysfunction[120] by increasing microvascular tone, endothelial cell adhesion molecule expression, cytokine expression, and parasitized erythrocyte sequestration.[121] These processes may cause varying degrees of functional obstruction and consequently reduce local delivery of oxygen and glucose. However, obstruction by infected erythrocytes does not generally produce neurologic sequelae akin to those that follow the physical occlusion in thrombotic stroke, as most patients with cerebral malaria who recover can do so rapidly within 48 hours and without such consequences. Systemic sequestration of metabolically active parasites, blood cells, and platelets likely contributes to the metabolic acidosis and thrombocytopenia commonly seen in severe malaria. Severe metabolic acidosis, hypoglycemia, hyperpyrexia, and nonconvulsive status epilepticus can contribute significantly to the cerebral malaria presentation, as suggested by the rapid clinical improvement of some patients after fluid resuscitation and blood transfusion, dextrose infusion, fever reduction, and anticonvulsants.[122-125]

HYPOGLYCEMIA

Hypoglycemia in malaria can cause coma and convulsions and contributes substantially to the morbidity and mortality associated with cerebral malaria.[43] The pathophysiologic mechanisms of hypoglycemia in children and adults seem to be different. In children, insulin levels are appropriate and hypoglycemia is associated with impaired hepatic gluconeogenesis and increased consumption of glucose by hypermetabolic peripheral tissues.[124,126-129] Large amounts of glucose are also consumed by intraerythrocytic parasites.[130] In adults, hypoglycemia is often associated with hyperinsulinemia,[131] which may result from pancreatic islet cell stimulation by parasite-derived factors and/or parenteral quinine or quinidine therapy.[132] Depletion of liver glycogen stores after decreased food intake during the prodromal period may also contribute to hypoglycemia.

ANEMIA

The pathophysiology of malarial anemia is multifactorial and complex.[133,134] The intravascular lysis and phagocytic removal of infected erythrocytes[135] contribute to anemia, but do not always account for the dramatic reductions in erythrocyte mass that can occur with acute *P. falciparum* malaria episodes. Additional processes have therefore been implicated in malarial anemia. Excess removal of noninfected erythrocytes may account for up to 90% of erythrocyte loss[136] and may be mediated by processes (e.g., oxidative stress) that enhance the senescence and impair the deformability of erythrocytes. The contribution of impaired bone marrow responses to malarial anemia is significant and probably involves general processes also found in other diseases. Release of inflammatory cytokines (e.g., TNF-α) are associated with impaired production of erythropoietin,[137,138] decreased responsiveness of erythroid progenitor cells to adequate levels of erythropoietin,[139,140] and increased erythrophagocytic activity.[141] These pathogenic processes account for normochromic/normocytic anemia seen in malaria, and explain the notable absence of a robust reticulocyte response. Although microcytosis and hypochromia are seen in malaria, these are often attributable to thalassemias and iron deficiency in endemic areas. Bacteremia, nutritional deficiencies (vitamins A and B12), concomitant infections (e.g., hookworm and *Schistosoma*), and genetic polymorphisms (G6PD deficiency) have also been associated with the level of anemia experienced during an acute malaria episode,[142] presumably by lowering the baseline from which hemoglobin levels acutely decline. In endemic areas where chloroquine resistance is prevalent, the inability of young children to clear their parasitemias with chloroquine contributes to their higher baseline prevalence of anemia when compared with children treated with more effective drugs.[143]

PULMONARY EDEMA AND RESPIRATORY DISTRESS

The most significant pulmonary manifestation directly attributable to *P. falciparum* is noncardiogenic pulmonary edema.[144,145] Sequestration of infected erythrocytes in the lungs is thought to initiate regional production of inflammatory cytokines that increase capillary permeability, leading sequentially to pulmonary edema, dyspnea, hypoxia, acute lung injury, and acute respiratory distress syndrome (ARDS).[146] Pulmonary edema is common with severe malaria in adults but infrequent in children, and it is not associated with pleural effusion. Iatrogenic fluid overload and acute renal failure may contribute to the development or worsening of pulmonary edema. Although pulmonary edema usually occurs after other features of severe disease (e.g., coma, acute renal failure) become manifest, it may occur at any time during the clinical course, even when the patient appears to be recovering on antimalarial therapy. Dyspnea and increased respiratory rate are features of impending pulmonary edema and often precede other clinical and radiologic signs (use of accessory muscles of respiration, generalized increase in interstitial markings).

Pulmonary manifestations of deep breathing and respiratory distress associated with severe malaria may also arise from metabolic acidosis,[44] severe acute respiratory infections,[128] sepsis-related ARDS, aspiration (especially with diminished consciousness or convulsions), and nosocomial pneumonia. Cerebral pathologic processes may result in abnormal breathing patterns including Cheyne-Stokes respirations and respiratory failure.[147]

METABOLIC (LACTIC) ACIDOSIS

Metabolic acidosis is a common feature of severe malaria and is associated with significant lactic acidemia in up to 85% of cases. Metabolic acidosis is principally caused by reduced delivery of oxygen to tissues, from the combined effects of anemia (decreased oxygen-carrying capacity), sequestration (microvascular obstruction), and hypovolemia (reduced perfusion) as a result of fluid losses caused by fever, decreased intake, vomiting, and diarrhea.[148] These effects produce a shift from aerobic to anaerobic metabolism and cause lactate levels to increase.[149] The following factors may also contribute to metabolic acidosis: production of lactate by anaerobic glycolysis in sequestered parasites,[150] reduction of hepatic blood flow leading to diminished lactate clearance,[151,152] induction of lactate production by TNF-α and other pro-inflammatory cytokines,[153] renal impairment,[151] and ingestion of exogenous acids (e.g., salicylate) or unknown constituents of traditional herbal remedies for fever.[154]

MALARIA OF PREGNANCY

Placental malaria results in maternal morbidity and mortality, intrauterine growth retardation, premature delivery, low birth weight, and increased newborn mortality.[2,155,156] Selective accumulation of mature parasites in the placenta involves their interaction with syncytiotrophoblastic CSA[78] possibly complemented by interactions with other molecules such as hyaluronic acid and immunoglobulins.[157-159] This is in contrast to the sequestration of infected erythrocytes in the systemic microvasculature, where CD36 is the major endothelial receptor. Parasites that accumulate in the placenta express PfEMP-1 variants that bind CSA[160,161] but not CD36.[89] Evidence suggests that women who experience a malaria episode from CSA-binding parasites during their first pregnancy lack immunity to the PfEMP-1 antigenic variants presented by these strains and, despite immunity to CD36-binding variants from previous infections, are highly susceptible to the new infection. Malaria in subsequent pregnancies is typically less severe than in the first pregnancy,[162] presumably because of a woman's previous experience with CSA-binding parasites.

The susceptibility of fetuses of first-time mothers to placental malaria may also be influenced by polymorphisms in the fms-like tyrosine kinase 1 (FLT1) gene, which were reported recently to be under natural selection pressure in malaria of pregnancy.[163] Maternal genotypes of increased FLT1 expression (SS genotypes of a 3′UTR dinucleotide sequence) were associated with prior fetal losses in first-time mothers with placental malaria, while SS genotypes in the newborns of first-time mothers were found to have higher occurrences of low birth weight. The placentas of SS newborns also showed greater inflammation as judged by histologic evaluations and transcript levels of IFN-γ and immunoglobulin heavy chain genes.[163]

PLASMODIUM VIVAX AND P. OVALE

Infections with P. vivax and P. ovale can be considered similar to each other from a clinical perspective. P. vivax infections can be tremendously debilitating and are sometimes associated with serious complications, including acute lung injury[164,165] and splenic rupture and associated pathologies.[166,167] Splenic rupture has been associated with acute and chronic infections and can occur spontaneously or with minor trauma, including manual examination of the spleen. Although more commonly associated with vivax malaria, splenic rupture has been associated with all four human malaria parasites. Anemia is

frequently observed as a consequence of acute or chronic infections, or as a result of repeated acute infections.[135] Suppressed erythrocyte production and hemolysis of both infected and noninfected erythrocytes have been implicated in the pathogenesis of vivax malarial anemia. Although not often fatal, P. vivax infections have recently been associated in Papua New Guinea and Papua Indonesia with severe disease manifestations including cerebral malaria, severe malarial anemia, and respiratory distress.[41,42]

In P. vivax malaria, merozoites are largely restricted to invasion of reticulocytes.[107] Since reticulocytes account for only a small proportion of the total erythrocyte mass, parasitemias in P. vivax infections are usually less than 1%. P. vivax and P. ovale do not exhibit sequestration as observed for P. falciparum and therefore are generally not associated with the extensive microvascular obstruction or regional and systemic inflammatory effects that characterize falciparum malaria. However, recent evidence suggests that P. vivax can cause lung injury by sequestering in the pulmonary microvasculature.[168] P. vivax parasites may avoid splenic entrapment by increasing rather than decreasing erythrocyte deformability.[169]

PLASMODIUM MALARIAE

The quartan malaria of P. malariae usually presents with fever and paroxysms similar to those of P. vivax but with a 3-day rather than 2-day periodicity. P. malariae often establishes parasitemias that are below levels of detection by microscopy. Patients can remain infected and asymptomatic for periods of many years before presenting with fevers, malaise, and splenomegaly decades after they have left an endemic area.[170] Chronic P. malariae infection can lead to nephrotic syndrome in young children living in endemic areas.[171,172] This complication has features of an immune complex–mediated glomerulonephritis.[173,174]

PLASMODIUM KNOWLESI

A large focus of human malaria caused by P. knowlesi was recently identified in Malaysia.[14] P. knowlesi is indistinguishable from P. malariae on blood smear examination, showing both immature and mature forms in the circulation. Unlike P. malariae, however, P. knowlesi produces acute illness and relatively high parasitemias. Indeed, the ability of P. knowlesi to replicate every 24 hours can cause daily fever spikes and rapidly produce hyperparasitemias that are life-threatening. In addition to hyperparasitemia, four fatal P. knowlesi malaria cases have been associated with abdominal pain, marked hepatorenal dysfunction, and refractory hypotension.[15]

Genetic Resistance

Life-threatening P. falciparum malaria has been a potent evolutionary force in shaping the human genome. Evidence for the natural selection of genetic polymorphisms can be found in the ethnic and geographic distributions of mutant hemoglobins, thalassemias, glucose-6-phosphate dehydrogenase (G6PD) deficiencies, erythrocyte membrane proteins, and cytokines and other mediators of inflammation and immunity.[175-179]

HEMOGLOBINS S, E, AND C

The geographic distributions of mutant hemoglobins overlap considerably with those of P. falciparum malaria.[180] Case-control and longitudinal cohort studies have associated malaria protection with hemoglobin S (HbS) heterozygosity (sickle cell trait), in which the 6th amino acid of the β-globin chain is mutated from glutamate to valine.[181-184] The genetic fitness of SS homozygosity (sickle cell disease) is very poor in sub-Saharan Africa, whereas the prevalence of AS heterozygotes can be 25% or more in some areas.[185] The HbS mutation thus exists as a balanced polymorphism: the malaria protective benefit afforded to AS heterozygotes offsets the childhood deaths of SS homozygotes. The mutation of HbC is in the same 6th position as the HbS mutation but differs in that the mutation is a glutamate to lysine substitution. A number of case-control studies in West Africa have associated HbC with malaria protection.[186-190]

Epidemiological studies have found similar parasite densities in AA and AS children, very high parasite densities in some AS children,[191] and occasional cases of severe malaria in AS children.[186,192] These observations are not fully explained by proposals that parasitized AS erythrocytes are more likely to sickle or support reduced parasite growth rates under conditions of low oxygen tension,[193-196] or by findings of enhanced phagocytosis of parasitized AS erythrocytes by macrophages.[197] Other mechanisms of protection that include additional genetic or environmental factors are likely operating in AS children. Malaria protection by HbC is also not associated with reduced parasite densities in vivo or significant impairment of parasite multiplication in vitro,[186,187,190,198] suggesting that HbC erythrocytes support normal invasion and development of *P. falciparum*.

In more recent studies of possible mechanisms of protection, parasitized AS and AC erythrocytes were found to be impaired in their adherence to microvascular endothelial cells and monocytes[198,199]—two interactions critical to the development of severe malaria. Abnormal display of the parasite's main virulence factor and cytoadherence ligand, PfEMP-1, on the surface of parasitized erythrocytes is one explanation for these findings. Reduced cytoadherence of parasitized AS and AC erythrocytes would still enable them to sequester in microvessels and reach appreciable parasite densities but would be expected to lessen the inflammatory consequences of cytoadherence, and thus reduce the chances of progressing to severe disease. It is also suggested that anti-PfEMP-1 antibodies acquired rapidly in endemic areas could synergize with HbS and HbC to further weaken cytoadherence interactions and ameliorate disease severity.[199]

HbE is another hemoglobin characterized by a single point mutation in the β-globin chain: a glutamate to lysine change at the 26th amino acid. This mutation also introduces an alternative splice site that reduces the amount of β-globin produced,[200] thereby conferring a thalassemia phenotype to HbE erythrocytes. Unlike HbS and HbC, HbE is found predominantly in Asia. Some epidemiologic studies have found HbE to protect against malaria,[201,202] while others have not.[203,204] Although HbE has been suggested to decrease the multiplication rate of *P. falciparum*,[205] parasite densities do not seem to differ between AA and HbE individuals with malaria.[202,204]

THALASSEMIAS

Thalassemia arises from deletion of one or more of the four genes encoding the α-globin chain or mutations or deletions in one of the two genes encoding the β-globin chain of hemoglobin. These conditions are generally benign in the heterozygous state and are associated with varying degrees of microcytic, hypochromic anemia. Further loss of expression in the homozygous state causes severe disease and can be incompatible with life. Mutations associated with thalassemias are protective against malaria and exist as balanced polymorphisms in populations.[206-208] Although *P. falciparum* development can be supported by thalassemic erythrocytes, some studies have demonstrated impaired growth, especially under conditions of oxidative stress.[209-211] Other studies have demonstrated that parasitized thalassemic erythrocytes bind increased amounts of antibody from both nonimmune and immune serum, which suggests the possibility of enhanced opsonization in vivo.[212,213] These mechanisms are difficult to reconcile with several recent studies from Africa, which show that both hetero- and homozygous α thalassemia protects against severe malaria without reducing parasite densities in vivo.[188,214-216] How heterozygous α thalassemia protects against severe malaria in Africa is uncertain. Increased microerythrocyte counts in α thalassemia homozygotes have been proposed to contribute to protection against severe malarial anemia in Papua New Guinea by a mechanism that reduces loss of erythrocytes and hemoglobin during infection.[217]

HEMOGLOBIN F

Hemoglobin F ($\alpha2/\gamma2$) is a normal hemoglobin expressed by the fetus in utero and during the first few months of life. The expression of HbF dramatically declines after the third month of life as HbA replaces it. The uncommon presentation of malaria in neonates younger than 6 months old led to the hypothesis that HbF contributes to malaria protection, along with maternal antibody. Proteases that are responsible for digesting host cell hemoglobin in the food vacuole of the parasite may work less efficiently on HbF than HbA.[218] Impaired antioxidant capacity of HbF-containing erythrocytes has also been proposed to contribute to malaria protection.[219]

GLUCOSE-6-PHOSPHATE DEHYDROGENASE DEFICIENCY

Glucose-6-phosphate dehydrogenase (G6PD) is a cytoplasmic enzyme that is essential for an erythrocyte's capacity to withstand oxidant stress, such as that exerted by the developing malaria parasite. The G6PD gene is located on the X-chromosome and is therefore present in only one copy in males. In heterozygous females carrying a mutant gene, mosaic populations of G6PD-deficient and G6PD-normal erythrocytes are produced from hematopoietic cells that have one or the other X-chromosome inactivated. G6PD deficiency is the most common enzymopathy in humans, with more than 300 allelic polymorphisms identified to date. The most common polymorphism in Africa (the A− allele, 10-50% enzyme activity) has been associated with malaria protection in children and pregnant women.[184,220,221]

In a large case-control study performed in populations of West and East Africa, male hemizygotes and female heterozygotes carrying the A− allele were reported to be 58% and 46% protected against severe malaria, respectively.[184] However, a more recent and larger study,[221] including reanalysis of data from the earlier study,[184] found that male hemizygotes but not female heterozygotes carrying the A− allele are protected against severe malaria. These findings agree with the facts that male hemizygotes carry erythrocytes uniformly deficient in G6PD, whereas female heterozygotes carry mosaic populations of G6PD-normal and G6PD-deficient erythrocytes. Enhanced phagocytosis of infected G6PD-deficient erythrocytes has been proposed to play a role in malaria protection.[222] While such phagocytosis is consistent with greater protection of males than females by G6PD deficiency, it does not account for the presence of similar parasite densities in G6PD-deficient males and females.[184,221] Alternative mechanisms of protection may therefore operate in vivo.

SOUTHEAST ASIAN OVALOCYTOSIS

A 27-bp deletion in band 3 (the major anion transporter in erythrocytes) causes Southeast Asian ovalocytosis (SAO) and leads to reduced membrane deformability.[223-225] These properties may be associated with reduced parasite invasion rates of ovalocytes in vitro and reduced parasitemias in heterozygous individuals.[226-229] How these findings relate mechanistically to the dramatic reduction in cerebral malaria episodes among SAO heterozygotes[230] has not yet been established.

ABO BLOOD GROUPS

Blood group O has recently been associated with protection against severe malaria,[231,232] a phenotype of parasitized erythrocytes that correlates with severe disease in Africa.[94-98] A mechanism of reduced rosetting in type O erythrocytes compared to type A, B, or AB erythrocytes has been associated with this protective effect.[231]

DUFFY ANTIGEN NEGATIVITY

Duffy antigen is an erythrocyte receptor for *P. vivax* merozoite invasion.[106,107] Erythrocytes lacking Duffy antigen are resistant to *P. vivax* invasion, which accounts for the extremely low incidence of vivax malaria in West Africa, where Duffy antigen negativity is highly prevalent.[233,234] Reduced Duffy antigen expression on erythrocytes has also been identified as a protective polymorphism against *P. vivax* malaria in Papua New Guinea.[235] Duffy antigen negativity does not protect against malaria from *P. falciparum*, *P. ovale*, or *P. malariae*.

Acquired Immunity and Antigenic Variation

Acquired immunity against malaria is not a sterilizing immunity against parasitemia. Instead, it is an immunity that ultimately prevents the development of symptomatic and severe disease despite the presence of malaria parasites in the bloodstream. It is an immunity that increases with age, cumulative number of episodes of malaria, and time spent living in an endemic area.[236] As individuals gain the experience of numerous infections in their lifetime, they can be chronically infected yet have only mild symptoms or none at all, that is, they develop disease-controlling immunity. In highly endemic areas, children have multiple bouts of malaria each year and suffer greatly under its morbidity and mortality when they are young, generally less than 5 to 10 years old, depending on the transmission level. Pregnant women, especially primagravidae, are an important exception to this general rule because of the ability of antigenically new CSA-binding parasites to sequester in the placenta (see earlier). Nonimmune individuals may develop high parasitemias (up to 80%) within a relatively short period of time.[237] Acquired immunity to malaria is believed to be short-lived without continual exposure to infection with different *P. falciparum* variants. While individuals who reside outside an endemic area for more than a year or two can develop symptomatic and/or severe malaria after their return,[238] one study found evidence that acquired immunity to *P. falciparum* malaria persists after several years of non-exposure in African immigrants living in France.[239]

Neonates appear to be fairly resistant to malaria during the first few months of life. This apparent immunity may be conferred by transplacentally acquired maternal IgG, although the presence of fetal hemoglobin within erythrocytes likely plays a role as well (see earlier).

Splenomegaly often accompanies malaria and is thought to indicate an important role of the spleen in parasite clearance. Removal of non-infected erythrocytes by the stimulated spleen, however, may contribute to anemia. In asplenic individuals, *P. falciparum* malaria can progress extremely rapidly to high parasitemias that include mature forms not usually found circulating in the bloodstream.[62,240,241]

The mechanism by which endemic populations acquire immunity to symptomatic and severe disease is not well understood.[242] Although antibodies and T-cell responses develop against a number of parasite antigens during natural infection, none of them have been found to be superior to age or parasite exposure as correlates of protective immunity.[243] Studies in which humans were infected with a single inoculum of *P. falciparum* in the use of malariotherapy for tertiary syphilis showed that erythrocyte infection peaks decreased in successive waves of parasitemia[244] (Fig. 275-5). Individuals who eventually cleared their infection were protected against subsequent reinfection by the same parasite strain but not protected against reinfection with a different *P. falciparum* strain.[245,246]

Antigen switching results in new waves of parasitemias that escape the antibody response already produced against previous waves. Waves of *P. falciparum* manifest clinically as recurrent or relapsing fevers reminiscent of those caused by *Borrelia recurrentis* relapsing fever or *Trypanosoma brucei rhodesiensis* African sleeping sickness, and may not be cleared for months to years.[247,248] An important component of the eventual acquisition of disease-controlling immunity (premunition) after repeated episodes of malaria is the development of an antibody repertoire that can recognize a full spectrum of PfEMP-1 variant antigens. Studies in endemic areas have shown that the ability of serum to recognize diverse heterologous parasite strains increases with age and that children tend to be infected with parasites against which they have no preexisting antibody.[249-252] The mechanisms by which variant-

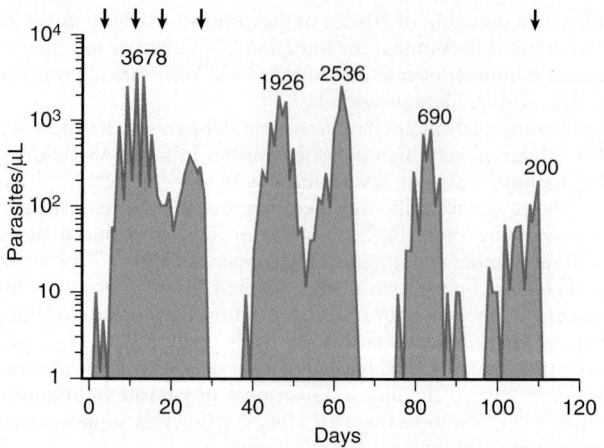

Figure 275-5 Premunition and antigenic variation. Parasitemia waves during recrudescence in a patient infected with *P. falciparum* as malariotherapy for tertiary syphilis. Although the individual had previously been infected with *P. falciparum*, drug treatments (*arrows*) were necessary to modify the primary attack and later for radical cure. Following subcurative drug treatments, four recrudescences occurred with parasite density peaks ultimately declining 10-fold. *(Adapted from Collins WE, Jeffery GM. A retrospective examination of sporozoite- and trophozoite-induced infections with Plasmodium falciparum: Development of parasitologic and clinical immunity during primary infection. Am J Trop Med Hyg. 1999;611 [Suppl]:4-19.)*

specific antibodies act in acquired immunity may include antibody-dependent cellular cytotoxicity, opsonization for uptake and destruction by splenic macrophages, and intereference with PfEMP-1–mediated cytoadherence interactions.

Epidemiology of Malaria

Malaria typically occurs in tropical regions of sub-Saharan Africa, Asia, Oceania, and Latin America (Fig. 275-6 and Fig. 328-2 in Ch. 328), but its distribution is continually changing. The CDC provides up-to-date information on the geographic distribution of malaria, including drug-resistant malaria, at *http://www.cdc.gov/malaria/travel* and in its publication, CDC Health Information for International Travel 2010, available on-line at *http://wwwn.cdc.gov/travel/contentYellowBook.aspx*.

Generally speaking, *P. falciparum* and *P. malariae* are found worldwide. *P. vivax* is infrequent in most of sub-Saharan Africa, but common elsewhere. *P. ovale* occurs in Africa and in foci within Asia and Oceania, and is often present with other *Plasmodium* species as a mixed infection.[253,254] Although most *P. knowlesi* infections of humans have been reported from Borneo and peninsular Malaysia,[14,15] cases have also been reported from other areas of Southeast Asia, including the Philippines, Singapore, Thailand, and Myanmar.[255]

Malaria is transmitted person to person by anopheline mosquitoes. Its transmission therefore requires competent mosquito vectors, a reservoir of infected humans, and conditions that bring them into proximity. The *Anopheles gambiae* complex of species and *A. funestus* transmit malaria with notoriously high efficiency and are the predominant vectors in sub-Saharan Africa, where environmental conditions favor their robust reproduction and transmission of parasites to large numbers of people. Malaria is transmitted predominantly during the wet season in endemic areas.

Malaria epidemics can result from the movement of people with no immunity into an endemic area (e.g., nomadic traders, seasonal forest laborers, and military personnel), the breakdown of control measures in areas under previously successful management programs, or unusually heavy rainfalls that can place indigenous populations at risk for higher than normal transmission.[256-258] Man-made environmental alterations (e.g., damming of rivers, deforestation) can lead to increases in malaria transmission by creating new mosquito habitats. Malaria

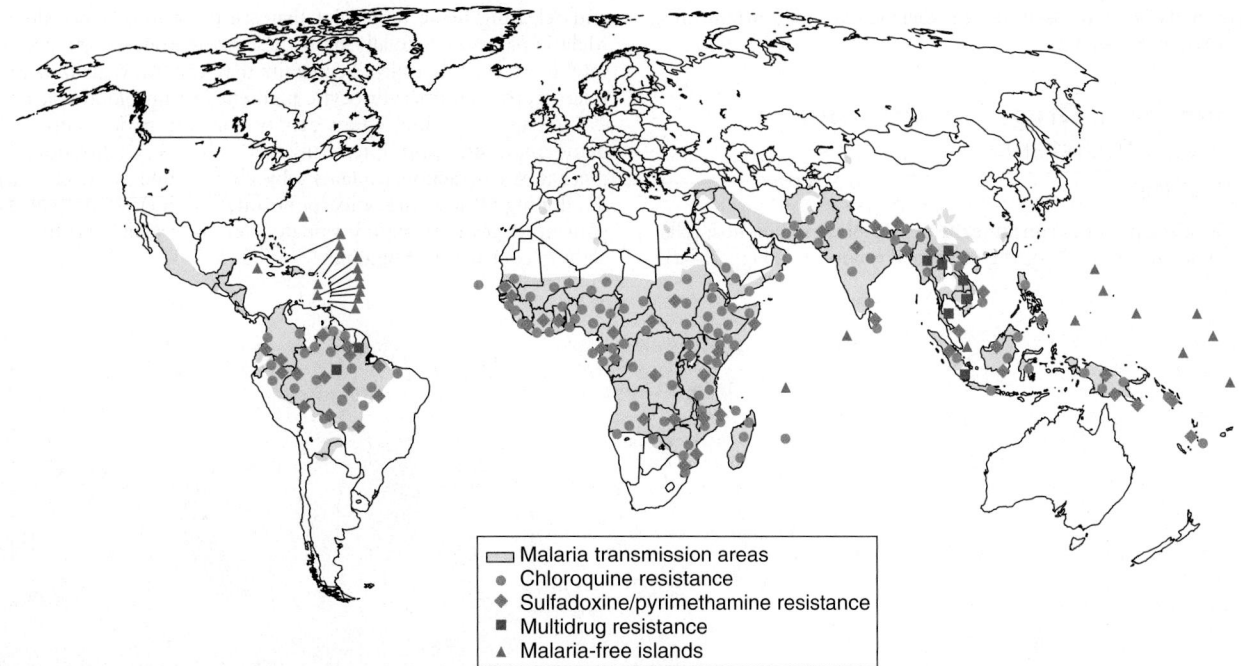

Figure 275-6 **Distribution of drug-resistant malaria.** *(From Wongsrichanalai C, Pickard AL, Wernsdorfer WH, Meshnick SR. Epidemiology of drug-resistant malaria. Lancet Infect Dis. 2002,2:209-218. Reprinted with permission from Elsevier. The CDC provides up-to-date information on the distribution of malaria and drug resistance at www.cdc.gov/travel.)*

may also arise in areas previously free of the disease as a result of immigration of populations from malaria-endemic areas (e.g., migrating workers, persons displaced by natural disasters or civil strife, resettlement of refugees).[259-262]

In the United States, changes including new agricultural and animal husbandry practices, improved housing with screens, water management with swamp drainage, and a radically altered landscape with urban developments led to a steady decline in malaria after the mid-19th century.[263] Final pockets of transmission were removed by the mid-20th century with the help of focused water management and insecticide spraying. Malaria diagnosed in the United States today is therefore almost always acquired in a malaria-endemic country by a returning traveler or immigrant. Because of parasite or host factors, immigrants may harbor parasites for months to years and not be recognized as possible sources of transmittable infection. Autochthonous transmission, although infrequent, typically occurs when parasitized individuals infect competent vectors (*A. albimanus, A. quadrimaculatus, A. freeborni*) that remain common in the United States.[264,265] "Airport malaria" occurs when infected mosquitoes arrive from an endemic country on an aircraft from which they escape to bite local residents.[266] Because mosquitoes travel short distances, infections of local residents tend to occur near airports.[267] The spraying of insecticide within aircraft leaving endemic areas reduces the incidence of airport malaria.[268] Malaria may also be acquired from needles shared among drug users; blood transfusion[269,270]; or solid organ kidney, heart, or liver transplantation.[271] These blood and organ donors are usually asymptomatic persons with low-level parasitemia from endemic areas. The incidence of transfusion-acquired malaria is reduced when returned travelers and immigrants are required to wait for periods of 3 years prior to donating blood (*http://www.fda.gov/cber/bldmem/072694.pdf*).[269]

Distribution of Drug Resistance

Chloroquine-resistant *P. falciparum* malaria is widespread in sub-Saharan Africa, Asia, and Latin America (see Fig. 275-6 and Fig. 328-2). It has also been reported in areas of the Middle East, including Iran, Yemen, Oman, and Saudi Arabia,[272-276] but not from Mexico, other regions of Central America west of the Panama Canal, Haiti, or the

Dominican Republic. High-grade resistance of *P. vivax* malaria to chloroquine has been reported in Oceania and parts of Southeast Asia.[277-279] Case reports of vivax malaria not responsive to chloroquine treatment have also been reported from Brazil, Guyana, Colombia, Peru, India, and Myanmar.[280-285] Chloroquine-resistant *P. malariae* has been reported in Sumatra, Indonesia.[286] In regions of Africa and China where chloroquine availability has ceased, chloroquine-sensitive *P. falciparum* strains have returned.[287,288]

Amodiaquine-resistant *P. falciparum* has been reported in several regions of Africa[289-293] and Asia.[294,295] Mefloquine-resistant *P. falciparum* malaria now occurs in Thailand, Cambodia, Myanmar, and Vietnam,[296-298] with scattered cases reported in the Amazon Basin[299] and Africa.[300]

Resistance to sulfadoxine-pyrimethamine (SP) is widespread through much of Southeast Asia,[301-303] the Amazon Basin,[304,305] and also occurs in sub-Saharan Africa.[306-308] The prevalence of SP resistance is highly variable in Africa, with some areas of West Africa showing relatively low rates of resistance.[309] Malaria strains resistant to cycloguanil (the active metabolite of proguanil) have been reported since the late 1940s[310-312] and can exhibit different degrees of cross-resistance to pyrimethamine.[313,314] Interindividual variations of conversion to cycloguanil may also contribute to clinical success or failure of proguanil treatment.[315-317]

Resistance to atovaquone-proguanil was previously reported only with its use in prophylaxis, but with increasing use for the treatment of uncomplicated malaria frank treatment failures have been reported from several countries.[318-322] Reduced susceptibility to quinine has been mostly reported in Southeast Asia[323] but also in sub-Saharan Africa and South America.[324,325]

Concerns about the emergence of resistance to artemisinin derivatives have increased recently with reports of treatment failures with artesunate-mefloquine and artemether-lumefantrine in Thai and Cambodian malaria control programs.[326] These failures may be associated with relatively slower elimination of parasites in response to artemisinin derivatives in vivo (prolonged clearance times), which invokes the specter of current artemisinin combination therapy (ACT) regimens becoming less effective. They also raise the possibility that rapid parasite clearance, a hallmark benefit of artemisinins in the treatment of severe malaria, may become less dependable after artemisinin dosing in Southeast Asia.[327]

Antimalarial Drugs: Mechanisms of Action and Resistance

CHLOROQUINE

Intraerythrocytic parasites consume the hemoglobin of their host cells, breaking it down within a large digestive food vacuole (see Fig. 275-4B)

and releasing heme molecules that are poisonous if not detoxified. Malaria parasites normally allow these heme molecules to polymerize into inert crystals called hemozoin that can be visualized by light microscopy as intraerythrocytic pigment in thin blood smears (Figs. 275-7E and H). Chloroquine acts by forming toxic complexes with heme molecules and interfering with their crystallization.[328] This mechanism of action explains why chloroquine is effective against developing intraerythrocytic trophozoites but ineffective against other parasite stages (i.e., mature gametocytes, liver schizonts) that do not actively consume hemoglobin.

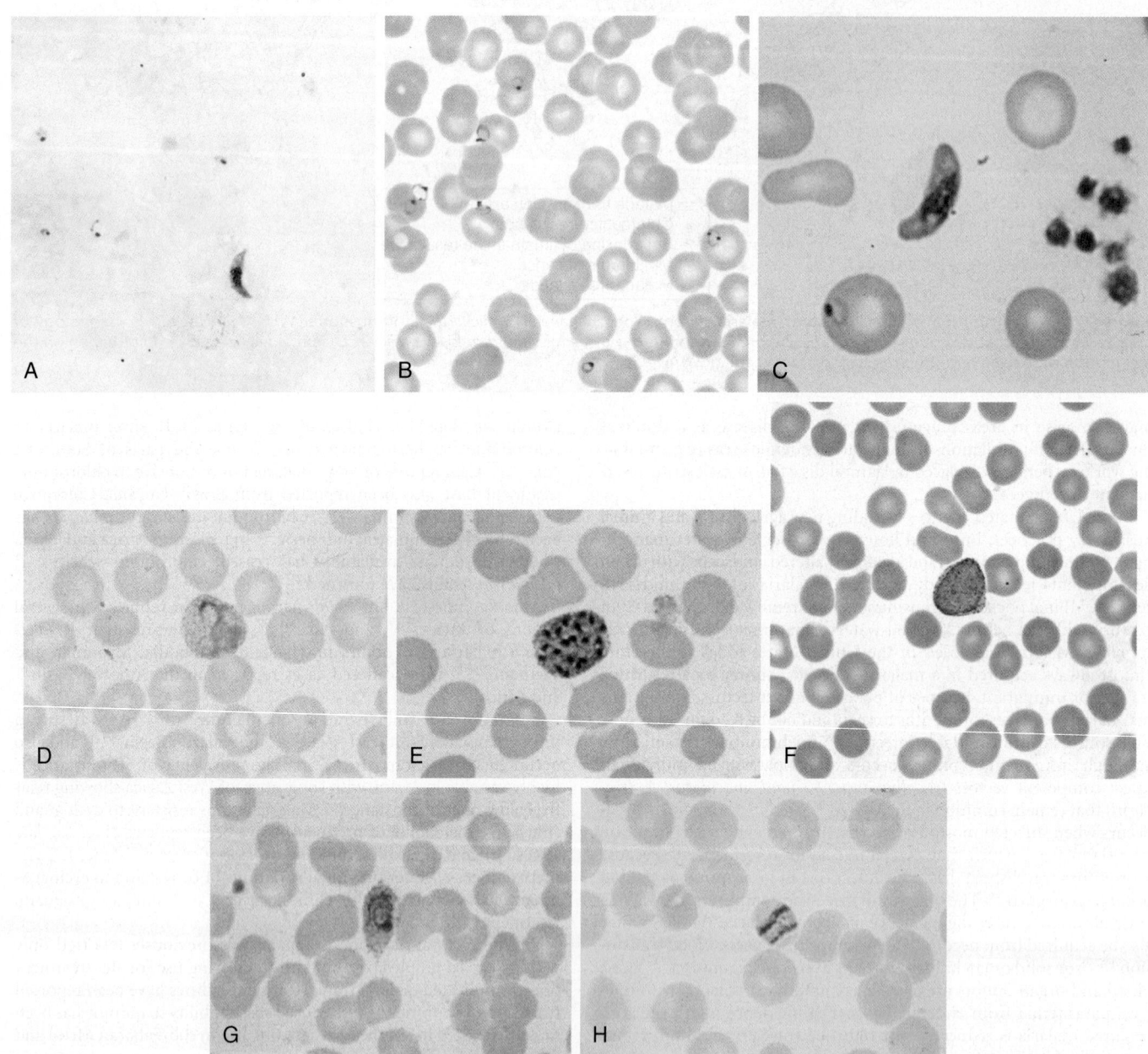

Figure 275-7 **Giemsa-stained thick (A) and thin (B-H) smears used for the diagnosis of malaria and the speciation of *Plasmodium* parasites.** **A,** Multiple signet-ring *P. falciparum* trophozoites, which are visualized outside erythrocytes in thick blood smear preparations. **B,** A multiply infected erythrocyte containing signet-ring *P. falciparum* trophozoites, including an accolade form positioned up against the inner surface of the erythrocyte membrane in fixed thin blood smear preparations. **C,** Banana-shaped gametocyte unique to *P. falciparum*. **D,** Ameboid trophozoite characteristic of *P. vivax*. Both *P. vivax*– and *P. ovale*–infected erythrocytes exhibit Schuffner's dots and tend to be enlarged compared with noninfected erythrocytes. **E,** *P. vivax* schizont. Mature *P. falciparum* parasites, by contrast, are rarely seen on blood smears because they sequester in the systemic microvasculature. **F,** *P. vivax* spherical gametocyte. **G,** *P. ovale* trophozoite. Note Schuffner's dots and ovoid shape of the infected erythrocyte. **H,** Characteristic band form trophozoite of *P. malariae*, containing intracellular pigment hemazoin. *(Images A, B, and F were kindly provided by DPDx [CDC's website for parasitology identification] at www.dpd.cdc.gov/dpdx/. Images C, D, E, G, and H were contributed by David Wyler, Newton, Massachusetts.)*

Chloroquine-resistant *P. falciparum* parasites reduce the amount of drug that accumulates in their digestive vacuoles.[329] The mechanism involves mutations in a conserved transport molecule of the digestive vacuole membrane termed PfCRT (*P. falciparum* chloroquine resistance transporter).[330-332] The mutations include a key change from lysine to threonine in the 76th amino acid (K76T) plus additional mutations that depend on their geographic origin.[330,333-335] Drug selection for mutant PfCRT is evident in the association of the K76T marker with increased plasma chloroquine levels[336] and with treatment failures in children receiving the drug.[337] Several lines of evidence now indicate that chloroquine resistance involves a specific interaction between chloroquine and the modified form of PfCRT[331] that promotes drug efflux from the digestive vacuole.[338-340]

While PfCRT is the central determinant of chloroquine resistance, other host and parasite factors also influence treatment outcomes. For example, clearance of phenotypically chloroquine-resistant parasites can occur after chloroquine treatment and becomes increasingly prevalent in children as they grow older, presumably owing to the immunity that develops from repeated episodes of malaria.[337,341] Parasite transport molecules in addition to PfCRT have also been proposed to modulate or contribute to the ability of chloroquine-resistant parasites to cope with the drug.[342,343]

SULFADOXINE-PYRIMETHAMINE

Dihydropteroate synthase (DHPS) and dihydrofolate reductase (DHFR) are sequentially involved in the folate pathway of nucleic acid synthesis. Pyrimethamine inhibits parasite DHFR and the production of tetrahydrofolate, an essential cofactor for one-carbon metabolism required for the synthesis of nucleic acids and certain amino acids. Point mutations in DHFR reduce its affinity for pyrimethamine. The substitution of asparagine for serine at position 108 in DHFR is critical for the initial development of pyrimethamine resistance, with additional mutations (Ile51, Arg59, Leu164) increasing the degree of pyrimethamine resistance.[344,345] Part of sulfadoxine's action is thought to be inhibition of parasite DHPS and point mutations in DHPS reduce its affinity for sulfadoxine.[346,347] Analysis of the mutant *dhfr* and *dhps* alleles in field studies supports conclusions that clinically significant resistance to pyrimethamine arises from multiple mutations in *dhfr* and *dhps* and that *dhps* mutations are likely selected after mutations in *dhfr* are already present.[348]

ATOVAQUONE-PROGUANIL (MALARONE)

Atovaquone binds cytochrome *b* and inhibits parasite mitochondrial electron transport, leading to collapse of the mitochondrial membrane potential.[349,350] This effect is potentiated by proguanil.[351] The substitution of serine for tyrosine at codon 268 of the cytochrome *b* gene is associated with resistance to atovaquone and the AP combination.[319,320,352,353] Cycloguanil, the active metabolite of proguanil, inhibits DHFR.[354] Point mutations in *dhfr* confer resistance to cycloguanil.[315,316,355,356]

DOXYCYCLINE

Doxycycline inhibits protein synthesis elongation by preventing binding of aminoacyl-tRNA to the ribosome 30S subunit. Resistance of human malaria parasites to this drug has not been described.

MEFLOQUINE, QUINIDINE, AND QUININE

Mefloquine, quinidine, and quinine are thought to form complexes toxic to the parasite by binding to heme. Mefloquine resistance may be associated in part with increases in expression and mutations in the P-glycoprotein homolog-1 gene *pfmdr1*.[342,357] Decreased quinine sensitivity is associated with resistance to other structurally related drugs such as mefloquine and halofantrine, suggesting that drug resistance mechanisms may share various genetic determinants.[358-360] Some studies have implicated *pfmdr1* mutations in mefloquine, quinine, and halofantrine resistance and *pfcrt* mutations in quinine and quinidine responses.[342,361,331,332,362] The different levels of quinine susceptibility among parasites and the relatively slow rate at which quinine resistance has spread throughout the world indicate that quinine resistance is a complex phenotype and is probably affected by other genes in addition to *pfmdr1* and *pfcrt*. The results of a linkage analysis and surveys of parasites from Southeast Asia, Africa, and South America support a model in which multiple genes can combine in different ways to produce similar phenotypes of reduced quinine response.[343,362]

ARTEMISININ DERIVATIVES

Although high level resistance to the artemisinin derivatives has not been found with clinical samples, successful selection of rodent malaria parasite strains with reduced susceptibility[363,364] and reports of *P. falciparum* strains with prolonged clearance times in vivo[327] raise concerns that strains of human malaria parasites with significant clinical resistance may evolve and spread. No molecular mechanism to account for artemisinin resistance has been established. An S769N mutation in an ATPase enzyme (PfATPase 6) was proposed as a possible determinant of artemisinin resistance,[365] and one study associated elevated IC50s with this mutation in strains of *P. falciparum* from French Guiana,[366] but resistance has not been associated with this mutation in field isolates elsewhere[327] nor has the mutation been found in rodent malaria parasites selected for resistance.[363]

Clinical Presentation and Diagnosis of Malaria

The malaria incubation period after an infective mosquito bite includes the time required for the parasites to progress through liver schizogony and produce symptoms by their propagation in the bloodstream. For primary attacks, this period is typically about 8 to 25 days but may be much longer depending on the immune status of the infected person, the strain as well as the species of *Plasmodium*, the dose of sporozoites, and the possible effects of partially effective chemoprophylaxis. Relapses from latent hypnozoites may develop months or years after mosquito bites. Late-onset or recrudescent *P. falciparum* malaria may also occur in individuals who have suppressed parasitemia of drug-resistant parasites with chemoprophylactic drugs[367] (see Fig. 275-2). Febrile patients presenting within 7 days of entering an endemic area are unlikely to have malaria, unless there has been earlier exposure to infective mosquito bites. As a general rule, and because of the dangers of acute *P. falciparum* infection, all travelers who have visited a malaria-endemic area in the 3 months prior to onset of fever or other suggestive symptoms should be considered to have malaria until proven otherwise. Even in patients beyond this time frame, it is wise to consider *P. falciparum* malaria, as illustrated, for example, in the recent report of a symptomatic presentation in an 18-year-old patient with sickle cell disease 4 years after visiting an endemic area.[248] Latent attacks from the reactivation of *P. vivax* or *P. ovale* hypnozoites usually occur within 3 years and are rare more than 5 years after exposure. Recrudescence of *P. malariae* symptoms in individuals with subclinical parasitemia has been reported decades after initial infection.[170,368,369]

HISTORY AND PHYSICAL EXAMINATION

Uncomplicated malaria typically presents as an undifferentiated febrile illness.[370] A series of 160 German nationals or residents with imported malaria presented to a travel clinic with the following symptoms: fever, 100%; headache, 100%; weakness, 94%; profuse night sweats, 91%; insomnia, 69%; arthralgias, 59%; myalgias, 56%; diarrhea, 13%; and abdominal cramps, 8%.[371] The bloodstream parasites of *P. falciparum* infections are often asynchronous and may produce continuous fever. In other infections, fever may be cyclical, recurring every 48 or 72 hours, depending on the species and synchrony of the replicating parasites. Parasite subpopulations on different cycles in the blood-stream may produce complicated fever patterns. Patients with cyclical fevers may be relatively asymptomatic during afebrile periods.

Particular elements from the history and physical examination, when considered together, may be suggestive of the diagnosis of malaria.[372-374] Cyclical paroxysms of chills and rigors, fever, and drenching sweats are characteristic although not necessarily specific for malaria. A travel history that reveals risk of exposure months to years before in an endemic region is an alert for malaria and should always be sought in presentations of fever. Findings on physical examination may include pallor and hepatosplenomegaly. Rarely, acute *Plasmodium* infections present with splenic rupture requiring surgery or conservative management.[375,376] Findings such as jaundice, diminished consciousness, or convulsions indicate severe malaria (see later). Rash, lymphadenopathy, and signs of pulmonary consolidation are distinctly uncommon.

THICK AND THIN BLOOD SMEARS

Light microscopy of Giemsa-stained blood smears is the accepted standard for malaria diagnosis. Thick and thin diagnostic blood smears should be *prepared and read immediately by experienced personnel* when the clinical presentation and travel history are compatible with malaria.[377] Preparation instructions and representative images from thick and thin smears are available from DPDx, the CDC's website for parasitological diagnosis: *http://www.dpd.cdc.gov/dpdx/HTML/Malaria.htm.*

Thick smears concentrate red cell layers approximately 40-fold and are used to screen a relatively large amount of blood for the presence of parasites. Because red cells are lysed in the process of staining in the thick smear technique, parasites are visualized *outside* red cells (see Fig. 275-7A). Assuming an average white cell count of 8000 per microliter, parasitemias can be estimated from thick smears by counting the number of parasites until 200 white cells have also been counted. This count, when multiplied by 40, gives an indication of the number of parasites per microliter of blood. The parasitemia percentage can then be calculated by dividing the parasite density by 4,000,000 (the average number of erythrocytes/μL in blood), and multiplying by 100.

Parasite density can be associated with disease severity and must be monitored during and after treatment to ensure adequate resolution of infection. Detectable parasitemia may lag behind aches, fevers, and chills, sometimes for many days; contrariwise, individuals with no antimalarial immunity may have severe manifestations of malaria even though parasites are very difficult to detect on blood smear. A *P. falciparum* infection also may not be apparent on an initial blood smear if the parasites are predominantly mature erythrocytic forms (i.e., trophozoites and schizonts) and are sequestering in the microvasculature. Therefore, if the initial blood smear is negative and malaria remains possible, the smear should be repeated every 12 hours until a diagnosis of malaria is made or ruled out. Before reading a thick blood smear as negative, at least 200 to 500 fields should be examined at ×1000 with an oil immersion objective lens; some experts recommend examining a thick smear for 20 minutes. Blood smear–positive cases of malaria diagnosed in the United States should be reported to the CDC using the Malaria Case Surveillance Form provided at *http://www.cdc.gov/malaria/clinicians.htm#case.*

Giemsa-stained thin smears are prepared from a much smaller amount of blood than thick smears and are used to determine the *Plasmodium* species (see Figs. 275-7B to H). Speciation of malaria parasites has important implications for treatment. *P. falciparum* infections are characterized by thin delicate rings that may be positioned against the inner surface of the red cell membrane (so-called accolade forms) (see Fig. 275-7B), multiply-infected cells containing signet-ring forms (see Fig. 275-7B), *absence* of trophozoites and schizonts because they are sequestered in the microvasculature, and banana-shaped gametocytes (see Fig. 275-7C). *P. vivax* and *P. ovale* are characterized by relatively thicker rings, ameboid trophozoites (see

Fig. 275-7D), and schizonts (see Fig. 275-7E) in the peripheral blood, and spherically shaped gametocytes (see Fig. 275-7F). Red cell enlargement and Schuffner's dots (see Fig. 275-7D and G) are common features of *P. vivax* and *P. ovale,* but not *P. falciparum* or *P. malariae. P. malariae* can be distinguished by its band forms, if present (see Fig. 275-7H). On blood smear examination, ring forms of *P. knowlesi* are indistiguishable from those of *P. falciparum,* and mature forms and gametocytes are indistinguishable from those of *P. malariae.*[14,255,378] Thin smear examination can yield additional useful information such as the presence of intraleukocytic pigment (a poor prognostic sign)[379] or other blood pathogens (e.g., filaria, *B. recurrentis*). *Babesia* species produce intraerythrocytic forms that may be confused with *Plasmodium* species,[380] but experienced personnel are able to distinguish between them.

RAPID DIAGNOSTIC TESTS

While evaluation of Giemsa-stained thick and thin smears remains the accepted standard for malaria diagnosis, rapid diagnostic tests have become increasingly useful.[381-385] In situations in which expert microscopic examination is delayed or difficult to obtain, medical decisions and management of malaria cases can benefit greatly from the appropriate use of rapid tests. Two types of rapid tests based on different detection schemes are presently available and are becoming more frequently used.

The first type is based on the detection of *Plasmodium* histidine-rich protein 2 (HRP-2).[386] In 556 travelers returning to France with suspected malaria, an FDA-approved commercial test based on HRP-2 had 96% sensitivity and 99% specificity for *Plasmodium* infection when compared with microscopy.[387] In 32 U.S. marines returning from Liberia with febrile illness, this test had a 100% sensitivity and a 100% specificity for *P. falciparum* infection when compared with microscopy.[388] Although HRP-2 tests are highly sensitive and specific for malaria diagnosis, they have certain limitations. First, they are of limited use to monitor therapeutic responses, as the tests are persistently positive up to 28 days after treatment. Second, HRP-2–based detection is limited to *P. falciparum,* so other antigen detection schemes are required for *P. vivax, P. ovale,* and *P. malariae.* These are generally less sensitive than is HRP-2 detection for *P. falciparum,*[387,389] making them less useful for the diagnosis of malaria in returned travelers who typically are infected with *P. vivax* at least as often as with *P. falciparum.* Third, the sensitivity of rapid detection tests for *P. falciparum* and *P. vivax* infections drops at parasite densities of less than 100-1000/μL,[389] making them less useful for the diagnosis of malaria in nonimmune returned travelers who may experience symptoms of malaria at low parasite densities. The World Health Organization provides a list of Malaria Rapid Diagnostic Test manufacturers and distributors along with various product specifications and company information (*http://www.wpro.who.int/sites/rdt/documents*).

The second type of rapid diagnostic test is based on detection of *P. falciparum*–specific lactate dehydrogenase (LDH) and pan-*Plasmodium* LDH.[390] These tests detect *Plasmodium* infections with sensitivity and specificity comparable with those of HRP-2 tests. In 556 travelers returning to France with suspected malaria, a parasite LDH test had 80% sensitivity and 98% specificity for *Plasmodium* infection when compared with microscopy.[387] Presently, a parasite LDH test commonly detects *P. vivax, P. ovale,* and *P. malariae* with less sensitivity than *P. falciparum* relative to expert microscopy.[387,391,392] For example, only 3 out of 12 (25%) *P. ovale* infections tested positive in French peacekeepers returning from Cote d'Ivoire with malaria.[393] A parasite LDH rapid diagnostic test detects *P. falciparum* and *P. vivax* infections with lower sensitivity when parasite densities are less than 100-1000/μL.[394] An advantage to parasite LDH detection is that the signal is proportional to *P. falciparum* parasitemia,[395] allowing for monitoring of therapeutic responses. Although this test is commercially available worldwide, it is currently provided only for research purposes in the United States.

OTHER LABORATORY TESTS

The results of routine laboratory tests are not specific for malaria, but may support its diagnosis. Some degree of anemia may be seen with malaria from all *Plasmodium* species. Decreases in hemoglobin, hematocrit, and haptoglobin and increases in lactic dehydrogenase may be marked with large *P. falciparum* parasite burdens. Microcytosis may be seen in patients from malaria-endemic areas but is often due to iron deficiency or thalassemia. Leukocyte counts may be high, normal, or low.[396] Platelet counts may be normal or slightly low,[397] but have been observed to be <70,000/µL in *P. falciparum* infection[398] and occasionally in *P. vivax* infection.[399] Sodium may be slightly low, possibly owing to syndrome of inappropriate antidiuretic hormone, excessive vomiting, or urinary losses.[400] Acidemia (pH less than 7.35), acidosis (bicarbonate < 15 mmol/L), and lactate levels >5 mmol/L can be seen in severe *P. falciparum* malaria (see later). Some degree of renal impairment is common in falciparum malaria and may be associated with increased creatinine, proteinuria, and hemoglobinuria.[401] Serum glucose is often low in children with falciparum malaria, but it is commonly normal in adults. In children with severe falciparum malaria, bacteremia/sepsis may be present at the time of initial clinical evaluation and blood cultures may be positive.[402,403]

SEVERE *P. FALCIPARUM* MALARIA

The World Health Organization (WHO) has established clinical and laboratory criteria for severe falciparum malaria that must be treated as an emergency with intensive medical care.[404] By WHO criteria, severe malaria is established by any of the criteria in Table 275-1 in the presence of *P. falciparum* parasitemia and with reasonable exclusion of an alternative diagnosis. Although these WHO criteria are largely based on the clinical presentation of severe malaria among young African children living in endemic areas, they are consistent with the clinical spectrum of severe malaria in travelers who might be encountered in nonendemic developed countries.[405] Nonimmune individuals who do not meet these criteria for severe malaria should be treated initially with antimalarial drugs as if they have it. In practice, because of the ability of *P. falciparum* infection to progress in just a few hours to severe and life-threatening complications, it is advisable to hospitalize all nonimmune individuals during their initial period of treatment. If blood smears or rapid diagnostic tests are negative but severe malaria is strongly suspected, patients should be treated for severe malaria while repeated thick smears and tests for other possible diseases are pursued for a definitive diagnosis.

Cerebral malaria is a syndrome characterized by diminished consciousness and/or seizures. In endemic areas, it typically occurs in young children and can manifest clinically as varying levels of consciousness, obtundation or coma, or seizures. The Blantyre coma scale is frequently used to measure the level of consciousness in children.[406] Seizures may be clinically inapparent, subtle motor, partial motor, generalized tonic-clonic, or partial motor with secondary generalization.[407] Multiple factors can contribute to cerebral malaria: hypoglycemia, acidosis, hyperpyrexia, the post-ictal state, and effects of anticonvulsant medication. In endemic areas, there may also be considerable overlap in the clinical presentations of cerebral malaria and other syndromes such as bacterial or viral meningitis, subdural hematoma, or sepsis.[110] Although cerebral malaria commonly resolves without neurological sequelae,[408] some children (especially those with status epilepticus) may develop psychosis, cerebellar ataxia, extrapyramidal rigidity, hemiplegia, or long-term cognitive and language impairment.[409-413]

Respiratory distress is characterized by dyspnea or deep breathing (Kussmaul's respiration), which may be accompanied by nasal flaring or intercostal retraction. In one study, deep breathing was 91% sensitive and 83% specific for the presence of severe metabolic acidosis (base excess less than or equal to −12), the underlying cause of respiratory distress.[44] *Prostration* from fluid and electrolyte depletion is determined by clinical judgement. If a child is 7 months of age or older, prostration may be defined as inability to sit unassisted. *Hyperparasitemia* is defined in endemic areas by WHO as parasite density greater than or equal to 500,000/mm³ (~10% parasitemia) and is associated with severe anemia, hypoglycemia, cerebral malaria, and renal failure. Although severity of disease is generally thought to correlate with parasite density, nonimmune individuals may present with severe malaria at any parasitemia, even at levels that may be difficult to detect by microscopy. *Severe anemia* is defined in endemic areas as hemoglobin ≤5 g/dL. Nonimmune individuals can present with signs and symptoms of severe anemia at hemoglobin levels significantly higher than 5 g/dL because of dehydration; with fluid repletion, rapid reductions from baseline hemoglobin levels can aggravate the symptoms of severe anemia. *Hypoglycemia* is defined as blood glucose ≤40 mg/dL and may contribute to diminished consciousness and seizures. *Hyperbilirubinemia* (manifesting as icterus or jaundice) is also an indicator of severe malaria, and may reflect underlying liver compromise. *Renal insufficiency* of severe malaria is defined in endemic areas as anuria for at least 24 hours. However, an infected nonimmune patient with any evidence of renal insufficiency, even that caused by hypovolemia and improved with fluid replacement, should be considered to have severe malaria. *Hemoglobinuria* manifests as dark (cola) colored urine ("blackwater fever"), distinct from the red appearance of hematuria. *Shock* of malaria is clinically indistinguishable from that of sepsis caused by Gram-negative bacteria. Special caution needs to be taken in the evaluation of shock, as concurrent sepsis is frequently present with parasitemia in severe malaria. In addition to potentiating hypoglycemia, *cessation of eating and drinking* contributes to hypovolemia and consequently to severe acidosis and respiratory distress. *Repetitive vomiting* also contributes to hypovolemia and may complicate oral treatment of severe malaria in resource-poor countries where parenteral therapy is not readily available. Medications used to treat malaria (e.g., chloroquine) may also cause vomiting, often warranting directly observed therapy. *Hyperpyrexia* is defined as axillary temperature ≥40°C and likely contributes to the severity of malaria through its association with febrile seizures.

Distinguishing Malaria from Other Illnesses with Similar Clinical Presentations

The differential diagnosis of the malaria presentation is broad and includes many febrile and influenza-like illnesses (Table 275-2). However, malaria should always lead the list in the differential diagnosis of fever in travelers or immigrants who have been in an endemic area within the previous 3 months and remain in consideration for years afterwards. Travelers and immigrants often present with common ailments and physicians must be alert to recognize and treat malaria to avoid a morbid or fatal outcome,[414-417] especially when they are working in temperate zones and do not often see malaria and other

TABLE 275-1	Diagnostic Features of Severe Malaria

Cerebral malaria (diminished consciousness, seizures)
Respiratory distress
Prostration
Hyperparasitemia
Severe anemia
Hypoglycemia
Jaundice/icterus
Renal insufficiency
Hemoglobinuria
Shock
Cessation of eating and drinking
Repetitive vomiting
Hyperpyrexia

TABLE 275-2	Differential Diagnosis of the Malaria Presentation: Selected Examples

Influenza
Enteric fever
Bacteremia/sepsis
Classic dengue fever
Acute schistosomiasis (Katayama fever)
Leptospirosis
African tick fever
East African trypanosomiasis (sleeping sickness)
Yellow fever

diseases of the tropics. It is estimated that 30 million travelers visit malaria-endemic regions each year. Cases of malaria acquired by international travelers probably number 25,000 annually, of which 10,000 are reported and 150 are fatal.[418]

Clinical criteria to distinguish malaria from other illnesses are critical because rapid diagnostic tests for those illnesses are often limited or not available, and definitive diagnoses often require non-routine methods of pathogen isolation or serological testing that rely on comparisons of acute and convalescent antibody titers 2 to 4 weeks later. The probabilities of specific diseases are affected by geographic area visited (e.g., yellow fever is not prevalent in Asia or India); type of travel (e.g., adventure travelers to Lake Malawi are more likely to acquire schistosomiasis or leptospirosis from fresh water contact than are visitors to Nairobi, Kenya); time of travel (e.g., dengue fever is much less likely to be acquired during the dry season, when mosquito transmission is markedly reduced); type of food and water ingested (e.g., enteric fever is relatively unlikely in persons eating only cooked food and bottled water); and vaccination history (e.g., the efficacy of yellow fever, hepatitis A and B vaccines makes these diseases unlikely if the patient is vaccinated). Self-reported compliance with mosquito repellents and malaria chemoprophylactic drugs, especially during the post-travel period should *not* be used to rule out malaria, as these reports are often inaccurate and no preventive regimen is 100% effective. Features of selected infectious diseases that may present like malaria are briefly summarized in the following paragraphs.

INFLUENZA

Like malaria, influenza may present with fever, headache, myalgias, and malaise. Prominent upper respiratory symptoms (rhinorrhea, sore throat, or dry cough) may help to distinguish influenza from malaria. The symptoms of many cases of malaria ultimately fatal to returned travelers in North America have been initially and mistakenly attributed to influenza.

ENTERIC FEVER

Salmonella typhi and *S. paratyphi* can be acquired in developing countries worldwide. Like malaria, enteric fever may present with fever, headache, nausea, malaise, anorexia, and myalgias. Prominent gastrointestinal symptoms (abdominal pain, constipation, or diarrhea), the findings of rose spots or relative bradycardia, and a history of unsanitary food or water consumption may help to support a diagnosis of enteric fever. A history of prior vaccination against *S. typhi* may not be useful in ruling out enteric fever because it is only 50% to 80% effective and does not protect against paratyphoidal illness.

BACTEREMIA/SEPSIS

The fever, hypotension, evidence of poor peripheral perfusion, altered mental status, and multiorgan dysfunction that characterizes bacteremia and sepsis can mimic severe malaria. One study found that bacteremia accompanied *P. falciparum* infection in 12% of young children who were admitted to hospital with the primary diagnosis of severe malaria.[312]

DENGUE FEVER

Patients with classic nonhemorrhagic dengue fever may present with fever, headache, nausea, malaise, or anorexia. Myalgias tend to be much more severe than those experienced during malaria episodes. Dengue fever may be distinguished from malaria by its centrifugal rash, petechiae, lymphadenopathy, conjunctival injection, pharyngeal erythema, and relative bradycardia. Although dengue virus is also transmitted by mosquitoes during the rainy season in tropical regions worldwide, its incubation period of 4 to 7 days is not at all typical of malaria.

ACUTE SCHISTOSOMIASIS (KATAYAMA FEVER)

Schistosoma trematodes are acquired from fresh water exposure (wading, swimming) in tropical regions worldwide. Patients with acute schistosomiasis may present 4 to 8 weeks after exposure with fever, headache, myalgias, malaise, and anorexia. Acute schistosomiasis can be distinguished from malaria by generalized urticaria and the findings of a pruritic rash at the site of cercarial penetration (usually on the legs), lymphadenopathy, and blood eosinophilia. Patients may present initially with focal neurologic signs as a result of egg dissemination to the central nervous system.

LEPTOSPIROSIS

Leptospira interrogans spirochetes are acquired from fresh water or soil exposure in tropical and temperate regions worldwide. Patients with leptospirosis usually present within 7 to 12 days of exposure with fever, headache, nausea, and myalgias. Leptospirosis can be distinguished from malaria by the findings of conjunctival suffusion or rash, but may progress to hepatic and renal insufficiency marked by hemorrhagic manifestations and pronounced hyperbilirubinemia (Weil's disease). This complication is similar to the severe malaria presentation, but extremely high bilirubin levels are more characteristic of Weil's disease.

AFRICAN TICK FEVER

Rickettsia africae is transmitted by tick bites, usually acquired during game hunting or safari travel to southern Africa between April and November. African tick fever may present with fever, headache, and myalgias, and can be differentiated from malaria by the findings of lymphadenitis or multiple inoculation eschars.

EAST AFRICAN TRYPANOSOMIASIS (SLEEPING SICKNESS)

Trypanosoma brucei rhodesiense causes the acute form of African sleeping sickness and is acquired from tsetse fly bites, typically in association with game and brush in eastern and southern Africa. Trypanosomiasis may present with fever, headache, myalgias, malaise, and anorexia, yet it may be differentiated from malaria by a red chancre at the bite site, posterior cervical lymphadenopathy, or rash. Like malaria, it may progress to involve multiple organs, including the central nervous system.

YELLOW FEVER

Yellow fever virus is acquired from mosquito bites in tropical regions worldwide. It is characterized by fever, headache, myalgias, nausea, anorexia, and jaundice. Yellow fever may be differentiated from malaria by the presence of conjunctival suffusion or relative bradycardia, and by its short incubation period (average 3 to 6 days). Yellow fever is extremely unlikely in patients who have been vaccinated against it within the previous 10 years. As with severe malaria, patients may appear acutely ill and progress to liver failure and hemorrhagic manifestations, multiorgan system failure, and death.

◼ Treatment (see also Ch. 44)

GENERAL PRINCIPLES

P. falciparum malaria can be fatal if not diagnosed and treated promptly and appropriately. This is especially true of nonimmune travelers returning from visits to malaria-endemic areas. Malaria is a disease of protean manifestations.[419] Its diagnosis can be delayed by the nonspecificity of the clinical presentation and routine laboratory tests, especially if blood smears (and, if available, a rapid detection test) are not examined. Life-threatening manifestations of malaria such as seizures, hypoglycemia, and pulmonary edema may develop rapidly in patients who appear relatively well at presentation or appear to respond initially to antimalarial drugs.

Although some patients with uncomplicated *P. falciparum* malaria can be treated successfully in an outpatient setting, patients with no immunity against the disease are at increased risk for sudden development of severe complications and should be hospitalized at least 48 hours to ensure adequate response to therapy, regardless of how well they appear at presentation. Hospitalization is likewise recommended for individuals from malaria-endemic countries but whose immune status nevertheless cannot be known with certainty.[420] Acute *P. falciparum* malaria in a nonimmune individual is always highly dangerous and unpredictable; even without adverse signs at presentation, a patient's condition may deteriorate dramatically after prompt hospitalization and apparently adequate treatment.[420] Contributing factors in such cases may include (1) replication of the parasites and their synchronous development into mature forms that sequester in the brain, leading to cerebral malaria, and (2) complications from the infection that lead to acute renal failure, lung injury, or hepatic insufficiency, even when the parasitemia is decreasing or the patient appears to be improving in other ways. Pregnant women, young children, and the elderly are at increased risk of morbidity and mortality and should be hospitalized regardless of their clinical state.[421-424]

Patients with *P. vivax*, *P. ovale*, or *P. malariae* malaria infrequently require hospitalization, though it is certainly necessary in cases with severe manifestations.[41,42,425] Patients with *P. knowlesi* malaria may require hospitalization as life-threatening manifestations of disease can develop rapidly.[15] Health care providers are encouraged to share their clinical experience with malaria patients by contacting the CDC at *nciddpdmalaria@cdc.gov*.

UNCOMPLICATED MALARIA

Treatment of falciparum malaria should always be initiated emergently, as the risk of its morbidity and mortality is increased with even short delays in medical care.[426] Uncomplicated malaria can be treated with oral medication as long as the patient is able to retain the drug; directly observed therapy may be appropriate in some cases to ensure adequate treatment. Drugs currently recommended for the treatment of uncomplicated malaria are listed in Table 275-3. Important adjunct treatment of malaria includes antipyretic, antiemetic, and anticonvulsant medications.

Because of the widespread patterns of drug resistance in the world today, no blanket recommendation suffices and alternatives must be considered when selecting an antimalarial drug. Chloroquine can be used to treat malaria acquired from those areas where chloroquine resistance has not been reported (Central America west of the Panama Canal, the Dominican Republic, and most regions of the Middle East). Chloroquine can also be used to treat *P. knowlesi* malaria acquired from Southeast Asia. Oral quinine *plus* doxycycline can be used for disease acquired in all areas and is particularly useful where chloroquine-resistant *P. falciparum* or *P. vivax* strains are present or where mefloquine-resistant *P. falciparum* strains are present (Thailand, Myanmar, Cambodia, and Vietnam). Atovaquone-proguanil (AP) is being used increasingly in the treatment of uncomplicated malaria, including in nonimmune individuals[427,428] although recrudes-

cence of parasitemia and failure of initial therapy with AP continue to be reported.[319-321,352,353,429]

If a patient cannot tolerate oral therapy, parenteral formulations of antimalarial drugs must be administered (see later). Up-to-date information on malaria treatment is available from the CDC's Malaria Hotline (770-488-7788, Monday-Friday, 8:00 AM-4:30 PM EST; 770-488-7100, after hours, weekends, holidays). Current guidelines for the treatment of malaria in the United States are also available at *http://www.cdc.gov/malaria/diagnosis_treatment/tx_clinicians.htm*.

CHLOROQUINE PHOSPHATE

Chloroquine is considered safe in pregnant women (all trimesters) and in children of all ages, including newborns.[430] It has a bitter taste and may cause nausea or vomiting (it can be taken with food to ameliorate gastrointestinal symptoms), headache, dizziness, blurred vision, or dysphoria. Chloroquine commonly produces a nonallergic pruritus in dark-skinned persons and may exacerbate psoriasis. It is associated with retinal toxicity at high doses taken chronically but not at doses used for malaria treatment. Acute chloroquine toxicity can produce convulsions, hypotension and shock, and cardiorespiratory arrest[431] and has also been reported to produce a psychosis resembling PCP psychosis.[432]

QUININE *PLUS* DOXYCYCLINE

The combination of quinine *plus* doxycycline is effective against multidrug-resistant parasites. Quinine has a bitter taste and may cause gastrointestinal upset and cinchonism (nausea, vomiting, dysphoria, tinnitus, and high-tone deafness). Hypoglycemia from quinine-induced insulin secretion can be an adverse event, particularly in pregnancy[431,433] and acute pulmonary edema has been reported in association with its use.[434] Doxycycline also causes gastrointestinal upset and commonly results in vaginal candidiasis, requiring concomitant use of antifungal suppositories. The requirement for multiple doses over 7 days and the gastrointestinal upset caused by both drugs may reduce the compliance and hence effectiveness of this regimen.[435] The use of all tetracyclines is contraindicated in children younger than 8 years old or in pregnant women because of adverse effects on tooth and bone development. In these cases, clindamycin may be a safe and effective substitute for doxycycline.[436-438]

MEFLOQUINE

Mefloquine can be used to treat most chloroquine-resistant parasites except for strains in areas such as Thailand, Myanmar, Cambodia, and Vietnam where resistance against this drug is present.[439,440] It may cause gastrointestinal upset, vomiting, dysphoria, dreams, mood changes, and neuropsychiatric reactions in a significant proportion of patients,[441-443] although there is no evidence for increased first-time diagnosis of depression with mefloquine relative to other commonly used antimalarials.[444] Mefloquine is cleared slowly as its elimination half-life is 2 to 3 weeks. Mefloquine may prolong the corrected QT interval and so it cannot be administered concurrently with quinine-like drugs (e.g., quinidine, quinine, halofantrine). Mefloquine should be used only with extreme caution or not at all in individuals with cardiac conduction diseases, as it can aggravate conduction abnormalities.

ATOVAQUONE-PROGUANIL (MALARONE, AP)

AP is used to treat multidrug-resistant parasites,[297,322,445] is well tolerated,[439,446] and has only rarely been associated with severe adverse reactions.[447,448] AP resistance is rare, being confined to a few case reports in nonimmune individuals in whom both recrudescence and initial treatment failure have been documented.[319,321,429,449]

TABLE 275-3	Malaria Treatment			
Drug	*Adult Dose*	*Pediatric Dose*******		*Precautions*
Uncomplicated malaria: *P. vivax, P. ovale, P. malariae, P. knowlesi*, or chloroquine-susceptible *P. falciparum*				
Chloroquine phosphate				
Supplied in 300-mg base (500-mg salt) tablets.	600 mg base (1000 mg salt), then 300 mg base (500 mg salt) at 6, 24, and 48 hours.	10 mg base/kg (max. 600 mg base), then 5 mg base/kg at 6, 24, and 48 hours.		None.
Uncomplicated malaria: chloroquine-resistant *P. falciparum* or chloroquine-resistant *P. vivax*				
Mefloquine%				
Supplied in 250-mg salt (228-mg base) tablets.	750 mg salt, followed by 500 mg 6-12 hours later.	<45 kg: 15 mg salt/kg, followed by 10 mg salt/kg 6-12 hours later.		Do not administer to individuals with cardiac conduction abnormalities, history of seizures, or serious psychiatric illnesses (e.g., psychosis, major depression). Do not use concomitantly with quinidine, quinine, or halofantrine.
Quinine sulfate *plus* doxycycline				
Quinine sulfate supplied in 325-mg salt tablets. Doxycycline supplied in 100-mg tablets.	Quinine 650 mg salt every 8 hours for 3 days* plus doxycycline 100 mg twice daily for 7 days.	Children 8-12 years old: Quinine 10 mg salt/kg every 8 hours for 3 days* plus doxycycline 2 mg/kg every 12 hours for 7 days. Children <8 years old: Quinine 10 mg salt/kg every 8 hours for 7 days.		Do not use doxycycline in children below the age of 8 years or in pregnant women.†
Atovaquone-proguanil (Malarone)				
Supplied in fixed-dose combination tablets containing 250 mg atovaquone and 100 mg proguanil (adult tablets) or 62.5 mg atovaquone and 25 mg proguanil (pediatric tablets).	Four adult tablets daily for 3 days (may be administered as 2 tablets twice daily).§	The number of *pediatric* or *adult* tablets taken daily for 3 days depends on patient's weight: 5-8 kg (2 pediatric tabs), 9-10 kg (3 pediatric tabs), 11-20 kg (1 adult tab), 21-30 kg (2 adult tabs), 31-40 kg (3 adult tabs), >40 kg (4 adult tabs).‡		Not recommended for chloroquine-resistant *P. vivax* due to inadequate efficacy data. Safety in pregnant or breastfeeding women is not established.
Artemether *plus* lumefantrine**				
Supplied in fixed-combination tablets containing 20 mg artemether and 120 mg lumefantrine.	6-dose regimen: 1st day: 4 tabs initially, then 4 tabs 8 hours later, 2nd day: 4 tabs twice daily, 3rd day: 4 tabs twice daily.	The number of tablets per dose taken according to adult time schedule depends on patient's weight: 5-14 kg (1 tab) 15-24 kg (2 tabs) 25-34 kg (3 tabs) ≥35 kg or ≥12 years of age (4 tabs).		Safety in pregnant or breastfeeding women is not established.
Severe *P. falciparum* malaria (or severe *P. knowlesi* malaria)				
Quinidine gluconate				
	Intravenous: 10 mg salt/kg loading dose (max. 600 mg) in normal saline infused slowly at a constant rate over 1-2 hours, followed by continuous infusion of 0.02 mg salt/kg/min for at least 24 hours and then until parasitemia <1% and oral therapy can be started.§	Intravenous: same dosing as for adult.		Do not administer as a bolus. Check blood glucose every 4-6 hours during first 24 hours of therapy. Administer 5%-10% dextrose along with quinidine to reduce risk of hypoglycemia. Monitor levels to keep between 3-8 μg/mL.
Artesunate				
Available in the United States from the CDC through an IND protocol.	Intravenous: artesunate 2.4 mg/kg, then 2.4 mg/kg at 12, 24, and 48 hours.¶	Intravenous: artesunate 2.4 mg/kg, then 2.4 mg/kg at 12, 24, and 48 hours.¶		None.
Quinine dihydrochloride				
Not available in the United States.	Intravenous: 20 mg/kg loading dose in 5% dextrose infused slowly at a constant rate over 4 hours, followed by maintenance dose 10 mg/kg over 3-4 hours at 8-hour intervals (max. 1800 mg/d) until oral therapy can be started.	Intravenous: 20 mg/kg loading dose in 5% dextrose infused slowly at a constant rate over 4 hours, followed by maintenance dose 10 mg/kg over 3-4 hours at 8-hour intervals (max. 1800 mg/d) until oral therapy can be started.		Do not administer as a bolus. Check blood glucose every 4-6 hours during first 24 hours of therapy. Administer 5%-10% dextrose along with quinine to reduce risk of hypoglycemia.
Artemether				
Not available in the United States.	Intramuscular: artemether 3.2 mg/kg on first day, then 1.6 mg/kg daily for 4 days.¶	Intramuscular: artemether 3.2 mg/kg on first day, then 1.6 mg/kg daily for 4 days.¶		None.
Prevention (terminal prophylaxis) of relapsing malaria: *P. vivax* or *P. ovale*				
Primaquine phosphate				
Supplied in 15-mg base (26.3-mg salt) tablets.	30 mg base once daily for 14 days after departure from malaria-endemic area.	0.5 mg base/kg daily for 14 days (max. 30 mg base/day) after departure from malaria-endemic area.		Test patient for G6PD deficiency and administer only if enzyme activity is normal.^^ Do not administer to pregnant women.***

%Mefloquine is recommended only if quinine *plus* doxycycline or atovaquone-proguanil cannot be used, due to the higher rates of neuropsychiatric reactions at treatment doses.
*For infections acquired in Southeast Asia, where reduced susceptibility to quinine has been reported, treat with quinine for 7 days.
†Doxycycline may be substituted by clindamycin 5 mg/kg (oral) every 8 hours for 7 days.
‡This regimen can also serve as presumptive self-treatment in travelers with febrile illness who do not have immediate access to medical care. This regimen is not recommended for self-treatment of individuals on atovaquone-proguanil prophylaxis.
§Complete therapy with quinine *plus* doxycycline regimen to complete a 7-day total course of therapy. In patients less than 8 years old, substitute clindamycin for doxycycline.
¶To prevent parasite recrudescence after artesunate treatment, complete therapy with a standard dose of atovaquone-proguanil, mefloquine, doxycycline, or clindamycin, given orally.
**In 2009, a formulation of artemether-lumefantrine received U.S. Food and Drug Administration approval.
***Pregnant women requiring terminal prophylaxis should receive chloroquine 300 mg base (500 mg salt) weekly until birth, and then primaquine after delivery if G6PD activity is normal.
****Pediatric doses should *never* exceed the recommended adult dose.
^^If G6PD activity is borderline, or as an alternative, administer primaquine 45 mg base weekly for 8 consecutive weeks. If G6PD activity is deficient, contact the CDC or an infectious diseases/tropical medicine specialist for advice.
Drug regimens adapted from: Advice for Travelers. *The Medical Letter.* April 15, 2002;1128;38-39; and Guidelines for Treatment of Malaria in the United States available at *http://www.cdc.gov/malaria/diagnosis_treatment/tx_clinicians.htm.*

ARTEMISININ COMBINATION THERAPY

Artemisinin and its derivatives (artesunate, artemether, dihydroartemisinin) are now commonly used in Africa and Southeast Asia for the treatment of uncomplicated malaria, including that caused by multidrug-resistant *P. falciparum*.[450] Parasite recrudescence weeks after therapy with artemisinins does occur, often the elimination of these drugs and recovery of parasitemia without selection of mutant parasites that are truly drug-resistant.[451] The addition of a partner drug (e.g., chloroquine, sulfadoxine-pyrimethamine, or mefloquine) to a 3-day course of an artemisinin derivative was shown in a meta-analysis to substantially reduce treatment failure and recrudescence.[452] For this reason and to reduce the risk that clinically significant resistance to artemisinin derivatives will emerge, the World Health Organization recommends use of artemisinin derivatives only in combination with partner drugs (i.e., artemisinin-based combination therapy; ACT).

Patterns of resistance to partner drugs determine which ACT should be used in particular geographic locations. Due to widespread resistance to chloroquine, ACT regimens that contain sulfadoxine-pyrimethamine, lumefantrine, or amodiaquine are used in Africa. Due to declining efficacy of mefloquine along the Thailand-Cambodia border,[429] artemisinin *plus* piperaquine is increasingly being recommended for use in Southeast Asia.[453-455] Artemether *plus* lumefantrine is now approved for use as a fixed-dose combination in the United States.

SELF-TREATMENT OF UNCOMPLICATED MALARIA IN TRAVELERS

Because treatment delay increases morbidity and mortality associated with malaria, travelers to isolated areas may benefit from standby therapy while they actively seek medical care.[456] Standby antimalarials in some cases might be advised to travelers for emergency self-treatment of fever or flu-like symptoms that occur at least 1 week after entering a malaria-endemic area. Drugs used for this purpose such as chloroquine, quinine *plus* doxycycline, atovaquone-proguanil, or mefloquine should be selected based on the resistance pattern of the area visited. Although self-treatment by travelers can be safe, effective, and potentially life-saving, no regimen is currently registered for this use in any country. No randomized controlled clinical trials have been or are likely to be performed owing to the high morbidity and mortality of untreated or inappropriately treated malaria in nonimmune individuals. Travelers should be discouraged from self-treatment using locally acquired products which may be of poor quality or outright fake.[457-460]

INTERMITTENT PRESUMPTIVE TREATMENT IN INFANTS AND PREGNANT WOMEN

In areas with intense transmission, infants 6 to 12 months of age suffer multiple episodes of malaria and are therefore at risk for life-threatening severe anemia.[461-463] Weekly chemoprophylaxis of infants protects against malarial fevers as well as anemia, but may compromise development of natural immunity.[464,465] Intermittent presumptive treatment (e.g., amodiaquine every 2 months for a total of 6 months; also known as intermittent preventative treatment) of infants can reduce malaria morbidity by 50% to 65% during the first year of life while still allowing sufficient exposure to parasites and development of immunity.[466,467] In areas of endemic transmission, malaria of pregnancy is associated with severe maternal anemia and low birth weight in newborns. Intermittent presumptive treatment has been shown to reduce the risk of severe anemia in women who received one to three doses of SP over the duration of their first pregnancy.[468]

SEVERE MALARIA

Successful treatment of patients with severe malaria requires frequent clinical monitoring and intensive nursing care and may demand sophisticated interventions such as continuous EKG or hemodynamic monitoring, mechanical ventilation, or hemodialysis. Replacement of blood and fluids may lead to rapid reductions in lactate, resolution of metabolic acidosis, improvement in renal function, and clinical improvement of critically ill patients.[469]

Quinidine gluconate is the only approved parenteral treatment for severe malaria in the United States, on the recommendation of the CDC in recognition of the impracticality of stocking quinine throughout the country.[470,471] However, hospital pharmacies may not carry quinidine on formulary and may not know how to obtain it readily from regional distributors. When the need for quinidine is more acute than can be met by the local or regional distributor, Eli Lilly Company (800-821-0538, Monday-Friday, 7:30 AM-4:15 PM EST; 317-276-2000, after hours, weekends, holidays) can arrange a rapid shipment of the drug. Assistance with the management of patients with severe malaria including the availability and use of quinidine can be obtained by contacting the CDC Malaria Hotline (770-488-7788, Monday-Friday, 8:00 AM-4:30 PM EST; 770-488-7100, after hours, weekends, holidays).

Outside the United States, artemisinin derivatives and quinine are widely used to treat severe malaria. In the United States, intravenous formulations of an artemisinin derivative are available from the CDC through an investigational new drug (IND) protocol (see later). In Canada, intravenous formulations of quinine are available through the Canadian Malaria Network, *http://www.hc-sc.gc.ca/pphb-dgspsp/tmp-pmv/quinine/pdf/quinine-cmn_e.pdf*. Antimalarial drug regimens used to treat severe malaria are presented in Table 275-3.

QUINIDINE GLUCONATE

Many physicians will be unfamiliar with quinidine as this drug has been largely supplanted with newer antiarrythmic agents. Quinidine has a narrow therapeutic window and must be used with extreme care in an intensive care unit.[470] Its use in consultation with a cardiologist or a physician with experience in treating malaria is advised. It is administered intravenously as an infusion until the patient improves clinically and can complete antimalarial treatment with oral medication. Quinidine levels should be monitored throughout the period of its administration (see Table 275-3). Quinidine is *never* administered as a bolus injection, which can lead to fatal hypotension. Potentially fatal adverse reactions can occur even at treatment doses. It can cause postural hypotension, so frequent blood pressure measurements should be made. Quinidine may cause prolongation of the corrected QT interval, putting the patient at risk for ventricular tachycardias (e.g., torsades de pointes), and should be administered with continuous ECG monitoring.[472] If QTc prolongation greater than 25% of baseline or hypotension unresponsive to fluid challenge develops, the infusion rate should be reduced or the infusion stopped. Since quinidine may cause hyperinsulinemic hypoglycemia, serum glucose must be monitored every 4 to 6 hours and with any acute neurological change (e.g., diminished consciousness, convulsions) that may arise from severe hypoglycemia. Administering 5% or 10% dextrose while infusing quinidine can reduce the incidence of hypoglycemia.

In patients taking medications that also prolong the QT interval, particularly when coadministered with drugs that suppress hepatic metabolism, the use of quinidine can be problematic. Although the initial loading dose of quinidine is not reduced in renal insufficiency, patients with malaria and acute renal failure may not clear quinidine effectively. Case reports illustrating the use of quinidine in the treatment of severe malaria have highlighted common clinical scenarios such as adjustment of infusion rates associated with elevated quinidine blood levels, prolonged QTc intervals, and arrhythmias as well as hypoglycemia, hypotension, and vomiting.[472] Quinidine levels should be maintained below 8 µg/mL, which may require reducing the dose by 30% to 50% to prevent drug accumulation in patients who remain seriously ill after 3 days of treatment. The response to quinidine is assessed by frequent blood smears every 6 to 8 hours to ensure rapid decrease in parasitemia. Once the patient improves and can take oral medications without vomiting, quinidine can be discontinued and a 7-day total course of treatment completed with a combination of quinine tablets and doxycycline.

ARTEMISININ DERIVATIVES

Artemisinin derivatives (artesunate, artemether, dihydroartemisinin) are derived from *Artemisia annua* (qing hao), an herbal plant used in China for millennia as therapy for fevers.[473] Artemisinin derivatives are consistently effective against multidrug-resistant parasites and result in rapid clearance of parasites and clinical improvement usually within 24 to 36 hours. They are well tolerated and safe in adults, children, and pregnant women.[474-476] Several million people have taken artemisinins to date with no significant adverse or treatment-limiting effects being reported.[477] Although neurotoxicity can occur with supraphysiologic doses in animals, it has not been documented in humans.[478] A review of 23 trials available in the Cochrane library found artemisinins were at least as effective as quinine for the treatment of severe malaria.[479]

In June 2007, the Walter Reed Army Institute for Research (WRAIR) and the CDC received FDA-approval for a collaborative IND protocol: "Intravenous Artesunate for Treatment of Severe Malaria in the United States." Artesunate is provided by the CDC to hospitals upon request and on an emergency basis to treat malaria patients who need IV treatment because of severe disease, who have high parasitemias, who are not able to take oral medications, who do not tolerate quinidine, who may have an adverse reaction to quinidine, or in those whom quinidine treatment has proven ineffective. To enroll a patient with severe malaria into this IND protocol, contact the CDC Malaria Hotline (770-488-7788, Monday-Friday, 8:00 AM-4:30 PM EST; 770-488-7100, after hours, weekends, holidays).

QUININE DIHYDROCHLORIDE

Quinine is the only readily available drug in some endemic areas for the parenteral treatment of patients with severe chloroquine-resistant malaria or patients with chloroquine-resistant uncomplicated malaria who cannot take oral medication because of vomiting. Quinine commonly causes hypoglycemia and the unpleasant side effects of cinchonism. Administration of quinine in a glucose infusion and frequent (every 4 to 6 hours) glucose checks help to avoid hypoglycemia, which in some cases can be life threatening. Quinine is much less cardiotoxic than quinidine, requiring no continuous ECG monitoring during its administration. IV formulations of quinine are not commercially available in the United States, nor can they be obtained from the CDC on an emergency basis.

SEPSIS IN SEVERE MALARIA

Broad-spectrum antibiotics should be administered while awaiting blood culture results to patients who present with a clinical picture consistent with sepsis syndrome. Bacteremia complicating severe malaria is not uncommon in infants and children and may cause any patient's clinical status to deteriorate abruptly.[402]

EXCHANGE TRANSFUSION IN SEVERE MALARIA

High parasitemias have been correlated with mortality in falciparum malaria, leading to the use of exchange transfusion (ET) as an adjunct therapeutic measure. ET may reduce parasite load, remove toxic substances, reduce microcirculatory sludging, and rapidly correct anemia. Although small case series claim beneficial effects of ET (including partial ET in young children),[480-484] a meta-analysis concluded that a randomized controlled trial is necessary to determine whether ET is

beneficial.[485] ET may be harmful and is associated with fluid overload, risk of transfusion reactions and related infections, and line sepsis. In addition, ET does not remove infected erythrocytes that are sequestered in deep tissue capillary beds, including those in the brain, and achieves only modest reductions in parasitemia.

NONFALCIPARUM MALARIA

All cases of malaria should be treated as falciparum malaria until proven otherwise because *P. falciparum* infections can rapidly become life-threatening. Infections with *P. vivax*, *P. ovale*, and *P. malariae* are treated with chloroquine, unless (1) they are acquired in geographic regions where these species are known or suspected to be chloroquine-resistant (Oceania and parts of Southeast Asia), or (2) any doubt exists as to the parasite species or if there is a mixed infection. Mixed infections consisting of two or more *Plasmodium* species may sometimes mask a *P. falciparum* subpopulation that can emerge during or after treatment. Non-falciparum infections likely to be chloroquine-resistant are treated with mefloquine or quinine *plus* doxycycline at doses listed in Table 275-3. The CDC does not recommend atovaquone-proguanil against nonfalciparum malaria due to insufficient evidence for its efficacy in treating *P. vivax* malaria. Infections with *P. knowlesi* can be treated with chloroquine unless severe manifestations are present, in which case parenteral treatment with quinine or an artemisinin derivative would be indicated.

Persistent liver stages (hypnozoites) of *P. vivax* and *P. ovale* may be treated with primaquine (see Table 275-3)[486-489] if there is no contraindication, but this treatment frequently fails due to noncompliance with the recommended 14-day regimen. After blood stage *P. vivax* and *P. ovale* infections are treated with chloroquine (a drug not effective against hypnozoites), primaquine is administered to prevent relapse. Taking primaquine with food ameliorates gastrointestinal side effects and improves compliance. Patients should be advised to discontinue the drug and seek medical evaluation if their urine becomes dark, as primaquine occasionally can cause some hemolysis in persons with mildly deficient or even normal G6PD activity. Primaquine causes methemoglobinemia in nearly all persons treated, but this is rarely clinically significant (bluish discoloration of mucous membranes may be observed).

Primaquine is contraindicated in persons with severe forms of G6PD deficiency (e.g., Mediterranean type) or methemoglobin reductase deficiency because of the danger of massive and potentially fatal hemolysis. Persons with less severe forms of G6PD deficiency have been treated with standard primaquine doses, but significant decreases in hematocrit levels were observed in some cases.[488] In such individuals, weekly dosing of primaquine for longer periods has been recommended.[490,491] Primaquine should not be administered to pregnant women, owing to the risk of hemolytic disease in the fetus. Individuals who do not receive primaquine (including pregnant women) should be monitored for relapses, and if these occur, they should be treated with blood-stage antimalarials. Primaquine should be administered to individuals who reside permanently in areas endemic for *P. vivax* or *P. ovale*, even if reinfection is likely. Primaquine is not administered to individuals who acquire infection by transfusion or transplantation, as hypnozoites develop only from mosquito-inoculated sporozoites. Primaquine is under evaluation for primary prophylaxis of *P. falciparum* and *P. vivax* malaria in travelers who are not pregnant and have normal G6PD activity levels.[492,493]

Prevention

RISK ASSESSMENT

The risk of acquiring malaria varies according to the geographic region visited, the travel destination within geographic areas (e.g., urban versus rural setting), type of accommodations (e.g., camping tent versus air-conditioned hotel), duration of stay (e.g., a less than 1-week business trip versus a 3-month travel adventure), time of travel (high versus low transmission season), altitude of destination (less than 2000 meters versus higher), and efficacy of and adherence to malaria prophylaxis measures.[494] Immigrants returning home to visit friends and relatives (so-called "VFR travelers") are at high risk for acquiring malaria because they often do not take prophylaxis, as they may not consider malaria a serious threat because of their previous experience with it, are unaware they have "lost" immunity to malaria and are now at risk for serious disease, do not realize the risks of traveling when pregnant or when taking young nonimmune children to malarious regions, or are medically underserved and therefore less likely to seek pretravel advice.

CHEMOPROPHYLAXIS

Lack of proper chemoprophylaxis continues to be associated with severe complications from malaria and death.[426,495-497] Malaria is effectively prevented in travelers and in pregnant women in endemic areas by the use of antimalarial drugs when prescribed and taken appropriately[498] (Table 275-4). In a 2006 report, 405 out of 602 (67.3%) U.S. civilians and 16 out of 17 (94.1%) pregnant travelers who acquired malaria in an endemic area did not properly follow a chemoprophylaxis regimen recommended by the CDC for their region of travel.[497]

Selection of an effective prophylactic regimen depends on geographic patterns of drug resistance, concomitant illnesses, and other factors that may affect compliance: number of pills, dosing interval (i.e., daily versus weekly), duration of travel, duration of pre- and posttravel medication, cost, and the reputation as well as the actual tolerability of side effects.[499] Chemoprophylaxis recommendations change frequently because of regional and temporal variability in malaria risk even within countries, the ongoing spread of drug-resistant parasites, and resurgence of malaria in areas previously free of the disease. Updates and information on outbreaks are reported by the CDC at *http://www.cdc.gov/malaria*. In April 2008, for example, the CDC recommended that travelers to Great Exuma, Bahamas, take chloroquine prophylaxis for *P. falciparum*. This recommendation was based on a confirmed malaria case in a person who traveled to Great Exuma in March 2008 and a history of two prior outbreaks of malaria there in 2006 and 2007. Information on the geographic risk of acquiring malaria can be found by using the CDC's Malaria Risk Map application at *http://www.cdc.gov/malaria/risk_map*.

P. VIVAX, P. OVALE, P. MALARIAE, AND CHLOROQUINE-SUSCEPTIBLE P. FALCIPARUM

Currently, chloroquine can be used in travelers to those limited areas where chloroquine-resistant *P. falciparum* has not been reported, such as some areas of Central America and the Caribbean. Although chloroquine has been associated with QT prolongation and hepatic insufficiency, these effects are unlikely to occur at the doses used for prophylaxis. Chloroquine may cause retinopathy and arrhythmias when it accumulates as a result of excessive or prolonged dosing. Periodic funduscopic examination is therefore recommended with long-term use. Chloroquine prophylaxis has been used extensively and safely in pregnant and breast-feeding women and in children of all ages, including newborns.[500] Chloroquine-containing combinations (e.g., chloroquine *plus* proguanil) are no longer recommended for malaria prophylaxis in areas with chloroquine resistance (this regimen was implicated in failure to protect in the death of an American traveler).[495] Travelers who are exposed to *P. vivax* or *P. ovale* and have normal G6PD activity can receive terminal prophylaxis with primaquine on their return, as discussed earlier.

CHLOROQUINE-RESISTANT P. FALCIPARUM

Mefloquine can be used in travelers to areas where chloroquine-resistant *P. falciparum* has been reported, *except* in areas where mefloquine

TABLE 275-4	Malaria Chemoprophylaxis			
Drug	**Adult Dose**	**Pediatric Dose**		**Precautions**
P. vivax, P. ovale, P. malariae, and chloroquine-susceptible P. falciparum				
Chloroquine phosphate				
Supplied in 300-mg base (500-mg salt) tablets.	300 mg base (500 mg salt) once weekly.*	5 mg base/kg (8.3 mg salt/kg base) once weekly, up to the adult dose of 300 mg base.*		Drug accumulation from prolonged use or inadvertent daily dosing may cause retinopathy.
Chloroquine-resistant P. falciparum				
Mefloquine**				
Supplied in 250-mg salt (228-mg base) tablets.	250 mg salt once weekly.†	Dosed according to body weight:* ≤9 kg: 5 mg salt/kg once weekly 10-19 kg: ¼ tab once weekly 20-30 kg: ½ tab once weekly 31-45 kg: ¾ tab once weekly >45 kg: 1 tab once weekly.		Do not use in individuals with cardiac conduction abnormalities, history of seizures, or serious psychiatric illnesses (e.g., psychosis, major depression). Do not use concomitantly with quinidine, quinine, or halofantrine. Do not use in first trimester of pregnancy.
Chloroquine- or mefloquine-resistant P. falciparum				
Doxycycline				
Supplied in 100-mg tablets.	100 mg once daily.‡	For children 8-12 years old: 2 mg/kg once daily, up to adult dose of 100 mg. For children >13 years old: 100 mg once daily.‡		Do not use doxycycline in children <8 years old or in pregnant women.
Atovaquone-proguanil				
Supplied in fixed combination tablets containing 250 mg atovaquone and 100 mg proguanil (adult tablets) or 62.5 mg atovaquone and 25 mg proguanil (pediatric tablets).	250 mg/100 mg (one adult tab) once daily.§	Dose per body weight§ 5-8 kg: ½ pediatric tab once daily 9-10 kg: ¾ pediatric tab once daily 11-20 kg: 1 pediatric tab once daily 21-30 kg: 2 pediatric tabs once daily 31-40 kg: 3 pediatric tabs once daily >40 kg: 1 adult tab once daily.§		Not recommended for children <5 kg, pregnant women, or women who are breastfeeding children <5 kg.

*Beginning 1-2 weeks before travel and continuing weekly for 4 weeks after leaving a malarious area.
†For travelers who will be at immediate high risk of malaria, a loading dose of mefloquine is usually well tolerated: 250 mg daily for 3 consecutive days, followed by weekly dosing as shown.
‡Beginning 1-2 days before travel and continuing daily for 4 weeks after leaving a malarious area.
§Beginning 1-2 days before travel and continuing daily for 7 days after leaving a malarious area.
**Travelers receiving a prescription for mefloquine should be provided a copy of the FDA Medication Guide, which can be found at *http://www.fda.gov/cder/foi/label/2003/19591s19lbl_Lariam.pdf*.
Drug regimens adapted from: Advice for Travelers. *The Medical Letter*. 2002;1128:38-39; and from the CDC at *http://wwwn.cdc.gov/travel/contentMalariaDrugsHC.aspx*.

resistance has also been reported, such as Thailand, Myanmar, Cambodia, and Vietnam.[501] Mefloquine may prolong the corrected QT interval and so cannot be given to individuals with cardiac conduction abnormalities and should also not be administered concurrently with other quinine-like drugs (quinidine, halofantrine), which can lead to sudden cardiac death. Mefloquine is also contraindicated in individuals with serious neuropsychiatric disorders (e.g., psychosis, major depression, or history of seizures). An estimated 5% of individuals report neuropsychologic events such as sleep disturbances, insomnia, nightmares, cognitive changes, anxiety, or depression that lead to drug discontinuation.[502,503] However, a systematic review of mefloquine prophylaxis trials available in the Cochrane Library yielded five randomized comparative studies that failed to demonstrate significant differences between the overall adverse event or discontinuation rates associated with mefloquine and other chemoprophylaxis regimens.[504] Although not approved for use during pregnancy, mefloquine prophylaxis has been reported safe and effective during the second and third trimesters[505-507] and possibly during the first trimester.[508] Because most adverse effects are noted within the first three doses, starting prophylaxis 3 weeks prior to travel enables travelers to test their tolerance of the drug before they depart.

CHLOROQUINE- OR MEFLOQUINE-RESISTANT P. FALCIPARUM

Doxycycline or atovaquone-proguanil (Malarone, AP) can be used in travelers to areas where mefloquine-resistant *P. falciparum* has been reported, or in those travelers who are at risk of acquiring chloroquine-resistant malaria but who cannot take mefloquine.[501,509-511] Failure of properly taken doxycycline prophylaxis is unlikely, as *Plasmodium* resistance has not been reported against this drug. Failures of AP *treatment* (not prophylaxis) have been documented against resistant *P. falciparum* and are being increasingly reported in the literature.[319,321,429,449]

Doxycycline frequently causes gastrointestinal upset (take with food) and may cause esophageal irritation and ulceration (take with water, sit up for 30 minutes), photosensitivity (use sunscreen), vaginal candidiasis (carry over-the-counter antifungal suppositories), and decreased effectiveness of hormonal contraceptive agents (use back-up method). Doxycycline should not be used by pregnant and breast-feeding women or children younger than 8 years old, owing to deleterious effects on bone and tooth development. In addition, doxycycline should not be taken with metal-containing antacids, which can decrease its absorption. Actual effectiveness of doxycycline may be slightly lower than that reported from some studies because of frequent noncompliance with its daily dosing requirement.

AP is safe, effective, and well tolerated in both short- and long-term nonimmune travelers and there are no contraindications to its use.[512-520] Its safety profile in pregnancy is currently unknown (Category C).

Most antimalarial drugs (chloroquine, mefloquine, and doxycycline) are taken for 4 weeks after the individual leaves a malarious area. This is to ensure that all liver stage *P. falciparum* parasites, against which these drugs have no or questionable activity, have entirely completed their development into merozoites and passed into the bloodstream, where they can be killed by the drugs. AP eradicates the liver stages of *P. falciparum* although not of *P. vivax*, so the current recommendation is to take this drug for only 7 days after leaving a malarious area.

In some areas, multiple species of *Plasmodium* are transmitted to travelers by mosquitoes and can include *P. falciparum*, *P. vivax*, *P. ovale*, *P. malariae*, and even *P. knowlesi*[378] in various combinations of risk. While the presence of chloroquine- or mefloquine-resistant *P. falciparum* might be used as the primary reason for selecting mefloquine, doxycycline or AP prophylaxis against malaria, these drugs are also effective in preventing primary *P. vivax* malaria.[520,521] However, these drugs will not kill hypnozoites in the liver, so terminal prophylaxis with primaquine is necessary.

MOSQUITO REPELLENT AND AVOIDANCE MEASURES

No chemoprophylactic regimen is 100% effective. Despite adequate serum mefloquine levels and other laboratory evidence of compliance, mefloquine prophylaxis has failed where mefloquine resistance is not thought to be common.[522] This example (as well as others) highlights the recommendation that measures to reduce mosquito bites should always accompany chemoprophylaxis.[523,524] Travelers can reduce mosquito bites by using N,N-diethyl-3-methylbenzamide (DEET)-containing insect repellents on exposed skin,[525-527] wearing permethrin-treated clothing, wearing clothes and footwear that cover as much skin as possible,[522] sleeping under insecticide-treated bed nets,[522,528,529] staying in housing with air-conditioning and well-screened areas cleared of mosquitoes, and refraining from outdoor activity during peak *Anopheles* biting hours from dusk to dawn.[530] For information on ordering insecticide-treated bed nets, see *http://www.travmed.com*.

VACCINATION

Currently, there is no malaria vaccine. Research progress has been made with vaccine candidates such as the Duffy-binding protein of *P. vivax*[531,532] and a PfEMP-1 molecule involved in *P. falciparum* malaria of pregnancy.[533,534] A vaccine based on a protein component (circumsporozoite protein) from the surface of *P. falciparum* sporozoites, RTSS/AS02, has proven safe, well tolerated, and immunogenic in clinical trials[535] and is now under advanced evaluations of efficacy. Some recent publications review important concepts in malaria vaccinology and discuss the state of research in the field.[536,537]

REFERENCES

1. Greenwood B. Malaria mortality and morbidity in Africa. *Bull World Health Organ*. 1999;77:617-618.
2. Guyatt HL, Snow RW. Malaria in pregnancy as an indirect cause of infant mortality in sub-Saharan Africa. *Trans R Soc Trop Med Hyg*. 2001;95:569-576.
3. Snow RW, Guerra CA, Noor AM, et al. The global distribution of clinical episodes of Plasmodium falciparum malaria. *Nature*. 2005;434:214-217.
4. World Health Organization. *World Malaria Report. Geneva: World Health Organization, 2008.*
5. Carter R, Mendis KN. Evolutionary and historical aspects of the burden of malaria. *Clin Microbiol Rev*. 2002;15:564-594.
6. Molineaux L, Gramiccia G. *The Garki Project: Research of the epidemiology and control of malaria in the Sudan savanna of West Africa.* World Health Organization Press; 1980.
7. Trape JF, Pison G, Preziosi MP, et al. Impact of chloroquine resistance on malaria mortality. *C R Acad Sci III*. 1998;321:689-697.
8. World Health Organization. *World Health Organization Tech Rep Ser*. 1990;805:1-141.
9. Zucker JR, Lackritz EM, Ruebush TK, 2nd, et al. Childhood mortality during and after hospitalization in western Kenya:

effect of malaria treatment regimens. *Am J Trop Med Hyg*. 1996;55:655-660.
10. Zucker JR, Ruebush TK, 2nd, Obonyo C, et al. The mortality consequences of the continued use of chloroquine in Africa: experience in Siaya, western Kenya. *Am J Trop Med Hyg*. 2003;68:386-390.
11. Wellems TE. Plasmodium chloroquine resistance and the search for a replacement antimalarial drug. *Science*. 2002;298:124-126.
12. Blackman MJ, Bannister LH. Apical organelles of Apicomplexa: biology and isolation by subcellular fractionation. *Mol Biochem Parasitol*. 2001;117:11-25.
13. Bruce-Chwatt LJ. Malaria as a zoonosis. *WHO/Zoon/66.90*, 1966;66:578.
14. Singh B, Kim Sung L, Matusop A, et al. A large focus of naturally acquired Plasmodium knowlesi infections in human beings. *Lancet*. 2004;363:1017-1024.
15. Cox-Singh J, Davis TM, Lee KS, et al. Plasmodium knowlesi malaria in humans is widely distributed and potentially life threatening. *Clin Infect Dis*. 2008;46:165-171.
16. Laveran A. Deuxieme note relative a un nouveau parasite trouve dan le sang des maladies atteints de la fievre palustre. *Bull Acad Med*. 1880;44:1346-1347.

17. Ross R. On some peculiar pigmented cells found in two mosquitoes fed on malarial blood. *Br Med J*. 1897:1786-1788.
18. Grassi B. Rapporti tra la malaria e peculiari insetti. *Atti R Accad Lincei*. 1898;7:163-172.
19. Shortt HE, Garnham PCC. The pre-erythrocytic development of *Plasmodium cynomolgi* and *Plasmodium vivax*. *Trans R Soc Trop Med Hyg*. 1948;41:785-795.
20. Sinnis P, Coppi A. A long and winding road: the Plasmodium sporozoite's journey in the mammalian host. *Parasitol Int*. 2007;56:171-178.
21. Sultan AA, Thathy V, Frevert U, et al. TRAP is necessary for gliding motility and infectivity of plasmodium sporozoites. *Cell*. 1997;90:511-522.
22. Lacroix C, Menard R. TRAP-like protein of Plasmodium sporozoites: linking gliding motility to host-cell traversal. *Trends Parasitol*. 2008;24:431-434.
23. Silvie O, Rubinstein E, Franetich JF, et al. Hepatocyte CD81 is required for Plasmodium falciparum and Plasmodium yoelii sporozoite infectivity. *Nat Med*. 2003;9:93-96.
24. Silvie O, Greco C, Franetich JF, et al. Expression of human CD81 differently affects host cell susceptibility to malaria sporozoites

depending on the Plasmodium species. *Cell Microbiol.* 2006;8: 1134-1146.

25. Yalaoui S, Huby T, Franetich JF, et al. Scavenger receptor BI boosts hepatocyte permissiveness to Plasmodium infection. *Cell Host Microbe.* 2008;4:283-292.
26. Rodrigues CD, Hannus M, Prudencio M, et al. Host scavenger receptor SR-BI plays a dual role in the establishment of malaria parasite liver infection. *Cell Host Microbe.* 2008;4:271-282.
27. Gilles HM, Warrell DA. *Bruce-Chwatt's Essential Malariaology.* 3rd ed. New York: Oxford University Press; 1993.
28. Blackman MJ. Malarial proteases and host cell egress: an 'emerging' cascade. *Cell Microbiol.* 2008;10:1925-1934.
29. Aikawa M, Miller LH, Johnson J, et al. Erythrocyte entry by malarial parasites. A moving junction between erythrocyte and parasite. *J Cell Biol.* 1978;77:72-82.
30. Aikawa M. *Fine structure of malaria parasites in the various stages of development.* Edinburgh, United Kingdom: Churchill Livingstone; 1988.
31. Sibley LD. Intracellular parasite invasion strategies. *Science.* 2004;304:248-253.
32. Cowman AF, Crabb BS. Invasion of red blood cells by malaria parasites. *Cell.* 2006;124:755-766.
33. Oh SS, Chishti AH. Host receptors in malaria merozoite invasion. *Curr Top Microbiol Immunol.* 2005;295:203-232.
34. Karunaweera ND, Grau GE, Gamage P, et al. Dynamics of fever and serum levels of tumor necrosis factor are closely associated during clinical paroxysms in Plasmodium vivax malaria. *Proc Natl Acad Sci U S A.* 1992;89:3200-3203.
35. Boyd MF. Historical review. In: Boyd MF, ed. *Malariology.* Philadelphia: Saunders; 1949;3-25.
36. Vijaykumar M, Naik RS, Gowda DC. Plasmodium falciparum glycosylphosphatidylinositol-induced TNF-alpha secretion by macrophages is mediated without membrane insertion or endocytosis. *J Biol Chem.* 2001;276:6909-6912.
37. Wijesekera SK, Carter R, Rathnayaka L, et al. A malaria parasite toxin associated with Plasmodium vivax paroxysms. *Clin Exp Immunol.* 1996;104:221-227.
38. Sachs J, Malaney P. The economic and social burden of malaria. *Nature.* 2002;415:680-685.
39. Breman JG. The ears of the hippopotamus: manifestations, determinants, and estimates of the malaria burden. *Am J Trop Med Hyg.* 2001;64:1-11.
40. *Malaria: Obstacles and Opportunities.* Washington, DC: National Academy Press, 1991.
41. Genton B, D'Acremont V, Rare L, et al. Plasmodium vivax and mixed infections are associated with severe malaria in children: a prospective cohort study from Papua New Guinea. *PLoS Med.* 2008;5:e127.
42. Tjitra E, Anstey NM, Sugiarto P, et al. Multidrug-resistant Plasmodium vivax associated with severe and fatal malaria: a prospective study in Papua, Indonesia. *PLoS Med.* 2008;5: e128.
43. Marsh K, Forster D, Waruiru C, et al. Indicators of life-threatening malaria in African children. *N Engl J Med.* 1995;332: 1399-1404.
44. English M, Waruiru C, Amukoye E, et al. Deep breathing in children with severe malaria: indicator of metabolic acidosis and poor outcome. *Am J Trop Med Hyg.* 1996;55:521-524.
45. Newbold C, Craig A, Kyes S, et al. Cytoadherence, pathogenesis and the infected red cell surface in Plasmodium falciparum. *Int J Parasitol.* 1999;29:927-937.
46. Sherman IW, Eda S, Winograd E. Cytoadherence and sequestration in Plasmodium falciparum: defining the ties that bind. *Microbes Infect.* 2003;5:897-909.
47. Chotivanich KT, Dondorp AM, White NJ, et al. The resistance to physiological shear stresses of the erythrocytic rosettes formed by cells infected with Plasmodium falciparum. *Ann Trop Med Parasitol.* 2000;94:219-226.
48. Kaul DK, Roth EF Jr, Nagel RL, et al. Rosetting of Plasmodium falciparum-infected red blood cells with uninfected red blood cells enhances microvascular obstruction under flow conditions. *Blood.* 1991;78:812-819.
49. Dondorp AM, Kager PA, Vreeken J, et al. Abnormal blood flow and red blood cell deformability in severe malaria. *Parasitol Today.* 2000;16:228-232.
50. Miller LH, Usami S, Chien S. Alteration in the rheologic properties of Plasmodium knowlesi–infected red cells. A possible mechanism for capillary obstruction. *J Clin Invest.* 1971;50: 1451-1455.
51. Pain A, Ferguson DJ, Kai O, et al. Platelet-mediated clumping of Plasmodium falciparum-infected erythrocytes is a common adhesive phenotype and is associated with severe malaria. *Proc Natl Acad Sci U S A.* 2001;98:1805-1810.
52. Chotivanich K, Sritabal J, Udomsangpetch R, et al. Platelet-induced autoagglutination of Plasmodium falciparum-infected red blood cells and disease severity in Thailand. *J Infect Dis.* 2004;189:1052-1055.
53. Luse SA, Miller LH. Plasmodium falciparum malaria. Ultrastructure of parasitized erythrocytes in cardiac vessels. *Am J Trop Med Hyg.* 1971;20:655-660.
54. Prommano O, Chaisri U, Turner GD, et al. A quantitative ultrastructural study of the liver and the spleen in fatal falciparum malaria. *Southeast Asian J Trop Med Public Health.* 2005;36:1359-1370.
55. MacPherson GG, Warrell MJ, White NJ, et al. Human cerebral malaria. A quantitative ultrastructural analysis of parasitized erythrocyte sequestration. *Am J Pathol.* 1985;119:385-401.
56. Oo MM, Aikawa M, Than T, et al. Human cerebral malaria: a pathological study. *J Neuropathol Exp Neurol.* 1987;46:223-231.
57. Pongponratn E, Riganti M, Punpoowong B, et al. Microvascular sequestration of parasitized erythrocytes in human falciparum malaria: a pathological study. *Am J Trop Med Hyg.* 1991;44: 168-175.
58. Nguansangiam S, Day NP, Hien TT, et al. A quantitative ultrastructural study of renal pathology in fatal Plasmodium falciparum malaria. *Trop Med Int Health.* 2007;12:1037-1050.
59. Wickramasinghe SN, Phillips RE, Looareesuwan S, et al. The bone marrow in human cerebral malaria: parasite sequestration within sinusoids. *Br J Haematol.* 1987;66:295-306.
60. Walter PR, Garin Y, Blot P. Placental pathologic changes in malaria. A histologic and ultrastructural study. *Am J Pathol.* 1982;109:330-342.
61. Pongponratn E, Turner GD, Day NP, et al. An ultrastructural study of the brain in fatal Plasmodium falciparum malaria. *Am J Trop Med Hyg.* 2003;69:345-359.
62. Pongponratn E, Viriyavejakul P, Wilairatana P, et al. Absence of knobs on parasitized red blood cells in a splenectomized patient in fatal falciparum malaria. *Southeast Asian J Trop Med Public Health.* 2000;31:829-835.
63. Langreth SG, Peterson E. Pathogenicity, stability, and immunogenicity of a knobless clone of Plasmodium falciparum in Colombian owl monkeys. *Infect Immun.* 1985;47:760-766.
64. Crabb BS, Cooke BM, Reeder JC, et al. Targeted gene disruption shows that knobs enable malaria-infected red cells to cytoadhere under physiological shear stress. *Cell.* 1997;89:287-296.
65. Yipp BG, Anand S, Schollaardt T, et al. Synergism of multiple adhesion molecules in mediating cytoadherence of Plasmodium falciparum-infected erythrocytes to microvascular endothelial cells under flow. *Blood.* 2000;96:2292-2298.
66. Craig A, Scherf A. Molecules on the surface of the Plasmodium falciparum infected erythrocyte and their role in malaria pathogenesis and immune evasion. *Mol Biochem Parasitol.* 2001; 115:129-143.
67. Su XZ, Heatwole VM, Wertheimer SP, et al. The large diverse gene family var encodes proteins involved in cytoadherence and antigenic variation of Plasmodium falciparum-infected erythrocytes. *Cell.* 1995;82:89-100.
68. Smith JD, Chitnis CE, Craig AG, et al. Switches in expression of Plasmodium falciparum var genes correlate with changes in antigenic and cytoadherent phenotypes of infected erythrocytes. *Cell.* 1995;82:101-110.
69. Baruch DI, Pasloske BL, Singh HB, et al. Cloning the P. falciparum gene encoding PfEMP1, a malarial variant antigen and adherence receptor on the surface of parasitized human erythrocytes. *Cell.* 1995;82:77-87.
70. Chen Q, Fernandez V, Sundstrom A, et al. Developmental selection of var gene expression in Plasmodium falciparum. *Nature.* 1998;394:392-395.
71. Deitsch KW, Calderwood MS, Wellems TE. Malaria. Cooperative silencing elements in var genes. *Nature.* 2001;412:875-876.
72. Gatton ML, Peters JM, Fowler EV, et al. Switching rates of Plasmodium falciparum var genes: faster than we thought? *Trends Parasitol.* 2003;19:202-208.
73. Roberts DJ, Craig AG, Berendt AR, et al. Rapid switching to multiple antigenic and adhesive phenotypes in malaria. *Nature.* 1992;357:689-692.
74. Roberts DD, Sherwood JA, Spitalnik SL, et al. Thrombospondin binds falciparum malaria parasitized erythrocytes and may mediate cytoadherence. *Nature.* 1985;318:64-66.
75. Cooke BM, Berendt AR, Craig AG, et al. Rolling and stationary cytoadhesion of red blood cells parasitized by Plasmodium falciparum: separate roles for ICAM-1, CD36 and thrombospondin. *Br J Haematol.* 1994;87:162-170.
76. Treutiger CJ, Heddini A, Fernandez V, et al. PECAM-1/CD31, an endothelial receptor for binding Plasmodium falciparum-infected erythrocytes. *Nat Med.* 1997;3:1405-1408.
77. Reeder JC, Cowman AF, Davern KM, et al. The adhesion of Plasmodium falciparum-infected erythrocytes to chondroitin sulfate A is mediated by P. falciparum erythrocyte membrane protein 1. *Proc Natl Acad Sci U S A.* 1999;96:5198-5202.
78. Fried M, Duffy PE. Adherence of Plasmodium falciparum to chondroitin sulfate A in the human placenta. *Science.* 1996;272: 1502-1504.
79. Montgomery J, Mphande FA, Berriman M, et al. Differential var gene expression in the organs of patients dying of falciparum malaria. *Mol Microbiol.* 2007;65:959-967.
80. Rottmann M, Lavstsen T, Mugasa JP, et al. Differential expression of var gene groups is associated with morbidity caused by Plasmodium falciparum infection in Tanzanian children. *Infect Immun.* 2006;74:3904-3911.
81. Kaestli M, Cockburn IA, Cortes A, et al. Virulence of malaria is associated with differential expression of Plasmodium falciparum var gene subgroups in a case-control study. *J Infect Dis.* 2006;193:1567-1574.
82. Jensen AT, Magistrado P, Sharp S, et al. Plasmodium falciparum associated with severe childhood malaria preferentially expresses PfEMP1 encoded by group A var genes. *J Exp Med.* 2004;199: 1179-1190.
83. Serghides L, Smith TG, Patel SN, et al. CD36 and malaria: friends or foes? *Trends Parasitol.* 2003;19:461-469.
84. Lindenthal C, Kremsner PG, Klinkert MQ. Commonly recognised Plasmodium falciparum parasites cause cerebral malaria. *Parasitol Res.* 2003;91:363-368.
85. Ockenhouse CF, Ho M, Tandon NN, et al. Molecular basis of sequestration in severe and uncomplicated Plasmodium falciparum malaria: differential adhesion of infected erythrocytes to CD36 and ICAM-1. *J Infect Dis.* 1991;164:163-169.
86. Turner GD, Morrison H, Jones M, et al. An immunohistochemical study of the pathology of fatal malaria. Evidence for widespread endothelial activation and a potential role for intercellular adhesion molecule-1 in cerebral sequestration. *Am J Pathol.* 1994;145:1057-1069.
87. Newbold C, Warn P, Black G, et al. Receptor-specific adhesion and clinical disease in Plasmodium falciparum. *Am J Trop Med Hyg.* 1997;57:389-398.
88. Biswas AK, Hafiz A, Banerjee B, et al. Plasmodium falciparum uses gC1qR/HABP1/p32 as a receptor to bind to vascular endothelium and for platelet-mediated clumping. *PLoS Pathog.* 2007; 3:1271-1280.
89. Gamain B, Smith JD, Miller LH, et al. Modifications in the CD36 binding domain of the Plasmodium falciparum variant antigen are responsible for the inability of chondroitin sulfate A adherent parasites to bind CD36. *Blood.* 2001;97:3268-3274.
90. Chen Q, Barragan A, Fernandez V, et al. Identification of Plasmodium falciparum erythrocyte membrane protein 1 (PfEMP1) as the rosetting ligand of the malaria parasite P. falciparum. *J Exp Med.* 1998;187:15-23.
91. Rowe JA, Moulds JM, Newbold CI, et al. *P. falciparum* rosetting mediated by a parasite-variant erythrocyte membrane protein and complement-receptor 1. *Nature.* 1997;388:292-295.
92. Barragan A, Kremsner PG, Wahlgren M, et al. Blood group A antigen is a coreceptor in Plasmodium falciparum rosetting. *Infect Immun.* 2000;68:2971-2975.
93. Cockburn IA, Mackinnon MJ, O'Donnell A, et al. A human complement receptor 1 polymorphism that reduces Plasmodium falciparum rosetting confers protection against severe malaria. *Proc Natl Acad Sci U S A.* 2004;101:272-277.
94. Heddini A, Pettersson F, Kai O, et al. Fresh isolates from children with severe Plasmodium falciparum malaria bind to multiple receptors. *Infect Immun.* 2001;69:5849-5856.
95. Treutiger CJ, Hedlund I, Helmby H, et al. Rosette formation in Plasmodium falciparum isolates and anti-rosette activity of sera from Gambians with cerebral or uncomplicated malaria. *Am J Trop Med Hyg.* 1992;46:503-510.
96. Carlson J, Helmby H, Hill AV, et al. Human cerebral malaria: association with erythrocyte rosetting and lack of anti-rosetting antibodies. *Lancet.* 1990;336:1457-1460.
97. Rowe A, Obeiro J, Newbold CI, et al. Plasmodium falciparum rosetting is associated with malaria severity in Kenya. *Infect Immun.* 1995;63:2323-2326.
98. Kun JF, Schmidt-Ott RJ, Lehman LG, et al. Merozoite surface antigen 1 and 2 genotypes and rosetting of Plasmodium falciparum in severe and mild malaria in Lambarene, Gabon. *Trans R Soc Trop Med Hyg.* 1998;92:110-114.
99. Ho M, Davis TM, Silamut K, et al. Rosette formation of Plasmodium falciparum-infected erythrocytes from patients with acute malaria. *Infect Immun.* 1991;59:2135-2139.
100. al-Yaman F, Genton B, Mokela D, et al. Human cerebral malaria: lack of significant association between erythrocyte rosetting and disease severity. *Trans R Soc Trop Med Hyg.* 1995; 89:55-58.
101. Field JW. Blood examination and prognosis in acute falciparum malaria. *Trans R Soc Trop Med Hyg.* 1949;43:33-48.
102. Chotivanich K, Udomsangpetch R, Simpson JA, et al. Parasite multiplication potential and the severity of Falciparum malaria. *J Infect Dis.* 2000;181:1206-1209.
103. Silamut K, White NJ. Relation of the stage of parasite development in the peripheral blood to prognosis in severe falciparum malaria. *Trans R Soc Trop Med Hyg.* 1993;87:436-443.
104. Amodu OK, Adeyemo AA, Olumese PE, et al. Intraleucocytic malaria pigment and clinical severity of malaria in children. *Trans R Soc Trop Med Hyg.* 1998;92:54-56.
105. Simpson JA, Silamut K, Chotivanich K, et al. Red cell selectivity in malaria: a study of multiple-infected erythrocytes. *Trans R Soc Trop Med Hyg.* 1999;93:165-168.
106. Miller LH, Mason SJ, Dvorak JA, et al. Erythrocyte receptors for (*Plasmodium knowlesi*) malaria: Duffy blood group determinants. *Science.* 1975;189:561-563.
107. Horuk R, Chitnis CE, Darbonne WC, et al. A receptor for the malarial parasite Plasmodium vivax: the erythrocyte chemokine receptor. *Science.* 1993;261:1182-1184.
108. Grau GE, Mackenzie CD, Carr RA, et al. Platelet accumulation in brain microvessels in fatal pediatric cerebral malaria. *J Infect Dis.* 2003;187:461-466.
109. Patnaik JK, Das BS, Mishra SK, et al. Vascular clogging, mononuclear cell margination, and enhanced vascular permeability in the pathogenesis of human cerebral malaria. *Am J Trop Med Hyg.* 1994;51:642-647.
110. Taylor TE, Fu WJ, Carr RA, et al. Differentiating the pathologies of cerebral malaria by postmortem parasite counts. *Nat Med.* 2004;10:143-145.
111. White VA, Lewallen S, Beare N, et al. Correlation of retinal haemorrhages with brain haemorrhages in children dying of cerebral malaria in Malawi. *Trans R Soc Trop Med Hyg.* 2001;95:618-621.
112. SenGupta SK, Naraqi S. The brain in cerebral malaria: a pathological study of 24 fatal cases in Papua New Guinea. *P N G Med J.* 1992;35:270-274.

113. Nagatake T, Hoang VT, Tegoshi T, et al. Pathology of falciparum malaria in Vietnam. *Am J Trop Med Hyg*. 1992;47:259-264.

114. Riganti M, Pongponratn E, Tegoshi T, et al. Human cerebral malaria in Thailand: a clinico-pathological correlation. *Immunol Lett*. 1990;25:199-205.

115. Grau GE, Taylor TE, Molyneux ME, et al. Tumor necrosis factor and disease severity in children with falciparum malaria. *N Engl J Med*. 1989;320:1586-1591.

116. Kern P, Hemmer CJ, Van Damme J, et al. Elevated tumor necrosis factor alpha and interleukin-6 serum levels as markers for complicated *Plasmodium falciparum* malaria. *Am J Med*. 1989;87:139-143.

117. Kwiatkowski D. Tumour necrosis factor, fever and fatality in falciparum malaria. *Immunol Lett*. 1990;25:213-216.

118. Dobbie MS, Hurst RD, Klein NJ, et al. Upregulation of intercellular adhesion molecule-1 expression on human endothelial cells by tumour necrosis factor-alpha in an in vitro model of the blood-brain barrier. *Brain Res*. 1999;830:330-336.

119. Wong D, Dorovini-Zis K. Upregulation of intercellular adhesion molecule-1 (ICAM-1) expression in primary cultures of human brain microvessel endothelial cells by cytokines and lipopolysaccharide. *J Neuroimmunol*. 1992;39:11-21.

120. Yeo TW, Lampah DA, Gitawati R, et al. Impaired nitric oxide bioavailability and L-arginine reversible endothelial dysfunction in adults with falciparum malaria. *J Exp Med*. 2007;204:2693-2704.

121. Weinberg JB, Lopansri BK, Mwaikambo E, et al. Arginine, nitric oxide, carbon monoxide, and endothelial function in severe malaria. *Curr Opin Infect Dis*. 2008;21:468-475.

122. Maitland K, Pamba A, Newton CR, et al. Response to volume resuscitation in children with severe malaria. *Pediatr Crit Care Med*. 2003;4:426-431.

123. Maitland K, Pamba A, English M, et al. Randomized trial of volume expansion with albumin or saline in children with severe malaria: preliminary evidence of albumin benefit. *Clin Infect Dis*. 2005;40:538-545.

124. White NJ, Miller KD, Marsh K, et al. Hypoglycaemia in African children with severe malaria. *Lancet*. 1987;1:708-711.

125. Ogutu BR, Newton CR. Management of seizures in children with falciparum malaria. *Trop Doct*. 2004;34:71-75.

126. Molyneux ME, Taylor TE, Wirima JJ, et al. Effect of rate of infusion of quinine on insulin and glucose responses in Malawian children with falciparum malaria. *BMJ*. 1989;299:602-603.

127. Krishna S, Waller DW, ter Kuile F, et al. Lactic acidosis and hypoglycaemia in children with severe malaria: pathophysiological and prognostic significance. *Trans R Soc Trop Med Hyg*. 1994;88:67-73.

128. English M, Punt J, Mwangi I, et al. Clinical overlap between malaria and severe pneumonia in Africa children in hospital. *Trans R Soc Trop Med Hyg*. 1996;90:658-662.

129. Dekker E, Hellerstein MK, Romijn JA, et al. Glucose homeostasis in children with falciparum malaria: precursor supply limits gluconeogenesis and glucose production. *J Clin Endocrinol Metab*. 1997;82:2514-2521.

130. Homewood CA. Carbohydrate metabolism of malarial parasites. *Bull World Health Organ*. 1977;55:229-235.

131. White NJ, Warrell DA, Chanthavanich P, et al. Severe hypoglycemia and hyperinsulinemia in falciparum malaria. *N Engl J Med*. 1983;309:61-66.

132. Phillips RE, Looareesuwan S, White NJ, et al. Hypoglycaemia and antimalarial drugs: quinidine and release of insulin. *Br Med J (Clin Res Ed)*. 1986;292:1319-1321.

133. Ekvall H. Malaria and anemia. *Curr Opin Hematol*. 2003;10:108-114.

134. Kai OK, Roberts DJ. The pathophysiology of malarial anaemia: where have all the red cells gone? *BMC Med*. 2008;6:24.

135. Selvam R, Baskaran G. Hematological impairments in recurrent Plasmodium vivax infected patients. *Jpn J Med Sci Biol*. 1996;49:151-165.

136. Jakeman GN, Saul A, Hogarth WL, et al. Anaemia of acute malaria infections in non-immune patients primarily results from destruction of uninfected erythrocytes. *Parasitology*. 1999;119(Pt 2):127-133.

137. Vedovato M, De Paoli Vitali E, Dapporto M, et al. Defective erythropoietin production in the anaemia of malaria. *Nephrol Dial Transplant*. 1999;14:1043-1044.

138. Burgmann H, Looareesuwan S, Kapiotis S, et al. Serum levels of erythropoietin in acute Plasmodium falciparum malaria. *Am J Trop Med Hyg*. 1996;54:280-283.

139. Verhoef H, West CE, Kraaijenhagen R, et al. Malarial anemia leads to adequately increased erythropoiesis in asymptomatic Kenyan children. *Blood*. 2002;100:3489-3494.

140. Burchard GD, Radloff P, Philipps J, et al. Increased erythropoietin production in children with severe malarial anemia. *Am J Trop Med Hyg*. 1995;53:547-551.

141. Abdalla SH. Hematopoiesis in human malaria. *Blood Cells*. 1990;16:401-416; discussion 17-9.

142. Calis JC, Phiri KS, Faragher EB, et al. Severe anemia in Malawian children. *N Engl J Med*. 2008;358:888-899.

143. Bloland PB, Lackritz EM, Kazembe PN, et al. Beyond chloroquine: implications of drug resistance for evaluating malaria therapy efficacy and treatment policy in Africa. *J Infect Dis*. 1993;167:932-937.

144. Charoenpan P, Indraprasit S, Kiatboonsri S, et al. Pulmonary edema in severe falciparum malaria. Hemodynamic study and clinicophysiologic correlation. *Chest*. 1990;97:1190-1197.

145. Feldman RM, Singer C. Noncardiogenic pulmonary edema and pulmonary fibrosis in falciparum malaria. *Rev Infect Dis*. 1987;9:134-139.

146. Taylor WR, White NJ. Malaria and the lung. *Clin Chest Med*. 2002;23:457-468.

147. Crawley J, English M, Waruiru C, et al. Abnormal respiratory patterns in childhood cerebral malaria. *Trans R Soc Trop Med Hyg*. 1998;92:305-308.

148. Maitland K, Levin M, English M, et al. Severe P. falciparum malaria in Kenyan children: evidence for hypovolaemia. *QJM*. 2003;96:427-434.

149. Agbenyega T, Angus BJ, Bedu-Addo G, et al. Glucose and lactate kinetics in children with severe malaria. *J Clin Endocrinol Metab*. 2000;85:1569-1576.

150. Vander Jagt DL, Hunsaker LA, Campos NM, et al. D-lactate production in erythrocytes infected with Plasmodium falciparum. *Mol Biochem Parasitol*. 1990;42:277-284.

151. Day NP, Phu NH, Mai NT, et al. The pathophysiologic and prognostic significance of acidosis in severe adult malaria. *Crit Care Med*. 2000;28:1833-1840.

152. Pukrittayakamee S, White NJ, Davis TM, et al. Hepatic blood flow and metabolism in severe falciparum malaria: clearance of intravenously administered galactose. *Clin Sci (Lond)*. 1992;82:63-70.

153. Tureen J. Effect of recombinant human tumor necrosis factor-alpha on cerebral oxygen uptake, cerebrospinal fluid lactate, and cerebral blood flow in the rabbit: role of nitric oxide. *J Clin Invest*. 1995;95:1086-1091.

154. English M, Marsh V, Amukoye E, et al. Chronic salicylate poisoning and severe malaria. *Lancet*. 1996;347:1736-1737.

155. Steketee RW, Wirima JJ, Hightower AW, et al. The effect of malaria and malaria prevention in pregnancy on offspring birthweight, prematurity, and intrauterine growth retardation in rural Malawi. *Am J Trop Med Hyg*. 1996;55:33-41.

156. Duffy PE, Fried M. Malaria in the pregnant woman. *Curr Top Microbiol Immunol*. 2005;295:169-200.

157. Beeson JG, Rogerson SJ, Cooke BM, et al. Adhesion of Plasmodium falciparum-infected erythrocytes to hyaluronic acid in placental malaria. *Nat Med*. 2000;6:86-90.

158. Flick K, Scholander C, Chen Q, et al. Role of nonimmune IgG bound to PfEMP1 in placental malaria. *Science*. 2001;293:2098-2100.

159. Beeson JG, Amin N, Kanjala M, et al. Selective accumulation of mature asexual stages of *Plasmodium falciparum*-infected erythrocytes in the placenta. *Infect Immun*. 2002;70:5412-5415.

160. Khattab A, Kun J, Deloron P, et al. Variants of *Plasmodium falciparum* erythrocyte membrane protein 1 expressed by different placental parasites are closely related and adhere to chondroitin sulfate A. *J Infect Dis*. 2001;183:1165-1169.

161. Khattab A, Kremsner PG, Klinkert MQ. Common surface-antigen var genes of limited diversity expressed by Plasmodium falciparum placental isolates separated by time and space. *J Infect Dis*. 2003;187:477-483.

162. van Eijk AM, Ayisi JG, ter Kuile FO, et al. Risk factors for malaria in pregnancy in an urban and peri-urban population in western Kenya. *Trans R Soc Trop Med Hyg*. 2002;96:586-592.

163. Muehlenbachs A, Fried M, Lachowitzer J, et al. Natural selection of FLT1 alleles and their association with malaria resistance in utero. *Proc Natl Acad Sci U S A*. 2008;105:14488-14491.

164. Carlini ME, White AC Jr, Atmar RL. Vivax malaria complicated by adult respiratory distress syndrome. *Clin Infect Dis*. 1999;28:1182-1183.

165. Torres JR, Perez H, Postigo MM, et al. Acute non-cardiogenic lung injury in benign tertian malaria. *Lancet*. 1997;350:31-32.

166. Oscherwitz SL. Chronic malaria with splenic rupture. *J Travel Med*. 2003;10:64-65.

167. Zingman BS, Viner BL. Splenic complications in malaria: case report and review. *Clin Infect Dis*. 1993;16:223-232.

168. Anstey NM, Handojo T, Pain MC, et al. Lung injury in vivax malaria: pathophysiological evidence for pulmonary vascular sequestration and posttreatment alveolar-capillary inflammation. *J Infect Dis*. 2007;195:589-596.

169. Suwanarusk R, Cooke BM, Dondorp AM, et al. The deformability of red blood cells parasitized by Plasmodium falciparum and P. vivax. *J Infect Dis*. 2004;189:190-194.

170. Vinetz JM, Li J, McCutchan TF, et al. *Plasmodium malariae* infection in an asymptomatic 74-year-old Greek woman with splenomegaly. *N Engl J Med*. 1998;338:367-371.

171. Okoro BA, Okafor HU, Nnoli LU. Childhood nephrotic syndrome in Enugu, Nigeria. *West Afr J Med*. 2000;19:137-141.

172. Abdurrahman MB. The role of infectious agents in the aetiology and pathogenesis of childhood nephrotic syndrome in Africa. *J Infect*. 1984;8:100-109.

173. Abdurrahman MB, Aikhionbare HA, Babaoye FA, et al. Clinicopathological features of childhood nephrotic syndrome in northern Nigeria. *Q J Med*. 1990;75:563-576.

174. Ward PA, Kibukamusoke JW. Evidence for soluble immune complexes in the pathogenesis of the glomerulonephritis of quartan malaria. *Lancet*. 1969;1:283-285.

175. McGuire W, Hill AV, Allsopp CE, et al. Variation in the TNF-alpha promoter region associated with susceptibility to cerebral malaria. *Nature*. 1994;371:508-510.

176. Knight JC, Udalova I, Hill AV, et al. A polymorphism that affects OCT-1 binding to the TNF promoter region is associated with severe malaria. *Nat Genet*. 1999;22:145-150.

177. Mangano VD, Luoni G, Rockett KA, et al. Interferon regulatory factor-1 polymorphisms are associated with the control of Plasmodium falciparum infection. *Genes Immun*. 2008;9:482.

178. Khor CC, Chapman SJ, Vannberg FO, et al. A Mal functional variant is associated with protection against invasive pneumococcal disease, bacteremia, malaria and tuberculosis. *Nat Genet*. 2007;39:523-528.

179. Cooke GS, Aucan C, Walley AJ, et al. Association of Fcgamma receptor IIa (CD32) polymorphism with severe malaria in West Africa. *Am J Trop Med Hyg*. 2003;69:565-568.

180. Flint J, Harding RM, Boyce AJ, et al. The population genetics of the haemoglobinopathies. *Baillieres Clin Haematol*. 1998;11:1-51.

181. Aidoo M, Terlouw DJ, Kolczak MS, et al. Protective effects of the sickle cell gene against malaria morbidity and mortality. *Lancet*. 2002;359:1311-1312.

182. Allison AC. Protection afforded by sickle-cell trait against subtertian malareal infection. *Br Med J*. 1954;1:290-294.

183. Willcox M, Bjorkman A, Brohult J, et al. A case-control study in northern Liberia of Plasmodium falciparum malaria in haemoglobin S and beta-thalassaemia traits. *Ann Trop Med Parasitol*. 1983;77:239-246.

184. Ruwende C, Khoo SC, Snow RW, et al. Natural selection of hemi- and heterozygotes for G6PD deficiency in Africa by resistance to severe malaria. *Nature*. 1995;376:246-249.

185. Fleming AF, Storey J, Molineaux L, et al. Abnormal haemoglobins in the Sudan savanna of Nigeria. I. Prevalence of haemoglobins and relationships between sickle cell trait, malaria, and survival. *Ann Trop Med Parasitol*. 1979;73:161-172.

186. Agarwal A, Guindo A, Cissoko Y, et al. Hemoglobin C associated with protection from severe malaria in the Dogon of Mali, a West African population with a low prevalence of hemoglobin S. *Blood*. 2000;96:2358-2363.

187. Modiano D, Luoni G, Sirima BS, et al. Haemoglobin C protects against clinical Plasmodium falciparum malaria. *Nature*. 2001;414:305-308.

188. May J, Evans JA, Timmann C, et al. Hemoglobin variants and disease manifestations in severe falciparum malaria. *JAMA*. 2007;297:2220-2226.

189. Mockenhaupt FP, Ehrhardt S, Cramer JP, et al. Hemoglobin C and resistance to severe malaria in Ghanaian children. *J Infect Dis*. 2004;190:1006-1009.

190. Mockenhaupt FP, Ehrhardt S, Otchwemah R, et al. Limited influence of haemoglobin variants on Plasmodium falciparum msp1 and msp2 alleles in symptomatic malaria. *Trans R Soc Trop Med Hyg*. 2004;98:302-310.

191. Achidi EA, Salimonu LS, Asuzu MC, et al. Studies on *Plasmodium falciparum* parasitemia and development of anemia in Nigerian infants during their first year of life. *Am J Trop Med Hyg*. 1996;55:138-143.

192. Olumese PE, Adeyemo AA, Ademowo OG, et al. The clinical manifestations of cerebral malaria among Nigerian children with the sickle cell trait. *Ann Trop Paediatr*. 1997;17:141-145.

193. Friedman MJ. Erythrocytic mechanism of sickle cell resistance to malaria. *Proc Natl Acad Sci U S A*. 1978;75:1994-1997.

194. Roth EF Jr, Friedman M, Ueda Y, et al. Sickling rates of human AS red cells infected in vitro with Plasmodium falciparum malaria. *Science*. 1978;202:650-652.

195. Luzzatto L, Nwachuku-Jarrett ES, Reddy S. Increased sickling of parasitised erythrocytes as mechanism of resistance against malaria in the sickle-cell trait. *Lancet*. 1970;1:319-321.

196. Pasvol G. The interaction between sickle haemoglobin and the malarial parasite Plasmodium falciparum. *Trans R Soc Trop Med Hyg*. 1980;74:701-705.

197. Ayi K, Turrini F, Piga A, et al. Enhanced phagocytosis of ring-parasitized mutant erythrocytes: a common mechanism that may explain protection against falciparum malaria in sickle trait and beta-thalassemia trait. *Blood*. 2004;104:3364-3371.

198. Fairhurst RM, Baruch DI, Brittain NJ, et al. Abnormal display of PfEMP-1 on erythrocytes carrying haemoglobin C may protect against malaria. *Nature*. 2005;435:1117-1121.

199. Cholera R, Brittain NJ, Gillrie MR, et al. Impaired cytoadherence of Plasmodium falciparum-infected erythrocytes containing sickle hemoglobin. *Proc Natl Acad Sci U S A*. 2008;105:991-996.

200. Orkin SH, Kazazian HH Jr, Antonarakis SE, et al. Abnormal RNA processing due to the exon mutation of beta E-globin gene. *Nature*. 1982;300:768-769.

201. Kitayaporn D, Nelson KE, Charoenlarp P, et al. Haemoglobin-E in the presence of oxidative substances from fava bean may be protective against Plasmodium falciparum malaria. *Trans R Soc Trop Med Hyg*. 1992;86:240-244.

202. Hutagalung R, Wilairatana P, Looareesuwan S, et al. Influence of hemoglobin E trait on the severity of Falciparum malaria. *J Infect Dis*. 1999;179:283-286.

203. Naka I, Ohashi J, Nuchnoi P, et al. Lack of Association of the HbE Variant with Protection from Cerebral Malaria in Thailand. *Biochem Genet*. 2008.

204. Oo M, Tin S, Marlar T, et al. Genetic red cell disorders and severity of falciparum malaria in Myanmar. *Bull World Health Organ*. 1995;73:659-665.

205. Chotivanich K, Udomsangpetch R, Pattanapanyasat K, et al. Hemoglobin E: a balanced polymorphism protective against

high parasitemias and thus severe P falciparum malaria. *Blood.* 2002;100:1172-1176.

206. Oppenheimer SJ, Hill AV, Gibson FD, et al. The interaction of alpha thalassaemia with malaria. *Trans R Soc Trop Med Hyg.* 1987;81:322-326.

207. Flint J, Hill AV, Bowden DK, et al. High frequencies of alpha-thalassaemia are the result of natural selection by malaria. *Nature.* 1986;321:744-750.

208. Weatherall DJ. Thalassaemia and malaria, revisited. *Ann Trop Med Parasitol.* 1997;91:885-890.

209. Pattanapanyasat K, Yongvanitchit K, Tongtawe P, et al. Impairment of Plasmodium falciparum growth in thalassemic red blood cells: further evidence by using biotin labeling and flow cytometry. *Blood.* 1999;93:3116-3119.

210. Senok AC, Li K, Nelson EA, et al. Invasion and growth of *Plasmodium falciparum* is inhibited in fractionated thalassaemic erythrocytes. *Trans R Soc Trop Med Hyg.* 1997;91:138-143.

211. Senok AC, Nelson EA, Li K, et al. Thalassaemia trait, red blood cell age and oxidant stress: effects on Plasmodium falciparum growth and sensitivity to artemisinin. *Trans R Soc Trop Med Hyg.* 1997;91:585-589.

212. Luzzi GA, Merry AH, Newbold CI, et al. Protection by alpha-thalassaemia against Plasmodium falciparum malaria: modified surface antigen expression rather than impaired growth or cytoadherence. *Immunol Lett.* 1991;30:233-240.

213. Luzzi GA, Merry AH, Newbold CI, et al. Surface antigen expression on Plasmodium falciparum-infected erythrocytes is modified in alpha- and beta-thalassemia. *J Exp Med.* 1991;173:785-791.

214. Williams TN, Wambua S, Uyoga S, et al. Both heterozygous and homozygous alpha+ thalassemias protect against severe and fatal *Plasmodium falciparum* malaria on the coast of Kenya. *Blood.* 2005;106:368-371.

215. Williams TN, Mwangi TW, Wambua S, et al. Negative epistasis between the malaria-protective effects of alpha+-thalassemia and the sickle cell trait. *Nat Genet.* 2005;37:1253-1257.

216. Wambua S, Mwangi TW, Kortok M, et al. The effect of alpha+-thalassaemia on the incidence of malaria and other diseases in children living on the coast of Kenya. *PLoS Med.* 2006;3:e158.

217. Fowkes FJ, Allen SJ, Allen A, et al. Increased microerythrocyte count in homozygous alpha(+)-thalassaemia contributes to protection against severe malarial anaemia. *PLoS Med.* 2008;5:e56.

218. Shear HL, Grinberg L, Gilman J, et al. Transgenic mice expressing human fetal globin are protected from malaria by a novel mechanism. *Blood.* 1998;92:2520-2526.

219. Friedman MJ. Oxidant damage mediates variant red cell resistance to malaria. *Nature.* 1979;280:245-247.

220. Mockenhaupt FP, Mandelkow J, Till H, et al. Reduced prevalence of Plasmodium falciparum infection and of concomitant anaemia in pregnant women with heterozygous G6PD deficiency. *Trop Med Int Health.* 2003;8:118-124.

221. Guindo A, Fairhurst RM, Doumbo OK, et al. X-linked G6PD deficiency protects hemizygous males but not heterozygous females against severe malaria. *PLoS Med.* 2007;4:e66.

222. Cappadoro M, Giribaldi G, O'Brien E, et al. Early phagocytosis of glucose-6-phosphate dehydrogenase (G6PD)-deficient erythrocytes parasitized by Plasmodium falciparum may explain malaria protection in G6PD deficiency. *Blood.* 1998;92:2527-2534.

223. Jarolim P, Palek J, Amato D, et al. Deletion in erythrocyte band 3 gene in malaria-resistant Southeast Asian ovalocytosis. *Proc Natl Acad Sci U S A.* 1991;88:11022-11026.

224. Mohandas N, Lie-Injo LE, Friedman M, et al. Rigid membranes of Malayan ovalocytes: a likely genetic barrier against malaria. *Blood.* 1984;63:1385-1392.

225. Liu SC, Palek J, Yi SJ, et al. Molecular basis of altered red blood cell membrane properties in Southeast Asian ovalocytosis: role of the mutant band 3 protein in band 3 oligomerization and retention by the membrane skeleton. *Blood.* 1995;86:349-358.

226. Dluzewski AR, Nash GB, Wilson RJ, et al. Invasion of hereditary ovalocytes by Plasmodium falciparum in vitro and its relation to intracellular ATP concentration. *Mol Biochem Parasitol.* 1992;55:1-7.

227. Foo LC, Rekhraj V, Chiang GL, et al. Ovalocytosis protects against severe malaria parasitemia in the Malayan aborigines. *Am J Trop Med Hyg.* 1992;47:271-275.

228. Cattani JA, Gibson FD, Alpers MP, et al. Hereditary ovalocytosis and reduced susceptibility to malaria in Papua New Guinea. *Trans R Soc Trop Med Hyg.* 1987;81:705-709.

229. Cortes A, Benet A, Cooke BM, et al. Ability of *Plasmodium falciparum* to invade Southeast Asian ovalocytes varies between parasite lines. *Blood.* 2004;104:2961-2966.

230. Allen SJ, O'Donnell A, Alexander ND, et al. Prevention of cerebral malaria in children in Papua New Guinea by southeast Asian ovalocytosis band 3. *Am J Trop Med Hyg.* 1999;60:1056-1060.

231. Rowe JA, Handel IG, Thera MA, et al. Blood group O protects against severe Plasmodium falciparum malaria through the mechanism of reduced rosetting. *Proc Natl Acad Sci U S A.* 2007;104:17471-17476.

232. Fry AE, Griffiths MJ, Auburn S, et al. Common variation in the ABO glycosyltransferase is associated with susceptibility to severe Plasmodium falciparum malaria. *Hum Mol Genet.* 2008;17:567-576.

233. Welch SG, McGregor IA, Williams K. The Duffy blood group and malaria prevalence in Gambian West Africans. *Trans R Soc Trop Med Hyg.* 1977;71:295-296.

234. Miller LH, Mason SJ, Clyde DF, et al. The resistance factor to Plasmodium vivax in blacks. The Duffy-blood-group genotype, FyFy. *N Engl J Med.* 1976;295:302-304.

235. Zimmerman PA, Woolley I, Masinde GL, et al. Emergence of FY*A(null) in a Plasmodium vivax-endemic region of Papua New Guinea. *Proc Natl Acad Sci U S A.* 1999;96:13973-13977.

236. Baird JK, Krisin, Barcus MJ, et al. Onset of clinical immunity to Plasmodium falciparum among Javanese migrants to Indonesian Papua. *Ann Trop Med Parasitol.* 2003;97:557-564.

237. Wichmann O, Loscher T, Jelinek T. Fatal malaria in a German couple returning from Burkina Faso. *Infection.* 2003;31:260-262.

238. Deloron P, Chougnet C. Is immunity to malaria really short-lived? *Parasitol Today.* 1992;8:375-378.

239. Bouchaud O, Cot M, Kony S, et al. Do African immigrants living in France have long-term malarial immunity? *Am J Trop Med Hyg.* 2005;72:21-25.

240. Chotivanich K, Udomsangpetch R, McGready R, et al. Central role of the spleen in malaria parasite clearance. *J Infect Dis.* 2002;185:1538-1541.

241. Grobusch MP, Borrmann S, Omva J, et al. Severe malaria in a splenectomised Gabonese woman. *Wien Klin Wochenschr.* 2003;115:63-65.

242. Artavanis-Tsakonas K, Tongren JE, Riley EM. The war between the malaria parasite and the immune system: immunity, immunoregulation and immunopathology. *Clin Exp Immunol.* 2003;133:145-152.

243. Marsh K, Otoo L, Hayes RJ, et al. Antibodies to blood stage antigens of *Plasmodium falciparum* in rural Gambians and their relation to protection against infection. *Trans R Soc Trop Med Hyg.* 1989;83:293-303.

244. Collins WE, Jeffery GM. A retrospective examination of sporozoite- and trophozoite-induced infections with Plasmodium falciparum: development of parasitologic and clinical immunity during primary infection. *Am J Trop Med Hyg.* 1999;61:4-19.

245. Collins WE, Jeffery GM. A retrospective examination of secondary sporozoite- and trophozoite-induced infections with *Plasmodium falciparum*: development of parasitologic and clinical immunity following secondary infection. *Am J Trop Med Hyg.* 1999;61:20-35.

246. Collins WE, Jeffery GM. A retrospective examination of sporozoite- and trophozoite-induced infections with *Plasmodium falciparum* in patients previously infected with heterologous species of *Plasmodium*: effect on development of parasitologic and clinical immunity. *Am J Trop Med Hyg.* 1999;61:36-43.

247. Sama W, Killeen G, Smith T. Estimating the duration of Plasmodium falciparum infection from trials of indoor residual spraying. *Am J Trop Med Hyg.* 2004;70:625-634.

248. Greenwood T, Vikerfors T, Sjoberg M, et al. Febrile Plasmodium falciparum malaria 4 years after exposure in a man with sickle cell disease. *Clin Infect Dis.* 2008;47:e39-41.

249. Bull PC, Kortok M, Kai O, et al. Plasmodium falciparum-infected erythrocytes: agglutination by diverse Kenyan plasma is associated with severe disease and young host age. *J Infect Dis.* 2000;182:252-259.

250. Ofori MF, Dodoo D, Staalsoe T, et al. Malaria-induced acquisition of antibodies to Plasmodium falciparum variant surface antigens. *Infect Immun.* 2002;70:2982-2988.

251. Tebo AE, Kremsner PG, Piper KP, et al. Low antibody responses to variant surface antigens of Plasmodium falciparum are associated with severe malaria and increased susceptibility to malaria attacks in Gabonese children. *Am J Trop Med Hyg.* 2002;67:597-603.

252. Bull PC, Lowe BS, Kortok M, et al. Parasite antigens on the infected red cell surface are targets for naturally acquired immunity to malaria. *Nat Med.* 1998;4:358-360.

253. Win TT, Lin K, Mizuno S, et al. Wide distribution of Plasmodium ovale in Myanmar. *Trop Med Int Health.* 2002;7:231-239.

254. Lysenko AJ, Beljaev AE. An analysis of the geographical distribution of Plasmodium ovale. *Bull World Health Organ.* 1969;40:383-394.

255. Cox-Singh J, Singh B. Knowlesi malaria: newly emergent and of public health importance? *Trends Parasitol.* 2008;24:406-410.

256. Jordan S, Jelinek T, Aida AO, et al. Population structure of Plasmodium falciparum isolates during an epidemic in southern Mauritania. *Trop Med Int Health.* 2001;6:761-766.

257. Tuck JJ, Green AD, Roberts KI. A malaria outbreak following a British military deployment to Sierra Leone. *J Infect.* 2003;47:225-230.

258. Das P. Ethiopia faces severe malaria epidemic. WHO predicts 15 million people could be infected. *Lancet.* 2003;362:2071.

259. Baomar A, Mohamed A. Malaria outbreak in a malaria-free region in Oman 1998: unknown impact of civil war in Africa. *Public Health.* 2000;114:480-483.

260. Schlagenhauf P, Steffen R, Loutan L. Migrants as a major risk group for imported malaria in European countries. *J Travel Med.* 2003;10:106-107.

261. Dar FK, Bayoumi R, al Karmi T, et al. Status of imported malaria in a control zone of the United Arab Emirates bordering an area of unstable malaria. *Trans R Soc Trop Med Hyg.* 1993;87:617-619.

262. Paxton LA, Slutsker L, Schultz LJ, et al. Imported malaria in Montagnard refugees settling in North Carolina: implications for prevention and control. *Am J Trop Med Hyg.* 1996;54:54-57.

263. Barber MA. The history of malaria in the United States. *Public Health Reports.* 1929;44:2575-2587.

264. Local transmission of Plasmodium vivax malaria–Palm Beach County, Florida, 2003. *MMWR Morb Mortal Wkly Rep.* 2003;52:908-911.

265. Zucker JR. Changing patterns of autochthonous malaria transmission in the United States: a review of recent outbreaks. *Emerg Infect Dis.* 1996;2:37-43.

266. Thang HD, Elsas RM, Veenstra J. Airport malaria: report of a case and a brief review of the literature. *Neth J Med.* 2002;60:441-443.

267. Lusina D, Legros F, Esteve V, et al. Airport malaria: four new cases in suburban Paris during summer 1999. *Euro Surveill.* 2000;5:76-80.

268. Gratz NG, Steffen R, Cocksedge W. Why aircraft disinsection? *Bull World Health Organ.* 2000;78:995-1004.

269. Mungai M, Tegtmeier G, Chamberland M, et al. Transfusion-transmitted malaria in the United States from 1963 through 1999. *N Engl J Med.* 2001;344:1973-1978.

270. Bruce-Chwatt LJ. Transfusion malaria revisited. *Trop Dis Bull.* 1982;79:827-840.

271. Chiche L, Lesage A, Duhamel C, et al. Posttransplant malaria: first case of transmission of Plasmodium falciparum from a white multiorgan donor to four recipients. *Transplantation.* 2003;75:166-168.

272. al Arishi HM, el Awad Ahmed F, al Bishi LA. Chloroquine-resistant Plasmodium falciparum malaria among children seen in a regional hospital, Tabuk, Saudi Arabia. *Trans R Soc Trop Med Hyg.* 2001;95:439-440.

273. Ghalib HW, Al-Ghamdi S, Akood M, et al. Therapeutic efficacy of chloroquine against uncomplicated, Plasmodium falciparum malaria in south-western Saudi Arabia. *Ann Trop Med Parasitol.* 2001;95:773-779.

274. Jafari S, Le Bras J, Asmar M, et al. Molecular survey of Plasmodium falciparum resistance in south-eastern Iran. *Ann Trop Med Parasitol.* 2003;97:119-124.

275. Al-Maktari MT, Bassiouny HK. Malaria status in Al-Hodeidah Governorate, Republic of Yemen. Part II: Human factors causing the persistence of chloroquine-resistant P. falciparum local strain. *J Egypt Soc Parasitol.* 2003;33:829-839.

276. Bayoumi RA, Dar FK, Tanira MO, et al. Effect of previous chloroquine intake on in vivo P. falciparum drug sensitivity. *East Afr Med J.* 1997;74:278-282.

277. Sumawinata IW, Bernadeta, Leksana B, et al. Very high risk of therapeutic failure with chloroquine for uncomplicated Plasmodium falciparum and P. vivax malaria in Indonesian Papua. *Am J Trop Med Hyg.* 2003;68:416-420.

278. Murphy GS, Basri H, Purnomo, et al. Vivax malaria resistant to treatment and prophylaxis with chloroquine. *Lancet.* 1993;341:96-100.

279. Baird JK, Wiady I, Fryauff DJ, et al. In vivo resistance to chloroquine by Plasmodium vivax and Plasmodium falciparum at Nabire, Irian Jaya, Indonesia. *Am J Trop Med Hyg.* 1997;56:627-631.

280. Soto J, Toledo J, Gutierrez P, et al. Plasmodium vivax clinically resistant to chloroquine in Colombia. *Am J Trop Med Hyg.* 2001;65:90-93.

281. Garavelli PL, Corti E. Chloroquine resistance in Plasmodium vivax: the first case in Brazil. *Trans R Soc Trop Med Hyg.* 1992;86:128.

282. Ruebush TK 2nd, Zegarra J, Cairo J, et al. Chloroquine-resistant Plasmodium vivax malaria in Peru. *Am J Trop Med Hyg.* 2003;69:548-552.

283. Marlar T, Myat Phone K, Aye Yu S, et al. Development of resistance to chloroquine by Plasmodium vivax in Myanmar. *Trans R Soc Trop Med Hyg.* 1995;89:307-308.

284. Garg M, Gopinathan N, Bodhe P, et al. Vivax malaria resistant to chloroquine: case reports from Bombay. *Trans R Soc Trop Med Hyg.* 1995;89:656-657.

285. Barrett JP, Behrens RH. Prophylaxis Failure Against Vivax Malaria in Guyana, South America. *J Travel Med.* 1996;3:60-61.

286. Maguire JD, Sumawinata IW, Masbar S, et al. Chloroquine-resistant Plasmodium malariae in south Sumatra, Indonesia. *Lancet.* 2002;360:58-60.

287. Laufer MK, Thesing PC, Eddington ND, et al. Return of chloroquine antimalarial efficacy in Malawi. *N Engl J Med.* 2006;355:1959-1966.

288. Wang X, Mu J, Li G, et al. Decreased prevalence of the Plasmodium falciparum chloroquine resistance transporter 76T marker associated with cessation of chloroquine use against P. falciparum malaria in Hainan, People's Republic of China. *Am J Trop Med Hyg.* 2005;72:410-414.

289. Mandi G, Mockenhaupt FP, Coulibaly B, et al. Efficacy of amodiaquine in the treatment of uncomplicated falciparum malaria in young children of rural north-western Burkina Faso. *Malar J.* 2008;7:58.

290. Holmgren G, Bjorkman A, Gil JP. Amodiaquine resistance is not related to rare findings of pfmdr1 gene amplifications in Kenya. *Trop Med Int Health.* 2006;11:1808-1812.

291. Dokomajilar C, Lankoande ZM, Dorsey G, et al. Roles of specific *Plasmodium falciparum* mutations in resistance to amodiaquine and sulfadoxine-pyrimethamine in Burkina Faso. *Am J Trop Med Hyg.* 2006;75:162-165.

292. Happi CT, Gbotosho GO, Folarin OA, et al. Association between mutations in Plasmodium falciparum chloroquine resistance transporter and P. falciparum multidrug resistance 1 genes and

in vivo amodiaquine resistance in P. falciparum malaria-infected children in Nigeria. *Am J Trop Med Hyg.* 2006;75: 155-161.

293. Zongo I, Dorsey G, Rouamba N, et al. Amodiaquine, sulfadoxine-pyrimethamine, and combination therapy for uncomplicated falciparum malaria: a randomized controlled trial from Burkina Faso. *Am J Trop Med Hyg.* 2005;73:826-832.

294. Marfurt J, Mueller I, Sie A, et al. Low efficacy of amodiaquine or chloroquine plus sulfadoxine-pyrimethamine against Plasmodium falciparum and P. vivax malaria in Papua New Guinea. *Am J Trop Med Hyg.* 2007;77:947-954.

295. Durrani N, Leslie T, Rahim S, et al. Efficacy of combination therapy with artesunate plus amodiaquine compared to monotherapy with chloroquine, amodiaquine or sulfadoxine-pyrimethamine for treatment of uncomplicated Plasmodium falciparum in Afghanistan. *Trop Med Int Health.* 2005;10:521-529.

296. Wongsrichanalai C, Sirichaisinthop J, Karwacki JJ, et al. Drug resistant malaria on the Thai-Myanmar and Thai-Cambodian borders. *Southeast Asian J Trop Med Public Health.* 2001;32:41-49.

297. Giao PT, De Vries PJ, Hung LQ, et al. Atovaquone-proguanil for recrudescent Plasmodium falciparum in Vietnam. *Ann Trop Med Parasitol.* 2003;97:575-580.

298. Nosten F, ter Kuile F, Chongsuphajaisiddhi T, et al. Mefloquine-resistant falciparum malaria on the Thai-Burmese border. *Lancet.* 1991;337:1140-1143.

299. Chia JK, Nakata MM, Co S. Smear-negative cerebral malaria due to mefloquine-resistant Plasmodium falciparum acquired in the Amazon. *J Infect Dis.* 1992;165:599-600.

300. Fryauff DJ, Owusu-Agyei S, Utz G, et al. Mefloquine treatment for uncomplicated falciparum malaria in young children 6-24 months of age in northern Ghana. *Am J Trop Med Hyg.* 2007; 76:224-231.

301. Maguire JD, Lacy MD, Sururi, et al. Chloroquine or sulfadoxine-pyrimethamine for the treatment of uncomplicated, Plasmodium falciparum malaria during an epidemic in Central Java, Indonesia. *Ann Trop Med Parasitol.* 2002;96: 655-668.

302. Mayxay M, Newton PN, Khanthavong M, et al. Chloroquine versus sulfadoxine-pyrimethamine for treatment of Plasmodium falciparum malaria in Savannakhet Province, Lao People's Democratic Republic: an assessment of national antimalarial drug recommendations. *Clin Infect Dis.* 2003;37:1021-1028.

303. Hurwitz ES, Johnson D, Campbell CC. Resistance of Plasmodium falciparum malaria to sulfadoxine-pyrimethamine ('Fansidar') in a refugee camp in Thailand. *Lancet.* 1981;1:1068-1070.

304. Aramburu Guarda J, Ramal Asayag C, Witzig R. Malaria reemergence in the Peruvian Amazon region. *Emerg Infect Dis.* 1999;5:209-215.

305. Vasconcelos KF, Plowe CV, Fontes CJ, et al. Mutations in Plasmodium falciparum dihydrofolate reductase and dihydropteroate synthase of isolates from the Amazon region of Brazil. *Mem Inst Oswaldo Cruz.* 2000;95:721-728.

306. Deloron P, Mayombo J, Le Cardinal A, et al. Sulfadoxine-pyrimethamine for the treatment of Plasmodium falciparum malaria in Gabonese children. *Trans R Soc Trop Med Hyg.* 2000;94:188-190.

307. Bijl HM, Kager J, Koetsier DW, et al. Chloroquine- and sulfadoxine-pyrimethamine-resistant Falciparum malaria in vivo—a pilot study in rural Zambia. *Trop Med Int Health.* 2000;5:692-695.

308. Gasasira AF, Dorsey G, Nzarubara B, et al. Comparative efficacy of aminoquinoline-antifolate combinations for the treatment of uncomplicated falciparum malaria in Kampala, Uganda. *Am J Trop Med Hyg.* 2003;68:127-132.

309. Landgraf B, Kollaritsch H, Wiedermann G, et al. Plasmodium falciparum: susceptibility in vitro and in vivo to chloroquine and sulfadoxine-pyrimethamine in Ghanaian schoolchildren. *Trans R Soc Trop Med Hyg.* 1994;88:440-442.

310. Chaudhuri RN, Rai Chaudhuri MN. Falciparum infection refractory to paludrine. *Indian Journal of Malaria.* 1949;3: 365-369.

311. Field JW, Edeson JFB. Paludrine-resistant falciparum malaria. *Transactions of the Royal Society of Tropical Medicine and Hygiene.* 1949;43:233-236.

312. Clyde DF. Field trials of repository antimalarial compounds. *J Trop Med Hyg.* 1969;72:81-85.

313. Peterson DS, Milhous WK, Wellems TE. Molecular basis of differential resistance to cycloguanil and pyrimethamine in *Plasmodium falciparum* malaria. *Proc Natl Acad Sci USA.* 1990; 87:3018-3022.

314. Foote SJ, Galatis D, Cowman AF. Amino acids in the dihydrofolate reductase-thymidylate synthase gene of Plasmodium falciparum involved in cycloguanil resistance differ from those involved in pyrimethamine resistance. *Proc Natl Acad Sci U S A.* 1990;87:3014-3017.

315. Helsby NA, Edwards G, Breckenridge AM, et al. The multiple dose pharmacokinetics of proguanil. *Br J Clin Pharmacol.* 1993;35:653-656.

316. Watkins WM, Chulay JD, Sixsmith DG, et al. A preliminary pharmacokinetic study of the antimalarial drugs, proguanil and chlorproguanil. *J Pharm Pharmacol.* 1987;39:261-265.

317. Yeo AE, Edstein MD, Shanks GD, et al. A statistical analysis of the antimalarial activity of proguanil and cycloguanil in human volunteers. *Ann Trop Med Parasitol.* 1994;88:587-594.

318. Wichmann O, Muehlen M, Gruss H, et al. Malarone treatment failure not associated with previously described mutations in the cytochrome b gene. *Malar J.* 2004;3:14.

319. Fivelman QL, Butcher GA, Adagu IS, et al. Malarone treatment failure and in vitro confirmation of resistance of Plasmodium falciparum isolate from Lagos, Nigeria. *Malar J.* 2002;1:1.

320. Schwartz E, Bujanover S, Kain KC. Genetic confirmation of atovaquone-proguanil-resistant Plasmodium falciparum malaria acquired by a nonimmune traveler to East Africa. *Clin Infect Dis.* 2003;37:450-451.

321. Rose GW, Suh KN, Kain KC, et al. Atovaquone-proguanil resistance in imported falciparum malaria in a young child. *Pediatr Infect Dis J.* 2008;27:567-569.

322. Krudsood S, Patel SN, Tangpukdee N, et al. Efficacy of atovaquone-proguanil for treatment of acute multidrug-resistant Plasmodium falciparum malaria in Thailand. *Am J Trop Med Hyg.* 2007;76:655-658.

323. Pukrittayakamee S, Supanaranond W, Looareesuwan S, et al. Quinine in severe falciparum malaria: evidence of declining efficacy in Thailand. *Trans R Soc Trop Med Hyg.* 1994;88:324-327.

324. Jelinek T, Schelbert P, Loscher T, et al. Quinine resistant falciparum malaria acquired in east Africa. *Trop Med Parasitol.* 1995;46:38-40.

325. Segurado AA, di Santi SM, Shiroma M. In vivo and in vitro Plasmodium falciparum resistance to chloroquine, amodiaquine and quinine in the Brazilian Amazon. *Rev Inst Med Trop Sao Paulo.* 1997;39:85-90.

326. Resistance to artemisinin derivatives along the Thai-Cambodian border. *Wkly Epidemiol Rec.* 2007;82:360.

327. White NJ. Qinghaosu (artemisinin): the price of success. *Science.* 2008;320:330-334.

328. Chou AC, Chevli R, Fitch CD. Ferriprotoporphyrin IX fulfills the criteria for identification as the chloroquine receptor of malaria parasites. *Biochemistry.* 1980;19:1543-1549.

329. Verdier F, Le Bras J, Clavier F, et al. Chloroquine uptake by Plasmodium falciparum-infected human erythrocytes during in vitro culture and its relationship to chloroquine resistance. *Antimicrob Agents Chemother.* 1985;27:561-564.

330. Fidock DA, Nomura T, Talley AK, et al. Mutations in the P. falciparum digestive vacuole transmembrane protein PfCRT and evidence for their role in chloroquine resistance. *Mol Cell.* 2000;6:861-871.

331. Cooper RA, Ferdig MT, Su XZ, et al. Alternative mutations at position 76 of the vacuolar transmembrane protein PfCRT are associated with chloroquine resistance and unique stereospecific quinine and quinidine responses in Plasmodium falciparum. *Mol Pharmacol.* 2002;61:35-42.

332. Sidhu AB, Verdier-Pinard D, Fidock DA. Chloroquine resistance in Plasmodium falciparum malaria parasites conferred by pfcrt mutations. *Science.* 2002;298:210-213.

333. Wootton JC, Feng X, Ferdig MT, et al. Genetic diversity and chloroquine selective sweeps in Plasmodium falciparum. *Nature.* 2002;418:320-323.

334. Nagesha HS, Casey GJ, Rieckmann KH, et al. New haplotypes of the Plasmodium falciparum chloroquine resistance transporter (pfcrt) gene among chloroquine-resistant parasite isolates. *Am J Trop Med Hyg.* 2003;68:398-402.

335. Chen N, Kyle DE, Pasay C, et al. pfcrt Allelic types with two novel amino acid mutations in chloroquine-resistant Plasmodium falciparum isolates from the Philippines. *Antimicrob Agents Chemother.* 2003;47:3500-3505.

336. May J, Meyer CG. Association of Plasmodium falciparum chloroquine resistance transporter variant T76 with age-related plasma chloroquine levels. *Am J Trop Med Hyg.* 2003;68: 143-146.

337. Djimde A, Doumbo OK, Cortese JF, et al. A molecular marker for chloroquine-resistant falciparum malaria. *N Engl J Med.* 2001;344:257-263.

338. Sanchez CP, Stein W, Lanzer M. Trans stimulation provides evidence for a drug efflux carrier as the mechanism of chloroquine resistance in Plasmodium falciparum. *Biochemistry.* 2003;42:9383-9394.

339. Krogstad DJ, Gluzman IY, Herwaldt BL, et al. Energy dependence of chloroquine accumulation and chloroquine efflux in Plasmodium falciparum. *Biochem Pharmacol.* 1992;43:57-62.

340. Bray PG, Martin RE, Tilley L, et al. Defining the role of PfCRT in Plasmodium falciparum chloroquine resistance. *Mol Microbiol.* 2005;56:323-333.

341. Djimde AA, Doumbo OK, Traore O, et al. Clearance of drug-resistant parasites as a model for protective immunity in Plasmodium falciparum malaria. *Am J Trop Med Hyg.* 2003;69: 558-563.

342. Reed MB, Saliba KJ, Caruana SR, et al. Pgh1 modulates sensitivity and resistance to multiple antimalarials in Plasmodium falciparum. *Nature.* 2000;403:906-909.

343. Mu J, Ferdig MT, Feng X, et al. Multiple transporters associated with malaria parasite responses to chloroquine and quinine. *Mol Microbiol.* 2003;49:977-989.

344. Peterson DS, Walliker D, Wellems TE. Evidence that a point mutation in dihydrofolate reductase-thymidylate synthase confers resistance to pyrimethamine in falciparum malaria. *Proc Natl Acad Sci U S A.* 1988;85:9114-9118.

345. Cowman AF, Morry MJ, Biggs BA, et al. Amino acid changes linked to pyrimethamine resistance in the dihydrofolate reductase-thymidylate synthase gene of *Plasmodium falciparum.* *Proc Natl Acad Sci U S A.* 1988;85:9109-9113.

346. Wang P, Read M, Sims PF, et al. Sulfadoxine resistance in the human malaria parasite *Plasmodium falciparum* is determined by mutations in dihydropteroate synthetase and an additional factor associated with folate utilization. *Mol Microbiol.* 1997; 23:979-986.

347. Triglia T, Menting JG, Wilson C, et al. Mutations in dihydropteroate synthase are responsible for sulfone and sulfonamide resistance in Plasmodium falciparum. *Proc Natl Acad Sci U S A.* 1997;94:13944-13949.

348. Plowe CV, Cortese JF, Djimde A, et al. Mutations in Plasmodium falciparum dihydrofolate reductase and dihydropteroate synthase and epidemiologic patterns of pyrimethamine-sulfadoxine use and resistance. *J Infect Dis.* 1997;176:1590-1596.

349. Srivastava IK, Morrisey JM, Darrouzet E, et al. Resistance mutations reveal the atovaquone-binding domain of cytochrome b in malaria parasites. *Mol Microbiol.* 1999;33:704-711.

350. Srivastava IK, Rottenberg H, Vaidya AB. Atovaquone, a broad spectrum antiparasitic drug, collapses mitochondrial membrane potential in a malarial parasite. *J Biol Chem.* 1997;272:3961-3966.

351. Srivastava IK, Vaidya AB. A mechanism for the synergistic antimalarial action of atovaquone and proguanil. *Antimicrob Agents Chemother.* 1999;43:1334-1339.

352. Schwobel B, Alifrangis M, Salanti A, et al. Different mutation patterns of atovaquone resistance to Plasmodium falciparum in vitro and in vivo: rapid detection of codon 268 polymorphisms in the cytochrome b as potential in vivo resistance marker. *Malar J.* 2003;2:5.

353. David KP, Alifrangis M, Salanti A, et al. Atovaquone/proguanil resistance in Africa: a case report. *Scand J Infect Dis.* 2003;35: 897-898.

354. Fidock DA, Nomura T, Wellems TE. Cycloguanil and its parent compound proguanil demonstrate distinct activities against Plasmodium falciparum malaria parasites transformed with human dihydrofolate reductase. *Mol Pharmacol.* 1998;54:1140-1147.

355. Basco LK, Ringwald P. Molecular epidemiology of malaria in Yaounde, Cameroon. VI. Sequence variations in the Plasmodium falciparum dihydrofolate reductase-thymidylate synthase gene and in vitro resistance to pyrimethamine and cycloguanil. *Am J Trop Med Hyg.* 2000;62:271-276.

356. Basco LK. Molecular epidemiology of malaria in Cameroon. XII. In vitro drug assays and molecular surveillance of chloroquine and proguanil resistance. *Am J Trop Med Hyg.* 2002; 67:383-387.

357. Pickard AL, Wongsrichanalai C, Purfield A, et al. Resistance to antimalarials in Southeast Asia and genetic polymorphisms in pfmdr1. *Antimicrob Agents Chemother.* 2003;47:2418-2423.

358. Basco LK, Le Bras J. In vitro activity of halofantrine and its relationship to other standard antimalarial drugs against African isolates and clones of Plasmodium falciparum. *Am J Trop Med Hyg.* 1992;47:521-527.

359. Brasseur P, Kouamouo J, Moyou-Somo R, et al. Multi-drug resistant falciparum malaria in Cameroon in 1987-1988. II. Mefloquine resistance confirmed in vivo and in vitro and its correlation with quinine resistance. *Am J Trop Med Hyg.* 1992;46:8-14.

360. Warsame M, Wernsdorfer WH, Payne D, et al. Susceptibility of Plasmodium falciparum in vitro to chloroquine, mefloquine, quinine and sulfadoxine/pyrimethamine in Somalia: relationships between the responses to the different drugs. *Trans R Soc Trop Med Hyg.* 1991;85:565-569.

361. Cowman AF, Galatis D, Thompson JK. Selection for mefloquine resistance in Plasmodium falciparum is linked to amplification of the pfmdr1 gene and cross-resistance to halofantrine and quinine. *Proc Natl Acad Sci U S A.* 1994;91:1143-1147.

362. Ferdig MT, Cooper RA, Mu J, et al. Dissecting the loci of low-level quinine resistance in malaria parasites. *Mol Microbiol.* 2004;52:985-997.

363. Afonso A, Hunt P, Cheesman S, et al. Malaria parasites can develop stable resistance to artemisinin but lack mutations in candidate genes atp6 (encoding the sarcoplasmic and endoplasmic reticulum Ca2+ ATPase), tctp, mdr1, and cg10. *Antimicrob Agents Chemother.* 2006;50:480-489.

364. Puri SK, Chandra R. Plasmodium vinckei: selection of a strain exhibiting stable resistance to arteether. *Exp Parasitol.* 2006;114: 129-132.

365. Eckstein-Ludwig U, Webb RJ, Van Goethem ID, et al. Artemisinins target the SERCA of Plasmodium falciparum. *Nature.* 2003;424:957-961.

366. Jambou R, Legrand E, Niang M, et al. Resistance of Plasmodium falciparum field isolates to in-vitro artemether and point mutations of the SERCA-type PfATPase6. *Lancet.* 2005;366:1960-1963.

367. Schwartz E, Parise M, Kozarsky P, et al. Delayed onset of malaria–implications for chemoprophylaxis in travelers. *N Engl J Med.* 2003;349:1510-1516.

368. Chadee DD, Tilluckdharry CC, Maharaj P, et al. Reactivation of Plasmodium malariae infection in a Trinidadian man after neurosurgery. *N Engl J Med.* 2000;342:1924.

369. Tsuchida H, Yamaguchi K, Yamamoto S, et al. Quartan malaria following splenectomy 36 years after infection. *Am J Trop Med Hyg.* 1982;31:163-165.

370. Kockaerts Y, Vanhees S, Knockaert DC, et al. Imported malaria in the 1990s: a review of 101 patients. *Eur J Emerg Med.* 2001;8: 287-290.

371. Jelinek T, Nothdurft HD, Loscher T. Malaria in Nonimmune Travelers: A Synopsis of History, Symptoms, and Treatment in 160 Patients. *J Travel Med.* 1994;1:199-202.
372. Hu KK, Maung C, Katz DL. Clinical diagnosis of malaria on the Thai-Myanmar border. *Yale J Biol Med.* 2001;74:303-308.
373. Casalino E, Le Bras J, Chaussin F, et al. Predictive factors of malaria in travelers to areas where malaria is endemic. *Arch Intern Med.* 2002;162:1625-1630.
374. van der Hoek W, Premasiri DA, Wickremasinghe AR. Early diagnosis and treatment of malaria in a refugee population in Sri Lanka. *Southeast Asian J Trop Med Public Health.* 1997;28:12-17.
375. Hamel CT, Blum J, Harder F, et al. Nonoperative treatment of splenic rupture in malaria tropica: review of literature and case report. *Acta Trop.* 2002;82:1-5.
376. Davies GR, Venkatesan P. Successful conservative management of splenic rupture in vivax malaria. *Trans R Soc Trop Med Hyg.* 2002;96:149-150.
377. Milne LM, Kyi MS, Chiodini PL, et al. Accuracy of routine laboratory diagnosis of malaria in the United Kingdom. *J Clin Pathol.* 1994;47:740-742.
378. Kantele A, Marti H, Felger I, et al. Monkey malaria in a European traveler returning from Malaysia. *Emerg Infect Dis.* 2008;14:1434-1436.
379. Nguyen PH, Day N, Pram TD, et al. Intraleucocytic malaria pigment and prognosis in severe malaria. *Trans R Soc Trop Med Hyg.* 1995;89:200-204.
380. Gutman JD, Kotton CN, Kratz A. Case records of the Massachusetts General Hospital. Weekly clinicopathological exercises. Case 29-2003. A 60-year-old man with fever, rigors, and sweats. *N Engl J Med.* 2003;349:1168-1175.
381. Jelinek T, Grobusch MP, Nothdurft HD. Use of dipstick tests for the rapid diagnosis of malaria in nonimmune travelers. *J Travel Med.* 2000;7:175-179.
382. Moody A. Rapid diagnostic tests for malaria parasites. *Clin Microbiol Rev.* 2002;15:66-78.
383. Craig MH, Sharp BL. Comparative evaluation of four techniques for the diagnosis of Plasmodium falciparum infections. *Trans R Soc Trop Med Hyg.* 1997;91:279-282.
384. Wongsrichanalai C, Barcus MJ, Muth S, et al. A review of malaria diagnostic tools: microscopy and rapid diagnostic test (RDT). *Am J Trop Med Hyg.* 2007;77:119-127.
385. Murray CK, Gasser RA Jr, Magill AJ, et al. Update on rapid diagnostic testing for malaria. *Clin Microbiol Rev.* 2008;21:97-110.
386. Beadle C, Long GW, Weiss WR, et al. Diagnosis of malaria by detection of Plasmodium falciparum HRP-2 antigen with a rapid dipstick antigen-capture assay. *Lancet.* 1994;343:564-568.
387. De Monbrison F, Gerome P, Chaulet JF, et al. Comparative diagnostic performance of two commercial rapid tests for malaria in a non-endemic area. *Eur J Clin Microbiol Infect Dis.* 2004;23:784-786.
388. Susi B, Whitman T, Blazes DL, et al. Rapid diagnostic test for Plasmodium falciparum in 32 Marines medically evacuated from Liberia with a febrile illness. *Ann Intern Med.* 2005;142:476-477.
389. Farcas GA, Zhong KJ, Lovegrove FE, et al. Evaluation of the Binax NOW ICT test versus polymerase chain reaction and microscopy for the detection of malaria in returned travelers. *Am J Trop Med Hyg.* 2003;69:589-592.
390. Singh N, Valecha N, Sharma VP. Malaria diagnosis by field workers using an immunochromatographic test. *Trans R Soc Trop Med Hyg.* 1997;91:396-397.
391. Grobusch MP, Hanscheid T, Zoller T, et al. Rapid immunochromatographic malarial antigen detection unreliable for detecting Plasmodium malariae and Plasmodium ovale. *Eur J Clin Microbiol Infect Dis.* 2002;21:818-820.
392. Ratsimbasoa A, Randriamanantena A, Raherinjafy R, et al. Which malaria rapid test for Madagascar? Field and laboratory evaluation of three tests and expert microscopy of samples from suspected malaria patients in Madagascar. *Am J Trop Med Hyg.* 2007;76:481-485.
393. Bigaillon C, Fontan E, Cavallo JD, et al. Ineffectiveness of the Binax NOW malaria test for diagnosis of Plasmodium ovale malaria. *J Clin Microbiol.* 2005;43:1011.
394. Soto Tarazona A, Solari Zerpa L, Mendoza Requena D, et al. Evaluation of the rapid diagnostic test OptiMAL for diagnosis of malaria due to Plasmodium vivax. *Braz J Infect Dis.* 2004;8:151-155.
395. Makler MT, Hinrichs DJ. Measurement of the lactate dehydrogenase activity of Plasmodium falciparum as an assessment of parasitemia. *Am J Trop Med Hyg.* 1993;48:205-210.
396. Ladhani S, Lowe B, Cole AO, et al. Changes in white blood cells and platelets in children with falciparum malaria: relationship to disease outcome. *Br J Haematol.* 2002;119:839-847.
397. Alfandari S, Santre C, Chidiac C, et al. Imported malaria: presentation and outcome of 111 cases. *Clin Microbiol Infect.* 1996;2:86-90.
398. Looareesuwan S, Davis JG, Allen DL, et al. Thrombocytopenia in malaria. *Southeast Asian J Trop Med Public Health.* 1992;23:44-50.
399. Oh MD, Shin H, Shin D, et al. Clinical features of vivax malaria. *Am J Trop Med Hyg.* 2001;65:143-146.
400. Ustianowski A, Schwab U, Pasvol G. Case report: severe acute symptomatic hyponatraemia in falciparum malaria. *Trans R Soc Trop Med Hyg.* 2002;96:647-648.
401. Eiam-Ong S. Malarial nephropathy. *Semin Nephrol.* 2003;23:21-33.
402. Berkley J, Mwarumba S, Bramham K, et al. Bacteraemia complicating severe malaria in children. *Trans R Soc Trop Med Hyg.* 1999;93:283-286.
403. Graham SM, Walsh AL, Molyneux EM, et al. Clinical presentation of non-typhoidal Salmonella bacteraemia in Malawian children. *Trans R Soc Trop Med Hyg.* 2000;94:310-314.
404. Severe falciparum malaria. World Health Organization, Communicable Diseases Cluster. *Trans R Soc Trop Med Hyg.* 2000;94(Suppl 1):S1-90.
405. Bruneel F, Hocqueloux L, Alberti C, et al. The clinical spectrum of severe imported falciparum malaria in the intensive care unit: report of 188 cases in adults. *Am J Respir Crit Care Med.* 2003;167:684-689.
406. Newton CR, Chokwe T, Schellenberg JA, et al. Coma scales for children with severe falciparum malaria. *Trans R Soc Trop Med Hyg.* 1997;91:161-165.
407. Crawley J, Smith S, Kirkham F, et al. Seizures and status epilepticus in childhood cerebral malaria. *QJM.* 1996;89:591-597.
408. Muntendam AH, Jaffar S, Bleichrodt N, et al. Absence of neuropsychological sequelae following cerebral malaria in Gambian children. *Trans R Soc Trop Med Hyg.* 1996;90:391-394.
409. Boivin MJ. Effects of early cerebral malaria on cognitive ability in Senegalese children. *J Dev Behav Pediatr.* 2002;23:353-364.
410. Carter JA, Neville BG, Newton CR. Neuro-cognitive impairment following acquired central nervous system infections in childhood: a systematic review. *Brain Res Brain Res Rev.* 2003;43:57-69.
411. Steele RW, Baffoe-Bonnie B. Cerebral malaria in children. *Pediatr Infect Dis J.* 1995;14:281-285.
412. van Hensbroek MB, Onyiorah E, Jaffar S, et al. A trial of artemether or quinine in children with cerebral malaria. *N Engl J Med.* 1996;335:69-75.
413. Bajiya HN, Kochar DK. Incidence and outcome of neurological sequelae in survivors of cerebral malaria. *J Assoc Physicians India.* 1996;44:679-681.
414. D'Acremont V, Landry P, Darioli R, et al. Treatment of imported malaria in an ambulatory setting: prospective study. *BMJ.* 2002;324:875-877.
415. Moore TA, Tomayko JF Jr, Wierman AM, et al. Imported malaria in the 1990s. A report of 59 cases from Houston, Tex. *Arch Fam Med.* 1994;3:130-136.
416. Humar A, Sharma S, Zoutman D, et al. Fatal falciparum malaria in Canadian travellers. *CMAJ.* 1997;156:1165-1167.
417. Kain KC, Harrington MA, Tennyson S, et al. Imported malaria: prospective analysis of problems in diagnosis and management. *Clin Infect Dis.* 1998;27:142-149.
418. Loutan L. Malaria: still a threat to travellers. *Int J Antimicrob Agents.* 2003;21:158-163.
419. Osler W. The study of fevers in the South. *JAMA.* 1896;26:999-1004.
420. Moore DA, Jennings RM, Doherty TF, et al. Assessing the severity of malaria. *BMJ.* 2003;326:808-809.
421. Hammerich A, Campbell OM, Chandramohan D. Unstable malaria transmission and maternal mortality—experiences from Rwanda. *Trop Med Int Health.* 2002;7:573-576.
422. Muhlberger N, Jelinek T, Behrens RH, et al. Age as a risk factor for severe manifestations and fatal outcome of falciparum malaria in European patients: observations from TropNetEurop and SIMPID Surveillance Data. *Clin Infect Dis.* 2003;36:990-995.
423. Luxemburger C, Ricci F, Nosten F, et al. The epidemiology of severe malaria in an area of low transmission in Thailand. *Trans R Soc Trop Med Hyg.* 1997;91:256-262.
424. Dondorp AM, Lee SJ, Faiz MA, et al. The relationship between age and the manifestations of and mortality associated with severe malaria. *Clin Infect Dis.* 2008;47:151-157.
425. Rifakis PM, Hernandez O, Fernandez CT, et al. Atypical Plasmodium vivax malaria in a traveler: bilateral hydronephrosis, severe thrombocytopenia, and hypotension. *J Travel Med.* 2008;15:119-121.
426. Greenberg AE, Lobel HO. Mortality from Plasmodium falciparum malaria in travelers from the United States, 1959 to 1987. *Ann Intern Med.* 1990;113:326-327.
427. Thybo S, Gjorup I, Ronn AM, et al. Atovaquone-proguanil (malarone): an effective treatment for uncomplicated Plasmodium falciparum malaria in travelers from Denmark. *J Travel Med.* 2004;11:220-223.
428. Hitani A, Nakamura T, Ohtomo H, et al. Efficacy and safety of atovaquone-proguanil compared with mefloquine in the treatment of nonimmune patients with uncomplicated P. falciparum malaria in Japan. *J Infect Chemother.* 2006;12:277-282.
429. Savini H, Bogreau H, Bertaux L, et al. First case of emergence of atovaquone-proguanil resistance in Plasmodium falciparum during treatment in a traveler in Comoros. *Antimicrob Agents Chemother.* 2008;52:2283-2284.
430. McGready R, Thwai KL, Cho T, et al. The effects of quinine and chloroquine antimalarial treatments in the first trimester of pregnancy. *Trans R Soc Trop Med Hyg.* 2002;96:180-184.
431. Taylor WR, White NJ. Antimalarial drug toxicity: a review. *Drug Saf.* 2004;27:25-61.
432. Collins GB, McAllister MS. Chloroquine psychosis masquerading as PCP: a case report. *J Psychoactive Drugs.* 2008;40:211-214.
433. Brasseur P, Guiguemde R, Diallo S, et al. Amodiaquine remains effective for treating uncomplicated malaria in west and central Africa. *Trans R Soc Trop Med Hyg.* 1999;93:645-650.
434. Everts RJ, Hayhurst MD, Nona BP. Acute pulmonary edema caused by quinine. *Pharmacotherapy.* 2004;24:1221-1224.
435. Fungladda W, Honrado ER, Thimasarn K, et al. Compliance with artesunate and quinine + tetracycline treatment of uncomplicated falciparum malaria in Thailand. *Bull World Health Organ.* 1998;76(Suppl 1):59-66.
436. McGready R, Cho T, Samuel, et al. Randomized comparison of quinine-clindamycin versus artesunate in the treatment of falciparum malaria in pregnancy. *Trans R Soc Trop Med Hyg.* 2001;95:651-656.
437. Pukrittayakamee S, Chantra A, Vanijanonta S, et al. Therapeutic responses to quinine and clindamycin in multidrug-resistant falciparum malaria. *Antimicrob Agents Chemother.* 2000;44:2395-2398.
438. Lell B, Kremsner PG. Clindamycin as an antimalarial drug: review of clinical trials. *Antimicrob Agents Chemother.* 2002;46:2315-2320.
439. Looareesuwan S, Wilairatana P, Chalermarut K, et al. Efficacy and safety of atovaquone/proguanil compared with mefloquine for treatment of acute Plasmodium falciparum malaria in Thailand. *Am J Trop Med Hyg.* 1999;60:526-532.
440. Marquino W, Huilca M, Calampa C, et al. Efficacy of mefloquine and a mefloquine-artesunate combination therapy for the treatment of uncomplicated Plasmodium falciparum malaria in the Amazon Basin of Peru. *Am J Trop Med Hyg.* 2003;68:608-612.
441. Ranque S, Parola P, Adehossi E, et al. Mefloquine versus 3-day oral quinine-clindamycin in uncomplicated imported falciparum malaria. *Travel Med Infect Dis.* 2007;5:306-309.
442. Matteelli A, Saleri N, Bisoffi Z, et al. Mefloquine versus quinine plus sulphalene-pyrimethamine (metakelfin) for treatment of uncomplicated imported falciparum malaria acquired in Africa. *Antimicrob Agents Chemother.* 2005;49:663-667.
443. Ranque S, Marchou B, Malvy D, et al. Treatment of imported malaria in adults: a multicentre study in France. *QJM.* 2005;98:737-743.
444. Meier CR, Wilcock K, Jick SS. The risk of severe depression, psychosis or panic attacks with prophylactic antimalarials. *Drug Saf.* 2004;27:203-213.
445. van Vugt M, Leonardi E, Phaipun L, et al. Treatment of uncomplicated multidrug-resistant falciparum malaria with artesunate-atovaquone-proguanil. *Clin Infect Dis.* 2002;35:1498-1504.
446. de Alencar FE, Cerutti C Jr, Durlacher RR, et al. Atovaquone and proguanil for the treatment of malaria in Brazil. *J Infect Dis.* 1997;175:1544-1547.
447. Emberger M, Lechner AM, Zelger B. Stevens-Johnson syndrome associated with Malarone antimalarial prophylaxis. *Clin Infect Dis.* 2003;37:e5-7.
448. Remich SA, Otieno W, Polhemus ME, et al. Bullous erythema multiforme after treatment with Malarone, a combination antimalarial composed of atovaquone and proguanil hydrochloride. *Trop Doct.* 2008;38:190-191.
449. Farnert A, Lindberg J, Gil P, et al. Evidence of Plasmodium falciparum malaria resistant to atovaquone and proguanil hydrochloride: case reports. *BMJ.* 2003;326:628-629.
450. Nosten F, White NJ. Artemisinin-based combination treatment of falciparum malaria. *Am J Trop Med Hyg.* 2007;77:181-192.
451. White NJ. The assessment of antimalarial drug efficacy. *Trends Parasitol.* 2002;18:458-464.
452. Adjuik M, Babiker A, Garner P, et al. Artesunate combinations for treatment of malaria: meta-analysis. *Lancet.* 2004;363:9-17.
453. Denis MB, Davis TM, Hewitt S, et al. Efficacy and safety of dihydroartemisinin-piperaquine (Artekin) in Cambodian children and adults with uncomplicated falciparum malaria. *Clin Infect Dis.* 2002;35:1469-1476.
454. Smithuis F, Kyaw MK, Phe O, et al. Efficacy and effectiveness of dihydroartemisinin-piperaquine versus artesunate-mefloquine in falciparum malaria: an open-label randomised comparison. *Lancet.* 2006;367:2075-2085.
455. Janssens B, van Herp M, Goubert L, et al. A randomized open study to assess the efficacy and tolerability of dihydroartemisinin-piperaquine for the treatment of uncomplicated falciparum malaria in Cambodia. *Trop Med Int Health.* 2007;12:251-259.
456. Nothdurft HD, Jelinek T, Pechel SM, et al. Stand-by treatment of suspected malaria in travellers. *Trop Med Parasitol.* 1995;46:161-163.
457. Rozendaal J. Fake antimalaria drugs in Cambodia. *Lancet.* 2001;357:890.
458. Bate R, Coticelli P, Tren R, et al. Antimalarial drug quality in the most severely malarious parts of Africa - a six country study. *PLoS ONE.* 2008;3:e2132.
459. Atemnkeng MA, De Cock K, Plaizier-Vercammen J. Quality control of active ingredients in artemisinin-derivative antimalarials within Kenya and DR Congo. *Trop Med Int Health.* 2007;12:68-74.
460. Tipke M, Diallo S, Coulibaly B, et al. Substandard anti-malarial drugs in Burkina Faso. *Malar J.* 2008;7:95.
461. Binka FN, Morris SS, Ross DA, et al. Patterns of malaria morbidity and mortality in children in northern Ghana. *Trans R Soc Trop Med Hyg.* 1994;88:381-385.

462. Kitua AY, Smith T, Alonso PL, et al. Plasmodium falciparum malaria in the first year of life in an area of intense and perennial transmission. *Trop Med Int Health.* 1996;1:475-484.
463. Cornet M, Le Hesran JY, Fievet N, et al. Prevalence of and risk factors for anemia in young children in southern Cameroon. *Am J Trop Med Hyg.* 1998;58:606-611.
464. Lemnge MM, Msangeni HA, Ronn AM, et al. Maloprim malaria prophylaxis in children living in a holoendemic village in north-eastern Tanzania. *Trans R Soc Trop Med Hyg.* 1997;91:68-73.
465. Menendez C, Kahigwa E, Hirt R, et al. Randomised placebo-controlled trial of iron supplementation and malaria chemoprophylaxis for prevention of severe anaemia and malaria in Tanzanian infants. *Lancet.* 1997;350:844-850.
466. Schellenberg D, Menendez C, Kahigwa E, et al. Intermittent treatment for malaria and anaemia control at time of routine vaccinations in Tanzanian infants: a randomised, placebo-controlled trial. *Lancet.* 2001;357:1471-1477.
467. Massaga JJ, Kitua AY, Lemnge MM, et al. Effect of intermittent treatment with amodiaquine on anaemia and malarial fevers in infants in Tanzania: a randomised placebo-controlled trial. *Lancet.* 2003;361:1853-1860.
468. Shulman CE, Dorman EK, Cutts F, et al. Intermittent sulphadoxine-pyrimethamine to prevent severe anaemia secondary to malaria in pregnancy: a randomised placebo-controlled trial. *Lancet.* 1999;353:632-636.
469. English M, Waruiru C, Marsh K. Transfusion for respiratory distress in life-threatening childhood malaria. *Am J Trop Med Hyg.* 1996;55:525-530.
470. Availability and use of parenteral quinidine gluconate for severe or complicated malaria. *MMWR Morb Mortal Wkly Rep.* 2000;49:1138-1140.
471. Treatment of severe Plasmodium falciparum malaria with quinidine gluconate: discontinuation of parenteral quinine from CDC drug service. *MMWR Morb Mortal Wkly Rep.* 1991; 40:240.
472. Bhavnani SM, Preston SL. Monitoring of intravenous quinidine infusion in the treatment of Plasmodium falciparum malaria. *Ann Pharmacother.* 1995;29:33-35.
473. van Agtmael MA, Eggelte TA, van Boxtel CJ. Artemisinin drugs in the treatment of malaria: from medicinal herb to registered medication. *Trends Pharmacol Sci.* 1999;20:199-205.
474. McGready R, Brockman A, Cho T, et al. Randomized comparison of mefloquine-artesunate versus quinine in the treatment of multidrug-resistant falciparum malaria in pregnancy. *Trans R Soc Trop Med Hyg.* 2000;94:689-693.
475. McGready R, Cho T, Keo NK, et al. Artemisinin antimalarials in pregnancy: a prospective treatment study of 539 episodes of multidrug-resistant Plasmodium falciparum. *Clin Infect Dis.* 2001;33:2009-2016.
476. Arnold K, Tran TH, Nguyen TC, et al. A randomized comparative study of artemisinine (qinghaosu) suppositories and oral quinine in acute falciparum malaria. *Trans R Soc Trop Med Hyg.* 1990;84:499-502.
477. Price R, van Vugt M, Phaipun L, et al. Adverse effects in patients with acute falciparum malaria treated with artemisinin derivatives. *Am J Trop Med Hyg.* 1999;60:547-555.
478. Hien TT, Turner GD, Mai NT, et al. Neuropathological assessment of artemether-treated severe malaria. *Lancet.* 2003;362:295-296.
479. McIntosh HM, Olliaro P. Artemisinin derivatives for treating severe malaria. Cochrane Database Syst Rev 2000:CD000527.
480. Rego SJ, Subba Rao SD, Hejmadi A, et al. Partial exchange transfusion as an adjunct to the treatment of severe falciparum malaria in children. *J Trop Pediatr.* 2001;47:118-119.
481. Looareesuwan S, Phillips RE, Karbwang J, et al. Plasmodium falciparum hyperparasitaemia: use of exchange transfusion in seven patients and a review of the literature. *Q J Med.* 1990;75: 471-481.
482. Miller KD, Greenberg AE, Campbell CC. Treatment of severe malaria in the United States with a continuous infusion of quinidine gluconate and exchange transfusion. *N Engl J Med.* 1989;321:65-70.
483. Burchard GD, Kroger J, Knobloch J, et al. Exchange blood transfusion in severe falciparum malaria: retrospective evaluation of 61 patients treated with, compared to 63 patients treated without, exchange transfusion. *Trop Med Int Health.* 1997;2: 733-740.
484. Hoontrakoon S, Suputtamongkol Y. Exchange transfusion as an adjunct to the treatment of severe falciparum malaria. *Trop Med Int Health.* 1998;3:156-161.
485. Riddle MS, Jackson JL, Sanders JW, et al. Exchange transfusion as an adjunct therapy in severe *Plasmodium falciparum* malaria: a meta-analysis. *Clin Infect Dis.* 2002;34:1192-1198.
486. Gogtay NJ, Desai S, Kamtekar KD, et al. Efficacies of 5- and 14-day primaquine regimens in the prevention of relapses in *Plasmodium vivax* infections. *Ann Trop Med Parasitol.* 1999; 93:809-812.
487. Rowland M, Durrani N. Randomized controlled trials of 5- and 14-days primaquine therapy against relapses of vivax malaria in an Afghan refugee settlement in Pakistan. *Trans R Soc Trop Med Hyg.* 1999;93:641-643.
488. Buchachart K, Krudsood S, Singhasivanon P, et al. Effect of primaquine standard dose (15 mg/day for 14 days) in the treatment of vivax malaria patients in Thailand. *Southeast Asian J Trop Med Public Health.* 2001;32:720-726.
489. Krudsood S, Tangpukdee N, Wilairatana P, et al. High-dose primaquine regimens against relapse of Plasmodium vivax malaria. *Am J Trop Med Hyg.* 2008;78:736-740.
490. Alving AS, Johnson CF, Tarlov AR, et al. Mitigation of the haemolytic effect of primaquine and enhancement of its action against exoerythrocytic forms of the Chesson strain of Piasmodium vivax by intermittent regimens of drug administration: a preliminary report. *Bull World Health Organ.* 1960;22:621-631.
491. Hill DR, Baird JK, Parise ME, et al. Primaquine: report from CDC expert meeting on malaria chemoprophylaxis I. *Am J Trop Med Hyg.* 2006;75:402-415.
492. Baird JK, Fryauff DJ, Hoffman SL. Primaquine for prevention of malaria in travelers. *Clin Infect Dis.* 2003;37:1659-1667.
493. Maguire JD, Llewellyn DM. Relapsing vivax malaria after 6 months of daily atovaquone/proguanil in Afghanistan: the case for expanded use of primaquine as a causal prophylactic. *J Travel Med.* 2007;14:411-414.
494. Moore DA, Grant AD, Armstrong M, et al. Risk factors for malaria in UK travellers. *Trans R Soc Trop Med Hyg.* 2004; 98:55-63.
495. Malaria deaths following inappropriate malaria chemoprophylaxis–United States, 2001. *MMWR Morb Mortal Wkly Rep.* 2001;50:597-599.
496. Muehlberger N, Jelinek T, Schlipkoeter U, et al. Effectiveness of chemoprophylaxis and other determinants of malaria in travellers to Kenya. *Trop Med Int Health.* 1998;3:357-363.
497. Mali S, Steele S, Slutsker L, et al. Malaria surveillance—United States, 2006. *MMWR Surveill Summ.* 2008;57:24-39.
498. Lobel HO, Baker MA, Gras FA, et al. Use of malaria prevention measures by North American and European travelers to East Africa. *J Travel Med.* 2001;8:167-172.
499. Freedman DO. Clinical practice. Malaria prevention in short-term travelers. *N Engl J Med.* 2008;359:603-612.
500. Cot M, Roisin A, Barro D, et al. Effect of chloroquine chemoprophylaxis during pregnancy on birth weight: results of a randomized trial. *Am J Trop Med Hyg.* 1992;46:21-27.
501. Ohrt C, Richie TL, Widjaja H, et al. Mefloquine compared with doxycycline for the prophylaxis of malaria in Indonesian soldiers. A randomized, double-blind, placebo-controlled trial. *Ann Intern Med.* 1997;126:963-972.
502. Weinke T, Trautmann M, Held T, et al. Neuropsychiatric side effects after the use of mefloquine. *Am J Trop Med Hyg.* 1991;45: 86-91.
503. Boudreau E, Schuster B, Sanchez J, et al. Tolerability of prophylactic Lariam regimens. *Trop Med Parasitol.* 1993;44:257-265.
504. Croft AM, Garner P. Mefloquine for preventing malaria in non-immune adult travellers. Cochrane Database Syst Rev 2000:CD000138.
505. Nosten F, ter Kuile F, Maelankiri L, et al. Mefloquine prophylaxis prevents malaria during pregnancy: a double-blind, placebo-controlled study. *J Infect Dis.* 1994;169:595-603.
506. Smoak BL, Writer JV, Keep LW, et al. The effects of inadvertent exposure of mefloquine chemoprophylaxis on pregnancy outcomes and infants of US Army servicewomen. *J Infect Dis.* 1997;176:831-833.
507. Vanhauwere B, Maradit H, Kerr L. Post-marketing surveillance of prophylactic mefloquine (Lariam) use in pregnancy. *Am J Trop Med Hyg.* 1998;58:17-21.
508. Phillips-Howard PA, Steffen R, Kerr L, et al. Safety of mefloquine and other antimalarial agents in the first trimester of pregnancy. *J Travel Med.* 1998;5:121-126.
509. Taylor WR, Richie TL, Fryauff DJ, et al. Malaria prophylaxis using azithromycin: a double-blind, placebo-controlled trial in Irian Jaya, Indonesia. *Clin Infect Dis.* 1999;28:74-81.
510. Sukwa TY, Mulenga M, Chisdaka N, et al. A randomized, double-blind, placebo-controlled field trial to determine the efficacy and safety of Malarone (atovaquone/proguanil) for the prophylaxis of malaria in Zambia. *Am J Trop Med Hyg.* 1999;60:521-525.
511. Shanks GD, Gordon DM, Klotz FW, et al. Efficacy and safety of atovaquone/proguanil as suppressive prophylaxis for Plasmodium falciparum malaria. *Clin Infect Dis.* 1998;27:494-499.
512. Petersen E. The safety of atovaquone/proguanil in long-term malaria prophylaxis of nonimmune adults. *J Travel Med.* 2003;10(Suppl 1):S13-S15; discussion S21.
513. Hogh B, Clarke PD, Camus D, et al. Atovaquone-proguanil versus chloroquine-proguanil for malaria prophylaxis in non-immune travellers: a randomised, double-blind study. Malarone International Study Team. *Lancet.* 2000;356:1888-1894.
514. Overbosch D, Schilthuis H, Bienzle U, et al. Atovaquone-proguanil versus mefloquine for malaria prophylaxis in nonimmune travelers: results from a randomized, double-blind study. *Clin Infect Dis.* 2001;33:1015-1021.
515. Kofoed K, Petersen E. The efficacy of chemoprophylaxis against malaria with chloroquine plus proguanil, mefloquine, and atovaquone plus proguanil in travelers from Denmark. *J Travel Med.* 2003;10:150-154.
516. Boggild AK, Parise ME, Lewis LS, et al. Atovaquone-proguanil: report from the CDC expert meeting on malaria chemoprophylaxis (II). *Am J Trop Med Hyg.* 2007;76:208-223.
517. Nakato H, Vivancos R, Hunter PR. A systematic review and meta-analysis of the effectiveness and safety of atovaquone proguanil (Malarone) for chemoprophylaxis against malaria. *J Antimicrob Chemother.* 2007;60:929-936.
518. van Genderen PJ, Koene HR, Spong K, et al. The safety and tolerance of atovaquone/proguanil for the long-term prophylaxis of plasmodium falciparum malaria in non-immune travelers and expatriates [corrected]. *J Travel Med.* 2007;14:92-95.
519. Camus D, Djossou F, Schilthuis HJ, et al. Atovaquone-proguanil versus chloroquine-proguanil for malaria prophylaxis in non-immune pediatric travelers: results of an international, randomized, open-label study. *Clin Infect Dis.* 2004;38:1716-1723.
520. Soto J, Toledo J, Luzz M, et al. Randomized, double-blind, placebo-controlled study of Malarone for malaria prophylaxis in non-immune Colombian soldiers. *Am J Trop Med Hyg.* 2006; 75:430-433.
521. Ling J, Baird JK, Fryauff DJ, et al. Randomized, placebo-controlled trial of atovaquone/proguanil for the prevention of Plasmodium falciparum or Plasmodium vivax malaria among migrants to Papua, Indonesia. *Clin Infect Dis.* 2002;35:825-833.
522. Wallace MR, Sharp TW, Smoak B, et al. Malaria among United States troops in Somalia. *Am J Med.* 1996;100:49-55.
523. Lillie TH, Schreck CE, Rahe AJ. Effectiveness of personal protection against mosquitoes in Alaska. *J Med Entomol.* 1988;25: 475-478.
524. Schoepke A, Steffen R, Gratz N. Effectiveness of personal protection measures against mosquito bites for malaria prophylaxis in travelers. *J Travel Med.* 1998;5:188-192.
525. Durrheim DN, Govere JM. Malaria outbreak control in an African village by community application of 'deet' mosquito repellent to ankles and feet. *Med Vet Entomol.* 2002;16:112-115.
526. Alexander B, Cadena H, Usma MC, et al. Laboratory and field evaluations of a repellent soap containing diethyl toluamide (DEET) and permethrin against phlebotomine sand flies (Diptera: Psychodidae) in Valle del Cauca, Colombia. *Am J Trop Med Hyg.* 1995;52:169-173.
527. Fradin MS. Mosquitoes and mosquito repellents: a clinician's guide. *Ann Intern Med.* 1998;128:931-940.
528. Lengeler C. Insecticide-treated bednets and curtains for preventing malaria. Cochrane Database Syst Rev 2000:CD000363.
529. Nevill CG, Some ES, Mung'ala VO, et al. Insecticide-treated bednets reduce mortality and severe morbidity from malaria among children on the Kenyan coast. *Trop Med Int Health.* 1996;1:139-146.
530. Kitchener S, Nasveld P, Russell B, et al. An outbreak of malaria in a forward battalion on active service in East Timor. *Mil Med.* 2003;168:457-459.
531. Chitnis CE, Sharma A. Targeting the Plasmodium vivax Duffy-binding protein. *Trends Parasitol.* 2008;24:29-34.
532. Grimberg BT, Udomsangpetch R, Xainli J, et al. Plasmodium vivax invasion of human erythrocytes inhibited by antibodies directed against the Duffy binding protein. *PLoS Med.* 2007;4: e337.
533. Avril M, Kulasekara BR, Gose SO, et al. Evidence for globally shared, cross-reacting polymorphic epitopes in the pregnancy-associated malaria vaccine candidate VAR2CSA. *Infect Immun.* 2008;76:1791-1800.
534. Oleinikov AV, Francis SE, Dorfman JR, et al. VAR2CSA domains expressed in Escherichia coli induce cross-reactive antibodies to native protein. *J Infect Dis.* 2008;197:1119-1123.
535. Aponte JJ, Aide P, Renom M, et al. Safety of the RTS,S/AS02D candidate malaria vaccine in infants living in a highly endemic area of Mozambique: a double blind randomised controlled phase I/IIb trial. *Lancet.* 2007;370:1543-1551.
536. Vekemans J, Ballou WR. Plasmodium falciparum malaria vaccines in development. *Expert Rev Vaccines.* 2008;7:223-240.
537. Saul A. Mosquito stage, transmission blocking vaccines for malaria. *Curr Opin Infect Dis.* 2007;20:476-481.

276

Leishmania Species: Visceral (Kala-Azar), Cutaneous, and Mucosal Leishmaniasis

ALAN J. MAGILL*

Introduction and General Principles

Leishmaniasis refers to a diverse spectrum of clinical syndromes caused by infection with protozoan parasites of the genus *Leishmania*. The clinical syndromes and manifestations of leishmaniasis vary widely but are often divided into the three clinically distinct syndromes of visceral leishmaniasis (VL), cutaneous leishmaniasis (CL), and mucosal leishmaniasis (ML). Although there are features common to all *Leishmania* infections, there is also much that is unique and specific to each syndrome. A single *Leishmania* species can produce more than one clinical syndrome, and each of the syndromes is caused by more than one species. The outcome in any one patient is a result of parasite factors (invasiveness, tropism, and pathogenicity) and the host's genetically determined cell-mediated immune responses. It is useful to view infection as leading to the leishmaniases, a heterogenous collection of clinical diseases, each with its own relatively unique geographic distribution, biology, ecology, local mammalian reservoir, and sandfly insect vector. Aspects that are shared across the spectrum are discussed initially followed by syndrome-specific information.

LIFE CYCLE

Leishmania spp. are diploid protozoa and have a dimorphic life cycle. A sexual stage has not yet been identified. The life cycle begins when the promastigote, an elongate, motile form (1.5-3.5 μm by 15-200 μm) of the parasite found in the sandfly digestive tract and proboscis, is transmitted into the skin of a mammalian host by the bite of small, delicate female sand flies when they take a blood meal. After inoculation by a sand fly, promastigotes are phagocytosed by macrophages in the dermis and transform into intracellular oval or round amastigotes (3-5 μm in length) that lack an exteriorized flagellum. Amastigotes are found inside phagolysosomes, where they multiply by simple binary division, eventually rupturing the cell and invading other reticuloendothelial (RE) cells. Released amastigotes go on to infect other mononuclear phagocytes. In Wright- and Giemsa-stained preparations, the amastigote cytoplasm appears blue, and the nucleus is relatively large, eccentrically located, and red. Amastigotes have a distinct, rod-shaped, red-staining structure called a kinetoplast, a specialized mitochondrial structure that contains a substantial amount of extranuclear DNA arranged as catenated minicircles and maxicircles. Visualization of the kinetoplast, which has a characteristic appearance under oil-immersion microscopy as seen in Fig. 276-1, confirms the diagnosis of leishmaniasis.

Additional mononuclear phagocytes are attracted to the site of the initial lesion and become infected. Amastigotes disseminate through regional lymphatics and the vascular system to infect mononuclear phagocytes throughout the reticuloendothelial system. The cycle is completed when female phlebotomine sand flies ingest parasitized cells. When in the digestive tract of the sand flies, *Leishmania* parasites develop through a series of flagellated intermediate stages to become infectious metacyclic promastigotes.

TAXONOMY AND CLASSIFICATION

The taxonomy of *Leishmania* parasites can be confusing and is constantly evolving. The genus *Leishmania* has been divided into two subgenera: *Viannia* and *Leishmania*. Species in the *Viannia* subgenus develop in the hindgut of the sand fly before migrating to the midgut and foregut (peripylaria), while those of the *Leishmania* subgenus develop in the midgut and foregut (suprapylaria).[1] Species of the *Viannia* subgenus are endemic in Central and South America. Members of the *Leishmania* subgenus are found throughout the world. Differences in the way parasites are characterized around the world and over time make the comparison of clinical correlates, treatment study outcomes, and prognosis challenging. The *Leishmania* spp. that infect humans, their geographic distributions, and the clinical syndromes they most commonly produce are summarized in Table 276-1.[1-4] Historically, *Leishmania* parasites have been divided into different species based on clinical, biologic, geographic, and epidemiologic criteria. For example, a parasite isolated from a patient with a typical "dry ulcer" in an urban setting in the Middle East was called *Leishmania tropica*.

Beginning in the early 1970s, intrinsic characteristics, such as biochemical and molecular markers, were identified and used to develop classification systems. Isoenzyme analysis by electrophoresis, developed in the 1970s, is widely used as a typing system and still valuable as a reference technique for parasite characterization. The taxonomic profile determined by isoenzyme electrophoresis is called a zymodeme. Isoenzyme analysis is most often successful with culture amplified parasites. It requires specialized laboratory expertise and usually cannot provide a result to the clinician in a meaningful time frame to affect the choice or duration of therapy. Further complicating isoenzyme interpretation, different research groups have adopted different techniques. The MON (for Montpellier, France) typing system, an authoritative standard from an acknowledged world reference center, uses 15 standardized isoenzyme loci analyzed by starch gel electrophoresis.[5] In contrast, American researchers more commonly use a system of three standardized isoenzyme loci identified by cellulose gel electrophoresis.[6] Intuitively, the use of more isoenzyme loci reveals greater differences between strains. The clinical implications of greater or lesser degrees of characterization are not clearly known but are likely to be important. For example, *Leishmania panamensis* and *Leishmania guyanensis*, considered different species in the past, may instead represent clusters within a spectrum of genetic diversity.[7]

From a clinician's perspective, a useful classification is one that accurately predicts natural history of infection and response to treatment. The use of polymerase chain reaction (PCR) assays using *Leishmania* spp.–specific oligonucleotide primers, other molecular and genetic information, and insights gained from the publication of the genomes of *Leishmania braziliensis*, *Leishmania major*, and *Leishmania infantum* will lead to an explosion of new knowledge.[8-10]

EPIDEMIOLOGY

The leishmaniases are widely distributed across the tropical, subtropical, and temperate regions in 88 countries, 72 of which are in developing areas of the world. More than 350 million women, men, and children are at risk in widely scattered areas. An estimated 12 million people suffer from leishmaniasis, with 500,000 new cases of VL per

*With the exception of any borrowed tables or figures, the content of this chapter is in the public domain. The opinions of the author do not represent the official views of the U.S. Department of Defense or the U.S. Army.

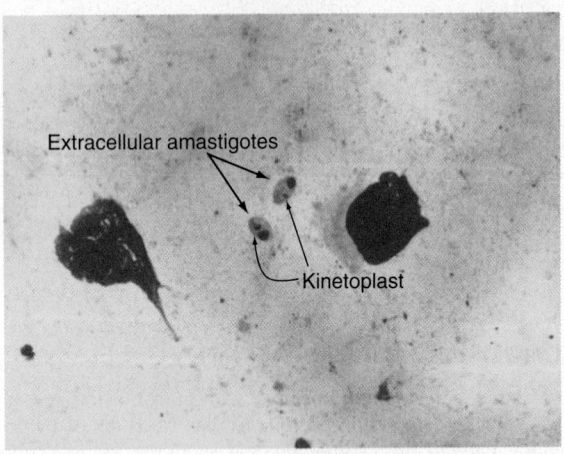

Figure 276-1 **Tissue smear obtained from a patient with cutaneous leishmaniasis caused by _Leishmania major._** Amastigotes, 3-4 μm in width and 4-5 μm in length are seen. Note the rod-shaped kinetoplast seen next to the nucleus. (Giemsa, original magnification ×1000.) *(Courtesy of Dr. Peter Weina, Bethesda, MD.)*

year and 1 to 1.5 million new cases of CL per year, with 2.4 million disability-adjusted life years (DALYs).[11] Approximately 90% of all cases of VL are found in three areas: the drainage basin of the Ganges River in eastern India and neighboring areas of southern Nepal (the "terai"), areas of Bangladesh that share the same ecology; the Sudan, where a large epidemic has occurred among displaced people[12-14]; and Brazil, where VL is endemic in rural areas and large periurban outbreaks have been reported from cities in the northeast.[15,16] VL has also emerged as an important opportunistic disease in persons with acquired immunodeficiency syndrome (AIDS) in southern Europe and other areas of the world where the two diseases coexist, in persons who have had organ transplants, and in association with other conditions in which cell-mediated immunity is compromised.

Approximately 90% of the world's CL cases occur in Iran, Saudi Arabia, and Syria in the Middle East; in Afghanistan in Central Asia; and in Brazil and Peru in Latin America.[11] CL is an important problem for residents, settlers, travelers, and military personnel visiting endemic areas. More than 2000 cases of CL have been reported among American troops serving in Iraq and Afghanistan since 2001. Other cases occur among North American civilians following exposure in endemic regions.[17] Finally, 90% of the cases of ML occur in three Latin American countries: Bolivia, Brazil, and Peru.

TABLE 276-1 *Leishmania* **Parasites, Major Clinical Syndromes, and Distribution**

Clinical Syndromes	Leishmania *Spp.*	*Location*
Visceral leishmaniasis (VL) (also known as kala-azar): generalized involvement of the reticuloendothelial system (spleen, bone marrow, liver, lymph nodes)	*Leishmania donovani* causes classic VL in Asia.	Major endemic/epidemic focus in Indian subcontinent (lowland terai region of southern Nepal, Bangladesh, Bihar province, and surrounding areas in India). Endemic/sporadic in China, Pakistan, Indian subcontinent.
	Leishmania infantum causes infantile VL in the Old World. *Leishmania chagasi/L. infantum* causes VL in the Americas.	Middle East, Mediterranean littoral, Balkans, Central and southwestern Asia, northern and western China, North and sub-Saharan Africa, Latin America
	Leishmania donovani/L.infantum	East Africa: Ethiopia, Kenya, Somalia, Sudan, Uganda
	Leishmania amazonensis is uncommon cause of atypical VL in the Americas.	Brazil (Bahia state)
	Leishmania tropica is rarely associated with VL syndrome, often atypical	Middle East, Saudi Arabia (U.S. troops), India, North Africa, Pakistan, Mediterranean littoral, Central and western Asia
Post–kala-azar dermal leishmaniasis	*L. donovani*	Indian subcontinent
	L. donovani/L. infantum	East Africa: Ethiopia, Kenya, Somalia, Sudan, Uganda
Old World cutaneous leishmaniasis: single or limited number of skin lesions	*Leishmania major* (also known as moist or rural oriental sore)	Middle East, India, Pakistan, Africa, Central and western Asia, northern and western China
	Leishmania tropica (also known as dry or urban oriental sore)	Mediterranean littoral, Middle East, North Africa, India, Pakistan, Central and western Asia
	Leishmania aethiopica	Ethiopian highlands, Kenya, Yemen
	L. infantum/L. chagasi (rare)	Middle East, Mediterranean littoral, Central Asia, northern and western China, North and sub-Saharan Africa
	L. donovani/L. infantum	East Africa: Ethiopia, Kenya, Somalia, Sudan, Uganda
New World cutaneous leishmaniasis: single or limited number of skin lesions	*Leishmania mexicana* (chiclero ulcer)	Central and South America, Texas
	L. amazonensis	Amazon Basin, neighboring areas, Bahia and other states of Brazil
	Leishmania pifanoi	Venezuela
	Leishmania garnhami	Venezuela
	Leishmania venezuelensis	Venezuela
	Leishmania (Viannia) braziliensis	Central and South America
	Leishmania (V.) guyanensis (forest yaws or pian bois)	Guyana, Surinam, northern Amazon Basin
	Leishmania (V.) peruviana (uta)	Peru (western Andes)
	Leishmania (V.) panamensis	Panama, Costa Rica, Colombia
	Leishmania (V.) colombiensis	Colombia and Panama
	L. infantum/L. chagasi	Central and South America
Leishmaniasis recidivans	*L. tropica*	North Africa, Afghanistan, and Middle East
Diffuse cutaneous leishmaniasis (DCL)	*L. amazonensis*	Amazon Basin, neighboring areas, Bahia and other states of Brazil
	L. pifanoi	Venezuela
	L. mexicana	Central and South America, Texas
	Leishmania spp.	Dominican Republic
	L. aethiopica	Ethiopian highlands, Kenya, Yemen
Disseminated leishmaniasis	*L. (V.) braziliensis* *L. (V.) amazonensis*	Brazil
American mucosal leishmaniasis	*L. (V.) braziliensis* (espundia)	Central and South America; most cases from Bolivia, Brazil, and Peru
	Other *Leishmania (V.)* spp. (*guyanensis, panamensis*) are rare.	Central and South America

Data from references 1-4.

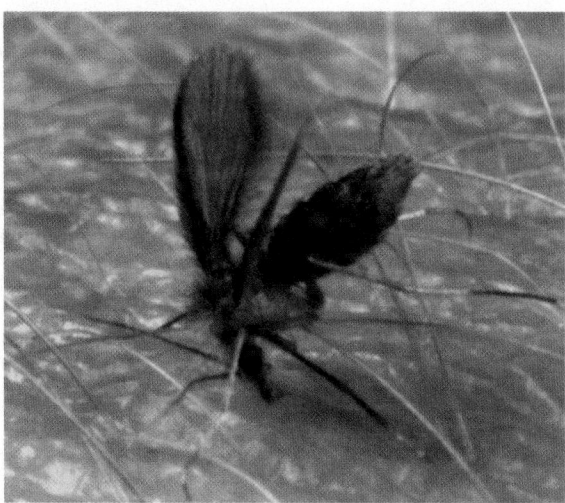

Figure 276-2 A female *Phlebotomus papatasi* sand fly taking a blood meal. Note the characteristic V shape of the wings at rest, the parallel veins, and the fine hairs on the trailing edge of the wings, allowing for silent flight.

Female sand flies of the genus *Lutzomyia* in the Americas and *Phlebotomus* elsewhere transmit *Leishmania* spp. (Fig. 276-2).[18] They are modified pool feeders. Sand flies breed in cracks in the walls of dwellings, in rubbish or rubble, or in rodent burrows. They are weak fliers and tend to remain close to the ground near their breeding sites. Promastigotes in the sand fly gut replicate and differentiate to metacyclic promastigotes over a period of approximately 1 week. Saliva from the sand fly enhances the infectivity of promastigotes through the effects of maxadilan, a potent vasodilator and immunomodulator, and possibly other factors.[19] Depending on the *Leishmania* species, the sand fly genus, and the geographic location, the major reservoirs are canines, rodents, or humans.[20]

Although most transmission is by sand fly bites, *Leishmania* can be transmitted by blood transfusions, sharing of needles by intravenous drug abusers, occupational exposures, congenital transmission, and rarely by sexual transmission.[21-25] Leucodepletion effectively reduces or eliminates transfusion-associated risk of *Leishmania* infction.[26]

PATHOGENESIS

Leishmaniasis can be thought of as a polar disorder similar to other intracellular infections such as leprosy (Fig. 276-3).[27] For example, the range of clinical features in CL parallels that of leprosy. At the polyparasitic end of the spectrum is diffuse cutaneous leishmaniasis (DCL), a relatively uncommon syndrome, in which there is little evidence of effective cell-mediated immune response. Heavily parasitized macrophages are abundant throughout the dermis, and few lymphocytes are present. Peripheral blood mononuclear cells neither proliferate nor produce INF-γ nor IL-2 in response to leishmanial antigens in vitro, and cutaneous delayed type hypersensitivity reactions are absent.[28] DCL has been compared to lepromatous leprosy in which there is a large number of mycobacteria in macrophages and no evidence of protective, Th1 cell–mediated immune responses.

At the oligoparasitic end of the spectrum lie leishmaniasis recidivans (LR), a hyperergic variant of CL caused by *L. tropica* infection in the Old World, in which chronic lesions slowly expand while healing at the center. Amastigotes are sparse, and a mononuclear cell infiltrate predominates. This is somewhat analogous to tuberculoid leprosy in which there is an intense mononuclear infiltrate with few mycobacteria. But CL and leprosy differ in important ways. Although the character and organization of the granuloma in leprosy are invariably characteristic of the position in the clinical spectrum, this is not true in simple cutaneous leishmaniasis in which lesions progress over time from a predominance of amastigote-containing macrophages and few lymphocytes to a granulomatous response with a predominance of lymphocytes and few parasites before healing.[29]

DIAGNOSIS

The diagnosis of all suspected *Leishmania* infections can be approached in three ways: clinical, parasitologic, and immunologic. A clinical diagnosis can have a very high pretest predictive probability in some settings. For example, a chronic ulcer present for many weeks with a typical appearance acquired in the jungles of Peru is very likely to be CL. Likewise, a person with fever, weight loss, pancytopenia, and hepatomegaly in known endemic areas of Bihar, India, is very likely to have VL.

Because of the toxicity of some of the drugs used to treat leishmaniasis and the prognostic importance of knowing the species causing CL, a confirmed parasitologic diagnosis is often desirable. A parasitologic diagnosis is confirmed by visualizing amastigotes in tissue or smears, promastigotes in culture, or amplifying *Leishmania*-specific DNA or RNA in a PCR. Knowing the infecting species may affect the choice to offer treatment, the choice of treatments, and the regimen or duration of chemotherapy. Immunologic diagnosis is an adjunct in most cases with various antibody tests, cell-mediated assays, and the use of skin tests where available to elicit delayed type hypersensitivity (DTH). The choice of the optimal diagnostic test or procedure depends on the parasite burden of the disease syndrome.

Understanding the likely parasite burden of the various *Leishmania* syndromes allows for the optimal choice of diagnostic testing (Fig. 276-3). Syndromes with very high parasite burdens (polyparasitic), such as VL and later-stage diffuse cutaneous leishmaniasis (DCL), are characterized by huge numbers of parasites, no cell-mediated immunity (anergy), and an easily detected antibody response. Syndromes with few or scanty numbers of parasites (oligoparasitic), such as ML and LR, are characterized by very few recognizable parasites, an exaggerated cell-mediated immune response, and a minimal antibody response. The utility of a relatively insensitive parasitologic test such as a Giemsa-stained smear in an oligoparasitic syndrome such as ML will be very low. A more appropriate parasitologic test in this syndrome would be PCR.[30]

TREATMENT

The diversity of *Leishmania* infections makes standard treatment recommendations impossible. Each region has different species complexes with a greater or lesser degree of genetic heterogeneity within

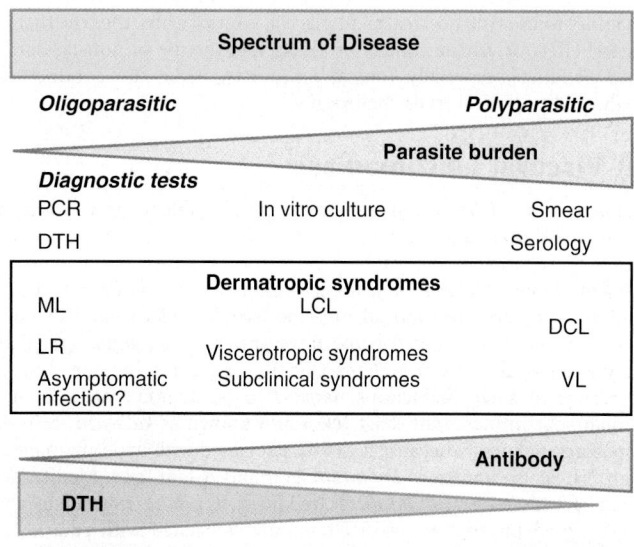

Figure 276-3 Spectrum of *Leishmania* infection and disease. DCL, diffuse cutaneous leishmaniasis; DTH, delayed type hypersensitivity; LCL, localized cutaneous leishmaniasis; LR, leishmaniasis recidivans; ML, mucosal leishmaniasis; PCR, polymerase chain reaction; VL, visceral leishmaniasis.

the complex. For example, *Leishmania donovani* in the Indian subcontinent[31] and *L. major* in the Old World[32] are relatively homogenous groupings, whereas *L. tropica*[33-35] and *L. braziliensis* are quite heterogenous.[36] These genetic differences may be reflected in variable natural history of infection and response to treatment. In addition, each geographic region has its own unique combination of sand fly vectors, mammalian reservoirs, and human hosts with different genetic backgrounds in varying zoonotic or anthroponotic cycles that leads to different disease outcomes and responses to treatment. A treatment regimen that is efficacious in one region may not work in another. For example, single-dose liposomal amphotericin B (AmBisome) leads to more than 95% efficacy in India[37] but requires a much higher total dose in the Sudan.[38,39]

The endpoints used in clinical trials include clinical cure, parasitologic cure, and immunologic cure. Clinical cure refers to the resolution of clinical symptoms and signs within a defined time period, such as resolution of fever, pancytopenia, and splenomegaly in VL, or complete epithelialization of an ulcer in CL. Parasitologic cure refers to the absence of parasites by smear, culture, or PCR after a treatment regimen. Immunologic cure can be demonstrated by a falling antibody titer or conversion of a skin test from negative to positive. Although current chemotherapy options result in a clinical cure, they seldom lead to true parasitologic cure. Persistence of *Leishmania* parasites in host tissue is the rule, not the exception, in spite of successful clinical cures.[40] Viable parasites can be cultured from old *Leishmania* scars in CL[41,42] and from lymph nodes following clinical cure in VL.[43] The persistence of *Leishmania* parasites following clinically successful chemotherapy is responsible for the reactivation and opportunistic infections in the immunocompromised.

It is not possible or useful to make standard or uniform treatment recommendations for the leishmaniasis syndromes worldwide.[44] Optimal drug treatment regimens for each geographic region and major syndrome are best defined in consideration of demonstrated regional efficacy, available resources, and risks and benefits assessments. In resource-rich countries, the efficacy, safety, and tolerability of drug regimens can be the primary factors influencing choice, whereas in developing countries and in endemic areas where resources are limited, several other factors, such as cost, local experience and preferences, and predictable availability, must be considered.

The design and reporting of clinical trials in CL, especially in the Old World,[45] are generally limited, making evidence-based treatment recommendations of low quality and strength. The confounding effects of a natural cure rate, marked interindividual variation, the inability to use true no-treatment placebo control arms, the true therapeutic effect of vehicle control products, and the use of nonstandardized products, especially topical ointments, make the conduct of high-quality clinical trials challenging.

Visceral Leishmaniasis

Parasites in the *L. donovani* complex are responsible for most cases of visceral leishmaniasis (see Table 276-1). *Leishmania chagasi*, once considered a separate species causing VL in the Americas, is now considered the same as *L. infantum*, which is endemic in the Mediterranean and was probably introduced into the New World by early explorers.[46,47] Continued debate on the taxonomy of *Leishmania* spp. that have been isolated from patients with VL continues, but the clinical relevance of such distinctions remains to be demonstrated. In the Indian subcontinent, late-stage VL is also known as *kala-azar* (Hindi for "black sickness") because it can be associated with hyperpigmentation. VL is also known as *Dumdum fever* and *Assam fever*. Mediterranean VL caused by *L. infantum* is also known as *infantile splenomegaly*. *Leishmania* spp. that are most commonly associated with cutaneous syndromes such as *Leishmania amazonensis* in Latin America[48,49] and *L. tropica* in Saudi Arabia, Kenya, Iran, and India are rarely isolated from patients with visceral syndromes.[50-53]

VL is a spectrum of symptoms and findings. At one extreme are persons with asymptomatic, inapparent, or self-resolving infections.

At the other are those with classic VL (kala-azar), who present with a characteristic pentad of prolonged fever, weight loss, hepatosplenomegaly, pancytopenia, and hypergammaglobulinemia (Fig. 276-4). Ratios of self-resolving infection to frank VL vary geographically, with a person's age (likely a partial surrogate for immunity) and the tests used to identify asymptomatic infection. Ratios of asymptomatic infection to VL cases are reported to range from 6.5:1 in children to 18:1 in adults with *L. infantum/L. chagasi* in northeastern Brazil.[54-56] Although many of those infected have no clinical manifestations, some experience mild symptoms or develop splenomegaly before either progressing to frank visceral leishmaniasis or undergoing spontaneous resolution. Persons who are immunocompromised by AIDS, neoplasm, malnutrition, or immunosuppressive therapy are at increased risk of developing progressive disease.

EPIDEMIOLOGY

VL occurs in widely dispersed areas of the world (see Table 276-1). Transmission depends on the sand fly vector, the presence of a suitable reservoir, and susceptible humans. In the Indian subcontinent, humans serve as the reservoir, and transmission is by *Phlebotomus argentipes* and other anthropophilic *Phlebotomus* spp. Persons with post–kala-azar dermal leishmaniasis (PKDL) may serve as the reservoir during interepidemic periods. VL caused by *L. infantum* also occurs in Central Asia and historically in southern China, where dogs and other canines are reservoirs.

In East Africa, VL occurs in Eritrea, Ethiopia, Kenya, Somalia, Sudan, and Uganda. *L. donovani* has been responsible for a very large epidemic among displaced persons in southern Sudan.[57-59] VL is

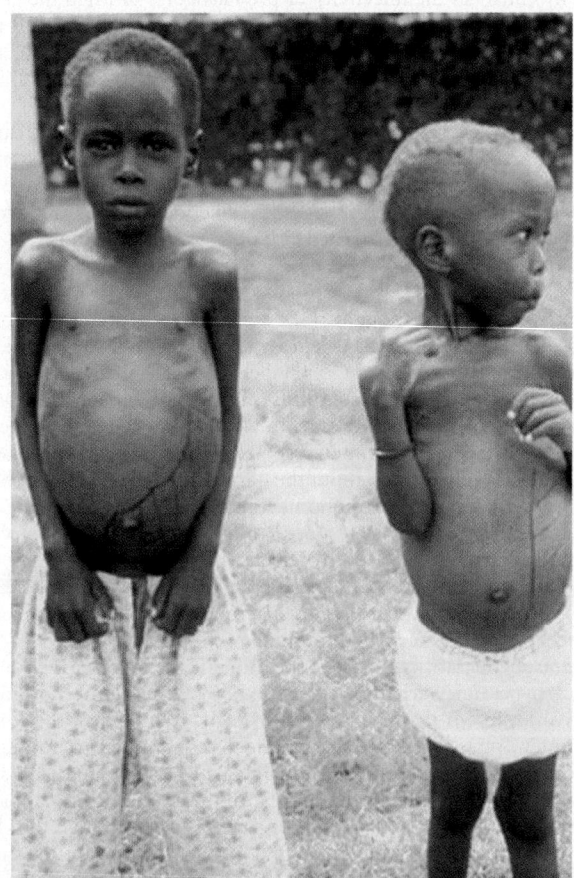

Figure 276-4 Children with visceral leishmaniasis in Kenya. Note signs of malnourishment and protruding abdomen with massive splenomegaly. *(Courtesy of Dr. Charles Oster, Washington, D.C.)*

endemic and sporadic in other areas of East Africa. Putative reservoirs include rats, gerbils, other rodents, and small carnivores. Humans may also be a reservoir during epidemics. The classification of visceralizing *Leishmania* parasites from East Africa remains unclear and disputed.[60]

VL occurs sporadically in the Mediterranean littoral and the Middle East, where rodents, such as the black rat, and dogs are reservoirs for *L. donovani* and *L. infantum,* respectively. Cases are typically encountered among infants, young children, and immunocompromised persons. VL emerged as an important opportunistic disease among persons with AIDS in southern Europe in Spain, France, and Italy.[61,62] Sharing of contaminated needles and syringes by intravenous drug users was implicated in artificial anthroponotic transmission of *Leishmania* in Spain.[63]

In Latin America *L. infantum/L. chagasi* is endemic and broadly distributed. Most areas have focal disease risk with a background of asymptomatic or subclinical infection with sporadic clinical cases in rural areas. The clustering of cases in households suggests that humans may also be reservoirs in these settings. Children are most frequently affected. *Lutzomyia longipalpis* is the major vector. Domestic dogs and wild foxes are reservoirs of infection.[54] Major periurban outbreaks of VL have been reported from cities in northeastern Brazil where suburbs have extended into endemic areas.[15,16,64]

Occasionally, *Leishmania* spp. that usually cause CL, such as *L. amazonensis, L. tropica,* or other *Leishmania* spp., are isolated from persons with visceral disease. For example, a small group of American military personnel who served in the Persian Gulf War acquired a "viscerotropic" form of *L. tropica* infection.[53]

PATHOGENESIS AND NATURAL HISTORY OF VISCERAL LEISHMANIASIS

Skin lesions at the site where promastigotes are inoculated are usually not apparent in persons with VL. Increasing numbers of amastigote-infected mononuclear phagocytes in the liver and spleen result in progressive hypertrophy of these organs, leading to clinically apparent hepatosplenomegaly. The spleen often becomes massively enlarged as splenic lymphoid follicles are replaced by parasitized mononuclear cells. In the liver there is a marked increase in the number and size of Kupffer cells, many of which contain amastigotes. Infected mononuclear phagocytes are also found in the bone marrow, lymph nodes, skin, and other organs in this disseminated disease.

The outcome of infection and the manifestations of disease are associated with genetically determined human immune responses, host nutritional status and immunocompetence, and environmental factors. There is evidence of both protective and disease-enhancing immune responses. Cytokines and chemokines play key roles in mediating the outcome of infection, but despite extensive studies in murine models and in naturally infected humans, the precise sequence of events that determines the outcome of infection has not been fully characterized.[65] Studies during an outbreak of VL in the Sudan showed that one locus on chromosome 22q12 and probably two loci on chromosome 2q22-23 control susceptibility to VL in this population.[66-72] Malnutrition has long been recognized as a risk factor for progression of infection to disease.[73-75]

Persons with self-resolving infection with *L. donovani* or *L. infantum/L. chagasi* and those who have undergone successful chemotherapy develop protective immune responses, but VL disease can develop years later if they become immunocompromised.

The resolution of infection and the development of immunity are associated with expansion of leishmania-specific Th1-type CD_4^+ T cells that secrete interferon-γ (INF-γ) and interleukin-2 (IL-2) in response to parasite antigens. IL-12 also plays an important early role in the development of protective immune responses. Evidence of leishmania-specific Th1 responses is missing in progressive disease. At the cellular level, INF-γ activates macrophages to kill amastigotes through L-arginine-dependent nitric oxide production, which follows induction of nitric oxide synthase and oxidative killing mechanisms. IL-1 and tumor necrosis factor-α (TNF-α) are prime macrophages for activation by INF-γ.

In persons with progressive infection who go on to develop VL, development of leishmania-specific Th1 responses is inhibited. Peripheral blood mononuclear cells neither proliferate nor produce INF-γ or IL-2 in response to leishmanial antigens in vitro. There is no evidence of delayed-type cutaneous hypersensitivity responses to leishmanial antigens. Paradoxically, antileishmanial antibodies are produced in high titer during progressive visceral leishmaniasis, but they are not protective. There is evidence of polyclonal B-cell activation. Progressive disease in humans is associated with production of IL-10 and transforming growth factor (TGF)-β. IL-10 is known to suppress the development of Th1 responses, and the activation of macrophages by INF-γ and TGF-β appears to play an important role early in infection.[76-84]

Why Th1 responses arise and dominate in some persons and not in others is not understood. The sequence of early cytokine responses; the manner in which leishmanial antigens are presented by macrophages and dendritic cells; parasite virulence factors; and the size of the infecting inoculum may all be important variables in identifying the precise sequence of events that leads to the development of immunity and identifying the immunogenetic determinants of human disease.

CLINICAL MANIFESTATIONS OF KALA-AZAR

The fully developed clinical manifestations of VL are similar in all endemic areas. The incubation period is typically several (2-8) months but has a wide range from as short as 10 days to more than a year. Knowing the exact time of exposure in endemic areas is not possible; incubation periods are often extrapolated from travelers with known exposure periods. Clinical disease may first become symptomatic years after exposure in persons who become immunocompromised. Immunocompromise secondary to a disease process, such as infection with human immunodeficiency virus (HIV) leading to AIDS; chronic use of immunosuppressive drugs such as corticosteroids, methotrexate, or the new class of TNF inhibitors; or use of immunosuppressive agents following solid organ transplantation, has been well described.[85-92] Anyone with a history of birth in, residence at, or travel to a *Leishmania*-endemic area is at risk of late reactivation if he or she becomes immunocompromised.

In cases with a subacute or chronic course, there is an insidious onset of fever, weakness, loss of appetite, weight loss, failure to thrive, and abdominal enlargement caused by hepatosplenomegaly. In endemic areas low-grade symptoms may persist for weeks to months before progressing to full-blown VL or resolving slowly. Because these symptoms may not be sufficiently severe to warrant medical attention in impoverished, endemic areas, patients may be called "subclinical" when they should be more appropriately called "oligosymptomatic." Fever may be intermittent, remittent with twice-daily temperature spikes (double quotidian), or, less commonly, continuous. Fever is relatively well tolerated, and older clinical references routinely noted that the patients were not acutely ill or "toxic" in appearance.

Acute presentations in persons without immunity are abrupt in onset, with high fever and chills and sometimes with a periodicity that suggests malaria.[93] Chills, but seldom rigors, accompany the temperature spikes. As time passes, the spleen can become massively enlarged. It is usually soft and nontender. The presence of a hard spleen suggests a hematologic disorder or another diagnosis such as schistosomiasis. The liver also enlarges; it usually has a sharp edge, soft consistency, and a smooth surface. Lymphadenopathy is common in patients in Sudan[59] but uncommon in other geographic areas. Elevated liver enzymes and bilirubin may be observed. Peripheral edema may be seen late in the disease, particularly in malnourished children. Hemorrhage can occur from one or more sites; epistaxis and gingival bleeding may be noted, as well as petechiae and ecchymoses on the extremities in late-stage disease. Many patients with visceral leishmaniasis become cachectic. This appears to be mediated in part by TNF-α and other cytokines that are known to have catabolic and anorectic effects.[94]

Secondary bacterial infections are common in persons with advanced VL. Patients can present with coinfection or acquire secondary bacterial infections as nosocomial pathogens during hospitalizations. It is important to recognize and treat clinically significant bacterial coinfections.[95-97] Death may result from pneumonia, septicemia, tuberculosis, dysentery, or measles, or it may be the consequence of malnutrition, severe anemia, or hemorrhage.

The laboratory findings include anemia, leukopenia, thrombocytopenia, and hypergammaglobulinemia. Anemia is almost always present and may be severe. It is usually normocytic and normochromic and appears to be due to a combination of factors including hemolysis, marrow replacement with leishmania-infected macrophages, hemorrhage, splenic sequestration of erythrocytes, hemodilution, and marrow-suppressive effects of cytokines such as TNF-α. Leukopenia is also prominent, with white blood cell counts occasionally as low as 1000/mm^3. It is not known whether the observed neutropenia is due to increased margination, splenic sequestration, an autoimmune process, or a combination of those factors. Eosinopenia (absence of eosinophils) is frequently observed. Of note, anemia and neutropenia have not been prominent in patients with VL who have undergone splenectomy. Hypergammaglobulinemia, circulating immune complexes, and rheumatoid factors are present in the sera of most patients with visceral leishmaniasis.[98,99] The globulin level may be as high as 9 g/dL; the ratio of globulin to albumin is typically high. The erythrocyte sedimentation rate is usually elevated.[100]

Renal involvement in VL is common. Acute renal failure, nephrotic syndrome, and proteinuria have been reported.[101-103] Acute glomerulonephritis,[101] proliferative glomerulonephritis,[103] collapsing focal segmental glomerulosclerosis,[104] acute interstitial nephritis,[103] and tubular cell necrosis and tubulitis[105] have all been described. In a recent retrospective study of 57 patients with VL caused by *L. infantum/chagasi* in Brazil, an elevated serum creatinine was seen in 26% of patients, and the only three deaths occurred in this group.[106] In a prospective study of 50 patients with VL caused by *L. infantum/chagasi* in another region of Brazil, abnormalities in glomerular filtration, urinary concentration, and acidification were consistently observed.[107]

VISCERAL LEISHMANIASIS IN PATIENTS WITH ACQUIRED IMMUNODEFICIENCY SYNDROME

Leishmania infection is persistent, and asymptomatic infections are not uncommon. When immunosuppression occurs in late-stage HIV infection, clinical VL can present as an opportunistic infection (OI). VL may be the presenting syndrome of AIDS or another late-stage OI in the terminal stages of disease. VL usually presents with typical combinations of fever, hepatomegaly, splenomegaly, weight loss, and pancytopenia when patients have CD4 counts of more than 50 cells/mm^3, but atypical presentations and localization of parasites are more common when CD4 cells are fewer than 50 cells/mm^3.[108] AIDS patients have extensive gastrointestinal tract involvement to include oral mucosa, esophagus, stomach, and small intestine and may present with chronic diarrhea.[62,109,110] Lung and pleural involvement presenting as pleural effusions and bone marrow involvement presenting as aplastic anemia also have been described.[111,112] The incidence of leishmanial OIs has decreased with the introduction of modern antiretroviral drug regimens,[113-116] but the number of cases of VL-HIV coinfection worldwide may increase dramatically as HIV infection continues to spread into *Leishmania*-endemic regions.[117-119] Although the incidence of VL as an OI decreased following the introduction of modern antiretroviral therapy, later relapse of VL remains problematic.[120]

VISCEROTROPIC LEISHMANIASIS

An unusual systemic syndrome associated with *L. tropica* infection, called *viscerotropic leishmaniasis*, was described in returning U.S. military personnel who served in the Persian Gulf War of 1990-1991.[52,53]

The symptoms included chronic low-grade fever, malaise, fatigue, and, in some cases, diarrhea. Mild splenomegaly was observed in some. None of the troops developed classical kala-azar or progressive visceral leishmaniasis. Subsequent studies failed to show an association between *L. tropica* infection and chronic fatigue and other symptoms associated with the Gulf War syndrome.[121] Similar oligosymptomatic syndromes have been reported in Brazil and Italy and likely are more common than those currently recognized because of the difficulty in making a parasitologic diagnosis.[55,122-124]

POST–KALA-AZAR DERMAL LEISHMANIASIS

Post–kala-azar dermal leishmaniasis (PKDL) follows the treatment of VL due to *L. donovani* in 5% to 10% of persons within 2 to 4 years following treatment in India and approximately 50% of persons within 6 months of treatment in the Sudan (Fig. 276-5).[125-128] PKDL is rarely seen following treatment of VL in Latin America or in the Mediterranean with *L. infantum/L. chagasi*, and, when reported, it has been in patients with concurrent AIDS.[129] PKDL is more commonly seen after treatment with pentavalent antimony compounds and appears to be less common after successful treatment with amphotericin B formulations,[130] although a definitive demonstration of this effect awaits a prospective clinical trial.

The skin lesions of PKDL are chronic and may persist for as long as 20 years in India, whereas in the Sudan they persist for only a few months to a year. The skin lesions consist of hyperpigmented or hypopigmented macules that progress to papules, nodules, and verrucous forms. They are found on the face, trunk, extremities, oral mucous membranes, and, occasionally, the genitals. They may be confused clinically and pathologically with leprosy. Patients generally feel well. The diagnosis is mainly clinical, but amastigotes can be detected in the skin in more than 80% of cases in the Sudan.

Antileishmanial treatment is generally indicated in Indian PKDL. In the Sudan, most cases cure spontaneously, but chronic or severe cases are treated. In a few instances in India, VL has recurred in patients

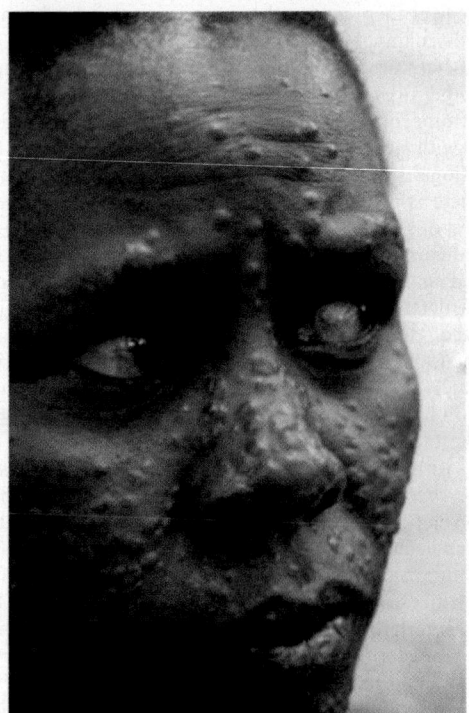

Figure 276-5 **Post–kala-azar dermal leishmaniasis (PKDL).** Papular lesions following the treatment of visceral leishmaniasis in Kenya. *(Courtesy of Dr. Tom Simpson, Baltimore, MD.)*

with PKDL. Patients with PKDL are thought to be infectious and serve as reservoirs for continued anthroponotic infection.[131] Treatment of PKDL patients, at least to render them noninfectious to sand flies, is likely an important part of a future successful control strategy.[132]

DIAGNOSIS

The positive predictive value of a clinical diagnosis of VL in a patient with the full pentad of prolonged fever, progressive weight loss, weakness, pronounced splenomegaly, hepatomegaly, cytopenias, and hypergammaglobulinemia from a known endemic area is very high. Clinical diagnosis without supporting parasitologic confirmation is unsatisfactory in patients with late-stage HIV infection or AIDS, returning travelers who may present with clinical symptoms months or years after exposure in low-transmission areas such as the Mediterranean, those with oligosymptomatic or viscerotropic syndromes, and those with atypical presentations.

The parasitologic diagnosis of VL can be confirmed by demonstrating amastigotes in tissue, isolating promastigotes in culture, or with a positive PCR. Splenic aspiration, liver biopsy, lymph node aspirates, and bone marrow aspirates have all been used with success. The spleen is the most sensitive location, and splenic aspiration to obtain a few drops of fluid for Wright- and Giemsa-stained smears, culture, and PCR is the most sensitive method for parasite identification.[133] Splenic aspirations are reported positive in over 95% of samples compared with bone marrow aspirations. The sensitivity of a bone marrow aspirate approaches that of a splenic aspirate when microscopists spend more time reviewing the smear.[134-136] A useful method for quantifying the parasite burden from splenic aspiration for staging of patients is widely used to stage patients and monitor response to treatment.[137] Splenic aspirations are routinely performed in some areas, but it can be associated with substantial hemorrhage, particularly in patients with advanced stages of disease who have undergone aspirations by inexperienced operators. The risk is lower when aspiration is performed quickly by an experienced person using a small-bore needle in patients with no laboratory evidence of coagulopathy.[133] Bone marrow aspiration is safer and preferred in nonendemic settings but is less sensitive. Amastigotes are seen in 40% to 90% of patients when compared with a positive splenic aspirate. The wide range reflects the stage of disease and the rigor of microscopic review because of the lower parasite burden in the bone marrow.

Liver biopsy is less likely to yield the diagnosis than is splenic puncture or bone marrow biopsy but occasionally is positive when bone marrow is negative.[138] Lymph node aspiration or biopsy may be diagnostic when enlarged nodes are present, as is often the case in Sudan. Amastigotes may also be seen within mononuclear cells in Wright- and Giemsa-stained smears of the buffy coat[139] or in biopsy specimens of various organs. The latter is particularly true in patients with AIDS in whom amastigotes in macrophages have been identified in bronchoalveolar lavage fluid, pleural effusions, or biopsy specimens of the oropharynx, stomach, or intestine. On occasion, parasites have been cultured from the buffy coat or blood. When the diagnosis of VL is suspected, parasitologic confirmation may require one than one technique and repeated procedures.[93]

Whenever possible, aspirates from the spleen, bone marrow, liver, or lymph nodes should be cultured. Specimens can be inoculated into one of several media [Schneider's modified media, Novy-MacNeal-Nicolle (NNN) media, and others] and maintained at ambient temperatures, 22° C to 26° C. Amastigotes must transform into motile promastigotes and then multiply in vitro to expand to a number that can be microscopically visualized. When the initial parasite inoculum is high, they may be seen in culture within a few days, but it may take several weeks for the concentration to reach the level of detection. Culturing parasites is an art and is unlikely to be performed in routine microbiology laboratories. In the United States, culture media and expert assistance are available from the Centers for Disease Control and Prevention (CDC). Isolates can be forwarded to the CDC or other WHO reference laboratories for speciation.

High-titer antileishmanial antibodies are typically present in immunocompetent patients with VL. A number of serologic tests using different antigens and assays are available. Currently, enzyme-linked immunosorbent assay (ELISA) and dipstick tests using *L. infantum/L. chagasi* recombinant k39 (rk39), a kinesin-like antigen,[140] have demonstrated excellent sensitivity and specificity for the diagnosis of VL in immunocompetent persons in India and Brazil but less so for those in East Africa.[141-143] Proper interpretation of rk39 test results requires an understanding of the antibody response. Titers to rk39 and other serologic tests remain elevated and detectable after successful treatment.[144] False-positive results may occur due to cross-reacting antibodies in patients with leprosy, Chagas' disease, cutaneous leishmaniasis,[145] and other infections. Antileishmanial antibodies may be absent or present at low titer in patients with AIDS, resulting in false-negative serological results. Other serologic test formats such as direct agglutination (DAT) and urine antigen detection have been used with variable success.[146,147] Each test format has its relative advantages and disadvantages depending on the intended use, resources, and cost considerations.

The sensitivity of a positive rK39 antibody dipstick test in individuals with suspected VL in India and with a therapeutic response to amphotericin B was shown to be 99% (119 of 120) in India.[148] The use of sensitive point of care diagnostic tests in patients with clinically suspect VL, along with the expected therapeutic response to a specific treatment such as amphotericin B, promises to restrict otherwise invasive procedures such as splenic aspiration only to those negative for rK39 or those who fail to improve with amphotericin B.

The leishmanin (Montenegro) skin test is negative in patients with active VL. It becomes positive in the majority of those in whom infection spontaneously resolves and in patients who have undergone successful chemotherapy. Although the skin test is useful in studies of the epidemiology, it has no value in the diagnosis of VL. The leishmanin skin test may be negative or positive in persons with PKDL, depending on the stage of disease.[125]

DIFFERENTIAL DIAGNOSIS

The differential diagnosis of late-stage VL with the full complement of symptoms and signs is limited to hematologic and lymphatic malignancies and occasionally disseminated histoplasmosis and tropical splenomegaly syndrome. Acute VL has a much broader differential to include malaria, enteric fevers, bacterial endocarditis, sarcoidosis, hemophagocytic syndromes, typhus, acute Chagas' disease (in Latin America), acute schistosomiasis, miliary tuberculosis, and amebic liver abscess. Subacute or chronic VL may be confused with brucellosis, prolonged *Salmonella* bacteremia, histoplasmosis, infectious mononucleosis, lymphoma, leukemia, myeloproliferative disease, hepatosplenic schistosomiasis, and chronic malaria. PKDL must be differentiated from leprosy, yaws, and syphilis.

▪ Cutaneous Leishmaniasis

CL is endemic in widely scattered areas throughout the world. The classic form of Old World CL is the "oriental sore," also known by a variety of colorful local expressions such as *bouton d'orient, bouton de Crete, bouton d'Alep, bouton de Biskra, Aleppo evil, Baghdad boil,* and *Dehli boil* in various regions of the Middle East, the Mediterranean littoral, Africa, India, and Asia. It is most frequently caused by *L. major, L. tropica,* or *Leishmania aethiopica,* but *L. donovani* and *L. infantum/L. chagasi* can also cause simple cutaneous leishmaniasis. The resulting skin lesions range from troublesome and unsightly to severe and complicated, but they generally are not life-threatening. Severe cases and facial lesions are very stigmatizing. Diffuse cutaneous leishmaniasis (DCL) due to *L. aethiopica* infection is reported from Ethiopia and adjacent areas of Africa.

American CL is endemic in widespread areas of Latin America. The causative species include *L. braziliensis, Leishmania mexicana, L. panamensis/L. guyanensis,* and many others (see Table 276-1). *L.*

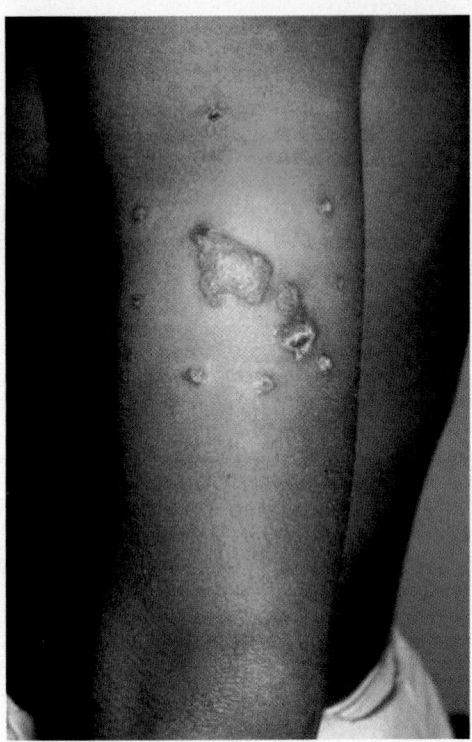

Figure 276-6 New World cutaneous leishmaniasis caused by *L. panamensis.* Note the plaquelike primary lesion with multiple satellite lesions.

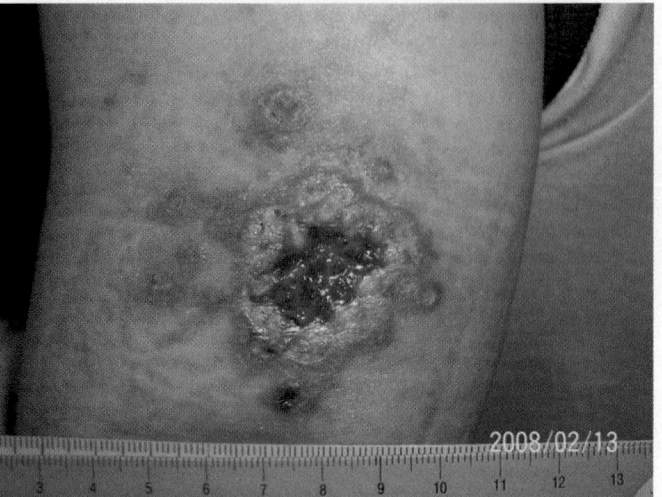

Figure 276-8 New World cutaneous leishmaniasis caused by *L. guyanensis.* *(Courtesy of Dr. Glenn Wortman, Washington, D.C.)*

infantum/L. chagasi is associated with simple nodular CL in Central America. Depending on the clinical presentation and geographic location, American CL is variously known as *pian bois* (bush yaws), *uta,* or *Chiclero's ulcer.*

The spectrum of New World CL disease includes single or multiple, localized, cutaneous ulcers (Figs. 276-6 to 276-9), diffuse cutaneous leishmaniasis, and mucosal disease (espundia) caused by *L. braziliensis* or, less commonly, other related *Leishmania* spp. (Fig. 276-10).

The spectrum of Old World CL disease includes single or multiple, localized, cutaneous ulcers (Figs. 276-11 and 276-12), diffuse cutaneous leishmaniasis, post–kala-azar dermal leishmaniasis (see Fig. 276-5), and leishmaniasis recidivans (Fig. 276-13).

EPIDEMIOLOGY

In the Old World, CL is usually a sporadic disease in endemic areas, but occasionally it occurs in an epidemic pattern, particularly when large groups of susceptible persons are exposed during road construction, refugee movements, or military activities.[149,150] *L. major* is an infection of desert rodents, primarily gerbils, and affects humans in arid and rural regions of the Middle East, North Africa, and central Asia. It has been a major problem for troops operating in endemic regions in the Middle East. The lesions tend to be larger and "wet" with an overlying exudate. *Phlebotomus papatasi* and other *Phlebotomus* spp. are the vectors.

L. tropica infects dogs and humans in urban areas of the Middle East such as Baghdad, Tehran, Kabul, and Damascus, as well as cities in the Mediterranean littoral, India, and Pakistan. The lesions tend to be crusted and "dry." The vectors include *Phlebotomus sergenti* and *P. papatasi.*

L. aethiopica is endemic in Ethiopia, Kenya, and southwest Africa. The primary reservoirs are the rock hyrax; rodents are secondary reservoirs. *Phlebotomus longipes* and *Phlebotomus pedifer* are the vectors. Occasionally *L. donovani* and *L. infantum/L. chagasi* cause simple CL.

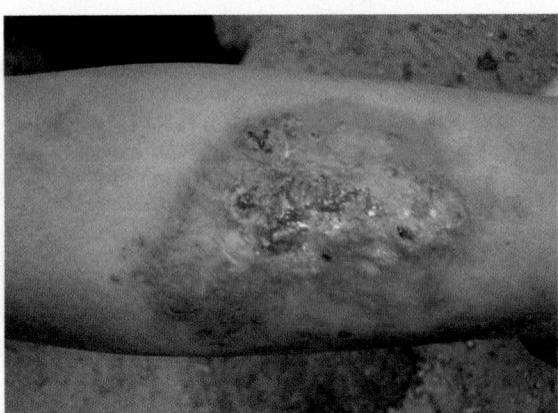

Figure 276-7 New World cutaneous leishmaniasis caused by *L. peruviana.* *(Courtesy of Dr. Alejandro Llanos-Cuentas, Lima, Peru.)*

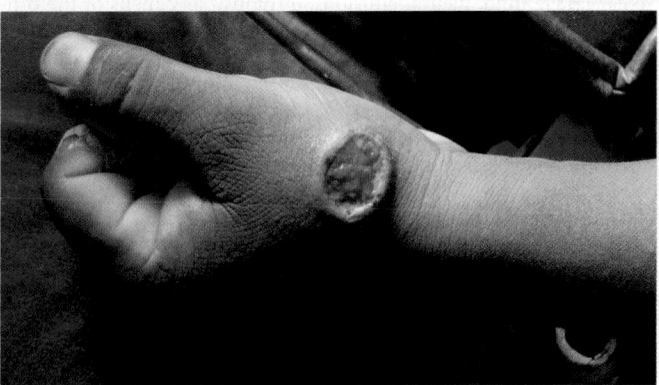

Figure 276-9 New World cutaneous leishmaniasis caused by *L. mexicana* acquired in Guatemala. Note the classic raised or rolled ulcer margin with surrounding induration. *(Courtesy of Dr. Byron Arana, Guatemala City, Guatemala.)*

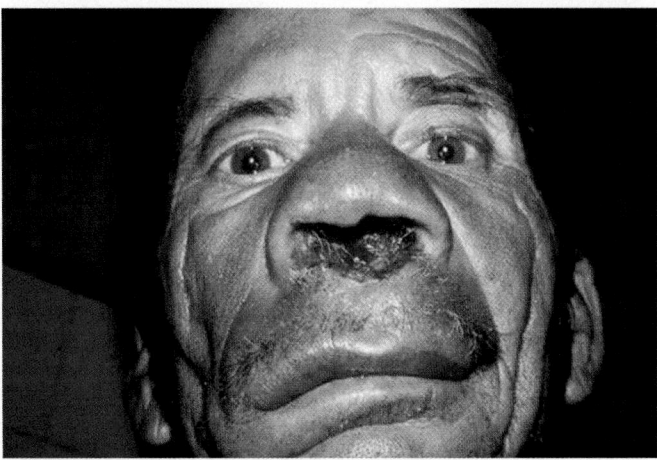

Figure 276-10   Mucosal leishmaniasis (espundia).

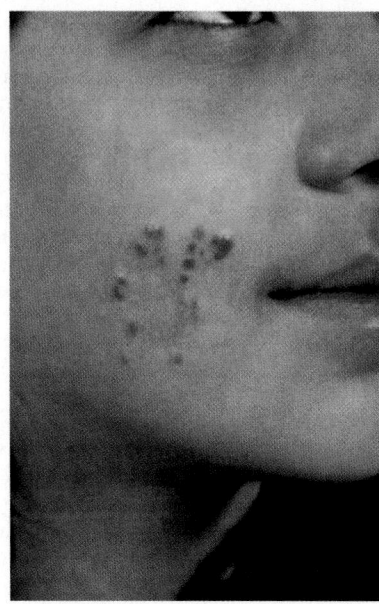

Figure 276-13   **Leishmaniasis recidivans.** A chronic oligoparasitic presentation of cutaneous leishmaniasis most commonly associated with *L. tropica* infection. Note the central scar from a previous primary ulcer surrounded by small papules. *(Courtesy of Dr. Jay Keystone, Toronto, Ontario, Canada.)*

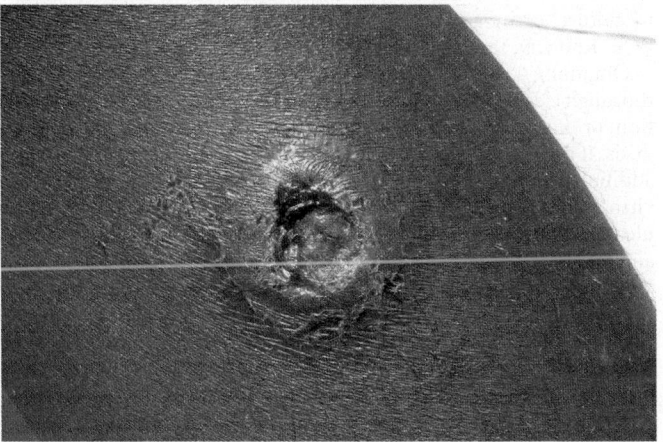

Figure 276-11   **Old World cutaneous leishmaniasis caused by *L. major.*** Note the classic raised or rolled ulcer margin with surrounding induration. *(Courtesy of Dr. Peter Weina, Bethesda, MD.)*

New World CL is usually a rural zoonosis.[3] The main reservoirs are forest rodents, except in the case of *Leishmania peruviana*, for which dogs are the primary reservoir. The vectors are ground-dwelling or arboreal *Lutzomyia* spp. Disease is common in persons working at the edge of the forest and among rural settlers. Outbreaks occur when areas of forest are cleared for roads, villages, or farms, or when military personnel or tourists enter endemic regions.

L. mexicana is responsible for American CL from northern Argentina to Texas, where a small number of autochthonous cases have been reported.[151,152] CL is an occupational hazard of gum, or chicle, collectors in Central America as well as persons living, working, or touring in endemic areas. Lesions typically appear on exposed areas of the extremities, the face, or the ears. A number of sylvatic rodents are reservoirs. *Lutzomyia* species are the vectors.

L. amazonensis produces a spectrum of disease in South America that includes simple cutaneous, diffuse cutaneous, and visceral leishmaniasis.[49] The vectors are *Lutzomyia* spp., and the reservoirs are forest animals.

L. braziliensis is found in widely scattered areas of Central and South America. It is responsible for cutaneous as well as mucosal leishmaniasis (ML). CL caused by *L. braziliensis* has been diagnosed among American tourists returning from Belize and other Latin American areas. *L. panamensis* is found in Panama and adjacent countries. It was an important problem for U.S. military personnel training in jungle areas of Panama. *L. guyanensis* is responsible for pian bois or bush yaws in the northern Amazon basin. *L. peruviana* is the cause of uta in Peru. It typically causes dry lesions.

PATHOGENESIS AND IMMUNOLOGY

The clinical manifestations of CL depend on the virulence factors of the infecting *Leishmania* spp. and the genetically determined immune responses of their human hosts. At the initial bite site, a papule forms, enlarges to a papulonodule, usually develops central ulceration, and slowly enlarges. Surrounding induration and raised borders are typical.[153]

CL is characterized by a mixed acute and chronic inflammatory infiltrate with infected and noninfected mononuclear phagocytes, lymphocytes, and plasma cells. There are areas of focal necrosis.[29] Early in infection, amastigote-containing macrophages dominate. Eventually, parasitized mononuclear phagocytes are eliminated, lymphocytes become prevalent, and a granulomatous response containing epithelioid cells and giant cells evolves. Lesions heal slowly, leaving a flat,

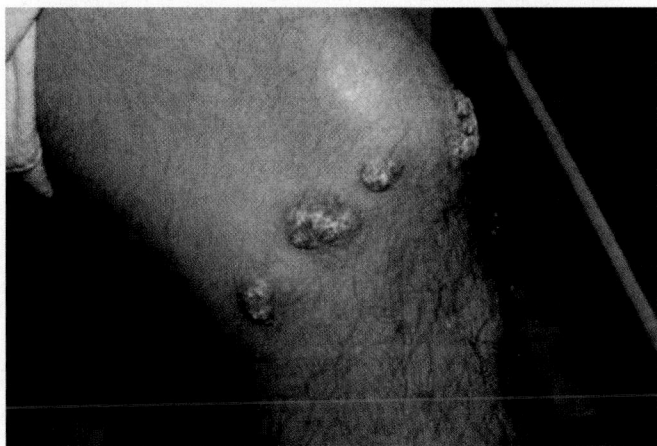

Figure 276-12   **Old World cutaneous leishmaniasis caused by *L. major.*** Note the atypical nodular or hyperkeratotic presentation that can be seen in 10% to 20% of patients.

atrophic, burnlike scar. Recovery is associated with a high level of resistance to reinfection by the homologous *Leishmania* spp.

Persons with cutaneous or mucosal leishmaniasis have evidence of both Th1 and Th2 lymphocytes in their lesions, but the systemic response is predominantly Th1. Their peripheral blood mononuclear cells proliferate and produce INF-γ and IL-2 in response to leishmanial antigens in vitro, and those infected exhibit delayed-type cutaneous hypersensitivity responses as evidenced by positive leishmanin skin tests in vivo. Complex chemokine and cytokine responses govern the tissue localization of effector cells and the resulting immune responses, but the precise sequence of events that results in skin necrosis and eventual healing has not yet been characterized.[154]

CLINICAL MANIFESTATIONS

The incubation period of CL typically varies from 2 weeks to several months, but it can be as long as several years. A wide variety of skin manifestations ranging from small papules, papulonodules, to dry, crusted lesions to large, deep, mutilating ulcers may be seen. Plaques, satellite lesions, psoriform, or verrucous lesions have all been described. The characteristics vary among *Leishmania* spp. and from one geographic area to another, but overlap occurs. Lesions with different characteristics may even be seen in the same patient. There may be a single lesion, multiple lesions, or widely disseminated disease with hundreds of smaller acneiform lesions. They are usually found on exposed areas of the body. No characteristic of the skin lesion is pathognomonic for CL or can be used to identify the causative *Leishmania* spp.

In general, *L. tropica* tends to cause "dry," crusted, slowly enlarging lesions that can persist for a year or more, whereas *L. major* and *L. braziliensis* are associated with "moist," exudative lesions that are larger, have a granulating base with overlying exudate, mature more rapidly, and typically heal after many months.

Ulcerative lesions are usually shallow and circular with well-defined, raised borders and a central bed of granulation tissue. They gradually increase in size and may develop a "pizza-like" appearance with a raised, circular outer margin, beefy red granulating base, and yellowish exudate on the surface. Satellite lesions may be present, and they may fuse with the original ulcer. Despite substantial tissue destruction, ulcers are usually not painful. The center of the granulating base of the ulcer may develop a hard excrescence, and a cutaneous horn may arise. Secondary staphylococcal or streptococcal cellulites can occur. After a variable period ranging from several months to longer than a year, ulcers heal, leaving flat, atrophic, depigmented, burnlike scars.

In *L. braziliensis* infection, regional lymphadenopathy may precede the development of cutaneous lesions by 1 to 12 weeks.[155,156] Patients may experience constitutional symptoms including malaise, anorexia, weight loss, and low-grade fever. As the skin ulcer develops, the lymphadenopathy and systemic symptoms subside. In *L. guyanensis,* and occasionally in *L. braziliensis* infection, a chain of nodules may develop along lymphatics proximal to the lesion, particularly if it is on an extremity, and mimic sporotrichosis.

DIFFUSE CUTANEOUS LEISHMANIASIS

The initial lesion in diffuse cutaneous leishmaniasis (DCL) starts as a localized papule that does not ulcerate. Satellite lesions develop around the initial papule, and organisms gradually spread in the skin, resulting in disseminated nodules primarily on the face and extremities. DCL has a protracted course and may last for the patient's lifetime.[157-160]

LEISHMANIASIS RECIDIVANS

Leishmaniasis recidivans (LR) is usually associated with *L. tropica* infection. It has been described across North Africa, the Middle East, Turkey, Southwest Asia, and Iran. The lesions are often on the face and consist of small papules that spread outward, leaving a scar at the center. The papules can wax and wane over many years. The chronic, nonhealing lesions can be especially problematic for young girls. LR is

a relapsing, tuberculoid form of CL characterized by very few parasites with an intense cell-mediated immune response. In nonendemic areas, it is most often seen in refugees or immigrants from endemic areas.

DISSEMINATED LEISHMANIASIS

Disseminated leishmaniasis (DL) is a syndrome characterized by hundreds of acneiform, papular, nodular, or ulcerated lesions in otherwise immunocompetent patients with *L. braziliensis* and *L. amazonensis* infections in Brazil.[161-163] Parasites are very few, and mucosal involvement is seen in 29% to 38%. The syndrome is most commonly observed in adult male agricultural workers in Brazil. Disseminated cutaneous lesions have also been observed in a limited number of patients with AIDS and in patients with organ transplants.[164]

DIAGNOSIS

One or more chronic skin lesions with the appropriate characteristics and a history of exposure in an endemic area suggest CL. A definite diagnosis is made by identifying amastigotes in tissue or promastigotes in culture, or by amplifying *Leishmania*-specific DNA or RNA in a PCR. Knowing the infecting species has relevance for chemotherapy.

Obtaining a specimen from an ulcer base requires meticulous and thorough cleaning and removal of exudate before the scraping, aspiration, or biopsy. Scrapings are often successful in confirming the diagnosis. If amastigotes are not seen on the initial smears, one can obtain additional scrapings, aspirates, or punch biopsies for more smears, in vitro culture, and PCR. Scrapings can be taken from any part of the ulcer that is clean and without exudate. Material obtained by scrapings and touch preparations made from biopsy samples are stained with a Wright-Giemsa preparation and examined under oil-immersion microscopy for amastigotes. A portion may also be used for histological examination and standard mycobacterial and fungal culture as clinically indicated. The diagnosis can also be made by tissue culture using nonbacteriostatic saline that has been injected and aspirated from the margin of the lesion.

The sensitivity of direct parasite identification and culture varies with the type and duration of the lesion and the infecting *Leishmania* sp. The combined sensitivity of these methods ranges from 50% to 90%.[165] When lymphadenopathy precedes or accompanies skin ulcers in *L. braziliensis* infection, the diagnosis can sometimes be made by aspirating an enlarged lymph node.[155,156]

Serologic assays are not generally helpful in the diagnosis of CL. Antileishmanial antibodies are detectable in the serum of only a minority of patients with CL, but actual sensitivity depends on the assay used, and the titers are usually low. The leishmanin skin test is usually positive in patients with simple CL.

The differential diagnosis includes sporotrichosis, blastomycosis, chromomycosis, lobomycosis, cutaneous tuberculosis, atypical mycobacterial infection, syphilis, yaws, leprosy, sarcoidosis, lupus vulgaris, and neoplasms of the skin. Rarely, lesions may assume a keloidal form and give the appearance of lobomycosis. In returning travelers, the competing diagnosis is tropical pyoderma, a chronic ulcerative lesion caused by typical gram-positive bacteria.

American Mucosal Leishmaniasis

About 2% to 5% of persons infected with *L. braziliensis,* or rarely a related *L. panamensis, L. guyanensis,* or *L. amazonensis,*[49,166] develop mucous membrane involvement of the nose, oral cavity, pharynx, or larynx months to years after their skin lesions have healed.[167,168] The percentage of patients infected with *L. braziliensis* who develop mucosal disease is relatively small. Mucosal involvement usually occurs following a resolved primary ulcer but occasionally is concurrent. The time between the primary lesion(s) and mucosal involvement may be as short as 1 month or as long as 2 decades.[167,170]

The initial symptoms of American mucosal leishmaniasis (ML) are often nasal stuffiness, discharge, discomfort, or epistaxis. Over time, a small nodule develops on the inferior turbinate or septum. Septal ulceration appears early and may progress to perforation and eventual destruction of the septum, resulting in nasal collapse, sometimes called a "tapir" nose because of the resemblance to the appearance of the South American tapir. Perforation can also occur through the soft palate. The upper lip may be involved in addition to the buccal, pharyngeal, or laryngeal mucosa, in that approximate order.[171] When hypertrophy predominates, resulting in a protuberant nose and lips, the condition is called *espundia*—a descriptive term likely derived from the Spanish word for "sponge" that was used to describe verrucous nasal lesions found in horses.[172] If ulceration predominates, there is severe mutilation. Any patient who complains of a change in voice or observed by others to have dysphonia requires a thorough examination of the epiglottis, vocal cords, and surrounding laryngal tissue. Occasionally severe inflammation can involve the epiglottis and threaten the airway. A plain lateral radiograph can demonstrate narrowing of the airway and soft tissue swelling as in any other presentation of epiglottis. In this setting, high-dose intravenous steroids must be given a day or two before the initiation of chemotherapy for ML. Acute airway obstruction can occur with the increase in inflammation that usually follows treatment of ML.[173] Rare involvement of the trachea as well as the genital mucosa has been reported. On rare occasions, mucosal lesions are so extensive or fibrosis so extensive that the individual is unable to eat or experiences fatal aspiration pneumonia.

Histopathologically, chronic mucosal lesions are characterized by an intense mononuclear cell infiltrate with few parasites. Persons with ML demonstrate strong systemic Th1 responses. Their peripheral blood mononuclear cells proliferate and produce INF-γ in response to leishmanial antigens in vitro, and their leishmanin skin tests are usually strongly positive.[174]

Various theories have been advanced to explain mucosal involvement. They include lower temperature, which favors parasite growth; failure of cell-mediated immune responses to be effective in mucosal tissue; local trauma; and capillary plexus trapping of amastigotes in the nose. Spontaneous cure of ML has been reported, but it is thought to be rare.[175] The lack of an appropriate animal model has hindered research on the immunopathology of the syndrome. Risk factors associated with the development of ML are male gender, young adult age, severe malnutrition, and duration of primary ulcer for more than 4 months.[176] Host immune response,[177] racial background,[178] parasite strain differences,[179] and familial clustering[180] are associated with increased risk of ML, but the associations are not seen in all studies. Although it is well known that the risk of ML associated with *L. braziliensis* is much higher in Bolivia, Brazil, and Peru, the distribution of the parasite extends from Mexico to Argentina.[181] ML is relatively uncommon in Middle America. Whether this difference is related to different parasite strains, host immune response differences, or even differences in sand fly vectors, such as components of sand fly saliva, awaits clarification.

Mucosal involvement is seen on occasion owing to the contiguous spread of cutaneous lesions caused by *L. tropica* or other *Leishmania* spp. In this setting it has been referred to as mucocutaneous leishmaniasis. ML has also been described in the Sudan associated with both *L. major* and *L. donovani*. In the Sudan, ML is sporadic, is found in VL areas, involves the upper respiratory tract and oral mucosa, is usually a primary disease but has been seen concurrent with or following VL, and may be caused by parasites that are genetically different from those associated with VL.[182-184] Mucosal involvement has also been described with *L. infantum* in the Mediterranean and is often associated with immunocompromised patients. Lesions are described as nodular or tumorlike masses.[185]

DIAGNOSIS

The clinical suspicion of ML is raised by visualizing abnormal mucosal lesions or when any nasal, oral, pharyngeal, or laryngeal symptoms are vocalized or elicited in a patient with a known past history of CL, a scar consistent with CL, or residence or travel to known endemic areas,

especially in the highest-risk countries of Bolivia, Brazil, and Peru. Parasitologic confirmation of ML occurs when amastigotes are identified in mucosal specimens obtained by snip biopsy or scraping and then visualized in touch preparations or tissue sections by Wright-Giemsa stains, when promastigotes are isolated in culture, or when parasite DNA is identified in a PCR reaction. ML is the prototypic oligoparasitic syndrome in the spectrum of *Leishmania*-related disease with a very low parasite burden, and traditional smear and culture have low sensitivity. In addition *L. braziliensis* is relatively difficult to grow and isolate in culture. Where available, PCR is the parasitologic diagnostic test of choice, with sensitivities of over 95% reported.[30] Validation of PCR testing to include specimen preparation, extraction, choice of primers, excluding inhibitors, and several other factors is very demanding, and no commercial assay is likely to be developed.[186] In addition to confirming *Leishmania* infection, use of subgenus (Viannia or not) and species-specific primers can provide species-level results prior to or just after the start of treatment may be used to aid management.[187]

A clinical diagnosis of ML can be made in an endemic area on the basis of typical clinical findings, a characteristic scar representing previous cutaneous infection, a positive leishmanin skin test result, or the presence of antileishmanial antibodies in serum (or a combination of any of these).[167,188] In general, mucosal disease caused by *L. braziliensis* is associated with higher antileishmanial antibody titers and stronger delayed-type hypersensitivity responses than simple cutaneous leishmaniasis. The leishmanin skin test is positive in 86% to 100% of cases. The sensitivity of tests for antileishmanial antibodies can vary widely with the assay and antigen used. There are no standardized, commercially available assays. Research centers often develop and use their own assays, making comparisons between sites impossible.

The differential diagnosis of ML includes paracoccidioidomycosis, syphilis, tertiary yaws, histoplasmosis, sarcoidosis, basal cell carcinoma, lethal midline granuloma, and T/NK cell lymphoma. The polyp-like nasal lesions that occur in some persons with ML may occasionally mimic rhinosporidiosis.

Treatment of Leishmaniasis

VISCERAL LEISHMANIASIS

Liposomal amphotericin B (AmBisome, Astellas Inc.) is the drug of choice for the treatment of VL in North America and any other setting where it can be safely administered and cost is not limiting. It is the only drug licensed for the treatment of VL in the United States,[44,189] and the approval was based on a review of treatment studies conducted in non-HIV and *Leishmania*/HIV-coinfected VL patients in the Mediterranean in the 1990s. The FDA-approved regimen for immunocompetent patients is 3.0 mg/kg of body weight per day on days 1 to 5, 14, and 21. A higher dose of 4.0 mg/kg of body weight per day on days 1 to 5, 10, 17, 24, 31, and 38 is recommended for immunocompromised patients. Cost and availability have limited its use in developing areas.[190] Different dose regimens have been tested worldwide, and efficacious regimens differ from one geographic location to another.[44] Shorter courses with higher daily doses have been used in studies in endemic areas with good results. Relapses can occur after liposomal amphotericin B and other forms of therapy in persons with AIDS, and an additional course(s) of liposomal amphotericin B may be necessary. Other lipid-associated amphotericin B preparations have been used in the treatment of VL, but the data to support their use in humans are much less extensive, and animal studies suggest liposomal preparations are superior.[191]

Pentavalent antimony (SbV) is still used for the treatment of VL in areas where *Leishmania* isolates remain susceptible and the cost of liposomal amphotericin B is prohibitive. It is no longer recommended in parts of India, where 40% of cases are now resistant.[192] The dose and regimen recommended for the treatment of VL is 20 mg of SbV/kg body weight daily for 28 days. Persons who respond slowly to the initial course of therapy or relapse may respond to a second course. Persons who fail to respond to SbV or acquire infection in areas where resistance is prevalent can be treated with liposomal amphotericin B, amphotericin B deoxycholate, or miltefosine in India. Primary failures and relapses are often observed in patients with concurrent AIDS.

Multiple preparations of SbV are manufactured and sold worldwide. Sodium stibogluconate (SSG; Pentostam, GSK), and meglumine antimoniate (MA; Glucantime, Sanofi Aventis) are the two best-known commercial products. Both are considered equivalent in efficacy and tolerability. One SSG generic formulation manufactured by Albert David Ltd. (Calcutta, India) was shown in direct comparative clinical trials to be equivalent to the branded products.[193,194] There are numerous other SbV products manufactured worldwide. These products can vary in total antimony content, the ratio of trivalent to pentavalent antimony (trivalent Sb is more toxic than SbV), and the physical and chemical characteristics of different lots of drug from the same manufacturer. Cardiac deaths have been associated with generic SbV with high osmolarity.[195,196] When used for VL, SbV can be given by intravenous (IV) or intramuscular (IM) route of administration. IM injections are painful and large volume. IV delivery is best with dilution of the daily dose at least 1:10 with 5% dextrose in water to reduce incidence of local thrombosis.

Side effects are common with SbV and include prominent gastrointestinal symptoms of anorexia, nausea, vomiting, and midepigastric pain likely associated with pancreatitis beginning early in the course of treatment. After the first week or so, myalgia and large-joint arthralgias sometimes appear and may become severe. Headache, asthenia, and malaise are common and occur early in treatment, but these complications seldom prevent completion of therapy. Elevated amylase and lipase occur in most recipients, but only a minority manifest clinically apparent pancreatitis. Persons with renal insufficiency seem to be at increased risk for this complication. Electrocardiographic changes are common and dose-dependent, and they include T-wave inversion and a prolonged QT interval.[197] Arrhythmias, sudden death, and torsades de pointes, especially with doses greater than 20 mg of SbV/kg of body weight per day, have been reported with SbV.[198,199] SbV should be used cautiously in the elderly and in patients with heart disease. Renal failure is a rare side effect. Mild nonspecific elevations (two- to fivefold) of AST and ALT are common, and a variety of cytopenias have been described. Rarely, angioedema and hypersensitivity reactions occur. SbV can be used in patients only with close medical supervision, periodically monitoring clinical symptoms and signs, complete blood counts, serum amylase, and lipase,[200] liver enzymes, renal function, and serial ECGs. Drug administration should be interrupted when laboratory values become modestly abnormal, especially when associated with symptoms. Deaths secondary to serious drug-related adverse events clearly occur.[201]

SbV should not be given during pregnancy, as a 57% spontaneous abortion rate was observed in one study.[39] In this same study, liposomal amphotericin B was used safely. SbV is a toxic and poorly tolerated drug, but it can be used with relative safety with close medical supervision.[202] The future role and place of SbV for the treatment of VL when amphotericin B or new combination regimens are readily available will likely diminish.[203]

A significant new drug for the treatment of Indian VL is miltefosine, an orally administered phosphocholine analogue now being used to treat patients in India, where SbV resistance is common.[204] Initially developed as an antineoplastic agent, miltefosine is associated with nausea, vomiting, and abdominal pain. Miltefosine was registered in India for the treatment of VL in 2002. Recently a postlicensure study was conducted among 1132 adult and pediatric VL patients in an outpatient setting. Compliance was good, with 1084 (95.5%) patients completing the full 28-day treatment course, and 971 (85.8%) patients returned for the final cure assessment at 6 months after treatment. The final cure rate was 82% by intention-to-treat analysis and 95% by per-protocol analysis (similar to the 94% cure rate in hospitalized patients). Treatment-related adverse events of common toxicity criteria grade 3 occurred in 3% of patients, including gastrointestinal toxicity and rise in liver transaminases, or serum creatinine levels, similar to previous

clinical experience.[205] Miltefosine is teratogenic, and its use in pregnancy is contraindicated. Adherence to a 28-day oral regimen with a drug that may cause gastrointestinal distress is problematic.[206] There is a real concern that subtherapeutic dosing of a single drug with a long half life could lead to the development of resistance.[207,208]

Other drugs used to treat VL include amphotericin B deoxycholate (Fungizone), pentamidine isethionate, and paromomycin. Amphotericin B deoxycholate must be given intravenously over prolonged periods of time and is associated with nephrotoxicity and other side effects.[209,210] Various doses and durations of therapy have been used; 1.0 mg per kg of body weight per day for 15 days or 1.0 mg per kg of body weight every other day for 30 days are two alternatives. Pentamidine isethionate is a toxic alternative with a number of side effects, including hypotension, life-threatening hypoglycemia caused by pancreatic β-cell injury, and later insulin-dependent diabetes mellitus. With availability of better drugs, its use for VL is no longer recommended.

Results of a randomized, controlled, phase III open-label study comparing injectable paromomycin, an aminoglycoside, with amphotericin B, the present standard of care in Bihar, India, in 667 patients was recently reported.[211] The paromomycin regimen studied was 11 mg/kg of body weight intramuscularly for 21 days. Paromomycin was shown to be noninferior to amphotericin B (final cure rate, 94.6% vs. 98.8%; difference, 4.2 percentage points; upper bound of the 97.5% confidence interval, 6.9; $P < .001$). Mortality rates in the two groups were less than 1%. Adverse events, which were more common among patients receiving paromomycin than among those receiving amphotericin B (6% vs. 2%, $P = .02$), included transient elevation of aspartate aminotransferase levels (>3 times the upper limit of the normal range); transient reversible ototoxicity (2% vs. 0, $P = .20$); and injection-site pain (55% vs. 0, $P < .001$). Adverse events more common in patients receiving amphotericin B, as compared with those receiving paromomycin, were nephrotoxicity (4% vs. 0, $P < .001$), fevers (57% vs. 3%), rigors (24% vs. 0, $P < .001$), and vomiting (10% vs. <1%, $P < .001$). Paromomycin was licensed for the treatment of VL in India in 2006, and phase IV evaluations are ongoing.

Treatment of VL in East Africa, the Mediterranean, and Latin America is predominantly with intramuscular SbV or amphotericin B deoxycholate. SbV remains efficacious in locations outside India and is usually the drug of choice to treat VL in East Africa and Latin America, with amphotericin B reserved for initial failures and relapses. In more resource-rich areas of the Mediterranean, liposomal amphotericin B is used as first-line treatment.

Patients with VL often have serious bacterial coinfections or tuberculosis that must be treated. They are also frequently malnourished. There are no parasitic or immunologic tests of cure, but patients do respond rather quickly to efficacious treatment with resolution of fever, improved sense of well-being, return of appetite within a week, and improving anemia and leukopenia in the second week. Splenomegaly may take weeks or longer to resolve. Relapses occur usually within 6 months of initial treatment success and are common in patients with AIDS. In addition to antileishmanial chemotherapy, patients with AIDS should receive highly active antiretroviral therapy. To prevent relapse, chronic suppressive antileishmanial therapy, symptom-based retreatment, and scheduled secondary prophylaxis have all been used, but the optimal drug and regimen have not been defined.

Chemotherapy of patients with PKDL is unsatisfactory. There are few controlled studies and only small case series. Also, clinical and parasitologic endpoints in PKDL are poorly defined. Severe PKDL in the Sudan is treated with SSG at 20 mg/kg of body weight per day for 2 to 3 months[212] and for up to 120 days in India with cure rates of 64% to 92% reported.[213] With the toxicity of SbV, especially in people who are otherwise not ill, and increasing SbV resistance in India, the future role of SbV in India is not clear. Amphotericin B deoxycholate and liposomal amphotericin B have been very promising when used in small numbers of patients in India[214] and the Sudan,[215] but additional studies are needed to define the role of amphotericin B in the treatment of PKDL.

Many now advocate combination chemotherapy regimens for VL with the same rationale that we use for tuberculosis and malaria. VL is a polyparasitic disease syndrome, and using two or more drugs may shorten overall regimens, decrease toxicity, and prevent the emergence of resistance. Single-dose liposomal amphotericin B plus short-course oral miltefosine is particularly attractive in India, and combination SSG and paromomycin has been used in the Sudan.[216,217] Several planned and ongoing clinical trials are comparing liposomal amphotericin B with miltefosine, liposomal amphotericin B and paromomycin, and miltefosine plus paromomycin sulfate.

CUTANEOUS LEISHMANIASIS

The treatment of CL syndromes is best approached by considering the extent and severity of lesions in each individual, the confirmed or most likely infecting parasite strain, the likelihood of natural healing, and the probability of late manifestations of ML following *L. braziliensis* infections. Because most cases of CL will eventually resolve and treatment, especially systemic, is not without risk, the first management decision in a patient with CL is whether to recommend specific treatment. Table 276-2 lists criteria that should be considered in making the initial treatment decision and the relative need for systemic versus a local treatment option. There are no licensed drugs for the treatment of CL or ML in the United States, but returning travelers can be offered a variety of options.[17]

Treatment of CL acquired in the Old World has recently been reviewed.[45] When systemic treatment is indicated, parenteral treatment is most often with intramuscular SbV in endemic countries and intravenous SbV in non-endemic countries. Although the optimal dosage and duration of therapy may vary from one geographic area to another, 20 mg of Sb/kg of body weight daily for 20 days is recommended. Healing of cutaneous lesions occurs slowly over a period of

weeks and is often incomplete at the end of the treatment course. Clinical trials demonstrating efficacy of parenteral SbV in *L. major* or *L. tropica* are lacking. In reality, intralesional SbV has been shown to give statistically higher cure rates, with lower systemic toxicity in studies of *L. major* in Saudi Arabia[218] and *L. tropica* in Afghanistan.[219] The toxicity associated with parenteral SbV, the need for parenteral administration over a prolonged period, and the lack of clear demonstrated clinical effects of parenteral SbV in Old World CL should factor in a careful risk benefit assessment of SbV use. Other parenteral systemic options such as amphotericin B have not been studied in Old World CL but could be considered as alternatives in individual cases.

Oral systemic treatment in Old World CL with several agents has been studied. Fluconazole, 200 mg daily for 6 weeks, cured 59% after 3 months, compared with 21% in a no-treatment control arm in persons with CL due to *L. major* in Saudi Arabia.[220] Modest beneficial effects have been seen with itraconazole, 200 mg orally daily for 6 to 8 weeks, with better outcome in *L. major* than *L. tropica*.[221-223] There is no demonstrated benefit of ketoconazole in Old World CL. Miltefosine given at 2.5 mg/kg daily for 28 days was shown to be at least as efficacious as IM SbV at 20 mg/kg daily for 14 days for the treatment of *L. major*, the national standard for the treatment of CL in Iran.[224]

Local therapies for Old World CL to include intralesional SbV, paromomycin-based topical creams and ointments, and hyperthermic and cryotherapy physical treatments have long been regional favorites, although they are less commonly used in nonendemic countries. The interpretation of clinical trial results with topical paromomycin-based products is confused by the use of the variety of formulations, but the combination of 15% paromomycin plus 12% methylbenzethonium chloride (MBCL) in soft white paraffin administered twice daily for 28 days is better than placebo in *L. major* infections but has no benefit in *L. tropica* infections.[45,225] Locally applied hyperthermic therapy administered with a ThermoMed device was compared with IM and IL SbV for the treatment of CL due to *L. tropica* in 401 patients with a single lesion in a randomized, controlled trial in Kabul, Afghanistan. Cure, defined as complete reepithelialization at 100 days after treatment initiation, was observed in 75 of 108 patients (69.4%) who received thermotherapy, 70 of 93 patients (75.3%) who received intralesional SSG, and 26 of 58 patients (44.8%) who received intramuscular SSG. The odds ratio for cure with thermotherapy was 2.80 (95% confidence interval [CI], 1.45-5.41), compared with intramuscular SSG treatment ($P = .002$). The time to cure was significantly shorter in the thermotherapy group (median, 53 days) than in the intralesional SSG or intramuscularly SSG group (median, 75 days and >100 days, respectively; $P = .003$).[219] The utility of a single application of heat treatment and the proven efficacy as compared to SbV for the treatment of *L. tropica* should favor hyperthermy. The practical limitation to single or a few lesions and access to a reliable and inexpensive delivery modality limit access and impact. There have been numerous reports of cures and therapeutic benefit with various combinations of local and topical treatments, often used clinically that have not been well studied, but many have been uncontrolled observations and lack any evidence base to support a recommendation for use.[45]

Treatment of CL acquired in the New World has also been recently reviewed.[226] Intramuscular SbV usually given at 20 mg/kg daily for 20 days is the most common medical treatment in the Americas and produced an overall cure rate of 76% (range 58% to 100%) in over 1000 patients entered into selected controlled trials.[226] Predicting who is most likely to respond to SbV treatment is much desired to prevent needless toxicity and save resources. Various clinical, epidemiologic, and laboratory criteria have been evaluated to find correlates of therapeutic success.[227-231] Young age (presumably reflecting a non- or less-immune status) and non-immunes (tourists and new immigrants to endemic locations), intrinsic SbV susceptibility, and geographic location (presumably reflecting *Leishmania* species or strain variations) have all been reported to correlate with therapeutic failure. Reported SbV efficacy tended to be lower in Brazil and higher in Colombia, and *L. braziliensis* and *L. peruviana* respond less well than *L. guyanensis*. Differing assay techniques may account for somewhat discrepant in vitro susceptibility testing of *Leishmania* parasites.

TABLE 276-2	Criteria to Consider When Deciding Initial Treatment Options in Patients with Cutaneous Leishmaniasis	
Criteria	*Favors No Treatment*	*Treatment Usually Indicated*
Age and direction of healing	Lesions clearly improving by patient history compared with a few weeks to a month prior	Lesions clearly getting worse by patient history compared to a few weeks to a month prior
Number of lesions	Single or just a few	Multiple (>5) and in different locations
Complexity	Uncomplicated	Complicated: restricts joint mobility, prevents wearing of clothes or shoes, nose and ear involvement
Size of lesion(s)	Small (<1 cm)	Very large (>5 cm)
Immune status	Immunocompetent	Immunocompromised
Mucosal involvement	None by history and exam	Yes
Location	Nonexposed skin	Exposed skin, especially facial
Leishmania braziliensis	*Leishmania* parasite isolated is not *L. braziliensis* or clearly acquired in geographic area without known *L. braziliensis* infection or with rare cases of mucosal leishmaniasis (Middle America)	*Leishmania* parasite isolated is characterized as *L. braziliensis* and acquired in geographic area with known risk of mucosal leishmaniasis*
How bothersome are lesions to patient and family?	No or little concern	Very concerned, preoccupied

*Patients with CL due to *L. braziliensis* acquired in Bolivia, Brazil, and Peru are at higher risk of developing mucosal leishmaniasis. Parenteral (systemic) treatment is usually recommended.

The efficacy of liposomal amphotericin B for New World CL has not yet been systematically accessed in a controlled study, but promising results have been reported in small series of nonimmune travelers.[232,233] The optimal dose and regimen is not defined for CL. Use of the FDA-approved regimen for VL of 3.0 mg/kg daily for days 1 through 5 and subsequent doses on day 14 and 21 (21 mg/kg total dose) is reasonable pending additional data. Where resources are less limiting, use of liposomal amphotericin B as a first choice for CL is appealing because the drug is available and approved by the U.S. FDA, and clinicians are familiar with its use. Liposomal amphotericin B is expensive and rarely used in endemic countries. However, amphotericin B deoxycholate is commonly used with good results in those who fail an initial course of SbV.

Pentamidine has a unique niche in the treatment of CL caused by *L. guyanensis* in French Guyana and Surinam. Cure rates as high as 90% are reported with just two intramuscular injections of 4 mg/kg.[234,235] Pentamidine is not efficacious in other geographic locations or in other *Leishmania* parasites.[226]

In the New World, ketoconazole, 600 mg daily for 28 days, cured 8 of 9 patients (89%) with *L. mexicana* in Guatemala[236] and 16 of 21 patients (76%) with *L. panamensis* in Panama.[87] Ketoconazole is not efficacious against *L. brasiliensis* in Guatemala.[236,237]

Efficacy of miltefosine in New Word CL was demonstrated in an open-label, dose escalation, phase I-II trial against *L. panamensis* in 72 male Colombian soldiers. A per-protocol cure rate for 50 to 100 mg per day of miltefosine was 66%. The per-protocol cure rate for 133 to 150 mg per day was 94%, similar to the historic per-protocol cure rate for parenteral SbV of 93%.[238] In a placebo-controlled study of miltefosine against CL in regions of Colombia where *L. panamensis* is common, the per-protocol cure rates for miltefosine and placebo were 91% (40 of 44 patients) and 38% (9 of 24).[239] In regions in Guatemala where *L. braziliensis* and *L. mexicana* are common, the per-protocol cure rates were 53% (20 of 38) for miltefosine and 21% (4 of 19) for placebo.[239] These results demonstrate miltefosine is a useful oral agent against CL caused by *L. panamensis* in Colombia, but unfortunately not against CL caused by *L. braziliensis* in Guatemala. More recently, in a randomized study of miltefosine and IM SbV in *L. braziliensis* in Bolivia, the per-protocol cure rates were 88% (36 of 41) for miltefosine and 94% (16 of 17) for IM SbV, not statistically different.[239a] The efficacy of miltefosine in the treatment of New World CL differs from region to region and must be evaluated in different settings to determine utility.[240] Miltefosine is not approved by the FDA, and it is not readily available in the United States.

Diffuse cutaneous leishmaniasis is relatively unresponsive to most forms of therapy. Miltefosine leads to an initial favorable response, but relapse follows. Immunotherapy with a combination of heat-killed *L. mexicana*, and viable BCG has been successful in Venezuela with minimal toxicity.[241]

In all forms of CL, attention should be directed to local wound care. CL is both a parasitic infection and an open wound. Antibiotics should be administered if there is evidence of cellulitis, painful or tender areas, or purulence.

AMERICAN MUCOSAL LEISHMANIASIS

SbV has been used for the treatment of American ML for decades, but the response is variable (51% to 88%) and relapses are common.[242] Early disease responds better than late-stage disease. Treatment regimens have varied, but a dose of 20 mg Sb /kg of body weight daily for 28 days is typically administered, with some patients requiring longer courses. There are no tests or rigid criteria to document cure. Those who do not respond or those who relapse can be treated with amphotericin B deoxycholate.[243-246] Depending on the patient's tolerance, 1.0 mg/kg of body weight is given intravenously daily or every other day for up to 30 days. Liposomal amphotericin B has been used successfully in a small number of cases.[247-249] The total dose is not well established, but ranges of 20 to 40 mg/kg have been reported.

Miltefosine, 2.5 mg/kg/day for 28 days, with follow-up for 12 months cured 83% (30 of 36) with mild disease (nasal mucosa) and 58% (21 of 36) with more extensive disease (palate, pharynx, and larynx) in an open, not randomized trial in Bolivian ML due to *L. braziliensis*.[250] Patients reportedly preferred the oral miltefosine and refused to be randomized to parenteral agents. For individuals who fail an initial course of SbV, miltefosine may be useful. The effectiveness of a long oral course of miltefosine if not given under directly observed therapy may be lower.

Other adjunctive approaches have been used with success. Oral pentoxifylline, an inhibitor of TNF-alpha, combined with SbV gave 100% cure (11 of 11) compared with a 58% cure (7 of 12) in the SbV only arm in Brazilian ML. Time to healing was sooner in the combination group as well.[250a] Immunotherapy with new-generation vaccines is also being tested.[251] Plastic surgery may be necessary to ameliorate the sequelae of mucosal leishmaniasis. It should be delayed for a year after successful therapy because grafts may be lost if relapse occurs.

Prevention

There are several approaches to prevention for individuals and communities as public health interventions. For the individual, there is no form of chemoprophylaxis or active (vaccine) or passive (immunoglobulin) immunoprophylaxis for travelers. Standard personal protective measures such as insect repellents that contain diethyltoluamide (DEET) and permethrin or other insecticides applied to clothing and insecticide-impregnated fine-mesh bed nets all provide protection against sand flies if used correctly.[252]

For community-based efforts in endemic areas, vector control and reservoir control are effective depending on local sand fly behavior and transmission dynamics. Residual insecticides applied in houses and other buildings have yielded good results in sites where peridomestic transmission occurs. Unfortunately, spraying is necessary at intervals, sand flies may become resistant, and there is concern about the environmental impact. Of note, the cessation of dichlorodiphenyltrichloroethane (DDT) spraying for malaria in Peru, India, Bangladesh, and southern Iran was followed by major epidemics and a resurgence of leishmaniasis.[253-257] In areas where transmission occurs away from dwellings, residual insecticides are obviously of no benefit. The efficacy of impregnated bed nets to reduce human–sand fly contact in at-risk populations living in endemic transmission areas is less certain and variable, with some studies showing an impact and others minimal or no impact.[258,259] The efficient use of bed nets to prevent leishmaniasis will depend on an understanding of both human behaviors and sand fly biology.[260]

Reservoir control is another option in areas with domestic animal or human reservoirs. In *L. infantum/L. chagasi* areas, domestic and wild dogs are thought to be the primary reservoir. Immunizing dogs, preventing infection through insecticide dog collars, and culling feral dogs should interrupt transmission and reduce human disease. In northeastern Brazil, infected domestic dogs have been identified by mass serologic testing and exterminated, but the efficacy of the program has been debated and it is poorly accepted. Recent studies suggest that insecticide-impregnated collars may protect dogs from sand fly bites and reduce the risk of human disease.[261,262] In sites where leishmaniasis is a zoonosis involving sylvatic mammals, reservoir control is rarely possible. In areas of anthroponotic (person–sand fly–person) transmission, case identification and treatment is important in control. Persons living in the same household as active cases and the existence of asymptomatic human infections in the community are a transmission risk.[263,264] In countries such as Spain where VL has been spread among intravenous drug users, needle exchange programs might limit transmission.

Although no commercial vaccine is currently available, there is a rationale to expect one in the future. The spontaneous resolution of human infection is associated with high-level immunity against the homologous infecting *Leishmania* spp.[265] Mothers living in endemic areas of the Middle East have exposed the buttocks of their children to sand flies to ensure that leishmanial infection occurs at an inconspicuous site, thus protecting them from later disfiguring facial lesions. Immunization with live parasites has been used for centuries, much like cowpox, by inoculating material from exudates of an active lesion into a covered part of the body.[266] In more recent years in Iran, Israel, and Uzbekistan, leishmanization has been performed by inoculating live *L. major* promastigotes taken from culture. Good results were obtained with the "Jericho" strain of *L. major*. Although this practice was effective in preventing naturally acquired disease, it was discontinued in Israel because some of the resulting lesions were slow to heal, others became secondarily infected, and parasites persisted at the site of inoculation even after the lesions healed. Leishmanization cannot be used on a large scale or in HIV endemic areas. Since *Leishmania* undergo biological changes in culture, lose their infectivity when subcultured, and cannot be lyophilized, they must be kept frozen in liquid nitrogen, and thus their delivery is impractical. The first generation of *Leishmania* vaccines included whole parasites with or without BCG as adjuvant.[267] These were used for prophylaxis or combined with antimonials for immunochemotherapy. Second-generation efforts have focused on identifying protective leishmanial immunogens—and effective adjuvants—and also on the development of genetically engineered, live, avirulent strains.[268-271] It is possible that an effective form of immunoprophylaxis will eventually come from one of these approaches.

In 2005, the governments of Bangladesh, India, and Nepal signed a memorandum of understanding to eliminate VL from the region. This ambitious elimination goal has five pillars: early diagnosis and complete treatment, integrated vector management and vector surveillance, effective disease surveillance through passive and active case detection, social mobilization and building partnerships, and clinical and operational research.[272] To be successful, this integrated approach will require sustained program implementation, coordination, and political will.

REFERENCES

1. Lainson R, Shaw J. Evolution, classification and geographic distribution. In: Peters W, Killick-Kendrick R, eds. *The Leishmaniases in Biology and Medicine*. Vol 1. London: Academic Press; 1987:1-120.
2. Banuls AL, Hide M, Prugnolle F. *Leishmania* and the leishmaniases: a parasite genetic update and advances in taxonomy, epidemiology and pathogenicity in humans. *Adv Parasitol*. 2007;64:1-109.
3. Grimaldi G Jr, Tesh RB, McMahon-Pratt D. A review of the geographic distribution and epidemiology of leishmaniasis in the New World. *Am J Trop Med Hyg*. 1989;41:687-725.
4. Peters W, Killick-Kendrick R, eds. *The Leishmaniases in Biology and Medicine*. London: Academic Press; 1987.
5. Tibayrenc M, Ayala FJ. Evolutionary genetics of Trypanosoma and *Leishmania*. *Microbes Infect*. 1999;1:465-472.
6. Kreutzer RD, Souraty N, Semko ME. Biochemical identities and differences among *Leishmania* species and subspecies. *Am J Trop Med Hyg*. 1987;36:22-32.
7. Banuls AL, Jonquieres R, Guerrini F, et al. Genetic analysis of *Leishmania* parasites in Ecuador: are *Leishmania* (Viannia) *panamensis* and *Leishmania* (V.) *guyanensis* distinct taxa? *Am J Trop Med Hyg*. 1999;61:838-845.
8. Peacock CS, Seeger K, Harris D, et al. Comparative genomic analysis of three *Leishmania* species that cause diverse human disease. *Nat Genet*. 2007;39:839-847.
9. Smith DF, Peacock CS, Cruz AK. Comparative genomics: from genotype to disease phenotype in the leishmaniases. *Int J Parasitol*. 2007;37:1173-1186.
10. Peacock CS. The practical implications of comparative kinetoplastid genomics. *SEB Exp Biol Ser*. 2007;58:25-45.
11. Desjeux P. Leishmaniasis: current situation and new perspectives. *Comp Immunol Microbiol Infect Dis*. 2004;27:305-318.
12. Kolaczinski JH, Hope A, Ruiz JA, et al. Kala-azar epidemiology and control, southern Sudan. *Emerg Infect Dis*. 2008;14:664-666.
13. Seaman J, Mercer AJ, Sondorp E. The epidemic of visceral leishmaniasis in western Upper Nile, southern Sudan: course and impact from 1984 to 1994. *Int J Epidemiol*. 1996;25:862-871.
14. Seaman J, Mercer AJ, Sondorp HE, et al. Epidemic visceral leishmaniasis in southern Sudan: treatment of severely debilitated patients under wartime conditions and with limited resources. *Ann Intern Med*. 1996;124:664-672.
15. Jeronimo SM, Duggal P, Braz RF, et al. An emerging peri-urban pattern of infection with *Leishmania chagasi*, the protozoan causing visceral leishmaniasis in northeast Brazil. *Scand J Infect Dis*. 2004;36:443-449.
16. Jeronimo SM, Oliveira RM, Mackay S, et al. An urban outbreak of visceral leishmaniasis in Natal, Brazil. *Trans R Soc Trop Med Hyg*. 1994;88:386-388.
17. Magill AJ. Cutaneous leishmaniasis in the returning traveler. *Infect Dis Clin North Am*. 2005;19:241-266, x-xi.
18. Lewis D, Ward R. Transmission and vectors. In: Peters W, Killick-Kendrick R, eds. *The Leishmaniasis in Biology and Medicine*. Vol 1. London: Academic Press; 1987:235-262.
19. Andrade BB, de Oliveira CI, Brodskyn CI, et al. Role of sand fly saliva in human and experimental leishmaniasis: current insights. *Scand J Immunol*. 2007;66:122-127.
20. Bates PA. Transmission of *Leishmania* metacyclic promastigotes by phlebotomine sand flies. *Int J Parasitol*. 2007;37:1097-1106.
21. Dey A, Singh S. Transfusion transmitted leishmaniasis: a case report and review of literature. *Indian J Med Microbiol*. 2006;24:165-170.
22. Cruz I, Canavate C, Rubio JM, et al. A nested polymerase chain reaction (Ln-PCR) for diagnosing and monitoring *Leishmania* infantum infection in patients co-infected with human immunodeficiency virus. *Trans R Soc Trop Med Hyg*. 2002;96:S185-S189.
23. Meinecke CK, Schottelius J, Oskam L, et al. Congenital transmission of visceral leishmaniasis (kala azar) from an asymptomatic mother to her child. *Pediatrics*. 1999;104:e65.
24. Magill AJ. Epidemiology of the leishmaniases. *Dermatol Clin*. 1995;13:505-523.
25. Symmers WS. Leishmaniasis acquired by contagion: a case of marital infection in Britain. *Lancet*. 1960;1:127-132.
26. Kyriakou DS, Alexandrakis MG, Passam FH, et al. Quick detection of *Leishmania* in peripheral blood by flow cytometry. Is prestorage leucodepletion necessary for leishmaniasis prevention in endemic areas? *Transfus Med*. 2003;13:59-62.
27. Silveira FT, Lainson R, Corbett CE. Clinical and immunopathological spectrum of American cutaneous leishmaniasis with special reference to the disease in Amazonian Brazil: a review. *Mem Inst Oswaldo Cruz*. 2004;99:239-251.
28. Barral A, Costa JM, Bittencourt AL, et al. Polar and subpolar diffuse cutaneous leishmaniasis in Brazil: clinical and immunopathologic aspects. *Int J Dermatol*. 1995;34:474-479.
29. Ridley DS. The pathogenesis of cutaneous leishmaniasis. *Trans R Soc Trop Med Hyg*. 1979;73:150-160.
30. Oliveira JG, Novais FO, de Oliveira CI, et al. Polymerase chain reaction (PCR) is highly sensitive for diagnosis of mucosal leishmaniasis. *Acta Trop*. 2005;94:55-59.
31. Alam MZ, Kuhls K, Schweynoch C, et al. Multilocus microsatellite typing (MLMT) reveals genetic homogeneity of *Leishmania* donovani strains in the Indian subcontinent. *Infect Genet Evol*. 2009;9:24-31.
32. Elfari M, Schnur LF, Strelkova MV, et al. Genetic and biological diversity among populations of *Leishmania* major from Central Asia, the Middle East and Africa. *Microbes Infect*. 2005;7:93-103.
33. Schwenkenbecher JM, Frohlich C, Gehre F, et al. Evolution and conservation of microsatellite markers for *Leishmania* tropica. *Infect Genet Evol*. 2004;4:99-105.
34. Schonian G, Schnur L, el Fari M, et al. Genetic heterogeneity in the species *Leishmania tropica* revealed by different PCR-based methods. *Trans R Soc Trop Med Hyg*. 2001;95:217-224.
35. Le Blancq SM, Peters W. *Leishmania* in the Old World: 2. Heterogeneity among L. tropica zymodemes. *Trans R Soc Trop Med Hyg*. 1986;80:113-119.
36. Saravia NG, Segura I, Holguin AF, et al. Epidemiologic, genetic, and clinical associations among phenotypically distinct populations of *Leishmania* (Viannia) in Colombia. *Am J Trop Med Hyg*. 1998;59:86-94.
37. Sundar S, Jha TK, Thakur CP, et al. Single-dose liposomal amphotericin B in the treatment of visceral leishmaniasis in India: a multicenter study. *Clin Infect Dis*. 2003;37:800-804.
38. Mueller M, Ritmeijer K, Balasegaram M, et al. Unresponsiveness to AmBisome in some Sudanese patients with kala-azar. *Trans R Soc Trop Med Hyg*. 2007;101:19-24.
39. Mueller M, Balasegaram M, Koummuki Y, et al. A comparison of liposomal amphotericin B with sodium stibogluconate for the treatment of visceral leishmaniasis in pregnancy in Sudan. *J Antimicrob Chemother*. 2006;58:811-815.
40. Aebischer T. Recurrent cutaneous leishmaniasis: a role for persistent parasites? *Parasitol Today*. 1994;10:25-28.
41. Mendonca MG, de Brito ME, Rodrigues EH, et al. Persistence of *Leishmania* parasites in scars after clinical cure of American cutaneous leishmaniasis: is there a sterile cure? *J Infect Dis*. 2004;189:1018-1023.
42. Schubach A, Marzochi MC, Cuzzi-Maya T, et al. Cutaneous scars in American tegumentary leishmaniasis patients: a site of *Leishmania* (Viannia) braziliensis persistence and viability eleven years after antimonial therapy and clinical cure. *Am J Trop Med Hyg*. 1998;58:824-827.
43. Dereure J, Duong Thanh H, Lavabre-Bertrand T, et al. Visceral leishmaniasis. Persistence of parasites in lymph nodes after clinical cure. *J Infect*. 2003;47:77-81.
44. Berman JD. U.S. Food and Drug Administration approval of AmBisome (liposomal amphotericin B) for treatment of visceral leishmaniasis. *Clin Infect Dis*. 1999;28:49-51.
45. Gonzalez U, Pinart M, Reveiz L, et al. Interventions for Old World cutaneous leishmaniasis. *Cochrane Database Syst Rev*. 2008:CD005067.
46. Mauricio IL, Stothard JR, Miles MA. The strange case of *Leishmania chagasi*. *Parasitol Today*. 2000;16:188-189.
47. Mauricio IL, Howard MK, Stothard JR, et al. Genomic diversity in the *Leishmania donovani* complex. *Parasitology*. 1999;119:237-246.
48. Aleixo JA, Nascimento ET, Monteiro GR, et al. Atypical American visceral leishmaniasis caused by disseminated *Leishmania amazonensis* infection presenting with hepatitis and adenopathy. *Trans R Soc Trop Med Hyg*. 2006;100:79-82.
49. Barral A, Pedral-Sampaio D, Grimaldi Junior G, et al. Leishmaniasis in Bahia, Brazil: evidence that *Leishmania* amazonensis produces a wide spectrum of clinical disease. *Am J Trop Med Hyg*. 1991;44:536-546.
50. Alborzi A, Rasouli M, Shamsizadeh A. *Leishmania* tropica-isolated patient with visceral leishmaniasis in southern Iran. *Am J Trop Med Hyg*. 2006;74:306-307.
51. Sacks DL, Kenney RT, Kreutzer RD, et al. Indian kala-azar caused by *Leishmania tropica*. *Lancet*. 1995;345:959-961.
52. Magill AJ, Grogl M, Johnson SC, et al. Visceral infection due to *Leishmania tropica* in a veteran of Operation Desert Storm who presented 2 years after leaving Saudi Arabia. *Clin Infect Dis*. 1994;19:805-806.
53. Magill AJ, Grogl M, Gasser RA Jr, et al. Visceral infection caused by *Leishmania tropica* in veterans of Operation Desert Storm. *N Engl J Med*. 1993;328:1383-1387.
54. Evans TG, Teixeira MJ, McAuliffe IT, et al. Epidemiology of visceral leishmaniasis in northeast Brazil. *J Infect Dis*. 1992;166:1124-1132.
55. Badaro R, Jones TC, Carvalho EM, et al. New perspectives on a subclinical form of visceral leishmaniasis. *J Infect Dis*. 1986;154:1003-1011.
56. Badaro R, Jones TC, Lorenco R, et al. A prospective study of visceral leishmaniasis in an endemic area of Brazil. *J Infect Dis*. 1986;154:639-649.
57. Zijlstra EE, Ali MS, el-Hassan AM, et al. Clinical aspects of kala-azar in children from the Sudan: a comparison with the disease in adults. *J Trop Pediatr*. 1992;38:17-21.
58. Zijlstra EE, Ali MS, el-Hassan AM, et al. Kala-azar in displaced people from southern Sudan: epidemiological, clinical and therapeutic findings. *Trans R Soc Trop Med Hyg*. 1991;85:365-369.
59. Zijlstra EE, el-Hassan AM. Leishmaniasis in Sudan. Visceral leishmaniasis. *Trans R Soc Trop Med Hyg*. 2001;95:S27-S58.
60. Jamjoom MB, Ashford RW, Bates PA, et al. *Leishmania donovani* is the only cause of visceral leishmaniasis in East Africa; previous descriptions of L. infantum and "L. archibaldi" from this region are a consequence of convergent evolution in the isoenzyme data. *Parasitology*. 2004;129:399-409.
61. Alvar J, Aparicio P, Aseffa A, et al. The relationship between leishmaniasis and AIDS: the second 10 years. *Clin Microbiol Rev*. 2008;21:334-359.
62. Alvar J, Canavate C, Gutierrez-Solar B, et al. *Leishmania* and human immunodeficiency virus coinfection: the first 10 years. *Clin Microbiol Rev*. 1997;10:298-319.
63. Cruz I, Morales MA, Noguer I, et al. *Leishmania* in discarded syringes from intravenous drug users. *Lancet*. 2002;359:1124-1125.

64. Nascimento EL, Martins DR, Monteiro GR, et al. Forum: geographic spread and urbanization of visceral leishmaniasis in Brazil. Postscript: new challenges in the epidemiology of *Leishmania chagasi* infection. *Cad Saude Publica.* 2008;24:2964-2967.
65. Wilson ME, Jeronimo SM, Pearson RD. Immunopathogenesis of infection with the visceralizing *Leishmania* species. *Microb Pathog.* 2005;38:147-160.
66. Jamieson SE, Miller EN, Peacock CS, et al. Genome-wide scan for visceral leishmaniasis susceptibility genes in Brazil. *Genes Immun.* 2007;8:84-90.
67. Miller EN, Fadl M, Mohamed HS, et al. Y chromosome lineage- and village-specific genes on chromosomes 1p22 and 6q27 control visceral leishmaniasis in Sudan. *PLoS Genet.* 2007;3:e71.
68. El-Safi S, Kheir MM, Bucheton B, et al. Genes and environment in susceptibility to visceral leishmaniasis. *C R Biol.* 2006;329:863-870.
69. Mohamed HS, Ibrahim ME, Miller EN, et al. SLC11A1 (formerly NRAMP1) and susceptibility to visceral leishmaniasis in The Sudan. *Eur J Hum Genet.* 2004;12:66-74.
70. Bucheton B, Abel L, El-Safi S, et al. A major susceptibility locus on chromosome 22q12 plays a critical role in the control of kala-azar. *Am J Hum Genet.* 2003;73:1052-1060.
71. Bucheton B, Abel L, Kheir MM, et al. Genetic control of visceral leishmaniasis in a Sudanese population: candidate gene testing indicates a linkage to the NRAMP1 region. *Genes Immun.* 2003;4:104-109.
72. Mohamed HS, Ibrahim ME, Miller EN, et al. Genetic susceptibility to visceral leishmaniasis in The Sudan: linkage and association with IL4 and IFNGR1. *Genes Immun.* 2003;4:351-355.
73. Anstead GM, Chandrasekar B, Zhao W, et al. Malnutrition alters the innate immune response and increases early visceralization following Leishmania donovani infection. *Infect Immun.* 2001;69:4709-4718.
74. Dye C, Williams BG. Malnutrition, age and the risk of parasitic disease: visceral leishmaniasis revisited. *Proc Biol Sci.* 1993;254:33-39.
75. Cerf BJ, Jones TC, Badaro R, et al. Malnutrition as a risk factor for severe visceral leishmaniasis. *J Infect Dis.* 1987;156:1030-1033.
76. Vinhas V, Andrade BB, Paes F, et al. Human anti-saliva immune response following experimental exposure to the visceral leishmaniasis vector, Lutzomyia longipalpis. *Eur J Immunol.* 2007;37:3111-3121.
77. Caldas A, Favali C, Aquino D, et al. Balance of IL-10 and interferon-gamma plasma levels in human visceral leishmaniasis: implications in the pathogenesis. *BMC Infect Dis.* 2005;5:113.
78. Caldas AJ, Costa JM, Silva AA, et al. Risk factors associated with asymptomatic infection by *Leishmania chagasi* in north-east Brazil. *Trans R Soc Trop Med Hyg.* 2002;96:21-28.
79. Barral A, Honda E, Caldas A, et al. Human immune response to sand fly salivary gland antigens: a useful epidemiological marker? *Am J Trop Med Hyg.* 2000;62:740-745.
80. Barral A, Teixeira M, Reis P, et al. Transforming growth factor-beta in human cutaneous leishmaniasis. *Am J Pathol.* 1995;147:947-954.
81. Karp CL, el-Safi SH, Wynn TA, et al. In vivo cytokine profiles in patients with kala-azar. Marked elevation of both interleukin-10 and interferon-gamma. *J Clin Invest.* 1993;91:1644-1648.
82. Holaday BJ, Pompeu MM, Jeronimo S, et al. Potential role for interleukin-10 in the immunosuppression associated with kala azar. *J Clin Invest.* 1993;92:2626-2632.
83. Holaday BJ, Pompeu MM, Evans T, et al. Correlates of *Leishmania*-specific immunity in the clinical spectrum of infection with *Leishmania chagasi. J Infect Dis.* 1993;167:411-417.
84. Nylén S, Sacks D. Interleukin-10 and the pathogenesis of human visceral leishmaniasis. *Trends Immunol.* 2007;28(9):378-384.
85. Tektonidou MG, Skopouli FN. Visceral leishmaniasis in a patient with psoriatic arthritis treated with infliximab: reactivation of a latent infection? *Clin Rheumatol.* 2008;27:541-542.
86. Oliveira RA, Silva LS, Carvalho VP, et al. Visceral leishmaniasis after renal transplantation: report of 4 cases in northeastern Brazil. *Transpl Infect Dis.* 2008;10:364-368.
87. Oliveira CM, Oliveira ML, Andrade SC, et al. Visceral leishmaniasis in renal transplant recipients: clinical aspects, diagnostic problems, and response to treatment. *Transplant Proc.* 2008;40:755-760.
88. Campos-Varela I, Len O, Castells L, et al. Visceral leishmaniasis among liver transplant recipients: an overview. *Liver Transpl.* 2008;14:1816-1819.
89. Antinori S, Cascio A, Parravicini C, et al. Leishmaniasis among organ transplant recipients. *Lancet Infect Dis.* 2008;8:191-199.
90. Agteresch HJ, van 't Veer MB, Cornelissen JJ, et al. Visceral leishmaniasis after allogeneic hematopoietic stem cell transplantation. *Bone Marrow Transplant.* 2007;40:391-393.
91. Pittalis S, Nicastri E, Spinazzola F, et al. *Leishmania infantum* leishmaniasis in corticosteroid–treated patients. *BMC Infect Dis.* 2006;6:177.
92. Fabre S, Gibert C, Lechiche C, et al. Visceral leishmaniasis infection in a rheumatoid arthritis patient treated with infliximab. *Clin Exp Rheumatol.* 2005;23:891-892.
93. Most H, Lavietes P. Kala-azar in American Military Personnel. *Medicine.* 1947;26:221-284.
94. Pearson RD, Cox G, Jeronimo SM, et al. Visceral leishmaniasis: a model for infection-induced cachexia. *Am J Trop Med Hyg.* 1992;47:8-15.
95. Barati M, Sharifi I, Daie Parizi M, et al. Bacterial infections in children with visceral leishmaniasis: observations made in Kerman province, southern Iran, between 1997 and 2007. *Ann Trop Med Parasitol.* 2008;102:635-641.
96. Kadivar MR, Kajbaf TZ, Karimi A, et al. Childhood visceral leishmaniasis complicated by bacterial infections. *East Mediterr Health J.* 2000;6:879-883.
97. Andrade TM, Carvalho EM, Rocha H. Bacterial infections in patients with visceral leishmaniasis. *J Infect Dis.* 1990;162:1354-1359.
98. Atta AM, Carvalho EM, Jeronimo SM, et al. Serum markers of rheumatoid arthritis in visceral leishmaniasis: rheumatoid factor and anti-cyclic citrullinated peptide antibody. *J Autoimmun.* 2007;28:55-58.
99. Pearson RD, de Alencar JE, Romito R, et al. Circulating immune complexes and rheumatoid factors in visceral leishmaniasis. *J Infect Dis.* 1983;147:1102.
100. Pagliano P, Rossi M, Rescigno C, et al. Mediterranean visceral leishmaniasis in HIV-negative adults: a retrospective analysis of 64 consecutive cases (1995-2001). *J Antimicrob Chemother.* 2003;52:264-268.
101. Duvic C, Nedelec G, Debord T, et al. [Important parasitic nephropathies: update from the recent literature]. *Nephrologie.* 1999;20:65-74.
102. Caravaca F, Munoz A, Pizarro JL, et al. Acute renal failure in visceral leishmaniasis. *Am J Nephrol.* 1991;11:350-352.
103. Dutra M, Martinelli R, de Carvalho EM, et al. Renal involvement in visceral leishmaniasis. *Am J Kidney Dis.* 1985;6:22-27.
104. Leblond V, Beaufils H, Ginsburg C, et al. Collapsing focal segmental glomerulosclerosis associated with visceral leishmaniasis. *Nephrol Dial Transplant.* 1994;9:1353.
105. Duarte MI, Silva MR, Goto H, et al. Interstitial nephritis in human kala-azar. *Trans R Soc Trop Med Hyg.* 1983;77:531-537.
106. Daher EF, Evangelista LF, Silva Junior GB, et al. Clinical presentation and renal evaluation of human visceral leishmaniasis (kala-azar): a retrospective study of 57 patients in Brazil. *Braz J Infect Dis.* 2008;12:329-332.
107. Lima Verde FA, Lima Verde FA, Lima Verde IA, et al. Evaluation of renal function in human visceral leishmaniasis (kala-azar): a prospective study on 50 patients from Brazil. *J Nephrol.* 2007;20:430-436.
108. Rosenthal E, Marty P, del Giudice P, et al. HIV and *Leishmania* coinfection: a review of 91 cases with focus on atypical locations of *Leishmania. Clin Infect Dis.* 2000;31:1093-1095.
109. Delsedime L, Coppola F, Mazzucco G. Gastric localization of systemic leishmaniasis in a patient with AIDS. *Histopathology.* 1991;19:93-95.
110. Datry A, Similowski T, Jais P, et al. AIDS-associated leishmaniasis: an unusual gastro-duodenal presentation. *Trans R Soc Trop Med Hyg.* 1990;84:239-240.
111. Chenoweth CE, Singal S, Pearson RD, et al. Acquired immunodeficiency syndrome-related visceral leishmaniasis presenting in a pleural effusion. *Chest.* 1993;103:648-649.
112. Grau JM, Bosch X, Salgado AC, et al. Human immunodeficiency virus (HIV) and aplastic anemia. *Ann Intern Med.* 1989;110:576-577.
113. ter Horst R, Collin SM, Ritmeijer K, et al. Concordant HIV infection and visceral leishmaniasis in Ethiopia: the influence of antiretroviral treatment and other factors on outcome. *Clin Infect Dis.* 2008;46:1702-1709.
114. Lopez-Velez R. The impact of highly active antiretroviral therapy (HAART) on visceral leishmaniasis in Spanish patients who are co-infected with HIV. *Ann Trop Med Parasitol.* 2003;97:143-147.
115. Fernandez Cotarelo MJ, Abellan Martinez J, Guerra Vales JM, et al. Effect of highly active antiretroviral therapy on the incidence and clinical manifestations of visceral leishmaniasis in human immunodeficiency virus-infected patients. *Clin Infect Dis.* 2003;37:973-977.
116. Tortajada C, Perez-Cuevas B, Moreno A, et al. Highly active antiretroviral therapy (HAART) modifies the incidence and outcome of visceral leishmaniasis in HIV-infected patients. *J Acquir Immune Defic Syndr.* 2002;30:364-366.
117. Mathur P, Samantaray JC, Vajpayee M, et al. Visceral leishmaniasis/human immunodeficiency virus co-infection in India: the focus of two epidemics. *J Med Microbiol.* 2006;55:919-922.
118. Rabello A, Orsini M, Disch J. *Leishmania*/HIV co-infection in Brazil: an appraisal. *Ann Trop Med Parasitol.* 2003;97:17-28.
119. Desjeux P, Alvar J. *Leishmania*/HIV co-infections: epidemiology in Europe. *Ann Trop Med Parasitol.* 2003;97:3-15.
120. Pasquau F, Ena J, Sanchez R, et al. Leishmaniasis as an opportunistic infection in HIV-infected patients: determinants of relapse and mortality in a collaborative study of 228 episodes in a Mediterreanean region. *Eur J Clin Microbiol Infect Dis.* 2005;24:411-418.
121. Hyams KC, Riddle J, Trump DH, et al. Endemic infectious diseases and biological warfare during the Gulf War: a decade of analysis and final concerns. *Am J Trop Med Hyg.* 2001;65:664-670.
122. Gama ME, Costa JM, Gomes CM, et al. Subclinical form of the American visceral leishmaniasis. *Mem Inst Oswaldo Cruz.* 2004;99:889-893.
123. Pampiglione S, Manson-Bahr PE, Giungi F, et al. Studies on Mediterranean leishmaniasis. 2. Asymptomatic cases of visceral leishmaniasis. *Trans R Soc Trop Med Hyg.* 1974;68:447-453.
124. Pampiglione S, La Placa M, Schlick G. Studies on mediterranean Leishmaniasis. I. An outbreak of visceral leishmaniasis in Northern Italy. *Trans R Soc Trop Med Hyg.* 1974;68:349-359.
125. Zijlstra EE, Musa AM, Khalil EA, et al. Post-kala-azar dermal leishmaniasis. *Lancet Infect Dis.* 2003;3:87-98.
126. Musa AM, Khalil EA, Raheem MA, et al. The natural history of Sudanese post-kala-azar dermal leishmaniasis: clinical, immunological and prognostic features. *Ann Trop Med Parasitol.* 2002;96:765-772.
127. Zijlstra EE, Khalil EA, Kager PA, et al. Post-kala-azar dermal leishmaniasis in the Sudan: clinical presentation and differential diagnosis. *Br J Dermatol.* 2000;143:136-143.
128. Thakur CP. Epidemiological, clinical and therapeutic features of Bihar kala-azar (including post kala-azar dermal leishmaniasis). *Trans R Soc Trop Med Hyg.* 1984;78:391-398.
129. Ridolfo AL, Gervasoni C, Antinori S, et al. Post-kala-azar dermal leishmaniasis during highly active antiretroviral therapy in an AIDS patient infected with *Leishmania infantum. J Infect.* 2000;40:199-202.
130. Thakur CP, Kumar A, Mitra G, et al. Impact of amphotericin-B in the treatment of kala-azar on the incidence of PKDL in Bihar, India. *Indian J Med Res.* 2008;128:38-44.
131. Addy M, Nandy A. Ten years of kala-azar in west Bengal, Part I. Did post-kala-azar dermal leishmaniasis initiate the outbreak in 24-Parganas? *Bull World Health Organ.* 1992;70:341-346.
132. Thakur CP, Kumar K. Post-kala-azar dermal leishmaniasis: a neglected aspect of kala-azar control programmes. *Ann Trop Med Parasitol.* 1992;86:355-359.
133. Kager PA, Rees PH, Manguyu FM, et al. Splenic aspiration; experience in Kenya. *Trop Geogr Med.* 1983;35:125-131.
134. Sarker CB, Alam KS, Jamal MF, et al. Sensitivity of splenic and bone marrow aspirate study for diagnosis of kala-azar. *Mymensingh Med J.* 2004;13:130-133.
135. Thakur CP. A comparison of intercostal and abdominal routes of splenic aspiration and bone marrow aspiration in the diagnosis of visceral leishmaniasis. *Trans R Soc Trop Med Hyg.* 1997;91:668-670.
136. Siddig M, Ghalib H, Shillington DC, et al. Visceral leishmaniasis in the Sudan: comparative parasitological methods of diagnosis. *Trans R Soc Trop Med Hyg.* 1988;82:66-68.
137. Chulay JD, Bryceson AD. Quantitation of amastigotes of *Leishmania donovani* in smears of splenic aspirates from patients with visceral leishmaniasis. *Am J Trop Med Hyg.* 1983;32:475-479.
138. Myles O, Wortmann GW, Cummings JF, et al. Visceral leishmaniasis: clinical observations in 4 US army soldiers deployed to Afghanistan or Iraq, 2002-2004. *Arch Intern Med.* 2007;167:1899-1901.
139. Lopez-Velez R, Laguna F, Alvar J, et al. Parasitic culture of buffy coat for diagnosis of visceral leishmaniasis in human immunodeficiency virus-infected patients. *J Clin Microbiol.* 1995;33:937-939.
140. Burns JM Jr, Shreffler WG, Benson DR, et al. Molecular characterization of a kinesin-related antigen of *Leishmania chagasi* that detects specific antibody in African and American visceral leishmaniasis. *Proc Natl Acad Sci U S A.* 1993;90:775-779.
141. Ritmeijer K, Melaku Y, Mueller M, et al. Evaluation of a new recombinant K39 rapid diagnostic test for Sudanese visceral leishmaniasis. *Am J Trop Med Hyg.* 2006;74:76-80.
142. Chappuis F, Rijal S, Soto A, et al. A meta-analysis of the diagnostic performance of the direct agglutination test and rK39 dipstick for visceral leishmaniasis. *BMJ.* 2006;333:723.
143. Braz RF, Nascimento ET, Martins DR, et al. The sensitivity and specificity of *Leishmania chagasi* recombinant K39 antigen in the diagnosis of American visceral leishmaniasis and in differentiating active from subclinical infection. *Am J Trop Med Hyg.* 2002;67:344-348.
144. De Almeida Silva L, Romero HD, Prata A, et al. Immunologic tests in patients after clinical cure of visceral leishmaniasis. *Am J Trop Med Hyg.* 2006;75:739-743.
145. Hartzell JD, Aronson NE, Weina PJ, et al. Positive rK39 serologic assay results in US servicemen with cutaneous leishmaniasis. *Am J Trop Med Hyg.* 2008;79:843-846.
146. Mandal J, Khurana S, Dubey ML, et al. Evaluation of direct agglutination test, rk39 Test, and ELISA for the diagnosis of visceral leishmaniasis. *Am J Trop Med Hyg.* 2008;79:76-78.
147. Boelaert M, El-Safi S, Hailu A, et al. Diagnostic tests for kala-azar: a multi-centre study of the freeze-dried DAT, rK39 strip test and KAtex in East Africa and the Indian subcontinent. *Trans R Soc Trop Med Hyg.* 2008;102:32-40.
148. Sundar S, Sahu M, Mehta H, et al. Noninvasive management of Indian visceral leishmaniasis: clinical application of diagnosis by K39 antigen strip testing at a kala-azar referral unit. *Clin Infect Dis.* 2002;35:581-586.
149. Giladi M, Danon YL, Greenblatt C, et al. Keziot—a new endemic site of cutaneous leishmaniasis in Israel. An epidemiological and clinical study of a non-immune population entering an endemic area. *Trop Geogr Med.* 1985;37:298-303.
150. Bienzle U, Ebert F, Dietrich M. Cutaneous leishmaniasis in Eastern Saudi Arabia. Epidemiological and clinical features in a nonimmune population living in an endemic area. *Tropenmed Parasitol.* 1978;29:188-193.
151. Wright NA, Davis LE, Aftergut KS, et al. Cutaneous leishmaniasis in Texas: A northern spread of endemic areas. *J Am Acad Dermatol.* 2008;58:650-652.

152. McHugh CP, Melby PC, LaFon SG. Leishmaniasis in Texas: epidemiology and clinical aspects of human cases. *Am J Trop Med Hyg.* 1996;55:547-555.
153. Herwaldt BL, Arana BA, Navin TR. The natural history of cutaneous leishmaniasis in Guatemala. *J Infect Dis.* 1992;165:518-527.
154. Ghersetich I, Menchini G, Teofoli P, et al. Immune response to *Leishmania* infection in human skin. *Clin Dermatol.* 1999;17:333-338.
155. Sousa Ade Q, Parise ME, Pompeu MM, et al. Bubonic leishmaniasis: a common manifestation of *Leishmania* (Viannia) braziliensis infection in Ceara, Brazil. *Am J Trop Med Hyg.* 1995;53:380-385.
156. Barral A, Guerreiro J, Bomfim G, et al. Lymphadenopathy as the first sign of human cutaneous infection by *Leishmania braziliensis.* *Am J Trop Med Hyg.* 1995;53:256-259.
157. Convit J, Pinardi ME, Rondon AJ. Diffuse cutaneous leishmaniasis: a disease due to an immunological defect of the host. *Trans R Soc Trop Med Hyg.* 1972;66:603-610.
158. Bryceson AD. Diffuse cutaneous leishmaniasis in Ethiopia. 3. Immunological studies. IV. Pathogenesis of diffuse cutaneous leishmaniasis. *Trans R Soc Trop Med Hyg.* 1970;64:380-393.
159. Bryceson AD. Diffuse cutaneous leishmaniasis in Ethiopia. II. Treatment. *Trans R Soc Trop Med Hyg.* 1970;64:369-379.
160. Bryceson AD. Diffuse cutaneous leishmaniasis in Ethiopia. I. The clinical and histological features of the disease. *Trans R Soc Trop Med Hyg.* 1969;63:708-737.
161. Turetz ML, Machado PR, Ko AI, et al. Disseminated leishmaniasis: a new and emerging form of leishmaniasis observed in northeastern Brazil. *J Infect Dis.* 2002;186:1829-1834.
162. Carvalho EM, Barral A, Costa JM, et al. Clinical and immunopathological aspects of disseminated cutaneous leishmaniasis. *Acta Trop.* 1994;56:315-325.
163. Costa JM, Marsden PD, Llanos-Cuentas EA, et al. Disseminated cutaneous leishmaniasis in a field clinic in Bahia, Brazil: a report of eight cases. *J Trop Med Hyg.* 1986;89:319-323.
164. Golino A, Duncan JM, Zeluff B, et al. Leishmaniasis in a heart transplant patient. *J Heart Lung Transplant.* 1992;11:820-823.
165. Weigle KA, de Davalos M, Heredia P, et al. Diagnosis of cutaneous and mucocutaneous leishmaniasis in Colombia: a comparison of seven methods. *Am J Trop Med Hyg.* 1987;36:489-496.
166. Osorio LE, Castillo CM, Ochoa MT. Mucosal leishmaniasis due to *Leishmania* (Viannia) panamensis in Colombia: clinical characteristics. *Am J Trop Med Hyg.* 1998;59:49-52.
167. Jones TC, Johnson WD Jr, Barretto AC, et al. Epidemiology of American cutaneous leishmaniasis due to *Leishmania braziliensis braziliensis.* *J Infect Dis.* 1987;156:73-83.
168. Marsden PD. Mucosal leishmaniasis ("espundia" Escomel, 1911). *Trans R Soc Trop Med Hyg.* 1986;80:859-876.
169. Reference not cited.
170. Walton BC, Chinel LV, Eguia y Eguia O. Onset of espundia after many years of occult infection with *Leishmania braziliensis.* *Am J Trop Med Hyg.* 1973;22:696-698.
171. Marsden P, Nonata R. Mucocutaneous leishmaniasis—a review of clinical aspects. *Rev Soc Bras Med Trop.* 1975;9:309-326.
172. Larson EE, Marsden PD. The origin of espundia. *Trans R Soc Trop Med Hyg.* 1987;81:880.
173. Costa JM, Netto EM, Marsden PD. Acute airway obstruction due to oedema of the larynx following antimony therapy in mucosal leishmaniasis. *Rev Soc Bras Med Trop.* 1986;19:109.
174. Bacellar O, Lessa H, Schriefer A, et al. Up-regulation of Th1-type responses in mucosal leishmaniasis patients. *Infect Immun.* 2002;70:6734-6740.
175. Marsden PD, Badaro R, Netto EM, et al. Spontaneous clinical resolution without specific treatment in mucosal leishmaniasis. *Trans R Soc Trop Med Hyg.* 1991;85:221.
176. Machado-Coelho GL, Caiaffa WT, Genaro O, et al. Risk factors for mucosal manifestation of American cutaneous leishmaniasis. *Trans R Soc Trop Med Hyg.* 2005;99:55-61.
177. Petzl-Erler ML, Belich MP, Queiroz-Telles F. Association of mucosal leishmaniasis with HLA. *Hum Immunol.* 1991;32:254-260.
178. Walton BC, Valverde L. Racial differences in espundia. *Ann Trop Med Parasitol.* 1979;73:23-29.
179. Saravia NG, Weigle K, Navas C, et al. Heterogeneity, geographic distribution, and pathogenicity of serodemes of *Leishmania viannia* in Colombia. *Am J Trop Med Hyg.* 2002;66:738-744.
180. Castellucci L, Cheng LH, Araujo C, et al. Familial aggregation of mucosal leishmaniasis in northeast Brazil. *Am J Trop Med Hyg.* 2005;73:69-73.
181. Grimaldi G Jr, Tesh RB. Leishmaniases of the New World: current concepts and implications for future research. *Clin Microbiol Rev.* 1993;6:230-250.
182. Mahdi M, Elamin EM, Melville SE, et al. Sudanese mucosal leishmaniasis: isolation of a parasite within the *Leishmania donovani* complex that differs genotypically from L. donovani causing classical visceral leishmaniasis. *Infect Genet Evol.* 2005;5:29-33.
183. el-Hassan AM, Zijlstra EE. Leishmaniasis in Sudan. Mucosal leishmaniasis. *Trans R Soc Trop Med Hyg.* 2001;95:S19-26.
184. el-Hassan AM, Meredith SE, Yagi HI, et al. Sudanese mucosal leishmaniasis: epidemiology, clinical features, diagnosis, immune responses and treatment. *Trans R Soc Trop Med Hyg.* 1995;89:647-652.
185. Aliaga L, Cobo F, Mediavilla JD, et al. Localized mucosal leishmaniasis due to *Leishmania* (Leishmania) infantum: clinical and microbiologic findings in 31 patients. *Medicine (Baltimore).* 2003;82:147-158.
186. Ovalle Bracho C, Porras de Quintana L, Muvdi Arenas S, et al. Polymerase chain reaction with two molecular targets in mucosal leishmaniasis' diagnosis: a validation study. *Mem Inst Oswaldo Cruz.* 2007;102:549-554.
187. Rodriguez-Gonzalez I, Marin C, Longoni SS, et al. Identification of New World *Leishmania* species from Peru by biochemical techniques and multiplex PCR assay. *FEMS Microbiol Lett.* 2007;267:9-16.
188. Cuba Cuba CA, Marsden PD, Barreto AC, et al. Parasitologic and immunologic diagnosis of American (mucocutaneous) leishmaniasis. *Bull Pan Am Health Organ.* 1981;15:249-259.
189. Meyerhoff A. U.S. Food and Drug Administration approval of AmBisome (liposomal amphotericin B) for treatment of visceral leishmaniasis. *Clin Infect Dis.* 1999;28:42-48; discussion 49-51.
190. Bern C, Adler-Moore J, Berenguer J, et al. Liposomal amphotericin B for the treatment of visceral leishmaniasis. *Clin Infect Dis.* 2006;43:917-924.
191. Yardley V, Croft SL. A comparison of the activities of three amphotericin B lipid formulations against experimental visceral and cutaneous leishmaniasis. *Int J Antimicrob Agents.* 2000;13:243-248.
192. Sundar S. Drug resistance in Indian visceral leishmaniasis. *Trop Med Int Health.* 2001;6:849-854.
193. Bermudez H, Rojas E, Garcia L, et al. Generic sodium stibogluconate is as safe and effective as branded meglumine antimoniate, for the treatment of tegumentary leishmaniasis in Isiboro Secure Park, Bolivia. *Ann Trop Med Parasitol.* 2006;100:591-600.
194. Veeken H, Ritmeijer K, Seaman J, et al. A randomized comparison of branded sodium stibogluconate and generic sodium stibogluconate for the treatment of visceral leishmaniasis under field conditions in Sudan. *Trop Med Int Health.* 2000;5:312-317.
195. Rijal S, Chappuis F, Singh R, et al. Sodium stibogluconate cardiotoxicity and safety of generics. *Trans R Soc Trop Med Hyg.* 2003;97:597-598.
196. Sundar S, Sinha PR, Agrawal NK, et al. A cluster of cases of severe cardiotoxicity among kala-azar patients treated with a high-osmolarity lot of sodium antimony gluconate. *Am J Trop Med Hyg.* 1998;59:139-143.
197. Chulay JD, Spencer HC, Mugambi M. Electrocardiographic changes during treatment of leishmaniasis with pentavalent antimony (sodium stibogluconate). *Am J Trop Med Hyg.* 1985;34:702-709.
198. Castello Viguer MT, Echanove Errazti I, Ridocci Soriano F, et al. [Torsades de pointes during treatment of leishmaniasis with meglumine antimoniate]. *Rev Esp Cardiol.* 1999;52:533-535.
199. Ortega-Carnicer J, Alcazar R, De la Torre M, et al. Pentavalent antimonial-induced torsade de pointes. *J Electrocardiol.* 1997;30:143-145.
200. Gasser RA Jr, Magill AJ, Oster CN, et al. Pancreatitis induced by pentavalent antimonial agents during treatment of leishmaniasis. *Clin Infect Dis.* 1994;18:83-90.
201. Ahasan HA, Chowdhury MA, Azhar MA, et al. Deaths in visceral leishmaniasis (kala-azar) during treatment. *Med J Malaysia.* 1996;51:29-32.
202. Winship KA. Toxicity of antimony and its compounds. *Adverse Drug React Acute Poisoning Rev.* 1987;6:67-90.
203. Thakur CP, Sinha GP, Pandey AK, et al. Do the diminishing efficacy and increasing toxicity of sodium stibogluconate in the treatment of visceral leishmaniasis in Bihar, India, justify its continued use as a first-line drug? An observational study of 80 cases. *Ann Trop Med Parasitol.* 1998;92:561-569.
204. Sundar S, Jha TK, Thakur CP, Bhattacharya SK, Rai M. Oral miltefosine for the treatment of Indian visceral leishmaniasis. *Trans R Soc Trop Med Hyg.* 2006;100:S26-S33.
205. Bhattacharya SK, Sinha PK, Sundar S, et al. Phase 4 trial of miltefosine for the treatment of Indian visceral leishmaniasis. *J Infect Dis.* 2007;196:591-598.
206. Sundar S, Olliaro PL. Miltefosine in the treatment of leishmaniasis: Clinical evidence for informed clinical risk management. *Ther Clin Risk Manag.* 2007;3:733-740.
207. Seifert K, Perez-Victoria FJ, Stettler M, et al. Inactivation of the miltefosine transporter, LdMT, causes miltefosine resistance that is conferred to the amastigote stage of *Leishmania donovani* and persists in vivo. *Int J Antimicrob Agents.* 2007;30:229-235.
208. Perez-Victoria FJ, Sanchez-Canete MP, Seifert K, et al. Mechanisms of experimental resistance of *Leishmania* to miltefosine: Implications for clinical use. *Drug Resist Updat.* 2006;9:26-39.
209. Sundar S, Chakravarty J, Rai VK, et al. Amphotericin B treatment for Indian visceral leishmaniasis: response to 15 daily versus alternate-day infusions. *Clin Infect Dis.* 2007;45:556-561.
210. Thakur CP, Sinha GP, Pandey AK, et al. Daily versus alternate-day regimen of amphotericin B in the treatment of kala-azar: a randomized comparison. *Bull World Health Organ.* 1994;72:931-936.
211. Sundar S, Jha TK, Thakur CP, et al. Injectable paromomycin for visceral leishmaniasis in India. *N Engl J Med.* 2007;356:2571-2581.
212. el Hassan AM, Ghalib HW, Zijlstra EE, et al. Post kala-azar dermal leishmaniasis in the Sudan: clinical features, pathology and treatment. *Trans R Soc Trop Med Hyg.* 1992;86:245-248.
213. Thakur CP, Kumar K, Sinha PK, et al. Treatment of post–kala-azar dermal leishmaniasis with sodium stibogluconate. *Br Med J (Clin Res Ed).* 1987;295:886-887.
214. Thakur CP, Narain S, Kumar N, et al. Amphotericin B is superior to sodium antimony gluconate in the treatment of Indian post–kala-azar dermal leishmaniasis. *Ann Trop Med Parasitol.* 1997;91:611-616.
215. Musa AM, Khalil EA, Mahgoub FA, et al. Efficacy of liposomal amphotericin B (AmBisome) in the treatment of persistent post–kala-azar dermal leishmaniasis (PKDL). *Ann Trop Med Parasitol.* 2005;99:563-569.
216. Sundar S, Rai M, Chakravarty J, et al. New treatment approach in Indian visceral leishmaniasis: single-dose liposomal amphotericin B followed by short-course oral miltefosine. *Clin Infect Dis.* 2008;47:1000-1006.
217. Melaku Y, Collin SM, Keus K, et al. Treatment of kala-azar in southern Sudan using a 17-day regimen of sodium stibogluconate combined with paromomycin: a retrospective comparison with 30-day sodium stibogluconate monotherapy. *Am J Trop Med Hyg.* 2007;77:89-94.
218. Alkhawajah AM, Larbi E, al-Gindan Y, et al. Treatment of cutaneous leishmaniasis with antimony: intramuscular versus intralesional administration. *Ann Trop Med Parasitol.* 1997;91:899-905.
219. Reithinger R, Mohsen M, Wahid M, et al. Efficacy of thermotherapy to treat cutaneous leishmaniasis caused by *Leishmania tropica* in Kabul, Afghanistan: a randomized, controlled trial. *Clin Infect Dis.* 2005;40:1148-1155.
220. Alrajhi AA, Ibrahim EA, De Vol EB, et al. Fluconazole for the treatment of cutaneous leishmaniasis caused by *Leishmania major.* *N Engl J Med.* 2002;346:891-895.
221. Nassiri-Kashani M, Firooz A, Khamesipour A, et al. A randomized, double-blind, placebo-controlled clinical trial of itraconazole in the treatment of cutaneous leishmaniasis. *J Eur Acad Dermatol Venereol.* 2005;19:80-83.
222. Dogra J, Saxena VN. Itraconazole and leishmaniasis: a randomised double-blind trial in cutaneous disease. *Int J Parasitol.* 1996;26:1413-1415.
223. al-Fouzan AS, al Saleh QA, Najem NM, et al. Cutaneous leishmaniasis in Kuwait. Clinical experience with itraconazole. *Int J Dermatol.* 1991;30:519-521.
224. Mohebali M, Fotouhi A, Hooshmand B, et al. Comparison of miltefosine and meglumine antimoniate for the treatment of zoonotic cutaneous leishmaniasis (ZCL) by a randomized clinical trial in Iran. *Acta Trop.* 2007;103:33-40.
225. Kim DH, Chung HJ, Bleys J, et al. Is paromomycin an effective and safe treatment against cutaneous leishmaniasis? A meta-analysis of 14 randomized controlled trials. *PLoS Negl Trop Dis.* 2009;3:e381.
226. Tuon FF, Amato VS, Graf ME, et al. Treatment of New World cutaneous leishmaniasis—a systematic review with a meta-analysis. *Int J Dermatol.* 2008;47:109-124.
227. Llanos-Cuentas A, Tulliano G, Araujo-Castillo R, et al. Clinical and parasite species risk factors for pentavalent antimonial treatment failure in cutaneous leishmaniasis in Peru. *Clin Infect Dis.* 2008;46:223-231.
228. Arevalo J, Ramirez L, Adaui V, et al. Influence of *Leishmania* (Viannia) species on the response to antimonial treatment in patients with American tegumentary leishmaniasis. *J Infect Dis.* 2007;195:1846-1851.
229. Yardley V, Ortuno N, Llanos-Cuentas A, et al. American tegumentary leishmaniasis: Is antimonial treatment outcome related to parasite drug susceptibility? *J Infect Dis.* 2006;194:1168-1175.
230. Rojas R, Valderrama L, Valderrama M, et al. Resistance to antimony and treatment failure in human *Leishmania* (Viannia) infection. *J Infect Dis.* 2006;193:1375-1383.
231. Lawn SD, Yardley V, Vega-Lopez F, et al. New World cutaneous leishmaniasis in returned travellers: treatment failures using intravenous sodium stibogluconate. *Trans R Soc Trop Med Hyg.* 2003;97:443-445.
232. Solomon M, Baum S, Barzilai A, et al. Liposomal amphotericin B in comparison to sodium stibogluconate for cutaneous infection due to *Leishmania braziliensis.* *J Am Acad Dermatol.* 2007;56:612-616.
233. Brown M, Noursadeghi M, Boyle J, et al. Successful liposomal amphotericin B treatment of *Leishmania braziliensis* cutaneous leishmaniasis. *Br J Dermatol.* 2005;153:203-205.
234. Lightburn E, Morand JJ, Meynard JB, et al. [Management of American cutaneous leishmaniasis. Outcome apropos of 326 cases treated with high-dose pentamidine isethionate]. *Med Trop (Mars).* 2003;63:35-44.
235. Lai AFEJ, Vrede MA, Soetosenojo RM, et al. Pentamidine, the drug of choice for the treatment of cutaneous leishmaniasis in Surinam. *Int J Dermatol.* 2002;41:796-800.
236. Navin TR, Arana BA, Arana FE, et al. Placebo-controlled clinical trial of sodium stibogluconate (Pentostam) versus ketoconazole for treating cutaneous leishmaniasis in Guatemala. *J Infect Dis.* 1992;165:528-534.
237. Saenz RE, Paz H, Berman JD. Efficacy of ketoconazole against *Leishmania braziliensis* panamensis cutaneous leishmaniasis. *Am J Med.* 1990;89:147-155.
238. Soto J, Toledo J, Gutierrez P, et al. Treatment of American cutaneous leishmaniasis with miltefosine, an oral agent. *Clin Infect Dis.* 2001;33:E57-61.
239. Soto J, Arana BA, Toledo J, et al. Miltefosine for new world cutaneous leishmaniasis. *Clin Infect Dis.* 2004;38:1266-1272.

239a. Soto J, Rea J, Balderrama M, et al. Efficacy of miltefosine for Bolivian cutaneous leishmaniasis. *Am J Trop Med Hyg*. 2008; 78(2):210-211.

240. Berman JJ. Treatment of leishmaniasis with miltefosine: 2008 status. *Expert Opin Drug Metab Toxicol*. 2008;4:1209-1216.

241. Convit J, Castellanos PL, Ulrich M, et al. Immunotherapy of localized, intermediate, and diffuse forms of American cutaneous leishmaniasis. *J Infect Dis*. 1989;160:104-115.

242. Amato VS, Tuon FF, Siqueira AM, et al. Treatment of mucosal leishmaniasis in Latin America: systematic review. *Am J Trop Med Hyg*. 2007;77:266-274.

243. Dedet JP, Melogno R, Cardenas F, et al. Rural campaign to diagnose and treat mucocutaneous leishmaniasis in Bolivia. *Bull World Health Organ*. 1995;73:339-345.

244. Crofts MA. Use of amphotericin B in mucocutaneous leishmaniasis. *J Trop Med Hyg*. 1976;79:111-113.

245. Prado JB. [Treatment of the mucosal forms of American leishmaniasis with amphotericin B.] *Rev Assoc Med Bras*. 1963;9:117-122.

246. Sampaio SA, Godoy JT, Paiva L, et al. The treatment of American (mucocutaneous) leishmaniasis with amphotericin B. *Arch Dermatol*. 1960;82:627-635.

247. Amato VS, Tuon FF, Campos A, et al. Treatment of mucosal leishmaniasis with a lipid formulation of amphotericin B. *Clin Infect Dis*. 2007;44:311-312.

248. Nonata R, Sampaio R, Marsden PD. Mucosal leishmaniasis unresponsive to glucantime therapy successfully treated with AmBisome. *Trans R Soc Trop Med Hyg*. 1997;91:77.

249. Sampaio RN, Marsden PD. [Treatment of the mucosal form of leishmaniasis without response to glucantime, with liposomal amphotericin B]. *Rev Soc Bras Med Trop*. 1997;30:125-128.

250. Soto J, Toledo J, Valda L, et al. Treatment of Bolivian mucosal leishmaniasis with miltefosine. *Clin Infect Dis*. 2007;44:350-356.

250a. Machado PR, Lessa H, Lessa M, et al. Oral pentoxifylline combined with pentavalent antimony: a randomized trial for mucosal leishmaniasis. *Clin Infect Dis*. 2007;44(6):788-793.

251. Badaro R, Lobo I, Munos A, et al. Immunotherapy for drug-refractory mucosal leishmaniasis. *J Infect Dis*. 2006;194:1151-1159.

252. Soto J, Medina F, Dember N, et al. Efficacy of permethrin-impregnated uniforms in the prevention of malaria and leishmaniasis in Colombian soldiers. *Clin Infect Dis*. 1995;21:599-602.

253. Davies CR, Llanos-Cuentas A, Canales J, et al. The fall and rise of Andean cutaneous leishmaniasis: transient impact of the DDT campaign in Peru. *Trans R Soc Trop Med Hyg*. 1994;88:389-393.

254. Elias M, Rahman AJ, Khan NI. Visceral leishmaniasis and its control in Bangladesh. *Bull World Health Organ*. 1989;67:43-49.

255. Mukhopadhyay AK, Chakravarty AK, Kureel VR, et al. Resurgence of Phlebotomus argentipes & Ph. papatasi in parts of Bihar (India) after DDT spraying. *Indian J Med Res*. 1987;85:158-160.

256. Seyedi-Rashti MA, Nadim A. Re-establishment of cutaneous leishmaniasis after cessation of anti-malaria spraying. *Trop Geogr Med*. 1975;27:79-82.

257. Nadim A, Amini H. The effect of antimalaria spraying on the transmission of zoonotic cutaneous leishmaniasis. *Trop Geogr Med*. 1970;22:479-481.

258. Dinesh DS, Das P, Picado A, et al. Long-lasting insecticidal nets fail at household level to reduce abundance of sandfly vector *Phlebotomus argentipes* in treated houses in Bihar (India). *Trop Med Int Health*. 2008;13:953-958.

259. Courtenay O, Gillingwater K, Gomes PA, et al. Deltamethrin-impregnated bednets reduce human landing rates of sandfly vector *Lutzomyia longipalpis* in Amazon households. *Med Vet Entomol*. 2007;21:168-176.

260. Dinesh DS, Ranjan A, Palit A, et al. Seasonal and nocturnal landing/biting behaviour of *Phlebotomus argentipes* (Diptera: Psychodidae). *Ann Trop Med Parasitol*. 2001;95:197-202.

261. Gavgani AS, Hodjati MH, Mohite H, et al. Effect of insecticide-impregnated dog collars on incidence of zoonotic visceral leishmaniasis in Iranian children: a matched-cluster randomised trial. *Lancet*. 2002;360:374-379.

262. Ashford DA, David JR, Freire M, et al. Studies on control of visceral leishmaniasis: impact of dog control on canine and human visceral leishmaniasis in Jacobina, Bahia, Brazil. *Am J Trop Med Hyg*. 1998;59:53-57.

263. Fakhar M, Motazedian MH, Hatam GR, et al. Asymptomatic human carriers of *Leishmania infantum*: possible reservoirs for Mediterranean visceral leishmaniasis in southern Iran. *Ann Trop Med Parasitol*. 2008;102:577-583.

264. Sakru N, Ozensoy Toz S, Korkmaz M, et al. The infection risk of visceral leishmaniasis among household members of active patients. *Parasitol Int*. 2006;55:131-133.

265. Lainson R, Shaw JJ. Leishmaniasis in Brazil: XII. Observations on cross-immunity in monkeys and man infected with *Leishmania mexicana mexicana, L. m. amazonensis, L. braziliensis braziliensis, L. b. guyanensis* and *L. b. panamensis*. *J Trop Med Hyg*. 1977;80(2):29-35.

266. Khamesipour A, Dowlati Y, Asilian A, et al. Leishmanization: use of an old method for evaluation of candidate vaccines against leishmaniasis. *Vaccine*. 2005;23:3642-3648.

267. Noazin S, Modabber F, Khamesipour A, et al. First generation leishmaniasis vaccines: a review of field efficacy trials. *Vaccine*. 2008;26:6759-6767.

268. Palatnik-de-Sousa CB. Vaccines for leishmaniasis in the forecoming 25 years. *Vaccine*. 2008;26:1709-1724.

269. Coler RN, Goto Y, Bogatzki L, et al. Leish-111f, a recombinant polyprotein vaccine that protects against visceral leishmaniasis by elicitation of CD4+ T cells. *Infect Immun*. 2007;75:4648-4654.

270. Coler RN, Reed SG. Second-generation vaccines against leishmaniasis. *Trends Parasitol*. 2005;21:244-249.

271. Skeiky YA, Coler RN, Brannon M, et al. Protective efficacy of a tandemly linked, multi-subunit recombinant leishmanial vaccine (Leish-111f) formulated in MPL adjuvant. *Vaccine*. 2002;20:3292-3303.

272. Joshi A, Narain JP, Prasittisuk C, et al. Can visceral leishmaniasis be eliminated from Asia? *J Vector Borne Dis*. 2008;45:105-111.

277

Trypanosoma Species (American Trypanosomiasis, Chagas' Disease): Biology of Trypanosomes

LOUIS V. KIRCHHOFF*

The genus *Trypanosoma* consists of several dozen species of protozoa.[1] Two of the three species that infect humans are pathogenic, and several other species cause severe and economically important diseases in domestic mammals. Broadly defined, the organisms belonging to this genus are protozoan flagellates of the family Trypanosomatidae, order Kinetoplastida, that pass through different morphologic stages (epimastigote, amastigote, and trypomastigote) in their vertebrate and invertebrate hosts. The criterion of three morphologic stages, however, is not fulfilled by each species in the genus. For example, only *Trypanosoma cruzi*, the etiologic agent of American trypanosomiasis, or Chagas' disease, and one other species, multiply in mammalian hosts as intracellular amastigotes similar to those seen in infections caused by organisms belonging to the genus *Leishmania*. In contrast, African trypanosomes, which cause sleeping sickness in humans and varying degrees of morbidity in wild and domestic mammals, do not have an intracellular form and multiply as trypomastigotes that circulate in the mammalian bloodstream and other extracellular spaces.

The trypomastigote form has a single flagellum originating near the kinetoplast, which is a DNA-containing structure located in the parasite's single, complex mitochondrion. The flagellum runs alongside the body of the parasite and is enveloped in an undulating membrane. It extends beyond the body as a free, threadlike structure. The undulating membrane and the free portion of the flagellum give the organism considerable motility.

According to their course of development in the vector, trypanosomes have been classified into two major groups:

1. *Stercoraria:* Multiplication in the mammalian host is discontinuous, taking place in the amastigote stage. Development in the vector (*Triatominae,* or kissing bugs) is completed in the hindgut (posterior station), and mammalian hosts become infected by contaminative transmission. The subgenus *Schizotrypanum* belongs to this group and includes *T. cruzi.*

2. *Salivaria:* Multiplication in the mammalian host is continuous, taking place in the trypomastigote stage. Development in the vector (*Glossina,* or tsetse fly) is completed in the salivary glands (anterior station), and inoculative transmission to the mammalian host occurs. The subgenus *Trypanozoon* belongs to this group and includes, among others, the subspecies *Trypanosoma brucei brucei,* which causes disease in animals but does not infect humans. *Trypanosoma brucei gambiense* and *Trypanosoma brucei rhodesiense,* the two causative agents of African sleeping sickness, or human African trypanosomiasis, are also found in this subgenus. As a group, these three subspecies are often referred to as the *T. brucei* complex. Endemic areas of Chagas' disease and African sleeping sickness do not overlap (Fig. 277-1). Moreover, there are such important differences in the transmission, pathogenesis, and clinical course of the two diseases that they have little in common except the genetic and morphologic similarities of the causative agents.

---

*All material in this chapter is in the public domain, with the exception of borrowed figures.

Chagas' Disease

LIFE CYCLE AND TRANSMISSION

T. cruzi, the causative agent of American trypanosomiasis, is transmitted by various species of bloodsucking triatomine insects, or kissing bugs (Fig. 277-2).[2,3] These vectors are found in large numbers in the wild, where they transmit the parasite among many mammalian species that constitute the natural reservoir, and in endemic areas they live in the nooks and crannies of substandard dwellings. The insects become infected by sucking blood from humans or other mammals that have circulating trypomastigotes (Fig. 277-3). The ingested parasites multiply in the midgut of the insects as epimastigotes, which are flagellates of a distinct morphologic type, and in the hindgut transform into infective metacyclic trypomastigotes that are discharged with the feces at the time of subsequent blood meals. Transmission to a second vertebrate host occurs when mucous membranes, conjunctivae, or breaks in the skin are contaminated with bug feces containing the infective forms. The parasites then enter a variety of host cell types and multiply in the cytoplasm after transformation into amastigotes. When multiplying amastigotes fill the host cell, they differentiate into trypomastigotes, and the cell ruptures. The parasites released invade local tissues or spread hematogenously to distant sites, thus initiating further cycles of multiplication, primarily in muscle cells, and maintaining a parasitemia infective for vectors.

Transmission of *T. cruzi* also occurs through blood transfusions[4-6] and typically takes place in cities when infected but asymptomatic migrants from endemic rural areas donate blood. Serologic screening of donated blood essentially has eliminated transmission by this route in most endemic areas. *T. cruzi* can also be transmitted by transplantation of organs obtained from chronically infected persons.[7-9] Roughly 5% of infants born to *T. cruzi*–infected women have congenital Chagas' disease. Although some of these infants have severe problems as a result of the infection, most are completely asymptomatic.[10-12] Finally, numerous laboratory accidents resulting in acute Chagas' disease have occurred as a consequence of the facility with which infective forms of the parasite can be produced in the laboratory.[13]

PATHOLOGY

In acute Chagas' disease, the inflammatory lesion caused by *T. cruzi* at the site of entry is called a *chagoma*.[14] Local histologic changes include intracellular parasitism of muscle and other subcutaneous tissues, interstitial edema, lymphocytic infiltration, and reactive hyperplasia of adjacent lymph nodes. Trypomastigotes released when host cells rupture often can be detected by microscopic examination of fresh blood. Muscles, including the myocardium, are the most heavily parasitized tissues. Myocarditis may develop in association with patchy areas of infected cells and necrosis.[15,16] The characteristic pseudocysts seen in sections of infected tissues are intracellular aggregates of amastigotes (Fig. 277-4). A lymphocytosis accompanies the high parasitemias of the acute illness, and mild elevation of transaminase levels is occasionally seen. In some patients, parasites may be found in the cerebrospinal fluid.[17]

Human Trypanosomiasis

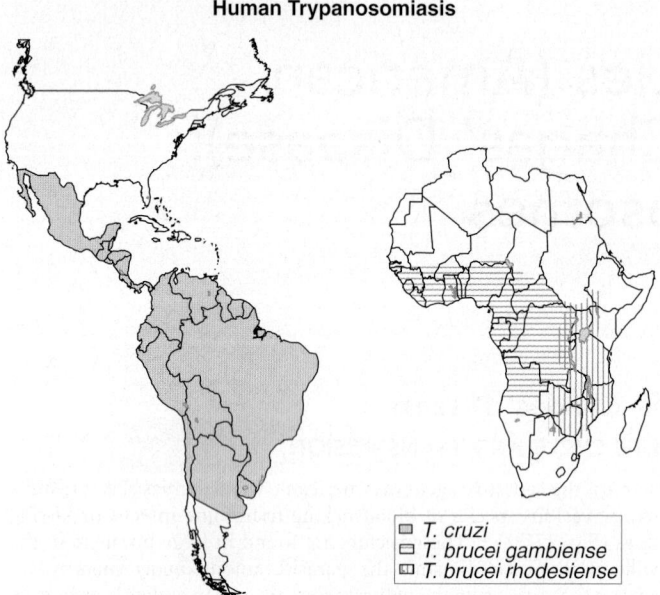

Figure 277-1 **Distribution of human trypanosomiasis.**

- ☐ *T. cruzi*
- ☐ *T. brucei gambiense*
- ☐ *T. brucei rhodesiense*

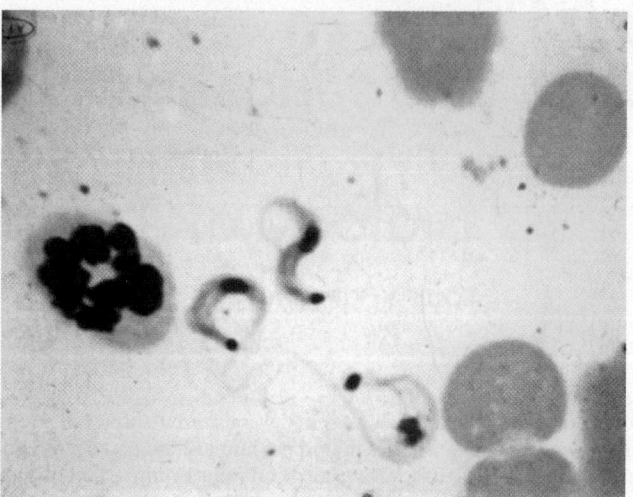

Figure 277-3 *Trypanosoma cruzi* **trypomastigotes in a smear of mouse blood (Giemsa, × 625).** *(Courtesy of Dr. Herbert B. Tanowitz, New York, NY.)*

The heart is the organ most commonly affected in chronic Chagas' disease. Gross examination of the hearts of chronic chagasic patients who died of heart failure reveals marked bilateral ventricular enlargement, often involving the right side of the heart more than the left. Thinning of the ventricular walls is common, as are apical aneurysms and mural thrombi. Widespread lymphocytic infiltration is present, accompanied by diffuse interstitial fibrosis and atrophy of myocardial cells. Parasites are rarely seen in stained sections of myocardial tissue, but studies using polymerase chain reaction (PCR) assays have demonstrated the presence of parasites in areas of focal inflammation.[18-20]

Pathologic changes are also common in the conduction system of chronic chagasic hearts and often correlate with premortem rhythm disturbances.[21] Dense fibrosis and chronic inflammatory lesions most frequently involve the right branch and the left anterior branch of the bundle of His, but lesions of this type are found in other parts of the conduction system as well.

The striking features apparent on gross examination of the esophagus or colon of a patient with chronic Chagas' disease of the digestive tract (megadisease) are the enormous dilation and muscular hypertro-

phy of the affected organs.[22,23] On microscopic examination, focal inflammatory lesions with lymphocytic infiltration are seen. A marked reduction in the number of neurons in the myenteric plexus is also apparent, and peri- and intraganglion fibrosis in the presence of Schwann cell proliferation and lymphocytosis is found. In most patients, the clinical effects of this parasympathetic denervation are confined to the esophagus or the colon, or both, but similar lesions have been observed in the biliary tree, the ureters, and other hollow viscera.

The pathogenesis of the cardiac and gastrointestinal lesions of chronic Chagas' disease has been debated for many years. In recent years convincing evidence has accumulated indicating that the persistence of parasites in heart muscle stimulates a chronic inflammatory process that often results in rhythm disturbances and cardiomyopathy.[24-26]

EPIDEMIOLOGY

T. cruzi infection is a zoonosis, and humans are merely unfortunate hosts whose involvement in the cycle of transmission is not necessary for the perpetuation of the parasite in nature. The triatomine vectors

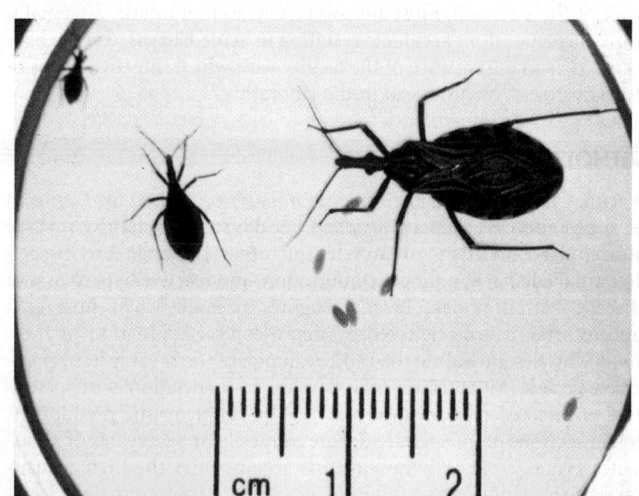

Figure 277-2 **Rhodnius prolixus, a common vector of *Trypanosoma cruzi.*** First- and second-stage nymphs, eggs, and adult.

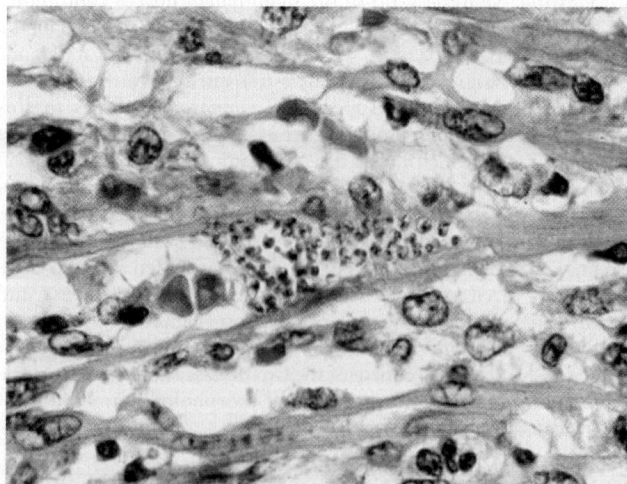

Figure 277-4 *Trypanosoma cruzi* **in the cardiac muscle of a child who died of acute Chagas' disease in Texas.** (H&E, × 900.)

necessary for natural transmission of *T. cruzi* are found in the Americas from the southern half of the United States to southern Argentina.[2] Infected insects have been found in uneven distributions throughout this range. Burrows, hollow trees, palm trees, and other animal shelters are sites where transmission of *T. cruzi* occurs among infected insects and nonhuman mammalian hosts. Vector transmission to humans generally occurs only in areas in which triatomine species that defecate during or immediately after blood meals are present. This limitation does not apply to the range of the infection in lower mammals, however, because they can acquire the infection by eating infected insects.[27,28] Interestingly, several outbreaks of acute Chagas' disease in humans in Brazil attributed to oral transmission through ingestion of food or drink contaminated with *T. cruzi*–infected vectors or their excreta have been reported.[29-32] In these incidents, many dozens of people became infected and some died of acute Chagas' disease. The occurrence of these outbreaks underscores the easy transmissability of the organism via the oral route and the need to keep vectors out of areas where food and drink are prepared and consumed.

T. cruzi has been isolated from more than 150 species of wild and domestic mammals. The ability of the parasite to adapt to such a wide variety of hosts, coupled with the long-term parasitemias in infected mammals, results in the presence of an enormous sylvatic and domestic reservoir in enzootic areas. Infected mammals have been found in the southern United States[33-35] and from there southward to central Argentina and Chile.[36]

Historically, humans become involved in the cycle of transmission when land is opened up for farming in enzootic areas where vector species adaptable to living in human dwellings, such as *Rhodnius prolixus* and *Triatoma infestans*, are prevalent. As the natural habitat of the vectors and mammalian hosts is disrupted, the insects take up residence in niches in the settlers' primitive wood, mud, and stone houses. In this way, the infected triatomine insects become domiciliary, and the domestic cycle of transmission is established to include domestic animals and humans.[37] Thus, human trypanosomiasis in Latin America is primarily a public health problem among poor persons who live in rural areas. Most new vector-borne infections occur in children younger than 10 years old. In a study of selected patients, the case fatality rate for untreated acute Chagas' disease was 12%,[38] but such a high rate likely reflects the fact that only seriously ill patients come to medical attention. The rate for all new infections is probably less than 1%.

It is currently estimated by the Pan American Health Organization that 8 million people are infected with *T. cruzi* and that up to 20,000 persons die each year of Chagas' disease.[39] In 2000 the total annual cost of the morbidity and death associated with Chagas' disease in all endemic countries was thought to be more than US$8 billion.[40] Despite this bleak picture, the current situation relating to the transmission of *T. cruzi* is much brighter. A major international control program in the Southern Cone nations of South America (Argentina, Bolivia, Brazil, Chile, Paraguay, and Uruguay), initiated in 1991, has achieved a marked reduction in transmission rates through education of at-risk populations and vector and blood bank control programs. Gradual reduction in prevalence rates in younger age groups and progressive reduction in the percentage of blood donors infected with *T. cruzi* stand as clear evidence of the success of the program.[41-43] Uruguay was certified as free of vector-borne transmission in 1997, and Chile followed in 1999. Brazil was declared transmission-free in 2006, and it is likely that Argentina will be be added to the list within a few years.[44] Similar control programs have been initiated in the Andean countries and also in Central America. In Mexico screening of donated blood for *T. cruzi* infection is likely to be mandated nationwide in the near future, although at the present time only 13% of the blood supply is screened serologically.[45] The barriers hindering the elimination of *T. cruzi* transmission to humans throughout the endemic range are economic and political, and no technical breakthroughs are necessary for its completion.

Only about 10% to 30% of persons with chronic *T. cruzi* infections will develop symptomatic Chagas' disease.[46] The age distribution of the onset of the two types of chronic diseases is broad. The relatively high frequency of sudden death in young adults observed in some regions in the past was attributed to the disturbances of cardiac rhythm associated with Chagas' disease, and many years ago in one highly endemic area in Brazil, chagasic cardiac disease was found to be the leading cause of death in young adults.[47] There is considerable geographic variation in the prevalence of symptomatic chronic Chagas' disease among infected persons. The prevalence of cardiac disease among persons who harbor the parasite chronically is lower in Venezuela, Colombia, Central America, and Mexico than in the rest of the endemic range. Similarly, megaesophagus and megacolon in association with *T. cruzi* infection are virtually unknown in the northern endemic range, whereas they reach 15% to 20% in the southern endemic regions. It is not known whether host factors or parasite strain differences are the primary determinants of this geographic variation in the patterns of clinical disease.[48]

Despite the presence of *T. cruzi*–infected triatomine vectors in many parts of the southern and western United States, only six autochthonous cases of Chagas' disease have been reported: three in Texas and one each in California, Tennessee, and Louisiana.[15,49,50] Moreover, screening of U.S. blood donors for Chagas' disease, which began in January 2007 and to date has involved testing of more than 15 million units, has only turned up a handful of donors who appear to have acquired *T. cruzi* infection here. The rarity of transmission of *T. cruzi* to humans in the United States probably results from our relatively high housing standards and the low overall vector density. In the past 30 years, about 15 laboratory-acquired and imported cases of acute Chagas' disease have been reported to the Centers for Disease Control and Prevention (CDC), but none in the latter group occurred in returning tourists. However, three instances of tourists returning to Europe from Latin America with acute *T. cruzi* infections have been reported.[51,52] Although the number of autochthonous and imported cases of acute *T. cruzi* infection that go unrecognized may be many times the number reported, the fact remains that acute Chagas' disease is extremely rare in the United States and there is no evidence whatsoever that the incidence is increasing.

In contrast, in recent decades the number of persons in the United States with chronic *T. cruzi* infections has grown considerably. It is estimated that 17 million persons born in countries in which Chagas' disease is endemic currently reside here. Roughly 11.5 million of these immigrants are from Mexico,[53] where the overall prevalnce of Chagas' disease likely is 0.5% to 1.0%. Moreover, a sizable proportion of these immigrants have come from Central America, a region in which the prevalence of *T. cruzi* infection generally is higher than it is in Mexico. A study of Salvadoran and Nicaraguan immigrants done 20 years ago in Washington, D.C., found a 5% prevalence of *T. cruzi* infection.[54] In a study of 300,000 donors in Los Angeles and Miami, the prevalence of *T. cruzi* infection was found to be 1 in 8800 in the general donor population and 1 in 710 among donors who had spent a month or more in an area in which Chagas' disease is endemic.[55,56] More recently, *T. cruzi* infection rates of 1 in 3285 and 1 in 5995 were found in blood donors in Los Angeles and Tucson,[57] and a *T. cruzi* prevalence of 0.7% was found among 500 Hispanic immigrants attending health fairs in Los Angeles (personal communication, Dr. Sheba Meymandi).

These findings and census data suggest that 100,000 *T. cruzi*–infected persons now reside in the United States. Prior to the implementation of donor screening, the presence of infected immigrants posed a risk of transfusion-associated transmission of *T. cruzi*, and seven such cases had been reported in the United States and Canada.[58] The confirmed rate of *T. cruzi* infection found in blood donors since the implementation of screening in January 2007 has been about 1 in 29,000.[6] The transplantation of organs obtained from three chronically infected immigrants resulted in five cases of acute Chagas' disease, one of which was fatal.[7,8]

Clinical Course

The clinical syndromes of acute *T. cruzi* infection and chronic Chagas' disease are quite different. The acute illness results from the first encounter of the host with the parasite, and chronic disease involves late sequelae.

Acute Chagas' disease[16] is usually an illness of children, but it can occur at any age. Only a small portion of acute infections caused by *T. cruzi* are recognized as such because of the mild and nonspecific nature of the symptoms in most patients and the lack of access to medical care. The first signs of illness occur at least a week after invasion by the parasites. When the parasite has entered through a break in the skin, a chagoma may appear, consisting of an indurated area of erythema and swelling accompanied by local lymph node involvement. Romaña's sign (Fig. 277-5), the classic sign of acute Chagas' disease, consists of painless edema of the palpebrae and periocular tissues and may appear when the conjunctiva is the portal of entry. These initial local signs can be followed by fever, malaise, anorexia, and edema of the face and lower extremities. Generalized lymphadenopathy and hepatosplenomegaly also may appear.

Overt central nervous system signs are not common, but meningoencephalitis develops in some patients and is associated with a very poor prognosis.[59] Severe myocarditis also develops in a small proportion of patients with acute disease, and most deaths are due to the resulting congestive heart failure.[15,16] Nonspecific electrocardiographic changes are seen, but the life-threatening arrhythmias that are frequent in chronic Chagas' disease generally do not occur. In untreated patients, symptoms resolve gradually over a period of weeks to months. Areas of local reaction around the eye or other sites of parasite entry can persist for several weeks, as can the lymphadenopathy and splenomegaly. After the spontaneous resolution of the acute illness, the patient enters what is called the indeterminate phase of Chagas' disease, which is characterized by asymptomatic and subpatent parasitemia and antibodies to a variety of *T. cruzi* antigens.

Chronic symptomatic Chagas' disease becomes apparent years or even decades after the initial infection. The heart is the organ most commonly involved, and symptoms reflect the rhythm disturbances, congestive heart failure, and thromboembolism that are characteristic of the chronic illness[60,61] (Fig. 277-6). Dizziness, syncope, and, less commonly, seizures result from a wide variety of arrhythmias. The cardiomyopathy that develops insidiously often primarily affects the right ventricle, and the classic signs of right-sided heart failure are frequently present. As in patients with arrhythmias, the progression of symptoms related to the cardiomyopathy may be gradual, and a vali-

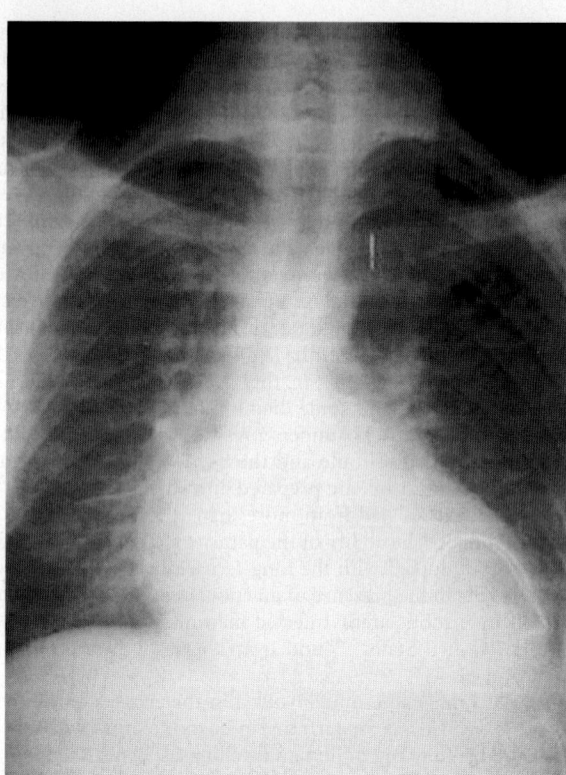

Figure 277-6 **Chest radiograph of a Bolivian patient with chronic *T. cruzi* infection, congestive heart failure, and rhythm disturbances (described in ref. 49).** Pacemaker wires are present in the area of the left ventricle.

dated risk-score assessment tool has been developed.[62] The clinical course is frequently complicated by emboli to the brain or other areas.

In patients with megaesophagus, symptoms are similar to those of idiopathic achalasia and may include dysphagia, odynophagia, chest pain, cough, and regurgitation[63,64] (Figs. 277-7 and 277-8). Hypersalivation and salivary gland hypertrophy have been observed. Aspiration can occur, especially during sleep, and in untreated patients repeated episodes of aspiration pneumonitis are common. Weight loss and even cachexia in patients with megaesophagus can combine with pulmonary infection to result in death. As in idiopathic achalasia, an increased incidence of cancer of the esophagus has been reported in patients with chagasic esophageal disease.

Patients with chagasic megacolon are plagued by chronic constipation and abdominal pain. Individuals with advanced disease can go for several weeks between bowel movements, and acute obstruction, occasionally with volvulus, can lead to perforation, septicemia, and death.

IMMUNOSUPPRESSION AND TRANSPLANTATION IN *T. CRUZI*–INFECTED PATIENTS

When persons who harbor *T. cruzi* chronically become immunosuppressed, reactivation of the infection can occur, sometimes with a severity that is greater than is typical of acute Chagas' disease in immunocompetent patients.[65-68] The incidence of reactivation in *T. cruzi*–infected patients who become immunosuppressed is not known. There have been several reports of reactivations of chronic *T. cruzi* infections after renal transplantation, and in two of these instances the central nervous system was involved. In my view, *T. cruzi* infection should not be a contraindication for kidney transplantation. In infected patients who do undergo the procedure, however, periodic monitoring for signs and symptoms of acute Chagas' disease should be carried out, and a specific search for *T. cruzi*, including careful neurologic evaluation, should be performed when acute illnesses occur postoperatively.

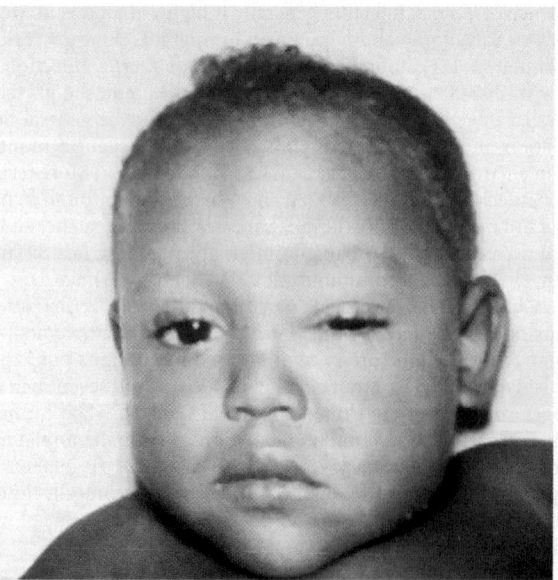

Figure 277-5 **Romaña's sign in an Argentinean child with acute Chagas' disease.** *(Courtesy of Dr. Humberto Lugones, Santiago del Estero, Argentina.)*

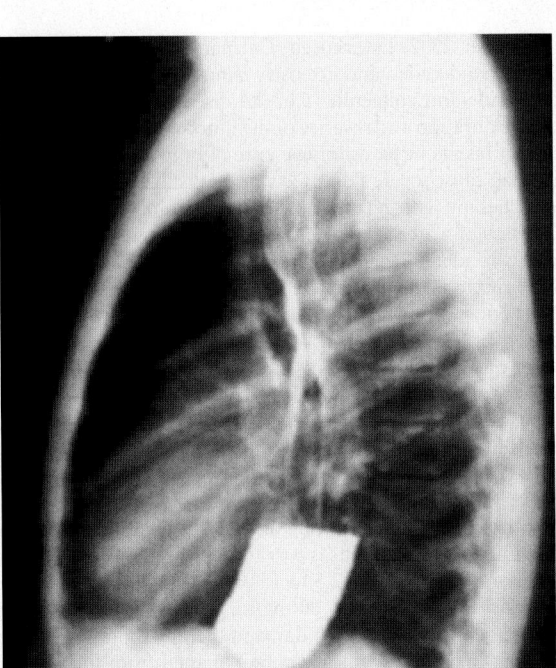

Figure 277-7 **Barium swallow radiographic study of a Brazilian patient with chronic *T. cruzi* infection and megaesophagus.** The markedly increased diameter of the esophagus as well as its failure to empty are typical findings in chagasic patients with megaesophagus. *(Courtesy of Dr. Franklin A. Neva, Bethesda, MD.)*

Immunosuppression caused by the human immunodeficiency virus (HIV) can also lead to recrudescence of chronic *T. cruzi* infection. To date, dozens of such patients have been described, one of whom was a Latin American immigrant living in the United States.[69-72] It is noteworthy that most of these patients developed *T. cruzi* brain abscesses, which do not occur in immunocompetent *T. cruzi*–infected patients. Interestingly, it has been observed that HIV viral loads increase in the context of reactivated acute Chagas' disease.[73] Calculations based on the epidemiologies of HIV and *T. cruzi* infections in Latin America

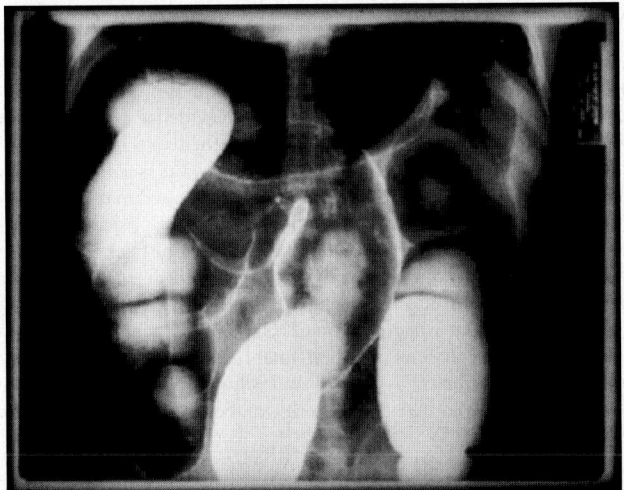

Figure 277-8 **Air-contrast barium enema of a constipated Bolivian patient with megacolon and chronic Chagas' disease.** The markedly increased diameters of the ascending, transverse, and sigmoid segments of the colon are readily apparent.

suggest that the incidence of brain abscesses caused by the latter in coinfected persons is extremely low.

Heart transplantation is an option in patients with end-stage Chagas' cardiac disease, and more than 100 *T. cruzi*–infected patients have undergone the procedure in Brazil and the United States.[74] When the procedure was first being done in Brazil, reactivated acute Chagas' disease occurred frequently as a consequence of the postoperative immunosuppression, but this has been less of a problem in recent years because reduced doses of cyclosporine have been used. An additional problem is the fact that the parasitologic approaches usually used to detect acute *T. cruzi* infections were not sensitive detectors of the reactivations.[75] Moreover, a higher than expected incidence of malignant neoplasm was observed in the Brazilian patients.[76,77] It is also noteworthy that patients who have had transplants for Chagas' heart disease occasionally develop cutaneous lesions containing large numbers of parasites,[78] as has been reported in Chagas' patients who received renal transplants,[66,79] and in coinfected persons with HIV/AIDS.[80] Despite these problems, the long-term survival of Chagas' patients with heart transplants is greater than that of persons transplanted for other reasons, probably because the pathology of chronic *T. cruzi* infection is often limited to the heart.[81]

DIAGNOSIS

The first consideration in the diagnosis of acute Chagas' disease is a history consistent with exposure to *T. cruzi*. This includes residence in an environment in which vector-borne transmission occurs, a recent transfusion in an endemic area where effective blood screening programs are not in place, birth of an infant to a *T. cruzi*–infected mother, or a laboratory accident involving the parasite. It is important to keep in mind, moreover, that, as noted, autochthonous *T. cruzi* infections in the United States are extremely rare and that imported cases among tourists returning to the United States have not been reported.

The diagnosis of acute Chagas' disease is made by detecting parasites, and testing for anti–*T. cruzi* immunoglobulin M (IgM) is not useful. Circulating parasites are motile and can often be seen in wet preparations of anticoagulated blood or buffy coat viewed under a cover slip or in microhematocrit tubes. In many cases, the parasites can also be seen in Giemsa-stained smears. In acutely infected immunocompetent patients, examination of blood preparations is the cornerstone of detecting *T. cruzi*. In immunocompromised patients suspected of having acute Chagas' disease, however, other specimens such as lymph node and bone marrow aspirates, pericardial fluid, and cerebrospinal fluid should be examined microscopically. When these methods fail to detect *T. cruzi* in a patient whose clinical and epidemiologic histories suggest that the parasite is present, as is often the case, efforts to grow the organism can be undertaken. This can be attempted by culturing blood or other specimens in liquid media[82] or by xenodiagnosis, which is a method involving laboratory-reared insect vectors. A major problem with the use of these two methods for diagnosing acute disease is the fact that they take at least several weeks to complete, and this is beyond the time at which decisions regarding drug treatment must be made. Furthermore, although it is thought that culture and xenodiagnosis are more sensitive than microscopic examination of blood and other specimens, their sensitivities may be no greater than 50%. In view of these considerations, it is obvious that improved methods for diagnosing acute *T. cruzi* infections are needed, and PCR assays may fulfill this role (see following). The diagnosis of congenital Chagas' disease must be parasitologic (microscopic examination of cord blood, or PCR) when done right after birth because of the presence of maternal anti–*T. cruzi* antibodies. Serologic testing for specific IgG should be done 6 to 9 months later if the initial parasitologic studies are negative.[10]

Chronic *T. cruzi* infection is usually diagnosed by detecting IgG antibodies that bind specifically to parasite antigens, and isolating the organism is not of primary importance. Currently more than 30 assays for serologic diagnosis of *T. cruzi* infection are available commercially. The majority are based on enzyme-linked immunosorbent assay, indirect hemagglutination, and indirect immunofluorescence formats, and they are used widely in Latin America for clinical testing and for screening donated blood.[83,84] Many of these conventional tests have sensitivities and specificities that are less than ideal, and false-positive reactions occur typically with specimens from patients having illnesses such as leishmaniasis, malaria, syphilis, and other parasitic and non-parasitic diseases. Because of these shortcomings, the Pan American Health Organization has recommended that samples be tested in two assays based on different formats before diagnostic decisions are made. Several assays based on mixtures of recombinant antigens are available or are in development and have shown promise for improved diagnostic accuracy.[85-88] Two assays have been cleared by the FDA for clinical testing in the United States (Chagas' Kit, Hemagen Diagnostics, Inc., Columbia, MD; Chagatest Recombinante, Laboratorios Wiener, Rosario, Argentina); only the Ortho *T. cruzi* Test System (Ortho-Clinical Diagnostics, Raritan, NJ), an ELISA based on a parasite lysate, has been cleared by the FDA for donor testing.[83] The Ortho assay is currently being used to test almost the entire U.S. supply of donated blood. A CLIA-approved radioimmune precipitation assay (Chagas' RIPA)[84,89] is being employed for confirmatory testing of donated units that are positive in the Ortho assay and is also available in my laboratory for testing clinical and research specimens.

The possibility of using PCR assays for detecting *T. cruzi* infection has been studied extensively. The numbers of parasites in the blood of patients with chronic *T. cruzi* infections is extremely low, but PCR assays have the potential for detecting such low numbers because the organisms have highly repetitive nuclear and kinetoplast DNA (kDNA) sequences that can be amplified by PCR. Two decades ago, Moser and colleagues[90] described a PCR test in which a 188–base pair nuclear repetitive DNA sequence is amplified (TCZ1-TCZ2 primers). Each parasite contains approximately 100,000 copies of this sequence, and in contrived experiments as little as 0.5% of the genome of a single parasite gave a positive result. Studies in mice with acute and chronic *T. cruzi* infections indicated clearly that this PCR assay is much more sensitive than microscopic examination of blood.[91] In a second PCR test, described at the same time by Sturm and coworkers,[92] a 330–base pair segment of the *T. cruzi* kinetoplast minicircle is amplified (S35-S36 primers). Each parasite is thought to have approximately 120,000 copies of this sequence, and in mixing experiments the authors were able to detect 0.1% of one parasite genome. In the only head-to-head comparisons of these two assays described to date, it appeared that the TCZ1-TCZ2 assay may have an edge in terms of sensitivity.[91,93]

Since the publication of these two original reports in 1989,[90,92] more than 100 articles have been published that deal with the detection of *T. cruzi* by PCR tests. Importantly, in a group of nine key human studies published in the 1990s, the sensitivities of the PCR assays ranged from 44.7% to 100%, with most results falling slightly over 90%.[82,94,95] More recent results indicate that the variable sensitivity of PCR assays for detecting *T. cruzi* continues to be a major issue.[96,97] Clearly this level of sensitivity is not high enough to allow use of these assays for confirmatory testing blood donations that are positive in screening assays. Nonetheless, PCR assays are useful for detecting *T. cruzi* in persons with borderline serology, in infected individuals who have received specific treatment, and in patients suspected of having acute or congenital Chagas' disease in whom parasites are not detected microscopically. In all such persons, only positive results can be taken as truly indicative of their infection status. A consortium of Latin American investigators recently met to standardize a PCR protocol for *T. cruzi* diagnosis with the goal of increasing the accuracy and comparability of results. The downside of such efforts, however, is that they may stifle innovation and impede progress. At the present time no PCR test for the detection of *T. cruzi* is available commercially.

TREATMENT

Current therapy for persons infected with *T. cruzi* is unsatisfactory. Two drugs are currently being used to treat patients infected with *T. cruzi*.[98,99] The first of these, the nitrofuran derivative nifurtimox

(Lampit, Bayer 2502, Leverkusen, Germany),[100] has been in use for more than two decades, and extensive clinical experience has accumulated. In acute and congenital Chagas' disease, nifurtimox markedly reduces the duration and severity of the illness and decreases mortality. However, it results in parasitologic cure in only about 70% of treated patients, can cause severe side effects, and must be taken for prolonged periods. Therapy with nifurtimox should be initiated as early as possible in cases of acute or congenital Chagas' disease. Moreover, when laboratory accidents occur in which there is a reasonable likelihood that *T. cruzi* infection will become established, therapy should be initiated without waiting for clinical or parasitologic indications of infection.

A large proportion of patients treated with nifurtimox experience adverse side effects. Gastrointestinal complaints include abdominal pain, nausea, vomiting, anorexia, and weight loss. Possible neurologic symptoms include restlessness, insomnia, twitching, paresthesias, and seizures. These symptoms generally disappear when the dosage is reduced or therapy is discontinued.

Nifurtimox is supplied as 30- and 120-mg tablets. The recommended oral dosage for adults is 8 to 10 mg/kg of body weight per day. The dose for adolescents is 12.5 to 15 mg/kg per day, and for children 1 to 10 years of age it is 15 to 20 mg/kg per day. The drug should be given in four divided doses each day, and therapy should be continued for 90 to 120 days. Nifurtimox can be obtained from the CDC Drug Service (404-639-3670).

Benznidazole (Rochagan, Roche 7-1051, São Paulo, Brazil),[101] a nitroimidazole derivative, is the second agent used to treat patients with Chagas' disease. The efficacy of this drug is similar to that of nifurtimox, with the exception that geographic differences in its efficacy have not been observed. Side effects include peripheral neuropathy, rash, and granulocytopenia. The recommended oral dosage of benznidazole is 5 mg/kg per day for 60 days. Benznidazole is used widely in Latin America, where it is viewed as the drug of choice by most specialists. It also can be obtained from the CDC Drug Service. There are no published data regarding the use of benznidazole and nifurtimox in pregnant women.

In terms of which groups of *T. cruzi*–infected persons should be given specific treatment, there is a broad consensus that infants with congenital Chagas' disease, all persons with acute *T. cruzi* infection, and chronically infected children 17 years old or younger should all be treated. This perspective is supported by clinical trial results that indicate clearly that treatment of such patients is useful in terms of the likelihood of parasitologic cure.[102-104]

The question of whether persons in the indeterminate or chronic symptomatic phases of *T. cruzi* infection should be treated with benznidazole or nifurtimox has been debated for many years. This is a thorny issue because these two drugs have to be taken for 2 to 4 months, frequently cause bothersome side effects, and have low parasitologic cure rates in persons with long-standing *T. cruzi* infections.[99,105] Moreover, there is no convincing evidence from properly controlled trials that treatment with either of the drugs is beneficial in such persons. The issue is complicated further by the lack of sensitivity of parasitologic assays, which by necessity must be used in trials to look for treatment failure since antibody titers can remain positive for years even when parasitologic cure has occurred. The ministries of health in Argentina and Brazil do not recommend treatment for persons in the indeterminate or chronic symptomatic phases of *T. cruzi* infection.[106] A panel of experts convened by the CDC in 2007 suggested that treatment be offered to persons with presumably long-standing indeterminate phase infections.[104] A major trial (the BENEFIT Multicentric Trial) designed to address the efficacy of benznidazole is currently under way.[107]

The usefulness of fluconazole, ketoconazole, itraconazole, posaconazole, and allopurinol has been studied extensively in laboratory animals and to a lesser extent in persons with Chagas' disease. None of these drugs has been shown to exert a level of anti–*T. cruzi* activity that warrants its use in humans. Most patients with acute Chagas' disease require no therapy other than benznidazole or nifurtimox because symptoms are generally self-limited even in the absence of drug treatment. The management of the occasional severely ill acute-phase patient with myocarditis or meningoencephalitis is largely supportive. The treatment of patients with chronic chagasic heart disease is also supportive. Chronically infected persons should have electrocardiograms performed every 6 months or so because pacemakers have been shown to be useful in the management of arrhythmias seen in chronic Chagas' disease. The congestive heart failure of cardiomyopathic Chagas' disease is generally treated with measures used in patients with cardiomyopathies due to other causes.[61,108,109]

Megaesophagus associated with Chagas' disease generally should be managed as is idiopathic achalasia.[64,110] The first approach to relieving symptoms is balloon dilation of the lower esophageal sphincter. Patients who fail to respond to repeated attempts at this approach are treated surgically. The procedure used most frequently is wide esophagocardiomyectomy of the anterior gastroesophageal junction, combined with valvuloplasty to reduce reflux. Patients with extreme megaesophagus are often treated with esophageal resection with reconstruction using an esophagogastroplasty. In industrialized countries, laparoscopic myotomy is being used with increasing frequency to treat idiopathic achalasia. This relatively simple procedure may become the approach of choice for both idiopathic achalasia and Chagas' megaesophagus. A possible role for the injection of botulinum toxin is being studied.[111]

Patients in the early stages of colonic dysfunction associated with chronic Chagas' disease can be managed with a high-fiber diet and occasional laxatives and enemas. Fecal impaction necessitating manual disimpaction may occur, as can toxic megacolon, which requires surgical treatment. Another complication of chagasic megacolon that requires immediate attention is volvulus. This usually occurs when the lengthened and enlarged sigmoid colon twists and folds on itself, causing a constellation of symptoms resulting from the obstruction. Endoscopic emptying can be performed initially in patients without radiographic, clinical, or endoscopic signs of ischemia in the affected area. Complicated cases should be treated with surgical decompression. In either event, however, surgical treatment of the megacolon is eventually necessary because of the high probability of recurrence of the volvulus. A number of surgical procedures have been used to treat advanced chagasic megacolon, and all include resection of the sigmoid colon as well as removal of part of the rectum.[112] The latter is performed to avoid recurrence of megacolon in the segment of the colon that is anastomosed to the rectum.

PREVENTION

In view of the possible serious consequences of chronic *T. cruzi* infection, I feel that all immigrants from endemic regions should be screened serologically. Identification of infected persons is important because the implantation of pacemakers has been shown to benefit some patients who develop rhythm disturbances. The possibility of congenital transmission is another justification for screening.

As noted earlier, to date seven cases of transfusion-associated transmission of *T. cruzi* have been reported in the United States and Canada. The courses of acute Chagas' disease in these patients were particularly fulminant because of immunosuppressive therapy they were receiving, and this certainly contributed to the definitive diagnoses. The question as to how best to avoid transmission of the parasite via transfusion in the United States has been debated for more than a decade, albeit prior to December 2006 in the context of a lack of an FDA-approved screening test. Common sense suggested that if serologic screening was warranted in the endemic countries from which the 17 million at-risk immigrants living here had come, then they should be screened when they presented for donation here. In the end, governmental and blood industry authorities embraced this view, and shortly after the FDA approved the Ortho *T. cruzi* ELISA Test System, widespread screening was implemented. Currently more than 90% of blood donated in the United States is tested for Chagas'. Selective testing schemes that focus on donors with relatively increased risk for harboring *T. cruzi* are being considered with the goal of decreasing the numbers of units tested and thus reduce costs.[113] Laboratory personnel should wear gloves and eye protection when working with *T. cruzi*, and suitable containment should be used when dealing with infected insects.[114,115] Persons traveling in endemic areas should avoid sleeping in dilapidated dwellings and should use insect repellent and bed nets to reduce exposure to vectors.[116,117] No vaccine is available for the prevention of transmission of *T. cruzi*. Special precautions for campers, hunters, and others engaging in outdoor activities in the United States are not warranted.

REFERENCES

1. Levine ND, Corliss JO, Cox FEG, et al. A newly revised classification of the protozoa. *J Protozool.* 1980;27:37-58.
2. Lent H, Wygodzinsky P. Revision of the Triatominae (Hemiptera, Reduviidae), and their significance as vectors of Chagas' disease. *Bull Am Museum Natural History.* 1979;163:123-520.
3. Tartarotti E, Azeredo-Oliveira MT, Ceron CR. Phylogenetic approach to the study of Triatomines (Triatominae, Heteroptera). *Braz J Biol.* 2006;66(2B):703-708.
4. Schmunis GA, Cruz JR. Safety of the blood supply in Latin America. *Clin Microbiol Rev.* 2005;18(1):12-29.
5. Kirchhoff LV, Paredes P, Lomeli-Guerrero A, et al. Transfusion-associated Chagas' disease (American trypanosomiasis) in Mexico: Implications for transfusion medicine in the United States. *Transfusion.* 2006;46(2):298-304.
6. Bern C, Montgomery SP, Katz L, et al. Chagas' disease and the US blood supply. *Curr Opin Infect Dis.* 2008;21(5):476-482.
7. Centers for Disease Control and Prevention. Chagas' disease after organ transplantation—United States, 2001. *MMWR.* 2002;51(10):210-212.
8. Centers for Disease Control and Prevention. Chagas' disease after organ transplantation—Los Angeles, California, 2006. *MMWR.* 2006;55(29):798-800.
9. Souza FF, Castro-E-Silva O, Marin Neto JA, et al. Acute chagasic myocardiopathy after orthotopic liver transplantation with donor and recipient serologically negative for *Trypanosoma cruzi*: a case report. *Transplant Proc.* 2008;40(3):875-878.
10. Freilij H, Altcheh J. Congenital Chagas' disease: diagnostic and clinical aspects. *Clin Infect Dis.* 1995;21(3):551-555.
11. Gurtler RE, Segura EL, Cohen JE. Congenital transmission of *Trypanosoma cruzi* infection in Argentina. *Emerging Infect Dis.* 2003;9(1):29-32.
12. Brutus L, Schneider D, Postigo J, et al. Congenital Chagas' disease: diagnostic and clinical aspects in an area without vectorial transmission, Bermejo, Bolivia. *Acta Trop.* 2008;106(3):195-199.
13. Herwaldt BL. Protozoa and helminths. In: Fleming DO, Hunt DL, eds. *Biological Safety: Principles and Practice.* 4th ed. Washington, DC: American Society for Microbiology; 2006:115-161.
14. Rassi A, Rassi Junior A, Rassi GG. Acute Chagas' disease. [Portuguese]. In: Brener Z, Andrade ZA, Barral-Netto M, eds. *Trypanosoma cruzi e Doença de Chagas.* Rio de Janeiro: Guanabara Koogan; 2000:231-245.
15. Ochs DE, Hnilica V, Moser DR, et al. Postmortem diagnosis of autochthonous acute chagasic myocarditis by polymerase chain reaction amplification of a species-specific DNA sequence of *Trypanosoma cruzi. Am J Trop Med Hyg.* 1996;34:526-529.
16. Parada H, Carrasco HA, Anez N, et al. Cardiac involvement is a constant finding in acute Chagas' disease: a clinical, parasitological and histopathological study. *Int J Cardiol.* 1997;60(1):49-54.
17. Hoff R, Teixeira RS, Carvalho JS, et al. *Trypanosoma cruzi* in the cerebrospinal fluid during the acute stage of Chagas' disease. *N Engl J Med.* 1978;298:604-606.
18. Jones EM, Colley DG, Tostes S, et al. Amplification of a *Trypanosoma cruzi* DNA sequence from inflammatory lesions in human Chagasic cardiomyopathy. *Am J Trop Med Hyg.* 1993;48:348-357.
19. Zhang L, Tarleton RL. Parasite persistence correlates with disease severity and localization in chronic Chagas' disease. *J Infect Dis.* 1999;180(2):480-486.
20. Benvenuti LA, Roggerio A, Freitas HF, et al. Chronic American trypanosomiasis: parasite persistence in endomyocardial biopsies is associated with high-grade myocarditis. *Ann Trop Med Parasitol.* 2008;102(6):481-487.
21. Andrade ZA, Andrade SG, Oliveira GB, et al. Histopathology of the conducting tissue of the heart in Chagas' myocarditis. *Am Heart J.* 1978;95:316-324.
22. Kirchhoff LV. American trypanosomiasis (Chagas' disease). *Gastroenterol Clinics N America.* 1996;25(3):517-533.
23. Rezende JM, Moreira H. Forma digestiva da doença de Chagas [Portuguese]. In: Brener Z, Andrade ZA, Barral-Netto M, eds. *Trypanosoma cruzi e Doença de Chagas.* 2nd ed. Rio de Janeiro: Guanabara Koogan; 2000:297-343.
24. Kierszenbaum F. Where do we stand on the autoimmunity hypothesis of Chagas' disease? *Trends Parasitol.* 2005;21(11):513-516.
25. Marin-Neto JA, Cunha-Neto E, Maciel BC, et al. Pathogenesis of chronic Chagas' heart disease. *Circulation.* 2007;115:1109-1123.
26. Bonney KM, Engman DM. Chagas' heart disease pathogenesis: one mechanism or many? *Curr Mol Med.* 2008;8(6):510-518.
27. Ryckman RE, Olsen LE. Epizootiology of *Trypanosoma cruzi* in Southwestern North America. Part VI. Insectivorous hosts of Triatominae—the perizootiological relationship to *Trypanosoma cruzi. J Med Entomol.* 1965;2:99-106.
28. Williams JT, Dick Jr EJ, Vandeberg JL, et al. Natural Chagas' disease in four baboons. *J Med Primatol* 2008;38:107-113.
29. Di Primio R. An outbreak of illness in Teutonia. *Trop Dis Bull.* 1968;65(4):400-401.
30. Shikanai-Yasuda MA, Marcondes CB, Guedes LA, et al. Possible oral transmission of acute Chagas' disease in Brazil. *Rev Inst Med Trop Sao Paulo.* 1991;33(5):351-357.
31. Dias JP, Bastos C, Araujo E, et al. Acute Chagas' disease outbreak associated with oral transmission. *Rev Soc Bras Med Trop.* 2008; 41(3):296-300.
32. Steindel M, Kramer PL, Scholl D, et al. Characterization of *Trypanosoma cruzi* isolated from humans, vectors, and animal reservoirs following an outbreak of acute human Chagas' disease in Santa Catarina State, Brazil. *Diagn Microbiol Infect Dis.* 2008; 60(1):25-32.
33. Bradley KK, Bergman DK, Woods JP, et al. Prevalence of American trypanosomiasis (Chagas' disease) among dogs in Oklahoma. *J Am Vet Med Assoc.* 2000;217(12):1853-1857.

34. Yabsley MJ, Brown EL, Roellig DM. Evaluation of the Chagas' Stat-Pak(TM) assay for detection of *Trypanosoma cruzi* antibodies in wildlife reservoirs. *J Parasitol.* 2008;1.

35. Kjos SA, Snowden KF, Craig TM, et al. Distribution and characterization of canine Chagas' disease in Texas. *Vet Parasitol.* 2008;152(3-4):249-256.

36. Roque AL, Xavier SC, da Rocha MG, et al. *Trypanosoma cruzi* transmission cycle among wild and domestic mammals in three areas of orally transmitted Chagas' disease outbreaks. *Am J Trop Med Hyg.* 2008;79(5):742-749.

37. Cohen JE, Gurtler RE. Modeling household transmission of American trypanosomiasis. *Science.* 2001;293(5530):694-698.

38. Laranja FS, Dias E, Nobrega G, et al. Chagas' disease: A clinical, epidemiologic, and pathologic study. *Circulation.* 1956;14:1035-1060.

39. Salvatella R. *Current status of Chagas' disease.* Washington, DC: Pan American Health Association; 2006.

40. Schmunis GA. American trypanosomiasis and its impact on public health in the Americas [Portuguese]. In: Brener Z, Andrade ZA, Barral-Netto M, eds. *Trypanosoma cruzi e Doença de Chagas.* 2nd ed. Rio de Janeiro: Guanabara Koogan; 2000:1-20.

41. Dias JC. Southern Cone Initiative for the elimination of domestic populations of *Triatoma infestans* and the interruption of transfusional Chagas' disease. Historical aspects, present situation, and perspectives. *Mem Inst Oswaldo Cruz.* 2007;102(suppl 1):11-18.

42. Sabino EC, Goncalez TT, Salles NA, et al. Trends in the prevalence of Chagas' disease among first-time blood donors in Sao Paulo, Brazil. *Transfusion.* 2003;43(7):853-856.

43. Schofield CJ, Jannin J, Salvatella R. The future of Chagas' disease control. *Trends Parasitol.* 2006;22:583-588.

44. Segura EL, Cura EN, Estani SA, et al. Long-term effects of a nationwide control program on the seropositivity for *Trypanosoma cruzi* infection in young men from Argentina. *Am J Trop Med Hyg.* 2000;62(3):353-362.

45. Anonymous. *La Salud en las Américas. Publicación Científica y Técnica No. 587 ed.* Washington, DC: Pan American Health Organization; 2002.

46. Mota EA, Guimaraes AC, Santana OO, et al. A nine-year prospective study of Chagas' disease in a defined rural population in Northeast Brazil. *Am J Trop Med Hyg.* 1990;42:429-440.

47. Amorim DS. Chagas' disease. *Progress in Cardiology.* 1979;235-279.

48. de Diego JA, Palau MT, Gamallo C, et al. Are genotypes of *Trypanosoma cruzi* involved in the challenge of chagasic cardiomyopathy? *Parasitol Res.* 1998;84(2):147-152.

49. Herwaldt BL, Grijalva MJ, Newsome AL, et al. Use of polymerase chain reaction to diagnose the fifth reported US case of autochthonous transmission of *Trypanosoma cruzi*, in Tennessee, 1998. *J Infect Dis.* 2000;181(1):395-399.

50. Dorn PL, Perniciaro L, Yabsley MJ, et al. Autochthonous transmission of *Trypanosoma cruzi*, Louisiana. *Emerg Infect Dis.* 2007;13(4):605-607.

51. Crovato F, Rebora A. Chagas' disease: a potential problem for Europe? *Dermatol.* 1997;195:184-185.

52. Lescure FX, Canestri A, Melliez H, et al. Chagas' disease, France. *Emerg Infect Dis.* 2008;14(4):644-646.

53. U.S. Census Bureau. *Foreign-Born Population by Place of Birth and Citizenship Status: 2006. Statistical Abstract of the United States: 2008.* Washington, DC: U.S. Department of Commerce; 2008.

54. Kirchhoff LV, Gam AA, Gilliam FC. American trypanosomiasis (Chagas' disease) in Central American immigrants. *Am J Med.* 1987;82:915-920.

55. Leiby DA, Read EJ, Lenes BA, et al. Seroepidemiology of *Trypanosoma cruzi*, etiologic agent of Chagas' disease, in U.S. blood donors. *J Infect Dis.* 1997;176:1047-1052.

56. Leiby DA, Herron RM Jr, Read EJ, et al. T*rypanosoma cruzi* in Los Angeles and Miami blood donors: impact of evolving donor demographics on seroprevalence and implications for transfusion transmission. *Transfusion.* 2002;42(5):549-555.

57. Centers for Disease Control and Prevention. Blood donor screening for Chagas disease—United States, 2006-2007. *MMWR.* 2007;56(07):141-143.

58. Young C, Losikoff P, Chawla A, et al. Transfusion-acquired *Trypanosoma cruzi* infection. *Transfusion.* 2007;47:540-544.

59. Kirchhoff LV. Trypanosomiasis of the central nervous system. In: Scheld WM, Marra CM, Whitely RJ, eds. *Infections of the Central Nervous System.* 3rd ed. 2004:777-789.

60. Carod-Artal FJ, Vargas AP, Horan TA, et al. Chagasic cardiomyopathy is independently associated with ischemic stroke in Chagas' disease. *Stroke.* 2005;36(5):965-970.

61. Pazin-Filho A, Romano MM, Gomes FR, et al. Left ventricular global performance and diastolic function in indeterminate and cardiac forms of Chagas' disease. *J Am Soc Echocardiogr.* 2007;20(12):1338-1343.

62. Rassi A Jr, Rassi A, Little WC, et al. Development and validation of a risk score for predicting death in Chagas' heart disease. *N Engl J Med.* 2006;355(8):799-808.

63. de Oliveira RB, Troncon LE, Dantas RO, et al. Gastrointestinal manifestations of Chagas' disease. *Am J Gastroenterol.* 1998;93(6):884-889.

64. Herbella FA, Oliveira DR, Del Grande JC. Are idiopathic and Chagasic achalasia two different diseases? *Dig Dis Sci.* 2004;49(3):353-360.

65. Riarte A, Luna C, Sabatiello R, et al. Chagas' disease in patients with kidney transplants: 7 years of experience 1989-1996. *Clin Infect Dis.* 1999;29(3):561-567.

66. Gallerano V, Consigli J, Pereyra S, et al. Chagas' disease reactivation with skin symptoms in a patient with kidney transplant. *Int J Dermatol.* 2007;46(6):607-610.

67. Campos SV, Strabelli TM, Amato NV, et al. Risk factors for Chagas' disease reactivation after heart transplantation. *J Heart Lung Transplant.* 2008;27(6):597-602.

68. Marchiori PE, Alexandre PL, Britto N, et al. Late reactivation of Chagas' disease presenting in a recipient as an expansive mass lesion in the brain after heart transplantation of chagasic myocardiopathy. *J Heart Lung Transplant.* 2007;(Nov):1091-1096.

69. Gluckstein D, Ciferri F, Ruskin J. Chagas' disease: another cause of cerebral mass in the acquired immunodeficiency syndrome. *Am J Med.* 1992;92:429-432.

70. Lambert N, Mehta B, Walters R, et al. Chagasic encephalitis as the initial manifestation of AIDS. *Ann Intern Med.* 2006 Jun 20;144(12):941-943.

71. Sartori AM, Ibrahim KY, Nunes Westphalen EV, et al. Manifestations of Chagas' disease (American trypanosomiasis) in patients with HIV/AIDS. *Ann Trop Med Parasitol.* 2007;101:31-50.

72. Cordova E, Boschi A, Ambrosioni J, et al. Reactivation of Chagas' disease with central nervous system involvement in HIV-infected patients in Argentina, 1992-2007. *Int J Infect Dis.* 2008;12(6):587-592.

73. Sartori AM, Caiaffa-Filho HH, Bezerra RC, et al. Exacerbation of HIV viral load simultaneous with asymptomatic reactivation of chronic Chagas' disease. *Am J Trop Med Hyg.* 2002;67(5):521-523.

74. Bocchi EA, Fiorelli A. The Brazilian experience with heart transplantation: a multicenter report. *J Heart Lung Transplant.* 2001;20(6):637-645.

75. Diez M, Favaloro L, Bertolotti A, et al. Usefulness of PCR strategies for early diagnosis of Chagas' disease reactivation and treatment follow-up in heart transplantation. *Am J Transplant.* 2007;7(6):1633-1640.

76. Bocchi EA, Higuchi ML, Vieira ML, et al. Higher incidence of malignant neoplasms after heart transplantation for treatment of chronic Chagas' heart disease. *J Heart Lung Transplant.* 1998;17(4):399-405.

77. Palma JH, Guilhen JC, Gaia DF, et al. Post-transplant lymphoproliferative disease presenting as a mass in the left ventricle in a heart transplant recipient at long-term follow-up. *J Heart Lung Transplant.* 2009;28(2):206-208.

78. Libow LF, Beltrani VP, Silvers DN, et al. Post-cardiac transplant reactivation of Chagas' disease diagnosed by skin biopsy. *Cutis.* 1991;48:37-40.

79. La Forgia MP, Pellerano G, las Mercedes PM, et al. Cutaneous manifestation of reactivation of Chagas' disease in a renal transplant patient: long-term follow-up. *Arch Dermatol.* 2003;139(1):104-105.

80. Sartori AM, Sotto MN, Braz LM, et al. Reactivation of Chagas' disease manifested by skin lesions in a patient with AIDS. *Trans R Soc Trop Med Hyg.* 1999;93(6):631-632.

81. Bocchi EA, Fiorelli A. The paradox of survival results after heart transplantation for cardiomyopathy caused by *Trypanosoma cruzi*. First Guidelines Group for Heart Transplantation of the Brazilian Society of Cardiology. *Ann Thor Surg.* 2001;71(6):1833-1838.

82. Castro AM, Luquetti AO, Rassi A, et al. Blood culture and polymerase chain reaction for the diagnosis of the chronic phase of human infection with *Trypanosoma cruzi*. *Parasitol Res.* 2002;88(10):894-900.

83. Gorlin J, Rossmann S, Robertson G, et al. Evaluation of a new *Trypanosoma cruzi* antibody assay for blood donor screening. *Transfusion.* 2008;48(3):531-540.

84. Otani MM, Vinelli E, Kirchhoff LV, et al. WHO comparative evaluation of serologic assays for Chagas' disease. *Transfusion.* 2009;49:1076-1082.

85. Oelemann W, Vanderborght BO, Verissimo Da Costa GC, et al. A recombinant peptide antigen line immunoassay optimized for the confirmation of Chagas' disease. *Transfusion.* 1999;39(7):711-717.

86. Chang CD, Cheng KY, Jiang L, et al. Evaluation of a prototype *Trypanosoma cruzi* antibody assay with recombinant antigens on a fully automated chemiluminescence analyzer for blood donor screening. *Transfusion.* 2006;46(10):1737-1744.

87. Cheng KY, Chang CD, Salbilla VA, et al. Immunoblot assay using recombinant antigens as a supplemental test to confirm antibodies to *Trypanosoma cruzi*. *Clinical and Vaccine Immunology.* 2007;14(4):355-361.

88. Houghton RL, Stevens YY, Hjerrild K, et al. A lateral flow immunoassay for diagnosis of *Trypanosoma cruzi* infection with high correlation to radioimmunoprecipitation assay. *Clin Vaccine Immunol.* 2009;16:515-520.

89. Kirchhoff LV, Gam AA, Gusmao RD, et al. Increased specificity of serodiagnosis of Chagas' disease by detection of antibody to the 72- and 90-kilodalton glycoproteins of *Trypanosoma cruzi*. *J Infect Dis.* 1987;155:561-564.

90. Moser DR, Kirchhoff LV, Donelson JE. Detection of *Trypanosoma cruzi* by polymerase chain reaction gene amplification. *J Clin Microbiol.* 1989;27:1744-1749.

91. Kirchhoff LV, Votava JR, Ochs DE, et al. Comparison of PCR and microscopic methods for detecting *Trypanosoma cruzi*. *J Clin Microbiol.* 1996;34(5):1171-1175.

92. Sturm NR, Degrave W, Morel C, et al. Sensitive detection and schizodeme classification of *Trypanosoma cruzi* cells by amplification of kinetoplast minicircle DNA sequences: use in diagnosis of Chagas' disease. *Mol Biochem Parasitol.* 1989;33:205-214.

93. Virreira M, Torrico F, Truyens C, et al. Comparison of polymerase chain reaction methods for reliable and easy detection of congenital *Trypanosoma cruzi* infection. *Am J Trop Med Hyg.* 2003;68(5):574-582.

94. Russomando G, de Tomassone MM, de Guillen I, et al. Treatment of congenital Chagas' disease diagnosed and followed up by the polymerase chain reaction. *Am J Trop Med Hyg.* 1998;59(3):487-491.

95. Gomes ML, Galvao LMC, Macedo AM, et al. Chagas' disease diagnosis: comparative analysis of parasitologic, molecular, and serologic methods. *Am J Trop Med Hyg.* 1999;60(2):205-210.

96. Portela-Lindoso AA, Shikanai-Yasuda MA. Chronic Chagas' disease: from xenodiagnosis and hemoculture to polymerase chain reaction [Portuguese]. *Revista de Saude Publica.* 2003;37(1):107-115.

97. Fitzwater S, Calderon M, Lafuente C, et al. Polymerase chain reaction for chronic *Trypanosoma cruzi* infection yields higher sensitivity in blood clot than buffy coat or whole blood specimens. *Am J Trop Med Hyg.* 2008;79(5):768-770.

98. Urbina JA. Chemotherapy of Chagas' disease. *Curr Pharm Des.* 2002;8(4):287-295.

99. Coura JR, de Castro SL. A critical review on Chagas' disease chemotherapy. *Mem Inst Oswaldo Cruz.* 2002;97(1):3-24.

100. Kirchhoff LV. Nifurtimox. In: Yu V, Weber R, Raoult D, eds. *Antimicrobial Therapy and Vaccines.* New York: Apple Trees Productions; 2004:867-868.

101. Kirchhoff LV. Benznidazole. In: Yu V, Weber R, Raoult D, eds. *Antimicrobial Therapy and Vaccines.* New York: Apple Trees Productions; 2004:762-763.

102. Schijman AG, Altcheh J, Burgos JM, et al. Aetiological treatment of congenital Chagas' disease diagnosed and monitored by the polymerase chain reaction. *J Antimicrob Chemother.* 2003;52(3):441-449.

103. Sosa-Estani S, Segura EL. Etiological treatment in patients infected by *Trypanosoma cruzi*: experiences in Argentina. *Curr Opin Infect Dis.* 2006;19:583-587.

104. Bern C, Montgomery SP, Herwaldt BL, et al. Evaluation and treatment of Chagas' disease in the United States: A systematic review. *JAMA.* 2007;298(18):2171-2181.

105. Lauria-Pires L, Nitz N, Vexenat AC, et al. The treatment of Chagas' disease patients with nitroderivative is unsatisfactory. *Rev Inst Med Trop Sao Paulo.* 2001;43(3):175-181.

106. Pinto Dias JC. The treatment of Chagas' disease (South American trypanosomiasis). *Ann Intern Med.* 2006;144:772-774.

107. Marin-Neto JA, Rassi A Jr, Morillo CA, et al. Rationale and design of a randomized placebo-controlled trial assessing the effects of etiologic treatment in Chagas' cardiomyopathy: the BENznidazole Evaluation For Interrupting Trypanosomiasis (BENEFIT). *Am Heart J.* 2008;156(1):37-43.

108. Rocha MO, Teixeira MM, Ribeiro AL. An update on the management of Chagas' cardiomyopathy. *Expert Rev Anti Infect Ther.* 2007;5(4):727-743.

109. Rassi A Jr, Rassi A, Rassi SG. Predictors of mortality in chronic Chagas' disease: a systematic review of observational studies. *Circulation.* 2007;115:1101-1108.

110. Herbella FA, Aquino JL, Stefani-Nakano S, et al. Treatment of achalasia: lessons learned with Chagas' disease. *Dis Esophagus.* 2008;21(5):461-467.

111. Brant C, Moraes-Filho JP, Siqueira E, et al. Intrasphincteric botulinum toxin injection in the treatment of chagasic achalasia. *Dis Esophagus.* 2003;16(1):33-38.

112. Garcia RL, de Matos BM, Feres O, et al. Surgical treatment of Chagas' megacolon. Critical analysis of outcome in operative methods. *Acta Cir Bras.* 2008;23(Suppl 1):83-92.

113. Wilson LS, Ramsey JM, Koplowicz YB, et al. Cost-effectiveness of implementation methods for ELISA serology testing of *Trypanosoma cruzi* in California blood banks. *Am J Trop Med Hyg.* 2008;79(1):53-68.

114. Hudson L, Grover F, Gutteridge WE, et al. Suggested guidelines for work with live *Trypanosoma cruzi*. *Trans R Soc Trop Med Hyg.* 1983;77:416-419.

115. *Biosafety in Microbiological and Biomedical Laboratories (BMBL).* 5th ed. Washington, DC: U.S. Department of Health and Human Services; 2007.

116. Kroeger A, Villegas E, Ordoñez-Gonzalez J, et al. Prevention of the transmission of Chagas' disease with pyrethroid-impregnated materials. *Am J Trop Med Hyg.* 2003;68(3):307-311.

117. Levy MZ, Quispe-Machaca VR, Ylla-Velasquez JL, et al. Impregnated netting slows infestation by *Triatoma infestans*. *Am J Trop Med Hyg.* 2008;79(4):528-534.

278

Agents of African Trypanosomiasis (Sleeping Sickness)

LOUIS V. KIRCHHOFF*

Parasites and Their Transmission

The agents of human African trypanosomiasis (sleeping sickness) are flagellated protozoan parasites that belong to the genus *Trypanosoma,* subgenus *Trypanozoon.*[1,2] A general description of the members of this genus and specific characteristics of the subgenus are presented in the introduction to Chapter 277. Three trypanosome subspecies, *T. brucei brucei, T. brucei rhodesiense,* and *T. brucei gambiense,* are considered here. They are indistinguishable morphologically, and as a group they are often referred to as the *T. brucei* complex. *T. b. brucei* is a parasite of wild and domestic animals that is not infectious to humans. In contrast, *T. b. rhodesiense,* which is primarily a parasite of wild game, can infect humans, and this difference in host specificity forms the basis of the distinction between the two subspecies. *T. b. gambiense* primarily infects humans, and infections of wild and domestic animals are of limited importance.

The members of the *T. brucei* complex are transmitted by various species of tsetse flies that belong to the genus *Glossina.*[3,4] These blood-sucking insects are found only in Africa, where their range covers millions of square kilometers of rain forest and savanna. The parasites undergo a developmental cycle in the insect vectors. Tsetse flies of both sexes become infected with trypanosomes when they ingest blood from infected mammalian hosts that contains trypomastigotes, the form of the parasite that circulates in the bloodstream. There are two forms of circulating trypomastigotes: long, slender organisms that are capable of dividing and short, stumpy forms thought to be nondividing parasites that are infective for the insect vectors (Fig. 278-1). Once in the midgut of the tsetse flies, stumpy trypomastigotes transform into relatively long, slender procyclic trypomastigotes. After many cycles of multiplication, the procyclic forms migrate to the salivary glands, where they differentiate into epimastigotes and continue to multiply. A final transformation occurs as the epimastigotes become nondividing metacyclic trypomastigotes. Transmission takes place when these infective forms are inoculated during a subsequent blood meal. The cycle is completed when the injected metacyclic forms become bloodstream trypomastigotes and begin to multiply in the blood or other extracellular spaces.

The capacity of African trypanosomes to multiply in the bloodstream of their mammalian hosts, where they are continually exposed to humoral defenses, constitutes a fundamental difference between the agents of sleeping sickness and *Trypanosoma cruzi,* the cause of Chagas' disease in the Americas. The African trypanosomes are able to evade immune destruction indefinitely because they undergo antigenic variation, a process in which they periodically change the antigenic structure of the coat of glycoproteins that covers the surface of the parasite. The molecular mechanisms that control this complex process have been studied intensively.[5-7] When epimastigotes transform into metacyclic trypomastigotes in the salivary glands of the tsetse fly, each parasite synthesizes a surface coat made up of one of about a dozen types of antigenic glycoproteins, called variant antigen types (VATs). Presumably, this occurs as a preadaptation to the relatively hostile environment of the mammalian host into which the metacyclics must be inoculated if they are to survive. After injection into a mammalian host, the parasites express metacyclic VATs for approximately 5 days, after which they switch to the expression of bloodstream VATs. Over time, the host sequentially mounts specific humoral responses directed against the predominantly expressed VATs. The population of parasites survives because an intrinsic rate of VAT switching provides an apparently endless supply of parasites that have surface glycoprotein coats to which the host has not been exposed previously.

Virtually all transmission of African trypanosomes to both wild and domestic animals, as well as to humans, takes place in the cyclic fashion just described. There is no evidence that these parasites can be transmitted by insects other than tsetse flies, and mechanical transmission by vectors is not important, although it may occur occasionally. Congenital transmission can occur, but in humans it is extremely rare,[8] as is transmission by blood transfusion. A small number of laboratory accidents resulting in infection with African trypanosomes have been reported.[9]

Pathogenesis and Pathology

The pathogenesis of African sleeping sickness is complex, and many aspects of the process are poorly understood.[10-12] The first sign of infection with African trypanosomes can be the acute inflammatory lesion (trypanosomal chancre) that appears a week or so after the bite of an infected tsetse fly and resolves spontaneously over several weeks. Interstitial multiplication of the trypanosomes takes place within the chancre, and there is an intense mononuclear cell reaction to the parasites, as well as edema and local tissue destruction.

After this initial local response, the infection evolves over weeks and months into a systemic hemolymphatic illness as the parasites disseminate widely through the lymphatics and the bloodstream. Systemic African trypanosomiasis without central nervous system (CNS) involvement is generally referred to as stage I disease. The parasites first travel from the site of inoculation to regional lymph nodes, where they proliferate and cause an inflammatory response. They then move through the lymphatics into the bloodstream, where multiplication continues. Egress of trypanosomes from vessels into interstitial spaces, where multiplication also takes place, is thought to be facilitated by increased vascular permeability.

In stage I trypanosomiasis, there is widespread lymphadenopathy and histiocytic proliferation, which may be followed by fibrosis. Morular cells (Mott cells) are also often present in tissue. These cells are plasmacytes with vacuolated cytoplasm and pyknotic nuclei that are thought to play a role in the production of immunoglobulin M (IgM).[13] The spleen may be enlarged, with generalized cellular proliferation, congestion, and focal necrosis. As the disease evolves, an endarteritis with perivascular infiltration of both parasites and lymphocytes may develop in lymph nodes and the spleen.

The heart is frequently involved in this stage of the disease, especially with *T. b. rhodesiense* infections. A pancarditis may develop involving all layers of the heart, including the mural and valvular endocardia.[14,15] The conduction system may also be affected, and involvement of the autonomic innervation of the heart has also been reported.[16] At the cellular level, pathologic changes include intense mononuclear infiltra-

---

*All material in this chapter is in the public domain, with the exception of a borrowed figure.

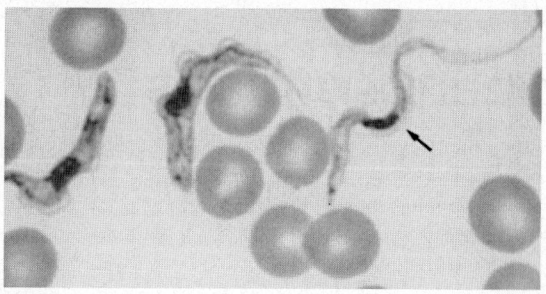

Figure 278-1   *Trypanosoma brucei rhodesiense* **trypomastigotes in rat blood.** The parasite indicated by the *arrow* is typical of the long, slender forms capable of multiplying in the mammalian host. The other two organisms represent the stumpy, nondividing forms infective for the insect vector. (Giemsa, ×1250.) *(Courtesy of Dr. G.A. Cook, Madison, WI.)*

tion consisting of lymphocytes, plasmacytes, and morular cells. As the infection progresses, myocytolysis and fibrosis may develop.

A number of hematologic manifestations accompany the development of stage I disease. Normocytic anemia is a regular feature in this phase of the illness and is usually accompanied by a brisk reticulocytosis. Several factors are thought to contribute to the anemia, and immune-mediated hemolysis may be important. Platelet counts are often reduced, especially in infections with *T. b. rhodesiense,* and disseminated intravascular coagulation before and during therapy has also been described. A moderate degree of leukocytosis is usually present, especially in the early months of the infection, and this is accompanied by polyclonal B-cell activation. High titers of immunoglobulins are a striking and constant feature of the illness. They consist primarily of polyclonal IgM that, for the most part, is not directed against specific parasite antigens. A number of other factors, including heterophile antibodies, rheumatoid factor, and anti-DNA antibodies, are often detectable. In addition, high levels of circulating antigen-antibody complexes are uniformly present, and these may play a role in the anemia, tissue damage, and increased vascular permeability that facilitate the dissemination of the parasites. Erythrocyte sedimentation rates are elevated, and hypocomplementemia has also been noted.

Stage II African trypanosomiasis involves invasion of the CNS. Parasites reach the brain and meninges via the bloodstream and cause meningoencephalitis or meningomyelitis, or both.[17] In the brain, they are found mainly in the frontal lobes, the pons, and the medulla, but other areas may be parasitized as well. Edema and hemorrhages may be evident on gross examination of affected areas at autopsy. Trypanosomes are present in perivascular areas, and nests of organisms can be found without apparent relation to blood vessels. The presence of parasites in the CNS is associated with infiltration of mononuclear cells that are predominantly lymphocytes, plasmacytes, and morular cells. The presence of parasites in the CNS is heralded by abnormal findings in the cerebrospinal fluid (CSF). The CSF may be under increased pressure, and the total protein concentration is elevated, with mononuclear cells predominating in addition to small numbers of morular cells and eosinophils. Trypanosomes are frequently present in the CSF as well.

Epidemiology

Sleeping sickness was a much greater problem in the past than it is at present.[18-20] The illness has undergone a resurgence in recent years, however, and major epidemics have occurred in the Sudan, Democratic Republic of Congo, Uganda, Angola, and several other endemic countries.[21-23] In some areas, wars and the resulting lack of control programs may be the important factors underlying the outbreaks. Approximately 50 to 60 million persons are at risk for acquiring the disease, and the total number of infected individuals is estimated to be around 300,000, although only 10,769 new cases were reported in

2007.[24] More exact figures are not available because the acquisition of reliable health statistics is difficult in the developing countries where the human trypanosomiases are endemic. West African (*gambiense*) trypanosomiasis and East African (*rhodesiense*) trypanosomiasis are epidemiologically distinct diseases. The general geographic distributions of these two illnesses are presented in Figure 277-1 of the previous chapter, and foci where transmission is known to occur are distributed throughout the indicated areas. Distinguishing epidemiologic and clinical features of the two diseases are presented in Table 278-1.

WEST AFRICAN TRYPANOSOMIASIS

West African trypanosomiasis is caused by *T. b. gambiense,* which is transmitted primarily by tsetse flies belonging to the *palpalis* group: *Glossina palpalis, Glossina tachinoides,* and *Glossina fuscipes.* These vectors inhabit forests and wooded areas along rivers, where conditions of temperature, moisture, and darkness favorable for them are combined with the availability of mammalian blood. This distribution of the vectors restricts the occurrence of human infection to the tropical rain forests of Central and West Africa. Despite the facts that these tsetse flies adapt to feeding on a variety of mammals and *T. b. gambiense* has been found in several wild animal species, infected humans likely constitute the only epidemiologically important reservoir of this subspecies.[25] The primary determinant of the risk of acquiring the infection is the frequency of contact with the vector. This risk increases during the dry season, when the density of both vectors and humans increases around limited numbers of water holes. Because of this pattern of transmission, West African trypanosomiasis is primarily a problem in rural populations, and tourists rarely become infected with *T. b. gambiense.* The course of the illness caused by *T. b. gambiense* is less severe than that caused by *T. b. rhodesiense,* although both forms eventually lead to death if not treated. In fact, many persons infected with *T. b. gambiense* are asymptomatic for long periods and continue to have contact with the vectors. This may be an important element in the persistence of the infection in the reservoir between epidemics.

EAST AFRICAN TRYPANOSOMIASIS

The etiologic agent of East African trypanosomiasis is *T. b. rhodesiense.* This subspecies is transmitted by tsetse flies of the *morsitans* group, principally *Glossina morsitans, Glossina pallidipes,* and *Glossina swynnertoni.* These vectors are widely distributed in savanna and woodland areas of Central and East Africa. Wild animals are the reservoir of this organism, principally antelope such as the bushbuck and hartebeest. These animals are trypanotolerant and generally do not suffer signifi-

TABLE 278-1	Comparisons of West African and East African Trypanosomiasis	
	West African (gambiense)	*East African* (rhodesiense)
Organism	*Trypanosoma brucei gambiense*	*Trypanosoma brucei rhodesiense*
Vectors	Tsetse flies (*palpalis* group)	Tsetse flies (*morsitans* group)
Primary reservoir	Humans	Antelope and cattle
Human illness	Chronic (late CNS disease)	Acute (early CNS disease)
Duration of illness	Months to years	<9 months
Lymphadenopathy	Prominent	Minimal
Parasitemia	Low	High
Diagnosis by rodent inoculation	No	Yes
Epidemiology	Rural populations	Tourists in game parks; workers in wild areas; rural populations

cant morbidity unless weakened by other illnesses. Cattle are the only domestic animals that can serve as a reservoir of *T. b. rhodesiense,* and infection with the parasite usually causes death if left untreated. Many other wild and domestic animals can be infected with this parasite, but their importance as reservoirs is minimal either because parasitemias are low or because they succumb quickly to the infection. The presence of the reservoir of *T. b. rhodesiense* and other trypanosome species in wild game in vast areas of Africa makes opening these lands for livestock difficult. Humans become infected with *T. b. rhodesiense* only incidentally, because for the most part risk results from contact with tsetse flies that principally feed on wild animals. Thus, the illness is an occupational hazard for persons such as game wardens who work in areas where infected wild animals and vectors are present. In addition, sporadic cases of *T. b. rhodesiense* infection occur among non-African tourists who visit game parks in East Africa.

The natural cycle of the African trypanosomes does not exist outside Africa, and human African trypanosomiasis in the United States and other nonendemic countries is limited to occasional imported cases, most of which are caused by *T. b. rhodesiense.*[26-28] During the past 25 years, roughly two dozen cases of imported African trypanosomiasis have been reported to the Centers for Disease Control and Prevention. Most of these cases were caused by *T. b. rhodesiense,* and several patients had CNS involvement. Despite the serious nature of the infection, all the patients were treated effectively.

Clinical Course

WEST AFRICAN TRYPANOSOMIASIS

An indurated, painful trypanosomal chancre may develop at the site where parasites were inoculated by an infected tsetse fly. This lesion usually appears 1 to 2 weeks after the bite of the infected fly and resolves spontaneously over several weeks. The chancre may ulcerate and reach a diameter of several centimeters; regional lymphadenopathy may also develop. However, the trypanosomal chancre is seldom seen in clinical practice. Thus, most patients develop systemic trypanosomiasis without experiencing the symptoms of localized disease.

The development of stage I (hemolymphatic) disease with dissemination of the parasites is marked by fever, which may appear weeks or months after the acquisition of the infection. The fever is characterized by intermittent bouts of high temperatures lasting for several days, and extended periods may intervene during which the patient is afebrile. As the chronic illness evolves, a wide variety of other signs and symptoms develop. Lymphadenopathy is a fairly constant feature of *gambiense* trypanosomiasis. The nodes are typically discrete, movable, rubbery, and nontender. With time they frequently become indurated as fibrosis develops. Supraclavicular and cervical nodes are often visibly discernible, and enlargement of the nodes of the posterior cervical triangle, or Winterbottom's sign, is a classic finding in persons infected with *T. b. gambiense.* Hepatosplenomegaly may be present as well.

Transient edema is a frequent sign during the hemolymphatic phase of the illness and can occur in the face as well as in the hands, feet, and other periarticular areas. Pruritus is common, and an irregular circinate rash is often present. The rash is typically located on the trunk, shoulders, buttocks, and thighs and consists of erythematous areas 5 to 10 cm in diameter with clear centers.[29] Other inconstant findings include malaise, headache, weakness, weight loss, arthralgias, and tachycardia. Amenorrhea and infertility in women as well as a loss of libido and impotence in men as a consequence of neuroendocrine dysfunction have been documented.[30,31]

Stage II (meningoencephalitic) disease is characterized by the insidious development of protean neurologic manifestations, accompanied by progressive alterations in the composition of the CSF.[17] In gambiense trypanosomiasis, CNS findings may develop months or even years after the initiation of the infection. Irritability, personality change, and loss of the ability to concentrate may develop before changes in the CSF become evident, and this underscores the some-

what arbitrary nature of the distinction between the hemolymphatic and CNS stages of the illness. A picture of progressive indifference develops, associated with daytime somnolence, sometimes alternating with restlessness and insomnia at night. Severe headache is common. The frequency and progressive nature of the somnolence result in the use of the term *sleeping sickness.* A listless gaze reflects a loss of spontaneity, and speech may become indistinct. Extrapyramidal signs often develop and may include choreiform movements of the trunk, neck, and extremities, tremors of the tongue and fingers, and fasciculations of a variety of muscle groups. Ataxia is a frequent sign, and the patient may appear to have Parkinson's disease, as a shuffling gait, hypertonia, tremors, and slurred speech develop. The final phase of the CNS disease is one of progressive neurologic impairment ending in coma and death.

Trypanosomiasis in children, which is relatively uncommon because they have less exposure to the vectors, does not differ greatly from the clinical illness seen in adults. However, the illness tends to run a more acute course, and the distinction between the hemolymphatic and CNS stages may be difficult to make.[32] Moreover, due to the protean nature of the symptoms and the lack of pathognomonic signs, the diagnosis is often missed in the early stages of the infection and is made only after neurologic impairment has developed.[33]

EAST AFRICAN TRYPANOSOMIASIS

The most striking general difference between West African and East African trypanosomiases is that the latter illness tends to follow a more acute course, presumably reflecting a relatively less effective adaptation of *T. b. rhodesiense* to humans.[34,35] The onset of symptoms usually occurs a few days after the patient has been bitten by an infected tsetse fly, but the incubation period may be as long as several weeks. Typically in tourists, systemic signs of infection such as fever, malaise, and headache appear before the end of the trip or shortly after their return home. As the illness progresses, the pattern of intermittent fever develops, and rash is a nearly constant feature of the early weeks of the illness. Lymph node swelling is not prominent in *rhodesiense* trypanosomiasis, and thus Winterbottom's sign is generally absent. Persistent tachycardia unrelated to the fevers is frequently present early in the course of the illness, and in some patients death may result from arrhythmias and congestive heart failure due to pancarditis even before CNS disease develops. In general, untreated rhodesiense trypanosomiasis usually leads to death in a matter of weeks to months, without a clear distinction between the hemolymphatic and CNS stages.

Diagnosis

Epidemiologic information and clinical findings often combine to suggest the diagnosis of African trypanosomiasis, and a high index of suspicion should be maintained with persons who have been in endemic areas. However, there are numerous other illnesses common in the tropics that cause symptoms similar to those seen in both the early and the late stages of sleeping sickness, and a definitive diagnosis of African trypanosomiasis requires demonstration of the parasite.[11,36,37]

If a chancre is present, fluid should be expressed and examined directly under light microscopy for the highly motile trypanosomes. Part of the specimen should be fixed and stained with Giemsa. Aspiration of soft lymph nodes early in the course of the infection can also be used to demonstrate the presence of parasites. This method is more effective in patients with West African trypanosomiasis because of the prominence of lymphadenopathy, but even in such patients, multiple aspirates are sometimes necessary before parasites are found. An enlarged node should be punctured and kneaded gently during aspiration, and the sample obtained should be examined directly and also after staining.

Examination of wet preparations and Giemsa-stained thin and thick smears of peripheral blood is also a sensitive method for detection of infection with African trypanosomes (see Fig. 278-1). This approach is more likely to be successful in the hemolymphatic stage of the illness, and it is much more useful in patients infected with *T. b. rhodesiense* because of the relatively high parasitemias. Because parasitemias may vary considerably from one day to the next, serial specimens should be examined. If parasites are not seen in blood from a patient whose history and clinical findings point to African trypanosomiasis as a possible diagnosis, efforts should be made to concentrate the organisms. This can be done by examining the buffy coat obtained by centrifuging 10 to 15 mL of anticoagulated blood microscopically as a wet preparation and after Giemsa staining. Miniature anion exchange columns, which retain blood cells but not trypanosomes, also can be useful in detecting parasites,[38,39] and PCR-based assays may be useful in some situations.[40-42]

Examination of the CSF is mandatory in all patients suspected of having African trypanosomiasis.[11] An increase in the CSF cell count is the first abnormality to be detected. Increased opening pressure of the fluid develops later, as do an elevated IgM level and total protein concentration. Examination of CSF processed by single or double centrifugation methods often reveals trypanosomes in patients with CNS involvement.[43,44] Any CSF abnormality in a patient in whom trypanosomes have been found in specimens from other sites must be viewed as indicative of CNS involvement, and this has implications for treatment that are discussed later. CSF cell counts and IgM levels may remain elevated for long periods after curative therapy.

An additional approach to patients in whom parasites cannot be demonstrated by the previously described methods is bone marrow aspiration. Trypanosomes may be found by careful examination of Giemsa-stained specimens. Moreover, material aspirated from the bone marrow can be inoculated into special liquid culture medium, as can blood, CSF, or lymph node aspirates obtained from the patient in whom trypanosomiasis is suspected.[45] Several serologic assays are available to aid in the diagnosis of African trypanosomiasis, but the variable sensitivity and specificity of these tests mandate that treatment decisions still be based on demonstration of the parasite. Nonetheless, these assays are useful in epidemiologic surveys. Detection of elevated serum IgM levels was used for many years as a screening procedure. Simple agglutination tests for trypanosomes performed on cards (CATT)[11,36,46] are available commercially and are easy to use under field conditions. These card assays are useful for screening populations at risk, after which parasitologic studies can be done on persons having positive results.

Treatment

Suramin, pentamidine, and organic arsenicals have been the mainstay for treating African trypanosomiasis for more than 50 years.[47] Eflornithine, which is effective in both the hemolymphatic and the CNS stages of West African trypanosomiasis, was added to the group in 1990. Therapy of gambiense and rhodesiense trypanosomiases must be individualized based on the absence or presence of CNS disease, side effects, and occasionally drug resistance of the infecting organisms. Suramin and pentamidine do not penetrate the CNS adequately. Thus, eflornithine can be used in patients with gambiense trypanosomiasis who have CNS disease, but because the response of *T. b. rhodesiense* to this drug has been variable,[48] patients with stage II rhodesiense trypanosomiasis must be treated with the arsenical melarsoprol, which is highly toxic (Table 278-2).[49] In the United States these drugs can be obtained from the Drug Service of the Centers for Disease Control and Prevention in Atlanta, Georgia. Currently recommended treatment protocols are summarized in a recent publication.[50]

Patients with the hemolymphatic stage of gambiense trypanosomiasis and normal CSF (stage I disease) should be treated with pentamidine isoethionate (Lomidine).[51] The dosage for both adults and children is 4 mg/kg, up to 300 mg/day, intravenously (IV) or intramuscularly (IM) for 10 days. Intramuscular injections of pentamidine are painful and may cause sterile abscesses. Immediate side effects of pentamidine can include nausea, vomiting, hypotension, and

TABLE 278-2	Drugs Recommended for Treatment of the African Trypanosomiases	
	Clinical Stage	
Causative Agent	**I**	**II**
Trypanosoma brucei gambiense	Pentamidine	Eflornithine
	Alt: Suramin	Alt: Melarsoprol
Trypanosoma brucei rhodesiense	Suramin	Melarsoprol

tachycardia. These reactions are generally transient and do not warrant discontinuation of therapy. Other side effects include nephrotoxicity, elevation of hepatic transaminases, neutropenia, rashes, and hypoglycemia.

Eflornithine (difluoromethylornithine [DFMO], Ornidyl) is highly effective in both the hemolymphatic and the CNS stages of gambiense trypanosomiasis.[52,53] This drug produces a dramatic reduction of symptoms and rapid clearing of parasites from blood and CSF. For adults the recommended dosage is 400 mg/kg per day IV in four divided doses for 14 days, and for children it is 500 to 600 mg/kg per day on the same schedule. Anemia, leukopenia, and thrombocytopenia are frequent in patients treated with eflornithine, but generally they are not clinically significant. Seizures and hearing loss have been reported rarely. Major disadvantages of eflornithine are the requirement that it be given intravenously, the amount of drug that must be given, and the duration of therapy. These factors, combined with the variable drug availability, make widespread use difficult, leaving pentamidine as the better choice for stage I gambiense disease. For patients with gambiense disease and CNS involvement, eflornithine is the drug of choice. It is as effective as melarsoprol but has far fewer side effects. The extent to which HIV coinfection affects the course of African trypanosomiasis and the efficacy of treatment is not clear and merits further investigation.[49,54]

Suramin (Bayer 205, Naphuride, Antrypol) is the first-choice drug for stage I rhodesiense trypanosomiasis. A 100- to 200-mg test dose is recommended, although anaphylactic reactions are rare. The treatment regimen for both adults and children, beginning 24 hours after the test dose, is 5 mg/kg on day 1, 10 mg/kg on day 3, and 20 mg/kg on days 5, 11, 17, 23, and 30. The exact spacing of the doses most likely is not important because suramin has a long half-life. The drug is administered by slow intravenous infusion of a freshly prepared 10% aqueous solution. Suramin causes a number of side effects and must be administered under the close supervision of a physician. Approximately 1 patient in 20,000 has an immediate, severe, and potentially fatal reaction to the drug consisting of nausea, vomiting, seizures, and shock. A number of less severe reactions can also occur, including fever, pruritus, photophobia, arthralgias, and skin eruptions. The most important side effect of suramin is renal damage. Transient proteinuria is often seen during treatment. Urinalysis should be done before giving each dose, and if proteinuria increases or casts and red cells appear in the urine sediment, the drug should be discontinued. Suramin should not be used in patients with renal insufficiency.

The drug of choice for rhodesiense trypanosomiasis with CNS involvement is the arsenical melarsoprol (mel B, Arsobal).[27,49,52,55] Melarsoprol cures both stages of the disease. Thus, it is also indicated for treatment of the hemolymphatic stage in patients in whom suramin or pentamidine has failed or could not be tolerated. However, it should never be the first choice for therapy of stage I trypanosomiasis because of its relatively high toxicity. In adults the drug is given in three courses of 3 days each. The recommended dosage is 2-3.6 mg/kg per day intravenously in three divided doses for 3 days, followed 1 week later by 3.6 mg/kg per day, also in three divided doses for 3 days. This latter course is then repeated 10 to 21 days later. In debilitated patients, treatment with suramin for 2 to 4 days before starting melarsoprol therapy and an 18-mg initial dose of the latter drug, followed by progressive drug increases, have been recommended. For pediatric patients, 18 to 25 mg/kg total should be given over 1 month. An initial dose of 0.36 mg/kg intravenously should be increased gradually to a maximum of 3.6 mg/kg at 1- to 5-day intervals for a total of 9 to 10 doses.

Melarsoprol is a highly toxic drug and should be administered with great care. The most important side effects involve the CNS. A substantial percentage of patients treated with melarsoprol develop reactive encephalopathy. The risk of this immune-mediated phenomenon and its associated mortality is reduced significantly by concomitant administration of prednisolone. Thus, all patients treated with melarsoprol should be given prednisolone at a dose of 1 mg/kg up to 40 mg per day, starting a day or two before initiation of melarsoprol therapy, continued through the period of treatment, and then tapered over several days.[56] Clinical indications of reactive encephalopathy include high fever, headache, tremor, impaired speech, seizures, and finally coma and death. Melarsoprol should be discontinued at the first sign of encephalopathy. It may be restarted cautiously with small doses a few days after the signs have resolved.

A number of other side effects are associated with melarsoprol therapy. Extravasation of the drug results in intense local reactions and, as with administration of other heavy metals, abdominal pain and vomiting are commonly observed. Jarisch-Herxheimer–type reactions have been reported, as have nephrotoxicity, abnormal liver function tests, and myocardial damage.

If a patient with gambiense CNS disease cannot tolerate eflornithine, or if the latter is not available, melarsoprol should be given at a dose of 2.2 mg/kg per day IV for 10 days. This compressed regimen for stage II gambiense disease has been shown in a randomized trial to be equally effective and no more toxic than the traditional regimen outlined previously.[57] Combination therapy for stage II disease with nifurtimox added to either eflornithine or melarsoprol has shown promise in early studies, and further trials of this approach are underway.[58-61]

Prevention

The trypanosomiases constitute complex public health and epizootic problems in many developing countries in Africa. Control programs that focus on eradication of vectors and drug treatment of infected humans and animals have been in operation in some regions for decades. Considerable progress has been made in a number of areas, but the lack of a consensus on the best approach to solving the overall problem of African trypanosomiasis, a paucity of resources, and political unrest stand in the way of effective control.[23,62] Individuals can reduce their risk of acquiring infections with trypanosomes by avoiding areas known to harbor infected insects, by wearing clothing that reduces the biting of the flies, and by using insect repellent. Chemoprophylaxis is not recommended because of the high toxicity of the drugs that are active against African trypanosomes, and no vaccine is available to prevent transmission of the parasites.

REFERENCES

1. Hoare CA. *The Trypanosomes of Mammals: A Zoological Monograph*. Oxford: Blackwell; 1972.
2. Hoare CA, Wallace FG. Developmental stages of trypanosomatid flagellates: a new terminology. *Nature*. 1966;212:1385-1386.
3. Aksoy S. Control of tsetse flies and trypanosomes using molecular genetics. *Vet Parasitol*. 2003;115:125-145.
4. Roditi I, Lehane MJ. Interactions between trypanosomes and tsetse flies. *Curr Opin Microbiol*. 2008;11:345-351.
5. Horn D. The molecular control of antigenic variation in *Trypanosoma brucei*. *Curr Mol Med*. 2004;4:563-576.
6. Pays E. Regulation of antigen gene expression in *Trypanosoma brucei*. *Trends Parasitol*. 2005;21:517-520.
7. Taylor JE, Rudenko G. Switching trypanosome coats: what's in the wardrobe? *Trends Genet*. 2006;22:614-620.
8. Mbala L, Matendo R, Kinkela T, et al. Congenital African trypanosomiasis in a newborn child with current neurologic symptomatology. *Trop Doct*. 1996;26:186-187.
9. Herwaldt BL. Protozoa and helminths. In: Fleming DO, Hunt DL, eds. *Biological Safety: Principles and Practice*. 4th ed. Washington, DC: American Society for Microbiology; 2006:115-161.
10. Poltera AA. Pathology of human African trypanosomiasis with reference to experimental African trypanosomiasis and infections of the central nervous system. *Br Med Bull*. 1985;41:169-174.
11. Kennedy PG. Diagnostic and neuropathogenesis issues in human African trypanosomiasis. *Int J Parasitol*. 2006;36:505-512.
12. Kennedy PG. Cytokines in central nervous system trypanosomiasis: cause, effect or both? *Trans R Soc Trop Med Hyg*. 2009;103:213-214.
13. Wery M, Mulumba PM, Lambert PH, et al. Hematologic manifestations, diagnosis, and immunopathology of African trypanosomiasis. *Semin Hematol*. 1982;19:83-92.
14. Poltera AA, Cox JN, Owor R. Pancarditis involving the conducting system and all valves in human African trypanosomiasis. *Br Heart J*. 1976;38:827-837.
15. Blum JA, Schmid C, Burri C, et al. Cardiac alterations in human African trypanosomiasis (*T.b. gambiense*) with respect to the disease stage and antiparasitic treatment. *PLoS Negl Trop Dis*. 2009;3:e383.
16. Poltera AA, Owor R, Cox JN. Pathological aspects of human African trypanosomiasis (HAT) in Uganda. A post-mortem survey of fourteen cases. *Virchows Arch Pathol Histol*. 1977;373:249-265.
17. Blum J, Schmid C, Burri C. Clinical aspects of 2541 patients with second stage human African trypanosomiasis. *Acta Trop*. 2006;97:55-64.
18. Jordan AM. *Trypanosomiasis Control and African Rural Development*. London: Longmans; 1986.
19. Hide G, Tait A, Maudlin I, et al. The origins, dynamics and generation of *Trypanosoma brucei rhodesiense* epidemics in East Africa. *Parasitol Today*. 1996;12:50-55.
20. Kennedy PG. The continuing problem of human African trypanosomiasis (sleeping sickness). *Ann Neurol*. 2008;64:116-126.
21. Lutumba P, Makieya E, Haw A, et al. Human African trypanosomiasis in a rural community, Democratic Republic of Congo. *Emerg Infect Dis*. 2007;13:248-254.
22. Fevre EM, Odiit M, Coleman PG, et al. Estimating the burden of *rhodesiense* sleeping sickness during an outbreak in Serere, eastern Uganda. *BMC Public Health*. 2008;8:96.
23. Simarro PP, Jannin J, Cattand P. Eliminating human African trypanosomiasis: where do we stand and what comes next? *PLoS Med*. 2008;5:e55.
24. Human African trypanosomiasis. World Health Organization. 3-10-2009.
25. Brun R, Balmer O. New developments in human African trypanosomiasis. *Curr Opin Infect Dis*. 2006;19:415-420.
26. Jelinek T, Bisoffi Z, Bonazzi L, et al. Cluster of African trypanosomiasis in travelers to Tanzanian national parks. *Emerging Infect Dis*. 2002;8:634-635.
27. Kumar N, Orenstein R, Uslan DZ, et al. Melarsoprol-associated multifocal inflammatory CNS illness in African trypanosomiasis. *Neurology*. 2006;66:1120-1121.
28. Darby JD, Huber MG, Sieling WL, et al. African trypanosomiasis in two short-term Australian travelers to Malawi. *J Travel Med*. 2008;15:375-377.
29. McGovern TW, Williams W, Fitzpatrick JE, et al. Cutaneous manifestations of African trypanosomiasis. *Arch Dermatol*. 1995;131:1178-1182.
30. Reincke M, Arlt W, Heppner C, et al. Neuroendocrine dysfunction in African trypanosomiasis. The role of cytokines. *Ann NY Acad Sci*. 1998;840:809-821.
31. Blum JA, Schmid C, Hatz C, et al. Sleeping glands? The role of endocrine disorders in sleeping sickness (*T.b. gambiense* human African trypanosomiasis). *Acta Trop*. 2007;104:16-24.
32. Buyst H. Sleeping sickness in children. *Ann Soc Belge Med Trop*. 1977;57:201-212.
33. Koko J, Dufillot D, Gahouma D, et al. Human African trypanosomiasis in children. A pediatrics service experience in Libreville, Gabon [French]. *Bull Soc Pathol Exot*. 1997;90:14-18.
34. Gear JHS, Miller B. The clinical manifestations of *rhodesiense* trypanosomiasis: An account of cases contracted in the Okavango swamps of Botswana. *Am J Trop Med Hyg*. 1986;35:1146-1152.
35. Odiit M, Kansiime F, Enyaru JC. Duration of symptoms and case fatality of sleeping sickness caused by *Trypanosoma brucei rhodesiense* in Tororo, Uganda. *East Afr Med J*. 1997;74:792-795.
36. Chappuis F, Loutan L, Simarro P, et al. Options for field diagnosis of human african trypanosomiasis. *Clin Microbiol Rev*. 2005;18:133-146.
37. Lutumba P, Meheus F, Robays J, et al. Cost-effectiveness of algorithms for confirmation test of human African trypanosomiasis. *Emerg Infect Dis*. 2007;13:1484-1490.
38. Truc P, Jamonneau V, N'Guessan P, et al. Parasitological diagnosis of human African trypanosomiasis: a comparison of the QBC and miniature anion-exchange centrifugation techniques. *Trans R Soc Trop Med Hyg*. 1998;92:288-289.
39. Chappuis F, Pittet A, Bovier PA, et al. Field evaluation of the CATT/*Trypanosoma brucei gambiense* on blood-impregnated filter papers for diagnosis of human African trypanosomiasis in southern Sudan. *Trop Med Int Health*. 2002;7:942-948.
40. Penchenier L, Simo G, Grebaut P, et al. Diagnosis of human trypanosomiasis, due to *Trypanosoma brucei gambiense* in central Africa, by the polymerase chain reaction. *Trans R Soc Trop Med Hyg*. 2000;94:392-394.
41. Jamonneau V, Solano P, Cuny G. [Use of molecular biology in the diagnosis of human African trypanosomiasis]. *Med Trop (Mars)*. 2001;61:347-354.
42. Jamonneau V, Solano P, Garcia A, et al. Stage determination and therapeutic decision in human African trypanosomiasis: value of polymerase chain reaction and immunoglobulin M quantification on the cerebrospinal fluid of sleeping sickness patients in Cote d'Ivoire. *Trop Med Int Health*. 2003;8:589-594.
43. Cattand P, Miezan BT, deRaadt P. Human African trypanosomiasis: use of double centrifugation of cerebrospinal fluid to detect trypanosomes. *Bull WHO*. 1988;66:83-86.
44. Miezan TW, Meda HA, Doua F, et al. Single centrifugation of cerebrospinal fluid in a sealed pasteur pipette for simple, rapid and sensitive detection of trypanosomes. *Trans R Soc Trop Med Hyg*. 2000;94:293.
45. Truc P, Aerts D, McNamara JJ, et al. Direct isolation *in vitro* of *Trypanosoma brucei* from man and other animals, and its potential value for the diganosis of gambian trypanosomiasis. *Trans R Soc Trop Med Hyg*. 1992;86:627-629.
46. Truc P, Lejon V, Magnus E, et al. Evaluation of the micro-CATT, CATT/*Trypanosoma brucei gambiense*, and LATEX/*T b gambiense* methods for serodiagnosis and surveillance of human African trypanosomiasis in West and Central Africa. *Bull WHO*. 2002;80:882-886.
47. Jannin J, Cattand P. Treatment and control of human African trypanosomiasis. *Curr Opin Infect Dis*. 2004;17:565-571.
48. Iten M, Mett H, Evans A, et al. Alterations in ornithine decarboxylase characteristics account for tolerance of *Trypanosoma brucei rhodesiense* to D,L-alpha-difluoromethylornithine. *Antimicrob Agents Chemother*. 1997;41:1922-1925.
49. Blum J, Nkunku S, Burri C. Clinical description of encephalopathic syndromes and risk factors for their occurrence and outcome during melarsoprol treatment of human African trypanosomiasis. *Trop Med Int Health*. 2001;6:390-400.
50. Anonymous. Drugs for parasitic infections. *Med Lett Drugs Ther*. 2007;(Suppl):1-15.
51. Doua F, Miezan TW, Sanon Singaro JR, et al. The efficacy of pentamidine in the treatment of early-late stage *Trypanosoma brucei gamnbiense* trypanosomiasis. *Am J Trop Med Hyg*. 1997;55:586-588.
52. Balasegaram M, Young H, Chappuis F, et al. Effectiveness of melarsoprol and eflornithine as first-line regimens for gambiense sleeping sickness in nine Medecins Sans Frontieres programmes. *Trans R Soc Trop Med Hyg*. 2009;103:280-290.
53. Priotto G, Pinoges L, Fursa IB, et al. Safety and effectiveness of first line eflornithine for *Trypanosoma brucei gambiense* sleeping sickness in Sudan: cohort study. *BMJ*. 2008;336:705-708.
54. Karp CL, Auwaerter PG. Coinfection with HIV and tropical infectious diseases. I. Protozoal pathogens. *Clin Infect Dis*. 2007;45:1208-1213.
55. Pepin J, Milord F, Khonde AN, et al. Risk factors for encephalopathy and mortality during melarsoprol treatment of *Trypanosoma brucei gambiense* sleeping sickness. *Trans R Soc Trop Med Hyg*. 1995;89:92-97.

56. Pepin J, Milord F, Guern C, et al. Trial of prednisolone for prevention of melarsoprol-induced encephalopathy in *gambiense* sleeping sickness. [Comment]. *Lancet.* 1989;1:1246-1250.

57. Burri C, Nkunku S, Merolle A, et al. Efficacy of new, concise schedule for melarsoprol in treatment of sleeping sickness caused by *Trypanosoma brucei gambiense*: a randomised trial. *Lancet.* 2000;355:1419-1425.

58. Bisser S, N'Siesi FX, Lejon V, et al. Equivalence trial of melarsoprol and nifurtimox monotherapy and combination therapy for the treatment of second-stage *Trypanosoma brucei gambiense* sleeping sickness. *J Infect Dis.* 2007;195:322-329.

59. Checchi F, Piola P, Ayikoru H, et al. Nifurtimox plus eflornithine for late-stage sleeping sickness in Uganda: A case series. *PLoS Negl Trop Dis.* 2007;1:e64.

60. Priotto G, Kasparian S, Ngouama D, et al. Nifurtimox-eflornithine combination therapy for second-stage *Trypanosoma brucei gambiense* sleeping sickness: a randomized clinical trial in Congo. *Clin Infect Dis.* 2007;45:1435-1442.

61. Croft SL. Kinetoplastida: new therapeutic strategies. *Parasite.* 2008;15:522-527.

62. Fevre EM, Picozzi K, Jannin J, et al. Human African trypanosomiasis: epidemiology and control. *Adv Parasitol* 2006;61:167-221.

279

Toxoplasma gondii

JOSÉ G. MONTOYA | JOHN C. BOOTHROYD | JOSEPH A. KOVACS

Although *Toxoplasma gondii* infects a large proportion of the world's human populations, it is an uncommon cause of disease. Certain individuals, however, are at high risk of severe or life-threatening disease due to this parasite. These include congenitally infected fetuses and newborns and immunologically impaired individuals. Congenital toxoplasmosis is the result of maternal infection acquired during gestation, an infection that is most often clinically inapparent. In immunodeficient patients, toxoplasmosis most often occurs in persons with defects in T cell–mediated immunity such as those receiving corticosteroids, anti–tumor necrosis factor (TNF) therapies, or cytotoxic drugs and those with hematologic malignancies, organ transplants, or acquired immunodeficiency syndrome (AIDS). In the vast majority of otherwise immunocompetent individuals, primary or chronic (latent) infection with *T. gondii* is asymptomatic; after the acute infection, a small percentage has chorioretinitis, lymphadenitis, or, even more rarely, myocarditis and polymyositis.[1]

T. gondii was first observed in the North African rodent (*Ctenodactylus gundi*) by Nicolle and Manceaux in 1908[2] and was recognized as a cause of human disease in an 11-month-old congenitally infected child by Janku in 1923.[3] It was reported as a cause of encephalitis by Wolf and colleagues,[4] who in 1939 observed it in a newborn who presented with seizures, intracranial calcifications, hydrocephalus, and chorioretinitis. Although relatively few cases of severe toxoplasmosis in adults were reported during the ensuing years, the remarkable report in 1968 by Vietzke and colleagues[5] from the National Cancer Institute of the National Institutes of Health highlighted *T. gondii* as a cause of life-threatening infection in patients with malignancy, predominantly in those with hematologic malignancies. Brain involvement with focal areas of encephalitis was the primary finding at autopsy in these patients. Since that time, several hundred cases in non-AIDS immunodeficient patients have been recorded in the literature.[6] In 1983, the first report of toxoplasmosis in AIDS patients appeared.[7] Toxoplasmic encephalitis (TE) subsequently was recognized as the major cause of space-occupying lesions in the brains of these patients, almost all of whom had serologic evidence of previous exposure to the parasite.[7] Despite the significant advances that have been achieved in the recent past, major challenges remain in the areas of prevention and management of the acute infection in pregnancy, the fetus, and the newborn[8] and in the understanding and treatment of toxoplasmic chorioretinitis[9] and infection in immunocompromised individuals.[1,6]

Etiology

T. gondii is a coccidian parasite of felids with humans and other warm-blooded animals serving as intermediate hosts. It belongs to the subphylum Apicomplexa, class Sporozoa and exists in nature in many forms: macro- and microgametes, the oocyst (which releases sporozoites), the tissue cyst (which contains and may release bradyzoites), and the tachyzoite (Fig. 279-1).[10]

Population genetic analysis has demonstrated that, at least within Europe and North America, most organisms isolated from both animals and humans can be grouped into one of three clonal genotypes (types I to III), which may identify clinically relevant biologic differences.[11] Clear differences have been observed in the frequency of parasite genotypes when *T. gondii* isolates from animals were compared with those of humans. Type III strains are common in animals but observed significantly less often in cases of human toxoplasmosis; most

cases in humans are caused by type II strains. Type II strains are significantly more often associated with reactivation of chronic infections and account for 65% of strains isolated from AIDS patients.[12] Both type I and II strains have been associated with human congenital toxoplasmosis.[12-14] Types II and III have to date not been detected in immunocompetent individuals with severe ocular disease.[15] Atypical and recombinant strains have been identified with increasing frequency in regions other than the United States and Europe and from animals other than humans and domestic animals; some of these strains appear to be associated with more severe disease, suggesting greater virulence, even in immunocompetent individuals.[16,17]

OOCYST

Cats eventually shed oocysts after they ingest any of the three forms of the parasite, at which time an enteroepithelial cycle begins. This sexual form of reproduction begins when the parasites penetrate the epithelial cells of the small intestine and initiate development of asexual and sexual (gametogony) forms of the parasite. Oocyst wall formation begins around the fertilized gamete, and when still immature, oocysts are discharged into the intestinal lumen by rupture of intestinal epithelial cells.[10] Unsporulated oocysts are subspherical to spherical and measure $10 \times 12 \, \mu m$ in diameter (Fig. 279-1A). Oocysts are formed in the small intestine only in felids and are excreted in the feces for periods varying from 7 to 20 days. As many as 10 million oocysts may be shed in the feces in a single day.[10] Sporulation, required for oocysts to become infectious, occurs outside the cat within 1 to 5 days, depending on temperature and the availability of oxygen. Sporulated oocysts contain two sporocysts (see Fig. 279-1A), each of which contains four sporozoites. Maturation is more rapid at warm temperatures (2 to 3 days at $24°C$ compared with 14 to 21 days at $11°C$).[10] Oocysts may remain viable for as long as 18 months in moist soil; this results in an environmental reservoir from which incidental hosts may be infected.

TACHYZOITE

The tachyzoite form (see Fig. 279-1B) is oval to crescentic in shape and measures 2 to 3 µm wide and 5 to 7 µm long; it requires an intracellular habitat to multiply despite having all the usual eukaryotic machinery necessary for reproduction. Tachyzoites are seen in both primary and reactivated infection; their presence is the hallmark of active infection. They reside and multiply within vacuoles in their host's cells, can infect virtually all phagocytic and nonphagocytic cell types,[10] and multiply approximately every 6 to 8 hours to form rosettes.[18] Continuous multiplication leads to cell disruption and release of organisms that go on to invade contiguous cells or are transported to other areas of the body by blood and lymph.[19] Tachyzoites appear to actively and rapidly migrate across epithelial cells and may travel to distant sites while extracellular.[20]

At the anterior end of the tachyzoite, there is a cone-shaped structure termed the *conoid*. It is protruded during the parasite's entry into host cells. *Rhoptries*, numbering four to eight, are club-shaped organelles that terminate within the conoid. The rhoptries, together with surrounding small, rod-shaped organelles (micronemes), have important secretory functions for parasitic invasion. *Dense granules* are organelles distributed throughout the cytoplasm. Their contents are released into a vacuole, termed the *parasitophorous vacuole*, that is

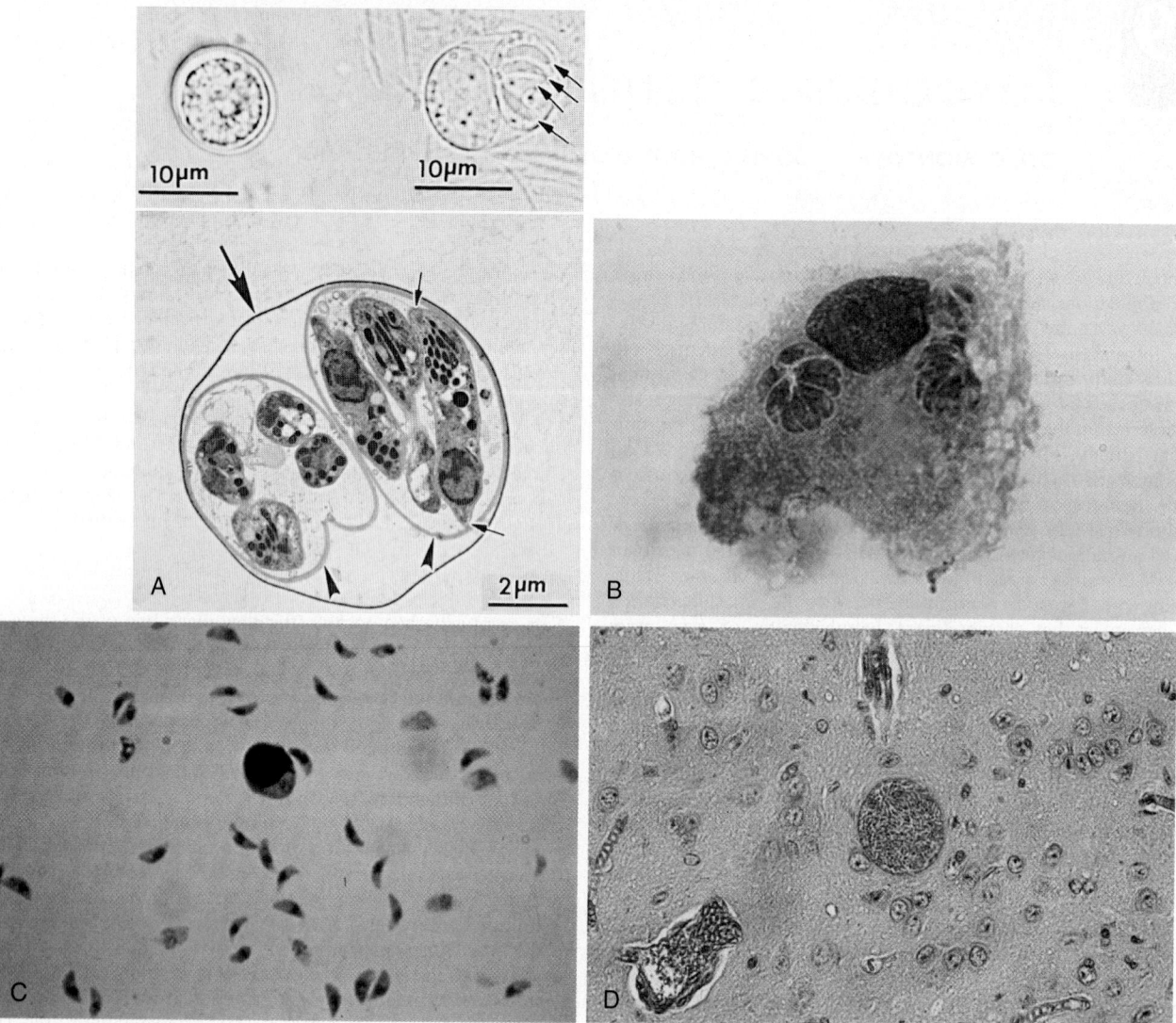

Figure 279-1 **The three forms of *Toxoplasma gondii* observed in nature. A,** Oocysts. Unsporulated oocyst (*top left*). Sporulated oocyst with two sporocysts (*top right*). Four sporozoites (*arrows*) are visible in one of the sporocysts. Transmission electron micrograph of a sporulated oocyst (*bottom*). Note the thin oocyst wall (*large arrow*), two sporocysts (*arrowheads*), and sporozoites, one of which is cut longitudinally (*small arrows*). (*Courtesy of Dr. J. P. Dubey, U.S. Department of Agriculture. Beltsville, MD.*) **B,** Giemsa stain demonstrating two rosettes of intracellular tachyzoites in a mouse bone marrow macrophage. **C,** Giemsa-stained smear of mouse peritoneal fluid demonstrating the tachyzoite form. **D,** Hematoxylin and eosin stain of the cyst form in the brain. (*B to D, Courtesy of Dr. Jack S. Remington, Stanford University and Palo Alto Medical Foundation.*)

formed around the parasite during entry into the cell and also into the external environment as excreted-secreted antigens.[10]

The rhoptries and micronemes produce a collection of proteins that are crucial for the invasion process.[21] These appear to mediate the attachment to the host cell including the moving junction, a ringlike point of contact between the parasite and host cell surface that migrates down the length of the parasite during invasion. The rhoptries also inject proteins into the host cell that are critical in manipulating the host cell, presumably to the advantage of the parasite.[22] These rhoptry proteins are very different (polymorphic) between different strains of *T. gondii* and seem to be responsible for many of the differences in virulence seen for types I, II, and III, as described previously.

Tachyzoites cannot survive desiccation, freezing and thawing, or extended exposure to gastric digestive juices.[23] They are propagated in the laboratory in the peritoneum of mice and in cultured cells. Tachyzoites can be visualized in sections stained with hematoxylin and eosin but are better visualized with Wright-Giemsa and immunoperoxidase stains.[24]

TISSUE CYST

Once the tachyzoite has invaded the target cell, it can undergo stage conversion into the bradyzoite form.[10] Tachyzoites and bradyzoites are structurally and phenotypically different. Tachyzoites multiply rapidly and synchronously, forming rosettes and lysing the cell, whereas the more slowly replicating bradyzoites form tissue cysts. Molecules are expressed in a stage-specific manner and are responsible for certain of the phenotypic differences between tachyzoites and bradyzoites. Interferon (IFN)-γ, nitric oxide (NO), heat shock proteins, pH, and temperature manipulations can trigger conversion of tachyzoites to bradyzoites in vitro and perhaps in vivo as well.[10]

Tissue cysts grow and remain within the host cell cytoplasm as the intracystic form wherein the bradyzoites continue to divide. Tissue cysts vary in size from younger ones that contain only a few bradyzoites to older tissue cysts that may contain several thousand bradyzoites and may reach more than 100 μm in size (see Fig. 279-1D). They appear spherical in the brain and conform to the shape of muscle fibers in heart and skeletal muscles. The central nervous system (CNS), eye, and skeletal, smooth, and heart muscles seem to be the most common sites of latent infection.[25] Because of their persistence in tissues, demonstration of tissue cysts in histologic sections does not necessarily mean that the infection was recently acquired or that it is clinically relevant. Tissue cysts stain well with periodic acid–Schiff, Wright-Giemsa, Gomori-methenamine silver, and immunoperoxidase stains. Tissue cysts in meat are rendered nonviable by γ-irradiation (0.4 kGy),[26] heating meat throughout to 67° C, or freezing to −20° C for 24 hours and then thawing,[27,28] but not by heating in a microwave.[29]

Although the tachyzoite form appears to be indiscriminate in the type of host cell parasitized, it has been suggested that in brain tissue, there is a predilection for tissue cyst formation to occur predominantly within neurons.[30,31] However, it has been shown that tissue cysts can form within astrocytes cultured in vitro.[32] In an electron microscopic study of the pathologic changes in brains of infected mice, tissue cysts were observed to remain intracellular throughout the period of study (22 months).[30] There is compelling evidence to suggest that bradyzoites can exit from intact tissue cysts and invade contiguous cells (where they convert to the tachyzoite form).[33] This is the likely explanation for the appearance of "daughter" cysts or clumps of cysts in the brain.

▣ Transmission and Epidemiology

T. gondii infection is a worldwide zoonosis. The organism infects herbivorous, omnivorous, and carnivorous animals, including birds.[34] Infection in humans most commonly occurs through the ingestion of raw or undercooked meat that contains tissue cysts, through the ingestion of water or food contaminated with oocysts, or congenitally through transplacental transmission from a mother who acquired her infection during gestation (Fig. 279-2). Less common are transmission by transplantation of an infected organ or transfusion of contaminated blood cells. Transmission has also occurred by accidental sticks[35] with contaminated needles or through exposing open lesions or mucosal surfaces to the parasite.[36] Coprophagous invertebrates, including cockroaches, filth flies, earthworms, snails, and slugs, may serve as transport hosts for oocysts to reach the gastrointestinal tract of animals or humans.

Because the sexual cycle of the parasite takes place in the small bowel of members of the cat family, cats play a significant role as powerful amplifiers of the infection in nature (see "Oocyst").[10] Epidemiologic surveys have revealed that in most areas of the world, the presence of cats is of primary importance for the transmission of the parasite. Excretion of oocysts has been reported to occur in approximately 1% of cats in diverse areas of the world.[36]

Although ingestion of raw or undercooked meat that contains viable *T. gondii* tissue cysts will result in infection, the relative frequency with which this occurs in relation to the frequency of infection due to ingestion of oocysts is unclear. For instance, in countries such as France, where eating undercooked meat is common and the prevalence of the infection is high, meat may be an important cause of the infection. (It was in Paris, France, that the meat-to-human hypothesis of the spread of *T. gondii* was proved.[37]) In contrast are countries such as those in Central America, where the prevalence of the infection in humans is high, but the ingestion of undercooked meat is uncommon.

Ingestion of tissue cysts in infected meat (primarily pork and lamb) is a major source of the infection in humans in the United States.[38] *T. gondii* infection is common in many animals used for food, especially sheep and pigs, with a lower prevalence in cattle, horses, and water buffaloes. Organisms may survive in tissue cysts in these animals for years and can be found in nearly all edible portions of an animal.[39] A seminal study on the prevalence of *T. gondii* in samples of meat used for human consumption (obtained from grocery stores) was performed in the United States in the 1960s.[40] The parasite was isolated from 32% of pork chops and 4% of lamb chops; there were no isolations from beef.[40] A recent polymerase chain reaction (PCR)–based study in England found 33% (19/57) of pork and 67% (6/9) of lamb samples positive for *T. gondii* DNA.[41]

Serologic surveys conducted in the past 20 years in the United States indicate that the prevalence of *T. gondii* in pigs is declining.[38] Seroprevalence in market weight pigs in North Carolina has been found to be as low as 0.58%.[42] This reduction in *T. gondii* prevalence has been attributed to changing management practices and consolidation of pig production into large-scale operations. However, although many pigs in the United States are raised in large-scale operations, there are still many isolated small swine farms and the prevalence of *T. gondii* in some of these pigs is high. Dubey and colleagues[38] reported that *T. gondii* was isolated from the tongue and hearts of 51 (92.7%) of 55 pigs destined for human consumption at a small farm in Massachusetts. Of note, meat for human consumption is not routinely inspected for *T. gondii* infection in the United States or elsewhere in the world.[38] Little is known about the prevalence of *T. gondii* infection in lambs. Although *T. gondii* infection of sheep is widely prevalent, the public health importance of this is unclear because in the United States, meat from adult sheep is not usually used for human consumption.[36] Reports of suspected transmission by unpasteurized goat's milk have appeared.[43,44] In addition to differences in how meat is cooked, the tendency for beef to harbor few if any cysts compared with lamb and pork may partly explain the differences in seroprevalence in the United States versus Europe; beef accounts for a much greater fraction of meat consumed in the United States compared with Europe, where lamb and pork are more popular.

T. gondii infection is also prevalent in game animals, especially black bears (80% infected) and white-tailed deer, as well as in raccoons (60% infected).[39] Infection in raccoons and bears is a good indicator of the prevalence of *T. gondii* in the environment because these animals are scavengers. Thus, wild animal meat can serve as a source of the infection for hunters and their families, especially when care is not taken while eviscerating and handling the game or when meat from these animals is served undercooked or uncooked.[39]

Although *T. gondii* tissue cysts may be found in edible tissues of chickens,[45] poultry products are probably not important in the transmission of *T. gondii* to humans because they are usually frozen for storage and thoroughly cooked to avoid diseases that could be caused by contamination by other organisms.[36] The parasite has been isolated from chicken eggs.[46]

The ingestion of vegetables and other food products contaminated with oocysts probably accounts for infection in seropositive vegetarians. Although isolation of tachyzoites from secretions of people with the acute infection has been claimed, human-to-human transmission of infection by this route has not been established. Outbreaks within families and other groups are common,[47-49] but there is no evidence of direct human-to-human transmission other than from mother to fetus.

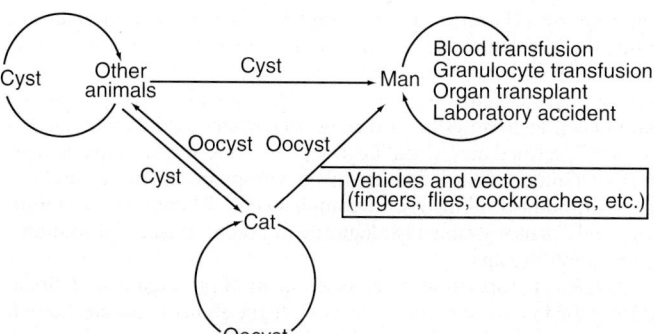

Figure 279-2 **Transmission and life cycle of *Toxoplasma gondii*.** *(From Knick JA, Remington JS. Toxoplasmosis in the adult: an overview. N Engl J Med 1978;298:550-553. Copyright © 1978 Massachusetts Medical Society. All rights reserved.)*

Recent epidemiologic studies have identified water as a potential source of *T. gondii* infection, in both humans and animals.[47,50,51] In vitro studies have demonstrated that oocysts can sporulate in seawater within 1 to 3 days, can survive in seawater for as long as 6 months, and can survive in water treated with sodium hypochlorite or ozone, but not ultraviolet radiation.[52-54] Population mapping studies of acutely infected individuals as well as case-control studies linked drinking unfiltered water (presumably contaminated with oocysts) to an outbreak of toxoplasmosis in a municipality in the western Canadian province of British Columbia[47] and to high endemic rates of toxoplasmosis in Rio de Janeiro state, Brazil.[51] In another Brazilian outbreak, *T. gondii* organisms were detected in water from an implicated reservoir by a variety of methods. Coastal freshwater runoff was observed to be a risk factor for *T. gondii* infection among southern sea otters along the California coast.[55]

In humans, the incidence of *T. gondii* antibodies increases with increasing age; the incidence does not vary significantly between sexes. The incidence tends to be less in cold regions, in hot and arid areas, and at high elevations. Slaughterhouse workers may have an increased risk of infection. The prevalence of antibody titers to *T. gondii* varies considerably among different geographic areas and also among individuals within a given population. These differences depend on a variety of factors including culinary habits and cleanliness of surroundings. A decrease in antibody prevalence over the past few decades has been observed in many countries. In the United States, the seroprevalence in U.S. military recruits decreased by one third between 1965 and 1989[56]; the crude seropositivity rate among recruits from 49 states was 9.5% in 1989 compared with 14.4% in 1965.[56] As another example, in the 1970s, 24% of women in the childbearing age group in the Palo Alto, California area were seropositive, whereas the rate in 2003 was 9%. Seroprevalence rates in the United States among such women range from 3% to greater than 35%, whereas rates higher than 50% are present in women of childbearing age in much of Western Europe, Africa, and South and Central America. The recent (1999 to 2004) overall age-adjusted seroprevalence of *T. gondii* infection in the United States, based on a study of 15,960 persons aged 6 to 49 years, was reported to be 10.8%, with a seroprevalence among women aged 15 to 44 years of 11%.[57] This study found an approximately 25% to 40% decline in seroprevalence compared with a similar survey a decade earlier. Although the prevalence of the infection appears to be declining in certain areas of the world such as Europe and the United States, this has not been the case or it has been documented to have increased in other geographic locales.[58] *T. gondii* may survive in citrated blood at 4°C for as long as 50 days, and infection has been transmitted through transfusion of whole blood or white blood cells. Leukocyte transfusions may pose a special risk.[59] The transmission of infection by organ transplantation has been documented and may result from the transplantation of an organ (e.g., heart) from a seropositive donor to a seronegative recipient.[60] In bone marrow transplant recipients, toxoplasmosis almost always is a result of recrudescence of a latent infection rather than from the transplant.[61,62]

The incidence of TE among human immunodeficiency virus (HIV)–infected individuals directly correlates with the prevalence of *T. gondii* antibodies among the general HIV-infected population, the degree of immunosuppression (best measured by the CD4 cell count),[63] the immunologic response to antiretroviral drugs, and the use of effective prophylactic treatment regimens against the development of TE.[64] AIDS-associated TE and toxoplasmosis involving other organs are usually due to reactivation of a chronic (latent) infection that results from the progressive immune dysfunction that develops in these patients.[65] It is estimated that 20% to 47% of AIDS patients who are infected with *T. gondii* but are not taking anti-*Toxoplasma* prophylaxis or antiretroviral drugs will ultimately develop TE.[63,65]

In recent years, a substantial decline in the incidence of TE[66] and toxoplasmosis-associated deaths[67] has been seen in HIV-infected patients who adhere to antiretroviral therapy and to effective anti-*Toxoplasma* prophylactic regimens.

In the United States, *T. gondii* seropositivity among HIV-infected patients varies from 10% to 45%[65] and directly correlates with the seropositivity in the general non-HIV–infected population. In contrast, the seroprevalence is approximately 50% to 78% in certain areas of Western Europe and Africa.[68,69] In a study in France, 1215 (72.2%) of 1683 HIV-infected patients had serologic evidence of exposure to *T. gondii*.[70] During the study period (1988 to 1995), the overall incidence of toxoplasmosis was estimated to be 1.53 per 100 patient-years, with an increase from 0.68 per 100 patient-years in 1988 to 2.1 per 100 patient-years in 1992 and a subsequent decline to 0.19 per 100 patient-years in 1995. Toxoplasmosis is rare in the HIV-infected pediatric population: 0.06 cases per 100 patient-years were reported in more than 3000 patients participating in clinical trials in the era before highly active antiretroviral therapy (HAART), but during a time when *Pneumocystis carinii* pneumonia (PCP) prophylaxis was recommended.

Of interest is the low reported incidence of TE in Africa despite *T. gondii* seroprevalence rates of 32% to 78%. The lack of autopsy data and of neuroimaging studies likely contributes to the low reported incidence. It has also been suggested that because of poor access to medical care, many HIV-infected patients in Africa die of infection by organisms such as *Mycobacterium tuberculosis* before the opportunistic infections associated with the advanced stage of HIV infection develop, including toxoplasmosis. However, in one autopsy series of 175 patients with AIDS-defining abnormalities from the Ivory Coast, the prevalence of TE was 21%.[71]

T. gondii infection may be acquired after the acquisition of HIV infection. Seroconversion rates between 2% and 5.5% have been reported in patients followed for periods as long as 28 months.[72]

Even before the emergence of AIDS, TE had been recognized as a cause of incapacitating disease and death among immunosuppressed patients,[6,73] especially in those whose underlying disease or therapy caused a deficiency in cell-mediated immunity. Patients with hematologic malignancies, especially those with Hodgkin's disease, are at a particularly higher risk of the development of recrudescence of the infection. Among organ transplant recipients, toxoplasmosis develops at a higher rate in those with heart, lung, kidney, and bone marrow transplants.

Pathogenesis and Immunity

T. gondii multiplies intracellularly at the site of invasion (the gastrointestinal tract is the major route for and the initial site of infection in nature); bradyzoites released from tissue cysts or sporozoites released from oocysts penetrate and multiply within intestinal epithelial cells. Organisms may spread first to the mesenteric lymph nodes and then to distant organs by invasion of lymphatics and blood. *T. gondii* infects virtually all cell types, and cell invasion occurs as an active process. Survival of tachyzoites is due to the formation of a parasitophorous vacuole that lacks host proteins necessary for fusion with lysosomes,[74] and consequently acidification does not occur. Active invasion of macrophages by tachyzoites does not trigger oxidative killing mechanisms. With the appearance of humoral and cellular immunity, only those parasites protected by an intracellular habitat or within tissue cysts survive. An effective immune response significantly reduces the number of tachyzoites in all tissues. Tachyzoites are killed by reactive oxygen intermediates,[75] acidification,[76] osmotic fluctuations, reactive nitrogen intermediates,[77] intracellular tryptophan depletion,[78] and specific antibody combined with complement.[79] Thereafter, tachyzoites are rarely demonstrable histologically in tissues of infected immunocompetent humans.

Tissue cyst formation takes place in multiple organs and tissues during the first week of infection. Despite the ability to isolate *T. gondii* from normal brains of chronically infected humans, the tissue cyst form is rarely observed in histologic preparations; it has been isolated from both brain and skeletal muscle in 10% of 52 *T. gondii*–seropositive patients who at autopsy had no clinical or pathologic evidence of the infection.[25] The tissue cyst form is responsible for residual (chronic or latent) infection and persists primarily in the brain, skeletal and heart muscle, and eye.[25,80]

In immunocompetent individuals, the initial infection and the resultant seeding of different organs lead to a chronic or latent infection without clinical significance. This chronic stage of the infection corresponds to the asymptomatic persistence of the tissue cyst form in multiple tissues. It is believed that periodically, bradyzoites are released from tissue cysts or that cysts "rupture"; cyst disruption in this setting is a clinically silent process effectively contained by the immune system and in the CNS likely results in small inflammatory nodules, with a limited degree of neuronal cell death and architectural damage.[33]

Whereas toxoplasmosis in severely immunodeficient individuals may be caused by primary infection, it most often is the result of recrudescence of a latent infection. It is widely held that reactivation is the result of disruption of the tissue cyst form followed by uncontrolled proliferation of organisms and tissue destruction. In individuals with deficient cell-mediated immunity, rapid, uncontrolled proliferation of *T. gondii* results in progressively enlarging necrotic lesions. It has been postulated that damage to any organ in these patients, including the brain, eye, heart, lung, skeletal muscle, gastrointestinal tract, and pancreas, can result directly from tissue cyst disruption in the parenchyma of the organ itself or from tissue cyst disruption elsewhere in the body followed by subsequent spread to that organ.[81] Hematogenous spread is supported by the observation of the development of simultaneous lesions in the brain and the presence of parasitemia in 14% to 38% of AIDS patients with TE.[82,83] Lymphocytes obtained from patients with AIDS have impaired production of IFN-γ[84] and interleukin (IL)-2[85] in response to stimulation with *T. gondii* antigens. Treatment of monocytes and monocyte-derived macrophages from AIDS patients with IFN-γ enhances their activity against *T. gondii*.[86] Coinfection with other opportunistic pathogens may predispose to reactivation; murine cytomegalovirus (CMV) induces reactivation of latent *T. gondii* infection in the lungs of experimental animals.[87]

Infection with *T. gondii* induces both humoral and cell-mediated immune responses. A well-orchestrated and effective systemic immune response is responsible for the early disappearance of *T. gondii* from peripheral blood during the acute infection and limits the parasite burden in other organs. Immunity in the immunocompetent host is lifelong. Exogenous reinfection, which has been demonstrated in laboratory animals, likely also occurs in humans but does not appear to result in clinically apparent disease.

T cells, macrophages, and type 1 cytokines (IFN-γ, IL-12) are crucial for control of *T. gondii* infection. Adoptive transfer and depletion experiments in murine models not only proved that T cells are essential for control of *T. gondii* infection but also demonstrated an interplay between CD4[+] and CD8[+] T cells in both the induction of resistance and the maintenance of latency. Additional studies revealed an expansion of both natural killer (NK) and γδ T cells early in infection that has been proposed to provide innate resistance while the adaptive response mediated through αβ CD4 and CD8 T cells develops. These different subsets of T cells and NK cells are likely to protect the host by secreting cytokines such as IFN-γ, IL-2, and TNF-α and apparently not by lysing *T. gondii*–infected cells.[88-90] Dendritic cells and neutrophils have also been shown to play an important role in control of acute infection, and the early production of IL-12 by these populations may determine the strong NK-cell and T-cell type 1 cytokine response triggered by the parasite.[91]

The costimulatory molecules CD28 and CD40 ligand are pivotal for the regulation of IL-12 and IFN-γ production in response to the parasite.[92] *T. gondii* infection of antigen-presenting cells such as dendritic cells and macrophages causes upregulation of the counterreceptors for CD28 and CD40L, CD80/CD86, and CD40.[92] Binding of CD80/CD86 to CD28 enhances production of IFN-γ by CD4[+] T cells. In addition, binding of CD40L to CD40 triggers IL-12 secretion, which in turn enhances production of IFN-γ. The relevance of CD40L in the immune response to *T. gondii* is supported by reports of TE and disseminated

toxoplasmosis in children with congenital defects in CD40L signaling (hyper-IgM syndrome).[93] Moreover, recent studies have demonstrated that expression of CD40L is defective on CD4[+] T cells from HIV-infected patients.[94] This deficiency may play a role in defective IL-12/IFN-γ production associated with HIV infection.

Cytokines play a critical role in defense against the infection and are important in the pathogenesis of toxoplasmosis and TE.[95] IL-12 enhances survival of T cell–deficient mice during *T. gondii* infection by stimulating the production of IFN-γ by NK cells[96] and is thought to also regulate the expression of the latter cytokine by T cells in immunocompetent mice.[97] IFN-γ has been shown to play a significant role in the prevention or development of TE in mice.[98] The administration of a monoclonal antibody against IFN-γ to chronically infected mice resulted in a dramatic worsening in the degree of encephalitis.[99] In mice with active TE, treatment with IFN-γ significantly reduced the inflammatory response and numbers of tachyzoites.[100]

Differences in IL-12 levels elicited during infection by different strains of the parasite may be responsible for some of the strain-specific differences in virulence.[101] These differences appear to be related to the activation (phosphorylation) of the transcription factor STAT3, which in turn is dependent on the particular allele of ROP16 injected by a given strain.[102]

TNF-α is another cytokine pivotal for control of *T. gondii* infection. TNF-α is required for triggering of IFN-γ–mediated activation of macrophages for *T. gondii*-cidal activity[103] and for NO (an inhibitor of *T. gondii* replication) production by macrophages.[104] The administration of TNF-α–neutralizing antibody to infected mice caused the death of the mice and an increase in the number of *T. gondii* tissue cysts in the brains of survivors.[105]

IL-10 has been shown to deactivate macrophages and result in reduced in vitro killing of *T. gondii*. IL-4 and IL-6, which are usually considered downregulatory cytokines, have been shown to be important in resistance against TE in the murine model.[106,107] IL-7 has also been shown to have a protective role against *T. gondii* in mice.[108] During the early stages of the infection, IL-12, IL-1, and TNF act in concert with IL-15 to stimulate NK cells to produce IFN-γ.[109]

IL-17[110] and IL-23[111,112] have also been implicated in the generation of a potent immune response but are not thought be essential for host resistance.

Several hypotheses have been proposed to explain the role of IFN-γ in host resistance to *T. gondii*. Involvement of reactive nitrogen intermediates (including NO) is suggested by the observation that NG-monomethyl-L-arginine, competitive analogue of L-arginine, simultaneously inhibits NO synthesis and intracellular tachyzoite killing by cytokine-activated peritoneal macrophages and microglial cells.[77,113,114] In addition, mice in which NO synthesis is impaired as a result of genetic disruptions of the IFN-γ or IFN regulatory factor-1 genes succumb to the acute infection.[115,116] Similar enhanced susceptibility was observed in mice treated with the reactive nitrogen intermediate inhibitor aminoguanidine[117] and in NO synthase-deficient mice.[118] The protective role of NO appears to be tissue specific rather than systemic.[118] Because control of the acute infection in vivo was unaffected by NO synthase deficiency, the major role of reactive nitrogen intermediates seems to be to maintain control of established infections in this mouse model.[118]

The IFN-γ–inducible p47 GTPases, IRGM3 (IGTP), and IRGM1 (LRG47) have been shown to be required for host control of *T. gondii* infection in the mouse,[119] and recent studies have linked IRGM3 with the autophagic destruction of *Toxoplasma*-containing vacuoles in IFN-γ–activated macrophages.[120,121]

Immunoglobulin (Ig) G, IgM, IgA, and IgE antibodies are produced in response to the infection. Extracellular tachyzoites are lysed by specific antibody when it is combined with complement. In mice, humoral immunity results in limited protection against less virulent strains of *T. gondii*, but not against virulent strains.[122]

Both astrocytes and microglia likely play important roles in the immune response against *T. gondii* within the CNS. In the early stages of TE in both humans and mice, there is a remarkable and widespread astrocytosis restricted to areas in which the parasite is detected.[95] Whereas *T. gondii* can invade, survive, and multiply within astrocytes, they are killed by activated microglia.[123]

Genetic Susceptibility

The observations in mice that genetic factors in the host contribute to the development and severity of TE[124-126] and the fact that not all HIV-infected patients with positive *T. gondii* serologic findings develop TE suggested the possibility that genetic factors may also play a role in the predisposition of AIDS patients for this disease.[127] The major histocompatibility complex class II gene *DQ3* (HLA-DQ3) has been significantly associated with the development of TE in North American white AIDS patients, whereas HLA-DQ1 was marginally protective.[127] HLA-DQ3 was also significantly associated with the development of hydrocephalus in children with congenital toxoplasmosis.[128] In the latter study, a mouse model transgenic for human major histocompatibility complex class II found higher organism burden with HLA-DQ3 than HLA-DQ1. In a South American white population, a study using a higher resolution typing method identified HLA-DQB*0402 and HLA-DRB1*08, which were in linkage disequilibrium, as risk factors for TE, whereas alleles of HLA-DQB3 were not.[129] Thus, further studies are needed to better define the contribution of various HLA alleles to susceptibility to TE. Another South American study identified an IL-10 promoter allele as a risk factor for toxoplasmic chorioretinitis.[130]

Pathology

Our knowledge of the pathology of infection in humans has come largely from autopsy studies in severely infected infants and immunodeficient patients. Data in immunocompetent adults are limited almost entirely to results obtained from lymph node biopsy specimens[131] and occasionally from myocardial or skeletal muscle tissue specimens.[132]

LYMPH NODE

The histopathologic changes in toxoplasmic lymphadenitis in immunocompetent individuals are frequently distinctive and often diagnostic (Fig. 279-3A).[131] There is a typical triad of findings: a reactive follicular hyperplasia, irregular clusters of epithelioid histiocytes encroaching on and blurring the margins of the germinal centers, and focal distention of sinuses with monocytoid cells (see Fig. 279-3A[133]). Langerhans giant cells, granulomas, microabscesses, and foci of necrosis are not typically seen. Rarely, tachyzoites or tissue cysts are demonstrable. *T. gondii* DNA has infrequently been amplified from lymph node tissue.[134]

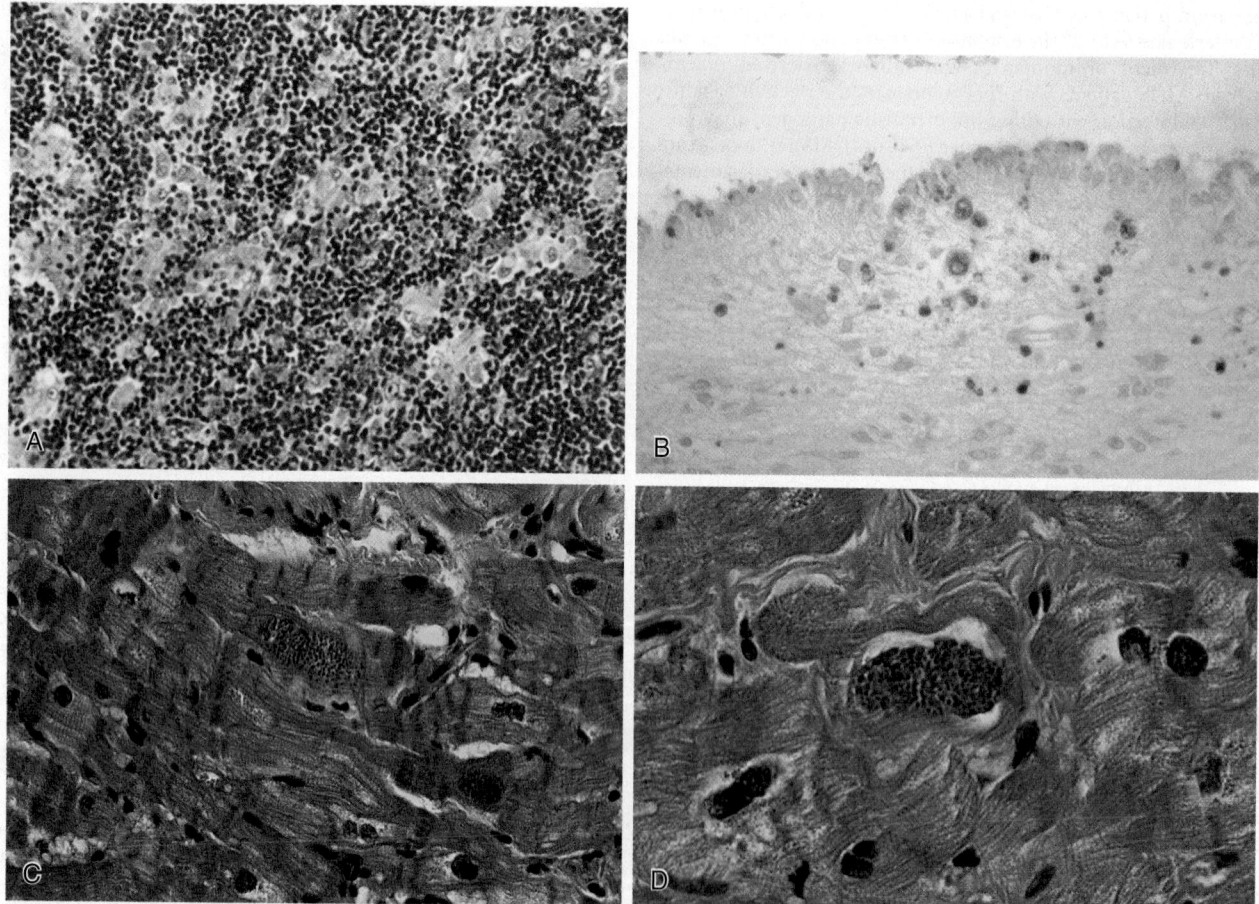

Figure 279-3 Histologic features of *Toxoplasma gondii* in humans. **A,** Hematoxylin and eosin stain of a lymph node biopsy specimen from an immunocompetent patient with toxoplasmic lymphadenitis. *(Courtesy of Dr. Henry Masur, Critical Care Medicine Department, NIH, Bethesda, MD.)* **B,** Positive immunoperoxidase stain of a brain biopsy specimen in a patient with acquired immunodeficiency syndrome and toxoplasmic encephalitis. **C,** Hematoxylin and eosin stain of a right ventricle endomyocardial biopsy specimen from a patient with toxoplasmic myocarditis. Organisms are seen within myocytes (see "Clinical Manifestations"). **D,** Hematoxylin and eosin stain of a right quadriceps muscle biopsy specimen depicting a tissue cyst from the same patient as shown in **C**. The patient also developed toxoplasmic polymyositis. *(**B** to **D,** Courtesy of Dr. Jack S. Remington, Stanford University and Palo Alto Medical Foundation.)*

CENTRAL NERVOUS SYSTEM

Damage to the CNS by *T. gondii* is characterized by multiple foci of enlarging necrosis and microglial nodules.[135] Necrosis is the most prominent feature of the disease because of vascular involvement by the lesions. In cases of congenital toxoplasmosis, necrosis of the brain is most intense in the cortex and basal ganglia and at times in the periventricular areas.[8,136] The necrotic areas may calcify and lead to striking radiographic findings suggestive but not pathognomonic of toxoplasmosis. Hydrocephalus may result from obstruction of the aqueduct of Sylvius or foramen of Monro. Tachyzoites and tissue cysts may be seen in and adjacent to necrotic foci, near or in glial nodules, in perivascular regions, and in cerebral tissue uninvolved by inflammatory change. The necrotic brain tissue autolyzes and is gradually shed into the ventricles. The protein content of such ventricular fluid may be in the range of grams per deciliter and has been shown to contain significant amounts of *T. gondii* antigens.

The presence of multiple brain abscesses is the most characteristic feature of TE in severely immunodeficient patients and is particularly characteristic in patients with AIDS.[6,137] Brain abscesses in AIDS patients are characterized by three histologic zones. The central area is avascular. Surrounding this is an intermediate hyperemic area with a prominent inflammatory infiltrate and perivascular cuffing by lymphocytes, plasma cells, and macrophages. Many tachyzoites and, at times, tissue cysts as well, appear at the margins of necrotic areas. An outer peripheral zone contains *T. gondii* tissue cysts.[138] In the areas around the abscesses, edema, vasculitis, hemorrhage, and cerebral infarction secondary to vascular involvement may also be present.[139] Important associated features in TE are the presence of arteritis, perivascular cuffing, and astrocytosis. Because these findings may also be present in patients with viral encephalitis, immunoperoxidase staining is important for differentiating these pathologic processes. Widespread, poorly demarcated, and confluent areas of necrosis with minimal inflammatory response are seen in some patients.[139] Identification of tachyzoites is pathognomonic of active infection, but their visualization may be difficult in hematoxylin and eosin–stained sections. The use of immunoperoxidase staining markedly improves the identification of both tissue cyst and tachyzoite forms and highlights the presence of *T. gondii* antigens (see Fig. 279-3B).[24] *T. gondii* DNA can be amplified from cerebrospinal fluid (CSF) or brain biopsy specimens of patients with TE.[140] Of note, positive PCR results in brain biopsy specimens need to be interpreted with caution. These results may be positive in patients chronically infected with the parasite whose CNS pathology can be explained by a diagnosis other than TE.

At autopsy in AIDS patients with TE, there is almost universal involvement of the cerebral hemispheres and a remarkable predilection for the basal ganglia.[65] In a consecutive autopsy study of 204 patients who died of AIDS, 46 (23%) had morphologic evidence of cerebral toxoplasmosis. In 38 (83%) of the 46 cases, histologic evidence of toxoplasmosis was restricted to the CNS. The cerebral hemispheres were affected in 91% of cases and the rostral basal ganglia in 78%.[139]

A diffuse form of TE has been described with histopathologic findings of widespread microglial nodules without abscess formation in the gray matter of the cerebrum, cerebellum, and brain stem.[141] In these patients, involvement by *T. gondii* was confirmed by immunoperoxidase stains that demonstrated tissue cysts and tachyzoites. In diffuse TE, the clinical course progresses rapidly to death. It has been postulated that in such cases, the lack of characteristic findings on computed tomography (CT) or magnetic resonance imaging (MRI) studies is due to insufficient time for abscesses to form before death occurs.

Leptomeningitis is infrequent and, when present, occurs over adjacent areas of encephalitis. Spinal cord necrotizing lesions are seen at autopsy in approximately 6% of patients with TE.[141] The differential diagnosis of TE lesions includes CNS lymphoma, progressive multifocal leukoencephalopathy, and infection caused by organisms such as CMV, *Cryptococcus neoformans*, *Aspergillus* spp., and *M. tuberculosis*. More than one agent may be present.

LUNG

Pulmonary toxoplasmosis in the immunodeficient patient may appear in the form of interstitial pneumonitis, necrotizing pneumonitis, consolidation, pleural effusion, or empyema, or all of these.[142] The pneumonitis is associated with the development of fibrinous or fibrinopurulent exudate. Tachyzoites may be found in alveolocytes, alveolar macrophages, pleural fluid, or extracellularly within alveolar exudate. *T. gondii* DNA may be demonstrated in bronchoalveolar lavage (BAL) fluid by PCR.[143]

EYE

Chorioretinitis in AIDS patients is characterized by segmental panophthalmitis and areas of coagulative necrosis associated with tissue cysts and tachyzoites.[144] Numerous organisms in the absence of remarkable inflammation may be seen around thrombosed retinal vessels adjacent to necrotic areas. Multiple and bilateral lesions may occur.[144] Amplification of parasite DNA in both aqueous humor and vitreous fluid has confirmed or supported the diagnosis of toxoplasmic chorioretinitis in patients with atypical retinal findings for ocular toxoplasmosis or who are immunocompromised.[145,146]

Eye infection in immunocompetent patients produces acute chorioretinitis characterized by severe inflammation and necrosis.[144] Granulomatous inflammation of the choroid is secondary to the necrotizing retinitis. There may be exudation into the vitreous or invasion of the vitreous by a budding mass of capillaries. Although rare, tachyzoites and tissue cysts may be demonstrated in the retina. The pathogenesis of recurrent chorioretinitis is controversial. One school proposes that rupture of tissue cysts releases viable organisms that induce necrosis and inflammation, whereas another school contends that chorioretinitis results from a hypersensitivity reaction triggered by unknown causes.[144] A recent study demonstrating the efficacy of trimethoprim-sulfamethoxazole (TMP-SMX) in preventing recurrences of chorioretinitis is consistent with the hypothesis that active organism replication is necessary for recurrence.[147]

Recent studies revealed a much higher incidence of ocular disease, which is often severe, among infected, immunocompetent people in South America than those in North America or Europe.[148-151] This difference seems most likely to be due to differences in the strains of *Toxoplasma* that predominate in these different regions.[16] This is consistent with observations in the United States where specific strains seemed to be associated with severe disease, although these studies involved relatively few patients and cannot be considered definitive.[152]

SKELETAL AND HEART MUSCLE

Myositis due to *T. gondii* has been reported in as many as 4% of HIV-infected patients who present with neuromuscular symptoms, and the same percentage has been observed in autopsy series of AIDS patients in whom a systematic histologic evaluation of the skeletal muscle was performed.[153] Successful isolation from skeletal muscle biopsy specimens has been reported.[154] Microscopy has revealed necrotic muscle fibers with a variable inflammatory reaction. Skeletal muscle involvement has also been reported in the non-AIDS immunodeficient patient.[6,132]

Toxoplasmic myocarditis is frequently noted at autopsy in AIDS patients but is usually clinically inapparent,[155] with CNS manifestations predominating.[156] Focal necrosis with edema and an inflammatory infiltrate is typical,[155] although abscesses may also be noted.[155,156] Similar histologic findings are seen in the non-AIDS immunodeficient population,[6] and in both groups, cardiac myocytes may be packed with tachyzoites (to produce pseudocysts) in the absence of an inflammatory response.

Biopsy-proven toxoplasmic myocarditis and polymyositis in the setting of acute toxoplasmosis have been reported in otherwise immunocompetent individuals and in patients taking corticosteroids (see Fig. 279-3C and D).[132]

OTHER ORGAN SYSTEMS

Extensive involvement of the gastrointestinal tract in AIDS patients may occur with tremendous variation in the inflammatory response.[157,158] Hemorrhagic gastritis and colitis have been described.[159] Other organs reported to be involved during toxoplasmosis include the liver,[160] pancreas,[161] seminiferous tubules,[162] prostate,[162] adrenals,[163] kidneys,[164] and bone marrow.[165]

Clinical Manifestations

Toxoplasmosis describes the clinical or pathologic disease caused by *T. gondii* and is distinct from *T. gondii* infection, which is asymptomatic in the vast majority of immunocompetent patients.

Toxoplasmosis is conveniently classified into five categories: (1) acquired in the immunocompetent patient, (2) acquired or reactivated in the immunodeficient patient, (3) ocular, (4) in pregnancy, and (5) congenital. In any category, the clinical presentations are not specific for toxoplasmosis, and a wide differential diagnosis must be considered for each clinical syndrome. Furthermore, methods of diagnosis and interpretation of test results may differ for each clinical category (e.g., serologic test results consistent with an infection acquired in the distant past for a nonimmunocompromised pregnant woman in the first half of her pregnancy are interpreted as no risk of congenital toxoplasmosis, whereas the same results for a patient about to undergo allogeneic hematopoietic stem cell or bone marrow transplantation are interpreted as high risk of life-threatening toxoplasmosis in the post-transplantation period, particularly if graft-versus-host disease develops in the patient).

TOXOPLASMOSIS IN THE IMMUNOCOMPETENT PATIENT

In the United States and Europe, only 10% to 20% of cases of *T. gondii* infection in immunocompetent adults and children are symptomatic.[166] Recent reports suggest that this proportion may be higher in other areas of the world such as Brazil and other countries in South America.[148,151] In addition, it seems that disease severity is also greater in countries outside Europe and the United States. For instance, a community outbreak of acute toxoplasmosis with an unusually severe clinical presentation was recently reported from the Surinamese village of Patam, near the French Guiana border.[167] Of 11 immunocompetent patients with toxoplasmosis, 8 had severe disseminated disease (including pneumonia and hepatitis) that resulted in three deaths, one adult, one newborn, and one fetus. Genotype analysis with 8 microsatellite markers revealed that a single strain was responsible for at least 5 of the 11 cases. The remarkable differences in clinical presentation of toxoplasmosis among patients from various regions of the world have significant implications when generating a differential diagnosis in travelers from the United States and Europe who become ill.

Most often, toxoplasmosis manifests as asymptomatic cervical lymphadenopathy, but any or all lymph node groups may be enlarged. On palpation, the nodes are usually discrete and nontender, rarely more than 3 cm in diameter, may vary in firmness, and do not suppurate.[168] However, the nodes may be tender or matted. Fever, malaise, night sweats, myalgias, sore throat, maculopapular rash, hepatosplenomegaly, or small numbers of atypical lymphocytes (<10%) may be present. The clinical picture may resemble infectious mononucleosis or CMV infection, but toxoplasmosis probably causes no more than 1% of "mononucleosis" syndromes.[169] Retroperitoneal or mesenteric lymphadenopathy may produce abdominal pain.

Toxoplasmic chorioretinitis as a manifestation of acute acquired infection is more common than previously recognized.[170-172] Chorioretinitis in the setting of acute acquired toxoplasmosis can occur either sporadically or in the context of an epidemic of acute toxoplasmosis.[171,173] For further discussion of this clinical entity, see "Ocular Toxoplasmosis in Immunocompetent Patients."

In most cases, the clinical course of toxoplasmosis in the immunocompetent patient is benign and self-limited. Symptoms, if present, usually resolve within a few months and rarely persist beyond 12 months. Lymphadenopathy may wax and wane for months and, in unusual cases, for 1 year or longer. Rarely, in an apparently healthy person, clinically overt disease develops (e.g., fever of unknown origin or potentially fatal disseminated disease, with myocarditis, pneumonitis, hepatitis, or encephalitis). These more aggressive forms of the disease have been more commonly reported from South America.[167] None of the clinical presentations of acquired toxoplasmosis is distinctive; the differential diagnosis of toxoplasmic lymphadenitis includes lymphoma, infectious mononucleosis, CMV, or human herpesvirus-6 "mononucleosis," cat-scratch disease, sarcoidosis, tuberculosis, tularemia, metastatic carcinoma, and leukemia. Acute acquired toxoplasmosis associated with multiple-organ involvement has been reported to mimic other causes of pneumonitis, hepatitis, myocarditis, polymyositis, or fever of unknown origin in apparently immunocompetent patients.[166]

T. gondii has been estimated to cause 3% to 7% of clinically significant lymphadenopathy.[168] The major diagnostic confusion with toxoplasmic lymphadenopathy occurs with Hodgkin's disease and the lymphomas. The diagnosis of recently acquired toxoplasmic lymphadenopathy is easily made serologically, but, unfortunately, physicians often do not consider this diagnosis in patients with lymphadenopathy. Serologic test titers diagnostic of acute *T. gondii* infection are often obtained after histologic examination of a node biopsy specimen has suggested the possibility of toxoplasmosis.[174]

Myocarditis as a manifestation of acute toxoplasmosis has been reported in relatively few patients.[132,175,176] It may occur clinically as an isolated disease process or as part of a variety of manifestations of the disseminated infection. Manifestations include arrhythmias, pericarditis, and heart failure.[132]

Myositis resembling polymyositis as a manifestation of acute toxoplasmosis has also been reported infrequently.[132,177,178] Dermatomyositis has been associated with toxoplasmosis, although a cause-and-effect relationship has not been proved.[179,180]

The clinical features of toxoplasmic myocarditis and polymyositis are illustrated by a case in which both were present in the same individual.[132] A 43-year-old woman presented with cardiogenic pulmonary edema followed by progressive sinus bradycardia and subsequent complete heart block; viral myocarditis was considered the most likely diagnosis. During the ensuing months, proximal muscle weakness developed while she was being treated with corticosteroids; the results of an endomyocardial biopsy (see Fig. 279-3C) and a quadriceps muscle biopsy (see Fig. 279-3D) revealed *T. gondii*.[132] Her symptoms improved on pyrimethamine-sulfadiazine. One year after her initial presentation with myocarditis, retinal lesions characteristic of toxoplasmic chorioretinitis were observed in her right eye. Serologic test results and follow-up were consistent with recently acquired toxoplasmosis.[132]

Several epidemiologic studies have suggested an association between infection with *T. gondii* and schizophrenia, but a definitive etiologic role of the parasite in psychiatric disorders has not been established.[181,182] Population-based studies that include large cohorts of patients followed since gestation will be necessary to clarify this potential association.

TOXOPLASMOSIS IN THE IMMUNODEFICIENT PATIENT

Whereas toxoplasmosis in otherwise normal individuals is usually benign, its protean clinical manifestations, unusual occurrence, and devastating consequences in immunocompromised individuals emphasize the need for clinical acumen in diagnosis and management of toxoplasmosis in these patients. The latter include those with hematologic malignancies (especially Hodgkin's disease and other lymphomas), organ transplant recipients, those with AIDS, and those receiving immunosuppressive therapy with corticosteroids, other immunomodulators such as anti-TNF-α therapy[183] and cytotoxic drugs. In immunodeficient patients, encephalitis, pneumonitis, and myocarditis reflect active infection in the most commonly involved organs.[6] Pneumonitis is a common and underrecognized manifestation of toxoplasmosis in these patients. Fever of unknown origin may be the sole manifestation of toxoplasmosis in the early stages of the disease. Disseminated infection with multiorgan involvement is not unusual; clinical manifestations may not necessarily reflect the extent and severity of the disseminated infection. Mortality approaches 100% if the infection is not treated or is treated only late in its course. Whereas serious toxoplasmosis in these patients often reflects recrudescence of a latent infection (from the cyst form of the organism) acquired in the distant past (e.g., in the setting of AIDS or bone marrow transplantation), it also results from recently acquired acute infection with the parasite, usually through the transplanted organ (e.g., solid organ transplants). Although clinical manifestations are similar in patients with different causes of their immunosuppression, additional considerations are provided here for the organ transplant recipient and patient with AIDS.

At present, TMP-SMX is used by most transplantation teams as prophylaxis against *Pneumocystis* pneumonia. Its use has also been shown to protect against toxoplasmosis. However, TMP-SMX is not protective in every case, and some patients are not able to tolerate the drug combination. In addition, in some patients sulfonamides may be contraindicated. Alternative drugs for prophylaxis are provided under "Treatment."

TOXOPLASMOSIS IN THE SOLID ORGAN TRANSPLANT PATIENT

Toxoplasmosis will most commonly develop in patients with solid organ transplants as a result of acquiring *T. gondii* infection through the transplanted organ when the allograft of a seropositive donor (D⁺) is given to a seronegative recipient (R⁻), resulting in a D⁺/R⁻ mismatch (Table 279-1). Toxoplasmosis can also be the result of reactivation of a previously acquired infection in the recipient regardless of the serologic status of the donor (D⁻/R⁺ or D⁺/R⁺) (see Table 279-1).

Knowledge of the overall prevalence of *Toxoplasma* antibodies in a population does not accurately predict the percentage of D⁺R⁻ *T. gondii* mismatches. Rather, this will depend on the prevalence of *T. gondii* antibodies in the age groups of the donor and recipient populations. For example, in a given geographic area, the prevalence of antibodies in young heart donors may be 3% to 10%, whereas in the older population of individuals who would more likely be recipients, it may be 15% to 30%. Testing for toxoplasma IgG antibodies should be performed in every organ transplant candidate before transplantation and on serum from every organ donor. This will allow for the identification of those recipients at greatest risk of the development of toxoplasmosis either because they were seronegative before transplantation and received an organ from a seropositive individual or because they were seropositive before transplantation and thus are at risk of reacti-

TABLE 279-1	Source of Toxoplasmosis in the Organ Transplant Patient
Transplant of an infected organ to a seronegative recipient (D⁺R⁻)	
Heart	
Heart-lung	
Kidney	
Liver and liver/pancreas	
Bone marrow (rare)	
Reactivation of latent infection in a seropositive recipient (D⁻R⁺ and D⁺R⁺)	
Bone marrow	
Hematopoietic stem cell	
Liver	
Kidney (rare)	

D, donor; R, recipient.

vation of their latent (chronic) toxoplasma infection. Unfortunately, toxoplasma serologies obtained in the early months post-transplantation frequently are not helpful, even in the presence of serious toxoplasmosis in these patients. This is especially true in bone marrow transplant patients in whom *T. gondii* antibodies demonstrable before transplantation might become negative, increase, or show no change post-transplantation despite life-threatening toxoplasmosis. Transfusion may further compound the difficulties encountered in serodiagnosis.

The actual incidence of toxoplasmosis among various organ transplant recipients is unknown. At present, there is no registry for these cases and many do not come to autopsy or are not published. There is especially a paucity of objective estimates of mortality due to toxoplasmosis in organ transplant recipients in whom the diagnosis was considered early and treatment begun promptly.

At autopsy, histopathologic evidence of multiorgan involvement by the parasite has been observed in organ transplant patients. The organs most commonly involved are the brain, heart, and lungs, but multiple other organs including eyes, liver, pancreas, adrenal, and kidney may also reveal the organism. Fever is often the first manifestation in transplant recipients, followed by signs referable to the brain and lungs.

Heart Transplantation

In a recent review of infections in cardiac transplant recipients at Stanford Medical Center from 1980 to 1996, results of serologic testing for *Toxoplasma* were available for 582 donors (35 [6%] had *T. gondii*–specific IgG antibodies) and 607 recipients (98 [16%] were positive).[184] Results of serologic testing for *Toxoplasma* were available for 575 D/R pairs; of these, 454 (79%) were D⁻/R⁻, 84 (14.6%) D⁻/R⁺, 32 (5.6%) D⁺/R⁻, and 5 (0.8%) D⁺/R⁺. Of the 32 D⁺/R⁻ patients, 16 were receiving TMP-SMX and/or pyrimethamine prophylaxis, and toxoplasmosis developed in none; however, in 4 (25%) of the 16 D⁺/R⁻ patients who were not taking either TMP-SMX or pyrimethamine toxoplasmosis developed, and all died of the infection. Clinical evidence of reactivation of the infection developed in none of the 98 patients who were seropositive for *T. gondii* preoperatively. The importance of prophylaxis is further evidenced in an earlier study at Papworth Hospital in England. Fatal or severe toxoplasmosis developed in 57% (4/7) of D⁺R⁻ mismatched heart transplant patients not receiving prophylaxis. Use of pyrimethamine, 25 mg/day for 6 weeks reduced the transmission rate to 14% (5/37). In those patients who received pyrimethamine and were infected by the donor heart, symptoms of the infection developed in only one (20%) in contrast to four of four (100%) who did not receive pyrimethamine prophylaxis. Subsequently prophylaxis with TMP-SMX (480/2400 mg PO twice daily for 1 year post-transplantation and when on oral prednisolone) was used in heart and lung transplant patients. Of those who were alive at 3 months post-transplantation, 28 (8.75%) were *T. gondii* mismatches; none had evidence of having acquired *Toxoplasma* infection. These investigators observed that use of prophylaxis might prolong the period before observation of seroconversion of donor-acquired infection in heart transplant patients for as long as 14 months post-transplantation.[185,186]

Thus, use of TMP-/SMX alone may be sufficient for prevention of toxoplasmosis in patients who are seronegative for *T. gondii* antibodies and who receive heart transplants from seropositive donors (i.e., D⁺/R⁻ patients). The optimal schedule for administration of TMP-SMX in heart transplant patients has not been defined. Physicians must decide whether a schedule of daily administration or administration three times weekly is to be followed. For HIV-infected patients, we routinely recommend daily use of TMP-SMX whenever feasible.

Toxoplasmosis in heart transplant recipients may simulate organ rejection. In such cases, toxoplasmosis has frequently been diagnosed by endomyocardial biopsy.

It is important to recognize that many heart transplant recipients with *T. gondii* antibodies before transplantation may show increases in *T. gondii*–specific antibodies (IgG and IgM). A clinical illness has not necessarily developed in these patients that can be attributed to toxoplasmosis.

Kidney Transplantation

In a review of 31 cases of toxoplasmosis in renal transplant patients, the majority occurred within the first 3 months after transplantation; 3 cases occurred more than 1 year after transplantation and 9 occurred during or immediately after a rejection episode.[187] The greatest risk was in D+R− mismatches. Fever, CNS signs, and pneumonia were the main clinical features. Chest x-rays showed bilateral pneumonia in most cases. The most common organs involved in the 15 cases diagnosed at autopsy were the brain, heart, and lungs. *T. gondii* was not demonstrable in the kidneys. Whereas the overall mortality rate was 64%, 10 of 11 treated patients survived, emphasizing the importance of early diagnosis and treatment. Acute toxoplasmosis in two recipients of renal allografts from the same donor has occurred.

Liver Transplantation

After orthotopic liver transplantation, toxoplasmosis most often results from activation of a latent infection in the allograft but also from activation of a quiescent pretransplantation infection in the recipient. In most published cases, clinical manifestations of toxoplasmosis appeared within the first 3 months post-transplantation. Fever was usually the first manifestation, and pneumonia, meningitis/encephalitis, and multiorgan failure were frequently observed. Retinochoroiditis requiring enucleation was observed in one patient.[188] Although it is a rare event, it is most often fatal.[189]

TOXOPLASMOSIS IN THE HEMATOPOIETIC STEM CELL TRANSPLANT AND BONE MARROW TRANSPLANT RECIPIENT

Stem cell transplantation is now done using stem cells harvested from the peripheral blood of the patient (autologous), matched (allogeneic) donor, or, less commonly, cord blood. More remotely, donor bone marrow was used as the source. To keep this literature separate, hematopoietic stem cell transplantation (HSCT) and bone marrow transplantation (BMT) are presented separately in this section. A recent report reviewed 41 cases of toxoplasmosis in patients who had undergone HSCT in 15 European transplantation centers from 1994 through 1998.[190] There were no cases among 6787 autologous HSCTs, whereas it occurred in 0.97% of 4231 allogeneic transplantations. The relatively low number of cases in their large survey is likely due to the use of TMP-SMX prophylaxis after engraftment in all allogenic BMTs in 91% of the institutions.[190] Of the patients with available serologies before transplant, 94% were seropositive for *T. gondii*. Graft–versus-host had developed before toxoplasmosis in 73%. Thirty (73%) had not received prophylaxis for toxoplasmosis, and only 3 were receiving it at the time of disease onset. The median day of onset was day 64 (range, 4 to 516 days). Fever with neurologic or pulmonary symptoms was seen most commonly; myocarditis was frequently seen at autopsy. Six patients had fever without evidence of organ involvement. Twenty-two (63%) died of toxoplasmosis. It is noteworthy that of the 23 patients who received specific therapy for toxoplasmosis for 6 days or longer, 11 (48%) had a complete response and 3 (13%) others improved. Survival in this setting is highest in patients with ocular and/or isolated cerebral toxoplasmosis, primarily when treatment is begun as soon as the diagnosis is suspected.[61,190] Survival in the presence of disseminated toxoplasmosis is rare in these HSCT patients.[61,190] Although reactivation of latent *Toxoplasma* infection in allogeneic HSCT patients most often occurs in the first 6 months post-transplantation (the majority occur in the first 30 to 90 days), late reactivation has been observed and must be considered in patients in whom late-onset (more than 6 months post-transplantation) graft-versus-host disease occurs.[191,192]

The incidence of toxoplasmosis in BMT ranged from 0.3% to 5% and was influenced by the prevalence of pretransplantation antibodies in the populations studied and whether toxoplasmosis prophylaxis was used. Major risk factors for toxoplasmosis included the presence of pretransplantation *T. gondii* antibodies in recipients and the occurrence of graft-versus-host disease. In a recent review of 110 published cases of toxoplasmosis after BMT,[61] 96% occurred after allogeneic BMT. Onset post-transplantation occurred on days 1 to 30 in 13%, on days 31 to 100 in 64%, and after day 100 in 23%. The infection occurred primarily in recipients who were seropositive pre-transplantation (88%), meaning that infection was more often reactivation in the recipient and not transplanted from the donor. The diagnosis was made antemortem in only 47% of the cases. Overall mortality was 80% (at a median 87 days post-transplantation), and in 66%, it was attributed to toxoplasmosis (at a median 74 days post-transplantation). Patients with isolated cerebral involvement had a better outcome (58% survival) than did patients with disseminated toxoplasmosis (20% survival); underlying disease was the only factor associated with clinical presentation, with acute leukemia being more common in patients with disseminated disease.

TMP-SMX prophylaxis, primarily used by transplantation teams to prevent *Pneumocystis* pneumonia, has been successful in preventing toxoplasmosis. In HSCT patients, this is usually begun after engraftment because of the potential of the drug combination for bone marrow suppression. The delay in instituting prophylaxis likely results in many more cases of toxoplasmosis than would be expected to occur if adequate prophylaxis was begun early after transplantation. This problem highlights the importance of identifying additional drugs for prophylaxis in these patients.

Toxoplasmosis in BMT patients frequently involves the lung (usually in the setting of multiorgan disease), with a high associated mortality (>90%). Most patients die within 7 days of onset of pulmonary symptoms and often have acute respiratory distress syndrome. In a review of 25 cases of pulmonary toxoplasmosis in BMT, onset of symptoms referable to the lungs occurred from 7 days to 1 year post-BMT; the majority occurred in the first 6 weeks.[193] Fever may be the first sign; if pulmonary infiltrates are observed, especially in the setting of rapid deterioration, immediate attempts at diagnosis must be made and empirical treatment begun. Undoubtedly, the high mortality in many instances has been due to the lack of early diagnosis and treatment. The organism can be observed on microscopic examination of BAL material. PCR performed on material obtained at BAL may be the diagnostic procedure of choice[193] PCR also can be performed on blood, serum, CSF, and bone marrow aspirates.

Ocular toxoplasmosis has been reported after allogeneic and autologous BMT and HSCT. In some cases, the ocular disease was due to reactivation of a previously observed toxoplasmic chorioretinitis, whereas in most, it was associated with disseminated infection. Definitive diagnosis has been made by direct observation of the parasite on histopathology sections, culture of tissue samples, or by PCR on vitreous fluid.

TOXOPLASMOSIS IN THE PATIENT WITH ACQUIRED IMMUNODEFICIENCY SYNDROME

Clinical manifestations of toxoplasmosis in AIDS patients commonly reflect encephalitis (i.e., TE), the lung (pneumonitis), and the eye (chorioretinitis).[137] Toxoplasmosis with multiorgan involvement manifesting with acute respiratory failure and hemodynamic abnormalities, similar to septic shock, has been reported, although septic shock has not been definitely proved to be due to *T. gondii*.[194] TE is the most common presentation of toxoplasmosis in AIDS patients[65] and is a frequent cause of focal CNS lesions in AIDS.[65] A wide range of clinical findings including altered mental state, seizures, weakness, cranial nerve disturbances, sensory abnormalities, cerebellar signs, meningismus, movement disorders, and neuropsychiatric manifestations are seen in TE. The characteristic presentation usually has a subacute onset with focal neurologic abnormalities in 58% to 89% of patients. However, in 15% to 25% of cases, the clinical presentation may be more abrupt, with seizures or cerebral hemorrhage. Most commonly, hemiparesis or abnormalities of speech, or both, are the major initial manifestations. Brain stem involvement often produces cranial nerve lesions, and many patients exhibit cerebral dysfunction with disorientation, altered mental state, lethargy, and coma. Less commonly, parkinsonism, focal dystonia, rubral tremor, hemichorea-hemiballismus, panhypopituitarism, diabetes insipidus, or the syndrome of inappropriate antidiuretic hormone secretion may dominate the clinical picture. In some patients, neuropsychiatric symptoms such as paranoid psychosis, dementia, anxiety, and agitation may be the major manifestations.

Diffuse TE[141] has been reported in relatively few AIDS patients; its actual incidence is unknown. This form of TE may manifest acutely and can be fatal rapidly; generalized cerebral dysfunction without focal signs is the most common manifestation, and CT scan findings may be within normal limits or reveal cerebral atrophy.

Spinal cord involvement by *T. gondii* in AIDS patients manifests as motor or sensory disturbances of single or multiple limbs, bladder or bowel dysfunctions, or both, and local pain. Patients may present with a clinical syndrome resembling a spinal cord tumor. Reports of cervical myelopathy,[195] thoracic myelopathy,[196] and conus medullaris syndrome[197] have been published.

Pulmonary disease due to toxoplasmosis has been reported in patients with AIDS, and the diagnosis may be made by demonstration of the parasite in BAL fluid.[198] In France, before HAART and the routine use of prophylaxis, the prevalence of pulmonary toxoplasmosis in patients dually infected with HIV and *T. gondii* was estimated to be approximately 5%.[199] Pulmonary toxoplasmosis occurs mainly in patients with advanced AIDS (mean CD4 count = 40 cells/µL ± 75 SD) and primarily presents as a prolonged febrile illness with cough and dyspnea,[198] which may be clinically indistinguishable from *Pneumocystis* pneumonia. Mortality, even with appropriate treatment, may be as high as 35%. Extrapulmonary disease may be present in approximately 50% of cases with toxoplasmic pneumonitis.[194] Often, pulmonary toxoplasmosis is not associated with TE; however, TE may develop after successful treatment of pulmonary toxoplasmosis when therapy is discontinued. The differential diagnosis of toxoplasmic pneumonitis includes *Pneumocystis* pneumonia and infection with *M. tuberculosis*, *C. neoformans*, *Coccidioides* spp., and *Histoplasma capsulatum*.

Toxoplasmic chorioretinitis is seen relatively infrequently in AIDS patients[200]; it commonly manifests with ocular pain and loss of visual acuity (Fig. 279-4). Funduscopic examination usually demonstrates necrotizing lesions that may be multifocal or bilateral.[200] Overlying vitreal inflammation is often present and may be extensive. The optic nerve may be involved in as many as 10% of cases. Toxoplasmic chorioretinitis in AIDS patients has been associated with concurrent TE in as many as 63% of patients. The differential diagnosis of toxoplasmic chorioretinitis in AIDS patients includes CMV retinitis, syphilis, herpes simplex, varicella zoster, and fungal infections. The diagnosis relies primarily on clinical findings and the response to anti–*T. gondii* therapy, although definitive diagnosis may be made by demonstration of the organism in retinal biopsy specimens,[200] isolation of the parasite from vitreous aspirates,[201] or amplification of the parasite DNA by PCR.[145]

Gastrointestinal involvement may result in abdominal pain, ascites (due to involvement of the stomach, peritoneum, or pancreas), or diarrhea. Acute hepatic failure due to *T. gondii* has been reported,[160] as has musculoskeletal involvement.[153]

Although the incidence of toxoplasmosis in HIV-infected patients began to decrease after the widespread use of TMP-SMX for PCP prophylaxis, the incidence decreased dramatically as a result of the immune reconstitution associated with HAART regimens. Approximately fourfold decreases in both incidence and deaths have been reported after the wide availability of HAART regimens.[66,67,202] Yet despite this, TE remains one of the most common HIV-related neurologic disorders, accounting for 26% of such cases in one recent study, with a 1-year estimated survival rate of 77%.[203] In contrast to mycobacterial and cryptococcal infections, immune reconstitution inflammatory syndrome after the initiation of HAART has been only rarely reported in association with toxoplasmosis.[204,205] In patients with CD4 counts that are sustained at levels higher than 200 cells/µL for 3 to 6 months while receiving HAART, prophylaxis regimens can be safely discontinued, although rare cases of disease can occur even in patients with well-controlled HIV infection.[206-209]

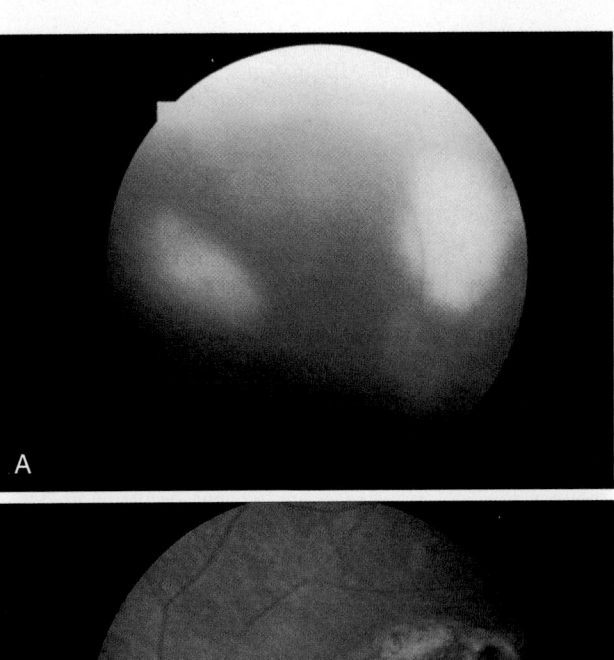

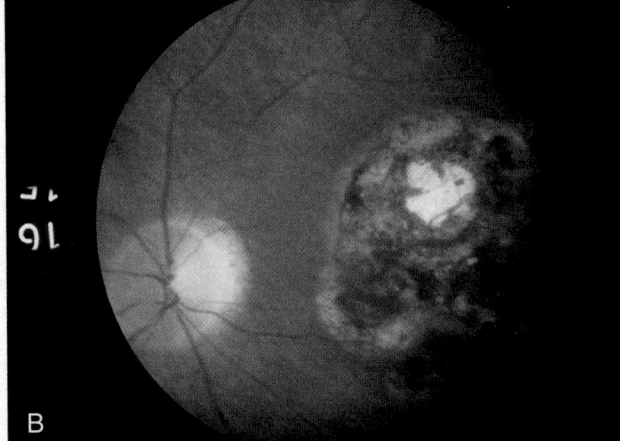

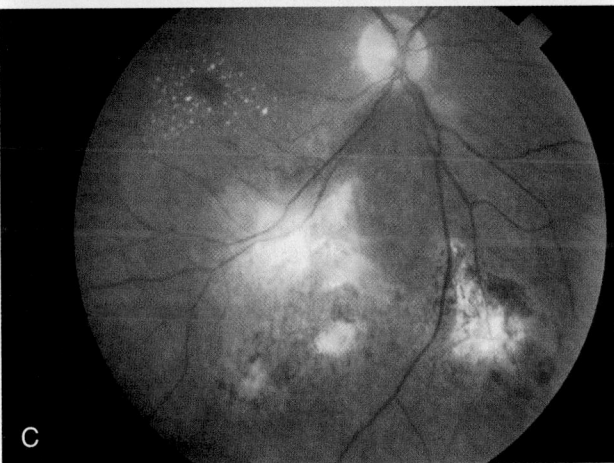

Figure 279-4 **Toxoplasmic chorioretinitis. A,** Active chorioretinitis with two lesions and vitreous haze in a patient infected with human immunodeficiency virus. **B,** A large inactive macular lesion typical of congenital disease. **C,** Active chorioretinitis in an immunocompetent patient from an endemic region in Brazil. There is an inactive lesion on the right. Note the macular star, which is due to an exudate around the macula. *(Courtesy of Dr. Robert Nussenblatt, National Eye Institute, Bethesda, MD; Dr. Claudio Silveira, Erechim, Brazil; and Dr. Rubens Belfort, São Paulo, Brazil.)*

There are no data on whether the strain of *T. gondii* affects the clinical outcome of infection in AIDS patients, and there are conflicting reports on whether a particular strain is more likely to cause infection in such patients.[12,210]

OCULAR TOXOPLASMOSIS IN IMMUNOCOMPETENT PATIENTS

T. gondii is one of the most frequently identified etiologies of uveitis and the most commonly identified pathogen to infect the retina of otherwise immunocompetent individuals.[9] Toxoplasmosis is responsible for more than 85% of posterior uveitis cases in southern Brazil, where in one study, typical lesions developed in 9.5% of 21 seroconverters and 8.3% of 131 seropositive patients without ocular involvement during 7 years of follow-up.[211-213] Chorioretinal lesions may result from congenital or postnatally acquired infection. In both these situations, lesions may occur during the acute or latent (chronic) stage of the infection.[171,214] Recurrences are frequent, occurring in 79% of patients followed for more than 5 years in one study, with a median time to recurrence of 2 years; they tend to occur immediately after an episode, are more common in patients older than 40 years old, are more common in the eye originally involved, and may be more common after cataract extraction.[215-217]

It is frequently difficult to determine whether the original infection was congenital or acquired in patients with recurrences of chorioretinitis.[172] Patients who present with chorioretinitis as a late sequela of the infection acquired in utero tend to have more severe disease and are more frequently in the second and third decades of life (it is rare after the age of 40 years); bilateral disease, old retinal scars, and involvement of the macula are hallmarks of the retinal disease in these cases as are recurrences (see Fig. 279-4).[218] By contrast, patients who present with toxoplasmic chorioretinitis in the setting of acute toxoplasmosis are more often between the fourth and sixth decades of life, most often have unilateral involvement, and have eye lesions that usually spare the macula and do not present with associated old scars.[171,172]

Whereas acquired *T. gondii* infection in otherwise healthy adults is most often subclinical, toxoplasmic chorioretinitis in these individuals may result in complete or partial loss of vision or in glaucoma and may necessitate enucleation.[144,218] Acute chorioretinitis may produce symptoms of blurred vision, scotoma, pain, photophobia, and epiphora. Impairment or a loss of central vision occurs when the macula is involved. As inflammation resolves, vision improves, frequently without complete recovery of visual acuity. In most cases, toxoplasmic chorioretinitis is diagnosed by ophthalmologic examination, and empirical therapy directed against the organism is often instituted based on clinical findings and serologic test results. Typical features of toxoplasmic chorioretinitis include intensely white focal lesions with an overlying, intense, vitreous inflammatory reaction (see Fig. 279-4). Focal necrotizing retinitis initially appears in the fundus as a yellowish-white, elevated cotton patch with indistinct margins, usually on the posterior pole. The lesions are often in small clusters, and individual lesions in the cluster may be of varied ages. With healing, the lesions become pale, atrophy, and develop black pigment (see Fig. 279-4). There can also be an associated secondary iridocyclitis and increased intraocular pressure.[144] The classic "headlight in the fog" appearance is due to the presence of active retinal lesions with severe vitreous inflammatory reaction. The choroid is secondarily inflamed. Recurrent lesions tend to occur at the borders of chorioretinal scars, and scars are often found in clusters. Panuveitis may accompany chorioretinitis, but isolated anterior uveitis has never been proven to occur.

Although the morphology of the lesions of acute toxoplasmic chorioretinitis in the setting of postnatally acquired disease may be indistinguishable from those observed in patients who have acute eye disease in later life due to a congenitally acquired infection, it is important to attempt to establish which type of the infection (postnatally acquired or congenital) is occurring in a given patient.[171] It seems that the congenitally acquired disease has a more guarded prognosis. From the public health perspective, it is important epidemiologically to establish whether the patient has acute acquired infection, to initiate efforts to identify the possible source of *T. gondii* infection, and to determine whether other individuals who may be at high risk of the development of severe, life-threatening disease (i.e., fetuses of serologically negative pregnant women or immunodeficient individuals) shared the same exposure as the individual with acute acquired toxoplasmic chorioretinitis. Serologic tests have been useful in establishing whether such patients have been infected recently.[170,171] In patients with chorioretinitis and IgG antibodies, additional serologic tests should be performed to determine whether the patient's infection is recently acquired.[171]

T. gondii chorioretinitis may resemble the posterior uveitis of tuberculosis, syphilis, leprosy, or presumed ocular histoplasmosis syndrome.

Atypical clinical and serologic manifestations of toxoplasmic chorioretinitis have been reported most commonly in elderly and in immunodeficient individuals.[145,219] Patients are considered to have atypical-appearing lesions when one or more of the following features are present: multiple foci of active retinitis, acute retinal necrosis syndrome (vitreitis, peripheral retinitis, retinal vasculitis), significant intraretinal hemorrhage, an absence of ophthalmoscopically visible chorioretinal scarring. In patients with atypical lesions or an inadequate clinical response to anti-*Toxoplasma* therapy or in whom other diagnostic procedures have not proved helpful, obtaining vitreous or aqueous fluid (in some cases, indicated for therapeutic reasons as well) for PCR should be considered early in the workup (see "Diagnosis").[146] In the future, it may be possible to determine which strain of the parasite is responsible for the infection and make a more accurate prognosis. Preliminary indications are that strain type may play an important role in determining the course of the infection,[151,152] and methods to distinguish strain type by looking for strain-specific antibodies using polymorphic peptides have shown some promise.[220]

TOXOPLASMOSIS DURING PREGNANCY

As in other immunocompetent individuals, acute *Toxoplasma* infection is asymptomatic in the majority of pregnant women. The most commonly recognized clinical manifestation of recent infection is regional lymphadenopathy. The primary concern is of transmission of infection to the fetus. The risk to the fetus does not correlate with whether the infection in the mother was symptomatic or asymptomatic during gestation. Transmission to the fetus has been limited almost solely to those women who acquire the infection during gestation. Otherwise healthy women who had *Toxoplasma* infection before becoming pregnant are protected from transmitting the infection to their fetuses. Rare exceptions to this dictum have been observed. In immunocompetent women infected with *T. gondii* shortly before conception, transmission to the fetus has occurred; in these very rare instances, the acute infection was acquired within 3 months of conception.[221-223] Transmission to the fetus has been rarely recognized as a consequence of reactivation of latent *T. gondii* infection in immunocompromised women infected with *T. gondii* before conception (chronic infection) (e.g., pregnant women coinfected with HIV and *T. gondii*,[224] patients with systemic lupus erythematosus who are being treated with corticosteroids). In addition, reinfection with a second, more aggressive strain of *T. gondii* of otherwise healthy pregnant women who are already chronically infected with the parasite has been proposed and documented as a possible mechanism of transmission to the fetus.[221]

CONGENITAL TOXOPLASMOSIS

Congenital infection may present in one of five forms: (1) ultrasound abnormalities consistent with toxoplasmosis or positive amniotic fluid PCR test results in the fetus; (2) neonatal disease; (3) disease (mild or severe) occurring in the first months of life; (4) sequelae or relapse of a previously undiagnosed infection during infancy, childhood, or adolescence; (5) subclinical infection.

Data accumulated from prospective studies indicate that the incidence and severity of congenital toxoplasmosis vary with the trimester during which the infection was acquired by the mother.[8] Moreover, there is an inverse relationship between the frequency of transmission and the severity of disease. Infants born of mothers who acquire their infection in the first or second trimester more frequently show severe congenital toxoplasmosis.[225] In contrast, the majority of children born of women who acquire their infection during the third trimester are born with the subclinical form of the infection. However, if left untreated, signs and symptoms of the disease develop in as many as 85% of these latter children, in most cases, chorioretinitis or delays in development.[226,227]

Infection acquired in the first trimester by women who were not treated with anti–*T. gondii* drugs resulted in congenital infection in 10% to 25% of cases.[225] For second- and third-trimester infections, the incidences of fetal infection ranged between 30% and 54% and 60% and 65%, respectively.[225] Early treatment of the mother with spiramycin seems to reduce the incidence of congenital infection by approximately 60%.[225,228-231] Maternal infection acquired around the time of conception and within the first 2 weeks of gestation and treated with spiramycin usually does not result in transmission.[230] Because of the high transmission rates observed in the late second trimester and during the third trimester, it is recommended that in patients in whom acute infection is highly suspected or confirmed of having occurred at 18 weeks of gestation or later, pyrimethamine-sulfadiazine be used. Recently, a group of European investigators suggested that the beneficial effects of the use of spiramycin or pyrimethamine-sulfadiazine during pregnancy on preventing vertical transmission or disease in the offspring by *T. gondii* need to be reevaluated with large randomized, placebo-controlled clinical trials (see "Treatment").

Frequency of transmission to the fetus and severity of disease in the offspring seem to be significantly affected by drug treatment with spiramycin and pyrimethamine-sulfadiazine, respectively. In cohorts in which most of the mothers were treated during gestation, transmission rates were low in the first trimester (i.e., 6% [95% confidence interval, 3% to 9%] at 13 weeks) and significantly increased as expected with advancing gestational age (i.e., 40% [95% confidence interval, 33% to 47% at 26 weeks and 72% [60% to 81%] at 36 weeks).[232] In contrast, clinical signs in the infected infant are more likely observed in offspring of women whose infection was acquired early in gestation. Depending on when during gestation the mother acquired her infection, the risk of severity of clinical manifestations in an infected fetus is 61% (95% confidence interval, 34% to 85%) at 13 weeks, 25% (95% confidence interval, 18% to 33%) at 26 weeks, and 9% (95% confidence interval, 4% to 17%) at 36 weeks.[232]

In addition to gestational age and treatment, transmission rates and severity of congenital disease are also likely to be affected by the strain of the parasite, parasite load,[233] and the immune status and genetics of the host.

Clinical manifestations of congenital toxoplasmosis vary. Most signs and clinical presentations are nonspecific and may mimic disease due to organisms such as herpes simplex virus, CMV, and rubella virus. Signs include chorioretinitis, strabismus, blindness, epilepsy, psychomotor or mental retardation, anemia, jaundice, rash, petechiae due to thrombocytopenia, encephalitis, pneumonitis, microcephaly, intracranial calcification, hydrocephalus, diarrhea, hypothermia, and nonspecific illness.[8] There may be no sequelae, or sequelae may develop or be evident at various times after birth. *T. gondii* infection is not known to cause fetal malformations by affecting the host's DNA.

A detailed examination by an experienced clinician may be necessary to detect signs of the infection.[8] In one prospective study,[234] 210 congenitally infected infants were identified: 2 patients (0.9%) died, 21 (10.9%) had severe disease, 71 (33.8%) were mildly afflicted, and 116 (54.4%) were without signs of the infection. More intensive examination of the latter 116 infants revealed abnormalities in 39; abnormal CSF was detected in 22 infants, chorioretinitis was seen in 17, and intracranial calcifications were found in 10. Premature infants often have CNS disease and ocular disease in the first 3 months of life. A milder disease frequently develops in full-term infants manifested by hepatosplenomegaly and lymphadenopathy that usually appears in the first 2 months of life. In these infants, disease reflecting damage to the CNS may occur later, and eye disease may occur months to years after birth.

Signs or symptoms of congenital toxoplasmosis subsequently develop in most infants with subclinical infection at birth.[227] In one study, clinical evaluation at a mean age of 8.3 years showed that 11 of the 13 infected children who had no signs of the disease after detailed examination in the newborn period experienced sequelae. Some of these children were treated with specific therapy in the newborn period. In each child, the initial manifestation was chorioretinitis, which appeared at a mean age of 3.7 years. Three children had unilateral blindness, whereas the other eight children had no loss of visual function. Neurologic sequelae developed in five children, including one child with delayed psychomotor development, microcephaly, and seizure disorder and two children with minor cerebellar signs. Sensorineural hearing loss occurred in 3 of 10 children evaluated. A study from The Netherlands[235] found that chorioretinitis developed in five of nine congenitally infected, untreated children followed for as long as 14 years. Information from prospective studies suggests that early initiation of specific therapy in those infants with congenital infection but without clinical signs will markedly reduce untoward sequelae.[236,237] In a recent study, in children who were diagnosed with toxoplasmic chorioretinitis only after their first year of life (and thus were not treated during their first year of life), new chorioretinal lesions were detected in more than 70% of the children when followed during their first decade of life.[238]

Among 108 congenitally infected children treated throughout their first year of life, at least one new chorioretinal lesion developed in 34 (31%); 14 (41%) of them had occurrences when they were 10 years or older, indicating that long-term follow-up is important in assessing the efficacy of treating toxoplasmosis during infancy.[239]

Uncommonly, latent *T. gondii* infection may reactivate in HIV-infected women and result in congenital transmission of the parasite. Congenital toxoplasmosis seems to occur more frequently in the offspring of women infected with both HIV and *T. gondii* than in those of women who are infected with *T. gondii* but not with HIV.[240] Infants with congenital toxoplasmosis born to HIV-infected mothers are also infected with HIV (suggesting that factors that predispose to the vertical transmission of HIV also favor the transmission of *T. gondii* or vice versa). Congenital toxoplasmosis in the HIV-infected infant seems to run a more rapid course than that in the non–HIV-infected infant, with the development of failure to thrive, fever, hepatosplenomegaly, chorioretinitis, and seizures. Most children have multiorgan involvement, including CNS, cardiac, and pulmonary disease.

It was recently reported that *T. gondii* causes more severe ocular disease in congenitally infected children in Brazil when compared with children in Europe.[149] This may be explained by the fact that pregnant women in Brazil are not routinely screened and treated for toxoplasmosis during gestation and possibly that more virulent genotypes of the parasite predominate in Brazil but are rarely found in Europe.

Congenital toxoplasmosis must be differentiated from rubella virus, CMV, herpes simplex virus, human herpesvirus 6, parvovirus B19, and lymphocytic choriomeningitis virus infections; syphilis, listeriosis, and other bacterial infections; other infectious encephalopathies; erythroblastosis fetalis; and sepsis. Herpes simplex virus, CMV, rubella virus, and syphilis may cause chorioretinitis; both CMV and rubella have been associated with hydrocephalus, microcephaly, and cerebral calcification. A markedly elevated CSF protein concentration is a hallmark of congenital toxoplasmosis.

T. gondii infection acquired during pregnancy has been implicated in spontaneous abortion, stillbirth, and premature births. On rare occasion, *T. gondii* has been isolated from the abortuses of women with chronic infection, but the frequency of *T. gondii* infection as a cause of abortion is unknown and controversial.

As with ocular disease, the strain of *T. gondii* may have an impact on the outcome of congenital infection. Studies in Europe have revealed conflicting data on whether type I strains, in particular, might be more likely to be responsible for congenital infection and/or serious disease.[13,14,241] As more accurate and sensitive tests for determining the genotype of an infecting strain are developed, this picture could change significantly.

Diagnosis

When considering toxoplasmosis in the differential diagnosis of a patient's illness, emphasis should not be placed on whether the patient has been exposed to cats. Transmission of oocysts virtually always occurs without knowledge of the patient and may be unrelated to direct exposure to a cat (e.g., transmission by contaminated vegetables or water). Patients with an indoor cat or cats that are fed only cooked food are not at risk of acquiring the infection from that cat. Serologic investigation of a cat to establish whether it is a potential source of the infection should be discouraged; the prevalence of *T. gondii* antibodies among cats in a given locale is usually similar to their prevalence in humans. Seropositivity does not predict shedding of oocysts.

Because the clinical manifestations of *T. gondii* infection may be protean and nonspecific, toxoplasmosis must be carefully considered in the differential diagnosis of a large variety of clinical presentations. The correct diagnostic tests must be performed and appropriately interpreted in light of the patient's clinical presentation. The usefulness of a given diagnostic method may differ considerably with the clinical entity, which can be toxoplasmosis in the immunocompetent or immunodeficient patient, ocular toxoplasmosis, toxoplasmosis in pregnancy, or congenital toxoplasmosis.[242]

Acute infection is diagnosed by the isolation of *T. gondii* or amplification of its DNA in blood or body fluids; demonstration of tachyzoites in histologic sections of tissue or in cytologic preparations of body fluids, the demonstration of a characteristic lymph node histologic appearance or of characteristic serologic test results, or demonstration of *T. gondii* tissue cysts in the placenta, fetus, or neonate.[8] Rarely, asymptomatic patients with latent infection have recurrent parasitemia.[243] Isolation of *T. gondii* from the tissues of older children or adults may only reflect the presence of tissue cysts. Finding numerous tissue cysts in tissue sections especially associated with inflammation suggests but does not prove the presence of active infection.

ISOLATION OF *TOXOPLASMA GONDII*

Isolation of *T. gondii* from blood or body fluids establishes that the infection is acute. In neonates, isolation of the organism from the placenta is highly suggestive of fetal involvement; isolation from fetal tissues is diagnostic of congenital infection.[8] Attempts at isolation of the parasite can be performed by mouse inoculation or inoculation of tissue cell cultures.[8] In tissue cell cultures, parasite-laden cells can be demonstrated with appropriate staining, and plaques are formed in which tachyzoites are easily recognized. Tissue cell culture has the advantage of widespread availability (e.g., virology laboratories) and yields results more rapidly (within 3 to 6 days) than does mouse inoculation. However, mouse inoculation is more sensitive.

HISTOLOGIC DIAGNOSIS

Demonstration of tachyzoites in tissue sections or smears of body fluid (e.g., CSF, amniotic fluid, BAL) establishes the diagnosis of acute infection.[8] It is often difficult to demonstrate tachyzoites in stained tissue sections. However, multiple tissue cysts near an inflammatory necrotic lesion probably establish the diagnosis.[244] Fluorescent antibody staining may be useful, but this method often yields nonspecific results.[245] The immunoperoxidase technique, which uses antisera to *T. gondii*, has proved both sensitive and specific; it has been used successfully in clinical settings to demonstrate the organisms in the CNS of patients with TE.[24] Both the fluorescent antibody and immunoperoxidase methods are applicable to unfixed or formalin-fixed, paraffin-embedded tissue sections.[24] Fluorescein-labeled monoclonal antibodies to *T. gondii* for

staining touch preparations of specimens[246] and rapid electron microscopy[247] have been used successfully to diagnose TE.

A rapid, technically simple, but underused method is the detection of *T. gondii* in air-dried, Wright-Giemsa–stained slides of centrifuged (e.g., cytocentrifuge) sediment of CSF or of brain aspirate or in impression smears of biopsy tissue.

Endomyocardial biopsy has been used successfully to diagnose toxoplasmosis in heart transplant recipients.[248] Characteristic histologic criteria alone are probably sufficient to establish the diagnosis of toxoplasmic lymphadenitis in older children and adults.[131]

POLYMERASE CHAIN REACTION

PCR amplification for the detection of *T. gondii* DNA in body fluids and tissues has successfully diagnosed congenital,[230,249] ocular,[145,146] cerebral, and disseminated toxoplasmosis.[250,251] PCR of amniotic fluid has revolutionized the diagnosis of intrauterine *T. gondii* infection by enabling an early diagnosis to be made, thereby avoiding the use of invasive procedures on the fetus.[8] PCR has also been successfully used on samples of CSF, blood, urine, placenta, and fetal tissues for the diagnosis of congenital infection.[8,252] The sensitivity of PCR in CSF varies between 11% and 77%, whereas the specificity is close to 100%.[251] PCR may also detect the parasite in buffy coat specimens of AIDS patients with TE.[251] The sensitivity of PCR on whole blood or buffy coat ranges from 15% to 85%. PCR on blood seems to be a valuable tool primarily in patients with disseminated disease; it is less sensitive in the detection of TE because a relatively low percentage of AIDS patients with TE have parasitemia.[253,254] Therapy for toxoplasmosis seems to influence the sensitivity of the method; sensitivity is higher in CSF or blood samples collected before or within the first week of therapy.[251]

Because there is no standardized PCR assay, performance characteristics will vary widely depending on the laboratory, gene target, primers, and sample preparation.[255] Primers targeting the multicopy *B1* gene seem to be the most sensitive and are the most widely used.[255,256] For maximum reliability, clinical samples should be sent to reference laboratories experienced in performing this assay.

SEROLOGIC TESTS FOR DEMONSTRATION OF ANTIBODY

The use of serologic tests for the demonstration of specific antibody to *T. gondii* is the primary method of diagnosis. A large number of tests have been described, some of which are available only in highly specialized laboratories. Different serologic tests often measure different antibodies that possess unique patterns of rise and fall with the time after infection.[242] However, initial serologic testing can be accomplished by simultaneously requesting IgG and IgM antibody tests. Commercial or nonreference laboratories can easily perform this task. Only positive results in IgM antibody tests need to be sent for confirmatory testing to reference laboratories (see later).

There is no single serologic test that can be used to support the diagnosis of acute or chronic infection by *T. gondii*. In most cases, a battery of tests is required to enable the distinction between acute and chronic infection. Which particular combination of tests is used depends on the specific clinical category of the patient (i.e., pregnant vs. immunodeficient patient, see "Clinical Manifestations"), the interval between acquisition of infection and sampling of sera,[174] and the question posed by the practitioner. The clinician must be familiar with these problems and consult reference laboratories if the need arises. A panel of tests consisting of the Sabin-Feldman dye test (IgG); IgM, IgA, and IgE enzyme-linked immunosorbent assays (ELISAs); differential agglutination test (measures IgG antibody and is also known as the AC/HS test); and the IgG avidity is used successfully by the Palo Alto Medical Foundation Toxoplasma Serology Laboratory (PAMF-TSL, 650-853-4828; http://www.pamf.org/serology/) to determine whether serologic test results are more likely consistent with infection acquired in the recent or more distant past.[132,171,174,257-259]

Immunoglobulin G Antibodies

The most widely used tests for the measurement of IgG antibody are the Sabin-Feldman dye test,[260] ELISA,[261,262] the indirect fluorescent antibody (IFA) test,[263] and the modified direct agglutination test.[264] In these tests, IgG antibodies usually appear within 1 to 2 weeks of acquisition of the infection, peak within 1 to 2 months, decrease at variable rates, and usually persist for life at relatively low titers.

Recent reports have shown that detecting antibodies to strain-specific peptides can reveal the genotype of the infecting strain, although this approach has yet to be developed into a reliable, clinically useful diagnostic method.[220]

Sabin-Feldman Dye Test

The Sabin-Feldman dye test is the reference serologic test against which other methods have been evaluated.[260] It is a sensitive and specific neutralization test. It measures primarily IgG antibodies that usually appear 1 to 2 weeks after the initiation of infection, reach peak titers in 6 to 8 weeks, and then gradually decline over 1 to 2 years.[8] Titers, usually at low levels, probably persist for life. This test is available in only a few reference laboratories, primarily because live organisms are required. A negative Sabin-Feldman dye test practically rules out previous exposure to *T. gondii* except in patients who have been infected very recently (e.g., within 1 to 2 weeks of exposure), are significantly immunocompromised (e.g., allogeneic bone marrow transplant patients), or have a primary immunodeficiency (e.g., congenital agammaglobulinemia). However, although rare, cases of documented TE and chorioretinitis have been reported in patients with negative dye test results.

Indirect Fluorescent Antibody Test

The IFA test seems to measure the same antibodies as the dye test, and its titers tend to parallel dye test titers.[8] False-positive results may occur with sera that contain antinuclear antibodies,[265] and false-negative results may occur in sera with low IgG antibody titers.

Agglutination Test

The agglutination test using formalin-preserved whole tachyzoites is available commercially (BioMérieux, Marcy-l'Etoile, France) and detects IgG antibody. The test is very sensitive to IgM antibody, and "natural" IgM antibody causes nonspecific agglutination in sera that yield negative results when tested using the dye test and the IFA test. This problem is avoided by including 2-mercaptoethanol in the test. The method is accurate, simple to perform, inexpensive, and excellent for screening purposes.[266] This method should not be used for the measurement of IgM antibodies.

When two different compounds (i.e., acetone and formalin) are used to fix parasites for use in the agglutination test, a "differential" agglutination test (AC/HS test) results because the different antigenic preparations vary in their ability to recognize sera obtained during the acute and chronic stages of the infection.[267] This test has proved useful in helping differentiate acute from chronic infections and is best used in combination with a battery of other tests.

Immunoglobulin G Enzyme-Linked Immunosorbent Assay

The IgG-ELISA method is now the most widely used for the demonstration of IgG antibodies to *T. gondii*. Most commercial IgG antibody test kits are accurate for the demonstration of IgG antibodies; however, it is important to recognize that one cannot use a single IgG titer, no matter what its level, to predict whether the infection was recently acquired or acquired in the distant past.

Immunoglobulin G Avidity Test

A number of tests for avidity of toxoplasma IgG antibodies have been introduced to help differentiate between recently acquired and distant infection.[268] This method is based on the observation that during acute *T. gondii* infection, IgG antibodies bind antigen weakly (i.e., have low avidity), whereas chronically infected patients have more strongly binding (high avidity) antibodies.[268] Protein-denaturing reagents, including urea, are used to dissociate the antibody-antigen complex. Low or equivocal avidity test results can persist for months to years after the primary infection,[268] and for this reason, a low or equivocal avidity test result must not be used to determine whether the infection was acquired recently. The time of conversion from low or equivocal to high avidity is highly variable among different individuals including pregnant women.[257,269,270] However, it has been demonstrated that once the avidity test result is high, the patient was infected at least 3 to 5 months earlier.[270] This timing depends on the method used. High avidity test results using the IgG VIDAS avidity test (VIDAS Toxoplasma IgG Avidity, BioMérieux), for example, have been essentially found only in pregnant women who have been infected for at least 4 months.[259,271]

At present, commercial avidity tests have not been released for marketing in the United States. The avidity test should only be used as an additional confirmatory diagnostic method in patients with positive and/or equivocal IgM test results or when the results of a battery of tests are equivocal or interpreted as consistent with the possibility of a recently acquired infection. Health care providers involved in the care of pregnant women should be aware that avidity testing is only a confirmatory test. It should not be used alone as a definitive test for decision making.

Immunoglobulin M Antibodies

IgM antibodies may appear earlier and decline more rapidly than IgG antibodies. IgM antibody tests have been widely used for the diagnosis of acute infection and to determine whether a pregnant woman has been infected during gestation or before conception. There has been a heightened awareness of the fact that titers in tests for IgM antibodies may persist for years after the acute infection and that the reliability of commercially available assays varies considerably.[272-274] Both the laboratory performing the test and the physician requesting the test should be aware of this problem. The U.S. Food and Drug Administration issued a health advisory to obstetricians, gynecologists, pediatricians, clinical pathologists, and infectious disease specialists warning about the use of *T. gondii* IgM commercial test kits as the sole determinant of recent infection in pregnant women.[275] At present, the decision to treat or undertake other medical interventions, including the termination of pregnancy, should be based on clinical evaluation and additional testing performed in reference or research laboratories with experience in the diagnosis of toxoplasmosis.[276] (For further discussion, see "*Toxoplasma gondii* Infection in Pregnancy.") The persistence of IgM antibodies for several years does not seem to have clinical significance.[8]

Indirect Fluorescent Antibody Test

IgM-IFA antibody appears within the first week of infection; titers increase rapidly, then decrease to low titers, and usually disappear within a few months. Low titers may persist for 1 year or longer.[277] Antinuclear antibodies and rheumatoid factor may cause false-positive results,[278] IgG-blocking antibodies can produce false-negative results in this test when IgG is not removed.[279]

Immunoglobulin M Enzyme-Linked Immunosorbent Assay

The double-sandwich IgM-ELISA for detection of IgM-specific antibodies to *T. gondii*[280-282] is currently the most widely used method for demonstration of IgM antibodies to *T. gondii* in adults, fetuses, and newborns.[218] In contrast to the conventional method in which the wells of microtiter plates are coated with antigen, the wells are coated with specific antibody to IgM. The double-sandwich IgM-ELISA is more sensitive than the IgM-IFA test for diagnosis of recently acquired infection, and serum samples that are negative on the dye test but that contain either antinuclear antibodies or rheumatoid factor and thus cause false-positive results of the IgM-IFA test are negative in the double-sandwich IgM-ELISA. This latter observation is attributed to the fact that serum IgM fractions are separated from IgG fractions during the initial step in the double-sandwich IgM-ELISA procedure.[218]

Despite the wide distribution of commercial test kits to measure IgM antibodies, these kits often have low specificity and the reported results are frequently misinterpreted. False-positive results and the problems associated with the persistence of positive titers even years after the initial infection remain major obstacles to correct interpretation of the results obtained with these tests.[273]

Immunoglobulin M Immunosorbent Agglutination Assay

The IgM-immunosorbent agglutination assay (ISAGA) (available from BioMérieux), which binds the patient's IgM to a solid surface and uses intact, killed tachyzoites to detect IgM antibodies, is highly sensitive.[283] The test is simple to perform, does not require the use of enzyme conjugate, and is read in the same manner as the agglutination test. Overall, it is more sensitive and specific than the IgM-IFA test. The presence of rheumatoid factor or antinuclear antibodies does not cause false-positive results in the IgM-ISAGA. In adults, it is more sensitive but much less specific than the double-sandwich IgM-ELISA method. In infants, the IgM-ISAGA is the most sensitive method and is used effectively for the diagnosis of congenital infection in infants 6 months of age or younger.[284] A positive IgM-ISAGA test result in the first 10 days of life should be repeated after 10 days to rule out the possibility of maternal contamination of IgM antibodies. The ISAGA method has also been used to detect IgA and IgE antibodies.

Immunoglobulin A Antibodies

IgA antibodies may be detected in sera of acutely infected adults and congenitally infected infants using ELISA or ISAGA.[285-287] As is true for IgM antibodies to the parasite, IgA antibodies may persist for many months or more than 1 year. For this reason, they are of little additional assistance for the diagnosis of the acute infection in the adult. In contrast, the increased sensitivity of IgA assays over IgM assays for the diagnosis of congenital toxoplasmosis represents a major advance in the serologic diagnosis of the infection in the fetus and newborn.[287] IgA antibodies are rarely detectable by ELISA in sera of AIDS patients with TE.[287] If IgA antibodies are detected in the newborn during the first 10 days of life, the test should be repeated 10 days after birth to make certain that what is being measured is not contaminating maternal IgA antibodies. The possibility that such contamination might occur is the reason that under most circumstances, peripheral blood rather than cord serum should be used to measure IgM, IgA, or IgE antibodies in the newborn.

Immunoglobulin E Antibodies

IgE antibodies are detectable by ELISA in sera of acutely infected adults,[288,289] congenitally infected infants,[288,289] and children with congenital toxoplasmic chorioretinitis.[290] The duration of IgE seropositivity is briefer than that with IgM or IgA antibodies and hence seems to be useful for identifying recently acquired infections.[174,289] T. gondii–specific IgE antibody has been detected in patients with TE and may be useful as a marker for TE in this population of patients.[289] Recently, an IgE-ELISA was assessed by studying 2036 sera from 792 subjects with and without toxoplasmosis.[291] IgE antibodies were present in 85.7% of asymptomatic seroconverters and in 100% of seroconverters with overt toxoplasmosis. For neonatal diagnosis of congenital toxoplasmosis, IgE was less sensitive than IgM and IgA, but simultaneous measurement of the three immunoglobulins at birth improved the diagnostic yield to 81%.[291] Emergence of specific IgE during postnatal treatment for congenital toxoplasmosis may indicate poor adherence or inadequate dosing.

RADIOLOGIC METHODS

Radiologic studies are of particular help in patients with toxoplasmosis of the CNS. The presence of calcifications in the brain of a newborn, detected by radiography, ultrasonography, or CT, should heighten the suspicion of T. gondii as the cause of the disease (Fig. 279-5A). In severely affected infants with congenital toxoplasmosis, unilateral or, more often, bilateral and symmetrical dilatation of the ventricles is a common finding.[218]

In the majority of immunodeficient patients with TE, CT scans show multiple bilateral cerebral lesions.[292] Although multiple lesions are more common in toxoplasmosis, they also may be solitary; a single lesion should not exclude TE as a diagnostic possibility. Clinicians should be aware that toxoplasmosis may manifest as an encephalitis that at autopsy is "diffuse," in which case, the neuroimaging study results may appear normal or reveal findings suggestive of HIV encephalopathy.[141]

CT scans in AIDS patients with TE reveal multiple ring-enhancing lesions in 70% to 80% of the cases.[137] In AIDS patients with detectable Toxoplasma IgG and multiple ring-enhancing lesions on CT or MRI who are not receiving appropriate antiretroviral treatment or anti-Toxoplasma prophylaxis, the predictive value for TE is approximately 80%.[293] Lesions tend to occur at the corticomedullary junction (frequently involving the basal ganglia) and are characteristically hypodense.[294,295] The number of lesions is frequently underestimated by CT, although delayed imaging after a double dose of intravenous contrast material may improve the sensitivity of this modality.[294-296] An enlarging hypodense lesion that does not enhance is a poor prognostic sign.[297] TE lesions on MRI studies appear as high signal abnormalities on T_2-weighted studies and reveal a rim of enhancement surrounding the edema on T_1-weighted contrast-enhanced images (see Fig. 279-5B and C). MRI has superior sensitivity (particularly if gadolinium is used for contrast) compared with CT and often demonstrates a lesion or lesions or more extensive disease not seen by CT.[296,298] Hence, MRI should be used as the initial study when feasible (or if a single lesion is demonstrated by CT). Nevertheless, even characteristic lesions on CT or MRI studies are not pathognomonic of TE. The major differential diagnosis of focal CNS lesions in AIDS patients is CNS lymphoma, which may manifest with multiple enhancing lesions in 40% of cases. The probability of TE decreases and the probability of lymphoma increases in the presence of single lesions on MRI.[292] A brain biopsy may therefore be required in the patient with a solitary lesion (especially if confirmed by MRI) to obtain a definitive diagnosis.[299]

In AIDS patients with TE, CT scan improvement is seen in as many as 90% of patients after 2 to 3 weeks of treatment.[292,294] Complete resolution takes from 6 weeks to 12 months; peripheral lesions resolve more rapidly than deeper ones. Smaller lesions usually resolve completely, as shown by MRI studies, within 3 to 5 weeks, but lesions with a mass effect tend to resolve more slowly and leave a small residual lesion.[300] A radiologic response to therapy lags behind the clinical response with better correlation between them observed by the end of acute therapy.[301]

CT and MRI in toxoplasmic myelopathy usually demonstrates localized enlargement of the spinal cord,[196,302] which may result in obstruction to dye flow on myelography.[196] Gadolinium enhancement of MRI studies usually highlights as an intramedullary lesion at the site of spinal cord enlargement.[302]

A variety of positron emission tomography scanning,[303] radionuclide scanning,[304] and magnetic resonance techniques[305] have been used to evaluate AIDS patients with focal CNS lesions, specifically to differentiate between toxoplasmosis and primary CNS lymphoma.[305] [18F]-Fluorodeoxyglucose positron emission tomography scanning is now widely used in the evaluation of patients with tumors. There is a significantly higher uptake of [18F]-fluorodeoxyglucose in patients with cerebral lymphoma than in patients with TE.[306] Radionuclide scanning has also been used to differentiate between CNS toxoplasmosis and lymphoma. Neoplasms usually demonstrate increased uptake of thallium-201 on both early and late scanning.[305] Although published studies suggest a high sensitivity and specificity of these studies, in practice, they often are not helpful, in part because of variability of uptake and in part because they are often used after an empirical trial of anti-Toxoplasma therapy. Thallium scans may have decreased diagnostic utility in the setting of HAART.[307]

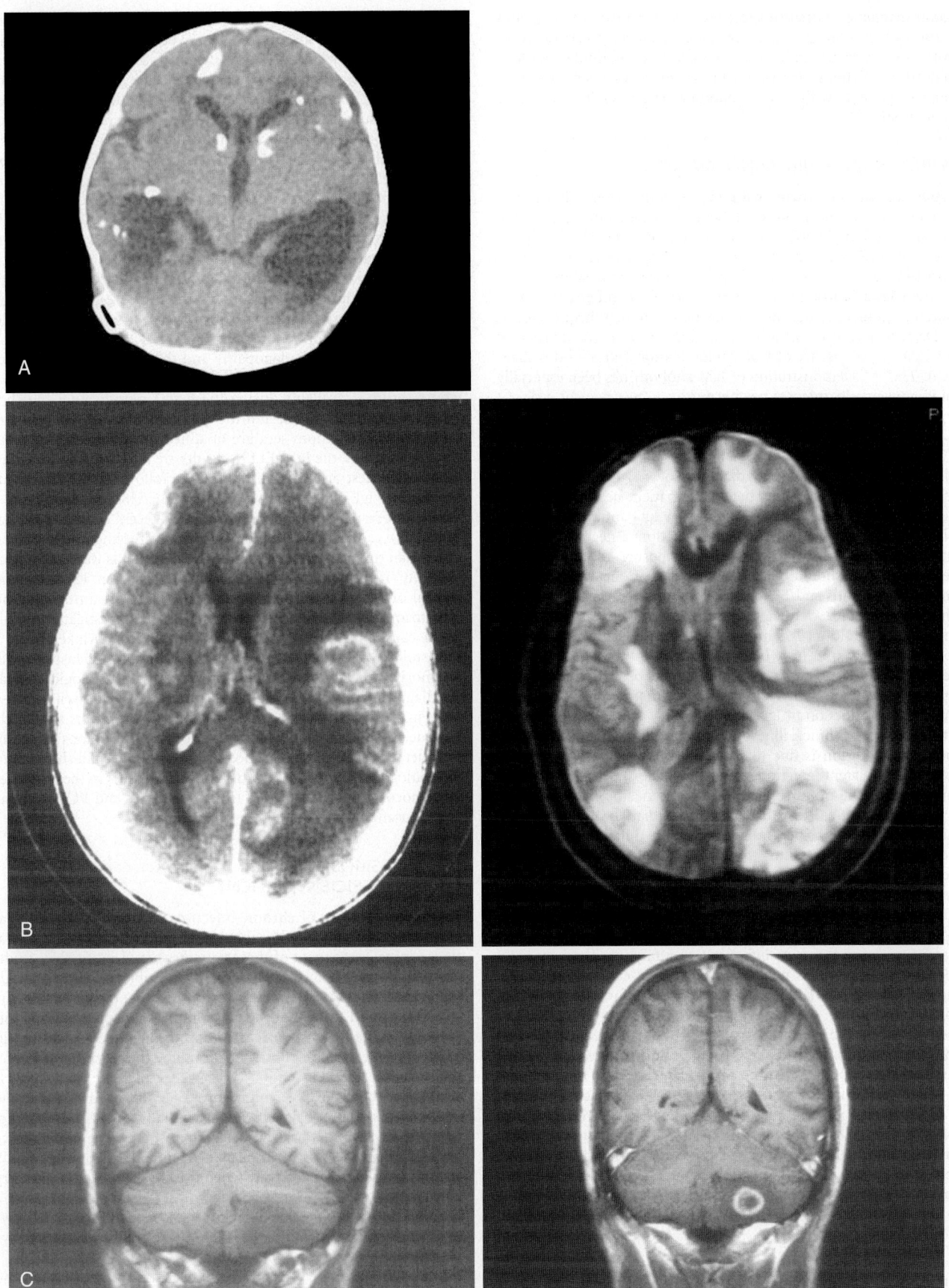

Figure 279-5 Imaging studies of central nervous system toxoplasmosis. A, Computed tomography scan of an infant born with congenital toxoplasmosis, illustrating the calcifications and hydrocephalus that are typically seen in the brain. **B,** Computed tomography scan with contrast enhancement (*left*) and T_2-weighted magnetic resonance imaging scan (*right*) of an acquired immunodeficiency syndrome patient with toxoplasmic encephalitis, demonstrating multiple lesions, which are more easily identified in the MRI scan. **C,** T_1-weighted magnetic resonance imaging scan, without (*left*) and with (*right*) contrast enhancement, of an acquired immunodeficiency syndrome patient with toxoplasmic encephalitis. Note the ring-enhancing lesion on the right.

Proton magnetic resonance spectroscopy to evaluate brain lesions has been used in a few patients. Magnetic resonance spectroscopy in patients with TE reveals an increase in the lactate and lipid contents[305] and a decrease in choline levels. In contrast, magnetic resonance spectroscopy in patients with CNS lymphoma reveals slightly increased levels of choline.[305]

CEREBROSPINAL FLUID ABNORMALITIES

CSF abnormalities in patients with TE are nonspecific; mild mononuclear pleocytosis and mild to moderate elevations in CSF protein are often observed; hypoglycorrhachia is uncommon.[165,308] Almost unique to infants with neonatal toxoplasmosis, however, is the very high protein content of the ventricular fluid. Although in some infants, the protein level is just slightly above normal, in others, it can be measured in grams per deciliter rather than in milligrams per deciliter.[218] Demonstration of intrathecal production of T. gondii–specific IgG or IgM in the absence of CSF contamination with blood is diagnostic of TE.[309,310] Demonstration of IgM antibody has been especially useful in congenitally infected newborns.[8]

DIAGNOSIS OF SPECIFIC CLINICAL ENTITIES

The initial step in pursuing the diagnosis of T. gondii infection or toxoplasmosis is to determine whether the patient has been exposed to the parasite. In virtually all cases, tests for IgG antibodies reliably establish the presence or absence of the infection; a negative IgG test essentially rules out previous or recent exposure to the parasite. However, clinicians should be aware that cases of documented toxoplasmic chorioretinitis and TE in adult patients have been observed in which IgG antibodies were not demonstrable; such cases are very uncommon. In addition, IgG antibodies may be absent in immunocompetent patients who have been tested within the first 2 weeks of the acute infection, in patients post-BMT despite being detectable pretransplantation, and in patients with severe primary immunodeficiencies involving production of IgG antibodies.

In the presence of clinical illness, it is important to establish whether the patient's condition is due to a recently acquired infection or to recrudescence of latent infection (chronic infection) or is unrelated to the infection. A true negative IgM test in an otherwise immunologically normal individual essentially rules out that the infection was recently acquired. A positive IgM test is more difficult to interpret correctly. One must not assume that a positive IgM test result is diagnostic of recently acquired infection. The presence of T. gondii–specific IgM antibodies can be interpreted as a true positive result consistent with recently acquired infection, a true positive result consistent with a chronic infection (IgM antibodies have been shown to persist for as long as 5 years after the acute infection), or a false-positive result. To establish which of these is most likely in a given case, confirmatory testing in a reference laboratory should be performed whenever feasible.[273,275]

The use of a combination or battery of tests has been useful for determining whether the patient has been recently infected or infected in the more distant past.[174,258] If the patient has received a blood transfusion, serologic tests may measure exogenously administered rather than endogenous antibody. The use of serologic tests to evaluate the response to therapy should be discouraged. The Toxoplasma Serology Laboratory at the Palo Alto Medical Foundation currently serves as a reference laboratory. Physicians in the Toxoplasma Serology Laboratory also offer interpretation of test results and consultation on treatment and patient management to clinicians in the United States and worldwide.

TOXOPLASMOSIS IN THE IMMUNOCOMPETENT PATIENT

Tests for IgG and IgM antibodies should be used for initial evaluation of immunocompetent patients. Testing of serial specimens obtained 3 weeks apart (in parallel) provides the best discriminatory power if the results in the initial specimen are equivocal. Negative results in both of these tests virtually rule out the diagnosis of toxoplasmosis. Early in infection, IgG antibodies may not be detectable, whereas IgM antibodies are present (hence, the need for both tests to be performed). Acute infection is supported by documented seroconversion of IgG or IgM antibodies or a greater than two-tube increase in antibody titer in sera run in parallel. A single high titer of any immunoglobulin antibodies is insufficient to make the diagnosis; IgG antibodies may persist at high titers for many years,[8] and IgM antibodies may be detectable for more than 12 months. When only a single serum sample is available, a battery or combination of tests is usually required in determining the likelihood that the infection is acute.

Toxoplasmosis should be considered in the differential diagnosis of lymphadenopathy, whether or not symptoms are present and especially in those patients without symptoms. Confirmatory serologic tests should be performed in such patients. The interval between the clinical onset of lymphadenopathy and the date that the specimen is drawn is critical for interpretation of the test results.[174] In patients whose serum is available during the first 3 months after the clinical onset, at least the IgG test and the IgM-ELISA results are positive. In those patients in whom sera are obtained more than 3 months after the clinical onset, the IgM-ELISA results are most likely to be negative, but the IgG test and at least one of the following tests are positive: IgA-ELISA, IgE-ELISA, IgE-ISAGA, or AC/HS test.[174] A high IgG avidity test result in an individual who has recent onset of lymphadenopathy (e.g., within 2 to 3 months of sera sampling) suggests a cause other than toxoplasmosis,[311] and further workup is warranted. A nonacute AC/HS pattern in an individual at less than 12 months after clinical onset of lymphadenopathy should suggest an etiology other than toxoplasmic lymphadenitis. In such cases, investigation for alternative causes, including malignancy, should be undertaken.[311]

Histologic diagnosis can be useful in some cases of suspected toxoplasmosis in the immunocompetent patient. The histologic criteria for the diagnosis of toxoplasmic lymphadenitis has been well established (see Fig. 279-3A) (see "Histologic Diagnosis").[131] In this setting, there is no need to visualize the parasite. Endomyocardial biopsy and biopsy of skeletal muscle have been successfully used to establish T. gondii as the etiologic agent of myocarditis and polymyositis in the rare cases in immunocompetent patients.[132] Isolation studies and PCR have rarely proved useful in immunocompetent patients.

TOXOPLASMOSIS IN THE IMMUNODEFICIENT PATIENT

Because reactivation of chronic infection is the most common cause of toxoplasmosis in patients with AIDS, malignancies, or organ transplants, initial assessment of these patients should routinely include an assay for T. gondii IgG antibodies. IgG antibody testing should be ideally performed as soon as it is established that the patient is immunocompromised or is about to be immunosuppressed. Those with a positive result are at risk of reactivation of the infection; those with a negative result should be instructed on how they can prevent becoming infected (see "Prevention"). Those at highest risk (e.g., HIV-infected patients not receiving appropriate antiretroviral therapy or anti-Toxoplasma prophylaxis) who are initially seronegative should be retested on an annual basis to determine whether they have seroconverted. Seronegative organ transplant recipients should be identified before transplantation to avoid, when feasible, their receiving an organ from a seropositive donor, particularly if it is a heart.[60]

In patients with AIDS and toxoplasmosis, the IgG titer may be relatively low, and tests for IgM, IgA, and IgE antibodies may be negative.[137]

In the early postoperative period in heart transplant recipients with pretransplantation Toxoplasma antibodies who present with a clinical illness, serologic test results may be misleading.[248,312] In these patients, results indicating apparent reactivation (increasing IgG and IgM titers) may be present in the absence of clinically apparent infection. In addition, serologic test results consistent with chronic infection may be seen in the presence of toxoplasmosis.[248,312] In heart transplant recipients in whom toxoplasmosis is suspected as a cause of altered myocardial function, endomyocardial biopsy has proved useful.[248] The parasite has been demonstrated in the myocardium of patients in whom the biopsy was performed because of a suspicion of rejection.[248] PCR testing of peripheral blood, BAL, CSF, vitreous fluid and other body fluids, or tissues may prove to be useful in patients with solid organ transplants who are suspected to have toxoplasmosis.

Diagnosis in the bone marrow transplant recipient often requires special consideration. It is critical in all BMT patients that a serum IgG titer be performed before the transplantation. Toxoplasmosis in these patients is almost always due to recrudescence of a latent infection. After BMT, the preexisting IgG antibody titer may increase, remain stable, decrease, or become negative. Thus, posttransplantation serology frequently is not helpful in this group of patients and emphasizes the need to know the patient's pretransplantation serologic status. Clinical evidence of encephalopathy, pneumonia, fever, or any other unexplained syndrome in BMT patients with preexisting *T. gondii* IgG antibodies must include toxoplasmosis in the differential diagnosis. The ultimate diagnosis of toxoplasmosis in these patients requires the use of histologic, DNA amplification, or isolation methods to detect the presence of the parasite. In patients with allogeneic hematopoietic stem cell transplants who are IgG antibody test positive for *T. gondii* before transplantation, routine PCR testing of peripheral blood specimens in the posttransplantation period has been proposed as an appropriate tool for guiding preemptive therapy. In one report of 106 patients, toxoplasmosis developed in 38% of those who had positive PCR results versus 0% in those who had negative results.[191]

Serologic tests in patients with hypo- or agammaglobulinemia may not be useful to diagnose toxoplasmosis; active infection can occur in these patients in the setting of negative IgG titers.

A definitive diagnosis of toxoplasmosis in the immunodeficient patient relies on histologic demonstration of the parasite (usually in association with an inflammatory process), detection of *T. gondii* DNA by PCR, or isolation of the parasite. PCR or attempts to isolate the parasite can be performed in essentially any body fluid or tissue that is clinically affected; peripheral blood testing by PCR (and in some instances for isolation) should be considered in immunocompromised patients suspected to have toxoplasmosis. The presence of tachyzoites is diagnostic of active infection. The presence of a solitary *T. gondii* tissue cyst may only reflect chronic infection unless it is associated with an area of inflammation (e.g., as seen in a myocardial biopsy specimen); however, visualization of several tissue cysts virtually always means that active infection is present.

When clinical signs suggest involvement of the CNS or spinal cord, the workup should include CT or MRI (see "Radiologic Methods") of the brain. These studies should be performed even if the neurologic examination does not reveal focal deficits.

Empirical anti–*T. gondii* therapy for patients with multiple ring-enhancing brain lesions (usually established by MRI), positive IgG antibody titers against *T. gondii*, and advanced immunodeficiency (e.g., AIDS patients with a CD4 count < 200 cells/μL or patients receiving intensive immunosuppressive therapy) is accepted practice; a clinical and radiologic response to specific anti–*T. gondii* therapy essentially confirms the diagnosis of TE (Fig. 279-6).

Brain biopsy should be considered in immunodeficient patients with presumed TE if a single lesion is seen on MRI, an IgG antibody test result is negative, or there is an inadequate clinical response (within a 2- to 3-week period) or progression during optimal therapy or in patients whom the physician considers have adhered to an effective prophylactic regimen against *T. gondii* (e.g., TMP-SMX). An impression smear of the brain biopsy specimen can be made and immediately examined for the presence of tachyzoites using the conventional Wright-Giemsa stain used for blood smears in most laboratories. The brain specimen should then be submitted to the pathology and microbiology departments for appropriate workup. In addition to hematoxylin and eosin staining, *T. gondii*–specific immunoperoxidase

staining should be performed. Because the amount of brain tissue obtained at aspiration or biopsy is usually small, sufficient tissue for mouse inoculation may not be available; however, this should be performed whenever feasible. A positive result may often be obtained with far less than 1 g of brain tissue. PCR has been used successfully in brain tissue to diagnose TE,[313] but a positive result should be interpreted with caution because it may not distinguish a patient with TE from one with latent infection (asymptomatic carrier of brain tissue cysts) who has CNS pathology due to a process other than toxoplasmosis.

If *T. gondii* serologic and radiologic study results are inconclusive or do not support a recommendation for empirical treatment and if brain biopsy is not feasible, a lumbar puncture should be considered if it is safe to perform; PCR can then be performed on the CSF specimen. CSF can also be sent for isolation studies. PCR examination of the CSF also can be used to detect Epstein-Barr virus, JC virus, or CMV DNA in patients in whom primary CNS lymphoma, progressive multifocal leukoencephalopathy, or CMV ventriculitis, respectively, have been entertained in the differential diagnosis. Especially in HIV-infected patients, a positive EBV PCR result is strongly suggestive of CNS lymphoma.[314] Demonstration of the intrathecal production of *T. gondii*–specific antibody within the CSF may help confirm the diagnosis.[310] Unless sufficient CSF is available, we suggest that the highest priority be for PCR and an attempt at isolation of the parasite.

In the appropriate clinical setting, it is important to include toxoplasmosis in the differential diagnosis of pulmonary symptoms, particularly in those individuals with interstitial infiltrates. Wright-Giemsa stain and PCR of BAL specimens are useful for the diagnosis of pulmonary toxoplasmosis.[143,315]

In patients with visual symptoms in whom toxoplasmic chorioretinitis is a possibility, PCR examination of vitreous or aqueous fluid can be considered and is particularly helpful in patients with atypical clinical features of toxoplasmic chorioretinitis.[146,219,316] Of note, PCR examination of the vitreous fluid can also be helpful when other etiologic agents such as herpes simplex virus, varicella-zoster virus, and CMV are considered in the differential diagnosis. The intraocular production of *T. gondii*–specific IgG antibodies (Goldmann-Witmer coefficient analysis of aqueous humor) has also been reported to be diagnostically useful in immunocompromised patients.[317]

PCR and isolation studies in peripheral blood can help establish *T. gondii* as the etiologic agent of a febrile syndrome or systemic symptoms of unclear cause.[251,318] These studies tend to have a higher yield early in the disease and before or shortly after specific anti–*T. gondii* therapy is initiated.[251]

In pursuing the diagnosis, histologic examination with the appropriate stains and mouse inoculation can be attempted in virtually any tissue suspected of being involved by *T. gondii*. Body fluids that should be considered for examination by PCR include CSF, blood, vitreous, aqueous, and BAL specimens. Reference laboratories should be contacted before diagnostic procedures to optimize the handling of the specimens and their yield.

OCULAR TOXOPLASMOSIS

Low titers of IgG antibody are usual in patients with active chorioretinitis due to reactivation of congenital *T. gondii* infection; IgM antibodies are not usually detected. When sera from such patients are examined in the dye test, they should be titered beginning with undiluted serum because, in some cases, the conventional initial dilution of 1 : 16 may be negative.

In most cases, toxoplasmic chorioretinitis is diagnosed by ophthalmologic examination, and empirical therapy directed against the organism is often instituted based on clinical findings and serologic test results. In a number of patients, the morphology of the retinal lesion or lesions may be nondiagnostic or, the response to treatment may be suboptimal or both. In such cases (unclear clinical diagnosis or inadequate clinical response or both), the detection of an abnormal *T. gondii*–antibody response in ocular fluids (Goldman-Witmer coefficient)[316,319] or demonstration of the parasite by isolation, histopatho-

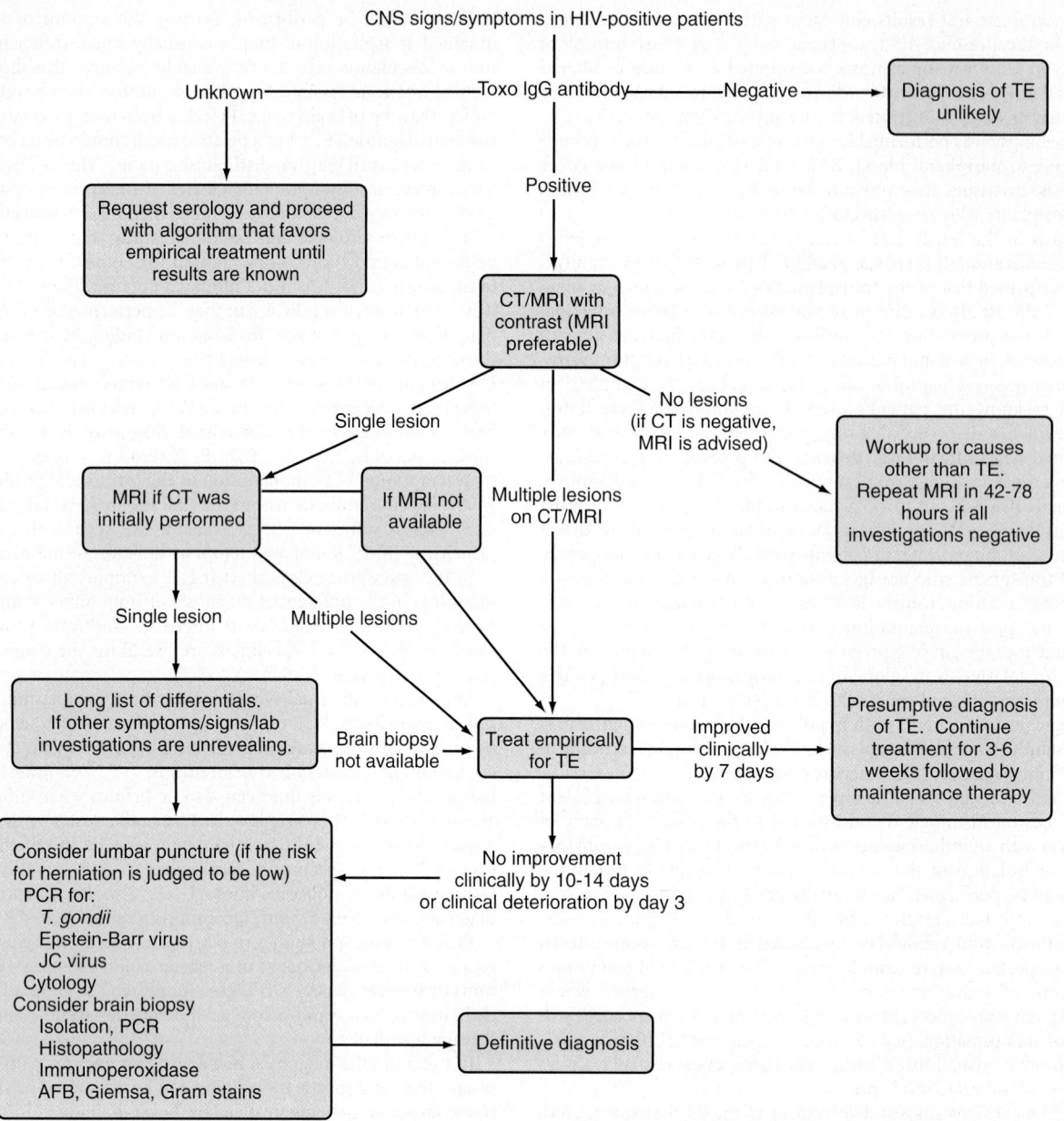

Figure 279-6 **Diagnostic approach and management algorithm for human immunodeficiency virus–infected patients with central nervous system symptoms or signs that might potentially be toxoplasmic encephalitis.** AFB, acid-fast bacilli; CT, computed tomography; MRI, magnetic resonance imaging; PCR, polymerase chain reaction; TE, toxoplasmic encephalitis.

logic examination, or PCR has been used successfully to establish the diagnosis.[144,320] PCR has been used in both vitreous and aqueous fluids in an attempt to support or confirm the diagnosis of *T. gondii* as the cause of the retinal lesions.[145,146,219,316] In patients in whom toxoplasmosis is considered in the differential diagnosis but in whom the presentation is atypical, PCR is a useful diagnostic aid. Vitreous biopsy is a potentially hazardous procedure, and its use should be considered only when other diagnostic measures have not revealed a cause.

TOXOPLASMA GONDII INFECTION IN PREGNANCY

Acute acquired *T. gondii* infection is diagnosed serologically by the same methods used for immunocompetent adults discussed earlier (Fig. 279-7).[276] Special care is taken to determine whether the infection was acquired before or after conception. This determination is frequently difficult because routine serologic screening is not conducted in pregnant women in the United States. Repeat serologic tests in a

pregnant woman who has been previously shown to have *T. gondii* antibodies are not helpful.

The diagnosis of acute *T. gondii* infection or toxoplasmosis ideally requires demonstration of an increase in titers in serial serum samples (either conversion from a negative to a positive titer or a significant increase from a low to a higher titer).[8] These specimens should be obtained at least 3 weeks apart and be tested in parallel. Because the diagnosis is frequently considered relatively late in the course of the patient's pregnancy, serologic test titers may already have reached their peak at the time that the first serum is obtained for testing. It therefore is often difficult to discriminate between infections acquired recently (possibly during pregnancy) and those acquired in the more distant past. Thus, the initial serum should be obtained as early as possible during gestation.

Initial screening of maternal serum involves testing for IgG and IgM antibodies; a lack of both Ig antibodies essentially excludes active infection but identifies the patient as being at risk of acquiring the infection

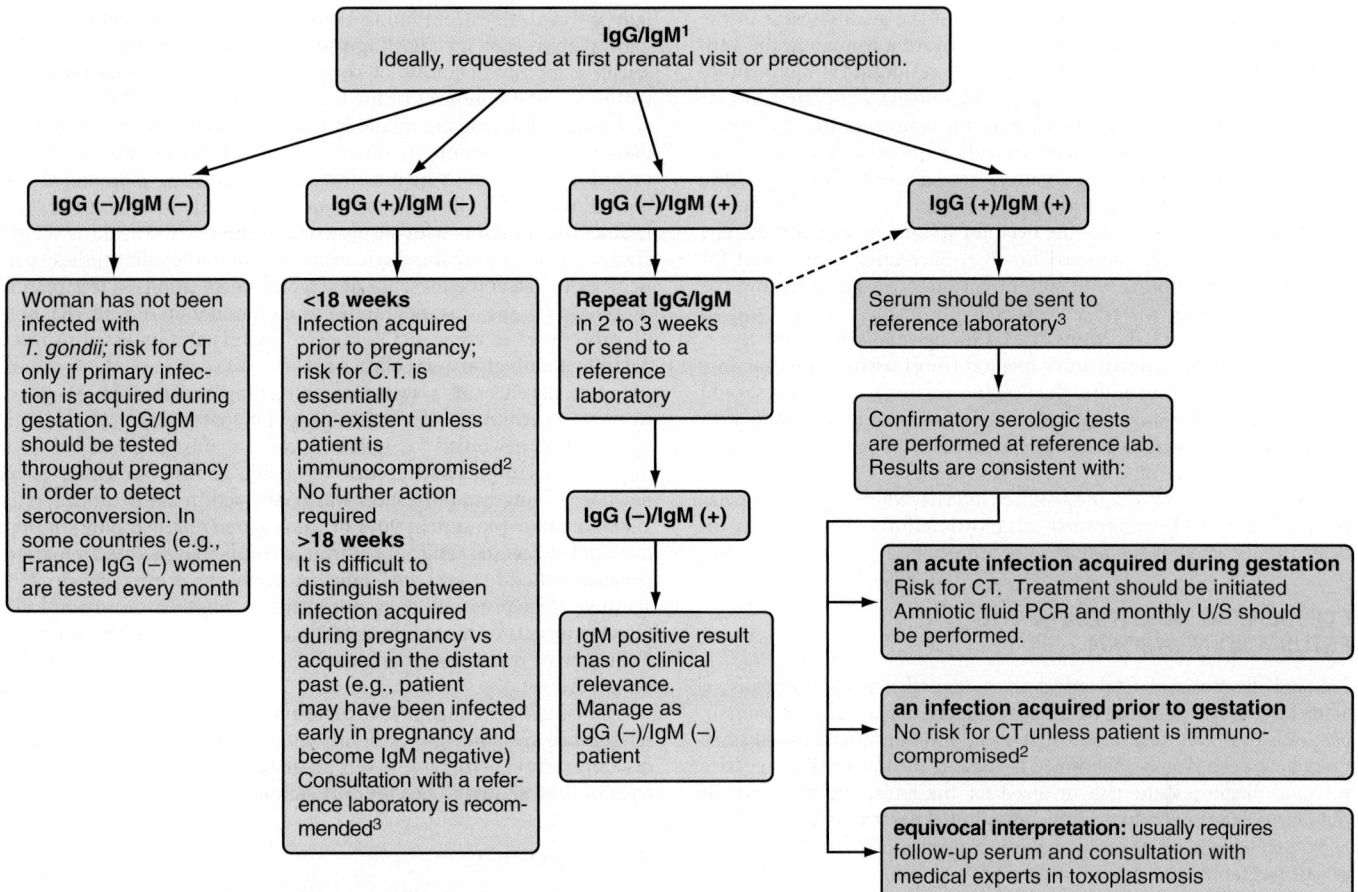

Figure 279-7 **Diagnostic approach and management algorithm of toxoplasmosis during pregnancy.** Most of the initial serologic screening can be accomplished by nonreference or commercial laboratories (*blue-shaded boxes*). Only positive immunoglobulin M results should be considered for additional testing and consultation with medical experts at a reference laboratory (*tan-shaded boxes*).

(and hence in need of instruction about primary prevention). The presence of IgG antibodies in the absence of IgM antibodies in the first two trimesters usually indicates chronic maternal infection with essentially no risk to the fetus (the exceptions are severely immunodeficient patients). In the third trimester, a negative IgM test titer is most likely consistent with a chronic maternal infection but does not exclude the possibility of an acute infection acquired early in pregnancy; this is especially true in those patients who exhibit a rapid decrease in their IgM titers during the acute infection. In these cases, the use of other serologic tests (e.g., IgA, IgE, AC/HS, avidity) may be particularly helpful.

A positive IgM test result requires further assessment with confirmatory testing at a reference laboratory (see also "Diagnosis of Specific Clinical Entities").[258,273,275,276] The use of confirmatory testing with a combination of serologic tests in a reference laboratory has proved helpful in discriminating between recently and more distantly acquired infections, and having an expert interpret the results to the patient's physician has been shown to reduce unnecessary induced abortions among pregnant women reported to have IgM antibodies.[258] Women who are informed that they have a positive IgM test

titer and that it signifies that their offspring will or might be infected often choose abortion. Unfortunately, a positive IgM test may not necessarily indicate infection acquired during gestation (a false-positive result or persistence of an IgM-positive result in the chronic stage of the infection), and thus an abortion may not be indicated. It is for this reason that confirmatory testing in a reference laboratory has been recommended by many experts and by the U.S. Food and Drug Administration.[275]

A number of tests for avidity of *Toxoplasma* IgG antibodies have been introduced to help differentiate between recently acquired and distant infection.[268,269,321] Studies of the kinetics of the avidity of IgG in pregnant women who have seroconverted during gestation have shown that women with high avidity test results have been infected with *T. gondii* for at least 3 to 5 months. Recently, it was demonstrated that, when used as a confirmatory test along with a battery of other tests in women in their first 16 weeks of gestation, detection of high-avidity IgG antibodies by the VIDAS IgG avidity test (BioMérieux), for example, can be a useful addition to the discriminatory power of a combination of tests in distinguishing recently acquired from chronic infection.[242,259]

It is critical to recognize that the value of the avidity test is in the first 3 to 5 months of gestation (i.e., the fetus of a woman in the 14th week of gestation with a positive IgM test result and a high-avidity result is not at risk of congenital toxoplasmosis).[259] Because low or equivocal avidity test results may persist for many months, their presence does not necessarily indicate recently acquired infection.

Confirmatory testing using a battery of tests and the VIDAS avidity method in pregnant women during their first 24 weeks of gestation has the potential to decrease the need for follow-up sera and thereby reduce costs, to make the need for PCR on amniotic fluid and for treatment of the mother with spiramycin unnecessary, to remove the pregnant woman's anxiety associated with further testing, and to decrease unnecessary abortions.[257-259] Although the avidity test represents an additional confirmatory method (most useful if high-avidity antibodies are detected within the first 16 weeks of gestation), it should not be used as the only confirmatory test for pregnant women with positive IgG and/or IgM antibodies because of the potential to misinterpret low or borderline avidity antibody results.

Once the diagnosis of acute acquired infection during pregnancy has been presumptively established, diagnostic efforts should focus on determining whether the fetus has been infected.

CONGENITAL INFECTION IN THE FETUS AND NEWBORN

Prenatal diagnosis of fetal infection is advised when a diagnosis of acute infection is established or highly suspected in a pregnant woman. Methods to obtain fetal blood such as periumbilical fetal blood sampling have been largely abandoned because of the rate of false-negative prenatal diagnoses, the risk involved for the fetus, and the delay in obtaining definitive results with conventional parasitologic tests.[230]

Prenatal diagnosis of congenital toxoplasmosis is currently based on ultrasonography and amniocentesis. PCR on amniotic fluid for the detection of T. gondii–specific DNA performed at 18 weeks of gestation or later is more sensitive, more rapid, and safer than conventional diagnostic procedures involving fetal blood sampling.[230] Amniotic fluid should be tested by PCR in all cases with serologic test results diagnostic of or highly suggestive of acute acquired infection during pregnancy and also if there is evidence of fetal damage on ultrasound examination (e.g., hydrocephalus and/or calcifications). In a recent prospective study conducted by three reference laboratories in France, congenital infection was ultimately documented in 75 of 270 cases. PCR on amniotic fluid had a sensitivity of 64%, specificity of 100%, positive predictive value of 100%, and negative predictive value of 88%.[322] Sensitivity was greatest when maternal infection occurred between 17 and 21 weeks of gestation. In those cases in which the approximate date of onset of infection is known, it has been suggested that amniocentesis be performed no earlier than 4 weeks thereafter, with the preferable time for amniocentesis being 17 to 21 weeks. However, in the United States, systematic monthly screening is not performed as it is in France; we suggest that, when feasible, amniocentesis be performed at 18 weeks of gestation. The reliability of PCR before 18 weeks of gestational age is unknown.[230]

Maternal IgG antibodies present in the newborn may reflect either past or recent infection in the mother. For this reason, tests for the detection of IgA and IgM antibodies are commonly used for the diagnosis of infection in the newborn (Fig. 279-8). It is essential to exclude maternal contamination of blood obtained at birth; serum samples obtained from peripheral blood and not from the umbilical cords are preferred. The demonstration of IgA antibodies seems to be more sensitive than the detection of IgM antibodies for establishing infection in the newborn.[287] If IgG antibodies are detected but serologic test results for IgM and IgA antibodies are negative and T. gondii is not isolated, follow-up serologic testing in suspected cases is indicated to attempt to establish the diagnosis. Maternally transferred antibodies usually decrease and disappear within 6 to 12 months. Studies using the Western blot technique have shown that maternal and infant sera may recognize different T. gondii antigens when the infant is congenitally infected.[323,324] Combining Western blot with conventional serologic analysis (i.e., IgG, IgM, IgA tests) has been reported to be more sensitive for the diagnosis of congenital toxoplasmosis at birth and within the first 3 months of life than either test alone.[324-326]

Additional diagnostic methods that have been used successfully to diagnose the infection in infants are direct demonstration of the organism by isolation in mice or cell culture (e.g., placental tissue, body fluid) and PCR on body fluids (e.g., CSF, blood, urine).[327-329] Evaluation of infants with suspected congenital toxoplasmosis should always include ophthalmologic examination, radiologic studies (particularly to detect the presence of cerebral calcifications; if feasible, CT is preferred over ultrasonography), and examination of CSF. Diagnostic procedures in congenitally infected infants are discussed in more detail by Remington and colleagues.[8]

In the absence of a systematic screening program for pregnant women, a secondary prevention program that consists of serologic testing of all newborns for IgM antibodies against T. gondii has been implemented in Massachusetts.[330,331] Using routine screening of all newborns, congenital infection was confirmed in approximately 1 in 12,000 infants. More than 90% of these were identified only through neonatal screening and not through initial clinical examination. Because testing for IgM antibodies in newborns is only 25% to 75% sensitive, this program does not detect a number of subclinically infected infants or those infected late in the third trimester (when the frequency of transmission is highest but antibody formation has not yet occurred).

In infants with congenital toxoplasmosis or congenital infection, a rebound in IgG and IgM antibody titers is frequently observed after discontinuation of therapy. In our experience, such a serologic rebound has not been shown to be clinically significant.[8]

Treatment

Currently recommended drugs against T. gondii act primarily against the tachyzoite form and thus do not eradicate the encysted form (bradyzoite). Pyrimethamine is considered the most effective anti-Toxoplasma agent and, if feasible, should always be included in drug regimens used against the parasite. Pyrimethamine is a folic acid antagonist. The most common side effect is dose-related suppression of the bone marrow, which may be decreased by concomitant administration of folinic acid (calcium leucovorin). It is not well established how often a blood count should be obtained; a reasonable strategy would be to check peripheral blood cell and platelet counts twice weekly until hematologic parameters have stabilized in a nontoxic range and then every 2 to 4 weeks. Folinic acid should be administered concomitantly to avoid bone marrow suppression. The parenteral form of folinic acid is well absorbed orally, and 5 to 10 mg of folinic acid (as much as 50 mg/day is used in AIDS patients) may be given orally (e.g., with orange juice at the same time as the pyrimethamine). Whereas folinic acid does not inhibit the action of pyrimethamine on tachyzoites, folic acid does and should not be used in patients being treated with pyrimethamine. Less serious side effects of pyrimethamine include gastrointestinal distress, rash, headaches, and a bad taste in the mouth.

Unless there are circumstances that preclude the use of more than one drug, there is no role for monotherapy in the treatment of toxoplasmosis. A second drug such as sulfadiazine or clindamycin should be added. Sulfadiazine acts synergistically with pyrimethamine; most other sulfonamides have inferior activity. The patient must maintain a good urine output to prevent crystalluria and oliguria. The most common side effects associated with sulfadiazine are skin rashes (which may be life-threatening)[332] and crystal-induced nephrotoxicity.[333] Worsening encephalopathy, hallucinations, or a new onset of psychiatric symptoms in patients with AIDS may be sulfadiazine induced and must be considered in the patient who is nonresponsive to otherwise appropriate anti-Toxoplasma treatment.[334] A drug rash with sulfonamide therapy does not necessarily preclude its use because successful desensitization protocols have been reported.[335,336] Clindamycin seems to act by targeting translation in the apicoplast of T. gondii.[337] Adverse

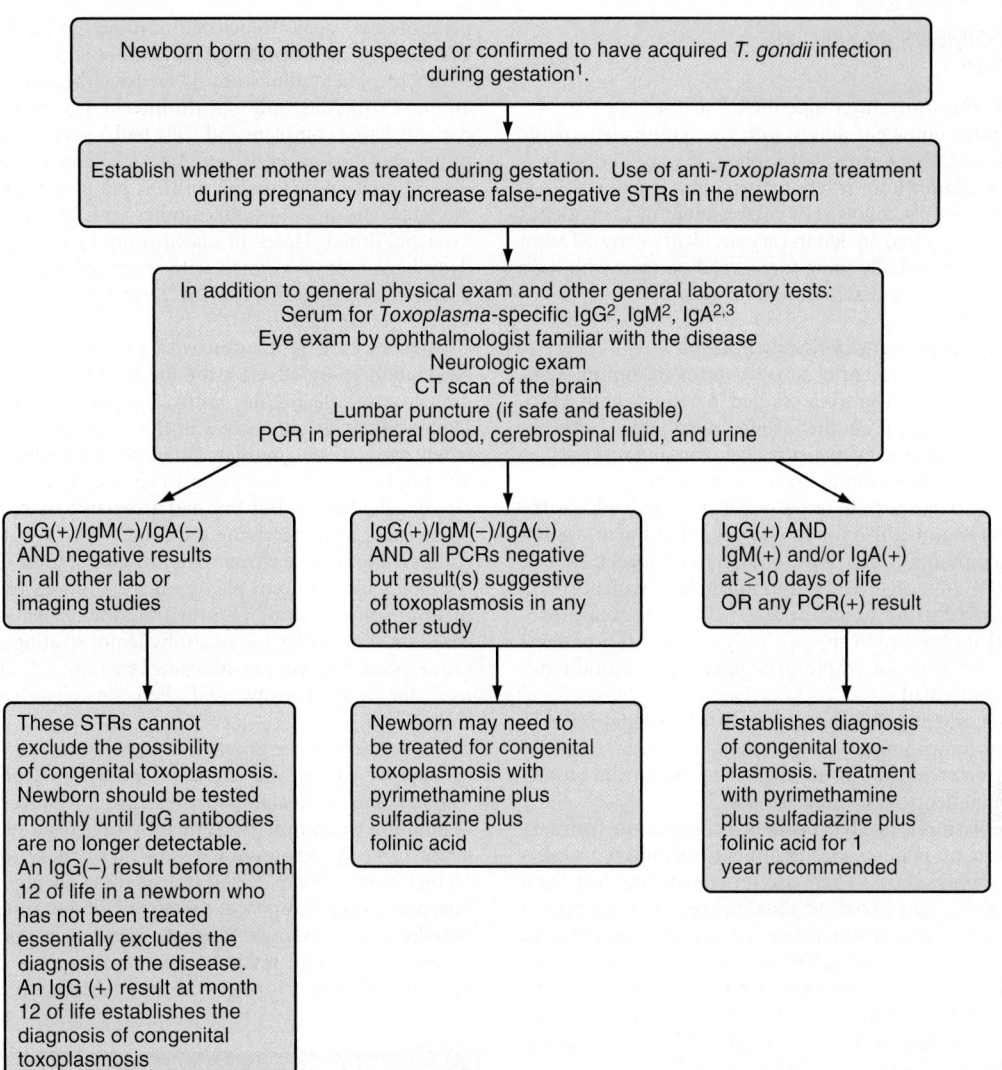

Newborn born to mother suspected or confirmed to have acquired *T. gondii* infection during gestation[1].		

Establish whether mother was treated during gestation. Use of anti-*Toxoplasma* treatment during pregnancy may increase false-negative STRs in the newborn

In addition to general physical exam and other general laboratory tests:
Serum for *Toxoplasma*-specific IgG[2], IgM[2], IgA[2,3]
Eye exam by ophthalmologist familiar with the disease
Neurologic exam
CT scan of the brain
Lumbar puncture (if safe and feasible)
PCR in peripheral blood, cerebrospinal fluid, and urine

IgG(+)/IgM(−)/IgA(−) AND negative results in all other lab or imaging studies	IgG(+)/IgM(−)/IgA(−) AND all PCRs negative but result(s) suggestive of toxoplasmosis in any other study	IgG(+) AND IgM(+) and/or IgA(+) at ≥10 days of life OR any PCR(+) result
These STRs cannot exclude the possibility of congenital toxoplasmosis. Newborn should be tested monthly until IgG antibodies are no longer detectable. An IgG(−) result before month 12 of life in a newborn who has not been treated essentially excludes the diagnosis of the disease. An IgG (+) result at month 12 of life establishes the diagnosis of congenital toxoplasmosis	Newborn may need to be treated for congenital toxoplasmosis with pyrimethamine plus sulfadiazine plus folinic acid	Establishes diagnosis of congenital toxo-plasmosis. Treatment with pyrimethamine plus sulfadiazine plus folinic acid for 1 year recommended

CT= computed tomography; lab = laboratory; PCR = polymerase chain reaction; STRs = serologic test results.
[1] Consider consultation with a physician expert in management of toxoplasmosis in the newborn and children, for example, the Palo Alto Medical Foundation Toxoplasma Serology Laboratory [PAMF-TSL], telephone number (650) 853-4828, http://www.toxoplasmosis.org/ or US [Chicago, IL] National Collaborative Treatment Trial Study, telephone number (773) 834-4152.
[2] At PAMF-TSL the dye test, the immunosorbent agglutination assay (ISAGA), and the ELISA methods are used for the detection of IgG, IgM, and IgA, respectively, in the newborn. These methods have been reported to have greater sensitivity than other techniques used for the detection of these antibodies.
[3] It is recommended to test for both IgM and IgA antibodies. Infected newborns can be positive for both or either one.

Figure 279-8 **Diagnostic approach and management algorithm of the newborn whose mother has been suspected or confirmed to have acquired toxoplasmosis during gestation.**

reactions to clindamycin include rash, nausea, vomiting, and diarrhea, which may be associated with *Clostridium difficile* infection. Myopathy with electromyographic abnormalities and elevated serum creatine phosphokinase levels have been described.[338]

Although clinical experience with TMP-SMX is more limited, this drug combination, which targets folate metabolism in a manner similar to pyrimethamine plus sulfadiazine, has documented activity and can be used in patients requiring parenteral therapy.[297] The role of other drugs including azithromycin, clarithromycin, atovaquone, and dapsone is less clear; they should only be used as alternatives to the regimens described previously and should be used in combination with pyrimethamine whenever possible.

Spiramycin has been used in pregnant women to attempt to reduce transmission to the fetus; it has not been shown to be effective for acute therapy, maintenance therapy, or primary prophylaxis of TE in AIDS patients. There is no evidence that spiramycin is teratogenic.

Although drugs used to treat toxoplasmosis in the setting of different clinical entities are basically the same, careful attention should be given to the dosing and dosing regimen. Recommended doses in immunocompromised patients are usually higher than those in immunocompetent patients. For instance, the recommended dose of pyrimethamine for patients with TE is 50 to 75 mg/day after a loading dose of 200 mg, whereas the dose to treat fetal infection during pregnancy is 25 to 50 mg/day after a loading dose of 100 mg in the mother.

TREATMENT REGIMENS IN SPECIFIC CLINICAL ENTITIES

Toxoplasmosis in the Immunocompetent Patient

Treatment of immunocompetent adults with the lymphadenopathic form is rarely indicated; this form is self-limited. If visceral disease is clinically overt or symptoms are severe or persistent, treatment may be indicated for 2 to 4 weeks, followed by reassessment of the patient's condition. Infections acquired by laboratory accident or transfusion of blood products are potentially more severe, and patients who have been infected in these ways probably should be treated.

Toxoplasmosis in the Immunodeficient Patient

Because experience with treatment of toxoplasmosis in immunodeficient patients has been most extensively studied in patients with AIDS, this section focuses primarily on this group of patients. However, information on treatment in AIDS patients likely can, in large part, be extrapolated directly to other immunodeficient patients.

If left untreated, toxoplasmosis in immunodeficient patients is often lethal. Treatment is recommended for 4 to 6 weeks after the resolution of all signs and symptoms (often for 6 months or longer). At one medical center, 80% of non-AIDS immunodeficient patients with toxoplasmosis improved with specific therapy.[339] This rate of improvement is similar to that observed in appropriately treated AIDS patients with TE.[301,340] Chronic (latent) asymptomatic infection in immunodeficient patients is not treated.

The exact dosing schedule for the treatment of toxoplasmosis in non-AIDS immunocompromised patients has not been defined.[5] However, useful information in this regard has resulted from studies performed in AIDS patients with toxoplasmosis.[99]

Therapy for toxoplasmosis in AIDS patients includes acute (primary or induction) treatment, maintenance treatment (secondary prophylaxis), and primary prophylaxis. There are no convincing data from prospective, carefully designed trials to allow the recommendation of monotherapy for induction, maintenance, or primary prophylaxis. Because relapse occurs in as many as 80% of cases[332] after the discontinuation of primary therapy, lifelong maintenance therapy is recommended unless the CD4 count increases to more than 200 cells/μL for at least 6 months in response to HAART (plasma HIV viral load will often be below detection limits during this period).[364]

Acute therapy should continue for at least 3 weeks,[65] and 6 weeks or more may be required for more severely ill patients in whom there has not been a complete response. Pyrimethamine combined with sulfadiazine and folinic acid is the therapy of choice for AIDS patients with toxoplasmosis and is the standard with which experimental regimens should be compared. This regimen is associated with clinical response in 68% to 95% of patients with TE.[340,341] Unfortunately, side effects from one or more of the drugs develop in as many as 40% of patients, requiring discontinuation of therapy.[165,292] Pyrimethamine-clindamycin and folinic acid seem comparable in efficacy to pyrimethamine-sulfadiazine,[340,342] but this combination also has substantial toxicity. TMP-SMX[343-345] (at 10 mg/kg/day of the trimethoprim component divided in two doses) has shown efficacy similar to that of the pyrimethamine/sulfadiazine regimen (with a more rapid radiologic response in the TMP-SMX group) in a randomized pilot trial in 77 patients with AIDS[346]; this provides an alternative regimen for situations in which parenteral therapy is required. Recently, an international, noncomparative study of atovaquone[347,348] (administered orally as a suspension) combined with either pyrimethamine or sulfadiazine as treatment for acute disease demonstrated 6-week response rates of 75% (21/28 patients) for atovaquone-pyrimethamine and 82% (9/11) for atovaquone-sulfadiazine.[349] Serum levels of atovaquone may predict response but are not commercially available.[348] TMP-SMX and atovaquone are both active against *Pneumocystis*, and thus anti-*Pneumocystis* prophylaxis does not need to be administered when these drugs are used. Because clindamycin-pyrimethamine treatment has no demonstrated anti-*Pneumocystis* activity, additional prophylaxis (e.g., aerosolized

pentamidine) needs to be coadministered if patients are at risk of the development of *Pneumocystis* pneumonia.

In a 13-patient pilot study of TE using the combination of pyrimethamine 75 mg/day and clarithromycin 1 g every 12 hours, 62% of patients had a complete and 23% had a partial clinical response; 15% of patients died by week 3 of therapy,[350] and adverse events resulted in discontinuation of therapy in 27%. No long-term follow-up data are available, and no additional studies with this drug combination have been published. Doses of clarithromycin higher than 500 mg twice daily have been associated with increased mortality in HIV-infected patients receiving therapy for *Mycobacterium avium* infection and should not be used.[351,352]

Dapsone in combination with pyrimethamine has been reported anecdotally to be effective for the treatment of TE when used in an oral dose of 100 mg/day with 25 mg/day of oral pyrimethamine.[353] Doxycycline has had success in the treatment of TE in a few patients when used at 300 mg/day IV in three divided doses.[354] A dose of 100 mg twice daily was given to six patients intolerant to pyrimethamine-sulfadiazine, but five had associated neurologic and radiologic recurrences while receiving the drug.[355] Further studies are needed to compare the relative efficacy and toxicity of these alternative regimens. Although azithromycin plus pyrimethamine is effective for the treatment of some cases of TE in AIDS patients, its use should be limited based on results of a recent study demonstrating an inferior response rate, especially during maintenance therapy.[356,357] Alternative regimens used for acute therapy and their dosing schedules are listed in Table 279-2.

Corticosteroids are often given to patients with TE for the reduction of cerebral edema and increased intracranial pressure. The clinical response and survival in patients with TE who received corticosteroids in addition to antimicrobial therapy have been reported to be no different from the response and survival of those who received antimicrobial agents alone.[301] The use of these agents may complicate the interpretation of empirical therapy of TE because partial clinical and radiologic improvement may be seen solely due to a reduction in cerebral edema and inflammation or a response of CNS lymphoma; moreover, they may further compromise the immune systems of these

TABLE 279-2	Guidelines for Acute/Primary Therapy of Toxoplasmic Encephalitis in Patients with Acquired Immunodeficiency Syndrome
Drug	**Dosing Schedule**
Standard Regimens	
Pyrimethamine	Oral 200 mg loading dose, then 50 (<60 kg) to 75 (>60 kg) mg PO qd
Folinic acid (leucovorin)* plus	10 to 20 mg PO, IV, or IM qd (up to 50 mg qd)
Sulfadiazine (preferred)	1000 (<60 kg) to 1500 mg (>60 kg) PO q6h
or	
Clindamycin	600 mg q6h PO or IV (up to 1200 mg IV) q6h
Possible Alternative Regimens	
a. Trimethoprim-sulfamethoxazole	5 mg/kg (trimethoprim component) PO or IV q12h (doses as high as 15-20 mg/kg/day of the trimethoprim component have been used)
b. Pyrimethamine and folinic acid plus one of the following†	As in standard regimens
Atovaquone	1500 mg q12h PO
Clarithromycin	500 mg q12h PO
Azithromycin	900-1200 mg qd PO
Dapsone	100 mg PO qd

*The dose of folinic acid can be titrated based on the hemogram to reduce pyrimethamine-associated myelotoxicity. As much as 50 mg/day has been used.

†These agents have been used in clinical studies with small numbers of patients and have response rates lower than those of the standard regimens (see text for references). They should be used only in patients who are intolerant of the standard regimens. Alternative agents must be used in combination with another antimicrobial agent (most frequently, pyrimethamine with folinic acid) that has proven clinical activity against *Toxoplasma gondii*.

already very immunodeficient patients. Therefore, their use should be limited to situations in which clinically significant edema or a mass effect is present.

Seizures occur in as many as 35% of patients with TE.[292] One retrospective study demonstrated a poorer outcome in those patients who received anticonvulsant therapy compared with those who did not.[332] Whether this result represents a true drug effect or a selection bias (given that those receiving anticonvulsant therapy are likely to be more severely ill) is unclear. Anticonvulsant agents may be responsible for numerous side effects and drug interactions; for instance, potentially serious interactions can occur between agents such as carbamazepine, phenobarbital, and phenytoin and other drugs used to treat HIV infection such as protease inhibitors. Anticonvulsant therapy is probably best administered when seizures have occurred.[332]

The time to clinical response in AIDS patients with TE who were receiving appropriate anti-*Toxoplasma* therapy has been evaluated in a study that included an objective, graded neurologic examination.[301] Of those with a response, 91% improved with respect to at least half of their baseline abnormalities by day 14.[301] AIDS patients with presumed TE had some degree of improvement within 7 to 10 days of the initiation of appropriate anti-*Toxoplasma* therapy. By contrast, a significant number of patients with an alternate diagnosis, including lymphoma, exhibited signs of clinical deterioration as early as 3 to 5 days after the initiation of the empirical regimen for presumed TE.[301] Headaches and seizures were insensitive indicators for a response to therapy. In some cases, toxoplasmosis has progressed to death despite the use of appropriate drug regimens.[340,342]

After successful primary therapy, drug doses are generally decreased for maintenance therapy. No single maintenance regimen that is efficacious with an acceptable adverse reaction profile has yet been identified. Relapse of TE occurs in approximately 20% to 30% of patients who are receiving maintenance therapy, in part because of nonadherence to and patient intolerance of the prescribed regimen.[165] Pyrimethamine (25 mg/day) plus sulfadiazine (500 mg four times daily) has been associated with the lowest relapse rate[340] and is recommended unless there are contraindications to its use. When daily therapy with pyrimethamine-sulfadiazine was compared with a twice-weekly regimen for the prevention of recurrence of TE, the latter was found to be less effective.[358,359] Although a subsequent trial by the same group found that three-times-weekly therapy was equivalent to daily therapy, the relapse rates for both groups (~14.5/100 patient-years) was higher than that seen with daily therapy (4.4/100 patient-years) in the earlier study.[359,360] Patients receiving the pyrimethamine-sulfadiazine combination do not require another regimen for PCP prophylaxis. Whereas PCP subsequently developed in 25% of patients receiving pyrimethamine-clindamycin,[361] PCP developed in no patients receiving pyrimethamine-sulfadiazine.[359,361] One 17-patient study demonstrated that TMP-SMX could be safely substituted for pyrimethamine-sulfadiazine after a median of 24 months of maintenance therapy in patients also receiving HAART; the major benefit was decreased pill burden.[362]

Because of drug toxicity, many patients are unable to continue taking the pyrimethamine-sulfadiazine combination for maintenance therapy. A higher relapse rate has been reported with the use of pyrimethamine-clindamycin compared with pyrimethamine-sulfadiazine for secondary prophylaxis of TE; hence, it is recommended that the clindamycin dose be 1800 mg/day if tolerated.[340,363,364] Encouraging results have been reported with other drug combinations. These include Fansidar (pyrimethamine-sulfadoxine), which has been used in a dose of one tablet twice weekly,[365] and pyrimethamine-dapsone administered on an intermittent schedule (two to three times weekly).[366-368] The long half-life of these agents allowed the longer dosing interval, but Fansidar may have an increased risk of severe cutaneous reactions, and the longer half-life results in slower drug clearance after discontinuation of therapy.[369] When pyrimethamine was used alone as maintenance therapy at 50 mg/day[370,371] and 100 mg/day,[370] the relapse rates were 10% to 28% and 5%, respectively. Atovaquone alone or in combination regimens also seems to have activity

based on uncontrolled trials; combination therapy (with sulfadiazine or pyrimethamine) should be used whenever possible.[347-349,372]

Primary prophylaxis against *T. gondii* in patients with AIDS has been shown to be effective in preventing acute TE.[373-375] In addition, the use of HAART in HIV-infected patients has had a profound effect in decreasing the incidence of TE in these patients.[66,67] Primary prophylaxis is recommended for patients who have detectable *Toxoplasma* IgG antibodies and whose lowest CD4$^+$ count has been less than 100/µL (many experts use <200/µL as the cutoff rather than 100/µL), regardless of the HIV RNA viral load.[364] TMP-SMX (one double-strength or single-strength tablet daily), dapsone (50 mg/day) plus pyrimethamine (50 mg/week), and Fansidar (twice weekly) have been reported to be effective in preventing the first episode of TE.[364,373,376,377]

Studies have demonstrated that it is safe to discontinue primary or secondary anti-*Toxoplasma* prophylaxis when recovery of a CD4$^+$ count to greater than 200 cells/µL is achieved and sustained in patients on HAART.[206-208,378,379] Current recommendations are to discontinue primary prophylaxis when the CD4 count has increased to more than 200 cells/µL for at least 3 months and secondary prophylaxis for at least 6 months.[364] It is important to recognize that in most of these studies, the median CD4 count was more than 300 cells/µL at enrollment and viral loads were below detection limits or reasonably controlled in most patients.

Roxithromycin administered at 900 mg once weekly (may be given in three divided doses)[380] was found in a small randomized trial to be effective for primary prophylaxis; roxithromycin is unavailable in the United States. Based on a number of clinical trials, pyrimethamine alone cannot be recommended for primary prophylaxis.[63,381,382] Clarithromycin[383] and spiramycin[384] have been ineffective for primary prophylaxis when they were used alone. In a randomized, placebo-controlled primary prophylaxis trial, clindamycin (600 mg/day) was associated with an unacceptably high rate of associated gastrointestinal disease, in particular diarrhea.[385]

It must be emphasized that in a number of studies of TMP-SMX,[373] pyrimethamine-dapsone,[376] and Fansidar[365] for primary prophylaxis, discontinuation of therapy as a result of adverse effects was reported in 29% to 39% of the patients. Thus, these regimens may not be satisfactory for a significant number of AIDS patients due to intolerance.

Data on the outcome of treatment of AIDS patients with toxoplasmosis outside the CNS are limited; available information on the therapy of ocular[200,386,387] and pulmonary[194,388] involvement indicates that these forms of toxoplasmosis are also responsive to treatment. Therapy was successful in 50% to 77% of patients with pulmonary toxoplasmosis.[194,388]

The hematologic toxicity associated with zidovudine and the high doses of pyrimethamine used for the treatment of TE are additive. Other drugs used in treating HIV-infected patients that cause myelosuppression include ganciclovir, flucytosine, trimethoprim, pentamidine, chemotherapy agents, and IFN-α.

OCULAR TOXOPLASMOSIS

The decision to treat active toxoplasmic chorioretinitis should be made based on a complete ophthalmologic evaluation. Treatment is most likely indicated in the following settings: any decrease in visual acuity, macular or peripapillary lesions, lesions greater than one optic disk diameter, lesions associated with a moderate to severe vitreous inflammatory reaction, the presence of multiple active lesions, the persistence of active disease for longer than 1 month, and any ocular lesions associated with recently acquired infection. Because the disease can be self-limited in immunocompetent patients, many clinicians may not treat small, peripheral retinal lesions that are not immediately vision threatening.[144,389-391]

The reported benefits of medical therapy are related primarily to the clinical presentation.[144,389] Because there is so much variation in the clinical manifestations of the retinal disease and because the disease may be self-limited even without treatment, the response to therapy is difficult to interpret. The combination of pyrimethamine (100 mg loading dose given over 24 hours, followed by 25 to 50 mg/day) and sulfadiazine (1 g given four times daily) for 4 to 6 weeks depending on the clinical response, which is considered classic therapy for ocular toxoplasmosis, is the most common drug combination used.[389] TMP-SMX showed responses similar to those with pyrimethamine-sulfadiazine in a recent randomized, single-blind trial, although the latter regimen was used at lower than standard doses.[392]

Clindamycin (300 mg PO every 6 hours for a minimum of 3 weeks) has also been used with favorable clinical results.[389] Other drugs that may have activity but have been inadequately studied include atovaquone and pyrimethamine plus azithromycin.[393,394] Systemic corticosteroids are indicated when lesions involve the macula, optic nerve head, or papillomacular bundle. Photocoagulation has been used for both the treatment of active lesions and prophylaxis against the spread of lesions because new lesions appear contiguous to old lesions.[389] In some patients, vitrectomy and lentectomy may be necessary.

Given the high relapse rate seen in some patients with ocular toxoplasmosis, prevention of recurrences would be highly desirable. A randomized, open-label trial of 124 patients found that TMP-SMX (1 double strength [160/800 mg] tablet every 3 days) was effective in decreasing the frequency of recurrences from 24% to 7% in a population at high risk of recurrences.[147] If confirmed in subsequent studies, such a regimen could be beneficial in patients with frequent or severe recurrences.

For the approach to ocular toxoplasmosis during pregnancy, see "Acute Acquired *Toxoplasma* Infection in Pregnant Women."

ACUTE ACQUIRED *TOXOPLASMA* INFECTION IN PREGNANT WOMEN

Treatment of the acutely infected pregnant woman does not eliminate but does seem to decrease the incidence of fetal infection. Because there is usually a delay between the acquisition of acute maternal infection, infection of the placenta, and subsequent infection of the fetus, identification of acute maternal infection necessitates immediate institution of treatment of the mother. Most experience of maternal treatment to prevent transmission to the fetus has been with spiramycin (1 g every 8 hours, obtainable in the United States from the U.S. Food and Drug Administration, telephone 301-796-1600). Spiramycin has been accepted by most investigators as being effective in reducing the frequency of maternal transmission of *T. gondii* to the fetus by approximately 60%.[228,276] Spiramycin is indicated for patients confirmed or suspected to have been infected before 18 weeks of gestation. It seems that its maximum efficacy is best achieved when given within 8 weeks of seroconversion.[231] Spiramcyin should be continued until delivery even if results of the amniotic fluid PCR are negative and ultrasound examinations are normal. If spiramycin cannot be used or is not available, it may be replaced by sulfadiazine (with appropriate precautions at term) or clindamycin alone. However, there are no data on the efficacy of sulfonamides, including sulfadiazine, or clindamycin when these drugs are used for this purpose.

Because spiramycin does not reliably cross the placenta,[395] if fetal infection is documented or highly suspected or maternal infection is confirmed or highly suspected of having been acquired at 18 weeks of gestation or later, the recommended therapeutic regimen is the combination of sulfadiazine (initial dose of 75 mg/kg, followed by 50 mg/kg every 12 hours [maximum, 4 g/day], pyrimethamine (50 mg every 12 hours for 2 days followed by 50 mg/day), and folinic acid (10 to 20 mg/day [during and 1 week after completion of pyrimethamine therapy]). Such treatment might be an alternative to the termination of pregnancy when abortion is not allowed by law or for women who desire to continue their pregnancy. Pyrimethamine should not be used in the first 12 to 14 weeks of pregnancy because of a concern for teratogenicity (in this circumstance, if indicated, we recommend that sulfadiazine be administered alone, although there are no data on its efficacy in this situation).[218] In addition, pyrimethamine-sulfadiazine

is also recommended for pregnant women in whom a recently acquired acute infection is highly suspected or confirmed during the late second or third trimester; this is due to the high rates of vertical transmission observed in those stages of gestation and should be recommended even though fetal infection may not yet have been confirmed.

A group of European investigators have reported that in their studies, a significant effect of prenatal treatment (in regard to type [i.e., spiramycin vs. pyrimethamine/sulfadiazine] and timing [delay in initiation of the drugs]) on the risk of mother-to-child transmission of toxoplasmosis was not detected.[396-399] These results are not surprising because the studies included very few untreated women in their analysis, and most untreated women were infected during the third trimester.[400] In their most recent study, this group reported evidence of an association between early treatment and reduced risk of congenital toxoplasmosis.[231]

The design of the studies performed to date has not permitted a definitive conclusion. The early studies suggested that spiramycin had a significant clinical benefit in the maternal transmission of the parasite to the fetus, whereas most of the recent studies could not find such benefit. Given that none of the studies have ruled out the possibility of a clinically significant benefit[400] and that the most recent study found benefit with early treatment, most authorities continue to recommend spiramycin or pyrimethamine-sulfadiazine for women with suspected or confirmed acute *T. gondii* infection acquired during gestation until studies definitively addressing this issue are performed.

Pregnant women with toxoplasmic chorioretinitis as a result of reactivation of chronic disease do not have a higher risk of transmitting the parasite to their offspring than do pregnant women who have been infected before pregnancy and do not have ocular disease. Their eye disease should be treated according to the indications discussed in the section "Ocular Toxoplasmosis." Pregnant women with toxoplasmic chorioretinitis thought to be a manifestation of recently acquired infection should be treated because of eye disease and the risk of transmission of the infection to their fetus.

CONGENITAL INFECTION

Detailed information on and recommendations for the postnatal treatment of congenital toxoplasmosis are reviewed elsewhere,[8] but we favor continuous sulfadiazine (50 mg/kg every 12 hours), pyrimethamine (loading dose: 1 mg/kg every 12 hours for 2 days; then beginning on day 3, 1 mg/kg/day for 2 or 6 months; then this dose every Monday, Wednesday, Friday), and folinic acid (10 mg three times weekly during and for 1 week after pyrimethamine therapy) for a minimum of 12 months.[237] Other groups have used pyrimethamine-sulfadiazine-folinic acid alternated with spiramycin (100 mg/kg/day).[8] Serial follow-up to gauge the response of the infant to therapy should include neuroradiology, ophthalmologic examinations, and CSF analysis, if indicated.[8]

For guidance on therapy in congenital cases, we recommend that physicians contact Dr. Rima McLeod at the University of Chicago, where a major study, the National Collaborative Treatment Trial, on the appropriate management of these cases is being performed (telephone 773-834-4152).[237] This study has shown that outcomes are substantially better for most, but not all, infants treated from the neonatal period for 12 months with pyrimethamine-sulfadiazine and leucovorin, compared with historical controls receiving no or short-course therapy.[237,401-403] Improvement in intellectual function, regression of retinal lesions, reduction in anticonvulsant drug requirements, and prevention of auditory sequelae seem to be the major benefits of such treatment, which was combined with CSF shunting, if required.[237] Signs of active infection resolved within weeks of initiation of treatment. In a significant number of treated children, cerebral calcifications decreased in size or resolved.[403] More recently, they also reported that new central chorioretinal lesions were uncommon (14%) in children with congenital toxoplasmosis who were treated during their first year of life, in contrast to historical reports of much higher rates (≥82%) for untreated children or those treated for only 1 month near birth.[239]

■ Prevention

GENERAL METHODS

Prevention is most important in seronegative pregnant women and immunodeficient patients. It is most readily accomplished through education of these patients by their personal physicians (Table 279-3). The goal is to avoid the ingestion of and contact with tissue cysts or sporulated oocysts. Tissue cysts in meat are made noninfectious by heating the meat to 66°C (meat should be cooked to "well done" with no pink meat visible in the center), or by freezing it to −20°C (which is not attainable in most home freezers). Meat that is smoked, cured in brine, or dried may still be infectious. Hands should be washed thoroughly after handling raw meat or vegetables, eggs should not be eaten raw, and unpasteurized milk (particularly milk from goats) should be avoided. Vectors such as flies and cockroaches should be controlled. Areas contaminated with cat feces should be avoided altogether. Disposable gloves should be worn while disposing of cat litter material, working in the garden, or cleaning a child's sandbox. Oocysts are killed if the cat litter pan is soaked in nearly boiling water for 5 minutes. If the litter pan is cleaned every day, oocysts will not have a chance to sporulate. Serologic testing of cats is unwarranted because testing does not demonstrate whether the infected cat is excreting oocysts. Untreated water has been shown to be an effective vehicle for the transmission of the parasite, and drinking water sources potentially contaminated with oocysts should be avoided.

SEROLOGIC SCREENING AND PROPHYLAXIS

Acute Toxoplasma gondii Infection or Toxoplasmosis in the Immunodeficient Patient

Transmission of *T. gondii* and death due to the infection have resulted from the transfusion of leukocyte-rich blood products and by organ transplantation in immunodeficient patients. Transmission of infection by these routes may occur frequently enough to warrant screening for antibody to *T. gondii* in leukocyte-rich blood product donors and possibly to exclude seropositive individuals as organ donors for seronegative potential recipients whenever feasible.

Primary prophylaxis can prevent toxoplasmosis in patients dually infected with HIV and *T. gondii* (see "Toxoplasmosis in the Immunodeficient Patient" under "Treatment"). Prophylactic treatment (pyrimethamine 25 mg/day PO for 6 weeks after transplantation) has been used with apparent success in seronegative recipients of hearts transplanted from seropositive donors.[404] However, TMP-SMX used for PCP prophylaxis in solid organ transplant patients is also effective as primary prophylaxis against *T. gondii* and can be used without the addition of pyrimethamine. Primary prophylaxis in BMT and HSCT patients is particularly challenging because TMP-SMX cannot safely be used early (i.e., before engraftment), whereas in patients with all other transplant organs, it can be used immediately after transplantation.

TABLE 279-3	Measures to Prevent Primary *Toxoplasma gondii* Infection
Avoid contact with materials potentially contaminated with cat feces, especially handling of cat litter and gardening. Gloves are advised when these activities are necessary. Because oocysts require 1 to 2 days to mature, dispose of all cat feces daily.	
Disinfect cat litter box with near-boiling water for 5 minutes before handling.	
Avoid mucous membrane contact when handling raw meat.	
Wash hands thoroughly after contact with raw meat.	
Kitchen surfaces and utensils that have come in contact with raw meat should be washed.	
Cook meat to 67°C (153°F) or "well done" (meat that is smoked or cured in brine may be infectious).	
Avoid ingestion of dried, smoked, or cured meat.	
Wash fruits and vegetables before consumption.	
Refrain from skinning animals.	
Avoid drinking water potentially contaminated with oocysts.	

Congenital Toxoplasma gondii Infection or Toxoplasmosis

Congenital toxoplasmosis is a preventable disease. It is therefore the responsibility of physicians who care for pregnant women to educate them on how they can prevent themselves from becoming infected (and thereby not place the fetus at risk). A lack of adoption of a systematic serologic screening program in the United States leaves education as the principal means of preventing this tragic disease. If physicians choose to screen their patients serologically, the appropriate tests must be used, the laboratory performing the tests must be competent, and the test results must be interpreted correctly. Nonreference laboratories can effectively accomplish the initial screening by simultaneously performing IgG and IgM antibody tests. Only IgM positive test results need to be sent to a reference laboratory for confirmatory testing (Palo Alto Medical Foundation Toxoplasma Serology Laboratory). In some countries (e.g., France and Austria), initially seronegative pregnant women are tested monthly during gestation; this schedule is optimal for detecting infection early enough to institute proper medical management. Women identified as possibly having acquired the infection during gestation can be considered for prenatal diagnosis (see "Congenital Infection in the Fetus and Newborn" under "Diagnosis of Specific Clinical Entities"). The appropriate use of prenatal diagnosis can markedly decrease the incidence of clinically significant congenital toxoplasmosis.[230,405,406]

Women with positive results in the initial IgG antibody test should have a test for IgM antibody performed on the same serum. If the IgM assay result is positive, the specimen should be sent to a reference laboratory for confirmatory testing (see "*Toxoplasma gondii* Infection in Pregnancy").[273,275] In patients with IgG antibodies at any titer, a negative IgM antibody test result in the first trimester, and no clinical signs of acute toxoplasmosis, no further testing would be necessary because the probability of acute acquired infection in these women is extremely low. Given the same circumstances in the second trimester of pregnancy, a negative IgM test result rules out, for practical purposes, recent acquisition of acute infection. A negative IgM test in the third trimester may occur in a patient who acquired the infection earlier in gestation.

The incidence of congenital toxoplasmosis has been shown to be lower in infants born of women who acquire the infection during gestation and are treated with spiramycin.[225,228,231] Results of a study in France[230] on the incidence of *T. gondii* infection in the fetuses of women whose date of acquiring the infection during the gestation was known and who were treated with spiramycin are shown in Table 279-4.

TABLE 279-4	Rates of Congenital Transmission in 270 Women and the Sensitivity and Negative Predictive Value of Amniotic Fluid Polymerase Chain Reaction for Prenatal Diagnosis of Congenital Toxoplasmosis, According to Gestational Age at Which Maternal Infection Was Acquired*†

Gestational Age at Maternal Infection (wk)*	No. of Infected Fetuses†/ Total (%)	Amniotic Fluid PCR Sensitivity (CI) (%)	NPV (CI) (%)
≤6	0/14 (0)	N/A	100 (78-100)
7-11	7/50 (14)	29 (8-65)	90 (81-98)
12-16	7/61 (11.5)	57 (21-94)	95 (86-98)
17-21	14/66 (21.2)	93 (68-99)	98 (90-99.7)
22-26	16/36 (44.4)	63 (39-86)	77 (61-93)
27-31	19/30 (63.3)	68 (48-89)	65 (42-87)
≥32	12/13 (92.3)	50 (22-78)	14 (3-52)
Total	75/270 (28)	N/A	N/A

The positive predictive value was 100%, regardless of gestational age. CI, confidence interval; N/A, not applicable; NPV, negative predictive value; PCR, polymerase chain reaction.

*Maternal infection was diagnosed by seroconversion in the 270 women; 261 (97%) were given treatment with spiramycin.

†Congenital infection was diagnosed by the persistence of *Toxoplasma* immunoglobulin G antibodies after 1 year of life.

Adapted from Montoya JG, Remington JS. Management of *Toxoplasma gondii* infection during pregnancy. *Clin Infect Dis.* 2008;47:554–566.

Recent studies suggested that prenatal treatment with spiramycin does not result in significantly lower rates of *T. gondii* vertical transmission.[396-399] These studies have serious limitations in their design including but not limited to small sample size, high variability in the method used to diagnose acute infection among different centers, lack of monitoring maternal drug compliance, and short follow-up of the cohort of infected children (see "Treatment"). The current policy for women with highly suspected or confirmed acute toxoplasmosis during the first or second trimester (before 18 weeks of gestation) is to receive spiramycin until delivery, unless a positive prenatal diagnosis is made, in which case pyrimethamine-sulfadiazine should be instituted until delivery. These studies provide no convincing evidence that these recommendations should be changed.[400]

In pregnant women infected with both HIV and *T. gondii*, we recommend that primary prophylaxis against *T. gondii* be introduced when their CD4 T-cell count decreases to less than 200/μL. If the patient is receiving TMP-SMX, additional prophylaxis is probably not necessary. Otherwise, spiramycin can be used at a dose of 3 g/day.

ACKNOWLEDGMENT

We gratefully acknowledge and thank Dr. Jack S. Remington, whose lifelong study of toxoplasmosis and authorship of previous editions of this chapter provided the foundation upon which the current chapter is based. We also thank Dr. Alan Sher for his review of the manuscript and helpful suggestions.

REFERENCES

1. Montoya JG, Liesenfeld O. Toxoplasmosis. *Lancet.* 2004; 363:1965-1976.
2. Nicolle C, Manceaux L. Sur une infection a corps de Leishman (ou organismes voisins) du gondi. *Compte rendu hebdomadaire des seances de l'Academie des sciences.* 1908;146:207-209.
3. Janku J. Pathogenesa a pathologicka anatomie tak nazvaneho vrozeneho kolobomu zlute skvrny v oku normalne velikem a mikrophthalmickem s nalezem parazitu v sitnici. *Cas Lek Ces.* 1923;62:1021-1027, 1054-1059, 1081-1085, 1111-1115, 1138-1144.
4. Wolf A, Cowen D, Paige BH. Toxoplasmic encephalomyelitis III. A new case of granulomatous encephalomyelitis due to a protozoon. *Am J Pathol.* 1939;15:657-694.
5. Vietzke WM, Gelderman AH, Grimley PM, et al. Toxoplasmosis complicating malignancy: experience at the National Cancer Institute. *Cancer.* 1968;21:816-827.
6. Israelski DM, Remington JS. Toxoplasmosis in the non-AIDS immunocompromised host. In: Remington J, Swartz M, eds. *Current Clinical Topics in Infectious Diseases.* Vol 13. London: Blackwell Scientific Publications; 1993:322-356.
7. Luft BJ, Conley F, Remington JS, et al. Outbreak of central-nervous-system toxoplasmosis in western Europe and North America. *Lancet.* 1983;1:781-784.
8. Remington JS, McLeod R, Thulliez P, et al. Toxoplasmosis. In: Remington JS, Klein JO, Wilson CB, Baker C, eds. *Infectious Diseases of the Fetus and Newborn Infant.* 6th ed. Philadelphia: Elsevier Saunders; 2006:947-1091.
9. Holland GN. Reconsidering the pathogenesis of ocular toxoplasmosis. *Am J Ophthalmol.* 1999;128:502-505.
10. Dubey JP, Lindsay DS, Speer CA. Structures of *Toxoplasma gondii* tachyzoites, bradyzoites, and sporozoites and biology and development of tissue cysts. *Clin Microbiol Rev.* 1998; 11:267-299.
11. Sibley LD, Boothroyd JC. Virulent strains of *Toxoplasma gondii* comprise a single clonal lineage. *Nature.* 1992;359:82-85.
12. Howe DK, Honore S, Derouin F, et al. Determination of genotypes of *Toxoplasma gondii* strains isolated from patients with toxoplasmosis. *J Clin Microbiol.* 1997;35:1411-1414.
13. Fuentes I, Rubio JM, Ramirez C, et al. Genotypic characterization of *Toxoplasma gondii* strains associated with human toxoplasmosis in Spain: direct analysis from clinical samples. *J Clin Microbiol.* 2001;39:1566-1570.
14. Ajzenberg D, Cogne N, Paris L, et al. Genotype of 86 *Toxoplasma gondii* isolates associated with human congenital toxoplasmosis, and correlation with clinical findings. *J Infect Dis.* 2002; 186:684-689.
15. Boothroyd JC, Grigg ME. Population biology of *Toxoplasma gondii* and its relevance to human infection: do different strains cause different disease? *Curr Opin Microbiol.* 2002;5:438-442.
16. Lehmann T, Marcet PL, Graham DH, et al. Globalization and the population structure of *Toxoplasma gondii*. *Proc Natl Acad Sci U S A.* 2006;103:11423-11428.
17. Darde ML. *Toxoplasma gondii*, "new" genotypes and virulence. *Parasite.* 2008;15:366-371.
18. Radke JR, Striepen B, Guerini MN, et al. Defining the cell cycle for the tachyzoite stage of *Toxoplasma gondii*. *Mol Biochem Parasitol.* 2001;115:165-175.
19. Dubey JP. Advances in the life cycle of *Toxoplasma gondii*. *Int J Parasitol.* 1998;28:1019-1024.
20. Barragan A, Sibley LD. Transepithelial migration of *Toxoplasma gondii* is linked to parasite motility and virulence. *J Exp Med.* 2002;195:1625-1633.
21. Carruthers V, Boothroyd JC. Pulling together: an integrated model of *Toxoplasma* cell invasion. *Curr Opin Microbiol.* 2007;10:83-89.
22. Boothroyd JC, Dubremetz JF. Kiss and spit: the dual roles of *Toxoplasma* rhoptries. *Nat Rev Microbiol.* 2008;6:79-88.
23. Dubey JP. Advances in the life cycle of *Toxoplasma gondii*. *Int J Parasitol.* 1998;28:1019-1024.
24. Conley FK, Jenkins KA, Remington JS. *Toxoplasma gondii* infection of the central nervous system: use of the peroxidase-antiperoxidase method to demonstrate *Toxoplasma* in formalin fixed, paraffin embedded tissue sections. *Hum Pathol.* 1981;12:690-698.
25. Remington JS, Cavanaugh EN. Isolation of the encysted form of *Toxoplasma gondii* from human skeletal muscle and brain. *N Engl J Med.* 1965;273:1308-1310.
26. Dubey J, Thayer D. Killing of different strains of *Toxoplasma gondii* tissue cysts by irradiation under defined conditions. *J Parasitol.* 1994;80:764-767.
27. Dubey J, Kotula A, Sharar A, et al. Effect of high temperature on infectivity of *Toxoplasma gondii* tissue cysts in pork. *J Parasitol.* 1990;76:201.
28. Jacobs L, Remington JS, Melton ML. The resistance of the encysted form of *Toxoplasma gondii*. *J Parasitol.* 1960;46:11-21.
29. El-Nawawi FA, Tawfik MA, Shaapan RM. Methods for inactivation of *Toxoplasma gondii* cysts in meat and tissues of experimentally infected sheep. *Foodborne Pathog Dis.* 2008;5: 687-690.
30. Ferguson DJP, Graham DI, Hutchinson WM. Pathological changes in the brains of mice infected with *Toxoplasma gondii*: a histological immunocytochemical and ultrastructural study. *Int J Exp Pathol.* 1991;72:463-474.
31. Sims TA, Hay J, Talbot IC. An electron microscope and immunohistochemical study of the intracellular location of *Toxoplasma* tissue cysts within the brains of mice with congenital toxoplasmosis. *Br J Exp Pathol.* 1989;70: 317-325.
32. Jones TC, Bienz KA, Erb P. In vitro cultivation of *Toxoplasma gondii* cysts in astrocytes in the presence of gamma interferon. *Infect Immun.* 1986;51:146-156.
33. Ferguson DJ, Hutchison WM, Pettersen E. Tissue cyst rupture in mice chronically infected with *Toxoplasma gondii*. *Parasitol Res.* 1989;75:599-603.
34. Dubey JP, Jones JL. *Toxoplasma gondii* infection in humans and animals in the United States. *Int J Parasitol.* 2008;38:1257-1278.
35. Neu HC. Toxoplasmosis transmitted at autopsy. *JAMA.* 1967;202:284-285.
36. Dubey J. Toxoplasmosis. *Am Vet Med Assoc.* 1994;205:1593-1598.
37. Desmonts G, Couvreur J, Alison F, et al. Etude epidemiologique sur la toxoplasmose: l'influence de la cuisson des viandes de boucherie sur la frequence de l'infection humaine. *Rev Fr Etud Clin Biol.* 1965;10:952-958.
38. Dubey JP, Gamble HR, Hill D, et al. P. High prevalence of viable *Toxoplasma gondii* infection in market weight pigs from a farm in Massachusetts. *J Parasitol.* 2002;88:1234-1238.
39. Hill D, Dubey JP. *Toxoplasma gondii*: transmission, diagnosis and prevention. *Clin Microbiol Infect.* 2002;8:634-640.
40. Remington JS. Toxoplasmosis and congenital infection. *Intrauterine Infect.* 1968;4:47-56.
41. Aspinall TV, Marlee D, Hyde JE, et al. Prevalence of *Toxoplasma gondii* in commercial meat products as monitored by polymerase chain reaction—food for thought? *Int J Parasitol.* 2002;32:1193-1199.
42. Davies PR, Morrow WE, Deen J, et al. Seroprevalence of *Toxoplasma gondii* and *Trichinella spiralis* in finishing swine raised in different production systems in North Carolina, USA. *Prev Vet Med.* 1998;36:67-76.
43. Riemann HP, Meyer ME, Theis JH, et al. Toxoplasmosis in an infant fed unpasteurized goat milk. *J Pediatr.* 1975;87: 573-576.
44. Sacks JJ, Roberto RR, Brooks NF. Toxoplasmosis infection associated with raw goat's milk. *JAMA.* 1982;248:1728-1732.
45. Dubey JP, Graham DH, Blackston CR, et al. Biological and genetic characterisation of *Toxoplasma gondii* isolates from chickens (*Gallus domesticus*) from Sao Paulo, Brazil: unexpected findings. *Int J Parasitol.* 2002;32:99-105.
46. Swartzberg JE, Remington JS. Transmission of *Toxoplasma*. *Am J Dis Child.* 1975;129:777-779.
47. Bowie WR, King AS, Werker DH, et al. Outbreak of toxoplasmosis associated with municipal drinking water. *Lancet.* 1997;350:173-177.
48. Luft BJ, Remington JS. Acute *Toxoplasma* infection among family members of patients with acute lymphadenopathic toxoplasmosis. *Arch Intern Med.* 1984;144:53-56.
49. Masur H, Jones TC, Lempert JA, et al. Outbreak of toxoplasmosis in a family and documentation of acquired retinochoroiditis. *Am J Med.* 1978;64:396-402.
50. Miller MA, Gardner IA, Kreuder C, et al. Coastal freshwater runoff is a risk factor for *Toxoplasma gondii* infection of southern sea otters (*Enhydra lutris nereis*). *Int J Parasitol.* 2002; 32:997-1006.
51. Bahia-Oliveira LM, Jones JL, Azevedo-Silva J, et al. Highly endemic, waterborne toxoplasmosis in north Rio de Janeiro state, Brazil. *Emerg Infect Dis.* 2003;9:55-62.
52. Dumetre A, Le Bras C, Baffet M, et al. Effects of ozone and ultraviolet radiation treatments on the infectivity of *Toxoplasma gondii* oocysts. *Vet Parasitol.* 2008;153:209-213.
53. Lindsay DS, Collins MV, Mitchell SM, et al. Sporulation and survival of *Toxoplasma gondii* oocysts in seawater. *J Eukaryot Microbiol.* 2003;50:687-688.
54. Wainwright KE, Miller MA, Barr BC, et al. Chemical inactivation of *Toxoplasma gondii* oocysts in water. *J Parasitol.* 2007;93:925-931.
55. Conrad PA, Miller MA, Kreuder C, et al. Transmission of *Toxoplasma*: clues from the study of sea otters as sentinels of *Toxoplasma gondii* flow into the marine environment. *Int J Parasitol.* 2005;35:1155-1168.
56. Smith KL, Wilson M, Hightower AW, et al. Prevalence of *Toxoplasma gondii* antibodies in U.S. military recruits in 1989: comparison with data published in 1965. *Clin Infect Dis.* 1996;23:1182-1183.
57. Jones JL, Kruszon-Moran D, Sanders-Lewis K, et al. *Toxoplasma gondii* infection in the United States, 1999-2004, decline from the prior decade. *Am J Trop Med Hyg.* 2007;77:405-410.
58. Rosso F, Les JT, Agudelo A, et al. Prevalence of infection with *Toxoplasma gondii* among pregnant women in Cali, Colombia, South America. *Am J Trop Med Hyg.* 2008;78:504-508.
59. Siegel SE, Lunde MN, Gelderman AH, et al. Transmission of toxoplasmosis by leukocyte transfusion. *Blood.* 1971;37: 388-394.
60. Ryning FW, McLeod R, Maddox JC, et al. Probable transmission of *Toxoplasma gondii* by organ transplantation. *Ann Intern Med.* 1979;90:47-49.
61. Mele A, Paterson PJ, Prentice HG, et al. Toxoplasmosis in bone marrow transplantation: a report of two cases and systematic review of the literature. *Bone Marrow Transplant.* 2002; 29:691-698.
62. Slavin MA, Meyers JD, Remington JS, et al. *Toxoplasma gondii* infection in marrow transplant recipients: a 20 year experience. *Bone Marrow Transplant.* 1994;13:549-557.
63. Leport C, Chêne G, Morlat P, et al. Pyrimethamine for primary prophylaxis of toxoplasmic encephalitis in patients with human immunodeficiency virus infection: a double-blind, randomized trial. *J Infect Dis.* 1996;173:91-97.
64. San-Andres FJ, Rubio R, Castilla J, et al. Incidence of acquired immunodeficiency syndrome-associated opportunistic diseases and the effect of treatment on a cohort of 1115 patients infected with human immunodeficiency virus, 1989-1997. *Clin Infect Dis.* 2003;36:1177-1185.
65. Luft BJ, Remington JS. Toxoplasmic encephalitis in AIDS (AIDS commentary). *Clin Infect Dis.* 1992;15:211-222.
66. Abgrall S, Rabaud C, Costagliola D. Incidence and risk factors for toxoplasmic encephalitis in human immunodeficiency virus-infected patients before and during the highly active antiretroviral therapy era. *Clin Infect Dis.* 2001;33:1747-1755.
67. Jones JL, Sehgal M, Maguire JH. Toxoplasmosis-associated deaths among human immunodeficiency virus-infected persons in the United States, 1992-1998. *Clin Infect Dis.* 2002;34: 1161.
68. Clumeck N. Some aspects of the epidemiology of toxoplasmosis and pneumocystosis in AIDS in Europe. *Eur J Clin Microbiol Infect Dis.* 1991;10:177-178.
69. Zumla A, Savva D, Wheeler RB, et al. *Toxoplasma* serology in Zambian and Ugandan patients infected with the human immunodeficiency virus. *Trans R Soc Trop Med Hyg.* 1991;85: 227-229.
70. Belanger F, Derouin F, Grangeot-Keros L, et al. Incidence and risk factors of toxoplasmosis in a cohort of human immunode-

ficiency virus-infected patients: 1988-1995. HEMOCO and SEROCO Study Groups. *Clin Infect Dis.* 1999;28:575-581.
71. Lucas S, Hounnou A, Peacock C, et al. The mortality and pathology of HIV infection in a West African city. *AIDS.* 1993; 7:1569-1579.
72. Wallace MR, Rossetti RJ, Olson PE. Cats and toxoplasmosis risk in HIV-infected adults. *JAMA.* 1993;269:76-77.
73. Ruskin J, Remington JS. Toxoplasmosis in the compromised host. *Ann Intern Med.* 1976;84:193-199.
74. Jones TC, Yeh S, Hirsch JG. The interaction between *Toxoplasma gondii* and mammalian cells. I. Mechanism of entry and intracellular fate of the parasite. *J Exp Med.* 1972;136: 1157-1172.
75. Murray HW, Nathans CF, Cohn ZA. Macrophages oxygen-dependent antimicrobial activity. IV. Role of endogenous scavengers of oxygen intermediates. *J Exp Med.* 1980;152: 1610-1624.
76. Sibley LD, Weidner E, Krahenbuhl JL. Phagosome acidification blocked by intracellular *Toxoplasma gondii*. *Nature.* 1985;315:416-419.
77. Adams LB, Hibbs Jr JB, Taintor RR, et al. Microbiostatic effect of murine-activated macrophages for *Toxoplasma gondii*. *J Immunol.* 1990;144:2725-2729.
78. Pfefferkorn ER. Interferon gamma blocks the growth of *Toxoplasma gondii* in human fibroblasts by inducing the host cells to degrade tryptophan. *Proc Natl Acad Sci U S A.* 1984;81:908-912.
79. Schreiber RD, Feldman HA. Identification of the activator system for antibody to *Toxoplasma* as the classical complement pathway. *J Infect Dis.* 1980;141:366-369.
80. Remington JS, Jacobs L, Kaufman HE. Studies on chronic toxoplasmosis: the relation of infective dose to residual infection and to the possibility of congenital transmission. *Am J Ophthalmol.* 1958;46:261-267.
81. Hofflin JM, Conley FK, Remington JS. Murine model of intracerebral toxoplasmosis. *J Infect Dis.* 1987;155:550-557.
82. Hofflin JM, Remington JS. Tissue culture isolation of *Toxoplasma* from blood of a patient with AIDS. *Arch Intern Med.* 1985;145:925-926.
83. Tirard V, Niel G, Rosenheim M, et al. Diagnosis of toxoplasmosis in patients with AIDS by isolation of the parasite from the blood. *N Engl J Med.* 1991;324:632.
84. Murray H, Rubin BY, Masur H, et al. Impaired production of lymphokines and immune (gamma) interferon in the acquired immunodeficiency syndrome. *N Engl J Med.* 1984;310:883-889.
85. Murray H, Welte K, Jacobs J, et al. Production and in vitro response to interleukin-2 in the acquired immunodeficiency syndrome. *J Clin Invest.* 1985;76:1959-1964.
86. Murray HW, Scavuzzo D, Jacobs JL, et al. In vitro and in vivo activation of human mononuclear phagocytes by interferon-gamma: studies with normal and AIDS monocytes. *J Immunol.* 1987;138:2457-2462.
87. Pomeroy C, Filice G, Hitt J, et al. Cytomegalovirus-induced reactivation of *Toxoplasma gondii* in mice: lung lymphocyte phenotypes and suppressor function. *J Infect Dis.* 1992; 166:677-681.
88. Hunter CA, Subauste C, Van Cleave V, et al. Production of gamma interferon by natural killer cells from *Toxoplasma gondii*-infected SCID mice: regulation by interleukin-10, interleukin-12, and tumor necrosis factor alpha. *Infect Immun.* 1994;62:2818-2824.
89. Khan I, Matsuura T, Kasper L. Interleukin-12 enhances murine survival against acute toxoplasmosis. *Infect Immun.* 1994; 62:1639-1642.
90. Yap GS, Sher A. Cell-mediated immunity to *Toxoplasma gondii*: initiation, regulation and effector function. *Immunobiology.* 1999;201:240-247.
91. Denkers EY, Butcher BA, Del Rio L, et al. Neutrophils, dendritic cells and *Toxoplasma*. *Int J Parasitol.* 2004;34:411-421.
92. Subauste CS, Wessendarp M, Sorensen RU, et al. CD40-CD40 ligand interaction is central to cell-mediated immunity against *Toxoplasma gondii*: patients with hyper IgM syndrome have a defective type 1 immune response that can be restored by soluble CD40 ligand trimer. *J Immunol.* 1999;162:6690-6700.
93. Levy J, Espanol-Boren T, Thomas C, et al. Clinical spectrum of X-linked hyper-IgM syndrome. *J Pediatr.* 1997;131:47-54.
94. Subauste CS, Wessendarp M, Smulian AG, et al. Role of CD40 ligand signaling in defective type 1 cytokine response in human immunodeficiency virus infection. *J Infect Dis.* 2001; 183:1722-1731.
95. Hunter CA, Remington JS. Immunopathogenesis of toxoplasmic encephalitis. *J Infect Dis.* 1994;170:1057-1067.
96. Gazzinelli R, Hieny S, Wynn T, et al. Interleukin 12 is required for the T-lymphocyte-independent induction of interferon g by an intracellular parasite and induces resistance in T-cell-deficient hosts. *Proc Natl Acad Sci U S A.* 1993;90:6115-6119.
97. Gazzinelli R, Wysocka M, Hayashi S, et al. Parasite-induced IL-12 stimulates early IFN-g synthesis and resistance during acute infection with *Toxoplasma gondii*. *J Immunol.* 1994; 153:2533-2543.
98. Suzuki Y, Orellana MA, Schreiber RD, et al. Interferon-γ: the major mediator of resistance against *Toxoplasma gondii*. *Science.* 1988;240:516-518.
99. Suzuki Y, Conley FK, Remington JS. Importance of endogenous IFN-γ for prevention of toxoplasmic encephalitis in mice. *J Immunol.* 1989;143:2045-2050.
100. Suzuki Y, Conley FK, Remington JS. Treatment of toxoplasmic encephalitis in mice with recombinant gamma interferon. *Infect Immun.* 1990;58:3050-3055.
101. Robben PM, Mordue DG, Truscott SM, et al. Production of IL-12 by macrophages infected with *Toxoplasma gondii* depends on the parasite genotype. *J Immunol.* 2004;172:3686-3694.
102. Saeij JP, Coller S, Boyle JP, et al. *Toxoplasma* co-opts host gene expression by injection of a polymorphic kinase homologue. *Nature.* 2007;445:324-327.
103. Sibley LD, Adams LB, Fukutomi Y, et al. Tumor necrosis factor-α triggers antitoxoplasmal activity of IFN-γ primed macrophages. *J Immunol.* 1991;147:2340-2345.
104. Langermans J, van der Hulst M, Nibbering P, et al. IFN-γ induced L-arginine-dependent toxoplasmastatic activity in murine peritoneal macrophages is mediated by endogenous tumor necrosis factor. *J Immunol.* 1992;148:568-574.
105. Chang H, Pechere J, Piguet P. Role of tumour necrosis factor in chronic murine *Toxoplasma gondii* encephalitis. *Immunol Infect Dis.* 1992;2:61-68.
106. Suzuki Y, Yang Q, Yang S, et al. IL-4 is protective against development of toxoplasmic encephalitis. *J Immunol.* 1996; 157:2564-2569.
107. Suzuki Y, Rani S, Liesenfeld O, et al. Impaired resistance to the development of toxoplasmic encephalitis in interleukin-6-deficient mice. *Infect Immun.* 1997;65:2339-2345.
108. Kasper LH, Matsuura T, Khan IA. IL-7 stimulates protective immunity in mice against the intracellular pathogen, *Toxoplasma gondii*. *J Immunol.* 1995;155:4798-4804.
109. Hunter CA, Neyer LA, Gabriel KE, et al. The role of CD28/B7 interaction in the regulation of NK cell responses during infection with *Toxoplasma gondii*. *J Immunol.* 1997;158:2285-2293.
110. Kelly MN, Kolls JK, Happel K, et al. Interleukin-17/interleukin-17 receptor-mediated signaling is important for generation of an optimal polymorphonuclear response against *Toxoplasma gondii* infection. *Infect Immun.* 2005;73:617-621.
111. Lieberman LA, Cardillo F, Owyang AM, et al. IL-23 provides a limited mechanism of resistance to acute toxoplasmosis in the absence of IL-12. *J Immunol.* 2004;173:1887-1893.
112. Stumhofer JS, Laurence A, Wilson EH, et al. Interleukin 27 negatively regulates the development of interleukin 17-producing T helper cells during chronic inflammation of the central nervous system. *Nat Immunol.* 2006;7:937-945.
113. Bohne W, Hessemann J, Gross U. Reduced replication of *Toxoplasma gondii* is necessary for induction of bradyzoite-specific antigens: a possible role for nitric oxide in triggering stage conversion. *Infect Immun.* 1994;62:1761-1767.
114. Chao C, Gekker G, Hu S, et al. Human microglial cell defense against *Toxoplasma gondii*. *J Immunol.* 1994;152:1246-1252.
115. Khan IA, Matssuura T, Fonseka S, et al. Production of nitric oxide (NO) is not essential for protection against acute *Toxoplasma gondii* infection in IRF-1$^{-/-}$ mice[1]. *J Immunol.* 1996; 156:636-643.
116. Scharton-Kersten TM, Wynn TA, Denkers EY, et al. In the absence of endogenous IFN-γ mice develop unimpaired IL-12 responses to *Toxoplasma gondii* while failing to control acute infection. *J Immunol.* 1996;157:4045-4054.
117. Hayashi S, Chan C, Gazzinelli R, et al. Contribution of nitric oxide to the host parasite equilibrium in toxoplasmosis. *J Immunol.* 1996;156:1476-1481.
118. Scharton-Kersten TM, Yap G, Magram J, et al. Inducible nitric oxide is essential for host control of persistent but not acute infection with the intracellular pathogen *Toxoplasma gondii*. *J Exp Med.* 1997;185:1261-1273.
119. Taylor GA, Feng CG, Sher A. Control of IFN-gamma-mediated host resistance to intracellular pathogens by immunity-related GTPases (p47 GTPases). *Microbes Infect.* 2007;9:1644-1651.
120. Martens S, Parvanova I, Zerrahn J, et al. Disruption of *Toxoplasma gondii* parasitophorous vacuoles by the mouse p47-resistance GTPases. *PLoS Pathog.* 2005;1:e24.
121. Ling YM, Shaw MH, Ayala C, et al. Vacuolar and plasma membrane stripping and autophagic elimination of *Toxoplasma gondii* in primed effector macrophages. *J Exp Med.* 2006; 203:2063-2071.
122. Pavia CS. Protection against experimental toxoplasmosis by adoptive immunotherapy. *J Immunol.* 1986;137:2985-2990.
123. Peterson P, Gekker G, Hu S, et al. Human astrocytes inhibit intracellular multiplication of *Toxoplasma gondii* by a nitric oxide-mediated mechanism. *J Infect Dis.* 1995;171:516-518.
124. Brown CR, McLeod R. Class I MHC genes and CD8^{+} T cells determine cyst number in *Toxoplasma gondii* infection. *J Immunol.* 1990;145:3438-3441.
125. Brown C, Hunter C, Estes R, et al. Definitive identification of a gene that confers resistance against *Toxoplasma* cyst burden and encephalitis. *Immunology.* 1995;85:419-428.
126. Suzuki Y, Joh K, Orellna MA, et al. A gene(s) within the H-2D region determines the development of toxoplasmic encephalitis in mice. *Immunology.* 1991;74:732-739.
127. Suzuki Y, Wong S-Y, Grumet FC, et al. Evidence for genetic regulation of susceptibility to toxoplasmic encephalitis in AIDS patients. *J Infect Dis.* 1996;173:265-268.
128. Mack D, Johnson J, Roberts F, et al. HLA-class II genes modify outcome of *Toxoplasma gondii* infection. *Int J Parasitol.* 1999;29:1351-1358.
129. Habegger de Sorrentino A, Lopez R, Motta P, et al. HLA class II involvement in HIV-associated toxoplasmic encephalitis development. *Clin Immunol.* 2005;115:133-137.
130. Cordeiro CA, Moreira PR, Andrade MS, et al. Interleukin-10 gene polymorphism (-1082G/A) is associated with toxoplasmic retinochoroiditis. *Invest Ophthalmol Vis Sci.* 2008;49: 1979-1982.
131. Dorfman RF, Remington JS. Value of lymph-node biopsy in the diagnosis of acute acquired toxoplasmosis. *N Engl J Med.* 1973;289:878-881.
132. Montoya JG, Jordan R, Lingamneni S, et al. Toxoplasmic myocarditis and polymyositis in patients with acute acquired toxoplasmosis diagnosed during life. *Clin Infect Dis.* 1997; 24:676-683.
133. Negri Gualdi C. [Infectious pseudomononucleosis in lymphomatous diseases]. *Minerva Med.* 1974;65:78-83.
134. Weiss L, Chen Y, Berry G, et al. Infrequent detection of *Toxoplasma gondii* genome in toxoplasmic lymphadenitis: a polymerase chain reaction study. *Hum Pathol.* 1992;23:154-158.
135. Montoya JG, Remington JS. Toxoplasmosis of the central nervous system. In: Peterson PK, Remington JS, eds. *In Defense of the Brain: Current Concepts in the Immunopathogenesis and Clinical Aspects of CNS Infections.* Boston: Blackwell Scientific; 1997:163-188.
136. Frenkel JK. Pathology and pathogenesis of congenital toxoplasmosis. *Bull N Y Acad Med.* 1974;50:182-191.
137. Liesenfeld O, Wong SY, Remington JS. Toxoplasmosis in the setting of AIDS. In: Bartlett JG, Merigan TC, Bolognesi D, eds. *Textbook of AIDS Medicine.* 2nd ed. Baltimore: Williams & Wilkins; 1999:225-259.
138. Post MJ, Chan JC, Hensley GT, et al. Toxoplasmosis encephalitis in Haitian adults with acquired immunodeficiency syndrome: a clinical-pathologic-CT correlation. *AJNR Am J Neuroradiol.* 1983;4:155-162.
139. Strittmatter C, Lang W, Wiestler OD, et al. The changing pattern of human immunodeficiency virus associated cerebral toxoplasmosis: a study of 46 postmortem cases. *Acta Neuropathol.* 1992;83:475-481.
140. Parmley SF, Goebel FD, Remington JS. Detection of *Toxoplasma gondii* DNA in cerebrospinal fluid from AIDS patients by polymerase chain reaction. *J Clin Microbiol.* 1992;30:3000-3002.
141. Gray F, Gherardi R, Wingate E, et al. Diffuse "encephalitic" cerebral toxoplasmosis in AIDS. *J Neurol.* 1989;236:273-277.
142. Mariuz P, Bosler EM, Luft BJ. *Toxoplasma* pneumonia. *Semin Respir Infect.* 1997;12:40-43.
143. Bretagne S, Costa J-M, Fleury-Feith J, et al. Quantitative competitive PCR with bronchoalveolar lavage fluid for diagnosis of toxoplasmosis in AIDS patients. *J Clin Microbiol.* 1995;33:1662-1664.
144. Holland GN, O'Connor GR, et al. Toxoplasmosis. In: Pepose JS, Holland GN, Wilhelmus KR, eds. *Ocular Infection and Immunity.* St. Louis: Mosby Yearbook; 1996:1183-1223.
145. Danise A, Cinque P, Vergani S, et al. Use of the polymerase chain reaction assays of aqueous humor in the differential diagnosis of retinitis in patients infected with human immunodeficiency virus. *Clin Infect Dis.* 1997;24:1100-1106.
146. Montoya JG, Parmley S, Liesenfeld O, et al. Use of the polymerase chain reaction for diagnosis of ocular toxoplasmosis. *Ophthalmology.* 1999;106:1554-1563.
147. Silveira C, Belfort Jr R, Muccioli C, et al. The effect of long-term intermittent trimethoprim/sulfamethoxazole treatment on recurrences of toxoplasmic retinochoroiditis. *Am J Ophthalmol.* 2002;134:41-46.
148. Jones JL, Muccioli C, Belfort Jr R, et al. Recently acquired *Toxoplasma gondii* infection, Brazil. *Emerg Infect Dis.* 2006; 12:582-587.
149. Gilbert RE, Freeman K, Lago EG, et al. Ocular sequelae of congenital toxoplasmosis in Brazil compared with Europe. *PLoS Negl Trop Dis.* 2008;2:e277.
150. de-la-Torre A, Lopez-Castillo CA, Gomez-Marin JE. Incidence and clinical characteristics in a Colombian cohort of ocular toxoplasmosis. *Eye.* 2009;23:1090-1093.
151. Vallochi AL, Muccioli C, Martins MC, et al. The genotype of *Toxoplasma gondii* strains causing ocular toxoplasmosis in humans in Brazil. *Am J Ophthalmol.* 2005;139:350-351.
152. Grigg ME, Ganatra J, Boothroyd JC, et al. Unusual abundance of atypical strains associated with human ocular toxoplasmosis. *J Infect Dis.* 2001;184:633-639.
153. Gherardi R, Baudrimont M, Lionnet F, et al. Skeletal muscle toxoplasmosis in patients with acquired immunodeficiency syndrome: a clinical and pathological study. *Ann Neurol.* 1992;32:535-542.
154. Calico I, Caballero E, Martinez O, et al. Isolation of *Toxoplasma gondii* from immunocompromised patients using tissue culture. *Infection.* 1991;19:340-342.
155. Roldan EO, Moskowitz L, Hensley GT. Pathology of the heart in acquired immunodeficiency syndrome. *Arch Pathol Lab Med.* 1987;111:943-946.
156. Adair OV, Randive N, Krasnow N. Isolated *Toxoplasma* myocarditis in acquired immune deficiency syndrome. *Am Heart J.* 1989;118:856-857.
157. Pauwels A, Meyohas MC, Eliaszewicz M, et al. *Toxoplasma* colitis in the acquired immunodeficiency syndrome. *Am J Gastroenterol.* 1992;87:518-519.
158. Smart PE, Weinfeld A, Thompson NE, et al. Toxoplasmosis of the stomach: a cause of antral narrowing. *Radiology.* 1990; 174:369-370.
159. Garcia LW, Hemphill RB, Marasco WA, et al. Acquired immunodeficiency syndrome with disseminated toxoplasmosis pre-

senting as an acute pulmonary and gastrointestinal illness. *Arch Pathol Lab Med.* 1991;115:459-463.
160. Brion J-P, Pelloux H, Le Marc'hadour F, et al. Acute *Toxoplasmic* hepatitis in a patient with AIDS. *Clin Infect Dis.* 1992; 15:183-184.
161. Bergin C, Murphy M, Lyons D, et al. *Toxoplasma* pneumonitis: fatal presentation of disseminated toxoplasmosis in a patient with AIDS. *Eur Respir J.* 1992;5:1018-1020.
162. Crider SR, Horstman WG, Massey GS. *Toxoplasma orchitis*: report of a case and a review of the literature. *Am J Med.* 1988;85:421-424.
163. Groll A, Schneider M, Althoff PH, et al. Morphology and clinical significance of AIDS-related lesions in the adrenals and pituitary. *Dtsch Med Wochenschr.* 1990;115:483-488.
164. Patrick AL, Roberts LA, Burton EN, et al. Focal and segmental glomerulosclerosis in the acquired immunodeficiency syndrome. *West Indian Med J.* 1986;35:200-202.
165. Renold C, Sugar A, Chave J-P, et al. *Toxoplasma* encephalitis in patients with the acquired immunodeficiency syndrome. *Medicine (Baltimore).* 1992;71:224-239.
166. Remington JS. Toxoplasmosis in the adult. *Bull N Y Acad Med.* 1974;50:211-227.
167. Demar M, Ajzenberg D, Maubon D, et al. Fatal outbreak of human toxoplasmosis along the Maroni River: epidemiological, clinical, and parasitological aspects. *Clin Infect Dis.* 2007; 45:e88-e95.
168. McCabe RE, Brooks RG, Dorfman RF, et al. Clinical spectrum in 107 cases of toxoplasmic lymphadenopathy. *Rev Infect Dis.* 1987;9:754-774.
169. Remington JS, Barnett CG, Meikel M, et al. Toxoplasmosis and infectious mononucleosis. *Arch Intern Med.* 1962;110:744-753.
170. Couvreur J, Thulliez P. Acquired toxoplasmosis with ocular or neurologic involvement [Toxoplasmose acquise à localisation oculaire ou neurologique]. *Presse Med.* 1996;25:438-442.
171. Montoya JG, Remington JS. Toxoplasmic chorioretinitis in the setting of acute acquired toxoplasmosis. *Clin Infect Dis.* 1996;23:277-282.
172. Delair E, Monnet D, Grabar S, et al. Respective roles of acquired and congenital infections in presumed ocular toxoplasmosis. *Am J Ophthalmol.* 2008;146:851-855.
173. Burnett AJ, Shortt SG, Isaac-Renton J, et al. Multiple cases of acquired toxoplasmosis retinitis presenting in an outbreak. *Ophthalmology.* 1998;105:1032-1037.
174. Montoya JG, Remington JS. Studies on the serodiagnosis of toxoplasmic lymphadenitis. *Clin Infect Dis.* 1995;20:781-790.
175. Cunningham T. Pancarditis in acute toxoplasmosis. *Am J Clin Pathol.* 1982;78:403-405.
176. Prado SP, Pacheco VC, Noemi IH, et al. [*Toxoplasma* pericarditis and myocarditis]. *Rev Chil Pediatr.* 1978;49:179-185.
177. Greenlee JE, Johnson Jr WD, Campa JF, et al. Adult toxoplasmosis presenting as polymyositis and cerebellar ataxia. *Ann Intern Med.* 1975;82:367-371.
178. Paspalaki PK, Mihailidou EP, Bitsori M, et al. Polymyositis and myocarditis associated with acquired toxoplasmosis in an immunocompetent girl. *BMC Musculoskelet Disord.* 2001; 2:8.
179. Palma S, Reyes H, Guzman L, et al. Dermatomyositis and toxoplasmosis. *Rev Med Chil.* 1984;111:164-167.
180. Pollock JL. Toxoplasmosis appearing to be dermatomyositis. *Arch Dermatol.* 1979;115:736-737.
181. Brown AS, Schaefer CA, Quesenberry Jr CP, et al. Maternal exposure to toxoplasmosis and risk of schizophrenia in adult offspring. *Am J Psychiatry.* 2005;162:767-773.
182. Niebuhr DW, Millikan AM, Cowan DN, et al. Selected infectious agents and risk of schizophrenia among U.S. military personnel. *Am J Psychiatry.* 2008;165:99-106.
183. Lassoued S, Zabraniecki L, Marin F, et al. Toxoplasmic chorioretinitis and antitumor necrosis factor treatment in rheumatoid arthritis. *Semin Arthritis Rheum.* 2007;36:262-263.
184. Montoya JG, Giraldo LF, Efron B, et al. Infectious complications among 620 consecutive heart transplant patients at Stanford University Medical Center. *Clin Infect Dis.* 2001;33:629-640.
185. Wreghitt TG, Gray JJ, Pavel P, et al. Efficacy of pyrimethamine for the prevention of donor-acquired *Toxoplasma gondii* infection in heart and heart-lung transplant patients. *Transpl Int.* 1992;5:197-200.
186. Wreghitt TG, McNeil K, Roth C, et al. Antibiotic prophylaxis for the prevention of donor-acquired *Toxoplasma gondii* infection in transplant patients [letter; comment]. *J Infect.* 1995; 31:253-254.
187. Renoult E, Georges E, Biava MF, et al. Toxoplasmosis in kidney transplant recipients: report of six cases and review. *Clin Infect Dis.* 1997;24:625-634.
188. Singer MA, Hagler WS, Grossniklaus HE. *Toxoplasma gondii* retinochoroiditis after liver transplantation. *Retina.* 1993; 13:40-45.
189. Botterel F, Ichai P, Feray C, et al. Disseminated toxoplasmosis, resulting from infection of allograft, after orthotopic liver transplantation: usefulness of quantitative PCR. *J Clin Microbiol.* 2002;40:1648-1650.
190. Martino R, Maertens J, Bretagne S, et al. Toxoplasmosis after hematopoietic stem cell transplantation. *Clin Infect Dis.* 2000;31: 1188-1195.
191. Martino R, Bretagne S, Einsele H, et al. Early detection of *Toxoplasma* infection by molecular monitoring of *Toxoplasma gondii* in peripheral blood samples after allogeneic stem cell transplantation. *Clin Infect Dis.* 2005;40:67-78.
192. Matsuo Y, Takeishi S, Miyamoto T, et al. Toxoplasmosis encephalitis following severe graft-vs.-host disease after allogeneic hematopoietic stem cell transplantation: 17 yr experience in Fukuoka BMT group. *Eur J Haematol.* 2007;79: 317-321.
193. Sing A, Leitritz L, Roggenkamp A, et al. Pulmonary toxoplasmosis in bone marrow transplant recipients: report of two cases and review. *Clin Infect Dis.* 1999;29:429-433.
194. Oksenhendler E, Cadranel J, Sarfati C, et al. *Toxoplasma gondii* pneumonia in patients with the acquired immunodeficiency syndrome. *Am J Med.* 1990;88:5-18N-15-21N.
195. Mehren M, Burns PJ, Mamani F, et al. Toxoplasmic myelitis mimicking intramedullary spinal cord tumor. *Neurology.* 1988;38:1648-1650.
196. Herskovitz S, Siegel SE, Schneider AT, et al. Spinal cord toxoplasmosis in AIDS. *Neurology.* 1989;39:1552-1553.
197. Overhage JM, Greist A, Brown DR. Conus medullaris syndrome resulting from *Toxoplasma gondii* infection in a patient with the acquired immunodeficiency syndrome. *Am J Med.* 1990;89:814-815.
198. Rabaud C, May T, Lucet JC, et al. Pulmonary toxoplasmosis in patients infected with human immunodeficiency virus: a French national study. *Clin Infect Dis.* 1996;23:1249-1254.
199. Derouin F, Sarfati C, Beauvais B, et al. Prevalence of pulmonary toxoplasmosis in HIV-infected patients. *AIDS.* 1990;4:1036.
200. Holland G, Engstrom Jr R, Glasgow B, et al. Ocular toxoplasmosis in patients with acquired immunodeficiency syndrome. *Am J Ophthalmol.* 1988;106:653-667.
201. Heinemann MH, Gold JM, Maisel J. Bilateral *Toxoplasma* retinochoroiditis in a patient with acquired immune deficiency syndrome. *Retina.* 1986;6:224-227.
202. Louie JK, Hsu LC, Osmond DH, et al. Trends in causes of death among persons with acquired immunodeficiency syndrome in the era of highly active antiretroviral therapy, San Francisco, 1994-1998. *J Infect Dis.* 2002;186:1023-1027.
203. Antinori A, Larussa D, Cingolani A, et al. Prevalence, associated factors, and prognostic determinants of AIDS-related toxoplasmic encephalitis in the era of advanced highly active antiretroviral therapy. *Clin Infect Dis.* 2004;39:1681-1691.
204. Ghosn J, Paris L, Ajzenberg D, et al. Atypical toxoplasmic manifestation after discontinuation of maintenance therapy in a human immunodeficiency virus type 1-infected patient with immune recovery. *Clin Infect Dis.* 2003;37:e112-e114.
205. Sendi P, Sachers F, Drechsler H, et al. Immune recovery vitreitis in an HIV patient with isolated toxoplasmic retinochoroiditis. *AIDS.* 2006;20:2237-2238.
206. Furrer H, Opravil M, Bernasconi E, et al. Stopping primary prophylaxis in HIV-1-infected patients at high risk of toxoplasma encephalitis. Swiss HIV Cohort Study. *Lancet.* 2000; 355:2217-2218.
207. Kirk O, Reiss P, Uberti-Foppa C, et al. Safe interruption of maintenance therapy against previous infection with four common HIV-associated opportunistic pathogens during potent antiretroviral therapy. *Ann Intern Med.* 2002;137:239-250.
208. Miro JM, Lopez JC, Podzamczer D, et al. Discontinuation of primary and secondary *Toxoplasma gondii* prophylaxis is safe in HIV-infected patients after immunological restoration with highly active antiretroviral therapy: results of an open, randomized, multicenter clinical trial. *Clin Infect Dis.* 2006; 43:79-89.
209. Stout JE, Lai JC, Giner J, et al. Reactivation of retinal toxoplasmosis despite evidence of immune response to highly active antiretroviral therapy. *Clin Infect Dis.* 2002;35:e37-e39.
210. Khan A, Su C, German M, et al. Genotyping of *Toxoplasma gondii* strains from immunocompromised patients reveals high prevalence of type I strains. *J Clin Microbiol.* 2005;43: 5881-5887.
211. Silveira C, Belfort Jr R, Burnier Jr M, et al. Acquired toxoplasmic infection as the cause of toxoplasmic retinochoroiditis in families. *Am J Ophthalmol.* 1988;106:362-364.
212. Glasner PD, Silveira C, Kruszon-Moran D, et al. An unusally high prevalence of ocular toxoplasmosis in Southern Brazil. *Am J Ophthalmol.* 1992;114:136-144.
213. Silveira C, Belfort Jr R, Muccioli C, et al. A follow-up study of *Toxoplasma gondii* infection in southern Brazil. *Am J Ophthalmol.* 2001;131:351-354.
214. Nussenblatt R, Belfort Jr R. Ocular toxoplasmosis. *JAMA.* 1994;271:302-307.
215. Bosch-Driessen LE, Berendschot TT, Ongkosuwito JV, et al. Ocular toxoplasmosis: clinical features and prognosis of 154 patients. *Ophthalmology.* 2002;109:869-878.
216. Bosch-Driessen LH, Plaisier MB, Stilma JS, et al. Reactivations of ocular toxoplasmosis after cataract extraction. *Ophthalmology.* 2002;109:41-45.
217. Holland GN, Crespi CM, ten Dam-van Loon N, et al. Analysis of recurrence patterns associated with toxoplasmic retinochoroiditis. *Am J Ophthalmol.* 2008;145:1007-1013.
218. Remington JS, McLeod R, Thulliez P, et al. Toxoplasmosis. In: Remington JS, Klein J, eds. *Infectious Diseases of the Fetus and Newborn Infant.* 5th ed. Philadelphia: WB Saunders; 2001:205-346.
219. Johnson MW, Greven CM, Jaffe GJ, et al. Atypical, severe toxoplasmic retinochoroiditis in elderly patients. *Ophthalmology.* 1997;104:48-57.
220. Kong JT, Grigg ME, Uyetake L, et al. Serotyping of *Toxoplasma gondii* infections in humans using synthetic peptides. *J Infect Dis.* 2003;187:1484-1495.
221. Gavinet MF, Robert F, Firtion G, et al. Congenital toxoplasmosis due to maternal reinfection during pregnancy. *J Clin Microbiol.* 1997;35:1276-1277.
222. Hennequin C, Dureau P, N'Guyen L, et al. Congenital toxoplasmosis acquired from an immune woman. *Pediatr Infect Dis.* 1997;16:75-76.
223. Vogel N, Kirisits M, Michael E, et al. Congenital toxoplasmosis transmitted from an immunologically competent mother infected before conception. *Clin Infect Dis.* 1996;23:1055-1060.
224. Minkoff H, Remington JS, Holman S, et al. Vertical transmission of *Toxoplasma* by human immunodeficiency virus-infected women. *Am J Obstet Gynecol.* 1997;176:555-559.
225. Desmonts G, Couvreur J. Congenital toxoplasmosis: a prospective study of the offspring of 542 women who acquired toxoplasmosis during pregnancy. In: Thalhammer O, Pollak A, Baumgarten K, eds. *Pathophysiology of Congenital Disease: Perinatal Medicine (6th European Congress, Vienna).* Stuttgart: Georg Thieme Publishers; 1979:51-60.
226. Koppe JG, Loewer-Sieger DH, De Roever-Bonnet H. Results of 20-year follow-up of congenital toxoplasmosis. *Am J Ophthalmol.* 1986;101:248-249.
227. Wilson CB, Remington JS, Stagno S, et al. Development of adverse sequelae in children born with subclinical congenital *Toxoplasma* infection. *Pediatrics.* 1980;66:767-774.
228. Forestier F. Fetal diseases, prenatal diagnoses and practical measures [Les foetopathies infectieuses—prevention, diagnostic prenatal, attitude pratique]. *Presse Med.* 1991;20:1448-1454.
229. Hohlfeld P, Daffos F, Thulliez P, et al. Fetal toxoplasmosis: outcome of pregnancy and infant follow-up after in utero treatment. *J Pediatr.* 1989;115:765-769.
230. Hohlfeld P, Daffos F, Costa J-M, et al. Prenatal diagnosis of congenital toxoplasmosis with polymerase-chain-reaction test on amniotic fluid. *N Engl J Med.* 1994;331:695-699.
231. Thiebaut R, Leproust S, Chene G, et al. Effectiveness of prenatal treatment for congenital toxoplasmosis: a meta-analysis of individual patients' data. *Lancet.* 2007;369:115-122.
232. Dunn D, Wallon M, Peyron F, et al. Mother-to-child transmission of toxoplasmosis: risk estimates for clinical counselling. *Lancet.* 1999;353:1829-1833.
233. Romand S, Chosson M, Franck J, et al. Usefulness of quantitative polymerase chain reaction in amniotic fluid as early prognostic marker of fetal infection with *Toxoplasma gondii. Am J Obstet Gynecol.* 2004;190:797-802.
234. Couvreur J, Desmonts G, Tournier G, et al. A homogeneous series of 210 cases of congenital toxoplasmosis in 0 to 11-month-old infants detected prospectively. *Ann Pediatr (Paris).* 1984;31:815-819.
235. De Roever-Bonnet H, Koppe JG, Loewer-Sieger DH. Follow-up of children with congenital *Toxoplasma* infection and children who become serologically negative after 1 year of age, all born in 1964-1965. In: Thalhammer O, Pollak A, Baumgarten K, eds. *Pathophysiology of Congenital Disease: Perinatal Medicine (6th European Congress, Vienna).* Stuttgart: Georg Thieme Publishers; 1979:61-75.
236. Labadie MD, Hazemann JJ. Contribution of health check-ups in children to the detection and epidemiologic study of congenital toxoplasmosis. *Ann Pediatr (Paris).* 1984;31:823-828.
237. McAuley J, Boyer KM, Patel D, et al. Early and longitudinal evaluations of treated infants and children and untreated historical patients with congenital toxoplasmosis: the Chicago Collaborative Treatment Trial. *Clin Infect Dis.* 1994;18:38-72.
238. Phan L, Kasza K, Jalbrzikowski J, et al. Longitudinal study of new eye lesions in children with toxoplasmosis who were not treated during the first year of life. *Am J Ophthalmol.* 2008;146:375-384.
239. Phan L, Kasza K, Jalbrzikowski J, et al. Longitudinal study of new eye lesions in treated congenital toxoplasmosis. *Ophthalmology.* 2008;115:553-559 e558.
240. Mitchell CD, Erlich SS, Mastrucci MT, et al. Congenital toxoplasmosis occurring in infants perinatally infected with human immunodeficiency virus 1. *Pediatr Infect Dis J.* 1990;9:512-518.
241. Nowakowska D, Colon I, Remington JS, et al. Genotyping of *Toxoplasma gondii* by multiplex PCR and peptide-based serological testing of samples from infants in Poland diagnosed with congenital toxoplasmosis. *J Clin Microbiol.* 2006;44:1382-1389.
242. Montoya JG. Laboratory diagnosis of *Toxoplasma gondii* infection and toxoplasmosis. *J Infect Dis.* 2002;185:S73-S82.
243. Miller MJ, Aronson WJ, Remington JS. Late parasitemia in asymptomatic acquired toxoplasmosis. *Ann Intern Med.* 1969;71:139-145.
244. Levy RM, Bredesen DE, Rosenblum ML. Opportunistic central nervous system pathology in patients with AIDS. *Ann Neurol.* 1988;23:S7-S12.
245. Frenkel JK, Piekarski G. The demonstration of *Toxoplasma* and other organisms by immunofluorescence: a pitfall [editorial]. *J Infect Dis.* 1978;138:265-266.
246. Sun T, Greenspan J, Tenenbaum M, et al. Diagnosis of cerebral toxoplasmosis using fluorescein-labeled antitoxoplasma monoclonal antibodies. *Am J Surg Pathol.* 1986;10:312-316.
247. Cerezo L, Alvarez M, Price G. Electron microscopic diagnosis of cerebral toxoplasmosis: case report. *J Neurosurg.* 1985;63: 470-472.
248. Luft BJ, Billingham M, Remington JS. Endomyocardial biopsy in the diagnosis of toxoplasmic myocarditis. *Transplant Proc.* 1986;18:1871-1873.
249. Grover CM, Thulliez P, Remington JS, et al. Rapid prenatal diagnosis of congenital *Toxoplasma* infection by using po-

lymerase chain reaction and amniotic fluid. *J Clin Microbiol.* 1990;28:2297-2301.
250. Cinque P, Scarpellini P, Vago L, et al. Diagnosis of central nervous system complications in HIV-infected patients: cerebrospinal fluid analysis by the polymerase chain reaction. *AIDS.* 1997;11:1-17.
251. Dupouy-Camet J, Lavareda de Souza L, Maslo C, et al. Detection of *Toxoplasma gondii* in venous blood from AIDS patients by polymerase chain reaction. *J Clin Microbiol.* 1993;31:1866-1869.
252. Fricker-Hidalgo H, Brenier-Pinchart MP, Schaal JP, et al. Value of *Toxoplasma gondii* detection in one hundred thirty-three placentas for the diagnosis of congenital toxoplasmosis. *Pediatr Infect Dis J.* 2007;26:845-846.
253. Dannemann BR, Israelski DM, Leoung GS, et al. *Toxoplasma* serology, parasitemia and antigenemia in patients at risk for toxoplasmic encephalitis. *AIDS.* 1991;5:1363-1365.
254. Pelloux H, Dupouy-Camet J, Derouin F, et al, group B-TS: a multicentre prospective study for the polymerase chain reaction detection of *Toxoplasma gondii* DNA in blood samples from 186 AIDS patients with suspected toxoplasmic encephalitis. *AIDS.* 1997;11:1888-1890.
255. Bastien P. Molecular diagnosis of toxoplasmosis. *Trans R Soc Trop Med Hyg.* 2002;96:S205-S215.
256. Jones CD, Okhravi N, Adamson P, et al. Comparison of PCR detection methods for B1, P30, and 18S rDNA genes of *T. gondii* in aqueous humor. *Invest Ophthalmol Vis Sci.* 2000;41:634-644.
257. Liesenfeld O, Montoya JG, Kinney S, et al. Effect of testing for IgG avidity in the diagnosis of *Toxoplasma gondii* infection in pregnant women: experience in a US reference laboratory. *J Infect Dis.* 2001;183:1248-1253.
258. Liesenfeld O, Montoya JG, Tathineni NJ, et al. Confirmatory serologic testing for acute toxoplasmosis and rate of induced abortions among women reported to have positive *Toxoplasma* immunoglobulin M antibody titers. *Am J Obstet Gynecol.* 2001;184:140-145.
259. Montoya JG, Liesenfeld O, Kinney S, et al. VIDAS test for avidity of *Toxoplasma*-specific immunoglobulin G for confirmatory testing of pregnant women. *J Clin Microbiol.* 2002;40:2504-2508.
260. Sabin AB, Feldman HA. Dyes as microchemical indicators of a new immunity phenomenon affecting a protozoan parasite (toxoplasma). *Science.* 1948;108:660-663.
261. Balsari A, Poli G, Molina V, et al. ELISA for *Toxoplasma* antibody detection: a comparison with other serodiagnostic tests. *J Clin Pathol.* 1980;33:640-643.
262. Walls KW, Bullock SL, English DK. Use of the enzyme-linked immunosorbent assay (ELISA) and its microadaptation for the serodiagnosis of toxoplasmosis. *J Clin Microbiol.* 1977;5:273-277.
263. Walton BC, Benchoff BM, Brooks WH. Comparison of the indirect fluorescent antibody test and methylene blue dye test for detection of antibodies to *Toxoplasma gondii. Am J Trop Med Hyg.* 1966;15:149-152.
264. Thulliez P, Remington JS, Santoro F, et al. A new agglutination test for the diagnosis of acute and chronic *Toxoplasma* infection. *Pathol Biol (Paris).* 1986;34:173-177.
265. Araujo FG, Barnett EV, Gentry LO, et al. False-positive anti-*Toxoplasma* fluorescent-antibody tests in patients with antinuclear antibodies. *Appl Microbiol.* 1971;22:270-275.
266. Desmonts G, Remington JS. Direct agglutination test for diagnosis of *Toxoplasma* infection: method for increasing sensitivity and specificity. *J Clin Microbiol.* 1980;11:562-568.
267. Dannemann BR, Vaughan WC, Thulliez P, et al. Differential agglutination test for diagnosis of recently acquired infection with *Toxoplasma gondii. J Clin Microbiol.* 1990;28:1928-1933.
268. Hedman K, Lappalainen M, Seppala I, et al. Recent primary *Toxoplasma* infection indicated by a low avidity of specific IgG. *J Infect Dis.* 1989;159:736-739.
269. Lappalainen M, Koskela P, Koskiniemi M, et al. Toxoplasmosis acquired during pregnancy: improved serodiagnosis based on avidity of IgG. *J Infect Dis.* 1993;167:691-697.
270. Montoya JG, Huffman HB, Remington JS. Evaluation of the immunoglobulin G avidity test for diagnosis of toxoplasmic lymphadenopathy. *J Clin Microbiol.* 2004;42:4627-4631.
271. Pelloux H, Brun E, Vernet G, et al. Determination of anti-*Toxoplasma gondii* immunoglobulin G avidity: adaptation to the VIDAS system (BioMerieux). *Diagn Microbiol Infect Dis.* 1998;32:69-73.
272. Bobic B, Sibalic D, Djurkovic-Djakovic O. High levels of IgM antibodies specific for *Toxoplasma gondii* in pregnancy 12 years after primary *Toxoplasma* infection. *Gynecol Obstet Invest.* 1991;31:182-184.
273. Liesenfeld O, Press C, Montoya JG, et al. False-positive results in immunoglobulin M (IgM) *Toxoplasma* antibody tests and importance of confirmatory testing: the Platelia toxo IgM test. *J Clin Microbiol.* 1997;35:174-178.
274. Wilson M, Ware DA, Walls KW. Evaluation of commercial serodiagnostic kits for toxoplasmosis. *J Clin Microbiol.* 1987;25:2262-2265.
275. FDA. Public Health Advisory: Limitations of *Toxoplasma* IgM commercial test kits. US Food and Drug Administration, Center for Devices and Radiological Health. Rockville, MD: The Center. Available at: URL: <http://www.fda.gov/cdrh/toxopha.html>; Accessed July 25, 1997.
276. Montoya JG, Remington JS. Management of *Toxoplasma gondii* infection during pregnancy. *Clin Infect Dis.* 2008;47:554-566.
277. Welch PC, Masur H, Jones TC, et al. Serologic diagnosis of acute lymphadenopathic toxoplasmosis. *J Infect Dis.* 1980;142:256-264.
278. Naot Y, Barnett EV, Remington JS. Method for avoiding false-positive results occurring in immunoglobulin M enzyme-linked immunosorbent assays due to presence of both rheumatoid factor and antinuclear antibodies. *J Clin Microbiol.* 1981;14:73-78.
279. Filice GA, Yeager AS, Remington JS. Diagnostic significance of immunoglobulin M antibodies to *Toxoplasma gondii* detected after separation of immunoglobulin M from immunoglobulin G antibodies. *J Clin Microbiol.* 1980;12:336-342.
280. Naot Y, Remington JS. An enzyme-linked immunosorbent assay for detection of IgM antibodies to *Toxoplasma gondii*: use for diagnosis of acute acquired toxoplasmosis. *J Infect Dis.* 1980;142:757-766.
281. Naot Y, Desmonts G, Remington JS. IgM enzyme-linked immunosorbent assay test for the diagnosis of congenital *Toxoplasma* infection. *J Pediatr.* 1981;98:32-36.
282. Siegel JP, Remington JS. Comparison of methods for quantitating antigen-specific immunoglobulin M antibody with a reverse enzyme-linked immunosorbent assay. *J Clin Microbiol.* 1983;18:63-70.
283. Remington JS, Eimstad WM, Araujo FG. Detection of immunoglobulin M antibodies with antigen-tagged latex particles in an immunosorbent assay. *J Clin Microbiol.* 1983;17:939-941.
284. Plantaz D, Goullier A, Jouk PS, et al. Value of the immunosorbent agglutination assay (ISAGA) in the early diagnosis of congenital toxoplasmosis. *Pediatrie.* 1987;42:387-391.
285. Decoster A, Slizewicz B, Simon J, et al. Platelia-toxo IgA, a new kit for early diagnosis of congenital toxoplasmosis by detection of anti-P30 immunoglobulin A antibodies. *J Clin Microbiol.* 1991;29:2291-2295.
286. Pinon JM, Thoannes H, Pouletty PH, et al. Detection of IgA specific for toxoplasmosis in serum and cerebrospinal fluid using a non-enzymatic IgA-capture assay. *Diagn Immunol.* 1986;4:223-227.
287. Stepick-Biek P, Thulliez P, Araujo FG, et al. IgA antibodies for diagnosis of acute congenital and acquired toxoplasmosis. *J Infect Dis.* 1990;162:270-273.
288. Pinon JM, Toubas D, Marx C, et al. Detection of specific immunoglobulin E in patients with toxoplasmosis. *J Clin Microbiol.* 1990;28:1739-1743.
289. Wong SY, Hadju M-P, Ramirez R, et al. The role of specific immunoglobulin E in diagnosis of acute *Toxoplasma* infection and toxoplasmosis. *J Clin Microbiol.* 1993;31:2952-2959.
290. Poirriez J, Toubas D, Marx-Chemia C, et al. Isotypic characterization of anti-*Toxoplasma gondii* antibodies in 18 cases of congenital toxoplasmic chorioretinitis. *Acta Ophthalmol (Copenh).* 1988;67:164-168.
291. Foudrinier F, Villena I, Jaussaud R, et al. Clinical value of specific immunoglobulin E detection by enzyme-linked immunosorbent assay in cases of acquired and congenital toxoplasmosis. *J Clin Microbiol.* 2003;41:1681-1686.
292. Porter SB, Sande M. Toxoplasmosis of the central nervous system in the acquired immunodeficiency syndrome. *N Engl J Med.* 1992;327:1643-1648.
293. Haverkos HW, Remington JS, Chan JC. Assessment of *Toxoplasma* encephalitis (TE) therapy: a cooperative study. *Am J Med.* 1987;82:907-914.
294. Levy RM, Rosenbloom S, Perrett LV. Neuroradiologic findings in AIDS: a review of 200 cases. *AJNR Am J Neuroradiol.* 1986;147:977-983.
295. Post MJ, Kursunoglu SJ, Hensley GT, et al. Cranial CT in acquired immunodeficiency syndrome: spectrum of diseases and optimal contrast enhancement technique. *AJR Am J Roentgenol.* 1985;145:929-940.
296. Levy RM, Mills CM, Posin JP, et al. The efficacy and clinical impact of brain imaging in neurologically symptomatic AIDS patients: a prospective CT/MRI study. *J Acquir Immune Defic Syndr.* 1990;3:461-471.
297. Post MJ, Chan JC, Hensley GT, et al. *Toxoplasma* encephalitis in Haitian adults with acquired immunodeficiency syndrome: a clinical-pathologic-CT correlation. *AJR Am J Roentgenol.* 1983;140:861-868.
298. Ciricillo SF, Rosenblum ML. Use of CT and MR imaging to distinguish intracranial lesions and to define the need for biopsy in AIDS patients. *J Neurosurg.* 1990;73:720-724.
299. Holloway RG, Mushlin AI. Intracranial mass lesions in acquired immunodeficiency syndrome: using decision analysis to determine the effectiveness of stereotactic brain biopsy. *Neurology.* 1996;46:1010-1015.
300. De La Paz R, Enzmann D. Neuroradiology of acquired immunodeficiency syndrome. In: Rosenblum ML, ed. *AIDS and the Nervous System.* New York: Raven Press; 1988:121-154.
301. Luft BJ, Hafner R, Korzun AH, et al. Toxoplasmic encephalitis in patients with the acquired immunodeficiency syndrome. *N Engl J Med.* 1993;329:995-1000.
302. Harris TM, Smith RR, Bognanno JR, et al. Toxoplasmic myelitis in AIDS: gadolinium-enhanced MR. *J Comput Assist Tomogr.* 1990;14:809-811.
303. O'Doherty MJ, Barrington SF, Campbell M, et al. PET scanning and the human immunodeficiency virus-positive patient. *J Nucl Med.* 1997;38:1575-1583.
304. Naddaf SY, Akisik MF, Aziz M, et al. Comparison between 201Tl-chloride and 99Tc(m)-sestamibi SPECT brain imaging for differentiating intracranial lymphoma from non-malignant lesions in AIDS patients. *Nucl Med Commun.* 1998;19:47-53.
305. Ramsey RG, Gean AD. Central nervous system toxoplasmosis. *Neuroimaging Clin North Am.* 1997;7:171-186.
306. Rosenfeld SS, Hoffman JM, Coleman RE, et al. Studies of primary central nervous system lymphoma with [18F]-fluorodeoxyglucose (FDG) PET. *J Nucl Med.* 1992;33:532-536.
307. Giancola ML, Rizzi EB, Schiavo R, et al. Reduced value of thallium-201 single-photon emission computed tomography in the management of HIV-related focal brain lesions in the era of highly active antiretroviral therapy. *AIDS Res Hum Retroviruses.* 2004;20:584-588.
308. Navia BA, Petito CK, Gold JW, et al. Cerebral toxoplasmosis complicating the acquired immune deficiency syndrome: clinical and neuropathological findings in 27 patients. *Ann Neurol.* 1986;19:224-238.
309. Orefice G, Carrieri PB, de Marinis T, et al. Use of the intrathecal synthesis of antitoxoplasma antibodies in the diagnostic assessment and in the follow-up of AIDS patients with cerebral toxoplasmosis. *Acta Neurol (Napoli).* 1990;12:79-81.
310. Potasman I, Resnick L, Luft BJ, et al. Intrathecal production of antibodies against *Toxoplasma gondii* in patients with toxoplasmic encephalitis and the acquired immunodeficiency syndrome (AIDS). *Ann Intern Med.* 1988;108:49-51.
311. Montoya JG, Berry A, Rosso F, et al. The differential agglutination test as a diagnostic aid in cases of toxoplasmic lymphadenitis. *J Clin Microbiol.* 2007;45:1463-1468.
312. Luft BJ, Naot Y, Araujo FG, et al. Primary and reactivated *Toxoplasma* infection in patients with cardiac transplants: clinical spectrum and problems in diagnosis in a defined population. *Ann Intern Med.* 1983;99:27-31.
313. Holliman RE, Johnson JD, Savva D. Diagnosis of cerebral toxoplasmosis in association with AIDS using the polymerase chain reaction. *Scand J Infect Dis.* 1990;22:243-244.
314. Bossolasco S, Cinque P, Ponzoni M, et al. Epstein-Barr virus DNA load in cerebrospinal fluid and plasma of patients with AIDS-related lymphoma. *J Neurovirol.* 2002;8:432-438.
315. Roth A, Roth B, Höffken G, et al. Application of the polymerase chain reaction to diagnosis of pulmonary toxoplasmosis in immunocompromised patients. *Eur J Clin Microbiol Infect Dis.* 1992;11:1177-1181.
316. Fardeau C, Romand S, Rao NA, et al. Diagnosis of toxoplasmic retinochoroiditis with atypical clinical features. *Am J Ophthalmol.* 2002;134:196-203.
317. Westeneng AC, Rothova A, de Boer JH, et al. Infectious uveitis in immunocompromised patients and the diagnostic value of polymerase chain reaction and Goldmann-Witmer coefficient in aqueous analysis. *Am J Ophthalmol.* 2007;144:781-785.
318. Bretagne S, Costa JM, Keuntz M, et al. Late toxoplasmosis evidenced by PCR in marrow transplant recipient. *Bone Marrow Transplant.* 1995;15:809-811.
319. Turunen HJ, Leinikki PO, Saari KM. Demonstration of intraocular synthesis of immunoglobulin G toxoplasma antibodies for specific diagnosis of toxoplasmic chorioretinitis by enzyme immunoassay. *J Clin Microbiol.* 1983;17:988-992.
320. Rothova A, de Boer JH, Ten Dam-van Loon NH, et al. Usefulness of aqueous humor analysis for the diagnosis of posterior uveitis. *Ophthalmology.* 2008;115:306-311.
321. Montoya JG, Huffman HB, Remington JS. Use of the VIDAS Toxo IgG avidity test for the diagnosis of toxoplasmic lymphadenopathy. Presented at the 40th Annual Meeting of the Infectious Diseases Society of America (IDSA). Chicago, IL, October 24-27, 2002.
322. Romand S, Wallon M, Franck J, et al. Prenatal diagnosis using polymerase chain reaction on amniotic fluid for congenital toxoplasmosis. *Obstet Gynecol.* 2001;97:296-300.
323. Remington JS, Araujo FG, Desmonts G. Recognition of different *Toxoplasma* antigens by IgM and IgG antibodies in mothers and their congenitally infected newborns. *J Infect Dis.* 1985;152:1020-1024.
324. Rilling V, Dietz K, Krczal D, et al. Evaluation of a commercial IgG/IgM Western blot assay for early postnatal diagnosis of congenital toxoplasmosis. *Eur J Clin Microbiol Infect Dis.* 2003;22:174-180.
325. Gallego-Marin C, Henao AC, Gomez-Marin JE. Clinical validation of a Western blot assay for congenital toxoplasmosis and newborn screening in a hospital in Armenia (Quindio) Colombia. *J Trop Pediatr.* 2006;52:107-112.
326. Tridapalli E, Capretti M, Farneti G, et al. Congenital toxoplasmosis: the importance of the Western blot method to avoid unnecessary therapy in potentially infected newborns. *Acta Paediatr.* 2008;97:1298-1300.
327. Cazenave J, Forestier F, Bessieres M, et al. Contribution of a new PCR assay to the prenatal diagnosis of congenital toxoplasmosis. *Prenat Diagn.* 1992;12:119-127.
328. Fuentes I, Rodriguez M, Domingo CJ, et al. Urine sample used for congenital toxoplasmosis diagnosis by PCR. *J Clin Microbiol.* 1996;34:2368-2371.
329. van de Ven E, Melchers W, Galama J, et al. Identification of *Toxoplasma gondii* infections by BI gene amplification. *J Clin Microbiol.* 1991;19:2120-2124.
330. Guerina N, Hsu H-W, Meissner H, et al. Neonatal serologic screening and early treatment for congenital *Toxoplasma gondii* infection. *N Engl J Med.* 1994;330:1858-1863.

331. Jara M, Hsu HW, Eaton RB, et al. Epidemiology of congenital toxoplasmosis identified by population-based newborn screening in Massachusetts. *Pediatr Infect Dis J*. 2001;20:1132-1135.
332. Cohn J, McMeeking A, Cohen W, et al. Evaluation of the policy of empiric treatment of suspected *Toxoplasma* encephalitis in patients with the acquired immunodeficiency syndrome. *Am J Med*. 1989;86:521-527.
333. Carbone LG, Bendixen B, Appel GB. Sulfadiazine-associated obstructive nephropathy occurring in a patient with the acquired immunodeficiency syndrome. *Am J Kidney Dis*. 1988;12:72-75.
334. Reboli AC, Mandler HD. Encephalopathy and psychoses associated with sulfadiazine in two patients with AIDS and CNS toxoplasmosis. *Clin Infect Dis*. 1992;15:556-557.
335. Leoung GS, Stanford JF, Giordano MF, et al. Trimethoprim-sulfamethoxazole (TMP-SMX) dose escalation versus direct rechallenge for *Pneumocystis carinii* pneumonia prophylaxis in human immunodeficiency virus-infected patients with previous adverse reaction to TMP-SMX. *J Infect Dis*. 2001;184:992-997.
336. Soffritti S, Ricci G, Prete A, et al. Successful desensitization to trimethoprim-sulfamethoxazole after allogeneic haematopoietic stem cell transplantation: preliminary observations. *Med Pediatr Oncol*. 2003;40:271-272.
337. Camps M, Arrizabalaga G, Boothroyd J. An rRNA mutation identifies the apicoplast as the target for clindamycin in *Toxoplasma gondii*. *Mol Microbiol*. 2002;43:1309-1318.
338. Coppola S, Angarano G, Monno L, et al. Adverse effects of clindamycin in the treatment of cerebral toxoplasmosis in AIDS patients. Presented at the VII International Conference on AIDS Florence, Italy, 1991.
339. Carey RM, Kimball AC, Armstrong D, et al. Toxoplasmosis: clinical experiences in a cancer hospital. *Am J Med*. 1973; 54:30-38.
340. Katlama C, De Wit S, O'Doherty E, et al. Pyrimethamine-clindamycin vs. pyrimethamine-sulfadiazine as acute and long-term therapy for toxoplasmic encephalitis in patients with aids. *Clin Infect Dis*. 1996;22:268-275.
341. Luft BJ, Remington JS. AIDS commentary: toxoplasmic encephalitis. *J Infect Dis*. 1988;157:1-6.
342. Dannemann BR, McCutchan JA, Israelski DA, et al. Treatment of toxoplasmic encephalitis in patients with AIDS: a randomized trial comparing pyrimethamine plus clindamycin to pyrimethamine plus sulfadiazine. *Ann Intern Med*. 1992;116:33-43.
343. Canessa A, Del Bono V, De Leo P, et al. Cotrimoxazole therapy of *Toxoplasma gondii* encephalitis in AIDS patients. *Eur J Clin Microbiol Infect Dis*. 1992;11:125-130.
344. Solbreux P, Sonnet J, Zech F. A retrospective study about the use of cotrimoxazole as diagnostic support and treatment of suspected cerebral toxoplasmosis in AIDS. *Acta Clin Belg*. 1990;45:85-96.
345. Torre D, Speranza F, Martegani R, et al. A retrospective study of treatment of cerebral toxoplasmosis in AIDS patients with trimethoprim-sulphamethoxazole. *J Infect*. 1998;37:15-18.
346. Torre D, Casari S, Speranza F, et al. Randomized trial of trimethoprim-sulfamethoxazole versus pyrimethamine-sulfadiazine for therapy of toxoplasmic encephalitis in patients with AIDS. Italian Collaborative Study Group. *Antimicrob Agents Chemother*. 1998;42:1346-1349.
347. Kovacs JA. Efficacy of atovaquone in treatment of toxoplasmosis in patients with AIDS. *Lancet*. 1992;340:637-638.
348. Torres R, Weinberg W, Stansell J, et al. Atovaquone for salvage treatment and suppression of toxoplasmic encephalitis in patients with AIDS. *Clin Infect Dis*. 1997;24:422-429.
349. Chirgwin K, Hafner R, Leport C, et al. Randomized phase II trial of atovaquone with pyrimethamine or sulfadiazine for treatment of toxoplasmic encephalitis in patients with acquired immunodeficiency syndrome: ACTG 237/ANRS 039 Study. AIDS Clinical Trials Group 237/Agence Nationale de Recherche sur le SIDA, Essai 039. *Clin Infect Dis*. 2002;34:1243-1250.
350. Fernandez-Martin J, Leport C, Morlat P, et al. Pyrimethamine-clarithromycin for therapy of acute *Toxoplasma* encephalitis in patients with AIDS. *Antimicrob Agents Chemother*. 1991;35:2049-2052.
351. Chaisson RE, Benson CA, Dube MP, et al. Clarithromycin therapy for bacteremic *Mycobacterium avium* complex disease: a randomized, double-blind, dose-ranging study in patients with AIDS. AIDS Clinical Trials Group Protocol 157 Study Team. *Ann Intern Med*. 1994;121:905-911.
352. Cohn DL, Fisher EJ, Peng GT, et al. A prospective randomized trial of four three-drug regimens in the treatment of disseminated *Mycobacterium avium* complex disease in AIDS patients: excess mortality associated with high-dose clarithromycin. Terry Beirn Community Programs for Clinical Research on AIDS. *Clin Infect Dis*. 1999;29:125-133.
353. Ward DJ. Dapsone/pyrimethamine for the treatment of toxoplasmic encephalitis. Presented at the VIII International Conference on AIDS, Amsterdam, The Netherlands, 1992.
354. Pope-Pegram L, Gathe J Jr, Bohn B, et al. Treatment of presumed central nervous system toxoplasmosis with doxycycline. Presented at the VII International Conference on AIDS, Florence, Italy, 1991.
355. Turett G, Pierone G, Masci J, et al. Failure of doxycycline in the treatment of cerebral toxoplasmosis. Presented at the Sixth International Conference on AIDS 1990; San Francisco, CA, 1990.
356. Saba J, Morlat P, Raffi F, et al. Pyrimethamine plus azithromycin for treatment of acute toxoplasmic encephalitis in patients with AIDS. *Eur J Clin Microbiol Infect Dis*. 1993;12:853-856.
357. Jacobson JM, Hafner R, Remington J, et al. Dose-escalation, phase I/II study of azithromycin and pyrimethamine for the treatment of toxoplasmic encephalitis in AIDS. *AIDS*. 2001;15:583-589.
358. Pedrol E, Gonzales-Clemente JM, Gatell JM, et al. Central nervous system toxoplasmosis in AIDS patients: efficacy of an intermittent maintenance therapy. *AIDS*. 1990;4:511-517.
359. Podzamczer D, Miró J, Bolao F, et al. Twice-weekly maintenance therapy with sulfadiazine-pyrimethamine to prevent recurrent toxoplasmic encephalitis in patients with AIDS. *Ann Intern Med*. 1995;123:175-180.
360. Podzamczer D, Miro JM, Ferrer E, et al. Thrice-weekly sulfadiazine-pyrimethamine for maintenance therapy of toxoplasmic encephalitis in HIV-infected patients. Spanish Toxoplasmosis Study Group. *Eur J Clin Microbiol Infect Dis*. 2000;19: 89-95.
361. Heald A, Flepp M, Chave J-P, et al. Treatment for cerebral toxoplasmosis protects against *Pneumocystis carinii* pneumonia in patients with AIDS. *Ann Intern Med*. 1991;115:760-763.
362. Duval X, Pajot O, Le Moing V, et al. Maintenance therapy with cotrimoxazole for toxoplasmic encephalitis in the era of highly active antiretroviral therapy. *AIDS*. 2004;18:1342-1344.
363. Remington JS, Vilde JL, Antunes F, et al. Clindamycin for toxoplasmosis encephalitis in AIDS. *Lancet*. 1991;338:1142-1143.
364. Guidelines for prevention and treatment of opportunistic infections in HIV-infected adults and adolescents: recommendations from CDC, the National Institutes of Health, and the HIV Medicine Association of the infectious Diseases Society of America. *MMWR Recomm Rep*. 2009 Apr 10;58(RR-4):1-207; quiz CE1-4.
365. Köppen S, Grunewald T, Jautzke G, et al. Prevention of *Pneumocystis carinii* pneumonia and toxoplasmic encephalitis in human immunodeficiency virus infected patients: a clinical approach comparing aerosolized pentamidine and pyrimethamine/sulfadoxine. *Clin Invest*. 1992;70:508-512.
366. Clotet B, Sirera G, Romeu J, et al. Twice-weekly dapsone-pyrimethamine for preventing PCP and cerebral toxoplasmosis. *AIDS*. 1991;5:601-602.
367. Opravil M, Hirschel B, Lazzarin A, et al. Once-weekly administration of dapsone/pyrimethamine vs. aerosolized pentamidine as a combined prophylaxis for *Pneumocystis carinii* pneumonia and toxoplasmic encephalitis in human immunodeficiency virus-infected patients. *Clin Infect Dis*. 1995;20:531-541.
368. Torres R, Barr M, Thorn M, et al. Randomized trial of dapsone and aerosolized pentamidine for the prophylaxis of *Pneumocystis carinii* pneumonia and toxoplasmic encephalitis. *Am J Med*. 1993;95:573-583.
369. Navin TR, Miller KD, Satriale RF, et al. Adverse reactions associated with pyrimethamine-sulfadoxine prophylaxis for *Pneumocystis carinii* infections in AIDS. *Lancet*. 1985;1:1332.
370. Maslo C, Matheron S, Saimot AG. Cerebral toxoplasmosis: assessment of maintenance therapy. Presented at: VIII International Conference on AIDS. Amsterdam, The Netherlands, 1992.
371. de Gans J, Portegies P, Reiss P, et al. Pyrimethamine alone as maintenance therapy for central nervous system toxoplasmosis in 38 patients with AIDS. *J AIDS*. 1992;5:137-142.
372. Katlama C, Mouthon B, Gourdon D, et al. Atovaquone as long-term suppressive therapy for toxoplasmic encephalitis in patients with AIDS and multiple drug intolerance. *AIDS*. 1996;10:1107-1112.
373. Carr A, Tindall B, Brew BJ, et al. Low-dose trimethoprim-sulfamethoxazole prophylaxis for toxoplasmic encephalitis in patients with AIDS. *Ann Intern Med*. 1992;117:106-111.
374. Bozzette S, Finkelstein D, Spector S, et al. A randomized trial of three antipneumocystis agents in patients with advanced human immunodeficiency virus infection. *N Engl J Med*. 1995;332: 693-699.
375. Podzamczer D, Salazar A, Jiménez J, et al. Intermittent trimethoprim-sulfamethoxazole compared with dapsone-pyrimethamine for the simultaneous primary prophylaxis of *Pneumocystis* pneumonia and toxoplasmosis in patients infected with HIV. *Ann Intern Med*. 1995;122:755-761.
376. Girard P-M, Landman R, Gaudebout C, et al. Dapsone-pyrimethamine compared with aerosolized pentamidine as a primary prophylaxis against *Pneumocystis carinii* pneumonia and toxoplasmosis in HIV infection. *N Engl J Med*. 1993; 328:1514-1520.
377. Schurmann D, Bergmann F, Albrecht H, et al. Effectiveness of twice-weekly pyrimethamine-sulfadoxine as primary prophylaxis of *Pneumocystis carinii* pneumonia and toxoplasmic encephalitis in patients with advanced HIV infection. *Eur J Clin Microbiol Infect Dis*. 2002;21:353-361.
378. Zeller V, Truffot C, Agher R, et al. Discontinuation of secondary prophylaxis against disseminated *Mycobacterium avium* complex infection and toxoplasmic encephalitis. *Clin Infect Dis*. 2002;34:662-667.
379. Mussini C, Pezzotti P, Govoni A, et al. Discontinuation of primary prophylaxis for *Pneumocystis carinii* pneumonia and toxoplasmic encephalitis in human immunodeficiency virus type I-infected patients: the changes in opportunistic prophylaxis study. *J Infect Dis*. 2000;181:1635-1642.
380. Durant J, Hazime F, Carles M, et al. Prevention of *Pneumocystis carinii* pneumonia and of cerebral toxoplasmosis by roxithromycin in HIV-infected patients. *Infection*. 1995;23:S33-S38.
381. Jacobson M, Besch C, Child C, et al. Primary prophylaxis with pyrimethamine for toxoplasmic encephalitis in patients with advanced human immunodeficiency virus disease: results of a randomized trial. *J Infect Dis*. 1994;169:384-394.
382. Klinker H, Langmann P, Richter E. Pyrimethamine alone as prophylaxis for cerebral toxoplasmosis in patients with advanced HIV infection. *Infection*. 1996;4:324-328.
383. Raffi F, Struillou L, Ninin E, et al. Breakthrough cerebral toxoplasmosis in patients with AIDS who are being treated with clarithromycin. *Clin Infect Dis*. 1995;20:1076-1077.
384. Leport C, Vilde JL, Katlama C, et al. Failure of spiramycin to prevent neurotoxoplasmosis in immunosuppressed patients. *Med Clin North Am*. 1986;70:677-692.
385. Jacobson M, Besch C, Child C, et al. Toxicity of clindamycin as prophylaxis for AIDS-associated toxoplasmic encephalitis. *Lancet*. 1992;339:333-334.
386. Cochereau-Massin I, LeHoang P, Lautier-Frau M, et al. Ocular *Toxoplasmosis* in human immunodeficiency virus-infected patients. *Am J Ophthalmol*. 1992;114:130-135.
387. Friedman AH, Orellana J, Gagliuso DJ, et al. Ocular toxoplasmosis in AIDS patients. *Trans Am Ophthalmol Soc*. 1990;88:63-88.
388. Schnapp L, Geaghan S, Campagna A, et al. *Toxoplasma gondii* pneumonitis in patients infected with the human immunodeficiency virus. *Arch Intern Med*. 1992;152:1073-1076.
389. Holland GN, Lewis KG. An update on current practices in the management of ocular toxoplasmosis. *Am J Ophthalmol*. 2002;134:102-114.
390. Holland GN. Ocular toxoplasmosis: a global reassessment. Part I: epidemiology and course of disease. *Am J Ophthalmol*. 2003; 136:973-988.
391. Holland GN. Ocular toxoplasmosis: a global reassessment. Part II: disease manifestations and management. *Am J Ophthalmol*. 2004;137:1-17.
392. Soheilian M, Sadoughi MM, Ghajarnia M, et al. Prospective randomized trial of trimethoprim/sulfamethoxazole versus pyrimethamine and sulfadiazine in the treatment of ocular toxoplasmosis. *Ophthalmology*. 2005;112:1876-1882.
393. Pearson PA, Piracha AR, Sen HA, et al. Atovaquone for the treatment of toxoplasma retinochoroiditis in immunocompetent patients. *Ophthalmology*. 1999;106:148-153.
394. Bosch-Driessen LH, Verbraak FD, Suttorp-Schulten MS, et al. A prospective, randomized trial of pyrimethamine and azithromycin vs pyrimethamine and sulfadiazine for the treatment of ocular toxoplasmosis. *Am J Ophthalmol*. 2002;134: 34-40.
395. Forestier F, Daffos F, Rainaut M, et al. Suivi therapeutique foetomaternel de la spiramycine en cours de grossesse. *Arch Fr Pediatr*. 1987;44:539-544.
396. Gilbert R, Gras L. Effect of timing and type of treatment on the risk of mother to child transmission of *Toxoplasma gondii*. *BJOG*. 2003;110:112-120.
397. Gilbert RE, Gras L, Wallon M, et al. Effect of prenatal treatment on mother to child transmission of *Toxoplasma gondii*: retrospective cohort study of 554 mother-child pairs in Lyon, France. *Int J Epidemiol*. 2001;30:1303-1308.
398. Gilbert R, Dunn D, Wallon M, et al. Ecological comparison of the risks of mother-to-child transmission and clinical manifestations of congenital toxoplasmosis according to prenatal treatment protocol. *Epidemiol Infect*. 2001;127:113-120.
399. Foulon W, Villena I, Stray-Pedersen B, et al. Treatment of toxoplasmosis during pregnancy: a multicenter study of impact on fetal transmission and children's sequelae at age 1 year. *Am J Obstet Gynecol*. 1999;180:410-415.
400. Thulliez P. Commentary: efficacy of prenatal treatment for toxoplasmosis: a possibility that cannot be ruled out. *Int J Epidemiol*. 2001;30:1315-1316.
401. McGee T, Wolters C, Stein L, et al. Absence of sensorineural hearing loss in treated infants and children with congenital toxoplasmosis. *Otolaryngol Head Neck Surg*. 1992;106: 75-80.
402. Mets MB, Holfels E, Boyer KM, et al. Eye manifestations of congenital toxoplasmosis. *Am J Ophthalmol*. 1996;122: 309-324.
403. Roizen N, Swisher CN, Stein MA, et al. Neurologic and developmental outcome in treated congenital toxoplasmosis. *Pediatrics*. 1995;95:11-20.
404. Wreghitt TG, Hakim M, Gray JJ, et al. Toxoplasmosis in heart and heart lung transplant recipients. *J Clin Pathol*. 1989; 42:194-199.
405. Daffos F, Forestier F, Capella-Pavlovsky M, et al. Prenatal management of 746 pregnancies at risk for congenital toxoplasmosis. *N Engl J Med*. 1988;318:271-275.
406. Desmonts G, Daffos F, Forestier F, et al. Prenatal diagnosis of congenital toxoplasmosis. *Lancet*. 1985;1:500-504.

280

Giardia lamblia

DAVID R. HILL | THEODORE E. NASH

Giardia lamblia, a flagellated enteric protozoan, is a common cause of endemic and epidemic diarrhea throughout the world. It is seen in waterborne outbreaks of diarrhea, in children who live in low-income countries, and occasionally in foodborne outbreaks. In the United States and Canada, it is the most commonly diagnosed enteric parasite.

Description of the Pathogen

Giardia has been recognized as an intestinal inhabitant since the late 1600s, when van Leeuwenhoek discovered it in his own stool. It was in the early 1900s that the parasite received the genus name *Giardia*. The designated species name for the human parasite has been *lamblia*, but *intestinalis* and *duodenalis* are also used. The genus *Giardia* falls under the category of intestinal flagellates in the division Protozoa.[1] On the basis of its small subunit ribosomal RNA sequence and the absence of many organelles such as mitochondria and a typical Golgi apparatus, it is one of the earliest branching eukaryotes, and it has been used as a model to understand the development of eukaryotic cells.[2,3] However, recent discovery of a mitosome that contains iron sulfur proteins indicates that *Giardia* was at one time endowed with mitochondria and only a remnant remains.[4,5]

The differentiation of *Giardia* into species has traditionally depended on morphology and the host of origin, with only a few species described: *G. lamblia* in humans, *Giardia muris* in mice, *Giardia agilis* in amphibians, *Giardia psittaci* in parakeets and *Giardia microti* in voles and muskrats (Table 280-1).[2] However, the understanding of *G. lamblia* has now moved to molecular typing,[6,7] as isolates from humans and many animals are morphologically indistinguishable. *G. lamblia* are divided into seven assemblages (or genotypes) from A to G (see Table 280-1). Assemblages A and B, which are associated with human infections, differ in phenotypic, biochemical, and molecular markers so that it is possible these two assemblages represent unique species. Parasites of assemblages A and B can also infect other mammalian hosts.[6-8] However, except for beaver,[9] no other animal species has been implicated in human *Giardia* outbreaks, suggesting that animals do not commonly serve as sources of infection.

The genome of the prototypic assemblage A isolate, WB, has been recently published (http://giardiadb.org).[10] The genome is approximately 11.7 megabase (Mb) distributed over five chromosomes; it is compact in structure and content. There is simplified DNA synthesis, transcription, RNA processing, and cell cycle machinery.

Giardia undergoes frequent antigenic variation; a single variant-specific surface protein (VSP) is expressed on the surface of *Giardia* and after several generations is replaced by another VSP.[11] This change of VSP can occur in the absence of an adaptive immune response. VSPs are a family of about 250 cysteine-rich proteins with similar motifs, general structure, and a conserved transmembrane carboxyl-terminal sequence.[10] Although all VSPs are transcribed, studies suggest that all but one are eliminated by RNAi mechanisms, leaving just one VSP expressed at any one time.[12] Antigenic variation occurs during infection of humans and animals, in vitro in culture, and during encystation.

The life cycle of *G. lamblia* is composed of two stages: the trophozoite, or freely living stage, and the cyst. The trophozoite is 9 to 21 μm long and 5 to 15 μm wide (Fig. 280-1A). It has a convex dorsal surface and a flat ventral surface containing the disk, which is often referred to as the *sucking* or *adhesive* disk. There are four pairs of posteriorly directed flagella that are involved in locomotion and perhaps attachment. Their intracytoplasmic projections are termed axonemes. The disk cytoskeleton is composed of a clockwise spiral array of microtubules joined by vertical microribbons.[13] Within these structural components are important antigens: tubulin within microtubules and giardins within microribbons. The disk also contains contractile proteins. The protozoan has two anteriorly placed nuclei, each with a prominent central karyosome and complete copies of the genome.[14] Each of the two *Giardia* nuclei maintain a high degree of homozygosity through fusion and exchange of DNA during encystation.[15]

On stained preparations, the nuclei create the characteristic facelike image. Median bodies—tight collections of microtubules—are placed transversely in a clawlike manner in *G. lamblia* and have been used to identify morphologically distinct types of *Giardia*.

Of the *Giardia* species, only *G. lamblia* has been successfully cultured in vitro.[16] Growth is enhanced by the presence of biliary lipids, a high concentration of cysteine, and low oxygen tension, thus helping to explain the predilection of *Giardia* for colonizing the upper small bowel. The trophozoite divides by longitudinal binary fission and has a doubling time in culture of 6 to 12 hours. It is an aerotolerant anaerobe and can scavenge oxygen to enhance survival.[17] *Giardia* uses glucose as the major source of carbohydrate energy, metabolizing it to the end products of acetate, ethanol, alanine, and carbon dioxide; adenosine triphosphate (ATP) is generated during this process.[2] The relative amounts of these end products depend on the oxygen tension in the environment.

Except for alanine, amino acids are taken up from the environment. Metabolism of arginine via the arginine dihydrolase pathway may be another mechanism for ATP generation. Phospholipids, fatty acids, cholesterol, and purine and pyrimidine nucleosides are also scavenged from the environment; there are no genes for purine and pyrimidine biosynthesis, and there are only enzymes sufficient for remodeling but not synthesis of lipid membrance components.[2,10]

G. lamblia trophozoites encyst to form smooth, oval, thin-walled cysts 8 to 12 μm long and 7 to 10 μm wide (see Fig. 280-1B). This process is well studied and a model system for vesicular transport and developmental biology.[18,19] Encystation can be induced in vitro by a number of methods such as cholesterol starvation or bile salt deprivation followed by alkaline pH and excess bile salts.[20] The process is complex and encompasses changes to many of *Giardia*'s basic processes including downregulation of trophozoite-specific genes and induction of encystation-specific genes.[21] The early phase is characterized by the formation of highly characteristic encystment vesicles (ESVs) in which cyst wall proteins (CWP) 1 through 3, as well as other proteins and a protease, are concentrated and processed.[18,22,23] Soluble CWPs can be detected in the stool and form the basis of many *Giardia* antigen diagnostic tests. The late phase of encystation consists of transport of the CWPs to the cell surface, their assembly with N-acetylgalactosamine (GalNAc) into the cyst wall, and then nuclear division and DNA replication without cell division, so that cysts are generated with a ploidy of 16N.[21] In vitro, the entire process takes about 16 hours.[24] On ultrastructural analysis, the cyst wall contains CWP and GalNAc polymer in insoluble fibrils. During encystation the disk is disassembled, stored as four fragments, and then rapidly reassembled into two new disks in the dividing, excysting parasite.[25]

Excystation is a highly coordinated process that is initiated when environmental stimuli such as gastric acid and pancreatic enzymes are detected across the cyst wall.[26] During this process, a parasite-derived cysteine protease is activated.[27] Because of the rapidity of excystation, cell-signaling events are likely to be important[28] in addition to new gene expression. An excyzoite containing four nuclei (4N each) is

TABLE 280-1	Typing of *Giardia* spp.	
Name	**Genotype**	**Host range**
Giardia agilis		Amphibians
Giardia ardeae		Birds
Giardia microti		Muskrats and voles
Giardia muris		Rodents
Giardia psittaci		Birds
Giardia lamblia	Assemblage A	Humans, primates, dogs, cats, cattle, sheep, deer, rodents
	Assemblage B	Humans, primates, dogs, cattle, horses, beaver
	Assemblage C	Dogs
	Assemblage D	Dogs
	Assemblage E	Cattle, goats, sheep, pig
	Assemblage F	Cats
	Assemblage G	Rodents

Adapted from Xiao L, Fayer R. Molecular characterisation of species and genotypes of *Cryptosporidium* and *Giardia* and assessment of zoonotic transmission. *Int J Parasitol.* 2008;38:1239-1255; Wielinga CM, Thompson RC. Comparative evaluation of *Giardia duodenalis* sequence data. *Parasitology.* 2007;134:1795-1821.

released; this divides twice without further DNA replication, resulting in four daughter trophozoites.[29]

Epidemiology

Giardia is distributed throughout the world. In the United States, *G. lamblia* has been demonstrated in 4% to 7% of stool specimens, making it the most commonly identified intestinal parasite. A U.S. epidemiologic survey of giardiasis from 2003 to 2005 found that 20,000 to 21,000 cases were reported annually, with the case rates in different states varying from 0.3 to 30.0 cases per 100,000 persons, and an overall mean of 7.[30] Because of underreporting, there may be 100,000 to 2.5 million cases annually. *Giardia* was most frequently reported in children 1 to 9 years old and adults 35 to 45 years old, and during the late summer and fall months; these findings are similar to those in Canada.[31] *Giardia* was the cause of diarrhea in 15% of children presenting to U.S. outpatient offices.[32]

In low-income regions of the world, *Giardia* is one of the first enteric pathogens to infect infants,[33-35] with peak prevalence rates of 15% to 30% occurring in children younger than 10 years.[36-40] Nearly all children in these settings become infected.

Acquisition of the parasite requires oral ingestion of *Giardia* cysts through contaminated water, or through person-to-person or foodborne transmission. The risk of giardiasis from drinking water in the U.S. has declined over the last 2 decades, as improved measures for water treatment have been implemented.[41] Although recreational water is also a risk for *Giardia*, *Cryptosporidium* is the most common cause of diarrhea in treated recreational water (e.g., swimming pools and interactive water fountains) and noroviruses, *Shigella* spp., and *Escherichia coli* O157:H7 are more common in untreated recreational water (e.g., lakes).[42,43] Surface water supplies can become contaminated by human or animal sources, and *Giardia* cysts survive well in the environment, particularly in cold water. Sampling of surface water demonstrates frequent contamination with *Giardia* cysts as well as those of *Cryptosporidium*. Backpackers who do not adequately treat water can become infected. In an epidemiologic survey from southwest England, swallowing water while swimming and drinking tap water (odds ratio of 1.3 for each additional glass per day) were associated with giardiasis.[44] Common to most waterborne outbreaks has been the use of untreated surface water or well water, or water treated by a faulty purification system or by inadequate chlorination and not also subjected to flocculation, sedimentation, and filtration.[43]

Person-to-person transmission occurs in groups with poor fecal-oral hygiene, such as young children in daycare centers and men who have sex with men. In children in daycare centers, the prevalence of

Giardia cyst passage has been as high as 20% to 50%.[45] Many young children are asymptomatic, but they can spread the infection within their homes and contribute to secondary spread within their communities.[46,47] The high North American prevalence of giardiasis in children aged 1 to 9 years would be consistent with this epidemiologic pattern.[30,31] Sexually active gay men have cyst passage rates as high as 20% and frequently report symptoms.[48] Reports that have documented the transmission of *Giardia* in commercial food establishments, corporate office settings, and small gatherings indicate that foodborne transmission may be more common than recognized.[49] Travelers who acquire *Giardia* have often visited countries in the Indian subcontinent and have traveled for a month or more.[50,51]

Molecular analysis and natural or experimental infection with parasites that are morphologically of the *G. lamblia* species have shown that many mammalian hosts can be infected; these include gerbils, mice, beavers, sheep, cattle, dogs, and cats.[6,7] In some regions, nearly all domestic cattle become infected, and *Giardia* is the most frequent intestinal parasite of domestic dogs in Australia.[52] However, most animal isolates are not in genetic groupings that infect humans (assemblages A and B), and have not been implicated as a source of human infection (see Table 280-1). An exception to this was a Canadian waterborne outbreak of giardiasis that was linked to beavers.[9] This emphasizes the importance of protecting water supplies that are used

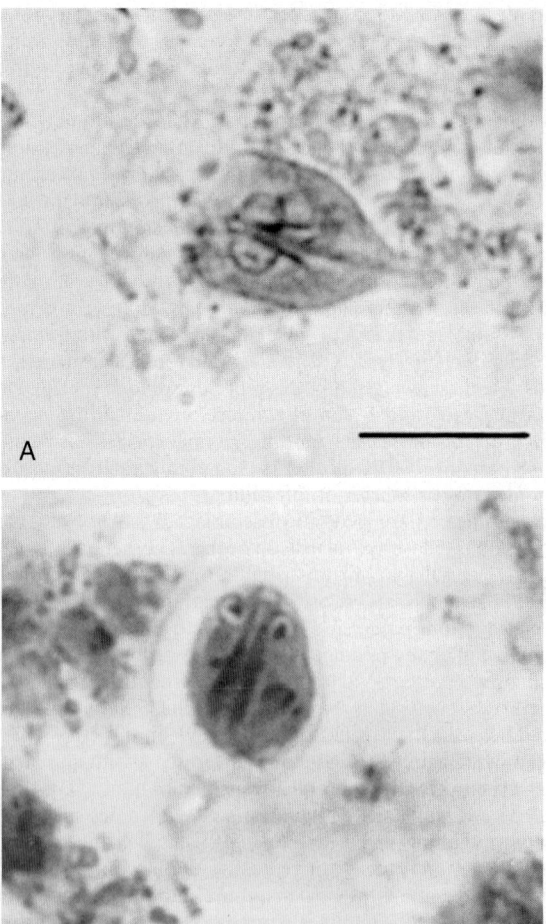

Figure 280-1 *Giardia lamblia* **trophozoite (A) and cyst (B) are demonstrated in a trichrome stain of fecal material.** Note the prominent nuclei in the trophozoite. In the cyst, the cytoplasm has separated from the cyst wall; centrally located axonemes, a clawlike median body, and two eccentrically located nuclei can be detected (bar = 10 μm).

for drinking from surface contamination, and of adequately purifying all public water supplies.

Pathogenesis and Immune Response

Giardia was once thought to be a harmless commensal, but its association with symptomatic diarrhea, malabsorption in children, and disease after waterborne outbreaks, travel, and experimental human infection[53] has clearly established its pathogenicity. The production of diarrhea, and occasionally malabsorption, is the result of a complex interaction of *Giardia* with the host, with the outcome related to the number and genotype of *Giardia* ingested and the host's previous experience with and immune response to the parasite.

Infection occurs after oral ingestion of as few as 10 to 25 cysts.[54] Although virulence characteristics of individual isolates have not been clearly determined, the ability to establish infection and to cause diarrhea varies between isolates and assemblages or genotypes.[2,53,55-57] After excystation, trophozoites colonize and multiply in the upper small bowel. Adherence of *G. lamblia* in the human gut is most likely via the ventral disk, with attachment at the brush border of enterocytes by either a suction or a clasping mechanism. Other specific adherence events have not been completely excluded.[58] The parasite may avoid being expelled by gut peristalsis by becoming trapped in intestinal mucus or between villi, or by adhering to enterocytes.[59]

Several pathogenic mechanisms have been postulated that rely on the effects of the parasites on the intestine: disruption of the intestinal epithelial brush border and function, mucosal invasion, and elaboration of an enterotoxin. Electron microscopy has documented disruption of the brush border in some patients, which could lead to the disaccharidase deficiencies commonly seen in giardiasis. Using in vitro, human, small intestine epithelial cell monolayers, *G. lamblia* can disrupt tight junctions, increase permeability, and induce apoptosis.[60-62] These effects are caspase-3 dependent.[60,61] The findings of epithelial barrier dysfunction and apoptosis have also been seen in duodenal biopsies from persons with giardiasis.[63] High levels of glucose with activation of the sodium-dependent glucose cotransporter can protect intestinal epithelial cells against *Giardia*-induced apoptosis.[64] *Giardia* have also been demonstrated to actively suppress the protective effect of intestinal nitric oxide[65] in mice by consuming arginine, which is used by epithelial cells to form nitric oxide.[66,67] Mucosal invasion is rare, and there is little reproducible evidence for the production of an enterotoxin. Simultaneous colonization of the small bowel with *Giardia* and *Enterobacteriaceae* or yeast may contribute to malabsorption in some patients by the deconjugation of bile salts.

The host immune response is the other important component of the host-parasite relationship.[29,68] Relatively little is known about protective responses in human giardiasis, and much of the information is extrapolated from mouse and gerbil models of infection with *G. muris* or *G. lamblia*. Even with these models there are differences in the response of mice to infection with a native parasite, *G. muris*, and a non-native parasite, *G. lamblia*. Nevertheless, host immunity plays a role in clearance of the parasite, in providing some protection against rechallenge, and, in certain instances, in production of disease. Several observations indicate that partially protective immunity can develop to *Giardia*. In rodent models of giardiasis, animals clear infection and develop partial resistance to reinfection. This experimental finding is supported by epidemiologic studies of human giardiasis; there were lower rates of symptomatic disease in long-term residents of endemic areas of North America than in visitors or short-term residents.[69,70] In contrast, reinfection is common, particularly in children in endemic settings,[35,38] and previously infected volunteers can be reinfected with the identical isolate after treatment.[53] Possible reasons for the ability to become reinfected are exposure to a different genotype, expression of a different VSP by an individual isolate, and age and nutritional status of the host.

Both B-cell and T-cell immunity appear to play essential roles in protective immunity.[29] Consideration of the importance of antibody has come from the increased susceptibility of patients with common

variable immunodeficiency to chronic giardiasis.[71] A systemic antibody response occurs in patients with *Giardia* and has been useful in seroprevalence studies.[72-75] Although serum immunoglobulin M (IgM) and IgG antibodies develop and with complement can be lethal to *Giardia* trophozoites, it is likely that gastrointestinal, secretory IgA antibodies play a more important role because of the luminal location of trophozoites.[76-78] In mice infected with *Giardia*, IgA has been the predominant antibody class detected in gut secretions: its development correlates temporally with control of the parasite, and its absence is associated with inability to resolve infection.[76,78,79] Inability to transport IgA across the epithelial membrane is also associated with the inability to clear *G. muris* infection.[80] The failure to develop IgA against specific *Giardia* antigens has been suggested to correlate with chronic giardiasis in humans.[81] The mechanism by which IgA prevents or helps to clear infection is probably by binding to trophozoites and preventing a critical adherence step; there is no evidence that IgA can kill trophozoites. *Giardia* species can produce an IgA protease.

Athymic, T-cell-deficient mice are unable to clear infection with *G. muris* or *G. lamblia* until the mice are reconstituted with lymphoid cells, particularly the CD4+ helper T lymphocyte.[79,82,83] After reconstitution, animals develop an abnormal intestinal histologic appearance that parallels the changes seen in some humans with giardiasis: flattening of villi, crypt hypertrophy, and a mononuclear cell infiltration of the submucosa.[84,85] B-cell-deficient mice were unable to clear infection with either *G. muris* or *G. lamblia,* and this effect went beyond just the failure of these mice to produce IgA.[78]

The contributions to the clearance of *Giardia* in murine models appear to be time dependent. Early, B-cell-independent mechanisms of control of *G. lamblia*-infected mice include interleukin (IL)-6.[86,87] This effect may be mediated via mast cells that produce IL-6 and contribute to increased intestinal motility that has been associated with improved clearance of parasites.[88,89] B-cell-mediated effects appear to be important later in the course of infection.[78]

The inflammatory response with damage to enterocytes could initiate a cytokine-mediated diarrhea, similar to the proposed mechanism for diarrhea production in adherent or minimally invasive coccidians such as *Cyclospora* and *Cryptosporidium*.[90] It could also stimulate increased epithelial cell turnover in the crypt region, changing the bowel's absorptive capacity.

Human milk can play a role in protection of the host against *Giardia*. Milk is cytotoxic to trophozoites when free fatty acids are released from milk triglycerides by the action of bile salt-stimulated lipase.[91] Both human and animal breast milk have been found to contain anti-*Giardia* antibodies, and several studies have demonstrated protection of breast-feeding infants from symptomatic infection.[92,93]

Predisposition to giardiasis has been documented in patients with common variable immunodeficiency and in children with X-linked agammaglobulinemia.[71] These patients have symptomatic disease with prolonged diarrhea, malabsorption, and marked changes on small bowel biopsy, which can include nodular lymphoid hyperplasia. On administration of anti-*Giardia* therapy, their symptoms improve and the histologic changes resolve. It remains unclear whether selective IgA deficiency is a predisposing factor.

Susceptibility to giardiasis has also been seen in patients with previous gastric surgery and reduced gastric acidity. There appears to be no association of giardiasis with blood group specificity. Patients with acquired immunodeficiency syndrome generally do not have more severe illness with *Giardia*; however, in some cases, the disease is refractory to treatment.[94]

Although it is clear that different *G. lamblia* isolates have different capacities for establishing infection and causing disease, the association of specific genotypes or assemblages with disease requires ongoing analysis of many isolates from multiple parts of the world.[2,53,55,56,95] Although *Giardia* organisms change their VSPs in vivo, the role that this plays in avoiding immune recognition and allowing persistent infection is speculative.[11,96]

Small bowel biopsy may demonstrate spruelike lesions or may be normal;[97] two studies have correlated the severity of diarrhea with the degree of histologic abnormality on biopsy.[85,98] The variation in the histologic appearance supports the multiple potential mechanisms for the production of diarrhea.

Clinical Manifestations

Infection with *G. lamblia* includes asymptomatic cyst passage, acute self-limited diarrhea, and a chronic syndrome of diarrhea, malabsorption, and weight loss. Of 100 people ingesting *Giardia* cysts, an estimated 5% to 15% become asymptomatic cyst passers, 25% to 50% become symptomatic with an acute diarrheal syndrome, and the remaining 35% to 70% have no trace of infection. Although many symptomatic patients spontaneously clear their infection, most develop a diarrheal syndrome lasting 1 week to several weeks and will end up being treated with antimicrobial therapy. For children in daycare centers, asymptomatic cyst passage has been documented to last as long as 6 months.

After the ingestion of *G. lamblia* cysts, there is an incubation period of 1 to 2 weeks before the onset of symptoms. The time from ingestion of cysts to detection of cysts in the stool may be longer than the incubation period.[53] Thus, a stool examination at the time of the onset of symptoms could be negative.

Symptomatic giardiasis is characterized by the acute onset of diarrhea, abdominal cramps, bloating, and flatulence (Table 280-2). The patient usually expresses feelings of malaise, nausea, and anorexia and may complain of sulfuric belching. Vomiting, fever, and tenesmus occur less commonly. Initially, stools may be profuse and watery, but later they are commonly greasy and foul smelling and may float. Gross blood, pus, and mucus are usually absent, and if examined microscopically, the stool is found to be free of polymorphonuclear cells. The presence of blood or polymorphonyclear cells suggests another diagnosis.

One of the most important distinguishing features is the prolonged duration of diarrhea with giardiasis. At the time of presentation, most patients have been symptomatic for more than 1 week to 10 days. Weight loss of about 10 pounds occurs more than 50% of the time and is another useful clinical feature.[48] Unusual associations include urticaria, reactive arthritis, biliary tract disease, and gastric infection. Gastric infection occurs exclusively in the presence of achlorhydria and has been seen in conjunction with *Helicobacter pylori*.[99]

Although most persons with giardiasis have a relatively benign course, some persons, particularly children younger than 5 years and pregnant women, can have severe illness characterized by volume depletion and require hospitalization.[100,101]

Patients who develop chronic diarrhea have profound malaise, lassitude, occasional headache, and diffuse abdominal and epigastric discomfort often exacerbated by eating. Stools may be greasy and foul smelling or frothy, yellowish, occurring in small volume, and frequently passed. Weight loss is usually present. Periods of diarrhea can be interrupted by periods of constipation or normal bowel habits, with the syndrome waxing and waning over months until therapy is given or spontaneous resolution occurs. Post-*Giardia* irritable bowel syndrome has been documented.[102]

Various degrees of malabsorption can be present. Children who present for evaluation for failure to thrive or with a spruelike illness have been found to have giardiasis.[98,103] Steatorrhea and malabsorption of vitamins A and B$_{12}$, protein, D-xylose, and iron have been documented.[104,105] The most common disaccharidase deficiency has been that of lactase, occurring in 20% to 40% of cases,[106] with post-*Giardia* lactose intolerance sometimes persisting for several weeks after treatment. This is often confused with relapse or reinfection.

The role that chronic infection with *Giardia* plays in the growth and development of children in the low-income regions of the world has been controversial. It is clear that high prevalence rates of *Giardia* exist in both symptomatic and asymptomatic children. Some studies point to a deleterious effect on growth and argue for the need to treat recurrent disease to allow catch-up growth.[35,104,107-109] Others emphasize the high prevalence of *Giardia* infection in asymptomatic children living in areas of poor sanitation and suggest that reinfection occurs so rapidly that repeated therapy is impractical and not indicated.[38,110,111,112] In addition, many children may be simultaneously infected with other bacterial, viral, and parasitic infections, making the contribution that *Giardia* makes to their illness less clear.

More recent studies have helped to clarify this issue. Evidence for stunting in Brazilian and Ecuadorian children infected with *Giardia*,[35,113] poor intestinal permeability in Nepali children,[114] low weight-for-age and height-for-age in Brazilian children with persistent symptomatic giardiasis,[37,115] significant wasting in Malaysian children,[36] and decreased cognitive function in Peruvian children with multiple episodes of giardiasis[34] point to a deleterious effect in children who already have a poor underlying nutritional state. These studies are in contrast to a longitudinal study in Bangladeshi children[116] and Peruvian children[38] that did not demonstrate effects on well-being or nutrition. In addition, well-nourished, asymptomatically infected children did not have signs of malnutrition.[117,118] Therefore, it is likely that prolonged episodes of giardiasis in children with underlying poor nutrition can have more deleterious effects than episodes in normal children. Why there are not uniform outcomes will require additional studies that examine the characteristics of the predominant *Giardia* isolates and underlying status of the hosts. Despite the conflicting findings, it remains important to maintain childhood nutrition and eliminate the risk factors for repeated episodes of diarrheal illness.

Diagnosis

The diagnosis of giardiasis should be considered in all patients with prolonged diarrhea, particularly that which is associated with malabsorption or weight loss. If there is a history of recent travel to an endemic area, the presence of small children in the home who attend daycare centers, or sexual risk factors, giardiasis is also more likely. Other diarrheal syndromes caused by viruses, noninvasive bacteria, and protozoans such as *Cryptosporidium* spp. and *Cyclospora cayetanensis*, as well as tropical sprue, should be considered in the differential diagnosis.

The traditional method of diagnosis has been to perform a stool examination for ova and parasites (O&P), looking for trophozoites or cysts. The O&P examination has been the assay with which other tests are compared. Parasites detected via immunofluorescence, and antigen detection using enzyme-linked immunosorbent assays (ELISAs) and nonenzymatic immunoassays are now commonly available.[119,120] For many laboratories they are the tests of choice because they are reproducible and rapid, and do not require a trained microscopist.[121]

In an O&P examination, the stool should be examined fresh and after preservation. A saline wet mount of fresh liquid stool obtained

TABLE 280-2	Symptoms of Giardiasis		
		Percentage	*Range*
Diarrhea		89	64-100
Malaise		84	72-97
Flatulence		74	35-97
Foul-smelling, greasy stools		72	57-79
Abdominal cramps		70	44-85
Bloating		69	42-97
Nausea		68	59-79
Anorexia		64	41-82
Weight loss		64	56-73
Vomiting		27	17-36
Fever		13	0-21
Urticaria		9	4-14
Constipation		9	0-17

From data reviewed in Hill DR. Giardiasis. Issues in diagnosis and management. *Infect Dis Clin North Am.* 1993;7:503-525.

in the acute stages of illness may yield motile trophozoites. In semi-formed stool, trophozoites are usually not found. These stools should be examined fresh for cysts after iodine staining or after preservation in 10% buffered formalin or polyvinyl alcohol and subsequent tri-chrome or iron hematoxylin staining. Formalin-ether or zinc sulfate flotation concentration techniques may increase the yield. *Giardia* should be identified 60% to 80% of the time after one stool, and some report over 90% identification after three stools.[48,122,123] Examination of a purged sample does not increase the yield.

Although antigen assays are used frequently for routine stool diagnostics, they are most helpful when giardiasis is the leading consideration, such as during an outbreak, when screening children in daycare, or when testing patients for cure after the completion of treatment. They are often less expensive than an O&P examination and are 85% to 98% sensitive and 90% to 100% specific.[119,120,124-129]

Because good results can be obtained with a carefully performed stool O&P examination or an antigen assay, sampling of the duodenal contents by string test or biopsy is generally not needed. However, in cases that are particularly difficult to diagnose, these procedures may be helpful. Three methods have been used: the string test, duodenal aspiration, and duodenal biopsy. The string test should yield bile-stained mucus from the duodenum that can be examined for trophozoites in a wet mount or after staining. Duodenal aspiration and biopsy are more invasive. Biopsies require touch preparations, Giemsa staining, and a careful search for trophozoites. An advantage of biopsy, particularly in patients infected with human immunodeficiency virus or persons with malabsorption, is the ability to identify a histologic abnormality that is not caused by giardiasis and to detect other pathogens. An aspirate can be sampled for small bowel overgrowth.

Testing for systemic anti-*Giardia* antibody is not generally available, but it has been useful in seroepidemiologic studies throughout the world.[72-75] IgG antibodies remain elevated for long periods, making them less helpful diagnostically in areas endemic for giardiasis. It is not clear if serum anti-*Giardia* IgM is useful in distinguishing current from past giardiasis.[130]

Although in vitro culture is available in research settings, it is not routinely used because of the difficulty of reproducibly isolating *Giardia* from patient samples.[16] Detection of *Giardia* nucleic acid by polymerase chain reaction or by gene probes is highly sensitive. It has been typically applied to the detection of parasites in water samples or to genotyping isolates from various mammalian hosts, although it is now being introduced for laboratory diagnostics.[6-8,131] The white blood cell count is usually normal, and eosinophilia is absent. Barium studies are generally nonspecific and show an increased transit time and irregular thickening of small bowel folds. These studies may interfere with the examination of stools.

Treatment

Routine isolation, culture, and susceptibility testing of *Giardia* have been difficult because of the variable success in establishing cultures from clinical specimens and the lack of standardization on sensitivity testing.[132] Drug resistance occurs for *Giardia* and can be induced in vitro,[133] but the clinical significance of this is not known because some isolates that appear clinically resistant are susceptible in vitro, and vice versa. Most information on drug efficacy, therefore, is provided by clinical experience.[132,134]

The drug of choice for the therapy of giardiasis in the United States is tinidazole (Tindamaz, Mission Pharmaceutical Company, San Antonio, TX) following its release in 2004 (Table 280-3).[135] Like metronidazole, it is a member of the nitroimidazole family. Prior to release, there was extensive experience with tinidazole for the treatment of giardiasis (as well as for amebiasis and trichomoniasis) outside of the United States.[132] It has high efficacy (approximately 90%), a favorable side effect profile, and, because of a longer half-life than metronidazole, can be given once daily. Although the U.S. Food and Drug Administration has never approved metronidazole for giardiasis, there are years of experience in using it against the parasite.

TABLE 280-3	Treatment of Giardiasis	
	Dosage	
Drug	*Adult*	*Pediatric*
Tinidazole	2 g, single dose	50 mg/kg, single dose (maximum, 2 g)
Metronidazole*	250 mg tid × 5-7 days	5 mg/kg tid × 7 days
Nitazoxanide	500 mg bid × 3 days	Age 12-47 mos: 100 mg bid × 3 days Age 4-11 yrs: 200 mg bid × 3 days
Albendazole*	400 mg qd × 5 days	15 mg/kg/day × 5-7 days (maximum, 400 mg)
Paromomycin*	500 mg tid × 5-10 days	30 mg/kg/day in 3 doses × 5-10 days
Quinacrine†	100 mg tid × 5-7 days	2 mg/kg tid × 7 days
Furazolidone†	100 mg qid × 7-10 days	2 mg/kg qid × 10 days

*Not a U.S. Food and Drug Administration–approved indication.
†No longer produced in the United States; may be obtained from some compounding pharmacies.

Tinidazole is effective as a single dose for both children and adults.[136] Metronidazole is given in divided doses for 5 to 7 days, with an efficacy of 80% to 95%. Adverse effects for tinidazole and metronidazole are similar: a metallic taste, nausea, dizziness, headache, and, rarely, reversible neutropenia, peripheral neuropathy or seizures. When taken with alcohol, they can produce a disulfiram-like effect. High-dose, short-course regimens of metronidazole have lower efficacy rates and may be poorly tolerated. There have been concerns about potential mutagenicity of metronidazole; however, this has not been documented in humans.[137]

The mechanism of action of metronidazole and presumably tinidazole is reductive activation of the nitro group by acceptance of electrons from parasite ferredoxins.[138,139] Once activated, it binds to parasite DNA, causing damage and trophozoite death. Metronidazole also inhibits parasite respiration. When resistance to metronidazole occurs, it correlates with decreased parasite pyruvate:ferredoxin oxidoreductase.[133]

Nitazoxanide (Alinia, Romark Pharmaceuticals, Tampa, FL) was approved in 2003 for use in pediatric giardiasis and cryptosporidiosis and more recently for giardiasis treatment in adults.[140] Whereas there is limited clinical experience with this drug compared with the nitroimidazoles, efficacy is in the range of 65% to 85% when a 3-day course of treatment is given.[141,142] Nitazoxanide has wide activity against a variety of intestinal parasites, some bacteria including *Clostridium difficile* and *H. pylori* and possibly rotavirus diarrhea.[141,143] Its mechanism of action is the inhibition of pyruvate:ferredoxin oxidoreductases, however, there does not appear to be cross-resistance with metronidazole-resistant parasites.[144] Its main side effect is gastrointestinal upset.

There is increasing experience with the benzimidazoles. Although efficacy with mebendazole is generally disappointing,[132,145] several studies have demonstrated success with albendazole in a single daily dose of 400 mg for 5 days.[132,146] The actual role of albendazole in therapy remains to be determined, but it is attractive because it has efficacy against many intestinal helminths and is used in low-income regions to decrease intestinal parasitism.

Quinacrine and furazolidone, a nitrofuran, and are no longer manufactured in the United States. Quinacrine has an efficacy of more than 90%, and if it can be obtained through alternative sources, it is given in divided doses for 5 to 7 days (see Table 280-3). The most common side effects are a bitter taste, nausea, vomiting, and abdominal cramping. Yellow discoloration of the skin, urine, and sclerae can occasionally occur, and exfoliative dermatitis is a rare side effect. Furazolidone has a success rate of about 80% to 85%, but may cause gastrointestinal side effects, turn urine brown, and cause mild hemolysis in glucose-6-phosphate dehydrogenase-deficient individuals.

For patients in whom one drug course fails or who infrequently relapse, a switch to a drug from a different class is generally effective.

For the unusual patient who is not cured with single-drug therapies, combination treatment, often with metronidazole and quinacrine, can be effective.[94,147,148] A randomized trial comparing metronidazole alone versus metronidazole plus the probiotic *Saccharomyces boulardii* demonstrated higher cure rates in the combination group.[149] Nitazoxanide may also be effective in patients with resistant giardiasis.[150] When refractory infection is suspected, it is important to establish true persistence by obtaining a repeat stool exam; for those patients who simply have post-*Giardia* lactose intolerance, further antiparasitic treatment is not needed.

For pregnant women with giardiasis, there is no consistently recommended therapy because of the theoretical adverse effects of anti-*Giardia* drugs on the fetus.[132] When the disease is mild and hydration and nutrition can be maintained, therapy can be delayed until after delivery, or at least until after the first trimester. If treatment is necessary, paromomycin, an oral aminoglycoside, can be tried. In limited clinical experience, it has an efficacy rate of 60% to 70%, but it has the advantage of not being measurably absorbed from the intestine in persons with normal renal function.[151] It is given in divided doses for 5 to 10 days (see Table 280-3). Metronidazole has been used extensively in pregnancy for the treatment of trichomoniasis. The teratogenic effect appears to be minimal and, if present, greatest during the first trimester, when both metronidzole and tinidazole should not be used.[132,135,151,152] If therapy cannot be avoided, then metronidazole can probably be used safely in the last two trimesters of pregnancy. High-dose, short-course regimens of metronidazole should not be used.

Prevention

The prevention of giardiasis requires proper handling and treatment of water used for communities, and good personal hygiene on an individual basis. Although chlorination alone is sufficient to kill *G. lamblia* cysts, important variables, such as water temperature, clarity, pH, and contact time, alter the efficacy of chlorine, and higher chlorine levels (4 to 6 mg/L) may be required.[41,153] Thus, in addition to chlorination, public water supplies should also be subjected to flocculation, sedimentation, and filtration.[30,41]

Travelers to low-income regions of the world or to wilderness areas should consider all water potentially contaminated because of the wide array of animal and human reservoirs of giardiasis. Bringing water to a boil is sufficient to kill all protozoal cysts; at high altitudes, boiling for a minute is reasonable. If boiling is impossible, halogenation is generally effective for *Giardia,* but *Cryptosporidium* is resistant,[154] and the sensitivity of *Cyclospora* is likely to be similar to that of *Cryptosporidium.* Chlorine-based (AquaClear; chlorine bleach: 5% to 6%, 2 to 4 drops/L) or iodine-based (Globaline, Potable-Aqua [tetraglycine hydroperiodide]; tincture of iodine: 2%, 5 drops/L) preparations can be used.[153] Contact time should be increased for water that is cold, and the concentration of halogen should be increased for turbid water. Small-volume personal water filters with pores of an "absolute" micron size of 0.2 to 1 μm can be used. Filtered water should also be halogenated to kill enteric viruses if they are considered a risk. Uncooked foods that may have been washed or prepared in contaminated water should be avoided.

The endemic foci present in daycare centers can be a major problem. It is not clear whether chronic, asymptomatic carriage of *Giardia* in otherwise well-nourished children is deleterious to their health.[117,118,155] For these reasons and because of potential side effects of treatment, some recommend that only symptomatic children be treated.[117,156] On the other hand, infected children transmit *Giardia* to parents and family members.[46,47] Because of these conflicting issues, each situation requires an individual decision. However, if strict hand washing and treatment of symptomatic children fail to control an outbreak of diarrhea, consideration can be given to treating all infected children.[157]

Venereal transmission of *Giardia* can be decreased by avoidance of oral-anal and oral-genital sex. Immunization of mice with CWP2 was immunogenic and partially protective against *G. lamblia* challenge.[158] There is a veterinary vaccine, but no vaccine for humans.[159]

REFERENCES

1. Garcia LS. Classification of human parasites, vectors, and similar organisms. *Clin Infect Dis.* 1999;29:734-736.
2. Adam RD. Biology of *Giardia lamblia. Clin Micro Rev.* 2001; 14:447-475.
3. Davis-Hayman SR, Nash TE. Genetic manipulation of *Giardia lamblia. Mol Biochem Parasitol.* 2002;122:1-7.
4. Lane S, Lloyd D. Current trends in research into the waterborne parasite *Giardia. Crit Rev Microbiol.* 2002;28:123-147.
5. Tovar J, Leon-Avila G, Sanchez LB, et al. Mitochondrial remnant organelles of *Giardia* function in iron-sulphur protein maturation. *Nature.* 2003;426:172-176.
6. Xiao L, Fayer R. Molecular characterisation of species and genotypes of *Cryptosporidium* and *Giardia* and assessment of zoonotic transmission. *Int J Parasitol.* 2008;38:1239-1255.
7. Wielinga CM, Thompson RC. Comparative evaluation of *Giardia duodenalis* sequence data. *Parasitol.* 2007;134:1795-1821.
8. Caccio SM, Ryan U. Molecular epidemiology of giardiasis. *Mol Biochem Parasitol.* 2008;160:75-80.
9. Baruch AC, Isaac-Renton J, Adam RD. The molecular epidemiology of *Giardia lamblia*: a sequence-based approach. *J Infect Dis.* 1996;174:233-236.
10. Morrison HG, McArthur AG, Gillin FD, et al. Genomic minimalism in the early diverging intestinal parasite *Giardia lamblia. Science.* 2007;317:1921-1926.
11. Nash TE. Surface antigenic variation in *Giardia lamblia. Mol Microbiol.* 2002;45:585-590.
12. Prucca CG, Slavin I, Quiroga R, et al. Antigenic variation in *Giardia lamblia* is regulated by RNA interference. *Nature.* 2008;456:750-754.
13. Elmendorf HG, Dawson SC, McCaffery JM. The cytoskeleton of *Giardia lamblia. Int J Parasitol.* 2003;33:3-28.
14. Yu LZ, Birky CW Jr, Adam RD. The two nuclei of *Giardia* each have complete copies of the genome and are partitioned equationally at cytokinesis. *Eukaryot Cell.* 2002;1:191-199.
15. Poxleitner MK, Carpenter ML, Mancuso JJ, et al. Evidence for karyogamy and exchange of genetic material in the binucleate intestinal parasite *Giardia intestinalis. Science.* 2008;319:1530-1533.
16. Clark CG, Diamond LS. Methods for cultivation of luminal parasitic protists of clinical importance. *Clin Microbiol Rev.* 2002;15:329-341.

17. Di Matteo A, Scandurra FM, Testa F, et al. The O2-scavenging flavodiiron protein in the human parasite *Giardia intestinalis. J Biol Chem.* 2008;283:4061-4068.
18. Lauwaet T, Davids BJ, Reiner DS, et al. Encystation of *Giardia lamblia*: a model for other parasites. *Curr Opin Microbiol.* 2007;10:554-559.
19. Elias EV, Quiroga R, Gottig N, et al. Characterization of SNAREs determines the absence of a typical golgi apparatus in the ancient eukaryote *Giardia lamblia. J Biol Chem.* 2008;283:35996-36010.
20. Gillin FD, Reiner DS, McCaffery JM. Cell biology of the primitive eukaryote *Giardia lamblia. Annu Rev Microbiol.* 1996;50:679-705.
21. Svard SG, Hagblom P, Palm JE. *Giardia lamblia*—a model organism for eukaryotic cell differentiation. *FEMS Microbiol Lett.* 2003;218:3-7.
22. Davids BJ, Reiner DS, Birkeland SR, et al. A new family of giardial cysteine-rich non-VSP protein genes and a novel cyst protein. *PLoS ONE.* 2006;1:e44.
23. DuBois KN, Abodeely M, Sakanari J, et al. Identification of the major cysteine protease of *Giardia* and its role in encystation. *J Biol Chem.* 2008;283:18024-18031.
24. Erlandsen SL, Macechko PT, van Keulen H, et al. Formation of the *Giardia* cyst wall: studies on extracellular assembly using immunogold labeling and high resolution field emission SEM. *J Eukaryot Microbiol.* 1996;43:416-429.
25. Palm D, Weiland M, McArthur AG, et al. Developmental changes in the adhesive disk during *Giardia* differentiation. *Mol Biochem Parasitol.* 2005;141:199-207.
26. Hetsko ML, McCaffery JM, Svard SG, et al. Cellular and transcriptional changes during excystation of *Giardia lamblia* in vitro. *Exp Parasitol.* 1998;88:172-183.
27. Ward W, Alvarado L, Rawlings ND, et al. A primitive enzyme for a primitive cell: the protease required for excystation of *Giardia. Cell.* 1997;89:437-444.
28. Reiner DS, Hetsko ML, Meszaros JG, et al. Calcium signaling in excystation of the early diverging eukaryote, *Giardia lamblia. J Biol Chem.* 2003;278:2533-2540.
29. Roxström-Lindquist K, Palm D, Reiner D, et al. *Giardia* immunity—an update. *Trends Parasitol.* 2006;22:26-31.
30. Yoder JS, Beach MJ. Giardiasis surveillance—United States, 2003-2005. *MMWR Surveill Summ.* 2007;56(SS-7):11-18.

31. Laupland KB, Church DL. Population-based laboratory surveillance for *Giardia* sp. and *Cryptosporidium* sp. infections in a large Canadian health region. *BMC Infect Dis.* 2005;5:72.
32. Caeiro JP, Mathewson JJ, Smith MA, et al. Etiology of outpatient pediatric nondysenteric diarrhea: a multicenter study in the United States. *Pediatr Infect Dis J.* 1999;18:94-97.
33. Fraser D, Dagan R, Naggan L, et al. Natural history of *Giardia lamblia* and *Cryptosporidium* infections in a cohort of Israeli Bedouin infants: a study of a population in transition. *Am J Trop Med Hyg.* 1997;57:544-549.
34. Berkman DS, Lescano AG, Gilman RH, et al. Effects of stunting, diarrhoeal disease, and parasitic infection during infancy on cognition in late childhood: a follow-up study. *Lancet.* 2002; 359:564-571.
35. Prado MS, Cairncross S, Strina A, et al. Asymptomatic giardiasis and growth in young children; a longitudinal study in Salvador, Brazil. *Parasitol.* 2005;131:51-56.
36. Al-Mekhlafi MS, Azlin M, Nor Aini U, et al. Giardiasis as a predictor of childhood malnutrition in Orang Asli children in Malaysia. *Trans R Soc Trop Med Hyg.* 2005;99:686-691.
37. Carvalho-Costa FA, Goncalves AQ, Lassance SL, et al. *Giardia lamblia* and other intestinal parasitic infections and their relationships with nutritional status in children in Brazilian Amazon. *Rev Inst Med Trop Sao Paulo.* 2007;49:147-153.
38. Hollm-Delgado MG, Gilman RH, Bern C, et al. Lack of an adverse effect of *Giardia intestinalis* infection on the health of Peruvian children. *Am J Epidemiol.* 2008;168:647-655.
39. Mahmud MA, Chappell C, Hossain MM, et al. Risk factors for development of first symptomatic *Giardia* infection among infants of a birth cohort in rural Egypt. *Am J Trop Med Hyg.* 1995;53:84-88.
40. Dib HH, Lu SQ, Wen SF. Prevalence of *Giardia lamblia* with or without diarrhea in South East, South East Asia and the Far East. *Parasitol Res.* 2008;103:239-251.
41. Yoder J, Roberts V, Craun GF, et al. Surveillance for waterborne disease and outbreaks associated with drinking water and water not intended for drinking—United States, 2005-2006. *MMWR Surveill Summ.* 2008;57(SS-9):39-62.
42. Yoder JS, Hlavsa MC, Craun GF, et al. Surveillance for waterborne disease and outbreaks associated with recreational water use and other aquatic facility-associated health events—United States, 2005-2006. *MMWR Surveill Summ.* 2008;57(SS-9):1-29.

43. Karanis P, Kourenti C, Smith H. Waterborne transmission of protozoan parasites: a worldwide review of outbreaks and lessons learnt. *J Water Health*. 2007;5:1-38.
44. Stuart JM, Orr HJ, Warburton FG, et al. Risk factors for sporadic giardiasis: a case-control study in southwestern England. *Emerg Infect Dis*. 2003;9:229-233.
45. Thompson SC. *Giardia lamblia* in children and the child care setting: a review of the literature. *J Paediatr Child Health*. 1994;30:202-209.
46. Overturf GD. Endemic giardiasis in the United States—role of the daycare center (editorial). *Clin Infect Dis*. 1994;18:764-765.
47. Katz DE, Heisey-Grove D, Beach M, et al. Prolonged outbreak of giardiasis with two modes of transmission. *Epidemiol Infect*. 2006;134:935-941.
48. Hill DR. Giardiasis. Issues in diagnosis and management. *Infect Dis Clin North Am*. 1993;7:503-525.
49. Mintz ED, Hudson-Wragg M, Mshar P, et al. Foodborne giardiasis in a corporate office setting. *J Infect Dis*. 1993;167: 250-253.
50. Jelinek T, Loscher T. Epidemiology of giardiasis in German travelers. *J Travel Med*. 2000;7:70-73.
51. Ekdahl K, Andersson Y. Imported giardiasis: impact of international travel, immigration, and adoption. *Am J Trop Med Hyg*. 2005;72:825-830.
52. Thompson RC, Palmer CS, O'Handley R. The public health and clinical significance of *Giardia* and *Cryptosporidium* in domestic animals. *Vet J*. 2008;177:18-25.
53. Nash TE, Herrington DA, Losonsky GA, et al. Experimental human infections with *Giardia lamblia*. *J Infect Dis*. 1987; 156:974-984.
54. Rendtorff RC. The experimental transmission of human intestinal protozoan parasites: II. *Giardia lamblia* cysts given in capsules. *Am J Hyg*. 1954;59:209-220.
55. Haque R, Roy S, Kabir M, et al. *Giardia* assemblage A infection and diarrhea in Bangladesh. *J Infect Dis*. 2005;192:2171-2173.
56. Kohli A, Bushen OY, Pinkerton RC, et al. *Giardia duodenalis* assemblage, clinical presentation and markers of intestinal inflammation in Brazilian children. *Trans R Soc Trop Med Hyg*. 2008;102:718-725.
57. Sahagun J, Clavel A, Goni P, et al. Correlation between the presence of symptoms and the *Giardia duodenalis* genotype. *Eur J Clin Microbiol Infect Dis*. 2008;27:81-83.
58. Jenkins M, O'Brien CN, Murphy C, et al. Antibodies to the ventral disc protein delta-giardin prevent in vitro binding of *Giardia lamblia* trophozoites. *J Parasitol*. In press.
59. Hernandez-Sanchez J, Linan RF, Salinas-Tobon M del R, et al. *Giardia duodenalis*: adhesion-deficient clones have reduced ability to establish infection in Mongolian gerbils. *Exp Parasitol*. 2008;119:364-372.
60. Chin AC, Teoh DA, Scott KG, et al. Strain-dependent induction of enterocyte apoptosis by *Giardia lamblia* disrupts epithelial barrier function in a caspase-3-dependent manner. *Infect Immun*. 2002;70:3673-3680.
61. Panaro MA, Cianciulli A, Mitolo V, et al. Caspase-dependent apoptosis of the HCT-8 epithelial cell line induced by the parasite *Giardia intestinalis*. *FEMS Immunol Med Microbiol*. 2007; 51:302-309.
62. Buret AG. Pathophysiology of enteric infections with *Giardia duodenalis*. *Parasite*. 2008;15:261-265.
63. Troeger H, Epple HJ, Schneider T, et al. Effect of chronic *Giardia lamblia* infection on epithelial transport and barrier function in human duodenum. *Gut*. 2007;56:328-335.
64. Yu LC, Huang CY, Kuo WT, et al. SGLT-1-mediated glucose uptake protects human intestinal epithelial cells against *Giardia duodenalis*–induced apoptosis. *Int J Parasitol*. 2008;38:923-934.
65. Ringqvist E, Palm JE, Skarin H, et al. Release of metabolic enzymes by *Giardia* in response to interaction with intestinal epithelial cells. *Mol Biochem Parasitol*. 2008;159:85-91.
66. Eckmann L, Laurent F, Langford TD, et al. Nitric oxide production by human intestinal epithelial cells and competition for arginine as potential determinants of host defense against the lumen-dwelling pathogen *Giardia lamblia*. *J Immunol*. 2000; 164:1478-1487.
67. Li E, Zhou P, Singer SM. Neuronal nitric oxide synthase is necessary for elimination of *Giardia lamblia* infections in mice. *J Immunol*. 2006;176:516-521.
68. Faubert G. Immune response to *Giardia duodenalis*. *Clin Micro Rev*. 2000;13:35-54.
69. Istre GR, Dunlop TS, Gaspard B, et al. Waterborne giardiasis at a mountain resort: evidence for acquired immunity. *Am J Public Health*. 1984;74:602-604.
70. Isaac-Renton JL, Lewis LF, Ong CS, et al. A second community outbreak of waterborne giardiasis in Canada and serological investigation of patients. *Trans R Soc Trop Med Hyg*. 1994;88: 395-399.
71. Oksenhendler E, Gerard L, Fieschi C, et al. Infections in 252 patients with common variable immunodeficiency. *Clin Infect Dis*. 2008;46:1547-1554.
72. Ljungström I, Castor B. Immune response to *Giardia lamblia* in a water-borne outbreak of giardiasis in Sweden. *J Med Micro*. 1992;36:347-352.
73. Soliman MM, Taghi-Kilani R, Abou-Shady AF, et al. Comparison of serum antibody response to *Giardia lamblia* of symptomatic and asymptomatic patients. *Am J Trop Med Hyg*. 1998;58: 232-239.
74. Isaac-Renton J, Blatherwick J, Bowie WR, et al. Epidemic and endemic seroprevalence of antibodies to *Cryptosporidium* and *Giardia* in residents of three communities with different drinking water supplies. *Am J Trop Med Hyg*. 1999;60:578-583.
75. Crump JA, Mendoza CE, Priest JW, et al. Comparing serologic response against enteric pathogens with reported diarrhea to assess the impact of improved household drinking water quality. *Am J Trop Med Hyg*. 2007;77:136-141.
76. Stäger S, Müller N. *Giardia lamblia* infections in B-cell-deficient transgenic mice. *Infect Immun*. 1997;65:3944-3946.
77. Rosales-Borjas DM, Diaz-Rivadeneyra J, Dona-Leyva A, et al. Secretory immune response to membrane antigens during *Giardia lamblia* infection in humans. *Infect Immun*. 1998;66: 756-759.
78. Langford TD, Housley MP, Boes M, et al. Central importance of immunoglobulin A in host defense against *Giardia* spp. *Infect Immun*. 2002;70:11-18.
79. Heyworth MF. Immunology of *Giardia* and *Cryptosporidium* infections. *J Infect Dis*. 1992;166:465-472.
80. Davids BJ, Palm JE, Housley MP, et al. Polymeric immunoglobulin receptor in intestinal immune defense against the lumen-dwelling protozoan parasite *Giardia*. *J Immunol*. 2006; 177:6281-6290.
81. Char S, Cervallos AM, Yamson P, et al. Impaired IgA response to *Giardia* heat shock antigen in children with persistent diarrhoea and giardiasis. *Gut*. 1993;34:38-40.
82. Singer SM, Nash TE. T-cell-dependent control of acute *Giardia lamblia* infections in mice. *Infect Immun*. 2000;68:170-175.
83. Scott KG, Logan MR, Klammer GM, et al. Jejunal brush border microvillous alterations in *Giardia muris*–infected mice: role of T lymphocytes and interleukin-6. *Infect Immun*. 2000;68: 3412-3418.
84. Ridley MJ, Ridley DS. Serum antibodies and jejunal histology in giardiasis. *J Clin Pathol*. 1976;29:30-34.
85. Duncombe VM, Bolin TD, Davis AE, et al. Histopathology in giardiasis: a correlation with diarrhea. *Aust N Z J Med*. 1978;8: 392-396.
86. Bienz M, Dai WJ, Welle M, et al. Interleukin-6-deficient mice are highly susceptible to *Giardia lamblia* infection but exhibit normal intestinal immunoglobulin A responses against the parasite. *Infect Immun*. 2003;71:1569-1573.
87. Zhou P, Li E, Zhu N, et al. Role of interleukin-6 in the control of acute and chronic *Giardia lamblia* infections in mice. *Infect Immun*. 2003;71:1566-1568.
88. Andersen YS, Gillin FD, Eckmann L. Adaptive immunity-dependent intestinal hypermotility contributes to host defense against *Giardia* spp. *Infect Immun*. 2006;74:2473-2476.
89. Li E, Zhao A, Shea-Donohue T, Singer SM. Mast cell–mediated changes in smooth muscle contractility during mouse giardiasis. *Infect Immun*. 2007;75:4514-4518.
90. Chen XM, Keithly JS, Paya CV, et al. Cryptosporidiosis. *N Engl J Med*. 2002;346:1723-1731.
91. Reiner DS, Wang CS, Gillin FD. Human milk kills *Giardia lamblia* by generating toxic lipolytic products. *J Infect Dis*. 1986; 154:825-832.
92. Mahmud MA, Chappell CL, Hossain MM, et al. Impact of breast-feeding on *Giardia lamblia* infections in Bilbeis, Egypt. *Am J Trop Med Hyg*. 2001;65:257-260.
93. Bilenko N, Ghosh R, Levy A, et al. Partial breastfeeding protects Bedouin infants from infection and morbidity: prospective cohort study. *Asia Pac J Clin Nutr*. 2008;17:243-249.
94. Nash TE. Treatment of *Giardia lamblia* infections. *Pediatr Infect Dis J*. 2001;20:193-195.
95. Perez Cordon G, Cordova Paz Soldan O, Vargas Vasquez F, et al. Prevalence of enteroparasites and genotyping of *Giardia lamblia* in Peruvian children. *Parasitol Res*. 2008;103:459-465.
96. Singer SM, Elmendorf HG, Conrad JT, et al. Biological selection of variant-specific surface proteins in *Giardia lamblia*. *J Infect Dis*. 2001;183:119-124.
97. Oberhuber G, Kastner N, Stolte M. Giardiasis: a histologic analysis of 567 cases. *Scand J Infect Dis*. 1997;32:48-51.
98. Hjelt K, Pœrregaard A, Krasilnikoff PA. Giardiasis causing chronic diarrhoea in suburban Copenhagen: incidence, physical growth, clinical symptoms and small intestinal abnormality. *Acta Pœdiatrica*. 1992;81:881-886.
99. Berney DM, Rampton D, van der Walt JD. Giardiasis of the stomach. *Postgrad Med J*. 1994;70:237-238.
100. Lengerich EJ, Addiss DG, Juranek DD. Severe giardiasis in the United States. *Clin Infect Dis*. 1994;18:760-763.
101. Robertson LJ. Severe giardiasis and cryptosporidiosis in Scotland, UK. *Epidemiol Infect*. 1996;117:551-561.
102. Morken MH, Lind RA, Valeur J, et al. Subjective health complaints and quality of life in patients with irritable bowel syndrome following *Giardia lamblia* infection: a case control study. *Scand J Gastroenterol*. 2009;44:308-313.
103. Behera B, Mirdha BR, Makharia GK, et al. Parasites in patients with malabsorption syndrome: a clinical study in children and adults. *Dig Dis Sci*. 2008;53:672-679.
104. Solomons NW. Giardiasis: nutritional implications. *Rev Infect Dis*. 1982;4:859-869.
105. Gillon J. Clinical studies in adults presenting with giardiasis to a gastrointestinal unit. *Scot Med J*. 1985;30:89-95.
106. Rana SV, Bhasin DK, Vinayak VK. Lactose hydrogen breath test in *Giardia lamblia*–positive patients. *Dig Dis Sci*. 2005;50: 259-261.
107. Gupta MC, Urrutia JJ. Effect of periodic antiascaris and antigiardia treatment on nutritional status of preschool children. *Am J Clin Nutr*. 1982;36:79-86.
108. Farthing MJG, Mata L, Urrutia JJ, et al. Natural history of *Giardia* infection of infants and children in rural Guatemala and its impact on physical growth. *Am J Clin Nutr*. 1986;43: 395-405.
109. Fraser D, Bilenko N, Deckelbaum RJ, et al. *Giardia lamblia* carriage in Israeli Bedouin infants: risk factors and consequences. *Clin Infect Dis*. 2000;30:419-424.
110. Sullivan PS, DuPont HL, Arafat RR, et al. Illness and reservoirs associated with *Giardia lamblia* infection in rural Egypt: the case against treatment in developing world environments of high endemicity. *Am J Epidemiol*. 1988;127:1272-1281.
111. Lunn PG, Erinoso HO, Northrop-Clewes CA, et al. *Giardia intestinalis* is unlikely to be a major cause of the poor growth of rural Gambian infants. *J Nutr*. 1999;129:872-877.
112. Goto R, Mascie-Taylor CG, Lunn PG. Impact of anti-*Giardia* and anthelminthic treatment on infant growth and intestinal permeability in rural Bangladesh: a randomised double-blind controlled study. *Trans R Soc Trop Med Hyg*. 2009;103: 520-529.
113. Sackey ME, Weigel MM, Armijos RX. Predictors and nutritional consequences of intestinal parasitic infections in rural Ecuadorian children. *J Trop Pediatr*. 2003;49:17-23.
114. Goto R, Panter-Brick C, Northrop-Clewes CA, et al. Poor intestinal permeability in mildly stunted Nepali children: associations with weaning practices and *Giardia lamblia* infection. *Br J Nutr*. 2002;88:141-149.
115. Newman RD, Moore SR, Lima AA, et al. A longitudinal study of *Giardia lamblia* infection in north-east Brazilian children. *Trop Med Int Health*. 2001;6:624-634.
116. Mondal D, Petri WA Jr, Sack RB, et al. *Entamoeba histolytica*–associated diarrheal illness is negatively associated with the growth of preschool children: evidence from a prospective study. *Trans R Soc Trop Med Hyg*. 2006;100:1032-1038.
117. Ish-Horowicz M, Korman SH, Shapiro M, et al. Asymptomatic giardiasis in children. *Pediatr Infect Dis J*. 1989;8:773-779.
118. Moya-Camarena SY, Sotelo N, Valencia ME. Effects of asymptomatic *Giardia intestinalis* infection on carbohydrate absorption in well-nourished Mexican children. *Am J Trop Med Hyg*. 2002;66:255-259.
119. Garcia LS, Shimizu RY. Evaluation of nine immunoassay kits (enzyme immunoassay and direct fluorescence) for detection of *Giardia lamblia* and *Cryptosporidium parvum* in human fecal specimens. *J Clin Microbiol*. 1997;35:1526-1529.
120. Aldeen WE, Carroll K, Robison A, et al. Comparison of nine commercially available enzyme-linked immunosorbent assays for the detection of *Giardia lamblia* in fecal specimens. *J Clin Microbiol*. 1998;36:1338-1340.
121. Church D, Miller K, Lichtenfeld A, et al. Screening for *Giardia/Cryptosporidium* infections using an enzyme immunoassay in a centralized regional microbiology laboratory. *Arch Pathol Lab Med*. 2005;129:754-759.
122. Hiatt RA, Markell EK, Ng E. How many stool examinations are necessary to detect pathogenic intestinal protozoa? *Am J Trop Med Hyg*. 1995;53:36-39.
123. Mank TG, Zaat JO, Deelder AM, et al. Sensitivity of microscopy versus enzyme immunoassay in the laboratory diagnosis of giardiasis. *Eur J Clin Microbiol Infect Dis*. 1997;16:615-619.
124. Boone JH, Wilkins TD, Nash TE, et al. TechLab and Alexon *Giardia* enzyme-linked immunosorbent assay kits detect cyst wall protein 1. *J Clin Microbiol*. 1999;37:611-614.
125. Zimmerman SK, Needham CA. Comparison of conventional stool concentration and preserved-smear methods with Merifluor Cryptosporidium/Giardia Direct Immunofluorescence Assay and ProSpecT Giardia EZ Microplate Assay for the detection of *Giardia lamblia*. *J Clin Microbiol*. 1995;33: 1942-1943.
126. Chan R, Chen J, York MK, et al. Evaluation of a combination rapid immunoassay for detection of *Giardia* and *Cryptosporidium* antigens. *J Clin Microbiol*. 2000;38:393-394.
127. Johnston SP, Ballard MM, Beach MJ, et al. Evaluation of three commercial assays for detection of *Giardia* and *Cryptosporidium* organisms in fecal specimens. *J Clin Microbiol*. 2003;41: 623-626.
128. Garcia LS, Garcia JP. Detection of *Giardia lamblia* antigens in human fecal specimens by a solid-phase qualitative immunochromatographic assay. *J Clin Microbiol*. 2006;44: 4587-4588.
129. Youn S, Kabir M, Haque R, Petri WA Jr. Evaluation of a screening test for detection of *Giardia* and *Cryptosporidium*. *J Clin Microbiol*. 2009;47:451-452.
130. Granot E, Spira DT, Fraser D, et al. Immunologic response to infection with *Giardia lamblia* in children: effect of different clinical settings. *J Trop Pediatr*. 1998;44:241-246.
131. Haque R, Roy S, Siddique A, et al. Multiplex real-time PCR assay for detection of *Entamoeba histolytica, Giardia intestinalis*, and *Cryptosporidium* spp. *Am J Trop Med Hyg*. 2007;76:713-717.
132. Gardner TB, Hill DR. Treatment of giardiasis. *Clin Micro Rev*. 2001;14:114-128.
133. Upcroft P, Upcroft JA. Drug targets and mechanisms of resistance in the anaerobic protozoa. *Clin Micro Rev*. 2001;14: 150-164.
134. Zaat JO, Mank T, Assendelft WJ. Drugs for treating giardiasis. *Cochrane Database Syst Rev*. 2000;CD000217.
135. Medical Letter. Tinidazole (Tindamax)—a new anti-protozoal drug. *Med Lett Drugs Ther*. 2004;46:70-72.
136. Speelman P. Single-dose tinidazole for the treatment of giardiasis. *Antimicrob Agents Chemother*. 1985;27:227-229.

137. Falagas ME, Walker AM, Jick H, et al. Late incidence of cancer after metronidazole use: a matched metronidazole user/nonuser study. *Clin Infect Dis.* 1998;26:384-388.

138. Samuelson J. Why metronidazole is active against both bacteria and parasites. *Antimicrob Agents Chemother.* 1999;43:1533-1541.

139. Upcroft J, Upcroft P. My favorite cell: *Giardia. Bioessays.* 1998;20:256-263.

140. Medical Letter. Nitazoxanide (*Alinia*)—a new anti-protozoal agent. *Med Lett Drug Ther.* 2003;45:29-31.

141. Anderson VR, Curran MP. Nitazoxanide: a review of its use in the treatment of gastrointestinal infections. *Drugs.* 2007;67:1947-1967.

142. Escobedo AA, Alvarez G, Gonzalez ME, et al. The treatment of giardiasis in children: single-dose tinidazole compared with 3 days of nitazoxanide. *Ann Trop Med Parasitol.* 2008;102:199-207.

143. Rossignol JF, Abu-Zekry M, Hussein A, et al. Effect of nitazoxanide for treatment of severe rotavirus diarrhoea: randomised double-blind placebo-controlled trial. *Lancet.* 2006;368:124-129.

144. Hoffman PS, Sisson G, Croxen MA, et al. Antiparasitic drug nitazoxanide inhibits the pyruvate oxidoreductases of *Helicobacter pylori*, selected anaerobic bacteria and parasites, and *Campylobacter jejuni. Antimicrob Agents Chemother.* 2007;51:868-876.

145. Canete R, Escobedo AA, Gonzalez ME, et al. Randomized clinical study of five days' therapy with mebendazole compared to quinacrine in the treatment of symptomatic giardiasis in children. *World J Gastroenterol.* 2006;12:6366-6370.

146. Alizadeh A, Ranjbar M, Kashani KM, et al. Albendazole versus metronidazole in the treatment of patients with giardiasis in the Islamic Republic of Iran. *East Mediterr Health J.* 2006;12:548-554.

147. Sawatzki M, Peter S, Hess C. Therapy-resistant diarrhea due to *Giardia lamblia* in a patient with common variable immunodeficiency disease. *Digestion.* 2007;75:101-102.

148. Morch K, Hanevik K, Robertson LJ, et al. Treatment-ladder and genetic characterisation of parasites in refractory giardiasis after an outbreak in Norway. *J Infect.* 2008;56:268-273.

149. Besirbellioglu BA, Ulcay A, Can M, et al. *Saccharomyces boulardii* and infection due to *Giardia lamblia. Scand J Infect Dis.* 2006;38:479-481.

150. Abboud P, Lemee V, Gargala G, et al. Successful treatment of metronidazole- and albendazole-resistant giardiasis with nitazoxanide in a patient with acquired immunodeficiency syndrome. *Clin Infect Dis.* 2001;32:1792-1794.

151. Rotblatt MD. Giardiasis and amebiasis in pregnancy. *Drug Intell Clin Pharm.* 1983;17:187-188.

152. Burtin P, Taddio A, Ariburnu O, et al. Safety of metronidazole in pregnancy: a meta-analysis. *Am J Obstet Gynecol.* 1995;172:525-529.

153. Backer HD. Water disinfection for international travelers. In: Keystone JS, Kozarsky PE, Freedman DO, et al, eds. *Travel Medicine.* Philadelphia, Elsevier, 2008:47-58.

154. Juranek DD. Cryptosporidiosis: sources of infection and guidelines for prevention. *Clin Infect Dis.* 1995;21(Suppl 1):S57-S61.

155. Nunez FA, Hernandez M, Finlay CM. Longitudinal study of giardiasis in three day care centres of Havana City. *Acta Trop.* 1999;73:237-242.

156. Pickering LK, Woodward WE, DuPont HL, et al. Occurrence of *Giardia lamblia* in children in day care centers. *J Pediatr.* 1984;104:522-526.

157. Bartlett AV, Englender SJ, Jarvis BA, et al. Controlled trial of *Giardia lamblia*: control strategies in day care centers. *Am J Public Health.* 1991;81:1001-1006.

158. Lee P, Abdul-Wahid A, Faubert GM. Comparison of the local immune response against *Giardia lamblia* cyst wall protein 2 induced by recombinant *Lactococcus lactis* and *Streptococcus gordonii. Microbes Infect.* 2008;11:20-28.

159. Olson ME, Ceri H, Morck DW. *Giardia* vaccination. *Parasitol Today.* 2000;16:213-217.

281

Trichomonas vaginalis

JANE R. SCHWEBKE

Trichomonas vaginalis is the causative agent of trichomoniasis, a common cause of vaginitis. In men, it may cause urethritis but is more commonly asymptomatic. Despite being a readily diagnosed and treatable sexually transmitted disease (STD), trichomoniasis is not a reportable infection, and control of the infection has received relatively little emphasis from public health STD control programs. More recently, however, appreciation of the high rates of disease and of associations of trichomoniasis in women with adverse outcomes of pregnancy and increased risk for HIV infection suggest a need for increased control efforts.

Taxonomy

T. vaginalis is a parasitic pear-shaped protozoan, with an average size of 10×7 μ. It has four free flagella and one recurrent, along the outer margin of the undulating membrane, a costa at the base of the undulating membrane, and an axostyle extending through the cell.[1] Unlike most eukaryotes, *T. vaginalis* lacks mitochondria and instead uses the hydrogenosome to accomplish fermentative carbohydrate metabolism, with hydrogen as the electron acceptor. The hydrogenosome appears to have a common ancestry with mitochondria based on similarities in protein import.[2] However, major differences exist between hydrogenosomes and mitochondria in that hydrogenosomes lack cytochromes, mitochondrial respiratory chain enzymes, and DNA.

Trichomonas tenax, found in oral gingival and tracheobronchial sites, and *Pentatrichomonas hominis*, isolated from the intestinal tract, are considered nonpathogenic and occur infrequently in humans. Each human species has specific tropism for its site of infection. *Tritrichomonas foetus* is perhaps the nonhuman trichomonad most similar to *T. vaginalis*. Aside from having three anterior flagella (versus four in *T. vaginalis*), there are few morphologic differences between the parasites, and *T. foetus* causes the sexually transmitted disease bovine trichomoniasis. *T. foetus* can be invasive to the fetus, having been demonstrated in the placenta, fetal lung, gut, and lymph nodes, and is a known cause of abortion in infected cattle.[3]

The life cycle of *T. vaginalis* is simple in that the trophozoite is transmitted through coitus and no cyst form is known. The trophozoite divides by binary fission and, in natural infections, gives rise to a population in the lumen and on the mucosal surfaces of the urogenital tracts of humans. There are estimated to be 10^1 to 10^5 protozoa/mL of vaginal fluid.[4] The organisms create microulcerations in the genital mucosa by direct contact, mediated by surface proteins.[5]

Our current understanding of immunity to *T. vaginalis* has come largely from observations of responses in human patients and experimentation using in vitro and animal models of the related species, *T. foetus*. Natural infection seems to produce immunity that is only partially protective, because reinfection of patients can be 30% on follow-up.[6] Infection in humans results in parasite-specific antibodies in the reproductive tract and, in most cases, circulating antibodies in the serum[7]; there is also evidence of lymphocyte priming, as detected by antigen-specific proliferation of peripheral blood mononuclear cells.[8] Thus, natural infection with *T. vaginalis* results in priming of acquired immune responses. A study of patients infected with *T. vaginalis* and HIV indicated no evidence of increased levels or longevity of parasite infection in these patients compared with those in patients infected with *T. vaginalis* but not HIV.[9] These observations may indicate that innate immunity involving chemotaxis and subsequent influx of neutrophils is much more important than acquired immunity in controlling infections with *T. vaginalis*, because neutrophils are often the most numerous leukocytes present in response to infection.[1]

The genome of *T. vaginalis* has been sequenced and provides considerable resources that may be used to define genes important in the pathogenesis of human trichomoniasis. The recent release of the 5X genome sequence data (http://www.tigr.org/tdb/e2k1/tvg/) makes the most comprehensive genomic sequence of this parasite available to date.[11]

Epidemiology

Humans are the only natural host of *T. vaginalis*. Trichomoniasis is an extremely common infection in the United States and worldwide. The prevalence of trichomoniasis in inner city U.S. STD clinics typically approaches 25% and may be higher in certain populations. In Los Angeles, for example, the prevalence among African American clients at a public clinic was 38%.[12] Among women aged 14 to 19 years, the overall prevalence of trichomonas in the United States was recently found to be 3.1%, but among African Americans the prevalence was 13.3%.[13] An estimate of the incidence of STDs in the United States estimated an annual incidence of trichomoniasis of 7.4 million new cases.[14] The World Health Organization has estimated that this infection accounts for almost 50% of all curable infections worldwide.[15] Studies of African populations have reported the prevalence of vaginal trichomoniasis to be between 11% and 25%. Laga and colleagues reported an incidence of 38% during a 4-month exposure interval among HIV-infected women in Zaire.[16]

Epidemiologically, *T. vaginalis* infections are commonly associated with other STDs and are a marker of high-risk sexual behavior. Trichomoniasis is frequently seen concomitantly with other STDs, particularly gonorrhea. Unlike other STDs, which have a higher prevalence among adolescents and young adults, the rates of trichomoniasis are more evenly distributed among sexually active women of all age groups, probably as a result of a lack of an organized disease control effort for this infection.[17] Although survival on fomites is documented, the organism is thought to be transmitted almost exclusively by sexual activity.[18]

Reported prevalence of urethral infection with *T. vaginalis* in males has varied, depending on the population studied and the diagnostic techniques used. In a series of sentinel studies using cultures of urine, urethra, coronal sulcus, and semen, Krieger and associates reported a prevalence of 11% in men attending an STD clinic.[19] Urethritis was present in half of the men with *Trichomonas* as the sole urethral pathogen. In a similar study conducted at an STD clinic in Denver, investigators found a prevalence rate of 2.8% by using urine sediment culture.[20] Among men attending an STD clinic in Birmingham, Alabama, *T. vaginalis* was detected by polymerase chain reaction (PCR) assay in 17% of men attending the clinic for a new-problem visit or screening. There was no significant difference in the detection of the organism between men with and without urethral symptoms (20% and 14.5%, respectively). Of men with nongonococcal urethritis, nearly as many had *T. vaginalis* detected as had chlamydia (19.9% and 25.2%, respectively).[21] Detection of *T. vaginalis* in men is increased if semen is tested in addition to urine and urethral specimens.[22]

Clinical Features

The organisms create microulcerations in the genital mucosa by direct contact, mediated by surface proteins.[5] In women, it is the squamous epithelium of the vagina that is infected. Interestingly, although 2% to 17% of newborn infant girls may have vaginal colonization if the mother is infected, the infection may not be sustained once the maternal effects of estrogen wear off and the vaginal pH becomes neutral.[23] Neonatal respiratory infections with *T. vaginalis* have also been reported.[24] Detection of trichomonas in older children should raise the suspicion of child abuse.[25]

The incubation period of this infection is unknown; however, in vitro studies suggest an incubation period of 4 to 28 days in women.[26] The clinical features of trichomoniasis in the female are summarized in Table 281-1. Symptoms in women include vaginal discharge, pruritus, and irritation. Signs of infection include vaginal discharge (42%), odor (50%), and edema or erythema (22 to 37%). The discharge is classically described as frothy, but it is actually frothy in only about 10% of patients (Fig. 281-1). The color of the discharge may vary. Colpitis macularis (strawberry cervix) is a specific clinical sign for this infection but is detected with reliability only by colposcopy and rarely during routine examination.[10] Other complaints may include dysuria and lower abdominal pain; the cause of the latter is unclear. The urethra is also infected in most women.[27] Almost 50% of all women with *T. vaginalis* are asymptomatic.[28] Therefore, if these women are not screened, the diagnosis will be missed. The extent of the inflammatory response to the parasite may determine the severity of the symptoms. Factors that influence the host inflammatory response are not well understood but may include hormonal levels, coexisting vaginal flora, and strain and relative concentration of the organisms present in the vagina. In men, the infection is usually asymptomatic, but some studies have suggested that it is a more common cause of nongonococcal urethritis (NGU) than previously recognized[19,21] and should certainly be considered as a diagnostic possibility in the man who fails initial therapy for NGU. Trichomoniasis in men may also rarely cause epididymitis, prostatitis, and superficial penile ulcerations.[29]

Diagnosis

Diagnosis of trichomoniasis in the female is usually accomplished via direct microscopic examination of the vaginal fluid; however, even for

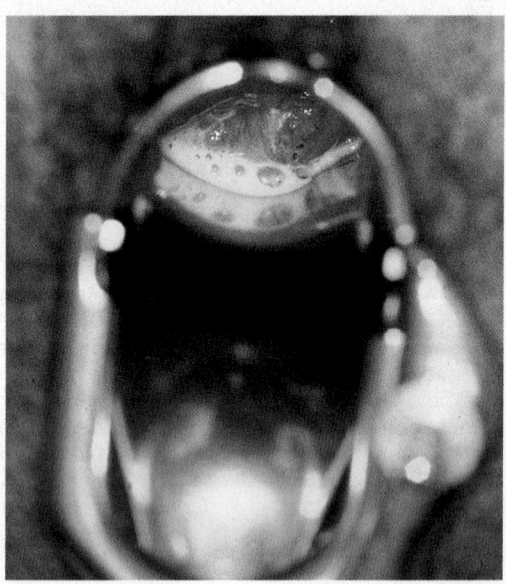

Figure 281-1   Vaginal discharge in a patient with trichomoniasis. Note the bubbles, which give the discharge a "frothy" appearance.

TABLE 281-1	Sensitivity of Clinical and Laboratory Features in Vaginal Trichomoniasis	
Parameter	*Clinical Feature*	*Percent Positive*
Symptoms	None	9-56
	Discharge	50-75
	Malodorous	~10
	Irritating, pruritic	23-82
	Dyspareunia	10-50
	Dysuria	30-50
	Lower abdominal discomfort	5-12
Signs	None	~15
	Vulvar erythema	10-20
	Excessive discharge	50-75
	Yellow, green	5-20
	Frothy	10-50
	Vaginal wall inflammation	40-75
	Strawberry cervix (direct visualization)	1-2
	Colpitis macularis (colposcope)	45
Laboratory findings	pH > 4.5	66-91
	Positive whiff test	~75
	Excess polymorphonuclear neutrophils on wet mount	~75

Data from Honigberg BM, ed. *Trichomonads Parasitic in Humans.* New York: Springer-Verlag; 1990; Bickley LS, Krisher KK, Punsalang Jr, et al. Comparison of direct fluorescent antibody, acridine orange, wet mount, and culture for detection of Trichomonas vaginalis in women attending a public sexually transmitted disease clinic. *Sex Transm Dis.* 1989;16:127-31; and Rein MF. Uncertainties and controversies in trichomoniasis. In: Sobel JD, ed. *Vulvovaginal Infections: Current Concepts in Diagnosis and Therapy.* New York: Academy Professional Information Services; 1990:73-85.

skilled diagnosticians, the sensitivity of this test is only 60% overall and may be less in asymptomatic women.[30] The presence of motile trichomonads is diagnostic. The pH of the vaginal fluid will usually be higher than 4.5 but can be normal (≤4.5). In these cases, the trichomonads are often sparser because they prefer a more alkaline pH. Neutrophils as well as altered vaginal bacterial flora are often seen. Culture media is commercially available and is currently the gold standard for diagnosis, but requires incubation.[31] Specimens have been shown to maintain viability in various transport media for up to 24 hours before inoculation into culture media. Other commercially available tests include an RNA probe semiautomated system, which also detects candidiasis and bacterial vaginosis, and a dipstick enzyme-linked immunosorbent assay (ELISA). Both of these tests are currently licensed only for vaginal specimens, can be used as point of care tests, and have sensitivities of about 80%.[32,33] They may be a good choice if microscopy is not available. Nucleic acid amplification tests (NAATs) are under development but have thus far shown variable results. Recently, a commercially available transcription-mediated amplification test became available in an analyte-specific reagent (ASR) format, and can be used with urine and genital specimens from men and women.[34] Diagnosis in general is much more difficult for males, with the best culture results obtained by combining urethral swabs and urine sediment for culture. Nonetheless, it is highly likely, as suggested by PCR results, that this approach lacks sensitivity.[35] Lack of a suitable screening test for males hampers public health control efforts of the disease. A commercially available NAAT would be of great importance in this regard.

Treatment

In most cases, the infection is easily treated with a single 2-g oral dose of metronidazole or tinidazole and, because it is an STD, sexual partners should be routinely treated.[36] The reported cure rates are 90% to 100%. Failure to treat the male sexual partner is likely the most common cause of recurrent disease in women and should be explored before assuming that the woman has a strain of *T. vaginalis* that is resistant to metronidazole. Metronidazole intravaginal gel has limited efficacy and should not be used. Although there continues to be some controversy about the safety of metronidazole in pregnancy, there has never been a documented case of fetal malformation attributed to its use, even when used in the first trimester.[37] Tinidazole has a plasma half-life twice that of metronidazole (12 to 14 hours for tinidazole vs.

6 to 7 hours for metronidazole)[38] and appears to be better tolerated, with fewer gastrointestinal side effects.

Resistance to metronidazole has been reported, estimated to be from 2.5% to 10% and less than 1% for tinidazole.[39] The mechanism of development of anaerobic resistance to metronidazole is controlled by hydrogenosomes, in that metronidazole competes for hydrogen as an electron acceptor. In metronidazole-resistant *T. vaginalis*, the expression levels of the hydrogenosomal enzymes pyruvate ferredoxin oxidoreductase, ferredoxin, malic enzyme, and hydrogenase are reduced dramatically, which probably eliminates the ability of the parasite to activate metronidazole.[40] Resistance is relative and can usually be overcome with higher doses of oral metronidazole. For example, marginal resistance, defined as an aerobic minimal lethal concentration (MLC) of metronidazole of 50 µg/mL, requires a total treatment dose of 10 g administered over several days for cure, whereas high-level resistance (MLC, 400 µg/mL) requires 40 g. IV formulations offer no advantage over the oral drug. Some authorities have recommended higher doses of oral medication in combination with pharmacy-prepared intravaginal preparations. Tinidazole, with its more favorable pharmacokinetics, may be the drug of choice when resistance is encountered. The Centers for Disease Control and Prevention (CDC) tested 195 metronidazole-resistant *T. vaginalis* clinical isolates submitted for MLC testing for both metronidazole and tinidazole. The mean aerobic metronidazole MLC was 400 µg/mL compared with an aerobic tinidazole MLC of 100 µg/mL.[41] Several clinical studies have evaluated various doses of tinidazole for treatment of metronidazole-resistant trichomoniasis. The largest series of patients was reported by Sobel and associates.[42] In this study, 20 patients with clinically refractory trichomoniasis (failure to respond to therapy with oral metronidazole, at least 500 mg twice daily for 7 days) were treated with high doses of oral and vaginal tinidazole (2 to 3 g PO, plus 1 to 1.5 g intravaginally for 14 days). The cure rate was 92% (22 of 24); no patients discontinued therapy because of side effects. Current CDC recommendations for patients failing a single 2-g dose of metronidazole are to treat next with metronidazole, 500 mg PO twice daily for 7 days, or a 2-g dose of tinidazole immediately. Failing that, treatment with tinidazole or metronidazole at 2 g PO for 5 days is suggested.[36] There are limited anecdotal reports of success with paromomycin cream; however, there may also be a high incidence of local side effects associated with this therapy.[43] Women with asymptomatic infection should be treated. If left untreated, they may later become symptomatic and continue to transmit the infection while untreated. Occasionally, patients are allergic to metronidazole. Because there is no effective alternative, desensitization is the only option.[44]

Complications

Long considered a minor STD, with few associated complications, infection with *T. vaginalis* has more recently been implicated as a cause of preterm delivery in several studies. In a large multicenter study, after adjusting for demographic, behavioral, and microbiological variables, *T. vaginalis* was significantly associated with low birth weight, premature rupture of membranes, and preterm delivery (relative risk, 1.4).[45] Similarly, Minkoff and co-workers[46] also documented a significant correlation between trichomoniasis and premature rupture of membranes. In that study, the incidence of this complication at term was 27.5% in women with *T. vaginalis* infection versus 12.8% in those without ($P = .03$).

Prospective studies of treatment of trichomoniasis during pregnancy for the prevention of preterm birth have yielded disappointing results. Among women with asymptomatic infection treated with metronidazole during the second and third trimesters of pregnancy, a trend toward increased preterm delivery was seen compared with the placebo group. However, the dose of metronidazole used was four times the recommended dose. In addition, the study was stopped prematurely because of a slow accrual of subjects and the trend for increased risk of preterm delivery in the treatment group.[47] A second study, conducted in Uganda, also found that treatment of trichomoniasis during pregnancy resulted in an increase in the incidence of preterm birth. However, this study was actually a subgroup analysis of a larger trial and was not properly designed to determine the effect of treatment of *T. vaginalis* during pregnancy on preterm birth.[48] Therefore, the question remains unanswered. Since the publication of these reports, the Centers CDC has not revised recommendations for treatment during pregnancy. Trichomoniasis has also been associated with vaginal cuff cellulitis following abdominal hysterectomy.[49]

Acquisition of HIV has been associated with trichomoniasis in several African studies, possibly as a result of the local inflammation often caused by the parasite. Leroy and collleagues[50] found a significant difference between the prevalence of trichomoniasis in a cohort of HIV-infected and noninfected pregnant women in Rwanda (20.2% and 10.9%, respectively; $P = .0007$). In a prospective study by Laga and associates,[16] the incidence of trichomoniasis was significantly associated with HIV seroconversion (odds ratio, 1.9) in a multivariate analysis of a cohort of women in Zaire. The associations between HIV and trichomoniasis, as well as other STDs, may relate to the following: (1) increased shedding of HIV as a result of the local inflammation produced by the STD; (2) increased susceptibility to HIV as a result of the macro- or microscopic breaks in mucosal barriers caused by the STD; (3) a higher prevalence of STDs among HIV-infected individuals as a result of common risk factors for both infections; and/or (4) an increased susceptibility to STDs as a result of the immunosuppression associated with HIV infection. Given the higher prevalence and incidence of trichomoniasis than most other treatable STDs in most studies to date, the attributable fraction of HIV acquisitions caused by trichomoniasis may eclipse the relative contribution of other STDs.[12] The RNA concentration of HIV in the seminal fluid of men with urethritis was significantly higher in men with trichomoniasis than in those with symptomatic urethritis with an unidentified cause.[51] In addition, successful treatment of trichomonal urethritis reduced the levels of HIV RNA so that they were similar to those seen in uninfected controls.[52]

REFERENCES

1. Honigberg B, King VM. Structure of *Trichomonas vaginalis* Donne. *J Parasitol.* 1964;50:345-364.
2. Dyall SD, Johnson PJ. Origins of hydrogenosomes and mitochondria: evolution and organelle biogenesis. *Curr Opin Microbiol.* 2000;3:404-411.
3. Burgess D, Knoblock KF. Identification of *Tritrichomonas foetus* in sections of bovine placental tissue with monoclonal antibodies. *J Parasitol.* 1989;75:977-980.
4. Phillip A, Carter-Scott P, Rogers C. An agar culture technique to quantitate *Trichomonas vaginalis* from women. *J Infect Dis.* 1987;155:304-308.
5. Arroyo R, Engbring J, Alderete J. Molecular basis of host epithelial cell recognition by *Trichomonas vaginalis*. *Molecular Microbiology.* 1992;6:853-862.
6. Niccolai L, Kopicko JJ, Kassie A, et al. Incidence and predictors of reinfection with *Trichomonas vaginalis* in HIV-infected women. *Sex Transm Dis.* 2000;27:284-288.
7. Honigberg B, Burgess DE. Trichomonads of importance in human medicine including *Dientamoeba fragilis*. In: Kreier JP, ed. *Parasitic Protozoa*, vol. 9. New York: Academic Press, 1994:1-109.
8. Mason P, Patterson BA. Proliferative response of human lymphocytes to secretory and cellular antigens of *Trichomonas vaginalis*. *J Parasitol.* 1985;71:265-268.
9. Cu-Uvin S, Ko H, Jamieson DJ, et al; HIV Epidemiology Research Study (HERS) Group. Prevalence, incidence, and persistence or recurrence of trichomoniasis among human immunodeficiency virus (HIV)-positive women and among HIV-negative women at high risk for HIV infection. *Clin Infect Dis.* 2002;34:1406-1411.
10. Wølner-Hanssen P, Krieger JN, Stevens CE, et al. Clinical manifestations of vaginal trichomoniasis. *JAMA.* 1989;261:571-576.
11. Carlton JM, Hirt RP, Silva JC, et al. Draft genome sequence of the sexually transmitted pathogen *Trichomonas vaginalis*. *Science.* 2007;315:207-212.
12. Sorvillo F, Kerndt P. *Trichomonas vaginalis* and amplification of HIV-1 transmission. *The Lancet.* 1998;351:213-214.
13. Sutton M, Sternberg M, Koumans EH, et al. The prevalence of *Trichomonas vaginalis* infection among reporoductive-age women in the United States, 2001-2004. *Clin Inf Dis.* 2007;45:1319-1326.
14. Weinstock H, Berman S, Cates W. Sexually transmitted diseases among American youth: Incidence and prevalence estimates, 2000. *Perspectives Sex Reprod Health.* 2004;36:6-10.
15. Cates W, American Social Health Association Panel. Estimates of the incidence and prevalence of sexually transmitted diseases in the United States. *Sex Transm Dis.* 1999;26:S2-S7.
16. Laga M, Manoka A, Kivuvu M, et al. Non-ulcerative sexually transmitted diseases as risk factors for HIV-1 transmission in women: Results from a cohort study. *AIDS.* 1993;7:95-102.
17. Lossick J. Epidemiology of urogenital trichomoniasis. In: Honigberg BM, ed. *Trichomonads Parasitic in Humans.* New York: Springer-Verlag, 1989:311-341.
18. Wilcox R. Epidemiological aspects of human trichomoniasis. *Br J Vener Dis.* 1960;36:167-174.
19. Krieger JN, Verdon M, Siegel N, et al. Natural history of urogenital trichomoniasis in men. *J Urol.* 1993;149:1455-1458.

20. Joyner J, Douglas J, Ragsdale S, et al. Comparative prevalence of infection with *Trichomonas vaginalis* among men attending a sexually transmitted diseases clinic. *Sex Transm Dis.* 2000;27:236-240.

21. Schwebke JR, Hook EW III. High rates of *Trichomonas vaginalis* among men attending a sexually transmitted diseases clinic: Implications for screening and urethritis management. *J Infect Dis.* 2003;188:465-468.

22. Seña AC, Miller WC, Hobbs MM, et al. *Trichomonas vaginalis* infection in male sexual partners: Implications for diagnosis, treatment, and prevention. *Clin Inf Dis.* 2007;44:13-22.

23. Danesh IS, Stephen JM, Gorbach J. Neonatal *Trichomonas vaginalis* infection. *J Emerg Med.* 1995;13:51-54.

24. al-Salihi FL, Curran JP, Wang J. Neonatal *Trichomonas vaginalis:* Report of three cases and review of the literature. *Pediatrics.* 1974;53:196-200.

25. Jones JG, Yamaguchi T, Lambert B. *Trichomonas vaginalis* infestations in sexually abused girls. *Am J Dis Child.* 1985;139:846-847.

26. Hesseltine H. Experimental human vaginal trichomoniasis. *J Infect Dis.* 1942;71:127.

27. Rein MF, Muller M. *Trichomonas vaginalis* and trichomoniasis. *Sex Trans Dis.* 1990;481-492.

28. Fouts AC, Kraus SJ. *Trichomonas vaginalis* reevaluation of its clinical presentation and laboratory diagnosis. *J Infect Dis.* 1980;177:167-174.

29. Krieger JN. Trichomoniasis in men: Old issues and new data. *Sex Transm Dis.* 1995;22:83-96.

30. Krieger JN, Tam MR, Stevens CE, et al. Diagnosis of trichomoniasis: Comparison of conventional wet-mount examination with cytologic studies, cultures, and monoclonal antibody staining of direct specimens. *JAMA.* 1988;259:1223-1227.

31. Draper D, Parker R, Patterson E, et al. Detection of *Trichomonas vaginalis* in pregnant women with the InPouch TV system. *J Clin Microbiol.* 1993;31:1016-1018.

32. Briselden AM, Hillier SL. Evaluation of Affirm VP microbial identification test for *Gardnerella vaginalis* and *Trichomonas vaginalis. J Clin Microbiol.* 1994;32:148-152.

33. Kurth A, Whittington WLH, Golden MR, et al. Performance of a new, rapid assay for *Trichomonas vaginalis. J Clin Microbiol.* 2004;42:2940-2943.

34. Nye MB, Schwebke JR, Body BA. Comparison of APTIMA *Trichomonas vaginalis* transcription-mediated amplification to wet mount microscopy, culture and PCR for diagnosis of trichomoniasis in men and women. *Am J Obstet Gynecol.* 2009;200: 188, e1-e7.

35. Schwebke J, Lawing L. Improved detection of *Trichomonas vaginalis* in males using DNA amplification. *J Clin Microbiol.* 2002; 3681-3683.

36. Centers for Disease Control and Prevention (CDC). Sexually transmitted diseases treatment guidelines. *MMWR Recomm Rep.* 2006;55(RR-11):49-56.

37. Roe F. Safety of nitroimidazoles. *Scand J Infect Dis Suppl.* 1985; 46:72-81.

38. Wood B, Monroe A. Pharmacokinetics of tinidazole and metronidazole after single large oral doses. *Br J Vener Dis.* 1975;51: 51-53.

39. Schwebke JR, Barrientes FJ. Prevalence of *Trichomonas vaginalis* isolates with resistance to metronidazole and tinidazole. *Antimicrob Agents Chemother.* 2006;50:4209-4210.

40. Land KM, Delgadillo-Correa MG, Tachezy J, et al. Targeted gene replacement of a ferredoxin gene in *Trichomonas vaginalis* does not lead to metronidazole resistance. *Mol Microbiol.* 2003; 51:115-122.

41. Crowell A, Sanders-Lewis KA, Secor WE. In vitro metronidazole and tinidazole activities against metronidazole-resistant strains of *Trichomonas vaginalis. Antimicrob Agents Chemother.* 2003;47: 1407-1409.

42. Sobel J, Nyirjesy P, Brown W. Tinidazole therapy for metronidazole-resistant vaginal trichomoniasis. *Clin Inf Dis.* 2001;33:1341-1346.

43. Sobel J, Nagappan V, Nyirjesy P. Metronidazole-resistant vaginal trichomoniasis—an emerging problem. *N Engl J Med.* 1999;341: 292-293.

44. Pearlman M, Yashar C, Ernst S, et al. An incremental dosing protocol for women with severe vaginal trichomoniasis and adverse reactions to metronidazole. *Am J Obstet Gynecol.* 1996;174:934-936.

45. Cotch MF, Pastorek JG, Nugent RP, et al. *Trichomonas vaginalis* associated with low birth weight and preterm delivery. *Sex Transm Dis.* 1997;24:361-362.

46. Minkoff H, Grunebaum AN, Schwarz RH, et al. Risk factors for prematurity and premature rupture of membranes: A prospective study of the vaginal flora in pregnancy. *Am J Obstet Gynecol.* 1984;150:965-972.

47. Klebanoff M, Carey J, Hauth J, et al. Failure of metronidazole to prevent preterm delivery among pregnant women with asymptomatic *Trichomonas vaginalis* infection. *N Engl J Med.* 2001;345:487-493.

48. Kigozi G, Brahmbhatt H, Wabwire-Mangen F, et al. Treatment of *Trichomonas* in pregnancy and adverse outcomes of pregnancy: A subanalysis of a randomized trial in Rakai, Uganda. *Am J Obstet Gynecol.* 2003;189:1398-1400.

49. Soper DE, Bump RC, Hurt WG. Bacterial vaginosis and trichomoniasis vaginitis are risk factors for cuff cellulitis after abdominal hysterectomy. *Am J Obstet Gynecol.* 1990;163:1016-1023.

50. Leroy V, De Clercq A, Ladner J, et al. Should screening of genital infections be part of antenatal care in areas of high HIV prevalence? A prospective cohort study from Kigali, Rwanda, 1992-1993. *Genitourin Med.* 1995;71:207-211.

51. Hobbs M, Kazembe P, Reed A, et al. *Trichomonas vaginalis* as a cause of urethritis in Malawian Men. *Sex Trans Dis.* 1999;26: 381-387.

52. Price Z, Zimba D, Hoffman IF, et al. Addition of treatment for trichomoniasis to syndromic management of urethritis in Malawi: A randomized clinical trial. *Sex Transm Dis.* 2003;30: 516-522.

53. Honigberg BM, ed. *Trichomonads Parasitic in Humans.* New York: Springer-Verlag, 1990:424.

54. Bickley LS, Krisher KK, Punsalang JR, et al. Comparison of direct fluorescent antibody, acridine orange, wet mount, and culture for detection of *Trichomonas vaginalis* in women attending a public sexually transmitted diseases clinic. *Sex Transm Dis.* 1989;16: 127-131.

55. Rein MF. Uncertainties and controversies in trichomoniasis. In: Sobel JD, ed. *Vulvovaginal Infection: Current Concepts in Diagnosis and Therapy.* New York: Academy Professional Information Services, 1990:73-85.

282

Babesia Species

JEFFREY A. GELFAND | EDOUARD G. VANNIER

Babesiosis is an emerging tick-borne infectious disease caused by protozoa of the genus *Babesia* that invade and eventually lyse erythrocytes. Wild and domestic animals are natural reservoir hosts for *Babesia* species. Only in the past 50 years has *Babesia* been recognized as a human pathogen. Typically a mild flulike illness in young and healthy individuals, babesiosis may develop into a life-threatening malaria-like syndrome in the asplenic or immunocompromised patient and in the elderly.

The first recorded reference to babesiosis is probably in Exodus 9:3, which describes the plague ("grievous murrain") visited upon the cattle of Pharaoh Ramses II. In 1888, while investigating the febrile hemoglobinuria and death of cattle in Romania, Viktor Babes, a Hungarian pathologist, observed an intraerythrocytic microorganism.[1] In 1893, Smith and Kilbourne described a similar piroplasm (from the Latin *pirum* for pear) in the erythrocytes of Texas cattle experiencing fever. Initially named *Pyrosoma*, this organism was later identified as *Babesia bigemina*. This was the seminal observation on the ability of hematophagous arthropods to transmit an infectious pathogen to a vertebrate host. The first well-documented case of human babesiosis was reported in 1957 by Skrabalo and Deanovic. A 33-year-old splenectomized herdsman had been grazing cattle on tick-infested pastures near Zagreb, Croatia. The infection was fulminant and fatal. Originally identified as *Babesia bovis*, the causative agent was later reported to be *Babesia divergens*. *B. divergens* is a parasite of cattle that is transmitted to humans by the tick *Ixodes ricinus*, a species endemic in Europe. Subsequent cases in Europe would confirm the importance of splenectomy to the severity of babesiosis caused by *B. divergens*. In 1969, a 59-year-old resident of Nantucket Island off the coast of Massachusetts presented with fever and headache. Unlike the European patients infected with *B. divergens*, this patient had an intact spleen. The causative agent was identified as *Babesia microti*, a parasite that infects white-footed mice and other microtine rodents. Spielman and colleagues subsequently identified the vector as the tick *Ixodes scapularis* (also known as *Ixodes dammini*). In the decades since, several thousands of cases have been reported in the United States alone. Once limited to the chain islands off the coast of New England, babesiosis caused by *B. microti* is now endemic on the northeastern mainland. In the upper Midwest, babesiosis may be caused by *B. microti* or *B. divergens*–like organisms. Although rare, cases of *Babesia duncani* infection are reported on the West Coast of the United States.

The Pathogen

Human babesiosis is a zoonotic disease that requires transmission of a *Babesia* species from a vertebrate reservoir to humans via an invertebrate vector. More than 100 species of *Babesia* have been reported to infect vertebrates, including mammals and birds.[2-5] Babesiae are protozoal parasites classified in the phylum Apicomplexa, class Aconoidasida, order Piroplasmidora, and family Babesiidae. In addition to Babesiidae, the order Piroplasmidora includes the family of Theileriidae. As for *Theileria* species, the intraerythrocytic form of *Babesia* species can present a pear-shape appearance, hence the name of piroplasm. Babesiidae also can be oval or round. Because of their ring conformation and peripheral location in the erythrocyte, *Babesia* organisms are frequently mistaken for *Plasmodium falciparum*. Babesial trophozoites undergo an asexual division (called merogony) in the vertebrate host erythrocyte. Once ingested by the tick (the invertebrate host), babesial gametocytes undergo sexual development that ulti-mately leads to the formation of sporozoites in the salivary glands of the tick.

EVENTS IN THE TICK

Although babesiosis may be acquired by blood transfusion,[6] *Babesia* organisms are most often transmitted during the blood meal of an infected hard-bodied tick of the genus *Ixodes*.[7,8] In Europe, *I. ricinus* is regarded as the main vector for transmission to humans of *B. divergens* (from cattle), *Babesia venatorum* (from roe deer), and *B. microti*.[9] *B. microti* is also found in *Ixodes trianguliceps*, but this tick rarely bites humans. In a case of *B. divergens*–like infection on the Canary Isles, *Ixodes ventalloi* is thought to be the vector. In the northeastern United States, *Ixodes scapularis* primarily feeds on white-tailed deer (*Odocoileus virginiamus*) and white-footed mice (*Peromyscus leucopus*) and occasionally transmits *B. microti* to humans. *I. scapularis* is also the vector for *Borrelia burgdorferi* and *Anaplasma phagocytophilum*, the causative agents of Lyme disease and human granulocytic anaplasmosis.[10] *B. divergens*–like organisms that cause babesiosis in the midwestern United States probably originate from cottontail rabbits[11] and may be transmitted by *Ixodes dentatus*. On the West Coast of the United States, the vector for transmission of *B. duncani* (previously referred to as WA1) is thought to be *Ixodes pacificus*. To date, the life cycles of *B. microti* and *I. scapularis* are best understood.[5,7]

The life cycle of *I. scapularis* has three active stages (larva, nymph, adult) and requires 2 years for completion (www.dpd.cdc.gov/dpdx/HTML/Babesiosis.htm). In the fall, adult stages primarily feed on the white-tailed deer. Deer are incompetent reservoirs for *B. microti*, but are essential for maintenance of *I. scapularis*. Adult ticks overwinter in an engorged state and lay eggs in the spring. Eggs hatch synchronously into larvae in late July. In August and September, larvae primarily feed on the mouse, *Peromyscus leucopeus*. Larvae overwinter and molt into nymphs in the spring. Nymphs feed on *P. leucopeus* from May through July and molt into adults in the fall. *I. scapularis* becomes infected as the larvae feeds on *B. microti*–infected *P. leucopeus*. In endemic areas such as Nantucket Island, approximately 40% of *P. leucopeus* mice are infected. Other reservoirs include chipmunks, meadow voles, shrews, bats, passerine, and raptorial birds. Once larvae have molted, nymphs remain infected with *B. microti* (trans-stadial transmission). There is no evidence of transovarial transmission of *B. microti* (as it occurs with *B. divergens*). Feeding of infected nymphs early in the summer results in the infection of naïve *P. leucopeus* mice that become a reservoir of *B. microti* for larvae that feed during late summer. This favors a high rate of transmission and therefore maintenance of *B. microti* in the enzootic cycle.

Larvae, nymphs, and adult ticks can all feed on humans, but the nymphal tick is the primary vector for transmission of *B. microti* to humans.[5] Over the past three decades, the white-tailed deer population has dramatically expanded in the northeastern United States. The increased number of deer reflects an increase in suitable deer habitat, usually secondary to revegetation of old farms and fields, and reduced hunting pressures in suburban areas. The expanding range of *I. scapularis* may be linked to long distance dispersal of this vector by coastal birds that undergo extensive seasonal migration. It is the presence of large numbers of deer, white-footed mice, and ticks that creates the conditions for infection of humans with *B. microti*. Cases of babesiosis increase during warmer months when both ticks and people are active and encroach on each other's territory. The small size of the nymph

(<2.5 mm), its pale gray ground color, inconspicuous feeding site, and benign local reaction to blood feeding together make the recollection of tick bites a rare finding.[12,13] Repletion of the tick with host blood requires at least 72 hours of attachment. Because sporogony is optimal as repletion with host blood is complete, prompt and careful removal of the tick decreases the likelihood of transmission.

Early after attachment of the tick, *B. microti*–infected erythrocytes accumulate in its gut.[5] A novel endocytic organelle, the cytostome, forms within the protozoan. Forty to 60 hours after attachment, microtubules accumulate at the anterior end of the organism to form a raylike structure known as "Strahlenkorper." On repletion of the feeding tick, these structures contribute to the fusion of gametes into a zygote. Using an arrowhead structure, zygotes penetrate the tick gut epithelium. The arrowhead structure dissociates, and the zygote translocates toward the basal lamina of the epithelium, enters the hemolymph, and becomes an ookinete. Ookinetes in turn invade the salivary acini of the tick. Once in the secretory or interstitial cells of the acinus, ookinetes undergo hypertrophy to become sporoblasts. Sporoblasts remain dormant while the larva overwinters. On attachment of the nymphal tick to the host, the temperature of the tick body rises, and sporogony is initiated. As the tick feeds, the sporoblast membrane folds. After 48 hours of feeding, micronemes and rhoptries appear. Cytoplasm starts to separate from the parent sporoblast, and nuclear division ensues. Thus, sporogony is a process of budding (not schizogony as in *Plasmodium*). A single sporoblast may generate as many as 10,000 sporozoites.

EVENTS IN VERTEBRATE HOSTS

During the last hours of feeding by the tick, a large number (as many as 100,000) of sporozoites is deposited in the dermis of the host.[5] Events that lead sporozoites from the feeding chamber in the dermis to the circulating erythrocytes remain poorly understood. Sporozoites from *Babesia* species do not undergo merogony in an exoerythrocytic compartment and instead invade erythrocytes. Variable merozoite surface antigens mediate the attachment of free sporozoites and merozoites to the erythrocyte.[1] The host membrane invaginates, leading to the formation of a parasitophorous vacuole that gradually disintegrates. The organism becomes a trophozoite moving freely in the host cytoplasm. The piroplasm undergoes binary fission, resulting in two or four merozoites (daughter cells; Fig. 282-1). Egress of merozoites leads to the loss of red blood cell membrane integrity. Because this asexual reproduction is asynchronous, massive hemolysis rarely occurs as it does with *Plasmodium* (synchronous schizogony).

MORPHOLOGIC AND PHYLOGENETIC CLASSIFICATIONS

Based on the size of the intraerythrocytic form (trophozoite), *Babesia* organisms have traditionally been classified into two groups. Small forms have a diameter of 1 to 3 μm and include *B. microti*, *B. duncani*, and *Babesia conradae*.[2,4,14] Large forms are 3 to 5 μm in diameter and include *B. bovis*, *B. canis*, and *Babesia odocoilei*.[7] Trophozoites of small *Babesia* species undergo two successive binary fissions to generate four merozoites arranged in a tetrad ("Maltese cross"). In contrast, trophozoites of large *Babesia* species bud into pairs of merozoites only. The size distinction is generally consistent with the phylogenetic classification based on the nuclear small subunit ribosomal RNA gene (18S rDNA), i.e., large *Babesia* species cluster into phylogenetic clades distinct from those containing small *Babesia* species. *B. divergens* and *Babesia gibsoni* are exceptions because they are small in diameter, but genetically related to the large *Babesia* species.[4,15] Phylogenetic analyses revealed that small *Babesia* species are more related to *Theileria* than to large *Babesia* species. This evolutionary link is in agreement with the lack of transovarial transmission of *Theileria* and small *Babesia* species in ticks.[7,8] In contrast, transovarial transmission is a characteristic of large *Babesia* species. Unlike small and large *Babesia* species, however, *Theileria* piroplasms undergo asexual division in lympho-

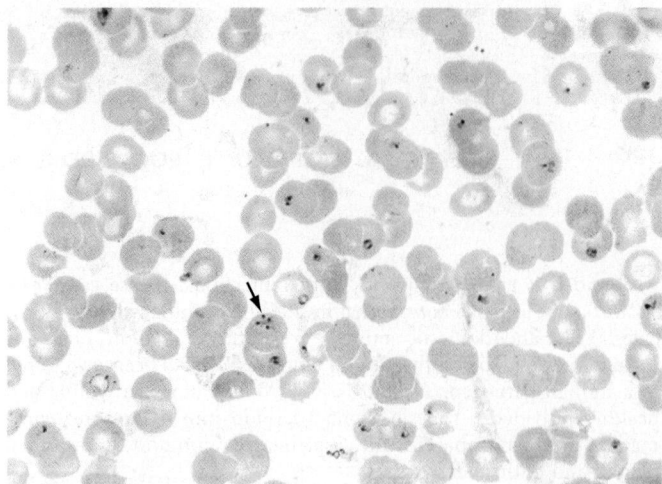

Figure 282-1   Giemsa stain of a thin blood film. A single trophozoite divides by intraerythrocytic merogony to generate four merozoites arranged in tetrads, also known as Maltese cross or quadruplet forms. Tetrads of merozoites are rare (*arrow*), but are pathognomonic of small *Babesia* spp. Tetrads are rarer in *Babesia microti* infection than in *Babesia duncani* infection. This case was found to be infected with *B. microti*. Note the nearby presence of ring forms, some with two chromatin dots. Ring forms have a peripheral location, as with *Plasmodium falciparum*, but their large clear central vacuole and the absence of brown pigment (hemozoin) are characteristic of *B. microti*. (*Courtesy from Dr. J. Vyas.*)

cytes before invading erythrocytes as merozoites. Babesiidae invade erythrocytes as sporozoites and do not exist in an exoerythrocytic form. The discovery of a lymphocytic exoerythrocytic stage of *Babesia equi* has led to the reclassification of this equine piroplasm as *Theileria equi*.

To date, based on phylogenetic analyses of the 18S rRNA gene, the β-tubulin gene, and the rRNA second internal transcribed spacer (ITS-2), piroplasms can be classified into five distinct clades.[2,4,9,11] The first clade contains *Babesia* spp. *sensu stricto* that infect ungulates but are rarely transmitted to humans. These include *B. bovis*, *B. bigemina*, and other *Babesia* species from cattle as well as *B. ovis*. The second clade contains bovine isolates of *B. divergens* from Europe, *B. divergens*–like organisms obtained from patients in the United States and Europe, *B. odocoilei* that infects white-tailed deer in the United States, the related *B. venatorum* identified in splenectomized patients in Europe, all *Babesia canis* subtypes, and *B. gibsoni* isolates obtained from dogs in Asia, Africa, and the midwestern United States. As for the first clade, piroplasms of the second clade are *Babesia* species *sensu stricto* as their transmission is trans-stadial and transovarial. The third clade contains *Theileria* species only, including *T. equi*. The fourth clade contains piroplasms found in the western United States, including *B. duncani* (WA1, CA5), *B. duncani*–type (WA2, CA6), and *B. duncani*–related (CA1-CA4) organisms, the main etiologic agents of human babesiosis on the Pacific coast; *B. conradae*, which infects dogs in California; and related piroplasms of wildlife mammals (deer, bighorn sheep) roaming in the same habitat. The fifth clade contains the *B. microti* species complex as well as *Babesia* species (*Babesia rodhaini*, *Babesia felis*, *Babesia leo*), which infect felines. The *B. microti* species complex itself can be divided in three clades.[14] The first clade contains *B. microti* isolates obtained from humans, ticks, or rodents in areas where human babesiosis is endemic (Massachusetts, Connecticut, Wisconsin) or rare or absent (coastal Maine, Switzerland, Russia). The Kobe strain isolated from a patient transfused with blood from a donor living on the Awaji Island near Kobe City is closely related to, but distinct from the zoonotic *B. microti* strains found in the United States.[9,14] Related to these zoonotic strains by a greater degree are the *B. microti* isolates from rodents in northern Japan (Hokkaido Island), eastern Siberia

(Vladivostok), and South Korea. The second clade groups piroplasms found in medium-sized carnivores, including the *B. microti*–like organism identified in Spanish dogs and tentatively termed *Theileria annae*. The third clade contains *B. microti* isolates obtained from rodents that live in areas where human babesiosis is absent (northern Maine, Alaska, Montana).

Epidemiology

UNITED STATES

Most babesial infections are caused by *B. microti* and are acquired by tick bite from May through September.[1] Three fourths of the cases are brought to medical attention in July and August.[12,13] The index case was identified in 1969 on Nantucket Island, off the coast of Massachusetts. As the number of cases on the island rapidly grew, the disease became known as "Nantucket fever."[16] Soon other areas of endemicity were identified, including Martha's Vineyard (Massachusetts), Block Island (Rhode Island), Shelter Island, eastern Long Island, and Fire Island (New York). Babesiosis is now endemic on the mainland, particularly from Cape Cod to the coastal counties of western Rhode Island and eastern Connecticut. Endemicity extends south to New Jersey. Isolated cases have been reported from upstate New York, Pennsylvania, Maryland, and Virginia. An asymptomatic infection has been reported from Georgia. As for Lyme disease, babesiosis caused by *B. microti* is endemic in the upper Midwest, particularly in Wisconsin and Minnesota.[17] To date, more than 300 cases of human babesiosis caused by *B. microti* have been documented in the literature. Although national notification is not required, babesiosis has become reportable in states with areas of endemicity. In New York State alone, more than 1500 cases have been notified since 1986, of which more than 1200 occurred in the past decade. Because the geographic range and the number of annual cases have steadily increased, babesiosis caused by *B. microti* is now considered an emerging infectious disease in the United States. Most cases present with a flulike illness, but those at risk of fulminant disease are immunosuppressed patients, asplenic individuals, and the elderly. Asymptomatic infection with *B. microti* may be more common than is recognized,[18] as suggested by the disparity between incidence of babesial disease and seroprevalence of antibodies against *B. microti* antigen.[19] Seroprevalence varies by year, study site, and sample population (community residents vs. blood donors), but has consistently been high in endemic areas, such as southern Connecticut (1.4% to 9%), Block Island (4.6% to 9%), and Shelter Island (4.3% to 6.9%).[6,19,20] Among blood donors on the South Fork in eastern Long Island, a highly endemic area, seroprevalence has even reached 15.8%. Although asymptomatic infection is considered the rule in many areas, on some sites such as Block Island, most babesial infections result in babesial disease.[19] Because asymptomatic infection may persist for many months without detectable parasitemia on blood smears and because two thirds of people with babesial infection do not recall a tick bite, blood transfusion is a mode of transmission. More than 50 transfusion-associated cases have been attributed to *B. microti*.[6,21] Blood products causing transfusion-associated cases are packed red blood cell (RBC) units, as well as platelet units because they typically contain small numbers of RBCs. Neonatal babesiosis is rare and has been acquired by tick bite, transfusion, or transplacental transmission.[22]

Babesiosis caused by *B. divergens*–like organisms is rare in the United States. The patients in all three documented cases were splenectomized. The first case was a 73-year-old man who had not traveled outside of Missouri in the previous 3 to 4 years.[23] The second case was a 56-year-old man from Kentucky.[24] The third case was an 82-year-old man from Washington state.[25] At admission, hallmarks were fever, marked thrombocytopenia, elevated creatinine, bilirubin, and lactate dehydrogenase. For each patient, intraerythrocytic organisms were noted on Giemsa-stained thin blood smears. Ring forms, pairs, and tetrads were observed. The accole position and the obtuse angle of the paired piriforms were suggestive of *B. divergens* organisms. Sera from the first and third cases showed a strong reactivity with *B. divergens* antigen, but no or mininal reactivity with *B. microti* and *B. duncani* antigens. No isolates were recovered by inoculation of patient blood in jirds and hamsters, although these hosts are highly suitable for *B. divergens*. Sequence analysis of the entire 18S rRNA gene revealed that the Missouri (MO1) and the Kentucky (KY) isolates are identical to babesial organisms obtained from eastern cottontail rabbits on Nantucket Island, but closely related to the *B. divergens* isolates from cattle (99.8% identity; 3-base pair difference) and to the isolate from the third case in Washington State (99.7% identity; 5-base pair difference).[11] Unlike *B. divergens*, isolates from eastern cottontail rabbits are not infectious to cattle. These differences in reservoir host (jird, hamster), infectivity for cattle, and 18S rRNA gene sequence indicate that *B. divergens* is not endemic in the United States and that at least two *B. divergens*–like organisms cause human babesiosis in the United States.

In the western United States, *B. duncani* and related babesial parasites are the major etiologic agents of human babesiosis. To date, nine such infections have been reported.[2] Seven were presumably acquired through tick bite, whereas two were transmitted during blood transfusion. The index case was a 41-year-old immunocompetent and normosplenic man from a rural forested area in south-central Washington State.[26] The initial diagnosis of malaria was changed to babesiosis when tetrads were noted on Giemsa-stained thin blood smears. Unlike *B. microti*, the isolate (WA1) was lethal to hamsters and jirds. Accordingly, the patient's serum failed to react with *B. microti* antigen. Four cases, all splenectomized men in their 20s to 40s, were subsequently reported from California.[27] All four patients initially presented with flulike symptoms characteristic of *B. microti* infection. Three (CA1, CA2, CA4) survived. Their sera failed to immunoreact with *B. microti*, but strongly immunoreacted with WA1. Sera from the WA1, CA1, CA2, and CA4 cases also reacted strongly with antigens from *B. conradae* (the canine small piroplasm from California), the BH1 strain of *Babesia* that infects the Californian desert bighorn sheep, and the MD1 strain of *Babesia* that infects the mule deer.[2] The first case of transfusion-acquired transmission involved a 76-year-old normosplenic man who had received multiple units of packed RBCs from a Washington State resident.[28] The second case was a premature male infant who received RBCs for anemia of prematurity.[29] The donor lived in the San Francisco Bay area and had recently traveled to a rural area in central Oregon. Babesial organisms were isolated from recipients (WA2, CA5) and donor (CA6). Analysis of the entire 18S rRNA gene revealed that WA1, WA2, CA5, and CA6 are phylogenetically indistinguishable and form a clade separate from *B. conradae* and from other piroplasms isolated from humans (CA1, CA3, CA4) and wild ungulates (MD1, BH1) in California. Among the California isolates, CA1, CA3, and MD1 are genotypically identical, and only differ from CA4 by 1 base pair and from BH1 by 5 base pairs. As mule deer and bighorn sheep are found at or near sites of probable transmission of babesiosis in California, these and other wild ungulates (fallow deer) may be the natural host reservoirs for the babesial piroplasms that infect people in California. Seroprevalence against *B. duncani* antigen ranges from 3.9% (among the enlisted men at the military fort where the CA1 case occurred; titers >1:320) and 4.8% (among neighbors of the WA1 case; titers >1/256) to 16.9% (south of the site where CA3 was acquired; titers >1/320). The incidence of *B. duncani* infection, however, remains unclear because there are too few clinical cases to validate the serologic test.

EUROPE

Since 1956 when the index case was diagnosed near Zagreb, Croatia, 39 cases have been reported in the literature.[9,15] Approximately two thirds have been attributed to *B. divergens*, although the 18S rRNA gene has been sequenced in only two cases. Because cattle is the definitive reservoir host for *B. divergens*, patients typically are residents of rural areas (farmers, foresters) or vacationers (campers, hikers, hunters) exposed to *I. ricinus* ticks as they work the land or recreate in the countryside. Most cases have been reported from France, Ireland, and Great Britain, particularly from regions with cattle. Cases occur between May and September or October, when *I. ricinus* ticks are active. Nearly all patients infected with *B. divergens* were splenectomized. Transfusion-associated babesiosis caused by *B. divergens* has never been reported.

Because most cases have been attributed to *B. divergens* based on morphology, seroreactivity, and infectivity, early studies may have overlooked piroplasms that are closely related to, but phylogenetically distinct from, *B. divergens*. Babesia EU1, provisionally named *B. venatorum*, is such a piroplasm. *B. venatorum* is most closely related to *B. odocoilei*, with which it forms a sister group to *B. divergens*.[3] *B. venatorum* was identified in the late 1990s as the etiologic agent of babesiosis in two asplenic men in their mid-fifties. The first lived in northern Italy and had chemotherapy for B-cell lymphoma. The second patient was from northeastern Austria. Babesiosis was mild in the Italian patient and moderately severe in the Austrian patient. A third case of *B. venatorum* infection has been reported from Germany.[30] The 63-year-old asplenic patient had been treated with rituximab for lymphoma. Although cases are few, splenectomy appears to be a risk factor for babesiosis caused by *B. venatorum*. The seroprevalence of asymptomatic infection in people remains unknown because the inoculation of jirds, hosts highly susceptible to *B. divergens*, has failed to amplify clinical isolates of *B. venatorum* and therefore to generate *B. venatorum* antigen.

Other *Babesia* spp. have been incriminated as the agents of babesiosis in Europe.[7-9] One case was attributed to *B. canis* and two others to *B. bovis*, including the index case in Croatia, but the evidence was unconvincing. The first case of *B. microti* infection was reported from Poland and most likely was imported from Brazil. A second case was possibly identified in Switzerland, but the evidence was inconclusive. In particular, *B. microti* DNA could not be amplified, despite the presence of babesial organisms on examination of Giemsa-stained blood smears. The first confirmed autochthonous case of *B. microti* infection was reported in 2007 from Thuringia, in eastern Germany.[31] A 42-year-old female patient diagnosed with acute myeloid leukemia (FAB M3) presented with fever and chest pain 1 week after her first cycle of chemotherapy. Six days before admission, she had received a platelet concentrate. Intraerythrocytic organisms were observed on Giemsa-stained blood smears. Sequencing of the 18S rRNA gene unequivocally identified the organism as *B. microti*. This case illustrates the importance of immunosuppression as a risk factor for clinical babesiosis. In support of the transmission of *B. microti* by contaminated blood products in Europe, serologic evidence of asymptomatic infection has emerged in midwestern Germany (1.7% among healthy blood donors; 11.5% among Lyme disease patients or asymptomatic patients with positive borreliosis serology), eastern Switzerland (1.5% among community residents), and eastern Croatia (1% among patients with a history of tick bite).[6]

REST OF THE WORLD

Sporadic cases have been documented around the world.[7-9] In Japan, a patient became ill in Kobe City after a transfusion of blood units obtained from an asymptomatic donor living on the nearby Awaji Island. The organism (Kobe type) was closely related to *B. microti*.[14] *B. microti*–like organisms have also been implicated in Taiwan (TW1) and in India. In South Korea, a case of transfusion-acquired babesiosis was caused by a large piroplasm (KO1) closely related to those found in sheep in China. On the African continent, cases of human babesiosis have been reported from South Africa, Mozambique, and Egypt. A *B. divergens*–like organism was isolated from a 34-year-old splenectomized resident of the Canary Islands, indicating that *Babesia* may not be limited to temperate zones. Because *Babesia* may be mistaken for *Plasmodium* in subtropical zones, babesiosis may be underdiagnosed in malaria endemic regions. Asymptomatic infections with *Babesia* spp. that typically infect domestic animals have been noted in Mexico (*B. bigemina*, *B. canis*) and Colombia (*B. bigemina*, *B. bovis*).

Clinical Manifestations

B. MICROTI INFECTION

In healthy individuals, infection may remain asymptomatic and undiagnosed.[18] When symptomatic, infection with *B. microti* often is mild to moderate.[16] The incubation period typically lasts 1 to 6 weeks after the bite of an infected tick and as long as 9 weeks if the infection is acquired by blood transfusion. The average time from onset of symptoms to diagnosis is 15 days.[12] Symptoms are nonspecific and consist of fatigue/weakness/malaise followed within days by fever (>38°C) and one or more of the following: shaking chills, sweats, headache, myalgia, arthralgia, and anorexia.[12,13,16,32] Fever is intermittent or persistent and may reach 41°C. Less common symptoms include neck stiffness, cough, sore throat, shortness of breath, weight loss, nausea, vomiting, diarrhea, and dark urine. Emotional lability, mild depression, transient hyperesthesia, photophobia, conjunctival injection, crampy abdominal pain, petechiae, and ecchymoses are occasionally noted. Malaise, myalgia, arthralgia, and shortness of breath differentiate babesiosis from other febrile illnesses.[12] Rash in the form of an erythema chronicum migrans may be observed, but is diagnostic of intercurrent Lyme disease.[32] In some patients, symptoms are so mild that no therapy is required. In others, symptoms resolve after single course of antimicrobial therapy. Symptoms usually abate within 2 weeks, sometimes within a few days. In some cases, however, symptoms such as fatigue and malaise persist for several months.[18] Other patients remain asymptomatic for months, if not years, despite the persistence of low-level parasitemia.[33] Infection may recrudesce after a malignancy develops or an immunosuppressive regimen is administered.[17,33]

On physical examination, fever is the salient feature.[12,13] Mild hepatomegaly and splenomegaly may be felt, but lymphadenopathy is absent. Jaundice, slight pharyngeal erythema, retinopathy with splinter hemorrhages, and retinal infarcts are rare.[1] Splenic infarcts may be revealed on computed tomography scans.[34] Splenic rupture without palpable splenomegaly has been reported.[35]

Parasitemia typically ranges from 1% to 20% in patients with an intact spleen and may be as high as 85% in asplenic patients.[1] Low hematocrit, low hemoglobin, elevated total bilirubin, depressed serum haptoglobin, and elevated reticulocyte counts are consistent with hemolytic anemia. The direct Coombs' test may be positive. Hemophagocytosis and increased erythropoiesis may be noted on bone marrow biopsy. Slightly increased liver enzymes (alkaline phosphatase, aspartate aminotransferase, alanine aminotransferase, lactic dehydrogenase) and thrombocytopenia differentiate babesiosis from other febrile illnesses. White blood cell counts are normal or slightly decreased. An increased erythrocyte sedimentation rate is compatible with an inflammatory process. Severe hemolysis is associated with hemoglobinuria and excess urobilinogen; blood urea nitrogen and serum creatinine levels may be elevated.

Although the number and duration of symptoms in people older than 50 years of age do not differ from those in younger adults, the rate of hospitalization is higher among older individuals.[19] The mean age on admission was 62 years in one study[13] and 53 years in another.[12] Previously healthy individuals hospitalized for babesiosis are generally older than patients with a significant medical history.[36] Severe babesiosis is frequent among asplenic individuals, patients coinfected with *B. burgdorferi* or human immunodeficiency virus (HIV) and patients immunosuppressed by therapies for cancer or transplantation. Approximately 40% of hospitalized patients have complications. Acute respiratory distress syndrome, disseminated intravascular coagulation, and congestive heart failure are most common.[12] Renal failure and myocardial infarction are less frequent. Severe anemia (hemoglobin <10 g/dL) and high parasitemia (>10%) are risk factors for complications. Alkaline phosphatase greater than 125 U/L, white blood cell counts greater than 5×10^9/L, and sex (male) are strong predictors of severe outcome defined by hospitalization longer than 2 weeks, stay in the ICU longer than 2 days, or death.[13] Death is the outcome in 5% to 9% of hospitalized cases and may occur despite parasitemia levels less than 1%.

INFECTION WITH OTHER *BABESIA* SPECIES

Most patients with symptomatic *B. divergens* infection are asplenic and experience a fulminant illness after an incubation period of 1 to 3 weeks.[15] Hemoglobinuria is the presenting symptom, followed by jaundice, persistent high fever (40° to 41°C), headache, shaking chills, drenching sweats, and myalgias. Parasitemia can reach 80%. Low hemoglobin levels (4 to 8 g/dL) are indicative of intense hemolysis. On physical examination, mild hepatomegaly may be noted. Without rapid treatment, a shocklike syndrome develops, with pulmonary edema and renal failure. The fatality rate is approximately 40%. Cases caused by *B. duncani* and by *B. venatorum* are few and are briefly presented in the "Epidemiology" section.

Pathogenesis

Because *Babesia* is an obligate parasite of erythrocytes, the pathogenesis of babesiosis results, in part, from the modification and rupture of these host cells by the pathogen. Asynchronous replication of *Babesia* explains the lack of periodicity in parasitemia and associated symptoms. Replication of *Babesia* creates an oxidative environment that results in structural modifications at the erythrocyte membrane.[37] Formation of neo-antigens is thought to create docking sites for autologous immunoglobulin G and complement factors, thereby promoting phagocytosis of *Babesia*-infected erythrocytes by macrophages in the red pulp of the spleen.[35] Splenomegaly has been attributed, in part, to the proliferation of these phagocytic cells. Egress of merozoites is accompanied by rupture of the host cell and release of hemoglobin into the bloodstream. Free hemoglobin is immediately complexed by haptoglobin and cleared by phagocytes. Because erythropoiesis is increased, severe anemia despite low-level parasitemia is best explained by the clearance of nonparasitized erythrocytes. Studies of *B. gibsoni* infection indicate that phagocytes are primed to produce reactive oxygen species, which, in turn, results in the oxidative damage of uninfected erythrocytes, thereby facilitating their opsonization and phagocytosis.[38] Erythrocytes infected with *B. microti* do not exhibit the "knob" structures found on erythrocytes harboring *P. falciparum* and formed by capping of parasite-derived antigens. The lack of "knobs" explains the lack of sequestration of erythrocytes in the microvasculature of *B. microti*–infected hosts.[34,39]

The host immune response is critical for resistance to babesiosis. In agreement with the severity of babesiosis in HIV patients,[40] studies in mice point to the central role of CD4[+] T cells in the resistance to *B. microti* infection.[41] This is corroborated by the susceptibility among elderly individuals who are known to experience a progressive contraction of their naïve CD4[+] T-cell compartment.[19,36] Although studies in mice failed to demonstrate a role for B cells,[42] recent studies on the persistence of *B. microti* infection in immunocompromised patients despite standard antimicrobial therapy suggest that B cells are necessary for clearance of *B. microti* parasitemia.[30,43] Interferon-γ plays a central role in the resistance to babesiosis, as revealed by mice infected with *B. duncani* or *B. microti*.[41,44] Natural killer cells are the main source of interferon-γ in the former infection, but CD4[+] T cells are in the latter. Interferon-γ, in synergy with inflammatory cytokines such as tumor necrosis factor-α, is known to activate an array of macrophage functions. The pathway by which macrophages destroy *Babesia* remains, however, unclear. Although cytokines are important to the unfolding of the immune response, they may also contribute to symptoms of babesiosis. Symptoms are those of virus-like illnesses and are suggestive of an inflammatory response involving pyrogenic cytokines such as TNF-α and interleukin-6. Both cytokines have been found in the blood of a symptomatic patient during the acute phase of infection with *B. microti*.[45] Monocytes are their likely sources. Cytokines may also contribute to complications. In mice infected with *B. duncani*, death results from pulmonary edema associated with intravascular margination of leukocytes. In this model, tumor necrosis factor-α is localized to the alveolar septa, and blockade of tumor necrosis factor activity prevents death.[46]

Diagnosis

Babesiosis typically is diagnosed by microscopic examination of Giemsa-stained thin blood smears.[1] When parasitemia is low, multiple blood smears may need to be examined over several days. *Babesia* spp. appear round, oval, or piriform (see Fig. 282-1). The ring form is most common, with one or a few red chromatic dots and a light blue cytoplasm. Tetrads of merozoites arranged in a Maltese cross are rare, but diagnostic of *B. microti* and *B. duncani*.[2] In case of severe infection, extracellular merozoites, either single or in clumps, can be observed. *Babesia* rings strongly resemble *P. falciparum* trophozoites, but lack the brownish pigment deposits (hemozoin) typical of older rings of *P. falciparum*. Gametes and schizonts typical of *Plasmodium* infections cannot be identified.

If parasites are not identified on blood smears, despite the presence of symptoms suggestive of babesiosis, a polymerase chain reaction assay is available.[1,7,8] When primers amplify a region of the 18S rRNA gene that greatly differs among *Babesia* spp., the organism is easily identified. Primers may also amplify a highly conserved region, allowing detection of several *Babesia* spp. The persistence of babesial DNA correlates with the persistence of symptoms and *B. microti* antibody titers.[33] In an untreated, asymptomatic patient, babesial DNA could be detected for as long as 17 months. Suspected cases of *B. microti* infection can be confirmed by inoculation of 1 mL of edetate-whole blood into the peritoneum of golden hamsters. *B. duncani* is lethal to hamsters and mice. *B. divergens* replicates readily in gerbils. Giemsa-stained blood smears will turn positive for the piroplasm 2 to 4 weeks after inoculation with human blood, if infected.

An indirect immunofluorescent antibody (immunoglobulin G only) test for *B. microti* is available through the Centers for Disease Control and Prevention. A serum titer of 1:64 or greater is diagnostic. Titers of 1:1024 or greater are indicative of active or recent infection.[1] Titers wane slowly over 8 to 12 months. Titers below 1:64 are generally considered indicative of previous infection. The caveat of serologic testing is that IgG titers are low during the acute phase of illness, at time of diagnosis, explaining why IgG titers poorly correlate with severity of symptoms. Serology is not practical for *B. divergens* infection as the incubation period is short and the infection fulminant.[15] Antibodies to *B. microti* antigen do not react with *B. divergens* or *B. duncani* antigen.[7,8] A synthetic peptide-based assay (enzyme-linked immunosorbent assay [EIA]) has been developed and uses immunodominant epitopes from two proteins secreted by *B. microti*.[6] EIA correlates well with the polymerase chain reaction and the immunofluorescent antibody test and may become valuable for high-throughput screening of blood samples in blood banks.

Treatment

B. MICROTI INFECTION

Asymptomatic individuals need not be treated, unless a *Babesia* species is detected on blood smear or by polymerase chain reaction for more than 3 months. Symptomatic patients should not be treated if blood smear and polymerase chain reaction results are negative. When *Babesia* is detected, symptomatic patients should be treated.[47]

Patients with severe *B. microti* infection should be given a combination of intravenous clindamycin plus oral quinine for 7 to 10 days.[47,48] Clindamycin may be given orally to less severe cases. Regimens for adults and children are provided in Table 282-1. Partial or complete RBC exchange transfusion is advised in cases of high parasitemia (>10%).[12,47,49] In these patients, exchange transfusions quickly and completely remove *Babesia*-infected erythrocytes as well as RBC debris and inflammatory mediators.[50] Although arbitrary levels of parasitemia (>10%) have been used to define the need for exchange transfusion, the degree of systemic illness should also be the indicator; acute respiratory distress syndrome or a syndrome resembling systemic inflammatory response syndrome is an indication for RBC exchange by apheresis.[51] Exchange transfusions also are recommended for patients with severe anemia (hemoglobin < 10 g/dL) or renal or hepatic compromise.

TABLE 282-1	Treatment of Human Babesiosis			
Organism	Severity	Adults	Children	
Babesia microti	Mild*	Atovaquone 750 mg q12h PO *plus* azithromycin 500-1000 mg/day PO on day 1, then 250 mg/day PO from day 2 on	Atovaquone 20 mg/kg q12h PO (maximum 750 mg/dose) *plus* azithromycin 10 mg/kg/day PO on day 1 (maximum 500 mg/dose), 5 mg/kg/day PO from day 2 on	
	Severe*	Clindamycin 300-600 mg q6h IV or 600 mg q8h PO *plus* quinine 650 mg q8h PO Consider RBC exchange transfusion	Clindamycin 7-10 mg/kg q6-8h IV or 7-10 mg/kg q6-8h PO (maximum 600 mg/dose) *plus* quinine 8 mg/kg q8h PO (maximum 650 mg/dose) Consider RBC exchange transfusion	
Babesia divergens†		Immediate complete RBC exchange transfusion *plus* clindamycin 600 mg q6-8h IV *plus* quinine 650 mg q8h PO	Immediate complete RBC exchange transfusion *plus* clindamycin 7-10 mg/kg q6-8h IV (maximum 600 mg/dose) *plus* quinine 8 mg/kg q8h PO (maximum 650 mg/dose)	

*Treatment for 7 to 10 days.
†Treatment for 7 to 10 days, but duration may vary. Note that, in asplenic individuals and in immunocompromised patients, therapy should be more than 6 weeks, including 2 weeks after parasites are no longer detected on blood smear.

In some instances, the clindamycin-quinine combination has failed. *B. microti* was cleared by the combination of azithromycin plus quinine in two patients refractory to clindamycin plus quinine. A patient with acquired immunodeficiency syndrome and infected with *B. microti* was successfully treated with a combination of clindamycin, doxycycline, and azithromycin after becoming allergic to quinine.[40] Because *B. microti* resembles *P. falciparum*, chloroquine has been administered but is ineffective. A number of other antimalarial and antiprotozoal therapies have likewise been largely unsuccessful, including primaquine, quinacrine, pyrimethamine, pyrimethamine-sulfadoxine, sulfadiazine, tetracycline, minocycline, pentamidine isethionate, and trimethoprim-sulfamethoxazole.

Patients with non–life-threatening *B. microti* infection should be given atovaquone plus azithromycin for 7 to 10 days.[47,52] This combination is as effective as clindamycin plus quinine in clearing parasitemia. Untoward drug reactions developed in 15% of patients given atovaquone plus azithromycin, but in 72% of patients given clindamycin plus quinine.[52] The atovaquone-azithromycin regimen has not been tested in patients with severe *B. microti* infection. Regimens for adults and children are provided in Table 282-1. For immunocompromised patients, higher doses of azithromycin (500-1000 mg/day) have been used. A patient with acquired immunodeficiency syndrome with persistent high-grade *B. microti* parasitemia was successfully treated with atovaquone-proguanil added to a regimen of exchange transfusion, azithromycin, atovaquone, clindamycin, and quinine; an asymptomatic recurrence was treated with atovaquone-proguanil monotherapy for 90 days.[53]

In patients with severe *B. microti* infection, hematocrit and parasitemia should be monitored daily or every other day until symptoms abate and parasitemia is less than 5%.[47] In patients with mild babesiosis, symptoms typically improve within the first 48 hours of therapy and should resolve within 3 months. Routine testing for babesial organisms is not needed for immunocompetent patients who have stayed asymptomatic for more than 3 months. In immunocompromised patients, the course of therapy should be prolonged beyond the standard period of 7 to 10 days. A recent series of 14 patients with persistent and relapsing *B. microti* infection highlights the need for a minimum of 6 weeks of therapy, with at least 2 weeks after the parasite is no longer seen on blood smear.[43] Multiple drug combinations were administered in these patients over the course of disease, but no particular combination was superior to another.

INFECTION WITH OTHER *BABESIA*

The combination of pentamidine with trimethoprim-sulfamethoxazole has been successful in the treatment of *B. divergens* infection in a splenectomized patient.[54] The standard regimen, however, is a complete blood exchange transfusion and medical therapy with intravenous clindamycin and oral quinine.[15]

In the United States, cases of *B. divergens*–like infections are treated with intravenous clindamycin and oral quinine or quinidine.[23-25] *B. duncani* infections also are treated with clindamycin plus quinine.[26,29] Two cases of *B. venatorum* infection in Europe were successfully treated with clindamycin, alone or in combination with quinine.[3] In a third patient who had previously been treated with rituximab, parasitemia relapsed. After several months of maintenance therapy with atovaquone, *B. venatorum* parasites were eventually cleared.[30]

▣ Prevention

The prevention of babesiosis requires avoidance of areas endemic for *I. scapularis* between May and September. This is especially important for splenectomized individuals and others who are immunocompromised. It is likely that babesiosis will become a greater problem in the future because patients with human immunodeficiency virus and those older than the age of 50 vacation and live in the ever-increasing geographic areas reporting babesial infection. Strategies for tick avoidance, tick removal, and a review of various acaricides can be found in Chapter 242 and at the Centers for Disease Control and Prevention website (http://www.cdc.gov/ticks/prevention.html).

To decrease transfusion-associated babesiosis, blood donors with a history of babesiosis are currently prohibited.[6,20] Screening of blood for *Babesia* organisms may be adopted in the near future and may decrease transfusion-associated babesiosis. Given the increasing confluence of the tick, the parasite, and susceptible people in ever-enlarging areas, clinicians should be increasingly alert to the possibility of this once arcane disease, babesiosis.

ACKNOWLEDGMENT
The authors are supported, in part, by NIA R01 AG19781.

REFERENCES

1. Vannier E, Gewurz BE, Krause PJ. Human babesiosis. *Infect Dis Clin North Am.* 2008;22:469-488.
2. Conrad PA, Kjemtrup AM, Carreno RA, et al. Description of *Babesia duncani* n.sp. (Apicomplexa: Babesiidae) from humans and its differentiation from other piroplasms. *Int J Parasitol.* 2006;36:779-789.
3. Herwaldt BL, Caccio S, Gherlinzoni F, et al. Molecular characterization of a non-*Babesia divergens* organism causing zoonotic babesiosis in Europe. *Emerg Infect Dis.* 2003;9:942-948.
4. Kjemtrup AM, Wainwright K, Miller M, et al. *Babesia conradae*, sp. Nov., a small canine *Babesia* identified in California. *Vet Parasitol.* 2006;138:103-111.
5. Telford III SR, Gorenflot A, Brasseur P, et al. Babesial infections in humans and wildlife. In: Kreier JP, ed. *Parasitic Protozoa.* San Diego: Academic Press; 1993:1-47.

6. Leiby DA. Babesiosis and blood transfusion: flying under the radar. *Vox Sang.* 2006;90:157-165.
7. Homer MJ, Aguilar-Delfin I, Telford SR 3rd, et al. Babesiosis. *Clin Microbiol Rev.* 2000;13:451-469.
8. Kjemtrup AM, Conrad PA. Human babesiosis: an emerging tick-borne disease. *Int J Parasitol.* 2000;30:1323-1337.
9. Hunfeld KP, Hildebrandt A, Gray JS. Babesiosis: recent insights into an ancient disease. *Int J Parasitol.* 2008;38:1219-1237.
10. Swanson SJ, Neitzel D, Reed KD, et al. Coinfections acquired from *Ixodes* ticks. *Clin Microbiol Rev.* 2006;19:708-727.
11. Holman PJ. Phylogenetic and biologic evidence that *Babesia divergens* is not endemic in the United States. *Ann N Y Acad Sci.* 2006;1081:518-525.

12. Hatcher JC, Greenberg PD, Antique J, et al. Severe babesiosis in Long Island: review of 34 cases and their complications. *Clin Infect Dis.* 2001;32:1117-1125.
13. White DJ, Talarico J, Chang HG, et al. Human babesiosis in New York State: review of 139 hospitalized cases and analysis of prognostic factors. *Arch Intern Med.* 1998;158:2149-2154.
14. Goethert HK, Telford SR 3rd. What is *Babesia microti*? *Parasitology.* 2003;127:301-309.
15. Zintl A, Mulcahy G, Skerrett HE, et al. *Babesia divergens*, a bovine blood parasite of veterinary and zoonotic importance. *Clin Microbiol Rev.* 2003;16:622-636.
16. Ruebush TK 2nd, Cassaday PB, Marsh HJ, et al. Human babesiosis on Nantucket Island: clinical features. *Ann Intern Med.* 1977;86:6-9.

17. Herwaldt BL, Springs FE, Roberts PP, et al. Babesiosis in Wisconsin: a potentially fatal disease. *Am J Trop Med Hyg.* 1995;53:146-151.

18. Ruebush TK 2nd, Juranek DD, Chisholm ES, et al. Human babesiosis on Nantucket Island: evidence for self-limited and subclinical infections. *N Engl J Med.* 1977;297:825-827.

19. Krause PJ, McKay K, Gadbaw J, et al. Increasing health burden of human babesiosis in endemic sites. *Am J Trop Med Hyg.* 2003;68:431-436.

20. McQuiston JH, Childs JE, Chamberland ME, et al. Transmission of tick-borne agents of disease by blood transfusion: a review of known and potential risks in the United States. *Transfusion.* 2000;40:274-284.

21. Gubernot DM, Lucey CT, Lee KC, et al. Babesia infection through blood transfusion: reports received by the US Food and Drug Administration, 1997-2007. *Clin Infect Dis.* 2009;48:25-30.

22. Fox LM, Wingerter S, Ahmed A, et al. Neonatal babesiosis: case report and review of the literature. *Pediatr Infect Dis J.* 2006;25:169-173.

23. Herwaldt B, Persing DH, Precigout EA, et al. A fatal case of babesiosis in Missouri: identification of another piroplasm that infects humans. *Ann Intern Med.* 1996;124:643-650.

24. Beattie JF, Michelson ML, Holman PJ. Acute babesiosis caused by Babesia divergens in a resident of Kentucky. *N Engl J Med.* 2002;347:697-698.

25. Herwaldt BL, de Bruyn G, Pieniazek NJ, et al. Babesia divergens-like infection, Washington State. *Emerg Infect Dis.* 2004;10:622-629.

26. Quick RE, Herwaldt BL, Thomford JW, et al. Babesiosis in Washington State: a new species of Babesia? *Ann Intern Med.* 1993;119:284-290.

27. Persing DH, Herwaldt BL, Glaser C, et al. Infection with a Babesia-like organism in northern California. *N Engl J Med.* 1995;332:298-303.

28. Herwaldt BL, Kjemtrup AM, Conrad PA, et al. Transfusion-transmitted babesiosis in Washington State: first reported case caused by a WA1-type parasite. *J Infect Dis.* 1997;175:1259-1262.

29. Kjemtrup AM, Lee B, Fritz CL, et al. Investigation of transfusion transmission of a WA1-type babesial parasite to a premature infant in California. *Transfusion.* 2002;42:1482-1487.

30. Haselbarth K, Tenter AM, Brade V, et al. First case of human babesiosis in Germany—clinical presentation and molecular characterisation of the pathogen. *Int J Med Microbiol.* 2007;297:197-204.

31. Hildebrandt A, Hunfeld KP, Baier M, et al. First confirmed autochthonous case of human Babesia microti infection in Europe. *Eur J Clin Microbiol Infect Dis.* 2007;26:595-601.

32. Krause PJ, Telford SR 3rd, Spielman A, et al. Concurrent Lyme disease and babesiosis: evidence for increased severity and duration of illness. *JAMA.* 1996;275:1657-1660.

33. Krause PJ, Spielman A, Telford SR 3rd, et al. Persistent parasitemia after acute babesiosis. *N Engl J Med.* 1998;339:160-165.

34. Florescu D, Sordillo PP, Glyptis A, et al. Splenic infarction in human babesiosis: two cases and discussion. *Clin Infect Dis.* 2008;46:e8-e11.

35. Kuwayama DP, Briones RJ. Spontaneous splenic rupture caused by Babesia microti infection. *Clin Infect Dis.* 2008;46:e92-e95.

36. Benach JL, Habicht GS. Clinical characteristics of human babesiosis. *J Infect Dis.* 1981;144:481.

37. Arese P, Turrini F, Schwarzer E. Band 3/complement-mediated recognition and removal of normally senescent and pathological human erythrocytes. *Cell Physiol Biochem.* 2005;16:133-146.

38. Otsuka Y, Yamasaki M, Yamato O, et al. The effect of macrophages on the erythrocyte oxidative damage and the pathogenesis of anemia in Babesia gibsoni-infected dogs with low parasitemia. *J Vet Med Sci.* 2002;64:221-226.

39. Clark IA, Budd AC, Hsue G, et al. Absence of erythrocyte sequestration in a case of babesiosis in a splenectomized human patient. *Malar J.* 2006;5:69.

40. Falagas ME, Klempner MS. Babesiosis in patients with AIDS: a chronic infection presenting as fever of unknown origin. *Clin Infect Dis.* 1996;22:809-812.

41. Igarashi I, Waki S, Ito M, et al. Role of CD4$^+$ T cells in the control of primary infection with Babesia microti in mice. *J Protozool Res.* 1994;4:164-171.

42. Clawson ML, Paciorkowski N, Rajan TV, et al. Cellular immunity, but not gamma interferon, is essential for resolution of Babesia microti infection in BALB/c mice. *Infect Immun.* 2002;70:5304-5306.

43. Krause PJ, Gewurz BE, Hill D, et al. Persistent and relapsing babesiosis in immunocompromised patients. *Clin Infect Dis.* 2008;46:370-376.

44. Aguilar-Delfin I, Wettstein PJ, Persing DH. Resistance to acute babesiosis is associated with interleukin-12- and gamma interferon-mediated responses and requires macrophages and natural killer cells. *Infect Immun.* 2003;71:2002-2008.

45. Shaio MF, Lin PR. A case study of cytokine profiles in acute human babesiosis. *Am J Trop Med Hyg.* 1998;58:335-337.

46. Hemmer RM, Ferrick DA, Conrad PA. Role of T cells and cytokines in fatal and resolving experimental babesiosis: protection in TNFRp55−/− mice infected with the human Babesia WA1 parasite. *J Parasitol.* 2000;86:736-742.

47. Wormser GP, Dattwyler RJ, Shapiro ED, et al. The clinical assessment, treatment, and prevention of Lyme disease, human granulocytic anaplasmosis, and babesiosis: clinical practice guidelines by the Infectious Diseases Society of America. *Clin Infect Dis.* 2006;43:1089-1134.

48. Wittner M, Rowin KS, Tanowitz HB, et al. Successful chemotherapy of transfusion babesiosis. *Ann Intern Med.* 1982;96:601-604.

49. Jacoby GA, Hunt JV, Kosinski KS, et al. Treatment of transfusion-transmitted babesiosis by exchange transfusion. *N Engl J Med.* 1980;303:1098-1100.

50. Dorman SE, Cannon ME, Telford SR 3rd, et al. Fulminant babesiosis treated with clindamycin, quinine, and whole-blood exchange transfusion. *Transfusion.* 2000;40:375-380.

51. Stowell CP, Gelfand JA, Shepard JA, et al. Case records of the Massachusetts General Hospital. Case 17-2007. A 25-year-old woman with relapsing fevers and recent onset of dyspnea. *N Engl J Med.* 2007;356:2313-2319.

52. Krause PJ, Lepore T, Sikand VK, et al. Atovaquone and azithromycin for the treatment of babesiosis. *N Engl J Med.* 2000;343:1454-1458.

53. Vyas JM, Telford SR, Robbins GK. Treatment of refractory Babesia microti infection with atovaquone-proguanil in an HIV-infected patient: case report. *Clin Infect Dis.* 2007;45:1588-1590.

54. Raoult D, Soulayrol L, Toga B, et al. Babesiosis, pentamidine, and cotrimoxazole. *Ann Intern Med.* 1987;107:944.

283

Cryptosporidium Species

A. CLINTON WHITE, JR

Protozoan parasites of the genus *Cryptosporidium* were first identified in the stomach of mice in 1907.[1] The species name *Cryptosporidium parvum* was proposed in 1912 to describe parasites identified in murine intestines.[2] Although *Cryptosporidium* was linked to gastrointestinal disease in turkeys in 1955 and to bovine diarrhea in 1971, the first human cases were described only in 1976.[3-6] Only a handful of cases had been reported before 1982. In the early 1980s, large numbers of cases were noted to be associated with the emerging epidemic of acquired immunodeficiency syndrome (AIDS).[7,8] Soon studies identified cases among animal handlers and children.[8,9] Shortly thereafter, *Cryptosporidium* was associated with waterborne outbreaks of diarrhea, including an outbreak in Milwaukee, Wisconsin, in 1993 that affected an estimated 403,000 persons.[10,11] Studies have now demonstrated that *Cryptosporidium* is an important cause of self-limited diarrhea in normal hosts worldwide, of persistent diarrhea in children in developing countries, and of chronic diarrhea in immunocompromised hosts including patients with AIDS.[12-14]

The Parasites

The genus *Cryptosporidium* consists of a group of protozoan parasites within the protist subphylum Apicomplexa (which also includes *Plasmodium* species). *Cryptosporidium* had been classified within the subclass Coccidiasina (coccidia), together with *Eimeria*, *Sarcocystis*, *Toxoplasma*, *Cyclospora*, and *Isospora*. Molecular biology studies, however, suggest that *Cryptosporidium* may have diverged earlier from the other apicomplexans and should be reclassified into a separate subclass.[15-18] The genomes of both *Cryptosporidium parvum* and *Cryptosporidium hominis* have been sequenced. Compared with other apicomplexan parasites, the genomes are relatively compact (9.1 and 9.2 Mb) with the loss of approximately 1400 genes compared with the *Plasmodium* parasites.[19-21] Many of these gene deletions may be due to the loss of the mitochondria and apicoplast, organelles found in most other apicomplexans, but not found in *Cryptosporidium* species. *Cryptosporidium* species also lack the genes for variable surface proteins contained in the *Plasmodium falciparum* genome (e.g., *var*, *rif*, and *stevor* genes). The metabolic pathways are also simplified (e.g., no Krebs cycle), but a number of transporters are present to scavenge molecules from the host.

Initially, species names were given based on the host species.[17,22] Most human isolates were thought to belong to a single species, *C. parvum*. Molecular studies have subsequently demonstrated that parasites previously termed *C. parvum* include a number of genotypes and occult species.[17,22] As of 2008, there are approximately 20 recognized *Cryptosporidium* species thought to be valid based on host specificity, morphology, and molecular biology studies and numerous other genotypes that may emerge as separate species.[17,23,24] The bovine genotype is commonly found in humans and bovines and is now designated by the species name *C. parvum*. It infects a wide range of mammalian hosts, including mice. By contrast, the human genotype, now termed *C. hominis*, is found mainly in humans and is rarely infectious for cattle or mice, but can infect gnotobiotic pigs and rarely other species.[25] In the gnotobiotic pig, the genotypes differ in lesion distribution and intensity of infection.[26] Based on these differences and comparative genomics, the species name *C. hominis* is now the accepted term for the human genotype.[17,22,25] Similarly, the *Cryptosporidium* parasite infecting dogs and humans has been reclassified as *Clostridium canis*.[17,22] Molecular biology studies have demonstrated that humans

can also be infected with *Clostridium meleagridis*, *Clostridium felis*, *Clostridium andersoni*, *Clostridium suis*, *Clostridium baylei*, and *Clostridium muris*.[17,27-34] The latter has been demonstrated to infect volunteers in experimental challenge studies (P. C. Okhuysen, personal communication, 2009). *Clostridium meleagridis*, formerly thought to mainly infect birds, has been identified in most large series and appears to cause approximately 1% of cases of human cryptosporidiosis. Other species have so far been noted to infect only reptiles, fish, birds, or nonhuman mammals.

Cryptosporidium species can complete their entire life cycle within a single host, including both asexual (merogony) and sexual (sporogony) reproductive cycles (Fig. 283-1). The life cycle begins with ingestion of the infectious oocyst. The infectious dose varies by several orders of magnitude from isolate to isolate.[35] For one bovine isolate, more than half of volunteers are infected with 10 oocysts.[35] *C. hominis* had a similar infectious dose for volunteers, with half getting diarrhea after a dose of 10 oocysts.[36] In the stomach and upper intestines, the oocysts are activated, producing serine and cysteine proteases and aminopeptidases, which allow the organisms to excyst, releasing four infective sporozoites.[37-41] Contact with the sialated carbohydrate surface of the epithelial cells may be an important trigger for excystation.[42] Each sporozoite contains an apical complex with specialized organelles involved in invasion including rhoptries, micronemes, and dense granules. The motile sporozoites bind to receptors on the surface of the intestinal epithelial cells. Several parasite ligands (including p30 [the galactose-*N*-acetylgalactosamine lectin]), the 1300-kDa circumsporozoite-like antigen, gp900, the thrombospondin-related adhesive protein of *Cryptosporidium*-1, the Cpgp40/15, and cp47) have been implicated in parasite attachment to the intestinal epithelium.[17,43-45] The parasites then induce actin polymerization and protrusion of the intestinal epithelial cell membrane, which is mediated by TKGFR, PI3kinase, and CDC42.[17,45-48] The membrane surrounds the sporozoite and fuses to form the parasitophorous vacuole, which remains in the microvillus layer on the surface of the epithelium.[49] A band of dense cytoskeletal elements separates the parasite from the host cytoplasm.[49] This band prevents free flow of materials between parasite and the host cell cytoplasm.[17,50] It also contains an adenosine triphosphate binding cassette, which likely functions as an efflux pump, contributing to the resistance of the organisms to chemotherapy.[51] Inside the parasitophorous vacuole, the parasites undergo asexual reproduction (merogony). They enlarge into trophozoite forms and divide to form type I meronts, which mature and rupture to release the motile merozoites. The merozoites bind to receptors on the epithelial cells and are engulfed by the cells. They then either repeat the process of merogony or undergo sexual differentiation. In that case, the merozoites differentiate into the micro- and macrogamonts. The microgamont releases the microgametes, which penetrate the cell infected with the macrogamont. The macrogamont and microgametes fuse to form the zygote form, which then undergoes meiosis to form the oocyst, containing four sporozoites. Two morphologic forms of the oocyst have been described. Thin-walled oocysts are thought to excyst within the same host in a process of self-infection.[52] The thick-walled oocysts are shed into the environment.

Epidemiology

Several factors define the epidemiology of cryptosporidiosis.[14,34,53] First, the oocysts are infectious when shed. Thus, parasites are readily

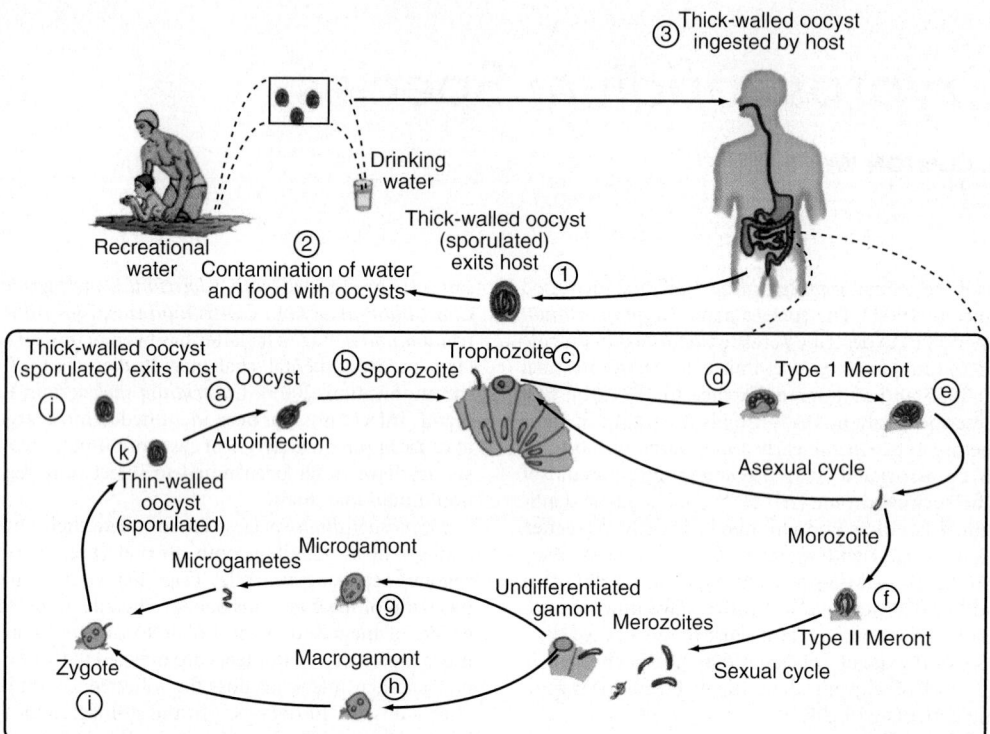

Figure 283-1 **Life cycle of *Cryptosporidium*.** Oocysts are excreted in the feces. Following ingestion, the sporozoites are released from the oocysts and attach to and invade intestinal epithelial cells (a, b). The cells engulf the parasites into a parasitophorous vacuole, where they enlarge to form the trophozoites (c), undergo asexual multiplication forming type I meronts (d, e), and release the motile merozoites (e). The merozoites reattach to epithelial cells. They may continue the asexual cycle or may undergo sexual multiplication producing type II meronts (f). The type II meronts differentiate into microgamonts (male, g) and macrogamonts (female, h). The microgametes fertilize the macrogametes to form the zygote (i). The zygotes develop into the oocysts. Two different types of oocysts are produced: the thick-walled oocyst, which is commonly excreted from the host (j), and the thin-walled oocyst (k), which is primarily involved in autoinfection. Oocysts are infective on excretion, thus permitting direct and immediate fecal-oral transmission. *(From the Centers for Disease Control DpDx: Cryptosporidiosis. http://www.dpd.cdc.gov/dpdx/HTML/Cryptosporidiosis. htm.)*

transmitted directly from person to person. Second, although *Cryptosporidium* does not multiply outside of the host, the infectious dose is low, facilitating transmission from sources with low-grade contamination, such as recreational water.[34,53,54] Third, the oocyst stage can survive for prolonged periods in the environment and resists disinfection, including chlorination. Its small size and resistance to chlorination facilitate waterborne transmission. Fourth, the host immune response limits the duration and severity of infection, such that disease is more commonly recognized in children (preimmune) or in compromised hosts, especially patients with AIDS. Finally, although some of the genotypes have important animal reservoirs, molecular studies demonstrate that most human infection is caused by species and subtypes that mainly affect humans. Hence, animal contact is associated with a minor component of transmission.

Cryptosporidium parasites have been found in every region of the world except Antarctica. Infection is generally more common in moist months.[34,54-61] For example, cases in the United States peak in July through September.[58] Most studies on the prevalence of infection have relied on detection of oocysts in fecal specimens submitted for parasitologic examination. Only 2426 to 3793 cases per year were reported in the United States from 1995 through 2002, but the number of reported cases increased to more than 8000 per year in 2005 through 2007 without other evidence suggesting more illness.[58] This increase coincided with the marketing of nitazoxanide and was thought to be the result of improved diagnosis. By contrast, estimates suggest that more than 300,000 persons in the United States are affected each year.[58,62] The difference stems from both underuse of diagnostic tests

for *Cryptosporidium* and underreporting.[54,58,63] Overall, older surveys not involving human immunodeficiency virus (HIV) patients documented oocysts in 1% to 3% of specimens from industrialized countries of Europe and North America (mean, 2.1%).[14] Most studies from developing countries document *Cryptosporidium* in 5% to 10% (mean, 6.1%).[14] With improving diagnostic techniques, more cases are being identified. For example, a survey from a large U.S. commercial laboratory documented oocysts in specimens from 121 of 2896 (4.2%) individuals.[64] Similarly, studies from England and the Netherlands showed that use of polymerase chain reaction (PCR) assays led to a doubling of the number of *Cryptosporidium* cases identified.[65,66] Studies from sub-Saharan Africa identified *Cryptosporidium* in 7.5% to 22.2% of cases when using microscopy.[67] However, a study from Uganda using a sensitive and specific PCR method documented *Cryptosporidium* in 444 of 1779 (25%) of cases of diarrhea, including 22% of acute diarrhea cases.[28] Similarly, oocysts were found in 83 of 445 (18.7%) children with diarrhea by direct immunofluorescence in a study from Brazil.[26] Recent studies have identified *Cryptosporidium* in 18% of children with diarrhea in South Africa, and 15% of cases of childhood diarrhea in India.[68,69] Studies using PCR assays on stool samples from AIDS patients with diarrhea have identified *Cryptosporidium* DNA in 18% to 74% of cases, significantly higher than with staining alone.[70-73] Thus, the prevalence is likely higher than suggested by earlier stool studies.

Serologic testing has also been used to determine the prevalence of cryptosporidiosis. Initial assays have used unfractionated oocyst antigens using enzyme-linked immunosorbent assay. Experimental challenge studies demonstrate that patients do not always seroconvert after infection, and some seronegative patients may be positive by immunoblot assay.[74-76] Most serosurveys have documented a seroprevalence of approximately 30% among U.S. adults, with higher rates associated with contact with contaminated water or animals.[77-80] In a study of 803 children in Oklahoma, 31% were seropositive, with rates increasing from 13% in those younger than 5 years old to 58% in those of ages 14 to 21.[81] Studies from the U.S.-Mexico border demonstrated seroprevalence rates of 82% in urban border communities and 89% among those in settlements lacking treated water.[82] That compares with rates of approximately 75% for children ages 11 to 13 in China and 64% for adults in urban Latin America.[78,83] By contrast, in a Brazilian shantytown and among Bedouins in Israel, more than 90% of children seroconverted during the first 2 years of life.[78,84] Studies comparing seroconversion and stool studies from birth cohorts in Peru and Israel suggest that serologic studies indicate that approximately half of infections are missed by stool examinations.[84,85]

A series of human challenge experiments were performed to determine the infectious dose of *Cryptosporidium* species. The initial studies were performed in seronegative volunteers with different strains of bovine genotype parasites. The studies discovered a low infectious dose, but considerable variability between isolates, with the dose infecting half of subjects ranging from approximately 1000 oocysts (UCP strain) to approximately 100 oocysts (Iowa strain) to fewer than 10 oocysts for a recent Texas isolate.[35,86] Based on these data, even a single oocyst should result in infection in a portion of those exposed.[87] When the volunteers were rechallenged, they had a higher infectious dose.[74] They also developed less severe manifestations in that they were less likely to shed organisms, but frequently developed symptomatic illness, with oocyst shedding detectable only by flow cytometry.[74] When volunteers who were seropositive were challenged, the infectious dose was 20- to 50-fold higher.[88] Subsequent studies have demonstrated similar infectious doses with a strain of *C. hominis*.[36] Because the infectious dose is low, transmission can readily occur from exposure to low doses, such as might be found in waterborne outbreaks.

Oocysts of *Cryptosporidium* are relatively resistant to environmental conditions. Oocysts can remain infectious for at least 6 months if kept moist, but viability decreases rapidly with dessication.[17,89-91] Oocyst viability does not decrease with storage at temperatures between 0 and 20°C. Viability decreases over a few hours with freezing (−20°C or lower). The oocysts can also be killed by heat including pasteurization.[17,89,92] Oocysts are highly resistant to chlorination. For example, 80 ppm chlorine only inactivated 90% of oocysts after 90 minutes incubation,[93] and the concentrations in tapwater (e.g., 5 ppm) had no effect.[94] The sensitivity of oocysts to chlorine is further decreased in the presence of fecal contamination.[95] Even incubation of oocysts for as long as 2 hours in household bleach failed to decrease infectivity.[96] By contrast, oocysts are sensitive to hydrogen peroxide, ozone, and ultraviolet radiation.[17] Sunlight decreased oocyst viability 40% after 24 hours.[97]

Surveys have demonstrated that most sources of drinking water were contaminated with oocysts before treatment.[98-100] Oocysts are more frequent and at higher densities in water contaminated with agricultural, sewage, or urban runoff. However, as many as 39% of apparently pristine sources were contaminated. Organisms found in the water include both *C. hominis* and *C. parvum* bovine genotype as well as animal species.[54,101-103] Even ground water is not infrequently contaminated.[98] Low-grade contamination has also been documented in samples of treated water, but this has been decreasing with improvements in water standards.[54,98,99,104]

More than 100 outbreaks of cryptosporidiosis have been linked to contaminated drinking water.[34,54,104] The first outbreak was reported in 1985 and was associated with unfiltered well water.[10] The largest documented waterborne outbreak of diarrhea occurred in Milwaukee in 1993.[11] One of two city water treatment plants was contaminated. More than 600 cases of *Cryptosporidium* infection were confirmed by parasitologic examination. Based on telephone surveys, diarrhea episodes were more widespread, with an estimated 403,000 people devel-

oping a diarrheal illness.[11] Interestingly, water quality never failed to meet the standards current at the time for turbidity and fecal coliform counts. Many of the waterborne outbreaks, including the outbreak in Milwaukee, have been caused by *C. hominis*.[34,54,105,106] Thus, the outbreaks are thought to result from fecal contamination of drinking water. Other outbreaks are associated with *C. parvum* (bovine genotype). In most cases, these can be tied to contamination of the watershed with agricultural runoff. For example, many of the outbreaks in England are associated with agricultural runoff from sheep farms.[34,54,106] Recent studies demonstrate a marked reduction in the number of outbreaks and cases associated with drinking water. For example, only a single outbreak of drinking water associated with illness due to *Cryptosporidium* was noted in the United States in 2005 and 2006.[100] Similarly, there has been a marked decrease in cryptosporidiosis in England and Wales associated with improved water standards.[34,54,104,106]

More than 100 outbreaks of cryptosporidiosis have been associated with contaminated recreational water just in the United States.[34,54,107-109] The number of outbreaks increased throughout the 1990s, and outbreaks continue to be common. *Cryptosporidium* is now the most common organism associated with waterborne-disease outbreaks associated with recreational water in the United States.[108,109] Swimming is one of the main risk factors for cryptosporidiosis.[58,110,111] Many outbreaks are associated with swimming pools and are tied to fecal accidents. Outbreaks have also involved water parks, lakes, rivers, beaches, and fountains.[34,54,107-109] The concentration of chlorine in pool water and limited filtration are often insufficient to disinfect the water. Not surprisingly, most outbreaks associated with fecal accidents are attributable to *C. hominis*.[34,54,107-109]

Foodborne infection occurs less frequently. Well-documented outbreaks have been tied to contaminated apple cider, unpasteurized milk, chicken salad, raw produce, and shellfish.[112-114] In developing countries, oocysts are commonly found on vegetables.[115] Oocysts have been frequently identified in shellfish from the Chesapeake Bay and in flies, but there is no good evidence of transmission to humans.[116,117]

Oocysts of *Cryptosporidium* are immediately infectious when shed. Thus, *Cryptosporidium* is associated with direct person-to-person spread. Person-to-person transmission was initially recognized in outbreaks associated with contact with daycare centers.[118-121] There are also documented cases of nosocomial transmission.[122-124] The risk of transmission from adult patients is small with standard precautions.[125] However, contact with a person ill with diarrhea or children in diapers remains a major risk factor for cryptosporidiosis.[110,111,126]

Secondary transmission within households is also common.[127] For example, in a study of household contacts of children with cryptosporidiosis in Brazil, Newman noted secondary cases in 18 of 31 households (58%) and involving 19% of household members.[125] In daycare-associated outbreaks, secondary transmission rates have ranged from 14% to 38%.[118,119] High rates of transmission were also noted in children during the Milwaukee outbreak, but only 5% of adult cases were associated with secondary transmission.[128]

Cryptosporidiosis is also associated with travel from developed to less developed countries.[34,54,111,126] This was first recognized in Finnish travelers to Russia and was thought to reflect contamination of drinking water.[129] *Cryptosporidium* was thought to cause approximately 2% of traveler's diarrhea cases.[130] However, in recent studies of travelers to Mexico using antigen-detection assays and PCR, the actual rates were as high as 6% of cases.[131] International travel remains a major risk factor for cryptosporidiosis in developed countries.[34,54,111,126,132] Most travel-associated cases are caused by *C. hominis*.[126]

Sexual transmission has been postulated to occur. Among HIV patients, cryptosporidiosis has been associated with homosexuality as an HIV risk factor.[133-135] Transmission is associated with anal-genital sex and the number of sex partners.[134,136]

C. parvum bovine was thought to infect primarily domestic animals with zoonotic transmission to humans. However, molecular studies have demonstrated that many of the human *C. parvum* infections are caused by subtype IIc, which typically only infects humans.[33,137] The first case series in immunocompetent individuals was associated with animal contact.[8] Numerous outbreaks have been tied to animal contact.[34,54] Animal contact is also associated with sporadic cryptosporisiosis.[111,126] In addition to cattle, sheep, pigs, and pets have also been implicated in zoonotic infection.[34,111,126,138-140]

The host immune response plays a key role in susceptibility. In studies from developing countries where there is heavy exposure, nearly all cases of cryptosporidiosis develop in young children, presumably owing to rapid development of immunity.[56,57,127,141,142] Human challenge studies document resistance to infection associated with previous challenge or prechallenge immunity (as documented by anti-*Cryptosporidium* antibodies).[74,88] There is also strong evidence of an increased frequency of infection in patients with altered cellular immunity.[143] Among HIV patients with diarrhea, *Cryptosporidium* was found in as many as three fourths of children with chronic diarrhea in developing countries.[14,70-73] In a waterborne outbreak affecting a drug treatment center, only 190 of 1392 (13.6%) HIV-negative patients developed cryptosporidiosis compared with 104 of 339 (30.6%) infected with HIV.[144] Among those with HIV, the infection rate varied with the CD4 cell count, ranging from 23% of those with CD4 cell counts greater than 1000 cells/µL to 46% of those with CD4 cell counts less than 100 cells/µL. However, infection was not more frequent in HIV patients during the Milwaukee outbreak.[145] Cryptosporidiosis has also been noted in other immunodeficient hosts including patients with primary immunodeficiencies, organ transplants, cancer, and diabetes.[143] There is an extremely high prevalence of cryptosporidiosis in the setting of X-linked immunodeficiency with hyperimmunoglobulin M because of a defect in the CD40 ligand.[146,147] In these two series, 26 of 109 (24%) cases were diagnosed with cryptosporidiosis. Furthermore, nearly half of cases developed biliary disease, primarily sclerosing cholangitis. Subsequent studies using PCR assays have demonstrated that most of these biliary tract infections were caused by *Cryptosporidium*.[148]

Pathology and Pathogenesis

Cryptosporidium organisms are found within parasitophorous vacuoles in the microvillus layer of epithelial cells (Fig. 283-2). In immunocompetent individuals, the organisms are localized primarily to the distal small intestines (e.g., terminal ileum) and proximal colon. However, in immunodeficient hosts, the parasites have been identified throughout the gut, in the biliary tract, and even in the respiratory tract.[149-151] Children with persistent cryptosporidiosis may have villous atrophy and a slight increase in lamina propria lymphocytes.[152] The distribution of parasites is limited and often spares the proximal small intestines. Heavier infection is associated with villous atrophy, crypt hyperplasia, and marked infiltration with lymphocytes, plasma cells,

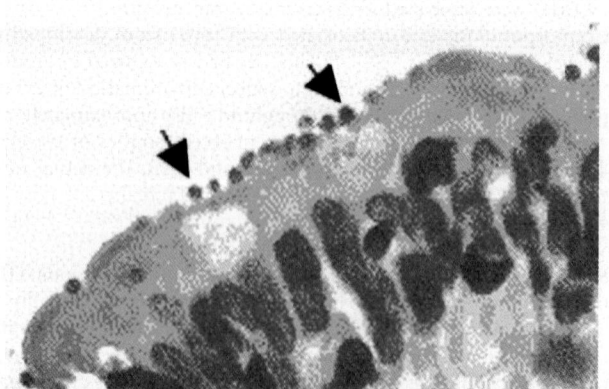

Figure 283-2 Intestinal biopsy specimen showing *Cryptosporidium* intracellular forms (*arrows*) along the surface of the intestinal epithelium. (*From Petri WA. Therapy of intestinal protozoa.* Trends Parasitol. *2003;19:523-526, with permission.*)

and even neutrophils[151,153-156] and is also associated with extraintestinal involvement.

Cryptosporidiosis is characterized clinically by watery diarrhea and malabsorption. The physiologic processes that are thought to account for these symptoms include sodium malabsorption, electrogenic chloride secretion, and increased intestinal permeability. The voluminous, watery diarrhea resembles that of toxin-mediated illnesses caused by cholera and toxogenic *Escherichia coli*. Some investigators claim to have identified enterotoxic activity in stools, but no secretory activity was detected in formal studies.[157,158]

Infection of intestinal epithelial cells leads to activation of nuclear factor kappa B.[159,160] Upstream signals may include TLR 2 and 4 signaling via MyD88.[161-163] Nuclear factor kappa B then activates anti-apoptotic mechanisms, but also leads to upregulation of a proinflammatory cascade. Murine models, human intestinal xenografts in severe combined immunodeficiency mice (SCID) mice, and both biopsy specimens and stool studies from human infection demonstrate increased expression of proinflammatory cytokines and markers of inflammation including tumor necrosis factor-α (TNF-α), interleukin (IL)-1β, IL-8, and lactoferrin.[164-172] Chemokines including IL-8 are produced by the infected epithelial cells.[172-177] The chemokines and cytokines recruit inflammatory and immune cells into the intestines. Infection also upregulates expression of cyclooxygenase-2, production of prostaglandins by the epithelial cells, and production of neuropeptides such as substance P by the inflammatory cells.[178-181] The physiologic consequences of infection include increased epithelial permeability, decreased sodium absorption, and chloride secretion.

Prostaglandins mediate decreased sodium in porcine and bovine cryptosporidiosis and are thought to also stimulate cyclic adenosine monophosphate–mediated chloride secretion.[164,178,180,182,183] In porcine models, diarrhea was induced by prostaglandins and controlled with cyclooxygenase inhibitors. Prostaglandin production was stimulated by TNF-α.[164] However, studies in volunteers and AIDS patients with chronic cryptosporidiosis did not demonstrate any correlation between expression or level of proinflammatory cytokines and symptoms.[167,184-186] Furthermore, prostaglandin inhibitors have not proven to be effective symptomatic therapy in human cryptosporidiosis.

More recently, neuropeptides have been implicated in the diarrhea. Robinson and colleagues[179] demonstrated a correlation between expression of the neuropeptide substance P and the presence and severity of diarrhea in volunteers challenged with *C. parvum* and AIDS patients with chronic cryptosporidiosis. In monkey models, *Cryptosporidium* infection is associated with increased expression of substance P and its receptor and substance P inhibitors blocked *Cryptosporidium*-induced intestinal permeability and chloride secretion.[181,187] Similarly, mice were protected against *C. parvum*–induced intestinal inflammation and illness by a substance P receptor antagonist.[188,189] Octreotide, a somatostatin analogue and substance P antagonist, partially suppresses diarrhea in chronic cryptosporidiosis and reverses altered intestinal function in vitro, suggesting a role for neuropeptides in diarrhea.[182,190]

Cryptosporidiosis is also characterized by defects in intestinal permeability. Increased permeability may result in decreased absorption of fluids and electrolytes as well as solute fluxes into the gut. Studies of AIDS patients with cryptosporidiosis have demonstrated a direct correlation between the severity of disease and altered intestinal permeability (as measured by ratios of excretion in the urine of lactulose and mannitol).[155,191,192] Similar defects have been noted in children with cryptosporidiosis.[193] *Cryptosporidium* infection directly induces defects in intestinal epithelial cell barrier function in vitro.[194-196] The latter can also be mimicked by treatment with proinflammatory cytokines such as interferon-γ (IFN-γ) and reversed by anti-inflammatory cytokines, such as transforming growth factor-β.[196] Substance P may be mediating the increased intestinal permeability and chloride secretion.[181,187]

Porcine and bovine cryptosporidiosis as well as infection in patients are associated with villous atrophy and crypt hyperplasia, thought to reflect epithelial cell turnover.[152,155,197-200] Although infection of epithelial cells stimulates anti-apoptotic mechanisms in infected cells, there is increased apoptosis in adjacent cells likely mediated by the interaction of FAS and FAS ligand.[159,160,201,202] Increased epithelial cell apoptosis has been demonstrated in biopsy specimens from infected intestines.[153] In vitro infection models show that infection initially stimulates anti-apoptotic signals, but after 24 hours of infection, pro-apoptotic molecules dominate.[203,204] Furthermore, as the organisms complete their cycle, they cause necrotic death of the infected cells.[195,205,206] The resultant loss of villous surface was, in turn, associated with decreased expression of glucose-stimulated sodium pumps.[183,200] Similarly, loss of villous surface area has been demonstrated in human infection as D-xylose malabsorption.[155,156,192,198] Studies of AIDS patients with severe cryptosporidiosis have also demonstrated malabsorption of bile acids, vitamin B_{12}, and fatty acids.[155,207,208] Metabolic studies of AIDS patients with chronic cryptosporidiosis demonstrate fat wasting with a decreased metabolic rate, consistent with decreased absorption.[209]

Host Response and Immunity

CD4$^+$ T cells play a key role in the control of human cryptosporidiosis.[172] In patients with HIV infection, cryptosporidiosis is self-limited in individuals with CD4 cell counts higher than 180/μL, chronic in patients with CD4 cell depletion to less than 100/μL, and fulminant in some of those with counts less than 50/μL.[133,210,211] Similarly, infection is chronic in mice without functional CD4 cells (anti-CD4 treatment, nude mice, SCID mice, major histocompatibility complex class II knockout mice).[212-215] These defects can be reversed by infusion of CD4$^+$ cells, particularly CD4$^+$ intraepithelial lymphocytes.[216-218] In support of the importance of MHC class II in human infection, Kirkpatrick and colleagues[219] noted an association between DQ alleles and susceptibility to infection. Furthermore, resolution of cryptosporidiosis among AIDS patients in response to effective antiretroviral therapy is associated with an influx of CD4 cells into the intestines.[220] The role of other cell populations has been less clear. CD8$^+$ cells are found at the site of infection in human and bovine infection.[165,221] Although major histocompatibility complex class I deficiency and CD8 depletion have little effect on murine cryptosporidiosis,[215,216] there are associations of MHC class I types in human infection. Also, CD8 cells produce IFN-γ in response to *Cryptosporidium* antigens.[172,219,222]

X-linked immunodeficiency with hyperimmunoglobulin M, caused by a defect in CD40 ligand (also termed CD154), is associated with increased frequency and severity of *Cryptosporidium* infection.[146,147] This syndrome is associated with profound defects in the ability of antigen-presenting cells to produce IL-12 and TNF-α and to stimulate production of IFN-γ.[223] SCID mice can resolve infection if given spleen cells that express CD40L.[224-227] This does not require cognate recognition because similar effects were seen with cells from RAG knockout mice with a transgenic ovalbumin-specific T-cell receptor.[226] Recovery required expression of CD40 on donor spleen cells, but not recipient epithelial cells.[227] Recent studies of infected human tissues noted that *Cryptosporidium* infection leads to upregulation of the TNF receptor family decoy receptor osteoprotegerin.[228] It was also detected in intestinal tissues after experimental infection. Its ligand, TRAIL, was able to eliminate infected cells in vitro, but this effect was reversed by osteoprotegerin, suggesting that TRAIL may be a key mediator of parasite clearance.[228]

Production of IFN-γ is a key mediator of the immune response to *Cryptosporidium*. In murine models, IFN-γ knockout mice develop chronic infection.[229,230] Furthermore, inactivation or depletion of IFN-γ causes further exacerbation of infection even beyond that noted with CD4 depletion.[231] IFN-γ is expressed in the intestines in both mice and cattle, peaking at the time of control of oocyst shedding.[232-234] Lymphocytes from people who have recovered from cryptosporidiosis produced IFN-γ after antigen stimulation in vitro, including HIV patients.[235,236] Approximately half of volunteers challenged with *C. parvum* express IFN-γ in the intestinal mucosa.[237] Treatment with IFN-γ can directly activate intestinal epithelial cell lines to partially clear *C. parvum* infection.[238] Similarly, inactivation of IL-12, the

major factor stimulating production of IFN-γ, causes chronic infection.[239,240]

Surprisingly, IFN-γ expression in normal volunteers was limited to the subset with evidence of previous exposure (either seropositive before challenge or demonstrating resistance to infection).[237] Similarly, IFN-γ production by cells from HIV patients during active cryptosporidiosis and from Haitian children with active cryptosporidiosis was very low, despite the fact that they had self-limited disease.[169,235] Thus, other factors appear to be involved in limiting human infection after initial exposure. In murine models, inactivation of IFN-γ expression resulted in only a mild chronic infection in BALB/c mice, but fatal infection in C57BL/6 mice.[230] Mild disease in BALB/c mice was associated with expression of IL-12, IL-4, and TNF-α.[168,241] In the absence of IFN-γ, IL-12 treatment only worsened cryptosporidiosis.[242] Similarly, treatment of AIDS patients with chronic cryptosporidiosis was associated with gastrointestinal side effects.[243] Although IL-4 synergizes with IFN-γ in eliminating infection of epithelial cells and IL-4 knockout mice displayed prolonged oocyst shedding, IL-4 treatment did not modulate infection in IFN-γ knockout mice.[242,244,245] By contrast, TNF-α limited infection in IFN-γ knockout mice, activated human epithelial cells to limit infection, and has been associated with control of infection in cattle.[165,168,238] In seronegative normal volunteers experimentally infected and AIDS patients recovering from cryptosporidiosis in response to antiretrovirals, control of infection was associated with expression of IL-15.[185,246] This effect is likely mediated by activation of natural killer cells. However, the role of natural killer cells in murine models has not been clearly demonstrated.[201-203] Another Th1 cytokine, IL-18, can limit cryptosporidiosis in IL-12 knockout mice and partially clear infection of epithelial cells in vitro.[247-249]

The role of antibody in the immune response to cryptosporidiosis is controversial.[172] Early studies noted cases of chronic cryptosporidiosis in patients with low antibody levels, but in most cases, studies were not performed to exclude coexisting T-cell dysfunction. In animal models, inactivation of B cells by antibody to the μ-chain or inactivation of the *muMT* gene did not affect clearance of cryptosporidiosis.[250,251] By contrast, treatment with high concentrations of anti-*Cryptosporidium* antibody did facilitate clearance.[252-256] Anecdotal reports suggested that hyperimmune bovine colostrums might improve cryptosporidiosis in AIDS, but a large randomized, controlled trial demonstrated no clinical benefit and decreases in oocyst shedding only at very high doses.[257] High levels of serum and fecal antibodies to *C. parvum* have been found in AIDS patients with chronic cryptosporidiosis.[258,259] Studies of the fecal antibody response in volunteers challenged with *C. parvum* demonstrated specific fecal antibody in most volunteers.[260] However, the presence and timing of antibody correlated with oocyst shedding rather than clearance or resistance to infection. Similarly, cytokines such as transforming growth factor-β that stimulate immunoglobulin A production often develop only after resolution of illness.[261] Thus, the role of antibody in cryptosporidiosis is at most modest. Nonimmune mechanisms may also be important in control of human cryptosporidiosis. For example, mannose-binding lectin levels have been shown to be low in AIDS patients and children with cryptosporidiosis. Mice with the mannose binding lectin gene inactivated are more susceptible to infection.[262-264] Beta defensins are induced in response to *Cryptosporidium* infection and can kill the parasites in vitro.[265,266]

Clinical Manifestations

Symptoms of cryptosporidiosis develop after a prepatent period during which the parasites invade the intestinal epithelium and proliferate. Studies of immunocompetent individuals with discrete exposures (e.g., travelers, point-source outbreaks, experimental infection) demonstrate a prepatent period of approximately 1 week.[11,35,267,268] There is, however, considerable variability, with a range of 1 to 30 days. This variability reflects in part strain differences between the organisms rather than dose.[26,35,268] Cryptosporidiosis is noted in both males and females. The age distribution varies considerably with the epidemiology of exposure. In developing countries, most cases occur among children younger than 5 years old. This is thought to reflect both high rates of fecal-oral exposure in children and the development of immunity in older children and adults. By contrast, in Finland, nearly all cases occur in adults, reflecting an association with foreign travel.[267] Waterborne epidemics in developed countries affect all ages.[58,128] Because *Cryptosporidium* infects primarily intestinal epithelial cells, it is not surprising that diarrhea is the most common clinical presentation. However, there are significant differences in the clinical presentation depending on the host and parasite population. The major groups include immunocompetent individuals in developed countries, children in developing countries, and immunocompromised hosts (primarily patients with AIDS).

IMMUNOCOMPETENT INDIVIDUALS IN DEVELOPED COUNTRIES

Most case series of immunocompetent individuals from developed countries have been associated with waterborne outbreaks, infection in travelers, animal contact, or infections of children in daycare and their contacts.[111,126] Most patients in outbreaks and among travelers are adults. Immunocompetent adults most commonly present with diarrhea. The diarrhea is usually described as watery, but may also be described as mucoid.[269] The median duration of illness in most case series is approximately 5 to 10 days. Accompanying symptoms are similar to those noted with other diarrheal illnesses including abdominal cramps, nausea, vomiting, and fever.[269] In comparative studies, cryptosporidiosis is less likely to cause vomiting than other causes of diarrhea. In one study, cryptosporidiosis was more frequently associated with respiratory symptoms.[270] As many as 40% of cases develop recurrent symptoms after initial resolution, which may lead to chronic symptoms similar to irritable bowel syndrome.[11,55,128,271,272] Relapses may follow a diarrhea-free period of several days to weeks. Clinical illness is more frequent and severe among the elderly.[273-275]

Several lines of evidence suggest that milder or even asymptomatic infection may also be very common. For example, seroconversion is more common than is clinically diagnosed disease in developed as well as developing countries.[81,84,85,276-278] During the large outbreak in Milwaukee, only a minority of the estimated 403,000 affected individuals presented for clinical care.[269,279] Patients identified by active case-finding or in children with negative stool studies were less severely ill and had a shorter duration of diarrhea than patients with cases confirmed by laboratory test results. Similarly, in a study of a waterborne outbreak involving a drug-treatment facility, immunocompetent cases had a mild illness, lasting only 4 days.[144] In addition, studies of normal volunteers challenged with *C. parvum* demonstrate that among those infected, most presented with a subclinical or mild illness only lasting for fewer than 5 days.[35,36,74,86,268] Many of the individuals with milder cases did not shed enough organisms to be detected by immunofluorescence, although, in some cases, infection was documented by flow cytometric analysis.[35]

CHILDHOOD DIARRHEA IN DEVELOPING COUNTRIES

Childhood diarrhea is the most common clinical manifestation of cryptosporidiosis in developing countries. Investigators in Asia, Africa, and Latin America have carefully studied cryptosporidial diarrheal illness among children.[28,29,33,55,68,123,127,169,280-285] These studies have demonstrated that cryptosporidiosis is common, causing at least 5% to 10% of cases of diarrhea. Most present with an acute diarrheal syndrome similar to that seen with other enteric pathogens with watery diarrhea, cramps, and abdominal pain. Less common features may include fever, shortness of breath, cough, and foul stools. Although most cases resolve quickly, as many as 45% of cases develop diarrhea persisting beyond 14 days.[127,286] Thus, *Cryptosporidium* is among the more common causes of persistent diarrhea in developing countries, causing approximately one third of cases.[28,29,55,141,286] It can also cause chronic diarrhea and malabsorption.[287,288] Furthermore, an episode of

persistent diarrhea, especially if caused by *Cryptosporidium*, is a marker for the onset of increased risk of recurrent episodes of diarrhea, weight loss, and premature death.[280,289-291] A long-term follow-up study of children with onset of cryptosporidiosis before age 1 year suggested an association with poorer physical fitness and poorer cognitive development that persists for years.[233] In a second study, long-term effects of early childhood malnutrition were noted, but there was no significant association with *Cryptosporidium* compared with other pathogens.[292] However, total duration of diarrhea is an important predictor of malnutrition. *Cryptosporidium* is more commonly associated with persistent diarrhea than other causes.[293] Molecular studies have demonstrated clinical differences between *Cryptosporidium* species and subtypes. In most studies, *C. hominis* is associated with more severe disease (more dehydration, longer duration, more oocysts shed) and *C. meleagridis* with milder disease.[33,271,283,285]

CRYPTOSPORIDIUM AND MALNUTRITION

Studies of childhood diarrhea in developing countries have consistently demonstrated an association between cryptosporidiosis and malnutrition. Case series and case-control studies noted that cryptosporidiosis was more severe in children with malnutrition.[28,55,123,141,143,291,294-296] For example, most deaths occur in malnourished children. These studies did not clearly distinguish the effects of cryptosporidiosis on nutritional status from the effects of malnutrition on cryptosporidiosis. Studies prospectively examining both nutritional status and *Cryptosporidium* infection in cohorts of children followed from birth demonstrated significant differences in nutritional status before *Cryptosporidium* infection.[280,297,298] Onset of cryptosporidiosis was associated with growth faltering, with a decrease of 300 to 400 g. Older children eventually recovered and experienced catch-up growth. In contrast, children infected before 1 year of age often never recovered.[280,297,298] In one study, children who were stunted at the time of *Cryptosporidium* infection also did not recover weight.[298] Furthermore, even asymptomatic infection (i.e., no diarrhea) was associated with mild growth faltering.[299] Thus, *Cryptosporidium* infection clearly causes acute malnutrition, and the long-term consequences of this interaction are likely to be worse in those infected in infancy or with previous malnutrition.

CRYPTOSPORIDIOSIS IN HUMAN IMMUNODEFICIENCY VIRUS INFECTION

HIV infection has been the most common host defense defect associated with cryptosporidiosis. Before the advent of effective antiretroviral combinations, most patients diagnosed with cryptosporidiosis had underlying HIV infection.[133] However, the incidence of cryptosporidiosis in HIV has dramatically decreased with improvements in antiretroviral therapy.[300,301] The clinical manifestations of cryptosporidiosis in HIV patients are variable. Among patients with CD4 cell counts greater than 150 cells/μL, most cases of cryptosporidiosis are self-limited, similar to those in normal hosts.[133,153,211,302] However, even these cases are more likely to relapse if the cellular immune response deteriorates. Surprisingly, in population-based studies, a substantial portion of *Cryptosporidium* infections in HIV patients are asymptomatic, and some cases are mild and self-limited, even in patients with advanced HIV infection. Other patients develop a chronic diarrheal illness. *Cryptosporidium* can be found in the stools of as many as three fourths of AIDS patients with diarrhea when stools are tested by PCR.[70-73] The chronic diarrhea is associated with frequent, foul-smelling, bulky stools. Most patients experience weight loss. Not surprisingly, studies have demonstrated nutrient malabsorption. Voluminous watery diarrhea or cholera-like illness develops in a minority of patients. The clinical picture is often confused by other concomitant opportunistic infections, including microsporidiosis, disseminated *Mycobacterium* infection, or cytomegaloviral colitis.[133,153] There may be slight differences in the clinical manifestations depending on the parasite species with milder disease caused by *C. meleagridis* and some *C. hominis* subtypes.[32,303]

Cryptosporidiosis in AIDS is also associated with extraintestinal disease, including involvement of the biliary and respiratory tract.[133,304-307] Respiratory tract involvement is often asymptomatic, but may also manifest as bilateral pulmonary infiltrates with dyspnea. Biliary tract involvement in cryptosporidiosis has been limited to patients with profound immunodeficiency. Biliary involvement correlated with a low CD4 cell count and a markedly shortened survival.[133,307] Patients may present with acalculous cholecystitis, sclerosing cholangitis, or pancreatitis.[133,307,308] Most patients present with right upper quadrant abdominal pain, which may be intermittent and colicky. Laboratory studies characteristically reveal elevated levels of alkaline phosphatase. Levels of bilirubin and transaminases are often elevated as well. In patients with associated pancreatitis, amylase and lipase are increased. Ultrasound examination may reveal dilation of the biliary duct and/or signs of gallbladder inflammation. However, most patients require an endoscopic retrograde cholecystopancreatographic evaluation to make the anatomic diagnosis. Biopsy specimens of the biliary ducts, staining of the bile, or stool studies may demonstrate the parasites. Most cases of biliary disease will reveal evidence of coinfection with cytomegalovirus or microsporidia as well.

Diagnosis

Parasites were first demonstrated by histologic staining of intestinal tissues. The organisms appear along the surface of the epithelial cells and may appear to be in the lumen (see Fig. 283-2). The intracellular forms stain purple with hematoxylin. Tissues are available only after invasive procedures, and the organisms are not consistently identified in biopsy specimens.

Like most intestinal parasites, *Cryptosporidium* infection is usually diagnosed by microscopic examination of stool. Generally, stools are preserved in 10% buffered formalin.[309,310] Fresh stools can also be tested, but are infectious to laboratory personnel.[310] Polyvinyl alcohol interferes with staining techniques and is not recommended. Frozen stools can be used for some immunoassays. Potassium dichromate (2.5%) can also be used to preserve organisms, but it does not decrease oocyst viability.

A number of concentration methods have been attempted. Formalin ether and formalin–ethyl acetate methods are commonly used in clinical laboratories. Either technique can improve the yield in cryptosporidiosis. However, oocysts may fail to sediment if centrifugation speeds or time are not increased.[309-311] Flotation methods (e.g., Sheather's sucrose flotation or sodium chloride) facilitate identification of the organisms. All are laborious and are used mainly in research laboratories. Immunomagnetic beads can be used to isolate and concentrate organisms and can dramatically improve sensitivity of stool examination.[26,309,312]

Wet mounts may be initially screened by direct or phase-contrast microscopy, which may allow rapid identification of heavy infection. However, the oocysts are small, 4 to 6 m in diameter, and similar in size and shape to yeast forms normally found in stool. They do not stain well with iodine or trichrome and cannot be differentiated from yeast forms by Giemsa staining. Thus, traditional approaches to stool examinations usually miss the organism. Many laboratories will not test for *Cryptosporidium* unless the tests are specifically requested.[63]

Differential staining was first noted with acid-fast stains. Oocysts stain pink or red, whereas yeast cells and fecal debris stain green or blue (Fig. 283-3). The most commonly used stain is a modification of the Ziehl-Neelsen stain.[309,310] A number of other modifications have been described including hot and cold techniques, incorporation of dimethyl sulfoxide, and use of the detergent Tergetol. The sensitivity of stool examination with acid-fast staining remains poor, requiring an oocyst concentration of greater than 500,000/mL in formed stools,[313] with fewer cases detected than with fluorescent methods.[314,315] Fluorescent stains (e.g., auramine O, auramine-rhodamine) can be read more quickly than other acid-fast stains and may have improved sensitivity (see Fig. 283-3).[316] However, these assays are plagued by false-positive results. All the acid-fast stains detect other parasites that may cause similar illnesses (e.g., *Isospora* and *Cyclospora*).

Immunofluorescent assays using oocyst-specific monoclonal antibodies are now commonly used to test for cryptosporidiosis. Immunofluorescent assay has been reported to be as sensitive[317-319] or as many as 10 times more sensitive than acid-fast staining.[314,315,320,321] Direct immunofluorescence using monoclonal antibodies is now the gold standard for stool examination. Some of the commercial immunofluorescent assays (Merifluor *Cryptosporidium/Giardia*, Meridian Diagnostics) are also sensitive and specific assays in giardiasis.[315,319]

Antigen-detection assays are being increasingly used for stool diagnosis. Commercial kits for *Cryptosporidium* are available in enzyme-linked immunosorbent assay and immunochromatographic formats. The enzyme-linked immunosorbent assay kits for *Cryptosporidium* have generally performed well for diagnosis of cryptosporidiosis with sensitivities ranging from 66% to 100% with excellent specificity.[309,310,317,319,322,323] Although the sensitivity has been poor in some studies,[315,318,324] most study results suggest improved sensitivity compared with microscopic methods. Quality control, however, may be an issue. For example, two kits were associated with pseudo-outbreaks stemming from false-positive results.[325,326] Some commercial enzyme-linked immunosorbent assay kits also test for *Giardia* and *Entamoeba* antigens.[321,322,327,328] The immunochromatographic tests are rapid tests

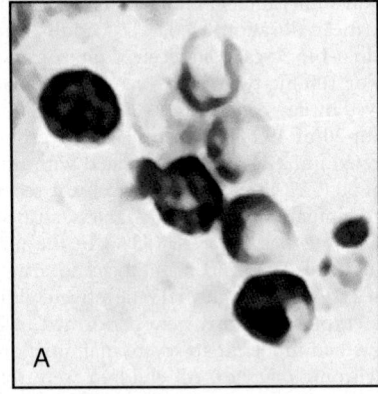 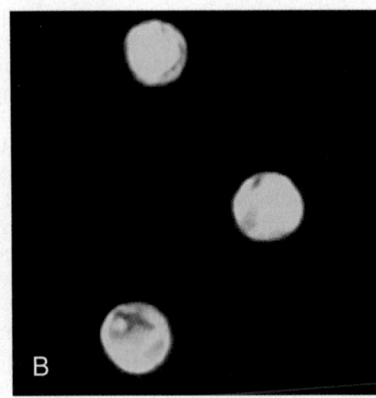 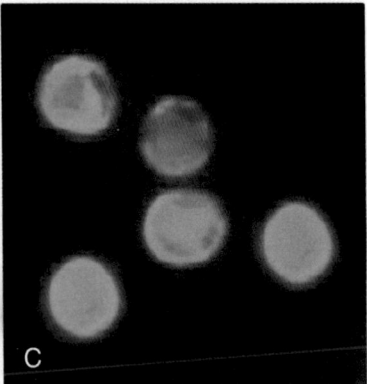

Figure 283-3 **Cryptosporidiosis is diagnosed by demonstration of organisms in stool samples.** This can be done with immunoassays for antigen or by microscopic demonstration of the organisms. Because the organisms are similar in size and shape to yeast normally found in stool, differential stains are required to identify the organism. These may include modified acid-fast stain (**A**) showing the oocysts are red organisms, fluorescent stains such as auramine-rhodamine (**B**), or immunofluorescence (**C**) (green organisms). *(From the Centers for Disease Control DpDx: Cryptosporidiosis. http://www.dpd.cdc.gov/dpdx/HTML/Cryptosporidiosis.htm.)*

for *Cryptosporidium* and *Giardia* antigen.[315,323,329] The sensitivity is similar to other assays, but the specificity is excellent and results are available in minutes.[315,323] Antigen assays as a group have the advantage of not requiring skills in microscopic identification of organisms.

PCR tests for *C. parvum* DNA have also been used to detect organisms. They also have increased sensitivity compared with microscopic studies of stool and nearly double the number of cases diagnosed compared with stool assays.[65,66,69,73,131] A recently developed commercial PCR enzyme-linked immunosorbent assay kit was able to detect 5 to 10 oocysts in spiked samples, suggesting that sensitive, standardized PCR assays may soon be available commercially.[330]

Management

Supportive therapy is a key component in the management of cryptosporidiosis. As is the case for all causes of diarrhea, replacement of fluids and electrolytes is a critically important first step in management. Oral rehydration is preferred, but severely ill patients may require parenteral fluids. Fluids should include sodium, potassium, bicarbonate, and glucose. Cryptosporidiosis is characterized by preferential loss of mature epithelial cells at the tips of the villi, and enzymes expressed on these cells including lactase are lost.[152] Thus, supportive care should include a lactose-free diet. In contrast to glucose-stimulated sodium pumps, which are expressed on the villus tips, glutamine-stimulated sodium absorption is not affected.[183,200] Glutamine supplementation, usually given in the form of alanyl-glutamine, may improve fluid absorption.[331-333] Although nutrition remains important, oral feeding is as effective as parenteral nutrition.[334]

Cryptosporidiosis is associated with increased intestinal transit, which could interfere with absorption of fluids, electrolytes, and drugs.[192,335] Thus, antimotility agents play a key role in therapy. Opiates are usually used as the initial antimotility agents. Loperamide and diphenoxylate/atropine combinations may ameliorate symptoms, but their efficacy is limited in severe disease. More potent opiates including tincture of opium may work in patients who have not responded. Octreotide, a synthetic peptide analogue of somatostatin, is approved by the U.S. Food and Drug Administration for the treatment of tumor-induced secretory diarrhea. Several trials have examined octreotide therapy in AIDS patients with diarrhea. Overall, octreotide was effective but not consistently more effective than other oral antidiarrheal agents.[336,337] Because of its high cost, its use is generally limited to refractory cases. The results of a single study suggested that the enkephalinase inhibitor acetorphan is more effective than somatostatin in AIDS-associated diarrhea.[338]

For immunodeficient patients, restoration of the immune response should be pursued. For AIDS patients with chronic cryptosporidiosis, effective antiretroviral therapy can result in dramatic improvement in diarrhea.[185,339-343] This should generally take the form of combinations of three or more potent antiretroviral drugs. The HIV protease inhibitors have anticryptosporidial activity in vitro and reduced infection by as much as 90% in an animal model.[344,345] Cryptosporidiosis can also cause malabsorption of antiretroviral medications, especially nucleoside reverse-transcriptase inhibitors.[331,335] With the data on their activity against *Cryptosporidium* and their higher genetic barrier to HIV resistance, I believe that HIV protease inhibitor–based combinations may have advantages over regimens based on non-nucleoside reverse-transcriptase inhibitors. Several recent studies have combined antiretroviral therapy with antiparasitic agents.[185,342,346] Although unproven, this approach should in theory improve the response to both treatments.

Biliary involvement in cryptosporidiosis usually requires specific interventions. Acalculous cholecystitis should be treated with cholecystectomy.[347] Patients with sclerosing cholangitis can usually be treated by endoscopic retrograde cholangiopancreatography. Sphincterotomy may result in temporary improvement. However, symptoms often recur unless a stent is placed.[133,348-350]

The role of antiparasitic therapy in cryptosporidiosis has been difficult to demonstrate. Attempts to screen drugs for anticryptosporidial

activity in vitro and in animal models have met with limited success.[351] In vitro screening of more than 200 agents failed to identify any highly effective agent. For some drugs, resistance is attributable to target insensitivity. For example, the *Cryptosporidium* dihydrofolate reductase-thymidylate synthetase contains novel amino acids at sites associated with antifolate resistance in other species.[352-355] A second reason for drug resistance stems from the unique location of the parasite within the host cell, but segregated in the parasitophorous vacuole, which does not communicate with the epithelial cell cytoplasm.[195]

No agent has proved reliably curative in severely immunocompromised patients. Because cryptosporidiosis is usually self-limited in immunocompetent hosts and can be variable in immunocompromised hosts, controlled trials are critically important. In compromised hosts, however, most trials have not been designed to detect partially active agents. Few studies of AIDS patients have rigorously excluded patients coinfected with *Mycobacteria*, microsporidia, or cytomegalovirus, all of which are common coinfections that may mask the effects of anticryptosporidial treatments.[356-358] Although a meta-analysis of seven randomized, controlled clinical trials found no clear evidence of efficacy of antiparasitic agents in the management of cryptosporidiosis in compromised hosts,[359] partially active drugs (which might prove useful in combination or in situations in which the patient's immune response can be boosted) may have been labeled as ineffective.

Nitazoxanide is a nitrothiazolyl-salicylamide, broad-spectrum antiparasitic drug.[360,361] Initial studies noted efficacy versus *Taenia saginata* and *Hymenolepis nana*. However, clinical development progressed only after antiprotozoal activity was demonstrated in the early 1990s. Nitazoxanide suspension was approved in the United States for treatment of cryptosporidiosis and giardiasis in children in 2002. Nitazoxanide is active against *Cryptosporidium* in vitro and in animal models. Nitazoxanide inhibits growth in vitro at concentrations of less than 10 μg/mL.[362,363] The metabolite tizoxanide is less active, but tizoxanide glucuronide is nearly as active as the parent compound. Nitazoxanide decreased parasite numbers, but was not curative in neonatal mice, immunosuppressed rats, and gnotobiotic pigs; it was not effective in SCID mice depleted of IFN-γ.[364-366]

Doumbo and colleagues[367] reported that 7 of 12 AIDS patients with cryptosporidiosis improved with a 7-day course of nitazoxanide, but diarrhea completely resolved in only 4 days. A randomized, controlled study of nitazoxanide in HIV patients with cryptosporidiosis performed in Mexico compared doses of 500 mg twice daily, 1 g twice daily, and placebo for 2 weeks.[368] Among HIV patients with CD4 cell counts greater than 50 cells/μL, 10 of 14 (71%) responded to 1 g/day and 9 of 10 (90%) to 2 g/day compared with 3 of 15 (20%) treated with placebo. By contrast, the response was no better than placebo for patients with CD4 cell counts of 50 cells/μL or less.

Three randomized trials were performed in patients with cryptosporidiosis who were not infected with HIV. An outpatient study was performed in Egypt on adults and children with cryptosporidiosis and prolonged diarrhea (mean duration, 13 days).[369] Adults, children 4 to 11 years old, or children 1 to 3 years old received nitazoxanide in doses of 500 mg, 200 mg, or 100 mg twice daily or matching placebo for 3 days. Diarrhea resolved by day 7 in 39 of 49 (80%) in the nitazoxanide group compared with 20 of 49 (41%) in the placebo group. Oocysts were no longer detected in 33 of 49 (67%) treated with nitazoxanide compared with 11 of 50 (22%) treated with placebo. A second trial of outpatients in Egypt compared nitazoxanide tablets, suspension, and placebo. The response rate was 27 of 28 (93%) in the nitazoxanide arms compared with 10 of 27 (37%) in the placebo arm.[370] Parallel randomized trials of HIV-infected and HIV-negative children hospitalized with chronic cryptosporidiosis were performed in Zambia.[287] Nearly all the subjects had moderate to severe malnutrition and persistent diarrhea or chronic diarrhea. All children were treated with nitazoxanide suspension (100 mg twice daily for 3 days) or matching placebo. In the trial of HIV-negative children, diarrhea had resolved by day 7 in 14 of 25 (56%) of those treated with nitazoxanide compared with 5 of 22 (23%) treated with placebo. Follow-up stool studies were free of oocysts in 13 of 25 (52%) children in the treatment group compared with 3 of 22 (14%) in the placebo group. Most of those who did not respond became well after a second course, given open label. Four HIV-negative children died; all were in the placebo group. Among the HIV-infected children, there were no significant differences in clinical and parasitologic responses or in mortality rate with nitazoxanide treatment.[287] An open-label study noted a response rate of 59% of AIDS patients treated with nitazoxanide.[371] Most were treated at doses of 1 g twice daily for at least 2 weeks. Thus, patients with severe defects of the cellular immune response may benefit from higher doses (e.g., 1 g twice daily), longer duration of treatment, or combined therapy with antiretroviral drugs and perhaps other antiparasitic agents.

Paromomycin is an orally administered nonabsorbable aminoglycoside originally approved in the 1960s as a luminal amebicide. Initial in vitro studies noted poor activity against *C. parvum*. However, when AIDS patients with cryptosporidiosis were treated with available antiparasitic drugs, some improved when treated with paromomycin.[133,351] Subsequently, in vitro studies demonstrated limited activity against *Cryptosporidium* with inhibitory concentrations in the range of 100 to 500 µg/mL.[351] Paromomycin is effective in animal models of cryptosporidiosis, but usually requires doses of 100 to 500 mg/kg/day.[351] Doses of approximately 25 to 35 mg/kg/day in two to four doses have been used in human trials, with estimated drug levels in the intestinal lumen barely more than the amount of drug needed to inhibit the organisms in cell culture.[372] The first 12 published case series of AIDS patients treated with paromomycin included more than 300 patients with a response rate of 67%.[133,373] Many of those with initial improvement later relapsed. Three randomized, controlled trials examined the effects of paromomycin in AIDS patients with cryptosporidiosis. Kanyok and colleagues[374] presented preliminary data from a small trial in 1993 demonstrating efficacy of paromomycin. In a small placebo-controlled trial incorporating quantitation of oocyst excretion, the paromomycin arm demonstrated a significant reduction in oocyst shedding (~70%), decreased stool frequency in those treated with paromomycin, but no cures.[356] Biliary tract involvement and *Mycobacteria* coinfection were common in those not responding. Hewitt and colleagues[375] compared paromomycin with placebo in a trial that included 35 AIDS patients. There was no difference between groups when analyzing those receiving treatment, but dropouts occurred only in the placebo arm. By intent-to-treat analysis with dropouts grouped with failures, the response rate was similar to that of previous trials with a trend favoring paromomycin over placebo.[358] The trial was prematurely terminated because of poor enrollment and was not powered to detect limited response rates. Limited efforts were made to exclude coinfections. Dose escalation demonstrated no further improvement with higher doses,[358] and higher doses have been associated with gastrointestinal and ototoxicity.[372] A meta-analysis of trials of antiparasitic drugs noted no clear evidence of efficacy.[359] However, this analysis has significant limitations, including the small numbers in trials and design flaws in the studies noted.

Macrolide antibiotics including spiramycin, azithromycin, roxithromycin, and clarithromycin have some activity against *Cryptosporidium*.[351] Spiramycin has been marketed in Europe for treatment of toxoplasmosis and respiratory tract infections. Sáez-Lloren and colleagues[376] reported shorter duration of symptoms and oocyst shedding when children were treated with 100 mg/kg/day spiramycin, but a second trial showed no effect.[377] The AIDS Clinical Trial Group (ACTG) conducted a randomized, controlled trial in 75 AIDS patients comparing spiramycin with placebo, but noted that spiramycin was not significantly better than placebo.[351] A trial of intravenous spiramycin was associated with significantly decreased oocyst shedding and a partial response in 75% of subjects.[351] However, there were high rates of adverse events including drug-associated intestinal injury.[378] Azithromycin has some activity against *Cryptosporidium* in vitro and in animal studies.[351] Case series note improvement in cryptosporidiosis among HIV and cancer patients treated with azithromycin.[379-381] In a placebo-controlled, multicenter trial, AIDS patients with cryptosporidiosis were randomly assigned to receive azithromycin 900 mg/day

PO or placebo. Overall, oocyst shedding, stool frequency, and weight loss were not significantly different.[351] A subsequent pilot trial of intravenous azithromycin also did not demonstrate changes in stool frequency or oocyst shedding.[351] Similar results were reported from another prospective study.[373] A pilot study in Egyptian schoolchildren suggested more rapid resolution with azithromycin treatment.[382]

Clarithromycin is also active in vitro and in animal studies.[383] There are only limited data on treatment of human cryptosporidiosis with clarithromycin. However, the drug may be useful in chemoprophylaxis (see later). Roxithromycin treatment was associated with improvement in AIDS-associated cryptosporidiosis in two uncontrolled studies.[384,385] Rifaximin, a nonabsorbable rifamycin, is approved by the U.S. Food and Drug Administration for the treatment of traveler's diarrhea. Although it has some activity against cryptosporidiosis in HIV patients, its efficacy has not been shown in rigorous trials.[386,387]

Anecdotal reports noted improvement in chronic cryptosporidiosis in patients treated with oral anti-*Cryptosporidium* immunoglobulin preparations.[388] However, two well-controlled trials examined oral bovine anti-*Cryptosporidium* immunoglobulin preparations in cryptosporidiosis. Bovine anti-*Cryptosporidium* immunoglobulin did not significantly decrease symptoms or oocyst shedding in experimental infection of volunteers.[389] In a large trial of bovine anti-*Cryptosporidium* immunoglobulin for cryptosporidiosis in AIDS patients, there was no effect on symptoms, and oocyst shedding decreased only slightly at a dose of 20 g/day.[257] At higher doses, oocyst excretion decreased, but the immunoglobulin preparation caused diarrhea.

Because individual drugs have limited activity, studies have investigated the effects of combinations. Smith and colleagues[357] conducted a pilot study of the combination of paromomycin combined with azithromycin in AIDS patients with chronic cryptosporidiosis. Overall, there was a 2-log decrease in oocyst shedding, but few patients were cured. Clinical failures were associated with biliary disease, coinfection with other enteric pathogens (especially cytomegalovirus), or side effects of the medications. Thus, combination therapy warrants further study.

▪ Prevention

Cryptosporidiosis is transmitted from person to person and via contaminated water and food. Water purification is an important public health measure. Because chlorination has little effect on the oocysts, water purification should generally involve flocculation and filtration.[98,99] Ultraviolet radiation or ozonation can disinfect contaminated water, but they are rarely used. Recreational waters, such as lakes, may pose a danger for compromised hosts, who should avoid untreated water.[390] Swimming pools are now an important source of infection. Contamination of treated recreational water, such as a fecal accident in a swimming pool, should prompt aggressive measures, including closing the pool temporarily.

Personal measures can be used to decontaminate infected or potentially infected water, such as in travel to developing countries, when the public water supply is contaminated, or as a routine in compromised hosts.[390] Water can be decontaminated by bringing it to a boil or by filtration using a filter with a pore size of 1 µm or smaller.[390,391]

Although cryptosporidiosis can be transmitted within health care facilities, risk is minimal with standard precautions.[125] Gloves should be worn and hands washed after handling material contaminated with fecal material. Instruments such as endoscopes need to be carefully disinfected between uses. Wearing gloves and handwashing can also prevent infection in daycare centers.

For patients with AIDS (CD4 cell counts less than 200 cells/µL), water should be boiled or filtered.[390] If HIV-infected persons travel in developing countries, they should be warned to meticulously avoid drinking tap water. They should avoid obvious sources of *Cryptosporidium* oocysts, such as people with diarrhea (particularly avoiding sexual practices that might involve exposure to feces), farm animals (particularly cattle), and domestic pets that are either very young (≤6 months) or have diarrhea. Chemoprophylaxis should also be considered. Two retrospective studies examined data from trials of prophylaxis of *Mycobacterium avium* for their effects on cryptosporidiosis. Holmberg and colleagues[392] compared the incidence of cryptosporidiosis in those given rifabutin, clarithromycin, or no drug for prevention of *M. avium* complex among patients in the HIV Outpatient Study cohort. The incidence of cryptosporidiosis was much lower in those treated with rifabutin and also lower in those treated with clarithromycin. Fichtenbaum and colleagues[393] analyzed patients enrolled in controlled trials of clarithromycin, rifabutin, both, or no drug for *M. avium* complex prophylaxis. They also noted a lower incidence of cryptosporidiosis than in groups treated with rifabutin. However, they could not confirm the efficacy of clarithromycin. However, the incidence of cryptosporidiosis was low in both studies. Rifaximin, a poorly absorbed rifamycin antibiotic approved by the U.S. Food and Drug Administration for treatment and commonly used to prevent traveler's diarrhea, may have some activity against *Cryptosporidium*, but the efficacy of therapy has not been addressed in vigorous trials.[386,387]

Experimental studies suggest that it may be possible to develop a vaccine to prevent cryptosporidiosis.[253,394-397] Vaccination would likely have to involve both human and animal hosts and would need to work against a number of species of parasites. Studies have so far not even demonstrated the feasibility of this approach.

REFERENCES

1. Tyzzer EE. A sporozoan found in peptic glands of the common mouse. *Proc Soc Exp Biol Med.* 1907;5:12-13.
2. Tyzzer EE. *Cryptosporidium parvum* (sp #nov) a coccidium found in the small intestine of the common mouse. *Arch Protistenkunde.* 1912;26:394-398.
3. Slavin D. *Cryptosporidium meleagridis* (sp nov). *J Comp Pathol.* 1955;65:262-266.
4. Pancier RJ, Thomassen RW, Garner FM. Cryptosporidial infection in a calf. *Vet Pathol.* 1971;8:479-484.
5. Nime FA, Burek JD, Page DL, et al. Acute enterocolitis in a human being infected with the protozoan *Cryptosporidium. Gastroenterology.* 1976;70:592-598.
6. Meisel JL, Perera DR, Meligro C, et al. Overwhelming watery diarrhea associated with a cryptosporidium in an immunosuppressed patient. *Gastroenterology.* 1976;70:1156-1160.
7. Cryptosporidiosis: assessment of chemotherapy of males with acquired immune deficiency syndrome (AIDS). *MMWR Morb Mortal Wkly Rep.* 1982;31:589-592.
8. Current WL, Reese NC, Ernst JV, et al. Human cryptosporidiosis in immunocompetent and immunodeficient persons: studies of an outbreak and experimental transmission. *N Engl J Med.* 1983;308:1252-1257.
9. Wolfson JS, Richter JM, Waldron MA, et al. Cryptosporidiosis in immunocompetent hosts. *N Engl J Med.* 1985;312:1278-1282.
10. D'Antonio RG, Win RE, Taylor JP, et al. A waterborne outbreak of cryptosporidiosis in normal hosts. *Ann Intern Med.* 1986;103: 886-888.
11. MacKenzie WR, Hoxie NJ, Proctor ME, et al. A massive outbreak of *Cryptosporidium* infection transmitted through the public water supply. *N Engl J Med.* 1994;331:161-167.
12. Kosek M, Alcantara C, Lima AA, et al. Cryptosporidiosis: an update. *Lancet Infect Dis.* 2001;1:262-269.
13. Chen XM, Keithly JS, Paya CV, et al. Cryptosporidiosis. *N Engl J Med.* 2002;346:1723-1731.
14. Bushen OY, Lima AA, Guerrant RL. Cryptosporidiosis. In: Guerrant RL, Walker DH, Weller PF, eds. *Tropical Infectious Diseases. Principle, Pathogens, and Practice.* Philadelphia: Churchill Livingstone, 2006:1003-1014.
15. Zhu G, Keithly JS, Philippe H. What is the phylogenetic position of *Cryptosporidium*? *Int J Syst Evol Microbiol.* 2000;50:1673-1681.
16. Barta JR, Thompson RC. What is *Cryptosporidium*? Reappraising its biology and phylogenetic affinities. *Trends Parasitol.* 2006;22:463-468.
17. Fayer R. General biology. In: Fayer R, Xiao L, eds. *Cryptosporidium and Cryptosporidiosis.* 2nd ed. Boca Raton, FL: CRC Press; 2008:1-42.
18. Kuo CH, Wares JP, Kissinger JC. The Apicomplexan whole-genome phylogeny: an analysis of incongruence among gene trees. *Mol Biol Evol.* 2008;25:2689-2698.
19. Xu P, Widmer G, Wang Y, et al. The genome of *Cryptosporidium hominis. Nature.* 2004;431:1107-1112.
20. Abrahamsen MS, Templeton TJ, Enomoto S, et al. Complete genome sequence of the apicomplexan, *Cryptosporidium parvum. Science.* 2004;304:441-445.
21. Kissinger JC. Genomics. In: Fayer R, Xiao L, eds. *Cryptosporidium and Cryptosporidiosis.* 2nd ed. Boca Raton, FL: CRC Press, 2008:43-56.
22. Xiao L, Fayer R, Ryan U, et al. *Cryptosporidium* taxonomy: recent advances and implications for public health. *Clin Microbiol Rev.* 2004;17:72-97.
23. Patel S, Pedraza-Diaz S, McLauchlin J, et al. Molecular characterisation of *Cryptosporidium parvum* from two large suspected waterborne outbreaks. Outbreak Control Team South and West Devon 1995, Incident Management Team and Further Epidemiological and Microbiological Studies Subgroup North Thames 1997. *Commun Dis Public Health.* 1998;1:231-233.
24. Robinson G, Elwin K, Chalmers RM. Unusual *Cryptosporidium* genotypes in human cases of diarrhea. *Emerg Infect Dis.* 2008;14:1800-1802.
25. Morgan-Ryan UM, Fall A, Ward LA, et al. *Cryptosporidium hominis* n. sp. (Apicomplexa: Cryptosporidiidae) from Homo sapiens. *J Eukaryot Microbiol.* 2002;49:433-440.
26. Pereira SJ, Ramirez NE, Xiao L, et al. Pathogenesis of human and bovine *Cryptosporidium parvum* in gnotobiotic pigs. *J Infect Dis.* 2002;186:715-718.
27. Pedraza-Diaz S, Amar CF, McLauchlin J, et al. *Cryptosporidium meleagridis* from humans: molecular analysis and description of affected patients. *J Infect.* 2001;42:243-250.
28. Tumwine JK, Kekitiinwa A, Nabukeera N, et al. *Cryptosporidium parvum* in children with diarrhea in Mulago Hospital, Kampala, Uganda. *Am J Trop Med Hyg.* 2003;68:710-715.
29. Gatei W, Wamae CN, Mbae C, et al. Cryptosporidiosis: prevalence, genotype analysis, and symptoms associated with infections in children in Kenya. *Am J Trop Med Hyg.* 2006;75: 78-82.
30. Muthusamy D, Rao SS, Ramani S, et al. Multilocus genotyping of *Cryptosporidium* sp. isolates from human immunodeficiency virus-infected individuals in South India. *J Clin Microbiol.* 2006;44:632-634.
31. Leoni F, Amar C, Nichols G, et al. Genetic analysis of *Cryptosporidium* from 2414 humans with diarrhoea in England between 1985 and 2000. *J Med Microbiol.* 2006;55:703-707.
32. Cama VA, Ross JM, Crawford S, et al. Differences in clinical manifestations among *Cryptosporidium* species and subtypes in HIV-infected persons. *J Infect Dis.* 2007;196:684-691.
33. Cama VA, Bern C, Roberts J, et al. *Cryptosporidium* species and subtypes and clinical manifestations in children, Peru. *Emerg Infect Dis.* 2008;14:1567-1574.
34. Nichols G. Epidemiology. In: Fayer R, Xiao L, eds. *Cryptosporidium and Cryptosporidiosis.* 2nd ed. Boca Raton, FL: CRC Press; 2008:79-118.
35. Okhuysen PC, Chappell CL, Crabb JH, et al. Virulence of three distinct *Cryptosporidium parvum* isolates for healthy adults. *J Infect Dis.* 1999;180:1275-1281.
36. Chappell CL, Okhuysen PC, Langer-Curry R, et al. *Cryptosporidium hominis*: experimental challenge of healthy adults. *Am J Trop Med Hyg.* 2006;75:851-857.
37. Forney JR, Yang S, Healey MC. Protease activity associated with excystation of *Cryptosporidium parvum* oocysts. *J Parasitol.* 1996;82:889-892.
38. Okhuysen PC, Chappell CL, Kettner C, et al. *Cryptosporidium parvum* metalloaminopeptidase inhibitors prevent in vitro excystation. *Antimicrob Agents Chemother.* 1996;40:2781-2784.
39. Wanyiri JW, O'Connor R, Allison G, et al. Proteolytic processing of the *Cryptosporidium* glycoprotein gp40/15 by human furin and by a parasite-derived furin-like protease activity. *Infect Immun.* 2007;75:184-192.
40. Feng X, Akiyoshi DE, Widmer G, et al. Characterization of subtilase protease in *Cryptosporidium parvum* and *C. hominis. J Parasitol.* 2007;93:619-626.
41. Na BK, Kang JM, Cheun HI, et al. Cryptopain-1, a cysteine protease of *Cryptosporidium parvum*, does not require the pro-domain for folding. *Parasitology.* 2009;136:149-157.
42. Choudhry N, Bajaj-Elliott M, McDonald V. The terminal sialic acid of glycoconjugates on the surface of intestinal epithelial cells activates excystation of *Cryptosporidium parvum. Infect Immun.* 2008;76:3735-3741.
43. Deng M, Templeton TJ, London NR, et al. *Cryptosporidium parvum* genes containing thrombospondin type 1 domains. *Infect Immun.* 2002;70:6987-6995.
44. Bhat N, Joe A, PereiraPerrin M, et al. *Cryptosporidium* p30, a galactose/N-acetylgalactosamine-specific lectin, mediates infection in vitro. *J Biol Chem.* 2007;282:34877-34887.
45. Borowski H, Clode PL, Thompson RC. Active invasion and/or encapsulation? A reappraisal of host-cell parasitism by *Cryptosporidium. Trends Parasitol.* 2008;24:509-516.
46. Chen XM, Huang BQ, Splinter PL, et al. Cdc42 and the actin-related protein/neural Wiskott-Aldrich syndrome protein network mediate cellular invasion by *Cryptosporidium parvum. Infect Immun.* 2004;72:3011-3021.
47. Chen XM, O'Hara SP, Huang BQ, et al. Localized glucose and water influx facilitates *Cryptosporidium parvum* cellular invasion by means of modulation of host-cell membrane protrusion. *Proc Natl Acad Sci U S A.* 2005;102:6338-6343.
48. O'Hara SP, Small AJ, Chen XM, et al. Host cell actin remodeling in response to *Cryptosporidium. Subcell Biochem.* 2008;47: 92-100.
49. Huang BQ, Chen XM, LaRusso NF. *Cryptosporidium parvum* attachment to and internalization by human biliary epithelia in vitro: a morphologic study. *J Parasitol.* 2004;90:212-221.
50. Griffiths JK, Balakrishnan R, Widmer G, et al. Paromomycin and geneticin inhibit intracellular *Cryptosporidium parvum* without trafficking through the host cell cytoplasm: implications for drug delivery. *Infect Immun.* 1998;66:3874-3883.
51. Perkins ME, Riojas YA, Wu TW, et al. CpABC, a *Cryptosporidium parvum* ATP-binding cassette protein at the host-parasite boundary in intracellular stages. *Proc Natl Acad Sci U S A.* 1999;96:5734-5739.
52. Hijjawi NS, Meloni BP, Morgan UM, et al. Complete development and long-term maintenance of *Cryptosporidium parvum* human and cattle genotypes in cell culture. *Int J Parasitol.* 2001;31:1048-1055.
53. Dillingham RA, Lima AA, Guerrant RL. Cryptosporidiosis: epidemiology and impact. *Microbes Infect.* 2002;4:1059-1066.
54. Nichols G, Chalmers R, Lake I, et al. Cryptosporidiosis: a report on the surveillance and epidemiology of *Cryptosporidium* infection in England and Wales: Foundation for Water Research, Marlow, Bucks, UK, 2006.
55. Newman RD, Sears CL, Moore SR, et al. Longitudinal study of *Cryptosporidium* infection in children in northeastern Brazil. *J Infect Dis.* 1999;180:167-175.
56. Perch M, Sodemann M, Jakobsen MS, et al. Seven years' experience with *Cryptosporidium parvum* in Guinea-Bissau, West Africa. *Ann Trop Paediatr.* 2001;21:313-318.
57. Bern C, Hernandez B, Lopez MB, et al. The contrasting epidemiology of *Cyclospora* and *Cryptosporidium* among outpatients in Guatemala. *Am J Trop Med Hyg.* 2000;63:231-235.
58. Yoder JS, Beach MJ. Cryptosporidiosis surveillance—United States, 2003-2005. *MMWR Surveill Summ.* 2007;56:1-10.
59. Semenza JC, Nichols G. Cryptosporidiosis surveillance and water-borne outbreaks in Europe. *Eur Surveill.* 2007;12:E13-E14.
60. Tuli L, Gulati AK, Sundar S, et al. Correlation between CD4 counts of HIV patients and enteric protozoan in different seasons—an experience of a tertiary care hospital in Varanasi (India). *BMC Gastroenterol.* 2008;8:36.
61. Muchiri JM, Ascolillo L, Mugambi M, et al. Seasonality of *Cryptosporidium* oocyst detection in surface waters of Meru, Kenya as determined by two isolation methods followed by PCR. *J Water Health.* 2009;7:67-75.
62. Mead PS, Slutsker L, Dietz V, et al. Food-related illness and death in the United States. *Emerg Infect Dis.* 1999;5:607-625.
63. Jones JL, Lopez A, Wahlquist SP, et al. Survey of clinical laboratory practices for parasitic diseases. *Clin Infect Dis.* 2004;38(Suppl 3):S198-S202.
64. Amin OM. Seasonal prevalence of intestinal parasites in the United States during 2000. *Am J Trop Med Hyg.* 2002;66:799-803.
65. Amar CF, East CL, Gray J, et al. Detection by PCR of eight groups of enteric pathogens in 4,627 faecal samples: re-examination of the English case-control Infectious Intestinal Disease Study (1993-1996). *Eur J Clin Microbiol Infect Dis.* 2007;26:311-323.
66. ten Hove R, Schuurman T, Kooistra M, et al. Detection of diarrhoea-causing protozoa in general practice patients in The Netherlands by multiplex real-time PCR. *Clin Microbiol Infect.* 2007;13:1001-1007.
67. Mor SM, Tzipori S. Cryptosporidiosis in children in sub-Saharan Africa: a lingering challenge. *Clin Infect Dis.* 2008;47:915-921.
68. Samie A, Bessong PO, Obi CL, et al. *Cryptosporidium* species: preliminary descriptions of the prevalence and genotype distribution among school children and hospital patients in the Venda region, Limpopo Province, South Africa. *Exp Parasitol.* 2006;114:314-322.
69. Ajjampur SS, Rajendran P, Ramani S, et al. Closing the diarrhoea diagnostic gap in Indian children by the application of molecular techniques. *J Med Microbiol.* 2008;57:1364-1368.
70. Houpt ER, Bushen OY, Sam NE, et al. Short report: asymptomatic *Cryptosporidium hominis* infection among human immunodeficiency virus-infected patients in Tanzania. *Am J Trop Med Hyg.* 2005;73:520-522.
71. Tumwine JK, Kekitiinwa A, Bakeera-Kitaka S, et al. Cryptosporidiosis and microsporidiosis in Ugandan children with persistent diarrhea with and without concurrent infection with the human immunodeficiency virus. *Am J Trop Med Hyg.* 2005;73:921-925.

72. Raccurt CP, Fouche B, Agnamey P, et al. Presence of *Enterocytozoon bieneusi* associated with intestinal coccidia in patients with chronic diarrhea visiting an HIV center in Haiti. *Am J Trop Med Hyg*. 2008;79:579-580.
73. Kaushik K, Khurana S, Wanchu A, et al. Evaluation of staining techniques, antigen detection and nested PCR for the diagnosis of cryptosporidiosis in HIV seropositive and seronegative patients. *Acta Trop*. 2008;107:1-7.
74. Okhuysen PC, Chappell CL, Sterling CR Jr, et al. Susceptibility and serologic response of healthy adults to reinfection with *Cryptosporidium parvum*. *Infect Immun*. 1998;66:441-443.
75. Frost F, de la Cruz AA, Moss DM, et al. Comparison of ELISA and Western blot assays for detection of *Cryptosporidium* antibody. *Epidemiol Infect*. 1998;121:205-211.
76. Moss DM, Bennett SM, Arrowood MJ, et al. Enzyme-linked immunotransfer blot analysis of a cryptosporidiosis outbreak on a United States Coast Guard cutter. *Am J Trop Med Hyg*. 1998;58:110-118.
77. Ungar BL, Mulligan M, Nutman TB. Serologic evidence of *Cryptosporidium* infection in US volunteers before and after Peace Corps service in Africa. *Arch Intern Med*. 1989;149:894-897.
78. Zu SX, Li JF, Barrett LJ, et al. Seroepidemiologic study of *Cryptosporidium* infection in children from rural communities of Anhui, China and Fortaleza, Brazil. *Am J Trop Med Hyg*. 1994;51:1-10.
79. Frost FJ, Muller T, Craun GF, et al. Serological evidence of endemic waterborne *Cryptosporidium* infections. *Ann Epidemiol*. 2002;12:222-227.
80. Lengerich EJ, Addiss DG, Marx JJ, et al. Increased exposure to cryptosporidia among dairy farmers in Wisconsin. *J Infect Dis*. 1993;167:1252-1255.
81. Kuhls TL, Mosier DA, Crawford DL, et al. Seroprevalence of cryptosporidial antibodies during infancy, childhood, and adolescence. *Clin Infect Dis*. 1994;18:731-735.
82. Leach CT, Koo FC, Kuhls TL, et al. Prevalence of *Cryptosporidium parvum* infection in children along the Texas-Mexico border and associated risk factors. *Am J Trop Med Hyg*. 2000;62:656-661.
83. Ungar BLP, Gilman RH, Lanata CF, et al. Seroepidemiology of *Cryptosporidium* infection in two Latin American populations. *J Infect Dis*. 1988;157:551-556.
84. Robin G, Fraser D, Orr N, et al. *Cryptosporidium* infection in Bedouin infants assessed by prospective evaluation of anticryptosporidial antibodies and stool examination. *Am J Epidemiol*. 2001;153:194-201.
85. Priest JW, Bern C, Roberts JM, et al. Changes in serum immunoglobulin G levels as a marker for *Cryptosporidium* sp. infection in Peruvian children. *J Clin Microbiol*. 2005;43:5298-5300.
86. DuPont H, Chappell C, Sterling C, et al. The infectivity of *Cryptosporidium parvum* in healthy volunteers. *N Engl J Med*. 1995;332:855-859.
87. Messner MJ, Chappell CL, Okhuysen PC. Risk assessment for *Cryptosporidium*: a hierarchical Bayesian analysis of human dose response data. *Water Res*. 2001;35:3934-3940.
88. Chappell CL, Okhuysen PC, Sterling CR, et al. Infectivity of *Cryptosporidium parvum* in healthy adults with pre-existing anti-*C. parvum* serum immunoglobulin G. *Am J Trop Med Hyg*. 1999;60:157-164.
89. Fayer R, Trout JM, Jenkins MC. Infectivity of *Cryptosporidium parvum* oocysts stored in water at environmental temperatures. *J Parasitol*. 1998;84:1165-1169.
90. Reinoso R, Becares E, Smith HV. Effect of various environmental factors on the viability of *Cryptosporidium parvum* oocysts. *J Appl Microbiol*. 2008;104:980-986.
91. Peng X, Murphy T, Holden NM. Evaluation of the effect of temperature on the die-off rate for *Cryptosporidium parvum* oocysts in water, soils, and feces. *Appl Environ Microbiol*. 2008;74:7101-7107.
92. Deng MQ, Cliver DO. Inactivation of *Cryptosporidium parvum* oocysts in cider by flash pasteurization. *J Food Prot*. 2001;64:523-527.
93. Korich DG, Mead JR, Madore MS, et al. Effects of ozone, chlorine dioxide, chlorine, and monochloramine on *Cryptosporidium parvum* oocyst viability. *Appl Environ Microbiol*. 1990;56:1423-1428.
94. Quinn CM, Betts WB. Longer term viability of chlorine-treated *Cryptosporidium* oocysts in tap water. *Biomed Lett*. 1993;48:315-318.
95. Carpenter C, Fayer R, Trout J, et al. Chlorine disinfection of recreational water for *Cryptosporidium parvum*. *Emerg Infect Dis*. 1999;5:579-584.
96. Fayer R. Effect of sodium hypochlorite exposure on infectivity of *Cryptosporidium parvum* oocysts for neonatal BALB/c mice. *Appl Environ Microbiol*. 1995;61:844-846.
97. Reinoso R, Becares E. Environmental inactivation of *Cryptosporidium parvum* oocysts in waste stabilization ponds. *Microb Ecol*. 2008;56:585-592.
98. Rose JB, Huffman DE, Gennaccaro A. Risk and control of waterborne cryptosporidiosis. *FEMS Microbiol Rev*. 2002;26:113-123.
99. Clancy JL, Hargy TM. Waterborne: drinking water. In: Fayer R, Xiao L, eds. *Cryptosporidium and Cryptosporidiosis*. 2nd ed. Boca Raton, FL: CRC Press; 2008:305-333.
100. Yoder J, Roberts V, Craun GF, et al. Surveillance for waterborne disease and outbreaks associated with drinking water and water not intended for drinking—United States, 2005-2006. *MMWR Surveill Summ*. 2008;57:39-62.
101. Ward PI, Deplazes P, Regli W, et al. Detection of eight *Cryptosporidium* genotypes in surface and waste waters in Europe. *Parasitology*. 2002;124:359-368.
102. LeChevallier MW, Di Giovanni GD, Clancy JL, et al. Comparison of method 1623 and cell culture-PCR for detection of *Cryptosporidium* spp. in source waters. *Appl Environ Microbiol*. 2003;69:971-979.
103. Xiao L, Alderisio KA, Jiang J. Detection of *Cryptosporidium* oocysts in water: effect of the number of samples and analytic replicates on test results. *Appl Environ Microbiol*. 2006;72:5942-5947.
104. Lake IR, Nichols G, Bentham G, et al. Cryptosporidiosis decline after regulation, England and Wales, 1989-2005. *Emerg Infect Dis*. 2007;13:623-625.
105. Sulaiman IM, Xiao L, Yang C, et al. Differentiating human from animal isolates of *Cryptosporidium parvum*. *Emerg Infect Dis*. 1998;4:681-685.
106. Leoni F, Mallon ME, Smith HV, et al. Multilocus analysis of *Cryptosporidium hominis* and *Cryptosporidium parvum* isolates from sporadic and outbreak-related human cases and *C. parvum* isolates from sporadic livestock cases in the United Kingdom. *J Clin Microbiol*. 2007;45:3286-3294.
107. Beach MJ. Waterborne: Recreational water. In: Fayer R, Xiao L, eds. *Cryptosporidium and Cryptosporidiosis*. 2nd ed. Boca Raton, FL: CRC Press; 2008:335-369.
108. Yoder JS, Hlavsa MC, Craun GF, et al. Surveillance for waterborne disease and outbreaks associated with recreational water use and other aquatic facility-associated health events—United States, 2005-2006. *MMWR Surveill Summ*. 2008;57:1-29.
109. Communitywide cryptosporidiosis outbreak—Utah, 2007. *MMWR Morb Mortal Wkly Rep*. 2008;57:989-993.
110. Robertson B, Sinclair MI, Forbes AB, et al. Case-control studies of sporadic cryptosporidiosis in Melbourne and Adelaide, Australia. *Epidemiol Infect*. 2002;128:419-431.
111. Roy SL, DeLong SM, Stenzel SA, et al. Risk factors for sporadic cryptosporidiosis among immunocompetent persons in the United States from 1999 to 2001. *J Clin Microbiol*. 2004;42:2944-2951.
112. Ortega YR, Cama VA. Foodborne transmission. In: Fayer R, Xiao L, eds. *Cryptosporidium and Cryptosporidiosis*. 2nd ed. Boca Raton, FL: CRC Press; 2008:289-304.
113. Gelletlie R, Stuart J, Soltanpoor N, et al. Cryptosporidiosis associated with school milk. *Lancet*. 1997;350:1005-1006.
114. Quiroz ES, Bern C, MacArthur JR, et al. An outbreak of cryptosporidiosis linked to a foodhandler. *J Infect Dis*. 2000;181:695-700.
115. Ortega YR, Roxas CR, Gilman RH, et al. Isolation of *Cryptosporidium parvum* and *Cyclospora cayetanensis* from vegetables collected in markets of an endemic region in Peru. *Am J Trop Med Hyg*. 1997;57:683-686.
116. Graczyk TK, Grimes BH, Knight R, et al. Detection of *Cryptosporidium parvum* and *Giardia lamblia* carried by synanthropic flies by combined fluorescent in situ hybridization and a monoclonal antibody. *Am J Trop Med Hyg*. 2003;68:228-232.
117. Graczyk TK, Lewis EJ, Glass G, et al. Quantitative assessment of viable *Cryptosporidium parvum* load in commercial oysters (Crassostrea virginica) in the Chesapeake Bay. *Parasitol Res*. 2007;100:247-253.
118. Alpert G, Bell LM, Kirkpatrick CE, et al. Outbreak of cryptosporidiosis in a day-care center. *Pediatrics*. 1986;77:152-157.
119. Heijbel H, Slaine K, Seigel B, et al. Outbreak of diarrhea in a day care center with spread to household members: the role of *Cryptosporidium*. *Pediatr Infect Dis J*. 1987;6:532-535.
120. Cordell RL, Addiss DG. Cryptosporidiosis in child care settings: a review of the literature and recommendations for prevention and control. *Pediatr Infect Dis J*. 1994;13:310-317.
121. Goncalves EM, da Silva AJ, Eduardo MB, et al. Multilocus genotyping of *Cryptosporidium hominis* associated with diarrhea outbreak in a day care unit in Sao Paulo. *Clinics*. 2006;61:119-126.
122. Koch KL, Phillips DJ, Aber RC, et al. Cryptosporidiosis in hospital personnel: evidence for person-to-person transmission. *Ann Intern Med*. 1984;102:593-596.
123. Sarabia-Arce S, Salazar-Lindo E, Gilman RH, et al. Case-control study of *Cryptosporidium parvum* infection in Peruvian children hospitalized for diarrhea: possible association with malnutrition and nosocomial infection. *Pediatr Infect Dis J*. 1990;9:627-631.
124. Navarrete S, Stetler HC, Avila C, et al. An outbreak of *Cryptosporidium* diarrhea in a pediatric hospital. *Pediatr Infect Dis J*. 1991;10:248-250.
125. Bruce BB, Blass MA, Blumberg HM, et al. Risk of *Cryptosporidium parvum* transmission between hospital roommates. *Clin Infect Dis*. 2000;31:947-950.
126. Hunter PR, Hughes S, Woodhouse S, et al. Sporadic cryptosporidiosis case-control study with genotyping. *Emerg Infect Dis*. 2004;10:1241-1249.
127. Newman RD, Zu SX, Wuhib T, et al. Household epidemiology of *Cryptosporidium parvum* infection in an urban community in northeast Brazil. *Ann Intern Med*. 1994;120:500-505.
128. MacKenzie WR, Schell WL, Blair KA, et al. Massive outbreak of waterborne *Cryptosporidium* infection in Milwaukee, Wisconsin: recurrence of illness and risk of secondary transmission. *Clin Infect Dis*. 1995;21:57-62.
129. Jokipii L, Pohjola S, Jokipii AM. Cryptosporidiosis associated with traveling and giardiasis. *Gastroenterology*. 1985;89:838-842.
130. Jelinek T, Lotze M, Eichenlaub S, et al. Prevalence of infection with *Cryptosporidium parvum* and *Cyclospora cayetanensis* among international travellers. *Gut*. 1997;41:801-804.
131. Nair P, Mohamed JA, DuPont HL, et al. Epidemiology of cryptosporidiosis in North American travelers to Mexico. *Am J Trop Med Hyg*. 2008;79:210-214.
132. Khalakdina A, Vugia DJ, Nadle J, et al. Is drinking water a risk factor for endemic cryptosporidiosis? A case-control study in the immunocompetent general population of the San Francisco Bay area. *BMC Public Health*. 2003;3:11.
133. Hashmey R, Smith NH, Cron S, et al. Cryptosporidiosis in Houston, Texas: a report of 95 cases. *Medicine (Baltimore)*. 1997;76:118-139.
134. Caputo C, Forbes A, Frost F, et al. Determinants of antibodies to *Cryptosporidium* infection among gay and bisexual men with HIV infection. *Epidemiol Infect*. 1999;122:291-297.
135. Khalakdina A, Tabnak F, Sun RK, et al. Race/ethnicity and other risk of factors associated with cryptosporidiosis as an initial AIDS-defining condition in California, 1980-99. *Epidemiol Infect*. 2001;127:535-543.
136. Hellard M, Hocking J, Willis J, et al. Risk factors leading to *Cryptosporidium* infection in men who have sex with men. *Sex Transm Infect*. 2003;79:412-414.
137. Hunter PR, Hadfield SJ, Wilkinson D, et al. Subtypes of *Cryptosporidium parvum* in humans and disease risk. *Emerg Infect Dis*. 2007;13:82-88.
138. Molbak K, Aaby P, Hojlyng N, et al. Risk factors for *Cryptosporidium* diarrhea in early childhood: a case-control study from Guinea-Bissau, West Africa. *Am J Epidemiol*. 1994;139:734-740.
139. Casemore DP. Sheep as a source of human cryptosporidiosis. *J Infect*. 1989;19:101-104.
140. Xiao L, Cama VA, Cabrera L, et al. Possible transmission of *Cryptosporidium canis* among children and a dog in a household. *J Clin Microbiol*. 2007;45:2014-2016.
141. Sallon S, el-Shawwa R, Khalil M, et al. Diarrhoeal disease in children in Gaza. *Ann Trop Med Parasitol*. 1994;88:175-182.
142. Bern C, Ortega Y, Checkley W, et al. Epidemiologic differences between cyclosporiasis and cryptosporidiosis in Peruvian children. *Emerg Infect Dis*. 2002;8:581-585.
143. Hunter PR, Nichols G. Epidemiology and clinical features of *Cryptosporidium* infection in immunocompromised patients. *Clin Microbiol Rev*. 2002;15:145-154.
144. Pozio E, Rezza G, Boshini A, et al. Clinical cryptosporidiosis and human immunodeficiency virus (HIV)-induced immunosuppression: findings from a longitudinal study of HIV-positive and HIV-negative former injection drug users. *J Infect Dis*. 1997;176:969-975.
145. Frisby HR, Addiss DG, Reiser WJ, et al. Clinical and epidemiologic features of a massive waterborne outbreak of cryptosporidiosis in persons with HIV infection. *J Acquir Immune Defic Syndr Hum Retrovirol*. 1997;16:367-373.
146. Hayward AR, Levy J, Facchetti F, et al. Cholangiopathy and tumors of the pancreas, liver, and biliary tree in boys with X-linked immunodeficiency with hyper-IgM. *J Immunol*. 1997;158:977-983.
147. Levy J, Espanol-Boren T, Thomas C, et al. Clinical spectrum of X-linked hyper-IgM syndrome. *J Pediatr*. 1997;131:47-54.
148. McLauchlin J, Amar CF, Pedraza-Diaz S, et al. Polymerase chain reaction-based diagnosis of infection with *Cryptosporidium* in children with primary immunodeficiencies. *Pediatr Infect Dis J*. 2003;22:329-335.
149. Kelly P, Makumbi FA, Carnaby S, et al. Variable distribution of *Cryptosporidium parvum* in the intestine of AIDS patients revealed by polymerase chain reaction. *Eur J Gastroenterol Hepatol*. 1998;10:855-858.
150. Goodwin TA. Cryptosporidiosis in the acquired immunodeficiency syndrome: a study of 15 autopsy cases. *Hum Pathol*. 1991;22:1215-1224.
151. Greenberg PD, Koch J, Cello JP. Diagnosis of *Cryptosporidium parvum* in patients with severe diarrhea and AIDS. *Dig Dis Sci*. 1996;41:2286-2290.
152. Phillips AD, Thomas AG, Walker-Smith JA. *Cryptosporidium*, chronic diarrhoea and the proximal small intestinal mucosa. *Gut*. 1992;33:1057-1061.
153. Lumadue JA, Manabe YC, Moore RD, et al. A clinicopathologic analysis of AIDS-related cryptosporidiosis. *AIDS*. 1998;12:2459-2466.
154. Genta RM, Chappell CL, White AC Jr, et al. Duodenal morphology and intensity of infection in AIDS-related cryptosporidiosis. *Gastroenterology*. 1993;105:1769-1775.
155. Goodgame RW, Kimball K, Ou C-N, et al. Intestinal function and injury in AIDS-related cryptosporidiosis. *Gastroenterology*. 1995;108:1075-1082.
156. Clayton F, Heller T, Kotler DP. Variation in the enteric distribution of *Cryptosporidia* in acquired immunodeficiency syndrome. *Am J Clin Pathol*. 1994;102:420-425.
157. Guarino A, Canani RB, Pozio E, et al. Enterotoxic effect of stool supernatants of *Cryptosporidium*-infected calves on human jejunum. *Gastroenterology*. 1994;106:28-34.
158. Guarino A, Canani RB, Casoli A, et al. Human intestinal cryptosporidiosis: secretory diarrhea and enterotoxic activity in Caco-2 cells. *J Infect Dis*. 1995;171:976-983.
159. McCole DF, Eckmann L, Laurent F, et al. Intestinal epithelial cell apoptosis following *Cryptosporidium parvum* infection. *Infect Immun*. 2000;68:1710-1713.

160. Chen XM, Levine SA, Splinter PL, et al. *Cryptosporidium parvum* activates nuclear factor kappaB in biliary epithelia preventing epithelial cell apoptosis. *Gastroenterology.* 2001;120:1774-1783.

161. Chen XM, O'Hara SP, Nelson JB, et al. Multiple TLRs are expressed in human cholangiocytes and mediate host epithelial defense responses to *Cryptosporidium parvum* via activation of NF-kappaB. *J Immunol.* 2005;175:7447-7456.

162. Chen XM, Splinter PL, O'Hara SP, et al. A cellular micro-RNA, let-7i, regulates Toll-like receptor 4 expression and contributes to cholangiocyte immune responses against *Cryptosporidium parvum* infection. *J Biol Chem.* 2007;282:28929-28938.

163. Rogers KA, Rogers AB, Leav BA, et al. MyD88-dependent pathways mediate resistance to *Cryptosporidium parvum* infection in mice. *Infect Immun.* 2006;74:549-556.

164. Kandil HM, Berschneider HM, Argenzio RA. Tumor necrosis factor α changes porcine intestinal ion transport through a paracrine mechanism involving prostaglandins. *Gut.* 1994;35:934-940.

165. Wyatt CR, Brackett EJ, Perryman LE, et al. Activation of intestinal intraepithelial T lymphocytes in calves infected with *Cryptosporidium parvum*. *Infect Immun.* 1997;65:185-190.

166. Seydel KB, Zhang T, Champion GA, et al. *Cryptosporidium parvum* infection of human intestinal xenografts in SCID mice induces production of human tumor necrosis factor alpha and interleukin-8. *Infect Immun.* 1998;66:2379-2382.

167. Robinson P, Okhuysen PC, Chappell CL, et al. Expression of tumor necrosis factor alpha and interleukin 1 beta in jejuna of volunteers after experimental challenge with *Cryptosporidium parvum* correlates with exposure but not with symptoms. *Infect Immun.* 2001;69:1172-1174.

168. Lacroix S, Mancassola R, Naciri M, et al. *Cryptosporidium parvum*-specific mucosal immune response in C57BL/6 neonatal and gamma interferon-deficient mice: role of tumor necrosis factor alpha in protection. *Infect Immun.* 2001;69:1635-1642.

169. Kirkpatrick BD, Daniels MM, Jean SS, et al. Cryptosporidiosis stimulates an inflammatory intestinal response in malnourished Haitian children. *J Infect Dis.* 2002;186:94-101.

170. Alcantara CS, Yang CH, Steiner TS, et al. Interleukin-8, tumor necrosis factor-alpha, and lactoferrin in immunocompetent hosts with experimental and Brazilian children with acquired cryptosporidiosis. *Am J Trop Med Hyg.* 2003;68:325-328.

171. Kirkpatrick BD, Noel F, Rouzier PD, et al. Childhood cryptosporidiosis is associated with a persistent systemic inflammatory response. *Clin Infect Dis.* 2006;43:604-608.

172. Pantenburg B, Dann SM, Wang HC, et al. Intestinal immune response to human *Cryptosporidium* sp. infection. *Infect Immun.* 2008;76:23-29.

173. Maillot C, Gargala G, Delaunay A, et al. *Cryptosporidium parvum* infection stimulates the secretion of TGF-beta, IL-8 and RANTES by Caco-2 cell line. *Parasitol Res.* 2000;86:947-949.

174. Laurent F, Eckmann L, Savidge TC, et al. *Cryptosporidium parvum* infection of human intestinal epithelial cells induces the polarized secretion of C-X-C chemokines. *Infect Immun.* 1997;65:5067-5073.

175. Lacroix-Lamande S, Mancassola R, Naciri M, et al. Role of gamma interferon in chemokine expression in the ileum of mice and in a murine intestinal epithelial cell line after *Cryptosporidium parvum* infection. *Infect Immun.* 2002;70:2090-2099.

176. Deng M, Lancto CA, Abrahamsen MS. *Cryptosporidium parvum* regulation of human epithelial cell gene expression. *Int J Parasitol.* 2004;34:73-82.

177. Wang HC, Dann SM, Okhuysen PC, et al. High levels of CXCL10 are produced by intestinal epithelial cells in AIDS patients with active cryptosporidiosis but not after reconstitution of immunity. *Infect Immun.* 2007;75:481-487.

178. Laurent F, Kagnoff MF, Savidge TC, et al. Human intestinal epithelial cells respond to *Cryptosporidium parvum* infection with increased prostaglandin H synthase 2 expression and prostaglandin E2 and F2alpha production. *Infect Immun.* 1998;66:1787-1790.

179. Robinson P, Okhuysen PC, Chappell CL, et al. Substance P expression correlates with severity of diarrhea in cryptosporidiosis. *J Infect Dis.* 2003;188:290-296.

180. Gookin JL, Duckett LL, Armstrong MU, et al. Nitric oxide synthase stimulates prostaglandin synthesis and barrier function in *C. parvum*-infected porcine ileum. *Am J Physiol Gastrointest Liver Physiol.* 2004;287:G571-G581.

181. Hernandez J, Lackner A, Aye P, et al. Substance P is responsible for physiological alterations such as increased chloride ion secretion and glucose malabsorption in cryptosporidiosis. *Infect Immun.* 2007;75:1137-1143.

182. Argenzio RA, Armstrong M, Rhoads JM. Role of the enteric nervous system in piglet cryptosporidiosis. *J Pharmacol Exp Ther.* 1996;279:1109-1115.

183. Cole J, Blikslager A, Hunt E, et al. Cyclooxygenase blockade and exogenous glutamine enhance sodium absorption in infected bovine ileum. *Am J Physiol Gastrointest Liver Physiol.* 2003;284:G516-G524.

184. Snijders F, van Deventer SJH, Bartelsman JFW, et al. Diarrhoea in HIV-infected patients: no evidence of cytokine-mediated inflammation in jejunal mucosa. *AIDS.* 1995;9:367-373.

185. Okhuysen PC, Robinson P, Nguyen MT, et al. Jejunal cytokine response in AIDS patients with chronic cryptosporidiosis and during immune reconstitution. *AIDS.* 2001;15:802-804.

186. Sharpstone DR, Rowbottom AW, Nelson MR, et al. Faecal tumour necrosis factor-alpha in individuals with HIV-related diarrhoea. *AIDS.* 1996;10:989-994.

187. Garza A, Lackner A, Aye P, et al. Substance P receptor antagonist reverses intestinal pathophysiological alterations occurring in a novel ex-vivo model of *Cryptosporidium parvum* infection of intestinal tissues derived from SIV-infected macaques. *J Med Primatol.* 2008;37:109-115.

188. Sonea IM, Palmer MV, Akili D, et al. Treatment with neurokinin-1 receptor antagonist reduces severity of inflammatory bowel disease induced by *Cryptosporidium parvum*. *Clin Diagn Lab Immunol.* 2002;9:333-340.

189. Robinson P, Martin Jr P, Garza A, et al. Substance P receptor antagonism for treatment of cryptosporidiosis in immunosuppressed mice. *J Parasitol.* 2008;94:1150-1154.

190. Guarino A, Canani R, Spagnuolo MI, et al. In vivo and in vitro efficacy of octreotide for treatment of enteric cryptosporidiosis. *Dig Dis Sci.* 1998;43:436-441.

191. Lima AA, Silva TM, Gifoni AM, et al. Mucosal injury and disruption of intestinal barrier function in HIV-infected individuals with and without diarrhea and cryptosporidiosis in northeast Brazil. *Am J Gastroenterol.* 1997;92:1861-1866.

192. Sharpstone D, Neild P, Crane R, et al. Small intestinal transit, absorption, and permeability in patients with AIDS with and without diarrhoea. *Gut.* 1999;45:70-76.

193. Zhang Y, Lee B, Thompson M, et al. Lactulose-mannitol intestinal permeability test in children with diarrhea caused by *Rotavirus* and *Cryptosporidium*. Diarrhea Working Group, Peru. *J Pediatr Gastroenterol Nutr.* 2000;31:16-21.

194. Adams RB, Guerrant RL, Zu S, et al. *Cryptosporidium parvum* infection of intestinal epithelium: morphologic and functional studies in an in-vitro model. *J Infect Dis.* 1994;169:170-177.

195. Griffiths JK, Moore R, Dooley S, et al. *Cryptosporidium parvum* infection of Caco-2 cell monolayers induces an apical monolayer defect, selectively increases transmonolayer permeability, and causes epithelial cell death. *Infect Immun.* 1994;62:4506-4514.

196. Roche JK, Martins CA, Cosme R, et al. Transforming growth factor beta1 ameliorates intestinal epithelial barrier disruption by *Cryptosporidium parvum* in vitro in the absence of mucosal T lymphocytes. *Infect Immun.* 2000;68:5635-5644.

197. Argenzio R, Liacos J, Levy M, et al. Villous atrophy, crypt hyperplasia, cellular infiltration, and impaired glucose-Na absorption in enteric porcine cryptosporidiosis of pigs. *Gastroenterology.* 1990;98:1129-1140.

198. Kotler DP, Francisco A, Clayton F, et al. Small intestinal injury and parasitic diseases in AIDS. *Ann Intern Med.* 1990;113:444-449.

199. Moore R, Tzipori S, Griffiths JK, et al. Temporal changes in permeability and structure of piglet ileum after site-specific infection by *Cryptosporidium parvum*. *Gastroenterology.* 1995;108:1030-1039.

200. Blikslager A, Hunt E, Guerrant R, et al. Glutamine transporter in crypts compensates for loss of villus absorption in bovine cryptosporidiosis. *Am J Physiol Gastrointest Liver Physiol.* 2001;281:G645-G653.

201. Motta I, Gissot M, Kanellopoulos JM, et al. Absence of weight loss during *Cryptosporidium* infection in susceptible mice deficient in Fas-mediated apoptosis. *Microbes Infect.* 2002;4:821-827.

202. Chen XM, Gores GJ, Paya CV, et al. *Cryptosporidium parvum* induced apoptosis in biliary epithelia by a Fas/Fas ligand-dependent mechanism. *Am J Physiol Gastrointest Liver Physiol.* 1999;277:G599-G608.

203. Mele R, Gomez Morales MA, Tosini F, et al. *Cryptosporidium parvum* at different developmental stages modulates host cell apoptosis in vitro. *Infect Immun.* 2004;72:6061-6067.

204. Liu J, Deng M, Lancto CA, et al. Biphasic modulation of apoptotic pathways in *Cryptosporidium parvum*-infected human intestinal epithelial cells. *Infect Immun.* 2009;77:837-849.

205. Chen XM, Levine SA, Tietz P, et al. *Cryptosporidium parvum* is cytopathic for cultured human biliary epithelia via an apoptotic mechanism. *Hepatology.* 1998;28:906-913.

206. Elliot DA, Clark DP. Host cell fate on *Cryptosporidium parvum* egress from MDCK cells. *Infect Immun.* 2003;71:5422-5462.

207. Sciarretta G, Bonazzi L, Furno A, et al. Bile acid malabsorption in AIDS-associated chronic diarrhea: a prospective 1-year study. *Am J Gastroenterol.* 1994;89:379-381.

208. Ribeiro Machado F, Gonzaga Vaz Coelho L, Chausson Y, et al. Fat malabsorption assessed by 14C-triolein breath test in HIV-positive patients in different stages of infection: is it an early event. *J Clin Gastroenterol.* 2000;30:403-408.

209. Sharpstone D, Phelan M, Gazzard B. Differential metabolic response in AIDS-related chronic protozoal diarrhoea. *HIV Med.* 2000;1:102-106.

210. Flanigan TP, Whalen C, Turner J, et al. *Cryptosporidium* infection and CD4 count. *Ann Intern Med.* 1992;116:840-842.

211. Blanshard C, Jackson A, Shanson D, et al. Cryptosporidiosis in HIV-seropositive patients. *Q J Med.* 1992;307/308:813-823.

212. Ungar BLP, Kao T-C, Burris JA, et al. *Cryptosporidium* infection in an adult mouse model. Independent roles for IFN-γ and CD4+ T lymphocytes in protective immunity. *J Immunol.* 1991;147:1014-1022.

213. McDonald V, Deer R, Uni S, et al. Immune responses to *Cryptosporidium muris* and *Cryptosporidium parvum* in adult immunocompetent and immunocompromised (nude and SCID) mice. *Infect Immun.* 1992;60:3325-3331.

214. Chen W, Harp JA, Harmsen AG. Requirement for CD4+ cells and gamma interferon in resolution of established *Cryptosporidium parvum* infection in mice. *Infect Immun.* 1993;61:3928-3932.

215. Aguirre SA, Mason PH, Perryman E. Susceptibility of major histocompatibility complex (MHC) class I and MHC class II-deficient mice to *Cryptosporidium parvum* infection. *Infect Immun.* 1994;62:697-699.

216. McDonald V, Robinson HA, Kelly JP, et al. *Cryptosporidium muris* in adult mice: adoptive transfer of immunity and protective roles of CD4 versus CD8 cells. *Infect Immun.* 1994;62:2289-2294.

217. Perryman LA, Mason PH, Chrisp CE. Effect of spleen cell populations in resolution of *Cryptosporidium parvum* infection in SCID mice. *Infect Immun.* 1994;62:1474-1477.

218. Culshaw RJ, Bancroft GJ, McDonald V. Gut epithelial lymphocytes induce immunity against *Cryptosporidium* infection through a mechanism involving gamma interferon production. *Infect Immun.* 1997;65:3074-3079.

219. Kirkpatrick BD, Haque R, Duggal P, et al. Association between *Cryptosporidium* infection and human leukocyte antigen class I and class II alleles. *J Infect Dis.* 2008;197:474-478.

220. Schmidt W, Wahnschaffe U, Schafer M, et al. Rapid increase of mucosal CD4 T cells followed by clearance of intestinal cryptosporidiosis in an AIDS patient receiving highly active antiretroviral therapy. *Gastroenterology.* 2001;120:984-987.

221. Abrabamsen MS. Bovine Ta cell responses to *Cryptosporidium parvum* infection. *Int J Parasitol.* 1998;28:1083-1088.

222. Preidis GA, Wang HC, Lewis DE, et al. Seropositive human subjects produce interferon gamma after stimulation with recombinant *Cryptosporidium hominis* gp15. *Am J Trop Med Hyg.* 2007;77:583-585.

223. Jain A, Atkinson TP, Lipsky PE, et al. Defects of T-cell effector function and post-thymic maturation in X-linked hyper-IgM syndrome. *J Clin Invest.* 1999;103:1151-1158.

224. Cosyns M, Tsirkin S, Jones M, et al. Requirement of CD40-CD40 ligand interaction for elimination of *Cryptosporidium parvum* from mice. *Infect Immun.* 1998;66:603-607.

225. Stephens J, Cosyns M, Jones M, et al. Liver and bile duct pathology following *Cryptosporidium parvum* infection of immunodeficient mice. *Hepatology.* 1999;30:27-35.

226. Lukin K, Cosyns M, Mitchell T, et al. Eradication of *Cryptosporidium parvum* infection by mice with ovalbumin-specific T cells. *Infect Immun.* 2000;68:2663-2670.

227. Hayward AR, Cosyns M, Jones M, et al. Marrow-derived CD40-positive cells are required for mice to clear *Cryptosporidium parvum* infection. *Infect Immun.* 2001;69:1630-1634.

228. Castellanos-Gonzalez A, Yancey LS, Wang HC, et al. *Cryptosporidium* infection of human intestinal epithelial cells increases expression of osteoprotegerin: a novel mechanism for evasion of host defenses. *J Infect Dis.* 2008;197:916-923.

229. Theodos CM, Sullivan KL, Griffiths JK, et al. Profiles of healing and nonhealing *Cryptosporidium parvum* infection in C57Bl/6 mice with functional B and T lymphocytes: the extent of gamma interferon modulation determines the outcome of infection. *Infect Immun.* 1997;65:4761-4769.

230. Mead JR, You X. Susceptibility differences to *Cryptosporidium parvum* infection in two strains of gamma interferon knockout mice. *J Parasitol.* 1998;84:1045-1048.

231. Tzipori S, Rand W, Theodos C. Evaluation of a two-phase scid mouse model preconditioned with anti-interferon-γ monoclonal antibody for drug testing against *Cryptosporidium parvum*. *J Infect Dis.* 1995;172:1160-1164.

232. Kapel N, Benhamou Y, Burand M, et al. Kinetics of mucosal gamma-interferon response during cryptosporidiosis in immunocompetent neonatal mice. *Parasitol Res.* 1996;82:664-6647.

233. Urban Jr JF, Fayer R, Sullivan C, et al. Local TH1 and TH2 responses to parasitic infection in the intestine: regulation by IFN-gamma and IL-4. *Vet Immunol Immunopathol.* 1996;54:337-344.

234. Fayer R, Gasbarre L, Pasquali P, et al. *Cryptosporidium parvum* infection in bovine neonates: dynamic clinical, parasitic and immunologic patterns. *Int J Parasitol.* 1998;28:49-56.

235. Gomez Morales MA, La Rosa G, Ludovisi A, et al. Cytokine profile induced by *Cryptosporidium* antigen in peripheral blood mononuclear cells from immunocompetent and immunosuppressed persons with cryptosporidiosis. *J Infect Dis.* 1999;179:967-973.

236. Kaushik K, Khurana S, Wanchu A, et al. Lymphoproliferative and cytokine responses to *Cryptosporidium parvum* in patients coinfected with *C. parvum* and human immunodeficiency virus. *Clin Vaccine Immunol.* 2009;16:116-121.

237. White AC, Robinson P, Okhuysen PC, et al. Interferon-gamma expression in jejunal biopsies in experimental human cryptosporidiosis correlates with prior sensitization and control of oocyst excretion. *J Infect Dis.* 2000;181:701-709.

238. Pollok RC, Farthing MJ, Bajaj-Elliott M, et al. Interferon gamma induces enterocyte resistance against infection by the intracellular pathogen *Cryptosporidium parvum*. *Gastroenterology.* 2001;120:99-107.

239. Urban JF, Fayer R, Chen S-J, et al. IL-12 protects immunocompetent and immunodeficient mice against infection with *Cryptosporidium parvum*. *J Immunol.* 1996;156:263-268.

240. Campbell LD, Stewart JN, Mead JR. Susceptibility to *Cryptosporidium parvum* infections in cytokine- and chemokine-receptor knockout mice. *J Parasitol.* 2002;88:1014-1016.

241. Smith LM, Bonafonte MT, Mead JR. Cytokine expression and specific lymphocyte proliferation in two strains of *Cryptospo-*

ridium parvum-infected gamma-interferon knockout mice. *J Parasitol.* 2000;86:300-307.

242. Smith LM, Bonafonte MT, Campbell LD, et al. Exogenous interleukin-12 (IL-12) exacerbates *Cryptosporidium parvum* infection in gamma interferon knockout mice. *Exp Parasitol.* 2001;98:123-133.
243. Okhuysen PC, Chappell CL, Lewis DE, et al. Treatment of chronic cryptosporidiosis in AIDS with rIL-12 induces an immune response associated with improvement but severe side-effects. *AIDS.* 2005;19:1333-1334.
244. Aguirre SA, Perryman LE, Davis WC, et al. IL-4 protects adult C57BL/6 mice from prolonged *Cryptosporidium parvum* infection: analysis of $CD4^+\alpha\beta^+IFN\text{-}\gamma^+$ and $CD4^+\alpha\beta$+IL-4^+ lymphocytes in gut-associated lymphoid tissue during resolution of infection. *J Immunol.* 1998;161:1891-1900.
245. Lean IS, McDonald SA, Bajaj-Elliott M, et al. Interleukin-4 and transforming growth factor beta have opposing regulatory effects on gamma interferon-mediated inhibition of *Cryptosporidium parvum* reproduction. *Infect Immun.* 2003;71:4580-4585.
246. Robinson P, Okhuysen PC, Chappell CL, et al. Expression of IL-15 and IL-4 in IFN-gamma-independent control of experimental human *Cryptosporidium parvum* infection. *Cytokine.* 2001;15:39-46.
247. McDonald V, Pollok RC, Dhaliwal W, et al. A potential role for interleukin-18 in inhibition of the development of *Cryptosporidium parvum. Clin Exp Immunol.* 2006;145:555-562.
248. Tessema TS, Schwamb B, Lochner M, et al. Dynamics of gut mucosal and systemic Th1/Th2 cytokine responses in interferon-gamma and interleukin-12p40 knock out mice during primary and challenge *Cryptosporidium parvum* infection. *Immunobiology.* 2009;214:454-466.
249. Ehigiator HN, McNair N, Mead JR. *Cryptosporidium parvum*: the contribution of Th1-inducing pathways to the resolution of infection in mice. *Exp Parasitol.* 2007;115:107-113.
250. Taghi-Kilani R, Sekla L, Hayglass KT. The role of humoral immunity in *Cryptosporidium* spp. infection: studies with B cell-depleted mice. *J Immunol.* 1990;145:1571-1576.
251. Chen W, Harp JA, Harmsen AG. *Cryptosporidium parvum* infection in gene-targeted B cell deficient mice. *J Parasitol.* 2003;89:391-393.
252. Arrowood MJ, Mead JR, Mahrt JL, et al. Effects of immune colostrum and orally administered antisporozoite monoclonal antibodies on the outcome of *Cryptosporidium parvum* infections in neonatal mice. *Infect Immun.* 1989;57:2283-2288.
253. Perryman LE, Kapil SJ, Jones ML, et al. Protection of calves against cryptosporidiosis with immune bovine colostrum induced by a *Cryptosporidium parvum* recombinant protein. *Vaccine.* 1999;17:2142-2149.
254. Sagodira S, Iochmann S, Mevelec MN, et al. Nasal immunization of mice with *Cryptosporidium parvum* DNA induces systemic and intestinal immune responses. *Parasite Immunol.* 1999;21:507-516.
255. Jenkins MC, O'Brien C, Trout J, et al. Hyperimmune bovine colostrum specific for recombinant *Cryptosporidium parvum* antigen confers partial protection against cryptosporidiosis in immunosuppressed adult mice. *Vaccine.* 1999;17:2453-2460.
256. Riggs MW. Recent advances in cryptosporidiosis: the immune response. *Microbes Infect.* 2002;4:1067-1080.
257. Fries L, Hillman K, Crabb J, et al. Clinical and microbiologic effects of bovine anti-*Cryptosporidium* immunoglobulin (BACI) on cryptosporidial diarrhea in AIDS [abstract M31]. In: *34th Interscience Conference on Antimicrobial Agents and Chemotherapy.* Orlando, FL: American Society for Microbiology; 1994.
258. Cozon G, Biron F, Jeannin M, et al. Secretory IgA antibodies to *Cryptosporidium parvum* in AIDS patients with chronic cryptosporidiosis. *J Infect Dis.* 1994;169:696-699.
259. Benhamou Y, Kapel N, Hoang C, et al. Inefficacy of intestinal secretory immune response to *Cryptosporidium* in the acquired immunodeficiency syndrome. *Gastroenterology.* 1995;108:627-635.
260. Dann SM, Okhuysen PC, Salameh BM, et al. Fecal antibodies to *Cryptosporidium parvum* in healthy volunteers. *Infect Immun.* 2000;68:5068-5074.
261. Robinson P, Okhuysen PC, Chappell CL, et al. Transforming growth factor beta1 is expressed in the jejunum after experimental *Cryptosporidium parvum* infection in humans. *Infect Immun.* 2000;68:5405-5407.
262. Kelly P, Jack DL, Naeem A, et al. Mannose-binding lectin is a component of innate mucosal defense against *Cryptosporidium parvum* in AIDS. *Gastroenterology.* 2000;119:1236-1242.
263. Kirkpatrick BD, Huston CD, Wagner D, et al. Serum mannose-binding lectin deficiency is associated with cryptosporidiosis in young Haitian children. *Clin Infect Dis.* 2006;43:289-294.
264. Petry F, Jakobi V, Wagner S, et al. Binding and activation of human and mouse complement by *Cryptosporidium parvum* (Apicomplexa) and susceptibility of C1q- and MBL-deficient mice to infection. *Mol Immunol.* 2008;45:3392-3400.
265. Tarver AP, Clark DP, Diamond G, et al. Enteric beta-defensin: molecular cloning and characterization of a gene with inducible intestinal epithelial cell expression associated with *Cryptosporidium parvum* infection. *Infect Immun.* 1998;66:1045-1056.
266. Zaalouk TK, Bajaj-Elliott M, et al. Differential regulation of beta-defensin gene expression during *Cryptosporidium parvum* infection. *Infect Immun.* 2004;72:2772-2779.
267. Jokipii L, Jokikii AMM. Timing of symptoms and oocyst excretion in human cryptosporidiosis. *N Engl J Med.* 1986;315:1643-1647.
268. Okhuysen PC, Rich SM, Chappell CL, et al. Infectivity of a *Cryptosporidium parvum* isolate of cervine origin for healthy adults and interferon-gamma knockout mice. *J Infect Dis.* 2002;185:1320-1325.
269. Mac Kenzie WR, Hoxie NJ, Proctor ME, et al. A massive outbreak in Milwaukee of *Cryptosporidium* infection transmitted through the public water supply. *N Engl J Med.* 1994;331:161-177.
270. Egger M, Mäusezahl D, Odermatt P, et al. Symptoms and transmission of intestinal cryptosporidiosis. *Arch Dis Child.* 1990;65:445-447.
271. Hunter PR, Hughes S, Woodhouse S, et al. Health sequelae of human cryptosporidiosis in immunocompetent patients. *Clin Infect Dis.* 2004;39:504-510.
272. Rees JR, Pannier MA, McNees A, et al. Persistent diarrhea, arthritis, and other complications of enteric infections: a pilot survey based on California FoodNet surveillance, 1998-1999. *Clin Infect Dis.* 2004;38(Suppl 3):S311-S317.
273. Gambhir IS, Jaiswal JP, Nath G. Significance of *Cryptosporidium* as an aetiology of acute infectious diarrhoea in elderly Indians. *Trop Med Int Health.* 2003;8:415-419.
274. Naumova EN, Egorov AI, Morris RD, et al. The elderly and waterborne *Cryptosporidium* infection: gastroenteritis hospitalizations before and during the 1993 Milwaukee outbreak. *Emerg Infect Dis.* 2003;9:418-425.
275. Neill MA, Rice SK, Ahmad NV, et al. Cryptosporidiosis: an unrecognized cause of diarrhea in elderly hospitalized patients. *Clin Infect Dis.* 1996;22:168-170.
276. Frost FJ, Fea E, Gilli G, et al. Serological evidence of *Cryptosporidium* infections in southern Europe. *Eur J Epidemiol.* 2000;16:385-390.
277. McDonald AC, Mac Kenzie WR, Addiss DG, et al. *Cryptosporidium parvum*-specific antibody responses among children residing in Milwaukee during the 1993 waterborne outbreak. *J Infect Dis.* 2001;183:1373-1379.
278. Priest JW, Bern C, Xiao L, et al. Longitudinal analysis of *Cryptosporidium* species-specific immunoglobulin G antibody responses in Peruvian children. *Clin Vaccine Immunol.* 2006;13:123-131.
279. Cicirello HG, Kehl KS, Addiss DG, et al. Cryptosporidiosis in children during a massive waterborne outbreak in Milwaukee, Wisconsin: clinical, laboratory and epidemiologic findings. *Epidemiol Infect.* 1997;119:53-60.
280. Agnew DG, Lima AA, Newman RD, et al. Cryptosporidiosis in northeastern Brazilian children: association with increased diarrhea morbidity. *J Infect Dis.* 1998;177:754-760.
281. Molbak K, Wested N, Hojlyng N, et al. The etiology of early childhood diarrhea: a community study from Guinea-Bissau. *J Infect Dis.* 1994;169:581-587.
282. Sallon S, el Showwa R, el Masri M, et al. Cryptosporidiosis in children in Gaza. *Ann Trop Paediatr.* 1991;11:277-281.
283. Ajjampur SS, Gladstone BP, Selvapandian D, et al. Molecular and spatial epidemiology of cryptosporidiosis in children in a semiurban community in South India. *J Clin Microbiol.* 2007;45:915-920.
284. Khan WA, Rogers KA, Karim MM, et al. Cryptosporidiosis among Bangladeshi children with diarrhea: a prospective, matched, case-control study of clinical features, epidemiology and systemic antibody responses. *Am J Trop Med Hyg.* 2004;71:412-419.
285. Bushen OY, Kohli A, Pinkerton RC, et al. Heavy cryptosporidial infections in children in northeast Brazil: comparison of *Cryptosporidium hominis* and *Cryptosporidium parvum. Trans R Soc Trop Med Hyg.* 2007;101:378-384.
286. Sodemann M, Jakobsen MS, Molbak K, et al. Episode-specific risk factors for progression of acute diarrhoea to persistent diarrhoea in West African children. *Trans R Soc Trop Med Hyg.* 1999;93:65-68.
287. Amadi B, Mwiya M, Musuku J, et al. Effect of nitazoxanide on morbidity and mortality in Zambian children with cryptosporidiosis: a randomised controlled trial. *Lancet.* 2002;360:1375-1380.
288. Behera B, Mirdha BR, Makharia GK, et al. Parasites in patients with malabsorption syndrome: a clinical study in children and adults. *Dig Dis Sci.* 2008;53:672-679.
289. Molbak K, Hojlyng N, Gottschau A, et al. Cryptosporidiosis in infancy and childhood mortality in Guinea Bissau, West Africa. *Br Med J.* 1993;307:417-420.
290. Lima AA, Moore SR, Barboza Jr MS, et al. Persistent diarrhea signals a critical period of increased diarrhea burdens and nutritional shortfalls: a prospective cohort study among children in northeastern Brazil. *J Infect Dis.* 2000;181:1643-1651.
291. Amadi B, Kelly P, Mwiya M, et al. Intestinal and systemic infection, HIV, and mortality in Zambian children with persistent diarrhea and malnutrition. *J Pediatr Gastroenterol Nutr.* 2001;32:550-554.
292. Guerrant DI, Moore SR, Lima AA, et al. Association of early childhood diarrhea and cryptosporidiosis with impaired physical fitness and cognitive function four-seven years later in a poor urban community in northeast Brazil. *Am J Trop Med Hyg.* 1999;61:707-713.
293. Checkley W, Buckley G, Gilman RH, et al. Multi-country analysis of the effects of diarrhoea on childhood stunting. *Int J Epidemiol.* 2008;37:816-830.
294. Macfarlane DE, Horner-Bryce J. Cryptosporidiosis in well-nourished and malnourished children. *Acta Paediatr Scand.* 1987;76:474-477.
295. Sallon S, Deckelbaum RJ, Schmid II, et al. *Cryptosporidium*, malnutrition, and chronic diarrhea. *Am J Dis Child.* 1988;142:312-315.
296. Javier Enriquez F, Avila CR, Ignacio Santos J, et al. *Cryptosporidium* infections in Mexican children: clinical, nutritional, enteropathogenic, and diagnostic evaluations. *Am J Trop Med Hyg.* 1997;56:254-257.
297. Molbak K, Andersen M, Aaby P, et al. *Cryptosporidium* infection in infancy as a cause of malnutrition: a community study from Guinea-Bissau, West Africa. *Am J Clin Nutr.* 1997;65:149-152.
298. Checkley W, Epstein LD, Gilman RH, et al. Effects of *Cryptosporidium parvum* infection in Peruvian children: growth faltering and subsequent catch-up growth. *Am J Epidemiol.* 1998;148:497-506.
299. Checkley W, Gilman RH, Epstein LD, et al. Asymptomatic and symptomatic cryptosporidiosis: their acute effect on weight gain in Peruvian children. *Am J Epidemiol.* 1997;145:156-163.
300. Kim LS, Hadley WK, Stansell J, et al. Declining prevalence of cryptosporidiosis in San Francisco. *Clin Infect Dis.* 1998;27:655-656.
301. Le Moing V, Bissuel F, Costagliola D, et al. Decreased prevalence of intestinal cryptosporidiosis in HIV-infected patients concomitant to the widespread use of protease inhibitors. *AIDS.* 1998;12:1395-1397.
302. Manabe YC, Clark DP, Moore RD, et al. Cryptosporidiosis in patients with AIDS: correlates of disease and survival. *Clin Infect Dis.* 1998;27:536-542.
303. Rao Ajjampur SS, Asirvatham JR, Muthusamy D, et al. Clinical features and risk factors associated with cryptosporidiosis in HIV infected adults in India. *Indian J Med Res.* 2007;126:553-557.
304. Lopez-Velez R, Tarazona R, Garcia Camacho A, et al. Intestinal and extraintestinal cryptosporidiosis in AIDS patients. *Eur J Clin Microbiol Infect Dis.* 1995;14:677-681.
305. Meynard JL, Meyohas MC, Binet D, et al. Pulmonary cryptosporidiosis in the acquired immunodeficiency syndrome. *Infection.* 1996;24:328-331.
306. Clavel A, Arnal AC, Sanchez EC, et al. Respiratory cryptosporidiosis: case series and review of the literature. *Infection.* 1996;24:341-346.
307. Vakil NB, Schwartz SM, Buggy BP, et al. Biliary cryptosporidiosis in HIV-infected people after the waterborne outbreak of cryptosporidiosis in Milwaukee. *N Engl J Med.* 1996;334:19-23.
308. Teare JP, Daly CA, Rodgers C, et al. Pancreatic abnormalities and AIDS related sclerosing cholangitis. *Genitourin Med.* 1997;73:271-273.
309. Smith HV. Diagnostics. In: Fayer R, Xiao L, eds. *Cryptosporidium and Cryptosporidiosis.* 2nd ed. Boca Raton, FL: CRC Press; 2008:173-208.
310. Cryptosporidiosis. Division of Parasitic Diseases, Centers for Disease Control and Prevention, <http://www.dpd.cdc.gov/dpdx/HTML/Cryptosporidiosis.htm>; Accessed January 15, 2009.
311. Clavel A, Arnal A, Sanchez E, et al. Comparison of 2 centrifugation procedures in the formalin-ethyl acetate stool concentration technique for the detection of *Cryptosporidium* oocysts. *Int J Parasitol.* 1996;26:671-672.
312. Webster KA, Smith HV, Giles M, et al. Detection of *Cryptosporidium parvum* oocysts in faeces: comparison of conventional coproscopical methods and the polymerase chain reaction. *Vet Parasitol.* 1996;61:5-13.
313. Weber R, Bryan R, Bishop H, et al. Threshold for detection of *Cryptosporidium* oocysts in human stool specimens: evidence for low sensitivity of current diagnostic methods. *J Clin Microbiol.* 1991;29:963-965.
314. Alles AJ, Waldron MA, Sierra LS, et al. Prospective comparison of direct immunofluorescence and conventional staining methods for detection of *Giardia* and *Cryptosporidium* spp. in human fecal specimens. *J Clin Microbiol.* 1995;33:1632-1634.
315. Johnston SP, Ballard MM, Beach MJ, et al. Evaluation of three commercial assays for detection of *Giardia* and *Cryptosporidium* organisms in fecal specimens. *J Clin Microbiol.* 2003;41:623-626.
316. Tortora GT, Malowitz R, Mendelsohn B, et al. Rhodamine-auramine O versus Kinyoun-carbolfuchsin acid-fast stains for detection of *Cryptosporidium* oocysts. *Clin Lab Sci.* 1992;5:568-569.
317. Dagan R, Fraser D, El-On J, et al. Evaluation of an enzyme immunoassay for the detection of *Cryptosporidium* spp. in stool specimens from infants and young children in field studies. *Am J Trop Med Hyg.* 1995;52:134-138.
318. Ignatius R, Eisenblatter M, Regnath T, et al. Efficacy of different methods for detection of low *Cryptosporidium parvum* oocyst numbers or antigen concentrations in stool specimens. *Eur J Clin Microbiol Infect Dis.* 1997;16:732-736.
319. Garcia LS, Shimizu RY. Evaluation of nine immunoassay kits (enzyme immunoassay and direct fluorescence) for detection of *Giardia lamblia* and *Cryptosporidium parvum* in human fecal specimens. *J Clin Microbiol.* 1997;35:1526-1529.
320. Balatbat AB, Jordan GW, Tang YJ, et al. Detection of *Cryptosporidium parvum* DNA in human feces by nested PCR. *J Clin Microbiol.* 1996;34:1769-1772.
321. Kehl KSC, Cicirello H, Havens PL. Comparison of four different methods for detection of *Cryptosporidium* species. *J Clin Microbiol.* 1995;33:416-418.

322. Garcia LS, Shimizu RY. Detection of *Giardia lamblia* and *Cryptosporidium parvum* antigens in human fecal specimens using the ColorPAC combination rapid solid-phase qualitative immunochromatographic assay. *J Clin Microbiol.* 2000;38:1267-1268.
323. Garcia LS, Shimizu RY, Novak S, et al. Commercial assay for detection of *Giardia lamblia* and *Cryptosporidium parvum* antigens in human fecal specimens by rapid solid-phase qualitative immunochromatography. *J Clin Microbiol.* 2003;41:209-212.
324. Newman RD, Jaeger KL, Wuhib T, et al. Evaluation of an antigen capture enzyme-linked immunosorbent assay for detection of *Cryptosporidium* oocysts. *J Clin Microbiol.* 1993;31:2080-2084.
325. Manufacturer's recall of rapid assay kits based on false positive *Cryptosporidium* antigen tests—Wisconsin, 2001-2002. *MMWR Morb Mortal Wkly Rep.* 2002;51:189.
326. Doing KM, Hamm JL, Jellison JA, et al. False-positive results obtained with the Alexon ProSpecT *Cryptosporidium* enzyme immunoassay. *J Clin Microbiol.* 1999;37:1582-1583.
327. Garcia LS, Shimizu RY, Bernard CN. Detection of *Giardia lamblia, Entamoeba histolytica/Entamoeba dispar*, and *Cryptosporidium parvum* antigens in human fecal specimens using the triage parasite panel enzyme immunoassay. *J Clin Microbiol.* 2000;38:3337-3340.
328. Youn S, Kabir M, Haque R, et al. Evaluation of a Screening Test for Detection of *Giardia* and *Cryptosporidium*. *J Clin Microbiol.* 2009;47:451-452.
329. Weitzel T, Dittrich S, Mohl I, et al. Evaluation of seven commercial antigen detection tests for *Giardia* and *Cryptosporidium* in stool samples. *Clin Microbiol Infect.* 2006;12:656-659.
330. Savin C, Sarfati C, Menotti J, et al. Assessment of cryptodiag for diagnosis of cryptosporidiosis and genotyping *Cryptosporidium* species. *J Clin Microbiol.* 2008;46:2590-2594.
331. Bushen OY, Davenport JA, Lima AB, et al. Diarrhea and reduced levels of antiretroviral drugs: improvement with glutamine or alanyl-glutamine in a randomized controlled trial in northeast Brazil. *Clin Infect Dis.* 2004;38:1764-1770.
332. Carneiro-Filho BA, Bushen OY, Brito GA, et al. Glutamine analogues as adjunctive therapy for infectious diarrhea. *Curr Infect Dis Rep.* 2003;5:114-119.
333. Lima NL, Soares AM, Mota RM, et al. Wasting and intestinal barrier function in children taking alanyl-glutamine-supplemented enteral formula. *J Pediatr Gastroenterol Nutr.* 2007;44:365-374.
334. Kotler DP, Fogleman L, Tierney AR. Comparison of total parenteral nutrition and an oral, semielemental diet on body composition, physical function, and nutrition-related costs in patients with malabsorption due to acquired immunodeficiency syndrome. *JPEN J Parenter Enteral Nutr.* 1998;22:120-126.
335. Brantley RK, Williams KR, Silva TM, et al. AIDS-associated diarrhea and wasting in Northeast Brazil is associated with subtherapeutic plasma levels of antiretroviral medications and with both bovine and human subtypes of *Cryptosporidium parvum*. *Braz J Infect Dis.* 2003;7:16-22.
336. Garcia Compean D, Ramos Jimenez J, Guzman de la Garza F, et al. Octreotide therapy of large-volume refractory AIDS-associated diarrhea: a randomized controlled trial. *AIDS.* 1994;8:1563-1567.
337. Simon DM, Cello JP, Valenzuela J, et al. Multicenter trial of octreotide in patients with refractory acquired immunodeficiency syndrome-associated diarrhea. *Gastroenterology.* 1995; 108:1753-1760.
338. Beaugerie L, Baumer P, Chaussade S, et al. Treatment of refractory diarrhoea in AIDS with acetorphan and octreotide: a randomized crossover study. *Eur J Gastroenterol Hepatol.* 1996; 8:485-489.
339. Carr A, Marriott D, Field A, et al. Treatment of HIV-1-associated microsporidiosis and cryptosporidiosis with combination antiretroviral therapy. *Lancet.* 1998;351:256-261.
340. Foudraine NA, Weverling GJ, van Grool T, et al. Improvement of chronic diarrhea in patients with advanced HIV-1 infection during potent antiretroviral therapy. *AIDS.* 1998;12:35-41.
341. Grube H, Ramratnam B, Ley C, et al. Resolution of AIDS associated cryptosporidiosis after treatment with indinavir. *Am J Gastroenterol.* 1997;92:726.
342. Maggi P, Larocca AM, Quarto M, et al. Effect of antiretroviral therapy on cryptosporidiosis and microsporidiosis in patients infected with human immunodeficiency virus type 1. *Eur J Clin Microbiol Infect Dis.* 2000;19:213-217.
343. Miao YM, Awad-El-Kariem FM, Franzen C, et al. Eradication of cryptosporidia and microsporidia following successful antiretroviral therapy. *J Acquir Immune Defic Syndr.* 2000;25:124-129.
344. Hommer V, Eichholz J, Petry F. Effect of antiretroviral protease inhibitors alone, and in combination with paromomycin, on the excystation, invasion and in vitro development of *Cryptosporidium parvum*. *J Antimicrob Chemother.* 2003;52:359-364.
345. Mele R, Gomez Morales MA, Tosini F, et al. Indinavir reduces *Cryptosporidium parvum* infection in both in vitro and in vivo models. *Int J Parasitol.* 2003;33:757-764.
346. Maggi P, Larocca AM, Ladisa N, et al. Opportunistic parasitic infections of the intestinal tract in the era of highly active antiretroviral therapy: is the CD4(+) count so important? *Clin Infect Dis.* 2001;33:1609-1611.
347. French AL, Beaudet LM, Benator DA, et al. Cholecystectomy in patients with AIDS—clinicopathologic correlations in 107 cases. *Clin Infect Dis.* 1995;21:852-858.
348. Bouche H, Housset C, Dumont JL, et al. AIDS-related cholangitis: diagnostic features and course in 15 patients. *J Hepatol.* 1993;17:34-39.
349. Cordero E, Lopez-Cortes LF, Belda O, et al. Acquired immunodeficiency syndrome-related cryptosporidial cholangitis: resolution with endobiliary prosthesis insertion. *Gastrointest Endosc.* 2001;53:534-535.
350. Yusuf TE, Baron TH. AIDS cholangiopathy. *Curr Treat Options Gastroenterol.* 2004;7:111-117.
351. Stockdale HD, Spencer JA, Blagburn BL. Prophylaxis and chemotherapy. In: Fayer R, Xiao L, eds. *Cryptosporidium and Cryptosporidiosis.* 2nd ed. Boca Raton, FL: CRC Press; 2008:255-287.
352. Vasquez JR, Gooze L, Kim K, et al. Potential antifolate resistance determinants and genotypic variation in the bifunctional dihydrofolate reductase-thymidylate synthase gene from human and bovine isolates of *Cryptosporidium parvum*. *Mol Biochem Parasitol.* 1996;79:153-165.
353. O'Neil RH, Lilien RH, Donald BR, et al. The crystal structure of dihydrofolate reductase-thymidylate synthase from *Cryptosporidium hominis* reveals a novel architecture for the bifunctional enzyme. *J Eukaryot Microbiol.* 2003;50(Suppl):555-556.
354. Anderson AC. Two crystal structures of dihydrofolate reductase-thymidylate synthase from *Cryptosporidium hominis* reveal protein-ligand interactions including a structural basis for observed antifolate resistance. *Acta Crystallogr Sect F Struct Biol Cryst Commun.* 2005;61:258-262.
355. Liu J, Bolstad DB, Bolstad ES, et al. Towards new antifolates targeting eukaryotic opportunistic infections. *Eukaryot Cell.* 2009;8:483-486.
356. White Jr AC, Chappell CL, Hayat CS, et al. Paromomycin for cryptosporidiosis in AIDS: a prospective, double-blind trial. *J Infect Dis.* 1994;170:419-424.
357. Smith NH, Cron S, Valdez LM, et al. Combination drug therapy for cryptosporidiosis in AIDS. *J Infect Dis.* 1998;178:900-903.
358. White Jr AC, Cron SG, Chappell CL. Paromomycin in cryptosporidiosis. *Clin Infect Dis.* 2001;32:1516-1517.
359. Abubakar I, Aliyu S, Arumugam C, et al. Prevention and treatment of cryptosporidiosis in immunocompromised patients. *Cochrane Database Syst Rev* 2007:CD004932.
360. White Jr AC. Nitazoxanide: a new broad spectrum antiparasitic agent. *Expert Rev Anti Infect Ther.* 2004;2:43-49.
361. Aslam S, Musher DM. Nitazoxanide: clinical studies of a broad-spectrum anti-infective agent. *Future Microbiol.* 2007;2: 583-590.
362. Theodos CM, Griffiths JK, D'Onfro J, et al. Efficacy of nitazoxanide against *Cryptosporidium parvum* in cell culture and in animal models. *Antimicrob Agents Chemother.* 1998;42: 1959-1965.
363. Gargala G, Delaunay A, Li X, et al. Efficacy of nitazoxanide, tizoxanide and tizoxanide glucuronide against *Cryptosporidium parvum* development in sporozoite-infected HCT-8 enterocystic cells. *J Antimicrob Chemother.* 2000;46:57-60.
364. Theodos CM. Innate and cell-mediated immune responses to *Cryptosporidium parvum*. *Adv Parasitol.* 1998;40:87-119.
365. Blagburn BL, Drain KL, Land TM, et al. Comparative efficacy evaluation of dicationic carbazole compounds, nitazoxanide, and paromomycin against *Cryptosporidium parvum* infections in a neonatal mouse model. *Antimicrob Agents Chemother.* 1998;42:2877-2882.
366. Li X, Brasseur P, Agnamey P, et al. Long-lasting anticryptosporidial activity of nitazoxanide in an immunosuppressed rat model. *Folia Parasitol (Praha).* 2003;50:19-22.
367. Doumbo O, Rossignol JF, Pichard E, et al. Nitazoxanide in the treatment of cryptosporidial diarrhea and other intestinal parasitic infections associated with acquired immunodeficiency syndrome in tropical Africa. *Am J Trop Med Hyg.* 1997;56: 637-639.
368. Rossignol JF, Hidalgo H, Feregrino M, et al. A double-'blind' placebo-controlled study of nitazoxanide in the treatment of cryptosporidial diarrhoea in AIDS patients in Mexico. *Trans R Soc Trop Med Hyg.* 1998;92:663-666.
369. Rossignol JF, Ayoub A, Ayers MS. Treatment of diarrhea caused by *Cryptosporidium parvum*: a prospective randomized, double-blind, placebo-controlled study of nitazoxanide. *J Infect Dis.* 2001;184:103-106.
370. Rossignol JF, Kabil SM, el-Gohary Y, et al. Effect of nitazoxanide in diarrhea and enteritis caused by *Cryptosporidium* species. *Clin Gastroenterol Hepatol.* 2006;4:320-324.
371. Rossignol JF. Nitazoxanide in the treatment of acquired immune deficiency syndrome-related cryptosporidiosis: results of the United States compassionate use program in 365 patients. *Aliment Pharmacol Ther.* 2006;24:887-894.
372. White Jr AC, Goodgame RW, Chappell CL. Paromomycin for cryptosporidiosis in AIDS-reply [letter]. *J Infect Dis.* 1995;171: 1071.
373. Blanshard C, Shanson DC, Gazzard BG. Pilot studies of azithromycin, letrazuril, and paromomycin in the treatment of cryptosporidiosis. *Int J STD AIDS.* 1997;8:124-129.
374. Kanyok TP, Novak RM, Danziger LH. Preliminary results of a randomized, blinded, control study of paromomycin vs placebo for treatment of *Cryptosporidium* diarrhea in AIDS patients. In: *IX International Conference on AIDS*. Berlin: London: Wellcome Foundation; 1993.
375. Hewitt RG, Yiannoutsos CT, Higgs ES, et al. Paromomycin: no more effective than placebo for treatment of cryptosporidiosis in patients with advanced human immunodeficiency virus infection. *Clin Infect Dis.* 2000;31:1084-1092.
376. Sáez-Llorens X, Odio CM, Umaña MA, et al. Spiramycin vs. placebo for treatment of acute diarrhea caused by *Cryptosporidium*. *Pediatr Infect Dis J.* 1989;8:136-140.
377. Wittenberg DF, Miller NM, van den Ende J. Spiramycin is not effective in treating *Cryptosporidium* diarrhea in infants: results of a double-blind randomized trial. *J Infect Dis.* 1989;159: 131-132.
378. Weikel C, Lazenby A, Belitsos P, et al. Intestinal injury associated with spiramycin therapy of *Cryptosporidium* infection in AIDS. *J Protozool.* 1991;38:147S.
379. Hicks P, Zwiener RJ, Squires J, et al. Azithromycin therapy for *Cryptosporidium parvum* infection in four children infected with human immunodeficiency virus. *J Pediatr.* 1996;129:297-300.
380. Nachbaur D, Kropshofer G, Feichtinger H, et al. Cryptosporidiosis after CD34-selected autologous peripheral blood stem cell transplantation (PBSCT): treatment with paromomycin, azithromycin and recombinant human interleukin-2. *Bone Marrow Transplant.* 1997;19:1261-1263.
381. Kadappu KK, Nagaraja MV, Rao PV, et al. Azithromycin as treatment for cryptosporidiosis in human immunodeficiency virus disease. *J Postgrad Med.* 2002;48:179-181.
382. Allam AF, Shehab AY. Efficacy of azithromycin, praziquantel and mirazid in treatment of cryptosporidiosis in school children. *J Egypt Soc Parasitol.* 2002;32:969-978.
383. Fayer R, Ellis W. Glycoside antibiotics alone and combined with tetracyclines for prophylaxis of experimental cryptosporidiosis in neonatal BALB/c mice. *J Parasitol.* 1993;79:553-558.
384. Sprinz E, Mallman R, Barcellos S, et al. AIDS-related cryptosporidial diarrhoea: an open study with roxithromycin. *J Antimicrob Chemother.* 1998;41(Suppl B):85-91.
385. Uip DE, Lima AL, Amato VS, et al. Roxithromycin treatment for diarrhoea caused by *Cryptosporidium* spp. in patients with AIDS. *J Antimicrob Chemother.* 1998;41(Suppl B):93-97.
386. Amenta M, Dalle Nogare ER, Colomba C, et al. Intestinal protozoa in HIV-infected patients: effect of rifaximin in *Cryptosporidium parvum* and *Blastocystis hominis* infections. *J Chemother.* 1999;11:391-395.
387. Gathe Jr JC, Mayberry C, Clemmons J, et al. Resolution of severe cryptosporidial diarrhea with rifaximin in patients with AIDS. *J Acquir Immune Defic Syndr.* 2008;48:363-364.
388. Greenberg PD, Cello JP. Treatment of severe diarrhea caused by *Cryptosporidium parvum* with oral bovine immunoglobulin concentrate in patients with AIDS. *J Acquir Immune Defic Syndr Hum Retrovirol.* 1996;13:348-354.
389. Okhuysen PC, Chappell CL, Crabb J, et al. Prophylactic effect of bovine anti-*Cryptosporidium* hyperimmune colostrum immunoglobulin in healthy volunteers challenged with *Cryptosporidium parvum*. *Clin Infect Dis.* 1998;26:1324-1329.
390. Masur H, Kaplan JE, Holmes KK, et al. Adult Prevention and Treatment of Opportunistic Infections Guidelines Working Group. Guidelines for Prevention and Treatment of Opportunistic Infections in HIV-Infected Adults and Adolescents [DRAFT]. June 18, 2008, 2008 <http://aidsinfo.nih.gov/content-files/Adult_OI.pdf>; Accessed January 25, 2009.
391. Addiss DG, Pond RS, Remshak M, et al. Reduction of risk of watery diarrhea with point-of-use water filters during a massive outbreak of waterborne *Cryptosporidium* infection in Milwaukee, Wisconsin, 1993. *Am J Trop Med Hyg.* 1996;54:549-553.
392. Holmberg SD, Moorman AC, Von Bargen JC, et al. Possible effectiveness of clarithromycin and rifabutin for cryptosporidiosis chemoprophylaxis in HIV disease. HIV Outpatient Study (HOPS) Investigators. *JAMA.* 1998;279:384-386.
393. Fichtenbaum CJ, Zackin R, Feinberg J, et al. Rifabutin but not clarithromycin prevents cryptosporidiosis in persons with advanced HIV infection. *AIDS.* 2000;14:2889-2893.
394. Sagodira S, Buzoni-Gatel D, Iochmann S, et al. Protection of kids against *Cryptosporidium parvum* infection after immunization of dams with CP15-DNA. *Vaccine.* 1999;17:2346-2355.
395. Jenkins MC. Present and future control of cryptosporidiosis in humans and animals. *Expert Rev Vaccines.* 2004;3:669-671.
396. He H, Zhao B, Liu L, et al. The humoral and cellular immune responses in mice induced by DNA vaccine expressing the sporozoite surface protein of *Cryptosporidium parvum*. *DNA Cell Biol.* 2004;23:335-339.
397. Ehigiator HN, Romagnoli P, Priest JW, et al. Induction of murine immune responses by DNA encoding a 23-kDa antigen of *Cryptosporidium parvum*. *Parasitol Res.* 2007;101:943-950.

284

Cyclospora cayetanensis, Isospora belli, Sarcocystis Species, Balantidium coli, and Blastocystis hominis

KATHRYN N. SUH | PHYLLIS KOZARSKY | JAY S. KEYSTONE

Coccidia Other Than Cryptosporidia

Cyclospora, *Isospora*, and *Sarcocystis* are coccidian parasites belonging to the phylum Apicomplexa, family Eimeriidae. Coccidian protozoan infections are now well recognized but still relatively uncommon causes of diarrheal disease. *Cryptosporidium parvum* and *Cyclospora cayetanensis*, two of the more commonly identified coccidian pathogens in diarrheal illness, accounted for only a small proportion of laboratory confirmed diarrheal disease reported to the Foodborne Diseases Active Surveillance Network (FoodNet) of the Centers for Disease Control and Prevention in 2006.[1] In 2007, the reported incidences of cryptosporidiosis and cyclosporiasis were 2.67 and 0.03 per 100,000 population, respectively, and seem high. However, such data need to be put into perspective when statistics show that *Salmonella* and *Campylobacter* occurred at a rate of 14.92 and 12.79 per 100,000, respectively, during the same time period.[2]

Cyclospora are genetically closely related to *Eimeria* and are more distantly related to *Isospora*, *Sarcocystis*, and *Toxoplasma*.[3] Although several species of *Cyclospora* have been identified, humans are the only known hosts for *C. cayetanensis*. Also, humans are the only recognized hosts for *Isospora belli*, and no other *Isospora* species has been confirmed to infect humans.

Clinical signs and symptoms do not distinguish disease caused by *Cyclospora*, *Cryptosporidia*, *Microsporidia*, *Isospora*, or other noninflammatory causes of diarrhea. However, knowledge of the occurrence of global outbreaks and the seasonal and geographic variation of diseases such as cyclosporiasis can help point to a particular pathogen. Infection with any of these agents can cause protracted and severe illness in immunocompromised hosts, in particular those with human immunodeficiency virus (HIV) infection, although the incidence of many coccidian infections seems to be decreasing since the introduction of highly active antiretroviral therapy.[4,5] *Cyclospora* in particular continues to be implicated in foodborne and waterborne outbreaks of diarrheal disease. In contrast, *Sarcocystis* infection is typically asymptomatic and rarely causes gastrointestinal symptoms.

CYCLOSPORA

Cyclosporiasis was first described in humans in Papua New Guinea in 1977. The organism was considered to be a blue-green alga but eluded accurate taxonomic classification until 1993, when Ortega and colleagues[6] in Peru succeeded in inducing sporulation and thus confirmed its genus, *Cyclospora*. It was named *C. cayetanensis* after the Universidad Peruana Cayetano Heredia in Lima, Peru, a major site of research on the infection.

Life Cycle

Cyclospora oocysts are spherical, measuring 8 to 10 μm in diameter. Ultrastructural studies of the unsporulated oocyst reveal an outer fibrillar coat and a cell wall and membrane. Unsporulated oocysts are excreted in the stool of infected individuals. Oocysts are quite resistant and can survive under diverse environmental conditions including freezing, 2% formalin, 2% potassium dichromate, and chlorination.

Sporulation is required for infectivity and requires at least 7 days of maturation outside of the human host; experimentally, in moderate temperatures, sporulation occurs within 7 to 13 days.[7] Each sporulated oocyst contains two sporocysts that each holds two sporozoites.

After ingestion of sporulated oocysts, excystation occurs in the proximal small bowel. Sporozoites penetrate the epithelial cells of the small intestine, where both asexual and sexual reproduction takes place. Although the asexual life cycle can continue endogenously within the intestinal epithelium, sexual reproduction leads to the development of zygotes. Zygotes mature into oocysts within the intestinal epithelium, which in turn are released in the stool after causing rupture of the host cells.

Epidemiology

Cyclospora infections occur worldwide, sporadically and in clusters, with a major increase in reported cases after its widespread recognition in the mid-1990s.[8] Cases have been reported from all regions of the world. The majority have been described in developing countries of the tropics and subtropics, where the disease seems to be endemic; cases in developed nations tend to be more frequently associated with recognized waterborne and foodborne outbreaks. Outbreaks in North America in the early and mid-1990s—notably, one outbreak among employees of a Chicago hospital that was attributed to ingestion of water from a contaminated water storage tank,[9] and a more widespread outbreak throughout the United States and Canada associated with consumption of contaminated raspberries imported from Guatemala[10]—brought considerable attention to this organism. Other produce including lettuce, basil, and snow peas has been implicated in foodborne outbreaks. Produce is presumably contaminated by washing or spraying with contaminated surface water.[8,11] Sporadic cases of disease also occur commonly in developed countries. Prevalence studies in stool samples from developed countries have identified *Cyclospora* in no more than 0.5% of samples.[8] *Cyclospora* has also been described as a cause of travelers' diarrhea,[12] although it is not one of the major causes of this illness. Finally, cyclosporiasis is a recognized opportunistic infection in those with HIV infection and other immunosuppressed conditions.

Humans are the only known hosts for *C. cayetanensis*. Transmission of *C. cayetanensis* occurs via the fecal-oral route, but direct person-to-person spread is unlikely due to the need for oocysts to sporulate in order to become infectious. The infectious dose has not been determined, but is presumed to be low.[13] Not surprisingly, in developing countries, infection is more common in children younger than 10 years of age,[14-16] with the risk of infection decreasing with increasing age. Infants may, however, be somewhat protected through breastfeeding. Infection occurs seasonally but varies according to geography, with the highest incidence in spring and summer (May through July) in the United States, in the warm season (April through June) in Peru,[14] before and during the monsoon season (May through October) in Nepal,[17] and during drier months (January through March) in Haiti.[18] Factors affecting seasonality and possible reservoirs during the off season have not yet been defined.

C. cayetanensis–like oocysts have been recovered from a variety of other animals including mice, rats, dogs, chickens, ducks, and nonhuman primates. Attempts to infect mammals and birds in the laboratory setting have been largely unsuccessful. It is unclear whether animals represent a source of human infection or whether the oocysts recovered from animal feces represent coprophagy or other zoonotic organisms that resemble *Cyclospora*. Oocysts have also been identified in sewage and vegetable washings.[11,19]

Clinical Manifestations

The clinical manifestations of *Cyclospora* infection are varied and differ according to the degree of endemnicity of the region in which infected individuals live. Asymptomatic infection is more common in the indigenous populations of developing countries, particularly in adults, suggesting that previous exposure may induce some degree of protective immunity among residents of these regions.[14] However, asymptomatic infection may occur in others, including those with HIV infection.[20]

Symptomatic disease occurs in both endemic and nonendemic regions. In developing countries, symptomatic disease is more likely to develop in the absence of previous exposure and is thus more common in children. After an incubation of 1 to 11 days (mean 7 days), illness begins abruptly. A flulike illness may precede the onset of diarrhea, which is invariably present with a median of six watery stools per day. Fatigue, anorexia, myalgia, abdominal cramps, flatus, and nausea occur frequently. Fever is present in approximately 25% of cases. Illness generally lasts from 1 to 7 weeks or longer and may result in dehydration and significant weight loss. Diarrhea can be cyclic or relapsing, especially in the absence of therapy. Disease may be life-threatening in immunocompromised patients; diarrhea tends to be more severe and prolonged and weight loss more common in patients with the acquired immunodeficiency syndrome (AIDS). Postinfectious fatigue can be profound in some individuals and may persist long after the resolution of other clinical symptoms. It is unknown whether the pathogenesis of disease is due to enterocyte dysfunction or whether toxins are secreted.

Extraintestinal complications of *Cyclospora* infection are exceedingly uncommon. Reiter syndrome[21] and Guillain-Barré syndrome[22] have both been reported after infection with *Cyclospora*. Biliary tract disease has been described in AIDS patients.[23,24]

Diagnosis

The diagnosis of cyclosporiasis generally relies on the microscopic identification of the oocysts in stool samples (Fig. 284-1A). Shedding of oocysts in stool can precede the onset of clinical illness, but the disappearance of symptoms and oocysts usually occurs simultaneously. Oocysts may be shed in low numbers during infection, and both concentration of stool specimens and collection of multiple specimens may be required to make the diagnosis.[8]

Although *Cyclospora* oocysts are approximately twice the size of *Cryptosporidia* oocysts, the two may be confused if oocysts are not measured. The organism is variably acid fast on modified Ziehl-Neelsen or Kinyoun stain (see Fig. 284-1B), and such techniques are superior to the examination of routine wet mounts, which require a trained eye for identification of the organism. Therefore, if cyclosporiasis is suspected, notification of the laboratory is prudent so that appropriate tests can be performed. If available, the demonstration of blue autofluorescence of the oocysts under ultraviolet epifluorescence microscopy is both rapid and sensitive, although not specific.[25] Additional stains including auramine,[26] safranin (see Fig. 284-1C),[27] and lactophenol cotton blue[28] can also be used.

Species-specific real-time polymerase chain reaction assays have been developed that are capable of detecting low concentrations of oocysts in stool.[29,30] Although polymerase chain reaction may be more sensitive than conventional diagnostic methods,[31] it is not widely available and requires additional validation in clinical settings. Flow cytometry has been proposed as an alternate method of diagnosis.[32] Antibodies to *Cyclospora* can be detected, but serologic tests are not commercially available.

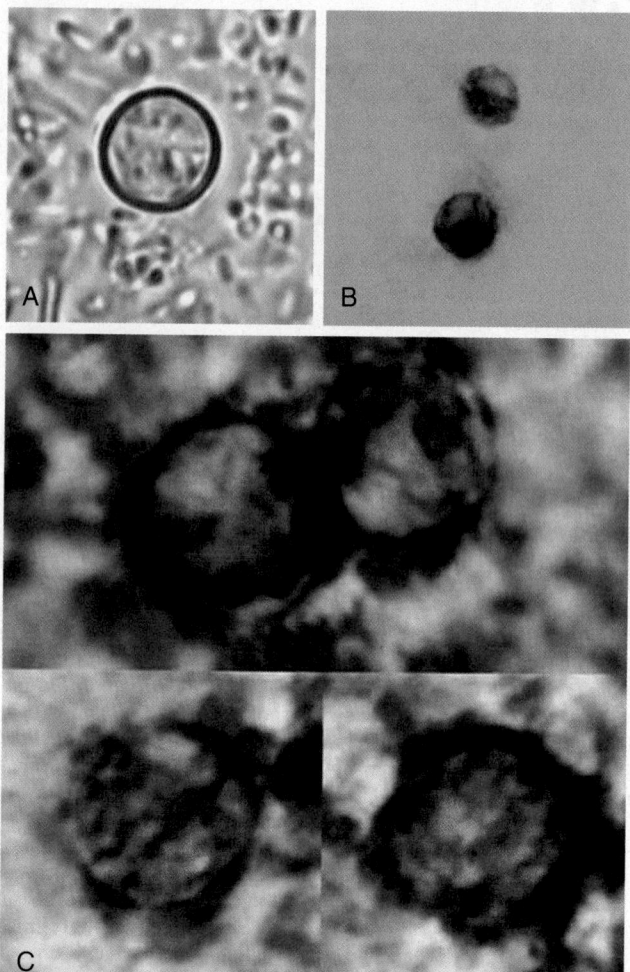

Figure 284-1 *Cyclospora* oocysts visualized with different staining methods. **A,** Wet mount. **B,** Variable staining with modified acid-fast stain. **C,** Uniform staining with modified safranin stain. Modification consists in heating in a microwave during staining. *(From DPDx Image Library, Centers for Disease Control and Prevention, Atlanta, GA.)*

The diagnosis may also be made by histopathologic or electron microscope examination of jejunal aspirates or biopsy specimens. Despite normal endoscopic findings, the histologic architecture of the small bowel is altered. Villous atrophy, acute and chronic inflammation in the lamina propria, and vascular dilatation may be seen microscopically. Routine hematoxylin and eosin staining of biopsy material may not permit adequate visualization of the organisms. Tissue sections may reveal *Cyclospora* in supranuclear locations within the cytoplasm, distinguishing them from *Cryptosporidia*, which are on the surface of the enterocytes.

Treatment

Trimethoprim-sulfamethoxazole (TMP-SMX) is the recommended treatment for cyclosporiasis. One double-strength tablet (160 mg trimethoprim/800 mg sulfamethoxazole) given twice daily is the usual dose for adults with normal renal function; for children, weight-based dosing (trimethoprim 5 mg/kg twice daily) should be used. Treatment is continued for 7 days in immunocompetent hosts[14,33] and for 7 to 10 days in patients with HIV infection.[34,35] Suppressive therapy with TMP-SMX (160/800 mg three times weekly) is recommended in HIV-infected patients due to the high rate of relapse of almost 50% in this population.[34]

Patients who cannot tolerate TMP-SMX may be treated with ciprofloxacin 500 mg twice daily for 7 days, based on a single study conducted in HIV-infected patients.[35] If suppressive therapy is indicated, a dose of 500 mg three times weekly may be used. Ciprofloxacin was, however, slightly less efficacious than TMP-SMX for both treatment and prophylaxis.[35] More recently, the thiazolide agent nitazoxanide, 500 mg twice daily for 7 days, has been used successfully to treat cyclosporiasis in an immunocompetent adult[36] and has been shown to be efficacious in the treatment of mixed parasitic infections (including cyclosporiasis) in children.[37] However, studies demonstrating its efficacy in the treatment of cyclosporiasis in HIV-infected patients are lacking.

ISOSPORA BELLI

I. belli was first described in 1915. It is the only one of more than 200 identified *Isospora* species that is known to cause human infection. Human infections previously attributed to *Isospora hominis* are more likely to have been caused by either *Sarcocystis* species or by misidentified *I. belli*.

Life Cycle

Immature *Isospora* oocysts, each containing a single sporoblast, are excreted in the stool of infected hosts. Oocysts can remain viable in the environment for months. Sporulation in the environment is required before oocysts become infectious. Sporulation generally requires 24 to 48 hours, but can occur within 16 hours in ideal conditions (30° to 37°C) and is hindered at temperatures below 20°C or above 40°C.[38] The single sporoblast divides in two, and each newly formed sporoblast subsequently matures into a sporocyst. The resulting infective elliptical oocyst (22 to 33 × 12 to 15 μm) contains two sporocysts, each with four sporozoites.

Ingestion of sporulated oocysts results in the release of sporozoites in the proximal small intestine. Sporozoites may develop into merozoites, with subsequent asexual reproduction occurring within enterocytes; over time, sexual reproduction follows, resulting in the development and passage of immature, unsporulated oocysts in feces. Rarely, some sporozoites can migrate out of the intestine to various tissues where they may remain dormant as cysts and later give rise to extraintestinal disease.[39,40]

Epidemiology

Isospora organisms are found worldwide but predominantly in tropical and subtropical climates, especially in South America, Africa, and Southeast Asia. In the United States, isosporiasis has been more commonly associated with HIV infection and other immunosuppressed conditions, immigration from Latin America, daycare centers, and psychiatric institutions. In patients with AIDS in the United States, *I. belli* infection accounted for approximately 2% to 3% of AIDS-defining illnesses in the 1980s, but this decreased to less than 0.1% in the late 1990s,[41] in large part because of the widespread use of TMP-SMX used to prevent *Pneumocystis jirovecii* pneumonia. In contrast, in developing countries, *I. belli* infections are frequently associated with chronic diarrhea in AIDS patients, occurring in 5% to 26% of these individuals.[42-44]

Isospora species other than *I. belli* have been found in a wide variety of animals, including cats and dogs. It is unclear whether most animals develop clinical disease or whether they merely act as paratenic hosts. Pigs are notable exceptions; *Isospora suis* can cause severe diarrheal disease and death in piglets and has been implicated in outbreaks of disease among nursing piglets.[38]

Clinical Manifestations

The pathogenesis of isosporiasis has not been determined, but may be the result of cell damage from direct consequences of parasite invasion, cell-mediated inflammation, or proteins and oxidants released from mast cells.

In immunocompetent hosts, *Isospora* infection is indistinguishable from other noninflammatory intestinal infections. After an incubation period of approximately 1 week, a self-limited diarrheal illness usually develops in patients that lasts 2 to 3 weeks and is characterized by malaise, anorexia, weight loss, abdominal cramps, and profuse watery diarrhea without blood. Fever is uncommon and if present is usually low grade. Oocyst shedding may persist for several weeks after recovery. Rarely, in the immunocompetent patient, chronic persistent or intermittent symptoms may continue for many years.[45]

In immunocompromised hosts, including those with HIV infection or malignancy and those receiving cytotoxic therapy, infection may result in protracted, severe diarrheal illness. Isosporiasis in HIV-infected patients generally occurs with CD4 counts less than 200 cells/mm³. Hemorrhagic colitis has been reported in the setting of HIV infection.[46] Disseminated extraintestinal disease has been reported in the setting of AIDS.[39,47,48] Other rare, atypical presentations reported in HIV-infected individuals include biliary tract disease[40,49] and reactive arthritis.[50]

Diagnosis

Typically, *I. belli* infection is diagnosed by identification of oocysts in stool in wet mounts (Fig. 284-2A) or modified acid-fast stained fecal smears (see Fig. 284-2B). Because *I. belli* parasites are shed intermittently in low numbers, multiple stool examinations may be required for diagnosis, and stool concentration (using flotation or sedimentation methods) may be required. Direct or concentrated wet mounts are preferable to permanent stain smears because oocysts are difficult to detect in preserved stool specimens. Auramine-rhodamine, lactophenol cotton blue, and safranin (see Fig. 284-2C) may also be used. Ultraviolet autofluorescence microscopy (see Fig. 284-2D) is a simple, rapid, and sensitive diagnostic method that is based on the detection of *Isospora* oocyst (blue) autofluorescence when a 330- to 380-nm ultraviolet filter is used.[51] Examination of small bowel specimens (e.g., duodenal aspirates) may be helpful if stool examination is negative. Peripheral blood eosinophilia and Charcot-Leyden crystals in stool, both unusual in other protozoan infections, have been reported.[52,53] Polymerase chain reaction can identify *I. belli* with high sensitivity and specificity,[54] but its use for routine diagnosis requires further study.

Histologic examination of the small bowel of infected patients is relatively nonspecific and reveals villous atrophy, crypt hyperplasia, and lamina propria infiltration with inflammatory cells, particularly eosinophils. Asexual and sexual stages of the parasite can be identified within parasitophorous vacuoles of enterocytes. In case reports of extraintestinal disease, intracellular cysts containing one to three trophozoites were identified in lymph nodes, liver, and spleen.[39,47,48]

Treatment

Treatment has been studied predominantly in HIV-infected patients. TMP-SMX (160 mg trimethoprim/800 mg sulfamethoxazole), the treatment of choice, is administered four times daily for 10 days. Patients with HIV infection usually respond to antimicrobial therapy within several days but have a 50% chance of relapse within 6 to 8 weeks if suppressive therapy is not administered.[55] TMP-SMX for this purpose is beneficial when taken either daily or three times weekly.[56]

Alternatives for treatment with sulfa intolerance include pyrimethamine (75 mg/day) together with folinic acid (10 to 25 mg/day),[57] or ciprofloxacin (500 mg twice daily for 7 days followed by suppressive therapy three times weekly).[35] Nitazoxanide has also been used successfully.[58,59] Other agents including diclazuril, roxithromycin, a combination of albendazole and ornidazole, metronidazole, quinacrine, and furazolidone may also be effective based on case reports.

SARCOCYSTIS SPECIES

Sarcocystis species, previously known as *Sarcosporidia*, are zoonotic protozoan parasites. Since the first report of sarcocystosis in mice in 1843, more than 120 species of *Sarcocystis* have been reported from a wide range of domestic and wild animals. Unlike many other coccidian parasites, *Sarcocystis* has an obligatory two-host cycle. Definitive and intermediate hosts are generally species specific, but have been identified for only half of all *Sarcocystis* species. Human sarcocystosis, often

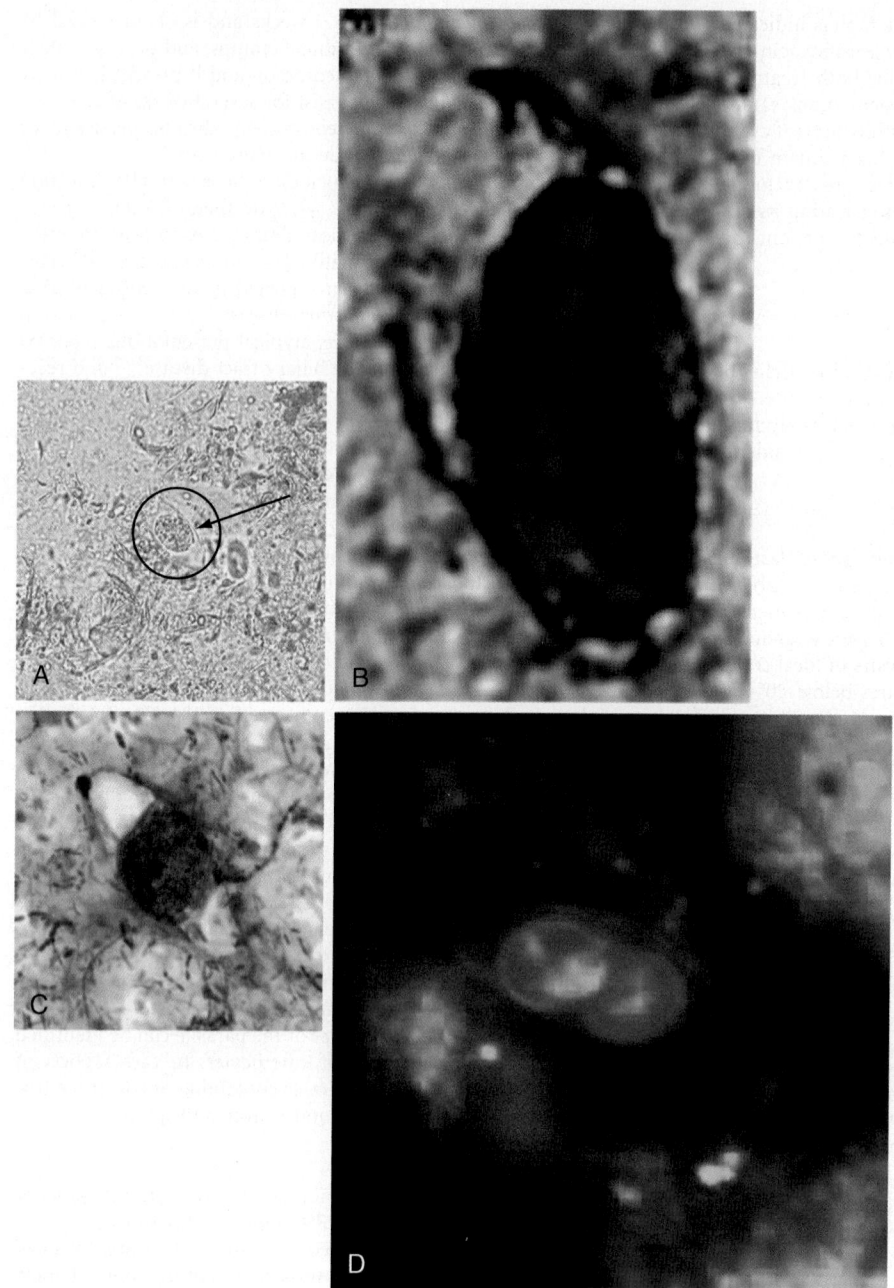

Figure 284-2 Immature oocysts of *Isospora belli*, each containing a single sporoblast. **A**, Wet mount. **B**, Modified acid-fast stain. **C**, Stained with safranin. **D**, Viewed under ultraviolet autofluorescence microscopy. *(From DPDx Image Library, Centers for Disease Control and Prevention, Atlanta, GA.)*

mistakenly attributed to *I. hominis* in the past, is caused by one of two species, *Sarcocystis hominis* or *Sarcocystis suihominis*.

Life Cycle

Humans may act as either definitive or intermediate hosts for *Sarcocystis*. Through the ingestion of poorly cooked or raw meat containing tissue cysts, humans may serve as definitive hosts for pork (*S. suihominis*) and cattle (*S. hominis*) *Sarcocystis*. Humans may also be incidental intermediate hosts when food or water contaminated with fecal sporocysts is ingested.

After consumption of tissue cysts by the definitive host (usually a carnivore), motile bradyzoites emerge from sarcocysts and enter the intestinal lamina propria. Bradyzoites mature into male and female forms, and sexual reproduction follows in the intestinal mucosa; mature oocysts, each of which contains two sporocysts, are formed. The thin walls of oocysts are readily disrupted, leading to shedding of both oocysts and infective sporocysts in the feces. Sporocysts in contrast are hardy, resisting treatment with bleach, chlorhexidine, and iodophores. Each sporocyst measures approximately 10 by 15 μm and contains four sporozoites.

After ingestion of sporocysts by the intermediate host (usually an herbivore), sporozoites are released, penetrate the intestinal epithelium, and migrate to vascular endothelium where they undergo cycles of asexual multiplication. Merozoites are released approximately 2 weeks after sporocysts are ingested. Merozoites are subsequently hematogenously disseminated and invade cardiac or striated muscle cells. Within muscle, the characteristic septate cysts (sarcocysts) containing bradyzoites develop. Sarcocysts become infectious only after they have matured, a process that may take 2 months or more depending on the species. The cycle is complete when mature muscle cysts are eaten by an appropriate definitive host.

Epidemiology

Although worldwide in distribution, most human cases of sarcocystis have been reported from tropical and subtropical climes, mainly Southeast Asia. Cases have been less commonly reported from other continents. Identification of *Sarcocystis* in stool or muscle or of antibodies in serum is most often an incidental finding. As many as 20% of residents in some endemic areas are seropositive, reflecting the sanitary conditions and dietary habits in these regions.[60]

Sarcocystis has been identified in many other animals including nonhuman primates, cattle, dogs, cats, rodents, and reptiles, among others.

Clinical Manifestations

Most individuals with sarcocystosis are asymptomatic. Naturally occurring gastrointestinal illness, when humans act as definitive hosts, is rare. In human volunteers who have ingested pork or beef containing *Sarcocystis* spp., a mild self-limited gastrointestinal illness has developed in some, whereas others have passed sarcocysts but remained asymptomatic. Symptoms induced by experimental challenge with infected meat include nausea, abdominal discomfort, and self-limited diarrhea, with symptom severity dependent on the amount of meat consumed.[61] Onset of diarrhea is generally rapid, within 48 hours of ingestion, and illness is typically brief and self-limited. Segmental eosinophilic and necrotizing enteritis attributed to sexual forms of *Sarcocystis* has been reported; however, causation in these cases was not definitely established.[62]

Muscular sarcocystosis is usually also asymptomatic. Symptoms were noted in only 10 of 52 persons with biopsy-confirmed muscle cysts described in the literature in one case series.[63] Muscle cysts vary greatly in size, ranging from 50 μm to 5 cm. Eosinophilic myositis has been reported, occurring in association with other symptoms including fever, bronchospasm, transient pruritic rashes, lymphadenopathy, subcutaneous nodules, and arthralgias.[63,64] Myocarditis seems to be rare.[63,65]

Systemic disease in one patient with AIDS, with organisms recovered from the stool, small bowel, liver, and blood, has also been reported.[66]

Diagnosis

Sarcocystosis can be suspected when compatible symptoms are present in conjunction with a history of recent consumption of raw or undercooked meat in an endemic area. Sporocysts may be identified in the stool of symptomatic (and asymptomatic) individuals. Oocysts (Fig. 284-3) are less commonly visualized in stool samples due to the fragility of their cell walls. Bright-field microscopy and fecal flotation wet mounts are optimal, using density gradient media rather than other sedimentation methods.[61] The Kato thick smear technique also has excellent sensitivity for diagnosis.[67] Speciation cannot be determined by microscopy.

For patients with symptoms suggestive of muscular disease, muscle biopsy using conventional histologic staining can demonstrate sarcocysts, although staining may be variable. Myositis and myonecrosis, tissue eosinophilia, and inflammatory changes may be seen in cases of eosinophilic myositis.[63]

Serology using Western blot is highly suggestive of previous exposure, but is not diagnostic for acute disease.[63]

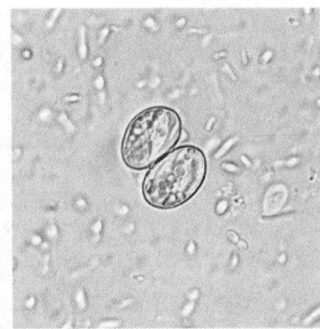

Figure 284-3 Mature oocyst of *Sarcocystis* **spp., containing two readily visualized sporocysts.** *(From DPDx Image Library, Centers for Disease Control and Prevention, Atlanta, GA.)*

Treatment

No specific treatment for *Sarcocystis* infection is known. Infection, if symptomatic, is generally self-limited. Albendazole suppressed symptoms in one human case but was not curative.[63] The efficacy of other antiparasitic agents in treating human disease is unknown. Corticosteroids may provide symptomatic relief in cases of eosinophilic myositis.

BALANTIDIUM COLI

Balantidium coli was identified in 1857. It is the largest protozoan and the only ciliate pathogen of humans.

Life Cycle

After ingestion of cysts via contaminated food or water, trophozoites are released in the small intestine. The oval trophozoite usually measures 30 to 150 μm in length and 25 to 120 μm in width, but may reach 200 μm in length. Its surface is covered with tiny cilia that propel it through the intestinal lumen. Trophozoites migrate to the large intestine where they multiply in the colon wall, and formation of cysts occurs. Cysts, which measure 40 to 60 μm in diameter, are the infective forms of the organism and survive well in the external environment.

Epidemiology

B. coli has a worldwide distribution, but is most frequently reported from Latin America, Southeast Asia, Papua New Guinea, and parts of the Middle East. Although *B. coli* is found in many mammals, domestic and wild pigs are considered to be the main reservoir for human infection, with prevalence rates of 40% to 100%.[68] In humans, the prevalence is usually less than 1%[69,70]; higher rates have been reported among individuals in hyperendemic areas and residential institutions. Human infection most often results from the ingestion of produce or water contaminated with pig excrement or from handling of the animal. Person-to-person transmission can also occur. However, humans are generally resistant to infection, and poor nutrition and underlying debility seem to be risk factors for disease.[68]

Clinical Manifestations

Most infections are asymptomatic. Clinical manifestations may include a chronic course characterized by intermittent diarrhea, abdominal pain, and weight loss. Rarely, a more fulminant colitis with blood and mucus in stools may occur; this may lead to intestinal perforation with subsequent peritonitis or extraintestinal disease.[71-73] A fatal case of *B. coli* pneumonia in a patient with cancer was reported,[74] and the organism has also been identified in the bladder of a patient with hematuria.[75]

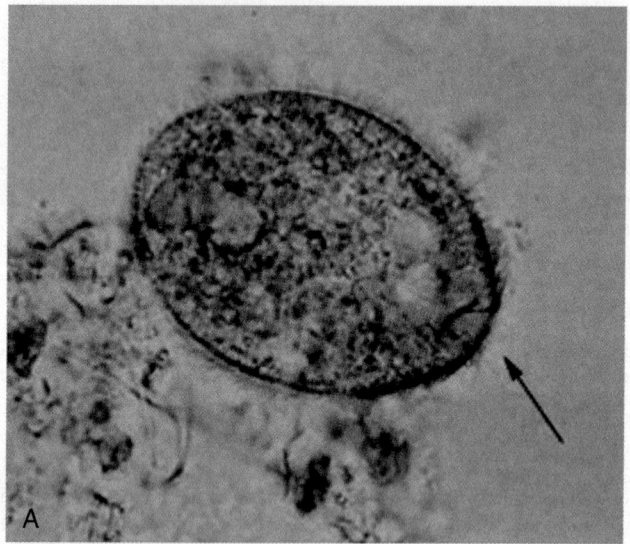

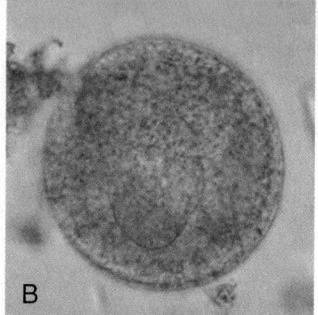

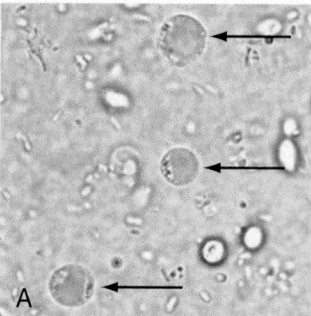

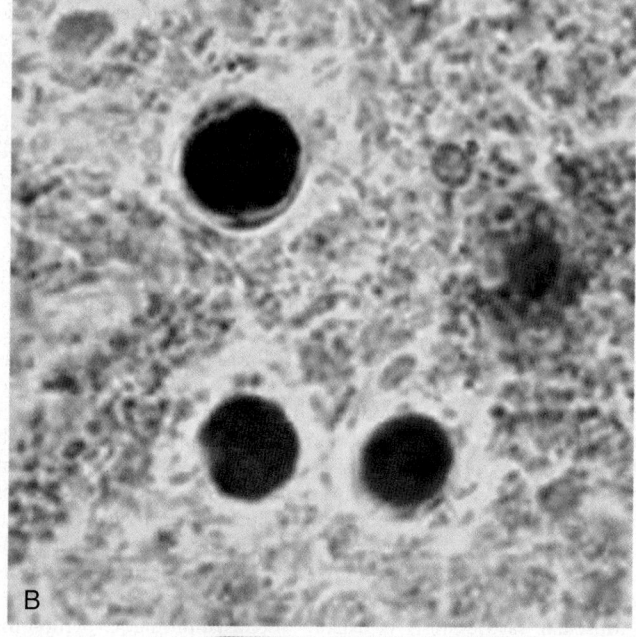

Figure 284-4 **A,** *Balantidium coli* trophozoite demonstrating cilia on the cell surface. A bean-shaped macronucleus is visible toward the left of the trophozoite. **B,** Wet mount of an unstained *B. coli* cyst. Cysts are infrequently visualized in stool. *(From DPDx Image Library, Centers for Disease Control and Prevention, Atlanta, GA.)*

Diagnosis and Treatment

Balantidiasis can be diagnosed by finding rapidly motile trophozoites (Fig. 284-4A) in fresh or preserved stool; cysts (see Fig. 284-4*B*) are infrequently detected. In invasive intestinal disease, endoscopic findings include necrosis and ulceration similar to those found in invasive amebiasis, bacterial dysentery, and inflammatory bowel disease; trophozoites may be recovered from scrapings of the periphery of ulcers detected on endoscopic examination. Pulmonary disease may be diagnosed by the identification of trophozoites in bronchoalveolar lavage specimens.

Tetracycline (500 mg four times daily for 10 days) is the treatment of choice, but other drugs such as iodoquinol (650 mg three times daily for 20 days) and metronidazole (750 mg three times daily for 5 days) are alternatives.[76] Nitazoxanide has also been used effectively.[77] Courses of therapy for as long as 20 days may be required for cure in HIV-infected persons.[78]

BLASTOCYSTIS HOMINIS

Despite its high prevalence throughout the world, major issues about *B. hominis* remain unresolved, including its taxonomy and pathogenicity. Sequences of the ssrURNA gene place *Blastocystis* in the stramenopiles, a diverse group of protist organisms that includes brown algae and diatoms[79]; under the six-kingdom classification, it is placed in the kingdom Chromista. Analysis of the elongation factor-1α gene, however, has indicated relatedness to *Entamoeba histolytica*.[80]

B. hominis exhibits considerable morphologic variability and karyotype diversity. At least 12 species from humans and animals have been

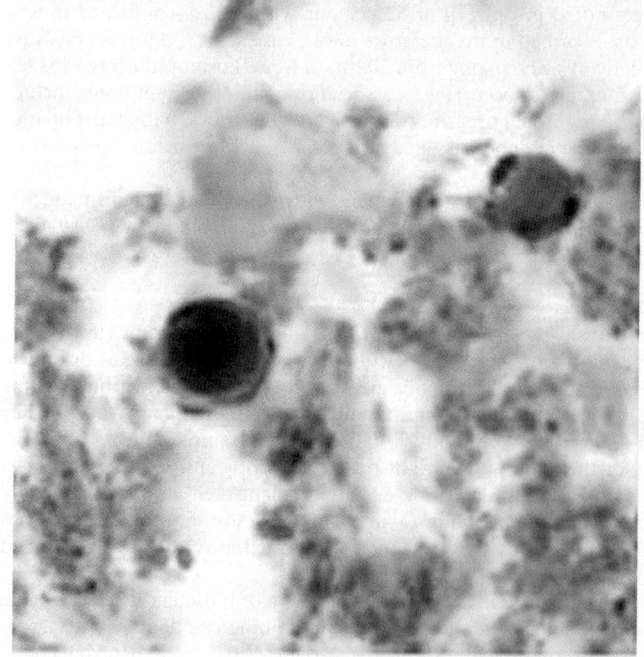

Figure 284-5 ***Blastocystis hominis* cysts. A,** Unstained wet mount. **B,** Stained with trichrome. Vacuoles vary from red to blue. *(From DPDx Image Library, Centers for Disease Control and Prevention, Atlanta, GA.)*

identified.[81] Humans are most commonly infected by subtype 3, a human subtype, but may also be infected by *Blastocystis* spp. of other primates, mammals, rodents, and birds.[82]

Life Cycle

Four major forms of *Blastocystis* predominate: vacuolar, granular, ameboid, and cystic forms. All four forms contain cytoplasm and organelles. The vacuolar form, with a central vacuole, usually measures between 4 and 15 μm but is highly variable in size and is the most frequently detected form in fecal specimens. The granular form is characterized by intracytoplasmic granules. The ameboid form is rarely visualized and has been suggested to be important in pathogenesis. More recently, cysts measuring 2 to 5 μm in size have been identified; they may be readily misidentified as fecal debris due to their small size. Multivacuolar and avacuolar forms have also been described.

Various life cycles have been proposed for *B. hominis*. Currently, it is believed that after ingestion of infective cysts, excystation occurs in the large intestine. Cysts then develop into vacuolar forms and undergo encystation before being excreted in stool.[82] Differentiation between the vacuolar and cystic forms has been observed using electron microscopy.[83] However, the methods of differentiation between the other forms of *B. hominis* remain unclear.

Epidemiology

B. hominis is distributed worldwide. The prevalence of blastocystosis in humans seems to be higher in developing countries (30% to 50%) than in developed countries (1.5% to 10%).[84] However, even within a given country, the reported prevalence rates vary greatly; in China, for example, the prevalence in four communities ranged from 1.9% to 32.6%.[85] Such variability may reflect differences not only in socioeconomic status, but also in local customs and living conditions.

Risk factors associated with infection include immune compromise, travel to and immigration from developing countries, and exposure to contaminated food and water.[82]

Clinical Manifestations

Clinical symptoms attributed to *B. hominis* include acute or chronic diarrhea, bloating, flatulence, abdominal cramps, and fatigue. Irritable bowel disease has been associated with *B. hominis*.[86,87] However, the role of *B. hominis* in causing disease remains controversial. It has been hypothesized that there may be virulent and avirulent strains of *B. hominis*, which could account for the variability in symptoms.

Evidence that *B. hominis* is causally linked to intestinal disease is based on numerous case reports and uncontrolled or retrospective series in which infection was associated with nonspecific gastrointestinal symptoms. In many studies that have included asymptomatic controls, neither the identification of *B. hominis* in stool samples nor the concentration of organisms in stool has been correlated with the presence of gastrointestinal symptoms.[88-91] However, observational studies of TMP-SMX therapy[92] and small placebo-controlled studies with metronidazole[93] and nitazoxanide[94] have all demonstrated symptomatic improvement coincident with reduction or elimination of the organism in stool and suggest that *B. hominis* may be pathogenic. The pathogenicity of the organism remains unclear because of the uncertainty that other causes of symptoms have been eliminated in case series and treatment trials and the inability of case-control studies to determine the association of a low-grade pathogen with disease.

Diagnosis

Diagnosis is based on demonstration of parasites in stool. Microscopic diagnosis may be challenging due to the variable forms and sizes of *B. hominis*. *B. hominis* may be visualized in wet mounts (Fig. 284-5A) and with a variety of routine staining techniques, but permanent smears are preferred for microscopic diagnosis. The trichrome stain (see Fig. 284-5B) seems to be the most sensitive for detection of *B. hominis*. Concentration methods that involve water washes can cause lysis of all recognized forms (in particular, vacuolar forms) of *B. hominis* and may be less sensitive than other microscopic techniques. The organism can also be identified by electron microscopy, although this is not a practical nor readily available technique.

In vitro cell cultivation in Jones' medium requires 48 to 72 hours for incubation, but has been shown to be more sensitive than microscopy and concentration methods, especially if small numbers of organisms are present.[95,96] Polymerase chain reaction is a highly sensitive and specific test[97] but is neither standardized nor widely available for routine diagnosis. Serology is not useful in diagnosing infection.

Treatment

Treatment of asymptomatic infections is unnecessary. Symptoms attributed to *B. hominis* infection are often self-limited, and therapy for "symptomatic" infections should be withheld until other causes of intestinal symptoms have been ruled out. Treatment of blastocystosis is unsatisfactory; metronidazole, TMP-SMX, and iodoquinol are the most commonly recommended therapies but are variably successful.[92,93,98] Nitazoxanide has been used with good effect in limited clinical studies.[37,94]

REFERENCES

1. Centers for Disease Control and Prevention. Preliminary FoodNet data on the incidence of infection with pathogens transmitted commonly through food—10 states, 2006. *MMWR Morb Mortal Wkly Rep.* 2007;56:336-339.
2. Centers for Disease Control and Prevention FoodNet—Foodborne Diseases Active Surveillance Network. <http://www.cdc.gov/foodnet/factsandfigures.htm>; Accessed November 21, 2008.
3. Franzen C, Muller A, Bialek R, et al. Taxonomic position of the human intestinal protozoan parasite *Isospora belli* as based on ribosomal RNA sequences. *Parasitol Res.* 2000;86:669-676.
4. Pozio E, Morales MA. The impact of HIV-protease inhibitors on opportunistic parasites. *Trends Parasitol.* 2005;21:58-63.
5. Lagrange-Xelot M, Porcher R, Sarfati C, et al. Isosporiasis in patients with HIV infection in the highly active antiretroviral therapy era in France. *HIV Med.* 2008;9:126-130.
6. Ortega YR, Sterling CR, Gilman RH, et al. *Cyclospora* species—a new protozoan pathogen of humans. *N Engl J Med.* 1993;328:1308-1312.
7. Ortega YR, Sterling CR, Gilman RH. *Cyclospora cayetanensis. Adv Parasitol.* 1998;40:399-418.
8. Herwaldt BL. *Cyclospora cayetanensis*: a review, focusing on the outbreaks of cyclosporiasis in the 1990s. *Clin Infect Dis.* 2000; 31:1040-1057.
9. Huang P, Weber JT, Sosin DM, et al. The first reported outbreak of diarrheal illness associated with *Cyclospora* in the United States. *Ann Intern Med.* 1995;123:409-414.
10. Herwaldt BL, Ackers M-L, *Cyclospora* Working Group: an outbreak in 1996 of cyclosporiasis associated with imported raspberries. *N Engl J Med.* 1997;336:1548-1556.

11. Sherchand JB, Cross JH, Jimba M, et al. Study of *Cyclospora cayetanensis* in health care facilities, sewage water and green leafy vegetables in Nepal. *Southeast Asian J Trop Med Public Health.* 1999;30:58-63.
12. Jelinek T, Lotze M, Eichenlaub S, et al. Prevalence of infection with *Cryptosporidium parvum* and *Cyclospora cayetanensis* among international travellers. *Gut.* 1997;41:801-804.
13. Sterling CR, Ortega YR. *Cyclospora*: an enigma worth unravelling. *Emerg Infect Dis.* 1999;5:48-53.
14. Madico G, McDonald J, Gilman RH, et al. Epidemiology and treatment of *Cyclospora cayetanensis* infection in Peruvian children. *Clin Infect Dis.* 1997;24:977-981.
15. Bern C, Hernandez B, Lopez MB, et al. The contrasting epidemiology of *Cyclospora* and *Cryptosporidium* among outpatients in Guatemala. *Am J Trop Med Hyg.* 2000;63: 231-235.
16. Kimura K, Rai SK, Rai G, et al. Study on *Cyclospora cayetanensis* associated with diarrheal disease in Nepal and Loa PDR. *Southeast Asian J Trop Med Public Health.* 2005;36:1371-1376.
17. Sherchand JB, Cross JH. Emerging pathogen *Cyclospora cayetanensis* infection in Nepal. *Southeast Asian J Trop Med Public Health.* 2001;32(Suppl 2):143-150.
18. Eberhard ML, Nace EK, Freeman AR, et al. *Cyclospora cayetanensis* infections in Haiti: a common occurrence in the absence of watery diarrhea. *Am J Trop Med Hyg.* 1999;60:584-586.
19. Ortega YR, Roxas CR, Gilman RH, et al. Isolation of *Cryptosporidium parvum* and *Cyclospora cayetanensis* from vegetables collected in markets of an endemic region in Peru. *Am J Trop Med Hyg.* 1997;57:683-686.

20. Schubach TM, Neves ES, Leite AC, et al. *Cyclospora cayetanensis* in an asymptomatic patient infected with HIV and HTLV-1. *Trans R Soc Trop Med Hyg.* 1997;91:175.
21. Connor BA, Johnson EJ, Soave R. Reiter syndrome following protracted symptoms of *Cyclospora* infection. *Emerg Infect Dis.* 2001;7:453-454.
22. Richardson RF Jr, Remler BF, Katirji B, et al. Guillain-Barre syndrome after *Cyclospora* infection. *Musc Nerve.* 1998;21: 669-671.
23. Sifuentes-Osornio J, Porras-Cortes G, Bendall RP, et al. *Cyclospora cayetanensis* infection in patients with and without AIDS: biliary disease as another clinical manifestation. *Clin Infect Dis.* 1995;21:1092-1097.
24. de Gorgolas M, Fortes J, Fernandez Guerrero ML. *Cyclospora cayetanensis* cholecystitis in a patient with AIDS. *Ann Intern Med.* 2001;134:166.
25. Berlin OGW, Peter JB, Gagne C, et al. Autofluorescence and the detection of *Cyclospora* oocysts. *Emerg Infect Dis.* 1998;4:127-128.
26. Hanscheid T, Cristino JM, Salgado MJ. Screening of auramine-stained smears of all fecal samples is a rapid and inexpensive way to increase the detection of coccidial infections. *Int J Infect Dis.* 2008;12:47-50.
27. Visvesvara GS, Moura H, Kovacs-Nace E, et al. Uniform staining of *Cyclospora* oocysts in fecal smears by a modified safranin technique with microwave heating. *J Clin Microbiol.* 1992;35: 730-733.
28. Parija SC, Shivaprakash MR, Jayakeerthi SR. Evaluation of lacto-phenol cotton blue (LPCB) for detection of *Cryptosporidium,*

Cyclospora and Isospora in the wet mount preparation of stool. Acta Trop. 2003;85:349-354.

29. Varma M, Hester JD, Schaefer FW III, et al. Detection of Cyclospora cayetanensis using a quantitative real-time PCR assay. J Microbiol Methods. 2003;53:27-36.

30. Chu DT, Sherchand MB, Cross JH, et al. Detection of Cyclospora cayetanensis in animal fecal isolates from Nepal using an FTA filter-base polymerase chain reaction method. Am J Trop Med Hyg. 2004;71:373-379.

31. Mundaca CC, Torres-Slimming PA, Araujo-Castillo RV, et al. Use of PCR to improve diagnostic yield in an outbreak of cyclosporiasis in Lima, Peru. Trans R Soc Trop Med Hyg. 2008;102:712-717.

32. Dixon BR, Bussey MJ, Parrington LJ, et al. Detection of Cyclospora cayetanensis oocysts in human fecal specimens by flow cytometry. J Clin Microbiol. 2005;43:2375-2379.

33. Hoge CW, Shlim DR, Ghirire M, et al. Placebo controlled trail of co-trimoxazole for Cyclospora infections among travellers and foreign residents in Nepal. Lancet. 1995;345:691-693.

34. Pape JW, Verdier RI, Boncy M, et al. Cyclospora infections in adults with HIV: clinical manifestations, treatment and prophylaxis. Ann Intern Med. 1994;121:654-657.

35. Verdier RI, Fitzgerald DW, Johnson WD, et al. Trimethoprim-sulfamethoxazole compared with ciprofloxacin for treatment and prophylaxis of Isospora belli and Cyclospora cayetanensis infection in HIV-infected patients: a randomized, controlled trial. Ann Intern Med. 2000;132:885-888.

36. Zimmer SM, Schuetz AN, Franco-Paredes C. Efficacy of nitazoxanide for cyclosporiasis in patients with sulfa allergy. Clin Infect Dis. 2007;44:466-467.

37. Diaz E, Mondragon J, Ramirez E, et al. Epidemiology and control of intestinal parasites with nitazoxanide in children in Mexico. Am J Trop Med Hyg. 2003;68:384-385.

38. Lindsay DS, Dubey JP, Blagburn BL. Biology of Isospora spp. from humans, nonhuman primates, and domestic animals. Clin Microbiol Rev. 1997;10:19-34.

39. Restrepo C, Macher AM, Radany EH. Disseminated extraintestinal isosporiasis in a patient with acquired immune deficiency syndrome. Am J Clin Pathol. 1987;87:536-542.

40. Bialek R, Overkamp D, Rettig I, et al. Case report: nitazoxanide treatment failure in chronic isosporiasis. Am J Trop Med Hyg. 2001;65:94-95.

41. Centers for Disease Control and Prevention. Surveillance for AIDS-defining opportunistic illnesses, 1992-1996. MMWR Surveill Summ. 1999;48:1-22.

42. Waywa D, Kongkriengdaj S, Chaidatch S, et al. Protozoan enteric infection in AIDS related diarrhea in Thailand. Southeast Asian J Trop Med Public Health. 2001;32(Suppl 2):151-155.

43. Lebbad M, Norrgren H, Naucler A, et al. Intestinal parasites in HIV-2 associated AIDS cases with chronic diarrhoea in Guinea-Bissau. Acta Trop. 2001;80:45-49.

44. Vignesh R, Balakrishnan AN, Shankar EM, et al. High proportion of isosporiasis among HIV-infected patients with diarrhea in southern India. Am J Trop Med Hyg. 2007;77:823-824.

45. Shaffer N, Moore L. Chronic travelers' diarrhea in a normal host due to Isospora belli. J Infect Dis. 1989;159:596-597.

46. Alfandari S, Ajana F, Senneville E, et al. Haemorrhagic ulcerative colitis due to Isospora belli in AIDS. Int J STD AIDS. 1995;6:216.

47. Michiels JF, Hofman P, Bernard E, et al. Intestinal and extraintestinal Isospora belli infection in an AIDS patient. Pathol Res Pract. 1994;190:1089-1093.

48. Bernard E, Delguidice P, Carles M, et al. Disseminated isosporiasis in an AIDS patient. Eur J Clin Microbiol Infect Dis. 1997;16:699-701.

49. Benator DA, French AL, Beaudet LM, et al. Isospora belli infection associated with acalculous cholecystitis in a patient with AIDS. Ann Intern Med. 1994;121:663-664.

50. Gonzalez-Dominguez J, Roldan R, Villanueva JL, et al. Isospora belli reactive arthritis in a patient with AIDS. Ann Rheum Dis. 1994;53:618-619.

51. Berlin OGW, Conteas CN, Sowerby TM. Detection of Isospora in the stools of AIDS patients using a new rapid autofluorescence technique. AIDS. 1996;10:442-443.

52. Trier JS, Moxey PC, Schimmel EM, et al. Chronic intestinal coccidiosis in man: intestinal morphology and response to treatment. Gastroenterology. 1974;66:923-935.

53. Brandborg LL, Goldberg SB, Breidenbach WC. Human coccidiosis—a possible cause of malabsorption. N Engl J Med. 1970;24:1306-1313.

54. ten Hove RJ, van Lieshout L, Brienen EAT, et al. Real-time polymerase chain reaction for detection of Isospora belli in stool samples. Diag Microbiol Infect Dis. 2008;61:280-283.

55. DeHovitz JA, Pape JW, Boncy M, et al. Clinical manifestations and therapy of Isospora belli infection in patients with acquired immunodeficiency syndrome. N Engl J Med. 1986;315:87-90.

56. Pape JW, Verdier RI, Johnson WD Jr. Treatment and prophylaxis of Isospora belli infection in patients with acquired immunodeficiency syndrome. N Engl J Med. 1989;320:1044-1047.

57. Weiss LM, Perlman D, Sherman J, et al. Isospora belli infection: treatment with pyrimethamine. Ann Intern Med. 1988;109:474-475.

58. Doumbo O, Rossignol JF, Pichard E, et al. Nitazoxanide in the treatment of cryptosporidial diarrhea and other intestinal parasitic infections associated with acquired immunodeficiency syndrome in tropical Africa. Am J Trop Med Hyg. 1997;56:637-639.

59. Romero Cabello R, Guerrero LR, Munoz Garcia MR, et al. Nitazoxanide for the treatment of intestinal protozoan and helminthic infections in Mexico. Trans R Soc Trop Med Hyg. 1997;91:701-703.

60. Kan SP, Pathmananthan R. Review of Sarcocystosis in Malaysia. Southeast Asian J Trop Med Public Health. 1991;22(Suppl):129-234.

61. Fayer R. Sarcocystis spp. in human infections. Clin Microbiol Rev. 2004;17:894-902.

62. Bunyaratvej S, Bunyawongwiroj P, Nitiyanant P. Human intestinal sarcosporidiosis: report of six cases. Am J Trop Med Hyg. 1982;31:36-41.

63. Arness MK, Brown JD, Dubey JP, et al. An outbreak of acute eosinophilic myositis attributed to human Sarcocystis parasitism. Am J Trop Med Hyg. 1999;61:548-553.

64. Van den Enden E, Praet M, Joos R, et al. Eosinophilic myositis resulting from sarcocystosis. J Trop Med Hyg. 1995;98:273-276.

65. Guarner J, Bhatnagar J, Shieh WJ, et al. Histopathologic, immunohistochemical, and polymerase chain reaction assays in the study of cases with fatal sporadic myocarditis. Hum Pathol. 2007;38:1412-1419.

66. Velasquez JH, Di Risio C, Etchart CB, et al. Systemic sarcocystosis in a patient with acquired immune deficiency syndrome. Hum Pathol. 2008;39:1263-1267.

67. Tungtrongchitr A, Chiworaporn C, Praewanich R, et al. The potential usefulness of the modified Kato thick smear technique in the detection of intestinal sarcocystosis during field surveys. Southeast Asian J Trop Med Public Health. 2007;38:232-238.

68. Schuster FL, Ramirez-Avila L. Current world status of Balantidium coli. Clin Microbiol Rev. 2008;21:626-638.

69. Borda CE, Rea MJ, Rosa JR, et al. Intestinal parasitism in San Cayetano, Corrientes, Argentina. Bull Pan Am Health Organ. 1996;30:227-233.

70. Esteban JG, Aguirre C, Angles R, et al. Balantidiasis in Aymara children from the northern Bolivian Altiplano. Am J Trop Med Hyg. 1998;59:922-927.

71. Dorfman S, Rangel O, Bravo LG. Balantidiasis: report of a fatal case with appendicular and pulmonary involvement. Trans R Soc Trop Med Hyg. 1984;78:833-834.

72. Ladas SD, Savva S, Frydas A, et al. Invasive balantidiasis presented as chronic colitis and lung involvement. Dig Dis Sci. 1989;34:1621-1623.

73. Ferry T, Bouhour D, de Monbrison F, et al. Severe peritonitis due to Balantidium coli acquired in France. Eur J Clin Microbiol Infect Dis. 2004;23:393-395.

74. Vasilakopoulou A, Dimarongona K, Samakovli A, et al. Balantidium coli pneumonia in an immunocompromised patient. Scand J Infect Dis. 2003;35:144-146.

75. Maleky F. Case report of Balantidium coli in human from south of Tehran, Iran. Indian J Med Sci. 1998;52:201-202.

76. Drugs for parasitic infections. Med Lett. 2007;5(Suppl):1-15.

77. Abaza H, El-Zayadi AR, Kabil SM, et al. Nitazoxanide in the treatment of patients with intestinal protozoan and helminthic infections: a report of 546 patients in Egypt. Curr Ther Res. 1998;59:116-121.

78. Clyti E, Aznar C, Couppie P, et al. A case of coinfection by Balantidium coli and HIV in French Guiana. Bull Soc Path Exotique. 1998;91:309-311.

79. Noel C, Peyronnet C, Gerbod D, et al. Phylogenetic analysis of Blastocystis isolates from different hosts based on the comparison of small-subunit rRNA gene sequences. Mol Biochem Parasitol. 2003;126:119-123.

80. Ho LC, Jeyaseelan K, Singh M. Use of the elongation factor-1 alpha gene in a polymerase chain reaction-based restriction-fragment-length polymorphism analysis of genetic heterogeneity among Blastocystis species. Mol Biochem Parasitol. 2001;112:287-291.

81. Noel C, Dufernez F, Gerbod D. Molecular phylogenies of Blastocystis isolates from different hosts: implications for genetic diversity, identification of species, and zoonosis. J Clin Microbiol. 2005;43:348-355.

82. Tan KSW. New insights on classification, identification, and clinical relevance of Blastocystis spp. Clin Microbiol Rev. 2008;21:639-665.

83. Moe KT, Singh M, Howe J, et al. Observations on the ultrastructure and viability of the cystic stage of Blastocystis hominis from human feces. Parasitol Res. 1996;82:439-449.

84. Stenzel DJ, Boreham PF. Blastocystis hominis revisited. Clin Microbiol Rev. 1996;563-584.

85. Li LH, Zhang XP, Lv S, et al. Cross-sectional surveys and subtype classification of human Blastocystis isolates from four epidemiological settings in China. Parasitol Res. 2007;102:83-90.

86. Giacometti A, Cirioni O, Fiorentini A, et al. Irritable bowel syndrome in patients with Blastocystis hominis infection. Eur J Clin Microbiol Infect Dis. 1999;18:436-439.

87. Yakoob J, Jafri W, Jafri N, et al. In vitro susceptibility of Blastocystis hominis isolated from patients with irritable bowel syndrome. Br J Biomed Sci. 2004;61:75-77.

88. Udkow MP, Markell EK. Blastocystis hominis: prevalence in asymptomatic versus symptomatic hosts. J Infect Dis. 1993;168:242-244.

89. Shlim DR, Hoge CW, Rajah R, et al. Is Blastocystis hominis a cause of diarrhea in travelers? A prospective controlled study in Nepal. Clin Infect Dis. 1995;21:97-101.

90. Kuo HY, Chiang DH, Wang CC, et al. Clinical significance of Blastocystis hominis: experience from a medical center in northern Taiwan. J Microbiol Immunol Infect. 2008;41:222-226.

91. Leder K, Hellard ME, Sinclair MI, et al. No correlation between clinical symptoms and Blastocystis hominis in immunocompetent individuals. J Gastroenterol Hepatol. 2005;20:1390-1394.

92. Ok UZ, Girginkardesler N, Balcioglu C, et al. Effect of trimethoprim-sulfamethaxazole in Blastocystis hominis infection. Am J Gastroenterol. 1999;94:3245-3247.

93. Nigro L, Larocca L, Massarelli L, et al. A placebo-controlled treatment trial of Blastocystis hominis infection with metronidazole. J Trav Med. 2003;10:128-130.

94. Rossignol JF, Kabil SM, Said M, et al. Effect of nitazoxanide in persistent diarrhea and enteritis associated with Blastocystis hominis. Clin Gastroenterol Hepatol. 2005;3:987-991.

95. Leelayoova S, Taamasri P, Rangsin R, et al. In-vitro cultivation: a sensitive method for detecting Blastocystis hominis. Ann Trop Med Parasitol. 2002;96:803-807.

96. Suresh K, Smith H. Comparison of methods for detecting Blastocystis hominis. Eur J Clin Microbiol Infect Dis. 2004;23:509-511.

97. Stensvold R, Brillowska-Dabrowskia A, Nielsen HV, et al. Detection of Blastocystis hominis in unpreserved stool specimens by using polymerase chain reaction. J Parasitol. 2006;92:1081-1087.

98. Grossman I, Weiss LM, Simon D, et al. Blastocystis hominis in hospital employees. Am J Gastroenterol. 1992;87:729-732.

Human Illness Associated with Harmful Algal Blooms

J. GLENN MORRIS, JR.

During the past several decades, the association of human health and environmental problems with harmful and toxic algae has been increasingly recognized,[1-3] as has awareness of the complex range of natural toxins (and toxin congeners) that can be produced by these microorganisms. Toxic species constitute a small percentage of the thousands of species of microscopic algae at the base of the marine food chain. However, when these species proliferate, they may cause massive killing of fish and shellfish, the death of marine mammals and seabirds, alterations in marine habitats, and, with specific exposure, human illness and death. Although blooms of certain species such as *Karenia brevis* (formerly known as *Gymnodinium breve*) may be manifested as "red tides," adverse events often occur in the absence of visible discoloration of water.

Harmful algal blooms are apparently increasing in frequency; in the United States, problems that in the past were confined to a few geographic locations are now being seen at multiple sites along the U.S. coastline (Fig. 285-1). The factors leading to this apparent increase in incidence are not well understood, although it has been postulated that human-related phenomena such as nutrient enrichment of waterways, climatic change, and disruption of ecosystems play a role.[1,2,4-7]

Eight clinical syndromes or illnesses are currently linked with harmful algal blooms (Table 285-1),[1] and as more research is done in this area, it is possible that other syndromes will be identified. Ciguatera fish poisoning, paralytic shellfish poisoning, and neurotoxic shellfish poisoning are also described in Chapter 99.

Ciguatera Fish Poisoning

Worldwide, ciguatera fish poisoning is the most common of the clinical syndromes associated with marine biotoxins. It is a major public health problem in the Caribbean and South Pacific regions, particularly in areas with tropical reefs.[8-10] Illness is caused by toxins (ciguatoxins, and others) that are passed up the marine food chain; large predatory reef fish (e.g., barracuda, jacks) have the greatest risk of being toxic. Toxins are produced by the dinoflagellate *Gambierdiscus toxicus*, the presence of which has been associated with disruption of normal reef ecology and reef communities.

Gastrointestinal symptoms—nausea, vomiting, and diarrhea—are the first manifestation of illness and usually occur within 24 hours of eating a toxic fish. In severe cases, patients may also be acutely bradycardic and hypotensive and, in rare instances (confined almost exclusively to cases in the Pacific region), may develop respiratory difficulties. The most characteristic symptoms are headache and dysesthesias: tingling sensations in the extremities and around the mouth, cold allodynia (cold objects feeling burning hot), burning sensation in the mouth, and aching pain around the teeth. These symptoms may persist for weeks to months[9-11] and may be linked with clinical depression. The diagnosis is clinical; other than identifying toxin in fish samples that may be left over from an implicated meal, there are no confirmatory tests. Treatment is symptomatic, including maintenance of adequate hydration, use of atropine for bradycardia, and administration of analgesics and antidepressants, as appropriate. Some literature suggests that intravenous mannitol alleviates acute symptoms, although no benefit was seen in one double-blind randomized clinical trial.[12] Anecdotal data suggest that tocainide helps alleviate neurologic symptoms.

Prevention is difficult, as toxic fish have a normal appearance and taste. In endemic areas, this may have major economic and nutritional impact, as local populations are often reluctant to eat locally caught fish because of the risk of ciguatera. Feeding of suspect fish to the family cat to see if symptoms result is a not uncommon practice prior to human consumption in such areas.

Paralytic Shellfish Poisoning

Paralytic shellfish poisoning is the most common cause of marine biotoxin–associated illness in the continental United States and Alaska.[13] Illness has traditionally been associated with eating clams and mussels that contain saxitoxins produced by *Alexandrium* spp. and related dinoflagellates, although a variety of other vehicles have been reported.[14] Unlike ciguatera poisoning, gastrointestinal symptoms are less prominent than neurologic manifestations: circumoral paresthesias and paresthesias of the extremities usually appear within 1 hour of ingesting toxic shellfish, and they may be accompanied by ataxia, dysphagia, and changes in mental status. Hypertension may occur and corresponds to the ingested dose, and, in the most severe cases, patients may proceed to respiratory paralysis, usually within the first 24 hours of illness. In experiments, saxitoxins can be identified in serum and urine samples from affected patients.[15] Treatment is symptomatic. Prevention is achieved through regular monitoring of shellfish populations for saxitoxin by public health authorities, with sampling data available on state health department web pages (e.g., the biotoxin web page of the Washington State Department of Health, http://www.doh.wa.gov/ehp/sf/BiotoxinProgram.htm).

Neurotoxic Shellfish Poisoning

Illness is caused by brevetoxins produced by *Karenia brevis*, a major cause of red tides along the Florida coast; other *Karenia* species have been implicated in illness in other parts of the world. Ingestion of shellfish containing the toxin causes nausea and vomiting, as well as circumoral paresthesias and paresthesias of the extremities. In more severe cases, patients may report ataxia, slurred speech, dizziness, and, in rare cases, mild respiratory distress.[16] Aerosolization of toxins by heavy wave action on the Atlantic coast of Florida can result in respiratory irritation and asthma-like symptoms in persons walking along affected beaches.[17] On an experimental basis, brevetoxin metabolites have been identified in urine samples from affected patients.[18] Treatment is symptomatic. The Florida Department of Health and other health authorities regularly monitor coastal areas for the presence of *K. brevis*, and they notify consumers accordingly. Data on occurrence of the organism in Florida waters are posed on the website of the Florida Department of Health (http://research.myfwc.com/features/view_article.asp?id=9670#Stata1).

Diarrhetic Shellfish Poisoning

Diarrhetic shellfish poisoning results from eating mussels, scallops, or clams that have been feeding on toxic *Dinophysis* or *Prorocentrum* species. Symptoms include diarrhea, nausea, vomiting, and abdominal pain (which may be quite severe). Although okadaic acid appears to be the primary toxin responsible for the observed clinical syndrome,

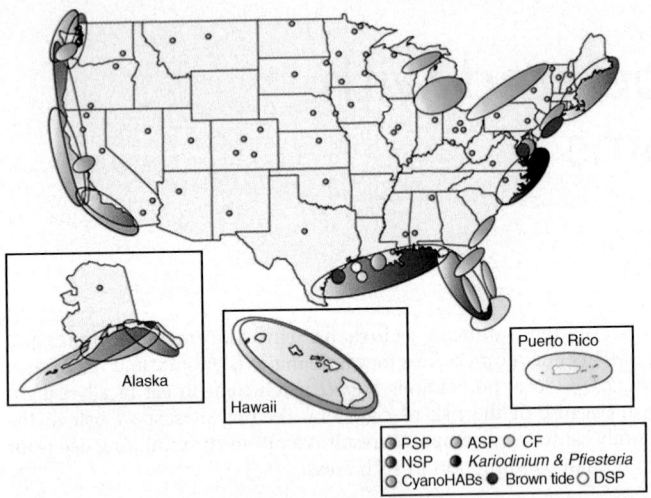

Figure 285-1 Sites and types of harmful algal blooms along the U.S. coast. ASP, amnesic shellfish poisoning; CF, ciguatera fish [poisoning]; cyanoHAB, cyanobacterial harmful algal bloom; DSP, diarrhetic shellfish poisoning; NSP, neurotoxic shellfish poisoning; PSP, paralytic shellfish poisoning. (*From The Harmful Algal Page. Available at www. whoi.edu/redtide/*)

other toxic compounds have been isolated from these species. Although case reports came initially from Japan, diarrhetic shellfish poisoning has now been reported from multiple locations in Europe, Asia, South America, and South Africa. One episode of diarrhetic shellfish poisoning has occurred in Nova Scotia in association with eating cultured mussels.[3] No U.S. cases have been confirmed, although the causative organisms have been identified in U.S. coastal waters.

Amnesic Shellfish Poisoning

Amnesic shellfish poisoning results from the ingestion of shellfish containing domoic acid, which is produced by the diatom *Pseudonitzschia*.[1] An outbreak of illnesses caused by this toxin was reported in the Atlantic provinces of Canada in 1987.[19] Symptoms included vomiting, abdominal cramps, diarrhea, headache, and loss of short-term memory. On neuropsychological testing several months after the acute intoxication, patients were found to have severe antegrade memory deficits with relative preservation of other cognitive functions; patients also had clinical and electromyographic evidence of pure motor or sensorimotor neuropathy or axonopathy. In four patients who died, neuropathologic studies demonstrated neuronal

necrosis and loss, predominantly in the hippocampus and amygdala.[20] Canadian authorities now analyze mussels and clams for domoic acid, and they close shellfish beds to harvesting when levels in shellish exceed 20 mg/g.

Domoic acid has been identified in the marine food web in multiple locations in the United States, including the Monterey Bay and Puget Sound areas. Elevated levels of domoic acid have been linked to neurologic illness and death in seabirds and sea lions[21] in these areas, possibly in relation to consumption of shellfish or anchovies. No cases of amnesic shellfish poisoning have been confirmed in the United States. However, a study in subsistence shellfish eating by Native American tribes in the Puget Sound area revealed that during years when high domoic acid levels were present in shellfish, infants born to shellfish-eating mothers had a significantly lower score on the Mental Developmental Index than did infants born in other years; children consuming shellfish during these "high-level" years also had poorer memory performance than did children who did not eat shellfish.[22] These data suggest that exposure to elevated domoic acid levels presents a health risk to infants and children, and they raise questions about the effect of chronic exposure to levels below the current limit of 20 mg/g.

Azaspiracid Shellfish Poisoning

In 1995, an outbreak of shellfish-associated illness that very closely resembled diarrhetic shellfish poisoning was reported in The Netherlands. Subsequent studies demonstrated that the implicated shellfish were contaminated not with okadaic acid (the cause of diarrhetic shellfish poisoning) but with what is now known as azaspiracid, a class of toxins linked with the dinoflagellate *Protoperidinium crassipes*. Toxic shellfish have subsequently been identified in multiple outbreaks of azaspiracid shellfish poisoning in western Europe and in Morocco.[23]

Lyngbya/Cyanobacteria Exposure Syndromes

Cyanobacterial species can produce thick, foul-smelling, high-biomass blooms (triggered, in many instances, by increasing nutrient flows) that have been linked to human illness, animal mortality, and adverse ecosystem and economic effects in the United States and worldwide. Microcystins, produced by cyanobacterial *Microcystis* species, are known to have toxic effects in animals; however, in a limited study of human recreational exposure to high microcystin levels in a small lake, no immediate human health effects were identified.[24] In contrast, *Lyngbya* species have been implicated in a series of studies as a cause of skin itching ("swimmers itch"), particularly in the inguinal region;

TABLE 285-1	Human Illness Associated with Harmful Algal Blooms		
Syndrome	*Causative Organisms*	*Toxin Produced*	*Clinical Manifestations*
Ciguatera fish poisoning	*Gambierdiscus toxicus* and others	Ciguatoxin	Acute gastroenteritis followed by paresthesias and other neurologic symptoms
Paralytic shellfish poisoning	*Alexandrium* spp. and others	Saxitoxins	Acute paresthesias and other neurologic manifestations; may progress rapidly to respiratory paralysis
Neurotoxic shellfish poisoning	*Karenia brevis*	Brevetoxins	Gastrointestinal and neurologic symptoms; formation of toxic aerosols by wave action can produce respiratory irritation and asthma-like symptoms
Diarrhetic shellfish poisoning	*Dinophysis* spp.	Okadaic acid and others	Acute gastroenteritis, abdominal pain
Amnesic shellfish poisoning	*Pseudo-nitzschia* spp.	Domoic acid	Gastroenteritis, followed by memory loss, neurologic manifestations; may progress to amnesia, coma, and death
Azaspiracid shellfish poisoning	*Protoperidinium crassipes*	Azaspiracid	Acute gastroenteritis, abdominal pain
Lyngbya or *Cyanobacteria* exposure syndromes	*Lyngbya* spp.	Lyngbyatoxin A, debromaplysiatoxin	"Swimmers' itch," particularly in inguinal area; sore eyes, ears; headache; possibly gastrointestinal symptoms (??)
	Microcystis spp.	Microcystins	
Pfiesteria-associated syndrome	*Pfiesteria* spp. (?)	Unidentified to date	Deficiencies in learning and memory; acute respiratory and eye irritation; acute confusional syndrome

sore eyes and ears; headache; and, in a small percentage of patients, abdominal pain and vomiting.[25]

Pfiesteria-Associated Syndrome

Pfiesteria was first isolated during the early 1990s as a suspected cause of massive fish killings in the New River and the Albemarle-Pamlico estuarine system of North Carolina.[26] Shortly after identifying the organism, laboratory investigators working with toxic *Pfiesteria* cultures began to note problems with respiratory irritation, skin rashes, and, most disturbing, cognition.[27] In subsequent studies conducted in the Chesapeake Bay region,[28] a significant association was found between the degree of exposure to waterways where *Pfiesteria* was known to be present and short-term deficiencies (of <6 months' duration) in learning, memory, and higher order cognitive function. Exposed persons also complained of headaches, skin lesions, and at times a burning sensation in water-exposed skin.[28,29] Although questions remain about the role of *Pfiesteria* spp. in the observed symptomatology, study results have suggested that bioactive material produced by the microorganism acts as an inhibitor of the N-methyl-D-aspartate (NMDA) neuroreceptor,[30] which appears to play a key role in learning and memory.

REFERENCES

1. The Harmful Algal Page. Available at ⟨http://www.whoi.edu/redtide⟩.
2. Todd ECD. Emerging diseases associated with seafood toxins and other water-borne agents. *Ann N Y Acad Sci.* 1994;740:77-94.
3. Morris JG Jr. *Pfiesteria*, "the cell from hell," and other toxic algal nightmares. *Clin Infect Dis.* 1999;28:1191-1198.
4. Ruff TA. Ciguatera in the Pacific: a link with military activities. *Lancet.* 1989;1:201-205.
5. Thomassin BA, Ali Halidi ME, Quod JP, et al. Evolution of *Gambierdiscus toxicus* populations in the coral reef complex of Mayotte Island (SW Indian Ocean) during the 1985-1991 period. *Bull Soc Pathol Exot.* 1992;85:449-452.
6. Tester PA. Harmful marine phytoplankton and shellfish toxicity: potential consequences of climatic change. *Ann N Y Acad Sci.* 1994;740:69-76.
7. Paul VJ. Global warming and cyanobacterial harmful algal blooms. *Adv Exp Med Biol.* 2008;619:239-257.
8. Morris JG Jr, Lewin P, Smith CW, et al. Ciguatera fish poisoning: epidemiology of the disease on St. Thomas, U.S. Virgin Islands. *Am J Trop Med Hyg.* 1982;31:574-578.
9. Chateau-Degat M-L, Dewailly E, Cerf N, et al. Temporal trends and epidemiological aspects of ciguatera in French Polynesia: a 10-year analysis. *Trop Med Intern Health.* 2007;12:485-492.
10. Lewis RJ. Ciguatera: Australian perspectives on a global problem. *Toxicon.* 2006;48:799-809.
11. Morris JG Jr, Lewin P, Hargrett NT, et al. Clinical features of ciguatera fish poisoning: a study of the disease in the U.S. Virgin Islands. *Arch Intern Med.* 1982;142:1090-1092.
12. Schnorf H, Taurarii M, Cundy T. Ciguatera fish poisoning: a double-blind randomized trial of mannitol therapy. *Neurology.* 2002;58:873-880.
13. Gessner BD, Middaugh JP. Paralytic shellfish poisoning in Alaska: a 20-year retrospective. *Am J Epidemiol.* 1995;141:766-770.
14. Deeds JR, Landsberg JH, Etheridge SM, et al. Non-traditional vectors for paralytic shellfish poisoning. *Mar Drugs.* 2008;6:308-348.
15. Gessner BD, Bell P, Doucette GJ, et al. Hypertension and identification of toxin in human urine and serum following a cluster of mussel-associated paralytic shellfish poisoning outbreaks. *Toxicon.* 1997;35:711-722.
16. Watkins SM, Reich A, Fleming LE, et al. Neurotoxic shellfish poisoning. *Mar Drugs.* 2008;6:431-455.
17. Fleming LE, Kirkpatrick B, Backer LC, et al. Aerosolized red-tide toxins (brevetoxins) and asthma. *Chest.* 2007;131:187-194.
18. Abraham A, Plakas SM, Flewelling LJ, et al. Biomarkers of neurotoxic shellfish poisoning. *Toxicon.* 2008;52:237-245.
19. Perl TM, Bedard L, Kosatsky T, et al. An outbreak of toxic encephalopathy caused by eating mussels contaminated with domoic acid. *N Engl J Med.* 1990;322:1775-1780.
20. Teitelbaum JS, Zatorre RJ, Carpenter S, et al. Neurologic sequelae of domoic acid intoxication due to ingestion of contaminated mussels. *N Engl J Med.* 1990;322:1781-1787.
21. Silvagni PA, Lowenstine LJ, Spraker T, et al. Pathology of domoic acid toxicity in California sea lions (*Zalophus californianus*). *Vet Pathol.* 2005;42:184-191.
22. Grattan LM, Lesoing M, Etesamypour-King A, et al. Potential health risks of domoic acid exposure to native American infants/toddlers and children in the Pacific Northwest: a pilot study [Abstract]. Presented at the Tenth International Conference on Harmful Algae, October 21-25, 2002, St. Pete Beach, FL.
23. Twiner MJ, Rehmann N, Hess P, et al. Azaspiracid shellfish poisoning: a review on the chemistry, ecology, and toxicology with an emphasis on human health impacts. *Mar Drugs.* 2008;6:39-72.
24. Backer LC, Carmichael W, Kirkpatrick B, et al. Recreational exposure to low concentrations of microcystins during an algal bloom in a small lake. *Mar Drugs.* 2008;6:389-406.
25. Osborne NJ, Shaw GR, Webb PM. Health effects of recreational exposure to Moreton Bay, Australia, waters during a *Lyngbya majuscula* bloom. *Environ Intern.* 2007;33:309-314.
26. Burkholder JM, Noga EJ, Hobbs CH, et al. New "phantom" dinoflagellate is the causative agent of major estuarine fish kills. *Nature.* 1992;358:407-410.
27. Glasgow HB Jr, Burkholder JM, Schmechel DE, et al. Insidious effects of a toxic estuarine dinoflagellate on fish survival and human health. *J Toxicol Environ Health.* 1995;46:501-522.
28. Grattan LM, Oldach D, Perl TM, et al. Learning and memory difficulties after environmental exposure to waterways containing toxin-producing *Pfiesteria* or *Pfiesteria*-like dinoflagellates. *Lancet.* 1998;352:532-539.
29. Haselow DR, Brown E, Tracy JK, et al. Gastrointestinal and respiratory tract symptoms following brief environmental exposure to aerosols during a *Pfiesteria*-related fish kill. *J Toxicol Environ Health A.* 2001;63:553-564.
30. El-Nabawi A, Quesenberry M, Saito K, et al. The N-methyl-D-aspartate neurotransmitter receptor is a mammalian brain target for the dinoflagellate *Pfiesteria piscicida* toxin. *Toxicol Appl Pharamacol.* 2000;169:84-93.

286

Introduction to Helminth Infections

JAMES H. MAGUIRE*

The helminthiases are among the most prevalent infections in the world and a leading cause of morbidity, particularly in developing areas. Literally billions of persons harbor at least one species of parasitic worm.[1] The helminths that parasitize humans include the nematodes (roundworms) and platyhelminths (flatworms); the latter group consists of cestodes (tapeworms) and trematodes (schistosomes and other flukes). Leeches, ectoparasites belonging to the phylum Annelida (segmented worms) are not discussed here (see Chapter 292). Some helminths are exclusively or primarily human parasites, whereas others parasitize both humans and various other mammals, and others are parasites of lower mammals and infect human beings incidentally.

Biology of Helminths

Helminths are multicellular organisms that range from less than 1 cm to more than 10 m in length. They are covered by a cuticle or tegument that protects them from digestion and environmental stresses. Reproductive organs take up a large part of the body regardless of whether the sexes are separate or the species is hermaphroditic, as is the case with cestodes and nonschistosomal trematodes. Neuromuscular, digestive, excretory, and secretory systems typically are smaller and less complex, in keeping with the parasitic state.

The life cycle of all worms includes an egg, one or more larval stages, and the adult. Transmission to humans occurs by ingestion of helminth eggs or larvae, penetration of intact skin by larvae, or inoculation of larvae by biting insects. Depending on the species, humans are the only host, the intermediate host (in which asexual reproduction takes place), or (when there are one or two intermediate hosts) the definitive host in which sexual reproduction occurs. Most helminths are unable to complete their life cycle within the human host, and development of eggs or larvae on soil, in water, or within a plant, arthropod, or other animal intermediate host is necessary. Hence the geographic distribution of these parasites reflects the environmental conditions necessary for development of eggs or larvae or for survival of intermediate hosts and vectors. The only way for the intensity of infection in a person to increase is by further exposure to the infective stage; in the absence of continued exposure, the infection lasts only as long as the life span of the adult worm. In contrast, a few species, most notably *Strongyloides stercoralis*, are able to reproduce and multiply in numbers within the definitive human host. In the case of *Strongyloides*, infectious larvae can be passed directly from one person to another, and transmission is possible in all geographic areas. Infection can persist for the life span of the host, and in the setting of immunosuppression, massive infections can result from distant exposure to even small numbers of infectious larvae.

Epidemiology

The prevalence of helminthic disease is highest in warm, developing areas, where climate, environment, and an abundance of vectors favor completion of the life cycle and where poverty leads to increased exposure to parasites because of poor sanitation, lack of clean water, and inadequate housing. Human activity can facilitate transmission,

as seen in the huge numbers of new cases of schistosomiasis and food-borne trematode infections resulting from water resource development projects for hydroelectric power, irrigation, and aquaculture.[2] Helminthic infections are less common in temperate and industrialized areas, where they have been imported after travel or residence in tropical areas or acquired locally from domestic or wild animals, via improperly prepared meat, fish, or vegetables, or from close personal contact, as in the case of pinworm infections.

Helminths produce large numbers of eggs or larvae and have a high reproductive capacity, which can lead to an extremely high prevalence of human infection when conditions are conducive to transmission, such as in rural areas in the tropics. Helminths are not uniformly distributed in human populations but are overdispersed, with most infected individuals harboring low worm burdens and only a small number harboring heavy infections.[3] The basis for aggregation of helminths in human populations may be related to the intrinsic biology of the parasites and density-dependent constraints on parasites such as competition for nutrients, parasite-induced pathology, and host factors including genetic susceptibility to infection, immunity, nutrition, and behavioral factors.

Pathogenesis and Host-Parasite Relationship

Most infected persons harbor few worms and have few or no signs or symptoms of disease, whereas a small proportion of persons with large numbers of worms are at risk of severe disease. Children with even moderate numbers of worms are at risk of malnutrition, impaired growth, and impaired intellectual development.[4] Polyparasitism is widespread throughout the tropics and subtropics, and infection with multiple species of helminths seems to have an additive or multiplicative effect on nutrition and pathology.[5] Although mortality rates attributable to helminthic infections are low, rates of chronic morbidity and debilitation are substantial.

Helminths produce disease by a variety of mechanisms, including mechanical effects such as intestinal obstruction (e.g., ascariasis), invasion of host cells or tissues with damage or loss of function (e.g., trichinellosis), or competition for nutrients (e.g., vitamin B_{12} deficiency from fish tapeworm infection). The host responses may lead to immunopathologic lesions such as schistosome egg granulomas, which contribute significantly to disease. Interactions with other pathogens or potential carcinogens may contribute to chronic sequelae, such as advanced liver disease associated with coinfection of hepatitis B or C with *Schistosoma mansoni* or bladder cancer associated with *Schistosoma haematobium*.[6]

Basic to understanding the pathogenesis of helminthiasis is an appreciation of the size of the organisms, the multiplicity of their antigens, and the chronicity of the infection. Host responses are composed of myriad immunologic and nonimmunologic factors, some of which contribute to disease. Sterilizing immunity to helminthic infections does not develop, and the extent to which previous infections with helminths lead to resistance to subsequent reinfection is not well defined. A degree of acquired immunity has been shown in infected individuals who were cured chemotherapeutically and then continued to live under the same conditions of exposure to infection.[7] These findings suggest that induction of resistance by vaccines may be a viable control strategy.

*This chapter is based in part on the chapter by Adel A.F. Mahmoud in the 5th edition. All material in this chapter is in the public domain, with the exception of any borrowed figures or tables.

Eosinophilia is a characteristic of many helminthic infections. Peripheral blood, bone marrow, and tissue eosinophilia is associated with the migration or presence of worms in tissues. Eosinophilia is not observed in infections with helminths that reside in the lumen of the human gut (e.g., tapeworms) or are contained in cystic structures (e.g., echinococcal cysts). Eosinophils seem to play a significant role in the killing of helminths and host resistance to helminthic infections and are responsible for a considerable amount of inflammatory pathology.[8] Chronic infection with worms typically leads to a constant state of immune activation characterized by a dominant Th2 type of cytokine profile and high immunoglobulin E levels, as well as proliferation and activation of eosinophils.[9] It is hypothesized that such an immune profile may have an adverse impact on the efficacy of vaccines against other classes of organisms[10] and progression of other infections such as malaria and human immunodeficiency virus/acquired immunodeficiency syndrome.[11,12] Helminth infections may affect the expression of allergic disease, and in some studies were associated with decreased risk of asthma and other atopic conditions, although other studies showed increased or no risk.[13,14]

Worms have successfully developed multiple strategies to evade host protective responses. Suggested mechanisms include encapsulation within a host fibrous reaction (hydatid cyst), intraluminal location (*Ascaris*), inhibition and modulation of the immune response (filariae, cysticerci), and acquisition of host antigens (schistosomes).

Diagnosis and Treatment of Helminthic Infections

Recognition of helminthic infections requires knowledge of their clinical presentation, geographic distribution, and epidemiologic risk factors. Persons with light infections may be asymptomatic, and the only clues to diagnosis may be a history of travel and potential exposure to the parasite as well as peripheral blood eosinophilia. It should be kept in mind, however, that eosinophilia may be absent, even in persons with invasive infections. The diagnosis of helminthic infections rests heavily on microscopic examination of stool, urine, blood, other body fluids, and tissue (Table 286-1).[15] When eggs or larvae are produced in abundance, microscopy can be extremely sensitive, but multiple examinations or concentration procedures may be necessary to detect light infections or infections with organisms such as *Strongyloides*, which often shed low numbers of larvae in the stool. Serologic tests may offer greater sensitivity than microscopic examination and

TABLE 286-1	Diagnosis of Major Helminthic Infections		
		Microscopic Diagnosis	
Parasite	*Stage*	*Specimen*	*Other Methods*
Roundworms (Nematodes)			
Intestinal Roundworms			
Ascaris lumbricoides (large intestinal roundworm)	Eggs	Feces	Identification of passed worm
Trichuris trichiura (whipworm)	Eggs	Feces	
Ancylostoma duodenale, Necator americanus (hookworm)	Eggs, larvae	Feces	
Strongyloides stercoralis (threadworm)	Larvae	Feces, duodenal fluid, sputum	Serology*
Enterobius vermicularis (pinworm)	Eggs	Swab of perianal skin; occasionally in feces	Cellophane tape test; identification of adult worms on skin
Tissue Roundworms			
Trichinella spiralis (trichinellosis)	Larvae	Muscle biopsy	Serology*
Dracunculus medinensis (guinea worm)			Identification of emergent adult worm
Wuchereria bancrofti, Brugia malayi (lymphatic filariasis)	Microfilariae	Blood, urine (in setting of chyluria)	Serology, antigen test (blood)
Loa loa (African eye worm)	Microfilariae	Blood	Identification of adult worm in eye, serology
Onchocerca volvulus (river blindness)	Microfilariae	Skin snip	Identification of adult worm in resected nodules
Ancylostoma braziliense, other species (creeping eruption)			Inspection of rash
Toxocara canis, Toxocara cati (visceral larva migrans)	Larvae	Biopsy of liver, other tissues (not recommended)	Serology* (preferred)
Flukes (Trematodes)			
Schistosoma mansoni, Schistosoma haematobium, Schistosoma japonicum, Schistosoma mekongi	Eggs	Feces, rectal snips, urine (*S. haematobium*)	Serology,* antigen test (serum and urine)
Fasciolopsis buski (intestinal fluke)	Eggs	Feces	
Heterophyes heterophyes (intestinal fluke)	Eggs	Feces	
Metagonimus yokogawai (intestinal fluke)	Eggs	Feces	
Clonorchis sinensis, Opisthorchis spp. (liver fluke)	Eggs	Feces, bile	Serology
Fasciola hepatica (liver fluke)	Eggs	Feces, bile	Serology
Paragonimus spp. (lung fluke)	Eggs	Sputum, feces	Serology*
Tapeworms (Cestodes)			
Intestinal Tapeworms			
Taenia saginata (beef tapeworm)	Eggs	Stool	Identification of passed proglottid (segment)
Hymenolepis nana (dwarf tapeworm)	Eggs	Stool	
Diphyllobothrium latum (fish tapeworm)	Eggs	Stool	Identification of passed proglottid
Taenia solium (pork tapeworm)	Eggs	Stool	Identification of passed proglottid; stool antigen test; serology
Larval Tapeworms			
Echinococcus granulosus (cystic hydatid disease)	Protoscolices, hooklets	Fluid from cyst	Serology,* CT, MRI, or US can be diagnostic
Echinococcus multilocularis (alveolar hydatid disease)	Larvae	Liver biopsy	Serology
Cysticercus (*T. solium*)	Larvae	Brain biopsy	Serology,* CT, or MRI or scan of head can be diagnostic

*Serologic test is available through Division of Parasitic Diseases, Centers for Disease Control and Prevention, Atlanta, GA.
CT, computed tomography; MRI, magnetic resonance imaging; US, ultrasonography.

may be the only way to avoid invasive diagnostic procedures for infections with tissue-invading helminths. Many serologic tests for helminths are available only from reference laboratories, and they may lack sensitivity or specificity and not distinguish between past and present infections. Assays to detect helminthic antigens and molecular diagnostic techniques are used mostly for research purposes and monitoring and evaluating control programs.

Excellent drugs are available for treating most helminthic infections. Because agents such as albendazole, mebendazole, praziquantel, and ivermectin are highly effective in single orally administered doses, as well as being safe and inexpensive, they are suitable for mass drug administration as well as individual treatment.[16] Heavy use of these drugs in control programs raises concerns for the emergence of resistance and the need for new drugs. A novel approach to treatment of individual persons with onchocerciasis and filariasis is the use of doxycycline to eliminate the endosymbiotic bacteria *Wolbachia* and thereby sterilize or kill the adult worms.[17] For infections such as cysticercosis, toxocariasis, and trichinellosis, anti-inflammatory agents are used to minimize tissue damage and symptoms caused by the host's response to the parasite.

Prevention and Control

Helminthic infections are prevented by (1) avoiding ingestion of infective eggs, larvae, or intermediate hosts infected with larvae; (2) preventing contact of bare skin with infective larvae; and (3) avoiding bites of infected vectors. At the personal level, these measures entail drinking safe water; properly cleaning, cooking, and otherwise preparing food; adequate hand washing and general hygiene; and using measures to avoid insect bites, among others. Communities can be protected by interventions such as provision of clean water and sanitation; enforcement of appropriate food-producing practices to prevent infection of fish, meat, and vegetables; vector control; and prevention or treatment of infections in domestic animals.

Global efforts to eradicate, eliminate, or reduce transmission of helminthic diseases are advancing as a result of partnerships among governments, international agencies, nongovernmental organizations, philanthropic institutions, and industry.[16] The guinea worm eradication program, which relies on community education and participation, provision of filters for drinking water, clean water sources, and case containment, is nearing its goal of zero cases globally.[18] The cornerstone of global programs to eliminate onchocerciasis and lymphatic filariasis and reduce disease due to schistosomiasis and intestinal helminths is periodic mass administration of anthelmintic drugs to populations at risk; attempts to lower costs and improve efficiency by integrating these different large-scale programs are progressing.[19] Ongoing research in support of these programs and to expand efforts to include other helminthic diseases focuses on the development of new drugs, diagnostic methods, control strategies, and novel tools such as anthelmintic vaccines.

REFERENCES

1. Crompton DWT, Savioli L. *Handbook of Helminthiases for Public Health*. Boca Raton: CRC Press-Taylor and Francis Group; 2007:3-24.
2. Fenwick A. Waterborne infectious diseases: could they be consigned to history? *Science*. 2005;313:1077-1081.
3. Anderson RM, May RM. *Infectious Diseases of Humans: Dynamics and Control*. New York: Oxford University Press; 1991: 433-606.
4. Hall A, Gillian H, Tuffrey V, et al. A review and meta-analysis of the impact of intestinal worms on child growth and nutrition. *Matern Child Nutr*. 2008;(Suppl 1):118-236.
5. Pullan R, Brooker S. The health impact of polyparasitism in humans: are we underestimating the burden of parasitic diseases? *Parasitology*. 2008;135;783-794.
6. Yosry A. Schistosomaisis and neoplasia. *Contrib Microbiol*. 2006;13:81-100.
7. Sturrock RF, Kimani R, Cottrell JB, et al. Observations on possible immunity to reinfection among Kenyan schoolchildren after treatment for *Schistosoma mansoni*. *Trans R Soc Trop Med Hyg*. 1983;77; 363-371.
8. Klion AD, Nutman TB. The role of eosinophils in host defense against helminth parasites. *J Allergy Clin Immunol*. 2004;113: 30-77.
9. Anthony RM, Rutitzky LI, Urban JF Jr, et al. Protective immune mechanisms in helminth infection. *Nat Rev Immunol*. 2007; 7:975-987.
10. Robinson TM, Nelson RG, Boyer JD. Parasitic infection and the polarized Th2 immune response can alter a vaccine-induced immune response. *DNA Cell Biol*. 2003;22: 421-430.
11. Hartgers FC, Yazdanbakhsh M. Co-infection of helminths and malaria: modulation of the immune responses to malaria. *Parasite Immunol*. 2006;28:497-506.
12. Walson JL, John-Stewart G. Treatment of helminth co-infection in HIV-1 infected individuals in resource-limited settings. Cochrane Database Syst Rev. 2008; CD006419;1-30.
13. van Riet E, Hartgers FC, Yazdanbakhsh M. Chronic helminth infections induce immunomodulation: consequences and mechanisms. *Immunobiology*. 2007;212:475-490.
14. Flohr C, Quinnell RJ, Britton J. Do helminths protect against atopy and allergic disease? *Clin Exp Allergy*. 2009;39:20-32.
15. Garcia LS. *Diagnostic Medical Parasitology*. 5th ed. Washington, DC: ASM Press; 2006:1202pp.
16. Molyneux D. Control of human parasitic diseases. *Adv Parasitol*. 2006;61:1-45.
17. Hoerauf A. Filariasis: new drugs and new opportunities for lymphatic filariasis and onchocerciasis. *Curr Opin Infect Dis*. 2008;21:673-681.
18. Update: progress toward global eradication of dracunculiasis. January 2007-June 2008. *MMWR Morb Mortal Wkly Rep*. 2008;57:1173-1176.
19. Lammie PJ, Fenwick A, Utzinger J. A blueprint for success: integration of neglected tropical disease control programmes. *Parasitol Today*. 2006;22:313-321.

Intestinal Nematodes (Roundworms)

JAMES H. MAGUIRE

There are 60 or more species of nematodes or roundworms that infect humans, approximately 80,000 species that infect other invertebrates, and nearly 500,000 free-living species, making the phylum Nematoda one of the largest in the animal kingdom.[1,2] Nematodes are the most common human parasites, with estimates indicating that greater than 1 billion people are infected with at least one of the four most important species—*Ascaris lumbricoides*, hookworm (*Necator americanus* and *Ancylostoma duodenale*), and *Trichuris trichiura*.[3,4] Infections by these four helminths constitute a major health burden in many areas of the world, particularly among the poorest people in developing countries. Many individuals harbor more than one of these four species as well as other helminths and protozoa throughout much of their lives.[5] Because of their profound negative effect on physical and intellectual growth, school attendance and performance, and future economic productivity, *Ascaris*, *Trichuris*, and hookworm are the targets of one the world's largest public health initiatives, namely, large-scale administration of anthelmintic drugs to school-aged children.[6]

All nematodes are nonsegmented, elongate, cylindrical organisms with a smooth cuticle and a body cavity that contains a tubular digestive tract, reproductive system, and other organs. Sexes are separate; and following mating, females produce eggs that give rise to larvae. The larvae then pass through four molts before reaching adulthood and sexual maturity.

Species of nematodes that live in the gut constitute the largest group of human helminths; other species live in or migrate through tissues, including those that are primarily parasites of lower animals. The most common intestinal nematodes—*Ascaris*, hookworm, and *Trichuris*—are also referred to as geohelminths because their eggs or larvae must develop on soil before becoming infective to humans (Table 287-1). Because of this requirement, these parasites cannot be transmitted directly from one person to another and cannot multiply in the host. In contrast, another geohelminth, *Strongyloides stercoralis*, is able to complete its life cycle entirely within the human host as well as on soil. Eggs of *Enterobius vermicularis*, the pinworm, become infective within 6 hours of release from the gravid female and exposure to oxygen. Like *Strongyloides*, pinworm can be transmitted directly from person to person.

The inability of the intestinal nematodes other than *Strongyloides* to replicate within the human host explains why they do not behave as opportunistic infections in people who have acquired immunodeficiency syndrome (AIDS) or who are receiving immunosuppressive medications. Although rapidly increasing numbers of adult *Strongyloides* and migrating larvae can overwhelm a person receiving corticosteroids, this complication is surprisingly rare in people with AIDS.[5] On the other hand, intestinal nematodes elicit a Th2 type of cytokine response that may lead to more rapid progression of human immunodeficiency virus (HIV) infection and progression to AIDS.[7-10] The efficacy of some vaccines against HIV infection is likely to be impaired by chronic helminthiasis.[11]

Ascariasis

Ascaris lumbricoides is the most common helminthic infection of humans, infecting more than one-fourth of the world's population.[3] Ascariasis is widely distributed throughout the world, and although most abundant in tropical countries, it also occurs in temperate areas. Most people infected with *Ascaris* are asymptomatic, but mortality is estimated to be 60,000 per year, and more than 15% of infected people experience some type of morbidity.[2,12-19]

LIFE CYCLE

The white or pinkish adult worms (15 to 35 cm in length) live and mate in the lumen of the small intestine, primarily the jejunum (Fig. 287-1). Each female worm has a daily output of 200,000 ova or more.[14] The fertile ovum is oval, has a thick shell with a mammillated albuminous covering, and is 50 to 70 μm × 40 to 50 μm (Fig. 287-2). When eggs in the single-cell stage are passed in the feces and reach a favorable environment, they become infective and contain a fully developed larva within 10 to 14 days at 30°C and within 6 weeks at 17°C.[14] Eggs ingested or inhaled and swallowed by humans hatch in the small intestine and release larvae that measure approximately 250 μm in length. The larvae then penetrate the intestinal wall and migrate via venous blood through the liver to the heart, reaching the lungs approximately 4 days after ingestion of the eggs. By 6 to 10 days later, they have attained a length of approximately 550 μm; they break into the alveoli and ascend the tracheobronchial tree. They are then swallowed and return to the intestines where they develop into mature worms, with egg production beginning approximately 2 months after ingestion of the eggs. Adult worms live approximately 10 to 24 months. Although the host mounts a response that includes production of various cytokines, specific and nonspecific immunoglobulin E (IgE) antibodies, and an expansion and mobilization of eosinophils, basophils, and mast cells, whatever protection is afforded is partial at best.[15] The ability of *Ascaris* to survive in the host is due in part to secretion of molecules that modulate lymphocyte proliferation and cytokine production and others that inhibit pepsin and protect maturing worms as they pass through the stomach to the small bowel.[4,15,16]

EPIDEMIOLOGY

The geographic distribution of ascariasis is determined by climate, sanitation, and human susceptibility to infection and behavior. Eggs embryonate and become infective only on soil in warm, humid environments, and transmission may be seasonal in areas where these conditions alternate with periods of extreme temperature and aridity. Children in impoverished rural areas who play on contaminated soil around homes are the most heavily infected and are constantly exposed to reinfection via hand-to-mouth transmission. Infection rates are also high among adults, especially in areas where human excrement ("night soil") or wastewater is used to fertilize crops.[17] In endemic areas, it is not unusual for more than 80% of the population to be infected.[12-18] The high prevalence of ascariasis worldwide is a consequence of the tremendous egg output from female worms and the remarkable ability of ova to resist unfavorable external environments. *Ascaris* eggs remain viable for up to 6 years in moist, loose soil, and they can survive freezing winter temperatures and short periods of desiccation.

In highly endemic communities, most people are infected with a small number of worms, and only a few people (usually children) have heavy infections. The latter group accounts for the bulk of the worms in the community and most of the eggs shed into the environment, and they are at highest risk of severe disease.[20]

Predisposition to infection and intensity of infection are determined by various factors, including the environment and human behavior, genetic predisposition, and host immunity.[21,22] Studies using human

TABLE 287-1	Features of Major Intestinal Nematodes					
Nematode	Transmission	Direct Person-to-Person Transmission	Geographic Distribution	Duration of Infection	Location of Adult Worm(s)	Treatment*
Ascaris lumbricoides	Ingestion of infective eggs	No	Warm, humid areas; temperate zones in warmer months	1-2 Years	Free in lumen of small bowel, primarily jejunum	Albendazole Mebendazole Pyrantel Ivermectin Levamisole Piperazine
Trichuris trichiura (whipworm)	Ingestion of infective eggs	No	Warm, humid areas; temperate zones in warmer months	1-3 Years	Anchored in superficial mucosa of cecum and colon	Albendazole Mebendazole
Necator americanus, Ancylostoma duodenale (hookworm)	Penetration of skin by filariform larvae	No	Warm, humid areas; temperate zones in warmer months	3-5 Years (*Necator*); 1 year (*Ancylostoma*)	Attached to mucosa of mid to upper portion of small bowel	Albendazole Mebendazole Levamisole Pyrantel
Strongyloides stercoralis	Penetration of skin or bowel mucosa by filariform larvae	Yes	Primarily warm, humid areas, but can be worldwide	Lifetime of host	Embedded in mucosa of duodenum, jejunum	Ivermectin† Albendazole Thiabendazole
Enterobius vermicularis (pinworm)	Ingestion of infective eggs	Yes	Worldwide	1 Month	Free in lumen of cecum, appendix, adjacent colon	Albendazole Mebendazole Pyrantel Ivermectin Levamisole Piperazine

*Nitazoxanide has been shown to be effective in the treatment of ascariasis, trichuriasis, and enterobiasis in several trials in Mexico.[59-61] Tribendimidine, which is licensed in China, was shown to be efficacious against *Ascaris* and had moderate efficacy against *Strongyloides* in a randomized trial.[62]
†Drug of choice.

genome scans have demonstrated that loci on three chromosomes account for a significant part of the individual variation in susceptibility to infection with *Ascaris*.[23]

Most cases of ascariasis in nonendemic regions occur among immigrants and travelers. These people lose their infections usually within a year of arrival, when the adult worms die. Occasionally, *Ascaris* infection is encountered in people who have never traveled. Imported farm produce contaminated with eggs was the source of infection in some cases. In others, infection was acquired locally by ingesting eggs that were shown by molecular studies to be eggs of the pig roundworm, *Ascaris suum*.[24,25]

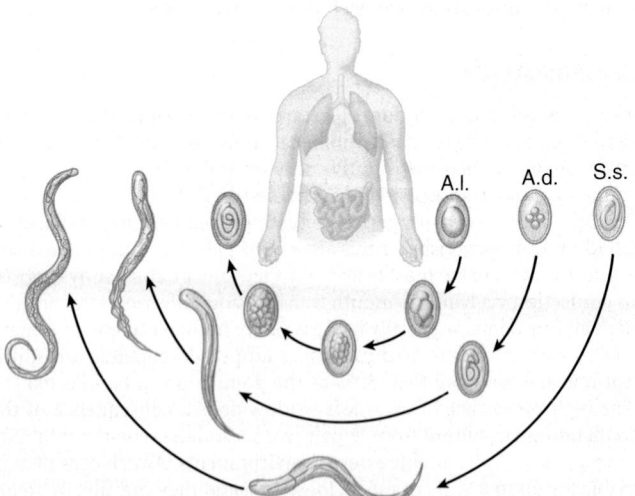

Figure 287-1 Life cycle of intestinal nematodes with a migratory phase through the lungs. Eggs are passed with stools in *Ascaris lumbricoides* (A.l.), *Necator americanus*, or *Ancylostoma duodenale* (A.d.), or they hatch in the lumen of the bowel in *Strongyloides stercoralis* (S.s.). *Ascaris* eggs mature in soil, and humans are infected upon ingestion of these eggs. With hookworm and strongyloidiasis, humans are infected via skin penetration by filariform larvae. In all three infections, larvae pass through a migratory phase via the lungs before reaching maturity at their final habitat in the small intestine.

CLINICAL SYNDROMES

Most people with *Ascaris* infections are asymptomatic. A small proportion of infected people develop pulmonary symptoms during the second week after ingestion of eggs, when larvae invade lung tissue and provoke an immune-mediated hypersensitivity response.[26] Symptoms include a nonproductive cough, chest discomfort, fever, and eosinophilia that disappears often by the time the worms reach maturity. In severe cases, patients develop dyspnea and an eosinophilic pneumonia (Löffler syndrome) with transient patchy infiltrates seen on radiographs. Seasonal outbreaks of pneumonitis have occurred in areas such as Saudi Arabia, where transmission of *Ascaris* is seasonal, whereas even isolated cases of pulmonary illness due to ascariasis are uncommon in areas where transmission is continuous.[27]

With most established infections, adult worms in the lumen of the small bowel provoke no symptoms or produce only mild abdominal discomfort, dyspepsia, loss of appetite, or nausea. Moderate and heavy infections, however, can impair the nutritional status of children, especially those living in areas where malnutrition due to other causes is common.[28-31] Infection with *Ascaris* has been shown to depress appetite and food intake by children, and it can interfere with absorption of proteins, fats, lactose, vitamin A, and iodine.[28] The impact on nutrition, intellectual development, cognitive performance, and growth is likely the most important health-related consequence of ascariasis worldwide.[29,30] Treatment of heavily infected children with anthelmintics has been shown to improve nutritional status, but provision of micronutrients, protein, and energy is necessary for underweight or stunted children to achieve catch-up growth.[29-32]

Other complications of chronic ascariasis, such as intestinal obstruction, obstruction of bile and pancreatic ducts, appendicitis, and intestinal perforation, are largely mechanical. Although the rate of serious complications among infected people is less than 0.1%, the huge number of infected people makes ascariasis a major cause of surgical admissions in the tropics.[33-35] Entanglement of a large number of adult worms in the lumen of the small bowel, usually near the ileocecal valve, provokes spasmodic contraction and obstruction, especially in children, who may harbor from 60 to more than 500 worms.[36] Obstruction may be partial or complete, and occasionally it is complicated by perforation, intussusception, volvulus, or death.[37] Intestinal obstruction due to ascariasis occurred in 1 of every 1000 infected children and was responsible for 25% of intestinal obstructions during a 10-year period

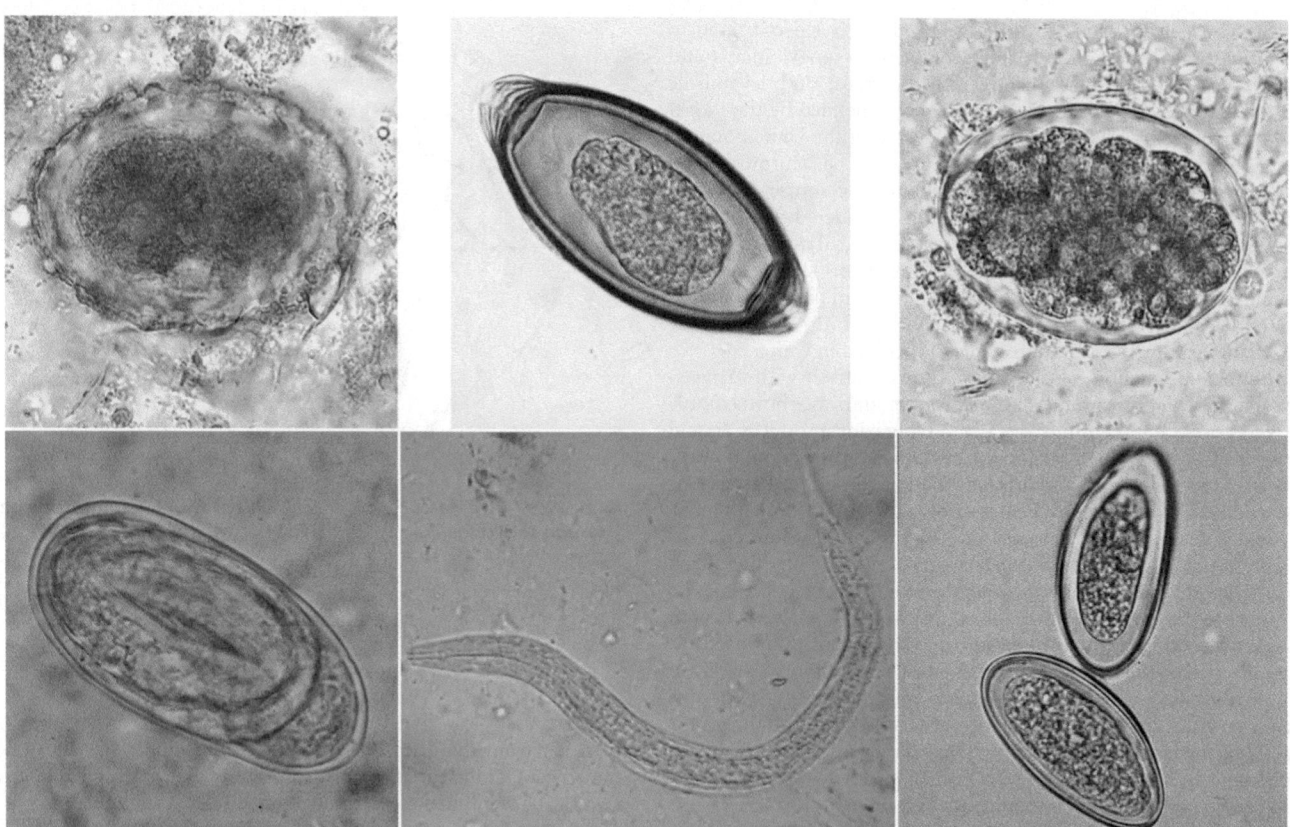

Figure 287-2   Eggs and larvae of common intestinal roundworms. Clockwise, beginning at upper left: *Ascaris lumbricoides; Trichuris trichiura;* hookworm; *Enterobius vermicularis; Strongyloides stercoralis;* and embryonated hookworm egg. *(From DPDx, Web site for laboratory diagnosis of parasitic diseases of the Division of Parasitic Diseases, National Centers for Zoonotic, Vector-borne, and Enteric Diseases, Centers for Disease Control and Prevention, Atlanta, GA [http://www.dpd.cdc.gov/DPDx/].)*

in Calabar, Nigeria.[33-37] It rarely occurs among adults, in whom the diameter of the bowel is greater than that of children, and travelers, in whom worm burdens typically are low.[38]

Individual worms have a tendency to enter and obstruct small orifices, most frequently the common bile duct, but also the pancreatic duct and appendix.[39,40] This complication is more common in adults than children, and it can result from increased migration of worms that occurs with general anesthesia, high fevers, fasting, or treatment with certain anthelmintic drugs such as mebendazole or albendazole. Compensatory dilatation of bile ducts following cholecystectomy or relaxation of the sphincter of Oddi due to high levels of progesterone during pregnancy increases the risk of biliary ascariasis.[41] Worms may exit the ductal system spontaneously without causing harm or may produce pyogenic cholangitis, liver abscess, hemorrhagic pancreatitis, or appendicitis, or they may die in situ and form the nidus of biliary stones.[42-44] In a series of 500 cases of biliary and pancreatic ascariasis from Kashmir, India, Khuroo et al. described biliary colic in 56% of people, acute cholangitis in 24%, acute cholecystitis in 13%, acute pancreatitis in 6%, and liver abscess in 1%.[40] Individual worms that wander aberrantly may perforate surgical wounds, Meckel's diverticulum, the appendix, and, rarely, portions of the bowel that appear otherwise normal.[44] Occasionally, passage of an adult worm per os, per rectum, or, less commonly, through the nose or a tear duct brings the patient to medical attention. Worms have been found escaping through umbilical and hernial fistulas, in the fallopian tubes and urinary bladder, and in the lungs and heart. *Ascaris* antigens are highly antigenic, and chronic ascariasis appears to increase the risk of asthma, although its effect on other atopic conditions is controversial.[45-48] Evidence is conflicting on whether ascariasis increases or decreases sus-

ceptibility to *Plasmodium falciparum* infection, the levels of parasitemia, and the occurrence of severe disease.[49,50]

DIAGNOSIS

Finding eggs in the feces establishes the diagnosis of ascariasis. Because of the enormous daily output of eggs by gravid female worms, microscopic examination of simple smears is often sufficient, and procedures to concentrate stool, such as the Kato-Katz thick smear or formalin-ethyl acetate sedimentation, may not be needed.[51] Larvae can be found in sputum or gastric aspirates during their migration through the lungs before eggs are present in the stool.[26] Adult worms passed through the mouth, anus, or nose are readily identified because of their large size and unsegmented cream-colored cuticle. Worms in a gas-filled loop of bowel can be seen on plain radiographs.[52] During barium studies, they appear as filling defects, and barium may fill the gut of the worm.[52] Ultrasonography, computed tomography, and endoscopic retrograde cholangiopancreatography (ERCP) readily demonstrate worms in the biliary tree and pancreatic duct.[53-55] Worms visualized in the biliary or pancreatic ducts during ERCP can be extracted with forceps.[56]

MANAGEMENT

All infections, including those that are light or asymptomatic, should be treated, preferably with oral albendazole (400 mg single dose), mebendazole (500 mg single dose or 100 mg twice daily for 3 days), or pyrantel pamoate (11 mg/kg single dose, maximum 1 g). All of these result in a high rate of cure or, in people not cured, a large reduction in worm burden, as estimated by egg output.[5,57] Ivermectin (150 to 200 μg/kg orally once), the drug of choice for strongyloidiasis and onchocerciasis, is effective for treating ascariasis, and levamisole (2.5 mg/kg once orally) is an alternative recommended by the World Health Organization (WHO) but not available in the United States.[5] Piperazine citrate, once the drug of choice, can be neurotoxic and hepatotoxic and is no longer available in many countries. Pyrantel pamoate and piperazine citrate have been considered safe for use during pregnancy for years. WHO also recommended use of albendazole and mebendazole during pregnancy based on safety data and concluded that these drugs may be used to treat children as young as 12 months.[5,58] Newer drugs that have activity against *Ascaris* include nitazoxanide and tribendimidine, which is licensed in China.[59-62]

Intestinal obstruction is best managed conservatively with nasogastric suction, repletion of fluids and electrolytes, and, once bowel motility is restored, anthelmintic therapy.[37] Piperazine produces flaccid paralysis of worms, which can help to relieve the obstruction. If available, the syrup is administered by instillation through a nasogastric tube. Indications for surgery include complete obstruction with inadequate decompression, lack of response within 24 to 48 hours, volvulus, intussusception, or perforation. Worms can frequently be milked into the large bowel at surgery, but enterotomy or resection may be necessary to relieve the obstruction. Conservative management with nasogastric suction, antispasmodics, analgesics, and intravenous fluids is usually effective in cases of biliary ascariasis.[39] Antibiotics are given if there is evidence of bacterial infection, and once acute symptoms subside an anthelmintic is given to prevent recurrence. Indications for endoscopic or surgical removal of worms include those that die or are trapped in ducts or invade the liver.[56] Patients with acute appendicitis or intestinal perforation also require surgical intervention.

Trichuriasis

An estimated 800 million or more people worldwide are infected with the whipworm *Trichuris trichiura*, primarily children living in poverty in the tropics and subtropics.[3,6,63] Its geographic distribution is similar to that of *A. lumbricoides*, and many people harbor infections with both *Trichuris* and *Ascaris*.

LIFE CYCLE

Pinkish gray adult worms measuring approximately 4 cm in length reside in the cecum and ascending colon and with heavy infections extend to the lower colon and rectum (Fig. 287-3). The thin whiplike anterior part of the parasite is embedded in a syncytial tunnel in the epithelium of the colon between the mouths of crypts; its thicker posterior extends into the lumen. After mating, the female worm each day produces 7000 to 20,000 barrel-shaped eggs measuring 50 × 20 μm, with a thick shell and a clear plug at each end (see Fig. 287-2). Eggs shed in the feces onto soil embryonate and become infective under optimal conditions of moisture and shade within 2 to 4 weeks. After the egg has been ingested, the larva emerges from the shell and penetrates mucosal crypts of the cecum. Here it undergoes a series of molts and then moves to the mouth of the crypts, where it secretes a protein that forms pores in lipid bilayers that allow the anterior end to become embedded in the epithelium.[6,64] Worms mature into adults and begin to oviposit within approximately 3 months; they live 1 to 3 years or longer.

EPIDEMIOLOGY

Trichuriasis is found in humid tropical environments and in temperate zones during warm and humid months. It is most common in poor rural communities and areas in which sanitary facilities are lacking and hands, food, and drink are easily contaminated. Most infected people harbor fewer than 20 worms, but a small proportion, usually children in the 5- to 15-year-old age group, harbor more than 200 worms.[63] In endemic communities, people with these heavy worm burdens typi-

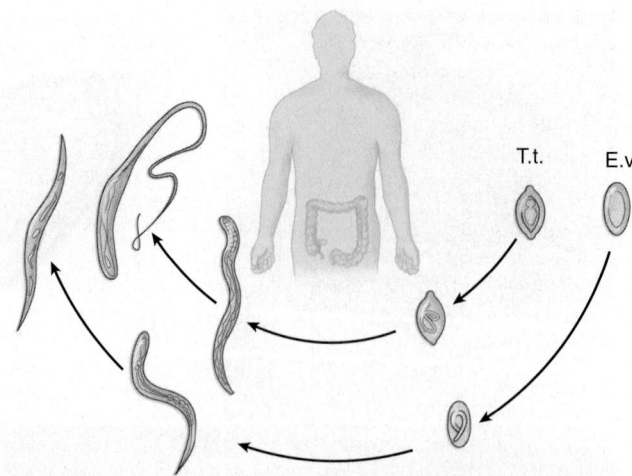

Figure 287-3 **Life cycle of nematodes without a migratory phase through the lungs.** *Trichuris trichiura* (T.t.) eggs are passed with stools; those of *Enterobius vermicularis* (E.v.) are deposited at the perianal region. They embryonate within a short time, and infection is acquired by ingestion. Eggs hatch in the intestine, and larvae migrate to their final habitat in the colon (T.t.) or cecum (E.v.).

cally represent less than 10% of the population and are the only ones to suffer from the disease.[20,65] Genetic studies indicate that approximately 25% of the variation in susceptibility to infection with *T. trichiura* can be attributed to genetic factors.[66,67]

CLINICAL SYNDROMES

Most people with trichuriasis have no symptoms or only peripheral blood eosinophilia. In people with heavy infections, the mucosa is inflamed, edematous, and friable, and there are increased numbers of macrophages in the lamina propria that produce tumor necrosis factor-α (TNF-α).[68] Children with chronic *Trichuris* colitis have chronic abdominal pain and diarrhea, iron deficiency anemia, growth retardation, and clubbing of the fingers.[69-72] They are at risk of developing the *Trichuris* dysentery syndrome, characterized by tenesmus and frequent passage of stools containing large amounts of mucus and often blood.[69,70] Recurrent rectal prolapse is common, and adult worms can been seen in the prolapsed mucosa.[72] In people with moderate or heavy infections, elevated systemic levels of TNF-α may contribute to growth retardation and impaired cognitive function.[68,73,74]

Trichuris has been shown to secrete molecules that induce anti-inflammatory cytokines.[16,75,76] It appears that infection with eggs of the porcine whipworm *Trichuris suis* may lead to improvement of inflammatory bowel disease.[77,78] There is understandable concern about the use of living zoonotic parasites for treating patients, but characterization of the responsible immunomodulatory molecules could lead to new therapeutic approaches.[79]

DIAGNOSIS

Trichuriasis is diagnosed by identifying the adult worms on the mucosa of the prolapsed rectum or at colonoscopy or by finding the lemon-shaped eggs in the stool.[63] Because the level of egg output is high (approximately 200 eggs/g of feces per worm pair), microscopic examination of a simple fecal smear is sufficient for diagnosis of symptomatic cases.

MANAGEMENT

Single doses of albendazole, mebendazole, and pyrantel pamoate cure less than 50% of people with whipworm infection, and the reduction in worm burden may be less than 60%.[57,80-82] Three days of albendazole

(400 mg orally daily) or mebendazole (100 mg twice daily) are more effective in light and moderate infections, but for heavy infections, courses of 5 to 7 days of albendazole or the combination of albendazole and ivermectin taken once yield higher rates of cure and a greater reduction in the intensity of the infection.[83-85]

Hookworm

Human infection with the two species of hookworm, *Ancylostoma duodenale* and *Necator americanus*, affects more than 10% of the world's population.[3,4,6,85] Iron-deficiency anemia from hookworm infection is a major health problem throughout the developing world and has especially severe consequences for growing children and women of childbearing age.[86,87] Hookworm infection occurs in tropical and subtropical zones between 45°N and 30°S latitude.[88] In 1909, the high prevalence of hookworm disease in the southern United States led to the establishment of the Rockefeller Commission and its highly successful control program, which contributed to the virtual elimination of transmission in the country today.[89]

LIFE CYCLE

Adult hookworms are small, cylindrical, grayish white nematodes measuring approximately 7 to 13 mm in length. They live chiefly in the upper small intestine, attached to the mucosa by their strong buccal capsules and biting plates or teeth. There are major differences between the two species.[88] *N. americanus* is shorter, removes less blood (0.03 ml/day vs. 0.20 ml/day), lives longer (3 to 5 years or more vs. 1 or 2 years), and produces fewer eggs (5000 to 10,000 vs. 10,000 to 25,000 per day) than *A. duodenale*. The ovoid, thin-shelled eggs of the two species measure $58 \times 36\ \mu m$ and are morphologically identical (see Fig. 287-1).

Under suitable conditions of humidity, temperature, and shade, eggs passed in the stool hatch on loamy soil within 1 or 2 days. The emergent rhabditiform larvae, which are noninfective, molt twice during the next 5 to 10 days and develop into filariform larvae, which are infective. Following contact of human skin with contaminated soil, filariform larvae penetrate through hair follicles and small fissures within minutes. The larvae are carried by the circulation to the lungs, penetrate the alveolar walls, and make their way up the trachea to be swallowed and carried to their final habitat in the small intestine. Gravid females start egg deposition 5 or 6 weeks after skin penetration. *A. duodenale* can be transmitted orally as well as percutaneously, and its larvae can undergo a period of arrested development in the host corresponding to times of the year when environmental conditions are unfavorable.[88] In order to evade the host immune response, hookworms secrete a variety of proteinases and other molecules that cleave immunoglobulins, break down chemokines that recruit eosinophils, and evoke release of interferon-γ from natural killer cells.[6,90]

EPIDEMIOLOGY

The distribution and prevalence of hookworm infections are limited by environmental conditions that include several months of warm weather (ideally 25° to 32°C) and a minimum annual rainfall of 50 to 60 inches. Larval development is susceptible to extremes of temperature, desiccation, and direct sunlight. Transmission within a community is limited to areas where people defecate and are then visited by people with bare feet or children playing on the ground. The intensity of infection rises during childhood and levels off during early adulthood. High rates of *A. duodenale* infection in children younger than age 1 year raise the possibility of transmammary or even transplacental transmission.[85,88]

CLINICAL SYNDROMES

Most people harbor light infections and are asymptomatic. Previously sensitized people may develop a pruritic maculopapular rash known as "ground itch" at the site of larval penetration. Migration of larvae through the lungs may provoke a transient pneumonitis, which occurs less frequently and is less severe than that caused by *Ascaris*. Previously unexposed people may develop epigastric pain, diarrhea, anorexia, and eosinophilia approximately 30 to 45 days after penetration as larvae begin attaching to the small bowel mucosa.[91] This syndrome has been recognized most commonly among military troops during operations in tropical zones and returning travelers who have had contact of skin with fecally contaminated soil.[92-94]

People infected with adult hookworms may experience chronic abdominal pain and persistent eosinophilia. The major manifestations of hookworm disease, however, are iron-deficiency anemia and protein energy malnutrition resulting from blood loss.[85,86] Adult worms draw mucosal plugs into their buccal cavity, secrete enzymes to expose underlying capillaries, and suck blood with powerful esophageal muscles. Bleeding is aggravated by anticoagulants and inhibitors of platelet activation produced by the worm, and it continues for some time after the feeding worm attaches to another site.[95-97] The development of anemia depends on the intensity and duration of the infection, the infecting species of worm, and iron stores, intake, and requirements.[86,87] Blood loss is gradual, allowing the body to adapt to the chronic anemic state. Features of hookworm-induced anemia include microcytic/hypochromic erythrocytes, pallor, weakness, lassitude, dyspnea, and edema due to hypoproteinemia, especially in malnourished children. Moderate infections and anemia can impair physical, cognitive, and intellectual growth in children, diminish productivity of workers, and threaten the outcome of pregnancy for both mother and child.[88,98,99] In the most severe cases, anemia caused by hookworms can lead to congestive heart failure and is directly responsible for approximately 60,000 deaths per year worldwide.[3,6] Infection of children with large numbers of hookworms and falciparum malaria leads to hemoglobin levels that are lower than those caused by either parasite alone.[100]

DIAGNOSIS

Direct fecal smear examination is adequate for diagnosis of clinically significant hookworm infections; concentration techniques are needed only for the lightest infections. For epidemiologic purposes, quantitative egg counts can be performed to determine the intensity of infection, and species can be identified by examining adult worms expelled after treatment or larvae obtained by fecal culture or by polymerase chain reaction (PCR)-based assays applied to samples of stool.

MANAGEMENT

Iron replacement alone can lead to restoration of a normal hemoglobin level in people with hookworm disease, but anemia recurs unless anthelmintic therapy is given. A single 400-mg dose of albendazole is the treatment of choice.[3,57] Mebendazole 100 mg twice daily for 3 days is more effective than a single dose of 500 mg, and several 11 mg/kg doses of pyrantel pamoate may be necessary to eliminate or reduce heavy infections.[57,101-103] Poor responses to mebendazole have been reported in areas where it had never been used before, as well as in areas where multiple rounds of community-based treatment had been carried out in the past.[101-103] The widespread practice of annual or semi-annual deworming of children and other groups has raised concerns about resistance developing to albendazole and mebendazole, and the need for new drugs or a vaccine. Indeed, resistance to different members of the benzimidazole class of anthelmintics, which are used widely in veterinary medicine, has been observed.[104,105] Although humans do not acquire protective immunity to hookworm infection, the success of experimental immunization of animals with larval vaccines or adult-stage antigens suggests that development of a human vaccine may be possible.[106] A candidate hookworm vaccine already in human trials is Na-ASP-2, which employs as antigen *Ancylostoma*-secreted protein (ASP), the target of protective immunity against the larval stage in canine infection.[106,107]

PREVENTION AND CONTROL OF ASCARIASIS, TRICHURIASIS, AND HOOKWORM INFECTION

Geohelminth infections are prevented by drinking safe water, properly cleaning and cooking food, hand washing, and wearing shoes. Because provision of safe water sources and adequate sanitation to protect entire communities is too expensive for many poor countries, WHO advocates administering anthelmintic drugs at regular intervals to populations at risk, with the intention of maintaining individual worm burdens at levels below those that cause morbidity and mortality.[3,4,18] This strategy is based on studies showing that regular deworming of children and other at-risk populations, including preschool children, pregnant women, and women of childbearing age, can prevent and reverse malnutrition, iron-deficiency anemia, impaired growth, poor school performance, and poor-outcome pregnancies.[3,18,108,109] The availability of effective broad-spectrum, safe, inexpensive single-dose drugs such as albendazole and others listed in Table 287-1 makes drug administration at the population level feasible. Efforts are under way to combine programs that focus on geohelminth infections with other programs directed at single diseases, including lymphatic filariasis, onchocerciasis, schistosomiasis, and malaria. This approach may lower the prevalence and intensity of geohelminth infections but is unlikely to eliminate transmission in the absence of sanitation, clean water supplies, and overall economic development. Major challenges to controlling geohelminthic infections at the population level include implementing and sustaining mass drug administration programs and preventing the emergence of drug resistance.[110]

Strongyloidiasis

Although estimates of the global prevalence of strongyloidiasis are imprecise and vary between 3 million and 100 million people infected, it is clear that infection with *Strongyloides stercoralis* is considerably less common than infections with other major intestinal nematodes.[3,111] Strongyloidiasis is found throughout the tropics and subtropics and in limited foci in areas of the United States and Europe. Its medical importance lies primarily in its ability to produce overwhelming infection in immunocompromised people, a consequence of its unique ability to replicate and increase in numbers without leaving its host.[111] A second species, *Strongyloides fuelleborni*, a parasite of primates, infects humans in areas of Africa and produces the life-threatening "swollen belly syndrome" with generalized edema and respiratory distress in infants approximately 2 months of age in Papua New Guinea.[112]

LIFE CYCLE

Semitransparent, colorless female worms measuring 2.2 mm in length live embedded in the mucosal epithelium of the upper small intestine, where they deposit their eggs. Eggs are produced by parthenogenesis because parasitic adult males do not exist.[111,113] The eggs hatch in the mucosa, and the emergent noninfectious rhabditiform larvae measuring 250 to 300 μm in length work their way into the lumen of the bowel (see Fig. 287-1). If excreted with feces onto soil in a warm, humid environment, they molt and develop into either infective filariform larvae measuring 550 μm or free-living adult males and females. The free-living adults mate and produce rhabditiform larvae, which can develop directly into infective filariform larvae or pass through a free-living cycle first. Filariform larvae penetrate human skin and undergo a migration similar to that of hookworms, which terminates 18 to 28 days later in the small bowel mucosa, where female adult worms begin producing eggs.

A key feature of the biology of *Strongyloides* is that small numbers of rhabditiform larvae develop into filariform larvae within the bowel, reenter the host through the colonic mucosa or perianal skin, and thus complete their life cycle without leaving the host. This process of autoinfection explains how the parasite can increase in numbers in the absence of exogenous reinfection, persist indefinitely in a single host,

and be transmitted directly from one person to another during close physical contact.[111]

EPIDEMIOLOGY

Transmission of *S. stercoralis* depends on the suitability of the soil, climatic conditions, sanitation, and human behavior. In addition to the tropics and subtropics, the parasite is endemic in small areas of Appalachia, the southeastern United States, Europe, Australia, and Japan.[111,114] Certain immigrant and refugee groups from endemic areas have high rates of infection: IgG antibodies to *Strongyloides* were found in 12% to 77% of refugees from three countries in Southeast Asia living in Canada and in 46% and 23% of Lost Boys and Girls of Sudan and Somali Bantu refugees, respectively, on arrival to the United States.[115,116] Person-to-person transmission accounts for other reports of strongyloidiasis outside of endemic areas in mental institutions and day care centers and among men who have sex with men.[117] Infections lasting more than 60 years have been documented in military veterans and immigrants who lived in endemic areas in the distant past.[1,118]

CLINICAL SYNDROMES

With acute infections, there may be a localized, pruritic, erythematous, papular rash soon after larval penetration. Pulmonary symptoms with eosinophilia may appear several days later, and diarrhea and abdominal pain develop several weeks after that and just before the appearance of larvae in the stool.[111] In chronic uncomplicated strongyloidiasis, host and parasite live in harmony, autoinfection is well regulated by the host's cell-mediated immunity, and the number of adult worms is low and stable. The immune response to *Strongyloides* infection is predominantly Th2, with high levels of interleukin (IL)-4, IL-5, IL-10, IL-13, serum IgE, and eosinophils in the peripheral blood.[119]

More than 50% of chronically infected people may be asymptomatic, and greater than 75% have a fluctuating eosinophilia, as high as 10% to 15%.[111] Some people develop recurrent maculopapular or urticarial rashes that involve primarily the buttocks, perineum, and thighs.[120] Migrating larvae may produce the pathognomonic larva currens, a serpiginous urticarial rash that advances as fast as 10 cm/hr. Adult worms and larvae traversing the upper small bowel mucosa may produce epigastric pain that resembles peptic ulcer pain, as well as nausea, diarrhea, and blood loss. Pulmonary symptoms are uncommon, and when present there is often underlying chronic obstructive lung disease.[111]

Severe, complicated strongyloidiasis, including the strongyloides hyperinfection and disseminated strongyloidiasis syndromes, results from increased generation of filariform larvae (accelerated autoinfection), typically when host immunity is impaired. In developed countries, the most common risk factor is use of corticosteroids; among reported cases, the mean daily dose was the equivalent of 52 mg of prednisone, and in 74% of cases the duration of corticosteroid therapy was greater than 1 month.[121,122] Other risk factors include use of TNF-α inhibitors and other immunosuppressive drugs, hematologic malignancies, impaired gut motility, hypochlorhydria, and diabetes or other debilitating chronic diseases.[122-124] Infection with human T-cell lymphotropic virus-1 (HTLV-1) is associated with impairment of Th2 immune responses and, consequently, increased susceptibility to infection with *Strongyloides*, higher rates of severe complicated strongyloidiasis, and poor response to treatment with frequent relapses.[119,122,125-127] There is controversy regarding the effect of strongyloidiasis on HTLV-1 viral load and progression to T-cell leukemia/lymphoma (see Chapter 168).[119]

Despite the undoubtedly large numbers of people infected with both *Strongyloides* and HIV worldwide, there have been relatively few case reports of hyperinfection among coinfected people with AIDS, and some of these people were also receiving corticosteroids.[6,128-130] The lack of association of HIV infection with severe strongyloidiasis may reflect a decrease in production of Th1 cytokines and increase in Th2 cytokines.[6,123] Complicated, severe strongyloidiasis and an immune reconstitution inflammatory syndrome with abdominal pain, vomiting, and anorexia have been reported after institution of antiretroviral therapy.[131,132]

With hyperinfection, increased numbers of larvae are found in the intestines and lungs, the organs involved in the normal autoinfection cycle.[111,122-124] With disseminated strongyloidiasis, larvae are also found in the central nervous system (CNS), kidneys, liver, and almost any other organ. Eosinophilia is usually absent. Gastrointestinal manifestations are common and include abdominal pain, nausea, vomiting, diarrhea, ileus, and edema of the bowel, which can lead to intestinal obstruction. The clinical picture may mimic that of ulcerative colitis.[133] Ulceration of the mucosa may produce massive hemorrhage, peritonitis, or bacterial sepsis. Larvae migrating beyond the gastrointestinal tract produce pneumonitis with cough, hemoptysis, and respiratory failure; diffuse interstitial infiltrates or consolidation may be seen on chest radiographs. Occasionally, sputum contains adult worms, rhabditiform larvae, and eggs in addition to the more usual filariform larvae.[111] CNS invasion may cause meningitis and brain abscesses, with larvae in the cerebrospinal fluid and tissue. Biopsy of linear rashes, petechiae, and purpura often shows larvae.[134] Gram-negative bacteria, *Bacteroides fragilis*, and other bacteria may gain access to the bloodstream through ulcers in the bowel or by transport on the surface and in the gut of migrating larvae; bacterial sepsis, meningitis, and pneumonia occur frequently.[121,122] The mortality associated with untreated disseminated strongyloidiasis approaches 100%, and even with treatment it may exceed 25%.[111,121,122,124]

DIAGNOSIS

Uncomplicated strongyloidiasis can be diagnosed by finding rhabditiform larvae on microscopic examination of the stool, either by direct smear, following concentration by the Baermann technique, or culture on agar plates, which is the most sensitive of the available concentration methods.[52,111,135] A short buccal cavity distinguishes *Strongyloides* larvae from hookworm larvae hatching in stool that is not examined promptly. Repeated stool examinations are often needed because the sensitivity of a single stool examination can be as low as 30% because of the small numbers of larvae that are shed. It may be necessary to sample duodenal fluid or obtain a small bowel biopsy to demonstrate organisms.[111] Serologic tests using crude larval antigens, such as the enzyme-linked immunoassay offered by the Centers for Disease Control and Prevention, have greater sensitivity and should be used to rule out *Strongyloides* infection when microscopic examinations are negative or not performed.[120,122] Such tests have a sensitivity that can exceed 95%, but specificity is lower because of cross-reactivity with other helminth infections.[120] An assay that utilizes luciferase immunoprecipitation systems to detect IgG antibodies to a recombinant *Strongyloides* antigen (NIE) and *S. stercoralis* immunoreactive antigen (SsIR) has sensitivity and specificity of 100%.[136] A real-time PCR to detect *Strongyloides* DNA in fecal samples also achieved 100% specificity and high sensitivity.[137] Hyperinfection and disseminated strongyloidiasis are readily diagnosed by examining stool, sputum, other body fluids, and tissues, which typically contain high numbers of filariform larvae.

MANAGEMENT

All people infected with S. *stercoralis* should be treated with the aim of eradicating the infection. Uncomplicated strongyloidiasis is treated with oral ivermectin 200 μg/kg once daily for 2 days, which is at least as effective but better tolerated than thiabendazole 25 mg/kg twice daily.[138,139] Albendazole 400 mg twice a day for 10 to 14 days is an alternative; shorter courses of albendazole are not as effective as ivermectin.[138-141]

Management of hyperinfection and disseminated strongyloidiasis includes prompt administration of anthelmintics and broad-spectrum antibiotics with activity against enteric organisms and, when possible,

discontinuation or reduction of immunosuppression. The drug of choice for severe, complicated strongyloidiasis is ivermectin, which should be given daily and continued for at least 7 days and until larvae are no longer detected in the stool, sputum, and urine.[138,141] In people with paralytic ileus, absorption of ivermectin may be impaired, even following administration by nasogastric tube.[142,143] Subcutaneous injection of a veterinary preparation of ivermectin yields serum levels of the drug significantly higher than those obtained by oral administration and has been successful when oral therapy has failed.[143,144] However, ivermectin is highly bound to serum proteins; in one fatal case, levels of free ivermectin were less than 1% of total, and 12 daily doses of subcutaneous ivermectin did not eliminate parasites.[145] Other approaches to therapy include rectal administration of ivermectin or thiabendazole,[142,146] combinations of albendazole and ivermectin,[143] and prolonged courses of albendazole or thiabendazole when ivermectin is not available.

Because eradication of infection is the goal for both uncomplicated and complicated strongyloidiasis, follow-up examinations are indicated and treatment should be repeated if larvae are identified in feces 2 weeks after completion of therapy.[143] Following successful treatment, IgG antibodies to *Strongyloides* have been shown to decline or disappear in 6 to 12 months.[147-149] Eosinophilia, if present, should resolve as well. In people with HTLV-1 infection or whose immunosuppression persists, two daily doses of ivermectin every 2 weeks may keep larvae suppressed.

PREVENTION OF HYPERINFECTION AND DISSEMINATED STRONGYLOIDIASIS

Immunosuppressed people, those about to receive immunosuppressive medications (especially corticosteroids), or people with HTLV-1 infection should be evaluated for possible strongyloidiasis if they have visited or lived in an endemic area, especially if there is a history of contact with potentially contaminated soil or beaches.[12,120] Those with potential exposure to *S. stercoralis* at any time during their lives should undergo serologic testing, even in the absence of symptoms or eosinophilia. A positive serologic test is an indication for treatment, even if multiple stool examinations are negative.

🔲 Enterobiasis

Enterobius vermicularis, or pinworm, is highly prevalent throughout the world. In the United States, it is the most common of all helminthic infections, with a prevalence estimated in the 1980s of 42 million cases; in several European countries, Peru, India, and Thailand, rates of pinworm infection among children exceeded 25%.[150-152] Pinworm infection is particularly common among children, institutionalized groups, and households; it is not associated with any specific socioeconomic level.[153]

LIFE CYCLE

E. vermicularis is a small white worm measuring 1 cm in length and inhabiting the cecum, appendix, and adjacent gut.[154] Gravid female worms containing an average of 10,000 ova migrate at night to the perianal and perineal regions, where they deposit their eggs and die; ova are infrequently deposited in the bowels. *Enterobius* ova are ovoid but flattened on one side and measure approximately 56×27 μm. The eggs embryonate within 6 hours and are transferred from the perianal region to nightclothes, bedding, and dust and air. The most common mode of transmission, however, is via the hands of the patient, particularly underneath the fingernails, through scratching or handling clothes and bed linen. Enterobiasis may be transmitted between sexual partners, especially those engaging in oral-anal sex. On ingestion, the embryos hatch in the duodenum, molt twice, and within 5 or 6 weeks develop into adult worms that live approximately 1 month.

EPIDEMIOLOGY

The prevalence of pinworm infection is lowest in infants and reaches its maximum in schoolchildren 5 to 14 years old.[154] The absence of an extended extracorporeal development stage favors both direct transmission to others and autoinfection. Eggs are infective within 6 hours of oviposition and may remain so for 20 days. Pinworm is primarily a familial or institutional infection associated with crowding. Because the life span of the worms is relatively brief, long-standing infections are due to continuous reinfection.[155]

CLINICAL SYNDROMES

Most pinworm infections are asymptomatic. When present, symptoms are related largely to perianal and perineal pruritus and scratching.[156] The most common complaints are local itching and restless sleep due to nocturnal anal pruritus. Dysuria, enuresis, vulvovaginitis, and vaginal discharge have been attributed to pinworm as well.[151,152] However, in a hospital-based study of children 2 to 12 years old, none of the signs and symptoms largely ascribed to enterobiasis was significantly more common in infected than in uninfected children.[157]

Occasionally, the migration of the parasite leads to ectopic disease, such as pelvic, cervical, vulvar, and peritoneal granulomas, which may be mistaken for other pelvic masses or may produce symptoms that mimic pelvic inflammatory disease.[158] The relationship between pinworm infection and appendicitis is unclear. In several studies, more normal than inflamed appendices removed at surgery for suspected appendicitis contained pinworms, suggesting that pinworms may cause symptoms resembling appendicitis without invading the mucosa.[159,160] Large numbers of larval pinworms, presumably from a single heavy exposure, have caused eosinophilic enterocolitis in adults and children.[161-163] Enterobiasis is usually not associated with significant eosinophilia or elevated serum IgE levels. There is evidence that the intestinal protozoan, *Dientamoeba fragilis*, is transmitted through ova of the pinworm.[164]

DIAGNOSIS

Although pinworms can be seen by the naked eye, they may be confused with bits of white thread or proglottids of *Dipylidium caninum*, a tapeworm of dogs and cats that occasionally infects children.[165] Pinworm eggs are usually not encountered in stool but are readily identified by microscopic examination of an adhesive cellophane tape pressed against the perianal region early in the morning.[154] A single examination detects 50% of infections, three examinations detect 90%, and five examinations detect 99%.

MANAGEMENT

Single doses of albendazole (400 mg), mebendazole (100 mg), ivermectin (200 μg/kg), or pyrantel pamoate (11 mg/kg up to 1 g) are highly effective. A second dose is given 2 weeks later because of the frequency of reinfection and autoinfection.[87] Other infected family members, classmates, or residents of long-term care facilities should be treated at the same time as the index case, but reinfections are common and repeated treatment courses may be needed.[154,166] Although personal cleanliness is a useful general principle, its role in the management of enterobiasis is minor, and overemphasis on cleanliness may enhance the psychological trauma and stigma associated with this infection.

REFERENCES

1. Muller R. The nematodes. In: *Worms and Human Disease*. 2nd ed. Wallingford, UK: CABI; 2002:109-235.
2. Coombs I, Crompton DWT. *A Guide to Human Helminths*. London: Taylor & Francis; 1991:1-4.
3. Crompton DWT, Savioli L. *Handbook of Helminthiases for Public Health*. Boca Raton, Fla: CRC Press; 2007:3-24, 203-245.
4. World Health Organization. *Deworming for Health and Development. Report of the Third Global Meeting of the Partners for Parasite Control*. Geneva: World Health Organization, 2005.
5. Viney ME, Brown M, Omoding NE, et al. Why does HIV infection not lead to disseminated strongyloidiasis? *J Infect Dis*. 2004;190:2175-2180.
6. Bethony J, Brooker S, Albonico M, et al. Soil-transmitted helminth infections: ascariasis, trichuriasis, and hookworm. *Lancet*. 2006;367:1521-1532.
7. Cooper PJ, Chico ME, Sandoval C, et al. Human infection with *Ascaris lumbricoides* is associated with a polarized cytokine response. *J Infect Dis*. 2000;182:1207-1213.
8. Fincham JE, Markus MB, Adams VJ. Could control of soil-transmitted helminthic infection influence the HIV/AIDS pandemic? *Acta Trop*. 2003;86:315-333.
9. Walson JL, Otieno PA, Mbuchi M, et al. Albendazole treatment of HIV-1 and helminth co-infection: a randomized, double-blind, placebo-controlled trial. *AIDS*. 2008;22:1601-1609.
10. Brown M, Kizza M, Watera C, et al. Helminth infection is not associated with faster progression of HIV disease in coinfected adults in Uganda. *J Infect Dis*. 2004;190:1869-1879.
11. Robinson TM, Nelson RG, Boyer JD. Parasitic infection and the polarized Th2 immune response can alter a vaccine-induced immune response. *DNA Cell Biol*. 2003;22:421-430.
12. Crompton DWT. Ascaris and ascariasis. *Adv Parasitol*. 2001;48:285-375.
13. DeSilva NR, Chan MS, Bundy DA. Morbidity and mortality due to ascariasis: reestimation and sensitivity analysis of global numbers at risk. *Trop Med Int Health*. 1997;2:519-528.
14. Crompton DWT, Nesheim MC, Pawlowski ZS, eds. *Ascariasis and Its Prevention and Control*. London: Taylor & Francis; 1989.
15. Anthony RM, Rutitzky LI, Urban JF Jr, et al. Protective immune mechanisms in helminth infection. *Nat Rev Immunol*. 2007;7:975-987.
16. Johnston MJG, MacDonald JA, McKay DM. Parasitic helminths: a pharmacopeia of anti-inflammatory molecules. *Parasitology*. 2009;136:125-147.
17. Esink JH, Blumenthal UJ, Brooker S. Wastewater quality and the risk of intestinal nematode infection in sewage farming families in Hyderabad, India. *Am J Trop Med Hyg*. 2008;79:561-567.

18. Albonico M, Montresor A, Crompton DWT, et al. Interventions for the control of soil-transmitted helminthiasis in the community. *Adv Parasitol*. 2006;61:311-348.
19. O'Lorcain P, Holland CV. The public health importance of *Ascaris lumbricoides*. *Parasitology*. 2000;121(Suppl):S51-S71.
20. Anderson RM, May RM. *Infectious Diseases of Humans: Dynamics and Control*. New York: Oxford University Press; 1991: 433-606.
21. Wakelin D, Farias SE, Bradley JE. Variation and immunity to intestinal worms. *Parasitology*. 2002;125(Suppl):S39-S50.
22. Quinell RJ. Genetics of susceptibility to human helminth infection. *Int J Parasitol*. 2003;33:1219-1231.
23. Williams-Blangero S, VandeBerg JL, Subedi J, et al. Localization of multiple qualitative trait loci influencing susceptibility to infection with *Ascaris*. *J Infect Dis*. 2008;197:66-71.
24. Anderson TJ. *Ascaris* infections in humans from North America: molecular evidence for cross-infection. *Parasitology*. 1995; 110:215-219.
25. Nejsum P, Parker ED Jr, Frydenberg J, et al. Ascariasis is a zoonosis in Denmark. *J Clin Microbiol*. 2005;43:1142-1148.
26. Gelpi AP, Mustafa A. *Ascaris* pneumonia. *Am J Med*. 1968;44:377-389.
27. Gelpi AP, Mustafa A. Seasonal pneumonitis with eosinophilia: a study of larval ascariasis in Saudi Arabs. *Am J Trop Med Hyg*. 1967;16:646-657.
28. Stephenson LS. The contribution of *Ascaris lumbricoides* to malnutrition in children. *Parasitology*. 1980;81:221-233.
29. Jardim-Botelho A, Brooker S, Geiger SM, et al. Age patterns in undernutrition and helminth infection in a rural area of Brazil: associations with ascariasis and hookworm. *Trop Med Int Health*. 2008;13:458-467.
30. Jardim-Botelho A, Raff S, Rodrigues R de A, et al. Hookworm, *Ascaris lumbricoides* infection and polyparasitism associated with poor cognitive performance in Brazilian schoolchildren. *Trop Med Int Health*. 2008;13:994-1004.
31. Hall A, Gillian H, Tuffrey V, et al. A review and meta-analysis of the impact of intestinal worms on child growth and nutrition. *Matern Child Nutr*. 2008;4(Suppl 1):118-236.
32. Hall A. Micronutrient supplements for children after deworming. *Lancet Infect Dis*. 2007;7:297-302.
33. Archibong AE, Ndoma-Egba R, Asindi AA. Intestinal obstruction in southeastern Nigerian children. *East Afr Med J*. 1994;71:286-289.
34. Blumenthal DS, Schultz MG. Incidence of intestinal obstruction in children infected with *Ascaris lumbricoides*. *Am J Trop Med Hyg*. 1975;24:801-805.
35. De Silva NR, Chan MS, Bundy DA. Morbidity and mortality due to Ascaris-induced intestinal obstruction. *Trans R Soc Trop Med Hyg*. 1997;91:31-36.

36. De Silva NR, Guyatt HL, Bundy DA. Worm burden in intestinal obstruction caused by *Ascaris lumbricoides*. *Trop Med Int Health*. 1997;2:189-190.
37. Wasadikar PP, Kulkami AB. Intestinal obstruction due to ascariasis. *Br J Surg*. 1997;84:410-412.
38. Teneza-Mora NC, Lavery EA, Chun HM. Partial small bowel obstruction in a traveler. *Clin Infect Dis*. 2006;43:214, 256-258.
39. Sandouk F, Haffar S, Zada M, et al. Pancreatic-biliary ascariasis: experience of 300 cases. *Am J Gastroenterol*. 1997;92:2264-2267.
40. Khuroo MS, Zargar SA, Mahajan R. Hepatobiliary and pancreatic ascariasis in India. *Lancet*. 1990;335:1503-1508.
41. Shah OJ, Showkat AZ, Robbani I. Biliary ascariasis: a review. *World J Surg*. 2006;30:1500-1506.
42. Javid G, Wani NA, Gulzar GM, et al. Ascaris-induced liver abscess. *World J Surg*. 1999;23:1191-1194.
43. Singh PA, Gupta SC, Agarawal R. *Ascaris lumbricoides* appendicitis in the tropics. *Trop Doct*. 1997;27:241.
44. Schulman A. Non-Western patterns of biliary stones and the role of ascariasis. *Radiology*. 1987;162:425-430.
45. Palmer LJ, Celedon JC, Weiss ST, et al. *Ascaris lumbricoides* infection is associated with increased risk of childhood asthma and atopy in rural China. *Am J Respir Crit Care Med*. 2002; 165:1489-1493.
46. Cooper PJ, Chico ME, Bland M, et al. Allergic symptoms, atopy, and geohelminth infections in a rural area of Ecuador. *Am J Respir Crit Care Med*. 2003;168:266-267.
47. Cooper PJ, Mitre E, Moncayo AL, et al. *Ascaris lumbricoides*-induced interleukin-10 is not associated with atopy in schoolchildren in a rural area of the tropics. *J Infect Dis*. 2008; 197:1333-1340.
48. Leonardi-Bee J, Pritchard D, Britton J, et al. Asthma and current intestinal parasite infection: systemic review and meta-analysis. *Am J Respir Crit Care Med*. 2006;174:514-523.
49. Brutus L, Wtier L, Briand V, et al. Parasitic co-infections: does *Ascaris lumbricoides* protect against *Plasmodium falciparum* infection? *Am J Trop Med Hyg*. 2006;75:194-198.
50. Hartgers FC, Yazdanbakhsh M. Co-infection of helminths and malaria: modulation of the immune responses to malaria. *Parasite Immunol*. 2006;28:497-506.
51. Garcia LS. *Diagnostic Medical Parasitology*. 5th ed. Washington, DC: ASM Press; 2006.
52. Reeder MM, Palmer PES. *The Radiology of Tropical Diseases*. 2nd ed. Berlin: Springer-Verlag; 2001:111-139.
53. Ng KK, Wong HF, Kong MS, et al. Biliary ascariasis: CT, MR cholangiopancreatography, and navigator endoscopic appearance—report of a case of acute biliary obstruction. *Abdom Imaging*. 1999;24:470-472.

54. Rocha MdeS, Costa NS, Costa JC, et al. CT identification of *Ascaris* in the biliary tract. *Abdom Imaging*. 1995;20: 317-319.
55. Ferreyra NP, Cerri GG. Ascariasis of the alimentary tract, liver, pancreas and biliary system: its diagnosis by ultrasonography. *Hepatogastroenterology*. 1998;45:932-937.
56. Valgaeren G, Duysburgh I, Fierens H, et al. Endoscopic treatment of biliary ascariasis: report of a case. *Acta Clin Belg*. 1996;51:97-100.
57. Keiser J, Utzinger J. Efficacy of current drugs against soil-transmitted helminth infections: systemic review and meta-analysis. *JAMA*. 2008;299:1937-1948.
58. Montresor A, Awasthi S, Crompton DW. Use of benzimidazoles in children younger than 24 months for the treatment of soil-transmitted helminthiasis. *Acta Trop*. 2003;86:223-232.
59. Galvan-Ramirez ML, Rivera N, Loeza ME, et al. Nitazoxanide in the treatment of *Ascaris lumbricoides* in a rural zone of Colima, Mexico. *J Helminthol*. 2007;81:255-259.
60. Romero R, Guerero LR, Munoz Garcia MR, et al. Nitazoxanide for the treatment of intestinal protozoan and helminthic infections in Mexico. *Trans R Soc Trop Med Hyg*. 1997;91: 701-703.
61. Diaz E, Mondragon J, Ramirez E, et al. Epidemiology and control of intestinal parasites with nitazoxanide in children in Mexico. *Am J Trop Med Hyg*. 2003;68:384-385.
62. Steinman P, Zhou X, Du Z, et al. Tribendimimidine and albendazole for treating soil-transmitted helminths, *Strongyloides stercoralis* and *Taenia* spp.: open-label, randomized trial. *PLoS Negl Trop Dis*. 2008;2:e322.
63. Cooper ES, Bundy DAP. Trichuriasis. *Clin Trop Med Comm Dis*. 1987;2:629-643.
64. Drake L, Korchev Y, Bashford L, et al. The major secreted protein of the whipworm, *Trichuris*, is a pore-forming protein. *Proc Biol Sci*. 1994;257:255-261.
65. Gilman RH, Chong UH, Davis C, et al. The adverse consequences of heavy *Trichuris* infection. *Trans R Soc Trop Med Hyg*. 1983;77:432-438.
66. Williams-Blangero S, McGarvey ST, Subedi J, et al. Genetic component to susceptibility to *Trichuris trichiura*: evidence from two Asian populations. *Genet Epidemiol*. 2002;22: 254-264.
67. Williams-Blangero S, Vandeberg JL, Subedi J, et al. Two quantitative trait loci influence whipworm (*Trichuris trichiura*) infection in a Nepalese population. *J Infect Dis*. 2008;197: 1198-1203.
68. MacDonald TT, Spencer J, Murch SH, et al. Immunoepidemiology of intestinal helminth infections: 3. Mucosal macrophages and cytokine production in the colon of children with *Trichuris trichiura* dysentery. *Trans R Soc Trop Med Hyg*. 1994; 88:265-268.
69. Ramdath DD, Simeon DT, Wong MS, et al. Iron status of school children with varying intensities of *Trichuris trichiura* infection. *Parasitology*. 1995;110:347-351.
70. MacDonald TT, Choy MY, Spencer J, et al. Histopathology and immunochemistry of the caecum in children with the *Trichuris* dysentery syndrome. *J Clin Pathol*. 1991;44:194-199.
71. Sandler M. Whipworm infestation in the colon and rectum simulating Crohn's disease. *Lancet*. 1981;2:210.
72. Jung RC, Beaver PC. Clinical observations on *Trichocephalus trichuris* (whipworm) infestation in children. *Pediatrics*. 1951; 8:548-557.
73. Cooper ES, Bundy DAP. *Trichuris* is not trivial. *Parasitol Today*. 1988;4:301-306.
74. Forrester JE, Bailar JC III, Esrey SA, et al. Randomized trial of albendazole and pyrantel in symptomless trichuriasis in children. *Lancet*. 1998;352:1103-1108.
75. Parthasarathy G, Mansfield LS. *Trichuris suis* excretory secretory products (ESP) elicit interleukin-6 (IL-6) and IL-10 secretion from intestinal epithelial cells (IPEC-1). *Vet Parasitol*. 2005; 131:317-324.
76. Wang LJ, Cao Y, Shi HN. Helminth infections and intestinal inflammation. *World J Gastroenterol*. 2008;7:5125-5132.
77. Summers RW, Elliott DE, Qadir K, et al. *Trichuris suis* seems to be safe and possibly effective in the treatment of inflammatory bowel disease. *Gastroenterology*. 2003;98:2034-2041.
78. Summers RW, Elliott DE. *Trichuris suis* therapy for active ulcerative colitis: randomized controlled trial. *Gastroenterology*. 2005;128:825-832.
79. Ruyssers NE, De Winter BY, De Man JG, et al. Worms and the treatment of inflammatory bowel disease: are molecules the answer? *Clin Dev Immunol*. 2008;2008:567314.
80. Olsen A, Namwanje H, Nejsum P, et al. Albendazole and mebendazole have low efficacy against *Trichuris trichiura* in school-age children in Kabale District, Uganda. *Trans R Soc Trop Med Hyg*. 2009;103:443-446.
81. Belizario VY, Amarillo ME, de Leon WU, et al. A comparison of the efficacy of single doses of albendazole, ivermectin, and diethylcarbamazine alone or in combinations against *Ascaris* and *Trichuris* spp. *Bull WHO*. 2003;81:35-42.
82. Sirivichayakul C, Pojjaroen-Anant C, Wisetsing P, et al. The effectiveness of 3, 5, or 7 days of albendazole for the treatment of *Trichuris trichiuria* infection. *Ann Trop Med Parasitol*. 2003;97:847-853.
83. Olsen A. Efficacy and safety of drug combinations in the treatment of schistosomiasis, soil-transmitted helminthiasis, lymphatic filariasis, and onchocerciasis. *Trans R Soc Trop Med Hyg*. 2007;101:747-758.
84. Reddy M, Gill SS, Kalkar SR, et al. Oral drug therapy for multiple neglected tropical diseases. *JAMA*. 2007;298:1911-1924.
85. Hotez PJ, Brooker S, Bethony JM, et al. Hookworm infection. *N Engl J Med*. 2004;351:799-807.
86. Gilles HM, Williams EJW, Ball PAJ. Hookworm infection and anemia: an epidemiological, clinical, and laboratory study. *Q J Med*. 1964;33:1-24.
87. Roche M, Layrisse M. The nature and causes of "hookworm anemia." *Am J Trop Med Hyg*. 1966;15:1032-1102.
88. Migasena S, Gilles HM. Hookworm infection. *Clin Trop Med Commun Dis*. 1987;2:617-627.
89. Wilcox LS. Worms and germs, drink and dementia: US health, society, and policy in the early 20th century. *Prev Chronic Dis*. 2008;5:1-12.
90. Johnston MJG, MacDonald JA, McKay DM. Parasitic helminths: a pharmacopeia of anti-inflammatory molecules. *Parasitology*. 2009;136:125-147.
91. Maxwell C, Hussain R, Nutman TB, et al. The clinical and immunological responses of normal human volunteers to low dose hookworm (*Necator americanus*) infection. *Am J Trop Med Hyg*. 1987;37:126-134.
92. Lawn SD, Grant AD, Wright SG. Case reports: acute hookworm infection; an unusual cause of profuse watery diarrhea in returned travellers. *Trans R Soc Trop Med Hyg*. 2003; 97:414-415.
93. Kelley PW, Takafuji ET, Wiener H, et al. An outbreak of hookworm infection associated with military operations in Grenada. *Milit Med*. 1989;154:55-59.
94. Bailey NS, Thomas R, Green AD, et al. Helminth infections in British troops following an operation in Sierra Leone. *Trans R Soc Trop Med Hyg*. 2006;100:842-846.
95. Capello M, Vlasuk GP, Bergum PW, et al. *Ancylostoma caninum* anticoagulant peptide: a hookworm-derived inhibitor of human coagulation factor Xa. *Proc Natl Acad Sci USA*. 1995;92:6152-6156.
96. Chadderdon RC, Cappello M. The hookworm platelet inhibitor: functional blockade of integrins GPIIb/IIIa (alphaIIb beta3) and GPIa/IIa (alpha2 beta1) inhibits platelet aggregation and adhesion in vitro. *J Infect Dis*. 1999;179:1235-1241.
97. Del Valle A, Jones BF, Harrison LM, et al. Isolation and molecular cloning of a secreted hookworm platelet inhibitor from adult *Ancylcostoma caninum*. *Mol Biochem Parasitol*. 2003;129: 167-177.
98. Sakti H, Nokes C, Hertanto WS, et al. Evidence for an association between hookworm infection and cognitive function in Indonesian school children. *Trop Med Int Health*. 1999; 4:322-334.
99. Christian P, Khatry SK, West KP Jr. Antenatal anthelmintic treatment, birthweight, and infant survival in rural Nepal. *Lancet*. 2004;364:981-983.
100. Verweij JJ, Brienen EA, Ziem J, et al. Simultaneous detection and quantification of *Ancylostoma duodenale, Necator americanus*, and *Oesophagostomum bifurcum* in fecal samples using multiplex real-time PCR. *Am J Trop Med Hyg*. 2007;77: 685-690.
101. Albonico M, Bickle Q, Ramsan M, et al. Efficacy of mebendazole and levamisole alone or in combination against intestinal nematode infections after repeated targetted mebendazole treatment in Zanzibar. *Bull World Health Organ*. 2003;81:343-352.
102. Sacko M, De Clercq D, Behnke JM, et al. Comparison of the efficacy of mebendazole, albendazole and pyrantel in treatment of human hookworm infections in the southern region of Mali, West Africa. *Trans R Soc Trop Med Hyg*. 1999;93: 195-203.
103. Carston F, Tuyen LN, Lewis S, et al. Low efficacy of mebendazole against hookworm in Vietnam: two randomized controlled trials. *Am J Trop Med Hyg*. 2007;76:732-736.
104. Geerts S, Gryseels B. Drug resistance in human helminths: current situation and lessons learned from livestock. *Clin Microbiol Rev*. 2000;13:207-222.
105. Geerts S, Gryseels B. Anthelmintic resistance in human helminths: a review. *Trop Med Int Health*. 2001;6:915-921.
106. Hotez PJ, Zhan B, Bethony JM, et al. Progress in the development of a recombinant vaccine for human hookworm and disease: the Human Hookworm Initiative. *Int J Parasitol*. 2003;33:1245-1258.
107. Diemert DJ, Bethony JM, Hotez PJ. Hookworm vaccines. *Clin Infect Dis*. 2008;46:282-288.
108. De Silva NR. Impact of mass chemotherapy on the morbidity due to soil-transmitted nematodes. *Acta Trop*. 2003;86: 197-214.
109. Stephenson LS. Optimising the benefits of anthelmintic treatment in children. *Paediatr Drugs*. 2001;3:495-508.
110. Lammie PJ, Fenwick A, Utzinger J. A blueprint for success: integration of neglected tropical disease control programmes. *Parasitol Today*. 2006;22:313-321.
111. Grove DI. Human strongyloidiasis. *Adv Parasitol*. 1996;38:251-309.
112. Ashford RW, Vince JD, Gratten MJ, et al. *Strongyloides* infection associated with acute infantile disease in Papua New Guinea. *Trans R Soc Trop Med Hyg*. 1978;72:554.
113. Viney ME, Lok JB. *Strongyloides* spp. *WormBook*. 2007;(May 23):1-15.
114. Kitchen LW, Tu KK, Kerns FT. *Strongyloides*-infected patients at Charleston area medical center, West Virginia, 1997-1998. *Clin Infect Dis*. 2000;31:E5-E6.
115. Gyorkos TW, Genta RM, MacLean JD. Seroepidemiology of *Strongyloides* infection in the Southeast Asian refugee population in Canada. *Am J Epidemiol*. 1990;132:257-264.
116. Posey DL, Blackburn BG, Weinberg M, et al. High prevalence and presumptive treatment of schistosomiasis and strongyloidiasis among African refugees. *Clin Infect Dis*. 2007;45:1310-1315.
117. Gatti S, Lopes R, Cevini C. Intestinal parasitic infections in an institution for the mentally retarded. *Ann Trop Med Parasitol*. 2000;94:453-460.
118. Genta RM, Weesner R, Douce RW, et al. Strongyloidiasis in US veterans of the Vietnam and other wars. *JAMA*. 1987;258: 49-52.
119. Carvalho EM, Porto DF. Epidemiological and clinical interaction between HTLV-1 and *Strongyloides stercoralis*. *Parasite Immunol*. 2004;26:487-497.
120. Siddiqui AS, Berl SL. Diagnosis of *Strongyloides stercoralis* infection. *Clin Infect Dis*. 2001;33:1040-1047.
121. Fardet L, Généreau T, Poirot JL, et al. Severe strongyloidiasis in corticosteroid-treated patients: case series and literature review. *J Infect*. 2007;54:18-27.
122. Marcos LA, Terashima A, DuPont HL, et al. *Strongyloides* hyperinfection syndrome: an emerging global infectious disease. *Tran R Soc Trop Med Hyg*. 2008;102:314-318.
123. Scowden EB, Schaffner W, Stone WJ. Overwhelming strongyloidiasis: an unappreciated opportunistic infection. *Medicine*. 1978;57:527-544.
124. Adedayo O, Grell G, Bellot P. Hyperinfective strongyloidiasis in the medical ward: review of 27 cases in 5 years. *South Med J*. 2002;95:711-716.
125. Porto AF, Neva FA, Bittencourt H. HTLV-1 decreases Th2 type of immune response in patients with strongyloidiasis. *Parasite Immunol*. 2001;23:503-507.
126. Porto AF, Oliveira Filho J, Neva FA, et al. Influence of human T-cell lymphocytotropic virus type 1 infection on serologic and skin tests for strongyloidiasis. *Am J Trop Med Hyg*. 2001;65: 610-613.
127. Terashima A, Alvarez H, Tello R, et al. Treatment failure in intestinal strongyloidiasis: an indicator of HTLV-I infection. *Int J Infect Dis*. 2002;6:28-30.
128. Gompels MM, Todd J, Peters BS, et al. Disseminated strongyloidiasis in AIDS: uncommon but important. *AIDS*. 1991; 5:329-332.
129. Torres JR, Isturiz R, Murillo J, et al. Efficacy of ivermectin in the treatment of strongyloidiasis complicating AIDS. *Clin Infect Dis*. 1993;17:900-902.
130. Siciliano RF, Mascheretti M, Gryschek RCB. Severe strongyloidiasis in AIDS: is steroid therapy guilty again? *J Acquir Immune Defic Syndr*. 2008;49:333-334.
131. Brown M, Cartledge JD, Miller RF. Dissemination of *Strongyloides stercoralis* as an immune restoration phenomenon in an HIV-1-infected man on antiretroviral therapy. *Int J STD AIDS*. 2006;17:560-561.
132. Lillie PJ, Barlow GD, Moss PJ, et al. Immune reconstitution syndrome to *Strongyloides stercoralis* infection. *AIDS*. 2007; 21:649-655.
133. Qu Z, Kundu UR, Abadeer RA, et al. *Strongyloides* colitis is a lethal mimic of ulcerative colitis: the key morphologic differential diagnosis. *Hum Pathol*. 2009;40:572-577.
134. Salluh JI, Bozza FA, Pinto TS, et al. Cutaneous periumbilical purpura in disseminated strongyloidiasis in cancer patients: a pathognomonic feature of potentially lethal disease? *Braz J Infect Dis*. 2005;9:419-424.
135. Hirata T, Nakamura H, Kinjo N, et al. Increased detection rate of *Strongyloides stercoralis* by repeated stool examination using the agar plate method. *Am J Trop Med Hyg*. 2007;77: 683-684.
136. Ramanathan R, Burbelo PD, Groot S, et al. A luciferase immunoprecipitation systems assay enhances the sensitivity and specificity of diagnosis of *Strongyloides stercoralis* infection. *J Infect Dis*. 2008;198:444-451.
137. Verweij JJ, Canales M, Polman K, et al. Molecular diagnosis of *Strongyloides stercoralis* in faecal samples using real-time PCR. *Trans R Soc Trop Med Hyg*. 2009;103:342-346.
138. Zaha O, Hirata T, Kinjo F, et al. Strongyloidiasis—progress in diagnosis and treatment. *Intern Med*. 2000;39:695-700.
139. Marti H, Haji HJ, Savioli L, et al. A comparative trial of a single-dose ivermectin versus three days of albendazole for treatment of *Strongyloides stercoralis* and other soil-transmitted infections in children. *Am J Trop Med Hyg*. 1996;55:477-481.
140. Suputtamongkol Y, Kungpanichkul N, Saowaluk S, et al. Efficacy and safety of a single-dose veterinary preparation of ivermectin versus 7-day high-dose albendazole for chronic strongyloidiasis. *Int J Antimicrob Agents*. 2008;31:46-49.
141. Lim S, Katz K, Krajden S, et al. Complicated and fatal *Strongyloides* infection in Canadians: risk factors, diagnosis and management. *Can Med Assoc J*. 2004;171:479-484.
142. Boken DJ, Leoni PA, Preheim LC. Treatment of *Strongyloides stercoralis* hyperinfection syndrome with thiabendazole administered per rectum. *Clin Infect Dis*. 1993;16:123-126.
143. Turner SA, Maclean JD, Fleckenstein L, et al. Parenteral administration of ivermectin in a patient with disseminated strongyloidiasis. *Am J Trop Med Hyg*. 2005;73:911-914.
144. Marty FM, Lowry CM, Rodriguez M, et al. Treatment of human disseminated strongyloidiasis with a parenteral veterinary formulation of ivermectin. *Clin Infect Dis*. 2005;41: e5-e6.

145. Leung V, Al-Rawahi GN, Grant J, et al. Case report: failure of subcutaneous ivermectin in treating *Strongyloides* hyperinfection. *Am J Trop Med Hyg.* 2008;79:853-855.
146. Tarr PE, Miele PS, Pergoy KS, et al. Case report: rectal administration of ivermectin to a patient with *Strongyloides* hyperinfection syndrome. *Am J Trop Med Hyg.* 2003;68:453-455.
147. Loutfy MR, Wilson M, Keystone JS, et al. Serology and eosinophil count in the diagnosis and management of strongyloidiasis in a non-endemic area. *Am J Trop Med Hyg.* 2002;66: 749-752.
148. Karunajeewa H, Heath K, Leslie D, et al. Parasite-specific IgG response and peripheral blood eosinophil count following albendazole treatment for presumed chronic strongyloidiasis. *J Travel Med.* 2006;13:84-89.
149. Page WA, Dempsey K, McCarthy JS. Utility of serological follow-up of chronic strongyloidiasis after anthelmintic chemotherapy. *Trans R Soc Trop Med Hyg.* 2006;100:1056-1062.
150. Wagner ED, Eby WC. Pinworm prevalence in California elementary school children, and diagnostic methods. *Am J Trop Med Hyg.* 1983;32:998-1001.
151. Burkhart CN, Burkhart CG. Assessment of frequency, transmission, and genitourinary complications of enterobiasis (pinworms). *Int J Dermatol.* 2005;44:837-840.

152. Gilman RH, Marquis GS, Miranda E. Prevalence and symptoms of *Enterobius vermicularis* in a Peruvian shanty town. *Am J Trop Med Hyg.* 1991;85:761-764.
153. Lohiya GS, Crinella FM, Lohiya S. Epidemiology and control of enterobiasis in a developmental center. *West J Med.* 2000;172:305-308.
154. Pawlowski ZS. Enterobiasis. *Clin Trop Med Commun Dis.* 1987;3:667-676.
155. Nunez FA, Hernandez M, Finlay CM. A longitudinal study of enterobiasis in three day care centers of Havana City. *Rev Inst Med Trop Sao Paulo.* 1996;38:129-132.
156. Weller TH, Sorenson CW. Enterobiasis: its incidence and symptomatology in a group of 505 children. *N Engl J Med.* 1941; 224:143-146.
157. Welsh NM. Recent insights into the childhood "social diseases"—gonorrhea, scabies, pediculosis, pinworms. *Clin Pediatr.* 1978;17:318-322.
158. Sun T, Schwartz NS, Sewell C, et al. *Enterobius* egg granuloma of the vulva and peritoneum: review of the literature. *Am J Trop Med Hyg.* 1991;45:249-253.
159. Dahlstrom JE, MacArthur EB. *Enterobius vermicularis*: a possible cause of symptoms resembling appendicitis. *Aust N Z J Surg.* 1994;64:692-694.

160. Sodergren MH, Jethwa P, Wilkonson S, et al. Presenting features of *Enterobius vermicularis* in the vermiform appendix. *Scand J Gastroenterol.* 2008;11:1-5.
161. Liu LX, Chi JY, Upton MP, et al. Eosinophilic colitis associated with larvae of the pinworm *Enterobius vermicularis. Lancet.* 1995;346:410-412.
162. Rajamanickam A, Usmani A, Suri S, et al. Chronic diarrhea and abdominal pain: pin the pinworm. *J Hosp Med.* 2009; 4:137-139.
163. Jardine M, Kokai G, Daizell AM. *Enterobius vermicularis* and colitis in children. *J Pediatr Gastroenterol Nutr.* 2006;43: 610-612.
164. Johnson EH, Windsor JJ, Clark GG. Emerging from obscurity: biological, clinical, and diagnostic aspects of *Dientamoeba fragilis. Clin Microbiol Rev.* 2004;17:553-570.
165. Samkari A, Kiska DL, Riddell SW, et al. *Dipylidium caninum* mimicking recurrent *Enterobius vermicularis* (pinworm) infection. *Clin Pediatr (Phila).* 2008;47:397-399.
166. Matsen JM, Turner JA. Reinfection in enterobiasis (pinworm infection): simultaneous treatment of family members. *Am J Dis Child.* 1969;118:576-581.

288

Tissue Nematodes, Including Trichinellosis, Dracunculiasis, and the Filariases

JAMES W. KAZURA

Tissue-dwelling nematode (roundworm) infections are widely distributed throughout the world. The health and socioeconomic impact of these infections is greatest in resource-poor settings in the tropics and subtropics, although populations in temperate and industrialized regions of the world continue to be at risk of infection and morbidity. Like all parasitic nematodes, the life cycle of these multicellular organisms includes five distinct stages: adult male or female worms and four larval stages distinguished from each other by a molting process that involves shedding of the parasite's surface cuticle and organ system differentiation dictated by developmentally regulated changes in gene expression. With the exception of *Trichinella* spp., which are transmitted directly to humans by ingestion of contaminated meat, infection involves obligatory development in and subsequent transmission by blood feeding invertebrate arthropods (the filariases) or swallowing of small freshwater crustaceans (copepods). Adult worms do not multiply in the human host and, therefore, the likelihood of developing a high enough worm burden to cause morbidity is directly related to the duration and intensity of exposure to vectors harboring infective larvae. Definitive diagnosis is made by microscopic visualization of parasites isolated from or present in host tissue, although this may be difficult or not indicated in all cases. Simple and inexpensive measures can be taken to avoid infection. Global efforts are under way to eliminate some tissue nematode infections as public health problems or even eradicate them by permanently stopping transmission. Effective anthelmintic drugs are available for the majority of these infections.

Infections acquired by eating contaminated meat and swallowing copepods harboring infective larvae are considered first. Filarial infections transmitted by blood feeding insects are described next.

Trichinellosis

Trichinellosis is acquired when undercooked meat of domestic pigs, horses, or game containing infective larvae of various *Trichinella* spp. is consumed. Symptomatic infections characterized by diarrhea, myositis, fever, and periorbital edema develop when large numbers of larvae are ingested.

THE PARASITE AND ITS LIFE CYCLE

Members of the *Trichinella* genus are zoonotic nematodes that infect carnivorous and omnivorous mammals in various ecologic and climatic settings.[1] Recent genomic and phylogenetic analyses indicate that of the 11 known species, there are 2 clades distinguished by the presence or absence of encapsulated third-stage larvae that have parasitized striated muscle cells[2,3] (Table 288-1). The 2 clades are estimated to have diverged from a common ancestor 15 to 20 million years ago. *Trichinella spiralis*, a species distributed throughout the world that infects pigs, rodents, and horses has historically been the most common cause of human infection. *Trichinella* spp. of wild game are of increasing importance in areas where food safety measures and livestock practices have led to a reduction in *T. spiralis*.[4]

The parasite life cycle commences with the enteral phase when meat containing infective third-stage larvae is eaten. Larvae of approximately 1 mm in length are liberated after digestion of the encapsulated cyst wall in the acid-pepsin environment of the stomach. These larvae pass rapidly to the lumen of the small intestine where they parasitize cells of the columnar epithelium. Four molts occur over 10 to 28 hours, culminating in the development of mature adult female and male worms in the epithelium of the small intestine. Fecund female worms produce and release first-stage (newborn) larvae that initiate the systemic phase of infection when they penetrate the gut wall, enter the lymphatics and eventually the blood circulation via the thoracic duct. Newborn larvae are dispersed in capillary beds throughout the body and ultimately parasitize striated muscle cells. After entering muscle, the larvae molt, encyst, and undergo development to become infective third-stage larvae within 15 days.[5] *T. spiralis* infective larvae encapsulated in collagenous cysts may remain viable for months to years. The cysts may calcify and be visible on radiographs.

EPIDEMIOLOGY

Trichinellosis historically has been associated with the consumption of undercooked pork products prepared from domestic swine. The epidemiologic significance of this source of infection has diminished over the latter part of the 20th century as the practice to feed pigs garbage containing *Trichinella*-infested meat scraps or rodents has been eliminated. Notably, outbreaks of *T. spiralis* infection associated with the consumption of pork from domestic swine has reemerged in several countries in Eastern Europe where veterinary public health and food production safety has been compromised coincidentally with economic hardship.[6] Consumption of meat from horses, wild game (boar, deer, bear, cougar, and walrus in areas where sylvatic trichinellosis is endemic) may also be the source of human infection. *T. spiralis* is the most common cause of human infection; *Trichinella brivoti*, *Trichinella pseudospiralis*, and *Trichinella murrelli* often underlie cases associated with consumption of wild game.

PATHOLOGIC CHARACTERISTICS

Pathologic manifestations of infection first appear in the gastrointestinal tract. Two to three weeks after ingestion of contaminated meat and establishment of adult worms in the upper small intestine, local villous atrophy, and mucosal and submucosal infiltration with neutrophils, eosinophils, and macrophages develop. However, the most characteristic pathologic change induced by the parasite is evident in skeletal muscle fibers. Histologically, edema and basophilic degeneration are present. Coiled worms, cyst walls resulting from parasitization of muscle cells, and infiltrates consisting of eosinophils and lymphocytes may be observed (Fig. 288-1). Although nonstriated muscle and other host tissues do not support the complete development of *Trichinella* to infective third-stage larvae, newborn larvae that disseminate to the myocardium, lung, and central nervous system in heavily infected individuals may cause local inflammation and tissue damage that have serious pathologic consequences (e.g., myocarditis, encephalitis, meningitis).

TABLE 288-1		Hosts and Geographic Distribution of Species of the Genus *Trichinella*		
Species	*Code*	*Common Hosts*	*Geographic Distribution*	*Encapsulated*
Trichinella spiralis	T1	Pigs, rodents, horses, bears, foxes	Worldwide	Yes
Trichinella nativa	T2	Bears, foxes, dogs	Arctic, sub-Arctic	Yes
Trichinella britova	T3	Dogs, cats, bears	Temperate areas, sub-Arctic	Yes
Trichinella pseudospiralis	T4	Birds, omnivorous mammals	Arctic, Tasmania	No
Trichinella murrelli	T5	Bears	North America	Yes
Not defined yet	T6	Bears	Sub-Arctic	Yes
Trichinella nelsoni	T7	Hyenas, cats	Tropical Africa	Yes
Not defined yet	T8	Lions, panthers	Southern Africa	Yes
Not defined yet	T9	Sylvatic carnivores	Japan	No

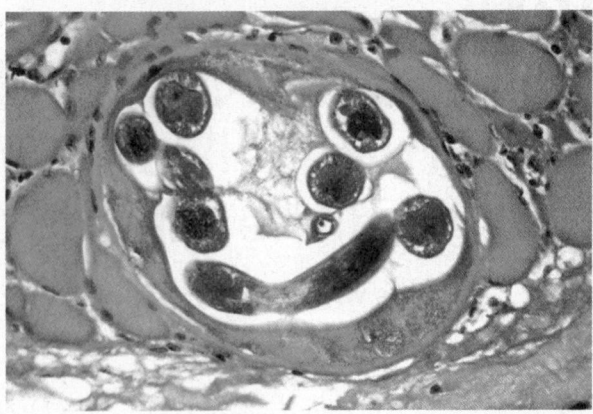

Figure 288-1 Coiled *Trichinella spiralis* larvae within a skeletal muscle cell. *(From McAdam AJ, Sharpe AH: Infectious diseases. In: Kumar V, ed. Robbins and Cotran Pathologic Basis of Disease, 8th ed. Philadelphia: Saunders; 2009.)*

CLINICAL FEATURES

Based on observations made under circumstances in which a common source of infested meat has been identified, the majority of infected individuals are asymptomatic. Morbidity is most likely to develop in persons who have ingested the highest parasite inocula. Watery diarrhea is the most common manifestation during the enteral phase of infection. Vomiting, abdominal discomfort, and nausea may also be observed. Prolonged diarrhea and other gastrointestinal symptoms in Native American adults who traditionally consume polar bear or walrus meat infested with *Trichinella nativa* have been suggested to reflect immunity acquired as a result of earlier infections. Facial and periorbital edema, fever, weakness, malaise, myalgia, urticarial rash, conjunctivitis, and conjunctival and subungual hemorrhages appear during the systemic phase when newborn larvae disseminate. These signs and symptoms are most severe and peak 2 to 4 weeks after ingestion of contaminated meat.[7-10] Weakness and myalgia appear first and are most severe in the extraocular, masseter, and neck muscles. Patients with high infection burdens may die of myocarditis, encephalitis, or pneumonia that becomes progressively severe after 4 to 8 weeks. It has been suggested that trichinellosis can lead to chronic muscle pain and weakness.

DIAGNOSIS

Trichinellosis should be considered in the differential diagnosis of patients presenting with myositis, eosinophilia, fever, elevated creatine phosphokinase and lactate dehydrogenase, and signs consistent with systemic dissemination of newborn larvae as described previously. Questioning regarding a history of consumption of undercooked meat from wild or farmed game, such as bear and boar or pigs raised in noncommercial and unregulated farms is informative. It is also helpful to determine whether a similar illness has developed in others who have consumed the same food. Antibodies to *Trichinella* spp. can be detected by a variety of techniques[11] (enzyme-linked immunosorbent assay is now used by the Centers for Disease Control and Prevention). Seroconversion usually occurs by approximately 3 weeks after ingestion of infective larvae. A biopsy specimen of painful muscle may reveal the presence of *Trichinella* spp., although this procedure is not recommended in most situations. It is useful to obtain a sample of the meat suspected to harbor the parasite because this can be used to confirm the origin of the infection. Various *Trichinella* spp. can be differentiated by DNA-based technologies such as polymerase chain reaction.[12]

The differential diagnosis of trichinellosis observed during the enteral phase of infection includes a wide variety of causes of gastro-

enteritis and diarrheal illnesses. During the systemic phase of infection, febrile illnesses including influenza and typhoid fever, connective tissue diseases such as dermatomyositis, and angioneurotic edema should be considered.

TREATMENT

There is currently no anthelmintic drug that has proved effective against newborn larvae or maturing first-stage larvae that cause myositis and other signs and symptoms that appear during the systemic phase of infection. Systemic corticosteroids in conjunction with mebendazole (see later) may be used in patients with severe illness, although proven benefit for this approach is lacking.

If the diagnosis is made during the enteral phase of infection (e.g., within 1 to 2 weeks of eating contaminated meat or when gastrointestinal signs and symptoms are present), mebendazole (200 to 400 mg PO three times daily for 3 days, then 400 to 500 mg PO three times daily for 10 days for all ages) may be used to eliminate adult worms from the small intestine.[13] Albendazole (400 mg PO twice daily for 8 to 14 days) may also be used.

PREVENTION

Awareness of and compliance with safety regulations prohibiting the use of garbage as a source of food for domestic animals, control of rodents, segregation of livestock from wild animals, and proper preparation of meat from wild animals will reduce the risk of infection with *Trichinella* spp. Inspection of meat for *Trichinella* is ideally done by direct digestion and visualization of encysted larvae.

Cooking meat to a temperature 55° C or higher (until pink fluid or flesh is not visible) kills *Trichinella* spp. Storage in a freezer (−15°C) for 3 or more weeks kills *T. spiralis* in pork, but this is not effective for *Trichinella* spp. larvae in horse and game meat. Drying, smoking as in the preparation of jerkies, and salting of meat should not be relied on to kill *Trichinella*.

Other Muscle Nematode Infections
HAYCOCKNEMA PERPLEXUM INFECTION

Haycocknema perplexum is a species of Muspiceoidia nematodes that has been observed in the tissues of Australian mammals and marsupials. Adult and larval stages of the nematode have been identified in muscle biopsy specimens of Australian patients from Tasmania and tropical northern Australia who present with chronic myositis, peripheral muscle weakness, and dysphagia accompanied by eosinophilia and elevated creatine phosphokinase.[14,15] Muscle weakness improved, and killing of parasites was observed after administration of multiple doses of albendazole. Corticosteroids are not indicated because this class of drugs may exacerbate muscle weakness and lead to a reduction of eosinophilia that misleads the clinician to conclude that a beneficial effect on a connective tissue disease such as polymyositis has occurred.

Dracunculiasis

Guinea worm disease or dracunculiasis is caused by the parasitic nematode *Dracunculus medinensis*. Once prevalent throughout southern Asia and parts of the Middle East, as of 2007 to 2008, indigenous infections were limited to focal areas of four countries in sub-Saharan Africa: Sudan, Ghana, Mali, and Niger.[16] The parasite causes debilitating skin lesions and secondary bacterial infections. Dracunculiasis has great socioeconomic impact in affected rural communities.

LIFE CYCLE

Humans are infected by swallowing fresh water from stagnant pools containing minute fresh water crustaceans (copepods) harboring infective larvae of *D. medinensis*. When the copepods are digested in the acid-pepsin environment of the stomach, larval forms are released from the body of the crustacean, after which they penetrate the wall of the small intestine and migrate through the thoracic musculature. Sexually mature male and female worms develop over 2 to 3 months. Gravid female worms mature over 10 to 14 months, migrate throughout the body, and ultimately reach the skin, particularly over the ankles, feet, and lower leg (Fig. 288-2). When skin comes into contact with water, the female worm (which may reach a length of 1 m) induces a local blister that eventually ruptures. Large numbers of larvae are released into the water when prolapsed loops of the uterine cavity

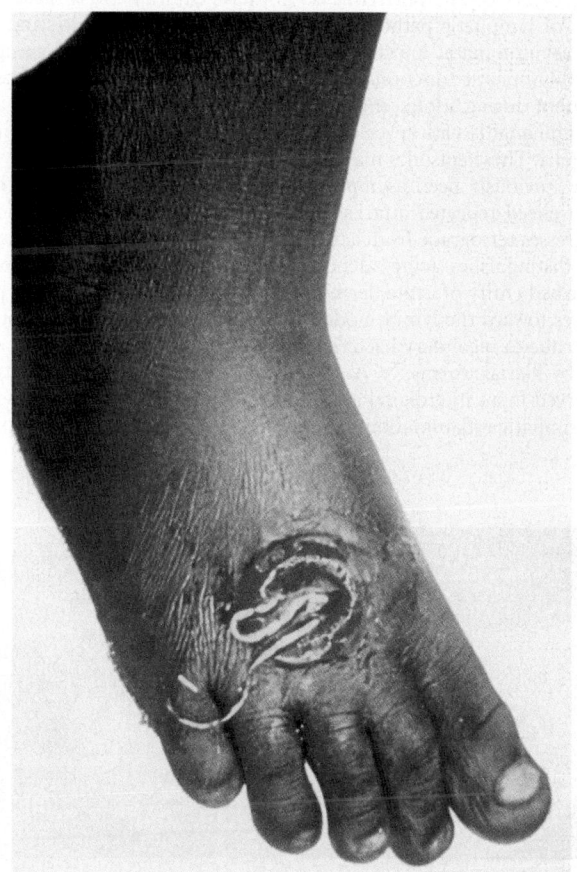

Figure 288-2 *Dracunculus medinensis* emerging from the skin over the foot.

contract. The motile free-swimming larvae infect copepods. *D. medinensis* larvae become infective for humans after further development in the intermediate copepod host over a 2-week period.[17]

EPIDEMIOLOGY

Clinical manifestations of *D. medinensis* infection appear approximately 1 year after ingestion of contaminated water and are highly seasonal as they coincide with the appearance of stagnant pools of surface water that vary according local climatic conditions. The prevalence of dracunculiasis is a strong indicator of socioeconomic development as communities are at highest risk where there is inadequate treatment of contaminated water, access to safe drinking water, and separation of bathing and drinking facilities.

CLINICAL FEATURES

Signs and symptoms of dracunculiasis appear approximately 1 year after infection when fecund adult female worms appear near the surface of the skin. The initial presentation is a painful papule that enlarges over hours to days to form a blister that allows a portion of the worm to emerge from the skin. The blister may be accompanied by local erythema, urticaria, fever, nausea, and pruritus. The entire worm may emerge over a period of several weeks. Complications include secondary bacterial infections that may lead to sepsis, local abscesses, and pyogenic arthritis. Affected individuals are incapacitated for approximately 8 weeks. The vast majority of worms emerge from the lower leg, ankle, and foot, although aberrant sites of emergence have been reported (e.g., head, neck, genitalia).

DIAGNOSIS AND TREATMENT

Dracunculiasis is diagnosed by the appearance of the skin blister and adult worm (see Fig. 288-2). There are no antihelmintic drugs known to be effective against *D. medinensis*. Application of wet compresses to the affected skin, administration of analgesics, and prevention of secondary bacterial infection by the use of topical antibiotics are recommended. Worms should be slowly and gently extracted over a period of several days using a small stick because breaking the worm can lead to allergic reactions and secondary bacterial infection.

CONTROL AND ERADICATION

The global effort to eradicate dracunculiasis commenced in 1986 when it was estimated that approximately 3.5 million cases occurred annually in 17 countries in Africa and in 3 countries in Asia. The program was closely linked with efforts to improve the safety of drinking water. Eradication is based on simple and cost-effective measures that include (1) filtration of drinking water through fine-meshed cloth to remove copepods, (2) killing copepods in sources of drinking water by application of Abate (temephos) larvicide, (3) provision of clean drinking water from boreholes or wells, and (4) educating residents of communities to avoid entering sources of drinking water if worms are emerging. The eradication effort has been remarkably successful. The total number of cases in the world was estimated to be 10,000 as of 2007.[18]

Filariases

Filarial parasites are threadlike nematodes transmitted to humans by obligatory bloodfeeding insect vectors. Pathology mainly involves the lymphatic system, skin, and eyes (Table 288-2). Repeated and long-duration exposure to insect vectors harboring infective larvae is generally necessary for humans to acquire these infections, although travelers to endemic areas occasionally become infected.[19,20] All filariae of medical significance except for *Loa loa* harbor rickettsia-like *Wolbachia* endosymbionts that are important in maintaining the reproductive capacity of adult female worms.

TABLE 288-2	Filarial Diseases and Infections of Humans			
Disease	**Genus Species of Filarial Pathogen**	**Major Clinicopathologic Manifestations**	**Areas of Endemicity**	**Insect Vectors**
Lymphatic filariasis	*Wuchereria bancrofti, Brugia malayi, Brugia timori*	Lymphedema of extremities and breasts, hydrocele, funiculitis, orchitis, tropical (pulmonary) eosinophilia	Sub-Saharan Africa, Southeast Asia, Oceania and western Pacific, Caribbean, limited areas of South America	*Anopheles, Culex, Aedes* spp. mosquitoes
Loiasis	*Loa loa*	Subcutaneous and conjunctival swelling	Western and central Africa	*Chrysops* spp. tabanid flies
Onchocerciasis	*Onchocerca volvulus*	Dermatitis, keratitis, chorioretinitis	Sub-Saharan Africa, Arabian peninsula, parts of Central and South America	*Simulium* spp. blackflies
Mansonellosis	*Mansonella ozzardi*	Rarely symptomatic	Caribbean, Central and South America	*Culicoides* spp. midges, *Simulium amazonicum* blackflies
	Mansonella perstans	Rarely symptomatic	Sub-Saharan Africa, northern coast of South America, Tunisia, Algeria	*Culicoides* spp.
	Mansonella streptocerca	Dermatitis, inguinal lymphadenopathy	Central and West Africa	*Culicoides grahamii*

LYMPHATIC FILARIASIS

Wuchereria bancrofti, Brugia malayi, and *Brugia timori* are the causative agents of bancroftian and brugian (sometimes referred to as Malayan) filariasis. Approximately 1 billion persons worldwide are at risk; 120 million residents of developing countries are currently estimated to be infected.[21,22] In contrast to many other mosquito-borne infections of medical significance, lymphatic filariae are transmitted by not just one but several genera of mosquitoes. These include *Anopheles, Culex,* and *Aedes* spp., which differ greatly in their efficiency of transmission (*Anopheles* and *Culex* spp. being the least and most efficient, respectively).[23,24] The major pathologic manifestations are acute transient episodes of fever accompanied by painful inflammation of the lymphatics of the extremities and male genitalia and chronic lymphatic dysfunction that leads to gross disfigurement of the male genitalia and progressive lymphedema and swelling of the legs, arms, or breasts.

Life Cycle

Infection is initiated when female mosquitoes release infective third-stage larvae into the puncture site of the skin created during bloodfeeding. These larvae pass rapidly through the dermis and enter local lymphatic vessels, where they molt to form fourth-stage larvae. Over 6 to 9 months, the parasites undergo another molt in afferent lymphatic vessels and eventually develop into sexually mature adult male and female worms. Adult worms largely reside in afferent lymphatic vessels of the upper and lower extremities and the lymphatics of the male genitalia, such as those draining the epididymis, testicles, and spermatic cord. Other areas of the body may also harbor adult worms, such as skin. Fecund female worms release as many as 10,000 first-stage larvae (commonly referred to as microfilariae) per day, which migrate from the lymphatics and enter the bloodstream. Microfilariae in peripheral blood are ingested by mosquitoes and undergo development to infective third-stage larvae after completing two molts in the mosquito over a period of 14 days. Adult worms are larger than microfilariae (100 × 0.25 mm and 150 × 7 μm, respectively; Fig. 288-3) and have a reproductive life span of 5 to 7 years. A characteristic feature of lymphatic filariasis in most endemic areas is the nocturnal periodicity of microfilaremia whereby peak levels of parasites appear in peripheral blood at night when the mosquito vectors are seeking a blood meal. During the day, microfilariae are sequestered in deep vascular beds and may not be detectable in peripheral blood.

Epidemiology

Lymphatic filariasis is endemic in South Asia, sub-Saharan Africa, and the Pacific. Countries with the highest prevalence include India, Indonesia, Papua New Guinea, Nigeria, Ghana, Kenya, and Tanzania. *Wuchereria bancrofti* is transmitted in nearly all endemic areas and constitutes 90% of cases worldwide. There is no animal reservoir for *W. bancrofti. B. malayi* is limited to southern and Southeast Asia and

parts of the Pacific and may infect cats and primates as well as humans. *B. timori* is found only in the islands of eastern Indonesia. The distribution of infection is heterogeneous within a given geographic region because the local spatial ecology is important in determining transmission and exposure to infective larvae (i.e., the proximity of mosquito breeding sites to human dwellings).[25] Because less than 1% of competent mosquito vectors contain infective larvae, intense exposure to mosquitoes is necessary to develop patent infection. Lymphatic filariasis has a profound detrimental effect on the economy and psychosexual health in societies where manual labor and subsistence agriculture are important in daily life.

Clinical Features

The vast majority of individuals with patent infections documented by the presence of microfilaremia do not have clinically overt manifestations of lymphatic pathology. Nevertheless, imaging studies indicate that asymptomatic infected adults and children may have compromised lymphatic function.[26-28] Overt pathologic sequelae first become apparent during adolescence and early adulthood, often as acute adenolymphangitis with fever and swelling of the leg, arm, or the male genitalia. These episodes may last for 4 to 7 days week in persons who have previously been asymptomatic or longer in persons who have experienced repeated attacks. The lymphatic inflammation typically progresses retrograde from axillary or inguinal lymph nodes, a feature that distinguishes acute adenolymphangitis from the more recently described entity of acute dermatolymphangioadenitis. The latter progresses toward the lymph node from a peripheral site and is thought to be due to secondary bacterial infection and not inflammation elicited by filarial worms.[29,30] A cut or entry wound of the skin may be observed in an interdigital area. So-called filarial fever in the absence of lymphatic inflammation may also be observed. In endemic popula-

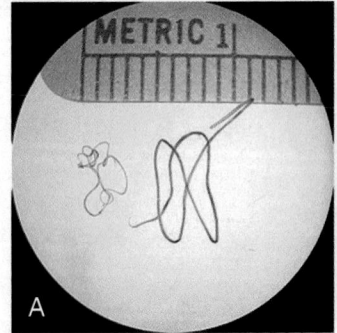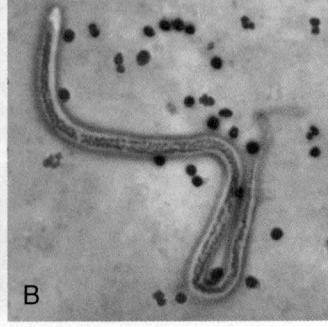

Figure 288-3 **Adult worms (A) and microfilariae (B) of** *Wuchereria bancrofti. (From DPDx Parasite Image Library collection, http://www. dpd.cdc.gov/dpdx/HTML/Image_Library.htm.)*

tions, filarial fevers may be difficult to distinguish from other common causes of acute febrile illness.

Repeated episodes of acute filarial disease often precede the development of chronic lymphatic pathology that includes lymphedema of the legs, arms, and breasts and chronic disfigurement of the male genitalia (Fig. 288-4). Male genital involvement is very common in *W. bancrofti* infection and uncommon in *Brugia* spp. infection. Chronic swelling of the legs and compromised lymphatic drainage may result in secondary bacterial infections and sclerosis and verrucous changes of the overlying skin. The most severe cases are sometimes referred to as elephantiasis. Male genital involvement includes hydrocele, funiculitis, epididymitis, and orchitis. There is a poor understanding of the pathogenesis of the various genital manifestations of lymphatic filariaisis.[31] Chyluria precipitated by the rupture of dilated lymphatic vessels into the genitourinary tract is an uncommon manifestation. Tropical pulmonary eosinophilia is described separately at the end of this section.

Pathogenesis

Adult worms residing in afferent lymphatic vessels and lymph nodes draining the legs, arms, male genitalia, and occasionally other anatomic sites presumably initiate the disease process when poorly characterized parasite mediators produce local lymphatic dilatation. Live motile worms exhibiting the "filarial dance" sign and nearby dilated lymphatic vessels can be detected by ultrasonography in the scrotum, inguinal lymph node, and breast[32,33] (videos can be viewed at http://www.filariajournal.com/content/2/1/3).

It is not clear why the majority of infected individuals remain asymptomatic while others develop acute or chronic manifestations of lymphatic filariasis. With respect to acute filarial pathology, the inten-sity of transmission and secondary bacterial infections may both be important in determining susceptibility.[34,35] The importance of worm burden as a determinant of chronic lymphatic pathology is controversial. Many persons with chronic lymphedema of the extremities have no evidence of active infection (particularly in India), whereas this is not the case in other *W. bancrofti* endemic areas such as Papua New Guinea. Adaptive T-cell responses, genetic susceptibility, worm burden, and innate immunity to the rickettsia-like *Wolbachia* endosymbiont of filarial parasites have been suggested to contribute to the complex clinical phenotypes of lymphedema and hydrocele, but a single unifying mechanism has not been defined.[36,37]

Diagnosis

Lymphatic filariasis is diagnosed by obtaining an appropriate history of exposure to mosquitoes in areas where the infection is endemic, observing clinical signs of pathology, and performing a variety of laboratory tests. As described previously, chronic lymphatic pathology such as lymphedema of an extremity or hydrocele primarily affects adults who are residents of endemic areas. A definitive diagnosis is made by microscopic detection of microfilaria in the blood or occasionally from other sites such as fluid aspirated from hydroceles. Blood to detect microfilaremia should generally be obtained at night when the peak density of parasitemia occurs. This is the case for most endemic areas except for *W. bancrofti* in some areas of Oceania. The sensitivity of detecting microfilaremia is enhanced by concentrating parasites by filtration of blood through polycarbonate (Nuclepore) filters that retain microfilariae. Polymerase chain reaction–based assays that detect as little as one microfilaria per milliliter of blood have been described.[38] An enzyme-linked immunosorbent assay–format antigen capture assay that detects antigen secreted by *W. bancrofti* adult worms has been an important diagnostic advance because this test allows documentation of active infection in the absence of microfilaremia.[39] An analogous test for *Brugia* spp. is not yet available. Biopsy of lymphatic tissues to identify adult worms is not justified. As described earlier, adult worms can be imaged in vivo by the use of Doppler ultrasonography.

Treatment

Persons with asymptomatic parasitemia should be treated with diethylcarbamazine at a dose of 6 mg/kg body weight/day divided into two or three doses over 14 days to a total of 72 mg/kg. The drug is highly effective at eliminating microfilariae but has only modest activity against adult worms. The filaricidal activity of diethylcarbamazine is greater against *W. bancrofti* than *B. malayi*. Side effects include fever and occasionally asthma-like symptoms in persons with high-level microfilaremia, and painful nodules that appear in the lymphatics, lymph nodes, skin, and male genitalia. The development of these nodules, usually less than 1 cm in diameter, is an inflammatory reaction to the death of adult worms or migrating larvae. They may appear days to weeks after taking antifilarial drugs, particularly diethylcarbamazine because it has greater macrofilaricidal activity than albendazole or ivermectin. Systemic posttreatment reactions are likely related to innate immune reactions to *Wolbachia* endosymbionts released by dying microfilariae. The severity of acute side effects may be reduced by initiating treatment with a lower dose of diethylcarbamazine (50 mg on day 1 followed by 50 mg three times on day 2 and 100 mg three times on day 3). Hydroceles may be repaired surgically, but prevention of recurrence is contingent on drug treatment.

It is not known whether diethylcarbamazine or other antifilarial drugs such as ivermectin and albendazole ameliorate preexisting lymphatic pathology because randomized clinical trials have not been performed. Some studies of mass drug treatment to control filariasis in endemic populations suggest that reducing transmission may decrease the incidence of chronic lymphatic pathology.[40]

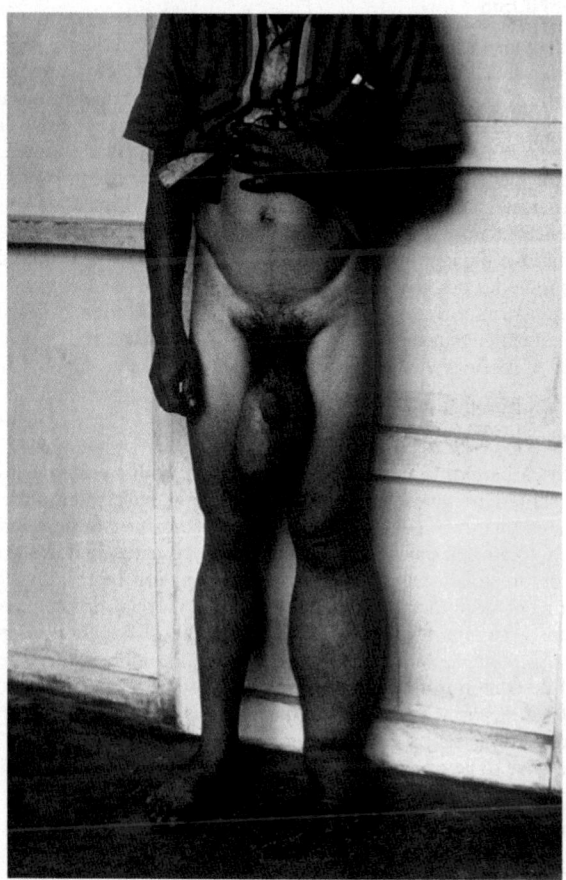

Figure 288-4 Man with inguinal lymphadenopathy, large bilateral hydroceles, marked edema of the lower left limb (particularly the leg and foot), and early signs of elephantiasis in the foot.

Prevention, Control, and Eradication

Lymphatic filariasis due to *W. bancrofti* has been targeted for elimination as a public health problem and for worldwide eradication by annual mass treatment with single-dose diethylcarbamazine combined with albendazole (in areas of the world where onchocerciasis and loiasis is not endemic) or ivermectin combined with albendazole (in areas where onchocerciasis and loiasis are endemic). *Brugia* spp. are less amenable to eradication because the parasite has an animal reservoir. It is currently believed that at least 5 years of annual mass treatment is necessary to stop transmission because this is the estimated reproductive life span of adult worms. Results of studies in Egypt indicate that this strategy will likely be successful in endemic areas where a good public health infrastructure exists.[41] It is not yet known whether similar success will be achieved in rural areas where population coverage with antifilarial drugs is suboptimal or vectors with greater transmission efficiency exist. The use of drugs that target the *Wolbachia* endosymbiont of filarial parasites (e.g., doxycycline) may provide added benefit as killing of these rickettsia-like bacteria reduces the fecundity and shortens the reproductive life span of adult worms.[42,43]

TROPICAL PULMONARY EOSINOPHILIA

This syndrome is associated with *W. bancrofti* and *B. malayi* infection. It is most commonly observed in south and southeast Asia and endemic areas of Brazil and Guyana. Patients are typically middle age males (male-to-female ratio, 4:1) who present with nocturnal asthma, cough, fever, weight loss, and fever. Microfilariae are not detectable in peripheral blood. High-level eosinophilia (>3000/μL blood) with elevated antifilarial antibodies and polyclonal immunoglobulin E are present. Chest x-rays typically show increased bronchovascular markings with a mottled appearance in the mid and lower lungs. Treatment with diethylcarbamazine leads to symptomatic improvement and reduces eosinophilia and immunoglobulin E levels. Retreatment may be necessary in some cases. If untreated, progressive interstitial fibrosis and restrictive lung disease may develop.[44]

▣ Loiasis

Adult worms of these nematodes migrate in subcutaneous tissue and occasionally the conjunctiva where they elicit transient painful swelling. The infection is endemic in central and West Africa.

LIFE CYCLE

Loa loa infective larvae are transmitted by female tabanid (red) flies (*Chrysops* spp.) that seek blood meals during the day. Adult worms measuring 30 to 70 × 0.3 mm develop over 6 to 12 months and migrate in subcutaneous tissues. Microfilariae released from fecund female worms migrate to the blood and have a diurnal periodicity. In contrast to other filarial pathogens of medical significance, *L. loa* do not harbor *Wolbachia* endosymbionts.

EPIDEMIOLOGY

Loiasis is endemic in coastal and rain forest regions of central and West Africa. The infection has been observed as far east as Uganda and Ethiopia. Infected individuals usually have a long history of residence in endemic areas with prolonged exposure to infected vectors; however, repeated short durations of intense exposure can also result in infection and morbidity, including expatriate nonresidents who travel to endemic areas.[45]

CLINICAL FEATURES

Most infected individuals are asymptomatic. The main clinical presentation is a Calabar swelling, which represents an angioedematous response to adult worms migrating through subcutaneous tissue. The 10- to 20-cm swelling lesions most commonly appear on the face and extremities and are preceded by itching and pain. Calabar swellings are transient and persist from several days to weeks. Adult worms may also

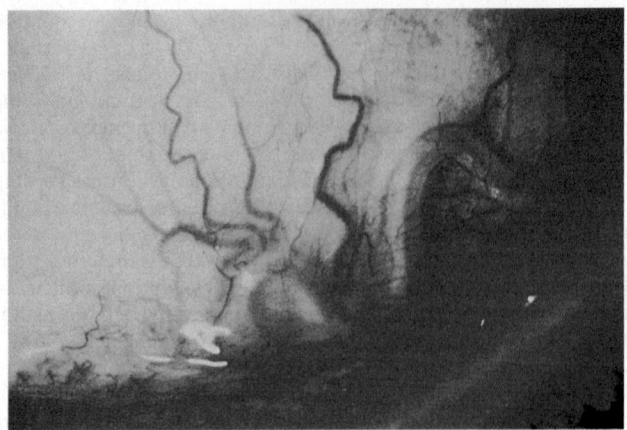

Figure 288-5 Serpentine adult *Loa loa* passing through the subconjunctiva.

migrate to the conjunctiva and produce an "eye worm" (Fig. 288-5). Other manifestations include renal complications (hematuria and proteinuria) and encephalitis, which are usually precipitated by treatment with the antifilarial drug diethylcarbamazine. In the case of encephalitis, persons with high-level microfilaremia (>2500 microfilariae/mL) are at high risk.[46] Precautions for treating such individuals are described later.

DIAGNOSIS

The diagnosis should be considered in persons who have resided in an endemic area and present with urticaria, an eye worm, or eosinophilia. Identification of microfilariae in the blood (which should be obtained during the day) or visualization of an adult worm in the conjunctiva confirms loiasis. Standardized and specific serologic tests for *L. loa* are not widely available outside the research laboratory setting. Polymerase chain reaction that detects multiple-copy *L. loa*–specific sequences is more sensitive than traditional filtration methods that rely on microscopic identification of microfilariae.[47] The differential diagnosis includes other causes of angioedema such as C1 inhibitor deficiency, worm infections such as onchocerciasis and mansonellosis (both of which may overlap in endemicity with loiasis), and the various causes of high-level eosinophilia.

TREATMENT

Diethylcarbamazine at a dose of 8 to 10 mg/kg body weight/day for 21 days should be given to persons who do not have microfilaremia. Repeated treatment courses with diethylcarbamazine may be necessary in 40% to 50% of patients. Calabar swelling, pruritus, and eye worms may be precipitated by treatment. Side effects can be minimized by concurrent administration of antihistamines or corticosteroids. In persons with high-level microfilaremia (>2500/mL), there is a significant risk of renal and central nervous system complications due the rapid destruction of large numbers of microfilariae. Options include withholding antihelmintic drugs, cytapheresis to remove microfilariae before administration of diethylcarbamazine, and administration of a single dose of ivermectin.[48]

PREVENTION AND CONTROL

Travelers who plan prolonged residence in endemic areas should take 300 mg diethylcarbamazine weekly as chemoprophylaxis.[49] There are currently no effective means to control the tabanid flies that transmit *L. loa*.

Onchocerciasis

Onchocerca volvulus is transmitted by blood feeding *Simulium* spp. black flies. Infection can cause dermatitis, subcutaneous nodules, keratitis, and chorioretinitis. The disease has a great socioeconomic impact because it causes reduced vision ("river blindness") and chronic skin disease in adults.

LIFE CYCLE

Infection is acquired when female *Simulium damnosum* sibling species (in Africa) and several other *Simulium* spp. (in the Americas and Arabian peninsula) take blood meals. Infective third-stage larvae migrate to subcutaneous tissue, undergo two molts, and eventually develop into threadlike sexually mature adult male (300 × 0.3 mm) or female worms (400 × 0.3 mm) over 6 to 12 months. Adult worms aggregate in nodules in subcutaneous tissue and muscle. Fecund female worms release unsheathed microfilariae (200 × 8 μm) that migrate to the dermis and eye.

EPIDEMIOLOGY

Onchocerciasis is endemic in West Africa, limited areas of central and northern South America, and the Arabian peninsula. An estimated 18 million persons are infected worldwide. The greatest number of infected individuals live in West Africa, particularly Nigeria and Congo.[50,51] Although there is great variability in the frequency of disease manifestations in various endemic areas, the majority of infected individuals are asymptomatic. Onchocerciasis in the Americas is characterized by low worm burden with little eye disease, whereas in savanna regions of West Africa, there is a much greater likelihood of reduced vision and blindness even though worm loads are only modestly greater. Onchocerciasis in rain forest regions of West Africa is also unlikely to cause blindness. Dermatologic manifestations of infection are common in areas of Africa outside either the rain forest or savanna.

PATHOLOGY AND CLINICAL FEATURES

Adult worms of both sexes reside in nonpainful vascularized fibrous nodules (0.5 × 3.0 cm) in a subcutaneous or intramuscular site. The lesions may be palpable. The major pathologic sequelae of clinical significance are due to inflammatory responses to microfilariae. In the skin, these include acute and chronic papular dermatitis, lichenified dermatitis, atrophy, and depigmentation.[52,53] Pruritus is usually the presenting symptom. In the eye, microfilariae that have migrated to the cornea initially elicit punctate keratitis. This can progress to a sclerosing keratitis that causes blindness. As described earlier, this outcome is most common in savanna forms of onchocerciasis in West Africa. Iridocyclitis and chorioretinitis are less common. *O. volvulus* infection may also cause inguinal lymph node fibrosis and atrophy of the overlying skin that leads to the appearance of hanging groin.

DIAGNOSIS

The diagnosis should be considered when the signs described above are present in an individual who has resided in an endemic area. Because transmission is inefficient, residence of months to years is usually (but not always) required to acquire *O. volvulus* infection. Identification of microfilariae in the skin or eye or adult worms in nodules is required for definitive diagnosis. Microfilariae in the skin are accessed by using a corneoscleral instrument to obtain a 1- to 2-mg biopsy specimen of the dermis overlying both scapulae, iliac crests, and calves. The skin snips are placed in microtiter plates containing saline held at 37°C for 60 minutes to 24 hours (depending on the microfilarial burden) to allow the parasites to emerge. The parasites are identified under low-power microscopy. Microfilariae in the eye can be identified by slit-lamp examination. In the research setting, polymerase chain reaction that detects a repetitive sequence in the *O. volvulus* genome can be used to identify persons with light infections that are not detectable by microscopy.[54] The differential diagnosis of onchocercal dermatitis includes scabies and the many other infectious and noninfectious causes of dermatitis. Eye disease may be mimicked by other infectious and noninfectious etiologies of chorioretinitis. Eye worms similar to those observed for loiasis do not occur because adult *O. volvulus* parasites do not migrate to the conjunctiva.

TREATMENT

Ivermectin, which is effective in killing microfilariae but not adult *O. volvulus* worms, is the drug of choice. The dose is 150 μg/kg body weight given as a single dose. A reduction in skin microfilariae is detectable within 2 weeks but may be incomplete. For expatriates who are more prone than lifelong residents of endemic areas to develop severe pruritus, more frequent treatment with ivermectin (e.g., every 3 months) may be necessary to control symptoms. Doxycycline, which kills the obligatory *Wolbachia* endosymbiont of *O. volvulus*, is highly effective in reducing microfilarial production by adult worms and may represent a novel strategy for reducing transmission in endemic areas.[55] However, there is no indication that this approach offers benefit for the treatment of the individual patient. In cases in which loiasis coexists with onchocerciasis (both infections are endemic in some areas of West Africa), the use of ivermectin carries a risk of precipitating encephalopathy in persons with high levels of *L. loa* microfilaremia. Cytapheresis may be used to reduce the level of *L. loa* microfilariae before treatment, but this is usually not an option in resource-poor settings.

PREVENTION AND CONTROL

Control of the *Simulium* vector by aerial dispersion of larvicides from 1974 to 2002 was highly successful in reducing blindness in 11 countries in west Africa where the savanna form of onchocerciasis was common. The African Program for Onchocerciasis Control, running since 1995 and scheduled to continue until 2009, is based on mass distribution of ivermectin in order to reduce and possibly stop transmission. A program to eliminate onchocerciasis from the Americas (Onchocerciasis Elimination Programme in the Americas) uses twice-yearly mass administration of ivermectin with the goal of eliminating onchocerciasis morbidity as a public health problem and interrupting transmission.[56-58]

Mansonellosis

These are poorly understood infections of humans that are asymptomatic in most individuals. Transmission is by bloodfeeding midges (*Culicoides* spp. for *Mansonella ozzardi*, *Mansonella perstans*, and *Mansonella streptocerca*) or black fly (*Simulium amazonicum* for *M. ozzardi*).

M. OZZARDI

The infection is endemic in northern South America, Central America, and some Caribbean islands. Unsheathed microfilariae circulate in the blood. Most infections are asymptomatic. Lymphadenopathy, urticaria, pruritus, pulmonary symptoms, and keratitis have been described. Ivermectin reduces microfilariae, but optimal treatment has not been defined.[59,60]

M. PERSTANS

The infection is endemic in parts of central and northern Africa, South America, and the Caribbean. Adult worms reside in serous cavities of the body and sheathed microfilariae circulate in the blood. Angioedema, urticaria, and pruritus have been attributed to the infection. Diethylcarbamazine lowers the level of microfilaremia. One report suggests that an intense course of oral albendazole may be more effective for lowering the microfilarial load and reducing symptoms.[60-62]

M. STREPTOCERCA

M. streptocerca is endemic in rain forest regions of central Africa and parts of Uganda.[63,64] Many infected individuals are asymptomatic, although some people develop inguinal lymphadenopathy and a chronic dermatitis with pruritus. The latter may be similar to that seen in persons with onchocerciasis. Microfilariae reside in the dermis and can be identified by obtaining a skin snip and identifying the parasite microscopically as described for onchocerciasis. *M. perstans* microfilariae are distinguished from those of *O. volvulus* by the hook-shaped tail of the former.[65] Treatment is with diethylcarbamazine at a dose similar to that described for lymphatic filariasis.

Zoonotic Filariae Reported to Cause Human Disease

Dirofilaria repens is a parasite of felids and canids transmitted by mosquitoes. Humans are nonpermissive hosts, but the parasite may undergo incomplete development in the eye. Subconjunctival, intraocular, and orbit lesions have been described. Treatment is by excision.[66] Subconjunctival infections with the canine parasite *Onchocerca lupi* in Europe[67] and *Setaria labiatopillosa* in Romania[68] have been reported.

REFERENCES

1. Pozio E. World distribution of *Trichinella* spp. Infections in animals and humans. *Vet Parasitol.* 2007;149:3-21.
2. Mitreva M, Jasmer DJ. Biology and genome of *Trichinella spiralis* (November 23, 2006), Wormbook, ed. The *C. elegans* Research Community, WormBook, doi/10.1895/wormbook.1.123.2, <http://www.wormbook.org>.
3. Zarlenga DS, Rosenthal BM, La Rosa G, et al. Post-Miocene expansion, colonization, and host switching drove speciation among extant nematodes of the archaic genus *Trichinella*. *Proc Nat Acad Sci U S A.* 2006;103:7345-7359.
4. McIntyre L, Pollock SL, Fyfe M, et al. Trichinellosis from consumption of wild game meat. *CMAJ.* 2007;176:449-451.
5. Bruschi F, Murrell KD. Trichinellosis. In: Guerrant RM, Walker DH, Weller PM, eds. *Tropical Infectious Diseases, Principles, Pathogens, and Practice.* 2nd ed. Philadelphia: Churchill Livingstone; 2006:1217-1224.
6. Pozio E. New patterns of *Trichinella* infection. *Vet Parasitol.* 2001:98:133-148.
7. Kocieka W. Trichinellosis: human disease, diagnosis and treatment. *Vet Parasitol.* 2000;93:365-383.
8. Ancelle T, Dupouy-Camet J, Desenclos JC, et al. A multifocal outbreak of trichinellosis linked to horse meat imported from North American to France in 1993. *Am J Trop Med Hyg.* 1998;59:615-619.
9. Barennes H, Sayasone S, Odermatt P, et al. A major trichinellosis outbreak suggesting a high endemicity of *Trichinella* infection in northern Laos. *Am J Trop Med Hyg.* 2008;78:40-44.
10. Schellenberg RS, Tan BJ, Irvine DJ, et al. An outbreak of trichinellosis in French hunters due to consumption of bear meat infected with *Trichinella nativa*, in 2 northern Saskatchewan communities. *J Infect Dis.* 2003;188:835-843.
11. Dupouy-Camet J, Kociecka W, Bruschi F, et al. Opinion on the diagnosis and treatment of human trichinellosis. *Expert Opin Pharmacother* 2002;3:1117-1130.
12. Zarlenga DS, Chute MB, Martin A, et al. A multiplex PCR for unequivocal differentiation of all encapsulated and non-encapsulated *Trichinella*. *Int J Parasitol* 1999;29:1859-1867.
13. Watt G, Saison D, Sacchi L, et al. Blinded, placebo-controlled trial of antiparasitic drugs for trichinosis myositis. *J Infect Dis.* 2000;182:371-374.
14. Dennet X, Siejka SJ, Andrews JR, et al. Polymyositis caused by a new genus of nematode. *Med J Aust.* 1998;226-227.
15. Bausroy R, Pennisi R, Robertson T, et al. Parasitic myositis in tropical Australia. *Med J Aust.* 2008;188:254-256.
16. Update: Progress toward global eradication of Dracunculiasis, January 2007-June 2008. *MMWR Morb Mortal Wkly Rep.* 2008;57:1173-1176.
17. Ruiz-Tiben E, Hopkins DR. Dracunculiasis. In: Guerrant RM, Walker DH, Weller PM, eds. *Tropical Infectious Diseases, Principles, Pathogens, and Practice.* 2nd ed. Philadelphia: Churchill Livingstone; 2006:1204-1208.
18. Voelker R. Persistence pays off in Guinea Worm fight. *JAMA.* 2007;298:1856-1857.
19. Klion AD. Filarial infections in travelers and immigrants. *Curr Infect Dis Rep.* 2008;10:50-57.
20. Lipner E, Law MA, Barnett E, et al. Filariasis in travelers presenting to the GeoSentinel Surveillance Network. *PLoS NTD.* 2008;1:e88.
21. Michael E, Bundy DA. Global mapping of lymphatic filariasis. *Parasitol Today.* 1997;13:472-476.
22. Michael E, Bundy DA, Grenfell BT. Re-assessing the global prevalence and distribution of lymphatic filariasis. *Parasitology.* 1996;112:409-428.
23. Gambhir M, Michael E. Complex ecological dynamics and eradicability of the vector borne macroparasitic disease, lymphatic filariasis. *PLoS ONE.* 2008;3:e2874.
24. Snow LC, Bockarie MJ, Michael E. Transmission dynamics of lymphatic filariasis: vector-specific density dependence in the development of *Wuchereria bancrofti* infective larvae in mosquitoes. *Med Vet Entomol.* 2006;20:261-272.
25. Rwegoshora RT, Simonsen PE, Meyrowitsch DW, et al. Bancroftian filariasis: house-to-house variation in the vectors and transmission—and the relationship to human infection—in an endemic community of coastal Tanzania. *Ann Trop Med Parasitol.* 2007;101:51-60.
26. Shenoy RK, Suma TK, Kumaraswami V, et al. Doppler ultrasonography reveals adult-worm nests in the lymph vessels of children with brugian filariasis. *Ann Trop Med Parasitol.* 2007;101:173-180.
27. Figueredo-Silva J, Dreyer G. Bancroftian filariasis in children and adolescents: clinical-pathological observations in 22 cases from an endemic area. *Ann Trop Med Parasitol.* 2005;99:759-769.
28. Fox LM, Furness BW, Haser JK, et al. Ultrasonographic examination of Haitian children with lymphatic filariasis: a longitudinal assessment in the context of antifilarial drug treatment. *Am J Trop Med Hyg.* 2005;72:642-648.
29. Dreyer G, Norões J, Figueredo-Silva J, et al. Pathogenesis of lymphatic disease in bancroftian filariasis: a clinical perspective. *Parasitol Today.* 2000;16:544-548.
30. Dreyer G, Medeiros Z, Netto MJ, et al. Acute attacks in the extremities of persons living in an area endemic for bancroftian filariasis: differentiation of two syndromes. *Trans R Soc Trop Med Hyg.* 1999;93:413-417.
31. Noroes J, Addiss D, Cedenho A, et al. Pathogenesis of filarial hydrocele: risk associated with intrascrotal nodules caused by death of adult *Wuchereria bancrofti*. *Trans R Soc Trop Med Hyg.* 2003;97:561-566.
32. Mand S, Debrah A, Batsa L, et al. Reliable and frequent detection of adult *Wuchereria bancrofti* in Ghanaian women by ultrasonography. *Trop Med Int Health.* 2004;9:1111-1114.
33. Mand S, Marfo-Debrekyei Y, Dittrich M, et al. Animated documentation of the filaria dance sign (FDS) in bancroftian filariasis. *Filaria J.* 2003;2:3.
34. Alexander ND, Perry RT, Dimber ZB, et al. Acute disease episodes in a *Wuchereria bancrofti*-endemic area of Papua New Guinea. *Am J Trop Med Hyg.* 1999;61:319-324.
35. Esterre P, Plichart C, Huin-Blondey MO, et al. Role of streptococcal infection in the acute pathology of lymphatic filariasis. *Parasite.* 2000;7:91-94.
36. Ottesen EA. Lymphatic filariasis: treatment, control and elimination. *Adv Parasitol.* 2006;61:395-441.
37. Rajan TV. Natural course of lymphatic filariasis: insights from epidemiology, experimental human infections, and clinical observations. *Am J Trop Med Hyg.* 2005;73:995-998.
38. Rao RU, Atkinson LJ, Ramzy RM, et al. A real-time PCR-based assay for detection of *Wuchereria bancrofti* DNA in blood and mosquitoes. *Am J Trop Med Hyg.* 2006;74:826-832.
39. Tisch DJ, Hazlett FE, Kastens W, et al. Ecologic and biologic determinants of filarial antigenemia in bancroftian filariasis in Papua New Guinea. *J Infect Dis.* 2001;184:898-904.
40. Bockarie MJ, Tisch DJ, Kastens W, et al. Mass treatment to eliminate filariasis in Papua New Guinea. *N Engl J Med.* 2002;347:1841-1848.
41. Ramzy RM, El Setouhy M, Helmy H, et al. Effect of yearly mass drug administration with diethylcarbamazine and albendazole on bancroftian filariasis in Egypt: a comprehensive assessment. *Lancet.* 2006;367:992-999.
42. Hoerauf A. Filariasis: new drugs and new opportunities for lymphatic filariasis and onchocerciasis. *Curr Opin Infect Dis.* 2008;21:673-681.
43. Mand S, Büttner DW, Hoerauf A. Bancroftian filariasis—absence of *Wolbachia* after doxycycline treatment. *Am J Trop Med Hyg.* 2008;78:854-855.
44. Vijayan VK. Tropical pulmonary eosinophilia: pathogenesis, diagnosis and management. *Curr Opin Pulm Med.* 2007;13:428-433.
45. Klion AD, Massougbodji A, Sadeler BC, et al. Loiasis in endemic and nonendemic populations: immunologically mediated differences in clinical presentation. *J Infect Dis.* 1991;163:1318-1325.
46. Carme B, Boulesteix J, Boutes H, et al. Five cases of encephalitis during treatment of loiasis with diethylcarbamazine. *Am J Trop Med Hyg.* 1991;44:684-690.
47. Touré FS, Kassambara L, Williams T et al. Human occult loiasis: improvement in diagnostic sensitivity by the use of a nested polymerase chain reaction. *Am J Trop Med Hyg.* 1998;59:144-149.
48. Boussinesq M. Loiasis. *Ann Trop Med Parasitol.* 2006;100:715-731.
49. Nutman TB, Miller KD, Mulligan M, et al. Diethylcarbamazine prophylaxis for human loiasis: results of a double-blind study. *N Engl J Med.* 1988;319:752-756.
50. Mathers CD, Ezzati M, Lopez AD. Measuring the burden of neglected tropical diseases: the global burden of disease framework. *PLoS Negl Trop Dis.* 2007;1:e114.
51. Hopkins DR, Richards Jr FO, Ruiz-Tiben E, et al. Dracunculiasis, onchocerciasis, schistosomiasis, and trachoma. *Ann N Y Acad Sci.* 2008;1136:45-52.
52. Freedman DO. Onchocerciasis. In: Guerrant RM, Walker DH, Weller PM, eds. *Tropical Infectious Diseases, Principles, Pathogens, and Practice.* 2nd ed. Philadelphia: Churchill Livingstone; 2006: 1176-1188.
53. Timmann C, Abraha RS, Hamelmann C, et al. Cutaneous pathology in onchocerciasis associated with pronounced systemic T-helper 2-type responses to *Onchocerca volvulus*. *Br J Dermatol.* 2003;149:782-787.
54. Zimmerman PA, Guderian RH, Aruajo E, et al. Polymerase chain reaction-based diagnosis of *Onchocerca volvulus* infection: improved detection of patients with onchocerciasis. *J Infect Dis.* 1994;169:686-689.
55. Hoerauf A, Specht S, Büttner M, et al. *Wolbachia endobacteria* depletion by doxycycline as antifilarial therapy has macrofilaricidal activity in onchocerciasis: a randomized placebo-controlled study. *Med Microbiol Immunol.* 2008;197:295-311.
56. Sauerbrey M. The Onchocerciasis Elimination Program for the Americas (OEPA). *Ann Trop Med Parasitol.* 2008;102(Suppl 1):25-29.
57. Thylefors B, Alleman M. Towards the elimination of onchocerciasis. *Ann Trop Med Parasitol.* 2006;100:733-746.
58. Brady MA, Hooper PJ, Ottesen EA. Projected benefits from integrating NTD programs in sub-Saharan Africa. *Trends Parasitol.* 2006;22:285-291.
59. Medeiros JF, Py-Daniel V, Barbosa UC, et al. Current profile of *Mansonella ozzardi* (Nematoda: Onchocercidae) in communities along the Ituxi river, Lábrea municipality, Amazonas, Brazil. *Mem Inst Oswaldo Cruz.* 2008;103:409-411.
60. Walther M, Muller R. Diagnosis of human filariases (except onchocerciasis). *Adv Parasitol.* 2003;53:149-193.
61. Asio SM, Simonsen PE, Onapa AW. A randomised, double-blind field trial of ivermectin alone and in combination with albendazole for the treatment of *Mansonella perstans* infections in Uganda. *Trans R Soc Trop Med Hyg.* 2009;103:274-279.
62. Asio SM, Simonsen PE, Onapa AW. *Mansonella perstans* filariasis in Uganda: patterns of microfilaraemia and clinical manifestations in two endemic communities. *Trans R Soc Trop Med Hyg.* 2009;10366-10373.
63. Fischer P, Tukesiga E, Büttner DW. Long-term suppression of *Mansonella streptocerca* microfilariae after treatment with ivermectin. *J Infect Dis.* 1999;180:1403-1405.
64. Bamuhiiga JT. *Mansonella streptocerca*: another filarial worm in the skin in Western Uganda. *Community Eye Health.* 1998;11:28.
65. Orihel TC. The tail of the *Mansonella streptocerca* microfilaria. *Am J Trop Med Hyg.* 1984;33:1278.
66. Gautam V, Rustagi IM, Singh S, et al. Subconjunctival infection with *Dirofilaria repens*. *Jpn J Infect Dis.* 2002;55:47-48.
67. Steter T, Szell Z, Egyed Z, et al. Subconjunctival zoonotic onchocerciasis in man: aberrant infection with *Onchocerca lupi*? *Ann Trop Med Parasitol.* 2002;96:497-502.
68. Panaitescu D, Freda A, Bain O, et al. Four cases of human filariosis due to *Setaria labiatopapillosa* found in Bucharest, Romania. *Roum Arch Microbiol Immunol.* 1999;58:203-207.

289

Trematodes (Schistosomes and Other Flukes)

JAMES H. MAGUIRE*

The trematode flatworms that infect humans include the schistosomes, which live in venules of the gastrointestinal or genitourinary tract, and other flukes, which inhabit the bile ducts, intestines, or lungs.[1] The geographic distribution of each species of trematode parallels the distribution of the specific freshwater snail that serves as its intermediate host (Table 289-1). Five species of schistosomes infect more than 200 million persons, and more than 65 species of other trematodes infect at least 40 million persons.[2-4]

Trematodes vary in length from 1 mm to more than 10 cm, are flattened dorsoventrally, and have an anterior and ventral sucker and a blind bifurcate intestinal tract. Schistosomes differ from other trematodes in several ways: the sexes of adult worms are separate, transmission is through penetration of skin by larvae, and there is only a single intermediate host, whereas other trematodes are hermaphroditic and are transmitted through ingestion of infected fish, crustaceans, or aquatic plants that serve as second intermediate hosts. Only a small proportion of persons with trematode infections harbor large numbers of worms and are at risk for severe disease; most are asymptomatic or experience subtle morbidity such as fatigue and cognitive or physical impairment.[3,5,6]

Schistosomes

Of an estimated 200 million persons infected with schistosomes in 74 countries and territories, about 120 million have symptoms, 20 million have severe disease, and 100,000 die each year.[1,2,4-6] Although control programs and socioeconomic development have nearly eliminated schistosomiasis in some parts of the world, progress has been slow elsewhere, especially in sub-Saharan Africa, where more than 80% of cases occur. Moreover, water resource development projects and population movements have spread the disease into regions where it was not previously endemic. Three main species, namely *Schistosoma mansoni, Schistosoma japonicum,* and *Schistosoma haematobium,* and two species with narrow geographic distribution, *Schistosoma mekongi* and *Schistosoma intercalatum,* cause human schistosomiasis or bilharziasis. A dozen or more other species of animal schistosomes can cause human infection, including schistosomes of birds and small mammals that cannot mature in the human host but die in the skin, where they cause a dermatitis.[5,7,8]

LIFE CYCLE

Adult worms measuring 1 to 2 cm in length and 0.3 to 0.6 mm in width live, mate, and feed on blood in the portal and mesenteric vessels (*S. japonicum, S. mekongi, S. mansoni, S. intercalatum*) or vesical plexus (*S. haematobium*).[7] The male worm folds around and encloses the female in its gynecophoral canal. Egg production varies from about 300 eggs per day for female *S. mansoni* and *S. haematobium* and 3000 eggs daily for *S. japonicum* (Fig. 289-1). Eggs, measuring 145 × 55 μm for *S. mansoni* and *S. haematobium* and 85 × 60 μm for *S. japonicum*

(Fig. 289-2), are deposited in the venules and make their way into the urine or feces and hatch in fresh water, where the miracidium, a 0.1-mm ciliated larva, emerges. The miracidium penetrates the body of the appropriate snail intermediate host and multiplies asexually. Within 4 to 6 weeks, thousands of motile, forked-tail cercariae 0.1 to 0.2 mm long emerge. On encountering human skin, the cercariae penetrate with the help of their glandular secretions, and within minutes, they lose their tails and change into schistosomula. This transformation from a freshwater environment to parasitic existence in the human host is associated with the unique formation of a heptalaminate membrane and other dramatic changes in cellular composition and function.[9] The schistosomula migrate to the lungs and liver, and in about 6 weeks, they mature to adult worms and descend through the venous system to their final habitat. Eggs appear in the feces or urine about 4 to 6 weeks after cercariae penetrate the skin. Adult schistosomes live on the average of 3 to 5 years but can survive for 30 years or more.[5-7]

EPIDEMIOLOGY

Transmission of schistosomiasis requires an appropriate snail intermediate host, fecal or urinary contamination of warm, slowly moving fresh water, and human entry into the snail-infested water. The snail host is specific for each species and strain of schistosome, which have a specific geographic distribution (see Table 289-1).[7] *S. mansoni* occurs in three South American countries, several Caribbean islands, and along with *S. haematobium,* in Africa and the Middle East, often in areas where the two species overlap.[2] *S. intercalatum* also can overlap with *S. haematobium* in parts of West and Central Africa but is less common. *S. japonicum* and *S. mekongi* occur in various Southeast Asian countries, and *S. japonicum* is found in China and the Philippines as well. Cattle, water buffaloes, pigs, dogs, and other mammals are naturally infected with *S. japonicum* and act as reservoir hosts, with a major role in transmission. Infections of rodents, sheep, primates, and other animals occur with *S. mansoni* and rarely *S. haematobium,* but they contribute little to maintenance of the life cycle.[5-7]

Transmission is focal in endemic countries and most intense in poor rural areas with inadequate sanitation and water supplies. The distribution of schistosomiasis is changing in many areas. The risk for infection is now nonexistent or negligible in previously highly endemic countries, including Japan, Morocco, Tunisia, Iran, Surinam, Venezuela, and the Caribbean countries.[2,4] Control programs have significantly reduced the incidence of infection and morbidity in Brazil, China, Saudi Arabia, Egypt, and the Philippines. Since 2000, strategies to reduce morbidity from schistosomiasis have been successfully implemented in several African countries, but in most of sub-Saharan Africa, high levels of endemicity persist, and dams and irrigation projects have led to major increases in the prevalence and extension of transmission to new areas.[4] Urban transmission now occurs in some large cities of Brazil and Africa.

In endemic communities, the distribution of the infection fits a negative binomial curve, with most infected persons harboring low worm burdens, and only a small proportion, usually children ages 8 to 12 years, have heavy infections.[5,6] Aggregation of the worm burden in a small proportion of infected individuals probably reflects a com-

---

*All material in this chapter is in the public domain, with the exception of any borrowed figures or tables.

TABLE 289-1	Features of Schistosomes and Other Important Trematodes				
Parasite	*Snail Intermediate Host (Genus)*	*Second Intermediate Host*	*Geographic Distribution*	*Location of Adult Worms*	*Treatment*
Schistosomes					
Schistosoma mansoni	*Biomphalaria*	None	South America, Africa, Caribbean, Arabian peninsula	Mesenteric venules	Praziquantel 40 mg/kg/day in 1 or 2 doses × 1 day Oxamniquine*
Schistosoma japonicum	*Onchomelania*	None	China, Philippines, Indonesia, Thailand	Mesenteric venules	Praziquantel 60 mg/kg/day in 3 doses × 1 day
Schistosoma mekongi	*Neotricula*	None	Cambodia, Laos	Mesenteric venules	Praziquantel 60 mg/kg/day in 3 doses × 1 day
Schistosoma intercalatum	*Bulinus*	None	Central and West Africa	Mesenteric venules	Praziquantel 40 mg/kg/day in 1 or 2 doses × 1 day
Schistosoma haematobium	*Bulinus*	None	Africa, Middle East	Venules of lower urinary tract	Praziquantel 40 mg/kg/day in 1 or 2 doses × 1 day Metriphonate*
Liver Flukes					
Clonorchis sinensis	*Bithynia, Parafossarulus*	Freshwater fish	China, Taiwan, Korea, Japan, Vietnam	Bile, pancreatic ducts	Praziquantel 75 mg/kg/day in 3 doses × 1-2 days Albendazole† 10 mg/kg/day × 10 days
Opisthorchis viverrini	*Bithynia*	Freshwater fish	Thailand, Laos, Cambodia	Bile, pancreatic ducts	Praziquantel 75 mg/kg/day in 3 doses × 1-2 days Albendazole† 10 mg/kg/day × 10 days
Opisthorchis felineus	*Bithynia*	Freshwater fish	Eastern Europe, former Soviet Union	Bile, pancreatic ducts	Praziquantel 75 mg/kg/day in 3 doses × 1-2 days Albendazole† 10 mg/kg/day × 10 days
Fasciola hepatica	*Lymnaea*	Watercress, other aquatic plants	Americas, Europe, Asia, western Pacific, North Africa	Bile ducts	Triclabendazole‡ 10 mg/kg × 1 day Bithionol* Nitazoxanide§
Intestinal Flukes					
Fasciolopsis buski	*Segmentina*	Aquatic plants	Far East, India	Small intestine	Praziquantel 25 mg/kg/day × 1 day Niclosamide† 40 mg/kg/day Triclabendazole§
Heterophyes heterophyes	*Pirenella, Cerithidea*	Freshwater fish	Far East, Egypt, Middle East, southern Europe	Small intestine	Praziquantel 25 mg/kg/day × 1 day Niclosamide† 1 g × 1 day Triclabendazole§
Metagonimus yokogawai	*Semisulcospira*	Freshwater fish	Far East, Russia, southern Europe	Small intestine	Praziquantel 25 mg/kg/day × 1 day Triclabendazole§
Lung Flukes					
Paragonimus westermani; other species	*Semisulcospira, Onchomelania, Thiara*	Freshwater crabs, crayfish	Far East, South Asia, Philippines, West Africa, South and Central America	Lungs	Praziquantel 75 mg/kg/day in 3 doses × 2 days Triclabendazole 10 mg/kg day × 3 days Bithionol*

*Not available or limited availability.
†Alternative drug.
‡In the United States, it is available for compassionate use from the manufacturer, Novartis; contact Victoria Pharmacy in Zurich, Switzerland.
§Limited data.

bination of factors, including the amount of water exposure, partial acquired immunity, age, and genetic susceptibility.[5,6,10,11] Because worms do not multiply in the host, the intensity of the infection depends on the number of cercariae encountered. Persons with heavy infections are at most risk for developing severe disease.

In the United States and other temperate areas, infection cannot be transmitted because of the absence of the appropriate snail intermediate host. Schistosomiasis is seen among immigrants from endemic areas and returning travelers, and sometimes it appears in small epidemics among persons engaging in adventure and nature tourism.[12-14]

PATHOGENESIS

The disease associated with schistosomiasis is largely due to the host's immune response to the larvae and eggs.[10,15-17] Mature adult worms evade the host's immune defenses by antigenic mimicry and other mechanisms mediated by the tegument, and thus contribute little to the immunopathology of the disease.[18] Different mechanisms are responsible for tissue injury during the stage of larval penetration, the acute stage, and the chronic infection.

In previously exposed persons, a protective response consisting primarily of specific immunoglobulin E (IgE) antibodies, eosinophils, and macrophages is directed against the schistosomula following cer-

carial penetration of the skin.[16] As a result, most organisms die in the skin and are surrounded by edema and massive cellular infiltrates in the dermis and epidermis that give rise to a papular dermatitis.

The syndrome of acute schistosomiasis occurs 2 to 12 weeks after a heavy first exposure to larvae during maturation and the initiation of egg deposition.[8,19,20] A febrile illness with features of serum sickness is thought to result from the formation of circulating immune complexes and production of high levels of proinflammatory cytokines. Acute disease develops primarily in previously unexposed persons and less commonly in heavy reinfections, usually due to *S. japonicum*. Symptomatic acute infections are rarely reported among persons who grow up in an endemic area, perhaps because they are not recognized or because of sensitization in utero as a result of maternal infection.[8]

Disease during the chronic stage of infection is due to the presence of eggs in host tissues and the immune response directed against the egg antigens.[10,16,17] Miracidia in the eggs secrete proteolytic enzymes through pores in the eggshell that facilitate passage of the eggs through blood vessel walls and tissues en route to the lumen of the intestinal or urinary tract. One third to one half of eggs reach the environment, with the remainder trapped in tissues or embolized to a distant site. The host response to toxic egg antigens and eggs retained in the tissues includes acute eosinophilic inflammation followed by granuloma formation, initially consisting of neutrophils, eosinophils, and mononuclear cells and later mostly lymphocytes, macrophages, multinucleated

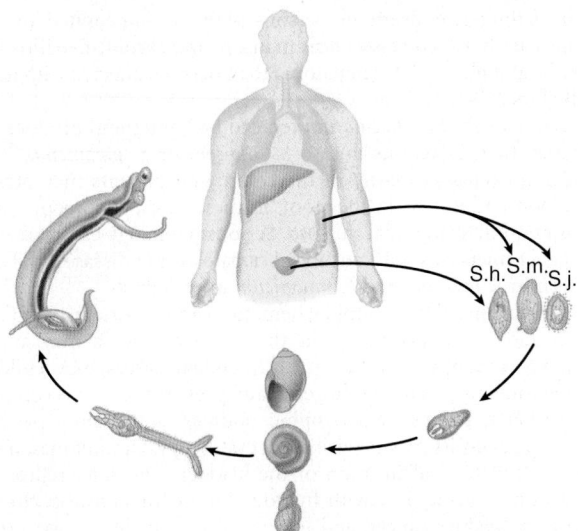

Figure 289-1 Life cycle of schistosomes. Eggs are passed in stools for *Schistosoma mansoni* (S.m.) and *Schistosoma japonicum* (S.j.) and in urine for *Schistosoma haematobium* (S.h.). The eggs hatch in fresh water, miracidia invade specific snail intermediate hosts, and in a few weeks forked-tail cercariae are liberated. These infective forms penetrate human skin, pass through a migratory phase in the lung and the liver, and then pass to their final habitat in the portal venous system (S.m. and S.j.) or the urinary bladder venous plexus (S.h.). Two other species infect humans, although less frequently. *Schistosoma intercalatum* produces terminal spined eggs that may be found in feces, whereas *Schistosoma mekongi* produces eggs similar to but smaller than those of *S. japonicum*, which may also be found in stools. These two species of schistosomes have characteristic snail intermediate hosts.

giant cells, and fibroblasts.[10,21-23] In *S. mansoni* and *S. haematobium* infections, the granulomatous response has been shown to be orchestrated by CD4+ T lymphocytes and is tightly regulated by various immunologic mechanisms.[17,19] They involve balanced Th1 and Th2 responses and the production of cytokines locally in the granulomas and systemically; these responses in turn are regulated by numerous other mediators and mechanisms.[10,23,24] In addition to destroying eggs, granulomas may mediate their passage into the lumen of the bowel or urinary tract. This hypothesis is supported by the finding of reduced egg output in persons with advanced human immunodeficiency virus (HIV) disease.[25]

Granulomas initiate tissue injury first through the inflammatory infiltrate and replacement of normal tissue and later through extensive collagen deposition and scarring.[10,15,17] Large granulomas and fibrosis cause the major pathologic lesions in chronic schistosomiasis. In the case of schistosomes that inhabit the mesenteric vessels, pathology is greatest in the intestines and the liver, the major site of egg embolism. With *S. haematobium* infection, the main system involved is the urinary tract. The result is inflammatory lesions and ulcerations of the mucosa, fibrotic scarring of the bowel, bladder, and lower ureteral walls, and obstruction of portal blood flow in the liver and urine flow through the ureters and bladder. During the early stages of schistosome infection, the granulomatous response is exuberant. Later, modulation of granulomatous hypersensitivity results in smaller granulomas and less fibrosis, which in turn probably play a significant role in limiting progression of the disease.[16,17,23]

The severity of disease in schistosomiasis is determined in part by the duration and intensity of the infection.[26-28] This relation is not exact, however, and other variables such as genetic susceptibility to disease, parasite strain, and coinfections with malaria, hepatitis viruses, HIV, and other infectious agents may be important.[25,29,30] Chronic schistosomiasis appears to be associated with a partial degree of resistance to reinfection directed against invading immature worms and mediated by antibodies and eosinophils.[31-34]

CLINICAL SYNDROMES

Schistosome Dermatitis

During penetration of cercariae, some previously exposed and unexposed persons experience a prickling sensation and may note urticaria followed by a macular rash several hours later.[6,8] In persons exposed for the first time, this rash disappears quickly, but in previously sensitized persons, it may persist and progress to a pruritic maculopapular rash that lasts for days. The rash is most severe in persons infected with schistosomes of birds or aquatic mammals, which die in the skin. This "swimmer's itch" is common in the Great Lakes region, New England, and other parts of the United States (see Chapter 291).

Figure 289-2 Life cycle of important parasitic flukes. Eggs are passed in stools for *Fasciola hepatica* (F.h.), *Clonorchis sinensis* (C.s.), and *Fasciolopsis buski* (F.b.) or in sputum for *Paragonimus westermani* (P.w.) infections. The next stage of multiplication occurs in specific snail intermediate hosts, followed by liberation of cercariae, which encyst on the second intermediate hosts (aquatic plants, fish, or crabs). These metacercariae represent the infective stage, and humans develop the infection after consumption of the second intermediate hosts. The final habitats of these flukes are the liver (F.h. and C.s.), intestines (F.b.), or lungs (P.w.).

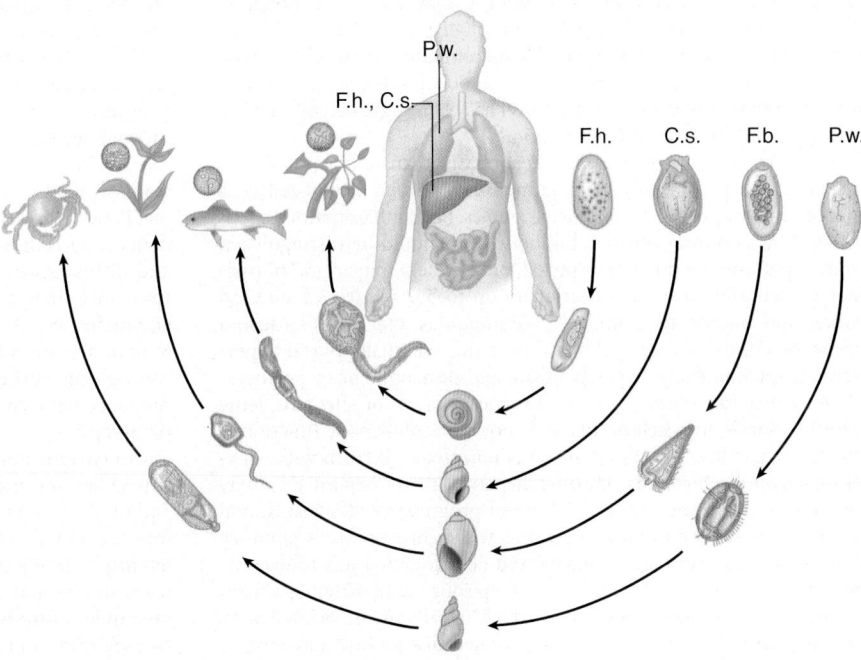

Acute Schistosomiasis

Previously uninfected persons from nonendemic areas may have no symptoms following first exposure or may develop symptoms of acute schistosomiasis (Katayama syndrome) 2 to 12 weeks after exposure, particularly to *S. japonicum* or *S. mansoni*.[6,8,19,20] The Katayama syndrome is unusual with *S. haematobium* and most severe with heavy infections, especially with *S. japonicum*. Onset of fever is often acute and accompanied by chills, fatigue, headache, myalgia, abdominal pain, diarrhea, and occasionally bloody stools. As many as 70% of patients develop nonproductive cough, dyspnea, chest pain, and diffuse infiltrates seen on chest radiography. The liver, spleen, and lymph nodes are often enlarged. Urticaria is common, and eosinophilia occurs in nearly all cases, but eggs may not be seen in the stools until late in the illness. Symptoms and signs usually disappear after 2 to 10 weeks, but persistent and more serious disease and even death may occur with heavy infections. Lesions of the central nervous system (CNS), genital tract, and skin due to aberrant migration of adult worms and ectopic deposition of eggs occurs in a small number of cases of acute infection, including in persons without systemic manifestations.[8,34] In some cases, eosinophil-mediated toxicity leading to vasculitis and small vessel thrombosis may be responsible for neurologic disease during acute infection.[35]

Chronic Schistosomiasis

Symptoms may be absent or mild in many patients who have light or moderate worm burdens. However, careful analysis of clinical and epidemiologic data has demonstrated subtle but important morbidity in persons with even light infections.[36] Chronic granulomatous inflammation and elevated levels of proinflamatory cytokines are believed to contribute to poor caloric intake, undernutrition, anemia of chronic inflammation, stunting, and impairment of work capacity and cognitive development in persons with chronic schistosomiasis.[35,36] Similar mechanisms, along with placental infection and inflammation, may be responsible for decreased birth weight and poor birth outcomes in infants born to mothers with chronic schistosomiasis.[37] When these previously underappreciated sequelae of infection have been taken into account, estimates of the disability asociated with schistosomiasis suggest a burden of disease as much as 50 times greater than previously reported.[38]

Eosinophilia is often present in persons with chronic schistosomiasis. Patients with light infections caused by the intestinal schistosomes *S. mansoni*, *S. japonicum*, and *S. mekongi* may complain of fatigue, intermittent abdominal pain, and diarrhea.[6,39,40] In heavy infections, blood loss from ulcerations or dysentery may lead to a moderate degree of anemia. Intestinal polyps have been observed, most commonly in Egypt, and strictures or large inflammatory masses may cause obstruction or mimic carcinoma.[41] An association between intestinal schistosomiasis and cancer of the bowel has been suggested but not yet demonstrated in a convincing fashion.[42]

An early sign of chronic schistosomiasis mansoni, japonica, or mekongi is hepatomegaly from granulomas around embolized eggs that become trapped in small portal venules. Such inflammatory hepatomegaly is common during childhood and should be distinguished from hepatomegaly due to periportal, or Symmers "pipestem," fibrosis that is seen after years of infection in up to 5% to 10% of infected young and middle-aged adults.[6,15] Granulomas and fibrosis cause a presinusoidal block to portal blood flow and eventually portal hypertension, splenomegaly, hypersplenism, and development of portosystemic collateral blood vessels. In most cases of hepatosplenic schistosomiasis, liver cell perfusion is not reduced, hepatic function is preserved, and liver function tests remain normal.[43] Persons with coexisting alcoholic cirrhosis, chronic hepatitis B, or hepatitis C may develop jaundice and ascites.[6,15] Natural progression of schistosomal disease occurs more rapidly in persons with schistosomiasis japonica than with schistosomiasis mansoni and occasionally leads to decompensated liver disease as well. Repeated episodes of hematemesis from bleeding esophageal varices occur, which usually are associated with low mortality in persons with compensated disease but may lead to

hepatic failure and death in persons with decompensated disease. Persons with both schistosomiasis mansoni and chronic hepatitis B or C may be at higher risk for hepatoma than persons infected with hepatitis B alone.[6,44]

Infections with *S. intercalatum* tend to be lighter and produce less pathology than infections due to *S. mansoni* or *S. japonicum*.[45] Egg deposition occurs primarily in the colon, and patients may present with blood and mucus in the stool; in these cases, endoscopy shows polyps and inflamed rectal mucosa. Serious pathology can be seen in *S. mekongi* infections with advanced hepatosplenic disease similar to that seen in *S. mansoni* and *S. japonicum* infections.[46]

In schistosomiasis haematobia, hematuria and dysuria from inflammation and small ulcerations in the bladder mucosa may appear within 3 to 4 months of infection.[47,48] In endemic areas, most children have microhematuria by age 10 years, and gross hematuria is common as well. Later, polyps, hypertrophic nodules, and "sandy patches" around egg deposits may be visible on cystoscopy. Granulomas, fibrosis, and ultimately calcification of the bladder wall cause reflux and obstruction of urine flow with hydroureter, hydronephrosis, chronic bacteriuria, bladder cancer, and in a small percentage of cases, renal failure. Deposition of *S. haematobium* eggs in the genital tract occurs in up to 75% of women and causes sandy patches with mucosal bleeding, abnormal blood vessels, and occasionally ulcerative, nodular, or papillomatous lesions of the vulva, perineum, and cervix.[49-51] These lesions increase the patient's susceptibility to HIV infection and other sexually transmitted diseases, and lesions of internal pelvic organs may cause bleeding and infertility. Hematospermia results from involvement of the prostate and seminal vesicles.[52] Associations have been demonstrated between *S. haematobium* infection, *Salmonella* urinary tract infections, and squamous cell carcinoma of the bladder; the latter has especially affected young and middle-aged men in Egypt.[47,53,54]

With schistosomiasis mansoni and japonica, eggs may bypass the liver through portosystemic collateral vessels and cause pulmonary disease; in schistosomiasis haematobia, eggs escape the vesical plexus and reach the lungs directly.[55,56] With severe cases, obstruction to pulmonary blood flow due to granulomatous inflammation and arteritis of small pulmonary arteries leads to cor pulmonale.[57] Subclinical glomerulonephritis is not uncommon in persons with chronic schistosomiasis; kidney biopsy has shown deposits of immune complexes containing schistosomal antigens in the glomerular basement membrane.[6,48] Ectopic egg deposition from aberrant migration of adult worms and embolization of eggs from distant sites are common with all species of schistosomes and can involve almost any organ. In most cases, the resulting lesions do not produce symptoms, but involvement of the CNS can cause serious cerebral and spinal cord disease.[34,58] CNS schistosomiasis is most common with *S. japonicum* infection, occurring in as many as 2% to 5% of infections and accounting for high rates of epilepsy in endemic areas. The brain is the usual site of CNS disease with schistosomiasis japonica, only occasionally with schistosomiasis mansoni, and virtually never with schistosomiasis haematobia. Patients present with focal or generalized seizures, focal neurologic deficits, signs of increased intracranial pressure due to the mass effect, and diffuse encephalitis. Computed tomography (CT) and magnetic resonance imaging (MRI) scans of the head show nodular and ring-enhancing lesions with surrounding edema. With *S. haematobium* and *S. mansoni* infections, eggs reach the lower spinal cord through Batson's plexus and produce either granulomatous lesions of the conus medullaris and cauda equina or transverse myelitis with back pain and paraplegia.

Concurrent infection with other organisms may affect the clinical course of schistosomiasis. Prolonged bacteremia with *Salmonella typhi* and other *Salmonella* species has been reported in persons chronically infected with *S. mansoni*, *S. japonicum*, *S. intercalatum*, and *S. haematobium*.[59] Unlike typhoid fever, the illness is indolent, with persistent fever, weight loss, and continuous bacteremia; and it can last months. Treatment of the bacterial infection without treating the schistosomiasis may result in relapse of bacteremia and symptoms. *Salmonella* can attach to the tegument and gut of schistosomes, and there is evidence that schistosomes and *Salmonella* share antigens that elicit immunologic tolerance to the bacterial infection.[6,15,59] Chronic *Salmonella* bacteriuria can complicate schistosomiasis haematobia. *Salmonella* bacteremia and bacteriuria have been associated with glomerulonephritis and nephrotic syndrome in persons with *S. haematobium* and *S. mansoni* infections.[48]

Chronic coinfection with hepatitis B or C worsens the prognosis of persons with hepatosplenic schistosomiasis, as already described.[6,15] The high rate of hepatitis C coinfection noted in Egypt probably reflects widespread transmission associated with parenteral antischistosomal treatment that was practiced until the 1980s.[60] HIV coinfection has been associated with decreased egg excretion in persons with *S. mansoni* and *S. haematobium* infections and decreased hematuria with *S. haematobium* infections because of impaired granuloma formation and increased trapping of eggs in tissue.[25,29] Treatment of schistosomiasis in persons with HIV coinfection has led to a decrease in HIV viral load, an increase in CD4+ T-cell counts, a decrease in schistosomal fecundity and egg excretion, but poor killing of adult worms.[61,62] An immune reconstitution phenomenon manifested by eosinophilic colitis with granulomas around dead and dying schistosome eggs followed antiretroviral treatment of an HIV-infected man with untreated chronic schistosomiasis.[63]

DIAGNOSIS

Schistosomiasis should be suspected in persons who have a history of freshwater exposure in endemic areas even in the absence of suggestive clinical findings or eosinophilia.[6,13] Hematuria is common with *S. haematobium* infections, and screening children for blood in their urine using dipsticks has provided reliable estimates of the prevalence of infection in areas of high endemicity.[6] Current diagnostic tests for schistosomiasis include serologic tests and microscopic examination of stool, urine, or tissue for eggs. Microscopy on a simple smear of feces or a drop of urine can detect heavy infections, but concentration procedures and repeated examinations are often needed because eggs may be passed intermittently or in small numbers. Several concentration procedures also allow quantification of egg output, such as the Kato-Katz technique, which uses 20 to 50 mg of fecal material, or filtration of a standard volume of urine through a Nucleopore membrane. Counts higher than 400 eggs per gram of feces or 10 mL of urine are considered heavy and are associated with an increased risk for complications. Microscopic examination of snips of rectal or bladder mucosa obtained at proctoscopy or cystoscopy may reveal eggs when the stool examination is negative. Because persons with inactive infections may continue to shed dead eggs into stool or urine for months, tests for egg viability such as egg hatching or microscopic examination of eggs for movement of flame cells should be performed. A reagent strip that uses monoclonal antibodies to detect somatic schistosome antigens in urine has a sensitivity of more than 85% and is suitable for use in the field.[64] A multiplex, real-time polymerase chain reaction (PCR) assay that detects and quantifies schistosome DNA in stool or urine has a sensitivity similar to that of microscopy of duplicate samples.[65]

Serologic tests for antibodies to schistosomes are available at the Centers for Disease Control and Prevention (CDC) in Atlanta, Georgia, and some commercial laboratories.[66] The CDC uses a combination of tests with purified adult worm antigens. Its Falcon assay screening test–enzyme-linked immunosorbent assay (FAST-ELISA) is 99% specific for all species and has a sensitivity of 99% for *S. mansoni* infection, 95% for *S. haematobium*, but less than 50% for *S. japonicum*. Because the FAST-ELISA may miss some *S. haematobium* and *S. japonicum* infections, immunoblots using species-specific antigens are performed in cases of potential exposure to these parasites. Serologic tests cannot distinguish active from past infections but are useful for screening previously unexposed travelers and expatriates.[12] In such persons, a positive serologic test is presumptive evidence of infection even if microscopic examination of stool or urine fails to reveal schistosome eggs. Serologic tests may turn positive before egg excretion during acute schistosomiasis, but otherwise the diagnosis rests on the epidemiologic history and clinical picture.[8]

Persons with confirmed schistosomiasis should be evaluated for evidence of disease. Urinalysis, urine culture, and serum creatinine determination are indicated for persons with *S. haematobium* infection. Any abnormality should prompt radiographic or other imaging study to detect complications such as thickening or calcification of the bladder wall, hydroureter, hydronephrosis, polyps, stones, or carcinoma of the bladder in persons with urinary schistosomiasis.[67] Evaluation of infections due to the intestinal schistosomes includes liver function tests and tests for chronic hepatitis B and C. Persons with evidence of liver disease or heavy infections should undergo imaging to document periportal fibrosis and signs of portal hypertension. Contrast studies, CT, MRI, and ultrasonography are sensitive means of detecting and evaluating urinary tract and hepatic pathology, although ultrasonography has become the preferred modality in endemic countries.[68,69] Standardized protocols have been developed by the World Health Organization (WHO) for ultrasonography in hospitals and the field. Esophageal varices are visualized by barium swallow or endoscopy.[6]

MANAGEMENT

Treatment is indicated for all persons with schistosomiasis. Cure of infection is desirable because even a single pair of worms may be responsible for a catastrophic neurologic complication such as transverse myelitis. In endemic areas where reinfection is inevitable, the goal is to reduce worm burdens to levels that are unlikely to produce disease.[4,70] Successful treatment not only prevents the development of complications, but if given early and reinfection is avoided, it also can cause partial or complete regression of intestinal lesions, urinary bladder wall thickening, bladder polyps, urinary obstruction, genital sandy patches, and periportal fibrosis.[4,71-73]

The drug of choice for treating all species of schistosomes is praziquantel (see Table 289-1), which affects membrane permeability in the parasite.[74] Paralysis and vacuolation of the tegument immobilize the worm and expose it to attack by the host immune system. After a single treatment of chronic infections, cure rates range from 65% to 90%; and in persons not cured, egg excretion is reduced by more than 90%.[4,6,8] Praziquantel does not affect developing schistosomula and may not abort an early infection.[74] Resistance to praziquantel has been documented in the laboratory, and there have been reports of decreased responsiveness in the field and anecdotal reports of returned travelers who required multiple courses of praziquantel to clear their infections.[75-79] Adverse effects, which are usually mild and last less than 24 hours, may be due to reactions to dying worms rather than drug toxicity. Patients may report headache, dizziness, or abdominal discomfort and less commonly nausea, vomiting, diarrhea, bloody stools, fever, and urticaria. WHO now recommends that praziquantel be given to pregnant and lactating women with schistosomiasis.[4,80] Persons with known or suspected cysticercosis should remain under observation during therapy because of the risk for seizures or other neurologic consequences of dying cysticerci. Persons with schistosomal disease of the CNS should also take corticosteroids to reduce the inflammation and edema around eggs.[33,34] Oxamniquine, an alternative for treatment of *S. mansoni* infections but with limited availability, is nearly as effective as praziquantel for infections acquired in the Western Hemisphere.[81] Higher doses are needed for strains of the parasite from Africa, and drug resistance has been documented. Metrifonate is effective only against urinary schistosomes; it requires three doses 2 weeks apart and is currently not available. The antimalarial drugs artemether and artesunate, active against all species of schistosomes, can kill schistosomula during the first 3 weeks of infection, and are synergistic with praziquantel in killing adult worms.[74,82,83] They are effective as prophylactic agents against *S. japonicum* and to a lesser extent other species when given every 2 weeks and have been approved for chemoprophylaxis in China.[74] A 3-day course of artesunate (combined with amodiaquine or pyrimethamine-sulfadoxine) cured more than 90% of *S. haematobium* infections in children receiving treatment for malaria.[84] Results of trials of artesunate in combination with praziquantel have shown superiority of the combination over praziquantel alone in several studies, but little difference in others.[74,85] More data are needed to determine whether combination therapy offers any advantages over monotherapy with praziquantel. Widespread use of artemisinin derivatives for treatment or prophylaxis in malaria-endemic areas should be avoided because of the risk for promoting artemisinin-resistant parasites.[6] The effectiveness of artemisinin compounds alone or with praziquantel for treatment of acute schistosomiasis is not known.[8] The symptoms of Katayama syndrome often require administration of corticosteroids to suppress the inflammatory process, but there is no consensus about proper anthelmintic treatment.[6,8,14,19,20] Some authorities administer praziquantel simultaneously with or shortly after administration of corticosteroids and treat *S. mansoni* and *S. haematobium* infections for up to 3 days and *S. japonicum* infections for up to 6 days in the doses listed in Table 289-1.[6,8] Other authors believe that praziquantel should not be used during the acute phase, because of its limited effectiveness against schistosomula, the lowering of serum levels by concomitant corticosteroid therapy, and the risk for reactions that develop in response to killing of parasites.[77,85,86] Treatment of asymptomatic persons 28 to 40 days after exposure prevented acute illness but not chronic infection, and treatment of persons within 10 to 15 days of exposure precipitated an acute illness, including severe complications such as bronchospasm and cerebral microinfarcts.[35,77,86] In all cases of acute schistosomiasis, a second course of therapy is recommended 4 to 6 weeks after the onset of symptoms. Stool or urine should be examined for eggs 6 to 8 weeks after symptoms subside, and persons who remain infected should receive a single dose of praziquantel, 40 to 60 mg/kg.[6,8,35] Because antischistosomal drugs may temporarily inhibit egg laying by adult worms, stool and urine should be examined for up to 6 months after completion of therapy for both acute and chronic infections. Eosinophilia, hematuria, or persistence of symptoms should prompt repeat parasitologic studies. Serologic tests may remain positive for several years after successful treatment.

PREVENTION AND CONTROL OF SCHISTOSOMIASIS

Travelers to areas where schistosomiasis is endemic should avoid contact with fresh water that may be infested with cercariae.[14] If contact is unavoidable, vigorous toweling of the skin may limit cercarial penetration after leaving the water, and medical follow-up should be sought after return from travel. Topical lotions and soaps have not reliably prevented infection after contact with cercariae, and further data are needed before recommending artemether for prophylaxis, which at any rate should not be used in malarious areas.

Control of schistosomiasis in endemic communities can be approached by providing sanitation and safe water supplies and eliminating snail intermediate hosts or their habitats. Because the cost of these interventions is beyond the reach of most poor countries, most schistosomiasis control programs are following the WHO-recommended strategy of regular administration of antischistosomal drugs (and drugs for soil-transmitted helminths) to populations at risk, primarily to maintain individual worm burdens at levels below those that cause morbidity and mortality, and secondarily to decrease transmission and prevalence of infection.[4,87,88] Because of difficulties in sustaining large-scale drug administration programs and the threat of selecting for drug-resistant organisms, this strategy is a temporary solution. Interruption of transmission in high-risk areas requires integrated and intensive strategies, as demonstrated in a highly successful community-based trial in China, which employed regular chemotherapy, removal of cattle from snail-infested grasslands, providing farmers with mechanized farm equipment, supplying tap water, building lavatories and latrines, providing boats with fecal-matter containers, and implementing an intensive health-education program.[89] Development of a vaccine to prevent heavy infections seems possible based on experimental studies in animals and evidence of acquired immunity in human populations.[90,91] Numerous vaccine candidates have been identified, and at least one antigen, the *S. haematobium* 28-kDA glutathione *S*-transferase, has entered into clinical trials.

Liver Flukes

The major liver flukes of humans are *Clonorchis sinensis* and several species of *Opisthorchis* (largely found in the Far East, Southeast Asia, and Russia), and *Fasciola hepatica*, which is widely distributed throughout the world (see Table 289-1).[3,92,93] Less common liver flukes include *Fasciola gigantica* in South America, Africa, and Southeast Asia; *Metorchis conjunctus* in North America; and *Opisthorchis guayaquilensis* in the Americas. All are infections of various lower animals and are transmitted through food. The lancet fluke, *Dicrocelium dendriticum*, which inhabits the biliary tree of ruminants and humans, is the exception: it is transmitted by eating infected ants, the second intermediate host.[94,95] Most commonly found in sheep-raising countries of the Mediterranean, it produces mild symptoms. False or spurious infections are detected when its eggs are shed in the stools of a person who ingested the liver of an infected animal.

CLONORCHIASIS AND OPISTHORCHIASIS

C. sinensis, Opisthorchis viverrini, and *Opisthorchis felineus* have similar life cycles, eggs, and capacity to produce disease; they differ primarily in their geographic distribution, the morphology of the adult worms, and the frequency with which the clinical syndromes occur.[3,96-98] *C. sinensis* is found primarily in eastern Asia, *O. viverrini* in Southeast Asia, and *O. felineus* in the former Soviet Union. Millions of persons are infected, and in some areas, it is not uncommon to find prevalence rates of 20% to 80%.

The hermaphroditic adult flukes are flat, elongated worms measuring 5 to 25 mm × 2 to 5 mm that inhabit the intrahepatic bile ducts (see Fig. 289-2). Their yellow-brown operculated eggs (30 × 12 μm) are fully embryonated when they pass out of the body in feces into fresh water (Fig. 289-3). The eggs are ingested by specific snails, inside of which they hatch into miracidia that develop and replicate to produce large numbers of cercariae. Cercariae are released into the water and penetrate susceptible freshwater fish, primarily carp, and then encyst as metacercariae. Several species of freshwater shrimp can also serve as the second intermediate host of *C. sinensis*.[97,99] Humans, cats, dogs, and other fish-eating mammals become infected by ingesting the metacercariae in raw or inadequately cooked fish; the metacercariae excyst in the duodenum and pass through the ampulla of Vater to the bile ducts, where adult worms mature and begin egg laying in about 3 to 4 weeks; they live as long as 30 years.

CLINICAL SYNDROMES

Most patients are asymptomatic but may have eosinophilia. An acute illness resembling acute schistosomiasis with fever, abdominal pain, hepatomegaly, urticaria, and eosinophilia occasionally develops 2 to 3 weeks after the initial exposure.[100,101] No gross changes are detected in the liver with mild or early infection, but irritation of bile duct walls by the suckers of the flukes and secreted metabolic products leads to inflammation and thickening of bile duct walls and localized obstruction in about 10% of persons with heavy chronic infections (1000 to 25,000 or more eggs per gram of stool). Patients complain of right upper quadrant discomfort, anorexia, and weight loss. On physical examination, the liver is palpable and firm. Pigment stones, recurring episodes of cholangitis with bacterial sepsis, cholecystitis, liver abscess, and occasionally pancreatitis occur in the most heavily infected persons.[102] An increased incidence of cholangiocarcinoma, an adenocarcinoma originating from hyperplastic biliary epithelium, has been associated most strongly with *O. viverrini* infection in Thailand but also with *C. sinensis* infections in China and elsewhere.[97,103,104]

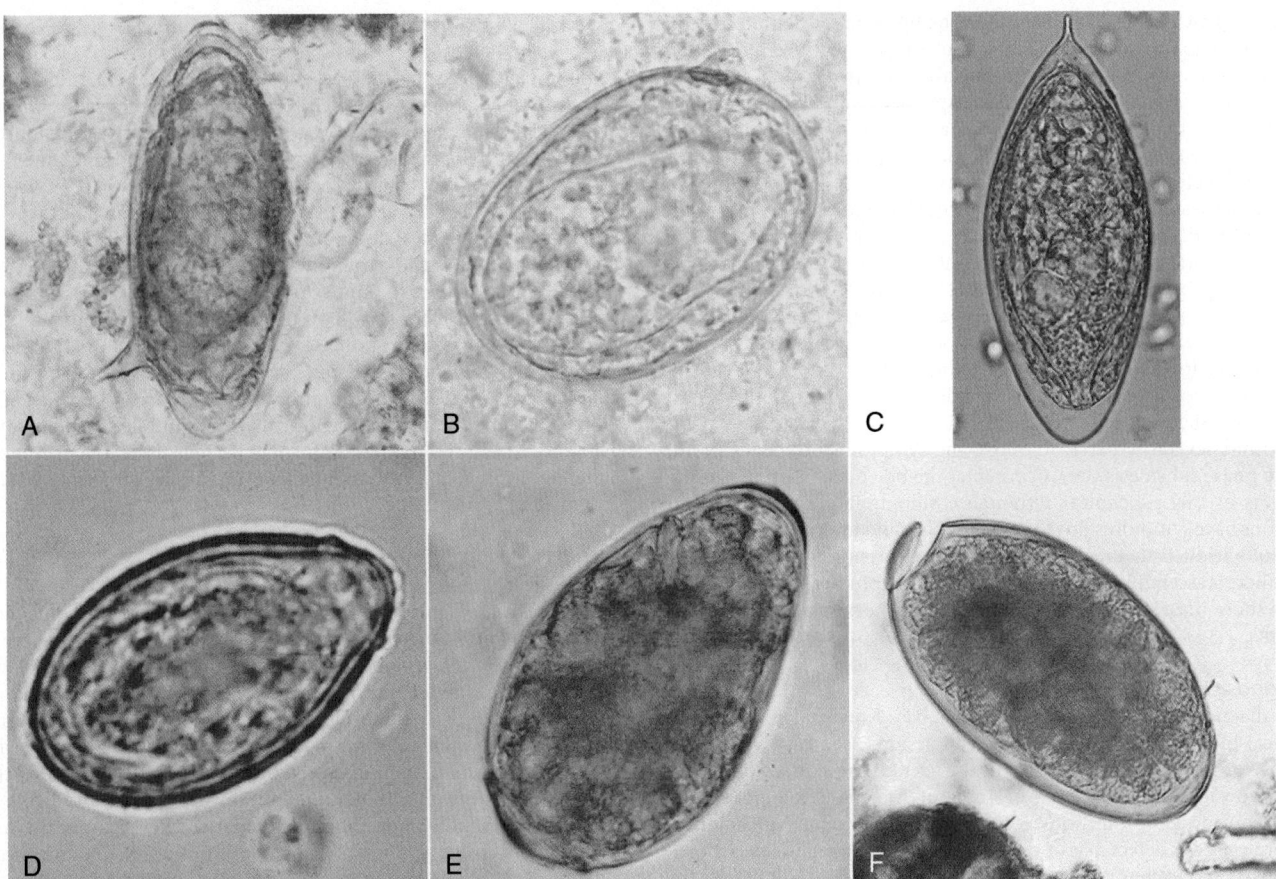

Figure 289-3 **Eggs of common human trematodes. A,** *Schistosoma mansoni;* **B,** *Schistosoma japonicum;* **C,** *Schistosoma haematobium;* **D,** *Clonorchis sinensis;* **E,** *Paragonimus westermani;* and **F,** *Fasciola hepatica* (note the partially open operculum). *(From DPDx, website for laboratory diagnosis of parasitic diseases of the Division of Parasitic Diseases, National Centers for Infectious Diseases, Centers for Disease Control and Prevention, Atlanta, GA [http://www.dpd.cdc.gov/DPDx/].)*

DIAGNOSIS AND MANAGEMENT

Liver fluke infection is diagnosed by finding eggs in the stool or by identifying adult worms during surgery or endoscopic retrograde cholangiopancreatography.[100,101,105] Eggs may not be found in the stool in infections with fewer than 20 adult flukes, and multiple examinations of concentrated specimens may be necessary. Serologic tests and antigen detection assays are under development but are not widely available outside of endemic areas. Ultrasonography, CT, or MRI can demonstrate dilation and stricture of bile ducts, thickening of the gallbladder wall, and stones.[105] Flukes within bile ducts are difficult to visualize and require high-resolution equipment, but flukes in the gallbladder are more readily seen.[105] M-mode ultrasonography may demonstrate moving worms, which appear as thin linear echoes in ducts or can be seen floating in the gallbladder.

A single course of praziquantel eradicates the infection in more than 85% of cases.[106,107] Albendazole in a dose of 10 mg/kg for 7 days may also be used.[95] Rarely, surgery is needed to relieve biliary tract obstruction.[102]

FASCIOLIASIS

Infection with the sheep liver fluke *Fasciola hepatica* results from ingesting uncooked watercress or other fresh aquatic vegetation in 61 countries worldwide, especially in sheep- and cattle-raising areas.[3,108-110] The global prevalence of human infection is in excess of 3 million. Infections have been reported from all continents except Antarctica, with the highest rates of infection in Bolivia, Peru, Egypt,

Iran, Portugal, and France. The ability of *F. hepatica* to adapt to new definitive hosts and new environments, such as the Bolivian Altiplano at 3800 to 4100 meters, accounts for its continued spread from its original European range.[108] Epidemics involving up to 100,000 persons have been reported in northwestern Iran.[108] A small number of cases, mostly imported, have been reported in the United States.[111,112] The closely related but larger *Fasciola gigantica* has a more limited distribution.

The hermaphroditic adult fluke is flat, brown, and leaf-shaped, and it measures about 3 × 1.5 cm. Mature worms in their natural hosts (mainly sheep and cattle) live in the common and hepatic bile ducts, where they deposit their eggs (see Fig. 289-2). The large oval, yellowish brown, operculate ova measuring 140 × 75 μm (see Fig. 289-3) pass to the intestines, are evacuated in the feces, and complete their development in fresh water. Within a few days miracidia hatch and invade their specific snail intermediate host, within which they undergo asexual replication, resulting in the release of cercariae that encyst as metacercariae on aquatic plants, including watercress, water caltrops, water lettuce, mint, and parsley. When swallowed, the infective metacercariae excyst, and the larvae penetrate the intestinal wall into the peritoneum, from whence they feed on liver parenchyma and pass through the liver capsule and tissues to the biliary tract.[3] About 3 to 4 months are needed from infection to oviposition in humans. Adult flukes can live as long as 10 years.

Clinical Syndromes

Infection with *F. hepatica* has two distinct clinical phases corresponding to the hepatic migratory phase of its life cycle and to the presence of the worms in their final habitat in the bile ducts.[92] Symptoms corresponding to migration of the larval fluke appear within 6 to 12 weeks of ingestion of metacercariae and can last 4 months or longer. Marked eosinophilia is seen in most infected persons, and abdominal pain, intermittent high fever, weight loss, and urticaria are common.[113] There may be tender hepatomegaly, jaundice, anemia, and elevation of liver function tests. Cough and chest pain occur in 10% to 15%, sometimes accompanied by a pleural effusion with eosinophils in the pleural fluid. Aberrant migration may produce migratory nodules in the skin, painful inflammation of the intestinal wall, and lesions in the lung, brain, genitourinary tract, or elsewhere. CT or MRI shows hypodense lesions measuring 1 cm or more in diameter that move to various parts of the liver over the course of several weeks.[105,114,115] Hypodense tortuous and branching linear tracks under the capsule correspond to necrosis, and eosinophilic inflammatory infiltrates are seen along the path of larval migration.[116,117]

Within several weeks to months, the symptoms and signs of the acute phase subside as the worms enter the bile ducts. Chronic fascioliasis is usually subclinical, although eosinophilia is common. Some persons have symptoms due to inflammation and intermittent obstruction of bile ducts that resemble biliary colic and cholecystitis; occasionally, there is ascending cholangitis. Ultrasonography or cholangiography may show masses in the common bile duct corresponding to adult worms.

Diagnosis and Management

The diagnosis during the acute stage is based on epidemiology, the clinical picture, and often characteristic lesions seen on CT or MRI. Biopsy of nodules on the surface of the liver, in the skin, or elsewhere may show inflammatory tracts or immature worms. Serologic tests are useful during acute infection because symptoms develop 1 to 2 months before eggs are detectable in the stool. Whole-worm antigens, coproantigens, and excretory-secretory proteins have been used in enzyme immunoassays and immunoblots; sensitivities of more than 90% are reported, but the specificity may be less owing to cross-reactivity with other helminths.[118] The definitive diagnosis is made by demonstrating eggs in samples of stool, bile, or duodenal aspirates or by recovering worms at surgery. Repeat examinations and concentration procedures may be necessary to detect eggs in the stool.

Unlike infections with other flukes, fascioliasis responds poorly to praziquantel. First-line treatment is with a single oral dose of triclabendazole, a well tolerated benzimidazole used in veterinary practice that is highly effective against mature and immature flukes.[106,119,120] Rates of cure are about 80%, and persons not cured with a single dose usually respond to a second dose. Treatment should be repeated if radiographic findings or eosinophilia fail to resolve or the titers of serologic tests do not decrease. Alternative therapy is with bithionol, which requires 10 to 15 doses and causes frequent side effects. Limited experience with nitazoxanide suggests cure rates of about 60%.[121] Artesunate has activity against *F. hepatica*, but cure rates are less than those with triclabendazole.[122]

Intestinal Flukes

More than 65 flukes are known to infect the human gastrointestinal tract.[1,3,123] Most are found in parts of Asia where the appropriate intermediate hosts and animal reservoirs are found. The best known intestinal flukes include *Fasciolopsis buski* and the heterophytid flukes *Heterophyes heterophyes* and *Metagonimus yokogawai*. *Nanophyetus salmincola*, which is transmitted in the Pacific Northwest of the United States, is discussed in Chapter 291.

FASCIOLOPSIS

Human infection with the large intestinal fluke *Fasciolopsis buski* occurs in the Far East, Southeast Asia, and southern Asia, where pigs are the major reservoir of infection.[4,108,124,125] The thick, fleshy adult worms range in length from 2 to 7.5 cm and in breadth from 0.8 to 2 cm. They inhabit the duodenum and jejunum, where they produce large operculated eggs (135 × 80 μm) (see Fig. 289-2). On reaching fresh water, the eggs hatch, releasing miracidia that penetrate a specific snail intermediate host in which they multiply and develop into free-living cercariae. The cercariae encyst into metacercariae on almost any aquatic plant. The metacercariae survive in most environments for up to 1 year. When raw or poorly cooked infected plants are ingested by humans, the metacercariae excyst in the intestines, and within 3 months, the parasites develop into mature worms that survive 6 months or more in the human host.

Adult flukes live in the upper portion of the small intestine, where they attach to the mucosa and produce local inflammation, ulceration, and abscesses. Fasciolopsiasis is mostly subclinical, although eosinophilia is marked in some persons.[92] In some cases, epigastric pain and diarrhea may be seen 1 or 2 months after exposure. With heavy infections, flukes may cause transient obstruction and ileus. Edema of the face and extremities may result from hypersensitivity to worm metabolites or from hypoalbuminemia due to malabsorption or protein-losing enteropathy.

HETEROPHYIASIS AND METAGONIMIASIS

There are at least 10 species of flukes in the family Heterophyidae, of which *Heterophyes heterophyes* and *Metagonimus yokogawai* are the most common. *H. heterophyes* is found primarily in the Nile delta region, Tunisia, and Turkey, whereas *M. yokogawai* is most prevalent in the Far East.[4,108,126] The adult flukes measure less than 2 mm in length and inhabit the small intestine of human, animal, or avian hosts, where they produce small operculate eggs (30 × 15 μm). The life cycle is similar to that of other trematodes and involves snails and fish living in fresh or brackish water. The metacercariae encyst under the scales of the fish. Infection is acquired by consumption of undercooked or salted fish. Adults begin producing eggs in about 9 days and live only a few months to less than 1 year.

Flukes attach to the small intestine wall, where they produce focal inflammation and ulcerations. Infected persons may experience colicky abdominal pain, dyspepsia, diarrhea, and eosinophilia. Flukes may penetrate the mucosa and deposit eggs that pass through lymphatics into the bloodstream. Eggs may embolize to the CNS, where they can cause myocarditis or focal lesions of the brain or spinal cord and occasionally death.

DIAGNOSIS AND MANAGEMENT

A definitive diagnosis depends on demonstration of eggs or adult worms in stools. Proper identification of the species by examining eggs is difficult because the morphology and size of eggs of different species are similar.[92] Eggs of *F. buski* can be confused with those of *F. hepatica*, and eggs of *H. heterophyes* and *M. yokogawai* can be confused with each other and with the eggs of *C. sinensis* and *Opisthorchis*. Species identification is best made by examining adult worms expelled after treatment.

The treatment of choice of all intestinal trematodes infections is praziquantel. Triclabendazole is also effective, and niclosamide is effective for treating *Fasciolopsis* and *Heterophyes* infections.[92,106]

Lung Flukes
PARAGONIMIASIS

More than 40 species of *Paragonimus* are recognized as parasites of mammals; however, only eight cause significant infections in humans.[1,3,127,128] *Paragonimus westermani*, the most important species infecting humans, is found in the Far East, principally Korea, Japan, Taiwan, China, and the Philippines. The other species are *Paragonimus miyazaki* (Japan), *Paragonimus skrjabini* and *Paragonimus hueitungensis* (China), *Paragonimus heterotrema* (China, Southeast Asia), *Paragonimus uterobilateralis* and *Paragonimus africanus* (Central and West

Africa), *Paragonimus mexicanus* (Central and South America), and *Paragonimus kellicotti* (North America).[129,130]

Reddish brown adult worms measuring 7 to 16 mm × 4 to 7 mm live in encapsulated cystic cavities in the parenchyma of the lung, usually close to bronchioles. Worms produce golden-brown operculate eggs (80 to 120 μm × 50 to 65 μm) that pass into the bronchioles and are coughed up; they are then either passed in sputum or swallowed and passed in feces (see Figs. 289-2 and 289-3). On reaching fresh water, they require 2 to 3 weeks to develop before miracidia hatch at 29° to 32° C. After 3 to 5 months of development and reproduction in the snail, stumpy-tailed cercariae emerge. They encyst in the muscles and viscera of crayfish and freshwater crabs. Human infection is initiated by consumption of these freshwater crustaceans if they are uncooked, partially cooked, salted, or pickled. Metacercariae excyst in the duodenum, penetrate the intestinal wall, and enter the peritoneal cavity. After several days, they migrate through the diaphragm to the pleural cavities and then into the lungs. A fibrous cyst wall develops around them, and egg deposition starts 5 to 6 weeks after infection. Worms may develop also in extrapulmonary sites including the liver, lymph nodes, skin, spinal cord, and brain. Adults may live as long as 20 to 25 years but generally are much shorter-lived.

CLINICAL SYNDROMES

At 2 to 15 days after ingestion of metacercariae, some persons develop abdominal pain and diarrhea followed by fever, chest pain, cough, urticaria, and eosinophilia. However, these initial symptoms are often absent, and light or moderate infections may remain undetected until first seen on a radiograph obtained for other reasons. The inflammatory reaction to adults encapsulated in the lungs and the shedding of eggs into the bronchial tree are responsible for chronic symptoms. Cough productive of brownish sputum with intermittent hemoptysis are the initial manifestations of chronic infection.[131] Later, the clinical picture resembles chronic bronchitis or bronchiectasis with profuse expectoration and pleuritic chest pain, dyspnea, chronic cough, chest pains, and occasional hemoptysis. Radiographs may be negative or show diffuse infiltration, cysts measuring about 4 cm in diameter, nodules, calcifications, pleural effusion, and pneumothorax. Pleural fluid is exudative and contains large numbers of eosinophils. The illness is often confused with pulmonary tuberculosis, but eosinophilia and the lack of fever suggest the true diagnosis.[128] The most commonly recognized form of extrapulmonary disease is involvement of the CNS, which is seen in as many as 25% of hospitalized cases. Parasite-induced meningitis may be the first manifestation, usually occurring within a year of pulmonary infection. Cerebral infections present as a space-occupying tumor, with seizures, headaches, visual disturbances, and motor or sensory deficits. Radiographs of the skull may show clusters of calcified cysts that resemble soap bubbles, and MRI and CT show aggregates of ring-enhancing lesions with surrounding edema.[132]

Other extrapulmonary infections include migratory allergic skin lesions similar to those seen with cutaneous larva migrans; these lesions are common during infections with *P. skrjabini* and other species in addition to infections with *P. westermani*. Flukes may also be found in the liver, spleen, peritoneum, intestinal wall, and intra-abdominal lymph nodes.

DIAGNOSIS AND MANAGEMENT

The diagnosis of paragonimiasis is established by identifying expectorated eggs in the sputum, swallowed eggs in the feces, or worms and eggs in biopsy specimens. Multiple examinations of stool and sputum may be necessary. Serologic tests are useful for diagnosing light or extrapulmonary infections.[133] Enzyme immunoassay tests are available, and an immunoblot assay performed at the CDC that uses a crude antigen extract of *P. westermani* has a sensitivity of 96% and a specificity of almost 100%.[134,135]

The treatment of choice for paragonimiasis is praziquantel. The alternative, triclabendazole, also has a high rate of cure.[106,128] Bithionol is used uncommonly because it has more frequent side effects. Because an inflammatory reaction to dying worms may precipitate seizures or other neurologic complications, corticosteroids should be used simultaneously with praziquantel for cerebral paragonimiasis.

Prevention of Food-Borne Fluke Infections

As aquaculture for production of freshwater fish and crustaceans continues to expand and provide a rapidly growing percentage of the supply for local and international markets, efforts to prevent and control nonschistosomal trematode infections are mandatory at all stages of the food chain. The focus is on food production and preparation because elimination of snail and animal hosts is neither desirable nor feasible. Educational interventions should also focus on preventing contamination of water sources with human and animal feces, especially ponds used for the cultivation of fish and aquatic plants. Education about proper preservation, cooking, or other preparation of food must take cultural practices and beliefs into account.

REFERENCES

1. Muller R. The nematodes. In: *Worms and Human Disease*. 2nd ed. Wallingford: CABI Publishing; 2002:109-235.
2. Engels D, Chitsulo L, Montresor A, et al. The global epidemiological situation of schistosomiasis and new approaches to control and research. *Acta Trop*. 2002;82:139-146.
3. Crompton DWT, Savioli L. *Handbook of Helminthiases for Public Health*. Boca Raton: CRC Press-Taylor and Francis Group; 2007:91-125.
4. Fenwick A, Rollinson D, Southgate V. Implementation of human schistosomiasis control: challenges and prospects. *Adv Parasitol*. 2006;61:567-616.
5. Jordan P, Webbe G, Sturrock RF. *Human Schistosomiasis*. Wallingford, UK: CAB International; 1993:1-465.
6. Gryssels B, Polman K, Clerinx J, et al. *Lancet*. 2006;368:1106-1118.
7. Sturrock RF. The schistosomes and their intermediate hosts. In: Mahmoud AAF, ed. *Schistosomiasis*. London: Imperial College Press; 2001:7-83.
8. Ross AG, Vickers D, Olds GR, et al. Katayama syndrome. *Lancet Infect Dis*. 2007;7:218-224.
9. Gobert GN, Moertel L, Brindley PJ, et al. Developmental gene expression profiles of the human pathogen *Schistosoma japonicum*. *BMC Genomics*. 2009;10:128-157.
10. Burke ML, Jones MK, Gobet GN, et al. Immunopathogenesis of human schistosomiasis. *Parasite Immunol*. 2009;31:163-176.
11. Kurtis JD, Friedman JF, Leenstra T, et al. Pubertal development predicts resistance to infection and reinfection with *Schistosoma japonicum*. *Clin Infect Dis*. 2006;42:1692-1698.

12. Corachan M. Schistosomiasis and international travel. *Clin Infect Dis*. 2002;35:446-450.
13. Nicolls DJ, Weld LH, Schwartz E, et al. Characteristics of schistosomiasis in travelers reported to the Geosentinel Surveillance Network 1997-2008. *Am J Trop Med Hyg*. 2008;79:729-734.
14. Leshem E, Maor Y, Meltzer E, et al. Acute schistosomiasis outbreak: clinical features and economic impact. *Clin Infect Dis*. 2008;47:1499-1506.
15. Von Lichtenberg F. Schistosomiasis. In: Connor DH, Chandler FW, Schwartz DA, et al, eds. *Pathology of Infectious Diseases*. Stamford, CT: Appleton & Lange; 1997:1537-1551.
16. Pearce EJ, MacDonald AS. The immunobiology of schistosomiasis. *Nat Rev Immunol*. 2002;2:499-511.
17. Wilson MS, Mentink-Kane MM, Pesce JT, et al. Immunopathology of schistosomiasis. *Immunol Cell Biol*. 2007;85:148-154.
18. Van Hellemond JJ, Retra K, Brouwers JFHM, et al. Functions of the tegument of schistosomes: clues from the proteome and lipidome. *Int J Parasitol*. 2006;36:691-699.
19. Doherty JF, Moody AH, Wright SG. Katayama fever: an acute manifestation of schistosomiasis. *BMJ*. 1996;313:1071-1072.
20. De Jesus AR, Silva A, Santana LB, et al. Clinical and immunological evaluation of 31 patients with acute schistosomiasis mansoni. *J Infect Dis*. 2002;185:98-105.
21. Warren KS, Domingo EO, Cowan RBT. Granuloma formation around schistosome eggs as a manifestation of delayed hypersensitivity. *Am J Pathol*. 1967;51:735-756.
22. Kassis AI, Warren KS, Mahmoud AAF. The *Schistosoma haematobium* egg granuloma. *Cell Immunol*. 1978;38:310-318.

23. Hoffmann KF, Wynn TA, Dunne DW. Cytokine-mediated host responses during schistosome infections: walking the fine line between immunological control and immunopathology. *Adv Parasitol*. 2002;52:265-307.
24. Johnston MJG, MacDonald JA, McKay DM. Parasitic helminths: a pharmacopeia of anti-inflammatory molecules. *Parasitology*. 2009;136:125-147.
25. Karanja DMS, Boyer AE, Strand M, et al. Studies on schistomiasis in western Kenya. I. Evidence for immune-facilitated excretion of schistosome eggs from patients with *Schistosoma mansoni* and human immunodeficiency virus coinfections. *Am J Trop Med Hyg*. 1997;56:515-521.
26. Cheever AW. A quantitative post-mortem study of schistosomiasis mansoni in man. *Am J Trop Med Hyg*. 1968;17:38-64.
27. Abdel Salam E, Abdel Fattah M. Prevalence and morbidity of *Schistosoma haematobium* in Egyptian children: a controlled study. *Am J Trop Med Hyg*. 1977;26:463-469.
28. Siongok TKA, Mahmoud AAF, Ouma JH, et al. Morbidity in schistosomiasis mansoni in relation to intensity of infection: study of a community in Machakos, Kenya. *Am J Trop Med Hyg*. 1976;25:273-284.
29. Karanja DMS, Hightower AW, Colley DG, et al. Resistance to reinfection with *Schistosoma mansoni* in occupationally exposed adults and effect of HIV-1 co-infection on susceptibility to schistosomiasis: a longitudinal study. *Lancet*. 2002;360:592-596.
30. Brooker S, Akhwale W, Pullan R, et al. Epidemiology of plasmodium-helminth co-infection in Africa: populations at risk,

potential impact on anemia and prospects for combining control. *Am J Trop Med Hyg*. 2007;77(6 Suppl.):88-98.
31. Kamal SM, Khalifa ES. Immune modulation by helminthic infections: worms and viral infections. *Parasite Immunol*. 2006;28:483-496.
32. Ellis MK, Zhao ZZ, Chen HG, et al. Analysis of the 5q31-33 locus shows an association between single nucleotide polymorphism variants in the IL-5 gene and symptomatic infection with the human blood fluke, *Schistosoma japonicum*. *J Immunol*. 2007; 179:8366–8371.
33. Secor WE. Immunology of human schistosomiasis: off the beaten path. *Parasite Immunol*. 2005;27:309-316.
34. Carod-Artal FJ. Neurological complications of *Schistosoma* infection. *Trans R S Trop Med Hyg*. 2008;102:107.
35. Jaureguiberry S, Ansart S, Perez L, et al. Acute neuroschistosomiasis: two cases associated with cerebral vasculitis. *Am J Trop Med Hyg*. 2007;76:964-966.
36. King CH, Dickman K, Tisch DJ. Reassessment of the cost of chronic helminthic infection: a meta-analysis of disability-related outcomes in endemic schistosomiasis. *Lancet*. 2005;365: 1561-1569.
37. Friedman JF, Mital P, Kanzaria HK, et al. Schistosomiasis and pregnancy. *Trends Parasitol*. 2007;23:159-164.
38. King CH, Dangerfield-Cha M. The unacknowledged impact of chronic schistosomiasis. *Chronic Illn*. 2008;4:65-79.
39. Prata A. Disease in schistosomiasis mansoni in Brazil. In: Mahmoud AAF, ed. *Schistosomiasis*. London: Imperial College Press; 2001:297-332.
40. Olveda RM. Disease in schistosomiasis japonica. In: Mahmoud AAF, ed. *Schistosomiasis*. London: Imperial College Press; 2001:361-390.
41. Lamyman MJ, Noble DJ, Narang S, et al. Small bowel obstruction secondary to intestinal schistosomiasis. *Trans R Soc Trop Med Hyg*. 2006;100:885-887.
42. Madbouly KM, Senagore AJ, Mukerjee A. Colorectal cancer in a population with endemic *Schistosoma mansoni*: is this an at-risk population. *Int J Colorectal Dis*. 2007;22:175-181.
43. Mies S, Neto OB, Beear A Jr. Systemic and hepatic hemodynamics in hepatosplenic Manson's schistosomiasis with and without propranolol. *Dig Dis Sci*. 1997;42:751-761.
44. Angelico M, Renganathan E, Gandin C, et al. Chronic liver disease in the Alexandria governorate, Egypt: contribution of schistosomiasis and hepatitis virus infection. *J Hepatol*. 1997;26: 236-243.
45. King CH. Disease due to *Schistosoma mekongi, S. intercalatum* and other schistosome species. In: Mahmoud AAF, ed. *Schistosomiasis*. London: Imperial College Press; 2001:391-412.
46. Urbani C, Sinoun M, Socheat D, et al. Epidemiology and control of mekongi schistosomiasis. *Acta Trop*. 2002;82:157-168.
47. King CH. Disease in schistosomiasis haematobia. In: Mahmoud AAF, ed. *Schistosomiasis*. London: Imperial College Press; 2001:265-295.
48. Barsoum RS. Schistosomiasis and the kidney. *Semin Nephrol*. 2003;23:34-41.
49. Kjetland EF, Ndhlovu PD, Mduluza T, et al. Simple clinical manifestations of genital *Schistosoma haematobium* infection in rural Zimbabwean women. *Am J Trop Med Hyg*. 2005;72: 311-319.
50. Kjetland EF, Ndhlovu PD, Mduluza T, et al. Genital schistosomiasis in women: a clinical 12-month in vivo study following treatment with praziquantel. *Trans R Soc Trop Med Hyg*. 2006;100:740-752.
51. Leutscher PD, Ramarokoto CE, Hoffmann S, et al. Coexistence of urogenital schistosomiasis and sexually transmitted infection in women and men living in an area where *Schistosoma haematobium* is endemic. *Clin Infect Dis*. 2008;47:775-782.
52. Schwartz E, Pick N, Shazberg G, et al. Hematospermia due to schistosome infection in travelers: diagnostic and treatment challenges. *Clin Infect Dis*. 2002;35:1420-1424.
53. Bedwani R, Renegenathan E, El Kwhsky F, et al. Schistosomiasis and the risk of bladder cancer in Alexandria, Egypt. *Br J Cancer*. 1998;77:1186-1189.
54. Badawi AF. Molecular and genetic events in schistosomiasis-associated human bladder cancer: role of oncogenes and tumor suppressor genes. *Cancer Lett*. 1996;105:123-138.
55. Moms W, Knaur CM. Cardiopulmonary manifestations of schistosomiasis. *Semin Respir Infect*. 1997;12:159-170.
56. Schwartz E. Pulmonary schistosomiasis. *Clin Chest Med*. 2002;23:433-443.
57. Butrous G, Ghofrani HA, Grimminger F. Pulmonary vascular disease in the developing world. *Circulation*. 2008;118: 1758-1766.
58. Pitella JE. Neuroschistosomiasis. *Brain Pathol*. 1997;7:649-662.
59. Young SW, Higashi G, Kamel R, et al. Interaction of salmonellae and schistosomes in host parasite relations. *Trans R Soc Trop Med Hyg*. 1973;67:797-802.
60. Frank C, Mohamed MK, Strickland GT, et al. The role of parenteral antischistosomal therapy in the spread of hepatitis C virus in Egypt. *Lancet*. 2000;355:887-891.
61. Kallestrup P, Zinyama R, Gomo E, et al. Schistosomiasis and HIV in rural Zimbabwe: effect of treatment of schistosomiasis on CD4 cell count and plasma HIV-1 RNA load. *J Infect Dis*. 2005;192:1956-1961.
62. Kallestrup P, Zinyama R, Gomo E, et al. Schistosomiasis and HIV in rural Zimbabwe: efficacy of treatment of schistosomiasis in individuals with HIV co-infection. *Clin Infect Dis*. 2006;42:1781-1789.
63. de Silva S, Walsh J, Brown M. Symptomatic *Schistosoma mansoni* infection as an immune restoration phenomenon in a patient receiving antiretroviral therapy. *Clin Infect Dis*. 2006;42:303-304.
64. Midzi N, Butterworth AE, Mduluza T, et al. Use of circulating cathodic antigen strips for the diagnosis of urinary schistosomiasis. *Trans R Soc Trop Med Hyg*. 2009;103:45-51.
65. ten Hove RJ, Verweij JJ, Vereecken K, et al. Multiplex real-time PCR for the detection and quantification of *Schistosoma mansoni* and *S. haematobium* infection in stool samples collected in northern Senegal. *Trans R Soc Trop Med Hyg*. 2008;102:179-185.
66. Tsang VC, Wilkins PP. Immunodiagnosis of schistosomiasis. *Immunol Invest*. 1997;26:175-186.
67. Medhat A, Zarzoura A, Nafeh M, et al. Evaluation of an ultrasonographic score for urinary bladder morbidity in *Schistosoma hematobium* infection. *Am J Trop Med Hyg*. 1997;57: 16-19.
68. Gerapacher-Lara R, Pinto-Silva RA, Rayes AA, et al. Ultrasonography of periportal fibrosis in schistosomiasis mansoni in Brazil. *Trans R Soc Trop Med Hyg*. 1997;91:307-309.
69. Thomas AK, Dittrich M, Kardorff R, et al. Evaluation of ultrasonographic staging systems for the assessment of *Schistosoma mansoni* induced hepatic involvement. *Acta Trop*. 1997;68: 347-356.
70. Fenwick A, Savioli L, Engels D, et al. Drugs for the control of parasitic diseases: current status and development in schistosomiasis. *Trends Parasitol*. 2003;19:509-515.
71. Berhe N, Myrvang B, Gundersen SG. Reversibility of schistosomal periportal thickening/fibrosis after praziquantel therapy: a twenty month follow-up study in Ethiopia. *Am J Trop Med Hyg*, 2008;78:228-234.
72. Richter J. The impact of chemotherapy on morbidity due to schistosomiasis. *Acta Trop*. 2003;86:161-183.
73. Kjetland EF, Ndhlovu PD, Kurewa EN, et al. Prevention of gynecologic contact bleeding and genital sandy patches by childhood anti-schistosomal treatment. *Am J Trop Med Hyg*. 2008;79: 79-83.
74. Caffrey, CR. Chemotherapy of schistosomiasis: Present and future. *Curr Opin Chem Biol*. 2007;11:433-439.
75. Ismail M, Metwally A, Fargholy A, et al. Characterization of isolates of *Schistosoma mansoni* from Egyptian villagers that tolerate high doses of praziquantel. *Am J Trop Med Hyg*. 1996;55:214-218.
76. Bennett JL, Dan T, Liang FT, et al. The development of resistance to antihelminthics: a perspective with an emphasis on the antischistosomal drug praziquantel. *Exp Parasitol*. 1997;87: 260-267.
77. Grandiere-Perez L, Ansart S, Paris L, et al. Efficacy of praziquantel during the incubation and invasive phase of *Schistosoma haematobium* schistosomiasis in 18 travellers. *Am J Trop Med Hyg*. 2006;74:814-818.
78. Ismail M, Botros S, Metwally A, et al. Resistance to praziquantel: direct evidence from *Schistosoma mansoni* isolated from Egyptian villagers. *Am J Trop Med Hyg*. 1999;60:932-935.
79. Alonso D, Munoz J, Gascon J, et al. Failure of standard treatment with praziquantel in two returned travelers with *Schistosoma haematobium* infection. *Am J Trop Med Hyg*. 2006;74:342-344.
80. Olds GR. Administration of praziquantel to pregnant and lactating women. *Acta Trop*. 2003;86:185-195.
81. Ferrari ML, Coelho PM, Antunes CM, et al. Efficacy of oxamniquine and praziquantel in the treatment of *Schistosoma mansoni* infection: a controlled trial. *Bull World Health Organ*. 2003;81:190-196.
82. Utzinger J, Shushua X, N'Goran EK, et al. The potential of artemether for the control of schistosomiasis. *Int J Parasitol*. 2001;31:1549-1562.
83. Utzinger J, Keiser J, Shuhua X, et al. Combination chemotherapy of schistosomiasis in laboratory studies and clinical trials. *Antimicrob Agents Chemother*. 2003;47:1487-1495.
84. Boulanger D, Dieng Y, Cisse B, et al. Antischistosomal efficacy of artusenate combination therapies administered as curative treatments for malaria attacks. *Trans R Soc Trop Med Hyg*. 2007;101:113-116.
85. Inyang-Etoh PC, Ejezie GC, Useh MF, et al. Efficacy of a combination of praziquantel and artesunate in the treatment of urinary schistosomiasis in Nigeria. 2009; *Trans R Soc Trop Med Hyg*. 2007;103:38-44.
86. Jaureguiberry S, Caumes E. Neurological involvement during Katayama syndrome. *Lancet Infect Dis*. 2008;8:9-10.
87. Utzinger J, Bergquist R, Shu-Hua X, et al. Sustainable schistosomiasis control—the way forward. *Lancet*. 2003;362:1932-1934.
88. Bergquist NR. Schistosomiasis: from risk assessment to control. *Trends Parasitol*. 2002;18:309-314.
89. Wang LD, Chen HG, Guo JG, et al. A strategy to control transmission of *Schistosoma japonicum* in China. *N Engl J Med*. 2009;360:121-128.
90. McManus DP, Loukas A. Current status of vaccines for schistosomiasis. *Clin Microbiol Rev*. 2008;21:225-242.
91. Siddiqui AA, Ahmad G, Damian RT, et al. *Parasitol Res*. 2008;102:825-833.
92. Liu LX, Harinasuta KT. Liver and intestinal flukes. *Gastroenterol Clin North Am*. 1996;25:627-636.
93. Kaewkes S. Taxonomy and biology of liver flukes. *Acta Trop*. 2003;88:177-186.
94. Haridy FM, Morsy TA, Ibrahim BB, et al. A preliminary study on dicrocoeliosis in Egypt, with a general review. *J Egypt Soc Parasitol*. 2003;33:85-96.
95. Sing A. On ants and men (an anthology). *Clin Infect Dis*. 2007;44:145-146.
96. Upatham ES, Viyanant V. *Opisthorchis viverrini* and opisthorchiasis: a historical review and future perspective. *Acta Trop*. 2003;88:171-176.
97. Chai J-Y, Murrell KD, Lymbery AJ. Fish-borne parasitic zoonoses: status and issues. *Int J Parasitol*. 2005;35:1233-1254.
98. Sithithaworn P, Haswell-Elkins M. Epidemiology of *Opisthorchis viverrini*. *Acta Trop*. 2003;88:187-189.
99. Lun ZR, Gasser RB, Lai DH. Clonorchiasis: a key foodborne zoonosis in China. *Lancet Infect Dis*. 2005;5:31-41.
100. Mairiang E, Mairiang P. Clinical manifestation of opisthorchiasis and treatment. *Acta Trop*. 2003;88:221-227.
101. Chan HH, Lai KH, Lo GH, et al. The clinical and cholangiographic picture of hepatic clonorchiasis. *J Clin Gastroenterol*. 2002;34:183-186.
102. Leung JW, Yu AS. Hepatolithiasis and biliary parasites. *Baillieres Clin Gastroenterol*. 1997;11:681-706.
103. Wutanapa P. Cholangiocarcinoma in patients with opisthorchiasis. *Br J Surg*. 1996;83:1062-1064.
104. Thuluvath PJ, Rai R, Venbrux AC, et al. Cholangiocarcinoma: a review. *Gastroenterologist*. 1997;5:306-315.
105. Lim JH, Kim SY, Park CM. Parasitic diseases of the biliary tract. *AJR Am J Roentgenol*. 2007;188:1596-1603.
106. Keiser J, Utzinger J. Food-borne trematodiasis: current chemotherapy and advances with artemisinins and synthetic trioxolanes. *Trends Parasitol*. 2007;23:605-612.
107. Pungpak S, Viravan C, Radomyos B, et al. *Opisthorchiasis viverrini* infection in Thailand: studies on the morbidity of the infection and resolution following praziquantel treatment. *Am J Trop Med Hyg*. 1997;56:311-314.
108. Mas-Coma S, Bargues MD, Valero MA. Fascioliasis and other plant-borne trematode zoonoses. *Int J Parasitol*. 2005;35: 1255-1278.
109. Esteban JG, Flores A, Angles R, et al. High endemicity of human fascioliasis between Lake Titicaca and La Paz Valley, Bolivia. *Trans R Soc Trop Med Hyg*. 1999;93:151-156.
110. Estaban JG, Gonzalez C, Curtale F, et al. Hyperendemic fascioliasis associated with schistosomiasis in villages in the Nile Delta of Egypt. *Am J Trop Med Hyg*. 2003;69:429-437.
111. MacLean JD, Graeme-Cook FM. Case records of the Massachusetts General Hospital: weekly clinicopathological exercises. Case 12-2002: a 50-year-old man with eosinophilia and fluctuating hepatic lesions. *N Engl J Med*. 2002;346:1232-1239.
112. Graham CS, Brodie SB, Weller PF. Imported *Fasciola hepatica* infection in the United States and treatment with triclabendazole. *Clin Infect Dis*. 2001;33:1-5.
113. Pulpeiro JR, Armesto V, Varela J, et al. Fascioliasis: findings in 15 patients. *Br J Radiol*. 1991;64:798-801.
114. Van Beers B, Pringot J, Geuber A, et al. Hepatobiliary fascioliasis: noninvasive imaging findings. *Radiology*. 1990;174: 809-810.
115. Han JK, Han D, Choi BL, et al. MR findings in human fascioliasis. *Trop Med Int Health*. 1996;1:367-372.
116. Cosme A, Ojeda E, Poch M, et al. Sonographic findings of hepatic lesions in human fascioliasis. *J Clin Ultrasound*. 2003;31:358-363.
117. Cevikol C, Karaali K, Senol U, et al. Human fascioliasis: MR imaging findings of hepatic lesions. *Eur Radiol*. 2003;13: 141-148.
118. Hillyer GV, De Galanes MS, Rodriguez Perez J, et al. Use of the Falcon assay screening test enzyme-linked immunosorbent assay (FAST-ELISA) and the enzyme-linked immunoelectrotransfer blot (EITB) to determine the prevalence of human fascioliasis in the Bolivian Altiplano. *Am J Trop Med Hyg*. 1992;46: 603-609.
119. Millan JC, Mull R, Freise S, et al. The efficacy and tolerability of triclabendazole in Cuban patients with latent and chronic *Fasciola hepatica* infection. *Am J Trop Med Hyg*. 2000;63:264-269.
120. Richter J, Freise S, Mull R, et al. Fascioliasis: sonographic abnormalities of the biliary tract and evolution after treatment with triclabendazole. *Trop Med Int Health*. 1999;4:774-781.
121. Favennec L, Jave Ortiz J, Gargala G, et al. Double-blind, randomized, placebo-controlled study of nitazoxanide in the treatment of fascioliasis in adults and children from northern Peru. *Aliment Pharmacol Ther*. 2003;17:265-270.
122. Hien TT, Truong NT, Minh NH, et al. A randomized controlled pilot study of artesunate versus triclabendazole for human fascioliasis in ventral Vietnam. *Am J Trop Med Hyg*. 2008;78: 388-392.
123. Fried B, Graczk TK, Tamang L. Food-borne intestinal trematode infections. *Parasitol Res*. 2004;93:159-170.
124. Waikagul J. Intestinal fluke infections in Southeast Asia. *Southeast Asian J Trop Med Public Health*. 1991;22(Suppl):158-162.
125. Graczyk TK, Gilman RH, Fried B. Fasciolopsiasis: is it a controllable food-borne disease? *Parasitol Res*. 2001;87:80-83.
126. Belizario VY Jr, Bersabe MJ, de Leon WU, et al. Intestinal heterophydiasis: an emerging food-borne parasitic zoonosis in southern Philippines. *Southeast Asian J Trop Med Public Health*. 2001;32(Suppl 2):36-42.
127. Blair D, Xu ZB, Agatsuma T. Paragonimiasis and the genus *Paragonimus*. *Adv Parasitol*. 1999;42:113-222.
128. Liu Q, Wei F, Liu, W, et al. Paragonimiasis: an important food-borne zoonosis in China. *Parasitol Today*. 2008;318-323.

129. DeFrain M, Hooker R. North American paragonimiasis: case report of a severe clinical infection. *Chest*. 2002;121:1368-1372.
130. Procop GW, Marty AM, Scheck DN, et al. North American paragonimiasis: a case report. *Acta Cytol*. 2000;44:75-80.
131. Kagawa FT. Pulmonary paragonimiasis. *Semin Respir Infect*. 1997;12:149-158.
132. Im JG, Chang KH, Reeder MM. Current diagnostic imaging of pulmonary and cerebral paragonimiasis with pathological correlation. *Semin Roentgenol*. 1997;32:301-324.
133. Mukae O, Taniguchi H, Ashitani J, et al. Case report: paragonimiasis westermani with seroconversion from immunoglobulin (Ig) M to IgG antibody with the clinical course. *Am J Trop Med Hyg*. 2001;65:837-839.
134. Slemenda SB, Maddison SE, Jong EC, et al. Diagnosis of paragonimiasis by immunoblot. *Am J Trop Med Hyg*. 1988;39:469-471.
135. Calvopina M, Guderian RH, Paredes W, et al. Treatment of human pulmonary paragonimiasis with triclabendazole: clinical tolerance and drug efficacy. *Trans R Soc Trop Med Hyg*. 1998;92:566-569.

290

Cestodes (Tapeworms)

CHARLES H. KING | JESSICA K. FAIRLEY

In humans, parasitic cestode infections occur in either of two forms: as mature tapeworms residing in the gastrointestinal tract or as one or more larval cysts (variously called hydatidosis, cysticercosis, coenurosis, or sparganosis) embedded in liver, lung, muscle, brain, eye, or other tissues.[1,2] The form taken by the infecting parasite depends on which cestode species causes the infection and, to a lesser extent, on the route by which the infection was acquired. Table 290-1 summarizes the common cestode parasites of humans, their typical vectors, and their usual symptoms.

This chapter begins with a discussion of parasite biology and the immunology of cestode infection followed by a description of individual parasite species: intestinal tapeworms (e.g., *Diphyllobothrium latum*, *Hymenolepis nana*, *Taenia saginata*, and *Taenia solium*) and invasive cestode parasites (cysticercosis [*T. solium*], hydatid and alveolar cyst disease [*Echinococcus* spp.], sparganosis, and coenurosis [*Taenia multiceps*]). Diagnosis and therapy, outlined briefly under the individual parasite headings, are discussed in greater detail at the end of each section.

Cestode Biology

PARASITE LIFE CYCLE

The parasitic cestodes discussed in this chapter are flatworms (platyhelminths) of the orders Pseudophyllidea (*Diphyllobothrium* and *Spirometra*) and Cyclophyllidea (other species), which divide their life cycle between two animal hosts (Fig. 290-1).[1,2] As mature tapeworms, these parasites reside in the intestinal tract of a definitive host, a carnivorous mammal. Depending on the parasite species, mature tapeworms vary in size from several millimeters (*Echinococcus* spp.) to 25 m (*Diphyllobothrium*).[1]

The tapeworm consists of several parts: a head (*scolex*), a neck, and a tail. The head has two or more suckers and in some cases a *rostellum*, or knob of small hooks, used to attach to the wall of the host's intestine (Fig. 290-2A).[3] The scolex is connected by a short neck to the lower portion of the tapeworm, the *strobila*, which is a ribbon-like chain of independent, but connected, segments called *proglottids* (see Fig. 290-2B). Each proglottid has both male and female sexual organs and is responsible for producing the parasite's eggs. Proglottids begin to develop in the neck region of the parasite and then mature and move downward in the strobila as new segments are added from above. The hermaphroditic proglottids become gravid and eventually break free of the tapeworm. Proglottids may degenerate in the stool, releasing eggs (thousands to millions per day) into the feces. Alternatively, intact proglottids may be passed in the stool, with egg release occurring outside the body. In some cases, a section of strobila may be passed in a single day, with no further release of proglottids for several days thereafter. In practical terms, this means that although the number of tapeworm eggs in the stool is usually high, detection of parasite eggs by standard stool examination may be sporadic. It therefore may require multiple stool samples, rectal swabs, and visual examination of stool and perineum for proglottids to detect a tapeworm infection. For some species of tapeworm (e.g., *T. saginata*), the proglottids are motile. They may migrate within the gastrointestinal tract, causing biliary or appendiceal obstruction, or out of the body, to be found in the perineum.

At the point at which eggs are released, two effective biotypes of parasite can be defined. If the eggs released from the parasite are partially developed, they are called *embryonated*. If the egg embryo has not yet begun its differentiation, the egg is referred to as *nonembryonated*. In biologic terms, the embryonated egg can immediately infect the next intermediate mammalian or insect host, typically a herbivore or omnivore, through ingestion of food containing the egg.[1] Such eggs, typical of *Echinococcus* spp., *Taenia* spp., and *H. nana*, may lie dormant in grazing areas or become scattered in the home environment and remain infectious for several months to years.[1,4] Once ingested, the egg hatches in the intermediate host's intestine, releasing an *oncosphere*, which penetrates the gut mucosa to reach the circulation. The oncosphere passes to any of several organs to form a parasite cyst, which is variously called a cysticercoid, cysticercus, alveolar cyst, or hydatid cyst, depending on its morphology. The life cycle of these parasites is completed when the carnivorous definitive host consumes the cyst-infected tissues of the intermediate host and the cyst develops into a mature tapeworm in the lumen of the definitive host's intestine.

For nonembryonated eggs, such as those of the fish tapeworm *D. latum*, initial development takes place outside the body in water, after which the eggs hatch to release a free-swimming *coracidium* larva.[5] In time, the coracidium is ingested by a small crustacean called a copepod and then develops into a procercoid larva within the copepod's tissues. When the copepod, in turn, is ingested by a fish or other intermediate host, the procercoid infects its musculature, developing into the next larval stage, the *plerocercoid* cyst, or *sparganum*. If an uncooked plerocercoid of *D. latum* is ingested by a human, its definitive host, it develops into a mature, intraluminal "fish tapeworm." However, if the fish containing the plerocercoid is ingested by another, larger fish, it does not become a tapeworm. It reencysts instead as a plerocercoid in the muscles of the second, larger fish.

Plerocercoid encystment or reencystment is significant in terms of human disease (as *sparganosis*) for cestode species for which humans cannot serve as the definitive host (e.g., *Spirometra mansonoides*, a tapeworm of dogs and felines). Plerocercoids can develop in human tissues if *Spirometra*-infested copepods are ingested in drinking water. Alternatively, human plerocercoid cysts may be acquired via the intestine from another intermediate host (e.g., tadpole, frog, and snake) if the meat of that aquatic host is eaten uncooked. Migrating plerocercoid cysts can also transfer directly into the skin or the eye if raw flesh of an aquatic intermediate host is used as a poultice in traditional healing.[5]

As a rule, humans are either definitive or intermediate hosts for a given cestode parasite, but not both. For example, humans are solely definitive hosts (i.e., with tapeworms) for *D. latum* (the fish tapeworm) and *T. saginata* ("beef tapeworm") and are solely intermediate hosts for *Echinococcus* spp. (hydatid cysts and alveolar cysts), *Spirometra* (sparganosis), and *T. multiceps* (coenurosis). There are two exceptions to this rule. The first is *T. solium*, which develops in humans as a cysticercus if ingested as an egg or as a tapeworm if ingested as a cysticercus in infected pork. It is thus possible for one patient to harbor both cyst and tapeworm forms of *T. solium*. Such dual infection is seen in approximately 25% of cysticercosis cases. The second exception is the dwarf tapeworm, *H. nana*, whose eggs after ingestion hatch in the gut and encyst within the wall of the human intestine. After 5 to 7 days, the cyst breaks open and the larva develops (within the same host) to become a mature tapeworm. The fertile eggs of this tapeworm may directly infect the mucosa, permitting a continued increase in the number of tapeworms in the affected host, without further exposure to environmental egg contamination. In this manner, humans serve as both intermediate and definitive hosts for *H. nana*. It should be stressed that single-host proliferation such as that of *H. nana* is highly

	TABLE 290-1	**Common Cestode Parasites of Humans, Their Typical Vectors, and Their Usual Symptoms**			
Parasite Species	*Developmental Stage Found in Humans*	*Common Name*	*Transmission Source*	*Symptoms Associated with Infection*	
Diphyllobothrium latum	Tapeworm	Fish tapeworm	Plerocercoid cysts in freshwater fish	Usually minimal; with prolonged or heavy infection, vitamin B_{12} deficiency	
Hymenolepis nana	Tapeworm, cysticercoids	Dwarf tapeworm	Infected humans	Mild abdominal discomfort	
Taenia saginata	Tapeworm	Beef tapeworm	Cysts in beef	Abdominal discomfort, proglottid migration	
Taenia solium	Tapeworm	Pork tapeworm	Cysticerci in pork	Minimal	
Taenia solium (Cysticercus cellulosae)	Cysticerci	Cysticercosis	Eggs from infected humans	Local inflammation, mass effect; if in CNS, seizures, hydrocephalus, arachnoiditis	
Echinococcus granulosus	Larval cysts	Hydatid cyst disease	Eggs from infected dogs	Mass effect leading to pain, obstruction of adjacent organs; less commonly, secondary bacterial infection, distal spread of daughter cysts	
Echinococcus multilocularis	Larval cysts	Alveolar cyst disease	Eggs from infected canines	Local invasion and mass effect leading to organ dysfunction; distal metastasis possible	
Taenia multiceps	Larval cysts	Coenurosis, bladder worm	Eggs from infected dogs	Local inflammation and mass effect	
Spirometra mansonoides	Larval cysts	Sparganosis	Cysts from infected copepods, frogs, snakes	Local inflammation and mass effect	

CNS, central nervous system.

unusual among human cestode infections and helminth infections in general. Normally, heavy cestode infections can be acquired only by repeated environmental exposure to eggs or infectious parasite cysts.

DISEASE PATHOGENESIS AND IMMUNOLOGY

Adult tapeworms in the intestinal tract generally cause minimal local pathology. Reduced nutrient absorption and alteration of gut motility have been described, but there is no firm association of adult tapeworm infection with specific bowel symptoms. An immune response to adult tapeworms provokes eosinophilia and immunoglobulin E (IgE) elevation in some patients, but the immune response does not appear to alter the course of an intraluminal tapeworm infection. In light of the limited range of potential hosts observed for most adult tapeworms, it has been suggested that host factors, including the presence or absence of specific immunoreactivity, may determine the success of parasite infections in various potential host species.[6]

The immune response to invasive cyst infection is more pronounced but is often unsuccessful in eradicating the cyst in susceptible hosts.

Infiltration with neutrophils and eosinophils is followed by local fibrosis, leading to cyst encapsulation and macrophage infiltration. Once the cyst is encapsulated, antigen release may be limited, leading to a reduction in the local inflammatory response. Specific antibody production remains detectable in the serum, however, and delayed-type hypersensitivity may be detected on skin testing. The immune response often increases later as the cyst begins to die and leak antigen or as it erodes into a body cavity, duct, or vessel, increasing local or systemic exposure to antigen. Experimentally, the anticyst immune response appears to limit dissemination of *Echinococcus* spp. after an initial infection.[6,7] Anticyst immunity is also likely to contribute to the spontaneous clearance of *H. nana* infection in older children. There is evidence of increased amounts of IgG subclasses as well as proinflammatory cytokines within the cerebrospinal fluid (CSF) of patients having severe neurocysticercosis.[8] It is unclear if this response contributes to the severity of the disease or is a consequence of severe infection; however, it does not effectively control the infection. Furthermore, symptomatic cysticercosis appears to be related to a depressed cellular immune response compared to the immune response of asymptomatic individuals.[8]

Intestinal Tapeworm Infections

DIPHYLLOBOTHRIUM LATUM

Diphyllobothrium latum, or fish tapeworm, is one of the pseudophyllidean cestodes transmitted via aquatic species.[5] Human infection with *D. latum* is acquired by eating uncooked freshwater fish containing the parasite's plerocercoid cysts. Some traditional modes of infection include consumption of dried or smoked fish, which may contain viable cysts if not further cooked, or tasting flavored freshwater fish (e.g., gefilte fish) before cooking. The enthusiasm for "raw bar" foods such as ceviche, sushi, and sashimi prepared from freshwater fish, especially salmon, has increased the transmission potential for *D. latum* in developed areas of North America.[9,10] Areas of the world in which *D. latum* is highly endemic (more than 2% prevalence) include specific lake and delta areas of Siberia, Europe (especially Scandinavia and other Baltic countries), North America, Japan, and Chile. In 2006, there was an outbreak in Lake Geneva, Switzerland, due to freshly caught raw perch served at a wedding.[11] Endemicity in rural areas is favored by stable zoonotic transmission through alternative nonhuman definitive hosts, including seals, cats, bears, minks, foxes, and wolves.

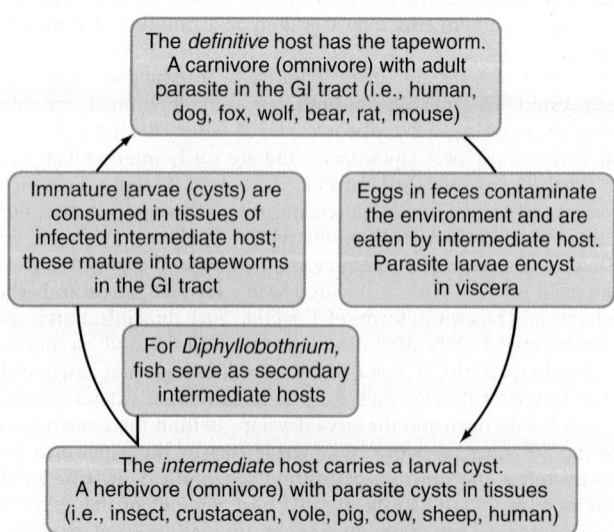

The *definitive* host has the tapeworm. A carnivore (omnivore) with adult parasite in the GI tract (i.e., human, dog, fox, wolf, bear, rat, mouse)

Immature larvae (cysts) are consumed in tissues of infected intermediate host; these mature into tapeworms in the GI tract

Eggs in feces contaminate the environment and are eaten by intermediate host. Parasite larvae encyst in viscera

For *Diphyllobothrium*, fish serve as secondary intermediate hosts

The *intermediate* host carries a larval cyst. A herbivore (omnivore) with parasite cysts in tissues (i.e., insect, crustacean, vole, pig, cow, sheep, human)

Figure 290-1 **Cestode parasites alternate larval and adult stages in two different hosts.**

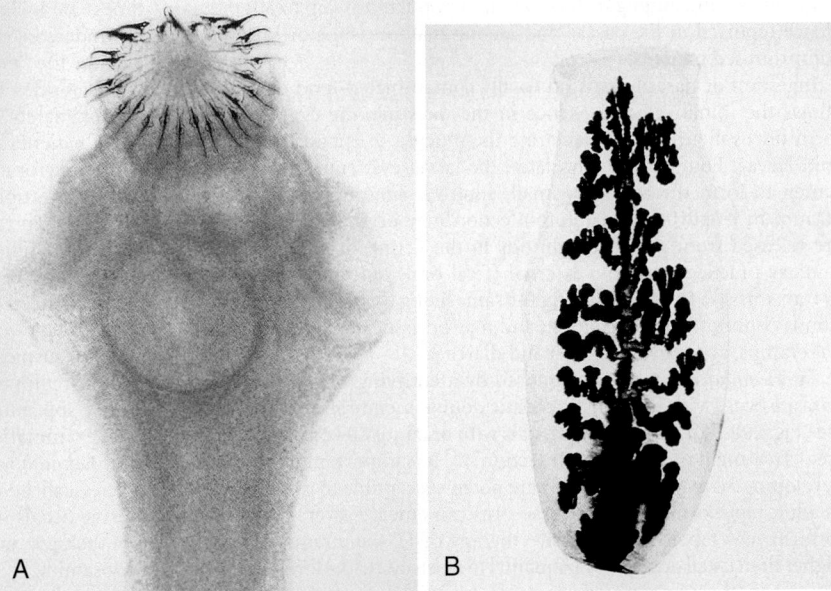

Figure 290-2 The scolex (**A**) and a proglottid (**B**) of the cestode *T. solium*. *(From Ash LR, Orihel TC. Atlas of Human Parasitology. 3rd ed. Chicago: ASCP; 1990.)*

Human *D. latum* tapeworms are large, reaching up to 25 m (3000 to 4000 proglottids) in length. It takes 3 to 6 weeks after exposure for the tapeworm to mature. Once established, a *D. latum* parasite may survive 30 years or more. Multiple tapeworms in the same patient are common. Normally, infection is asymptomatic, but a proportion of infected individuals report nonspecific symptoms of weakness (66%), dizziness (53%), salt craving (62%), diarrhea (22%), and intermittent abdominal discomfort.[5]

Prolonged (more than 3 or 4 years) or heavy *D. latum* infection may lead to megaloblastic anemia caused by vitamin B_{12} deficiency. The vitamin B_{12} deficiency is a consequence of two factors: parasite-mediated dissociation of the vitamin B_{12}–intrinsic factor complex in the gut lumen (making vitamin B_{12} unavailable to the host) and heavy vitamin uptake and use by the parasite. Megaloblastic anemia may be worsened by concurrent folate deficiency, which also occurs as a consequence of *D. latum* infection. Vitamin B_{12} deficiency may be sufficiently severe to cause injury to the nervous system, including peripheral neuropathy and severe combined degeneration of the central nervous system (CNS).

For diagnosis, tapeworm infection may first be suspected based on the patient's history or when contrast studies of the intestine show an intraluminal, ribbon-like filling defect. Definitive diagnosis of *D. latum* infection is made by detection of 45 × 65-mm operculated parasite eggs on stool examination (Fig. 290-3A and B). Recovery of proglottids (with a characteristic central uterus) also establishes the diagnosis.

Treatment is with a single course of niclosamide or praziquantel (see "Treatment of Tapeworm Infection").[12] Mild vitamin B_{12} deficiency is reversed by eradicating the tapeworm. Severe vitamin B_{12} deficiency should be treated with parenteral vitamin injections. If a patient presents with B_{12} deficiency and epidemiologic risk factors for fish tapeworm infection, one should maintain a high index of suspicion for possible infection.

HYMENOLEPIS NANA

Hymenolepis nana, also known as dwarf tapeworm, is a cyclophyllidean tapeworm with embryonated eggs.[5] It is probably the most prevalent tapeworm worldwide, and it is the only tapeworm that can be transmitted directly from human to human. Areas of endemicity (up to 26% prevalence) include Asia, southern and eastern Europe, Central and South America, and Africa. In North America, infection is most

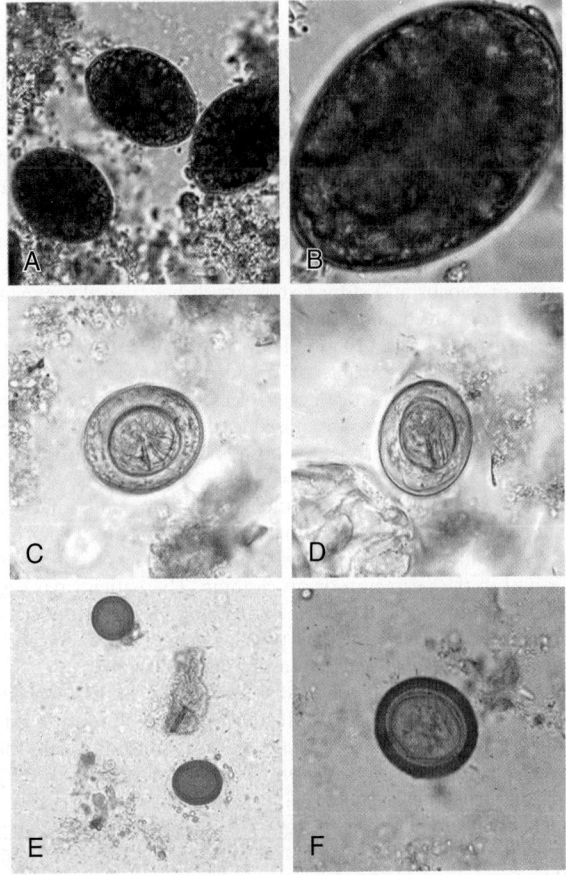

Figure 290-3 **A** and **B,** Eggs of *D. latum* (55 to 75 μm × 40 to 50 μm) in an iodine-stained wet mount. Note the knob at the abopercular end in **B. C** and **D,** Eggs of *H. nana* (30 to 50 μm) in an unstained wet mount. Note the presence of hooks in the oncosphere and polar filaments within the space between the oncosphere and outer shell. **E** and **F,** *Taenia* spp. eggs (30 to 35 μm) in unstained wet mounts. The eggs of *T. solium* and *T. saginata* are indistinguishable from each other, as well as from other members of the Taeniidae.

frequently found among institutionalized populations (up to 8% prevalence reported in the past)[13] and among malnourished or immunocompromised patients.

Ingestion of parasite eggs on fecally contaminated food or fomites allows the initial infection. Once in the intestine, the eggs hatch to form oncospheres, which penetrate the mucosa to encyst as cysticercoid larvae. Four or five days later, the larval cyst ruptures into the lumen to form the relatively small, adult *H. nana* tapeworm (15 to 50 mm in length). Internal autoinfection may occur as parasite eggs are released from gravid proglottids in the ileum. In addition, poor sanitary practices promote external (fecal-oral) autoinfection as well as transmission to others sharing the same living quarters. Heavy infection is common among children and may be associated with abdominal cramps, anorexia, dizziness, and diarrhea.

An *H. nana* infection is diagnosed by identifying the 30 × 47-mm parasite eggs (with their characteristic double membrane) in the stool (see Fig. 290-3C and D). Treatment is with praziquantel or niclosamide (see "Treatment of Tapeworm Infection").[12] It is important to note that developing *H. nana* cysticercoids are not as susceptible to drug therapy as adult tapeworms. Because these cysts can emerge several days later to form new tapeworms, effective therapy of *H. nana* requires either higher than usual doses of praziquantel to reach cysticidal levels or more prolonged therapy with niclosamide (to eliminate emerging tapeworms) for a period of 5 to 7 days. Nitazoxanide has also been used to treat infection, appears to be highly effective, and has been used as an alternative therapy after treatment failures with niclosamide.[14]

TAENIA SAGINATA

Taenia saginata, known as the beef tapeworm, is transmitted to humans in the form of infectious larval cysts found in the meat of cattle, which serve as the parasite's usual intermediate host.[1,5] The *T. saginata* tapeworm is common in cattle-breeding areas of the world. The areas with the highest prevalence (up to 27%) are in central Asia, the Near East, and Central and East Africa. Areas of lower prevalence (<1%) are found in Europe, Southeast Asia, Central America, and South America. Consumption of "measly" (i.e., cyst-infected) uncooked or undercooked beef is the usual means of transmission. Rare steak or kebabs and steak tartare are dishes typically associated with *T. saginata* infection. In the definitive human host, adult *T. saginata* tapeworms are large (10 m in length) and can contain more than 1000 proglottids, each capable of producing thousands of eggs. If, through poor sanitary practices, eggs released in the feces are allowed to reach grazing areas, cattle are subsequently infected with *T. saginata* cysticerci. Alternative intermediate hosts include llamas, buffalo, and giraffes.

Symptoms are absent in most patients with *T. saginata* infection. A small number report mild abdominal cramps or malaise. The proglottids of *T. saginata* are motile and occasionally migrate out of the anus, to be found in the perineum or on clothing. The patient may report seeing moving segments in the feces or passing several feet of strobila at one time. These events are often psychologically distressing and are associated with significant anxiety-associated symptoms.

Specific diagnosis of *T. saginata* infection can be established by recovery of parasite proglottids.[1,5] If only eggs are found in the stool, it is important to note that *T. saginata* eggs are morphologically indistinguishable from those of *T. solium* (see Fig. 290-3E and F). With *T. solium* tapeworms there is potential for autoinfection with cysticercosis; therefore, if any *Taenia* spp. eggs are detected, treatment should be given without delay for further speciation. Effective oral treatment for either *Taenia* spp. is obtained with praziquantel or niclosamide (see "Treatment of Tapeworm Infection").[12]

TAENIA SOLIUM

Humans can serve as either intermediate or definitive hosts for *T. solium*. Individuals who ingest *T. solium* eggs develop tissue infection with parasite cysts, a condition known as cysticercosis (details of this illness are included under "Cysticercosis"). Patients who consume raw or undercooked pork containing infectious larval cysts (cysticerci) acquire the "pork tapeworm"—that is, the adult form of *T. solium*, which resides in the intestinal tract.[1,5] These tapeworms develop to approximately 2 to 8 m in length and may survive for 10 to 20 years. Some patients harbor both cysticerci and *T. solium* tapeworms, and it is possible for a tapeworm-carrying individual to develop cysticercosis by autoinfection. Areas in which *T. solium* infection is endemic include Mexico, Central America, South America, Africa, Southeast Asia, India, the Philippines, and southern Europe.

Infection with *T. solium* tapeworms is generally asymptomatic unless cysticercosis, caused by autoinfection with parasite eggs, supervenes. If tapeworm infection is diagnosed, one should also have a high index of suspicion for concomitant cysticercosis. The proglottids of *T. solium* are not motile (unlike those of *T. saginata*) and do not migrate. *Taenia* spp. infection is readily diagnosed by detecting eggs during stool examination, but *T. solium* eggs are indistinguishable from those of *T. saginata* (see Fig. 290-3E and F). If a proglottid is recovered, the species can be identified based on the characteristic features of the uterine canals in the segment.[1,3] Species identification is not required for therapy, which can be achieved with either praziquantel or niclosamide.[12]

Other Species Causing Tapeworm Infection in Humans

Human tapeworm infection may also be caused by *Dipylidium caninum*, a more frequent parasite of dogs and cats, or by *Hymenolepis diminuta*, a tapeworm that usually infects rats.[1,5] Such infections are acquired by consumption of insects (fleas or beetles) containing the larval cysticercoids of these species and are most commonly seen among children. Human infection with tapeworm species related to *D. latum*—*Diphyllobothrium klebanovskii*, *Diphyllobothrium dendriticum*, *Diphyllobothrium ursi*, and *Diphyllobothrium dalliae*—has been described in the Arctic and areas of Siberia. *Diphyllobothrium nihonkainse*, common in Japan, is another related fish tapeworm that can cause infections in humans, and it has been reported in isolated cases in Europe after ingestion of imported fish.[15] *Taenia asiatica*, described in 1993 and confused with *T. saginata* in the past, is found in some countries of Southeast Asia. In contrast to *T. saginata* and *T. solium*, this parasite is viscerotropic and is transmissible through ingestion of visceral organs from pigs rather than from muscle.[16] Rarely, other tapeworm species infect humans, particularly individuals with unusual dietary habits, such as the consumption of uncooked animal viscera. Infection is diagnosed by identifying characteristic parasite eggs in the stool. Effective treatment is obtained with praziquantel or niclosamide.

Diagnosis of Tapeworm Infection

Because mature tapeworm infection is strictly an intraluminal intestinal infection, the most practical approach to diagnosis is examination of the feces for parasite eggs or proglottids. As discussed under "Cestode Biology," egg release in the stool may be variable because of an irregular rate of proglottid detachment and degeneration. Thus, examination of stool samples taken on several different days may be required to establish a diagnosis. Sensitivity for egg detection may be improved by formyl ethyl acetate or other concentration techniques. Because cestode eggs are relatively heavy, sedimentation procedures (not flotation) provide a more efficient means to isolate tapeworm eggs. When handling specimens, it is important to remember that *T. solium* eggs are infective for humans and cause cysticercosis. For this reason, precautions should be taken to avoid any potential contamination of fingers or clothing with parasite eggs.

In some cases, intact proglottids are passed in the stool. This is most common with *D. latum*, *T. saginata*, *T. solium*, and *D. caninum*. Expelled proglottids tend to degenerate over time, so fixation and staining of specimens are recommended to allow effective microscopic speciation. Although species identification is not essential for treatment, identification of *T. solium* infection is significant and should prompt consideration of possible cysticercosis in the index patient or among his or her household contacts.[17] Proglottids of *D. latum* (fish tapeworm) often pass as short chains of grayish white connected segments, each 11 × 3 mm, with a central uterine structure.[5] Proglottids of the pork tapeworm, *T. solium*, are 11 × 5 mm, with a lateral genital pore and 7 to 13 branches on either side of the central uterine canal. Proglottids of *T. saginata*, the beef tapeworm, have a similar appearance but may be distinguished by the larger number of lateral uterine branches (15 to 20) in the proglottid. *T. saginata* proglottids are motile and may emerge spontaneously from the anus to be found on the perineum, on the legs, or on clothing. Proglottids of *D. caninum* (23 × 8 mm) are also motile and may be described by the patient (or parent) as whitish, moving cucumber seedlike objects in the stool. *D. caninum* proglottids may also become adherent to perianal hairs and then dry to form a whitish yellow object resembling a small grain of rice. Recently, detection of specific coproantigens in the stool has improved diagnosis of *Taenia* infection and is genus specific. It carries a specificity of up to 95% to 98%. Newer polymerase chain reaction-based tests also show potential to identify infection at a species level.[18,19]

Treatment of Tapeworm Infection

Tapeworm infection should be treated whenever diagnosed. Safe, effective treatment of intestinal tapeworm infection may be achieved with either praziquantel or niclosamide. Both are well-tolerated oral agents that have direct parasiticidal effects on intraluminal cestode parasites. Although both agents are usually effective and considered first-line, there have been reports of treatment failure, likely secondary to resistance. In some cases, nitazoxanide has been used as an alternative drug and has been found to be safe and effective.[20]

NICLOSAMIDE

Niclosamide is a poorly absorbed, narrow-spectrum anthelmintic that is available as 500-mg chewable tablets (Yomesan, Bayer).[12] However, it is no longer commercially available in the United States. The drug is normally taken as a 2-g (four-tablet) single dose for adults, as a 1.5-g (three-tablet) dose for children weighing more than 34 kg (75 pounds), or as a 1-g (two-tablet) dose for children weighing 11 to 34 kg (25 to 75 pounds). A single treatment is effective for *D. latum*, *T. saginata*, *D. caninum*, and *T. solium* tapeworms.

Eradication of *H. nana* tapeworm infection requires a more prolonged course of therapy (repeat daily doses for 1 week) because of concomitant infection with maturing *H. nana* cysts, which are not affected by the drug. It is normally recommended that after the first dose, subsequent doses for *H. nana* (i.e., days 2 through 7) be reduced to 1 g daily for adults and large children (>34 kg) and to 0.5 g daily for small children. These follow-up doses are intended to kill any newly emerging *H. nana* tapeworms and should completely eliminate the infection. Nevertheless, it is appropriate to rescreen the patient's stool for parasite eggs 1 and 3 months after therapy to ensure cure. A repeated cycle of standard dosing (as just outlined) is usually sufficient to eliminate persistent infection.

Niclosamide must be thoroughly chewed before swallowing to obtain the maximal anthelmintic effect. Because the drug is poorly absorbed, the typical side effects of niclosamide are mild, occurring at a rate of approximately 10%.[12] They include malaise, mild abdominal pain, and nausea on the day of administration. High doses of niclosamide have not been shown to have mutagenic effects in animals, and the drug has been placed in Food and Drug Administration (FDA) Pregnancy Category B. Normally, treatment should be delayed until after pregnancy, but with *T. solium* there is concern that patients may develop cysticercosis through autoinfection with parasite eggs. Considering the relative risks and benefits, it may be appropriate to treat pregnant women who have *T. solium* tapeworms at the time of diag-

nosis and not delay therapy. Concern has also been raised about the possibility of internal autoinfection during *T. solium* therapy because of the release and possible retrograde intestinal movement of eggs during therapy. Although such autoinfection has not been documented, some experts recommend a mild laxative 1 or 2 hours after niclosamide treatment to avoid this possibility in *T. solium*-infected patients.

PRAZIQUANTEL

Praziquantel is a broad-spectrum anthelmintic used to treat both trematode and cestode infections.[12] It is available as a scored, 600-mg coated tablet (Biltricide, Bayer); it has excellent activity against all tapeworms and is given as a single dose of 5 to 10 mg/kg for both children and adults. The exception to this regimen is *H. nana* infection, for which a higher dose of 25 mg/kg is recommended. If the *H. nana* infection is heavy, it is recommended that the dose be repeated 1 week after the initial therapy. Follow-up stool screening is recommended at 1 and 3 months to ensure eradication of infection.

Mild side effects occur in 10% to 50% of those treated, depending on the population. They include transient dizziness, headache, malaise, abdominal pain, and nausea. Moderate side effects, including sedation, vomiting, diarrhea, urticaria, rash, fever, and mild transaminitis, are not as common (<10%) and are also transient. Like niclosamide, praziquantel is classified in FDA Pregnancy Category B and should be used during pregnancy only if clearly needed. Praziquantel is well absorbed from the gastrointestinal tract and enters breast milk. Because the safety of praziquantel in children younger than 4 years is not established, women who are breast-feeding infants should not allow them to nurse for 24 hours after treatment is given.

Invasive Cestode Infections

CYSTICERCOSIS

Cysticercosis is a tissue infection with larval cysts of the cestode *T. solium* in which the patient serves as an intermediate host for the parasite. Infection is acquired by consumption of *T. solium* eggs by fecal-oral transmission from a *T. solium* tapeworm carrier. Prevalence is high wherever *T. solium* tapeworms are common (i.e., Mexico, Central America, South America, the Philippines, and Southeast Asia), and the World Health Organization estimates that there are more than 50,000 deaths per year from neurocysticercosis.[21] Infected subjects normally harbor multiple cysts in many parts of the body. In areas of endemicity, the cumulative infection risk increases with age, frequent consumption of pork, and poor household hygiene.[22] Symptoms may develop because of local inflammation at the site of involvement; however, apart from CNS and cardiac involvement, serious disease is rare. Neurologic symptoms are the most prominent.

Neurocysticercosis is the term used for human CNS involvement with *T. solium* cysts.[23] Infection may involve any part of the CNS, but symptomatic disease is most often related to intracerebral lesions (causing mass effects, seizures, or both) (Fig. 290-4), intraventricular cysts (causing hydrocephalus), subarachnoid lesions (causing chronic meningitis), and spinal cord lesions (causing cord compression syndrome or meningitis). Seizures, occurring in up to 70% of patients with neurocysticercosis, and intracranial hypertension are the most common clinical features.[21] Intraparenchymal cerebral cysts typically enlarge slowly, causing minimal symptoms until years or decades after the onset of infection, when the cysts begin to die. At this point, cysts may lose osmoregulation and begin to swell. They may also leak antigenic material that provokes a severe inflammatory response (cerebritis and meningitis). Both processes contribute to symptoms of focal or generalized seizures, sensorimotor deficits, intellectual impairment, psychiatric disorders, and symptoms of hydrocephalus. In regions where *T. solium* is endemic, as many as 30% to 50% of patients with seizures have antibodies to *T. solium*, compared with the 2% to 11% prevalence in the general population, suggesting the likelihood that

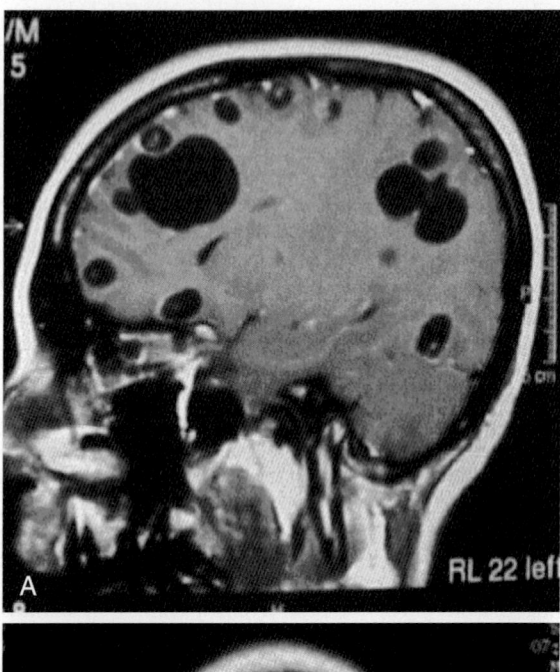

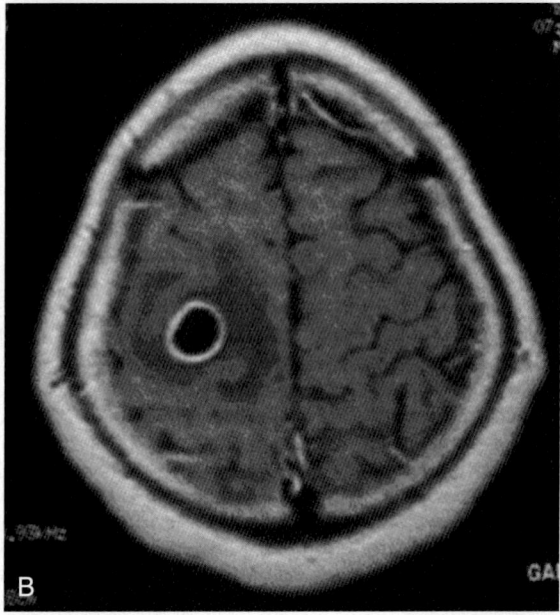

Figure 290-4 Magnetic resonance images of (**A**) massive cysticercosis and (**B**) "colloidal" cyst defined by early signs of inflammation around the cysticercus. *(From Garcia HH, Del Brutto OH. Imaging findings in neurocysticercosis. Acta Tropica. 2003;87:71-78.)*

neurocysticercosis is an underlying cause of their disease.[23] Further studies using computed tomography in areas of Guatemala, Mexico, Ecuador, and Honduras have shown that up to 20% of the general population have asymptomatic brain calcifications.[24]

Because of their critical location, intraventricular cysts and basilar cysts tend to cause symptoms early during the course of the infection. The symptoms are due to obstruction of CSF flow or local meningeal irritation, which leads to injury to local blood vessels, cranial nerves, or the brain stem.[23] An aggressive form of basilar neurocysticercosis, called *racemose cysticerosis*, has been described in which cysts proliferate at the base of the brain, resulting in mental deterioration, coma, and death. Intraparenchymal spinal cord lesions are often symptomatic early because of direct local pressure effects. When spinal column cysts develop outside the cord itself, the onset of symptoms may be more gradual. The slow onset of external cord compression, arach-

noiditis, or radiculopathy may result in a confusing progression of symptoms. In the CNS, multiple cysticerci are the rule, and active symptoms may refer to one or several locations.

Diagnosis and treatment of cysticercosis depend on the site of involvement and the symptoms experienced. Travel to or residence in an endemic area significantly increases the likelihood of the diagnosis, although transmission has been documented to occur within the United States in people living in the same household as a *T. solium*-infected immigrant. Cysts outside the CNS tend not to be symptomatic. These cysts eventually die and calcify, to be detected incidentally on plain radiographs of the limbs. Although symptomatic cardiac cysticercosis is rarely reported, autopsy reports of cysticercosis patients have shown cysts involving the heart in up to 23% of cases. Symptoms of cardiac cysticercosis can include heart failure or conduction abnormalities.[25]

For symptomatic cysts outside the CNS, the optimal approach is surgical resection. Medical therapy with praziquantel or albendazole may also be employed.[12,23] Deep tissue and CNS lesions are more difficult to diagnose and treat surgically. Lesions may involve critical organs, making surgical removal technically not feasible. Presenting symptoms often suggest a tumor, and a specific diagnosis of cysticercosis is often first suspected on the basis of imaging studies (computed tomography [CT] or magnetic resonance imaging [MRI]), which show multiple enhancing and nonenhancing unilocular cysts.[23] Cerebral cysts are usually multiple (an average of 7 to 10 per patient). CSF examination may show lymphocytic or eosinophilic pleocytosis, hypoglycorrhachia, and elevated protein levels. A suspected diagnosis may be strengthened by serology that is available commercially or through the Centers for Disease Control and Prevention (CDC) in Atlanta, Georgia. The serology indicates prior exposure to *T. solium* antigens. Patients infected with other helminths, particularly other cestodes, may have circulating antibodies that cross react with antigens of *T. solium* in some assays.[27] However, immunoblotting techniques with the purified glycoprotein fraction of cyst fluid appear to offer a sensitive and specific diagnosis.[26,27] The sensitivity of antibody testing tends to be high for patients with multiple cysts (94%) but substantially lower for patients with single cysts or calcified cysts (as low as 28%).[28] CT and MRI remain the most effective means of diagnosis, however, and in the presence of a characteristic scan, negative serology should not exclude the diagnosis of cysticercosis.[23]

The utility of drug therapy for neurocysticercosis has been a controversial topic. Initially, a number of nonrandomized case series (each involving a small number of treated patients compared with historical control subjects) suggested that both praziquantel and albendazole hastened the clearance of cysticercal lesions seen on CT or MRI.[29] Following those initial reports, small, concurrently controlled, randomized trials had indicated that anthelmintic therapy given with corticosteroids was not superior to corticosteroid therapy alone for long-term control of seizures or resolution of *intraparenchymal* CNS cysticerci.[23] However, two larger, more recent randomized controlled trials have attempted to resolve the controversy and have shown some benefit of antihelminthic therapy. The first trial, performed in Peru, entailed a trial of placebo alone versus albendazole with corticosteroids for treatment of patients with seizures and viable parenchymal cysts (i.e., those cysts with little or no surrounding enhancement). Patients in the treatment arm showed reductions in generalized seizures and faster resolution of the cysts.[30] The second trial, performed in Ecuador, included patients with both parenchymal and extraparenchymal cysts and compared corticosteroid therapy alone versus albendazole given with corticosteroids. The trial showed a faster resolution of active (or viable) cysts (as opposed to degenerating cysts) in the albendazole arm at 1 to 6 months, with no additional benefit beyond this time. However, this study did not show any benefit in seizure reduction.[31] Neither study showed significant increases in adverse effects with antiparasite therapy, apart from a slight increase in seizures early in treatment. In addition, the second trial confirmed previous studies indicating that treatment of purely calcified cysts did not provide benefit. Another study of treatment for single active cysts, as well as a recent meta-analysis, provide supporting data for the use of cystidal agents in the treatment of parenchymal disease.[32,33] However, concerning case reports have indicated that anthelmintic therapy may exacerbate obstruction of CSF flow, enhance eye inflammation in ocular disease, and increase the risk of pericystic vasculitis, with increased risk of stroke.[34,35] Thus, although data from recent clinical trials appear to show benefits with low risk of adverse outcomes, apparently favoring antiparasitic treatment for parenchymal neurocysticercosis, some controversy and clinical concerns remain, and individual treatment decisions should be discussed with experienced practitioners. Furthermore, despite the reported benefits of treatment, there are still a significant number of people who remain with symptoms after treatment, highlighting the need for further research on treatment modalities.

Still, randomized, well-controlled trials have not yet evaluated the treatment of other forms of neurocysticercosis (i.e., intraventricular, subarachnoid/basilar, and spinal cysticercosis), and the true value of drug treatment for these forms of the disease is not known.[23] However, because drug treatment of *intraventricular* cysts may prove efficacious and because of the higher risk for disease progression, therapy for this form of the disease is currently recommended by experienced groups. Likewise, due to the progression and degree of complications of disease with subarachnoid or sylvian fissure cysts, treatment with cystidal medications is generally recommended, with close attention to the management of intracranial hypertension.[21] Antihelminthic treatment for extensive infections, such as encephalitis, is generally not recommended given the potential adverse effects due to treatment-induced inflammation.

If, on the basis of a review of the latest literature, the decision is made to treat an individual patient with complicated neurocysticercosis medically, treatment should generally be high doses of praziquantel (50 to 100 mg/kg/day for 15 to 30 days divided in three doses)[12,29,36] or albendazole (10 to 15 mg/kg/day divided in two doses, with maximum of 800 mg per day, for 8 days),[13] with the goal of achieving drug levels sufficient to kill any remaining living cysts. As noted previously, cyst death is often accompanied by increased local inflammation, leading to an increase in symptoms. Before, during, and after drug therapy, seizures should be controlled with appropriate antiepileptic medications, and symptomatic hydrocephalus should be relieved by shunting. Shunt complications caused by blockage and bacterial infection are common in patients with neurocysticercosis.[37] CNS inflammation can be reduced by concurrent administration of pharmacologic doses of corticosteroids (dexamethasone)[38]; however, corticosteroids do not necessarily eliminate the risk of serious complications, such as infarction[35,39] or intracranial pressure elevation.[40] Limited pharmacologic evidence suggests that concurrent corticosteroid therapy lowers serum praziquantel levels. In contrast, corticosteroid therapy (variably) increases the circulating levels of albendazole and its active metabolites in some patients. On this basis, and also based on a recent meta-analysis favoring albendazole over praziquantel, many experts now favor the use of albendazole for medical treatment of neurocysticercosis.[40,41]

A poor response to either surgical or drug therapy is more common with intraventricular or cisternal cysts and with racemose neurocysticercosis.[29] For these lesions, the drug levels achieved in the CSF and cyst during medical therapy are likely to be lower than for parenchymal CNS cysts, making drug failure more likely, often necessitating a longer duration of anticystidal treatment and multiple courses of treatment. Surgical approaches to these areas are difficult, and local inflammation may prevent easy removal of the cyst, although endoscopic removal of ventricular cysts has shown promising results and its use continues to expand.[21] Retained cyst material may result in postoperative recurrence. Nevertheless, successful therapy of ventricular and basilar cysts has been achieved in a small number of patients by either medical or surgical means.[42,43] Individualized therapy, possibly including a combined surgical-medical approach, is recommended in such cases.[23,36]

ECHINOCOCCOSIS (HYDATID AND ALVEOLAR CYST DISEASE)

When humans serve as inadvertent intermediate hosts for cestodes of *Echinococcus* spp., which are carried as tapeworms by canines such as dogs, wolves, and foxes, disease may result from the development of expanding parasite cysts in visceral organs.[2,44] This condition, termed *echinococcosis*, has two forms: hydatid or unilocular cyst disease, caused by *Echinococcus granulosus*, and alveolar cyst disease, caused by *Echinococcus multilocularis*. In addition, polycystic or "neotropical" echinococcosis is caused by either *Echinococcus vogeli* or the much less common *Echinococcus oligarthrus*, both found in Central or South America. *E. vogeli* infections are similar to alveolar cyst disease, whereas *E. oligarthrus* infections appear less aggressive.[45] Sheep, goats, camels, and horses are among the usual intermediate hosts for *E. granulosus*, but because *E. granulosus* is transmitted by domestic dogs in livestock-raising areas, hydatid disease is prevalent worldwide (Africa, Middle East, southern Europe, Latin America, and southwestern United States). *E. multilocularis* infections (found in northern forest areas of Europe, Asia, and North America and in the Arctic regions) and *E. vogeli* infections (found in South American highlands) are transmitted by wild canines and are much less common.

Humans acquire echinococcosis by ingesting viable parasite eggs with their food.[2,44] The parasite eggs are distributed via local environmental contamination by the feces of tapeworm-infected canines. Eggs are partially resistant to desiccation and remain viable for many weeks,[4] allowing delayed transmission to individuals with no direct contact with vector animals. Once in the intestinal tract, the eggs hatch to form oncospheres that penetrate the mucosa and enter the circulation. Oncospheres then encyst in host viscera, developing over time to form mature larval cysts (Fig. 290-5).

Infection with *E. granulosus*, cystic echinococcosis, is estimated to occur in up to 2% to 6% of endemic populations, and the annual incidence in Europe is on the rise in some areas. Risk factors include unsanitary living conditions, slaughter of livestock in close proximity to humans and dogs, and uncontrolled dog populations. Sheep raising, in particular, is associated with a high prevalence of disease.[18,46] The hydatid cysts of *E. granulosus* tend to form in the liver (50% to 70% of patients) or lung (20% to 30%) but may be found in any organ of the body, including brain, heart, and bones (<10%). They grow to 5 to 10 cm in size within the first year and can survive for years or even decades. Symptoms are often absent, and in many cases infection is

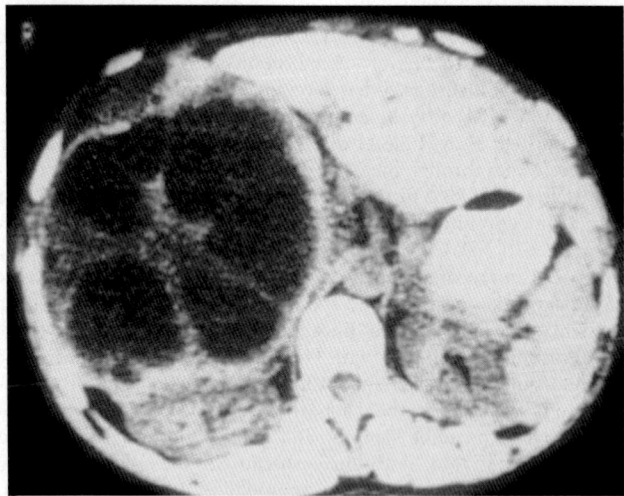

Figure 290-5 Hydatid cysts of the liver detected on computed tomographic scan. Note the well-demarcated wall and characteristic septate internal structures (daughter cysts).

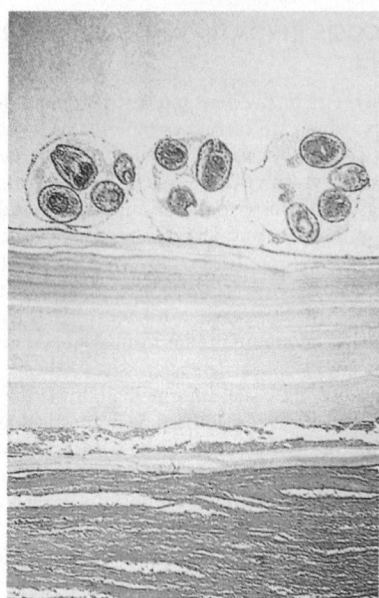

Figure 290-6 Daughter cyst formation from the germinal membrane of a hydatid cyst. *(From Ash LR, Orihel TC. Atlas of Human Parasitology. 3rd ed. Chicago: ASCP; 1990.)*

detected only incidentally by imaging studies. When symptoms do occur, they are usually due to the mass effect of the enlarging cyst in a confined space. Hydatid cysts contain a germinal layer that allows asexual budding to form "daughter" cysts within the primary cyst (Fig. 290-6). If a cyst erodes into the biliary tree or a bronchus, the cyst contents, including daughter cysts, may enter the lumen and cause obstruction or postobstructive bacterial infection. Bacteria may enter the cyst, causing pyogenic abscess formation in the cyst. Cyst leakage or rupture may be associated with a severe allergic reaction to parasite antigens; in the most extreme cases, patients may have anaphylactoid reactions, including hypotension, syncope, and fever, after cyst rupture. A dangerous complication of cyst rupture is secondary seeding of daughter cysts into other areas of the body. Their subsequent enlargement may be associated with critical failure of one or more organs, which is associated with significant morbidity and mortality. Fewer than 10% of patients develop such complications; and because the infection is normally self-limited, it is likely that most infections never come to medical attention.[47] Nevertheless, symptomatic cysts should be treated and asymptomatic cysts carefully observed for a number of years to avert complications of infection.

Infection that is suspected based on imaging studies (ultrasonography, CT, and MRI) may be confirmed by a specific enzyme-linked immunosorbent assay (ELISA) and Western blot serology (available in the United States through the CDC), confirming exposure to the parasite.[48,49] Serology is 80% to 100% sensitive and 88% to 96% specific for liver cyst infection but less sensitive for lung (50% to 56%) or other organ (25% to 56%) involvement. Additional assays continue to be developed using recombinant *Echinococcus* antigens and may provide better diagnostic sensitivity and specificity.[48,49,50] Eosinophilia is not a consistent or reliable finding. Imaging remains more sensitive (90% with ultrasound and higher with CT and MRI) than serodiagnostic techniques, and a characteristic scan in the presence of negative serologic results still suggests the diagnosis of echinococcosis.[47,51]

Optimal treatment of symptomatic cysts is surgical resection to remove the cyst in toto. Traditionally, because of the risk of spreading infection due to cyst rupture, the recommended approach has been to visualize the cyst, remove a fraction of the fluid, and instill a cysticidal agent (hypertonic [30%] saline, cetrimide, or 70% to 95% ethanol) to kill the germinal layer and daughter cysts before resection.[2] Thirty minutes after instillation, the cyst is totally removed. A number of

drains are left in the cyst bed to limit the risk of secondary bacterial infection.

Although time-honored, the efficacy of this open surgical approach has not been validated in clinical trials, and given the availability of effective perioperative drug therapy to limit spread, some experts have questioned the need to instill cysticidal agents during surgery.[2] Laparoscopic surgery for cyst removal has been done in less advanced cases (in which spillage of contents is not as likely to occur). In this type of case, the minimally invasive approach may have fewer complications with approximately equal efficacy, although its role in treatment still needs to be fully defined.[51]

Certainly, cysts communicating with the biliary tree or branches should not have a cysticidal agent instilled because of the risk of postoperative sclerosing cholangitis.[44,52] It may be more prudent to treat the patient perioperatively with an anthelmintic agent active against *Echinococcus* cysts (albendazole and mebendazole)[53-55] to limit the risk of intraoperative dissemination of daughter cysts. Preoperative treatment with abendazole for 1 to 3 months has been shown to significantly reduce the number of viable cysts found on surgery.[51] Medical therapy for inoperative cysts with albendazole or mebendazole has provided improvement in most patients (55% to 79%) and cure in a smaller number (29%).[53-55] The preferred agent is albendazole because of its greater absorption from the gastrointestinal tract and higher plasma levels. It is given for three or more cycles at a dose of 400 mg twice a day for 4 weeks (for those less than 60 kg: 15 mg/kg/day divided in two doses), followed by a 2-week rest without therapy. The alternative agent, mebendazole, is poorly absorbed and must be taken at higher doses (50 to 70 mg/kg/day) for several months to achieve a therapeutic effect.[55]

The response to drug therapy depends on the cyst size and location.[55,56] Unfortunately, bone cysts, which are frequently not amenable to surgery, respond less well to drug treatment than other cysts. The response to drug therapy is best monitored by serial imaging studies; cyst disappearance or shrinkage along with increasing cyst density is thought to indicate a positive response.

An intermediate intervention for inoperable cysts has been developed, known as the PAIR procedure (puncture, aspiration, injection, reaspiration).[44,56-58] While the patient is receiving anthelmintics to reduce the risk of cyst dissemination, the hydatid cyst may be aspirated with a thin needle under CT guidance. Approximately 30% of the cyst fluid volume is removed. Detection of protoscolices in the cyst fluid allows confirmation of cyst viability. An equal volume of 95% ethanol or other scolicidal agent (e.g., 0.5% cetrimide) is then instilled into the cyst cavity and allowed to react for 30 minutes before removing the needle. Results indicate arrest or involution of cysts after treatment. A modified technique uses a special catheter system to simultaneously evacuate the cyst contents while infusing the scolicidal agent. The PAIR procedure has several specific indications, and the overall experience with PAIR is relatively limited compared to traditional treatment methods. However, there is some evidence, based on meta-analysis, that there are fewer complications and lower recurrence rates with PAIR compared to standard surgery. More studies are needed to confirm this finding.[51]

Alveolar cyst disease caused by *E. multilocularis* is relatively more aggressive. It is much less common in humans, with an incidence in endemic countries ranging from 0.02 to 1.4 per 100,000. However, increasing fox populations, with a noted increase in prevalence of parasite infection among foxes, may pose an increasing health concern for humans.[18] For example, in Europe, with the development of an effective rabies vaccine program, fox populations began to increase after the 1980s. In concert, the incidence of alveolar echinococcosis doubled from 2001 to 2005 compared to previous years.[59] *E. multilocularis* cysts reproduce asexually by lateral budding. Their gradual invasion of adjacent tissue is tumor-like, and sections of the parasite may "metastasize" to distal parts of the body.[2,44] Symptoms are usually of gradual onset, referring to the organ involved, which is most commonly the liver. Complications include biliary tract disease, portal hypertension, and Budd-Chiari syndrome. Consequently, there is higher morbidity and mortality compared to those for cystic (hydatid) echinococcosis. Initial imaging studies are usually highly suspicious for carcinoma or sarcoma, and biopsy may provide the first indication of infection. Serology, available from the CDC, is highly sensitive and specific, and when combined with characteristic imaging studies it offers an alternative means of establishing the diagnosis.[48] For operable cases, wide surgical resection (e.g., hepatic lobectomy or liver transplantation) is recommended to ensure total removal of the cyst.[54,60] Adjuvant albendazole therapy to reduce cyst size before surgery or limit intraoperative spread has been reported to be beneficial in case series.[2,61] For inoperable cases, drug therapy with mebendazole or albendazole has provided arrest or cure of disease in some patients.[2,54] The efficacy of surgical or drug therapy may be monitored by serial imaging and serology.

OTHER INVASIVE CESTODES

Human tissue infection with plerocercoid cysts of several cestode species is referred to, collectively, as *sparganosis*. These parasites, like *D. latum*, pass through several developmental stages in copepods and vertebrates.[1] The definitive hosts for tapeworms of these species are usually canines or felines. Humans acquire inadvertent parasite infection by ingesting copepods (in water) or by consumption of or prolonged exposure to uncooked meat of plerocercoid-infected animals.[62-64]

Sparganosis has been reported in South America, Japan, China, and other areas of Asia in association with traditional use of frog- or snake-meat poultices. Infection has rarely been reported from Europe and North America. Sparganosis may be the proliferating or nonproliferating type. Infection acquired in the United States is usually due to the species *Spirometra mansonoides*, which is nonproliferating. In other areas of the world, proliferating forms are more common. These forms branch by lateral division and may detach to spread to other, distal areas of the body.[62] Clinical presentation typically involves local inflammation at the site of invasion (skin and eye are the most common sites for poultice application). Cerebral sparganosis is a rare and severe complication. There is local lymphocytic and eosinophilic inflammation surrounding the parasite(s). Tissue injury may be particularly severe in the eye. Diagnosis is usually by biopsy, although serologic testing has been used in some areas.[5] Treatment is by injection with ethanol, surgical resection, or both. Medical therapy with various anthelmintics has not produced a beneficial effect.

Coenurosis is human cyst infection with the cestodes *T. multiceps*, *Taenia crassiceps*, and *Taenia serialis*, which cause tapeworms in dogs.[65] The cysts are unilocular, with multiple protoscolices, but do not contain daughter cysts. Symptomatic disease is usually associated with involvement of the eye or the CNS. Clinically, the cysts may be difficult to distinguish from cysticercosis or hydatid disease. Basal arachnoiditis and hydrocephalus are common. There is no reliable serologic test. Surgical resection is the recommended mode of therapy.[65]

Prevention of Cestode Infection

Prevention of cestode infection depends on interrupting the parasite life cycle. Transmission of human tapeworm infection can be reduced or eliminated by the following sanitary measures: (1) careful disposal of human sewage to limit environmental spread of parasite eggs; (2) limitation of forage areas and use of safe feed for vector animals such as cattle or swine that serve as common intermediate hosts; (3) meat inspection before marketing to exclude cyst-infested carcasses; and (4) prolonged freezing (at less than ~18° C), thorough cooking of meat (at more than 50° C), or both to kill any cysts in the tissues. Control of fish tapeworm is more difficult to achieve because the infected fish can range freely, and there are nonhuman reservoirs for the tapeworm (e.g., bear and seals) that can continue to infect fish despite the presence of good human sanitation.

Prevention of invasive cestode infection is more complex. Because this form of human infection results from egg ingestion and the eggs may have been spread throughout an area by free-ranging definitive hosts such as dogs or humans, infection may be difficult to avoid. It is significant that half of the patients with hydatid cysts do not recall specific exposure to dogs, although they may have resided in or visited an area of endemicity. Successful control of *E. granulosus* transmission has been achieved by regular screening and treatment of dogs in areas of endemicity in New Zealand, Tasmania, and the British Isles[66] to eliminate adult tapeworm carriage and local release of eggs. Similar programs to treat rural dogs and foxes have been proposed for control of *E. multilocularis* transmission.[67] Treatment of human carriers in areas in which *T. solium* is endemic, as well as health education campaigns focusing on self-recognition of human tapeworm carriers and the corralling of pigs, has proved effective in controlling transmission of cysticercosis.[24,68,69] However, many barriers, particularly involving socioeconomic factors, still exist. Field trials also indicate that anti-*Echinococcus* and anti-cysticercus vaccines can significantly reduce infection in farm animals (sheep and pigs), which may further lower the level of peridomestic transmission.[70]

In areas of good sanitation (e.g., the United States), autochthonous transmission of cysticercosis is rare but can occur in settings in which a *T. solium* tapeworm-carrying individual shares living or cooking quarters with susceptible individuals.[18,65] Screening of immigrants from *T. solium*-endemic areas and treatment of identified tapeworm infections would eliminate the risk of cysticercosis transmission to nontravelers.

REFERENCES

1. Wittner M, White, C, Tanowitz HB. Introduction to tapeworm infections. In: Guerrant RL, Walker DH, Weller PF, eds. *Tropical Infectious Diseases: Principles, Pathogens & Practice.* Philadelphia: Churchill Livingstone; 2006:1286-1287.
2. Schantz PM, Kern P, Brunetti E. Echinococcosis. In: Guerrant RL, Walker DH, Weller PF, eds. *Tropical Infectious Diseases: Principles, Pathogens & Practice.* Philadelphia: Churchill Livingstone; 2006:1304-1324.
3. Ash LR, Orihel TC. *Atlas of Human Parasitology.* 3rd ed. Chicago: ASCP; 1990.
4. Wachira TM, Macpherson CN, Gathuma JM. Release and survival of *Echinococcus* eggs in different environments in Turkana, and their possible impact on the incidence of hydatidosis in man and livestock. *J Helminthol.* 1991;65:55-61.
5. Wittner M, Tanowitz HB. *Taenia* and other tapeworms. In: Guerrant RL, Walker DH, Weller PF, eds. *Tropical Infectious Diseases: Principles, Pathogens & Practice.* Philadelphia: Churchill Livingstone; 2006:1337-1339.
6. Vuitton DA. The ambiguous role of immunity in echinococcosis: protection of the host or of the parasite? *Acta Trop.* 2003;85:119-132.
7. Rau ME, Tanner CE. BCG suppresses growth and metastasis of hydatid infections. *Nature.* 1975;256:318-319.
8. Chavarría A, Fleury A, García E, et al. Relationship between the clinical heterogeneity of neurocysticercosis and the immune-inflammatory profiles. *Clin Immunol.* 2006;116:271-278.
9. Deardorff TL, Kent ML. Prevalence of larval *Anisakis* simplex in pen-reared and wild-caught salmon (Salmonidae) from Puget Sound, Washington. *J Wildl Dis.* 1989;25:416-419.
10. Durborow RM. Health and safety concerns in fisheries and aquaculture. *Occup Med.* 1999;14:373-406.
11. Jackson Y, Pastore R, Sudre P, et al. *Diphyllobothrium latum* outbreak from marinated raw perch, Lake Geneva, Switzerland. *Emerg Infect Dis.* 2007;13:1957-1958.
12. Drugs for parasitic infections. *Med Lett Drugs Ther.* 〈www.medletter.com〉; 2002.
13. Yoeli M, Most H, Hammond J, et al. Parasitic infections in a closed community: results of a 10-year survey in Willowbrook State School. *Trans R Soc Trop Med Hyg.* 1972;66:764-766.
14. Chero JC, Saito M, Bustos JA, et al. *Hymenolepis nana* infection: symptoms and response to nitazoxanide in field conditions. *Trans R Soc Trop Med Hyg.* 2007;101:203-205.
15. Wicht B, de Marval F, Peduzzi R. *Diphyllobothrium nihonkaiense* (Yamane et al. 1986) in Switzerland: First molecular evidence and case reports. *Parasitol Int.* 2007;56:195-199.
16. Eom KS. What is Asian *Taenia*? *Parasitol Int.* 2006;55: S137-S141.
17. Kruskal BA, Moths L, Teele DW. Neurocysticercosis in a child with no history of travel outside the continental United States. *Clin Infect Dis.* 1993;16:290-292.
18. Schantz PM. Progress in diagnosis, treatment, and elimination of echinococcosis and cysticercosis. *Parasitol Int.* 2006;55: S7-S13.
19. Craig P, Ito A. Intestinal cestodes. *Curr Opin Infect Dis.* 2007;20:524-532.
20. Lateef M, Zargar SA, Khan AR, et al. Successful treatment of niclosamide- and praziquantel-resistant beef tapeworm infection with nitazoxanide. *Int J Infect Dis.* 2008;12:80-82.
21. Garcia HH, Del Brutto OH. Neurocysticercosis: updated concepts about an old disease. *Lancet Neurol.* 2005;4:653-661.
22. Sarti E, Schantz PM, Plancarte A, et al. Prevalence and risk factors for *Taenia solium* taeniasis and cysticercosis in humans and pigs in a village in Morelos, Mexico. *Am J Trop Med Hyg.* 1992;46:677-685.
23. Carpio A. Neurocysticercosis: an update. *Lancet Infect Dis.* 2002;2:751-762.

24. Garcia HH, Gonzalez AE, Del Brutto OH, et al. Strategies for the elimination of taeniasis/cysticercosis. *J Neurol Sci.* 2007;262: 153-157.
25. Eberly MD, Soh EK, Bannister SP, et al. Isolated cardiac cysticercosis in an adolescent. *Pediatr Infect Dis J.* 2008;27:369-371.
26. Diaz JF, Verastegui M, Gilman RH, et al. Immunodiagnosis of human cysticercosis (*Taenia solium*): a field comparison of an antibody-enzyme-linked immunosorbent assay (ELISA), an antigen-ELISA, and an enzyme-linked immunoelectrotransfer blot (EITB) assay in Peru; the Cysticercosis Working Group in Peru (CWG). *Am J Trop Med Hyg.* 1992;46:610-615.
27. Tsang VCW, Brand JA, Boyer AE. An enzyme-linked immunoelectrotransfer blot assay and glycoprotein antigens for diagnosing human cysticercosis (*Taenia solium*). *J Infect Dis.* 1989;159:50-59.
28. Wilson M, Bryan RT, Fried JA, et al. Clinical evaluation of the cysticercosis enzyme-linked immunoelectrotransfer blot in patients with neurocysticercosis. *J Infect Dis.* 1991;164:1007-1009.
29. Del Brutto OH, Sotelo J. Neurocysticercosis: an update. *Rev Infect Dis.* 1988;10:1075-1087.
30. Garcia HH, Pretell EJ, Gilman RH, et al. A trial of antiparasitic treatment to reduce the rate of seizures due to cerebral cysticercosis. *N Engl J Med.* 2004;350:249-258.
31. Carpio A, Kelvin EA, Bagiella E, et al. Effects of abendazole treatment on neurocysticercosis: a randomised controlled trial. *J Neurol Neurosurg Psychiatry.* 2008;79:1050-1055.
32. Thussu A, Chattopadhyay A, Sawhney IMS, et al. Albendazole therapy for single enhancing CT lesions (SSECTL) in the brain in epilepsy. *J Neurol Neurosurg Psychiatry.* 2008;79: 272-275.
33. Del Brutto OH, Roos KL, Coffey CS, et al. Meta-analysis: cystidal drugs for neurocysticercosis: albendazole and praziquantal. *Ann Intern Med.* 2006;145:43-51.
34. Evans C, Garcia HH, Gilman RH, et al. Controversies in the management of cysticercosis. *Emerg Infect Dis.* 1997;3:403-405.
35. Bang OY, Heo JH, Choi SA, et al. Large cerebral infarction during praziquantel therapy in neurocysticercosis. *Stroke.* 1997;28:211-213. [See comment by Del Brutto OH. *Stroke.* 1997;28:1088.]
36. Garcia HH, Evans CA, Nash TE, et al. Current consensus guidelines for treatment of neurocysticercosis. *Clin Microbiol Rev.* 2002;15:747-756.
37. Sotelo J, Marin C. Hydrocephalus secondary to cysticercotic arachnoiditis: a long-term follow-up review of 92 cases. *J Neurosurg.* 1987;66:686-689.
38. DeGhetaldi LD, Norman RM, Douville AW. Cerebral cysticercosis treated biphasically with dexamethasone and pranziquantel. *Ann Intern Med.* 1983;99:179-181.

39. Woo E, Yu YL, Huang CY. Cerebral infarct precipitated by praziquantel in neurocysticercosis: a cautionary note. *Trop Geogr Med.* 1988;40:143-146.
40. Takayangui OM, Jardim E. Therapy for neurocysticercosis: comparison between albendazole and pranziquantel. *Arch Neurol.* 1992;49:290-294.
41. Matthaiou DK, Panos G, Adamidi ES, et al. Albendazole versus praziquantel in the treatment of neurocysticercosis: a meta-analysis of comparative trials. *PLoS Negl Trop Dis.* 2008;2: e194.
42. Del Brutto OH, Sotelo J. Albendazole therapy for subarachnoid and ventricular cysticercosis: a case report. *J Neurosurg.* 1990;72:816-817.
43. Cuetter AC, Garcia-Bobadilla J, Guerra LG, et al. Neurocysticercosis: focus on intraventricular disease. *Clin Infect Dis.* 1997;24:157-164.
44. Ammann RW, Eckert J. Cestodes: Echinococcus. *Gastroenterol Clin North Am.* 1996;25:655-689.
45. Eckert J, Deplazes P. Biological, epidemiological, and clinical aspects of echinococcosis, a zoonosis of increasing concern. *Clin Microbiol Rev.* 2004;17:107-135.
46. Gavidia CM, Gonzalez AE, Zhang W, et al. Diagnosis of cystic echinococcosis, central Peruvian Highlands. *Emerg Infect Dis.* 2008;14:260-266.
47. MacPherson CNL, Milner R. Performance characteristics and quality control of community based ultrasound surveys for cystic and alveolar echinococcosis. *Acta Trop.* 2003;85:203-209.
48. Zhang W, McManus DP. Concepts of immunology and diagnosis of hydatid disease. *Clin Microbiol Rev.* 2003;16:18-36.
49. Ortona E, Rigano R, Butarri B, et al. An update on immunodiagnosis of cystic echinococcosis. *Acta Trop.* 2003;85:165-171.
50. Hernandez-Gonzalez A, Muro A, Barrera I, et al. Usefulness of four different *Echinococcus granulosus* recombinant antigens for serodiagnosis of unilocular hydatid disease (UHD) and postsurgical follow-up of patients treated for UHD. *Clin Vaccine Immunol.* 2008;15:147-153.
51. Filippou D, Tselepis D, Filippou G, et al. Advances in liver echinococcosis: diagnosis and treatment. *Clin Gastroenterol Hepatol.* 2007;5:152-159.
52. Teres J, Gomez J, Bouguera M, et al. Sclerosing cholangitis after surgical treatment of hepatic echinococcal cysts: report of three cases. *Am J Surg.* 1984;148:694-697.
53. Ammann RW. Improvement of liver resectional therapy by adjuvant chemotherapy in alveolar hydatid disease; Swiss Echinococcosis Study Group (SESG). *Parasitol Res.* 1991;77:290-293.
54. World Health Organization. Guidelines for treatment of cystic and alveolar echinococcosis in humans. *Bull WHO.* 1996;74: 231-242.

55. El-On J. Benzimidazole treatment of cystic echinococcosis. *Acta Trop.* 2003;85:243-252.
56. Todorov T, Mechkov G, Vutova K, et al. Factors influencing the response to chemotherapy in human cystic *Echinococcus. Bull WHO.* 1992;70:347-358.
57. Filice C, Di Perri G, Strosselli M, et al. Parasitologic findings in percutaneous drainage of human hydatid liver cysts. *J Infect Dis.* 1990;161:1290-1295.
58. Mawhorter S, Temeck B, Chang R, et al. Nonsurgical therapy for pulmonary hydatid cyst disease. *Chest.* 1997;112:1432-1436.
59. Schweiger A, Ammann RW, Candinas D, et al. Human alveolar echinococcosis after fox population increase, Switzerland. *Emerg Infect Dis.* 2007;13:878-882.
60. Mboti B, Van de Stadt J, Carlier Y, et al. Long-term disease-free survival after liver transplantation for alveolar echinococcosis. *Acta Chir Belg.* 1996;96:229-232.
61. Wilson JF, Rausch RL, McMahon BJ, et al. Albendazole therapy in alveolar hydatid disease: a report of favorable results in two patients after short-term therapy. *Am J Trop Med Hyg.* 1987;37:162-168.
62. Kim DG, Paek SH, Chang KH, et al. Cerebral sparganosis: clinical manifestations, treatment and outcome. *J Neurosurg.* 1996;85: 1066-1071.
63. Kron MA, Guderian R, Guevara A, et al. Abdominal sparganosis in Ecuador: a case report. *Am J Trop Med Hyg.* 1991;44: 146-150.
64. Nakamura T, Hara M, Matsuoka M, et al. Human proliferative sparganosis: a new Japanese case. *Am J Clin Pathol.* 1990;94: 224-228.
65. Garcia HH, Wittner M, Coyle CM, et al. Cysticercosis. In: Guerrant RL, Walker DH, Weeler PF, eds. *Tropical Infectious Diseases: Principles, Pathogens & Practice.* Philadelphia: Churchill Livingstone; 2006:1289-1303.
66. Gemmell MA. Australasian contributions to an understanding of the epidemiology and control of hydatid disease caused by *Echinococcus granulosus*: past, present and future. *Int J Parasitol.* 1990;20:431-456.
67. Craig PS, McManus DP, Lightowlers MW, et al. Prevention and control of cystic echinococcosis. *Lancet Infect Dis.* 2007;7: 385-394.
68. Cruz M, Davis A, Dixon H, et al. Operational studies on the control of *Taenia solium* taeniasis/cysticercosis in Ecuador. *Bull WHO.* 1989;67:401-407.
69. Flisser A, Gyorkos TW. Contribution of immunodiagnostic tests to epidemiological/intervention studies of cysticercosis/taeniosis in Mexico. *Parasite Immunol.* 2007;29:637-649.
70. Lightowlers MW, Flisser A, Gauci CG, et al. Vaccination against cysticercosis and hydatid disease. *Parisitol Today.* 2000;16: 191-196.

291

Visceral Larva Migrans and Other Unusual Helminth Infections

THEODORE E. NASH*

Most helminths that infect humans are relatively host-specific to humans, undergo characteristic migration and development, and are found in typical anatomic locations. However, these helminths sometimes undergo atypical or aborted migrations and cause symptoms or signs because of their unusual or ectopic location. A good example of this is the deposition of schistosomal ova and the subsequent granulomatous inflammatory lesions in the spinal cord or brain. In addition, some helminths of animals can also infect humans. Examples are *Echinococcus granulosus* and *Trichinella spiralis,* which commonly infect humans, migrate and develop normally, and reside in locations similar to those in the animal host. In contrast, other helminths of animals are unable to develop or migrate normally. Commonly, they undergo prolonged aberrant migrations or locate abnormally in the tissues as underdeveloped larvae and incite an eosinophilic inflammation that is responsible for many of the symptoms and signs of these infections. Although a large number of animal parasites may infect humans, most do so rarely. In contrast, some helminths of animals infect humans more commonly and cause distinctive clinical syndromes (Table 291-1), sometimes associated with characteristic epidemiology, exposure history, and geographic locations. More often than not, similar clinical syndromes are caused by a group of related parasites. The diagnosis is suggested on clinical and epidemiologic grounds. Although pathologic examination of tissue can sometimes establish the diagnosis, the detection of larvae is commonly unrewarding. Serologic tests are sometimes helpful (see "Visceral Larva Migrans [Toxocariasis]") but usually are not fully evaluated, are experimental, or are unavailable.

The diagnostic procedures used to detect infections differ for each parasite, so a clear idea of the potential causes is essential. The physician must understand the sensitivity of the diagnostic procedures and the abilities of the laboratory personnel performing them. For example, intestinal *Ascaris* infections are readily detected in the stool. On the other hand, the number of *Strongyloides* larvae or *Schistosomia mansoni* ova present in the feces may be difficult to detect, and special stool concentration methods may be needed. Patients may present during the prepatent period before the parasite can be detected, such as with ascariasis or schistosomiasis. Repeated stool examinations eventually diagnose both infections. The usefulness of serologic testing varies, but serologic tests can be helpful for suggesting diagnoses and ruling out infections. Few serologic tests for parasitic infections have been standardized, so the sensitivity and specificity may differ from published values and from laboratory to laboratory.

▣ Visceral Larva Migrans (Toxocariasis)

Visceral larva migrans (VLM) is a syndrome characterized in its most florid state by eosinophilia, fever, and hepatomegaly. It is caused primarily by infection with *Toxocara canis* but also by *Toxocara cati* and other helminths less frequently.[1-3]

LIFE CYCLE IN THE DOG

Toxocara canis infects dogs and related mammals by a number of mechanisms.[1] Most commonly, ingested eggs hatch in the small intes-

tine and the resulting larvae migrate to the liver, lung, and trachea. They are then swallowed and mature in the lumen of the small intestine, where eggs are shed. Other larvae migrate to and remain dormant in the muscles but are capable of development even years after the primary infection, particularly in pregnant bitches. During pregnancy, larvae again develop and infect the pups transplacentally and transmammarily. Not uncommonly, infective larvae are found in the feces of the pups. Eggs are not infectious when passed in the feces and take 3 to 4 weeks to develop. They are hardy and often remain viable for months. Large numbers of viable eggs contaminate the environment because of the high prevalence of infection in dogs and the ability of eggs to survive relatively harsh environmental conditions. Humans become infected mostly from ingesting viable ova that contaminate the soil where dogs defecate. Ingestion of raw organs containing larvae, which is common in some regions is another means of infection.[4]

INFECTION IN HUMANS

Prevalence

Toxocariasis is prevalent wherever dogs or cats are found and *Toxocara* eggs are able to survive. The prevalence of infection or disease in humans is not known, but seroepidemiologic studies show wide differences in prevalence, depending on the population tested. In the United States, seropositivity ranged from 2.8%[5] in an unselected population, to 23.1%[6] in a kindergarten population in the southern United States, to 54%[7] in a selected rural community. None of the seropositive persons had recognizable disease.

Clinical Manifestations

Visceral larva migrans occurs most commonly in children younger than 6 years, frequently after ingestion of contaminated soil.[3,5] Disease manifestations vary and range from asymptomatic infection to fulminant disease and death, but it is increasingly appreciated that most infections are asymptomatic. Those who come to medical attention most commonly complain of cough, fever, wheezing, and other generalized symptoms.[6-8] The liver is the organ most frequently involved, and hepatomegaly is a common finding, although almost any organ can be affected. Splenomegaly occurs in a small number of patients, and lymphadenopathy has been noted. Lung involvement with radiologic findings has been documented in 32% to 44% of patients, but respiratory distress occurs rarely. Skin lesions such as urticaria and nodules have also been described. Seizures have been noted to occur with increased frequency in VLM, but severe neurologic involvement is infrequent.[9] Eye involvement in VLM is unusual but has been documented (see later, "Ocular Larva Migrans"). Eosinophilia, usually accompanied by leukocytosis, is the hallmark of VLM. Laboratory findings include hypergammaglobulinemia and elevated isohemagglutinin titers to A and B blood group antigens, which are caused by the host's immune response to cross-reacting antigens on the surface of *T. canis* or *T. cati* larvae.

Diagnosis

The diagnosis of VLM is usually suggested clinically by the presence of eosinophilia, leukocytosis, or both in a young child also presenting with hepatomegaly or signs and symptoms of other organ involvement. A history of pica and exposure to puppies is common. In the United States, patients are more commonly black and from rural areas.

---

*All material in this chapter is in the public domain, with the exception of any borrowed figures or tables.

TABLE 291-1	Clinical Syndromes Associated with Unusual Helminth Infections in Humans	
Clinical Syndrome	*Parasite*	*Usual Host*
Visceral larva migrans	*Toxocara canis*	Canines
	Toxocara cati	Felines
	Baylisascaris procyonis	Raccoons
Eosinophilic gastroenteritis	*Anisakis* spp.	Sea mammals
	Phocanema spp.	Sea mammals
	Ancylostoma caninum	Canines
Cutaneous larva migrans	*Ancylostoma braziliense*	Canines, felines
	Ancylostoma caninum	Canines, felines
	Uncinaria stenocephala	Canines, felines
Eosinophilic meningitis	*Angiostrongylus cantonensis*	Rats
	Gnathostoma spinigerum	Felines, other mammals
Pulmonary or cutaneous nodules	*Dirofilaria* spp.	Canines, other mammals
Abdominal angiostrongyliasis	*Angiostrongylus costaricensis*	Cotton rats
Capillariasis	*Capillaria philippinensis*	Birds
Diarrhea	*Nanophyetus salmincola*	Mammals, birds
Swimmer's itch	*Trichobilharzia* spp.	Birds

The diagnosis is definitively confirmed by finding larvae in the affected tissues by histologic examination or by digestion of tissue; however, larvae are frequently not found. CT scans have demonstrated ill-defined hypodense round lesions in the liver of VLM patients, the basis of which is not clear.[4] The enzyme-linked immunosorbent assay (ELISA) using extracts of excretory or secretory products of *T. canis* larvae appears specific and useful for confirming the clinical diagnosis.[10] However, *Toxocara* antibody titers in populations without clinically apparent VLM vary dramatically, and elevated titers cannot definitively establish the diagnosis.

Differential Diagnosis

Eosinophilia, fever, and hepatomegaly are frequently caused by helminths that migrate through the body. *Baylisascaris procyonis* (an ascarid of raccoons) is a recognized cause of larval migrans in the United States.[11] Others are acute schistosomiasis, *Fasciola hepatica* infections, *Ascaris lumbricoides* abscess of the liver, acute liver fluke infections (*Clonorchis sinensis*, *Opisthorchis viverrini*), complications from *Echinococcus* infection of the liver, *Capillaria hepatica*, and other invasive helminths. Diseases not caused by parasitic infections should also be considered. Children with mild disease may manifest only eosinophilia.

Treatment and Management

Most patients recover without specific therapy. Treatment with anti-inflammatory or anthelmintic drugs may be considered for those with severe complications usually caused by involvement of the brain, lungs, or heart. There is no proven effective therapy, although albendazole, thiabendazole, mebendazole, diethylcarbamazine, and other anthelmintics have been used. Indeed, injury to the parasite may provoke an intense inflammatory response leading to worsening of the clinical picture. Corticosteroids have been used with and without specific antilarval therapy, with some reports of improvement.

Prevention

Visceral larva migrans can be easily prevented by a number of simple but effective measures that prevent *T. canis* or *T. cati* eggs from contaminating the environment and children from ingesting eggs. Dogs, particularly puppies, should be periodically tested and treated for *Toxocara* and other worms. Pica should be prevented. Sandboxes in which young children play should be covered when not in use to prevent defecation by dogs and cats.

Ocular Larva Migrans

Ocular larva migrans is caused primarily by an infection of the eye with *T. canis* larvae.[12] Although a present or past history of clinically recog-

nized VLM has occasionally been noted, almost all patients present with unilateral eye visual loss without a past history or present systemic symptoms or signs. Presumably, a larva becomes entrapped in the eye by chance, resulting in an eosinophilic inflammatory mass. Children are most commonly affected and, on the average, are older (mean, 8.6 years in one study) than those diagnosed with VLM. Although the most common lesion is a chorioretinal granuloma in the posterior pole or, occasionally more peripherally, diffuse panuveitis may also be seen. Retinal detachment may occur. This entity was first recognized after examining eyes enucleated for the treatment of presumed retinoblastoma, and remains the most important distinction that ophthalmologists must make in children with subretinal lesions.[12]

Eosinophilia, hepatomegaly, and other signs and symptoms of VLM are usually lacking. The diagnosis is established clinically. Although the serum titers to *Toxocara* larvae are higher than those of a control population,[13] many patients with ocular larva migrans have low or negative titers. However, elevated vitreous[14] and aqueous fluid titers[15] to *Toxocara* larvae compared with serum levels appear useful for establishing the diagnosis. There is no specific therapy.

A characteristic clinically recognizable syndrome, diffuse unilateral subacute neuroretinitis, is caused by infection with helminth larvae of *B. procyonis* and *Toxocara* spp.[16] and other unidentified nematodes.[17,18] A motile larva is commonly found in or below the retina. Photocoagulation is curative. Anthelmintic therapy such as albendazole or thiabendazole may be effective.

Baylisascariasis

Baylisascaris procyonis, an ascarid of raccoons, is a recognized cause of visceral larval migrans in humans and many other animals.[19-22] The life cycle is similar to that of dog and cat ascarids, and infection occurs after ingestion of ova excreted in raccoon feces that subsequently contaminates soil and the environment. Although the clinical manifestations are similar to those caused by dog and cat ascarids, severe and commonly fatal eosinophilic meningoencephalitis occurs in more than half the cases. Eye involvement is common and is one of the known causes of diffuse unilateral subacute neuroretinitis.[16,17] The diagnosis is established by detecting typical larvae in tissues; an experimental serologic examination has been reported but is not routinely available. There is no proven therapy. Of the available drugs, albendazole and corticosteroids are most commonly tried.[17]

Anisakiasis

Anisakiasis is caused by the accidental infection of humans by larvae found in saltwater fish and squid. Definitive hosts are marine mammals. The clinical syndrome is caused by penetration of larvae into the stomach or small intestine. It is characterized by upper or lower abdominal symptoms, or both. The diagnosis is suggested by a history of ingesting raw, salted, pickled, smoked, or poorly cooked fish.

LIFE CYCLE IN MARINE MAMMALS

Larvae of the family Anisakidae, including *Anisakis*, *Pseudoterranova*, and occasionally other genera, can accidentally infect humans.[1,23-25] The adults are found in the stomach of marine mammals. The eggs, passed in the feces, hatch as free-swimming larvae, are ingested by certain crustaceans, and are eaten by fish and squid. When ingested by appropriate marine mammals, such as dolphins, seals, and whales, the larvae burrow head first into the stomach. When consumed by humans, the larvae attempt and many times succeed in burrowing into the stomach or intestine, resulting in typical symptoms.

CLINICAL SYNDROME

Anisakiasis occurs after ingesting raw or improperly cooked marine fish. The disease, initially recognized in the Netherlands after the ingestion of raw herring, is most frequently reported from Japan, where raw fish is commonly eaten. In the United States, infection is still uncommon but is now more frequently recognized because of increased ingestion of raw fish, particularly Pacific salmon. Cod, halibut, pollock, greenling, herring, anchovies, hake, tuna, sardines, and mackerel are other fish that have been implicated.

Clinical manifestations are caused by penetration of worms into the gastrointestinal tract, usually the stomach but also the lower small intestine, most commonly the ileum.[24-26] Occasionally, throat irritation is followed by coughing up the characteristic worm. Initial invasion is associated with acute symptoms, whereas the presence of worms for longer periods causes chronic symptoms. The location of the worms and symptoms depend somewhat on the genus, with *Pseudoterranova* commonly associated with infection of the stomach and *Anisakis* with the intestine. Symptoms usually occur within 48 hours after ingestion, but this pattern is variable. With gastric anisakiasis, patients complain of intense abdominal pain, nausea, and vomiting. Small intestinal involvement is less common and results in lower abdominal pain and signs of obstruction mimicking those of appendicitis. Symptoms may be chronic, sometimes lasting for months and, rarely, years. These symptoms are associated with intestinal masses containing the parasite and are sometimes confused with a tumor, regional enteritis, or diverticulitis. Worms are occasionally located ectopically outside the gastrointestinal tract. *Anisakis* larvae in seafood have been implicated as a cause of acute allergic manifestations such as urticaria, angioedema, and anaphylaxis, with or without accompanying abdominal gastrointestinal symptoms in patients who ingest raw fish.[27-31] In vitro studies and skin tests indicate that sensitization to *Anisakis* antigen is common in this population, whereas sensitization to fish is uncommon.[25,29-31]

LABORATORY FINDINGS

Eosinophilia is usually not present in patients with gastric or intestinal anisakiasis. Leukocytosis is not consistently present with acute anisakiasis but has been noted in almost two thirds of the patients with intestinal involvement in one series.

DIAGNOSIS

Anisakiasis should be considered in anyone with a history of ingesting raw marine fish and suggestive abdominal symptoms. A definitive diagnosis can be established by endoscopy, radiographic studies, or pathologic examination of tissue. In the upper gastrointestinal tract, worms are found partially embedded in any area of the stomach and may be associated with localized mucosal edema, erosions, or mass lesions.[32,33] Upper gastrointestinal radiographic studies may reveal the outline of a worm associated with mucosal edema or tumor formation. Removing the worm during endoscopy definitively establishes the diagnosis and is curative.[26] Intestinal anisakiasis is diagnosed clinically. Varied degrees of thickening of the walls and narrowing of the lumen of the ileum or jejunum are found on radiographic studies. High-resolution ultrasonography has demonstrated small intestinal wall thickening and localized ascites around the involved section of bowel. Examination of aspirated ascites has revealed a preponderance of eosinophils.[34] Lesions resolve within 2 to 3 weeks. Occasionally, removal of the intestinal mass is required to establish the diagnosis and effectively treat the patient. Tissues show inflammatory masses, many eosinophils, and the characteristic helminth. Serologic tests are not generally available but may be useful, particularly in patients whose symptoms have lasted longer than 1 week.[35]

TREATMENT

Symptoms diminish spontaneously in most patients without specific therapy, although the process is hastened by removing worms lodged in the stomach during endoscopy. In one series of intestinal anisakiasis, all 12 patients became asymptomatic by 2 weeks.[32] A report of treatment with albendazole in a case diagnosed only by serology is, at best, suggestive of efficacy.[36] One Japanese investigator has commonly prescribed antacids after removing the stomach worms.

PREVENTION

Larvae resist heating up to 50°C as well as pickling, salting, and some methods of smoking. Infection can be prevented by cooking or freezing fish for 24 hours before ingestion.

CUTANEOUS LARVA MIGRANS (CREEPING ERUPTION)

Cutaneous larva migrans is characterized as serpiginous, reddened, elevated, pruritic skin lesions usually caused by the dog or cat hookworms *Ancylostoma braziliense*, *Ancylostoma caninum*, or *Uncinaria stenocephala*.[1,37] Other animal hookworms including *Bunostomum phlebotomum*, the human hookworms, *Strongyloides stercoralis*, *Gnathostoma spinigerum* and, rarely, insect larvae, can cause a similar picture.

Like human hookworms, *A. braziliense* larvae infect dogs and cats by burrowing through the skin. The adults reside in the intestine and shed eggs, which undergo development into infectious larvae outside the body in places protected from desiccation and temperature extremes, such as sandy shady areas around beaches or under houses. Infections are most common in warm climates, such as the southeastern United States, and occur in children more commonly than in adults. Larvae penetrate the skin, causing tingling followed by itching, vesicle formation, and typically raised, reddened, serpiginous tracks that mark the route of the parasite.[1,38] With severe infections, persons may have hundreds of tracks. Little further development of the parasite occurs. Usually, there are few, if any, systemic symptoms, although some reports have documented lung infiltrates and, rarely, severe lung dysfunction and recovery of parasites in the sputum. Eosinophilia has been noted with some infections. The skin lesions are readily recognized, and the diagnosis is made clinically. Biopsy specimens usually show an eosinophilic inflammatory infiltrate, but the migrating parasite is usually not identified. Therefore, biopsies are usually not indicated to establish the diagnosis.

Without treatment, skin lesions gradually disappear[39] but commonly cause severe itching. Ivermectin given once or twice if needed at 200 µg/kg is the treatment of choice. Albendazole (400 to 800 mg/day PO for 3 to 5 days) is an effective alternative treatment.[40,41]

Eosinophilic Meningitis

Infection of humans with larvae of *Angiostrongylus cantonensis*, the rat lung worm, is characterized by invasion of the brain, leading to signs and symptoms of meningitis and encephalitis associated with an eosinophilic pleocytosis in the cerebrospinal fluid (CSF) and peripheral eosinophilia.[36] The adults of *A. cantonensis* reside in the lungs of rats.[1] Eggs hatch in the lungs and the larvae are swallowed, expelled in the feces, and seek an appropriate molluscan intermediate host, where the parasite develops into infective third-stage larvae. Infective larvae are found in a number of mollusks including slugs, land snails, and a land planarian; they are also found in a number of unrelated animals, including freshwater prawns, land and coconut crabs, and frogs. After ingestion by rats, the infective larvae migrate to the pulmonary arteries and then the lung, enter the blood vessels, and thereby migrate to the brain. Eventually, they return to the lungs via the vasculature. In humans, migration of the larvae to the brain causes eosinophilic meningitis, encephalitis, or both.

Epidemics and sporadic infections occur most commonly in the South Pacific,[42] Southeast Asia,[43] and Taiwan,[44] but more recently have been recognized in Jamaica,[45] Cuba,[46] Egypt,[47] Hawaii, and other regions. The most commonly recognized sources of human infection are raw or undercooked snails, prawns, or crabs. Contamination of foods such as leafy vegetables by larvae deposited by slugs or snails may also occur. Caesar salad was implicated in one epidemic.[45]

Clinical manifestations vary and, although fatalities occur, particularly with massive infections, most patients have a relatively uncomplicated course.[42-44,48] During one well-characterized epidemic, the incubation period ranged from 1 to 6 days after ingestion of infected snails.[42] Symptoms include headache, stiff neck, fever, rash, pruritus, abdominal pain, constitutional complaints, nausea, and vomiting. Neurologic involvement varies from no complaints to paresthesias and pain, weakness, various focal neurologic findings (sixth and fourth cranial nerve palsies are frequently noted), coma, and death. In general, the patients do not appear to be as ill as those who have bacterial meningitis. Signs of meningitis are frequent, but nonspecific. CSF leukocytosis with more than 10% eosinophils is frequent. CSF glucose levels are usually normal, but depressed values have been noted.

The diagnosis is usually established clinically, although serology, if available, is useful.[45] Occasionally, a characteristic larva is found in the CSF at the time of lumbar puncture. A history of travel or being in an endemic region and ingestion of raw or partially cooked implicated foods should be sought. In severe cases, magnetic resonance imaging (MRI) shows meningeal enhancement, tracts in the brain or spinal cord (or both), increased abnormal subcortical and periventricular T2-weighted MRI signals, and enhancing subcortical lesions.[49,50] A heavy worm burden increases the probability of brain involvement. Analysis of the antibody responses by Western blots has shown the development of a characteristic 31-kDa band in infected patients and therefore appears to be a helpful test. However, the lack of availability of the parasite antigen is likely to limit the usefulness of this assay.[45,51]

Symptomatic therapy includes corticosteroids, which have been shown to decrease the duration of headaches in a randomized trial.[52] One well-designed trial compared albendazole treatment alone with placebo and found a marginally significant decrease in headache in the experimental group.[53] However, others have suggested that albendazole does not improve the clinical results compared with corticosteroids alone.[54]

Repeated CSF lumbar punctures appear to be helpful for treating associated headaches, presumably by decreasing CSF pressure. Recovery usually occurs by 2 months, although prolonged symptoms and signs are occasionally noted.

Gnathostomiasis

A characteristic syndrome of intermittent, nonpitting edematous swellings of subcutaneous tissues associated with eosinophilia is caused by migration throughout the body of larvae from a number of species of helminths of the genus *Gnathostoma* (most commonly, *G. spinigerum* in Southeast Asia).[55-57] Although cutaneous symptoms are frequent, any organ may be involved, and the most serious manifestations involve migration of larvae into the brain or spinal cord. Most of these infections occur in Southeast Asia, but large numbers have been recognized in Mexico.[58] Endogenous human infections have also been documented in Spain, Peru, Ecuador, India, China, Japan, Bangladesh, and other areas.

LIFE CYCLE

The adult worms reside in tumorous burrows in the stomachs of a large number of mammals, including cats of various types, dogs, opossums, and raccoons.[1,59] Eggs are shed in the feces, hatch after about 1 week, and are subsequently ingested by small crustaceans called *Cyclops*. These crustaceans are subsequently ingested by a variety of other animals including fish, frogs, and snakes, where they encyst in the muscles as infectious larvae. When eaten by the appropriate definitive host, larvae migrate through the body and eventually invade the stomach, where they mature, mate, and release eggs in the feces. The spectrum of animals that spread infections to humans has broadened considerably because infectious larvae can be passed unaltered from animal to animal after ingestion (paratenic carriage). Most infections occur after eating undercooked freshwater fish, chicken, or pork.

However, infectious larvae can also burrow through the skin, or infections may occur after ingesting *Cyclops* in contaminated water. Rarely, prenatal transmission has been documented.

CLINICAL MANIFESTATIONS

Acute signs and symptoms such as nausea, vomiting, gastrointestinal pain, and fever may occur shortly after ingestion and likely are caused by the initial invasion of the infecting larva into and out of the intestines.[57,60] The most prominent signs, which occur as early as 3 to 4 weeks after ingestion, are intermittent migratory subcutaneus swellings. They may occur anywhere. They are usually nonpitting, often erythematous, and occasionally pruritic and painful. They may also occur as nodules or abscesses or resemble classic cutaneous larva migrans. Eosinophilia is usually present and may be extreme. Migrating larvae may invade any tissue and give rise to symptoms related to specific organs such as the eye, intestines, spinal cord, and brain. Involvement of the latter results in the most serious complication, eosinophilic encephalomyelitis.[55,56] Although gnathostomiasis is a less frequent cause of encephalomyelitis compared to *A. cantonensis,* it tends to result in permanent neurologic deficits and death because there is more invasion of the brain substance. Consistent with this, the CSF has an increased number of red blood cells.

DIAGNOSIS

In some areas of Southeast Asia, gnathostomiasis is a common illness. The diagnosis is suggested when there is a history of intermittent subcutaneous swelling in the presence of eosinophilia and a history of ingesting raw fish or other implicated foods from endemic areas. Serology is helpful and supports or suggests the diagnosis in cryptic cases but is not easily available in nonendemic regions.[61] Occasionally, the worms can be isolated from the migratory swellings or from lesions that develop following treatment, but attempts at parasite recovery are mostly unsuccessful.

DIFFERENTIAL DIAGNOSIS

The syndrome is relatively distinctive. *Loa loa* may present with Calabar swellings and eosinophilia, but the epidemiology is distinctive, and the swellings are not erythematous and do not resemble larval migrans. Cutaneous larval migrans is usually not accompanied by eosinophilia, and there is a distinctive epidemiology. Strongyloidiasis is not commonly associated with swellings and eosinophilia and can be distinguished by the presence of positive serology for *Strongyloides* and/or a positive stool examination.

TREATMENT

Both ivermectin (200 µg/kg for one dose) and albendazole (400 mg/day for 21 days) give cure rates of better than 90%.[62,63]

PREVENTION

Avoiding uncooked pickled fish and other implicated foods prevents infection in most individuals.

Abdominal Angiostrongyliasis

Clinical manifestations of human infections of *Angiostrongylus costaricensis* are caused by penetration and development of the parasite in the lower small bowel and adjacent colon. They are characterized by abdominal pain, vomiting, and a right lower quadrant mass.[64] In the normal host, the rat, adult parasites reside in the arteries and arterioles of the ileocecal area of the intestine. Eggs deposited in the tissue hatch, and the larvae migrate through the intestinal wall into the lumen and are excreted in the feces. Larvae are then ingested by the intermediate host (the slug) and, after further development, become infectious for rats after ingestion. Most likely, the larvae undergo a systemic migration, mature in the intestinal lymphatics, and penetrate the arterioles and arteries in the ileocecal area of the rat, where they reside as adults. In humans, the parasite follows a similar pattern of migration, except that eggs are retained in the tissues and larvae do not appear in the feces. Adult parasites are found most commonly in the arteries and arterioles around the ileocecum and deposit eggs there. Both the eggs and worms provoke an inflammatory response, which results in occluded vessels, an accompanying vasculitis, and an eosinophilic, granulomatous, edematous mass.

Infection of humans, most commonly children, has been recognized in Central and South America, occasionally the Caribbean and, rarely, Africa and other areas. The manner of human infection is not usually known, but it may occur after accidental ingestion of infected slugs or of foods contaminated with larvae deposited in the mucous slime trail of slugs. Mint was implicated in one small epidemic.[65]

Patients are mildly to moderately ill and complain of abdominal pain and tenderness, vomiting, and fever; a right lower quadrant mass is noted in about 50% of cases.[66] Surgery reveals that the cecum, ascending colon, ileum, and appendix are involved to varied degrees. The syndrome resembles appendicitis, except for the usual presence of eosinophilia and leukocytosis in angiostrongyliasis. Perforation occurs uncommonly, and the worms may be found ectopically in extraintestinal sites.[66]

The diagnosis is suspected clinically and confirmed by examination of biopsied or excised specimens. Radiographic findings are nonspecific and show filling defects and spasticity of the ileum, cecum, or colon. Serologic tests have been described that are relatively sensitive and specific, but they are not widely available.[67]

Most patients undergo laparotomy with removal of the inflamed areas; the natural history of infected children is unclear. It is not known if specific anthelmintic therapy is effective, but some clinically diagnosed children have been treated with diethylcarbamazine and thiabendazole (25 mg/kg PO twice daily for 3 days; maximum 3 g/day, which may be toxic) without undergoing surgery. An alternative treatment is mebendazole, 200 to 400 mg three times daily for 10 days.

Massive ascaris infections may present with intestinal masses and may be confused with infections caused by *Angiostrongylus costaricensis*. Infections can be prevented by treating potentially contaminated vegetables with 1.5% bleach at room temperature for 15 minutes.[68]

Eosinophilic Gastroenteritis

One cause of eosinophilic gastroenteritis is infection of humans with *Ancylostoma caninum*, a hookworm of dogs.[69-71] This syndrome is apparently limited to Northern Australia, although the conditions for human infection are likely present in many regions. After invading the skin, the usually single larva migrates to the ileum, and to the colon to a lesser degree, where there is an intense focal response to the worm including ulceration, inflammatory nodules, inflammation, thickening, and stricture formation. Gastrointestinal pain, nausea, vomiting, diarrhea, and bowel obstruction are common and almost always are accompanied by eosinophilia and leukocytosis. Ova are not produced, but the adult worm can sometimes be seen by endoscopy. Patients respond to a standard course of mebendazole 100 mg three times daily for 3 days.

Dirofilariasis

Accidental human infections with *Dirofilaria* result most commonly in a lung nodule or subcutaneous mass. Two groups of parasites of the genus *Dirofilaria* accidentally infect humans.[1] The clinical presentations are generally different, which reflects the final location of the adults in the usual animal host. The adult worms of *Dirofilaria immitis*, the dog heartworm and the only important parasite in the first group, reside in the right side of the heart and the right pulmonary vessels; they are most commonly located in the lungs in humans but may also occur in other areas, mostly the subcutaneous tissues.

Dirofilaria immitis is transmitted by a mosquito to its most common host, the domesticated dog, and other related mammals. After development in subcutaneous tissues, the parasites migrate as young adults to the right side of the heart and the right pulmonary vessels. In humans, the immature filariae migrate similarly but do not fully develop and die, which causes a local vasculitis leading to pulmonary infarcts. Histologic examination usually reveals a dead worm in an infarct with vasculitis and with granulomatous and occasionally eosinophilic inflammation.

Most infections occur in the southeastern United States through infections and transmission to dogs and by accidental transmission to humans. Persons are asymptomatic in more than 50% of the infections and show a coin lesion on a routine chest radiograph.[72,73] Others complain of cough, chest pain, or hemoptysis, most likely caused by pulmonary infarction. In some cases, lung infiltrates are noted that resolve into nodules.[74] Eosinophilia occurs in less than 15% of cases.

The diagnosis is made with certainty only by biopsy. Although serologic tests are available, their sensitivity and specificity are not adequate to rule out other potential life-threatening conditions, such as a tumor.

Adults of the second group of filariae (subgenus *Nochtiella*) reside in the subcutaneous tissues of various mammals and usually cause inflammatory subcutaneous masses in humans.[75] These parasites include *D. tenuis* (raccoon), *D. ursi* (bear), *D. subdermata* (porcupine), and *D. repens* (dogs and cats in Europe and Asia). Conjunctival infection with *D. repens* has been increasingly reported. Patients present with inflammatory subcutaneous masses containing increased numbers of eosinophils. As in infections with *D. immitis,* there are few if any systemic symptoms, and eosinophilia is not usually present. The diagnosis is established by biopsy. However, careful inspection of the entire tissue may be needed to find the parasite. Other filariae of animals such as *Brugia* sp. have also been found in lymphoid or other tissues of humans.

Capillariasis

Capillaria philippinensis inhabits the small bowel of humans, causing diarrhea and malabsorption.[76] Infections have been recognized mostly in the Philippines but also in Thailand, Taiwan, Japan, Korea, Egypt, China, Indonesia, and Iran. The life cycle is incompletely understood, although freshwater fish contain larvae infectious for humans and birds.[77] The latter may be an important reservoir host. After raw freshwater fish are eaten, the larvae invade the jejunum and ileum, and the resulting adults produce both eggs and larvae. Unlike almost all helminths that infect humans, with the exception of *Strongyloides stercoralis*, the parasite multiplies in the gut. This process is known as autoinfection and results in an overwhelming infection. In fulminant cases, autopsies reveal a thickened, edematous small bowel with a flattened mucosa containing a mononuclear infiltrate. Numerous adults, larvae, and eggs are present in both the lumen and mucosa. Larvae infectious for birds, humans, and other mammals develop in certain freshwater fish after ingestion of eggs. Almost all the signs and symptoms are related to progressive diarrhea and malabsorption. Patients complain of borborygmi, abdominal pain, vomiting, weight loss, and malaise resulting in wasting, abdominal distention, and edema. Fever and eosinophilia are uncommon, although eosinophilia has been noted after therapy. Laboratory examinations document the typical findings of protein-losing enteropathy, fat, mineral, and vitamin malabsorption, and electrolyte loss. The diagnosis is established by detecting the characteristic *Trichuris trichiura*–like ova or larvae in the stool. No serologic tests are available.

In untreated patients, mortality rates of up to 33% have been documented, but specific anthelmintic therapy is effective and life-saving. Therapy with mebendazole, 200 mg orally twice daily for 20 days, or albendazole[77] is effective. Relapses are treated with prolonged courses of therapy. Infection is prevented by eating only properly cooked freshwater fish.

Nanophyetiasis

Human infections with *Nanophyetus salmincola*, a diminutive small intestine–dwelling trematode, have been increasingly recognized in the Pacific Northwest of the United States.[78] Humans and other mammals and birds become infected after ingesting raw or undercooked freshwater fish (most commonly salminoid fish) or their eggs.

Gastrointestinal symptoms, including diarrhea, abdominal pain, and gas or bloating with accompanying eosinophilia, suggest the diagnosis. However, asymptomatic infections are common. The diagnosis is established by finding the characteristic small, operculated unembryonated ova in the feces. Praziquantel, 20 mg/kg three times for 1 day, is effective treatment.

Swimmer's Itch

This is also known as schistosomal dermatitis, cercarial dermatitis, and clam digger's itch. Cercariae, the infective form of a large number of blood flukes of birds, such as avian schistosomes (commonly *Trichobilharzia*), those in nonhuman mammals, and less commonly human schistosomes, can cause a characteristic dermatitis in humans associated with penetration of the cercariae into the skin.[1] They are produced and then released by various species of mollusks, which are the intermediate hosts. The clinical manifestations in humans are almost always limited to the skin.[79] Infections are frequent in many areas of the world but are particularly common in persons exposed to the freshwater lakes of the northern United States. However, infections also occur after exposure to saltwater (clam digger's itch).

Although the clinical manifestations vary after the initial exposure, symptoms are typically mild and sometimes go unnoticed.[80,81] The patient complains of itching followed by the appearance of macules at the site of penetration of the cercariae. By 24 hours, the macules have disappeared and begin to be replaced by papules. After repeated exposures, reactions occur earlier than 24 hours after exposure and are more severe. Papules are larger and associated with erythema, itching, and edema. The symptoms subside by 4 to 7 days, but in severe cases they may last weeks.

Control of infection can be obtained by ridding bathing areas of the molluscan intermediate host or the definitive host, or by avoiding infected bodies of water. Treatment is symptomatic. There is no specific anthelmintic therapy.

REFERENCES

1. Beaver PC, Jung RC, Cupp EW. *Clinical Parasitology*. Philadelphia: Lea & Febiger; 1984.
2. Beaver PC, Snyder CH, Carrera GM, et al. Chronic eosinophilia due to visceral larva migrans: Report of three cases. *Pediatrics*. 1952;9:7.
3. Huntley CC, Costas MC, Lyerly BS. Visceral larva migrans syndrome: Clinical characteristics and immunologic studies in 51 patients. *Pediatrics*. 1965;36:523.
4. Chang S, Lim JH, Choi D, et al. Hepatic visceral larva migrans of *Toxocara canis*: CT and sonographic findings. *AJR Am J Roentgenol*. 2006;187:W622.
5. Glickman LT, Schantz PM. Epidemiology and pathogenesis of zoonotic toxocariasis. *Epidemiol Rev*. 1981;3:230.
6. Worley G, Green JA, Frothingham TE, et al. Toxocara canis infection: Clinical and epidemiological associations with seropositivity in kindergarten children. *J Infect Dis*. 1984;159:591.
7. Jones WE, Schantz PM, Foreman K, et al. Human toxocariasis in a rural community. *Am J Dis Child*. 1980;134:967.
8. Mok CH. Visceral larva migrans: A discussion based on review of the literature. *Clin Pediatr*. 1968;7:565.
9. Finsterer J, Auer H. Neurotoxocarosis. *Rev Inst Med Trop Sao Paulo*. 2007;49:279.
10. Glickman L, Schantz P, Dombroske R, et al. Evaluation of serodiagnostic tests for visceral larva migrans. *Am J Trop Med Hyg*. 1978;27:492.
11. Cunningham CK, Kazacos KR, McMillan JA, et al. Diagnosis and management of Baylisascaris procyonis infection in an infant with nonfatal meningoencephalitis. *Clin Infect Dis*. 1994;18:868.
12. Wilder HC. Nematode endophthalmitis. *Trans Am Acad Ophthalmol Otolaryngol*. 1950;55:99.
13. Schantz PM, Meyer D, Glickman LT. Clinical, serologic, and epidemiologic characteristics of ocular toxocariasis. *Am J Trop Med Hyg*. 1979;28:24.
14. Biglan AW, Glickman LT, Lobes LA. Serum and vitreous Toxocara antibody in nematode endophthalmitis. *Am J Ophthalmol*. 1979;88:898.
15. Felberg NT, Shields JA, Federman JL. Antibody to *Toxocara canis* in the aqueous humor. *Arch Ophthalmol*. 1981;99:1563.
16. Gass JD, Braunstein RA. Further observations concerning the diffuse unilateral subacute neuroretinitis syndrome. *Arch Ophthalmol*. 1983;101:1689-1697.
17. De Souza EC, Nakashima Y. Diffuse unilateral subacute neuroretinitis: Report of transvitreal surgical removal of a subretinal nematode. *Ophthalmology*. 1995;102:1183.
18. Gass JD, Callanan DG, Bowman CB. Oral therapy in diffuse unilateral subacute neuroretinitis. *Arch Ophthalmol*. 1992;110:675.
19. Fox AS, Kazacos KR, Gould NS. Fatal eosinophilic meningoencephalitis and visceral larva migrans caused by the raccoon ascarid *Bayliscaris procyonis*. *N Engl J Med*. 1985;312:1619.
20. Park SY, Glaser C, Murray WJ, et al. Raccoon roundworm (*Baylisascaris procyonis*) encephalitis: Case report and field investigation. *Pediatrics*. 2000;106:E56.
21. Rowley HA, Uht RM, Kazacos KR, et al. Radiologic-pathologic findings in raccoon roundworm (*Baylisascaris procyonis*) encephalitis. *Am J Neuroradiol*. 2000;21:415.
22. Gavin PJ, Kazacos KR, Shulman ST. Baylisascariasis. *Clin Microbiol Rev*. 2005;18:703.
23. Smith JW, Wootten R. Anisakis and anisakiasis. In: Lumsden WHR, Muller R, Baker JR, eds. *Advances in Parasitology*, vol 16. London: Academic Press; 1978:93-163.
24. Van Thiel PH, Kuipers FC, Roskam RTH. A nematode parasitic to herring, causing acute abdominal syndromes in man. *Trop Geogr Med*. 1960;2:97.
25. Yokogawa N, Yoshimura H. Clinicopathologic studies of larval anisakiasis in Japan. *Am J Trop Med Hyg*. 1967;16:723.
26. Sugimachi K, Inokuchi K, Ooiwa T, et al. Acute gastric anisakiasis: Analysis of 178 cases. *JAMA*. 1985;253:1012.
27. Montoro A, Perteguer MJ, Chivato T, et al. Recidivous acute urticaria caused by *Anisakis simplex*. *Allergy*. 1997;52:985.
28. Alonso A, Daschner A, Moreno-Ancillo A. Anaphylaxis with *Anisakis simplex* in the gastric mucosa. *N Engl J Med*. 1997;337:350.
29. Del Pozo MD, Audicana M, Diez JM, et al. Anisakis simplex, a relevant etiologic factor in acute urticaria. *Allergy*. 1997;52:576.
30. Moreno-Ancillo A, Caballero MT, Cabanas R, et al. Allergic reactions to Anisakis simplex parasitizing seafood. *Ann Allergy Asthma Immunol*. 1997;79:246.
31. Daschner A, Alonso-Gomez A, Cabanas R, et al. Gastroallergic anisakiasis: Borderline between food allergy and parasitic disease: Clinical and allergologic evaluation of 20 patients with confirmed acute parasitism by *Anisakis simplex*. *J Allergy Clin Immunol*. 2000;105:176.
32. Matsui T, Iida M, Murakami M, et al. Intestinal anisakiasis: Clinical and radiologic features. *Radiology*. 1985;157:299.
33. Kusuhara T, Watanabe K, Fukuda M. Radiographic study of acute gastric anisakiasis. *Gastrointest Radiol*. 1984;9:305.
34. Shirahama M, Koga T, Ishibashi H, et al. Intestinal anisakiasis: US in diagnosis. *Radiology*. 1991;185:789.
35. Ishikura H, Kikuchi K, Nagasawa K, et al. *Anisakidae* and anisakiosis. *Prog Clin Parasitol*. 1993;3:4.
36. Moore DA, Girdwood RW, Chiodini PL. Treatment of anisakiasis with albendazole. *Lancet*. 2002;360:54.
37. Heukelbach J, Feldmeier H. Epidemiological and clinical characteristics of hookworm-related cutaneous larva migrans. *Lancet Infect Dis*. 2008;8:302-309.
38. Hitch JM. Systemic treatment of creeping eruption. *Arch Dermatol Syph*. 1947;55:664.
39. Katz R, Ziegler J, Blank H. The natural course of creeping eruption and treatment with thiabendazole. *Arch Dermatol*. 1965;91:420.
40. Caumes E. Treatment of cutaneous larva migrans and Toxocara infection. *Fundam Clin Pharmacol*. 2003;17:213.
41. Bouchaud O, Houze S, Schiemann R, et al. Cutaneous larva migrans in travelers: A prospective study, with assessment of therapy with ivermectin. *Clin Infect Dis*. 2000;31:493.
42. Kliks MM, Kroenke K, Hardman JM. Eosinophilic radiculomyeloencephalitis: An angiostrongyliasis outbreak in American Samoa related to ingestion of *Achatina fulica* snails. *Am J Trop Med Hyg*. 1982;31:1114.
43. Punyagupta S, Juttijudata P, Bunnag T. Eosinophilic meningitis in Thailand: Clinical studies of 484 typical cases probably caused by *Angiostrongylus cantonensis*. *Am J Trop Med Hyg*. 1975;24:921.
44. Yii CY. Clinical observations on eosinophilic meningitis and meningoencephalitis caused by *Angiostrongylus cantonensis* in Taiwan. *Am J Trop Med Hyg*. 1976;25:233.
45. Slom TJ, Cortese MM, Gerber SI, et al. An outbreak of eosinophilic meningitis caused by *Angiostrongylus cantonensis* in travelers returning from the Caribbean. *N Engl J Med*. 2002;346:668.
46. Martinez-Delgado JF, Gonzalez-Cortinas M, Tapanes-Cruz TR, et al. Eosinophilic meningoencephalitis in Villa Clara (Cuba): A study of 17 patients. *Rev Neurol*. 2000;31:417.
47. Brown FM, Mohareb EW, Yousif F, et al. Angiostrongylus eosinophilic meningitis in Egypt. *Lancet*. 1996;348:964.
48. Rosen L, Chappell R, Laqueur GL, et al. Eosinophilic meningoencephalitis caused by a metastrongylid lungworm of rats. *JAMA*. 1962;179:620.
49. Kanpittaya J, Jitpimolmard S, Tiamkao S, et al. MR findings of eosinophilic meningoencephalitis attributed to *Angiostrongylus cantonensis*. *AJNR Am J Neuroradiol*. 2000;21:1090.
50. Jin EH, Ma Q, Ma DQ, et al. Magnetic resonance imaging of eosinophilic meningoencephalitis caused by *Angiostrongylus cantonensis* following eating freshwater snails. *Chin Med J*. 2008;12167.
51. Nuamtanong S. The evaluation of the 29- and 31-kDa antigens in female *Angiostrongylus cantonensis* for serodiagnosis of human angiostrongyliasis. *Southeast Asian J Trop Med Public Health*. 1996;27:291.
52. Chotmongkol V, Sawanyawisuth K, Thavornpitak Y. Corticosteroid treatment of eosinophilic meningitis. *Clin Infect Dis*. 2000;31:660.
53. Jitpimolmard S, Sawanyawisuth K, Morakote N, et al. Albendazole therapy for eosinophilic meningitis caused by *Angiostrongylus cantonensis*. *Parasitol Res*. 2007;100:1293.
54. Sawanyawisuth K, Sawanyawisuth K. Treatment of angiostrongyliasis. *Trans R Soc Trop Med Hyg*. 2008;102:990.
55. Chitanondh H, Rosen L. Fatal eosinophilic encephalomyelitis caused by the nematode *Gnathostoma spinigerum*. *Am J Trop Med Hyg*. 1967;16:638.
56. Punyagupta S, Juttijudata P. Two fatal cases of eosinophilic myeloencephalitis, a newly recognized disease caused by *Gnathostoma spinigerum*. *Trans R Soc Trop Med Hyg*. 1968;62:801.
57. Rusnak JM, Lucey DR. Clinical gnathostomiasis: Case report and review of the English-language literature. *Clin Infect Dis*. 1993;16:33.
58. Diaz-Camacho SP, Zazueta-Ramos M, Ponce-Torrecillas E, et al. Clinical manifestations and immunodiagnosis of gnathostomiasis in Culiacan, Mexico. *Am J Trop Med Hyg*. 1998;59:908.
59. Miyazaki I. On the genus *Gnathostoma* and human gnathostomiasis, with special reference to Japan. *Exp Parasitol*. 1960;9:338.
60. Migasena S, Pitisuttithum P, Desakorn V. Gnathostoma larva migrans among guests of a New Year party. *Southeast Asian J Trop Med Public Health*. 1991;22(Suppl):225.
61. Dharmkrong-at A, Migasena S, Suntharasamai P, et al. Enzyme-linked immunosorbent assay for detection of antibody to *Gnathostoma* antigen in patients with intermittent cutaneous migratory swelling. *J Clin Microbiol*. 1986;23:847.
62. Kraivichian P, Kulkumthorn M, Yingyourd P, et al. Albendazole for the treatment of human gnathostomiasis. *Trans R Soc Trop Med Hyg*. 1992;86:418.
63. Nontasut P, Bussaratid V, Chullawichit S, et al. Comparison of ivermectin and albendazole treatment for gnathostomiasis. *Southeast Asian J Trop Med Public Health*. 2000;31:374.
64. Morera P, Cepedes R. Angiostrongylus costaricensis n. sp. (Nematoda: metastrongyloidea), a new lungworm occurring in man in Costa Rica. *Rev Biol Trop*. 1971;18:173.
65. Kramer MH, Greer GJ, Quinonez JF, et al. First reported outbreak of abdominal angiostrongyliasis. *Clin Infect Dis*. 1998;26:365.
66. Loria-Cortes R, Lobo-Sanahuga JF. Clinical abdominal angiostrongylosis: A study of 116 children with intestinal eosinophilic granuloma caused by Angiostrongylus costaricensis. *Am J Trop Med Hyg*. 1980;29:538.

67. Geiger SM, Laitano AC, Sievers-Tostes C, et al. Detection of the acute phase of abdominal angiostrongyliasis with a parasite-specific IgG enzyme linked immunosorbent assay. *Mem Inst Oswaldo Cruz.* 2001;96:515.

68. Zanini GM, Graeff-Teixeira C. Inactivation of infective larvae of *Angiostrongylus costaricensis* with short-time incubations in 1.5% bleach solution, vinegar or saturated cooking salt solution. *Acta Trop.* 2001;78:17.

69. Provic P, Croese J. Human eosinophilic enteritis caused by dog hookworm *Ancylostoma caninum. Lancet.* 1990;335:1299.

70. Croese J, Loukas A, Opdebeeck J, et al. Human enteric infection with canine hookworms. *Ann Intern Med.* 1994;120:369.

71. Croese TJ. Eosinophilic enteritis: A recent North Queensland experience. *Aust N Z J Med.* 1988;18:848.

72. Orihel TC, Eberhard ML. Zoonotic filariasis. *Clin Microbiol Rev.* 1998;11:366.

73. Cifferri F. Human pulmonary dirofilariasis in the United States: A critical review. *Am J Trop Med Hyg.* 1982;31:302.

74. Kochar AS. Human pulmonary dirofilariasis: Report of three cases and brief review of the literature. *Am J Clin Pathol.* 1985;84:19.

75. Beaver PC, Wolfson JS, Waldron MA. *Dirofilaria ursi*-like parasites acquired by humans in the northern United States and Canada: Report of two cases and brief review. *Am J Trop Med Hyg.* 1987;37:357.

76. Whalen GE, Strickland GT, Cross HJ, et al. Intestinal capillariasis: A new disease in man. *Lancet.* 1969;1:13.

77. Cross JH. Intestinal capillariasis. *Clin Microbiol Rev.* 1992;5:120.

78. Fritsche TR, Eastburn RL, Wiggens LH, et al. Praziquantel for treatment of human *Nanophyetus salmincola* (*Troglotrema salmincola*) infection. *J Infect Dis.* 1989;160:896.

79. Horak P, Kolarova L, Adema CM. Biology of the schistosome genus *Trichobilharzia. Adv Parasitol.* 2002;52:155.

80. Olivier L. Schistosome dermatitis, a sensitization phenomenon. *Am J Hyg.* 1949;49:290.

81. MacFarlane MV. Schistosome dermatitis in New Zealand. Part II. Pathology and immunology of cercarial lesions. *Am J Hyg.* 1949;50:152.

SECTION K ECTOPARASITIC DISEASES

292

Introduction to Ectoparasitic Diseases

JAMES H. DIAZ

Ectoparasites infest the skin and its appendages, such as the hair and sebaceous glands, and most external orifices, especially the ears, nares, and orbits. Like endoparasites, ectoparasites may be obligatory parasites, programmed to feed on human hosts to complete their life cycles, or facultative parasites, preferring to feed on nonhuman hosts, infesting humans only as accidental or dead-end hosts. Over the past 2 decades, there have been several reports of significant outbreaks of ectoparasitic diseases, principally myiasis, scabies, and tungiasis, both in indigenous populations and in travelers returning from developing nations and even exclusive tropical beach resorts.[1,2] Many common ectoparasites, such as head lice and scabies mites, are also developing increasing resistances to medical therapies, including the safest topical insecticides.[3-6] Other ectoparasites, such as the New World human botfly, *Dermatobia hominis*, and the jigger or chigoe flea, *Tunga penetrans*, are resistant to systemic and topical antiparasitics, and can only be treated surgically.

Ectoparasitic diseases have reemerged as unusual, but not uncommon, infectious diseases worldwide, especially in high-risk populations. Indigenous populations of ectoparasite-endemic tropical nations often suffer from recurrent infestations and superinfestations that can result in severe disfigurement from facial cavitary myiasis or permanent disability from tungiasis-associated autoamputations.

Taxonomy of Ectoparasites

The phylum Arthropoda is the largest phylum of the animal kingdom and includes the subphylum Crustacea and the classes Insecta and Arachnida. All the medically important ectoparasites, including fleas, flies, lice, mites, and ticks, are members of the phylum Arthropoda and have chitinous exoskeletons, segmented bodies, and jointed appendages. Fleas, flies, and lice are six-legged members of the class Insecta, which also includes the mosquitoes and true bugs (order Hemiptera). Mites, including chigger and scabies mites, and ticks are the eight-legged members of the class Arachnida, subclass Acari. The arthropod ectoparasites of medical importance are stratified by taxonomic classes and distinguishing external anatomic characteristics in Table 292-1.

Epidemiology of Ectoparasitic Diseases

Ectoparasitic diseases share many of the general characteristics of emerging infectious diseases. Commonly shared characteristics of ectoparisitoses and emerging infectious diseases include the following: (1) origination as zoonoses, with disease establishment dependent on arthropod vector competency; (2) introduction into new, susceptible host populations; (3) infection by endemic agents given selective advantages by changing ecologic or socioeconomic conditions; and (4) recent movement from rural to urban endemic areas, often following migrating human host populations seeking better economic opportunities.[7-9]

To assess the potential combined impact of increasing international travel and the relaxation of quarantine regulations for imported animals in the United Kingdom (UK) on arthropod-induced ectoparasitic dermatoses, McGarry and colleagues have analyzed 73 insect specimens removed from symptomatic patients and submitted to their laboratory for identification at the Liverpool School of Tropical Medicine during the years 1994 to 2000.[10] Of the 73 specimens identified, there were 27 ticks, 24 flies, 15 miscellaneous insects, and 7 mites. Most of the arthropod dermatoses originated in the UK ($n = 46$, 63%), and were caused by tick bites ($n = 18$), principally *Ixodid ricinus* (the common sheep tick), an important European vector of Lyme disease and neuroborreliosis. Myiasis cases predominated in returning travelers ($n = 18$, 67%), principally furuncular myiasis from larval infestation by *Cordylobia anthropophaga* ($n = 9$), the Tumbu fly, or *Dermatobia hominis* ($n = 4$), the human botfly. Among the arthropod dermatoses caused by miscellaneous arthropods, most were pediculosis pubis caused by infestation with *Phthirus pubis*, the pubic louse ($n = 7$), or hemorrhagic, bullous bite groupings caused by *Cimex lectularius*, the common bedbug ($n = 3$). The authors concluded that exotic ectoparasitic infestations, particularly myiasis, predominated in returning travelers from Africa and Latin America; pubic lice were domestic, likely sexually transmitted, infestations; and bedbug infestations were domestically and internationally acquired, often by fomites on bedding and luggage.

Mechanisms of Ectoparasite-Borne Diseases and Injuries

The arthropod ectoparasites can threaten human health directly by burrowing into, feeding, dwelling, and reproducing in human skin and orifices (mites, fleas, flies), or by blood or tissue juice sucking (fleas, lice, mites, ticks). The arthropod ectoparasites can also threaten human health indirectly by infectious disease transmission (fleas, mites, ticks). Ticks are the most versatile ectoparasitic arthropods and can transmit a variety of infectious diseases (viral, bacterial, and protozoan) and even inject paralytic toxins (tick paralysis) during their prolonged blood meals. Unlike other ectoparasites, ticks can be infective as males and females and throughout all stages of their development. The most commonly encountered arthropod ectoparasites, excluding ticks, and the major clinical manifestations of their infestations are featured in Table 292-2.

Conclusions

Recent epidemiologic evidence now supports the endemicity of several ectoparasitic diseases and their arthropod vectors (Table 292-3) and human and animal reservoir hosts throughout the developing world and in many parts of the developed world, including Europe and the United States. Ectoparasitic diseases have also reemerged in regions where they were once effectively controlled. Ectoparasitic diseases will continue to reemerge in the developed world for several reasons, including the following: (1) the globalization of trade and commerce with ectoparasites and their human and animal hosts traveling worldwide on airplanes and container ships; (2) mass movements of populations from rural to urban areas and from developing to developed nations; (3) the worldwide legitimate and illegal trade of exotic animals and animal hides and skins; (4) the accidental and intentional introduction of exotic animal species into new regions with welcoming ecosystems; and (4) the growing populations of susceptible, and often immunocompromised human hosts, living in long-term care facilities and in crowded and impoverished periurban communities.

TABLE 292-1	Taxonomy of Arthropods (Phylum Arthropoda) of Major Medical Importance*	
Phylum and Class	*Common Names*	*No. of Legs, No. of Body Segments, Other Identifying Anatomic Features*
Phylum Arthopoda, Class Insecta		
Order Culicinae	Mosquitoes	Six, three, wings
Order Diptera	Flies*	Six, three, wings
Order Hemiptera	True bugs (e.g., bedbugs, reduviid bugs)	Six, three, ± wings
Order Hymenoptera	Ants, bees, wasps	Six, three, ± wings
Order Phthiraptera	Lice*	Six, three, no wings
Order Siphonaptera	Fleas*	Six, three, no wings
Phylum Arthropoda, Class Arachnida		
Subclass Acari	Mites and ticks*	Eight, one globose body, no distinct heads†, no wings
Order Araneae	Spiders	Eight, two, no wings
Order Scorpiones	Scorpions	Eight, two, abdomens with terminal stingers

*The arthropod ectoparasites of major medical importance by taxonomic order and distinctive anatomic features.
†Mouthparts visible dorsally only in ixodid (hard) ticks.

TABLE 292-2	Common Arthropod Ectoparasites (excluding ticks) and Clinical Manifestations of Ectoparasitoses		
Representative Species of Infesting Arthropod Ectoparasites	*Common Names of Infesting Arthropod Ectoparasite*	*Geographic Distribution*	*Major Clinical Manifestations of Ectoparasitoses*
Class Insecta, Order Phtiraptera, Suborder Anoplura	Lice		
Pediculus humanus corporis	Body louse	Worldwide	Pediculosis corporis
Pediculus humanus capitis	Head louse	Worldwide	Pediculosis capitis
Phthirus pubis	Crab (pubic) louse	Worldwide	Pediculosis pubis (phthiriasis)
Order Diptera	Flies		
Family Calliphoridae	Screwworms		
Auchmeromyia senegalensis	Congo floor-maggot fly	Sub-Saharan Africa, Cape Verde Islands	Larvae are nocturnal blood feeders, no myiasis (tissue invasion); wound (cutaneous) myiasis
Callitroga americana	American screwworm	North and Central America	Cavitary (invasive) myiasis
Chrysomyia bezziana	Old World screwworm	Tropical Africa, Asia, Indonesia	Cavitary (invasive) myiasis
Cochliomyia hominivorax	New World screwworm	Central and South America	Furuncular myiasis
Cordylobia anthropophaga	Tumbu (mango) fly	Africa	Furuncular myiasis
Family Oestridae	Botflies		
Cuterebra spp.	Rodent botfly	North and Central America	Furuncular myiasis
Dermatobia hominis	Human botfly	Central and South America	Furuncular myiasis
Order Siphonaptera	Fleas		
Ctenocephalides spp.	Cat (Chlamydophila felis) and dog fleas (C. canis)	Worldwide	Bite groupings (mechanical vectors of dog and rat tapeworms)
Pulex irritans	Human flea	Worldwide	Bite groupings (plague vector in Chilean Andes)
Tunga penetrans	Chigoe (jigger) flea	Central and South America, Africa, Europe, Asia	Tungiasis
Xenopsylla cheopis	Oriental rat flea	Africa, Americas	Most efficient bubonic plague vector
Class Arachnida	Spiders, mites, ticks	Worldwide	
Subclass Acari	Mites and ticks		
Sarcoptes scabiei	Itch (scabies) mite	Worldwide	Scabies, crusted (Norwegian) scabies
Eutrombicula alfreddugesi	Common chigger (redbug chigger)	Worldwide	Chiggers
Leptotrombidium akamushi	Japanese-Asian rodent chigger	Japan, India, Australia	Potential scrub typhus (Tsutsugamushi disease) vector
Leptotrombidium deliensis	Indian-Asian rodent chigger	Eurasia-Eastern Asia, Southeast Asia, India, Australia, Indo-Pacific Islands	Potential scrub typhus (Tsutsugamushi disease) vector

TABLE 292-3	Selected Diseases Transmitted by Arthropods	

Infectious Disease	Vector
Anaplasmosis (human granulocytotropic)	Hard ticks
Arbovirus diseases (including yellow fever, dengue fever, encephalitis)	Mosquitoes and ticks
Babesiosis	Hard ticks
Boutonneuse fever (tick bite fever; *Rickettsia conorii*)	Hard ticks
Chagas disease	Triatome (kissing) bugs
Colorado tick fever	Hard ticks
Ehrlichiosis, monocytotropic and ewingii	Hard ticks
Endemic relapsing fever (*Borrelia duttonii*)	Soft ticks
Epidemic relapsing fever (*Borrelia recurrentis*)	Human body lice
Epidemic typhus (*Rickettsia prowazekii*)	Human body lice
Filariasis (*Wuchereria bancrofti, Brugia malayi*)	Mosquitoes
Leishmaniasis (*Leishmania* spp.)	Lutzomyia sandfly in the Americas, phlebotomid flies elsewhere
Loiasis (*Loa loa*)	Tabanid flies
Lyme disease (*Borrelia burgodorferi*)	Hard ticks
Malaria (*Plasmodium* spp.)	Mosquitoes
Murine typhus (*Rickettsia mooseri*)	Rat fleas, lice
Onchocerciasis (*Onchocerca volvulus*)	Black flies
Plague (*Yersinia pestis*)	Rat fleas
Q fever (*Coxiella burnetii*)	Hard ticks, fleas
Rickettsialpox (*Rickettsia akari*)	Mouse mites
Rocky Mountain spotted fever (*Rickettsia rickettsii*)	Hard ticks
Scrub typhus (*Rickettsia tsutsugamushi*)	Mites (chiggers)
Trypanosomiasis, African sleeping sickness	Glossina (tsetse) flies
West Nile fever	Mosquitoes

REFERENCES

1. Heukelbach J, Mencke N, Feldmeier H. Cutaneous larva migrans and tungiasis: The challenge to control zoonotic ectoparasitoses associated with poverty. *Trop Med Int Health*. 2002;7:907-910.
2. Heukelbach J, Gomide M, Araujo F Jr, et al. Cutaneous larva migrans and tungiasis in international travelers exiting Brazil: An airport survey. *J Travel Med*. 2007;14:374-380.
3. Roberts RJ. Head lice. *N Engl J Med*. 2002;346:1645-1650.
4. Meinking TL, Serrano L, Hard B, et al. Comparative in vitro pediculicidal efficacy of treatments in a resistant head lice population in the United States. *Arch Dermatol*. 2002;138:220-224.
5. Lebwohl M, Clark L, Levitt J. Therapy for head lice based on life cycle, resistance, and safety considerations. *Pediatrics*. 2007;119:965-974.
6. Chosidow O. Scabies. *N Engl J Med*. 2006;354:1718-1727.
7. Walker DH, Barbour AG, Oliver JH, et al. Emerging zoonotic and vector-borne diseases: Ecological and epidemiological factors. *JAMA*. 1996;275:463-469.
8. McFee RB. Global infections: Avian influenza and other significant emerging pathogens. *Dis Mon*. 2007;53:343-347.
9. Marano N, Arguin PM, Pappaioanou M. Impact of globalization and animal trade on infectious disease ecology. *Emerg Infect Dis*. 2007;13:1807-1809.
10. McGarry JW, McCall PJ, Welby S. Arthropod dermatoses acquired in the UK and overseas. *Lancet*. 2001;357:2105-2106.

293

Lice (Pediculosis)

JAMES H. DIAZ

Pediculosis is a complex of three different human infestations with two species of blood-sucking lice of the insect order Phthiraptera, suborder Anoplura: (1) *Pediculus humanus* and (2) *Phthirus pubis*. Sometime after early humans began to wear clothes, *P. humanus* evolved into two clinically distinct ectoparasitic variants, *P. humanus* var. *corporis*, the body louse (Fig. 293-1), and *P. humanus* var. *capitis*, the head louse (Fig. 293-2). Although morphologically indistinct, these human louse variants do not interbreed, prefer unique anatomic niches on human hosts, and are now considered distinct species. Specifically, head lice (*P. humanus capitis*) leave their hair shaft nests for blood meals on the scalp and body lice (*P. humanus corporis*) leave their clothes seams nests for blood meals on the body. *Phthirus pubis*, the crab or pubic louse (Fig. 293-3), is morphologically distinct from the two *P. humanus* species, has a crab-shaped body, prefers to dwell in the hair-bearing areas of the pubic and inguinal areas, but may also infest the hairy areas of the axillae, chest, and abdomen and even the eyelashes (phthiriasis palpebrum). Pubic lice remain relatively stationary, unless mating or egg laying, anchored to the bases of hair shafts while blood feeding.

Epidemiology

Pediculosis capitis, or head lice, is the most common of the three types of human pediculoses, afflicting millions of people annually, mostly school-aged children, in developing and industrialized nations. Body lice infestations, or pediculosis corporis, are associated with poor hygiene and low socioeconomic status and primarily infest the indigent, institutionalized, homeless, refugees from civil unrest, and immunocompromised. Body and head lice are transmitted by direct contact between infested individuals and, much less commonly, by indirect contact with fomites, such as bedding, clothing, headgear, combs and brushes. Pubic lice infestations, or phthiriasis, are caused by *P. pubis*, the pubic or crab louse. Pubic lice are more often transmitted during sexual rather than fomite contacts and often coexist with crusted (Norwegian) genital scabies and other sexually transmitted diseases.

Unlike head lice and pubic lice, body lice can transmit several bacterial diseases. Homeless, immunocompromised, and refugee populations are at greatest risks of body lice infestations and epidemics of louse-borne bacterial diseases, including the following: (1) relapsing fever caused by *Borrelia recurrentis*, (2) trench fever caused by *Bartonella quintana*, (3) epidemic typhus caused by *Rickettsia prowazekii*, (4) bacillary angiomatosis caused by *Bartonella henselae* and *Bartonella quintana*, and (5) subacute bacterial endocarditis caused by *Bartonella elizabethae*. *Bartonella* (formerly *Rochalimaea*) *elizabethae* and *B. quintana* have extensive domestic and wild animal zoonotic reservoirs. They have been recognized as infectious organisms of high importance, not only in displaced populations in evacuee and refugee camps, but also in immunocompromised subjects, particularly homeless individuals with the acquired immunodeficiency syndrome (AIDS).[1-3]

Diagnosis of Lice Infestations

Lice infestations are diagnosed by demonstrating live adult lice, nymphs, and viable eggs, or nits, in their precise human ecologic niches. Adult lice are flattened dorsoventrally and are 1 mm (pubic lice) to 3 mm (head and body lice) in length, have three pairs of legs ending in powerful claws that can grip hair shafts, and exhibit a reddish-brown hue after blood feeding (see Figs. 293-2 and 3). Females can live on their hosts for up to 3 months, lay up to 300 nits in a lifetime, and die within 24 hours when separated from hosts (see Fig. 293-2). Nits are oval in shape, less than 1 mm in diameter, grayish-white in color, and fluoresce in ultraviolet or Wood's light, when viable (Fig. 293-4). Nits are deposited on hair shafts at the skin surface, and hatch nymphs within 6 to 10 days (see Fig. 293-4). Nymphs resemble miniature adults and grow to adulthood within 10 days. Empty egg cases remain attached to hair shafts after hatching, and are not diagnostic of active infection.[4] Head lice and their viable nits are often attached to hairs close to the scalp, especially in occipital and postauricular locations. Because body lice only visit their human hosts to feed on blood, adults, nymphs, and nits are found in clothing, usually aligned along inner seams (Fig. 293-5). Pubic lice and their nits may be found in the pubic, perianal, and inguinal areas, in axillary and chest hair, and even in the eyelashes (phthiriasis palpebrum), especially in children acquiring pubic lice infestations from parents (Fig. 293-6).[5]

Clinical Manifestations and Differential Diagnosis

HEAD LICE

The clinical manifestations of pediculosis capitis range from asymptomatic infestations to severe pruritus, with self-inflicted, often secondarily infected, excoriations with impetigo and postoccipital lymphadenopathy. The differential diagnosis of pediculosis capitis includes eczema, lichen simplex chronicus, dandruff, seborrheic dermatitis, and bacterial impetigo.

BODY LICE

Despite the fact that body lice reside in clothing, often along seams, and not on the body like head lice, pediculosis corporis infestation is often much more symptomatic than pediculosis capitis and causes severe pruritus, with extensive self-inflicted excoriations (see Fig. 293-5). The sites of blood feeding are often present as erythematous macules, papules, or areas of papular urticaria with a central hemorrhagic punctum. The differential diagnosis includes eczematous dermatitis, lichen simplex chronicus, and scabies.

CRAB LICE (PEDICULOSIS PUBIS)

Infestation with pediculosis pubis (phthiriasis), or crab lice, is less symptomatic compared with pediculosis capitis. These organisms affect all hair–bearing regions, most commonly the pubic and perianal areas, but also the upper eyelashes and the hairy areas of the axillae, chest, and abdomen. More extensive infestations usually occur in males with more body hair–bearing regions than females. Pubic lice may appear as 1- to 2-mm brownish-gray specks in infested hairy areas, where they remain stationary for days with claws grasping hair shafts and mouth parts embedded in the skin (see Fig. 293-3). The average life span for *Phthirus pubis* is 17 days for females and 22 days for males. Females deposit grayish-white eggs or nits at the skin-hair junctions. The egg incubation period is 7 to 8 days, and the life cycle from egg to adult is 22 to 27 days. Clinical manifestations include papular urticaria and self-inflicted, often infected, excoriations at blood feeding sites, and regional, usually inguinal, lymphadenopathy

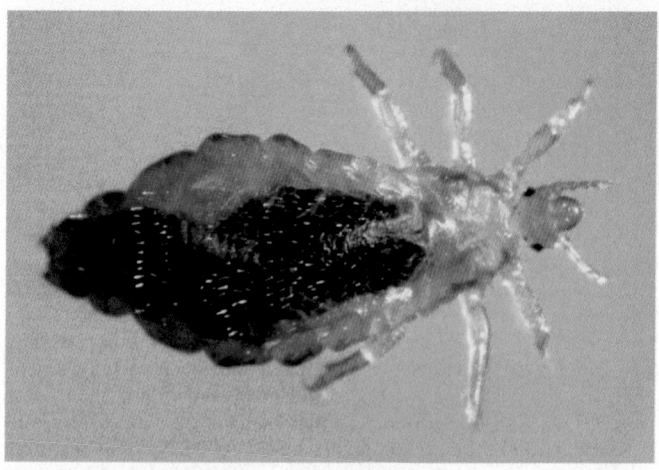

Figure 293-1 **Dorsal view of a female body louse, *Pediculus humanus* var. *corporis*.** *(From Centers for Disease Control and Prevention [CDC], Atlanta, GA. CDC Public Health Image Library, image 9204.)*

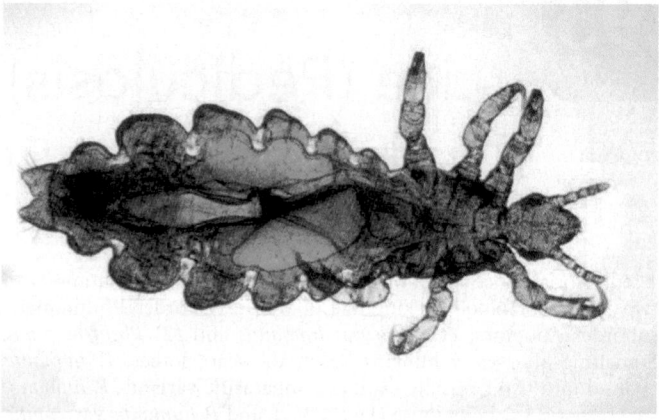

Figure 293-2 **Dorsal view of a female head louse, *Pediculus humanus* var. *capitis*, containing eggs or nits.** *(From Centers for Disease Control and Prevention [CDC], Atlanta, GA. CDC Public Health Image Library, image 377.)*

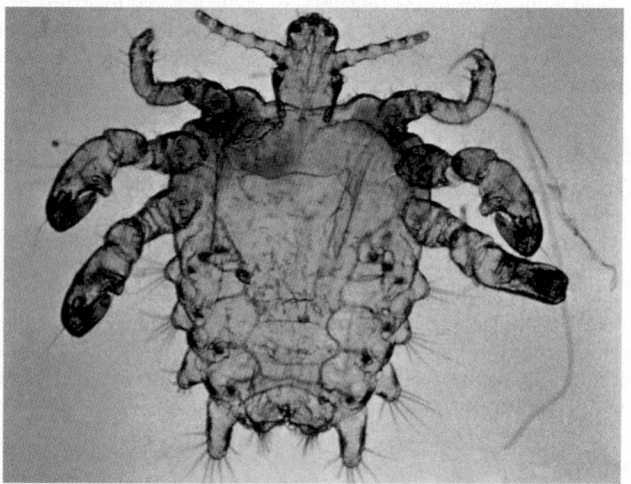

Figure 293-3 **Enlarged ventral image of a pubic or crab louse, *Phthirus pubis*.** *(From Centers for Disease Control and Prevention [CDC], Atlanta, GA. CDC Public Health Image Library, image 4077.)*

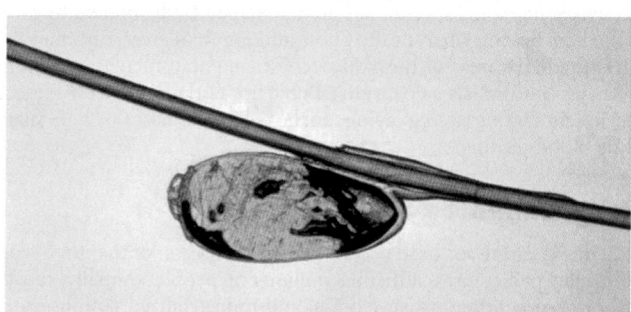

Figure 293-4 **The unhatched nit or egg of the head louse, *Pediculus humanus* var. *capitis*, attached to a hair shaft.** Note the red eye spots of the developing nymph embryo. *(From Centers for Disease Control and Prevention [CDC], Atlanta, GA. CDC Public Health Image Library, image 378.)*

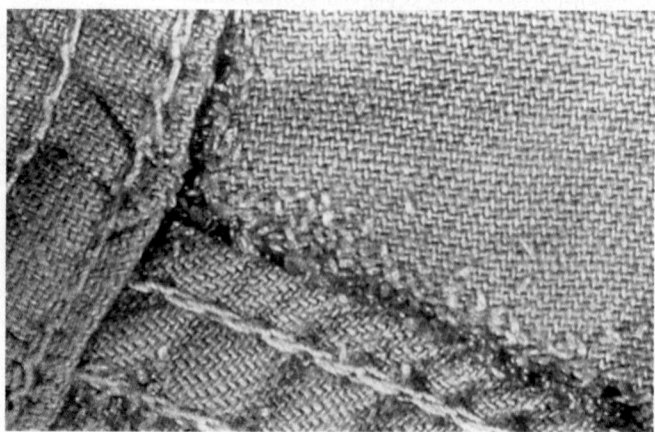

Figure 293-5 **Live eggs from the body louse, *Pediculus humanus* var. *corporis*, lining the seams of clothing.** *(From Centers for Disease Control and Prevention [CDC], Atlanta, GA. CDC Public Health Image Library, image 5270.)*

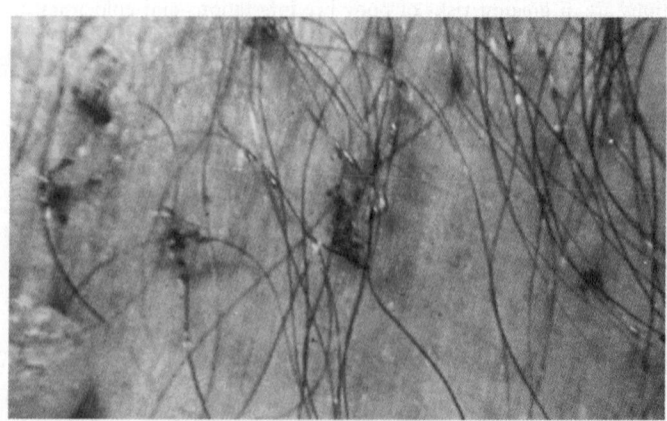

Figure 293-6 **Erythematous lesions seen in the pubic region of a patient in response to the bites of blood-feeding crab or pubic louse, *Phthirus pubis*.** *(From Centers for Disease Control and Prevention [CDC], Atlanta, GA. CDC Public Health Image Library, image 4078.)*

TABLE 293-1	Recommended Pediculicide Treatments for Pediculosis Capitis*				
Pediculicide	Trade Names	Therapeutic Efficacy (Ovicidal, Pediculicidal)	Safety Profile	Contraindications
0.33% pyrethrins + 4% piperonyl butoxide shampoo	A-200 (OTC) RID (OTC)	95% ovicidal; no residual activity; increasing drug resistance	Excellent	Chrysanthemum and daisy (plant family Compositae) allergies possible contraindications
1%-5% permethrin cream rinse	Acticin (OTC) (Rx) Nix (OTC)	2-wk residual activity; increasing drug resistance	Excellent	Prior allergic reactions
0.5% malathion lotion, 1% malathion shampoo	Ovide (Rx)	95% ovicidal; rapid (5 min) killing; good residual activity; increasing drug resistance	Flammable 78% isopropyl alcohol vehicle stings eyes, skin, mucosa; increasing drug resistance; organophosphate poisoning risks with overapplication and ingestion	Infants and children <6 mo of age; pregnancy; breast-feeding
1% lindane lotion and shampoo	Generic (Rx)	95% ovicidal; no residual activity; increasing drug resistance	Potential for CNS toxicity from organochlorine poisoning, usually manifesting as seizures, with overapplication and ingestion	Preexisting seizure disorder; infants and children <6 mo of age; pregnancy; breast-feeding
Ivermectin, 200 μg/kg single PO dose, repeated in 10 days. 0.8% shampoo (off-label use)	Stromectol (Rx); not ovicidal; second dose recommended	Excellent	Excellent, but not in widespread use; nausea and vomiting possible; take on empty stomach with water only	Safety in pregnancy uncertain; not recommended for children weighing <5 kg; not FDA-approved for pediculosis in United States

*Carbaryl (Sevin), a carbamate pesticide, is not currently approved or available as a human topical preparation for use for pediculosis in the United States. Carbaryl is, however, prescribed for pediculosis in Europe and elsewhere. Ectoparasite resistance to carbaryl has not been reported.

CNS, central nervous system; FDA, U.S. Food and Drug Administration; OTC, over-the-counter availability; Rx, available by prescription only.

(see Fig. 293-6). Pathognomonic findings may include maculae ceruleae (*taches bleues*), bluish-gray irregularly shaped macules, 0.5 to 1 cm in diameter, scattered over the lower abdominal wall, buttocks, and upper thighs.[6] *Maculae ceruleae* may be caused by subcutaneous tissue staining from heme pigments altered by louse saliva and digestion. The differential diagnosis of crab lice includes eczematous dermatitis, seborrheic dermatitis, tinea cruris, folliculitis, molluscum contagiosum, and scabies, which frequently coexists with phthiriasis. Management includes initial bathing with soap and water, followed by two topical or systemic treatments with pediculicides, 7 to 10 days apart (Table 293-1).

Therapy

Both *Pediculus humanus* species (head and body lice) and *Phthirus pubis* (the crab or pubic louse) have now demonstrated high levels of resistance worldwide to the safest topical pediculicides, specifically the natural pyrethrins and synthetic pyrethroids (permethrin, phenothrin).[4,7-11] In addition, resistance to lindane, an organochlorine insecticide, and malathion, an organophosphate insecticide, both alone and combined with pyrethroids, has been reported in the United Kingdom and elsewhere.[4,7] In a randomized comparison of wet combing versus 0.5% malathion shampoos for head lice in the United Kingdom, Roberts and colleagues reported a 78% cure rate for malathion shampoo versus 38% for wet combing.[9] In an in vitro pediculicidal efficacy comparison of five pediculicides available in the United States, Meinking and associates reported the following results: (1) there were significant differences in the pediculicidal efficacies of the five pesticides tested; (2) malathion was the only tested pesticide in their study that had not become less effective as a pediculicide; (3) the ranked order of therapeutic effectiveness from most to least effective was 0.5% malathion, undiluted natural pyrethrins with piperonyl butoxide, 1% permethrin, diluted natural pyrethrins with piperonyl butoxide, and 1% lindane; and (4) some head lice in the United States had become resistant to most pediculicides.[10]

The increasing resistance of head lice to the pyrethrins and pyrethroids has led to the increasing use of more toxic pesticides, specifically lindane, malathion, and carbaryl (not approved by the U.S. Food and Drug Administration [FDA] in the United States), in treating pyrethroid-resistant pediculosis capitis worldwide.[7,10,11] Lindane is being inappropriately overprescribed, especially for recurrent infestations with lindane-resistant head lice.[4,6] Lindane is an organochlorine insecticide that bioaccumulates in adipose and nerve tissue with overapplication and can cause seizures, especially in children, or if ingested.[4,8] Although malathion, an organophosphate pesticide, has demonstrated the greatest therapeutic efficacy against head lice in the United States, it is an irreversible acetylcholinesterase inhibitor that can cause a cholinergic toxidrome and fatal neuromuscular paralysis following overapplication or ingestion.[10] Carbaryl, a carbamate pesticide, highly effective against both head lice and scabies, is being increasingly prescribed for *pediculosis capitis* outside the United States, especially in the United Kingdom and Europe.[11] Carbaryl is a reversible (nonaging) acetylcholinesterase inhibitor, closely related to the organophosphate pesticides that can also cause a cholinergic (muscarinic and nicotinic) toxidrome following overapplication or ingestion.

Unfortunately, all the topical pesticides used to treat ectoparasitic infections share the same three characteristics as the three most commonly ingested childhood poisons[12]: (1) prescribed, often over-the counter (OTC), medications, (2) household products, and (3) pesticides.[12] As the prevalence of ectoparasitic infections with pesticide-resistant ectoparasites increases, alternative pesticides, more toxic than pyrethrins and pyrethroids, will be prescribed for ectoparasitic infestations, medications will continue to be administered in households, and household accidental overapplication or ingestion of more toxic pesticide formulations for pediculosis may increase without enhanced public health education measures.[13]

TREATMENT OF PEDICULOSIS CAPITIS INFESTATION

Management of pediculosis capitis includes two topical or systemic treatments with pediculocides, 7 to 10 days apart, and removal of all viable nits by carefully combing wet hair. Olive oil, petroleum jelly, or HairClean 1-2-3 are preferred hair-wetting agents, and plastic combs are preferred over metal combs. Unfortunately, the ideal pediculicide with 100% killing activity against lice and nits does not exist. Table 293-1 presents the most commonly used pediculicides for lice infestations. As noted, drug resistance is increasing against the safest pediculicides, the pyrethrins and synthetic pyrethroids, and even lindane and malathion, an effective ovicidal insecticide with 95% efficacy against viable nits.[4,7,8]

TREATMENT OF BODY LICE INFESTATION

Management includes initial bathing with soap and water, followed by two topical or systemic treatments with pediculicides, 7 to 10 days apart (see Table 293-1). Topical medications should be applied to clean affected areas, allowed to dry, and not rinsed for 8 (malathion) to 24 (pyrethrins, pyrethroids) hours.

Prevention

Prevention strategies for head lice include combinations of sanitizing the environment and, more importantly, eliminating all human reservoirs of head lice in households, apartments, housing complexes, classrooms, and schools. Some common preventive interventions include the following: (1) avoiding contact with potentially contaminated items, such as hats, head sets, clothing, towels, combs, brushes, bedding, and upholstery; (2) soaking all combs and brushes in isopropyl alcohol or 2% Lysol solution; (3) sanitizing the household environment by high heat cycle washing and drying of all bedding, clothing, and headgear; and (4) inspecting high-risk schoolchildren for active head lice, viable nits, and nymphs. Lebwohl and co-workers have recommended that "no-nit policies" in schools be abandoned.[4] As noted, nonviable nits are simply empty egg cases and do not indicate active infestation.

Prevention and control strategies for pediculosis corporis should include the following:

1. Hot cycle washing and drying of all clothing and bedding
2. Clothing and body delousing with 1% permethrin dusting powder, especially in outbreak situations with potential for bacterial disease transmission
3. Institution of basic personal hygiene and sanitation measures, including showering, body washing, and clean clothing changes

Prevention strategies for pubic lice are similar to the prevention strategies for body lice and should include the following:

1. Hot cycle washing and drying of all clothing and bedding
2. Institution of basic personal hygiene and sanitation measures
3. Treatment of sexual contacts with active infestations
4. Examination and laboratory testing of patients and their sexual contacts for other sexually transmitted diseases, especially crusted scabies and AIDS.

REFERENCES

1. Pape M, Kollaras P, Mandraveli K, et al. Occurrence of *Bartonella henselae* and *Bartonella quintana* among human immunodeficiency virus-infected patients. *Ann N Y Acad Sci.* 2005;1063: 299-301.
2. Loutit JS. *Bartonella* infections: Biverse and elusive. *Hosp Pract (Minneap).* 1998;33:37-38.
3. Maurin M, Birtles R, Raoult D. Current knowledge of *Bartonella* species. *Eur J Clin Microbiol.* 1997;16:487-506.
4. Lebwohl M, Clark L, Levitt J. Therapy for head lice based on life cycle, resistance, and safety considerations. *Pediatrics.* 2007; 119:965-974.
5. Downs AM, Stafford KA, Harvey I, et al. Evidence for double resistance to permethrin and malathion in head lice. *Br J Dermatol.* 1999;141:508-511.
6. Burkhart CG. Relationship of treatment-resistant head lice to the safety and efficacy of pediculicides. *Mayo Clin Proceed.* 2004;79: 661-666.
7. Roberts RJ, Casey D, Morgan DA, et al. Comparison of wet combing with malathion for treatment of head lice in the UK: A pragmatic randomized controlled trial. *Lancet.* 2000;356:540-544.
8. Meinking TL, Serrano L, Hard B, et al. Comparative in vitro pediculicidal efficacy of treatments in a resistant head lice population in the United States. *Arch Dermatol.* 2002;138:220-224.
9. Hill N. Control of head lice: past present, and future. *Exp Rev Antiinfect Ther.* 2006;4:887-894.
10. Uziel Y, Adler A, Aharonowitz G, et al. Unintentional childhood poisonings in the Sharon area in Israel: A prospective 5-year study. *Ped Emerg Care.* 2005;21:248-251.
11. Diaz JH. Increasing pesticide-resistant ectoparasitic infections may increase pesticide poisoning risks in children. *J La State Med Soc.* 2008;160:210-220.
12. Burkhart CN. Oral ivermectin therapy for phthiriasis palpebrum. *Arch Ophthalmol.* 2008;118:134-135.
13. Chapel TA, Katta T, Kusmar T, et al. Pediculosis pubis in a clinic for sexually transmitted diseases. *Sex Transm Dis.* 1979;6:257-260.

294

Scabies

JAMES H. DIAZ

Scabies, an infestation by the itch or scabies mite, *Sarcoptes scabiei* var. *hominis*, has remained a major public health problem throughout the developing world (Fig. 294-1). Scabies has now become a significant reemerging ectoparasitosis in its most severe form, crusted or Norwegian scabies (Fig. 294-2), in the developed world, especially among the homeless, institutionalized older adults, mentally retarded, and immunocompromised.[1]

Epidemiology

The worldwide annual prevalence of scabies has been estimated to be about 300 million cases.[2] Although more often associated with crowding, homelessness, and institutionalization, scabies occurs worldwide in both genders, at all ages, and among all ethnic and socioeconomic groups. In the United Kingdom (UK), scabies is more prevalent in women and children living in urban areas and occurs more often during winter than summer.[3] In a 2008 prospective survey in Ghent, Belgium, Lapeere and colleagues reported a crude incidence for scabies of 28 cases/100,000 inhabitants/year.[4] The highest annual incidence of scabies was noted in immigrants (88/100,000) and in those older than 75 years (51/100,000). Scabies is hyperendemic throughout the developing world, especially in sub-Saharan Africa (13% annual prevalence rate), India, the Aboriginal regions of northern Australia, and the South Pacific Islands, especially the Solomon Islands.[2,5,6]

Scabies infestations and superinfestations with crusted (Norwegian) scabies are more prevalent among several specific high-risk groups, including the following: (1) men who have sex with men; (2) patients treated in sexually transmitted disease clinics; (3) homeless patients with the acquired immunodeficiency syndrome (AIDS); and (4) patients with human T-cell lymphotropic virus type 1 (HTLV-1) infection.[1,7,8] Many experts now recommend evaluating all high-risk patients with crusted scabies for human immunodeficiency virus (HIV) and HTLV-1 infection.[9] In a prospective study of 23 patients with crusted scabies in Peru, HTLV-1 infection was diagnosed in 16 patients (69.6%) by enzyme-linked immunosorbent assay (ELISA) and confirmed by Western immunoblot analysis.[8] In addition to HTLV-1 infection, other significant comorbid features for crusted scabies in the Peruvian study included corticosteroid therapy (8.6%), malnutrition (8.6%), and Down syndrome (4.3%).

Transmission

Unlike ectoparasitic fleas and flies, scabies mites cannot jump or fly, but can crawl at a rate of 2.5 cm/min on warm, moist skin (see Fig. 294-1).[2] They can survive for 24 to 36 hours at room temperature and average humidity and remain capable of infesting humans.[10] Scabies is most easily transmitted by skin-to-skin contact, as with sex partners, children playing, or even health providers examining highly infectious patients with crusted scabies. High-risk sexual behaviors for contracting scabies include sporadic sexual contacts and men who have sex with men.[4] Scabies mites have not been demonstrated to transmit HIV, HTLV-1, or any other infectious agent. The more mites there are on a human host, the greater the risks of transmission by close direct contact, more so than by indirect contact with fomites, such as shared bedding and clothing. Although rare, the indirect transmission of scabies occurs and is more common among immunocompromised hosts with AIDS, family members of an index atypical (crusted) case, and within the institutional settings described.[1]

Several nonhuman species of sarcoptid mites can cause animal scabies with itching, inflammation, and hair loss. Animal scabies occurs commonly in domestic pets and animals, especially in cats, dogs, pigs, horses, and camels. Immunocompromised individuals may also contract animal scabies from domestic animals, usually dogs, with sarcoptic mange. Animal scabies mites are facultative ectoparasites in humans and cannot effectively complete their life cycles in human dead-end hosts. Infestations are usually self-limited in humans, but can be treated successfully, if indicated, with 5% permethrin lotion, 10% crotamiton cream or lotion, or oral ivermectin.

Clinical Manifestations

The human scabies mite is an obligate parasite and completes its entire life cycle on its human hosts as females burrow intradermally to lay eggs and larvae emerge and mature to reinfest the same or new hosts. Female mites burrow preferentially into the thinner areas of the epidermis by dissolving the stratum corneum with proteolytic secretions. Burrows are usually no deeper than the stratum granulosum. Female mites then lay their eggs at the end of tunneled burrows 5 to 10 mm long, and larvae hatch 2 to 3 days after eggs are laid. The entire incubation period from eggs to full-grown mites lasts about 14 to 15 days.[11] The human incubation period from initial infestation to symptom development is 3 to 6 weeks in initial infestations and as short as 1 to 3 days in reinfestations as a result of prior sensitization to mite antigens.[2]

Classic or typical scabies presents as generalized, intense nocturnal itching in a characteristic topographic distribution as 10 to 15 fertile female mites are transferred from infected patients to new hosts. The skin eruptions in reinfestations and atypical forms of scabies are considered consequences of infestation and hypersensitivity reactions to mite antigens.[2]

In classic scabies, the preferred distribution of skin eruptions includes hairless areas with a thin stratum corneum, such as the sides and interdigital web spaces of fingers and toes, popliteal fossae, flexor surfaces of the wrists, buttocks, and female breasts (Fig. 294-3).[2] Although inflammatory pruritic papules are present at most infested sites, the pathognomonic linear to serpiginous intradermal burrows, 5 to 10 mm long, dotted with fecal lithes (pellets) or scybala, and terminating in raised papules hiding ovipositing females, may be absent. Nonspecific secondary lesions occur commonly as the result of scratching and secondary infection and include self-inflicted excoriations, eczematization, lichenification, and impetigo.

Scabies may also present in three atypical forms, especially in high-risk institutionalized or immunocompromised patients with HIV or HTLV-1 infections. The atypical forms of scabies include (1) scalp scabies in infants, (2) crusted (Norwegian) scabies in institutionalized and immunocompromised patients, and (3) sexually transmitted nodular scabies. Scabietic nodules will develop in 7% to 10% of patients with scabies infestations, usually in males on the penis and scrotum, and appear as darkened, tender nodules 5 to 20 mm in diameter, often with a raised female mite burrow on top (Fig. 294-4). The atypical forms of scabies are compared with classic scabies and stratified by high-risk human host populations, presenting clinical manifestations, and differential diagnoses in Table 294-1.

Diagnosis

Although newer diagnostic methods are under investigation, the diagnosis of scabies is made predominantly by epidemiologic considerations and clinical observations. A clinical diagnosis may be confirmed by low-power microscopic examination of a burrow skin scraping that

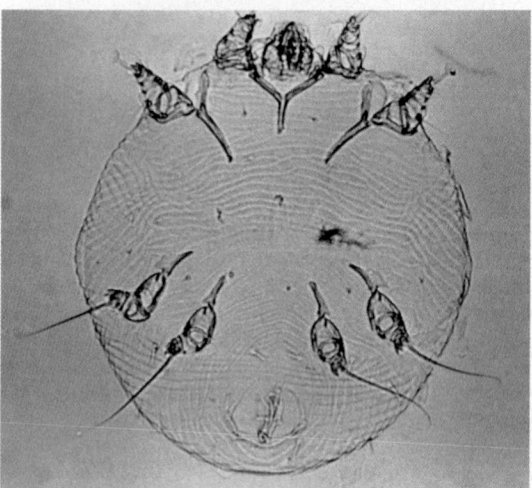

Figure 294-1 **Micrograph of a cleared and slide-mounted scabies mite, *Sarcoptes scabiei* (ventral view).** *(From Centers for Disease Control and Prevention [CDC], Atlanta, GA. CDC Public Health Image Library, image 6301.)*

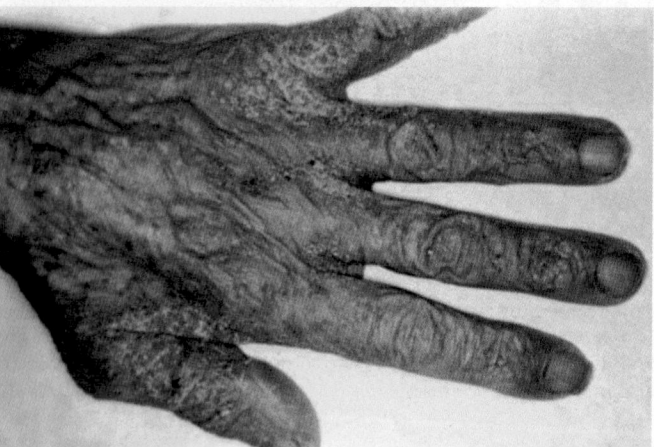

Figure 294-3 **Dorsal view of an older patient's hand demonstrating a crusted scabies infestation by the scabies mite, *Sarcoptes scabiei.*** Note the localized crusting in the interdigital web spaces. *(From Centers for Disease Control and Prevention [CDC], Atlanta, GA. CDC Public Health Image Library, image 4800.)*

excavates the female mite, 0.2 to 0.5 mm in length, translucent with brown legs, and too small to be seen with the naked eye. Eggs (0.02 to 0.03 mm in diameter), smaller eggshell fragments, and fecal lithes or pellets may also be identified in microscopic specimens of burrow scrapings (see Fig. 294-1).[2] Potassium hydroxide should not be used to mount the burrow scrapings because it can dissolve mite fecal lithes. As noted, the failure to identify pathognomonic burrows and to find mites is common, particularly in initial cases with low parasite burdens, and does not rule out scabies.

In atypical scabies cases, skin biopsy may help confirm the diagnosis.[2] Although untested in controlled trials in large study populations, newer diagnostic methods for scabies now under investigation include enhanced microscopic techniques (e.g., epiluminescence microscopy, noncomputed dermoscopy), immunologic detection of specific scabies antibodies by enzyme-linked immunosorbent assay (ELISA), and molecular identification of scabies DNA by polymerase chain reaction (PCR) assay.[12-14]

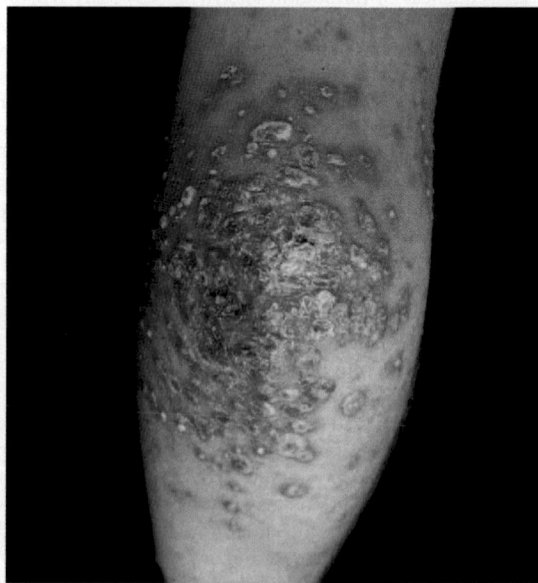

Figure 294-2 **Crusted (Norwegian) scabies on the extensor surface of the elbow secondarily infected with *Staphylococcus aureus.*** Note the confluence of the crusts and pustules and the similarity of the lesion to psoriasis, both in its hyperkeratotic appearance and in its location on an extensor surface. Risk factors for crusted scabies include immunocompromise by advanced age, prolonged glucocorticoid therapy, cancer chemotherapy, and human immunodeficiency virus or human T-cell lymphotropic virus type 1 infection. *(From Fitzpatrick TB, Johnson RA, Wolff K, Suurmond D. Color Atlas and Synopsis of Clinical Dermatology. 4th ed. New York: McGraw-Hill; 2001:841.)*

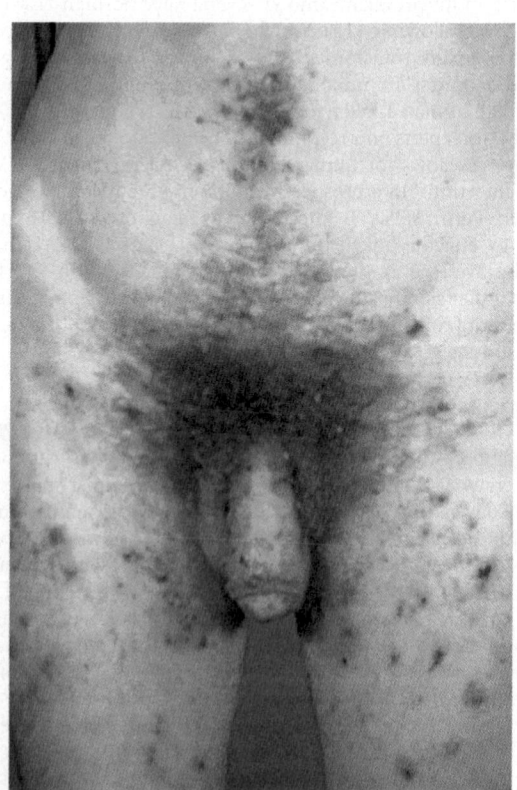

Figure 294-4 **Sexually transmitted nodular scabies infestation in a male caused by the scabies mite, *Sarcoptes scabiei.*** Note the nodular pustular lesions clustered around the umbilicus and inner thighs. *(From Centers for Disease Control and Prevention [CDC], Atlanta, GA. CDC Public Health Image Library, image 6538.)*

TABLE 294-1	Different Presenting Forms of Scabies		
Presenting Forms of Scabies	Specific High-Risk Populations	Clinical Manifestations	Limited Differential Diagnoses
Classic scabies (scabies vulgaris)	Infants and children; sexually active adults; men who have sex with men	Intense generalized pruritus, worse at night; inflammatory pruritic papules localized to finger webs, flexor aspects of wrists, elbows, axillae, buttocks, genitalia, female breasts; lesions and pruritus spare the face, head, and neck; secondary lesions include eczematization, excoriation, impetigo	Dermatitis herpetiformis, drug reactions, eczema, pediculosis corporis, lichen planus, pityriasis rosea
Scalp scabies	Infants and children; institutionalized older adults; AIDS patients; patients with preexisting crusted scabies	Atypical crusted papular lesions of the scalp, face, palms, and soles	Dermatomyositis, ringworm, seborrheic dermatitis
Crusted scabies (Norwegian scabies, scabies norvegica, scabies crustosa)	Institutionalized older adults; institutionalized developmentally disabled (Down syndrome); homeless, especially HIV-positive; all immunocompromised patients, particularly those with AIDS-, HIV-, HTLV-1–positive; transplant recipients; patients on prolonged systemic steroids and chemotherapy	Psoriasiform hyperkeratotic papular lesions of the scalp, face, neck, hands, feet, with extensive nail involvement; eczematization and impetigo common	Contact dermatitis, drug reactions, eczema, erythroderma, ichthyosis, psoriasis
Nodular scabies	Sexually active adults; men who have sex with men; HIV-positive men > HIV-positive women	Violaceous pruritic nodules localized to male genitalia, groin, axillae, representing hypersensitivity reaction to mite antigens	Acropustulosis, atopic dermatitis, Darier's disease, lupus erythematosus, lymphomatoid papulosis, papular urticaria, necrotizing vasculitis, secondary syphilis

AIDS, acquired immunodeficiency syndrome; HIV, human immunodeficiency virus; HTLV-1, human T-cell lymphotropic virus type 1.

Treatment

Topical or oral scabicides should be used to treat infested persons and their close personal contacts simultaneously, regardless of the presence of symptoms.[2] Currently recommended treatment options for scabies are listed in Table 294-2. In a review on the treatment of scabies, Strong and Johnstone noted that both topical 5% permethrin and oral ivermectin appear most effective for individual infections, more research would be needed to compare the effectiveness of malathion with permethrin for individual infections, and there was insufficient evidence to recommend specific miticides to control community and institutional outbreaks of scabies at present.[15] The most effective topical treatments for scabies are 5% permethrin cream and 1% lindane cream or lotion, with permethrin safer and slightly more effective than lindane, an organochlorine pesticide capable of causing seizures and sudden death caused by overapplication or accidental ingestions.[16,17] The other topical treatments for scabies include 10% to 25% benzoyl benzoate lotions (not available in the United States), 10% crotamiton cream or lotion, 2% to 10% sulfur in petrolatum ointments, and 0.8% ivermectin lotion (not available in the United States; see Table 294-2).

The topical treatments for scabies may not be well accepted or tolerated by some patients for many reasons, including severe burning and stinging (with benzyl benzoate and 5% permethrin) in cases of secondarily excoriated or eczematous infestations, and in demented or disabled patients, who may not be able to comply with application regimens. In such cases, a single oral dose of ivermectin, 200 μg/kg, may offer a more acceptable and equally effective alternative. In a 2007 prospective trial, Sule and Thacher compared the effectiveness of oral ivermectin, 200 μg/kg, with topical 25% benzoyl benzoate and monosulfiram soap in 210 Nigerian patients aged 5 to 65 years with scabies.[18] Subjects with persistent lesions received a second course of therapy after 2 weeks. The investigators observed resolution of all lesions in 77 of 98 subjects (79%) treated with ivermectin and in 60 of 102 subjects (59%) treated topically (P = .003). The scabies cure rate at 4 weeks was 95% in the ivermectin group and 86% in the topical treatment group (P = .04). It was concluded that oral ivermectin is as effective as topical treatment with benzyl benzoate and monosulfiram in scabies and leads to more rapid improvement. Ivermectin, however, is not ovicidal, and a second course of oral treatment at adult mite maturation time of 14 to 15 days is now recommended.[2,19]

In a prospective trial comparing oral ivermectin with topical 5% permethrin in scabies, Usha and Gopalakrishnan Nair reported a 70% cure rate with a single dose of ivermectin compared with a 95% cure rate with topical 5% permethrin (P < .003), but a second dose of ivermectin, 200 μg/kg, taken 2 weeks later, increased the cure rate to 95%.[19] Nevertheless, the Centers for Disease Control and Prevention (CDC) recommends topical 5% permethrin cream or lotion as first-line therapy for scabies, especially in initial classic infestations.[20] Unfortunately, scabies mite drug resistance to both topical 5% permethrin preparations and oral ivermectin have now emerged in severe outbreaks of crusted scabies and in the hyperendemic regions noted.[21]

Prevention

Prevention and control strategies for scabies include the following: (1) aggressive treatment of infested patients and all close household, institutional, and sexual contacts, especially in cases of highly infectious crusted scabies; (2) disposal of or hot wash-dry sterilization of all index case–contaminated clothing and bedding by machine washing and drying at 60°C or higher; (3) provision of improved access for personal hygiene and health care for all displaced, homeless, or institutionalized persons; and (4) aggressive control of outbreaks of zoonotic scabies with the potential for human transmission caused by the sarcoptid mites of various domestic animals, especially cats, dogs, camels, pigs, and horses.[2,22]

Conclusions

All patients with scabies and their close household, institutional, and sexual contacts should be informed that scabies is a transmissible ectoparasitic infestation and that several topical treatments and an effective oral treatment are now readily available and highly effective (see Table 294-2). Precise diagnosis should be confirmed, if possible, by microscopic, immunologic, or molecular methods. Topical 5% permethrin preparations remain reasonable first-line therapies for classic scabies, and are recommended by the CDC. Topical benzoyl benzoate preparations are equally effective alternative choices. Oral ivermectin, 200 μg/kg initially and repeated in 2 weeks, may be preferred for patients who cannot tolerate topical therapies or who are unable to adhere to topical application schedules, or who have atypical or topical drug-resistant scabies. Sexually active patients with nodular scabies

TABLE 294-2	Currently Recommended Treatment for Scabies				
Scabicides	FDA Approved?	Pregnancy Category*	Dosing Schedule	Safety Profile	Contraindications
5% permethrin cream (Actin, Nix, Elimite)	Yes	B	Apply from neck down; wash off after 8-14 hr; good residual activity, but second application recommended after 1 wk	Excellent; itching and stinging on application	Prior allergic reactions; infants <2 mo of age; breast-feeding
1% lindane lotion or cream	Yes	B	Apply 30-60 mL from neck down; wash off after 8-12 hr; no residual activity; increasing drug resistance	Potential for CNS toxicity from organochloride poisoning, usually manifesting as seizures, with overapplication and ingestions	Preexisting seizure disorder; infants and children <6 mo of age; pregnancy; breast-feeding
10% crotamiton cream or lotion (Eurax)	Yes	C	Apply from neck down on two consecutive nights; wash off 24 hr after second application	Excellent; not very effective; exacerbates pruritus	None
2%-10% sulfur in petrolatum ointments	No	C	Apply for 2-3 days, then wash	Excellent; not very effective	Preexisting sulfur allergy
10%-25% benzoyl benzoate lotion	No	None	Two applications for 24 hr with 1-day to 1-wk interval	Irritant; exacerbates pruritus; can induce contact irritant dermatitis and pruritic cutaneous xerosis	Preexisting eczema
0.5% malathion lotion (Ovide), 1% malathion shampoo (unavailable in the United States)	No	B	95% ovicidal; rapid (5 min) killing; good residual activity Increasing drug resistance	Flammable 78% isopropyl alcohol vehicle stings eyes, skin, mucosa Increasing drug resistance; organophosphate poisoning risk with overapplication and ingestions	Infants and children <6 mo of age; pregnancy; breast-feeding
Ivermectin (Stromectol), 0.8% lotion (unavailable in the United States)	Yes	C	200-µg/kg single PO dose, may be repeated in 14-15 days; not ovicidal, second dose highly recommended on day 14 or 15; recommended for endemic or epidemic scabies in institutions and refugee camps	Excellent; may cause nausea and vomiting; take on empty stomach with water	Safety in pregnancy uncertain; probably safe during breast-feeding; not recommended for children weighing <15 kg

*U.S. Food and Drug Administration (FDA) safety in pregnancy categories: A, safety established; B, presumed safe; C, uncertain safety; D, unsafe; X, highly unsafe.
CNS, central nervous system.

should be screened for other sexually transmitted diseases. Serious consideration should be given to screening patients with crusted scabies for HIV and HTLV-1 infections, particularly in scabies and HTLV-1 hyperendemic regions of the world and in homeless shelter outbreaks of crusted scabies. Future molecular investigations of scabies mite biology and genetic drug resistance are needed to permit the development of better diagnostic tools and treatment strategies for human scabies, especially atypical scabies.

REFERENCES

1. Tijoe M, Vissers WH. Scabies outbreaks in nursing homes for the elderly: Recognition, treatment options and control of reinfestation. *Drugs Aging.* 2008;25:299-306.
2. Chosidow O. Scabies. *N Engl J Med.* 2006;354:1718-1727.
3. Downs AMR, Harvey I, Kennedy CTC. The epidemiology of head lice and scabies in the UK. *Epidemiol Infect.* 1999;122:471-477.
4. Lapeere H, Naeyaert JM, DeWeert J, et al. Incidence of scabies in Belgium. *Epidemiol Infect.* 2008;136:395-398.
5. Mahé A, Faye O, N'Diaye HT, et al. Definition of an algorithm for the management of common skin diseases at primary health care level in sub-Saharan Africa. *Trans R Soc Trop Med Hyg.* 2005;99:39-47.
6. Lawrence G, Leafasia J, Sheridan J, et al. Control of scabies, skin sores and haematuria in children in the Solomon Islands: Another role for ivermectin. *Bull World Health Organ.* 2005;83: 34-42.
7. Otero L, Varela JA, Espinosa E, et al. *Sarcoptes scabiei* in a sexually transmitted infections unit: A 15-year study. *Sex Transm Dis.* 2004;31:761-765.
8. Blas M, Bravo F, Wenceslao C, et al. Norwegian scabies in Peru: The impact of human T cell lymphotropic virus type 1 infection. *Am J Trop Med Hyg.* 2005;72:855-857.
9. Del Guidice P, Sainte Marie D, Gerard Y, et al. Is crusted (Norwegian) scabies a marker of adult T cell leukemia/lymphoma in human T-lymphotropic virus type 1-seropositive patients? *J Infect Dis.* 1997;176:1090-1092.
10. Arlian LG, Runyan RA, Achar S, et al. Survival and infectivity of *Sarcoptes scabiei* var. *canis* and var. *hominis.* *J Am Acad Dermatol.* 1984;11:210-215.
11. Walton SF, Holt DC, Currie BJ, et al. Scabies: New future for a neglected disease. *Adv Parasitol.* 2004;57:309-376.
12. Argenziano G, Fabbrocini G, Delfino M. Epiluminescence microscopy: A new approach to in vivo detection of *Sarcoptes scabiei.* *Arch Dermatol.* 1997;133:751-753.
13. Prins C, Stucki L, French L, et al. Dermoscopy for the in vivo detection of *Sarcoptes scabiei.* *Dermatology.* 2004;208:241-243.
14. Walton SF, McBroom J, Mathews JD, et al. Crusted scabies: A molecular analysis of *Sarcoptes scabiei* variety *hominis* populations from patients with repeated infestations. *Clin Infect Dis.* 1999;29:1226-1230.
15. Strong M, Johnstone PW. Interventions for treating scabies. Cochrane Database Syst Rev. 2007(3):CD000320.
16. Singal A, Thami GP. Lindane neurotoxicity in childhood. *Am J Ther.* 2006;13:277-280.
17. Sudakin DL. Fatality after a single dermal application of lindane lotion. *Arch Environ Occup Health.* 2007;62:201-203.
18. Sule HM, Thacher TD. Comparison of ivermectin and benzyl benzoate lotion for scabies in Nigerian patients. *Am J Trop Med Hyg.* 2007;76:392-395.
19. Usha V, Gopalakrishnan Nair TV. A comparative study of oral ivermectin and topical permethrin cream in the treatment of scabies. *J Am Acad Dermatol.* 2000;42:236-240.
20. Centers for Disease Control and Prevention (CDC). Scabies. 2008. Available at <http://www.cdc.gov/scabies>.
21. Mounsey KE, Holt DC, McCarthy J, et al. Scabies: Molecular perspectives and therapeutic implications in the face of emerging drug resistance. *Future Microbiol.* 2008;3:57-66.
22. Arlian LG, Estes SA, Vyszenski-Moher DL. Prevalence of *Sarcoptes scabiei* in the homes and nursing homes of scabietic patients. *J Am Acad Dermatol.* 2002;46:794-796.

295

Myiasis and Tungiasis

JAMES H. DIAZ

Flies and fleas are mostly bothersome biting nuisances of humans and animals that can also transmit infectious diseases and deeply invade living tissues, causing amputation, disfigurement and, rarely, death. Flies can serve as mechanical vectors of shigellosis, and rat fleas can transmit bubonic plague and murine typhus. Flies may lay their eggs on human flesh and their developing larvae, or maggots, can invade subcutaneous tissues, and penetrate external body cavities, such as the orbits, ears, and nares. Flea larvae can also burrow into subcutaneous tissues to feed, mature, and promote secondary infections with incapacitating sequelae, including autoamputation of toes and fingers, especially in impoverished tropical communities plagued by endemic jigger fleas (*Tunga penetrans*).

Myiasis

Myiasis is an ectoparasitic infestation of viable or necrotic tissues by the dipterous larvae of higher flies and may be broadly classified as obligatory or facultative myiasis. In obligatory myiasis, maggots must live and feed on human or animal hosts as part of their life cycle. In facultative myiasis, normally free-living maggots that preferentially feed on carrion and decaying matter will attack and feed on the necrotic sores and wounds of living human and animal hosts. Maggot therapy with blowfly larvae is still used today to débride necrotic wounds.

Myiasis may be further stratified clinically as furuncular (subcutaneous) myiasis, wound (superficial cutaneous) myiasis, cavitary (atrial or invasive) myiasis, intestinal myiasis, urinary myiasis, and vaginal myiasis. Furuncular myiasis is the most common clinical manifestation of myiasis and occurs when one or more larvae penetrate the skin, causing pustular lesions that resemble boils or furuncles. Larval maggots can also infest external orifices, sores, or open wounds, causing cavitary and wound myiasis. Cavitary myiasis is usually caused by screwworm larvae that can penetrate festering wounds or invade the orbits, nostrils, or external ear canals (Figs. 295-1 and 295-2). Intestinal myiasis is uncommon, usually caused by the accidental ingestion of maggot-contaminated food, and is characterized by self-limited nausea, vomiting, and diarrhea. Genitourinary myiasis is also uncommon and may present as dysuria, hematuria, and pyuria, following larval invasion of the urethra (urinary myiasis) and/or vagina (vaginal myiasis).

Although there are many families of dipterous flies (order Diptera), flies from three families cause most human and animal myiasis: (1) Oestridae, or botflies; (2) Calliphoridae, screwworms and blowflies; and (3) Sarcophagidae, carrion-feeding flies. The most common myiasis-causing fly species are classified taxonomically and stratified by clinical type of myiasis infestation in Table 295-1.

EPIDEMIOLOGY

In a 2007 retrospective epidemiologic study in Rio de Janeiro, Marquez and colleagues described 71 patients with furuncular and cavitary myiasis during the period 1999 to 2003.[1] Myiasis was more prevalent among adults older than 51 years (42%) and children younger than 10 years (34%). Most of the population was male (61%) and impoverished (62%). The predominant causative agent of furuncular myiasis was *Dermatobia hominis*, the New World human botfly, and the predominant causative agent of cavitary myiasis was *Cochliomyia macellaria*, an indigenous species of New World screwworm.

The authors concluded that myiasis is an opportunistic infestation of disadvantaged vulnerable populations living in nonhygienic conditions. In a similar retrospective collective analysis, Jiang described 54 cases of human myiasis in China from 1995 to 2001.[2] Although the Chinese cases were equally distributed between genders, most cases occurred in infants and children (72%) and were described as either hypodermic-invasive (*n* = 31) or ocular (*n* = 12). In another collective review in 2002, Schwartz and Gur reported 12 cases of furuncular myiasis caused by *Dermatobia hominis*, the human botfly, in 12 Israeli travelers returning from four South American countries in the Amazon Basin.[3] In 2003, Tamir and associates reported two cases of furuncular myiasis caused by *Cordylobia rodhani*, Lund's fly, in Israeli travelers returning from Ghana.[4] In addition to *D. hominis* and *Cordylobia* spp., *Cuterebra* species of botflies can also cause furuncular myiasis in North America, as well as throughout Africa and Asia (Fig. 295-3). Shorter and co-workers reported two cases of *Cuterebra* species botfly-induced furuncular myiasis in New England in children (see Fig. 295-3).

CLINICAL MANIFESTATIONS

The most common forms of human myiasis worldwide are furuncular myiasis and cavitary (invasive) myiasis. Furuncular myiasis is most often caused by subcutaneous larval invasion by the Tumbu fly, *Cordylobia anthropophaga*, in Africa and the New World human botfly, *Dermatobia hominis*, in the subtropical and tropical areas of the Americas (see Table 295-1). Cavitary myiasis is usually caused by zoonotic screwworm larval deposition in open wounds or external orifices, such as the nares, ears, and orbits, and may be characterized by deep tissue larval invasion, with secondary infection and extensive tissue necrosis. *Cochliomyia hominivorax*, the New World screwworm, is a common cause of cavitary myiasis in the Americas and *Chrysomyia bezziana*, the Old World screwworm, is a common cause of cavitary myiasis in Africa, Asia, and Indonesia.[5] Cavitary myiasis must be managed aggressively with surgical débridement and antibiotic therapy of secondary infections to limit tissue damage and disfigurement (see Figs. 295-1 and 295-2).

Although the clinical manifestations, treatments, and prevention strategies are similar in furuncular myiasis, the mechanisms of larval fly invasion are often different. The gravid female Tumbu fly deposits its eggs on moist sandy soil or on wet clothing (e.g., cloth diapers) hung outside to dry. When the human victim dons egg-infested clothing, larvae emerge and rapidly burrow into the skin with sharp mandibles for further development. On the other hand, the female botfly captures blood-feeding insects, usually mosquitoes, in midflight and attaches her eggs to the undersurface of the insect.[6] The intermediate biting vector then delivers the botfly eggs to its blood meal victims, where the eggs hatch immediately and release their larvae to feed on warm-blooded hosts. Human botfly larvae then rapidly burrow into the skin with sharp mandibles to begin their developmental instar stages, which can last 6 to 12 weeks.[4]

In addition to travel history in endemic regions, the mechanisms of larval fly invasion also assist in differentiating the cause of furuncular myiasis. In Tumbu fly (*Cordylobia anthropophaga*) myiasis, lesions are usually located on body regions covered by clothing, such as the buttocks and trunk. In New World human botfly (*Dermatobia hominis*) myiasis, lesions are usually located on exposed areas, such as the scalp, face, and extremities.

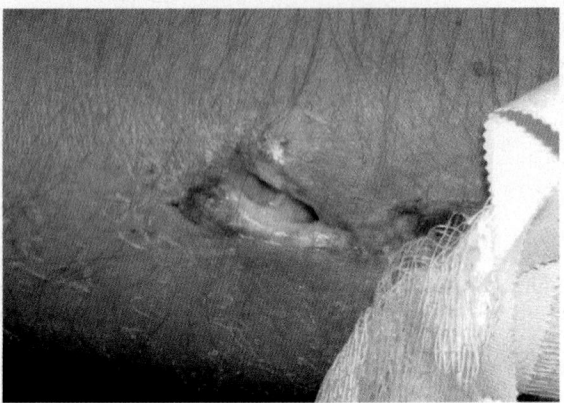

Figure 295-1 Forearm exit site wound of a third stage (instar) New World screwworm fly larva or maggot, *Cochliomyia hominivorax.* *(From Centers for Disease Control and Prevention [CDC], Atlanta, GA. CDC Public Health Image Library, image 1427.)*

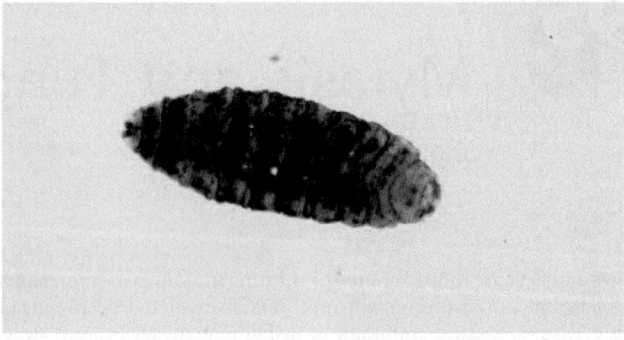

Figure 295-2 16-mm long third-stage (instar) New World screwworm fly larva or maggot, *Cochliomyia hominivorax.* This had just emerged from a forearm exit wound (see Fig. 295-1) after tissue feeding in a traumatic wound for 9 days. *(From Centers for Disease Control and Prevention [CDC], Atlanta, GA. CDC Public Health Image Library, image 1427.)*

After completing three instar stages, the final larval forms of the Tumbu fly and human botfly will wriggle out of their draining, boil-like, 1- to 2-cm furuncular swellings, drop to the ground, and pupate into adult flies within 9 to 14 days. Victims may recall a flying insect bite that preceded human botfly-induced furuncular myiasis.[6] While developing in their furuncles, larvae are active, protrude intermittently through draining wounds, and maintain surface contact for respiration with their posterior, paired spiracles.[7] Anterior hooklets anchor the maggots in place subcutaneously, making manual removal, even with forceps, difficult (see Fig. 295-3).[8]

TREATMENT

Management strategies for furuncular myiasis include coaxing embedded larvae from furuncles by smothering their respiratory spiracles, often visible in lesions, with occlusive coatings of Vaseline (petroleum) ointment, clear fingernail polish, tobacco tar, pork fat, raw beefsteak, or bacon strips.[7] The injection of lidocaine into draining lesions has also been recommended as a successful extraction technique.[9] Nevertheless, unsuccessful occlusive therapy may asphyxiate larvae and necessitate their surgical or vacuum extraction.[10] Along with larval removal, myiasis wounds should be cleansed and conservatively débrided, tetanus prophylaxis administered, and bacterial secondary infections treated with antibiotics. Although *Clostridium tetani* infections of penetrating wounds does occur, tetanus has not been reported in myiasis but has been reported following ectoparasitic infestations with *Tunga penetrans*, the chigoe (jigger) flea, in Africa and South America.[11]

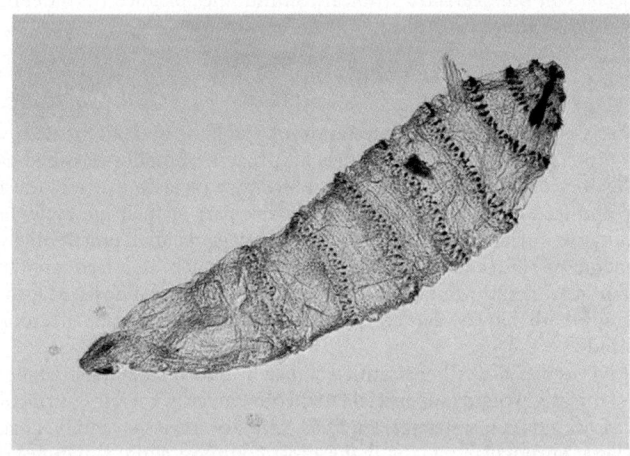

Figure 295-3 First-stage (instar) larva of a *Cuterebra* spp. botfly native to North America. Note the rows of anterior hooklets that can anchor the feeding larva to the dermis. *(From Centers for Disease Control and Prevention [CDC], Atlanta, GA. CDC Public Health Image Library, image 1427.)*

PREVENTION AND CONTROL

Prevention and control strategies for myiasis include the following: (1) control of domestic and livestock animal larval infestations; (2) sanitary disposal of animal carcasses and offal to deny flies their preferred breeding grounds; (3) proper management of any open human

TABLE 295-1	Myiasis-Causing Flies			
Family (Common Family Name)	**Taxonomic Classification**	**Common Name**	**Geographic Distribution**	**Type of Myiasis Infestation**
Oestridae (botflies)	*Dermatobia hominis*	New World botfly	Caribbean, Central and South America	Furuncular
	Cuterebra spp.	Rodent and rabbit botflies	North America, northern Central America	Furuncular
Calliphoridae (screwworm flies, blowflies)	*Cordylobia anthropophaga*	Tumbu fly	Africa	Furuncular
	Cordylobia rodhani	Lund's fly	Africa	Furuncular
	Auchmeromyia senegalensis	Congo floor mat fly	Africa	Superficial cutaneous (no tissue invasion)
	Cochliomyia hominivorax	New World screwworm	Southern North America, Central and South America	Wound, cavitary
	Chrysomyia bezziana			Wound, cavitary
	Lucilia spp.	Old World screwworm	Africa, Asia	Wound, cavitary
	Calliphora spp.	Greenbottle blowflies	Worldwide	Wound (used for maggot therapy)
		Bluebottle blowflies	Worldwide	Wound (used for maggot therapy)
Sarcophagidae (carrion flies)	*Sarcophaga carnaria*		Africa	Wound, cavitary, gastrointestinal
	Wohlfahrtia magnifica		Africa	Wound, cavitary, gastrointestinal

		Flea Vector			
Infectious Disease	*Causative Agent*	*(Common Name)*	*Animal Reservoir*	*Major Clinical Manifestations*	*Treatment*

TABLE 295-2 Flea-Transmitted Infectious Diseases

Infectious Disease	*Causative Agent*	*Flea Vector (Common Name)*	*Animal Reservoir*	*Major Clinical Manifestations*	*Treatment*
Bubonic plague	*Yersinia pestis*	*Xenopsylla cheopis* (rat flea); *Oropsylla montana* (squirrel flea)	Rodents (rats, prairie dogs, squirrels); domestic animals (cats > dogs)	Headache, fever, chills, regional lymphadenopathy—draining buboes, pneumonitis (secondary plague pneumonia), septicemia, meningitis; case fatality rate, 14%	Antibiotic therapy recommended within 24 hr with any of the following effective antibiotics: tetracyclines, gentamicin, streptomycin, chloramphenicol
Murine typhus	*Rickettsia typhi*	*Xenopsylla cheopis* (rat flea); *Nosopsyllus fasciatus* (northern rat flea); *Oropsylla montana* (squirrel flea)	Rodents (rats and mice)	Fever, headache, maculopapular rash, thrombocytopenia, rarely pneumonitis and encephalitis	Doxycycline, 100 mg bid × 7-10 days
Flea-borne spotted fever	*Rickettsia felis*	*Ctenocephalides felis* (cat flea)	Rodents (rats, mice, opossums)	Nonspecific fever, headache, maculopapular rash	Tetracyclines (doxycycline)
Cat-scratch fever (disease)	*Bartonella henselae*	*Ctenocephalides felis* (cat flea)	Feral cats (kittens)	Low-grade fever, malaise, regional and rarely multifocal lymphadenopathy, endocarditis; complications more common in HIV and include bacillary angiomatosis, peliosis hepatitis, neuroretinitis, encephalopathy	Doxycycline and macrolides (azithromycin) effective; add rifampin for complications
Tungiasis—portal of entry for *Clostridium tetani*	Ectoparasite	*Tunga penetrans* (chigoe or jigger flea)	Humans; domestic animals (dogs > cats and pigs)	Painful white papules with central black pits discharging eggs and feces with lateral pressure, especially on dorsal aspects of toes under toenails and on heels	Surgical extraction of gravid female fleas; ivermectin ineffective in humans and only partially effective in dogs for jigger flea management

wounds or cutaneous infections; (4) cementing floors to deny floor maggot flies' preferred egg-laying surfaces; (5) sleeping on raised beds or cots in screened huts or tents; (6) wearing long-sleeved shirts and pants, which can be pyrethrin- or pyrethroid-impregnated; (7) spraying exposed skin with diethyl toluamide (*N,N*-diethyl-meta-toluamide [DEET])–containing repellents; and (8) ironing all clothes and diapers left outside to dry in Tumbu fly habitats.

Flea Infestations

Fleas of the insect order Siphonaptera are a small group of morphologically similar wingless ectoparasites of warm-blooded animals, including humans, which are not only biting nuisances, but also competent vectors of infectious diseases, most notably *Yersinia pestis* and murine typhus (Table 295-2). Although fleas are often classified by host specificity (or presence of head combs), all fleas can rapidly adapt from animal to nearby human hosts, especially if preferred hosts are exterminated by disease or pesticides. Fleas undergo complete metamorphosis from egg to adult stages, with larvae, pupae, and adults exhibiting different morphologies and preferred habitats. Signaled by vibrations and locally rising carbon dioxide levels, adult fleas emerge from egg cases within weeks, leap onto the closest mammalian hosts, and begin blood feeding and reproducing.

Tungiasis

A currently reemerging, combless, ectoparasitic flea, *Tunga penetrans*, the chigoe or jigger sand flea, is endemic in the Caribbean and South America, where it originated, and in sub-Saharan Africa, where it was introduced. Tungiasis, a painful, cutaneous infestation with the gravid female jigger flea, is now hyperendemic in underprivileged communities in Africa, South America, and the Caribbean, has successfully reemerged in Mexico and Central America, and has been increasingly

reported in travelers returning from subtropical and tropical areas worldwide.[12-14]

EPIDEMIOLOGY

In travelers returning to accessible health care infrastructures in developed nations, tungiasis is an exotic infestation, with a minimal parasite burden and a simple surgical cure. However, in the impoverished and underserved communities of developing tropical nations, tungiasis is a recurrent infestation with a high parasite burden causing significant morbidity. In a 2003 descriptive study in over 90% of a population of a poor fishing village in Brazil, Muehlen and colleagues found a 51.3% point prevalence of tungiasis with more males (54%) infested than females, and prevalence peaks in children aged 5 to 9 years and adults aged 60 years and older.[15] In a 2007 point prevalence study in another poor community in northeastern Brazil, Ariza and associates examined 142 persons with jigger flea superinfestations and counted a total of 3445 lesions on feet (median, 17 lesions; maximum, 18 lesions).[16] More than 70% of patients presented with foot pain, 59% complained of difficulty walking, 46% had toenail loss, 42% had foot abscesses, and 25% had deformed toes. In a regional prevalence study of five towns in southwestern Trinidad, Chadee found the prevalence of tungiasis to range from 15.7% to 17.9%, with feet more often infected than other anatomic regions, males more likely infested than females, and higher parasite burdens in males (5.44 ± 2.54 fleas) than females (2.38 ± 2.00 fleas).[17] In a 2007 cross-sectional study of 142 households in a rural community in western Nigeria, Ugbomoiko and associates reported a 45.2% point prevalence of tungiasis, with 95% of the lesions on the feet, no gender difference in prevalence, but prevalence peaks between ages 6 and 14 years and at age 60 years and older.[18] Ectopic lesions of the elbows and hands occurred in 10% of the population. In a study of the ectopic localization of tungiasis among 1184 residents of a poor community in northeastern Brazil with a 33.6% point prevalence of

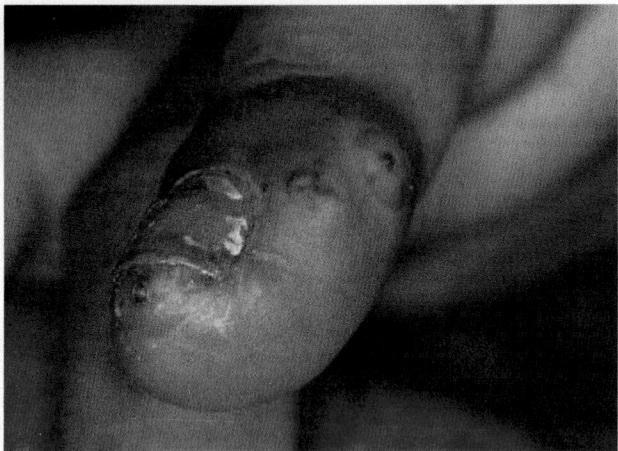

Figure 295-4 Three periungual lesions of tungiasis on the index finger of a 6-year-old girl. These were caused by tissue-feeding gravid female jigger fleas, *Tunga penetrans*. (*From Feldmeier H, Eisele M, Sabóia-Moura RC, Heukelbach J. Severe tungiasis in underprivileged communities: Case series from Brazil. Emerg Infect Dis. 2003;9: 949-955.*)

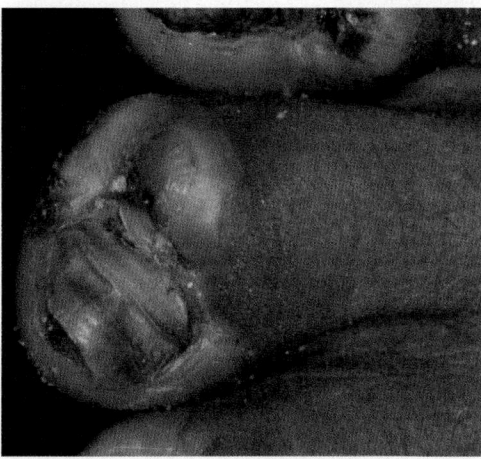

Figure 295-5 Periungual lesion of tungiasis on the fourth toe of a 50-year-old woman. This was caused by a tissue-feeding gravid female jigger flea, *Tunga penetrans*. Note the elevation of the nail bed by the lesion. (*From Feldmeier H, Eisele M, Sabóia-Moura RC, Heukelbach J. Severe tungiasis in underprivileged communities: Case series from Brazil. Emerg Infect Dis. 2003;9:949-955.*)

tungiasis, Heukelbach and co-workers reported that 6% of all lesions presented at sites other than feet, most commonly on the hands (5.5%) but also on the buttocks, elbows, and thighs (Fig. 295-4).[19]

In French Guiana and Brazil, the most important zoonotic reservoir of flea-transmitted tungiasis was in domestic and stray dogs.[20,21] In a comparison of the prevalence of tungiasis in animals and humans in an impoverished Brazilian community, Pilger and colleagues reported a human prevalence of 39%, a combined domestic cat and dog prevalence of 59%, and a higher prevalence (42%) of tungiasis in households with infested dogs and cats.[21] By comparison, Sanushi and associates, in a review of 14 cases of tungiasis in travelers returning to the United States, reported that patients manifested at most two lesions and complained only of local pain and itching.[22]

CLINICAL MANIFESTATIONS

Tungiasis is caused by the dermal penetration of the gravid female jigger (chigoe) flea to feed on blood and tissue juices, usually on the feet (or heels), under or near the toenails, or in the interdigital web spaces (Fig. 295-5).[12] Although the smallest of flea species (1 mm long or shorter), the gravid female will swell with hundreds of developing eggs within days to 2000 times its size, expelling eggs over a period of 3 weeks or less, and then dying and leaving its shriveled carcass in a contaminated wound track. Initially, the embedded jigger flea will produce a subcutaneous papule or vesicle 6 to 8 mm in diameter, with a central black dot pinpointing the exteriorized segments, including the anus, genital opening, and breathing spiracles (see Figs. 295-4 and 295-5). The papule darkens with intralesional hemorrhage and, if squeezed, will extrude eggs, feces, and internal organs through exteriorized posterior abdominal segments. The differential diagnosis of tungiasis includes bacterial skin infections (impetigo), bacterial and fungal paronychia, cercarial dermatitis, fire ant bites, folliculitis, and scabies. The complications of tungiasis include septicemia, abscesses, fissures, toenail (fingernail) loss, necrotic ulcers, osteomyelitis, and eventual autoamputation of toes and, less often, fingers (Fig. 295-6). Tungiasis has been associated with lethal tetanus in nonvaccinated individuals and was identified as the place of entry for 10% of tetanus cases in Sao Paulo in a 1991 study.[11,23]

TREATMENT

Management strategies for tungiasis include extracting all embedded fleas immediately with sterile needles or curettes, administering tetanus

prophylaxis, and treating secondary wound infections with appropriate topical and/or oral antibiotics. Other than surgical extraction, there are no other therapeutic options for tungiasis. There remains a definite need for an effective antiparasitic drug treatment option for tungiasis, especially in superinfestations.[24] In a double-blinded, randomized, placebo-controlled trial, Heukelbach and co-workers have shown that a single dose of oral ivermectin, 300 µg/kg repeated at 24 hours, shows no clinical efficacy compared with placebo as measured by parasite signs of viability or death.[24]

PREVENTION AND CONTROL

In addition to wearing shoes, which can be sprayed with pyrethroid or diethyl toluamide–containing solutions, and not sitting naked on bare ground, other preventive strategies for tungiasis include the following: (1) insecticide treatment of flea-infested domestic and stray animals and pets with 10% pyrethrin or pyrethroid sprays, or 1% to 4% mala-

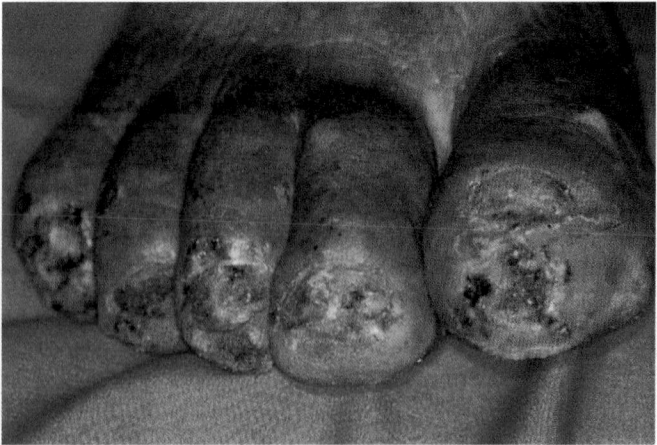

Figure 295-6 The right foot of a 50-year-old man suffering from recurrent tungiasis. Note that all nails have been lost in the recurrent infestations and nonhealing wounds remain on all toes. The patient had chronic pain and could only wear slippers and walk with difficulty. (*From Feldmeier H, Eisele M, Sabóia-Moura RC, Heukelbach J. Severe tungiasis in underprivileged communities: Case series from Brazil. Emerg Infect Dis. 2003;9:949-955.*)

thion powder; (2) foot bathing of domestic and stray dogs and pigs with insecticide solutions, such as 2% trichlorfon (Neguvon); and (3) spraying or dusting households, especially those with dirt floors, with 1% to 4% malathion. Other strategies for the environmental control of jigger fleas include improved stray animal control, especially for cats and dogs; providing cement foundation or slab flooring for dirt-floored homes or building raised homes with solid floors; discouraging stray dogs and cats and other domestic animals, especially pigs, as indoor pets; and spraying rodent and stray animal runways and paths and household unpaved walkways and dirt floors with solutions containing kerosene, fuel oil, 1% lindane, 1% to 4% malathion, or 2% trichlorfon.

REFERENCES

1. Marquez AT, Mattos Mda S, Nascimento SB. Myiasis associated with some socioeconomic factors in five urban areas of the State of Rio de Janeiro. *Rev Soc Brasil Med Trop.* 2007;40:175-180.
2. Jiang C. A collective analysis of 54 cases of human myiasis in China from 1995-2001. *Chinese Med J.* 2002;115:1445-1447.
3. Schwartz E, Gur H. *Dermatobia hominis* myiasis: An emerging disease among travelers to the Amazon Basin of Bolivia. *J Travel Med.* 2002;9:97-99.
4. Tamir J, Haik J, Schwartz E. Myiasis with Lund's fly (*Cordylobia rodhani*) in travelers. *J Travel Med.* 2003;10:293-295.
5. Seppännen M, Virolainen-Julkunen A, Kakko I, et al. Myiasis during adventure sports race. *Emerg Infect Dis.* 2004;10:137-139.
6. Sloop GD, Lopez FA. Furuncular myiasis. *J LA State Med Soc.* 2006;158:14-16.
7. Liebert PS, Madden RC. Human botfly larva in a child's scalp. *J Ped Surg.* 2004;39:629-630.
8. Shorter N, Werninghaus K, Mooney D, et al. Furuncular cuterebrid myiasis. *J Ped Surg.* 1997;32:1511-1513.
9. Lui H, Buck HW. Cutaneous myiasis: A simple and effective technique for extraction of *Dermatobia hominis* larvae. *Int J Dermatol.* 1992;31:657-679.
10. Boggild AK, Keystone JS, Kain KC. Furuncular myiasis: A simple and rapid method for extraction of intact *Dermatobia hominis* larvae. *Clin Infect Dis.* 2002;35:336-338.
11. Obengui P. La tungose et le tétanus au C.H. U. de Brazzaville. [Tungiasis and tetanus at the University Hospital Center in Brazzaville.] *Dakar Med.* 1989;34:44-48.
12. Feldmeier H, Eisele M, Sabóia-Moura RC, et al. Severe tungiasis in underprivileged communities: Case series from Brazil. *Emerg Infect Dis.* 2003;9:949-955.
13. Ibanez-Bernal S, Velasco-Castrejon O. New records of tungiasis in Mexico (Siphonaptera: Tungidae). *J Med Entomol.* 1996;33:988-989.
14. Heukelbach J, Gomide M, Araújo F Jr, et al. Cutaneous larva migrans and tungiasis in international travelers exiting Brazil: An airport survey. *J Travel Med.* 2007;14:374-380.
15. Muehlen M, Heukelbach J, Wilcke T, et al. Investigations on the biology, epidemiology, pathology and control of *Tunga penetrans* in Brazil. II. Prevalence, parasite load and topographic distribution of lesions in a population of a traditional fishing village. *Parasitol Res.* 2003;90:449-453.
16. Ariza L, Seidenschwang M, Buckendahl J, et al. Tungiasis: A neglected disease causing severe morbidity in a shantytown in Fortaleza, State of Ceara. *Rev Soc Brasil Med Trop.* 2007;40:63-67.
17. Chadee DD. Tungiasis among five communities in south-western Trinidad, West Indies. *Ann Trop Med Parasitol.* 1998;92:107-113.
18. Ugbomoiko US, Ofoezie IE, Heukelbach J. Tungiasis: High prevalence, parasite load, and morbidity in a rural community in Lagos State, Nigeria. *Int J Dermatol.* 2007;46:475-481.
19. Heukelbach J, Wilcke T, Eisele M, et al. Ectopic localization of tungiasis. *Am J Trop Med Hyg.* 2002;67:214-216.
20. Rietschel W. Observations of the sand flea (*Tunga penetrans*) in humans and dogs in French Guiana. *Tierarztliche Praxis.* 1989;17:189-193.
21. Pilger D, Schwalfenberg S, Heukelbach J, et al. Investigations on the biology, epidemiology, pathology and control of *Tunga penetrans* in Brazil. II. The importance of animal reservoirs for human infestation. *Parasitol Res.* 2008;102:875-880.
22. Sanushi ID, Brown EB, Shepard TG, et al. Tungiasis: Report of one case and review of the 14 reported cases in the United States. *J Am Acad Dermatol.* 1989;20:941-944.
23. Litvoc J, Leite RM, Katz G. Aspectos epidemiológicos do tétano no estado de São Paulo (Brasil). [Epidemiology of tetanus in São Paulo State (Brazil).] *Rev Inst Med Trop São Paulo.* 1991;33:447-484.
24. Heukelbach J, Franck S, Feldmeier H. Therapy of tungiasis: A double-blinded trial randomized controlled trial with oral ivermectin. *Mem Inst Oswaldo Cruz, Rio de Janeiro.* 2004;99:873-876.

Mites, Including Chiggers

JAMES H. DIAZ

Mites, including chigger and scabies mites, are among the smallest arthropods with most barely visible without magnification. Only about 25 species of the over 3000 species of chigger, animal, plant, and scabies mites are of any medical importance, and most of these are simply biting nuisances and do not transmit infectious diseases.[1] Mites are closely related to ticks, but not as prodigious at blood-feeding. They also do not transmit as broad a range of infectious microbial diseases as ticks. The most serious diseases transmitted by mites are scrub typhus and rickettsialpox.

Only biting larvae of Asian scrub typhus chiggers (*Leptotrombidium* species) can transmit scrub typhus caused by *Orientia tsutsugamushi* (formerly *Rickettsia tsutsugamushi*), and only biting house-mouse mites (*Liponyssoides sanguineus*) can transmit rickettsialpox caused by *Rickettsia akari*. Both scrub typhus mites and house-mouse mites are, like ticks, capable of inheriting bacterial infections by transovarial transmission, and maintaining infections in several mite generations as bacteria are passed from adult to juvenile stages (nymphs and larvae) by transstadial transmission. Originally considered vectors of a rodent zoonosis, scrub typhus chiggers are the main environmental reservoirs of *O. tsutsugamushi* in endemic regions with much smaller secondary reservoirs in wild rodents.[1] Common house mice are the zoonotic reservoirs of *R. akari*, not only in crowded urban apartment buildings in the United States, but also in mice-infested buildings, such as sheds and barns, in more rural locations worldwide.[2]

Mite Taxonomy and Ecology

Mites may be commonly classified as scabies mites (see Chapter 294), trombiculid or chigger mites (also called chiggers, red bugs, and itch mites), human follicle mites, dust mites, and a variety of animal and plant mites (Table 296-1). All mite species develop close generational associations with their ecosystems and zoonotic reservoirs, often referred to as mite islands.[1] Mite islands usually border cleared land and scrub bush and have several habitat requirements including grassy vegetation with warm soil temperatures and high humidity, frequently visiting rodent hosts to feed larvae and sufficient, small insect fauna to feed nymphs and reproducing adults. Humans stumbling onto mite islands are at significantly higher risks of larval chigger bites or trombidiosis worldwide or scrub typhus in the endemic regions of Eurasia and Asia.

Epidemiology and Outcomes of Mite Infestations

Among the trombiculid chiggers (Trombiculidae family), including the scrub typhus-transmitting *Leptotrombidium* species, only the larvae are human and animal ectoparasites. The larger chigger nymphs and adults are free-living and feed on small insects and their eggs. All trombiculid larvae exhibit a unique method of feeding on their human hosts and transmitting salivary secretions, which may contain *O. tsutsugamushi* in endemic regions. When larval mites have selected a human host, they will congregate where the skin is soft, warm, and moist; particularly where clothing is tight against the skin, such as under waistbands, undergarment bands, and socks. Initially painless, chigger bites cluster in these regions on the genitalia, perineum, thighs, buttocks, waists, and ankles, and become symptomatic in 3 to 6 hours (Fig. 296-1). Larvae pierce the skin with sharp mouthparts and inject tissue-dissolving saliva to create a pool of lymph, other body fluids, and dissolved epithelial cells to drink from (see Fig. 296-1). Unlike ticks, mites are not blood-feeders, but tissue-juice feeders. The repeated injection of saliva into the bite wound induces a host reaction that forms a strawlike hollow tube, known as a hypostome or stylostome, which extends downward into the host's skin, anchoring the mite firmly.[1,3] Some trombiculid larvae remain attached to and feeding on human hosts for up to a month, but the larval vectors of scrub typhus feed only for 2 to 10 days before dropping to the ground engorged, and ready to mature into free-ranging nymphs.

All of the noninfectious chigger larvae can cause scrub itch or trombidiosis, with the American chigger mite (*Eutrombicula alfreddugesi*) being the most common culprit in the United States; the European harvest mite, *Neotrombicula autumnalis*, is the most common culprit in Europe and the Asian chigger, *Eutrombicula sarcina*, the most common culprit in Asia. Among the scrub typhus-carrying *Leptotrombidium* larval chigger mites, *Leptotrombidium deliense*, the Asian rodent chigger, is a principal vector throughout eastern Asia and Eurasia.

Following *O. tsutsugamushi*–infected *Leptotrombidium* chigger bites, there is an 8- to 10-day incubation period before the onset of classic clinical manifestations of scrub typhus with bite eschar, regional lymphadenopathy, conjunctival injection, hearing loss, and centrifugal rash (Fig. 296-2).[4] Many cases are nonclassic with nonspecific clinical manifestations and go undiagnosed, especially when serologic tests are unavailable. In the temperate regions of Eurasia, there is a definite scrub typhus seasonal transmission cycle determined by peaking temperatures and humidity during weeks of marked seasonal change between spring and summer and fall and winter; in the tropics, scrub typhus transmission occurs year-round. Fatal complications may include adult respiratory distress syndrome (ARDS), especially in older patients, hypotensive shock, acute renal failure, encephalomyelitis, and disseminated intravascular coagulation.[4]

The house-mouse mite, *Liponyssoides sanguineus*, maintains a rickettsial zoonosis in its preferred house-mouse (*Mus musculus*) reservoir, and can transmit rickettsialpox caused by *R. akari* through its bites.[1,3] Although initially described in clusters in crowded apartment complexes in large U.S. cities, including New York, Boston, Cleveland, Philadelphia, and Pittsburgh, rickettsialpox has now been reported in rural areas of the United States and eastern Europe. Many experts feel that rickettsialpox is underreported and more widely distributed in silent sylvan cycles worldwide. The incubation period and initial clinical manifestations of rickettsialpox mirror those of scrub typhus with eschar formation at the bite site within 10 to 12 days, followed by fever, chills, severe headache, conjunctival injection, and truncal maculopapular then vesicular rash.[2,5] Hearing loss does not occur, and regional lymphadenopathy is uncommon (Table 296-2). Unlike scrub typhus, complications are rare, but may include thrombocytopenia and interstitial pneumonia.[2,5]

Dermatophagoides species dust mites have highly allergenic exoskeletons, body fragments, and feces; all of which can be easily aerosolized during bed-making and pillow-fluffing. Allergens from living and dead dust mites frequently cause allergic rhinitis and asthmatic bronchitis in predisposed, atopic persons. The American house dust mite, *Dermatophagoides farinae*, is now distributed worldwide, as is the European house dust mite, *Dermatophagoides pteronyssinus*.[3] House dust mites prefer to live in bedrooms year-round, especially in mattresses and carpets in warm, humid homes. They exhibit maximum growth and reproduction during seasonal warming cycles at ambient temperatures at or above 25°C and relative humidity at or above 75%.[3]

TABLE 296-1	Mites of Medical Importance				
Family Genus, species	**Common Names (Plant or Animal Mite)**	**Geographic Distribution**	**Maintenance in Nature**	**Clinical Manifestations**	**Infectious Disease Transmission**
Sarcoptidae					
Sarcoptes scabiei var. *hominis*	Scabies (itch) mite (human mite)	Worldwide	Obligate ectoparasite of man, human reservoir	Classical scabies Atypical scabies	None
Trombiculidae					
Neotrombicula autumnalis	European harvest mite (animal mite)	Europe	Free-living ectoparasites of small mammals and birds	Scrub itch (trombidiosis)	None
Eutrombicula alfreddugesi	American chigger mite (animal mite)	Western hemisphere	Free-living ectoparasites of small mammals and birds	Scrub itch (trombidiosis)	None
E. sarcina	Asian chigger mite (animal mite)	Asia, Australia	Free-living ectoparasites of small mammals and birds	Scrub itch (trombidiosis)	None
Leptotrombidium deliense	Asian rodent chigger (animal mite)	Southeast Asia, Japan, Philippines, South Pacific, Australia	Free-living ectoparasites of rodents and insectivores, transovarial-transstadial passage of ID agent	Scrub typhus (tsutsugamushi disease)	*Orientia tsutsugamushi* (formerly *Rickettsia tsutsugamushi*), causative agent of scrub typhus
L. akamushi, L. pallidum, and *L. scutellaris*	Japanese rodent chiggers (animal mites)	Japan	Same	Same	Same
L. arenicola and *L. fletcheri*	Malaysian rodent chiggers (animal mites)	Malaysia	Same	Same	Same
L. pavlovskyi	Russian rodent chigger (animal mite)	Far east of former Soviet Union	Same	Same	Same
Demodicidae					
Demodex folliculorum	Hair follicle mite	Worldwide	Obligate ectoparasite of man, human host reservoir in hair follicles	Benign follicular (scaling) dermatitis Chronic blepharitis (demodecidosis)	None
Demodex brevis	Sebaceous gland mite	Worldwide	Obligate ectoparasite of man, human host reservoir in sebaceous glands	May potentiate granulomatous acne	None
Pyroglyphidae					
Dermatophagoides pteronyssinus	European house dust mite (human mite)	Worldwide	Free-living ectoparasites of man; live in human bedrooms, especially in mattresses; feed on human skin detritus	House dust mite allergies and asthma	None
D. farinae	American house dust mite (human mite)	Same	Same	None	
Dermanyssidae					
Liponyssoides sanguineus (formerly *Allodermanyssus sanguineus*)	House mouse mite	North America, Northern Europe and Asia, Africa	Free-living ectoparasites of field mice, transovarial-transstadial passage of ID agent	Rickettsialpox	Yes (*Rickettsia akari*)
Dermanyssus gallinae	Red poultry (chicken) mite	Worldwide	Free-living ectoparasites of domestic and wild birds	Poultry workers' dermatitis of hands	None
Macronyssidae					
Ornithonyssus bacoti	Tropical rat mite	Temperate and tropical regions worldwide	Free-living ectoparasites of large rodents: *Rattus rattus, Rattus norvegicus*	Urticarial papulovesicular to pustular dermatitis	None
O. bursa	Tropical fowl mite	Same	Free-living ectoparasites of domestic and wild birds	Pruritic papules in a scabietic distribution: finger webs, axillae, groin, buttocks	None
Laelapidae					
Laelaps echidnina	Spiny rat mite	Worldwide, the most prevalent rodent mite species in the U.S.	Free-living ectoparasites of large rodents: *Rattus rattus, Rattus norvegicus*	Nonspecific mite-bite dermatitis	None
Pyemotidae					
Pyemotes tritici (formerly *Pediculoides ventricosus*)	Grain (straw) itch mite	Worldwide	Free-living ectoparasites of straw-, hay-, grain-, and rice-eating moths, beetles, weevils	Grain workers' pruritic vesicular eruption	None
Peymotes herfsi	Oak leaf gall mite	Europe, introduced into the U.S.	Free-living ectoparasites of gall-making larvae of oak trees	Pruritic, erythematous, vesicular eruptions of limbs, face, and neck	None

TABLE 296-1	Mites of Medical Importance—cont'd				
Family Genus, species	Common Names (Plant or Animal Mite)	Geographic Distribution	Maintenance in Nature	Clinical Manifestations	Infectious Disease Transmission
Acaridae*					
Carpoglyphus lactis	Cheese and dried fruit mites	Worldwide	Free-living ectoparasites of cheeses and dried fruits	Cheese and fruit workers' dermatitis	None
Tyrophagus putrescentiae	Copra (dried coconut meat or kernel) mite	Copra (dried coconut meat or kernel) growing areas	Free-living ectoparasites of coconut copra	Copra itch	None
Glycyphagidae*					
Glycyphagus domesticus	Grocer's mite	Worldwide	Free-living ectoparasites of fruits and vegetables	Grocer's itch	None
G. destructor	Hay mite	Worldwide	Free-living ectoparasites of cut hay	Hay workers' and hayriders' allergy, asthma, rhinitis, conjunctivitis	None

*The acarid and glycyphagid plant mites may *rarely* enter the gastrointestinal tract if swallowed with food and cause intestinal distress (gastrointestinal acariasis). They may also be inhaled in aerosols and cause bronchial irritation and respiratory distress (respiratory acariasis). They may crawl into the urethra to cause dysuria (urinary acariasis). The mites can be recovered from feces, sputum, and urine. Treatment is supportive. Although they may *rarely* infest humans, plant mites are all free-living and do not reproduce in human dead-end hosts.

Scabies and follicle mites are the only exclusively human ectoparasitic mites and cannot transmit infectious diseases. Less serious, but more common than scabies, is infestation with the human follicle mites, *Demodex folliculorum*, which inhabit hair follicles, and *Demodex brevis*, which inhabit sebaceous glands. These diminutive (0.1 to 0.4 mm in length) human mites feed on sebum and exfoliated skin, while lodged in human hair follicles or sebaceous gland pores. *Demodex* mites will cluster in follicles on the nose, eyelids, and nasolabial folds, and have even been found living in earwax. All of the developmental stages of *Demodex* mites occur over an egg-to-egg cycle of 13 to 15 days entirely within hair follicles or sebaceous glands, especially in females overusing cream-based facial cosmetics. Other than causing comedones or "blackheads," *Demodex* infestations cause few adverse symptoms, and rarely need treatment, unless infestations are associated with acne, blepharitis, impetigo, rosacea, or seborrheic dermatitis.[1,3]

Although of limited clinical significance, a number of plant and animal mite species can cause bothersome erythematous papulovesicular eruptions if encountered. Bites from the red chicken or poultry mite, *Dermanyssus gallinae*, can cause a pruritic dermatitis usually on the backs of the hands and forearms in poultry workers (Fig. 296-3).[6] Both St. Louis encephalitis virus and western equine encephalitis virus have been isolated from naturally infected red chicken mites, but they are not preferred vectors for these mosquito-borne arboviruses (see Fig. 296-3).[6] Bites from the rat mite, *Ornithonyssus bacoti*, ubiquitous in the temperate areas of Europe and the Americas, can cause a papulovesicular dermatitis in stockyard and warehouse workers. The rat mite can also transmit *Rickettsia typhi*, the agent of murine typhus from rat to rat, maintaining the rodent zoonosis, but is incapable of human transmission.[6] The bird mite, *Ornithonyssus bursa*, is a common ectoparasite of pigeons worldwide and a frequent cause of mite infestations with maculopapular dermatitis of the finger webs and axillae in pigeon-breeders and fanciers.[7]

The plant mites are common causes of annoying infestations with pruritic, erythematous maculopapular rashes on the limbs and face of arborists, landscapers, and campers. The North American grain or straw itch mite, *Pyemotes tritici* (formerly *Pediculoides ventricosus*),

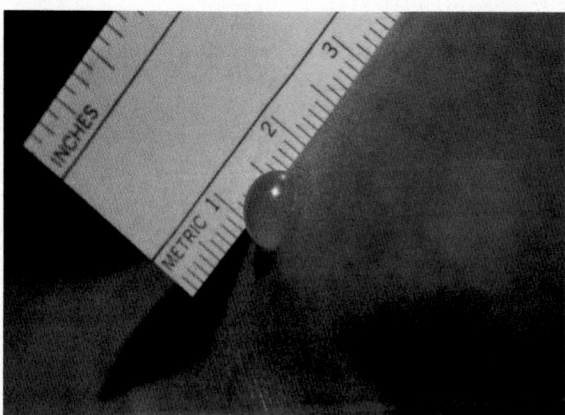

Figure 296-1 **An intensely pruritic red bleb 24 hours after a bite inflicted by a larval trombiculid species chigger mite.** Although these species of lymph-sucking mites do not transmit infectious diseases in the United States, many species of larval trombiculids will transmit scrub typhus or tsutsugamushi disease, caused by the rickettsial microorganism, *Orientia* (formerly *Rickettsia*) *tsutsugamushi*, throughout Southeast Asia and the western Pacific regions. *(From U.S. Department of Health and Human Services, Centers for Disease Control and Prevention, Atlanta, GA. CDC Public Health Image Library, PHIL ID # 3806.)*

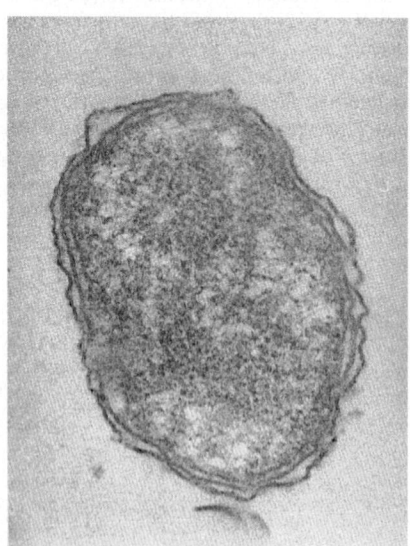

Figure 296-2 **A transmission electron micrograph of an extracellular *Orientia tsutsugamushi* rickettsial microorganism, the causative agent of scrub typhus or tsutsugamushi disease throughout Southeast Asia and the Western Pacific region.** During World War II, scrub typhus was second only to malaria as a cause of hospitalization among U.S. troops in the Pacific theater of operations.[1] *(From U.S. Department of Health and Human Services, Centers for Disease Control and Prevention, Atlanta, GA. CDC Public Health Image Library, PHIL ID # 8730.)*

TABLE 296-2 The Presentation, Diagnosis, Differential Diagnosis, and Management of Mite-Transmitted Scrub Typhus vs. Rickettsialpox		
The Major Mite-Transmitted Infectious Diseases	*Scrub Typhus*	*Rickettsialpox*
Bacterial agent	*Orientia* (formerly *Rickettsia*) *tsutsugamushi**	*Rickettsia akari*
Mite vector	Larvae of *Leptotrombidium* species of Asian rodent chigger mites	Common house-mouse mites, *Liponyssoides sanguineus*
Incubation period	8-10 days (range 8-20 days)	10-12 days
Mite-bite site	Painless initial bite, eschar at bite site (50%)	Painless initial bite, eschar at bite site
Presenting constitutional symptoms	Fever, chills, headaches, myalgia, pathognomonic hearing loss (30%)	Fever, chills, severe headache, myalgia
Conjunctival injection	Present	May be present
Regional lymphadenopathy	Present regionally and tender	Usually absent
Associated rash exanthema	Delayed truncal onset, erythematous macules, then maculopapules that spread peripherally	Abrupt truncal onset, erythematous macules that develop central vesicles in crops
Chest findings	Cough, tachypnea, dyspnea, bibasilar rales	Asymptomatic bibasilar rales
Chest x-ray findings	Infiltrates common	Usually normal
Potential complications	Adult respiratory distress syndromes, acute renal failure, disseminated intravascular coagulation, encephalomyelitis	Thrombocytopenia
Differential diagnoses	Infectious mononucleosis, leptospirosis, tularemia, anthrax, spotted fever rickettsioses	Chickenpox, tick-bite eschar
Diagnostic methods	Screening: rapid dipstick recombinant 56-kDa protein antigen test Serodiagnostic: indirect immunofluorescent antibody tests, immunoperoxidase assays Confirmatory: microscopic isolation of agent from blood or tissues, polymerase chain reaction for agent DNA (or RNA)	Serodiagnostic: immunofluorescent antibody assay for IgG to both *R. akari* and *R. rickettsia*, with follow-up cross-adsorption testing for predominant antibodies Confirmatory: isolation from skin biopsy
Recommended treatments	Tetracycline 500 mg orally 4 × daily × 1 wk, or doxycycline 100 mg twice daily × 1 wk, or IV chloramphenicol, 50-75 mg/kg/day × 1 wk (only for complicated cases) In childhood and pregnancy, consider the macrolides: azithromycin, clarithromycin, or roxithromycin	Doxycycline 100 mg orally twice daily × 7-10 days
Outcomes = Case fatality rates (%)	1-15%	< 1%

*Although initially classified among the *Rickettsia*, the causative agent of scrub typhus, *Orientia tsutsugamushi* (originally *Rickettsia tsutsugamushi*) has now been reclassified into a separate genus, *Orientia*, based on molecular evidence that its cell wall differs significantly from *Rickettsia* both ultrastructurally and in its component proteins.[4]

feeds preferentially on the larvae of insects that infest hay and straw (and some grains), and can burrow superficially into the skin, causing a papulovesicular dermatitis, especially in persons sleeping on straw mattresses or riding on hay wagons (Fig. 296-4).[3,6] In the summer of 2004, a relative of the straw itch mite, the oak leaf gall mite (*Peymotes herfsi*), which feeds on insect larvae within galls in pin oak trees, caused an outbreak of plant itch dermatitis in Kansas. Galls are irregular plant growths, particularly rolled leaves, caused by chemical reactions between feeding insects and reacting plant hormones. Approximately 300 residents of Pittsburg, Kansas, sought medical attention for an intensely pruritic, erythematious, papular rash clustering on the face,

neck, and limbs (Fig. 296-5). The lesions healed within days following topical treatment with antihistamines and steroids. Investigators determined that the rashes resulted from multiple bites from oak leaf gall mites dropping from trees and floating in the wind after feeding in pin oak trees.[8]

ACARINA > PEDICULOIDIDAE

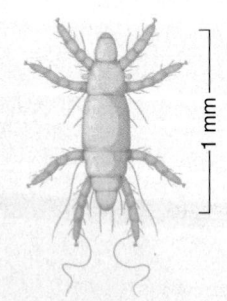

Pyemotes ventricosus
(Newport)
(female, dorsal aspect)

ACARINA > DERMANYSSIDAE

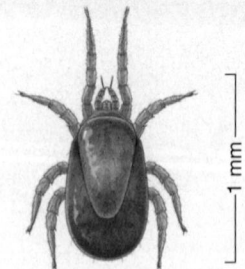

Dermanyssus gallinae (DeGeer)
(female, dorsal aspect)

Figure 296-3 An illustration of the dorsal aspect of the female red chicken (poultry) mite, *Dermanyssus gallinae*, which is a common cause of poultry workers' and pigeon breeders' dermatitis worldwide. *(From U.S. Department of Health and Human Services, Centers for Disease Control and Prevention, Atlanta, GA. CDC Public Health Image Library, PHIL ID # 5482.)*

Figure 296-4 An illustration of the dorsal aspect of the female grain (straw) itch mite, *Pyemotes tritici* (formerly *Pyemotes ventricosus*), which is a common cause of highly pruritic and papulovesicular rashes among hay threshers, hay wagon riders, outdoor yard workers, and campers during late summers worldwide. A similar plant mite, *Pyemotes herfsi*, the European oak leaf gall mite, caused an outbreak of pruritic, erythematous papulovesicular rashes causing 300 residents of Pittsburg, Kansas, to seek medical care in late August 2004.[8] *(From U.S. Department of Health and Human Services, Centers for Disease Control and Prevention, Atlanta, GA. CDC Public Health Image Library, PHIL ID # 5482.)*

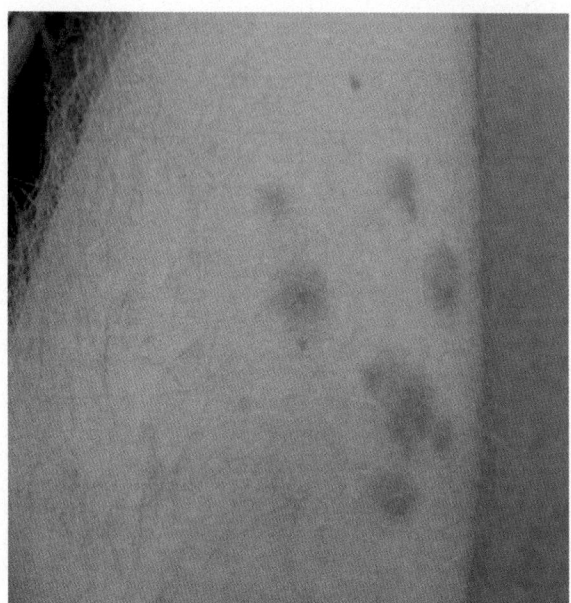

Figure 296-5 Close-up photograph of the pruritic, erythematous papulovesicular bite lesions inflicted by the European oak leaf gall mite on a resident of Pittsburg, Kansas, in late August 2004.[8] *(From U.S. Department of Health and Human Services, Centers for Disease Control and Prevention, Atlanta, GA; CDC MMWR. Outbreak of pruritic reaches associated with mites—Kansas, 2004. MMWR 2005;54(38); 952-955. Photo courtesy A. Broce, L. Zurek, Kansas State University. Available at http://www.cdc.gov/mmwr/preview/mmwrhtml/mm5438a3. htm.)*

Diagnosis and Management of Mite Infestations

All larval chigger bites will cluster where clothing is tight against the skin, especially the genitalia, thighs, buttocks, waists, and ankles, and generally not create itching and discomfort until the larvae have withdrawn their mouthparts and departed. Forcibly removing feeding chiggers often decapitates larvae leaving mouthparts embedded to cause further inflammation.[1] Untested strategies for removing feeding, engorged chiggers intact have included painting chigger bite sites with colloidion, clear fingernail polish, or Liquid Skin and then drying the sites with a hair dryer and peeling the coated and dried chiggers off the skin intact. Intense itching will commence within 3 to 6 hours after bites, which will then be followed by intensely pruritic, erythematous papules (10-12 hours), and crusting and healing (24-48 hours; see Fig. 296-1).[1,3] Treatment is supportive with soap and water cleansing, warm water soaks, and topical, local anesthetics and antihistamines. Impetigo and secondary infections are potential complications that would necessitate antibiotic treatment.

Follicle mite infestations on the face usually require no treatment other than soap and water washing to reduce infestations.[1,3,6] Scalp and eyelash infestations will respond to washes with 0.5% selenium or 10% sulfur-containing creams, lotions, or shampoos, with care to avoid ocular instillation. Chronic follicle mite infestations (demodecidosis) with blepharitis and rosacea-like dermatitis may require treatment with a single oral dose of ivermectin, 200 µg/kg, especially in immunocompromised patients. Most animal and plant mite bites can also be managed symptomatically with topical agents, unless active infestations are present, which can be controlled with topical 10% crotamiton, 25% benzyl benzoate, or topical 1% lindane or 1% malathion preparations. House dust mite allergies may be managed by immunotherapy with house dust mite extracts.

Although initially classified among the *Rickettsia*, the causative agent of scrub typhus, *O. tsutsugamushi* (originally *R. tsutsugamushi*) has now been reclassified into a separate genus, *Orientia*, based on molecular evidence that its cell wall differs significantly from *Rickettsia* both ultrastructurally and in its component proteins (see Fig. 296-2). Nevertheless, mite-transmitted scrub typhus and rickettsialpox present clinically in a similar fashion; both infections respond to treatment with oral tetracycline, oral doxycycline, or IV chloramphenicol, which is not recommended due to its bone marrow toxicity (see Table 296-2 for comparison of the presenting clinical manifestations, diagnostic methods, differential diagnosis, treatment strategies, and outcomes for scrub typhus and rickettsialpox).[4]

Prevention of Mite Infestations and Mite-Transmitted Infectious Diseases

Prevention and control strategies for mite ectoparasites include: (1) household and campsite spraying of pyrethrin and pyrethroid-containing insecticides; (2) spraying or impregnating pyrethrin and pyrethroid-containing repellants on clothing; (3) applying diethyl toluamide-containing insect repellants (N, N-diethyl-methyl-toluamide, abbreviated DEET) to exposed skin; (4) gently washing exposed or infested areas of the body with soap and water to remove stylosome-attached mites without decapitating them; (5) improving rodent reservoir control in campgrounds, homes, apartments, barns, sheds, and, especially, in crowded public housing; (6) treating straw beds, straw mattresses, and hayride wagons with pyrethrin and pyrethroid-containing insecticides; and (7) vacuuming bedrooms and mattresses and washing bed linens regularly, and covering mattresses and pillows with plastic covers to minimize house dust mite levels. There are no vaccines for scrub typhus or rickettsialpox. Weekly doses of 200 mg of doxycycline can prevent *O. tsutsugamushi* infections.[4]

Conclusion

In summary, mites are ubiquitous and bothersome pests and of these, most are trombiculid larvae (chiggers) and animal and plant mites, which do not transmit infectious diseases. Only about 20 species are of medical importance: the Asian and Eurasian *Leptotrombidium* species of trombiculid larvae (chiggers) can transmit scrub typhus in endemic regions, and the house-mouse mite can transmit rickettsialpox from a mouse zoonosis in urban and rural settings, which is more widespread than initially thought.

REFERENCES

1. Service MW. Scrub typhus mites (Trombiculidae). In: Service MW, ed. *Medical Entomology for Students.* London: Chapman and Hall; 1996:256-262.
2. Krusell A, Comer JA, Sexton DJ. Rickettsialpox in North Carolina: a case report. *Emerg Infect Dis.* 2002;8:727-728.
3. Goddard J. Mites. In: Goddard J, ed. *Physician's Guide to Arthropods of Medical Importance.* 4th ed. Boca Raton, FL: CRC Press; 2002:229-246.
4. Watt G, Walker DH. Scrub typhus. In: Guerrant RL, Walker DH, Weller PF, eds. *Tropical Infectious Diseases: Principles, Pathogens and Practice.* 2nd ed. Philadelphia: Churchill Livingston; 2006: 557-562.
5. Ozturk MK, Gunes T, Kose ET, et al. Rickettsialpox in Turkey. *Emerg Infect Dis.* 2003;9:1498-1499.
6. Neva FA, Brown HW. Class Arachnida—ticks, mites, spiders, scorpions. In: Neva FA, Brown HW, eds. *Basic Clinical Parasitol-* ogy. East Norwalk, CT: Appleton and Lange; 1994:300-311.
7. Kong TK, To WK. Bird-mite infestation. *N Engl J Med.* 2006; 354:1728.
8. Hansen G, Taylor C, Goedeke J, et al. Outbreak of pruritic rashes associated with mites—Kansas, 2004. *MMWR Morb Mortal Weekly Rep.* 2005;54:952-955.

297

Ticks, Including Tick Paralysis

JAMES H. DIAZ

Ticks are the most competent and versatile of all arthropod vectors of zoonotic infectious diseases for several reasons. First, ticks are not afflicted by most of the microorganisms that they may transmit or the paralytic salivary toxins that they may transfer during blood feeding. Second, and unlike mosquitoes, ticks can transmit the broadest range of infectious microbes among all arthropods, including bacteria, viruses, and parasites. Third, ticks can vertically transmit infectious microorganisms congenitally to their offspring of both genders (trans-ovarian transmission) and then disseminate carrier state infections among all generational growth stages (trans-stadial transmission). Fourth, ticks have capitalized on many competitive advantages afforded them by evolving changes in climate and human lifestyle including the following: wider geographic distributions and longer active breeding and blood-feeding seasons as a result of increases in global mean temperatures and humidity; greater abundance of wild animal reservoir hosts no longer effectively controlled, particularly deer, medium-sized mammals, and rodents; greater residential construction in recently cleared woodlands adjacent to pastures and yards preferred by domestic animal and human hosts; and more vacation and leisure time activities enjoyed by humans and their pets during prolonged tick host-questing and blood-feeding seasons from earlier springs through later falls and milder winters.[1] In short, ticks of all ages and both genders may remain infectious for generations without having to reacquire infections from host reservoirs, and environmental and behavioral changes now place humans and ticks together outdoors for longer periods for tick breeding, blood feeding, and infectious disease transmission.

Tick Biology, Behavior, and Taxonomy

With the exception of toothed hypostomes for blood feeding and claw-less palps, adult ticks resemble large mites with eight legs and disk-shaped bodies.[2] There are four stages in the tick life cycle—egg, six-legged larva, nymph, and adult. Ticks are classified into three families: the Ixodidae, or hard ticks; the Argasidae, or soft ticks; and the Nuttalliellidae, a much lesser known family, with characteristics of both hard and soft ticks.[2] Ixodid ticks have a hard dorsal plate or scutum, which is absent in the soft-bodied, argasid ticks. Ixodid ticks also exhibit more sexual dimorphism than argasid ticks, with both genders looking alike. However, all blood-fed ticks, especially females, are capable of enormous expansion, and engorged ixodid females are often confused with engorged argasid females. Although ticks from all families may serve as disease vectors, the ixodid or hard ticks are responsible for most tick-borne diseases in the United States.

Ixodid ticks have mouth parts that are attached anteriorly and visible dorsally. They live in open exposed environments, such as woodlands, grasslands, meadows, and scrub brush areas. Argasid ticks are leathery and have subterminally attached mouth parts that are not visible dorsally. Agrasid ticks prefer to live in more sheltered environments, such as animal nests, caves, and crevices. All ticks feed by cutting a small hole in the host's epidermis with their chelicerae and then inserting their hypostomes into the cut, with blood flow maintained by salivary anticoagulants.[2] Ticks are attracted to warm-blooded hosts by vibration and exhaled CO_2. Ixodid ticks will actually "quest" for hosts by climbing onto vegetation with their forelegs outstretched, waiting to embrace passing hosts (Fig. 297-1). Ticks spend relatively short periods of their lives mating and blood feeding on hosts, with soft ticks feeding rapidly for hours and then dropping off, whereas

hard ticks blood-feed for days (6 to 12) before dropping off for egg laying.

Epidemiology of Tick-borne Infectious Diseases

Tick-borne infectious diseases have challenged researchers and physicians since Dr. Howard T. Ricketts identified the wood tick, *Dermacentor andersoni*, as the vector of Rocky Mountain spotted fever (RMSF) in 1906 and firmly established the insect vector theory of infectious disease transmission.[3] The emergence of Lyme disease in the early 1970s, whose causative agent, the spirochete *Borrelia burgdorferi*, was not identified until 1982, sparked renewed interest in tick-borne diseases in the United States and Europe (Fig. 297-2).[4]

By the early 1990s, Lyme borreliosis had become the most common arthropod-borne infectious disease in the United States and Europe.[5] Since the 1970s, every decade now describes emerging or rediscovered tick-borne infectious disease and new vectors for previously described tick-borne diseases, such as RMSF.[6] These latest discoveries have been spawned by new immunodiagnostic technologies, especially by nucleic acid identification technologies, particularly the polymerase chain reaction (PCR) assay.

By the 1980s and 1990s, the causative agents of the ehrlichioses were stratified as newly emerging, rickettsia-like species, and later (2001) were completely reorganized into separate genera, *Ehrlichia* and *Anaplasma*.[7,8] In 1997, Kirkland and coauthors described a new erythema migrans–like rash illness in North Carolina, a nonendemic region for Lyme disease, transmitted by the lone star tick, *Amblyomma americanum* (see Fig. 297-1). This new borreliosis would soon be named the southern tick–associated rash illness (STARI) or Master's disease, but its causative agent, *B. lonestari*, a new *Borrelia* species, would not be identified until 2004 (see Fig. 297-2).[10]

By 2004, ticks were recognized as the most common vectors of all arthropod-borne infectious diseases in Europe, five new spotted fever–causing rickettsiae were described, four new subspecies of the Lyme disease–causing *B. burgdorferi* complex were identified, a new relapsing fever borreliosis species was isolated, and anaplasmosis was exported to Europe from the United States.[11] In a seemingly unending era of new discoveries in tick-transmitted diseases, another new and unanticipated vector for RMSF, *Rhipicephalus sanguineus*, the brown dog tick, was identified in the United States in 2005 (Fig. 297-3).[12]

Because most tick-borne diseases are caused by obligate intracellular organisms, many of which infect erythrocytes, granulocytes, or vascular endothelial lining cells, many tick-borne infections may also be transmitted by blood product transfusions and by organ transplants. Blood product–transmitted infections have now been described for the tick-borne rickettsial diseases (including Q fever), babesiosis, and ehrlichiosis. In 2008, the Centers for Disease Control and Prevention (CDC) reported the first case in which transfusion transmission of *Anaplasma phagocytophilum*, the tick-borne causative agent of anaplasmosis (formerly human granulocytic ehrlichiosis [HGE]) was confirmed microscopically and serologically by testing of both the recipient and donor.[13]

Today, the seroprevalence of tick-borne diseases is increasing significantly among blood and organ donors in the United States, combined tick-transmitted infections have been described in regional U.S. populations, and an unexplained increase in the virulence of

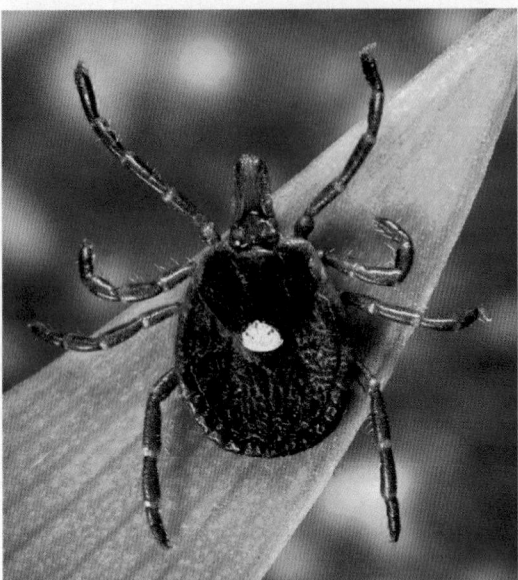

Figure 297-1 *Amblyomma americanum*, **the lone star tick, "quest-ing" for a host.** Shown is the dorsal view of a female lone star tick, the vector of southern tick-associated rash illness (STARI) caused by the spirochete *Borrelia lonestari*. Note the "lone star" mark located in the center of the dorsal surface. *(From Centers for Disease Control and Prevention [CDC], Atlanta, GA. Public Health Image Library, image 8683.)*

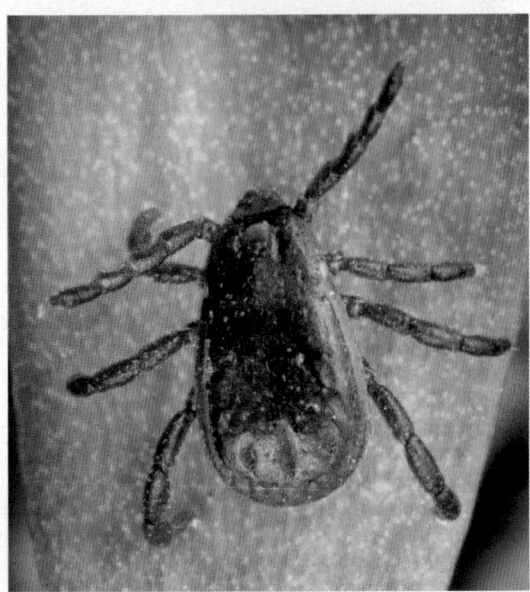

Figure 297-3 *Rhipicephalus sanguineus*, **the brown dog tick, "questing" for a host.** This is a dorsal view of a male tick, a new and unanticipated vector for Rocky Mountain spotted fever (RMSF) in addi-tion to the historical vectors, *Dermacentor andersoni*, the Rocky Moun-tain wood tick, and *Dermacentor variabilis*, the American dog tick. *(From Centers for Disease Control and Prevention [CDC], Atlanta, GA. Public Health Image Library, image 7646.)*

tick-borne infectious diseases has been described in the United States (RMSF), Europe, and North Africa (Mediterranean spotted fever) and Australia (Queensland tick typhus). Several tick-borne infectious dis-eases have now been reclassified by the CDC as potential biologic terrorism agents, including the following: *Francisella tularensis* (tula-remia), a category A agent (highly likely microorganism to be weapon-ized); *Coxiella burnetii* (Q fever), a category B agent (less likely to be weaponized); and the tick-borne encephalitis and hemorrhagic fever viruses, category C agents (least likely to be weaponized). In the future, the tick-transmitted infectious diseases will increase in prevalence over wider distributions at higher altitudes in a warmer world. Unexpected tick vectors of emerging infections caused by obligate intracellular microorganisms will continue to be discovered as people spend more leisure times outdoors in temperate climates in tick-preferred ecosystems.

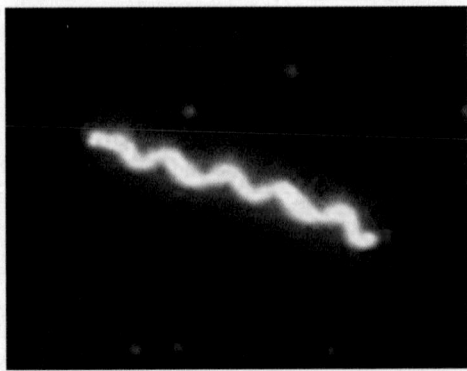

Figure 297-2 *Borrelia burgdorferi*, **the causative bacterium of Lyme disease.** Note the characteristic coiled spring appearance of a spirochete (peripheral blood smear, immunofluorescent stain under dark-field microscopy, ×1000). *(From Centers for Disease Control and Prevention [CDC], Atlanta, GA. Public Health Image Library. Courtesy of Dr. Robert D. Gilmore.)*

Tick-borne Bacterial Infections

SPIROCHETAL INFECTIONS (BORRELIOSES)

The borrelioses are a large group of tick-borne spirochetal diseases caused by several species of *Borrelia*, with unique geographic distribu-tions, tick vectors, and host animal reservoirs (Table 297-1). The bor-relioses are stratified into three separate epidemiologic and clinical presentations—Lyme borreliosis, STARI, and the tick-borne relapsing fevers (Table 297-2).

Lyme borreliosis (LB) or Lyme disease is now the most common tick-borne infectious disease in the northern hemisphere and the most common arthropod-borne infectious disease in the United States.[5,14] In the United States, LB is caused by *Borrelia burgdorferi* (*sensu stricto*), first identified as a novel bacterial spirochete in 1982, and transmitted to humans by *Ixodes* spp. hard ticks in U.S. regional pockets, specifi-cally the Northeast (*I. scapularis*), upper Midwest (*I. scapularis*), and Pacific Coast (*I. pacificus*; Fig. 297-4; see Fig. 297-2). Although *B. burgdorferi* is the sole agent of LB in the United States and has been exported to Europe, most cases of LB in Europe and northern Asia are caused by *B. afzelii* and *B. garinii* (see Table 297-1). Collectively, the three *Borrelia* species are often referred to as *B. burgdorferi* (*sensu lato*). Ticks usually acquire *Borrelia* infections as larvae or nymphs by blood-feeding on small reservoir hosts, most commonly birds and rodents, and may transmit LB to humans during blood feeding, which may go unnoticed (see Fig. 297-4). *Borrelia* organisms are further maintained in nature as infected adult *Ixodes* ticks blood-feed on larger mammals, such as deer.

Unlike argasid or soft ticks, *Ixodes* ticks prefer temperate ecotonal zones of canopied forests abutting cleared scrub or grasslands, and transmit *B. burgdorferi* to humans during outdoor exposures in such habitats. Because *Borrelia* spirochetes must migrate from the tick's midgut to the salivary gland during blood feeding, tick attachments for less than 24 hours rarely result in LB in humans.[15] After an incuba-tion period of 1 to 2 weeks, the hallmark of spirochete transmission manifests as solitary erythema migrans, a maculopapular erythema-tous rash with a bull's eye pattern, at the site of tick attachment (Fig.

TABLE 297-1	**Tick-borne Spirochetal Borrelioses**			
Borrelia Species	**Tick-borne Diseases**	**Geographic Distribution**	**Tick Vectors**	**Wild Animal Reservoirs**
B. afzelii	European Lyme borreliosis (LB)	Europe, Scandinavia	Ixodes ricinus	Mammals—deer, rodents
B. burgdorferi	American LB	North America, specifically U.S. Northeast, Midwest, Pacific Northwest; Europe	I. scapularis (eastern United States), I. pacificus (western United States)	Mammals—deer, rodents (preferred by nymphs)
B. crocidurae	North African tick-borne relapsing fever (TBRF)	North Africa, Mediterranean Basin	Ornithodoros erraticus	Mammals—rodents, birds
B. duttonii	East African TBRF	East, Central, and South Africa	O. moubata	Humans are main reservoir
B. garinii	European LB	Northern Europe, Russia, Asia	I. ricinus (Europe), I. persulcatus (Asia)	Mammals—rodents, birds
B. hermsii	American TBRF	Western United States and Canada	O. hermsii	Mammals—rodents, chipmunks, squirrels
B. hispanica	Hispano-African TBRF	Iberian peninsula—Spain, Portugal; northwestern Africa—Algeria, Morocco, Tunisia	O. marocanus	Mammals—rodents
B. latyschewii	White TBRF	Russian Caucasus regions (Tajikistan, Uzbekistan), Central Asia	O. tartakovskyi	Mammals—rodents
B. lonestari	Southern tick-associated rash illness (STARI), or Master's disease	Southeastern United States from southeastern Atlantic coast west to Central Texas, Oklahoma, Missouri	Amblyomma americanum	Mammals—rodents, cattle, other domestic animals; some reptiles, especially lizards
B. mazzottii	Southern TBRF	Southern United States, Mexico, Central America, South America	O. talaje	Mammals—rodents
B. parkeri	Western TBRF	Southwest and south central United States, Mexico	O. parkeri	Mammals—rodents
B. persica	Asiatic-African TBRF	Middle East (Egypt, Iran), Central Asia, Western China, Northern India	O. tholozani	Mammals—rodents
B. turicatae	American Southwestern TBRF	Southwest and south central United States, Mexico, Central America	O. turicata	Mammals—rodents, armadillos, opossums, pigs, and monkeys (Panama)
B. venezuelensis	Venezuelan TBRF	Central and South America	O. rudis	Mammals—rodents, opossums, armadillos, monkeys (Panama, Colombia)

297-5). Erythema migrans also occurs in STARI at the site of *Amblyomma americanum* or lone star tick attachment, and results from the subcutaneous centrifugal movement of the spirochetes from the bite sites to the central circulation and target organs (see Fig. 297-5).

In a meta-analysis of 53 longitudinal studies of LB in the United States and Europe, Tibbles and Edlow have reported that many patients do not recall a tick bite (74% in the United States, 36% in Europe), constitutional symptoms of low grade fever (lower than 39°C) and headache are common but nausea and vomiting are rare, and a solitary erythema migrans lesion is the most common initial presentation of LB (81% in the United States, 88% in Europe).[16] Although deaths from LB are rare, the greatest morbidity from target organ damage in LB

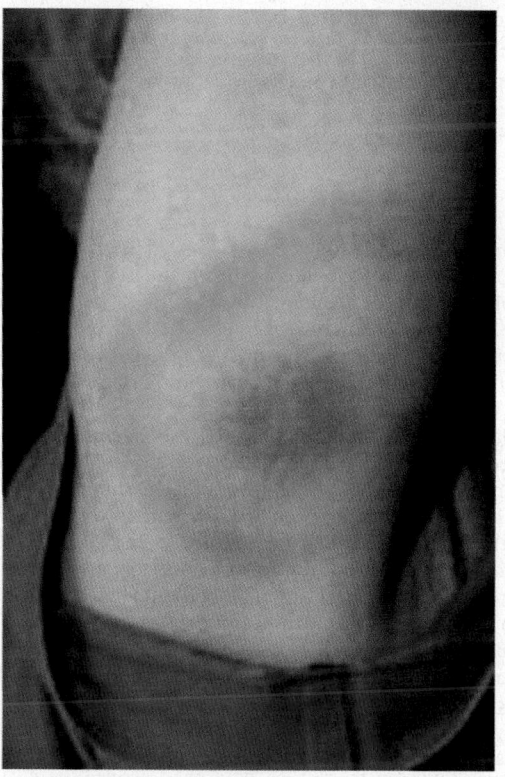

Figure 297-5 Erythema migrans. Shown is the pathognomonic "bull's eye" rash at the bite sites of *Borrelia burgdorferi* or *B. lonestari*–infected ixodid ticks, tick vectors of Lyme disease and southern tick–associated rash illness (STARI), respectively, in endemic regions of the United States. *(From Centers for Disease Control and Prevention [CDC], Atlanta, GA. Public Health Image Library, image 9875.)*

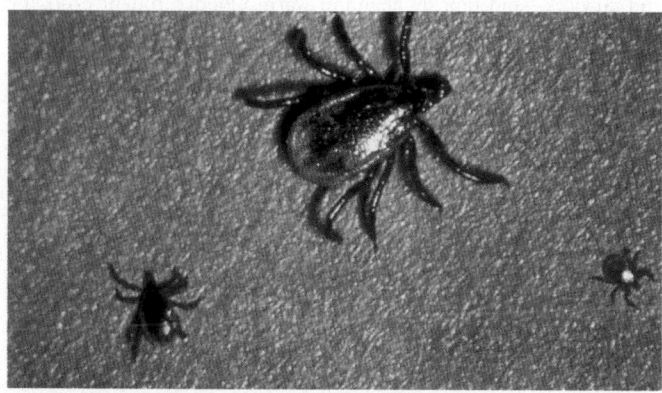

Figure 297-4 *Ixodes scapularis*. Shown are the black-legged deer tick, adult female and nymphs. These are arthropod vectors of babesiosis and Lyme disease, especially nymphs, whose bites are most often unnoticed. *(From Centers for Disease Control and Prevention [CDC], Atlanta, GA. Public Health Image Library, image 1205.)*

TABLE 297-2	Clinicopathophysiologic Comparison of Lyme Borreliosis, Southern Tick-associated Rash Illness (STARI), and Tick-borne Relapsing Fever		
Infectious Disease Characteristics	**Lyme Borreliosis**	**Southern Tick-associated Rash Illness**	**Tick-borne Relapsing Fever**
Microbial agents	*Borrelia burgdorferi* (United States, Europe), *B. afzelii* (Europe, Asia), *B. garinii* (Europe, Asia)	*Borrelia lonestari*—has now been isolated from a skin biopsy of patient with STARI and cultured in vitro from infected *Amblyomma americanum* ticks	Many *Ornithodoros* species of soft ticks (see Table 297-1)
Preferred tick vectors	*Ixodes* spp. hard ticks	*A. americanum*	*Ornithodoros* spp. soft ticks
Preferred animal reservoirs	Rodents—nymphs Deer, birds—adults	Lizards	Rodents—nymphs; humans—*B. duttoni* only; deer, birds—adults
Endemicity	Highly endemic in United States and Europe	Southeastern United States	Highly endemic among vector-populated regions worldwide
Fever ≥39° C	Very uncommon	Absent; low-grade grade fever may occur rarely	Present in relapsing episodes 1-3 days each; may reach 43°C
Relapsing fevers	Not present	Not present	Present
Erythema migrans, or other rash	Present as annular or target-like maculopapular rash (mean diameter, 7 cm); more common on extremities	Present and mimics that of Lyme disease but with a smaller mean diameter of 4.5 cm; more common on trunk	Absent
Arthritis	May be present in untreated (up to 60%) late, or "chronic" infections, manifesting as oligoarthritis	Arthralgias, myalgias, and neck stiffness may occur less commonly than with Lyme disease; no chronic arthritic complications	Neck stiffness, arthralgias, myalgias common, not arthritis
Neurologic manifestations	May be present in up to 15% of cases; includes headache, cranial nerve (CN) VII neuritis—Bell's palsy	Dizziness, headache, memory loss, concentration difficulty may occur; no chronic neurologic complications	Common—meningitis, meningoencephalitis; neuritis of CN VII—Bell's palsy; CN VIII—deafness, myelitis, radiculopathy
Other presenting clinical manifestations	Myocarditis, conduction defects in late-onset and "chronic" cases in up to 8% of cases	Regional lymphadenopathy may occur; chronic complications have not been described	Splenomegaly in most, hepatomegaly in 10% of cases; myocarditis manifesting as prolonged QTc interval
Best screening serodiagnostics	Giemsa- or Wright-stained peripheral smear, phase contrast, or dark-field microscopy for spirochetes; ELISA, IFA	Epidemiologic and clinical presentation; no presently available screening serodiagnostics; Lyme disease ruled out by ELISA, IFA, Western immunoblot	Giemsa- or Wright-stained peripheral smear, phase contrast, or dark-field microscopy for spirochetes; ELISA, IFA
Best confirmatory diagnostics	In vitro cultivation, Western immmunoblot, PCR assay	PCR assay on skin biopsy; in vitro cultivation	In vitro cultivation (not recommended; biosafety level 3 laboratory required), rodent inoculation, PCR assay
Recommended antibiotic therapy	Doxycycline, 100 g PO bid, or amoxicillin, 500 mg PO tid, for 14-21 days; parenteral therapy for CNS involvement	Doxycycline, 100 g PO bid, or amoxicillin, 500 mg PO tid, for 14-21 days	Tetracycline, 500 mg or 12.5 mg/kg PO qid, or doxycycline, 100 mg PO bid, or erythromycin, 500 mg or 12.5 mg/kg PO qid for 10 days; parenteral therapy with penicillin G or ceftriaxone recommended for CNS involvement

CNS, central nervous system; ELISA, enzyme-linked immunosorbent assay; IFA, immunofluorescence assay; PCR, polymerase chain reaction.

occurs in patients with prolonged or untreated infections with approximately 5% to 8% developing cardiac manifestations, 15% to 20% developing neurologic manifestations, and 40% to 60% developing chronic arthritis.[15-17] However, if LB is recognized and treated early in the erythema migrans stage, cure rates will exceed 90%, late manifestations will be avoided, and outcomes will be excellent (see Table 297-2).

The Jarisch-Herxheimer reaction (JHR), an inflammatory cytokine-mediated reaction to dying spirochetes with a worsening of presenting symptoms, vasodilatation, and myocardial dysfunction, may occur during antibiotic treatment for LB, but is more common following antibiotic therapy for tick-borne relapsing fevers. There have been no reported deaths from JHR during antibiotic therapy for LB, and the very rare case fatalities from LB have been attributed to cardiac conduction abnormalities from myocarditis in untreated cases. There is substantial risk and little to no benefit associated with additional antibiotic treatment of patients with any chronic sequelae of LB after appropriate initial treatment.[15,17]

First recognized in 1998, STARI manifests initially as erythema migrans, as in LB, but occurs in regions in which *B. burgdorferi* is not endemic and follows the prolonged attachment of blood-feeding lone star ticks, *Amblyomma americanum*, more abundant in the southeast and south central United States (see Figs. 297-1 and 297-5).[9,18] STARI may be difficult to distinguish from LB, causes fewer and milder constitutional symptoms than LB, and is not associated with target organ damage or chronic or late manifestations. STARI should be treated initially with oral doxycycline or amoxicillin following the same regimen as for LB (see Table 297-2).

The tick-borne relapsing fevers (TBRFs) comprise a worldwide group of serious bacterial infections by *Borrelia* spirochetes following brief, painless, and usually unnoticed bites by *Ornithodoros* spp. argasid soft ticks. These ticks prefer indoor living—in cabins, caves, and crevices—and quickly abandon warm-blooded rodent hosts for egg laying (see Table 297-1).[19,20] Unlike the ixodid ticks, *Ornithodoros* ticks feed very briefly, usually for less than 30 minutes, and at night.[15] Adults can live for as long as 15 to 20 years and survive without blood meals for several years. Transovarian transmission of the TBRF spirochetes occurs commonly among all species and, unlike LB-causing *Borrelia* species, TBRF spirochetes are already present in the salivary glands at the onset of blood feeding and do not need time to migrate from the gut to the mouth parts. The wild animal host reservoirs of TBRF are maintained in birds and several mammals, most commonly rodents. The bite of a TBRF-infected tick is painless and the bite site is marked after a few days by a small red to violaceous papule, with a central eschar.[21] One spirochete is sufficient to initiate TBRF, and the infection rate after a single bite by an infected tick is over 50%. The incubation period to onset of the first febrile episode is 3 to 12 days.

TBRF is defined clinically by the sudden onset of two or more episodes of high fever (more than 39°C) spaced by afebrile periods of 4 to 14 days, with the first febrile episode lasting 3 to 6 days and the relapsing episodes lasting 1 to 3 days each.[15,20,21] The first episode ends with a 15 to 30 minute "crisis" with tachycardia, hypertension, hyperpyrexia (as high as 43°C), and rigors, followed by diaphoresis and defervescence.[19-21] All febrile episodes are accompanied by nausea, headache, neck stiffness, myalgia, and arthralgia. The relapsing febrile episodes result from the growth of new spirochete populations in the blood to replace those killed by macrophages and cytokines. Most patients will have splenomegaly, 10% will have hepatomegaly, and most will have elevated transaminase levels, unconjugated bilirubin, and prolonged prothrombin and partial thromboplastin times. Direct neurologic involvement is more common than in LB and may include cranial nerve neuritis (especially cranial nerves VII and VIII), radiculopathy, and myelopathy. Myocarditis is also more common than in LB, may be complicated by adult respiratory distress syndrome (ARDS), pulmonary edema, and cardiomegaly, and is often fatal. Diagnostic and treatment strategies for TBRF are outlined in Table 297-2.

The JHR is much more common, although rarely fatal, during treatment for TBRF than during treatment for LB and occurs in 30% to 40% of patients with TBRF.[15] At present, no prophylactic strategies to reduce the severity of the JHR have proven beneficial or have been adequately tested in multiple clinical trials, including therapy with antipyretics, corticosteroids, or naloxone. Treatment with penicillin instead of tetracycline has a slightly lower risk of causing JHR during antibiotic therapy for TBRF.

SPOTTED FEVER GROUP RICKETTSIAL INFECTIONS

The family Rickettsiaceae contains two genera, the spotted fever–causing genus *Rickettsia* and the typhus-causing genus *Orientia* (see Chapters 187 and 192). The rickettsiae may be further stratified clinically into the tick-borne spotted fever group and mouse mite–transmitted rickettsialpox caused by *R. akari* (see Chapter 188). The rickettsiae are obligate intracellular, gram-negative bacteria that thrive in ixodid tick salivary glands and are transmitted during blood feeding. Once injected into the host, rickettsiae are initially distributed regionally via lymphatics with some species causing marked regional lymphadenopathy (*Rickettsia slovaca*). Within 2 to 14 days (mean, 7 days) rickettsiae are disseminated hematogenously to vascular endothelial lining cells of target organs, including the central nervous system (CNS), lungs, and myocardium. Rickettsiae gain entry into host endothelial cells in a Trojan horse–like manner by using outer membrane proteins (OmpA and OmpB) to stimulate endocytosis. Once within phagosomes, rickettsiae escape to enter the cytosol or nucleus for rapid replication by binary fission, safe from host immune attack. The tick-borne rickettsial diseases that cause spotted fevers (SFs) are compared in a descending order of clinical severity of infection by preferred tick vectors and wild animal reservoirs in Table 297-3.

The global epidemiology of the tick-borne SF-causing rickettsiae has dramatically evolved since the transmission cycle of RMSF was first described by Ricketts in 1906 with the following: emerging new strains and diseases (*R. slovaca*–associated lymphadenopathy); greater understanding of the highly conserved genome of several related species (*R. africae-R. parkeri* and the *R. conorii* subspecies); wider geographic distribution and greater virulence of existing strains (*R. rickettsia, R. conorii* subspecies, *R. australis*); unanticipated new tick vectors for some SFs (*Rhipicephalus sanguineus* for RMSF in the United States); cluster outbreaks of tick-borne rickettsioses in returning travelers (*R. africae* causing African tick bite fever); and regional clusters and epidemic cycles of more severe SFs worldwide (RMSF in the United States, Mediterranean SF [MSF] in Europe, and Queensland tick typhus [QTT] in Australia).[3,4,12,22-26] The reasons for such changes in rickettsial SF epidemiology are unclear and may include warming temperatures and increasing humidity, more frequent drought-rain cycles, residential development in preferred tick ecosystems, more competent tick vectors given competitive advantages by environmental and genetic changes, more frequent contact between ticks and humans outdoors, and international trade and travel distributing tick vectors and their preferred animal hosts quickly and widely.

The tick-borne SF rickettsioses share many common features in clinical presentations including incubation periods of approximately 1 week, flulike prodromes of fever, headache, myalgia, nausea, vomiting, and abdominal pain (that may mimic acute appendicitis in RMSF), spotty rashes within 3 to 5 days of fever onset, and necrotic eschars at tick bite sites (Fig. 297-6). Some SF rickettsial diseases may be "spotless," including RMSF in 10% to 15% of cases, complicating early differential diagnosis.[22] The tick-borne rickettsial infections that can cause spotty rashes include *R. rickettsii* (RMSF), *R. conorii* (MSF), *R. australis* (QTT), and *R. africae-R. parkeri* (African–North American tick bite fever) in about 50% of cases (see Fig. 297-6).[25,26] The tick-borne rickettsial infections that are associated with one or more necrotic eschars at tick bite sites include *R. conorii, R. australis, R. africae-R. parkeri, R. japonica, R. slovaca, R. aeschlimannii,* and *R. honei.* The SF rickettsioses may vary in severity from causing multisystem organ failure (RMSF, MSF) to painful lymphadenopathy (*R. africae-R. parkeri, R. slovaca*) to mild to subclinical disease (*R. aeschlimannii*).[24]

After an average incubation period of 1 week, RMSF starts with a flulike, febrile prodrome followed by a characteristic maculopapular

TABLE 297-3	Spotted Fever Group of Tick-borne Rickettsioses				
Rickettsia *Species*	*Tick-borne Diseases*	*Geographic Distribution*	*Tick Vectors*	*Wild Animal Reservoirs (Mammals)*
R. rickettsii	Rocky Mountain spotted fever (SF), Brazilian SF	Continental United States, Central America (Costa Rica, Mexico, Panama), South America (Argentina, Brazil)	*Amblyomma, Dermacentor, Rhipicephalus* spp.	Ungulates, rodents
R. conorii	Boutonneuse fever, Mediterranean SF, Israeli SF, Astrakhan SF, Indian tick typhus, Kenyan tick typhus	Mediterranean basin, Africa, Middle East, Asia	*Rhipicephalus* spp.	Ungulates, rodents
R. sibirica	North Asian tick typhus (Siberian tick typhus)	Africa (Niger, Mali, South Africa), Asia (Russia, China, Mongolia, Pakistan, Kazakhstan, Kirgizia, Tajikistan), Europe (France)	*Dermacentor, Haemaphysalis, Hyalomma* spp.	Ungulates, rodents
R. japonica	Japanese SF	Japan and China	*Haemaphysalis* spp., *Ixodes ovatus*	Ungulates, rodents
R. australis	Queensland tick typhus	Eastern Australian seaboard from Cairns, Queensland, to Gippsland, Victoria	*Ixodes* spp., especially *I. holocyclus*	Rodents
R. honei	Flinders Island SF	Southern Australia, Thailand	*Aponomma* spp.	Rodents
R. africae and *R. parkeri*	African tick bite fever	Sub-Saharan Africa, North America, South America, Caribbean	*Amblyomma* spp.	Rodents
R. slovaca	Tick-borne lymphadenopathy; *Dermacentor*-borne eschar, lymphadenopathy, or necrosis	Europe	*Dermacentor* spp.	Ungulates, rodents
R. aeschlimannii	Not named at present	Southern Europe, Africa	*Hyalomma* spp.	Ungulates, rodents

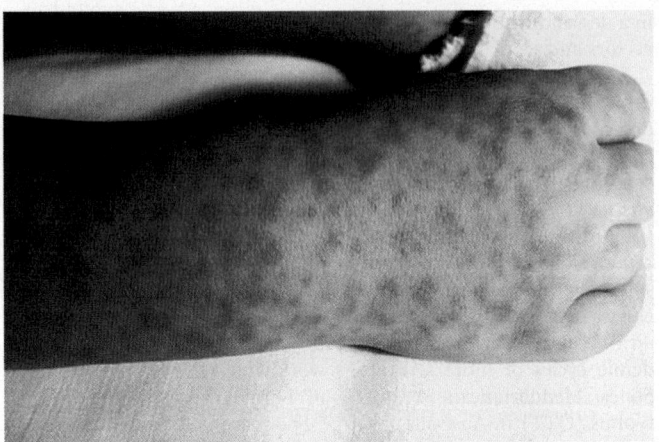

Figure 297-6 **Characteristic initial distal maculopapular-petechial rash of Rocky Mountain spotted fever (RMSF).** This is on the dorsal aspect of a child's right hand and wrist. *(From Centers for Disease Control and Prevention [CDC], Atlanta, GA. Public Health Image Library, image 1962.)*

evolving to petechial rash in 85% to 90% of cases in 3 to 5 days.[22] The pathognomonic rash starts distally on the wrists and ankles and then spreads centripetally up the limbs (see Fig. 297-6). The pathophysiologic mechanisms of petechial rashes and target organ system damage (CNS, lungs, heart) in the SF rickettsioses include vascular endothelial cell damage by microbial replication, vascular inflammation (vasculitis), and increased widespread vascular permeability, which may result in hypovolemic shock, oliguric prerenal failure from acute tubular necrosis, cerebral edema, and noncardiogenic pulmonary edema. Distal, digital skin necrosis may occur in severe cases of RMSF and QTT from hypoperfusion. Cardiac vasculitis may manifest as myocarditis with intraventricular conduction blocks. Aside from petechial rash and thrombocytopenia, other hemorrhagic manifestations in RMSF and other SFs are rare. CNS complications in RMSF and other severe SF infections may include ataxia, photophobia, transient deafness, focal neurologic deficits, meningismus, meningoencephalitis, seizures, and coma. Pulmonary complications may include cough, alveolar infiltrates, interstitial pneumonitis, pleural effusions, pulmonary edema, and ARDS.[24-26]

Initially, MSF caused by *R. conorii*, was thought to be a more benign disease than RMSF. In 1981, severe cases of MSF with multiple eschars and multisystem disease similar to RMSF with CNS, renal, and pulmonary complications were first reported, and now appear to be increasing across Europe. In a 1997 outbreak of MSF in Portugal, case-fatality rates (CFRs) of 32% were recorded and exceeded those of untreated RMSF of 23%.[24] QTT, African tick bite fever (ATBF), and *R. slovaca*–associated lymphadenopathy are generally milder diseases than RMSF and MSF. However, severe cases of QTT with RMSF-like complications, including renal insufficiency and pulmonary infiltrates, were recently reported from Australia.[26]

Although ATBF caused by *R. africae*, a similar tick bite fever in North America caused by *R. parkeri*, and *R. slovaca* infections may all cause multiple necrotic eschars and painful regional lymphadenopathy, these SF infections are often spotless (≥50% or more) and follow typical rickettsial SF prodromes.[25,26] A history of tick bites, eschars, and painful regional lymphadenopathy help establish the correct diagnosis, especially in the absence of adequate diagnostic laboratory services. The precise laboratory diagnosis of tick-borne rickettsial SFs may be established by microbiologic isolation of the causative organisms from skin biopsies or blood cultures, nonspecific immunofluorescent antibody tests that cross react with many SF antigens, other immunocytologic techniques to demonstrate intracellular rickettsiae, and PCR assay to identify and speciate rickettsial DNA or RNA.

Antibiotic treatment mainstays for the tick-borne rickettsial SFs remain the tetracyclines for most cases and chloramphenicol for severe multisystem disease and during pregnancy.[22] Although the quinolones, azithromycin, and clarithromycin may be as effective as tetracyclines and chloramphenicol for rapidly managing some SFs, they are not recommended for initial therapy at this time. Although short, 1- to 2-day courses of doxycycline have been reported to be as successful as 10-day courses in some SF infections (e.g., MSF), such treatment strategies have not been tested in randomized controlled trials in other SF infections, and are also not recommended at this time. Most authorities now recommend that tetracycline, chloramphenicol, or ciprofloxacin for tetracycline-allergic patients be continued for a minimum or 7 days or until the patient has been afebrile for at least 48 hours and is improving clinically.

Q FEVER

Q (query) fever was first described in Australia in 1935 and its causative organism, *Coxiella burnetii*, was isolated shortly thereafter.[27] *C. burnetii* is a gram-negative, intracellular, spore-forming bacterium that is the sole species of its genus. *C. burnetii* is genetically related to *Legionella pneumophila* and, like *L. pneumophila*, *C. burnetii* is usually transmitted to humans by inhalation of contaminated aerosols. Q fever is a zoonosis with worldwide distribution and extensive domestic animal (cattle, sheep, goats, cats, dogs), wild animal (birds, rabbits, reptiles), and arthropod (ticks) reservoirs. In most cases, humans are not infected by tick bites, but by the inhaling spores or bacteria in aerosols contaminated with infectious particles in dried animal feces, milk, or products of conception.[28] Q fever may also be transmitted by ingestion of contaminated milk, by vertical transmission from mother to fetus, by contaminated blood product transfusion, and even percutaneously by crushing infected ticks near breaks in the skin barrier.

C. burnetii is reactivated during pregnancy and multiplies extensively in the placenta, exposing abattoir workers, veterinarians, researchers (especially those working with parturient sheep), and domestic pet owners (especially of cats) to highly infectious aerosols during delivery.[27,28] Recently, several cases of Q fever were reported among U.S. military personnel deployed to Iraq and Afghanistan and in travelers returning from Asia, Latin America, and sub-Saharan Africa.[29] *C. burnetii* has long been considered as a potential bioterrorism weapon for several reasons, including its environmental stability, spore-forming capability, ease of aerosolized dispersal, and high pathogenicity, with an ability to initiate infection with a single microorganism.

After an average 2-week incubation period (range, 2 to 29 days), Q fever may manifest as a wide variety of illnesses in humans, including the following: acute Q fever, a self-limited febrile illness with severe headache, retro-orbital pain, and nonproductive cough; Q fever pneumonia with consolidated opacities, pleural effusions, and hilar lymphadenopathy on chest radiographs; Q fever granulomatous hepatitis, usually following ingestion of contaminated milk; CNS Q fever with protean manifestations ranging from aseptic meningoencephalitis and transient behavioral and sensory disturbances to cranial nerve palsies and hemifacial pain mimicking trigeminal neuralgia; and chronic Q fever endocarditis, especially in predisposed patients with congenital valvulopathies, prosthetic heart valves, aortic aneurysms, or vascular grafts.[27-29] Patients who are immunocompromised by pregnancy, congenital immunodeficiency disorders, cancer, HIV-AIDS, organ transplant antirejection therapy, renal dialysis, or prolonged corticosteroid therapy are at greater risk of acquiring more severe and chronic Q fever infections.[28]

Because the isolation of *C. burnetii* requires biosafety containment level 3, most diagnostic laboratory strategies for Q fever rely on microscopic detection on Giemsa-stained smears of blood or sputum or tissue biopsies (liver, excised heart valves), on antibody detection by immunofluorescent assays, or on DNA detection by PCR assay.[27,28] The prognosis is usually excellent in the acute Q fever illnesses, and mortality is rare after appropriate antibiotic therapy with tetracyclines (doxycycline is preferred—100 mg PO twice daily for 14 days) or fluoroquinolones. Chronic Q fever endocarditis will require prolonged treatment with two antibiotics, either rifampin (300 mg PO twice daily) and ciprofloxacin (750 mg PO twice daily) for 3 years, or doxycycline (100 mg PO twice daily) and hydroxychloroquine (200 mg PO three times daily) for at least 18 months. Such combined therapies will require close monitoring for drug toxicities, especially hepatotoxicity from rifampin and oculotoxicity from hydroxychloroquine. In addition, all patients with Q fever endocarditis should undergo screening transesophageal echocardiography for underlying valvulopathies. Chronically infected heart valves and vascular grafts will require surgical replacement.

TULAREMIA

Tularemia, also known as rabbit fever or deer fly fever, was first described as a zoonosis in squirrels in Tulare County, California, in 1911. Its causative agent, *Francisella tularensis*, was later identified as a gram-negative coccobacillus by Dr. Edward Francis during an investigation of deer fly fever in Utah in 1921.[30] Tularemia occurs in regional pockets worldwide, has a very large wild and domestic animal reservoir, and is seasonally transmitted to humans by ixodid tick and deerfly bites and by contact with infected animals, especially rabbits and muskrats. The primary tick vector of tularemia in the United States is the American dog tick, *Dermacentor variabilis* (Fig. 297-7). Tick-transmitted tularemia is most commonly reported during the spring and summer (May to August) worldwide. Infected animal contact–transmitted tularemia occurs more often during the fall through hunting and trapping seasons, especially among male hunters who field-clean infected animal carcasses. *F. tularensis* is an extremely stable microorganism in nature, surviving in soil, water, and animal carcasses for months to years. In addition to fecal or vomit contamination of tick bites and direct inoculation of intact skin or mucosal surfaces when crushing ticks or skinning animals, tularemia may also be transmitted by ingesting raw or undercooked infected game or bush meats, drinking contaminated water, or inhaling aerosolized microorganisms.[31-33]

In 2000, a cluster outbreak of primary pneumonic tularemia in 11 patients (1 fatality) was reported from Martha's Vineyard, Massachusetts. A case-control investigation of the outbreak implicated aerosolized exposure to *F. tularensis* during summertime brush cutting and lawn mowing as significant (odds ratio [OR], 9.2; 95% confidence interval [CI], 1.6 to 68.0) risk factors for pneumonic tularemia.[34] Concerns about inhalation transmission and potential biologic weaponization of *F. tularensis* led to the reinstatement of tularemia as a nationally notifiable infectious disease in 2000.[31,32] The CDC reported a total of 1368 cases of tularemia from 44 states from 1990 to 2000 (period prevalence, 124 cases/year; range, 86-93 cases/year), with most cases

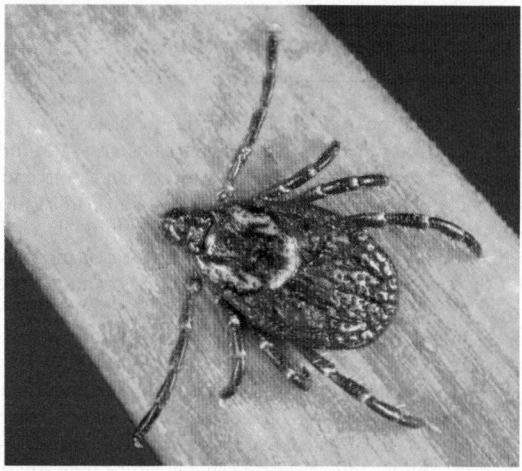

Figure 297-7 **"Questing" female American dog tick, *Dermacentor variabilis*.** This is a vector of tick paralysis in the southeastern United States and Pacific Northwest and a vector of Rocky Mountain spotted fever (RMSF) in addition to the Rocky Mountain wood tick, *Dermacentor andersoni*, in the western United States. *(From Centers for Disease Control and Prevention [CDC], Atlanta, GA. Public Health Image Library, image 170.)*

occurring in males during May to August in regional pockets including Arkansas and Missouri, eastern Oklahoma and Kansas, southern Montana and South Dakota, and Martha's Vineyard.[31]

There are two biovars of *F. tularensis* with biovar A (*F. tularensis* biogroup *tularensis*) causing 60% to 90% of tularemia cases in North America, and biovar B (*F. tularensis* biogroup *palearctica*) causing a milder disease throughout Europe and Asia.[32,33,35] The presenting clinical manifestations of infection will depend on the virulence of the biovars (A > B), route of entry of microorganisms, multisystem infections, and immunocompetence of infected hosts.

The portal of entry of *F. tularensis* has historically been used to classify the clinical manifestations of tularemia, with untreated pneumonic tularemia having the highest CFRs of 30% to 60% (Table 297-4).[31-35] The differential diagnosis of ulceroglandular tularemia, the most common presentation, is extensive and includes other arthropod bites, bacterial and viral infections, and fungal diseases capable of causing skin ulcers with painful regional lymphadenopathy. Diagnostic strategies for tularemia include the following: microscopic identification or culture in biosafety level (BSL) 3 facilities of microorganisms from blood, sputum, gastric lavage fluid, lung biopsy, or lymph node aspirates (sensitivity, 10% to 25%); acute and convalescent serology

TABLE 297-4	Clinical Classification of Tularemia Based on the Portal of Entry		
Clinical Classification of Tularemia Cases	**Case Definition by Clinical Presentation**	**Portals of Entry of Francisella tularensis**	**Case Frequency, United States (%)**
Ulceroglandular	Malaise, fever, bite eschars or ulcers, painful regional lymphadenopathy	Tick or deer-fly bite, or direct inoculation across intact dermis	80
Glandular	Malaise, fever, suppurative lymphadenopathy	Direct inoculation across intact dermis	15
Oropharyngeal	Malaise, fever, sore throat, dysphagia, painful cervical lymphadenopathy	Ingestion of raw or undercooked infected game or bush meats	<5
Oculoglandular	Malaise, fever, ocular infection, regional facial lymphadenopathy	Ocular inoculation of infectious fluids or animal danders, or autoinoculation from bite eschar or ulcers	1
Typhoidal	Malaise, fever, abdominal pain, mesenteric lymphadenopathy, mimics typhoid fever	Ingestion of contaminated water	Rare
Pneumonic	Malaise, fever, pneumonia with multiple ill-defined infiltrates, hilar lymphadenopathy; mimics inhalation anthrax	Inhalation of contaminated aerosols, aerosolized bioweapon exposures, or hematogenous spreading from glandular or typhoidal infections	Rare, except on Martha's Vineyard following aerosolized exposures during mechanized bush trimming and lawn mowing

comparing antibody titers (sensitivity more than 85%); direct immunofluorescent antibody testing; and antigen detection by PCR (sensitivity, 50% to 73%). Frequently accompanying laboratory abnormalities in tularemia include significant elevations in the erythrocyte sedimentation rate (ESR), significant leukocytosis (higher than 10,000/μL), often with normal differential counts, and thrombocytosis. The recommended treatment strategies for tularemia have evolved considerably from historic treatments with painful IM injections of streptomycin to oral therapy with the aminoglycosides and fluoroquinolones, which are effective in 86% of cases and may result in resolution of ulcers within 72 hours. Most cases in adults, including pneumonic tularemia, may be managed with fluoroquinolones alone (ciprofloxacin, 400 mg IV or 500 mg PO twice daily for 7 to 14 days, or levofloxacin, 500 mg IV or PO twice daily for 7 to 14 days), with aminoglycosides (gentamicin or amikacin, 3 to 5 mg/kg/day for 10 to 14 days) reserved for pediatric infections and widely disseminated systemic infections. Relapse rates are highest with oral tetracyclines, including doxycycline, and chloramphenicol, which may still be indicated for cases with CNS dissemination, despite its potential for bone marrow toxicity.

TICK-BORNE EHRLICHIOSES AND ANAPLASMOSIS

The human ehrlichioses and anaplasmosis (formerly known as human monocytic and human granulocytic ehrlichiosis, respectively) are classic examples of emerging tick-borne infectious diseases. Since 1986, four new tick-borne bacterial species have been identified and classified into a new family, Anaplasmataceae. The four genera of Anaplasmataceae are all obligate, intracellular, gram-negative bacteria, closely related genetically to the family Rickettsiaceae. The Anaplasmataceae include two genera that are synergistic parasites of flat worms (*Neorickettsia sennetsu*) and filarial worms (*Wolbachia* spp.) and two genera that are tick-borne bacterial infections of many mammals, including humans, *Ehrlichia* and *Anaplasma* (Fig. 297-8).[36,37] Like rickettsiae, the Anaplasmataceae attach to molecular ligands on phagocytic cells to gain Trojan horse–like entry into leukocytes and then trick intracellular phagosomes into releasing them into the cytosol for replication (see Fig. 297-8).[38]

The tick-borne Anaplasmataceae are now endemic in the United States and have preferred geographic distributions, tick vectors, and wild and domestic animal reservoirs (Table 297-5). They spread from the infected tick's gut to its salivary gland, are inoculated over 24 to

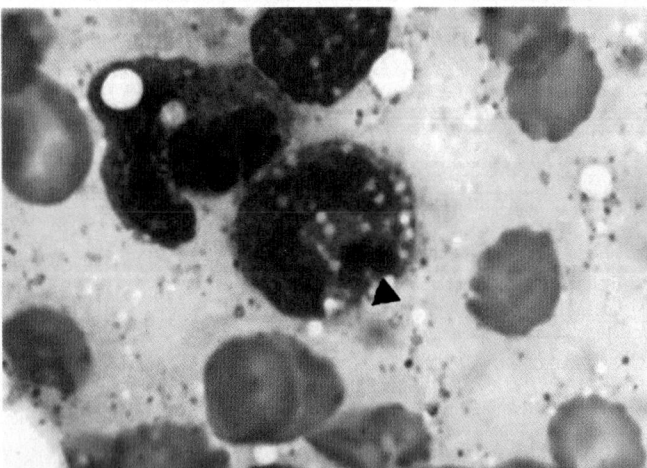

Figure 297-8 *Ehrlichia chaffeensis* morula (*arrowhead*) within a monocyte. (Peripheral blood smear, Wright's stain, ×1000.) (*From Safdar N, Love RB, Maki DG. Severe* Ehrlichia chaffeensis *infection in a lung transplant recipient: A review of ehrlichiosis in the immunocompromised patient. Emerg Infect Dis. 2002;8:320-323.*)

36 hours into the host's dermis, and cause subclinical (especially in children) to severe and potentially fatal infections (especially in immunocompromised adults) within 1 to 4 weeks. Because transovarian transmission in ticks has not been observed, the major reservoirs of the Anaplasmataceae in nature are wild and domestic animals.[36,37] Although the presenting clinical manifestations are similar among Anaplasmataceae infections, the potential multisystem complications and resulting CFRs from these diseases are ultimately determined by the immunocompetence of human hosts (see Table 297-5). The human Anaplasmataceae are resistant to fluoroquinolones, but remain susceptible to tetracyclines, which are now recommended for children and adults. Because there are no vaccines for the tick-borne ehrlichioses and anaplasmosis, the best preventive measures are tick avoidance and control and rapid removal of blood-feeding ticks by 36 hours or less.[38]

Tick-borne Protozoal Infections

BABESIAL INFECTIONS

Babesiosis is a tick-borne, malaria-like zoonosis that usually causes subclinical infections with prolonged parasitemias in humans, and can be transmitted vertically in utero and horizontally by blood product transfusion.[38-42] Babesiosis was initially described in cattle with red water (hemoglobinuric) fever in 1888, when Victor Babes observed inclusions within bovine erythrocytes. Theobald Smith later identified the causative agent of bovine red water fever in 1893 as *Babesia bigemina*, accurately described the parasite's life cycle, and demonstrated for the first time the arthropod-borne transmission of an infectious disease. Although more than 100 species of *Babesia* have now been identified as zoonoses in domestic and wild mammals, only a few species can cause babesiosis in man, a disease characterized by fever, intravascular hemolysis, and hemoglobinuria (Table 297-6). In severe cases, usually in immunocompromised or splenectomized human hosts, massive hemoglobinuria may be associated with severe anemia, jaundice, acute renal failure, and increased CFRs. Babesiosis is now reemerging as an arthropod-borne parasitic disease, as confirmed by increasing numbers of reported cases in the northeast United States and increasing seroprevalence rates there and in California.

Human babesiosis may be divided into two epidemiologic and clinical patterns based on the causative *Babesia* species, their regional endemicity, and the immunocompetence of their human dead-end hosts (see Table 297-6). The first pattern is caused by *Babesia divergens* and related species or subspecies and occurs in immunocompromised, and often splenectomized, human hosts. It includes *B. divergens* babesiosis, first in Eastern and now in Western Europe, a *B. divergens*–like babesiosis in the Midwest caused by a *Babesia* species designated MO-1, and a babesiosis along the Pacific Coast caused by *B. divergens*–like species designated as WA-1 and as CA types (e.g., CA-1, CA-2).[38-42] The *B. divergens*–related species are maintained in tick vectors by transovarial and trans-stadial transmission of the parasites, and most infections are transmitted by diminutive and usually unidentified and unnoticed nymphal ticks.[43] The human *B. divergens*–like cases occur primarily in cattle ranching regions during the summer months, when tick vectors are most active and the incidence of bovine red water fever is greatest. These are the more severe cases of babesiosis, with hemolytic anemia, hemoglobinuria, and renal failure, usually in the splenectomized.

The second and more common pattern of babesiosis in the United States occurs in regional pockets on the northeast coast (New York, Massachusetts, Rhode Island, Connecticut, New Jersey, and offshore islands [Block Island, Long Island, Nantucket]) and upper Midwest (Minnesota, Wisconsin) and is caused by *Babesia microti*, a rodent *Babesia* species transmitted to humans by the same ixodid ticks (black-legged deer ticks) that transmit Lyme disease (see Fig. 297-4).[38] Thus, *B. microti* babesiosis in the United States parallels the distribution of Lyme disease and its tick vectors, occurs in clusters in the same regional pockets as Lyme disease, and may coexist with Lyme disease in an

TABLE 297-5	Human Ehrlichioses and Anaplasmosis		
	Currently Preferred Disease Nomenclature		
Parameter	*Human Monocytotropic Ehrlichiosis*	*Human Granulocytotropic Ehrlichiosis (HME)*	*Human Granulocytotropic Anaplasmosis*
Former disease nomenclature	Human monocytic ehrlichiosis	Human granulocytic ehrlichiosis	Human granulocytic ehrlichiosis
Causative agent(s)	*Ehrlichia chaffeensis*	*Ehrlichia ewingii, Ehrlichia cani*—one asymptomatic human case reported in Venezuela	*Anaplasma phagocytophilum*
Leukocyte targets	Monocytic cell phagosomes	Neutrophil phagosomes	Granulocyte-neutrophil phagosomes
Tick vectors	*Amblyomma americanum* (lone star ticks)	*Amblyomma americanum* (lone star ticks), *Dermacentor variabilis* (American dog ticks)	*Ixodes persulcatus* complex (American deer ticks)—*I. scapularis, I. ricinus, I. pacificus*
Animal reservoirs	White-tailed deer, coyotes, dogs	White-tailed deer, dogs	Rodents, deer, ruminants, horses
U.S. regional distribution	Southeastern and south central United States	South central United States	Northeast United States, upper Midwest, northern California
U.S. regional prevalence	2-5 cases/100,000	Up to 10% of presumed HME cases have *E. ewingii* infections in south central United States	50-60 cases/100,000; high seroprevalence rates in children (>20%) who have had subclinical infections
Seasonal occurrences	April-September, peaking in July	Spring-fall	May-July
Incubation periods (wk)	1-4	1-4	1-4
Modes of transmission	Tick bite, blood product transfusion	Tick bite, blood product transfusion	Tick bite, blood product transfusion, nosocomial
Frequently presenting clinical manifestations	Fever, malaise, headache, myalgias, rash in <40%	Same initial manifestations, but much milder, except in immunocompromised individuals	Fever, malaise, headache, myalgias; rarely rash
Laboratory abnormalities	Leukopenia, thrombocytopenia, transaminitis	Leukopenia, thrombocytopenia, transaminitis	More pronounced and prolonged leukopenia, thrombocytopenia, transaminitis
Potential complications, especially in immunocompromised individuals	Meningoencephalitis, acute renal and respiratory failure, hepatitis, myocarditis	Milder and less likely. except in patients immunocompromised by HIV/AIDS, organ transplantation, prolonged corticosteroid therapy	May be significant in immunocompromised patients with high fevers, seizures, confusion, hemorrhagic diathesis, rhabdomyolysis, shock, acute tubular necrosis, adult respiratory distress syndrome; some specific CNS complications may include eighth nerve palsy, brachial plexopathy, demyelinating polyneuropathy
Case-fatality rate (CFR)	3%, higher in immunocompromised individuals	No deaths reported	0.5%, higher CFR in immunocompromised individuals
Recommended confirmatory diagnostic tests	Wright-stained peripheral blood smears with characteristic intracytoplasmic morulae in monocytes, DNA detection by PCR assay, culture	Wright-stained peripheral blood smears with characteristic intracytoplasmic morulae in neutrophils, DNA detection by PCR	Wright-stained peripheral blood smears with characteristic intracytoplasmic aggregates in neutrophils, DNA detection by PCR assay, increased immunofluorescent antibodies in initial and paired serum samples
Current antibiotic resistance	Fluoroquinolones	Fluoroquinolones	Fluoroquinolones
Currently recommended antibiotic therapy, adults	Doxycycline, 100 mg PO bid, or tetracycline, 250-500 mg PO qid, for minimum of 3 days postdefervescence to maximum of 14-21 days	Doxycycline, 100 mg PO bid, or tetracycline, 250-500 mg PO qid, for minimum of 3 days postdefervescence to maximum of 14-21 days	Doxycycline, 100 mg PO bid, or tetracycline, 250-500 mg PO qid for minimum of 3 days postdefervescence to maximum of 14-21 days
Currently recommended antibiotic therapy, children	Doxycycline, 4.4 mg/kg PO bid, or tetracycline, 25-50 mg/kg PO qid, for minimum of 3 days postdefervescence to maximum of 14-21 days	Doxycycline, 4.4 mg/kg PO bid, or tetracycline, 25-50 mg/kg PO qid, for minimum of 3 days postdefervescence to maximum of 14-21 days	Doxycycline, 4.4 mg/kg PO bid, or tetracycline, 25-50 mg/kg PO qid, for minimum of 3 days postdefervescence to maximum of 14-21 days

HIV/AIDS, human immunodeficiency virus infection/acquired immunodeficiency syndrome; PCR, polymerase chain reaction.

increasing number of cases.[44,45] *B. microti*–induced babesiosis occurs during the warmest months, with 80% of cases reported between May and August, when deer ticks are most active.[39] Humans are usually infected by unnoticed bites by nymphal deer ticks from rodent reservoirs in mice, especially the white-footed mouse (*Peromyscus leucopus*), rather than deer.

Diagnostic strategies for babesiosis include the demonstration of characteristic intra- and extraerythrocytic organisms on Giemsa-stained thin smears and subinoculation of human blood samples into hamsters for suspected *B. microti* infections, or into gerbils for suspected *B. divergens*–related infections (Fig. 297-9).[38,41,42] The serologic methods, especially useful when microscopic methods fail in low parasitemias, include indirect immunofluorescent antibody testing for specific IgM antibodies in acute infections and PCR-based assays to detect *Babesia* DNA and species-specific DNA sequences.

Quinine (650 mg orally three times daily) and clindamycin (1.2 g IV twice daily or 600 mg orally three times daily), continued for 1 week or until parasitemias are in remission, can be used to treat babesiosis

caused by all species.[38] Quinine and clindamycin are preferred therapies for WA-1 babesiosis and for severe *B. microti* infections, especially in older adults and splenectomized or immunosuppressed individuals.[42] For non–life-threatening *B. microti* infections, a 2-week course of oral atovaquone (750 mg twice daily) and azithromycin (500 mg on day 1, followed by 250 to 600 mg/day for 1 week) cleared parasitemias as effectively as quinine and clindamycin, with fewer side effects. For coinfections with *B. burgdorferi*, patients should be treated specifically for Lyme disease with doxycycline (200 mg orally twice daily for 2 weeks) and with antimalarials for babesiosis.[44,45]

Tick-borne Viral Infections

TICK-BORNE VIRAL ENCEPHALITIDES

The tick-borne viral infections are caused primarily by flaviviruses and may be divided into two separate clinical presentations, each with preferred tick vectors and wild animal reservoirs—the viral encepha-

TABLE 297-6 Causal Agents and Clinical Manifestations of Babesiosis					
Babesia *species*	*Geographic Distribution*	*Tick Vectors*	*Animal Reservoirs*	*Epidemiology*	*Clinical Manifestations*
Babesia divergens	UK, Western Europe, Eastern Europe, Sweden, Russia. Not reported in the United States	*Ixodes ricinus*	Cattle Reindeer	Incubation 1-4 weeks Occurs during summer months in cattle-raising regions Targets splenectomized or immunocompromised patients primarily	Fulminant course with high case-fatality rate Fever, rigors, headache, myalgia, jaundice, hemoglobinuria, hemolytic anemia, acute renal failure, multi-organ failure
Babesia microti	Parallels the U.S. Northeast endemic regions for *Borrelia burgdorferi*, especially the islands off NY, MA, CT, and RI and focal areas in CT, NJ, WI, and MN	Deer ticks: *Ixodes dammini* and *Ixodes scapularis*	White-footed mouse (*Peromyscus leucopus*)	Incubation 1-4 weeks following tick bites or 4-9 weeks following blood transfusions Transmission primarily by nymphal ticks Targets older, not necessarily immunocompromised patients—particularly severe in those immunocompromised by HIV infection, advanced age, co-infections with *B. burgdorferi* Seasonality parallels tick nymph activity; 80% of cases occur May-August	Often asymptomatic in young, healthy patients Self-limited influenza-like febrile illness with onset of anorexia, malaise, lethargy, followed in 1 week by high fever, diaphoresis, myalgias; mild splenomegaly, rarely hepatomegaly Later hemolysis, hemolytic anemia, thrombocytopenia, jaundice, acute renal failure, especially in the splenectomized, elderly, or the immunocompromised Complications include ARDS and DIC Case-fatality rate 5%
MO-1 (a relative or subspecies of B. divergens)	Rural Missouri and Kentucky	*Ixodes dentatus* (rabbit tick)	Rabbits Birds	Incubation 1-4 weeks following tick bites Spring to autumn seasonality Targets the splenectomized, like *B. divergens*	Same as above—often asymptomatic, except in the splenectomized, who will develop high parasitemias and multi-organ failure
WA-1 (a relative or subspecies of B. gibsoni)	Rural Washington state	Ixodid ticks, including *Ixodes dentatus*	Unknown— wild canids and ungulates suspected	Incubation 1-4 weeks Targets the splenectomized, elderly, immunocompromised, premature infants May be transmitted by blood transfusion	Same as above—often asymptomatic, except in the splenectomized, who will develop high parasitemias and multi-organ failure
CA-1, CA-2, etc. subspecies (relatives or subspecies of mule deer and bighorn sheep *Babesia* species)	U.S. Pacific coast, primarily rural and semirural areas of California	Ixodid ticks	Unknown— mule deer and bighorn sheep suspected	Incubation 1-4 weeks Targets the splenectomized, elderly, immunocompromised, and premature infants	Same as above—often asymptomatic, except in the splenectomized, who will develop high parasitemias and multi-organ failure

ARDS, acute respiratory distress syndrome; DIC, disseminated intravascular coagulation.

litides and viral hemorrhagic fevers (Table 297-7). The tick-borne viral infections share several common clinical and epidemiologic characteristics including the following: incubation periods of approximately 1 week; biphasic illnesses separated by symptom-free periods beginning with flulike viremic stages, and ending with CNS or hemorrhagic

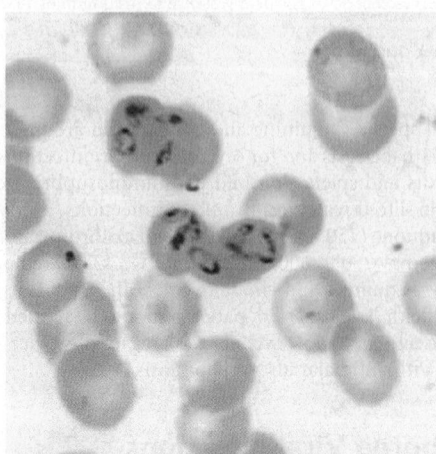

Figure 297-9 *Babesia microti.* Note the vacuolated intra-erythrocytic ring forms (*arrows*) and the clumped extra-erythrocytic forms (thin blood smear, Giemsa stain, ×1000). *(From Centers for Disease Control and Prevention [CDC], Atlanta, GA: DPDx Image Library. Available at http://www.cdc.gov/dpdx/HTML/Babesiosis.htm.)*

manifestations with increased CFRs; nonspecific serodiagnosis by comparing acute and convalescent sera for increased antibody titers or by hemagglutination inhibition; specific serodiagnosis by enzyme-linked immunosorbent assay (ELISA) and antigen detection from blood or cerebrospinal fluid (CSF) by reverse transcriptase (RT)-PCR; no specific treatments other than supportive therapy; and significantly increased postinfection morbidity.[46]

From a global distribution perspective, the tick-borne encephalitis viruses (TBEVs) are separated into the Old World (Eastern Hemisphere) and New World (Western Hemisphere) strains, with the Old World strains having significantly higher CFRs (20% to 40%) and permanent neurologic morbidity rates (28% to 30%) than the New World strains (CFR, 10% to 15%; morbidity rate <10%).[46] Although additional Old World flaviviral strains have now been discovered in sheep reservoirs, the most common Old World TBEVs have been further stratified regionally into three major subtypes—European or Central European (TBEV-Eu), Siberian or Russian Spring-Summer (TBEV-Sib), and Far Eastern (TBEV-FE; see Table 297-7). Except for the Old World TBEVs with sheep reservoirs, all the TBEVs are transmitted by the injection of infected saliva from viremic ixodid ticks. During blood feeding, viruses in tick saliva will increase up to 10-fold and render early removal of the feeding tick ineffective in preventing disease. The preferred wild animal reservoirs for TBEVs include rodents, insectivores, medium-sized mammals, deer and other ungulates, birds, and less often, domestic animals (see Table 297-7).

Powassan (POW) encephalitis, first isolated in 1958, typifies a New World TBEV with a confined regional distribution in the New England states and Eastern Canada, several ixodid tick vectors, primarily *Ixodes* spp., an extensive wild animal reservoir in rodents and medium-sized

TABLE 297-7	**Representative Tick-borne Viral Encephalitides and Hemorrhagic Fevers**				
Virus Name	*Viral Syndrome*	*Family Taxonomy*	*Geographic Distribution*	*Tick Vectors*	*Wild Animal Reservoirs*
Central European tick-borne encephalitis (TBEV-Eu)	TBE	Flaviviridae	Europe, except Iberian Peninsula	Ixodid ticks, especially *Dermacentor marginatus*, *Ixodes persulcatus*, and *I. ricinus*	Mammals—especially rodents, including hedgehogs, wood mice, and voles; deer and other ungulates, birds, domestic livestock, especially goats
Powassan encephalitis	TBE	Flaviviridae	Canada, Northeastern United States, Far Eastern Russia	*Ixodes* spp., particularly *I. cookei*, *Dermacentor andersoni*	Mammals—rodents, skunks, other medium-sized mammals, especially woodchucks
Langat	TBE	Flaviviridae	Malaysia	Ixodid ticks	Mammals—monkeys, rodents
Louping Ill	TBE	Flaviviridae	United States, Scotland	Ixodid ticks	Sheep
Russian (Siberian) spring-summer encephalitis (TBEV-Sib)	TBE	Flaviviridae	Russia	*Ixodes* spp., *I. persulcatus*, *I. ricinus*	Mammals—rodents including hedgehogs, wood mice, voles; also birds, deer, other ungulates, domestic livestock, especially goats
Far Eastern TBE (TBEV-FE)	TBE	Flaviviridae	Eastern Russia, China to Far Eastern Japan	*I. persulcatus*	Mammals—rodents, including hedgehogs, wood mice, voles; also birds, deer, other ungulates, domestic livestock, especially goats
Turkish sheep encephalitis	TBE	Flaviviridae	Turkey	Ixodid ticks	Sheep
Crimean-Congo hemorrhagic fever (HF)	HF	Bunyaviridae	Asia, Eastern Europe, Africa, Middle East	*Hyalomma marginatum*, *Hyalomma anatolicum*	Mammals—many domestic animals (buffalo, camels, cattle, goats, sheep), rabbits, rodents (hedgehogs), birds
Kyasanur Forest disease	HF	Flaviviridae	Western India	*Haemaphysalis spinigera*	Mammals, especially monkeys, domestic livestock (cattle, goats, sheep), rodents, insectivores
Omsk HF	HF	Flaviviridae	Western Siberia	*Dermacentor reticulatus*, *Ixodes apronophorus*	Mammals—rodents, especially muskrats, water voles

mammals, especially woodchucks and skunks, and a seasonal occurrence.[47] Cases occur from May to December and peak during June to September, when ticks are most active. Patients with POW will present with somnolence, headache, confusion, high fever, weakness, ataxia, and CSF lymphocytosis. Transient improvement may be followed by neurologic deterioration, evidence of ischemia or demyelination on magnetic resonance imaging (MRI), and slow recovery, often with permanent deficits including memory loss, weakness, ophthalmoplegia, and lower extremity paraparesis. Unlike the Old World TBEVs, POW is uncommon, with only 31 confirmed cases reported by the CDC from 1958 to 2001. Because there is no vaccine or specific therapy for POW, the best means of prevention is protection from tick bites.

The Old World TBEVs remain common causes of permanent neurologic morbidity from Scandinavia to Eastern Japan, with more than 10,000 cases reported per year, a third of which will result in permanent neurologic deficits.[46] In addition to tick bites, the Old World TBEVs may occasionally be transmitted by ingestion of unpasteurized milk products from viremic livestock (especially goats), breast-feeding, and slaughter of viremic animals. Old World TBE is typically biphasic in over 70% of cases, with an initial febrile flulike presentation followed by a 1-week (range, 1 to 21 days) symptom-free interval. This honeymoon or recovery period is followed by meningoencephalitis with CSF pleocytosis, with or without myelitis, and a poliomyelitis-like flaccid paralysis that targets the arms, neck, and shoulders. MRI and electroencephalographic abnormalities are common but nonspecific. Other acute neurologic complications may include altered consciousness, seizure activity, cranial nerve palsies, and an often fatal bulbar syndrome with cardiorespiratory failure. Because no specific treatments other than supportive therapy exist, tick avoidance and immunization remain the best preventive measures. Effective vaccines have now been developed for the three subtypes of Old World TBEVs, and some have been shown to even provide cross-protection among the subtypes in experimentally infected animals.

TICK-BORNE VIRAL HEMORRHAGIC FEVERS

The tick-borne hemorrhagic fever (TBHF) viruses are maintained in nature in extensive wild and domestic animal reservoirs and are trans-mitted by infected ixodid tick bites, squashing infected ticks, creating infective aerosols, direct contact with blood or tissues from infected animals or humans, or nosocomial spread among medical personnel.[48] TBHFs may be caused by flaviviruses and bunyaviruses, which are distributed throughout Eastern Europe, Africa, and Asia. They are characterized clinically by biphasic illnesses that present with febrile flulike symptoms and end with hepatomegaly and hemorrhagic manifestations (petechiae, purpura, subconjunctival, and pharyngeal hemorrhage, thrombocytopenia, cerebral hemorrhage, disseminated intravascular coagulation [DIC]) separated by a few afebrile days. CFRs range from 10% to over 50%, with most deaths occurring within 5 to 14 days of symptom onset during hemorrhagic stages. Diagnoses may be confirmed by immunologic techniques, such as antibody increases in paired sera and ELISA, and by molecular techniques, such as RT-PCR. Although ribavirin can inhibit Crimean-Congo hemorrhagic fever (CCHF) virus replication in animal models, it has not been tested in clinical trials in humans with CCHF. Nevertheless, if TBHF is suspected in the tropics and laboratory confirmation is unavailable, IV ribavirin (30 mg/kg initially, followed by 16 mg/kg four times daily for 4 days, and then 8 mg/kg three times daily for 6 days) is recommended for severe cases, and oral ribavirin is recommended for high-risk contacts. All patients with TBHFs should be placed in isolation and strict universal precautions should be practiced by all medical personnel. A mouse brain–derived CCHF vaccine has been developed in Bulgaria, but is not available elsewhere. In the absence of a universal vaccine, the best preventive measures for the TBHFs are tick avoidance and control, rapid burial of dead animals, and personal protective equipment for abattoir workers and medical personnel.

TICK-BORNE COLTIVIRUSES

The tick-borne coltiviruses of the family Reoviridae are all double-stranded RNA viruses of the genus *Coltivirus* and include Colorado tick fever virus (CTFV), endemic in the United States and Canadian Rocky Mountain regions, the California tick fever virus (TFV) of rabbits (CTFV-Ca), the Salmon River virus (SRV) of Idaho, a serotype of the CTFVs, and the European Eyach virus (EYAV).[49] The ixodid or hard ticks are the only vectors of the coltiviruses with *Dermacentor* ticks (mainly *D. andersoni*) being the principal vectors of CTFV and SRV in the Rocky Mountains and *Ixodes* ticks (*I. ricinus*, *I. ventalloi*) being the only vectors of EYAV throughout Europe. CTFV has the widest host range among the coltiviruses, which includes squirrels, other rodents, rabbits, porcupines, marmots, deer, elk, sheep, and coyotes. The remaining coltiviruses have fewer, more specific wild animal hosts, including the black-tailed jackrabbit (*Lepus californicus*) for CTFV-Ca and primarily the European rabbit (*Oryctolagus cunniculus*) but also rodents, deer, domestic goats, and sheep for EYAV. The coltiviruses are maintained in nature by ixodid ticks that blood-feed on wild animal hosts with prolonged viremias and then transmit coltiviruses trans-stadially, but not transovarially. Infected nymphs hibernate over winter, and previously infected nymphs and newly infected adults will then transmit coltiviruses to human dead-end hosts during spring-summer blood feeding. CTFV has also been transmitted by blood transfusion and congenitally.

Both CTFV and SRV can cause biphasic to triphasic febrile illnesses that mimic mild cases of RMSF without rash. Leukopenia and thrombocytopenia are common laboratory manifestations of coltivirus infections.[49] Complications are rare but may include meningoencephalitis, orchitis, hemorrhagic fever, pericarditis, and myocarditis. EYAV infections are more often complicated by CNS manifestations than American strain coltivirus infections. The most common differential diagnoses for the tick-borne coltiviruses are other tick-borne febrile diseases, most commonly RMSF in North America, which may be distinguished from CTF and SRV infections by its characteristic rash and leukocytosis. Serologic diagnostic methods to detect anticoltivirus antibodies include complement fixation, seroneutralization assay, immunofluorescence assay, ELISA, and Western immunoblot. The most specific and confirmatory laboratory diagnostic methods include RT-PCR assays to identify CTFV-RNA (or the RNA of its cross-reacting serotypes, CTFV-Ca and SRV), or the isolation of coltiviruses following intracerebral inoculation of infected human blood into suckling mice. Treatment for all tick-borne coltivirus infections is entirely supportive, and long-term complications are rare in uncomplicated cases.

Tick Paralysis

First described in 1912 in Australia, Canada, and the United States, tick paralysis is a rare regional and seasonal cause of acute ataxia and ascending paralysis with an incubation period of 4 to 7 days following female tick attachment, mating, and blood feeding.[50-53] Although 43 species of ticks have been implicated in tick paralysis cases worldwide, most cases occur in the United States and Canadian Pacific Northwest (Washington state and British Columbia) and in Australia. In the U.S. Pacific Northwest, tick paralysis is caused by the American dog tick, *D. variabilis*, or the Rocky Mountain wood tick, *Dermacentor andersoni*, during April through June, when *Dermacentor* ticks emerge from hibernation to mate and to seek blood meals (see Fig. 297-7).[53-55] The mechanism of neurotoxic paralysis in *Dermacentor* tick paralysis is unknown, but neuroelectrophysiologic studies have suggested that sodium flux across axonal membranes is blocked at the nodes of Ranvier, leaving neuromuscular transmission unimpeded.[56] In Australia, the marsupial ixodid tick, *Ixodes holocyclus*, can cause a more severe form of ascending neuromuscular paralysis by producing a botulinum-like neurotoxin that blocks neuromuscular transmission by inhibiting the presynaptic release of acetylcholine.[57]

Most cases of tick paralysis in North America have occurred sporadically in young girls with long hair concealing ticks feeding on the scalp or neck.[55] However, a four-patient cluster of *Dermacentor* tick paralysis, including a 6-year-old girl with a tick on her hairline, and three adults with ticks on the neck (*n* = 1) and back (*n* = 2), was reported from Colorado in 2006.[53]

Although botulism causes a descending neuromuscular paralysis with a preserved sensorium, tick paralysis, Guillain-Barré syndrome, acute poliomyelitis, and spinal cord tumors may all cause acute ascending paralysis with preserved mental status and must be differentiated from each other (Table 297-8).[53-55] Because poliomyelitis has been nearly eradicated by vaccination worldwide, tick paralysis is frequently misdiagnosed as Guillain-Barré syndrome and the correct diagnosis is made accidentally by finding an engorged, usually female, tick on the scalp, head, or neck during hair combing, or when applying electroencephalography (EEG) electrodes (see Table 297-8). Without tick removal, the CFR for tick paralysis is approximately 10%. Postmortem examinations of persons who died suddenly of unexplained paralytic illnesses have demonstrated attached ticks on their heads and necks.[58]

The treatment of *Dermacentor* tick paralysis simply requires removing the tick with forceps (or tweezers) to restore neuromuscular function within 24 hours. Although *I. holocyclus* tick paralysis is also treated by tick removal, transient neuromuscular deterioration may occur for 24-48 hours following tick removal.[55,57] The administration of *I. holocyclus* antitoxin prior to tick removal and prolonged observation for hypoventilation have been recommended.

TABLE 297-8	Clinical Differential Diagnosis of Tick Paralysis versus Ascending Neuromuscular Paralysis with Preserved Sensorium			
Presenting Clinical Features	*Tick Paralysis*	*Guillain-Barré Syndrome*	*Cervical Spinal Cord Lesion*	*Poliomyelitis*
Onset of ascending paralysis	Acute, rapid, within 24-48 hr	Slower onset, days to weeks	Abrupt to gradual	Days to weeks
Ataxia	Present	Absent	Absent	Absent
Deep tendon reflexes	Hyporeflexia progressing to areflexia	Hyporeflexia progressing to areflexia	Variable	Hyporeflexia progressing to areflexia
Babinski sign	Absent	Absent	Present	Absent
Sensory loss	None	Mild	Present	None
Meningeal signs	Absent	Rarely present	Absent	Present
Fever	Absent	Rarely present	Absent	Present
CSF findings				
Protein levels (mg/dL)	Normal	High (≥40)	Normal to high	High
White cells per mm³	<10	<10		>10
Differential counts	Normal	<10 mononuclear cells/mm³	Variable	Lymphocytosis
Nerve conduction studies	↑ Latency in distal motor nerves ↓ Nerve conduction velocity ↓ Amplitude of motor and sensory nerve action potentials	Similar	Similar	Similar
Time to neurologic recovery	Rapid, ≤24 hr after tick removal	Weeks to months	Variable	Months to years
Permanent neurologic deficits	None after tick removal	Permanent paresis possible	Permanent paresis possible	Permanent paresis possible

CSF, cerebrospinal fluid.

Prevention and Control of Tick-Borne Infectious Diseases and Paralytic Poisonings

There are a number of strategies that can be used in the prevention and control of tick-borne infectious diseases, including immunization, personal protective measures, landscape management, and wildlife management. In the 1990s, a Lyme disease vaccine was developed for the United States, but was withdrawn from the market in 2002 because of poor sales. Immunization strategies to prevent tick-borne infectious diseases have proved far more effective in Europe and Asia than in the United States, where neurologic complications from TBEVs are second only to Japanese encephalitis as causes of permanent paraparesis.[46] Current immunization programs for tick-borne viral diseases now provide primary prevention of TBEV-Eu in Europe, TBEV-Sib in Russia and the Middle East, TBEV-FE in China and the Far East, and CCHF in Bulgaria. A canine antitoxin for *I. holocyclus*–induced tick paralysis has been used to reverse tick paralysis in animals and humans in Australia.[55,57]

In addition to immunization, antibiotics following presumed ixodid tick bites with erythema migrans have been recommended as prophylactic therapeutic strategies for the primary prevention of some tick-borne infections. A randomized clinical trial found that a single 200-mg dose of doxycycline administered within 72 hours of a tick bite was 87% effective in preventing Lyme disease.[59]

Finally, because most tick-borne infectious diseases may also be transmitted by blood product transfusions, screening blood product donors in high seroprevalence areas for Lyme disease and other borrelioses, babesiosis, ehrlichioses, and anaplasmosis would eliminate transfusion-transmitted cases. Physicians are encouraged to order leukocyte-reduced blood components for blood product transfusions potentially to reduce the risks of ehrlichiosis and anaplasmosis, especially in regions that are highly endemic for leukocytotropic tick-borne infectious diseases.[13]

Personal protective measures to prevent tick-transmitted diseases include wearing appropriate clothing, using insect repellents, and performing regular tick checks. Wearing long pants tucked into socks, long-sleeved shirts, and light-colored clothing can help keep ticks off the skin and make them easier to spot on clothing. Impregnating clothing with permethrin, routinely performed by the military on maneuvers, is a highly effective repellent against ticks and other insects. The topical application of insect repellents containing 20% to 50% formulations of *N,N*-diethyl-meta-toluamide (DEET) directly on the skin is another effective and recommended measure.

Most patients with Lyme disease, TBRF, babesiosis, ehrlichioses, and anaplasmosis will not recall tick bites because these diseases are often transmitted by diminutive nymphal ticks. Nevertheless, tick localization and removal as soon as possible, preferably within 36 hours, remain recommended strategies to prevent the rickettsial and viral ixodid tick-borne diseases and to reverse tick paralysis. Ticks should always be removed with forceps (or tweezers), not fingers (because squashing ticks can transmit several tick-borne diseases across dermal barriers or create infectious aerosols), and in contiguity with their feeding mouth parts, rather than burning ticks with spent matches or painting embedded ticks with adhesives or nail polishes.

Landscape management strategies to prevent tick-borne diseases include widespread application of acaricides over tick-preferred ecosystems, removal of vegetation and leaf litter near homes and recreation sites, and creation of dry barriers of gravel, stone, or wood chips between forested areas and yards or playgrounds. Wildlife management strategies to prevent tick-borne diseases include encouraging the development of better veterinary vaccines for tick-borne diseases with large domestic animal reservoirs, applying acaricides actively to domestic animals and passively to deer and cattle at baited feeding and watering stations or salt licks, and setting out acaricide-baited rodent houses for rodents to occupy or acaricide-baited cotton balls for rodents to adopt as nesting materials, especially in crawl spaces under homes and near playgrounds.

Conclusions

Most emerging infectious diseases today, such as West Nile virus and severe acute respiratory syndrome (SARS), arise from zoonotic reservoirs, and many are transmitted by arthropod vectors. Because ticks are the most common insect vectors of zoonotic diseases, ticks have become common arthropod vectors of emerging zoonotic diseases, including Lyme disease, ehrlichiosis, and anaplasmosis. Ticks are highly competent and versatile vectors of infectious diseases because ticks of all ages and both genders may remain infectious for generations, without having to reacquire infections from host reservoirs. Finally, recent environmental changes and human behaviors now place humans and ticks together outdoors for longer periods in welcoming ecosystems for breeding, blood feeding, and infectious disease transmission. Better prevention and treatment strategies for tick-borne diseases are indicated now, before the highly conserved genomes of tick-transmitted microorganisms reassort their nucleic acids with their hosts and develop antimicrobial resistance (especially to tetracyclines) or superpathogen capabilities, either by nature's own design or human terrorist intent.

REFERENCES

1. Suss J, Klaus C, Gerstengarbe FW, et al. What makes ticks tick? Climate change, ticks, and tick-borne diseases. *J Travel Med.* 2008;15:39-45.
2. Goddard J. Ticks. In: Goddard J. *Physician's Guide to Arthropods of Medical Importance.* 4th ed. Boca Raton, FL: CRC Press; 2003:327-386.
3. Dumler JS, Walker DH. Rocky mountain spotted fever—changing ecology and persisting vigilance. *N Engl J Med.* 2005; 353:551-553.
4. Parola P, Raoult D. Tick-borne bacterial diseases emerging in Europe. *Clin Microbial Infect Dis.* 2001;7:80-83.
5. Centers for Disease Control and Prevention (CDC). Lyme disease—United States, 1994. *MMWR Morb Mortal Wkly Rep.* 1995;44:459-462.
6. Telford SR III, Goethert HK. Emerging tick-borne infections: Rediscovered and better characterized, or truly "new"? *Parasitology.* 2004;129(Suppl 3):1-27.
7. Dumler JS, Walker DH. Ehrlichiosis and anaplasmosis. In: Guerrant RL, Walker DH, Weller PF, eds. *Tropical Infectious Diseases: Principles, Pathogens, and Practice.* 2nd ed. Philadelphia: Elsevier Churchill Livingstone; 2006:564-573.
8. Dumler JS, Barbet AF, Bekker CP, et al. Reorganization of genera in the families Rickettsiaceae and Anaplasmataceae in the order Rickettsiales: Unification of some species of *Ehrlichia* with *Anaplasma*, *Cowdria* with *Ehrlichia*, and *Ehrlichia* with *Neorickettsia*, descriptions of six new species combinations and designation of *Ehrlichia equi* and HGE agent as subjective synonyms of *Ehrlichia phagocytophila. Int J Syst Evol Microbiol.* 2001;51:2145-2165.
9. Kirkland KB, Klimko TB, Meriweather RA, et al. Erythema migrans-like rash at a camp in North Carolina: A new tick-borne disease? *Arch Int Med.* 1997;157:2635-2641.
10. Varela AS, Luttrell MP, Howerth EW, et al. First culture isolation of *Borrelia lonestari*, putative agent of southern tick-associated rash illness. *J Clin Microbiol.* 2004;42:1163-1169.
11. Parola P. Tick-borne rickettsial diseases: Emerging risks in Europe. *Comp Immunol Microbiol Infect Dis.* 2004;27:297-304.
12. Demma LJ, Traeger MS, Nicholson WL, et al. Rocky Mountain spotted fever from an unexpected tick vector in Arizona. *N Engl J Med.* 2005;353:587-594.
13. Centers for Disease Control and Prevention (CDC). *Anaplasma phagocytophilum* transmitted through blood transfusion—Minnesota, 2007. *MMWR Morb Mortal Wkly Rep.* 2008;57:1145-1148.
14. Blanton L, Keith B, Brzezinski W. Southern tick-associated rash illness: Erythema migrans is not always Lyme disease. *So Med J.* 2008;101:759-760.
15. Barbour AG. Relapsing fever and other *Borrelia* diseases. In: Guerrant RL, Walker DH, Weller PF, eds. *Tropical Infectious Diseases: Principles, Pathogens, and Practice.* 2nd ed. Philadelphia: Elsevier Churchill Livingstone; 2006:499-510.
16. Tibbles CD, Edlow JA. Does this patient have erythema migrans? *JAMA.* 2007;297:2617-2627.
17. Feder HM Jr, Johnson BJB, O'Connell S, et al. A critical appraisal of "chronic Lyme disease." *N Engl J Med.* 2007;357:1422-1430.
18. Masters EJ, Grigery CN, Masters RW. STARI, or Masters disease—tick-vectored Lyme-like illness. *Infect Dis Clin North Am.* 2008;22:361-376.
19. Dworkin MS, Anderson DE Jr, Schwan TG, et al. Tick-borne relapsing fever in the northwestern United States and southwestern Canada. *Clin Infect Dis.* 1998;26:122-131.
20. Dworkin MS, Schoemaker PC, Fritz CL, et al. The epidemiology of tick-borne relapsing fever in the United States. *Am J Trop Med Hyg.* 2002;54:289-293.
21. Centers for Disease Control and Prevention (CDC). Acute respiratory distress syndrome in persons with tickborne relapsing fever—three states, 2004-2005. *MMWR Morb Mortal Wkly Rep.* 2007;56:1073-1076.
22. Sexton DJ, Walker DH. Spotted fever group rickettsioses. In: Guerrant RL, Walker DH, Weller PF, eds. *Tropical Infectious Diseases: Principles, Pathogens, and Practice.* 2nd ed. Philadelphia: Elsevier Churchill Livingstone; 2006:539-547.
23. Walker DH. Targeting rickettsia. *N Engl J Med.* 2006;354:1418-1420.
24. Rovery C, Bourqui P, Raoult D. Questions on Mediterranean spotted fever a century after its discovery. *Emerg Infect Dis.* 2008;14:1360-1367.
25. Tsai YS, Wu YH, Kao PT, et al. African tick bite fever. *J Formos Med Assoc.* 2008;107:73-76.
26. McBride WJH, Hanson JP, Miller R, et al. Severe spotted group rickettsiosis in Australia. *Emerg Infect Dis.* 2007;13:1742-1744.
27. Marrie TJ. Q fever. In: Guerrant RL, Walker DH, Weller PF, eds. *Tropical Infectious Diseases: Principles, Pathogens, and Practice.*

2nd ed. Philadelphia: Elsevier Churchill Livingstone; 2006: 574-577.

28. Hartzell JD, Wood-Morris RN, Martinez LJ, et al. Q fever: Epidemiology, diagnosis, and treatment. *Mayo Clin Proc.* 2008; 83:574-579.

29. Ta TH, Jimenez B, Navarro M, et al. Q fever in returned febrile travelers. *J Travel Med.* 2008;15:126-129.

30. Francis E. Tularemia: Francis 1921. The occurrence of tularemia in nature as a disease of man. *Public Health Rep.* 1921;36: 1731-1738.

31. Centers for Disease Control and Prevention (CDC). Tularemia—United States, 1990-2000. *MMWR Morb Mortal Wkly Rep.* 2002;51:181-184.

32. Guffey MB, Dalzell A, Kelly DR, et al. Ulceroglandular tularemia in a nonendemic area. *So Med J.* 2007;100:304-308.

33. Amsden JR, Warmack S, Gubbins PO. Tick-borne bacterial, rickettsial, spirochetal, and protozoal infectious diseases in the United States: A comprehensive review. *Pharmacotherapy.* 2002;25:191-210.

34. Feldman KA, Enscore RE, Lathrop SL, et al. An outbreak of primary pneumonic tularemia on Martha's Vineyard. *N Engl J Med.* 2001;345:1601-1606.

35. Kantardjiev T, Ivanov I, Velinov T, et al. Tularemia outbreak, Bulgaria, 1997-2005. *Emerg Infect Dis.* 2006;12:678-680.

36. Dumler JS, Madigan JE, Pusterla N, et al. Ehrlichioses in humans: Epidemiology, clinical presentation, diagnosis, and treatment. *Clin Infect Dis.* 2007;45(Suppl 1):S45-S51.

37. Dumler JS, Walker DH. Ehrlichioses and anaplasmosis. In: Guerrant RL, Walker DH, Weller PF, eds. *Tropical Infectious Diseases: Principles, Pathogens, and Practice.* 2nd ed. Philadelphia: Elsevier Churchill Livingstone; 2006:564-573.

38. Telford SR III, Maguire JH. Babesiosis. In: Guerrant RL, Walker DH, Weller PF, eds. *Tropical Infectious Diseases: Principles, Pathogens, and Practice.* 2nd ed. Philadelphia: Elsevier Churchill Livingstone; 2006:1063-1071.

39. Fritz CL, Kjemtrup AM, Conrad PA, et al. Seroepidemiology of emerging tickborne infectious diseases in a northern California community. *J Infect Dis.* 1997;175:1432-1439.

40. New DL, Quinn JB, Quereshi MZ, et al. Vertically transmitted babesiosis. *J Pediatr.* 1997;131:163-164.

41. Herwaldt BL, Kjemtrup AM, Conrad PA, et al. Transfusion-transmitted babesiosis in Washington state: First reported case caused by a WA1-type parasite. *J Infect Dis.* 1997;175:1259-1262.

42. Kjemtrup AM, Lee B, Fritz CL, et al. Investigation of transfusion transmission of a WA1-type babesial parasite to a premature infant in California. *Transfusion.* 2002;42:1482-1487.

43. Goethert HK, Telford SR III. Enzootic transmission of *Babesia divergens* among cottontail rabbits on Nantucket island, Massachusetts. *Am J Trop Med Hyg.* 2003;69:455-460.

44. Krause PJ, Spielman A, Telford SR III, et al. Persistent parasitemia after acute babesiosis. *N Engl J Med.* 1998;339:160-165.

45. Belongia EA. Epidemiology and impact of coinfections from *Ixodes* ticks. *Vector Borne Zoonotic Dis.* 2002;2:265-273.

46. Lindquist L. Tick-borne encephalitis. *Lancet.* 2008;371:1861-1871.

47. Centers for Disease Control and Prevention (CDC). Outbreak of Powassan encephalitis—Maine and Vermont, 1999-2001. *MMWR Morb Mortal Wkly Rep.* 2001;50:761-764.

48. Watts DM, Flick R, Peters CJ, et al. Bunyaviral fevers: Rift Valley fever and Crimean-Congo hemorrhagic fever. In: Guerrant RL, Walker DH, Weller PF, eds. *Tropical Infectious Diseases: Principles, Pathogens, and Practice.* 2nd ed. Philadelphia: Elsevier Churchill Livingstone; 2006:756-761.

49. Attoui H, Jaafar FM, de Micco P, et al. Coltiviruses and seadornaviruses in North America, Europe, and Asia. *Emerg Infect Dis.* 2005;11:1673-1679.

50. Temple IU. Acute ascending paralysis, or tick paralysis. *Med Sentinel.* 1912;20:507-514.

51. Todd JL. Tick bite in British Columbia. *Can Med Assoc J.* 1912;2:1118-1119.

52. Cleland JB. Injuries and diseases of man in Australia attributable to animals (except insects). *Australas Med Gaz.* 1912;32:295-299.

53. Centers for Disease Control and Prevention (CDC). Cluster of tick paralysis cases—Colorado, 2006. *MMWR Morb Mortal Wkly Rep.* 2006;55:933-935.

54. Gordon BM, Giza CC. Tick paralysis presenting in an urban environment. *Ped Neurol.* 2004;30:122-124.

55. Felz MW, Smith CD, Swift TR. A six-year-old girl with tick paralysis. *N Engl J Med.* 2000;342:90-94.

56. Swift TR, Ignacio OJ. Tick paralysis: Electrophysiologic studies. *Neurology.* 1975;25:1130-1133.

57. Grattan-Smith PJ, Morris JG, Johnston JG, et al. Clinical and neurophysiological features of tick paralysis. *Brain.* 1997;120: 1975-1987.

58. Rose I. A review of tick paralysis. *Can Med Assoc J.* 1954; 70:175-176.

59. Nadelman RB, Nowakowski J, Fish D, et al. Prophylaxis with single dose doxycycline for the prevention of Lyme disease after an *Ixodes scapularis* tick bite. *N Engl J Med.* 2001;345:79-84.

298

Kawasaki Syndrome

FRANK T. SAULSBURY

Kawasaki syndrome is an acute systemic vasculitis that affects primarily infants and young children. It was first reported in the Japanese literature in 1967 by Dr. Tomisaku Kawasaki.[1] The initial reports in the English literature appeared in the 1970s under the designation of "mucocutaneous lymph node syndrome." Kawasaki syndrome is not a new disease; earlier descriptions of infantile periarteritis nodosa almost certainly represented examples of Kawasaki syndrome.

Epidemiology

Although Kawasaki syndrome is recognized throughout the world, it is particularly common in Japan, with an incidence of 112/100,000 children younger than 5 years.[2] In the United States, the incidence of Kawasaki syndrome is approximately 17/100,000 children younger than 5 years.[3] In the United States, the disease is more common in children of Asian ancestry.[3] Kawasaki syndrome has been reported in a few adults, but it is overwhelmingly a disease of young children. The peak age of onset is 1 to 2 years, and 80% of patients are younger than 5 years of age. The male-to-female ratio is 1.5:1.

Kawasaki syndrome occurs sporadically and in mini-epidemics. Both endemic and epidemic cases occur more commonly in late winter and spring. Person-to-person spread has not been documented, and secondary cases in contacts of affected patients are unusual. Nevertheless, Kawasaki syndrome occurs in siblings (especially twins) of affected patients more frequently than in the general population.[4] More than half of the secondary cases in siblings develop within 10 days after the first case, suggesting a common exposure to an infectious agent.

Clinical Features

The diagnosis of Kawasaki syndrome is established by the presence of the clinical criteria listed in Table 298-1.[5] Fever is usually the initial feature of Kawasaki syndrome. It is characteristically high, spiking, and prolonged, and it persists for 1 to 2 weeks in untreated patients. Bilateral nonpurulent conjunctivitis ensues shortly after the onset of fever and lasts 1 to 2 weeks in untreated patients. The conjunctival involvement is characterized by hyperemia and injection of the bulbar conjunctivae (Fig. 298-1). Changes of the oropharyngeal mucosa, consisting of (1) erythema progressing to fissuring, cracking, and bleeding of the lips; (2) strawberry tongue; and (3) diffuse erythema of the oropharynx, are prominent during the acute febrile period (see Fig. 298-1).

Changes of the extremities include erythema of the palms and soles accompanied by firm, indurative edema. The swollen extremities may be painful. During recovery, 2 to 3 weeks after the onset of fever, a distinctive pattern of skin desquamation develops. Desquamation begins in the periungual region and often extends to involve the entire palms and soles. The erythematous rash of Kawasaki syndrome usually appears shortly after the onset of fever and persists during the febrile period. Most often, the rash is a raised, deep red, plaquelike eruption (Fig. 298-2). A morbilliform maculopapular rash with multiforme-like target lesions, a scarlatiniform erythroderma, and, rarely, a fine pustular eruption have also been observed in Kawasaki syndrome. Typically, there is widespread involvement of the trunk and extremities, with accentuation in the perineal area.

Cervical lymphadenopathy is the least common of the principal diagnostic criteria. At least one lymph node measuring more than 1.5 cm in diameter is necessary to fulfill the criterion for this finding. Usually, there is enlargement of a single cervical lymph node; the nodes are firm, nonfluctuant, and only moderately tender.

In addition to the clinical features that constitute the diagnostic criteria, there are a wide variety of associated findings in Kawasaki syndrome. Some of the more common features are listed in Table 298-2.[6]

Up to 10% of patients do not fulfill the requisite clinical criteria and are designated as having incomplete Kawasaki syndrome. Incomplete disease is especially common in infants younger than 12 months. Patients with incomplete Kawasaki syndrome are at risk for coronary artery aneurysms.[7] Indeed, finding coronary artery aneurysms may be the only way to diagnose incomplete Kawasaki syndrome definitively.

The clinical course of untreated Kawasaki syndrome is triphasic. The acute febrile phase, lasting 7 to 14 days, is dominated by the features comprising the diagnostic criteria. Irritability, anorexia, aseptic meningitis, and hepatic dysfunction are also prominent features of the acute phase. During the subacute phase, which lasts 2 to 4 weeks, fever, rash, and lymphadenopathy resolve, but irritability and conjunctival injection may persist. Arthritis and desquamation of the fingers and toes occur during the subacute phase. Thrombocytosis, often reaching very high levels, is seen during the subacute phase. This is when patients are at greatest risk of coronary artery thrombosis. The convalescent phase of Kawasaki syndrome begins when all clinical signs have disappeared, and it continues until the sedimentation rate and platelet count return to normal, usually 6 to 10 weeks after the onset of illness.

Recurrent Kawasaki syndrome after apparent resolution is rare, occurring in only 1% to 3% of patients.[6] Most recurrences develop within a few weeks of the original episode.

Cardiac Involvement

Although carditis is not included in the diagnostic criteria, cardiac involvement is the hallmark of Kawasaki syndrome and is the major source of morbidity and mortality. During the acute phase, up to 50% of patients have myocarditis manifested by tachycardia and gallop rhythms. Occasionally, myocarditis is severe enough to produce overt congestive heart failure. Pericarditis, conduction disturbances, and regurgitation of the mitral and aortic valves are less frequent manifestations of cardiac involvement during the acute phase.[5]

The most serious complication of Kawasaki syndrome is coronary arteritis, with damage to the intima and media of the proximal coronary arteries. When compared with norms based on body surface area, up to 50% of patients have transient dilatation of the coronary arteries and 20% develop coronary artery aneurysms.[5,8] Dilatation of the proximal coronary arteries may be detected as early as 7 days after the onset of fever, with a peak frequency of coronary aneurysm formation occurring within 2 to 4 weeks of the onset of illness. If unrecognized and untreated, the coronary aneurysms are prone to clot during the subacute phase of the illness, when the patients are hypercoagulable because of the extreme thrombocytosis. Sudden death from coronary thrombosis and myocardial infraction occurs in 1% to 2% of untreated patients.

The coronary aneurysms regress within 1 to 2 years in most patients.[9] However, even with echocardiographic resolution of the aneurysms, there may be persistent coronary artery stenosis and cardiac ischemia in some patients. The long-term consequences of coronary arteritis are unclear, but ischemic heart disease, myocardial infarction, and sudden

TABLE 298-1	Diagnostic Criteria for Kawasaki Syndrome

A. Fever of at least 5 days' duration (100%)
B. Presence of at least four of the following five conditions*:
  1. Bilateral conjunctivitis (85%)
  2. Changes in the lips and oral mucosa (90%)
    Dry, red, fissured lips
    "Strawberry tongue"
    Oropharyngeal erythema
  3. Changes in the extremities (75%)
    Erythema of palms and soles
    Edema of hands and feet
    Periungual desquamation
  4. Polymorphous rash (80%)
  5. Cervical lymphadenopathy (70%)
C. Illness not explained by other known disease processes

*Kawasaki syndrome may be diagnosed in patients with fever and fewer than the required four of five other criteria in the presence of coronary artery abnormalities.

TABLE 298-2	Associated Features of Kawasaki Syndrome

1. Cardiac disease
   Coronary artery aneurysms
   Myocarditis
   Pericarditis
   Mitral or aortic regurgitation
   Arrhythmias
2. Irritability
3. Arthralgia, arthritis
4. Aseptic meningitis
5. Urethritis with sterile pyuria
6. Hepatitis
7. Hydrops of the gallbladder
8. Pancreatitis
9. Pneumonitis
10. Anterior uveitis
11. Sensorineural hearing loss
12. Peripheral ischemia

death have been reported in young adult survivors of childhood Kawasaki syndrome.[10]

Laboratory Features

The laboratory features of Kawasaki syndrome are nonspecific and nondiagnostic. Most patients have a moderate leukocytosis with a left shift. The sedimentation rate and C-reactive protein concentration are almost universally elevated during the acute febrile period. Patients with prolonged fever often have anemia and hypoalbuminemia. Sterile pyuria and elevated alanine aminotransferase levels are present in approximately 50% of patients. The platelet count, which is normal in the first few days of Kawasaki syndrome, begins to rise in the second week of the illness and may ultimately exceed 1,000,000/μL in untreated patients. Tests for antinuclear antibody and rheumatoid factor are routinely negative.

Differential Diagnosis

The diagnostic criteria for Kawasaki syndrome are not entirely sensitive or specific. Moreover, there is no diagnostic laboratory test for Kawasaki syndrome. Thus, it is necessary to consider other conditions in the differential diagnosis of Kawasaki syndrome. Some of these conditions are presented in Table 298-3.[6]

TABLE 298-3	Differential Diagnosis of Kawasaki Syndrome

Infections

Measles
Scarlet fever
Staphylococcal or streptococcal toxic shock syndrome
Rocky Mountain spotted fever
Parvovirus B19 infection
Leptospirosis
Adenovirus infection
Enterovirus infection

Other Conditions

Rheumatic fever
Stevens-Johnson syndrome
Systemic juvenile rheumatoid arthritis
Polyarteritis nodosa
Reiter's syndrome
Drug reaction

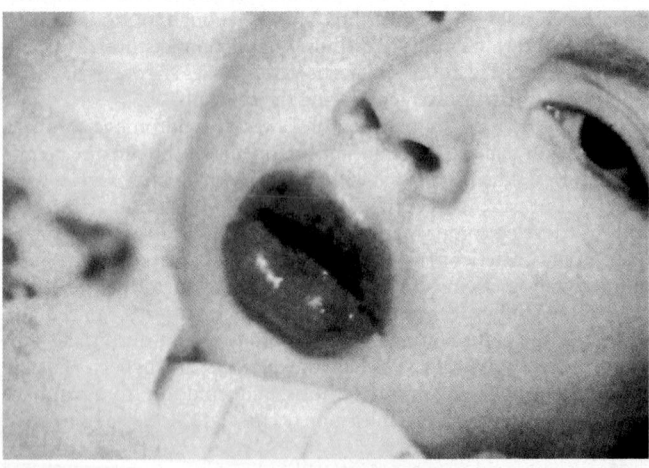

Figure 298-1 Conjunctival injection, lip edema, and erythema in a 2-year-old boy on the sixth day of illness. (*From Council on Cardiovascular Disease in the Young; Committee on Rheumatic Fever, Endocarditis, and Kawasaki Disease; American Heart Association. Diagnostic guidelines for Kawasaki disease. Circulation. 2001;103:335-336.*)

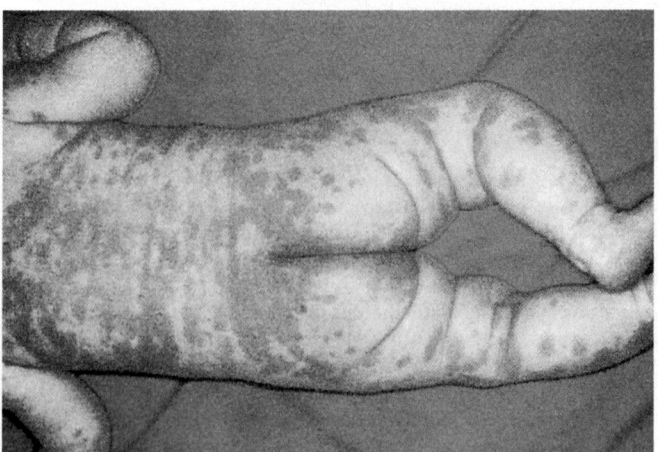

Figure 298-2 Rash of Kawasaki disease in a 7-month-old boy on the fourth day of illness. (*From Council on Cardiovascular Disease in the Young; Committee on Rheumatic Fever, Endocarditis, and Kawasaki Disease; American Heart Association. Diagnostic guidelines for Kawasaki disease. Circulation. 2001;103:335-336.*)

Pathology

Kawasaki syndrome is a generalized vasculitis involving small and medium-sized arteries, with a predilection for the coronary arteries. Histologically, Kawasaki syndrome is characterized by endothelial cell necrosis, leukocyte infiltration of the media and adventitia, medial disruption, aneurysmal dilatation, and intraluminal thrombosis.

Etiology and Pathogenesis

The clinical and epidemiologic features of Kawasaki syndrome clearly suggest an infectious cause. However, intensive efforts during the past 40 years have failed to identify a single verifiable infectious cause of Kawasaki syndrome. Some evidence has suggested that Kawasaki syndrome may be caused by superantigen bacterial toxins.[11] Superantigens stimulate large populations of T cells expressing particular T-cell receptor β-chain variable region gene products. The immunologic consequences of superantigen stimulation include massive proliferation and expansion of the target T cells with resultant production of proinflammatory cytokines.

A number of toxins produced by *Staphylococcus aureus* and *Streptococcus pyogenes* are known to have superantigen properties. Several lines of evidence support a role for staphylococcal or streptococcal superantigen toxins in the pathogenesis of Kawasaki syndrome. First, skewed distribution of the Vβ repertoire of T cells in the peripheral blood and tissues of patients with Kawasaki syndrome provides indirect evidence of exposure to superantigens.[11-16] Second, staphylococci and streptococci elaborating superantigen toxins (toxic shock syndrome toxin-1 and streptococcal pyrogenic exotoxin, respectively) have been cultured from patients with Kawasaki syndrome.[17] Third, infants with Kawasaki syndrome develop antibodies to a number of staphylococcal and streptococcal superantigen toxins.[18] However, other studies have not confirmed the skewed Vβ repertoire of T cells in the peripheral blood of patients with Kawasaki syndrome, and these studies suggest that conventional antigens rather than superantigens are involved in the etiology of Kawasaki syndrome.[19-22] Moreover, culture and serologic data have disputed the role of staphylococcal or streptococcal superantigen toxins in the pathophysiology of Kawasaki syndrome.[23,24]

Regardless of the inciting agent, Kawasaki syndrome is characterized by intense activation of the immune system, marked production of inflammatory cytokines, and recruitment of endothelial cells into the inflammatory process.[25,26] Cytokine-induced production of vascular endothelial growth factor and matrix metalloproteinases appear to be the final common pathway in the development of coronary artery aneurysms.[27-30]

The increased incidence of Kawasaki syndrome in children of Asian ancestry and in siblings of affected children suggests a genetic contribution to the risk of the disease. Early attention focused on major histocompatibility complex (MHC) associations. To date, no clear, consistent MHC class I or II associations with Kawasaki syndrome have been demonstrated.[31] Some studies have suggested that genes involved in the inflammatory response or the innate immune system may be associated with Kawasaki syndrome.[32-34] Nevertheless, definitive information concerning the genetic susceptibility to Kawasaki syndrome is lacking.

Therapy

Despite incomplete knowledge about the etiology and pathogenesis, there has been effective therapy for Kawasaki syndrome for more than 20 years. Randomized studies have demonstrated that high-dose IV immune globulin (IVIG) is extremely effective therapy for Kawasaki syndrome.[35,36] The use of IVIG has resulted in a substantial decrease in the morbidity and mortality associated with Kawasaki syndrome. IVIG produces rapid resolution of fever and other clinical manifestations of the acute febrile phase and reverses the laboratory indices of systemic inflammation. More importantly, IVIG reduces the incidence of coronary artery aneurysms to 3% to 4% compared with 20% in untreated patients.[35,36] A number of dosage schedules have been studied, but the most effective regimen is a single infusion of IVIG in a dosage of 2 g/kg given over 10 hours.[36] Treatment should be initiated within the first 10 days of the illness, and preferably within 7 days. Administration of IVIG before day 5 of the illness provides no benefit in preventing coronary abnormalities.[37,38] Morover, early treatment has been associated with an increased risk of IVIG treatment failure and the need for re-treatment.

Approximately 10% to 15% of patients have persistent fever or recrudescence of fever more than 48 hours after initiation of IGIV therapy. These patients are at increased risk for the development of coronary artery aneurysms, and should be re-treated with 2 g/kg of IVIG.[39,40] Age younger than 12 months, a platelet count less than 300,000/μL, C-reactive protein concentration higher than 8 mg/dL, and an elevated alanine aminotransferase level represent risk factors for failure of initial IVIG treatment.[41-43]

The optimal management of patients who remain febrile despite repeated IVIG infusions remains unclear. Emerging data suggest that corticosteroid therapy is effective in resolving the disease in patients who are refractory to IVIG.[44-46] More recently, infliximab, a monoclonal antibody to tumor necrosis factor-α (TNF-α), has also been used successfully in patients resistant to IVIG therapy.[47] Unfortunately, most patients who have received corticosteroids or infliximab for IVIG resistance already had coronary aneurysms by the time these agents were used.

Although corticosteroids are the mainstay of treatment for almost all forms of vasculitis, Kawasaki syndrome has been the exception. Several small prospective studies have shown that patients treated with IVIG plus corticosteroids have a shorter duration of fever and more rapid resolution of the acute-phase reactants compared with patients treated with IVIG alone,[48-50] but none of the studies were sufficiently powered to show a difference in the incidence of coronary abnormalities. More recently, two large prospective studies of corticosteroids plus IVIG in the initial treatment of Kawasaki syndrome produced somewhat conflicting results. One study used IVIG 2 g/kg plus prednisone in a dose of 2 mg/kg/day until the C-reactive protein was normal, then tapered the dose over 2 weeks, compared with IVIG alone. The corticosteroid-treated patients had a significantly shorter duration of fever, shorter time to normalization of the C-reactive protein level, decreased incidence of coronary artery abnormalities, and decreased need for IVIG retreatment.[51] Another study used IVIG 2 g/kg plus methylprednisolone in a dose of 30 mg/kg IV as a single dose compared with IVIG alone. With this regimen, there was no difference in the duration of fever, incidence of coronary abnormalities, or need for IVIG retreatment.[52] Thus, current evidence suggests that corticosteroids should be used with IVIG in patients who have failed initial IVIG treatment.[5] In addition, emerging data suggest that corticosteroids are useful as adjunctive therapy to IVIG in the initial management of Kawasaki syndrome. The addition of corticosteroids should be strongly considered in the initial treatment of patients who have risk factors for IVIG failure.[41-43]

The mechanisms whereby IVIG produces dramatic beneficial effects remain unclear. IVIG is a powerful immunomodulating agent and may directly reverse a number of the immunologic abnormalities associated with Kawasaki syndrome. The rapidity with which IVIG works suggests toxin neutralization as a possible mechanism of action.

Aspirin is used as adjunctive therapy in Kawasaki syndrome. Traditionally, aspirin is administered in anti-inflammatory dosages (80 to 100 mg/kg/day) until the patient is afebrile or until day 14 of the illness. The dosage is then reduced to 3 to 5 mg/kg/day to provide an antiplatelet effect during the period of thrombocytosis, when patients are at risk for clotting coronary artery aneurysms.[5] Because IVIG therapy aborts the acute phase of the illness so rapidly, treatment with low-dose aspirin from the outset seems reasonable, but this regimen has not been studied prospectively. Nevertheless, a meta-analysis of published data and a retrospective study has found no significant difference between the incidence of coronary artery disease in patients treated with IVIG plus high-dose aspirin and those treated with IVIG and low-dose aspirin.[53,54] In patients with no evidence of coronary artery disease, low-dose aspirin is continued for 6 to 8 weeks. In patients with coronary aneurysms despite IVIG therapy, low-dose aspirin should be continued indefinitely or until the aneurysms resolve.

Echocardiography at the time of diagnosis provides valuable baseline information. All patients should have repeat echocardiography 3 to 6 weeks after therapy to guide the duration of aspirin therapy. Patients with coronary artery abnormalities should receive long-term monitoring of cardiac function.

REFERENCES

1. Kawasaki T. Acute febrile mucocutaneous syndrome with lymphoid involvement with specific desquamation of the fingers and toes in children: Clinical observations of 50 cases. *Jpn J Allergy*. 1967;16:178-222.
2. Yanagawa H, Nakamura Y, Yashiro M, et al. Incidence survey of Kawasaki disease in 1997 and 1998 in Japan. *Pediatrics*. 2001;107:e33.
3. Holman RC, Curns AT, Belay ED, et al. Kawasaki syndrome hospitalizations in the United States, 1997 and 2000. *Pediatrics*. 2003;112:495-501.
4. Fugita Y, Kakamura Y, Sakata K, et al. Kawasaki disease in families. *Pediatrics*. 1989;84:666-669.
5. Newburger JW, Takahashi M, Gerber MA, et al. Diagnosis, treatment and long-term management of Kawasaki disease. *Circulation*. 2004;110:2747-2771.
6. Mason WH, Takahashi M. Kawasaki syndrome. *Clin Infect Dis*. 1999;28:169-187.
7. Fukushige J, Takahashi N, Ueda Y, et al. Incidence and clinical features of incomplete Kawasaki disease. *Acta Paediatr*. 1994;83:1057-1060.
8. deZori A, Colan SD, Gauvreau K, et al. Coronary artery dimensions may be misclassified as normal in Kawasaki disease. *J Pediatr*. 1998;133:254-258.
9. Kato H, Ichinose E, Yoshioka F, et al. Fate of coronary aneurysms in Kawasaki disease: A serial coronary angiography and long-term follow-up study. *Am J Cardiol*. 1982;49:1758-1766.
10. Burns JC, Shike H, Gordon JB, et al. Sequelae of Kawasaki disease in adolescents and young adults. *J Am Coll Cardiol*. 1996;28:253-257.
11. Matsubara K, Fukaya T. The role of group A streptococcus and *Staphylococcus aureus* in Kawasaki disease. *Curr Opin Infect Dis*. 2007;20:298-303.
12. Abe J, Kotzin BL, Jujo K, et al. Selective expansion of T cells expressing T-cell receptor variable regions V beta 2 and V beta 8 in Kawasaki disease. *Proc Natl Acad Sci U S A*. 1992;89:4066-4070.
13. Brogan PA, Shah V, Klein N, et al. T cell Vβ repertoires in childhood vasculitides. *Clin Exp Immunol*. 2003;131:517-527.
14. Yoshioka T, Matsutani T, Iwagami S, et al. Polyclonal expansion of TCRBV2 and TCRBV6 bearing T cells in patients with Kawasaki disease. *Immunology*. 1999;96:465-472.
15. Leung DYM, Giorno RC, Kazemi LV, et al. Evidence for superantigen involvement in cardiovascular injury due to Kawasaki syndrome. *J Immunol*. 1995;155:5018-5021.
16. Yamashiro Y, Nagata S, Oguchi S, et al. Selective increase of Vβ2+ T cells in the small intestinal mucosa in Kawasaki disease. *Pediatr Res*. 1996;39:264-266.
17. Leung DYM, Meissner HC, Fulton DR, et al. Toxic shock syndrome toxin-secreting *Staphylococcus aureus* in Kawasaki syndrome. *Lancet*. 1993;342:1385-1388.
18. Matsubara K, Fukaya T, Miwa K, et al. Development of serum IgM antibodies against superantigens of *Staphylococcus aureus* and *Streptococcus pyogenes* in Kawasaki disease. *Clin Exp Immunol*. 2006;143:427-434.
19. Pietra BA, De Inocencio J, Giannini EH, et al. TCR Vβ family repertoire and T cell activation markers in Kawasaki disease. *J Immunol*. 1994;153:1881-1888.
20. Jason J, Montana E, Donald JF, et al. Kawasaki disease and the T cell antigen receptor. *Hum Immunol*. 1998;59:29-38.
21. Mancia L, Wahlstrom J, Schiller B, et al. Characterization of the T-cell receptor V-β repertoire in Kawasaki disease. *Scand J Immunol*. 1998;48:443-449.
22. Rowley AH, Shulman ST, Spike BT, et al. Oligoclonal IgA response in the vascular wall in acute Kawasaki disease. *J Immunol*. 2001;166:1334-1343.
23. Morita A, Imada Y, Igarashi H, et al. Serologic evidence that streptococcal superantigens are not involved in the pathogenesis of Kawasaki disease. *Microbiol Immunol*. 1997;41:895-900.
24. Leung DYM, Meissner HC, Shulman ST, et al. Prevalence of superantigen-secreting bacteria in patients with Kawasaki disease. *J Pediatr*. 2002;140:742-746.
25. Yeung RSM. Pathogenesis and treatment of Kawasaki's disease. *Curr Opin Rheumatol*. 2005;17:617-623.
26. Wittkowski H, Hirono K, Ichida F, et al. Acute Kawasaki disease is associated with reverse regulation of soluble receptor for advance glycation end products and its proinflammatory ligand S100A12. *Arthritis Rheum*. 2007;56:4174-4181.
27. Hamamichi Y, Ichida F, Yu X, et al. Neutrophils and mononuclear cells express vascular endothelial growth factor in acute Kawasaki disease: Its possible role in progression of coronary artery lesions. *Pediatr Res*. 2001;49:74-80.
28. Freeman AF, Crawford SE, Cornwall ML, et al. Angiogenesis in fatal acute Kawasaki disease coronary artery and myocardium. *Pediatr Cardiol*. 2005;26:578-584.
29. Gavin PJ, Crawford SE, Shulman ST, et al. Systemic arterial expression of matrix metalloproteinases 2 and 9 in acute Kawasaki disease. *Arterioscler Thromb Vasc Biol*. 2003;23:576-581.
30. Lau AC, Rosenberg H, Duong TT, et al. Elastolytic matrix metalloproteinases and coronary outcome in children with Kawasaki disease. *Pediatr Res*. 2007;61:710-715.
31. Barron KS, Silverman ED, Gonzales JC, et al. Major histocompatibility complex class II alleles in Kawasaki syndrome: Lack of consistent correlation with disease or cardiac involvement. *J Rheumatol*. 1992;19:1790-1793.
32. Quasney MW, Bronstein DE, Cantor RM, et al. Increased frequency of alleles associated with elevated tumor necrosis factor-alpha levels in children with Kawasaki disease. *Pediatr Res*. 2001;49:685-690.
33. Ouchi K, Suzuki Y, Shirakawa T, et al. Polymorphism of SLC11A1 (formerly NRAMP1) gene confers susceptibility to Kawasaki disease. *J Infect Dis*. 2003;187:326-329.
34. Biezeveld MH, Kuipers IM, Geissler J, et al. Association of mannose-binding lectin genotype with cardiovascular abnormalities in Kawasaki disease. *Lancet*. 2003;361:1268-1270.
35. Newburger JW, Takahashi M, Burns JC, et al. The treatment of Kawasaki syndrome with intravenous gamma globulin. *N Engl J Med*. 1986;315:341-347.
36. Newburger JW, Takahashi M, Beiser AS, et al. A single intravenous infusion of gamma globulin as compared with four infusions in the treatment of acute Kawasaki syndrome. *N Engl J Med*. 1991;324:1633-1639.
37. Fong NC, Hui YW, Li CK, et al. Evaluation of the efficacy of treatment of Kawasaki disease before day 5 of illness. *Pediatr Cardiol*. 2004;25:31-34.
38. Muta H, Ishii M, Egami K, et al. Early intravenous gamma-globulin treatment for Kawasaki disease: the nationwide surveys in Japan. *J Pediatr*. 2004;144:496-499.
39. Burns JC, Capparelli EV, Brown JA, et al. Intravenous gamma-globulin treatment and retreatment in Kawasaki disease. *Pediatr Infect Dis J*. 1998;17:1144-1148.
40. Durongpisitkul K, Soongswang J, Laohaprasitiporn D, et al. Immunoglobulin failure and retreatment in Kawasaki disease. *Pediatr Cardiol*. 2003;24:145-148.
41. Egami K, Muta H, Ishii M, et al. Prediction of resistance to intravenous immunoglobulin treatment in patients with Kawasaki disease. *J Pediatr*. 2006;149:237-240.
42. Kobayashi T, Inoue Y, Takenchi K, et al. Prediction of intravenous immunoglobulin unresponsiveness in patients with Kawasaki disease. *Circulation*. 2006;113:2606-2612.
43. Sano T, Kurotobi S, Matsuzaki K, et al. Prediction of non-responsiveness to standard high-dose gamma-globulin therapy in patients with acute Kawasaki disease before starting initial treatment. *Eur J Pediatr*. 2007;166:131-137.
44. Hashino K, Ishii M, Iemura M, et al. Re-treatment for immune globulin-resistant Kawasaki disease: a comparative study of additional immune globulin and steroid pulse therapy. *Pediatr Int*. 2001;43:211-217.
45. Takeshita S, Kawamura Y, Nakatani K, et al. Standard-dose and short-term corticosteroid therapy in immunoglobulin-resistant Kawasaki disease. *Clin Immunol*. 2005;44:423-426.
46. Lang BA, Yeung RSM, Oen KG, et al. Corticosteroid treatment of refractory Kawasaki disease. *J Rheumatol*. 2006;33:803-809.
47. Burns JC, Mason WH, Hauger SB, et al. Infliximab treatment for refractory Kawasaki syndrome. *J Pediatr*. 2005:146:662-667.
48. Sundel RP, Baker AL, Fulton DR, et al. Corticosteroids in the initial treatment of Kawasaki disease: report of a randomized trial. *J Pediatr*. 2003;142:611-616.
49. Okada Y, Shinohara M, Kobayashi T, et al. Effect of corticosteroids in addition to intravenous gamma globulin therapy on serum cytokine levels in the acute phase of Kawasaki disease in children. *J Pediatr*. 2003;143:363-367.
50. Jibiki T, Terai M, Kurosaki T, et al. Efficacy of intravenous immune globulin therapy combined with dexamethasone for the initial treatment of acute Kawasaki disease. *Eur J Pediatr*. 2004;163:229-233.
51. Inoue Y, Okada Y, Shinohara M, et al. A multicenter prospective randomized trial of corticosteroids in primary therapy for Kawasaki disease: Clinical course and coronary artery outcome. *J Pediatr*. 2006;149:336-341.
52. Newburger JW, Sleeper LA, McCrindle BW, Randomized trial of pulsed corticosteroid therapy for primary treatment of Kawasaki disease. *N Engl J Med*. 2007;356:663-675.
53. Terai M, Shulman ST. Prevalence of coronary artery abnormalities is highly dependent on gamma globulin dose but independent of salicylate dose. *J Pediatr*. 1997;131:888-893.
54. Saulsbury FT. Comparison of high-dose and low-dose aspirin plus intravenous immunoglobulin in the treatment of Kawasaki syndrome. *Clin Pediatr*. 2002;41:597-601.

Special Problems

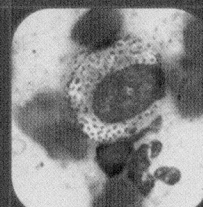

299

Organization for Infection Control

MICHAEL B. EDMOND | RICHARD P. WENZEL

Infection control as a formal discipline in the United States developed during the late 1950s, primarily to address the problem of nosocomial staphylococcal infections. Over the next 50 years, the field of infection control developed incrementally in response to medical advances by incorporating the science of epidemiology to elucidate risk factors for health care–associated infections (HAIs), so that interventions to prevent HAIs could be tested and implemented. However, in the past decade, three pivotal events signaled the beginning of a new era in health care epidemiology—the Institute of Medicine's report on errors in health care,[1] which included HAIs; the Chicago Tribune expose on HAIs,[2] which was the beginning of the mainstream media's interest in this topic; and the publication of dramatic reductions in bloodstream infection rates by simply standardizing the process of catheter insertion.[3,4] This new era in health care epidemiology is characterized by increasing scrutiny and regulation, and consumer demands for more transparency and accountability, along with calls for rapid reductions in HAI rates.[5]

The primary role of an infection-control program is to reduce the risk of hospital-acquired infection, thereby protecting patients, employees, health care students, and visitors. HAIs develop in 1.7 million patients yearly in the United States[6] and account for approximately 100,000 deaths. Two-thirds of the deaths are due to pneumonia and bloodstream infection. Given the associated morbidity, mortality, and cost of HAIs, the value of infection control is obvious.

Each hospital should develop an infection control plan that outlines the scope of the infection control program, the overarching and specific goals, along with the metrics used to assess progress towards those goals. Periodically throughout the year, the plan should be reviewed and updated as goals are met and new issues develop. At the end of each year, a more formal infection control risk assessment should be conducted and the findings reflected in the infection control plan for the upcoming year.

The functions of a hospital epidemiology program vary from institution to institution but can generally be divided into the following areas: (1) surveillance, (2) outbreak investigation, (3) education, (4) employee health, (5) the monitoring and management of institutional antibiotic use and antibiotic resistance, (6) the development of infection-control policies and procedures, (7) environmental hygiene, and (8) new-product evaluation. In some hospitals, quality improvement is also undertaken through the hospital epidemiology program. In the academic setting, additional functions of the program may include research and the provision of consultative services to other acute care and long-term care facilities, public health agencies, and the university campus. The major functions of the effective hospital epidemiology program are listed in Table 299-1, some of which are discussed in further detail here.

Surveillance

The first aim of surveillance is to determine endemic rates of infection. Once these rates have been established, an outbreak can be identified when its rate of occurrence is significantly higher than the endemic rate. The importance of surveillance was demonstrated by the Study on the Efficacy of Nosocomial Infection Control, which found a 32% reduction in nosocomial infections in hospitals with active surveillance programs compared with hospitals without such programs.[7] Data from hospitals in the National Nosocomial Infection Surveillance System (NNIS) demonstrated that from 1990 to 1999, nosocomial blood-stream infections decreased by 44% in medical intensive care units (ICUs), 32% in pediatric ICUs, and 31% in surgical ICUs.[8] As hospitals gain experience in standardization of patient care processes (e.g., central venous catheter insertion, head of bed elevation), further reductions in HAIs have been observed. Over the past several years, many hospitals have begun to monitor compliance with process measures, because feedback to health care workers on compliance with best practices more forcefully drives compliance than simply providing feedback on infection rates.[9,10]

Surveillance for HAIs has generally targeted areas of the hospital where the highest rates of infection, highest impact of infection, and antibiotic resistance are likely to be found. These areas include ICUs, cardiothoracic surgery units, and hematology and oncology units. However, with the current scrutiny on HAIs, hospital-wide surveillance (i.e., concurrent surveillance throughout the hospital) is becoming more prevalent and has been mandated in some states. As more hospitals implement electronic medical records, hospital-wide surveillance has become less daunting from a resource perspective. For example, collection of device days (denominator data), which previously required a daily review of patients, often by an infection control nurse, can now be accomplished via extraction of data entered into the electronic record by the bedside nurse as part of the daily patient nursing assessment. Hospitals with sophisticated information systems may be able to streamline surveillance through the development of computer-based algorithms that identify patients at highest risk of a HAI. Surveillance for some infections (e.g., bloodstream infections or infections with antimicrobial-resistant organisms) is primarily microbiology-based; therefore, hospital-wide surveillance for targeted infections can be implemented relatively easily.

The highest quality surveillance methodology for HAIs was developed by the Centers for Disease Control and Prevention (CDC) and is unit-based, infection site-specific, and risk-adjusted (i.e., expressed in terms of device-specific denominators). Because the National Healthcare Safety Network (NHSN) methodology is the most widely accepted, hospitals that use it are able to compare their institutional rates to those of a large group of hospitals across the country.

Unit-based surveillance trends should periodically be reported back to the health care workers in the unit. It is important that the data be delivered with clarity in a nonconfrontational manner. Although HAI rates (e.g., bloodstream infections per 1000 catheter days) are useful for interhospital comparisons and the analysis of institutional long-term trends, feedback to frontline providers is more meaningful when expressed as a raw number of infections (e.g., four central line associated bloodstream infections in the past 3 months).

Infectious diseases of public health importance should be reported to public health agencies, whose requirements vary by state. Increasingly, states are mandating surveillance for HAIs with public reporting.[11] Many states have required that hospitals join NHSN to ensure standardization of infection definitions, data collection, and analysis. This has resulted in rapid growth in NHSN from approximately 300 hospitals to nearly 2000.

Outbreak Investigation

Data accumulated by ongoing surveillance allow detection of nosocomial outbreaks. When the monthly rate for a particular infection exceeds the 95% confidence interval based on the previous years' rates for that month, the possibility of an outbreak exists and an investiga-

TABLE 299-1	Functions that May Fall under the Purview of the Epidemiology Unit

Surveillance for health care–associated infections
Outbreak detection and management
Education of patients and health care workers
Occupational health program for health care workers
   Postexposure prophylaxis for health care workers exposed to pathogens in the work setting
   Management of the infected health care worker (restriction from work or particular activities)
   Respiratory protection program
Antimicrobial usage monitoring and control, and formulary decisions
Development and implementation of policy to decrease the risk of health care associated infection
Patient safety program
Environmental monitoring for hygiene and infectious hazards
   Construction infection control (via design process and monitoring of infectious hazards associated with demolition, renovation, and construction)
   Infectious waste management
New product evaluation
Quality assessment
Bioterrorism preparedness
Sterilization and disinfection of medical instruments and devices
Regulatory compliance

tion is warranted. At other times, an astute observation of a potential cluster of infections by physicians, nurses, or the microbiology laboratory technologists should prompt at least an initial investigation.

When the cluster involves a common organism, hospitals with the capability of performing rapid molecular typing may do so first. If the cluster appears to be polyclonal, it is most likely due to antimicrobial usage patterns, a technical problem, or an importation of strains; a formal case-control study may not be necessary. A clonal outbreak suggests a point source or nosocomial transmission, in which case a case-control study may be warranted.

The primary investigating team should include the hospital epidemiologist, the director of employee health, the infection-control professionals, and in some cases, the director of the microbiology laboratory. External consultants are necessary in some cases. The steps of an outbreak investigation are summarized in Table 299-2.

Education

A substantial role for the infection-control professional is to educate hospital personnel in the areas of communicable disease control, sterilization, disinfection, and institutional infection-control policies. In many hospitals, the epidemiology team is responsible for blood-borne pathogen training and in some hospitals for airborne-isolation–mask training and fit testing. Some hospitals have successfully established an infection-control liaison program, whereby each hospital unit appoints a nurse who attends educational sessions periodically and helps disseminate infection-control information to colleagues.

Hospital Employee Health

The hospital epidemiology program must work closely with the employee health service. Issues such as the management of exposure to blood-borne pathogens and other communicable diseases (e.g., varicella, influenza, meningococcal disease, tuberculosis) require a concerted effort by the two groups. In addition, the employee health service is responsible for ensuring that health care workers are fit for duty and free of communicable diseases. At the time of employment, workers should be reviewed to ensure that they have adequate immunity against illnesses such as rubella, measles, mumps, pertussis, tetanus, hepatitis B, and varicella. In addition, baseline and periodic skin testing for tuberculosis should be performed, as well as postexposure testing. The employee health service should proactively and creatively devise delivery systems that encourage compliance with and remove barriers to annual influenza vaccination by all health care workers.

Antimicrobial Use

Nearly 60% of hospitalized patients receive antimicrobial agents, and antimicrobial usage varies widely across hospitals.[12] The hospital epidemiology program should monitor the antimicrobial susceptibility profiles produced by the microbiology laboratory on a regular basis to observe for trends in the development of antimicrobial resistance. The results should be correlated with the antimicrobial agents currently used in the institution. The best data are obtained if nosocomial isolates are distinguished from community-acquired isolates, if only bloodstream isolates are tested (true pathogens with high mortality), and if only one isolate per patient is counted in the numerator and denominator.

Efforts should be made to optimize antimicrobial prophylaxis for operative procedures, optimize the choice and duration of empiric antimicrobial therapy, and improve antimicrobial prescribing practices. A variety of approaches can be undertaken, including educational, administrative (e.g., formulary restrictions), and direct interventions by a team that manages antimicrobial use in real time.[13]

Policy Development

The primary administrative function of the infection-control program is to develop, implement, and continually evaluate policies and procedures designed to minimize the risk of HAIs. Some policies are designed to be implemented institution-wide, whereas others apply to specific areas of the hospital. Policies are generally developed by the infection-control committee after a review of data generated in-house, as well as information available from the medical literature. Recommendations from the infection-control committee may then need to be forwarded to other committees for review and approval before disseminating the new policy.

Environmental Hygiene

As the hospitalized population has become more immunosuppressed, the importance of environmental hygiene has significantly increased. Technical issues regarding air handling, construction, demolition, water supply, pest control, and medical waste management may require collaboration with engineers, architects, and other nonmedical

TABLE 299-2	Steps for Investigating an Outbreak

1. Contact the microbiology laboratory so all isolates can be saved for further analysis.
2. Develop a case definition.
3. Using the case definition, show statistically that current rates are significantly higher than pre-outbreak rates.
4. Review the relevant medical literature.
5. Plot an epidemic curve with the number of cases on the y-axis and time on the x-axis.
6. Review the charts of case patients and develop line lists containing demographic data (dates of admission and procedures, ward locations, dates) and exposure to potential risk factors.
7. Plot a time line with data for all common events. The number of cases is plotted on the y-axis, and the time interval between infection and potential risk factor (e.g., procedure, medication, contact with potentially infected patient or health care worker) is plotted on the x-axis.
8. Formulate a hypothesis regarding the source of infection and mechanism of transmission.
9. Perform a case-control study, comparing infected patients of the same age, gender, and service with exposure to potential risk factors.
10. Institute temporary infection-control measures.
11. Obtain cultures of suspected common sources.
12. Perform molecular typing to determine relatedness of isolates.
13. Continue surveillance to document the efficacy of control measures.
14. Summarize the findings of the investigation in a report for the infection-control committee.
15. The infection-control committee should review infection-control policies related to the outbreak and revise if necessary.

professionals, including external consultants. The CDC has produced a document on environmental infection control[14] that is an excellent resource for hospital epidemiologists on these issues.

New-Product Evaluation

A large number of new medical products are marketed each year. These products may be introduced into the hospital setting with few data to support their efficacy or their advantage over existing products. Often the new products are significantly more costly. The hospital epidemiology program should play an active role in evaluating data on new products designed to reduce infections or protect health care workers and then make recommendations regarding their introduction to the hospital. It is helpful if hospitals maintain a log of all newly accepted products and their dates of initial use. Such information could suggest the source of a new rise in infections.

Quality Assessment

The components of quality monitoring include data collection, data analysis using epidemiologic and other methods, data interpretation, interventions implemented to improve performance, and verification that these interventions have actually improved quality.[15] Optimally, the assessment of quality should occur at every stage of health care delivery, from access to the hospital through hospitalization and post-discharge follow-up. The determinants of the quality of medical care and the assessment of quality have been categorized into structure, process, and outcome.[16] Process refers to the set of actions required to provide care to the patient, and outcome is the result of those actions. Although assessment of outcome usually is the most meaningful, it is also the most difficult; and Donabedian has argued that case-mix adjustment methodology is not yet sophisticated enough to allow assessment of quality on the basis of outcomes only.[16] Efforts to monitor and improve quality should focus on high-volume diagnoses and procedures as well as high-cost procedures. The use of administrative data sets to assess quality should be avoided, as these data are collected for billing purposes and often utilize imprecise definitions of conditions, a situation that can lead to misclassification of cases.

Historically, the division of labor between hospital quality improvement programs and infection control programs was based on whether the problem was infectious or noninfectious. More recently, however, the dividing line has blurred as national quality improvement projects have begun to address the issue of HAIs.

ORGANIZATION OF THE EPIDEMIOLOGY PROGRAM

The organizational structure for infection control should be tailored to meet the demands of the hospital and to use available resources optimally. Large hospitals with a high proportion of tertiary care patients require a more complex system to meet their needs.

Hospital Epidemiologist

The hospital epidemiologist occupies a unique position. He or she must interface with many hospital departments, hospital administrators and extramural agencies, directly supervise the infection-control program, and in some hospitals direct the quality assessment program. In areas where subspecialists are available, the position is generally held by a physician who is trained in infectious diseases. Unfortunately, however, many of these physicians have little or no training in the discipline of epidemiology.

Before assuming the position of hospital epidemiologist, the physician should meet with key hospital administrators to discuss the responsibilities and expectations of the position and to negotiate the human and material resources, including the salary support that will be made available to implement the infection-control program. An excellent review of resources necessary to operate an infection-control program is found in the Society for Healthcare Epidemiology of America position paper on infrastructure for infection control.[17]

Infection-Control Professionals

Talented infection-control professionals (ICPs) are essential for the operation of an excellent infection-control program. These individuals are usually registered nurses with clinical experience or medical technologists with experience in microbiology. The effective ICP must have a working knowledge of epidemiologic principles and basic microbiology and a sound understanding of the operations of the health care institution.

During the 1980s, the CDC recommended that hospitals have one ICP for every 250 beds.[7] Since that time, the number of hospital beds has decreased, the severity of illness of hospitalized patients has markedly increased, with a corresponding increase in the number of critical care beds, infection control issues in the ambulatory setting have increased, and many new duties have been assumed by infection control programs. In response, the Society for Healthcare Epidemiology of America has recommended that the CDC ratio is no longer valid.[17] In a survey of University Health System Consortium hospitals, a median of one ICP full-time equivalent per 137 occupied beds was documented.[18] A study utilizing the Delphi method determined that for acute care hospitals the optimal ratio is one ICP per 100 to 125 beds.[19]

Infection-Control Committee

A multidisciplinary infection control committee that meets at least quarterly is recommended. This committee should include representatives from the medical and nursing staffs, hospital administration, and the person or persons directly responsible for management of the infection-control program. The committee also typically includes the infection-control professionals and representatives from the microbiology laboratory, pharmacy, operating room, and departments of employee health, housekeeping, central services, and engineering and maintenance. The ideal characteristics of committee members include the following: (1) an interest in infection control, (2) representation of a large group within the hospital, (3) authority in their given specialty, (4) tact, and (5) charisma.

Over the past few decades, controlling HAIs has become highly technical. Therefore the bulk of the committee's work is best accomplished by a core of experts that includes the hospital epidemiologist, infection-control professionals, a microbiologist, and the director of employee health. Policy formulations should be developed by this subgroup and, after thoughtful consideration, brought to the entire committee for review, ratification, and support from political and administrative standpoints. Thus, the full infection-control committee functions to educate key hospital administrators, provide the political support that allows the core members to implement policy, and disseminate new policy.

The meeting's agenda should be well planned and circulated to committee members before the meeting. In addition, the committee members should receive all policies to be reviewed before the meeting to allow adequate time for review by individual committee members and to improve the efficiency of the meeting.

The agenda should begin with an approval of the minutes of the previous meeting. This is followed by brief reports by representatives of the pharmacy, employee health department, the clinical microbiology laboratory, and the local public health department. In addition, all communicable disease exposure workups from the previous month are summarized. Ideally, old business is kept to a minimum. The monthly or quarterly infection rates and trends should be reviewed. The focus of the meeting then turns to more in-depth reports of a few current issues, including outbreak investigations. Invited guests may discuss various aspects of these issues. It is also helpful to review, update, and reapprove a few existing policies at each meeting on an ongoing basis.

HOSPITAL ACCREDITATION

In order for hospitals to receive reimbursement from the Center for Medicare & Medicaid Services (CMS), it must demonstrate via an accreditation process that it is in compliance with the conditions of participation. Infection control is an integral part of this process. Accreditation can be accomplished via routine surveys by a state survey agency. However, most hospitals seek accreditation via an alternative agency, The Joint Commission (TJC; formerly The Joint Commission on Accreditation of Healthcare Organizations). In the past few years, TJC has shifted its emphasis from policy and procedure to demonstration of compliance by reviewing the continuum of care delivered to randomly chosen patients (*tracer methodology*). TJC has been a powerful force because Medicare funding is vitally important to most hospitals. Recently, CMS approved a second accreditation agency, Det Norske Veritas Healthcare (DNVH), the first alternative to TJC in 40 years.

Future Challenges

Increasing costs in the provision of medical care with concurrent decreases in reimbursement have created enormous financial pressures on health care institutions. Implementation of a prospective payment system for medical services placed an emphasis on the avoidance of complications that prolong hospital stays, including HAIs, and provides an economic impetus for focusing on the quality of medical care. More recently, Medicare implemented a new policy, no longer upgrading payment associated with some HAIs, and some commercial payers have enacted similar policies. Coupled with the recent attention on HAIs by the media and consumer advocacy organizations, the policy has propelled infection control programs into a new era of much greater scrutiny and a demand for higher accountability.

Despite the increasing severity of illness of hospitalized patients, the greater prevalence of invasive technologies, and a higher prevalence of immunosuppressed patients, hospital epidemiologists are now expected to achieve the goal of eliminating HAIs (*getting to zero*). Importantly, the infection control community must acknowledge that most HAIs are preventable and respond with a strong commitment to decrease HAIs to the irreducible minimum. Obviously patients with severely depressed immune systems at risk for infections from their own flora will pose continuing challenges.

The hospital epidemiologist as a steward of scarce resources and unfunded mandates must decide how best to appropriate resources within his or her purview but must also justify the cost of the marginal benefits gained by enhanced infection-control activities in light of the impact on other programs with different goals in the health system. Infection control programs should adopt the approach of interventional epidemiology, which examines issues from a more global perspective. Such an approach focuses on and integrates clinical outcomes, economic impact, and customer (health care provider and patient) satisfaction to balance quality and cost.[20]

Emerging infectious diseases and the threat of bioterrorism require infection control programs to be able to respond more quickly to protect patients and health care workers, even in some cases with few data on the mechanism of disease transmission. Protecting the health care worker with a chronic blood-borne infection and his or her patients remains a challenge, as does the protection of immunosuppressed patients and health care workers from environmental pathogens.

Lastly, and perhaps most importantly, it remains the responsibility of the hospital epidemiologist to evaluate the medical literature and newly collected data critically when making decisions that affect the safety of patients and health care workers. Ensuring that all decisions are evidence-based and free of ideology, politics, or coercion of any form should be a deeply implanted ethic for all involved in this field.

REFERENCES

1. Kohn LT, Corrigan JM, Donaldson MS, eds. *To err is human: Building a safer health system.* Washington, D.C: National Academy Press; 1999.
2. Berens MJ: Unhealthy hospitals. *Chicago Tribune.* July 21, 2002.
3. Berenholtz SM, Pronovost PJ, Lipsett PA, et al. Eliminating catheter-related bloodstream infections in the intensive care unit. *Crit Care Med.* 2004;32:2014-2020.
4. Pronovost P, Needham D, Berenholtz S, et al. An intervention to decrease catheter-related bloodstream infections in the ICU. *N Engl J Med.* 2006;355:2725-2732.
5. Edmond M, Eickhoff TC. Who is steering the ship? External influences on infection control programs. *Clin Infect Dis.* 2008;46:1746-1750.
6. Klevens RM, Edwards JR, Richards CL Jr, et al. Estimating health care-associated infections and deaths in U.S. hospitals, 2002. *Public Health Rep.* 2007;122:160-166.
7. Haley RW, Culver DH, White JW, et al. The efficacy of infection surveillance and control programs in preventing nosocomial infections in US hospitals. *Am J Epidemiol.* 1985;121:182-205.
8. Centers for Disease Control and Prevention. Monitoring hospital-acquired infections to promote patient safety—United States, 1990-1999. *MMWR Morb Mortal Wkly Rep.* 2000;49:149-153.
9. Berhe M, Edmond MB, Bearman GM. Practices and an assessment of health care workers' perceptions of compliance with infection control knowledge of nosocomial infections. *Am J Infect Control.* 2005;33:55-57.
10. Assanasen S, Edmond M, Bearman G. Impact of 2 different levels of performance feedback on compliance with infection control process measures in 2 intensive care units. *Am J Infect Control.* 2008;36:407-413.
11. Edmond MB, Bearman GM. Mandatory public reporting in the USA: An example to follow? *J Hosp Infect.* 2007;65(Suppl 2):182-188.
12. MacDougall C, Polk RE. Variability in rates of use of antibacterials among 130 US hospitals and risk-adjustment models for inter-hospital comparison. *Infect Control Hosp Epidemiol.* 2008;29:203-211.
13. MacDougall C, Polk RE. Antimicrobial stewardship programs in health care systems. *Clin Microbiol Rev.* 2005;18:638-656.
14. Schulster L, Chinn RY, CDC. Guidelines for environmental infection control in health-care facilities: Recommendations of CDC and the Healthcare Infection Control Practices Advisory Committee (HICPAC). *MMWR Recomm Rep.* 2003;52:1-42.
15. Donabedian A. Contributions of epidemiology to quality assessment and monitoring. *Infect Control Hosp Epidemiol.* 1990;11:117-121.
16. Donabedian A. *An Introduction to Quality Assurance in Health Care.* Bashshur R, ed. Oxford, UK: Oxford University Press; 2003:46-57.
17. Scheckler WE, Brimhall D, Buck AS, et al. Requirements for infrastructure and essential activities of infection control and epidemiology in hospitals: A consensus panel report. *Infect Control Hosp Epidemiol.* 1998;19:114-124.
18. Friedman C, Chenoweth C. A survey of infection control professional staffing patterns at University Health System Consortium Institutions. *Am J Infect Control.* 1998;26:239-244.
19. O'Boyle C, Jackson M, Henly SJ. Staffing requirements for infection control programs in U.S. health care facilities: Delphi project. *Am J Infect Control.* 2002;30:321-333.
20. Garcia R, Bernard B, Kennedy V. The fifth evolutionary era in infection control: Interventional epidemiology. *Am J Infect Control.* 2000;28:30-43.

300

Isolation

MICHAEL B. EDMOND | RICHARD P. WENZEL

The purpose of isolating patients is to prevent the transmission of microorganisms from infected or colonized patients to other patients, hospital visitors, and health care workers, who may subsequently transmit them to other patients or become infected or colonized themselves. Although isolation guidelines are based on current understanding of the mechanisms of the transmission of organisms, few well-controlled studies have been performed to demonstrate their efficacy. Because health care–associated infections (HAIs) are relatively uncommon events, any study designed to demonstrate efficacy requires sample sizes that are often prohibitively large. Thus, studies evaluating the efficacy of infection control measures often lack the power to allow one to conclude confidently that there has been a lack of effect (i.e., such studies have a high probability of type II error).

Because the process of isolating patients is expensive, time-consuming, often uncomfortable for patients, and may impede care, it should be implemented only when necessary. Conversely, failure to isolate a patient with a transmissible disease may lead to morbidity and mortality, and may ultimately be expensive when one considers the direct costs of an investigation of an outbreak and excess length of stay and the indirect costs of lost productivity. The practice of isolating patients has moved from the requirement for separate infectious disease hospitals to separate wards for these patients, and ultimately to providing precautions in the general hospital environment. In 2006, the American Institute of Architects, in its Guidelines for Design and Construction of Health Care Facilities, made single-patient rooms the standard.[1] Hospitals that have single-patient rooms exclusively are able to isolate patients with transmissibile diseases without disrupting patient flow.[2] However, existing facilities often have a significant proportion of double-patient rooms.

In 2007, the Centers for Disease Control and Prevention (CDC) and the Healthcare Infection Control Practices Advisory Committee issued a revision of the recommended guidelines for isolation.[3] These guidelines outlined a two-tiered approach: standard precautions, which apply to all patients, and transmission-based precautions, which apply to patients with documented or suspected infection or colonization with certain microorganisms. These guidelines are summarized in Table 300-1.

Standard Precautions

Standard precautions are based on the assumption that all patients may potentially be colonized or infected with organisms that can be transmitted wherever health care is provided. Therefore, standard precautions stipulate that gloves should be worn to touch any of the following: blood, all body fluids, secretions, and excretions, except sweat, regardless of whether they are visibly bloody, nonintact skin, and mucous membranes.[3] Hands should be washed immediately after gloves are removed, before and after patient contact, and after contact with items in the patient's environment that may be contaminated.

For procedures that are likely to generate splashes or sprays of body fluid, a mask with eye protection or a face shield to protect the mucosa of the eyes, nose and mouth, as well as a gown, should be worn. Disposable gowns should be made of an impervious material to prevent penetration and subsequent contamination of the skin or clothing. Needles and syringes should be used only once and, when possible single-dose medication vials should be used. Needles should not be recapped, bent, or broken but should be disposed of in puncture-resistant containers.

Two new elements were added to Standard Precautions in 2007.[3] The first is the requirement for health care workers performing procedures involving lumbar puncture to wear masks to prevent contamination of the spinal needle or the procedure site with the oral flora of the operator, which may occur when the operator is talking. The second new element is respiratory hygiene, which includes instructing patients to cover their nose and mouth with a tissue when coughing or sneezing, using hand hygiene after contact with respiratory secretions, placing a surgical mask on the coughing patient in common areas, and spatially separating patients with respiratory infections from other patients when feasible.

HAND HYGIENE

Because most HAIs are transmitted by contact, primarily via the hands of health care workers,[4] hand washing remains the single most important means to prevent transmission of nosocomial pathogens. Nonetheless, most observational studies in intensive care units (ICUs) have found that hand-washing compliance by health care workers is less than 50%.[5] Currently, higher rates of compliance are more likely because of the increased attention focused on HAIs and the Joint Commission's mandate to measure hand hygiene via the National Patient Safety Goals program. It has been estimated that an increase in hand-washing compliance by 1.5- to 2.0-fold would result in a 25% to 50% decrease in the incidence of HAIs,[6] but most studies designed to improve hand-washing compliance have not demonstrated a lasting positive effect.

The microorganisms on hands can be divided into transient flora and resident flora.[7] The resident flora include organisms of low virulence (e.g., coagulase-negative staphylococci, *Micrococcus, Corynebacterium*) that are rarely transmitted to patients except when introduced by invasive procedures.[8] They are not easily removed through hand washing. The transient flora, however, are important causes of HAIs. These organisms are acquired primarily by contact, are loosely attached to the skin, and are easily washed off. Thus, the purpose of hand washing in the hospital is to remove the transient flora recently acquired by contact with patients or environmental surfaces.[8] In addition, HAIs have been attributed to bacterial contamination of artificial fingernails; therefore, they should not be worn by health care workers.

Alcohol-based hand rubs have become the recommended agents for hand hygiene in the health care setting.[5] In situations in which the hands are visibly soiled, washing with soap (antimicrobial or nonantimicrobial) and water is recommended. In addition, when caring for patients with *Clostridium difficile* diarrhea, the CDC suggests that soap and water be used because of the poor sporicidal activity of alcohols.[3] Hand decontamination should be performed before and after contact with patients and immediately after removing gloves.[5]

Wall-mounted dispensers with medicated, alcohol-based, waterless hand rubs should be installed in all hospital and outpatient rooms. In areas in which this is not feasible, individual health care workers should carry small containers of waterless agents.

GLOVES

Gloves should be worn by health care workers to prevent contamination of the hands with microorganisms, to prevent exposure of the health care worker to blood-borne pathogens, and to reduce the risk of transmission of microorganisms from the hands of the health care

TABLE 300-1	Essential Elements of Isolation Precautions				
			Transmission Based Precautions		
Elements	**Standard Precautions**	**Airborne**	**Droplet**	**Contact**	
Room		Negative pressure, single patient room required with air exhausted to outside or through HEPA filters; door must be closed	Single-patient room preferred; door may remain open	Single-patient room preferred; door may remain open; use disposable, noncritical, patient care equipment or dedicate to a single patient	
Mask		N95 or portable respirator for those entering room; place surgical mask on patient if transport out of room required	Surgical mask for those entering room; place surgical mask on patient if transport out of room required		
Eye, mouth, nose protection	For any activity likely to generate a splash, spray, or aerosol				
Gowns	For any activity likely to generate a splash or spray			For entering the room	
Gloves	For contact with any body fluid, mucous membrane, or nonintact skin			For entering the room	
Hand hygiene	Before and after patient contact; after contact with any body fluid, mucous membrane, or nonintact skin; after contact with inanimate objects in the immediate vicinity of the patient				

worker to the patient. However, gloves do not replace the need for hand hygiene. In addition, gloves should be changed during the care of a patient when moving from a contaminated body site (e.g., wound or perineal care) to a clean body site. Contamination of the hands can occur with organisms on the surface of the gloves when they are removed, and some gloves have small perforations that may allow organisms to contaminate the hands. Thus, gloves should be viewed as an adjunctive protective barrier but not as a substitute for hand hygiene.

Transmission-Based Precautions

Transmission-based precautions apply to selected patients based on a suspected or confirmed clinical syndrome, a specific diagnosis, or colonization or infection with epidemiologically important organisms. It is important to note that transmission-based precautions are always implemented in conjunction with standard precautions. Three types of transmission-based precautions have been developed for the major modes of transmission of infectious agents in the health care setting—airborne, droplet, and contact.[3] A few diseases (e.g., varicella, severe acute respiratory syndrome [SARS]) require more than one isolation category. Essential elements of each category are outlined in Table 300-1, and indications for implementation are delineated in Table 300-2.

AIRBORNE PRECAUTIONS

Airborne precautions are designed to prevent the transmission of diseases by droplet nuclei (particles smaller than 5 μm) or dust particles containing the infectious agent.[3] These particles can remain suspended in the air and travel long distances. If the particles are inhaled, a susceptible host may develop infection. Airborne precautions are indicated for patients with documented or suspected tuberculosis (pulmonary or laryngeal), measles, varicella, or disseminated zoster. Patients who are infected with, or at high risk for infection with, human immunodeficiency virus (HIV), with fever, cough, and a pulmonary infiltrate, should be empirically placed under airborne precautions until tuberculosis can be ruled out.[3] Although open tuberculous skin wounds are uncommon, they have been presumptively associated with nosocomial transmission after manipulation of the wound (surgical débridement, dressing changes, irrigation).[9-11] Therefore, such patients should be placed under airborne

precautions. Patients with nontuberculous (atypical) mycobacterial pulmonary disease need not be isolated because person-to-person transmission does not occur.

Under airborne precautions, patients should be placed in a private room with monitored negative air pressure in relation to surrounding areas, and the room air must undergo at least six, but preferably 12, exchanges per hour.[12] The door to the isolation room must remain closed. Air from the isolation room should be exhausted directly to the outside, away from air intakes, and not recirculated. If outdoor exhaust is not possible, air should be exhausted through high-efficiency filters before it is returned to the general ventilation system.[12]

All persons entering the room of patients with suspected or confirmed tuberculosis must wear a personal respirator that filters 1-μm particles with an efficiency of at least 95% (N95 mask). These special masks must fit different facial sizes and characteristics, be fit-tested so that there is leakage of 10% or less, and be able to be checked for fit each time the health care worker puts on the mask. The Occupational Safety and Health Administration (OSHA) requires that health care workers who manage patients with tuberculosis undergo fit testing and training for self-fit checking.[12] In 2008, OSHA began enforcing a requirement for annual fit testing of health care workers.[13] Transporting the patient from the isolation room should be limited, and the patient should be fitted with a standard surgical mask before leaving the room.[3] Before transport, hospital personnel in the area receiving the patient should be notified so that proper precautions can be implemented. Gowns and gloves are used as dictated by standard precautions.

Any patient with confirmed or suspected tuberculosis should be instructed to cover his or her mouth and nose with a tissue when coughing or sneezing. Patients should remain in isolation until tuberculosis can be ruled out. Patients with confirmed tuberculosis who are receiving effective antituberculous therapy, are clinically improving with decreased cough frequency, and have three consecutive sputum smears each at least 8 hours apart, with no detectable acid-fast bacilli, can be released from isolation.[12] Patients with multidrug-resistant disease should remain in isolation for the duration of their hospital stay. Patients with active tuberculosis who require surgery present a special problem because operating rooms are typically at positive pressure. Thus, special precautions are necessary. Hospitalization is unwarranted solely to provide isolation for clinically stable patients who are compliant with antituberculous therapy and agree to stay in their homes.

TABLE 300-2	Indications for Transmission-Based Precautions	
Airborne Precautions	*Droplet Precautions*	*Contact Precautions*
Situations Requiring Empirical Implementation of Precautions		
Vesicular rash*	Meningitis	Acute diarrhea with likely infectious cause in incontinent or diapered patient
Maculopapular rash with cough, coryza and fever	Petechial or ecchymotic rash with fever	Vesicular rash*
Cough, fever, upper lobe pulmonary infiltrate	Paroxysmal or severe persistent cough during periods of pertussis activity	Respiratory infections in infants and young children
Cough, fever, any pulmonary infiltrate in an HIV-infected patient (or at high risk for HIV infection)		History of infection or colonization with MDR organisms
		Skin, wound, or urinary tract infection in a patient with recent hospital or nursing home stay in facility where MDR organisms are prevalent
Cough, fever, any pulmonary infiltrate, recent travel to regions with oubreaks of SARS or avian influenza*		Abscess or draining wound that cannot be covered
		Cough, fever, any pulmonary infiltrate and recent travel to regions with oubreaks of SARS, avian influenza*
Known or Suspected Diseases or Pathogens		
Measles	Adenovirus pneumonia*; conjunctivitis*	Adenovirus pneumonia*; conjunctivitis*
Monkeypox*	Diphtheria, pharyngeal	*Burkholderia cepacia* pneumonia in cystic fibrosis
Tuberculosis, pulmonary, laryngeal; draining lesion (e.g., from osteomyelitis)*	*Haemophilus influenzae* meningitis, epiglottitis; pneumonia (infants, children)	*Clostridium difficile* diarrhea
SARS*	Influenza	Conjunctivitis, acute viral
Smallpox*	Meningococcal infections	Decubitus ulcer, infected, drainage not contained
Varicella*	Mumps	Diarrhea, infectious, in diapered or incontinent patient
Zoster (disseminated; immunocompromised patient until dissemination ruled out)*	*Mycoplasma* pneumonia	Diphtheria, cutaneous
	Parvovirus B19	Enteroviral infections (infants, young children)
	Pertussis	Furunculosis (infants, young children)
	Plague, pneumonic	Hepatitis A, E (diapered or incontinent patient)
	Rhinovirus*	HSV (neonatal, disseminated, severe primary mucocutaneous)
	Rubella	Human metapneumovirus
	SARS*	Impetigo
	Streptococcal (group A) pneumonia; serious invasive disease; major skin, wound, or burn infection*; pharyngitis, scarlet fever (infants or young children)	Lice
		MDR bacteria (e.g., MRSA, VRE, VISA, VRSA, ESBLs, resistant *S. pneumoniae*) infection or colonization
	Viral hemorrhagic fevers*	Monkeypox*
		Parainfluenza infection (infants, children)
		Rhinovirus*
		Rotavirus
		RSV infection (infants, children, immunocompromised)
		Rubella, congenital
		SARS*
		Scabies
		Smallpox*
		Staphylococcus aureus major skin, wound or burn infection
		Streptococcal (group A) major skin, burn, or wound infection*
		Tuberculous draining lesion
		Vaccinia: fetal, generalized, progressive, eczema vaccinatum
		Varicella*
		Viral hemorrhagic fevers*
		Zoster (disseminated; immunocompromised until dissemination ruled out)*

*Condition requires two types of precaution.

ESBLs, extended-spectrum β-lactamases; HIV, human immunodeficiency virus; HSV, herpes simplex virus; MDR, multidrug-resistant; MRSA, methicillin-resistant *Staphylococcus aureus*; RSV, respiratory syncytial virus; SARS, severe acute respiratory syndrome; VISA, vancomycin-intermediate *Staphylococcus aureus*; VRE, vancomycin-resistant enterococci; VRSA, vancomycin-resistant *Staphylococcus aureus*.

Patients with known or suspected measles, varicella, or disseminated zoster require airborne isolation. Nonimmune health care workers should avoid entering the rooms of these patients when possible and, if they are required to enter the room, should wear an N95 mask.[3]

DROPLET PRECAUTIONS

Droplet precautions are used to prevent transmission by large-particle (droplet) aerosols. Unlike droplet nuclei, droplets are larger, do not remain suspended in the air, and do not travel long distances. They are produced when the infected patient talks, coughs, or sneezes and during some procedures (e.g., suctioning, bronchoscopy). A susceptible host may become infected if the infectious droplets land on the mucosal surfaces of the nose, mouth, or eye.

Droplet precautions require patients to be placed in a private room, but no special air handling is necessary.[3] Alternatively, patients with the same disease can be placed in the same room with the privacy curtain between beds drawn if a private room is not available. Because droplets do not travel long distances (usually no more than 3 feet, although occasionally 6 to 10 feet), the door to the room may remain open. Health care workers should wear a standard surgical mask when entering the room. Gowns and gloves should be worn when dictated

by standard precautions. When transported out of the isolation room, the patient should be fitted with a standard surgical mask.[3]

Some illnesses that require droplet precautions include invasive *Haemophilus influenzae* type b and meningococcal infections, *Mycoplasma pneumoniae* pneumonia, pertussis, mumps, rubella, and parvovirus B19 infections. Although influenza is generally transmitted via droplets, on rare occasions airborne transmission has occurred.

CONTACT PRECAUTIONS

Contact precautions are implemented to prevent the transmission of epidemiologically important organisms from an infected or colonized patient through direct contact (touching the patient) or indirect contact (touching contaminated objects or surfaces in the patient's environment). Patients with contact precautions should be placed in a private room, although patients infected with the same organism may be placed in the same room when private rooms are not available.[3] Multidrug-resistant organisms, such as vancomycin-resistant enterococci and methicillin-resistant *Staphylococcus aureus* (MRSA) contaminate the environment (surfaces and items) in the vicinity of the infected or colonized patient. Therefore, barrier precautions to prevent contamination of exposed skin and clothing should be used. Gowns and gloves should be worn when entering the patient's room and removed before leaving it. Gowns should be removed before leaving the isolation room, and care must be taken to prevent contamination of clothing while removing the gown.[3] After removing gloves, the hands must be decontaminated immediately with a medicated hand-washing agent or an alcohol-based hand rub, and care should be taken to prevent recontamination of the hands before leaving the room.

Numerous studies have documented contamination of noncritical patient care equipment (e.g., stethoscopes, blood pressure cuffs) with vancomycin-resistant enterococci and MRSA. These items should remain in the isolation room and not be used for other patients. If the items must be shared, they should be cleaned and disinfected before reuse. Transport of the patient from the isolation room should be kept to a minimum.

Contact precautions are indicated for patients infected or colonized with multidrug-resistant bacteria (e.g., MRSA, vancomycin-resistant enterococci, multidrug-resistant gram negative bacilli).[3] Other indications include *Clostridium difficile* enteritis, infections transmitted by the fecal-oral route (e.g., *Shigella*, rotavirus, hepatitis A virus infections) in patients who are diapered or incontinent, and acute diarrheal diseases likely to be infectious in origin. Infants and young children with respiratory syncytial virus, parainfluenza, or enteroviral infection and patients with neonatal, disseminated, or severe primary mucocutaneous herpes simplex virus infection should also be placed under contact precautions. Ectoparasitic infestations (lice and scabies) are additional indications. Patients with varicella or disseminated zoster require both contact and airborne precautions.

REFERENCES

1. American Institute of Architects, Facilities Guidelines Institute. *Guidelines for Design and Construction of Health Care Facilities.* Washington, DC: The American Institute of Architects Press, 2006.
2. Detsky ME, Etchells E. Single-patient rooms for safe patient-centered hospitals. JAMA. 2008;300:954-956.
3. Seigel JD, Rhinehart E, Jackson M, et al. 2007 *Guideline for Isolation Precautions: Preventing Tranmission of Infectious Agents in Healthcare Settings.* Available at http://www.cdc.gov/ncidod/dhqp/pdf/isolation2007.pdf.
4. Bauer TM, Ofner E, Just HM, et al. An epidemiological study assessing the relative importance of airborne and direct contact transmission of microorganisms in a medical intensive care unit. J Hosp Infect. 1990;15:301-309.
5. Boyce JM, Pittet D. Healthcare Infection Control Practices Advisory Committee, Society for Healthcare Epidemiology of America, Association for Professionals in Infection Control, Infectious Diseases Society of America Hand Hygiene Task Force. Guideline for hand hygiene in health-care settings: Recommendations of the Healthcare Infection Control Practices Advisory Committee and the HICPAC/SHEA/APIC/IDSA Hand Hygiene Task Force. Infect Control Hosp Epidemiol. 2002;23(Suppl 12):S3-S40.
6. Doebbeling BN, Stanley GL, Sheetz CT, et al. Comparative efficacy of alternative hand-washing agents in reducing nosocomial infections in intensive care units. N Engl J Med. 1992;327:88.
7. Price PB. The bacteriology of normal skin: A new quantitative test applied to a study of the bacterial flora and the disinfectant action of mechanical cleaning. J Infect Dis. 1938;63:301.
8. Steere AC, Mallison GF. Handwashing practices for the prevention of nosocomial infections. Ann Intern Med. 1975;83:683-690.
9. Framptom MW. An outbreak of tuberculosis among hospital personnel caring for a patient with a skin ulcer. Ann Intern Med. 1992;117:312-313.
10. Hutton MD, Stead WW, Cauthen GM, et al. Nosocomial transmission of tuberculosis associated with a draining abscess. J Infect Dis. 1990;161:286-295.
11. Stead WW. Skin ulcers and tuberculosis outbreaks. Ann Intern Med. 1993;118:474.
12. Jensen PA, Lambert LA, Iademarco MF, et al. Guidelines for preventing the transmission of *Mycobacterium tuberculosis* in health-care settings, 2005. MMWR Morb Mortal Wkly Rep. 2005;54(RR17):1-141.
13. Occupational Safety and Health Administration. *Standard Interpretations: Tuberculosis and Ressiratory Protection Enforcement.* Available at http://www.osha.gov/pls/oshaweb/owadisp.show_document?p_table=Interpretations&p_id=26013.

301

Disinfection, Sterilization, and Control of Hospital Waste

WILLIAM A. RUTALA | DAVID J. WEBER

Each year in the United States, approximately 46.5 million surgical procedures and an even larger number of invasive medical procedures are performed.[1] For example, at least 10 million gastrointestinal endoscopies are performed per year.[2] Each of these procedures involves contact by a medical device or surgical instrument with a patient's sterile tissue or mucous membranes. A major risk of all such procedures is the introduction of infection. Failure to properly disinfect or sterilize equipment carries not only the risk associated with breach of the host barriers but the additional risk of person-to-person transmission (e.g., of hepatitis B virus) and transmission of environmental pathogens (e.g., *Pseudomonas aeruginosa*).

Achieving disinfection and sterilization through the use of disinfectants and sterilization practices is essential for ensuring that medical and surgical instruments do not transmit infectious pathogens to patients. Because it is unnecessary to sterilize all items involved in patient care, health care policies must identify whether cleaning, disinfection, or sterilization is indicated primarily on the basis of the items' intended use.

Multiple studies in many countries have documented lack of compliance with established guidelines for disinfection and sterilization.[3,4] Failure to comply with scientifically based guidelines has led to numerous outbreaks.[4-8] In this chapter, a pragmatic approach to the judicious selection and proper use of disinfection and sterilization processes is based on well-designed studies assessing the efficacy (through laboratory investigations) and effectiveness (through clinical studies) of disinfection and sterilization procedures. In addition, we briefly review the management of medical waste in health care facilities.

Definition of Terms

Sterilization is the complete elimination or destruction of all forms of microbial life and is accomplished in health care facilities by either physical or chemical processes. Steam under pressure, dry heat, ethylene oxide (ETO) gas, hydrogen peroxide gas plasma, ozone, and liquid chemicals are the principal sterilizing agents used in health care facilities. Sterilization is intended to convey an absolute meaning, not a relative one. Unfortunately, some health professionals, as well as the technical and commercial literature, refer to "disinfection" as "sterilization" and items as "partially sterile." When chemicals are used for the purposes of destroying all forms of microbiologic life, including fungal and bacterial spores, they may be called *chemical sterilants*. The same germicides used for shorter exposure periods may also be part of the disinfection process (i.e., high-level disinfection).

Disinfection is a process that eliminates many or all pathogenic microorganisms on inanimate objects, with the exception of bacterial spores. Disinfection is usually accomplished with the use of liquid chemicals or wet pasteurization in health care settings. The efficacy of disinfection is affected by a number of factors, each of which may nullify or limit the efficacy of the process. Some of the factors that affect both disinfection and sterilization efficacy are the prior cleaning of the object; the organic and inorganic load present; the type and level of microbial contamination; the concentration of and exposure time to the germicide; the nature of the object (e.g., crevices, hinges, and lumens); the presence of biofilms; the temperature and pH of the disinfection process; and, in some cases, the relative humidity of the sterilization process (e.g., with ETO).

By definition, therefore, disinfection differs from sterilization by its lack of sporicidal property, but this is an oversimplification. A few disinfectants kill spores with prolonged exposure times (e.g., 3 to 12 hours) and are called *chemical sterilants*. At similar concentrations but with shorter exposure periods (e.g., 20 minutes for 2% glutaraldehyde), the same disinfectants kill all microorganisms except large numbers of bacterial spores and are called *high-level disinfectants. Low-level disinfectants* may kill most vegetative bacteria, some fungi, and some viruses in a practical period of time (≤10 minutes), whereas *intermediate-level disinfectants* may kill mycobacteria, vegetative bacteria, most viruses, and most fungi but do not necessarily kill bacterial spores. The germicides differ markedly among themselves, primarily in the antimicrobial spectrum and rapidity of action, as described in Table 301-1.

Cleaning, in comparison, is the removal of visible soil (e.g., organic and inorganic material) from objects and surfaces, and it is normally accomplished by manual or mechanical means through the use of water with detergents or enzymatic products. Thorough cleaning is essential before high-level disinfection and sterilization, because inorganic and organic materials that remain on the surfaces of instruments interfere with the effectiveness of these processes. Also, if the soiled materials become dried or baked onto the instruments, the removal process becomes more difficult, and the disinfection or sterilization process is less effective or ineffective. Surgical instruments should be presoaked or rinsed to prevent drying of blood and to soften or remove blood from the instruments. *Decontamination* is a procedure that removes pathogenic microorganisms from objects so that they are safe to handle, use, or discard.

Terms with a suffix "-cide" or "-cidal" for killing action also are commonly used. For example, a *germicide* is an agent that can kill microorganisms, particularly pathogenic organisms ("germs"). Germicides include both antiseptics and disinfectants. *Antiseptics* are germicides applied to living tissue and skin, whereas *disinfectants* are antimicrobials applied only to inanimate objects. In general, antiseptics are used only on the skin and not for surface disinfection, and disinfectants are rarely used for skin antisepsis because they may cause injury to skin and other tissues. Other words with the suffix "-cide" (e.g., *virucide, fungicide, bactericide, sporicide,* and *tuberculocide*) can kill the type of microorganism identified by the prefix. For example, a bactericide is an agent that kills bacteria.[9-14]

A Rational Approach to Disinfection and Sterilization

In the late 1960s, Earle H. Spaulding[10] devised a rational approach to disinfection and sterilization of items or equipment used in patient care. This classification scheme is so clear and logical that it has been retained, refined, and successfully used by infection control professionals and others in planning methods for disinfection or sterilization.[9,11,13,15-17] Spaulding believed that the nature of disinfection could be understood more readily if instruments and items for patient care were divided into three categories on the basis of degree of risk of infection involved in the use of the items. The three categories he described were *critical, semicritical,* and *noncritical.*

TABLE 301-1	Methods of Sterilization and Disinfection				
	Sterilization		**Disinfection**		
	Critical Items (Enter Tissue or Vascular System or Blood Flows Through Them)		*High-Level (Semicritical Items; Contact with Mucous Membrane or Nonintact Skin [Except Dental])*	*Intermediate-Level (Some Semicritical Items* and Noncritical Items)*	*Low-Level (Noncritical Items; Contact with Intact Skin)*
Object	PROCEDURE	EXPOSURE TIME	PROCEDURE (EXPOSURE TIME, 12-30 MIN AT ≥20°C)[†,‡]	PROCEDURE (EXPOSURE TIME, ≥1 MIN)[§]	PROCEDURE (EXPOSURE TIME, ≥1 MIN)[§]
Smooth, hard surface*,‖	Heat sterilization	Manufacturer's recommendations	Glutaraldehyde-based formulations; 1.12% glutaraldehyde with 1.93% phenol/phenate; 3.4% glutaraldehyde with 26% isopropanol	Ethyl or isopropyl alcohol (70%-90%)	Ethyl or isopropyl alcohol (70%-90%)
	Ethylene oxide gas	Manufacturer's recommendations	Ortho-phthalaldehyde ≥0.55%	Sodium hypochlorite[¶]	Sodium hypochlorite
	Hydrogen peroxide gas plasma and ozone	Manufacturer's recommendations	Hydrogen peroxide 7.5%	Phenolic germicidal detergent solution	Phenolic germicidal detergent solution
	Glutaraldehyde-based formulations; 1.12% glutaraldehyde with 1.93% phenol/phenate; 3.4% glutaraldehyde with 26% isopropanol	10 hr at 20°-25°C	Hydrogen peroxide plus peracetic acid	Iodophor germicidal detergent solution	Iodophor germicidal detergent solution
	Hydrogen peroxide 7.5%	6 hr	Wet pasteurization at 70°C for 30 min with detergent cleaning**		Quaternary ammonium germicidal detergent solution
	Peracetic acid	12 min at 50°-56°C	Hypochlorite, single-use chlorine generated on site by electrolyzing saline containing >650-675 active free chlorine		Accelerated hydrogen peroxide, 0.5%
	Hydrogen peroxide plus peracetic acid	3-8 hr			
Rubber tubing and catheters‡,‖	Heat sterilization	Manufacturer's recommendations	Glutaraldehyde-based formulations; 1.12% glutaraldehyde with 1.93% phenol/phenate; 3.4% glutaraldehyde with 26% isopropanol		
	Ethylene oxide gas	Manufacturer's recommendations	Ortho-phthalaldehyde ≥0.55%		
	Hydrogen peroxide gas plasma and ozone	Manufacturer's recommendations	Hydrogen peroxide 7.5%		
	Glutaraldehyde-based formulations; 1.12% glutaraldehyde with 1.93% phenol/phenate; 3.4% glutaraldehyde with 26% isopropanol	10 hr at 20°-25°C	Hydrogen peroxide plus peracetic acid		
	Hydrogen peroxide 7.5%	6 hr	Wet pasteurization at 70°C for 30 min with detergent cleaning**		
	Peracetic acid	12 min at 50°-56°C	Hypochlorite, single-use chlorine generated on site by electrolyzing saline containing >650-675 active free chlorine		
	Hydrogen peroxide plus peracetic acid	3-8 hr			

Note: The selection and use of disinfectants in the health-care field is dynamic, and products not in existence when this chapter was written may become available. As newer disinfectants become available, persons or committees responsible for selecting disinfectants and sterilization processes should be guided by products cleared by the U.S. Food and Drug Administration (FDA) and the U.S. Environment Protection Agency (EPA), as well as by information in the scientific literature.

For heat sterilization, including steam or hot air, see manufacturer's recommendations (steam sterilization processing time, 3-30 minutes).

For ethylene oxide gas, see manufacturer's recommendations (generally 1-6 hours' processing time plus aeration time of 8-12 hours at 50°-60°C).

For hydrogen peroxide gas plasma, see manufacturer's recommendations for internal diameter and length restrictions (processing time, 28-72 minutes); for ozone, see manufacturer's recommendations for internal diameter and length restrictions.

In glutaraldehyde-based formulations (≥2% glutaraldehyde), caution should be exercised with all glutaraldehyde formulations when further in-use dilution is anticipated. One glutaraldehyde-based product has a high-level disinfection claim of 5 minutes at 35°C.

Hydrogen peroxide 7.5% will corrode copper, zinc, and brass.

For peracetic acid, the concentration is variable, but 0.2% or greater is sporicidal. Peracetic acid immersion system operates at 50°-56°C.

Hydrogen peroxide plus peracetic acid are in the following combinations: 7.35% hydrogen peroxide plus 0.23% peracetic acid; 8.3% hydrogen peroxide plus 7.0% peracetic acid; 1% hydrogen peroxide plus 0.08% peracetic acid (will corrode metal instruments).

Hypochlorite will corrode metal instruments.

Sodium hypochlorite is 5.25%-6.15% household bleach diluted to 1:500; this provides >100 ppm of available chlorine.

For phenolic germicidal detergent solution, iodophor germicidal detergent solution, and quaternary ammonium germicidal detergent solution, follow product label for dilution for use.

For accelerated hydrogen peroxide, 0.5%, follow product label.

NA, Not applicable.

Modified from Rutala,[13,16] Simmons,[11] and Rutala et al.[17]

| TABLE 301-1 | Methods of Sterilization and Disinfection—cont'd |

	Sterilization		Disinfection		
	Critical Items (Enter Tissue or Vascular System or Blood Flows Through Them)		*High-Level (Semicritical Items; Contact with Mucous Membrane or Nonintact Skin [Except Dental])*	*Intermediate-Level (Some Semicritical Items* and Noncritical Items)*	*Low-Level (Noncritical Items; Contact with Intact Skin)*
Object	PROCEDURE	EXPOSURE TIME	PROCEDURE (EXPOSURE TIME, 12-30 MIN AT ≥20° C)[†,‡]	PROCEDURE (EXPOSURE TIME, ≥1 MIN)[§]	PROCEDURE (EXPOSURE TIME, ≥1 MIN)[§]
Polyethylene tubing[‡‡]	Heat sterilization	Manufacturer's recommendations	Glutaraldehyde-based formulations; 1.12% glutaraldehyde with 1.93% phenol/phenate; 3.4% glutaraldehyde with 26% isopropanol		
	Ethylene oxide gas	Manufacturer's recommendations	Ortho-phthalaldehyde ≥0.55%		
	Hydrogen peroxide gas plasma and ozone	Manufacturer's recommendations	Hydrogen peroxide 7.5%		
	Glutaraldehyde-based formulations; 1.12% glutaraldehyde with 1.93% phenol/phenate; 3.4% glutaraldehyde with 26% isopropanol	10 hr at 20°-25° C	Hydrogen peroxide plus peracetic acid		
	Hydrogen peroxide 7.5%	6 hr	Wet pasteurization at 70° C for 30 min with detergent cleaning**		
	Peracetic acid	12 min at 50°-56° C	Hypochlorite, single-use chlorine generated on-site by electrolyzing saline containing >650-675 active free chlorine		
	Hydrogen peroxide plus peracetic acid	3-8 hr			
Thermometers (oral and rectal)[††]				Ethyl or isopropyl alcohol (70%-90%)[††]	
Hinged instruments[‖]	Heat sterilization	Manufacturer's recommendations	Glutaraldehyde-based formulations; 1.12% glutaraldehyde with 1.93% phenol/phenate; 3.4% glutaraldehyde with 26% isopropanol		
	Ethylene oxide gas	Manufacturer's recommendations	Ortho-phthalaldehyde ≥0.55%		
	Hydrogen peroxide gas plasma and ozone	Manufacturer's recommendations	Hydrogen peroxide 7.5%		
	Glutaraldehyde-based formulations; 1.12% glutaraldehyde with 1.93% phenol/phenate; 3.4% glutaraldehyde with 26% isopropanol	10 hr at 20°-25° C	Hydrogen peroxide plus peracetic acid		
	Hydrogen peroxide 7.5%	6 hr	Wet pasteurization at 70° C for 30 min with detergent cleaning**		
	Peracetic acid	12 min at 50°-56° C	Hypochlorite, single-use chlorine generated on-site by electrolyzing saline containing >650-675 active free chlorine		
	Hydrogen peroxide plus peracetic acid	3-8 hr			

*See text for discussion of hydrotherapy.

†The longer the exposure to a disinfectant, the more likely it is that all microorganisms will be eliminated. Ten-minute exposure is not adequate to disinfect many objects, especially those that are difficult to clean because they have narrow channels or other areas that can harbor organic material and bacteria. At 20°C, 20-minute exposure is the minimum time needed to reliably kill *Mycobacterium tuberculosis* and nontuberculous mycobacteria with a 2% glutaraldehyde. With the exception of >2% glutaraldehydes, follow the FDA-cleared high-level disinfection claim. Some high-level disinfectants have a reduced exposure time (e.g., ortho-phthalaldehyde [OPA] for 12 minutes at 20°C) because of their rapid activity against mycobacteria or reduced exposure time because of increased mycobactericidal activity at elevated temperature (e.g., 2.5% glutaraldehyde for 5 minutes at 35°C; 0.55% OPA for 5 minutes at 25°C in automated endoscope reprocessor).

‡Tubing must be completely filled for high-level disinfection and liquid chemical sterilization; care must be taken to avoid entrapment of air bubbles during immersion.

§By law, all applicable label instructions on EPA-registered products must be followed. If the user selects exposure conditions that differ from those on the EPA-registered products label, the user assumes liability from any injuries resulting from off-label use and is potentially subject to enforcement action under the Federal Insecticide, Fungicide, and Rodenticide Act (FIFRA).

‖Material compatibility should be investigated when appropriate.

¶A concentration of 1000 ppm available chlorine should be considered when cultures or concentrated preparations of microorganisms have spilled (5.25% to 6.15% household bleach diluted 1:50 provides >1000 ppm available chlorine). This solution may corrode some surfaces.

**Pasteurization (washer-disinfector) of respiratory therapy or anesthesia equipment is a recognized alternative to high-level disinfection. Some data challenge the efficacy of some pasteurization units.

††Do not mix rectal and oral thermometers at any stage of handling or processing.

‡‡Thermostability should be investigated when appropriate.

CRITICAL ITEMS

Critical items are so called because of the high risk of infection if such items are contaminated with any microorganism, including bacterial spores. Thus, objects that enter sterile tissue or the vascular system absolutely must be sterile because any microbial contamination could result in disease transmission. This category includes surgical instruments, cardiac and urinary catheters, implants, and ultrasound probes used in sterile body cavities. Most of the items in this category should be purchased as sterile or be subjected to steam sterilization if possible. If heat-sensitive, an object may be treated with ETO, hydrogen peroxide gas plasma, ozone, or liquid chemical sterilants if other methods are unsuitable. Table 301-1 lists several germicides categorized as chemical sterilants. These include more than 2.4% glutaraldehyde-based formulations, 0.95% glutaraldehyde with 1.64% phenol/phenate, 3.4% glutaraldehyde with 26% isopropanol, 7.5% stabilized hydrogen peroxide, 7.35% hydrogen peroxide with 0.23% peracetic acid, 8.3% hydrogen peroxide with 7.0% peracetic acid, 0.2% peracetic acid, more than 0.55% ortho-phthalaldehyde (OPA), and 0.08% peracetic acid with 1.0% hydrogen peroxide. Liquid chemical sterilants can be relied upon to produce sterility only if cleaning, to eliminate organic and inorganic material, precedes treatment, and if proper guidelines regarding concentration, contact time, temperature, and pH are met.

SEMICRITICAL ITEMS

Semicritical items are those that come in contact with mucous membranes or nonintact skin. Respiratory therapy and anesthesia equipment, some endoscopes, laryngoscope blades, esophageal manometry probes, endocavitary probes, anorectal manometry catheters, and diaphragm fitting rings are included in this category. These medical devices should be free of all microorganisms, although small numbers of bacterial spores may safely be present. Intact mucous membranes, such as those of the lungs or the gastrointestinal tract, generally are resistant to infection by common bacterial spores but susceptible to other organisms such as bacteria, mycobacteria, and viruses. Semicritical items minimally require high-level disinfection with chemical disinfectants. Glutaraldehyde, hydrogen peroxide, OPA, and peracetic acid with hydrogen peroxide are cleared by the U.S. Food and Drug Administration (FDA) and are dependable high-level disinfectants if the factors influencing germicidal procedures are met (Table 301-2; see also Table 301-1). When a disinfectant is selected for use with certain items used in patient care, the chemical compatibility after extended use with the items to be disinfected also must be considered.

The complete elimination of all microorganisms in or on an instrument, except for small numbers of bacterial spores, is the traditional definition of high-level disinfection. The FDA's definition of high-level disinfection is a sterilant used for a shorter contact time to achieve a

TABLE 301-2	Summary of Advantages and Disadvantages of Chemical Agents Used as Chemical Sterilants* or as High-Level Disinfectants	
Sterilization Method	*Advantages*	*Disadvantages*
Peracetic acid plus hydrogen peroxide	No activation required Odor or irritation not significant	Concerns about compatibility with materials (lead, brass, copper, zinc), both cosmetic and functional Limited clinical experience Potential for eye and skin damage
Glutaraldehyde	Numerous studies on use have been published Relatively inexpensive Excellent compatibility with materials	Respiratory irritation from glutaraldehyde vapor Pungent and irritating odor Relatively slow mycobactericidal activity Coagulates blood and fixes tissue to surfaces Allergic contact dermatitis Glutaraldehyde vapor monitoring recommended
Hydrogen peroxide	No activation required May enhance removal of organic matter and organisms No disposal issues No odor or irritation issues Does not coagulate blood or fix tissues to surfaces Inactivates *Cryptosporidium* organisms Studies on its use have been published	Concerns about compatibility with materials (brass, zinc, copper, and nickel/silver plating), both cosmetic and functional Serious eye damage with contact
Ortho-phthalaldehyde	Fast-acting high-level disinfectant No activation required Odor not significant Excellent compatibility with materials is claimed Is claimed not to coagulate blood or fix tissues to surfaces	Stains skin, mucous membranes, clothing, and environmental surfaces Repeated exposure may result in hypersensitivity in some patients with bladder cancer More expensive than glutaraldehyde Eye irritation with contact Slow sporicidal activity
Peracetic acid	Rapid sterilization cycle time (30-45 min) Sterilization possible by low-temperature (50°-55°C) liquid immersion Environmentally friendly by-products (acetic acid, O₂, H₂O) Fully automated Single-use system eliminates need for concentration testing Standardized cycle May enhance removal of organic material and endotoxin No adverse health effects to operators under normal operating conditions Compatible with many materials and instruments Sterilant flows through scope, facilitating removal of salt, protein, and microbes Rapidly sporicidal Provides procedure standardization (constant dilution, perfusion of channel, temperatures, exposure)	Potential incompatibility with materials (e.g., aluminum anodized coating becomes dull) Used only for immersible instruments Biologic indicator may not be suitable for routine monitoring Only one scope or a small number of instruments can be processed in a cycle More expensive (endoscope repairs, operating costs, purchase costs) than high-level disinfection Serious eye and skin damage (concentrated solution) with contact Point-of-use system, no sterile storage

*All products listed are effective in presence of some organic soil, are relatively easy to use, and have a broad spectrum of antimicrobial activity (bacteria, fungi, viruses, bacterial spores, and mycobacteria). These characteristics are documented in the literature; contact the manufacturer of the instrument and sterilant for additional information. All products listed are cleared by the U.S. Food and Drug Administration (FDA) as chemical sterilants except ortho-phthalaldehyde, which is an FDA-cleared high-level disinfectant.
Modified from Rutala WA, Weber DJ. Disinfection of endoscopes: review of new chemical sterilants used for high-level disinfection. *Infect Control Hosp Epidemiol.* 1999;20:69-76.

6-log$_{10}$ killing of an appropriate mycobacterial species. Cleaning followed by high-level disinfection should eliminate sufficient pathogens to prevent transmission of infection.[18,19]

Ideally, laparoscopes and arthroscopes entering sterile tissue should be sterilized between patients. However, they sometimes undergo only high-level disinfection between patients in the United States.[20-22] As with flexible endoscopes, these devices may be difficult to clean and perform high-level disinfection and sterilization because of intricate device design (e.g., long narrow lumens, hinges). Meticulous cleaning must precede any high-level disinfection and sterilization process. Newer models of these instruments can withstand steam sterilization that for critical items would be preferable to high-level disinfection.

Semicritical items should be rinsed with sterile water after high-level disinfection, to prevent their contamination with organisms that may be present in tap water, such as nontuberculous mycobacteria,[8-23] Legionella,[24-25] or gram-negative bacilli such as Pseudomonas organisms.[13,15,26-28] In circumstances in which rinsing with sterile water rinse is not feasible, a tap water or filtered water (0.2-μm filter) rinse should be followed by an alcohol rinse and forced-air drying.[20,28,29] Forced-air drying markedly reduces bacterial contamination of stored endoscopes, probably by removing the wet environment favorable for bacterial growth.[29] After rinsing, items should be dried and stored (e.g., packaged) in a manner that protects them from recontamination.

Some items that may come in contact with nonintact skin for a brief period of time (e.g., hydrotherapy tanks, bed side rails) are usually considered noncritical surfaces and are disinfected with low- or intermediate-level disinfectants (e.g., phenolic, iodophor, alcohol, chlorine).[30] Because hydrotherapy tanks have been linked to spread of infection, some facilities have chosen to disinfect them with recommended levels of chlorine.[30]

NONCRITICAL ITEMS

Noncritical items are those that come in contact with intact skin but not mucous membranes. Intact skin acts as an effective barrier to most microorganisms; therefore, the sterility of items coming in contact with intact skin is "not critical." Examples of noncritical items are bedpans, blood pressure cuffs, crutches, bed rails, bedside tables, furniture, and floors. In contrast to critical and some semicritical items, most noncritical reusable items may be decontaminated where they are used and do not need to be transported to a central processing area. There is virtually no documented risk of transmitting infectious agents to patients through noncritical items[27] when they are used as noncritical items and do not contact nonintact skin or mucous membranes. However, these items (e.g., bedside tables, bed rails) could potentially contribute to secondary transmission by contaminating the hands of health care workers or by contact with medical equipment that will subsequently come in contact with patients.[9,31-34] Table 301-1 lists several low-level disinfectants that may be used for noncritical items. The exposure time listed in Table 301-1 is 1 minute or longer. Most U.S. Environmental Protection Agency (EPA)–registered disinfectants have a 10-minute label claim. However, multiple investigators have demonstrated the effectiveness of these disinfectants against vegetative bacteria (e.g., Listeria organisms, Escherichia coli, Salmonella organisms, vancomycin-resistant enterococci [VRE], methicillin-resistant Staphylococcus aureus [MRSA]), yeasts (e.g., Candida), mycobacteria (e.g., Mycobacterium tuberculosis), and viruses (e.g. poliovirus) at exposure times of 30 to 60 seconds.[31-43] Thus, it is acceptable to disinfect noncritical medical equipment (e.g., blood pressure cuff) and noncritical surfaces (e.g., bedside table) with an EPA-registered disinfectant or a disinfectant or detergent at the proper use-dilution and a contact time of at least 1 minute.[44] Because the typical drying time for a germicide on a surface is 1 to 3 minutes (unless the product contains alcohol [e.g., a 60% to 70% alcohol solution will dry in about 30 seconds]; N. Omidbakhsh, written communication) one application of the germicide on all surfaces to be disinfected is recommended.

Mops (microfiber and cotton-string), reusable cleaning cloths, and disposable wipes are regularly used to achieve low-level disinfection.[45,46] However, they are commonly not kept adequately cleaned and disinfected, and if the water-disinfectant mixture is not changed regularly (e.g., after every three to four rooms, at intervals no longer than 60 minutes), the mopping procedure may actually spread heavy microbial contamination throughout the health care facility.[47] In one study, standard laundering provided acceptable decontamination of heavily contaminated mop heads, but chemical disinfection with a phenolic solution was less effective.[47] The frequent (e.g., daily) laundering of cotton-string mops is, therefore, recommended.

Disinfection of Health Care Equipment

A great number of disinfectants are used alone or in combinations (e.g., hydrogen peroxide and peracetic acid) in the health care setting. These include alcohols, chlorine and chlorine compounds, formaldehyde, glutaraldehyde, OPA, hydrogen peroxide, iodophors, peracetic acid, phenolics, and quaternary ammonium compounds. With some exceptions (e.g., ethanol or bleach), commercial formulations based on these chemicals are considered unique products and must be registered with the EPA or cleared by the FDA. In most instances, a given product is designed for a specific purpose and is to be used in a certain manner. Therefore, the label should be read carefully to ensure that the right product is selected for the intended use and applied in an efficient manner. In addition, caution must be exercised to avoid hazards with using cleaners and disinfectants on electronic medical equipment. Problems associated with inappropriate use of liquids on electronic medical equipment have included equipment fires, equipment malfunctions, and burns of health care workers.[48]

Disinfectants are not interchangeable and an overview of the performance characteristics of each is provided in the following sections so the user has sufficient information to select an appropriate disinfectant for any item and use it in the most efficient way. Excessive costs may be attributed to incorrect concentrations and inappropriate disinfectants. Finally, occupational diseases among cleaning personnel have been associated with the use of several disinfectants such as formaldehyde, glutaraldehyde, and chlorine, and precautions (e.g., gloves, proper ventilation) should be used to minimize exposure.[49] Asthma and reactive airway disease may occur in sensitized individuals exposed to any airborne chemical, including germicides. Clinically important asthma may occur at levels below ceiling levels regulated by the Occupational Safety and Health Administration (OSHA) or recommended by the National Institute for Occupational Safety and Health (NIOSH). The preferred method of control is to eliminate the chemical (through engineering controls or substitution) or relocate the worker.

CHEMICAL DISINFECTANTS

Alcohol

In the health care setting, "alcohol" refers to two water-soluble chemical compounds whose germicidal characteristics are generally underrated: ethyl alcohol and isopropyl alcohol.[50] These alcohols are rapidly bactericidal rather than bacteriostatic against vegetative forms of bacteria; they also are tuberculocidal, fungicidal, and virucidal but do not destroy bacterial spores. Their lethal activity drops sharply when they are diluted to less than 50% concentration; the optimum bactericidal concentration is in the range of 60% to 90% solutions in water (volume/volume).[51,52]

Alcohols are not recommended for sterilizing medical and surgical materials, principally because of their lack of sporicidal action and their inability to penetrate protein-rich materials. Fatal postoperative wound infections with Clostridium organisms have occurred when alcohols were used to sterilize surgical instruments contaminated with bacterial spores.[53] Alcohols have been used effectively to disinfect oral and rectal thermometers, hospital pagers, scissors, mannequins used for cardiopulmonary resuscitation (CPR), external surfaces of equipment (e.g., ventilator), and stethoscopes.[54] Alcohol towelettes have been used for years to disinfect small surfaces such as rubber stoppers of multiple-dose medication vials or vaccine bottles.

Alcohols are flammable and consequently must be stored in a cool, well-ventilated area. They also evaporate rapidly and this makes extended exposure time difficult to achieve unless the items are immersed.

Chlorine and Chlorine Compounds

Hypochlorites are the most widely used of the chlorine disinfectants and are available in a liquid form (e.g., sodium hypochlorite) or a solid form (e.g., calcium hypochlorite). The most prevalent chlorine products in the United States are aqueous solutions of 5.25% to 6.15% sodium hypochlorite, which usually are called "household bleach." They have a broad spectrum of antimicrobial activity (i.e., bactericidal, virucidal, fungicidal, mycobactericidal, sporicidal), do not leave toxic residues, are unaffected by water hardness, are inexpensive and fast acting,[55] remove dried or fixed organisms and biofilms from surfaces,[56] and have a low incidence of serious toxicity.[57,58] Sodium hypochlorite at the concentration used in domestic bleach (5.25% to 6.15%) may produce ocular irritation or oropharygeal, esophageal, and gastric burns.[49,59,60] Other disadvantages of hypochlorites include corrosiveness to metals in high concentrations (>500 ppm), inactivation by organic matter, discoloring or "bleaching" of fabrics, release of toxic chlorine gas when mixed with ammonia or acid (e.g., household cleaning agents),[61] and relative stability.[62]

Researchers have examined the microbicidal activity of a new disinfectant, "superoxidized water." The concept of electrolyzing saline to create a disinfectant or antiseptics is appealing because the basic materials of saline and electricity are cheap and the end product (i.e., water) is not damaging to the environment. The main products of this water are hypochlorous acid (e.g., at a concentration of about 144 mg/L) and chlorine. As with any germicide, the antimicrobial activity of superoxidized water is strongly affected by the concentration of the active ingredient (available free chlorine).[63] Data have shown that freshly generated superoxidized water is rapidly effective (<2 minutes) in achieving a 5-log$_{10}$ reduction of pathogenic microorganisms (i.e., M. tuberculosis, Mycobacterium chelonae, poliovirus, human immunodeficiency virus [HIV], MRSA, E. coli, Candida albicans, Enterococcus faecalis, P. aeruginosa) in the absence of organic loading. However, the biocidal activity of this disinfectant was substantially reduced in the presence of organic material (5% horse serum).[64,65]

Hypochlorites are widely used in health care facilities in a variety of settings.[55] Inorganic chlorine solution is used for disinfecting tonometer heads[66] and for spot disinfection of countertops and floors. A 1:10 to 1:100 dilution of 5.25% to 6.15% sodium hypochlorite (i.e., household bleach)[67-70] or an EPA-registered tuberculocidal disinfectant[13] has been recommended for decontaminating blood spills. For small spills of blood (i.e., drops of blood) on noncritical surfaces, the area can be disinfected with a 1:100 dilution of 5.25% to 6.15% sodium hypochlorite or an EPA-registered tuberculocidal disinfectant. Because hypochlorites and other germicides are substantially inactivated in the presence of blood,[43,71] large spills of blood necessitate cleaning of the surface before an EPA-registered disinfectant or a 1:10 (final concentration) solution of household bleach is applied. If a sharps injury is possible, there should be an initial decontamination,[49,72] followed by cleaning and terminal disinfection (1:10 final concentration).[43] Extreme care should always be employed to prevent percutaneous injury. At least 500 ppm available chlorine for 10 minutes is recommended for decontamination of CPR training mannequins. In health care, hypochlorite is also used as an irrigating agent in endodontic treatment and for disinfecting laundry, dental appliances, hydrotherapy tanks,[30] regulated medical waste before disposal,[55] applanation tonometers,[73] and the water distribution system in hemodialysis centers and hemodialysis machines.[54] Disinfection with a 1:10 dilution of concentrated sodium hypochlorite (i.e., bleach) has been shown to be effective in reducing environmental contamination in patient rooms and in reducing Clostridium difficile infection rates in hospital units where there is a high endemic C. difficile infection rate or in an outbreak setting.[17,74,75]

Chlorine has long been favored as the preferred disinfectant in water treatment. Hyperchlorination of a Legionella-contaminated hospital water system[30] resulted in a dramatic decrease (30% to 1.5%) in the isolation of Legionella pneumophila from water outlets and a cessation of health care–associated legionnaires' disease in the affected unit.[76,77] Chloramine T and hypochlorites have been used in disinfecting hydrotherapy equipment.[54]

Hypochlorite solutions in tap water at a pH greater than 8 stored at room temperature (23°C) in closed, opaque plastic containers may lose up to 40% to 50% of their free available chlorine level over a period of 1 month. Thus, if a user wished to have a solution containing 500 ppm of available chlorine at day 30, a solution containing 1000 ppm of chlorine should be prepared at time 0. There is no decomposition of sodium hypochlorite solution after 30 days when it is stored in a closed brown bottle.[62]

Glutaraldehyde

Glutaraldehyde is a saturated dialdehyde that has been widely accepted as a high-level disinfectant and chemical sterilant.[78] Aqueous solutions of glutaraldehyde are acidic and, in general in this state, are not sporicidal. Only when the solution is "activated" (made alkaline) by use of alkalinizing agents to a pH of 7.5 to 8.5 does the solution become sporicidal. Once "activated," these solutions have a shelf life of minimally 14 days because of the polymerization of the glutaraldehyde molecules at alkaline pH levels. This polymerization blocks the active sites (aldehyde groups) of the glutaraldehyde molecules that are responsible for its biocidal activity.

Novel glutaraldehyde formulations (e.g., glutaraldehyde-phenol-sodium phenate, potentiated acid glutaraldehyde, stabilized alkaline glutaraldehyde) produced since the mid-1960s have overcome the problem of rapid loss of activity (e.g., usefulness now lasts 28 to 30 days) while generally maintaining excellent microbicidal activity.[54,79,80] However, their antimicrobial activity is dependent not only on age but also on use conditions such as dilution and organic stress. The use of glutaraldehyde-based solutions in health care facilities is common because they have excellent biocidal properties; they are active in the presence of organic matter (20% bovine serum); and they do not corrode endoscopic equipment, thermometers, rubber, or plastic equipment. The advantages, disadvantages, and characteristics of glutaraldehyde are listed in Table 301-2.

The in vitro inactivation of microorganisms by glutaraldehydes has been extensively investigated and reviewed.[81] Several investigators showed that 2% or higher aqueous solutions of glutaraldehyde, buffered to a pH of 7.5 to 8.5 with sodium bicarbonate, were effective in killing vegetative bacteria in less than 2 minutes; M. tuberculosis, fungi, and viruses in less than 10 minutes; and spores of Bacillus and Clostridium species in 3 hours.[81,82] Spores of C. difficile are more rapidly killed by 2% glutaraldehyde than are spores of other species of Clostridium and Bacillus.[83,84] There have been reports of microorganisms with relative resistance to glutaraldehyde, including some mycobacteria (M. chelonae, Mycobacterium avium-intracellulare, Mycobacterium xenopi),[85,86] Methylobacterium mesophilicum,[87] Trichosporon organisms, fungal ascospores (e.g., Microascus cinereus, Chaetomium globosum), and Cryptosporidium organisms.[88] M. chelonae persisted in a 0.2% glutaraldehyde solution used to store porcine prosthetic heart valves.[89]

During use, glutaraldehyde commonly becomes diluted, and studies have revealed a glutaraldehyde concentration decline after a few days of use in an automatic endoscope washer.[90] This occurs because instruments are not thoroughly dried and water is carried in with the instrument, which increases the solution's volume and dilutes its effective concentration. Therefore, semicritical equipment must be disinfected with an acceptable concentration of glutaraldehyde. Data suggest that 1.0% to 1.5% glutaraldehyde is the minimum effective concentration for higher than 2% glutaraldehyde solutions used as high-level disinfectants.[90-92] Chemical test strips or liquid chemical monitors are available for determining whether the concentration of glutaraldehyde is effective despite repeated use and dilution. The frequency of testing should be based on how frequently the solutions are used (e.g., if it is used daily, test daily; if it is used weekly, test before use; if it is used 30 times per day, test each 10th use) but the strips should not be used to extend its life beyond the expiration date. Data suggest that the chemicals in the test strip deteriorate over time,[93] and a manufacturer's expiration date should be placed on the bottles. The bottle of test strips should be dated when opened and used for the period of time indicated on the bottle (e.g., 120 days). The results of test strip monitoring should be documented. The glutaraldehyde test kits have been preliminarily evaluated for accuracy and range,[93] but their reliability has been questioned.[94] The concentration should be considered unacceptable or unsafe when the test result indicates a dilution below the product's minimum effective concentration (generally to 1.0% to 1.5% glutaraldehyde or lower); this result is shown by the indicator's not changing color.

Glutaraldehyde is used most commonly as a high-level disinfectant for medical equipment such as endoscopes.[72] Glutaraldehyde does not corrode metal and does not damage lensed instruments, rubber, or plastics. The FDA-cleared labels for high-level disinfection with higher than 2% glutaraldehyde at 25°C range from 20 to 90 minutes, depending on the product. However, multiple scientific studies and professional organizations support the efficacy of higher than 2% glutaraldehyde for 20 minutes at 20°C.[13] At minimum, this latter recommendation should be followed. Glutaraldehyde should not be used for cleaning noncritical surfaces because it is too toxic and expensive.

Colitis is sometimes believed to be caused by glutaraldehyde exposure from residual disinfecting solution in the endoscope solution channels; it is preventable by careful endoscope rinsing.[49] One study revealed that residual glutaraldehyde levels were higher and more variable after manual disinfection (<0.2 to 159.5 mg/L) than after automatic disinfection (0.2 to 6.3 mg/L).[95] Similarly, keratopathy and corneal decompensation were caused by ophthalmic instruments that were inadequately rinsed after soaking in 2% glutaraldehyde.[96]

Glutaraldehyde exposure should be monitored to ensure a safe work environment. In the absence of an OSHA permissible exposure limit, if the glutaraldehyde level is higher than the American Conference of Governmental Industrial Hygienists (ACGIH) ceiling limit of 0.05 ppm, it would be prudent to take corrective action and repeat monitoring.[97]

Hydrogen Peroxide

The literature contains several accounts of the properties, germicidal effectiveness, and potential uses for stabilized hydrogen peroxide in the health care setting. Published reports ascribe good germicidal activity to hydrogen peroxide and attest to its bactericidal, virucidal, sporicidal, and fungicidal properties.[98-101] The advantages, disadvantages, and characteristics of hydrogen peroxide are listed in Table 301-2. As with other chemical sterilants, dilution of the hydrogen peroxide must be monitored by regularly testing the minimum effective concentration (i.e., 7.5% to 6.0%). In compatibility testing, Olympus America found that both cosmetic changes (e.g., discoloration of black anodized metal finishes)[72] and functional changes with the tested endoscopes were caused by the 7.5% hydrogen peroxide (Olympus America, written communication, October 15, 1999).

Commercially available 3% hydrogen peroxide is a stable and effective disinfectant when used on inanimate surfaces. It has been used in concentrations of 3% to 6% for the disinfection of soft contact lenses (e.g., 3% for 2 to 3 hours),[98,102] tonometer biprisms, ventilators, fabrics,[103] and endoscopes.[104] Hydrogen peroxide was effective in spot-disinfecting fabrics in patients' rooms.[103] Corneal damage from a hydrogen peroxide-soaked tonometer tip that was not properly rinsed has been reported.[105]

An accelerated hydrogen peroxide–based technology has been used for disinfection of noncritical environmental surfaces and equipment used in patient care[106] and for high-level disinfection of semicritical equipment such as endoscopes.[107] The product is claimed to have excellent antimicrobial performance and a favorable safety profile. Another hydrogen peroxide–based method has also been used for equipment cleaning.[108]

Iodophors

Iodine solutions or tinctures have long been used by health professionals, primarily as antiseptics on skin or tissue. An iodophor is a combination of iodine and a solubilizing agent or carrier; the resulting complex provides a sustained-release reservoir of iodine and releases small amounts of free iodine in aqueous solution. The FDA has not cleared any liquid chemical sterilants or high-level disinfectants whose main active ingredient is an iodophor. However, iodophors have been used both as antiseptics and disinfectants. The best known and most widely used iodophor is povidone-iodine, a compound of polyvinylpyrrolidone with iodine. This product and other iodophors retain the germicidal efficacy of iodine but, unlike iodine, are generally nonstaining and are relatively nontoxic and nonirritating.[109]

Several reports have documented intrinsic microbial contamination of antiseptic formulations of povidone-iodine and poloxamer-iodine.[110,111] "Free" iodine (I_2) was found to contribute to the bactericidal activity of iodophors, and dilutions of iodophors have been shown to demonstrate more rapid bactericidal action than does a full-strength povidone-iodine solution. Therefore, iodophors must be diluted according to the manufacturers' directions to achieve antimicrobial activity.

Published studies on the in vitro antimicrobial efficacy of iodophors have demonstrated that iodophors are bactericidal, mycobactericidal, and virucidal but may require prolonged contact times to kill certain fungi and bacterial spores.[10,112-115]

Besides their use as antiseptics, iodophors have been used for the disinfection of blood culture bottles and medical equipment such as hydrotherapy tanks and thermometers. Antiseptic iodophors are not suitable for use as hard-surface disinfectants because of concentration differences. Iodophors formulated as antiseptics contain less free iodine than do those formulated as disinfectants.[116] Iodine and iodine-based antiseptics should not be used on silicone catheters because the silicone tubing may be adversely affected.[117]

Ortho-phthalaldehyde

OPA is a high-level disinfectant that received FDA clearance in October 1999. It contains at least 0.55% 1,2-benzenedicarboxaldehyde, and it has supplanted glutaraldehyde as the most commonly used high-level disinfectant in the United States. OPA solution is a clear, pale-blue liquid with a pH of 7.5. The advantages, disadvantages, and characteristics of OPA are listed in Table 301-2.

Studies have demonstrated excellent microbicidal activity in in vitro studies,[54,72,88,118-123] including superior mycobactericidal activity (5 $\log_{10}$ reduction in 5 minutes) in comparison with glutaraldehyde. Walsh and colleagues also found OPA effective (>5-$\log_{10}$ reduction) against a wide range of microorganisms, including glutaraldehyde-resistant mycobacteria and *Bacillus atrophaeus* spores.[121]

OPA has several potential advantages over glutaraldehyde. It has excellent stability over a wide pH range (pH of 3 to 9), is not known to irritate the eyes and nasal passages, does not require exposure monitoring, has a barely perceptible odor, and requires no activation. OPA, like glutaraldehyde, has excellent compatibility with materials. A potential disadvantage of OPA is that it stains proteins gray (including unprotected skin) and thus must be handled with caution.[72] However, skin staining would indicate improper handling, which necessitates additional training, personal protective equipment (gloves, eye and mouth protection, fluid-resistant gowns), or both. OPA residues remaining on inadequately water-rinsed transesophageal echocardiogram probes may leave stains in the patient's mouth. Meticulous cleaning, with the correct OPA exposure time (e.g., 12 minutes), and copious rinsing of the probe with water should obviate this problem. OPA has been linked to several episodes of anaphylaxis after cystoscopy[124]; therefore, the instructions for its use have been modified, and its use as a disinfectant is contraindicated in the reprocessing of all urologic instrumentation for patients with a history of bladder cancer. Health care workers should wear personal protective equipment when handling contaminated instruments, equipment, and chemicals.[119] In addition, equipment must be thoroughly rinsed to prevent discoloration of a patient's skin or mucous membranes.

Peracetic Acid

Peracetic acid, or peroxyacetic acid, is characterized by very rapid action against all microorganisms. Special advantages of peracetic acid are its lack of harmful decomposition products (i.e., acetic acid, water, oxygen, hydrogen peroxide), its enhancement of the removal of organic material,[125] and the fact that it leaves no residue. It remains effective in the presence of organic matter and is sporicidal even at low temperatures. Peracetic acid can corrode copper, brass, bronze, plain steel, and galvanized iron, but these effects can be reduced by additives and pH modifications. The advantages, disadvantages, and characteristics of peracetic acid are listed in Table 301-2.

Peracetic acid inactivates gram-positive and gram-negative bacteria, fungi, and yeasts in less than 5 minutes at less than 100 ppm. In the presence of organic matter, 200 to 500 ppm is required. For viruses, the dosage range is wide (12-2250 ppm); poliovirus is inactivated in yeast extract in 15 minutes with 1500 to 2250 ppm. An automated machine in which peracetic acid is used to chemically sterilize medical instruments (e.g., endoscopes, arthroscopes) and surgical instruments is available in the United States.[126,127] The sterilant, 35% peracetic acid, is diluted to 0.2% with filtered water at a temperature of 50°C. Simulated-use trials have demonstrated excellent microbicidal activity,[127-131] and three clinical trials have demonstrated both excellent microbial killing and no clinical failures that have led to infection.[132-134] In three clusters of infection in which the automated endoscope reprocessor was used with peracetic acid, the infections were linked to inadequately processed bronchoscopes when inappropriate channel connectors were used with the system.[135,136] These clusters highlight the importance of training, proper model-specific endoscope connector systems, and quality control procedures to ensure compliance with endoscope manufacturer's recommendations and professional organization guidelines. An alternative high-level disinfectant available in the United Kingdom contains 0.35% peracetic acid. Although this product is rapidly effective against a broad range of microorganisms,[137,138] it tarnishes the metal of endoscopes and is unstable, which results in only a 24-hour use life.[138]

Peracetic Acid with Hydrogen Peroxide

Three chemical sterilants that have been cleared by the FDA contain peracetic acid plus hydrogen peroxide (0.08% peracetic acid plus 1.0% hydrogen peroxide, 0.23% peracetic acid plus 7.35% hydrogen peroxide, and 8.3% hydrogen peroxide plus 7.0% peracetic acid). The advantages, disadvantages, and characteristics of peracetic acid with hydrogen peroxide are listed in Table 301-2.

The bactericidal properties of peracetic acid plus hydrogen peroxide have been demonstrated.[139] The manufacturer's data demonstrated that this combination inactivated all microorganisms except bacterial spores within 20 minutes. The 0.08% peracetic acid plus 1.0% hydrogen peroxide product was effective in inactivating a glutaraldehyde-resistant mycobacteria.[140]

The combination of peracetic acid and hydrogen peroxide has been used for disinfecting hemodialyzers.[141] The percentage of dialysis centers using a disinfectant of peracetic acid with hydrogen peroxide for reprocessing dialyzers increased from 5% in 1983 to 62% in 2001.[142]

Phenolics

Phenol has occupied a prominent place in the field of hospital disinfection since its initial use as a germicide by Sir Joseph Lister in his pioneering work on antiseptic surgery during the 19th century. Since the 1960s, however, work has been concentrated on the numerous phenol derivatives, or phenolics, and their antimicrobial properties. Phenol derivatives are formed when a functional group (e.g., alkyl,

phenyl, benzyl, halogen) replaces one of the hydrogen atoms on the aromatic ring. Two phenol derivatives commonly found as constituents of hospital disinfectants are ortho-phenylphenol and ortho-benzyl-para-chlorophenol.

Published reports on the antimicrobial efficacy of commonly used phenolics showed that they were bactericidal, fungicidal, virucidal, and tuberculocidal.[10,42,54,112,143-147]

Many phenolic germicides are registered by the EPA as disinfectants for use on environmental surfaces (e.g., bedside tables, bed rails, laboratory surfaces) and noncritical medical devices. Phenolics are not cleared by the FDA as high-level disinfectants for use with semicritical items but could be used to preclean or decontaminate critical and semicritical devices before terminal sterilization or high-level disinfection.

The use of phenolics in nurseries has been questioned because of the occurrence of hyperbilirubinemia in infants placed in bassinets on which phenolic detergents were used.[148] In addition, Doan and coworkers demonstrated increases in bilirubin level in infants exposed to phenolics in comparison with infants not exposed to phenolics when the phenolic was prepared according to the manufacturers' recommended dilution.[149] If phenolics are used to clean nursery floors, they must be diluted according to the recommendation on the product label. Phenolics (and other disinfectants) should not be used to clean infant bassinets and incubators while occupied. If phenolics are used to terminally clean infant bassinets and incubators, the surfaces should be rinsed thoroughly with water and dried before the infant bassinets and incubators are reused.[13]

Quaternary Ammonium Compounds

The quaternary ammonium compounds are widely used as surface disinfectants. There have been some reports of infections linked to contaminated quaternary ammonium compounds used to disinfect supplies or equipment used in patient care, such as cystoscopes or cardiac catheters.[150,151] As with several other disinfectants (e.g., phenolics, iodophors), gram-negative bacteria have been found to survive or grow in them.[152]

Results from manufacturers' data sheets and from published scientific literature indicate that the quaternary ammonium compounds sold as hospital disinfectants are generally fungicidal, bactericidal, and virucidal against lipophilic (enveloped) viruses; they are not sporicidal and generally not tuberculocidal or virucidal against hydrophilic (nonenveloped) viruses.[10,38,39,41,42,112,153-155] Best and colleagues[38] and Rutala and associates[112] demonstrated the poor mycobactericidal activities of quaternary ammonium compounds.

These compounds are commonly used in ordinary environmental sanitation of noncritical surfaces such as floors, furniture, and walls. The use of EPA-registered quaternary ammonium compounds is appropriate in disinfecting medical equipment that comes into contact with intact skin (e.g., blood pressure cuffs).

Pasteurization

Pasteurization is not a sterilization process; its purpose is to destroy all pathogenic microorganisms except bacterial spores. The time-temperature relation for hot-water pasteurization is generally greater than 70°C (158°F) for 30 minutes. The water temperature and time should be monitored as part of a quality assurance program.[156] Pasteurization of equipment used in respiratory therapy[157,158] and of anesthesia equipment[159] is a recognized alternative to chemical disinfection.

■ Sterilization

Most medical and surgical devices used in health care facilities are made of materials that are heat stable, and thus they are sterilized by heat, primarily steam sterilization. However, since 1950, there has been an increase in medical devices and instruments made of materials (e.g., plastics) that require only low-temperature sterilization. ETO gas has been used since the 1950s for heat- and moisture-sensitive medical devices. Since the early 1990s, a number of new, low-temperature sterilization systems (e.g., hydrogen peroxide gas plasma, peracetic acid immersion, ozone, vaporized hydrogen peroxide) have been developed and are being used to sterilize medical devices. This section reviews sterilization technologies used in health care and makes recommendations for their optimal performance in the processing of medical devices.[14,15,17,160-167]

Sterilization destroys all microorganisms on the surface of an article or in a fluid to prevent disease transmission associated with the use of that item. Although the use of inadequately sterilized critical items carries a high risk of transmitting pathogens, documentation of such transmission is exceedingly rare.[168,169] This is probably because the sterilization processes used in health care facilities are highly safe. What constitutes "sterile" is measured as a probability of sterility for each item to be sterilized, commonly referred to as the sterility assurance level (SAL) of the product. The SAL is defined as the probability of a single viable microorganism occurring on a product after sterilization. SAL is normally expressed as 10^{-n}. For example, if the probability of a spore surviving were one in 1 million, the SAL would be 10^{-6}.[170,171] In short, a SAL is an estimate of lethality of the entire sterilization process and is a conservative calculation. Dual SALs (e.g., 10^{-3} SAL for blood culture tubes and drainage bags; 10^{-6} SAL for scalpels and implants) have been used in the United States for many years, and the choice of a 10^{-6} SAL was strictly arbitrary and not associated with any adverse outcomes (e.g., infections in patients).[170]

Medical devices that have contact with sterile body tissues or fluids are considered critical items. These items should be sterile when used because any microbial contamination could result in disease transmission. Such items include surgical instruments, biopsy forceps, and implanted medical devices. If these items are heat resistant, the recommended sterilization process is steam sterilization because it has the largest margin of safety as a result of its reliability, consistency, and lethality. However, reprocessing heat- and moisture-sensitive items necessitates use of a low-temperature sterilization technology (e.g., ETO, hydrogen peroxide gas plasma, peracetic acid, ozone).[172] A summary of the advantages and disadvantages for commonly used sterilization technologies is presented in Table 301-3.

STEAM STERILIZATION

Of all the methods available for sterilization, moist heat in the form of saturated steam under pressure is the most widely used and the most dependable. Steam sterilization is nontoxic, inexpensive,[173] rapidly microbicidal, and sporicidal, and steam rapidly heats and penetrates fabrics (see Table 301-3).[174] Like all sterilization processes, steam sterilization has some deleterious effects on some materials, including corrosion and combustion of lubricants used with dental handpieces[175]; reduction in ability to transmit light used with laryngoscopes[176]; and increased hardening time (5.6-fold) with plaster cast.[177]

The basic procedure of steam sterilization, as accomplished in an autoclave, is to expose each item to direct steam contact at the required temperature and pressure for the specified time. Thus, steam sterilization entails four parameters: steam, pressure, temperature, and time.

TABLE 301-3	Summary of Advantages and Disadvantages of Commonly Used Sterilization Technologies	
Sterilization Method	**Advantages**	**Disadvantages**
Steam	Nontoxic to patient, staff, and environment Cycle easy to control and monitor Rapidly microbicidal Least affected by organic/inorganic soils among sterilization processes listed Rapid cycle time Penetrates medical packing, device lumens	Deleterious to heat-sensitive instruments Microsurgical instruments may be damaged by repeated exposure May leave instruments wet, causing them to rust Potential for burns
Hydrogen peroxide gas plasma	Safe for the environment Leaves no toxic residuals Cycle time is 28-75 min (varies with model type) and no aeration is necessary Used for heat- and moisture-sensitive items, inasmuch as process temperature <50°C Simple to operate, install (208-V outlet), and monitor Compatible with most medical devices Requires only electrical outlet	Cellulose (paper), linens, and liquids cannot be processed Sterilization chamber size, 1.8-9.4 cubic feet total volume (varies with model type) Some endoscopes or medical devices with long or narrow lumens cannot be processed at this time in the United States (see manufacturer's recommendations for internal diameter and length restrictions) Requires synthetic packaging (polypropylene wraps, polyolefin pouches) and special container tray Hydrogen peroxide may be toxic at levels greater than 1 ppm time-weighted average
100% Ethylene oxide (ETO)	Penetrates packaging materials, device lumens Single-dose cartridge and negative-pressure chamber minimize the potential for gas leak and ETO exposure Simple to operate and monitor Compatible with most medical materials	Aeration time necessary to remove ETO residue Sterilization chamber size, 4.0-7.9 cubic feet total volume (varies with model type) ETO is toxic, carcinogenic, and flammable ETO emission is regulated by states, but catalytic cell removes 99.9% of ETO and converts it to CO_2 and H_2O ETO cartridges should be stored in flammable liquid storage cabinet Lengthy cycle and aeration time
ETO mixtures • 8.6% ETO/91.4% HCFC • 10% ETO/90% HCFC • 8.5% ETO/91.5% CO_2	Penetrates medical packaging and many plastics Compatible with most medical materials Cycle easy to control and monitor	Some states (e.g., California, New York, Michigan) require ETO emission reduction of 90%-99.9% CFC (inert gas that eliminates explosion hazard) banned in 1995 Potential hazards to staff and patients Lengthy cycle/aeration time ETO is toxic, carcinogenic, and flammable
Peracetic acid	Rapid cycle time (30-45 min) Low temperature (50°-55°C liquid immersion sterilization) Environmentally friendly by-products Sterilant flows through endoscope, which facilitates removal of salt, protein, and microbe	Point-of-use system, no sterile storage Biologic indicator may not be suitable for routine monitoring Used for only immersible instruments Incompatibility with some materials (e.g., aluminum anodized coating becomes dull) Only one scope or a small number of instruments processed in a cycle Potential for serious eye and skin damage (concentrated solution) with contact

CFC, chlorofluorocarbon; HCFC, hydrochlorofluorocarbon.
Modified from Rutala WA, Weber DJ. Clinical effectiveness of low-temperature sterilization technologies. *Infect Control Hosp Epidemiol.* 1998;19:798-804.

The ideal steam for sterilization is dry saturated steam and entrained water (dryness fraction, ≥97%).[162] Pressure serves as a means to obtain the high temperatures necessary to quickly kill microorganisms. Specific temperatures must be obtained to ensure the microbicidal activity. The two common steam-sterilizing temperatures are 121°C (250°F) and 132°C (270°F). These temperatures (and other high temperatures) must be maintained for a minimal time to kill microorganisms. Recognized minimum exposure periods for sterilization of wrapped health care supplies are 30 minutes at 121°C (250°F) in a gravity displacement sterilizer and 4 minutes at 132°C (270°C) in a prevacuum sterilizer. At constant temperatures, sterilization times vary, depending on the type of item (e.g., metal vs. rubber, plastic, items with lumens), whether the item is wrapped or unwrapped, and the type of sterilizer.

The two basic types of steam sterilizers (autoclaves) are the gravity displacement autoclave and the high-speed prevacuum sterilizer. In the former, steam is admitted at the top or the sides of the sterilizing chamber, and because the steam is lighter than air, it forces air out the bottom of the chamber through the drain vent. The gravity displacement autoclaves are used primarily to process laboratory media, water, pharmaceutical products, regulated medical waste, and nonporous articles whose surfaces have direct steam contact. With gravity displacement sterilizers, the penetration time into porous items is prolonged because of incomplete air elimination. The high-speed prevacuum sterilizers are similar to the gravity displacement sterilizers except that they are fitted with a vacuum pump (or ejector) to ensure air removal from the sterilizing chamber and load before the steam is admitted. The advantage of using a vacuum pump is that there is nearly instantaneous steam penetration even into porous loads.

Like other sterilization systems, the steam cycle is monitored by mechanical, chemical, and biologic monitors. Steam sterilizers usually are monitored through the use of a printout (or graphically) to measure temperature, the time at the temperature, and pressure. Typically, chemical indicators are affixed to the outside and incorporated into the device to monitor the temperature or time and temperature. The effectiveness of steam sterilization is monitored with a biologic indicator containing spores of *Geobacillus stearothermophilus* (formerly known as *Bacillus stearothermophilus*). Positive spore test results are relatively rare and can be attributed to operator error, inadequate steam delivery,[178] or equipment malfunction.

Portable steam sterilizers are used in outpatient, dental, and rural clinics. These sterilizers are designed for small instruments, such as hypodermic syringes and needles and dental instruments. The ability of the sterilizer to reach physical parameters necessary to achieve sterilization should be monitored by mechanical, chemical, and biologic indicators.

Steam sterilization should be used whenever possible on all critical and semicritical items that are heat and moisture resistant (e.g., steam-sterilizable equipment for respiratory therapy and for anesthesia), even when it is not essential to prevent pathogen transmission. Steam sterilizers also are used in health care facilities to decontaminate microbiologic waste and sharps containers,[179] but additional exposure time is required in the gravity displacement sterilizer for these items.

FLASH STERILIZATION

"Flash" steam sterilization was originally defined by Underwood and Perkins as sterilization of an unwrapped object at 132°C (270°F) for 3 minutes at 27 to 28 pounds (12.3 to 12.7 kg) of pressure in a gravity displacement sterilizer.[180] Currently, the time required for flash sterilization depends on the type of sterilizer and the type of item (i.e., porous vs. nonporous items). For example, the minimum flash sterilization cycle time for nonporous items only (i.e., routine metal instruments, no lumens) at 132°C (270°F) in a prevacuum sterilizer is 3 minutes. Although the wrapped method of sterilization is preferred for the reasons listed below, correctly performed flash sterilization is an effective process for the sterilization of critical medical devices.[181,182] Flash sterilization is a modification of conventional steam sterilization

(either gravity or prevacuum) in which the flashed item is placed in an open tray or is placed in a specially designed, covered, rigid container to allow for rapid penetration of steam. Historically, it is not recommended as a routine sterilization method because of the lack of timely biologic indicators to monitor performance, absence of protective packaging after sterilization, possibility for contamination of processed items during transportation to the operating rooms, and the sterilization cycle parameters (i.e., time, temperature, pressure) are minimal. To address some of these concerns, many health care facilities have the following protocol in place: placing equipment for flash sterilization close to operating rooms to facilitate aseptic delivery to the point of use (usually the sterile field in an ongoing surgical procedure); extending the exposure time to ensure lethality comparable with that of sterilized wrapped items (e.g., 4 minutes at 132°C [270°F])[183,184]; using biologic indicators that provide results in 1 hour for flash-sterilized items[183,184]; and using protective packaging that enables steam penetration.[161,166,167,182] Furthermore, some rigid, reusable sterilization container systems have been designed and validated by the container manufacturer for use with flash cycles. When sterile items are open to air, they eventually become contaminated. Thus, the longer a sterile item is exposed to air, the greater the number of microorganisms that will settle on it.

Surgical site infections as a consequence of flash sterilization have rarely, if ever, been reported. The only report of possible infections was an abstract describing an increased incidence of neurosurgical infections; the investigators noted that surgical instruments were flash sterilized between cases and two of three craniotomy infections involved plate implants that were flash sterilized.[185] However, no details were provided on the sterilization parameters (e.g., temperature, time, chemical indicators) or other conditions that might have increased the risk of infection. A report of two patients who received burns during surgery from instruments that had been flash sterilized reinforced the need to develop policies and educate staff to prevent the use of instruments hot enough to cause clinical burns.[186] Staff should use precautions to prevent burns with potentially hot instruments (e.g., transport tray using heat-protective gloves). Patient burns may be prevented by either air-cooling the instruments or immersion in sterile liquid (e.g., saline).

Flash sterilization is considered acceptable for processing cleaned items used in patient care that cannot be packaged, sterilized, and stored before use. It is also used when there is insufficient time to sterilize an item by the preferred package method. The current recommendations are that flash sterilization not be used for reasons of convenience, as an alternative to purchasing additional instrument sets, or to save time.[166] Because of the potential for serious infections, flash sterilization is not recommended for implantable devices (i.e., devices placed into a surgically or naturally formed cavity of the human body); however, flash sterilization may be unavoidable for some devices (e.g., orthopedic screw, plates). If flash sterilization of an implantable device is unavoidable, record keeping (e.g., load identification, patient's name or hospital identifier, biologic indicator result) is essential for epidemiologic tracking (e.g., of surgical site infection, for tracing results of biologic indicators to patients who received the item to document sterility) and for an assessment of the reliability of the sterilization process (e.g., evaluation of biologic monitoring records and sterilization maintenance records noting preventive maintenance and repairs, with dates).

ETHYLENE OXIDE GAS STERILIZATION

ETO is a colorless gas that is flammable and explosive. The four essential parameters (operational ranges) are gas concentration (450 to 1200 mg/L); temperature (37° to 63°C [98.6° to 145°F]); relative humidity (40% to 80%; water molecules carry ETO to reactive sites); and exposure time (1 to 6 hours). These parameters influence the effectiveness of ETO sterilization.[163,187,188] Within certain limitations, an increase in gas concentration and in temperature may shorten the time necessary for achieving sterilization.

The main disadvantages associated with ETO are the lengthy cycle time, the cost, and its potential hazards to patients and staff; the main advantage is that it can sterilize heat- or moisture-sensitive medical equipment without deleterious effects on the material used in the medical devices (see Table 301-3). Acute exposure to ETO may result in irritation (e.g., to skin, eyes, gastrointestinal or respiratory tract) and central nervous system depression.[49] Chronic inhalation has been linked to the formation of cataracts, cognitive impairment, neurologic dysfunction, and disabling polyneuropathies.[49] Occupational exposure in health care facilities has been linked to hematologic changes and an increased risk of spontaneous abortions and various cancers.[49] ETO should be considered a known human carcinogen.[189]

The use of ETO evolved when few alternatives existed for sterilizing heat- and moisture-sensitive medical devices; however, favorable properties (see Table 301-3) account for its continued widespread use.[190] Two ETO gas mixtures are available to replace ETO-chlorofluorocarbon (CFC) mixtures for large-capacity, tank-supplied sterilizers. The ETO-carbon dioxide (CO_2) mixture consists of 8.5% ETO and 91.5% CO_2. This mixture is less expensive than ETO-hydrochlorofluorocarbon (HCFC), but a disadvantage is the need for pressure vessels rated for steam sterilization, because higher pressures (28-psi gauge) are required. The other mixture, which is a drop-in CFC replacement, is ETO mixed with HCFC. HCFCs are approximately 50-fold less damaging to the earth's ozone layer than are CFCs. The EPA will begin regulation of HCFCs in 2015 and will terminate production in 2030. ETO-HCFC mixtures are provided by companies as a drop-in replacement for CFC-12; one mixture consists of 8.6% ETO and 91.4% HCFC, and the other mixture is composed of 10% ETO and 90% HCFC.[190] An alternative to the pressurized mixed-gas ETO systems is 100% ETO. The 100% ETO sterilizers in which unit-dose cartridges are used eliminate the need for external tanks.

The excellent microbicidal activity of ETO has been demonstrated in several studies[130,131,191-194] and summarized in published reports.[195] ETO inactivates all microorganisms, although bacterial spores (especially *B. atrophaeus*) are more resistant than other microorganisms. For this reason, *B. atrophaeus* is the recommended biologic indicator.

Like all sterilization processes, the effectiveness of ETO sterilization can be altered by lumen length, lumen diameter, inorganic salts, and organic materials.[130,131,192-194,196] For example, although ETO is not used commonly for reprocessing endoscopes,[20] several studies have shown failure of ETO in inactivating contaminating spores in endoscope channels[196] or lumen test units[130,192,194] and residual ETO levels averaging 66.2 ppm even after the standard degassing time.[104] Failure of ETO also has been observed when dental handpieces were contaminated with *Streptococcus mutans* and exposed to ETO.[197] It is recommended that dental handpieces be steam sterilized.

ETO is used in health care facilities to sterilize critical items (and sometimes semicritical items) that are moisture or heat sensitive and cannot be sterilized by steam.

HYDROGEN PEROXIDE GAS PLASMA

New sterilization technology based on gas plasma was patented in 1987 and marketed in the United States in 1993. Gas plasmas have been referred to as the fourth state of matter (i.e., liquids, solids, gases, and gas plasmas). Gas plasmas are generated in an enclosed chamber under deep vacuum; radiofrequency or microwave energy is used to excite the gas (i.e., hydrogen peroxide) molecules and produce charged particles, many of which are in the form of free radicals (e.g., hydroxyl and hydroperoxyl). The biologic indicator used with this system is *G. stearothermophilus* spores.

This process has the ability to inactivate a broad range of microorganisms, including resistant bacterial spores. Studies have been conducted against vegetative bacteria (including mycobacteria), yeasts, fungi, viruses, and bacterial spores.[130,193,194,198-204] Like all sterilization processes, the effectiveness can be altered by lumen length, lumen diameter, inorganic salts, and organic materials.[130,193,194,196,198,199]

Materials and devices that cannot tolerate high temperatures and humidity, such as some plastics, electrical devices, and corrosion-susceptible metal alloys, can be sterilized by hydrogen peroxide gas plasma. This method has been compatible with most (>95%) medical devices and materials tested.[205,206]

OZONE

Ozone has been used for years as a disinfectant of drinking water. Ozone is produced when O_2 is energized and split into two monatomic (O_1) molecules. The monatomic oxygen molecules then collide with O_2 molecules to form ozone, which is O_3. Thus, ozone consists of O_2 with a loosely bonded third oxygen atom that is readily available to attach to, and oxidize, other molecules. This additional oxygen atom makes ozone a powerful oxidant that destroys microorganisms but is highly unstable (i.e., it has a half-life of 22 minutes at room temperature).

A sterilization process in which ozone is used as the sterilant was cleared by the FDA in August 2003 for processing reusable medical devices. The sterilizer creates its own sterilant internally from United States Pharmacopeia (USP)–grade oxygen, steam-quality water, and electricity; the sterilant is converted back to oxygen and water vapor at the end of the cycle by passing through a catalyst before its exhaust is expelled into the room. The duration of the sterilization cycle is about 4 hours and 15 minutes, and it occurs at 30° to 35°C (86° to 95°F). Microbial efficacy has been demonstrated by achieving a SAL of 10^{-6} with a variety of microorganisms to include the most resistant microorganism, *G. stearothermophilus*.[207]

The ozone process is compatible with a wide range of commonly used materials, including stainless steel, titanium, anodized aluminum, ceramic, glass, silica, polyvinyl chloride, Teflon, silicone, polypropylene, polyethylene, and acrylic. In addition, rigid lumen devices of the following diameters and lengths can be processed: internal diameter > 2 mm, length ≤ 25 cm; internal diameter > 3 mm, length ≤ 47 cm; and internal diameter > 4 mm, length ≤ 60 cm.

The process should be safe for use by the operator because there is no handling of the sterilant, no toxic emissions, and no residue to aerate, and because operating temperature is low, there is no danger of an accidental burn. The cycle is monitored through a self-contained biologic indicator and a chemical indicator. The sterilization chamber is small, about 4 cubic feet (S. Dufresne, written communication, July 2004).

A gaseous ozone generator was investigated for decontamination of rooms used to house patients colonized with MRSA. The results demonstrated that the device tested would be inadequate for the decontamination of a hospital room.[208]

PERACETIC ACID STERILIZATION

Peracetic acid is a highly biocidal oxidizer that maintains its efficacy in the presence of organic soil. Peracetic acid removes surface contaminants (primarily protein) on endoscopic tubing.[125,126] An automated machine in which peracetic acid was used to sterilize medical, surgical, and dental instruments chemically (e.g., endoscopes, arthroscopes) was introduced in 1988. This microprocessor-controlled, low-temperature sterilization method is commonly used in the United States.[78] Interchangeable trays are available to enable the processing of up to three rigid endoscopes or one flexible endoscope. Connectors are available for most types of flexible endoscopes for the irrigation of all channels by directed flow. Rigid endoscopes are placed within a lidded container, and the sterilant fills the lumens either by immersion in the circulating sterilant or by use of channel connectors to direct the flow into the lumen or lumens (the importance of channel connectors is discussed later). As with any sterilization process, the system can sterilize only surfaces that can be contacted by the sterilant. For example, bronchoscopy-related infections occurred when bronchoscopes were processed with the wrong connector.[135,136] The importance of channel connectors to achieve sterilization was also demonstrated for rigid lumen devices.[193,209]

The manufacturers suggest the use of biologic monitors (*G. stearothermophilus* spore strips) both at the time of installation and routinely to ensure effectiveness of the process. The manufacturer's clip must be used to hold the strip in the designated spot in the machine, because a broader clamp will not allow the sterilant to reach the spores trapped under it.[210] The processor is equipped with a conductivity probe that automatically aborts the cycle if the buffer system is not detected in a fresh container of the peracetic acid solution. A chemical monitoring strip that detects that the active ingredient is greater than 1500 ppm is available for routine use as an additional process control.

Peracetic acid will inactivate gram-positive and gram-negative bacteria, fungi, and yeasts in less than 5 minutes at less than 100 ppm. In the presence of organic matter, 200 to 500 ppm is required. For viruses, the dosage range is wide (12 to 2250 ppm); poliovirus is inactivated in yeast extract in 15 minutes with 1500 to 2250 ppm. Bacterial spores in suspension are inactivated in 15 seconds to 30 minutes with 500 to 10,000 ppm (0.05% to 1%).[99]

OSHA Blood-Borne Pathogen Standard

In December 1991, OSHA published a standard, "Occupational Exposure to Bloodborne Pathogens," for eliminating or minimizing occupational exposure to blood-borne pathogens.[211] One component of this requirement is that all equipment and all environmental and working surfaces be cleaned and decontaminated with an appropriate disinfectant after contact with blood or other potentially infectious materials. Although the OSHA standard does not specify the type of disinfectant or procedure, the original OSHA compliance document[212] suggested that a germicide must be tuberculocidal to kill the hepatitis B virus (HBV) (e.g., phenolic, chlorine). However, in February 1997, OSHA amended its policy[213] and stated that EPA-registered disinfectants that are labeled as effective against HIV and HBV would be considered as appropriate disinfectants "... provided such surfaces have not become contaminated with agent(s) or volumes of or concentrations of agent(s) for which higher level disinfection is recommended." For cases in which blood-borne pathogens other than HBV or HIV are of concern, OSHA continues to require the use of EPA-registered tuberculocidal disinfectants or hypochlorite solution (diluted 1:10 or 1:100 with water).[68,213] Studies have demonstrated that, in the presence of large blood spills, a 1:10 final dilution of EPA-registered hypochlorite solution should initially be used to inactivate blood-borne viruses[43,214] to minimize risk of disease to the health care worker from percutaneous injury during the clean-up process.

EMERGING PATHOGENS

Emerging pathogens are of growing concern to the general public and infection control professionals. Relevant pathogens include *Cryptosporidium parvum*, *Helicobacter pylori*, *E. coli* O157:H7, rotavirus, human papillomavirus, norovirus, severe acute respiratory syndrome (SARS), coronavirus, avian influenza virus, Creutzfeldt-Jacob disease (CJD), and multidrug-resistant bacteria such as VRE and MRSA. The susceptibility of each of these pathogens to chemical disinfectants and sterilants has been studied. With the exceptions discussed as follows, all of these emerging pathogens are susceptible to currently available chemical disinfectants and sterilants.[215]

Cryptosporidium is resistant to chlorine at concentrations used in potable water. *C. parvum* is not completely inactivated by most disinfectants used in health care, including ethyl alcohol,[88] glutaraldehyde,[88,216] 5.25% hypochlorite,[88] peracetic acid,[88] OPA,[88] phenol,[88,216] povidone-iodine,[88,216] and quaternary ammonium compounds.[88] The only chemical disinfectants and sterilants able to inactivate greater than 3 $\log_{10}$ of *C. parvum* organisms were 6% and 7.5% hydrogen peroxide.[88] Sterilization methods—including steam,[88] ETO,[88,217] and hydrogen peroxide gas plasma—fully inactivate *C. parvum*.[88] Although

most disinfectants are ineffective against *C. parvum*, current cleaning and disinfection practices appear satisfactory to prevent health care–associated transmission. For example, endoscopes are unlikely to represent an important vehicle for the transmission of *C. parvum* because, according to the results of bacterial studies, mechanical cleaning removes approximately 10^4 organisms, and drying rapidly results in loss of *C. parvum* viability (e.g., at 30 minutes, there is a 2.9 $\log_{10}$ decrease, and at 60 minutes, a 3.8 $\log_{10}$ decrease).[88]

Chlorine at approximately 1 ppm has been found capable of eliminating approximately 4 $\log_{10}$ of *E. coli* O157:H7 organisms within 1 minute in a suspension test.[218] Electrolyzed oxidizing water at 23°C was effective in 10 minutes in producing a 5 $\log_{10}$ decrease in *E. coli* O157:H7 organisms inoculated onto kitchen cutting boards.[219] The following disinfectants eliminated more than 5 $\log_{10}$ of *E. coli* O157:H7 within 30 seconds: a quaternary ammonium compound, a phenolic, a hypochlorite (1:10 dilution of 5.25% bleach), and ethanol.[37]

Data on the susceptibility of *H. pylori* to disinfectants are available. Using a suspension test, Akamatsu and colleagues assessed the effectiveness of a variety of disinfectants against nine strains of *H. pylori*.[220] Ethanol (80%) and glutaraldehyde (0.5%) killed all strains within 15 seconds; chlorhexidine gluconate (0.05% and 1.0%), benzalkonium chloride (0.025% and 0.1%), alkyldiaminoethylglycine hydrochloride (0.1%), povidone-iodine (0.1%), and sodium hypochlorite (150 ppm) killed all strains within 30 seconds. In the presence of organic matter, both ethanol (80%) and glutaraldehyde (0.5%) retained similar bactericidal activity, but the other disinfectants had reduced bactericidal activity. In particular, the bactericidal activity of povidone-iodine (0.1%) and sodium hypochlorite (150 ppm) was markedly decreased in the presence of dried yeast solution: killing times increased to 5 to 10 minutes and 5 to 30 minutes, respectively. Disinfection of experimentally contaminated endoscopes with 2% glutaraldehyde (10-, 20-, and 45-minute exposure times) or with the peracetic acid system (with and without active peracetic acid) has been demonstrated to be effective in eliminating *H. pylori*.[221] Epidemiologic investigations of patients who had undergone endoscopy with endoscopes mechanically washed and disinfected with 2.0% to 2.3% glutaraldehyde have revealed no evidence of person-to-person transmission of *H. pylori* infection.[222,223]

An outbreak of health care–associated rotavirus gastroenteritis on a pediatric unit has been reported.[224] Person-to-person transmission via the hands of health care workers was proposed as the mechanism of spread. Prolonged survival of rotavirus on environmental surfaces (90 minutes to more than 10 days at room temperature) and hands (>4 hours) has been demonstrated. Rotavirus suspended in feces can survive for a longer time.[225,226] Vectors for this infection have included air, hands, fomites, water, and food.[226] Products with demonstrated efficacy (>3 $\log_{10}$ reduction in virus) against rotavirus within 1 minute include 95% ethanol, 70% isopropanol, some phenolics, 2% glutaraldehyde, 0.35% peracetic acid, and some quaternary ammonium compounds.[41,227-229] In a human challenge study, a disinfectant spray (0.1% ortho-phenylphenol and 79% ethanol), sodium hypochlorite (800 ppm free chlorine), and a phenol-based product (14.7% phenol diluted 1:256 in tap water) was sprayed onto contaminated stainless steel disks; this was effective in interrupting the transfer of a human rotavirus from stainless steel disk to finger pads of volunteers after an exposure time of 3 to 10 minutes. A quaternary ammonium product (7.05% quaternary ammonium compound diluted 1:128 in tap water) and tap water allowed transfer of virus.[36]

Data on the inactivation of human papillomavirus by disinfectants are limited because in vitro replication of complete virions has not been achieved. However, studies with the bovine papillomavirus have shown a 99.9% inactivation with a 0.3% povidone-iodine solution.[230] The effect of chlorine on the H5N1 subtype of the avian influenza virus was evaluated. Free chlorine concentrations typically used in drinking water treatment (0.52 to 1.08 ppm) were sufficient to inactivate the virus by more than 3 $\log_{10}$ with an exposure time of 1 minute.[231]

More is known about the inactivation of norovirus (members of the family *Caliciviridae* and important causes of gastroenteritis in humans) even though they cannot be grown in tissue culture. Improper disinfection of environmental surfaces contaminated by the feces or vomitus of infected patients is believed to play a role in the spread of noroviruses in some settings.[232,233] Prolonged survival of a norovirus surrogate (i.e., feline calicivirus [FCV], a closely related cultivable virus) has been demonstrated (e.g., at room temperature, FCV in a dried state survived 18 to 21 days).[155] Inactivation studies with FCV have shown the effectiveness of chlorine, glutaraldehyde, and iodine-based products, whereas a quaternary ammonium compound, detergent, and ethanol were less effective.[155] Sattar[234] also evaluated the effectiveness of several disinfectants against FCV and found that bleach, diluted to 1000 ppm of available chlorine, reduced infectivity of FCV by 4.5 logs in 1 minute. Other effective (>10,000 fold reduction in virus) disinfectants included accelerated hydrogen peroxide, 5000 ppm (3 minutes); chlorine dioxide, 1000 ppm chlorine (1 minute); a mixture of four quaternary ammonium compounds, 2470 ppm (10 minutes); 79% ethanol with 0.1% quaternary ammonium compound (3 minutes); and 75% ethanol (10 minutes).[234] Gehrke and coworkers showed that 70% ethanol and 70% 1-propanol reduced FCV by 3 to 4 $\log_{10}$ in 30 seconds.[235]

The CDC announced that a previously unrecognized coronavirus in humans is the cause of SARS.[236] Two coronaviruses that are known to infect humans causes approximately one third of common colds and may cause gastroenteritis. The virucidal efficacy of chemical germicides against coronavirus has been investigated. Sattar and colleagues,[237] investigating the activity of disinfectants against coronavirus 229E, found that several disinfectants were effective after a 1-minute contact time: sodium hypochlorite (at a free chlorine concentration of 1000 ppm and 5000 ppm), 70% ethyl alcohol, and povidone-iodine (1% iodine). Saknimit and coworkers[238] showed that 70% ethanol, 50% isopropanol, 0.05% benzalkonium chloride, 50 ppm iodine in iodophor, 0.23% sodium chlorite, 1% cresol soap, and 0.7% formaldehyde inactivated more than 3 logs of two animal coronaviruses (mouse hepatitis virus, canine coronavirus) after a 10-minute exposure time. Sizun and associates demonstrated the activity of povidone-iodine against human coronaviruses 229E and OC43.[239] Because the SARS coronavirus is stable in feces and urine at room temperature for at least 1 to 2 days,[239a] surfaces may be a possible source of contamination and lead to infection with the SARS coronavirus; therefore, they should be disinfected. Until more precise information is available, the environment in which SARS patients are housed is assumed to be heavily contaminated, and the room and equipment should be thoroughly disinfected daily and after the patient is discharged. EPA-registered disinfectants or 1:100 dilution of household bleach and water should be used for surface disinfection and disinfection on noncritical equipment used in patient care. High-level disinfection and sterilization of semicritical and critical medical devices, respectively, do not need to be altered for patients with known or suspected SARS.

The prions of CJD and other transmissible spongiform encephalopathies exhibit an unusual resistance to conventional chemical and physical decontamination methods. Because the CJD agent is not readily inactivated by conventional disinfection and sterilization procedures and because of the invariably fatal outcome of CJD, the procedures for disinfection and sterilization of the CJD prion have been both cautious and controversial for many years. For disinfection and sterilization of prion-contaminated medical devices, instruments should be kept wet or damp until they are decontaminated, and they should be decontaminated as soon as possible after use. Dried films of tissue are more resistant to prion inactivation by steam sterilization than are tissues that were kept moist. This may be because of the rapid heating that occurs in the film of dried material in comparison with the bulk of the sample and the rapid fixation of the prion protein in the dried film.[240] It also appears that prions in the dried portions of the brain macerates are less efficiently inactivated than those in undisturbed tissue. For high-risk tissues (brain, spinal cord, and eyes), high-risk patients known or suspected to be infected with CJD, and critical or semicritical medical devices, recommendations are to clean the device and sterilize it by one of four methods, with a combination of sodium hydroxide and autoclave as recommended by the World Health Organization[241] (option 1 or 2) or use of the autoclave as recommended in the scientific literature[242] (option 3 or 4):

1. Immerse in a solution of 40 g NaOH in 1 L of water for 1 hour; remove and rinse in water, then transfer to an open pan and put in autoclave [121°C gravity displacement or 134°C porous or prevacuum sterilizer] for 1 hour.
2. Immerse instruments in 40 g of NaOH in 1 L of water for 1 hour and heat in a gravity displacement sterilizer at 121°C for 30 minutes. (However, the combination of sodium hydroxide and steam sterilization may be deleterious to surgical instruments, sterilizers, as well as harmful to sterilizer operators who would be breathing vaporized chemicals unless engineering controls or use of personal protective equipment prevents exposure.[243])
3. Place in autoclave at 134°C for 18 minutes in a prevacuum sterilizer.
4. Place in autoclave at 132°C (270°F) for 1 hour in a gravity displacement sterilizer.

The temperature should not exceed 134°C (273°F) because under certain conditions, the effectiveness of the autoclave actually declines as the temperature is increased (e.g., 136°C [277°F] or 138°C [280°F]).[244] Prion-contaminated medical devices that are impossible or difficult to clean should be discarded. Flash sterilization should not be used for reprocessing. To minimize environmental contamination, noncritical environmental surfaces should be covered with plastic-backed paper; when the paper is contaminated with high-risk tissues, it should be properly discarded. Environmental surfaces (noncritical) contaminated with high-risk tissues (e.g., laboratory surfaces) should be cleaned and then spot decontaminated with a 1:10 dilution of hypochlorite solutions.

Neurosurgical instruments may be contaminated during procedures performed on patients in whom CJD is later diagnosed. To minimize the possibility that these instruments will be reused, health care facilities should consider using the sterilization guidelines outlined above for neurosurgical instruments used during brain biopsy in patients in whom a specific lesion has not been demonstrated (e.g., by magnetic resonance imaging or computerized tomographic scans). Alternatively, neurosurgical instruments used in such patients could be disposable[242] or quarantined until the pathologic review of the brain biopsy rules out CJD.

No data have shown that antibiotic-resistant bacteria are less sensitive to the liquid chemical germicides than are antibiotic-sensitive bacteria at currently used germicide contact conditions and concentrations.[245] Several studies have revealed antibiotic-resistant hospital strains of common health care–associated pathogens (e.g., *Enterococcus* species, *P. aeruginosa*, *Klebsiella pneumoniae*, *E. coli*, *Staphylococcus aureus*, and *Staphylococcus epidermidis*) to be equally susceptible to disinfectants as are antibiotic-sensitive strains.[37,246-248] The susceptibility of glycopeptide-intermediate *S. aureus* was similar to vancomycin-susceptible MRSA.[249] On the basis of these data, routine disinfection and housekeeping protocols do not need to be altered, because of antibiotic resistance provided the disinfection method is effective.[250,251] In evaluating the efficacy of selected cleaning methods (e.g., quaternary ammonium compound–sprayed cloth, and quaternary ammonium compound–immersed cloth) for eliminating VRE, Rutala and associates found that currently used disinfection processes are probably highly effective in eliminating VRE. Despite the in vitro effectiveness of disinfectants, it is critical that the disinfectant have contact with the contaminated surface in order to remove or inactivate the pathogen.[250]

Inactivation of Bioterrorist Agents

Concern about the potential for biologic terrorism has escalated.[252,253] The CDC has categorized several agents as "high priority" because they can be easily disseminated or transmitted person to person, cause high rates of mortality, and are likely to cause public panic and social disruption.[254] These agents include *Bacillus anthracis* (anthrax), *Yersinia pestis* (plague), variola major (smallpox), *Clostridium botulinum* toxin (botulism), *Francisella tularensis* (tularemia), filoviruses (Ebola hemorrhagic fever, Marburg hemorrhagic fever); and arenaviruses (Lassa [Lassa fever], Junin [Argentine hemorrhagic fever]).[254]

A few comments regarding the role of sterilization and disinfection of potential agents of bioterrorism can be made. First, the susceptibility of these agents to germicides in vitro is similar to that of other related pathogens. For example, variola is similar to vaccinia[113] and *B. anthracis* is similar to *B. atrophaeus* (a close relative of *Bacillus subtilis*).[255] Thus, the susceptibility of genetically similar organisms can be extrapolated from the larger database available. Second, many of the potential bioterrorist agents are stable enough in the environment that contaminated environmental surfaces or fomites could lead to transmission of agents such as *B. anthracis*, *F. tularensis*, variola major, *C. botulinum* toxin, and *Coxiella burnetii*.[256] Third, data suggest that current disinfection and sterilization practices are appropriate for the management of equipment used in patient care and of environmental surfaces when potentially contaminated patients are evaluated or admitted in a health care facility after exposure to a bioterrorist agent. For example, sodium hypochlorite may be used for surface disinfection (see U.S. Environmental Protection Agency [EPA] fact sheet[256a]). In instances in which the health care facility is the site of a bioterrorist attack, environmental decontamination may require special decontamination procedures (e.g., chlorine dioxide gas for anthrax spores[256b]). Use of disinfectants for decontamination after a bioterrorist attack requires crises exemption from the EPA.[256c] Of only theoretical concern is the possibility that a bioterrorist agent could be engineered to be less susceptible to disinfection and sterilization processes.

Current Issues in Disinfection and Sterilization

As mentioned, the Spaulding classification scheme enables categorization of medical devices on the basis of risk of infection involved with use. The categories of medical devices are critical, semicritical, and noncritical. Several issues in disinfection and sterilization are discussed in the appropriate risk category.

For critical items (which enter sterile tissue) that require sterilization, two new sterilization processes are likely to be integrated into health care for sterilization of heat-sensitive medical materials and devices. One involves nonthermal plasma (Plasma-Sol), which is produced at atmospheric temperature and pressure, generates sterilants that kill concentrations of microorganisms, and inactivates viruses during a 10-minute exposure.[257] The other new sterilization process involves vaporized hydrogen peroxide (Amsco V-PRO 1). It has also shown to be effective in killing a wide range of microorganisms[258] and is intended for use as a low-temperature sterilization process of properly prepared reusable metal and nonmetal medical devices. In addition, a new EPA rule requires the following actions: make sure to run full loads in ETO sterilizers; run partial loads if it is medically necessary; and when loads are not full, note the medical reasons and who authorized the partial load.

Several issues affect the reprocessing of semicritical items (which touch mucous membranes), such as endoscopes, endocavitary probes, and laryngoscopes. First, new high-level disinfectants include a solution of 2% accelerated hydrogen peroxide,[107] one of 8.3% hydrogen peroxide with 7.0% peracetic acid, and one of 3.4% glutaraldehyde with 26% isopropanol.[259] Second, because breaches of high-level disinfection and sterilization guidelines are not uncommon, a 14-step protocol was developed to aid infection control professionals in the evaluation of potential disinfection and sterilization failures.[260] Third, to prevent disease transmission associated with laryngoscopes, prostate biopsy probes, and endoscopes, reprocessing of the device must be adequate. Several writers have reviewed the recommendations for reprocessing semicritical medical devices that have been associated with disease transmission.[261-264]

With regard to the disinfection of noncritical items such as environmental surfaces, there are several noteworthy observations. First, and of importance, Carling and colleagues used an invisible fluorescent targeting method that assessed whether frequently touched objects in a patient's room were cleaned as part of terminal disinfection procedure.[265] They found that of a standardized set of 14 objects, 50% were not cleaned at all. This information should be used to develop focused administrative and educational interventions that incorporate ongoing feedback to the environmental services staff to improve cleaning and disinfection practices. For example, health care facilities may need to introduce the use of checklists or other tools (e.g., invisible fluorescent dyes) to ensure complete cleaning of all potentially contaminated surfaces. The inadequacy of terminal room disinfection probably explains why admission to a room previously occupied by an MRSA-positive patient or a VRE-positive patient significantly increased the odds of acquisition for MRSA and VRE.[266] These observations highlight the importance of cleaning all surfaces and all accessible equipment each time cleaning is done in patient rooms. Second, health care facilities have started to use microfiber mops, rather than conventional cotton string mops, to clean floors. The microfiber mops demonstrated superior microbial removal over cotton string mops when used with a detergent cleaner.[46] Third, an accelerated hydrogen peroxide product (0.5%) that reportedly has virucidal, bactericidal, fungicidal, and tuberculocidal activity has been introduced into the United States for disinfection of noncritical environmental surfaces and equipment.[106]

CONTROL OF HOSPITAL WASTE

Health care facilities that generate medical, chemical, or radiologic waste have a moral and legal obligation to dispose of this waste in a manner that poses minimal potential hazard to the environment or public health. The proper disposal of this waste requires a dynamic waste management plan that conforms to federal, state, and local regulations and has adequate personnel and financial resources to ensure implementation.

Medical waste disposal has been a major problem in the United States since the 1970s. The problem accelerated as a result of both medical waste's washing ashore in some coastal states in 1987 and 1988 and the perceived threat of acquiring HIV infection through this waste. This has led to restrictive rules governing the disposal of medical waste in many states and an increase in the volume of waste defined as regulated medical waste. Coincidentally, with an increase in volume of regulated medical waste (formerly called *infectious waste*), the options for medical waste treatment and disposal are diminishing because of space and environmental concerns. This section reviews some of the principles of medical waste management, but a more detailed description of collection, storage, processing, transporting, treatment, and public health implications of medical waste may be found elsewhere.[267-271]

Despite the attention given to medical waste by the public, the media, and all levels of government, the terms *hospital waste*, *medical waste*, *regulated medical waste*, and *infectious waste* are often used as synonyms. Hospital waste is all biologic and nonbiologic waste that is discarded and not intended for further use. Medical waste is materials generated as a result of patient diagnosis, immunization, or treatment, such as soiled dressings or intravenous tubing. Infectious waste is the portion of medical waste that could potentially transmit an infectious disease. The U.S. Congress and the EPA used the term *regulated medical waste* rather than *infectious waste* in the Medical Waste Tracking Act of 1988 in deference to the remote possibility of disease transmission associated with this waste. Thus, "medical waste" is a subset of "hospital waste," and "regulated medical waste" (which is synonymous with "infectious waste" from a regulatory perspective) is a subset of "medical waste."[267]

As stated, regulated medical waste (infectious waste) is capable of producing an infectious disease. This definition requires a consideration of the factors necessary for disease induction, which include dose, host susceptibility, presence of a pathogen, virulence of a pathogen, and the most commonly absent factor, a portal of entry. For a waste to be infectious, therefore, it must contain pathogens with sufficient virulence and quantity so that a susceptible host's exposure to the waste could result in an infectious disease. Because there are no tests that allow infectious waste to be identified objectively, responsible agencies (such as the CDC, EPA, or states) define waste as infectious when it is suspected to contain pathogens in sufficient number to cause disease. Not only does this subjective definition result in conflicting opinions from the CDC, EPA, and state agencies on what constitutes infectious waste and how it should be treated but it also unduly emphasizes the mere presence of pathogens.

Guidelines produced by the CDC have designated five types of hospital waste as regulated medical waste (i.e., microbiology laboratory waste, pathology and anatomy waste, contaminated animal carcasses, blood, and sharps).[30] According to the EPA guidelines, the same types of waste are infectious or regulated medical waste but communicable disease isolation waste is also designated.[270] In the Medical Waste Tracking Act, the EPA modified its position on "communicable disease isolation waste" by including only certain "highly" communicable disease waste such as class 4 (e.g., Marburg, Ebola, and Lassa viruses) as regulated medical waste[272] (Table 301-4). In a systematic random survey of all U.S. hospitals conducted in July 1987 and January 1988, the rates of overall compliance with the CDC and EPA recommendations were 82% and 75%, respectively. Not only were the majority of hospitals in compliance but also the hospitals frequently treated other hospital waste as infectious, including contaminated laboratory waste (87%), surgery waste (78%), dialysis waste (69%), items contacting secretions (63%), intensive care waste (37%), and emergency room waste (41%).[267]

A key component in evaluating the impact of a medical waste management program is the quantity of waste produced per patient. Hospitalized patients generate about 7 kg (15 pounds) of hospital waste per day. The amount of hospital waste generated by U.S. hospitals is more than 6 million kilograms ($\approx$ 6700 tons) per day. U.S. hospitals designate approximately 15% of the total hospital waste by weight as infectious (more than 900,000 kg [about 1000 tons] of infectious waste per day).[267] Not surprisingly, the percentage of medical waste treated as infectious increases with the number and types of medical waste

TABLE 301-4	Types of Medical Waste Designated as Infectious and Recommended Disposal or Treatment Methods: CDC and EPA*				
Source or Type of Medical Waste	**Centers for Disease Control and Prevention (CDC)**[30]		**U.S. Environmental Protection Agency (EPA)**[270]		*Medical Waste Tracking Act*[272]*: Infectious Waste*[†]
	Infectious Waste Methods	*Disposal/Treatment*	*Infectious Waste Methods*	*Disposal/Treatment*	
Microbiologic (e.g., stocks and cultures of infectious agents)	Yes	Steam sterilization Incineration	Yes	Steam sterilization Incineration Thermal inactivation Chemical disinfection for liquids only	Yes
Blood and blood products	Yes	Steam sterilization Incineration Sanitary sewer (EPA requires secondary treatment)	Yes	Steam sterilization Incineration Sanitary sewer (EPA requires secondary treatment) Chemical disinfection for liquids only	Yes
Pathologic (e.g., tissue, organs)	Yes	Incineration	Yes	Incineration Steam sterilization with incineration or grinding Cremation or burial by mortician	Yes
Sharps (e.g., needles)	Yes	Steam sterilization Incineration	Yes	Steam sterilization Incineration	Yes[‡]
Communicable disease isolation	No	—	Yes	Steam sterilization Incineration	Yes[‡]
Contaminated animal carcasses, body parts, and bedding	Yes	Steam sterilization Incineration (carcasses)	Yes	Incineration Steam sterilization with incineration or grinding (not bedding)	Yes
Contaminated laboratory wastes	No	—	Optional[§]	If considered infectious waste, use steam sterilization or incineration	No
Surgery and autopsy wastes	No	—	Optional	If considered infectious waste, use steam sterilization or incineration	No
Dialysis unit	No	—	Optional	If considered infectious waste, use steam sterilization or incineration	No
Contaminated equipment	No	—	Optional	If considered infectious waste, use steam sterilization or incineration	No

*The Joint Commission for the Accreditation of Healthcare Organizations requires the presence of a hazardous waste system designed and operated in accordance with applicable law and regulations.
[†]The Act went into effect on June 22, 1989, and expired June 22, 1991. It affected only four states (New Jersey, New York, Connecticut, and Rhode Island). The Act required both treatment (any method, technique, or process designed to change the biologic character or composition of medical waste so as to eliminate or reduce its potential for causing disease) and destruction (waste is ruined, torn apart, or mutilated so that it is no longer generally recognizable as medical waste).
[‡]Medical Waste Tracking Act specified used and unused sharps. The Act regulated wastes from persons with highly communicable diseases such as those caused by class 4 etiologic agents (e.g., Marburg, Ebola, Lassa).
[§]The EPA stated that the decision to handle optional infectious waste as infectious should be made by a responsible, authorized person or committee at the individual facility.
From Rutala WA, Mayhall CG, Society of Hospital Epidemiology of America. Position paper: medical waste. *Infect Control Hosp Epidemiol.* 1992;13;38-48.

classified as infectious. For example, about 6% of hospital waste would be treated as infectious waste if the CDC guidelines are followed, but 45% of hospital waste could be considered infectious waste under the Medical Waste Tracking Act.[267,273]

Most U.S. hospitals designate and treat microbiologic, pathologic, isolation, blood, and sharp waste as infectious.[267] In the late 1980s, treatment of infectious waste by U.S. hospitals was most commonly accomplished by incineration (64% to 93%, depending on type of waste), but emission regulations that limit air pollutants has reduced the number and the use of incineration for medical waste. For example, in September 1997, there were an estimated 2373 medical waste incinerators in the United States, but in 2003, there were 115 medical waste incinerators (F. L. Porter, written communication, 2003). Autoclaves or steam sterilizers have become the primary nonincineration technology used by hospital to process their regulated medical waste (except pathology waste) (E. Krisiunas, written communication, 2008). Several other nonincineration alternatives have been proposed for treating regulated medical waste (e.g., mechanical and chemical disinfection, microwave decontamination, steam disinfection, and compacting).[271] Nonregulated medical waste is generally discarded in a properly sited and operated sanitary landfill because this is a safe and inexpensive disposal method (e.g., landfill disposal costs $0.02 to $0.05 per pound, whereas contract incinerators cost $0.20 to $0.60 per pound).

The conflicting opinions of state and federal regulations are related to the paucity of microbiologic and epidemiologic evidence that medical waste represents a threat to the public health. First, with the exception of "sharps" such as needles, which have caused disease only in an occupational setting, there is no scientific evidence that medical waste has caused disease in the hospital or the community. Second, data demonstrate that household waste contains, on average, 100 times as many microorganisms with pathogenic potential for humans as

does medical waste.[274] Third, detailed reports of the beach wash-ups revealed that most waste on beaches was debris (about 99%) such as wood, plastic, and paper, not medical waste. EPA documents acknowledged that much of the medical waste that washed ashore in the summer of 1988 was syringe related (65%) and had been used in home health care and illegal drug use. Fourth, studies have shown that most U.S. hospitals are in compliance with the CDC infectious waste guidelines. Fifth, although the principal purpose of the Medical Waste Tracking Act was to reduce medical waste on beaches, its intended benefit has not been demonstrated. The relative number of syringes on the beaches in states affected by the Medical Waste Tracking Act was significantly greater during implementation of the Act (17.23%) than before the Act went into effect (3.2%).[273] If regulatory control were based on epidemiologic, microbiologic, and environmental data, only two types of medical waste would require special handling and treatment: sharps and microbiologic waste.

Federal medical waste regulations have been promulgated by the Department of Transportation (DOT) and OSHA. The DOT regulation involves the transport of infectious substances and medical waste and went into effect January 1996.[275] The OSHA Bloodborne Pathogen Standard requires labeling to designate waste that poses a health threat in the workplace. The OSHA definition of regulated waste is not intended to designate waste that must be treated. In fact, if the OSHA definition of regulated waste (rather than state regulations) is applied to designate infectious waste for treatment by incineration or other means, additional expenses may be incurred unintentionally.[211]

Conclusion

When properly used, disinfection and sterilization can ensure the safe use of invasive and noninvasive medical devices. However, current disinfection and sterilization guidelines must be strictly followed.

REFERENCES

1. Centers for Disease Control and Prevention. *Ambulatory and inpatient procedures in the United States, 1996.* Atlanta, GA: Centers for Disease Control and Prevention; 1998:1-39.
2. American Society for Gastrointestinal Endoscopy. Position statement: reprocessing of flexible gastrointestinal endoscopes. *Gastrointest Endosc.* 1996;43:541-546.
3. Uttley AH, Simpson RA. Audit of bronchoscope disinfection: a survey of procedures in England and Wales and incidents of mycobacterial contamination. *J Hosp Infect.* 1994;26:301-308.
4. Spach DH, Silverstein FE, Stamm WE. Transmission of infection by gastrointestinal endoscopy and bronchoscopy. *Ann Intern Med.* 1993;118:117-128.
5. Weber DJ, Rutala WA. Lessons from outbreaks associated with bronchoscopy. *Infect Control Hosp Epidemiol.* 2001;22:403-408.
6. Weber DJ, Rutala WA, DiMarino AJ Jr. The prevention of infection following gastrointestinal endoscopy: the importance of prophylaxis and reprocessing. In: DiMarino AJ Jr, Benjamin SB, eds. *Gastrointestinal Diseases: An Endoscopic Approach.* Thorofare, NJ: Slack Inc.; 2002:87-106.
7. Meyers H, Brown-Elliott BA, Moore D, et al. An outbreak of *Mycobacterium chelonae* infection following liposuction. *Clin Infect Dis.* 2002;34:1500-1507.
8. Lowry PW, Jarvis WR, Oberle AD, et al. *Mycobacterium chelonae* causing otitis media in an ear-nose-and-throat practice. *N Engl J Med.* 1988;319:978-982.
9. Favero MS, Bond WW. Chemical disinfection of medical and surgical materials. In: Block SS, ed. *Disinfection, Sterilization, and Preservation.* 5th ed. Philadelphia: Lippincott Williams & Wilkins; 2001:881-917.
10. Spaulding EH. Chemical disinfection of medical and surgical materials. In: Lawrence C, Block SS, eds. *Disinfection, Sterilization, and Preservation.* Philadelphia: Lea & Febiger; 1968:517-531.
11. Simmons BP. CDC guidelines for the prevention and control of nosocomial infections. Guideline for hospital environmental control. *Am J Infect Control.* 1983;11:97-120.
12. Block SS, ed. *Disinfection, Sterilization, and Preservation.* 5th ed. Philadelphia: Lippincott Williams & Wilkins; 2001.
13. Rutala WA, 1994, 1995, and 1996 APIC Guidelines Committee. APIC guideline for selection and use of disinfectants. Association for Professionals in Infection Control and Epidemiology, Inc. *Am J Infect Control.* 1996;24:313-342.
14. Rutala WA. Disinfection, sterilization and waste disposal. In: Wenzel RP, ed. *Prevention and Control of Nosocomial Infections.* Baltimore: Williams & Wilkins; 1997:539-593.

15. Garner JS, Favero MS. CDC guideline for handwashing and hospital environmental control, 1985. *Infect Control.* 1986;7:231-243.
16. Rutala WA. APIC guideline for selection and use of disinfectants. *Am J Infect Control.* 1990;18:99-117.
17. Rutala WA, Weber DJ, Healthcare Infection Control Practices Advisory Committee. Guideline for disinfection and sterilization in healthcare facilities, 2008. cdc.gov/ncidod/dhqp/pdf/guidelines/Disinfection_Nov_2008.pdf.
18. Foliente RL, Kovacs BJ, Aprecio RM, et al. Efficacy of high-level disinfectants for reprocessing gastrointestinal endoscopes in simulated-use testing. *Gastrointest Endosc.* 2001;53:456-462.
19. Kovacs BJ, Chen YK, Kettering JD, et al. High-level disinfection of gastrointestinal endoscopes: are current guidelines adequate? *Am J Gastroenterol.* 1999;94:1546-1550.
20. Rutala WA, Clontz EP, Weber DJ, et al. Disinfection practices for endoscopes and other semicritical items. *Infect Control Hosp Epidemiol.* 1991;12:282-288.
21. Phillips J, Hulka B, Hulka J, et al. Laparoscopic procedures: the American Association of Gynecologic Laparoscopists' membership survey for 1975. *J Reprod Med.* 1977;18:227-232.
22. Muscarella LF. Current instrument reprocessing practices: results of a national survey. *Gastrointest Nurs.* 2001;24:253-260.
23. Wallace RJ Jr, Brown BA, Griffith DE. Nosocomial outbreaks/pseudo-outbreaks caused by nontuberculous mycobacteria. *Annu Rev Microbiol.* 1998;52:453-490.
24. Meenhorst PL, Reingold AL, Groothuis DG, et al. Water-related nosocomial pneumonia caused by *Legionella pneumophila* serogroups 1 and 10. *J Infect Dis.* 1985;152:356-364.
25. Atlas RM. *Legionella*: from environmental habitats to disease pathology, detection and control. *Environ Microbiol.* 1999;1:283-293.
26. Rutala WA, Weber DJ. Water as a reservoir of nosocomial pathogens. *Infect Control Hosp Epidemiol.* 1997;18:609-616.
27. Weber DJ, Rutala WA. Environmental issues and nosocomial infections. In: Wenzel RP, ed. *Prevention and Control of Nosocomial Infections.* Baltimore: Williams & Wilkins; 1997:491-514.
28. Society of Gastroenterology Nurses and Associates. Standards for infection control and reprocessing of flexible gastrointestinal endoscopes. *Gastroenterol Nurs.* 2000;23:172-179.
29. Gerding DN, Peterson LR, Vennes JA. Cleaning and disinfection of fiberoptic endoscopes: evaluation of glutaraldehyde exposure time and forced-air drying. *Gastroenterology.* 1982;83:613-618.

30. Centers for Disease Control and Prevention. Guidelines for environmental infection control in health-care facilities, 2003. *MMWR.* 2003;52(No. RR-10):1-44.
31. Sattar SA, Lloyd-Evans N, Springthorpe VS, et al. Institutional outbreaks of rotavirus diarrhoea: potential role of fomites and environmental surfaces as vehicles for virus transmission. *J Hyg (Lond).* 1986;96:277-289.
32. Weber DJ, Rutala WA. Role of environmental contamination in the transmission of vancomycin-resistant enterococci. *Infect Control Hosp Epidemiol.* 1997;18:306-309.
33. Ward RL, Bernstein DI, Knowlton DR, et al. Prevention of surface-to-human transmission of rotaviruses by treatment with disinfectant spray. *J Clin Microbiol.* 1991;29:1991-1996.
34. Sattar SA, Jacobsen H, Springthorpe VS, et al. Chemical disinfection to interrupt transfer of rhinovirus type 14 from environmental surfaces to hands. *Appl Environ Microbiol.* 1993;59:1579-1585.
35. Gwaltney JM Jr, Hendley JO. Transmission of experimental rhinovirus infection by contaminated surfaces. *Am J Epidemiol.* 1982;116:828-833.
36. Sattar SA, Jacobsen H, Rahman H, et al. Interruption of rotavirus spread through chemical disinfection. *Infect Control Hosp Epidemiol.* 1994;15:751-756.
37. Rutala WA, Barbee SL, Aguiar NC, et al. Antimicrobial activity of home disinfectants and natural products against potential human pathogens. *Infect Control Hosp Epidemiol.* 2000;21:33-38.
38. Best M, Sattar SA, Springthorpe VS, et al. Efficacies of selected disinfectants against *Mycobacterium tuberculosis. J Clin Microbiol.* 1990;28:2234-2239.
39. Best M, Kennedy ME, Coates F. Efficacy of a variety of disinfectants against *Listeria* spp. *Appl Environ Microbiol.* 1990;56:377-380.
40. Best M, Springthorpe VS, Sattar SA. Feasibility of a combined carrier test for disinfectants: studies with a mixture of five types of microorganisms. *Am J Infect Control.* 1994;22:152-162.
41. Springthorpe VS, Grenier JL, Lloyd-Evans N, et al. Chemical disinfection of human rotaviruses: efficacy of commercially-available products in suspension tests. *J Hyg (Lond).* 1986;97:139-161.
42. Sattar SA, Springthorpe VS. Survival and disinfectant inactivation of the human immunodeficiency virus: a critical review. *Rev Infect Dis.* 1991;13:430-447.
43. Weber DJ, Barbee SL, Sobsey MD, et al. The effect of blood on the antiviral activity of sodium hypochlorite, a phenolic, and a

quaternary ammonium compound. *Infect Control Hosp Epidemiol.* 1999;20:821-827.

44. Pentella MA, Fisher T, Chandler S, et al. Are disinfectants accurately prepared for use in hospital patient care areas? *Infect Control Hosp Epidemiol.* 2000;21:103.
45. Rutala WA, White MS, Gergen MF, et al. Bacterial contamination of keyboards: efficacy and functional impact of disinfectants. *Infect Control Hosp Epidemiol.* 2006;27:372-377.
46. Rutala WA, Gergen MF, Weber DJ. Microbiologic evaluation of microfiber mops for surface disinfection. *Am J Infect Control.* 2007;35:569-573.
47. Westwood JC, Mitchell MA, Legace S. Hospital sanitation: the massive bacterial contamination of the wet mop. *Appl Microbiol.* 1971;21:693-697.
48. U.S. Food and Drug Administration. *Public health notification from FDA, CDC, EPA and OSHA: avoiding hazards with using cleaners and disinfectants on electronic medical equipment.* Washington, DC: Department of Health & Human Services; 2007.
49. Weber DJ, Rutala WA. Occupational risks associated with the use of selected disinfectants and sterilants. In: Rutala WA, ed. *Disinfection, Sterilization, and Antisepsis in Healthcare.* Champlain, NY: Polyscience Publications; 1998:211-226.
50. Spaulding EH. Alcohol as a surgical disinfectant. *AORN J.* 1964;2:67-71.
51. Morton HE. The relationship of concentration and germicidal efficiency of ethyl alcohol. *Ann N Y Acad Sci.* 1950;53:191-196.
52. Ali Y, Dolan MJ, Fendler EJ, et al. Alcohols. In: Block SS, ed. *Disinfection, Sterilization, and Preservation.* 5th ed. Philadelphia: Lippincott Williams & Wilkins; 2001:229-254.
53. Nye RN, Mallory TB. A note on the fallacy of using alcohol for the sterilization of surgical instruments. *Boston Med Surg J.* 1923;189:561-563.
54. Rutala WA, Weber DJ. Selection and use of disinfectants in healthcare. In: Mayhall CG, ed. *Infection Control and Hospital Epidemiology.* Philadelphia: Lippincott Williams & Wilkins; 2004:1473-1522.
55. Rutala WA, Weber DJ. Uses of inorganic hypochlorite (bleach) in health-care facilities. *Clin Microbiol Rev.* 1997;10:597-610.
56. Merritt K, Hitchins VM, Brown SA. Safety and cleaning of medical materials and devices. *J Biomed Mater Res.* 2000;53:131-136.
57. Jakobsson SW, Rajs J, Jonsson JA, et al. Poisoning with sodium hypochlorite solution. Report of a fatal case, supplemented with an experimental and clinico-epidemiological study. *Am J Forensic Med Pathol.* 1991;12:320-327.
58. Heidemann SM, Goetting MG. Treatment of acute hypoxemic respiratory failure caused by chlorine exposure. *Pediatr Emerg Care.* 1991;7:87-88.
59. French RJ, Tabb HG, Rutledge LJ. Esophageal stenosis produced by ingestion of bleach: report of two cases. *South Med J.* 1970;63:1140-1144.
60. Ingram TA. Response of the human eye to accidental exposure to sodium hypochlorite. *J Endod.* 1990;16:235-238.
61. Mrvos R, Dean BS, Krenzelok EP. Home exposures to chlorine/chloramine gas: review of 216 cases. *South Med J.* 1993;86:654-657.
62. Rutala WA, Cole EC, Thomann CA, et al. Stability and bactericidal activity of chlorine solutions. *Infect Control Hosp Epidemiol.* 1998;19:323-327.
63. Sampson MN, Muir AV. Not all super-oxidized waters are the same [Comment]. *J Hosp Infect.* 2002;52:228-229.
64. Selkon JB, Babb JR, Morris R. Evaluation of the antimicrobial activity of a new super-oxidized water, Sterilox®, for the disinfection of endoscopes. *J Hosp Infect.* 1999;41:59-70.
65. Shetty N, Srinivasan S, Holton J, et al. Evaluation of microbicidal activity of a new disinfectant: Sterilox® 2500 against *Clostridium difficile* spores, *Helicobacter pylori,* vancomycin resistant *Enterococcus* species, *Candida albicans* and several *Mycobacterium* species. *J Hosp Infect.* 1999;41:101-105.
66. Nagington J, Sutehall GM, Whipp P. Tonometer disinfection and viruses. *Br J Ophthalmol.* 1983;67:674-676.
67. Centers for Disease Control. Acquired immune deficiency syndrome (AIDS): precautions for clinical and laboratory staffs. *MMWR Morb Mortal Wkly Rep.* 1982;31:577-580.
68. Centers for Disease Control. Recommendations for prevention of HIV transmission in health-care settings. *MMWR Morb Mortal Wkly Rep.* 1987;36(Suppl. 2):1S-18S.
69. Centers for Disease Control. Guidelines for prevention of transmission of human immunodeficiency virus and hepatitis B virus to health-care and public-safety workers. *MMWR Morb Mortal Wkly Rep.* 1989;38(Suppl. 6):1-37.
70. Garner JS, Simmons BP. Guideline for isolation precautions in hospitals. *Infect Control.* 1983;4:245-325.
71. Bloomfield SF, Miller EA. A comparison of hypochlorite and phenolic disinfectants for disinfection of clean and soiled surfaces and blood spillages. *J Hosp Infect.* 1989;13:231-239.
72. Rutala WA, Weber DJ. Disinfection of endoscopes: review of new chemical sterilants used for high-level disinfection. *Infect Control Hosp Epidemiol.* 1999;20:69-76.
73. Rutala WA, Peacock JE, Gergen MF, et al. Efficacy of hospital germicides against adenovirus 8, a common cause of epidemic keratoconjunctivitis in health care facilities. *Antimicrob Agents Chemother.* 2006;50:1419-1424.
74. Gerding DN, Muto CA, Owens RC Jr. Measures to control and prevent *Clostridium difficile* infection. *Clin Infect Dis.* 2008;46(Suppl. 1):S43-S49.
75. Perez J, Springthorpe S, Sattar SA. Activity of selected oxidizing microbicides against spores of *Clostridium difficile:* relevance to environmental control. *Am J Infect Control.* 2005;33:320-325.
76. Helms CM, Massanari RM, Zeitler R, et al. Legionnaires' disease associated with a hospital water system: a cluster of 24 nosocomial cases. *Ann Intern Med.* 1983;99:172-178.
77. Helms C, Massanari R, Wenzel R, et al. Control of epidemic nosocomial legionellosis: a 5 year progress report on continuous hyperchlorination of a water distribution system. In: Abstracts of 27th Interscience Conference on Antimicrobial Agents and Chemotherapy. October 1987;349:158.
78. Cheung RJ, Ortiz D, DiMarino AJ Jr. GI endoscopic reprocessing practices in the United States. *Gastrointest Endosc.* 1999;50:362-368.
79. Miner NA, McDowell JW, Willcockson GW, et al. Antimicrobial and other properties of a new stabilized alkaline glutaraldehyde disinfectant/sterilizer. *Am J Hosp Pharm.* 1977;34:376-382.
80. Pepper RE. Comparison of the activities and stabilities of alkaline glutaraldehyde sterilizing solutions. *Infect Control.* 1980;1:90-92.
81. Scott EM, Gorman SP. Glutaraldehyde. In: Block SS, ed. *Disinfection, Sterilization, and Preservation.* 5th ed. Philadelphia: Lippincott Williams & Wilkins; 2001:361-381.
82. Russell AD. Glutaraldehyde: current status and uses. *Infect Control Hosp Epidemiol.* 1994;15:724-733.
83. Rutala WA, Gergen MF, Weber DJ. Inactivation of *Clostridium difficile* spores by disinfectants. *Infect Control Hosp Epidemiol.* 1993;14:36-39.
84. Dyas A, Das BC. The activity of glutaraldehyde against *Clostridium difficile. J Hosp Infect.* 1985;6:41-45.
85. van Klingeren B, Pullen W. Glutaraldehyde resistant mycobacteria from endoscope washers. *J Hosp Infect.* 1993;25:147-149.
86. Griffiths PA, Babb JR, Bradley CR, et al. Glutaraldehyde-resistant *Mycobacterium chelonae* from endoscope washer disinfectors. *J Appl Microbiol.* 1997;82:519-526.
87. Webster E, Ribner B, Streed LL, et al. Microbial contamination of activated 2% glutaraldehyde used in high-level disinfection of endoscopes [Abstract]. *Am J Infect Control.* 1996;24:153.
88. Barbee SL, Weber DJ, Sobsey MD, et al. Inactivation of *Cryptosporidium parvum* oocyst infectivity by disinfection and sterilization processes. *Gastrointest Endosc.* 1999;49:605-611.
89. Laskowski LF, Marr JJ, Spernoga JF, et al. Fastidious *Mycobacteria* grown from porcine prosthetic-heart-valve cultures. *N Engl J Med.* 1977;297:101-102.
90. Mbithi JN, Springthorpe VS, Sattar SA, et al. Bactericidal, virucidal, and mycobactericidal activities of reused alkaline glutaraldehyde in an endoscopy unit. *J Clin Microbiol.* 1993;31:2988-2995.
91. Cole EC, Rutala WA, Nessen L, et al. Effect of methodology, dilution, and exposure time on the tuberculocidal activity of glutaraldehyde-based disinfectants. *Appl Environ Microbiol.* 1990;56:1813-1817.
92. Collins FM, Montalbine V. Mycobactericidal activity of glutaraldehyde solutions. *J Clin Microbiol.* 1976;4:408-412.
93. Overton D, Burgess JO, Beck B, et al. Glutaraldehyde test kits: evaluation for accuracy and range. *Gen Dent.* 1989;37:126, 128.
94. Cooke RPD, Goddard SV, Chatterley R, et al. Monitoring glutaraldehyde dilution in automated washer/disinfectors. *J Hosp Infect.* 2001;48:242-246.
95. Farina A, Fievet MH, Plassart F, et al. Residual glutaraldehyde levels in fiberoptic endoscopes: measurement and implications for patient toxicity. *J Hosp Infect.* 1999;43:293-297.
96. Dailey JR, Parnes RE, Aminlari A. Glutaraldehyde keratopathy. *Am J Ophthalmol.* 1993;115:256-258.
97. Newman MA, Kachuba JB. Glutaraldehyde: a potential health risk to nurses. *Gastroenterol Nurs.* 1992;14:296-300 [discussion, Gastroenterol Nurs. 1992;14:300-301].
98. Turner FJ. Hydrogen peroxide and other oxidant disinfectants. In: Block SS, ed. *Disinfection, Sterilization, and Preservation.* 3rd ed. Philadelphia: Lea & Febiger; 1983:240-250.
99. Block SS. Peroxygen compounds. In: Block SS, ed. *Disinfection, Sterilization, and Preservation,* 5th ed. Philadelphia: Lippincott Williams & Wilkins; 2001:185-204.
100. Sattar SA, Springthorpe VS, Rochon M. A product based on accelerated and stabilized hydrogen peroxide: evidence for broad-spectrum germicidal activity. *Can J Infect Control.* 1998(Winter):123-130.
101. Rutala WA, Gergen MF, Weber DJ. Sporicidal activity of chemical sterilants used in hospitals. *Infect Control Hosp Epidemiol.* 1993;14:713-718.
102. Silvany RE, Dougherty JM, McCulley JP, et al. The effect of currently available contact lens disinfection systems on *Acanthamoeba castellanii* and *Acanthamoeba polyphaga. Ophthalmology.* 1990;97:286-290.
103. Neely AN, Maley MP. The 1999 Lindberg Award. 3% hydrogen peroxide for the gram-positive disinfection of fabrics. *J Burn Care Rehabil.* 1999;20:471-477.
104. Vesley D, Norlien KG, Nelson B, et al. Significant factors in the disinfection and sterilization of flexible endoscopes. *Am J Infect Control.* 1992;20:291-300.
105. Levenson JE. Corneal damage from improperly cleaned tonometer tips. *Arch Ophthalmol.* 1989;107:1117.
106. Omidbakhsh N, Sattar SA. Broad-spectrum microbicidal activity, toxicologic assessment, and materials compatibility of a new generation of accelerated hydrogen peroxide-based environmental surface disinfectant. *Am J Infect Control.* 2006;34:251-257.
107. Omidbakhsh N. A new peroxide-based flexible endoscope-compatible high-level disinfectant. *Am J Infect Control.* 2006;34:571-577.
108. Alfa MJ, Jackson M. A new hydrogen peroxide-based medical-device detergent with germicidal properties: comparison with enzymatic cleaners. *Am J Infect Control.* 2001;29:168-177.
109. Gottardi W. Iodine and iodine compounds. In: Block SS, ed. *Disinfection, Sterilization, and Preservation.* 5th ed. Philadelphia: Lippincott Williams & Wilkins; 2001:159-184.
110. Craven DE, Moody B, Connolly MG, et al. Pseudobacteremia caused by povidone-iodine solution contaminated with *Pseudomonas cepacia. N Engl J Med.* 1981;305:621-623.
111. Berkelman RL, Lewin S, Allen JR, et al. Pseudobacteremia attributed to contamination of povidone-iodine with *Pseudomonas cepacia. Ann Intern Med.* 1981;95:32-36.
112. Rutala WA, Cole EC, Wannamaker NS, et al. Inactivation of *Mycobacterium tuberculosis* and *Mycobacterium bovis* by 14 hospital disinfectants. *Am J Med.* 1991;91:267S-271S.
113. Klein M, DeForest A. The inactivation of viruses by germicides. Chem *Specialists Manuf Assoc Proc.* 1963;49:116-118.
114. Berkelman RL, Holland BW, Anderson RL. Increased bactericidal activity of dilute preparations of povidone-iodine solutions. *J Clin Microbiol.* 1982;15:635-639.
115. Wallbank AM, Drulak M, Poffenroth L, et al. Wescodyne: lack of activity against poliovirus in the presence of organic matter. *Health Lab Sci.* 1978;15:133-137.
116. Favero MS, Bond WW. Chemical disinfection of medical and surgical materials. In: Block SS, ed. *Disinfection, Sterilization, and Preservation,* 4th ed. Philadelphia: Lea & Febiger; 1991:617-641.
117. Medcomp frequently asked questions. Available at http://www.medcompnet.com/faq/index.html.
118. Gordon MD, Ezzell RJ, Bruckner NI, et al. Enhancement of mycobactericidal activity of glutaraldehyde with α,β-unsaturated and aromatic aldehydes. *J Indust Microbiol.* 1994;13:77-82.
119. Rutala WA, Weber DJ. New disinfection and sterilization methods. *Emerg Infect Dis.* 2001;7:348-353.
120. Gregory AW, Schaalje GB, Smart JD, et al. The mycobactericidal efficacy of ortho-phthalaldehyde and the comparative resistances of *Mycobacterium bovis, Mycobacterium terrae,* and *Mycobacterium chelonae. Infect Control Hosp Epidemiol.* 1999;20:324-330.
121. Walsh SE, Maillard JY, Russell AD. Ortho-phthalaldehyde: a possible alternative to glutaraldehyde for high level disinfection. *J Appl Microbiol.* 1999;86:1039-1046.
122. Alfa MJ, Sitter DL. In-hospital evaluation of orthophthalaldehyde as a high level disinfectant for flexible endoscopes. *J Hosp Infect.* 1994;26:15-26.
123. Roberts CG, Chan-Myers HB, Favero MS. Virucidal activity of ortho-phthalaldehyde solutions against hepatitis B and C viruses. *Am J Infect Control.* 2008;36:223-226.
124. Sokol WN. Nine episodes of anaphylaxis following cytoscopy caused by Cidex OPA (ortho-phthalaldehyde) high-level disinfectant in 4 patients after cystoscopy. *J Allergy Clin Immunol.* 2004;114:392-397.
125. Tucker RC, Lestini BJ, Marchant RE. Surface analysis of clinically used expanded PTFE endoscopic tubing treated by the STERIS PROCESS. *ASAIO J.* 1996;42:306-313.
126. Malchesky PS. Medical applications of peracetic acid. In: Block SS, ed. *Disinfection, Sterilization, and Preservation,* 5th ed. Philadelphia: Lippincott Williams & Wilkins; 2001:979-996.
127. Mannion PT. The use of peracetic acid for the reprocessing of flexible endoscopes and rigid cystoscopes and laparoscopes. *J Hosp Infect.* 1995;29:313-315.
128. Bradley CR, Babb JR, Ayliffe GA. Evaluation of the Steris System 1 Peracetic Acid Endoscope Processor. *J Hosp Infect.* 1995;29:143-151.
129. Duc DL, Ribiollet A, Dode X, et al. Evaluation of the microbicidal efficacy of Steris System I for digestive endoscopes using GERMANDE and ASTM validation protocols. *J Hosp Infect.* 2001;48:135-141.
130. Alfa MJ, Olson N, Degagne P, et al. New low temperature sterilization technologies: microbicidal activity and clinical efficacy. In: Rutala WA, ed. *Disinfection, Sterilization, and Antisepsis in Healthcare.* Champlain, NY: Polyscience Publications; 1998:67-78.
131. Alfa MJ, DeGagne P, Olson N, et al. Comparison of liquid chemical sterilization with peracetic acid and ethylene oxide sterilization for long narrow lumens. *Am J Infect Control.* 1998;26:469-477.
132. Fuselier HA Jr, Mason C. Liquid sterilization versus high level disinfection in the urologic office. *Urology.* 1997;50:337-340.
133. Seballos RJ, Walsh AL, Mehta AC. Clinical evaluation of a liquid chemical sterilization system for flexible bronchoscopes. *J Bronchol.* 1995;2:192-199.
134. Wallace CG, Agee PM, Demicco DD. Liquid chemical sterilization using peracetic acid. An alternative approach to endoscope processing. *ASAIO J.* 1995;41:151-154.
135. Centers for Disease Control and Prevention. Bronchoscopy-related infections and pseudoinfections—New York, 1996 and 1998. *MMWR Morb Mortal Wkly Rep.* 1999;48(26):557-560.
136. U.S. Food and Drug Administration, Centers for Disease Control and Prevention. *FDA and CDC Public Health Advisory: Infections from Endoscopes Inadequately Reprocessed by an Automated Endoscope Reprocessing System.* Rockville, MD: U.S. Food and Drug Administration; 1999.

137. Middleton AM, Chadwick MV, Gaya H. Disinfection of bronchoscopes, contaminated in vitro with *Mycobacterium tuberculosis, Mycobacterium avium-intracellulare* and *Mycobacterium chelonae* in sputum, using stabilized, buffered peracetic acid solution ("Nu-Cidex"). *J Hosp Infect.* 1997;37:137-143.
138. Holton J, Shetty N. In-use stability of Nu-Cidex. *J Hosp Infect.* 1997;35:245-248.
139. Alasri A, Roques C, Michel G, et al. Bactericidal properties of peracetic acid and hydrogen peroxide, alone and in combination, and chlorine and formaldehyde against bacterial water strains. *Can J Microbiol.* 1992;38:635-642.
140. Stanley P. Destruction of a glutaraldehyde-resistant mycobacterium by a per-oxygen disinfectant [Abstract]. *Am J Infect Control.* 1998;26:185.
141. Fleming SJ, Foreman K, Shanley K, et al. Dialyser reprocessing with Renalin. *Am J Nephrol.* 1991;11:27-31.
142. Tokars JI, Finelli L, Alter MJ, et al. National surveillance of dialysis-associated diseases in the United States, 2001. *Semin Dialysis.* 2004;17:310-319.
143. Rutala WA, Cole EC. Ineffectiveness of hospital disinfectants against bacteria: a collaborative study. *Infect Control.* 1987;8:501-506.
144. Prindle RF. Phenolic compounds. In: Block SS, ed. *Disinfection, Sterilization, and Preservation,* 3rd ed. Philadelphia: Lea & Febiger; 1983:197-224.
145. Cole EC, Rutala WA, Samsa GP. Disinfectant testing using a modified use-dilution method: collaborative study. *J Assoc Off Anal Chem.* 1988;71:1187-1194.
146. Goddard PA, McCue KA. Phenolic compounds. In: Block SS, ed. *Disinfection, Sterilization, and Preservation,* 5th ed. Philadelphia: Lippincott Williams & Wilkins; 2001:255-281.
147. Sagripanti JL, Eklund CA, Trost PA, et al. Comparative sensitivity of 13 species of pathogenic bacteria to seven chemical germicides. *Am J Infect Control.* 1997;25:335-339.
148. Wysowski DK, Flynt JW Jr, Goldfield M, et al. Epidemic neonatal hyperbilirubinemia and use of a phenolic disinfectant detergent. *Pediatrics.* 1978;61:165-170.
149. Doan HM, Keith L, Shennan AT. Phenol and neonatal jaundice. *Pediatrics.* 1979;64:324-325.
150. Shickman MD, Guze LB, Pearce ML. Bacteremia following cardiac catheterization. *N Engl J Med.* 1959;260:1164-1166.
151. Ehrenkranz NJ, Bolyard EA, Wiener M, et al. Antibiotic-sensitive *Serratia marcescens* infections complicating cardiopulmonary operations: contaminated disinfectant as a reservoir. *Lancet.* 1980;2:1289-1292.
152. Weber DJ, Rutala WA, Sickbert-Bennett EE. Outbreaks associated with contaminated antiseptics and disinfectants. *Antimicrob Agents Chemother.* 2007;51:916-919.
153. Mbithi JN, Springthorpe VS, Sattar SA. Chemical disinfection of hepatitis A virus on environmental surfaces. *Appl Environ Microbiol.* 1990;56:3601-3604.
154. Petrocci AN. Surface active agents: quaternary ammonium compounds. In: Block SS, ed. *Disinfection, Sterilization, and Preservation.* 3rd ed. Philadelphia: Lea & Febiger; 1983:309-329.
155. Doultree JC, Druce JD, Birch CJ, et al. Inactivation of feline calicivirus, a Norwalk virus surrogate. *J Hosp Infect.* 1999; 41:51-57.
156. Cefai C, Richards J, Gould FK, et al. An outbreak of respiratory tract infection resulting from incomplete disinfection of ventilatory equipment. *J Hosp Infect.* 1990;15:177-182.
157. Gurevich I, Tafuro P, Ristuccia P, et al. Disinfection of respirator tubing: a comparison of chemical versus hot water machine-assisted processing. *J Hosp Infect.* 1983;4:199-208.
158. Rutala WA, Weber DJ, Gergen MF, et al. Efficacy of a washer-pasteurizer for disinfection of respiratory-care equipment. *Infect Control Hosp Epidemiol.* 2000;21:333-336.
159. Jette LP, Lambert NG. Evaluation of two hot water washer disinfectors for medical instruments. *Infect Control Hosp Epidemiol.* 1988;9:194-199.
160. Association for the Advancement of Medical Instrumentation. *Good Hospital Practice: Steam Sterilization and Sterility Assurance.* Arlington, VA: Association for the Advancement of Medical Instrumentation; 1993.
161. Association for the Advancement of Medical Instrumentation. *Flash Sterilization: Steam Sterilization of Patient Care Items for Immediate Use.* Arlington, VA: AAMI; 1996.
162. Association for the Advancement of Medical Instrumentation. *Steam Sterilization and Sterility Assurance in Health Care Facilities.* Arlington, VA: ANSI/AAMI ST46; 2002.
163. Association for the Advancement of Medical Instrumentation. *Ethylene Oxide Sterilization in Health Care Facilities: Safety and Effectiveness.* Arlington, VA: AAMI; 1999.
164. Association of Operating Room Nurses. Recommended Practices for Sterilization in Perioperative Practice Settings. *2000 Standards, Recommended Practices, and Guidelines.* Denver, CO: Association of Operating Room Nurses; 2000: 347-358.
165. Association for Peri-operative Registered Nurses. Recommended practices for cleaning and caring for surgical instruments and powered equipment. *AORN J.* 2002;75:727-741.
166. Mangram AJ, Horan TC, Pearson ML, et al. Guideline for prevention of surgical site infection, 1999. Hospital Infection Control Practices Advisory Committee. *Infect Control Hosp Epidemiol.* 1999;20:250-278.
167. Education Design. *Best practices for the prevention of surgical site infection.* Denver, CO: Education Design; 1998.
168. Singh J, Bhatia R, Gandhi JC, et al. Outbreak of viral hepatitis B in a rural community in India linked to inadequately sterilized needles and syringes. *Bull World Health Organ.* 1998;76:93-98.
169. Eickhoff TC. An outbreak of surgical wound infections due to *Clostridium perfringens. Surg Gynecol Obstet.* 1962;114:102-108.
170. Favero MS. Sterility assurance: concepts for patient safety. In: Rutala WA, ed. *Disinfection, Sterilization and Antisepsis: Principles and Practices in Healthcare Facilities.* Washington, DC: Association for Professionals in Infection Control and Epidemiology; 2001:110-119.
171. Oxborrow GS, Berube R. Sterility testing-validation of sterilization processes, and sporicide testing. In: Block SS, ed. *Disinfection, Sterilization, and Preservation.* 4th ed. Philadelphia: Lea & Febiger; 1991:1047-1057.
172. Rutala WA, Weber DJ. Clinical effectiveness of low-temperature sterilization technologies. *Infect Control Hosp Epidemiol.* 1998; 19:798-804.
173. Adler S, Scherrer M, Daschner FD. Costs of low-temperature plasma sterilization compared with other sterilization methods. *J Hosp Infect.* 1998;40:125-134.
174. Joslyn L. Sterilization by heat. In: Block SS, ed. *Disinfection, Sterilization, and Preservation.* 5th ed. Philadelphia: Lippincott Williams & Wilkins; 2001:695-728.
175. Silverstone SE, Hill DE. Evaluation of sterilization of dental handpieces by heating in synthetic compressor lubricant. *Gen Dent.* 1999;47:158-160.
176. Bucx MJ, Veldman DJ, Beenhakker MM, et al. The effect of steam sterilisation on light intensity provided by fibrelight Macintosh laryngoscopes. *Anaesthesia.* 2000;55:185-186.
177. Gilbert JA, Phillips HO. The effect of steam sterilization on plaster casting material. *Clinical Orthopaed Rel Res.* 1984: 241-244.
178. Bryce EA, Roberts FJ, Clements B, et al. When the biological indicator is positive: investigating autoclave failures. *Infect Control Hosp Epidemiol.* 1997;18:654-656.
179. Rutala WA, Stiegel MM, Sarubbi FA Jr. Decontamination of laboratory microbiological waste by steam sterilization. *Appl Environ Microbiol.* 1982;43:1311-1316.
180. Rutala WA. Disinfection and flash sterilization in the operating room. *J Ophthal Nurs Technol.* 1991;10:106-115.
181. Maki DG, Hassemer CA. Flash sterilization: carefully measured haste. *Infect Control.* 1987;8:307-310.
182. Barrett T. Flash sterilization: what are the risks? In: Rutala WA, ed. *Disinfection, Sterilization and Antisepsis: Principles and Practices in Healthcare Facilities.* Washington, DC: Association for Professionals in Infection Control and Epidemiology; 2001:70-76.
183. Vesley D, Langholz AC, Rohlfing SR, et al. Fluorimetric detection of a *Bacillus stearothermophilus* spore-bound enzyme, α-D-glucosidase, for rapid identification of flash sterilization failure. *Appl Environ Microbiol.* 1992;58:717-719.
184. Rutala WA, Gergen MF, Weber DJ. Evaluation of a rapid readout biological indicator for flash sterilization with three biological indicators and three chemical indicators. *Infect Control Hosp Epidemiol.* 1993;14:390-394.
185. Hood E, Stout N, Catto B. Flash sterilization and neurosurgical site infections: guilt by association. *Am J Infect Control.* 1997;25:156.
186. Rutala WA, Weber DJ, Chappell KJ. Patient injury from flash-sterilized instruments. *Infect Control Hosp Epidemiol.* 1999;20:458.
187. Ernst RR, Doyle JE. Sterilization with gaseous ethylene oxide: a review of chemical and physical factors. *Biotech Bioeng.* 1968;10:1-31.
188. Joslyn L. Gaseous chemical sterilization. In: Block SS, ed. *Disinfection, Sterilization, and Preservation.* 5th ed. Philadelphia: Lippincott Williams & Wilkins; 2001:337-360.
189. National Toxicology Program. Home page available at <http://ntp-server.niehs.nih.gov/>
190. Ethylene oxide sterilization: how hospitals can adapt to the changes. *Health Devices.* 1994;23:485-492.
191. Ries MD, Weaver K, Beals N. Safety and efficacy of ethylene oxide sterilized polyethylene in total knee arthroplasty. *Clin Orthop Relat Res.* 1996(331):159-163.
192. Alfa MJ, DeGagne P, Olson N. Bacterial killing ability of 10% ethylene oxide plus 90% hydrochlorofluorocarbon sterilizing gas. *Infect Control Hosp Epidemiol.* 1997;18:641-645.
193. Rutala WA, Gergen MF, Weber DJ. Comparative evaluation of the sporicidal activity of new low-temperature sterilization technologies: ethylene oxide, 2 plasma sterilization systems, and liquid peracetic acid. *Am J Infect Control.* 1998;26:393-398.
194. Alfa MJ, DeGagne P, Olson N, et al. Comparison of ion plasma, vaporized hydrogen peroxide and 100% ethylene oxide sterilizers to the 12/88 ethylene oxide gas sterilizer. *Infect Control Hosp Epidemiol.* 1996;17:92-100.
195. Parisi AN, Young WE. Sterilization with ethylene oxide and other gases. In: Block SS, ed. *Disinfection, Sterilization, and Preservation,* 4th ed. Philadelphia: Lea & Febiger; 1991:580-595.
196. Holler C, Martiny H, Christiansen B, et al. The efficacy of low temperature plasma (LTP) sterilization, a new sterilization technique. *Zentralbl Hyg Umweltmed.* 1993;194:380-391.
197. Parker HH, Johnson RB. Effectiveness of ethylene oxide for sterilization of dental handpieces. *J Dent.* 1995;23:113-115.
198. Borneff M, Ruppert J, Okpara J, et al. Efficacy testing of low-temperature plasma sterilization (LTP) with test object models simulating practice conditions. *Zentr Steril.* 1995;3:361-371.
199. Borneff-Lipp M, Okpara J, Bodendorf M, et al. Validation of low-temperature-plasma (LPT) sterilization systems: comparison of two technical versions, the Sterrad 100, 1.8 and the 100S. *Hyg Mikrobiol.* 1997;3:21-28.
200. Jacobs PT, Lin SM. Sterilization processes utilizing low-temperature plasma. In: Block SS, ed. *Disinfection, Sterilization, and Preservation,* 5th ed. Philadelphia: Lippincott Williams & Wilkins; 2001:747-763.
201. Rutala WA, Gergen MF, Weber DJ. Sporicidal activity of a new low-temperature sterilization technology: the Sterrad 50 sterilizer. *Infect Control Hosp Epidemiol.* 1999;20:514-516.
202. Roberts C, Antonoplos P. Inactivation of human immunodeficiency virus type 1, hepatitis A virus, respiratory syncytial virus, vaccinia virus, herpes simplex virus type 1, and poliovirus type 2 by hydrogen peroxide gas plasma sterilization. *Am J Infect Control.* 1998;26:94-101.
203. Kyi MS, Holton J, Ridgway GL. Assessment of the efficacy of a low temperature hydrogen peroxide gas plasma sterilization system. *J Hosp Infect.* 1995;31:275-284.
204. Borneff-Lipp M, Kaetzke A, Durr M. Evaluation of low temperature hydrogen peroxide plasma sterilization. *Zentr Steril.* 2008;16:35-42.
205. Feldman LA, Hui HK. Compatibility of medical devices and materials with low-temperature hydrogen peroxide gas plasma. *Med Device Diagn Indust.* 1997;19:57-62.
206. Jacobs PT, Smith D. The new Sterrad 100S sterilization system: features and advantages. *Zentr Steril.* 1998;6:86-94.
207. Dufresne S, Leblond H, Chaunet M. Relationship between lumen diameter and length sterilized in the 125L ozone sterilizer. *Am J Infect Control.* 2008;36:291-297.
208. Berrington AW, Pedler SJ. Investigation of gaseous ozone for MRSA decontamination of hospital side-rooms. *J Hosp Infect.* 1998;40:61-65.
209. Rutala WA, Weber DJ. Importance of lumen flow in liquid chemical sterilization. *Am J Infect Control.* 1999;20:458-459.
210. Gurevich I, Qadri SMH, Cunha BA. False-positive results of spore tests from improper clip use with the Steris chemical sterilant system. *Infect Control Hosp Epidemiol.* 1992;21:42-43.
211. Occupational Safety and Health Administration. Occupational exposure to bloodborne pathogens; final rule. *Fed Regist.* 1991;56:64003-64182.
212. Occupational Safety and Health Administration. *OSHA Instruction CPL 2-2.44C.* Washington, DC: Office of Health Compliance Assistance; 1992.
213. Occupational Safety and Health Administration. *OSHA Memorandum from Stephen Mallinger. EPA-Registered Disinfectants for HIV/HBV.* Washington, DC: Occupational Safety and Health Administration; 1997.
214. Payan C, Cottin J, Lemarie C, et al. Inactivation of hepatitis B virus in plasma by hospital in-use chemical disinfectants assessed by a modified HepG2 cell culture. *J Hosp Infect.* 2001;47:282-287.
215. Rutala WA, Weber DJ. Infection control: the role of disinfection and sterilization. *J Hosp Infect.* 1999;43:S43-S55.
216. Wilson JA, Margolin AB. The efficacy of three common hospital liquid germicides to inactivate *Cryptosporidium parvum* oocysts. *J Hosp Infect.* 1999;42:231-237.
217. Fayer R, Graczyk TK, Cranfield MR, et al. Gaseous disinfection of *Cryptosporidium parvum* oocysts. *Appl Environ Microbiol.* 1996;62:3908-3909.
218. Rice EW, Clark RM, Johnson CH. Chlorine inactivation of *Escherichia coli* O157:H7. *Emerg Infect Dis.* 1999;5:461-463.
219. Venkitanarayanan KS, Ezeike GO, Hung YC, et al. Inactivation of *Escherichia coli* O157:H7 and *Listeria monocytogenes* on plastic kitchen cutting boards by electrolyzed oxidizing water. *J Food Prot.* 1999;62:857-860.
220. Akamatsu T, Tabata K, Hironga M, et al. Transmission of *Helicobacter pylori* infection via flexible fiberoptic endoscopy. *Am J Infect Control.* 1996;24:396-401.
221. Cronmiller JR, Nelson DK, Jackson DK, et al. Efficacy of conventional endoscopic disinfection and sterilization methods against *Helicobacter pylori* contamination. *Helicobacter.* 1999;4:198-203.
222. Wu MS, Wang JT, Yang JC, et al. Effective reduction of *Helicobacter pylori* infection after upper gastrointestinal endoscopy by mechanical washing of the endoscope. *Hepatogastroenterology.* 1996;43:1660-1664.
223. Shimada T, Terano A, Ota S, et al. Risk of iatrogenic transmission of *Helicobacter pylori* by gastroscopes. *Lancet.* 1996;347: 1342-1343.
224. Chapin M, Yatabe J, Cherry JD. An outbreak of rotavirus gastroenteritis on a pediatric unit. *Am J Infect Control.* 1983; 11:88-91.
225. Keswick BH, Pickering LK, DuPont HL, et al. Survival and detection of rotaviruses on environmental surfaces in day care centers. *Appl Environ Microbiol.* 1983;46:813-816.
226. Ansari SA, Spingthorpe S, Sattar SA. Survival and vehicular spread of human rotaviruses: possible relation to seasonality of outbreaks. *Rev Infect Dis.* 1991;13:448-461.
227. Sattar SA, Raphael RA, Lochnan H, et al. Rotavirus inactivation by chemical disinfectants and antiseptics used in hospitals. *Can J Microbiol.* 1983;29:1464-1469.
228. Lloyd-Evans N, Springthorpe VS, Sattar SA. Chemical disinfection of human rotavirus–contaminated inanimate surfaces. *J Hyg (Lond).* 1986;97:163-173.
229. Tan JA, Schnagl RD. Inactivation of a rotavirus by disinfectants. *Med J Aust.* 1981;1:19-23.

230. Sokal DC, Hermonat PL. Inactivation of papillomavirus by low concentrations of povidone-iodine. *Sex Transm Dis.* 1995;22: 22-24.

231. Rice EW, Adcock NJ, Sivaganesan M, et al. Chlorine inactivation of highly pathogenic avian influenza virus (H5N1). *Emerg Infect Dis.* 2007;13:1568-1570.

232. Green J, Wright PA, Gallimore CI, et al. The role of environmental contamination with small round structured viruses in a hospital outbreak investigated by reverse-transcriptase polymerase chain reaction assay. *J Hosp Infect.* 1998;39:39-45.

233. Evans MR, Meldrum R, Lane W, et al. An outbreak of viral gastroenteritis following environmental contamination at a concert hall. *Epidemiol Infect.* 2002;129:355-360.

234. Sattar SA. Microbicides and the environmental control of nosocomial viral infections. *J Hosp Infect.* 2004;56(Suppl.): S64-S69.

235. Gehrke C, Steinmann J, Goroncy-Bermes P. Inactivation of feline calicivirus, a surrogate of norovirus (formerly Norwalk-like viruses), by different types of alcohol in vitro and in vivo. *J Hosp Infect.* 2004;46:55-60.

236. Centers for Disease Control and Prevention. Update: severe acute respiratory syndrome—United States, May 14, 2003. *MMWR Morb Mortal Wkly Rep.* 2003;52:436-438.

237. Sattar SA, Springthorpe VS, Karim Y, et al. Chemical disinfection of non-porous inanimate surfaces experimentally contaminated with four human pathogenic viruses. *Epidemiol Infect.* 1989;102:493-505.

238. Saknimit M, Inatsuki I, Sugiyama Y, et al. Virucidal efficacy of physico-chemical treatments against coronaviruses and parvoviruses of laboratory animals. *Jikken Dobutsu.* 1988;37: 341-345.

239. Sizun J, Yu MW, Talbot PJ. Survival of human coronaviruses 229E and OC43 in suspension and after drying on surfaces: a possible source of hospital-acquired infections. *J Hosp Infect.* 2000;46:55-60.

239a. World Health Organization. *First Data on Stability and Resistance of SARS Coronavirus Compiled by Members of WHO Laboratory Network.* Geneva: World Health Organization; 2003. Available at <http://www.who.int/csr/sars/survival_2003_05_04/en/index.html>

240. Taylor DM. Inactivation of transmissible degenerative encephalopathy agents: a review. *Vet J.* 2000;159:10-17.

241. World Health Organization. WHO Infection Control Guidelines for Transmissible Spongiform Encephalopathies. Available at <http://www.who.int/csr/resources/publications/bse/whocdscsraph2003.pdf>.

242. Rutala WA, Weber DJ. Creutzfeldt-Jakob disease: recommendations for disinfection and sterilization. *Clin Infect Dis.* 2001;32: 1348-1356.

243. Brown SA, Merritt K. Use of containment pans and lids for autoclaving caustic solutions. *Am J Infect Control.* 2003;31: 257-260.

244. Taylor DM. Inactivation of prions by physical and chemical means. *J Hosp Infect.* 1999;43(Suppl.):S69-S76.

245. Weber DJ, Rutala WA. Use of germicides in the home and health care setting: is there a relationship between germicide use and antimicrobial resistance? *Infect Control Hosp Epidemiol.* 2006;27:1107-1119.

246. Rutala WA, Stiegel MM, Sarubbi FA, et al. Susceptibility of antibiotic-susceptible and antibiotic-resistant hospital bacteria to disinfectants. *Infect Control Hosp Epidemiol.* 1997;18: 417-421.

247. Anderson RL, Carr JH, Bond WW, et al. Susceptibility of vancomycin-resistant enterococci to environmental disinfectants. *Infect Control Hosp Epidemiol.* 1997;18:195-199.

248. Sakagami Y, Kajimura K. Bactericidal activities of disinfectants against vancomycin-resistant enterococci. *J Hosp Infect.* 2002;50: 140-144.

249. Sehulster LM, Anderson RL. Susceptibility of glycopeptide-intermediate resistant *Staphylococcus aureus* (GISA) to surface disinfectants, hand washing chemicals, and a skin antiseptic [Abstract Y-3]. Presented at the 98th General Meeting of American Society for Microbiology, Atlanta, May 1998.

250. Rutala WA, Weber DJ, Gergen MF. Studies on the disinfection of VRE-contaminated surfaces. *Infect Control Hosp Epidemiol.* 2000;21:548.

251. Byers KE, Durbin LJ, Simonton BM, et al. Disinfection of hospital rooms contaminated with vancomycin-resistant *Enterococcus faecium. Infect Control Hosp Epidemiol.* 1998;19:261-264.

252. Leggiadro RJ. The threat of biological terrorism: a public health and infection control reality. *Infect Control Hosp Epidemiol.* 2000;21:53-56.

253. Henderson DA. The looming threat of bioterrorism. *Science.* 1999;283:1279-1282.

254. Biological and chemical terrorism: strategic plan for preparedness and response. Recommendations of the CDC Strategic Planning Work Group. *MMWR Recomm Rep.* 2000;49(RR-4): 1-14.

255. Brazis AR, Leslie JE, Kabler PW, et al. The inactivation of spores of *Bacillus globigii* and *Bacillus anthracis* by free available chlorine. *Appl Microbiol.* 1958;6:338-342.

256. Weber DJ, Rutala WA. Risks and prevention of nosocomial transmission of rare zoonotic diseases. *Clin Infect Dis.* 2001;32:446-456.

256a. U.S. Environmental Protection Agency. Anthrax Spore Decontamination Using Bleach (Sodium Hypochlorite). Available at <http://www.epa.gov/pesticides/factsheets/chemicals/bleachfactsheet.htm>.

256b. U.S. Environmental Protection Agency. Anthrax Spore Decontamination Using Chlorine Dioxide. Available at <http://www.epa.gov/pesticides/factsheets/chemicals/chlorinedioxidefactsheet.htm>.

256c. U.S. Environmental Protection Agency. Pesticide Emergency Exemptions. Available at <http://www.epa.gov/opprd001/section18/>.

257. Venezia RA, Orrico M, Houston E, et al. Lethal activity of nonthermal plasma sterilization against microorganisms. *Infect Control Hosp Epidemiol.* 2008;29:430-436.

258. Klapes NA, Vesley D. Vapor-phase hydrogen peroxide as a surface decontaminant and sterilant. *Appl Environ Microbiol.* 1990;56:503-506.

259. U.S. Food and Drug Administration. FDA-cleared sterilants and high-level disinfectants with general claims for processing reusable medical and dental devices, March, 2009. <www.fda.gov/cdrh/ode/germlab.html>.

260. Rutala WA, Weber DJ. How to assess disease transmission when there is a failure to follow recommended disinfection and sterilization principles. *Infect Control Hosp Epidemiol.* 2007; 28:519-524.

261. Rutala WA, Gergen MF, Weber DJ. Disinfection of a probe used in ultrasound-guided prostate biopsy. *Infect Control Hosp Epidemiol.* 2007;28:916-919.

262. Nelson DB, Jarvis WR, Rutala WA, et al. Multi-society guideline for reprocessing flexible gastrointestinal endoscopes. *Infect Control Hosp Epidemiol.* 2003;24:532-537.

263. American Society for Gastrointestinal Endoscopy Standards of Practice Committee. Infection control during GI endoscopy. *Gastrointest Endosc.* 2008;67:781-790.

264. Muscarella LF. Prevention of disease transmission during flexible laryngoscopy. *Am J Infect Control.* 2007;35:536-544.

265. Carling PC, Parry MF, Von Beheren SM, et al. Identifying opportunities to enhance environmental cleaning in 23 acute care hospitals. *Infect Control Hosp Epidemiol.* 2008;29: 1-7.

266. Huang SS, Datta R, Platt R. Risk of acquiring antibiotic-resistant bacteria from prior room occupants. *Arch Int Med.* 2006;166: 1945-1951.

267. Rutala WA, Odette RL, Samsa GP. Management of infectious waste by United States hospitals. *JAMA.* 1989;262:1635-1640.

268. Rutala WA, Sarubbi FA. Management of infectious waste from hospitals. *Infect Control.* 1983;4:198-204.

269. Agency for Toxic Substances and Disease Registry. *The Public Health Implications of Medical Waste: A Report to Congress.* Washington, DC: U.S. Department of Health and Human Services; 1990.

270. U.S. Environmental Protection Agency. *EPA Guide for Infectious Waste Management.* Washington, DC: U.S. Environmental Protection Agency; 1986.

271. Office of Technology Assessment (OTA-0-459). *Finding the Rx for Managing Medical Wastes.* Washington, DC: U.S. Government Printing Office; 1990.

272. U.S. Environmental Protection Agency. Standards for the tracking and management of medical waste; interim final rule and request for comments. *Fed Regist.* 1989;54:12326-12395.

273. Rutala WA, Weber DJ. Infectious waste: mismatch between science and policy. *N Engl J Med.* 1991;325:578-582.

274. Rutala WA, Mayhall CG, Society for Hospital Epidemiology of America. SHEA position paper: medical waste. *Infect Control Hosp Epidemiol.* 1992;13:38-48.

275. U.S. Department of Transportation. Infectious substances; final rule. *Fed Regist.* 1995;60:48779-48787.

Infections Caused by Percutaneous Intravascular Devices

SUSAN E. BEEKMANN | DAVID K. HENDERSON*

The relentless progress of medical science and technology has been accompanied by the development of a host of new diagnostic and therapeutic medical devices, each of which is associated with its own complications. Included in the list of devices and the complications of their use to be discussed in this chapter are peripheral and central intravenous catheters, including nontunneled central catheters and tunneled (Hickman or Broviac) catheters with or without the Groshong tip (which remains closed unless the catheter is in use), peripherally inserted central venous catheters (PICCs), totally implanted intravascular access devices (ports), pulmonary artery catheters, and arterial lines.

As early as 1977, Maki suggested that more than 25,000 patients develop device-related bacteremia in the United States each year.[1] More recently, the Centers for Disease Control and Prevention (CDC) has estimated that approximately 80,000 central line–associated bloodstream infections (CLABSIs) currently occur in intensive care units (ICUs) each year.[2] The burgeoning use of an ever-expanding array of vascular access devices in medicine has resulted in even more complications associated with their use. Rates of bacteremia associated with the use of intravascular devices increased significantly into the early 2000s. Recent data suggest that the rates of CLABSIs may be decreasing, perhaps as a result of prevention programs implemented in many hospitals since 2001.[3] An intense focus on prevention of health care-associated infections, including CLABSIs, and requirements for the incorporation of performance measures into regulatory and financial reimbursement systems has the potential to significantly reduce these infections.[4,5]

Such device-associated infections occur as sporadic cases as well as in case clusters caused by the same organism. Vascular catheters have become an increasingly important source of bacteremias, increasing from 3% in the mid-1970s to 19% in the early 1990s.[6] Primary bacteremias (i.e., no apparent local infection elsewhere caused by the same organism), including intravascular catheter sources, now account for approximately one half of all ICU-related bacteremias.[7,8] In cancer patients, 56% of all bloodstream infections from 1999 to 2000 were CLABSIs.[9] The problem of iatrogenic, device-associated bacteremia is not unique to the United States; in one prospective study of bacteremia from Australia, nosocomial bacteremias accounted for 40% of all cases of bacteremia, and half of the nosocomial cases were device associated.[10] Although most data on CLABSI rates are derived from studies in ICUs, Marshall and colleagues reported that the incidence of CLABSIs in non-ICU, general medical patients was comparable to the rate in ICU patients.[11]

Both local and systemic infection may result from contamination of intravascular devices. Local cellulitis, abscess formation, septic thrombophlebitis, device-associated bacteremia, and endocarditis all occur as complications of intravascular therapy and monitoring.

Pathogenesis

For intravascular device-related bacteremia to occur, microorganisms must gain access to the extraluminal or intraluminal surface of the device. Microbial adherence and incorporation into biofilms then occurs, resulting first in infection and then, in some instances, in hematogenous dissemination.[12] Figure 302-1 illustrates the potential points of access to an intravascular device, each of which has been associated with both sporadic cases and case clusters of nosocomial bacteremia. Whereas the skin entry site has long been thought to be the most important portal of entry for invading microorganisms, the catheter hub–lumen has also been shown to be a major contributor to catheter-related bacteremia.[13,14] The most common point of access appears to vary, depending on the duration of time the catheter has been in place. Each of the three major sources of intravenous device-related bacteremia is discussed in the following sections.

CONTAMINATION OF THE INFUSATE

Contamination of the fluid administered through the device is a major cause of epidemic intravenous device-related bacteremias. Nonetheless, infusate contamination is a rare cause of bacteremia. Infusion-related sepsis has been reviewed in detail,[15] and both manufacture-related[16] and in-use[17] contamination of infusate have been documented as causes of device-associated sepsis.

Another factor influencing the pathogenesis of infusate-associated infection is the composition of the fluid. Different infusion fluids support the growth of differing pathogens. The microbiology of outbreaks of infusate-related sepsis is somewhat monotonous; pathogens such as *Enterobacter*, *Citrobacter*, and *Serratia* predominate. No infusate is entirely free of risk; even sterile water for injection can support the growth of *Burkholderia cepacia*.[18] Parenteral nutrition solutions are superb substrates for the growth of certain microorganisms.[19] Casein hydrolysate solutions support the growth of many bacteria and fungi.[20] Lipid emulsions support bacterial growth extremely well,[21] and their use has also been associated with a risk for fungemia caused by the lipid-dependent yeast *Malassezia furfur*, although not with contaminated infusates.[22] This risk has been primarily identified in the neonatal intensive care setting and has been less commonly seen in adults.[22] The risk for coagulase-negative staphylococcal bacteremia in neonates has been directly linked to the administration of lipid infusions.[23] Several additional outbreaks of bacteremias have been linked to compounding pharmacies that adhere to different quality-control standards.[24,25] One national outbreak of *Serratia marcescens* bacteremias occurred as a result of contaminated magnesium sulfate solution,[25] and a second outbreak of *Pseudomonas putida* and *Stenotrophomonas maltophilia* was associated with contaminated heparin catheter-lock solution.[24]

Parenteral nutrition solutions may also become contaminated during compounding in the hospital pharmacy.[26,27] Two similar outbreaks of *Candida parapsilosis* infections were linked to the backflow of yeasts into parenteral nutrition solution because vacuum pumps were used improperly.[26,27]

The composition of the infusate also influences the degree of irritation of the vascular intima at the site of infusion. Fluids that are not isotonic, those at nonphysiologic pH, and those containing particulates all may irritate the vascular wall, thus provoking thrombus formation. Such thrombi may be seeded with microbes—either hematogenously or by direct extension.

---

*All material in this chapter is in the public domain, with the exception of any borrowed figures or tables.

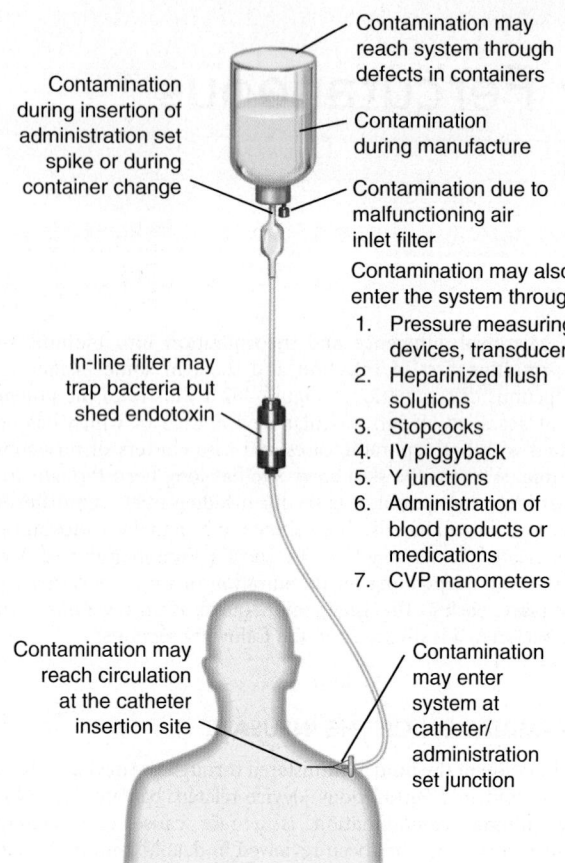

Contamination during insertion of administration set spike or during container change

Contamination may reach system through defects in containers

Contamination during manufacture

Contamination due to malfunctioning air inlet filter

Contamination may also enter the system through
1. Pressure measuring devices, transducers
2. Heparinized flush solutions
3. Stopcocks
4. IV piggyback
5. Y junctions
6. Administration of blood products or medications
7. CVP manometers

In-line filter may trap bacteria but shed endotoxin

Contamination may reach circulation at the catheter insertion site

Contamination may enter system at catheter/administration set junction

Figure 302-1 Points of access for microbial contamination in infusion therapy.

CONTAMINATION OF THE CATHETER HUB AND LUMEN

Contamination of the catheter hub–infusion tubing junction as a significant contributor to device-associated infection has been championed by Sitges-Serra and colleagues.[14,28-30] These investigators suggested that endemic coagulase-negative staphylococcal bacteremias often arise as a result of contamination of the catheter hub with these organisms. A randomized study examining the effects of a redesigned protective hub found these hubs to be associated with a significantly lower rate of catheter sepsis and culture-positive catheter hubs,[31] suggesting that the hub is a common portal of entry for bacteria. Other investigators have incriminated the hub–tubing junction (particularly when it does not allow a good fit) in the pathogenesis of epidemics of coagulase-negative staphylococcal infection.[32,33] Maki and Ringer found hub contamination to be the second most heavily weighted risk factor for catheter-associated infection in a large, prospective study.[34] Salzman and colleagues noted that more than 50% of episodes of central venous catheter-related sepsis occurring in a neonatal ICU were preceded by colonization of the catheter hub with the incriminated organism.[35] In a subsequent experimental study, these investigators found that swabbing the catheter hub with disinfectant substantially reduced the hub's microbial burden and that preparations containing 70% ethanol were both more effective and more likely to be safer for the patient than preparations containing chlorhexidine.[36] Sherertz estimated that the hub, lumen, or both contributed two thirds of the microorganisms that infected long-term catheters and that one fourth of the microorganisms were from the skin.[37] Finally, several outbreaks of bacteremia have been traced to contaminated medications—either those added directly to the system or those piggybacked into a side

port.[38,39] Clusters of infection also have been linked to flushing catheters with fluids from a contaminated common source.[40]

Conversely, some new technologies may be associated with increased risks for catheter-associated infection. Whereas the implementation of needleless intravenous admixture systems provided a safer workplace environment for health care providers, some data suggest that use of these devices may be associated with increased risk for device-associated infection.[41] Multiple investigations of bacteremia outbreaks associated with needleless devices have suggested that the mechanism for bacteremia may involve contamination from the end cap.[42-46] Interestingly, different studies have paradoxically found either increased or decreased risk with the same needleless system (e.g., the Interlink device [Baxter, Deerfield, IL]),[43,44] leading to the conclusion that the primary risk associated with these devices is related to how the systems are used (e.g., frequency of changing end caps and adherence to recommended infection control procedures) rather than factors intrinsic to the system.[44] Appropriate staff education regarding use of these devices and ensuring compliance with the manufacturer's recommendations is recommended to prevent device-related bacteremia.

CONTAMINATION OF SKIN AT THE DEVICE INSERTION SITE

Many authorities believe that the catheter insertion tract provides the major avenue for the ingress of microbial invaders.[1,10,14,15,32,34,47,48] Several studies have focused on microbial colonization around the catheter insertion site as a significant risk factor for catheter-associated infection.[49] Supporting this contention are the studies of Cooper and Hopkins that demonstrated organisms on the exterior surface of catheters rather than within the catheter lumen.[50] In the prospective study of Maki and Ringer, colonization around the catheter insertion site was the most strongly associated risk factor for local catheter infection.[34] Similarly, Safdar determined that most catheter-related bacteremias occurring with short-term noncuffed central catheters were extraluminally acquired and derived from the cutaneous microflora.[51] Skin appears to be the primary source of intravenous device-related bacteremia for short-term catheters, placed for an average duration of less than 8 days.[52-54]

Skin colonization is a dynamic process. Atela and co-workers conducted a prospective study to assess the turnover of superficial skin colonization by performing serial quantitative cultures of skin and the catheter hub.[47] Strains recovered from the targeted superficial skin sites demonstrated a poor correlation both with strains from previous skin cultures and with catheter tip isolates.[47] Herwaldt and colleagues examined the source of coagulase-negative staphylococcal bacteremias in hematology-oncology patients and found that the same strain was identified in both skin and blood cultures in only 6 of 20 episodes.[55] The matching strain was isolated only from other sites (primarily nares) in the remaining 70% of episodes, leading these investigators to the conclusion that mucous membranes might be a reservoir for strains of coagulase-negative staphylococci causing bacteremia in immunocompromised patients. Importantly, these investigators were unable to identify colonization with the same strain for the majority of bacteremias; only 4 of the 21 nosocomial bloodstream infections were preceded by colonization with the same strain. Most nosocomial coagulase-negative staphylococcal bacteremias in this study appeared to result from extrinsic introduction of the organism.

Epidemiology

Rates of central venous catheter-associated bacteremia have been reported by the CDC's National Nosocomial Infection Surveillance (NNIS) system since 1970; however, this system has effectively been replaced by the National Healthcare Safety Network. In 2006, rates of CLABSIs ranged from 1.5 (in inpatient medical/surgical wards) to 6.8 (in burn ICUs) bacteremias per 1000 central venous catheter days.[3] Previous NNIS rates from 1992 to June 2004[56] were higher: The previous medical ICU rate was 5.0 compared to 2.9 in the current report, perhaps indicating an actual reduction in the number of bacteremias.

Intravenous device-related bacteremia rates are influenced by patient-related parameters, catheter-related parameters, and hospital-related parameters (Table 302-1). Because of methodologic difficulties in performing appropriate scientific studies to characterize relative risk, many of these risk factors have been identified either retrospectively or in the epidemic setting. Still, each of the patient-related factors identified in Table 302-1 has been associated with an increased risk of device-associated infection.[57] Alteration of the patient's skin flora, either as a result of antimicrobial therapy or by colonization with an epidemic strain carried on the hands of hospital personnel, is a common event preceding catheter site infection. In addition, certain therapeutic devices (e.g., semipermeable membrane dressings) may actually increase the cutaneous microbial burden surrounding the catheter insertion site.[58,59] Failure of hospital personnel to perform appropriate hand hygiene procedures, particularly in the ICU setting, has been well documented.[60-62] Numerous epidemics of device-associated bacteremia have been linked to hospital personnel carrying an epidemic strain on their hands. Manipulating the system for repositioning, for obtaining a sample, or for any other reason increases the likelihood that the catheter may become contaminated.[63] This point has been best illustrated in studies of infectious complications associated with catheters used for parenteral nutrition (discussed later).

Several catheter characteristics or properties have been suggested to be associated with an increased risk for catheter-associated infection. Catheters that irritate the vascular intima and provoke thrombogenesis and catheters that are made of materials that are intrinsically thrombogenic are likely to be associated with an increased risk for device-associated infection.[64] Older studies suggest that stiff catheters were associated with higher infection rates.[65] Such catheters are likely to be more mobile in the insertion tract and are thought to be more thrombogenic. A clear association has been established between the thrombogenicity of a catheter and the risk for device-associated infection.[66,67]

TABLE 302-1	Risk Factors for Device-Associated Bacteremia

Granulocytopenia
Immunosuppressive chemotherapy
Loss of skin integrity (e.g., burns, psoriasis)
Severity of underlying illness
Active infection at other site
Alteration in patient's cutaneous microflora
Failure of health care provider to wash hands
Contaminated ointment or cream
Catheter composition/construction
  Flexibility/stiffness
  Thrombogenicity[64]
  Microbial adherence properties and biofilm production[77]
Size of catheter
Number of catheter lumens[73]
Catheter function/use
Catheter management strategies—number of entries into the system
Type of catheter (plastic > steel)
Location of catheter (central > peripheral[335]; jugular > femoral > subclavian[53,93,400]; lower extremity sites > upper extremity sites)
Type of placement (cutdown > percutaneous)[171,183,335]
Duration of placement (at least 72 hr > less than 72 hr)[34,171,222,335*]
Emergent placement > elective
Skill of venipuncturist (others > IV team)[89,222]
Type/use of catheter (balloon-tipped, flow-directed > percutaneously placed central venous > implanted central venous)[249]
Nursing staffing variables (nurse-to-patient ratio[95]; lower regular registered nurse-to-patient ratio and higher float pool registered nurse-to-patient ratio)[96,97,396]

*Although several studies support this precept, another has questioned it.[173]

Despite differences in thrombogenicity, some authorities believe that all catheters become coated with a fibrin sheath soon after placement.[68] Currently, the majority of catheters are manufactured with antithrombogenic polymers, such as polyurethane.

Catheter composition may influence the risk for infection in another way. Sheth and co-workers have shown that certain microorganisms, most notably staphylococci, are able to adhere better to a catheter made from polyvinyl chloride than to a Teflon catheter.[69] Rotrosen and colleagues demonstrated increased adherence of *Candida* spp. to polyvinyl chloride catheters compared with Teflon catheters.[70] In a rabbit model, silicon catheters are easier to infect with *Staphylococcus aureus* than are those made of polyurethane, Teflon, or polyvinyl chloride.[71] One might hypothesize that materials that facilitate microbial adherence may be associated with an increased risk for device-associated infection. Newer therapeutic interventions have focused on diminishing adherence to the catheter by a variety of different mechanisms.

The physical size of the catheter (and therefore the size of the defect in the skin's intrinsic host defenses) is also likely to be correlated with increased risk. Similarly, increasing the number of lumens in a catheter has been suggested to increase the risk for catheter-associated infections. Several studies have suggested that the use of multiple lumen catheters is associated with an increased risk for catheter-associated infection compared with the use of single-lumen catheters.[44,72,73] Not all studies have found this difference.[74,75]

The presence of distant infection resulting in hematogenous seeding of the intravascular device has been incriminated in the pathogenesis of device-associated infection in some series.[49,76] Several factors may influence the risk for catheter seeding, including catheter composition, local thrombus formation at the catheter insertion site, intensity of bacteremia, the infecting pathogen, duration of catheterization, duration of bacteremia, and the patient's ability to mount an immunologic response to the infection.

Formation of a bacterial biofilm is now thought to be a virtually universal phenomenon following insertion of intravascular devices.[77] Microorganisms then embed themselves in and under the biofilm layer and become the source of intraluminal colonization and, eventually, the sources of CLABSIs.[78] Certain chelators, including ethylenediamine-tetraacetic acid (EDTA) and sodium citrate, inhibit bacterial growth and fibrin formation.[79] The presence of fibrin deposits may explain the difficulty in treating totally implanted venous access port bacteremias without removal of the device.[80,81] Antibiotic concentrations should be 100 to 1000 times greater to kill sessile bacteria within a biofilm than for planktonic bacteria.[82-85]

Finally, the manner in which the catheter is used may influence risk. For example, risks for infection with pulmonary artery catheters may be higher because of the manner in which they are used.[86] In critically ill patients, these catheters are used intensively (although now somewhat less frequently than in the recent past): They are frequently repositioned to obtain accurate readings, they are used to obtain samples for the measurement of cardiac output, and they can be used to obtain mixed venous blood to measure oxygen and carbon dioxide tensions.

Catheter management, including both insertion and maintenance, also may influence risk for infection. Several studies have shown that catheters placed by less experienced personnel are at increased risk for infection.[87,88] Another study analyzed the efficacy of using a skilled team for the placement of peripheral intravenous catheters.[89] In this study, an intravenous therapy team significantly reduced both local and bacteremic complications associated with the placement of peripheral intravenous catheters, in part related to the timely replacement of the catheters. Two studies suggest that insertion of central venous catheters with less than maximal sterile barriers increases the risk of catheter-related infection.[53,90] Several studies have suggested that the number of times the system is entered also influences the risk for infection.[63,91,92] More than a single attempt to insert the catheter has also been found to be a risk factor for bacteremia.[75] Insertion at a subclavian rather than a femoral site is clearly associated with a lesser risk of both infectious and thrombotic complications.[73,93,94] In addition to the factors outlined previously, the risk of developing catheter-associated bacteremia is related to the patient and his or her intrinsic host defense mechanisms, as well as to factors related to the patient's hospital environment or therapy (see Table 302-1). The physician cannot alter most such patient-related factors; however, these data can be used when evaluating the risks associated with, the necessity for, and the duration of intravenous therapy.

In addition to patient-related risk factors, several hospital-related risk factors for CLABSIs have been either identified or proposed (see Table 302-1). In contraposition to the patient-related factors, such hospital-related factors can often be altered for patient benefit. Nurse staffing variables, including nurse-to-patient ratio, level of training, and permanent assignment to the unit ("float" nurse vs. regular unit staff nurse), have been shown to affect bacteremia rates.[95-97] As noted previously, the level of experience of the individual inserting the catheter (i.e., the number of previous catheter insertions) was also found to affect catheter-related bacteremia rates.[98] In addition, a number of studies have found that an education program focusing on risk factors and practice modifications is associated with decreased rates of CLABSIs.[99,100]

Microbiology

Staphylococci continue to predominate as the most frequently encountered pathogens in device-related infections. Although *S. aureus* is a frequent cause of device-associated infection, the coagulase-negative staphylococci have become the most common causes of these infections in the past two decades, especially in immunocompromised patients and those in whom long-term central venous access is required.[101,102] Nonetheless, the incidence of *S. aureus* bacteremia is increasing, driven largely by the blossoming epidemic of community-associated methicillin-resistant strains.[103]

Although there are some minor microbiologic differences among the devices or therapies under discussion, as a genus, staphylococci account for two thirds to 90% of the episodes of bacteremia associated with these devices.[6,104] Studies suggest that coagulase-negative staphylococci may be able to adhere to plastic catheters more aggressively than can other organisms.[105] This property would result in a selective advantage for coagulase-negative staphylococci in causing device-associated infections.

Other commonly encountered isolates are listed in Table 302-2. Some institutions have observed a recent increase in catheter-associated infection caused by gram-negative bacilli.[106,107] One study of patients with hematologic malignancies with Hickman catheters identified a predominance of gram-negative organisms (68%) causing catheter-related bacteremias in this nonneutropenic population.[108] Raad and colleagues reported that gram-negative bloodstream infections in cancer patients with solid tumors were most likely catheter related.[9] The past decade has witnessed an increasing occurrence of CLABSIs caused by multiply resistant gram-negative rods, most notably *Acinetobacter baumannii*.[109] CLABSIs caused by *A. baumannii* often occur in critically ill, immunosuppressed, highly antimicrobial agent–experienced patients who can ill afford any bacteremia, let alone one caused by multiply drug-resistant bacteria.[110]

Patients with femoral catheters in one study had higher rates of gram-negative bacteremias and yeast-related fungemias.[111] The occurrence of some of the more unusual isolates (e.g., *Enterobacter* spp., *Burkholderia cepacia* complex, and *Citrobacter freundii*) as a clear cause of the device-associated infection should at least suggest the possibility of a contaminated infusion product or an aqueous environmental reservoir for these pathogens.[40,112-114]

Other organisms may cause such infections (e.g., *Flavobacterium* and *Acinetobacter* spp.); however, such organisms have been infrequently associated with either infusion-related or cannula-related infections.[17] Concomitant with the increasing empirical use of broad-spectrum antimicrobials in severely immunosuppressed patients, cases of device-associated bloodstream infection caused by a variety of unusual bacterial, mycobacterial, and fungal pathogens have been reported with increasing frequency.[10,115-122]

Diagnosis

Clinical detection of catheter-associated septicemia is sometimes difficult. Clinical markers show a poor correlation with intravenous device-related bacteremia.[123] Serum procalcitonin has been studied extensively as a marker of sepsis, and one meta-analysis concluded that it differentiated bacterial from noninfected cases of systemic inflammation with greater accuracy than did C-reactive protein (CRP).[124] Nonetheless, currently available assays often do not provide definitive results; many patients with bacteremia have indeterminate levels of procalcitonin.[124] A more sensitive, second-generation assay might allow daily monitoring in patients with intravascular catheters in order to predict the onset of bacteremia.[125] The presence of fever has a high sensitivity for bacteremia but poor specificity, and local inflammation has better specificity but poor sensitivity. In addition to the presence of an indwelling intravascular device, several clinical features should alert the physician to the possibility of device-associated bacteremia. Salient features of device-associated sepsis that help distinguish it from other bacteremic syndromes are listed in Table 302-3. Generally, blood

TABLE 302-2	Microbiology of Device-Associated Bacteremia

Coagulase-negative staphylococci including *Staphylococcus epidermidis**
Staphylococcus aureus
Enterococcus spp.
Serratia marcescens†
Candida albicans‡
Candida tropicalis‡
Pseudomonas aeruginosa§
Klebsiella spp.†
Enterobacter spp.†
Citrobacter freundii†
Corynebacterium (especially *C. jeikeium*)‖
Acinetobacter (especially *A. baumannii*)¶
Burkholderia cepacia complex§

*Most common pathogen for long-term lines; also associated with lipid infusions in neonates.
†Frequently associated with contaminated infusate.
‡Most often associated with total parenteral nutrition; usually along the catheter path but occasionally as a result of contaminated infusate.
§May arise from a water source (e.g., infusate) or may reflect cutaneous colonization.
‖*C. jeikeium* bacteremia occurs almost exclusively in severely immunosuppressed patients who are or have been receiving broad-spectrum antibiotics and who have indwelling intravascular devices.
¶*A. baumannii* (often multiply drug-resistant) is becoming increasingly prevalent as a pathogen in ICUs, especially among critically ill patients who require life support interventions (e.g., ventilator support) and those who have received multiple courses of antimicrobials.

TABLE 302-3	Factors Differentiating Device-Associated Bacteremia from Other Septic Syndromes

Local phlebitis, inflammation, or both at catheter insertion site

Lack of other source for bacteremia

Sepsis occurring in a patient not otherwise at high risk for bacteremia

Localized embolic disease distal to cannulated artery[131,300]

Hematogenous *Candida* endophthalmitis in patients receiving total parenteral nutrition[216,217]

Presence of ≥15 colonies of bacteria on semiquantitative culture of the catheter tip[126-128]

Sepsis apparently refractory to "appropriate" antimicrobial therapy

Resolution of febrile syndrome after device removal

Typical (*S. aureus*, *S. epidermidis*, or other coagulase-negative staphylococci) or unusual (*B. cepacia* complex, *Enterobacter agglomerans*, *E. cloacae*) microbiology

Clustered infections caused by infusion-related organisms

culture results positive for coagulase-negative staphylococci, *S. aureus*, or *Candida* spp., in the absence of any other identifiable source of infection, increase the possibility of intravenous device-related bacteremia.[123] Although none of these criteria specifically identifies the intravascular device as the source of sepsis, the presence of these clinical findings should at least raise the possibility of device-associated bacteremia.

Cultures of the catheter tip have been reported to be of variable value. Before the development of the semiquantitative culturing technique reported by Maki and colleagues,[126,127] most clinical microbiology laboratories used broth culture of catheter tips to attempt to detect contaminated catheters. This technique yielded results that were highly variable and unreliable.[126-128] Catheter tip cultures should not be performed for diagnosis of bacteremia related to subcutaneous venous ports; instead, culture of the material inside the port reservoir is more sensitive.[80,129,130]

Using the semiquantitative culture technique, which defines a positive catheter tip culture as yielding 15 or more colonies,[126,127] in combination with a relatively strict definition of catheter-associated sepsis, Maki and colleagues reported a specificity in short peripheral catheters ranging between 76% and 96% and a positive predictive value of a positive catheter tip culture ranging between 16%[127] and 31%[126] in four studies.[126,127,131,132] Data regarding the sensitivity of the semiquantitative culture technique are not available because the authors incorporated having a positive catheter tip culture as part of their definition of both local catheter infection and catheter-acquired bacteremia.[126,127,131,132] The cutoff point of 15 colonies per catheter as a definition for "infection" appears to have been somewhat arbitrary in these studies. The authors noted that most infected catheters yield confluent growth when using the semiquantitative technique. These original studies from the late 1970s found that *S. aureus*, rather than coagulase-negative staphylococci, *Candida* spp., and *Enterococcus* spp., were the predominate microorganisms causing bacteremia, and short peripheral catheters (5.7 cm) or steel needles comprised most of the catheters studied. Given the current differences in microbiology and in intravascular devices now in use, these studies may be somewhat less relevant in the 21st century than they were 30 years ago.[133]

Several investigators have tried to modify Maki's technique to improve the predictability of the procedure. Cleri and co-workers reported a technique for quantitatively culturing catheters in broth.[134] This system, which is slightly more cumbersome for the laboratory, was considered by these authors to have three advantages over the system described by Maki and colleagues: (1) the ability to detect organisms within the lumen of the insert, (2) the ability to evaluate relative numbers of organisms from different catheter segments, and (3) the ability to compare relative numbers of organisms present in mixed infections.[134] Brun-Buisson and colleagues used a simplified quantitative broth dilution tip culture to evaluate catheters as potential sources for infection and found this technique to be 97.5% sensitive and 88% specific for the diagnosis of device-associated bacteremia, using a strict clinical definition.[135] Subsequently, Gutierrez and co-workers found a modified broth dilution technique to be only slightly more sensitive, but substantially more labor-intensive, than the semiquantitative technique.[136] The latter authors advocated the use of semiquantitative cultures because of the ease with which this test is performed. Hnatiuk and co-workers demonstrated a substantial increase in sensitivity for the semiquantitative technique when the catheter tip cultures are plated at the patient's bedside rather than cutting the tip into a sterile tube and sending the tip to the laboratory for culture.[137]

Farr and co-workers conducted a meta-analysis of catheter culturing techniques and suggested that the accuracy increases for catheter segment cultures with increasing quantitation (i.e., qualitative < semiquantitative < quantitative).[128] The increase in accuracy is primarily due to the increased specificity of the more quantitative tests. They found that quantitative catheter segment culture was the only method associated with sensitivity and specificity higher than 90%.[128] Similarly,

Shertz and associates suggested that the common practice of culturing a single segment of a central vascular catheter is inadequate.[138] Safdar and colleagues also found that qualitative culture of the catheter segment was the least accurate of the tests they studied, primarily because of poor specificity.[139]

Although the relative merits of these various procedures remain to be definitively delineated, the ease of performing the semiquantitative technique described by Maki and co-workers[126,127] has kept this procedure in widespread clinical use. Attempts to culture newer catheters with antimicrobial coating used for prevention of CLABSIs may lead to false-negative results.[140,141] Specific inhibitors are available to inhibit the effect for silver sulfadiazine–chlorhexidine-coated catheters,[140] but no inhibitors have been identified for minocycline–rifampin-coated catheters.

Other investigators have suggested alternative techniques for diagnosing catheter-associated infections.[128,142-144] Acridine orange leukocyte cytospin testing of blood drawn through the catheter has been studied as a method of diagnosing infection while maintaining the catheter.[145,146] A meta-analysis concluded that this test offers rapid diagnosis of catheter-related bacteremia with good accuracy but lower sensitivity.[139] Although some experience is being gained with the direct Gram stain, none of these newer techniques appear to be effective enough to supplant the semiquantitative method. One group has published a description of an endoluminal brush method,[143] suggesting that this procedure can be employed without sacrificing the intravascular line. These authors suggest that the procedure is substantially more sensitive and more specific than the semiquantitative technique. Presumably because this procedure is slightly cumbersome, it has not been widely embraced. Others have reported that endoluminal catheter colonization is invariably present in cases of catheter-related bacteremia.[33] Some authors have recommended a combination of direct and microbiologic techniques.[128,142]

Mosca and co-workers emphasized the benefits of obtaining blood cultures by using the Isolator system (Isolator, Wampole Laboratories, Cranbury, NJ), which allows for a quantitative estimate of microbial burden in the specimen.[147] Whereas several additional studies have underscored the usefulness of the Isolator system, one study has suggested that results obtained with traditional blood cultures may be complementary to those obtained with the Isolator system and that, whenever feasible, both approaches should be used.[148] Paired quantitative blood cultures have been studied by several groups.[129,149] This technique involves drawing one set of cultures through the device and another set percutaneously; catheter-related infection is diagnosed when cultures are positive from both sites and the concentration of microorganisms in the culture from the device is three- to fivefold higher than in the peripheral culture.

Maki and colleagues performed a meta-analysis to determine the most accurate diagnostic methods for intravenous device-related bacteremia.[139] They determined that quantitative or semiquantitative culture of the catheter combined with two blood cultures (one peripheral and one through the catheter) is most accurate for short-term central catheters.[139] Paired quantitative blood culture was determined to be the most accurate diagnostic method for long-term devices, including tunneled and totally implanted catheters. These authors specifically recommend, as does the CDC,[2,123] that vascular catheters not be cultured if no signs of infection are present. As noted previously, several studies have recommended a differential comparison of quantitative cultures obtained peripherally and quantitative cultures obtained by drawing blood back through the suspected catheter to document the occurrence of catheter-acquired sepsis.[9,150-152] Some authors have suggested that paired quantitative blood cultures (as described previously) obviate the need to remove the catheter and include culture of the tip in the diagnostic algorithm.[153] Because of the complexity of the epidemiology of device-associated bacteremia and the increased technical complexity of the differential blood culturing procedure, the broad applicability of these and the earlier findings nonetheless remains unclear. In addition, despite the evidence that quantitative blood cultures are useful in diagnosing intravascular catheter bacteremias, many clinical microbiology laboratories do not offer this service because of the cost and complexity.

Recently, interest has focused on a method that is based on differential time to positivity of qualitative blood cultures drawn simultaneously from both a catheter and peripherally.[154-158] Blot and colleagues suggested that the speed with which bacterial isolates can be detected in the microbiology laboratory may distinguish catheter-associated from non–catheter-associated infection.[154] Presumably because of a higher bacterial concentration, the blood cultures drawn through an infected central venous catheter often demonstrate growth much more rapidly than those drawn peripherally.[156] Other groups have determined that this differential time to positivity (between cultures drawn through the catheter and peripherally) compares favorably with quantitative blood cultures for the diagnosis of CLABSIs.[157-159] This same differential time to positivity was examined in a group of cancer patients[160] and in critically ill patients[161] and was found not to be useful for many clinical presentations, leaving the validity of this factor undetermined for clinical use. Safdar and colleagues examined this methodology in a meta-analysis and concluded that although paired quantitative blood cultures were the most accurate diagnostic method, using the differential time to positivity provides comparable sensitivity and acceptable specificity.[139]

The usefulness of "through-the-line" cultures has been questioned repeatedly because these cultures may become contaminated easily. Tonnesen and associates reported that blood drawn through venous or arterial catheters gave concordant results with cultures obtained by peripheral venipuncture in 92% of cases.[162] In 5% of cases, results of catheter "pull-back" cultures were considered to represent false positives (most were *Staphylococcus epidermidis*), and in an additional 2%, catheter-drawn cultures were reported to be falsely negative.[162] Similar results were reported by Felices and co-workers,[163] who compared the results of cultures obtained by peripheral venipuncture with cultures obtained through central venous catheters. A subsequent study reported that rates of contamination for venipuncture versus cultures drawn through the catheter were not significantly different.[164] The incidence of false-positive drawback cultures may greatly depend on the type of intravenous device used to draw the cultures and the care taken in obtaining the specimen. If the details of the method used to obtain the culture are unknown, relying entirely on cultures obtained by drawing blood through an indwelling catheter may be imprudent. In well-defined circumstances in which device-associated bacteria is an important consideration in the patient's differential diagnosis, however, these cultures may provide valuable information.[134-136,147,148,150-152,165,166] As reported by DesJardin and colleagues, culture of blood drawn through either a central catheter or a peripheral vein shows excellent negative predictive value.[167] Blood cultures drawn through a central catheter have a lower positive predictive value than do blood cultures drawn percutaneously, but drawing blood through a catheter may be an acceptable method for ruling out bacteremia. We recommend drawing at least two sets of blood cultures when device-related bacteremia is suspected, with at least one set drawn percutaneously.

Occasionally, intracellular bacteria may be identified in routine differential blood smears. The finding of intracellular bacteria in such routine studies on a central venous catheter blood specimen often indicates active infection. In one study, six such patients were asymptomatic at the time bacteria were detected on their differential blood smears; nonetheless, all six had blood cultures positive for coagulase-negative staphylococci.[168] The identification of intracellular bacteria on differential blood smears from patients who have vascular access devices should prompt consideration for catheter removal, even if the patient is asymptomatic.[168]

During the past 15 years, molecular methods have begun to play an increasingly prominent role in the diagnostic microbiology laboratory. Linares and co-workers summarized the importance of molecular techniques in the laboratory.[28] Examples of the usefulness of these techniques include the use of randomly amplified polymorphic DNA analysis for the rapid fingerprinting of coagulase-negative staphylococci,[169] the use of other molecular typing methods (e.g., pulsed-field electrophoresis and localization and/or probing the vicinity of the *mecA* gene),[28,170] and the molecular identification of antimicrobial resistance even before speciation can be completed. These molecular techniques are particularly valuable in epidemiologic investigations.

Device-Specific Issues

PERIPHERAL INTRAVENOUS CANNULIZATION

In general, peripheral catheters are associated with much lower infection risks than are central catheters. Steel needles have been associated with lower rates of local infections, bacteremic infections, and local phlebitis than have plastic catheters.[171] Tully and associates, however, demonstrated that steel catheters placed by an intravenous team nurse were associated with significantly less phlebitis but significantly more episodes of infiltration than were Teflon catheters.[172] In this study, all catheters were removed in less than 72 hours; infection rates for both catheter types were extremely low, and there were no differences in local or systemic infection rates between the two groups.[172] Approximately 20 years later, Bregenzer and colleagues demonstrated that the risks for catheter-related complications—phlebitis, catheter-related infections, and mechanical complications—did not increase during extended (i.e., longer than 72 hours) catheterization.[173] These authors suggested that the CDC's recommendation for routine replacement of peripheral intravenous catheters be reevaluated, particularly considering the additional costs associated with routine catheter replacement, as well as the additional discomfort for the patient.[173] Lai showed similar rates of phlebitis in peripheral catheters left in place for 72 versus 96 hours.[174] Other studies have similarly demonstrated that prolonged duration of cannulation was not associated with increased risk for phlebitis.[175,176] The CDC now recommends that peripheral catheters be replaced every 72 to 96 hours in adults to prevent phlebitis.[2] A variety of factors including the development of new materials for catheter construction, as well as new dressing and catheter care techniques, likely explain some of these differences. Peripheral catheters should not be routinely replaced in children unless phlebitis or infiltration occurs.

The location of catheter placement also may influence subsequent infection rates. Catheters placed in the lower extremities, particularly those placed in the femoral veins, are associated with increased risk for many complications, including infection.[171,172,177-181] Martin and co-workers evaluated axillary vein cannulation as an alternative to the internal jugular insertion site and found that the rates of catheter-related infection and other complications were similar to those observed after internal jugular vein catheterization.[182]

Catheters placed percutaneously are associated with lower infection rates than are those placed by cutdown.[171,183] Catheters placed emergently are also at higher risk for infection, presumably as a result of breaks in technique at the time of placement.[184] Several authors have suggested that catheters placed by members of an intravenous therapy team are associated with lower complication rates than are those placed by other health care professionals.[89,185]

Techniques for the placement and care of indwelling venous cannulas have been reviewed in detail.[171] Several aspects of catheter maintenance and care have been controversial, although more definitive studies have answered some questions. These issues are discussed further in the section titled "Prevention of Device-Associated Bacteremia."

Finally, two studies have demonstrated that routinely changing intravenous administration sets at 48 rather than 24 hours was not associated with a significant increase in the infusion-related bacteremia rate.[186,187] Snydman and co-workers[188] and Maki and colleagues[189] compared the relative safety of changing administration sets at 72-hour intervals with changing them at 48 hours. Neither study identified an increased risk with the 72-hour interval.

Thus, inserting a peripheral catheter, dressing it, hooking up the administration set, and changing all three at 72- to 96-hour intervals now seems both safe and practical and reasonable.

CENTRAL VENOUS CATHETERS: SHORT-TERM AND PARENTERAL NUTRITION ISSUES

Because central venous catheters frequently remain in place longer than peripheral catheters, certain problems either occur with more frequency or are unique to these catheters. In addition, because of the placement of these catheters in the great veins, complications of placement such as infective endocarditis and suppurative thrombophlebitis of the great veins represent life-threatening events.

Michel and colleagues studied 390 catheters placed into the subclavian vein by identical technique, in an attempt to determine risk factors associated with microbial colonization.[190] In this study, the presence of distant infection, bacteremia, or tracheostomy was associated with an increased risk for catheter colonization.[190] Unfortunately, these authors chose to culture the catheters by using the broth culture technique, which, as noted previously, yields notoriously unreliable results.[171]

The presence of either intraluminal or extraluminal fibrin has been proposed as predisposing to the development of catheter-associated infection.[66-68,191-194] Stillman and colleagues studied 94 central catheters and found that all 11 catheters categorized as infected in their study and 30 of 83 not found to be either infected or colonized had gross visible evidence of either intraluminal or surface thrombin at the time of removal.[66] Lloyd and co-workers failed to find a deleterious effect associated with the so-called fibrin sheath when evaluating a rat model of device-associated bacteremia.[195] Another rat model found that catheter colonization decreases with the decrease in fibrin within the pericatheter sheath.[196]

Routine replacement of central venous catheters is not necessary and exposes the patient to the increased risks of catheter manipulation and mechanical complications with new sites.[197] The CDC has recommended against routine replacement of central venous catheters, PICCs, hemodialysis catheters, or pulmonary artery catheters to prevent catheter-related infections.[2] The issue of whether central catheters should be changed over a guidewire remains controversial. Use of a guidewire obviates the need for a second percutaneous puncture of the great veins and may be preferable for catheter exchanges judged routine or mandated by some reason other than suspected infection. Little scientific evidence supports guidewire use if catheter-associated infection is suspected. Maher and colleagues used this technique successfully for catheter exchange in situations assessed as "low risk for infection."[198] Two additional studies suggest that guidewire exchange may not be particularly useful if device-associated infection is suspected.[199,200] In one of these two studies, guidewire catheter exchange was associated with an increased risk of bloodstream infection but a lower risk of mechanical complications.[200] In one experimental study, replacement of a biofilm-colonized central venous catheter over a guidewire was associated with an increased risk for colonization of the new catheter, as well as an increased risk for production of detached, slime-enclosed, antibiotic-resistant aggregates that may disseminate the infection to other sites.[151]

Whereas guidewire exchange of central venous catheters may be associated with a greater risk for catheter-related infection, this technique may result in many fewer mechanical complications than would be the case for repuncture.[201] Specifically, exchange over a guidewire is associated with lower risks for some complications (e.g., bleeding and pneumothorax).[199,200] If a guidewire is to be used for catheter exchange, culture of the removed or "old" catheter tip should be performed. In addition, blood cultures should be drawn through the old line before removal. If either of these cultures becomes positive, the most conservative approach would be to remove the "replacement" catheter and perform appropriate cultures. If central access is still desired, a third catheter should be placed at a new puncture site. In situations in which the catheter is being removed for suspected sepsis, in our opinion, exchange over a guidewire should not be attempted. Conversely, one study suggested a possible benefit of guidewire exchange for patients who have catheter-associated candidemia.[202]

The umbilical vein catheter that is commonly used for vascular access in neonates presents some unique problems. Because of the extensive microbiologic flora of the umbilical stump, these catheters are at high risk for both colonization and infection.[203,204] Although high rates of umbilical catheter-associated infection have been reported in several studies,[203,204] not all centers report such high rates.[205] One study reported a much lower incidence of infectious complications when the umbilical artery (rather than the umbilical vein) was cannulated for infusion.[206]

Thrombosis of the great veins, with the attendant risk for suppurative thrombophlebitis, is a major complication of central catheter placement.[180] Thrombosis occurs with increased frequency in patients with malignancies[178] (particularly those who have mediastinal lymphadenopathy) and in patients with sickle cell disease.[207] In instances in which central catheters are placed in patients with these underlying illnesses, thrombotic and infectious complications should be anticipated, prevented (when possible), diagnosed early, and treated aggressively.

Additional issues relating to catheter composition and effectiveness of subcutaneous tunneling of catheters and risks associated with electronic monitoring devices are discussed later.

Several aspects of the delivery of parenteral nutrition separate this mode of intravascular therapy from others. First, the composition of the infusate supports the growth of different microorganisms, most notably certain of the *Candida* spp.[19,20,208] Patients receiving parenteral nutrition in one study had an increased incidence of polymicrobial and multidrug-resistant bacteremias.[209] Second, catheters used to deliver parenteral nutrition are often required to remain in place much longer than either peripheral or other central venous cannulas. For this reason, problems with catheter contamination become much more of a concern. Third, the hypertonicity of the solution causes irritation of the vascular intima, which in turn may cause thrombosis. Thrombosis provides a nidus for, and an increased risk for, infection. Fourth, because patients who require parenteral nutrition are frequently severely ill as a result of neoplasms, trauma, or inflammatory bowel disease, the risk for bacteremia is higher. Therefore, the potential for hematogenous seeding of the catheter is high. Several studies have found an association between use of parenteral nutrition and an increased risk of death.[210,211] One study found that use of total parenteral nutrition declined significantly from 2000 to 2005 in critical care trauma patients, and this decrease was associated with fewer complications, including bacteremia and sepsis.[210]

For these and other reasons, the placement, management, and care of catheters used for parenteral nutrition have received a great deal of attention. Ryan and colleagues, in a prospective study of 200 catheters, documented that the risk of catheter-associated infection increased significantly when the integrity of the delivery system was interrupted.[91] Snydman and colleagues subsequently found that the occurrence of so-called line violations was highly associated with the development of catheter-associated sepsis.[92] For these reasons, the CDC has recommended that the administration of parenteral nutrition be supervised and conducted by members of a team (Table 302-4).[212] In their study, Snydman and colleagues also attempted to correlate the results of twice-weekly 1-mL pour-plate blood cultures with the subsequent development of catheter colonization and sepsis. Similar to the previously cited studies,[162,163] although concordance was high among blood cultures, catheter tip cultures, and peripheral blood cultures, cultures obtained through the catheter demonstrated a reasonably high incidence of false positivity, primarily as a result of *S. epidermidis* contamination.[213] A recent study found that increased parenteral caloric intake is an independent risk factor for bacteremia, and that this association is unrelated to hyperglycemia.[214]

Candida infection has been a particular problem in patients receiving parenteral nutrition.[215-218] Curry and Quie reported a 16% incidence of candidemia among patients receiving parenteral nutrition in a prospective study in a hospital that did not have a dedicated team.[215] In another prospective study of 131 postoperative patients who were receiving parenteral nutrition, 13 patients were detected as developing

TABLE 302-4	Prevention of Infusion-Related Infection in Parenteral Nutrition (TPN)

Administration of TPN should be under the supervision of a team of health care professionals (usually a nurse, pharmacist, and physician). Both the decision regarding appropriateness of TPN therapy and protocols for insertions, maintenance, and delivery of TPN should be under the responsibility of this team.

TPN solution should be prepared using sterile or aseptic technique when possible in a laminar flow hood. Once prepared, the solution should be infused immediately or stored at 4°C.

Placement of the catheter should be performed by using maximal sterile barrier precautions, including mask, sterile gown and gloves, large sterile drape, and appropriate skin preparation preferably with chlorhexidine.[326-328]

Once placed, the catheter should be anchored to avoid movement, which may result in local irritation of the insertion site or transport of organisms along the insertion path.

If possible, the system should be kept closed, avoiding unnecessary entry for blood drawing and administration of other fluids or blood products via the TPN line.

If multiple lumens/ports are present, one lumen/port should be designated as the parenteral nutrition site.

Other aspects of TPN administration are either of empirical or theoretical value, have shown equivocal or borderline results in studies, have shown conflicting results in studies, or have been demonstrated to be of value in small studies. Definitive studies to document the merit of these techniques are needed before they are routinely implemented; these include the following:
- Routine application of antiseptic cream at the site of catheter insertion (either at the time of venipuncture or at routine dressing change)
- Routine dressing changes and skin defatting with acetone
- Routine use of semipermeable dressing materials. A meta-analysis of data from several studies suggests that these dressings may actually play a detrimental role in catheter infections.[336]
- Routine use of in-line membrane filters (no benefit demonstrated)
- Use of silicone or other less traumatic, nonthrombogenic catheters; use of heparin-bonded catheters; use of low-dose heparin infusions
- Tunneling the catheter subcutaneously to increase the anatomic distance between catheter insertion site and the point at which the catheter enters the vessel (appears to be useful in several small studies)
- Routine use of antibiotic lock prophylaxis with heparin plus vancomycin

Modified from Goldman D, Maki D. Infection control in total parenteral nutrition. *JAMA.* 1973;223:1360-1364.

chorioretinal lesions consistent with hematogenous *Candida* endophthalmitis; 7 of the patients had positive blood cultures for *Candida*.[216] Although most of these infections are presumed to arise as a result of yeast contamination at the catheter entry site, occasional outbreaks of *Candida* infection resulting from parenteral nutrition solution that was intrinsically contaminated have been reported.[26,27] Because of the risk of intrinsic as well as in-use contamination of parenteral nutrition solutions with *Candida* or other microorganisms, some authorities have recommended the routine use of an in-line membrane filter to prevent infusion-related sepsis.[219] Such filters have been implicated as a cause of device-associated infection or device-associated endotoxemia, however, and the risk-to-benefit ratio for their use has not been established.

Because the catheter frequently must be left in place for an extended period of time and because of the increased thrombogenicity of parenteral nutrition fluid, several modifications of the delivery system of the catheter have been advocated. Among the suggested mechanisms for decreasing infections in this situation are (1) either bonding heparin or a heparin-like substance to the catheter or infusing heparin with the infusate in an attempt to minimize fibrin sheath formation[194,220]; (2) constructing the catheter of a more flexible substance, thereby producing less trauma to the vascular endothelium[221]; and (3) tunneling the catheter under the skin in an attempt to decrease access of pathogens to the circulation.[221]

A final and often difficult issue is deciding when to remove a parenteral nutrition catheter for suspected sepsis. In the past, most authorities recommended the removal of a catheter whenever infection was suspected. In separate studies, Ryan and co-workers[91] and Maher and associates[198] suggested that nearly 70% of catheters removed for suspected sepsis are apparently removed unnecessarily. Thus, the

parenteral nutrition team is often faced with the dilemma of whether or not to remove the catheter from a patient in whom the evidence for infection is equivocal. Such a patient may have many reasons for fever; therefore, the diagnosis of infection may be difficult. Often, patients are severely immunosuppressed, thrombocytopenic, or both, and the risks associated with catheter replacement may be quite high. Several clinical features may help the physician decide how to manage the catheter.[191,222] The presence of positive blood cultures (particularly for *Candida* or coagulase-negative staphylococci) in the absence of another source for the infection or in the presence of hemodynamic instability, embolic phenomena, leukocytosis, or profound leukopenia may herald the onset of catheter-associated sepsis. In addition, the development of new glucose intolerance in a parenteral nutrition patient whose carbohydrate metabolism had been previously well regulated may be an early subtle sign of bacteremia.[191,216]

CENTRAL VENOUS CATHETERS: LONG-TERM ISSUES

In 1973, Broviac and colleagues reported their initial experience with the use of a chronic indwelling right atrial catheter for the delivery of long-term parenteral nutrition.[223] Venous access also has long been a problem for patients receiving chemotherapy for malignancy. Hickman and colleagues modified the Broviac catheter, which has a smaller lumen, for use in patients undergoing bone marrow transplantation.[224] This catheter can be used for the administration of intensive chemotherapy, the administration of other medicines and fluids, transfusion, and phlebotomy. These catheters spare the patient both physical and psychological trauma. In the ensuing years, a number of additional modifications of these catheters have been devised, including the Groshong valve.[225] These modified catheters and implanted infusion ports, which were introduced in 1982, represent a major step forward in the management of all patients who require long-term central venous access but have been especially useful in the management of immunosuppressed patients and particularly in immunosuppressed children in whom venous access is frequently problematic. Use of these devices in a variety of clinical settings has become the standard of care during the past several decades.

Several centers have reported their experiences using these catheters, and many series report remarkably low rates of infection. Initial reports suggested that the rate of catheter infection in nonneutropenic patients was approximately one infection per 5.5 patient years.[226] Press and colleagues summarized 1088 catheter placements from 18 studies in their literature review. In their summary data, these authors reported approximately 0.14 infections per 100 catheter days.[227] Table 302-5 presents a similar summary, including several published studies evaluating infection and bacteremia risks associated with the use of implanted catheters and infusion ports.[102,228-243] The slightly elevated rate of all infections (0.15 infections for each 100 catheter days), as well as the elevated risk for bacteremia (0.11 infections for each 100 catheter days), may be more of a reflection of the severity of the patients' illnesses, the increasing immunosuppression associated with their therapies, and the increasingly invasive care provided to critically ill patients. The differences noted between implanted ports and Hickman/Broviac catheters may also be a reflection of the populations being treated.

Several centers have reported remarkable success—few infections and few other complications as well—with totally implantable access ports.[244-248] In one of the earliest of these studies, the rate of infections for each 100 catheter days was 0.43—comparable to rates of other implantable catheters.[245] Subsequent studies have demonstrated even lower infection risks.[231,235,237,239,240,243,246,247,249] One epidemiologic study found in multiple logistic regression analysis that the only factor associated with risk for infection of these devices was the number of times the system was entered.[250] Another study concluded that infections are the primary reason for late-term complications and port removal.[251] This group determined that patients with recurrent device implantation and with ongoing chemotherapy are significantly more likely to need device removal.[251]

| TABLE 302-5 | Infectious Complications Associated with Implanted, Long-Term Catheters |

Authors	Number of Patients	Type of Catheter	Exit Site/Tunnel/Pocket Infections (%)	CLABSIs (%)	Duration of Catheterization (Range)	All Infections per 100 Catheter Days	CLABSIs per 100 Catheter Days
Blacklock et al.[226]	25	H	14 (56)	2 (8)	70 (5-256)	0.91	0.11
Larson et al.[236]	34	H	4 (11.8)	4 (11.8)	110.3 (3-355)	0.23	0.12
Wade et al.[102]	51	H	5 (9.8)	3 (5.9)	91 (4-457)	0.17	0.06
Rizzari et al.[238]	125	H/B	3 (2.4)	106 (85)	134 (6-488)	0.53	0.51
Viscoli et al.[242]	145	B	6 (4.1)	57 (39)	171 (2-647)	0.26	0.19
Hogan and Pulito[232]	84	B	6 (7.1)	9 (10.7)	33.4 (2-119)	0.39	0.29
Alurkar et al.[228]	91	H/B	6 (6.6)	31 (34)	74.6 (NG)	0.54	0.41
Wacker et al.[243]	44	B	NG	15 (34)	236 (15-806)	NG	0.06
	33	P	NG	6 (18)	316 (12-1294)	NG	0.10
Johnson et al.[234]	64	B	25 (39)	33 (51.6)	251 (NG)	0.28	0.19
Lokich et al.[237]	92	P	6 (6.5)	2 (2.2)	127 (7-450)	0.06	0.02
Shulman et al.[240]	31	P	1 (3.2)	4 (12.9)	232 (14-607)	0.07	0.05
Cairo et al.[229]	46	H/B	14 (30)	23 (50)	163 (9-365)	0.48	0.30
Hockenberry et al.[231]	82	P	8 (10)	4 (4.9)	168 (7-1030)	0.06	0.02
van Hoff et al.[401]	59	H/B	7 (12)	30 (51)	220 (NG)	0.28	0.23
Ulz et al.[241]	111	H/B	3 (2.7)	63 (57)	81 (1-167)	0.69	0.66
Kappers-Klunne et al.[235]	23	H	0 (0)	19 (83)	166 (1-605)	0.50	0.50
	20	P	2 (10)	9 (45)	164 (1-971)	0.33	0.27
Ross et al.[239]	39	H/B	11 (28)	4 (10)	365 (30-426)	0.13	0.03
	49	P	7 (14)	0 (0)	350 (7-395)	0.07	0.00
Biffi et al.[402]	175	P	1 (0.6)	4 (2.2)	180 (4-559)	0.02	0.003
Elishoov et al.[230]	242	H/B	28 (12)	46 (19)	40 (7-187)	0.79	0.52
Schwarz et al.[403]	680	P	31	31	310 (2-1960)	0.02	0.01
Chang et al.[218]	572	P	11 (1.9)	21 (3.7)	358 (1-1742)	0.015	0.01
Subtotal (by catheter type)	**1183**	**H/B**	**132 (11)**	**445 (38)**	**147 (1-806)**	**0.40**	**0.26**
	1734	**P**	**67 (3.9)**	**81 (4.7)**	**231 (1-1960)**	**0.12**	**0.08**
Total	**2917**	**–**	**199 (6.8)**	**526 (18.0)**	**147 (1-1960)**	**0.15**	**0.11**

B, Broviac; CLABSIs, central line–associated bloodstream infections; H, Hickman; NG, not given; P, totally implantable port (e.g., Port-A-Cath, Infus-A-Port, and Mediport).

Pocket infections, defined as the spread of infection into the subcutaneous pocket of a totally implanted intravascular device,[123] are considered an absolute reason for device removal because of the poor response to antimicrobial therapy by bacteria inside the biofilms on the port inner surface.[123,252] Pocket infections remain among the most difficult infectious complications associated with implanted ports. Evidence from studies of intravascular cardiac device infections suggests that risk of local device infections, including pocket infections, in these devices is increasing at a faster rate than the corresponding increase in device implantations.[253,254]

During the past decade, the use of PICC lines for intermediate and long-term access has increased dramatically in both home care and hospital settings.[255-258] These catheters have several advantages over some of the other long-term access devices: PICCs may be inserted at the bedside[255] by nonphysician providers[259,260]; they are placed into children and neonates under fluoroscopy with relative ease[75,256]; and they are useful for administration of chemotherapy, antimicrobial agents, and parenteral nutrition,[256,257,261] particularly in pediatric patients requiring long-term nutritional support.[257,261] Skilled interventional radiology is needed for difficult insertions, for catheter salvage, and to ensure that the catheter is not misplaced or misdirected.[255] A major problem is device failure, with as many as 10%[261] to 27%[262] of these catheters developing mechanical malfunction. One group suggested that PICC lines may be less cost-effective than currently believed because of the more difficult insertion into some patients and higher thrombophlebitis rates.[259] Another group determined that PICC lines are more likely to develop mechanical complications and have a shorter survival time than central venous catheters.[262] Many institutions, including ours, have elected to develop a skilled team approach to the insertion and management of these catheters.

Intraluminal contamination may represent the most important route of infection for implanted catheters and ports, further suggesting that strategies aimed at decreasing the risks for intraluminal contamination could substantially lower infection rates with these types of intravascular devices.

Several issues regarding the care and maintenance of these catheters remain unsettled. Among these issues are (1) whether a dressing should be placed over the exit site (and if so, what dressing materials should be used and how frequently should the dressing be changed); (2) whether the system should be routinely flushed (and if so, how frequently and with what); (3) whether blood cultures obtained through the catheter are reliable indicators of catheter contamination; and (4) what are the indications for catheter removal, and can either or both local infection and bacteremia be treated with the catheter in place?

Although definitive answers to these questions remain elusive, at the National Institutes of Health Clinical Center, a sterile dry gauze dressing or a semipermeable membrane is kept in place over the exit site. These dressings are changed at least twice weekly. We also use an every-other-day heparin flush (5 mL of 100 units/mL) to attempt to keep the catheters patent. Higher heparin concentrations are associated with an increased risk for anticoagulating the patient. The CDC guidelines suggest that well-healed exit sites might not require dressings.[2]

The issue of pull-back blood cultures was discussed previously. Repeated isolation of the same organism from cultures drawn through the catheter indicates a need for therapy. Individual positive cultures and sporadic positive cultures are difficult to interpret in the absence of clinical or laboratory correlates. As noted previously, some groups believe that quantitative cultures may prove particularly helpful in establishing a diagnosis in this setting.

The problem of how best to treat an infection in a patient with a long-term venous access catheter in place is a difficult one. Hiemenz and colleagues reported success in treating 90% of proven bacteremias while leaving the catheter in place.[263] Some organisms (e.g., *Bacillus* spp. and *Candida* spp.) may be difficult to eradicate,[264] although Hartman and Shuchat had some success in treating *Candida* infections.[265] Guidelines for managing these infections have been published jointly by the Infectious Diseases Society of America, the Society of Critical Care Medicine, and the Society for Healthcare Epidemiology of America.[123] Several studies have advocated the use of thrombolytic agents (e.g., urokinase or tissue plasminogen activator) in combination with appropriate antimicrobials to treat both thrombosis and infections associated with implanted catheters.[192,266,267] These studies suggest that eradicating the fibrin sheath that forms around the catheter may make therapy of a catheter-associated infection much more likely to succeed.

A number of studies have shown that instilling antimicrobials into a catheter and leaving the solution to dwell (i.e., antimicrobial catheter lock) is effective in treating some catheter-related bacteremias.[268-272] Benoit and colleagues suggested more than a decade ago that intraluminal antibiotic treatment was effective in treatment of bacteremia in a small uncontrolled study.[268] These investigators also found that intraluminal therapy with amphotericin B also may suppress, but not eradicate, *Candida* infections in tunneled catheters.[268] Similarly, McCarthy and co-workers successfully treated gram-positive catheter infections by instilling teicoplanin daily into "infected" central catheters for 4 to 9 days and allowing the drug to dwell in the lumen of the catheter.[269] Three recent studies suggested that antibiotic lock therapy in combination with appropriate systemic antimicrobials was effective in clearing the bacteremia and allowing retention of the catheter in 67%,[271] 84%,[270] and 93%[272] of patients. Bacteremias caused by coagulase-negative staphylococci may be particularly amenable to antibiotic lock therapy,[123,270] whereas at least one group has suggested that routine vancomycin antibiotic lock therapy is not appropriate for patients with *S. aureus* catheter-related bacteremia.[273] Another group suggested that liposomal amphotericin B lock therapy may successfully eradicate fungemia secondary to several *Candida* species without the need for catheter removal.[274] Raad and colleagues reported that daptomycin, minocycline, and tigecycline may be more effective in eradicating methicillin-resistant *S. aureus* embedded in biofilms than linezolid or vancomycin,[275] and they further suggested that minocycline-EDTA in 25% ethanol is highly effective at rapidly eradicating *S. aureus* and *Candida parapsilosis* embedded in biofilm.[276] Several groups also have reported that use of an ethanol catheter lock in combination with systemic antimicrobials may be relatively effective in treatment of CLABSIs.[277-279] Thus, additional experience has suggested that, perhaps with the exception of true tunnel and pocket infections, many, if not most, infections of indwelling central catheters may be amenable to therapy with the device left in place. Patients should be carefully evaluated for evidence of complicated device-related infections, including tunnel infection, pocket infections of ports, bloodstream infection that continues despite 72 hours or more of antimicrobial therapy to which the infecting organisms are susceptible, septic emboli, septic thrombosis, endocarditis, and osteomyelitis. The device/catheter should be removed for any of these conditions.

Use of catheters placed for long-term central venous access has also fostered some new kinds of complications. For example, use of these catheters has been associated with the rare complication of septic thrombosis of the atrium.[280,281]

PULMONARY ARTERY CATHETERS

The use of indwelling, balloon-tipped pulmonary artery catheters[282] revolutionized the management of hemodynamically unstable, critically ill patients. Despite an ongoing controversy about the safety of and benefit associated with the use of these catheters,[283,284] approximately 1.5 million are used each year in the United States alone.[285] The placement of such a catheter in one of the great veins, across the tricuspid and pulmonic valves, and into the pulmonary vasculature is not without complications, however. Michel and co-workers demonstrated that 29 of 153 pulmonary artery catheter tips produced microbial growth in thioglycolate broth.[286] Although no patient in this study

was considered to develop sepsis secondary to the contaminated catheter, other studies have suggested a reasonably high rate of contamination with occasional episodes of catheter-related sepsis and nosocomial endocarditis.[287] The majority of these catheters are heparin bonded, which reduces catheter thrombosis and microbial adherence to the catheter.

Katz and colleagues retrospectively studied complications associated with the placement of 392 balloon-tipped catheters; of these, 17 (4.2%) were assessed to be associated with bacteremia.[287] Maki estimated that 3% to 5% of these catheters kept in place for more than 72 hours will result in CLABSIs[222] and concluded that efforts should be made to limit the duration of pulmonary artery catheters to no more than 4 days.[288] A study of 1000 patients randomized to receive either pulmonary artery catheters or central venous catheters found similar rates of infection in both groups (five CLABSIs in the pulmonary artery catheter group vs. three CLABSIs in the central venous catheter group).[283] Another group found that 4 of 215 (1.9%) patients undergoing pulmonary artery catheterization developed infection compared to no infections in the control group.[289] One study evaluated complications associated with the use of a "hands-off" pulmonary artery catheter that is completely shielded during balloon testing, preparation, and insertion[290]; use of this catheter was associated with a substantial reduction in systemic infections related to the catheter.[290]

Another problem relatively unique to the flow-directed, balloon-tipped pulmonary artery catheter is that such catheters may traumatize the right-sided heart valves and the right-sided endocardium. In a study of 102 consecutive autopsies of patients who died in the hospital, 26 (25.5%) had had an indwelling intracardiac catheter inserted before death.[291] Six of these patients were excluded from analysis (4 patients died 48 hours or less after catheter placement; 2 patients had permanent transvenous pacemakers in place for many years with the anticipated endocardial fibrosis). Of the remaining 20 patients, 6 had vegetations present, and 88% of the patients had some evidence of intracardiac damage.[291] One patient had infective endocarditis on the tricuspid valve. Other studies have reported slightly lower but significant incidences of right-sided heart vegetations among monitored patients coming to autopsy.[292] Greene and colleagues noted a 10-fold increase in the incidence of valvular vegetations when they compared a period of time before the introduction of balloon-tipped pulmonary artery catheters with a time in which the catheters were in wide use.[292] Severely burned patients may be at even higher risk for this complication.[293] Nosocomial endocarditis is increasing in frequency: In one study, 9.3% of cases of endocarditis diagnosed in a referral hospital were both nosocomial in origin and unrelated to prior cardiac surgery.[294] Two studies found that between 28%[295] and 33%[296] of cases of endocarditis were nosocomial in origin, with the majority from line-related sepsis. Hemodialysis patients, in particular, are at increased risk of nosocomial or health care–associated endocarditis.[297,298]

No prospective study has addressed risk factors associated with infection of these catheters, nor have studies assessed the efficacy of devices designed to decrease the risk of catheter-associated infection (e.g., leaving the introducer sheath in the vein to protect the catheter).[286] Changing these catheters over a guidewire may present a major risk factor for infection. A study in cardiac surgery patients found that greater than 4 days of catheterization was the single variable associated with increased risk of pulmonary artery catheter colonization.[299] CDC guidelines currently recommend that pulmonary artery catheters need not be changed more frequently than every 7 days.[2] Infection risks associated with other aspects of monitoring equipment (e.g., transducer domes and heparin flush solution) are discussed next.

ARTERIAL LINES, TRANSDUCERS, AND TRANSDUCER DOMES

The widespread use of arterial lines for blood pressure monitoring or for obtaining arterial samples for blood gas determinations has yielded yet another source of device-associated infection. In addition, the technical electronic equipment used for hemodynamic monitoring—

transducers and their associated paraphernalia—has also been cited as a source of device-associated infection.

Stamm and colleagues reported an outbreak of *Flavobacterium* bacteremia among monitored patients in an ICU.[17] Ultimately, these organisms were cultured from in-use radial artery catheters, from stopcocks, and from ice used to cool syringes for blood gas determinations.[17] Adams and colleagues reported a series of 147 radial artery cannulations in infants in whom umbilical artery cannulation failed.[300] In this series, there were two episodes of catheter-related sepsis. Band and Maki used the semiquantitative catheter tip culture technique to study 130 arterial catheters in 95 patients.[131] In their series, 23 catheters were classified as showing "local infection" (e.g., >15 colonies per semiquantitative culture), and there were five episodes of sepsis.[131] Factors associated with increased risk for infection were (1) duration of catheterization (especially longer than 96 hours), (2) placement by cutdown rather than percutaneously, and (3) clinical signs of local inflammation. Femoral placement of arterial catheters also has been associated with higher rates of colonization and catheter infection than other placement sites.[301,302]

Maki and Hassemer reported a prospective study designed to assess the endemic rate of bacteremia associated with arterial monitoring.[303] Transducer chamber fluid was demonstrated to be contaminated in nearly 12% of the cases. There were eight cases of bacteremia—four definitely related and four possibly related to the extrinsic contamination.[303] Maki also suggested an increased risk for infection of arterial catheters associated with replacing the catheter using a guidewire. In another study, Maki and colleagues reviewed 14 studies of arterial catheters used for hemodynamic monitoring, and they determined that the pooled mean rate of arterial catheter-related bacteremia per 100 catheters was 0.8 (95% confidence interval, 0.6 to 1.1) and the pooled mean rate of arterial catheter-related bacteremia per 1000 catheter-days was 1.7 (95% confidence interval, 1.2 to 2.3), a rate approaching that of short-term central venous catheters.[249] Koh and colleagues found similar incidence densities of arterial and central venous catheter colonization but more than twofold increased rates of bacteremic infection with central venous catheters compared to arterial catheters.[301] Mermel noted in an editorial that if 6 million arterial catheters are used each year in the United States and the risk of bacteremia is 0.8,[249] then there are approximately 48,000 arterial catheter-related bloodstream infections each year.[304]

Several epidemics of infection resulting from improper sterilization of reusable transducer domes have been reported.[187,305] However, with the introduction of disposable transducer domes, one might assume that these problems would be overcome. Buxton and colleagues reported an epidemic of *Enterobacter* infections that was associated with the contamination of disposable transducer domes during their initial setup.[187] The chambers and domes were apparently contaminated by the hands of hospital personnel who had handled heavily contaminated transducer heads.[187] West and colleagues also reported *Serratia* sepsis resulting from transducer dome cracks.[306] In this study, supposedly disposable transducer domes were being resterilized, with resultant cracks or breaks in the dome membrane.

Another potential reservoir for nosocomial bacteremia is the heparin flush solution used to irrigate certain intravascular devices continually. This fluid has been implicated as a reservoir for outbreaks of device-associated bacteremia in several instances.[40]

Several authors have made recommendations regarding the prevention of infection associated with intravascular monitoring devices.[2,131,303,305] A summary of these recommendations is presented in Table 302-6.

Prevention of Device-Associated Bacteremia

A number of reports have suggested that CLABSIs can be prevented using simultaneous implementation of an array of practice improvements (i.e., "bundles").[307-311] Evidence of improved outcomes following multifaceted interventions, along with the emergence of prevention of health care–associated infections as a national priority,[4,5,312] resulted in the publication of a compendium of strategies to prevent CLABSIs by the Society for Healthcare Epidemiology of America and the Infectious Diseases Society of America Standards and Practice Guidelines Committee[11,313] that supplement existing, more detailed guidelines.[2] The recent limitation of additional reimbursement by the Centers for Medicare and Medicaid Services for a diagnosis of vascular catheter-associated infection[4] will provide additional financial incentives for health care facilities to prevent these infections.

BEFORE INSERTION OF VASCULAR CATHETERS

Education of health care personnel regarding standardized catheter insertion, care, and prevention of infection has been shown to reduce the incidence of catheter-associated infections.[88,100,314-316] All health care personnel involved in catheter insertion and maintenance should complete an educational program regarding catheter-associated infections prior to performing these duties.[11] Engaging hospital leadership and allowing for flexibility in implementation have been suggested as key components to maximize the benefits of these programs.[317] In a meta-analysis, Safdar and Abad concurred that educational interventions can reduce rates of health care–associated infections.[318] They also concluded that additional studies with clearly described, easily reproducible, and widely generalizable educational tools that had been validated were needed, particularly in general hospital wards rather than ICUs.[318]

Catheter insertion checklists to ensure adherence to infection control practices have been used as part of the practice improvement bundle in a number of studies.[307,309,310] Use of these checklists should be accompanied by standardized catheter insertion kits/carts containing all necessary items for insertion.[11,307]

AT INSERTION

Hand hygiene prior to catheter insertion or manipulation is an absolute requirement[319] and has been shown to be successful in reducing health care–associated infections.[316,320-322] Maximal sterile barrier precautions, including a mask, cap, sterile gown and gloves, and a large sterile drape to cover the patient, have also been shown to reduce central venous catheter-associated infections.[90,323,324] This tenet was confirmed by a prospective study that demonstrated that use of maximal sterile barrier precautions had an independent and significant association with a decrease in the risk of catheter infection of more than fivefold.[325] This same group performed a multivariate logistic

TABLE 302-6	Prevention of Infection Associated with Hemodynamic Monitoring
Place arterial lines, central venous lines, and flow-directed, balloon-tipped catheters by using sterile technique. Maximal sterile barrier precautions should be used. The skin should be prepared with an effective antiseptic solution (e.g., chlorhexidine).[326,397,404]	
Place the catheters percutaneously and anchor well to avoid catheter movement. Dress the insertion site appropriately.	
Use heparinized saline (not dextrose-containing solutions or parenteral nutrition) for continuous-flush solutions.	
Do not reuse transducer domes; sterilize reusable part of transducer setup according to manufacturer's instructions between patients.	
Replace transducers, tubing, and continuous-flow devices every 96 hours[2,405]; do not routinely replace peripheral arterial catheters to prevent infection.	
Use sterile fluid to fill the chamber dome; use aseptic technique in the assembly.	
Avoid placing unnecessary junctions or stopcocks into the apparatus; minimize manipulation of the system.	
Whenever possible, avoid exchanging arterial catheters over guidewires; use of guidewire exchange technique for arterial catheters is associated with increased infection risk.	

regression analysis to determine that wearing a mask alone had a statistically significant association with a reduced infection rate.[325]

Techniques used for skin preparation, prior to catheter insertion, also appear to influence the risk for infection. In one study, skin preparation and decontamination with 0.5% chlorhexidine gluconate in 70% isopropyl alcohol was more effective than 10% povidone-iodine in preventing colonization of peripheral catheters in neonates.[326] Chlorhexidine-containing antiseptics have been shown to be effective in diminishing rates of catheter colonization, and they have shown varying efficacy in reducing intravenous device-related bacteremias.[327] A 2002 meta-analysis determined that chlorhexidine gluconate significantly reduces the incidence of bacteremia in patients with central venous catheters compared to povidone-iodine for insertion-site skin disinfection.[328] A comparison of 10% aqueous povidone iodine, 2% aqueous chlorhexidine gluconate, and 0.5% alcoholic chlorhexidine gluconate determined that both chlorhexidine solutions were similarly effective in preventing colonization of central venous and arterial catheters.[329] Small and colleagues found that 2% chlorhexidine gluconate in 70% isopropyl alcohol was more effective in reducing the number of peripheral venous catheters that were colonized or contaminated than 70% isopropyl alcohol alone.[330] Likewise, Mimoz and co-workers recommended use of chlorhexidine-based solutions rather than povidone-iodine.[331] However, hypersensitivity reactions to chlorhexidine have been reported.[332,333] The CDC guidelines recommend disinfecting skin before catheter insertion and during dressing changes using tincture of iodine and iodophors, 70% alcohol, or, preferably, a 2% chlorhexidine-based preparation.[2] Recently, an alcoholic chlorhexidine solution containing a concentration of chlorhexidine gluconate greater than 0.5% has been recommended for skin preparation in patients older than 2 months of age.[11] The antiseptic solution must be allowed to dry before making the skin puncture.

AFTER INSERTION

Even with the most stringent application of strategies to decrease catheter-associated infections, the presence of a vascular catheter remains a clear risk factor for infection. Thus, the need for continued vascular access should be assessed at least daily,[11] and all nonessential catheters should be removed immediately.

Contamination of catheter hubs, needleless connectors, and injection ports is a major risk factor for catheter-associated infection, and disinfection has been determined to reduce microbial burden.[35,36,46,334] Recent guidelines recommend cleaning all catheter hubs and injection ports with an alcoholic chlorhexidine preparation or 70% alcohol to reduce contamination.[11] Older guidelines recommend cleaning injection ports with 70% alcohol or an iodophor before accessing the system; access ports for needleless intravascular devices should be wiped with an appropriate antiseptic.[2] We agree that thorough disinfection of all catheter hubs and injection ports prior to access seems prudent and reasonable.

Authorities have recommended placing a sterile dressing over the catheter entry site.[2,171,335] Maki and colleagues studied standard tape and gauze dressings in comparison with two transparent polyurethane dressings.[288] They concluded that polyurethane dressings appear to be safe and may be left on for up to 5 days.[288] Hoffmann and co-workers performed a meta-analysis of studies attempting to assess the use of semipermeable membrane dressing materials at catheter insertion sites.[336] These investigators found a significantly increased risk of catheter-tip colonization when transparent compared with gauze dressings were used to dress either central or peripheral catheter insertion sites. In addition, they found a trend (although not statistically significant in their meta-analysis) toward an increased risk for bacteremia and catheter sepsis associated with the use of semipermeable dressings as insertion-site dressings for central venous catheters.[336] The CDC guidelines suggest that because the risk for catheter-related bacteremias did not differ between the groups,[336] choice of dressings can be a matter of preference.[2] A chlorhexidine gluconate-impregnated dressing has been studied by several groups.[326,337-339] This dressing was as

effective as 10% povidine-iodine skin scrub and transparent polyurethane dressing in neonates, and redressing the site every 3 to 7 days was required.[326] Another study of children determined that the chlorhexidine gluconate-impregnated sponge significantly reduced the rates of central venous catheter colonization.[338] A third group studied this chlorhexidine dressing with tunneled catheters in adults and concluded that it reduced the incidence of exit site/tunnel infections without prolonging catheter survival in neutropenic patients.[337] This same dressing used in adults with short-term central venous catheters undergoing chemotherapy was found to significantly reduce the incidence of bloodstream infection.[339]

The data on frequency of dressing changes are not conclusive. Randomized clinical trials have most often concluded that increasing time to dressing changes with transparent dressings does not affect site colonization.[340-342] Anecdotal data of institutional experiences with these issues suggest that increased time intervals between dressing changes and perhaps transparent dressings themselves are associated with increased bacteremia rates.[343] The increased ease of visual inspection and savings on nursing personnel time related to less frequent dressing changes likely do affect dressing choices in at least some institutions. One study of 55 hospitals' practices found that two thirds used transparent, semipermeable dressings.[344] Nonetheless, no definitive data exist to determine the best dressing methodology. The CDC has recommended changing the site dressing when it becomes damp, loosened, or soiled, and at least every 7 days for transparent dressings for adults. When gauze dressings are used for short-term central venous catheters, those dressings should be replaced every 2 days.[2]

Use of topical antibiotic or antiseptic ointments at the insertion site of catheters is currently not recommended by U.S. authorities[2,345] except in the case of hemodialysis catheter insertion sites in patients with a history of recurrent S. aureus CLABSIs.[11] Several studies examining the use of povidone-iodine ointment have produced conflicting results. Results of topical mupirocin ointment application have been more promising,[346] but mupirocin resistance has been documented.[347] In addition, ointments without fungicidal activity have been associated with increased rates of catheter colonization with Candida spp.[52] The clinical utility of these ointments is questionable, and we do not recommend their routine use except as an adjunct for extremely high-risk hemodialysis patients with recurrent CLABSIs. Rhame and colleagues reviewed the composite experience of six different studies that were designed to address this issue.[335] In five of these studies, there were no differences between topical antimicrobial agents and placebo. In the smallest series in this review (a study of 78 catheter insertions), there were three infections in the placebo group and none in the therapy group.[335] Maki and Band[348] prospectively studied the following three regimens of catheter care: (1) application of polymyxin-neomycin-bacitracin ointment at insertion and every 48 hours, (2) application of iodophor ointment at insertion and every 48 hours, or (3) no ointment. In their study of 827 random catheter insertions, there were no differences in either catheter-acquired sepsis (two cases in each group) or local inflammation (38.9% vs. 41.9% vs. 41.7%, respectively). The only difference noted was in semiquantitative cultures of catheter tips.[348] In the polymyxin-neomycin-bacitracin ointment group there were 6 positive cultures, in the iodophor group there were 10, and in the control group there were 18. This difference was greatest in catheters that were left in place for more than 4 days. Thus, information regarding the efficacy of these antimicrobial ointments or creams for intravascular cannulas is contradictory and confusing, and the clinical utility of these compounds remains questionable.

The use of in-line membrane filters has also been advocated as a mechanism for reducing the incidence of catheter-acquired infection.[219] Because, as noted previously, the major points of entry are the skin insertion site and the catheter hub, one might suspect that such devices would be of limited usefulness in preventing most catheter-acquired septicemias. No investigators have recommended the routine inclusion of such filters in all intravenous setups, nor has any study demonstrated conclusive evidence that the routine use of such filters results in a lowering of the infusion-related bacteremia rate. In isolated situations (e.g., if particulate matter is present in the infusate, if the solution must hang for an extended period of time, or perhaps in a situation in which an infusate such as parenteral nutrition solution supports the growth of microorganisms extremely well), the addition of these filters to the system is of theoretical value. However, even in cases in which the infusion fluid is contaminated, organisms trapped on the filter may shed endotoxins into the patient's circulation.[349]

SPECIAL APPROACHES FOR THE PREVENTION OF CLABSIS

Antimicrobial Prophylaxis

Some investigators have advocated using prophylactic antimicrobials in specific, defined circumstances to prevent catheter-associated infection. For example, Baier and colleagues found that prophylactic treatment of neonates with central catheters with vancomycin effectively prevented coagulase-negative staphylococcal bacteremia associated with the use of these catheters.[350] The use of continuous-infusion vancomycin for low-birth-weight infants has been shown to decrease rates of coagulase-negative staphylococci bacteremia.[351] Unfortunately, prolonged low levels of vancomycin, such as result from this form of prophylaxis, could predispose to vancomycin resistance. Raad and co-workers have used novobiocin and rifampin to attempt to prevent catheter-associated infections in patients receiving interleukin-2 (IL-2).[352] Although the antimicrobial prophylaxis was poorly tolerated (and had to be discontinued in nearly one third of patients), the regimen was thought to be successful.[352] Others have reported success in preventing catheter-associated infections in IL-2 recipients without using antimicrobial prophylaxis. Systemic antimicrobial prophylaxis is strongly discouraged.[2,11]

Antimicrobial Lock Prophylaxis

The use of antimicrobial lock solutions, in which an antibiotic or other antimicrobial is injected into the catheter lumen and the solution is left to dwell within the lumen for periods of some hours or days, has been examined as a method of preventing catheter infection during the past several years.[353-358] Antibiotic lock therapy in combination with systemic antibiotic is now recommended for uncomplicated bacteremias related to tunneled central venous catheters or implantable devices when the catheter is not removed and the infection is due to coagulase-negative staphylococci, *S. aureus*, or gram-negative bacilli.[123] Currently, antimicrobial locks for prevention of CLABSIs or other catheter-related infections are not recommended for use in all patients with central venous catheters.[11] This technique has been shown in four meta-analyses to help prevent CLABSIs among hemodialysis patients.[355-357,359] Similar results have been found in patients with malignancy.[358] Four of five studies in hematology-oncology patient populations demonstrated efficacy of vancomycin plus heparin as antibiotic lock prophylaxis[353,360-362]; a fifth study found no significant difference in bacteremia rates or time to the first episode of bacteremia when heparin flush was compared with a heparin plus vancomycin flush solution.[363] Although neither vancomycin[361] nor ciprofloxacin[360] could be detected in the blood after flushing with either antibiotic, concern about development of vancomycin-resistant organisms following widespread use of small amounts of vancomycin has limited use of this prophylactic technique. Safdar and Maki performed a meta-analysis examining the use of vancomycin-containing locks in preventing bloodstream infection in patients with long-term central venous access devices.[364] They concluded that use of vancomycin lock solution in high-risk patient populations, including patients with malignancy, with long-term central catheters reduces the risk of bloodstream infection. These authors also acknowledge the concern regarding promotion of antimicrobial resistance with use of antibiotic lock solutions, and they suggest that anti-infective solutions should be studied that have broad-spectrum anti-infective activity but that do not select for resistance.[364] Such agents include taurolidine,[365-367] minocycline-EDTA,[368,369] and ethanol.[370,371] Antimicrobial locks are currently recommended for use in preventing CLABSIs for two groups of patients:

(1) those with limited venous access and a history of recurrent CLABSIs and (2) those with heightened risk for severe sequelae from CLABSIs.[11]

Antimicrobial Catheters

Another approach that has been advocated to reduce the risk for central venous catheter-associated infection is bonding of an antimicrobial agent or antiseptic to the device or by the addition of a subcutaneous catheter cuff impregnated with an antiseptic or antimicrobial. First-generation antiseptic catheters are coated on the external surface with chlorhexidine and sulfadiazine silver; second-generation catheters are impregnated with chlorhexidine and sulfadiazine silver on both external and internal surfaces. The antibiotic-coated catheter approved in the United States is impregnated on both internal and external surfaces with minocycline and rifampin. The third catheter type currently is impregnated with silver, platinum, and carbon and releases topical silver ions. A 2005 review of these catheters concluded that 40% of intravascular device-related bloodstream infections are preventable with the use of antimicrobial-impregnated central venous catheters.[372] These authors also emphasized that based on the results of 19 randomized, controlled trials, three meta-analyses, and two cost-benefit analyses, the overwhelming preponderance of evidence concerning the use of antimicrobial catheters suggests efficacy.[372] A recent systematic review examined 32 trials of various types of antimicrobial central venous catheters and concluded that the pooled results for all catheters suggest a statistically significant advantage in reducing CLABSIs with an odds ratio of 0.45.[373] This review also found that the pooled results of nine studies examining catheters treated only externally showed a nonsignificant effect on decreasing CLABSIs.[373] Another review of 34 studies concluded that first-generation chlorhexidine–silver sulfadiazine catheters reduce the risk of CLABSIs, and that minocycline-rifampin catheters are significantly more effective relative to these first-generation chlorhexidine–silver sulfadiazine catheters.[374] The second-generation chlorhexidine–silver sulfadiazine catheters showed nonsignificant reductions in risk of CLABSIs compared with uncoated catheters,[374] although microbial colonization of the catheters appears to be reduced.[375]

Minocycline-rifampin coating, compared with first-generation chlorhexidine–silver sulfadiazine catheters, appears to have superior and more prolonged activity against staphylococci.[376] Several subsequent studies have shown that these minocycline-rifampin catheters significantly decrease the risk of CLABSIs.[377-381] In vitro and in vivo data suggest that the efficacy of the minocycline-rifampin catheters may be prolonged beyond that of chlorhexidine–silver sulfadiazine catheters[379,382]; first-generation chlorhexidine–silver sulfadiazine catheters are known to be efficacious only when the average insertion time is less than 8 days.[383] The efficacy of the minocycline-rifampin catheters when kept in situ for longer periods of time has been assessed in one study.[380] In this study, the minocycline-rifampin silicone catheters had a mean dwell time of 68.2 days and were associated with a significant decrease in CLABSIs.[380] These antibiotic-impregnated catheters are associated with a theoretical risk of increased antimicrobial resistance,[384] and one in vitro study found that second-generation chlorhexidine–silver sulfadiazine catheters appear to be more resistant to colonization with rifampin-resistant *Staphylococcus epidermidis* than minocycline-rifampin catheters.[385]

Chlorhexidine–silver sulfadiazine catheters have been shown to be cost-effective in patients at high risk of intravenous device–related bacteremia. Another cost-effectiveness analysis suggested that the clinical and economic benefits of minocycline-rifampin catheters increase with days of catheterization.[386] For patients with central venous catheters in situ for 8 days, minocycline-rifampin catheters were more beneficial than chlorhexidine–silver sulfadiazine catheters, and cost savings accrued in patients catheterized for at least 13 days. Another review examined 11 randomized studies comparing patients with central venous catheters impregnated with antimicrobial agents with control patients receiving nonimpregnated central venous catheters.[387] These authors concluded that the efficacy of antimicrobial-impregnated central venous catheters in preventing catheter-related bacteremias is questionable, and that routine use of these catheters must be reevaluated. Halton and Graves reviewed a series of cost-effectiveness studies in 2007 and concluded that use of antibiotic-coated catheters compared with use of either antiseptic-coated or standard catheters was both clinically effective and cost-saving.[388] Another study suggests that only patients receiving parenteral nutrition may benefit from antiseptic-impregnated central venous catheters.[97] Recent guidelines suggest that use of antimicrobial-impregnated catheters should be reserved for locations or patient populations, or both, that have unacceptably high CLABSI rates despite implementation of the basic prevention strategies, including education, use of maximal sterile barriers, and use of chlorhexidine antisepsis of skin prior to catheter insertion.[11] None of these antimicrobial catheters were, alone, capable of reducing CLABSI rates to zero. We believe that anti-infective catheters should be implemented only as part of a comprehensive nosocomial bacteremia prevention strategy, which also includes education of staff and adequate skin antisepsis. Institutions can choose to implement one of these catheters after review of both their current and their goal intravenous device-associated bacteremia rates. Further research is needed to define the actual effect of these catheters on bacteremia rates, as well as the most efficacious catheters for different durations of catheterization and different subpopulations of patients.

Use of heparin or other anticoagulants has also been advocated as a method for reducing both thrombotic and infectious complications of central venous catheterization. One study found a clear benefit of covalently bonding heparin to catheters.[389] In this study, the use of catheters to which heparin had been covalently bonded decreased bacterial colonization in vitro and also decreased the device-associated infection rate in vivo.[389] Randolph and co-workers concluded that heparin administration effectively reduces thrombus formation and may reduce catheter-related infections in patients who have central venous and pulmonary artery catheters in place.[390] Several anticoagulants have been suggested for use in this setting, and Randolph and co-workers noted that cost-effectiveness comparisons of these several preparations (e.g., unfractionated heparin, low-molecular-weight heparin, and warfarin) are needed.[390] Goey and colleagues ascribed the relatively low incidence of thrombosis and infection in their large series of catheters placed in patients receiving IL-2 infusions (a population of patients known to be at substantially increased risk for catheter-associated infection) to the use of tunneled catheters and prophylactic heparin.[391] Several reviews of various anticoagulants used in the prevention of CLABSIs all conclude that these agents, including urokinase,[392] tissue plasminogen activator,[393] and heparin-bonded catheters,[394] may be effective but underscore the fact that more adequately powered clinical trials are needed. Currently, we do not recommend routine use of urokinase or other thrombolytic agents as adjunctive therapy in patients with catheter-related bacteremia.

OTHER PREVENTION ISSUES

The role of appropriate nurse staffing in preventing catheter-associated infection deserves attention. In one study, nursing staff reductions during a period of increased use of parenteral nutrition were directly associated with an increase in catheter-associated bacteremias in a surgical ICU.[95] Robert and colleagues reported in 2000 that bacteremias in surgical ICU patients increased when nurse staffing changed to include fewer "regular" registered nurses and more pool/agency nurses.[96] "Float" nurses (usually assigned elsewhere in the hospital or from an agency) were associated with an increased risk of CLABSIs in ICU patients in another study,[97] suggesting that an increased proportion of nurses with less than 1 year of experience in the ICU can lead to increased risk of CLABSIs.[395] Adequate nurse staffing has been identified as one factor integral to preventing bacteremia.[396] In this era of increased focus on preventing these infections, the impact of staffing reductions on untoward outcomes is deserving of careful scrutiny.[95]

New scientific approaches are needed to help establish optimal techniques for catheter management,[59,189,397,398] and further technologic advances such as bonding antimicrobial and antiseptic agents to the intravascular device may also reduce risks for device-associated infection. A survey of use of CLABSI prevention practices in 516 U.S. hospitals found that fewer than half of non-Veterans Affairs hospitals reported concurrent use of maximal sterile barrier precautions, chlorhexidine gluconate, and avoidance of routine central line changes.[399] Wider use of recommended prevention practices, including the bundling of complementary strategies, is needed to reach the desired outcome of zero CLABSIs. Increased attention to such details can significantly lower the endemic rate of device-associated infection as well as decrease the number of epidemics of such infections.

REFERENCES

1. Maki D. *Sepsis Arising from Extrinsic Contamination of the Infusion and Measures for Control.* Lancaster, UK: MTP Press; 1977.
2. O'Grady NP, Alexander M, Dellinger EP, et al. Guidelines for the prevention of intravascular catheter-related infections. *Infect Control Hosp Epidemiol.* 2002;23:759-769.
3. Edwards JR, Peterson KD, Andrus ML, et al. National Healthcare Safety Network (NHSN) Report, data summary for 2006, issued June 2007. *Am J Infect Control.* 2007;35:290-301.
4. Centers for Medicare and Medicaid Services. Hospital-Acquired Conditions (Present on Admission Indicator). Available at http://www.cms.hhs.gov/HospitalAcqCond/06_Hospital-Acquired_Conditions.asp#TopOfPage. Accessed October 10, 2008.
5. The Joint Commission. 2009 National Patient Safety Goals Hospital Program. Available at http://www.jointcommission.org/PatientSafety/NationalPatientSafetyGoals/09_hap_npsgs.htm. Accessed October 10, 2008.
6. Weinstein MP, Towns ML, Quartey SM, et al. The clinical significance of positive blood cultures in the 1990s: a prospective comprehensive evaluation of the microbiology, epidemiology, and outcome of bacteremia and fungemia in adults. *Clin Infect Dis.* 1997;24:584-602.
7. Hugonnet S, Harbarth S, Ferriere K, et al. Bacteremic sepsis in intensive care: temporal trends in incidence, organ dysfunction, and prognosis. *Crit Care Med.* 2003;31:390-394.
8. Renaud B, Brun-Buisson C; ICU-Bacteremia Study Group. Outcomes of primary and catheter-related bacteremia: a cohort and case-control study in critically ill patients. *Am J Respir Crit Care Med.* 2001;163:1584-1590.
9. Raad I, Hachem R, Hanna H, et al. Sources and outcomes of bloodstream infections in cancer patients: the role of central venous catheters. *Eur J Clin Microbiol Infect Dis.* 2007;26:549-556.
10. McGregor AR, Collignon PJ. Bacteraemia and fungaemia in an Australian general hospital—associations and outcomes. *Med J Aust.* 1993;158:671-674.
11. Marschall J, Mermel LA, Classen D, et al. Strategies to prevent central line-associated bloodstream infections in acute care hospitals. *Infect Control Hosp Epidemiol.* 2008;29:S22-S30.
12. Marrie T, Costerton JW. Scanning and transmission electron microscopy of in situ bacterial colonization of intravenous and intraarterial catheters. *J Clin Microbiol.* 1984;19:687-693.
13. Cheesbrough JS, Finch RG, Burden RP. A prospective study of the mechanisms of infection associated with hemodialysis catheters. *J Infect Dis.* 1986;154:579-589.
14. Linares J, Sitges-Serra A, Garau J, et al. Pathogenesis of catheter sepsis: a prospective study with quantitative and semiquantitative cultures of catheter hub and segments. *J Clin Microbiol.* 1985;21:357-360.
15. Maki D. Nosocomial bacteremia: an epidemiologic overview. *Am J Med.* 1981;70:719-732.
16. Maki D, Rhame F, Mackel D, et al. Nationwide epidemic of septicemia caused by contaminated intravenous products: I. Epidemiologic and clinical features. *Am J Med.* 1976;60:471-485.
17. Stamm W, Colella J, Anderson M, et al. Indwelling arterial catheters as a source of nosocomial bacteremia: an outbreak caused by *Flavobacterium* species. *N Engl J Med.* 1975;292:1099-1102.
18. Douce RW, Zurita J, Sanchez O, et al. Investigation of an outbreak of central venous catheter-associated bloodstream infection due to contaminated water. *Infect Control Hosp Epidemiol.* 2008;29:364-366.
19. Goldmann D, Martin W, Worthington J. Growth of bacteria and fungi in total parenteral nutrition solutions. *Am J Surg.* 1973;126:314-318.
20. Maki D. Growth properties of microorganisms in infusion fluid and method of detection. In: Phillips I, ed. *Microbiologic Hazards of Intravenous Therapy.* Lancaster, UK: MTP Press; 1977:13-47.
21. Jarvis W, Highsmith A. Bacterial growth and endotoxin production in lipid emulsion. *J Clin Microbiol.* 1984;19:17-20.
22. Dankner W, Spector S, Fierer J. *Malassezia* fungemia in neonates and adults: complication of hyperalimentation. *Rev Infect Dis.* 1987;9:743-837.
23. Avila-Figueroa C, Goldmann DA, Richardson DK, et al. Intravenous lipid emulsions are the major determinant of coagulase-negative staphylococcal bacteremia in very low birth weight newborns. *Pediatr Infect Dis J.* 1998;17:10-17.
24. Souza Dias MB, Habert AB, Borrasca V, et al. Salvage of long-term central venous catheters during an outbreak of *Pseudomonas putida* and *Stenotrophomonas maltophilia* infections associated with contaminated heparin catheter-lock solution. *Infect Control Hosp Epidemiol.* 2008;29:125-130.
25. Sunenshine RH, Tan ET, Terashita DM, et al. A multistate outbreak of *Serratia marcescens* bloodstream infection associated with contaminated intravenous magnesium sulfate from a compounding pharmacy. *Clin Infect Dis.* 2007;45:527-533.
26. Plouffe J, Brown D, Silva J, et al. Nosocomial outbreak of *Candida parapsilosis* fungemia related to intravenous infusions. *Arch Intern Med.* 1977;137:1686-1689.
27. Solomon S, Khabbaz R, Parker R, et al. An outbreak of *Candida parapsilosis* bloodstream infections in patients receiving parenteral nutrition. *J Infect Dis.* 1984;149:98-102.
28. Linares J, Dominguez MA, Martin R. Current laboratory techniques in the diagnosis of catheter-related infections. *Nutrition.* 1997;13:10S-14S.
29. Sitges-Serra A, Hernandez R, Maestro S, et al. Prevention of catheter sepsis: the hub. *Nutrition.* 1997;13:30S-35S.
30. Sitges-Serra A, Puig P, Jaurrieta E, et al. Hub colonization as the initial step in an outbreak of catheter-related sepsis due to coagulase negative staphylococci during parenteral nutrition. *J Parenter Enteral Nutr.* 1984;8:668-672.

31. Segura M, Alvarez-Lerma F, Tellado JM, et al. A clinical trial on the prevention of catheter-related sepsis using a new hub model. *Ann Surg.* 1996;223:363-369.
32. Pemberton L, Lyman B, Mandal J, et al. Outbreak of *Staphylococcus epidermidis* nosocomial infections in patients receiving total parenteral nutrition. *J Parenter Enteral Nutr.* 1984;8:325-326.
33. Dobbins BM, Kite P, Kindon A, et al. DNA fingerprinting analysis of coagulase negative staphylococci implicated in catheter related bloodstream infections. *J Clin Pathol.* 2002;55:824-828.
34. Maki D, Ringer M. Evaluation of dressing regimens for prevention of infection with peripheral intravenous catheters: gauze, a transparent polyurethane dressing, and an iodophor-transparent dressing. *JAMA.* 1987;258:2396-2403.
35. Salzman MB, Isenberg HD, Shapiro JF, et al. A prospective study of the catheter hub as the portal of entry for microorganisms causing catheter-related sepsis in neonates. *J Infect Dis.* 1993;167:487-490.
36. Salzman M, Isenberg H, Rubin L. Use of disinfectants to reduce microbial contamination of hubs of vascular catheters. *J Clin Microbiol.* 1993;31:475-479.
37. Sheretz RJ. Pathogenesis of vascular catheter-related infections. In: Seifert H, Jansen B, Farr BM, eds. *Catheter-Related Infections.* New York: Marcel Dekker; 1997:1-29.
38. Grohskopf LA, Roth VR, Feikin DR, et al. *Serratia liquefaciens* bloodstream infections from contamination of epoetin alfa at a hemodialysis center. *N Engl J Med.* 2001;344:1491-1497.
39. Ostrowsky BE, Whitener C, Bredenberg HK, et al. *Serratia marcescens* bacteremia traced to an infused narcotic. *N Engl J Med.* 2002;346:1529-1537.
40. van Laer F, Raes D, Vandamme P, et al. An outbreak of *Burkholderia cepacia* with septicemia on a cardiology ward. *Infect Control Hosp Epidemiol.* 1998;19:112-113.
41. Rupp ME, Sholtz LA, Jourdan DR, et al. Outbreak of bloodstream infection temporally associated with the use of an intravascular needleless valve. *Clin Infect Dis.* 2007;44:1408-1414.
42. Cookson ST, Ihrig M, O'Mara EM, et al. Increased bloodstream infection rates in surgical patients associated with variation from recommended use and care following implementation of a needleless device. *Infect Control Hosp Epidemiol.* 1998;19:23-27.
43. Danzig LE, Short LJ, Collins K, et al. Bloodstream infections associated with a needleless intravenous infusion system in patients receiving home infusion therapy. *JAMA.* 1995;273:1862-1864.
44. Do AN, Ray BJ, Banerjee SN, et al. Bloodstream infection associated with needleless device use and the importance of infection-control practices in the home health care setting. *J Infect Dis.* 1999;179:442-448.
45. McDonald LC, Banerjee SN, Jarvis WR. Line-associated bloodstream infections in pediatric intensive-care-unit patients associated with a needleless device and intermittent intravenous therapy. *Infect Control Hosp Epidemiol.* 1998;19:772-777.
46. Casey AL, Worthington T, Lambert PA, et al. A randomized, prospective clinical trial to assess the potential infection risk associated with the PosiFlow needleless connector. *J Hosp Infect.* 2003;54:288-293.
47. Atela I, Coll P, Rello J, et al. Serial surveillance cultures of skin and catheter hub specimens from critically ill patients with central venous catheters: molecular epidemiology of infection and implications for clinical management and research. *J Clin Microbiol.* 1997;35:1784-1790.
48. Salzman MB, Rubin LG. Relevance of the catheter hub as a portal for microorganisms causing catheter-related bloodstream infections. *Nutrition.* 1997;13:15S-17S.
49. Bjornson H, Colley R, Bower R, et al. Association between microorganism growth at the catheter insertion site and colonization of the catheter in patients receiving total parenteral nutrition. *Surgery.* 1982;92:720-727.
50. Cooper G, Hopkins C. Rapid diagnosis of intravascular catheter-associated infection by direct Gram-staining of catheter segments. *N Engl J Med.* 1985;18:1142-1150.
51. Safdar N, Maki DG. The pathogenesis of catheter-related bloodstream infection with noncuffed short-term central venous catheters. *Intensive Care Med.* 2004;30:62-67.
52. Flowers RH, Schwenzer KJ, Kopel RF, et al. Efficacy of an attachable subcutaneous cuff for the prevention of intravascular catheter-related infection. *JAMA.* 1989;261:878-883.
53. Mermel LA, McCormick RD, Springman SR, et al. The pathogenesis and epidemiology of catheter-related infection with pulmonary artery Swan-Ganz catheters: a prospective study utilizing molecular subtyping. *Am J Med.* 1991;91:197S-205S.
54. Mer M, Duse AG, Galpin JS, et al. Central venous catheterization: a prospective, randomized, double-blind study. *Clin Appl Thromb Hemost.* 2008;15:19-26.
55. Herwaldt LA, Hollis RJ, Boyken LD, et al. Molecular epidemiology of coagulase-negative staphylococci isolated from immunocompromised patients. *Infect Control Hosp Epidemiol.* 1992;13:86-92.
56. Centers for Disease Control and Prevention, National Nosocomial Infections Surveillance System. National Nosocomial Infections Surveillance (NNIS) System report, data summary from January 1992 to June 2004, issued October 2004. *Am J Infect Control.* 2004;32:440-485.
57. Safdar N, Kluger DM, Maki DG. A review of risk factors for catheter-related bloodstream infection caused by percutane-
ously inserted, noncuffed central venous catheters: implications for preventive strategies. *Medicine.* 2002;81:466-479.
58. Craven D, Lichtenberg A, Kunches L, et al. A randomized study comparing a transparent polyurethane dressing to a dry gauze dressing for peripheral intravenous catheter sites. *Infect Control.* 1985;6:361-366.
59. Kelsey M, Gosling M. A comparison of the morbidity associated with occlusive and non-occlusive dressings applied to peripheral intravenous devices. *J Hosp Infect.* 1984;5:313-321.
60. Albert R, Condie F. Hand-washing patterns in medical intensive care units. *N Engl J Med.* 1981;304:1465-1466.
61. Preston G, Larson E, Stamm W. The effect of private isolation rooms on patient care practices, colonization, and infection in an intensive care unit. *Am J Med.* 1981;70:641-645.
62. Haas JP, Larson EL. Compliance with hand hygiene guidelines: where are we in 2008? *Am J Nurs.* 2008;108:40-4445.
63. Lucas JW, Berger AM, Fitzgerald A, et al. Nosocomial infections in patients with central catheters. *J Intraven Nurs.* 1992;15:44-48.
64. Raad I, Luna M, Khalil SA, et al. The relationship between the thrombotic and infectious complications of central venous catheters. *JAMA.* 1994;271:1014-1016.
65. Welch G, McKeel D Jr, Silverstein P, et al. The role of catheter composition in the development of thrombophlebitis. *Surg Gynecol Obstet.* 1974;138:421-424.
66. Stillman R, Soliman S, Garcia L, et al. Etiology of catheter associated sepsis. *Arch Surg.* 1977;112:1497-1499.
67. Linder L, Curelaru I, Gustavsson B, et al. Material thrombogenicity in central venous catheterization: a comparison between soft, antebrachial catheters of silicone elastomer and polyurethane. *J Parenter Enteral Nutr.* 1984;8:399-406.
68. Bozzetti F. Central venous catheter sepsis. *Surg Gynecol Obstet.* 1985;161:293-301.
69. Sheth N, Franson T, Rose H, et al. Colonization of bacteria on polyvinyl chloride and Teflon intravascular catheter in hospitalized patients. *J Clin Microbiol.* 1983;18:1061-1063.
70. Rotrosen D, Calderone R, Edwards J Jr. Adherence of *Candida* species to host tissues and plastic surfaces. *Rev Infect Dis.* 1986;8:73-85.
71. Sherertz R, Carruth WA, Marosok RD, et al. Contribution of vascular catheter material to the pathogenesis of infection: the enhanced risk of silicone in vivo. *J Biomater Res.* 1995;29:634-645.
72. Yeung C, May J, Hughes R. Infection rate for single-lumen vs. triple-lumen subclavian catheters. *Infect Control Hosp Epidemiol.* 1988;9:154-158.
73. Templeton A, Schlegel M, Fleisch F, et al. Multilumen central venous catheters increase risk for catheter-related bloodstream infection: prospective surveillance study. *Infection.* 2008;36:322-327.
74. Kelly C, Ligas J, Smith C, et al. Sepsis due to triple-lumen central venous catheters. *Surg Gynecol Obstet.* 1986;163:14-16.
75. Tan LH, Hess B, Diaz LK, et al. Survey of the use of peripherally inserted central venous catheters in neonates with critical congenital cardiac disease. *Cardiol Young.* 2007;17:196-201.
76. Kovalevich D, Faubion W, Bender J, et al. Association of parenteral nutrition catheter sepsis with urinary tract infections. *J Parenter Enteral Nutr.* 1986;10:639-641.
77. Raad II, Fang X, Keutgen XM, et al. The role of chelators in preventing biofilm formation and catheter-related bloodstream infections. *Curr Opin Infect Dis.* 2008;21:385-392.
78. Donlan RM, Costerton JW. Biofilms: survival mechanisms of clinically relevant microorganisms. *Clin Microbiol Rev.* 2002;15:167-193.
79. Shanks RM, Sargent JL, Martinez RM, et al. Catheter lock solutions influence staphylococcal biofilm formation on abiotic surfaces. *Nephrol Dial Transplant.* 2006;21:2247-2255.
80. Longuet P, Douard MC, Arlet G, et al. Venous access port-related bacteremia in patients with acquired immunodeficiency syndrome or cancer: the reservoir as a diagnostic and therapeutic tool. *Clin Infect Dis.* 2001;32:1776-1783.
81. del Pozo JL, Serrera A, Martinez-Cuesta A, et al. Biofilm related infections: is there a place for conservative treatment of port-related bloodstream infections? *Int J Artif Organs.* 2006;29:379-386.
82. Guggenbichler JP, Berchtold D, Allerberger F, et al. In vitro and in vivo effect of antibiotics on catheters colonized by staphylococci. *Eur J Clin Microbiol Infect Dis.* 1992;11:408-415.
83. Kropec A, Huebner J, Wursthorn M, et al. In vitro activity of vancomycin and teicoplanin against *Staphylococcus aureus* and *Staphylococcus epidermidis* colonizing catheters. *Eur J Clin Microbiol Infect Dis.* 1993;12:545-548.
84. Pascual A, Ramirez de Arellano E, Martinez Martinez L, et al. Effect of polyurethane catheters and bacterial biofilms on the in-vitro activity of antimicrobials against *Staphylococcus epidermidis.* *J Hosp Infect.* 1993;24:211-218.
85. Simon VC, Simon M. Antibacterial activity of teicoplanin and vancomycin in combination with rifampicin, fusidic acid or fosfomycin against staphylococci on vein catheters. *Scand J Infect Dis Suppl.* 1990;72:14-19.
86. Hampton A, Sheretz R. Vascular-access infections in hospitalized patients. *Surg Clin North Am.* 1988;68:57-71.
87. Armstrong C, Mayhall C, Miller K, et al. Prospective study of catheter replacement and other risk factors for infection of hyperalimentation catheters. *J Infect Dis.* 1986;154:808-816.
88. Eggimann P, Harbarth S, Constantin MN, et al. Impact of a prevention strategy targeted at vascular-access care on incidence
of infections acquired in intensive care. *Lancet.* 2000;355:1864-1868.
89. Soifer NE, Borzak S, Edlin BR, et al. Prevention of peripheral venous catheter complications with an intravenous therapy team: a randomized controlled trial. *Arch Intern Med.* 1998;158:473-477.
90. Raad I, Hohn DC, Gilbreath BJ, et al. Prevention of central venous catheter-related infections by using maximal sterile barrier precautions during insertion. *Infect Control Hosp Epidemiol.* 1994;15:231-238.
91. Ryan J, Abel R, Abbott W, et al. Catheter complications in total parenteral nutrition: a prospective study of 200 consecutive patients. *N Engl J Med.* 1974;290:757-761.
92. Snydman D, Murray S, Kornfeld S, et al. Total parenteral nutrition-related infections: prospective epidemiologic study using semiquantitative methods. *Am J Med.* 1982;73:695-699.
93. Merrer J, De Jonghe B, Golliot F, et al. Complications of femoral and subclavian venous catheterization in critically ill patients: a randomized controlled trial. *JAMA.* 2001;286:700-707.
94. Hamilton HC, Foxcroft DR. Central venous access sites for the prevention of venous thrombosis, stenosis and infection in patients requiring long-term intravenous therapy. *Cochrane Database Syst Rev.* 2007:CD00484.
95. Fridkin SK, Pear SM, Williamson TH, et al. The role of understaffing in central venous catheter-associated bloodstream infections. *Infect Control Hosp Epidemiol.* 1996;17:150-158.
96. Robert J, Fridkin SK, Blumberg HM, et al. The influence of the composition of the nursing staff on primary bloodstream infection rates in a surgical intensive care unit. *Infect Control Hosp Epidemiol.* 2000;21:12-17.
97. Alonso-Echanove J, Edwards JR, Richards MJ, et al. Effect of nurse staffing and antimicrobial-impregnated central venous catheters on the risk for bloodstream infections in intensive care units. *Infect Control Hosp Epidemiol.* 2003;24:916-925.
98. Kritchevsky SB, Braun BI, Kusek L, et al. The impact of hospital practice on central venous catheter associated bloodstream infection rates at the patient and unit level: a multicenter study. *Am J Med Qual.* 2008;23:24-38.
99. Rosenthal VD, Guzman S, Pezzotto SM, et al. Effect of an infection control program using education and performance feedback on rates of intravascular device-associated blood stream infections in intensive care units in Argentina. *Am J Infect Control.* 2003;31:405-409.
100. Warren DK, Zack JE, Mayfield JL, et al. The effect of an education program on the incidence of central venous catheter-associated bloodstream infection in a medical ICU. *Chest.* 2004;126:1612-1618.
101. Schulin T, Voss A. Coagulase-negative staphylococci as a cause of infections related to intravascular prosthetic devices: limitations of present therapy. *Clin Microbiol Infect.* 2001;7:1-7.
102. Wade JC, Schimpff SC, Newman KA, et al. *Staphylococcus epidermidis:* an increasing cause of infection in patients with granulocytopenia. *Ann Intern Med.* 1982;97:503-508.
103. Saginur R, Suh KN. *Staphylococcus aureus* bacteraemia of unknown primary source: where do we stand? *Int J Antimicrob Agents.* 2008;32:S21-S25.
104. Diekema DJ, Beekmann SE, Chapin KC, et al. Epidemiology and outcome of nosocomial and community onset bloodstream infection. *J Clin Microbiol.* 2003;41:3655-3660.
105. Christensen G, Simpson A, Bisno A, et al. Adherence of slime-producing strains of *Staphylococcus epidermidis* to smooth surfaces. *Infect Immun.* 1982;37:318-326.
106. Castagnola E, Conte M, Venzano P, et al. Broviac catheter-related bacteraemias due to unusual pathogens in children with cancer: case reports with literature review. *J Infect.* 1997;34:215-218.
107. Castagnola E, Garaventa A, Viscoli C, et al. Changing pattern of pathogens causing Broviac catheter-related bacteraemias in children with cancer. *J Hosp Infect.* 1995;29:129-133.
108. Chee L, Brown M, Sasadeusz J, et al. Gram-negative organisms predominate in Hickman line-related infections in non-neutropenic patients with hematological malignancies. *J Infect.* 2008;56:227-233.
109. Marchaim D, Zaidenstein R, Lazarovitch T, et al. Epidemiology of bacteremia episodes in a single center: increase in Gram-negative isolates, antibiotics resistance, and patient age. *Eur J Clin Microbiol Infect Dis.* 2008;27:1045-1051.
110. Shih MJ, Lee NY, Lee HC, et al. Risk factors of multidrug resistance in nosocomial bacteremia due to *Acinetobacter baumannii:* a case-control study. *J Microbiol Immunol Infect.* 2008;41:118-123.
111. Lorente L, Jimenez A, Santana M, et al. Microorganisms responsible for intravascular catheter-related bloodstream infection according to the catheter site. *Crit Care Med.* 2007;35:2424-2427.
112. Goetz AM, Rihs JD, Chow JW, et al. An outbreak of infusion-related *Klebsiella pneumoniae* bacteremia in a liver transplantation unit. *Clin Infect Dis.* 1995;21:1501-1503.
113. Henderson DK, Baptiste RF, Parrillo J, et al. Indolent epidemic of *Pseudomonas cepacia* bacteremia and pseudobacteremia in an intensive care unit traced to a contaminated blood gas analyzer. *Am J Med.* 1988;84:75-81.
114. Pegues DA, Carson LA, Anderson RL, et al. Outbreak of *Pseudomonas cepacia* bacteremia in oncology patients. *Clin Infect Dis.* 1993;16:407-411.

115. Ashkenazi S, Leibovici L, Samra Z, et al. Risk factors for mortality due to bacteremia and fungemia in childhood. *Clin Infect Dis.* 1992;14:949-951.
116. D'Antonio D, Pizzigallo E, Iacone A, et al. Occurrence of bacteremia in hematologic patients. *Eur J Epidemiol.* 1992;8:687-692.
117. Lecciones JA, Lee JW, Navarro EE, et al. Vascular catheter-associated fungemia in patients with cancer: analysis of 155 episodes. *Clin Infect Dis.* 1992;14:875-883.
118. Leibovici L, Konisberger H, Pitlik SD, et al. Bacteremia and fungemia of unknown origin in adults. *Clin Infect Dis.* 1992;14:436-443.
119. Rello J, Quintana E, Mirelis B, et al. Polymicrobial bacteremia in critically ill patients. *Intensive Care Med.* 1993;19:22-25.
120. Walsh TJ, Gonzalez C, Roilides E, et al. Fungemia in children infected with the human immunodeficiency virus: new epidemiologic patterns, emerging pathogens, and improved outcome with antifungal therapy. *Clin Infect Dis.* 1995;20:900-906.
121. Hawkins C, Qi C, Warren J, et al. Catheter-related bloodstream infections caused by rapidly growing nontuberculous mycobacteria: a case series including rare species. *Diagn Microbiol Infect Dis.* 2008;61:187-191.
122. Sulpher J, Desjardins M, Lee BC. Central venous catheter-associated *Leifsonia aquatica* bacteremia in a hemodialysis-dependent patient. *Diag Microbiol Infect Dis.* 2008;61:64-66.
123. Mermel LA, Farr BM, Sherertz RJ, et al. Guidelines for the management of intravascular catheter-related infections. *J Intraven Nurs.* 2001;24:180-205.
124. Simon L, Gauvin F, Amre DK, et al. Serum procalcitonin and C-reactive protein levels as markers of bacterial infection: a systematic review and meta-analysis. *Clin Infect Dis.* 2004;39:206-217.
125. Becker KL, Snider R, Nylen ES. Procalcitonin assay in systemic inflammation, infection, and sepsis: clinical utility and limitations. *Crit Care Med.* 2008;36:941-952.
126. Maki D, Jarrett F, Sarafin H. A semiquantitative method for identification of catheter-related infection in the burn patient. *J Surg Res.* 1977;22:513-520.
127. Maki D, Weise C, Sarafin H. A semiquantitative method for identifying intravenous-catheter-related infection. *N Engl J Med.* 1977;296:1305-1309.
128. Siegman-Igra Y, Anglim AM, Shapiro DE, et al. Diagnosis of vascular catheter-related bloodstream infection: a meta-analysis. *J Clin Microbiol.* 1997;35:928-936.
129. Douard MC, Arlet G, Longuet P, et al. Diagnosis of venous access port-related infections. *Clin Infect Dis.* 1999;29:1197-1202.
130. Whitman ED, Boatman AM. Comparison of diagnostic specimens and methods to evaluate infected venous access ports. *Am J Surg.* 1995;170:665-670.
131. Band J, Maki D. Infections caused by arterial catheters used for hemodynamic monitoring. *Am J Med.* 1979;67:735-741.
132. Band JD, Alvarado CJ, Maki DG. A semiquantitative culture technique for identifying infection due to steel needles used for intravenous therapy. *Am J Clin Pathol.* 1979;72:980-984.
133. Dooley DP, Garcia A, Kelly JW, et al. Validation of catheter semiquantitative culture technique for nonstaphylococcal organisms. *J Clin Microbiol.* 1996;34:409-412.
134. Cleri D, Corrado M, Seligman S. Quantitative culture of intravenous catheters and other intravascular inserts. *J Infect Dis.* 1980;141:781-786.
135. Brun-Buisson C, Abrouk F, Legrand P, et al. Diagnosis of central venous catheter-related sepsis: critical level of quantitative tip cultures. *Arch Intern Med.* 1987;147:873-877.
136. Gutierrez J, Leon C, Matamoros R, et al. Catheter-related bacteremia and fungemia: reliability of two methods for catheter culture. *Diagn Microbiol Infect Dis.* 1992;15:575-578.
137. Hnatiuk O, Pike J, Stolzfus D, et al. Value of bedside plating of semiquantitative cultures for diagnosis of central venous catheter-related infections in ICU patients. *Chest.* 1993;103:896-899.
138. Sherertz RJ, Heard SO, Raad II. Diagnosis of triple-lumen catheter infection: comparison of roll plate, sonication, and flushing methodologies. *J Clin Microbiol.* 1997;35:641-646.
139. Safdar N, Fine JP, Maki DG. Meta-analysis: methods for diagnosing intravascular device-related bloodstream infection. *Ann Intern Med.* 2005;142:451-466.
140. Schierholz JM, Bach A, Fleck C, et al. Measurement of ultrasonic-induced chlorhexidine liberation: correlation of the activity of chlorhexidine-silver-sulfadiazine-impregnated catheters to agar roll technique and broth culture. *J Hosp Infect.* 2000;44:141-145.
141. Schmitt SK, Knapp C, Hall GS, et al. Impact of chlorhexidine-silver sulfadiazine-impregnated central venous catheters on in vitro quantitation of catheter-associated bacteria. *J Clin Microbiol.* 1996;34:508-511.
142. Collignon P, Chan R, Munro R. Rapid diagnosis of intravascular catheter-related sepsis. *Arch Intern Med.* 1987;147:1609-1612.
143. Kite P, Dobbins BM, Wilcox MH, et al. Evaluation of a novel endoluminal brush method for in situ diagnosis of catheter related sepsis. *J Clin Pathol.* 1997;50:278-282.
144. McGeer A, Righter J. Improving our ability to diagnose infections associated with central venous catheters: value of Gram's staining and culture of entry site swabs. *Can Med Assoc J.* 1987;137:1009-1015.
145. Bong JJ, Kite P, Ammorei BJ, et al. The use of a rapid in situ test in the detection of central venous catheter-related bloodstream infection: a prospective study. *J Parenter Enteral Nutr.* 2003;27:146-150.
146. Kite P, Dobbins BM, Wilcox MH, et al. Rapid diagnosis of central-venous-catheter-related bloodstream infection without catheter removal. *Lancet.* 1999;354:1504-1507.
147. Mosca R, Curtas S, Forbes B, et al. The benefits of isolator cultures in the management of suspected catheter sepsis. *Surgery.* 1987;102:718-723.
148. Ascher DP, Shoupe BA, Robb M, et al. Comparison of standard and quantitative blood cultures in the evaluation of children with suspected central venous line sepsis. *Diagn Microbiol Infect Dis.* 1992;15:499-503.
149. Flynn PM, Shenep JL, Barrett FF. Differential quantitation with a commercial blood culture tube for diagnosis of catheter-related infection. *J Clin Microbiol.* 1988;26:1045-1046.
150. Capdevila JA, Planes AM, Palomar M, et al. Value of differential quantitative blood cultures in the diagnosis of catheter-related sepsis. *Eur J Clin Microbiol Infect Dis.* 1992;11:403-407.
151. Olson IE, Lam K, Bodey GP, et al. Evaluation of strategies for central venous catheter replacement. *Crit Care Med.* 1992;20:797-804.
152. Wing E, Norden C, Shadduck R, et al. Use of quantitative bacteriologic techniques to diagnose catheter-related sepsis. *Arch Intern Med.* 1979;139:482-488.
153. Quilici N, Audibert G, Conroy MC, et al. Differential quantitative blood cultures in the diagnosis of catheter-related sepsis in intensive care units. *Clin Infect Dis.* 1997;25:1066-1070.
154. Blot F, Schmidt E, Nitenberg G, et al. Earlier positivity of central-venous- versus peripheral-blood cultures is highly predictive of catheter-related sepsis. *J Clin Microbiol.* 1998;36:105-109.
155. Bouza E, Alvarado N, Alcala L, et al. A randomized and prospective study of 3 procedures for the diagnosis of catheter-related bloodstream infection without catheter withdrawal. *Clin Infect Dis.* 2007;44:820-826.
156. Raad I, Hanna HA, Alakech B, et al. Differential time to positivity: a useful method for diagnosing catheter-related bloodstream infections. *Ann Intern Med.* 2004;140:18-25.
157. Seifert H, Cornely O, Seggewiss K, et al. Bloodstream infection in neutropenic cancer patients related to short-term nontunnelled catheters determined by quantitative blood cultures, differential time to positivity, and molecular epidemiological typing with pulsed-field gel electrophoresis. *J Clin Microbiol.* 2003;41:118-123.
158. Acuna M, O'Ryan M, Cofre J, et al. Differential time to positivity and quantitative cultures for noninvasive diagnosis of catheter-related blood stream infection in children. *Pediatr Infect Dis J.* 2008;27:681-685.
159. Catton JA, Dobbins BM, Kite P, et al. In situ diagnosis of intravascular catheter-related bloodstream infection: a comparison of quantitative culture, differential time to positivity, and endoluminal brushing. *Crit Care Med.* 2005;33:787-791.
160. Malgrange VB, Escande MC, Theobald S. Validity of earlier positivity of central venous blood cultures in comparison with peripheral blood cultures for diagnosing catheter-related bacteremia in cancer patients. *J Clin Microbiol.* 2001;39:274-278.
161. Rijnders BJ, Verwaest C, Peetermans WE, et al. Difference in time to positivity of hub-blood versus non hub-blood cultures is not useful for the diagnosis of catheter-related bloodstream infection in critically ill patients. *Crit Care Med.* 2001;29:1399-1403.
162. Tonnesen A, Peuler M, Lockwood W. Cultures of blood drawn by catheters vs. venipuncture. *JAMA.* 1976;235:1877.
163. Felices F, Hernandez J, Ruiz J, et al. Use of the central venous pressure catheter to obtain blood cultures. *Crit Care Med.* 1979;7:78-79.
164. Souvenir D, Anderson DE Jr, Palpant S, et al. Blood cultures positive for coagulase-negative staphylococci: antisepsis, pseudobacteremia, and therapy of patients. *J Clin Microbiol.* 1998;36:1923-1926.
165. Pettigren R, Lang D, Haycock D, et al. Catheter-related sepsis in patients on intravenous nutrition: a prospective study of quantitative catheter cultures and guideline changes for suspected sepsis. *Br J Surg.* 1985;72:52-55.
166. Chatzinikolaou I, Hanna H, Darouiche R, et al. Prospective study of the value of quantitative culture of organisms from blood collected through central venous catheters in differentiating between contamination and bloodstream infection. *J Clin Microbiol.* 2006;44:1834-1835.
167. DesJardin J, Falagas ME, Ruthazer R, et al. Clinical utility of blood cultures drawn from indwelling central venous catheters in hospitalized patients with cancer. *Ann Intern Med.* 1999;131:641-647.
168. Torlakovic E, Hibbs JR, Miller JS, et al. Intracellular bacteria in blood smears in patients with central venous catheters. *Arch Intern Med.* 1995;155:1547-1550.
169. Bingen E, Barc MC, Brahimi N, et al. Randomly amplified polymorphic DNA analysis provides rapid differentiation of methicillin-resistant coagulase-negative staphylococcus bacteremia isolates in pediatric hospital. *J Clin Microbiol.* 1995;33:1657-1659.
170. Dominguez MA, Linares J, Pulido A, et al. Molecular tracking of coagulase-negative staphylococcal isolates from catheter-related infections. *Microb Drug Resist.* 1996;2:423-429.
171. Maki D, Goldmann D, Rhame F. Infection control in intravenous therapy. *Ann Intern Med.* 1973;79:867-887.
172. Tully J, Friedland G, Baldini M, et al. Complications of intravenous therapy with steel needles and Teflon catheters. *Am J Med.* 1981;70:702-706.
173. Bregenzer T, Conen D, Sakmann P, et al. Is routine replacement of peripheral intravenous catheters necessary? *Arch Intern Med.* 1998;158:151-156.
174. Lai KK. Safety of prolonging peripheral cannula and i.v. tubing use from 72 hours to 96 hours. *Am J Infect Control.* 1998;26:66-70.
175. Cornely OA, Bethe U, Pauls R, et al. Peripheral Teflon catheters: factors determining incidence of phlebitis and duration of cannulation. *Infect Control Hosp Epidemiol.* 2002;23:249-253.
176. Webster J, Clarke S, Paterson D, et al. Routine care of peripheral intravenous catheters versus clinically indicated replacement: randomised controlled trial. *BMJ.* 2008;337:a339.
177. Crane D. Venous interruption for septic thrombophlebitis. *N Engl J Med.* 1962;262:947-951.
178. De Cicco M, Matovic M, Balestreri L, et al. Central venous thrombosis: an early and frequent complication in cancer patients bearing long-term silastic catheter: a prospective study. *Thromb Res.* 1997;86:101-113.
179. Harden JL, Kemp L, Mirtallo J. Femoral catheters increase risk of infection in total parenteral nutrition patients. *Nutr Clin Pract.* 1995;10:60-66.
180. Khan EA, Correa AG, Baker CJ. Suppurative thrombophlebitis in children: a ten-year experience. *Pediatr Infect Dis J.* 1997;16:63-67.
181. Munster A. Septic thrombophlebitis: a surgical disorder. *JAMA.* 1974;230:1010-1011.
182. Martin C, Bruder N, Papazian L, et al. Catheter-related infections following axillary vein catheterization. *Acta Anaesthesiol Scand.* 1998;42:52-56.
183. Moran J, Atwood R, Rowe M. A clinical and bacteriologic study of infections associated with venous cutdowns. *N Engl J Med.* 1965;272:554-560.
184. Pujol M, Hornero A, Saballs M, et al. Clinical epidemiology and outcomes of peripheral venous catheter-related bloodstream infections at a university-affiliated hospital. *J Hosp Infect.* 2007;67:22-29.
185. Maki DG. Improving the safety of peripheral intravenous catheters. *BMJ.* 2008;337:a630.
186. Band J, Maki D. Safety of changing intravenous delivery systems at longer than 24-hour intervals. *Ann Intern Med.* 1979;91:173-178.
187. Buxton A, Anderson R, Klimek J, et al. Failure of disposable domes to prevent septicemia from contaminated pressure transducers. *Chest.* 1978;74:508-513.
188. Snydman D, Reidy M, Perry L, et al. Safety of changing intravenous (IV) administration sets containing burettes at longer than 48 hour intervals. *Infect Control.* 1987;8:113-116.
189. Maki D, Boiticelli J, LeRoy M, et al. Prospective study of replacing administration sets for intravenous therapy at 48 vs. 72 hour intervals: 72 hours is safe and cost-effective. *JAMA.* 1987;258:1777-1781.
190. Michel L, McMichan J, Bachy J. Microbial colonization of indwelling central venous catheters: statistical evaluation of potential contaminating factors. *Am J Surg.* 1979;137:745-748.
191. Henderson D, Myers R, Laniak J. Catheter-acquired infection in total parenteral nutrition. *Nat Intraven Ther Assoc J.* 1982;5:62-68.
192. Jones GR, Konsler GK, Dunaway RP, et al. Prospective analysis of urokinase in the treatment of catheter sepsis in pediatric hematology-oncology patients. *J Pediatr Surg.* 1993;28:350-355.
193. Peters W, Bush W, McIntyre R, et al. The development of fibrin sheath on indwelling venous catheters. *Surg Gynecol Obstet.* 1973;137:43-47.
194. Ruggiero R, Aisenstein T. Central catheter fibrin sleeve; heparin effect. *J Parenter Enteral Nutr.* 1983;7:270-273.
195. Lloyd DA, Shanbhogue LK, Doherty PJ, et al. Does the fibrin coat around a central venous catheter influence catheter-related sepsis? *J Pediatr Surg.* 1993;28:345-348.
196. Keller JE, Hindman JW, Mehall JR, et al. Enoxaparin inhibits fibrin sheath formation and decreases central venous catheter colonization following bacteremic challenge. *Crit Care Med.* 2006;34:1450-1455.
197. Timsit JF. Scheduled replacement of central venous catheters is not necessary. *Infect Control Hosp Epidemiol.* 2000;21:371-374.
198. Maher M, Henderson D, Brennan M. Central venous catheter exchange in cancer patients during total parenteral nutrition. *Nat Intraven Ther Assoc J.* 1982;5:54-60.
199. Bach A, Böhrer H, Geiss HK. Safety of a guidewire technique for replacement of pulmonary artery catheters. *J Cardiothorac Vasc Anesth.* 1992;6:711-714.
200. Cobb DK, High KP, Sawyer RG, et al. A controlled trial of scheduled replacement of central venous and pulmonary-artery catheters. *N Engl J Med.* 1992;327:1062-1068.
201. Cook D, Randolph A, Kernerman P, et al. Central venous catheter replacement strategies: a systematic review of the literature. *Crit Care Med.* 1997;25:1417-1424.
202. Anaissie EJ, Rex JH, Uzun O, et al. Predictors of adverse outcome in cancer patients with candidemia. *Am J Med.* 1998;104:238-245.
203. Anagnostakis D, Kamba A, Petrochilou V, et al. Risk of infection associated with umbilical vein catheterization: a prospective study in 75 newborn infants. *J Pediatr.* 1973;86:759-765.

204. Balagtas R, Bell C, Edwards L, et al. Risk of local and systemic infections associated with umbilical vein catheterization: a prospective study in 86 newborn patients. *Pediatrics.* 1971;48:359-367.
205. Munson D, Thompson T, Johnson D, et al. Coagulase-negative staphylococcal septicemia: experience in a newborn intensive care unit. *J Pediatr.* 1982;101:602-605.
206. Symansky M, Fox H. Umbilical vessel catheterization: indications, management, and evaluation of the technique. *J Pediatr.* 1972;80:820-826.
207. McCready CE, Doughty HA, Pearson TC. Experience with the Port-A-Cath in sickle cell disease. *Clin Lab Haematol.* 1996;18:79-82.
208. Paganini H, Rodriguez Brieshcke T, Santos P, et al. Risk factors for nosocomial candidaemia: a case-control study in children. *J Hosp Infect.* 2002;50:304-308.
209. Marra AR, Opilla M, Edmond MB, et al. Epidemiology of bloodstream infections in patients receiving long-term total parenteral nutrition. *J Clin Gastroenterol.* 2007;41:19-28.
210. Rhee P, Hadjizacharia P, Trankiem C, et al. What happened to total parenteral nutrition? The disappearance of its use in a trauma intensive care unit. *J Trauma.* 2007;63:1215-1222.
211. Elke G, Schadler D, Engel C, et al. Current practice in nutritional support and its association with mortality in septic patients—results from a national, prospective, multicenter study. *Crit Care Med.* 2008;36:1762-1767.
212. Goldmann D, Maki D. Infection control in total parenteral nutrition. *JAMA.* 1973;223:1360-1364.
213. Syndman D, Murray S, Kornfield S, et al. Total parenteral nutrition-related infections: prospective epidemiologic study using semiquantitative methods. *Am J Med.* 1982:695-699.
214. Dissanaike S, Shelton M, Warner K, et al. The risk for bloodstream infections is associated with increased parenteral caloric intake in patients receiving parenteral nutrition. *Crit Care.* 2007;11:R114.
215. Curry C, Quie P. Fungal septicemia in patients receiving parenteral hyperalimentation. *N Engl J Med.* 1971;285:1221-1225.
216. Henderson D, Edwards J Jr, Montgomerie J. Hematogenous *Candida* endophthalmitis in patients receiving parenteral hyperalimentation fluids. *J Infect Dis.* 1981;143:655-661.
217. Montgomerie J, Edwards J Jr. Association of infection due to *Candida albicans* with intravenous hyperalimentation. *J Infect Dis.* 1978;127:197-201.
218. Chang L, Tsai JS, Huang SJ, et al. Evaluation of infectious complications of the implantable venous access system in a general oncologic population. *Am J Infect Control.* 2003;31:34-39.
219. Wilmore D, Dudrick S. An in-line filter for intravenous solutions. *Arch Surg.* 1969;99:462-463.
220. Bailey M. Reduction of catheter-associated sepsis in parenteral nutrition using low-dose intravenous heparin. *Br Med J.* 1979;1:1671-1673.
221. Mitchell A, Atkins S, Royle G, et al. Reduced catheter sepsis and prolonged catheter life using a tunnelled silicone rubber catheter for total parenteral nutrition. *Br J Surg.* 1982;69:420-422.
222. Maki D. Epidemic nosocomial bacteremias. In: Wenzel R, ed. *Handbook of Hospital Acquired Infections.* Boca Raton, Florida: CRC Press; 1981:371-512.
223. Broviac J, Cole J, Scribner B. A silicone rubber atrial catheter for prolonged parenteral alimentation. *Surg Gynecol Obstet.* 1973;136:602-606.
224. Hickman R, Buckner C, Clift R, et al. A modified right atrial catheter for access to the venous system in marrow transplant recipients. *Surg Gynecol Obstet.* 1979;148:871-875.
225. Delmore JE, Horbelt DV, Jack BL, et al. Experience with the Groshong long-term central venous catheter. *Gynecol Oncol.* 1989;34:216-218.
226. Blacklock H, Hill R, Clarke A, et al. Use of modified subcutaneous right-atrial catheter for venous access in leukaemic patients. *Lancet.* 1980;1:993-995.
227. Press O, Ramsey P, Larson E, et al. Hickman catheter infections in patients with malignancies. *Medicine (Baltimore).* 1984;63:189-200.
228. Alurkar SS, Dhabhar BN, Pathak AB, et al. Long-term right atrial catheters in patients with malignancies: an Indian experience. *J Surg Oncol.* 1992;51:183-187.
229. Cairo MS, Spooner S, Sowden L, et al. Long-term use of indwelling multipurpose silastic catheters in pediatric cancer patients treated with aggressive chemotherapy. *J Clin Oncol.* 1986;4:784-788.
230. Elishoov H, Or R, Strauss N, et al. Nosocomial colonization, septicemia, and Hickman/Broviac catheter-related infections in bone marrow transplant recipients: a 5-year prospective study. *Medicine (Baltimore).* 1998;77:83-101.
231. Hockenberry MJ, Schultz WH, Bennett B, et al. Experience with minimal complications in implanted catheters in children. *Am J Pediatr Hematol Oncol.* 1989;11:295-299.
232. Hogan L, Pulito AR. Broviac central venous catheters inserted via the saphenous or femoral vein in the NICU under local anesthesia. *J Pediatr Surg.* 1992;27:1185-1188.
233. Holloway RW, Orr JW. An evaluation of Groshong central venous catheters on a gynecologic oncology service. *Gynecol Oncol.* 1995;56:211-217.
234. Johnson PR, Decker MD, Edwards KM, et al. Frequency of Broviac catheter infections in pediatric oncology patients. *J Infect Dis.* 1986;154:570-578.
235. Kappers-Klunne MC, Degener JE, Stijnen T, et al. Complications from long-term indwelling central venous catheters in hematologic patients with special reference to infection. *Cancer.* 1989;64:1747-1752.
236. Larson EB, Wooding M, Hickman RO. Infectious complications of right atrial catheters used for venous access in patients receiving intensive chemotherapy. *Surg Gynecol Obstet.* 1981;153:369-373.
237. Lokich JJ, Bothe A Jr, Benotti P, et al. Complications and management of implanted venous access catheters. *J Clin Oncol.* 1985;3:710-717.
238. Rizzari C, Palamone G, Corbetta A, et al. Central venous catheter-related infections in pediatric hematology-oncology patients: role of home and hospital management. *Pediatr Hematol Oncol.* 1992;9:115-123.
239. Ross MN, Haase GM, Poole MA, et al. Comparison of totally implanted reservoirs with external catheters as venous access devices in pediatric oncologic patients. *Surg Gynecol Obstet.* 1988;167:141-144.
240. Shulman RJ, Rahman S, Mahoney D, et al. A totally implanted venous access system used in pediatric patients with cancer. *J Clin Oncol.* 1987;5:137-140.
241. Ulz L, Petersen FB, Ford R, et al. A prospective study of complications in Hickman right-atrial catheters in marrow transplant patients. *J Parenter Enteral Nutr.* 1990;14:27-30.
242. Viscoli C, Garaventa A, Boni L, et al. Role of Broviac catheters in infections in children with cancer. *Pediatr Infect Dis J.* 1988;7:556-560.
243. Wacker P, Bugmann P, Halperin DS, et al. Comparison of totally implanted and external catheters in paediatric oncology patients. *Eur J Cancer.* 1992;28A:841.
244. Becton D, Kletzel M, Golladay E, et al. An experience with an implanted port system in 66 children with cancer. *Cancer.* 1988;61:376-378.
245. Brothers T, VanMoll L, Niederhuber J, et al. Experience with subcutaneous infusion ports in three hundred patients. *Surg Gynecol Obstet.* 1988;166:295-301.
246. Poorter RL, Lauw FN, Bemelman WA, et al. Complications of an implantable venous access device (Port-a-Cath) during intermittent continuous infusion of chemotherapy. *Eur J Cancer.* 1996;32A:2262-2266.
247. Puig-la Calle J Jr, Lopez Sanchez S, Piedrafita Serra E, et al. Totally implanted device for long-term intravenous chemotherapy: experience in 123 adult patients with solid neoplasms. *J Surg Oncol.* 1996;62:273-278.
248. Ozyuvaci E, Kutlu F. Totally implantable venous access devices via subclavian vein: a retrospective study of 368 oncology patients. *Adv Ther.* 2006;23:574-581.
249. Maki DG, Kluger DM, Crnich CJ. The risk of bloodstream infection in adults with different intravascular devices: a systematic review of 200 published prospective studies. *Mayo Clin Proc.* 2006;81:1159-1171.
250. Duthoit D, Devleeshouwer C, Paesmans M, et al. Infection of totally implantable chamber catheters in cancer patients: multivariate analysis of risk factors. Paper presented at the 33rd Interscience Conference on Antimicrobial Agents and Chemotherapy, New Orleans, Louisiana, 1993.
251. Fischer L, Knebel P, Schroder S, et al. Reasons for explantation of totally implantable access ports: a multivariate analysis of 385 consecutive patients. *Ann Surg Oncol.* 2008;15:1124-1129.
252. Vescia S, Baumgartner AK, Jacobs VR, et al. Management of venous port systems in oncology: a review of current evidence. *Ann Oncol.* 2008;19:9-15.
253. Corey GR, Lalani T. Risk of intravascular cardiac device infections in patients with bacteraemia: impact on device removal. *Int J Antimicrob Agents.* 2008;32:S26-S29.
254. Sohail MR, Uslan DZ, Kahan AH, et al. Management and outcome of permanent pacemaker and implantable cardioverter-defibrillator infections. *J Am Coll Cardiol.* 2007;49:1851-1859.
255. Cardella JF, Cardella K, Bacci N, et al. Cumulative experience with 1,273 peripherally inserted central catheters at a single institution. *J Vasc Interv Radiol.* 1996;7:5-13.
256. Chait PG, Ingram J, Phillips-Gordon C, et al. Peripherally inserted central catheters in children. *Radiology.* 1995;197:775-778.
257. Yeung CY, Lee HC, Huang FY, et al. Sepsis during total parenteral nutrition: exploration of risk factors and determination of the effectiveness of peripherally inserted central venous catheters. *Pediatr Infect Dis J.* 1998;17:135-142.
258. Safdar N, Maki DG. Risk of catheter-related bloodstream infection with peripherally inserted central venous catheters used in hospitalized patients. *Chest.* 2005;128:489-495.
259. Cowl CT, Weinstock JV, Al-Jurf A, et al. Complications and cost associated with parenteral nutrition delivered to hospitalized patients through either subclavian or peripherally-inserted central catheters. *Clin Nutr.* 2000;19:237-243.
260. Horattas MC, Trupiano J, Hopkins S, et al. Changing concepts in long-term central venous access: catheter selection and cost savings. *Am J Infect Control.* 2001;29:32-40.
261. Loughran SC, Borzatta M. Peripherally inserted central catheters: a report of 2506 catheter days. *J Parenter Enteral Nutr.* 1995;19:133-136.
262. Hussain S, Gomez MM, Wludyka P, et al. Survival times and complications of catheters used for outpatient parenteral antibiotic therapy in children. *Clin Pediatr.* 2007;46:247-251.
263. Hiemenz J, Robichaud K, Johnston M, et al. Bacteremia in patients with indwelling silastic catheters. *Proc Am Soc Clin Oncol.* 1982;1:57.
264. Hiemenz J, Skelton J, Pizzo P. Perspective on the management of catheter-related infections in cancer patients. *Pediatr Infect Dis.* 1987;5:6-11.
265. Hartman G, Shuchat S. Management of septic complications associated with silastic catheters in childhood malignancies. *Pediatr Infect Dis J.* 1987;6:1042-1047.
266. Ascher DP, Shoupe BA, Maybee D, et al. Persistent catheter-related bacteremia: clearance with antibiotics and urokinase. *J Pediatr Surg.* 1993;28:627-629.
267. Onder AM, Chandar J, Simon N, et al. Treatment of catheter-related bacteremia with tissue plasminogen activator antibiotic locks. *Pediatr Nephrol.* 2008;23:457-464.
268. Benoit JL, Carandang G, Sitrin M, et al. Intraluminal antibiotic treatment of central venous catheter infections in patients receiving parenteral nutrition at home. *Clin Infect Dis.* 1995;21:1286-1288.
269. McCarthy A, Byrne M, Breathnach F, et al. "In-situ" teicoplanin for central venous catheter infection. *Ir J Med Sci.* 1995;164:125-127.
270. Fortun J, Grill F, Martin-Davila P, et al. Treatment of long-term intravascular catheter-related bacteraemia with antibiotic-lock therapy. *J Antimicrob Chemother.* 2006;58:816-821.
271. Rijnders BJ, Van Wijngaerden E, Vandecasteele SJ, et al. Treatment of long-term intravascular catheter-related bacteraemia with antibiotic lock: randomized, placebo-controlled trial. *J Antimicrob Chemother.* 2005;55:90-94.
272. Viale P, Pagani L, Petrosillo N, et al. Antibiotic lock—technique for the treatment of catheter-related bloodstream infections. *J Chemother.* 2003;15:152-156.
273. Maya ID, Carlton D, Estrada E, et al. Treatment of dialysis catheter-related *Staphylococcus aureus* bacteremia with an antibiotic lock: a quality improvement report. *Am J Kidney Dis.* 2007;50:289-295.
274. Buckler BS, Sams RN, Goei VL, et al. Treatment of central venous catheter fungal infection using liposomal amphotericin-B lock therapy. *Pediatr Infect Dis J.* 2008;27:762-764.
275. Raad I, Hanna H, Jiang Y, et al. Comparative activities of daptomycin, linezolid, and tigecycline against catheter-related methicillin-resistant *Staphylococcus* bacteremic isolates embedded in biofilm. *Antimicrob Agents Chemother.* 2007;51:1656-1660.
276. Raad I, Hanna H, Dvorak T, et al. Optimal antimicrobial catheter lock solution, using different combinations of minocycline, EDTA, and 25-percent ethanol, rapidly eradicates organisms embedded in biofilm. *Antimicrob Agents Chemother.* 2007;51:78-83.
277. Broom J, Woods M, Allworth A, et al. Ethanol lock therapy to treat tunnelled central venous catheter-associated blood stream infections: results from a prospective trial. *Scand J Infect Dis.* 2008;40:399-406.
278. Dannenberg C, Bierbach U, Rothe A, et al. Ethanol-lock technique in the treatment of bloodstream infections in pediatric oncology patients with Broviac catheter. *J Pediatr Hematol Oncol.* 2003;25:616-621.
279. Onland W, Shin CE, Fustar S, et al. Ethanol-lock technique for persistent bacteremia of long-term intravascular devices in pediatric patients. *Arch Pediatr Adolesc Med.* 2006;160:1049-1053.
280. Hollingsed MJ, Morales JM, Roughneen PT, et al. Surgical management of catheter tip thrombus: surgical therapy for right atrial thrombus and fungal endocarditis (*Candida tropicalis*) complicating paediatric sickle-cell disease. *Perfusion.* 1997;12:197-201.
281. Schleman KA, Tullis G, Blum R. Intracardiac mass complicating *Malassezia furfur* fungemia. *Chest.* 2000;118:1828-1829.
282. Swan H, Ganz W, Forrester J. Catheterization of the heart in a man with the use of a flow-directed balloon-tipped catheter. *N Engl J Med.* 1970;283:447-451.
283. Wheeler AP, Bernard GR, Thompson BT, et al. Pulmonary-artery versus central venous catheter to guide treatment of acute lung injury. *N Engl J Med.* 2006;354:2213-2224.
284. Harvey SE, Welch CA, Harrison DA, et al. Post hoc insights from PAC-Man—the U.K. pulmonary artery catheter trial. *Crit Care Med.* 2008;36:1714-1721.
285. Frazier SK, Skinner GJ. Pulmonary artery catheters: state of the controversy. *J Cardiovasc Nurs.* 2008;23:113-121.
286. Michel L, Marsh M, McMichan J, et al. Infection of pulmonary artery catheters in critically ill patients. *JAMA.* 1981;245:1032-1036.
287. Katz J, Cronan L, Barash P, et al. Pulmonary artery flow-guided catheters in the perioperative period. *JAMA.* 1977;237:2832-2834.
288. Maki DG, Stolz SS, Wheeler S, et al. A prospective, randomized trial of gauze and two polyurethane dressings for site care of pulmonary artery catheters: implications for catheter management. *Crit Care Med.* 1994;22:1729-1737.
289. Shah MR, Hasselblad V, Stevenson LW, et al. Impact of the pulmonary artery catheter in critically ill patients: meta-analysis of randomized clinical trials. *JAMA.* 2005;294:1664-1670.
290. Cohen Y, Fosse JP, Karoubi P, et al. The "hands-off" catheter and the prevention of systemic infections associated with pulmonary artery catheter: a prospective study. *Am J Respir Crit Care Med.* 1998;157:284-287.
291. Ford S, Manley P. Indwelling cardiac catheters: an autopsy study of associated endocardial lesions. *Arch Pathol Lab Med.* 1982;106:314-317.

292. Greene J Jr, Fitzwater J, Clemmer T. Septic endocarditis and indwelling pulmonary artery catheters. *JAMA*. 1975;233:891-892.
293. Ehrie M, Morgan A, Moore F, et al. Endocarditis with the indwelling balloon-tipped pulmonary artery catheter in burn patients. *J Trauma*. 1978;18:664-666.
294. Fernandez-Guerrero ML, Verdejo C, Azofra J, et al. Hospital-acquired infectious endocarditis not associated with cardiac surgery: an emerging problem. *Clin Infect Dis*. 1995;20:16-23.
295. Cheng A, Athan E, Appelbe A, et al. The changing profile of bacterial endocarditis as seen at an Australian provincial centre. *Heart Lung Circ*. 2002;11:26-31.
296. Hill EE, Herijgers P, Claus P, et al. Infective endocarditis: changing epidemiology and predictors of 6-month mortality: a prospective cohort study. *Eur Heart J*. 2007;28:196-203.
297. Nucifora G, Badano LP, Viale P, et al. Infective endocarditis in chronic haemodialysis patients: an increasing clinical challenge. *Eur Heart J*. 2007;28:2307-2312.
298. Ribot S, Siddiqi SW, Chen C. Right heart complications of dual lumen tunneled venous catheters in hemodialysis patients. *Am J Med Sci*. 2005;330:204-208.
299. Kac G, Durain E, Amrein C, et al. Colonization and infection of pulmonary artery catheter in cardiac surgery patients: epidemiology and multivariate analysis of risk factors. *Crit Care Med*. 2001;29:971-975.
300. Adams J, Speer M, Rudolph A. Bacterial colonization of radial artery catheters. *Pediatrics*. 1980;65:94-97.
301. Koh DB, Gowardman JR, Rickard CM, et al. Prospective study of peripheral arterial catheter infection and comparison with concurrently sited central venous catheters. *Crit Care Med*. 2008;36:397-402.
302. Lorente L, Santacreu R, Martin MM, et al. Arterial catheter-related infection of 2949 catheters. *Crit Care*. 2006;10:R83.
303. Maki D, Hassemer C. Endemic rate of fluid contamination and related septicemia in arterial pressure monitoring. *Am J Med*. 1981;70:733-738.
304. Mermel LA. Arterial catheters are not risk-free spigots. *Crit Care Med*. 2008;36:620-622.
305. Weinstein R, Stamm W, Kramer L, et al. Pressure monitoring devices: overlooked source of nosocomial infection. *JAMA*. 1976;236:936-938.
306. West C, Wayle B, Touneson A, et al. Nosocomial *Serratia marcescens* bacteremia associated with reuse of disposable monitoring domes. Paper presented at the Seventeenth Interscience Conference on Antimicrobial Agents and Chemotherapy, New York, 1977.
307. Berenholtz SM, Pronovost PJ, Lipsett PA, et al. Eliminating catheter-related bloodstream infections in the intensive care unit. *Crit Care Med*. 2004;32:2014-2020.
308. Costello JM, Morrow DF, Graham DA, et al. Systematic intervention to reduce central line-associated bloodstream infection rates in a pediatric cardiac intensive care unit. *Pediatrics*. 2008;121:915-923.
309. Muto C, Herbert C, Harrison E, et al. Reduction in central line-associated bloodstream infections among patients in intensive care units—Pennsylvania, April 2001-March 2005. *MMWR Morb Mortal Wkly Rep*. 2005;54:1013-1016.
310. Pronovost P, Needham D, Berenholtz S, et al. An intervention to decrease catheter-related bloodstream infections in the ICU. *N Engl J Med*. 2006;355:2725-2732.
311. Warren DK, Cosgrove SE, Diekema DJ, et al. A multicenter intervention to prevent catheter-associated bloodstream infections. *Infect Control Hosp Epidemiol*. 2006;27:662-669.
312. Institute for Healthcare Improvement. 5 Million Lives Campaign: Prevent Central Line-Associated Bloodstream Infections. Available at http://www.ihi.org/IHI/Programs/Campaign/CentralLineInfection.htm. Accessed October 10, 2008.
313. Yokoe DS, Mermel LA, Anderson DJ, et al. Executive summary: a compendium of strategies to prevent healthcare-associated infections in acute care hospitals. *Infect Control Hosp Epidemiol*. 2008;29:S12-S21.
314. Coopersmith CM, Rebmann TL, Zack JE, et al. Effect of an education program on decreasing catheter-related bloodstream infections in the surgical intensive care unit. *Crit Care Med*. 2002;30:59-64.
315. Sherertz RJ, Ely EW, Westbrook DM, et al. Education of physicians-in-training can decrease the risk for vascular catheter infection. *Ann Intern Med*. 2000;132:641-648.
316. Yilmaz G, Caylan R, Aydin K, et al. Effect of education on the rate of and the understanding of risk factors for intravascular catheter-related infections. *Infect Control Hosp Epidemiol*. 2007;28:689-694.
317. Kidd KM, Sinkowitz-Cochran RL, Giblin TB, et al. Barriers to and facilitators of implementing an intervention to reduce the incidence of catheter-associated bloodstream infections. *Infect Control Hosp Epidemiol*. 2007;28:103-105.
318. Safdar N, Abad C. Educational interventions for prevention of healthcare-associated infection: a systematic review. *Crit Care Med*. 2008;36:933-940.
319. Occupational Safety and Health Administration. Regulations (Standards—29 CFR) Bloodborne pathogens. -1910.1030. Available at http://www.osha.gov/pls/oshaweb/owadisp.show_document?p_table=STANDARDS&p_id=10051. Accessed October 10, 2008.
320. Pessoa-Silva CL, Hugonnet S, Pfister R, et al. Reduction of health care associated infection risk in neonates by successful hand hygiene promotion. *Pediatrics*. 2007;120:e382-e390.
321. Rosenthal VD, Guzman S, Safdar N. Reduction in nosocomial infection with improved hand hygiene in intensive care units of a tertiary care hospital in Argentina. *Am J Infect Control*. 2005;33:392-397.
322. Doebbeling BN, Stanley GL, Sheetz CT, et al. Comparative efficacy of alternative hand-washing agents in reducing nosocomial infections in intensive care units. *N Engl J Med*. 1992;327:88-93.
323. Hu KK, Lipsky BA, Veenstra DL, et al. Using maximal sterile barriers to prevent central venous catheter-related infection: a systematic evidence-based review. *Am J Infect Control*. 2004;32:231-238.
324. Young EM, Commiskey ML, Wilson SJ. Translating evidence into practice to prevent central venous catheter-associated bloodstream infections: a systems-based intervention. *Am J Infect Control*. 2006;34:503-506.
325. Lee DH, Jung KY, Choi YH. Use of maximal sterile barrier precautions and/or antimicrobial-coated catheters to reduce the risk of central venous catheter-related bloodstream infection. *Infect Control Hosp Epidemiol*. 2008;29:947-953.
326. Garland JS, Buck RK, Maloney P, et al. Comparison of 10% povidone-iodine and 0.5% chlorhexidine gluconate for the prevention of peripheral intravenous catheter colonization in neonates: a prospective trial. *Pediatr Infect Dis J*. 1995;14:510-516.
327. Humar A, Ostromecki A, Direnfeld J, et al. Prospective randomized trial of 10% povidone-iodine versus 0.5% tincture of chlorhexidine as cutaneous antisepsis for prevention of central venous catheter infection. *Clin Infect Dis*. 2000;31:1001-1007.
328. Chaiyakunapruk N, Veenstra DL, Lipsky BA, et al. Chlorhexidine compared with povidone-iodine solution for vascular catheter-site care: a meta-analysis. *Ann Intern Med*. 2002;136:792-801. [Summary for patients in *Ann Intern Med*. 2002;136:I26.]
329. Valles J, Fernandez I, Alcaraz D, et al. Prospective randomized trial of 3 antiseptic solutions for prevention of catheter colonization in an intensive care unit for adult patients. *Infect Control Hosp Epidemiol*. 2008;29:847-853.
330. Small H, Adams D, Casey AL, et al. Efficacy of adding 2% (w/v) chlorhexidine gluconate to 70% (v/v) isopropyl alcohol for skin disinfection prior to peripheral venous cannulation. *Infect Control Hosp Epidemiol*. 2008;29:963-965.
331. Mimoz O, Villeminey S, Ragot S, et al. Chlorhexidine-based antiseptic solution vs alcohol-based povidone-iodine for central venous catheter care. *Arch Intern Med*. 2007;167:2066-2072.
332. Aalto-Korte K, Makinen-Kiljunen S. Symptoms of immediate chlorhexidine hypersensitivity in patients with a positive prick test. *Contact Dermatitis*. 2006;55:173-177.
333. Garvey LH, Kroigaard M, Poulsen LK, et al. IgE-mediated allergy to chlorhexidine. *J Allergy Clin Immunol*. 2007;120:409-415.
334. Oto J, Nishimura M, Morimatsu H, et al. Comparison of contamination between conventional three-way stopcock and needleless injection device: a randomized controlled trial. *Med Sci Monit*. 2007;13:CR417-CR421.
335. Rhame F, Maki D, Bennett J. *Intravenous Cannula-Related Infections*. Boston, Mass: Little, Brown; 1979.
336. Hoffmann KK, Weber DJ, Samsa GP, et al. Transparent polyurethane film as an intravenous catheter dressing: a meta-analysis of the infection risks. *JAMA*. 1992;267:2072-2076.
337. Chambers ST, Sanders J, Patton WN, et al. Reduction of exit-site infections of tunnelled intravascular catheters among neutropenic patients by sustained-release chlorhexidine dressings: results from a prospective randomized controlled trial. *J Hosp Infect*. 2005;61:53-61.
338. Levy I, Katz J, Solter E, et al. Chlorhexidine-impregnated dressing for prevention of colonization of central venous catheters in infants and children: a randomized controlled study. *Pediatr Infect Dis J*. 2005;24:676-679.
339. Ruschulte H, Franke M, Gastmeier P, et al. Prevention of central venous catheter related infections with chlorhexidine gluconate impregnated wound dressings: a randomized controlled trial. *Ann Hematol*. 2008;88:267-272.
340. Giles Y, Aksoy M, Tezelman S. What really affects the incidence of central venous catheter-related infections for short-term catheterization? *Acta Chir Belg*. 2002;102:256-258.
341. Rasero L, Degl'Innocenti M, Mocali M, et al. Comparison of two different time interval protocols for central venous catheter dressing in bone marrow transplant patients: results of a randomized, multicenter study. *Haematologia*. 2000;85:275-279.
342. Benhamou E, Fessard E, Com-Nougue C, et al. Less frequent catheter dressing changes decrease local cutaneous toxicity of high-dose chemotherapy in children, without increasing the rate of catheter-related infections: results of a randomised trial. *Bone Marrow Transplant*. 2002;29:653-658.
343. Curchoe RM, Powers J, El-Daher N. Weekly transparent dressing changes linked to increased bacteremia rates. *Infect Control Hosp Epidemiol*. 2002;23:730-732.
344. Braun BI, Kritchevsky SB, Wong ES, et al. Preventing central venous catheter-associated primary bloodstream infections: characteristics of practices among hospitals participating in the Evaluation of Processes and Indicators in Infection Control (EPIC) study. *Infect Control Hosp Epidemiol*. 2003;24:926-935.
345. Crnich CJ, Maki DG. The promise of novel technology for the prevention of intravascular device-related bloodstream infection: I. Pathogenesis and short-term devices. *Clin Infect Dis*. 2002;34:1232-1242.
346. Johnson DW, MacGinley R, Kay TD, et al. A randomized controlled trial of topical exit site mupirocin application in patients with tunnelled, cuffed haemodialysis catheters. *Nephrol Dial Transplant*. 2002;17:1802-1807.
347. Miller MA, Dascal A, Portnoy J, et al. Development of mupirocin resistance among methicillin-resistant *Staphylococcus aureus* after widespread use of nasal mupirocin ointment. *Infect Control Hosp Epidemiol*. 1996;17:811-813.
348. Maki D, Band J. A comparative study of polyantibiotic and iodophor ointments in prevention of vascular catheter-related infection. *Am J Med*. 1981;70:739-744.
349. Rusmin S, DeLuca P. Effect of antibiotics and osmotic change on the release of endotoxin by bacteria retained on intravenous in-line filters. *Am J Hosp Pharm*. 1975;32:378-380.
350. Baier RJ, Bocchini JA Jr, Brown EG. Selective use of vancomycin to prevent coagulase-negative staphylococcal nosocomial bacteremia in high risk very low birth weight infants. *Pediatr Infect Dis J*. 1998;17:179-183.
351. Kacica MA, Horgan MJ, Ochoa L, et al. Prevention of gram-positive sepsis in neonates weighing less than 1500 grams. *J Pediatr*. 1994;125:253-258.
352. Raad II, Hachem RY, Abi-Said D, et al. A prospective crossover randomized trial of novobiocin and rifampin prophylaxis for the prevention of intravascular catheter infections in cancer patients treated with interleukin-2. *Cancer*. 1998;82:403-411.
353. Carratala J, Niubo J, Fernandez-Sevilla A, et al. Randomized, double-blind trial of an antibiotic-lock technique for prevention of gram-positive central venous catheter-related infection in neutropenic patients with cancer. *Antimicrobial Agents Chemother*. 1999;43:2200-2204.
354. Messing B, Peitra-Cohen S, Debure A, et al. Antibiotic-lock technique: a new approach to optimal therapy for catheter-related sepsis in home-parenteral nutrition patients. *J Parenter Enteral Nutr*. 1988;12:185-189.
355. James MT, Conley J, Tonelli M, et al. Meta-analysis: antibiotics for prophylaxis against hemodialysis catheter-related infections. *Ann Intern Med*. 2008;148:596-605.
356. Jaffer Y, Selby NM, Taal MW, et al. A meta-analysis of hemodialysis catheter locking solutions in the prevention of catheter-related infection. *Am J Kidney Dis*. 2008;51:233-241.
357. Labriola L, Crott R, Jadoul M. Preventing haemodialysis catheter-related bacteraemia with an antimicrobial lock solution: a meta-analysis of prospective randomized trials. *Nephrol Dial Transplant*. 2008;23:1666-1672.
358. van de Wetering MD, van Woensel JB. Prophylactic antibiotics for preventing early central venous catheter Gram positive infections in oncology patients. *Cochrane Database Syst Rev*. 2007:CD003295.
359. Yahav D, Rozen-Zvi B, Gafter-Gvili A, et al. Antimicrobial lock solutions for the prevention of infections associated with intravascular catheters in patients undergoing hemodialysis: systematic review and meta-analysis of randomized, controlled trials. *Clin Infect Dis*. 2008;47:83-93.
360. Henrickson KJ, Axtell RA, Hoover SM, et al. Prevention of central venous catheter-related infections and thrombotic events in immunocompromised children by the use of vancomycin/ciprofloxacin/heparin flush solution: a randomized, multicenter, double-blind trial. *J Clin Oncol*. 2000;18:1269-1278.
361. Schwartz C, Henrickson KJ, Roghmann K, et al. Prevention of bacteremia attributed to luminal colonization of tunneled central venous catheters with vancomycin-susceptible organisms. *J Clin Oncol*. 1990;8:1591-1597.
362. Barriga FJ, Varas M, Potin M, et al. Efficacy of a vancomycin solution to prevent bacteremia associated with an indwelling central venous catheter in neutropenic and non-neutropenic cancer patients. *Med Pediatr Oncol*. 1997;28:196-200.
363. Rackoff WR, Weiman M, Jakobowski D, et al. A randomized, controlled trial of the efficacy of a heparin and vancomycin solution in preventing central venous catheter infections in children. *J Pediatr*. 1995;127:147-151.
364. Safdar N, Maki DG. Use of vancomycin-containing lock or flush solutions for prevention of bloodstream infection associated with central venous access devices: a meta-analysis of prospective, randomized trials. *Clin Infect Dis*. 2006;43:474-484.
365. Betjes MG, van Agteren M. Prevention of dialysis catheter-related sepsis with a citrate-taurolidine-containing lock solution. *Nephrol Dial Transplant*. 2004;19:1546-1551.
366. Bradshaw JH, Puntis JW. Taurolidine and catheter-related bloodstream infection: a systematic review of the literature. *J Pediatr Gastroenterol Nutr*. 2008;47:179-186.
367. Simon A, Ammann RA, Wiszniewsky G, et al. Taurolidine-citrate lock solution (TauroLock) significantly reduces CVAD-associated grampositive infections in pediatric cancer patients. *BMC Infect Dis*. 2008;8:102.
368. Bleyer AJ, Mason L, Russell G, et al. A randomized, controlled trial of a new vascular catheter flush solution (minocycline-EDTA) in temporary hemodialysis access. *Infect Control Hosp Epidemiol*. 2005;26:520-524.
369. Chatzinikolaou I, Zipf TF, Hanna H, et al. Minocycline-ethylenediaminetetraacetate lock solution for the prevention of implantable port infections in children with cancer. *Clin Infect Dis*. 2003;36:116-119.
370. Crnich CJ, Halfmann JA, Crone WC, et al. The effects of prolonged ethanol exposure on the mechanical properties of polyurethane and silicone catheters used for intravascular access. *Infect Control Hosp Epidemiol*. 2005;26:708-714.

371. Sanders J, Pithie A, Ganly P, et al. A prospective double-blind randomized trial comparing intraluminal ethanol with heparinized saline for the prevention of catheter-associated bloodstream infection in immunosuppressed haematology patients. *J Antimicrob Chemother.* 2008;62:809-815.

372. Crnich CJ, Maki DG. Are antimicrobial-impregnated catheters effective? When does repetition reach the point of exhaustion? *Clin Infect Dis.* 2005;41:681-685.

373. Hockenhull JC, Dwan K, Boland A, et al. The clinical effectiveness and cost-effectiveness of central venous catheters treated with anti-infective agents in preventing bloodstream infections: a systematic review and economic evaluation. *Health Technol Assess.* 2008;12:1-154.

374. Ramritu P, Halton K, Collignon P, et al. A systematic review comparing the relative effectiveness of antimicrobial-coated catheters in intensive care units. *Am J Infect Control.* 2008; 36:104-117.

375. Rupp ME, Lisco SJ, Lipsett PA, et al. Effect of a second-generation venous catheter impregnated with chlorhexidine and silver sulfadiazine on central catheter-related infections: a randomized, controlled trial. *Ann Intern Med.* 2005;143:570-580.

376. Raad I, Darouiche R, Hachem R, et al. The broad-spectrum activity and efficacy of catheters coated with minocycline and rifampin. *J Infect Dis.* 1996;173:418-424.

377. Chatzinikolaou I, Finkel K, Hanna H, et al. Antibiotic-coated hemodialysis catheters for the prevention of vascular catheter-related infections: a prospective, randomized study. *Am J Med.* 2003;115:352-357.

378. Darouiche RO, Berger DH, Khardori N, et al. Comparison of antimicrobial impregnation with tunneling of long-term central venous catheters: a randomized controlled trial. *Ann Surg.* 2005;242:193-200.

379. Darouiche RO, Raad II, Heard SO, et al. A comparison of two antimicrobial-impregnated central venous catheters. *N Engl J Med.* 1999;340:1-8.

380. Hanna H, Benjamin R, Chatzinikolaou I, et al. Long-term silicone central venous catheters impregnated with minocycline and rifampin decrease rates of catheter-related bloodstream infection in cancer patients: a prospective randomized clinical trial. *J Clin Oncol.* 2004;22:3163-3171.

381. Raad I, Darouiche R, Dupuis J, et al. Central venous catheters coated with minocycline and rifampin for the prevention of catheter-related colonization and bloodstream infections: a randomized, double-blind trial: the Texas Medical Center Catheter Study Group. *Ann Intern Med.* 1997;127:267-274.

382. Yorganci K, Krepel C, Weigelt JA, et al. In vitro evaluation of the antibacterial activity of three different central venous catheters against gram-positive bacteria. *Eur J Clin Microbiol Infect Dis.* 2002;21:379-384.

383. Walder B, Pittet D, Tramer MR. Prevention of bloodstream infections with central venous catheters treated with anti-infective agents depends on catheter type and insertion time: evidence from a meta-analysis. *Infect Control Hosp Epidemiol.* 2002;23:748-756.

384. Falagas ME, Fragoulis K, Bliziotis IA, et al. Rifampicin-impregnated central venous catheters: a meta-analysis of randomized controlled trials. *J Antimicrob Chemother.* 2007;59:359-369.

385. Sampath LA, Tambe SM, Modak SM. In vitro and in vivo efficacy of catheters impregnated with antiseptics or antibiotics: evaluation of the risk of bacterial resistance to the antimicrobials in the catheters. *Infect Control Hosp Epidemiol.* 2001;22: 640-646.

386. Marciante KD, Veenstra DL, Lipsky BA, et al. Which antimicrobial impregnated central venous catheter should we use? Modeling the costs and outcomes of antimicrobial catheter use. *Am J Infect Control.* 2003;31:1-8.

387. McConnell SA, Gubbins PO, Anaissie EJ. Do antimicrobial-impregnated central venous catheters prevent catheter-related bloodstream infection? *Clin Infect Dis.* 2003;37:65-72.

388. Halton K, Graves N. Economic evaluation and catheter-related bloodstream infections. *Emerg Infect Dis.* 2007;13:815-823.

389. Appelgren P, Ransjo U, Bindslev L, et al. Surface heparinization of central venous catheters reduces microbial colonization in vitro and in vivo: results from a prospective, randomized trial. *Crit Care Med.* 1996;24:1482-1489.

390. Randolph AG, Cook DJ, Gonzales CA, et al. Benefit of heparin in central venous and pulmonary artery catheters: a meta-analysis of randomized controlled trials. *Chest.* 1998;113: 165-171.

391. Goey SH, Verweij J, Bolhuis RL, et al. Tunnelled central venous catheters yield a low incidence of septicaemia in interleukin-2-treated patients. *Cancer Immunol Immunother.* 1997;44: 301-304.

392. Kethireddy S, Safdar N. Urokinase lock or flush solution for prevention of bloodstream infections associated with central venous catheters for chemotherapy: a meta-analysis of prospective randomized trials. *J Vasc Access.* 2008;9:51-57.

393. Ragni MV, Journeycake JM, Brambilla DJ. Tissue plasminogen activator to prevent central venous access device infections: a systematic review of central venous access catheter thrombosis,

infection and thromboprophylaxis. *Haemophilia.* 2008;14: 30-38.

394. Shah PS, Shah N. Heparin-bonded catheters for prolonging the patency of central venous catheters in children. *Cochrane Database Syst Rev.* 2007:CD005983.

395. Sherertz RJ, Jarvis WR. Vascular catheters inserted in the trenches versus guideline documents: can the discrepancies be resolved? *Infect Control Hosp Epidemiol.* 2003;24:887-889.

396. Jackson M, Chiarello LA, Gaynes RP, et al. Nurse staffing and health care-associated infections: proceedings from a working group meeting. *Am J Infect Control.* 2002;30:199-206.

397. Maki D. Pathogenesis and strategies for prevention. Paper presented at the 33rd Interscience Conference on Antimicrobial Agents and Chemotherapy, New Orleans, Louisiana, 1993.

398. Maki D, McCormack K. Defatting catheter insertion sites in total parenteral nutrition is of no value as an infection control measure. *Am J Med.* 1987;83:833-840.

399. Krein SL, Hofer TP, Kowalski CP, et al. Use of central venous catheter-related bloodstream infection prevention practices by US hospitals. *Mayo Clin Proc.* 2007;82:672-678.

400. Richet H, Hubert B, Nitemberg G, et al. Prospective multicenter study of vascular-catheter-related complications and risk factors for positive central-catheter cultures in intensive care unit patients. *J Clin Microbiol.* 1990;28:2520-2525.

401. van Hoff J, Berg AT, Seashore JH. The effect of right atrial catheters on the infectious complications of chemotherapy in children. *J Clin Oncol.* 1990;8:1255.

402. Biffi R, Corrado F, de Braud F, et al. Long-term, totally implantable central venous access ports connected to a Groshong catheter for chemotherapy of solid tumours: experience from 178 cases using a single type of device. *Eur J Cancer.* 1997;33:1190-1194.

403. Schwarz RE, Groeger JS, Coit DG. Subcutaneously implanted central venous access devices in cancer patients: a prospective analysis. *Cancer.* 1997;79:1635-1640.

404. Sheehan G, Leicht K, O'Brien M, et al. Chlorhexidine versus povidone-iodine as cutaneous antisepsis for prevention of vascular catheter infections. Paper presented at the 33rd Interscience Conference on Antimicrobial Agents and Chemotherapy, New Orleans, Louisiana, 1993.

405. Luskin RL, Weinstein RA, Nathan C, et al. Extended use of disposable pressure transducers: a bacteriologic evaluation. *JAMA.* 1986;255:916-920.

303

Nosocomial Pneumonia

DONALD E. CRAVEN | ALEXANDRA CHRONEOU

Hospital-acquired pneumonia (HAP) is defined as an infection that occurs in a patient who has been hospitalized more than 48 hours, and ventilator-associated pneumonia (VAP) is an infection that occurs in an intensive care unit (ICU) patient more than 48 hours after endotracheal intubation and mechanical ventilation.[1,2] Despite recent advances in antimicrobial therapy, better supportive care, and a wide range of prevention measures, HAP and VAP remain significant causes of patient morbidity and mortality as well as health care costs.[1-3]

This chapter highlights the changing epidemiology, pathogenesis, diagnosis, principles for antibiotic treatment, and current evidence-based prevention strategies for HAP and VAP. Emphasis is placed on bacterial pathogens in immunocompetent adults. Readers are referred to recent reviews, guidelines, and chapters for more detail due to our text and reference limitations.[2]

Epidemiology

Rates of HAP have varied between 5 and 10 episodes per 1000 hospital admissions and tend to be higher in university versus nonteaching hospitals. By comparison, rates of VAP have a pooled mean of 7.3/1000 ventilator days for medical ICU patients versus 13.2/1000 ventilator days for surgical ICU patients, but these rates have most likely decreased due to better prevention efforts.[1-3] Crude rates of VAP are dynamic and may vary by patient population, severity of disease, and method of diagnosis.[1-3] Rates of VAP are related to the duration of mechanical ventilation and have been estimated to be 3% per day during the first 5 days and 2% per day thereafter.[4]

Crude mortality rates for HAP estimates are approximately 10% and are higher for VAP with a range of 20% to 60% depending on the patient, severity of disease, specific pathogen isolated, and management.[1-3,5] Unfortunately, data are limited on short- and long-term morbidity, but clinical observations suggest that HAP and VAP may significantly alter quality of life for survivors.

Prevention strategies for HAP and VAP reduce patient mortality, morbidity, and health care costs.[1,2,6,7] An average episode of VAP has been estimated to increase hospitalization by 12 days, ventilator days by 6 days, ICU stay by 6 days, and hospital costs from $12,000 to $40,000 per episode.[1-3]

Etiology

Etiologic agents causing HAP and VAP include a wide spectrum of bacteria shown in Table 303-1. Over the past 20 years, there has been a dramatic increase in health care–associated respiratory infections due to antibiotic-resistant or multidrug resistant (MDR) pathogens.[1] Bacteria causing HAP and VAP may originate from the patient's endogenous flora, other patients, hospital staff, contaminated devices, or the inanimate environment.[8,9] The spectrum of bacterial pathogens in the ICU are dynamic and may vary with time, by hospital, type of ICU, and specific patient population, emphasizing the importance of up-to-date surveillance data.[1-3,10-12] Early-onset HAP (occurring during the first 5 days of the hospital stay) is more likely to be caused by antibiotic-sensitive pathogens, such as Streptococcus pneumoniae, Moraxella catarrhalis, Haemophilus influenzae, anaerobic bacteria, or Legionella pneumophila.[1,3]

Predisposing factors for patient colonization and infection with MDR pathogens that require a different spectrum of initial, empirical antibiotic therapy include recent hospitalization, residence in a long-term health care facility, the presence of significant chronic disease, debility, and recent antibiotic therapy.[13,14] MDR pathogens of concern include gram-negative bacilli (extended-spectrum β-lactamase–producing Klebsiella pneumoniae, Acinetobacter baumannii, Pseudomonas aeruginosa) or methicillin-resistant Staphylococcus aureus (MRSA).[1] P. aeruginosa, the most common MDR gram-negative pathogen causing VAP, and some isolates that are pan-resistant (sensitive only to polymyxin) or having exotoxin III have been associated with increased patient mortality.[15] Also, outbreaks of VAP due to other MDR gram-negative bacilli, especially A. baumannii, have been reported over the past decade and have been difficult to control and eradicate.[1,16,17]

Gram-negative bacilli have been implicated in more than 60% of reported episodes of HAP and VAP, but pneumonia due to S. aureus now accounts for 20% to 40% of episodes, most of which are now MRSA.[1-3] HAP and VAP due to hospital-acquired MRSA have been increasing worldwide for the past 10 years, and there is now evidence that community-acquired MRSA is also a cause of HAP and VAP.[16] In contrast to the hospital-MRSA strains, community-acquired MRSA isolates are genetically distinct and almost uniformly carry the Panton-Valentine leukocidin and factors that seem to increase damage to lung tissue.[16] In addition, increasing or creeping resistance to vancomycin and identification of glycopeptide or vancomycin intermediate–resistant S. aureus isolates seem to be emerging worldwide.[18] Of greater concern is the lack of detection of these isolates with the techniques currently used in many microbiology laboratories.

Pathogenesis

The outcome of HAP and VAP depends on the number and types of colonizing pathogen(s) that enter the lower respiratory tract and the host's mechanical, cellular, and humoral defenses (Fig. 303-1).[1,2,7] For HAP, microaspiration is the primary route of bacterial entry into the lower respiratory tract; risk factors include sedation, intubation for operative procedures, vomiting, and impaired swallowing.[1,2] For VAP, leakage of bacteria and oral secretions around the endotracheal cuff, inhalation of contaminated aerosols, or reflux of contaminated ventilator tubing condensate are the primary routes of bacterial entry into the lower respiratory tract (Fig. 303-2).[7] Local trauma and inflammation from the endotracheal tube increase tracheal colonization and reduce clearance of organisms from the lower respiratory tract. Not widely appreciated is the impact of biofilm-encased bacteria in the endotracheal tube lumen. These bacteria increase over time and may be transported into the distal lung alveoli after routine suctioning or bronchoscopy. These biofilm-encased bacteria are protected against killing by antibiotics and host mechanical, cellular, and humoral defenses.[19,20] The outcome of the pathogen-host battle determines whether the outcome will be tracheal colonization, tracheobronchitis, or HAP/VAP.

In intubated patients, lower respiratory tract colonization may progress to ventilator-associated tracheobronchitis (VAT), which may be a precursor to VAP or, in selected patients, difficult to distinguish from VAP.[21,22] Nseir and colleagues[21] define VAT as the presence of clinical signs of lower respiratory tract infection (fever, leukocytosis, and purulent sputum), with a quantitative endotracheal sputum sample having a respiratory tract pathogen at a concentration of more than 10^6 organisms per milliliter and the absence of a new or progressive infiltrate on chest x-ray. Others may prefer different quantitative

TABLE 303-1	Summary of Current Guidelines for Initial Appropriate Therapy for Hospital-Acquired Pneumonia and Ventilator-Associated Pneumonia, Based on the Identification of Risk Factors for Colonization and Infection with Multidrug-Resistant Bacterial Pathogens Requiring Broader Spectrum, Empirical Antibiotic Therapy

Non-MDR Pathogens	Antibiotic Therapy (Doses Based on Normal Renal Function)	Clinical Comments (Selected References)
Streptococcus pneumoniae	Levofloxacin 750 mg/day IV/PO, moxifloxacin 400 mg/day IV/PO, or gemifloxacin 320 mg/day PO *or*	Beginning in 2008, *S. pneumoniae* penicillin susceptibility is defined as ≤2 μg/mg. The older definition was ≤0.06 μg/mL. • Nearly all pneumococci in the U.S. are sensitive to levoquin and ceftriaxone. • Data suggest that pneumococcal bacteremia treated with two drugs had better outcomes than those treated with a single antibiotic.
Haemophilus influenzae	Ceftriaxone 1 g/day IV *or*	
Anaerobes	Ampicillin-sulbactam 3 g q6h IV ±	Anaerobic coverage provided by moxifloxacin, ampicillin-sulbactam
Non-ESBL+GNR	Azithromycin 500 mg/day IV, then 250 mg/day IV	
Legionella pneumophila		For suspected *L. pneumophila*, use a fluoroquinolone or azithromycin

MDR Pathogens	Antibiotic Therapy (Doses Based on Normal Renal Function)	Clinical Comments (Selected References)
Methicillin-resistant *Staphylococcus aureus* (MRSA)	Vancomycin 15 mg/kg q12h. (Target vancomycin blood trough level = 15-20 μg/mL) *or* Linezolid 600 mg q12h IV/PO	• Hospital-acquired MRSA and community-acquired MRSA clones (US 300/400) are emerging in hospitals.[16] • High doses of vancomycin are recommended due to treatment failures possibly related to inadequate dosing.[1,58,59] • High doses of vancomycin may cause greater renal toxicity in the severely ill, those with renal failure, or those on therapy with other nephrotoxic medications.[60] • Linezolid achieves high concentrations in lung fluid, inhibits toxin production, and may be useful in patients with renal failure or lack of response to vancomycin.[61,62] • Increasing resistance to vancomycin (MICs 2 μg/mL) or vancomycin intermediate-resistant *S. aureus* (MIC 4-8 μg/mL) are associated with poorer outcomes and may be missed with current microbiologic methods.[18,59]
Pseudomonas aeruginosa	Cephalosporins 3rd/4th generation: (e.g., cefepime 2 g q8-12h IV *or* ceftazidime 2 g q8h IV) *or* carbapenem (e.g., imipenem 1 g q8h, *or* meropenem 1 g q8h) *or* e.g., piperacillin-tazobactam 4.5 g q6h IV or 3.375 g 6 hr over 4-hr infusion *plus* Aminoglycoside (e.g., amikacin 15 mg/kg/day IV, gentamicin 5-7 mg/kg/day IV, *or* tobramycin 5-7 mg/kg/day IV) *or* Antipseudomonal fluoroquinolone (e.g., ciprofloxacin 400 mg q8h IV) *or* levofloxacin 750 mg qd IV)	• *P. aeruginosa* has the capacity to develop resistance to all antibiotics except polymyxin.[1,18] • Automated in vitro susceptibility testing for β-lactam antibiotic may have a high rate of false susceptibility and resistance compared with disk diffusion and E tests.[31] • Extended infusion of piperacillin-tazobactam improves time above the MIC and may reduce mortality.[33] • The use of combination therapy (β-lactam + an aminoglycoside) vs. monotherapy does not reduce resistance or improve patient outcomes.[63,64] If *P. aeruginosa* is suspected, combination therapy should be used until antibiotic sensitivity is available.[1] • Caution is advised for empirical use of fluoroquinolones due to excessive prescribing, greater resistance, and risk of MRSA.[65]
Acinetobacter species	Carbapenem (imipenem, meropenem) See doses above *plus* Aminoglycoside (amikacin, gentamicin, or tobramycin), see doses above *or* Polymyxin B or Colistin (see Ch. 32 for dose)	• Treatment options for *Acinetobacter* ventilator-associated pneumonia are limited due to widespread antibiotic resistance.[66] • There are reports of discordance between in vitro susceptibility testing and clinical responses to carbapenems and other antibiotics.[66] • Initial antibiotic therapy for highly resistant isolates may be limited to polymyxin E (Colistin)[67,68] plus aminoglycosides or rifampin (10 mg/kg q12h). • Aerosolized polymyxin has been advocated as adjunctive therapy for treating ventilator-associated pneumonia due to MDR gram-negative bacilli.[17,68]
ESBL+ *Klebsiella pneumoniae* or *Escherichia coli* or *Enterobacter* species	Carbapenem (imipenem, meropenem), see doses above ± Aminoglycoside (amikacin, gentamicin, or tobramycin), see doses above	• ESBL-positive strains are rapidly evolving and carbapenems are the surest agents for therapy (for ESBL-positive organisms), although carbapenem resistance is beginning to increase.[17,69] • Concerns have been raised about the accuracy of in vitro antibiotic sensitivity testing for detecting ESBL-positive isolates.[8,64,69] • The hallmark of ESBL-positive *K. pneumoniae* and *E. coli* is a variable response to cephalosporins, and thus 3rd- and 4th-generation agents should be avoided as monotherapy.[17,69] • A most reliable empirical choice is a carbapenem ± an aminoglycoside.[17,69] • 3rd- and 4th-generation cephalosporins should not be used for treatment of *Enterobacter* spp. ventilator-associated pneumonia because of the high frequency of resistance of this pathogen to this therapy.[17,70]

ESBL, extended-spectrum β-lactamase; GNR, gram-negative rods; MDR, multidrug resistant; MIC, minimal inhibitory concentration.

Adapted in part from Niederman MS, Craven DE, Bonten MJ. American Thoracic Society and Infectious Diseases Society of America (ATS/IDSA): Guideline for the Management of Adults with Hospital-acquired, Ventilator-associated, and Healthcare-associated Pneumonia. *Ann J Respir Crit Care Med.* 2005;171:388-416, and Craven DE, Chroneou A, Zias N, et al. Ventilator-associated tracheobronchitis (VAT): the impact of targeted antibiotic therapy on patient outcomes. *Chest.* 2009;135:521-528.

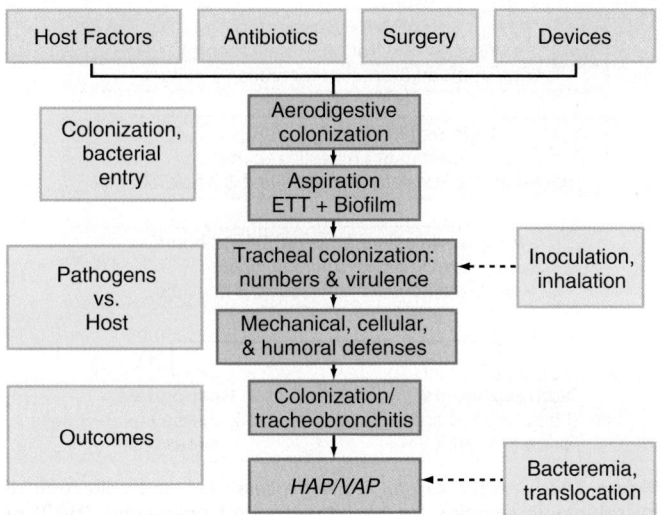

Figure 303-1 **Pathogenesis of hospital-acquired pneumonia (HAP) and ventilator-associated pneumonia (VAP).** The "battlefield" between the pathogens entering the lower respiratory tract and the host defenses determines possible outcomes: colonization, tracheobronchitis or HAP/VAP. ETT, endotracheal tube.

thresholds or use of a semiquantitative endotracheal aspirate having moderate to heavy growth of a respiratory tract pathogen.

Diagnosis

The best diagnostic sensitivity (identifying patients with pneumonia) and specificity (accuracy of the diagnosis) combine clinical signs and symptoms with microbiologic sputum smear (Gram stain) and bacterial culture.[2,3] Clinical signs and symptoms suggesting HAP and VAP

include at least two of three clinical features (temperature >38°C or hypothermia), leukocytosis, leukopenia, increased immature neutrophils ("bandemia") or purulent respiratory secretions, and the presence of a new or progressive radiographic infiltrate. Blood cultures may be helpful, but positive cultures are uncommon, except in patients with pneumococcal and *S. aureus* pneumonia. The clinical pulmonary infection score, used in some ICUs, gives points for clinical, radiographic, physiologic, and microbiologic data for a single numerical result. The ratio of alveolar partial pressure of oxygen (Pao_2) to the fractional inhaled oxygen partial pressure of oxygen (Fio_2) is a key physiologic parameter. A clinical pulmonary infection score of more than 6 correlates well with the presence of clinical pneumonia.[1-3]

The major route of bacteria into and out of the lung is via the trachea. The presence of bacteria and polymorphonuclear cells on sputum Gram stain and a sputum culture having significant growth of a bacterial pathogen by semiquantitative or quantitative bacteriologic techniques help to confirm the clinical suspicion of pneumonia or tracheobronchitis.[1,22] In patients with HAP, it may be more difficult to obtain and interpret sputum samples than in VAP patients. The diagnosis of VAP has greater specificity than HAP, but can be limited by increased bacterial colonization in the endotracheal aspirates or the presence of VAT that may mimic VAP, especially in patients with previous or increasing pulmonary infiltrates due to congestive heart failure, adult respiratory distress syndrome, pulmonary emboli, or atelectasis.

Examination of endotracheal aspirates by Gram stain allows rapid insight into the number and types of bacteria, as well as the number of polymorphonuclear leukocytes and macrophages that are suggestive of inflammation and infection. The presence of bacteria on Gram stain (smear) correlates with cultures of approximately 10^5 bacteria per milliliter of sputum and also provides a clue to the offending bacteria (i.e., gram-positive cocci in clusters suggest *S. aureus* and gram-negative bacilli may suggest *Klebsiella* spp., *Escherichia coli*, or *P. aeruginosa*). Endotracheal aspirate cultures, using the semiquantitative endotracheal aspirates, are reported as moderate or heavy growth of a pathogen, which helps to confirm a diagnosis of VAP or VAT. Endotracheal

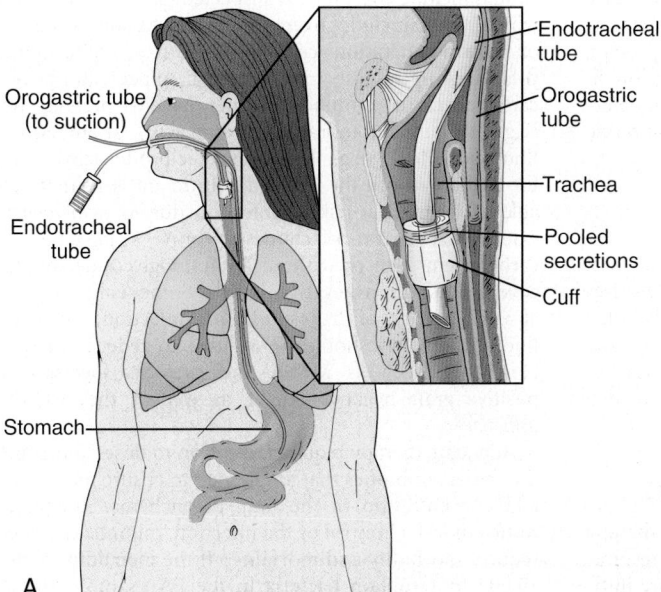

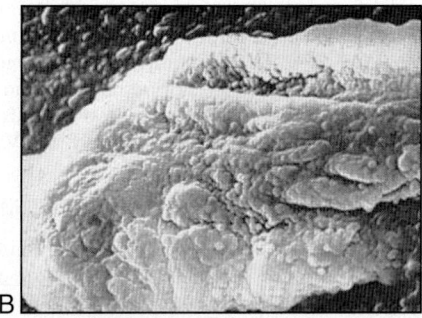

Figure 303-2 **A,** Diagram of a patient on mechanical ventilation with an orogastric tube for gastric suction. Oropharyngeal secretions containing millions of bacteria per milliliter have pooled above the cuff and are not removed by suctioning through the tube. When the patient is treated with antimicrobial agents, bacteria in these secretions may become increasingly resistant to the antibiotics being administered to the patient. When the cuff is deflated or moved, these secretions have greater access to the tracheobronchial tree and the alveoli. **B,** Scanning micrograph of a biofilm that forms inside the endotracheal tube after a few days. Organisms from this biofilm are aspirated into the alveoli and become an increasing part of the bacteria grown from cultures of endotracheal aspirates. These biofilm organisms are resistant to antimicrobial agents in secretions that reach them and are not accessible to the host's immune system.

aspirate growth reported as rare or few probably represents tracheal colonization. Some microbiology laboratories report quantitative endotracheal aspirates in which a pathogen growth of more than 10^{5-6} colony-forming units per milliliter (CFU/mL) is consistent with a diagnosis of VAP.

Quantitative distal airway samples obtained by bronchoscopic bronchoalveolar lavage (BAL) ($>10^4$ CFU/mL) or protective specimen brush ($>10^3$ CFU/mL), or nonbronchoscopic BAL or protective specimen brush have good diagnostic sensitivity and probably a higher specificity than endotracheal aspirate samples, but these techniques are not widely available, are more expensive, and require expertise.[1-3,23] Clearly, samples should be collected before antibiotics are initiated or changed and, ideally, should not significantly delay the initiation of empirical antibiotic therapy.[1,3,23]

The advantages of using semiquantitative or quantitative endotracheal aspirates versus distal lung parenchyma sampling by BAL/protective specimen brush for the diagnosis of VAP remain controversial. Most hospitals in the United States use semiquantitative endotracheal aspirates for the diagnosis of VAP. In one large, prospective, randomized trial of VAP diagnosis, patients having bronchoscopic BAL or protective specimen brush diagnosis had a significantly lower 14-day mortality rate (16.2% vs. 25.8%; 95% confidence interval [CI]: −17.4 to −1.8; P = .02), less mean sepsis-related organ failure at day 3 (6.1 vs. 7.0; P = .03) and day 7 (4.9 vs. 5.8; P = .04), and a decreased mean number of antibiotic-free days (5.0 vs. 2.2; P < .001) than patients having a clinical diagnosis and sputum endotracheal aspirates.[23] In contrast, in a recent randomized study by a Canadian Critical Care Trials group, patients were randomly assigned to undergo bronchoscopic BAL versus semiquantitative endotracheal aspirates and also to receive empirical combination antibiotic therapy or monotherapy. The BAL group and the endotracheal aspiration group also had similar rates of targeted therapy (74.2% and 74.6%, respectively; P = .90), similar number of days alive without antibiotics (10.4 vs. 10.6, P = not significant), and maximum organ dysfunction scores (mean ± standard deviation, 8.3 vs. 8.6; P = not significant). The two groups did not differ significantly in the length of hospital or ICU stay.[24]

Biologic markers, such as procalcitonin and soluble triggering receptor expressed on myeloid cells, may be helpful adjuncts for the diagnosis and management of VAP.[25,26] Although they both have greater diagnostic accuracy than most commonly used clinical parameters and other biomarkers of infection, such as C-reactive protein, they can be increased in noninfectious conditions or remain low in patients with true infection.[27] Furthermore, these assays cannot determine the causative organisms and associated patterns of antibiotic susceptibility.

Principles of Antibiotic Therapy

The basic principles of antibiotic management of HAP and VAP emphasized in the American Thoracic Society and Infectious Diseases Society of America Guideline include (1) selection of an initial antibiotic regimen (Fig. 303-3), (2) de-escalation of initial antibiotic therapy when possible, (3) stopping antibiotics in responders, and (4) further evaluation of nonresponders. Other guidelines have also provided similar recommendations for management of HAP and VAP.[1,28,29]

INITIAL EMPIRICAL ANTIBIOTIC THERAPY REGIMENS

Data suggest that delays in initiating appropriate antibiotic therapy increase patient morbidity and mortality.[1] Blood cultures and respiratory sputum samples should be collected before antibiotics are initiated to ensure proper therapy and to provide better de-escalation of antibiotics 36 to 48 hours later.[1]

The initial empirical antibiotic regimen should be appropriate (pathogen is sensitive to the antibiotic in vitro), based on the presence or absence of risk factors for MDR bacterial pathogens that have been emerging over the past two decades, and be administered without delay (see Table 303-1). Risk factors for MDR pathogens include previ-

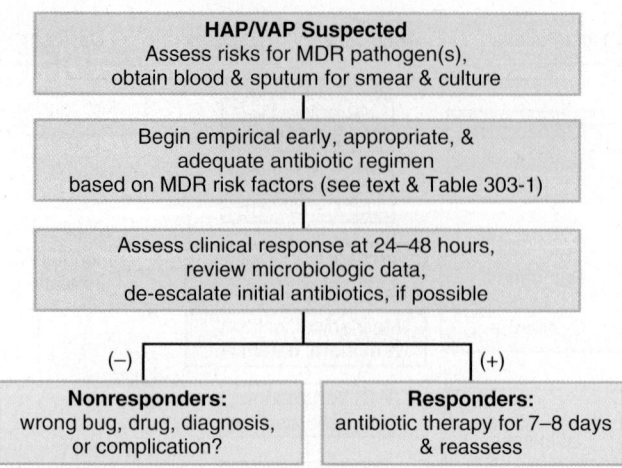

Figure 303-3 After careful clinical assessment and collection of microbiologic samples for hospital-acquired pneumonia (HAP) or ventilator-associated pneumonia (VAP), patients should be started on early, appropriate, and adequate antibiotic therapy to cover suspected pathogens (see text and Table 303-1). Based on the clinical response and microbiologic data 24 to 48 hours later, the initial, empirical antibiotic regimen should be de-escalated, if possible. In responders, antibiotics should be discontinued after 7 total days of therapy and responders should be reevaluated. MDR, multidrug resistant.

ous antibiotic therapy or recent hospitalization, late-onset HAP and VAP, residents of long-term health care facilities, immunocompromised patients, and exposure to resident ICU MDR pathogens. Many experts also believe that severity of the patient's disease (i.e., presence of shock or hypotension) should also be considered to ensure coverage for all suspected pathogens. If the pathogen has been identified, targeted antibiotic therapy can be used.

Initial empirical therapy for patients with MDR risk factors for VAP should include coverage for suspected pathogens endemic in the ICU, which should include coverage for gram-negative bacilli; either a third- or fourth-generation cephalosporin (e.g., ceftazidime, cefepime), β-lactam/β-lactamase inhibitor (e.g., piperacillin-tazobactam) or a carbepenem (e.g., imipenem, meropenem) plus an aminoglycoside (e.g., gentamicin, tobramycin, amikacin) or an anti-pseudomonal fluoroquinolone (e.g., levofloxacin, ciprofloxacin) is recommended for 48 hours until the sputum culture and sensitivity data are available.[1] If there is a risk of infection due to *Acinetobacter* species or extended-spectrum β-lactamase–positive *K. pneumoniae* or *E. coli*, a carbepenem with or without an aminoglycoside should be used for coverage of gram-negative bacilli. Some data suggest that in the absence of risk of *L. pneumophila* infection, initial coverage with fluoroquinolones should be avoided to reduce emergence of MDR pathogens, such as MRSA and extended-spectrum β-lactamase–positive gram-negative bacilli, as well as the risk of *Clostridium difficile*.[30]

Adequate therapy requires attention to doses and administration of the initial antibiotics that are needed to ensure maximum penetration and concentration in the lung parenchyma. Adequate dosing also results in faster control of the infection, minimizes tissue damage, and reduces morbidity and mortality.[1] If the inoculum in the lung is from 10,000 to 1 million bacteria in the BAL sample, the total bacterial burden in the lung would be several logs higher, which underscores the importance of administering early, appropriate, and adequate antibiotic therapy. In contrast to other tissues, the lung is similar to a sponge that has many air pockets and may become filled with pus and bacteria that could be perceived as microabscesses. In addition, penetration of antibiotics may also be impaired in patients who experience biofilm-encased bacteria aspirated from the endotracheal tube.

Ideally, concentrations of antibiotics should remain above the minimal inhibitory concentration (MIC) of the pathogen as long as possible to have maximal effect in reducing the bacterial burden in the lung.[1] The MIC of the pathogen is also important. It is not widely appreciated that the MICs performed in vitro in the microbiology laboratory on agar are crude surrogates and may not reflect in vivo MICs and also do not take into consideration concentrations of lung bacteria. For some pathogens, there have also been concerns about the accuracy of the antibiotic sensitivity pattern by different automated methods.[31] There can also be other variables in vivo, such as the impact of necrotic tissue, abscess formation, inflammation, blood supply, and the presence of a foreign body (endotracheal tube with biofilm-encased bacteria), that can alter the efficiency of bacterial killing.

For all these concerns, the administration of and initial dose of the antibiotic needed to achieve maximal time above the MIC of the specific pathogen(s) are important targets, but may vary from patient to patient.[32] Lodise and colleagues,[33] in a nonrandomized trial, reported that mortality rates in patients who were treated with 3.375 g of piperacillin-tazobactam given as a 4-hour infusion every 8 hours were significantly lower (12.2% vs. 31.6%, respectively; $P = .04$) than rates in patients given the same dose as a 30-minute infusion every 4 to 6 hours. Also, the median duration of hospital stay after collection of samples for culture was significantly shorter for patients who received extended-infusion therapy than for patients who received intermittent-infusion therapy (21 days vs. 38 days; $P = .02$). Similar concepts of dosing may apply to other antibiotics, such as the carbapenems and cefepime.[32]

Narrowing the Spectrum and Limiting the Duration of Therapy

Although initial antibiotic coverage should be liberal and sufficiently broad to cover all suspected pathogens, narrowing the spectrum or streamlining antibiotic therapy at 24 or 48 hours should be based on the patient's clinical response (fever, oxygenation, leukocyte count, appearance, and vital signs) and microbiologic data (Gram stain, culture, and antibiotic sensitivity data).[1]

Narrowing the spectrum improves patient outcomes by minimizing the complications of broad-spectrum antibiotic use, such as *C. difficile*, selection of MDR pathogens, and superinfection.[1,34,35] Evidence-based data indicate that the use of combination therapy for HAP and VAP due to *P. aeruginosa*, does not improve outcomes of infections and may increase the risk of adverse effects.[1] In patients without evidence of VAP, further evaluation may be needed to search for other sources of infection or potential causes of fever or leukocytosis.

Evidence-based data support limiting the total duration of antibiotic therapy to 7 days in responders who do not have other complications, such as empyema or bacteremia with MRSA that may seed other tissues.[1,36] In a large trial, patients with VAP randomized to 7 days of antibiotic therapy were compared with patients treated for 15 days; there was no difference in mortality or recurrent infections, but patients on the shorter therapy course had significantly more mean antibiotic-free days (13.1 vs. 8.7 days, $P < .001$). There was a trend toward higher rates of recurrence in patients with VAP due to *P. aeruginosa* in the 7-day treatment group, but no significant differences were noted in mortality or other important clinical response parameters.[36] The American Thoracic Society and Infectious Diseases Society of America Guideline recommended 7 days of therapy for uncomplicated HAP or VAP with close follow-up for any signs of relapse in patients with HAP or VAP due to *P. aeruginosa*.[1]

Serum markers such as procalcitonin may also be helpful to guide antibiotic treatment.[37] The use of procalcitonin levels and changes in oxygenation may provide important clues for patients who are more likely to relapse or need a longer duration of antibiotic therapy.[27] Luyt and colleagues[38] conducted a prospective, observational study and found that serum procalcitonin levels decreased during the clinical course of VAP but were significantly higher from day 1 to day 7 in patients with unfavorable outcomes.[9] A serum procalcitonin threshold of more than 0.5 ng/mL on day 7 was the strongest independent marker of unfavorable outcome with an odds ratio of 64.2. Therefore, in the future, procalcitonin kinetics could serve as a novel marker of prognosis for patients with VAP.

EVALUATION OF CLINICAL NONRESPONDERS

In most patients, clinical improvement takes 24 to 48 hours.[1] Therefore, the selected antimicrobial regimen should not be changed during this time unless there is evidence of progressive deterioration. Possible causes for clinical deterioration or failure to improve include wrong diagnosis (pulmonary embolism with infarction, atelectasis, pulmonary hemorrhage, neoplastic or connective tissue disease, acute respiratory distress syndrome with diffuse alveolar damage, other source of infection); wrong therapy (drug-resistant pathogen, inadequate dosing, wrong antimicrobial agent); wrong pathogen (tuberculosis; fungal, parasitic, viral infection; or *Legionella* infection), complication (empyema or lung abscess, *C. difficile* infection, drug fever); or a bacterial superinfection.[1]

▣ Prevention

BASIC TARGETS

Tremendous progress has been made in reducing health care–associated infections in the past 5 years.[1,3,6,39,40] Prevention in the ICU has become a high priority. It is now a "team sport" that requires leadership, organization, goals, clearly defined roles, checklists, quality improvement targets, and data feedback at multidisciplinary staff meetings.[6,41] An overview of selected prevention strategies taken from detailed evidence-based national guidelines and review articles is summarized in Table 303-2.[1,2,41,42]

Effective prophylaxis of VAP should begin with a team armed with evidence-based goals, targeted interventions, adequate nurse staffing ratios, and education of all ICU staff. In one study, use of a self-study module, with in-service teaching programs, fact sheets, and posters resulted in a 58% reduction in VAP and cost savings of $425,000 to more than $4,000,000.[43] Proper isolation and effective infection control practices with adequate environmental cleaning are other cornerstones for VAP prevention.[1,2,6,41,42] Unfortunately, staff compliance with proven infection control measures, such as hand hygiene, remains inconsistent and needs greater attention in many hospitals. Antibiotic stewardship programs play an important role in reducing the risk of all health care–associated infections and reduce the risk of colonization with MDR pathogens and complications such as *C. difficile* infections.[1,2,6]

The use of the Institute for Healthcare Improvement "bundles" has been credited with increased awareness, goals, monitoring methods, and feedback that have helped reduce VAP and other health care–associated infection rates nationwide. The Institute for Healthcare Improvement "bundle" recommendations for VAP include maintaining patients in a semiupright position (avoiding supine patient positioning) and sedation vacations that facilitate earlier extubation.[2,6,41,44] Because VAP rates may need to be reported in many states and hospital reimbursements may be tied to VAP, additional prevention strategies that target endotracheal tube and bacterial colonization are discussed here and presented in Table 303-2.

TARGETING THE ENDOTRACHEAL TUBE AND BIOFILM ISSUES

The endotracheal tube is a primary target for prevention strategies because it facilitates bacterial entry into the lower respiratory tract and limits effective removal of secretions from the lower respiratory tract by cough.[1-3] In addition, the endotracheal tube may have biofilm-encased bacteria that are sheltered from killing by antibiotics and host cellular defenses. These bacteria may be embolized to the distal lung during suctioning.[1,2,19]

TABLE 303-2	Summary of Prevention Strategies for Hospital-Acquired Pneumonia and Ventilator-Associated Pneumonia
Basics for Prevention	**Comments (Reference)**
Model: multidisciplinary team, with a "champion" to lead, setting goals; use of "bundles," checklists, monitoring and data feedback	Use of evidence-based data, goals, checklists, and feedback of data suggested Benchmarks should be discussed and reevaluated regularly.[2,6,41,42]
Staff education and proper ICU staffing for nurses and respiratory therapists	Staff education programs for physicians, nurses, and respiratory therapists to improve awareness; provide current data[43] Proper staffing and patient nurse ratios critical for patient safety Adherence to guidelines, protocols, and infection control standards[71]
Infection control	Data support effective hand hygiene to reduce spread of multidrug resistant pathogens[1,2] Environmental cleaning needed Surveillance of MDR pathogens, outbreaks, data feedback changes Screening for MRSA suggested and debated
Antibiotic control	Antibiotic stewardship reduces inappropriate antibiotic use, costs, and risk of infection with MDR pathogens Designated pharmacist, infectious disease consultant, or computer program to assess antibiotic use and dosing are beneficial[1,2]
Prevention of aspiration for HAP	Check speech and swallow studies to prevent recurrent aspiration[2] Check sedation, head of the bed after extubation, avoid reintubation, check diet
Vaccination	Before discharge, assess need for vaccinations such as influenza and pneumococcal vaccines and acellular pertussis vaccine boosts, if indicated
Smoking cessation	Smoking cessation programs strongly recommended[1,2]
Nutritional counseling and physical therapy	Counsel for malnutrition and obesity and provide early physical therapy[2]
Control of hyperglycemia with insulin therapy	Use of intensive insulin therapy to lower blood sugar to levels of 80-110 mg/dL was effective in reducing mortality, infections, and length of mechanical ventilation in surgical ICU patients[72] Results were not as good with medical ICU patients, and there have been concerns about the risk of hypoglycemia with these blood sugar target values[41]
VAP Prevention Strategies	
Use of ICU "bundles"	Use of Institute for Healthcare Improvement and other team bundles to reduce risk of VAP[40,71] (semiupright patient positioning, stress bleeding prophylaxis, deep venous thrombosis prophylaxis, sedation vacation)
Semiupright position (avoiding supine positioning)	Maintain patient semiupright (>30 degrees, if possible)[1,2] Do not keep patient supine, especially when receiving enteral nutrition[1,2,41]
Oral care	Oral care is widely used to prevent VAP[2] but does not reach the subglottic area Effective in comparative, nonrandomized trials[73]
Enteral feedings	Enteral feeding preferred to parenteral nutrition Protocols help standardize implementation and monitoring[1,2]
Selective digestive decontamination (SDD)	Combinations of antibiotics given orally (through the nasogastric tube) ± systemically in randomized, controlled trials demonstrate reduced rates of lower respiratory tract infections compared with controls; decreased mortality noted in SDD patients receiving systemic antibiotics[54] SDD should be used selectively in the US due to widespread presence of MDR pathogens; more widely used in Europe[1,2]
Endotracheal Tube Targets	
Sedation vacation with awakening and breathing trials	Implement standard protocols to limit sedation, assess use of continuous sedation, and enhance awakening to reduce duration of intubation[1-3,19] Use of spontaneous awakening and breathing trials that increase earlier extubation, reduce length of stay and mortality[44]
Noninvasive positive-pressure ventilation (NIPPV)	NIPPV to prevent intubation is supported by several clinical trials to reduce pneumonia and improve patient outcomes[45] NIPPV especially important for patients with chronic obstructive pulmonary disease and congestive heart failure[1,2,45]
Continuous aspiration of subglottic secretions (CASS)	CASS significantly decreased VAP in several randomized clinical trials[50,74] Requires more staff time and cost
Silver-coated endotracheal tube (s-ETT)	In a randomized VAP trial, colloidal s-ETT reduced microbiologically confirmed VAP by 36% overall ($P < .02$) and 48% ($P < .005$) in first 10 days No difference was noted in secondary outcomes: mortality, length of hospital stay, and antibiotic use[51]
Early tracheostomy	Three randomized trials suggest possible benefit from early tracheostomy; some methodologic concerns, but may be helpful in critically ill patients who will probably need long-term intubation and later tracheostomy[75]

HAP, hospital-acquired pneumonia; ICU, intensive care unit; MDR, multidrug resistant; MRSA, methicillin-resistant *Staphylococcus aureus*; VAP, ventilator-acquired pneumonia.
Taken in part from guidelines and reviews.[1,2,6,41,56]

Noninvasive Positive-Pressure Ventilation

Noninvasive positive-pressure ventilation provides ventilatory support without the need for intubation and is an effective alternative for patients with acute exacerbations of chronic obstructive pulmonary disease or acute hypoxemic respiratory failure. Noninvasive positive-pressure ventilation is associated with decreased rates of pneumonia, antibiotic use, and patient mortality.[1,2,45] A recent Cochrane review reported that invasive positive-pressure ventilation decreased mortal-

ity (relative risk, 0.41; 95% CI: 0.22 to 0.76), lowered the rates of VAP (relative risk, 0.28; 95% CI: 0.90 to 0.85), and decreased the length of ICU and hospital stays.[46]

Sedation and Weaning Protocols

Limiting the use of continuous sedation and paralytic agents that depress cough coupled with sedation vacations and weaning protocols that facilitate removal of the endotracheal tube are strongly recommended to reduce days of mechanical ventilation and lower rates of VAP.[44,47-49] In a recent study, patients randomized to a spontaneous awakening trial alone or in combination with a spontaneous breathing trial had significantly reduced mechanical ventilator days (14.7 vs. 11.6; 95% CI: 0.7 to 5.6; $P = .02$), ICU days (median time, 9.1 vs. 12.9; $P = .01$), and lower mortality (hazard ratio, 0.68; 95% CI: 0.50 to 0.92; $P = .01$).[44] Some investigators have suggested early tracheostomy in patients with respiratory failure who will need long-term mechanical ventilation (see Table 303-2).

Continuous Subglottic Secretion Drainage
Continuous aspiration of subglottic secretions through use of specially designed endotracheal tubes with a wider elliptical hole helps facilitate drainage of subglottic secretions and bacteria entering the trachea. A recent meta-analysis demonstrated that continuous aspiration of subglottic secretions reduced the incidence of VAP by half (risk ratio, 0.51; 95% CI: 1.7 to 2.3), shortened ICU stay by 3 days (95% CI: 2.1 to 3.9), and delayed the onset of VAP by 6 days. Continuous aspiration of subglottic secretions was also cost-effective, saving $4992 per episode of VAP prevented or $1872 per patient; but mortality was not affected.[50] Limitations may be tube cost, identifying early the patients who will need to be intubated for more than 48 hours, and the need for increased staff time.

Silver-Coated Endotracheal Tube
The North American Silver-Coated Endotracheal Tube (NASCENT) Study was a randomized study comparing a colloidal silver-coated-endotracheal tube with a control endotracheal tube.[51] The incidence of VAP, using microbiologic confirmation by BAL with more than 10^4 organisms per milliliter, was significantly lower in the silver-coated endotracheal tube group (4.8% vs. 7.5%, $P = .03$), with a relative risk reduction for VAP of 36%. The silver-coated endotracheal tube group had a delayed onset of VAP, had its greatest effect noted in patients ventilated for more than 48 hours, and was effective against both *P. aeruginosa* and MRSA. No significant differences were noted between patients in terms of length of hospital stay, antibiotic use, and mortality.

TARGETING AIRWAY COLONIZATION

Oral Care and Oral Antiseptics
The oral antiseptic chlorhexidine has demonstrated efficacy in reducing VAP, especially in cardiac surgery patients.[52] In a recent multicenter, double-blind, randomized clinical trial of VAP outcomes, subjects treated with 2% chlorhexidine paste were compared with patients randomized to 2% chlorohexidine plus 2% colistin (paste) or placebo.[53] Although the risk of VAP was reduced by 65% in the chlorhexidine group ($P = .01$), no difference was noted in ventilator days, length of hospital stay, or mortality.

Antibiotic Prophylaxis
Modulation of oropharyngeal colonization by combinations of oral antibiotics, with or without systemic therapy, or selective decontamination of the digestive tract is effective in preventing VAP, but data are difficult to assess because of methodologic study quality, spectrum of regimens used, and differences in study populations.[1,2] Clinical evidence of the efficacy of selective decontamination of the digestive tract was recently reported in a Cochrane review[54] and demonstrated a reduction in respiratory tract infections and overall mortality without an increase in antibiotic resistance in adult patients receiving intensive care. Because of increased concerns over rapid increases in MDR pathogens and *C. difficile* diarrhea in hospitals in the United States, recent guidelines have suggested that selective decontamination of the digestive tract should be limited to selected ICU patient populations and not used routinely for widespread VAP prevention.[1,2,53]

Targeting Ventilator-Associated Tracheobronchitis to Prevent Ventilator-Associated Pneumonia
Accurate diagnosis of VAP is limited by the lack of a common diagnostic gold standard.[55] Intubated patients have ready access to lower airway sputum, which can be evaluated by smear and microbiologic culture. We suggest routine use of serial quantitative microbiologic cultures to assess lower airway colonization, to increase the clinical suspicion for VAP, and to help clinicians distinguish between colonization and infection, VAT, and VAP.[21,56]

VAT seems to be a risk factor for and precursor of VAP and a potential target for prophylaxis.[21,56] Nseir and co-workers[21] used serial, quantitative, endotracheal aspirates to follow levels of bacterial colonization to identify patients with VAT having a bacterial pathogen greater than 10^6 organisms per milliliter who would be eligible for a randomization trial of targeted antibiotic therapy versus no therapy. Patients randomized to targeted antibiotic therapy for VAT had a significant decrease in VAP ($P < .02$), more mechanical ventilation–free days ($P < .001$), as well as lower ICU mortality and shorter length of hospital stay ($P < .05$). Of note is that VAP occurred in 41% of the control group versus none of the antibiotic-treated patients. If confirmed, these data suggest a potential, new paradigm for managing VAT, may also help in preventing VAP, and could provide a microbiologic benchmark for assessing rates of lower respiratory tract infections.

Summary

There has been tremendous progress in our understanding of HAP and VAP pathogenesis, antibiotic management, and implementation of prevention strategies.[29] HAP and VAP are dynamic and complex diseases with associated morbidity and mortality that will require constant surveillance and efforts to improve therapy and prophylaxis. Antibiotic management of HAP and VAP should start a careful clinical assessment and collection of appropriate blood and sputum samples followed by the use of early, appropriate, and adequate antibiotic therapy. In our opinion, liberal use of initial antibiotics is most important for patients who are elderly, severely ill, or debilitated or have ultimately or rapidly fatal underlying diseases. At 24 to 48 hours, the patient's clinical progress, cultures, and antibiotic sensitivities should be assessed and the initial broad-spectrum antibiotic regimen streamlined or de-escalated to conserve antibiotics and reduce secondary complications from antibiotic therapy. Finally, the duration of therapy should be limited to 7 days in responders to reduce the risk of *C. difficile* infection and colonization or superinfection with MDR pathogens. Each patient will also require careful follow-up after antibiotics are discontinued.

Investing in prevention is cost-effective and the key to reduced mortality and morbidity. The Institute for Healthcare Improvement has been a force for "sowing seeds of change,"[40] but other methods of prevention may be needed to further reduce VAP in high-risk populations. All efforts to reduce intubation and removal of the device as soon as possible are important in VAP prevention strategies. This could be accomplished by limiting oversedation, effective weaning protocols, use of noninvasive positive-pressure ventilation, or early tracheostomy in selected patients. Furthermore, the use of continuous aspiration of subglottic secretions or a silver-coated endotracheal tube or VAT as a target for intervention should be considered for VAP prevention.

Quite simply, "an ounce of prevention is definitely worth more than a pound of cure," especially if the Centers for Medicare and Medicaid Services consider HAP and VAP "medical errors" or "never events" that will reduce hospital reimbursement. Proper implementation of effective HAP and VAP prevention measures will take teamwork, thought, investment, and change in culture that will reduce, but will not eliminate them. In addition, spreading these "seeds of change" to long-term care rehabilitation facilities and nursing homes would be a logical step because, according to an old African proverb, "the best time to plant a tree is 20 years ago, the second best time is now."

REFERENCES

1. Niederman MS, Craven DE, Bonten MJ. American Thoracic Society and Infectious Diseases Society of America (ATS/IDSA): Guideline for the Management of Adults with Hospital-acquired, Ventilator-associated, and Healthcare-associated Pneumonia. *Am J Respir Crit Care Med.* 2005;171:388-416.
2. Tablan OC, Anderson LJ, Besser R, et al. Guidelines for preventing health-care–associated pneumonia, 2003: recommendations of CDC and the Healthcare Infection Control Practices Advisory Committee. *MMWR Recomm Rep.* 2004;53:1-36.
3. Chastre J, Fagon JY. Ventilator-associated pneumonia. *Am J Respir Crit Care Med.* 2002;165:867-903.
4. Cook DJ, Walter SD, Cook RJ, et al. Incidence of and risk factors for ventilator-associated pneumonia in critically ill patients. *Ann Intern Med.* 1998;129:433-440.
5. Fagon JY, Chastre J, Domart Y, et al. Mortality due to ventilator-associated pneumonia or colonization with *Pseudomonas* or *Acinetobacter* species: assessment by quantitative culture of samples obtained by a protected specimen brush. *Clin Infect Dis.* 1996;23:538-542.
6. Kollef MH. Prevention of hospital-associated pneumonia and ventilator-associated pneumonia. *Crit Care Med.* 2004;32:1396-1405.
7. Craven DE, Steger KA. Nosocomial pneumonia in mechanically ventilated adult patients: epidemiology and prevention in 1996. *Semin Respir Infect.* 1996;11:32-53.
8. Safdar N, Crnich CJ, Maki DG. The pathogenesis of ventilator-associated pneumonia: its relevance to developing effective strategies for prevention. *Respir Care.* 2005;50:725-739.
9. Bonten MJ, Weinstein RA. Infection control in intensive care units and prevention of ventilator-associated pneumonia. *Semin Respir Infect.* 2000;15:327-335.
10. National Nosocomial Infections Surveillance (NNIS) System Report, data summary from January 1992 through June 2004, issued October 2004. *Am J Infect Control.* 2004;32:470-485.
11. Rello J, Ollendorf DA, Oster G, et al. Epidemiology and outcomes of ventilator-associated pneumonia in a large US database. *Chest.* 2002;122:2115-2121.
12. Rello J, Lorente C, Diaz E, et al. Incidence, etiology, and outcome of nosocomial pneumonia in ICU patients requiring percutaneous tracheotomy for mechanical ventilation. *Chest.* 2003;124:2239-2243.
13. Trouillet JL, Chastre J, Vuagnat A, et al. Ventilator-associated pneumonia caused by potentially drug-resistant bacteria. *Am J Respir Crit Care Med.* 1998;157:531-539.
14. Kollef MH, Shorr A, Tabak YP, et al. Epidemiology and outcomes of health-care-associated pneumonia: results from a large US database of culture-positive pneumonia. *Chest.* 2005;128:3854-3862.
15. Roy-Burman A, Savel RH, Racine S, et al. Type III protein secretion is associated with death in lower respiratory and systemic *Pseudomonas aeruginosa* infections. *J Infect Dis.* 2001;183:1767-1774.
16. Popovich KJ, Weinstein RA, Hota B. Are community-associated methicillin-resistant *Staphylococcus aureus* (MRSA) strains replacing traditional nosocomial MRSA strains? *Clin Infect Dis.* 2008;46:787-794.
17. Jacoby GA, Munoz-Price LS. The new beta-lactamases. *N Engl J Med.* 2005;352:380-391.
18. de Lassence A, Hidri N, Timsit JF, et al. Control and outcome of a large outbreak of colonization and infection with glycopeptide-intermediate *Staphylococcus aureus* in an intensive care unit. *Clin Infect Dis.* 2006;42:170-178.
19. Prince AS. Biofilms, antimicrobial resistance, and airway infection. *N Engl J Med.* 2002;347:1110-1111.
20. Inglis TJ, Lim EW, Lee GS, et al. Endogenous source of bacteria in tracheal tube and proximal ventilator breathing system in intensive care patients. *Br J Anaesth.* 1998;80:41-45.
21. Nseir S, Favory R, Jozefowicz E, et al. Antimicrobial treatment for ventilator-associated tracheobronchitis: a randomized controlled multicenter study. *Crit Care.* 2008;12:R62.
22. Craven DE. Ventilator-associated tracheobronchitis (VAT): questions, answers and a new paradigm? *Crit Care.* 2008;12:157.
23. Fagon JY, Chastre J, Wolff M, et al. Invasive and noninvasive strategies for management of suspected ventilator-associated pneumonia: a randomized trial. *Ann Intern Med.* 2000;132:621-630.
24. The Canadian Clinical Trial Group. A randomized trial of diagnostic techniques for ventilator-associated pneumonia. *N Engl J Med.* 2006;355:2619-2630.
25. Gibot S, Cravoisy A, Levy B, et al. Soluble triggering receptor expressed on myeloid cells and the diagnosis of pneumonia. *N Engl J Med.* 2004;350:451-458.
26. Ramirez P, Garcia MA, Ferrer M, et al. Sequential measurements of procalcitonin levels in diagnosing ventilator-associated pneumonia. *Eur Respir J.* 2008;31:356-362.
27. Chastre J, Luyt CE, Trouillet JL, et al. New diagnostic and prognostic markers of ventilator-associated pneumonia. *Curr Opin Crit Care.* 2006;12:446-451.
28. Song JH. Treatment recommendations of hospital-acquired pneumonia in Asian countries: first consensus report by the Asian HAP Working Group. *Am J Infect Control.* 2008;36:S83-S92.
29. Masterton RG, Galloway A, French G, et al. Guidelines for the management of hospital-acquired pneumonia in the UK: report of the working party on hospital-acquired pneumonia of the British Society for Antimicrobial Chemotherapy. *J Antimicrob Chemother.* 2008;62:5-34.
30. Nseir S, Di Pompeo C, Soubrier S, et al. First-generation fluoroquinolone use and subsequent emergence of multiple drug-resistant bacteria in the intensive care unit. *Crit Care Med.* 2005;33:283-289.
31. Sader HS, Fritsche TR, Jones RN. Accuracy of three automated systems (MicroScan WalkAway, VITEK, and VITEK 2) for susceptibility testing of *Pseudomonas aeruginosa* against five broad-spectrum beta-lactam agents. *J Clin Microbiol.* 2006;44:1101-1104.
32. Lodise TP, Lomaestro BM, Drusano GL. Application of antimicrobial pharmacodynamic concepts into clinical practice: focus on beta-lactam antibiotics: insights from the Society of Infectious Diseases Pharmacists. *Pharmacotherapy.* 2006;26:1320-1332.
33. Loise TP Jr, Lomaestro B, Drusano GL. Piperacillin-tazobactam for *Pseudomonas aeruginosa* infection: clinical implications of an extended-infusion dosing strategy. *Clin Infect Dis.* 2007;44:357-363.
34. Alvarez-Lerma F, Alvarez B, Luque P, et al. Empiric broad-spectrum antibiotic therapy of nosocomial pneumonia in the intensive care unit: a prospective observational study. *Crit Care.* 2006;10:R78.
35. Niederman MS. The importance of de-escalating antimicrobial therapy in patients with ventilator-associated pneumonia. *Semin Respir Crit Care Med.* 2006;27:45-50.
36. Chastre J, Wolff M, Fagon JY, et al. Comparison of 8 vs 15 days of antibiotic therapy for ventilator-associated pneumonia in adults: a randomized trial. *JAMA.* 2003;290:2588-2598.
37. Christ-Crain M, Jaccard-Stolz D, Bingisser R, et al. Effect of procalcitonin-guided treatment on antibiotic use and outcome in lower respiratory tract infections: cluster-randomised, single-blinded intervention trial. *Lancet.* 2004;363:600-607.
38. Luyt CE, Guerin V, Combes A, et al. Procalcitonin kinetics as a prognostic marker of ventilator-associated pneumonia. *Am J Respir Crit Care Med.* 2005;171:48-53.
39. Craven DE, Steger Craven K, Duncan RA. *Hospital-Acquired Pneumonia.* Boston: Little Brown; 2007.
40. Resar R, Pronovost P, Haraden C, et al. Using a bundle approach to improve ventilator care processes and reduce ventilator-associated pneumonia. *Jt Comm J Qual Patient Saf.* 2005;31:243-248.
41. Craven DE. Preventing ventilator-associated pneumonia in adults: sowing seeds of change. *Chest.* 2006;130:251-260.
42. Eggimann P, Pittet D. Infection control in the ICU. *Chest.* 2001;120:2059-2093.
43. Zack JE, Garrison T, Trovillion E, et al. Effect of an education program aimed at reducing the occurrence of ventilator-associated pneumonia. *Crit Care Med.* 2002;30:2407-2412.
44. Girard TD, Kress JP, Fuchs BD, et al. Efficacy and safety of a paired sedation and ventilator weaning protocol for mechanically ventilated patients in intensive care (Awakening and Breathing Controlled trial): a randomised controlled trial. *Lancet.* 2008;371:126-134.
45. Burns KE, Adhikari NK, Meade MO. A meta-analysis of noninvasive weaning to facilitate liberation from mechanical ventilation. *Can J Anaesth.* 2006;53:305-315.
46. Burns K. Noinvasive positive pressure ventilation as a weaning strategy for intubated adults with respiratory failure. In: Adhikari N, ed. *The Cochrane Collaboration Issue 1*, 2006:1-25.
47. Schweickert WD, Gehlbach BK, Pohlman AS, et al. Daily interruption of sedative infusions and complications of critical illness in mechanically ventilated patients. *Crit Care Med.* 2004;32:1272-1276.
48. Kress JP, Pohlman AS, O'Connor MF, et al. Daily interruption of sedative infusions in critically ill patients undergoing mechanical ventilation. *N Engl J Med.* 2000;342:1471-1477.
49. Marelich GP, Murin S, Battistella F, et al. Protocol weaning of mechanical ventilation in medical and surgical patients by respiratory care practitioners and nurses: effect on weaning time and incidence of ventilator-associated pneumonia. *Chest.* 2000;118:459-467.
50. Dezfulian C, Shojania K, Collard HR, et al. Subglottic secretion drainage for preventing ventilator-associated pneumonia: a meta-analysis. *Am J Med.* 2005;118:11-18.
51. Kollef MH, Afessa B, Anzueto A, et al. Silver-coated endotracheal tubes and incidence of ventilator-associated pneumonia. The NASCENT trial. *JAMA.* 2008;300:805-813.
52. Chlebicki MP, Safdar N. Topical chlorhexidine for prevention of ventilator-associated pneumonia: a meta-analysis. *Crit Care Med.* 2007;35:595-602.
53. Koeman M, van der Ven AJ, Hak E, et al. Oral decontamination with chlorhexidine reduces the incidence of ventilator-associated pneumonia. *Am J Respir Crit Care Med.* 2006;173:1348-1355.
54. Liberati A, D'Amico R, Pifferi M, et al. Antibiotic prophylaxis to reduce respiratory tract infections and mortality in adults receiving intensive care. *Cochrane Database Syst Rev.* 2004:CD000022.
55. Klompas M. Does this patient have ventilator-associated pneumonia? *JAMA.* 2007;297:1583-1593.
56. Craven DE, Chroneou A, Zias N, et al. Ventilator-associated tracheobronchitis (VAT): the impact of targeted antibiotic therapy on patient outcomes. *Chest.* 2009;135:521-528.
57. Mandell LA, Wunderink RG, Anzueto A, et al. Infectious Diseases Society of America/American Thoracic Society consensus guidelines on the management of community-acquired pneumonia in adults. *Clin Infect Dis.* 2007;44(Suppl 2):S27-S72.
58. Moise PA, Forrest A, Bhavnani SM, et al. Area under the inhibitory curve and a pneumonia scoring system for predicting outcomes of vancomycin therapy for respiratory infections by *Staphylococcus aureus*. *Am J Health Syst Pharm.* 2000;57(Suppl 2):S4-S9.
59. Deresinski S. Counterpoint: vancomycin and *Staphylococcus aureus*—an antibiotic enters obsolescence. *Clin Infect Dis.* 2007;44:1543-1548.
60. Hidayat LK, Hsu DI, Quist R, et al. High-dose vancomycin therapy for methicillin-resistant *Staphylococcus aureus* infections: efficacy and toxicity. *Arch Intern Med.* 2006;166:2138-2144.
61. Conte JE Jr, Golden JA, Kipps J, et al. Intrapulmonary pharmacokinetics of linezolid. *Antimicrob Agents Chemother.* 2002;46:1475-1480.
62. Stevens DL, Ma Y, Salmi DB, et al. Impact of antibiotics on expression of virulence-associated exotoxin genes in methicillin-sensitive and methicillin-resistant *Staphylococcus aureus*. *J Infect Dis.* 2007;195:202-211.
63. Paul M, Benuri-Silbiger I, Soares-Weiser K, et al. Beta lactam monotherapy versus beta lactam-aminoglycoside combination therapy for sepsis in immunocompetent patients: systematic review and meta-analysis of randomised trials. *Br Med J.* 2004;328:668.
64. Bliziotis IA, Samonis G, Vardakas KZ, et al. Effect of aminoglycoside and beta-lactam combination therapy versus beta-lactam monotherapy on the emergence of antimicrobial resistance: a meta-analysis of randomized, controlled trials. *Clin Infect Dis.* 2005;41:149-158.
65. Nseir S, Ader F, Marquette CH, et al. Impact of fluoroquinolone use on multidrug-resistant bacteria emergence. *Pathol Biol (Paris).* 2005;53:470-475.
66. Munoz-Price LS, Weinstein RA. *Acinetobacter* infection. *N Engl J Med.* 2008;358:1271-1281.
67. Manikal VM, Landman D, Saurina G, et al. Endemic carbapenem-resistant *Acinetobacter* species in Brooklyn, New York: citywide prevalence, interinstitutional spread, and relation to antibiotic usage. *Clin Infect Dis.* 2000;31:101-106.
68. Linden PK, Paterson DL. Parenteral and inhaled colistin for treatment of ventilator-associated pneumonia. *Clin Infect Dis.* 2006;43(Suppl 2):S89-S94.
69. Paterson DL, Ko WC, Von Gottberg A, et al. Antibiotic therapy for *Klebsiella pneumoniae* bacteremia: implications of production of extended-spectrum beta-lactamases. *Clin Infect Dis.* 2004;39:31-37.
70. Chow JW, Fine MJ, Shlaes DM, et al. *Enterobacter* bacteremia: clinical features and emergence of antibiotic resistance during therapy. *Ann Intern Med.* 1991;115:585-590.
71. Fox MY. Toward a zero VAP rate: personal and team approaches in the ICU. *Crit Care Nurs Q.* 2006;29:108-114; quiz 115-1126.
72. van den Berghe G, Wouters P, Weekers F, et al. Intensive insulin therapy in the critically ill patients. *N Engl J Med.* 2001;345:1359-1367.
73. Mori H, Hirasawa H, Oda S, et al. Oral care reduces incidence of ventilator-associated pneumonia in ICU populations. *Intensive Care Med.* 2006;32:230-236.
74. Lorente L, Blot S, Rello J. Evidence on measures for the prevention of ventilator-associated pneumonia. *Eur Respir J.* 2007;30:1193-1207.
75. Griffiths J, Barber VS, Morgan L, et al. Systematic review and meta-analysis of studies of the timing of tracheostomy in adult patients undergoing artificial ventilation. *Br Med J.* 2005;330:1243.

Nosocomial Urinary Tract Infections

THOMAS M. HOOTON

Nosocomial urinary tract infection (UTI) refers to UTI that is acquired in a hospital, but the term is often used to refer to UTI acquired in any institutional setting providing health care. The Centers for Disease Control and Prevention uses the more generic term, *health care-associated*, instead of *nosocomial*[1] that can also be used in reference to infections that are related to health care activities that take place anywhere, including the home. The vast majority of nosocomial UTIs occur in patients whose urinary tracts are currently or recently catheterized. The focus of this chapter is on catheter-associated bacterial UTIs occurring in adults in hospitals and long-term–care facilities (LTCFs). Candiduria, the most common type of nosocomial fungal UTI, is discussed in a separate section of the chapter.

There are major differences in the epidemiology, pathogenesis, treatment, and prevention of nosocomial UTI and uncomplicated UTI which are shown in Table 304-1.

UTI is a non-specific term that generally refers to bacterial or fungal infection of the bladder or kidney, or both, in a patient, without regard to the presence or absence of urinary symptoms. In this chapter, catheter-associated (CA) bacteriuria is defined as the presence of significant bacteriuria (quantity of bacteria in the urine suggestive of infection rather than contamination) without regard to the presence or absence of urinary symptoms, CA-asymptomatic bacteriuria (ASB) as the presence of significant bacteriuria in a patient without symptoms referable to the urinary tract, and CA-UTI as the presence of significant bacteriuria in a patient with symptoms or signs referable to the urinary tract. Unfortunately, CA-bacteriuria is a non-specific term frequently used in the urinary catheter literature rather than the more specific terms, CA-ASB and CA-UTI. CA-bacteriuria is comprised mostly of CA-ASB, but in most papers one cannot discern what proportion of patients have CA-UTI.

The relationship between CA-ASB and CA-UTI and other clinical outcomes remains unclear and complicates our assessment of the importance of CA-ASB. The vast majority of patients with CA-ASB do not progress to CA-UTI, and factors that trigger a symptomatic event in patients with ASB are not known. Thus, even though the presence of CA-ASB is presumably necessary for the development of CA-UTI, the development of urinary symptoms must require some facilitating event(s), such as tissue invasion, that we don't yet understand. On the other hand, even if CA-ASB itself is benign, there are several reasons that may justify efforts to prevent it. For example, it may predispose one to CA-UTI through a common pathogenic pathway, in which case interventions that prevent CA-ASB would be expected to prevent CA-UTI. Additionally, CA-bacteriuria (mostly CA-ASB) is the source of most episodes of nosocomial bacteremia, and may be associated with increased mortality,[2,3] although this latter point is controversial. In hospitals and LTCFs, CA-ASB represents a large reservoir of antimicrobial-resistant urinary pathogens in patients that increases the risk of cross-infection among catheterized patients. CA-ASB also provides an ubiquitous infection for physicians who have a low threshold for using antimicrobials (inappropriately). Almost no studies evaluate the effect of preventing CA-ASB on outcomes other than CA-UTI, but the relationships between CA-ASB and these clinical outcomes, including CA-UTI, are difficult to demonstrate in most studies, given the large sample sizes needed to demonstrate such a benefit.

Therefore, even though treatment of ASB is not recommended except in certain circumstances, such as pregnancy,[4] it is possible that prevention of CA-ASB might lead to fewer episodes of CA-UTI, bacteremia, fever episodes, cross-infection and inappropriate antimicrobial use. In fact, the greatest impact of effective CA-UTI-prevention interventions may be to prevent large numbers of episodes of CA-ASB, and their sequelae, rather than the few episodes of CA-UTI that occur in these patients. This seems unlikely to be determined in clinical trials any time soon, given the need for complex study designs and large sample sizes.

■ Epidemiology

INCIDENCE AND PREVALENCE

Nosocomial UTIs (comprised mostly of ASB), up to 97% of which are associated with instrumentation of the urinary tract,[5,6] are the most common nosocomial infection worldwide[7] and account for up to 40% of nosocomial infections in U.S. hospitals each year.[8,9] UTI is also the leading cause of infection in LTCFs and most of these are also catheter-associated.[10,11]

Urinary catheterization is very prevalent in hospitals and LTCFs and its use appears to be increasing, at least in hospitals.[12] Approximately 15% to 25% of patients in general hospitals have a catheter inserted at some time during their stay,[8,13] mainly to assist with accurate monitoring of urine output during acute illness or following surgery, to treat urinary retention, and for investigative purposes. Most of these patients are catheterized for only 2 to 4 days.[14] About 5% to 10% of LTCF residents are managed with urethral catheterization, in some cases for years, and it is estimated that more than 100,000 patients in U.S. LTCFs have a urethral catheter in place at any given time,[11,14-17] most commonly for incontinence in women and bladder outlet obstruction in men. The incidence of bacteriuria associated with indwelling urethral catheterization with a closed drainage system is approximately 3% to 8% per day[13,18,19] and, thus, many patients catheterized for short periods of time and almost all those catheterized for a month or more will have CA-bacteriuria, compared with only 3.1% of those with *in-and-out* catheterization and 1.4% of noncatheterized hospital patients.[8] One month is a convenient dividing line between short-term and long-term catheterization,[14] and it is used as such in this chapter, except where stated otherwise.

RISK FACTORS

The duration of catheterization is the most important risk factor for the development of CA-bacteriuria.[14,20,21] Other risk factors for CA-bacteriuria include the lack of systemic antimicrobial therapy, female sex, meatal colonization with uropathogens, microbial colonization of the drainage bag, catheter insertion outside the operating room, catheter care violations, absence of use of a drip chamber, rapidly fatal underlying illness, older age, diabetes, and elevated serum creatinine at the time of catheterization.[13,21-23] Risk factors in patients with nosocomial UTIs not associated with catheterization include other forms of instrumentation of the urinary tract. Many noncatheterized patients with nosocomial UTI are probably also at increased risk for UTI in the community, due to host behavioral or genetic factors associated with increased risk for UTI.[24]

COMPLICATIONS

Most episodes of CA-bacteriuria occur in asymptomatic patients, with studies showing that less than one quarter of patients with CA-bacteriuria develop UTI symptoms.[25-28] In one study of 235 new cases of nosocomial CA-bacteriuria, more than 90% of the infected patients

TABLE 304-1	**Comparison of Uncomplicated Urinary Tract Infection and Nosocomial Urinary Tract Infection**	
	Uncomplicated	*Nosocomial*
Age	Younger	Older
Sex	Female, rare in males	Male and female, female predominance
Main risk factor	Intercourse	Urinary catheter
Pathogenesis	Fecal organisms ascend urethra to bladder	Extraluminal: fecal organisms ascend catheter-urethra interface to bladder.
		Intraluminal: fecal or exogenous (cross-infection) organisms enter drainage system that has been disconnected, ascend through catheter to bladder
Uropathogen virulence	More virulent: pyelo > cystitis > ASB or fecal	Less virulent than in uncomplicated UTI
Microbiology	Single pathogen, usually *E. coli*; yeast rare	Single (short-term catheter) to multiple (long-term catheter) organisms; diverse flora with gram-negatives, gram-positives, *Candida* sp.
Clinical	ASB in about 5% of women, but prevalence a function of culture frequency; transient, benign.	CA-bacteriuria in about 5% per day of catheter; >90% is CA-ASB, usually persistent, most do not progress to CA-UTI.
	Cystitis: dysuria, frequency and/or urgency.	CA-UTI: fever, altered mental status, other non-specific signs/symptoms, usually no lower tract symptoms
	Pyelonephritis: fever, back pain/tenderness	
Diagnosis	ASB: ≥10^5 CFU/mL	CA-ASB: ≥10^5 CFU/mL
	Cystitis/pyelonephritis: ≥10^3 CFU/mL	CA-UTI: ≥10^3 CFU/mL
Resistance	Common but predictable; fluoroquinolone resistance rare	Multidrug resistance common and less predictable; fluoroquinolone resistance not rare
Treatment	3-day regimen	5-14 day regimen, depending on severity
Prevention	Abstinence; antimicrobial prophylaxis	Reduce urinary catheterization; condom, intermittent or suprapubic catheter vs. indwelling urethral catheter; strict closed system with indwelling urethral catheter
Public health	Strains spread via food chain and within family units	Large reservoir of multidrug-resistant uropathogens; cross-infection a concern

ASB, asymptomatic bacteriuria; CA, catheter acquired; UTI, urinary tract infection.

were asymptomatic and afebrile.[28] In another study of catheterized and bacteriuric female patients in a LTCF, the incidence of febrile episodes of possible urinary origin was only 1.1 episodes per 100 catheterized patient-days, and most of these episodes were low grade, lasted for less than a day, and resolved without antibiotic treatment.[29]

However, as noted previously, there are significant consequences of CA-bacteriuria, which is usually associated with an inflammatory response in both short-term and long-term catheterized patients. Bacteremia complicates CA-bacteriuria in up to 4% of cases,[28,30,31] and about 15% of episodes of nosocomial bacteremia are attributable to the urinary tract.[30] Additionally, CA-bacteriuria is the most common source of gram-negative bacteremia in hospitalized patients.[32] However, one recent study of hospitalized patients found that only 1 of the 235 episodes of CA-bacteriuria was unequivocally associated with secondary bloodstream infection.[28] The low risk of bacteremia associated with CA-bacteriuria may be due in part to its being primarily comprised of ASB, which likely is associated with low tissue invasiveness, the low prevalence of *Escherichia coli* in episodes of CA-bacteriuria (compared with uncomplicated UTI), and the low prevalence of bacterial virulence factors, such as P fimbriae in *E. coli* strains causing nosocomial UTI.[33]

Nosocomial UTI is also the most common source of bacteremia in LTCFs, accounting for 40% to 55% of bacteremias,[34,35] and bacteremia is often polymicrobial in these patients.

Patients undergoing long-term indwelling catheterization, in addition to almost universal polymicrobial bacteriuria, may develop symptomatic lower and upper UTI, bacteremia, frequent febrile episodes, catheter obstruction, renal and bladder stone formation associated with urease-producing uropathogens, local genitourinary infections, fistula formation, incontinence and bladder cancer.[14] Chronic renal inflammation and pyelonephritis is often found at autopsy in patients who had been on long-term urinary catheterization, many of whom were afebrile at the time of death.[36] Catheter blockage can be a recurrent problem in long-term catheterized patients, and results from encrustation formed by urease-producing organisms, especially *Proteus mirabilis*, which hydrolyze urea to ammonia with formation of struvite and apatite crystals in the catheter lumen.

The effect of CA-bacteriuria on mortality remains controversial. One prospective study of 1458 hospitalized patients with indwelling bladder catheterizations showed that mortality was approximately 3 times higher in those with CA-bacteriuria compared with those who were not infected,[2] and another showed that the degree of reduction in CA-bacteriuria with use of bladder catheters with preconnected sealed junctions corresponded closely with the degree of mortality reduction.[3] Increased mortality has also been reported in residents of LTCFs with chronic indwelling catheters—presumably most of these patients were bacteriuric, but bacteriuria was not assessed in this study.[37] However, others have not shown an increased mortality risk associated with CA-bacteriuria,[38-40] and the association may be explained by confounding as catheterized patients tend to be sicker and more functionally impaired.[41,42]

One important consequence of CA-bacteriuria is that it comprises a large reservoir of antibiotic-resistant organisms that may be transmitted between patients who have urinary catheters or other invasive devices.[21,43-46] Another is that CA-bacteriuria is a frequent target for antimicrobial therapy, often inappropriate, which contributes to the problem of antimicrobial resistance in hospitals and LTCFs. For example, in one recent prospective study of inpatients with an indwelling catheter and CA-ASB, 15 (52%) of 29 patients were treated with antimicrobials inappropriately.[47]

MICROBIOLOGY

Unlike the narrow and predictable spectrum of causative agents in uncomplicated UTI,[48] a broad range of bacteria can cause nosocomial UTI, and many are resistant to multiple antimicrobial agents.[42] Most episodes of bacteriuria in short-term catheterized patients are caused by single organisms, mostly enterococci and gram-negative bacilli.[28] *E. coli* causes most episodes of CA-bacteriuria,[42] although it is not as prevalent as in uncomplicated UTI.[48] Other Enterobacteriaceae, such as *Klebsiella* spp., *Serratia* spp., *Citrobacter* spp., and *Enterobacter* spp., nonfermenters such as *Pseudomonas aeruginosa*, and gram-positive cocci, including coagulase negative staphylococci and *Enterococcus* spp., cause most of the other infections.[42] Funguria, mostly candiduria, is reported in 3% to 32% of patients catheterized for short periods of time.[28,42] In a study of 7574 uropathogens isolated in patients with nosocomial UTIs in medical-surgical ICUs reported in the U.S. National Nosocomial Infection Surveillance System from 1992 to 1998, *Candida albicans* constituted 15.3% and all fungal isolates 31.2% of all urinary isolates compared with 18.5% for *E. coli*, 14.3% for enterococcus and 10.3% for *P. aeruginosa.*[6] Fungi were more commonly reported in UTIs in catheterized patients than in noncatheterized patients (32% vs. 21%).

Bacteriuria in long-term catheterized patients is usually polymicrobial and, in addition to the pathogens commonly seen in short-term catheterized patients, commonly includes less familiar species such as *P. mirabilis, Providencia* spp., and *Morganella morganii.*[42] In these patients, new episodes of infection often occur periodically in the presence of existing infection with organisms that may persist for months.[49,50] A urine culture obtained from a patient whose catheter has a biofilm may not accurately reflect the status of bacteriuria in the bladder,[51,52] and it is recommended that urine cultures from chronically catheterized patients be obtained from a freshly placed catheter.

PATHOGENESIS

In noncatheterized patients, the usual origin of uropathogens is their own fecal microflora which colonizes the periurethral area and ascends to the bladder, resulting in bacteriuria with or without symptoms. In the mouse model of UTI, inoculation of *E. coli* into the bladder is followed by invasion of the superficial bladder cells and the formation of large intracellular bacterial colonies that, in response to infection, exfoliate and are removed with the flow of urine.[53] To avoid clearance by exfoliation, these intracellular uropathogens can reemerge and eventually establish a persistent, quiescent bacterial reservoir within the bladder mucosa that may serve as a source for recurrent acute infections.[53] Although internalization of uropathogenic *E. coli* into bladder and renal epithelial cells has been observed in vitro and in vivo,[54] there is only sparse evidence that this phenomenon occurs in humans,[55,56] and only indirect evidence that the intracellular bacterial colonies observed in the mouse occur in humans.[57] It is possible that invasion of uropathogens into uroepithelial cells is the trigger for urinary symptoms, but an inflammatory response is not sufficient to cause urinary symptoms since pyuria often accompanies ASB in both catheterized and noncatheterized patients.

Strains of *E. coli* associated with symptomatic lower or upper tract infection in healthy hosts are more likely to have certain putative virulence determinants, such as P fimbriae, compared with colonic strains and those causing ASB.[58,59] However, many symptomatic UTIs are caused by *E. coli* with a virulence profile similar to that in strains causing ASB, and these putative virulence factors can be found in strains causing ASB, or in colonic flora.

Symptomatic UTI in healthy women is facilitated by sexual intercourse and alterations of vaginal microflora, such as that caused by diaphragm and spermicide use, antimicrobial use or estrogen deficiency, and in healthy men by anal or vaginal intercourse with a colonized partner, or lack of circumcision.[24,60] Risk factors for ASB in healthy women are similar to those for symptomatic UTI, suggesting a common pathogenic pathway. In postmenopausal women, anatomical and functional characteristics of the genitourinary tract are more strongly associated with UTI risk than in younger women.[60] In addition, there is mounting evidence for a genetic predisposition to UTI.[24,61]

Several host defense mechanisms are thought to have a role in protecting individuals from UTI. These include, in addition to the innate and adaptive immune response, the physical barrier of the urethral mucosa, especially in the male, removal of bladder bacteriuria by micturition, intrinsic antibacterial properties of the bladder, an antiadherence glycosaminoglycan secreted by bladder epithelium, exfoliation of bladder epithelial cells, and properties of urine itself, including very high or low urine osmolality, a high urea concentration, a high organic acid concentration, and a low pH.[58,62] However, the importance of these host defense mechanisms in preventing UTI is unknown since few studies have compared host characteristics between patients prone to UTI and those not prone.[63]

The most important predisposing factor for nosocomial UTI is urinary catheterization which perturbs host defense mechanisms and provides easier access of uropathogens to the bladder. The indwelling urethral catheter introduces an inoculum of bacteria into the bladder at the time of insertion, facilitates ascension of uropathogens from the meatus to the bladder via the catheter-mucosa interface, provides a pool of organisms in the drainage bag, if the closed system is not maintained, which can ascend intraluminally to the bladder, compromises complete voiding, and constitutes a frequently manipulated foreign body on which pathogens are deposited via the hands of personnel. Indwelling urinary catheters provide a surface for the attachment of host cell binding receptors that are recognized by bacterial adhesins, thus enhancing microbial adhesion, as well as disrupting the uroepithelial mucosa to expose new binding sites for bacterial adhesins.[54] Bacteria attached to the catheter surface form exopolysaccharides that entrap bacteria, which replicate and form microcolonies that mature into biofilms on the inner and outer surfaces of the catheter.[22,54] These biofilms protect uropathogens from antibiotics and the host immune response and facilitate transfer of antibiotic resistance genes.[54] Some uropathogens in biofilms, such as *Proteus* sp., have the ability to hydrolyze urea to free ammonia and raise the urinary pH, which facilitates precipitation of minerals such as hydroxyapatite or struvite, creating encrustations that can block catheter flow.[22,54]

The source of uropathogens in catheterized patients includes patients' endogenous flora, health care personnel, or inanimate objects.[22,43,64,65] Not unexpectedly, uropathogen virulence determinants such as P fimbriae appear to be of much less importance in the pathogenesis of nosocomial UTIs compared with uncomplicated UTIs.[33,58,59] Approximately two-thirds (79% for gram-positive cocci and 54% for gram-negative bacilli) of the uropathogens causing CA-bacteriuria in patients with indwelling urethral catheters are extraluminally acquired (ascension along the catheter-urethral mucosa interface) and one-third are intraluminally acquired,[66] although in some trials the proportion of strains originating from the drainage bag is much less. Rectal and periurethral colonization with the infecting strain often precedes CA-bacteriuria, especially in women.[65] The relative importance of the intraluminal pathway has much to do with the frequency with which closed drainage systems are breached, which has been shown to be associated with UTI. The negative impact of the catheter is demonstrated by the finding that, despite the continuous drainage of urine through the catheter, in patients with catheter urine colony counts as low as 3 to 4 CFU/mL who are not given antibiotics, the level of bacteriuria or candiduria uniformly rises to greater than 10^5 CFU/mL within 24 to 48 hours in those who remain catheterized.[67]

Diagnosis

SIGNIFICANT BACTERIURIA

Significant bacteriuria is the level of bacteriuria that suggests bladder bacteriuria rather than contamination, and is based on growth from a urine specimen collected in a manner to minimize contamination and transported to the laboratory in a timely fashion to limit bacterial growth. The preferred method of obtaining a urine culture in patients with short-term catheterization is by sampling through the catheter port or, if a port is not present, puncturing the catheter tubing with a needle and syringe.[42] In those with long-term indwelling catheters, the catheter urine may be unreliable,[51,52] so a urine specimen should be obtained from a freshly placed catheter. Cultures should not be obtained from the drainage bag.

The level of bacteriuria considered significant in an asymptomatic noncatheterized woman is derived from studies in which colony counts in voided urine specimens were compared with paired catheter or suprapubic aspirate specimens.[68] In these studies, a bacterial count of greater than or equal to 10^5 CFU/mL in a catheterized specimen was confirmed by a repeat catheterized specimen in more than 95% of cases. On the other hand, greater than or equal to 10^5 CFU/mL in a voided urine specimen was confirmed in a second voided specimen in only 80% of cases. However, two consecutive positive voided urine cultures predicted a third positive voided urine culture with 95% confidence. Therefore, two consecutive voided specimens with greater than or equal to 10^5 CFU/mL predict bladder bacteriuria with the same degree of accuracy as a single urine specimen obtained through a catheter. Nevertheless, for practical purposes and cost containment, a single urine specimen with greater than or equal to 10^5 CFU/mL is often used to define significant bacteriuria in clinical practice and many studies.[4] Microbiologic criteria for diagnosis of ASB in noncatheterized men are not as well validated. The finding of a single voided urine specimen with greater than or equal to 10^5 CFU/mL of an Enterobacteriaceae was reproducible in 98% of asymptomatic ambulatory men when the culture was repeated within 1 week.[69] Thus, a single, clean-catch voided urine specimen with greater than or equal to 10^5 CFU/mL identifies ASB in men.[4] Based on a comparison of voided urine specimens (from freshly applied condom catheters) and paired catheter specimens, greater than or equal to 10^5 CFU/mL is also the appropriate quantitative criterion for ASB in a man with a condom catheter.[70]

In symptomatic noncatheterized men and women, lower colony counts have been shown to be significant. For example, in women with uncomplicated cystitis, bacterial colony counts in voided urine as low as 10^2 CFU/mL have been shown to reflect bladder infection.[71] In men with urinary symptoms, a quantitative count of greater than or equal to 10^3 CFU/mL in a voided specimen best differentiates sterile from infected bladder urine.[72]

In urine specimens obtained by urethral catheterization from symptomatic or asymptomatic men and women, periurethral contamination is less of a problem, and lower quantitative counts of greater than or equal to 10^2 CFU/mL are considered to be significant in both men and women.[4,73] The significance of this colony-count threshold was demonstrated in the study previously mentioned, showing that the level of bacteriuria or candiduria rapidly increases from small quantities to greater than 10^5 CFU/mL in catheterized individuals.[67]

Most clinical laboratories do not routinely quantify urine cultures to 10^2 CFU/mL, so it is reasonable to use a quantitative count of greater than or equal to 10^3 CFU/mL in a symptomatic person, whether catheterized or not, as an indicator of CA-UTI, because this threshold is a reasonable compromise between sensitivity in detecting bladder bacteriuria and feasibility for the microbiology laboratory in quantifying organisms. On the other hand, greater than or equal to 10^5 CFU/mL is a reasonable criterion for the diagnosis of ASB in women and men, even though lower counts probably represent true bladder bacteriuria, at least when found in catheter specimens, since increased specificity is desirable. In this regard, CA-ASB should not be screened for except in research studies and in selected clinical situations such as pregnant women or pending urologic surgery.[4]

PYURIA

Pyuria is evidence of inflammation in the genitourinary tract and is present in almost all persons with symptomatic UTIs. It is also common in persons with ASB,[4] including 30% to 75% of bacteriuric patients with short-term indwelling urethral catheters and 50% to 100% of individuals with long-term indwelling catheters. In 761 newly catheterized patients in a university hospital, the specificity of pyuria for CA-bacteriuria (>10^5 CFU/mL—almost all were asymptomatic) was 90%, but the sensitivity was only 47%.[74] In a longitudinal study of patients with long-term urinary catheters, bacteriuria and pyuria were common, even during asymptomatic periods, and did not change during symptomatic UTI episodes.[75] Thus, in the catheterized patient, the presence or absence or degree of pyuria alone does not, by itself, differentiate CA-ASB from CA-UTI, but in a symptomatic patient its absence suggests that CA-UTI is not the cause of the symptoms.

SYMPTOMS AND SIGNS

The majority of patients with CA-bacteriuria lack symptoms, as demonstrated in a study of 1497 newly catheterized patients who were followed prospectively with daily urine cultures, urine leukocyte counts and symptom assessment.[28] Only 8% of 194 patients with CA-bacteriuria (defined as >10^3 CFU/mL; 85% of patients had >10^5 in at least one culture) who could respond to symptom assessment reported symptoms referable to the urinary tract, although bacteriuria and pyuria had been present in most for many days. Additionally, there were no significant differences between catheterized patients with and without CA-bacteriuria in signs or symptoms commonly associated with UTI—fever, dysuria, urgency, or flank pain—or in leukocytosis. The lack of an association between fever and CA-bacteriuria has also been convincingly demonstrated in other studies.[29,41] Thus, in the presence of an indwelling urinary catheter, symptoms referable to the urinary tract, fever, or peripheral leukocytosis have little predictive value for the diagnosis of CA-UTI. Likewise, no studies have demonstrated that odorous or cloudy urine in a catheterized individual has clinical significance.

Nevertheless, catheterized patients with symptoms or signs compatible with UTI that are not explainable by another condition after a thorough evaluation warrant treatment. Signs and symptoms compatible with CA-UTI include new onset or worsening of fever, altered mental status, flank pain, costovertebral angle tenderness, rigors, pelvic discomfort, new or worsening incontinence, malaise, or lethargy. In patients with spinal cord injury (SCI), increased spasticity, autonomic dysreflexia or sense of unease are also compatible with CA-UTI. Patients with CA-UTI usually do not manifest the classic symptoms of dysuria, frequency, and urgency.

Prevention

Prevention of symptomatic CA-UTI is the main objective of prevention strategies in patients for whom urinary catheterization is being considered or has been performed. However, there may also be benefits to preventing CA-ASB in such patients, although, as noted previously, such benefits have usually not been evaluated as end points in clinical trials. In the discussion that follows, the impact of interventions on CA-ASB and CA-UTI will be mentioned when data are available, but most studies use CA-bacteriuria (comprised mostly of CA-ASB) as the outcome of interest.

The following text discusses in detail those practices for which published data suggest that they should be implemented, those for which there are some positive data but not enough to warrant routine implementation, and those which do not warrant routine implementation based on interpretation of currently available data.

PREVENTION STRATEGIES THAT SHOULD BE ROUTINE

Prevention Components of Infection Control Programs
Intensive infection surveillance and control programs in U.S. hospitals are strongly associated with reductions in rates of nosocomial UTI.[76] Updated, evidence-based comprehensive guidelines have been recently published for prevention and surveillance of CA-UTIs in hospitalized patients.[77] UTI-prevention strategies in this guideline that are strongly recommended for hospitals to incorporate into their infection control programs are shown in Table 304-2.

Although cross-infection of bacteriuria in catheterized patients is common and many episodes of nosocomial bacteriuria occur in clusters,[43] the data are conflicting as to whether segregation of patients with urinary catheters from noncatheterized patients reduces the risk of CA-bacteriuria.[78,79] However, this practice seems reasonable in institutions in which it is feasible. In addition, periodic performance feedback of CA-bacteriuria rates to staff members may be effective in reducing CA-bacteriuria rates,[80,81] presumably by resulting in improved compliance with infection control measures.

Residents of LTCFs have a risk of developing health care-associated infections that approaches that seen in acute care hospital patients, and in the United States almost as many such infections occur annually in LTCFs as in hospitals.[11] To address this problem, guidelines for infection prevention and control in LTCFs have been recently published.[11] There has been less research on the efficacy of infection control strategies in LTCFs compared with hospitals, but guidelines for prevention

TABLE 304-2	Catheter-Associated Urinary Tract Infection Prevention and Monitoring Strategies Strongly Recommended for Acute Care Hospitals

Develop and implement written guidelines for use of urinary catheters
Ensure that supplies necessary for aseptic-technique catheter insertion are available
Implement a medical record documentation system for catheter use
Ensure sufficient trained personnel and resources for surveillance of catheter use and outcomes
Perform surveillance of CA-UTI in high-risk groups or units, using valid methodology
Educate health care personnel about CA-UTI prevention techniques
Insert urinary catheters only when necessary and remove them when appropriate
Consider alternatives, such as condom or in-and-out catheterization, when appropriate
Practice hand hygiene upon insertion and any manipulation of the catheter and site
Insert catheters using aseptic technique and sterile equipment
Use gloves, a drape, and sponges; a sterile or antiseptic solution for cleaning the urethral meatus; and a single-use packet of sterile lubricant jelly for insertion
Properly secure catheter to prevent movement
Maintain a sterile, continuously closed drainage system
Do not disconnect the catheter and drainage tubes unless the catheter must be irrigated
To examine urine, aspirate a small sample from the sampling port with sterile syringe
Collect larger volumes of urine for special analyses aseptically from the drainage bag
Maintain unobstructed urine flow
Empty collecting bag regularly, use separate collecting container for each patient
Keep the collecting bag below the level of the bladder at all times
Routine hygiene is appropriate for cleaning the meatal area
In locations or populations with unacceptably high CA-UTI rates despite the above:
  • Implement a program to identify and remove catheters that are no longer necessary
  • Develop a protocol for management of postoperative urinary retention
  • Establish a system for analyzing and reporting data on catheter use and adverse events

CA-UTI, catheter-associated urinary tract infection.
Adapted from Lo E, Nicolle L, Classen D, et al. Strategies to prevent catheter-associated urinary tract infections in acute care hospitals. *Infect Control Hosp Epidemiol.* 2008;29:S41-S50.

of CA-UTIs in hospitalized patients are thought to be generally applicable to catheterized residents in LTCFs.[11]

Saint and colleagues recently conducted a national study of U.S. hospitals to ascertain the practices used to prevent nosocomial UTI.[82] Overall, 56% of hospitals did not have a system for monitoring which patients had urinary catheters placed, and 74% did not monitor catheter duration. Additionally, there was no strategy that appeared to be widely used to prevent nosocomial UTI. It remains to be seen whether the Centers for Medicare & Medicaid Services modification of the hospital reimbursement system designed to eliminate payments previously provided to hospitals for treatment of CA-UTI will be an impetus for U.S. hospitals to direct more resources to prevention of CA-UTI.[83] It must be noted, however, that our ability to prevent CA-ASB or CA-UTI in patients who have appropriate indications for catheterization is quite limited, especially in those requiring long-term bladder drainage, with currently available infection prevention techniques.

Reduction of Unnecessary Catheterization
Reducing unnecessary catheterization is the most effective way to prevent CA-ASB and CA-UTI. Studies have repeatedly documented that urinary catheters are often inserted for inappropriate reasons or remain in place longer than necessary. In studies of hospitalized patients with urinary catheters, the initial indication for catheter use was judged inappropriate in up to 50% of cases, and continued catheterization inappropriate for almost half of catheter-days.[27,84-86] Additionally, the reason for catheter placement is often not stated and orders for catheterization are often not written.[87] In the medical intensive care unit, many unjustified catheter days are due to monitoring of urine output when it is no longer indicated, and on medical wards,

urinary incontinence is a major reason for unjustified initial and continued urinary catheterization. One problem is that clinicians are often unaware that their patients are catheterized. In one study, providers were unaware of patient catheterization for 28% of the 319 provider-patient observations—21% for students, 22% for interns, 27% for residents, and 38% for attending physicians.[88] For patients who were inappropriately catheterized, providers were unaware of catheter use for 41% of the 108 provider-patient observations.

Several strategies have been demonstrated to be effective in reducing inappropriate insertion of catheters and duration of catheterization. Strategies shown to reduce inappropriate insertion of catheters include education and use of a catheter indication sheet in the emergency department,[89] use of a multifaceted intervention restricting urinary catheterization in the operating room and post-anesthesia care unit and expedited catheter removal on the postoperative surgical ward,[90] use of an ultrasound bladder scanner to assess bladder volumes following surgery,[91] and use of in-and-out catheterization rather than short-term indwelling catheterization in postoperative patients with urinary retention.[92] Use of portable bladder ultrasound devices to reduce unnecessary catheterization warrants further study in the care of oliguric patients.[93,94]

Strategies shown to reduce the duration of indwelling urethral catheterization, and in some cases better documentation in the medical record and a reduction in CA-UTI, include physician reminders by the nursing staff or computer prompts to remove unnecessary catheters after admission, prewritten orders for the removal of urinary catheters if predetermined criteria are not met,[95-100] and earlier removal of the catheter following treatment for urethral strictures, acute retention of urine, and various surgical procedures, than is commonly done in practice.[101]

Hospitals and LTCFs should develop institution-specific indications for inserting indwelling urinary catheters, monitor adherence to use of such indications in catheterizing patients, and implement reminder systems for nurses and physicians as to which patients are catheterized. Generally accepted indications for use of indwelling urinary catheters include perioperative use for selected surgical procedures, use during prolonged surgical procedures with general or spinal anesthesia, urine output monitoring in critically ill patients, management of acute urinary retention and urinary obstruction, temporary relief or longer term drainage of clinically significant urinary retention if surgical correction is not indicated, assistance in pressure ulcer healing for incontinent patients, and, as an exception, at a patient's request to improve comfort.[20,77,84]

Alternatives to Indwelling Urethral Catheterization
Although comparative studies are sparse, the consensus is that indwelling urethral catheterization places the patient at the greatest risk for CA-bacteriuria and other complications, and that alternative bladder drainage modalities should be used when appropriate.[102] Alternatives to indwelling urethral catheterization include the use of external collection devices, including condom catheters, intermittent catheterization, or suprapubic catheterization. Each of these catheterization methods has been shown in selected populations to reduce the risk of CA-bacteriuria over the short term. However, there are limitations to the use of all such urinary catheterization alternatives.

Condom Catheterization. In non-randomized studies, use of condom catheters has been shown to result in a lower incidence of CA-bacteriuria compared with indwelling urethral catheters.[20] These impressions were confirmed in a recent prospective, randomized trial of 75 men at a Veterans Administration hospital in which patients without dementia who had an indwelling catheter were about five times as likely to develop CA-bacteriuria, CA-UTI or to die (CA-bacteriuria was the predominant outcome in this combined outcome variable) as those with appropriately sized condom catheters.[103] No difference was seen in those patients with dementia, which may have to do with the increased risk of CA-bacteriuria in patients who manipulate their condom catheters.[20] Thus, in men with low post-void residual volume who are not cognitively impaired, condom catheters are preferable to indwelling urethral catheters for short-term catheterization and probably for long-term catheterization. Some men may not be able to wear a condom catheter, such as those with a small or ulcerated penis. There is currently no satisfactory external catheter suitable for use by women.

Intermittent Catheterization. Intermittent catheterization is a technique in which the bladder is drained of urine by catheterization by oneself or a caregiver usually every 4 to 6 hours, so that the amount of urine obtained with each collection is generally no more than 500 mL.[102] The schedule of intermittent catheterization is tailored for each individual to minimize the number of catheterizations while not allowing the bladder to become overdistended. Guttman and Frankel in 1966 described intermittent catheterization using sterile technique,[104] and Lapides and colleagues later demonstrated that the clean (non-sterile) technique was safe, and associated with a low incidence of complications in patients with neurogenic bladders.[105] Intermittent catheterization is widely viewed to be associated with fewer complications than indwelling catheterization, including CA-bacteriuria, hydronephrosis, bladder and renal calculi, bladder cancer, and autonomic dysreflexia,[102,106] and it has become the standard of care for appropriate women and men with SCIs. It is also a commonly used alternative in patients without SCI who need long-term assistance with voiding.[42,107] However, there are no randomized controlled trials that have compared intermittent urethral, indwelling urethral, suprapubic or condom catheterization in patients on long-term catheterization, including those with neurogenic bladders.[108] On the other hand, a meta-analysis of trials comparing catheterization methods in patients (mostly post-surgical) undergoing short-term catheterization found that indwelling urethral catheterization was associated with more CA-bacteriuria than intermittent catheterization (relative risk [RR] 2.90; 95% confidence interval [CI] 1.44 to 5.84), even though indwelling catheterization was less costly.[109] Nevertheless, intermittent catheterization is not commonly used for short-term catheterization because of the educational, motivational, and staff-time requirements necessary for its implementation.

Among patients undergoing long-term intermittent catheterization, randomized controlled studies in adults in hospitals, LTCFs and outpatient settings with or without neurogenic bladders have shown no difference in risk of CA-ASB or CA-UTI with use of sterile technique compared with clean (non-sterile) technique, with use of sterile catheters versus multiple-use catheters with the clean technique, or with daily or weekly replacement of multiple-use catheters.[107,110] Different techniques have been studied to reduce the microbial contamination of multiple-use catheters, including rinsing with tap water, air-drying, and keeping it dry until reuse, microwaving or soaking the catheter in disinfectants, but there are no published trials evaluating the effectiveness of these methods in preventing CA-bacteriuria. Although there are no data that re-use of catheters increases infection risk, it is inconvenient for many patients who find it difficult to clean their catheters away from home and others find it non-aesthetic.

Complications associated with long-term intermittent catheterization, although apparently less common than with indwelling urethral catheterization, include CA-bacteriuria, prostatitis, epididymitis, urethritis, urethral trauma with bleeding and subsequent urethral strictures and false passages.[102,106] Hydrophilic catheters, compared with standard catheters, reduce the friction of catheter insertion and urethral inflammation and are associated with improved patient satisfaction, and some studies suggest a reduction in CA-bacteriuria. These catheters have been widely used in Europe for many years in patients on intermittent catheterization. However, currently available data do not support the routine use of hydrophilic catheters to prevent CA-bacteriuria or sequelae of urethral trauma in patients managed with intermittent catheterization.[110,111] Larger well-designed studies of the hydrophilic catheter are warranted.

Limitations to intermittent catheterization include limited staff to perform the procedure or educate patients, inability or unwillingness of patients to perform frequent catheterizations, or abnormal urethral anatomy such as stricture, false passages, or bladder neck obstruction. Upper extremity impairment due to cervical SCI or other abnormality, obesity, and spasticity also make intermittent catheterization challenging for both males and females.

Suprapubic Catheterization. Potential advantages of suprapubic catheters in patients who need bladder drainage, compared with indwelling urethral catheters, include lower risk of CA-bacteriuria because abdominal skin is less likely to be colonized with uropathogens compared with the urethra, reduced risk of urethral trauma and stricture, less interference with sexual activity, and, in those undergoing short-term catheterization, ability to more easily assess the appropriate time for catheter removal. A meta-analysis of randomized trials in patients undergoing short-term catheterization found that indwelling urethral catheterization, compared to suprapubic catheterization, was associated with more CA-bacteriuria (RR 2.60; 95% CI 2.12-3.18), recatheterization (RR 4.12; 95% CI 2.94-7.56), and discomfort (RR 2.98; 95% CI 2.31-3.85).[109] A review of randomized, controlled trials comparing indwelling urethral and suprapubic catheters in patients undergoing colorectal surgery had similar conclusions.[112] Suprapubic catheters appear to be commonly used in gynecologic surgery in some centers, but their use is limited, presumably because their insertion is an invasive procedure, they are harder to change when necessary, and they still can leak. As mentioned previously, different catheterization methods have not been compared in patients with neurogenic bladders,[108] or other patient groups on long-term catheterization. Comparisons of intermittent urethral catheterization, suprapubic catheterization, and indwelling urethral catheterization are needed in such patient groups.

Techniques for Catheter Insertion and Maintenance

Although use of aseptic technique for inserting indwelling urethral catheters is widely recommended,[77] few data exist to support such a recommendation. Some studies have shown that catheter insertion outside the operating room (where adherence to aseptic technique may be less than optimal) is associated with a higher risk of CA-bacteriuria.[66] However, no significant difference in risk of CA-bacteriuria was found in a study of 156 patients undergoing preoperative urethral catheterization who were randomized to sterile versus clean technique for catheter insertion.[113] Moreover, in patients managed with intermittent catheterization who are catheterized multiple times daily, there appears to be no difference in infection risk with non-sterile compared with sterile technique. Nevertheless, given the ubiquity of multi-drug resistant pathogens in the health care environment, it seems prudent to use aseptic technique for inserting indwelling urethral catheters in patients in the hospital or LTCF.[77]

Introduction of the closed catheter drainage system, in which the collecting bag is attached to the distal end of the collecting tube, was perhaps the most important advance in prevention of CA-bacteriuria.[14,18,20] In patients managed with catheter drainage into open containers, 95% of patients develop CA-bacteriuria by 96 hours.[114] By comparison, about 50% of patients managed with closed drainage systems develop CA-bacteriuria by 14 days of continuous catheterization.[18] Based on such historical comparisons, closed systems have become the standard for bladder drainage. However, it is important that closed drainage systems remain closed, since disconnections at the catheter-collecting tube junctions have been shown to increase the risk of CA-bacteriuria.[3,13,115] Diagnostic urine samples should be aspirated using aseptic technique through ports in the distal catheter and larger volumes of urine for special analyses should be collected aseptically from the drainage bag with care not to contaminate the end of the drainage tube from potentially contaminated measuring containers.[64] The catheter should be properly anchored to minimize movement, since movement of urethral catheters may cause urethral trauma and may facilitate the ascension of organisms up the urethral-catheter interface. Importantly, the drainage tube should not be allowed to move above the level of the bladder or below the level of the collection bag.[21]

PREVENTION STRATEGIES WITH POSSIBLE BENEFIT

Although these practices might have benefit, they are not recommended for routine use.

Antimicrobial Coated Catheters

In vitro studies have shown anti-adherence or antimicrobial activity associated with silver-, minocycline and rifampin-, and nitrofurazone-coated catheters.[116-118] A meta-analysis of randomized trials comparing types of indwelling urinary catheters in hospitalized adults undergoing short-term catheterization found that use of silver alloy catheters, but not silver oxide catheters, compared with standard catheters, significantly reduced the incidence of CA-ASB in patients catheterized up to 2 weeks.[119] Other meta-analyses have also concluded that silver alloy-coated, but not silver oxide-coated, catheters are protective against CA-bacteriuria in patients catheterized short-term, but with no clear effect on significant clinical endpoints including CA-UTI, morbidity, secondary bloodstream infection, other health care–associated infections, and cost savings in any patient population.[120,121] Moreover, it has been proposed recently that the purported benefits of silver alloy in preventing CA-bacteriuria are attributable to the different catheters (silicone vs. latex) used in previous trials, rather than the silver alloy.[122,123] Antibiotic-coated catheters have also been evaluated in clinical trials. In one study, patients randomized to catheters impregnated with minocycline and rifampicin had significantly lower rates of CA-gram-positive bacteriuria, but not with CA-gram-negative bacteria or CA-candiduria, than those in the control group up to 2 weeks after catheter insertion.[124] In another study of nitrofurazone-coated catheters in adult trauma patients, CA-bacteriuria and candiduria (there were few episodes of CA-candiduria) occurred less frequently in the nitrofurazone catheter group than in the control group, with the reduction apparent after only a few days and lasting throughout the first 30 days of catheterization.[125] There are no data to show that antimicrobial-coated catheters are beneficial in patients managed with long-term catheterization (>30 days).[126] Resistance to catheter antimicrobials, particularly antibiotics, has not been demonstrated in published clinical trials, but this remains a concern and needs further study. In summary, although antimicrobial-coated urinary catheters appear to have some benefit in the prevention of CA-ASB in some trials of short-term catheterized patients, questions remain about their safety and effectiveness and, thus, available data do not support their routine use to prevent CA-bacteriuria.

Prophylaxis with Antimicrobial Agents

Systemic Antibiotics. Systemic antibiotic drug therapy has been shown repeatedly in prospective and retrospective studies to prevent CA-bacteriuria, although the protective effect appears to be transient and development of antimicrobial resistance has been noted in some studies.[14,20,65] A meta-analysis of randomized, controlled trials in surgical and non-surgical patients undergoing short-term catheterization found that prophylaxis with antibiotics such as trimethoprim-sulfamethoxazole or ciprofloxacin reduces the rate of CA-bacteriuria and, in some studies, CA-UTI, but that concerns about selection for antimicrobial resistance have not been adequately addressed.[127] Systemic antimicrobials, including fluoroquinolones, nitrofurantoin, and trimethoprim-sulfamethoxazole, also appear to reduce CA-bacteriuria and CA-UTI in long-term catheterized patients,[128] but antimicrobial resistance has been demonstrated in several trials in this population. For example, one study comparing norfloxacin and placebo in elderly nursing home patients with indwelling urethral catheters demonstrated a highly significant reduction of CA-UTI, but 25% of strains in placebo patients vs. 90% of strains in norfloxacin patients were resistant to norfloxacin at the end of the prophylaxis period.[129]

Because of the potential for the development of antimicrobial resistance and adverse effects and cost, routine use of systemic antimicrobial agents to prevent CA-bacteriuria or CA-UTI should be discouraged. Some authorities have suggested a possible role for prophylactic systemic antimicrobial agents in short-term catheterized patients who may be at high risk for complications if UTI occurs, such as patients who are granulocytopenic, undergo urologic or gynecologic surgery, or undergo surgery involving a foreign body.[14,21,130] However, no studies of prophylactic antibiotics have been performed in catheterized persons in these groups.

Unfortunately, as many as 60% to 80% of hospitalized, catheterized patients receive antimicrobials for a variety of reasons,[18,131] and not controlling for this important variable in the analyses of many intervention trials may explain why some interventions have not been shown to be effective in preventing CA-bacteriuria.

Methenamine Salts. Methenamine salts (methenamine mandelate and methenamine hippurate) are hydrolyzed to ammonia and formaldehyde, which is responsible for the antibacterial activity of methenamine. Antimicrobial activity in urine is correlated with urinary concentrations of formaldehyde, and the urinary concentration of formaldehyde is dependent on the concentration of methenamine in the urine and the urine pH.[132] Maintaining a low urinary pH (below 6) is necessary to achieve bactericidal concentrations of formaldehyde, but the association between therapeutic efficacy and low urinary pH has not been confirmed consistently.[132] In addition, the optimal method to acidify the urine in a patient on methenamine is not known. Ascorbic acid is often used to acidify the urine, but up to 4 g per day has shown no significant effect on mean urinary pH, and doses as high as 12 g per day may be required to adequately acidify the urine.[132]

Methenamine salts have been shown to prevent uncomplicated cystitis in young women,[132-134] but are not as effective or convenient as currently available regimens for prevention of UTI. In addition, methenamine salts are generally considered to have limited effectiveness in preventing CA-UTI in patients with indwelling catheters for whom the time for hydrolysis to formaldehyde is limited.[20,132] However, a meta-analysis of randomized, controlled studies of methenamine hippurate in patients undergoing short-term catheterization following gynecologic surgery found that CA-bacteriuria and CA-UTI were significantly reduced in the methenamine group compared to the control group.[135] This unexpected benefit may have been due in part to the administration of methenamine for several days after the catheters had been removed in some cases.[136] Methenamine does not appear to prevent CA-bacteriuria or CA-UTI in SCI patients with neurogenic bladders irrespective of the method of bladder management.[137,138] There are no published data on the use of methenamine in patients using condom catheterization.

Overall, the data are unconvincing that methenamine is effective in reducing the risk of CA-bacteriuria or CA-UTI in patients managed with long-term indwelling catheterization—patients most in need of an effective agent that does not select for antimicrobial resistance. Methenamine does appear to be effective in post-gynecologic surgery patients undergoing short-term catheterization, and its use in this situation may be considered, although this group suffers limited morbidity from CA-bacteriuria. It may also be reasonable to consider a trial use of methenamine in noncatheterized patients who have recurrent nosocomial UTI or patients on intermittent catheterization who have recurrent episodes of CA-UTI, even though its benefit in such patients is unproven. Methenamine is likely to be most effective in situations where the urine pH is low and there is time for hydrolysis of methenamine to achieve sufficient concentrations of formaldehyde. If used, the recommended dose of methenamine hippurate is 1 g twice daily and that for methenamine mandelate is 1 g four times daily, and the urinary pH should be maintained below 6.0.

PREVENTION STRATEGIES WITH LITTLE BENEFIT

These strategies have little or no demonstrated benefit and are not recommended for routine use.

Enhanced Meatal Care

Reducing meatal colonization would seem to be a reasonable measure to reduce the risk of CA-UTI, given that ascension of uropathogens along the catheter-urethral interface is the predominant source of CA-bacteriuria.[66] However, results of large randomized trials have shown no significant reduction in CA-bacteriuria in men or women, compared with usual care (debris removal at daily baths), with one or more times daily meatal cleansing using non-antiseptic green soap or applications of povidone-iodine solution and ointment, poly-antibiotic ointment or cream, or silver sulfadiazine 1% cream.[14,19,20,65] Likewise, simultaneous interventions to block bacterial entry at the urethral insertion site, catheter drainage tube junction, and outflow tube of the drainage bag were not effective in preventing CA-bacteriuria.[19] Possible reasons why enhanced meatal care has not been effective in reducing CA-bacteriuria include the negative effect of increased catheter manipulation associated with the interventions, inadequate residual antiseptic activity of the topical agent, and lack of effect on the intraluminal route of infection.

Cranberry Products

There is some evidence from randomized, controlled trials that cranberry products may be effective in reducing the risk of symptomatic UTIs in women with recurrent UTI, but its effectiveness for elderly men and women or people requiring catheterization is less certain.[139] Randomized, placebo-controlled studies of cranberry in doses up to 2 g daily to prevent CA-bacteriuria or CA-UTI in patients with neurogenic bladders are mostly negative.[137,139] The routine use of cranberry products for prevention of nosocomial UTI should be discouraged due to lack of clearly demonstrated efficacy in preventing CA-ASB or CA-UTI, problems of tolerance with long-term use, and cost. There are no published data on the use of cranberry products for prevention of CA-ASB or CA-UTI in catheterized adults without neurogenic bladder.

Bladder Irrigation with Antimicrobials or Saline

Bladder irrigation with povidone-iodine or chlorhexidine has been effective in preventing CA-bacteriuria in some studies of orthopedic and urologic patients undergoing short-term catheterization.[140,141] Overall, however, bladder irrigation with agents such as povidone-iodine, chlorhexidine, neomycin, or polymyxin B sulfate has shown little overall benefit in the era of closed urinary drainage.[14,20] In one demonstrative study, 187 adult patients who required short-term urinary catheterization were randomized to closed drainage with a triple-lumen, neomycin-polymyxin irrigated system, or a double-lumen non-irrigated catheter system.[115] There was no significant difference in the rates of CA-bacteriuria between the two groups, but uropathogens isolated from irrigated patients were significantly more resistant to the irrigating antibiotic than those in the non-irrigated group. In summary, catheter irrigation does not appear to be effective in preventing or eradicating CA-bacteriuria in the majority of patients with short-term or long-term indwelling catheterization, is time consuming, and may select for antimicrobial-resistant organisms.

Catheter irrigation also does not appear to be beneficial in reducing the risk of catheter blockage resulting from encrustation formed by urease-producing organisms in the catheter biofilm. In a randomized crossover trial of 32 long-term catheterized and bacteriuric women in whom 10 weeks of once-daily normal saline irrigation was compared with 10 weeks of no irrigation, the incidence of catheter obstructions and febrile episodes, including those that appeared to be of urinary origin, were similar.[142]

Antimicrobial Drugs in the Drainage Bag

Once the drainage bag becomes contaminated, subsequent CA-bacteriuria occurs in almost all patients who remain catheterized,[13] and positioning of the drainage tube above the level of the bladder or below the level of the collection bag is a predictor for an increased risk of CA-bacteriuria.[21] Studies suggest an intraluminal source, presumably secondary to contaminated catheter drainage bags, is the origin of CA-bacteriuria in approximately one third of cases,[66] although one large study showed that bag contamination with the same organism responsible for CA-bacteriuria preceded infection in only 7% of

patients who developed bacteriuria.[79] Investigators have attempted to prevent CA-bacteriuria by sterilizing the drainage bag, but results of randomized trials evaluating the addition of chlorhexidine, hydrogen peroxide, or povidone-iodine to the bag suggest that this intervention is not effective.[14,20,65,79] Such a strategy would not be expected to be effective if the integrity of the closed drainage system is carefully maintained, as that should minimize bacterial entry into the drainage bag.

Routine Catheter Change

Urinary catheters readily develop biofilms on their inner and outer surfaces once they are inserted, and these biofilms protect uropathogens from antibiotics and the host immune response.[54] In long-term catheterized patients, catheters are often changed routinely at periodic intervals (e.g., monthly) to reduce the risk of CA-bacteriuria as well as for aesthetic reasons but, surprisingly, there are no published clinical trials that have evaluated this practice. Moreover, it has been recommended that patients who experience repeated early catheter blockage should have their catheters changed every 7 to 10 days to avoid obstruction,[143] but this practice also has not been evaluated in clinical trials. The practice of routine catheter change with the purpose of preventing infection or blockage, or both, is unlikely to change in the absence of data to address this issue.

Prophylactic Antimicrobials at Catheter Removal or Replacement

Fever and bacteremia can occur at the time of removal or replacement of a urethral catheter, and prophylactic antibiotics are sometimes used to prevent such events. Among catheterized and bacteriuric women in LTCFs, transient fever is twice as common within 24 hours of catheter replacement, compared with other days.[29] Studies in chronically catheterized and bacteriuric men and women have shown that bacteremia occurs in 4% to 10% of patients after urethral catheter removal or replacement, but episodes are transient and asymptomatic.[144-146] Randomized, controlled trials with oral ciprofloxacin or bladder irrigation with povidone-iodine administered prior to catheter removal have shown no benefit in preventing CA-bacteriuria,[147,148] but the effect of antimicrobial prophylaxis on prevention of bacteremia is unknown. Nevertheless, based on these observations, prophylactic antimicrobials are not routinely recommended for catheter removal or replacement. This recommendation is also supported by the low rate of serious complications in the large number of patients undergoing long-term intermittent catheterization with clean technique in the setting of chronic bacteriuria.

STRATEGIES FOR FURTHER INVESTIGATION

Intraurethral devices that are easily inserted at cystoscopy can remain in place for months (migration often occurs), and are well tolerated. The devices have been developed to relieve urinary retention without use of a urethral catheter in men with prostatic hypertrophy.[149-151] A magnetic controlled urethral prosthesis for the management of chronic urinary retention in women has shown some promise.[152] In patients with SCI and neurogenic bladders, devices or techniques other than catheterization in use or under development include artificial urethral sphincters, urethral stents, intraurethral pumps, electrical stimulation of the sacral root, intraspinal microstimulation, urethral afferent stimulation, and injectable microstimulators.[153] It remains to be seen whether these catheter-avoiding techniques will reduce the risk of CA-bacteriuria.

Strategies to induce bacterial interference to reduce the risk of CA-UTI in patients on long-term catheterization by inoculating organisms of low virulence into the bladder hold promise, based on small pilot trials,[154] and are under current investigation.

Strategies to inhibit biofilm formation are under investigation. Treatment of abiotic surfaces with group II capsular polysaccharides has been shown to drastically reduce both initial adhesion and biofilm development by important nosocomial pathogens, which may lead to new strategies to limit biofilm formation on medical indwelling devices.[155]

Nosocomial Asymptomatic Bacteriuria

ROUTINE SCREENING AND TREATMENT

Screening and treatment of ASB have not been shown to be beneficial, select for antimicrobial resistance and are not recommended, except in pregnant women and patients who undergo traumatic genitourinary procedures associated with mucosal bleeding.[4,156] Populations that have been extensively studied and for whom these recommendations apply include premenopausal, nonpregnant women; diabetic women; older people living in the community; elderly, institutionalized subjects; persons with SCI; and catheterized patients.[4] For example, in 35 patients undergoing long-term catheterization, a prospective, randomized trial of cephalexin or no antibiotic therapy for episodes of CA-ASB caused by susceptible organisms reported no differences between the two groups in incidence and prevalence of CA-bacteriuria, CA-UTI, or obstructed catheters in patients followed up to 44 weeks.[157] In addition, 47% of reinfecting organisms in the cephalexin group compared with 26% in the control group were highly resistant to cephalexin. Even if treatment of CA-ASB was found to be useful, one study in which daily catheter urine cultures were obtained found that 60% of 25 episodes of CA-UTI occurred on the same day that CA-bacteriuria was first detected,[26] complicating attempts at preemptive therapy. Moreover, when CA-UTIs do occur, they generally respond promptly to treatment.[158] It is not known whether eradication of CA-ASB might be beneficial in reducing cross-infection or inappropriate antimicrobial usage; this has not been studied.

A prospective, randomized, placebo-controlled trial of antimicrobial treatment of CA-ASB persisting 48 hours after removal of short-term catheters in hospitalized women reported significantly improved microbiologic and clinical outcomes at 14 days in treated women.[159] Seven (17%) of 42 women randomized to receive no therapy developed CA-UTI by 14 days, whereas no women in the treatment group became symptomatic. Nevertheless, the long term benefit of screening for and eradicating post-catheterization CA-ASB to prevent CA-UTI warrants further study,[14] and this approach is currently not recommended.

Management of Nosocomial Urinary Tract Infection

Bacteriuria in a catheterized person with symptoms or signs compatible with a UTI (usually fever) in the absence of another obvious cause of the symptoms or signs should be treated with antimicrobials. Even when another potential source of fever is identified, it is often appropriate to ensure antimicrobial coverage of the urinary organism, especially in sick patients. The wide variety of underlying conditions, diverse spectrum of possible etiologic agents, and paucity of controlled clinical trials with stratification according to specific complicating factors make generalizing about antimicrobial therapy difficult for nosocomial CA-UTI. Antibiotics alone may not be successful, if underlying anatomic, functional or metabolic defects are not corrected. However, urinary catheterization itself should not complicate eradication of bacteriuria, although it predisposes to early recurrence.

URINE CULTURE AND CATHETER REPLACEMENT BEFORE TREATMENT

Nosocomial UTIs, especially in patients with long-term catheterization, are often polymicrobial and caused by multiple-drug–resistant uropathogens, so urine cultures should be obtained prior to treatment to confirm that the empiric regimen provides appropriate coverage and to allow tailoring of the regimen based on antimicrobial susceptibility data.[42,130] The culture should be obtained from a freshly placed catheter if the catheter has been in place for a few days, because the catheter biofilm may result in spurious culture results.[51,52] Moreover, clinical outcomes are improved if the catheter is replaced, as shown in a prospective randomized controlled trial in elderly nursing home residents with long-term indwelling catheters and CA-UTI. This study demonstrated that patients whose catheters had been in place for longer than 2 weeks and who underwent catheter replacement before antimicrobial treatment had significantly shorter time to improved clinical status and significantly lower rates of polymicrobic CA-bacteriuria and CA-UTI after therapy, compared with those who did not undergo catheter replacement.[160] These study findings support replacing the catheter and obtaining a urine culture from a freshly placed catheter prior to antibiotic treatment for CA-UTI if the catheter has been in place for at least 2 weeks and cannot be removed.

CHOICE OF ANTIBIOTIC

The choice of antibiotic agent for empiric treatment should be based on available information, including the urine Gram-stain results, previous urine culture results, or the antimicrobial sensitivity patterns of urinary pathogens isolated in the patient's hospital or LTCF.[42,130] The likelihood of multi-drug resistance is much greater in patients with nosocomial UTIs acquired in a medical or surgical ICU or LTCF compared with a patient on a general ward who has had little previous exposure to the hospital or LTCF. Depending on the antimicrobial susceptibility patterns in the hospital or LTCF, patients with mild-to-moderate illness without alterations in mental status or hemodynamic status may be treated with a urinary fluoroquinolone, such as ciprofloxacin or levofloxacin, or a broad-spectrum cephalosporin such as ceftriaxone or cefepime. Potential concerns with these choices include the increasing prevalence of resistance to fluoroquinolones in institutional settings and the frequency of enterococcal infections.[42] If the patient has evidence of pyelonephritis or urosepsis, one should consider a broader-spectrum drug such as piperacillin-tazobactam or a carbapenem for empiric treatment. If the urine Gram stain shows gram-positive cocci (most likely enterococci or staphylococci), treatment with vancomycin is reasonable. The antimicrobial regimen should be tailored as appropriate when the infecting strain has been identified and antimicrobial susceptibilities are known.

DURATION

The optimal duration of antibiotic treatment for CA-UTI is not known. Reviews of complicated UTI have recommended treatment durations from 7 to 10 days,[14] 7 to 14 days,[42] and 7 to 21 days,[130] depending on the severity of the infection. However, it is desirable to limit the duration of treatment, especially for milder infections, to reduce the selection pressure for drug-resistant flora, especially in patients on long-term catheterization. Few studies have been performed that evaluate duration of treatment in populations with CA- or other complicated UTIs. In one small trial of women with lower tract CA-UTI, cure rates were comparable with a single dose and 10-day regimen of trimethoprim-sulfamethoxazole.[159] However, single-dose therapy was ineffective in eradicating bacteriuria in institutionalized, elderly men.[161] In a randomized, double-blind, placebo-controlled trial comparing 3-day and 14-day regimens of ciprofloxacin for the treatment of mild CA-UTI in 60 patients with SCI, there was no difference in clinical outcomes at long-term follow-up.[162] Most recently, clinical and microbiologic success rates following treatment were almost identical in a noninferiority study of 619 patients with acute pyelonephritis or complicated UTI treated with a 5-day course of levofloxacin or a 10-day course of ciprofloxacin.[163] These data suggest that a 7-day regimen is reasonable for most patients with CA-UTI, depending on their clinical response, and shorter regimens, such as a 5-day regimen of a urinary fluoroquinolone, are likely to be sufficient in those patients who are less severely ill, infected with uropathogens susceptible to the antibiotic used, and have a rapid response to treatment.

Fungal Urinary Tract Infection

Candida species cause the vast majority of fungal infections of the urinary tract and account for 10% to 15% of nosocomial UTIs,[164] and most hospitalized patients with candiduria are outside the ICU.[165] In a prospective multicenter surveillance study of 861 hospitalized patients with funguria, *C. albicans* was found in 52% and *Candida glabrata* in 16%.[166] In patients with nosocomial UTIs in medical-surgical ICUs reported in the U.S. National Nosocomial Infection Surveillance System from 1992 to 1998, *C. albicans* constituted 15.3% and all fungal isolates 31.2% of all urinary isolates.[6] In medical ICUs, *C. albicans* was the most commonly reported urinary isolate (21%) and all fungal isolates constituted 39% of all isolates.[167] The proportion of isolates represented by fungi were almost double that for the period 1986 to 1989.[167] *Candida parapsilosis*, a common cause of candidemia in adults and neonates, is uncommonly isolated from urine of adults.[168]

Among patients with nosocomial funguria enrolled in a multicenter prospective surveillance study, 85% had concomitant nonfungal infections, 90% previous exposure to antimicrobial agents, 83% urinary tract drainage devices, 39% diabetes, 38% urinary tract abnormalities, and 22% a malignancy—only 11% had no obvious underlying illness.[166] Although only 1.3% of the 530 patients with candiduria followed for 12 weeks had documented candidemia, the importance of comorbid conditions was reflected in the 20% mortality rate.

Determination of the clinical significance of candiduria can be problematic, as it can represent contamination of a voided specimen, colonization of catheters or stents, bladder infection, ascending kidney infection, or kidney infection associated with candidemia. Hematogenous dissemination is relatively much more likely to be the source of candiduria than is found with bacteriuria.[168] Unlike bacteriuria, there are no established colony count thresholds to help distinguish contamination from bladder infection. The presence of pseudohyphae in the urine is also not helpful in distinguishing contamination from infection. In noncatheterized women with candiduria, a catheter specimen may be indicated to rule out contamination with perineal flora.[168] In the catheterized patient, pyuria is a nonspecific finding, but its absence suggests that candiduria is not causing tissue invasion. Most nosocomial candiduria occurs in catheterized patients, and most episodes are asymptomatic. In the large prospective study of nosocomial funguria mentioned earlier, only 2% to 4% of patients had urinary symptoms,[166] although comorbidities and urinary catheterization may complicate assessment of symptoms.

Ascending infection of the kidney and disseminated candidiasis are rarely associated with candiduria and usually occur in the setting of obstruction of the urinary tract. In a retrospective study of 26 cases of candidemia associated with a well-defined urinary tract source, urinary tract abnormalities, mostly obstruction, were present in 88%, and 73% had undergone urinary tract procedures before the onset of candidemia.[169] Episodes of candidemia were brief and low-grade in intensity, although 2 of 5 in-hospital deaths were attributable to candidiasis. Paired urine and blood strains of *Candida*, however, may not be the same strain, as demonstrated in a case-control study in which 52% of paired strains were different by molecular typing.[170] Other complications associated with fungal infections of the genitourinary tract include fever, fungus balls in the bladder or renal pelvis, renal and perirenal abscesses, emphysematous pyelitis or pyelonephritis, and papillary necrosis—many of these complication are more likely to occur in diabetics.

Few treatment studies have been performed in patients with candiduria,[164] and there remain questions as to whom to treat, when to treat, and how long to treat. Asymptomatic nosocomial candiduria rarely requires treatment, because it often resolves spontaneously, morbidity is low and treatment is often followed by rapid recurrence and may select out for resistant organisms.[171,172] In the large prospective observational study mentioned previously, funguria cleared in 76% of 155 patients who had no specific therapy for funguria and in 35% of 116 patients who had their catheter removed as the only treatment.[166] Other studies have shown spontaneous clearance rates of candiduria ranging from 29% to 62%.[166] In a randomized, placebo-controlled trial of 316 hospitalized patients with asymptomatic or minimally symptomatic candiduria, a 2-week course of fluconazole resulted in signifi-

cantly higher eradication rates than placebo at 2 weeks of treatment (50% vs. 29%), but there was no significant difference in candiduria rates 2 weeks after completion of treatment.[172] In placebo recipients who had their catheters removed, 41% had eradication of candiduria compared with only 20% who had their catheters replaced. Pyelonephritis, candidemia, and fungus-related death were not observed in this study. Thus, treatment of asymptomatic candiduria is not generally indicated, but the contributing cause of candiduria should be addressed, such as changing or removing the indwelling catheter or stent and discontinuing inappropriate antibiotic therapy.

Candiduria should be treated in symptomatic patients, and those with systemic signs or symptoms should be evaluated for disseminated infection with imaging and blood cultures. Treatment is also indicated in patients with neutropenia, infants with low birth weight, and patients who will undergo urologic manipulations, because these conditions have a higher association with upper tract infection or dissemination.[168,171] Recent data have raised questions as to whether asymptomatic candiduria in patients with renal transplants warrants treatment.[173] Treatment strategies tried over the past few decades include bladder irrigation with amphotericin B, intravenous amphotericin B, oral flucytosine, and fluconazole. The treatment regimen should be tailored according to the identified Candida species and whether localized or disseminated infection is present. Oral fluconazole is the most commonly used regimen; of note, doses adjusted for renal insufficiency may result in subtherapeutic concentrations.[164] Systemic amphotericin B deoxycholate is no more effective than fluconazole for susceptible strains, and bladder irrigation with amphotericin B deoxycholate is rarely used. Echinocandins such as caspofungin are minimally excreted and voriconazole is not excreted in the urine and they should not be considered first line agents for candiduria. However, these drugs achieve appropriate tissue levels and would be appropriate in patients with invasive infections involving the renal or bladder parenchyma. Case reports suggest that caspofungin and micafungin may be effective in patients with *C. glabrata*-associated UTI.[174,175] Even with apparently successful local or systemic antifungal therapy for candiduria, relapse is frequent, and this likelihood is increased by continued use of a urinary catheter. Persistent candiduria, especially in immunocompromised patients, warrants radiologic imaging of the kidneys to evaluate for hydronephrosis, bezoars, or perinephric abscesses associated with ascending infection.

Summary

Nosocomial bacteriuria and candiduria are very common, mostly associated with urinary catheterization, and usually asymptomatic. Whereas any symptomatic UTI should be treated, published data do not support routine screening to detect nosocomial bacteriuria or candiduria in asymptomatic patients, because treatment does not appear to alter the natural course of infection and an increase in antimicrobial resistance often results. However, among asymptomatic patients with bacteriuria or funguria, we need a better understanding as to who has upper tract involvement or tissue invasion, how these affect the clinical course, and thus, who, if any, might benefit from screening and treatment. The quality of clinical trials needs to be improved, as many are nonrandomized, underpowered, and use nonspecific terminology and poorly described methodology. Studies of interventions to prevent CA bacterial infections need to address whether they prevent not only CA-UTI (which many have not), but also whether prevention of CA-ASB reduces inappropriate antimicrobial use and cross-infection. Safe, effective and tolerable external urine collection devices for women are needed.

Strategies that are effective for prevention of CA-bacteriuria are likely to also prevent CA-candiduria. The most effective way to reduce nosocomial UTIs is to reduce urinary catheterization by restricting use to patients who have clear indications and by removing the catheter as soon as it is no longer needed. Implementation of strategies to reduce catheterization is likely to have more impact on CA-bacteriuria than implementation of other strategies addressed in this guideline.

However, use of multiple infection control techniques and strategies simultaneously (called *bundling*) likely offers the best opportunity to reduce the morbidity and mortality associated with nosocomial infections.[176] Hopefully, research into better alternatives to catheterization and methods to prevent or limit biofilm formation will eventually provide relief to patients who do require urinary catheterization.

REFERENCES

1. Horan TC, Andrus M, Dudeck MA. CDC/NHSN surveillance definition of health care-associated infection and criteria for specific types of infections in the acute care setting. *Am J Infect Control.* 2008;36:309-332.
2. Platt R, Polk BF, Murdock B, et al. Mortality associated with nosocomial urinary-tract infection. *N Engl J Med.* 1982;307:637-642.
3. Platt R, Polk BF, Murdock B, et al. Reduction of mortality associated with nosocomial urinary tract infection. *Lancet.* 1983;1:893-897.
4. Nicolle LE, Bradley S, Colgan R, et al. Infectious Diseases Society of America guidelines for the diagnosis and treatment of asymptomatic bacteriuria in adults. *Clin Infect Dis.* 2005;40:643-654.
5. Bronsema DA, Adams JR, Pallares R, et al. Secular trends in rates and etiology of nosocomial urinary tract infections at a university hospital. *J Urol.* 1993;150:414-416.
6. Richards MJ, Edwards JR, Culver DH, et al. Nosocomial infections in combined medical-surgical intensive care units in the United States. *Infect Control Hosp Epidemiol.* 2000;21:510-515.
7. Tambyah PA. Catheter-associated urinary tract infections: Diagnosis and prophylaxis. *Int J Antimicrob Agents.* 2004;24(Suppl 1):S44-S48.
8. Haley RW, Hooton TM, Culver DH, et al. Nosocomial infections in U.S. hospitals, 1975-1976: estimated frequency by selected characteristics of patients. *Am J Med.* 1981;70:947-959.
9. Haley RW, Culver DH, White JW, et al. The nationwide nosocomial infection rate. A new need for vital statistics. *Am J Epidemiol.* 1985;121:159-167.
10. Nicolle LE, Strausbaugh LJ, Garibaldi RA. Infections and antibiotic resistance in nursing homes. *Clin Microbiol Rev.* 1996;9:1-17.
11. Smith PW, Bennett G, Bradley S, et al. SHEA/APIC guideline: Infection prevention and control in the long-term care facility. *Infect Control Hosp Epidemiol.* 2008;29:785-814.
12. Weinstein JW, Mazon D, Pantelick E, et al. A decade of prevalence surveys in a tertiary-care center: Trends in nosocomial infection rates, device utilization, and patient acuity. *Infect Control Hosp Epidemiol.* 1999;20:543-548.
13. Garibaldi RA, Burke JP, Dickman ML, et al. Factors predisposing to bacteriuria during indwelling urethral catheterization. *N Engl J Med.* 1974;291:215-219.
14. Warren JW. Catheter-associated urinary tract infections. *Infect Dis Clin North Am.* 1997;11:609-622.
15. Warren JW, Steinberg L, Hebel JR, et al. The prevalence of urethral catheterization in Maryland nursing homes. *Arch Intern Med.* 1989;149:1535-1537.
16. Garibaldi RA, Brodine S, Matsumiya S. Infections among patients in nursing homes: Policies, prevalence, problems. *N Engl J Med.* 1981;305:731-735.
17. Warren JW. Catheter-associated bacteriuria in long-term care facilities. *Infect Control Hosp Epidemiol.* 1994;15:557-562.
18. Kunin CM, McCormack RC. Prevention of catheter-induced urinary-tract infections by sterile closed drainage. *N Engl J Med.* 1966;274:1155-1161.
19. Classen DC, Larsen RA, Burke JP, et al. Prevention of catheter-associated bacteriuria: Clinical trial of methods to block three known pathways of infection. *Am J Infect Control.* 1991;19:136-142.
20. Saint S, Lipsky BA. Preventing catheter-related bacteriuria: Should we? Can we? How? *Arch Intern Med.* 1999;159:800-808.
21. Maki DG, Tambyah PA. Engineering out the risk for infection with urinary catheters. *Emerg Infect Dis.* 2001;7:342-347.
22. Saint S, Chenoweth CE. Biofilms and catheter-associated urinary tract infections. *Infect Dis Clin North Am.* 2003;17:411-432.
23. Platt R, Polk BF, Murdock B, et al. Risk factors for nosocomial urinary tract infection. *Am J Epidemiol.* 1986;124:977-985.
24. Finer G, Landau D. Pathogenesis of urinary tract infections with normal female anatomy. *Lancet Infect Dis.* 2004;4:631-635.
25. Saint S. Clinical and economic consequences of nosocomial catheter-related bacteriuria. *Am J Infect Control.* 2000;28:68-75.
26. Garibaldi RA, Mooney BR, Epstein BJ, et al. An evaluation of daily bacteriologic monitoring to identify preventable episodes of catheter-associated urinary tract infection. *Infect Control.* 1982;3:466-470.
27. Hartstein AI, Garber SB, Ward TT, et al. Nosocomial urinary tract infection: A prospective evaluation of 108 catheterized patients. *Infect Control.* 1981;2:380-386.
28. Tambyah PA, Maki DG. Catheter-associated urinary tract infection is rarely symptomatic: A prospective study of 1,497 catheterized patients. *Arch Intern Med.* 2000;160:678-682.
29. Warren JW, Damron D, Tenney JH, et al. Fever, bacteremia, and death as complications of bacteriuria in women with long-term urethral catheters. *J Infect Dis.* 1987;155:1151-1158.
30. Bryan CS, Reynolds KL. Hospital-acquired bacteremic urinary tract infection: Epidemiology and outcome. *J Urol.* 1984;132:494-498.
31. Krieger JN, Kaiser DL, Wenzel RP. Urinary tract etiology of bloodstream infections in hospitalized patients. *J Infect Dis.* 1983;148:57-62.
32. Kreger BE, Craven DE, Carling PC, et al. Gram-negative bacteremia. III. Reassessment of etiology, epidemiology and ecology in 612 patients. *Am J Med.* 1980;68:332-343.
33. Ikäheimo R, Siitonen A, Kärkkäinen U, et al. Virulence characteristics of Escherichia coli in nosocomial urinary tract infection. *Clin Infect Dis.* 1993;16:785-791.
34. Muder RR, Brennen C, Wagener MM, et al. Bacteremia in a long-term-care facility: a five-year prospective study of 163 consecutive episodes. *Clin Infect Dis.* 1992;14:647-654.
35. Rudman D, Hontanosas A, Cohen Z, et al. Clinical correlates of bacteremia in a Veterans Administration extended care facility. *J Am Geriatr Soc.* 1988;36:726-732.
36. Warren JW, Muncie HL Jr, Hebel JR, et al. Long-term urethral catheterization increases risk of chronic pyelonephritis and renal inflammation. *J Am Geriatr Soc.* 1994;42:1286-1290.
37. Kunin CM, Douthitt S, Dancing J, et al. The association between the use of urinary catheters and morbidity and mortality among elderly patients in nursing homes. *Am J Epidemiol.* 1992;135:291-301.
38. Laupland KB, Bagshaw SM, Gregson DB, et al. Intensive care unit-acquired urinary tract infections in a regional critical care system. *Crit Care.* 2005;9:R60-R65.
39. Bueno-Cavanillas A, Delgado-Rodriguez M, Lopez-Luque A, et al. Influence of nosocomial infection on mortality rate in an intensive care unit. *Crit Care Med.* 1994;22:55-60.
40. Clec'h C, Schwebel C, Francais A, et al. Does catheter-associated urinary tract infection increase mortality in critically ill patients? *Infect Control Hosp Epidemiol.* 2007;28:1367-1373.
41. Kunin CM, Chin QF, Chambers S. Morbidity and mortality associated with indwelling urinary catheters in elderly patients in a nursing home—confounding due to the presence of associated diseases. *J Am Geriatr Soc.* 1987;35:1001-1006.
42. Nicolle LE. Catheter-related urinary tract infection. *Drugs Aging.* 2005;22:627-639.
43. Schaberg DR, Haley RW, Highsmith AK, et al. Nosocomial bacteriuria: A prospective study of case clustering and antimicrobial resistance. *Ann Intern Med.* 1980;93:420-424.
44. Jarlier V, Fosse T, Philippon A. Antibiotic susceptibility in aerobic gram-negative bacilli isolated in intensive care units in 39 French teaching hospitals (ICU study). *Intensive Care Med.* 1996;22:1057-1065.
45. Bjork DT, Pelletier LL, Tight RR. Urinary tract infections with antibiotic resistant organisms in catheterized nursing home patients. *Infect Control.* 1984;5:173-176.
46. Wagenlehner FM, Krcmery S, Held C, et al. Epidemiological analysis of the spread of pathogens from a urological ward using genotypic, phenotypic and clinical parameters. *Int J Antimicrob Agents.* 2002;19:583-591.
47. Dalen DM, Zvonar RK, Jessamine PG. An evaluation of the management of asymptomatic catheter-associated bacteriuria and candiduria at The Ottawa Hospital. *Can J Infect Dis Med Microbiol.* 2005;16:166-170.
48. Hooton TM, Stamm WE. Diagnosis and treatment of uncomplicated urinary tract infection. *Infect Dis Clin North Am.* 1997;11:551-581.
49. Warren JW, Tenney JH, Hoopes JM, et al. A prospective microbiologic study of bacteriuria in patients with chronic indwelling urethral catheters. *J Infect Dis.* 1982;146:719-723.
50. Rahav G, Pinco E, Silbaq F, et al. Molecular epidemiology of catheter-associated bacteriuria in nursing home patients. *J Clin Microbiol.* 1994;32:1031-1034.
51. Bergqvist D, Bronnestam R, Hedelin H, et al. The relevance of urinary sampling methods in patients with indwelling Foley catheters. *Br J Urol.* 1980;52:92-95.
52. Tenney JH, Warren JW. Bacteriuria in women with long-term catheters: Paired comparison of indwelling and replacement catheters. *J Infect Dis.* 1988;157:199-202.
53. Mulvey MA, Schilling JD, Hultgren SJ. Establishment of a persistent *Escherichia coli* reservoir during the acute phase of a bladder infection. *Infect Immun.* 2001;69:4572-4579.
54. Jacobsen SM, Stickler DJ, Mobley HL, et al. Complicated catheter-associated urinary tract infections due to Escherichia coli and Proteus mirabilis. *Clin Microbiol Rev.* 2008;21:26-59.
55. Elliott TSJ, Reed L, Slack RCB, et al. Bacteriology and ultrastructure of the bladder in patients with urinary tract infections. *J Infect.* 1985;11:191-199.
56. Elliott TSJ, Slack RCB, Bishop MC. Scanning electron microscopy of human bladder mucosa in acute and chronic urinary tract infection. *Br J Urol.* 1984;56:38-43.
57. Rosen DA, Hooton TM, Stamm WE, et al. Detection of intracellular bacterial communities in human urinary tract infection. *PLoS Med.* 2007;4:e329.
58. Warren JW, Mobley HLT, Donnenberg MS. Host-parasite interactions and host defense mechanisms. In: Schrier RW, ed. *Diseases of the Kidney and Urinary Tract.* 7th ed. Philadelphia: Lippincott Williams & Wilkins; 2001:903-921.
59. Johnson JR. Microbial virulence determinants and the pathogenesis of urinary tract infection. *Infect Dis Clin North Am.* 2003;17:261-278.
60. Hooton TM. Pathogenesis of urinary tract infections: An update. *J Antimicrob Chemother.* 2000;46(Suppl 1):1-7.
61. Lundstedt AC, Leijonhufvud I, Ragnarsdottir B, et al. Inherited susceptibility to acute pyelonephritis: A family study of urinary tract infection. *J Infect Dis.* 2007;195:1227-1234.
62. Sobel JD. New aspects of pathogenesis of lower urinary tract infections. *Urology.* 1985;26(5 Suppl):11-16.
63. Hooton TM, Stapleton AE, Roberts PL, et al. Perineal anatomy and urine-voiding characteristics of young women with and without recurrent urinary tract infections. *Clin Infect Dis.* 1999;29:1600-1601.
64. Rutala WA, Kennedy VA, Loflin HB, et al. Serratia marcescens nosocomial infections of the urinary tract associated with urine measuring containers and urinometers. *Am J Med.* 1981;70:659-663.
65. Stamm WE. Catheter-associated urinary tract infections: Epidemiology, pathogenesis, and prevention. *Am J Med.* 1991;91:65S-71S.
66. Tambyah PA, Halvorson KT, Maki DG. A prospective study of pathogenesis of catheter-associated urinary tract infections. *Mayo Clin Proc.* 1999;74:131-136.
67. Stark RP, Maki DG. Bacteriuria in the catheterized patient. What quantitative level of bacteriuria is relevant? *N Engl J Med.* 1984;311:560-564.
68. Norden CW, Kass EH. Bacteriuria of pregnancy—a critical appraisal. *Annu Rev Med.* 1968;19:431-470.
69. Gleckman R, Esposito A, Crowley M, et al. Reliability of a single urine culture in establishing diagnosis of asymptomatic bacteriuria in adult males. *J Clin Microbiol.* 1979;9:596-597.
70. Nicolle LE, Harding GK, Kennedy J, et al. Urine specimen collection with external devices for diagnosis of bacteriuria in elderly incontinent men. *J Clin Microbiol.* 1988;26:1115-1119.
71. Stamm WE, Counts GW, Running KR, et al. Diagnosis of coliform infection in acutely dysuric women. *N Engl J Med.* 1982;307:463-468.
72. Lipsky BA, Ireton RC, Fihn SD, et al. Diagnosis of bacteriuria in men: Specimen collection and culture interpretation. *J Infect Dis.* 1987;155:847-854.
73. The prevention and management of urinary tract infections among people with spinal cord injuries. National Institute on Disability and Rehabilitation Research Consensus Statement. January 27-29, 1992. *J Am Paraplegia Soc.* 1992;15:194-204.
74. Tambyah PA, Maki DG. The relationship between pyuria and infection in patients with indwelling urinary catheters: A prospective study of 761 patients. *Arch Intern Med.* 2000;160:673-677.
75. Steward DK, Wood GL, Cohen RL, et al. Failure of the urinalysis and quantitative urine culture in diagnosing symptomatic urinary tract infections in patients with long-term urinary catheters. *Am J Infect Control.* 1985;13:154-160.
76. Haley RW, Culver DH, White JW, et al. The efficacy of infection surveillance and control programs in preventing nosocomial infections in US hospitals. *Am J Epidemiol.* 1985;121:182-205.
77. Lo E, Nicolle L, Classen D, et al. Strategies to prevent catheter-associated urinary tract infections in acute care hospitals. *Infect Control Hosp Epidemiol.* 2008;29(Suppl 1):S41-S50.
78. Fryklund B, Haeggman S, Burman LG. Transmission of urinary bacterial strains between patients with indwelling catheters—nursing in the same room and in separate rooms compared. *J Hosp Infect.* 1997;36:147-153.
79. Thompson RL, Haley CE, Searcy MA, et al. Catheter-associated bacteriuria. Failure to reduce attack rates using periodic instillations of a disinfectant into urinary drainage systems. *JAMA.* 1984;251:747-751.
80. Goetz AM, Kedzuf S, Wagener M, et al. Feedback to nursing staff as an intervention to reduce catheter-associated urinary tract infections. *Am J Infect Control.* 1999;27:402-404.

81. Rosenthal VD, Guzman S, Safdar N. Effect of education and performance feedback on rates of catheter-associated urinary tract infection in intensive care units in Argentina. *Infect Control Hosp Epidemiol.* 2004;25:47-50.
82. Saint S, Kowalski CP, Kaufman SR, et al. Preventing hospital-acquired urinary tract infection in the United States: A national study. *Clin Infect Dis.* 2008;46:243-250.
83. Wald HL, Kramer AM. Nonpayment for harms resulting from medical care: Catheter-associated urinary tract infections. *JAMA.* 2007;298:2782-2784.
84. Jain P, Parada JP, David A, et al. Overuse of the indwelling urinary tract catheter in hospitalized medical patients. *Arch Intern Med.* 1995;155:1425-1429.
85. Munasinghe RL, Yazdani H, Siddique M, et al. Appropriateness of use of indwelling urinary catheters in patients admitted to the medical service. *Infect Control Hosp Epidemiol.* 2001;22: 647-649.
86. Gardam MA, Amihod B, Orenstein P, et al. Overutilization of indwelling urinary catheters and the development of nosocomial urinary tract infections. *Clin Perform Qual Health Care.* 1998;6:99-102.
87. Gokula RR, Hickner JA, Smith MA. Inappropriate use of urinary catheters in elderly patients at a midwestern community teaching hospital. *Am J Infect Control.* 2004;32:196-199.
88. Saint S, Wiese J, Amory JK, et al. Are physicians aware of which of their patients have indwelling urinary catheters? *Am J Med.* 2000;109:476-480.
89. Gokula RM, Smith MA, Hickner J. Emergency room staff education and use of a urinary catheter indication sheet improves appropriate use of foley catheters. *Am J Infect Control.* 2007;35:589-593.
90. Stephan F, Sax H, Wachsmuth M, et al. Reduction of urinary tract infection and antibiotic use after surgery: A controlled, prospective, before-after intervention study. *Clin Infect Dis.* 2006;42:1544-1551.
91. Slappendel R, Weber EW. Non-invasive measurement of bladder volume as an indication for bladder catheterization after orthopaedic surgery and its effect on urinary tract infections. *Eur J Anaesthesiol.* 1999;16:503-506.
92. Lau H, Lam B. Management of postoperative urinary retention: A randomized trial of in-out versus overnight catheterization. *ANZ J Surg.* 2004;74:658-661.
93. Kunin C. Nosocomial urinary tract infections and the indwelling catheter. What is new and what is true? *Chest.* 2001;120: 10-12.
94. Stevens E. Bladder ultrasound: Avoiding unnecessary catheterizations. *Medsurg Nurs.* 2005;14:249-253.
95. Huang WC, Wann SR, Lin SL, et al. Catheter-associated urinary tract infections in intensive care units can be reduced by prompting physicians to remove unnecessary catheters. *Infect Control Hosp Epidemiol.* 2004;25:974-978.
96. Apisarnthanarak A, Thongphubeth K, Sirinvaravong S, et al. Effectiveness of multifaceted hospitalwide quality improvement programs featuring an intervention to remove unnecessary urinary catheters at a tertiary care center in Thailand. *Infect Control Hosp Epidemiol.* 2007;28:791-798.
97. Saint S, Kaufman SR, Thompson M, et al. A reminder reduces urinary catheterization in hospitalized patients. *Jt Comm J Qual Patient Saf.* 2005;31:455-462.
98. Cornia PB, Amory JK, Fraser S, et al. Computer-based order entry decreases duration of indwelling urinary catheterization in hospitalized patients. *Am J Med.* 2003;114: 404-407.
99. Topal J, Conklin S, Camp K, et al. Prevention of nosocomial catheter-associated urinary tract infections through computerized feedback to physicians and a nurse-directed protocol. *Am J Med Qual.* 2005;20:121-126.
100. Loeb M, Hunt D, O'Halloran K, et al. Stop orders to reduce inappropriate urinary catheterization in hospitalized patients: a randomized controlled trial. *J Gen Intern Med.* 2008;23: 816-820.
101. Griffiths R, Fernandez R. Strategies for the removal of short-term indwelling urethral catheters in adults. *Cochrane Database Syst Rev.* 2007(2):CD004011.
102. Bladder management for adults with spinal cord injury: A clinical practice guideline for health-care providers. *J Spinal Cord Med.* 2006;29:527-573.
103. Saint S, Kaufman SR, Rogers MA, et al. Condom versus indwelling urinary catheters: A randomized trial. *J Am Geriatr Soc.* 2006;54:1055-1061.
104. Guttman L, Frankel H. The value of intermittent catheterization in the early management of traumatic paraplegia and tetraplegia. *Paraplegia.* 1966;4:63-84.
105. Lapides J, Diokno AC, Silber SJ, et al. Clean, intermittent self-catheterization in the treatment of urinary tract disease. *J Urol.* 1972;107:458-461.
106. Wyndaele JJ. Complications of intermittent catheterization: Their prevention and treatment. *Spinal Cord.* 2002;40:536-541.
107. Duffy LM, Cleary J, Ahern S, et al. Clean intermittent catheterization: Safe, cost-effective bladder management for male residents of VA nursing homes. *J Am Geriatr Soc.* 1995; 43:865-870.
108. Jamison J, Maguire S, McCann J. Catheter policies for management of long term voiding problems in adults with neurogenic bladder disorders. *Cochrane Database Syst Rev.* 2004(2): CD004375.
109. Niel-Weise BS, van den Broek PJ. Urinary catheter policies for short-term bladder drainage in adults. *Cochrane Database Syst Rev.* 2005(3):CD004203.
110. Moore KN, Fader M, Getliffe K. Long-term bladder management by intermittent catheterisation in adults and children. *Cochrane Database Syst Rev.* 2007(4):CD006008.
111. Hedlund H, Hjelmås K, Jonsson O, et al. Hydrophilic versus non-coated catheters for intermittent catheterization. *Scand J Urol Nephrol.* 2001;35:49-53.
112. Branagan GW, Moran BJ. Published evidence favors the use of suprapubic catheters in pelvic colorectal surgery. *Dis Colon Rectum.* 2002;45:1104-1108.
113. Carapeti EA, Andrews SM, Bentley PG. Randomised study of sterile versus non-sterile urethral catheterisation. *Ann R Coll Surg Engl.* 1996;78:59-60.
114. Kass EH. Asymptomatic infections of the urinary tract. *Trans Assoc Am Physicians.* 1956;69:56-64.
115. Warren JW, Platt R, Thomas RJ, et al. Antibiotic irrigation and catheter-associated urinary-tract infections. *N Engl J Med.* 1978;299:570-573.
116. Ahearn DG, Grace DT, Jennings MJ, et al. Effects of hydrogel/silver coatings on in vitro adhesion to catheters of bacteria associated with urinary tract infections. *Curr Microbiol.* 2000;41: 120-125.
117. Darouiche RO, Safar H, Raad II. In vitro efficacy of antimicrobial-coated bladder catheters in inhibiting bacterial migration along catheter surface. *J Infect Dis.* 1997;176:1109-1112.
118. Johnson JR, Delavari P, Azar M. Activities of a nitrofurazone-containing urinary catheter and a silver hydrogel catheter against multidrug-resistant bacteria characteristic of catheter-associated urinary tract infection. *Antimicrob Agents Chemother.* 1999;43:2990-2995.
119. Schumm K, Lam TB. Types of urethral catheters for management of short-term voiding problems in hospitalised adults. *Cochrane Database Syst Rev.* 2008(2):CD004013.
120. Drekonja DM, Kuskowski MA, Wilt TJ, et al. Antimicrobial urinary catheters: A systematic review. *Expert Rev Med Devices.* 2008;5:495-506.
121. Johnson JR, Kuskowski MA, Wilt TJ. Systematic review: antimicrobial urinary catheters to prevent catheter-associated urinary tract infection in hospitalized patients. *Ann Intern Med.* 2006;144:116-126.
122. Srinivasan A, Karchmer T, Richards A, et al. A prospective trial of a novel, silicone-based, silver-coated foley catheter for the prevention of nosocomial urinary tract infections. *Infect Control Hosp Epidemiol.* 2006;27:38-43.
123. Crnich CJ, Drinka PJ. Does the composition of urinary catheters influence clinical outcomes and the results of research studies? *Infect Control Hosp Epidemiol.* 2007;28:102-103.
124. Darouiche RO, Smith JA Jr, Hanna H, et al. Efficacy of antimicrobial-impregnated bladder catheters in reducing catheter-associated bacteriuria: A prospective, randomized, multicenter clinical trial. *Urology.* 1999;54:976-981.
125. Stensballe J, Tvede M, Looms D, et al. Infection risk with nitrofurazone-impregnated urinary catheters in trauma patients: A randomized trial. *Ann Intern Med.* 2007;147:285-293.
126. Jahn P, Preuss M, Kernig A, et al. Types of indwelling urinary catheters for long-term bladder drainage in adults. *Cochrane Database Syst Rev.* 2007(3):CD004997.
127. Niel-Weise BS, van den Broek PJ. Antibiotic policies for short-term catheter bladder drainage in adults. *Cochrane Database Syst Rev.* 2005(3):CD005428.
128. Niël-Weise BS, van den Broek PJ. Urinary catheter policies for long-term bladder drainage. *Cochrane Database Syst Rev.* 2005;(1):CD004201.
129. Rutschmann OT, Zwahlen A. Use of norfloxacin for prevention of symptomatic urinary tract infection in chronically catheterized patients. *Eur J Clin Microbiol Infect Dis.* 1995;14:441-444.
130. Stamm WE, Hooton TM. Management of urinary tract infections in adults. *N Engl J Med.* 1993;329:1328-1334.
131. Hustinx WN, Mintjes-de Groot AJ, Verkooyen RP, et al. Impact of concurrent antimicrobial therapy on catheter-associated urinary tract infection. *J Hosp Infect.* 1991;18:45-56.
132. Gleckman R, Alvarez S, Joubert DW, et al. Drug therapy reviews: methenamine mandelate and methenamine hippurate. *Am J Hosp Pharm.* 1979;36:1509-1512.
133. Cronberg S, Welin CO, Henriksson L, et al. Prevention of recurrent acute cystitis by methenamine hippurate: double blind controlled crossover long term study. *Br Med J (Clin Res Ed).* 1987;294:1507-1508.
134. Harding GK, Ronald AR. A controlled study of antimicrobial prophylaxis of recurrent urinary infection in women. *N Engl J Med.* 1974;291:597-601.
135. Lee BB, Simpson JM, Craig JC, et al. Methenamine hippurate for preventing urinary tract infections. *Cochrane Database Syst Rev.* 2007(4):CD003265.
136. Schiotz HA, Guttu K. Value of urinary prophylaxis with methenamine in gynecologic surgery. *Acta Obstet Gynecol Scand.* 2002;81:743-746.
137. Lee BB, Haran MJ, Hunt LM, et al. Spinal-injured neuropathic bladder antisepsis (SINBA) trial. *Spinal Cord.* 2007;45:542-550.
138. Kuhlemeier KV, Stover SL, Lloyd LK. Prophylactic antibacterial therapy for preventing urinary tract infections in spinal cord injury patients. *J Urol.* 1985;134:514-517.
139. Jepson RG, Craig JC. Cranberries for preventing urinary tract infections. *Cochrane Database Syst Rev.* 2008(1):CD001321.
140. van den Broek PJ, Daha TJ, Mouton RP. Bladder irrigation with povidone-iodine in prevention of urinary-tract infections associated with intermittent urethral catheterisation. *Lancet.* 1985;1:563-565.
141. Ball AJ, Carr TW, Gillespie WA, et al. Bladder irrigation with chlorhexidine for the prevention of urinary infection after transurethral operations: A prospective controlled study. *J Urol.* 1987;138:491-494.
142. Muncie HL Jr, Hoopes JM, Damron DJ, et al. Once-daily irrigation of long-term urethral catheters with normal saline. Lack of benefit. *Arch Intern Med.* 1989;149:441-443.
143. Kunin CM, Chin QF, Chambers S. Indwelling urinary catheters in the elderly. Relation of "catheter life" to formation of encrustations in patients with and without blocked catheters. *Am J Med.* 1987;82:405-411.
144. Jewes LA, Gillespie WA, Leadbetter A, et al. Bacteriuria and bacteraemia in patients with long-term indwelling catheters—a domiciliary study. *J Med Microbiol.* 1988;26:61-65.
145. Polastri F, Auckenthaler R, Loew F, et al. Absence of significant bacteremia during urinary catheter manipulation in patients with chronic indwelling catheters. *J Am Geriatr Soc.* 1990;38:1203-1208.
146. Bregenzer T, Frei R, Widmer AF, et al. Low risk of bacteremia during catheter replacement in patients with long-term urinary catheters. *Arch Intern Med.* 1997;157:521-525.
147. Wazait HD, Patel HR, van der Meulen JH, et al. A pilot randomized double-blind placebo-controlled trial on the use of antibiotics on urinary catheter removal to reduce the rate of urinary tract infection: The pitfalls of ciprofloxacin. *BJU Int.* 2004;94:1048-1050.
148. Schneeberger PM, Vreede RW, Bogdanowicz JF, et al. A randomized study on the effect of bladder irrigation with povidone-iodine before removal of an indwelling catheter. *J Hosp Infect.* 1992;21:223-229.
149. Sassine AM, Schulman CC. Intraurethral catheter in high-risk patients with urinary retention: 3 years of experience. *Eur Urol.* 1994;25:131-134.
150. Kaplan SA, Merrill DC, Mosely WG, et al. The titanium intraprostatic stent: The United States experience. *J Urol.* 1993;150:1624-1629.
151. Ozgür GK, Sivrikaya A, Bilen R, et al. The use of intraurethral prostatic spiral in high risk patients for surgery with benign prostatic hyperplasia. *Int Urol Nephrol.* 1993;25:65-70.
152. Mazouni C, Karsenty G, Bladou F, et al. Urethral device in women with chronic urinary retention: an alternative to self-catheterization? *Eur J Obstet Gynecol Reprod Biol.* 2004; 115:80-84.
153. Gaunt RA, Prochazka A. Control of urinary bladder function with devices: Successes and failures. *Prog Brain Res.* 2006;152:163-194.
154. Darouiche RO, Thornby JI, Cerra-Stewart C, et al. Bacterial interference for prevention of urinary tract infection: A prospective, randomized, placebo-controlled, double-blind pilot trial. *Clin Infect Dis.* 2005;41:1531-1534.
155. Valle J, Da Re S, Henry N, et al. Broad-spectrum biofilm inhibition by a secreted bacterial polysaccharide. *Proc Natl Acad Sci U S A.* 2006;103:12558-12563.
156. Screening for asymptomatic bacteriuria in adults: U.S. Preventive Services Task Force reaffirmation recommendation statement. *Ann Intern Med.* 2008;149:43-47.
157. Warren JW, Anthony WC, Hoopes JM, et al. Cephalexin for susceptible bacteriuria in afebrile, long-term catheterized patients. *JAMA.* 1982;248:454-458.
158. Lewis RI, Carrion HM, Lockhart JL, et al. Significance of asymptomatic bacteriuria in neurogenic bladder disease. *Urology.* 1984;23:343-347.
159. Harding GK, Nicolle LE, Ronald AR, et al. How long should catheter-acquired urinary tract infection in women be treated? A randomized controlled study. *Ann Intern Med.* 1991; 114:713-719.
160. Raz R, Schiller D, Nicolle LE. Chronic indwelling catheter replacement before antimicrobial therapy for symptomatic urinary tract infection. *J Urol.* 2000;164:1254-1258.
161. Nicolle LE, Bjornson J, Harding GK, et al. Bacteriuria in elderly institutionalized men. *N Engl J Med.* 1983;309:1420-1425.
162. Dow G, Rao P, Harding G, et al. A prospective, randomized trial of 3 or 14 days of ciprofloxacin treatment for acute urinary tract infection in patients with spinal cord injury. *Clin Infect Dis.* 2004;39:658-664.
163. Peterson J, Kaul S, Khashab M, et al. A double-blind, randomized comparison of levofloxacin 750 mg once-daily for five days with ciprofloxacin 400/500 mg twice-daily for 10 days for the treatment of complicated urinary tract infections and acute pyelonephritis. *Urology.* 2008;71:17-22.
164. Lundstrom T, Sobel J. Nosocomial candiduria: A review. *Clin Infect Dis.* 2001;32:1602-1607.
165. Shay AC, Miller LG. An estimate of the incidence of candiduria among hospitalized patients in the United States. *Infect Control Hosp Epidemiol.* 2004;25:894-895.
166. Kauffman CA, Vazquez JA, Sobel JD, et al. Prospective multicenter surveillance study of funguria in hospitalized patients. The National Institute for Allergy and Infectious Diseases (NIAID) Mycoses Study Group. *Clin Infect Dis.* 2000;30:14-18.
167. Richards MJ, Edwards JR, Culver DH, et al. Nosocomial infections in medical intensive care units in the United States. *Crit Care Med.* 1999;27:887-892.

168. Kauffman CA. Candiduria. *Clin Infect Dis*. 2005;41:S371-S376.
169. Ang BS, Telenti A, King B, et al. Candidemia from a urinary tract source: Microbiological aspects and clinical significance. *Clin Infect Dis*. 1993;17:662-666.
170. Binelli CA, Moretti ML, Assis RS, et al. Investigation of the possible association between nosocomial candiduria and candidaemia. *Clin Microbiol Infect*. 2006;12:538-543.
171. Pappas PG, Kauffman CA, Andes D, et al. Clinical practice guidelines for the management of candidiasis: 2009 update by the Infectious Diseases Society of America. *Clin Infect Dis*. 2009;48:503-535.
172. Sobel JD, Kauffman CA, McKinsey D, et al. Candiduria: a randomized, double-blind study of treatment with fluconazole and placebo. The National Institute of Allergy and Infectious Diseases (NIAID) Mycoses Study Group. *Clin Infect Dis*. 2000;30:19-24.
173. Safdar N, Slattery WR, Knasinski V, et al. Predictors and outcomes of candiduria in renal transplant recipients. *Clin Infect Dis*. 2005;40:1413-1421.
174. Sobel JD, Bradshaw SK, Lipka CJ, et al. Caspofungin in the treatment of symptomatic candiduria. *Clin Infect Dis*. 2007;44:e46-49.
175. Lagrotteria D, Rotstein C, Lee CH. Treatment of candiduria with micafungin: A case series. *Can J Infect Dis Med Microbiol*. 2007;18:149-150.
176. Curtis LT. Prevention of hospital-acquired infections: review of non-pharmacological interventions. *J Hosp Infect*. 2008;69:204-219.

305

Nosocomial Hepatitis and Other Transfusion- and Transplantation-Transmitted Infections

KENT A. SEPKOWITZ | MATTHEW J. KUEHNERT

▦ Nosocomial Hepatitis

The potential for blood-borne transmission of hepatitis B first was noted in 1885, when Lurman described jaundice in factory workers who had received smallpox vaccine prepared from "human lymph."[1] More reports appeared in the subsequent decades as use of vaccines derived from human serum became more common.[2] In addition, more frequent use of phlebotomy equipment,[3] insulin therapy,[4] and intramuscular injection of antibiotics all led to small outbreaks of jaundice, which were ascribed to a transmissible "icterogenic" agent.

By the late 1940s, studies to clarify the modes of transmission were undertaken. Central to these was the use of human volunteers, who were given putatively infectious material intradermally, intranasally, or by ingestion of feces and then observed for development of jaundice.[2,5-10] From these landmark reports arose our current understanding of the basic principles of transmission of infectious hepatitis (hepatitis A) and serum hepatitis (hepatitis B).

The first report of occupational disease in health care workers (HCWs) was provided by Leibowitz and colleagues,[11] who described jaundice in a blood bank nurse with numerous needle pricks on her hands and fingers. A spate of similar reports followed, describing occupationally acquired hepatitis among nurses, blood bank workers, phlebotomists, house staff, and others.[12-14] Soon, the workers' compensation boards of certain states ruled that viral hepatitis was a compensible occupational hazard. Improved understanding of routes of transmission, more comprehensive and rigorous infection control including needle disposal, and, for hepatitis B, vaccination of workers at risk have helped to decrease, but not eliminate, this occupational risk. A corollary risk, that of transmission of infection from infected HCWs, particularly surgeons, to non-immune patients, has been described for hepatitis B[15,16] and hepatitis C.[17]

FECAL-ORAL TRANSMISSION

Hepatitis A

Most series suggest that hepatitis A does not represent an occupational risk for HCWs.[18] Although they are rare, nosocomial outbreaks have been reported from blood transfusion or fecal-oral exposure. Most reports are from pediatric or neonatal intensive care units.[19-21] Adults with[22,23] and without[24] diarrhea have transmitted disease to HCWs and to other patients.

Interruption of transmission through administration of intramuscular immune globulin to contacts has been used effectively for many years[18] (Table 305-1). Broad-scale vaccination also may help interrupt nosocomial spread. Current Centers for Disease Control and Prevention (CDC) and Advisory Committee on Immunization Practices (ACIP) recommendations consider that hepatitis A vaccination "is or might be" indicated for HCWs, but it is not recommended.[18,25] Few employee health services routinely provide the vaccine. Only HCWs who work with hepatitis A virus (HAV) in the laboratory or with HAV-infected primates should routinely be vaccinated.[26,27]

Hepatitis E

Outbreaks of hepatitis E have occurred in developing countries, but nosocomial transmission has not been described in the West. In Pakistan, an outbreak of hepatitis E affected up to 18 people (7 confirmed and 11 possible cases). Assessment of the outbreak suggested that spread occurred due to improper sharing of intravenous equipment sets among patients.[28]

BLOOD-BORNE TRANSMISSION

Hepatitis B

Epidemiology. Hepatitis B was the first blood-borne disease recognized to pose an occupational hazard.[11-14] An early review found a preponderance of cases among pathologists, laboratory workers, and blood bank workers, demonstrating the risk of blood exposure.[12] Vaccine to prevent hepatitis B virus (HBV) infection became available in the United States in 1982, although acceptance of this initial human plasma–derived product was limited. Acceptance of the currently used recombinant HBV vaccine is much higher.

In 1987, growing attention to the potential for occupational acquisition of the human immunodeficiency virus (HIV) led the U.S. Department of Labor, in conjunction with Department of Health and Human Services, to recommend Universal Precautions to protect against exposure to body fluids.[18,25,29] Four years later, the Occupational Safety and Health Administration published the Federal Blood Borne Pathogens Standard, which went into effect in early 1992.[30] This mandated that HCWs with potential exposure to blood or other potentially infectious materials either be offered the hepatitis B vaccine series free of charge, demonstrate immunity to hepatitis B, or formally decline vaccination.[30] Compliance with this recommendation has resulted in a 95% reduction of occupationally acquired hepatitis B,[31,32] although rare cases continue to occur.

Seroprevalence. Dentists, physicians, laboratory workers, dialysis workers, cleaning service employees, employees of facilities for the mentally handicapped, and nurses are the HCW groups with the highest prevalence.[33-36] The extent of exposure to blood has a greater effect on risk than does frequency of contact with patients.

Incidence after Exposure. Before the availability of vaccine, the incidence of hepatitis B was 5 to 10 times greater among physicians and dentists and more than 10 times greater among surgeons, dialysis workers, those caring for the mentally handicapped, and laboratory workers with blood exposure, compared with the general population.[29,36] The risk of transmission from a single needlestick exposure varies according to the hepatitis B e antigen (HBeAg) status of the source case. It ranges from 1% to 6% for HBeAg-negative blood to 22% to 31% for HBeAg-positive blood[37] (see Table 305-1). Not all cases of hepatitis B transmission are explained by specific exposures, suggesting that other modes of spread exist. Infection related to environmental contamination is suggested by high HBV seroprevalence among unvaccinated dialysis patients and personnel.[33,38]

TABLE 305-1	Nosocomial Hepatitis: Transmission Rates and Interventions		
Hepatitis	Rate* (%)	Prevention	Comment
A	10-30	Vaccine not given routinely to HCWs; immune globulin in outbreak setting	ACIP advises vaccine "is or might be" indicated for HCWs.
B	HBeAg⁻ source: 3 HBeAg⁺ source: 22-31	HBV vaccination	HCWs with previous response to vaccine need no additional postexposure treatment regardless of level of exposure. HCWs with no history of vaccination or no or unknown response to vaccine should receive HBIG; vaccination also should be considered. The role of antivirals (e.g., lamivudine) is not defined.
C	1-10	Immunoglobulin not recommended; peg-INF for acute disease	Ribavirin with peg-INF has not been studied for this indication but may be effective.
Delta	Unknown; outbreaks described only in dialysis units	HBV vaccination	Segregate HBsAg⁺ dialysis patients by delta antibody status
E	Unknown	Standard precautions	

*Rate of transmission from outbreak or needlestick exposure.

ACIP, Advisory Committee on Immunization Practices; HBeAg, HB e antigen; HBIG, hepatitis B immune globulin; HBsAg, hepatitis B surface antigen; HBV, hepatitis B virus; HCWs, health care workers; peg-INF, pegylated interferon.

Reported Transmissions.
Worker-to-Patient Transmission. Over the last several decades, dozens of episodes involving HCW-to-patient transmission of hepatitis B have been described, resulting in hundreds of secondary cases (range, 1 to 55 secondary cases per source case)[15,39-44] In a series of 10 clusters reported from the United Kingdom, the transmission rate ranged from 0.3% to 9%.[42,43] At least 42 of the 47 HCWs involved were dentists or surgeons. No cases of transmission from dentists to others have been reported since 1987, demonstrating the effectiveness of Universal Precautions.[43] Lack of clustering may delay recognition of transmission.[44] In response to these concerns, in 1991, the CDC promulgated recommendations for preventing transmission of HIV and HBV to patients during exposure-prone invasive procedures.[45] Some have thought the recommendations too restrictive.[46]

In one outbreak, 19 (13%) of 144 susceptible patients operated on by an HBeAg-positive thoracic surgery resident developed acute hepatitis B infection despite appropriate infection control.[15] Thirteen available isolates, including the surgeon's, were identical when compared by molecular analysis. Examination of the resident's surgical technique suggested that small cuts in his fingers, sustained by tying suture, resulted in entry of his blood into patients' wounds. Ironically, the surgeon had declined hepatitis B vaccine 2 years earlier and then had become infected as the result of an occupational exposure.

In most but not all of the reported instances, the source worker was HBeAg-positive. However, in one series, four HBeAg-negative surgeons each transmitted disease.[16] The cases occurred in England, where restriction of HBeAg-positive surgeons (principally cardiothoracic, gynecologic, orthopedic, and abdominal) is strictly enforced. Confirmation of transmission was aided by HBV DNA sequencing of both the putative source and secondary cases. Since these reports, inquiry into all newly diagnosed cases of hepatitis B includes a determination

of whether the patient had undergone surgery in the previous 6 months.

Patient-to-Worker Transmission. Widespread transmission from a single patient to several HCWs is rare. In one instance, a patient in the preclinical window period for hepatitis B sustained severe trauma and underwent several surgeries.[47] At least four HCWs, including nurses and physicians, developed acute hepatitis temporally consistent with transmission from this patient.

Dialysis Setting. For many years, dialysis patients and staff were at high risk for occupational acquisition of hepatitis B, given their high frequency of sharp injury or mucocutaneous exposure (5 instances per 10,000 dialysis procedures[48]), the high titers of HBV in blood ($\geq 10^9$/mL), and the ability of HBV to survive well in the environment.[49] However, with segregation of patients by room, staff, and machine according to surface antigen (HBsAg) status; institution of active vaccination programs; monthly serologic testing of susceptible patients; and attention to disinfection, equipment, and cleaning procedures, this rate has decreased sharply.[38,49] When rates were compared from a classic study conducted before the availability of vaccine,[38,50] the incidence of new HBsAg among patients was found to have decreased from 3% to 0.05%, and the prevalence from 7.8% to 0.9%. During the same period, vaccination coverage of staff increased to 88% and HCW HBV incidence decreased from 2.6% to less than 0.5%.

Despite these gains, outbreaks continue in centers that fail to identify HBV-infected patients, that share staff and equipment, or that fail to vaccinate susceptible patients.[49] A recent CDC-led survey found that the incidence of HBV among dialysis patients was higher in centers where injectable medications were prepared on a medication cart or area, rather than in a dedicated medication room.[38]

Other Nosocomial Transmissions. In some countries, nosocomial transmission continues to account for a substantial proportion of overall hepatitis B cases.[51,52] In addition, transmission related to spring-loaded finger-stick devices,[53,54] endomyocardial biopsy,[55] endoscopy equipment,[56] acupuncture needles,[57] multidose medication vials,[58] diabetic care,[59] and jet injections[60] has been reported. In developing countries, re-use of needles may contribute substantially to risk.[52] In addition, patients (so-called medical tourists) who for financial or other reasons receive care in countries with a high prevalence of HBV may unknowingly invite the additional risk of virus acquisition.[61]

Interventions and Management. Management in exposed or susceptible workers has been well summarized elsewhere[37,62] (see Table 305-1 and Chapter 146). Treatment should be given within 24 hours after exposure. Intramuscular hepatitis B immune globulin (HBIG) was the original intervention for postexposure prophylaxis.[63] It is still used, in conjunction with initiation of a vaccine series, for management after exposure in unvaccinated HCWs and vaccine nonresponders. Vaccine nonresponders should receive a second dose 1 month later (HBIG dose, 0.06 mL/kg).[18] Vaccine and HBIG may be given at the same time but should be administered with separate needles and syringes and at different anatomic sites. Plain immune globulin does not contain sufficient titers of HBIG and should not be given.[18] The role of antiviral agents such as lamivudine and adefovir in the management of nosocomial exposure has not been determined.

The durability of hepatitis B vaccine–induced immunity is not known.[64] Vaccine-induced antibody predictably wanes in many initial responders. However, in longitudinal reports, persons with waning antibody (to <10 mIU/mL) have not developed clinical hepatitis.[65] Rather, those newly infected typically develop core antibody (HBcAb) with subclinical disease. Therefore, the CDC does not recommend routine revaccination of HCWs or patients, except for dialysis patients. Dialysis patients should have their antibody level determined annually and be revaccinated when the level drops to less than 10 mIU/mL.[66]

Because of the cost, determination of antibody to HBV prior to vaccination is not recommended.[25] Postvaccination testing should be routinely provided to all HCWs with an anticipated risk of occupational exposure. Knowledge of serostatus assists management of subsequent exposures.[25,37] For vaccine responders, no postexposure intervention is required, regardless of the HBsAg or HBeAg status of the source. Vaccinated HCWs with an unknown response to vaccine should have their antibody titer checked immediately after exposure and be treated according to the result (see Table 305-1). Vaccine is generally well tolerated.

The best long-term management for the hepatitis B vaccine nonresponder is not known. This is of particular importance because up to 10% of vaccinated persons do not seroconvert.[67] Risk factors for a suboptimal response include cigarette smoking, increasing age, obesity, and, in some series, male sex.[67] Persons who do not seroconvert after the initial three-dose series should be evaluated for HBsAg carrier state and, if negative, receive a second three-dose series.[37] Among those receiving a second course, up to half seroconvert. A third series for nonresponders is not recommended. Strategies to increase the likelihood of eventual vaccine response include intradermal vaccination[68,69] and double-dose vaccination in a standard three-dose series of combined hepatitis A and hepatitis B vaccine.[70] Neither approach has been approved.

Vaccine Acceptance Rates. A series of CDC-led articles on HCW vaccination has demonstrated steadily rising acceptance. A 1995 report[31] found a 51% acceptance rate, whereas, most recently, examination of rates among employees in 2002-2003 revealed that 75% of all HCWs, or 2.5 million people, had completed the vaccine series, with the highest rates (approximately 80%) among nurses and doctors.[71] However, coverage remains incomplete, even in those groups at highest risk.[72] In U.S. dialysis centers in 2002, 56% of patients and 90% of staff had been vaccinated.[38]

Hepatitis C
Seroprevalence. Most[48,73,74] series suggest that those HCWs who are at increased risk for hepatitis B, including dialysis workers, laboratory workers, surgeons, nurses, and workers with the mentally impaired, have no increase in HCV seroprevalence. A 2000 survey of U.S. dialysis staff demonstrated 1.7% seroprevalence, similar to the overall prevalence in the United States (1% to 2%).[38] Only 40% of centers routinely determined the HCV serostatus of staff, however.[38] Older studies had suggested that dentists, particularly oral surgeons, might have an elevated risk.[75,76]

Incidence after Exposure. Seroconversion occurs in 0% to 10% of nonimmune HCWs who sustain needlesticks from a source case with hepatitis C.[25,48,77-79] Maternal-fetal transmission rates are similar (5% to 9%). Rates may vary because of differences in the diagnostic test used (antibody or hepatitis C virus [HCV] RNA). The highest transmission rate (10%) was from a study in which HCV RNA was used to detect infection in exposed workers.[78] This high rate has not been duplicated, and most studies have placed the transmission rate at less than 3%. A correlation between HCV RNA quantitative level in the source patient and risk of transmission has not been established.

A report of simultaneous transmission of HCV and HIV from a single needlestick was remarkable for the delayed time to seroconversion against each virus and the fulminantly fatal course of the HCV infection.[80] The frequency of this phenomenon is not known.

Reported Transmissions.
Worker-to-Patient Transmission. A cardiac surgeon transmitted HCV to at least five patients who underwent valve replacement.[17] Molecular analysis showed significant homology between the surgeon's and the patients' virus. The surgeon was treated with interferon-alfa-2b and ribavirin until his HCV RNA level became undetectable. At that point, he was allowed to resume performing surgery. In a case of transmission from an anesthesiologist to a surgical patient, no cause was elucidated.[81] A thoracic surgeon[82] and an anesthesiologist in a gynecology clinic[83] also were demonstrated to have transmitted HCV to patients. Transmission from a patient to an anesthesiology assistant and subsequently to five different patients has been described.[84]

Dialysis Setting. Despite improvements, transmission of HCV remains a substantial problem for dialysis centers throughout the world.[38,85-87] In most series, HCV seroprevalence among dialysis patients is 2- to 10-fold higher than in the general population. The CDC reported regularly on dialysis-associated diseases in the United States through 2002. Their last survey, which included 96% of all U.S. centers representing more than 260,000 patients and 58,000 staff members, 63% of the institutions routinely tested patients for HCV, an increase from 39% in 1995.[38] The prevalence of HCV infection among dialysis patients was 7.8%; in the year 2000, the prevalence among staff at these centers was 1.7%.[38] HCV incidence across the centers was 0.34%. Seroprevalence is even higher in many European and Asian centers, exceeding 40% in some cities. Incidence estimates have ranged from 0.6% to 2%.[38,88] The prevalence of HCV among peritoneal dialysis patients, in contrast, is not elevated.[86,89]

Because of their compromised immune response, dialysis patients may fail to mount a significant antibody response to HCV. This was particularly apparent with the first-generation test, because only about half of dialysis patients subsequently shown to have HCV were seropositive. The sensitivity of second- and third-generation tests is much improved, although one study found HCV RNA in 28% of dialysis patients who had negative second-generation HCV enzyme-linked immunosorbent assay tests.[90] Routine use of HCV RNA has therefore been advocated by some.[90] However, this is mitigated by the substantial cost and the difficulties of performing the test and reproducing the result. Regular surveillance of serum alanine aminotransferase (ALT) levels has been recommended as a less costly, more reproducible approach for screening dialysis patients for incident HCV.[90]

Early reports demonstrated that nosocomial spread was caused by overt interruptions in infection control,[91] and one more recent report suggested that HCV was transmitted by contaminated hands of HCWs, demonstrating that the problem persists.[92,93] In most newer studies, however, obvious breaches of infection control in dialysis centers and elsewhere[94] have not been identified, suggesting that either subtle interruptions are responsible for spread or HCV transmission is incompletely understood. Supporting the latter interpretation, some studies utilizing genotypic analysis have not demonstrated spread among persons treated in the same or adjacent beds; rather, linked cases have been located throughout the dialysis center, suggesting widely dispersed transmission by an uncertain mechanism.[95]

Recognized risk factors for acquisition of HCV include blood transfusion and duration of dialysis time,[94] with the latter being more significant. The frequency and therefore the risk of blood transfusion has been reduced by the use of erythropoietin.[85] Possible explanations for the association with duration of dialysis include sharing of dialysis machines by HCV-infected and uninfected patients and reprocessing of dialyzers from HCV-infected patients.[96,97] In U.S. dialysis centers, the incidence was significantly higher among those that used nondisposable rather than disposable containers for priming the dialyzer.[38]

Some researchers have advocated keeping HCV-infected dialysis patients together, similar to the successful approach taken with HBV-infected patients. The CDC, however, does not advocate this approach[80] because of the lack of sensitivity of the anti-HCV test, which means that not all infectious persons would be isolated, and because of the risk of superinfection for those already infected.[86]

Solid Tumor Transplantation. Transplantation of HCV-infected organs into HCV-infected or uninfected hosts is an area of increasing concern.[86] Almost all susceptible recipients of HCV-positive organs eventually develop HCV infection,[98] which may be severe.[98,99] In most series, however, no adverse effect on overall survival of patients or grafts has been found, although recipients of HCV-positive organs had a higher rate of liver-related morbidity and mortality.[98,99] Many organ banks now avoid using organs from HCV-positive donors except for lifesaving procedures such as heart, lung, and liver transplantation.[86] Transmission of HCV to eight organ or tissue recipients from a single, seronegative, and nucleic acid amplification test (NAT)-positive organ donor has been described.[100] The donor died early in the HCV "window period."

Other Nosocomial Transmissions. In recent years, more reports have described clustering of hepatitis C cases around various health-care-related exposures, including transmissions related to endoscopy,[101,102] retrograde cholangiogram,[103] computed tomography scanning,[104] re-use of needles and syringes,[105] use of multidose vials,[106,107] use of a spring-loaded finger-stick device,[108] and sclerotherapy for varicose veins.[109] In addition, transmission has been described related to assisted conception,[110] immunoadsorption therapy in hemophilia,[111] and, perhaps, razor sharing between two residents of a psychiatric hospital.[112] Transmission also may occur in nonhospital health care settings.[112a]

In a recent, highly publicized report from Las Vegas, Nevada, several patients seen at one endoscopy clinic were found to have hepatitis C. The infection was thought to be related to inappropriate re-use of syringes and use of medication vials intended for single use on multiple persons.[101] In other reports from endoscopy clinics, the transmission may have occurred due to inadequate cleaning of the biopsy suction channel of the colonoscope or failure to autoclave some equipment, such as biopsy forceps.[113]

Several reports have suggested an association between development of HCV infection and hospitalization on an oncology or bone marrow transplant floor,[114,115] or on a urology,[116] liver,[117] or generalized[118] ward. Although some studies are from relatively resource-poor countries, where re-use of needles may be the cause, others remain puzzling. Prolonged hospitalization often is a risk in these reports, and, in one large U.S. outbreak, transmission was thought to be related to shared saline bags contaminated through syringe re-use.[114] Detection of HCV by the second-generation test was lower among immunocompromised cancer patients than expected for normal hosts, leading the authors to suggest adding additional testing, such as NAT, to screen compromised hosts.[119]

Management. The CDC recommends determining the HCV serostatus of the source patient after any exposure.[37,80] For the exposed HCW, baseline and 6-month follow-up testing for HCV antibody (second-generation test) and ALT should be obtained. Between 5% and 10% of infections are not detected by enzyme immunoassay but may be identified with NAT screening for viral RNA. This technique is routine for blood banks (see later discussion) and could be used in the occupational exposure setting as well.

Optimal management of a needlestick exposure is unknown, but immune globulin is not recommended.[80] Immediate prospects for an effective vaccine are limited. Interferon-alfa may have a role in early infection: in one study, HCV resolved in all 14 HCWs who were treated with interferon soon after acute infection.[120]

Hepatitis D

Delta virus is a defective RNA virus that requires the presence of active HBV infection (acute HBV or HBsAg carrier state) to infect the liver. In a report of transmission of the delta agent from a dialysis center,[121] a dually infected source patient regularly shared a dialysis machine with an asymptomatic HBsAg carrier. The latter patient subsequently developed acute delta hepatitis. A surgeon may also have become dually infected after a deep needlestick sustained while operating on the same source patient. Review identified several additional possible instances of delta hepatitis transmission in dialysis centers. This led to the current recommendation that patients and staff be vaccinated against HBV and that dialysis patients be separated according to delta virus status. Specifically, delta-positive, HBsAg-positive patients should receive dialysis in a separate room from delta-negative, HBsAg-positive patients.

▪ Transfusion-Associated Infections

Beeson reported the first cases of transfusion-associated infection in 1943, describing seven patients who developed hepatitis 33 to 119 days after receiving a red blood cell (RBC) or plasma transfusion.[122] The advent of the acquired immunodeficiency syndrome (AIDS) epidemic in the 1980s, followed by recognition of transfusion transmission of hepatitis C, and, most recently, documentation of the association of the West Nile virus (WNV) epidemic with transfusion-transmitted infection, have continued to draw attention to the safety of the blood supply, particularly the potential risk from emerging infectious agents.[123-125]

Although infections with HCV and WNV have been the most publicized, a wide spectrum of other organisms, including bacteria, parasites, and prions, have been transmitted by transfusion.[126] Of these, bacteria transmitted by transfusion, often associated with platelets, occurs most commonly and may cause sepsis and death.[127] Recognition of the threat of *Trypanosoma cruzi* transmission via transfusion and the availability of suitable testing have led to screening for this pathogen, which is the cause of Chagas' disease. Tick-borne agents also are recognized to pose an increasing risk to transfusion safety, including transmission of babesiosis and, most recently, anaplasmosis. Transmission of variant Creutzfeldt-Jakob disease (vCJD) via transfusion has occurred in the United Kingdom.

An ongoing dilemma of the blood-banking community is a mandate to ensure a maximally safe blood supply while giving consideration to the cost of such measures. Pathogen reduction of blood components, using methods that inactivate the nucleic material present in most viruses and bacteria, has been proposed to obviate the ever-increasing list of needed screening tests, but no such technology has been approved for use in the United States. The current questions for screening donors that have been adopted by most blood banks are presented in Figure 305-1, and the laboratory screening measures currently in place are listed in Table 305-2. Pathogens or diseases screened solely through donor interview include babesiosis, malaria, and vCJD.

SCOPE OF BLOOD TRANSFUSION

According to estimates from the World Health Organization (WHO), more than 80 million units of blood are collected in the world annually. Less than 45% of donated blood is collected in developing and transitional countries, which are home to about 80% of the world's population. Of the 150 countries providing data to WHO, 31 were not able to screen all of their donated blood for one or more of the four infections (HIV, HBV, HCV, and syphilis) that are most widely

TABLE 305-2	Laboratory Screening Performed for Pathogens or Diseases by Blood Collection Centers in the United States

Mandated by U.S. Food and Drug Administration
Hepatitis B surface antigen (HBsAg)
Hepatitis B core antibody (anti-HBcAb)
Hepatitis C virus antibody (anti-HCV)
HIV-1 and HIV-2 antibody (anti-HIV-1 and anti-HIV-2)
HIV p24 antigen
HTLV-I and HTLV-II antibody (anti-HTLV-I and anti-HTLV-II)
Serologic test for syphilis
NAT for HIV and HCV
Additionally Required by Accrediting Organizations*
Platelet screening for bacterial contamination[†]
Performed Voluntarily
NAT for West Nile virus
Serologic test for *Trypanosoma cruzi*
Serologic test for CMV (on request)
Available
NAT for hepatitis B virus

*Including AABB (formerly known as the American Association of Blood Banks) and the College of American Pathologists.
[†]Generally, liquid culture media for apheresis units and pH or glucose indicators for whole blood–derived pooled units.
CMV, cytomegalovirus; HIV, human immunodeficiency virus; HTLV, human T-cell lymphotropic virus; NAT, nucleic acid amplification testing.

Full-Length Donor History Questionnaire

	Yes	No
Are you		
1. Feeling healthy and well today?	❑	❑
2. Currently taking an antibiotic?	❑	❑
3. Currently taking any other medication for an infection?	❑	❑
Please read the Medication Deferral List.		
4. Are you now taking or have you ever taken any medications on the Medication Deferral List?	❑	❑
5. Have you read the educational materials?	❑	❑
In the past **48 hours**		
6. Have you taken aspirin or anything that has aspirin in it?	❑	❑
In the past **6 weeks**		
7. Female donors: Have you been pregnant or are you pregnant now? (Males: check "I am male.")	❑	❑	❑ I am male
In the past **8 weeks have you**		
8. Donated blood, platelets or plasma?	❑	❑
9. Had any vaccinations or other shots?	❑	❑
10. Had contact with someone who had a smallpox vaccination?	❑	❑
In the past **16 weeks**		
11. Have you donated a double unit of red cells using an apheresis machine?	❑	❑
In the past **12 months have you**		
12. Had a blood transfusion?	❑	❑
13. Had a transplant such as organ, tissue, or bone marrow?	❑	❑
14. Had a graft such as bone or skin?	❑	❑
15. Come into contact with someone else's blood?	❑	❑
16. Had an accidental needle-stick?	❑	❑
17. Had sexual contact with anyone who has HIV/AIDS or has had a positive test for the HIV/AIDS virus?	❑	❑
18. Had sexual contact with a prostitute or anyone else who takes money or drugs or other payment for sex?	❑	❑
19. Had sexual contact with anyone who has ever used needles to take drugs or steroids, or anything <u>not</u> prescribed by their doctor?	❑	❑
20. Had sexual contact with anyone who has hemophilia or has used clotting factor concentrates?	❑	❑
21. Female donors: Had sexual contact with a male who has ever had sexual contact with another male? (Males: check "I am male.")	❑	❑	❑ I am male
22. Had sexual contact with a person who has hepatitis?	❑	❑
23. Lived with a person who has hepatitis?	❑	❑
24. Had a tattoo?	❑	❑
25. Had ear or body piercing?	❑	❑

v.1.2   eff February 2007

Figure 305-1 AABB Blood Donor History Questionnaire, Version 1.2, February 2007. Available at http://www.aabb.org/Documents/Donate_Blood/Donor_History_Questionnaire/udhqfullv1-2.pdf (accessed April 2009).

recognized to be transmitted through blood and are recommended by WHO to be screened at donation.[128,129]

Surveys to determine blood product use in the United States, led by the National Heart and Lung Institute (now called the National Heart, Lung and Blood Institute), began in 1971.[130] In the United States, surveys have reported the frequency of blood collection and utilization since the late 1980s, most recently through the Nationwide Blood Collection and Utilization Survey (NCBUS), which has been conducted biannually since 1998.[130-133] In the 2007 NCBUS report, reflecting data collected in 2006, there were approximately 14.5 million whole-blood and 12.5 million apheresis collections, with more than 30 million blood components transfused.[133] Each recipient received an average of 3 units of blood. In 1997, 14.7 million whole-blood and RBC units, 4.0 million units of fresh-frozen plasma, 10.4 million units of platelets (i.e., both pooled and apheresis units), and 1.0 million units of cryoprecipitate were given.[133] The number of RBC transfusions has slowly increased after reaching a nadir in the late 1990s. The number of transfused platelets also has slowly increased, but this is due entirely to platelets collected by apheresis, because the amount of whole blood–derived or pooled platelets has declined dramatically in the same interval. In addition to contributions from the voluntary donor pool, 12 million units of plasma are collected annually from paid donors and

Full-Length Donor History Questionnaire—cont'd

	Yes	No
26. Had or been treated for syphilis or gonorrhea?	☐	☐
27. Been in juvenile detention, lockup, jail, or prison for more than 72 hours?	☐	☐
In the past three years have you		
28. Been outside the United States or Canada?	☐	☐
From 1980 through 1996,		
29. Did you spend time that adds up to three (3) months or more in the United Kingdom? (Review list of countries in the UK)	☐	☐
30. Were you a member of the U.S. military, a civilian military employee, or a dependent of a member of the U.S. military?	☐	☐
From 1980 to the present, did you		
31. Spend time that adds up to five (5) years or more in Europe? (Review list of countries in Europe.)	☐	☐
32. Receive a blood transfusion in the United Kingdom or France? (Review list of countries in the UK.)	☐	☐
From 1977 to the present, have you		
33. Received money, drugs, or other payment for sex?	☐	☐
34. Male donors: had sexual contact with another male, even once? (Females: check "I am female.")	☐	☐
Have you EVER		
35. Had a positive test for the HIV/AIDS virus?	☐	☐
36. Used needles to take drugs, steroids, or anything not prescribed by your doctor?	☐	☐
37. Used clotting factor concentrates?	☐	☐
38. Had hepatitis?	☐	☐
39. Had malaria?	☐	☐
40. Had Chagas' disease?	☐	☐
41. Had babesiosis?	☐	☐
42. Received a dura mater (or brain covering) graft?	☐	☐
43. Had any type of cancer, including leukemia?	☐	☐
44. Had any problems with your heart or lungs?	☐	☐
45. Had a bleeding condition or a blood disease?	☐	☐
46. Had sexual contact with anyone who was born in or lived in Africa?	☐	☐
47. Been in Africa?	☐	☐
48. Have any of your relatives had Creutzfeldt-Jakob disease?	☐	☐

(Question 34: ☐ I am female)

v.1.2   eff February 2007

Figure 305-1, con't.

are used to prepare immunoglobulin, albumin, and various other plasma-derived products.[133]

By 1987, the cost of collecting, processing, and transfusing patients exceeded $3 billion; since then, costs have increased steadily with the addition of new screening tests and the implementation of leukoreduction.[130] In 2006, the average price paid by a hospital was $213.94 for a unit of leukocyte-reduced RBCs, $59.84 for fresh-frozen plasma, $84.25 for whole blood–derived platelets, and $528.72 for apheresis platelets, so current costs are likely to exceed $5 billion annually.[133]

It has been estimated that the annual likelihood of an individual's receiving a transfusion is about 0.89% and increases dramatically with age; in 2006, the transfusion rate in the U.S. population was 49 units per 1000 people.[133,134] Because of concern about contracting an infectious disease, there has been a shift toward autologous and donor-directed blood donation over the past decade. However, donor-directed units, usually given by family members for a specific patient, have been shown to have higher rates of various infectious agents. Recently, there has been movement away from donor-directed donation and toward building a dedicated, voluntary repeat donor population.[132,133] Viral infections are much less common among repeat donors compared with first-time whole-blood donors, and they may be even less common among donors associated with apheresis collection.[135,136]

About 50% of blood components transfused in the United States are leukocyte-reduced, a modification that is performed to filter out the majority of white blood cells. Leukoreduction is performed to reduce nonhemolytic transfusion reactions, but it may also reduce the risk of infectious disease transmission through removal of infected white blood cells, particularly for cell-associated agents such as cytomegalovirus (discussed later).[137]

In 2006, only about 33,000 units, or 0.9% of the donated allogeneic blood supply, were discarded on testing, usually because of detection of a potentially transmissible infection.[133] This reflects a dramatic decrease in units discarded due to testing, perhaps reflecting improved accuracy of screening tests and retention of repeat donors. The incidence of viral markers in donated units was increased among volunteers who donated after September 11, 2001, primarily due to a large cohort of first-time and infrequent repeat donors.[138]

BLOOD-BORNE PATHOGENS: HIV, HTLV, AND HEPATITIS VIRUSES

Historically, transfusion-associated transmission risk has persisted for HIV, HBV, HCV, and human T-cell lymphotropic virus type I (HTLV-I) for two distinct reasons: (1) the incomplete sensitivity of the available serologic screening tests, which ranges from about 95% for HCV to more than 99% for HIV, and (2) the "window" period, which is defined as the period between acute infection (and potential infectivity) and the time when available tests can reliably detect infection.

The recent development and implementation of routine NAT has transformed blood bank screening for viral pathogens.[139-142] NAT can detect viral RNA within the first 10 to 14 days, narrowing the window period by 7 to 10 days for HIV and by 50 to 60 days for HCV. Additional NAT tests that have been developed for blood donor screening, including tests for WNV, HBV, and parvovirus B19; of these, only the WNV test has been uniformly adopted for use in screening.[143]

With introduction of NAT, the risk of acquiring HIV or HCV per unit of blood transfused has plummeted from approximately 1 per 500,000 for HIV and 1 per 100,000 for HCV before NAT to a current rate of 1 per 2 million for both viruses. Detected cases are so unusual that the incidence has to be estimated statistically.[144] As remarkable as this advance is, a small window period remains, meaning that the risk of receiving one of these viruses in a unit of blood is not zero. Three cases of HIV and many more cases of HCV transmission through transfusion have been recognized since NAT was implemented; the modeling data estimate more cases than the number reported, so some cases likely go unrecognized.

The advent of NAT also has had a substantial impact on the choice of serologic tests. In addition to sensitivity, blood bankers seek optimal specificity: false-positive or indeterminant tests exclude otherwise appropriate donors from subsequent donations and create anxiety due to incorrect diagnosis of infection. The introduction of an extremely sensitive test such as NAT allows blood banks to focus on the specificity of other screening tests, thereby limiting the number of persons potentially excluded from the donor pool because of misleading test results. An example of this potential benefit is found with the enzyme immunoassay tests used for HCV. Although sensitivity varies little between the second- and third-generation antibody tests, the third-generation assay has superior specificity, decreasing the proportion of persons with indeterminant antibody tests for HCV.[145] The introduction of HBV NAT could have similar potential, but thus far the test has not been adopted for blood screening.

Human Immunodeficiency Virus Type 1

More than 8000 persons in the United States have developed AIDS from receipt of blood or tissue.[146] In addition, at least 50% of all hemophiliacs in the United States and Europe became infected with HIV from 1978 to 1985, most from receipt of infected plasma factors, with the highest incidence in 1982, when there were 22 infections per 100 person-years.[147] The first HIV screening test was introduced in 1985, and since 1987 few new infections among hemophiliacs have been reported.[147] As noted, the introduction of NAT screening has substantially lowered the risk of HIV transmission, with the last reported case occurring in 2002.

Redundant methods of testing also have been useful in confirming the status of infection for blood donor follow-up. Polymerase chain reaction (PCR) for HIV RNA detection has been useful in clarifying the HIV serostatus of persons with indeterminate results of Western blot tests.[148] These reactions occur in about 1 of every 5000 donations and usually represent false-positive tests.[149]

Human Immunodeficiency Virus Type 2

In June 1992, the U.S. Food and Drug Administration (FDA) mandated screening for HIV-2.[150] Since then, few HIV-2–positive donors have been identified, and no cases of transmission have occurred in the United States, although transfusion-related HIV-2 cases have occurred elsewhere.[151,152]

Human T-Cell Lymphotropic Virus Types I and II

HTLV-I and HTLV-II, unlike HIV-1 and HIV-2, are cell associated and therefore predominantly transmissible only with blood component transfusions.[153] Screening for both types is done with a single test. The rate of transmission of HTLV-I decreased almost 10-fold (from 1 per 8500 to 1 per 69,000) after introduction of the screening test.[154] Transplantation of solid organs from an HTLV-I–infected donor resulted in rapid progression to subacute myelopathy in three recipients; this phenomenon has not been described in transfusion recipients.[155]

Hepatitis B and D Viruses

HBV remains the most common blood-borne viral pathogen in the donor population and the one with the highest residual risk despite screening; HBV is transmitted in approximately 1 of every 205,000 transfusions.[156] Risk persists both because the screening test is incompletely sensitive (transmission from HBsAg-negative donors has long been recognized) and because of the prolonged window period of about 2 months. In countries that screen for HBcAb, most transmissions derive from the window period, whereas in those that do not check HBcAb status, half derive from the window period and the others are due to the insensitivity of HBsAg as a screening test.[128]

NAT for HBV was developed for blood screening but to date has been implemented only for investigational use, because there have been arguments against a favorable cost-benefit ratio. With current sensitivity, NAT would shorten the window period modestly, from 59 to 49 days. This in turn might result in only a small reduction in risk, from about 1 in 220,000 to 1 in 250,000.[157] However, data suggest that the residual risk reduction may be higher. In Central Europe, where NAT has been used since 1997, routine screening identified 6 additional infected donors out of 3.6 million tests.[158] This yielded a residual transmission risk of about 1 per 350,000 transfusions. More sensitive screens are particularly needed in HBV-endemic areas, such as Taiwan, where HBcAb testing is not routinely performed and transfusion-acquired HBV is a relatively frequent event.[159] Testing for HBcAb, in addition to HBsAg, remains important; in some cases, it more sensitive than NAT, so implementation of new testing does not obviate the use of these other tests for donor HBV infection.[160] Increasing use of hepatitis B vaccination may further reduce the risk of transmission.

Screening of donors for HBsAg excludes most, but not all, carriers of delta virus.[161] Identification of donors with antibody to the delta agent is not done routinely, so there is a residual risk of transmission of delta virus to HBsAg-positive recipients.

Hepatitis C Virus

Hepatitis C, historically known as "non-A, non-B hepatitis," was transmitted to as many as 7% to 10% of transfusion recipients in the late 1970s and early 1980s.[162] The transmission rate of hepatitis C has decreased with improved screening tests to identify the virus, providing an excellent example of how implementation of each new generation of screening technology has improved blood safety. More than 90% of recipients of HCV-contaminated blood products develop HCV infection.[163] An older survey using the second-generation test found that 3.6 per 1000 U.S. donors were positive for HCV,[164] a prevalence lower than that in the U.S. population, which is about 10 to 20 per 1000 donors. HCV infection in blood donors usually is the result of intravenous drug use, although other risks have been identified.[115]

Before any testing, 0.45% of all transfusions transmitted HCV. With the introduction in 1986 of surrogate marker testing (ALT and HBcAb), the rate decreased to 0.19%, and with the introduction of the first-generation antibody test for HCV in 1990, the rate fell to 0.03%. The second-generation test lowered the rate even further, mostly by identifying chronic infections more accurately (i.e., increasing sensitivity) rather than by shortening the window period. The introduction of

NAT reduced the transmission risk to about 1 in 1.5 to 2 million transfusions.[140,141,144]

Administration of intravenous immune globulin (IVIG) previously was associated with transmission of HCV[166]; however, the FDA now requires a heat inactivation step as part of the preparation of all IVIG products. In addition, all immunoglobulin products, even those given by intramuscular injection (which have never been associated with transmission of any infectious agent), are now screened for HCV.

West Nile Virus
WNV has been transmitted by blood transfusion to at least 32 persons since this route of transmission was first recognized during the summer of 2002.[125] In addition, it has been transmitted by organ transplantation.[167] In response to this emerging threat, a NAT test for WNV was quickly developed and implemented by 2003 and is now in routine use for blood donor screening; thousands of WNV-infected donations have been interdicted.[142,143] Because of the logistic and financial burden of individual testing, WNV screening assays test pools of 6 or 16 donations (i.e., minipools), with follow-up screening of positive minipools by individual sample NAT. However, "break-through" cases of WNV transfusion transmission still occur, because minipool testing is not as sensitive as individual sample NAT. In response, blood banks are using strategies to trigger a switch from minipool to individual NAT in areas with high epidemic activity during seasonal peaks.[168] Clinicians should suspect WNV in recently transfused or transplanted individuals who develop unexplained encephalitis or flaccid paralysis.[169]

Herpesviruses
Human herpesvirus 8 (HHV-8), the cause of Kaposi's sarcoma, is thought to be primarily white cell associated, suggesting a low risk of transmission, and few cases of transmission have been documented. The low rate of recognized transmission may reflect, in part, the difficulty in test performance and the high positive background rate, but studies have suggested a link.[170,171] One epidemiologic study completed in Uganda estimated the rate of transmission to be 2.8% for non-leukoreduced RBC units, with excess risk associated with storage times shorter than 4 days.[172] Further studies are needed to determine whether leukoreduction can mitigate this risk. Transmission of HHV-8 resulting in Kaposi's sarcoma has been described more frequently in recipients of solid organ transplants.[173]

The transmission risk for cytomegalovirus (CMV) has been well summarized.[174] CMV, similar to HHV-8, is highly cell associated and can be transmitted with white blood cells that persist in RBC or platelet transfusions. Transmission of CMV from fresh-frozen plasma or cryoprecipitate has not been reported. The insensitivity of the serologic test has resulted in a residual risk of transmission of 0% to 6%, even when CMV-seronegative donors are used.[174] Because the demand for CMV-seronegative blood outstrips the supply, approaches such as leukocyte filtration of CMV-seropositive blood are often used, although the two approaches may not be equivalent in reducing CMV transmission risk.[137]

Screening for Epstein-Barr virus is not performed routinely, despite reports of transfusion-associated transmission.

Parvovirus B19
Parvovirus B19 has been transmitted in coagulation factor concentrates. The risk of transmission to cryoprecipitate recipients may persist despite treating with solvent and detergent and heating to 100°C after lyophilization.[175] An epidemiologic study showed a significant correlation between receipt of treatment products, B19 seropositivity, and joint range-of-motion limitations.[176]

Hepatitis A and E Viruses
Transmission of HAV via transfusion has been described with RBCs, particularly in infants,[177,178] and with factor VIII concentrate.[179] Donors with early, asymptomatic infection may transmit HAV.[180] Factor VIII–

associated transmission has occurred despite appropriate use of organic solvent and detergent to inactivate the virus. The lack of a lipid envelope around HAV may have contributed to incomplete virus killing during preparation of the concentrate. Because of this small but persistent risk, vaccination for hepatitis A has been recommended for chronic recipients of products made from pooled plasma.[181] Review of all cases of hepatitis from 1998 to 2002 in the United States among persons with bleeding disorders revealed no acquisition of HAV via factor concentrates.[182]

Hepatitis E virus, which is endemic in many developing countries and has similar epidemiology to HAV, has been implicated in transfusion transmission worldwide but has not yet been reported in the United States.[183]

Non–A-E Hepatitis
The search for the cause of non–A-E hepatitis has yielded many contenders but no indisputable etiology to date. Hepatitis G virus (HGV) has been found in 1% to 7% of donors and can be transmitted by transfusion.[184] The risk of transmission is in the range of 5.3 per 10,000 units.[185] However, HGV has been shown not to be a cause of non–A-E hepatitis, and the clinical implications of HGV infection remain undetermined.[184]

Two, somewhat related, single-stranded, unencapsulated DNA viruses, called transfusion-transmitted virus (TTV) and SEN virus (designating the initials of the first patient investigated) have been considered as causes of non–A-E hepatitis.[186,187] Both viruses are present worldwide and are often found in the blood of persons with post-transfusion non–A-E hepatitis. However, after initial interest, no causal association was established.

BACTERIAL PATHOGENS

Infusion of blood products contaminated by bacteria is a relatively frequent and potentially lethal risk of blood transfusion.[126,188] As the risk of transfusion-transmitted viral infection has decreased dramatically, the frequency of transfusion-transmitted bacterial infection has remained unchanged. A possible exception to this persistent risk is transfusion transmission of *Treponema pallidum*, the etiologic agent of syphilis, which has not been reported to have occurred for decades, presumably because of poor spirochete survival under current storage conditions.[189-191]

Bacterial contamination may arise from donation, processing, storage, or transfusion and can result in transfusion-transmitted sepsis and death. Because platelets are stored at room temperature, they are at higher risk for bacterial growth than RBCs, which are stored at refrigerated temperatures. Bacterial contamination of blood components has been the most frequent cause of transfusion-related fatalities reported to the FDA after hemolytic reactions, accounting for more than 10% of transfusion-associated fatalities between 1985 and 1999. Although visual inspection can sometimes reveal a significantly contaminated unit, this is not always the case (Fig. 305-2).

Based on culturing, estimates have placed the rate of bacterial contamination at 1 per 2000 to 3000 units for platelets and 1 per 30,000 units for RBCs.[192-195] Estimates of the rate of clinically evident reactions after transfusion of bacterially contaminated blood products vary more widely, from 1 in 5000 to 1 in 100,000, although it is generally agreed that pooled platelets confer a greater risk per therapeutic dose than do platelets collected by apheresis.[196] A national study, The Assessment of the Frequency of Blood Component Bacterial Contamination Associated with Transfusion (BaCon), was designed to identify severe reactions that resulted in confirmed transfusion-transmitted sepsis through passive reporting. Over a 3-year period, there were 56 reports and 34 confirmed cases, principally from contaminated platelets. Although *Staphylococcus* and other gram-positive organisms were most frequently associated with transfusion-transmitted sepsis, gram-negative organisms, such as

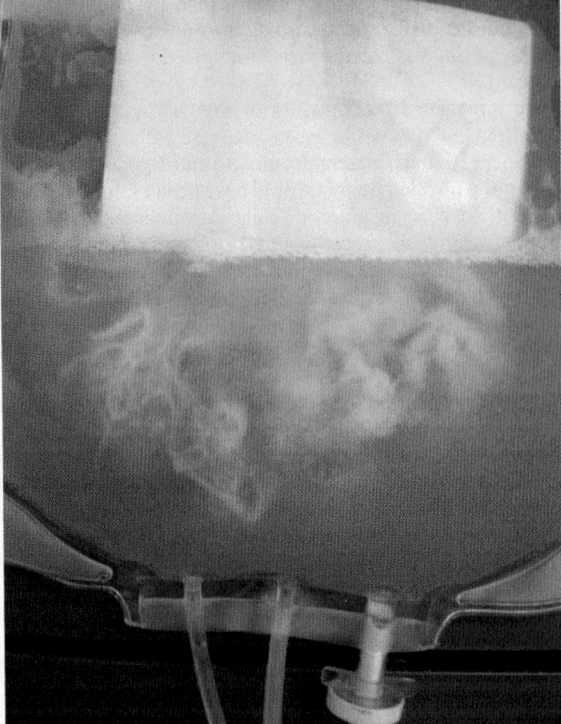

Figure 305-2 Pooled platelet unit containing *Klebsiella pneumoniae* (quantitative culture, 6.5 colony-forming units [CFUs] per milliliter), showing fibrinous coagulation 4 days after laboratory inoculation. *(From Hay S, Brecher M. Egg drop soup platelets: Gross bacterial contamination of a platelet product.* Transfusion. *2007;47:1335-1336.)*

Escherichia coli and *Serratia* spp., were statistically associated with fatal outcome. Nine persons (26.5%) died from the transmitted infection. The BaCon study estimates of transfusion-transmitted sepsis were 1 in 100,000 units for platelets and 1 in 5 million for RBCs, reflecting the difficulty of recognition and confirmation of these poorly appreciated clinical events.[127,197]

For both RBCs and platelets, longer storage time is well established as a risk factor for bacterial contamination. However, gram-negative organisms can be fast growing and can result in lethal endotoxin levels in 3-day-old platelets. Further shortening of the current 5-day platelet storage times is not feasible, because it would probably result in discarding too many uninfected units, exacerbating the nation's chronic blood supply shortage. In addition, contamination may occur during production and packaging of blood bags.[198] Recently, AABB required members to use a method to detect bacterial contamination in platelets; in apheresis platelets, liquid culture media methods are typically used by the blood collection centers, whereas for pooled platelets, the methods are varied and not well validated. This has resulted in a risk that is significant reduced but still present. The American Red Cross has described a decrease in risk of septic reactions due to apheresis platelets from 1 in 33,000 to 1 in 75,000; the risk from pooled platelets is presumably unchanged.[199] Other approaches to risk reduction are being actively pursued in the United States and have already been implemented in other countries. These include avoidance by improved skin preparation and diversion of the initial 15 to 30 mL of the blood draw; optimization of volume and storage time before culture; development of point-of-use tests at the time of transfusion; and pathogen reduction methods, including inactivation by photochemical treatment of units.[126]

Investigation of the potentially immunosuppressive consequences of blood transfusion is ongoing, but several reports suggest that blood

transfusion, particularly of units with longer storage times, can lead to increased risk of infection and adverse outcome.[200]

Red Blood Cells

Gram-negative bacteria, including *Yersinia enterocolitica, Pseudomonas fluorescens, Serratia marcescens*, and *Serratia liquefaciens*, accounted for most of the reported cases of transfusion-transmitted infection caused by contaminated RBCs historically[192,201] (Table 305-3). Transmission of bacterial infection through RBCs is less common than through platelets, because RBCs are stored at refrigerated temperatures, allowing a longer shelf life. Storage of RBCs may extend 35 to 42 days depending on the type of additive used. Almost all instances of infection are associated with erythrocytes stored longer than 9 days and appear to derive from enhanced growth of certain organisms at cold storage (4°C) temperatures. This was best exemplified by a case of transfusion-associated *Y. enterocolitica* in an autologous blood donor, who became bacteremic after receiving his own stored blood 41 days after donation.[202]

Donors with *Y. enterocolitica* infection are typically symptom free at the time of blood donation, although many recall having had a diarrheal illness about 1 month before donation. Although diarrhea may indicate exposure to contaminated food, a donor question regarding diarrheal illness has not been adopted into the standard questionnaire because of lack of specificity of the complaint. If it were used as a screening question, up to 10% of donors would be excluded.[192] Despite its suggestion of an association with *Y. enterocolitica*–contaminated products, the BaCon Study detected only one case of transfusion-transmitted sepsis caused by *Y. enterocolitica* and heralded replacement of this organism in RBC contamination with other gram-negative organisms, such as *E. coli* and unusual *Pseudomonas* and *Serratia* spp.[201] Patient bacteremia with *P. fluorescens* or *S. liquefaciens* should prompt a thorough search for a potential nosocomial source, such as contaminated transfusion or infusion products. Unlike platelets, there are no current laboratory-based screening measures in place to reduce the risk of bacterial contamination in RBCs, although development of a rapid endotoxin test is underway.

Platelets

A different spectrum of bacteria is associated with transfusion of platelets.[203,204] The most commonly recovered organisms are *Staphylococci* and streptococcal species. Gram-negative bacteria, including the Enterobacteriaceae (*E. coli, S. marcescens, Enterobacter* spp.) are less common but may be associated with rapid growth, production of endotoxin, and death[127] (see Table 305-3).

In past years, patients received pooled platelets from 6 to 10 donors, any one of which might be contaminated, thereby increasing the risk per transfusion. A large shift to use of single-donor platelets (via apheresis) may decrease this risk.[196]

As with RBCs, contaminated platelets tend to be older (e.g., 4 or 5 days of storage).[205] Because of this, the FDA, in 1985, shortened the acceptable storage time for platelets from 7 days to the current

TABLE 305-3	Organisms Implicated in Fatal Blood Transfusion-Transmitted Bacteremia, Including Association with Endotoxin (Results from BaCon Study)*
Platelets	
Group B streptococcus	
Escherichia coli	
*Pseudomonas rettgeri**	
*Serratia marcescens**	
Red Blood Cell Units	
Staphylococcus epidermidis	
*Serratia liquefaciens**	

*Associated with 9090 to 273,500 endotoxin-forming units per milliliter.
From Kuehnert MJ, Roth VR, Haley NR, et al. Transfusion-transmitted bacterial infection in the United States, 1998 through 2000. *Transfusion*. 2001;41:1493-1499.

5 days. Apheresis platelets are typically stored for a briefer period, further reducing risk associated with use of this product. A study to extend the shelf life of apheresis platelets from 5 to 7 days was halted due to an unacceptable number of organisms cultured from screened units.[206]

OTHER AGENTS TRANSMITTED THROUGH BLOOD COMPONENTS

Tick-borne Bacteria

Anaplasmosis and other tick-borne diseases, including human ehrlichiosis and Rocky Mountain spotted fever, represent a potential risk for transmission via blood transfusion in the United States.[207] Screening for a recent history of tick bite is unlikely to identify high-risk donors, because this exposure is unlikely to be recalled.[207] As the incidence of tick-borne diseases increases, physician vigilance for possible transmission of these agents via transfusion also should increase.

Anaplasma phagocytophilum, the causative agent of human granu-locytic ehrlichiosis, has been reported to have been transmitted by transfusion of RBCs.[208] Rickettsiae, including the etiologic agent of Rocky Mountain spotted fever, also may rarely be transmitted by blood transfusion.[207] Because rickettsia infect white blood cells, leuko-reduction techniques would be expected to reduce the risk of transmission through cellular components. Although Lyme disease has long been postulated to be transmitted by transfusion, no single case of transmission through blood components has yet been recognized; this may be due to lack of survival of the etiologic spirochete under blood component storage conditions. Possible infection with tick-borne agents should be suspected if transfusion recipients develop acute thrombocytopenia or hemolytic anemia after transfusion, especially if accompanied by fever. Simultaneous infection with multiple tick-borne agents (e.g., *Babesia* and *Anaplasma* spp.) should also be considered.[208]

Parasites

T. cruzi, which causes Chagas' disease, is endemic in certain areas of South America and Central America. Rare cases of *T. cruzi* trans-mitted by blood transfusion have been reported by U.S. investiga-tors.[209] Up to 100,000 persons with *T. cruzi* infection reside in the United States. In Los Angeles and Miami, where immigration from endemic areas is high, a study found that 7.3% and 14.3% of all blood donors, respectively, had a risk of *T. cruzi* by history. Of these, 1 in 7500 to 9000 had detectable antibody. Lookback did not find seropositivity or disease in 18 recipients of the units from seroposi-tive donors, but the data were limited.[210] Although prevalence of the disease among donors is low overall, the availability of a blood antibody test resulted in voluntary adoption of screening by multiple blood centers, constituting the majority of the blood supply.[211] An estimated 1 in 30,000 donors had *T. cruzi* infection on initial screen-ing and confirmation testing; the most frequent positive results were reported from California and Florida, although there was a nation-wide distribution, reflecting immigration broadly from endemic countries.[211] Lookback studies in progress indicate that the transmis-sion rate may be as low as 10%, but treatment of the hundreds of infected donors recognized on screening is a difficult issue.[212,213] The number of donors with evidence of past infection who have no clear risk factors has also raised the possibility that there may be more autochthonous cases of Chagas' disease than currently appreciated.[214]

At least 70 cases of transfusion-associated babesiosis have been recognized since 1979, and many more are suspected, because the disease currently is not nationally notifiable.[215,216] Most investigated cases are found to be due to *Babesia microti*, found mostly in the Northeastern and upper Midwestern states. However, other species, such as *Babesia duncani* (previously known as WA-1), have also been implicated, and because blood products are transported outside endemic areas, transfusion-transmitted babesiosis can occur any-where in the United States. Patients who are immunocompromised

or asplenic are at particular risk for increased disease severity. Blood donor screening for babesiosis is performed by questionnaire only. Because the incidence of transfusion transmission of babesiosis appears to be increasing, the need for effective screening becomes more urgent.[216]

Transfusion-related transmission of malaria has long been recog-nized. In the United States between 1963 and 1999, 93 cases of trans-fusion-associated malaria were diagnosed, and 10 patients died.[217] The majority of the infected donors would have been excluded had current deferral criteria been in place, or fully implemented, at the time of donation. Transfusion transmission of malaria has continued to decline, with the few cases recognized being associated with a history of malaria or with residence in a malarious area, rather than an isolated history of brief travel.[218]

Prions

The risk of transmission of sporadic Creutzfeldt-Jakob disease via transfusion is unknown, although no cases have been recognized.[219] In contrast, vCJD, which is acquired from eating beef and beef prod-ucts contaminated with the agent that causes bovine spongiform encephalopathy, has been documented to be transmitted by transfu-sion. Between 2003 and 2007, there were four reports, all in the United Kingdom, of individuals who acquired the vCJD agent through RBC transfusions. Two of the RBC recipients developed vCJD and died from the disease; the third died of an unrelated illness but had evi-dence of infection, and the fourth affected individual was still alive as of 2007.[220,221] These cases were unlikely to have been detected without a robust system operating in the United Kingdom for follow-up of health care outcomes in transfusion recipients. Before cases were reported, considerable concern in the United States led to exclusion of blood donors from Britain and of those with prolonged stays in western Europe. Although significant donor deferrals resulted, the precautionary measures appeared to be justified.[222]

Infectious Diseases Transmitted through Transplantation of Solid Organs and Other Tissues

Advances in health care technology have led to a proliferation in bio-logic products collected to sustain and improve the quality of life; more than 25,000 solid organs and 1.5 million tissue allografts are trans-planted each year. However, the proliferation of these products also has increased the opportunities for transmission of infectious patho-gens, including viruses, bacteria, and parasites. One organ and tissue donor could potentially transmit disease, including infection or malig-nancy, to as many as 100 recipients. Transmission of disease through solid organ and tissue transplantation is both a public health issue and a patient safety issue, because events can result in serious illness and death in recipients.

Examples of diseases or organisms transmitted through transplanta-tion of organs or other tissues include HIV, HCV, WNV, rabies, lym-phocytic choriomeningitis virus (LCMV), tuberculosis, malaria, babesiosis, and *T. cruzi* (Chagas' disease). For WNV, rabies, and LCMV, recognition of meningoencephalitis or unusual autopsy find-ings in multiple recipients at the same institution led to linkage to a common donor, who was found on further investigation to be infected.[167,223,224]

Recent efforts from mandated reporting have led to estimates that infectious diseases or malignancies may be transmitted to as many as 1% of all solid organ transplant recipients, in many of whom transmis-sion goes unrecognized, with illness instead attributed to organ rejec-tion or reactivated disease.[225] It is critical for health care providers to recognize unusual outcomes in these patients and to communicate information on suspected transmission in such cases as quickly as possible, so that public health authorities can investigate and help initi-ate prevention measures.

REFERENCES

1. MacCallum FO, Bauer DJ. Homologous serum jaundice: Transmission experiments with human volunteers. *Lancet*. 1944;5:622-627.
2. Seeff LB, Beebe GW, Hoofnagle JH, et al. A serologic follow-up of the 1942 epidemic of post-vaccination hepatitis in the United States Army. *N Engl J Med*. 1987;16:965-970.
3. Mendelssohn K, Witts LJ. Transmission of infection during withdrawal of blood. *Br Med J*. 1945;5:625-626.
4. Droller J. An outbreak of hepatitis in a diabetic clinic. *Br Med J*. 1945;5:623-625.
5. Neefe JR, Stokes J, Gellis SS. Homologous serum hepatitis and infectious (epidemic) hepatitis: Experimental study of immunity and cross immunity in volunteers, a preliminary report. *Am J Med Sci*. 1945;210:561-575.
6. MacCallum FO, Bradley WH. Transmission of infective hepatitis to human volunteers. *Lancet*. 1944;2:228-231.
7. Neefe JR, Stokes J Jr, Reinhold JG, et al. Hepatitis due to the injection of homologous blood products in human volunteers. *J Clin Invest*. 1944;23:836-853.
8. Neefe JR, Stokes J Jr, Reinhold JG. Oral administration to volunteers of feces from patients with homologous serum hepatitis and infectious (epidemic) hepatitis. *Am J Med Sci*. 1945;210:29-32.
9. Paul JR, Havens WP Jr, Sabin AB. Transmission experiments in serum jaundice and infectious hepatitis. *JAMA*. 1945;128:911-915.
10. Rosenbaum JR, Sepkowitz KA. Infectious disease experimentation involving human volunteers. *Clin Infect Dis*. 2002;34:963-971.
11. Liebowitz S, Greenwald L, Cohen I, Litwins J. Serum hepatitis in a blood bank worker. *JAMA*. 1949;140:1331-1333.
12. Trumbull ML, Greiner DJ. Homologous serum jaundice: An occupational hazard to medical personnel. *JAMA*. 1951;145:965-967.
13. Kuh C, Ward WE. Occupational virus hepatitis: An apparent hazard for medical personnel. *JAMA*. 1950:143:631-635.
14. Byrne EB. Viral hepatitis: An occupational hazard of medical personnel. *JAMA*. 1966;195:362-364.
15. Harpaz R, Von Seidlein L, Averhoff FM, et al. Transmission of hepatitis B virus to multiple patients from a surgeon without evidence of inadequate infection control. *N Engl J Med*. 1996;334:549-554.
16. The Incident Investigation Teams. Transmission of hepatitis B to patients from four infected surgeons without hepatitis B e antigen. *N Engl J Med*. 1997;336:178-184.
17. Esteban JI, Gomez J, Martell M, et al. Transmission of hepatitis C virus by a cardiac surgeon. *N Engl J Med*. 1996;334:555-560.
18. Centers for Disease Control and Prevention. Immunization of health-care workers: Recommendations of the Advisory Committee on Immunization Practices (ACIP) and the Hospital Infection Control Practices Advisory Committee (HICPAC). *MMWR Morb Mortal Wkly Rep*. 1997;46(RR-18):1-42.
19. Noble RC, Kane MA, Reeves SA, et al. Posttransfusion hepatitis A in a neonatal intensive care unit. *JAMA*. 1984;252:2711-2715.
20. Drusin LM, Sohmer M, Groshen SL, et al. Nosocomial hepatitis A infection in a paediatric intensive care unit. *Arch Dis Child*. 1987;62:690-695.
21. Doebbeling BN, Li N, Wenzel RP. An outbreak of hepatitis A among health care workers: Risk factors for transmission. *Am J Public Health*. 1993;83:1679-1684.
22. Goodman RA, Carder CC, Allen JR, et al. Nosocomial hepatitis A transmission by an adult patient with diarrhea. *Am J Med*. 1982;73:220-226.
23. Baptiste R, Koziol D, Henderson DK. Nosocomial transmission of hepatitis A in an adult population. *Infect Control*. 1987;8:364-370.
24. Jensenius M, Ringertz SH, Berild D, et al. Prolonged nosocomial outbreak of hepatitis A arising from an alcoholic with pneumonia. *Scand J Infect Dis*. 1998;30:119-123.
25. Bolyard EA, Tablan OC, Williams WW, et al. Guideline for infection control in healthcare personnel, 1998. Hospital Infection Control Practices Advisory Committee. *Infect Control Hosp Epidemiol*. 1998;19:407-463.
26. Recommended adult immunization schedule—United States, October 2007-September 2008. *MMWR Morb Mortal Wkly Rep*. 2007;56:Q1-A4. Available at http://www.cdc.gov/mmwr/preview/mmwrhtml/mm5641-Immunizational.htm (accessed April 2009).
27. Prevention of hepatitis A through active or passive immunization: Recommendations of the Advisory Committee on Immunization Practices (ACIP). *MMWR Morb Mortal Wkly Rep*. 2006;55(RR-07):1-23. Available at http://www.cdc.gov/mmwr/preview/mmwrhtml/rr5507a1.htm (accessed April 2009).
28. Siddiqui AR, Jooma RA, Smego RA Jr. Nosocomial outbreak of hepatitis E in Pakistan with possible parenteral transmission. *Clin Infect Dis*. 2005;40:908-909.
29. Mahoney FJ, Stewart K, Hu H, et al. Progress toward the elimination of hepatitis B virus transmission among health care workers in the United States. *Arch Intern Med*. 1997;157:2601-2605.
30. Occupational Safety and Health Administration. Occupational exposure to bloodborne pathogens: Final rule. *Fed Regist*. 1991;56:64175-64182.
31. Agerton TB, Mahoney FJ, Polish LB, et al. Impact of the bloodborne pathogens standard on vaccination of healthcare workers with hepatitis B vaccine. *Infect Control Hosp Epidemiol*. 1995;16:287-291.
32. Centers for Disease Control and Prevention. Hepatitis B vaccination—United States, 1982-2002. *MMWR Morb Mortal Wkly Rep*. 2002;51:549-552, 563.
33. Mast EE, Alter MJ. Prevention of hepatitis B virus infection among health-care workers. In: Ellis RE, ed. *Hepatitis B Vaccines in Clinical Practice*. New York: Marcel Dekker; 1993:295-307.
34. Lewis TL, Alter HJ, Chalmers TC, et al. A comparison of the frequency of hepatitis-B antigen and antibody in hospital and nonhospital personnel. *N Engl J Med*. 1973;289:647-651.
35. Feldman RE, Schiff ER. Hepatitis in dental professionals. *JAMA*. 1975;232:1228-1230.
36. Gibas A, Blewett DR, Schoenfeld DA, et al. Prevalence and incidence of viral hepatitis in health workers in the prehepatitis B vaccination era. *Am J Epidemiol*. 1992;136:603-610.
37. Centers for Disease Control and Prevention. Updated U.S. Public Health Service guidelines for the management of occupational exposures to HBV, HCV, and HIV and recommendations for postexposure prophylaxis. *MMWR Morb Mortal Wkly Rep*. 2001;50(RR-11):1-52.
38. Finelli L, Miller JT, Tokars JI, et al. National surveillance of dialysis-associated diseases in the United States, 2002. *Semin Dial*. 2005;18:52-61.
39. Garibaldi RA, Rasmussen CM, Holmes AW, et al. Hospital-acquired serum hepatitis: Report of an outbreak. *JAMA*. 1972;219:1577-1580.
40. Gerety RJ. Hepatitis B transmission between dental or medical workers and patients. *Ann Intern Med*. 1981;95:229-231.
41. Lettau LA, Smith JD, Williams D, et al. Transmission of hepatitis B with resultant restriction of surgical practice. *JAMA*. 1986;255:934-937.
42. Weber DJ, Hoffmann KK, Rutala WA. Management of the healthcare worker infected with human immunodeficiency virus: Lessons from nosocomial transmission of hepatitis B virus. *Infect Control Hosp Epidemiol*. 1991;12:625-630.
43. Bell DM, Shapiro CN, Ciesielski CA, et al. Preventing bloodborne pathogen transmission from health-care workers to patients: The CDC perspective. *Surg Clin North Am*. 1995;75:1189-1203.
44. Spijkerman IJ, van Doorn LJ, Janssen MH, et al. Transmission of hepatitis B virus from a surgeon to his patients during high-risk and low-risk surgical procedures during 4 years. *Infect Control Hosp Epidemiol*. 2002;23:306-312.
45. Recommendations for preventing transmission of human immunodeficiency virus and hepatitis B virus to patients during exposure-prone invasive procedures. *AORN J*. 1991;54:576-582.
46. Gerberding JL. The infected health care provider. *N Engl J Med*. 1996;334:594-595.
47. Shanson DC. Hepatitis B outbreak in operating-theatre and intensive care staff (Letter). *Lancet*. 1980;2:596.
48. Petrosillo N, Puro V, Jagger J, et al. The risks of occupational exposure and infection by human immunodeficiency virus, hepatitis B virus, and hepatitis C virus in the dialysis setting. Italian Multicenter Study on Nosocomial and Occupational Risk of Infections in Dialysis. *Am J Infect Control*. 1995;23:278-285.
49. Centers for Disease Control and Prevention. Outbreaks of hepatitis B virus infection among hemodialysis patients—California, Nebraska, and Texas, 1994. *MMWR Morb Mortal Wkly Rep*. 1996;45:285-289.
50. Alter MJ, Favero MS, Maynard JE. Impact of infection control strategies on the incidence of dialysis-associated hepatitis in the United States. *J Infect Dis*. 1986;153:1149-1151.
51. Narendranathan M, Philip M. Reusable needles: A major risk factor for acute virus B hepatitis. *Trop Doct*. 1993;23:64-66.
52. Hutin YJ, Harpaz R, Drobeniuc J, et al. Injections given in healthcare settings as a major source of acute hepatitis B in Moldova. *Int J Epidemiol*. 1999;28:782-786.
53. Polish LB, Shapiro CN, Bauer F, et al. Nosocomial transmission of hepatitis B virus associated with the use of a spring-loaded finger-stick device. *N Engl J Med*. 1992;326:721-725.
54. De Schrijver K, Maes I, Van Damme P, et al. An outbreak of nosocomial hepatitis B virus infection in a nursing home for the elderly in Antwerp (Belgium). *Acta Clin Belg*. 2005;60:63-69.
55. Rosenheim M, Cadranel JF, Stuyver L, et al. Nosocomial transmission of hepatitis B virus associated with endomyocardial biopsy. *Gastroenterol Clin Biol*. 2006;30:1274-1280.
56. Morris IM, Cattle DS, Smits BJ. Endoscopy and transmission of hepatitis B (Letter). *Lancet*. 1975;2:1152.
57. Kent GP, Brondum J, Keenlyside RA, et al. A large outbreak of acupuncture-associated hepatitis B. *Am J Epidemiol*. 1988;127:591-598.
58. Oren I, Hershow RC, Ben-Porath E, et al. A common-source outbreak of fulminant hepatitis B in a hospital. *Ann Intern Med*. 1989;110:691-698.
59. Khan AJ, Cotter SM, Schulz B, et al. Nosocomial transmission of hepatitis B virus infection among residents with diabetes in a skilled nursing facility. *Infect Control Hosp Epidemiol*. 2002;23:313-318.
60. Canter J, Mackey K, Good LS, et al. An outbreak of hepatitis B associated with jet injections in a weight reduction clinic. *Arch Intern Med*. 1990;150:1923-1927.
61. Harling R, Turbitt D, Millar M, et al. Passage from India: An outbreak of hepatitis B linked to a patient who acquired infection from health care overseas. *Public Health*. 2007;121:734-741.
62. Centers for Disease Control and Prevention. A comprehensive immunization strategy to eliminate transmission of hepatitis B virus infection in the United States. *MMWR Morb Mortal Wkly Rep*. 2006;55(RR-16):1-25. Available at http://www.cdc.gov/mmwr/preview/mmwrhtml/rr5516a1.htm (accessed April 2009).
63. Beasley RP, Hwang LY, Stevens CE, et al. Efficacy of hepatitis B immune globulin for prevention of perinatal transmission of the hepatitis B virus carrier state: Final report of a randomized double-blind, placebo-controlled trial. *Hepatology*. 1983;3:135-141.
64. McMahon BJ, Bruden DL, Petersen KM, et al. Antibody levels and protection after hepatitis B vaccination: Results of a 15-year follow-up. *Ann Intern Med*. 2005;142:333-341.
65. Wainwright RB, Bulkow LR, Parkinson AJ, et al. Protection provided by hepatitis B vaccine in a Yupik Eskimo population: Results of a 10-year study. *J Infect Dis*. 1997;175:674-677.
66. Centers for Disease Control and Prevention. Recommendations for identification and public health management of persons with chronic hepatitis B virus infection. *MMWR Morb Mortal Wkly Rep*. 2008;57(RR-08):1-20. Available at http://www.cdc.gov/mmwr/preview/mmwrhtml/rr5708a1.htm (accessed April 2009).
67. Roome AJ, Walsh SJ, Cartter ML, et al. Hepatitis B vaccine responsiveness in Connecticut public safety personnel. *JAMA*. 1993;270:2931-2934.
68. Playford EG, Hogan PG, Bansal AS, et al. Intradermal recombinant hepatitis B vaccine for healthcare workers who fail to respond to intramuscular vaccine. *Infect Control Hosp Epidemiol*. 2002;23:87-90.
69. Ghebrehewet S, Baxter D, Falconer M, Paver K. Intradermal recombinant hepatitis B vaccination (IDRV) for nonresponsive healthcare workers (HCWs). *Hum Vaccine*. 2008;4:280-285.
70. Cardell K, Akerlind B, Sällberg M, et al. Excellent response rate to a double dose of the combined hepatitis A and B vaccine in previous nonresponders to hepatitis B vaccine. *J Infect Dis*. 2008;198:299-304.
71. Simard EP, Miller JT, George PA, et al. Hepatitis B vaccination coverage levels among healthcare workers in the United States, 2002-2003. *Infect Control Hosp Epidemiol*. 2007;28:783-790.
72. Halpern SD, Asch DA, Shaked A, et al. Inadequate hepatitis B vaccination and post-exposure evaluation among transplant surgeons: Prevalence, correlates, and implications. *Ann Surg*. 2006;244:305-309.
73. Centers for Disease Control and Prevention. Recommendations for follow-up of health-care workers after occupational exposure to hepatitis C virus. *MMWR Morb Mortal Wkly Rep*. 1997;46:603-606.
74. Zuckerman J, Clewley G, Griffiths P, et al. Prevalence of hepatitis C antibodies in clinical health-care workers. *Lancet*. 1994;343:1618-1620.
75. Klein RS, Freeman K, Taylor PE, et al. Occupational risk for hepatitis C virus infection among New York City dentists. *Lancet*. 1991;338:1539-1542.
76. Thomas DL, Gruninger SE, Siew C, et al. Occupational risk of hepatitis C infections among general dentists and oral surgeons in North America. *Am J Med*. 1996;100:41-45.
77. Lanphear BP, Linnemann CC, Cannon CG, et al. Decline of clinical hepatitis B in workers at a general hospital: Relation to increasing vaccine-induced immunity. *Clin Infect Dis*. 1993;16:10-14.
78. Mitsui T, Iwano K, Masuko K, et al. Hepatitis C virus infection in medical personnel after needlestick accident. *Hepatology*. 1992;16:1109-1114.
79. Puro V, Petrosillo N, Ippolito G, et al. Occupational hepatitis C virus infection in Italian health care workers. Italian Study Group on Occupational Risk of Bloodborne Infections. *Am J Public Health*. 1995;85:1272-1275.
80. Ridzon R, Gallagher K, Ciesielski C, et al. Simultaneous transmission of human immunodeficiency virus and hepatitis C virus from a needle-stick injury. *N Engl J Med*. 1997;336:919-922.
81. Cody SH, Hainan OV, Garfein RS, et al. Hepatitis C virus transmission from an anesthesiologist to a patient. *Arch Intern Med*. 2002;162:345-350.
82. Stark K, Hänel M, Berg T, et al. Nosocomial transmission of hepatitis C virus from an anesthesiologist to three patients: Epidemiologic and molecular evidence. *Arch Virol*. 2006;151:1025-1030.
83. Cardell K, Widell A, Frydén A, et al. Nosocomial hepatitis C in a thoracic surgery unit: Retrospective findings generating a prospective study. *J Hosp Infect*. 2008;68:322-328.
84. Ross RS, Viazov S, Gross T, et al. Transmission of hepatitis C virus from a patient to an anesthesiology assistant to five patients. *N Engl J Med*. 2000;343:1851-1854.
85. Simon N, Courouce AM, Lemarrec N, et al. A twelve year natural history of hepatitis C virus infection in hemodialyzed patients. *Kidney Int*. 1994;46:504-511.

86. Pereira BJ, Levey AS. Hepatitis C virus infection in dialysis and renal transplantation. *Kidney Int.* 1997;51:981-999.
87. Fabrizi F, Martin P. Hepatitis C virus infection in dialysis: An emerging clinical reality. *Int J Artif Organs.* 2001;24:123-130.
88. Fabrizi F, Martin P, Dixit V, et al. Acquisition of hepatitis C virus in hemodialysis patients: A prospective study by branched DNA signal amplification assay. *Am J Kidney Dis.* 1998;31:647-654.
89. Puttinger H, Vychytil A. Hepatitis B and C in peritoneal dialysis patients. *Semin Nephrol.* 2002;22:351-360.
90. Caramelo C, Bartolome J, Albalate M, et al. Undiagnosed hepatitis C virus infection in hemodialysis patients: Value of HCV RNA and liver enzyme levels. *Kidney Int.* 1996;50:2027-2031.
91. Niu MT, Alter MJ, Kristensen C, et al. Outbreak of hemodialysis-associated non-A, non-B hepatitis and correlation with antibody to hepatitis C virus. *Am J Kidney Dis.* 1992;19:345-352.
92. Savey A, Simon F, Izopet J, et al. A large nosocomial outbreak of hepatitis C virus infections at a hemodialysis center. *Infect Control Hosp Epidemiol.* 2005;26:752-760.
93. Girou E, Chevaliez S, Challine D, et al. Determinant roles of environmental contamination and noncompliance with standard precautions in the risk of hepatitis C virus transmission in a hemodialysis unit. *Clin Infect Dis.* 2008;47:627-633.
94. Hardy NM, Sandroni S, Danielson S, et al. Antibody to hepatitis C virus increases with time on hemodialysis. *Clin Nephrol.* 1992;38:44-48.
95. Forns X, Fernandez-Llama P, Pons M, et al. Incidence and risk factors of hepatitis C virus infection in a haemodialysis unit. *Nephrol Dial Transplant.* 1997;12:736-740.
96. Hayashi H, Okuda K, Yokosuka O, et al. Adsorption of hepatitis C virus particles onto the dialyzer membrane. *Artif Organs.* 1997;21:1056-1059.
97. Rahnavardi M, Hosseini Moghaddam SM, Alavian SM. Hepatitis C in hemodialysis patients: Current global magnitude, natural history, diagnostic difficulties, and preventive measures. *Am J Nephrol.* 2008;28:628-640.
98. Pereira BJ, Milford EL, Kirkman RL, et al. Transmission of hepatitis C virus by organ transplantation. *N Engl J Med.* 1991;325:454-460.
99. Pereira BJ, Milford EL, Kirkman RL, et al. Prevalence of hepatitis C virus RNA in organ donors positive for hepatitis C antibody and in the recipients of their organs. *N Engl J Med.* 1992;327:910-915.
100. Tugwell BD, Patel PR, Williams IT, et al. Transmission of hepatitis C virus to several organ and tissue recipients from an antibody-negative donor. *Ann Intern Med.* 2005;143:648-654.
101. Centers for Disease Control and Prevention. Acute hepatitis C virus infections attributed to unsafe injection practices at an endoscopy clinic—Nevada, 2007. *MMWR Morb Mortal Wkly Rep.* 2008;57;513-517. Available at http://www.cdc.gov/mmwr/preview/mmwrhtml/mm5719a2.htm (accessed April 2009).
102. Muscarella LF. Recommendations for preventing hepatitis C virus infection: Analysis of a Brooklyn endoscopy clinic's outbreak. *Infect Control Hosp Epidemiol.* 2001;22:669.
103. Tennenbaum R, Colardelle P, Chochon M, et al. Hepatitis C after retrograde cholangiography (in French). *Gastroenterol Clin Biol.* 1993;17:763-764.
104. Pañella H, Rius C, Caylà JA, Barcelona Hepatitis C Nosocomial Research Working Group. Transmission of hepatitis C virus during computed tomography scanning with contrast. *Emerg Infect Dis.* 2008;14:333-336.
105. Comstock RD, Mallonee S, Fox JL, et al. A large nosocomial outbreak of hepatitis C and hepatitis B among patients receiving pain remediation treatments. *Infect Control Hosp Epidemiol.* 2004;25:576-583.
106. Krause G, Trepka MJ, Whisenhunt RS, et al. Nosocomial transmission of hepatitis C virus associated with the use of multidose saline vials. *Infect Control Hosp Epidemiol.* 2003;24:122-127.
107. Germain JM, Carbonne A, Thiers V, et al. Patient-to-patient transmission of hepatitis C virus through the use of multidose vials during general anesthesia. *Infect Control Hosp Epidemiol.* 2005;26:789-792.
108. Desenclos JC, Bourdoil-Razes M, Rolin B, et al. Hepatitis C in a ward for cystic fibrosis and diabetic patients: Possible transmission by spring-loaded finger-stick devices for self-monitoring of capillary blood glucose. *Infect Control Hosp Epidemiol.* 2001;22:701-707.
109. de Lédinghen V, Trimoulet P, Mannant PR, et al. Outbreak of hepatitis C virus infection during sclerotherapy of varicose veins: Long-term follow-up of 196 patients (4535 patient-years). *J Hepatol.* 2007;46:19-25.
110. Lesourd F, Izopet J, Mervan C, et al. Transmissions of hepatitis C virus during the ancillary procedures for assisted conception. *Hum Reprod.* 2000;15:1083-1085.
111. Kaiser R, Geulen O, Matz B, et al. Risk of hepatitis C after immunoadsorption. *Infect Control Hosp Epidemiol.* 2002;23:342-343.
112. Sawayama Y, Hayashi J, Kakuda K, et al. Hepatitis C virus infection in institutionalized psychiatric patients: Possible role of transmission by razor sharing. *Dig Dis Sci.* 2000;45:351-356.
112a. Thompson ND, Perz JF, Moorman AC, Holmberg SD. Nonhospital health care–associated hepatitis B and C virus transmission: United States, 1998-2008. *Ann Intern Med.* 2009;150:33-39.
113. Karmochkine M, Carrat F, Dos Santos O, et al. A case-control study of risk factors for hepatitis C infection in patients with unexplained routes of infection. *J Viral Hepat.* 2006;13:775-782.
114. Macedo de Oliveira A, White KL, Leschinsky DP, et al. An outbreak of hepatitis C virus infections among outpatients at a hematology/oncology clinic. *Ann Intern Med.* 2005;142:898-902.
115. Sepkowitz KA. Risk to cancer patients from nosocomial hepatitis C virus. *Infect Control Hosp Epidemiol.* 2004;25:599-602.
116. Pekova LM, Teocharov P, Sakarev A. Clinical course and outcome of a nosocomial outbreak of hepatitis C in a urology ward. *J Hosp Infect.* 2007;67:86-91.
117. Forns X, Martínez-Bauer E, Feliu A, et al. Nosocomial transmission of HCV in the liver unit of a tertiary care center. *Hepatology.* 2005;41:115-122.
118. Martínez-Bauer E, Forns X, Armelles M, et al. for Spanish Acute HCV Study Group. Hospital admission is a relevant source of hepatitis C virus acquisition in Spain. *J Hepatol.* 2008;48:20-27.
119. Macedo de Oliveira A, White KL, Beecham BD, et al. Sensitivity of second-generation enzyme immunoassay for detection of hepatitis C virus infection among oncology patients. *J Clin Virol.* 2006;35:21-25.
120. Jaeckel E, Cornberg M, Wedemeyer H, et al. Treatment of acute hepatitis C with interferon alfa-2b. *N Engl J Med.* 2001;345:1452-1457.
121. Lettau LA, Alfred HJ, Glew RH, et al. Nosocomial transmission of delta hepatitis. *Ann Intern Med.* 1986;104:631-635.
122. Beeson PB. Jaundice occurring one to four months after transfusion of blood or plasma. *JAMA.* 1943;121:1332-1334.
123. Chamberland ME. Emerging infectious agents: Do they pose a risk to the safety of transfused blood and blood products? *Clin Infect Dis.* 2002;34:797-805.
124. Busch MP, Kleinman SH, Nemo GJ. Current and emerging infectious risks of blood transfusions. *JAMA.* 2003;289:959-962.
125. Pealer LN, Marfin AA, Petersen LR, et al. Transmission of West Nile virus through blood transfusion in the United States, 2002. *N Engl J Med.* 2003;349:1236-1245.
126. Blajchman MA, Vamvakas EC. The continuing risk of transfusion transmitted infections. *N Engl J Med.* 2006;355:1303-1305.
127. Kuehnert MJ, Roth VR, Haley NR, et al. Transfusion-transmitted bacterial infection in the United States, 1998 through 2000. *Transfusion.* 2001;41:1493-1499.
128. Glynn SA, Kleinman SH, Wright DJ, et al. International application of the incidence rate/window period model. *Transfusion.* 2002;42:966-972.
129. World Health Organization update: Blood safety and donation. June 2008. Available at http://www.who.int/mediacentre/factsheets/fs279/en/ (accessed April 2009).
130. Surgenor DM, Wallace EL, Hao SHS, et al. Collection and transfusion of blood in the United States, 1982-1988. *N Engl J Med.* 1990;322:1646-1651.
131. Sullivan MT, McCullough J, Schreiber GB, et al. Blood collection and transfusion in the United States in 1997. *Transfusion.* 2002;42:1253-1260.
132. National Blood Data Resource Center. *Comprehensive Report on Blood Collection and Transfusion in the United States in 2001: Executive Summary.* Bethesda, MD: NBDRC; 2003.
133. U.S. Department of Health and Human Serices. The 2007 National Blood Collection and Utilization Survey Report. Available at http://www.hhs.gov/ophs/bloodsafety/2007nbcus_survey.pdf (accessed April 2009).
134. Vamvakas EC, Taswell HF. Epidemiology of blood transfusion. *Transfusion.* 1994;34:464-470.
135. Williams AE, Thomson RA, Schreiber GB, et al. Estimates of infectious disease risk factors in US blood donors. Retrovirus Epidemiology Donor Study. *JAMA.* 1997;277:967-972.
136. Glynn SA, Schreiber GB, Busch MP, et al. Demographic characteristics, unreported risk behaviors, and the prevalence and incidence of viral infections: A comparison of apheresis and whole-blood donors. The Retrovirus Epidemiology Donor Study. *Transfusion.* 1998;38:350-358.
137. Bowden RA, Slichter SJ, Sayers M, et al. A comparison of filtered leukocyte-reduced and cytomegalovirus (CMV) seronegative blood products for the prevention of transfusion-associated CMV infection after marrow transplant. *Blood.* 1995;86:3598-3603.
138. Glynn SA, Busch MP, Schreiber GB. Effect of a national disaster on blood supply and safety: The September 11 experience. *JAMA.* 2003;289:2246-2253.
139. Busch MP, Kleinman SH, Nemo GJ. Current and emerging infectious risks of blood transfusions. *JAMA.* 2003;289:959-962.
140. Stramer SL, Glynn SA, Kleinman SH, et al. Detection of HIV-1 and HCV infections among antibody-negative US blood donors by nucleic acid amplification testing. *N Engl J Med.* 2004;351:760-768.
141. Dodd RY, Notari EP, Stramer SL. Current prevalence and incidence of infectious disease markers and estimated window-period risk in the American Red Cross blood donor population. *Transfusion.* 2002;42:975-979.
142. Stramer SL, Fang CT, Foster GA, et al. West Nile virus among blood donors in the United States, 2003 and 2004. *N Engl J Med.* 2005;353:451-459.
143. Busch, MP, Caglioti S, Robertson EF, et al. Screening the blood supply for West Nile virus RNA by nucleic acid amplification testing. *N Engl J Med.* 2005;353;460-467.
144. Busch MP, Glynn SA, Stramer SL, et al. A new strategy for estimating risks of transfusion-transmitted viral infections based on rates of detection of recently infected donors. *Transfusion.* 2005;45:254-264.
145. Sharma UK, Stramer SL, Wright DJ, et al. Impact of changes in viral marker screening assays. Retrovirus Epidemiology Donor Study. *Transfusion.* 2003;43:202-214.
146. Centers for Disease Control and Prevention. HIV/AIDS surveillance report. *MMWR Morb Mortal Wkly Rep.* 1997;9:10.
147. Kroner BL, Rosenberg PS, Aledort LM, et al. HIV-1 infection incidence among persons with hemophilia in the United States and western Europe, 1978-1990. Multicenter Hemophilia Cohort Study. *J Acquir Immune Defic Syndr.* 1994;7:279-286.
148. Leitman SF, Klein HG, Melpolder JJ, et al. Clinical implications of positive tests for antibodies to human immunodeficiency virus type 1 in asymptomatic blood donors. *N Engl J Med.* 1989;321:917-924.
149. Busch MP, Kleinman SH, Williams AE, et al. Frequency of human immunodeficiency virus (HIV) infection among contemporary anti-HIV-1 and anti-HIV-1/2 supplemental test–indeterminate blood donors. The Retrovirus Epidemiology Donor Study. *Transfusion.* 1996;36:37-44.
150. Centers for Disease Control and Prevention. Update: HIV-2 infection among blood and plasma donors—United States, June 1992-June 1995. *MMWR Morb Mortal Wkly Rep.* 1995;44:603-606.
151. Sullivan, MT, Guido, EA, Metler, RP, et al. Identification and characterization of an HIV-2 antibody-positive blood donor in the United States. *Transfusion.* 1998;38:189.
152. Gomes P, Abecasis A, Almeida M, et al. Transmission of HIV-2. *Lancet Infect Dis.* 2003;3:683-684.
153. Chamberland M, Khabbaz RF. Emerging issues in blood safety. *Infect Dis Clin North Am.* 1998;12:217-229.
154. Vrielink H, Zaaijer HL, Reesink HW. The clinical relevance of HTLV type I and II in transfusion medicine. *Transfus Med Rev.* 1997;11:173-179.
155. Toro C, Rodes B, Poveda E, et al. Rapid development of subacute myelopathy in three organ transplant recipients after transmission of human T-cell lymphotropic virus type I from a single donor. *Transplantation.* 2003;75:102-104.
156. Hollinger FB, Dodd RY. Hepatitis B virus traceback and lookback: Factors to consider. *Transfusion.* 2009;49:176-184.
157. Kleinman SH, Strong DM, Tegtmeier GG, et al. Hepatitis B virus (HBV) DNA screening of blood donations in minipools with the COBAS AmpliScreen HBV test. *Transfusion.* 2005;45:1247-1257.
158. Roth WK, Weber M, Petersen D, et al. NAT for HBV and anti-HBc testing increase blood safety. *Transfusion.* 2002;42:869-875.
159. Wang JT, Lee CZ, Chen PJ, et al. Transfusion-transmitted HBV infection in an endemic area: The necessity of more sensitive screening for HBV carriers. *Transfusion.* 2002;42:1592-1597.
160. Kleinman SH, Kuhns MC, Todd DS, et al. Frequency of HBV DNA detection in US blood donors testing positive for the presence of anti-HBc: Implications for transfusion transmission and donor screening. *Transfusion.* 2003;43:696-704.
161. Rosina F, Saracco G, Rizzetto M. Risk of post-transfusion infection with the hepatitis delta virus: A multicenter study. *N Engl J Med.* 1985;312:1488-1491.
162. Alter HJ, Purcell RH, Holland PV, et al. Donor transaminase and recipient hepatitis: Impact on blood transfusion services. *JAMA.* 1981;246:630-634.
163. Goldman M, Juodvalkis S, Gill P, et al. Hepatitis C lookback. *Transfus Med Rev.* 1998;12:84-93.
164. Murphy EL, Bryzman S, Williams AE, et al. Demographic determinants of hepatitis C virus seroprevalence among blood donors. *JAMA.* 1996;275:995-1000.
165. Conry-Cantilena C, VanRaden M, Gibble J, et al. Routes of infection, viremia, and liver disease in blood donors found to have hepatitis C virus infection. *N Engl J Med.* 1996;334:1691-1696.
166. Bresee JS, Mast EE, Coleman PJ, et al. Hepatitis C virus infection associated with administration of intravenous immune globulin: A cohort study. *JAMA.* 1996;276:1563-1567.
167. Iwamoto M, Jernigan DB, Guasch A, et al. Transmission of West Nile virus from an organ donor to four transplant recipients. *N Engl J Med.* 2003;29:348:2196-2203.
168. Centers for Disease Control and Prevention. West Nile virus transmission through blood transfusion—South Dakota, 2006. *MMWR Morb Mortal Wkl Rep.* 2007;56:76-79.
169. Centers for Disease Control and Prevention. West Nile virus infections in organ transplant recipients—New York and Pennsylvania, August-September, 2005. *MMWR Morb Mortal Wkly Rep.* 2005;54:1021-1023.
170. Pellett PE, Wright DJ, Engels EA, et al. Multicenter comparison of serologic assays and estimation of human herpesvirus 8 seroprevalence among US blood donors. *Transfusion.* 2003;43:1260-1268.
171. Dollard SC, Nelson KE, Ness PM, et al. Possible transmission of human herpesvirus-8 by blood transfusion in a historical United States cohort. *Transfusion.* 2005;45:500-503.
172. Hladik W, Dollard SC, Mermin J, et al. Transmission of human herpesvirus 8 by blood transfusion. *N Engl J Med.* 2006;355:1331-1338.

173. Barozzi P, Luppi M, Facchetti F, et al. Post-transplant Kaposi sarcoma originates from the seeding of donor-derived progenitors. *Nat Med.* 2003;9:554-561.

174. Bowden RA. Transfusion-transmitted cytomegalovirus infection. *Hematol Oncol Clin North Am.* 1995;9:155-166.

175. Santagostino E, Mannucci PM, Gringeri A, et al. Transmission of parvovirus B19 by coagulation factor concentrates exposed to 100 degrees C heat after lyophilization. *Transfusion.* 1997;37:517-522.

176. Soucie JM, Siwak EB, Hooper WC, et al. Universal Data Collection Project Working Group. Human parvovirus B19 in young male patients with hemophilia A: Associations with treatment product exposure and joint range-of-motion limitation. *Transfusion.* 2004;44:1179-1185.

177. Sherertz RJ, Russell BA, Reuman PD. Transmission of hepatitis A by transfusion of blood products. *Arch Intern Med.* 1984;144:1579-1580.

178. Giacoia GP, Kasprisin DO. Transfusion-acquired hepatitis A. *South Med J.* 1989;82:1357-1360.

179. Mannucci PM, Gdovin S, Gringeri A, et al. Transmission of hepatitis A to patients with hemophilia by factor VIII concentrates treated with organic solvent and detergent to inactivate viruses. The Italian Collaborative Group. *Ann Intern Med.* 1994;120:1-7.

180. Diwan AH, Stubbs JR, Carnahan GE. Transmission of hepatitis A via WBC-reduced RBCs and FFP from a single donation. *Transfusion.* 2003;43:536-540.

181. Centers for Disease Control and Prevention. Prevention of hepatitis A through active or passive immunization: Recommendations of the Advisory Committee on Immunization Practices (ACIP). *MMWR Morb Mortal Wkly Rep.* 1999;48(RR-12):1-37.

182. Centers for Disease Control and Prevention. Blood safety monitoring among persons with bleeding disorders—United States, May 1998-June 2002. *MMWR Morb Mortal Wkly Rep.* 2003;51:1152-1154.

183. Dalton HR, Bendall R, Ijaz S, et al. Hepatitis E: An emerging infection in developed countries. *Lancet Infect Dis.* 2008;8:698-709.

184. Alter HJ, Nakatsuji Y, Melpolder J, et al. The incidence of transfusion-associated GB virus infection and its relation to liver disease. *N Engl J Med.* 1997;336:747-754.

185. Prati D, Zanella A, Bosoni P, et al. The incidence and natural course of transfusion-associated GB virus C/hepatitis G virus infection in a cohort of thalassemic patients. The Cooleycare Cooperative Group. *Blood.* 1998;91:774-777.

186. Shibata M, Wang RY, Yoshiba M, et al. The presence of a newly identified infectious agent (SEN virus) in patients with liver diseases and in blood donors in Japan. *J Infect Dis.* 2001;184:400-404.

187. Yzebe D, Xueref S, Baratin D, et al. TT virus: A review of the literature. *Panminerva Med.* 2002;44:167-177.

188. Jacobs MR, Palavecino E, Yomtovian R. Don't bug me: The problem of bacterial contamination of blood components—Challenges and solutions. *Transfusion.* 2001;41:1331-1334.

189. Gardella C, Marfin AA, Kahn RH, et al. Persons with early syphilis identified through blood or plasma donation screening in the United States. *J Infect Dis.* 2002;185:545-549.

190. van der Sluis JJ, Onvlee PC, Kothe FC, et al. Transfusion syphilis, survival of *Treponema pallidum* in donor blood. I: Report of an orientating study. *Vox Sang.* 1984;47:197-204.

191. Orton SL, Liu H, Dodd RY, et al. ARCNET Epidemiology Group. Prevalence of circulating *Treponema pallidum* DNA and RNA in blood donors with confirmed-positive syphilis tests. *Transfusion.* 42:94-99, 2002.

192. Wagner SJ, Friedman LI, Dodd RY. Transfusion-associated bacterial sepsis. *Clin Microbiol Rev.* 1994;7:290-302.

193. Klein HG, Dodd RY, Ness PM, et al. Current status of microbial contamination of blood components: Summary of a conference. *Transfusion.* 1997;37:95-101.

194. Reading FC, Brecher ME. Transfusion-related bacterial sepsis. *Curr Opin Hematol.* 2001;8:380-386.

195. Blajchman MA, Goldman M. Bacterial contamination of platelet concentrates. *Semin Hematol.* 2001;38(Suppl 11):20-26.

196. Ness P. Single-donor platelets reduce the risk of septic platelet transfusion reactions. *Transfusion.* 2001;41:857-861.

197. Yomtovian R. A prospective microbiologic surveillance program to detect and prevent the transfusion of bacterially contaminated platelets. *Transfusion.* 1993;33:902-909.

198. Heltberg O, Skov F, Gerner-Smidt P, et al. Nosocomial epidemic of *Serratia marcescens* septicemia ascribed to contaminated blood transfusion bags. *Transfusion.* 1993;33:221-227.

199. Eder AF, Kennedy JM, Dy BA, et al. American Red Cross Regional Blood Centers. Bacterial screening of apheresis platelets and the residual risk of septic transfusion reactions: The American Red Cross experience (2004-2006). *Transfusion.* 2007;47:1134-1142.

200. Koch CG, Liang L, Sessler DI, et al. Duration of red-cell storage and complications after cardiac surgery. *N Engl J Med.* 2008;358:1229-1239.

201. Roth VR, Arduino MJ, Nobiletti J, et al. Transfusion-related sepsis due to Serratia liquefaciens in the United States. *Transfusion.* 2000;40:931-935.

202. Richards C, Kolins J, Trindade CD. Autologous transfusion–transmitted *Yersinia enterocolitica* (Letter). *JAMA.* 1992;268:1541-1542.

203. Buchholz DH, Young VM, Friedman NR, et al. Bacterial proliferation in platelet products stored at room temperature: Transfusion-induced *Enterobacter* sepsis. *N Engl J Med.* 1971;285:429-433.

204. Morrow JF, Braine HG, Kickler TS, et al. Septic reactions to platelet transfusions: A persistent problem. *JAMA.* 1991;266:555-558.

205. Leiby DA, Kerr KL, Campos JM, et al. A retrospective analysis of microbial contaminants in outdated random-donor platelets from multiple sites. *Transfusion.* 1997;37:259-263.

206. Kleinman S, Dumont LJ, Tomasulo P, et al. The impact of discontinuation of 7-day storage of apheresis platelets (PASSPORT) on recipient safety: An illustration of the need for proper risk assessments. *Transfusion.* 2009, Jan 5 [Epub ahead of print].

207. McQuiston JH, Childs JE, Chamberland ME, et al, for the Working Group on Transfusion Transmission of Tick-borne Diseases. Transmission of tick-borne agents of disease by blood transfusion: A review of known and potential risks in the United States. *Transfusion.* 2000;40:274-284.

208. Centers for Disease Control and Prevention. *Anaplasma phagocytophilum* transmitted through blood transfusion—Minnesota, 2007. *MMWR Morb Mortal Wkly Rep.* 2008;57:1145-1148.

209. Young C, Losikoff P, Chawla A, et al. Transfusion-acquired Trypanosoma cruzi infection. *Transfusion.* 2007;47:540-544.

210. Leiby DA, Herron RM Jr, Read EJ, et al. *Trypanosoma cruzi* in Los Angeles and Miami blood donors: Impact of evolving donor demographics on seroprevalence and implications for transfusion transmission. *Transfusion.* 2002;42:549-555.

211. Centers for Disease Control and Prevention. Blood donor screening for Chagas disease—United States, 2006-2007. *MMWR Morb Mortal Wkly Rep.* 2007;56:141-143.

212. Stramer S, Foster G, Townsend R, et al. *Trypanosoma cruzi* antibody screening in US blood donors: One year experience at the American Red Cross (Abstract P5-020A). AABB Annual Meeting, Montreal, October 2008.

213. Bern C, Montgomery SP, Herwaldt BL, et al. Evaluation and treatment of Chagas disease in the United States: A systematic review. *JAMA.* 2007;298:2171-2181.

214. Jett P, Cantey P, Hand S, et al. Chagas disease in Mississippi: Investigation of suspected autochthonous infections in the United States (Abstract S40-020E). AABB Annual Meeting, Montreal, October 2008.

215. Herwaldt BL, Neitzel DF, Gorlin JB, et al. Transmission of *Babesia microti* in Minnesota through four blood donations from the same donor over a 6-month period. *Transfusion.* 2002;42:1154-1158.

216. Gubernot DM, Lucey CT, Lee KC, et al. Babesia infection through blood transfusions: Reports received by the US Food and Drug Administration, 1997-2007. *Transfusion.* 2009;48:25-30.

217. Mungai M, Tegtmeier G, Chamberland M, et al. Transfusion-transmitted malaria in the United States from 1963 through 1999. *N Engl J Med.* 2001;344:1973-1978.

218. Centers for Disease Control and Prevention. Malaria Surveillance—United States, 2006. *MMWR Morb Mortal Wkly Rep.* 2008;57(SS05):24-39.

219. Zou S, Fang CT, Schonberger LB. Transfusion transmission of human prion diseases. *Transfus Med Rev.* 2008;22:58-69.

220. Peden A, Head MW, Ritchie DL, et al. Preclinical vCJD after blood transfusion in a PRNP codon 129 heterozygous patient. *Lancet.* 2004;364:527-531.

221. UK Health Protection Agency. Variant CJD and blood. http://www.hpa.ogr.uk/webw/HPAweb&Page&HPAwebAutoListName/Page/1225960597236?p=1225960597236; Last reviewed Jan 21 2009. Accessed June 5 2009.

222. Murphy EL, Connor JD, McEvoy P, et al. Estimating blood donor loss due to the variant CJD travel deferral. *Transfusion.* 2004;44:645-650.

223. Srinivasan A, Burton EC, Kuehnert MJ, et al.; and the Rabies in Transplant Recipients Investigation Team. Transmission of rabies virus from an organ donor to four transplant recipients. *N Engl J Med.* 2005;352:1103-1111.

224. Fischer SA, Graham MB, Kuehnert MJ, et al. Transmission of lymphocytic choriomeningitis virus by organ transplantation. *N Engl J Med.* 2006;354:2235-2249.

225. Ison MG, Hager J, Blumberg E, et al. Donor-derived disease transmission events in the US: Data reviewed by the OPTN/UNOS Disease Transmission Advisory Committee. *Am J Transplant.* (in press).

306

Human Immunodeficiency Virus in Health Care Settings

DAVID K. HENDERSON*

The risk for transmission of blood-borne pathogens in the health care setting has become a matter of substantial concern to health care providers since the late 1980s. Despite the fact that hospital-associated transmission of hepatitis had been identified as a problem since the late 1940s,[1] the epidemic of human immunodeficiency virus (HIV) infection in the United States in the early 1980s focused the attention of health care providers and regulators on this important issue. Since then, researchers have learned that HIV can be transmitted from patient to health care worker, from health care worker to patient, and from one patient to another in health care settings.[2] Thus, occupational HIV infection occurs uncommonly, iatrogenic infection is even more rare, and carefully designed interventions to prevent exposures (and to manage exposures when they occur) can reduce the risk of transmission in either direction. This chapter describes the epidemiology of HIV infections acquired in health care settings, methods to prevent these infections, and the principles of management for health care–associated exposures.

■ Occupational HIV Transmission from Infected Patients to Health Care Personnel

REPORTED CASES OF OCCUPATIONAL HIV INFECTION

As of December 2008, 57 instances of occupational HIV transmission to health care workers in the United States had been reported to the Centers for Disease Control and Prevention (CDC) (Denise Cardo, personal communication, December 2008; Fig. 306-1).[3] In all but one of these cases, occupational transmission was documented by demonstrating HIV antibody seroconversions that occurred after discrete HIV exposures. In the single exception, occupational infection in a scientific laboratory worker was documented by demonstrating that the HIV genetic sequence of the worker's virus isolate was nearly identical to that of the laboratory strain with which the individual was working.

In addition to the 57 documented cases of occupational infection in the United States, "possible" occupational infections in 138 health care providers have been reported to the CDC, and 100 more such cases have been reported worldwide.[3,4] Baseline HIV serologic tests were not performed in these individuals at the time of known or potential exposures to HIV, and so the temporal relationship between exposure and seroconversion could not be confirmed. However, none of the individuals reported nonoccupational behaviors associated with risk for HIV infection, and all recalled at least one exposure to blood or body fluids before their HIV infections were diagnosed. The demographics of this population suggest that some but not all of these individuals probably had confounding community-based risks.[5]

MECHANISMS OF OCCUPATIONAL HIV INFECTION

Most of the occupational HIV infections that have been documented in the United States have been associated with parenteral injuries

inflicted by hollow-bore needles that had been used in veins or arteries, but other sharp instruments have also been involved in transmission. Six instances of HIV infection have occurred after either exposure of breaks in the skin to HIV-contaminated fluids or exposure of mucous membranes to HIV-contaminated materials. Each of these six instances involved a large-volume exposure, an extended duration of exposure, or both. In one case of mucous membrane exposure in Europe, the inoculum was smaller.[6] One reported case was associated with several exposures, over an extended period.[7] To date, contamination of intact skin with blood or other infectious material, close personal contact with infected patients, and contact with contaminated environmental surfaces or fomites have not been linked to occupational HIV transmission. Aerosolization of blood can occur during dental, pathologic, laboratory, and surgical procedures, and conventional surgical masks do not prevent inhalation of aerosols. Nonetheless, to date, no data indicate that aerosol exposure is a route of HIV transmission in any setting.

Exposures to blood from HIV-infected patients account for all but 4 of the 57 documented occupational infections in the United States. Of those four, one occupational HIV infection resulted from exposure to bloody pleural fluid, and two involved exposure to concentrated preparations of HIV in scientific laboratories; for the fourth, the source material was not reported.

DEFINITION OF OCCUPATIONAL HIV EXPOSURE

The instances of documented occupational HIV transmission have been helpful in developing a definition of what constitutes an exposure that is associated with a risk for HIV transmission. As noted in the previous section, exposure routes implicated in occupational HIV transmission include (1) percutaneous injury (e.g., needle puncture or cut caused by a needle or other sharp object); (2) mucous membrane contamination; and (3) contamination of nonintact skin (e.g., skin that is chapped, abraded, or afflicted with dermatitis).[8] Even though HIV-infected blood contamination of intact skin has not been implicated in occupational infection, exposures of intact skin to contaminated blood for extended periods (several minutes or longer) or exposures involving extensive areas of skin should be considered potentially infective, largely because unrecognized areas of inadequate skin integrity could serve as portals of entry for the virus.

Sources of HIV that may pose a risk of transmission through these routes include blood; visibly bloody fluids; tissues; and other body fluids, including semen, vaginal secretions, and cerebrospinal, synovial, pleural, peritoneal, pericardial, and amniotic fluids.[7] In addition, any direct cutaneous or mucosal contact (i.e., without barrier protection) to concentrated HIV in a scientific or research laboratory or production facility should be considered an exposure.

Although nonoccupational episodes of HIV transmission have been attributed to contact with blood-contaminated saliva, these incidents were not analogous to the contact with saliva that occurs during dental or medical care.[8] In the absence of visible blood in the saliva, exposure to saliva from a person infected with HIV is not thought to pose a risk for HIV transmission. Exposure to products that are not visibly bloody (tears, sweat, urine, or feces) from infected patients does not constitute exposure to HIV. Whereas human breast milk has been implicated in perinatal transmission of HIV, this route of transmission is not analogous to occupational exposure, and contact with breast milk from a

---

*All material in this chapter is in the public domain, with the exception of any borrowed figures or tables.

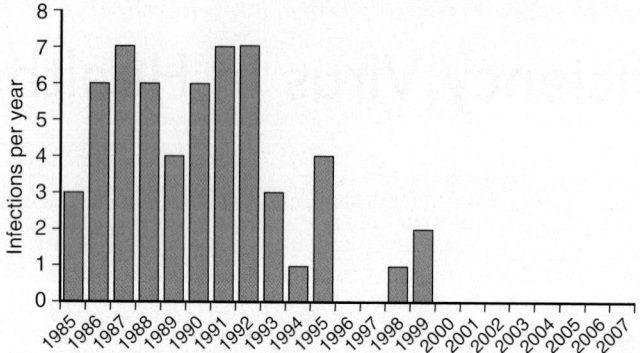

Figure 306-1 Occupational human immunodeficiency virus (HIV) infections in U.S. health care workers reported to the Centers for Disease Control and Prevention, by year of report, 1985 to 2001. *(Modified from Henderson DK, Gerberding JL. Healthcare worker issues, including occupational and nonoccupational postexposure management. In: Dolin RM, Masur H, Saag MS, eds. AIDS Therapy. 2nd ed. New York: Churchill Livingstone; 2002:327; and Do AN, Ciesielski CA, Metler RP, et al. Occupationally acquired human immunodeficiency virus [HIV] infection: national case surveillance data during 20 years of the HIV epidemic in the United States. Infect Control Hosp Epidemiol. 2003;24:86.)*

patient infected with HIV does not constitute an occupational exposure.[8]

OCCUPATIONAL HIV EXPOSURE TRANSMISSION RISK

Assessing Infection Risk in Populations of Exposed Health Care Personnel

Worldwide, more than 20 prospective studies helped quantify the transmission risk associated with discrete occupational HIV exposures (summarized by Henderson and Gerberding[2] and by Ippolito and associates[9]). In each of these studies, health care workers who sustained occupational HIV exposures were tested for HIV antibody at the baseline (i.e., at the time of exposure) and periodically thereafter, at regular follow-up intervals, to detect new infections.

Pooled data from these studies suggest that the average risk of HIV transmission associated with percutaneous exposures to blood-contaminated sharp objects that have been used on HIV-infected individuals is 0.32% (21 infections associated with 6498 exposures; 95% confidence interval of 0.18% to 0.46% [summarized by Henderson and Gerberding[2]]). The estimated risk of mucocutaneous transmission is 0.03% (1 infection associated with 2885 HIV exposures involving mucous membranes or nonintact skin), but this estimate may be biased because the single transmission event was actually reported before prospective data were collected from the involved institution.[10] The risk of infection, if any, in association with intact skin exposure to HIV is too low to be detected in these studies.[11]

Factors Associated with HIV Infection Risk

The average risk of transmission derived from prospective studies is helpful in evaluating populations of exposed persons but does not necessarily reflect the risk associated with the specific exposure experienced by an individual health care worker. Many factors are either known or suspected to affect the infection risk in specific cases, including the route of transmission (see earlier discussion), the inoculum of infectious virus, and the exposed worker's immunologic response to the exposure.

The inoculum of virus is related both to the volume of material involved in the exposure and the titer of virus in that material. Laboratory models of needlestick exposure demonstrate that exposure volume increases with needle size and depth of penetration and that hollow needles generally transmit more blood than do suture needles of com-

parable size.[12,13] In one model, when the needle passed through one or more layers of latex or vinyl gloves before contacting the skin, the volume of blood transferred to the skin was reduced by more than 50% for hollow needles and more than 80% for suture needles.[13] However, in all experimental conditions, the blood volume transferred to skin varied by a single order of magnitude. Large volumes of blood—with or without prolonged duration of contact and a portal of entry—are common features in the reported cases of infection through mucosal surfaces or skin, but the number of cases is too small to identify and quantify risk factors associated with increasing risk for mucocutaneous infection.

The amount of infectious virus present in the source material may vary by several logarithms, depending on the patient's stage and severity of HIV infection and the effect of antiretroviral treatments. Thus, viral titer is probably a very important predictor of transmission risk.[14-16] In general, the titer of HIV circulating in the blood compartment is highest at the time of seroconversion and during advanced stages of acquired immunodeficiency syndrome (AIDS). Both cell-free and cell-associated virus circulate in the blood of HIV-infected individuals. Tests to quantify cell-free HIV RNA (viral load) in plasma are in widespread use and provide a convenient and reasonably accurate measure of virus replication. However, these tests do not determine what proportion of the plasma virus titer is actually infectious. Quantifying cell-associated virus is much more difficult, although HIV DNA in peripheral blood monocytes can be quantified in a few specialized laboratories. In some studies, higher viral load has been associated with an increased risk for perinatal transmission.[17,18] Conversely, HIV transmission from persons with plasma viral loads below the limits of quantification (based on the assays in use at the time the data were collected) has been reported in instances of mother-to-infant transmission[17,18] and in one occupational infection.[19] As a general tenet, the amounts of cell-free and cell-associated virus present in the circulation of any given patient are highly correlated, but more data are needed to determine which component is more important in predicting transmission risk.

To define factors associated with transmission risk, the CDC conducted a retrospective case-control study of percutaneous exposure to HIV among health care personnel.[20] In this study, deep injuries, visibly bloody sharp devices, and devices that had been used in blood vessels were independent predictors of HIV transmission. Each of these factors is probably an indirect measure of the size of the viral inoculum. In this same study, the odds of acquiring infection after percutaneous exposure were six times higher when the source patient had preterminal AIDS (defined as death within 2 months) than when the source patient had earlier stages of infection (Table 306-1). This difference may also be simply a reflection of higher viral inocula. Patients who have advanced HIV disease often have very high titers of circulating HIV. However, the virus strains found in these patients have both phenotypic characteristics (e.g., syncytium induction, macrophage tropism) and genotypic characteristics (e.g., large numbers of HIV quasispecies) that may also contribute to the increased transmission risk associated with advanced HIV disease. The fact that most cases of documented occupational transmission involved exposure to patients who had advanced HIV infection is consistent with the hypothesis that the quantitative or qualitative differences present in these patients do increase the risk. However, patients who have advanced disease are also more likely to be hospitalized and are also, therefore, more likely to undergo procedures that pose an exposure risk to health care personnel.

The immunologic responses of the exposed health care workers also appear to affect the probability of HIV transmission. At least three outcomes are believed to follow HIV exposure: (1) infection (HIV antibody seroconversion and long-term systemic infection); (2) no infection, no immunologic response; and (3) "aborted infection" (limited cellular infection detected by T-cell response to HIV antigens, no long-term systemic infection, no HIV antibody seroconversion). Immunologic evidence supporting the concept of "aborted infection" comes from studies of uninfected prostitutes,[21,22] from studies of sexual

Logistic-Regression Analysis of Risk Factors for HIV Transmission after Percutaneous Exposure to HIV-Infected Blood				
	U.S. Cases*		**All Cases†**	
Risk Factor	**Odds Ratio**	**95% Confidence Interval‡**	**Odds Ratio**	**95% Confidence Interval‡**
Deep injury	13	4.4-42	15	6.0-41
Visible blood on injuring device	4.5	1.4-16	6.2	2.2-21
Injuring device used in artery or vein	3.6	1.3-11	4.3	1.7-12
Terminal illness in source patient§	8.5	2.8-28	5.6	2.0-16
Postexposure use of zidovudine	0.14	0.03-0.47	0.19	0.06-0.52

*All were significant at $P < .02$.

†All were significant at $P < .01$.

‡Adjusted odds ratios (95% confidence interval) reflect the odds of seroconversion after exposure in workers with the risk factor, as opposed to those without it.

§Terminal illness was defined as disease leading to death of the source patient from acquired immunodeficiency syndrome within 2 months after the health care worker's exposure.

HIV, human immunodeficiency virus.

From Cardo DM, Culver DH, Ciesielski CA, et al. A case-control study of HIV seroconversion in health care workers after percutaneous exposure. Centers for Disease Control and Prevention Needlestick Surveillance Group. N Engl J Med. 1997;337:1485-1490. Copyright © 1997 Massachusetts Medical Society. All rights reserved.

partners of infected persons,[23-26] from studies of children born to HIV-infected mothers,[27] from patients inadvertently exposed to blood from infected patients during the provision of health care who remain uninfected,[28] and from studies of occupationally exposed, but uninfected, health care workers.[29-32]

In the study of the exposed but uninfected hospitalized patients who had a point-source exposure to blood from a patient known to be infected with both HIV and hepatitis B, the investigators were able to obtain postexposure lymphocytes from three of the five patients identified as acquiring hepatitis B in the potential outbreak. Cryopreserved lymphocytes from three exposed patients were tested for interferon-γ release in response to stimulation with peptides from structural and nonstructural HIV proteins. The investigators also were able to identify circulating HIV-specific CD8 cells by using tetramer staining. T cells from these individuals released interferon-γ in response to stimulation with HIV peptides, demonstrating that the cells had been primed in vivo with HIV antigens. These data demonstrate an HIV-specific cell-mediated immune response in patients who did not develop HIV infection, despite a documented intravenous point-source exposure to replicating HIV that was significant enough to transmit hepatitis B. None of these patients developed antibody responses to HIV-associated antigens.

Similarly, T lymphocytes derived from the peripheral blood of some uninfected health care workers who were exposed to HIV through needle-related injuries can be stimulated to proliferate and secrete cytokines when exposed to HIV antigens in vitro.[29-31] The precise role of the cellular immune response in host defense against HIV infection is not delineated, and it is not known why some individuals appear to be able to clear or abort the infection. Nonetheless, the observation is consistent with the hypothesis that the cellular immune system is one important determinant of exposure outcome.

Characteristics Associated with Exposures Resulting in HIV Seroconversion in Health Care Workers

For the 51 instances of occupational infection for which data concerning the characteristics and timing of HIV seroconversion have been reported to CDC, 81% were associated with illnesses compatible with primary HIV infection (i.e., the seroconversion illness) a median of 25 days after exposure.[8,33] The clinical syndrome occurring in health care workers who were seroconverters was indistinguishable from that observed in persons with primary HIV infection acquired through

nonoccupational exposures. The median interval from exposure to documentation of a positive result of an HIV antibody test was 46 days (mean, 65 days). This estimate was limited by the fact that testing is performed at variable intervals after exposure and the precise date of seroconversion is often not known with certainty. Overall, of health care workers who become infected as a result of occupational exposures, 95% are expected to undergo seroconversion within 6 months of the exposure.[33] This estimate is basically identical to that for infection associated with other exposure routes.

Three cases of delayed HIV seroconversion among health care workers have been reported.[19,33-35] For each of these health care workers, the result of HIV antibody testing was negative 6 months after an occupational exposure, but it became positive sometime in the ensuing 1 to 7 months. For one of these cases, DNA sequencing confirmed that the infection was occupationally acquired. Interestingly, two of these health care workers were also infected with hepatitis C virus (HCV) as a result of the index needlestick exposure. In both instances, HCV infection was unusually severe; in one case, the disease course was rapidly fatal. It is not clear whether coinfection with these two viruses directly influences the timing or severity of either HIV or HCV infection. Nonetheless, most experts agree that until more data are available, if health care workers are exposed to both viruses and develop serologic evidence of HCV infection 6 weeks to 9 months after occupational exposure, they should be carefully monitored for late HIV seroconversion up to a year after exposure.

IATROGENIC HIV TRANSMISSION FROM INFECTED HEALTH CARE PERSONNEL TO PATIENTS

Case Reports of HIV Transmission from Infected Providers to Patients

Since the onset of the AIDS epidemic in the early 1980s, only four instances of HIV transmission from infected health care workers to one or more patients have been reported.[36-42] Of these instances of transmission, one occurred in the United States in 1990[38-41]; two were reported from France[36,42,43]; and the fourth was reported from Spain.[37]

The episode in the United States involved a cluster of six patients whose HIV infections were linked epidemiologically and through DNA sequencing to a dentist who had AIDS. Although the investigation indicated that HIV transmission occurred in the dentist's office and probably represented transmission from dentist to patient rather than from patient to patient, the precise mechanisms of transmission were not determined. Although the dentist was a patient in his own practice, no deficiency of infection control that would readily explain HIV transmission to the six patients could be identified. The dentist did not report occupational injuries that could have created an opportunity for cross-contamination, nor was it proved that the infections were intentionally transmitted. The extremely high rate of transmission in this situation remains unexplained.

The second episode of iatrogenic HIV transmission involved an orthopedic surgeon in France whose HIV transmission to one patient was confirmed through DNA sequence analysis of viral isolates obtained from the surgeon and the patient.[36,43] The surgeon in this case probably became infected as a result of an occupational injury sustained during a surgical procedure performed in 1983. The surgeon was not aware of his infection until AIDS was diagnosed in 1994. Investigators initiated a retrospective investigation of the 3004 patients who had undergone at least one invasive procedure that was performed by the infected surgeon since 1983. Investigators were able to contact 2458 of these 3004 patients and were able to assess the HIV infection status of 983 of these 2458 patients. One patient, who had a negative result of an HIV antibody test before undergoing the first of three procedures performed by the index surgeon, was found to be infected with HIV when she underwent preoperative testing before a third procedure. Although the precise mechanism of transmission is unknown, the duration of the initial procedure (10 hours) and a presumably high viral titer in the surgeon were hypothesized as contributing factors to the transmission event. No breaches in recommended infection-control practices were identified. In the third instance, also in France, the virus was thought to have been transmitted from an infected nurse to a patient (according to the phylogenetic analysis of the isolates from the patient and the nurse), although no route of transmission could be identified.[42] In a subsequent retrospective study of the 7580 patients of the infected nurse, investigators were able to notify 5308 of the patients concerning the potential for exposure.[44] No additional HIV infections were detected in the 2293 (of these 5308 patients) who were tested. The nurse who was identified as the probable source of the patient's infection was coinfected with HCV and was found to have both a high HIV viral burden, as well as advanced HCV-induced hepatic disease, including clotting abnormalities.

In the fourth case of iatrogenic transmission of HIV (about which only limited information has been published), in Spain,[37] a woman was infected with HIV by her gynecologist, presumably during the conduct of a cesarian section. Spanish officials conducted a retrospective study in which 250 of 275 of the gynecologist's patients were tested; no additional infections were identified.[37]

Investigations of Patients Treated by HIV-Infected Health Care Personnel

Several investigators have evaluated the risk of HIV transmission for patients of clinical practitioners identified as being HIV-infected by studying patients who underwent procedures performed by the infected practitioner (summarized by Henderson and Gerberding[2]). In March 1992, the CDC developed a database to monitor the results of retrospective investigations of health care workers infected with HIV to assess the risk for this mode of HIV transmission. Excluding the patients (discussed earlier) from the Florida dental practice, as of December 1998, the CDC has obtained information from the investigations of 66 HIV-infected health care workers in the United States.[45,46] The health care workers included 29 dentists and dental students, 7 physicians and medical students, 16 surgeons and obstetricians, and 1 podiatrist. HIV test results were available from patients of 53 of these 66 HIV-infected health care workers. In total, 22,759 patients of these health care workers were tested. No HIV infections were reported among 13,667 tested from the practices of 40 of these HIV-infected health care providers. For the remaining 13 HIV-infected providers (7 dentists and 6 surgeons and obstetricians), 9108 patients were tested, and 113 were identified with HIV infection. Of these 113 infected patients, follow-up investigations have been completed for all but 3. To date, no infections have been linked to the infected health care provider. Genetic sequence analysis was performed on HIV strains from 3 of the infected clinicians and 30 of their patients who were infected with HIV, including 3 of the 5 patients who had no identified risk for HIV infection. In no instances were the viral strains of patients and the infected workers genetically related (Table 306-2). These retrospective studies have important limitations; most notable is the fact that in virtually all the studies,

follow-up evaluation and testing were incomplete. Despite these limitations, these data are consistent with previous assessments that the risk of HIV transmission from infected health care personnel to patients is extremely low.

Iatrogenic Transmission Detected in the CDC's HIV/AIDS Surveillance Database

In the United States, persons who have AIDS or, in some states, those infected with HIV who are reported to state and local health departments with no identified risk for HIV infection are studied to determine the likely mode of HIV acquisition.[47] These studies include a review of medical records, contact with health care providers, and interviews with the patients. Of persons who are identified as having no reported risk for HIV infection, approximately 10% cannot be contacted for follow-up, have died, or are otherwise unable to be interviewed. For the remainder, investigations are successful in identifying established modes of infection for more than 95%. With the exception of the Florida dental investigation discussed in detail previously, no cases of HIV transmission from an infected health care provider have been identified through the CDC's nationwide HIV/AIDS surveillance system.

Provider-to-Patient Transmission Risk Assessment

In general, three conditions are necessary to create a risk for provider-to-patient HIV transmission:

1. The health care provider must be infected with HIV and have infectious HIV circulating in the bloodstream.
2. The provider must be injured or have a condition (e.g., weeping dermatitis) that provides some other source for direct exposure to infected blood or body fluids for a patient.
3. The injury mechanism or condition must present an opportunity for the provider's blood or body fluids to contact a patient's mucous membranes, wound, or traumatized tissue directly (i.e., "recontact").

There is currently no mechanism for reliably estimating the infectivity of individuals infected with HIV, and, at least for now, all infected persons are assumed to be infectious (condition 1), although in time, the circulating viral burden may provide an important "proxy" for condition 1. At present, data are inadequate for establishing a threshold or cutoff for infectivity. Most infected health care personnel pose no risk to patients because they neither perform procedures in which they risk penetrating injuries nor have dermatologic conditions that are a potential conduit of exposure of patients to infected body fluids (condition 2). In addition, most health care providers do not perform the kind of invasive procedures, such as surgical or obstetric interventions, in which an injury could expose the patient to infected blood (condition 3).

The risk of blood-borne pathogen transmission to patients during recontacts is not known but is believed to be lower than that associated with most occupational exposures. Most provider injuries potentially associated with blood exposure to the patient that have been reported in observational studies involved the penetration of a surgeon's glove by a solid sharp (e.g., suture needle, bone spicule).[48,49] In most of these observed cases, no wound or bleeding was evident at the site of the provider's injury. Many such injuries were not associated with a detectable perforation in the provider's glove, as measured by the water distention leak test.[48] The "recontact" transmission risk may be even lower than is currently perceived, inasmuch as suture needle punctures transfer a smaller volume than do hollow-bore needles, and inasmuch as this blood inoculum may be reduced even further when the needle passes through glove material.[13]

After years of experience managing HIV infections in the health care setting, physicians now have a substantial body of epidemiologic evidence that demonstrates the risk of nosocomial HIV transmission to patients from an infected provider to be extremely low, even when all three of the conditions associated with transmission risk are present. Furthermore, the already low risk to patients can be reduced further by adherence to standard infection-control practices, prevention of

TABLE 306-2	Epidemiologic and Laboratory Follow-up of Patients of Health Care Workers Infected with HIV, January 1995			
Characteristic		Total	Number with Viral Strains Sequenced	Number with Sequences Related to Those of the Health Care Worker's Virus
Infected before treatment		28	0	—
Established risk factors		62	14	0
Other potential for exposure to HIV		15	13	0
No identified risk		5	3	0
Investigation incomplete		3	0	—
Total		113	30	0

HIV, human immunodeficiency virus.
From Robert LM, Chamberland ME, Cleveland JL, et al. Investigations of patients of health-care workers infected with HIV. *Ann Intern Med.* 1995;22:654.

percutaneous injuries during invasive procedures, and changes in surgical practice (see "Primary Prevention").[50,51] Guidelines for managing infected providers are discussed in more detail in a later section (see "Management of Infected Health Care Providers").

NOSOCOMIAL HIV TRANSMISSION FROM INFECTED PATIENTS TO OTHER PATIENTS

Episodes of nosocomial HIV transmission from one patient to another have most frequently involved breaches in proper infection-control practices and disinfection procedures. Reuse or improper sterilization of blood-contaminated injection needles or syringes has been linked to HIV transmission to hospitalized children in Russia,[52] Libya,[52,53] Romania,[52,54-56] several countries in Africa,[57-61] and India[62] and probably in other developing countries. Medical errors in three institutions (two in the United States and one in The Netherlands) resulted in inadvertent exposures of patients to HIV, as a result of injection of blood from HIV-infected patients during nuclear medicine procedures.[63] Contamination of multidose vials frequently has been incriminated as a vehicle for transmission of HIV and other blood-borne pathogens in several instances in both industrialized and developing countries.[59,64-67]

Five patients in Australia who underwent minor outpatient surgical procedures necessitating local anesthesia that were performed on the same day by an HIV-negative surgeon were subsequently found to be HIV positive.[68] The first infected patient had known risk factors for HIV and was the probable source of infection for the other four patients. The exact mode of patient-to-patient transmission in this practice has not been elucidated. No cases of patient-to-patient transmission of HIV have been reported from hemodialysis centers in the United States. Conversely, HIV transmission to at least nine patients in a hemodialysis center in Colombia has been reported and was attributed to inadequate disinfection and reuse of contaminated access needles; similar cases have been reported from Argentina and Egypt.[69-73]

Primary Prevention

STANDARD (UNIVERSAL) PRECAUTIONS

In 1985 the CDC recommended that the blood of all persons be regarded as infectious, because identification of all patients carrying blood-borne pathogen infections was not possible.[74-76] In 1987 the term *universal precautions* was coined to communicate this concept. Universal precautions were designed to prevent direct contact with blood, bloody body fluids, and certain other fluids (amniotic fluid, semen, vaginal fluid, cerebrospinal fluid, serous transudates and exudates, and inflammatory exudates) that were either known or likely to be associated with blood-borne pathogen transmission. Central to universal precautions is the appropriate use of barriers, such as gloves for procedures associated with a risk of contact with these fluids, tissues, and materials; the use of masks and protective eyewear when the health care worker anticipates the possibility of splash or splatter; and the use of gowns or other protective garments whenever the practitioner identifies a likelihood of soiling of clothing. *Body substance isolation* (or *body substance precautions*) is a highly similar, alternative system of infection control that is practiced by many institutions.[77] In accordance with the body substance isolation approach, the health care worker's decision about the use of barrier protection is based on the degree of anticipated contact with all body fluids and tissues, irrespective of the patient's diagnosis. Both universal precautions and body substance isolation include measures to prevent needle-related injuries. In 1996, the CDC recommended the adoption of an infection control system, *standard precautions,* that effectively merged the most beneficial aspects of the universal precautions and body substance isolation approaches.[78] Whereas universal precautions were designed primarily to reduce the risk for patient to provider transmission of blood-borne pathogens, standard precautions are designed to reduce the risk for bidirectional transmission of infectious diseases in the health care setting. Standard precautions apply to *all* patients and require the use of gloves, protective clothing, and other barriers, as needed, to prevent direct contact with all body fluids (except sweat). As is the case for all of these isolation systems, percutaneous injury prevention is a key component of standard precautions. These guidelines also include standards for the cleaning and reprocessing of equipment used in patient care.

In 1987 the Occupational Safety and Health Administration (OSHA) issued a Joint Advisory Notice designed to enforce compliance with universal precautions for health care personnel.[79] In 1991, the U.S. Department of Labor and OSHA implemented a federal standard designed to enforce compliance with universal precautions.[80] In addition, many states enacted legislation requiring that universal precautions be implemented as a condition of funding for the health care institutions. The 1991 standard presented a hierarchy of control measures that institutions should incorporate into their blood-borne pathogen exposure control plan. These measures included engineering controls (use of equipment and devices designed to be inherently safer), work practice controls (safety procedures), and personal protective equipment.

In several studies that evaluated the efficacy of universal precautions in preventing blood contact, implementation and enforcement resulted in a significant reduction in exposure frequency.[81-84] Factors associated with efficacy of these programs in reducing exposures include training, enforcement, and feedback about exposure mechanisms to managers and front-line workers. Implementation of universal precautions has also been associated with a reduction in the frequency of percutaneous injuries caused by needles and other sharp instruments. The fact that reducing occupational exposure will necessarily reduce occupational infection seems intuitively clear; however, because the frequency of occupational HIV infection is so low, the effect of implementing universal precautions or any other intervention program on the incidence of occupational HIV infection cannot be measured. What is known, however, is that occupational HIV infections have been decreasing in frequency in the United States beginning in the 1990s (Denise Cardo, personal communication, December 2008; see Fig. 306-1).[2,3] Several factors probably have contributed to the observed decrease in occupational infections: possible decreased reporting of occupational infections to the CDC; less aggressive case finding; fewer exposures because of the effective use of universal and standard precautions (i.e., primary prevention); and efficacy of highly active antiretroviral therapy in lowering infected patients' viral burdens, in reducing the need for hospitalization of HIV-infected patients, and in decreasing the numbers and types of procedures required by HIV-infected patients,[85] as well as with regard to the presumed efficacy of antiretroviral postexposure prophylaxis (i.e., secondary prevention, discussed later).

INJURY PREVENTION DURING ROUTINE PATIENT CARE

Needle punctures are the most frequent cause of occupational HIV infection, and priority for their prevention is highest. All health care workers, including those who actually perform or assist with procedures, those employed as housekeepers and laundry workers, and other nonclinicians, are at risk for injury and infection. For this reason, prevention efforts must incorporate strategies that prevent injuries while the needle is being used for its intended purpose, as well as strategies that decrease the risk for injuries after use or disposal of the device.

One component of injury prevention that may be overlooked is avoidance of unnecessary needle use. Phlebotomy is a common indication for using needles and is also the procedure most commonly associated with occupational HIV infection. To reduce opportunities for injury, health care workers should avoid "routine" blood drawing that does not contribute to patient care; use better planning to minimize the number of phlebotomies necessary to obtain the necessary blood tests; and use needleless vascular access ports for blood withdrawal and injection of medication. Similarly, avoiding unnecessary placement of intravenous catheters when alternative routes are available for administering therapy will decrease the opportunity for needle-related injuries.

Implementation of needleless or protected-needle infusion systems can reduce the frequency of needle-related injuries.[86-89] The effect of this intervention on disease transmission is less certain because most needles used for intravenous infusion are not contaminated with blood. Not every institution that has implemented one of these systems has found it to be effective in preventing disease transmission or cost-effective.[90] Needles used for heparin flushes and those in contact with ports close to the site of intravenous line insertion are more likely to be contaminated with blood and hence are more hazardous. In reality, determining whether an infusion needle is or has been contaminated is often difficult, if not impossible. Preventing injuries associated with intravenous infusions is therefore an important component of risk management, even though such injuries may be substantially less likely to transmit infection. Of most importance is that improving worker safety must not increase the risk of infection or complications among patients; results of several studies have suggested an increased risk for device-associated bacteremia in association with the use of needleless intravenous systems.[91-93]

Safer needle devices that have been engineered to retract, cover, or blunt the needle are now in widespread use. Some of these devices have safety features that are activated while the needle is being used for its intended purpose. Other safety features are activated after withdrawal from the patient. The most effective devices are passive (do not require the user to activate the safety feature), do not require extensive training, and are cost-effective. A multicenter study conducted and reported by the CDC demonstrated that implementing safer needle devices for phlebotomy procedures is an effective strategy for preventing percutaneous injuries.[94-96] Improved product design and lower cost may lead to even more effective programs for protecting workers during procedures that require the use of needles.

All needles and other sharp instruments, with or without safety features, should be discarded in puncture-resistant containers. Such containers should be located as close as possible to the point of use in emergency rooms, in operating rooms, and in other areas of patient care. Proper disposal also prevents injuries caused by needles that have been carelessly discarded. Needle disposal programs can significantly reduce the incidence of injury. Rates of needle-related injury can probably be reduced by ensuring that needle disposal containers are available at all points of needle use and by ensuring that infection-control staff provide feedback about the exposure risks to concerned staff.

Finally, some investigators have suggested that employees who have certain personality profiles associated with risk-taking may have increased risks for occupational exposures to blood.[97]

INJURY PREVENTION DURING INVASIVE SURGICAL, OBSTETRIC, DENTAL, AND RADIOLOGIC PROCEDURES

Preventing intraoperative and intraprocedural injuries that confer a risk of blood exposure is an important priority for preventing HIV transmission among health care providers and their patients. For operative procedures, data from observational studies indicate that the risk of provider injury is highest during procedures lasting longer than 2.5 to 3.0 hours, when intraoperative blood loss exceeds 250 to 300 mL, and during certain categories of major procedures (e.g., intra-abdominal gynecologic procedures, vaginal hysterectomies, major vascular procedures, and orthopedic procedures).[49,98-106]

Prevention priorities in the operating room are based on the same principles used in other health care settings.[107-113] The least invasive surgical approach that will achieve the desired patient outcome is preferable. For example, fiber-optic techniques usually pose a lower risk of injury and blood exposure than do more invasive surgical approaches. Similarly, when patient safety allows, alternatives to needles and other sharp implements (e.g., use of adhesive tape, staples,

and tissue glue rather than sutures; electrocautery rather than scalpels) should be used.

Suture needles are the most frequent cause of injuries in operating and delivery rooms. Curved suture needles with blunted tips are now available and appear to be an acceptable replacement of standard curved suture needles for suturing many types of tissue.[114-119] Use of these needles is effective in preventing intraoperative injuries. In one multicenter study, 1.9 injuries per 1000 curved suture needles used were observed during gynecologic surgery, but no injuries were associated with the use of blunted suture needles.[114] The estimated odds of sustaining an injury with a curved suture needle were reduced by 87% when 50% of the suture needles used during a procedure were blunted. Use of blunted suture needles is also associated with a lower incidence of glove perforation. Surgeons involved in these studies were overall accepting of the blunted needle, and no adverse outcomes in patients were noted.

Another approach that has been advocated to reduce risk for percutaneous exposures during the conduct of invasive procedures is the so-called "no-touch" technique. Aspects of this technique include using instruments, rather than hands, for retracting and exploring tissue; avoiding the simultaneous presence of the hands of two or more operators in the procedural field; avoiding hand-to-hand passage of sharp instruments by using a "neutral zone" (e.g., emesis basin, Mayo stand, or magnetic pad); and announcing the transfer of sharp instruments from person to person.

Gloves provide an important barrier between potentially infectious materials and health care providers. Sterile surgical gloves prevent microbial contamination of patient wounds and sterile instruments and also protect surgical personnel from cutaneous blood contact. Surgical gloves do not provide a barrier to sharp object penetration, but they may reduce the volume of blood transferred to the skin and hence decrease the risk of infection by a blood-borne pathogen.

Unfortunately, glove perforation is extremely common, especially during major surgical procedures of long duration. Breakdown in glove integrity can cause contamination of exposed tissue and blood contamination of the provider's hands, and if the provider sustains an injury that results in bleeding (needle puncture) or tissue trauma (suture-induced "shear injury"), the patient may be exposed to the provider's blood or interstitial fluids. Double gloving is one strategy that may attenuate these problems. Without exception, in all studies of double gloving, the prevalence of inner glove perforation was significantly lower than that of the outer glove.[120-130] In addition, double gloving reduces the frequency of visible blood contamination of providers' hands.

Overall, the thumb, index, and middle fingers of the nondominant hand are the most common glove perforation sites.[49,131,132] Reinforcement of these areas is one approach to prevent perforation.[107,133-136] The use of gloves that increase the thickness of the barrier between a patient and the provider creates concern about manual dexterity and tactile sensitivity.[134,136,137] In a study that measured two-point discrimination and the ability to tie surgical knots, double gloving did not affect performance. Some measures of tactile sensitivity are reduced, but not the ability to discriminate between suture pairs. In a subjective assessment, surgeons reported that double gloving did impair comfort, sensitivity, and dexterity, but acceptance was better if the inner glove was larger than the outer glove.[137]

The benefit of double gloving, glove reinforcement, and new glove materials in preventing disease transmission has not been proved. Nevertheless, double gloving greatly decreases perforation of the inner glove and reduces blood contamination of the operator's hands. Most authorities now recommend routine double gloving during invasive surgical and obstetric procedures.[51,138]

As emphasized previously, preventing intraoperative injuries to surgical care providers is the most important strategy for preventing the transmission of HIV and other blood-borne pathogens to patients. In two studies of intraoperative provider injuries, 11.4% to 29% of the sharp objects that injured the provider subsequently recontacted the patient.[48,49] These exposures are preventable by immediately replacing the contaminated suture needle or other sharp object before reuse. Recontacts can also occur when the provider is injured by bone spicules or materials permanently embedded in the patient's body.[48,49] These sources of potential exposure might be prevented by the use of reinforced gloves,[139,140] liners, or other devices or materials to protect the provider's hands.[107,134-136,139,141] Gloves constructed of monofilament polymers or other materials resistant to tears have become available for use when manipulation of bone fragments or of suture wires is needed, but as noted previously, their use is not universal because of the associated decrease in tactile sensation.

The frequency of blood exposure among dental personnel has declined since the 1990s. Surveys conducted at annual meetings of the American Dental Association revealed that the mean number of injuries involving blood or body fluid contact reported by dentists decreased from 12.0 to 2.2 per year between 1986 and 1993.[142] This impressive decline may be the result of the widespread implementation of universal precautions in dental practices, safer instrumentation, and educational programs for dental professionals and patients. Nonetheless, a significant number of exposures continue to occur in the dental health care setting.[143]

Specific practices designed to prevent injuries include use of the one-handed "scoop" technique and mechanical devices for recapping needles used to administer local anesthetic; restricting the use of fingers during suturing and administration of anesthetic; controlling the placement of sharp instruments (such as scalers and laboratory knives); and improvements in the ergonomic design of dental operatories.[144] Safer devices such as self-sheathing anesthetic needles, dental units designed to shield burs in handpieces, and plastic finger guards might also contribute to safer dental care.

Today, most injuries to dental personnel actually occur outside the patient's mouth, involve very small amounts of blood, and are unlikely to pose a risk to patients.[142,144-146] In a 7-month observational study of dentists and of oral and maxillofacial surgical residents in two New York City teaching hospitals, injuries were observed during 0.1% of dental procedures, and 86% of these injuries occurred outside the patient's mouth.[145] Only one needle puncture was observed during 16,000 anesthetic injections.

Low exposure rates have been observed during outpatient oral surgical procedures as well. However, oral procedures performed in the operating room are associated with injuries caused by surgical wires during fracture reduction.[121,147,148] The use of small plates instead of wires during the surgical treatment of some mandibular fractures, as well as reinforced gloves, may help prevent some of these injuries.

Interventional radiologists, stimulated by increasing awareness of blood-borne pathogen risks, have developed similar approaches to risk aversion in the interventional radiology suite,[149-151] a venue in which particular attention must be paid to the risk for splashes, spattering, and mucous membrane exposures.[152]

Management of Occupational Exposures to HIV in the Health Care Setting

INITIAL EXPOSURE MANAGEMENT

Exposure Reporting

Employers of health care workers and other employees at risk for occupational HIV exposure and infection are required to provide a system for reporting exposure and prompt access to medical care.[79,80] Many institutions have developed "needlestick hotlines" or other rapid-response systems to direct exposed persons to triage and to initiate immediate treatment.[153] However, even in facilities with excellent reporting mechanisms and on-site clinical expertise, many exposures are not reported. In fact, underreporting remains a problem in myriad clinical settings and in health care institutions around the world.[154-161] All persons at risk must be informed of the importance of immediate exposure reporting to ensure that preventive care can be initiated in time to be effective.

Exposure Site Management

Wounds and skin sites that have been in contact with blood or body fluids should be washed with soap and water.[8,162] Exposed mucous membranes should be flushed with tap water. Eyes should be flushed with sterile water or a commercial eye irrigant when available or else with clean tap water. Antiseptics can be used to flush the wound, but they are not known to reduce the incidence of infection, and decontamination should not be delayed until they are obtained.

Counseling and Triage

The emotional impact of a known or suspected HIV exposure is usually significant, especially in the first hours to days after the episode.[163,164] During this time, it is helpful to have access to supportive counseling by experienced clinicians who are familiar with the special medical and psychological needs of exposed persons. The clinician must function as an effective translator. Objective information about exposure risk and the pros and cons of chemoprophylaxis must be communicated to an individual who is usually preoccupied with very subjective emotions.[153,165] Although trying to talk an exposed worker out of "irrational" fear when objective data indicate that the risk is low may seem intuitively tempting, such reassurance is rarely successful. To the worker, the exposure risk may feel like 100%, and no amount of epidemiologic data is likely to change this impression in the short run. The most important initial messages to communicate are probably empathy (e.g., "I can see how frightening this is for you"), validation (e.g., "Most people in your situation feel the way you do now"), and reassurance (e.g., "This is difficult, but I'll help you get through it"). Because the exposed individual is very likely to be preoccupied, the counselor should be patient and prepared to answer the same questions repeatedly.

Health care workers who are too upset or confused to make a decision about chemoprophylaxis can sometimes be helped by suggesting that treatment be started immediately, with the option to stop it later (e.g., "Start treatment now, and then tomorrow we can decide whether continuing is your best option"). Buying some time in this manner alleviates the additional pressure to make an immediate decision about initiating the full 4-week course of treatment; empowers workers to be able to change their minds about treatment when they are able to evaluate the risks and benefits more objectively; and (on the basis of animal data) provides the best opportunity for therapeutic efficacy.[153,165,166]

Several points must be emphasized for any health care worker who is facing a decision about postexposure chemoprophylactic treatment: (1) Most persons exposed to HIV are not infected, even if no treatment is administered; (2) treatment can be stopped at any time; (3) data about the efficacy and safety of chemoprophylactic regimens are incomplete; (4) to date, zidovudine is the only drug for which there are any data suggestive of efficacy in preventing HIV transmission; and (5) no data prove that combination treatment is more effective than single-drug therapy for HIV prevention.

Health care workers who sustain exposure to HIV should be counseled to avoid transmission to others during the follow-up period, especially during the first 6 to 12 weeks after exposure, when seroconversion is most likely to occur.[8] Recommended practices to avoid transmission include sexual abstinence or the use of condoms to prevent sexual transmission, as well as the avoidance of blood and organ donation. If the exposed person is breast-feeding, discontinuation of breast-feeding should be considered, especially for high-risk exposures. It is not necessary, however, to modify an exposed health care worker's responsibilities for patient care to prevent transmission to patients.

Counselors should also provide reassurance, review information about the degree of risk present, and inform the worker about procedures to protect the confidentiality of the exposure medical records. As noted earlier, the most important message to communicate to most workers is that occupational HIV transmission is very unlikely; 99.7% of exposures do not result in HIV infection, even if chemoprophylaxis is not administered. Continued reassurance from a supportive clinician, coupled with practical advice about measures to prevent future exposure, enables the worker to cope successfully with the exposure and its aftermath. Counselors should also be alert to the concerns of sexual partners, co-workers, family, and friends of the exposed worker. Referral for ongoing supportive therapy during the follow-up interval is helpful for the minority of exposed persons who experience difficulty in adjusting to the stress inherent in waiting the 6 months for testing to be complete. Finally, adherence to the chemoprophylaxis regimen may be enhanced if skilled counselors provide advice to the drug recipients. In the San Francisco Post Exposure Prevention Project, the frequency of side effects was similar to those in the health care worker studies; however, nearly 80% of participants completed the 4 weeks of therapy. The authors ascribed this success largely to the intensive, skilled counseling that enrollees received.[167,168]

EXPOSURE HISTORY

When an exposure is reported, the first priority is to evaluate the risk of infection and the need for immediate wound care and prophylactic treatment. After these issues have been addressed and the exposed worker is calm enough to engage in a more detailed discussion, the interviewer can elicit additional details about the exposure. A thorough exposure history can help troubleshoot problems that led to the exposure and, in aggregate form, monitor trends relevant to ongoing exposure prevention efforts. I recommend that institutions systematically collect information about all such exposures to look for common circumstances or flawed processes that may be modified to reduce these risks further.

If exposure to HIV (or hepatitis B or C virus infection [see Chapter 305]) has occurred, the risk of transmission for any or each of the pathogens to which the individual is exposed should be assessed. If the source patient is known to be infected with HIV, the interviewer should determine the stage of illness, recent results of viral load testing (if available), and recent antiretroviral treatment history.[8,153,165] If the source patient's HIV status is not known, information relevant to the probability of infection (e.g., presence or absence of risk behaviors by the source patient), as well as clinical and epidemiologic clues that suggest undiagnosed HIV infection, should be recorded and should be considered when recommendations for follow-up management are made.

For needle punctures or similar percutaneous injuries, information about the source material and exposure characteristics known to be associated with an increased risk of HIV transmission (deep injury, visibly bloody device, device used in an artery or vein) should be carefully collected and recorded.[8,20] In addition, the practitioner should also inquire about factors likely to increase the risk of transmission (e.g., injection of a volume of blood, exposure to hollow-bore needle, exposure to large-gauge needle, visible blood on the device, device used in a vascular channel, device used on a source patient who is known to have high viral burden or progressive disease).

For mucosal exposure, the body fluid or material involved and the exposed site, volume of material, and duration of contact before decontamination should be recorded. In addition to these data, for reported skin contacts, the condition of the skin at the site of contact should be evaluated to detect lesions that could provide a portal of entry and influence the risk of infection. For intact skin exposures without an obvious portal of entry, infection is so unlikely that further evaluation and treatment are not necessary unless the contact is prolonged or involves a large area of intact skin. Even then, the risk of HIV infection is extremely small.[11]

Human bites rarely transmit HIV (see later discussion).[169-172] The person who inflicted the bite may sustain a mucosal blood exposure to HIV, but only if the skin was penetrated, the bite wound bled, or both. The person who is bitten is usually not at risk for HIV infection unless blood or visibly bloody saliva was in direct contact with the bite wound. Penetrating bite wounds do pose a risk for bacterial wound infection, and appropriate wound care and antibacterial prophylaxis should be provided, when indicated (see Chapter 319).

When the exposure risk has been assessed and urgent treatment has been provided, and when the health care worker is able and willing to cooperate, the individual providing care should obtain a more detailed history about the exposure. Information should be recorded about when, where, and how the exposure occurred, the type of device involved, the presence or absence of safety features (and, if present, their state of activation), and when in the course of handling the device the exposure occurred (e.g., during use, after use, during disposal). As noted previously, each institution should pool these data and should periodically evaluate them systematically to identify opportunities to improve processes to reduce health care workers' risks and to increase patients' and workers' safety.

EVALUATING THE SOURCE OF EXPOSURE

An individual who is known to be the source of an occupational exposure should be evaluated for HIV and hepatitis B and C virus infections (see Chapter 305).[8] The medical record is a useful source of information, but interviewing the source patient often provides the most accurate data about infection risks. If the HIV infection status of the source patient is unknown, he or she should be asked to consent to testing for HIV antibodies (and other blood-borne pathogens). If consent is not obtained, further evaluation of HIV status should comply with applicable state laws and local policies.[2] The privacy of the source patient should be protected, irrespective of either the decision to test or the test result.

HIV testing of the source patient should be performed as soon as possible. In many facilities, conventional HIV tests (e.g., enzyme immunoassay) can be completed very quickly. A rapid HIV antibody test approved by the U.S. Food and Drug Administration is an acceptable alternative, especially if conventional tests cannot be completed within 24 to 48 hours. This rapid testing technology has been improved significantly since it was first introduced (see Chapter 119). In general, repeatedly reactive results of enzyme immunoassay or a rapid test are highly suggestive of infection, but false-positive results do occur.[153] Reactive test results should be confirmed by Western blot or immunofluorescent antibody before disclosure to the exposure source. A negative conventional enzyme immunoassay is sufficient to exclude a diagnosis of HIV, unless the source patient has clinical evidence of primary HIV infection or HIV-related disease. A negative result of a rapid test is also very reliable in ruling out infection, but false-negative findings have been reported, especially from laboratories that have little experience with older test kits. Institutions using the newest technology have found false-negative results to be far less frequent occurrences.

If the source patient cannot be tested, the "pretest" probability of blood-borne pathogen infection should be assessed by using available clinical, epidemiologic and laboratory information, and most importantly, common sense.[8,153,165] A similar approach applies to situations when the exposure source is not known. HIV testing of needles, syringes, or other sharp instruments associated with exposures is dangerous and is not recommended.

EVALUATING THE EXPOSED HEALTH CARE WORKER

Health care personnel who report occupational exposure should be evaluated for susceptibility to infection by blood-borne pathogens.[2] Baseline testing (i.e., testing to establish infection status at the time of exposure) for HIV antibody should be performed. If the source patient is seronegative for HIV, baseline testing or further follow-up of the worker is not normally necessary unless the source patient has clinical evidence of primary HIV infection. Without a negative result of a baseline HIV test, it is extremely difficult to prove that infection was temporally related to the exposure event. In some instances, demonstrating close genetic similarity in virus sequences obtained from the source patient and the infected health care provider has confirmed the source of exposure, but these studies are expensive and difficult to obtain, and sometimes the results are difficult to interpret. The evaluation should also include information about the use of medications and underlying medical conditions or circumstances (e.g., pregnancy, breast-feeding) that could influence the choice of antiretroviral drugs used for prophylaxis. Pregnancy testing should be offered to all women of childbearing age. Testing for other blood-borne viral infections should not be overlooked.

The Role of HIV Testing in Preventing Occupational and Nosocomial HIV Infection

HIV testing of patients is not recommended as an infection-control procedure, because current standards of practice are designed to prevent the transmission of blood-borne pathogens from all patients, regardless of whether HIV infection is known. No data have demonstrated that preprocedural identification of infected patients reduces the chance of exposure; in one study, the exposure risk was not affected by knowledge of the patient's HIV infection status.[131] Researchers at Johns Hopkins University—an institution in which undiagnosed HIV infection is highly prevalent among patients in the emergency department—evaluated preoperative testing of elective surgical patients.[173] More than 4000 consecutive patients were tested for HIV, and 18 were found to be infected. Of these patients, 10 were aware of their HIV status before the preoperative test was performed, and all 13 provided histories of risk factors for infection. The authors concluded that the prevalence of HIV infection was too low to justify routine preoperative testing in this institution, and the practice was abandoned.[173] The improvement in the reliability and accuracy of rapid HIV tests may allow reliable preoperative screening of patients who require emergency surgery. However, this practice cannot be recommended unless it is demonstrated to result in reduced exposure risk without adverse outcomes in patients.

Although HIV testing is not a useful strategy for preventing occupational and nosocomial HIV transmission, clinicians should address HIV risk in the context of clinical care of their patients. Some patients at risk for HIV infection lack access to HIV testing in the community, and because they have no access to testing, their HIV infections may remain undiagnosed until they have advanced complications. HIV risk assessment should be conducted as a routine component of patient care, even in the emergency department and acute care settings. Patients who relate histories of risk behaviors for HIV infection should be encouraged to consent to HIV counseling and testing. If the responsible clinician is not prepared to offer prevention counseling at the time that testing is requested, an appropriate counseling referral should be arranged.

Routine HIV testing of health care personnel is not recommended. Health care personnel who sustain blood exposures, including those who perform invasive procedures, are advised to be aware of their blood-borne pathogens infection statuses and to seek postexposure testing for HIV and other blood-borne pathogens when indicated by the exposure circumstances, as outlined previously.

MANAGEMENT OF INFECTED HEALTH CARE PROVIDERS

In 1991, the CDC recommended that invasive surgical and dental procedures that had been implicated in hepatitis B virus transmission from infected health care workers to patients be considered "exposure-prone."[174] The characteristics of these procedures included digital palpation of a needle tip in a body cavity or the simultaneous presence of a clinician's fingers and a needle or other sharp object in a poorly visualized or highly confined anatomic site. The CDC also recommended that invasive procedures associated with an increased risk for provider injury in observational studies be considered exposure prone. These and other exposure-prone procedures were to be identified by medical, surgical, and dental organizations, with input

from the institutions where these procedures were performed. Ultimately, efforts to create a consensus regarding a list of exposure-prone procedures were not successful. Infections in health care personnel who performed exposure-prone procedures were to be reviewed by an advisory panel to determine under what circumstances, if any, the personnel would be allowed to practice.[174] In addition, allowed procedures could be performed only after informed consent was obtained from the patient.

All states were required by Congress to implement these (or equivalent) recommendations. Because of the difficulty in implementing the guidelines, Dr. William Roper, then CDC director, noted in a 1992 letter to state health departments that the states, not the CDC, would certify the equivalency of their guidelines and further stated that "...exposure-prone procedures are best determined on a case-by-case basis, taking into consideration the specific procedure, as well as the skill, technique, and possible impairment of the infected health-care worker." Thus, as a result, substantial variability in the state-by-state interpretation and implementation of these guidelines has emerged, and the role of the expert review panel is underscored. In turn, decisions about managing infected health care workers are often inconsistent and are more likely to be influenced by court decisions rather than by science.

Updated guidelines are clearly warranted, specifically guidelines that take into consideration information developed since the previous guidelines were published. For example, new guidelines could be based on the role of cirulating viral DNA or viral burden, or both, in transmission; the impact of highly active antiretroviral therapy on providers' viral burdens; and the contribution of new safety devices and precautions (i.e., primary prevention) in reducing risks for exposure. Most experts agree that until new guidelines are developed, practice restrictions are appropriate when an infected health care worker is found to be impaired and cannot safely practice, when a pattern of substandard infection-control practice is demonstrated, or when HIV transmission to a patient has occurred or is suspected.[51] Despite the very small magnitude of risk for transmission of HIV from provider to patient, most national guidelines still recommend that HIV-infected providers be prevented from performing exposure-prone, invasive procedures.[174,175] If transmission is documented or suspected, the state or local health department should be contacted for consultation about the need for additional investigation.

Secondary HIV Prevention: Postexposure Prophylaxis in Health Care Settings

In January 1990, the CDC issued the first set of guidelines that included considerations regarding the use of antiretroviral agents for postexposure prophylaxis after occupational HIV infections.[176] By June 1996, a U.S. Public Health Service interagency working group, with input from other experts, published recommendations for providing antiretroviral treatment after occupational HIV exposure to prevent infection.[177] These recommendations and two subsequent sets of updated recommendations[8,178] were based on data from several sources that strongly suggested that in some instances, antiretroviral treatment soon after occupational exposure to HIV could prevent infection. In effect, these recommendations established a standard of care for managing occupational HIV exposure among health care personnel that includes access to postexposure antiretroviral chemoprophylaxis. Specific recommendations for managing provider-to-patient HIV exposures were not included in these guidelines. This section is a discussion of treatment recommendations and exposure management advice relevant to occupational exposure in health care workers. Whereas these recommendations focus on the management of occupational exposures for health care providers, the same principles and approach also apply to nosocomial or iatrogenic exposures to HIV for patients.

RATIONALE FOR ANTIRETROVIRAL CHEMOPROPHYLAXIS FOR OCCUPATIONAL EXPOSURES TO HIV

The rationale for postexposure chemoprophylaxis is based on (1) the current understanding of the early events in the pathogenesis of HIV infection; (2) the biologic plausibility of pharmacologic intervention in this process of HIV pathogenesis; (3) studies of the safety and efficacy of antiretroviral prophylaxis in animal models of retroviral infection; (4) clinical trials demonstrating the efficacy of HIV chemoprophylaxis in animal studies and other human clinical settings; (5) epidemiologic data from studies of exposed health care personnel; and (6) clinical experience with these drugs in this setting since the 1980s.[165,179,180] Together, these types of data provide support for the prophylactic administration of antiretroviral drugs after HIV exposures associated with a transmission risk in health care settings. Each of these classes of information is considered in more detail in the following paragraphs.

Biologic Plausibility of Antiretroviral Chemoprophylaxis

The hypothesis underlying the administration of antiretroviral chemoprophylaxis is that postexposure treatment provided during a "window of opportunity" will attenuate initial HIV replication and prevent systemic HIV infection. Dendritic cells in the mucosa and skin are believed to be the initial target for HIV infection or capture.[181,182] Dendritic cells also play a role in initiating HIV infection of CD4+ T cells in regional lymph nodes.[183] In a primate model of simian immunodeficiency virus (SIV) infection, SIV remained localized in association with dendritic cells underlying the site of vaginal inoculation for the first 24 hours after exposure to cell-free virus.[184] Within 24 to 48 hours, these cells appeared to migrate to regional lymph nodes and present SIV to T lymphocytes. Cell-free and cell-associated SIV was detected in the peripheral blood within 5 days after inoculation.

Additional in vitro studies have further characterized the earliest events in HIV exposure and infection of dendritic cells. "Immature" dendritic cells in the skin and mucous membranes function to capture and process foreign antigens.[185] These cells also express important HIV co-receptors (e.g., CD4 and CCR5). Conversely, these immature dendritic cells lack surface molecules (CD40, CD54, CD86) that are required for efficient activation of T cells. As dendritic cells "mature," they begin expressing these latter receptors. Immature dendritic cells can support replication of HIV in vitro; however, mature cells do not permit replication, unless T cells are present in the milieu. Granelli-Piperno and colleagues suggested that mature dendritic cells in the presence of (and perhaps even in direct contact with) T cells undergo a single round of HIV replication that enables infection of T cells, which in turn enable HIV to replicate rapidly.[185] In this in vitro system, zidovudine treatment cannot prevent either HIV replication in dendritic cells or HIV transfer from dendritic cells to T cells; however, zidovudine does prevent productive T-cell infection in this system.

Blauvelt and colleagues demonstrated that viral capture by, and productive infection of, dendritic cells are mediated through separate pathways; they also proposed that in designing strategies to block transmission of HIV, researchers should consider interfering with both these processes (i.e., both viral capture and infection).[186] Blauvelt and colleagues also demonstrated that productive HIV infection of Langerhans cells is regulated by surface expression of CD4 and CCR5 and that viral capture is mediated through a newly described C-type lectin, DC-SIGN. Dendritic cells that have captured virus through DC-SIGN (but not HIV-infected dendritic cells) facilitate infection of T cells in chronically infected individuals. Blauvelt and colleagues hypothesized that blocking DC-SIGN–mediated HIV capture may represent a new approach to antiviral therapy.[187]

These and other experiments support the concept that productive HIV infection occurs in a sequence of events involving initial capture or infection, or both, of dendritic target cells near the exposure site with subsequent transmission of HIV to susceptible T cells in regional lymph nodes. Each step in this sequence is a potential target for chemoprophylactic intervention. Early antiretroviral treatment appears most likely to prevent infection by blocking the infection of T cells, presumably in the regional lymph nodes. Unfortunately, the available data do not enable prediction of either the maximum time interval after exposure in which prophylaxis might work or the factors that might affect the timing of these events in individual cases. Interrupting or delaying the productive infection of T cells could also allow time for the development of specific cellular immunity directed against HIV in the exposed health care worker.

Animal studies provide evidence for an important role for the cellular immune system in postexposure prophylaxis against HIV infection. Ruprecht and Bronson demonstrated in a mouse retroviral model that successful postexposure prophylaxis requires intact cellular immunity.[188] Putkonen and co-workers demonstrated robust specific cellular responses in macaques in which SIV infection was successfully prevented by postexposure prophylaxis.[189] In the latter study, the macaques developed a strong enough immune response that a second challenge with the same viral inoculum resulted in either no or significantly limited infection.[189] In a second similar study, challenge with different SIV isolates after successful antiretroviral chemoprophylaxis also produced either no or significantly limited infection.[190]

Together, all these data suggest that antiretroviral chemoprophylaxis administered soon after an occupational exposure, in concert with a cellular immune response, may prevent or inhibit systemic HIV infection. This preventive effect theoretically is caused by limiting the proliferation of virus in dendritic cells in the skin or in T cells in regional lymph nodes during a period of time in which the virus remains relatively localized, and this effect may be bolstered by a robust cellular immune response.

Some investigators have suggested that administration of antiretroviral chemoprophylaxis may prevent or diminish cellular responses to HIV antigens. D'Amico and associates demonstrated that only one of seven health care workers treated with zidovudine developed HIV envelope-specific cytotoxic T-lymphocyte responses, in comparison, of 13 workers who did not receive prophylaxis, 6 developed these responses.[191] Conversely, some investigators have suggested that certain antiretroviral agents may also have beneficial immunomodulatory effects. For example, Zidek and colleagues found that the nucleotide analogue phenoxymethylpropyladenine stimulates macrophage secretion of interleukin-1β, interleukin-10, and tumor necrosis factor-α, in addition to promoting the production of the chemokines RANTES (regulated on activation, normal T expressed and secreted) and macrophage inflammatory protein 1α in both macrophages and lymphocytes.[192]

Efficacy of Antiretroviral Chemoprophylaxis in Animal Retroviral Infections

Antiretroviral chemoprophylaxis is effective in many murine and feline models of retrovirus infection, but these models may or may not be relevant to human HIV infection.[193] The earliest studies of chemoprophylactic safety and efficacy in mice and cats demonstrated limited, if any, benefit.[194,195] Similarly, most early studies designed to evaluate the efficacy of antiretroviral chemoprophylaxis of SIV infection in nonhuman primates demonstrated limited protection.[193,196] Virtually all of these early experiments entailed intravenous injection of very high inocula of HIV type 2 or SIV (to ensure infection in 100% of control animals). This exposure route that would bypass the cellular events that occur at an occupational or mucosal exposure site (described in detail previously), and these inoculum sizes were far in excess of what might reasonably be anticipated in an occupational exposure.

Benefits associated with postexposure prophylaxis in more recent experiments in animal models include (1) delay or complete suppression of viremia; (2) inhibition of viral replication and development of a long-lasting, protective cellular immune response; and (3) complete protection (i.e., true chemoprophylactic efficacy).[190,197-202]

In general, postexposure prophylaxis is most likely to be effective in animal models in which the exposure inoculum is relatively low, when treatment is started soon after exposure (usually within 24 hours), and when treatment is continued for at least several days to weeks after inoculation.[193,199] In one study of SIV in macaques, all the animals that received postexposure treatment for 28 days remained uninfected; only half the animals that were treated for 10 days remained uninfected; and none of the animals that received only 3 days of treatment were protected.[199] Similarly, delay in initiating prophylaxis was detrimental in this model. All of the animals that were treated within 24 hours of intravenous SIV infection remained uninfected, whereas only 50% of the animals that received treatment beginning 48 hours after infection and only 25% of the animals that received treatment beginning 72 hours after exposure were protected. Otten and colleagues demonstrated similar findings in a macaque study assessing postexposure prophylaxis after vaginal inoculation with HIV type 2. All animals treated within 48 hours were protected, whereas only some of the animals that received the antiretroviral agent 72 hours after inoculation remained uninfected.[203] If these animal models are relevant to occupational HIV transmission prevention, the current recommendations for postexposure management should maximize the potential for postexposure treatment to be an effective prevention strategy.

Clinical Trials Relevant to Postexposure Chemoprophylaxis

In a randomized, controlled, prospective trial (AIDS Clinical Trial Group, protocol 076), zidovudine or placebo was administered to HIV-infected pregnant women during the second and third trimesters of pregnancy and to newborns for 6 weeks after birth (see Chapter 126).[204] The infection rate among infants receiving treatment was 67% lower than that observed in the placebo recipients. In this study, less than 20% of the protective effect of zidovudine was attributable to a reduction in maternal HIV viral load, which suggests that additional mechanisms contributed to the observed benefit of therapy.[17,18] In two subsequent studies, treatment of newborns of infected mothers who did not receive any antiretroviral therapy before delivery was also effective in preventing perinatal infection, an observation that strongly supports a direct postexposure prophylactic effect of antiretroviral treatment in this clinical context.[205,206]

Because of the very low risk for infection per exposure (i.e., 0.3%; see previous discussion), assessing the efficacy of postexposure chemoprophylaxis in a prospective clinical trial of health care workers sustaining occupational exposures to HIV is not feasible. Between 1987 and 1989, the Burroughs-Wellcome Company sponsored a prospective placebo-controlled clinical trial that was designed to evaluate the efficacy of zidovudine chemoprophylaxis for health care workers after they sustained occupational exposures.[207,208] This trial was terminated prematurely because of inadequate enrollment. In view of the data just described that implies at least a direct benefit of postexposure prophylaxis, justifying the conduct of a placebo-controlled trial of postexposure antiretroviral chemoprophylaxis would now be problematic.

Epidemiologic and Clinical Evidence for and against the Efficacy of Postexposure Chemoprophylaxis

In the CDC's retrospective case-control study of health care workers (see Table 306-1), postexposure treatment with zidovudine was associated with an 81% reduction in the odds of infection (95% confidence interval: 43% to 94%) after adjustment for relevant exposure risk factors.[20,209] This relatively small study was not designed to evaluate treatment; thus, the effect of the drug regimen (dose, time to initiation, duration) on efficacy could not be determined. The study did not prove that treatment was effective, and limitations inherent in the design, including the small number of cases and the fact that cases and controls were not from the same cohort, must be considered.[210] Nevertheless, this study provided very suggestive epidemiologic evidence that zidovudine afforded some protection to exposed health care workers.

Antiretroviral chemoprophylaxis for occupational exposures to HIV has been in use in the United States since the late 1980s.[180] The numbers of occupational infections with HIV that have been reported to CDC

have decreased steadily. Figure 306-1 stratifies the cases of occupational infections reported to CDC from 1992 through 2007 and demonstrates a decrease in the number of cases of occupational HIV infections reported to CDC over time (Denise Cardo, personal communication, December 2008).[3] Several factors are probably contributing to this decrease, including reduced reporting to CDC as the epidemic matures; less aggressive case finding by the CDC and other local and state public health officials; the use of primary exposure prevention strategies, which results in fewer exposures; the efficacy of highly active antiretroviral therapy in lowering the viral burden in HIV-infected source patients, in reducing the likelihood of hospitalization of health care workers, and in decreasing the need for, and numbers of, invasive procedures that place health care workers at risk for exposure[85]; and the use of postexposure antiretroviral chemoprophylaxis for occupational exposures.

Two anecdotal case reports also suggest postexposure treatment efficacy. The first of these reports was about a child who had received a transfusion of HIV-infected blood from a donor in the "window" (i.e., before the donor became HIV antibody positive, but at a time when the donor probably had high titers of HIV RNA in his circulation); the child remained uninfected after aggressive postexposure treatment with antiretroviral agents.[211] Transfusion of HIV-infected blood has been associated with nearly 100% risk for subsequent infection in the transfusion recipient.[212] The second of these anecdotal reports described a health care worker who sustained an occupational HIV exposure; subsequently, while the worker received three-drug postexposure prophylaxis, HIV RNA was detected by polymerase chain reaction in two separate samples (14 and 18 days after exposure). The worker remained uninfected (as assessed by serial nucleic acid tests and antibody determinations more than 1 year after exposure) but did produce a robust HIV-specific cellular immune response.[32]

Prophylaxis failures have been documented in at least 22 instances.[8,178] In more than 75% of the instances of failure, zidovudine was used as a single agent. Only six instances of failure have been reported in association with the use of multiple-agent prophylaxis regimens (two reported failures of two-drug regimens, four failures of three-drug regimens, and one failure of a four-drug regimen).[8,178,213-215] In 14 of the 22 instances of postexposure prophylaxis failure, the source patient for the exposure had previously been treated with one or more antiretroviral agents; thus, it is possible that antiretroviral resistance may explain, at least in part, the chemoprophylaxis failure.[8] However, several additional factors may have contributed to these failures: exposure to high HIV inocula; delayed initiation of prophylaxis; failure to achieve adequate drug concentrations; inadequate treatment duration; and a variety of other variables that may have affected either the health care worker's immune responsiveness or the infectivity of the viral strain to which the worker was exposed. Finally, not all failures are what they appear. Both Lucey and associates[216] and Jochimsen and co-workers[217] reported the details of instances of putative occupational infections that, on further detailed investigation, were shown to be unrelated to the occupational exposures.

ANTIRETROVIRAL DRUGS FOR CHEMOPROPHYLAXIS

Choosing a Treatment Regimen

Several factors influence the selection of antiretroviral drugs for prophylaxis regimen: (1) the type of exposure and the estimated risk of HIV transmission associated with the exposure; (2) the probability that drug-resistant virus strains are currently circulating in the source patient and are likely to be present in the exposure inoculum; (3) the safety profile and likelihood of the health care worker's adherence to the proposed treatment regimens; and (4) the cost of the agents. Several antiretroviral agents belonging to at least seven classes of drugs are available for the treatment of HIV disease.[8,218-220] These agents include nucleoside reverse transcriptase inhibitors, nucleotide reverse transcriptase inhibitors, non-nucleoside reverse transcriptase inhibitors, protease inhibitors, and fusion inhibitors.

TABLE 306-3	Current Recommendations by the CDC and U.S. Public Health Service for Chemoprophylaxis of Occupational Exposures to HIV*		
HIV exposures associated with a recognized transmission risk	"Basic regimens"	Zidovudine (ZDV) *plus either* lamivudine (3TC) *or* emtricitabine (FTC)
		Tenofovir (TDF) *plus either* lamivudine (3TC) *or* emtricitabine (FTC)
	Alternative "basic regimens"	Stavudine (d4T) *plus* lamivudine (3TC)
		Stavudine (d4T) *plus* emtricitabine (FTC)†
HIV exposures for which the nature of the exposure is suggestive of elevated risk of transmission‡	Expanded regimen (i.e., "basic regimen" plus)	Lopinavir/ritonavir (Kaletra)
	Alternative expanded regimens: "basic regimen" plus one or more of the agents listed on the right	Atazanavir Fosamprenavir§ Indinavir‖ *plus* ritonavir Saquinavir *plus* ritonavir Efavirenz†

*The role of newer agents (e.g., integrase inhibitors, CCR5 inhibitors) remains undetermined.
†Agent is not recommended for use during pregnancy.
‡Elevated risk is associated with "deep" injury, injury with a device that has been used in an HIV-infected patient's artery or vein, injuries involving large-volume blood loss, and blood containing a high titer of HIV.
§Toxic effects have been reported[238] (see text).
‖Medication should be taken on an empty stomach, and daily fluid consumption should be increased (e.g., six 8-oz glasses of water daily).
CDC, Centers for Disease Control and Prevention; HIV, human immunodeficiency virus.
Modified from Panlilio AL. Updated U.S. Public Health Service guidelines for the management of occupational exposures to HIV and recommendations for postexposure prophylaxis. *MMWR Recomm Rep.* 2005;54(RR-9):1-17.

The "basic regimen" currently recommended by the CDC for treatment after occupational HIV exposures that confer an infection risk includes (1) a combination of zidovudine with either lamivudine or emtricitabine or (2) a combination of tenofovir with either lamivudine or emtricitibine (Table 306-3).[178] Combinations of antiretroviral drugs are more effective than single agents for treating established HIV infection; however, no data demonstrate that combinations of drugs are more effective for prophylaxis than is zidovudine (or any other agent) used alone. The rationale for including lamivudine as a second drug in the basic regimen is that zidovudine resistance is increasing among patients with HIV infection.[7,221-226] The most recent guidelines list a combination of stavudine (d4T) and either lamivudine or emtricitabine as acceptable alternative "basic regimens."[178]

The CDC recommends an "expanded regimen" that includes a protease inhibitor or a non-nucleoside reverse transcriptase inhibitor in addition to the basic regimen described previously. The regimen is recommended for exposures for which the risk of HIV infection is increased (i.e., high volume of inoculum or exposure to materials containing a high HIV titer).[20,178] In the most recent set of recommendations, the lopinavir/ritonavir (Kaletra) combination is listed as the preferred choice for an expanded regimen, with atazanavir, fosamprenavir, the indinavir/ritonavir combination, the saquinavir/ritonavir combination, and efavirenz all listed as acceptable alternatives.[178] With regard to Kaletra, the CDC issued a notification of dose modification for the combination because the manufacturer stopped marketing one formulation of the product.[227] The previous regimen for the capsule formulation (no longer available) was three capsules twice daily. The product is now available only in tablet form; each tablet contains 200 mg of lopinavir and 50 mg of ritonavir. Thus, to achieve the same recommended daily amount of the agents, the dosing regimen has been modified to two tablets, twice daily. The previously used dosing regimen should *not* be used because it is probably not as well tolerated and could result in increased toxicity.

In September 2007, the manufacturer of nelfinavir issued a warning that the product contained high levels of ethyl methane mesylate, a known carcinogen, mutagen, and teratogen. The CDC issued a warning

about including it in postexposure prophylaxis regimens.[227] In addition, in late 2007, Pavel and colleagues reported severe hepatotoxicity in association with a regimen of zidovudine, lamivudine, and fosamprenavir/ritonavir.[228] In this report, patients received postexposure prophylaxis with this regimen, and 54% had grade 1 or 2 toxic effects; 11.5% had moderately severe rash; and two patients experienced grade 4 hepatic toxicity, with liver enzymes elevated more than 10-fold.

Efavirenz is the only non-nucleoside reverse transcriptase inhibitor that, to date, has been specifically recommended for use in the expanded regimen. This agent should not be used when the health care worker is, or might be, pregnant. Efavirenz affects the metabolism and blood levels of protease inhibitors in the body (particularly indinavir, saquinavir, and amprenavir); for this reason, guidelines for dosing the available protease inhibitors with efavirenz have been developed (see Chapter 128). The role of non-nucleoside reverse transcriptase inhibitors, and specifically of nevirapine, which has been used by some clinicians in the postexposure setting, is less clear. Nevirapine has been used commonly in some settings, and its use for postexposure prophylaxis has been associated with serious and sometimes life-threatening toxic effects that appear to be more probable than the infection risk associated with most exposures.[229-232] Nevirapine is not included as a recommended agent in the two most recent iterations of the CDC guidelines.[8,178] The U.S. Public Health Service (USPHS) probably will continue to modify its list of agents recommended for use in this setting, as additional agents are marketed and as physicians learn more about the unanticipated toxic effects associated with already marketed agents.

The basic and expanded drug regimens described by the CDC are good choices when the source patient is unlikely to harbor virus isolates that are resistant to the drugs included in the chosen regimen. Resistance to all antiretroviral drugs has been reported, and transmission of resistant strains can occur.[213,222,224-226,233] Drug resistance is most likely to be present among patients with high viral loads who are not responding to treatment or do not adhere to the treatment regimen. Unfortunately, clinical predictions about drug resistance are neither sensitive nor specific. Special genotypic and phenotypic tests to detect HIV resistance are not readily available to provide support for prophylactic treatment decisions. When drug resistance is suspected, empirical prophylactic treatment regimens should be based on the same principles used to select drugs for HIV-infected patients in whom treatment is failing.[234] Many experts recommend the use of at least two drugs that the source patient has not taken in the recent past (i.e., preceding 30 days). For example, treatment with tenofovir and emtricitabine (with or without a protease inhibitor) may be appropriate when treatment with zidovudine plus lamivudine is failing. The combination of didanosine and stavudine should not be administered to pregnant patients. Similarly, stavudine plus lamivudine (or emtricitabine) is a reasonable choice when zidovudine therapy is failing or when the patient is deemed likely to have had a predominance of zidovudine-resistant strains circulating in the blood stream at the time that exposure occurred.[235] If the resistance is likely to involve an entire class of antiretroviral drugs (e.g., protease inhibitors), including one or more agents from other classes makes implicit sense.[234,235]

In view of all the complexities inherent in selecting antiretroviral drugs, consultation with an expert in HIV treatment is recommended when exposure to drug-resistant HIV is a concern. However, treatment should not be delayed to obtain such consultation. One approach is immediately to begin the basic or expanded regimen and then seek help from an expert about modifying the regimen. If local expertise is not available, clinicians in the United States who need consultative assistance concerning prophylaxis for occupational HIV exposure can also contact the National Clinicians' Post-exposure Hotline (PEP-Line) (Table 306-4).

Adverse Effects Associated with Postexposure Chemoprophylaxis

Adverse effects have been associated with all agents and regimens used for postexposure prophylaxis (summarized by the CDC[227] and other

TABLE 306-4	Management of HIV Exposure and Chemoprophylactic Treatment: HIV Postexposure Prophylaxis Resources and Registries
National HIV/AIDS Clinicians' Consultation Center: Postexposure Prophylaxis Hotline	Phone: 888-448-4911 Web site: http://www.nccc.ucsf.edu/Hotlines/PEPline.html
Antiretroviral Pregnancy Registry	Phone (US and Canada): 800-258-4263 or 800-800-1052 Phone (International): 910-256-0238 Web site: http://www.apregistry.com Fax (International): 910-256-0637 Address: Research Park, 1011 Ashes Drive, Wilmington, NC 28405
U.S. Food and Drug Administration (reporting unusual or severe toxicity to antiretroviral agents—MedWatch)	Phone: 800-332-1088 Web site: www.fda.gov/medwatch
Reporting to the CDC HIV seroconversions in health care workers who received postexposure prophylaxis	Phone: 888-448-4911

AIDS, acquired immunodeficiency syndrome; CDC, Centers for Disease Control and Prevention; HIV, human immunodeficiency virus.

investigators[228,236-242]). The frequency, severity, duration, and reversibility of side effects are important considerations in formulating a prophylactic treatment regimen. Unusual or serious and unexpected toxic effects of antiretroviral drugs should be reported to the manufacturer and the U.S. Food and Drug Administration (see Table 306-4). Despite the fact that the use of these drugs in the postexposure setting has become the standard of care, no agent has been approved or labeled for postexposure chemoprophylaxis for HIV exposures; therefore, all such use must be considered "off-label."

Most of the information about prophylactic treatment side effects was derived from studies of health care workers who took zidovudine alone, usually at doses of 1000 to 1200 mg/day (i.e., doses higher than the currently recommended dose; summarized by Lee and Henderson[237]). More than 50% of those treated reported at least one side effect, and about 30% stopped treatment because of their symptoms. Use of nucleoside analogues for postexposure prophylaxis has been associated with bone marrow suppression (e.g., decreases in hemoglobin and absolute neutrophil counts), nausea, vomiting, diarrhea, abdominal pain, headache, neuropathies, myalgias, lassitude, malaise, and insomnia. In a few instances, more severe toxic effects have been reported, including cases of severe rash with hepatic dysfunction and seizures. Subjective side effects are especially common in the population of health care workers receiving postexposure chemoprophylaxis. Use of protease inhibitors in chemoprophylaxis regimens has been associated with nausea, vomiting, diarrhea, abdominal pain, hyperglycemia, hyperlipidemia, hypercholesterolemia, galactorrhea,[238] hyperprolactinemia,[238] cholestatic jaundice,[240] headache, anorexia, altered taste sensation, and paresthesias.[237] In addition, the literature contains a few instances of nephrolithiasis[241] and lipodystrophy[243] associated with protease inhibitor administration for postexposure prophylaxis. Health care workers who took regimens that included two or more antiretroviral drugs experienced frequent side effects (summarized by Lee and Henderson[237]). In almost every instance, side effects ceased when treatment was stopped.

Although non-nucleoside reverse transcriptase inhibitors are not primary choices for prophylaxis in most published guidelines,[8,178] these agents (most frequently nevirapine) are used in some settings for postexposure chemoprophylaxis.[244] The rash that occurs commonly with the non-nucleoside agents can easily be confused with the HIV seroconversion illness. On occasion, the rash associated with these agents is severe; the literature contains two case reports of possible Stevens-Johnson syndrome in health care workers taking nevirapine as postexposure chemoprophylaxis.[229] Fever and gastrointestinal symptoms have also been reported to occur commonly when non-nucleoside reverse transcriptase inhibitors were used for postexposure therapy.

Perhaps of most concern is the report of two instances of severe hepatic dysfunction (one of which necessitated liver transplantation) and 10 additional cases of moderate hepatic toxicity in health care workers who took nevirapine as part of a chemoprophylaxis regimen.[229-232] Another report described a single instance of severe ototoxicity that occurred in a health care worker who received a postexposure prophylaxis regimen composed of stavudine, lamivudine, and nevirapine.[245] As noted earlier, the non-nucleoside reverse transcriptase inhibitor efavirenz is included in the list of acceptable alternative agents in the most recent USPHS guidelines.[178]

Side effects associated with HIV chemoprophylaxis are similar to those observed in HIV-infected patients, and most can be managed symptomatically (e.g., acetaminophen for headache and myalgia; prochlorperazine for nausea; antimotility drugs for diarrhea). Nephrolithiasis and urinary tract obstruction associated with indinavir can be prevented by increasing fluid intake to at least six 8-oz glasses of water per day. Because drug interactions are especially common with protease inhibitors, practitioners providing care should carefully evaluate all other drugs currently being taken by an exposed health care worker. Protease inhibitors can inhibit the metabolism of nonsedating antihistamines and other hepatically metabolized drugs. Some of these agents (e.g., nelfinavir, ritonavir) accelerate the clearance of certain drugs, including oral contraceptives. Women taking these protease inhibitors should be encouraged to use alternative or additional contraceptive measures.

Chemoprophylaxis in Pregnancy

Pregnant women who sustain occupational exposures should be offered postexposure antiretroviral chemoprophylaxis.[165,166,178,235] The decision to offer treatment should be based on the same considerations that apply to other health care personnel sustaining these exposures. In counseling the exposed health care worker who is pregnant, the counselor must address the potential risks and benefits both for the worker and her fetus. Specifically, the counselor should provide detailed information about what is known about the risk of HIV transmission to the mother and the fetus, the issue of teratogenicity in the context of the stages of pregnancy, and what is known about the pharmacokinetics, the safety, and the tolerability of antiretroviral drugs during pregnancy.[165,166,178,235,237,246,247] In addition, the prescribing practitioner must be aware that antiretroviral drugs may cause or exacerbate conditions that are especially serious during pregnancy (e.g., nausea, nephrolithiasis, hyperbilirubinemia, and hyperglycemia). In view of these complexities, input from experts in managing antiretroviral drugs during pregnancy may be helpful both to the exposed health care worker and to her physician.

The risk to the fetus of administering a 28-day course of postexposure prophylaxis with antiretroviral agents remains undefined. My colleagues and I use several principles to guide the administration of postexposure prophylaxis in pregnancy. The decision of whether to take postexposure prophylaxis can be made only by the pregnant worker. She must be provided with accurate, thorough, unbiased counseling.

All available antiretroviral agents have the potential for carcinogenicity, teratogenicity, or mutagenicity, or a combination of these. In premarketing studies in animals, some agents have been shown to be mutagenic. In studies in which zidovudine was administered to animals at a dosage 35 times higher than the label-indication dosage in humans for 18 to 22 months, the risk for certain hepatic tumors was increased.[176] The relevance of such studies to administration of this agent to pregnant health care workers who have sustained occupational exposures is unclear. Similarly, in studies of efavirenz given to cynomolgus monkeys at drug levels similar to those produced in human dosing, teratogenic effects were demonstrated. Because of the potential relevance of these studies, most authorities do not recommend that pregnant patient take efavirenz.

Limited safety data address the risk of administering antiretrovirals to HIV-uninfected pregnant women or the pharmacologic actions of the drugs in this setting. Evaluations of the efficacy of antiretrovirals in preventing vertical HIV provide useful, but not directly comparable, information about the use of these drugs in the postexposure setting. A large French study identified fetal neurologic/mitochondrial toxicity associated with administration of nucleoside analogues during pregnancy.[248] Two infant deaths and six additional instances of probable mitochondrial toxicity were identified in HIV-uninfected offspring of HIV-infected mothers in this large trial. Both deaths were associated with mitochondrial toxicity that led to progressive neurologic disease.[248] Interestingly, no fetal deaths attributable to, or associated with, antiretroviral-induced mitochondrial toxicity have been identified among several large vertical transmission studies that have been conducted in the United States. The differences between the French and U.S. experiences are currently not well understood and remain the subject of substantial controversy.[249,250]

Treatment of HIV-infected pregnant women with the didanosine/stavudine (ddI/d4T) combination has also been associated with increased risk. Several instances of severe pancreatitis and lactic acidosis have been reported, and in some instances, this syndrome has been associated with maternal death, fetal death, or both.[251,251a] To my knowledge, this severe complication has not been observed in pregnant individuals taking ddI/d4T postexposure prophylaxis; however, because of the adverse experience with these agents in the treatment of HIV infection during pregnancy, this combination is not recommended for postexposure management in pregnant health care workers sustaining occupational HIV exposures.

The Antiretroviral Pregnancy Registry was designed to help evaluate the safety of administering antiretroviral agents during pregnancy and to detect evidence suggestive of teratogenicity or other serious adverse events. To date, the Antiretroviral Pregnancy Registry has not detected an increased risk of birth defects in infants with in utero exposure to zidovudine. Less information is available for other antiretroviral drugs, although a similar safety profile appears to be developing with regard to the use of lamivudine during pregnancy.[247]

INDICATIONS FOR CHEMOPROPHYLAXIS

Current USPHS guidelines for postexposure chemoprophylaxis reflect a balance between the estimated risk of HIV transmission associated with specific exposures and the potential risks associated with treatment.[178] In general, chemoprophylaxis is recommended for exposures known to confer a transmission risk, should be considered for exposures with a "negligible risk," and *may not* be warranted for exposures that do not pose a known transmission risk.[178] In this framework, treatment is recommended for all percutaneous exposures to HIV and for large-volume or long-duration mucosal and nonintact skin exposures that involve high titers of HIV (e.g., blood from patients with advanced HIV disease, high viral load, or low CD4+ counts). Treatment should be considered for small-volume, short-duration mucosal and nonintact skin exposure if the source patient is known or suspected to have a high circulating viral burden. Treatment is not indicated for most intact skin contacts.

The actual risk associated with a specific exposure to HIV is impossible to predict. Because the efficacy of chemoprophylaxis may never be demonstrated definitively in a clinical trial, and because the agents involved are associated with substantial toxic effects, postexposure prophylaxis must, in every instance, be implemented with caution. Current USPHS guidelines are based on exposures to blood or other potentially infectious materials known to contain HIV, not materials of uncertain HIV status. Unfortunately, the guidelines have been interpreted to imply that antiretroviral chemoprophylaxis should be started for all blood exposures, unless HIV infection is specifically ruled out by a negative result of a test on a source patient.

"Source Unknown" Exposures
Decisions about treatment when the source material is not known to contain HIV should be based on a careful risk assessment, including a determination of (1) the probability of HIV infection in the source patient; (2) the type of exposure and the associated risk of HIV trans-

mission with such an exposure, if HIV was, in fact, present; and (3) the risks associated with treatment for the health care worker. In many "source unknown" exposures, the risk of transmission is negligible, and treatment is simply not indicated. Only if the assessment suggests that the risk of HIV transmission outweighs the risk of treatment is it reasonable to initiate the basic treatment regimen until test results or other data become available.

Postexposure Chemoprophylaxis for Nonoccupational HIV Exposures
The use of antiretroviral chemoprophylaxis for nonoccupational exposures has been investigated intensively.[167,168,252-260] The Committee on Pediatric AIDS of the American Academy of Pediatrics published detailed guidelines for managing the often unique exposures experienced by children and adolescents.[252] Management of sexual exposures is discussed elsewhere in this text (see Chapter 128). The rationale for providing postexposure chemoprophylaxis in select cases of nonoccupational or community HIV exposure is no different from that for providing prophylaxis for occupational exposures. Nonetheless, because of the toxicity and risk associated, both occupational and nonoccupational chemoprophylaxis should always be provided cautiously and only in the context of a comprehensive program designed to prevent subsequent exposures. In providing postexposure chemoprophylaxis for nonoccupational exposures, clinicians should evaluate the circumstances of each exposure, provide counseling about the risks for infection and secondary transmission, and provide up-to-date information about the risks and benefits of antiretroviral chemotherapy. In many instances, the care provider's primary role is one of reassurance, inasmuch as the risk for transmission associated with many such community exposures may be quite small. Several reports describe instances in which HIV transmission has been associated with human bites.[169-172,261-263] Evaluation of the bitten individual should include baseline testing for preexisting HIV infection, an offer of postexposure prophylaxis if the patient is exposed to HIV, and follow-up identical to that described for other parenteral HIV exposures. Another nonoccupational setting in which postexposure chemoprophylaxis is frequently administered is after sexual assault.[254,256,257,264-267] Individuals providing counseling for victims of sexual assault must carefully consider the extreme physical and psychological trauma that such patients have experienced.

TIMING AND DURATION OF CHEMOPROPHYLAXIS

Treatment should be initiated as soon as possible after exposure. In most animal studies, efficacy is reduced when treatment is delayed for more than 24 hours,[199] but the relevance of this observation to low-inoculum transcutaneous and transmucosal occupational exposures to HIV is not known. Nonetheless, occupational exposures to HIV should be regarded as urgent medical concerns. When indicated, chemoprophylaxis should be started as soon as practical (i.e., within a few hours rather than days). When consultation is needed to select the best regimen, beginning the basic or expanded regimen until additional information is available may be the best course of action, rather than delaying the start of treatment. In cases in which the risk of transmission is very high, treatment even after a long delay (e.g., 1 to 2 weeks) should still be considered. Even if infection is not prevented, early treatment of acute HIV infection may be beneficial. The optimal duration of chemoprophylaxis is not known. A 4-week regimen is currently recommended, primarily on the basis of clinical experience.[165,166,178,235]

FOLLOW-UP FOR OCCUPATIONAL HIV EXPOSURES

Postexposure Medical Evaluation and HIV Testing
In addition to baseline HIV testing, serologic testing for a documented occupational HIV exposure is usually performed 6 weeks, 3 months, and 6 months after exposure.[178] Sequential testing is useful in allaying fears, in documenting seronegativity, and, in rare instances, in diag-

nosing HIV infection. Testing for more than 6 months is not routinely recommended, although some institutions test at 1 year after exposure if the health care worker who sustained the exposure requests testing.[165,166] Several types of exposures may be associated with increased risk for transmission. For example, if a high volume of blood was injected or if the injury simultaneously exposed the health care worker to HIV and HCV (particularly if HCV was transmitted in the exposure), extending the testing interval for several more months is recommended.

Symptoms of acute retroviral infection (fever, lymphadenopathy, pharyngitis, rash, headache, profound fatigue) have been associated with approximately 80% of reported occupational infections, even when chemoprophylaxis was administered (see Chapter 121).[34] For this reason, all HIV-exposed persons should be advised to return for evaluation and HIV testing if an illness suggestive of the acute retroviral syndrome occurs. Conversely, not every fever and rash is indicative of acute HIV infection; drug reactions or other intercurrent illnesses can mimic primary HIV infection. HIV antibody tests may be negative or indeterminate during the early phases of the seroconversion illness. Immunoblot, viral load tests (quantitative HIV RNA polymerase chain reaction), or viral cultures may be more sensitive methods for detecting early infection (see Chapter 119). Whereas these latter tests may be of value in differentiating seroconversion from other illnesses, these latter tests are *not* indicated in the routine management of occupational HIV exposures.

Ongoing Monitoring for Individuals Receiving Postexposure Chemoprophylaxis

Health care workers who elect to receive chemoprophylaxis after HIV exposure should return 48 to 72 hours after initiation of treatment for routine evaluation for signs and symptoms of drug toxicity and to make certain that all questions and concerns are addressed. The exposed patient should next be seen no later than 2 weeks after initiation of therapy (some practitioners prefer weekly evaluations for the first month). The clinician evaluating the patient should obtain a careful history, perform a focused physical examination, and obtain relevant laboratory tests appropriate to the drug regimen. As a general rule, a complete blood cell count and renal and hepatic chemical function tests are usually indicated. A random blood glucose measurement and a lipid profile should be included whenever protease inhibitor therapy is included in the regimen.[8,178,239,240]

Exposed health care workers who choose to receive chemoprophylaxis should be advised of the importance of completing the prescribed regimen. They should be provided information about potential drug interactions and what medications not to take with the prophylactic drug regimen; the side effects of the drugs that have been prescribed and measures to minimize these effects; and methods of clinical monitoring for toxicity during the follow-up period. They should be alerted to the need for immediate evaluation of symptoms of the seroconversion illness and of symptoms suggestive of serious toxicity (e.g., back or abdominal pain, pain on urination or blood in the urine, and symptoms of hyperglycemia, such as increased thirst or frequent urination).

Health care workers who do not complete the recommended regimen often stop because of the side effects (e.g., nausea and diarrhea). Without changing the regimen, clinicians can often manage these symptoms by prescribing antimotility and antiemetic agents or other medications that target the specific symptoms. In other situations, modifying the dose interval (e.g., giving a drug more frequently throughout the day in lower doses, as recommended by the manufacturer) may also promote adherence to the regimen.

REFERENCES

1. Leibowitz S, Greenwald L, Cohen I, et al. Serum hepatitis in a blood bank worker. *JAMA.* 1949;140:1331-1333.
2. Henderson DK, Gerberding JL. Healthcare worker issues, including occupational and nonoccupational postexposure management. In: Dolin R, Masur H, Saag MS, eds. *AIDS Therapy.* 2nd ed. New York: Churchill Livingstone; 2002: 327-346.
3. Do AN, Ciesielski CA, Metler RP, et al. Occupationally acquired human immunodeficiency virus (HIV) infection: national case surveillance data during 20 years of the HIV epidemic in the United States. *Infect Control Hosp Epidemiol.* 2003;24: 86-96.
4. Tomkins S, Ncube F. Occupationally acquired HIV: international reports to December 2002. *Eur Surveill.* 2005;10: E050310-E050312.
5. Beekmann SE, Fahey BJ, Gerberding JL, et al. Risky business: using necessarily imprecise casualty counts to estimate occupational risks for HIV-1 infection. *Infect Control Hosp Epidemiol.* 1990;11:371-379.
6. Eberle J, Habermann J, Gurtler LG. HIV-1 infection transmitted by serum droplets into the eye: a case report. *AIDS.* 2000;14: 206-207.
7. Beltrami EM, Kozak A, Williams IT, et al. Transmission of HIV and hepatitis C virus from a nursing home patient to a health care worker. *Am J Infect Dis.* 2003;31:168-175.
8. Centers for Disease Control and Prevention. Updated U.S. Public Health Service guidelines for the management of occupational exposures to HBV, HCV, and HIV and recommendations for postexposure prophylaxis. *MMWR Morb Mortal Wkly Rep.* 2001;50(RR-11):1-52.
9. Ippolito G, Puro V, Heptonstall J, et al. Occupational human immunodeficiency virus infection in health care workers: worldwide cases through September 1997. *Clin Infect Dis.* 1999;28: 365-383.
10. Gioananni P, Sinicco A, Cariti G, et al. HIV infection acquired by a nurse. *Eur J Epidemiol.* 1988;4:119-120.
11. Fahey BJ, Koziol DE, Banks SM, et al. Frequency of nonparenteral occupational exposures to blood and body fluids before and after universal precautions training. *Am J Med.* 1991;90: 145-153.
12. Bennett NT, Howard RJ. Quantity of blood inoculated in a needlestick injury from suture needles. *J Am Coll Surg.* 1994;178:107-110.
13. Mast ST, Woolwine JD, Gerberding JL. Efficacy of gloves in reducing blood volumes transferred during simulated needlestick injury. *J Infect Dis.* 1993;168:1589-1592.
14. Daar ES, Moudgil T, Meyer RD, et al. Transient high levels of viremia in patients with primary human immunodeficiency virus type 1 infection. *N Engl J Med.* 1991;324:961-964.
15. Ho DD, Moudgil T, Alam M. Quantitation of human immunodeficiency virus type 1 in the blood of infected persons. *N Engl J Med.* 1989;321:1621-1625.
16. Saag MS, Crain MJ, Decker WD, et al. High-level viremia in adults and children infected with human immunodeficiency virus: relation to disease stage and CD4+ lymphocyte levels. *J Infect Dis.* 1991;164:72-80.
17. Cao Y, Krogstad P, Korber BT, et al. Maternal HIV-1 viral load and vertical transmission of infection: the Ariel Project for the prevention of HIV transmission from mother to infant. *Nat Med.* 1997;3:549-552.
18. Sperling RS, Shapiro DE, Coombs RW, et al. Maternal viral load, zidovudine treatment, and the risk of transmission of human immunodeficiency virus type 1 from mother to infant. Pediatric AIDS Clinical Trials Group Protocol 076 Study Group. *N Engl J Med.* 1996;335:1621-1629.
19. Henderson DK, Gerberding JL. Human immunodeficiency virus in the healthcare setting. In: Mandell GL, Dolin R, Bennett JE, eds. *Principles and Practice of Infectious Diseases.* 6th ed. Philadelphia: Churchill-Livingstone; 2004:3391-3409.
20. Cardo DM, Culver DH, Ciesielski CA, et al. A case-control study of HIV seroconversion in health care workers after percutaneous exposure. *N Engl J Med.* 1997;337:1485-1490.
21. Rowland-Jones S, Dong T, Krausa P, et al. The role of cytotoxic T-cells in HIV infection. *Dev Biol Stand.* 1998;92: 209-214.
22. Rowland-Jones S, Sutton J, Ariyoshi K, et al. HIV-specific cytotoxic T-cells in HIV-exposed but uninfected Gambian women. *Nat Med.* 1995;1:59-64.
23. Clerici M, Giorgi JV, Chou CC, et al. Cell-mediated immune response to human immunodeficiency virus (HIV) type 1 in seronegative homosexual men with recent sexual exposure to HIV-1. *J Infect Dis.* 1992;165:1012-1019.
24. Kelker HC, Seidlin M, Vogler M, et al. Lymphocytes from some long-term seronegative heterosexual partners of HIV-infected individuals proliferate in response to HIV antigens. *AIDS Res Hum Retroviruses.* 1992;8:1355-1359.
25. Mazzoli S, Trabattoni D, Lo Caputo S, et al. HIV-specific mucosal and cellular immunity in HIV-seronegative partners of HIV-seropositive individuals. *Nat Med.* 1997;3:1250-1257.
26. Ranki A, Mattinen S, Yarchoan R, et al. T-cell response towards HIV in infected individuals with and without zidovudine therapy, and in HIV-exposed sexual partners. *AIDS.* 1989;3: 63-69.
27. Cheynier R, Langlade-Demoyen P, Marescot MR, et al. Cytotoxic T lymphocyte responses in the peripheral blood of children born to human immunodeficiency virus-1-infected mothers. *Eur J Immunol.* 1992;22:2211-2217.
28. Missale G, Papagno L, Penna A, et al. Parenteral exposure to high HIV viremia leads to virus-specific T cell priming without evidence of infection. *Eur J Immunol.* 2004;34:3208-3215.
29. Clerici M, Levin JM, Kessler HA, et al. HIV-specific T-helper activity in seronegative health care workers exposed to contaminated blood. *JAMA.* 1994;271:42-46.
30. Pinto LA, Landay AL, Berzofsky JA, et al. Immune response to human immunodeficiency virus (HIV) in healthcare workers occupationally exposed to HIV-contaminated blood. *Am J Med.* 1997;102(Suppl. 5B):21-24.
31. Pinto LA, Sullivan J, Berzofsky JA, et al. ENV-specific cytotoxic T lymphocyte responses in HIV seronegative health care workers occupationally exposed to HIV-contaminated body fluids. *J Clin Invest.* 1995;96:867-876.
32. Puro V, Calcagno G, Anselmo M, et al. Transient detection of plasma HIV-1 RNA during postexposure prophylaxis. *Infect Control Hosp Epidemiol.* 2000;21:529-531.
33. Busch MP, Sattem GA. Time course of viremia and antibody seroconversion following human immunodeficiency virus exposure. *Am J Med.* 1997;102(Suppl. 5B):117-124.
34. Ciesielski CA, Metler RP. Duration of time between exposure and seroconversion in healthcare workers with occupationally acquired infection with human immunodeficiency virus. *Am J Med.* 1997;102(Suppl. 5B):115-116.
35. Ridzon R, Gallagher K, Ciesielski C, et al. Simultaneous transmission of human immunodeficiency virus and hepatitis C virus from a needle-stick injury. *N Engl J Med.* 1997;336: 919-922.
36. Blanchard A, Ferris S, Chamaret S, et al. Molecular evidence for nosocomial transmission of human immunodeficiency virus from a surgeon to one of his patients. *J Virol.* 1998;72:4537-4540.
37. Bosch X. Second case of doctor-to-patient HIV transmission. *Lancet Infect Dis.* 2003;3:261.
38. Centers for Disease Control. Possible transmission of human immunodeficiency virus to a patient during an invasive dental procedure. *MMWR Morb Mortal Wkly Rep.* 1990;39:489-493.
39. Centers for Disease Control. Update: Transmission of HIV infection during an invasive dental procedure—Florida. *MMWR Morb Mortal Wkly Rep.* 1991;40:21-33.
40. Ciesielski CA, Bell DM, Marianos DW. Transmission of HIV from infected health-care workers to patients. *AIDS.* 1991;5(Suppl. 2):S93-S97.
41. Ciesielski CA, Marianos DW, Schochetman G, et al. The 1990 Florida dental investigation. The press and the science. *Ann Intern Med.* 1994;121:886-888.
42. Goujon CP, Schneider VM, Grofti J, et al. Phylogenetic analyses indicate an atypical nurse-to-patient transmission of human immunodeficiency virus type 1. *J Virol.* 2000;74:2525-2532.

43. Lot F, Seguier JC, Fegueux S, et al. Probable transmission of HIV from an orthopedic surgeon to a patient in France. *Ann Intern Med.* 1999;130:1-6.
44. Astagneau P, Lot F, Bouvet E, et al. Lookback investigation of patients potentially exposed to HIV type 1 after a nurse-to-patient transmission. *Am J Infect Control.* 2002;30:242-245.
45. Centers for Disease Control. Update: investigations of persons treated by HIV-infected health-care workers—United States. *MMWR Morb Mortal Wkly Rep.* 1993;42:329-331, 337.
46. Robert LM, Chamberland ME, Cleveland JL, et al. Investigations of patients of health care workers infected with HIV: the Centers for Disease Control and Prevention database. *Ann Intern Med.* 1995;122:653-657.
47. Castro KG, Lifson AR, White CR, et al. Investigations of AIDS patients with no previously identified risk factors. *JAMA.* 1988;259:1338-1342.
48. Gerberding JL, Rose DA, Ramiro NZ, et al. Intraoperative provider injuries and potential patient recontacts at San Francisco General Hospital. *Infect Control Hosp Epidemiol.* 1994;15:20.
49. Tokars JI, Bell DM, Culver DH, et al. Percutaneous injuries during surgical procedures. *JAMA.* 1992;267:2899-2904.
50. Gerberding JL. Provider-to-patient HIV transmission: how to keep it exceedingly rare. *Ann Intern Med.* 1999;130:64-65.
51. Henderson DK, The AIDS/Tuberculosis Subcommittee of the Society for Healthcare Epidemiology of America. Management of healthcare workers infected with hepatitis B virus, hepatitis C virus, human immunodeficiency virus, or other bloodborne pathogens. AIDS/TB Committee of the Society for Healthcare Epidemiology of America. *Infect Control Hosp Epidemiol.* 1997; 18:349-363.
52. Gisselquist DP. Estimating HIV-1 transmission efficiency through unsafe medical injections. *Int J STD AIDS.* 2002;13: 152-159.
53. Yerly S, Quadri R, Negro F, et al. Nosocomial outbreak of multiple bloodborne viral infections. *J Infect Dis.* 2001;184: 369-372.
54. Injection practices among nurses—Valcea, Romania, 1998. *MMWR Morb Mortal Wkly Rep.* 2001;50:59-61.
55. Hersh BS, Popovici F, Jezek Z, et al. Risk factors for HIV infection among abandoned Romanian children. *AIDS.* 1993;7:1617-1624.
56. Patrascu IV, Dumitrescu O. The epidemic of human immunodeficiency virus infection in Romanian children. *AIDS Res Hum Retroviruses.* 1993;9:99-104.
57. Deuchert E, Brody S. The evidence for health-care transmission of HIV in Africa should determine prevention priorities. *Int J STD AIDS.* 2007;18:290-291.
58. Ekwueme DU, Weniger BG, Chen RT. Model-based estimates of risks of disease transmission and economic costs of seven injection devices in sub-Saharan Africa. *Bull World Health Organ.* 2002;80:859-870.
59. Gisselquist D, Rothenberg R, Potterat J, et al. HIV infections in sub-Saharan Africa not explained by sexual or vertical transmission. *Int J STD AIDS.* 2002;13:657-666.
60. Priddy F, Tesfaye F, Mengistu Y, et al. Potential for medical transmission of HIV in Ethiopia. *AIDS.* 2005;19:348-350.
61. Whitworth JA, Biraro S, Shafer LA, et al. HIV incidence and recent injections among adults in rural southwestern Uganda. *AIDS.* 2007;21:1056-1058.
62. Tahir M, Sharma SK, Smith-Rohrberg D. Unsafe medical injections and HIV transmission in India. *Lancet Infect Dis.* 2007;7:178-179.
63. Centers for Disease Control. Patient exposures to HIV during nuclear medicine procedures. *MMWR Morb Mortal Wkly Rep.* 1992;41:575-578.
64. Gisselquist D, Upham G, Potterat JJ. Efficiency of human immunodeficiency virus transmission through injections and other medical procedures: evidence, estimates, and unfinished business. *Infect Control Hosp Epidemiol.* 2006;27:944-952.
65. Hutin YJ, Goldstein ST, Varma JK, et al. An outbreak of hospital-acquired hepatitis B virus infection among patients receiving chronic hemodialysis. *Infect Control Hosp Epidemiol.* 1999;20: 731-735.
66. Katzenstein TL, Jorgensen LB, Permin H, et al. Nosocomial HIV-transmission in an outpatient clinic detected by epidemiological and phylogenetic analyses. *AIDS.* 1999;13:1737-1744.
67. Kidd-Ljunggren K, Broman E, Ekvall H, et al. Nosocomial transmission of hepatitis B virus infection through multiple-dose vials. *J Hosp Infect.* 1999;43(1):57-62.
68. Chant K, Lowe D, Rubin G, et al. Patient-to-patient transmission of HIV in private surgical consulting rooms. *Lancet.* 1993;342:1548-1549.
69. Centers for Disease Control and Prevention. HIV transmission in a dialysis center—Colombia, 1991-1993. *MMWR Morb Mortal Wkly Rep.* 1995;44:404-405, 411-412.
70. El Sayed NM, Gomatos PJ, Beck-Sague CM, et al. Epidemic transmission of human immunodeficiency virus in renal dialysis centers in Egypt. *J Infect Dis.* 2000;181:91-97.
71. Hassan NF, el Ghorab NM, Abdel Rehim MS, et al. HIV infection in renal dialysis patients in Egypt. *AIDS.* 1994;8:853.
72. Velandia M, Fridkin SK, Cardenas V, et al. Transmission of HIV in dialysis centre. *Lancet.* 1995;345:1417-1422.
73. Zuckerman M. Surveillance and control of blood-borne virus infections in haemodialysis units. *J Hosp Infect.* 2002;50:1-5.
74. Centers for Disease Control. Recommendations for protection against viral hepatitis. *MMWR Morb Mortal Wkly Rep.* 1985;34: 313-324, 329-335.
75. Centers for Disease Control. Recommendations for prevention of HIV transmission in health-care settings. *MMWR Morb Mortal Wkly Rep.* 1987;36(Suppl 2):1S-18S.
76. Centers for Disease Control. Update: universal precautions for prevention of transmission of human immunodeficiency virus, hepatitis B virus, and other bloodborne pathogens in health-care settings. *MMWR Morb Mortal Wkly Rep.* 1988;37:377-382; 387-378.
77. Lynch P, Jackson MM, Cummings MJ, et al. Rethinking the role of isolation practices in the prevention of nosocomial infections. *Ann Intern Med.* 1987;107:243-246.
78. Garner JS. Guideline for isolation precautions in hospitals. The Hospital Infection Control Practices Advisory Committee. *Infect Control Hosp Epidemiol.* 1996;17:53-80.
79. Department of Labor, Department of Health and Human Services. Joint Advisory Notice: Protection against occupational exposure to hepatitis B virus (HBV) and human immunodeficiency virus (HIV). *Fed Regist.* 1987;52:41818-41824.
80. Department of Labor OSHA. Occupational exposure to bloodborne pathogens; final rule. *Fed Regist.* 1991;56:64175-64182.
81. Beekmann SE, Vlahov D, Koziol DE, et al. Temporal association between implementation of universal precautions and a sustained, progressive decrease in percutaneous exposures to blood. *Clin Infect Dis.* 1994;18:562-569.
82. Haiduven DJ, DeMaio TM, Stevens DA. A five-year study of needlestick injuries: significant reduction associated with communication, education, and convenient placement of sharps containers. *Infect Control Hosp Epidemiol.* 1992;13: 265-271.
83. Kristensen MS, Wernberg NM, Anker-Møller E. Healthcare workers' risk of contact with body fluids in a hospital: the effect of complying with the universal precautions policy. *Infect Control Hosp Epidemiol.* 1992;13:719-724.
84. Wong ES, Stotka JL, Mayhall CG, et al. Cost-efficacy of hospital infection control before and after the implementation of universal precautions [Abstract 786]. Presented at the 29th Interscience Conference on Antimicrobial Agents and Chemotherapy. Houston TX, September 1989.
85. De Carli G, Puro V, Petrosillo N, et al. "Side" effects of HAART: decreasing and changing occupational exposure to HIV-infected patients. *J Biol Regul Homeost Agents.* 2001;15:235-237.
86. Jagger J, Hunt EH, Brand-Elnaggar J, et al. Rates of needle-stick injury caused by various devices in a university hospital. *N Engl J Med.* 1988;319:284-288.
87. Mendelson MH, Short LJ, Schechter CB, et al. Study of a needleless intermittent intravenous-access system for peripheral infusions: analysis of staff, patient, and institutional outcomes. *Infect Control Hosp Epidemiol.* 1998;19:401-406.
88. Skolnick R, LaRocca J, Barba D, et al. Evaluation and implementation of a needleless intravenous system: making needlesticks a needless problem. *Am J Infect Control.* 1993;21:39-41.
89. Yassi A, McGill ML, Khokhar JB. Efficacy and cost-effectiveness of a needleless intravenous access system. *Am J Infect Control.* 1995;23:57-64.
90. MacPherson J. The interlink needleless intravenous system did not reduce the number of needlestick injuries in Christchurch hospital operating theatres. *N Z Med J.* 1996;109:387-388.
91. Casey AL, Elliott TS. Infection risks associated with needleless intravenous access devices. *Nurs Stand.* 2007;22:38-44.
92. Maragakis LL, Bradley KL, Song X, et al. Increased catheter-related bloodstream infection rates after the introduction of a new mechanical valve intravenous access port. *Infect Control Hosp Epidemiol.* 2006;27:67-70.
93. Rupp ME, Sholtz LA, Jourdan DR, et al. Outbreak of bloodstream infection temporally associated with the use of an intravascular needleless valve. *Clin Infect Dis.* 2007;44:1408-1414.
94. Alvarado-Ramy F, Beltrami EM, Short LJ, et al. A comprehensive approach to percutaneous injury prevention during phlebotomy: results of a multicenter study, 1993-1995. *Infect Control Hosp Epidemiol.* 2003;24:97-104.
95. Centers for Disease Control and Prevention. Evaluation of safety devices for preventing percutaneous injuries among health-care workers during phlebotomy procedures—Minneapolis–St. Paul, New York City, and San Francisco, 1993-1995. *MMWR Morb Mortal Wkly Rep.* 1997;46:21-25.
96. Mendelson MH, Lin-Chen BY, Solomon R, et al. Evaluation of a safety resheathable winged steel needle for prevention of percutaneous injuries associated with intravascular-access procedures among healthcare workers. *Infect Control Hosp Epidemiol.* 2003;24:105-112.
97. Rabaud C, Zanea A, Mur JM, et al. Occupational exposure to blood: search for a relation between personality and behavior. *Infect Control Hosp Epidemiol.* 2000;21:564-574.
98. Folin AC, Nordstrom GM. Accidental blood contact during orthopedic surgical procedures. *Infect Control Hosp Epidemiol.* 1997;18:244-246.
99. Gerberding JL, Littell C, Brown A, et al. Cumulative risk of HIV and hepatitis B among health care workers: longterm serologic followup and gene amplification for latent HIV infection. Presented at the 30th Interscience Conference on Antimicrobial Agents and Chemotherapy. (Abstract 959). Atlanta, GA, October 1990.
100. Lynch P, White MC. Perioperative blood contact and exposures: a comparison of incident reports and focused studies. *Am J Infect Control.* 1993;21:357-363.
101. Panlilio AL, Foy DR, Edwards JR, et al. Blood contacts during surgical procedures. *JAMA.* 1991;265:1533-1537.
102. Panlilio AL, Welch BA, Bell DM, et al. Blood and amniotic fluid contact sustained by obstetric personnel during deliveries. *Am J Obstet Gynecol.* 1992;167:703-708.
103. Popejoy SL, Fry DE. Blood contact and exposure in the operating room. *Surg Gynecol Obstet.* 1991;172:480-483.
104. Quebbeman EJ, Telford GL, Hubbard S, et al. Risk of blood contamination and injury to operating room personnel. *Ann Surg.* 1991;214:614-620.
105. Robert L, Short L, Chamberland M, et al. Percutaneous injuries sustained during gynecologic surgery. *Infect Control Hosp Epidemiol.* 1994;15:349.
106. White MC, Lynch P. Blood contact and exposures among operating room personnel: a multicenter study. *Am J Infect Control.* 1993;21:243-248.
107. Akduman D, Kim LE, Parks RL, et al. Use of personal protective equipment and operating room behaviors in four surgical subspecialties: personal protective equipment and behaviors in surgery. *Infect Control Hosp Epidemiol.* 1999;20:110-114.
108. American Academy of Orthopedic Surgeons Task Force on AIDS and Orthopedic Surgery. *Recommendations for the Prevention of Human Immunodeficiency Virus (HIV) Transmission in the Practice of Orthopedic Surgery.* Park Ridge, IL; 1989.
109. Davis JM, Demling RH, Lewis FR, et al. The Surgical Infection Society's policy on human immunodeficiency virus and hepatitis B and C infection. The Ad Hoc Committee on Acquired Immunodeficiency Syndrome and Hepatitis. *Arch Surg.* 1992; 127:218-221.
110. Hester RA, Nelson CL, Harrison S. Control of contamination of the operative team in total joint arthroplasty. *J Arthroplasty.* 1992;7:267-269.
111. Lewis FR Jr, Short LJ, Howard RJ, et al. Epidemiology of injuries by needles and other sharp instruments. Minimizing sharp injuries in gynecologic and obstetric operations. *Surg Clin North Am.* 1995;75:1105-1121.
112. Loudon MA, Stonebridge PA. Minimizing the risk of penetrating injury to surgical staff in the operating theatre: towards sharp-free surgery. *J R Coll Surg Edinb.* 1998;43:6-8.
113. Tobias AM, Chang B. Pulsed irrigation of extremity wounds: a simple technique for splashback reduction. *Ann Plast Surg.* 2002;48:443-444.
114. Centers for Disease Control and Prevention. Evaluation of blunt suture needles in preventing percutaneous injuries among health-care workers during gynecologic surgical procedures—New York City, March 1993–June 1994. *MMWR Morb Mortal Wkly Rep.* 1997;46:25-29.
115. Hartley JE, Ahmed S, Milkins R, et al. Randomized trial of blunt-tipped versus cutting needles to reduce glove puncture during mass closure of the abdomen. *Br J Surg.* 1996;83:1156-1157.
116. Miller SS, Sabharwal A. Subcuticular skin closure using a "blunt" needle. *Ann R Coll Surg Engl.* 1994;76:281.
117. Mingoli A, Sapienza P, Sgarzini G, et al. Influence of blunt needles on surgical glove perforation and safety for the surgeon. *Am J Surg.* 1996;172:512-516.
118. Montz FJ, Fowler JM, Farias-Eisner R, et al. Blunt needles in fascial closure. *Surg Gynecol Obstet.* 1991;173:147-148.
119. Wright KU, Moran CG, Briggs PJ. Glove perforation during hip arthroplasty. A randomised prospective study of a new taper-point needle. *J Bone Joint Surg Br.* 1993;75:918-920.
120. Aarnio P, Laine T. Glove perforation rate in vascular surgery—a comparison between single and double gloving. *Vasa.* 2001; 30:122-124.
121. Avery CM, Taylor J, Johnson PA. Double gloving and a system for identifying glove perforations in maxillofacial trauma surgery. *Br J Oral Maxillofac Surg.* 1999;37:316-319.
122. Chapman S, Duff P. Frequency of glove perforations and subsequent blood contact in association with selected obstetric surgical procedures. *Am J Obstet Gynecol.* 1993;168:1354-1357.
123. Cohen MS, Do JT, Tahery DP, et al. Efficacy of double gloving as a protection against blood exposure in dermatologic surgery. *J Dermatol Surg Oncol.* 1992;18:873-874.
124. Gerberding JL, Littell C, Tarkington A, et al. Risk of exposure of surgical personnel to patients' blood during surgery at San Francisco General Hospital. *N Engl J Med.* 1990;322:1788-1793.
125. Hollaus PH, Lax F, Janakiev D, et al. Glove perforation rate in open lung surgery. *Eur J Cardiothorac Surg.* 1999;15:461-464.
126. Kovavisarach E, Jaravechson S. Comparison of perforation between single and double-gloving in perineorrhaphy after vaginal delivery: a randomized controlled trial. *Aust N Z J Obstet Gynaecol.* 1998;38(1):58-60.
127. Kovavisarach E, Seedadee C. Randomised controlled trial of glove perforation in single and double-gloving methods in gynaecologic surgery. *Aust N Z J Obstet Gynaecol.* 2002;42: 519-521.
128. Kovavisarach E, Vanitchanon P. Perforation in single- and double-gloving methods for cesarean section. *Int J Gynaecol Obstet.* 1999;67:157-161.
129. Laine T, Aarnio P. How often does glove perforation occur in surgery? Comparison between single gloves and a double-gloving system. *Am J Surg.* 2001;181:564-566.
130. Naver LP, Gottrup F. Incidence of glove perforations in gastrointestinal surgery and the protective effect of double gloves: a prospective, randomised controlled study. *Eur J Surg.* 2000;166:293-295.
131. Gerberding JL, Ramiro N, Perlman J, et al. Intraoperative blood exposures at San Francisco General Hospital: provider injuries and patient recontacts. Presented at the 31st Annual Meeting of

the Infectious Diseases Society of America. New Orleans, 1993.

132. Quebbeman EJ, Telford GL, Wadsworth K, et al. Double gloving. Protecting surgeons from blood contamination in the operating room. *Arch Surg.* 1992;127:213-216.
133. Gerberding JL, Quebbeman EJ, Rhodes RS. Hand protection. *Surg Clin North Am.* 1995;75:1133-1139.
134. Leslie LF, Woods JA, Thacker JG, et al. Needle puncture resistance of surgical gloves, finger guards, and glove liners. *J Biomed Mater Res.* 1996;33:41-46.
135. Salkin JA, Stuchin SA, Kummer FJ, et al. The effectiveness of cut-proof glove liners: cut and puncture resistance, dexterity, and sensibility. *Orthopedics.* 1995;18:1067-1071.
136. Woods JA, Leslie LF, Drake DB, et al. Effect of puncture resistant surgical gloves, finger guards, and glove liners on cutaneous sensibility and surgical psychomotor skills. *J Biomed Mater Res.* 1996;33(1):47-51.
137. Wilson SJ, Sellu D, Uy A, et al. Subjective effects of double gloves on surgical performance. *Ann R Coll Surg Engl.* 1996;78:20-22.
138. Gerberding JL. Procedure-specific infection control for preventing intraoperative blood exposures. *Am J Infect Control.* 1993;21:364-367.
139. Alrawi SJ, Houshan I, Zanial SA, et al. Cardiac surgical procedures and glove reinforcements. *Heart Surg Forum.* 2002;5:66-68.
140. Weber LW. Evaluation of the rate, location, and morphology of perforations in surgical gloves worn in urological operations. *Appl Occup Environ Hyg.* 2003;18:65-73.
141. Bebbington MW, Treissman MJ. The use of a surgical assist device to reduce glove perforations in postdelivery vaginal repair: a randomized controlled trial. *Am J Obstet Gynecol.* 1996;175(4 Pt 1):862-866.
142. Cleveland JL, Gooch BF, Lockwood SA. Occupational blood exposures in dentistry: a decade in review. *Infect Control Hosp Epidemiol.* 1997;18:717-721.
143. Cleveland JL, Barker L, Gooch BF, et al. Use of HIV postexposure prophylaxis by dental health care personnel: an overview and updated recommendations. *J Am Dent Assoc.* 2002;133:1619-1626.
144. Ramos-Gomez F, Ellison J, Greenspan D, et al. Accidental exposures to blood and body fluids among health care workers in dental teaching clinics: a prospective study. *J Am Dent Assoc.* 1997;128:1253-1261.
145. Cleveland JL, Lockwood SA, Gooch BF, et al. Percutaneous injuries in dentistry: an observational study. *J Am Dent Assoc.* 1995;126:745-751.
146. Siew C, Gruninger SE, Miaw CL, et al. Percutaneous injuries in practicing dentists. A prospective study using a 20-day diary. *J Am Dent Assoc.* 1995;126:1227-1234.
147. Carlton JE, Dodson TB, Cleveland JL, et al. Percutaneous injuries during oral and maxillofacial surgery procedures. *J Oral Maxillofac Surg.* 1997;55:553-556.
148. Gooch BF, Siew C, Cleveland JL, et al. Occupational blood exposure and HIV infection among oral and maxillofacial surgeons. *Oral Surg Oral Med Oral Pathol Oral Radiol Endod.* 1998;85:128-134.
149. Hall FM. Double gloving during interventional procedures. *AJR Am J Roentgenol.* 1993;161:678.
150. Hansen ME, McIntire DD, Miller GL 3rd, et al. Use of universal precautions in interventional radiology: results of a national survey. *Am J Infect Control.* 1994;22:1-5.
151. Wall SD, Olcott EW, Gerberding JL. AIDS risk and risk reduction in the radiology department. *AJR Am J Roentgenol.* 1991;157:911-917.
152. McWilliams RG, Blanshard KS. The risk of blood splash contamination during angiography. *Clin Radiol.* 1994;49:59-60.
153. Gerberding JL. Post-exposure prophylaxis for human immunodeficiency virus at San Francisco General Hospital. *Am J Med.* 1997;102:85-89.
154. Beltrami EM, Williams IT, Shapiro CN, et al. Risk and management of blood-borne infections in health care workers. *Clin Microbiol Rev.* 2000;13:385-407.
155. Benítez Rodríguez E, Ruiz Moruno AJ, Córdoba Doña JA, et al. Underreporting of percutaneous exposure accidents in a teaching hospital in Spain. *Clin Perform Qual Health Care.* 1999;7:88-91.
156. Burke S, Madan I. Contamination incidents among doctors and midwives: reasons for non-reporting and knowledge of risks. *Occup Med (Lond).* 1997;47:357-360.
157. Hamory BH. Underreporting of needlestick injuries in a university hospital. *Am J Infect Control.* 1983;11:174-177.
158. Mangione CM, Gerberding JL, Cummings SR. Occupational exposure to HIV: frequency and rates of underreporting of percutaneous and mucocutaneous exposures by medical housestaff. *Am J Med.* 1991;90:85-90.
159. Radecki S, Abbott A, Eloi L. Occupational human immunodeficiency virus exposure among residents and medical students: an analysis of 5-year follow-up data. *Arch Intern Med.* 2000;160:3107-3111.
160. Shiao JS, McLaws ML, Huang KY, et al. Prevalence of nonreporting behavior of sharps injuries in Taiwanese health care workers. *Am J Infect Control.* 1999;27:254-257.
161. Tandberg D, Stewart KK, Doezema D. Under-reporting of contaminated needlestick injuries in emergency health care workers. *Ann Emerg Med.* 1991;20:66-70.
162. Gerberding JL, Henderson DK. Design of rational infection control policies for human immunodeficiency virus infection. *J Infect Dis.* 1987;156:861-864.
163. Armstrong K, Gorden R, Santorella G. Occupational exposure of health care workers (HCWs) to human immunodeficiency virus (HIV): stress reactions and counseling interventions. *Soc Work Health Care.* 1995;21:61-80.
164. Dilley JW. Counseling health care workers after accidental exposures. *Focus.* 1990;5:3-4.
165. Henderson DK. HIV postexposure prophylaxis in the 21st century. *Emerg Infect Dis.* 2001;7:254-258.
166. Henderson DK. Postexposure chemoprophylaxis for occupational exposures to the human immunodeficiency virus. *JAMA.* 1999;281:931-936.
167. Kahn JO, Martin JN, Roland ME, et al. Feasibility of postexposure prophylaxis (PEP) against human immunodeficiency virus infection after sexual or injection drug use exposure: the San Francisco PEP Study. *J Infect Dis.* 2001;183:707-714.
168. Roland ME, Martin JN, Grant RM, et al. Postexposure prophylaxis for human immunodeficiency virus infection after sexual or injection drug use exposure: identification and characterization of the source of exposure. *J Infect Dis.* 2001;184:1608-1612.
169. Khajotia RR, Lee E. Transmission of human immunodeficiency virus through saliva after a lip bite. *Arch Intern Med.* 1997;157:1901.
170. Pretty IA, Anderson GS, Sweet DJ. Human bites and the risk of human immunodeficiency virus transmission. *Am J Forensic Med Pathol.* 1999;20:232-239.
171. Richman KM, Rickman LS. The potential for transmission of human immunodeficiency virus through human bites. *J Acquir Immune Defic Syndr.* 1993;6:402-406.
172. Vidmar L, Poljak M, Tomazic J, et al. Transmission of HIV-1 by human bite. *Lancet.* 1996;347:1762.
173. Charache P, Cameron JL, Maters AW, et al. Prevalence of infection with human immunodeficiency virus in elective surgery patients. *Ann Surg.* 1991;214:562-568.
174. Centers for Disease Control. Recommendations for preventing transmission of human immunodeficiency virus and hepatitis B virus to patients during exposure-prone invasive procedures. *MMWR Morb Mortal Wkly Rep.* 1991;40(RR-8):1-9.
175. U.S. Department of Health. HIV-infected health care workers: guidance on management and patient notification [Best Practice Guidance]. Available at http://www.dh.gov.uk/en/Publicationsandstatistics/Publications/PublicationsPolicyAndGuidance/DH_4116415 (accessed February 8, 2007).
176. Centers for Disease Control. Public Health Service statement on management of occupational exposure to human immunodeficiency virus, including considerations regarding zidovudine postexposure use. *MMWR Morbid Mortal Wkly Rep.* 1990;39(RR-1):1-14.
177. Centers for Disease Control and Prevention. Update: provisional Public Health Service recommendations for chemoprophylaxis after occupational exposure to HIV. *MMWR Morb Mortal Wkly Rep.* 1996;45:468-480.
178. Panlilio AL, Cardo DM, Grohskopf LA, et al. Updated U.S. Public Health Service guidelines for the management of occupational exposures to HIV and recommendations for postexposure prophylaxis. *MMWR Recomm Rep.* 2005;54(RR-9):1-17.
179. Gerberding JL, Katz MH. Post-exposure prophylaxis for HIV. *Adv Exp Med Biol.* 1999;458:213-222.
180. Henderson DK, Gerberding JL. Prophylactic zidovudine after occupational exposure to the human immunodeficiency virus: an interim analysis. *J Infect Dis.* 1989;160:321-327.
181. Blauvelt A. The role of skin dendritic cells in the initiation of human immunodeficiency virus infection. *Am J Med.* 1997;102 (Suppl. 5B):16-20.
182. Blauvelt A, Clerici M, Lucey DR, et al. Functional studies of epidermal Langerhans cells and blood monocytes in HIV-infected persons. *J Immunol.* 1995;154:3506-3515.
183. Blauvelt A, Glushakova S, Margolis LB. HIV-infected human V-infected human Langerhans cells transmit infection to human lymphoid tissue ex vivo. *AIDS.* 2000;14:647-651.
184. Spira AI, Marx PA, Patterson BK, et al. Cellular targets of infection and route of viral dissemination after an intravaginal inoculation of simian immunodeficiency virus into rhesus macaques. *J Exp Med.* 1996;183:215-225.
185. Granelli-Piperno A, Finkel V, Delgado E, et al. Virus replication begins in dendritic cells during the transmission of HIV-1 from mature dendritic cells to T cells. *Curr Biol.* 1999;9:21-29.
186. Blauvelt A, Asada H, Saville MW, et al. Productive infection of dendritic cells by HIV-1 and their ability to capture virus are mediated through separate pathways. *J Clin Invest.* 1997;100:2043-2053.
187. Piguet V, Blauvelt A. Essential roles for dendritic cells in the pathogenesis and potential treatment of HIV disease. *J Invest Dermatol.* 2002;119:365-369.
188. Ruprecht RM, Bronson R. Chemoprevention of retroviral infection: success is determined by virus inoculum strength and cellular immunity. *DNA Cell Biol.* 1994;13:59-66.
189. Putkonen P, Mäkitalo B, Böttiger D, et al. Protection of human immunodeficiency virus type 2–exposed seronegative macaques from mucosal simian immunodeficiency virus transmission. *J Virol.* 1997;71:4981-4984.
190. Tsai CC, Emau P, Sun JC, et al. Post-exposure chemoprophylaxis (PECP) against SIV infection of macaques as a model for protection from HIV infection. *J Med Primatol.* 2000;29:248-258.
191. D'Amico R, Pinto LA, Meyer P, et al. Effect of zidovudine post-exposure prophylaxis on the development of HIV-specific cytotoxic T-lymphocyte responses in HIV-exposed healthcare workers. *Infect Control Hosp Epidemiol.* 1999;20:428-430.
192. Zidek Z, Frankova D, Holy A. Activation by 9-(R)-[2-(phosphonomethoxy)propyl]adenine of chemokine (RANTES, macrophage inflammatory protein 1α) and cytokine (tumor necrosis factor α, interleukin-10 [IL-10], IL-1β) production. *Antimicrob Agents Chemother.* 2001;45:3381-3386.
193. Black RJ. Animal studies of prophylaxis. *Am J Med.* 1997;102(Suppl. 5B):39-44.
194. Ruprecht RM, O'Brien LG, Rossoni LD, et al. Suppression of mouse viraemia and retroviral disease by 3′-azido-3′deoxythymidine. *Nature.* 1986;323:467-469.
195. Tavares L, Roneker C, Johnston K, et al. 3′-Azido-3′deoxythymidine in feline leukemia virus–infected cats: a model for therapy and prophylaxis of AIDS. *Cancer Res.* 1987;47:3190-3194.
196. Fazely F, Haseltine WA, Rodger RF, et al. Postexposure chemoprophylaxis with ZDV or ZDV combined with interferon-alpha: failure after inoculating rhesus monkeys with a high dose of SIV. *J Acquir Immune Defic Syndr.* 1991;4:1093-1097.
197. Böttiger D, Johansson NG, Samuelsson B, et al. Prevention of simian immunodeficiency virus, SIVsm, or HIV-2 infection in cynomolgus monkeys by pre- and postexposure administration of BEA-005. *AIDS.* 1997;11:157-162.
198. Böttiger D, Putkonen P, Oberg B. Prevention of HIV-2 and SIV infections in cynomolgus macaques by prophylactic treatment with 3′-fluorothymidine. *AIDS Res Hum Retroviruses.* 1992;8:1235-1238.
199. Tsai CC, Emau P, Follis KE, et al. Effectiveness of postinoculation (R)-9-(2-phosphonylmethoxypropyl) adenine treatment for prevention of persistent simian immunodeficiency virus SIVmne infection depends critically on timing of initiation and duration of treatment. *J Virol.* 1998;72:4265-4273.
200. Tsai CC, Follis KE, Sabo A, et al. Prevention of SIV infection in macaques by (R)-9-(2-phosphonylmethoxypropyl)adenine. *Science.* 1995;270:1197-1199.
201. Van Rompay KK, Dailey PJ, Tarara RP, et al. Early short-term 9-[2-(R)-(phosphonomethoxy)propyl]adenine treatment favorably alters the subsequent disease course in simian immunodeficiency virus–infected newborn Rhesus macaques. *J Virol.* 1999;73:2947-2955.
202. Van Rompay KK, Marthas ML, Ramos RA, et al. Simian immunodeficiency virus (SIV) infection of infant rhesus macaques as a model to test antiretroviral drug prophylaxis and therapy: oral 3′-azido-3′-deoxythymidine prevents SIV infection. *Antimicrob Agents Chemother.* 1992;36:2381-2386.
203. Otten RA, Smith DK, Adams DR, et al. Efficacy of postexposure prophylaxis after intravaginal exposure of pig-tailed macaques to a human-derived retrovirus (human immunodeficiency virus type 2). *J Virol.* 2000;74:9771-9775.
204. Connor EM, Sperling RS, Gelber R, et al. Reduction of maternal-infant transmission of human immunodeficiency virus type 1 with zidovudine treatment. Pediatric AIDS Clinical Trials Group Protocol 076 Study Group. *N Engl J Med.* 1994;331:1173-1180.
205. Bulterys M, Orloff S, Abrams E, et al. Impact of zidovudine post-perinatal exposure prophylaxis on vertical HIV-1 transmission: a prospective cohort study in four US cities [Abstract 15]. Presented at Global Strategies for the Prevention of HIV Transmission from Mothers to Infants. Toronto, ON, Canada, September 1-6, 1999.
206. Wade NA, Birkhead GS, Warren BL, et al. Abbreviated regimens of zidovudine prophylaxis and perinatal transmission of the human immunodeficiency virus. *N Engl J Med.* 1998;339:1409-1414.
207. LaFon SW, Lehrman SN, Barry DW. Prophylactically administered Retrovir in health care workers potentially exposed to the human immunodeficiency virus. *J Infect Dis.* 1988;158:503.
208. LaFon SW, Mooney BD, McMullen JP. A double-blind, placebo-controlled study of the safety and efficacy of Retrovir (zidovudine) as a chemoprophylactic agent in health care workers exposed to HIV [Abstract]. Presented at the 30th Interscience Conference on Antimicrobial Agents and Chemotherapy. Atlanta, October, 1990.
209. Centers for Disease Control and Prevention. Case-control study of HIV seroconversion in health-care workers after percutaneous exposure to HIV-infected blood—France, United Kingdom, and United States, January 1988–August 1994. *MMWR Morb Mortal Wkly Rep.* 1995;44:929-933.
210. Henderson DK. Postexposure treatment of HIV—taking some risks for safety's sake. *N Engl J Med.* 1997;337:1542-1543.
211. Katzenstein TL, Dickmeiss E, Aladdin H, et al. Failure to develop HIV infection after receipt of HIV-contaminated blood and postexposure prophylaxis. *Ann Intern Med.* 2000;133:31-34.
212. Ward JW, Deppe DA, Samson S, et al. Human immunodeficiency virus infection from blood donors who later developed the acquired immunodeficiency syndrome. *Ann Intern Med.* 1987;106:61-62.
213. Beltrami EM, Luo CC, de la Torre N, et al. Transmission of drug-resistant HIV after an occupational exposure despite post-exposure prophylaxis with a combination drug regimen. *Infect Control Hosp Epidemiol.* 2002;23:345-348.

214. Hawkins DA, Asboe D, Barlow K, et al. Seroconversion to HIV-1 following a needlestick injury despite combination post-exposure prophylaxis. *J Infect.* 2001;43:12-15.

215. Perdue B, Wolderufael D, Mellors J, et al. HIV-1 transmission by a needle-stick injury despite rapid initiation of four-drug postexposure prophylaxis. Presented at the 6th Conference on Retroviruses and Opportunistic Infections. Chicago, January 31–February 4, 1999.

216. Lucey D, Milum S, Lindquist C, et al. Pseudofailure of zidovudine prophylaxis after a human immunodeficiency virus–positive needlestick. *J Infect Dis.* 1990;162:1211-1212.

217. Jochimsen EM, Luo CC, Beltrami JF, et al. Investigations of possible failures of postexposure prophylaxis following occupational exposures to human immunodeficiency virus. *Arch Intern Med.* 1999;159:2361-2363.

218. Gulick RM. New antiretroviral drugs. *Clin Microbiol Infect.* 2003;9:186-193.

219. Lalezari JP, Henry K, O'Hearn M, et al. Enfuvirtide, an HIV-1 fusion inhibitor, for drug-resistant HIV infection in North and South America. *N Engl J Med.* 2003;348:2175-2185.

220. Mechai F, Quertainmont Y, Sahali S, et al. Post-exposure prophylaxis with a maraviroc-containing regimen after occupational exposure to a multi-resistant HIV-infected source person. *J Med Virol.* 2008;80:9-10.

221. Beltrami EM, Cheingsong R, Heneine WM, et al. Antiretroviral drug resistance in human immunodeficiency virus–infected source patients for occupational exposures to healthcare workers. *Infect Control Hosp Epidemiol.* 2003;24:724-730.

222. Grant RM, Hecht FM, Warmerdam M, et al. Time trends in primary HIV-1 drug resistance among recently infected persons. *JAMA.* 2002;288:181-188.

223. Little SJ, Holte S, Routy JP, et al. Antiretroviral-drug resistance among patients recently infected with HIV. *N Engl J Med.* 2002;347:385-394.

224. Liu L, May S, Richman DD, et al. Comparison of algorithms that interpret genotypic HIV-1 drug resistance to determine the prevalence of transmitted drug resistance. *AIDS.* 2008;22:835-839.

225. Mayers DL. Prevalence and incidence of resistance to zidovudine and other antiretroviral drugs. *Am J Med.* 1997;102(Suppl. 5B):S70-S75.

226. Truong HM, Grant RM, McFarland W, et al. Routine surveillance for the detection of acute and recent HIV infections and transmission of antiretroviral resistance. *AIDS.* 2006;20:2193-2197.

227. Centers for Disease Control and Prevention. Notice to readers: updated information regarding antiretroviral agents used as HIV postexposure prophylaxis for occupational HIV exposures. *MMWR Morbid Mortal Wkly Rep.* 2007;56:1291-1292.

228. Pavel S, Burty C, Alcaraz I, et al. Severe liver toxicity in postexposure prophylaxis for HIV infection with a zidovudine, lamivudine, and fosamprenavir/ritonavir regimen. *AIDS.* 2007;21:268-269.

229. Centers for Disease Control and Prevention. Serious adverse events attributed to nevirapine regimens for postexposure prophylaxis after HIV exposures—worldwide, 1997-2000. *MMWR Morb Mortal Wkly Rep.* 2001;49:1153-1156.

230. Johnson AA, Ray AS, Hanes J, et al. Toxicity of antiviral nucleoside analogs and the human mitochondrial DNA polymerase. *J Biol Chem.* 2001;276:40847-40857.

231. Johnson S, Chan J, Bennett CL. Hepatotoxicity after prophylaxis with a nevirapine-containing antiretroviral regimen. *Ann Intern Med.* 2002;137:146-147.

232. Sha BE, Proia LA, Kessler HA. Adverse effects associated with use of nevirapine in HIV postexposure prophylaxis for 2 health care workers. *JAMA.* 2000;284:2723.

233. Leigh Brown AJ, Frost SD, Mathews WC, et al. Transmission fitness of drug-resistant human immunodeficiency virus and the prevalence of resistance in the antiretroviral-treated population. *J Infect Dis.* 2003;187:683-686.

234. Panel on Antiretroviral Guidelines for Adults and Adolescents. Guidelines for the use of antiretroviral agents in HIV-1–infected adults and adolescents. Washington, DC: U.S. Department of Health and Human Services. Available at http://www.aidsinfo.nih.gov/ContentFiles/AdultandAdolescentGL.pdf (accessed November 3, 2008).

235. Gerberding JL. Clinical practice. Occupational exposure to HIV in health care settings. *N Engl J Med.* 2003;348:826-833.

236. Garcia F, Plana M, Mestre G, et al. Metabolic and immunological effects of antiretroviral agents in healthy individuals receiving post-exposure prophylaxis. *Antivir Ther.* 2002;7:195-197.

237. Lee LM, Henderson DK. Tolerability of postexposure antiretroviral prophylaxis for occupational exposures to HIV. *Drug Saf.* 2001;24:587-597.

238. Luzzati R, Crosato IM, Mascioli M, et al. Galactorrhoea and hyperprolactinemia associated with HIV postexposure chemoprophylaxis. *AIDS.* 2002;16:1306-1307.

239. Rabaud C, Bevilacqua S, Beguinot I, et al. Tolerability of postexposure prophylaxis with zidovudine, lamivudine, and nelfinavir for human immunodeficiency virus infection. *Clin Infect Dis.* 2001;32:1494-1495.

240. Trape M, Barnosky S. Nelfinavir in expanded postexposure prophylaxis causing acute hepatitis with cholestatic features: two case reports. *Infect Control Hosp Epidemiol.* 2001;22:333-334.

241. Wang SA, Panlilio AL, Doi PA, et al. Experience of healthcare workers taking postexposure prophylaxis after occupational HIV exposures: findings of the HIV Postexposure Prophylaxis Registry. *Infect Control Hosp Epidemiol.* 2000;21:780-785.

242. Wang SA, Puro V. Toxicity of post-exposure prophylaxis for human immunodeficiency virus. In: Panlilio L, ed. Balliere's Clinical Infectious Diseases. Vol 5. London, UK: Balliere-Tindall; 1999:349-363.

243. Spenatto N, Viraben R. Early lipodystrophy occurring during post-exposure prophylaxis. *Sex Transm Infect.* 1998;74:455.

244. Benn PD, Mercey DE, Brink N, et al. Prophylaxis with a nevirapine-containing triple regimen after exposure to HIV-1. *Lancet.* 2001;357:687-688.

245. Rey D, L'Heritier A, Lang JM. Severe ototoxicity in a health care worker who received postexposure prophylaxis with stavudine, lamivudine, and nevirapine after occupational exposure to HIV. *Clin Infect Dis.* 2002;34:418-419.

246. Centers for Disease Control and Prevention. Public Health Service Task Force recommendations for the use of antiretroviral drugs in pregnant women infected with HIV-1 for maternal health and for reducing perinatal HIV-1 transmission in the United States. *MMWR Morb Mortal Wkly Rep.* 1998;47 (RR-2):1-30.

247. Culnane M, Fowler MG, Lee S, et al. Evaluation for late effects of in utero (IU) ZDV exposure among uninfected infants born to HIV+ women enrolled in ACTG 076 and 210 [Abstract 485]. *Clin Infect Dis.* 1997;25:445.

248. Blanche S, Tardieu M, Rustin P, et al. Persistent mitochondrial dysfunction and perinatal exposure to antiretroviral nucleoside analogues. *Lancet.* 1999;354:1084-1089.

249. Foster C, Lyall H. HIV and mitochondrial toxicity in children. *J Antimicrob Chemother.* 2008;61:8-12.

250. Thorne C, Newell ML. Safety of agents used to prevent mother-to-child transmission of HIV: is there any cause for concern? *Drug Saf.* 2007;30:203-213.

251. U.S. Food and Drug Administration. 2001 Safety alerts for drugs, biologics, medical devices, and dietary supplements [MedWatch]. Available at http://www.fda.gov/medwatch/safety/2001/safety01.htm#zerit.

251a. U.S. Food and Drug Administration. FDA/Bristol Myers Squibb issues caution for HIV combination therapy with Zerit and Videx in pregnant women [FDA Talk Paper]. Available at http://www.fda.gov/bbs/topics/ANSWERS/ANS01063.html.

252. Havens PL. Postexposure prophylaxis in children and adolescents for nonoccupational exposure to human immunodeficiency virus. *Pediatrics.* 2003;111(6 Pt 1):1475-1489.

253. Katz MH, Gerberding JL. Management of occupational and nonoccupational postexposure HIV prophylaxis. *Curr Infect Dis Rep.* 2002;4:543-549.

254. Limb S, Kawsar M, Forster GE. HIV post-exposure prophylaxis after sexual assault: the experience of a sexual assault service in London. *Int J STD AIDS.* 2002;13:602-605.

255. Lurie P, Miller S, Hecht F, et al. Postexposure prophylaxis after nonoccupational HIV exposure: clinical, ethical, and policy considerations. *JAMA.* 1998;280:1769-1773.

256. Wiebe ER, Comay SE, McGregor M, et al. Offering HIV prophylaxis to people who have been sexually assaulted: 16 months' experience in a sexual assault service. *CMAJ.* 2000;162:641-645.

257. Neu N, Heffernan-Vacca S, Millery M, et al. Postexposure prophylaxis for HIV in children and adolescents after sexual assault: a prospective observational study in an urban medical center. *Sex Transm Dis.* 2007;34:65-68.

258. Poynten IM, Smith DE, Cooper DA, et al. The public health impact of widespread availability of nonoccupational postexposure prophylaxis against HIV. *HIV Med.* 2007;8:374-381.

259. Roland ME. A model for communitywide delivery of postexposure prophylaxis after potential sexual exposure to HIV. *Sex Transm Dis.* 2007;34:294-296.

260. Roland ME. Postexposure prophylaxis after sexual exposure to HIV. *Curr Opin Infect Dis.* 2007;20:39-46.

261. Disability. Officer who contracted HIV through bite is granted benefits. *AIDS Policy Law.* 2004;19:7.

262. Andreo SM, Barra LA, Costa LJ, et al. HIV type 1 transmission by human bite. *AIDS Res Hum Retroviruses.* 2004;20:349-350.

263. Bartholomew CF, Jones AM. Human bites: a rare risk factor for HIV transmission. *AIDS.* 2006;20:631-632.

264. Babl FE, Cooper ER, Kastner B, et al. Prophylaxis against possible human immunodeficiency virus exposure after nonoccupational needlestick injuries or sexual assaults in children and adolescents. *Arch Pediatr Adolesc Med.* 2001;155:680-682.

265. Bamberger JD, Waldo CR, Gerberding JL, et al. Postexposure prophylaxis for human immunodeficiency virus (HIV) infection following sexual assault. *Am J Med.* 1999;106:323-326.

266. Lamba H, Murphy SM. Sexual assault and sexually transmitted infections: an updated review. *Int J STD AIDS.* 2000;11:487-491.

267. Merchant RC, Keshavarz R. Human immunodeficiency virus postexposure prophylaxis for adolescents and children. *Pediatrics.* 2001;108:E38.

Nosocomial Herpesvirus Infections

TARA N. PALMORE | DAVID K. HENDERSON*

Eight herpesviruses commonly infect humans. The two herpes simplex viruses (HSV-1 and HSV-2) and varicella-zoster virus (VZV) are neurotropic and cause skin lesions and neurologic disease. Cytomegalovirus (CMV) and Epstein-Barr virus (EBV) cause mononucleosis in normal hosts and severe systemic morbidity in immunocompromised persons. Human herpesvirus 6 (HHV-6) and human herpesvirus 7 (HHV-7) cause a spectrum of illness, from the acute childhood febrile illness roseola infantum (exanthem subitum) to demyelinating disease, lymphoproliferative syndromes, and systemic infections in immunocompromised patients.[1-8] Human herpesvirus 8 (HHV-8), most similar in biology to EBV, is implicated in the occurrence of primary effusion lymphomas, multicentric Castleman's disease, and Kaposi's sarcoma.[5,9,10] A ninth herpesvirus, *Herpesvirus simiae,* is a rare cause of human infection (see Chapter 142). With the clear exception of VZV and the possible exceptions of HHV-6 and HHV-7, the remaining herpesviruses that infect humans apparently require close personal contact for person-to-person spread and are therefore not classified as highly contagious.

Two properties shared by members of this family of viruses are important to emphasize: (1) All of these viruses can, after causing a primary infection, persist in a latent state in the body and subsequently cause recrudescent or reactivation infection; and (2) differentiation of recrudescent infection from primary infection is often difficult and makes identification of true nosocomial infections problematic. Historically, this distinction has often been made on the basis of serologic evidence, the reliability of which may be questionable. Because recrudescent infections are common among immunosuppressed patients, they are discussed in detail in the chapters of this book dealing with each of the different viruses.

Herpesviruses have become important nosocomial pathogens for several reasons, including the presence of some of these agents in blood, blood products, and organ transplants, as well as the high prevalence of these infections in the population at large. The purpose of this chapter is to discuss the risk of nosocomial transmission of each of these agents and to discuss appropriate techniques to be used to prevent transmission of these agents to patients and personnel in the hospital.

Herpes Simplex Viruses

RISK OF NOSOCOMIAL TRANSMISSION

Transmission of HSV-1 and HSV-2 from infected patients to staff has been well documented.[11-18] Both HSV-1 and HSV-2 have been associated with the occurrence of herpetic whitlow. Primary HSV-1 infection has also been reported after mouth-to-mouth resuscitation.[14]

Similarly, Amir and colleagues reported primary oral HSV infections in four pediatric care providers that occurred, at least apparently, as a result of occupational exposures.[19] The investigators argued that these infections were likely acquired in the workplace, although no point source was identified and molecular techniques were not used to assess whether all were infected with similar isolates. Although a great deal of attention has been focused on the problem of HSV-2 infection in obstetric and neonatal intensive care unit (NICU) settings, HSV-1 has also been associated with outbreaks of infection in hospital personnel and their families.[20] Once in a nursery or a NICU, for example, an infant with HSV infection may serve as a reservoir for

transmission to other infants, although the risk of such transmission appears to be small.[21] Whereas HSV infection occurring as a result of the infant acquiring infection during delivery has been well documented, postpartum acquisition of HSV has been much less common and more difficult to document, and the diagnosis has been made most often on empirical grounds.[22,23]

Suspected transmission of HSV-1 from staff to patients has also been reported in decades-old studies. Linnemann and colleagues used restriction enzyme analysis to demonstrate that two cases of HSV-1 infection in neonates in the same nursery were caused by viruses with identical restriction endonuclease patterns.[23] Sakaoka and colleagues reported two clusters of HSV-1 infections at two separate hospitals.[21] Both clusters involved three neonates, and in both instances all three infants had HSV-1 isolates that produced virtually identical endonuclease cleavage profiles. Although not proved definitively, an environmental reservoir (radiant warmer) was incriminated in one cluster. In the other, three infants born at one hospital approximately 1 year apart were infected with strains of HSV-1 that yielded identical restriction endonuclease patterns. The researchers postulated that health care workers providing care for these infants developed periodic reactivation of HSV-1 infection resulting in transmission to the infants. Despite these anecdotal reports and despite the fact that the risk has not yet been measured, the risk of iatrogenic transmission of HSV to susceptible patients, including neonates, appears to be quite small.

MECHANISM OF NOSOCOMIAL TRANSMISSION

The frequent occurrence of whitlow in ICU personnel, respiratory care personnel, and dentists argues for a primary role for cutaneous inoculations of HSV-1 from oral secretions of infected patients directly into the skin of health care providers. Although many, if not most, whitlows represent primary infection with HSV, reactivation infection or recrudescence can occur,[11,12,24] and one experimental study has demonstrated the possibility for reinfection.[25]

Oral lesions caused by HSV-1 contain large quantities of virus and represent a potential reservoir for nosocomial transmission. For this reason, dental practitioners are at increased risk for occupational infections.[15,25] In one study oral lesions were found to have an average of greater than 10^8 plaque-forming units per milliliter of vesicular fluid.[26] Moreover, high titers of virus remained in lesions of severely immunocompromised patients for 3 weeks or longer. Turner and colleagues demonstrated that HSV-1 could be cultured from the hands of six of nine adults who had oral lesions.[27] In addition, in the same study HSV-1 isolates were shown to survive drying on skin, plastic, and cloth for up to 4 hours. Both patients and hospital personnel can harbor inapparent reactivation infections. In one prospective study, 9.6% of asymptomatic staff members of an obstetric hospital were found to have HSV in saliva.[28]

HSV-contaminated breast milk has been inferentially incriminated in one case as being responsible for the postpartum transmission of HSV[29]; however, HSV infection of either mother or child is not a contraindication to breast-feeding unless there are active HSV lesions around the nipple.[30]

PREVENTION OF NOSOCOMIAL TRANSMISSION

Use of Universal or Standard Precautions[31] should minimize the risk for transmission of HSV-1. Patients who have extensive oral, genital, or cutaneous disease may require more stringent isolation precautions.

---

*All material in this chapter is in the public domain, with the exception of any borrowed figures or tables.

All personnel having direct contact with an HSV-infected patient should practice careful handwashing. Personnel performing procedures involving oral or genital secretions (e.g., suctioning, placement of an oral airway, dental work, irrigation of a Foley catheter, dressing changes) should wear gloves. Such patients are a reservoir for whitlow but probably represent minimal risk to other patients, with only the following few exceptions. Patients who have disseminated HSV lesions should not be roomed with immunocompromised patients or with patients who have severe atopic histories[32] or defects in skin integrity (e.g., burn patients,[33] persons with eczema). Alternatively, in a nursery, a neonatal ICU, or a burn ward, such patients are optimally managed using strict isolation or, when possible, cohort nursing.

A special problem arises when the mother of a newborn has active, nongenital HSV infection. The newborn and mother should be placed on contact isolation, and, in the case of maternal orolabial infection, the mother should wear gloves and a mask when feeding or handling the infant. Mothers with active HSV lesions around the nipples should not breastfeed.[30,34,35] Treatment with acyclovir or other effective antiviral agents may hasten the clearing of the lesions.

Management of parturient mothers with genital HSV and babies exposed to mothers with genital infections is discussed in detail in the literature.[30,36-42] Optimal care of infants born to infected mothers includes placing the infant in a "special" nursery during hospitalization (for up to 14 days). Such infants should be evaluated frequently for signs of HSV infection. Depending on the stage of the mother's disease (i.e., primary versus secondary) and the extent of disease at delivery (i.e., modest versus extensive), empirical, antiviral treatment of the newborn may be appropriate. Many authorities empirically treat infants exposed to the birth canal of a mother who has active HSV infection acquired late in the course of her pregnancy with acyclovir.[36,40,43]

Because the efficacy of antiviral therapy in the setting of neonatal infection is increased when therapy is administered early in the course of the infection,[36,43] caregivers must maintain a high index of suspicion for neonatal HSV infection in children born to both symptomatic and asymptomatic mothers. Strikingly, neonatal HSV infection frequently occurs in infants born to mothers who had negative histories for past or recent genital HSV infection.[44] Brown and colleagues demonstrated that the approximately one third of women who shed HSV in early labor have recently acquired genital HSV. Infants of mothers who have recently acquired infection were found to be 10 times more likely to develop neonatal HSV infection than infants of women who have asymptomatic reactivation.[38]

Infants developing signs or symptoms of active infection should initially be managed using Standard Precautions; if more extensive disease develops, strict isolation or cohort nursing in a private room or in an isolation room in the NICU may be more effective. If such a room is not available, the infant should be separated from other infants in the nursery or NICU. Placing the infant in an incubator or isolette may raise the consciousness of the staff regarding the potential for transmission.[35,45]

Mothers who have active genital lesions should be allowed to feed or handle infants; however, before handling her baby, the mother should cover all lesions, carefully wash her hands, and put on clean hospital garb. If an infant is restricted to a NICU or nursery for life-support purposes, the mother may visit that area if all lesions are crusted over and covered. In addition, in the circumstance in which vaginal delivery by a mother known or suspected of having active genital HSV infection is attempted, fetal scalp monitoring should not be performed because of the risk of infection caused by inoculation.[37]

MANAGEMENT OF INFECTED OR EXPOSED PERSONNEL

Hospital personnel who have active oral or other cutaneous infection should not be permitted to care for high-risk patients until the lesions are entirely crusted and dry. Examples of such high-risk patients include premature infants, newborns, severely immunocompromised patients, burn patients, and patients with diseases affecting skin integrity. In the event that an infected individual must work to provide adequate care in a high-risk area, the provider should ensure that dressings (or a mask) cover all lesions. When practical, gloves should be worn. Particularly in situations in which the health care provider has active lesions on the hands, double-gloving may further reduce the risk for exposure. Most important, frequent glove changes and strict handwashing techniques (and/or use of alcohol-based hand disinfectants) should be used.

Varicella-Zoster Virus

RISK OF TRANSMISSION

Of the members of the herpesvirus family, VZV is by far the most contagious. For this reason, most adults have been exposed to the virus and have a prior history of chickenpox (varicella). The risk of transmission is highest in pediatric populations. Among adults, patients and staff from rural areas and locales where the incidence of VZV infection is lower (e.g., Pacific Islands, tropical climates) are at highest risk for acquisition.[46-49]

The major problems with nosocomial transmission of VZV infection occur in areas housing potentially susceptible immunosuppressed patients (e.g., pediatric oncology units). In immunocompetent patients, both primary infections (varicella) and recrudescent VZV infections (herpes zoster) are usually benign, self-limited infections, although varicella is more severe in adults than in children.[50] Effective antiviral therapy has reduced substantially the risks for severe morbidity and mortality caused by VZV infection for patients who are immunosuppressed, yet both primary and recrudescent VZV infections continue to be associated with increased morbidity and the potential for mortality for immunosuppressed patients. Finally, varicella occurring during pregnancy is associated with increased severity (see also Chapter 137).[51,52] The extent to which immunocompromised patients who have had chickenpox are at risk for exogenous reinfection is a matter of some controversy. Several investigators have suggested that immunocompromised patients may be at risk of acquiring exogenous reinfection with VZV, either in the form of a second case of chickenpox[53,54] or as atypical generalized zoster, a syndrome reported to resemble disseminated zoster without an antecedent dermatome.[55,56] Whereas primary VZV infection generally produces lifetime protection against exogenous reinfection, rare instances of reinfection, some caused by alterations in host defense, have been documented in the literature,[53,54,57] and may be more common than previously thought.[57]

MECHANISMS OF TRANSMISSION

Nosocomial transmission of VZV infection does occur. Several studies have clearly demonstrated airborne transmission from an index case with varicella to susceptible children.[58-60] A susceptible patient or staff member also may acquire primary infection as a result of direct contact with lesions from a patient with dermatomal zoster.[60] Person-to-person transmission of VZV from patients who have dermatomal zoster has been documented.[54,60-64] In two reports, patients with localized zoster were identified as the index cases in health care–associated outbreaks of varicella.[54,61] In both outbreaks, transmission of VZV may have occurred via the airborne route, environmental contamination, or the hands of health care workers. Although it is less contagious than primary varicella, one report suggests localized zoster may be a more frequent cause of nosocomial infection than varicella.[65]

Garnett and Grenfell have argued that the presence of varicella in the community may reduce the incidence of zoster among individuals who have latent infection, presumably as a result of an immunologic "boosting" phenomenon arising from the exposure to patients who have varicella.[66] Widespread childhood vaccination has reduced the circulating VZV and lessened the contribution of natural boosting. However, an increasing number of adults older than 60 are being vaccinated with the zoster vaccine, newly recommended by the Centers for Disease Control and Prevention (CDC),[67] and eventual widespread vaccination may serve this function.

PREVENTION OF NOSOCOMIAL TRANSMISSION

Because VZV is highly contagious and because VZV infection may be life threatening, particularly in severely immunosuppressed patient populations, several sets of recommendations regarding techniques to be used to prevent nosocomial transmission of VZV infection have been published.[31,50,59,68-72] Whenever practical, patients who have active VZV infections should not be hospitalized. If patients with active infections must be hospitalized, most authorities recommend that patients with dermatomal zoster be managed with appropriate barriers (e.g., gloves when touching the patient or the patient's lesions) and that the patient's door be labeled with a sign warning people who have not had chickenpox not to enter the patient's room. Use of the so-called Standard Precautions has been considered adequate for managing patients who have localized zoster.[31] Severely immunocompromised patients who develop dermatomal zoster (i.e., those with hematologic or reticuloendothelial malignancies, those with the acquired immunodeficiency syndrome [AIDS], and those receiving high-dose corticosteroids or multidrug chemotherapy) should be started on antiviral therapy and placed on strict isolation until it is clear that dissemination is not occurring. If new lesions stop occurring and few are outside the dermatome, the patients may be managed with simple barrier (i.e., standard) precautions.[31] Patients with varicella or disseminated zoster should be placed on strict isolation precautions because of high transmissibility. Because of the potential for airborne transmission of VZV, Gustafson and colleagues have recommended that hospitalized patients with varicella be placed downwind from other potentially susceptible patients.[58] Use of a negative-pressure isolation room is optimal. Anderson and co-workers documented the absence of VZV transmission over a 1-year period in a pediatrics hospital using negative pressure ventilation rooms.[73]

If a susceptible immunocompromised patient is exposed to a person with VZV infection, transmission of the infection can be prevented (or the severity of infection reduced) by the administration of hyperimmune globulin (varicella-zoster immunoglobulin [VariZIG]). To be effective, VariZIG should be administered as soon as possible after exposure. The CDC recommends that VariZIG be given within 96 hours of exposure.[74] VariZIG must be given intramuscularly, which is a problem for anticoagulated or thrombocytopenic patients. The dose is one vial (125 units) per 10 kg body weight up to a maximum of five vials, about 8 to 9 mL. As VZV immune globulin has not been proved to be uniformly efficacious, some centers use high-dose antiviral drugs in addition to VariZIG as postexposure prophylaxis.[75] The role of VariZIG in prophylaxis for recipients of stem cell transplantation who were previously immune is unclear; a handful of reports document reinfection with VZV in such patients despite previous seropositivity. Current expert opinion is that selected VZV-seropositive patients should receive prophylaxis with antiviral drugs but not immune globulin.[75] For immunocompromised patients unable to take VariZIG or who are more than 72 hours postexposure, a course of high-dose antiviral therapy through day 22 after exposure can be considered.

VZV infections are common, and, in spite of good infection control procedures, VZV is frequently introduced into the hospital environment in an uncontrolled fashion. Over the past several years, the use of antiviral agents (e.g., acyclovir) has been shown to be of benefit in patients who have primary or recrudescent VZV infection (reviewed in detail in references 76-79). Especially in immunocompromised patients, acyclovir should be initiated as early as the first symptoms of infection arise. In addition to being a proven benefit to the infected patient,[80-82] antiviral therapy may reduce the risk for nosocomial spread of this airborne pathogen. Because of the urgency involved in identifying exposed, susceptible, immunosuppressed patients, an organized approach to a potential outbreak is advisable. We have developed a flow chart to manage potential nosocomial outbreaks of VZV infection (Fig. 307-1).[70] Others have used a similar approach.[68]

A number of published reports document transmission of the varicella vaccine strain of VZV from recently vaccinated persons to household or other close contacts, including residents of a long-term care facility.[83-85] Nearly all cases have involved vaccinees with vesicular rashes. Transmission of the Oka vaccine strain from health care providers recently immunized with the varicella vaccine to VZV-naïve or immunocompromised patients is a theoretical possibility, but only if the vaccinee has skin lesions. The benefits of vaccinating health care workers far outweigh these risks. Although no cases of secondary transmission have been reported following vaccination of health care workers, we recommend that providers who develop vesicular lesions after varicella vaccination be furloughed until all lesions are crusted. The same concerns about transmission may not apply to the zoster vaccine, as it is not known to elicit vesicular lesions. This vaccine also uses the Oka strain of VZV, but there are no documented cases of secondary transmission from zoster vaccinees.

INVESTIGATING NOSOCOMIAL EXPOSURE TO VARICELLA-ZOSTER VIRUS

Cases of VZV infection are identified by routine ward rounds, routine surveillance activities, and by referrals from patient care areas. Once a suspected case is identified, the diagnosis is confirmed, either by hospital epidemiology service staff members or by staff of the clinical virology laboratory. First and foremost, the diagnosis of VZV should be confirmed, preferably by direct fluorescent antibody-stained smear of vesical fluid. If the suspected diagnosis is incorrect, the investigation is aborted. Once the diagnosis is confirmed, the investigation is divided into two separate areas: (1) the patient-related epidemiologic investigation and (2) the staff-related epidemiologic investigation. Because of the necessity for administering passive immunoglobulin prophylaxis to exposed, susceptible, immunocompromised children within 96 hours of exposure to be effective, the initial focus of the investigation is on patients. Similarly, if antiviral prophylaxis is chosen, prompt administration of the agent is important to success. In the event that immunosuppressed staff are potentially exposed, they should be managed in the same expeditious manner as immunosuppressed patients.

An in-hospital "travel history" is first obtained from the index case. As in-hospital exposures may take place in any of a number of patient-related areas, several diverse areas must be considered in history taking (see Fig. 307-1). When any of these areas are included in the patient's travel history, the departmental records from that area should be examined. Patients documented to be in that area at the same time as the index case should be included in the population at risk.

The second component of the patient-related investigation is the direct identification of patients at high risk for severe complications of primary VZV infection (see Fig. 307-1). We use three methods to identify such patients: (1) compiling a computer list of all hospitalized pediatric, oncology, and transplant patients; (2) compiling a list of all ambulatory care patients, including those children and severely immunosuppressed adults who might be staying outside the hospital but returning daily for chemotherapy, phlebotomy, and/or other infusions or treatments; and (3) questioning the inpatient pediatrics, oncology, and transplant staff.

Once the population at risk has been identified, the immunologic status of all patients on the list is assessed. If a patient is found to be potentially immunosuppressed (i.e., hematologic malignancy receiving chemotherapy, high-dose steroid therapy, congenital or acquired immunodeficiency), the patient and the medical staff are questioned regarding the potential for exposure and for a prior history of chickenpox or prior varicella immunization. If the patient is potentially exposed and has a negative or equivocal history of VZV infection, a baseline serology is drawn and VariZIG is administered.[74,86] In immunocompetent patients up to 120 hours from exposure, varicella vaccination should be considered.[31] If a patient is determined to have had

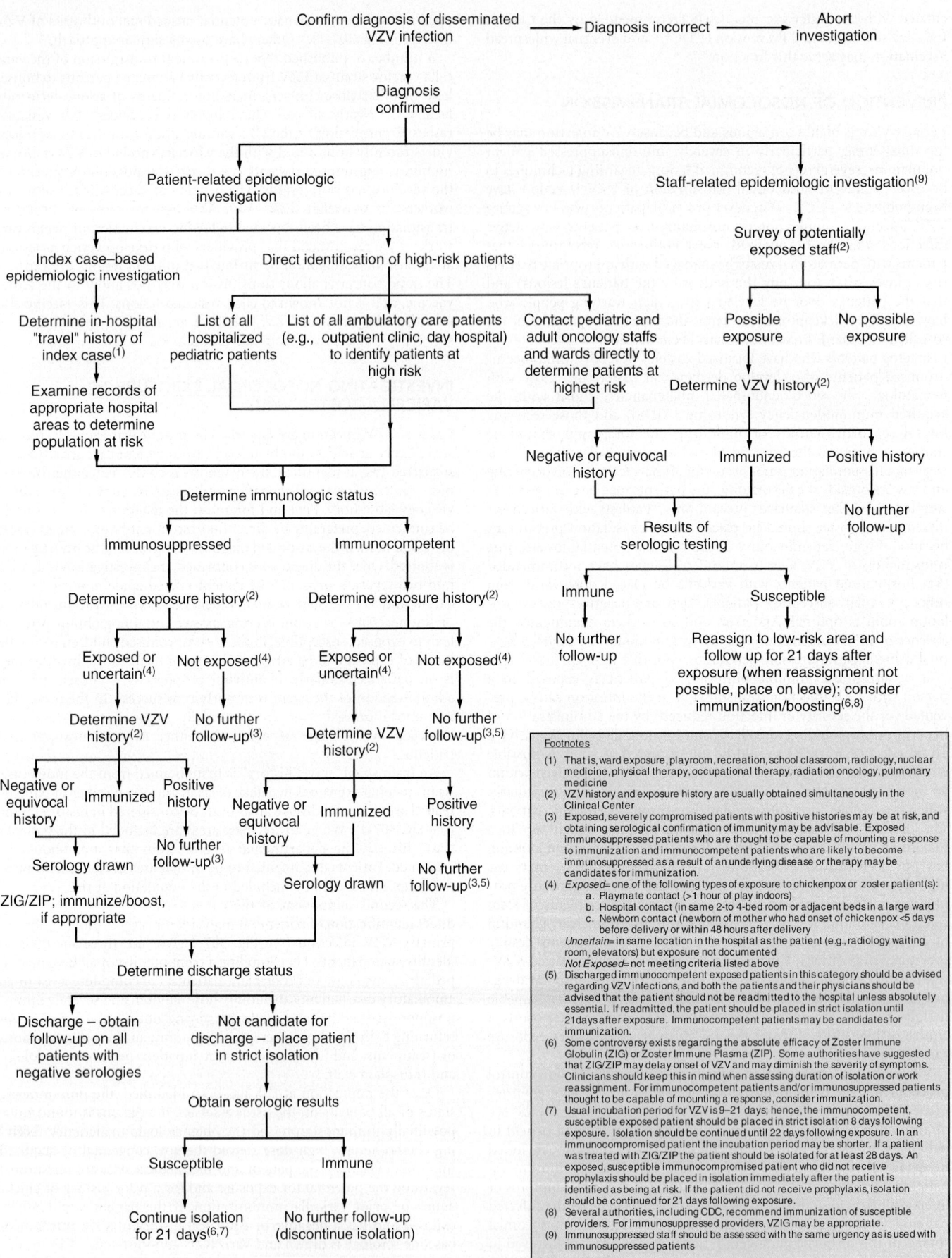

Figure 307-1 Algorithm for the evaluation of a potential nosocomial outbreak of VZV infection.

primary VZV infection or is determined not to have been exposed, no further follow-up is needed.

If patients on the potentially exposed list are found to be immunocompetent, exposure and VZV histories are obtained after work-up of immunocompromised patients. Exposed, susceptible immunocompetent patients have serologies drawn and, when possible, are discharged. In general, those with negative exposure histories or positive histories of prior VZV infection need no further follow-up.

If patients must remain hospitalized, serologic determination of immunity using a sensitive technique, such as fluorescent antimembrane antibody assay (FAMA),[87] immune adherence hemagglutination inhibition assay (IAHIA),[88] or enzyme-linked immunosorbent assay (ELISA),[89] may help determine which exposed patients are susceptible. Less sensitive tests, such as complement fixation, are not reliable indicators of immunity.

Exposed, susceptible, immunocompetent patients should be placed in strict isolation from 9 days after the first possible exposure until 21 days after the last possible exposure. Exposed, susceptible, immunosuppressed patients (even those receiving VariZIG or prophylactic acyclovir) should be placed in strict isolation at the time the patient is identified as being at risk until at least 21 days after the last possible exposure. Some studies have suggested that administration of zoster immune plasma or earlier preparations of VariZIG to exposed, susceptible, immunosuppressed patients actually lengthened the incubation period for such patients up to 28 days. Although instances of lengthened incubation periods have not been reported with VariZIG, physicians responsible for care of such patients should be mindful of this possibility when planning extended in-hospital care for these patients.[74] As noted earlier, acyclovir should be administered to susceptible, exposed immunosuppressed patients at the first suggestion of clinical illness caused by VZV,[77,80-82] and many investigators have argued for its prophylactic use in susceptible individuals from days 3 to 22 or, if the patient has received VariZig, days 3 to 38. A substantial literature exists describing the use of this agent as treatment in immunocompetent patients as well, particularly for adolescents and adults who develop varicella (see Chapter 137).[50,90-93]

MANAGEMENT OF INFECTED OR EXPOSED PERSONNEL

The other major aspect of the work-up of a potential nosocomial outbreak of VZV infection is the assessment of potentially exposed staff (see Fig. 307-1). Exposure and VZV histories are taken from all potentially exposed staff. Potentially exposed staff who relate negative or equivocal histories of VZV infection should have serologic assessment of immunity using a sensitive test (discussed earlier). Immunocompromised employees should be managed with the same sense of urgency that is used for immunosuppressed patients.

In our view, exposed, susceptible employees should be reassigned to a low-risk area or be placed on administrative leave from 8 days after the first possible exposure until 21 days after the last possible exposure (although some have advocated a more liberal approach).[94] If employees desiring to work in an area with a high prevalence of VZV infection are found to be susceptible on the basis of assessment of humoral[87-89] and, possibly, cell-mediated[95] immunity to VZV, such employees may be candidates for the varicella vaccine.[50,71,96-99]

Employees who develop primary VZV infection or zoster should not care for or be in the same area with patients until the last lesion is crusted over (usually 7 or 8 days after the appearance of the last lesion). Employees who have zoster should be reassigned so that they also not work in high-risk areas until all lesions have crusted over.

▦ Cytomegalovirus

RISK FOR NOSOCOMIAL TRANSMISSION

The nosocomial epidemiology of CMV infection is incompletely understood. Part of the difficulty in assessing the magnitude of risk for

nosocomial transmission lies in the difficulty in discriminating between endogenous reactivation infection and exogenous reinfection (i.e., infection with a second strain of CMV). The term *secondary infection* is used here to encompass both possibilities. In several settings, the risk of an individual patient acquiring CMV infection, either in the hospital or as a result of iatrogenic intervention, appears to be quite high. Premature infants and infants in newborn nurseries are at increased risk for CMV acquisition.[100-103] Studies have suggested that from 14% to 30% of infants residing in a neonatal ICU for longer than 1 month acquire CMV infection.[102-104]

Recipients of organ transplants are also at high risk for both primary and secondary CMV infection. As immunosuppressive regimens have become more powerful, secondary CMV infections have become increasingly more common. One strategy employed to attempt to reduce the incidence of CMV infection in this population is to use newer immunosuppressive regimens in combination with appropriate antiviral chemoprophylaxis.[105] A summary of 12 studies that used various techniques to assess CMV infection in renal transplant recipients demonstrated that 53% of seronegative transplant recipients acquired infection and 85% of seropositive transplant recipients either shed virus or developed a fourfold rise in anti-CMV antibody titer.[106] Because these results include some studies that used only complement fixation to document infection, these numbers probably represent conservative estimates of the risk of a renal transplant recipient acquiring CMV infection. Heart transplant recipients are also at high risk for CMV infection. In an early study 62% of seronegative heart transplant patients seroconverted post-transplant, and 60% of patients who were seropositive before heart transplantation developed fourfold rises in antibody titer after transplantation.[107] Recipients of allogeneic stem cell transplants are also at increased risk for CMV reactivation, particularly if graft-versus-host disease is present.[108,109] In one study published in 1982, 39% of all seronegative stem cell transplant recipients acquired primary infection, and 61% of seropositive bone marrow recipients developed evidence of secondary CMV infection.[108] With current stem cell transplantation techniques, transmission of CMV from donor to seronegative recipient is uncommon.

Recipients of granulocyte transfusions have also been demonstrated to be at risk for acquiring CMV infection. In the study cited in the preceding paragraph,[108] 48% of seronegative bone marrow recipients who received granulocyte transfusions seroconverted, compared with 33% of seronegative recipients who did not receive granulocyte transfusions, although the results may have been confounded by receipt of platelet and red cell transfusions that were not matched for CMV status.[110] In an earlier study, Winston and colleagues demonstrated that 61% of patients receiving granulocyte transfusions developed evidence of CMV seroconversion, but not disease, compared with 26% of age- and disease-matched recipients.[111]

Several studies have suggested that the transfusion of fresh whole blood is also implicated in the transmission of CMV. The risk for acquisition of CMV has been shown to be associated with increasing numbers of units transfused. With older techniques, the risk of acquiring CMV infection was estimated to be between 2.4% and 2.7% per unit of transfused whole blood.[112,113] High-risk recipients now receive either whole blood from a seronegative donor or blood that has been filtered to deplete leukocytes, decreasing CMV transmission to 1% to 4% (see Chapter 311). Although the risk for CMV transmission by parenteral exposure seems clear, the issue of whether hospital patients or hospital personnel are at risk for acquiring CMV by nonparenteral routes of exposure is less clear. Although apparently uncommon, nonparenteral transmission of CMV from patient to patient has been reasonably well documented.[114,115] Breast milk has been implicated as a source of primary neonatal infection.[115-118] One study definitively documented nonparenteral spread of CMV among three infants in a neonatal ICU by using restriction endonuclease analysis.[115] The investigator concluded, however, that such common-source outbreaks are apparently uncommon. In a similar study, Aitken and colleagues evaluated a cluster of five CMV infections in a special-care nursery, concluding that the infections were not epidemiologically linked.[119] In a study using similar technology, Demmler and coworkers demonstrated patient-to-patient transmission of a single strain of CMV in a busy chronic care pediatrics hospital.[114] The researchers isolated CMV from patients' hands, health care workers' hands, and hospitalized infants' diapers.

The issue of whether hospital personnel are at risk for acquiring CMV infection is a controversial one. Some investigators have suggested that hospital personnel are at slightly higher risk for seroconversion than are age-matched controls who do not have patient contact.[120] Conversely, the intensive studies by Ahlfors in Sweden found little evidence that nurses were at greater risk of acquiring CMV infection than other age-matched Swedish women.[121] A study using restriction enzyme analysis of CMV DNA demonstrated no correlation between the CMV strain infecting a neonate and the strain of CMV found to be infecting a nurse who cared for the infant.[122] In a second study using similar technology, significant differences were found in DNA from CMV isolates obtained from a physician who became infected while caring for a CMV-infected child and the isolate from the child.[123] In both studies, the health care professionals were pregnant, and both elected to have abortions. CMV with identical restriction patterns to the maternal isolates was grown from each of the infected fetuses.

Several additional studies have suggested minimal or negligible risk for patient-to-staff transmission of CMV.[114,124-126] Balfour and Balfour compared CMV infection rates in three groups of nurses—those working in neonatal ICUs, those working in renal transplant/dialysis units, and student nurses—with age-matched blood donors.[125] No association was found between prevalence of infection among patients and CMV seroconversion, so the authors of this study concluded that nurses were no more likely to develop CMV infection than were the age-matched blood donor controls.

Demmler and colleagues also found no association between CMV seroconversion and occupational exposure to CMV in two pediatric hospitals in Texas.[114] This study also found no correlation between prevalence of infection in patients and seroconversion in health care providers. Adler and co-workers used restriction endonucleases to evaluate CMV isolates from 34 hospitalized newborn infants and from the one seronegative health care worker who developed primary CMV infection during a 3-year study period.[124] No two isolates were identical. Balcarek and colleagues found a rate of CMV seroconversion among employees of a children's hospital similar to that in the general population.[127]

Finally, because patients who are infected with the human immunodeficiency virus (HIV) (particularly those who have AIDS) are known to harbor and shed large quantities of herpesviruses, Gerberding and associates evaluated health care workers who provided care for HIV-1–infected patients for serologic evidence of CMV infection and failed to find an elevated rate of CMV acquisition.[126]

Conversely, other investigators, although failing to demonstrate patient-to-staff transmission of CMV, have postulated that the risk for transmission is likely to be higher for personnel working with patients who have a high prevalence of CMV infection.[128,129] Although such a hypothesis seems plausible, to our knowledge no direct evidence supports this contention.

At this time no instances of patient-to-staff transmission of CMV have been linked by molecular analysis of the CMV isolates. One investigator has, however, used endonuclease analysis to document apparent nonparenteral transmission of CMV from an infected infant to his seronegative mother.[115] Thus, the magnitude of the risk of patient-to-staff transmission of CMV, especially when appropriate isolation procedures are observed, would appear to be small.

MECHANISMS OF NOSOCOMIAL TRANSMISSION

In instances in which primary infection with CMV is documented to have occurred in the hospital setting, the parenteral route of transmission has almost always been implicated.

Most primary infections in the NICU can be traced to the transfusion of whole blood contaminated with CMV.[100,102,103,112,113] Consumption of breast milk contaminated with CMV has been suggested to be an important nonparenteral mechanism of postnatal transmission of CMV to neonates.[115-118,130] The possibility also has been raised, but not to our knowledge documented, that fomites or health care professionals may be vectors for nonparenteral transmission of CMV in unusual circumstances.

Renal transplant recipients can acquire primary CMV infection from blood transfusions, from leukocyte infusions,[131] or from the transplanted organ itself.[132] Recipients of bone marrow allografts can acquire CMV infection through receipt of an infected allograft, through transfused blood or platelets, or through infected leukocyte infusions.[102,133-135] If nonparenteral transmission is occurring in the hospital, it occurs uncommonly and, if it occurs, would likely be due to exposure of susceptible individuals (patients or employees) to contaminated excreta or secretions, presumably via the oral or respiratory routes.

PREVENTION OF NOSOCOMIAL TRANSMISSION

Several measures can be implemented to minimize the risk of CMV transmission in a high-risk setting in the hospital. Choosing organ and stem cell donors who are CMV seronegative for transplant recipients who are also CMV seronegative is an effective way to minimize the risk for subsequent CMV infection in the recipient. Betts was among the first to advocate using the donor's serologic status as a major determinant in selecting a donor kidney for a seronegative recipient.[136] Winston and co-workers have suggested that seronegative donors be given priority as potential leukocyte donors, because of the evidence that CMV is leukocyte associated and because the development of CMV infection in recipients of leukocytes is often a serious problem.[111]

Transfusing patients at high risk for CMV infection with either leukocyte-depleted blood[137-139] or with washed, frozen red cells[140] is being used routinely to reduce the risk of CMV transmission, although one paper has suggested that neither is as effective as using CMV-seronegative donors.[141] Thus, the risk for transfusion-associated CMV disease can be reduced substantially by using CMV-seronegative donors; by using frozen, deglycerolized red blood cells; and by using products that have the leukocytes removed with filters. Viremia in blood donors with active, subclinical CMV infection, however, may be one reason for the incomplete efficacy of leukoreduction.[142] The relative efficacy of these three approaches remains somewhat controversial; however, efficacy of all three approaches has been demonstrated. Some investigators have suggested that adding back potentially cytotoxic donor T lymphocytes a month or more following transplantation may help control graft-versus-host disease, help preserve a graft-versus-leukemia effect, and help reduce the risk for serious CMV infections in allogeneic bone marrow transplantation patients.[143-146] The use of specific anti-CMV immunoglobulin has been associated with a reduction in CMV-associated morbidity in solid organ transplant recipients and patients at risk for CMV disease.[147-149]

Prophylactic or preemptive treatment, or both, with antivirals, particularly with ganciclovir, has also been used to reduce risks for infection, reactivation, or severe sequelae of CMV infection, particularly in transplant recipients. In one such study, preemptive therapy with ganciclovir prevented all except one case of CMV disease before day 100 after transplantation after detection of CMV antigenemia.[141] Several studies have demonstrated the benefit of combinations of antiviral and immunoglobulin prophylaxis in the prevention of CMV disease in the transplantation setting.[139-141,149-153]

Because most pregnant women secreting CMV in cervical mucus and breast milk are asymptomatic, and (unlike infection with the herpes simplex viruses) because perinatal infection with CMV is rarely associated with symptomatic illness in the newborn, no precautions are advocated for mothers known to be secreting CMV at delivery.

Immunosuppressed patients who are infected with CMV (e.g., patients with AIDS, transplant recipients, or babies with congenital infection) excrete large quantities of virus in many different body fluids. Appropriate precautions for such patients should include gloves for contact with wounds or lesions or for contact with blood, secretions, or excreta. Also, infected patients in the neonatal ICU should be segregated from noninfected babies. Other precautions advisable in caring for such patients include handling linens and other reusable patient care items as isolation materials and emphasizing hand hygiene after each patient contact. In general, strict adherence to Standard Precautions should minimize the already small risk for occupational or nosocomial infection with CMV.[31]

MANAGEMENT OF INFECTED, EXPOSED, AND POTENTIALLY EXPOSED PERSONNEL

The risk for staff-to-patient transmission of CMV has received little attention in the literature. To our knowledge, only one study has attempted to assess this risk. Demmler and colleagues found no evidence of CMV transmission among patients cared for by four CMV-shedding health care workers.[114] These investigators concluded that, although a theoretical possibility, the risk of staff-to-patient transmission of CMV was sufficiently small to allow infected health care workers to continue working.[114] Based on currently available evidence regarding the transmission and transmissibility of CMV, such an approach seems entirely reasonable.

The issue of limiting exposure of pregnant health care workers to CMV-infected patients remains somewhat controversial. Although, as noted earlier, data documenting CMV transmission from patient to staff are nonexistent, a commonsense approach to the care of infected patients is appropriate. In an earlier edition of this text,[154] one of us recommended that pregnant health care workers be restricted from taking care of patients with CMV infection. Several factors subsequently caused our Hospital Infections Committee to reassess this difficult and controversial issue.

First, a number of additional articles (see "Risk for Nosocomial Transmission," earlier) have been published further documenting that the risk for occupational or nosocomial infection with CMV is quite small. Because the number of seroconversions in these studies is small, a very large study would be required to measure the magnitude of the small risk of CMV transmission to health care workers precisely. Nonetheless, the expanded, consistent database is reassuring.

Second, numerous investigators have pointed out that many patients who excrete CMV (e.g., immunosuppressed patients, AIDS patients, dialysis patients, transplant recipients) have no signs or symptoms of CMV infection. Such patients are frequently not identified as being infected or infectious during the course of hospitalization. In fact, most patients shedding CMV who are hospitalized will not be specifically identified as having CMV infection; for this reason a broader approach to our patient population seems prudent.

Third, because the magnitude of risk to pregnant health care workers is currently below the limits of detection, the administrative problems associated with a more restrictive policy may not be justified (i.e., if pregnant health care workers are restricted, how should one manage health care workers who "think they might be" or "are trying to become" or "are not trying to prevent" becoming pregnant?).

Fourth, adherence to Universal/Standard Precautions guidelines issued by the CDC[155] and mandated by the U.S. Department of Labor's Occupational Safety and Health Administration[156] should reduce the already small risk for CMV transmission from patients to health care workers.

An initial clarification of the Universal Precautions policy noted that these precautions do not apply to feces, urine, saliva, sweat, sputum, or tears.[157] In this update, the CDC emphasized that Universal Precautions are supplementary or baseline precautions and that these new precautions are not designed to replace standard infection control policy. Specifically, this update notes that prior CDC guidelines recommended wearing gloves to prevent gross microbial contamination of hands. This latter recommendation deserves careful consideration when handling urine from any patient. Although Universal Precautions do not apply to saliva, the previous recommendation for wearing gloves before performing digital examination of mucous membranes

remains in effect. The subsequent issuance of the Standard Precautions guidelines by the CDC underscores the importance of using barriers for contact with all body fluids.

These new recommendations also allow the health care worker to use judgment in deciding whether barriers (such as gloves) are needed. These new guidelines emphasize the importance of hand hygiene, which, if practiced appropriately, should minimize the risk for occupational CMV infection.

Finally, the issue of routine screening of health care workers for antibody to CMV is also controversial. Whereas several articles have addressed this complex issue,[158-160] the lack of consensus is apparent. The CDC does not advocate routine screening.[159] Conversely, Adler[158] and Plotkin[160] support periodic serologic testing for "potentially pregnant" employees whose jobs entail exposure to CMV-infected patients. Onorato and colleagues argue that no data indicate that routine testing will have any impact on the risk of congenital CMV infection.[159] Our Hospital Infections Committee and Occupational Medical Service have decided not to offer routine screening of employees. Because the risk of patient-to-staff transmission is, as yet, unmeasurable and because adherence to Universal Precautions will further reduce this risk, we do not recommend reassignment of pregnant health care workers. Rather, we have chosen to educate staff aggressively regarding CMV and other occupational risks and to emphasize the importance of good hygiene and Universal/Standard Precautions during pregnancy. For all these reasons, we do not recommend reassignment of pregnant health care workers.

Epstein-Barr Virus
RISK FOR NOSOCOMIAL TRANSMISSION

The risk of nosocomial transmission of EBV appears to be very small. Several instances of nosocomial transmission of EBV to patients have been identified.[161-172] Secondary infections (the majority of which appear to be reactivation of latent infection in the immunosuppressed transplant recipient) may be associated with a lymphoproliferative disorder (reviewed in references 173-175). As the overwhelming majority of these infections represent recrudescence, rather than acquired infection, they are discussed in more detail in Chapter 139.

Transmission of EBV from patient to staff or staff to patient has not been described, although Ginsburg and colleagues have described an outbreak of infectious mononucleosis in personnel working in an outpatient clinic,[165] and Chang and colleagues have described the apparent transmissibility of EBV in a relatively crowded nursery providing domiciliary care.[162] One epidemiologic study found a possible risk for occupational acquisition of EBV among dentists and dental students.[176]

MECHANISMS OF TRANSMISSION

Patients who have been shown to have acquired nosocomial EBV infection have been recipients of blood or plasma transfusions,[161,163,164,166-168,170-172] solid organ transplants,[177] and bone marrow allografts[169,178] apparently infected with EBV. In addition, one study has demonstrated evidence of EBV DNA in breast milk.[179] EBV appears to be one of the least contagious of the herpesviruses, and most authorities believe that intravenous inoculation or intimate contact is required for transmission of the virus.

PREVENTION OF NOSOCOMIAL TRANSMISSION

Patients known to have EBV in their secretions may be a reservoir for infection if health care workers follow extremely poor hygiene practices. In 1975, the CDC recommended that patients with infectious mononucleosis be placed on secretion precautions.[180] In more recent recommendations, the CDC stated that isolation precautions are unnecessary.[31] Adherence to Universal/Standard Precautions, use of appropriate barriers, and attention to hand hygiene will further reduce the risk for occupational infection. As is the case for CMV infection in transplantation, some investigators have found a benefit of infusing donor-specific lymphocytes as "adoptive immunotherapy" to treat the EBV-associated lymphoproliferative disorders.[173,181-183]

MANAGEMENT OF INFECTED OR EXPOSED PERSONNEL

Staff who acquire an EBV infection (e.g., infectious mononucleosis) may excrete virus much longer than symptoms persist,[184] but if good hygienic practices are followed (e.g., hand hygiene) personnel presumably represent an extremely small risk for transmittal of the infection.

Human Herpesvirus 6 and Human Herpesvirus 7
RISK FOR NOSOCOMIAL TRANSMISSION

HHV-6 and HHV-7 are somewhat similar, β-subgroup herpesviruses that are most closely related to CMV. HHV-6 (first called human B-lymphotropic virus[7]) was identified as a human pathogen in the mid- and late 1980s.[6] Subsequently, this virus has been shown to be a cause of roseola infantum (exanthem subitum) (see Chapter 140).[185] This childhood exanthem is reasonably contagious and may present a risk for nosocomial transmission, particularly in pediatric hospitals. Acute HHV-6 infection has also been associated with both a mononucleosis-like syndrome, as well as a self-limited hepatitis.[186] A clear association between HHV-6 infection and acute febrile seizures has now been established, as well.[187] In addition, HHV-6 has been associated with several less common syndromes, including encephalitis, disseminated infection, and perhaps pneumonia. This virus also may complicate solid organ transplantation as well as bone marrow transplantation. HHV-6 has also been found (presumably as an opportunist) in peripheral blood of AIDS patients.[6]

HHV-7 was identified initially in 1990.[188] Initial studies failed to name a disease process associated with HHV-7 infection.[189,190] HHV-7 is frequently found in human saliva,[190] and, similar to HHV-6, is a T-lymphotropic virus. Although HHV-7 infection has clearly been associated with febrile syndromes in young children and with a syndrome similar to roseola (usually occurring in children older than 2 years of age), studies have yet to identify a definitive syndrome in most children infected with this herpesvirus.

MECHANISMS OF TRANSMISSION

Although HHV-6 and HHV-7 DNA have been detected in several body fluids,[191-193] the principal route of infection is likely salivary,[194-196] and salivary glands may serve as a viral reservoir.[197,198] Outbreaks of HHV-6 infection have been reported in daycare centers.[199,200] The nosocomial epidemiology of infection with HHV-6 remains indistinct, but a conservative approach to the management of this infection in the hospital seems prudent. As is suggested by the Standard Precautions guidelines, secretions (particularly oral secretions) from all patients should be considered potentially infectious, and pediatric care providers should pay special attention to the potential for cross-contamination in nurseries. Most care providers are likely to be immune to HHV-6 infection because of prior infection.

PREVENTION OF NOSOCOMIAL TRANSMISSION

Virtually nothing is known about the nosocomial epidemiology of HHV-6 and HHV-7. Because of the apparent contagiousness of roseola, hospitalized patients who have roseola should be treated similarly to patients with VZV infection (see "Prevention of Nosocomial Transmission" in the earlier Varicella-Zoster Virus section). Until definitive data are available to address the nosocomial transmissibility of HHV-6, using the VZV (i.e., airborne) model for prevention seems reasonable. Techniques for establishing the diagnosis of HHV-7 infection are in their infancy and are not generally available.

In the unusual instance in which the diagnosis of HHV-7 is established, use of Standard Precautions for such patients seems prudent. Based on the fact that children who acquire HHV-7 infection are generally older than those who acquire HHV-6 infection, HHV-7 appears to be less transmissible than HHV-6. At a minimum, in the absence of defined infection syndromes associated with HHV-7 infection, use of Standard Precautions for these patients should provide adequate protection.

Human Herpesvirus 8
RISK FOR NOSOCOMIAL TRANSMISSION

HHV-8 is a gamma herpesvirus that is most closely related to EBV. HHV-8 has been closely associated with Kaposi's sarcoma and (in combination with EBV) body-cavity lymphoma in patients who are infected with HIV. HHV-8 was identified initially in 1994.[201,202] The viral DNA sequence has been isolated from patients who have Kaposi's sarcomas that are both HIV-related and unrelated to HIV infection or infection risk (i.e., patients who have classic Mediterranean Kaposi's sarcoma). Little is known about the epidemiology of HHV-8, and almost nothing is known about the potential for nosocomial transmission. Initial data suggest that the virus is most likely acquired during or after adolescence. By analogy, the epidemiology of HHV-8 may be similar to that of EBV. There is evidence that HHV-8 may be transmissible via several routes, including sexual contact,[203-206] blood products,[203,207,208] and salivary shedding.[209,210] Based on these preliminary data, Standard Precautions should also be an effective management strategy for patients infected with HHV-8. Optimal management of needlestick exposures to source patients known to harbor HHV-8 remains undefined.

REFERENCES

1. Black JB, Pellett PE. Human herpesvirus 7. *Rev Med Virol.* 1999;9:245-262.
2. Caserta MT, Mock DJ, Dewhurst S. Human herpesvirus 6. *Clin Infect Dis.* 2001;33:829-833.
3. Clark DA. Human herpesvirus 6. *Rev Med Virol.* 2000;10:155-173.
4. Clark DA, Griffiths PD. Human herpesvirus 6: relevance of infection in the immunocompromised host. *Br J Haematol.* 2003;120:384-395.
5. Lee LM, Henderson DK. Emerging viral infections. *Curr Opin Infect Dis.* 2001;14:467-480.
6. Lopez C, Pellett P, Steward J, et al. Characterizations of human herpesvirus-6. *J Infect Dis.* 1988;157:1271-1273.
7. Salahuddin SZ, Ablashi DV, Markham PD, et al. Isolation of a new virus, HBLV, in patients with lymphoproliferative disorders. *Science.* 1986;234:596-601.
8. Ward KN. Human herpesviruses-6 and -7 infections. *Curr Opin Infect Dis.* 2005;18:247-252.
9. Hengge UR, Ruzicka T, Tyring SK, et al. Update on Kaposi's sarcoma and other HHV8 associated diseases. Part 1: epidemiology, environmental predispositions, clinical manifestations, and therapy. *Lancet Infect Dis.* 2002;2:281-292.
10. Hengge UR, Ruzicka T, Tyring SK, et al. Update on Kaposi's sarcoma and other HHV8 associated diseases. Part 2: pathogenesis, Castleman's disease, and pleural effusion lymphoma. *Lancet Infect Dis.* 2002;2:344-352.
11. Crane L, Lerner A. Herpetic whitlow: A manifestation of primary infection with herpes simplex virus type 1 or type 2. *J Infect Dis.* 1978;137:855-856.
12. Gill M, Arlette J, Buchan K. Herpes simplex virus infections of the hand. A profile of 79 cases. *Am J Med.* 1988;84:89-93.
13. Gunbay T, Gunbay S, Kandemir S. Herpetic whitlow. *Quintessence Int.* 1993;24:363-364.
14. Hendricks A, Shapiro E. Primary herpes simplex infection following mouth-to-mouth resuscitation. *JAMA.* 1980;243:257-259.
15. Lewis MA. Herpes simplex virus: an occupational hazard in dentistry. *Int Dent J.* 2004;54:103-111.
16. Perl TM, Haugen TH, Pfaller MA, et al. Transmission of herpes simplex virus type 1 infection in an intensive care unit. *Ann Intern Med.* 1992;117:584-586.
17. Rosato F, Rosato E, Plotkin S. Herpetic paronychia—an occupational hazard of medical personnel. *N Engl J Med.* 1964;270:979-982.
18. Stern H, Eleck S, Millar D, et al. Herpetic whitlow: A form of cross-infection in hospitals. *Lancet.* 1959;2:871-874.
19. Amir J, Nussinovitch M, Kleper R, et al. Primary herpes simplex virus type 1 gingivostomatitis in pediatric personnel. *Infection.* 1997;25(5):310-312.
20. Adams G, Stover B, Keenlyside R, et al. Nosocomial herpetic infections in a pediatric intensive care unit. *Am J Epidemiol.* 1981;113:126-132.
21. Sakaoka H, Saheki Y, Uzuki K, et al. Two outbreaks of herpes simplex virus type 1 nosocomial infection among newborns. *J Clin Microbiol.* 1986;24:36-40.
22. Light I. Postnatal acquisition of herpes simplex virus by the newborn infant: A review of the literature. *Pediatrics.* 1979;63:480-482.

23. Linnemann CC Jr, Buchman TG, Light IJ, et al. Transmission of herpes simplex virus, type 1 in a nursery for the newborn: Identification of viral isolates by DNA fingerprinting. *Lancet.* 1978;1:964-966.
24. Haburchak D. Recurrent herpetic whitlow due to herpes simplex virus type 2. *Arch Intern Med.* 1978;138:1418-1419.
25. Blank H, Haines H. Experimental reinfection with herpes simplex virus. *J Invest Dermatol.* 1973;61:223-225.
26. Daniels C, LeGoff S. Shedding of infectious virus/antibody complexes from vesicular lesions of patients with recurrent herpes labialis. *Lancet.* 1975;2:524-528.
27. Turner R, Shehab Z, Osborne K, et al. Shedding and survival of herpes simplex virus from "fever blisters." *Pediatrics.* 1982; 70:547-549.
28. Hatherly L, Hayes K, Jack I. Herpes virus in an obstetric hospital: II. Asymptomatic virus excretion in staff members. *Med J Aust.* 1980;2:273-275.
29. Dunkle L, Schmidt R, O'Connor D. Neonatal herpes simplex infection possibly acquired via maternal breast milk. *Pediatrics.* 1979;63:250-251.
30. American College of Obstetrics and Gynecology. ACOG Practice Bulletin: Management of Herpes in Pregnancy. *Obstet Gynecol.* 2007;109:1489-1498.
31. Siegel JD, Rhinehart E, Jackson M, et al. 2007 Guidelines for isolation precautions: Preventing transmission of infectious agents in health care settings. *Am J Infect Control.* 2007;35(Suppl 2):S65-164.
32. Bussmann C, Peng WM, Bieber T, et al. Molecular pathogenesis and clinical implications of eczema herpeticum. *Expert Rev Mol Med.* 2008;10:e21.
33. McGill SN, Cartotto RC. Herpes simplex virus infection in a paediatric burn patient: case report and review. *Burns.* 2000;26: 194-199.
34. Aitken C, Jeffries DJ. Nosocomial spread of viral disease. *Clin Microbiol Rev.* 2001;14:528-546.
35. Kibrick S. Herpes simplex infection at term: What to do with mother, newborn, and nursery personnel. *JAMA.* 1980;243: 157-160.
36. Baker DA. Issues and management of herpes in pregnancy. *Int J Fertil Womens Med.* 2002;47:129-135.
37. Brown Z. Preventing herpes simplex virus transmission to the neonate. *Herpes.* 2004;11(Suppl 3):175A-186A.
38. Brown ZA, Selke S, Zeh J, et al. The acquisition of herpes simplex virus during pregnancy. *N Engl J Med.* 1997;337: 509-515.
39. Brown ZA, Wald A, Morrow RA, et al. Effect of serologic status and cesarean delivery on transmission rates of herpes simplex virus from mother to infant. *JAMA.* 2003;289:203-209.
40. Enright AM, Prober CG. Neonatal herpes infection: diagnosis, treatment and prevention. *Semin Neonatol.* 2002;7:283-291.
41. Eskild A, Jeansson S, Stray-Pedersen B, et al. Herpes simplex virus type-2 infection in pregnancy: no risk of fetal death: results from a nested case-control study within 35,940 women. *BJOG Brit J Obstet Gynecol.* 2002;109:1030-1035.
42. Money D, Steben M. Guidelines for the management of herpes simplex virus in pregnancy. *J Obstet Gynaecol Can.* 2008;30: 514-526.
43. Whitley RJ, Kimberlin DW. Treatment of viral infections during pregnancy and the neonatal period. *Clin Perinatol.* 1997;24: 267-283.
44. Garland SM. Neonatal herpes simplex: Royal Women's Hospital 10-year experience with management guidelines for herpes in pregnancy. *Aust N Z J Obstet Gynaecol.* 1992;32:331-334.
45. Gibbs RS, Mead PB. Preventing neonatal herpes—current strategies. *N Engl J Med.* 1992;326:946-947.
46. Apisarnthanarak A, Kitphati R, Tawatsupha P, et al. Outbreak of varicella-zoster virus infection among Thai healthcare workers. *Infect Control Hosp Epidemiol.* 2007;28:430-434.
47. Mandal BK, Mukherjee PP, Murphy C, et al. Adult susceptibility to varicella in the tropics is a rural phenomenon due to the lack of previous exposure. *J Infect Dis.* 1998;178(Suppl 1):S52-S54.
48. Nassar NT, Touma HC. Brief report: Susceptibility of Filipino nurses to the varicella zoster virus. *Infect Control.* 1986;7: 71-72.
49. Richard VS, John TJ, Kenneth J, et al. Should health care workers in the tropics be immunized against varicella? *J Hosp Infect.* 2001;47:243-245.
50. Marin M, Guris D, Chaves SS, et al. Prevention of varicella: recommendations of the Advisory Committee on Immunization Practices (ACIP). *MMWR Recomm Rep.* 2007;56(RR-4): 1-40.
51. Gardella C, Brown ZA. Managing varicella zoster infection in pregnancy. *Cleve Clin J Med.* 2007;74:290-296.
52. Harger JH, Ernest JM, Thurnau GR, et al. Risk factors and outcome of varicella-zoster virus pneumonia in pregnant women. *J Infect Dis.* 2002;185:422-427.
53. Gershon A, Steinberg S, Gelb L. Clinical reinfection with varicella zoster virus. *J Infect Dis.* 1984;149:137-142.
54. Lopez AS, Burnett-Hartman A, Nambiar R, et al. Transmission of a newly characterized strain of varicella-zoster virus from a patient with herpes zoster in a long-term-care facility, West Virginia, 2004. *J Infect Dis.* 2008;197:646-653.
55. Morens D, Bregman D, West M, et al. An outbreak of varicella-zoster virus infection among cancer patients. *Ann Intern Med.* 1980;93:414-419.
56. Schimpff S, Serpick A, Stoler B, et al. Varicella-zoster infection in patients with cancer. *Ann Intern Med.* 1972;76:241-254.
57. Hall S, Maupin T, Seward J, et al. Second varicella infections: are they more common than previously thought? *Pediatrics.* 2002;109:1068-1073.
58. Gustafson T, Lavely G, Brawner E, et al. An outbreak of airborne nosocomial varicella. *Pediatrics.* 1982;70:550-556.
59. Leclair J, Zaia J, Levin M, et al. Airborne transmission of chickenpox in a hospital. *N Engl J Med.* 1980;302:450-453.
60. Wreghitt TG, Whipp PJ, Bagnall J. Transmission of chickenpox to two intensive care unit nurses from a liver transplant patient with zoster. *J Hosp Infect.* 1992;20:125-126.
61. Asano Y, Iwayama S, Miyata T, et al. Spread of varicella in hospitalized children having no direct contact with an indicator zoster case and its prevention by a live vaccine. *Biken J.* 1980; 23:157-161.
62. Berlin B, Campbell T. Hospital-acquired herpes zoster following exposure to chickenpox. *JAMA.* 1970;211:1831-1833.
63. Feinstein A, Trau H, Schewach-Millet M. Herpes zoster in a husband and wife. *Int J Dermatol.* 1980;19:514-516.
64. Josephson A, Gombert ME. Airborne transmission of nosocomial varicella from localized zoster. *J Infect Dis.* 1988;158: 238-241.
65. Wreghitt TG, Whipp J, Redpath C, et al. An analysis of infection control of varicella-zoster virus infections in Addenbrooke's Hospital Cambridge over a 5-year period, 1987-92. *Epidemiol Infect.* 1996;117:165-171.
66. Garnett GP, Grenfell BT. The epidemiology of varicella-zoster virus infections: the influence of varicella on the prevalence of herpes zoster. *Epidemiol Infect.* 1992;108:513-528.
67. Harpaz R, Ortega-Sanchez IR, Seward JF. Prevention of herpes zoster: recommendations of the Advisory Committee on Immunization Practices (ACIP). *MMWR Recomm Rep.* 2008;57(RR-5):1-30; quiz CE32-CE34.
68. Hayden G, Meyers J, Dixon R. Nosocomial varicella: II. Suggested guidelines for management. *West J Med.* 1979;130: 300-303.
69. Josephson A, Karanfil L, Gombert ME. Strategies for the management of varicella-susceptible healthcare workers after a known exposure. *Infect Control Hosp Epidemiol.* 1990;11:309-313.
70. Laniak J, Myers R, Henderson D. Algorithm for the control of nosocomial varicella zoster virus infections. Paper presented at: Proceedings of the 82nd Annual Meeting of the American Society for Microbiology, 1982; Washington, D.C.
71. Sepkowitz KA. Occupationally acquired infections in health care workers. Part I. *Ann Intern Med.* 1996;125:826-834.
72. Weber D, Rutala W, Parnam C. Impact and costs of varicella prevention in a university hospital. *Am J Public Health.* 1988; 78:19-23.
73. Anderson J, Bonner M, Scheifele D, et al. Lack of nosocomial spread of varicella in a pediatric hospital with negative pressure ventilated rooms. *Infect Control.* 1985;6:120-121.
74. Centers for Disease Control and Prevention. A new product (VariZIG) for postexposure prophylaxis of varicella available under an investigational new drug application expanded access protocol. *MMWR Morb Mortal Wkly Rep.* 2006;55:209-210.
75. Weinstock DM, Boeckh M, Boulad F, et al. Postexposure prophylaxis against varicella-zoster virus infection among recipients of hematopoietic stem cell transplant: Unresolved issues. *Infect Control Hosp Epidemiol.* 2004;25:603-608.
76. Arvin AM. Management of varicella-zoster virus infections in children. *Adv Exp Med Biol.* 1999;458:167-174.
77. Arvin AM. Antiviral therapy for varicella and herpes zoster. *Semin Pediatr Infect Dis.* 2002;13:12-21.
78. Dwyer DE, Cunningham AL. 10: Herpes simplex and varicella-zoster virus infections. *Med J Aust.* 2002;177:267-273.
79. Waugh SM, Pillay D, Carrington D, et al. Antiviral prophylaxis and treatment (excluding HIV therapy). *J Clin Virol.* 2002;25: 241-266.
80. Balfour HH Jr. Intravenous acyclovir therapy for varicella in immunocompromised children. *J Pediatr.* 1984;104:134-136.
81. Nyerges G, Meszner Z, Gyarmati E, et al. Acyclovir prevents dissemination of varicella in immunocompromised children. *J Infect Dis.* 1988;157:309-313.
82. Prober CG, Kirk LE, Keeney RE. Acyclovir therapy of chickenpox in immunosuppressed children—a collaborative study. *J Pediatr.* 1982;101:622-625.
83. Grossberg R, Harpaz R, Rubtcova E, et al. Secondary transmission of varicella vaccine virus in a chronic care facility for children. *J Pediatr.* 2006;148:842-844.
84. Sharrar RG, LaRussa P, Galea SA, et al. The postmarketing safety profile of varicella vaccine. *Vaccine.* 2000;19:916-923.
85. Tsolia M, Gershon AA, Steinberg SP, et al. Live attenuated varicella vaccine: evidence that the virus is attenuated and the importance of skin lesions in transmission of varicella-zoster virus. National Institute of Allergy and Infectious Diseases Varicella Vaccine Collaborative Study Group. *J Pediatr.* 1990;116: 184-189.
86. Balfour H, Groth K, McCullough J, et al. Prevention or modification of varicella using zoster immune plasma. *Am J Dis Child.* 1977;131:693-696.
87. Williams V, Gershon A, Brunell P. Serologic response to varicella-zoster membrane antigens measured by indirect immunofluorescence. *J Infect Dis.* 1974;130:669-672.
88. Gershon A, Kalter Z, Steinberg S. Detection of antibody to varicella-zoster virus by immune adherence hemagglutination. *Proc Soc Exp Biol Med.* 1976;151:762.
89. Stanley J, Myers M, Edmond B, et al. An enzyme-linked immunosorbent assay for detection of antibody to varicella zoster virus. *J Clin Microbiol.* 1982;15:205-211.
90. Balfour HJ, Kelly JM, Suarez CS, et al. Acyclovir treatment of varicella in otherwise healthy children. *J Pediatr.* 1990;116:633-639.
91. Balfour HJ, Rotbart HA, Feldman S, et al. Acyclovir treatment of varicella in otherwise healthy adolescents. The Collaborative Acyclovir Varicella Study Group. *J Pediatr.* 1992;120:627-633.
92. Ogilvie MM. Antiviral prophylaxis and treatment in chickenpox. A review prepared for the UK Advisory Group on Chickenpox on behalf of the British Society for the Study of Infection. *J Infect.* 1998;36(Suppl 1):31-38.
93. Wallace MR, Bowler WA, Murray NB, et al. Treatment of adult varicella with oral acyclovir. A randomized, placebo-controlled trial. *Ann Intern Med.* 1992;117:358-363.
94. Rado J, Tako J, Geder L, et al. Herpes zoster house epidemic in steriod-treated patients. *Arch Intern Med.* 1965;116:329-335.
95. Gershon A, Steinberg S, Smith M. Cell-mediated immunity to varicella zoster virus demonstrated by viral inactivation with human leukocytes. *Infect Immun.* 1976;13:1549-1553.
96. Lussier N, Weiss K, Laverdiere M. Varicella-zoster screening and management programs in healthcare facilities in Canada. *Infect Control Hosp Epidemiol.* 1999;20:562-563.
97. O'Neill J, Buttery J. Varicella and paediatric staff: current practice and vaccine cost-effectiveness. *J Hosp Infect.* 2003;53:117-119.
98. Qureshi M, Gordon SM, Yen-Lieberman B, et al. Controlling varicella in the healthcare setting: barriers to varicella vaccination among healthcare workers. *Infect Control Hosp Epidemiol.* 1999;20:516-518.
99. Weber DJ, Rutala WA, Hamilton H. Prevention and control of varicella-zoster infections in healthcare facilities. *Infect Control Hosp Epidemiol.* 1996;17:694-705.
100. Ballard R, Drew L, Hufnagle K, et al. Acquired cytomegalovirus infection in preterm infants. *Am J Dis Child.* 1979;133: 482-485.
101. Spector S, Edwards D, Coen R. Association of acquired cytomegalovirus infections and bronchopulmonary dysplasia in premature infants. *Pediatr Res.* 1982;16:309.
102. Spector S, Schmidt W, Ticknor W, et al. Cytomegaloviruria in older infants in intensive care units. *J Pediatr.* 1979;59:444-446.
103. Yeager A, Grumet F, Hufleigh E, et al. Prevention of transfusion-acquired cytomegalovirus infections in newborn infants. *J Pediatr.* 1981;98:281-287.
104. Spector S, Spector D. Molecular epidemiology of cytomegalovirus infection in premature twin infants and their mother. *Pediatr Infect Dis.* 1982;1:405-409.
105. Singh N. Antiviral drugs for cytomegalovirus in transplant recipients: advantages of preemptive therapy. *Rev Med Virol.* 2006;16:281-287.
106. Glenn J. Cytomegalovirus infections following renal transplantation. *Infect Dis.* 1981;3:1151-1178.
107. Pollard R, Arvin A, Gamberg P, et al. Specific cell-mediated immunity and infections with herpes viruses in cardiac transplant recipients. *Am J Med.* 1982;73:679-687.
108. Hersman J, Meyers J, Thomas E, et al. The effect of granulocyte transfusions on the incidence of cytomegalovirus infection after allogeneic marrow transplantation. *Ann Intern Med.* 1982;96:149-152.
109. Serody JS, Shea TC. Prevention of infections in bone marrow transplant recipients. *Infect Dis Clin North Am.* 1997;11: 459-477.
110. Vij R, DiPersio JF, Venkatraman P, et al. Donor CMV serostatus has no impact on CMV viremia or disease when prophylactic granulocyte transfusions are given following allogeneic peripheral blood stem cell transplantation. *Blood.* 2003;101:2067-2069.
111. Winston D, Winston S, Howell C, et al. Cytomegalovirus infections associated with leukocyte transfusions. *Ann Intern Med.* 1980;93:671-675.
112. Armstrong J, Tarr G, Youngblood L, et al. Cytomegalovirus infection in children undergoing open heart surgery. *Yale J Biol Med.* 1976;49:83-91.
113. Prince A, Szmuness W, Millian S, et al. A serologic study of cytomegalovirus infections associated with blood transfusions. *N Engl J Med.* 1971;284:1125-1132.
114. Demmler G, Yow M, Spector S, et al. Nosocomial cytomegalovirus infections within two hospitals caring for infants and children. *J Infect Dis.* 1987;156:9-16.
115. Spector S. Transmission of cytomegalovirus among infants in hospital documented by restriction-endonuclease-digestion analyses. *Lancet.* 1983;1:378-381.
116. Bryant P, Morley C, Garland S, et al. Cytomegalovirus transmission from breast milk in premature babies: does it matter? *Arch Dis Child Fetal Neonatal Ed.* 2002;87:F75-F77.
117. Hayes K, Danks D, Gibas H. Brief recordings: Cytomegalovirus in human milk. *N Engl J Med.* 1972;287:177-178.
118. Stiehm ER, Keller MA. Breast milk transmission of viral disease. *Adv Nutr Res.* 2001;10:105-122.
119. Aitken C, Booth J, Booth M, et al. Molecular epidemiology and significance of a cluster of cases of CMV infection occurring on a special care baby unit. *J Hosp Infect.* 1996;34:183-189.
120. Yeager A. Longitudinal, serological study of cytomegalovirus infections in nurses and in personnel without patient contact. *J Clin Microbiol.* 1975;2:448-452.

121. Ahlfors K. Epidemiological studies of congenital cytomegalovirus infection. *Scand J Infect Dis.* 1982;34(Suppl):1-36.

122. Yow M, Lakeman A, Stagno S, et al. Use of restriction enzymes to investigate the source of a primary cytomegalovirus infection in a pediatric nurse. *Pediatrics.* 1982;70:713-716.

123. Wilfert C, Huang E, Stagno S. Restriction endonuclease analysis of cytomegalovirus deoxyribonucleic acid as an epidemiologic tool. *Pediatrics.* 1982;70:717-721.

124. Adler S, Baggett J, Wilson M, et al. Molecular epidemiology of cytomegalovirus in a nursery: Lack of evidence for nosocomial transmission. *Pediatr.* 1986;108:117-123.

125. Balfour C, Balfour H Jr. Cytomegalovirus is not an occupational risk for nurses in renal transplant and neonatal units. Results of a prospective surveillance study. *JAMA.* 1986;256:1909-1914.

126. Gerberding J, Bryant-LeBlanc C, Nelson K, et al. Risk of transmitting the human immunodeficiency virus, cytomegalovirus, and hepatitis B virus to health-care workers exposed to AIDS patients and AIDS-related conditions. *J Infect Dis.* 1987; 156:1-8.

127. Balcarek KB, Bagley R, Cloud GA, et al. Cytomegalovirus infection among employees of a children's hospital. No evidence for increased risk associated with patient care. *JAMA.* 1990;263: 840-844.

128. Dworsky M, Welch K, Cassady G, et al. Occupational risk for primary cytomegalovirus infection among pediatric health-care workers. *N Engl J Med.* 1983;309:950-953.

129. Pass R. Epidemiology and transmission of cytomegalovirus. *J Infect Dis.* 1985;152:243-248.

130. Takahashi R, Tagawa M, Sanjo M, et al. Severe postnatal cytomegalovirus infection in a very premature infant. *Neonatology.* 2007;92:236-239.

131. Lang D, Ebert P, Rodgers B, et al. Reduction of post-transfusion cytomegalovirus infection following use of leukocyte-depleted blood. *Transfusion.* 1977;17:391-395.

132. Ho M, Suwausirikul S, Dowling J, et al. The transplanted kidney as a source of cytomegalovirus infection. *N Engl J Med.* 1975;293:1109-1112.

133. Bowden RA. Transfusion-transmitted cytomegalovirus infection. *Hematol Oncol Clin North Am.* 1995;9:155-166.

134. Bowden RA, Slichter SJ, Sayers M, et al. A comparison of filtered leukocyte-reduced and cytomegalovirus (CMV) seronegative blood products for the prevention of transfusion-associated CMV infection after marrow transplant [see comments]. *Blood.* 1995;86:3598-3603.

135. Ho M. Epidemiology of cytomegalovirus infections. *Rev Infect Dis.* 1990;12(Suppl 7):S701-S710.

136. Betts R. Cytomegalovirus vaccine in renal transplants. *Ann Intern Med.* 1979;91:780-782.

137. Preiksaitis JK, Sandhu J, Strautman M. The risk of transfusion-acquired CMV infection in seronegative solid-organ transplant recipients receiving non–WBC-reduced blood components not screened for CMV antibody (1984 to 1996): experience at a single Canadian center. *Transfusion.* 2002;42:396-402.

138. Roback JD. CMV and blood transfusions. *Rev Med Virol.* 2002;12:211-219.

139. Sullivan KM, Dykewicz CA, Longworth DL, et al. Preventing opportunistic infections after hematopoietic stem cell transplantation: the Centers for Disease Control and Prevention, Infectious Diseases Society of America, and American Society for Blood and Marrow Transplantation Practice Guidelines and beyond. *Hematology (Am Soc Hematol Educ Program).* 2001: 392-421.

140. Brady M, Milan J, Anderson D, et al. Use of deglycerolized red blood cells to prevent post-transfusion infection with cytomegalovirus in neonates. *J Infect Dis.* 1984;150:334-339.

141. Nichols WG, Price TH, Gooley T, et al. Transfusion-transmitted cytomegalovirus infection after receipt of leukoreduced blood products. *Blood.* 2003;101:4195-4200.

142. Ziemann M, Krueger S, Maier AB, et al. High prevalence of cytomegalovirus DNA in plasma samples of blood donors in connection with seroconversion. *Transfusion.* 2007;47:1972-1983.

143. Barrett AJ, Mavroudis D, Tisdale J, et al. T cell–depleted bone marrow transplantation and delayed T cell add-back to control acute GVHD and conserve a graft-versus-leukemia effect. *Bone Marrow Transplant.* 1998;21:543-551.

144. Couriel D, Canosa J, Engler H, et al. Early reactivation of cytomegalovirus and high risk of interstitial pneumonitis following T-depleted BMT for adults with hematological malignancies. *Bone Marrow Transplant.* 1996;18:347-353.

145. Dazzi F, Goldman JM. Adoptive immunotherapy following allogeneic bone marrow transplantation. *Annu Rev Med.* 1998;49: 329-340.

146. Mavroudis DA, Read EJ, Molldrem J, et al. T cell–depleted granulocyte colony-stimulating factor (G-CSF) modified allogenic bone marrow transplantation for hematological malignancy improves graft CD34⁺ cell content but is associated with delayed pancytopenia. *Bone Marrow Transplant.* 1998;21:431-440.

147. Falagas ME, Snydman DR, Ruthazer R, et al. Cytomegalovirus immune globulin (CMVIG) prophylaxis is associated with increased survival after orthotopic liver transplantation. The Boston Center for Liver Transplantation CMVIG Study Group. *Clin Transplant.* 1997;11(5 Pt 1):432-437.

148. Kocher AA, Bonaros N, Dunkler D, et al. Long-term results of CMV hyperimmune globulin prophylaxis in 377 heart transplant recipients. *J Heart Lung Transplant.* 2003;22:250-257.

149. Morales E, Andres A, Gonzalez E, et al. Prophylaxis of cytomegalovirus disease with ganciclovir or anti-CMV immunoglobulin in renal transplant recipients who receive antilymphocytic antibodies as induction therapy. *Transplant Proc.* 2002;34:73-74.

150. Nakamura R, Cortez K, Solomon S, et al. High-dose acyclovir and pre-emptive ganciclovir to prevent cytomegalovirus disease in myeloablative and non-myeloablative allogeneic stem cell transplantation. *Bone Marrow Transplant.* 2002;30:235-242.

151. Valantine HA, Luikart H, Doyle R, et al. Impact of cytomegalovirus hyperimmune globulin on outcome after cardiothoracic transplantation: a comparative study of combined prophylaxis with CMV hyperimmune globulin plus ganciclovir versus ganciclovir alone. *Transplantation.* 2001;72:1647-1652.

152. van der Bij W, Speich R. Management of cytomegalovirus infection and disease after solid-organ transplantation. *Clin Infect Dis.* 2001;33(Suppl 1):S32-S37.

153. Zamora MR. Use of cytomegalovirus immune globulin and ganciclovir for the prevention of cytomegalovirus disease in lung transplantation. *Transpl Infect Dis.* 2001;3(Suppl 2):49-56.

154. Henderson D. Nosocomial herpesvirus infections. In: Mandell G, Douglas R, Bennett J, eds. *Principles and Practice of Infectious Diseases.* New York: Churchill Livingstone; 1985:1630-1637.

155. Centers for Disease Control. Recommendation for prevention of HIV transmission in health-care settings. *MMWR.* 1987;36(Suppl 2):1-18.

156. Department of Labor (OSHA). Occupational exposure to bloodborne pathogens; final rule. *Federal Register.* 1991;56: 64175-64182.

157. Centers for Disease Control. Update: Universal precautions for prevention of transmission of human immunodeficiency virus, hepatitis B virus, and other bloodborne pathogens in health care settings. *MMWR.* 1988;37:277-282, 287-278.

158. Adler S. Nosocomial transmission of cytomegalovirus. *Pediatr Infect Dis.* 1986;5:239-246.

159. Onorato I, Morens D, Martone W, et al. Epidemiology of cytomegalovirus infections: Recommendations for prevention and control. *Rev Infect Dis.* 1985;7:479-497.

160. Plotkin S. Cytomegalovirus in hospitals. *Pediatr Infect Dis.* 1986;5:177-178.

161. Blacklow N, Watson B, Miller G, et al. Mononucleosis with heterophil antibodies: Epstein-Barr virus infection acquisition by an elderly patient in hospital. *Am J Med.* 1971;51:549-552.

162. Chang R, Rosen L, Kapikian A. Epstein-Barr virus infections in a nursery. *Am J Epidemiol.* 1981;113:22-29.

163. Corey L, Stamm W, Feorino P, et al. HBsAg-negative hepatitis in a hemodialysis unit: Relation of Epstein-Barr virus. *N Engl J Med.* 1975;293:1273-1278.

164. Gerber P, Walsh J, Rosenblum E, et al. Association of Epstein-Barr infection with the post-perfusion syndrome. *Lancet.* 1969;1:593-595.

165. Ginsburg C, Henle G, Henle W. An outbreak of infectious mononucleosis among the personnel in an outpatient clinic. *Am J Epidemiol.* 1976;104:571-575.

166. Henle W, Henle G, Harrison F, et al. Antibody responses to the Epstein-Barr virus and cytomegalovirus after open-heart and other surgery. *N Engl J Med.* 1970;282:1068-1074.

167. Purtilo D, Paquin L, Sakamota K, et al. Persistent transfusion-associated infectious mononucleosis with transient acquired immunodeficiency. *Am J Med.* 1980;68:437-440.

168. Solem J, Jorgensen W. Accidentally transmitted infectious mononucleosis: Report of a case. *Acta Med Scand.* 1969;186: 433-437.

169. Sullivan J, Wallen W, Johnson F. Epstein-Barr virus infection following bone-marrow transplantation. *Int J Cancer.* 1978;22: 132-135.

170. Tattevin P, Cremieux AC, Descamps D, et al. Transfusion-related infectious mononucleosis. *Scand J Infect Dis.* 2002;34: 777-778.

171. Turner A, MacDonald R, Cooper B. Transmission of infectious mononucleosis by transfusion of pre-illness plasma. *Ann Intern Med.* 1972;77:751-753.

172. Virolainen M, Anderson L, Lalla M, et al. T-lymphocyte proliferation in mononucleosis. *Clin Immunol Immunopathol.* 1973; 2:114-120.

173. Cohen JI. Benign and malignant Epstein-Barr virus–associated B-cell lymphoproliferative diseases. *Semin Hematol.* 2003;40: 116-123.

174. Patel R, Paya CV. Infections in solid-organ transplant recipients. *Clin Microbiol Rev.* 1997;10:86-124.

175. Yachie A, Kanegane H, Kasahara Y. Epstein-Barr virus–associated T-/natural killer cell lymphoproliferative diseases. *Semin Hematol.* 2003;40:124-132.

176. Herbert AM, Bagg J, Walker DM, et al. Seroepidemiology of herpes virus infections among dental personnel. *J Dent.* 1995; 23:339-342.

177. Cen H, Breinig MC, Atchison RW, et al. Epstein-Barr virus transmission via the donor organs in solid organ transplantation: polymerase chain reaction and restriction fragment length polymorphism analysis of IR2, IR3, and IR4. *J Virol.* 1991;65:976-980.

178. Epstein JB, Phillips K, Sherlock CH. Viral serology after bone marrow transplantation. *Viral Immunol.* 1991;4:133-137.

179. Junker AK, Thomas EE, Radcliffe A, et al. Epstein-Barr virus shedding in breast milk. *Am J Med Sci.* 1991;302:220-223.

180. Centers for Disease Control. *Isolation Techniques for Use in Hospitals.* 2nd ed. Washington, D.C.: Government Printing Office; 1975.

181. Heslop HE, Rooney CM. Adoptive cellular immunotherapy for EBV lymphoproliferative disease. *Immunol Rev.* 1997;157: 217-222.

182. Little RF, Yarchoan R. Treatment of gammaherpesvirus-related neoplastic disorders in the immunosuppressed host. *Semin Hematol.* 2003;40(Apr):163-171.

183. O'Reilly RJ, Lacerda JF, Lucas KG, et al. Adoptive cell therapy with donor lymphocytes for EBV-associated lymphomas developing after allogeneic marrow transplants. *Important Adv Oncol.* 1996:149-166.

184. Miller G, Niederman J, Andrews L. Prolonged oropharyngeal excretion of Epstein-Barr virus after infectious mononucleosis. *N Engl J Med.* 1973;288:229-232.

185. Yamanishi K, Shiraki K, Kondo T, et al. Identification of human herpesvirus-6 as a causal agent for *Exanthem subitum. Lancet.* 1988;1:1065-1067.

186. Irving WL, Chang J, Raymond DR, et al. *Roseola infantum* and other syndromes associated with acute HHV6 infection. *Arch Dis Child.* 1990;65:1297-1300.

187. Hall CB, Long CE, Schnabel KC, et al. Human herpesvirus-6 infection in children. A prospective study of complications and reactivation. *N Engl J Med.* 1994;331:432-438.

188. Frenkel N, Schirmer EC, Wyatt LS, et al. Isolation of a new herpesvirus from human CD4⁺ T cells. *Proc Natl Acad Sci U S A.* 1990;87:748-752.

189. Frenkel N, Wyatt LS. HHV-6 and HHV-7 as exogenous agents in human lymphocytes. *Dev Biol Stand.* 1992;76:259-265.

190. Wyatt LS, Frenkel N. Human herpesvirus-7 is a constitutive inhabitant of adult human saliva. *J Virol.* 1992;66:3206-3209.

191. Baillargeon J, Piper J, Leach CT. Epidemiology of human herpesvirus 6 (HHV-6) infection in pregnant and nonpregnant women. *J Clin Virol.* 2000;16:149-157.

192. Caserta MT, Hall CB, Schnabel K, et al. Human herpesvirus (HHV)-6 and HHV-7 infections in pregnant women. *J Infect Dis.* 2007;196:1296-1303.

193. Fujisaki H, Tanaka-Taya K, Tanabe H, et al. Detection of human herpesvirus 7 (HHV-7) DNA in breast milk by polymerase chain reaction and prevalence of HHV-7 antibody in breast-fed and bottle-fed children. *J Med Virol.* 1998;56:275-279.

194. Cone RW, Huang ML, Ashley R, et al. Human herpesvirus 6 DNA in peripheral blood cells and saliva from immunocompetent individuals. *J Clin Microbiol.* 1994;32:2633.

195. Pereira CM, Gasparetto PF, Correa ME, et al. Human herpesvirus 6 in oral fluids from healthy individuals. *Arch Oral Biol.* 2004;49(Dec):1043-1046.

196. Takahashi Y, Yamada M, Nakamura J, et al. Transmission of human herpesvirus 7 through multigenerational families in the same household. *Pediatr Infect Dis J.* 1997;16:975-978.

197. Di Luca D, Mirandola P, Ravaioli T, et al. Human herpesviruses 6 and 7 in salivary glands and shedding in saliva of healthy and human immunodeficiency virus positive individuals. *J Med Virol.* 1995;45:462-468.

198. Yadav M, Nambiar S, Khoo SP, et al. Detection of human herpesvirus 7 in salivary glands. *Arch Oral Biol.* 1997;42:559-567.

199. Freitas RB, Monteiro TA, Linhares AC. Outbreaks of human-herpes virus 6 (HHV-6) infection in day-care centers in Belem, Para, Brazil. *Rev Inst Med Trop Sao Paulo.* 2000;42:305-311.

200. Okuno T, Mukai T, Baba K, et al. Outbreak of exanthem subitum in an orphanage. *J Pediatr.* 1991;119:759-761.

201. Ambroziak JA, Blackbourn DJ, Herndier BG, et al. Herpes-like sequences in HIV-infected and uninfected Kaposi's sarcoma patients. *Science.* 1995;268:582-583.

202. Chang Y, Cesarman E, Pessin MS, et al. Identification of herpesvirus-like DNA sequences in AIDS-associated Kaposi's sarcoma. *Science.* 1994;266:1865-1869.

203. Cannon MJ, Dollard SC, Smith DK, et al. Blood-borne and sexual transmission of human herpesvirus 8 in women with or at risk for human immunodeficiency virus infection. *N Engl J Med.* 2001;344:637-643.

204. Dukers NH, Renwick N, Prins M, et al. Risk factors for human herpesvirus 8 seropositivity and seroconversion in a cohort of homosexual men. *Am J Epidemiol.* 2000;151:213-224.

205. Martin JN, Ganem DE, Osmond DH, et al. Sexual transmission and the natural history of human herpesvirus 8 infection. *N Engl J Med.* 1998;338:948-954.

206. Melbye M, Cook PM, Hjalgrim H, et al. Risk factors for Kaposi's sarcoma–associated herpesvirus (KSHV/HHV-8) seropositivity in a cohort of homosexual men, 1981-1996. *Int J Cancer.* 1998; 77:543-548.

207. Blackbourn DJ, Ambroziak J, Lennette E, et al. Infectious human herpesvirus 8 in a healthy North American blood donor. *Lancet.* 1997;349:609-611.

208. Engels EA, Eastman H, Ablashi DV, et al. Risk of transfusion-associated transmission of human herpesvirus 8. *J Natl Cancer Inst.* 1999;91:1773-1775.

209. Cattani P, Capuano M, Cerimele F, et al. Human herpesvirus 8 seroprevalence and evaluation of nonsexual transmission routes by detection of DNA in clinical specimens from human immunodeficiency virus–seronegative patients from central and southern Italy, with and without Kaposi's sarcoma. *J Clin Microbiol.* 1999;37:1150-1153.

210. Pauk J, Huang ML, Brodie SJ, et al. Mucosal shedding of human herpesvirus 8 in men. *N Engl J Med.* 2000;343:1369-1377.

308

Infections in the Immunocompromised Host: General Principles

J. PETER DONNELLY | NICOLE M. A. BLIJLEVENS | BEN E. De PAUW

An intact defense system offers protection against most microbial aggressors through a complex interrelationship of protecting surfaces, cells, and soluble factors. Optimal nutritional status and normal organ function, together with granulocytes, macrophages, antibodies, complement, and other components of the cellular and humoral immune system, provide protection against potentially pathogenic microorganisms. The resident flora normally does not cause infection or alert the immune system, and it may protect against pathogens by competing for binding sites on the surfaces and for the available nutrients.

Infection is a principal cause of morbidity and mortality of immunocompromised patients. Hence, a comprehensive understanding of the possible causes of infectious complications and the predisposing factors involved, as well as a comprehensive anti-infective strategy, is imperative when offering these patients care. The physician attending to immunocompromised patients has to be particularly aware of all potential risk factors for infection, including those related to the underlying disease and its treatment, because although susceptibility to infection is increased, timely diagnosis is difficult.

Deficiencies in Components of Host Defenses

Appreciation of the predisposing risk factors is an essential but perplexing exercise in that it suggests that each individual component plays an independent role. Certain organisms infect patients with specific defects, and these associations should be taken into account when selecting therapy. However, this is by no means always predictable. Theoretically, a specific deficiency increases the patient's susceptibility to the very pathogens that are eradicated by that particular host defense mechanism (Table 308-1). Although a basic pattern is recognizable, the types and severity of infectious complications are often unpredictable. Single, isolated deficiencies are infrequently encountered, and malfunction of one part of the system often influences several other components. Moreover, therapeutic interventions and the underlying disease will perturb a range of defense mechanisms. Although the risks associated with granulocytopenia are well-known, other toxicities, especially those affecting the mucosal barrier, are considered to be of greater importance than was previously the case. The advent of aggressive treatments has altered the classic concept of specific defects of host defense mechanisms in the various types of diseases because the effects of antineoplastic chemotherapy and irradiation are now seen as the primary factors determining the nature and extent of the defect. Also, transplantation (especially stem cells) can cause defects in host immunity via graft-versus-host interactions as well as immune suppressive chemotherapy. Patients with impaired humoral immunity as manifested by defective opsonization and phagocytosis of bacteria will also be exposed to chemotherapy-induced neutropenia or deficient cellular immunity as a result of treatment with purine analogues or monoclonal antibodies for treating malignancies.

GRANULOCYTES

In normal circumstances, neutrophils, sometimes accompanied by eosinophils, congregate at the site of inflammation and are followed by macrophages. Formation of this inflammatory exudate is the result of activation of humoral factors and normal function of the vascular endothelium (see Chapter 8). Meanwhile, in the peripheral blood, granulocytosis evolves as a consequence of release of the marrow reserve and increased granulocytopoiesis, which is regulated by hematopoietic growth factors such as interleukin (IL)-3, granulocyte-macrophage colony-stimulating factor, and granulocyte colony-stimulating factor.

Virtually all cytotoxic drugs used in the treatment of malignant diseases have a deleterious effect on the proliferation of normal hematopoietic progenitor cells. Therefore, after obliteration of the mitotic pool and depletion of the marrow pool reserve, granulocytopenia ensues. Likewise, therapeutic radiation can induce clinically important granulocytopenia, depending on the dose rate, total dose given, and irradiated area of the body. Total body irradiation, as used to prepare for a hematopoietic stem cell (HSC) transplant, is the most obvious illustration of the possible negative impact of irradiation. Thus, profound neutropenia is an unavoidable consequence of the treatment of malignancy and may persist for 3 or 4 weeks or even longer. Granulocytopenia or a treatment-related decrease in the granulocyte count is probably the most important primary risk factor for infection. Fever develops in nearly all cases of profound granulocytopenia (i.e., a granulocyte count $<100/mm^3$ for more than 3 weeks), whereas only one fifth of the febrile episodes in cancer patients occur when granulocyte counts are normal.[1] Moreover, during iatrogenic granulocytopenia, the risk of infection and infection-related mortality increases proportionally with time.

Granulocytes that accumulate at the site of infection are of little use if they are unable to function normally. Antineoplastic drugs and irradiation each interfere with these nonproliferating cells and their function, resulting in decreased chemotaxis, diminished phagocytic capacity, and defective intracellular killing by granulocytes. Glucocorticosteroids seem to enhance granulocytopoiesis and mobilize the marginal and the marrow pool reserve, but these putative positive effects on neutrophilic granulocytes are offset by numerous disadvantages. These drugs curb the accumulation of neutrophils at the site of inflammation by reducing their adherent capacity and diminishing their chemotactic activity. Furthermore, they decrease phagocytosis and intracellular killing of microorganisms. The lack of functioning neutrophils deprives the host of a primary defense mechanism against invading microorganisms, which are consequently able to readily establish themselves, initiate local infection, disseminate unhindered, and eventually lead to fulminant sepsis and death unless treated promptly and effectively.

CELLULAR AND HUMORAL IMMUNITY

The host defense against pathogenic microorganisms encompasses innate and acquired immunity. The innate immune system comprises both cellular components, including monocytes, neutrophils, and natural killer cells, and humoral components, including complement, some antibodies ("natural" antibodies, perhaps directed against normal flora), and lysozyme. This mechanism is very effective in dealing with the vast majority of infectious agents. It has become clear that the innate immune system not only specifically recognizes various classes of microorganisms via pattern recognition receptors (pathogen-associated-molecular patterns) that sense conserved structures of the invading microorganisms but also initiates and modulates the

TABLE 308-1	Immunodeficiencies and Associated Prevalent Pathogens
Defect	**Pathogen**
Granulocytopenia	Gram-positive cocci
	Staphylococcus aureus
	Coagulase-negative staphylococci (*epidermidis, haemolyticus, hominis*)
	Viridans group streptococci (*mitis, oralis*)
	Granulicatella and *Abiotrophia* species (formerly nutritionally variant streptococci)
	Enterococci (*faecalis, faecium*)
	Gram-negative bacilli
	Escherichia coli
	Pseudomonas aeruginosa
	Klebsiella pneumoniae
	Enterobacter and *Citrobacter* species
Damaged integument	
Skin–central venous catheter related	Coagulase-negative staphylococci (*epidermidis, haemolyticus, hominis*)
	Staphylococcus aureus
	Stenotrophomonas maltophilia
	Pseudomonas aeruginosa
	Acinetobacter species
	Corynebacteria
	Candida species (*albicans, parapsilosis*)
	Rhizopus species
Oral mucositis	Viridans group streptococci (*mitis, oralis*)
	Abiotrophia and *Granulicatella* species (nutritionally variant streptococci)
	Capnocytophaga species
	Fusobacterium species
	Rothia mucilaginosa
	Candida species (*albicans, tropicalis, glabrata*)
	Herpes simplex virus
Gut mucosal barrier injury	*Escherichia coli*
	Pseudomonas aeruginosa
	Coagulase-negative staphylococci
	Enterococci (*faecalis, faecium*)
	Candida species
Neutropenic enterocolitis	*Clostridium* species (*septicum, tertium*)
	Staphylococcus aureus
	Pseudomonas aeruginosa
Impaired cellular immunity	Herpesviruses
	Cytomegalovirus
	Respiratory viruses
	Listeria monocytogenes
	Nocardia species
	Mycobacterium tuberculosis
	Nontuberculous mycobacteria
	Pneumocystis jirovecii
	Aspergillus species
	Cryptococcus species
	Histoplasma capsulatum
	Coccidioides species
	Penicillium marneffei
	Toxoplasma gondii
Impaired humoral immunity	*Streptococcus pneumoniae*
	Haemophilus influenzae
Compromised organ function	
Spleen	*Streptococcus pneumoniae*
	Haemophilus influenzae
	Neisseria meningitidis
Deferoxamine for iron overload	*Rhizopus* species

subsequent adaptive responses delivered by T cells and B cells by their interaction with antigen-presenting cells (especially dendritic cells).

Normal macrophages have a limited capacity for killing ingested microorganisms, and various organisms are able to survive and replicate inside the cell, unless the macrophage becomes activated. Activation of macrophages is a complex process primarily under the control of cytokines. Both antigen-specific and antigen-nonspecific cells contribute to the development of cellular immunity. The antigen-specific branch of cell-mediated immunity can be divided into two major categories. One category involves cytotoxic effector cells, which are able to lyse virus-infected or foreign lymphocytes and macrophages. The second category involves subpopulations of T cells that mediate delayed-type hypersensitivity reactions after antigen recognition when an antigen is displayed together with the major histocompatibility complex on the surface of specialized antigen-presenting cells.

This fine-tuned system can easily be deregulated by congenital defects or defects acquired as a result of a disease or its treatment. Long-term cytotoxic therapy, extensive irradiation, and immunosuppressive drugs such as corticosteroids, azathioprine, cyclosporine, tacrolimus, sirolimus, and everolimus suppress cellular immunity. Some monoclonal antibodies, such as alemtuzumab and rituximab, are being used as antitumor and immunosuppressive agents and can exert profound and prolonged effects on cellular immunity. Purine analogues, including fludarabine and cladribine, are particularly detrimental to cellular immunity and create a situation similar to acquired immunodeficiency syndrome. Likewise, malignant lymphomas, particularly Hodgkin's disease, are associated with impaired cellular immunity. Allogeneic HSC transplantation brings about a long-lasting dysfunction of T and B cells, especially in association with graft-versus-host disease and its treatment (Table 308-2). The coordination of cellular immunity is often lost, and when aided and abetted by suppressed humoral immunity, the paracrine mediators released go on to induce the sepsis cascade, which may culminate in multiorgan failure instead of arresting infection.[2]

The humoral branch of the immune system, which is primarily responsible for clearing extracellular bacteria, involves the interaction of B cells with antigen and their subsequent proliferation and differentiation into antibody-secreting plasma cells (see Chapter 6). An important difference in antigen recognition by T cells and B cells is that the latter can recognize some antigens without the help of an antigen-presenting cell. The humoral system can identify a plethora of bacterial or viral microorganisms, as well as the soluble proteins that they release. When challenged by an antigen, immunoglobulins are produced that bind to the antigen. The specific functions of immunoglobulin G and immunoglobulin M (IgM) include neutralization of the antigen as well as complement activation and opsonization—that is, enhancement of phagocytosis of the antigen by neutrophils and macrophages. Secretory immunoglobulin A (IgA), which is found on mucosal surfaces, is not an opsonin but nonetheless inhibits the motility of bacteria and prevents them from adhering to epithelial cells. The production of immunoglobulins is decreased in lymphoproliferative disorders such as chronic lymphocytic leukemia and multiple myeloma, whereas humoral immunity is generally well preserved in patients with acute leukemia. However, intensive radiotherapy and chemotherapy will lead not only to neutropenia but also ultimately to hypogammaglobulinemia.

The spleen is the principal organ for eliminating microbes that are not opsonized, such as encapsulated bacteria. Macrophages that occupy strategic positions within the organ are able to remove them. The primary immunoglobulin response also takes place in the spleen. Spleen-produced specific opsonizing antibodies are necessary for efficient phagocytosis of encapsulated bacteria. Splenectomy may result in a reduced level of the complement factor properdin and thereby lead to suboptimal opsonization,[3] a decrease in functional tuftsin, and low levels of circulating IgM.[4] The lack of opsonizing antibodies in serum against common encapsulated bacteria impairs the activity of all phagocytic cells, including granulocytes, monocytes, and macrophages. As a consequence, infections with *Streptococcus pneumoniae*

TABLE 308-2	Sequence of Infective Events in Relation to the Phases of Allogeneic Stem Cell Transplantation		
	Early Phase	Mid-recovery Phase	Late Phase
Host Defense Mechanisms without Graft-versus-Host Disease			
Phagocytes	Absent	Deficient	Normal
Integument			
Skin	Damaged	Damaged	Intact
Mucous membranes	Severely damaged	Damaged	Intact
Cellular immunity	Slightly impaired	Impaired	Impaired
Humoral immunity	Normal	Impaired	Severely impaired
Host Defense Mechanisms with Graft-versus-Host Disease			
Phagocytes	Absent	Deficient	Normal
Integument			
Skin	Damaged	Damaged	Damaged
Mucous membranes	Damaged	Severely damaged	Damaged
Cellular immunity	Slightly impaired	Severely impaired	Severely impaired
Humoral immunity	Normal	Impaired	Severely impaired
Prevalent Infections			
Mucosa	Herpes simplex virus	Herpes simplex virus	Herpes simplex virus
	Viridans streptococci	*Candida* species	*Candida* species
	Coagulase-negative staphylococci		
Lung	Gram-negative bacilli	Cytomegalovirus	*Streptococcus pneumoniae*
	Aspergillus species	*Aspergillus* species	Viruses
			Pneumocystis jirovecii
Blood	Viridans streptococci	Staphylococci	
	Staphylococci	*Streptococcus pneumoniae*	
	Gram-negative bacilli	*Candida* species	*Neisseria meningitidis*
	Candida species		

and *Haemophilus influenzae* are often more severe in splenectomized patients, as well as in those who have received an HSC transplant and are functionally asplenic.

PHYSICAL BARRIERS: THE INTEGUMENT

The skin, the respiratory tract (including the nasal cavity), the ears and conjunctiva, the alimentary tract, and the genitourinary tract are in contact with the environment (Fig. 308-1) and provide a first line of defense against microbial invasion. The skin and the mucosal surfaces of the alimentary and respiratory tracts form principal barriers against microbial invasion. These surfaces are normally colonized with a variety of microorganisms, including many different genera of bacteria and yeast that have an intimate association with a particular ecologic niche and help maintain the function and integrity of this first line of defense. When intact and healthy, both the mucosa and the skin are capable of resisting colonization with the allochthonous organisms found in the immediate environment, as long as an ecologic balance is maintained within the indigenous microbial flora. Acidity plays a crucial role both in disinfecting the stomach and in regulating the microbial milieu of the vagina. The integrity of the mucosa, production of saliva and mucus, peristalsis, bile acids, digestive enzymes, and levels of defensins, trefoil factors, and secretory IgA also play an important role in maintaining a favorable microecology.[5,6] Elimination of an inoculum is achieved by sneezing and coughing of microbes trapped in mucus, whereas flushing of the mouth and esophagus by saliva, as well as micturition and peristalsis, inhibits continuous intimate contact between a given surface area and unattached invasive microorganisms.

The Skin

Healthy skin provides an effective barrier against invasion by microorganisms, mainly by remaining intact. Desquamation helps limit the opportunities for transient organisms to establish residence. Normally, very little water is present on the skin surface. Colonization with organisms sensitive to desiccation, such as gram-negative bacilli, is not favored. The skin also forms an acid mantle with a pH of 5.0 to 6.0, and its surface temperature is on average approximately 5° C lower than the core body temperature.[7] Besides containing secretory IgA, sweat also possesses sufficient salt to create a high osmotic pressure. Organisms that can withstand these conditions and compete successfully for binding sites and nutrients include staphylococci, corynebacteria, and the lipophilic yeast *Malassezia furfur*.[7] These organisms further modulate the microecology of the skin by releasing fatty acids from sebaceous secretions to produce a hydrophobic milieu as well as lactic and propionic acids, which help maintain a low pH. Many of the bacteria also elaborate bacteriocins that inhibit other microorganisms.

The composition of the skin microflora is influenced by general factors including climate, body location, age, sex, race, and occupation, as well as by the use of soaps, detergents, and disinfectants. Antibiotics secreted in sweat disturb the balance within the commensal flora and leave the surface vulnerable to colonization by exogenous gram-negative bacilli. Antibiotics also exert selective pressure on the skin flora and cause resistance to emerge, as has been observed during treatment with ciprofloxacin.[8] Moreover, ciprofloxacin is excreted in sweat and induces resistance among skin staphylococci within a few days of exposure.[9,10] β-Lactam antibiotics, including ceftazidime, ceftriaxone, cefuroxime, benzylpenicillin, and phenoxymethylpenicillin (penicillin V), can also be found in sweat, which might explain the ready selection of resistant staphylococci.[11] Chemotherapy and irradiation can bring about radical changes in healthy skin that cause hair loss, dryness, and loss of sweat production.

Needle punctures and catheters provide a ready means of access for microorganisms through the stratum corneum and into the bloodstream. When the skin is broken, the release of fibronectin is thought to assist colonization with *Staphylococcus aureus*, whereas other changes facilitate colonization with gram-negative bacilli such as *Acinetobacter baumannii* and enteric bacteria. Abraded skin can lead to local infection, which can be a reservoir that promotes further spread to entry sites of intravenous catheters. When the balance is lost between

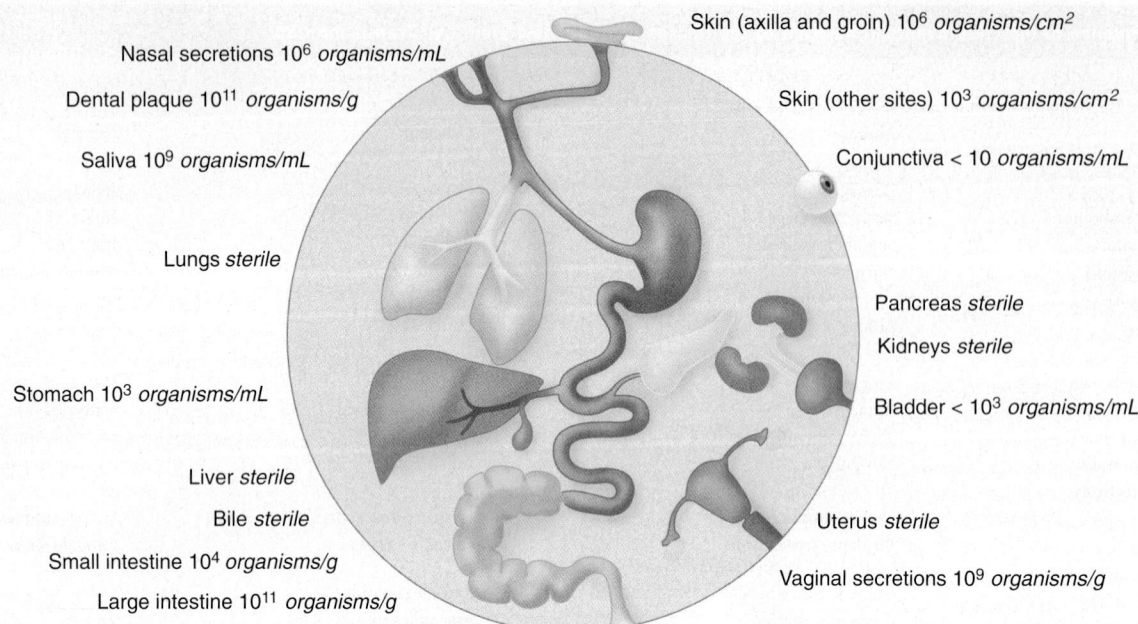

Nasal secretions 10^6 *organisms/mL*

Dental plaque 10^{11} *organisms/g*

Saliva 10^9 *organisms/mL*

Lungs *sterile*

Stomach 10^3 *organisms/mL*

Liver *sterile*

Bile *sterile*

Small intestine 10^4 *organisms/g*

Large intestine 10^{11} *organisms/g*

Skin (axilla and groin) 10^6 *organisms/cm²*

Skin (other sites) 10^3 *organisms/cm²*

Conjunctiva < 10 *organisms/mL*

Pancreas *sterile*

Kidneys *sterile*

Bladder < 10^3 *organisms/mL*

Uterus *sterile*

Vaginal secretions 10^9 *organisms/g*

Figure 308-1 **Body surfaces and their resident microbial flora.** The integument comprises the skin, the respiratory tract (including the nasal cavity, ears, and conjunctivae), the alimentary tract, and the genitourinary tract and provides the first line of defense against microbial invasion. These body surfaces are normally colonized with a variety of microorganisms, including many different genera of bacteria and yeasts, but the range, number of species, and microbial biomass associated with the mucosal surfaces of the alimentary tract far exceed those of the skin. *(From Noskin GA, ed. Management of Infectious Complications in Cancer Patients. Boston: Kluwer Academic; 1998.)*

host defenses and commensal flora around hair follicles, the follicles can become inflamed and necrotic and form a potential nidus of infection. Clinical infection therefore results from breaks in the skin, loss of local immunity, and disturbances within the resident flora.

Vascular devices have gained widespread acceptance as a relatively safe form of long-term venous access, but regular use is associated with a marked increase in the incidence of bacteremia with coagulase-negative staphylococci, which frequently colonize the catheter lumen.[12,13] These staphylococci are commonly resistant to aminoglycosides, trimethoprim-sulfamethoxazole, and penicillinase-resistant penicillins and may also be resistant to fluoroquinolones.[14] Unless the catheter ends in an implanted port, skin commensal flora have potential access into the bloodstream. The hub is the most likely source of contamination leading to catheter colonization,[15] and the risk increases with use.[16] Infections related to the external surface of the catheter (exit-site infections and tunnel infections) can result in serious soft tissue infection, most notably by *S. aureus.* Exit-site infections occur much less frequently than does intraluminal contamination. The latter may be caused by a variety of bacteria, many of which have relatively low virulence. Once established, these infections can be very difficult to treat without removing the device, particularly those caused by *Bacillus* spp., *Candida* spp., and *Pseudomonas aeruginosa.*[17-20]

The Alimentary Tract

Microbial Flora. Anaerobic bacteria predominate among the resident flora of the oral cavity and large intestine population and play a crucial role in maintaining a healthy commensal flora by providing the facility to withstand the establishment of exogenous organisms, which is known as colonization resistance.[21] However, the microbial flora is not the only participant in the establishment and maintenance of colonization resistance.

Many antibiotics also exert a negative influence on the commensal flora. Very susceptible bacteria such as the oral *Neisseria* spp. are suppressed by a wide range of antimicrobial agents, whereas oral viridans streptococci of the *mitis* group, such as *Streptococcus mitis* and *Streptococcus oralis,*[22] and other unusual oral commensal flora such as

Rothia mucilaginosa and *Capnocytophaga* spp. are likely to be selected by antimicrobial agents, to which the bacteria are only marginally susceptible, if at all. In particular, penicillins, rifampin, clindamycin, macrolides, bacitracin, and vancomycin significantly impair colonization resistance, probably because they inhibit the gram-positive nonsporulating, lactic acid-producing bacilli such as bifidobacteria.[23] Certain cephalosporins are also detrimental, whereas trimethoprim-sulfamethoxazole and the quinolones have been declared "friendly"; hence their frequent use as prophylaxis.[23] Unexpectedly, imipenem used at higher doses led to an increase in diarrhea caused by *Clostridium difficile.*[24] Newer antibiotics such as tigecycline with activity against anaerobic gram-positive bacteria may lead to increases in the numbers of *Candida.* This change usually reflects marked perturbations of the gut ecology.[25] However, this effect does not increase the risk of infection due to *C. difficile.*[26] Chlorhexidine mouthwashes used to minimize plaque and gingivitis also influence the microflora.[27-29]

Because the normal commensal flora attach to the surfaces of the epithelium, their loss creates an ecologic vacuum that allows other organisms to establish colonization by occupying the vacant cell surfaces or by taking advantage of the surfeit of nutrients. Collapse of the ecology is invariably manifested by yeast overgrowth and colonization with nosocomial bacteria such as *Klebsiella pneumoniae* and *P. aeruginosa*[30-33] and failure to detect viable anaerobes directly or indirectly.[30,31] Examples of infectious complications associated with disturbance of the normal microbial equilibrium include the selection of previously uncommon species such as *Enterococcus faecium* and *Clostridium septicum.*

Dyspepsia is sufficiently commonplace for antacids such as H2 blockers and proton pump inhibitors to be regularly prescribed. Reduced gastric acidity inadvertently destroys the natural barrier that prevents gastric and intestinal colonization by oral commensal flora, many of which are resistant to most of the antimicrobial agents used for prophylaxis in impaired hosts. When patients swallow large amounts of mucus as a result of severe mucositis, any oral commensal flora may survive passage to the bowel. Loss of the gastric barrier therefore effectively extends the area of potential sites for colonization to the full length of the alimentary tract, which may explain the pathogenesis of α-hemolytic (viridans group) streptococcal bacteremia.[34-36] Viridans streptococci, usually *S. mitis*, can cause infections associated with life-threatening complications, including septic shock and pneumonitis and acute respiratory distress syndrome. High-dose cytarabine predisposes to these.[35,37-39] Finally, the ecology of the bowel flora is markedly altered by diarrhea induced by treatment with certain cytostatic agents such as cytarabine,[40] by graft-versus-host disease,[41] and by total body irradiation.[42] Various coagulase-negative staphylococci, including *Staphylococcus epidermidis*, are also present in the endogenous oral flora and gastrointestinal tract of neutropenic patients. Plasmid pattern analysis of coagulase-negative staphylococcal bloodstream isolates has shown that the mucosa is the origin of bacteremia in 70% of patients managed in a hematology ward of one center.[43] Others have found that vascular catheters were the most likely source of coagulase-negative *Staphylococcus* bacteremia in patients with hematologic malignancies (see Chapter 302). However, there is clear evidence that the coagulase-negative staphylococci responsible for bacteremia can originate from both the mucosa of the oral cavity and gut, as well as the catheter.[44,45]

Mucosal Barrier Injury. Injury to the mucosal barrier induced by chemotherapy and radiation therapy is probably the most substantial and earliest breach in the host defenses against infecting microorganisms. The process is more complex than just the direct effect of cytotoxic therapy on cells with a high mitotic index, such as epithelial cells of the mouth and gastrointestinal tract, and the indirect effect of local infections associated with evolving neutropenia. Sonis[46] postulated that the pathobiology of mucositis involved five sequential but overlapping phases (Fig. 308-2), culminating in tissue damage that mani-

fests clinically as mucositis. The initiation phase involves free radical generation and induction of apoptotic cell death induced by both DNA and non-DNA damage. The primary damage response phase occurs next, during which the master transcription factor, nuclear factor kappa B (NF-κB), leads to the upregulation of several genes resulting in the production of the proinflammatory cytokines (tumor necrosis factor-α, IL-1β, and IL-6) and then signal amplification. The net result is the ulceration phase, in which microorganisms and their cell wall products peptidoglycan and lipopolysaccharide can translocate the damaged physical barrier more easily and are able to activate tissue macrophages to produce more proinflammatory cytokines, thereby exacerbating the damage. Last, the healing phase occurs and is to a certain extent dependent on the rate of recovery of stem cells that are capable of repopulating the epithelium. Cytostatic chemotherapy regimens and irradiation injury induce varying degrees of mucosal barrier injury with differing dynamics, although the progression and decline of signs may be similar.[47] Individual patients are also likely to vary in their susceptibility to mucosal damage, suggesting that there are genetic differences in the expression of proinflammatory cytokines or proteins that control stem cell apoptosis (e.g., p53 and bcl-2 along the gastrointestinal tract).[48,49]

There is extensive gastrointestinal-associated lymphoid tissue in which lymphocytes and macrophages are located and that responds to irradiation and chemotherapy with inflammation.[50,51] Moreover, gut epithelial cells actively participate in the innate and adaptive immune response. They are capable of producing and secreting proinflammatory cytokines and upregulating the production of major histocompatibility complex class II molecules and other adhesion molecules after sensing specific pathogen-associated molecular patterns, such as endotoxin, muramyl dipeptide, and other bacterial antigens.[50] Muramyl dipeptide is sensed by NOD2, an intracytosolic pattern-recognition receptor expressed in Paneth cells, dendritic cells, neutrophils, and monocytes. NOD2/CARD15 polymorphisms result in uncontrolled inflammation of gut mucosa in Crohn's disease and gut graft-versus-host disease after allogeneic HSC transplantation.[52] Mucositis is the clinical manifestation of mucosal barrier injury and is characterized by functional complaints such as pain and difficulty in swallowing (dysphagia), and anatomic changes such as edema, erythema, ulceration, pseudomembrane formation, and alterations in mucus consistency with changes in saliva production (xerostomia). Mucositis results in significant morbidity and markedly lowers the quality of life for several weeks following cytotoxic chemotherapy and irradiation. Modern remission induction cytostatic chemotherapy and conditioning regimens for HSC transplantation often induce substantial injury to the mucosa. Combinations containing melphalan, etoposide, methotrexate, cytarabine, and idarubicin have all been shown to induce mucositis,[53,54] which can be very severe when anthracyclines are combined with total body irradiation and cyclophosphamide to condition patients for HSC transplantation or reinfusion.[55] Systemic drug exposure is the key determinant driving severe mucositis risk in high-dose chemotherapy-treated recipients of autologous transplants.[53] Patients receiving a melphalan dose of 70 mg/m^2 or greater had a 23-fold increased risk of developing mucositis compared with those receiving lower doses.[56] The duration and incidence of fever, parenteral narcotic use, total parenteral nutrition, antibiotic therapy, and the length of stay in a hospital are all correlated with the severity of mucositis, as is the risk of significant infections and mortality.[53,57,58] Oral viridans streptococcal infections are related to mucosal barrier injury of the upper part of the digestive tract, particularly the oral cavity, whereas enteric gram-negative bacillary infections and neutropenic enterocolitis are related to the lower part of the digestive tract.

It is likely that severe mucositis leads to a commensurate increase in the number of unusual bacteria causing infection by providing them with a portal of entry, which may explain the increase in bacteremia caused by oral commensal gram-positive cocci such as the viridans streptococci, *Rothia mucilaginosa*, and *Capnocytophaga* spp.[34,59-63] Besides damage to the oropharyngeal, esophageal, and gastric mucosa, chemotherapy and irradiation impair gut function and lead to rapid

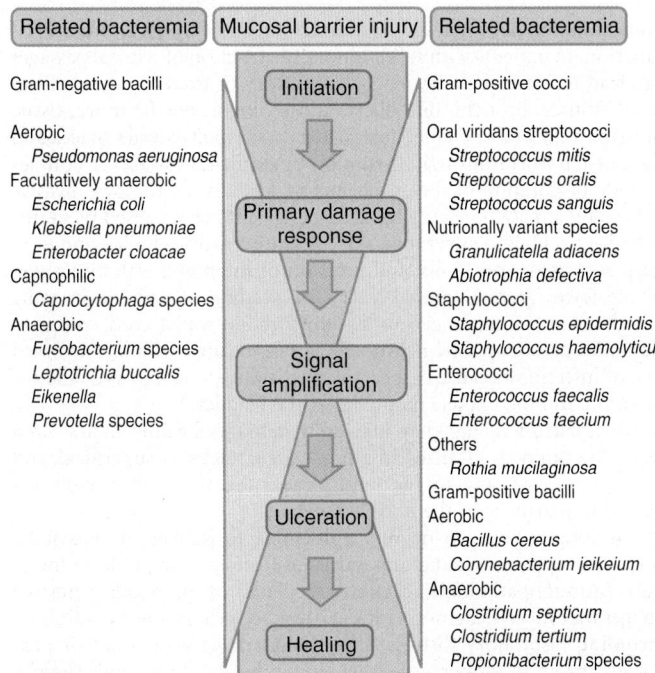

Figure 308-2 Mucosal barrier injury induced by cytostatic chemotherapy and irradiation is believed to occur in five more or less sequential phases. The process elicits a local and systemic inflammatory response, which may be accompanied by signs and symptoms of oral mucositis and gut dysfunction and even sepsis. Infection may be local but often involves dissemination via the bloodstream to distant sites. Bacteremia can be caused by a variety of normally commensal resident flora found on the skin and mucous membranes of the alimentary tract as well as potential pathogens acquired exogenously.

alterations in permeability. The increased absorption of sugars such as rhamnose, mannose, and lactulose and the decreased uptake of xylose after chemotherapy, irradiation, or a combination of both indicate a loss of integrity and damage to tight junctions.[54,64,65] Perturbed gut function has been shown to be one of the factors that, together with antibiotic usage and colonization with *Candida* spp., predisposes patients with leukemia to invasive candidiasis, and it also appears to be a risk factor for neutropenic enterocolitis.[64] Impaired gut function and integrity may also facilitate translocation, particularly translocation of gram-negative bacilli such as *P. aeruginosa*, into the bloodstream of patients colonized with the organism.[66] Gut toxicity has also been shown to be responsible for the reduced absorption of quinolones[67,68] and has been implicated in the erratic bioavailability of the antifungal agents itraconazole and posaconazole.[69,70] Finally, a dysfunctional gut will have a marked effect on the nutritional status of the patient not least by the diminished release of citrulline, the nitrogen transporter of the human body, by a reduced number of functioning enterocytes.[71]

The Oral Cavity. The oral cavity is a complex region providing other likely portals of entry besides mucositis, which essentially affects the nonkeratinous areas of the inner lips, buccal mucosa, underside of the tongue, and roof of the mouth. These surfaces may become erythematous, inflamed, and swollen and thus limit the intake of both food and drink, with the risk of malnutrition and catabolism.[72] Moreover, mucosal changes normally progress to a peak severity coinciding independently with the nadir of bone marrow aplasia and then begin to recover as hematopoiesis returns.[29,55,72] Extensive mucosal damage is often accompanied by a decline in saliva production leading to a dry mouth. Any mucus produced may be extremely viscous and difficult to either swallow or cough up.[73,74] Periodontal disease may be exacerbated, and minor oral cuts and abrasions may become inflamed and ulcerated.

The health of the periodontium probably also plays a role. For instance, organisms found in periodontal pockets, including viridans streptococci, appeared in the bloodstream of 13 (43%) of 20 patients soon after probing.[75] Toothbrushing[76-79] as well as more invasive procedures, including tooth extraction and periodontal and endodontic treatment, can also lead to transient bacteremia.[80-82] Not surprisingly, the origin of several different species of bacteria-causing bacteremia has been traced to the oral cavity, and not all can be explained by mucositis. These include the oral viridans group streptococci[83] but also *Fusobacterium* species and the related *Leptotrichia* species,[84-86] and even *S. epidermidis*.[44,45]

The Gastrointestinal Tract. The gastrointestinal tract has long been implicated as the principal origin of infections caused by the enteric gram-negative bacilli, including *Escherichia coli*, *K. pneumoniae*, and *Enterobacter* species,[87] providing the motivation for adopting prophylaxis with fluoroquinolones.[88-90] More recently, the role of neutropenic enterocolitis or typhlitis, a severe form of mucosal damage of the gut induced by cytotoxic therapy, has also become clearer in providing a portal of entry for various toxin-producing bacteria, including *S. aureus*, *P. aeruginosa*, various *Clostridium* species, and even *Bacillus cereus*.[91-94] This illustrates how the delicate balance between the host and the resident microflora can be disturbed in the setting of mucosal barrier injury and prolonged exposure to antibiotics. Colonization by *Candida* species of the mucosal surfaces appears to be a prerequisite for local mucosal infection and subsequent invasive disease.[95] Mucosal barrier injury, including neutropenic enterocolitis, is also an independent risk factor for invasive candidiasis among patients receiving cytotoxic chemotherapy.[54,64] Mucosal barrier injury and exposure to antimicrobial agents may explain the emergence of most infections arising in neutropenic patients and perhaps others (Fig. 308-3). Urinary tract infections, although rare in the absence of a Foley catheter, can be initiated through hematogenous spread from the gut as well as via perianal or vaginal contamination.

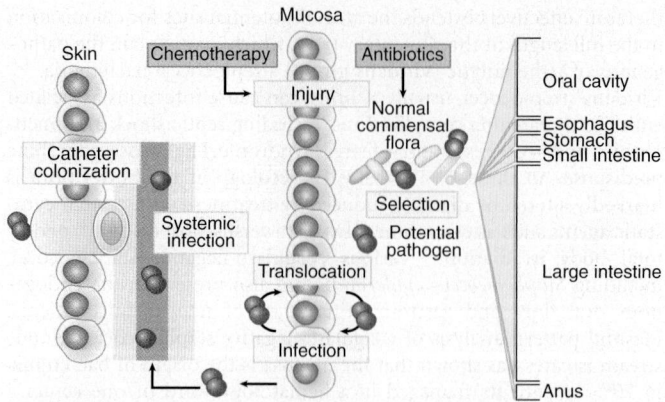

Figure 308-3 **Model to explain the origins of infection in neutropenic patients.** Chemotherapy induces injury to the mucosal barrier. At the same time, antimicrobial agents used for prophylaxis (e.g., fluoroquinolones) exert selective pressure on the ecology whereby more resistant members of the resident flora (e.g., viridans streptococci, staphylococci, gram-negative bacilli, and yeasts) increase in number. The gastric acid barrier of the stomach is usually breached by the use of drugs such as the histamine type 2 antagonists (e.g., ranitidine) and proton pump inhibitors (e.g., omeprazole) so that microorganisms that are ingested pass onward to the small intestine and beyond. Any colonization occurring on damaged mucosa would allow translocation from the alimentary tract or local infection, either of which can lead to bloodstream invasion and ultimately to systemic infection. In the case of the coagulase-negative staphylococci (e.g., *Staphylococcus epidermidis*), the alimentary tract might be the original source of bacteremia leading to colonization of the lumen of a vascular catheter.

OTHER ORGAN DYSFUNCTION

Tumors themselves may predispose to infection by local organ dysfunction. In patients with solid tumors, obstruction of natural passages can lead to inadequate drainage of secretory or excretory fluids from nasal sinuses, bronchi, bile ducts, and so forth. Furthermore, tissue invasion may create connections between normally sterile spaces and the outside world through disruption of epithelial surfaces. Examples include perforation of the esophagus by mediastinal tumors, invasive gynecologic malignancies with local pelvic abscesses caused by gram-negative bacilli and anaerobes, skin ulceration with cellulitis and even deep soft tissue infections, and invasion of the bowel wall by tumors of the lower gastrointestinal tract with seeding of bacteria into the bloodstream. Central nervous system tumors, spinal cord compression, and paraneoplastic neuropathy are associated with an increased risk of infection because of a diminished ability to cough and swallow or vomit and incomplete emptying of the bladder.[96]

Treatment of malignancy inevitably damages healthy tissue. Even when the tumor is localized in a single area, relatively superficial, and readily removed, any surgery and local irradiation will nonetheless extend impairment of the normal defenses.

The lung appears to be very vulnerable to damage by cytostatic chemotherapy and irradiation and is exquisitely susceptible to infection. Immunopathologic reactions mediated by pulmonary macrophages that survive chemotherapy can lead to various other syndromes, including respiratory distress. Lung hemorrhage as a result of profound thrombocytopenia further imperils the lung and thereby increases the risk of infection. Inhalation of spores of *Aspergillus* spp. and other molds may lead to infection of the sinuses, bronchi, and lungs.

Herpesviruses may play a role in this process not only as direct pathogens but also because infection leads to impaired lymphocyte function and, in the case of herpes simplex virus, damage to mucosal surfaces.[97] Dead or dying tissue alters the local microbial ecology and thereby creates a nidus for infection. Resident flora such as *Candida* spp. can establish a superficial infection marked by the presence of pseudomembranes over the ulcerated tissue, but they can also initiate local invasion and progressive spread to the esophagus and gastrointestinal tract, culminating in disseminated candidiasis. In a healthy host, these conditions rarely prove fatal, are usually readily apparent and relatively short lived, and can generally be managed simply. However, when hypoplastic bone marrow is present at the same time, the lack of neutrophils allows any potential pathogen that has invaded the tissues or translocated to the bloodstream to disseminate readily. Consequently, the transition from colonization to disseminated infection is likely to require fewer steps and involve much lower inocula than is necessary in patients whose immunity is not so comprehensively compromised. The trend toward more intensive chemotherapy and the increasing use of allogeneic and autologous HSC transplantation augments the number of patients who will experience the double jeopardy of profound neutropenia and damage to the natural barriers of the skin and mucosa.

PLATELETS

The protective role of platelets in healthy individuals is often underestimated but becomes obvious during treatment of a malignant disease. Thrombocytopenia is an almost inevitable repercussion of intensive chemotherapy and irradiation, but decreased thrombocyte function is a similar matter of concern. Thrombocytopathy is either disease related or caused by concurrent medication. The consequences of both increased susceptibility to infection and decreased capacity to repair damaged tissues can be considerable and may have an impact on the eventual outcome of a treatment episode. Thrombocytopenia also appears to be an independent risk factor for bacteremia,[98,99] and the incidence of major hemorrhage at autopsy of patients who die with or of an infection is striking.

NUTRITIONAL STATUS

Patients who weigh less than 75% of their ideal body weight or who have experienced rapid weight loss and have hypoalbuminemia are severely nutritionally deficient, which correlates inversely with survival. Poor nutritional status endangers the integrity of host defenses because of the catabolic state induced by cachexia and the malnutrition that results from anorexia, therapy-induced nausea and vomiting, gastrointestinal obstruction, altered permeability, mucositis, and metabolic derangements. A state of iron deficiency reduces the microbicidal capacity of neutrophils and T-lymphocyte function in vitro. Nutrition may be given parenterally or via a nasogastric tube to redress the balance, but neither is entirely without risk because each introduces yet another breach in the normal barriers and increases the risk of aspiration, particularly when consciousness is impaired.

CONCURRENT ILLNESSES

Psychological stress is thought to suppress host defense mechanisms. This general assumption has been corroborated by observations that psychological stress has a negative influence on the function of T cells and natural killer cells. Indeed, stress appears to be connected with an increased risk of acute viral respiratory illness, a risk that was related to the amount of stress, most likely mediated by endogenous opioids, hormones from the hypothalamic-pituitary-adrenal axis, catecholamines, and cytokines. Concomitant chronic illnesses enhance the risk of infection. Patients with a preexistent immune disturbance, such as a congenital immunodeficiency syndrome, are doubly jeopardized. The negative impact of smoking on patients with primary lung tumors is obvious and due to colonization of their airways with virulent encapsulated microorganisms and impaired clearance of secretions. Patients with diabetes mellitus are prone to genitourinary tract and wound infections, and they frequently suffer from concurrent vascular disease and neuropathy. The proclivity to infection in patients with poorly controlled diabetes mellitus is not difficult to explain in view of aberrations such as impaired opsonization and decreased chemotactic

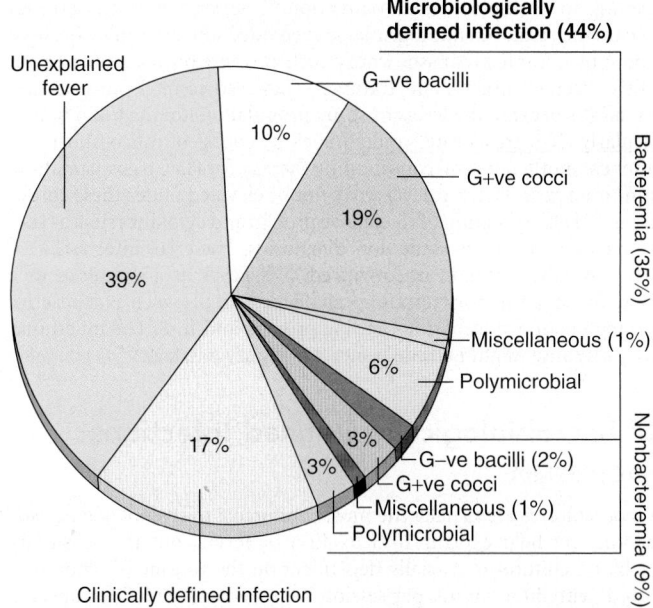

Figure 308-4 **Causes of infection in 968 episodes of fever and neutropenia.** *(Unpublished data derived from the study of De Pauw BE, Deresinski SC, Feld R, et al. Ceftazidime compared with piperacillin and tobramycin for the empiric treatment of fever in neutropenic patients with cancer: A multicenter randomized trial. Ann Intern Med. 1994; 120:834-844.)*

activity of granulocytes and monocytes. Diabetes mellitus also predisposes to infections such as malignant external otitis caused by *P. aeruginosa*.[94] Treatment of iron overload with deferoxamine predisposes to rhinocerebral and pulmonary mucormycosis by providing the fungus with an available source of iron.[98,99]

Origin of Fever and Infections

An infectious origin of a fever can be confirmed microbiologically or clinically in only 30% to 50% of all febrile neutropenic patients (Fig. 308-4). Infectious complications usually arise insidiously in these patients because of a muted inflammatory response and the lack of pus, which can be attributed to the absence of granulocytes; even the presence of chills or rigors does not always correspond with bacteremia.[100] However, foci of infections can also remain undetected because the physical examination was too cursory, specimens were either inappropriate or not collected at all, or the microbiologic investigations were incomplete or too insensitive. Obtaining a careful recent medical history and examining the patient thoroughly for any evidence of inflammation or infection should be considered obligatory, but getting a proper specimen is much more difficult because aspiration or biopsy is usually required, which is ill-advised for thrombocytopenic patients. Besides, even when a specimen is obtained from a normally sterile site, the yield is generally low. Consequently, failure to undertake an adequate physical examination and to obtain appropriate samples will result in fever being unexplained. Yet the fact that most patients without any proven infection improve clinically after treatment with broad-spectrum antibacterial agents suggests the presence of an occult bacterial infection in many cases.

THE SYSTEMIC INFLAMMATORY RESPONSE SYNDROME AND SEPSIS

Although neutropenic patients cannot mount a normal host response to tissue injury, the systemic inflammatory response syndrome and sepsis can and do develop when inflammation is uncontrolled and proinflammatory substances spread to other distant sites, ultimately leading to multiple organ dysfunction.[101] Sepsis syndromes are not always the result of endotoxemia or even infection and can be brought about by noninfective tissue injury such as severe burns, acute pancreatitis, elective surgery, and trauma.[2] They also result from extensive mucositis because the levels of some proinflammatory cytokines, particularly IL-6, are elevated and parallel the course of mucosal damage after chemotherapy and conditioning therapy for HSC transplantation; tumor necrosis factor-α levels may not be elevated under these conditions.[102] Determination of C-reactive protein and cytokines such as IL-6 is recommended by some for diagnosing bacterial infection,[103-106] whereas others remain unconvinced.[107,108] Fever as a symptom of a systemic inflammatory response can be measured, as well as C-reactive protein, lipopolysaccharide-binding protein, and IL-8. The inflammatory response might precede bacteremia by several days.[109]

Microbiologically Defined Infections

BACTEREMIA

Blood cultures are usually the most productive microbiologic investigation and help explain 10% to 40% of fevers, but the sensitivity of blood cultures is crucially dependent on the volume of blood cultured, with 30 to 40 mL per session being recommended for optimal results.[110-114] It has become common practice to draw at least 10 mL of blood for culture by venipuncture when investigating fever immediately before starting empirical therapy, together with at least 10 mL through each lumen of a central vascular catheter when one is present. During the past decade, a change from gram-negative to gram-positive bacteria has occurred,[115,116] but virtually any microorganism can cause infection in severely immunosuppressed patients. Infusion of the appropriate antibiotic through catheter ports that are culture positive may be helpful in clearing colonized catheters.[115,117] Once therapy is started, the value of further blood cultures is small if the patient is responding clinically. Patients with catheter-acquired sepsis who remain febrile with positive blood cultures usually need their catheters removed. In recent years, at least in clinical trials, blood cultures have been repeated 3 or 4 days after starting empirical therapy as a means of detecting persistent bacteremia.

Bacteremia Related to Intravascular Catheters

Coagulase-negative staphylococci are the most common cause of catheter-acquired sepsis,[12,14] but they are also recovered from catheter blood in circumstances suggesting that they are not causing the fever that prompted the blood culture. It is always easier to interpret the results of culturing of blood drawn from a peripheral vein. Simultaneous quantitative blood cultures from the catheter and a peripheral vein have been advocated but have not convincingly discriminated between catheter-acquired sepsis, sepsis from another source, asymptomatic intraluminal colonization of the catheter, and accidental contamination while drawing blood from the catheter hub. Others have adopted the differential time to positivity of blood cultures drawn through a catheter lumen in relation to those drawn simultaneously by venopuncture to distinguish "true bacteremia" from catheter-related bacteraemia.[118-120] In all cases, the decision to treat is based not just on the blood culture but also on the clinical findings.

Bacteremia Related to Damaged Mucosa

With the increasing importance of mucositis, several investigators have drawn attention to the significance of viridans streptococci,[121] especially in patients who prophylactically receive oral quinolones, which enhance the survival of these bacteria on damaged mucous membranes.[34,35,37-39,61] However, the signs and symptoms of viridans streptococcal infection might be inconspicuous to completely absent. In view of the direct correlation between the rate of positive blood cultures and the severity of damage to the mucosal surface, the normal habitat for these organisms, it is questionable whether viridans streptococci are true pathogens in all cases or whether they represent only an epiphenomenon.[5,122] In fact, during the course of a normal day, the acts of chewing and toothbrushing lead to transient bacteremia caused mainly by viridans streptococci. In view of the extent of the damage in many cases, it is not surprising that next to streptococci, *Clostridium perfringens* and *Clostridium septicum* septicemia, classically with massive hemolysis and diffuse intravascular coagulation, can arise during mucositis. In patients with profuse diarrhea and severe abdominal pain in combination with virtually absent audible bowel sounds, recovery of *C. septicum* from the blood may confirm the diagnosis of typhlitis.[123]

Other Infections

Oral Cavity

Oral infections are difficult to diagnose by appearance in patients with mucositis. Culture of oral lesions for herpes simplex virus and smears of scrapings for *Candida* pseudohyphae can be helpful.

Respiratory Tract Including Lung

Apparently trivial complaints such as a persistent dry cough may prove to be an early sign of impending pneumonia from *Aspergillus* spp.,[124] respiratory syncytial virus, or influenza virus. Thoracic computed tomographic scans are more sensitive in detecting pulmonary infiltrates compatible with aspergillosis than are plain chest radiographs.[125] Bronchoalveolar lavage specimens from patients with pulmonary infiltrates should have a battery of tests that usually includes smears for *Pneumocystis jerovecii* (formerly *carinii*), the acid-fast bacilli and *Nocardia* spp., bacteria, and molds, as well as culture for fungi and bacteria, including *Legionella* spp., *Mycobacterium* spp., *Nocardia* spp., and respiratory viruses (influenza and parainfluenza viruses, adenovirus, respiratory syncytial virus, and cytomegalovirus). *Aspergillus* antigen can also be detected in bronchoalveolar specimens, although the sensitivity and specificity of the test on respiratory specimens are unclear.[125-128] Rapid assays by enzyme-linked immunosorbent assay, direct fluorescent antibody, or dot blot are also available for influenza virus, respiratory syncytial virus, and adenovirus. Nasopharyngeal swabs in children and nasopharyngeal washes in adults are useful in culturing respiratory viruses in patients with upper respiratory symptoms. With current techniques, results are available in 24 to 48 hours (see Chapter 17). Testing for *Legionella* antigen in the urine of patients with pneumonia is also useful.

Skin

Identifying the cause of skin and underlying soft tissue infections is equally difficult because culturing swabs of lesions rarely discriminates between pathogens and commensal flora. As an exception, Gram stain and culture from pus expressed from a catheter exit site can be useful. Culture and histologic examination of skin punch biopsy specimens is very helpful in the diagnosis of isolated maculopapular or ulcerated lesions. Disseminated infections by *Candida* spp., *Trichosporon* spp., and *Fusarium* spp. in a neutropenic patient may be manifested by skin lesions while blood cultures remain negative. Skin lesions may be the source of *Fusarium* fungemia.[129] Ecthyma gangrenosum from *P. aeruginosa* may be accompanied by positive blood cultures, but lesions with the same appearance in a neutropenic patient can be caused by *Aspergillus* spp. or the agents of mucormycosis. These fungal lesions require biopsy for diagnosis. Aspiration of skin lesions is seldom successful unless pus is present.

Vascular Devices

Infections associated with intravenous catheters are assumed to mostly originate from contamination of the catheter hub. Bacteria, typically coagulase-negative staphylococci, can be cultured from the blood drawn back through intravenous catheters, and yet the patient's condition does not appear septic when the culture becomes positive. The contaminated catheter may have already been removed since the culture was obtained, or the culture may have been contaminated at the time that blood was withdrawn. In afebrile patients, repeating blood cultures may be all that is indicated. In other cases, the organism can be cultured repeatedly from blood drawn through the same catheter port but not from blood drawn peripherally, thus suggesting that the organism has not yet been able to cause sepsis but has colonized the catheter. Removing the device or administering antibiotics through the same port may be indicated to circumvent future sepsis.[117]

Gastrointestinal Tract

It is difficult to diagnose enteric infection, especially when nausea, vomiting, diarrhea, bowel cramps, and melena can all be due to toxicity related to chemotherapy, irradiation, or graft-versus-host disease. Endoscopy can be critical in the diagnosis of herpes simplex, *Candida* spp., and cytomegalovirus mucosal lesions. Detection of herpes simplex virus and cytomegalovirus in intestinal biopsy can be enhanced if both culture and immunoperoxidase staining of the tissue are done. The bowel flora can become the major reservoir of vancomycin-resistant enterococci, *Candida albicans*, *K. pneumoniae*, and *P. aeruginosa*. Organisms can be spread from the bowel onto the skin and, by the fecal-oral route, into the mouth. Skin organisms can be spread to other patients by the hands of health care workers and, through intravenous catheters, into the patient's bloodstream. Oral flora can be aspirated into the airway, particularly when the patient is intubated. Passage of bowel organisms into the bloodstream can occur through chemotherapy-induced ulcers. Fever in the presence of diarrhea or abdominal pain should prompt a cytotoxicity assay on stool for *C. difficile* toxin. The enzyme immunoassay for toxin is less sensitive. Neutropenic patients with right lower quadrant pain may have typhlitis, the diagnosis of which can be supported by an edematous colonic wall on abdominal computed tomography with oral contrast. Recovery of *C. septicum* from the bloodstream usually portends neutropenic enterocolitis.

Urinary Tract

Urine should be obtained for standard culture when there are signs or symptoms of a urinary tract infection but not otherwise. Urine from HSC transplant recipients with hemorrhagic cystitis should be tested for adenovirus by culture or antigen detection.

Sequential Infective Events

The sequence of risk factors (Fig. 308-5) determines to a large extent the order of infectious events in granulocytopenic cancer patients, which means that the types of infection occurring early in the granulocytopenic period differ from late infectious complications. Profound granulocytopenia and mucosal damage usually ensue approximately 10 days after initiating a course of chemotherapy and are followed by fever and bacteremia within a few days when toxicity is at its most pronounced. Clinically defined infections usually lag behind by a few days. Invasive pulmonary aspergillosis develops in a few patients early in the course of granulocytopenia.[130] Infections related to central venous catheters have to be considered approximately 10 days after their insertion, with the risk increasing with the length of time that the catheter is left in place.[12]

The initial risk period resolves with recovery of the granulocyte count. Very intensively treated patients are still at risk because of granulocytopathy, deficient cell-mediated immunity, and hypogammaglobulinemia. The kind of infectious complications for such

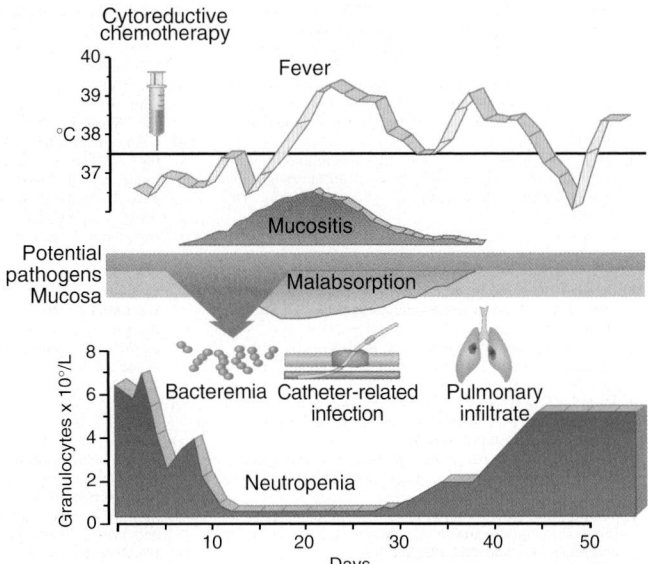

Figure 308-5 The sequence of events during neutropenia. Profound granulocytopenia and mucosal damage usually develop approximately 1 week after the start of cytoreductive chemotherapy. Thereafter, infectious and other complications tend to coincide with one another, placing the patient at most risk. Fever develops approximately 1 week later, and if there is bacteremia, it mostly occurs at this time. The risk of infections related to the central venous catheter increases with the length of time that the catheter is left in place, but signs and symptoms usually manifest themselves during the first few days of fever—that is, during the third week after starting chemotherapy. Infectious complications related to the lung tend to occur a few days later, often being recognized only after 5 or 6 days of fever. The period of risk of bacterial and fungal infection diminishes with recovery of the granulocytes when the clinical manifestations of tissue infections may be temporarily exacerbated before finally resolving.

patients is determined by the pace of reconstitution of these other components of the immune system. The major factor that influences immunologic reconstitution after allogeneic HSC transplantation is acute graft-versus-host disease and its treatment.[131] Cytomegalovirus, adenovirus, and fungi, including *P. jirovecii*, constitute the major pathogens during this episode. A third major risk period in these patients begins approximately 3 months after the procedure, at the time that chronic graft-versus-host disease develops. Sinopulmonary infections and cutaneous infections are common and probably related to the IgA deficiency with or without sicca syndrome and severely impaired cellular immunity. Varicella-zoster is probably the most frequent cutaneous infection, and pulmonary infections caused by cytomegalovirus and *P. jirovecii* are regularly encountered. Months, if not years, after successful engraftment or recovery from other very aggressive treatment, encapsulated organisms can cause rapidly fatal bacteremia and severe respiratory infections because of the lack of opsonizing antibodies.

REFERENCES

1. Bodey GP, Buckley M, Sathe YS, et al. Quantitative relationships between circulating leukocytes and infection in patients with acute leukemia. *Ann Intern Med.* 1966;64:328-340.
2. Bone RC. The pathogenesis of sepsis. *Ann Intern Med.* 1991;115:457-469.
3. Carlisle H, Saslaw S. Properdin levels in splenectomized persons. *Proc Soc Exp Biol Med.* 1959;102:150-155.
4. Van der Meer J. Defects in host defense mechanisms. In: Rubin R, Young LS, eds. *Current Approaches to Infection in the Compromised Host.* New York: Plenum Medical; 1994:33-66.

5. Donnelly JP. Chemoprophylaxis for the prevention of bacterial and fungal infections. *Cancer Treat Res.* 1995;79:45-81.
6. Van der Waaij D. Effect of antibiotics on colonization resistance. In: Easmon CS, ed. *Medical Microbiology.* London: Academic Press; 1984:227-237.
7. Roth RR, James WD. Microbial ecology of the skin. *Ann Rev Microbiol.* 1988;42:441-464.
8. Kotilainen P, Nikoskelainen J, Huovinen P. Emergence of ciprofloxacin-resistant coagulase-negative staphylococcal skin flora in immunocompromised patients receiving ciprofloxacin. *J Infect Dis.* 1990;161:41-44.

9. Høiby N, Jarløv JO, Kemp M, et al. Excretion of ciprofloxacin in sweat and multiresistant *Staphylococcus epidermidis*. *Lancet.* 1997;349:167-169.
10. Høiby N, Johansen HK. Ciprofloxacin in sweat and antibiotic resistance. *Lancet.* 1995;346:1235.
11. Hoiby N, Pers C, Johansen HK, et al. Excretion of beta-lactam antibiotics in sweat—a neglected mechanism for development of antibiotic resistance? *Antimicrobial Agents Chemother.* 2000;44:2855-2857.
12. Raad II, Bodey GP. Infectious complications of indwelling vascular catheters. *Clin Infect Dis.* 1992;15:197-208.

13. Weightman NC, Simpson EM, Speller DCE, et al. Bacteraemia related to indwelling central venous catheters: prevention, diagnosis and treatment. *Eur J Clin Microbiol Infect Dis.* 1988;7:125-129.
14. Hedin G, Hambraeus A. Multiply antibiotic-resistant *Staphylococcus epidermidis* in patients, staff and environment—a one-week survey in a bone marrow transplant unit. *J Hosp Infect.* 1991;17:95-106.
15. Salzman MB, Isenberg HD, Shapiro JF, et al. A prospective study of the catheter hub as the portal of entry for microorganisms causing catheter-related sepsis in neonates. *J Infect Dis.* 1993;167:487-490.
16. Groeger JS, Lucas AB, Thaler HT, et al. Infectious morbidity associated with long-term use of venous access devices in patients with cancer. *Ann Intern Med.* 1993;119:1168-1174.
17. De Pauw BE, Novakova IR, Donnelly JP. Options and limitations of teicoplanin in febrile granulocytopenic patients. *Br J Haematol.* 1990;2:1-5.
18. Lecciones JA, Lee JW, Navarro EE, et al. Vascular catheter-associated fungemia in patients with cancer: analysis of 155 episodes. *Clin Infect Dis.* 1992;14:875-883.
19. Morrison VA, Haake RJ, Weisdorf DJ. Non-*Candida* fungal infections after bone marrow transplantation: risk factors and outcome. *Am J Med.* 1994;96:497-503.
20. Weems JJ. *Candida* parapsilosis: epidemiology, pathogenicity, clinical manifestations and antibiotic susceptibility. *Clin Infect Dis.* 1992;14:756-766.
21. Van der Waaij D. The ecology of the human intestine and its consequences for overgrowth by pathogens such as *Clostridium difficile*. *Ann Rev Microbiol.* 1989;43:69-87.
22. Facklam R. What happened to the streptococci: overview of taxonomic and nomenclature changes. *Clin Microbiol Rev.* 2002;15:613-630.
23. Donnelly JP, Maschmeyer G, Daenen S. Selective oral antimicrobial prophylaxis for the prevention of infection in acute leukaemia—ciprofloxacin versus co-trimoxazole plus colistin. The EORTC-Gnotobiotic Project Group. *Eur J Cancer.* 1992; 28:873-878.
24. Freifeld AG, Walsh T, Marshall D, et al. Monotherapy for fever and neutropenia in cancer patients: A randomized comparison of ceftazidime versus imipenem. *J Clin Oncol.* 1995;13: 165-176.
25. Samonis G, Maraki S, Barbounakis E, et al. Effects of vancomycin, teicoplanin, linezolid, quinupristin-dalfopristin, and telithromycin on murine gut colonization by *Candida albicans*. *Med Mycol.* 2006;44:193-196.
26. Wilcox MH. Evidence for low risk of *Clostridium difficile* infection associated with tigecycline. *Clin Microbiol Infect.* 2007;13:949-952.
27. Ferretti GA, Ash RC, Brown AT, et al. Chlorhexidine for prophylaxis against oral infections and associated complications in patients receiving bone marrow transplants. *J Am Dent Assoc.* 1987;114:461-467.
28. Meurman JH, Laine P, Murtomaa H, et al. Effect of antiseptic mouthwashes on some clinical and microbiological findings in the mouths of lymphoma patients receiving cytostatic drugs. *J Clin Periodontol.* 1991;18:587-591.
29. Weisdorf DJ, Bostrom B, Raether D, et al. Oropharyngeal mucositis complicating bone marrow transplantation: prognostic factors and the effect of chlorhexidine mouth rinse. *Bone Marrow Transpl.* 1989;4:89-95.
30. Louie TJ, Chubb H, Bow EJ, et al. Preservation of colonization resistance parameters during empiric therapy with aztreonam in febrile neutropenic patient. *Rev Infect Dis.* 1985;7:S747-S761.
31. Meijer-Severs GJ, Van Santen E. Short-chain fatty acids and succinate in feces of healthy human volunteers and their correlation with anaerobic cultural counts. *J Gastroenterol.* 1987;22: 672-676.
32. Schimpff SC. Infection prevention during profound granulocytopenia: new approaches to alimentary canal microbial suppression. *Ann Intern Med.* 1980;93:358-361.
33. Van Der Waaij D. The colonization resistance of the digestive tract of man and animals. In: Fliedner TM, Heit H, Niethammer D, Pflieger H, eds. *Clinical and Experimental Gnotobiotics*. New York: Gustav Fischer Verlag; 1979.
34. Bochud PY, Calandra T, Francioli P. Bacteremia due to viridans streptococci in neutropenic patients: a review. *Am J Med.* 1994;97:256-264.
35. Elting LS, Bodey GP, Keefe BH. Septicemia and shock syndrome due to viridans streptococci: a case-control study of predisposing factors. *Clin Infect Dis.* 1992;14:1201-1207.
36. Van der Lelie H, Van Ketel RJ, Von dem Borne AEGK, et al. Incidence and clinical epidemiology of streptococcal septicemia during treatment of acute myeloid leukemia. *Scand J Infect Dis.* 1991;23:163-168.
37. Dompeling EC, Donnelly JP, Raemaekers JM, et al. Pre-emptive administration of corticosteroids prevents the development of ARDS associated with *Streptococcus mitis* bacteremia following chemotherapy with high-dose cytarabine. *Ann Hematol.* 1994;69:69-71.
38. Dybedal I, Lamvik J. Respiratory insufficiency in acute leukemia following treatment with cytosine arabinoside and septicemia with *Streptococcus viridans*. *Eur J Haematol.* 1989;42:405-406.
39. Kern W, Kurrle E, Schmeiser T. Streptococcal bacteremia in adult patients with leukemia undergoing aggressive chemotherapy: a review of 55 cases. *Infection.* 1990;18:138-145.
40. Peters WG, Willemze R, Colly LP, et al. Side effects of intermediate- and high-dose cytosine arabinoside in the treatment of refractory or relapsed acute leukaemia and non-Hodgkin's lymphoma. *Netherlands J Med.* 1987;30:64-74.
41. Guiot HFL, Biemond J, Klasen E, et al. Protein loss during acute graft-versus-host disease: diagnostics and clinical significance. *Eur J Haematol.* 1987;38:187-196.
42. Callum JL, Brandwein JM, Sutcliffe SB, et al. Influence of total body irradiation on infections after autologous bone marrow transplantation. *Bone Marrow Transpl.* 1991;8:245-251.
43. Herwaldt LA, Hollis RJ, Boyken LD, et al. Molecular epidemiology of coagulase-negative staphylococci isolated from immunocompromised patients. *Infect Control Hosp Epidemiol.* 1992;13:86-92.
44. Costa SF, Miceli MH, Anaissie EJ. Mucosa or skin as source of coagulase-negative staphylococcal bacteraemia? *Lancet Infect Dis.* 2004;4:278-286.
45. Kennedy HF, Morrison D, Kaufmann ME, et al. Origins of *Staphylococcus epidermidis* and *Streptococcus oralis* causing bacteraemia in a bone marrow transplant patient. *J Med Microbiol.* 2000;49:367-370.
46. Sonis ST. The pathobiology of mucositis. *Nature Rev.* 2004;4:277-284.
47. Sonis ST, Elting LS, Keefe D, et al. Perspectives on cancer therapy-induced mucosal injury: pathogenesis, measurement, epidemiology, and consequences for patients. *Cancer.* 2004;100:1995-2025.
48. Kim JM, Eckmann L, Savidge TC, et al. Apoptosis of human intestinal epithelial cells after bacterial invasion. *J Clin Invest.* 1998;102:1815-1823.
49. Potten CS, Wilson JW, Booth C. Regulation and significance of apoptosis in the stem cells of the gastrointestinal epithelium. *Stem Cells.* 1997;15:82-93.
50. Blijlevens NM, Donnelly JP, De Pauw BE. Mucosal barrier injury: biology, pathology, clinical counterparts and consequences of intensive treatment for haematological malignancy: an overview. *Bone Marrow Transpl.* 2000;25:1269-1278.
51. Xun CQ, Thompson JS, Jennings CD, et al. Effect of total body irradiation, busulfan-cyclophosphamide, or cyclophosphamide conditioning on inflammatory cytokine release and development of acute and chronic graft-versus-host disease in H-2-incompatible transplanted SCID mice. *Blood.* 1994;83: 2360-2367.
52. Holler E, Rogler G, Herfarth H, et al. Both donor and recipient NOD2/CARD15 mutations associate with transplant-related mortality and GvHD following allogeneic stem cell transplantation. *Blood.* 2004;104:889-894.
53. Blijlevens N, Schwenkglenks M, Bacon P, et al. Prospective oral mucositis audit: oral mucositis in patients receiving high-dose melphalan or BEAM conditioning chemotherapy—European Blood and Marrow Transplantation Mucositis Advisory Group. *J Clin Oncol.* 2008;26:1519-1525.
54. Bow EJ, Loewen R, Cheang MS, et al. Cytotoxic therapy-induced D-xylose malabsorption and invasive infection during remission-induction therapy for acute myeloid leukemia in adults. *J Clin Oncol.* 1997;15:2254-2261.
55. Donnelly JP, Muus P, Schattenberg A, et al. A scheme for daily monitoring of oral mucositis in allogeneic BMT recipients. *Bone Marrow Transpl.* 1992;9:409-413.
56. Kuhne A, Sezer O, Heider U, et al. Population pharmacokinetics of melphalan and glutathione S-transferase polymorphisms in relation to side effects. *Clin Pharmacol Ther.* 2008;83:749-757.
57. Sonis ST, Oster G, Fuchs H, et al. Oral mucositis and the clinical and economic outcomes of hematopoietic stem-cell transplantation. *J Clin Oncol.* 2001;19:2201-2205.
58. Fanning SR, Rybicki L, Kalaycio M, et al. Severe mucositis is associated with reduced survival after autologous stem cell transplantation for lymphoid malignancies. *Br J Haematol.* 2006;135:374-381.
59. Bilgrami S, Bergstrom SK, Peterson DE, et al. *Capnocytophaga* bacteremia in a patient with Hodgkin's disease following bone marrow transplantation: case report and review. *Clin Infect Dis.* 1992;14:1045-1049.
60. Classen DC, Burke JP, Ford CD, et al. *Streptococcus mitis* sepsis in bone marrow transplant patients receiving oral antimicrobial prophylaxis. *Am J Med.* 1990;89:441-446.
61. De Pauw BE, Donnelly JP, De Witte T, et al. Options and limitations of long-term oral ciprofloxacin as antibacterial prophylaxis in allogeneic bone marrow transplant recipients. *Bone Marrow Transpl.* 1990;5:179-182.
62. McWhinney PHM, Gillespie SH, Kibbler CC, et al. *Streptococcus mitis* and ARDS in neutropenic patients. *Lancet.* 1991;337: 429.
63. Weers-Pothoff G, Novakova IR, Donnelly JP, et al. Bacteraemia caused by *Stomatococcus mucilaginosus* in a granulocytopenic patient with acute lymphocytic leukaemia. *Netherlands J Med.* 1989;35:143-146.
64. Bow EJ, Loewen R, Cheang MS, et al. Invasive fungal disease in adults undergoing remission-induction therapy for acute myeloid leukemia: the pathogenetic role of the antileukemic regimen. *Clin Infect Dis.* 1995;21:361-369.
65. Keefe DM, Cummins AG, Dale BM, et al. Effect of high-dose chemotherapy on intestinal permeability in humans. *Clin Sci.* 1997;92:385-389.
66. Tancrede CH, Andremont AO. Bacterial translocation and gram-negative bacteremia in patients with hematological malignancies. *J Infect Dis.* 1985;152:99-103.
67. Brown NM, White LO, Blundell EL, et al. Absorption of oral ofloxacin after cytotoxic chemotherapy for haematological malignancy. *J Antimicrob Chemother.* 1993;32:117-122.
68. Johnson EJ, MacGowan AP, Potter MN, et al. Reduced absorption of oral ciprofloxacin after chemotherapy for haematological malignancy. *J Antimicrob Chemother.* 1990;25:837-842.
69. Prentice AG, Warnock DW, Johnson SA, et al. Multiple dose pharmacokinetics of an oral solution of itraconazole in autologous bone marrow transplant recipients. *J Antimicrob Chemother.* 1994;34:247-252.
70. Gubbins PO, Krishna G, Sansone-Parsons A, et al. Pharmacokinetics and safety of oral posaconazole in neutropenic stem cell transplant recipients. *Antimicrob Agents Chemother.* 2006;50: 1993-1999.
71. Blijlevens NM, Lutgens LC, Schattenberg AV, et al. Citrulline: a potentially simple quantitative marker of intestinal epithelial damage following myeloablative therapy. *Bone Marrow Transpl.* 2004;34:193-196.
72. Raemaekers J, De Witte T, Schattenberg A, et al. Prevention of leukaemic relapse after transplantation with lymphocyte-depleted marrow by intensification of the conditioning regimen with a 6-day continuous infusion of anthracyclines. *Bone Marrow Transpl.* 1989;4:167-171.
73. McGuire DB, Altomonte V, Peterson DE, et al. Patterns of mucositis and pain in patients receiving preparative chemotherapy and bone marrow transplantation. *Oncol Nursing Forum.* 1993;20:1493-1502.
74. Kolbinson DA, Schubert MM, Fluornoy N, et al. Early oral changes following bone marrow transplantation. *Oral Surg Oral Med Oral Pathol.* 1988;66:130-138.
75. Daly C, Mitchell D, Grossberg D, et al. Bacteraemia caused by periodontal probing. *Aust Dent J.* 1997;42:77-80.
76. Bhanji S, Williams B, Sheller B, et al. Transient bacteremia induced by toothbrushing: a comparison of the Sonicare toothbrush with a conventional toothbrush. *Pediatr Dent.* 2002;24:295-299.
77. Kennedy HF, Morrison D, Tomlinson D, et al. Gingivitis and toothbrushes: potential roles in viridans streptococcal bacteraemia. *J Infect.* 2003;46:67-70.
78. Lucas V, Roberts GJ. Odontogenic bacteremia following tooth cleaning procedures in children. *Pediatr Dent.* 2000;22: 96-100.
79. Schlein RA, Kudlick EM, Reindorf CA, et al. Toothbrushing and transient bacteremia in patients undergoing orthodontic treatment. *Am J Orthod Dentofacial Orthop.* 1991;99:466-472.
80. Debelian GJ, Olsen I, Tronstad L. Systemic diseases caused by oral microorganisms. *Endodont Dent Traumatol.* 1994;10: 57-65.
81. Lucas VS, Omar J, Vieira A, et al. The relationship between odontogenic bacteraemia and orthodontic treatment procedures. *Eur J Orthodont.* 2002;24:293-301.
82. Takai S, Kuriyama T, Yanagisawa M, et al. Incidence and bacteriology of bacteremia associated with various oral and maxillofacial surgical procedures. *Oral Surg Oral Med Oral Pathol Oral Radiol Endodont.* 2005;99:292-298.
83. Bochud PY, Eggiman P, Calandra T, et al. Bacteremia due to viridans streptococcus in neutropenic patients with cancer—clinical spectrum and risk factors. *Clin Infect Dis.* 1994;18:25-31.
84. Baquero F, Fernandez J, Dronda F, et al. Capnophilic and anaerobic bacteremia in neutropenic patients: an oral source. *Rev Infect Dis.* 1990;12(Suppl 2):S157-S160.
85. Fanourgiakis P, Georgala A, Vekemans M, et al. Bacteremia due to *Stomatococcus mucilaginosus* in neutropenic patients in the setting of a cancer institute. *Clin Microbiol Infect.* 2003;9: 1068-1072.
86. Landsaat PM, van der Lelie H, Bongaerts G, et al. *Fusobacterium nucleatum*, a new invasive pathogen in neutropenic patients? *Scand J Infect Dis.* 1995;27:83-84.
87. Schimpff SC. Gram-negative bacteremia. *Support Care Cancer.* 1993;1:5-18.
88. Cruciani M, Rampazzo R, Malena M, et al. Prophylaxis with fluoroquinolones for bacterial infections in neutropenic patients: a meta-analysis. *Clin Infect Dis.* 1996;23:795-805.
89. Engels EA, Lau J, Barza M. Efficacy of quinolone prophylaxis in neutropenic cancer patients: a meta-analysis. *J Clin Oncol.* 1998;16:1179-1187.
90. Gafter-Gvili A, Paul M, Fraser A, et al. Effect of quinolone prophylaxis in afebrile neutropenic patients on microbial resistance: systematic review and meta-analysis. *J Antimicrob Chemother.* 2007;59:5-22.
91. Coleman N, Speirs G, Khan J, et al. Neutropenic enterocolitis associated with *Clostridium tertium*. *J Clin Pathol.* 1993;46: 180-183.
92. Gomez L, Martino R, Rolston KV. Neutropenic enterocolitis: spectrum of the disease and comparison of definite and possible cases. *Clin Infect Dis.* 1998;27:695-699.
93. Pouwels MJ, Donnelly JP, Raemaekers JM, et al. *Clostridium septicum* sepsis and neutropenic enterocolitis in a patient treated with intensive chemotherapy for acute myeloid leukemia. *Ann Hematol.* 1997;74:143-147.
94. Ginsburg AS, Salazar LG, True LD, et al. Fatal *Bacillus cereus* sepsis following resolving neutropenic enterocolitis during the treatment of acute leukemia. *Am J Hematol.* 2003;72:204-208.
95. Nucci M, Anaissie E. Revisiting the source of candidemia: skin or gut? *Clin Infect Dis.* 2001;33:1959-1967.

96. McGeer A, Feld R. Epidemiology of infection in immunocompromised oncological patients. In: Glauser M, Calandra T, eds. *Ballière's Clinical Infectious Diseases*. London: Ballière Tindall; 1994:415-438.

97. Bergmann OJ. Oral infections in haematological patients—pathogenesis and clinical significance. *Danish Med Bull*. 1992;39:15-29.

98. Alexander J, Limaye AP, Ko CW, et al. Association of hepatic iron overload with invasive fungal infection in liver transplant recipients. *Liver Transpl*. 2006;12:1799-1804.

99. Maertens J, Demuynck H, Verbeken EK, et al. Mucormycosis in allogeneic bone marrow transplant recipients: report of five cases and review of the role of iron overload in the pathogenesis. *Bone Marrow Transpl*. 1999;24:307-312.

100. Sickles EA, Greene WH, Wiernik PH. Clinical presentation of infection in granulocytopenic patients. *Arch Intern Med*. 1975;135:715-719.

101. Soto A, Evans TJ, Cohen J. Proinflammatory cytokine production by human peripheral blood mononuclear cells stimulated with cell-free supernatants of viridans streptococci. *Cytokine*. 1996;8:300-304.

102. Pechumer H, Wilhelm M, Zieglerheitbrock HWL. Interleukin-6 (IL-6) levels in febrile children during maximal aplasia alter bone marrow transplantation (BMT) are similar to those in children with normal hematopoiesis. *Ann Hematol*. 1995;70:309-312.

103. De Bel C, Gerritsen E, De Maaker G, et al. C-reactive protein in the management of children with fever after allogeneic bone marrow transplantation. *Infection*. 1991;19:92-96.

104. Manian FA. A prospective study of daily measurement of C-reactive protein in serum of adults with neutropenia. *Clin Infect Dis*. 1995;21:114-121.

105. Rintala E, Irjala K, Nikoskelainen J. Value of measurement of C-reactive protein in febrile patients with hematological malignancies. *Eur J Clin Microbiol Infect Dis*. 1992;11: 973-978.

106. Santolaya ME, Cofre J, Beresi V. C-reactive protein: a valuable aid for the management of febrile children with cancer and neutropenia. *Clin Infect Dis*. 1994;18:589-595.

107. Ligtenberg PC, Hoepelman IM, Oude Sogtoen GAC, et al. C-reactive protein in the diagnosis and management of infections in granulocytopenic and non-granulocytopenic patients. *Eur J Clin Microbiol Infect Dis*. 1991;10:25-31.

108. Riikonen P, Saarinen UM, Teppo AM, et al. Cytokine and acute-phase reactant levels in serum of children with cancer admitted for fever and neutropenia. *J Infect Dis*. 1992;166: 432-436.

109. Blijlevens NM, Donnelly JP, DePauw BE. Inflammatory response to mucosal barrier injury after myeloablative therapy in allogeneic stem cell transplant recipients. *Bone Marrow Transpl*. 2005;36:703-707.

110. Falagas ME, Kazantzi MS, Bliziotis IA. Comparison of utility of blood cultures from intravascular catheters and peripheral veins: a systematic review and decision analysis. *J Med Microbiol*. 2008;57:1-8.

111. Lee A, Mirrett S, Reller LB, et al. Detection of bloodstream infections in adults: how many blood cultures are needed? *J Clin Microbiol*. 2007;45:3546-3548.

112. Penack O, Rempf P, Eisenblatter M, et al. Bloodstream infections in neutropenic patients: early detection of pathogens and directed antimicrobial therapy due to surveillance blood cultures. *Ann Oncol*. 2007;18:1870-1874.

113. Mermel LA, Maki DG. Detection of bacteremia in adults: consequences of culturing an inadequate volume of blood. *Ann Intern Med*. 1993;119:270-272.

114. Lamy B, Roy P, Carret G, et al. What is the relevance of obtaining multiple blood samples for culture? A comprehensive model to optimize the strategy for diagnosing bacteremia. *Clin Infect Dis*. 2002;35:842-850.

115. Safdar A, Rodriguez GH, Balakrishnan M, et al. Changing trends in etiology of bacteremia in patients with cancer. *Eur J Clin Microbiol Infect Dis*. 2006;25:522-526.

116. The EORTC International Antimicrobial Therapy Cooperative Group. Gram-positive bacteraemia in granulocytopenic cancer patients. *Eur J Cancer*. 1990;26:569-574.

117. Mermel LA, Farr BM, Sherertz RJ, et al. Guidelines for the management of intravascular catheter-related infections. *J Intraven Nurs*. 2001;24:180-205.

118. Blot F, Nitenberg G, Chachaty E, et al. Diagnosis of catheter-related bacteraemia: a prospective comparison of the time to positivity of hub-blood versus peripheral-blood cultures. *Lancet*. 1999;354:1071-1077.

119. Germanakis I, Christidou A, Galanakis E, et al. Qualitative versus quantitative blood cultures in the diagnosis of catheter-related bloodstream infections in children with malignancy. *Pediatr Blood Cancer*. 2005;45:939-944.

120. Rijnders BJ, Verwaest C, Peetermans WE, et al. Difference in time to positivity of hub-blood versus nonhub-blood cultures is not useful for the diagnosis of catheter-related bloodstream infection in critically ill patients. *Crit Care Med*. 2001;29:1399-1403.

121. Villablanca JG, Steiner M, Kersey J, et al. The clinical spectrum of infections with viridans streptococci in bone marrow transplant patients. *Bone Marrow Transpl*. 1990;5:387-393.

122. Donnelly JP, Muus P, Horrevorts AM, et al. Failure of clindamycin to influence the course of severe oromucositis associated with streptococcal bacteraemia in allogeneic bone marrow transplant recipients. *Scand J Infect Dis*. 1993;25:43-50.

123. Johnson S, Driks MR, Tweten RK, et al. Clinical courses of seven survivors of *Clostridium septicum* infection and their immunologic responses to α-toxin. *Clin Infect Dis*. 1994;19:761-764.

124. Novakova IR, Donnelly JP, De Pauw B. Potential sites of infection that develop in febrile neutropenic patients. *Leukemia Lymphoma*. 1993;10:461-467.

125. Caillot D, Casasnovas O, Bernard A, et al. Improved management of invasive pulmonary aspergillosis in neutropenic patients using early thoracic computed tomographic scan and surgery. *J Clin Oncol*. 1997;15:139-147.

126. Seyfarth HJ, Nenoff P, Winkler J, et al. *Aspergillus* detection in bronchoscopically acquired material: significance and interpretation. *Mycoses*. 2001;44:356-360.

127. Becker MJ, Lugtenburg EJ, Cornelissen JJ, et al. Galactomannan detection in computerized tomography-based broncho-alveolar lavage fluid and serum in haematological patients at risk for invasive pulmonary aspergillosis. *Br J Haematol*. 2003;121: 448-457.

128. Denning DW, Kibbler CC, Barnes RA. British Society for Medical Mycology proposed standards of care for patients with invasive fungal infections. *Lancet Infect Dis*. 2003;3:230-240.

129. Musa MO, Al Eisa A, Halim M, et al. The spectrum of *Fusarium* infection in immunocompromised patients with haematological malignancies and in non-immunocompromised patients: a single institution experience over 10 years. *Br J Haematol*. 2000;108:544-548.

130. Gerson SL, Talbot GH, Hurwitz S, et al. Prolonged granulocytopenia: the major risk factor for invasive pulmonary aspergillosis in patients with acute leukemia. *Ann Intern Med*. 1984;100:345-351.

131. Meyers JD. Infection in bone marrow transplant recipients. *Am J Med*. 1986;81:27-38.

309

Prophylaxis and Empirical Therapy of Infection in Cancer Patients

CLAUDIO VISCOLI | ELIO CASTAGNOLA

Cancer patients probably represent the best example of how both a disease and its treatment can impair the complex immunologic network in charge of maintaining the integrity of our body and defend it from infection from both the external and the internal environment. Local factors in host defense, including the mucosal and skin barriers to infection, are discussed in Chapter 308.[1,2] This chapter focuses on the critical role of bone marrow function in cancer patients. It has been known for decades that a granulocyte count less than 500 cells/mm^3 (and even more so with a count <100 cells/mm^3) is associated with an increased risk of severe bacterial and fungal infectious complications.[3,4] There is also evidence that patients with a granulocyte count between 500 and 1000 cells/mm^3, especially if rapidly decreasing, are also at high risk of infection because neutropenia is not a static but, rather, a dynamic concept. However, a survey on fever during neutropenia in children with cancer[5] showed the presence of severe infectious complications (e.g., bacteremia or invasive mycosis) in patients with a polymorphonuclear (PMN) count that never dropped below 50 cells/mm^3, suggesting the presence of a "gray zone" that should be carefully monitored.

As shown in Table 309-1, the clinical approach to a cancer patient with signs and symptoms of infection is multifactorial. Before planning a rational management intervention, physicians should be able to answer several crucial questions about the type and stage of the underlying disease and the clinical presentation.

Infections in cancer patients have often been considered nosocomial infections, despite the fact that these patients are often cared for as outpatients or even on a home-care basis. For this reason, a new terminology (health care–associated infections) has been proposed that seems to fit better with the current situation in the cancer management field. In fact, a study on infectious complications in 113 adults receiving treatment for acute hematologic malignancies showed that 91% of 223 infectious episodes were actually associated with the type of care patients had received, but only 42% of the episodes were truly "nosocomial" in origin.[6] In the following sections, we describe the epidemiology and management principles of infection in cancer patients. We do not deal specifically with risk factors and clinical presentations of specific infections because they are presented in chapters focused on individual infectious agents. Similarly, infections in recipients of allogeneic hematopoietic stem cell transplant (HSCT) are discussed elsewhere (see Chapter 311).

Epidemiology

Knowing the incidence of febrile episodes and documented infections in a given group of cancer patients is mandatory for the implementation of management strategies, especially prophylaxis. Unfortunately, epidemiologic data about these patients are rarely generated by ad hoc surveillance studies but are usually extrapolated from studies of empirical antibiotic therapy or prophylaxis, in which patients are selected according to inclusion and exclusion criteria. As a consequence, these studies are partially inadequate to describe the actual epidemiologic situation in the general patient population. In addition, little information is available about nonneutropenic patients. In general, epidemiologic data about the clinical impact of infection are mainly reported as percentages of events over a given number of patients or treatment courses, without adjusting for the duration of periods at risk. This is probably a mistake because the duration of the risk exposure is crucial to understand the real impact of a given phenomenon, whose incidence rate should be reported as number of events over the period at risk (usually 1000 days). Tables 309-2 and 309-3 report the epidemiology of febrile episodes, bacteremias, and invasive mycoses in cancer patients as derived from papers published after the year 2000.[5,7-22] Table 309-4 reports the incidence of fungal infections in studies published during the same period.[5,7,8,12,19,22-30] All these data clearly show that the incidence (rates and percentages) of infectious complications is strictly related to the intensity of antineoplastic chemotherapy. Patients with acute leukemia or non-Hodgkin's lymphoma and those undergoing autologous HSCT have a higher risk of infectious complications compared to those treated for solid tumors. In addition to the intensity of chemotherapy, differences in rates of infectious complications have also been observed according to the status of the neoplastic disease. An active disease was associated with a rate of 12.9/1000 days at risk in acute leukemias and 8.2/1000 days in solid tumors, whereas in patients in complete remission the rate was 5.7/1000 days at risk in acute leukemias and 6.0/1000 days in solid tumors.[31] The state of remission or presence/progression of the underlying disease is also an important factor for the prognosis of severe infectious complications, including invasive aspergillosis. The rate of infection in cancer has also been evaluated according to specific risk factors. For example, in 1993 Carlisle and co-workers[32] analyzed the rates of nosocomial infections in neutropenic cancer patients and reported an overall rate of 46.3 episodes/1000 neutropenic days, with rates of 12.9 for bacteremias and 2.92 for invasive mycoses. Recently, a study conducted in children and adults undergoing HSCT showed an overall rate of 38.9 infections/1000 days at risk (39.4 in children and 38.4 in adults), with a rate of 14.7 infections/1000 days for bacteremia (11.0 in children and 19.2 in adults).[33] Another study in children, using the cutoff of 1000 PMN/mm^3 for the definition of neutropenia, showed a rate of 25.1 episodes/1000 days at risk, with only 34% of neutropenic episodes complicated by fever.[5] Incidence rates varied according to the intensity of chemotherapy, with values of 37.7/1000 neutropenic days in acute leukemia, non-Hodgkin's lymphoma, or conditioning regimens for HSCT (64% of neutropenic periods complicated by fever). Incidence of infection was slightly lower in patients receiving aggressive treatment for solid tumors: 24.7/1000 neutropenic days (32% of neutropenic periods complicated by fever). Incidence of infection in all other treatments excluding maintenance was 13.7/1000 neutropenic days (24% of neutropenic periods complicated by fever). During maintenance treatment for acute leukemia and non-Hodgkin's lymphoma, the incidence was 5.0/1000 neutropenic days (9% of neutropenic periods complicated by fever). This study also showed that the majority of primary febrile episodes occurred soon after the onset of neutropenia (median, 3 days).

In addition to neutropenia, other factors such as the severity of mucosal barrier injury may have an impact on rates of infection. Indeed, it has been demonstrated that in patients receiving HSCT, the severity of mucosal barrier injury is strictly related to fever, independently from the severity and duration of myelosuppression. Genetic aspects might also be important and are increasingly reported as able to influence rate and severity of infection. For example, in nonleukemic patients receiving less intensive chemotherapy, decreased levels of mannose-binding protein were associated with an increased risk of

TABLE 309-1	Clinical Approach to Cancer Patients with Signs and Symptoms of infection
Question about	*Rationale for the Question*
The underlying disease • Acute leukemia? Solid tumor? Lymphoma? Other? • Active disease? In remission? Not evaluable?	The incidence of infectious complications is different according to the underlying disease and consequent intensity of chemotherapy. The stage of disease may influence type and risk of infection.
Did the patient recently (within 1 month) receive chemotherapy? • Yes or no? • Which drugs and which schedule? • How many days ago? • Autologous HSCT? • Monoclonal antibodies (anti-CD20, CD52, etc.)?	Different drugs may give different types of immunosuppression and favor different infectious complications.
White blood cell count • Is the patient neutropenic (PMN < 500/mm³ or <1000/mm³ but rapidly decreasing)? • Was the patient granulocytopenic in the previous 30 days?	The presence of neutropenia significantly increases the risk of infection.
Central venous access • Yes or no? • Has the catheter been manipulated (including infusions) within a few hours before occurrence of fever?	The central venous access may be an important source of infection.
Administration of prophylaxis (No? Yes? Which prophylaxis?) Was the patient compliant? Is there the possibility of lack of absorption or drug interactions? • Antibacterial • Antifungal • Antiviral • Other (*Pneumocystis jirovecii*, etc.)	Breakthrough infections are always possible and fever during prophylaxis is failure of prophylaxis, unless otherwise proven. However, the occurrence of a bacterial/fungal/viral infection during specific prophylaxis may influence the choice of empirical therapy, depending on the drug used for prophylaxis. A resistant pathogen should be suspected in every case, unless the patient was clearly noncompliant and/or there is the possibility of poor absorption, increased metabolism, or drug interaction (e.g., azoles such as itraconazole, voriconazole, and posaconazole). Knowledge of local epidemiology, including susceptibility pattern, is mandatory for correct diagnostic and therapeutic management.
Past history of infection (both before and after the diagnosis of tumor)	It may suggest the etiology and drive the therapeutic choice (e.g., tuberculosis, toxoplasmosis, and other endemic or opportunistic fungal infections).
Country of origin	Specific endemic infections can reactivate (Chagas' disease, strongyloidiasis, tuberculosis, and endemic mycoses).
The clinical picture	It may suggest the etiology and drive the therapeutic choice.

HSCT, hematopoietic stem cell transplant; PMN, polymorphonuclear.

TABLE 309-2	Rates of Infectious Complications in Cancer Patients in Studies Published after 2000			
		Episodes/1000 Days at Risk		
Patient Population	*Type of Disease*	*Any Type of Infection or Febrile Episode*	*Bacteremia*	*Invasive Mycosis*
Adults[9]	Hematologic malignancies, not analyzed in detail	19.2	4.7	0.7
Children[10]	Solid tumors, not analyzed in detail	13.7	—	—
Children[20]	Malignancies, not analyzed in detail	13.3	2.8	0.49
Children[11]	Hematologic malignancies, not analyzed in detail	18.1	5.7	0.27
Children[21]	Malignancies, not analyzed in detail	—	8.2	
Children[18]	Malignancies, not analyzed in detail	13.0	—	—
Children[12]	ALL, aggressive treatment	—	1.9	0.3
	ALL, less aggressive treatment	—	0.9	0.1
	AnLL, aggressive treatment	—	2.7	0.5
Children[10]	ALL	27.1	—	—
	AnLL	12.0	—	—
	NHL	18.0	—	—
Children[8]	Solid tumors not analyzed in detail, aggressively treated	—	1.1	0.1
	Solid tumors not analyzed in detail, less aggressively treated	—	0.2	0
Children[7]	Aggressive treatment for neuroblastoma	—	1.7	0.1
	Autologous HSCT for neuroblastoma	—	4.3	0
Children[3]	Neutropenic AL/NHL, aggressive treatment	31.1	5.1	2.1
	Neutropenic AL/NHL, not aggressive treatment	12.8	1.1	0
	Neutropenic ST, aggressive treatment	24.7	1.5	0.1
	Neutropenic ST, not aggressive treatment	14.7	0.9	0.6
	Neutropenic autologous HSCT	37.8	5.1	0.7
Adults[13]	Neutropenic autologous HSCT	—	18.9	—
Adults[14]	Malignancies not analyzed in detail, with MBL deficit	—	7.7	—
	Malignancies not analyzed in detail, without MBL deficit	—	7.1	—

—, Data not reported; AL, acute leukemia; ALL, acute lymphocytic leukemia; AnLL, acute nonlymphocytic leukemia; HSCT, hematopoietic stem cell transplant; MBL, mannose-binding ligand; NHL, non-Hodgkin's lymphoma; ST, solid tumor.

TABLE 309-3	Proportions of Infectious Complications in Cancer Patients in Studies Published after 2000			
		Percentage of Patients or Episodes with Infectious Complications*		
Patient Population	Type of Disease	Any Type of Infectious or Febrile Episode	Bacteremia	Invasive Mycosis
Adults and children[15]	Malignancies, not analyzed in detail	62	35	—
Adults[14]	Malignancy or autologous HSCT, not analyzed in detail	—	18	—
Children[11]	Hematologic malignancies, not analyzed in detail	8	3	0.1
Adults[16]	High risk AL	78	30	—
	High risk NHL or HSCT in solid tumors	73	23	—
Adults[9]	Hematologic malignancies, not analyzed in detail	45	11	1.7
Adults[26]	Acute promyelocytic leukemia	59	22	1.6
	Other AnLL	—	37	3.8
Adults[22]	AnLL	—	38	9
Children[24]	AnLL	94	25	1.6
Children[12]	ALL, aggressive treatment	—	30	5
	ALL, less aggressive treatment	—	17	2
	AnLL, aggressive treatment	—	34	6
Adults[17]	Low risk solid tumors, not analyzed in detail	12	0.4	—
Children[8]	Aggressive treatment for solid tumor, not analyzed in detail	—	27	1.3
	Autologous HSCT	—	21	0.8
	Less aggressive treatment for solid tumors, not analyzed in detail	—	3	0
Children[7]	Aggressive treatment for neuroblastoma	—	31	4
	Autologous HSCT for neuroblastoma	—	16	0
Children	Neutropenic AL/NHL, aggressive treatment	48	25	10
	Neutropenic AL/NHL, not aggressivel treatment	21	8	0
	Neutropenic ST, aggressive treatment	32	6	0.4
	Neutropenic ST, not aggressive treatment	22	7	4
	Neutropenic postautologous HSCT	58	14	2
Children	Neutropenic with AML, receiving G-CSF	61	14	2
	Neutropenic with AML, not receiving G-CSF	56	11	0

*Percentages of events over enrolled patients.

—, Data not reported; AL, acute leukemia; ALL, acute lymphocytic leukemia; AnLL, acute nonlymphocytic leukemia; G-CSF, granulocyte colony-stimulating factor; HSCT, hematopoietic stem cell transplant; NHL, non-Hodgkin's lymphoma; ST, solid tumor.

infection (49.9 vs. 29.6/1000 days at risk, $P = 0.01$), although this effect was less evident in the context of prolonged neutropenia.[14]

Central venous catheters (CVCs) are another well-known factor facilitating infection in cancer patients (see Chapter 302). Table 309-5 reports the incidence of catheter-related complications in cancer patients.[20,34-49] These complications are more frequently observed in partially implanted than in totally implanted devices and also in double-lumen compared to single-lumen devices. Bacteremia represents the most frequent infectious complications, whereas exit site, tunnel, and other types of CVC-related infections are less frequently reported. The number of CVC manipulations, which are related with the aggressiveness of antineoplastic chemotherapy and the consequent need of supportive care, represents the most important risk factor for the development of these infections. In recent years, monoclonal antibodies targeting immunologically active cells and cytokines have become very popular in hematology, especially those originating in the lymphatic tissues, and for the management of graft-versus-host disease in HSCT recipients. Unfortunately, the impact of these agents on the development of infectious complications cannot be fully appreciated because clinical trials of immunomodulating drugs have not used clear definitions of infection and, in some cases, have not reported infections at all. In addition, because these drugs are frequently administered with other antineoplastic compounds, it is difficult to disentangle the effect of any single drug. The majority of available data concern the use of alemtuzumab, a monoclonal antibody directed against CD52-positive lymphocytes. Studies show that nearly 50% of patients treated with alemtuzumab in combination with other drugs (e.g., purine analogues) developed severe bacterial, fungal, protozoal, and viral infections, both from exogenous sources and, possibly more frequently,

from endogenous reactivation.[50] Less clinical evidence is available on rituximab, a monoclonal antibody to CD20 lymphocytes, although both bacterial and viral infections seem to be increased in these patients, probably because of hypogammaglobulinemia. Patients with solid tumors frequently undergo surgical procedures before or after cycles of chemotherapy and/or radiotherapy. Although very little controlled data are available, it seems that surgical and intensive care unit-related factors are more important than previous antineoplastic chemotherapy in determining the risk of infection. Recent data on patients with peritoneal carcinomatosis undergoing peritonectomy and intraperitoneal hyperthermic chemotherapy indicate that the proportion of infectious complications is high, varying from 24% to 36%,[51-53] with more than two infectious episodes per patient.[51] Both personal experience and published data indicate that bacteremia, usually associated with surgical site infection and deep organ abscess, is not uncommon in urologic, gynecologic, and abdominal surgery.[51,53] In breast cancer, surgical site infection is a complication in 4% to 8% of cases, especially if immediate breast reconstruction is performed, and it occurs more often in patients who have received previous chemotherapy.[54,55] In one study, the incidence of surgical site infection in elective colon and rectal surgery was 9% and 18%, respectively.[56] A similar infectious rate (9.5%) has been reported for orthopedic surgery in patients without known preoperative infections.[57] Interestingly, in this study the use of an implant or allograft did not represent a risk factor for infectious complications. Finally, postoperative respiratory infections have been reported in nearly 4% of patients undergoing surgery for lung cancer, and they occur more frequently in the presence of advanced age, impaired respiratory function, advanced pathologic stage, and induction therapy.

TABLE 309-4	Incidence of Invasive Fungal Infections in Patients Receiving Antineoplastic Chemotherapy in Studies Published after 2000				
		Number of Patients or Therapeutic Procedures	Episodes of Invasive Mycoses		
			Proven or Probable		
Study Population	Underlying Diseases and/or Phases of Treatment		Yeasts	Molds	Possible
Adults with hematologic malignancies[25]	AnLL	3012	134 (4%)	239 (8%)	—
	ALL	1173	26 (2%)	51 (5%)	—
	Other	7617	32 (0.4%)	59 (0.7%)	—
Adults with hematologic malignancies[26]	Less aggressive treatment for AnLL	308	3 (3%)	1 (0.3%)	13 (4%)
	Aggressive treatment for AnLL	436	16 (4%)	1 (0.2%)	—
Adults with malignancies[23]	Autologous HSCT	1979	7 (0.3%)	7 (0.3%)	—
Adults with hematologic malignancies[22]	Induction/consolidation/reinduction/ HSCT for AnLL	42	9 (21%)	5 (12%)	—
Adults with hematologic malignancies[30]	AnLL	1596	96 (6%)	174 (11%)	—
Children with hematologic malignancies[24]	AnLL	304	2 (0.6%)	5 (1.6%)	6 (2%)
Children with hematologic malignancies[12]	AnLL	111	0	7 (6%)	2 (1.8%)
	ALL, aggressive treatment	213	2 (0.9%)	3 (1.4%)	5 (2.3%)
	ALL, less aggressive treatment	138	0	0	3 (2.2%)
Children with solid tumors[8]	Solid tumors, aggressive treatment (including autologous HSCT)	691	7 (1%)	4 (0.5%)	—
	Solid tumors, less aggressive treatment	311	0	0	—
Children with high-risk neuroblastoma[7]	Aggressive treatment	104	3 (3%)	1 (1%)	0
	Autologous HSCT	88	0	0	0
Neutropenic children[3]	AL/NHL, aggressive treatment	252	4 (1.6%)	3 (1.2%)	4 (1.6%)
	AL/NHL, not aggressive treatment	260	2 (0.8%)	0	0
	ST, aggressive treatment	727	1 (0.1%)	1 (0.1%)	0
	ST, not aggressive treatment	201	1 (0.5%)	1 (0.5%)	0
	Autologous HSCT	171	1(0.6%)	1 (0.6%)	0
Neutropenic children with AML[19]	Receiving G-CSF	161	3 (1.8%)	1 (0.6%)	—
	Not receiving G-CSF	156	0	0	—
Review data in adults[23]	Neutropenic postautologous HSCT	4747	—	25 (0.5%)	—
Review data in pediatrics[29]	Autologous HSCT	260	16 (6%)	4 (1.5%)	—
Empirical antifungal therapy in adults (multicenter)[27,28]	Different types	987	21 (2%)	27 (3%)	—
		1035	57 (5%)	52 (5%)	—

—, Data not reported; AL, acute leukemia; ALL, acute lymphocytic leukemia; AML, acute myelocytic leukemia; AnLL, acute nonlymphocytic leukemia; HSCT, hematopoietic stem cell transplant; NHL, non-Hodgkin's lymphoma; ST, solid tumor.

Etiology

Surveillance studies on pathogens causing infection in cancer patients are of the utmost importance for the implementation of management strategies. Large-scale studies are obviously crucial because they can provide information about worldwide trends, but single-center surveillance studies are just as important because every center may have peculiarities related to the type of patient, type of care, and local antibiotic policies. As previously mentioned, etiologic data should be obtained from ad hoc surveillance studies and not be extrapolated from clinical trials, from which many patients or episodes tend to be excluded based on enrollment criteria. Most of the available information concerns bacterial and fungal pathogens isolated in bloodstream infection, whereas the impact of viral infections is much more difficult to ascertain from published reports.

BACTERIAL INFECTIONS AND RESISTANCE TO ANTIBIOTICS

As shown in Figures 309-1 and 309-2, published data indicate that gram-positive bacteria, mainly coagulase-negative staphylococci, usually represent the most frequent pathogens isolated in bloodstream infections.[5,7,8,10,12,16,20-22,24,26,58-64] Other gram-positives include enterococci and viridans streptococci. At least in some centers, enterococcal infections are increasing with the emergence of *Enterococcus faecium*. For example, in the HSCT unit at "S. Martino" Hospital, Genoa, Italy, during the period from 2004 to 2007 there were 168 bloodstream infections in 132 patients, with isolation of 182 pathogens. Of 103 gram-positive bacteria, 44% were staphylococci (almost all coagulase-negative

staphylococci), 39% enterococci, and 11% viridans streptococci. Staphylococcal bacteremias decreased sharply during the observation period from 54% (37/68) in 2004 and 2005 to 23% (8/35) in 2006 and 2007 ($P = .002$), whereas the rate of enterococcal isolates per year remained stable. However, *E. faecium* replaced *Enterococcus faecalis* as the predominant enterococcal species, with an *E. faecalis*-to-*E. faecium* ratio decreasing from 4.5 in 2004 to 0.3 in 2007 ($P = .006$).[65] In many centers, gram-negative bacteria are increasing with respect to gram-positive cocci, both in neutropenic and in nonneutropenic patients, especially in nonbacteremic episodes or in the presence of extensive

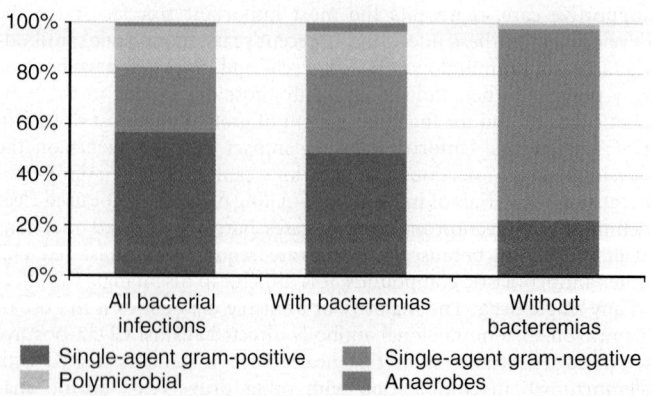

Figure 309-1 Etiology of bacterial infections. (*Data from references 4, 7, 8, 10, 12, 16, 20-22, 24, 26, 58, and 64.*)

TABLE 309-5	Percentages and Rates (Mean Values) of Infectious Complications Related to the Presence of Venous Access in Cancer Patients				
Type of Infection	*Type of Device*	*Infections/ 100 Devices*	*Infections/ 1000 Device-Days*	*Notes*
Any type	HB	14.5	0.6	Single-lumen catheters[34]
		34.6	1.40	Double-lumen catheters[34]
	HB with PASV	31	0.84	[34]
	PICC	26	8	[42]
	Hohn catheter	—	1.3	[45]
Bacteremias	HB	—	4.8	[48]
		—	3.3	[20]
		22.5	1.6	Review (all patients, mainly hematology and oncology patients)[35]
	HB with Groshong valve	21	0.98	[41]
	TIVAD	8	0.09	[38]
		—	1.8	[20]
		—	0.7	[48]
		3.6	0.1	Review (all patients, mainly hematology and oncology patients)[35]
	TIVAD with Groshong valve	2.4	0.12	[40]
	Peripheral TIVAD	4.0	0.1	Review (all patients, including hematology and oncology patients); few specific data for cancer patients[35]
	PICC	10	0.63	[47]
		1.5	2.2	[43]
		3.1	1.1	Review (all patients, including hematology and oncology patients); few specific data for cancer patients[35]
	Hohn catheter	8	1.1	[44]
	Nontunneled CVC	—	5.2	[20]
		4.4	2.7	Review (all patients, including hematology and oncology patients); few specific data for cancer patients[35]
	Midline	0.4	0.2	
	Medicated chlorhexidine/silver sulfadiazine CVC	2.6	1.6	
	Peripheral plastic catheter	2.0	8.6	
Bacteremia following catheter malfunction	HB	1	—	3% of bacteremias were followed by malfunctioning events; survey of 418 catheters[36]
Exit site/tunnel	HB	1.6	—	[37]
		11	—	Review[49]
	HB with Groshong valve	6	0.18	[41]
	PICC	1.6	0.1	[47]
Pocket	TIVAD	1.9	0.02	[38]
		4	—	Review (all patients, mainly hematology and oncology patients)[35]
	TIVAD with Groshong valve	0.56	0.03	[40]
Surgical site (within 30 days from catheter insertion)	HB	1.4	0.48	[37]
	TIVAD	1	—	[39]
		3.7	1.34	[46]
	HB/TIVAD	—	0.19	Type of infected catheter not specified[20]

—, Data not available; CVC, central venous catheter; HB, Hichman-Broviac; PASV, pressure-activated safety valve; PICC, peripherally inserted central catheter; TIVAD, totally implanted venous access device (port).

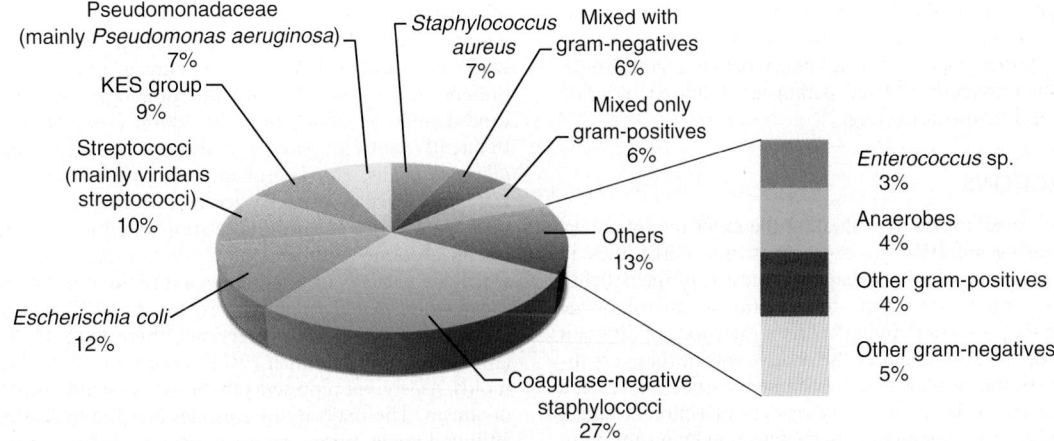

Figure 309-2 **Etiology of bacteremias.** (Data from references 4, 7, 8, 10, 12, 16, 20-22, 24, 26, 58, and 64.)

surgery. In the study performed at "S. Martino" Hospital, the overall number of gram-negative bacteremias per year remained stable during the study period, whereas the number of bacteremias due to gram-positive cocci decreased.[65] Therefore, the relative rate of gram-negative bacteremias increased from 28% in 2004 to 48% in 2007. The gram-positive/gram-negative ratio decreased significantly from 2.4 in 2004 to 1 in 2007 ($P = .043$) and from 2 in 2004 and 2005 to 1 in 2006 and 2007 ($P = .029$).

Anaerobic bacteria are isolated in less than 1% of positive blood cultures in cancer patients, but the proportion increases to 3% in abdominal oncologic surgery.[51] Anaerobes are usually isolated in polymicrobial bacteremias, especially with gram-negative rods,[66] with a rate that seems to be higher than that observed in nononcologic patients undergoing similar surgery (0.597/1000 hospital days vs. 0.033/1000 hospital days, respectively). Having an active hematologic malignancy, receiving aggressive chemotherapy or HSCT, or undergoing extended abdominal surgery are the most important risk factors for developing anaerobic or polymicrobial bacteremia. Catheter-related bacteremias are generally due to gram-positive cocci (especially coagulase-negative staphylococci) that are actually isolated in more than 50% of the episodes. Gram-negative rods can also cause catheter-related bacteremias, in a proportion of cases varying from 25% to 40% of the episodes, although the source of infection may be different because gram-positive cocci usually come from skin or hub contamination, whereas gram-negative rods (especially *Klebsiella, Enterobacter, Citrobacter, Achromobacter, Serratia,* and *Pseudomonas* non-*aeruginosa*) are more likely related to catheter management. Polymicrobial infections are not rare (8% to 49% of the episodes), with a predominance of gram-negative bacteria, whereas fungi (mainly *Candida* sp.) are usually isolated in no more than 10% of catheter-related bloodstream infections.[20,34-49] Bacterial gastroenteritis by classic enteric pathogens (*Salmonella* and *Shigella*) is a rare event in patients with acute leukemia, involving less than 1% of acute enteritis following chemotherapy.[67] *Clostridium difficile* and *Helicobacter pylori* have also been described as possible causes of gastrointestinal disease, with different degrees of severity in cancer patients. The recently described new strain of *C. difficile* with a previously rare toxin gene variant has the potential to cause severe problems in cancer patients as well (see Chapter 96). *Mycoplasma pneumoniae* and *Chlamydia* have been rarely described as a cause of pneumonia in cancer patients, but it is possible that their incidence is underreported. *Mycobacterium tuberculosis* is an increasing problem in many developed countries, with a high incidence in the population that is either increasing slightly or not decreasing any more. In cancer patients, tuberculosis is probably underestimated and underdiagnosed, although there are data showing that the rate approximates 90 cases/100,000 people (i.e., ninefold higher than in the general population in developed countries).[68] Immigrants from high-endemicity countries and people belonging to racial and ethnic minorities account for most of the cases. On the contrary, infections due to nontubercular mycobacteria are extremely rare. Finally, disseminated tuberculosis caused by *Mycobacterium bovis* may occur in patients receiving Calmette-Guérin bacillus immunotherapy. Interestingly, in nonneutropenic febrile cancer patients, gram negatives are the most frequently isolated pathogens, followed by gram positives, yeasts, and filamentous fungi.[69]

FUNGAL INFECTIONS

There are several uncertainties in evaluating the exact role of fungal organisms in causing infection in cancer patients. Difficulties in obtaining an accurate microbiologic diagnosis because of the patient's critical condition, poor sensitivity of traditional microbiologic methods, and the frequent overlapping between infections of different etiology have made the assessment of the relative role of these organisms problematic. In the past few years, a number of studies have been performed for the diagnosis of invasive mycoses by detection of fungal antigens. *Aspergillus* galactomannan antigen detection by means of an enzyme-linked immunoassay test is now widely used for the diagnosis

of invasive aspergillosis in cancer patients (see Chapter 258). An index greater than 0.7 in a single test (static cutoff) or greater than 0.5 in two consecutive samples (dynamic cutoff) is suggestive in high-risk patients of probable invasive aspergillosis. The specificity of the test may approximate 92% for documented aspergillosis in hematologic malignancies.[70] The detection of the galactomannan antigen in bronchoalveolar lavage or cerebrospinal fluid has been reported to be diagnostic of pulmonary and cerebral invasive aspergillosis, respectively. False-positive results occur with the concomitant administration of some antibiotics (especially piperacillin-tazobactam and amoxicillin-clavulanate) or some pediatric formulas (see Chapter 258). Other studies have shown that $(1\rightarrow3)$ β-D-glucan (a component of the fungal cell wall) may be an important tool in the diagnosis of fungal infections. The test is positive in many fungal infections, excluding cryptococcosis and mucormycosis (see Chapters 259 and 263). At least four commercial kits are available. Depending on the method used, cutoff levels between 60 and 120 pg/mL in at least one sample or 7 pg/mL or greater in two consecutive samples have been proposed.[71-73] False-positive results have been observed with the glucan test as well. Antibiotics (amoxicillin-clavulanate), bacterial infections (*Alcaligenes faecalis, Streptococcus pneumoniae,* and *Pseudomonas aeruginosa*), albumin, blood products prepared with cellulose filters, hemodialysis (cellulose membranes), intravenous treatment with immunoglobulins, and exposure to gauzes and other glucan-containing materials have all been associated with false-positive glucan tests. In addition, excess manipulation of a sample can result in glucan contamination and therefore cause a false-positive result. New advances are expected in the near future from biomolecular methods, although so far the use of the polymerase chain reaction for the diagnosis of bacterial and fungal infections in cancer patients must be considered as an experimental, nonstandardized procedure (see Chapter 17).

Another important advance toward the goal of clarifying the exact role of fungal infections in cancer patients has been an initiative carried out by the European Organization for Research and Treatment of Cancer (EORTC) and the Mycoses Study Group with the preparation of a set of shared definitions. The idea has been to establish three levels of diagnostic certainty, as "proven," "probable," and "possible" invasive mycoses. Although designed for epidemiologic purposes or clinical trial design, there is a trend to use the definitions in the everyday clinical practice. Proven fungal infection requires a positive culture from a sterile site and/or histopathologic evidence or, only for disseminated cryptococcosis, the presence of cryptococcal antigen in the cerebrospinal fluid. The definition of probable infection is determined by the concomitant presence of a host factor, a clinical criterion, and a mycologic criterion. The host factor is a characteristic by which individuals predisposed to acquire invasive fungal diseases can be recognized. The clinical criteria must be consistent with the fungal disease and must be temporally related to the current episode. Mycologic criteria include the presence of molds in sputum or bronchoalveolar lavage (culture, smear, or cytology) or a positive test for the detection of constituents of the fungal cell wall, such as galactomannan or β-D-glucan. Finally, the definition of "possible" invasive mycosis includes cases in which host factors and clinical criteria are concomitantly present, in the absence of any microbiologic confirmation. In proven candidemias, as shown in Table 309-4, *Candida* species is the most frequently isolated yeast, and there is an increasing role for non-*albicans* strains. This is probably due to the extensive use of prophylactic fluconazole, which has led to a striking reduction in the number of infections due to susceptible strains and to a relative increase (but not in absolute numbers) of *Candida krusei* and *Candida glabrata,* which are partially or totally resistant to fluconazole and sometimes to other azoles as well. In our experience in HSCT, among 182 pathogens isolated in bloodstream infections, there were 11 fungal organisms (9%), almost all of which (9/11) were non-*albicans* strains.[65] Among molds, *Aspergillus* represents the most frequently isolated or suspected organism. The majority of episodes are due to *Aspergillus fumigatus,* although some centers report infections due to *Aspergillus flavus* and *Aspergillus terreus.* *Aspergillus* species are ubiquitous molds whose primary ecologic niche is represented by decomposing vegetable material, including potted plant soil, flowers, and carpets. In healthy individuals, *Aspergillus* conidia are trapped in the upper respiratory tract and only a small proportion of them enter the lower airways, where *Aspergillus* can play a pathogenic role as an allergen. In immunocompromised patients, especially those with hematologic malignancies and allogeneic transplants, spores can germinate and cause invasive disease. Hospital sources have been reported to include dust from building construction or renovation and potable water supplies. Aspergillosis can be a nosocomial infection, although strains isolated from patients and from the hospital environment have rarely been shown to be genetically identical. In addition, patients can become colonized after hospital discharge or arrive at the hospital already colonized. Therefore, invasive aspergillosis in patients with malignancy or receiving HSCT should be considered an endemic disease that is usually community acquired, with occasional epidemic outbreaks possibly associated with massive environmental exposures (in and outside the hospital).

Concerning the incidence of aspergillosis in hematologic malignancies, in a multicenter study performed in Italy from 1999 to 2003 on 11,802 adults, Pagano and co-workers found invasive aspergillosis in 2.6% of patients.[25] The incidence varied according to the underlying disease (and therefore the aggressiveness and intensity of chemotherapy): 7.9% in acute nonlymphoblastic leukemia; 4.3% in acute lymphoblastic leukemia; 2.3% in chronic myelogenous leukemia; and less than 1% in chronic lymphocytic leukemia, Hodgkin's disease, non–Hodgkin's lymphoma, and multiple myeloma. *A. fumigatus* was identified in 53% of documented cases. The frequency in autologous HSCT was low at 0.3% (7/1979). This observation is consistent with those of other reports describing a 0.5% to 2% incidence of invasive aspergillosis after autologous HSCT,[74-76] observed during neutropenia preceding the engraftment. Other fungi can cause disease in immunocompromised cancer patients. In some centers, there have been increasing reports of mucormycosis. However, it is unclear whether this represents a general emerging problem, whether it relies on local factors, or whether these diseases are simply diagnosed more often due to increased clinical and diagnostic awareness. Other fungi, such as *Cryptococcus*, *Blastoschizomyces*, *Scedosporium*, *Fusarium*, and *Trichosporon*, have been reported, although sporadically. *Pneumocystis jirovecii* is a well-known cause of pneumonia in cancer patients not receiving specific prophylaxis, with attack rates varying from 6.5% to 43% in acute lymphoblastic leukemia, 4% to 25% in rhabdomyosarcomas, and nearly 1% in Hodgkin's disease and primary or metastatic central nervous system tumors. Some cases have also been described after autologous HSCT.[77]

VIRAL INFECTIONS

Viruses are not frequently reported as a cause of infectious complications in cancer patients unless they are undergoing allogeneic transplantation, even in the presence of neutropenia.[5] For example, a positive pp65 antigenemia for cytomegalovirus (CMV) has been reported in 9% of non-HSCT recipients and in 12% of patients undergoing autologous HSCT[78] without necessarily being accompanied by CMV disease. CMV is an unusual cause of pneumonia in patients with leukemia or lymphoma or following autologous HSCT, and the risk seems to be higher among patients receiving monoclonal antibodies, especially alemtuzumab. Respiratory viruses are not an infrequent cause of pulmonary complications in cancer patients and are probably underestimated as a cause of fever, whereas viral gastroenteritis may be a frequent complication in pediatric oncology. Both adenoviruses and parvovirus B19 have been reported as causes of severe disease in cancer patients. Finally, the reactivation of hepatotropic viruses (HBV and HCV) may represent important problems in endemic areas (for HBV) or in the presence of inadequate pretransfusion blood screening (both HBV and HCV), or both. These aspects must be kept in mind in developed countries in an era of increasing immigration.

OTHER PATHOGENS

The risk of unusual infections or reinfections due to endemic fungi (histoplasmosis, coccidioidomycosis, and others), protozoa (South American trypanosomiasis and malaria), helminths (strongyloidiasis), and other tropical diseases should be considered in endemic areas and in immigrants.

Chemoprophylaxis

Considering the remarkable mortality and morbidity associated with infection in cancer patients, prevention has always been considered a desirable goal. However, this is not true in absolute terms because every prophylactic protocol should be weighed against the efficacy of prophylaxis, the frequency of the complications, the cost, toxicity, and impact on the development of resistance.

Table 309-6 summarizes the different regimes for primary prophylaxis that have been considered appropriate in cancer patients based on clinical trials and guidelines. In the following sections, we delineate the advantages and disadvantages of the different approaches.

ANTIBACTERIAL PROPHYLAXIS

Chemoprophylaxis for the prevention of bacterial infections was first proposed in clinical practice based on the discovery that 80% of the bacterial pathogens causing infection in neutropenic cancer patients were originating from the patient's endogenous flora, but that approximately half of them were acquired during the hospital stay. Therefore, the first approach relied on the administration of nonabsorbable antibiotics aimed at totally (including anaerobes) or partially (excluding anaerobes) suppressing the intestinal bacterial flora and preventing the acquisition of exogenous organisms. Intestinal decontamination was often employed for patients confined to laminar airflow rooms and in conjunction with other protective measures (total protective isolation). Gentamicin, vancomycin, and nystatin were used as nonabsorbable drugs to suppress intestinal flora. Trimethoprim-sulfamethoxazole, called co-trimoxazole, usually given in combination with oral nystatin or amphotericin B, was a popular drug for prophylaxis because the antifungal provided a topical effect on colonic *Candida* and the cotrimoxazole provided systemic prophylaxis. Subsequently, co-trimoxazole was replaced by the quinolones. Practice changed and patients were no longer confined in laminar airflow rooms but instead placed in rooms with HEPA-filtered air and protective isolation.

For patients with chemotherapy-induced cytopenia, it is not clear whether protective isolation (reverse) in hospitals or attempts at equivalent procedures at home have an impact on infectious complications. Moreover, low bacterial diet seems not to offer additional benefit as an infection preventive compared to normal diet.

Before 2005, clinical evidence supported a positive effect of fluoroquinolones only on the incidence of gram-negative infections, but without any effect on the incidence of fever during neutropenia, gram-positive infections, or survival. Guidelines for the management of febrile neutropenia discouraged the widespread use of prophylaxis in neutropenic cancer patients or suggested a selective and careful use. A meta-analysis published in 2005[15] showed that prophylaxis during neutropenia with absorbable drugs, especially quinolones, significantly reduced the risk of death and the rates of both unexplained fever and documented bacterial infections. No significant increase in the rate of fluoroquinolone resistance was found, although no study was designed to evaluate the impact on microbial ecology. Other limitations were the poor quality of some studies included in the meta-analyses. Soon after this study was performed, the Gruppo Italiano Malattie Ematologiche Maligne dell'Adulto (GIMEMA) group published a randomized clinical trial of 760 consecutive patients with acute leukemia or lymphoma who received either levofloxacin or placebo for the prophylaxis of fever and infection during single episodes of neutropenia. Lymphoma patients were included only if receiving autologous HSCT.[16]

TABLE 309-6	Suggested Prophylaxis for Infections in Cancer Patients		
	Drug	*Schedule*	*Patient Population*
Antibacterial	Ciprofloxacin	500 mg, bid	Adults receiving chemotherapy for acute leukemia or autologous HSCT
	Levofloxacin	500 mg, once daily	Patients with solid tumor at the first cycle of chemotherapy and in subsequent cycles only if this prophylaxis failed
			Starting with chemotherapy and continuing until resolution of neutropenia or initiation of empirical antibacterial therapy for febrile neutropenia
	Amoxicillin-clavulanate	25 mg/kg (maximum 1000 mg), bid	Children receiving chemotherapy for acute leukemia or non-Hodgkin's lymphoma
Antifungal	Posaconazole	200 mg tid, orally with a (fatty) meal	Patients receiving chemotherapy for acute leukemia or myelodisplastic syndrome
	Fluconazole	400 mg, once daily	Patients receiving chemotherapy for acute myelogenous leukemia with cytarabine plus anthracycline regimens (administered for 7 and 3 days, respectively) and high-dose cytarabine-containing regimens
	Different drugs		Secondary prophylaxis according to isolated pathogen and/or clinical picture
Pneumocystis jirovecii	Trimethoprim-sulfamethoxazole	25 mg/kg of TMP-SMX (5 mg/kg of TMP), maximum 1920 mg (two double-strength capsules) in two divided doses for 3 consecutive days per week (daily administration of single-strength TMP-SMX has also been demonstrated effective)	All patients receiving chemotherapy with steroids, including those with solid tumors (e.g., brain cancer)
	Dapsone	2 mg/kg/day (maximum 100 mg), on alternate days three times a week	In patients who cannot tolerate TMP-SMX
	Aerosolized pentamidine	300 mg once a month with nebulizer	In patients who cannot tolerate TMP-SMX; effective but more difficult to administer
	Atovaquone	1500 mg in two divided doses	In patients who cannot tolerate TMP-SMX
Antiviral	Acyclovir	Adults more than 40 kg: 800 mg PO twice daily, or 250 mg/M^2 IV every 12 hr	In patients with positive anti-HSV antibodies
	Valacyclovir	500 mg PO twice daily	In patients with positive anti-HSV antibodies
	Valacyclovir	1 g PO three times daily	In patients in contact with chickenpox who did not receive prompt administration of specific immunoglobulins
	Lamivudine	100 mg/day	In HBV-positive patients
Tuberculosis	Isoniazid	300 mg once daily	Efficacy not specifically evaluated in cancer patients
CVC	None	Good skin preparation and the use of sterile techniques at time of device insertion	All patients with indwelling central venous catheter
		Good maintenance procedures	
Others	Growth factors	5 µg/kg/day either subcutaneously or as an IV infusion over at least 1 hr or pegylated filgrastim 6 mg once	For the prevention of febrile neutropenia in patients who have a high risk of this complication based on age, medical history, disease characteristics, and myelotoxicity of the chemotherapy regimen
			Secondary prophylaxis with CSF is recommended for patients who experienced a neutropenic complication from a prior cycle of chemotherapy (for which primary prophylaxis was not received), in which a reduced dose may compromise disease-free or overall survival or treatment outcome
			Efficacy not fully demonstrated for pegylated filgrastim
	Immunoglobulins	Polyclonal immunoglobulins: 400 mg/kg every 21-28 days	Patients with chronic lymphocytic leukemia after the second episode of severe bacterial infection
			Patients with leukemia or lymphoma with hypogammaglobulinemia (<400 mg/dL) and severe bacterial infections (reasonable, but not proven)
		Specific anti-VZV (VariZIG)125 IU every 10 kg of body weight (maximum 625 IU)	In high-risk contact with a negative history of varicella within 72-96 hr of the at-risk contact

CSF, colony-stimulating factor; CVC, central venous catheter; HBV, hepatitis B virus; HSCT, hematopoietic stem cell transplant; HSV, herpes simplex virus; TMP-SMX, trimethoprim-sulfamethoxazole.

Only one episode per patient was included. Patients in the active drug group had far lower relative risks for developing bacterial infections and febrile neutropenia than those in the placebo group. As expected, almost all pathogens isolated in documented infections in the active drug group were resistant to quinolones. Both overall and infection-related mortality rates were low (4% and 3%, respectively) and were similar in the two groups, although there was a trend favoring the active intervention group. By extrapolating from the first meta-analysis using only studies on high-risk patients and pooling these data with the GIMEMA data, the effect of prophylaxis on the overall mortality became statistically significant.[79] The proportion of resistant strains did not change over time when comparing two studies performed by the same group 10 years apart.[16,80] The authors argued that the selective pressure exerted by the use of fluoroquinolone prophylaxis might be counterbalanced by the decreased need to use empirical antibacterial therapy, thus limiting the risk of emergence of resistance to the drugs used for empirical therapy. The problem of inducing resistance was also addressed in the meta-analysis,[15,79] which concluded that in trials reporting resistance data, patients who received fluoroquinolones developed no more infections due to resistant pathogens than did patients receiving placebo (relative risk, 1.04; 95% confidence interval, 0.73 to 1.5). For institutions using fluoroquinolone prophylaxis, careful monitoring for an increase in the isolation of resistant strains was highly recommended.

The issue of prophylaxis was also addressed in low-risk patients undergoing standard chemotherapy for solid tumors.[17] In a very large trial (1565 patients), chemoprophylaxis was administered throughout the duration of chemotherapy and data regarding several chemotherapy cycles were analyzed. Statistically significant differences were found in the number of patients who had at least one febrile episode (11% and 15% in the levofloxacin and placebo groups, respectively) and in the need for hospitalization, whereas no difference was demonstrated in the incidence of more objective endpoints, such as severe infections and both infection-related and overall mortality. These results cannot be taken as definitive because of several methodological problems, including some confusion regarding endpoints, definitions, and outcome-related variables. Despite the favorable results of this study, it is generally not recommended that patients with solid tumors be given quinolones for prophylaxis. Rather, the drug should be reserved for therapeutic purposes.

In reading publications about clinical trials, it is worth remembering that (1) randomized clinical trials (and obviously meta-analyses derived from them) cannot be used for epidemiologic purposes because they do not collect data on infections occurring after the end of the study and in patients not enrolled in the trial; (2) patients are entered only once in clinical trials of prophylaxis,[15,79] so there is no information about its efficacy after repeated chemotherapy and prophylactic cycles; (3) meta-analyses are almost always performed on old data, not reflecting the current situation; (4) there are unequivocal data showing that increased quinolone resistance may be observed in patients who did not receive these drugs but who were affected by the use of quinolone prophylaxis in the institution; and (5) the widespread use of fluoroquinolones has been associated with the emergence of bacteria displaying cross-resistance to fluoroquinolones, β-lactams, and aminoglycosides.

In conclusion, the use of antibacterial prophylaxis of febrile neutropenia has advantages and disadvantages. Antibacterial prophylaxis has no indication, at least routinely, in low-risk patients, such as those receiving chemotherapy for solid tumors or lymphomas. In high-risk patients, the use of fluoroquinolones should be weighed against the risk of resistance, and an anti-*Pseudomonas* drug should always be part of the empirical regimen in case of fever and suspected infection under prophylaxis. If this strategy is chosen, the number of patients who need to receive antibacterial prophylaxis for preventing various outcomes (the number needed to treat) may be different according to the type of underlying disease and the incidence of the complication. Quinolone prophylaxis should not be started or used before cyclophosphamide because this has resulted in significantly lower exposure to 4-hydroxy-cyclophosphamide (the active metabolite of cyclophosphamide) in patients with non-Hodgkin's lymphoma.[81]

ANTIFUNGAL CHEMOPROPHYLAXIS

Primary Prophylaxis

Invasive mycoses are severe complications of antineoplastic chemotherapy, especially in patients with acute leukemia, and their role has increased in recent years. Although fungal infections usually represent no more than 10% of all infections (Tables 309-2 through 309-4), their associated mortality is very high. Therefore, preventing invasive fungal infections has always been considered a desirable approach. Until recently, no single randomized clinical trial had demonstrated a positive effect of antifungal prophylaxis on mortality (both overall and fungal related) but only reductions of some specific infections (candidiasis, but not aspergillosis). These results were confirmed by a large meta-analysis[82] demonstrating that prophylaxis reduced overall mortality compared with placebo or no drug with a number needed to treat of 43 to prevent one death. This effect was statistically significant for autologous and allogeneic HSCT recipients, borderline statistically significant for patients with acute leukemia (mostly undergoing induction chemotherapy), and nonsignificant for other malignancies. Antifungal prophylaxis reduced the risk for what was categorized as fungal-related death, any diagnosis of invasive mycosis (proven, probable, and possible), and the use of empirical antifungal therapy. All

types of prophylaxis reduced the incidence of *Candida* infections (*albicans* and non-*albicans*), but in patients receiving fluconazole there was a trend toward increased risk of invasive aspergillosis. This meta-analysis also included a randomized clinical trial in adults receiving multiple cycles of chemotherapy for hematologic malignancies in which the administration of posaconazole determined a statistically significant advantage in terms of mortality and a 6% absolute reduction in the relative risk of invasive mycosis, from 8% to 2% (primary endpoint), with a significant reduction also in the cumulative risk of infection compared with standard prophylaxis (fluconazole or itraconazole).[83] Given this reduction in the incidence of fungal infections and the incidence observed in the control group, the number needed to prevent one proven/probable invasive mycosis was 16, and the number needed to prevent one fungal infection-related death was 27.[84] However, with lower infection and mortality rates, the number needed to prevent one infection or one death would be higher. This underlines the need for every center to obtain accurate information on the local epidemiology of invasive mycosis and therefore tailor the results of clinical trials at every local situation. In addition, posaconazole is only available as an oral solution and absorption is highly variable, depending heavily on ingestion of a fatty meal with the drug, and gastrointestinal side effects are not unusual. The prolonged and widespread administration of antifungal prophylaxis with triazoles has been linked, with some uncertainty, to an increased risk of bacteremia, selection of natively resistant species, and the possible induction of resistance in previously susceptible *Candida* strains. Included in the list of putatively induced resistant species is *C. krusei* and *C. glabrata* from fluconazole use, agents of mucormycosis from voriconazole use, and *Aspergillus* from use of fluconazole.

Secondary Prophylaxis

Patients with a history of invasive mycosis may be at high risk of reactivation when undergoing further chemotherapy. In these patients, secondary antifungal prophylaxis is recommended. The recurrence of invasive aspergillosis has been attributed to less than 1 month of antifungal therapy before transplant and with persistence of radiologic abnormalities after treatment.[85] The role of secondary prophylaxis in preventing relapses has not been systematically studied, even though a longer duration of antifungal therapy before HSCT has been associated with a better outcome. The drug for secondary prophylaxis should be chosen according to the etiology of the infection, the localization, the drugs available and their formulations, and risks of interactions with other therapies, especially those for the treatment of the underlying disease.

Prophylaxis against *Pneumocystis jirovecii*

The risk of *P. jirovecii* pneumonia is particularly high in patients with acute lymphoblastic leukemia treated with standard chemotherapy or undergoing autologous transplants. Other patients at risk for this complication are those with solid tumors, especially of the central nervous system (mainly those with primary or secondary brain tumors receiving high-dose steroids for prolonged periods of time). The duration of risk after treatment discontinuation is not known, nor is the exact dose and duration of steroid therapy that is sufficient to predispose to the infection. Several drugs affecting cell-mediated immunity have also been associated with the risk of *P. jirovecii* pneumonia, including fludarabine, ara-C (cytarabine), methotrexate, D-actinomycin, bleomycin, and L-asparaginase. An absolute CD4+ lymphocyte count of 200/mm³ or less, or 15% or less (or similar age-related values for children), has been suggested as an indication for prophylaxis, at least in bone marrow transplants. One double-strength tablet of trimethoprim-sulfamethoxazole, given three times a week, remains the drug of choice, provided the patient is strictly compliant with the prescription. Other drugs have demonstrated efficacy in patients who cannot tolerate co-trimoxazole (see Chapter 270).

ANTIVIRAL PROPHYLAXIS

No primary antiviral chemoprophylaxis is currently recommended for patients with solid tumors, lymphomas, or acute or chronic leukemias. Secondary prophylaxis can be an option in patients who experienced recurring viral infection in previous chemotherapy cycles. Herpes simplex virus (HSV) reactivation is frequent in HSV-seropositive patients, particularly in hematopoietic stem cell transplant recipients, and it may increase the severity of oral mucositis. The recommended dose for prophylaxis against HSV for adults weighing more than 40 kg is twice-daily administration of one of these three: acyclovir 800 mg PO, acyclovir 250 mg/M^2 IV, or valacyclovir 500 mg PO. It has been postulated, but never proven, that acyclovir prophylaxis, by reducing the severity of oral stomatitis, may also reduce the incidence of bacterial infections originating from the oral flora. Varicella may represent a severe complication in patients receiving antineoplastic chemotherapy. The intravenous administration of specific immunoglobulin (VariZIG) within 72 to 96 hours of the contact represents the recommended prophylactic approach, although protection is far from absolute. If VariZIG is not available or in case of delayed notification of the contact at risk, valacyclovir 1 g three times daily for adults weighing more than 40 kg is an alternative, although efficacy is not established. Prophylactic therapy should be started on the third day after contact and continued for 22 days after exposure. If VariZIG is given, valacyclovir is continued for 28 days postexposure.

Lamivudine, started 4 weeks before chemotherapy (when possible) and continued for at least 6 months after chemotherapy has been completed, should be offered to patients with HBV infection, possibly including those negative for HbsAg and anti-HbsAg but positive for HBV DNA and HBcAb. As previously mentioned, alemtuzumab is a potent reactivator of latent intracellular pathogens, including CMV. For this reason, all patients included in alemtuzumab clinical trials have received antiviral prophylaxis (acyclovir 200 mg three times a day, famciclovir 500 mg two times a day, or valacyclovir 500 mg two times a day) for at least 2 months after completion of therapy.

PROPHYLAXIS OF TUBERCULOSIS

Latent tuberculosis may reactivate during immunosuppression following antineoplastic chemotherapy. Although no specific study in cancer patients has been performed, data from other immunocompromised patients show that isoniazid should probably be used for 6 to 9 months to prevent tuberculosis in immunocompromised patients with probable latent infection,[86] and it should be considered for patients with a positive history of tuberculosis, a positive skin test, positive interferon-γ test (enzyme-linked immunosorbent spot or quantiFERON), household exposure, previous Calmette-Guérin bacillus immunotherapy, or history of an inadequately treated tuberculosis.

THE ROLE OF COLONY-STIMULATING FACTORS IN PROPHYLAXIS

Colony-stimulating factors are used with the aim of facilitating more dose-intense treatments and decreasing treatment-related complications. In solid tumors, studies using prophylactic granulocyte colony-stimulating factor (G-CSF) have consistently demonstrated a decrease in the length and severity of neutropenia and a decrease in the incidence of febrile neutropenia.[87] On the contrary, in patients with hematologic malignancies, CSF significantly reduced the duration of severe neutropenia, but there was no significant reduction in febrile complications (even the most severe), duration of hospitalization, and patient outcome.[88,89]

THE ROLE OF IMMUNOGLOBULINS IN PROPHYLAXIS

Many neoplastic diseases, especially chronic lymphocytic leukemia, are associated with reduced production of immunoglobulins. Because maintenance of normal levels is important to prevent infections in patients with primary immunodeficiency, the same approach has been used in patients with secondary, iatrogenic defects. Studies performed on chronic leukemias have shown a reduction of infectious episodes occurring in patients with less than 600 mg/dL of immunoglobulin G (IgG), with monthly administration of immunoglobulin, provided the treatment could be given for at least 6 months.[90] This treatment reduced bacterial infections but had no effect on viral and fungal diseases. Therefore, because there are many controversial issues regarding immunoglobulin treatment, especially concerning cost, scarce availability, and optimum dosage, it seems reasonable to recommend immunoglobulins only in patients with a marked reduction of serum IgG and with more than two recent severe infections.

Treatment of Unexplained Fever in Neutropenic Patients

Fever during neutropenia has always been considered a medical emergency and should always be considered as due to infection, unless proven otherwise. Febrile episodes during the course of neutropenia are classified according to the presence or absence of a microbiologic or clinical documentation of infection. On this basis, febrile complications in neutropenic cancer patients are classified as (1) microbiologically documented infections (MDIs) with bacteremia (isolation of a significant pathogen from one or more blood cultures); (2) MDIs without bacteremia (isolation of a significant pathogen from a well-defined site of infection, usually urine; respiratory secretions obtained with sterile procedures or abscess aspiration); (3) clinically documented infections in the presence of a clinical picture clearly and objectively infectious in nature but without microbiologic proof; and (4) unexplained fever or fever of unknown origin, when clinical and microbiologic proof is lacking, but the clinical course is compatible with an infection. The development of fever or signs of infection without fever or even hypothermia in a neutropenic cancer patient must always raise the suspicion of an infection that must receive prompt empirical antibacterial treatment. The reliability of empirical therapy is clearly demonstrated by data on infection-related mortality in bacteremic cancer patients in the 1960s compared to data from present times. Fifty years ago, when empirical therapy was not routinely used, mortality was as high as 90% in some series of bacteremic neutropenic patients.[91-93] In the following years, with the adoption of the empirical antibacterial therapy approach, the availability of new antibiotics, and the general improvement of supportive care, mortality decreased dramatically. Although these data should be considered with some caution because they are derived from clinical trials and not from ad hoc epidemiologic studies, it is nevertheless impressive that in the EORTC trials of empirical therapy from 1978 to 1995, among nearly 800 documented bacteremias, the overall mortality rate decreased from 21% to 7%. In particular, the 30-day mortality rate from any cause in cancer patients with gram-negative and gram-positive bacteremia is currently as low as 10% and 6%, respectively.[94] Pure epidemiologic studies including all patients, not just those eligible to enter a clinical trial, show slightly higher but still acceptable rates (5% for gram positives, 18% for gram negatives, and 13% for polymicrobial bacteremias),[64] considering the increased intensity of chemotherapeutic regimens. Recent experience at "S. Martino" Hospital[65] in bacteremic patients undergoing HSCT showed a crude overall mortality rate at 7 and 30 days after each bloodstream infection episode of 11% and 20%, respectively. The early (7 days) mortality rate was 7%, 17%, 22%, and 14% in single gram-positive, single gram-negative, fungal (*Candida*), and polymicrobial bacteremias, respectively. *Pseudomonas aeruginosa* (7/17, 41%) was the pathogen with the highest associated 7-day mortality rate.

THE LOW-RISK PATIENT

An important change in the natural history of infections in cancer patients has been the increasing number of patients with solid tumors who are treated with high-dose chemotherapy and therefore develop neutropenia and fever. This has led several investigators to realize that not all neutropenic cancer patients are the same and that there are patients in whom the clinical course of fever during neutropenia seems to be particularly favorable. Indeed, even if treated with intensive regimens, patients with solid tumors rarely remain neutropenic for more than 8 to 10 days. In most cases, these patients are clinically stabilized within 48 hours after the first appearance of fever and are without fever within 3 or 4 days. According to this concept, the empirical therapy of febrile neutropenia in cancer patients should not be the same in every situation and in every patient but, rather, should be modulated according to individual risk factors. On the basis of this concept, several studies have been performed with the aim of identifying a priori, in a scientific way and not empirically, the patient populations at low risk. In the Multinational Association for Supportive Care in Cancer (MASCC) study,[95] factors associated with good prognosis in febrile neutropenic cancer adults were the "burden of the illness," indicating mild or moderate clinical symptoms at presentation; the absence of hypotension; the absence of chronic obstructive pulmonary disease; the presence of solid tumor or, in patients with hematologic malignancies, the absence of previous fungal infection; outpatient status; the absence of dehydration; and age younger than 60 years. Each factor was weighted and a score was given. In the validation set, a risk index score higher than 21 identified low-risk patients, with positive and negative predictive values of 91% and 36%, respectively. At this threshold, sensitivity and specificity were 71% and 68%, respectively, for a 30% misclassification rate. A similar score has also been elaborated and validated in children (Table 309-7).[60] The MASCC and the pediatric scores have been applied successfully in clinical practice. If low-risk patients can be reliably identified, the next logical step would be to try to discharge these patients early or even to treat them as outpatients or provide home management. Advances allowing outpatient management include long-term intravenous access with peripherally inserted central catheters, tunneled catheters, and totally implanted lines coupled with programmable pumps; intravenous antibiotics with a long half-life that can be safely administered once daily; oral antibiotics with reliable bioavailability and expanded spectrum of action; and the presence of nurse and doctor teams for home care. Obviously, the home environment must be clean and stable; have basic necessities such as a telephone, heating and refrigeration, and running water; and should not be too far from the hospital. In addition, someone in the patient's family should be skillful enough to provide basic assistance and to manage the central catheter and intravenous infusions. In principle, the antibiotic regimens for outpatient management should include not only a broad spectrum of action and good tolerability but also favorable pharmacokinetics, allowing single daily dosing for drugs with intravenous administration or good oral absorption. Of course, the choice of strategy should be balanced with the type of pathogens involved and the degree of antibiotic resistance. A first approach that was shown to be safe, reliable, and comparable with a classic cephalosporin plus aminoglycoside combination was single-daily intravenous ceftriaxone plus amikacin administered in an outpatient setting. The second step was to test oral versus intravenous therapy. Two studies showed ciprofloxacin plus amoxicillin-clavulanate to be as effective as standard intravenous combination therapy, although with some gastrointestinal side effects. The third approach was to test extended-spectrum moxifloxacin as single-drug oral therapy, and this treatment had a favorable result. Finally, the approach of starting with intravenous therapy cephalosporin and then switching to an oral cephalosporin was tested and shown to be effective and safe in children with cancer. Switching therapy from intravenous to oral ciprofloxacin has also been demonstrated to be a safe practice in adults not receiving this drug because prophylaxis and similar results have been obtained with oral ciprofloxacin administered after one dose of intravenous ceftriaxone plus amikacin.

THE HIGH-RISK PATIENT

The specific composition of the regimen for empirical therapy of febrile neutropenia in high-risk patients remains controversial and subject to change. Although the results of clinical trials play a pivotal role in the choice, other factors should be considered as well, including local antibiotic policies, bacteriologic statistics, resistance patterns, antibiotic toxicity, and cost. In addition, a number of patient-related factors should be taken into account, such as clinical presentation, organ failure, and status of the underlying disease and expected dura-

TABLE 309-7 Factors Associated with Low Risk of Severe Infection or an Uncomplicated Clinical Course in Febrile Neutropenic Cancer Patients*

	MASCC Score		Pediatric Score
	Clinical Parameter	*Score*	*Clinical Parameter*
Clinical data available at onset of febrile neutropenia or soon after admission	Burden of illness: no or mild symptoms	5	Hypotension
	No hypotension	5	
	No chronic obstructive pulmonary disease	4	Relapse of leukemia
	Solid tumor or no previous fungal infection	4	
	No dehydration	3	≤7 days since receipt of chemotherapy
	Outpatient status	3	
	Burden of illness: moderate symptoms	3	
	Patient's age <60 years	2	
Laboratory data available after admission			Platelets ≤50,000/μL C-reactive protein ≥90 mg/L
Notes and risk evaluation	Points attributed to the variable "burden of illness" are not cumulative. The maximum theoretical score is therefore 26.	Low-risk patient: score ≥ 21	**Low-Risk Patient** Absence of all the parameters Presence of only one of the following parameters: ≤7 days since receipt of chemotherapy *or* Platelets ≤50,000/μL **High-Risk Patient** Presence of one of the following parameters: Hypotension Relapse of leukemia C-reactive protein ≥90 mg/L *or* Concomitant presence of two or more of the identified parameters

*The MASCC score and the pediatric score are derived from prospective studies and validated with independent data sets.
MASCC, Multinational Association for Supportive Care in Cancer study.

tion of neutropenia. Currently, escalation therapy (i.e., starting with a relatively narrow-spectrum coverage and then adjusting therapy if necessary) seems appropriate in the majority of cases. Monotherapy with an anti-*Pseudomonas* β-lactam antibiotic (ceftazidime, cefepime, or piperacillin-tazobactam) probably represents the most rational approach in centers without evidence of increased resistance phenomena,[96] with the carbapenems used as second-line therapy in failing patients with documented infections. Antibiotics should be administered at the maximum dosage and according to their best infusion schedule, as from pharmacokinetic/pharmacodynamic parameters. In a standard clinical situation, combining an aminoglycoside with a β-lactam is not deemed necessary because of more toxicity and no clinical advantage. This was clearly shown by a double-blind placebo-controlled clinical trial comparing piperacillin-tazobactam with placebo versus the same drug with amikacin. Currently, the use of amikacin in front-line empirical antibacterial therapy can be recommended only in association with ceftriaxone to ensure some kind of anti-*Pseudomonas* coverage. The empirical use of an anti-gram-positive antibiotic such as vancomycin, teicoplanin, linezolid, or daptomycin is not recommended by any guideline, either as initial therapy or in nonresponding patients, unless a resistant pathogen is isolated.[97] However, data suggest that antibiotic resistance may soon have an impact in hematologic and oncologic wards. For example, in the aforementioned experience at "S. Martino" Hospital, we observed an increase in the incidence of bacteremias due to methicillin-resistant *S. aureus*, ampicillin-resistant enterococci, and ciprofloxacin-resistant and extended-spectrum β-lactamase–producing gram negatives. These results led us to change the empirical therapy approach, with a diversified deescalating approach tailored to the clinical presentation: Meropenem plus vancomycin represents the empirical therapy in patients presenting with severe sepsis, septic shock, or suspected bacterial pneumonia in order to avoid inadequate treatment of bacteremia possibly caused by extended-spectrum β-lactamase–producer gram-negative rods and to provide adequate treatment for enterococci and methicillin-resistant staphylococci. Then, vancomycin is discontinued within 3 days, if not necessary. Colistin is considered as second-line therapy if a multidrug-resistant gram negative is isolated, whereas linezolid is used in case of staphylococcal or enterococcal pneumonia. In less severe conditions (i.e., fever, no pneumonia, and stable hemodynamic conditions), the escalating approach is still used, with piperacillin-tazobactam as first-line empirical monotherapy. Using amikacin in combination might be an option in some instances, although nephrotoxicity is a serious problem in high-risk populations.

Table 309-8 summarizes the possible major antibiotic regimens being used for empirical therapy of febrile neutropenia in different settings according to randomized clinical trials and guidelines. It must again be stressed that every patient is a single human and clinical entity and that every decision should be based on clinical, microbiologic, patient-related, and epidemiologic grounds.

ANTIBACTERIAL TREATMENT MODIFICATION

Frequent therapeutic changes are common in cancer patients with persistent fever and granulocytopenia. Microbiologically documented infections should be treated with antibiotics to which the isolated pathogen is susceptible in vitro, even if the patient's clinical condition improves spontaneously. It is also appropriate when clear signs of treatment failure are evident (Table 309-9) or in the presence of a clinical picture suggestive of a specific etiology that is likely not covered by the allocated antibiotics (e.g., catheter-related infection, perianal cellulitis, and abdominal typhlitis). More controversial is what to do when the patient remains febrile in the absence of evident signs of

TABLE 309-8	Empirical Therapies during Febrile Neutropenia				
Patient Type	Drug	Route of Administration	Daily Pediatric Dosage (mg/kg)	Daily Adult Dosage (mg)	Number of Daily Divided Doses
High risk	Piperacillin-tazobactam	IV	300 (as piperacillin)	12,000 (as piperacillin)	3
	Ceftazidime	IV	100	6,000	3
	Cefepime	IV	100	4,000-6,000	3
	Meropenem	IV	60	3,000	3
	Imipenem cylastatin	IV	60-100 (as imipenem)	2,000-3,000 (as imipenem)	3-4
	Ciprofloxacin	IV	15-30	1,200-1,500	2
	Ceftriaxone	IV	80	2,000	1
	Amikacin	IV	20	1,000-1,500	1
	Presence of skin lesions or suspect CVC infection				
	Vancomycin	IV	40	2,000	2
	Teicoplanin	IV	10 (a loading dose of 10 mg/kg bid must be administered on the first day of treatment)	600-1,200 (a loading dose of 600 mg bid must be administered on the first day of treatment)	1 (2 doses must be administered on the first day of treatment)
Non–high risk	Association				
	Amoxicillin clavulanate +	Oral	60 (as amoxicillin)	1,500-3,000 (as amoxicillin)	3
	Ciprofloxacin	Oral	30	1,500	2
	Switch therapy				
	Cefixime *or*	Oral	8	400	2
	Ciprofloxacin	Oral	30	1,500	2
Empirical or preemptive antifungal therapy	Amphotericin B deoxycholate*	IV	0.5-1	0.5-1 mg/kg	1
	Liposomal amphotericin B	IV	3	3 mg/kg	1
	Amphotericin B lipid complex	IV	5	5 mg/kg	1
	Caspofungin	IV	50 mg/m² for age <12 years	70 on first day, 50 on the following days	1
	Voriconazole	IV	7 mg/kg q12h for age <12 years	6 mg/kg q12h ×2, then 4 mg/kg q12h	2
	Fluconazole†	IV	6-10	400	1

*Contraindicated in the presence of risk factors for renal toxicity (e.g., impaired renal function at baseline, nephrotoxic co-medication including aminoglycoside antibiotics, and history of previous toxicity).
†In patients at low risk of invasive mold infection.
CVC, central venous catheter.

TABLE 309-9	Proposed Definition of Failure of Empirical Antibacterial Therapy Derived from the Experience of EORTC-IATG Studies

- Persistence of fever (>39°C) and chills after 24-48 hr of therapy
- Relapse of fever (>38°C) after at least 24 hr of defervescence
- Progression of sepsis syndrome toward organ failure
- Development of disseminated intravascular coagulation, acute respiratory distress syndrome, and multiple organ failure
- Persistence of positive cultures from site of infection or blood after 24 hr of therapy
- Relapse of the primary infection
- Appearance of a new infection

EORTC, European Organization for Research and Treatment of Cancer; IATG, International Antimicrobial Therapy Group.

clinical deterioration but also in the absence of any microbiologic or clinical documentation of infection (unexplained fever or fever of unknown origin) or in documented infections due to pathogens that are sensitive to the initial empirical regimen in vitro. In general, good clinical practice in infectious diseases suggests that persistence of fever does not necessarily mean failure of a given antibiotic regimen, especially if the patient is otherwise clinically stable. A febrile and neutropenic patient with bacteremia might require 2 to 7 days to defervescence, even if the isolated pathogen is sensitive to the allocated antibiotic regimen. Therefore, it is likely that in patients with fever but who are otherwise in good clinical condition, the best clinical option should be watchful waiting and nothing else. There is little evidence that a planned, progressive succession of antibiotic therapy in cancer patients can be recommended for widespread use.

EMPIRICAL OR PREEMPTIVE ANTIFUNGAL THERAPY

The empirical antifungal therapy consists of administering an antifungal drug in a persistently febrile and neutropenic cancer patient after a variable period of empirical antibacterial therapy, in the absence of any clinical, microbiologic, or radiologic documentation of a fungal infection.[98] The rationale for this practice is based on old autopsy studies showing fungal infections undetected during life and on two randomized studies that enrolled less than 200 patients total. These studies were not double blind or placebo controlled, and they did not conclude an unequivocal advantage for empirical antifungal therapy. In both studies, the statistical power of the observed results was very small, especially for subgroup analyses. Nevertheless, empirical antifungal therapy in persistently febrile and granulocytopenic cancer patients without documented infections has become common practice in many cancer centers worldwide, and many drugs have been tested for this indication. Except for the first studies, which used as the main endpoint persistence of fever and survival, most studies have used a very controversial composite clinical endpoint, which included five criteria (defervescence, no discontinuation for toxicity, treatment of baseline fungal infections, prevention of breakthrough fungal infections, and survival). In general, no drug was significantly more effective than the control one, and differences were only based on lower toxicity. Awareness has grown that the empirical approach has resulted in a tremendous overtreatment of just a symptom (fever). This realization and recent advances in diagnosis are making the practice of empirical therapy more problematic and have encouraged development of a preemptive approach. Briefly, preemptive therapy is aimed at treating a fungal disease when suggestive but not definitive diagnosis is present. The requirement for initiating preemptive therapy hinges on either a radiologic result (lung computed tomography scan) or a microbiologic result (Aspergillus galactomannan in serum or bronchoalveolar lavage [BAL] fluid and cytologic detection of fungal hyphae or positive culture on sputum or BAL fluid). Whether or not a pulmonary infiltrate is enough or typical radiologic signs are required to start an antifungal is a matter of debate. Similarly, some centers start an antifungal when both radiologic signs and laboratory confirmations are available, whereas others prefer to be more conservative and start when a positive galactomannan is found or an infiltrate is detected, whichever occurs first. Despite these differences in interpretation, some sort of preemptive therapy is becoming the rule, at least in European centers and at least in those centers in which these diagnostic procedures are available and well organized. This approach reduces the number of patients unnecessarily exposed to an antifungal drug. Table 309-8 reports drugs indicated for empirical or preemptive antifungal therapy. Drugs approved for empirical therapy include liposomal amphotericin B, caspofungin, and itraconazole, whereas the drug approved for treatment of invasive aspergillosis is voriconazole, followed closely by liposomal amphotericin B, with caspofungin as an alternative, especially when lack of toxicity is pivotal. No drug has been approved for preemptive therapy.

INITIAL MANAGEMENT OF A NEUTROPENIC PATIENT WITH A SITE OF INFECTION

The Patient with a Catheter-Related Infection

Empirical therapy for a suspected indwelling CVC-related infection in patients with febrile neutropenia is practiced in some centers despite recommendations from guideline committees that this not be done without specific reasons, including septic shock, rapidly progressive infection, infection at the exit or tunnel site, or blood culture results indicating a catheter source (see Chapter 302). Another exception to the use of monotherapy is in institutions with frequent catheter sepsis from methicillin-resistant *Staphylococcus aureus*, vancomycin-resistant enterococci, or other pathogens resistant to the usual monotherapy for neutropenic patients. Although initial treatment may not cover coagulase-negative staphylococci, these bacteria grow rapidly in blood culture and cause generally more indolent infection. The choice of the antibiotic regimen for suspected catheter sepsis should be based on the epidemiology of CVC-related infections in each individual center and on the renal function and other characteristics of the individual patient. In contrast, the empirical inclusion of an antifungal drug seems not to be appropriate in light of the relatively low incidence of candidemia in this clinical setting. After the causative pathogen has been identified, treatment should be tailored according to its susceptibility pattern. For more specific therapeutic options, see Chapter 302.

The Febrile Cancer Patient with Pulmonary Infiltrates

The choice of the empirical therapy in neutropenic patients with a pulmonary infiltrate should be based on the type of infiltrate and the time of appearance with respect to onset of fever and epidemiologic or anamnestic data. For example, viridans streptococci are a frequent cause of adult respiratory distress syndrome (ARDS) in neutropenic patients with severe oral mucositis. If this is a likely possibility, a penicillin in combination with a glycopeptide is the most logical choice. If the pneumonia is part of the initial clinical presentation of febrile neutropenia, it is likely that the infecting pathogen is an opportunistic agent typical of neutropenic patients (*S. aureus*, *Klebsiella*, or *P. aeruginosa*). Therefore, the same antibiotic regimen commonly used for febrile neutropenia in high-risk patients should be used, although a severe and complicated clinical course should be expected. On the contrary, if pneumonia apparently occurs as a breakthrough infection in a patient already receiving broad-spectrum antibiotics, a fungal etiology is likely and antifungal therapy is logical, although a resistant bacterial pathogen, including *Legionella* or *M. pneumoniae*, is also a possibility. Interstitial pneumonia is relatively rare during neutropenia, but it does occur. In this case, CMV, influenza virus, *P. jirovecii*, and *Mycoplasma pneumoniae* are the likely etiologies. The appropriate diagnostic measures should be implemented, and treatment should be tailored accordingly.

The Febrile Cancer Patient with Abdominal Symptoms

Febrile neutropenic patients may present with gastrointestinal signs and symptoms such as abdominal pain, nausea, vomiting, and diarrhea in addition to fever. In these patients, an initial conservative management with bowel rest, intravenous fluids, total parenteral nutrition, and broad-spectrum antibiotics with antianaerobic activity is first choice. In some cases (3% to 6%) of patients receiving aggressive treatment for acute leukemia, full-blown neutropenic enterocolitis develops, which is a severe clinical syndrome characterized by fever, severe abdominal pain, and sometimes hemorrhagic diarrhea evolving to acute abdomen and septic shock. In centers with a high incidence of *C. difficile* infection, antibiotic treatment directed toward this pathogen should also be considered in the initial therapeutic approach (see Chapter 96). Surgical intervention is usually not indicated but may be recommended in the setting of obstruction, perforation, persistent gastrointestinal bleeding despite correction of thrombocytopenia and coagulopathy, and clinical deterioration.

OTHER TREATMENTS

Granulocyte Transfusions

Granulocyte transfusions from donors stimulated with growth factors have been proposed in desperate cases of life-threatening bacterial and fungal infections in patients with persistent neutropenia unlikely to recover promptly. The evidence for clinical efficacy is limited to that of case reports and small series, and the results are not uniform.[99] In any case, the average number of collected granulocytes for adults should be greater than 1×10^{10}.

Use of Colony-Stimulating Factors

Many case reports have suggested the effectiveness of growth factors in the treatment of severe, life-threatening bacterial or fungal infections. However, a meta-analysis published in 2002 suggested the lack of efficacy of systematic, widespread use of G-CSF for therapy of febrile neutropenia.[100] In any case, the use of G-CSF (5 μg/kg/day) may be an option in patients with fever and neutropenia who are at high risk for infection-associated complications or who have prognostic factors that are predictive of poor clinical outcomes, such as prolonged (>10 days) and profound ($<0.1 \times 10^9$/L) neutropenia, age older than 65 years, uncontrolled primary disease, pneumonia, hypotension, and multiorgan dysfunction (sepsis syndrome). It should also be remembered that in patients with pulmonary aspergillosis, a (too) rapid recovery of the granulocyte count may be associated with the development of severe complications such as pneumothorax or fatal hemoptysis.

Use of Steroids

The use of steroids in septic shock is still a matter of debate even though low dosages have been suggested as effective adjuvant therapy in patients with septic syndrome. However, in neutropenic patients with bacteremia and ARDS (in these cases, viridans streptococci are the leading etiologic agents) or in the presence of *P. jirovecii* pneumonia, corticosteroids have been advocated as a useful therapeutic option.

REFERENCES

1. Sonis ST, Oster G, Fuchs H, et al. Oral mucositis and the clinical and economic outcomes of hematopoietic stem-cell transplantation. *J Clin Oncol.* 2001;19:2201-2205.
2. van der Velden WJFM, Blijlevens NMA, Feuth T, et al. Febrile mucositis in haematopoietic SCT recipients. *Bone Marrow Transpl.* 2009;43:55-60.
3. Bodey GP, Buckley M, Sathe YS, et al. Quantitative relationships between circulating leukocytes and infection in patients with acute leukemia. *Ann Intern Med.* 1966;64:328-340.
4. Sickles EA, Greene WH, Wiernik PH. Clinical presentation of infection in granulocytopenic patients. *Arch Intern Med.* 1975;135:715-719.
5. Castagnola E, Fontana V, Caviglia I, et al. A prospective study on the epidemiology of febrile episodes during chemotherapy-induced neutropenia in children with cancer or after hemopoietic stem cell transplantation. *Clin Infect Dis.* 2007;45:1296-1304.
6. Chehata S, Grira C, Legrand P, et al. Applying the concept of healthcare-associated infections to hematology programs. *Haematologica.* 2006;91:1414-1417.
7. Castagnola E, Conte M, Parodi S, et al. Incidence of bacteremias and invasive mycoses in children with high risk neuroblastoma. *Pediatr Blood Cancer.* 2007;49:672-677.
8. Haupt R, Romanengo M, Fears T, et al. Incidence of septicaemias and invasive mycoses in children undergoing treatment for solid tumours: a 12-year experience at a single Italian institution. *Eur J Cancer.* 2001;37:2413-2419.
9. Engelhard D, Cordonnier C, Shaw PJ, et al. Early and late invasive pneumococcal infection following stem cell transplantation: a European Bone Marrow Transplantation survey. *Br J Haematol.* 2002;117:444-450.
10. Urrea M, Rives S, Cruz O, et al. Nosocomial infections among pediatric hematology/oncology patients: results of a prospective incidence study. *Am J Infect Control.* 2004;32:205-208.
11. Simon A, Fleischhack G, Hasan C, et al. Surveillance for nosocomial and central line-related infections among pediatric hematology-oncology. *Infect Control Hosp Epidemiol.* 2000;21:592-596.
12. Castagnola E, Caviglia I, Pistorio A, et al. Bloodstream infections and invasive mycoses in children undergoing acute leukaemia treatment: a 13-year experience at a single Italian institution. *Eur J Cancer.* 2005;41:1439-1445.
13. Dettenkofer M, Wenzler-Röttele S, Babikir R, et al. Surveillance of nosocomial sepsis and pneumonia in patients with a bone marrow or peripheral blood stem cell transplant: a multicenter project. *Clin Infect Dis.* 2005;40:926-931.
14. Vekemans M, Robinson J, Georgala A, et al. Low mannose-binding lectin concentration is associated with severe infection in patients with hematological cancer who are undergoing chemotherapy. *Clin Infect Dis.* 2007;44:1593-1601.
15. Gafter-Gvili A, Fraser A, Paul M, et al. Meta-analysis: antibiotic prophylaxis reduces mortality in neutropenic patients. *Ann Intern Med.* 2005;142:979-995.
16. Bucaneve G, Micozzi A, Menichetti F, et al. Levofloxacin to prevent bacterial infection in patients with cancer and neutropenia. *N Engl J Med.* 2005;353:977-987.
17. Cullen M, Steven N, Billingham L, et al. Antibacterial prophylaxis after chemotherapy for solid tumors and lymphomas. *N Engl J Med.* 2005;353:988-998.
18. Simon A, Bode U, Fleischhack G, et al. Surveillance of nosocomial infections in pediatric cancer patients. *Am J Infect Control.* 2005;33:611.
19. Lehrnbecher T, Zimmermann M, Reinhardt D, et al. Prophylactic human granulocyte colony-stimulating factor after induction therapy in pediatric acute myeloid leukemia. *Blood.* 2007;109:936-943.
20. Simon A, Ammann RA, Bode U, et al. Healthcare-associated infections in pediatric cancer patients: results of a prospective surveillance study from university hospitals in Germany and Switzerland. *BMC Infect Dis.* 2008;8:70.
21. Paulus SC, van Saene HK, Hemsworth S, et al. A prospective study of septicaemia on a paediatric oncology unit: a three-year experience at the Royal Liverpool Children's Hospital, Alder Hey, UK. *Eur J Cancer.* 2005;41:2132-2140.
22. Madani TA. Clinical infections and bloodstream isolates associated with fever in patients undergoing chemotherapy for acute myeloid leukemia. *Infection.* 2000;28:367-373.
23. Pagano L, Caira M, Nosari A, et al. Fungal infections in recipients of hematopoietic stem cell transplants: results of the SEIFEM B-2004 study—Sorveglianza Epidemiologica Infezioni Fungine Nelle Emopatie Maligne. *Clin Infect Dis.* 2007;45:1161-1170.
24. Lehrnbecher T, Varwig D, Kaiser J, et al. Infectious complications in pediatric acute myeloid leukemia: analysis of the prospective multi-institutional clinical trial AML-BFM 93. *Leukemia.* 2004;18:72-77.
25. Pagano L, Caira M, Candoni A, et al. The epidemiology of fungal infections in patients with hematologic malignancies: the SEIFEM-2004 study. *Haematologica.* 2006;91:1068-1075.
26. Girmenia C, Lo Coco F, Breccia M, et al. Infectious complications in patients with acute promyelocytic leukaemia treated with the AIDA regimen. *Leukemia.* 2003;17:925-930.
27. Walsh TJ, Pappas P, Winston DJ, et al. Voriconazole compared with liposomal amphotericin B for empirical antifungal therapy in patients with neutropenia and persistent fever. *N Engl J Med.* 2002;346:225-234.
28. Walsh TJ, Teppler H, Donowitz GR, et al. Caspofungin versus liposomal amphotericin B for empirical antifungal therapy in patients with persistent fever and neutropenia. *N Engl J Med.* 2004;351:1391-1402.
29. Castagnola R, Faraci M, Moroni C, et al. Invasive mycoses in children receiving hemopoietic SCT. *Bone Marrow Transplant.* 2008;41:S107-S111.
30. Caira M, Girmenia C, Fadda RM, et al. Invasive fungal infections in patients with acute myeloid leukemia and in those submitted to allogeneic hemopoietic stem cell transplant: who is at highest risk? *Eur J Haematol.* 2008;81:242-243.
31. Auletta JJ, O'Riordan MA, Nieder ML. Infections in children with cancer: a continued need for the comprehensive physical examination. *J Pediatr Hematol Oncol.* 1999;21:501-508.
32. Carlisle PS, Gucalp R, Wiernik PH. Nosocomial infections in neutropenic cancer patients. *Infect Control Hosp Epidemiol.* 1993;14:320-324.
33. Laws HJ, Kobbe G, Dilloo D, et al. Surveillance of nosocomial infections in paediatric recipients of bone marrow or peripheral blood stem cell transplantation during neutropenia, compared with adult recipients. *J Hosp Infect.* 2006;62:80-88.
34. Fratino G, Molinari AC, Parodi S, et al. Central venous catheter-related complications in children with oncological/hematological diseases: an observational study of 418 devices. *Ann Oncol.* 2005;16:648-654.
35. Maki DG, Kluger DM, Crnich CJ. The risk of bloodstream infection in adults with different intravascular devices: a systematic review of 200 published prospective studies. *Mayo Clin Proc.* 2006;81:1159-1171.
36. Castagnola E, Fratino G, Valera M, et al. Correlation between "malfunctioning events" and catheter-related infections in pediatric cancer patients bearing tunneled indwelling central venous catheter: results of a prospective observational study. *Support Care Cancer.* 2005;13:757-759.
37. Castagnola E, Molinari AC, Giacchino M, et al. Incidence of catheter-related infections within 30 days from insertion of Hickman-Broviac catheters. *Pediatr Blood Cancer.* 2007;48:35-38.
38. Hengartner H, Berger C, Nadal D, et al. Port-A-Cath infections in children with cancer. *Eur J Cancer.* 2004;40:2452-2458.
39. Povoski SP. A prospective analysis of the cephalic vein cutdown approach for chronic indwelling central venous access in 100 consecutive cancer patients. *Ann Surg Oncol.* 2000;7:496-502.
40. Biffi R, Corrado F, de Braud F, et al. Long-term, totally implantable central venous access ports connected to a Groshong catheter for chemotherapy of solid tumours: experience from 178 cases using a single type of device. *Eur J Cancer.* 1997;33:1190-1194.
41. Cogliati AA, Dell'Utri D, Picardi A, et al. Central venous catheterization in pediatric patients affected by hematological malignancies. *Haematologica.* 1995;80:448-450.
42. Cheong K, Perry D, Karapetis C, et al. High rate of complications associated with peripherally inserted central venous catheters in patients with solid tumours. *Intern Med J.* 2004;34:234-238.
43. Harter C, Ostendorf T, Bach A, et al. Peripherally inserted central venous catheters for autologous blood progenitor cell transplantation in patients with haematological malignancies. *Support Care Cancer.* 2003;11:790-794.
44. Openshaw KL, Picus D, Hicks ME, et al. Interventional radiologic placement of Hohn central venous catheters: results and complications in 100 consecutive patients. *J Vasc Interv Radiol.* 1994;5:111-115.
45. Raad I, Davis S, Becker M, et al. Low infection rate and long durability of nontunneled silastic catheters: a safe and cost-effective alternative for long-term venous access. *Arch Intern Med.* 1993;153:1791-1796.
46. Penel N, Neu JC, Clisant S, et al. Risk factors for early catheter-related infections in cancer patients. *Cancer.* 2007;110:1586-1592.
47. Abedin S, Kapoor G. Peripherally inserted central venous catheters are a good option for prolonged venous access in children with cancer. *Pediatr Blood Cancer.* 2008;51:251-255.

48. Allen RC, Holdsworth MT, Johnson CA, et al. Risk determinants for catheter-associated blood stream infections in children and young adults with cancer. *Pediatr Blood Cancer.* 2008;51:53-58.

49. Beekmann SE, Henderson DK. Infections caused by percutaneous intravascular devices. In: Mandell GL, Bennett JE, Doolin R, eds. *Principles and Practice of Infectious Diseases.* Philadelphia: Churchill Livingstone; 2005:3347-3362.

50. Koo S, Baden LR. Infectious complications associated with immunomodulating monoclonal antibodies used in the treatment of hematologic malignancy. *Natl Compr Canc Netw.* 2008;6:202-213.

51. Capone A, Valle M, Proietti F, et al. Postoperative infections in cytoreductive surgery with hyperthermic intraperitoneal intraoperative chemotherapy for peritoneal carcinomatosis. *J Surg Oncol.* 2007;96:507-513.

52. Glehen O, Kwiatkowski F, Sugarbaker PH, et al. Cytoreductive surgery combined with perioperative intraperitoneal chemotherapy for the management of peritoneal carcinomatosis from colorectal cancer: a multi-institutional study. *J Clin Oncol.* 2004;22:3284-3292.

53. Sugarbaker PH, Alderman R, Edwards G, et al. Prospective morbidity and mortality assessment of cytoreductive surgery plus perioperative intraperitoneal chemotherapy to treat peritoneal dissemination of appendiceal mucinous malignancy. *Ann Surg Oncol.* 2006;13:635-644.

54. Mortenson MM, Schneider PD, Khatri VP, et al. Immediate breast reconstruction after mastectomy increases wound complications: however, initiation of adjuvant chemotherapy is not delayed. *Arch Surg.* 2004;139:988-991.

55. Penel N, Yazdanpanah Y, Chauvet M, et al. Prevention of surgical site infection after breast cancer surgery by targeted prophylaxis antibiotic in patients at high risk of surgical site infection. *J Surg Oncol.* 2007;96:124-129.

56. Konishi T, Watanabe T, Kishimoto J, et al. Elective colon and rectal surgery differ in risk factors for wound infection results of prospective surveillance. *Ann Surg.* 2006;244:758-763.

57. Morris CD, Sepkowitz K, Fonshell C, et al. Prospective identification of risk factors for wound infection after lower extremity oncologic surgery. *Ann Surg Oncol.* 2003;10:778-782.

58. Kamana M, Escalante C, Mullen CA, et al. Bacterial infections in low-risk, febrile neutropenic patients: over a decade of experience at a comprehensive cancer center. *Cancer.* 2005;104: 422-426.

59. Del Favero A, Menichetti F, Martino P, et al. A multicenter, double-blind, placebo-controlled trial comparing piperacillin-tazobactam with and without amikacin as empiric therapy for febrile neutropenia. *Clin Infect Dis.* 2001;33:1295-1301.

60. Santolaya ME, Alvarez AM, Avilés CL, et al. Prospective evaluation of a model of prediction of invasive bacterial infection risk among children with cancer, fever, and neutropenia. *Clin Infect Dis.* 2002;35:678-683.

61. Santolaya ME, Alvarez AM, Becker A, et al. Prospective, multicenter evaluation of risk factors associated with invasive bacterial infection in children with cancer, neutropenia, and fever. *J Clin Oncol.* 2001;19:3415-3421.

62. Wisplinghoff H, Seifert H, Wenzel RP, et al. Current trends in the epidemiology of nosocomial bloodstream infections in patients with hematological malignancies and solid neoplasms in hospitals in the United States. *Clin Infect Dis.* 2003;36:1103-1110.

63. Reich G, Cornely OA, Sandherr M, et al. Empirical antimicrobial monotherapy in patients after high-dose chemotherapy and autologous stem cell transplantation: a randomised, multicentre trial. *Br J Haematol.* 2005;130:265-270.

64. Klastersky J, Ameye L, Maertens J, et al. Bacteraemia in febrile neutropenic cancer patients. *Int J Antimicrob Agents.* 2007;30: S51-S59.

65. Mikulska M, Del Bono V, Raiola AM, et al. Blood stream infections in allogeneic hematopoietic stem cell transplant recipients: reemergence of gram-negative rods and increasing antibiotic resistance. *Biol Blood Marrow Transplant.* 2009;15:47-53.

66. Zahar JR, Farhat H, Chachaty E, et al. Incidence and clinical significance of anaerobic bacteraemia in cancer patients: a 6-year retrospective study. *Clin Microbiol Infect.* 2005;11: 724-729.

67. Gorschlüter M, Hahn C, Ziske C, et al. Low frequency of enteric infections by *Salmonella, Shigella, Yersinia* and *Campylobacter* in patients with acute leukemia. *Infection.* 2002;30:22-25.

68. Libshitz HI, Pannu HK, Elting LS, et al. Tuberculosis in cancer patients: an update. *J Thorac Imaging.* 1997;12:41-46.

69. Jagarlamudi R, Kumar L, Kochupillai V, et al. Infections in acute leukemia: an analysis of 240 febrile episodes. *Med Oncol.* 2000;17:111-116.

70. Pfeiffer CD, Fine JP, Safdar N. Diagnosis of invasive aspergillosis using a galactomannan assay: a meta-analysis. *Clin Infect Dis.* 2006;42:1417-1427.

71. Odabasi Z, Mattiuzzi G, Estey E, et al. Beta-D-glucan as a diagnostic adjunct for invasive fungal infections: validation, cutoff development, and performance in patients with acute myelogenous leukemia and myelodysplastic syndrome. *Clin Infect Dis.* 2004;39:199-205.

72. Pazos C, Ponton J, Del Palacio A. Contribution of (1-3)-β-D-glucan chromogenic assay to diagnosis and therapeutic monitoring of invasive aspergillosis in neutropenic adult patients: a comparison with serial screening for circulating galactomannan. *J Clin Microbiol.* 2005;43:299-305.

73. Senn L, Robinson JO, Schmidt S, et al. 1,3-β-D-Glucan antigenemia for early diagnosis of invasive fungal infections in neutropenic patients with acute leukemia. *Clin Infect Dis.* 2008;46:878-885.

74. Cornet M, Fleury L, Maslo C, et al. Epidemiology of invasive aspergillosis in France: a six-year multicentric survey in the Greater Paris area. *J Hosp Infect.* 2002;51:288-296.

75. Morgan J, Wannemuehler KA, Marr KA, et al. Incidence of invasive aspergillosis following hematopoietic stem cell and solid organ transplantation: interim results of a prospective multicenter surveillance program. *Med Mycol.* 2005;43:S49-S58.

76. Zaoutis TE, Heydon K, Chu JH, et al. Epidemiology, outcomes, and costs of invasive aspergillosis in immunocompromised children in the United States, 2000. *Pediatrics.* 2006;117: e711-e716.

77. Rodriguez M, Fishman JA. Prevention of infection due to *Pneumocystis* spp. in human immunodeficiency virus-negative immunocompromised patients. *Clin Microbiol Rev.* 2004;17: 770-782.

78. Han XY. Epidemiologic analysis of reactivated cytomegalovirus antigenemia in patients with cancer. *J Clin Microbiol.* 2007;45: 1126-1132.

79. Leibovici L, Paul M, Cullen M, et al. Antibiotic prophylaxis in neutropenic patients: new evidence, practical decisions. *Cancer.* 2006;107:1743-1751.

80. Anonymous. Prevention of bacterial infection in neutropenic patients with hematologic malignancies: a randomized, multicenter trial comparing norfloxacin with ciprofloxacin. The GIMEMA Infection Program. Gruppo Italiano Malattie Ematologiche Maligne dell'Adulto. *Ann Intern Med.* 1991;115: 7-12.

81. Bucaneve G, Castagnola E, Viscoli C, et al. Quinolone prophylaxis for bacterial infections in afebrile high risk neutropenic patients. *Eur J Cancer Suppl.* 2007;5:5-12.

82. Robenshtok E, Gafter-Gvili A, Goldberg A, et al. Antifungal prophylaxis in cancer patients after chemotherapy or hematopoietic stem-cell transplantation: systematic review and meta-analysis. *J Clin Oncol.* 2007;34:5471-5489.

83. Cornely OA, Maertens J, Winston DJ, et al. Posaconazole vs. fluconazole or itraconazole prophylaxis in patients with neutropenia. *N Engl J Med.* 2007;356:348-359.

84. Cornely OA, Ullmann AJ. Numbers needed to treat with posaconazole prophylaxis to prevent invasive fungal infection and death. *Clin Infect Dis.* 2008;46:1626-1628.

85. Sipsas NV, Kontoyiannis DP. Clinical issues regarding relapsing aspergillosis and the efficacy of secondary antifungal prophylaxis in patients with hematological malignancies. *Clin Infect Dis.* 2006;42:1584-1591.

86. Hernández-Cruz B, Ponce-de-León-Rosales S, Sifuentes-Osornio J, et al. Tuberculosis prophylaxis in patients with steroid treatment and systemic rheumatic diseases: a case-control study. *Clin Exp Rheumatol.* 1999;17:81-87.

87. Timmer-Bonte JN, Tjan-Heijnen VC. Febrile neutropenia: highlighting the role of prophylactic antibiotics and granulocyte colony-stimulating factor during standard dose chemotherapy for solid tumors. *Anticancer Drugs.* 2006;17:881-889.

88. Levenga TH, Timmer-Bonte JNH. Review of the value of colony stimulating factors for prophylaxis of febrile neutropenic episodes in adult patients treated for haematological malignancies. *Br J Haematol.* 2007;138:146-152.

89. Wittman B, Horan J, Lyman GH. Prophylactic colony-stimulating factors in children receiving myelosuppressive chemotherapy: a meta-analysis of randomized controlled trials. *Cancer Treat Rev.* 2006;32:298-303.

90. Molica S, Musto P, Chiurazzi F, et al. Prophylaxis against infections with low-dose intravenous immunoglobulins (IVIG) in chronic lymphocytic leukemia: results of a crossover study. *Haematologica.* 1996;81:121-126.

91. DuPont HL, Spink WW. Infections due to gram-negative organisms: an analysis of 860 patients with bacteremia at the University of Minnesota Medical Center, 1958-1966. *Medicine (Baltimore).* 1969;48:307-332.

92. Bodey GP, Rodriguez V, Chang HY, et al. Fever and infection in leukemic patients: a study of 494 consecutive patients. *Cancer.* 1978;41:1610-1622.

93. Chang HY, Rodriguez V, Narboni G, et al. Causes of death in adults with acute leukemia. *Medicine (Baltimore).* 1976; 55:259-268.

94. Viscoli C. EORTC International Antimicrobial Therapy Group. Management of infection in cancer patients: studies of the EORTC International Antimicrobial Therapy Group (IATG). *Eur J Cancer.* 2002;38:S82-S87.

95. Klastersky J, Paesmans M, Rubenstein EB, et al. The Multinational Association for Supportive Care in Cancer risk index: a multinational scoring system for identifying low-risk febrile neutropenic cancer patients. *J Clin Oncol.* 2000;18:3038-3051.

96. Drgona L, Paul M, Bucaneve G, et al. The need for aminoglycosides in combination with beta-lactams for high-risk, febrile neutropenic patients with leukaemia. *Eur J Cancer Suppl.* 2007;5:13-22.

97. Cometta A, Marchetti O, Calandra T. Empirical use of anti–gram-positive antibiotics in febrile neutropenic cancer patients with acute leukaemia. *Eur J Cancer Suppl.* 2007;5:23-31.

98. Marchetti O, Cordonnier C, Calandra T. Empirical antifungal therapy in neutropaenic cancer patients with persistent fever. *Eur J Cancer Suppl.* 2007;5:32-42.

99. van de Wetering MD, Weggelaar N, Offringa M, et al. Granulocyte transfusions in neutropaenic children: a systematic review of the literature. *Eur J Cancer.* 2007;4:2082-2092.

100. Berghmans T, Paesmans M, Lafitte JJ, et al. Therapeutic use of granulocyte and granulocyte-macrophage colony-stimulating factors in febrile neutropenic cancer patients: a systematic review of the literature with meta-analysis. *Support Care Cancer.* 2002;10:181-188.

310

Risk Factors and Approaches to Infections in Transplant Recipients

J. STEPHEN DUMMER | LORA D. THOMAS

Successful clinical organ transplantation dates from 1954, when the immunologic barrier to transplantation was ingeniously circumvented in a few patients with kidney failure by using organs from donors who were identical twins with the patients.[1] Subsequently, transplantation of organs from genetically different individuals was attempted with lymphoid irradiation to suppress the recipient's immune response to the allograft, but these efforts met with only occasional success. In the early 1960s, immunosuppressive regimens employing azathioprine and corticosteroids were introduced. These provided more effective control of allograft rejection that not only was sustainable but could be adjusted according to an individual patient's circumstances. This development catapulted kidney transplantation beyond the experimental stage, and both living-related and cadaveric renal transplantation became part of regular clinical practice. Attempts at heart and liver transplantation proved more challenging, and these clinical efforts remained limited to a few dedicated programs for more than a decade. The next major watershed in the development of transplantation was the introduction of cyclosporine in the early 1980s. This development ushered in a marked expansion of heart and liver transplantation, promoted further growth of renal transplantation, and made lung transplantation possible. Currently, more than 28,000 solid organ transplantations are performed yearly in the United States, and most patients retain the grafts and survive many years after transplantation.[2] As a result, patients with various types of transplants are now routinely encountered in general practice.

Except for issues related to the function and rejection of the transplanted organ, infections are the most important problem after transplantation. The clinical manifestations of infection are variable and depend on the infecting pathogen, the prior immune status of the host, the type of transplantation, the time after transplantation, and the level of pharmacologic immunosuppression. With this complexity in mind, it is useful to address some general principles that may aid in the diagnosis, management, and understanding of infections after transplantation.

The occurrence of infection requires a susceptible host and an available pathogen. Transplant recipients are not equally susceptible to all pathogens. For instance, most enteroviruses do not appear to infect transplant recipients with greater frequency or severity than they do normal hosts. A transplant recipient also may be quite susceptible to a given pathogen but may have a low risk of infection because of lack of exposure. For example, tuberculosis is rarely encountered at most transplantation centers in developed countries, but it can be a major problem in transplant recipients in parts of the world and in clinical settings in which infection cannot be avoided.[3] Likewise, transplant recipients with no past exposure to cytomegalovirus (CMV) who receive organs from CMV-seronegative donors are at low risk for CMV infection, whatever their level of immunosuppression. In clinical practice, the clinician can and should use this sort of information to assess each patient's individual susceptibility to important pathogens.

Infections are most frequent and most varied during the first 6 months after transplantation.[4] During this period, patients have all the risk factors for infection (Table 310-1): They may still be affected—either directly or indirectly—by their underlying disease; because they have undergone major surgery and been in the intensive care unit, they are at risk for wound and other nosocomial infections; and because

they have received large doses of immunosuppressive drugs, the allograft may be malfunctioning as a result of rejection or other factors. This early period also covers the time of highest risk for infection by opportunistic microorganisms such as CMV and *Nocardia*, *Aspergillus*, *Pneumocystis*, or *Toxoplasma* organisms. These pathogens received much attention in the early literature on transplantation-related infections; more recently, their clinical impact has been diminished by the widespread use of antimicrobial prophylactic regimens early after transplantation.[5] These regimens have virtually eliminated some infectious complications, such as *Pneumocystis* pneumonia, and have provided substantial but still imperfect control of others, such as CMV disease. With time—usually about 6 to 9 months after transplantation—the risk of infection tends to decrease. The level of vigilance may therefore be reduced, except for individual patients whose risk has remained high because of continued requirement for high doses of immunosuppression.

Host Factors of Infection

Underlying chronic diseases of the transplant recipient may persist or even worsen after transplantation (see Table 310-1). The basic disease that led to transplantation may be cured by the procedure, but on occasion, it is not. Patients undergoing transplantation because of fulminant hepatitis B virus (HBV) infection usually clear the virus, but chronic infection with HBV or hepatitis C virus (HCV) persists in most patients after transplantation.[6] The end-organ effect of diabetes mellitus on blood vessels and nerves continues to be a major problem in diabetic patients with renal transplants and predisposes such patients to the development of infections of soft tissue and the urinary tract.[7] Single-lung transplant recipients are at risk for infection in their native lung as a result of structural problems caused by the underlying pulmonary disease.[8] Other preexisting medical conditions such as gallbladder disease or diverticulosis may be clinically quiescent before transplantation and first become manifest in the post-transplantation period, when their detection and management is complicated by chronic immunosuppressive therapy.

Along with the patient's underlying condition, medications, particularly antibiotics and immunosuppressive agents, have an effect on the type and severity of infections in the early post-transplantation period. For example, liver transplant recipients who receive antibiotics or corticosteroids before transplantation may be more likely to develop systemic *Candida* infections after transplantation.[9] Lung transplantation candidates who have received corticosteroids and other immunosuppressive medications to treat pulmonary fibrosis may reactivate asymptomatic CMV infection before they receive the transplant and may be at higher risk for disease caused by CMV after transplantation.[10]

Effect of Type of Transplantation

The type of transplantation is an important determinant of the type of infections occurring after transplantation. Sites of major surgery are vulnerable to bacterial and fungal infection. The transplanted organ has to survive outside the body and then must reestablish an adequate vascular supply to regain its functional integrity. Allograft reactions of

<table>
<tr><td colspan="2">TABLE 310-1 | Factors That Contribute to Infection after Transplantation</td></tr>
</table>

Category	Examples and Comments
Pretransplantation Host Factors	
Underlying medical conditions and chronic infections	Conditions that persist or recur (hepatitis B virus, hepatitis C virus, diabetes mellitus)
	Conditions that exacerbate (chronic bronchitis, gallbladder disease)
Lack of specific immunity	Conducive to important primary infections (e.g., cytomegalovirus, Epstein-Barr virus, varicella-zoster virus, toxoplasmosis)
Prior colonization	Nosocomial gram-negative bacilli, *Candida* organisms, staphylococci, vancomycin-resistant enterococci
Prior latent or cryptic infection	Reactivation produces clinical infection (tuberculosis, cytomegalovirus, herpes simplex virus, varicella-zoster virus, *Trypanosoma cruzi* and possibly *Pneumocystis*)
Prior medications	Immunosuppressive agents and antibiotics influence post-transplantation susceptibility to infection
Transplantation Factors	
Type of organ transplanted	Site of transplantation and allograft are most common sites of infection
	Allograft may transmit infection or be more susceptible to infection as a result of ischemic injury or allograft reactions
Trauma of surgery	Surgical stress, duration of surgery
Immunosuppression	
Immunosuppressive agents	Corticosteroids, azathioprine and other cytotoxic agents, cyclosporine, tacrolimus, rapamycin, polyclonal and monoclonal antilymphocyte serums
Infective immunosuppression	Primary cytomegalovirus infection and chronic hepatitis C virus infection are associated with more bacterial and fungal infection
Allograft Reactions	
Graft-versus-host reaction	Affects all areas of immunity and is a major factor in bacterial, viral, and fungal infection in stem cell transplantation
Host-versus-graft reaction	Possible cofactor in allograft infection

a higher risk for fungal infection.[16] Lymphoceles resulting from interruption of lymphatic drainage after kidney transplantation may become superinfected with bacteria. In transplantation of the lung, peritracheal or peribronchial infection may follow breakdown of the airway anastomosis. Anastomotic infections may also predispose to infections of the transplanted lung, either directly or secondarily to obstruction after placement of a bronchial stent.[8]

The susceptibility of the grafted organ to invasion by CMV and other viruses is a striking example of the vulnerability of allografts to infection. Data collected in Pittsburgh in the 1980s on the frequency of CMV infection and disease in different groups of transplant recipients showed that the frequency of CMV pneumonia was 4 to 16 times higher in heart-lung transplant recipients than in patients with other types of transplants.[12-15] The vulnerability of the transplanted lung to infection extends to other viruses. Lung recipients also are susceptible to severe infections with adenovirus and paramyxoviruses, such as respiratory syncytial virus.[17] The reason the transplanted lung is so vulnerable to viral infections has not been elucidated. It may be related to the presence in the allograft of a cytokine milieu favorable to viral replication or to the inability of cytotoxic CD8+ T cells to effectively kill cells with differing human leukocyte antigen (HLA) types. The transplanted liver is also more susceptible than a native liver to viral infections, including CMV, HBV, HCV, herpes simplex virus (HSV), and possibly adenovirus.[6,18,19]

Immunosuppression

Of all the factors contributing to the occurrence of infections in transplant recipients, the most obvious and probably the most consequential is iatrogenic immunosuppression. The effects of immunosuppressive agents have become more apparent as surgical techniques have improved and surgical infections have declined. Despite significant broadening availability of immunosuppressive agents after the introduction of cyclosporine in 1983, tacrolimus in 1994, mycophenolate mofetil in 1995, and rapamycin in 1999, the ideal suppressive regimen that prevents rejection but preserves antimicrobial immunity remains elusive.

The major immunosuppressive agents may be divided into several categories. Corticosteroids broadly inhibit immune responses, including innate inflammatory responses, cellular immunity, and, to a lesser extent, antibody formation.[20] Although corticosteroids are inadequate

the host-versus-graft or graft-versus-host type may occur (see Table 310-1). These reactions are known to reduce resistance to infection by viruses and to contribute to the graft's being a *locus minoris resistentiae*.[11] Data collected in the 1980s showed that the most common site of infection in recipients of solid organ transplants was the site of transplantation.[12-15] Recipients of bone marrow transplant do not have surgical sites, but they are unique because, in addition to depressed T-cell immunity common to other types of transplantation, leukopenia and depressed humoral immunity occur. This leads to a heightened vulnerability to many varieties of infection.

The contribution of surgical factors to infection is best illustrated by hepatic transplantation.[15,16] With this type of surgery, the function of the biliary and vascular anastomoses in the porta hepatis is most vulnerable. For example, most abscesses in the transplanted liver result either from liver ischemia caused by hepatic artery thrombosis or from obstruction to bile flow from biliary strictures.[15] There is also a striking correlation between the total hours that liver recipients spend in the operating room and the mean number of episodes of infection per patient (Fig. 310-1).[15] The duration of these operations is undoubtedly a reflection of many individual risk factors, including surgical stress, loss of blood and body fluids, direct tissue damage, and the various metabolic derangements that may occur during a prolonged operation. By the mid-1990s, improvements in anesthesia and surgical technique led to a decrease in the average length of liver transplantation surgery to 6 to 7 hours, but longer operations were still associated with

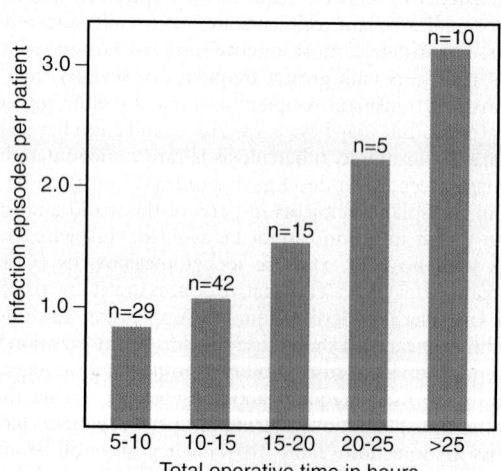

Figure 310-1 **Frequency of severe infections in relation to time spent in liver transplant surgery.** *(Data from reference 2.)*

as single agents to sustain graft survival, they have remained a part of most immunosuppressive regimens. High doses of prednisone and hyperglycemia were found to be significant factors in the frequency of infections and deaths from infection in kidney transplant recipients.[21] In an effort to free patients from the undesirable side effects of corticosteroid therapy, more transplantation centers have been prescribing early steroid withdrawal and steroid avoidance regimens, particularly in recipients of abdominal organ transplants.[22] In a meta-analysis of randomized trials in which steroid-free regimens were compared with steroid-based immunosuppression regimens in liver transplant recipients, no difference in overall risk of infection was revealed. However, the analysis revealed that steroid avoidance might reduce the risk of CMV infection and HCV recurrence.[23]

The introduction of cytotoxic drugs, such as methotrexate, cyclophosphamide, and azathioprine, was a major advance in immunosuppression that made transplantation across HLA barriers feasible. All the cytotoxic drugs interfere with DNA synthesis, thereby suppressing the bone marrow and reducing peripheral blood cell counts. In addition to marrow suppression, azathioprine may cause pancreatitis, a reversible hepatitis, rash, and gastrointestinal disturbances. Azathioprine was once the mainstay of immunosuppression for transplanted organs, but its use has declined sharply since the introduction of cyclosporine and other more potent immunosuppressive medications.[22]

Cyclosporine was approved in 1983. It is an unusual cyclic peptide, consisting of 11 amino acids, whose main action is to inhibit the normal production of cytokines when CD4[+] T cells are exposed to foreign antigens.[24] The primary cytokine inhibited is interleukin-2. Suppressor cells and B cells are relatively spared. Concentrations of the drug as low as 100 ng/mL effectively inhibit mixed lymphocyte reactions. Patients treated with cyclosporine alone for various autoimmune diseases show very low rates of clinical infection, which is suggestive of the importance of corticosteroids and other cofactors for infection in transplant recipients (see Table 310-1). Most studies, whether randomized or historically controlled, have demonstrated that the introduction of cyclosporine led to lower rates of infection in transplant recipients.[15,25,26]

Hofflin and colleagues compared the rates of infectious morbidity and mortality between cohorts of heart transplant recipients receiving immunosuppressive regimens based on either azathioprine or cyclosporine.[26] Patients receiving cyclosporine had lower rates of infection (71% vs. 89%) and a lower infectious mortality rate (11% vs. 39%). The rates of infection have not been compared in liver recipients receiving azathioprine- versus cyclosporine-based regimens. However, most early deaths in liver transplant recipients are linked to infection, and the substantial decline in mortality rates among liver transplant recipients that occurred after cyclosporine was introduced implies an associated reduction in infectious mortality.[12,13,15]

Tacrolimus was approved in 1994. It is a macrolide produced by *Streptomyces tsukubaensis*. Despite some differences in the pathway of action, its mode of action is strikingly similar to that of cyclosporine in that it inhibits production of interleukin-2 and other cytokines by CD4[+] T cells.[27] It is about 10 to 100 times more potent than cyclosporine. Randomized trials have demonstrated that tacrolimus-based immunosuppression results in lower rates of acute rejection and graft loss than does cyclosporine-based therapy, particularly in kidney and liver transplant recipients. However, tacrolimus is linked to higher rates of neurologic and gastrointestinal symptoms and with development of diabetes mellitus.[28,29] Use of tacrolimus as primary immunosuppressive therapy has not been shown convincingly to either increase or decrease the risk of infection.[30]

Mycophenolate mofetil was approved in 1995 for renal transplant recipients and in 1997 for heart transplant recipients. It is a cytotoxic drug with an antiproliferative effect on T and B lymphocytes. It is not intended to replace cyclosporine or tacrolimus as primary immunosuppressive therapy; rather, it is meant to replace azathioprine in triple-drug regimens.[31] A blinded, randomized, three-arm study in renal transplant recipients revealed superiority of mycophenolate mofetil over azathioprine; biopsy-proven rejection occurred in 38% of aza-

thioprine recipients, in comparison with 19.8% and 17.5% in the two mycophenolate mofetil conditions.[32] In this study, the numbers of patients developing infections were similar across the three groups. The main side effects of mycophenolate mofetil are marrow depression and diarrhea. The use of mycophenolate mofetil may also increase the risk of CMV disease.[31]

Rapamycin (also known as sirolimus) was released in 1999. Rapamycin interferes with cell cycle proliferation and blocks intracellular signaling mechanisms initiated by cytokines by inhibiting a regulatory kinase, mammalian target of rapamycin (mTOR).[31] Everolimus is another mTOR inhibitor that has been used in transplant recipients, but it is not yet approved in the United States. Unlike cyclosporine and tacrolimus, mTOR inhibitors have no direct nephrotoxicity. They frequently cause hyperlipidemia and occasionally cause myelosuppression. They also have been linked to delayed wound healing, oral ulcerations, and a rare drug-induced interstitial pneumonitis. Some data suggest that rapamycin use is associated with reduced rates of post-transplantation malignancy and CMV disease.[33,34]

Table 310-2 is a list of commercially available polyclonal and monoclonal antibody preparations used for immunosuppression in transplant recipients. These antibodies are used either to treat rejection refractory to corticosteroids or as "induction therapy."[22] Induction therapy, administered in the immediate post-transplantation period, is aimed at providing a high early level of immunosuppression while avoiding nephrotoxicity from calcineurin inhibitors. Each antibody has its own individual adverse effects and provides a variable, but usually long, duration of immunosuppression.[31,35-41] Mason and colleagues demonstrated a significant increase in infection rates during the first 3 months after use of polyclonal antithymocyte globulin for treatment of rejection of the heart.[38]

Many reports have also testified to the enhancing role of antithymocyte globulin and monoclonal OKT3 antibodies on CMV disease and post-transplantation lymphoproliferative disease in transplant recipients.[35,39-41] Antithymocyte globulins are raised in rabbits or horses by immunization with human thymocytes. Because they are foreign proteins, they may cause a serum sickness in the transplant recipient that typically begins about 10 days after administration. OKT3 is a

TABLE 310-2	Antibody Preparations Used to Prevent or Treat Rejection
Agent	*Adverse Effects*[31,35-41]
Polyclonal Antibodies	
Antithymocyte globulins* • Anti–human thymocyte immune globulin (rabbit) (Thymoglobulin) • Lymphocyte immune globulin, antithymocyte (equine) (Atgam)	Serum sickness, thrombocytopenia, lymphopenia (can last up to 2-3 years with Thymoglobulin), increased risk of CMV, PTLD
Monoclonal Antibodies	
Anti-CD25 (IL-2 receptor) antibodies[†] • Basiliximab (Simulect) • Daclizumab (Zenapax)	Hypersensitivity reactions, infection risk not significantly increased
Anti-CD20 antibody[‡] • Rituximab (Rituxan)	Infusion reactions, HBV reactivation
Anti-CD52 antibody[§] • Alemtuzumab (Campath)	Infusion reactions, increased risk of CMV, *Pneumocystis jirovecii* pneumonia, invasive fungal infections, immunosuppression effects that can last up to 12 months
Anti-CD3 antibody[‖] • Muromonab-CD3 (Orthoclone OKT3)	Aseptic meningitis, cytokine release syndrome, pulmonary edema, increased risk of CMV, PTLD

*Used for induction and rejection.
[†]Used for induction, not used for rejection.
[‡]Used primarily for humoral rejection, blood type (ABO) mismatch, and recipients with a positive crossmatch (off-label use).
[§]Used for induction and rejection (off-label use).
[‖]Used for rejection, not used frequently for induction.
CMV, cytomegalovirus; HBV, hepatitis B virus; PTLD, post-transplantation lymphoproliferative disease.

monoclonal mouse antibody directed against the CD3 receptor on T cells. OKT3 does not cause serum sickness, because immunosuppression can be achieved with milligram quantities of the drug. However, OKT3 antibodies can stimulate cytokine release from T cells and lead to pulmonary edema and a sepsis-like syndrome during the first 2 to 3 days of administration. Another poorly understood, but well-documented adverse effect of OKT3 is aseptic meningitis.

Alemtuzumab is an anti-CD52 monoclonal antibody and is currently approved for the treatment of B-cell chronic lymphocytic leukemia. It is increasingly being used in transplant recipients for either induction therapy or treatment for acute rejection unresponsive to corticosteroids. This agent targets a cell surface molecule (CD52) common to many immune cells and causes significant reduction in CD4+ and CD8+ T cells, natural killer cells, and CD19+ B cells. This effect may last 12 months or longer after administration.[36] In contrast to agents that affect only T cells, its use has not been associated with an increased rate of post-transplantation lymphoproliferative disease, probably because its action against B cells suppresses Epstein-Barr virus (EBV) infection. The infectious risk of alemtuzumab is reported to be significantly higher when it is used as salvage treatment for acute rejection than when it is used as induction therapy.[42]

Infecting Microbial Agents

The most important pathogens infecting transplant recipients are listed in Table 310-3. There are two types of endogenous organisms. One type represents endogenous flora that colonize the mucous membranes of the gastrointestinal tract, including the oropharynx, the nares, and the skin adjacent to the oral and anal orifices. These are among the most important potential pathogens and are represented by the common gram-negative and gram-positive bacteria listed in Table 310-3. These organisms produce local infections by contaminating adjacent wound sites, or they may infect systemically by invading blood vessels or lymphatic vessels. They may be transmitted from one site to another in the same patient by a surgical procedure or on contaminated instruments and hands. They can also be transmitted from organ donors to recipients.

Candida spp. are a normal component of gastrointestinal tract flora and represent the most frequent and consequential fungal pathogens.[9] Superficial mucosal infections with *Candida* spp., such as thrush and *Candida* vaginitis, may be seen in all types of transplantation. Candidemia and visceral *Candida* infections are common after liver and pancreatic transplantation and occur occasionally in recipients of other types of transplants in an intensive care setting. Although *Candida albicans* remains the most commonly encountered species, some large transplantation centers are reporting increasing rates of invasive candidiasis with non-*albicans* species such as *Candida glabrata* and *Candida tropicalis*.[43]

Other colonizing organisms that received attention in the 1990s include antibiotic-resistant gram-positive cocci, such as vancomycin-resistant enterococci (VRE) and methicillin-resistant *Staphylococcus aureus* (MRSA). VRE has become a particular problem in liver transplant recipients, who have many risk factors for colonization, such as the prolonged use of broad-spectrum antibiotics.[44] One large liver transplantation center documented that nearly 15% of liver transplant recipients and candidates had rectal colonization with VRE, and this colonization was independently associated with an increased risk of VRE infection and death.[45] There is no current consensus on whether transplant recipients or candidates should be actively screened for MRSA or VRE colonization.

Another type of endogenous organism is found in latent tissue infection. Such infections are generally not detectable at the time of transplantation, but the microbial agents may reactivate and proliferate when the patient becomes immunosuppressed. The existence of this type of flora is best demonstrated by herpesviruses, *Toxoplasma* organisms, and the tubercle bacillus. Their latency may be detected indirectly by serologic or immunologic tests. The situation is less clear in the case of *Pneumocystis jirovecii*, but the remarkable frequency of *Pneumocystis*

TABLE 310-3	Common Microbial Agents Causing Infection after Transplantation	
Bacteria		
Gram-negative bacteria		This group of organisms can cause superficial wound infections or infections of the blood and deeper tissues of the urinary tract, lung, thorax, and abdomen. Despite a succession of highly effective antibiotics, these remain among the most frequent causes of bacterial infection.
• Enteric bacteria (*Escherichia coli*, other Enterobacteriaceae)		
• *Pseudomonas*		
• *Acinetobacter*		
• *Serratia*		
• *Bacteroides* and other anaerobes		
• *Legionella*		Nosocomial from water supply.
Gram-positive aerobes		
• *Staphylococcus aureus*		Infections with *S. epidermidis* and methicillin-resistant *S. aureus* have increased in frequency
• *Staphylococcus epidermidis*		
• *Streptococcus* spp.		
• *Enterococcus* spp.		Vancomycin-resistant enterococci are major pathogens in liver transplant recipients
• *Pneumococcus* spp.		
• *Listeria monocytogenes*		*Listeria* organisms are an occasional cause of severe meningitis
• *Nocardia* spp.		
Gram-negative coccobacilli		Infection often seen with underlying lung disease
• *Haemophilus influenzae*		
• *Moraxella* spp.		
Fungi		
Candida spp.		*Candida* spp. are the most common endogenous fungi; deep *Candida* infection is a particular problem after liver transplantation
Aspergillus spp.		
Cryptococcus spp.		
Agents of mucormycosis		
Histoplasma capsulatum		Encountered primarily in endemic areas
Coccidioides spp.		Encountered primarily in the southwestern United States
Pneumocystis jirovecii		Probably latent in humans
Viruses		
Herpesvirus group		Herpesvirus infection is common after transplantation because many subjects are latently infected with one or more species that reactivate. Donor transmission is an important source of CMV and EBV
• Herpes simplex (HSV)		
• Cytomegalovirus (CMV)		
• Varicella-zoster virus		
• Epstein-Barr virus (EBV)		
• Human herpesvirus-6 and -7		
• Human herpesvirus-8		Highly associated with Kaposi's sarcoma
Human immunodeficiency virus type 1 (HIV-1)		Increasing numbers of organs are being transplanted in HIV-positive individuals with well-controlled infection
Adenovirus		Pediatric, only occasional in adults
Rotavirus		Primarily pediatric
Respiratory syncytial virus		During community outbreaks
Influenza A and B viruses		
Parainfluenza viruses		
West Nile virus		Donor transmission documented
Hepatitis B virus		
Hepatitis C virus		
Polyomavirus		BK virus causes nephropathy in kidney transplant recipients. JC virus causes progressive leukoencephalopathy.
Papillomavirus		
Parvovirus		Severe hypoproliferative anemia
Mycoplasmas		
Mycoplasma hominis		Can cause wound infection after transplantation, as well as other types of systemic infection, including arthritis, meningitis, and peritonitis
Ehrlichia Organisms		
Ehrlichia chafeensis		Endemic areas
Ehrlichia ewingii		
Anaplasma phagocytophilum		
Protozoa and Parasites		
Toxoplasma gondii		Usually a primary infection in solid organ transplantation
Trypanosoma cruzi		May be reactivated in a previously infected recipient or be acquired from donor
Strongyloides stercoralis		Prior infection may intensify during immunosuppression

pneumonia in patients with the acquired immunodeficiency syndrome (AIDS) suggests that latent infection by this organism is common, if not ubiquitous.

A number of organisms are transmitted through the air from the physical environment, particularly fungi such as *Aspergillus, Coccidioides, Histoplasma*, and *Cryptococcus*. *Aspergillus*, cryptococcal, and nocardial infections are seen in all geographic regions, but post-transplantation coccidioidomycosis is a problem uniquely of certain endemic regions, such as the arid deserts of the southwestern United States, and most reported cases of histoplasmosis after transplantation have also occurred in endemic areas.[46,47]

The most frequent source of infectious agents in the patient's environment is still other human beings. In the postoperative period, nosocomial transmission of respiratory viruses and common gram-positive and gram-negative organisms occurs through contaminated hands of hospital personnel or through inanimate objects such as respiratory equipment, endoscopes, intravascular lines, and urinary catheters that have been handled by such personnel. This equipment may at times amplify the agent if organisms are permitted to grow in reservoirs such as water baths and humidifiers.

Some bacteria listed in Table 310-3 probably have exogenous sources, but these are often undefined. *Pseudomonas* organisms may come from environmental water sources or raw vegetables. *Listeria* may arise from contaminated food sources, but a source is rarely identified in the sporadic cases of meningitis that are seen in populations of transplant recipients.[48] The *Legionella* organisms, including *Legionella pneumophila* and *Legionella micdadei*, are well-described causes of pneumonia in transplant recipients.[49] Hot-water reservoirs have been demonstrated to be a common source of nosocomial legionellosis. Identification and treatment of these contaminated water sources is an important infection control practice in hospitals with endemic *Legionella* infection.[49,50]

Transfused blood products and donated organs have been documented sources of infection in transplant recipients.[51,52] Although transmission of some agents such as HCV and CMV has declined as a result of improved blood-banking practices, the reports of transmission of West Nile virus, rabies virus, and arenaviruses by transplanted organs have highlighted the threat of receiving blood and organs from other individuals.[53-56] It has also created a difficult and currently unresolved challenge to organ procurement agencies to develop laboratory tests that can prove a potential donor is free of these uncommon infections.[53] Another emerging agent is human herpesvirus-8. Donor transmission of this virus has not been recognized in the United States, but it has been demonstrated in Europe and shown to lead to clinical cases of Kaposi's sarcoma.[57] The major agents transmitted by allografts are listed in Table 310-4. Of these pathogens, CMV is most frequently transmitted by organs. It would be desirable to use only CMV-seronegative donors to transplant organs into CMV-seronegative transplant recipients.[11] However, such selection is not the usual practice because of the short supply of donor organs, the varying rate of morbidity from CMV infection after transplantation, and the availability of effective antiviral treatment. In order to prevent blood-borne transmission, CMV-seronegative transplant recipients are given blood transfusions from CMV-seronegative blood donors, or filters are used to deplete the blood of white blood cells, the component in the blood that carries the latent virus.

Toxoplasma organisms have been transmitted by seropositive heart donors, but transmission by other organs is rare.[58] HSV infections have occasionally been transmitted from kidney donors to HSV-seronegative recipients, and it is likely that EBV-seropositive donors are a major source of primary EBV infection in seronegative recipients.[59,60] The risk of HCV transmission is high (≈50%) when the donor is serologically positive for HCV, even in nonliver transplant recipients.[61] Organs from HCV-seropositive donors, however, are sometimes used in recipients who are severely ill or already seropositive for the virus. The risk of transmission of HBV is greatest if the organ donor has clear evidence of active infection, usually indicated by either a positive surface antigen (HBsAg) or core immunoglobulin M antibody (HBcIgM). The risk

TABLE 310-4	Major Infective Agents Transmitted by Donated Tissues, Blood, and Blood Products
Type of Tissue	*Infective Agent*
Kidney, heart, liver, lung, bone marrow	Cytomegalovirus[11,41,52]
Heart, kidney	Toxoplasmosis[58]
Heart	*Trypanosoma cruzi*[54]
Kidney, liver	Herpes simplex virus[59]
Kidney	Human herpesvirus-8[57]
Kidney, heart, liver	HIV-1, hepatitis B virus, hepatitis C virus, West Nile virus[61]
Kidney, liver, lung	Lymphocytic choriomeningitis virus, Old World arenavirus[55,56]
Kidney, liver, cornea	Rabies[54]
Blood*	Cytomegalovirus, Epstein-Barr virus, HIV-1, hepatitis B virus, hepatitis A virus, delta hepatitis virus, hepatitis C virus, human T-cell lymphotropic virus 1[51]
	West Nile virus[55]
Leukocytes	Cytomegalovirus, HIV-1[51]

*On rare occasions, *T. cruzi* malaria, babesiosis, and syphilis have been transmitted by blood transfusion.[51]

HIV, human immunodeficiency virus.

associated with receiving a graft from a donor who is seropositive for immunoglobulin G antibody to core antigen (HBcIgG) but seronegative for HBsAG and HBcIgM is less clear; however, it can be predicted partially on the basis of the organ that is transplanted and the immune status of the recipient. Approximately half of all liver transplant recipients eventually acquire HBV infection from an HBcIgG-positive donor, whereas the transmission rate is low (≤3%) for nonliver transplant recipients.[61] Preexisting immunity to HBV in the recipient, either by vaccination or by previous infection, appears to reduce but not totally eliminate the risk of transmission. Donors, whose only marker of HBV infection is a positive surface antibody (HBsAB), are considered to represent a low risk for transmission. Donor transmission of HBV has been successfully managed in recipients by treatment with lamivudine and hepatitis B immune globulin.[62]

Human immunodeficiency virus type 1 (HIV-1) is efficiently transmitted through donor organs, tissues, and blood products.[61,63] There is a consensus that organs from donors seropositive for HIV-1 should not be transplanted. The Centers for Disease Control and Prevention has developed guidelines mandating that organ procurement personnel obtain a history of any risk factors for HIV-1 infection that could signal the possibility of transmission of HIV-1 despite negative results of antibody tests. The mandate includes the responsibility of sharing any relevant information with the intended recipient and family.[64] In 2007, four organ recipients acquired HIV-1 and HCV from a donor who was seronegative for both viruses.[64] Cases like these have sparked interest in utilizing nucleic acid testing to identify infected donors during early infection when viremia is present, but antibodies have not yet developed. Such methods could potentially reduce the window period for detecting acute donor infections to 1 to 2 weeks.[65]

Evaluation before Transplantation

Evaluation of the patient for infectious risks before transplantation has proved extremely valuable, and all transplantation centers have some formal screening mechanisms.[66] The first goal of such screening should be to detect the presence of any active infection in the candidate that might amplify and become a major problem after transplantation. Examples are a history of chronic bronchitis and the presence of active dental infection. Most patients with cystic fibrosis who undergo lung transplantation have pulmonary infections with resistant organisms such as *Pseudomonas aeruginosa* and MRSA. The perioperative antibiotic prophylaxis for these patients is usually targeted to cover the most recent isolates from the sputum.[8]

The second step in a pretransplantation evaluation is to document a history of exposure. The patient should be questioned about occupational exposures and hobbies, and a brief history of travel and residence should be obtained to explore possible exposure to tropical illnesses or endemic mycoses. This history should include past documentation of tuberculosis, previous tuberculin skin test results, and any exposure that might have placed the patient at risk of acquiring tuberculosis, such as extended travel in developing countries or incarceration in a prison. Third, a battery of tests to screen for infectious disease should be performed, as outlined in Table 310-5. The results establish the presence of chronic viral pathogens (HIV-1, HCV, HBV) and help assess susceptibility to reactivation or new infection by key transplant pathogens such as the herpesviruses and *Toxoplasma gondii*. Tuberculin skin testing should be performed for all patients unless they have had a definitely positive test result in the past. Coccidioidomycosis complement fixation antibody tests are also recommended for individuals with residence or significant exposure over the preceding 2 years in known endemic areas. Patients with residence outside the United States may require specialized testing for *Trypanosoma cruzi*, malaria, luminal parasites such as strongyloides, or human herpesvirus-8.[54]

The most useful tests before transplantation are the herpesvirus serologic profiles, because they predict whether the patient is at risk for reactivation or primary infection with these viruses. An example is knowledge of a patient's varicella serologic status: Few patients are seronegative, but these few are at high risk of potentially fatal varicella infection after transplantation. Knowledge of risk status allows for intensive counseling and immunization of these patients.[67] Seropositive patients, in contrast, can be told that they are at no risk from exposure to chickenpox or shingles and require no intervention after exposure. CMV antibody testing before transplantation provides the best way to stratify risk for CMV disease after transplantation. Many transplantation centers modify their management of high-risk CMV-seronegative patients who have seropositive donors by instituting closer follow-up or giving more aggressive antiviral prophylaxis.

The incidence of active tuberculosis is 30 to 50 times higher in transplant recipients than in the general population.[3] The risk of hepa-

totoxicity from isoniazid prophylaxis appears to be low in transplant recipients without preexisting liver disease.[68] We believe that most patients with positive tuberculin skin tests should be treated with isoniazid, but assessment of risks and benefits in individual patients is also important, and the optimal timing of prophylaxis should be considered. For instance, in liver transplant candidates with decompensated liver disease, isoniazid prophylaxis might be delayed until after liver transplantation, when the risk for tuberculosis is higher and the patient is more clinically stable.

HIV-positive patients with end-stage organ disease were previously denied access to organ transplantation: Because of the immunosuppression required for transplantation, HIV progression often accelerated. Now that highly active antiretroviral therapy can provide very effective virological suppression of HIV, more transplantation centers are offering organ transplantation to HIV-positive patients with well-controlled infection. Such transplantations, however, may be complicated by difficult drug interactions between the transplant immunosuppression regimen and antiretroviral therapy. So far, studies of kidney transplantation in selected HIV-infected patients show early term (1- to 3-year) survival of patients and grafts that are comparable to outcomes in renal recipients without HIV infection.[69,70] Surprisingly high rates of acute cellular rejection have been seen in HIV-positive renal recipients in some studies. This has been variously attributed to drug interactions between immunosuppressive agents and antiretroviral drugs or dysregulation of the immune system caused by HIV infection.[69] HIV-infected liver recipients may have worse survival than liver recipients without HIV infection, particularly if they are coinfected with HCV.[71] HIV-positive transplant recipients may be particularly susceptible to the immunosuppressive effect of anti-T cell antibodies, In one study of 11 HIV-positive renal recipients who received thymoglobulin, CD4$^+$ T cell counts remained below 200 cells/μL for an average of 342 days after drug administration, despite adequate suppression of HIV.[72]

Monitoring for Infection

Routine surveillance for bacterial infection is of limited benefit in most recipients of solid organ transplants. One possible exception might be the routine surveillance of respiratory secretions of lung recipients who are intubated in the intensive care unit. These patients are at risk for both pneumonia and transplant rejection, and it may be easier to assess changes in pulmonary status when serial sputum results are available. Surveillance for fungi is also a common practice after lung transplantation, because of the high risk for infection with *Aspergillus* and other molds.[8,73]

Many transplantation programs monitor for CMV infection in patients during the first 3 to 6 months after transplantation. Viral load assays such as blood antigenemia or quantitative polymerase chain reaction (PCR) testing for CMV have replaced conventional and shell vial cultures as the virus tests of choice. These tests are more rapid and sensitive than cultures. They provide quantitative information on viral load that is correlated with the development of symptomatic infection.[74] Routine virologic testing for CMV has enabled a preemptive approach to antiviral treatment and successfully prevented progression to overt CMV disease both in patients with stem cell transplants and in those with solid organ transplants.[74-76] Monitoring of the viral load by quantitative PCR has also been studied for other viral infections in transplant recipients. Some studies have correlated the presence of high viral loads of EBV in blood samples from transplant recipients with the later development of EBV-related lymphoproliferative disease.[77] The viral loads of HBV and HCV have predictive power for the course of these infections after transplantation, and their measurement is essential for monitoring the response to treatment.[62,78] According to preliminary evidence, quantitative PCR screening of renal transplant recipients for infection with BK virus (a polyomavirus) and the use of these results to adjust levels of immunosuppression may be an effective way to reduce the incidence of polyomavirus nephropathy.[79]

TABLE 310-5	Routine Laboratory Studies before and after Transplantation	
Before Transplantation*	**After Transplantation**
Cytomegalovirus immunoglobulin G (IgG) antibody	Viral load monitoring for cytomegalovirus
Epstein-Barr virus IgG antibody	Antibody studies (as clinically indicated)
Herpes simplex (types 1 and 2) antibody	
Varicella-zoster IgG antibody	
Toxoplasma IgG antibody (heart transplant recipients)	
Hepatitis B screen†	
Hepatitis C enzyme immunoassay‡	
Human immunodeficiency virus antibody	
Tuberculin skin test	
Stool for ova and parasites§	

*For serologic studies, it is most important to collect serum before transplantation. Studies may then be done as clinically indicated.

†Should include at least surface antigen, core antibody, and surface antibody.

‡Second- or third-generation test. Liver candidates and patients with laboratory or clinical evidence of liver disease should also undergo a polymerase chain reaction assay for hepatitis C.

§Primarily useful for former or current residents of tropical and subtropical regions. The incidence of strongyloidiasis after transplantation has fallen dramatically since the mid-1980s.

IgG, immunoglobulin G.

Prophylactic Measures

Prophylactic regimens are frequently used to prevent infection in transplant recipients. Immunization is potentially the most cost-effective way to prevent infection. Although trials large enough to demonstrate clinical effectiveness of vaccines have not been performed with transplant populations, numerous smaller studies of antibody responses have been conducted. The response of renal recipients to booster doses of tetanus and diphtheria toxoids appears to be adequate, although reduced in comparison with the response in immunocompetent persons.[80] Transplant recipients also respond to pneumococcal vaccine but have lower peak antibody titers and a less durable response than do healthy controls.[81] The seroconversion rates of transplant recipients to influenza vaccine are generally inferior to those of control populations.[82]

There is an understandable reluctance to use live vaccines in transplant recipients. Measles and varicella vaccines have been used safely in small groups of transplant recipients with seroconversion rates of 73% and 65%, respectively,[83] but more studies need to be done before live vaccines can be recommended for general use after transplantation. We advocate that transplant candidates update their immunizations and receive vaccines—including pneumococcal, influenza, and HBV vaccines—that are recommended for patients in the general population who have chronic diseases. Transplant candidates should also be offered varicella immunization if they are seronegative for this virus, and liver transplant candidates should receive immunization for hepatitis A if they lack immunity. After transplantation, patients should finish any incomplete immunization series before transplantation and continue to receive other established inactivated vaccines on schedule.[84] In practice, we often postpone immunization when the patient is heavily immunosuppressed (e.g., during the first 3 months after solid organ transplantation) because the response is likely to be poor in this setting. Concerns in the transplant community that vaccines may cause rejection have not been substantiated.[84]

Antimicrobial agents commonly used for prophylaxis are listed in Table 310-6. Transplant surgeons routinely administer perioperative intravenous antibiotics to prevent intraoperative sepsis and wound infections. The type of antibiotics used varies greatly, and the optimal durations have not been established by studies or consensus. Oral antibiotics to prevent infection are also widely used. The most commonly used prophylactic antimicrobial agent is trimethoprim-sulfamethoxazole (TMP-SMX). TMP-SMX provides superior prophylaxis against *P. jirovecii* pneumonia in all populations that have been studied. It has now become part of standard care at transplantation centers. Dosages as low as two to three double-strength tablets (160/800 mg per tablet) a week are effective. Daily dosing of TMP-SMX in the first few months after transplantation also reduces urinary tract and other bacterial infections in renal transplant recipients.[85] In one study, patients taking TMP-SMX had 25% higher serum creatinine levels than patients not taking TMP-SMX, but this was fully reversible on discontinuation of the TMP-SMX. It is claimed, but not proved, that TMP-SMX prophylaxis also decreases the rate of infections caused by some serious opportunistic pathogens, including *Legionella*, *Nocardia*, and *Listeria*.

Prophylactic quinolones are used at some stem cell transplantation centers. They have been shown to reliably decrease the rate of fever and gram-negative bacteremias during the neutropenic phase of chemotherapy.[86] No effect on mortality has been demonstrated. Antiviral prophylaxis is desirable in transplant recipients because of the clinical importance of herpesvirus infections. Acyclovir is effective in preventing HSV infection in the early post-transplantation period. It is indicated in HSV-seropositive liver and lung transplant recipients because they have a risk of visceral disease caused by HSV in the transplanted organ.[8,18,67] Acyclovir is also commonly used to prevent mucocutaneous HSV infection in other solid organ recipients. Although acyclovir has marginal therapeutic activity against CMV, controlled studies have revealed that it does provide some protection against CMV disease when given prophylactically in high doses.[87] Ganciclovir has been

TABLE 310-6	Antimicrobial Prophylactic Regimens in Transplantation
Pathogen	*Prophylactic Agents*
Protozoa	
Toxoplasmosis	TMP-SMX
	Pyrimethamine
Virus	
Herpes simplex	Acyclovir*
Cytomegalovirus	Ganciclovir†
	Acyclovir
	Immunoglobulin
	Foscarnet‡
Influenza	Oseltamivir
Fungus	
Candida	Fluconazole
	Nystatin
	Clotrimazole
Aspergillus	Itraconazole
	Voriconazole
	Posaconazole
	Liposomal amphotericin B
Pneumocystis	TMP-SMX
	Dapsone
	Inhaled pentamidine
Bacteria	
Wound infection	Variable
Urinary tract infection	TMP-SMX
Neutropenic infection	Quinolones
Tuberculosis	Isoniazid
Pneumococcus	Penicillin (stem cell transplants)

*Includes oral and intravenous acyclovir and valacyclovir.
†Includes oral and intravenous ganciclovir and valganciclovir.
‡Used mostly in bone marrow recipients who have low blood cell counts.
TMP-SMX, trimethoprim-sulfamethoxazole.

favored by many clinicians as the prophylactic antiviral agent of choice because it has greater intrinsic activity than acyclovir against CMV, while remaining active against HSV. When given to marrow recipients for 100 days after neutrophil engraftment, intravenous ganciclovir reduced CMV disease in the first 6 months by 72%, but its use was associated with excess neutropenia and increased bacterial infections.[88] Merigan and co-workers studied the use of intravenous ganciclovir prophylaxis for 4 weeks after heart transplantation and demonstrated a significant reduction in CMV disease in CMV-seropositive heart recipients.[89] The regimen was not effective in CMV-seronegative recipients who received organs from seropositive donors. By extending prophylaxis with intravenous ganciclovir prophylaxis to 100 days after transplantation in liver recipients, Winston and colleagues were able to achieve impressive reductions in CMV disease in all CMV serogroups.[90]

Large placebo-controlled trials of CMV prophylaxis with oral regimens have also demonstrated positive results. In a randomized trial in which oral ganciclovir (1 g three times daily) for 12 weeks was compared with placebo in liver transplant recipients, CMV disease was significantly reduced (from 17% to 4%) in the treatment group.[91] The cases of CMV disease in the patients taking oral ganciclovir consisted only of CMV syndromes and mild CMV hepatitis. Valacyclovir, a prodrug of acyclovir that yields serum levels of acyclovir similar to those achieved with intravenous dosing, was compared with placebo in 616 renal recipients.[92] The frequency of CMV disease among those taking valacyclovir was reduced from 5% to 1% in CMV-seropositive patients and from 39% to 14% in CMV-seronegative recipients with seropositive donors. Only 1% of patients developed CMV disease while taking valacyclovir.

Valganciclovir is an oral prodrug of ganciclovir that has 60% bioavailability and provides drug exposure similar to that provided by intravenous infusions. In one randomized trial, valganciclovir was compared with oral ganciclovir for CMV prophylaxis in 371 CMV-seronegative recipients of solid organ transplants who had CMV-seropositive donors; CMV disease occurred at equivalent rates in both groups during the first post-transplantation year. Almost all cases of CMV disease in the trial occurred more than 100 days after transplantation, after the prophylactic regimens were stopped.[93]

To prevent CMV disease, an alternative to CMV prophylaxis is to monitor patients with viral load testing for some months after transplantation and administer preemptive antiviral treatment when the viral load reaches a predetermined threshold. Potential advantages of preemptive therapy are lesser toxic effects and lower costs for antiviral drugs. Also, most cases of CMV disease being managed by preemptive therapy occur early after transplantation, when patients are still being closely monitored at the transplantation center.[94] Available data suggest that prophylaxis and preemptive therapy provide similar control of CMV disease.[88,94-96] There is some evidence, however, that long-term graft function may be superior when prophylaxis is employed.[87,92,95] Whether prophylaxis or preemptive therapy is the best approach has not been fully elucidated. Preemptive therapy is more widely used than prophylaxis in stem cell transplantation because of the concern for marrow toxicity in this population.[75,88] In solid organ transplantation, prophylaxis appears to have more advocates, but the evidence is still too unclear to force a consensus on which strategy is best.

Immune control is another available modality in CMV prophylaxis. Intravenous immune globulin has been widely studied for the prophylaxis of CMV disease after stem cell transplantation. The results of these studies have been mixed, and this approach is no longer strongly advocated for CMV control in this population. Although the results of studies of immune globulin prophylaxis for CMV in solid organ transplantation are also mixed, a systematic review of 11 randomized trials concluded that the use of immune globulin prophylaxis led to a reduction in both CMV disease and mortality.[97] None of the cited trials included prophylactic use of ganciclovir in its intravenous or oral formulations in either the treatment or control population. Thus, it remains unclear whether immune globulin adds any additional benefits beyond that achieved with modern antiviral approaches to CMV management.

The decision on how to manage CMV infection in transplant recipients is complex and is best made after careful consideration of the efficacy, side effects, and cost of the regimens under consideration, as well as the transplant type and the estimated risk of severe CMV disease in the intended recipient. Balancing and weighing these factors inevitably brings the values and philosophy of the treating physicians into play.

Transplant recipients are at risk for thrush and other forms of mucocutaneous candidiasis, but these are effectively prevented by treatment with oral nystatin or clotrimazole troches. Oral systemic azoles are also effective and should be preferred in intubated patients because topical preparations cannot reliably be delivered to the pharynx and esophagus. Prophylaxis can usually be discontinued when prednisone doses drop to 20 mg/day or less, but it may need to be restarted during treatment of rejection with high-dose steroids or intercurrent antibiotic use. Prophylaxis for systemic fungal infection is now being used in many centers for patients at high risk, such as stem cell, liver, and lung recipients. Intravenous and oral azoles have been the most widely used prophylactic agents. Controlled trials of antifungal prophylaxis in solid organ transplantation have largely been confined to studies in liver recipients. Fluconazole has been established as an effective agent; its use in liver recipients has produced a 75% reduction in invasive fungal infections but no improvement in mortality rates.[98] Limited data suggest that itraconazole and liposomal amphotericin may have similar efficacy, but both these drugs have more side effects than does fluconazole. Candida spp. are the major fungal pathogen in liver transplant recipients.[8,9,15] Lung recipients, in contrast, suffer from a high rate of infection with Aspergillus and other molds, and this has prompted lung transplantation centers to administer antifungal prophylaxis with agents active against molds, such as oral itraconazole and inhaled amphotericin, despite the lack of controlled antifungal trials in this patient group.[73]

In the early 1990s, large randomized studies in bone marrow recipients established fluconazole (400 mg/day) as a safe and effective drug for fungal prophylaxis.[99] Fluconazole's lack of activity against molds,

however, is a definite shortcoming in allogeneic stem cell transplantation, because invasive mold infections are highly lethal in these patients and affect 10% or more of the population. A number of newer antifungal agents have been studied in large, controlled trials in stem cell transplant recipients, but a clear choice for a new prophylactic antifungal standard has not yet emerged. Because of their intrinsic activity, tolerability, oral availability, and the rigor and size of the supporting studies, voriconazole and posaconazole currently seem the most attractive candidates.[100] Both agents appear to reduce the incidence of invasive aspergillosis, but neither drug has been shown to reduce overall mortality rates.[101,102] With both, issues with variable serum levels arise: With posaconazole, absorption is limited and unpredictable; with voriconazole, metabolism varies. Pharmacokinetic monitoring may be needed to achieve optimal results with these compounds.[100]

Another form of prophylaxis that has been proposed is pyrimethamine (25 mg/day, together with folinic acid, 5 to 10 mg/day, for 6 weeks) for heart recipients who are seronegative for Toxoplasma and receive an organ from a Toxoplasma-seropositive donor.[103] However, the widespread use of TMP-SMX for Pneumocystis prophylaxis appears to provide excellent protection against Toxoplasma infection, and it is unclear whether the addition of pyrimethamine provides any further benefit.[104] Some stem cell transplantation centers also administer long-term oral penicillin prophylaxis to allogeneic transplant recipients because of the significant occurrence of severe pneumococcal infection late after transplantation.

Liver transplantation involves the breach of a potentially colonized upper gastrointestinal tract. Some groups have advocated decontamination of the gut as a method of decreasing bacterial and fungal sepsis in this population. Selective decontamination is usually accomplished with the oral administration of nonabsorbable antibiotics such as polymyxin E, gentamicin, and nystatin in the perioperative period.[105] The merits of gut decontamination remain uncertain, despite available clinical trials.

Prevention of Exposure to Infection

One way of decreasing infectious episodes in transplant recipients would be to prevent exposure to potential pathogens. Most transplantation centers have developed policies that are designed to reduce the chance of patients' encountering microbial pathogens. The recommendations usually target infections that are known to be important in transplant recipients and are based on the best current understanding of transmission and pathogenesis. Table 310-7 lists some recommendations found in recent publications.[66,106] The list gives some general guidelines and is not meant to be exhaustive. These recommendations also do not account for differences in susceptibility among patients. For instance, the risk for aspergillosis is not uniform among transplant recipients and is a concern mostly after allogeneic stem cell and lung transplantation or in patients who are receiving high doses of corticosteroids. Similarly, lung transplant recipients are known to have greater difficulty with respiratory viral infections than are kidney, heart, or liver recipients.[17] Clinicians can and should modify their recommendations on the basis of this differential susceptibility to infection, reserving the strictest recommendations for the patients at highest risk. Some pathogens such as Mycobacterium tuberculosis or Coccidioides immitis are relatively virulent, even in immunocompetent hosts, and it is probably not prudent for any transplant recipient, even one who is healthy and on low doses of immunosuppressive drugs, to work as a prison guard or participate in an archeological excavation outside of Tucson, Arizona.

Approach to Fever in the Transplant Recipient

Although immunosuppressive drugs can blunt the febrile response to infection, most transplant recipients with clinical infections have temperature elevations; often this is the first indication that something is awry. Patients should be told to monitor their temperature if they feel

TABLE 310-7	Prevention of Exposure to Pathogens
Type of Exposure	*Intervention*
Hospital Exposures	
Nosocomial bacteria	Use standard precautions, particularly hand washing before and after patient exposures
Respiratory viruses	Restrict access to visitors and staff with colds If contact cannot be restricted, use masks and gloves
Airborne molds	Remove patients from areas of construction, or erect barriers around construction Use masks for patient transport through high-risk areas Use HEPA-filtered air (only for stem cell transplant recipients)
Legionella infection	If nosocomial legionellosis is present, test water supply and decontaminate it, if possible Supply bottled water for oral use, and prevent exposure to aerosolized water, as in showers
Outpatient Exposures	
Enteric pathogens	Cook meat thoroughly, wash fresh fruit and vegetables, wash hands after cooking, avoid certain soft cheeses (e.g., brie, feta) Advise patient to avoid the following: • Drinking water from lakes, streams, and untested wells • Contact with human and animal feces • Unpasteurized milk and juices, raw eggs, and products made with raw eggs
Respiratory viruses	Advise patient to avoid small children or crowded public places or to wash hands after contact Immunize patient and family members against influenza yearly Provide pharmacologic prophylaxis for influenza (in selected patients)
Varicella	Advise varicella-zoster virus–seronegative patient to avoid contact with patients who have shingles or chickenpox
Zoonoses	Advise patient of the following: • To avoid changing litter boxes, cleaning bird cages, or cleaning aquaria • To wear gloves if such cleaning is unavoidable • To avoid jobs that involve frequent animal contact
Airborne molds	Advise patient to avoid closed spaces with high risks of fungal exposure (barns, silos, chicken coops, attics, caves) or high-risk activities (e.g., archeological excavation, especially in southwestern United States)
Legionella infection	Advise patient to avoid water aerosols (whirlpools and commercial displays) and hospital or other institutional tap water that is not tested or treated
Sexually transmitted diseases	Advise patient to use safe sexual practices
Exotic and tropical infections	Advise patient to confer with infectious disease specialist before international travel outside of North America and western Europe

HEPA, high-efficiency particulate air (filter).

ill and to call their physician if the temperature is elevated. For a febrile patient, the physician's first task is to identify possible sites and sources of infection and assess the severity of illness. Patients with typical upper respiratory tract infections and low-grade fevers (less than 38.0° C) can generally be observed clinically. If the patient has a temperature higher than 38.0° C and the cause is not apparent, a medical evaluation should be undertaken. If the patient has symptoms suggestive of a serious localized infection, the patient should be evaluated even in the absence of demonstrable fever.

The most important parts of this workup are a thorough history and a careful physical examination. A chest radiograph should be obtained to establish whether there is evidence for infection in the lungs. Patients with acute pulmonary infiltrates or with persistent fevers higher than 38.5° C usually need to be hospitalized for further workup. Most patients who cannot go about their normal daily activities should probably be evaluated in the hospital, unless the cause of their dysfunction is apparent and can be managed at home. Initial evaluation should include blood and urine cultures, examination of respiratory secretions (if pneumonia is suspected), white blood cell count and differ-

ential, liver function tests, and microscopic examination of the urine. Viral screening tests should be ordered if the patient is still in the high-risk early post-transplantation period (1 to 4 months) or has recently been treated for rejection or if the clinical findings are strongly suggestive of CMV disease. Delayed manifestations of CMV disease are not uncommon in CMV-seronegative patients with seropositive donor transplants who have received antiviral prophylaxis. The manifestations usually occur about 4 to 8 weeks after the antiviral prophylaxis is discontinued.[93] Antibiotics can often be withheld from patients who appear well and in whom no source of infection has been identified in the preliminary workup. A lumbar puncture need not be a routine part of the initial workup of febrile transplant recipients, but a sample of spinal fluid should be obtained from patients with headache or other neurologic complaints.

In a patient with a clear site of infection, evaluation should focus on quickly obtaining adequate samples for culture and smears from that site. Persistent fever (≥7 days) without positive culture findings or an apparent site of infection is a diagnostic and therapeutic problem.

Relatively few clinical entities appear to account for the majority of these fevers of unknown origin (FUOs), the most frequent of which are viral syndromes caused by CMV or occasionally by EBV. Human herpesvirus-6 has also emerged as an occasional cause of FUO in the early post-transplantation period.[107] Other infections that may manifest in this manner are parvovirus infection, systemic toxoplasmosis, and smoldering *Pneumocystis* infection manifesting with a normal-appearing chest radiograph. Deep tissue abscesses generally occur in or near the anatomic site of a recent operation. Disseminated candidiasis usually occurs early after transplantation in patients who are neutropenic or have stayed in the intensive care unit. These patients almost always have received broad-spectrum antibiotics and have central intravenous catheters. The risk for invasive candidiasis is highest in liver recipients; moderate in pancreas, lung, and heart-lung recipients; and low in kidney and heart recipients. Disseminated coccidioidomycosis and histoplasmosis may cause FUO; most of these cases occur in patients who reside in or have recently traveled to endemic areas. Tuberculosis, although uncommon, should always be considered a potential cause of FUO, especially if there is a history of exposure or of extensive residence or travel in developing countries. Whenever an unusual clinical syndrome is associated with fever in the early post-transplant period, clinicians should always consider the possibility of transmission of an unusual infection by the donor organ. Although donor-transmitted infections are uncommon, it may be helpful to look at the medical records of the donor and investigate whether other recipients of organs from the same donor are also ill. Clinicians should keep an open mind to potential causes because new agents are constantly being implicated in donor transmission.[53-56]

Not all fevers are caused by infections. Two important causes of noninfectious fevers in transplant recipients are drug reactions (especially reactions to anti–T-cell antibodies) and transplant rejection. Rejection is most likely to cause fever when it is severe and occurs early after transplantation. Fever caused by transplant rejection is most common in lung recipients, less common in kidney and liver recipients, and rare in heart recipients. Other noninfectious causes of fever are venous or arterial thrombosis, organ ischemia resulting from infarction or inadequate preservation, lymphoproliferative tumors, and hemolytic reactions.

Finally, it must also be conceded that infections in transplant recipients may occur without any fever. Fever sometimes appears to be suppressed by the use of high-dose corticosteroids; at other times, severe organ failure (heart, liver, or kidney) appears to be implicated. Some infections, such as progressive multifocal leukoencephalopathy, polyomavirus infections, or giardiasis, never cause fever, and others frequently do not. *Pneumocystis* pneumonia may manifest with only cough and dyspnea. Fungal infections, particularly focal fungal infections confined to the lung, are frequently afebrile. Even cryptococcal meningitis may manifest with only chronic headache and subtle neurologic symptoms. A good caveat for the physician is always to consider infection a possible cause of any new symptom or sign.

REFERENCES

1. Murray JE. Human organ transplantation: Background and consequences. *Science.* 1992;256:1411.
2. United Network for Organ Sharing. 2007 *Annual Report of the U.S. Organ Procurement and Transplantation Network and the Scientific Registry of Transplant Recipients: Transplant Data 1997-2006.* Health Resources and Services Administration, Healthcare Systems Bureau, Rockville MD, Division of Transplantation. The data and analyses in the 2007 Annual Report of the U.S. Organ Procurement and Transplantation Network and the Scientific Registry of Transplant Recipients have been supplied by the United Network for Organ Sharing (UNOS) and the University Renal Research and Education Association (URREA) under contract with the U.S. Department of Health and Human Services. The authors alone are responsible for the reporting and interpretation of the data.
3. Munoz P, Rodriguez C, Bouza E. *Mycobacterium tuberculosis* infection in recipients of solid organ transplants. *Clin Infect Dis.* 2005;40:581.
4. Fishman JA,. Infection in solid-organ-transplant recipients. *N Engl J Med.* 2007;357:2601.
5. Soave R. Prophylaxis strategies for solid-organ transplantation. *Clin Infect Dis.* 2001;33(Suppl. 1):S26.
6. Riediger C, Berberat PO, Sauer P, et al. Prophylaxis and treatment of recurrent viral hepatitis after liver transplantation. *Nephrol Dial Transplant.* 2007;22(Suppl. 8):viii37-viii46.
7. Tolkoff-Rubin NE, Rubin RH. The infectious disease problems of the diabetic renal transplant recipient. *Infect Dis Clin North Am.* 1995;9:117.
8. Speich R, Van der Bij W. Epidemiology and management of infections after lung transplantation. *Clin Infect Dis.* 2001;33 (Suppl. 1):S58-S65.
9. Wajszczuk CP, Dummer JS, Ho M, et al. Fungal infections in liver transplant recipients. *Transplantation.* 1985;40:347.
10. Milstone AP, Brumble LM, Loyd JE, et al. Active CMV infection before lung transplantation: risk factors and clinical implications. *J Heart Lung Transplant.* 2000;19:744.
11. Ho M. *Cytomegalovirus: Biology and Infection.* 2nd ed. New York: Plenum Press; 1991:249.
12. Dummer JS, Hardy A, Poorsattar A, et al. Early infections in kidney, heart, and liver transplant recipients on cyclosporine. *Transplantation.* 1983;36:259.
13. Ho M, Wajszczuk CP, Hardy A, et al. Infections in kidney, heart, and liver transplant recipients on cyclosporine. *Transplant Proc.* 1983;15:2768.
14. Dummer JS. Infectious complications. In: Cooper DKC, Novitzky D, eds. *The Transplantation and Replacement of Thoracic Organs.* Lancaster, UK: Kluwer Academic Publishers; 1990: 325.
15. Kusne S, Dummer JS, Singh N, et al. Infections after liver transplantation: an analysis of 101 consecutive cases. *Medicine (Baltimore).* 1988;67:132.
16. Hadley S, Samore MH, Lewis WD, et al. Major infectious complications after orthotopic liver transplantation and comparison of outcomes in patients receiving cyclosporine or FK506 as primary immunosuppression. *Transplantation.* 1995;59:851.
17. Billings JL, Hertz MI, Wendt CH. Community respiratory virus infections following lung transplantation. *Transpl Infect Dis.* 2001;3:138-148.
18. Kusne S, Schwartz M, Breinig MK, et al. Herpes simplex virus hepatitis after solid organ transplantation in adults. *J Infect Dis.* 1991;163:1001.
19. Michaels MG, Green M, Wald ER, et al. Adenovirus infection in pediatric liver transplant recipients. *J Infect Dis.* 1992;165: 170.
20. Meuleman J, Katz P. The immunologic effects, kinetics, and use of glucocorticoids. *Med Clin North Am.* 1985;69:805.
21. Anderson RJ, Schafer LA, Olin DB, et al. Infectious risk factors in the immunosuppressed host. *Am J Med.* 1973;54:453.
22. Meier-Kriesche HU, Li S, Gruessner RW, et al. Immunosuppression: evolution in practice and trends, 1994-2004. *Am J Transplant.* 2006;6:1111
23. Segev DL, Sozio SM, Shin EJ, et al. Steroid avoidance in liver transplantation: meta-analysis and meta-regression of randomized trials. *Liver Transpl.* 2008;14:512.
24. Kahan BD. Cyclosporine. *N Engl J Med.* 1989;321:1725.
25. Najarian JS, Fryd DS, Strand M, et al. A single institution, randomized, prospective trial of cyclosporin versus azathioprine–antilymphocyte globulin for immunosuppression in renal allograft recipients. *Ann Surg.* 1985;201:142.
26. Hofflin JM, Potasman I, Baldwin JC, et al. Infectious complications in heart transplant patients receiving cyclosporine and corticosteroids. *Ann Intern Med.* 1987;106:209.
27. Spencer CM, Goa KL, Gillis JC. Tacrolimus: an update of its pharmacology and clinical efficacy in the management of organ transplantation. *Drugs.* 1997;54:925.
28. Webster A, Woodroffe RC, Taylor RS, et al. Tacrolimus versus cyclosporine as primary immunosuppression for kidney transplant recipients. *Cochrane Database Syst Rev.* 2005(4): CD003961.
29. Haddad EM, McAlister VC, Renouf E, et al. Cyclosporin versus tacrolimus for liver transplanted patients. *Cochrane Database Syst Rev.* 2006(4):CD005161.
30. Pirsch JD. Cytomegalovirus infection and posttransplant lymphoproliferative disease in renal transplant recipients: results of the U.S. multicenter FK506. Kidney Transplant Study Group. *Transplantation.* 1999;68:1203.
31. Halloran PF. Immunosuppressive drugs for kidney transplantation. *N Engl J Med.* 2004;351:2715.
32. Sollinger HW. Mycophenolate mofetil for the prevention of acute rejection in primary cadaveric renal allograft recipients. US Renal Transplant Mycophenolate Mofetil Study Group. *Transplantation.* 1995;60:225.
33. Campistol JM, Eris J, Oberbauer R, et al. Sirolimus therapy after early cyclosporine withdrawal reduces the risk for cancer in adult renal transplantation. *J Am Soc Nephrol.* 2006;17: 581.
34. Demopoulos L, Polinsky M, Steele G, et al. Reduced risk of cytomegalovirus infection in solid organ transplant recipients treated with sirolimus: a pooled analysis of clinical trials. *Transplant Proc.* 2008;40:1407.
35. Charpentier B, Rostaing L, Berthoux F, et al. A three-arm study comparing immediate tacrolimus therapy with antithymocyte globulin induction therapy followed by tacrolimus or cyclosporine A in adult renal transplant recipients. *Transplantation.* 2003;75:844.
36. Koo S, Baden LR. Infectious complications associated with immunomodulating monoclonal antibodies used in the treatment of hematologic malignancy. *J Natl Compr Canc Netw.* 2008;6:202.
37. Garcia-Rodriguez MJ, Canales MA, Hernandez-Maraver D, et al, Late reactivation of resolved hepatitis B virus infection: an increasing complication post rituximab-based regimens treatment? *Am J Hematol.* 2008;83:673.
38. Mason JW, Stinson EB, Hunt SA, et al. Infections after cardiac transplantation: relation to rejection therapy. *Ann Intern Med.* 1976;85:69.
39. Bieber CP, Heberling RL, Jamieson SW, et al. Lymphoma in cardiac transplant recipients: association with use of cyclosporin A, prednisone and antithymocyte globulin (ATG). In: Purtilo DT, ed. *Immune Deficiency and Cancer.* New York: Plenum Press; 1984:309.
40. Swinnen LJ, Costanzo-Nordin MR, Fisher SG, et al. Increased incidence of lymphoproliferative disorder after immunosuppression with the monoclonal antibody OKT3 in cardiac-transplant recipients. *N Engl J Med.* 1990;323:1723.
41. Singh N, Dummer JS, Kusne S, et al. Infections with cytomegalovirus and other herpesviruses in 121 liver transplant recipients: transmission by donated organ and the effect of OKT3 antibodies. *J Infect Dis.* 1988;158:124.
42. Peleg AY, Husain S, Kwak EJ, et al. Opportunistic infections in 547 organ transplant recipients receiving alemtuzumab, a humanized monoclonal CD-52 antibody. *Clin Infect Dis.* 2007; 44:204
43. Husain S, Tollemar J, Dominguez EA, et al. Changes in the spectrum and risk factors for invasive candidiasis in liver transplant recipients: prospective, multicenter, case-controlled study. *Transplantation.* 2003;75:2023.
44. Linden PK, Pasculle AW, Manez R, et al. Differences in outcomes for patients with bacteremia due to vancomycin-resistant *Enterococcus faecium* or vancomycin-susceptible *E. faecium*. *Clin Infect Dis.* 1996;22:663.
45. Russell DL, Flood A, Zaroda TE, et al. Outcomes of colonization with MRSA and VRE among liver transplant candidates and recipients. *Am J Transplant.* 2008;8:1737.
46. Cohen IM, Galgiani JN, Potter D, et al. Coccidioidomycosis in renal replacement therapy. *Arch Intern Med.* 1982;142:489.
47. Wheat LJ, Smith EJ, Sathapatayavongs B, et al. Histoplasmosis in renal allograft recipients: two large urban outbreaks. *Arch Intern Med.* 1983;143:703.
48. Dummer JS, Allos GM. Gastrointestinal infections in transplant patients. In: Blaser MJ, Smith PD, Ravidin JI, et al, eds. *Infections of the Gastrointestinal Tract.* Philadelphia: Lippincott Williams & Wilkins; 2002:457.
49. Stout JE, Yu VL. Legionellosis. *N Engl J Med.* 1997;337:682.
50. Sabria M, Yu VL. Hospital acquired legionellosis: solutions for a preventable infection. *Lancet Infect Dis.* 2002;2:368.
51. Simon TL, Dzik WH, Snyder EL, et al. *Rossi's Principles of Transfusion Medicine.* 3rd ed. Philadelphia: Lippincott Williams & Wilkins; 2002.
52. Gottesdiener KM. Transplanted infections: donor-to-host transmission with the allograft. *Ann Intern Med.* 1989;110:1001.
53. Humar A, Fishman JA. Donor-derived infection: old problem, new solutions? *Am J Transplant.* 2008;8:1087.
54. Martin-Davila P, Fortun J, Lopez-Velez R, et al. Transmission of tropical and geographically restricted infections during solid-organ transplantation. *Clin Microbiol Rev.* 2008;21:60.
55. Iwamoto M, Jernigan DB, Guasch A, et al. Transmission of West Nile virus from an organ donor to four transplant recipients. *N Engl J Med.* 2003;348:2196.
56. Centers for Disease Control and Prevention. Brief report: lymphocytic choriomeningitis virus transmitted through solid organ transplantation: Massachusetts, 2008. *MMWR Morb Mortal Wkly Rep.* 2008;57:799.
57. Regamey N, Tamm M, Wernli M, et al. Transmission of human herpesvirus-8 infection from renal transplant donors to recipients. *N Engl J Med.* 1998;339:1358.
58. Luft BJ, Naot Y, Araujo FG, et al. Primary and reactivated *Toxoplasma* infection in patients with cardiac transplants: clinical spectrum and problems in diagnosis in a defined population. *Ann Intern Med.* 1983;99:27.
59. Dummer JS, Armstrong J, Somers J, et al. Transmission of infection with herpes simplex virus by renal transplantation. *J Infect Dis.* 1987;155:202.
60. Cen H, Breinig MC, Atchison RW, et al. Epstein-Barr virus transmission via the donor organs in solid organ transplantation: polymerase chain reaction and restriction fragment length polymorphism analysis of IR2, IR3, and IR4. *J Virol.* 1991;65:976.
61. Delmonico FL. Cadaver organ donor screening for infectious agents in solid organ transplantation. *Clin Infect Dis.* 2000;31:781
62. Coffin CS, Terrault NA. Management of hepatitis B in liver transplant recipients. *J Viral Hepatitis.* 2007;14(Suppl. 1):37.
63. Erice A, Rhame FS, Heussner RC, et al. Human immunodeficiency virus infection in patients with solid-organ transplants: report of five cases and review. *Rev Infect Dis.* 1991;13:537.
64. Halpern SD, Shaked A, Hasz RD, et al. Informing candidates for solid-organ transplantation about donor risk factors. *N Engl J Med.* 2008;358:2832.
65. Fishman JA, Greenwald MA, Kuehnert MT. Enhancing transplant safety: a new era in the microbiological evaluation of organ donors? *Am J Transplant.* 2007;7:2562.
66. Patel R, Paya CV. Infections in solid-organ transplant recipients. *Clin Microbiol Rev.* 1997;10:86.
67. Miller GG, Dummer JS. Herpes simplex and varicella zoster viruses: forgotten but not gone. *Am J Transplant.* 2007;7:741.
68. Antony SJ, Ynares C, Dummer JS. Isoniazid hepatotoxicity in renal transplant recipients. *Clin Transplant.* 1997;11:34.
69. Roland ME, Barin B, Carlson L, et al. HIV-infected liver and kidney transplant recipients: 1- and 3-year outcomes. *Am J Transplant.* 2008;8:355.
70. Gruber SA, Doshi MD, Cincotta E, et al. Preliminary experience with renal transplantation in HIV+ recipients: low acute rejection and infection rates. *Transplantation.* 2008;86:269.
71. Mindikoglu AL, Regev A, Magder LS. Impact of human immunodeficiency virus on survival after liver transplantation: analysis of United Network for Organ Sharing database. *Transplantation.* 2008;85:359.
72. Carter JT, Melcher ML, Carlson LL, et al. Thymoglobulin-associated Cd4[+] T-cell depletion and infection risk in HIV-infected renal transplant recipients. *Am J Transplant.* 2006;6:753.
73. Dummer JS, Lazariashvilli N, Barnes J, et al. A survery of antifungal management in lung transplantation. *J Heart Lung Transplant.* 2004;23:1376.
74. Piparinen H, Helantera I, Suni J, et al. Quantitative PCR in the diagnosis of CMV infection and the monitoring of viral load during the antiviral treatment in renal transplant patients. *J Med Virol.* 2005;76:367.
75. Einsele H, Ehninger G, Hebart H, et al. Polymerase chain reaction monitoring reduces the incidence of cytomegalovirus disease and the duration and side effects of antiviral therapy after bone marrow transplantation. *Blood.* 1995;86:2815.
76. Singh N, Yu VL, Mieles L, et al. High dose acyclovir compared with short course preemptive ganciclovir therapy to prevent cytomegalovirus disease in liver transplant recipients: a randomized trial. *Ann Intern Med.* 1994;120:375.
77. Bingler MA, Feingold R, Miller SA, et al. Chronic high Epstein-Barr virus load state and risk for late-onset posttransplant lymphoproliferative disease/lymphoma in children. *Am J Transplant.* 2008;8:442.
78. Roche B, Samuel D. Risk factors for hepatitis C recurrence after liver transplantation. *J Viral Hepat.* 2007;14(Suppl. 1):89.
79. Brennan DC, Agha I, Bohl DL, et al. Incidence of BK with tacrolimus versus cyclosporine and impact of preemptive immunosuppression reduction. *Am J Transplant.* 2005;582.
80. Huzly D, Neifer S, Reinke P, et al. Routine immunizations in adult renal transplant recipients. *Transplantation.* 1997;63:839.
81. Kumar D, Welsh S, Siegal D, et al. Immunogenicity of pneumococcal vaccine in renal transplant recipients—three year follow-up of a randomized trial. *Am J Transplant.* 2007;7:633.
82. Blumberg EA, Albano C, Pruett T, et al. The immunogenicity of influenza virus vaccine in solid organ transplant recipients. *Clin Infect Dis.* 1996;22:295.
83. Khan S, Ehrlichman J, Rand EB. Live-virus immunization after orthotopic liver transplantation. *Pediatr Transplant.* 2006;10:78.
84. Sester M, Gärtner BC, Girndt M, Sester U. Vaccination of the solid organ transplant recipient. *Transplant Rev (Orlando).* 2008;22:274-284.
85. Fox BC, Sollinger HW, Belzer FO, et al. A prospective, randomized, double-blind study of trimethoprim-sulfamethoxazole for prophylaxis of infection in renal transplantation: clinical efficacy, absorption of trimethoprim-sulfamethoxazole, effects on the microflora, and the cost-benefit of prophylaxis. *Am J Med.* 1990;89:255.
86. Bucaneve G, Micozzi A, Menichetti F, et al. Levofloxacin to prevent bacterial infection in patients with cancer and neutropenia. *N Engl J Med.* 2005;353:977.
87. Kalil AC, Levitsky J, Lyden E et al. Meta-analysis: the efficacy of strategies to prevent organ disease by cytomegalovirus in solid organ transplant recipients. *Ann Intern Med.* 2005;143:870.
88. Goodrich JM, Bowden RA, Fisher L, et al. Ganciclovir prophylaxis to prevent cytomegalovirus disease after allogeneic marrow transplant. *Ann Intern Med.* 1993;118:173.

89. Merigan TC, Renlund DG, Keay S, et al. A controlled trial of ganciclovir to prevent cytomegalovirus disease after heart transplantation. *N Engl J Med.* 1992;326:1182.
90. Winston DJ, Wirin D, Shaked A, et al. Randomised comparison of ganciclovir and high-dose acyclovir for long-term cytomegalovirus prophylaxis in liver-transplant recipients. *Lancet.* 1995;346:69.
91. Gane E, Saliba F, Valdecasas GJ, et al. Randomised trial of efficacy and safety of oral ganciclovir in the prevention of cytomegalovirus disease in liver-transplant recipients. *Lancet.* 1997;350:1729.
92. Lowance D, Neumayer H-H, Legendre CM, et al. Valacyclovir for the prevention of cytomegalovirus disease after renal transplantation. *N Engl J Med.* 1999;340:1462.
93. Paya C, Humar A, Dominguez E, et al. Efficacy and safety of valganciclovir vs. oral ganciclovir for prevention of cytomegalovirus disease in solid organ transplant recipients. *Am J Transplant.* 2004;4:611.
94. Sun H-Y, Wagener MM, Singh N, et al. Prevention of posttransplant cytomegalovirus disease and related outcomes with valganciclovir: A systematic review. *Am J Transplant.* 2008; 8:2111-2118.
95. Khoury JA, Storch GA, Bohl DL, et al. Prophylactic versus preemptive oral valanciclovir for the management of cytomegalovirus infection in adult renal transplant recipients. *Am J Transplant.* 2006;6:2134.
96. Miller GG, Kaplan B. Prophylaxis versus preemptive protocols for CMV: do they impact graft survival? *Am J Transplant.* 2008;8:913.
97. Bonaros N, Mayer B, Schachner T, et al. CMV-hyperimmune globulin for preventing cytomegalovirus infection and disease in solid organ transplant recipients: a meta-analysis. *Clin Transplant.* 2008;22:89.
98. Playford EG, Webster AC, Sorrell TC, et al. Systematic review and meta-analysis of antifungal agents for preventing fungal infections in liver transplant recipients. *Eur J Clin Microbiol Infect Dis.* 2006;25:549.
99. Goodman JL, Winston DJ, Grenfield RA, et al. A controlled trial of fluconazole to prevent fungal infections in patients undergoing bone marrow transplantation. *N Engl J Med.* 1992;326:845.
100. Marr K. Primary antifungal prophylaxis in hematopoietic stem cell transplant recipients: clinical implications of recent studies. *Curr Opin Infect Dis.* 2008;21:409.
101. Ullmann A, Lipton J, Vesole D, et al. Posaconazole or fluconazole for prophylaxis in severe graft-versus-host disease. *New Engl J Med.* 2007;356:335.
102. Wingard J, Carter S, Walsh T, et al. Results of a randomized, double-blind trial of fluconazole (FLU) vs. voriconazole (Vori) for the prevention of invasive fungal infection in 600 allogeneic blood and marrow (BMT) patients. Presented at the 49th annual meeting of the American Society of Hematology. Atlanta, December 2007.
103. Wreghitt TG, Gray JJ, Pavel P, et al. Efficacy of pyrimethamine for the prevention of donor-acquired *Toxoplasma gondii* infection in heart and heart-lung transplant patients. *Transpl Int.* 1992;5:197.
104. Baden LR, Katz JT, Franck L, et al. Successful toxoplasmosis prophylaxis after orthotopic cardiac transplantation with trimethoprim-sulfamethoxazole. *Transplantation.* 2003;75:339.
105. Hellinger WC, Yao JD, Alvarez S, et al. A randomized, prospective, double-blinded evaluation of selective bowel decontamination in liver transplantation. *Transplantation.* 2002;73: 1904.
106. Strategies for safe living following solid organ transplantation. *Am J Transplant.* 2004;4(Suppl. 10):156.
107. Ljungman P, Singh N. Human herpesvirus-6 infection in solid organ and stem cell transplant recipients. *J Clin Virol.* 2006;37 (Suppl 1):S87.

311

Infections in Recipients of Hematopoietic Cell Transplantation

JO-ANNE H. YOUNG | DANIEL J. WEISDORF

The clinical approach to infections in patients undergoing hematopoietic cell transplantation (HCT) involves an understanding of basic transplantation techniques, clinical syndromes, host defense defects at different times after transplantation, the natural history of individual infections, and the mechanisms underlying reconstitution of the immune system after transplantation. In general, the dominant elements of infectious risks for bacterial, viral, fungal, and parasitic infections after HCT depend on the pretransplantation exposure history (viral serostatus), whether the transplant is from an autologous or an allogeneic donor source, and the day after transplantation under consideration. The distinguishing determinant of infectious risk between autologous and allogeneic grafts is the associated risk incurred by ongoing immunosuppression from graft-versus-host disease (GVHD) and its therapy; differing tempos of humoral and cellular immune reconstitution also affect the risk. The time period after transplantation defines eras of differing transplantation complications and the evolution of the slowly resolving post-transplantation immunodeficiency: cutaneous and mucosal barrier breakdown, neutropenia, lymphopenia, hypogammaglobulinemia, or a combination of these. Many post-transplantation complications mimic infectious processes, and multiple infections may occur in the same patient at the same time. Therefore, the patient undergoing HCT should be examined in the context of pretransplantation infections, serologic profiles to document infection latency, conditioning regimen, available culture data from mucosal surfaces, contemporaneous transplantation complications in the patient's institution, current antimicrobial prophylaxis, and the current degree and duration of neutropenia and lymphopenia.

Basic Transplantation Techniques

HCT involves the intravenous delivery of hematopoietic stem cells to a recipient whose hematopoietic and immune systems have been ablated or altered by a cytotoxic preparative regimen, commonly referred to as the *conditioning regimen,* given over the 4 to 10 days before transplantation. Hematopoietic stem cells are obtained from bone marrow, peripheral blood, or umbilical cord blood.[1,2] HCT is an option in treatment for disorders of bone marrow failure (aplastic anemia, Fanconi anemia), malignancies (acute and chronic leukemias), lymphomas, multiple myeloma, hemoglobinopathies, severe immunodeficiency syndromes, inborn errors of metabolism (osteopetrosis, chronic granulomatous disease, Hurler's syndrome, inherited leukodystrophies, other lysosomal disorders), and high-risk solid tumors (neuroblastoma, germ cell tumors). It is currently used investigationally in treatment of diseases such as epidermolysis bullosa, and autoimmune disorders (scleroderma).[3,4]

Autologous HCT is used in the treatment of multiple myeloma, neuroblastoma, and certain lymphomas; morbidity and mortality arise from regimen-related toxic effects and early infections. Allogeneic HCT is used for the remaining diseases listed previously, with the additional issue of GVHD. Substantial improvements in the supportive care of severely immunosuppressed patients have evolved since the 1980s. As outcomes with transplantation improve, the determination of transplantation as an option depends less on the availability of certain donor sources (i.e., whether there is a matched sibling) than in prior decades. Unrelated adult volunteer donors are available for more

than half the general population and umbilical cord blood is used increasingly as a source of stem cells for transplantation.[5] Umbilical cord blood has been shown to be an effective alternative for patients who lack a suitable adult donor, but its use is limited by success in finding an umbilical cord blood unit with an adequate cell dose. Newer strategies such as transplanting with two umbilical cord blood units has enabled transplantation in adults.[6]

The conditioning regimen used to prepare the host is a major determinant of outcome because of variable host tissue injury and the potential for induction of prolonged immunodeficiency. Conditioning regimens may include immunosuppressive and cytotoxic chemotherapy alone or in combination with radiation. Conditioning can damage mucosal surfaces, facilitating transmucosal origin of bloodstream infections.[7] The infectious risks of the patient undergoing HCT are affected by transplantation complications, including the direct effects of this high-dose cytoreductive therapy, such as mucositis, hemorrhagic cystitis, diarrhea, and hepatic veno-occlusive disease (VOD); GVHD; and relapse of the underlying hematologic or oncologic disease.

CHEMOTHERAPY

Busulfan and melphalan are commonly used alkylating agents that are toxic to myeloid stem cells. Cyclophosphamide-containing regimens predispose patients to hemorrhagic cystitis. Fludarabine is less cytotoxic but intensely immunosuppressive and is often included in reduced-intensity or nonmyeloablative conditioning regimens.[8] Antithymocyte globulin, which alters the function of or eliminates T lymphocytes, is used for the conditioning regimen for aplastic anemia and, at times, for GVHD treatment.[9] Chills and fever commonly occur among patients receiving antithymocyte globulin and can be managed by symptomatic treatment and slowing of the infusion. Serum sickness—a syndrome of fever, arthralgia, and rash—can occur with subsequent antithymocyte globulin doses; it is treated with corticosteroid therapy. Antilymphoid antibodies, including alemtuzumab or rituximab, can induce prolonged and profound lymphopenia. Some GVHD prevention strategies include ex vivo graft manipulation (CD34+ or CD3− selection) for T-lymphocyte depletion. While lessening the risks of GVHD, these maneuvers may also delay immune recovery, particularly in haploidentical or human leukocyte antigen (HLA)–mismatched HCT.

IRRADIATION

Total body irradiation may be administered as a single dose or fractionated in multiple doses given over several days. Diarrhea occurs in virtually all treated patients in the first week after irradiation; it may be treated symptomatically while stool culture is pending to rule out infectious causes. Severe oral mucositis occurs in many irradiated patients and is aggravated by prolonged neutropenia and the use of methotrexate for GVHD prophylaxis.[7] As long as bleeding and oral inflammation do not compromise the patient's airway, mucositis is treated symptomatically. Keratinocyte growth factor has proven activity in the prevention of oral and intestinal mucositis.[10,11] Its use to limit mucositis may be of benefit in patients receiving highly toxic conditioning and GVHD prophylaxis regimens, including high-dose total body irradiation, high-dose melphalan, or post-HCT methotrexate.[12] Reduction in infections or mortality has not been demonstrated.[13,14] Lower dose, nonmyeloablative conditioning regimens may be intensely immunosuppressive but less cytotoxic, resulting in less mucosal, enteric, and hepatic injury in the early weeks after transplantation.

HUMAN LEUKOCYTE ANTIGEN MATCHING

In general, engraftment is most rapid, and thus neutropenia is briefest, when the patient and allogeneic donor are completely matched at all genetic HLA loci. Similarly, identical twin (syngeneic) transplantations or those in which hematopoietic stem cells collected from the recipient (autologous) are used lead to prompt neutrophil recovery. Allogeneic HCT (sibling or unrelated donor) has the highest chance of success when fully HLA-matched sibling donor transplants are used, but fewer than 30% of intended recipients have a matched sibling donor available.[15-17] Greater HLA mismatch augments risks of rejection, GVHD, and prolonged immunodeficiency.[18]

NONMYELOABLATIVE TRANSPLANT PREPARATION

Reduced-intensity, or nonmyeloablative, regimens have been developed with the goal of permitting donor-derived hematopoietic and immunologic reconstitution.[19] These regimens provide a somewhat weaker anticancer effect and rely on the graft-versus-tumor effects to eradicate underlying malignancies. Doses of total body irradiation are usually not more than 2 Gy, in comparison with 12 to 14 Gy in fully ablative transplants. Fludarabine, antithymocyte globulin, or lower doses of cytotoxic drugs may be used with induction of extended immune suppression.[20] This approach is often used for older patients or those with significant medical comorbid conditions.

PREVENTION OF INFECTION

Preventive strategies include protective isolation for reduced exposure to pathogens,[21] enhancement of host immune reconstitution with hematopoietic growth factors, prophylaxis during high-risk periods with targeted antimicrobial chemotherapy,[22-24] and suppression of subclinical infection with preemptive therapy. Prophylaxis or preemptive strategies are more effective than treatment after infection is established, and the mortality rate among patients with established infections continues to be high despite available therapy. After mucositis has cleared and oral alimentation has resumed, oral therapy is preferred for prophylaxis.

◼ Clinical Syndromes Unique to the Hematopoietic Cell Transplantation Recipient

HEMORRHAGIC CYSTITIS

Hemorrhagic cystitis is a common complication that can lead to gross hematuria, clots, urinary retention, and impairment of renal function. Cystitis that occurs within 1 week after marrow infusion usually is noninfectious in origin, caused instead by the administration of high-dose cyclophosphamide or busulfan in the conditioning regimen.[25] Prophylactic measures include mesna, forced diuresis, and continuous bladder irrigation; supportive care for established cystitis may also necessitate transfusions, intravesical instillations (e.g., prostaglandins, epidermal growth factor, cauterizing vesicants), hyperbaric oxygen,[26,27] and, in rare instance, cystostomy or cystectomy. Later in the posttransplantation period, GVHD and infection are contributing causes of cystitis. The majority of infectious agents are viral, usually either the polyomavirus BK or adenovirus; herpes simplex virus (HSV), cytomegalovirus (CMV), the polyomavirus JC, human herpesvirus type 6 (HHV-6), and *Strongyloides* infections occur in lower frequencies.[28-30] Polyomaviruses are shed in the urine in many HCT patients without clinical symptoms (see Chapter 145).[31] Higher viral loads of BK virus may indicate a risk for hemorrhagic cystitis.[32] No standard antiviral treatment is currently available for viruria caused by BK virus or adenovirus, although intravesicular cidofovir can be used when hemorrhage persists despite continuous bladder irrigation.[33]

VENO-OCCLUSIVE DISEASE

VOD is a syndrome of liver toxicity that occurs at any time after the onset of the high-dose conditioning regimen, usually before days 20 to 30. It is characterized by painful hepatomegaly, 5% or more weight gain, and hyperbilirubinemia (bilirubin levels >2 mg/dL).[34] Severe VOD (sometimes called *sinusoidal obstruction syndrome*), with marked jaundice or ascites, leads to multiorgan failure involving the kidneys, heart, and lungs.[35] Sometimes effective anticoagulant or antithrombolytic therapy can be initiated before serious organ failure. Approximately 5% to 10% of patients with VOD die. Defibrotide, which stabilizes endothelium and limits microvascular thrombosis, may be very effective in VOD, but definitive, controlled data are unavailable. It has strong promise as a potent new treatment option.[36,37]

Clinical predictors of severe VOD include cytoreductive therapy at high doses, the presence of hepatitis before cytoreductive therapy, persistent fever during cytoreductive therapy, previous radiation therapy to the liver, and the presence of schistosomal hepatic periportal fibrosis. Conditions that may mimic VOD include cholestasis in patients with septicemia, hepatic infiltration secondary to infection or tumor, pericardial tamponade, CMV, hepatitis, and intra-abdominal disease such as pancreatitis, peritonitis, or cholecystitis. In addition, early GVHD and cyclosporine-induced cholestasis are noninfectious causes of liver toxicity that may coexist with or mimic VOD. Diagnosis of VOD may be difficult, and ultrasound assessment of hepatic portal venous flow may yield normal findings. On occasion, liver biopsy with immunohistochemical staining and culture to rule out infectious causes may be indicated, although risk of hemorrhage is markedly increased. Hepatotoxic and nephrotoxic drugs should be avoided in patients with VOD. Genetic polymorphisms in drug metabolism may modify risks of VOD, but their clinical predictive value is under study.

GRAFT-VERSUS-HOST DISEASE

GVHD is a major, life-threatening complication, developing in 40% to 80% of patients after allogeneic transplantation.[38] The risk of developing GVHD is higher in older patients and with partially matched or unrelated donor HCT.[39] Donor T lymphocytes mount an immune attack against the recipient's tissues. Clinical manifestations of acute GVHD include rash, cholestatic hepatitis, nausea, vomiting, and diarrhea. Cyclosporine or tacrolimus, usually given with methotrexate, are effective immunosuppressive agents for the prevention of GVHD and are usually started before transplantation. GVHD itself can compound and prolong post-HCT immunodeficiency. The corticosteroids or other immunosuppressive drugs used for treatment of GVHD may impair phagocytic function and directly worsen lymphopenia and cellular immune deficiency.[40-42] Patients with acute and chronic GVHD have splenic dysfunction and thus an added risk for infection with encapsulated bacteria such as *Streptococcus pneumoniae, Neisseria meningitidis,* and *Haemophilus influenzae.* T cell depletion is less associated with GVHD but more with CMV and aspergillosis infections[43] and sometimes with very delayed immune recovery.

HEPATITIS

Clinical hepatitis in HCT recipients can range from fever accompanied by abdominal pain to fulminant illness. Infectious hepatitis must be distinguished from several common noninfectious causes, including liver dysfunction related to the conditioning regimen (i.e., VOD), acute GVHD, cholestatic liver injury related to sepsis, and chemical hepatitis related to either drugs or hyperalimentation.[44]

Clinically important viral hepatitis syndromes that occur after transplantation include acquisition or reactivation of infection with hepatitis B virus (HBV), hepatitis C virus (HCV), varicella-zoster virus (VZV), adenovirus, HSV, CMV, and HHV-6.[45] Reactivation of HBV is more likely than HCV to result in fulminant hepatitis, although this occurs in only a minority of infected patients. Disseminated VZV and adenovirus infections may manifest with elevations in serum aminotransferase levels; these elevations can precede the appearance of other disease manifestations by several days. In rare cases, liver biopsy with viral culture and polymerase chain reaction (PCR) may be needed to establish a diagnosis of severe hepatitis in the early postengraftment period. Viruses such as hepatitis G virus and transfusion-transmitted viruses are not known to influence the outcome of HCT.

HBV (surface antigen, surface antibody, and core antibody) and HCV serologic profiles are tested in donor and recipient before HCT. Pretransplantation imaging studies or liver biopsy may be needed to evaluate HCV-seropositive patients with abnormal liver enzyme levels or tender hepatomegaly. Donors and recipients with positivity for HBV surface antigen should be tested for viral load with PCR studies for HBV DNA before transplantation, because the risk of HBV hepatitis can be reduced by treatment to lower a detectable viral load. Lamivudine, adefovir, and tenofovir are commonly used to suppress HBV replication (see Chapter 146).[46]

A transplant from an HBV-infected individual can be used as donor material if no alternative donor is available or if the intended recipient is already seropositive. HBV can be transmitted from a surface antigen–positive (or, less likely, core antibody–positive) donor to a recipient who is either HBV-naive or surface antibody–positive but core antibody–negative. The risk of transmission is low when an HBV-positive donor has an undetectable viral load. If the recipient is HBV-naive before transplantation, the subsequent infection is more likely to have clinical consequences. If the transplant can be delayed, then HBV vaccination of the recipient or use of HBV immune globulin may reduce the likelihood of hepatitis after transplantation. HBV immunity can be transferred from a surface antibody–positive donor to an HBV-naive recipient. Through adoptive immunity transfer, HBV infection can be cleared by transplant from a surface antibody–positive donor to a surface antigen–positive recipient.

After transplantation, the following recipients should be monitored periodically with PCR testing of HBV DNA viral load: (1) those with liver enzyme elevation suggestive of activation of HBV from latency; (2) those with transplants from HBV-infected donors; and (3) those with known infection before transplantation. High HBV viral load ($>10^5$ copies/mL) is the most important risk factor for clinically apparent reactivation in recipients positive for surface antigen.[47] Among recipients in whom PCR studies of HBV DNA yield positive results persistently after transplantation despite treatment, the risk of fatal liver disease may be up to 12%.

HCV-positive donors and recipients should undergo RNA viral load testing. An HCV-infected individual can serve as a donor. In contrast to HBV, however, the rate of transmission of HCV from a HCV RNA-positive donor approaches 100%. Interferon can be used to suppress HCV replication in donors,[48] but its limited efficacy, systemic and hematologic toxicity, and delayed response may not correct active HCV to render a donor suitable for donation.

Because the cellular immune system must be functioning in order for HCV to produce hepatitis, few clinical consequences are recognizable in the recipient early after HCT. HCV infection does not increase the incidence of VOD. Beyond 10 years, the long-term complication of HCV infection is cirrhosis.[49] No data have demonstrated a correlation between hepatitis C genotype and type or severity of liver disease after transplantation. Because of the myelosuppressive effects of interferon and other antiviral agents, their use in the treatment of hepatitis C after HCT is limited.

PNEUMONIA SYNDROMES

Infectious pneumonias must be distinguished from noninfectious pulmonary complications after HCT, which can include pulmonary edema, pleural effusion, alveolar hemorrhage, radiation injury (pneumonitis or fibrosis), drug reactions, adult respiratory distress syndrome, idiopathic pneumonia syndrome, cytolytic thrombi (causing multiple peripheral lung nodules), bronchiolitis obliterans, bronchiolitis obliterans with organizing pneumonia, and chronic GVHD.[50] Management of noninfectious pneumonias requires that lower respiratory tract infection be ruled out. Their pathophysiologic processes may be distinct: some syndromes may be more likely to respond therapeutically to high-dose corticosteroids.

Diffuse alveolar hemorrhage begins with dyspnea and alveolar infiltrates and is distinguished from other noninfectious pneumonias by progressively bloody return during bronchoscopic examination and alveolar lavage.[51,52] The syndrome usually occurs in the second and third weeks after HCT. Thrombocytopenia, rapid neutrophil recovery, infection, toxic effects of drugs and of radiation, intensely cytotoxic regimens, and solid malignancy have been implicated as risk factors. Corticosteroids are recommended but improve chances of survival only infrequently.

Idiopathic pneumonia syndrome is a process of widespread alveolar injury that is characterized clinically by diffuse interstitial infiltrates and varying degrees of respiratory failure in the absence of active lower respiratory tract infection. It is thought to be related to the chemotherapy or total body irradiation, or both, used as part of the conditioning regimen, which induces proinflammatory cytokine release and increasing alveolar capillary permeability. Idiopathic pneumonia syndrome occurs in 8% to 17% of patients but may be more frequent after allogeneic than autologous transplantation. Mortality rates are 60% to 80%. Idiopathic pneumonia syndrome occurs classically in two peaks: one in the first few weeks and the other in the second and third month after transplantation. Steroids and sometimes etanercept may yield a clinical response.[53]

DIARRHEA

Diarrhea after transplantation is primarily a result of noninfectious causes such as regimen-related gut mucosal toxicity and GVHD. Diarrhea is associated with infection in fewer than 20% of cases.[54,55] The list of infectious agents responsible for diarrhea includes *Clostridium difficile*, adenovirus, rotavirus, enterovirus, coxsackievirus, HHV-6, *Escherichia coli*, and *Salmonella*, *Giardia*, *Strongyloides*, *Cryptosporidium*, and *Campylobacter* spp. Infection with *C. difficile* occurs with increasing frequency.[56] Outbreaks of diarrhea have been reported for *Cryptosporidium* and enterovirus. From other countries, reports of diarrhea have been associated with *Trichostrongylus* spp.

Typhlitis, or neutropenic enterocolitis, is an anaerobic infectious syndrome that is relatively common and may be associated with diarrhea during neutropenia.[57] Typhlitis is preceded by fever, abdominal pain, and right lower quadrant tenderness that may be accompanied by rebound. Computed tomographic scanning of the abdomen reveals right-sided colonic enlargement and inflammation with thickening of the mucosa. Therapy against anaerobic bacteria should be added to the medical regimen.

RASH

Skin eruptions are often noninfectious, occurring as a direct result of radiation effect from conditioning therapy or secondary to GVHD or drug allergy.[58] Rashes from conditioning regimens can result in the sudden onset of marked erythema over large areas of the body and blistering on the hands and feet. A skin biopsy can assist in distinguishing infectious from noninfectious causes of rash. For all lesions suspected to be infectious, samples should be submitted for culture or biopsy. The most common infectious causes are VZV, catheter-related exit site or tunnel infections, primary cutaneous fungal infections, and secondary cutaneous manifestations of disseminated bacterial or fungal infections.[59] Focal areas of bacterial cellulitis may occur on the lower extremities in the setting of edema from heart failure, VOD, lymphedema, and impaired venous return.

OSTEOMYELITIS

Osteomyelitis is uncommon after HCT. The spectrum of organisms can include atypical mycobacteria, yeasts, and molds, in addition to bacteria.[60,61] In rare instances, osteomyelitis follows marrow aspiration from the sternum or marrow harvest from the iliac crest.[62,63] When prolonged pain and fever occur after bone marrow harvest, osteomyelitis caused by *Staphylococcus aureus* should be considered.

▣ Patterns of Immunosuppression at Different Times after Myeloablative Hematopoietic Cell Transplantation

Historically, three risk periods of immunologic deficiency occur predictably in recipients of HCT (Fig. 311-1). They are the preengraftment period, the early postengraftment period (until day 100), and the late postengraftment period (after day 100). An understanding of the immune deficiencies in each risk period and the period of peak risk for individual infections that are observed with standard infection prophylaxis helps the clinician recognize uncommon manifestations of these infectious pathogens (Table 311-1).[64]

PREENGRAFTMENT RISK PERIOD

The preengraftment risk period begins with the onset of conditioning therapy and continues until approximately days 20 to 40 after transplantation. By definition, graft failure occurs if there is no neutrophil recovery by day 42. Pretransplantation neutropenia is associated with increased infection-related mortality.[65] Bacterial infections are common during this time of profound neutropenia and lymphopenia, necessitating prophylactic and promptly administered empirical systemic antibiotic therapy (see Chapter 309).[66] Prophylactic systemic antibiotics (often a fluoroquinolone such as levofloxacin) can be administered when the neutrophil count drops to less than 500/mm³ and continued until the neutrophil count recovers to prevent bacterial infection (see Chapter 310). Gastrointestinal decontamination with nonabsorbable antibiotics was used in the past but is now rarely performed.

TABLE 311-1 Infections after Hematopoietic Cell Transplantation (HCT), in Order of Occurrence

Organism	Peak Time Period of Risk (Weeks after HCT)	Usual Prophylaxis	Incidence
Preengraftment Risk Period (1-4 Weeks)			
Herpes simplex virus (seropositive)[70,137-139]	1-2	Acyclovir or valacyclovir	5%-9%
Gram-positive bacteremia (most commonly coagulase-negative staphylococci, viridans-group streptococci, and enterococci)[100,103,104,110-112,114]	1-4	Prophylactic broad-spectrum antibiotics	20%-30%
Gram-negative bacteremia[66,67,105]	1-4	Prophylactic broad-spectrum antibiotics	5%-10%
Candida[71-74,81,208,219,222,223]	1-4	Fluconazole, micafungin, voriconazole	Systemic infection: <5% Colonization: 30%
Aspergillus and other molds[74,79,81,209,212,226]	1-4	HEPA air filtration Itraconazole, voriconazole, micafungin, or low-dose amphotericin	<5%
Respiratory viruses[176,178,180,182-186,188,189]	2-5	Isolation, hand washing	15%
Idiopathic pneumonia syndrome[50]	2-4	—	8%-17%
Early Postengraftment (4-26 Weeks) and Late Postengraftment (26-52 Weeks) Risk Periods			
Cytomegalovirus (seropositive)[43,90,92,97,142-145]	7-26	Ganciclovir or foscarnet	<5% (end organ disease) up to 40% (antigenemia/viremia)
Varicella-zoster virus (seropositive)[158,159]	4-52	—*	≤50%
Aspergillus and other molds[79,80,210,212,226]	4-26	Itraconazole, posaconazole, or voriconazole	10%-15%
BK virus[31]	—	—	≤50% (shedding)
Adenovirus[170-172]	—	—	4%-5%
Pneumocystis jirovecii[82,84,215]	4-104	Trimethoprim-sulfamethoxazole	<1%
Toxoplasma gondii (seropositive)[278,280,281]	2-8	—†,‡	2%-7%
Infrequent Infections (May Span Multiple Risk Periods)			
Herpes simplex virus (seronegative)	—	—	<2%
Cytomegalovirus (seronegative)[135,140,141]	—	Blood product screening or filtration	1%-4%
Varicella-zoster virus (seronegative)	—	—	<3%
Streptococcus pneumoniae[106]§	—	Vaccination, penicillin‖¶	<1%
Haemophilus influenzae[290,291]§	—	Vaccination, penicillin‖¶	—
Neisseria meningitidis[290,291]§	—	Penicillin¶	—
Human herpesvirus-6[199,201,202]	—	Ganciclovir or foscarnet	<2%
Epstein-Barr virus[194-196]	—	—	<1% (disease)
Nocardia spp.[131]	—	—‡	<1%
Legionella spp.[127-130]	—	—	<1%
Mycobacterium spp.[115,116,124,125]	—	Screening, then prophylaxis	<1%
Listeria monocytogenes[132-134]	—	—	<1%

*Antiviral medications used to prevent other viral infections may be acting as prophylaxis against reactivation of varicella-zoster virus.
†Prophylaxis with pyrimethamine-sulfadoxine may be used for seropositive patients in countries with a high rate of seroprevalence.[188]
‡The sulfa component of *Pneumocystis* prophylaxis may be acting as prophylaxis against *Toxoplasma* or *Nocardia* infection.
§Risk is increased in patients with chronic graft-versus-host disease.
‖Efficacy in transplant recipients is undetermined.
¶Increasing penicillin resistance may indicate a need for macrolides or extended-spectrum quinolones.
HEPA, high-efficiency particulate air (filter).

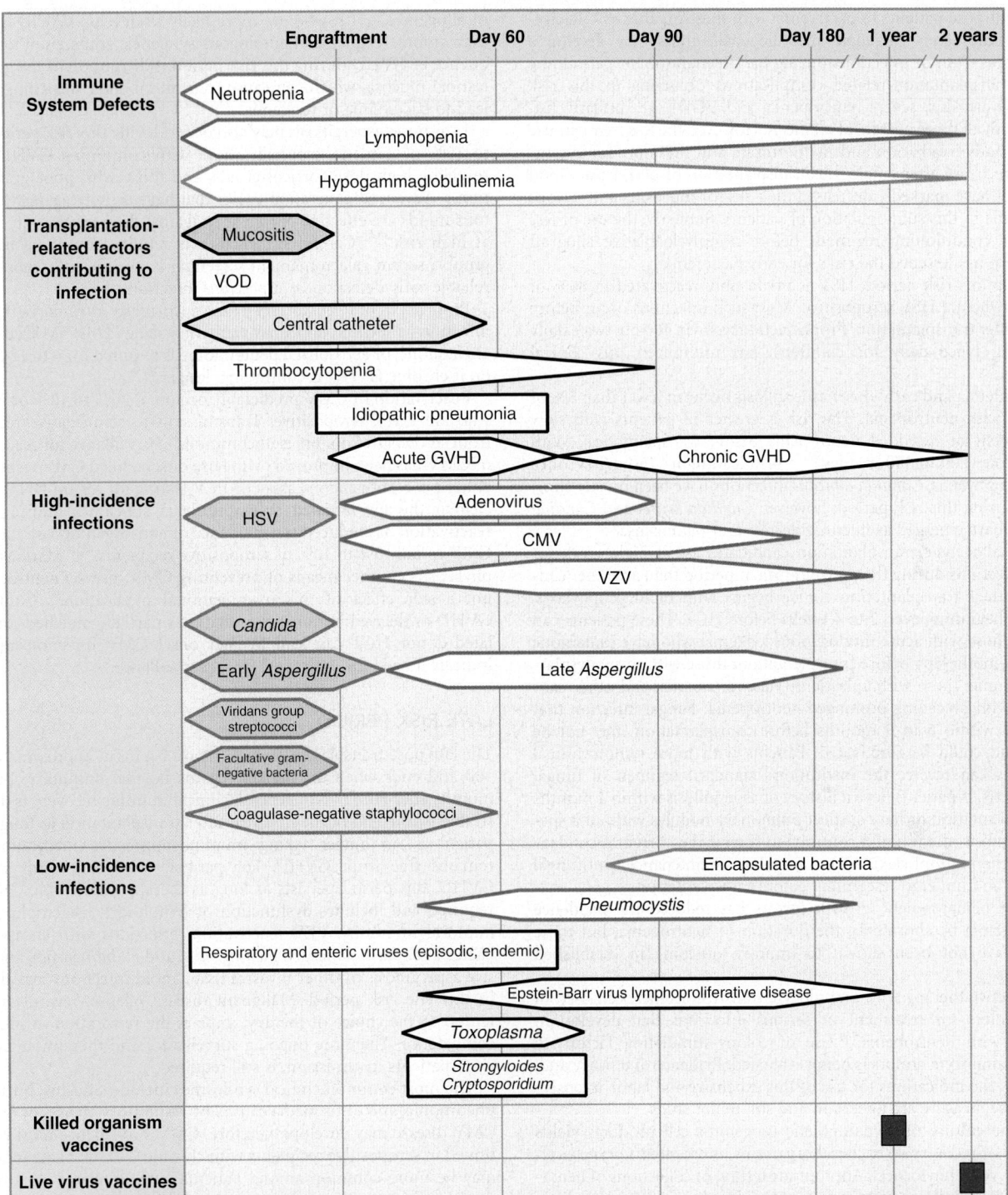

Figure 311-1. Phases of predictable opportunistic infections among patients undergoing hematopoietic cell transplantation (HCT). Immune defects predisposing to infection are bordered by color (*pink*, neutropenia; *blue*, lymphopenia; *green*, hypogammaglobulinemia). Barrier defects predisposing to infection are shaded in color (*yellow*, mucosal breakdown; *silver*, skin breakdown). Contribution of defects to infections occurring with high incidence are designated by border color (for immune defects) or shading (for barrier defects) or both. CMV, cytomegalovirus; GVHD, graft-versus-host disease; HSV, herpes simplex virus; VOD, veno-occlusive disease; VZV, varicella-zoster virus. (*Adapted from Van Burik J-AH, Freifeld AG. Infection in the severely immunocompromised host. In: Abeloff MD, Armitage JO, Niederhuber JE, et al, eds. Clinical Oncology. 3rd ed. Philadelphia: Churchill Livingstone; 2004:942.*)

Prophylactic antibiotic use has shifted the spectrum of gastrointestinal flora to potentially pathogenic organisms such as *C. difficile*, and the etiologic agents of bacteremia have shifted to more gram-positive organisms; in particular, coagulase-negative staphylococci and viridans-group streptococci are more often isolated from febrile neutropenic HCT recipients.[67] Mechanical barrier defects caused by mucositis and central catheters predispose patients to bloodstream infections by allowing access for skin-colonizing organisms and gastrointestinal mucosal flora to otherwise sterile body sites.[68] Colonization with vancomycin-resistant enterococci or other multidrug-resistant pathogens may predispose patients to bacteremia with these organisms.[69] Recipients of autologous-syngeneic and allogeneic grafts may develop a similar spectrum of infections during the preengraftment period; the major transplantation-related complications occurring in this risk period (mucositis, severe neutropenia, and VOD) are similarly frequent with all types of transplantations. However, the less frequent use of total body irradiation and methotrexate and the more rapid neutrophil recovery after autologous transplantation of peripheral blood stem cells have markedly decreased the risks for mucositis and serious bacteremia in this subpopulation of patients. Similarly, the use of less intensive conditioning regimens before nonmyeloablative allograft placement has lessened the risks for early bacteremia.

During this risk period, HSV is predictably reactivated in 80% of patients who are HSV seropositive. Most such infections occur before week 4 after transplantation. Prophylactic acyclovir, 400 mg twice daily (5 mg/kg twice daily for children), has minimized this clinical infection.[70]

Candidemia and early-onset aspergillosis occur in fewer than 5% of patients with neutropenia. The risk is greater in patients with slow engraftment or extended neutropenia before transplantation. With fluconazole (200 to 400 mg/day)[71-73] or micafungin[74] (50 mg IV once daily) prophylaxis, *Candida albicans* infections have been mostly eliminated during this risk period; however, *Candida krusei* and *Candida glabrata* have emerged as fluconazole-resistant pathogens.[75]

Some allogeneic transplantation candidates are at higher risk for mold infections during the preengraftment period than are other candidates; their transplantation course begins with mold prophylaxis, possibly beginning even 2 to 4 weeks before HCT. These patients can include those with acute myelogenous leukemia who have undergone serial chemotherapy before transplantation; those with myelodysplastic syndrome; those with aplastic or Fanconi anemia; and other candidates with preceding prolonged neutropenia. Fungal infection that occurred within 6 to 9 months before transplantation may not be cured and could be reactivated. Patients with more remote fungal infections can receive the institution's standard regimen of fungal prophylaxis. If patients have a history of aspergillosis within 4 months of transplantation or have suspect pulmonary nodules without a specific diagnosis, they should continue to receive the current secondary fungal chemoprophylaxis (i.e., ongoing maintenance antifungal therapy) and undergo rescanning before transplantation.

Use of hematopoietic growth factors has reduced the incidence of bacteremia by shortening the duration of neutropenia, but these agents have not been shown to improve outcome in established infections.

Adjunctive therapy with granulocyte transfusions has been used in some centers for treatment of serious infections that develop in patients with neutropenia.[76] Use of colony-stimulating factors to prime granulocyte donors is being evaluated. Evidence of efficacy and, therefore, the indications for use of this expensive and labor-intensive supportive measure are uncertain and still under study.

Routine culture of hematopoietic progenitor cell products yields low rates of recovery of bacterial organisms, most often *Corynebacterium* spp. or staphylococci. Appropriate testing of collections of hematopoietic stem cell products includes routine culture of hematopoietic progenitor cells before HCT, but patients receiving culture-positive harvests usually do so without clinically adverse outcomes.[77,78]

POSTENGRAFTMENT RISK PERIOD

The postengraftment period begins with neutrophil recovery and continues until day 100, when early B- and T-lymphocyte functional recovery may be initially apparent. Reconstituted T lymphocytes have abnormal function for approximately 18 months, as evidenced by CD4 deficiency and by in vitro antigen and mitogen proliferative responses. However, T-lymphocyte reconstitution may be blunted by the effects of GVHD or CMV and their attendant treatments (corticosteroids, cyclosporine, anti–T-lymphocyte therapy, and ganciclovir). As a result, the rate of infection during this risk period is higher among recipients

of allogeneic grafts, who are more likely to develop GVHD or CMV, than among recipients of autologous-syngeneic grafts. Another consequence of GVHD during this risk period is disruption of the gastrointestinal mucosa, which can cause transmural entry of pathogens and lead to bacteremia or fungemia.

Late-onset aspergillosis may also occur during this risk period in up to 10% of patients, especially those with continuing GVHD, those receiving high-dose corticosteroids, and those with poor graft function.[79] Advanced-generation azoles that have activity against filamentous molds are effective prophylaxis against deep mycoses in patients at high risk.[80,81] Careful surveillance is required for these high-risk groups; serum galactomannan screening is insufficiently sensitive for reliable early detection of *Aspergillus* infections.[22]

Prophylaxis of *Pneumocystis jirovecii* (formerly *Pneumocystis carinii*) infection with trimethoprim-sulfamethoxazole (TMP-SMX), dapsone, atovaquone, or aerosolized pentamidine is required for 6 to 12 months or, if chronic GVHD is continuing, longer.[82-86]

Reactivation of CMV predictably occurs in 20% to 40% of patients who are CMV seropositive. Transmission to seronegative recipients from seropositive donors is uncommon.[43] Surveillance for reactivation of CMV has been improved by the use of scheduled CMV testing with either pp65 antigenemia assay or PCR testing for serum DNA.[87] Ganciclovir therapy initiated preemptively at subclinical indications of reactivation has reduced the incidence of end-organ disease caused by CMV to only 5% to 10% of seropositive recipients.[88,89] Maribavir prophylaxis is another means of preventing CMV disease; neutropenia is not a side effect of this investigational medication.[90] Continuing GVHD or delayed immune recovery after partially matched- or unrelated-donor HCT can lead to later onset CMV infection and may indicate a need for prolonged CMV surveillance.

LATE RISK PERIOD

The late post-transplantation risk period begins at approximately day 100 and ends when the patient regains normal immunity, 18 to 36 months after HCT.[91-95] In general, clinical immune recovery is demonstrable by the end of the first year after transplantation as long as the patient is no longer taking immunosuppressive medication and remains free from GVHD. For patients with continuing chronic GVHD, this period persists as long as therapy for chronic GVHD is required and includes dysfunction of lymphocyte, macrophage, and humoral immunity. VZV reactivation, infections with encapsulated bacteria (*S. pneumoniae*, *N. meningitidis*, and *H. influenzae*), and invasive aspergillosis or other invasive tissue mold infections may develop in this late risk period. Malignant disease relapse, regardless of its tempo or the choice of therapy, impairs the restoration of immunocompetence. Therefore ongoing surveillance and therapy, as in post-HCT patients in remission, is still required.

The most common clinical syndromes include sinusitis, bronchitis, pneumonia, and otitis media caused by respiratory viruses or bacteria. CMV disease may develop; therefore, CMV surveillance must be continued in seropositive recipients with chronic GVHD.[92] Late infections may be more common among patients with unrelated donors than among patients whose donors were family members, even in the absence of GVHD. Approximately 50% of late pneumonias in patients with ongoing chronic GVHD are caused by noninfectious interstitial pneumonitis. Lung histopathologic studies reveal obliterative bronchitis that may respond to corticosteroid therapy.

Immunosuppression after Nonmyeloablative Hematopoietic Cell Transplantation

Nonmyeloablative HCT is associated with less disruption of mucosal barriers, shorter periods of severe neutropenia, fewer episodes of bacteremia in the first 30 days, and a trend toward fewer episodes of bacteremia during the first 100 days after HCT.[96] However, this type of transplantation can still be associated with severe GVHD, often necessitating high-dose corticosteroid treatment. It is often used for older patients and those with compromised organ function and poor performance status. GVHD, CMV disease, and invasive fungal infection may be delayed 1 to 2 months, but the overall incidences of these conditions are similar to those with conventional HCT during the first year after transplantation.[96-98] Patients undergoing nonmyeloablative HCT should receive surveillance for CMV and fungal infections well beyond day 100, as well as preemptive or prophylactic treatment similar to that for myeloablative HCT recipients between day 100 and 1 year after HCT.

Measures to Reduce Risks of Infection

Protective measures that should be discussed before HCT and reinforced during the recovery period involve travel, crowds, and pets. With regard to travel, there are no particular restrictions, but strategies to minimize transmission of infectious diseases have been summarized.[21,22] Some social situations, such as sitting in a crowded movie theater or classroom, may increase the risk of acquiring a viral respiratory illness. Turning away from individuals who are coughing or sneezing, or even quickly donning a mask, may be helpful in preventing transmission of airborne infection. Patients need instruction to remember to augment infection prevention by washing their hands as soon as possible after being close to someone with a cold. Because outbreaks of noroviruses have involved cruise ships, and because other types of outbreaks (e.g., *Staphylococcus*) are commonly associated with the close living quarters of this type of vacation, cruise ships may be unwise vacation choices.

Healthy dogs and cats are considered acceptable pets. However, immunosuppressed patients should not be responsible for scooping cat litter because of potential *Toxoplasma* cyst exposure. Similarly, such patients should not play in sandboxes because these areas are concentrated sites that outdoor cats may use as litter boxes. Because reptiles of many sorts have been reported to be infected with *Salmonella*, such patients should not touch these animals or their aquarium homes. The heated water of tropical fish tanks may carry *Mycobacterium marinum*. *Chlamydophila psittaci* can be transmitted from psittacine birds.

Hand washing or the use of alcohol-based hand rub disinfectant is the mainstay of infection prevention in the hospital or clinic.[99] Persons entering the patient's room to perform examination or touch the patient (including visitors, as well as health care workers) should wash or disinfect their hands outside the room.[21] During respiratory virus season, infection control personnel will often add extra signage to doorways and other places on the wards to remind visitors of the importance of hand washing. Staff and visitors with respiratory viral infections should not be permitted to have direct contact with the patient. Routine use of gown, gloves, or masks, or a combination of these, is not required in the presence of a neutropenic transplant recipient, but ongoing caution to prevent interperson or nosocomial transmission is essential.

Natural History of Individual Infections after Hematopoietic Cell Transplantation

With advances in infection prevention strategies, the risk periods for some infections are changing. It is important to understand the natural history of individual infections as they occur in the HCT recipient and how it may be distinct from that in other immunocompromised patient populations. Infections that occur with a high incidence among HCT recipients justify prophylaxis during the applicable risk period or empirical treatment during the course of infection (see Table 311-1).[24]

BACTERIAL INFECTIONS

Gram-positive organisms account for half of bacteremias occurring after HCT.[100-102] Although the skin has been thought to be the primary reservoir for these organisms, colonization of the gastrointestinal tract may be an additional source. *Staphylococcus epidermidis* (i.e., coagulase-negative *Staphylococcus*) is the species most commonly recovered in culture from the skin and nose. Oropharyngeal organisms include *Streptococcus pyogenes*, *Streptococcus mitis*, and *Enterococcus* spp. (vancomycin-sensitive and vancomycin-resistant). Unlike catheter-associated infections with *S. aureus*, *Candida* spp., or some gram-negative bacilli, most gram-positive bacteremias can be managed successfully without removal of the intravascular device.[103,104] Methicillin-resistant *S. aureus* (MRSA), which had been rare in neutropenic infections, is becoming more frequent. If the patient does not respond to initial antibiotic management, or if there is tenderness or erythema along the tunnel tract, the catheter should be removed. In rare cases, adjunctive surgical débridement of the skin tunnel is needed. Catheter removal and surgical débridement are often required when a tunnel infection is caused by rapidly growing mycobacteria.

Gram-negative organisms are the second most frequent cause of bloodstream infection. The incidence of infection with *Pseudomonas* spp. is low, in part because of the use of antipseudomonal antibiotics for prophylaxis against, and initial empirical therapy for, neutropenic fever. Although bacteremias have historically occurred during the neutropenic period, bacteremias continue to develop in patients with long-term central intravenous catheters, in patients with ongoing immunosuppression resulting from GVHD or its therapy, and in those with neutropenia secondary to graft failure or drug-related marrow suppression (e.g., ganciclovir).[105]

Encapsulated Bacteria

For patients who experience chronic GVHD or are otherwise asplenic, the risk for life-threatening bacterial sepsis with encapsulated organisms is increased. Invasive pneumococcal infection may occur months to years after HCT. The annual incidence is 8 per 1000 allogeneic HCT recipients and higher (21 per 1000) among those with chronic GVHD.[106] Penicillin or macrolide prophylaxis may be indicated until immunosuppression is discontinued.[94,107] Reports of penicillin-resistant pneumococcal infections have prompted a change in prophylaxis from penicillin to a quinolone in some centers.[108,109]

Viridans-Group Streptococci

Viridans-group streptococcal bacteremias, mostly caused by *S. mitis*, may carry a high mortality rate early after HCT.[110-113] Poor dental hygiene is a risk factor for *S. mitis* bacteremia in HCT patients.[114] Normally antibiotic sensitive, these organisms may be resistant to norfloxacin, ciprofloxacin, and penicillin in patients receiving prophylactic antibiotics. Vancomycin is the drug of choice for HCT patients. Oral ulcerations caused by HSV reactivation during conditioning are thought to be an entry point, corroborated by a decreased incidence of viridans-group streptococcal septicemia after active prophylaxis of HSV infections with acyclovir.[111]

Mycobacteria

Mycobacteria are an infrequent cause of infection after HCT, but it is important to identify them because treatment requires medication that would not be used empirically. The rapidly growing nontuberculous mycobacteria are responsible for catheter exit site infections, tunnel infections, bacteremia (with waterborne *Mycobacterium mucogenicum*), or pneumonia.[115,116] Infection with *Mycobacterium tuberculosis* occurs predominantly in countries with high endemic rates; the number of cases may be increasing worldwide as transplantation becomes available globally.[117-121] Transplantation candidates and donors who are at risk for reactivation of latent tuberculosis can be readily identified during the pretransplantation evaluation on the basis of residence in endemic areas or close contact with another person with known or suspected tuberculosis. Screening is recommended with tuberculin skin testing or an ex vivo interferon-γ release assay, such as QuantiFERON-TB Gold.[122-125] Clinically significant infection can be prevented by antituberculous prophylaxis when positive QuantiFERON-TB Gold assays or reactive tuberculin skin testing yields positive results. Potential transplantation patients and donors should also receive screening if they have a history of abnormal chest radiographic findings before transplantation, have recently traveled to a foreign country for longer than 3 months, have been employed in an institution with tuberculous clients, have a history of alcoholism or intravenous drug use, or are seropositive for human immunodeficiency virus (HIV). QuantiFERON-TB Gold has 96% to 99% specificity that is unaffected by the vaccine for bacille Calmette-Guérin.[126] For patients with a positive result of a screening test but no signs of active tuberculosis and no previous antituberculous therapy, a chest radiograph and liver function studies should be obtained, in addition to peritransplantation and 9-month post-transplantation therapy with isoniazid and pyridoxine.

Intracellular Bacteria

Legionellosis[127-130] and nocardiosis[131] are uncommon, but both can manifest as pneumonia or lung nodules in the HCT patient. Detection of *Legionella* by direct fluorescent antibody (DFA) assays has proved unreliable in the HCT setting because of false-positive results and because it does not detect a high proportion of disease caused by *Legionella* species. These species include *Legionella feeleii*, *Legionella micdadei*, and *Legionella bozemanae*.[130] Infection can persist or relapse after 3 weeks of appropriate antimicrobial therapy, which suggests that prolonged antibiotic treatment is indicated for HCT recipients with legionellosis.[129] Medical therapies for nocardiosis often consist of administration of sulfonamide in combination with a synergistic agent; adjunctive surgical débridement may be useful for catheter-related infections with this organism. The role of other intracellular bacterial agents as pathogens has not been well defined, but *Listeria monocytogenes* infection may manifest as bacteremia or meningitis.[132-134]

VIRAL INFECTIONS

Certain viral infections are preventable. Administration of acyclovir for HSV-seropositive patients during the preengraftment period is widely accepted. CMV-safe (serologically screened or filtered) blood product transfusions for CMV-seronegative patients have proved especially effective in preventing transfusion-acquired CMV infections.[135,136] Periodic (e.g., weekly) CMV diagnostic surveillance for CMV-seropositive patients during the postengraftment period and prompt institution of antiviral therapy are essential. CMV-seronegative patients are at comparatively low risk; therefore, diagnostic monitoring continues for only 6 to 10 weeks. Scrupulous hand washing and avoidance of crowds to prevent transmission of respiratory viral and other infections (in the hospital or ambulatory clinic) remain the mainstay of effective infection control practice for this vulnerable population.[21]

Herpes Simplex Virus

Among HSV-seropositive recipients during the first month after transplantation, the incidence of HSV reactivation can be reduced from 80% to less than 5% through the use of acyclovir or valacyclovir, initiated at the time of conditioning and continued until mucositis has diminished.[70,137,138] The majority of postengraftment HSV infections are confined to the oropharynx, although the infection occasionally extends directly to squamous epithelial surfaces in the esophagus, larynx, or skin in the perioral or perianal areas. Patients who do not respond to acyclovir after engraftment, and particularly those who have received prolonged or repeated courses of acyclovir, may have acyclovir-resistant HSV. Foscarnet or cidofovir may be beneficial in that setting. In uncommon cases, HSV infection causes Bell's palsy, hepatitis, or encephalitis. Valacyclovir achieves predictably higher drug levels than does acyclovir after oral administration.[138,139]

TABLE 311-2	Weekly Screening Schedule for Initiation of Preemptive Cytomegalovirus (CMV) Therapy after Hematopoietic Cell Transplantation		
CMV Serostatus of Recipient	CMV Serostatus of Donor	Blood Products	Duration of Weekly Surveillance
Seronegative	Seronegative	CMV safe*	Weeks 2 to 12
Seronegative	Seropositive	CMV safe*	Weeks 2 to 12
Seronegative	None	CMV safe*	Weeks 2 to 5
Seropositive	Seronegative or seropositive	CMV untested	Weeks 2 to 12, then every 2-4 weeks until week 26†
Seropositive	None	CMV untested	Weeks 2 to 5

*Blood filtered to remove neutrophils or from seronegative donor.
†Possible indications for testing beyond week 26 include high risk for late CMV disease (e.g., in patients treated with steroids for GVHD).

Cytomegalovirus

The historical incidence rate of primary CMV infection among the CMV-seronegative HCT recipient can be reduced from 40% toward 4% or less by use of CMV-safe blood products during transfusions.[140,141] The incidence of CMV reactivation, traditionally 70% in CMV-seropositive patients with allogeneic transplants and 45% among patients with autologous transplants, can be reduced to between 20% and 40% by the use of preemptive or prophylactic antiviral therapy with ganciclovir or foscarnet.[88,142-145] Results with acyclovir and valacyclovir have varied.[146-148] With the current practice of preemptive early ganciclovir, the median time of onset of CMV end-organ disease has been delayed from 1 to 2 months toward 4 to 6 months after HCT; this indicates that CMV surveillance must be longer in groups at high risk.[92]

Weekly screening enables identification of patients who might benefit most from preemptive therapy with ganciclovir (Table 311-2). CMV pp65 leukocyte antigen and quantitative DNA PCR testing are excellent methods for early CMV detection, although antigen testing is unreliable during neutropenia. Once CMV is identified by an early detection method, most patients are treated with 7 to 14 days of induction ganciclovir therapy (5 mg/kg intravenously twice daily), followed by maintenance therapy (ganciclovir, 5 mg/kg intravenously once daily, or valganciclovir, 900 mg orally once daily), for several weeks beyond negative CMV test results (Table 311-3). Maintenance therapy may need to be continued for patients with persistent detection of virus or those with profound immunosuppression caused by active GVHD.

Oral valganciclovir is a safe and effective ganciclovir prodrug, with the valine ester cleaved during the first pass through the liver, and it can be considered for the patient who needs long-term maintenance and is otherwise taking oral medications without difficulty. A valganciclovir dosage of 900 mg once per day produces blood-level drug exposure similar to those produced by an intravenous 5 mg/kg dose of ganciclovir.

Foscarnet can be used empirically for patients who have marrow suppression from ganciclovir, who fail to respond to ganciclovir, or who have concurrent HHV-6 viremia. Foscarnet is administered in doses of 90 mg/kg intravenously every 12 hours for induction and 90 mg/kg intravenously every 24 hours for maintenance. Good urine flow can minimize irritation of the urethra and labia by foscarnet. The serum biochemical abnormalities (chelation of calcium and phosphate) accompanying foscarnet therapy necessitates hospital observation and very careful electrolyte monitoring at least through the initial days of its use.

End-organ manifestations of CMV disease include pneumonia (63%), enteritis (26%), and, in rare cases, retinitis (5%).[89] CMV pneumonia occurs in fewer than 5% of CMV-seropositive allogeneic patients who receive ganciclovir preemptive therapy during the first 100 days.[89] Among patients with CMV pneumonitis, the mortality rate is as high as 50%, even when prompt treatment is combined with intravenous immune globulin (IVIG) or CMV-specific immune glob-

TABLE 311-3	Suggestions for Management of Possible Cytomegalovirus (CMV) Infection after Hematopoietic Cell Transplantation (HCT)	
Indication	*Strategy**	*Comment*
Prevention		
Allogeneic Transplant		
Seropositive recipient	Ganciclovir[†] induction, 5 mg/kg bid for 7-14 days, followed by 5 mg/kg daily until the end of maintenance *or* Ganciclovir prophylaxis at engraftment	Some cases of CMV disease may occur shortly after ganciclovir discontinuation CMV reactivation might be delayed, occurring later after HCT
Seronegative recipient with seropositive donor	Ganciclovir induction, 5 mg/kg bid for 7-14 days, followed by 5 mg/kg daily until the end of maintenance *and* Seronegative or filtered blood products	Prophylaxis at engraftment is not recommended because of the low incidence of post-transplantation infection
Seronegative recipient with seronegative donor	Seronegative or filtered blood products	
Autologous Transplant		
Seropositive recipient	Early ganciclovir induction, 5 mg/kg ganciclovir bid for 7 days, followed by 5 mg/kg daily for 14 days of maintenance	Because of the very low risk in some settings, monitoring is not uniformly advocated
Seronegative recipient	Seronegative or filtered blood products	
Treatment of Disease		
CMV pneumonia	Ganciclovir induction, 5 mg/kg bid for 14-21 days, followed by 5 mg/kg daily for at least 3-4 weeks of maintenance *plus* IVIG every other day for the duration of induction	Extended maintenance throughout periods of severe immunosuppression (i.e., GVHD treatment) may be considered
Gastrointestinal disease	Ganciclovir induction, 5 mg/kg bid for 14-21 days, followed by 5 mg/kg daily for at least 3-4 wk of maintenance *plus* IVIG weekly for 3 weeks	If deep ulcerations are present, maintenance may be required for a longer time
Marrow failure	Foscarnet, 90 mg/kg bid for 14 days, followed by 90 mg/kg daily for 2 weeks *plus* G-CSF	Ganciclovir plus IVIG has also been used
Retinitis	Ganciclovir, 5 mg/kg bid for 14-21 days, followed by 5 mg/kg daily for at least 3-4 weeks	Extended maintenance may be required

*Regimens should be accompanied by weekly monitoring with antigenemia or PCR-based nucleic acid testing.

[†]Oral 900-mg doses of valganciclovir produce blood levels that are similar to those for the standard intravenous dose (5 mg/kg) of ganciclovir.

G-CSF, granulocyte colony-stimulating factor; GVHD, graft-versus-host disease; IVIG, intravenous immune globulin; PCR, polymerase chain reaction.

ulin.[149] CMV viremia and pneumonitis are rare before engraftment.[150,151] Anorexia, nausea, vomiting, and sometimes diarrhea characterize CMV gastroenteritis; the diagnosis is made by endoscopy and biopsy with immunoperoxidase staining of CMV-infected cells.[152,153] CMV disease of the gastrointestinal tract is often associated with GVHD of the specific organ.[153] Response to therapy is not assured,

even with ganciclovir and IVIG. Although CMV retinitis is common among patients infected with HIV, it is quite uncommon among HCT recipients.[154]

Once an end organ has established disease from CMV, the infection is difficult to treat. CMV pneumonitis is treated with a combination of ganciclovir at induction doses for 14 to 21 days and IVIG (500 mg/kg every other day for the duration of induction, 14 to 21 days) and then with maintenance ganciclovir. Standard IVIG is generally used because CMV-specific immune globulin is scarce and has not been shown to improve outcome. CMV enteritis is treated with ganciclovir at induction doses for 3 weeks or longer without IVIG.[155] Treatment of protracted CMV enteritis might include ganciclovir and IVIG or a longer duration of ganciclovir maintenance therapy to facilitate gastrointestinal healing.[153]

Development of a CMV-specific cytotoxic T-lymphocyte response is critical for the reconstitution of normal immunity and protection from late CMV disease.[156] Long-term IVIG delays recovery of CMV immunity. For patients who remain at risk for late disease, CMV monitoring should be continued beyond day 100. Patients who are treated with acyclovir followed by ganciclovir or those treated with serial ganciclovir courses may be at increased risk of developing genotypic resistance. Clinical resistance episodes should be treated with foscarnet (or cidofovir) until assays for mutations in the UL97 or UL54 gene are able to confirm virologic resistance.[157] Extended ganciclovir therapy appears to delay recovery of cytotoxic T-lymphocyte activity, either by a direct effect on lymphocytes or by limitation of the amount of antigen exposure to lymphocytes. This immunodeficiency can be reversed when cytotoxic T lymphocytes are given adoptively, but this technology is available only at some tertiary centers.[156]

Varicella-Zoster Virus

VZV infection is a primary occurrence (5% of occurrences) or a reactivation (95%) in 40% of patients at any time in the first year after transplantation.[158,159] VZV can be effectively prevented with acyclovir prophylaxis,[160] but VZV prophylaxis is not employed at all transplantation centers because only 30% to 50% of adult patients and 25% of pediatric patients develop this infection during the first year after transplantation. The median time of onset is 5 months after transplantation. Prolonged antiviral prophylaxis may delay the onset of VZV but is not associated with rebound VZV.[160] Localized zoster may manifest atypically with a few vesicles, or skin lesions may appear as atypical vesicles; therefore, laboratory confirmation of VZV reactivation is recommended.

Manifestations of VZV disease are most often dermatomal shingles but may include hemorrhagic pneumonia, hepatitis, abdominal pain, central nervous system disease, thrombocytopenia, and retinal necrosis.[161-165] Disseminated or visceral varicelliform zoster may manifest as low back pain or acute abdominal pain before the appearance of skin lesions. GVHD is a strong predictor of VZV dissemination, which involves visceral organs in 20% to 40% of patients.[161,166] Most fatal cases of disseminated or abdominal zoster occur in patients who were treated with suboptimal doses of acyclovir or for whom therapy was initiated relatively late in the course of infection. High-dose acyclovir (10 mg/kg IV every 8 hours) has been the treatment of choice for disseminated VZV infection. Valacyclovir and famciclovir can be used as stepdown treatment after intravenous acyclovir or as initial treatment of localized infection. Patients who are already seropositive can acquire a second primary VZV infection. VZV vaccination is recommended at the 2-year anniversary visit for patients who have been free of immunosuppressive medications for several months, unless the underlying hematologic or oncologic disease is in relapse.[167,168] The vaccine used should be the lower plaque-forming unit version (Varivax) used for prevention of chickenpox among children, not the higher titer (Zostavax) vaccine used for immunocompetent older adults.

VZV is a fastidious virus and may not withstand the time required to transport the specimen to the diagnostic laboratory. By scraping the base of a vesicle and examining the cells by DFA with VZV-specific monoclonal antibodies, clinicians can best diagnose lesions of herpes zoster and chickenpox. The Tzanck smear is less sensitive and is no longer recommended. Tissue diagnosis can be made through histologic examination, immunohistochemical techniques, or culture.

When a VZV-seronegative patient receives a significant exposure to a person with active or incubating chickenpox, a course of acyclovir with or without varicella-zoster immune globulin (VariZIG) is recommended to prevent chickenpox.[169] Acyclovir in the usual treatment doses of 10 mg/kg intravenously every 8 hours for 3 to 22 days after exposure seems appropriate. For a VZV-seropositive patient living in the same dwelling as someone with an index case of active chickenpox or shingles, acyclovir is reported to be useful in preventing new infection. VariZIG is usually not given to seropositive patients, but antiviral prophylaxis is often recommended, depending on the exposure, the length of time since the transplantation, and the level of immunosuppression. For lower risk patients, valacyclovir, 1 g orally three times daily, may be appropriate, although the efficacy in this situation is unknown. Patients already receiving empirical ganciclovir for CMV reactivation do not need further antiviral drugs.

Adenovirus
Adenovirus infection reactivates in approximately 12% of allogeneic and approximately 6% of autologous HCT patients.[170,171] Chronic shedding can occur in the absence of clinical disease, but adenovirus can also be acquired from respiratory droplet transmission. In its most common clinical manifestation in this setting, adenovirus is a cause of hemorrhagic cystitis.[28] Systemic infection in the lungs, liver, gastrointestinal tract, and kidneys occurs in 18% to 20% of infected patients. GVHD is a risk factor for the occurrence of adenovirus infection after HCT.[172] In addition, allogeneic patients who do not receive ganciclovir (seronegative for CMV or seropositive without need for ganciclovir) are at higher risk for developing adenovirus infection than are patients who did receive ganciclovir, even though ganciclovir has no activity against adenovirus.[170] Immunofluorescence, shell vial, or conventional tube culture of blood, urine, stool, or tissue can be used to diagnose adenovirus. PCR testing may also be helpful in diagnosis.[173] No effective therapy is available for adenoviral infections, although cidofovir has been used in patients able to tolerate the nephrotoxicity.[174,175]

Respiratory Viruses
Patients who have undergone HCT and develop a respiratory viral infection typically present with rhinorrhea and nasal congestion and may also have fever, cough, throat pain, headache, or myalgias.[176] The common pathogens in such patients include respiratory syncytial virus, parainfluenza virus, and, to a lesser extent, influenza virus and rhinovirus.[176-186] Human metapneumovirus infections may be culture negative.[187] Current methods allow detection of respiratory syncytial virus, parainfluenza, and influenza in respiratory specimens within 48 hours (see Chapter 17). Respiratory virus infections commonly occur during the winter season and cause pneumonia in up to 50% of patients. In contrast, parainfluenza 3 virus infections may occur throughout the year,[184,185] and nosocomial outbreaks of respiratory syncytial virus have occurred outside the established winter season. Influenza, most often type A, infrequently progresses to pneumonia. Prophylactic or early initiation of oseltamivir therapy during outbreaks seems reasonable, although evidence of efficacy in immunosuppressed hosts is not available.

Respiratory syncytial virus and parainfluenza are associated with a high incidence of progression from upper to lower tract disease among infected patients. Upper respiratory tract illness with parainfluenza usually resolves without serious sequelae. Lower tract infection has a mortality rate of 80% for respiratory syncytial virus and 30% to 35% for parainfluenza virus.[178,188,189] Therapy with aerosolized ribavirin or a combination of ribavirin and IVIG or monoclonal antibody (palivizumab [Synagis]) has been used for respiratory syncytial virus.[176,190] The survival rate appears to be higher when treatment is initiated before significant hypoxia is present, and aerosolized ribavirin may help to decrease the viral burden.[190,191] There are only anecdotal case reports regarding the effectiveness of ribavirin for treatment of respiratory viruses other than respiratory syncytial virus, including parainfluenza, adenovirus, and influenza. Preemptive therapy with aerosolized ribavirin in patients with positive nasopharyngeal cultures for respiratory syncytial virus appears promising. Patients who develop respiratory viral pneumonia before engraftment have poorer outcomes. Aerosolized ribavirin (Virazole) is administered by a face mask to adults through a small particle aerosol generator. This device can be used for patients on a ventilator. Although there are no data on what dose may be effective, 6 g (one vial) per 12 hours once daily, is one schedule. Contamination of the patient's room with this possibly teratogenic agent is of concern to pregnant hospital staff.

Prevention of exposure is critical because treatment is not very effective. Protection involves the use of frequent hand washing by hospital staff and isolation of patients with cold symptoms. In addition, family members and health care workers with upper respiratory tract symptoms should be separated from patients. Vaccination of family members, health care workers, and other close contacts against influenza may help control exposures. Amantadine or rimantadine prophylaxis has limited usefulness because of the widespread development of resistance. Oseltamivir provides useful prophylaxis against both influenza A and B and appeared useful when used in a housing facility for HCT recipients.[192] Immune globulin prophylaxis with respiratory syncytial virus–specific polyclonal or monoclonal antibody, which is useful in infants at high risk, has not been sufficiently evaluated in the HCT setting.[193] During the respiratory virus season, all patients with respiratory symptoms should have a sample taken from the nasopharynx to be evaluated for respiratory viruses with DFA staining and shell vial or conventional tube culture.

Epstein-Barr Virus
The majority of Epstein-Barr virus (EBV) reactivation is subclinical and requires no therapy. The incidence of EBV-related complications may be higher (7%) among recipients of umbilical cord blood transplants with a nonmyeloablative preparative regimen than among recipients of HLA-matched, unrelated-donor marrow myeloablative transplants (3%). In addition, the incidence of EBV-related complications is significantly higher in a subset of patients treated with antithymocyte globulin (21%).[194] HLA-mismatched (especially haploidentical) or T-depleted grafts may lead to prolonged T-lymphopenia and augment the risk of EBV reactivation. Quantitative diagnostic testing of EBV viral load is not standardized across institutions, although future multiplexing of EBV into CMV monitoring assays may lead to new monitoring algorithms. EBV is a cause of a posttransplantation lymphoproliferative disorder (PTLD) that arises when anti–T-lymphocyte immunosuppressive therapy is ongoing.[195] In most cases, high viral loads are associated with progression to PTLD.[196] Infusions of rituximab or nonirradiated donor leukocytes may be effective treatment for allograft recipients with high-titer EBV viremia or PTLD.[194,197,198]

Human Herpesvirus-6
HHV-6 has been implicated as a possible cause of bone marrow suppression, fatal meningoencephalitis, and interstitial pneumonitis in fewer than 2% of HCT patients.[199] Recipients of umbilical cord blood may have more viremia than do other populations.[200] HHV-6 appears to reactivate commonly, occurring in 46% of HCT patients according to culture diagnosis and as many as 100% of patients according to PCR of blood.[201] Many episodes of reactivation detected by DNA PCR may be asymptomatic, and the value of therapy for subclinical viremia is unknown. Most strains of HHV-6 identified after HCT appear to be caused by the B variant in blood or urine, although the A variant has been correlated with pneumonitis.[202] HHV-6 has 60% DNA homology with CMV, and treatment of documented infection is usually initiated with induction doses of ganciclovir or foscarnet. Responses to antiviral therapy are not universal, and benefits of ganciclovir versus foscarnet have not been determined.[203]

Parvovirus

Parvovirus B19 is a rare cause of refractory anemia with erythroid hypoplasia after HCT.[204-207] Antibody or PCR tests detect parvovirus, although PCR may yield positive findings for months after the acute infection. Use of single-patient rooms on HCT wards may be preventing transmission of this contagious virus to other patients undergoing HCT, and the administration of IVIG for other reasons may be treating subclinical infections.

FUNGAL INFECTIONS

Invasive fungal infections are important causes of morbidity and mortality. The major causes of invasive fungal disease include *Candida* spp., *Aspergillus* spp., and, less frequently, the non-*Aspergillus* filamentous molds. Patients undergoing allogeneic transplantation are at 10-fold increased risk for invasive fungal infection in comparison with patients receiving an autologous graft. Systemic fluconazole prophylaxis or low-dose amphotericin B (0.1 to 0.3 mg/kg daily) can decrease the incidence of deep candidiasis.[71-73,208,209] Advanced-generation azoles and micafungin prophylaxis extend the spectrum of organisms covered to include molds, but their general value or cost-effectiveness for all allograft recipients has not been shown.[74,81,210-212] Empirical therapy of febrile neutropenic patients is discussed in Chapter 310.

Pneumocystis

P. jirovecii infection[213] usually manifests as pneumonia with dyspnea, cough, fever, and bilateral infiltrates in the majority of infected patients.[82] It can occur after both autologous and allogeneic transplantation, although the frequency is lower for the former. Before the use of routine prophylaxis, *Pneumocystis* infection occurred in approximately 7% of patients who underwent allogeneic HCT, at a median of 1 to 3 months after transplantation, and was associated with a 5% risk of death.[214,215] Prophylaxis with TMP-SMX has resulted in negligible rates of infection. For patients who do not tolerate medications containing sulfa, prophylaxis options include desensitization with TMP-SMX, use of dapsone,[86,216] atovaquone,[217] and inhaled pentamidine.[83,218] The treatment of choice for *P. jirovecii* infection is TMP-SMX.[82,84]

Candida

Candidiasis is an infection acquired from endogenous organisms colonizing the gastrointestinal tract; it usually manifests as fungemia or visceral candidiasis (see Chapter 257). Before fluconazole prophylaxis, the onset of candidiasis occurred at a median of 2 to 3 weeks after transplantation, and *Candida* spp. were second in frequency to *Aspergillus* spp. as the cause of brain abscess after HCT.[219,220] The current cumulative incidence rate of invasive candidiasis during the first year after HCT is probably less than 5%.[221] Risk factors for invasive candidiasis include neutropenia, breakdown of the normal mucosal barriers, and the use of broad-spectrum antibiotics or corticosteroids. *C. albicans* infections are successfully prevented when fluconazole is given as prophylaxis from the time of conditioning until either engraftment or day 75 after HCT. The strategy of prolonged therapy has been associated with improved survival rates, although the mechanism of the observed benefits is uncertain.[73,222,223] The benefit of fluconazole prophylaxis is less clear for autologous transplants, for which the degree of mucositis is less.

With the use of fluconazole since the 1990s, the number of *Candida* infections has decreased.[208] The spectrum of colonizing and infecting *Candida* organisms has shifted from *C. albicans* and *Candida tropicalis* to include *C. krusei*, *C. glabrata*, and *Candida parapsilosis*.[75] *C. krusei* is innately resistant to fluconazole.

Aspergillus

Aspergillus and other mold infections are acquired exogenously, by inhalation of spores into the respiratory tract from the environment, and may occur with higher frequency during the summer in some localities.[79] Common sites of initial infection include the lung and sinuses, although contiguous or hematogenous extension to the central nervous system or other internal organs may occur. With the use of fluconazole prophylaxis during the preengraftment period, invasive aspergillosis emerged as the leading fungal infection found at autopsy among patients who underwent HCT.[208] Preengraftment prophylaxis with micafungin or voriconazole is now being used for patients who may have *Aspergillus* incubating at the time of transplantation. Postengraftment prophylaxis with posaconazole or voriconazole has led to a decrease in mortality among patients with a high risk of invasive aspergillosis.[80,224]

The incidence of invasive aspergillosis among patients undergoing HCT ranges from 4% to 15%.[79,225,226] The onset of *Aspergillus* infection after HCT occurs in a bimodal distribution, with the first peak at 2 to 3 weeks (during neutropenia) and the second at 3 to 4 months after HCT, usually in conjunction with persisting GVHD.[79] Postengraftment aspergillosis can occur after 6 months, again alongside chronic GVHD but also with CMV. Older age is associated with the acquisition of aspergillosis during either the preengraftment or postengraftment risk periods. Donor type, male gender, and summer season are specific risk factors for preengraftment aspergillosis, whereas construction in the vicinity of the hospital, GVHD and the attendant corticosteroid therapy, lymphopenia, CMV, respiratory virus infection, and multiple myeloma are significant risk factors for the development of postengraftment aspergillosis.[79,227] Early aspergillosis is temporally associated with neutropenia; therefore, infection among autologous HCT patients is rare after engraftment. The estimated 1-year survival rate among patients with invasive aspergillosis is 7% to 30%, although more aggressive, prolonged, or combination antifungal therapies may be improving these outcomes a bit.

Preventive strategies should focus on reducing both environmental and host risk factors. The use of high-efficiency particulate air (HEPA)–filtered air systems or laminar airflow rooms during the preengraftment risk period aid in the prevention of infection, particularly for allograft recipients. HEPA filters are capable of removing particles greater than 0.2 μm in diameter, such as mold spores. The patient's room is continuously maintained at positive pressure in relation to the corridor, which enhances the barrier effect. For transport out of HEPA-filtered rooms or after discharge, tight-fitting face masks reproduce this barrier and are sometimes used, at least for the early post-HCT period.

Patients might ask whether portable HEPA filters should be purchased for use after the hospitalization. This extra measure can be implemented on an individual basis, if units are obtained for each of the rooms that the patient will occupy during the day and night and if each unit is sized for the room it will be placed in. There is no evidence of the clinical efficacy of these filters out of the hospital in preventing acquisition of airborne mold infections, and for outpatients, they are probably of little value and considerable expense.

Other prevention strategies, including nasal and aerosolized amphotericin B, have not been studied in controlled trials.

The availability of accurate early diagnostic tests for invasive fungal infections lags behind those for other types of infections. The most promising diagnostic assay, the *Aspergillus* galactomannan test,[228-230] is most useful for patients not already taking antifungal therapy that includes coverage for molds, which is a minority of allogeneic recipients.[231] Other antigen- and nucleic acid–based diagnostic tests have been studied for early diagnosis of invasive tissue mold infection, but they have not been routinely adopted in clinical laboratories. Most have not been tested in large numbers of clinical samples from HCT recipients. Blood cultures for molds rarely yield positive findings of mold organisms, except in the case of *Fusarium*.

A high index of suspicion in persistently febrile neutropenic patients and timely computed tomography of the chest to detect new infiltrates are important for early detection of invasive pulmonary aspergillosis. A small "ground-glass" halo around the lung lesion or pleura-based or nodular infiltrates on computed tomography scans are highly suggestive of aspergillosis or other mold infection in this setting. Bronchoscopy with culture of lavage fluid for fungi, as well as other organisms common to immunocompromised hosts, is important. A lack of clinical or radiographic response during empirical antifungal therapy may necessitate tissue sampling. Minimally invasive surgery (video-assisted thoracoscopic surgery) is associated with less morbidity than is open lung biopsy.

Patients who have undergone HCT and have suspected invasive mold infections should begin taking a mold-active antifungal agent while diagnostic procedures are being arranged. Advanced-generation azole agents and echinocandins have less nephrotoxicity than do lipid preparations of amphotericin B. A lack of clinical or radiographic response during proven infection may necessitate a switch to an agent from a different class[232] or to combination therapy.[233] Combination treatment of fungal infections with echinocandins, azoles, and polyene agents is becoming increasingly common, although results of randomized clinical trials are not available. Echinocandin agents may be fungistatic, rather than fungicidal, in the case of mold infections because their interruption of cell wall synthesis is limited to certain areas of growing hyphae.

For documented invasive tissue mold infection, therapy is usually continued until some weeks (4 to 6) after lesions are resolved or stable, immunosuppression has decreased, and the patient is afebrile. Although amphotericin B had been the gold standard antifungal since the 1960s, voriconazole produced superior outcomes in treatment for aspergillosis in 53% of patients, in contrast to 32% of patients treated with amphotericin B (followed by other antifungal therapy).[234] Treatment of central nervous system mold infections should include voriconazole, which (on the basis of a small number of samples) attains cerebrospinal fluid levels approximately 50% of plasma levels and central nervous system tissue levels approximately 200% of plasma levels.

After initial control of an aspergillosis infection, subsequent maintenance therapy for the duration of immunosuppression has been advocated to reduce the risk of reactivation. Multiple drug-drug interactions occur with the azoles, and adjustments may be required for immunosuppressive agents. Transient visual disturbances or hallucinations are common with voriconazole. Difficulty in achieving therapeutic plasma drug levels complicates the administration of itraconazole. Itraconazole solution has improved oral bioavailability over the capsule and can be used, although blood level monitoring may be needed to ensure adequate absorption. Posaconazole has good anti-mold activity, but its oral absorption requires high fat intake, which may not be feasible in patients with GVHD or other enteric complications.

Other Yeasts

Malassezia furfur causes tinea versicolor and catheter-related fungemia.[235] Response to either topical or systemic therapy is slow; recovery of granulocyte counts is usually associated with resolution.[236] Catheter removal and discontinuation of intravenous lipids are important for a successful outcome in cases of fungemia. Trichosporonosis has manifested as fungemia, skin lesions, pneumonitis, and arthritis.[237-239] Fungemia, usually acquired via an intravenous catheter, has been reported with *Trichosporon* and *Rhodotorula* spp., *Cryptococcus laurentii*, and *Hansenula anomala*. Meningitis with *Cryptococcus neoformans* is unusual, in contrast to its frequent occurrence among patients infected with HIV. Widespread anti-*Candida* prophylaxis with fluconazole may contribute to the low frequency of these infections.

Other Molds

Non-*Aspergillus* molds such as *Alternaria*, *Penicillium*, *Neosartorya*, *Microascus*, and *Phialophora* spp. are infrequent causes of invasive tissue infections whose clinical appearance is similar to that of *Aspergillus* infection. They are indistinguishable from *Aspergillus* hyphae in tissue sections; thus, culture is required for identification. Disseminated fusariosis is generally a fatal infection for patients who have undergone HCT, manifesting as positive blood cultures, skin lesions, or endophthalmitis.[240] Successful resolution is usually associated with

neutrophil recovery in addition to antifungal therapy.[241] In the case of fusarial endophthalmitis, enucleation of the affected eye may be required.

Mucormycosis is uncommon after HCT, but it mimics aspergillosis and may occur long after HCT.[242,243] The cause of one hepatic infection included over-the-counter herbal medication.[244] Patients receiving voriconazole prophylaxis are at risk for breakthrough infection with invasive mucormycosis, but the risk of such breakthrough infections appears low.[245-248] Posaconazole may be an effective maintenance treatment for infections caused by certain species of *Mucorales* after response to amphotericin B.[249] Clinically significant infections caused by the dimorphic fungi, including coccidioidomycosis, histoplasmosis, and blastomycosis, are unusual even in hyperendemic areas of the United States.

PARASITIC INFECTIONS

Parasitic infection after HCT usually manifests as reactivation of toxoplasmosis,[250] although Chagas' disease,[251-255] malaria,[256-261] strongyloidiasis,[262] schistosomiasis,[263] *Clonorchis* infection,[264] giardiasis,[265,266] cryptosporidiosis,[265,267-270] pulmonary microsporidiosis,[271-273] and *Acanthamoeba* and *Trichomonas* meningoencephalitis[274-277] have also been reported. Routine blood smears before HCT cannot be used to rule out malarial transmission. In Hong Kong, *Clonorchis sinensis* infection was identified in only 1% of screening stool examinations performed 7 days before HCT.[264] None of the patients had symptoms related to clonorchiasis; patients received praziquantel (25 mg/kg orally three times for 1 day) before HCT, and subsequent stool examinations did not reveal the presence of ova.

Toxoplasmosis is infrequent after HCT, occurring in 2% to 7% of patients who are seropositive before transplantation.[278-281] Although the parasite can be transmitted as a primary infection through marrow, blood products, or donor solid organs, toxoplasmosis in patients who have undergone HCT is almost always the result of reactivation of prior infection. GVHD is a risk factor relating to the suppression of cell-mediated immunity that is critical for host defense against *Toxoplasma gondii*.[282] The clinical presentation includes fever, encephalitis with focal cerebral lesions, pneumonitis, or myocarditis. One postmortem diagnosis of disseminated toxoplasmosis was associated with hemophagocytic syndrome.[283] Parasitemia is a feature of reactivation that may be identified in tissue culture, although many diagnoses are now made with PCR.[284,285] Stereotactic brain biopsy is also useful in diagnosis of the infection.[286] The identifiable risk period is 2 to 8 weeks after HCT. Seropositive patients not receiving TMP-SMX are at risk for breakthrough toxoplasmosis.[287] For these patients, *Toxoplasma* reactivation can be monitored through PCR during the first 1 to 3 months after HCT.[288] In countries with a high prevalence of seropositivity, prophylaxis seems logical and justifies the use of pyrimethamine-sulfadoxine among seropositive HCT recipients.[289] However, in countries where the prevalence is low, routine prophylaxis is not justified.

Methods of Immune System Reconstitution after Hematopoietic Cell Transplantation

VACCINATION

Patients undergoing autologous or allogeneic HCT eventually lose immunity to the common childhood diseases and should be reimmunized 1 and 2 years after transplantation (Table 311-4; see Fig. 311-1).[168] The efficacy of vaccination is influenced by the time elapsed since transplantation, the nature of the hematopoietic graft, the presence of GVHD, and the use of serial immunization.[290] There have been no reports of exacerbation of GVHD after immunization of patients who underwent HCT. A national survey of HCT immunization prac-

TABLE 311-4	Suggested Schedule for Vaccination after Hematopoietic Cell Transplantation (HCT)		
	Time Period for Immunization after HCT		
Vaccine	*12 Months*	*14 Months*	*24 Months*
Inactivated Vaccines			
Diphtheria, tetanus, acellular pertussis	X	X	X
Haemophilus influenzae serotype B conjugate	X	X	X
Hepatitis B	X	X	X
Pneumococcal	X (7-valent conjugated)		X* (7-valent conjugated)
Inactivated polio	X	X	X
Influenza	Lifelong, seasonal administration of inactivated vaccine, beginning before HCT and resuming ≥6 mo after HCT, is recommended		
Hepatitis A	Routine administration is not indicated. If hepatitis A vaccination is given, two doses, given 6-12 months apart, are required		
Meningococcal conjugate	Routine administration is not indicated		
Human papillomavirus	Administration is recommended for women younger than 27 years		
Rabies	Routine administration is not indicated; any decision to use should be individualized		
Live Replication Competent Vaccines			
Measles-mumps-rubella:	Administration is not indicated		X*,†
Varicella-zoster (Varivax)	Administration is not indicated		X*,†
Yellow fever virus	Routine administration is not indicated; any decision to use should be individualized		

*Optional.
†In patients with no active graft-versus-host disease or immunosuppressive therapy.

tices revealed that vaccines were underutilized and schedules for revaccination varied.[291] All transplant recipients should be immunized on the same schedule, regardless of cell source.[292]

All indicated nonlive vaccines should be administered to patients who have undergone HCT, regardless of transplant type or presence of GVHD. Such patients should be revaccinated every 10 years with the combined tetanus-diphtheria toxoid, absorbed. No data are available on safety and immunogenicity of pertussis vaccination in such patients. At 1 year, they should also be immunized against polio by the inactivated intramuscular vaccine, *H. influenzae* type B, hepatitis B, and *S. pneumoniae*. If the patient was previously immunized, only one dose of hepatitis B vaccine should be given. Postvaccine titers of hepatitis B virus should be documented to ensure response and adequate protection, even when the vaccine is given at the specified time interval after HCT.[293] At 2 years, a second dose of pneumococcal vaccine is optional; it provides a second opportunity to vaccinate persons who failed to respond to the first dose, especially patients with chronic GVHD. Lifelong, seasonal administration of influenza vaccine should begin before HCT and resume by 2 to 6 months after HCT. Children younger than 9 years who are receiving influenza vaccination for the first time require two doses yearly. Influenza vaccine for HCT ward employees, clinical health care workers, and household contacts may be especially necessary within the first year or for patients with ongoing GVHD, in whom protective responses may be impaired.

Live virus vaccines such as measles-mumps-rubella and varicella should not be given to transplant recipients with active GVHD or ongoing immunosuppressive therapy; the first doses are given to trans-

plant recipients more than 24 months after HCT who are taking no immunosuppressive medications and are presumed immunocompetent. A second measles-mumps-rubella dose should be given 6 to 12 months later; however, the benefit of a second dose in this population has not been evaluated.

Vaccination with live-attenuated VZV vaccine (Varivax, not Zostavax) is used for VZV-seronegative patients who no longer require immunosuppressive therapy and are free of GVHD, but no controlled study has demonstrated its safety in the HCT setting. Therefore, use of varicella vaccine in patients who have undergone HCT should be restricted to research protocols for patients more than 24 months after HCT and who are presumed immunocompetent. When varicella vaccination is given to persons older than 13 years, two doses, given 4 to 8 weeks apart, are required. Susceptible family members should receive VZV vaccine to minimize chickenpox exposure for VZV-seronegative transplant recipients.

Routine administration of hepatitis A, meningococcal, and rabies vaccines is not indicated. Hepatitis A vaccine is recommended for transplant recipients with chronic liver disease, including hepatitis C infection or chronic GVHD, or who live in hepatitis A–endemic areas or in areas experiencing outbreaks. If given, hepatitis A vaccination requires two doses, given 6 to 12 months apart. For transplant recipients with potential occupational exposure to rabies, preexposure rabies vaccination should be delayed until at least 12 months, if not 24 months, after HCT.

IMMUNOGLOBULIN REPLACEMENT

The major defect in humoral immunity is the absence of specific antibody production. Antibody levels in the first year after HCT are affected primarily by pretransplantation levels in the recipient and, to a lesser degree, in the donor.[294] Among patients with chronic GVHD, reduced production of opsonizing antibody and of all classes of immunoglobulin G and immunoglobulin A antibodies is seen.[295] This immunodeficiency is further complicated by poor splenic function and is associated with recurrent pneumococcal infections and episodes of bronchitis or pneumonia. IVIG does not prevent infections when given weekly during the preengraftment or late risk periods, but it does reduce rates of septicemia and localized infection when given in the postengraftment risk period after transplantation.[296-298] It may modulate the severity of GVHD.[299] Replacement IVIG (200 to 500 mg/kg every 1 to 2 weeks) may be beneficial for patients with immunoglobulin G levels lower than 400 mg/dL; however, in one prospective trial, its routine use delayed recovery of antigen (viral)–specific immunity.[297]

The role of hyperimmune globulin for prevention of specific infections is less clear. High-titer CMV globulin for prevention of CMV infection and treatment of end-organ CMV disease has proved to be of clear benefit in comparison with IVIG. However, antiviral drugs are effective in providing protection against CMV disease. Therefore, because of its limited availability, as well as cost considerations, the use of CMV-specific globulin has decreased at many transplantation centers. Hyperimmune respiratory syncytial virus globulin provided only a very modest increase in neutralizing antibody when given in the first 6 weeks after HCT.[193] The use of virus-specific monoclonal antibodies as preventive measures against respiratory syncytial virus and CMV is currently under investigation. Hepatitis B, human rabies, and tetanus immune globulin should be used as needed in the event of exposures. VariZIG is a human polyclonal immunoglobulin G available for intramuscular or intravenous administration under an expanded access program through Cangene Corporation for patients at high risk within the first 72 hours of exposure. VariZIG administration may extend the varicella incubation period from 10 days to as much as 28 days, is expensive, and is not uniformly effective in preventing chickenpox in patients who have undergone HCT.

REFERENCES

1. Grewal SS, Barker JN, Davies SM, et al. Unrelated donor hematopoietic cell transplantation: marrow or umbilical cord blood? *Blood.* 2003;101:4233-4244.
2. Brown JA, Boussiotis VA. Umbilical cord blood transplantation: basic biology and clinical challenges to immune reconstitution. *Clin Immunol.* 2008;127:286-297.
3. Dvorak CC, Cowan MJ. Hematopoietic stem cell transplantation for primary immunodeficiency disease. *Bone Marrow Transplant.* 2008;41:119-126.
4. Burt RK, Loh Y, Pearce W, et al. Clinical applications of blood-derived and marrow-derived stem cells for nonmalignant diseases. *JAMA.* 2008;299:925-936.
5. Brunstein CG, Wagner JE. Umbilical cord blood transplantation and banking. *Annu Rev Med.* 2006;57:403-417.
6. Brunstein CG, Wagner JE. Cord blood transplantation for adults. *Vox Sang.* 2006;91:195-205.
7. Filicko J, Lazarus HM, Flomenberg N. Mucosal injury in patients undergoing hematopoietic progenitor cell transplantation: new approaches to prophylaxis and treatment. *Bone Marrow Transplant.* 2003;31:1-10.
8. Chaudhury S, Auerbach AD, Kernan NA, et al. Fludarabine-based cytoreductive regimen and T-cell–depleted grafts from alternative donors for the treatment of high-risk patients with Fanconi anaemia. *Br J Haematol.* 2008;140:644-655.
9. Macmillan ML, Couriel D, Weisdorf DJ, et al. A phase 2/3 multicenter randomized clinical trial of ABX-CBL versus ATG as secondary therapy for steroid-resistant acute graft-versus-host disease. *Blood.* 2007;109:2657-2662.
10. Tsirigotis P, Triantafyllou K, Girkas K, et al. Keratinocyte growth factor is effective in the prevention of intestinal mucositis in patients with hematological malignancies treated with high-dose chemotherapy and autologous hematopoietic SCT: a video-capsule endoscopy study. *Bone Marrow Transplant.* 2008; 42:337-343.
11. Stiff P. Mucositis associated with stem cell transplantation: current status and innovative approaches to management. *Bone Marrow Transplant.* 2001;27(Suppl. 2):S3-S11.
12. Spielberger R, Stiff P, Bensinger W, et al. Palifermin for oral mucositis after intensive therapy for hematologic cancers. *N Engl J Med.* 2004;351:2590-2598.
13. Levine JE, Blazar BR, DeFor T, et al. Long-term follow-up of a phase I/II randomized, placebo-controlled trial of palifermin to prevent graft-versus-host disease after related donor allogeneic hematopoietic cell transplantation. *Biol Blood Marrow Transplant.* 2008;14:1017-1021.
14. Blazar BR, Weisdorf DJ, Defor T, et al. Phase 1/2 randomized, placebo-control trial of palifermin to prevent graft-versus-host disease after allogeneic hematopoietic stem cell transplantation. *Blood.* 2006;108:3216-3222.
15. Petersdorf EW, Hansen JA, Martin PJ, et al. Major-histocompatibility-complex class I alleles and antigens in hematopoietic-cell transplantation. *N Engl J Med.* 2001;345:1794-1800.
16. Rubinstein P. HLA matching for bone marrow transplantation—how much is enough? *N Engl J Med.* 2001;345:1842-1844.
17. Majhail NS, Weisdorf DJ, Wagner JE, et al. Comparable results of umbilical cord blood and HLA-matched sibling donor hematopoietic stem cell transplantation after reduced-intensity preparative regimen for advanced Hodgkin lymphoma. *Blood.* 2006;107:3804-3807.
18. Anasetti C, Amos D, Beatty PG, et al. Effect of HLA compatibility on engraftment of bone marrow transplants in patients with leukemia or lymphoma. *N Engl J Med.* 1989;320:197-204.
19. Majhail NS, Brunstein CG, Tomblyn M, et al. Reduced-intensity allogeneic transplant in patients older than 55 years: unrelated umbilical cord blood is safe and effective for patients without a matched related donor. *Biol Blood Marrow Transplant.* 2008;14:282-289.
20. Niederwieser D, Maris M, Shizuru JA, et al. Low-dose total body irradiation and fludarabine followed by hematopoietic cell transplantation from HLA-matched or mismatched unrelated donors and postgrafting immunosuppression with cyclosporine and mycophenolate mofetil can induce durable complete chimerism and sustained remissions in patients with hematological diseases. *Blood.* 2003;101:1620-1629.
21. Dykewicz CA. Hospital infection control in hematopoietic stem cell transplant recipients. *Emerg Infect Dis.* 2001;7:263-267.
22. Dykewicz CA. Summary of the guidelines for preventing opportunistic infections among hematopoietic stem cell transplant recipients. *Clin Infect Dis.* 2001;33:139-144.
23. Dykewicz CA. Guidelines for preventing opportunistic infections among hematopoietic stem cell transplant recipients: focus on community respiratory virus infections. *Biol Blood Marrow Transplant.* 2001;7(Suppl):19S-22S.
24. Sullivan KM, Dykewicz CA, Longworth DL, et al. Preventing opportunistic infections after hematopoietic stem cell transplantation: the Centers for Disease Control and Prevention, Infectious Diseases Society of America, and American Society for Blood and Marrow Transplantation Practice guidelines and beyond. *Hematology.* 2001;1:392-421.
25. Korkmaz A, Topal T, Oter S. Pathophysiological aspects of cyclophosphamide and ifosfamide induced hemorrhagic cystitis; implication of reactive oxygen and nitrogen species as well as PARP activation. *Cell Biol Toxicol.* 2007;23:303-312.
26. Focosi D, Maggi F, Pistolesi D, et al. Hyperbaric oxygen therapy in BKV-associated hemorrhagic cystitis refractory to intravenous and intravesical cidofovir: case report and review of literature. *Leuk Res.* 2009;33:556-560.
27. Yoshida T, Kawashima A, Ujike T, et al. Hyperbaric oxygen therapy for radiation-induced hemorrhagic cystitis. *Int J Urol.* 2008;15:639-641.
28. Akiyama H, Kurosu T, Sakashita C, et al. Adenovirus is a key pathogen in hemorrhagic cystitis associated with bone marrow transplantation. *Clin Infect Dis.* 2001;32:1325-1330.
29. Dropulic LK, Jones RJ. Polyomavirus BK infection in blood and marrow transplant recipients. *Bone Marrow Transplant.* 2008; 41:11-18.
30. Childs R, Sanchez C, Engler H, et al. High incidence of adeno- and polyomavirus-induced hemorrhagic cystitis in bone marrow allotransplantation for hematological malignancy following T cell depletion and cyclosporine. *Bone Marrow Transplant.* 1998;22:889-893.
31. Priftakis P, Bogdanovic G, Kokhaei P, et al. BK virus quantification in urine samples of bone marrow transplanted patients is helpful for diagnosis of hemorrhagic cystitis, although wide individual variations exist. *J Clin Virol.* 2003;26:71-77.
32. Leung AY, Mak R, Lie AK, et al. Clinicopathological features and risk factors of clinically overt haemorrhagic cystitis complicating bone marrow transplantation. *Bone Marrow Transplant.* 2002; 29:509-513.
33. Bridges B, Donegan S, Badros A. Cidofovir bladder instillation for the treatment of BK hemorrhagic cystitis after allogeneic stem cell transplantation. *Am J Hematol.* 2006;81:535-537.
34. Litzow MR, Repoussis PD, Schroeder G, et al. Veno-occlusive disease of the liver after blood and marrow transplantation: analysis of pre- and post-transplant risk factors associated with severity and results of therapy with tissue plasminogen activator. *Leuk Lymphoma.* 2002;43:2099-2107.
35. McDonald GB, Hinds MS, Fisher LD, et al. Veno-occlusive disease of the liver and multiorgan failure after bone marrow transplantation: a cohort study of 355 patients. *Ann Intern Med.* 1993;118:255-267.
36. Ho VT, Revta C, Richardson PG. Hepatic veno-occlusive disease after hematopoietic stem cell transplantation: update on defibrotide and other current investigational therapies. *Bone Marrow Transplant.* 2008;41:229-237.
37. Kornblum N, Ayyanar K, Benimetskaya L, et al. Defibrotide, a polydisperse mixture of single-stranded phosphodiester oligonucleotides with lifesaving activity in severe hepatic veno-occlusive disease: clinical outcomes and potential mechanisms of action. *Oligonucleotides.* 2006;16:105-114.
38. Weisdorf D. Graft vs. host disease: pathology, prophylaxis and therapy GVHD overview. *Best Pract Res Clin Haematol.* 2008;21: 99-100.
39. Weisdorf D. Should all unrelated donors for transplantation be matched? *Best Pract Res Clin Haematol.* 2008;21:79-83.
40. Perales MA, Ishill N, Lomazow WA, et al. Long-term follow-up of patients treated with daclizumab for steroid-refractory acute graft-vs-host disease. *Bone Marrow Transplant.* 2007;40:481-486.
41. Kim SS. Treatment options in steroid-refractory acute graft-versus-host disease following hematopoietic stem cell transplantation. *Ann Pharmacother.* 2007;41:1436-1444.
42. Fraser CJ, Scott Baker K. The management and outcome of chronic graft-versus-host disease. *Br J Haematol.* 2007;138:131-145.
43. van Burik J-AH, Carter SL, Freifeld AG, et al. Higher-risk of cytomegalovirus and aspergillus infections in recipients of T cell depleted unrelated bone marrow: analysis of infectious complications in patients treated with T cell depletion versus immune suppressive therapy to prevent graft-versus-host disease. *Biol Blood Marrow Transplant.* 2007;13:1487-1498.
44. Levitsky J, Sorrell MF. Hepatic complications of hematopoietic cell transplantation. *Curr Gastroenterol Rep.* 2007;9:60-65.
45. Arai S, Lee LA, Vogelsang GB. A systematic approach to hepatic complications in hematopoietic stem cell transplantation. *J Hematother Stem Cell Res.* 2002;11:215-229.
46. Lau GK, He ML, Fong DY, et al. Preemptive use of lamivudine reduces hepatitis B exacerbation after allogeneic hematopoietic cell transplantation. *Hepatology.* 2002;36:702-709.
47. Lau GK, Leung YH, Fong DY, et al. High hepatitis B virus DNA viral load as the most important risk factor for HBV reactivation in patients positive for HBV surface antigen undergoing autologous hematopoietic cell transplantation. *Blood.* 2002;99:2324-2330.
48. Vance EA, Soiffer RJ, McDonald GB, et al. Prevention of transmission of hepatitis C virus in bone marrow transplantation by treating the donor with alpha-interferon. *Transplantation.* 1996; 62:1358-1360.
49. Peffault de Latour R, Levy V, Asselah T, et al. Long-term outcome of hepatitis C infection after bone marrow transplantation. *Blood.* 2004;103:1618-1624.
50. Khurshid I, Anderson LC. Non-infectious pulmonary complications after bone marrow transplantation. *Postgrad Med J.* 2002; 78:257-262.
51. Majhail NS, Parks K, Defor TE, et al. Diffuse alveolar hemorrhage and infection-associated alveolar hemorrhage following hematopoietic stem cell transplantation: related and high-risk clinical syndromes. *Biol Blood Marrow Transplant.* 2006;12: 1038-1046.
52. Majhail NS, Ness KK, Burns LJ, et al. Late effects in survivors of Hodgkin and non-Hodgkin lymphoma treated with autologous hematopoietic cell transplantation: a report from the Bone Marrow Transplant Survivor Study. *Biol Blood Marrow Transplant.* 2007;13:1153-1159.
53. Yanik GA, Ho VT, Levine JE, et al. The impact of soluble tumor necrosis factor receptor etanercept on the treatment of idiopathic pneumonia syndrome after allogeneic hematopoietic stem cell transplantation. *Blood.* 2008;112:3073-3081.
54. Kamboj M, Mihu CN, Sepkowitz K, et al. Work-up for infectious diarrhea after allogeneic hematopoietic stem cell transplantation: single specimen testing results in cost savings without compromising diagnostic yield. *Transpl Infect Dis.* 2007; 9:265-269.
55. van Kraaij MG, Dekker AW, Verdonck LF, et al. Infectious gastro-enteritis: an uncommon cause of diarrhoea in adult allogeneic and autologous stem cell transplant recipients. *Bone Marrow Transplant.* 2000;26:299-303.
56. Chakrabarti S, Lees A, Jones SG, et al. *Clostridium difficile* infection in allogeneic stem cell transplant recipients is associated with severe graft-versus-host disease and non-relapse mortality. *Bone Marrow Transplant.* 2000;26:871-876.
57. Davila ML. Neutropenic enterocolitis. *Curr Opin Gastroenterol.* 2006;22:44-47.
58. Canninga-Van Dijk MR, Sanders CJ, Verdonck LF, et al. Differential diagnosis of skin lesions after allogeneic haematopoietic stem cell transplantation. *Histopathology.* 2003;42:313-330.
59. van Burik J-A, Colven R, Spach D. Cutaneous aspergillosis. *J Clin Microbiol.* 1998;36:3115-3121.
60. Ferra C, Doebbeling BN, Hollis RJ, et al. *Candida tropicalis* vertebral osteomyelitis: a late sequela of fungemia. *Clin Infect Dis.* 1994;19:697-703.
61. Miyakis S, Velegraki A, Delikou S, et al. Invasive *Acremonium strictum* infection in a bone marrow transplant recipient. *Pediatr Infect Dis J.* 2006;25:273-275.
62. Barasch A, Mosier KM, D'Ambrosio JA, et al. Postextraction osteomyelitis in a bone marrow transplant recipient. *Oral Surg Oral Med Oral Pathol.* 1993;75:391-396.
63. Shah M, Watanakunakorn C. *Staphylococcus aureus* sternal osteomyelitis complicating bone marrow aspiration. *South Med J.* 1978;71:348-349.
64. Centers for Disease Control and Prevention; the Infectious Disease Society of America; American Society of Blood and Marrow Transplantation. Guidelines for preventing opportunistic infections among hematopoietic stem cell transplant recipients. *MMWR Recomm Rep.* 2000;49(RR-10):1-125, CE1-7.
65. Scott BL, Park JY, Deeg HJ, et al. Pretransplant neutropenia is associated with poor-risk cytogenetic features and increased infection-related mortality in patients with myelodysplastic syndromes. *Biol Blood Marrow Transplant.* 2008;14:799-806.
66. Sepkowitz KA. Antibiotic prophylaxis in patients receiving hematopoietic stem cell transplant. *Bone Marrow Transplant.* 2002;29:367-371.
67. Collin BA, Leather HL, Wingard JR, et al. Evolution, incidence, and susceptibility of bacterial bloodstream isolates from 519 bone marrow transplant patients. *Clin Infect Dis.* 2001;33:947-953.
68. Marena C, Zecca M, Carenini ML, et al. Incidence of, and risk factors for, nosocomial infections among hematopoietic stem cell transplantation recipients, with impact on procedure-related mortality. *Infect Control Hosp Epidemiol.* 2001;22:510-517.
69. Oliveira AL, de Souza M, Carvalho-Dias VM, et al. Epidemiology of bacteremia and factors associated with multi-drug–resistant gram-negative bacteremia in hematopoietic stem cell transplant recipients. *Bone Marrow Transplant.* 2007;39:775-781.
70. Wade JC, Newton B, Flournoy N, et al. Oral acyclovir for prevention of herpes simplex virus reactivation after marrow transplantation. *Ann Intern Med.* 1984;100:823-828.
71. Goodman JL, Winston DJ, Greenfield RA, et al. A controlled trial of fluconazole to prevent fungal infections in patients undergoing bone marrow transplantation. *N Engl J Med.* 1992; 326:845-851.
72. MacMillan ML, Goodman JL, DeFor TE, et al. Fluconazole to prevent yeast infections in bone marrow transplantation patients: a randomized trial of high versus reduced dose, and determination of the value of maintenance therapy. *Am J Med.* 2002;112:369-379.
73. Slavin MA, Osborne B, Adams R, et al. Efficacy and safety of fluconazole prophylaxis for fungal infections after marrow transplantation—a prospective, randomized, double-blind study. *J Infect Dis.* 1995;171:1545-1552.
74. van Burik JA, Ratanatharathorn V, Stepan DE, et al. Micafungin versus fluconazole for prophylaxis against invasive fungal infections during neutropenia in patients undergoing hematopoietic stem cell transplantation. *Clin Infect Dis.* 2004;39:1407-1416.
75. Hachem R, Hanna H, Kontoyiannis D, et al. The changing epidemiology of invasive candidiasis: *Candida glabrata* and *Candida krusei* as the leading causes of candidemia in hematologic malignancy. *Cancer.* 2008;112:2493-2499.

76. Hübel K, Carter R, Liles W, et al. Granulocyte transfusion therapy for infections in candidates and recipients of hematopoietic cell transplantation: a comparative analysis of feasibility and outcome of community donors versus related donors. *Transfusion*. 2002;42:1414-1421.
77. Lazarus HM, Magalhaes-Silverman M, Fox RM, et al. Contamination during in vitro processing of bone marrow for transplantation: clinical significance. *Bone Marrow Transplant*. 1991;7:241-246.
78. Nasser RM, Hajjar I, Sandhaus LM, et al. Routine cultures of bone marrow and peripheral stem cell harvests: clinical impact, cost analysis, and review. *Clin Infect Dis*. 1998;27:886-888.
79. Wald A, Leisenring W, van Burik JA, et al. Epidemiology of *Aspergillus* infections in a large cohort of patients undergoing bone marrow transplantation. *J Infect Dis*. 1997;175:1459-1466.
80. Ullmann AJ, Lipton JH, Vesole DH, et al. Posaconazole or fluconazole for prophylaxis in severe graft-versus-host disease. *N Engl J Med*. 2007;356:335-347.
81. Wingard J, Carter S, Walsh T, et al. Results of a randomized, double-blind trial of fluconazole vs. voriconazole for the prevention of invasive fungal infections in 600 allogeneic blood and marrow transplant patients [Abstract no. 163]. *Blood*. 2007;110:11.
82. Tuan IZ, Dennison D, Weisdorf DJ. *Pneumocystis carinii* pneumonitis following bone marrow transplantation. *Bone Marrow Transplant*. 1992;10:267-272.
83. Link H, Vohringer HF, Wingen F, et al. Pentamidine aerosol for prophylaxis of *Pneumocystis carinii* pneumonia after BMT. *Bone Marrow Transplant*. 1993;11:403-406.
84. Souza JP, Boeckh M, Gooley TA, et al. High rates of *Pneumocystis carinii* pneumonia in allogeneic blood and marrow transplant recipients receiving dapsone prophylaxis. *Clin Infect Dis*. 1999;29:1467-1471.
85. Fishman JA. Prevention of infection caused by *Pneumocystis carinii* in transplant recipients. *Clin Infect Dis*. 2001;33:1397-1405.
86. Sangiolo D, Storer B, Nash R, et al. Toxicity and efficacy of daily dapsone as *Pneumocystis jirovecii* prophylaxis after hematopoietic stem cell transplantation: a case-control study. *Biol Blood Marrow Transplant*. 2005;11:521-529.
87. Yakushiji K, Gondo H, Kamezaki K, et al. Monitoring of cytomegalovirus reactivation after allogeneic stem cell transplantation: comparison of an antigenemia assay and quantitative real-time polymerase chain reaction. *Bone Marrow Transplant*. 2002;29:599-606.
88. Boeckh M, Gooley TA, Myerson D, et al. Cytomegalovirus pp65 antigenemia-guided early treatment with ganciclovir versus ganciclovir at engraftment after allogeneic marrow transplantation: a randomized double-blind study. *Blood*. 1996;88:4063-4071.
89. Walker CM, van Burik JA, DeFor TE, et al. Cytomegalovirus infection after allogeneic transplantation: comparison of cord blood with peripheral blood and marrow graft sources. *Biol Blood Marrow Transplant*. 2007;13:1106-1115.
90. Winston DJ, Young JA, Pullarkat V, et al. Maribavir prophylaxis for prevention of cytomegalovirus infection in allogeneic stem cell transplant recipients: a multicenter, randomized, double-blind, placebo-controlled, dose-ranging study. *Blood*. 2008;111:5403-5410.
91. Sullivan KM, Mori M, Sanders J, et al. Late complications of allogeneic and autologous marrow transplantation. *Bone Marrow Transplant*. 1992;10(Suppl. 1):127-134.
92. Boeckh M, Leisenring W, Riddell SR, et al. Late cytomegalovirus disease and mortality in recipients of allogeneic hematopoietic stem cell transplants: importance of viral load and T-cell immunity. *Blood*. 2003;101:407-414.
93. Ochs L, Shu XO, Miller J, et al. Late infections after allogeneic bone marrow transplantations: comparison of incidence in related and unrelated donor transplant recipients. *Blood*. 1995;86:3979-3986.
94. Roy V, Ochs L, Weisdorf D. Late infections following allogeneic bone marrow transplantation: suggested strategies for prophylaxis. *Leuk Lymphoma*. 1997;26:1-15.
95. Robin M, Porcher R, De Castro Araujo R, et al. Risk factors for late infections after allogeneic hematopoietic stem cell transplantation from a matched related donor. *Biol Blood Marrow Transplant*. 2007;13:1304-1312.
96. Junghanss C, Marr KA, Carter RA, et al. Incidence and outcome of bacterial and fungal infections following nonmyeloablative compared with myeloablative allogeneic hematopoietic stem cell transplantation: a matched control study. *Biol Blood Marrow Transplant*. 2002;8:512-520.
97. Junghanss C, Boeckh M, Carter RA, et al. Incidence and outcome of cytomegalovirus infections following nonmyeloablative compared with myeloablative allogeneic stem cell transplantation, a matched control study. *Blood*. 2002;99:1978-1985.
98. Hagen EA, Stern H, Porter D, et al. High rate of invasive fungal infections following nonmyeloablative allogeneic transplantation. *Clin Infect Dis*. 2003;36:9-15.
99. Boyce JM, Pittet D. Guideline for hand hygiene in health-care settings: recommendations of the Healthcare Infection Control Practices Advisory Committee and the HICPAC/SHEA/APIC/IDSA Hand Hygiene Task Force. *Infect Control Hosp Epidemiol*. 2002;23(12 Suppl.):S3-S40.
100. Elishoov H, Or R, Strauss N, et al. Nosocomial colonization, septicemia, and Hickman/Broviac catheter–related infections in bone marrow transplant recipients. A 5-year prospective study. *Medicine (Baltimore)*. 1998;77:83-101.
101. Engelhard D, Elishoov H, Strauss N, et al. Nosocomial coagulase-negative staphylococcal infections in bone marrow transplantation recipients with central vein catheter. A 5-year prospective study. *Transplantation*. 1996;61:430-434.
102. Toor AA, van Burik JA, Weisdorf DJ. Infections during mobilizing chemotherapy and following autologous stem cell transplantation. *Bone Marrow Transplant*. 2001;28:1129-1134.
103. Schots R, Trullemans F, Van Riet I, et al. The clinical impact of early gram-positive bacteremia and the use of vancomycin after allogeneic bone marrow transplantation. *Transplantation*. 2000;69:1511-1514.
104. Arns da Cunha C, Weisdorf D, Shu XO, et al. Early gram-positive bacteremia in BMT recipients: impact of three different approaches to antimicrobial prophylaxis. *Bone Marrow Transplantation*. 1998;21:173-180.
105. Hakki M, Limaye AP, Kim HW, et al. Invasive *Pseudomonas aeruginosa* infections: high rate of recurrence and mortality after hematopoietic cell transplantation. *Bone Marrow Transplant*. 2007;39:687-693.
106. Engelhard D, Cordonnier C, Shaw PJ, et al. Early and late invasive pneumococcal infection following stem cell transplantation: a European Bone Marrow Transplantation survey. *Br J Haematol*. 2002;117:444-450.
107. Schutze GE, Mason EO Jr, Wald ER, et al. Pneumococcal infections in children after transplantation. *Clin Infect Dis*. 2001;33:16-21.
108. Haddad PA, Repka TL, Weisdorf DJ. Penicillin-resistant *Streptococcus pneumoniae* septic shock and meningitis complicating chronic graft versus host disease: a case report and review of the literature. *Am J Med*. 2002;113:152-155.
109. Tauro S, Dobie D, Richardson G, et al. Recurrent penicillin-resistant pneumococcal sepsis after matched unrelated donor transplantation for refractory T cell lymphoma. *Bone Marrow Transplant*. 2000;26:1017-1019.
110. Steiner M, Villablanca J, Kersey J, et al. Viridans streptococcal shock in bone marrow transplantation patients. *Am J Hematol*. 1993;42:354-358.
111. Ringden O, Heimdahl A, Lonnqvist B, et al. Decreased incidence of viridans streptococcal septicaemia in allogeneic bone marrow transplant recipients after the introduction of acyclovir. *Lancet*. 1984;314:744.
112. Razonable RR, Litzow MR, Khaliq Y, et al. Bacteremia due to viridans group streptococci with diminished susceptibility to levofloxacin among neutropenic patients receiving levofloxacin prophylaxis. *Clin Infect Dis*. 2002;34:1469-1474.
113. Almyroudis NG, Fuller A, Jakubowski A, et al. Pre- and post-engraftment bloodstream infection rates and associated mortality in allogeneic hematopoietic stem cell transplant recipients. *Transpl Infect Dis*. 2005;7:11-17.
114. Graber CJ, de Almeida KN, Atkinson JC, et al. Dental health and viridans streptococcal bacteremia in allogeneic hematopoietic stem cell transplant recipients. *Bone Marrow Transplant*. 2001;27:537-542.
115. Gaviria JM, Garcia PJ, Garrido SM, et al. Nontuberculous mycobacterial infections in hematopoietic stem cell transplant recipients: characteristics of respiratory and catheter-related infections. *Biol Blood Marrow Transplant*. 2000;6:361-369.
116. Roy V, Weisdorf D. Mycobacterial infections following bone marrow transplantation: a 20 year retrospective review. *Bone Marrow Transplantation*. 1997;19:467-470.
117. Maeda T, Kusumi E, Kami M, et al. Disseminated tuberculosis following reduced-intensity cord blood transplantation for adult patients with hematological diseases. *Bone Marrow Transplant*. 2005;35:91-97.
118. Lee J, Lee MH, Kim WS, et al. Tuberculosis in hematopoietic stem cell transplant recipients in Korea. *Int J Hematol*. 2004;79:185-188.
119. George B, Mathews V, Srivastava V, et al. Tuberculosis among allogeneic bone marrow transplant recipients in India. *Bone Marrow Transplant*. 2001;27:973-975.
120. Budak-Alpdogan T, Tangun Y, Kalayoglu-Besisik S, et al. The frequency of tuberculosis in adult allogeneic stem cell transplant recipients in Turkey. *Biol Blood Marrow Transplant*. 2000;6:370-374.
121. Ip MSM, Yuen KY, Woo PCY, et al. Risk factors for pulmonary tuberculosis in bone marrow transplant recipients. *Am J Respir Crit Care Med*. 1998;158:1173-1177.
122. Pai M, Zwerling A, Menzies D. Systematic review: T-cell–based assays for the diagnosis of latent tuberculosis infection: an update. *Ann Intern Med*. 2008;149:177-184.
123. Menzies D, Pai M, Comstock G. Meta-analysis: new tests for the diagnosis of latent tuberculosis infection: areas of uncertainty and recommendations for research. *Ann Intern Med*. 2007;146:340-354.
124. Mazurek GH, Jereb J, Lobue P, et al. Guidelines for using the QuantiFERON-TB Gold test for detecting *Mycobacterium tuberculosis* infection, United States. *MMWR Recomm Rep*. 2005;54(RR-15):49-55.
125. Kobashi Y, Obase Y, Fukuda M, et al. Clinical reevaluation of the QuantiFERON TB-2G test as a diagnostic method for differentiating active tuberculosis from nontuberculous mycobacteriosis. *Clin Infect Dis*. 2006;43:1540-1546.
126. Lee SS, Liu YC, Huang TS, et al. Comparison of the interferon-gamma release assay and the tuberculin skin test for contact investigation of tuberculosis in BCG-vaccinated health care workers. *Scand J Infect Dis*. 2008;40:373-380.
127. Kugler JW, Armitage JO, Helms CM, et al. Nosocomial Legionnaires' disease. Occurrence in recipients of bone marrow transplants. *Am J Med*. 1983;74:281-288.
128. Oren I, Zuckerman T, Avivi I, et al. Nosocomial outbreak of *Legionella pneumophila* serogroup 3 pneumonia in a new bone marrow transplant unit: evaluation, treatment and control. *Bone Marrow Transplant*. 2002;30:175-179.
129. Harrington RD, Woolfrey AE, Bowden R, et al. Legionellosis in a bone marrow transplant center. *Bone Marrow Transplant*. 1996;18:361-368.
130. Schwebke JR, Hackman R, Bowden R. Pneumonia due to *Legionella micdadei* in bone marrow transplant recipients. *Rev Infect Dis*. 1990;12:824-828.
131. van Burik J-A, Hackman R, Nadeem S, et al. Nocardiosis after bone marrow transplantation: a retrospective study. *Clin Infect Dis*. 1997;24:1154-1160.
132. Martino R, Lopez R, Pericas R, et al. Listeriosis in bone marrow transplant recipient. *Clin Infect Dis*. 1996;23:419-420.
133. Chang J, Powles R, Mehta J, et al. Listeriosis in the bone marrow transplant recipient. *Clin Infect Dis*. 1995;21:1289-1290.
134. Long SG, Leyland MJ, Milligan DW. *Listeria* meningitis after bone marrow transplantation. *Bone Marrow Transplant*. 1993;12:537-539.
135. Ljungman P, Larsson K, Kumlien G, et al. Leukocyte depleted, unscreened blood products give a low risk for CMV infection and disease in CMV seronegative allogeneic stem cell transplant recipients with seronegative stem cell donors. *Scand J Infect Dis*. 2002;34:347-350.
136. Bowden RA, Slichter SJ, Sayers MH, et al. Use of leukocyte-depleted platelets and cytomegalovirus-seronegative red blood cells for prevention of primary cytomegalovirus infection after marrow transplant. *Blood*. 1991;78:246-250.
137. Saral R, Burns WH, Laskin OL, et al. Acyclovir prophylaxis of herpes simplex virus infections. A randomized, double-blind, controlled trial in bone marrow transplant recipients. *N Engl J Med*. 1981;305(2):63-67.
138. Dignani MC, Mykietiuk A, Michelet M, et al. Valacyclovir prophylaxis for the prevention of herpes simplex virus reactivation in recipients of progenitor cells transplantation. *Bone Marrow Transplant*. 2002;29:263-267.
139. Liesveld JL, Abboud CN, Ifthikharuddin JJ, et al. Oral valacyclovir versus intravenous acyclovir in preventing herpes simplex virus infections in autologous stem cell transplant recipients. *Biol Blood Marrow Transplant*. 2002;8:662-665.
140. Nichols WG, Price TH, Gooley T, et al. Transfusion-transmitted cytomegalovirus infection after receipt of leukoreduced blood products. *Blood*. 2003;101:4195-4200.
141. Bowden RA, Slichter SJ, Sayers M, et al. A comparison of filtered leukocyte-reduced and cytomegalovirus seronegative blood products for the prevention of transfusion-associated CMV infection after marrow transplant. *Blood*. 1995;86:3598-3603.
142. Goodrich JM, Mori M, Gleaves CA, et al. Early treatment with ganciclovir to prevent cytomegalovirus disease after allogeneic bone marrow transplantation. *N Engl J Med*. 1991;325:1601-1607.
143. Reusser P, Einsele H, Lee J, et al. Randomized multicenter trial of foscarnet versus ganciclovir for preemptive therapy of cytomegalovirus infection after allogeneic stem cell transplantation. *Blood*. 2002;99:1159-1164.
144. Goodrich JM, Bowden RA, Fisher L, et al. Ganciclovir prophylaxis to prevent cytomegalovirus disease after allogeneic marrow transplant. *Ann Intern Med*. 1993;118:173-178.
145. Winston DJ, Ho WG, Bartoni K, et al. Ganciclovir prophylaxis of cytomegalovirus infection and disease in allogeneic bone marrow transplant recipients. Results of a placebo- controlled, double-blind trial. *Ann Intern Med*. 1993;118:179-184.
146. Prentice HG, Gluckman E, Powles RL, et al. Impact of long-term acyclovir on cytomegalovirus infection and survival after allogeneic bone marrow transplantation. European Acyclovir for CMV Prophylaxis Study Group. *Lancet*. 1994;343:749-753.
147. Burns LJ, Miller W, Kandaswamy C, et al. Randomized clinical trial of ganciclovir vs acyclovir for prevention of cytomegalovirus antigenemia after allogeneic transplantation. *Bone Marrow Transplant*. 2002;30:945-951.
148. Winston DJ, Yeager AM, Chandrasekar PH, et al. Randomized comparison of oral valacyclovir and intravenous ganciclovir for prevention of cytomegalovirus disease after allogeneic bone marrow transplantation. *Clin Infect Dis*. 2003;36:749-758.
149. Reed EC, Bowden RA, Dandliker PS, et al. Treatment of cytomegalovirus pneumonia with ganciclovir and intravenous cytomegalovirus immunoglobulin in patients with bone marrow transplants. *Ann Intern Med*. 1988;109:783-788.
150. Limaye AP, Bowden RA, Myerson D, et al. Cytomegalovirus disease occurring before engraftment in marrow transplant recipients. *Clin Infect Dis*. 1997;24:830-835.
151. Limaye AP, Huang ML, Leisenring W, et al. Cytomegalovirus DNA load in plasma for the diagnosis of CMV disease before engraftment in hematopoietic stem-cell transplant recipients. *J Infect Dis*. 2001;183:377-382.
152. Hackman RC, Wolford JL, Gleaves CA, et al. Recognition and rapid diagnosis of upper gastrointestinal cytomegalovirus infection in marrow transplant recipients. A comparison of seven virologic methods. *Transplantation*. 1994;57:231-237.

153. van Burik JA, Lawatsch EJ, DeFor TE, et al. Cytomegalovirus enteritis among hematopoietic stem cell transplant recipients. *Biol Blood Marrow Transplant.* 2001;7:674-679.

154. Crippa F, Corey L, Chuang EL, et al. Virological, clinical, and ophthalmologic features of cytomegalovirus retinitis after hematopoietic stem cell transplantation. *Clin Infect Dis.* 2001;32: 214-219.

155. Reed EC, Shepp DH, Dandliker PS, et al. Ganciclovir treatment of cytomegalovirus infection of the gastrointestinal tract after marrow transplantation. *Bone Marrow Transplant.* 1988;3:199-206.

156. Walter EA, Greenberg PD, Gilbert MJ, et al. Reconstitution of cellular immunity against cytomegalovirus in recipients of allogeneic bone marrow by transfer of T-cell clones from the donor. *N Engl J Med.* 1995;333:1038-1044.

157. Erice A, Borrell N, Li W, et al. Ganciclovir susceptibilities and analysis of UL97 region in cytomegalovirus isolates from bone marrow recipients with CMV disease after antiviral prophylaxis. *J Infect Dis.* 1998;178:531-534.

158. Arvin AM. Varicella-zoster virus: pathogenesis, immunity, and clinical management in hematopoietic cell transplant recipients. *Biol Blood Marrow Transplant.* 2000;6:219-230.

159. Steer CB, Szer J, Sasadeusz J, et al. Varicella-zoster infection after allogeneic bone marrow transplantation: incidence, risk factors and prevention with low-dose aciclovir and ganciclovir. *Bone Marrow Transplant.* 2000;25:657-664.

160. Erard V, Guthrie KA, Varley C, et al. One-year acyclovir prophylaxis for preventing varicella-zoster virus disease after hematopoietic cell transplantation: no evidence of rebound varicella-zoster virus disease after drug discontinuation. *Blood.* 2007;110:3071-3077.

161. David DS, Tegtmeier BR, O'Donnell MR, et al. Visceral varicella-zoster after bone marrow transplantation: report of a case series and review of the literature. *Am J Gastroenterol.* 1998;93: 810-813.

162. Schiller GJ, Nimer SD, Gajewski JL, et al. Abdominal presentation of varicella zoster infection in recipients of allogeneic bone marrow transplantation. *Bone Marrow Transplant.* 1991;7:489-491.

163. Tenenbaum T, Kramm CM, Laws HJ, et al. Pre-eruptive varicella zoster virus encephalitis in two children after haematopoietic stem cell transplantation. *Med Pediatr Oncol.* 2002;38:288-289.

164. Verdonck LF, Cornelissen JJ, Dekker AW, et al. Acute abdominal pain as a presenting symptom of varicella zoster virus infection in recipients of bone marrow transplants. *Clin Infect Dis.* 1993;16:190-191.

165. Austin R. Clinical review. Progressive outer retinal necrosis syndrome: a comprehensive review of its clinical presentation, relationship to immune system status, and management. *Clin Eye Vision Care.* 2000;12:119-129.

166. Han CS, Miller W, Haake R, et al. Varicella zoster infection after bone marrow transplantation: incidence, risk factors and complications. *Bone Marrow Transplant.* 1994;13:277-283.

167. Sauerbrei A, Prager J, Hengst U, et al. Varicella vaccination in children after bone marrow transplantation. *Bone Marrow Transplant.* 1997;20:381-383.

168. Guidelines for preventing infectious complications among hematopoietic cell transplant recipients: a global perspective recommendations of the Center for International Blood and Marrow Transplant Research (CIBMTR®), the National Marrow Donor Program (NMDP), the European Blood and Marrow Transplant Group (EBMT), the American Society of Blood and Marrow Transplantation (ASBMT), the Canadian Blood and Marrow Transplant Group (CBMTG), the Infectious Disease Society of America (IDSA), the Society for Healthcare Epidemiology of America (SHEA), the Association of Medical Microbiology and Infectious Diseases Canada (AMMI), the Centers for Disease Control and Prevention (CDC), and the Health Resources and Services Administration (HRSA). *Biol Blood Marrow Transplant.* (in press).

169. Weinstock DM, Boeckh M, Boulad F, et al. Postexposure prophylaxis against varicella-zoster virus infection among recipients of hematopoietic stem cell transplant: unresolved issues. *Infect Control Hosp Epidemiol.* 2004;25:603-608.

170. Bruno B, Gooley T, Hackman RC, et al. Adenovirus infection in hematopoietic stem cell transplantation: effect of ganciclovir and impact on survival. *Biol Blood Marrow Transplant.* 2003;9:341-352.

171. Symeonidis N, Jakubowski A, Pierre-Louis S, et al. Invasive adenoviral infections in T-cell–depleted allogeneic hematopoietic stem cell transplantation: high mortality in the era of cidofovir. *Transpl Infect Dis.* 2007;9:108-113.

172. Shields AF, Hackman RC, Fife KH, et al. Adenovirus infections in patients undergoing bone marrow transplantation. *N Engl J Med.* 1985;312:529-533.

173. Erard V, Huang ML, Ferrenberg J, et al. Quantitative real-time polymerase chain reaction for detection of adenovirus after T cell–replete hematopoietic cell transplantation: viral load as a marker for invasive disease. *Clin Infect Dis.* 2007;45:958-965.

174. Fanourgiakis P, Georgala A, Vekemans M, et al. Intravesical instillation of cidofovir in the treatment of hemorrhagic cystitis caused by adenovirus type 11 in a bone marrow transplant recipient. *Clin Infect Dis.* 2005;40:199-201.

175. Ljungman P, Ribaud P, Eyrich M, et al. Cidofovir for adenovirus infections after allogeneic hematopoietic stem cell transplantation: a survey by the Infectious Diseases Working Party of the European Group for Blood and Marrow Transplantation. *Bone Marrow Transplant.* 2003;31:481-486.

176. Small TN, Casson A, Malak SF, et al. Respiratory syncytial virus infection following hematopoietic stem cell transplantation. *Bone Marrow Transplant.* 2002;29:321-327.

177. Chakrabarti S, Collingham KE, Marshall T, et al. Respiratory virus infections in adult T cell-depleted transplant recipients: the role of cellular immunity. *Transplantation.* 2001;72:1460-1463.

178. Nichols WG, Gooley T, Boeckh M. Community-acquired respiratory syncytial virus and parainfluenza virus infections after hematopoietic stem cell transplantation: the Fred Hutchinson Cancer Research Center experience. *Biol Blood Marrow Transplant.* 2001;7(Suppl):11S-15S.

179. Chakrabarti S, Avivi I, Mackinnon S, et al. Respiratory virus infections in transplant recipients after reduced-intensity conditioning with Campath-1H: high incidence but low mortality. *Br J Haematol.* 2002;119:1125-1132.

180. Veys P, Owens C. Respiratory infections following haemopoietic stem cell transplantation in children. *Br Med Bull.* 2002;61: 151-174.

181. Gutman JA, Peck AJ, Kuypers J, et al. Rhinovirus as a cause of fatal lower respiratory tract infection in adult stem cell transplantation patients: a report of two cases. *Bone Marrow Transplant.* 2007;40:809-811.

182. Kim YJ, Boeckh M, Englund JA. Community respiratory virus infections in immunocompromised patients: hematopoietic stem cell and solid organ transplant recipients, and individuals with human immunodeficiency virus infection. *Semin Respir Crit Care Med.* 2007;28:222-242.

183. Peck AJ, Englund JA, Kuypers J, et al. Respiratory virus infection among hematopoietic cell transplant recipients: evidence for asymptomatic parainfluenza virus infection. *Blood.* 2007;110:1681-1688.

184. Nichols WG, Corey L, Gooley T, et al. Parainfluenza virus infections after hematopoietic stem cell transplantation: risk factors, response to antiviral therapy, and effect on transplant outcome. *Blood.* 2001;98:573-578.

185. Lewis VA, Champlin R, Englund J, et al. Respiratory disease due to parainfluenza virus in adult bone marrow transplant recipients. *Clin Infect Dis.* 1996;23:1033-1037.

186. Ison MG, Hayden FG, Kaiser L, et al. Rhinovirus infections in hematopoietic stem cell transplant recipients with pneumonia. *Clin Infect Dis.* 2003;36:1139-1143.

187. Englund JA, Boeckh M, Kuypers J, et al. Brief communication: fatal human metapneumovirus infection in stem-cell transplant recipients. *Ann Intern Med.* 2006;144:344-349.

188. Harrington RD, Hooton TM, Hackman RC, et al. An outbreak of respiratory syncytial virus in a bone marrow transplant center. *J Infect Dis.* 1992;165:987-993.

189. Wendt CH, Weisdorf DJ, Jordan MC, et al. Parainfluenza virus respiratory infection after bone marrow transplantation. *N Engl J Med.* 1992;326:921-926.

190. Whimbey E, Champlin RE, Englund JA, et al. Combination therapy with aerosolized ribavirin and intravenous immunoglobulin for respiratory syncytial virus disease in adult bone marrow transplant recipients. *Bone Marrow Transplant.* 1995;16:393-399.

191. Boeckh M, Englund J, Li Y, et al. Randomized controlled multicenter trial of aerosolized ribavirin for respiratory syncytial virus upper respiratory tract infection in hematopoietic cell transplant recipients. *Clin Infect Dis.* 2007;44:245-249.

192. Vu D, Peck AJ, Nichols WG, et al. Safety and tolerability of oseltamivir prophylaxis in hematopoietic stem cell transplant recipients: a retrospective case-control study. *Clin Infect Dis.* 2007;45:187-193.

193. Cortez K, Murphy BR, Almeida KN, et al. Immune-globulin prophylaxis of respiratory syncytial virus infection in patients undergoing stem-cell transplantation. *J Infect Dis.* 2002;186:834-838.

194. Brunstein CG, Weisdorf DJ, DeFor T, et al. Marked increased risk of Epstein-Barr virus–related complications with the addition of antithymocyte globulin to a nonmyeloablative conditioning prior to unrelated umbilical cord blood transplantation. *Blood.* 2006;108:2874-2880.

195. Loren AW, Porter DL, Stadtmauer EA, et al. Post-transplant lymphoproliferative disorder: a review. *Bone Marrow Transplant.* 2003;31:145-155.

196. van Esser JW, van der Holt B, Meijer E, et al. Epstein-Barr virus reactivation is a frequent event after allogeneic stem cell transplantation and quantitatively predicts EBV-lymphoproliferative disease following T-cell–depleted SCT. *Blood.* 2001;98:972-978.

197. Clave E, Agbalika F, Bajzik V, et al. Epstein-Barr virus reactivation in allogeneic stem cell transplantation: relationship between viral load, EBV-specific T-cell reconstitution and rituximab therapy. *Transplantation.* 2004;77:76-84.

198. van Esser JW, Niesters HG, van der Holt B, et al. Prevention of Epstein-Barr virus–lymphoproliferative disease by molecular monitoring and preemptive rituximab in high-risk patients after allogeneic stem cell transplantation. *Blood.* 2002;99:4364-4369.

199. Zerr DM, Corey L, Kim HW, et al. Clinical outcomes of human herpesvirus 6 reactivation after hematopoietic stem cell transplantation. *Clin Infect Dis.* 2005;40:932-940.

200. Sashihara J, Tanaka-Taya K, Tanaka S, et al. High incidence of human herpesvirus 6 infection with a high viral load in cord blood stem cell transplant recipients. *Blood.* 2002;100:2005-2011.

201. Boutolleau D, Fernandez C, Andre E, et al. Human herpesvirus-6 and HHV-7: two closely related viruses with different infection profiles in stem cell transplantation recipients. *J Infect Dis.* 2003;187:179-186.

202. Cone RW, Hackman RC, Huang ML, et al. Human herpesvirus 6 in lung tissue from patients with pneumonitis after bone marrow transplantation. *N Engl J Med.* 1993;329:156-161.

203. Zerr DM, Gupta D, Huang ML, et al. Effect of antivirals on human herpesvirus 6 replication in hematopoietic stem cell transplant recipients. *Clin Infect Dis.* 2002;34:309-317.

204. Eid AJ, Brown RA, Patel R, et al. Parvovirus B19 infection after transplantation: a review of 98 cases. *Clin Infect Dis.* 2006;43: 40-48.

205. Solano C, Juan O, Gimeno C, et al. Engraftment failure associated with peripheral blood stem cell transplantation after B19 parvovirus infection. *Blood.* 1996;88:1515-1517.

206. Cohen BJ, Beard S, Knowles WA, et al. Chronic anemia due to parvovirus B19 infection in a bone marrow transplant patient after platelet transfusion. *Transfusion.* 1997;37:947-952.

207. Azzi A, Fanci R, Ciappi S, et al. Human parvovirus B19 infection in bone marrow transplantation patients. *Am J Hematol.* 1993; 44:207-209.

208. van Burik J-A, Leisenring W, Myerson D, et al. The effect of prophylactic fluconazole on the clinical spectrum of fungal diseases in bone marrow transplant recipients with special attention to hepatic candidiasis: an autopsy study of 355 patients. *Medicine (Baltimore).* 1998;77:246-254.

209. Riley DK, Pavia AT, Beatty PG, et al. The prophylactic use of low-dose amphotericin B in bone marrow transplant patients. *Am J Med.* 1994;97:509-514.

210. Marr KA, Crippa F, Leisenring W, et al. Itraconazole versus fluconazole for prevention of fungal infections in patients receiving allogeneic stem cell transplants. *Blood.* 2004;103:1527-1533.

211. Winston DJ, Emmanouilides C, Bartoni K, et al. Elimination of *Aspergillus* infection in allogeneic stem cell transplant recipients with long-term itraconazole prophylaxis: prevention is better than treatment. *Blood.* 2004;104:1581.

212. Winston DJ, Maziarz RT, Chandrasekar PH, et al. Intravenous and oral itraconazole versus intravenous and oral fluconazole for long-term antifungal prophylaxis in allogeneic hematopoietic stem cell transplant recipients. A multicenter, randomized trial. *Ann Intern Med.* 2003;138:705-713.

213. Stringer JR, Beard CB, Miller RF, et al. A new name (*Pneumocystis jirovecii*) for *Pneumocystis* from humans. *Emerg Infect Dis.* 2002;8:891-896.

214. Lyytikainen O, Ruutu T, Volin L, et al. Late onset *Pneumocystis carinii* pneumonia following allogeneic bone marrow transplantation. *Bone Marrow Transplant.* 1996;17:1057-1059.

215. Saito T, Seo S, Kanda Y, et al. Early onset *Pneumocystis carinii* pneumonia after allogeneic peripheral blood stem cell transplantation. *Am J Hematol.* 2001;67:206-209.

216. Maltezou HC, Petropoulos D, Choroszy M, et al. Dapsone for *Pneumocystis carinii* prophylaxis in children undergoing bone marrow transplantation. *Bone Marrow Transplant.* 1997;20:879-881.

217. Colby C, McAfee S, Sackstein R, et al. A prospective randomized trial comparing the toxicity and safety of atovaquone with trimethoprim/sulfamethoxazole as *Pneumocystis carinii* pneumonia prophylaxis following autologous peripheral blood stem cell transplantation. *Bone Marrow Transplant.* 1999;24:897-902.

218. Milstone AM, Balakrishnan SL, Foster CB, et al. Failure of intravenous pentamidine prophylaxis to prevent *Pneumocystis* pneumonia in a pediatric hematopoietic stem cell transplant (HSCT) patient. *Pediatr Blood Cancer.* 2006;47:859-860.

219. Goodrich JM, Reed EC, Mori M, et al. Clinical features and analysis of risk factors for invasive candidal infection after marrow transplantation. *J Infect Dis.* 1991;164:731-740.

220. Hagensee ME, Bauwens JE, Kjos B, et al. Brain abscess following marrow transplantation: experience at the Fred Hutchinson Cancer Research Center, 1984-1992. *Clin Infect Dis.* 1994;19:402-408.

221. Fukuda T, Boeckh M, Carter RA, et al. Invasive fungal infections in recipients of allogeneic hematopoietic stem cell transplantation after nonmyeloablative conditioning: risks and outcomes. *Blood.* 2003;10:10.

222. Marr KA, Seidel K, Slavin MA, et al. Prolonged fluconazole prophylaxis is associated with persistent protection against candidiasis-related death in allogeneic marrow transplant recipients: long-term follow-up of a randomized, placebo-controlled trial. *Blood.* 2000;96:2055-2061.

223. Marr KA, Seidel K, White TC, et al. Candidemia in allogeneic blood and marrow transplant recipients: evolution of risk factors after the adoption of prophylactic fluconazole. *J Infect Dis.* 2000;181:309-316.

224. Upton A, Kirby KA, Carpenter P, et al. Invasive aspergillosis following hematopoietic cell transplantation: outcomes and prognostic factors associated with mortality. *Clin Infect Dis.* 2007;44:531-540.

225. Marr KA, Carter RA, Crippa F, et al. Epidemiology and outcome of mould infections in hematopoietic stem cell transplant recipients. *Clin Infect Dis.* 2002;34:909-917.

226. Marr KA, Carter RA, Boeckh M, et al. Invasive aspergillosis in allogeneic stem cell transplant recipients: changes in epidemiology and risk factors. *Blood.* 2002;100:4358-4366.

227. Garcia-Vidal C, Upton A, Kirby KA, et al. Epidemiology of invasive mold infections in allogeneic stem cell transplant recip-

ients: biological risk factors for infection according to time after transplantation. *Clin Infect Dis.* 2008;47:1041-1050.

228. Maertens J, Theunissen K, Verbeken E, et al. Prospective clinical evaluation of lower cut-offs for galactomannan detection in adult neutropenic cancer patients and haematological stem cell transplant recipients. *Br J Haematol.* 2004;126:852-860.

229. Maertens J, Van Eldere J, Verhaegen J, et al. Use of circulating galactomannan screening for early diagnosis of invasive aspergillosis in allogeneic stem cell transplant recipients. *J Infect Dis.* 2002;186:1297-1306.

230. Maertens J, Verhaegen J, Lagrou K, et al. Screening for circulating galactomannan as a noninvasive diagnostic tool for invasive aspergillosis in prolonged neutropenic patients and stem cell transplantation recipients: a prospective validation. *Blood.* 2001;97:1604-1610.

231. Foy PC, van Burik JA, Weisdorf DJ. Galactomannan antigen enzyme-linked immunosorbent assay for diagnosis of invasive aspergillosis after hematopoietic stem cell transplantation. *Biol Blood Marrow Transplant.* 2007;13:440-443.

232. Bowden R, Chandrasekar P, White MH, et al. A double-blind, randomized, controlled trial of amphotericin B colloidal dispersion versus amphotericin B for treatment of invasive aspergillosis in immunocompromised patients. *Clin Infect Dis.* 2002;35:359-366.

233. Denning DW, Marr KA, Lau WM, et al. Micafungin (FK463), alone or in combination with other systemic antifungal agents, for the treatment of acute invasive aspergillosis. *J Infect.* 2006; 53:337-349.

234. Herbrecht R, Denning DW, Patterson TF, et al. Voriconazole versus amphotericin B for primary therapy of invasive aspergillosis. *N Engl J Med.* 2002;347:408-415.

235. Morrison VA, Weisdorf DJ. The spectrum of *Malassezia* infections in the bone marrow transplant population. *Bone Marrow Transplant.* 2000;26:645-648.

236. Bufill JA, Lum LG, Caya JG, et al. *Pityrosporum* folliculitis after bone marrow transplantation. Clinical observations in five patients. *Ann Intern Med.* 1988;108:560-563.

237. Jahagirdar BN, Morrison VA. Emerging fungal pathogens in patients with hematologic malignancies and marrow/stem-cell transplant recipients. *Semin Respir Infect.* 2002;17:113-120.

238. Goodman D, Pamer E, Jakubowski A, et al. Breakthrough trichosporonosis in a bone marrow transplant recipient receiving caspofungin acetate. *Clin Infect Dis.* 2002;35(3):E35-E36.

239. Grauer ME, Bokemeyer C, Bautsch W, et al. Successful treatment of a *Trichosporon beigelii* septicemia in a granulocytopenic patient with amphotericin B and granulocyte colony-stimulating factor. *Infection.* 1994;22:283-286.

240. Blazar BR, Hurd DD, Snover DC, et al. Invasive *Fusarium* infections in bone marrow transplant recipients. *Am J Med.* 1984;77:645-651.

241. Nucci M, Marr KA, Queiroz-Telles F, et al. *Fusarium* infection in hematopoietic stem cell transplant recipients. *Clin Infect Dis.* 2004;38:1237-1242.

242. Maertens J, Demuynck H, Verbeken EK, et al. Mucormycosis in allogeneic bone marrow transplant recipients: report of five cases and review of the role of iron overload in the pathogenesis. *Bone Marrow Transplant.* 1999;24:307-312.

243. Morrison VA, McGlave PB. Mucormycosis in the BMT population. *Bone Marrow Transplant.* 1993;11:383.

244. Oliver MR, Van Voorhis WC, Boeckh M, et al. Hepatic mucormycosis in a bone marrow transplant recipient who ingested naturopathic medicine. *Clin Infect Dis.* 1996;22:521-524.

245. Siwek GT, Dodgson KJ, de Magalhaes-Silverman M, et al. Invasive zygomycosis in hematopoietic stem cell transplant recipients receiving voriconazole prophylaxis. *Clin Infect Dis.* 2004;39:584-587.

246. Marty FM, Cosimi LA, Baden LR. Breakthrough zygomycosis after voriconazole treatment in recipients of hematopoietic stem-cell transplants. *N Engl J Med.* 2004;350:950-952.

247. Ustun C, Farrow S, DeRemer D, et al. Early fatal *Rhizopus* infection on voriconazole prophylaxis following allogeneic stem cell transplantation. *Bone Marrow Transplant.* 2007;39:807-808.

248. Kontoyiannis DP, Lionakis MS, Lewis RE, et al. Zygomycosis in a tertiary-care cancer center in the era of *Aspergillus*-active antifungal therapy: a case-control observational study of 27 recent cases. *J Infect Dis.* 2005;191:1350-1360.

249. van Burik JA, Hare RS, Solomon HF, et al. Posaconazole is effective as salvage therapy in zygomycosis: a retrospective summary of 91 cases. *Clin Infect Dis.* 2006;42(7):e61-e65.

250. Martino R, Maertens J, Bretagne S, et al. Toxoplasmosis after hematopoietic stem cell transplantation. *Clin Infect Dis.* 2000; 31:1188-1195.

251. Villalba R, Fornes G, Alvarez MA, et al. Acute Chagas' disease in a recipient of a bone marrow transplant in Spain: case report. *Clin Infect Dis.* 1992;14:594-595.

252. Altclas J, Jaimovich G, Milovic V, et al. Chagas' disease after bone marrow transplantation. *Bone Marrow Transplant.* 1996;18:447-448.

253. Pasternak J, Amato Neto V, Hammerschlack N. Chagas' disease after bone marrow transplantation. *Bone Marrow Transplant.* 1997;19:958.

254. Dictar M, Sinagra A, Veron MT, et al. Recipients and donors of bone marrow transplants suffering from Chagas' disease: management and preemptive therapy of parasitemia. *Bone Marrow Transplant.* 1998;21:391-393.

255. Fores R, Sanjuan I, Portero F, et al. Chagas disease in a recipient of cord blood transplantation. *Bone Marrow Transplant.* 2007; 39:127-128.

256. Dharmasena F, Gordon-Smith EC. Transmission of malaria by bone marrow transplantation. *Transplantation.* 1986;42: 228.

257. Lefrere F, Besson C, Datry A, et al. Transmission of *Plasmodium falciparum* by allogeneic bone marrow transplantation. *Bone Marrow Transplant.* 1996;18:473-474.

258. Salutari P, Sica S, Chiusolo P, et al. *Plasmodium vivax* malaria after autologous bone marrow transplantation: an unusual complication. *Bone Marrow Transplant.* 1996;18:805-806.

259. O'Donnell J, Goldman JM, Wagner K, et al. Donor-derived *Plasmodium vivax* infection following volunteer unrelated bone marrow transplantation. *Bone Marrow Transplant.* 1998;21:313-314.

260. Raina V, Sharma A, Gujral S, Kumar R. *Plasmodium vivax* causing pancytopenia after allogeneic blood stem cell transplantation in CML. *Bone Marrow Transplant.* 1998;22:205-206.

261. Tran VB, Lin KH. Malaria infection after allogeneic bone marrow transplantation in a child with thalassemia. *Bone Marrow Transplant.* 1997;19:1259-1260.

262. Steiner B, Riebold D, Wolff D, et al. *Strongyloides stercoralis* eggs in a urethral smear after bone marrow transplantation. *Clin Infect Dis.* 2002;34:1280-1281.

263. Mahmoud HK. Schistosomiasis as a predisposing factor to veno-occlusive disease of the liver following allogeneic bone marrow transplantation. *Bone Marrow Transplant.* 1996;17:401-403.

264. Woo PC, Lie AK, Yuen K, et al. Clonorchiasis in bone marrow transplant recipients. *Clin Infect Dis.* 1998;27:382-384.

265. Blakey JL, Barnes GL, Bishop RF, et al. Infectious diarrhea in children undergoing bone-marrow transplantation. *Aust N Z J Med.* 1989;19:31-36.

266. Bromiker R, Korman SH, Or R, et al. Severe giardiasis in two patients undergoing bone marrow transplantation. *Bone Marrow Transplant.* 1989;4:701-703.

267. Faraci M, Cappelli B, Morreale G, et al. Nitazoxanide or CD3+/CD4+ lymphocytes for recovery from severe *Cryptosporidium* infection after allogeneic bone marrow transplant? *Pediatr Transplant.* 2007;11:113-116.

268. Muller CI, Zeiser R, Grullich C, et al. Intestinal cryptosporidiosis mimicking acute graft-versus-host disease following matched unrelated hematopoietic stem cell transplantation. *Transplantation.* 2004;77:1478-1479.

269. Dimicoli S, Bensoussan D, Latger-Cannard V, et al. Complete recovery from *Cryptosporidium parvum* infection with gastroenteritis and sclerosing cholangitis after successful bone marrow transplantation in two brothers with X-linked hyper-IgM syndrome. *Bone Marrow Transplant.* 2003;32:733-737.

270. Nachbaur D, Kropshofer G, Feichtinger H, et al. Cryptosporidiosis after CD34-selected autologous peripheral blood stem cell transplantation. Treatment with paromomycin, azithromycin and recombinant human interleukin-2. *Bone Marrow Transplant.* 1997;19:1261-1263.

271. Kelkar R, Sastry PS, Kulkarni SS, et al. Pulmonary microsporidial infection in a patient with CML undergoing allogeneic marrow transplant. *Bone Marrow Transplant.* 1997;19:179-182.

272. Orenstein JM, Russo P, Didier ES, et al. Fatal pulmonary microsporidiosis due to *Encephalitozoon cuniculi* following allogeneic bone marrow transplantation for acute myelogenous leukemia. *Ultrastruct Pathol.* 2005;29:269-276.

273. Teachey DT, Russo P, Orenstein JM, et al. Pulmonary infection with microsporidia after allogeneic bone marrow transplantation. *Bone Marrow Transplant.* 2004;33:299-302.

274. Feingold JM, Abraham J, Bilgrami S, et al. *Acanthamoeba* meningoencephalitis following autologous peripheral stem cell transplantation. *Bone Marrow Transplant.* 1998;22:297-300.

275. Peman J, Jarque I, Frasquet J, et al. Unexpected postmortem diagnosis of *Acanthamoeba* meningoencephalitis following allogeneic peripheral blood stem cell transplantation. *Am J Transplant.* 2008;8:1562-1566.

276. Castellano-Sanchez A, Popp AC, Nolte FS, et al. *Acanthamoeba castellani* encephalitis following partially mismatched related donor peripheral stem cell transplantation. *Transpl Infect Dis.* 2003;5:191-194.

277. Okamoto S, Wakui M, Kobayashi H, et al. *Trichomonas foetus* meningoencephalitis after allogeneic peripheral blood stem cell transplantation. *Bone Marrow Transplant.* 1998;21:89-91.

278. Derouin F, Devergie A, Auber P, et al. Toxoplasmosis in bone marrow-transplant recipients: report of seven cases and review. *Clin Infect Dis.* 1992;15:267-270.

279. Mele A, Paterson PJ, Prentice HG, et al. Toxoplasmosis in bone marrow transplantation: a report of two cases and systematic review of the literature. *Bone Marrow Transplant.* 2002;29:691-698.

280. Martino R, Cordonnier C. Toxoplasmosis following allogeneic hematopoietic stem cell transplantation. *Bone Marrow Transplant.* 2003;31:617-618.

281. Slavin MA, Meyers JD, Remington JS, et al. *Toxoplasma gondii* infection in marrow transplant recipients: a 20 year experience. *Bone Marrow Transplant.* 1994;13:549-557.

282. Matsuo Y, Takeishi S, Miyamoto T, et al. Toxoplasmosis encephalitis following severe graft-vs.-host disease after allogeneic hematopoietic stem cell transplantation: 17 yr experience in Fukuoka BMT group. *Eur J Haematol.* 2007;79: 317-321.

283. Duband S, Cornillon J, Tavernier E, et al. Toxoplasmosis with hemophagocytic syndrome after bone marrow transplantation: diagnosis at autopsy. *Transpl Infect Dis.* 2008;10:372-374.

284. Lewis JS Jr, Khoury H, Storch GA, et al. PCR for the diagnosis of toxoplasmosis after hematopoietic stem cell transplantation. *Expert Rev Mol Diagn.* 2002;2:616-624.

285. Martino R, Bretagne S, Einsele H, et al. Early detection of *Toxoplasma* infection by molecular monitoring of *Toxoplasma gondii* in peripheral blood samples after allogeneic stem cell transplantation. *Clin Infect Dis.* 2005;40:67-78.

286. Cibickova L, Horacek J, Prasil P, et al. Cerebral toxoplasmosis in an allogeneic peripheral stem cell transplant recipient: case report and review of literature. *Transpl Infect Dis.* 2007;9:332-335.

287. Megged O, Shalit I, Yaniv I, et al. Breakthrough cerebral toxoplasmosis in a patient receiving atovaquone prophylaxis after a hematopoietic stem cell transplantation. *Pediatr Transplant.* 2008;12:902-905.

288. Bretagne S, Costa JM, Foulet F, et al. Prospective study of *Toxoplasma* reactivation by polymerase chain reaction in allogeneic stem-cell transplant recipients. *Transpl Infect Dis.* 2000;2: 127-132.

289. Foot AB, Garin YJ, Ribaud P, et al. Prophylaxis of toxoplasmosis infection with pyrimethamine/sulfadoxine (Fansidar) in bone marrow transplant recipients. *Bone Marrow Transplant.* 1994; 14:241-245.

290. Singhal S, Mehta J. Reimmunization after blood or marrow stem cell transplantation. *Bone Marrow Transplant.* 1999;23:637-646.

291. Henning KJ, White MH, Sepkowitz KA, et al. A national survey of immunization practices following allogeneic bone marrow transplantation. *JAMA.* 1997;277:1148-1151.

292. Gandhi MK, Egner W, Sizer L, et al. Antibody responses to vaccinations given within the first two years after transplant are similar between autologous peripheral blood stem cell and bone marrow transplant recipients. *Bone Marrow Transplant.* 2001; 28:775-781.

293. Jaffe D, Papadopoulos EB, Young JW, et al. Immunogenicity of recombinant hepatitis B vaccine in recipients of unrelated or related allogeneic hematopoietic cell transplants. *Blood.* 2006; 108:2470-2475.

294. Storek J, Viganego F, Dawson MA, et al. Factors affecting antibody levels after allogeneic hematopoietic cell transplantation. *Blood.* 2003;101:3319-3324.

295. Witherspoon RP, Storb R, Ochs HD, et al. Recovery of antibody production in human allogeneic marrow graft recipients: influence of time posttransplantation, the presence or absence of chronic graft-versus-host disease, and antithymocyte globulin treatment. *Blood.* 1981;58:360-368.

296. Sullivan KM, Kopecky KJ, Jocom J, et al. Immunomodulatory and antimicrobial efficacy of intravenous immunoglobulin in bone marrow transplantation. *N Engl J Med.* 1990;323:705-712.

297. Sullivan KM, Storek J, Kopecky KJ, et al. A controlled trial of long-term administration of intravenous immunoglobulin to prevent late infection and chronic graft-vs.-host disease after marrow transplantation: clinical outcome and effect on subsequent immune recovery. *Biol Blood Marrow Transplant.* 1996;2:44-53.

298. Wolff SN, Fay JW, Herzig RH, et al. High-dose weekly intravenous immunoglobulin to prevent infections in patients undergoing autologous bone marrow transplantation or severe myelosuppressive therapy. A study of the American Bone Marrow Transplant Group. *Ann Intern Med.* 1993;118:937-942.

299. Winston DJ, Antin JH, Wolff SN, et al. A multicenter, randomized, double-blind comparison of different doses of intravenous immunoglobulin for prevention of graft-versus-host disease and infection after allogeneic bone marrow transplantation. *Bone Marrow Transplant.* 2001;28:187-196.

312

Infections in Solid Organ Transplant Recipients

J. STEPHEN DUMMER | NINA SINGH

After the introduction of cyclosporine as a major immunosuppressive agent, there was a marked increase in the transplantation of solid organs. Graft and patient survival rates improved for recipients of all types of organs, and liver, heart, and lung transplantation advanced from being quasi-experimental procedures to established and accepted therapies. Table 312-1 shows the most recent data available on graft and patient survival released by the United Network for Organ Sharing (UNOS).[1] The best results are for living-related kidney transplantation: 98% of recipients are alive and 95% have functioning allografts 1 year after transplantation. The greatest progress may have been in liver transplantation, in which the 1-year survival rate before the use of cyclosporine was only 32%, compared with a 3-year survival rate of 79% in the current era. The survival rates for lung, heart-lung, and intestinal transplant recipients have lagged behind the other groups, but these procedures were only introduced in the 1980s, and experience has been gained slowly because of the limited number of operations performed.

Improvements in graft and patient survival have been paralleled by a decline in mortality from infections.[2,3] For instance, the risk of death from infection in heart recipients transplanted in Pittsburgh fell significantly between 1981 and 1990 (Fig. 312-1A). In the last group of patients studied, mortality from infectious causes during the first 3 years after transplantation was only about 4.5%.[2] Likewise, the early post-transplantation mortality rate from infection in liver recipients in Pittsburgh decreased significantly, from 47% in the early 1980s[4] to 23% in the late 1980s[5] and 7% in the early 1990s.[6] More recent data on infectious causes of death after transplantation are limited, but one study suggested that infection-related mortality in heart transplantation may no longer be improving. In this multi-institutional analysis of mortality in 7290 heart recipients transplanted between 1990 and 2000, the 3-year infection-related mortality rate was unchanged at 4.5% to 5.0% throughout the decade. By contrast, the mortality rate from rejection and graft vasculopathy fell significantly during the same period (see Fig. 312-1B).[7]

Time of Occurrence of Infections after Transplantation

The risk of infection is highest during the first few months after transplantation, when the patient is still under close medical surveillance. The kinds of infections seen within this high-risk period are not uniform but follow a typical time schema.[8] Common infections during the first month after transplantation are those that might be seen after any surgical procedure: respiratory, urinary tract, wound, and intravascular catheter infections caused by nosocomial bacteria. Except for the reactivation of herpes simplex virus (HSV), infections related to deficient T-cell immunity are not encountered. After 1 month, surgical infections decline in importance, and typical opportunistic infections associated with the immunosuppressed state emerge. These include *Pneumocystis* pneumonia, opportunistic fungal infections, nocardiosis, and, most importantly, cytomegalovirus (CMV) infection. This time schema of infections was first described in renal transplantation but is applicable to other types of transplantation with a few alterations. In liver transplant recipients, for instance, postsurgical infection may

extend into the second and third month because of retransplantation or reoperation for technical complications.[5] Also, opportunistic fungal infections occur during the first month in liver and lung transplant recipients because of their high susceptibility.[5,9,10]

Figure 312-2 illustrates the incidence of severe infections documented at various times after liver transplantation.[5] The figure excludes minor infections such as afebrile cystitis or localized HSV infection. It is apparent that the frequency of severe infections was quite high during the first and second months. Bacterial and fungal infections were most common in the first month and viral infections (mostly CMV) in the second month. The "protozoal" infections were mostly *Pneumocystis* pneumonia and are no longer seen today because of the effectiveness of trimethoprim-sulfamethoxazole (TMP-SMX) prophylaxis. After 6 months, the rate of severe infections declined to about 1 infection for every 4 patient-years. These late infections were all caused by bacteria or fungi. This rate of late infection is similar to the frequency of severe, late infections seen in heart transplant recipients.[11]

The most frequent infections that occur more than 6 months after transplantation are simply the common infections found in any population.[2,8] Community-acquired pneumonia, diverticulitis, and cholecystitis are not unique for transplant recipients, but because of immune suppression these infections may manifest in an altered fashion or result in more severe sequelae.[2,8] Other late manifestations may represent reactivated or chronic viral infections. Eruptions of herpes zoster may occur at any time after transplantation.[12] Subacute or chronic hepatitis, particularly that caused by hepatitis C virus (HCV), may become manifest many years after transplantation.[13] A number of tumors related to viral infection may also occur late, the most frequent being warts (verruca vulgaris). Also, some lymphomas and lymphoproliferative syndromes related to Epstein-Barr virus (EBV) occur after more than 1 year.[14] A third type of late infection relates to chronic graft dysfunction. Lung transplant recipients with chronic rejection develop obliterative bronchiolitis and are susceptible to recurrent bacterial bronchitis and pneumonia.[15] Liver transplant recipients may have recurrent cholangitis, often in association with biliary stricture.[5]

Finally, the risk for "opportunistic" infection declines, but never completely disappears. Infection due to endemic fungi such as cryptococcus or histoplasma often manifests late and without any apparent inciting event or change in immunosuppression.

Types of Transplants and Characteristic Infections

Table 312-2 presents the type, severity, and characteristic sites of infections in 315 kidney, heart, heart-lung, and liver transplant recipients observed during the first year after transplantation.[5,11,16-18] These data were collected at the University of Pittsburgh on patients who received similar immunosuppressive regimens, before the advent of the complex prophylactic antimicrobial regimens used today. Therefore, the differences between the groups should reflect intrinsic differences in the epidemiology of infections in the different organ groups rather than variations in environment or medical management.

As can be seen from the table, the type and frequency of infections and the infection-related mortality rate varied widely with the organ

TABLE 312-1	Overall Graft and Patient Survival Rates by Organ Transplanted			
	Graft Survival (%)		**Patient Survival (%)**	
Organ	*1 yr*	*3 yr*	*1 yr*	*3 yr*
Kidney—living donor	95	89	98	95
Kidney—deceased donor	90	79	95	88
Pancreas (with kidney)	86	80	95	91
Heart	87	79	88	80
Liver—deceased donor	82	74	87	79
Intestine	73	54	81	67
Lung	82	65	84	68
Heart-lung	75	55	75	56

Adapted from *The 2007 Annual Report of the U.S. Organ Procurement and Transplantation Network and the Scientific Registry of Transplant Recipients: Transplant Data 1997-2006.* Rockville, MD: Health Resources and Services Administration, Healthcare Systems Bureau, Division of Transplantation, 2007.

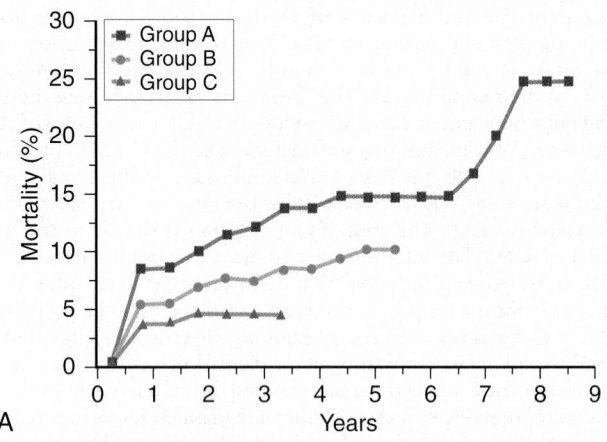

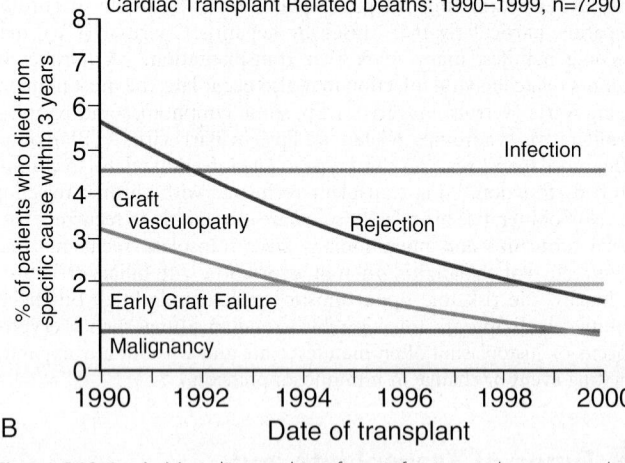

Figure 312-1 **A,** Mortality resulting from infections in heart transplant recipients in three different time periods: group A, 1980-1985 (179 patients); group B, 1985-1987 (179 patients); group C, 1987-1990 (180 patients). Group A versus group C, *P* = 0.015. Mortality from other causes has been censored. **B,** Proportion of patients dying of specific causes during the first 3 years after heart transplantation from 1990 to 2000 in a multicenter analysis of 7290 patients. Over the decade deaths due to infection stayed constant, but deaths due to rejection and graft vasculopathy declined. (**A,** *Data from Dummer JS. Antibiotic prophylaxis and management of infectious complications. In: Kaye MP, O'Connell JB, eds. Heart and Lung Transplantation 2000. Austin, TX: R.G. Landes; 1993:78.* **B,** *Data from Kirklin JK, Naftel DC, Bourge RC, et al. Evolving trends in risk profiles and causes of death after heart transplantation: A ten-year multi-institutional study. J Thorac Cardiovasc Surg. 2003;125:881.*)

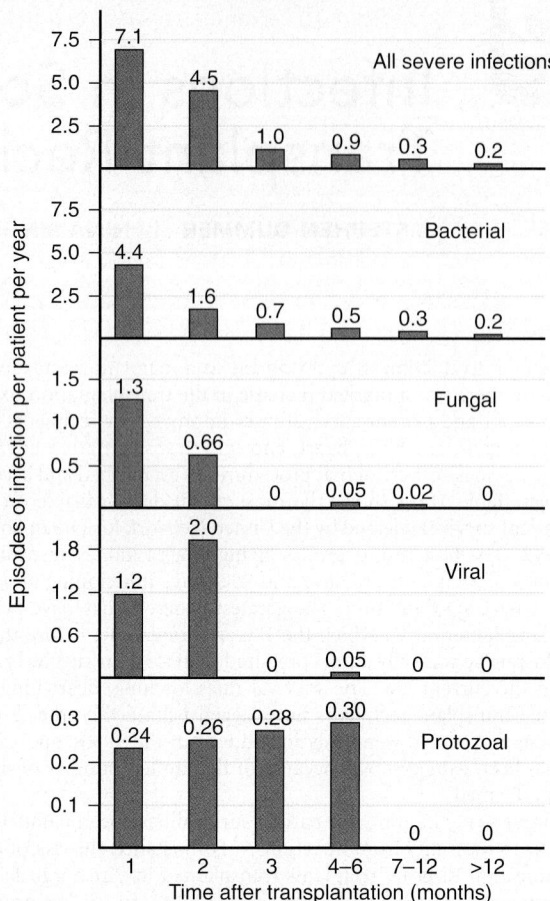

Figure 312-2 **Incidence and timing of severe infections after liver transplantation, expressed in episodes of infection per liver transplant patient per year.** Data on all severe, bacterial, fungal, viral, and "protozoal" (mostly *Pneumocystis*) infections are included.

or organs transplanted. The number of episodes of infection per patient was lowest in the renal group, and none of these patients died of infection. The heart-lung recipients, by contrast, had more than three times the number of infections and the largest number of deaths associated with infection (45%). The liver transplant group also had a high mortality rate and almost five times the rate of bacteremia of the renal group. Invasive fungal infections were frequent in liver and heart-lung recipients, intermediate in heart recipients, and absent in renal recipients. It is particularly striking how much better the outcome was for heart recipients than for heart-lung recipients, even though they were managed by the same medical team and received the same immunosuppressive regimen. Finally, Table 312-2 shows that the most common sites of infection after transplantation were closely related to the site of surgery.

KIDNEY TRANSPLANT RECIPIENTS

The most common site of infection in renal transplant recipients is the urinary tract, and most bacteremias in renal recipients arise from the urinary tract.[19] By 3 years after transplantation, more than half of all renal recipients will have been diagnosed with upper or lower urinary tract infection.[20] Many infections are uncomplicated cystitis, but Giral and colleagues documented graft pyelonephritis in 13% of 1387 renal recipients over a 13-year interval.[21] In their study, pyelonephritis occurring in the first 3 months was associated with reduced graft survival, but later infections were not. However, a larger, multivariate analysis of more than 28,000 kidney recipients in the Medicare data-

TABLE 312-2	Frequency, Severity, and Type of Infections Occurring in the First Year after Transplantation							
Type of Transplant	N	Infections per Patient	Infection-Related Mortality (%)	Bacteremia (%)	CMV Disease (%)*	Deep Fungal Infection (%)	Most Common Site	Proportion of All Infections (%)
Renal	64	0.98	0	5	8 (5)	0	Urinary tract	41
Heart	119	1.36	15	13	16 (5)	8	Lung	27
Heart-lung	31	3.19	45	19	39 (32)	23	Lung	57
Liver	101	1.86	23	23	22 (5)	16	Abdomen and biliary tract	23

*Numbers in parentheses indicate percentage of all patients with cytomegalovirus (CMV) pneumonia.
Data are from the University of Pittsburgh experience, 1983-1990, compiled from references 5, 11, and 16-18.

base showed that a diagnosis of upper or lower urinary tract infection after 6 months was associated with worse long-term graft function and survival.[20] Chronic and recurrent urinary tract infections remain problematic. Abnormalities such as ureteral reflux, strictures at the ureterovesical junction, or neurogenic bladder should be sought in patients with recurrent infections. Avoidance of surgical complications and use of primary antimicrobial prophylaxis after surgery are the most important means of decreasing the frequency of urinary infection. Despite the importance of urinary infection and graft pyelonephritis in this population, there are no controlled trial data on which to base decisions regarding treatment type and duration, and conventional treatment is recommended in most cases. Administering an extended course of antibiotics (≥4 weeks) or considering a course of secondary antibiotic prophylaxis is reasonable in patients who have severe graft pyelonephritis or recurrent infections with the same organism.[22]

The clinician also should be alert to the possible occurrence of unusual urinary pathogens. We have seen urinary tract tuberculosis that arose from a focus in the native kidney during the first 2 weeks after transplantation. *Mycoplasma hominis* infection of the urinary tract may cause a breakdown of the ureterovesical anastomosis with subsequent graft loss.[23] Histoplasmosis may involve the transplanted kidney and cause renal failure.[24]

Historically, pneumonia occurred in 25% to 30% of renal transplant recipients and was the most common infectious cause of death.[25] In the past, bacteria were a less prominent cause of transplantation-associated pneumonia than CMV and opportunists such as fungi, *Nocardia*, and *Pneumocystis*. More recently, CMV and other opportunistic infections have come under better control, and conventional bacterial pathogens have become relatively more common in transplant populations.[8,26]

Wound infections are relatively infrequent but may be a serious problem, particularly if they involve the perinephric space. A study of 2013 kidney recipients transplanted in Minnesota between 1984 and 1998 showed a combined superficial and deep wound infection rate of 4.8%.[27] Risk factors for infection in order of relative risk were a body mass index greater than 30 kg/m^2, post-transplantation urinary leak, reoperation through the transplant incision, use of mycophenolate mofetil for immunosuppression, and presence of diabetes mellitus.

Although Table 312-2 lists no deaths from infection in renal transplant recipients, some such deaths may be expected. In a survey of 604 renal transplant recipients in Minnesota, patients with infection had a 3-year survival rate of 88%, compared with 92% in patients without infection, revealing a small but significant increase in mortality.[28]

Some renal transplant recipients continue to have frequent problems with infection even after the first 6 months. These patients often have received excess immunosuppression or have chronic dysfunction of the allograft or other major organs. A few suffer from chronic viral infections such as HCV.[29]

HEART TRANSPLANT RECIPIENTS

Heart transplant recipients have more infections and are more affected by them than are kidney transplant recipients.[11,18] In a survey of 620 heart transplant recipients at Stanford University, infections were the most common cause of death.[30] The most common infections were

bacterial pneumonias, urinary infections, herpesvirus infections, and invasive fungal infections. Most pneumonias in heart and other transplant recipients are caused by common pathogenic bacteria (Table 312-3).[3,11,30] Although the incidence of pneumonia is highest during the first few months after transplantation, bacterial pneumonias occur sporadically in the late post-transplantation period, after the patient has recovered from the immediate effects of surgery.

Mediastinitis and sternal wound infections are postoperative complications unique to heart and heart-lung transplant recipients. The pathogens seen are similar to those observed in other patients undergoing cardiothoracic surgery, with *Staphylococcus aureus* and *Staphylococcus epidermidis* predominating. The incidence of mediastinitis in two large transplant series was quite similar: 2.5% (9/361) and 2.9% (18/620).[30,31] The initial clinical presentation may be subtle, with low-grade fever or an elevated leukocyte count being the only manifestation. Later, more specific signs develop, such as erythema, tenderness, or drainage along the sternal incision. One must also be alert to the possible presence of unusual pathogens. Mediastinitis and sternal wound infections in heart recipients have been caused by *M. hominis*, *Legionella pneumophila*, *Aspergillus*, and *Nocardia*.[23,30] It may be necessary to include special media in the microbiologic workup of these infections. Factors that are thought to predispose to mediastinitis in this population are repeat operations for hemorrhage, use of antirejection therapy, and the presence of diabetes mellitus.[31] Surgical drainage appears to be crucial to the successful treatment of mediastinitis in the transplant patient. There is considerable controversy regarding the best mode of drainage.

Mechanical left-ventricular assist devices with an external power source are now widely used as a bridge to transplantation.[32] Infections of these devices are common and fall into distinct types: infections of the driveline, which are often limited to the exit site; deep infections

TABLE 312-3	Microbial Causes of Pneumonia in Transplant Recipients	
Early Pneumonia (≤30 days)		Late Pneumonia (>30 days)
Common Causes		
Gram-negative enteric bacilli		Pneumococcus
Staphylococcus aureus		*Haemophilus influenzae*
Aspiration		No cause identified
Less Common Causes		
Aspergillus		*Pneumocystis*
Herpes simplex virus		*Nocardia*
Legionella		*Legionella*
Toxoplasma gondii		*Aspergillus*
		Gram-negative enteric bacilli
		Staphylococcus aureus
		Aspiration
		Cytomegalovirus
		Varicella-zoster virus
		Paramyxoviruses
		Tuberculosis
		Coccidioidomycosis
		Histoplasmosis

in the pocket surrounding the actual device; and bacterial or fungal bloodstream infections, which may be associated with internal infection of the device. Management of these infections is very challenging and beyond the scope of this chapter. In many cases, the infection can be controlled well enough to permit transplantation[32] (see Chapter 79).

A number of other infections are more commonly reported in heart recipients than in patients receiving other types of transplants. These include toxoplasmosis, nocardiosis, and Chagas' disease.[33-35] Toxoplasma-seronegative heart recipients are at increased risk for toxoplasmosis because the infection can be acquired from organisms encysted in the heart muscle of toxoplasma-seropositive donors. Clinical toxoplasmosis usually occurs a few weeks to a few months after transplantation and is manifested by necrotizing pneumonitis, myocarditis, and encephalitis. Clinical toxoplasmosis is now uncommon in heart recipients, apparently because of the protection provided by the use of TMP-SMX for *Pneumocystis* prophylaxis.[30]

Symptomatic reactivation of *Trypanosoma cruzi* infection may be seen in immunocompromised patients, including transplant recipients. About one fourth of patients who undergo heart transplantation for cardiomyopathy caused by chronic *T. cruzi* infection have relapses of acute Chagas' disease, with clinical manifestations of fever, myocarditis, and skin lesions.[33] The disease can usually be controlled with chemotherapy. A recent large series from Brazil reported excellent overall outcomes in 117 patients transplanted for Chagas' disease, with only two deaths occurring from *T. cruzi* infection.[33] Detection of parasite DNA sequences in blood samples appears to be a useful way to monitor patients for reactivation after transplantation.[36]

Nocardia infections have also been more frequently reported in heart and lung transplant recipients than in recipients of kidney or liver transplants, but the biologic reason for this increased rate of nocardiosis is unknown.[30,35] The doses of TMP-SMX used for *Pneumocystis* prophylaxis do not provide reliable protection against *Nocardia* infection.

Heart recipients frequently suffer trauma to the tricuspid valve and right ventricular endocardium from repeated endomyocardial biopsies, a common post-transplantation practice. Endocarditis appears to be somewhat more common in heart transplant populations than in immunocompetent persons. Most cases occur during the first year after transplantation and may be caused by unusual organisms such as *Aspergillus* or *Legionella* species.[37]

LUNG AND HEART-LUNG TRANSPLANT RECIPIENTS

As a result of the shortage of suitable donors, the field of lung and heart-lung transplantation has progressed at a slower rate than other transplant specialties. In many respects, lung and heart-lung transplant recipients have infectious problems similar to those of heart transplant recipients, but the infections are more frequent and more severe. Reports of lung and heart-lung transplantation emphasize the high rate of bacterial lung infections, especially during the first few weeks after transplantation.[10,16,38] These patients also have higher rates of mediastinitis, invasive fungal infections, and CMV pneumonia than comparable heart recipients.[16,39]

Heart-lung and lung transplant recipients develop invasive pulmonary aspergillosis more frequently than do patients with other types of organ transplants.[40] A unique form of aspergillosis involving the airway mucosa, called tracheobronchial aspergillosis, is observed almost exclusively in lung and heart-lung recipients. The airway lesions of this disease can be directly visualized and diagnosed during bronchoscopy. This form of aspergillosis has a better prognosis than does aspergillosis invading the lung parenchyma.[40] The predisposition of lung recipients to invasive aspergillosis has led lung transplant centers to commonly employ antifungal prophylaxis active against molds. Oral azoles and inhaled amphotericin are the most widely used agents.

The heightened vulnerability of the transplanted lung to infection is probably multifactorial. In addition to mechanical factors related to decreased mucociliary clearance, diminished lymphatic drainage, and ablation of the cough reflex, allograft reactions appear to play an important, if poorly understood, role.[38] In the late post-transplant period, up to two thirds of patients develop obliterative bronchiolitis.[41] This process is the main pathologic manifestation of chronic rejection of the lung and has been associated with recurrent pulmonary infections.[15] The lung allograft is also particularly susceptible to viral infection, as has been documented for CMV, HSV, paramyxovirus, and adenovirus infections.[11,15,16,39,42,43] Accordingly, lung transplant centers often utilize aggressive regimens for prophylaxis of herpesvirus infections and include diagnostic tests for respiratory viruses in the workup of patients who present with acute chest infections.

The first success in transplanting lungs was achieved with combined heart-lung transplantation. Single- and double-lung transplantation have now largely replaced heart-lung transplantation as the procedures of choice for most patients with end-stage lung disease. Heart-lung transplantation is now usually reserved for patients who have Eisenmenger's syndrome and whose cardiac abnormalities cannot be surgically repaired. Single- and double-lung procedures also leave the donor heart available for another patient with end-stage heart disease. The types of infections seen in lung transplant recipients are similar to those in heart-lung recipients, although the overall survival rate is better.[1,10] A unique aspect of single-lung transplantation is the occurrence of infections in the native lung. This lung may be predisposed to infection because of defects of ventilation or perfusion caused by the underlying lung disease.[38,44]

Prospective donors for lung transplantation are intubated in intensive care units. Therefore, the airways of these donors are often colonized with microorganisms, and occult parenchymal infection may be present.[38,44] Before implantation of the lungs, it is customary to obtain cultures and Gram stains of the donor airways to guide antibiotic therapy. Initial antibiotic prophylaxis should be aimed at common nosocomial pathogens encountered in the intensive care unit, including methicillin-resistant *S. aureus* and enteric gram-negative bacilli. Another problem unique to lung transplantation has been dehiscence of the airway anastomosis. This occurs during the first few weeks after transplantation. It is frequently associated with bacterial or fungal infection at the anastomotic site. The incidence of this complication appears to be declining.[44]

LIVER TRANSPLANT RECIPIENTS

Liver transplant recipients have higher rates of infection than renal or heart transplant recipients, and most deaths are associated with infection, either as a primary or as a secondary cause. Despite a decline in the mortality rate in recent years, infections have remained a major threat.[5,6] Bacteria are the most common pathogens causing serious infection after liver transplantation. The reported incidence in larger series has varied from 59% to 68%.[5,45] About half of these infections occur within 2 weeks after the transplant operation.[45] Identified risk factors include a prolonged duration of surgery, transfusion of large quantities of blood, use of a choledochojejunostomy (Roux-en-Y procedure) for bile drainage, repeat transplantation, and CMV infection.[5,45] The most important sites of infection are the abdomen and biliary tract, the surgical wound, the lungs, and the bloodstream, with or without associated catheter infection.

Liver transplant recipients have a higher rate of fungal infections than do other solid organ transplant recipients. The reported incidence has been 15% to 42%, with a case-fatality rate of 25% to 82%.[4,5,46,47] Eighty percent of fungal infections occur during the first month and 90% during the first 2 months after transplantation.[4] Risk factors for invasive fungal infections include elevated serum creatinine, longer operative time, retransplantation, hepatic iron overload, and colonization with *Candida* at the time of transplantation.[47,48] Other risk factors identified in various studies were administration of steroids before or after operation, duration of broad-spectrum antibiotic use, and CMV infection.[4,5,47]

Candida is the predominant pathogen, causing 62% to 88% of the invasive fungal infections in this population, although it has declined in relative importance compared to *Aspergillus,* other molds, and *Cryp-*

tococcus.[49] Almost one third of candidal infections in liver transplant recipients are caused by non-*albicans* species.[50] Fluconazole prophylaxis was found to be a risk factor for the emergence of non-*albicans Candida* species as pathogens in liver transplant recipients.[50] Invasive candidiasis contributes significantly to mortality after liver transplantation. In a case-controlled study, liver transplant recipients with invasive candidiasis had a 36% mortality rate, compared with 2% in the control patients.[50]

Invasive aspergillosis occurs in 1% to 8% of liver transplant recipients. Major risk factors for invasive aspergillosis in liver transplantation include retransplantation, fulminant hepatic failure as an indication for transplantation, renal dysfunction and hemodialysis, and poor allograft function.[40,51] Invasive aspergillosis typically develops in the early post-transplantation period.[51,52] Recently, however, *Aspergillus* infections have been reported to occur more than 90 days after transplantation, a possible consequence of improved early management and delayed occurrence of risk factors such as CMV infection.[51,53] Liver transplant recipients are uniquely predisposed to disseminated invasive aspergillosis, which occurs in 50% to 60% of cases.[54] The mortality rate from invasive aspergillosis in liver transplant recipients ranges from 65% to 90%; requirement of dialysis and CMV infection constitute independent predictors of mortality.[53]

Abdominal Infections in Liver Transplant Recipients

Transplantation of the liver differs from other transplant operations in the length and difficulty of the surgery and the frequency of bleeding problems. In addition, many liver transplant recipients have poor nutrition and severe metabolic difficulties. Abdominal infections after liver transplantation are often related to technical aspects and complications of the operation.[5,55] For example, anastomosis of the biliary duct to a Roux-en-Y loop of jejunum is associated with more intra-abdominal infections, especially invasive fungal infections, than is primary anastomosis of the donor's to the recipient's common bile duct.[5,47]

Most *liver abscesses* in the transplanted liver are related to surgical problems such as biliary stricture or hepatic artery thrombosis.[5] The abscesses may be either solitary or multiple. They manifest as a febrile illness with bacteremia and leukocytosis. The organisms responsible are gram-negative enteric bacilli, enterococci, and anaerobes. The diagnosis is made by ultrasonography or computed tomography. Treatment with drainage and intravenous antibiotics is usually successful, provided the source is biliary infection and any structural abnormalities can be corrected. If hepatic artery thrombosis is the predisposing factor, the infectious symptoms can usually be controlled with antibiotics, but retransplantation may ultimately be necessary.

Cholangitis after liver transplantation also results from technical problems. The most common predisposing problem is biliary stricture. Patients with strictures may have periodic bouts of cholangitis. Some patients improve after dilatation procedures or stent placement, but in others operative repair is necessary. It may not be easy to make a firm diagnosis of cholangitis, because many patients do not manifest the classic Charcot triad of fever, abdominal pain, and jaundice. The clinical presentation may resemble hepatic rejection. The diagnosis is more reliable if bacteremia is present or if a liver biopsy indicates pericholangitis with aggregates of neutrophils around bile ducts. Empirical treatment for cholangitis should include antibiotics to cover gram-negative enteric bacilli, enterococci, and anaerobes. Procedures such as T-tube cholangiography and endoscopic retrograde cholangiopancreatography may be followed by cholangitis and occasionally by bacteremia. Therefore, a single dose of a prophylactic antibiotic is recommended.

Peritonitis can accompany other intra-abdominal infections and frequently complicates biliary leaks or disruption of an abdominal viscus. Bile peritonitis may occur after extraction of a T-tube. It is often well tolerated and may resolve by itself, but occasionally the leak persists and the chemical peritonitis becomes secondarily infected. The most common organisms involved in peritonitis are enterococci and aerobic enteric gram-negative rods, but staphylococcal and candidal

infections are not infrequent. Treatment of established peritonitis requires prolonged antibiotic therapy, together with drainage of associated abscesses and repair of technical problems such as biliary leaks.

Abdominal abscesses are usually found in patients who have had frequent or lengthy abdominal operations.[5] Only about one third of abdominal abscesses are associated with bacteremia. The location is frequently in the subhepatic space, but splenic, pericolic, and pelvic abscesses are also seen. Most patients with abscesses have undergone an abdominal operation within the preceding 30 days.[5] One third of abscesses are polymicrobial. Although common enteric organisms cause most abscesses, coagulase-positive or coagulase-negative staphylococci are also seen. Imaging studies (computed tomography, ultrasound) usually define the location of the abscess. As with any other abscesses, the appropriate treatment is a combination of drainage and antibiotics directed against the responsible pathogens. Fever is part of the clinical presentation in most cases, but some abscesses, especially those caused by *Candida,* may not cause significant fever.

PANCREAS TRANSPLANT RECIPIENTS

About 1300 pancreas transplant operations are performed in the United States annually, or approximately 1 for every 10 renal transplantations.[1] Current patient and graft survival rates are similar to those for kidney transplantation alone, but infection-related morbidity is higher.[1,56] A formal comparison of infections after isolated kidney and combined kidney-pancreas transplantation showed more wound complications and CMV disease among the patients receiving combined organs.[56]

The postoperative infection rate and the causative pathogens depend primarily on the technique used for drainage of exocrine secretions of the pancreas. In recent years, the practice of draining these secretions into the small bowel (enteric drainage) has gained precedence over the previous practice of drainage into the bladder.[57] Enteric drainage has been associated with lower rates of urinary tract infection.[58] However, intra-abdominal infections remain a significant complication of enteric drainage procedures, and aerobic and anaerobic enteric flora predominate in abscesses associated with enteric drainage.[59] The microorganisms found in infections in which the viscus has not been opened are usually from the skin flora.[60] *Candida,* however, is a common pathogen in all types of surgical site infections, including those using bladder drainage.

SMALL BOWEL TRANSPLANT RECIPIENTS

Although small bowel transplantation has been practiced for more than 2 decades, it remains a complex and technically challenging procedure that is performed only at a few centers and in fewer than 200 patients annually. It is used in patients who are dependent on parenteral nutrition for survival because of congenital or acquired intestinal disease or short-gut syndrome after intestinal resection.[61] Current 1-year graft and patient survival rates of 73% and 81%, respectively, appear to be acceptable. However, many patients have slow return of bowel function after the procedure, resulting in prolonged hospitalizations. Rejection episodes cause mucosal injury and may lead to breakdown of the "bowel-blood" barrier with subsequent septic syndromes that may be fatal.[62] This form of transplantation may also be complicated by graft-versus-host disease, presumably as a result of the large amount of lymphoid tissue transplanted with the gut.

More than 90% of small bowel transplant recipients develop significant infections, and the reported rates of infection are higher than in other transplant groups.[61,62] Intra-abdominal pyogenic infections and bloodstream infections predominate, but the transplanted gut, like the transplanted lung, is very susceptible to CMV infection, including a tendency to relapse after successful antiviral treatment.[64] Multivisceral transplant recipients and those undergoing colonic segment transplantation with small bowel transplantation are more likely to develop infections.[63] It is noteworthy that small bowel transplant recipients also remain very susceptible to infections in the late post-transplantation period (i.e., >6 months after operation).[63] The incidence of EBV-associated lymphoproliferative disorders approaches 10%, and the tumors often involve the gut.[61]

Sites and Types of Infection

INFECTIONS OF THE SKIN AND WOUND INFECTIONS

Infections of the skin are common after transplantation but are rarely life-threatening. They constitute a significant nuisance to the transplant recipient, and they may indicate the presence of serious systemic infection. The most important pathogens are listed in Table 312-4.

All solid organ transplant recipients are at risk for wound infections. The reported incidence of wound infections varies from center to center and among types of transplantation; it is highest in liver and pancreas transplant recipients, intermediate in lung and heart-lung recipients, and lowest in heart and renal transplant recipients.[4,5,11,16,27,31,38,57] The most common isolate is *S. aureus,* but infections with gram-negative enteric bacteria, *S. epidermidis, Candida* spp., and *M. hominis* may also be seen. Rarely, mucormycosis can cause a surgical wound infection in a transplant recipient.[4] In such cases, the wound is typically black from tissue infarction caused by fungal invasion of the blood vessels. Tissue biopsy is required for a definitive diagnosis, and therapy should include wide surgical débridement.

The most common cutaneous viral infections are those caused by HSV and varicella-zoster virus (discussed later). Warts are a common problem and may be extensive in patients who survive more than 1 decade after transplantation. They usually are treated with surgery, including electrosurgery or cryosurgery, or by the application of chemical agents such as podophyllin.

Dermatophyte infections usually respond to topical antifungals, but systemic therapy may be required for severe cases. Subcutaneous infections caused by *Alternaria, Exophiala,* and other darkly pigmented or dematiaceous fungi are encountered occasionally.[65] They manifest as mildly tender nodular lesions. Most infections spread locally without dissemination. Biopsy with fungal culture is required for a specific diagnosis. Therapy must be individualized, but a combination of resection and therapy with an oral azole such as itraconazole is often effective.[65]

Mycobacterium chelonae causes pigmented nodular skin lesions that occur singly or in groups, often on the extremities. About half of the cases are multifocal at presentation.[66] The skin is also a target organ for many systemic infections. Systemic bacterial, fungal, nocardial, mycobacterial, and CMV infections may include skin manifestations. As a rule, one should aggressively investigate any new and unusual skin lesion with a biopsy.

INFECTIONS OF THE URINARY TRACT

Urinary tract infections were discussed earlier, in the section on kidney transplant recipients.

INFECTIONS OF THE BLOODSTREAM

The basic approach to bacteremia is the same whether or not the patient has undergone transplantation. The first step is to ascertain the source of the bacteremia. Common sites producing bacterial bloodstream infections are the lung, the urinary tract, the abdomen (includ-

ing the biliary tract), soft tissues, and intravenous catheters. The inability to pinpoint a source is not rare, especially in liver transplant recipients.[5,25] In one large study of bacteremia in multiple transplant groups at a single institution, the overall mortality rate was 23%.[25] Mortality was highest among heart recipients and lowest among kidney recipients. Risk factors for mortality were the presence of a gram-negative or polymicrobial infection, onset of infection early after transplantation, the presence of pneumonia, and impaired kidney and liver function.

The source of bacteremia varies with the type of transplantation and is most commonly related to the transplantation site (see Table 312-2). For example, 41% to 50% of the bacteremias in kidney recipients come from the urinary tract or from perinephric sources.[25] Bacteremia in kidney recipients is relatively uncommon in the very early post-transplantation period (14 days) but relatively more common in the late post-transplantation period.

Among 101 liver recipients monitored for longer than 1 year, 33 bacteremias occurred in 26 patients.[5] Thirty-six percent of the bacteremias had a fatal outcome. The most common source was the abdomen (33%), followed by the urinary tract (21%), the surgical wound (9%), intravenous catheters (6%), and the lung (6%). Twenty-one percent of the bacteremias had no documented source, but most of these probably originated in the abdomen. Gram-negative enteric bacilli were the most common isolates in this and another contemporaneous series.[45] In recent years, bacteremia has continued to be a major problem, but the spectrum of bloodstream isolates has shifted, and resistant gram-positive organisms, such as methicillin-resistant staphylococci and vancomycin-resistant enterococci, now predominate.[67]

Hofflin and colleagues noted a decline in the incidence of bacteremia from 29% to 15% in heart transplant patients at Stanford University after a change to cyclosporine-based immunosuppression.[3] The isolates were equally divided between gram-negative and gram-positive bacteria. In subsequent years, the incidence of bacteremia continued to decline. In a later survey of infections among heart transplant recipients from the same institution, only 38 bacteremias were documented in 620 patients. There was also a shift in the type of organism isolated: 80% of bacteremias in the later study were caused by gram-positive organisms, with a predominance of staphylococcal species.[30]

Bacteremia was documented in 56 lung recipients at four transplant centers over 3½ years. The incidence was 11.5% among the 305 patients who received their transplants during the study interval. Infection in the lung or in a vascular catheter accounted for 88% of the bacteremias. Almost half of the isolates, whether gram-positive or gram-negative, exhibited resistance to multiple antibiotics.[68] The overall mortality rate was 25%, and mortality was associated with concurrent mechanical ventilation and altered mental status.

INFECTIONS IN THE CHEST

The usual microbial causes of pneumonia in the transplant recipient are listed in Table 312-3. They are subdivided according to whether the pneumonia occurs during the first month after transplantation or later and whether the cause is common or less common. The key to the management of lung infections in transplant recipients is rapid identification of the responsible pathogen and initiation of specific therapy. Patients with a brief duration of symptoms (3 days) who have a focal chest infiltrate and are producing sputum with neutrophils on Gram stain are likely to have a routine bacterial pneumonia. Empirical therapy to cover common typical and atypical bacterial pathogens can be started while culture results are awaited. Patients who have an illness lasting longer than 7 days, who have a nonproductive cough, or who have diffuse infiltrates or nodular lesions on chest imaging are more likely to be infected with an unusual or opportunistic pathogen, and consideration should be given to the use of invasive techniques to make the diagnosis. Invasive workup is also indicated for patients who are deteriorating rapidly or appear to have a conventional pneumonia but are not responding to treatment.

TABLE 312-4	Skin Pathogens in Solid Organ Transplant Recipients	
Staphylococcus aureus	*Mycobacterium chelonae*
Herpes simplex virus	*Candida* spp.
Varicella-zoster virus	Dematiaceous fungi
Papillomavirus	Dermatophytes

The reported frequency of *Legionella* infection varies widely, depending on its endemicity in the hospital and the sensitivity of diagnostic methods.[69] Even if *Legionella* organisms are absent from the nosocomial environment, sporadic community-acquired cases can occur among transplant recipients, because *Legionella* infection accounts for 2% to 15% of community-acquired pneumonias.[69] The radiographic presentation is variable and may include focal infiltrates spreading to multiple lobes, globular pleural-based lesions, lung abscess, pleural effusion, or pericardial effusion. Any one of the serotypes of *L. pneumophila* or *L. micdadei* may be responsible. Legionellosis in transplant patients should be treated with azithromycin or a quinolone antibiotic.[69]

Infections caused by *Aspergillus, Nocardia,* or endemic mycoses may be relatively common in some localities. The environmental factors determining these occurrences are poorly understood. *Aspergillus* infections usually are diagnosed in patients who have recently received high doses of corticosteroids, but *Nocardia* infections and endemic mycoses often occur in patients receiving baseline levels of immunosuppression. Community-acquired respiratory viruses such as respiratory syncytial virus (RSV) may cause pneumonia in transplant recipients. They are a greater problem for lung recipients than for patients with other types of solid organ transplants.[42-44]

ABDOMINAL AND GASTROINTESTINAL INFECTIONS

Intra-abdominal infections in liver transplant recipients have already been discussed. These infections also occur at increased frequency among recipients of pancreas and small bowel transplants.[55,56,63] They are less common after transplant operations that do not involve the abdomen. When they do occur, they are usually related to preexisting medical conditions, such as biliary stones or diverticulosis.

Studies in developing countries show that transplant recipients are very susceptible to *Salmonella* infection, but infections caused by *Shigella* or *Campylobacter* do not appear to be increased in frequency.[70] *Clostridium difficile* colitis has emerged as one of the most common causes of diarrhea in transplant recipients who are heavily treated with antibiotics.[70-72] Toxic megacolon may develop in 5% to 12%, and recurrent colitis in approximately 22% of organ transplant recipients who have *C. difficile* colitis. *Helicobacter* infection has been associated with the occurrence of a low-grade gastric lymphoma, called MALToma, in a small number of transplant recipients.[73] Most of these tumors have regressed after reduction of immunosuppression and use of antibiotic therapy to treat the *Helicobacter* infection.

Hyperinfection and disseminated infection with *Strongyloides stercoralis* were substantial problems in the past but appear to have virtually disappeared.[8] Universal pretransplantation screening of stools for *Strongyloides* is probably not cost-effective, but vigilance for this infection should be maintained for patients from endemic areas.

Hepatitis

The most important causes of hepatitis in transplant recipients are hepatitis B virus (HBV), HCV, and CMV. In many respects, CMV is the least important cause of hepatitis, because the infection is usually mild and never leads to chronic hepatitis. Liver transplant candidates with chronic HBV infection routinely reinfect their allografts. In the 1980s, survival rate 5 years after transplantation for such patients was only about 50%.[74] Reinfection rates after transplantation have been lower and outcomes better in patients with fulminant hepatitis B infection and in those with hepatitis D coinfection, but these represent only a minority of the patients with HBV infection. In the past, many transplant centers considered chronic hepatitis B infection to be a contraindication to liver transplantation.[75]

In the current era, the outlook for patients at risk for recurrent HBV infection after liver transplantation has been greatly improved by the availability of agents able to prevent or treat this recurrence and the development of quantitative molecular techniques to measure the hepatitis B viral load in the blood. The first advance occurred in the late 1980s, when it was shown that regular infusions of hepatitis B

immunoglobulin (HBIG) after liver transplantation in HBV-infected patients substantially reduced their rate of HBV recurrence, to approximately 30%, and improved mortality.[75] The addition of an antiviral agent active against HBV to the HBIG regimen further reduced the rate of HBV recurrence, to less than 10%, and brought the long-term survival of HBV-infected patients in line with that of patients without HBV infection.[74]

How best to manage HBV infection in liver transplantation remains an area of active research, but the main issue now is not whether to give preventive therapy but how to simplify the HBIG and antiviral regimens and reduce costs.[74,75] Lamivudine is an attractive choice for antiviral treatment because of its tolerability and relatively low cost. When used alone, it has been associated with a 25% to 50% rate of resistance development related to mutations in the YMDD motif of the DNA polymerase, but the rates of resistance are much lower when lamivudine is used with HBIG. For patients who do develop resistance to lamivudine, there has been a proliferation of other antiviral agents active against HBV. Adefovir is the best studied of these agents, and it is active against lamivudine-resistant mutants, but entecavir, tenofovir, emtricitabine, and telbivudine are also active and will likely play an increasing role in the future.[74,75] Whatever agents are used, it is important to monitor HBV viral loads after transplantation to detect breakthrough infection before clinical consequences develop. It has been recommended that antiviral therapy against HBV be modified whenever a persistent elevation of the viral load (>3 log copies/mL) is detected.[74]

The presence of chronic HBV infection was also shown in a recently published meta-analysis to adversely influence long-term outcomes after kidney transplantation.[76] This appeared to be due, in part, to a higher rate of death from underlying cirrhosis and hepatocellular carcinoma in the HBV-infected patients.[76] This finding underscores the importance of carefully evaluating hepatitis serology and liver function in patients presenting as candidates for transplantation of organs other than the liver.

HCV infection occurs in all transplant groups, but the prevalence is highest among liver and kidney transplant recipients.[13,77] A small number (4% to 7%) of HCV-infected transplant recipients (of all organ types) develop progressive fatal cholestatic liver disease during the first year after transplantation. These cases are marked by a high viral load, and liver biopsies show severe hepatocyte dropout with minimal parenchymal inflammation.[78] The long-term outcome of other HCV-infected patients depends to some extent on the organ transplanted. Liver transplant candidates who have HCV viremia before transplantation almost always reinfect their liver grafts after transplantation, and 46% to 97% develop hepatitis during the first 2 to 3½ years after transplantation.[13] This ongoing HCV infection leads to graft cirrhosis in up to 30% of patients by 5 years after transplantation. Findings from the National Institute of Diabetes and Digestive and Kidney Diseases (NIDDK) liver transplantation database have shown that long-term outcomes (>5 years) after liver transplantation for HCV are similar to those after liver transplantation for other indications.[78] However, a retrospective analysis of more than 10,000 liver recipients in the UNOS database showed that medium-term survival of HCV-infected patients was inferior to that of uninfected patients.[79] Longitudinal studies in kidney transplant populations have also shown that chronic HCV infection has an adverse impact on survival, but this effect is not clearly discernible until the second decade after transplantation.[80] Excess deaths are due not only to the direct effects of liver disease, but also to a higher rate of sepsis.[81]

There is great interest in discovering factors that predict the progression of liver disease due to HCV infection in transplant recipients. Some of the implicated factors in liver transplantation are the degree of immunosuppression, the use of antirejection therapy, high viral loads before or early after transplantation, older donor age, CMV infection, and, in some studies, infection with HCV type 1b.[82] Although the choice of a calcineurin inhibitor and use of mycophenolate mofetil have not been conclusively shown to have an effect on HCV recurrence rates, higher cumulative exposure to corticosteroids is associated with increased mortality and more severe histologic recurrence of HCV.[82]

Antiviral treatment of recurrent HCV infection after liver transplantation is under active investigation. Interferon-alfa monotherapy produces end-of-treatment responses in only 12% to 36% of liver recipients with HCV infection, but very few patients have sustained responses 6 months later.[13] The use of combination therapy with long-acting pegylated interferons and ribavirin has led to sustained virologic response rates of 26% to 50%.[13] Based on these data, pegylated interferon with or without ribavirin is the treatment of choice for histopathologically documented hepatitis C recurrence, but there are differences of opinion on optimal timing and selection of patients for treatment.[13,82] In actual practice, interferon and ribavirin have side effects that make them difficult to administer to liver transplant recipients, so that only a small proportion of the patients are actually able to benefit from their use.

Hepatitis E virus (HEV) is endemic in many developing countries of the world. The virus is a small, non-enveloped RNA virus that is transmitted by the fecal-oral route and was thought to cause only an acute hepatitis. Recently, however, acute HEV infection was shown to progress to a chronic hepatitis in 8 of 14 organ transplant recipients.[83] Currently, there are no effective preventive or therapeutic options for HEV infection.

INFECTIONS OF THE CENTRAL NERVOUS SYSTEM

Infections of the central nervous system (CNS) in transplant patients require prompt evaluation and diagnosis and early, appropriate therapy. Table 312-5 lists the most important agents.[84] Notably absent from the list are pyogenic bacteria and HSV, which are otherwise common pathogens in transplant patients at sites outside the nervous system. The highest risk for opportunistic CNS infection is from 1 to 6 months after transplantation; an exception is cryptococcal meningitis, which is often a "late" event.[85]

Listeria monocytogenes is a motile, gram-positive rod that typically causes bacteremia, meningitis, and, at times, cerebritis in immunosuppressed transplant recipients.[86] The Gram stain of the cerebrospinal fluid (CSF) is negative in more than half of the cases. Usually, the diagnosis is made by culturing the organism from CSF or blood. All patients with *Listeria* bacteremia should undergo lumbar puncture, even in the absence of CNS signs, because the mortality rate is much higher when CNS disease is present.[86] This infection responds well to antibiotic therapy, but relapses may occur, and a prolonged course of therapy (3 weeks) is recommended.

Aspergillus fumigatus is a ubiquitous fungus that is an important cause of CNS infection in immunocompromised patients. The most common portal of entry is the lung; invasive sinus infection also occurs but is less common. Patients with *Aspergillus* infection usually have been recently transplanted and are receiving high doses of corticosteroids. The type of transplant is also important: lung and liver transplant recipients are more susceptible than other transplant patients.[9,84,40] *Aspergillus* is an angiotropic mold, and hematogenous spread to the brain can occur early in the course of the infection. *Aspergillus* is the most common cause of infectious brain lesions in the early post-transplantation period.[84] Computed tomography scans of the brain reveal single or multiple low-density lesions with a predilection for the gray-white junction. In the past, the mortality rate of CNS aspergillosis was almost 100% (see Chapter 258).[40] The recent introduction of new

antifungal agents with enhanced activity against *Aspergillus* may help to improve the dismal prognosis of invasive CNS aspergillosis.

Other fungi that have caused parenchymal brain infections in transplant recipients include *Candida* spp, *Mucorales,* and dematiaceous fungi such as *Cladophialophora*.[65,84] The lesions caused by *Candida* usually occur in patients with disseminated candidiasis or candidemia. The overall mortality rate is high in patients with CNS infection caused by *Mucorales* or dematiaceous fungi, and therapy with a combination of antifungal medication and surgical resection is generally recommended.[65,84]

Cryptococcal meningitis usually occurs in the late post-transplantation period and has a subacute course. Pulmonary disease caused by *Cryptococcus* coexists in about 40%, and fungemia is present in 33% to 35% of the cases.[87] A lumbar puncture should be performed in any patient with cryptococcosis, even in the absence of CNS signs. The spinal fluid usually has less than 500 white blood cells per milliliter with lymphocyte predominance and a positive cryptococcal antigen test.[84,85] India ink preparations reveal positive findings in 40% to 50% of patients. Serum cryptococcal antigen is positive in 88% to 98% of transplant recipients with CNS cryptococcosis.[85,87-90]

Up to 33% of the patients with CNS cryptococcosis have CNS lesions due to *Cryptococcus* on neuroimaging.[87] New lesions developing after initiation of antifungal therapy may represent immune reconstitution syndrome, an inflammatory tissue response that results from improvement in cellular immunity after reduction or cessation of immunosuppression and reversal of *Cryptococcus*-associated immunosuppression.[90] Overall mortality in solid organ transplant recipients with cryptococcosis in the current era is approximately 15% to 20%.[88] In a case series of 28 solid organ transplant recipients with cryptococcal meningitis, mortality correlated with altered mental status, absence of headache, and liver failure, with the latter factor being an independent predictor for death.[85] More recently, receipt of calcineurin inhibitors has been shown to be independently associated with a lower mortality rate in transplant recipients with cryptococcosis.[88] These improved outcomes may be attributable in part to the synergistic interactions of calcineurin inhibitors with antifungal azoles.[88]

Toxoplasma gondii is a protozoan that can cause a nonspecific encephalopathy, diffuse meningoencephalitis, or progressive single or multiple brain lesions.[84] *Toxoplasma* infection has been reported in all types of solid organ transplantation but has most often been described in cardiac transplantation, because the organism can become encysted in cardiac muscle after primary infection. The donor heart can then become a source of infection to a non-immune cardiac recipient.[34] Serology should be performed on cardiac donors and recipients to identify patients at risk for disease transmitted by the allograft. The fatality rate is high, and often the diagnosis is not established until autopsy. The treatment of choice is pyrimethamine (50 to 75 mg/day) and sulfadiazine (4 to 6 g/day). Folinic acid (5 to 15 mg/day) is usually added to the regimen to prevent marrow suppression.

Nocardia asteroides is a gram-positive, beaded, branching rod that may cause single or multiple brain abscesses or, less commonly, meningitis. For unknown reasons, the incidence of pulmonary nocardiosis varies considerably among centers.[86] The primary portal of infection is pulmonary, with metastatic spread to bone, skin, and CNS. *Nocardia* brain abscesses may benefit from stereotactic biopsy and surgical drainage in addition to long-term (9- to 12-month) antimicrobial therapy. Sulfonamides are the mainstay of treatment, because they penetrate the CNS well and most isolates are susceptible. In the presence of disseminated disease, it may be prudent to use more than one drug and to perform susceptibility testing on isolates. Agents such as amikacin, imipenem, and cefotaxime have shown good activity in animal models, with more rapid killing than sulfonamides.[91]

Specific Problems of Virus Infections

This section covers most issues related to viral infections in transplant recipients. Hepatitis viruses were discussed earlier, in the section on abdominal and gastrointestinal infections. The complex topics of anti-

TABLE 312-5	Pathogens of the Central Nervous System in Solid Organ Transplant Recipients
Listeria monocytogenes	Dematiaceous fungi
Nocardia spp.	*Toxoplasma gondii*
Cryptococcus neoformans	Varicella-zoster virus
Aspergillus spp.	Polyomavirus (JC virus)
Agents of mucormycosis	Human herpesvirus-6
Candida spp.	

viral prophylaxis and the pretransplantation evaluation of candidate recipients and donors are discussed in Chapter 310.

Human herpesvirus-6 (HHV-6) is a recently described cause of fever and leukopenia in transplant recipients.[92] This virus is the etiologic agent of roseola and is associated with febrile seizures in children. Evidence of prior HHV-6 infection has been documented in 87% to 91% of solid organ transplant recipients. Therefore, most HHV-6 disease in transplant recipients is considered to be caused by reactivation infection. Overall, 38% to 55% of renal, 22% to 54% of liver, and 36% to 57% of the heart or heart-lung transplant recipients develop HHV-6 infection.[92,93] Most patients with HHV-6 infection are asymptomatic, but a few develop fever and leukopenia.

HERPES SIMPLEX VIRUS AND VARICELLA-ZOSTER VIRUS INFECTIONS

HSV reactivates after transplantation in approximately 60% of recipients not given antiviral prophylaxis.[11,12,17,18] About half of these persons develop symptomatic oral or genital lesions. Genital herpes may become clinically evident for the first time after transplantation and can be very distressing for the patient. Reactivation of HSV usually occurs during the first 1 to 2 weeks after transplantation. Visceral infection caused by HSV has been reported in a small number of patients; most cases have been HSV hepatitis after liver transplantation or HSV pneumonia after lung transplantation.[10,12] A rare event is primary HSV infection occurring early after transplantation; the donor organ has been shown to be the source in a few patients.[12] These primary HSV infections may produce a severe septic syndrome with hypotension and disseminated intravascular coagulation.[12]

Most cases of reactivated HSV infection are easily diagnosed and respond well to antiviral therapy. Use of antiviral prophylaxis prevents HSV infection; it is a reasonable approach and is preferred in patients who are at risk for visceral HSV infection, such as lung or liver transplant recipients. Low-dose acyclovir (400 mg twice daily) for the first 3 to 4 weeks after transplantation is usually sufficient.

Herpes zoster is reported in 7% to 18% of patients.[11,12,17,30,94] Induction therapy with T cell antibodies was an independent predictor for the development of herpes zoster in one study.[94] Antiviral therapy is indicated, because healing is often slow, and transplant recipients occasionally develop neurologic complications or disseminated infection. Oral therapy with acyclovir, valacyclovir, or famciclovir suffices for dermatomal zoster. If the patient has ophthalmic zoster or there is evidence of dissemination, intravenous acyclovir is used initially. Chickenpox in a transplant patient also usually requires admission to the hospital and treatment with intravenous acyclovir, although some pediatric heart transplant recipients on low doses of immunosuppression have been successfully treated for chickenpox with oral valacyclovir.[95] Obtaining serology results for varicella-zoster virus before transplantation identifies patients at risk for chickenpox, so that they can be considered for vaccination and counseled to avoid (and report) exposures.[12] Varicella-seronegative transplant recipients who are exposed to chickenpox may benefit from the use of varicella-zoster immune globulin if it can be given within 96 hours (see Chapter 307).[12]

CYTOMEGALOVIRUS INFECTIONS

In the absence of any form of preventive therapy, CMV infection (evidence of culturable virus or viral proteins or nucleic acid) occurs in 36% to 100% and symptomatic disease in 11% to 72% of solid organ transplant recipients. Primary infections occurring in seronegative recipients with a seropositive donor are more likely to be symptomatic.[17,96,97] The proportion of infected patients who become symptomatic is also a function of the intensity of immunosuppression.

The most common and least serious type of CMV disease is a mononucleosis syndrome characterized by fever, frequently of prolonged duration, with few or no focal symptoms. Abnormalities may be found on liver function tests, although jaundice rarely occurs, and leukopenia is often present. Tissue-invasive disease may manifest as pneumonitis,

gastrointestinal disease, or hepatitis. In this era when prolonged antiviral prophylaxis is routinely employed, CMV disease in organ transplant recipients often is a late manifestation, and up to 60% of these cases have tissue-invasive disease.[97] Interstitial pneumonia is the most serious complication of CMV infection and is present in most fatal cases. Fever, dyspnea, hypoxemia, and diffuse infiltrates on chest radiographs are typical findings but are not pathognomonic, and bronchoalveolar lavage or lung biopsy is required for diagnosis. CMV pneumonia may coexist with other pathogens in the lung, particularly *Pneumocystis*.

One of the more troublesome manifestations of CMV disease is ulcerations in the gastrointestinal tract. These ulcerations are often multiple. They may be found anywhere from the esophagus to the rectum.[70,98] Severe complications such as bleeding or perforation occur in some patients. CMV disease should be considered in the differential diagnosis of transplant recipients who have fever and acute or subacute abdominal symptoms, especially if transplantation occurred within the last 4 to 6 months or there was a recent intensification of immunosuppression. The exact frequency with which CMV causes gastrointestinal disease is difficult to determine, because a definite diagnosis depends on endoscopy, and CMV may involve inaccessible parts of the bowel.[70]

CMV hepatitis occurs in up to 17% of liver transplant recipients and is more common with primary than with reactivation infection.[99] The pathologic finding is microabscesses scattered around the liver lobule. CMV inclusion bodies may be easy to find or scant. The disease is typically mild and may be an incidental finding in asymptomatic patients undergoing liver biopsy to evaluate elevation of their liver enzymes.[99]

Intravenous ganciclovir is the preferred agent for the treatment of symptomatic CMV disease in transplant recipients. The duration of therapy is usually about 2 weeks, but this may be extended to 3 weeks or longer in patients with severe disease or primary infection. In patients with CMV disease and viremia, therapy should be continued until resolution of CMV viremia, because the risk of relapse is lower in patients who do not have detectable CMV DNA after ganciclovir therapy. Although ganciclovir is proven to be effective, its administration requires parenteral access. A large, randomized, multicenter trial (the VICTOR study) demonstrated that oral valganciclovir is safe and has long-term outcomes comparable to those of intravenous ganciclovir for the treatment of CMV disease in organ transplant patients.[100] Foscarnet and cidofovir are also active against CMV but are used infrequently in solid organ recipients because of their side effects. These agents may be effective alternatives to ganciclovir in patients with ganciclovir-resistant CMV.

The greatest advance in regard to CMV infection in transplantation in recent years has been the development of accurate and reproducible quantitative methods to assess viral load and the implementation of effective prophylactic and preemptive regimens to prevent disease caused by CMV. These topics are discussed in Chapter 310.

RESPIRATORY VIRAL INFECTIONS

Respiratory viral infections received little mention in early reports of infections after solid organ transplantation but are now recognized to be important pathogens.[42,43,101] The recent availability of polymerase chain reaction (PCR) techniques to detect viruses is playing an important role in helping to diagnose and study these infections.[102,103] Most reports of severe respiratory virus infection are from pediatric transplant populations or lung transplant recipients.[42,43,101-103] Adenoviruses may cause asymptomatic infection, but they also can cause diffuse pneumonia, necrotizing hepatitis, and hemorrhagic cystitis.[43,101] In one series of pediatric liver transplant recipients, the mortality rate of invasive adenovirus infection was 45%.[101] Antiviral agents such as ribavirin and cidofovir have been used to treat adenovirus infection, but their effectiveness remains uncertain.

Infections with paramyxoviruses, such as RSV, should be considered in the differential diagnosis whenever a transplant recipient has a respiratory tract illness, particularly if the patient has preceding upper respiratory symptoms, the physical examination shows prominent airway findings such as wheezing and rhonchi, and no definite bacterial etiology can be established. Most cases occur between November and April, but parainfluenza virus type 3 infections occur year round. Ribavirin is active against RSV, and the aerosolized preparation has been well tolerated when used to treat RSV lung infection in stem cell and lung transplant populations. Available studies suggest that it may be a helpful agent, but conclusive proof of efficacy is lacking.[42,104]

Influenza has been documented frequently in transplant patients in recent studies. At one center, influenza was 10 to 20 times more common among lung recipients than recipients of other transplants.[105] Influenza was very morbid but usually was not fatal. Influenza pneumonia appears to be rare, and the main threat, as in immunocompetent patients, is bacterial superinfection. Transplant patients and their household contacts should be given yearly immunizations against influenza. Consideration should also be given to providing antiviral prophylaxis to high-risk patients during outbreaks of influenza.[105]

POLYOMAVIRUS INFECTIONS AND NEPHROPATHY

Polyomavirus infection of the urinary tract was first described in a renal transplant recipient almost 40 years ago, and subsequent studies have shown that polyomaviruses can be detected in up to 60% of renal transplant patients.[106] For more than 2 decades after the discovery of these viruses, they were occasionally associated with transient renal dysfunction or ureteral stenosis. In the last 15 years, polyomaviruses have emerged as important pathogens and have been shown to cause an infectious nephropathy, in 2% to 8% of renal transplant recipients, that frequently leads to graft failure.[107] In almost all cases, the responsible polyomavirus has been BK virus. JC virus and SV40 have been detected as a cause of nephropathy in a few patients, but their pathogenic role is less well established.[108]

It is not known why BK nephropathy has emerged only recently. The usual explanation is the introduction of new, very potent, immunosuppressive medications.[106] BK virus primarily infects renal tubular cells, producing intranuclear "ground-glass" inclusions accompanied by an interstitial nephritis.[106,108] Despite this inflammatory nephritis, patients with polyomavirus nephropathy do not have fever or any other symptoms of infection and present with only a rising serum creatinine concentration.[106] Polyomaviruses may be detected in the patient's urine by a variety of techniques, including culture, cytology, electron microscopy, and PCR. Mere detection of virus in the urine, however, has low specificity for the presence of polyomavirus nephropathy.[106-108]

The specificity of PCR diagnosis can be enhanced substantially by looking for the virus in plasma and by performing quantitative PCR.[107] Even with these refinements, however, a definite diagnosis of polyomavirus nephropathy requires a renal biopsy.[106] Figure 312-3 illustrates the typical light microscopic appearance of polyomavirus nephropathy, with enlarged, virally infected tubular cells and an associated interstitial infiltrate.

The renal dysfunction associated with polyomavirus infection often improves or stabilizes if immunosuppression is decreased, but between one third and one half of patients still progress to kidney failure.[108] Some transplant centers monitor patients for polyomavirus and preemptively reduce immunosuppression if viral levels are high. In one well-conducted, prospective study, this appeared to be an effective way to prevent nephropathy, but follow-up was limited to the first year after transplantation.[109] Antiviral agents such as cidofovir and leflunomide have been reported to be useful therapies in anecdotal reports, but solid evidence that these agents are effective is lacking.[106]

Progressive multifocal leukoencephalopathy (PML) occurs in patients with impairment of T-cell immunity and is caused by JC virus.[108] Unlike the situation in acquired immunodeficiency syndrome (AIDS), in which PML occurs in 4% to 5% of patients with very low CD4 counts, PML is a rare occurrence after transplantation. Patients develop profound neurologic deficits that can include various motor, sensory, visual, or cognitive findings occurring over a subacute course of weeks to months. A brain biopsy is required for a definitive diag-

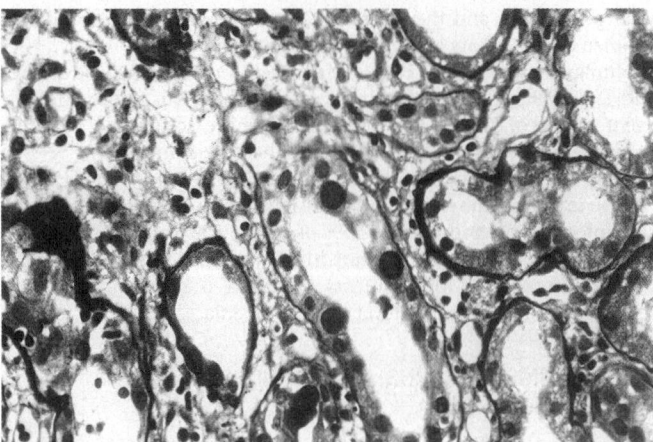

Figure 312-3 Characteristic histologic appearance of BK nephropathy in the kidney. The tubular cells have smudgy, basophilic intranuclear inclusions, and there is a pleomorphic cellular infiltrate of lymphocytes, plasma cells, and occasional neutrophils in the interstitium. (Jones silver stain; ×400). (*Courtesy of Agnes B. Fogo, MD.*)

nosis, but the diagnosis is strongly suggested by the finding of characteristic white matter changes on magnetic resonance imaging (MRI) and JC virus DNA by PCR in the CSF.[108]

HUMAN HERPESVIRUS-8 AND KAPOSI'S SARCOMA

Unlike other herpesviruses, HHV-8 infection is relatively geographically restricted. The highest seroprevalence for HHV-8 is found in central and southern Africa, the Middle East, and European countries bordering the Mediterranean.[110] HHV-8 infection has been strongly linked to the occurrence of Kaposi's sarcoma after transplantation, and most cases occur in patients who are seropositive before transplantation. Current estimates are that about 15% of HHV-8–seropositive patients develop Kaposi's sarcoma during the first 3 years after transplantation.[110] Transmission of HHV-8 by organ donation with subsequent development of Kaposi's sarcoma has also been documented but accounts for fewer cases.[111] Almost all transplant recipients with Kaposi's sarcoma present with mucocutaneous lesions; gastrointestinal lesions are seen in about 50% of patients, and lung or lymph node involvement occurs in about 20%.[110]

Up to one half of transplant patients with Kaposi's sarcoma experience regression of their tumors after their doses of immunosuppressive drugs are substantially reduced. Switching immunosuppression from a calcineurin inhibitor to sirolimus has also been associated with tumor regression.[110] Patients who do not respond to a change in immunosuppression require chemotherapy. Mortality ranges from 10% to 60% depending on the degree of visceral involvement.

LYMPHOPROLIFERATIVE DISEASE AND EPSTEIN-BARR VIRUS INFECTION

Primary EBV infection occurs in about three fourths of seronegative pediatric or adult transplant recipients.[112-114] Reactivation infection, defined by a serologic rise to EBV viral capsid antigen, is detected in about one third of seropositive transplant recipients. Most infections occur within the first 4 months after transplantation.[114] The most important disease associated with EBV infection in transplant recipients is post-transplantation lymphoproliferative disorder (PTLD). Most patients with PTLD (80% to 90%) have evidence of EBV infection. by serologic rises or by measurement of EBV viral load in saliva or peripheral blood.[113,115] The risk for PTLD is 10- to 76-fold higher in transplant recipients who are EBV-seronegative before transplantation than in patients who are seropositive.[113] For instance, we found that

35% of 40 adult EBV-seronegative liver transplant recipients developed PTLD during follow-up.[14] This compares with a PTLD rate of only 2% in EBV-seropositive adult liver transplant recipients and underscores the importance of assessing pretransplantation serology for EBV.[112,113] The other major risk factor for PTLD is the use of high doses of immunosuppression, especially polyclonal or monoclonal antibody formulations directed against T cells.[113] The detection of high viral loads of EBV in the blood by PCR has been associated with a high risk for PTLD in some studies, but the predictive power of this finding needs to be validated in larger, prospective studies.[113]

PTLD is very variable in its presentation.[113,114] It may resemble infectious mononucleosis without evidence of tissue involvement except in tonsils and peripheral lymph nodes. A second manifestation is a diffuse polymorphous B-cell infiltration in many visceral organs. This type may be preceded by a mononucleosis-like episode that either evolves directly into the tissue infiltrative process or is temporally separated from it. The third clinical presentation is the appearance of localized extranodal lymphomas in the gastrointestinal tract, thorax, or other parts of the body, including the brain. These are mostly B-cell lymphomas and usually contain EBV genome detectable by nucleic acid hybridization or EBV-specific antigens detectable by immunohistochemistry. The tumors may be either monoclonal or oligoclonal, as determined by immunoglobulin G (IgG) light-chain phenotype or immunoglobulin gene rearrangement studies.[116]

Antiviral medications such as acyclovir and ganciclovir inhibit the lytic phase of EBV infection and virion production, but they are not able to affect the replication of cells latently infected with EBV.[113] There is no definite evidence that the use of antiviral medications provides any benefit in treating or preventing PTLD, but theoretical considerations and data from some retrospective studies suggest that post-transplantation antiviral prophylaxis may decrease the overall incidence of PTLD.[113,117] Reduction or elimination of immunosuppression may lead to regression of PTLD in about one half of cases.[113,116] Regression is more likely with tumors that appear during the first year after transplantation and with those that are polymorphous in appearance or contain tumor cells that are polyclonal by laboratory studies.[113,116] However, there is no prognostic indicator that is entirely reliable. Treatment of PTLD by infusion of monoclonal antibodies directed against surface antigens of B cells is a theoretically attractive approach and has achieved initial remissions in about two thirds of patients with PTLD.[113] Tumors with more malignant phenotypes require chemotherapy. The infusion of human leukocyte antigen (HLA)-compatible, EBV-specific cytotoxic T lymphocytes (CTLs) has been found to be an effective treatment in cases of PTLD occurring in marrow recipients.[113] Autologous EBV-specific CTLs have also been expanded in vitro from solid organ transplant recipients with PTLD, but clinical experience using these cells for therapy is still very limited.[118]

REFERENCES

1. United Network for Organ Sharing. *The 2007 Annual Report of the U.S. Organ Procurement and Transplantation Network and the Scientific Registry of Transplant Recipients: Transplant Data 1997-2006.* Rockville, MD: Health Resources and Services Administration, Healthcare Systems Bureau, Rockville, MD, Division of Transplantation; 2007.*
2. Dummer JS. Antibiotic prophylaxis and management of infectious complications. In: Kaye MP, O'Connell JB, eds. *Heart Lung Transplant 2000.* Austin, TX: R.G. Landes; 1993:78.
3. Hofflin JM, Potasman I, Baldwin JC, et al. Infectious complications in heart transplant patients receiving cyclosporine and corticosteroids. *Ann Intern Med.* 1987;106:209.
4. Wajszczuk CP, Dummer JS, Ho M, et al. Fungal infections in liver transplant recipients. *Transplantation.* 1985;40:347.
5. Kusne S, Dummer JS, Singh N, et al. Infections after liver transplantation: An analysis of 101 consecutive cases. *Medicine (Baltimore).* 1988;67:132.
6. Kusne S, Fung J, Alessiani M, et al. Infections during a randomized trial comparing cyclosporine to FK 506 immunosuppression in liver transplantation. *Transplant Proc.* 1992;24:429.
7. Kirklin JK, Naftel DC, Bourge RC, et al. Evolving trends in risk profiles and causes of death after heart transplantation: A ten-year multi-institutional study. *J Thorac Cardiovasc Surg.* 2003; 125:881.
8. Fishman JA. Infection in solid-organ transplant recipients. *N Engl J Med.* 2007;357:2601.
9. Kusne S, Torre-Cisneros J, Manez R, et al. Factors associated with invasive lung aspergillosis and the significance of positive *Aspergillus* culture after liver transplantation. *J Infect Dis.* 1992; 166:1379.
10. Maurer JR, Tullis E, Grossman RF, et al. Infectious complications following lung transplantation. *Chest.* 1992;101:1056.
11. Dummer JS. Infectious complications of transplantation. *Cardiovasc Clin.* 1990;20:163.
12. Miller GG, Dummer JS. Herpes simplex and varicella zoster viruses: Forgotten but not gone. *Am J Transplant.* 2007;7:741.
13. Berenguer M. Management of hepatitis C virus in the transplant patient. *Clin Liver Dis.* 2007;11:355.
14. Manez R, Breinig MC, Linden P, et al. Posttransplant lymphoproliferative disease in primary Epstein-Barr virus infection after liver transplantation: The role of cytomegalovirus disease. *J Infect Dis.* 1997;176:1462.
15. Duncan AJ, Dummer JS, Paradis IL, et al. Cytomegalovirus infection and survival in lung transplant recipients. *J Heart Lung Transplant.* 1991;10:638.
16. Dummer JS. Infectious complications of heart-lung recipients. In: Cooper DKC, Novitzky D, eds. *The Transplantation and Replacement of Thoracic Organs.* Lancaster, England: Kluwer; 1990:325.
17. Singh N, Dummer JS, Kusne S, et al. Infections with cytomegalovirus and other herpesviruses in 121 liver transplant recipients: Transmission by donated organ and the effect of OKT3 antibodies. *J Infect Dis.* 1988;158:124.
18. Ho M, Wajszczuk CP, Hardy A, et al. Infections in kidney, heart, and liver transplant recipients on cyclosporine. *Transplant Proc.* 1983;15:2768.
19. Wagener MM, Yu VL. Bacteremia in transplant recipients: A prospective study of demographics, etiologic agents, risk factors and outcomes. *Am J Infect Control.* 1992;20:239.
20. Abbott KC, Swanson SJ, Richter ER, et al. Late urinary infection after renal transplantation in the United States. *Am J Kidney Dis.* 2004;44:353
21. Giral M, Pascuariello G, Karam G, et al. Acute graft pyelonephritis and long-term kidney allograft dysfunction. *Kidney Int.* 2002;61:1880.
22. Tolkoff-Rubin NE, Rubin RH. Urinary tract infection in the immunocompromised host: Lessons from kidney transplantation and the AIDS epidemic. *Infect Dis Clin North Am.* 1997; 11:707.
23. McMahon DK, Dummer JS, Pasculle AW, et al. Extragenital *Mycoplasma hominis* infections in adults. *Am J Med.* 1990;89: 275.
24. Superdock KR, Dummer JS, Koch MO, et al. Disseminated histoplasmosis presenting as urinary tract obstruction in a renal transplant recipient. *Am J Kidney Dis.* 1994;23:600.
25. Ramsey PG, Rubin RH, Tolkoff-Rubin NE, et al. The renal transplant patient with fever and pulmonary infiltrates: Etiology, clinical manifestations, and management. *Medicine (Baltimore).* 1980;59:206.
26. Chang FY, Singh N, Gayowski T, et al. Fever in liver transplant recipients: Changing spectrum of etiologic agents. *Clin Infect Dis.* 1998;26:59.
27. Humar A, Ramcharan T, Denny R, et al. Are wound complications after a kidney transplant more common with modern immunosuppression? *Transplantation.* 2001;72:1920.
28. Brayman KL, Stephanian E, Matas AJ, et al. Analysis of infectious complications occurring after solid-organ transplantation. *Arch Surg.* 1992;127:38.
29. Rubin RH. Infection in the organ transplant patient. In: Rubin RH, Young LS, eds. *Clinical Approach to Infection in the Immunocompromised Host.* 4th ed. New York: Springer; 2002:573.
30. Montoya JG, Giraldo LF, Efron B, et al. Infectious complications among 620 consecutive heart transplant patients at Stanford University. *Clin Infect Dis.* 2001;33:629.
31. Baldwin RT, Radovancevic B, Sweeney MS, et al. Bacterial mediastinitis after heart transplantation. *J Heart Lung Transplant.* 1992;11:545.
32. Goldstein DJ, Oz MC, Rose EA. Medical progress: Implantable left ventricular assist devices. *N Engl J Med.* 1998;329:1522.
33. Bocchi EA, Fiorelli A. The paradox of survival results after heart transplantation for cardiomyopathy caused by *Trypanosoma cruzi.* First Guidelines Group for Heart Transplantation of the Brazilian Society of Cardiology. *Ann Thoracic Surg.* 2001;71:1833.
34. Luft BJ, Naot Y, Araujo FG, et al. Primary and reactivated toxoplasma infection in patients with cardiac transplants: Clinical spectrum and problems in diagnosis in a defined population. *Ann Intern Med.* 1983;99:27.
35. Peleg AY, Husain S, Qureshi ZA, et al. Risk factors, clinical characteristics and outcome of *Nocardia* infection in organ transplant recipients: A matched case-control study. *Clin Infect Dis.* 2007;44:1307
36. Diez M, Favaloro L, Bertolotti A, et al. Usefulness of PCR strategies for early diagnosis of Chagas' disease reactivation and treatment follow-up in heart transplantation, *Am J Transplant.* 2007;7:1633.
37. Paterson DL, Dominguez EA, Chang FY, et al. Infective endocarditis in solid organ transplant recipients. *Clin Inf Dis.* 1998;26:689.
38. Thomas LD, Dummer JS. Bacterial infections and *Pneumocystis* infection. In: Lynch JP, Ross D, eds. *Lung and Heart-Lung Transplantation.* New York: Marcel Dekker; 2006:587.
39. Kramer MR, Marshall SE, Starnes VA, et al. Infectious complications in heart-lung transplantation: Analysis of 200 episodes. *Arch Intern Med.* 1993;153:2010.
40. Singh N, Paterson DL. *Aspergillus* infections in transplant recipients. *Clin Microbiol Rev.* 2005;18:44.
41. Estenne M, Hertz MI. Bronchiolitis obliterans after human lung transplantation. *Am J Respir Crit Care Med.* 2002;166: 440.
42. Englund JA, Piedra PA, Whimbey E. Prevention and treatment of respiratory syncytial virus and parainfluenza viruses in immunocompromised patients. *Am J Med.* 1997;102(Suppl 3A):61.
43. Bridges ND, Spray TL, Colins MH, et al. Adenovirus infection in the lung results in graft failure after transplantation. *J Thorac Cardiovasc Surg.* 1998;116:617.
44. Speich R, van der Bij W. Epidemiology and management of infections after lung transplantation. *Clin Infect Dis.* 2001;33 (Suppl 1):S58.
45. George DL, Arnow PM, Fox AS, et al. Bacterial infection as a complication of liver transplantation: Epidemiology and risk factors. *Rev Infect Dis.* 1991;13:387.
46. Castaldo P, Stratta R, Wood P. Clinical spectrum of fungal infections complicating liver transplantation. *Arch Surg.* 1991;126:149.
47. Collins LA, Samore MH, Roberts MS, et al. Risk factors for invasive fungal infections complicating orthotopic liver transplantation. *J Infect Dis.* 1994;170:644.
48. Alexander J, Limaye AP, Ko CW, et al. Association of hepatic iron overload with invasive fungal infection in liver transplant recipients. *Liver Transpl.* 2006;12:1799.
49. Singh N, Wagener MM, Marino IR, et al. Trends in invasive fungal infections in liver transplant recipients: Correlation with evolution in transplantation practices. *Transplantation.* 2002;73:63.
50. Husain S, Tollemar J, Dominguez EA, et al. Changes in the spectrum and risk factors for invasive candidiasis in liver

*The data and analyses in The 2007 Annual Report of the U.S. Organ Procurement and Transplantation Network and the Scientific Registry of Transplant Recipients have been supplied by UNOS and Arbor Research under contract with HHS. The authors alone are responsible for the reporting and interpretation of the data; the views expressed herein are those of the authors and not necessarily those of the U.S. Government.

transplant recipients: Prospective, multicenter, case-controlled study. *Transplantation*. 2003;75:2023.
51. Fortun J, Martin-Davila P, Moreno S, et al. Risk factors for invasive aspergillosis in liver transplant recipients. *Liver Transpl*. 2002;8:1065.
52. Paya CV. Fungal infections in solid-organ transplantation. *Clin Infect Dis*. 1993;16:677.
53. Singh N, Avery RK, Munoz P, et al. Trends in risk profiles for and mortality associated with invasive aspergillosis among liver transplant recipients. *Clin Infect Dis*. 2003;36:46.
54. Singh N, Limaye AP, Forrest G, et al. Combination of voriconazole and caspofungin as primary therapy for invasive aspergillosis in solid organ transplant recipients: A prospective, multicenter, observational study. *Transplantation*. 2006;81:302.
55. Lebeau G, Yanaga K, Marsh JW, et al. Analysis of surgical complications after 397 hepatic transplantations. *Surg Gynecol Obstet*. 1990;170:317.
56. Rosen CB, Frohnert PP, Velosa JA, et al. Morbidity of pancreas transplantation during cadaveric renal transplantation. *Transplantation*. 1991;51:123.
57. Auchincloss H, Shaffer D. Pancreas transplantation. In: Ginns LC, Cosimi AB, Morris PJ, eds. *Transplantation*. Malden, MA: Blackwell Science; 1999:395.
58. Pirsch JD, Odorico JS, D'Allesandro AM, et al. Posttransplant infection in enteric- versus bladder-drained simultaneous pancreas-kidney transplant recipients. *Clin Transplant*. 1998;66:1746.
59. Berger N, Guggenbichler S, Steurer W, et al. Bloodstream infection following 217 consecutive systemic-enteric drained pancreas transplants. *BMC Infect Dis*. 2006;6:127.
60. Lumbreras C, Fernandez I, Velosa J, et al. Infectious complications following pancreatic transplantation: Incidence, microbiological and clinical characteristics, and outcome. *Clin Infect Dis*. 1995;20:514.
61. Grant D. Intestinal transplantation: Report of the international registry 1997. *Transplantation*. 1999;67:1061.
62. Loinaz C, Kato T, Nishida S, et al. Bacterial infections after intrestine and multivisceral transplantation: The experience of the University of Miami (1994-2001). *Hepatogastroenterology*. 2006;53:234.
63. Kusne S, Furukawa H, Abu-Elmagd K, et al. Infectious complications after small bowel transplantation in adults: An update. *Transplant Proc*. 1996;28:2761.
64. Kusne S, Manez R, Frye BL, et al. Use of DNA amplification for diagnosis of cytomegalovirus enteritis after intestinal transplantation. *Gastroenterology*. 1997;112:1121.
65. Singh N, Feng YC, Gayowski T, et al. Infections due to dematiaceous fungi in organ transplant recipients: Case report and review. *Clin Infect Dis*. 1997;24:369.
66. Wallace RJJ, Brown BA, Onyi GO. Skin, soft tissue and bone infections due to *Mycobacterium chelonae chelonae:* Importance of prior corticosteroid therapy, frequency of disseminated infections and resistance to antimicrobials other than clarithromycin. *J Infect Dis*. 1992;166:405.
67. Newell KA, Millis JM, Arnow PM, et al. Incidence and outcome of infection by vancomycin-resistant *Enterococcus* following orthotopic liver transplantation. *Transplantation*. 1998;65:439.
68. Husain S, Chan KM, Palmer SM, et al. Bacteremia in lung transplant recipients in the current era. *Am J Transplant*. 2006;6:3000.
69. Stout JE, Yu VL. Legionellosis. *N Engl J Med*. 1997;337:682.
70. Dummer JS, Mishu, B. Gastrointestinal infections in organ transplant recipients. In Blaser M, Smith PD, Ravidin JI, et al, eds. *Infections of the Gastrointestinal Tract*. 2nd ed. Philadelphia: Lippincott Williams & Wilkins; 2002:457.
71. Keven K, Basu A, Re L, et al. *Clostridium difficile* colitis in patients after kidney and pancreas-kidney transplantation. *Transpl Infect Dis*. 2004;6:10.
72. Stelzmueller I, Goegele H, Biebl M, et al. *Clostridium difficile* colitis in solid organ transplantation: A single-center experience. *Dig Dis Sci*. 2007;52:3231.
73. Aull MJ, Buell JF, Peddi VR, et al. MALToma: A *Helicobacter pylori*-associated malignancy in transplant patients. A report from the Israel Penn International Transplant Tumor Registry with a review of published literature. *Transplantation*. 2003;75:225.
74. Coffin CS, Terrault NA. Management of hepatitis B in liver transplant recipients. *J Viral Hepatitis*. 2007;14(Suppl 1):37.
75. Roche B, Samuel D. Treatment of hepatitis B and C after liver transplantation. Part 1: Hepatitis B. *Transpl Int*. 2005;17:746.
76. Fabrizi F, Martin P, Dixit V, et al. HBsAg seropositive status and survival after renal transplantation: Meta-analysis of observational studies. *Am J Transplant*. 2005;5:2913.
77. Kliem V, van den Hoff U, Brunkhorst R, et al. The long-term course of hepatitis C after kidney transplantation. *Transplantation*. 1996;62:1417.
78. Charlton M, Ruppert K, Belle SH, et al. Long-term results and modeling to predict outcomes in recipients with HCV infection: Results of the NIDDK liver transplantation database. *Liver Transpl*. 2004;10:1120.
79. Forman LM, Lewis JD, Berlin JA, et al. The association between hepatitis C infection and survival after liver transplantation. *Gastroenterology*. 2002;122:689.
80. Gane E, Pilmore H. Management of chronic viral hepatitis before and after renal transplantation. *Transplantation*. 2002; 74:427.
81. Legendre C, Garrigue V, Le Bihan C, et al. Harmful long-term impact of hepatitis C virus infection in kidney transplant recipients. *Transplantation*. 1998;65:667-670.
82. Charlton M. Natural history of hepatitis C and outcomes following liver transplantation. *Clin Liver Dis*. 2003;7:585.
83. Kamar N, Selves J, Mansuy JM, et al. Hepatitis E virus and chronic hepatitis in organ-transplant recipients. *N Engl J Med*. 2008;358:811.
84. Singh N, Husain S. Infections of the central nervous system in transplant recipients. *Transplant Infect Dis*. 2000;2:101.
85. Wu G, Vilchez RA, Eidelman B, et al. Cryptococcal meningitis: An analysis among 5,521 consecutive organ transplant recipients. *Transpl Infect Dis*. 2002;4:183.
86. Dummer JS. Other bacterial infections after hematopoietic stem cell or solid organ transplantation. In: Bowden R, Paya CV, Ljungman P, Engelhard D, eds. *Transplant Infections*. 2nd ed. Philadelphia: Lippincott Williams & Wilkins; 2003:259-276.
87. Husain S, Wagener MM, Singh N. *Cryptococcus neoformans* infection in organ transplant recipients: Variables influencing clinical characteristics and outcome. *Emerg Infect Dis*. 2001;7:375.
88. Singh N, Alexander BD, Lortholary O, et al. *Cryptococcus neoformans* in organ transplant recipients: Impact of calcineurin-inhibitor agents on mortality. *J Infect Dis*. 2007;195:756
89. Singh N, Lortholary O, Dromer F, et al. Central nervous system cryptococcosis in solid organ transplant recipients: Prognostic implications of cryptococcal antigen assay and abnormal neuroimaging findings. *Transplantation*. 2008;86:647.
90. Singh N, Lortholary O, Alexander BD, et al. An "immune reconstitution syndrome"-like entity associated with *Cryptococcus neoformans* infection in organ transplant recipients. *Clin Infect Dis*. 2005;40:1756.
91. Gombert ME, Aulicino TM, duBouchet L, et al. Therapy of experimental cerebral nocardiosis with imipenem, amikacin, trimethoprim-sulfamethoxazole, and minocycline. *Antimicrob Agents Chemother*. 1986;30:270.
92. Ljungman P, Singh N. Human herpesvirus-6 infection in solid organ and stem cell transplant recipients. *J Clin Virol*. 2006;37:S87.
93. Seeley WW, Marty FM, Holmes TM, et al. Post-transplant acute limbic encephalitis clinical features and relationship to HHV-6. *Neurology*. 2007;69:156.
94. Gourishankar S, McDermid JC, Jhangri GS, et al. Herpes zoster infection folowing solid organ transplantation: Incidence, risk factors and outcomes in the current immunosuppressive era. *Am J Transplant*. 2004;4:108.
95. Dodd DA, Burger J, Edwards KM, et al. Varicella in a pediatric heart transplant population on nonsteroid immunosuppression. *Pediatrics*. 2001;108:E80.
96. Ho M. *Cytomegalovirus: Biology and Infection*. 2nd ed. New York: Plenum Press; 1991:249-256.
97. Sun HY, Wagener MM, Singh N. Prevention of posttransplant cytomegalovirus disease and related outcomes with valganciclovir: A systematic review. *Am J Transplant*. 2008;8:2111.
98. Dummer JS, White LT, Ho M, et al. Morbidity of cytomegalovirus infection in recipients of heart or heart-lung transplants who received cyclosporine. *J Infect Dis*. 1985;152:1182.
99. Paya CV, Hermans PE, Wiesner RH, et al. Cytomegalovirus hepatitis in liver transplantation: Prospective analysis of 93 consecutive orthotopic liver transplantations. *J Infect Dis*. 1989;160:752.
100. Asberg A, Humar A, Rollag H. Oral valganciclovir is noninferior to intravenous ganciclovir for the treatment of cytomegalovirus disease in solid organ transplant recipients *Am J Transplant*. 2007;7:2106.
101. Michaels MG, Green M, Wald ER, et al. Adenovirus infection in pediatric liver transplant recipients. *J Infect Dis*. 1992;165:170.
102. Garbino J, Gerbase MW, Wunderli W, et al. Lower respiratory viral illnesses: Improved diagnosis by molecular methods and clinical impact, *Am J Respir Crit Care Med*. 2004;170:1197.
103. Milstone AP, Brumble LM, Barnes J, et al. A single season prospective study of respiratory viral infections in lung transplant recipients. *Eur Respir J*. 2006;28:131.
104. McCurdy LH, Milstone A, Dummer S. Clinical features and outcomes of paramyxoviral infection in lung transplant recipients treated with ribavirin. *J Heart Lung Transpl*. 2003;22:745
105. Vilchez RA, Fung J, Kusne S. The pathogenesis and management of influenza virus infection in organ transplant recipients. *Transplant Infect Dis*. 2002;4:177.
106. Randhawa P, Brennan DC. BK virus infection in transplant recipients: An overview and update. *Am J Transplant*. 2006;6:2000.
107. Hirsch HH, Knowles W, Dickenmann M, et al. Prospective study of polyoma type BK replication and nephropathy in renal-transplant recipients. *N Engl J Med*. 2002;347:488.
108. Kwak EJ, Vilchez RA, Randhawa P, et al. Pathogenesis and management of polyomavirus infection in transplant patients. *Clin Infect Dis*. 2002;35:1081.
109. Brennan DC, Agha I, Bohl DL, et al. Incidence of BK with tacrolimus versus cyclosporine and impact of pre-emptive immunosuppression reduction. *Am J Transplant*. 2005;5:582.
110. Lebbe C, Legendre C, Frances C, et al. Kaposi sarcoma in transplantation. *Transpl Rev (Orlando)*. 2008;22:252.
111. Regamey N, Tamm M, Wernli M, et al. Transmission of human herpesvirus-8 infection from renal transplant donors to recipients. *N Engl J Med*. 1998;339:1358-1363.
112 Ho M, Jaffe R, Miller G, et al. The frequency of Epstein-Barr virus infection and associated lymphoproliferative syndrome after transplantation and its manifestations in children. *Transplantation*. 1988;45:719.
113. Preiksaitis JK, New developments in the diagnosis and management of posttransplantation lymphoproliferative disorders in solid organ transplant recipients. *Clin Inf Dis*. 2004;39:1016.
114. Breinig MK, Zitelli B, Starzl TE, et al. Epstein-Barr virus, cytomegalovirus and other viral infections in children after liver transplantation. *J Infect Dis*. 1987;156:273.
115. Rowe DT, Qu L, Reyes J, et al. Use of quantitative competitive PCR to measure Epstein-Barr virus genome load in the peripheral blood of pediatric transplant patients with lymphoproliferative disorders. *J Clin Microbiol*. 1997;35:2852.
116. Starzl TE, Nalesnik MA, Porter KA, et al. Reversibility of lymphomas and lymphoproliferative lesions developing under cyclosporin-steroid therapy. *Lancet*. 1984;1:583.
117. Funch DP, Walker AM, Schneider G, et al. Ganciclovir and acyclovir reduce the risk of post-transplant lymphoproliferative disorder in renal transplant recipients. *Am J Transplant*. 2005;5:2894.
118. Khanna R, Bell S, Sherritt M, et al. Activation and adoptive transfer of Epstein-Barr virus-specific cytotoxic T cells in solid organ transplant patients with posttransplant lymphoproliferative disease. *Proc Natl Acad Sci. U S A*. 1999;96:10391.

Infections in Patients with Spinal Cord Injury

RABIH O. DAROUICHE

Much has changed since ancient Egyptians viewed spinal cord injury as "an ailment not to be treated."[1] By the beginning of the 20th century, however, little was changed, because 80% of United States soldiers who fought in World War I died within the first 2 weeks after sustaining spinal cord injury (SCI).[2] The first signs of important progress became apparent in the 1940s, when comprehensive medical programs were constructed to treat the casualties of World War II.[2] Since then, the management of SCI patients has dramatically improved, resulting in almost normal life expectancy at the present time.

More than 250,000 Americans currently suffer from the consequences of SCI and, with an annual incidence of 40 cases/million population, over 11,000 new cases of SCI occur in the United States each year.[3] Because the most common infectious cause of SCI is spinal epidural abscess,[4] the rising incidence of this infection has contributed to the expanding population of SCI patients.[5] Not only can infection cause SCI, but it frequently occurs subsequent to the injury and can result in major morbidity and mortality. Urinary tract infection is the most common infectious complication after both traumatic and nontraumatic SCI.[6]

Most infections that occur in SCI patients also affect able-bodied patients, but the frequency and clinical characteristics of infections vary between these populations. Whereas urinary tract infections are the most common,[7] pneumonia has the highest infection-associated mortality,[8] and infections of pressure sores and underlying bone are probably the most difficult to manage.[9] Although SCI patients are particularly predisposed to infection in the acute setting of the injury, the vast majority of infections occur much later in this population, whose life expectancy is almost similar to that of able-bodied subjects. This chapter addresses the factors that predispose to infection, analyzes the challenges in evaluating patients for infection, discusses the most prominent infections in this population, and assesses multiresistant organisms in the SCI setting.

Factors That Predispose to Infection

SCI does not depress general host immunity. Uninfected individuals with SCI have a normal function of T and B lymphocytes. Although patients with SCI usually have higher levels of inflammatory markers, including C-reactive protein and cytokines such as interleukin-6 and tumor necrosis factor-α, than able-bodied cohorts,[10,11] this difference can be attributed to undetected inflammation or occult infection. However, SCI patients may suffer from complicating conditions (including stress, malnutrition, and renal failure) or receive medications (e.g., high-dose glucocorticosteroids in the acute setting of SCI) that can impair the immune response to infection. More importantly, SCI patients possess unique factors that predispose them to infection of specific body organ systems.

For example, most patients have a neurogenic bladder and suffer from frequent episodes of urinary tract infection attributed to urinary stasis and bladder catheterization. Urinary stasis greatly impairs the naturally protective mechanisms of the urinary tract, such as the washout effect of voiding and the phagocytic capacity of bladder epithelial cells. Even though some techniques of bladder catheterization are safer than others, none can be carried out without the potential risk of introducing organisms into the urinary tract. Both paralytic ileus and abnormal state of consciousness caused by associated head injury and/or illicit drug ingestion can predispose to aspiration pneu-

monia in the acute stage of SCI. In persons with cervical or high thoracic cord lesions, weakness of the diaphragmatic and intercostal muscles impairs the capacity to clear respiratory secretions. Skin breakdown in anesthetic areas, immobility, disuse-induced muscle atrophy, urinary leakage, and fecal contamination predispose to infection of pressure sores.

Frequent insertion in SCI patients of urologic, vascular, orthopedic, respiratory, gastrointestinal, and neurosurgical devices predispose to various prosthesis-related infections. This helps explain why hospital-acquired infections most commonly affect the urinary tract, bloodstream, and musculoskeletal system.[12] Patients with SCI generally have a higher rate of hospital-acquired infections than other groups of patients. About one third of SCI patients develop infection during hospitalization, with an overall incidence of 35 episodes of hospital-acquired infection/1000 hospital-days.

Challenges in Evaluating Patients for Infection

A number of unique challenges can be encountered when attempting to establish diagnosis and provide treatment of infections in the SCI population (Table 313-1). Infection frequently manifests differently in the SCI population than in able-bodied individuals. Altered or absent sensations constitute the single most important impediment to the diagnosis of infection in this population. For example, dysuria, frequency, and urgency, symptoms that are regularly present in able-bodied patients who suffer from urinary tract infection, rarely exist in infected SCI patients. The diagnosis of perinephric abscess is particularly challenging in patients with high sensory levels who do not appreciate flank pain or tenderness.[13] The inability to recognize the signs and symptoms of cord damage contributes to the delay in diagnosing spinal epidural abscess below the level of injury.[5] The diagnostic dilemma caused by the paucity of clinical findings can be heightened by the presence of neurogenic or referred pain that may not be related to the infection. Furthermore, multiple infections occur concurrently in up to 20% of SCI patients. Even more problematic than identifying the source of an infection is discerning whether fever is caused by an infection or noninfectious conditions that may closely mimic infections and cause almost one fifth of episodes of fever in SCI patients.

A diagnostic conundrum may exist when unique thermoregulatory and autonomic disturbances cause fever in SCI patients. Because of the imbalance between heat production and heat loss, patients with an SCI above T8 may not be able to maintain a normal body temperature in response to heating or cooling (poikilothermia).[14] This phenomenon of altered thermoregulation is attributed to the loss of sweating and muscular activity below the spinal cord lesion. These factors may contribute to the occurrence of self-limited febrile episodes in SCI patients that resolve spontaneously within hours to days. However, neither alterations in environmental temperature nor changes in a subject's sweating and muscular activity may explain the occurrence of prolonged fever in recently injured quadriplegic patients who have no identifiable focus of infection.[15] This unique syndrome, so-called quadriplegia fever, lasts weeks to months and is problematic because it may incite repeated evaluation for infection and multiple courses of antibiotics, but to no avail. Rarely, fever may occur in the context of autonomic dysreflexia, a paroxysmal syndrome characterized mainly

TABLE 313-1	Challenges in Evaluating Spinal Cord–Injured Patients for Infection

General Factors

Altered or absent sensations
Interference of neurogenic pain with localization of source of infection
Coexistence of multiple infections
Mimicry of infection by noninfectious conditions
Thermoregulatory and autonomic disturbances
Need for adjusted dosing of vancomycin and aminoglycosides

Infection-Specific Factors

Urinary tract infection
  Almost universal prevalence of bacteriuria
  Value of pyuria as indicator of infection
  Nonspecific manifestations of symptomatic infection
  Investigation of urine cultures growing several bacterial species
Pneumonia
  Impact of ineffective cough on determining microbial cause
  Defective perception of dyspnea and need to evaluate gas exchange
  Eligibility for and efficacy of immunization
Infections of pressure sores
  Limitations of history provided by patient
  Supreme importance of physical findings in diagnosing ulcer infection
  Universal bacterial colonization of pressure sores and unreliability of swab cultures
  Potential reasons for failure to respond to therapy
  Deceptive appearance of sinus tract
Osteomyelitis
  Representative nature of cultured samples
  Possible variations of findings from bones beneath different sores
  Significance of organisms growing from cultures of bone
  Poor predictive value of clinical evaluation
  Appropriateness of imaging studies for diagnosis and for follow-up

by hypertension, sweating, facial flushing, and headache. Occasionally, bradycardia may also be present and can help differentiate febrile episodes of autonomic dysreflexia from infection. This type of autonomic hyperactivity is seen only in patients with SCI above T6 and is usually triggered by distention of viscera (bladder and rectum), cutaneous stimulation (e.g., ingrown toenails), or even infection.

Treatment of infection in SCI patients also poses special challenges. For example, two opposing factors resulting from changes in body composition following SCI can alter the disposition of systemically administered antibiotics, such as vancomycin[16] and aminoglycosides.[17] On the one hand, patients with SCI have an expanded extracellular volume attributed to retention of extracellular water as subclinical edema and replacement of decreased skeletal muscle mass by extracellular water. As a result, these patients have a larger weight-adjusted volume of distribution of drugs and may require larger weight-adjusted loading and maintenance doses than able-bodied counterparts to achieve similar antibiotic concentrations. This potential effect on antibiotic concentration can be counteracted, at least in part, by the frequent overestimation of creatinine clearance when using formulas that were originally devised for non-SCI individuals to predict creatinine clearance in patients with chronic SCI who have low serum creatinine levels.[18] The misapplication of such formulas has prompted the evaluation of modified methods for proper administration of vancomycin and other antibiotics in the SCI population.

Urinary Tract Infections

This is the most common infection in patients with SCI and occurs at a rate of 2.5 episodes/patient/year.[7] In patients with chronic indwelling bladder catheters (transurethral or suprapubic), bacteriuria is almost universal (culture of a randomly obtained urine sample is positive in almost 98% of cases). These SCI patients have a higher rate of bacteriuria than those who rely on intermittent bladder catheterization (98% vs. 70%). A longer interval between intermittent bladder catheterizations may be associated with a higher incidence of bacteriuria. Although outpatients may find it more practical to use clean reusable rather than sterile catheters for intermittent bladder catheterization, there is conflicting evidence regarding the value of clean versus sterile bladder catheterization.[19]

Asymptomatic bladder colonization may progress to symptomatic urinary tract infection, but often does not.[20] Typical manifestations of urinary tract infection (including dysuria, urgency, frequency, suprapubic discomfort and, in patients with pyelonephritis, costovertebral angle tenderness) are rarely present in SCI patients. Instead, change in voiding habits, increase in the residual volume of urine in the bladder, foul-smelling urine, worsening of muscular spasticity, and/or aggravation of autonomic dysreflexia are often the only clinical clues to the presence of urinary tract infection. Because of the nonspecificity of these clinical manifestations, other causes should be excluded before diagnosing urinary tract infection. Although the lack of pyuria reasonably predicts the absence of urinary tract infection in SCI patients, pyuria is a nonspecific finding that is also observed in uninfected individuals who have inflammation of the urinary tract caused by catheter manipulations, renal calculi, and interstitial nephritis. Other commonly reported abnormal laboratory findings in the urine, including nitrite and leukocyte esterase, are also not specific for infection.[21] Another diagnostic limitation is that about two fifths of SCI patients incorrectly attribute their bouts of illness to a urinary tract infection (UTI).[22] As with other patient populations who require bladder catheterization, quantification of bacteriuria in SCI patients may not help differentiate between asymptomatic bladder colonization and symptomatic urinary tract infection. As few as 10^2 colony-forming units (CFU)/mL of urine from catheter-dependent patients or 10^4 CFU/mL of urine from catheter-free males using external condoms can be associated with symptomatic UTI.[23]

Most cases of urinary tract infection in SCI patients are caused by commensal organisms of the bowel and perineum, particularly gram-negative bacilli and enterococci.[24] The patient's gender and level of injury may affect the microbiology of organisms residing in the bladder. For example, *Escherichia coli* and *Enterococcus* spp. have been reported to cause more than two thirds of cases of UTI in female patients undergoing intermittent catheterization.[25] In contrast, *Klebsiella pneumoniae* is one of the most common causes of UTI in hospitalized SCI patients,[20] with particularly high prevalence of bacterial strains that exhibit strong type 1 fimbrial-mediated adherence to uroepithelial cells.[26] In that regard, *E. coli* strains that cause urinary tract infection in adult SCI patients may exhibit more virulence factors (e.g., hemolysis and D-mannose–resistant hemagglutination of human erythrocytes) than strains that asymptomatically reside in the bladder of SCI patients or the rectum of healthy volunteers.[27]

The finding of polymicrobial bacteriuria is particularly problematic in SCI patients. Almost half of positive urine cultures in SCI patients grow more than one organism,[28] and polymicrobial bacteriuria can be more prevalent in patients who have chronic indwelling urethral catheters. Although isolation of multiple bacterial species in the general population is often viewed as indicative of contamination, a similar finding in catheter-dependent SCI patients should not be disregarded. Isolation of several uropathogens can be associated with a UTI that fails to respond to antibiotic therapy directed against only one or some of the organisms but is eradicated after providing additional antimicrobial coverage against other isolated organisms. Although most urine cultures are obtained from patients with only lower UTI and in whom the yield of blood cultures is extremely low, the detection of concurrent bacteremia confirms the pathogenicity of organisms isolated from urine culture. Even in patients who have pyelonephritis in association with polymicrobial bacteriuria, isolation of only one organism from blood cultures may not negate the role of other bacteria in causing urinary tract infection. Because it is difficult to differentiate accurately among organisms found in culture that are causing infection and those that are asymptomatic colonizers. it may be reasonable to treat all potentially pathogenic organisms grown from urine cultures in patients diagnosed with infection.

Not since the advent of closed urinary drainage almost a half-century ago have we found a preventive approach that dramatically protects against UTIs. Optimizing urinary drainage and switching, whenever feasible, from indwelling bladder catheter to intermittent bladder catheterization, or even external condom-based drainage, remain the cornerstone of prevention.[9,29] The incidence of bladder stones, a condition associated with UTIs, is also lower in patients who rely on intermittent bladder catheterization versus indwelling bladder catheters.[30] The potential impact of varying the frequency of exchanging indwelling bladder catheters on the incidence of urinary tract infection is yet to be established.[31] The use of a catheter securement device was shown in a prospective, randomized, multicenter clinical trial in SCI patients to reduce catheter-related UTI as compared with traditional catheter care.[32] This benefit was theoretically attributed to limiting the injury to the uroepithelium caused by movement of the indwelling catheter, Although there exist clinical data regarding the ability of some antimicrobial-modified, short-term, indwelling bladder catheters to reduce the rate of bacteriuria in non-SCI patients, there is no evidence, so far, that such catheters can prevent UTIs in SCI patients with long-term indwelling bladder catheters.

Because asymptomatic bacteriuria can progress to symptomatic infection, a number of approaches have been designed to prevent or eradicate asymptomatic bacteriuria. Although the use of antiseptics or antibiotics for prophylaxis in SCI patients could decrease the rate of urinary tract infection caused by organisms susceptible to the administered antimicrobials, the overall incidence of infection caused by all organisms (including organisms susceptible or resistant to the used antimicrobial) is not significantly altered.[33,34] Because of the lack of overall efficacy, drug adverse events, and emergence of antibiotic resistance, prophylactic use of systemic antimicrobials is generally not recommended. Possible exceptions include the presence of struvite urinary stones in association with urea-splitting organisms such as *Proteus mirabilis*[35] and clinical scenarios in which asymptomatic bacteriuria might be associated with complications, as is the case in pregnant patients and those embarking on urologic procedures.[36]

The limited clinical success of traditional preventive measures has prompted the interest in exploring innovative approaches, particularly bacterial interference using a nonpathogenic strain of *E. coli* 83972.[37] Intentional colonization of the neurogenic bladder with a nonpathogenic strain of *E. coli* has been reported in both a prospective open-label[38] and randomized, placebo-controlled, double-blind[39] pilot clinical trials to be safe and protective against the development of UTI. Another potentially protective approach that was recently studied is the use of cranberry dietary supplement in an attempt to inhibit bacterial adherence to the uroepithelium and reduce the biofilm formation by urinary pathogens without altering the urine pH.[40] However, the clinical efficacy of this approach in patients with SCI remains rather controversial because some studies have demonstrated benefit,[40] whereas others did not.[41]

Asymptomatic bacteriuria in catheter-dependent patients should not be treated with systemic antibiotics[42] or bladder irrigation.[43] Optimal management of symptomatic UTI depends on the location of infection and the condition of the host. Analysis of urine samples obtained by ureteral catheterization, the definitive procedure for distinguishing between upper and lower urinary tract infection, is not practical in the clinical setting. Sequential analysis of urine specimens after irrigation of the bladder (bladder washout technique) is not reliable for localizing the site of urinary tract infection because of the frequent occurrence of vesicoureteral reflux in SCI patients. Despite the absence of adequate support in the literature, most physicians suspect pyelonephritis in the presence of high fever, chills, systemic toxicity, or leukocyte casts in urinary sediment.

Results of studies in otherwise healthy individuals indicating that short courses of oral antibiotics (a single large dose or a 3-day course) are efficacious in eradicating uncomplicated lower UTI should not be extrapolated to the SCI population. A prospective, randomized, double-blind, placebo-controlled trial has shown a significantly better response to a 14- versus 3-day course of ciprofloxacin for treatment of lower UTI in SCI patients, but that study excluded subjects with long-term indwelling bladder catheters.[44] In the absence of supportive clinical trials, most catheter-related infections of the neurogenic bladder are treated with a 10-day course of antibiotics. In SCI patients with vesicoureteral reflux, pyelonephritis is likely to occur and is usually treated with a 2-week course of antibiotics. A longer duration of antibiotic therapy (4 to 6 weeks) is advocated for patients with persistent infection, documented relapse of infection, or prostatitis.

In patients with persistent infection, documented relapse of infection (by the same bacterial strain), or frequent reinfections (by different organisms), the urinary tract should be investigated for anatomic abnormalities (e.g., stone, abscess, stricture) and functional alterations (including vesicoureteral reflux and high residual volume of urine in bladder). Although pyuria regresses to normal values (less than 10^4 white blood cells/mL of uncentrifuged urine) after the completion of successful treatment of UTI in SCI patients with intermittent bladder catheterization, above-normal levels of pyuria may persist after treatment of infection associated with indwelling bladder catheters.[45]

Pneumonia

Although generally much less frequent than UTIs, pneumonia is the most common pulmonary complication in the immediate postinjury period[46] and is particularly likely to occur in the first few months after cervical or high thoracic SCI and in quadriplegics and those at least 55 years of age.[8] The relatively high mortality associated with pneumonia makes it the leading cause of death caused by infection in this population.[8] Pneumonia in acutely injured patients is associated with prolonged length of stay and escalated hospital costs.[47] In patients who aspirate gastric contents, pneumonia is usually caused by gram-negative and/or anaerobic bacteria. As is the case in able-bodied persons, bacterial community-acquired pneumonia in SCI patients is mostly caused by *Streptococcus pneumoniae*, *Haemophilus influenzae*, and *Branhamella catarrhalis*.[48] *Staphylococcus aureus* (mostly methicillin-resistant *S. aureus* [MRSA]) and *Pseudomonas aeruginosa* commonly cause pneumonia in mechanically ventilated patients and in those with tracheostomy tubes. Because of defective sensations of respiratory muscle fatigue and altered perceptions of dyspnea, SCI patients with pneumonia may progress to respiratory failure in an unpredictable fashion. Therefore, evaluation of gas exchange, preferably by analysis of arterial blood gases, is strongly recommended when treating pneumonia. Transcutaneous measurement of oxygen saturation may also be used, but with caution, because heated electrodes can produce burns on anesthetized skin.

A number of noninfectious conditions can clinically mimic pneumonia. For example, atelectasis, like pneumonia, commonly occurs because of retained pulmonary secretions early after injury to the cervical or high thoracic cord. In such patients, with altered or absent sensations of chest pain and dyspnea and ineffective cough, the only clinical clues that suggest the diagnosis of pneumonia may include tachypnea, tachycardia, fever, and leukocytosis. However, atelectasis may also be accompanied by an element of low-grade fever and leukocytosis. The site of pulmonary involvement may not help differentiate atelectasis from pneumonia because both conditions predominantly involve the left lung because of the difficulty in suctioning the left main stem bronchus, which branches off at a more acute angle than the right bronchus. Occasionally, bronchoscopy is required for diagnostic and therapeutic purposes.

Another condition that can be clinically confused with pneumonia is pulmonary embolism, which occurs in about 5% of SCI patients, frequently without an identifiable thrombotic source. Although pulmonary embolism can ordinarily be diagnosed by a ventilation-perfusion lung scan, the observed defects on scanning may be uninterpretable in patients who also have atelectasis. In such cases, a pulmonary angiogram may be required for definitive diagnosis. A negative D-dimer test in the blood would reasonably rule out pulmonary embolism. In the acute stage of SCI, associated fracture of a long bone can lead to fat embolism, which may or may not present with the clinical stigmata of petechiae and cerebral dysfunction. Aspiration of gastric contents in the presence of paralytic ileus and an ineffective cough reflex can lead to chemical pneumonitis that mimics bacterial pneumonia; evaluation of an adequate sample of respiratory secretions may help differentiate between these two clinical entities. Finally, pulmonary contusion can be mistaken for pneumonia in the acute setting of SCI.

Because patients with SCI may be at a greater risk of developing pneumonia than able-bodied subjects, it is important to assess the immunization status in such patients. By virtue of age (older than 50 years), chronic respiratory disease, or residence in chronic care facilities, or all of these, almost two thirds of SCI patients are eligible for vaccination against *S. pneumoniae* and influenza viruses. The antibody response to pneumococcal[49] and influenza[50] vaccination of SCI patients is adequate. Notwithstanding the lack of studies that examine the clinical benefit of these vaccinations in this population, it may be justifiable to administer pneumococcal and influenza vaccines to all SCI patients.

Pneumonia in SCI patients is usually treated with a 10- to 14-day course of antibiotic therapy. A quinolone or combination of a macrolide and cephalosporin are adequate for empirical treatment of community-acquired respiratory infections in the absence of aspiration or respiratory devices.[51,52] Coverage for anaerobes, gram-negative bacteria, and MRSA is required for therapy of hospital-acquired aspiration pneumonia. Agents active against MRSA and *P. aeruginosa* should be empirically considered in patients with infections associated with respiratory devices. The reported observation that most antibiotics prescribed for acute respiratory conditions in SCI patients are considered unnecessary underscores the essential role of education in preventing antibiotic abuse.[53]

Infections of Pressure Sores

Local factors that contribute to infection of pressure sores include breaks in the integrity of the skin barrier, pressure-induced changes, and contamination from contiguous dirty areas. Accordingly, pressure sores frequently become infected with staphylococci, streptococci, or gram-negative and/or anaerobic bacteria. Most pressure sores in SCI patients develop in areas adjacent to the ischium, sacrum, and greater trochanter. In paralyzed individuals who cannot directly visualize the ulcers, their history is usually incomplete and the infection is already advanced by the time they seek medical care. Patients with SCI are more likely than the general population to develop Fournier gangrene, the most fearsome necrotizing fasciitis that affects the perineal and genital regions and usually results from polymicrobial infection.[54] Because of the inadequacy of sensations, physical findings, including fever, purulent drainage, and surrounding inflammatory changes such as erythema, swelling, and warmth, are usually relied on to diagnose infection.

Because pressure sores are universally colonized by bacteria, samples for culture should not be obtained unless infection is clinically evident. In patients with seemingly infected pressure ulcers, biopsy of deep tissue may constitute the most reliable means for determining the infectious cause. Cultures of swab specimens from the ulcer or the sinus tract are generally unreliable, and cultures of material obtained by needle aspiration tend to overestimate the number of bacterial isolates. If cellulitis is recognized adjacent to a decubitus ulcer, the challenge to the clinician is to discern the infecting organism(s). Biopsy of deep soft tissue is the most reliable means for determining the microbiologic cause of infection.

A combined medical-surgical approach is often required to establish cure of the infection. The continuous application of negative pressure to deep ulcers by using a vacuum-assisted closure device (VAC) can enhance wound healing in selective patients by removing excessive edema, promoting granulation, and stimulating angiogenesis. Although it is possible that this technique can also facilitate delivery of systemically administered antibiotics to the infected area, the potential benefit of a vacuum-assisted closure device as an adjunct to antibiotic therapy is still unclear.[55] Surgery is done to débride nonviable tissue and drain infected material. A lack of response of infected ulcers to therapy may be the result of inadequate antibiotic therapy, unrecognized soft tissue abscess, communication of the ulcer with an infected bone or joint, or a fistula communicating with the gastrointestinal or urinary tract. The appearance of newly isolated bacterial

species soon after initiating antibiotic therapy probably indicates colonization, and unless there has been an initial response followed by recurrence of fever, these organisms may be ignored. Even in patients with apparently healed ulcers, deep soft tissue abscesses may exist, sometimes causing fever or even bacteremia.

Although the sensitivity of nuclear scans for detecting soft tissue abscesses is generally very high, this test can also be positive in SCI patients who have an infected pressure sore without an associated abscess. Soft tissue abscess in association with an infected sore can be more accurately diagnosed by computed tomography or magnetic resonance imaging than by nuclear scans. Because pressure necrosis affects subcutaneous tissues and muscles more than the skin, the opening of a sinus tract onto the skin may appear deceptively small. Although potentially helpful, probing may not reveal the full depth of the tract. Sinography delineates the full depth of the tract and the potential communication with bone, joint, intra-abdominal abscess, or visceral organs. Injection of dye into the intestines or bladder may also help establish fistulous connections.

Osteomyelitis

Most cases of osteomyelitis in SCI patients occur beneath pressure sores. Less common forms include prosthesis-related, postoperative, hematogenous, and vertebral osteomyelitis. In general, it is difficult to determine whether bone beneath a decubitus ulcer is infected and, if infected, which organisms(s) is responsible. Cultures of a swab specimen from the ulcer are of little value in predicting the causative organisms of osteomyelitis. The definitive diagnosis of osteomyelitis beneath pressure sores requires histopathologic examination of bone tissue.[9] Histopathologic examination of bone specimens obtained by percutaneous needle biopsy demonstrates osteomyelitis beneath about one fifth to one third of pressure sores. Because osteomyelitis is likely to be a focal process and percutaneous bone biopsy may fail to sample infected foci, bone infection can be documented more frequently in patients in whom intraoperative bone biopsy is performed. In patients with multiple pressure ulcers, histopathologic evaluation of a bone specimen from one site may not necessarily reflect the same findings beneath the other ulcers. In addition, even if pathologic findings are similar, bone cultures from various sites may grow different organisms.

Because of the high frequency of bacterial colonization of fibrotic tissue adherent to bone, cultures of bone specimens are positive in most patients in whom histopathologic examination of bone tissue is not compatible with osteomyelitis.[9] Moreover, quantitative bone cultures do not differentiate osteomyelitis from colonization or infection of overlying soft tissue. Therefore, in patients with histopathologic evidence of osteomyelitis, it may be reasonable to direct antibiotic treatment against all organisms that grow from cultures of bone, except those that are usual colonizers, such as *Staphylococcus epidermidis* and diphtheroids. Most cases of osteomyelitis beneath pressure sores are caused by two or more bacterial species, including gram-positive cocci (mainly *S. aureus* and streptococci), gram-negative bacilli (including *P. aeruginosa* and Enterobacteriaceae group), and anaerobes (particularly *Bacteroides* and *Fusobacterium* spp.).

Clinical evaluation poorly predicts the presence of osteomyelitis beneath nonhealing deep pressure sores. In particular, clinical information (duration of ulcer, bone exposure, purulent drainage, fever), laboratory data (e.g., white blood cell count, erythrocyte sedimentation rate), and radiologic findings (plain roentgenograms and technetium bone scans) do not correlate well with the likelihood of finding histopathologic evidence of infection of bone. Nuclear scans are extremely sensitive but poorly specific for diagnosing osteomyelitis beneath pressure sores.[9,56] This low specificity is attributed to the capacity of the injected agent to concentrate in areas of bone in which pressure-induced changes exist or in foci of heterotopic ossification. The most desired finding of a bone scan is a negative result, which would essentially exclude the diagnosis of osteomyelitis beneath pressure sores and obviate the need for bone biopsy. Although magnetic resonance imaging has been successfully used to identify osteomyelitis as the cause of nonhealing pressure ulcers,[57] this diagnostic tool should be used judiciously.

Although failure of decubitus ulcers to heal can result from underlying osteomyelitis,[9] it is more likely to result from noninfectious causes such as pressure-related changes, spasticity, malnutrition, and heterotopic bone ossification. The latter entity can mimic osteomyelitis clinically and radiologically. Heterotopic bone ossification evolves in up to half of SCI patients, particularly those who are completely paralyzed or have pressure sores; usually in the first year after injury there are other inciting phenomena, such as infection or surgery. It can cause warm erythematous swelling of soft tissues, primarily in areas adjacent to the hip and knee. Although the serum alkaline phosphatase level can be elevated early, it is not diagnostic of heterotopic bone ossification because many other proliferative bone processes may also cause an abnormal elevation. Roentgenographic changes are often absent for 1 to 2 weeks after clinical signs appear, but by then a technetium bone scan should reveal increased uptake.

Patients with SCI who have osteomyelitis beneath pressure sores are usually treated with antibiotics and, when indicated, surgery. Even though the ideal duration of antibiotic therapy is not clear, most patients receive at least 4 to 6 weeks of antibiotic therapy. If all infected bone is excised at the time of surgery, which should be confirmed with histopathology, a shorter course of antibiotics may suffice. Although parenteral antibiotics have traditionally been used, oral administration of effective drugs may be preferred. Musculocutaneous flap surgery is preferable to débridement alone because the transposition of a well-vascularized muscle allows more extensive removal of devitalized tissue, enhances the host's defense against infection, and provides a better vascular supply to facilitate bone healing. Diligent care should be given to prevent postoperative flap wound infections that could impair the vitality of the musculocutaneous flap. Patients with improperly treated osteomyelitis may develop deep abscesses and a sinus tract after reconstructive surgery.[58] In patients with recurrent infection or very extensive disease, hemipelvectomy may be considered.[59] Changes on plain roentgenograms and bone scans may persist after what clinically seems to be successful treatment of osteomyelitis.[9]

Other Considerations

BACTEREMIA

Infections of the urinary tract, pressure sores, lungs, and vascular access are the most common identifiable sources of bacteremia in patients with SCI.[60] In bacteremic patients without an apparent source, an occult deep-seated abscess may be the culprit. Bacteremia associated with infections of the urinary tract and long-term hemodialysis access are mostly caused by gram-negative bacilli, whereas staphylococci are the most frequent isolates from blood cultures in patients with infection of pressure sores or short-term vascular access.[61] Because

vascular catheter-related bacteremia is several-fold more likely to be caused by gram-negative bacteria in SCI patients than in the general population,[62] gram-negative coverage should be considered when initiating empirical antibiotic therapy.

INTRA-ABDOMINAL INFECTION

The most common intra-abdominal infections in SCI patients affect the gallbladder or present as abscesses. Cholelithiasis occurs more commonly in SCI patients than in the general population. Although most gallstones may remain asymptomatic, some may cause cholecystitis or migrate down the common bile duct to cause cholangitis or pancreatitis. A ruptured viscus or, less commonly, a fistulous connection with a pressure sore can result in the formation of intra-abdominal abscesses. Intra-abdominal infections may be misdiagnosed, particularly in patients with high cord lesions, because they frequently manifest with abdominal distention, diffuse spasm of abdominal wall musculature, and rigidity on palpation, but no localized abdominal pain or tenderness. Ultrasound examination or computed tomography of the abdomen should help establish the correct diagnosis. Nasogastric tube placement and impaired sinus drainage in the supine position predispose SCI patients to occult maxillary sinusitis.[63]

MULTIRESISTANT ORGANISMS IN THE SCI SETTING

The multiresistant bacteria that have a predilection to affect SCI units more than general nursing wards include MRSA, vancomycin-resistant *Enterococcus* (VRE), gram-negative bacilli that produce extended-spectrum beta lactamase (ESBL), and *Clostridium difficile*. Roommate contacts of patients colonized or infected by any of these multiresistant bacteria are at increased risk for acquiring those organisms.[64]

Of these multiresistant organisms, MRSA is the most common; it is responsible for a large share of both hospital- and community-acquired infections.[65] Although routine decolonization is not necessary, hospital surveillance and strict adherence to infection control practices can blunt the spread of MRSA.[66] Unlike MRSA, which could exist in almost every body organ, VRE is cultured mostly from the urine, particularly in catheter-dependent patients. Although most episodes of growth of VRE from urine cultures represent asymptomatic bacteriuria and do not require antibiotic treatment, VRE colonization and residence in a long-term facility increase the risk for subsequent bacteremia.[67] Catheter-dependent SCI patients are predisposed to develop urinary tract infection caused by ESBL-producing multiresistant gram-negative bacilli, such as *E. coli*, and *Klebsiella pneumoniae*.[68] The frequent administration of antibiotics and relatively inadequate hygiene in SCI patients help explain the high risk of clinical infection by *C. difficile*.[69] In patients with neurogenic bowel and defective sensation, *C. difficile*–associated gastrointestinal disease can remain clinically undetected until a catastrophe such as toxic megacolon or bowel perforation evolves.

REFERENCES

1. Hughes JT. The Edwin Smith Surgical Papyrus: An analysis of the first case reports of spinal cord injuries. *Paraplegia.* 1988;26:71-82.
2. Tulsky D. The impacts of the model SCI system: Historical perspective. *J Spinal Cord Med.* 2002;25:310-315.
3. National Spinal Cord Injury Statistical Center. Spinal cord facts and figures, June 2006 update. *J Spinal Cord Med.* 2007;30:539-540.
4. McKinley W, Merrell C, Meade M, et al. Rehabilitation outcomes after infection-related spinal cord disease: A retrospective analysis. *Am J Phys Med Rehabil.* 2008;87:275-280.
5. Darouiche RO. Spinal epidural abscess. *N Engl J Med.* 2006;355:2012-2020.
6. Tauqir SF, Mirza S, Gul S, et al. Complications in patients with spinal cord injuries sustained in an earthquake in Northern Pakistan. *J Spinal Cord Med.* 2007;30:373-377.
7. Siroky MB. Pathogenesis of bacteriuria and infection in the spinal cord injured patient. *Am J Med.* 2002;113(Suppl. 1A):67S-79S.
8. DeVivo MJ, Kartus PL, Stover SL, et al. Cause of death for patients with spinal cord injuries. *Arch Intern Med.* 1989;149:1761-1766.

9. Darouiche RO, Landon GC, Klima M, et al. Osteomyelitis associated with pressure sores. *Arch Intern Med.* 1994;154:753-758.
10. Davies AI, Hayes KC, Dekaban GA. Clinical correlates of elevated serum concentrations of cytokines and autoantibodies in patients with spinal cord injury. *Arch Phys Med Rehabil.* 2007;88:1384-1393.
11. Wang TD, Wang YH, Huang TS, et al. Circulating levels of markers of inflammation and endothelial activation are increased in men with chronic spinal cord injury. *J Formos Med Assoc.* 2007;106:919-928.
12. Evans CT, LaVela SL, Weaver FM, et al. Epidemiology of hospital-acquired infections in veterans with spinal cord injury and disorder. *Infect Control Hosp Epidemiol.* 2008;29:234-242.
13. Deck AJ, Yang CC. Perinephric abscesses in the neurologically impaired. *Spinal Cord.* 2001;39:477-481.
14. Colachis S, Otis S. Occurrence of fever associated with thermoregulation dysfunction after acute spinal cord injury. *Am J Phys Rehabil.* 1995;74:114-119.
15. Sugarman B. Fever in recently injured quadriplegic persons. *Arch Phys Med Rehabil.* 1982;63:639-640.

16. Griver AR, Prince RA, Darouiche RO. A simple method for administering vancomycin in the spinal cord–injured population. *Arch Phys Med Rehabil.* 1997;78:459-462.
17. Gilman TM, Brunnemann SR, Segal JL. Comparison of population pharmacokinetic models for gentamicin in spinal cord–injured and able-bodied patients. *Antimicrob Agents Chemother.* 1993;37:93-99.
18. Mirahmadi MK, Byrne C, Barton C, et al. Prediction of creatinine clearance from serum creatinine in spinal cord injury patients. *Paraplegia.* 1983;21:23-29.
19. Shekelle PG, Morton SC, Clark KA, et al. Systematic review of risk factors for urinary tract infection in adults with spinal cord dysfunction. *J Spinal Cord Med.* 1999;22:258-272.
20. Darouiche R, Cadle R, Zenon G, et al. Progression from asymptomatic to symptomatic urinary tract infection in patients with SCI: A preliminary study. *J Am Paraplegia Soc.* 1993;16:221-226.
21. Hoffman JM, Wadhwani R, Kelly E, et al. Nitrite and leukocyte dipstick testing for urinary tract infection in individuals with spinal cord injury. *J Spinal Cord Med.* 2004;27:128-132.

22. Linsenmeyer TA, Oakley A. Accuracy of individuals with spinal cord injury at predicting urinary tract infections based on their symptoms. *J Spinal Cord Med.* 2003;26:352-357.

23. National Institute on Disability and Rehabilitation Research (NIDRR) Consensus Statement. The prevention and management of urinary tract infection among people with spinal cord injuries. *J Am Paraplegia Soc.* 1992;15:194-207.

24. Waites KB, Canupp KC, DeVivo MJ. Microbiology of the urethra and perineum and its relationship to bacteriuria in community-residing men with spinal cord injury. *J Spinal Cord Med.* 2004; 27:448-452.

25. Bennett CJ, Young MN, Darrington H. Differences in urinary tract infection in male and female spinal cord injury patients on intermittent catheterization. *Paraplegia.* 1995;33:69-72.

26. Kil KS, Darouiche RO, Hull RA, et al. Identification of a *Klebsiella pneumoniae* strain associated with nosocomial urinary tract infection. *J Clin Microbiol.* 1997;35:2370-2374.

27. Hull RA, Rudy DC, Wieser IE, et al. Virulence factors of *Escherichia coli* isolates from patients with symptomatic and asymptomatic bacteriuria and neuropathic bladders due to spinal cord and brain injuries. *J Clin Microbiol.* 1998;36:115-117.

28. Darouiche RO, Priebe M, Clarridge JE. Limited vs full microbiological investigation for the management of symptomatic polymicrobial urinary tract infection in adult spinal cord-injured patients. *Spinal Cord.* 1997;35:534-539.

29. Esclarin De Ruz A, Garcia Leoni E, Herruzo Cabrera R. Epidemiology and risk factors for urinary tract infection in patients with spinal cord injury. *J Urol.* 2000;164:1285-1289.

30. Weld KJ, Dmochowski RR. Effect of bladder management on urological complications in spinal cord-injured patients. *J Urol.* 2000;163:768-772.

31. Ho CH, Kirshblum S, Linsenmeyer TA, et al. Effects of the routine change of chronic indwelling Foley catheters in persons with spinal cord injury. *J Spinal Cord Med.* 2001;24:101-104.

32. Darouiche RO, Goetz L, Kaldis T, et al. Impact of StatLock securing device on symptomatic catheter-related urinary tract Infection: A prospective, randomized, multicenter clinical trial. *Am J Infect Control.* 2006;34:555-560.

33. Morton SC, Shekelle PG, Adams JL, et al. Antimicrobial prophylaxis for urinary tract infection in persons with spinal cord dysfunction. *Arch Phys Med Rehabil.* 2002;83:129-138.

34. Salomon J, Denys P, Merle C, et al. Prevention of urinary tract infection in spinal cord-injured patients: Safety and efficacy of a weekly oral cyclic antibiotic (WOCA) programme with a 2-year follow-up—an observational prospective study. *J Antimicrob Chemother.* 2006;57:784-788.

35. Hung EW, Darouiche RO, Trautner BW. Proteus bacteriuria is associated with significant morbidity in spinal cord injury. *Spinal Cord.* 2007;45:616-620.

36. Pannek J, Nehiba M. Morbidity of urodynamic testing in patients with spinal cord injury: Is antibiotic prophylaxis necessary? *Spinal Cord.* 2007;45:771-774.

37. Hull R, Rudy D, Donovan W, et al. Urinary tract infection prophylaxis using *Escherichia coli* 83972 in spinal cord-injured patients. *J Urol.* 2000;163:872-877.

38. Darouiche RO, Donovan WH, Del Terzo M, et al. Pilot trial of bacterial interference for preventing urinary tract infection. *Urology.* 2001;58:339-344.

39. Darouiche RO, Thornby JI, Cerra-Stewart C, et al. Bacterial interference for prevention of urinary tract infection: A prospective, randomized, placebo-controlled, double-blind pilot trial. *Clin Infect Dis.* 2005;41:1531-1534.

40. Hess MJ, Hess PE, Sullivan MR, et al. Evaluation of cranberry tablets for the prevention of urinary tract infections in spinal cord injured patients with neurogenic bladder. *Spinal Cord.* 2008;46: 622-626.

41. Lee B, Haran MJ, Hunt LM, et al. Spinal-injured neuroptahic bladder antisepsis (SINBA) trial. *Spinal Cord.* 2007;45:542-550.

42. Nicolle LE, Bradley S, Colgan R, et al. Infectious Diseases Society of America guidelines for the diagnosis and treatment of asymptomatic treatment in adults. *Clin Infect Dis.* 2005;40:643-654.

43. Waites KB, Canupp KC, Roper JF, et al. Evaluation of three methods of bladder irrigation to treat bacteriuria in persons with neurogenic bladder. *J Spinal Cord Med.* 2006;29:217-226.

44. Dow G, Rao P, Harding G, et al. A prospective, randomized trial of 3 or 14 days of ciprofloxacin treatment for acute urinary tract infection in patients with spinal cord injury. *Clin Infect Dis.* 2004;39:658-664.

45. Joshi A, Darouiche RO. Regression of pyuria during the treatment of symptomatic urinary tract infection in patients with spinal cord injury. *Spinal Cord.* 1996;34:742-744.

46. Burns SP. Acute respiratory infections in persons with spinal cord injury. *Phys Med Rehabil Clin North Am.* 2004;42:450-458.

47. Winslow C, Bode RK, Felton D, et al. Impact of respiratory complications on length of stay and hospital costs in acute cervical spine injury. *Chest.* 2002;121:1548-1554.

48. Chang HT, Evans CT, Weaver FM, et al. Etiology and outcomes of veterans with spinal cord injury and disorders hospitalized with community-acquired pneumonia. *Arch Phys Med Rehabil.* 2005;86:262-267.

49. Darouiche RO, Groover J, Rowland J, et al. Pneumococcal vaccination for patients with spinal cord injury. *Arch Phys Med Rehabil.* 1993;74:1354-1357.

50. Trautner BW, Atmar RL, Hulstrom A, et al. Inactivated influenza vaccination for people with spinal cord injury. *Arch Phys Med Rehabil.* 2004;85:1886-1889.

51. Buns SP, Weaver FM, Parada JP, et al. Management of community-acquired pneumonia in persons with spinal cord injury. *Spinal Cord.* 2004; 42:450-458.

52. Lodise TP, Kwa A, Cosler L, et al. Comparison of beta-lactam and macrolide combination therapy versus fluoroquinolone monotherapy in hospitalized Veterans Affairs patients with community-acquired pneumonia. *Antimicrob Agents Chemother.* 2007; 51:3977-3982.

53. Evans CT, Smith B, Parada JP, et al. Trends in antibiotic prescribing for acute respiratory infection in veterans with spinal cord injury and disorder. *J Antimicrob Chemother.* 2005;55:1045-1049.

54. Nambiar PK, Lander S, Midha M, et al. Fournier gangrene in spinal cord injury: A case report. *J Spinal Cord Med.* 2005;28: 121-124.

55. Ford CN, Reinhard ER, Yeh D, et al. Interim analysis of a prospective, randomized trial of vacuum-assisted closure versus the health point system in the management of pressure ulcers. *Ann Plast Surg.* 2002;49:55-61.

56. Melkun ET, Lewis VL Jr. Evaluation of (111) indium-labeled autologous leukocyte scintigraphy for the diagnosis of chronic osteomyelitis in patients with grade IV pressure ulcers, as compared with a standard diagnostic protocol. *Ann Plast Surg.* 2005;54:633-636.

57. Ruan CM, Escobedo E, Harrison S, et al. Magnetic resonance imaging of nonhealing pressure ulcers and myocutaneous flaps. *Arch Phys Med Rehabil.* 1998;79:1080-1088.

58. Han H, Lewis VL Jr, Wiedrich TA, et al. The value of Jamshidi core needle bone biopsy in predicting postoperative osteomyelitis in grade IV pressure ulcer patients. *Plast Reconstr Surg.* 2002;110: 118-122.

59. Chan JW, Virgo KS, Johnson FE. Hemipelvectomy for severe decubitus ulcers in patients with previous spinal cord injury. *Am J Surg.* 2003;185:69-73.

60. Mylotte JM, Graham R, Kahler L, et al. Epidemiology of nosocomial infection and resistant organisms in patients admitted for the first time to an acute rehabilitation unit. *Clin Infect Dis.* 2000;30:425-432.

61. Wall BM, Mangold T, Huch KM, et al. Bacteremia in the chronic spinal cord injury population: Risk factors for mortality. *J Spinal Cord Med.* 2003;26:248-253.

62. Hussain R, Cevallos ME, Darouiche RO, et al. Gram-negative intravascular catheter-related bacteremia in patients with spinal cord injury. *Arch Phys Med Rehabil.* 2008;89:339-342.

63. Lew HL, Han J, Robinson LR, et al. Occult maxillary sinusitis as a cause of fever in tetraplegia: 2 case reports. *Arch Phys Med Rehabil.* 2002;83:430-432.

64. Zhou Q, Moore C, Eden S, et al; Mount Sinai Hospital Infection Control Team. Factors associated with acquisition of vancomycin-resistant enterococci (VRE) in roommate contacts of patients colonized or infected with VRE in a tertiary care hospital. *Infect Control Hosp Epidemiol.* 2008;29:398-403.

65. Kappel C, Widmer A, Geng V, et al. Successful control of methicillin-resistant *Staphylococcus aureus* in a spinal cord injury center: A 10-year prospective study including molecular typing. *Spinal Cord.* 2008;46:438-444.

66. Mylotte JM, Kahler L, Graham R, et al. Prospective surveillance for antibiotic-resistant organisms in patients with spinal cord injury admitted to an acute rehabilitation unit. *Am J Infect Control.* 2000;28:291-297.

67. Olivier CN, Blake RK, Steed LL, et al. Risk of vancomycin-resistant enterococcus (VRE) bloodstream infection among patients colonized with VRE. *Infect Control Hosp Epidemiol.* 2008;29:404-409.

68. Apisarnthanarak A, Bailey TC, Fraser VJ. Duration of stool colonization in patients infected with extended-spectrum beta-lactamase-producing *Escherichia coli* and *Klebsiella pneumoniae.* *Clin Infect Dis.* 2008;46:1322-1323.

69. Marciniak C, Chen D, Stein AC, et al. Prevalence of *Clostridium difficile* colonization at admission to rehabilitation. *Arch Phys Med Rehabil.* 2006; 87:1086-1090.

Infections in the Elderly

KENT B. CROSSLEY* I PHILLIP K. PETERSON

The extremes of age are appreciated as periods of increased susceptibility to infection. In the elderly (which we define as people 65 years of age or older), there are many reasons for more frequent infection. These include impairment of cell-mediated and humoral immunity[1] and reduced physiologic functions such as cough reflex, circulation, and wound healing.[2] Increased prevalence of many chronic illnesses associated with infection, use of immunosuppressive drugs, and communal living probably are also partly responsible for the increased frequency of infection in the elderly. It is well established that many infections are both more frequent (e.g., herpes zoster, listeriosis, urinary tract infection) and more often associated with mortality (e.g., bacteremia, meningitis, malaria[3]) in older individuals. Conversely, some infections (e.g., sexually transmitted diseases) are less common in the elderly.

The elderly are a large and increasing segment of the population worldwide. It is estimated that, of all human beings who have ever lived to be 65 years or older, half are currently alive.[4] In 1900, only 15 million people were age 65 years or older (1% of the global population). In 1992, 342 million people were in this age group (6.2% of the world population), and by the year 2050 this number is projected to expand to 2.5 billion (about 20% of the world population). In the United States the number of people over 65 is expected to double between 2000 and 2030.[5]

A high proportion of lifetime health care costs are expended in the last few months before death. Older patients have more frequent admissions, longer hospital stays, higher mortality, and higher total hospital costs than younger patients.[1,2,6] Infections are one of the most common reasons for the elderly to be transferred from a nursing home to an acute care hospital.[7] Transfers are also associated with an increased risk of adverse effects.[3] Developing better ways to treat infections in elderly patients in long-term care facilities (thus avoiding transfer to an acute care institution) could potentially both improve the quality of their care and save substantial amounts of money.

In this chapter, we discuss infections that are disproportionately common in the elderly. Many infections in the aged share a common denominator of muted clinical signs and symptoms. It is key to remember that most physiologic responses to infection are blunted in the aged.[8] Peak temperatures, maximal white blood cell counts, and intensity of many clinical symptoms and signs are less marked in the elderly.[4] Understanding this is crucial to adequately caring for elderly individuals.

Urinary Tract Infections

Urinary tract infections (UTIs) are more common in women than men until advanced age. The incidence of asymptomatic bacteriuria (defined as the presence of greater than 10^5 organisms per mL of urine in the absence of symptoms) in women increases by about 1% per decade so that women 70 to 80 years old have a 7% to 8% annual incidence of bacteriuria. In men, bacteriuria becomes increasingly prevalent with age, largely as a result of urethral obstruction caused by prostatic hypertrophy. The prevalence of bacteriuria in the elderly is about 10% in men and 20% in women.[9] In residents of nursing homes and in the hospitalized elderly, bacteriuria is more common, and the frequencies in men and women become similar.[10] Bacteriuria often disappears spontaneously in the aged without any intervention.[11]

Asymptomatic bacteriuria in the elderly does not require antibiotic therapy.[6] Functionally disabled elderly individuals are more prone to

have bacteriuria, and they are also more apt to die from the cause of their primary disability.[12] Controlled studies of antibiotic treatment of elderly bacteriuric men and women have not shown decreased survival in the untreated population. Nicolle and colleagues[13] demonstrated that treatment of bacteriuria in elderly men or women usually results in only transient clearing and is often complicated by drug-related side effects. Even though the majority of elderly institutionalized women with asymptomatic bacteriuria may have upper tract involvement, there is no good evidence that treatment is associated with any benefit.[14]

The etiology of symptomatic UTIs in the elderly largely depends on where the infection was acquired. Among individuals living in the community, the distribution of organisms causing infection in the elderly is similar to that seen in younger persons. In institutionalized elderly individuals, there is a marked change in pathogens, with one third of cases of UTI or bacteriuria caused by *Escherichia coli* and about as many caused by *Proteus* spp. There is more than a sixfold increase in the frequency of *Klebsiella* spp. and *Pseudomonas aeruginosa* compared with that in noninstitutionalized persons. Up to 25% of these infections may be polymicrobial.[11] A significant excess of gram-positive infections in elderly men with UTIs has also been observed.[12] In several studies, bacteriuria has been reported to be transient and the responsible organisms to change frequently.[11,15-19] The common use of antibiotics in long-term care institutions is undoubtedly one factor altering the etiology of these infections. Both the organisms recovered and the antibiotic susceptibility of the isolates may be a function of the patient's exposure to antibiotics.

Pyuria is not a reliable marker for bacteriuria. In the studies of Baldassarre and Kaye,[12] 60.9% of 133 women with pyuria did not have bacteriuria. Of 184 women who did not have pyuria, in contrast, only 4.3% were bacteriuric.[12] Absence of pyuria in women is a strong predictor of absence of infection.

Symptomatic UTI should always be treated in older individuals. Antibiotic selection should be guided by a Gram-stained specimen of urine and the patient's history. Residence in a nursing home, recent hospital stays, previous antibiotic therapy, and a history of multiple UTIs are all associated with more resistant organisms. Enterococci and *Staphylococcus aureus* cause a significant minority of infections in older patients. Because many drugs used to treat gram-negative infection are not active against these organisms, it is important to exclude them by the urine Gram stain.

For elderly patients with apparent acute upper tract disease, hemodynamic instability is more common than in younger patients,[20-21] and parenteral antimicrobial therapy and hospitalization are often appropriate. If gram-positive organisms are present in urine, vancomycin is probably the best empirical therapy. For gram-negative infection, a third-generation cephalosporin or another β-lactam (e.g., ticarcillin-clavulanate) or ciprofloxacin is a good initial choice. Patients at high risk of having resistant organisms are best treated initially with a broad-spectrum β-lactam or a carbapenem and an aminoglycoside, beginning with a low dose (e.g., 1 mg/kg/day) until blood aminoglycoside levels can be obtained. With both gram-negative and gram-positive infections, final therapy should be guided by susceptibility studies. As with younger patients, failure of symptoms (e.g., chills or fever) to resolve, persisting back pain, or continuing positive urine cultures require careful evaluation to exclude obstruction or a perinephric abscess.

Prevention of recurrent UTIs in elderly women has been evaluated in three studies. Raz and Stamm[22] found that intravaginal estriol in postmenopausal women results in decreased colonization with Enterobacteriaceae and fewer infections. Ouslander and colleagues found no

---

*All material in this chapter is in the public domain, with the exception of any borrowed figures or tables.

3857

effect on the incidence of bacteriuria in a placebo-controlled trial when elderly institutionalized women were given oral estrogen-progestin for 6 months.[23] Raz and coworkers compared estriol-containing vaginal pessaries with oral nitrofurantoin for prevention of recurrent UTI in elderly women.[24] The pessary was significantly less effective than nitrofurantoin in the prevention of infection. A recent Cochrane review concluded that regular ingestion of cranberry juice reduced the incidence of UTI in women with recurrent infection.[25] Studies in the elderly have shown cranberry juice reduces the incidence of bacteriuria[26] but not the development of UTI.[27]

Urinary catheters are a significant cause of UTI in the elderly.[28] These devices should be avoided whenever possible. Virtually all patients with indwelling catheters in place for 30 days or longer are bacteriuric, but only a small percentage of these patients develop symptomatic infection. Conversely, about two thirds of febrile illnesses in elderly patients with indwelling catheters are the result of UTI.[29] Warren and coworkers[30] have shown that infection-related mortality in elderly bacteriuric women is limited to severely debilitated patients. When symptomatic infections develop in patients with indwelling catheters, they should be treated empirically as described previously. Although catheter removal is usually recommended, there is little evidence that it is needed as part of the treatment of a catheter-associated UTI. It is also unclear whether intermittent catheterization is associated with a reduction in the frequency of either bacteriuria or symptomatic infections.[31,32] Condom catheters are less likely to be associated with bacteriuria or symptomatic UTI than indwelling catheters.[33]

Cystitis (manifested by dysuria, urgency, and frequency in a patient who is usually afebrile) is probably best managed with short-course (3-day) antibiotic therapy. Although more data about the efficacy of short-course therapy of lower UTIs in the elderly are needed, cost and complications are reduced and cure rates appear to be similar to those achieved with longer periods of therapy.[34,35] Single-dose therapy is less effective than 3- to 6-day treatment but associated with greater patient acceptance.[35] Short-course therapy is only for women; men (because of the potential of a prostatic focus of infection) should be treated for at least 10 to 14 days.[10] A recent prospective randomized study in men found that 2 weeks of oral ciprofloxacin (500 mg twice daily) was as effective as 4 weeks. Two thirds of subjects were older than 50 years of age.[36] Appropriate drugs include trimethoprim-sulfamethoxazole and one of the quinolones for cystitis.

Pneumonia

The association between aging and pneumonia has been recognized for many years. Sir William Osler (who himself was to die of bacterial pneumonia) described the disease in his textbook as "a friend of the elderly."[37] Marrie[38] reported that community-acquired pneumonia occurred 50 times as frequently in individuals older than 75 than in 15- to 19-year-olds. Hospitalization rates for pneumonia have also increased significantly over the last 15 years.[39] Among elderly residents of long-term-care facilities, the frequency of pneumonia is sixfold to tenfold higher than among community-dwelling elderly.[40] In addition to their significant associated mortality, pneumonic infections are more expensive to treat in the aged because of increased length of hospital stay.[41] Moreover, they often herald the approach of death. In one study, half of elderly patients with community-acquired pneumonia died in the next year.[42]

Streptococcus pneumoniae, gram-negative enteric bacilli, *Haemophilus influenzae* and *S. aureus* are the most commonly identified bacterial pathogens in recent studies of elderly individuals hospitalized with pneumonia.[43] Although most studies of the etiology of pneumonia in the elderly are limited by the use of expectorated sputum as the source of culture, in general, in both community and institutional settings, the risk of gram-negative and *S. aureus* pulmonary infection appears to be increased in the elderly.[43]

Non-bacterial causes of pneumonia are increasingly being recognized in the aged. Respiratory syncytial virus (RSV) has been recently recognized as a relatively common cause of pneumonia in older individuals.[44,45] These infections, which occur primarily in nursing homes, are often of rapid onset and may be clinically very similar to influenza virus infection.[46]

Some studies have recognized that rhinoviruses may be associated with lower respiratory tract disease in the elderly, but their overall importance is uncertain.[47] Human metapneumovirus has also been reported to cause lower respiratory tract infection in elderly patients.[48] The organism was recovered from 4% of 193 consecutive adults hospitalized with pneumonia.[49] *Chlamydophila pneumoniae* has been noted to cause an outbreak of respiratory infection in a nursing home.[50]

As with other infections in the aged, the clinical presentation of pneumonia is usually muted. Temperatures of patients with bacteremic pneumococcal pneumonia who are elderly are lower than those of younger individuals, and cough and fever may be absent in elderly patients with pneumonia.[51] Very elderly patients (>80 years) are more likely to be afebrile or have changed mental status and less likely to complain of pleuritic chest pain, headache, or myalgia than younger patients.[52]

It is important to culture the blood and sputum of elderly patients with apparent pneumonia. However, sputum is often difficult to collect, and in some seriously ill elderly individuals, it may be appropriate to attempt to obtain a specimen for culture that does not pass through the oropharynx (e.g., by bronchoalveolar lavage or by use of a covered brush). These invasive procedures for obtaining sputum are generally used when microorganisms other than common bacterial pathogens are being considered.

Empirical management of pneumonia in elderly individuals requires treatment with an antimicrobial agent that is effective against a broad range of possible causative organisms.[53] One of the third-generation cephalosporins that has good activity against *S. pneumoniae*, *S. aureus*, *H. influenzae*, and common gram-negative organisms (e.g., cefotaxime or ceftriaxone) is appropriate for community-acquired infections in hospitalized patients. Addition of azithromycin or using a fluoroquinolone for coverage of atypical bacteria, such as *Legionella pneumophila* and *C. pneumoniae*, is recommended by the guidelines set forth by the Infectious Diseases Society of America/American Thoracic Society (IDSA-ATS Guidelines).[54]

Among hospitalized patients, those older than 65 develop pneumonia twice as often as younger patients.[55] Risk factors for nosocomial pneumonia included poor nutrition, endotracheal intubation, and neuromuscular disease. Interestingly, mortality of patients with respiratory disease in intensive care units is not predictable on the basis of age alone but requires examination of comorbid conditions.[56] In hospital-acquired infections, initial broad-spectrum coverage that includes *P. aeruginosa* (e.g., a carbapenem or a broad-spectrum β-lactam with an aminoglycoside) is appropriate. Although published data from studies of the elderly are limited so far, the broad-spectrum quinolones are promising agents for nursing home–acquired pneumonia. Improved clinical outcome may result from treatment that avoids hospital transfer.[57]

Efforts to prevent pneumonia are very important, particularly in the frail elderly. These should include immunization with the pneumococcal polysaccharide vaccine and influenza vaccine.[58] Both of these immunizations are being used with greater frequency in recent years. A 1999 study of U.S. adults 65 years of age or older found that 66.9% had received an influenza immunization in the prior year and 54.1% a pneumococcal immunization at some time.[59]

Data that support the use of influenza vaccine in the aged have accumulated rapidly. Cohort studies of elderly members of managed care organizations have demonstrated substantial decline in the incidence of both hospitalization and death among those immunized against influenza.[60,61] Greatest reductions were among the high-risk elderly. Studies have also found reductions in mortality from causes other than influenza (e.g., cardiac disease and stroke) among immunized elderly.[62,63] Two recent studies reach divergent conclusions about the impact of influenza immunization on the frequency of community-acquired pneumonia in the aged.[64,65]

Methods to control influenza during an outbreak should include limiting contact between elderly individuals and people with symptoms of respiratory illness. Use of amantadine, rimantadine, or oseltamivir may reduce the duration of influenza virus infection and may prevent the development of influenza when given as prophylaxis to patients in nursing homes.[66]

The evidence that pneumococcal polysaccharide vaccine reduces morbidity and mortality from disease caused by *S. pneumoniae* in the elderly is less clear.[67] One recent study of a cohort of 47,000 individuals 65 years of age or older found that the risk of pneumococcal bacteremia was reduced by immunization but the risk of pneumococcal pneumonia was not.[68] A review of meta-analyses reached the same conclusion.[69] Data from the Centers for Disease Control and Prevention (CDC) indicate a decline in invasive pneumococcal disease among the elderly in the years from 1996 through 2001. This is thought to be due to the use of the protein-polysaccharide vaccine among young children, with subsequent benefit to elderly individuals who come into contact with young children.[70]

Tuberculosis

Tuberculosis is the most common reportable disease among persons older than 65 years.[71] Some 19% of tuberculosis cases in the United States in 2007 were in patients in this age group.[72] Among elderly in the community, the incidence is twice that in the general population, and in residents of nursing homes, the incidence is four times that in the community.

Usually development of disease in the elderly is thought to reflect reactivation of infection acquired at a younger age and is due to declining cellular immunity associated with aging. In addition, poor nutrition, the increased occurrence of diabetes and other diseases common to the elderly and use of corticosteroid therapy may further exacerbate immunodeficiency and increase the risk of reactivation of *Mycobacterium tuberculosis* infection.

Tuberculin testing is commonly required on admission to long-term care facilities. Testing should be done using intradermal (the Mantoux technique) administration of purified protein derivative. Because regular skin testing is done in long-term care facilities, the use of a two-step technique is recommended in their residents.[73] For individuals who have positive purified protein derivative tests, chest roentgenograms should be obtained and then repeated on a regular basis. Follow-up tuberculin testing and chest roentgenograms are recommended at a frequency determined by the prevalence of tuberculous disease in the community (typically at 6- to 24-month intervals). Tuberculin-positive patients need to be closely followed.[74] Unexplained weight loss or fever, pulmonary symptoms, unexplained lymphadenopathy, or changes in renal function should be clues to the possible presence of active tuberculosis.

The key to diagnosing tuberculosis in the elderly is to maintain a high index of suspicion. The tuberculin skin test may be more often negative in older patients with active tuberculosis than in younger individuals.[75] It is also imperative to remember that some manifestations may be atypical.[76] A recent meta-analysis found that fever, night sweats, and hemoptysis were all significantly less common in patients older than 60.[75] Three of four elderly patients with tuberculosis have pulmonary involvement, although cavitation is less common than in younger patients.[77,78]

Guidelines for therapy of latent tuberculosis with isoniazid are not age-specific.[79] Toxicity from this drug in the aged is uncommon and should not be a reason to withhold treatment with isoniazid (INH).[74] See Chapter 250 for additional information about the therapy of tuberculosis.

Pressure Sores and Skin Infections

Pressure sores are most common in the seriously disabled elderly and are typically quite difficult to treat. Among elderly nursing home residents studied recently in Baltimore, 26.2% had pressure ulcers at the time of hospitalization.[80] The incidence increases as a function of age.[81] Pressure sores occur primarily in individuals with impaired mobility, and the usual cause is skin necrosis resulting from ischemia.[82] The ulcer that develops may be associated with a number of infectious complications. In order of decreasing frequency, these are local infection, cellulitis of surrounding tissue, contiguous osteomyelitis, and bacteremia.[83]

Guidelines for prevention of pressure lesions in adults have been published by several groups including the American Geriatric Society.[84] Key components include monitoring patients who are at risk, reducing exposure of the skin to pressure, maintaining the skin in a clean and dry condition, and promoting good nutritional status.

Most pressure ulcers in the elderly yield multiple organisms when cultured. Aerobes that are commonly recovered include staphylococci, enterococci, *Proteus mirabilis*, *E. coli*, and *Pseudomonas* spp. In addition, anaerobic *Peptostreptococcus*, *Bacteroides fragilis*, and *Clostridium* spp. are frequently isolated from these infections. Making an accurate bacteriologic diagnosis is difficult. Many of the issues involved in determining the bacteriology of an infected pressure sore are similar to those confronted in the assessment of infected diabetic foot ulcers. Swabbing the wound often yields organisms that are colonizers and not actually causes of infection. It may be most appropriate to aspirate material from the margin or base of the ulcer, directing the needle through intact skin.

Therapy of pressure ulcers should include pressure relief, appropriate nutrition, and débridement.[85] A variety of treatments have been used and there is no clear evidence to favor one over another.[86] Topical antimicrobial agents have not been shown to be effective. Systemic antibiotic therapy should be reserved for infected ulcers.

A variety of empirical antibiotic regimens have been suggested for patients with pressure ulcer–associated cellulitis, osteomyelitis, or bacteremia. Bacteremia in this situation is usually caused by *P. mirabilis*, *S. aureus*, or *B. fragilis*.[83] In general, any regimen that is active against the majority of organisms that are usually causal is appropriate. Although a 10- to 14-day course is commonly prescribed, no studies have carefully defined the duration of therapy. While advanced inanition is the most common cause of failure of these lesions to heal, osteomyelitis needs to be ruled out by physical examination and roentgenography. If osteomyelitis is present, a more extended course of therapy is needed. A comprehensive review of the management of infected pressure sores has been published.[87]

Some common types of cellulitis may be more severe and associated with increased mortality in elderly individuals compared with younger patients. In particular, outbreaks of skin infection caused by group A β-hemolytic streptococci associated with bacteremia have been reported in nursing homes in the United States.[88,89] Invasive Group B streptococcal disease is most frequent in the elderly and the incidence of these infections has increased in recent years.[90] Because many of these infections are fatal and because of the high costs of inpatient management, cutaneous infections in elderly patients need to be treated promptly. Skin and soft tissue infections are common in the nursing home setting; In a recent Swedish study of infections in a group of 58 nursing homes, 16% involved skin and soft tissue.[91] Herpes zoster is also particularly common in the elderly and often associated with severe and protracted pain. Pathogenesis and therapy of this disease are discussed elsewhere in this volume (see Chapter 137).

Bacteremia

Probably because of the increased prevalence of chronic diseases in older individuals, bacteremic illnesses are more frequent and more often associated with death in the elderly.[92,93] In both the hospital and the community, bacteremia is more common in the aged.[94] In one study based on the National Hospital Discharge Survey, patients older than 65 had a 13-fold increase in the frequency of sepsis.[92]

A number of studies have pointed out the blunted clinical responses to bacteremia in elderly patients. It is clear that elderly patients may be bacteremic and remain afebrile.[95] Also, a significant proportion of patients may not have neutrophilia.[96] Weakness and altered mental status may be the presenting symptoms.

The main sources of community-acquired bacteremia in the elderly, in order of decreasing frequency, are the urinary tract, intra-abdominal sites, and lungs.[97] In long-term care facilities, the urinary tract is the most frequent source, followed by the respiratory tract.[98] Organisms most commonly recovered from patients with bacteremia associated with skin sources are *S. aureus, Staphylococcus epidermidis,* gram-negative enteric bacteria, and anaerobes.[97] Bacteria from the urinary tract are usually gram-negative enterics or enterococci; from the biliary tract, gram-negative enterics or anaerobes; and from the respiratory tract, *H. influenzae, S. pneumoniae,* group B streptococci, or gram-negative enterics. Group G streptococcal bacteremia (usually from a cutaneous source) is especially common in the aged. In one recent review, the median age of cases was 72 years.[99]

Because of their increased risk of complications and higher mortality, elderly patients should be treated as soon as a presumptive diagnosis of bacteremia is considered. Selection of a proper antibiotic regimen is guided by the same principles as for younger individuals. It is important to remember that elderly patients eliminate most antibiotics more slowly than younger individuals; dosages should be adjusted accordingly. Aminoglycosides, because of the increasing potential for toxicity with age, are best used with caution.[100]

Infective Endocarditis

Infective endocarditis is especially common in elderly individuals. In many studies of endocarditis, more than 50% of patients are 60 or more years of age.[101-103] The increased incidence of endocarditis in the elderly seems to be related to prolonged survival of patients with cardiac valvular disease and the use of prosthetic heart valves, intravascular monitoring devices, and surgically implanted materials.

The diagnosis of infective endocarditis may be particularly difficult in the elderly. Often, presenting signs and symptoms are nonspecific, and development of weakness, malaise, weight loss, confusion, and so on may be the only evidence of infection. A recent study noted that Osler's nodes are less common in the elderly than in younger patients.[104] In one study, more than two thirds of cases of endocarditis in elderly patients were misdiagnosed at the time of admission.[105] Musculoskeletal manifestations are often mistakenly ascribed to primary rheumatologic disorders, and heart murmurs are considered benign or thought to result from calcific lesions associated with aging.

Several studies suggest that older patients have an increased frequency of endocarditis caused by gram-positive organisms.[101,102,104] These include *Enterococcus faecalis* (usually from the urinary tract) and *Streptococcus bovis* (usually from a colonic source).[104,105] It is important to remember the association of *S. bovis* with gastrointestinal carcinoma. In individuals with prosthetic valves, the likelihood is high that the infection is caused by staphylococci or enterococci.

Although the therapy of infective endocarditis in an elderly individual is not different from that in a younger person (see Chapter 77), two points need to be emphasized. First, because of less rapid elimination of many antimicrobials in elderly patients, care needs to be taken in dosing and monitoring levels of potentially toxic drugs. Second, because elderly patients do not tolerate long hospital stays well, every effort should be made to administer parenteral therapy on an outpatient basis. As in younger patients, careful observation is required for possible complications, including recurrent episodes of fever and congestive heart failure.

In the elderly, cardiac complications of endocarditis such as congestive heart failure are increased by nonvalvular causes of decompensation such as myocardial infarction, conduction abnormalities, arrhythmias, myocarditis, or myocardial abscess. Elderly persons are prone to arterial embolization, the second most common complication of infective endocarditis. The mortality associated with infective endocarditis is substantially greater in elderly than in younger patients,

and permanent disability and a need for long-term care are common outcomes.[104,105]

Antibiotic prophylaxis to prevent development of endocarditis is important in older individuals. This topic has been reviewed in a statement regarding prevention published by the American Heart Association[106] (see Chapter 80).

Infectious Diarrhea

Diarrhea is a significant cause of morbidity and mortality in the elderly. One study found that 51% of deaths caused by diarrhea over a 9-year period occurred in individuals older than 74.[107] A disproportionate share of diarrheal deaths occurred in elderly nursing home residents.[10]

Older patients may be at increased risk for *Salmonella* infections because of achlorhydria, decreased intestinal motility associated with medications, other coexistent gastrointestinal diseases, and more frequent use of antibiotics. Some authors have suggested that patients older than 50 should be considered for antibiotic therapy for uncomplicated *Salmonella* gastroenteritis. This assumes that older patients may not tolerate these infections well and that, if bacteremic, they may be at increased risk for vascular infection caused by salmonellae. The quinolones have assumed an important role in the empirical therapy of acute gastroenteritis when a bacterial etiology is suspected, and this class of agents is usually active against *Salmonella* spp.

Because antibiotics shorten the duration of *Shigella* gastroenteritis, therapy is indicated to reduce the risk of fluid and electrolyte imbalance in the elderly. Antibiotic therapy is also recommended for diarrhea caused by *Campylobacter jejuni,* invasive *E. coli, Vibrio parahaemolyticus,* and *Yersinia enterocolitica* (see Chapter 93).

In the nursing home setting, outbreaks of diarrhea occur relatively commonly during the winter months. Both noroviruses and rotaviruses have been implicated in these episodes.[108] Noroviruses, the most common non-bacterial cause of gastroenteritis in the community, are a frequent cause of outbreaks of diarrhea and vomiting in long-term care institutions. Transmission of the viruses—which are infectious in low inoculum and relatively resistant to commonly used disinfectants—is by the fecal-oral route, by airborne transmission from vomitus, and by food. The median time of viral shedding was recently shown in a study of elderly volunteers to be 28.7 days.[109] While the median duration of illness in health care settings is three days, one study found 40% of patients at least 85 years of age remained symptomatic after four days.[110] Fatalities in aged long-term care residents have been documented.[111] Shared bathroom facilities, persisting excretion of the virus, incontinent residents and limited handwashing facilities all favor the occurrence of norovirus outbreaks in residential facilities.

There are also substantial data associating *Clostridium difficile* diarrhea with residence in a long-term care institution.[112] This organism is increasingly recognized as a cause of sporadic cases of diarrhea in the elderly. It is the most common reportable cause of diarrhea in the elderly in Great Britain.[113] The mean age of patients with *C. difficile* was 67.6 years in one recent national study. Mortality increased dramatically with increasing age; rates in patients older than 80 were twice that in patients in their 50s.[114]

Enterohemorrhagic *E. coli* (O157:H7) has been reported to cause outbreaks of gastroenteritis in long-term care institutions.[115] *Cryptosporidium* is also newly appreciated as a cause of diarrhea in the aged.[116] A recent study suggests that this organism may be associated with more severe disease, a shorter incubation period, and a higher risk of secondary transmission in the aged.[117] Although *Candida* spp. have been implicated as a cause of diarrhea in elderly patients,[118] isolation of this fungus from stool, even in high colony counts, appears to indicate colonization and not infection. Microsporidia have recently been documented as a cause of chronic diarrhea in the elderly.[119] A study from China suggests that severity of hookworm infestation correlates with age.[120]

Central Nervous System Infections

MENINGITIS

As is true of other serious infections in the aged, the case-fatality ratio of meningitis is higher than in younger individuals.[121] In a recent study of pneumococcal meningitis, mortality in patients older than 60 was twice that of younger patients (36.7% vs. 17.5%).[122]

It is well established that the organisms that cause meningitis in elderly individuals differ from the distribution of bacteria seen in younger adults.[123] The major causes of meningitis in the aged are *S. pneumoniae, Listeria monocytogenes,* gram-negative bacilli, and *Streptococcus agalactiae.* Disease caused by *Neisseria meningitidis* and *H. influenzae* is uncommon in elderly patients.[124,125] As suggested in a number of studies, viral meningitis is also relatively uncommon in the elderly.

The signs and symptoms of bacterial meningitis in the elderly are muted. Nuchal rigidity is often found on examination of elderly patients who do not have bacterial meningitis.[126,127] Usually, these patients have coexistent neurologic deficits. Elderly patients who have nuchal rigidity in the absence of other neurologic problems should not be dismissed as having "osteoarthritis of the cervical spine" but should be intensively investigated for possible meningitis. Other symptoms suggestive of the diagnosis include change in mental status and fever.[128] In one recent study, the combination of fever, neck stiffness, and altered mental status was more common in the elderly than among younger patients.[123]

Several reviews of meningitis suggest that the laboratory findings for elderly people do not differ from those for younger individuals. Complications, however, are more frequent in older individuals.[123-126] Gorse and coworkers[125] found that the frequency of complications (including neurologic complications, pneumonia, and UTIs) was approximately twice as high in patients older than 65 as in younger patients.

The empirical treatment of meningitis in elderly patients needs to cover *S. pneumoniae, L. monocytogenes,* and gram-negative bacilli. Because *L. monocytogenes* is not susceptible to cephalosporins, an appropriate empirical regimen includes ampicillin with cefotaxime or ceftriaxone. In areas where cephalosporin-resistant *S. pneumoniae* have been encountered, vancomycin should be used empirically until culture and antibiotic susceptibility results are known.

ARBOVIRAL INFECTIONS

West Nile virus infection was first recognized in the United States in 1999 and in subsequent years has become widely distributed throughout the United States and Canada (see Chapter 153). It is clear that this virus has a major predilection for causing serious infections in older individuals. In the initial outbreak in 1999 in New York City, 88% of hospitalized patients were 50 years of age or older; the median age in this population was 71 years.[127]

Most cases of the disease are not apparent, perhaps not even symptomatic. Fever is the only manifestation in perhaps half the symptomatic cases. In one study of these patients, only 23% were older than or equal to 65 years of age.[128] Data from the 1999 outbreak in New York City suggested that the frequency of severe neurologic disease, compared with patients from birth to 19 years of age, was 10 times greater in individuals 50 to 59, and 43 times higher in those at least 80 years of age. The same outbreak data suggested that persons 75 years and older were nine times more likely to die of their illness than younger individuals.[129] The basis for this increased severity of infection in the elderly is unknown and contrasts sharply with other arbovirus infections. A recent study has reported a prolonged time to recovery (>1 year) among elderly with meningoencephalitis.[130] Focal neurological injury may not be more common in aged patients.[131]

Septic Arthritis

In one recent study, 61% of persons with septic arthritis were older than 60.[132] The mortality in the elderly is higher, and recovery of joint function is less satisfactory. Septic arthritis is commonly associated with preexisting rheumatoid arthritis, prosthetic joints, or degenerative arthritis.[133] These associations, as well as with diseases such as diabetes mellitus and malignancy and with cytotoxic or systemic corticosteroid therapy, suggest that immunologic defects may play an important role in the pathogenesis of septic arthritis in the elderly.

The knee joint is most frequently involved, followed by the wrist and shoulder joint. Although most elderly patients with septic arthritis complain of a painful, swollen joint, in contrast to younger patients, they are seldom totally immobilized by pain and muscle spasm is infrequent. Gavet and colleagues reported that half of cases did not have a leukocytosis.[132] As in younger patients, the most commonly isolated organism is *S. aureus,* but gram-negative bacilli are also frequent causes in the elderly. In addition, septic arthritis is associated more frequently with osteomyelitis in the older patient.

Fever and Fever of Undetermined Origin

Many elderly persons appear to have lower body temperatures than are traditionally accepted as normal and consequently have a diminished febrile response to infection.[134,135] In elderly individuals, an oral temperature of greater than 99°F should be considered elevated. However, 95% of elderly patients who have infection show some febrile response.[136] One study examined the importance of fever in 470 consecutive elderly patients with temperatures of 100.0°F or greater who were seen in an emergency room.[137] Three quarters of these patients were classified by the authors as seriously ill. The most frequent diagnoses included pneumonia (24%), UTI (21.7%), and septicemia (12.8%). Many of these patients did not have high fever, tachycardia, leukocytosis, or tachypnea.

Two recent reviews of fever of undetermined origin (FUO) in the elderly have been published.[138,139] Both point out that non-infectious inflammatory processes (i.e., rheumatic diseases) are as frequent as infections as a cause of FUO in the aged. Temporal arteritis and polymyalgia rheumatica are the two most frequent rheumatic conditions among the elderly. Tuberculosis was the most frequent infection in recent studies. Tumors accounted for about one-eighth of cases and drug-related fever for about 6%. In some 13% of FUO cases, no diagnosis was made.

Antimicrobial Considerations

Although the elderly are the group most likely to receive antibiotic therapy when hospitalized and in nursing homes, most information about the effects of aging on the pharmacokinetics and toxicity of antimicrobial agents is relatively recent.[140,141] Physiologic changes that accompany advanced age may significantly affect the absorption, distribution, plasma protein binding, metabolism, and elimination of many antibiotics. The risk of toxicity of some antimicrobials is also increased in the elderly. Newer antibiotics have been studied more extensively in older patients. The phenomenon of *polypharmacy,* which is so common in this age group, greatly increases the chances of drug interactions. Extensive information about the use of antibiotics in nursing homes—and programs to improve usage—has been published.[142-144]

Few studies have considered the relationship between age and prevalence of infections caused by antibiotic-resistant organisms. Recent U.S. data document a marked increase in fluoroquinolone use in older individuals.[145] One Japanese study points to a marked increase in prevalence of fluoroquinolone resistance with increasing age.[146] Given the common usage of fluoroquinolones in the treatment of UTI and pneumonia in the elderly, one can predict that emergence of resistance of *S. pneumoniae* and other pathogens to this class of antibiotics will first be seen as a major problem in this age group. Initiation of a fluoroquinolone reduction policy in Ontario did not result in an overall increase in hospitalizations among the elderly for infection.[147] However, admissions for urinary tract infections did significantly increase over predicted numbers ($P < .01$).

Infection, and the need for antibiotic therapy, is common among elderly patients as the end of life approaches. Whether to prescribe antibiotics in these situations is an issue that has not been extensively examined. The role of ethical considerations in the management of these patients has recently been reviewed.[148]

Immunizations

Important information about several travel-related immunization issues in the elderly has recently been reviewed. The most important of these considerations are highlighted here. As noted, many vaccines have not been evaluated in elderly individuals.[149] In general, antibody response to most vaccines is muted in elderly individuals, most likely reflecting the waning of immune responses associated with aging.

Hepatitis A and B Vaccines. Data suggest that antibody titers with these vaccines (separately or as a combined vaccine) are lower in the elderly. One recent review suggested post-vaccination antibody testing in elderly travellers.[150]

Yellow Fever Vaccine. A study from the CDC found that elderly individuals immunized for the first time have a fourfold to sixfold higher risk of severe illness after yellow fever vaccination than do younger individuals.[151] The mechanism and incidence of this reaction are not yet known. Data from the Vaccine Adverse Event Reporting System also suggest that these reactions occur with increasing frequency with increasing age.[152]

Rabies Vaccine. Two studies suggest that rabies vaccine antibody titers are substantially lower in older subjects. As is true with hepatitis immunizations, the significance of this is unknown.[153,154]

Zoster Vaccine. The Advisory Committee on Immunization Practices has endorsed the use of a live attenuated strain vaccine for all individuals older than or at 60 years of age.[155] The vaccine is recommended for all individuals including those with a previous episode of zoster and with chronic medical conditions. The vaccine reduces the incidence of zoster and of pain and postherpetic neuralgia.

Prevention

A number of studies suggest that age per se is not an independent risk factor for many types of infection. Whereas many studies of infections in elderly populations comprise patients who have suffered the consequences of age-related physiologic impairment (i.e., senescence), a majority of elderly people are healthy and living independently at home. Of Americans who are in the age group 65 to 74, 89% are fully functioning and robust. Of those 75 to 84 years of age, 73% enjoy this health status, and 40% of individuals 85 years of age or older continue to have aged successfully.[4]

Prevention of infection in the aged is increasingly viewed as a need to prevent comorbidities and nutritional deficiencies that contribute to the pathogenesis of infection. In addition to immunizations (with influenza, pneumococcal, and tetanus vaccines), mounting evidence supports the value of adequate nutrition, exercise, social engagement, and continued involvement in productive activities in the attainment of a long and qualitatively rich life.[4]

REFERENCES

1. Curns AT, Holman RC, Sejvar JJ, et al. Infectious disease hospitalizations among older adults in the United States from 1990 through 2002. *Arch Intern Med.* 2005;165:2514-2520.
2. Greenberg S. *A profile of older Americans: 2007.* Department of Health and Human Services Administration on Aging.
3. Boockvar KS, Gruber-Baldini AL, Burton L, et al. Outcomes of infection in nursing home residents with and without early hospital transfer. *J Am Geriatr Soc.* 2005;53:590-596.
4. Meyer KC. Lung infections and aging. *Ageing Res Rev.* 2004;3:55-67.
5. Crossley K, Peterson PK. Infections in the elderly—New developments. In: Remington JS, Swartz MN, eds. *Current Clinical Topics in Infectious Diseases.* Malden, Mass.: Blackwell Science; 1998:75-100.
6. Nicolle LE, Bradley S, Colgan R, et al. Infectious diseases society of America guidelines for the diagnosis and treatment of asymptomatic bacteriuria in adults. *Clin Infect Dis.* 2005;40:643-654.
7. Irvine PW, Van Buren N, Crossley K. Causes for hospitalization of nursing home residents: The role of infection. *J Am Geriatr Soc.* 1984;32:103-107.
8. Norman DC, Toledo SD. Infections in elderly persons. *Clin Geriatr Med.* 1992;8:713-719.
9. Sobel JD, Kaye D. Urinary tract infections. In: Mandell GL, Douglas RG Jr, Bennett JE, eds. *Principles and Practice of Infectious Diseases.* 3rd ed. New York: Churchill Livingstone; 1990:582-611.
10. Lipsky BA. Urinary tract infections in men: Epidemiology, pathophysiology, diagnosis, and treatment. *Ann Intern Med.* 1989;110:138-150.
11. Nicolle LE. Asymptomatic bacteriuria in the elderly. *Infect Dis Clin North Am.* 1997;11:647-662.
12. Baldassarre JS, Kaye D. Special problems of urinary tract infection in the elderly. *Med Clin North Am.* 1991;75:375-390.
13. Nicolle LE, Bjornson J, Harding GK, et al. Bacteriuria in elderly institutionalized men. *N Engl J Med.* 1983;309:1420-1425.
14. Nicolle LE, Mayhew WJ, Bryan L. Prospective randomized comparison of therapy and no therapy for asymptomatic bacteriuria in institutionalized elderly women. *Am J Med.* 1987;83:27-33.
15. Mims AD, Norman DC, Yamamura RH, et al. Clinically inapparent (asymptomatic) bacteriuria in ambulatory elderly men: Epidemiological, clinical, and microbiological findings. *J Am Geriatr Soc.* 1990;38:1209-1214.
16. Boscia JA, Kobasa WD, Knight RA, et al. Epidemiology of bacteriuria in an elderly ambulatory population. *Am J Med.* 1986;80:208-214.
17. Gleckman RA. Urinary tract infection. *Clin Geriatr Med.* 1992;8:793-819.
18. Kasviki-Charvati P, Drolette-Kefakis B, Papanayiotou PC, et al. Turnover of bacteriuria in old age. *Age Ageing.* 1982;11:169-174.
19. Sourander LB, Kasanen A. A 5-year follow-up of bacteriuria in the aged. *Gerontol Clin.* 1972;14:274-281.
20. Gleckman R, Blagg N, Hibert D, et al. Acute pyelonephritis in the elderly. *South Med J.* 1982;75:551-554.
21. Tal S, Guller V, Levi S, et al. A. Profile and prognosis of febrile elderly patients with bacteremic urinary tract infection. *J Infect.* 2005;50:296-305.
22. Raz R, Stamm WE. A controlled trial of intravaginal estriol in postmenopausal women with recurrent urinary tract infections. *N Engl J Med.* 1993;329:753-756.
23. Ouslander JG, Greendale GA, Uman G, et al. Effects of oral estrogen and progestin on the lower urinary tract among female nursing home residents. *J Am Geriatr Soc.* 2001;49:803-807.
24. Raz R, Colodner R, Rohana Y, et al. Effectiveness of estriol-containing vaginal pessaries and nitrofurantoin macrocrystal therapy in the prevention of recurrent urinary tract infection in postmenopausal women. *Clin Infect Dis.* 2003;36:1362-1368.
25. Jepson RG, Craig JC. Cranberries for preventing urinary tract infections. Cochrane Database Syst Rev 2008(1):CD001321.
26. Avorn J, Monane M, Gurwitz JH, et al. Reduction of bacteriuria and pyuria after ingestion of cranberry juice. *JAMA.* 1994;271:751-754.
27. McMurdo ME, Bissett LY, Price RJ, et al. Does ingestion of cranberry juice reduce symptomatic urinary tract infections in older people in hospital? A double-blind, placebo-controlled trial. *Age Aging.* 2005;34:256-261.
28. Warren HW. Catheter-associated urinary tract infections. *Infect Dis Clin North Am.* 1997;11:609-622.
29. Ouslander JG, Schapira M, Schnelle JF, et al. Pyuria and asymptomatic bacteriuria in elderly ambulatory women. *Ann Intern Med.* 1989;110:404-405.
30. Warren JW, Damron D, Tenney JH, et al. Fever, bacteremia, and death as complications of bacteriuria in women with long-term urethral catheters. *J Infect Dis.* 1987;155:1151-1158.
31. Nicolle LE. Prevention and treatment of urinary catheter-related infections in older patients. *Drugs Aging.* 1994;4:379-391.
32. Tang MW, Kwok TC, Hui E, et al. Intermittent versus indwelling urinary catheterization in older female patients. *Maturitas.* 2006;53:274-281.
33. Saint S, Kaufman SR, Rogers MA, et al. Condom versus indwelling urinary catheters: A randomized trial. *J Am Geriatr Soc.* 2006;54:1055-1061.
34. Vogel T, Verreault R, Gourdeau M, et al. Optimal duration of antibiotic therapy for uncomplicated urinary tract infection in older women: A double-blind randomized controlled trial. *CMAJ.* 2004;170:469-473.
35. Lutters M, Vogt N. Antibiotic duration for treating uncomplicated, symptomatic lower urinary tract infections in elderly women. Cochrane Database Syst Rev 2002(3):CD001535.
36. Ulleryd P, Sandberg T. Ciprofloxacin for 2 or 4 weeks in the treatment of febrile urinary tract infection in men: A randomized trial with a 1 year follow-up. *Scand J Infect Dis.* 2003;35:34-39.
37. Osler W, ed. *The Principles and Practice of Medicine.* 3rd ed. New York: Appleton; 1898:109.
38. Marrie TJ. Epidemiology of community-acquired pneumonia in the elderly. *Semin Respir Infect.* 1990;5:260-268.
39. Fry AM, Shay DK, Holman RC, et al. Trends in hospitalizations for pneumonia among persons aged 65 years or older in the United States, 1988-2002. *JAMA.* 2005;294:2712-2719.
40. Marrie TJ. Pneumonia in the long-term-care facility. *Infect Control Hosp Epidemiol.* 2002;23:159-164.
41. Marston BJ, Plouffe JF, File TM Jr, et al. Incidence of community-acquired pneumonia requiring hospitalization. Results of a population-based active surveillance study in Ohio. The community-based pneumonia incidence study group. *Arch Intern Med.* 1997;157:1709-1718.
42. Kaplan V, Clermont G, Griffin MF, et al. Pneumonia: Still the old man's friend? *Arch Intern Med.* 2003;163:317-323.
43. Janssens JP, Krause KH. Pneumonia in the very old. *Lancet Infect Dis.* 2004;4:112-124.
44. Falsey AR. Respiratory syncytial virus infection in adults. *Semin Respir Crit Care Med.* 2007;28:171-181.
45. Falsey AR, Walsh EE. Viral pneumonia in older adults. *Clin Infect Dis.* 2006;42:518-524.
46. Walsh EE, Peterson DR, Falsey AR. Is clinical recognition of respiratory syncytial virus infection in hospitalized elderly and high-risk adults possible? *J Infect Dis.* 2007;195:1046-1051.
47. Nicholson KG, Kent J, Hammersley V, et al. Risk factors for lower respiratory complications of rhinovirus infections in elderly people living in the community: Prospective cohort study. *BMJ.* 1996;313:1119-1123.
48. Falsey AR. Human metapneumovirus infection in adults. *Pediatr Infect Dis J.* 2008;27(10 suppl):S80-S83.
49. Johnstone J, Majumdar SR, Fox JD, et al. Viral infection in adults hospitalized with community acquired pneumonia: Prevalence, pathogens and presentation. *Chest.* 2008;134:1141-1148.
50. Nakashima K, Tanaka T, Kramer MH, et al. Outbreak of chlamydia pneumoniae infection in a Japanese nursing home, 1999-2000. *Infect Control Hosp Epidemiol.* 2006;27:1171-1177.

51. Bentley DW. Bacterial pneumonia in the elderly: Clinical features, diagnosis, etiology, and treatment. *Gerontology*. 1984;30: 297-307.
52. Fernandez-Sabe N, Carratala J, Roson B, et al. Community-acquired pneumonia in very elderly patients: Causative organisms, clinical characteristics, and outcomes. *Medicine (Baltimore)*. 2003;82:159-169.
53. Norman DC. Pneumonia in the elderly: Empiric antimicrobial therapy. *Geriatrics*. 1991;46:26-32.
54. Mandell LA, Wunderink RG, Anzueto A, et al. Infectious diseases society of America/American thoracic society consensus guidelines on the management of community-acquired pneumonia in adults. *Clin Infect Dis*. 2007;44:S27-S72.
55. Hanson LC, Weber DJ, Rutala WA, et al. Risk factors for nosocomial pneumonia in the elderly. *Am J Med*. 1992;92: 161-166.
56. Heuser MD, Case LD, Ettinger WH. Mortality in intensive care patients with respiratory disease: Is age important? *Arch Intern Med*. 1992;152:1683-1688.
57. Fried TR, Gillick MR, Lipsitz LA. Short-term functional outcomes of long-term care residents with pneumonia treated with and without hospital transfer. *J Am Geriatr Soc*. 1997;45: 302-306.
58. Monto AS, Terpenning MS. The value of influenza and pneumococcal vaccines in the elderly. *Drugs Aging*. 1996;6: 445-451.
59. Centers for Disease Control and Prevention. Influenza and pneumococcal vaccination levels among persons aged ≥ 65 years—United States, 1999. *MMWR Morb Mortal Wkly Rep*. 2001;50:532-537.
60. Hak E, Nordin J, Wei F, et al. Influence of high-risk medical conditions on the effectiveness of influenza vaccination among elderly members of 3 large managed-care organizations. *Clin Infect Dis*. 2002;35:370-377.
61. Voordouw BC, van der Linden PD, Simonian S, et al. Influenza vaccination in community-dwelling elderly: Impact on mortality and influenza-associated morbidity. *Arch Intern Med*. 2003;163:1089-1094.
62. Nichol KL, Nordin J, Mullooly J, et al. Influenza vaccination and reduction in hospitalizations for cardiac disease and stroke among the elderly. *N Engl J Med*. 2003;348:1322-1332.
63. Christenson B, Lundbergh P, Hedlund J, et al. Effects of a large-scale intervention with influenza and 23-valent pneumococcal vaccines in adults aged 65 years or older: A prospective study. *Lancet*. 2001;357:1008-1011.
64. Skull SA, Andrews RM, Byrnes GB, et al. Prevention of community-acquired pneumonia among a cohort of hospitalized elderly: Benefit due to influenza and pneumococcal vaccination not demonstrated. *Vaccine*. 2007;25:4631-4640.
65. Voordouw BC, Sturkenboom MC, Dieleman JP, et al. Annual influenza vaccination in community-dwelling elderly individuals and the risk of lower respiratory tract infections or pneumonia. *Arch Intern Med*. 2006;166:1980-1985.
66. Arden NH, Patriarca PA, Fasano MB, et al. The roles of vaccination and amantadine prophylaxis in controlling an outbreak of influenza A (H3N2) in a nursing home. *Arch Intern Med*. 1988;148:865-868.
67. Artz AS, Ershler WB, Longo DL. Pneumococcal vaccination and revaccination of older adults. *Clin Microbiol Rev*. 2003;16: 308-318.
68. Jackson LA, Neuzil KM, Yu O, et al. Effectiveness of pneumococcal polysaccharide vaccine in older adults. *N Engl J Med*. 2003;348:1747-1755.
69. Melegaro A, Edmunds WJ. The 23-valent pneumococcal polysaccharide vaccine. Part I. Efficacy of PPV in the elderly: A comparison of meta-analyses. *Eur J Epidemiol*. 2004;19:353-363.
70. Whitney CG, Farley MM, Hadler J, et al. Decline in invasive pneumococcal disease after the introduction of protein-polysaccharide conjugate vaccine. *N Engl J Med*. 2003;348: 1737-1746.
71. Centers for Disease Control and Prevention. Ten leading nationally notifiable infectious diseases—United States, 1995. *MMWR Morb Mortal Wkly Rep*. 1996;45:883-884.
72. Centers for Disease Control and Prevention. *Reported tuberculosis in the United States, 2007*. Atlanta, Ga.: U.S. Department of Health and Human Services, CDC; 2008.
73. Stead WW, Dutt AK. Tuberculosis in elderly persons. *Annu Rev Med*. 1991;42:267-276.
74. Dutt AK, Stead WW. Tuberculosis. *Clin Geriatr Med*. 1992;8: 761-775.
75. Perez-Guzman C, Vargas MH, Torres-Cruz A, et al. Does aging modify pulmonary tuberculosis?: A meta-analytical review. *Chest*. 1999;116:961-9670.
76. Davies P. Tuberculosis in the elderly: Epidemiology and optimal management. *Drugs Aging*. 1996;8:436-444.
77. Rajagopalan S. Tuberculosis and aging: A global health problem. *Clin Infect Dis*. 2001;33:1034-1039.
78. Perez-Guzman C, Torres Cruz A, Villarreal-Velarde H, et al. Progressive age-related changes in pulmonary tuberculosis images and the effect of diabetes. *Am J Respir Crit Care Med*. 2000;162:1738-1740.
79. Centers for Disease Control and Prevention. Targeted tuberculin testing and treatment of latent tuberculosis infection. *MMWR Morb Mortal Wkly Rep*. 2000;49:1-54.
80. Keelaghan E, Margolis D, Zhan M, et al. Prevalence of pressure ulcers in hospital admission among nursing home residents transferred to the hospital. *Wound Repair Regen*. 2008;16:331-336.
81. Margolis DJ, Bilker W, Knauss J, et al. The incidence and prevalence of pressure ulcers among elderly patients in general medical practice. *Ann Epidemiol*. 2002;12:321-325.
82. Kertesz D, Chow AW. Infected pressure and diabetic ulcers. *Clin Geriatr Med*. 1992;8:835-852.
83. Bryan CS, Dew CE, Reynolds KL. Bacteremia associated with decubitus ulcers. *Arch Intern Med*. 1983;143:2093-2095.
84. AGS Clinical Practice Committee. Pressure ulcers in adults: Prediction and prevention. *J Am Geriatr Soc*. 1996;44:1118-1119.
85. European Pressure Ulcer Advisory Panel. European guidelines for pressure ulcer treatment. 〈http://www.epuap.org/gltreatment.html〉.
86. Reddy M, Gill SS, Kalkar SR, et al. Treatment of pressure ulcers: a systematic review. *JAMA*. 2008;300:2647-2662.
87. Livesley NJ, Chow AW. Infected pressure ulcers in elderly individuals. *Clin Infect Dis*. 2002;35:1390-1396.
88. Auerbach SB, Schwartz B, Williams D, et al. Outbreak of invasive group A streptococcal infections in a nursing home: Lessons on prevention and control. *Arch Intern Med*. 1992;152:1017-1022.
89. Rainbow J, Jewell B, Danila RN, et al. Invasive group a streptococcal disease in nursing homes, Minnesota 1995-2006. *Emerg Infect Dis*. 2008;14:772-777.
90. Phares CR, Lynfield R, Farley MM, et al. Active Bacterial Core Surveillance / Emerging Infections Program Network. Epidemiology of invasive group B streptococcal disease in the United States, 1999-2005. *JAMA*. 2008;299:2056-2065.
91. Petterson E, Vernby A, Molstad S, et al. Infections and antibiotic prescribing in Swedish nursing homes: A cross-sectional study. *Scand J Infect Dis*. 2008;40:393-398.
92. Martin GS, Mannino DM, Moss M. The effect of age on the development and outcome of adult sepsis. *Crit Care Med*. 2006;34:15-21.
93. Meyers BR, Sherman E, Mendelson MH, et al. Bloodstream infections in the elderly. *Am J Med*. 1989;86:379-384.
94. McBean M, Rajamani S. Increasing rates of hospitalization due to septicemia in the US elderly population, 1986-1997. *J Infect Dis*. 2001;183:596-603.
95. Gleckman R, Hibert D. Afebrile bacteremia: A phenomenon in geriatric patients. *JAMA*. 1982;248:1478-1481.
96. Chassagne P, Perol M-B, Doucet J, et al. Is presentation of bacteremia in the elderly the same as in younger patients? *Am J Med*. 1996;100:65-70.
97. Leibovici L. Bacteraemia in the very old. *Drugs Aging*. 1995;6: 456-464.
98. Mylotte JM, Tayara A, Goodnough S. Epidemiology of bloodstream infection in nursing home residents: Evaluation in a large cohort from multiple homes. *Clin Infect Dis*. 2002;35:1484-1490.
99. Lewthwaite P, Parsons HK, Bates CJ, et al. Group G streptococcal bacteraemia: An opportunistic infection associated with immune senescence. *Scand J Infect Dis*. 2002;34:83-87.
100. Morike K, Schwab M, Klotz U. Use of aminoglycosides in elderly patients. *Drugs Aging*. 1997;10:259-277.
101. Terpenning MS, Buggy BP, Kauffman CA. Infective endocarditis: Clinical features in young and elderly patients. *Am J Med*. 1987;83:626-634.
102. Watanakunakorn C, Burkert T. Infective endocarditis at a large community teaching hospital, 1980-1990: A review of 210 episodes. *Medicine (Baltimore)*. 1993;72:90-102.
103. Tleyjeh IM, Steckelberg JM, Murad HS, et al. Temporal trends in infective endocarditis: a population-based study in Olmsted county, Minnesota. *JAMA*. 2005;293:3022-3028.
104. Di Salvo G, Thuny F, Rosenberg V, et al. Endocarditis in the elderly: Clinical, echocardiographic, and prognostic features. *Eur Heart J*. 2003;24:1576-1583.
105. Barrau K, Boulamery A, Imbert G, et al. Causative organisms of infective endocarditis according to host status. *Clin Microbiol Infect*. 2004;10:302-308.
106. Wilson W, Taubert KA, Gewitz M, et al. Prevention of infective endocarditis: A guideline from the American Heart Association Rheumatic Fever, Endocarditis, and Kawasaki Disease Committee, Council on Cardiovascular Disease in the Young, and the Council on Clinical Cardiology, Council on Cardiovascular Surgery and Anesthesia, and the Quality of Care and Outcomes Research Interdisciplinary Working Group. *Circulation*. 2007; 116:1736-1754.
107. Lew JF, Glass RI, Gangarosa RE, et al. Diarrheal deaths in the United States, 1979 through 1987. *JAMA*. 1991;265:3280-3284.
108. Augustin AK, Simor AE, Shorrock C, et al. Outbreaks of gastroenteritis due to Norwalk-like virus in two long-term care facilities for the elderly. *Can J Infect Control*. 1995;10:111-113.
109. Tu ET, Bull RA, Kim MJ, et al. Norovirus excretion in an aged-care setting. *J Clin Microbiol*. 2008;46:2119-2121.
110. Lopman BA, Reacher MH, Vipond IB, et al. Clinical manifestation of norovirus gastroenteritis in health care settings. *Clin Infect Dis*. 2004;39:318-324
111. Centers for Disease Control and Prevention (CDC). Norovirus activity—United States, 2006-2007. *MMWR Morb Mortal Wkly Rep*. 2007;56:842-846.
112. Bentley DW. *Clostridium difficile*-associated disease in long-term care facilities. *Infect Control Hosp Epidemiol*. 1990;11:434-438.
113. Wilcox MH. Cleaning up *Clostridium difficile* infection. *Lancet*. 1996;348:767-769.
114. Ricciardi R, Rothenberger DA, Madoff RD, et al. Increasing prevalence and severity of Clostridium difficile colitis in hospitalized patients in the United States. *Arch Surg*. 2007;142:624-631.
115. Ryan CA, Tauxe RV, Hosek GW, et al. *Escherichia coli* O157:H7 diarrhea in a nursing home: Clinical, epidemiological, and pathological findings. *J Infect Dis*. 1986;154:631-638.
116. Neill MA, Rice SK, Ahmad NV, et al. Cryptosporidiosis: An unrecognized cause of diarrhea in elderly hospitalized patients. *Clin Infect Dis*. 1996;22:168-170.
117. Naumova EN, Egorov AI, Morris RD, et al. The elderly and waterborne *Cryptosporidium* infection: Gastroenteritis hospitalizations before and during the 1993 Milwaukee outbreak. *Emerg Infect Dis*. 2003;9:418-425.
118. Danna PL, Urban C, Bellin E, et al. Role of *Candida* in pathogenesis of antibiotic-associated diarrhoea in elderly inpatients. *Lancet*. 1991;337:511-514.
119. Lores B, Lopez-Miragaya I, Arias C, et al. Intestinal microsporidiosis due to *Enterocytozoon bieneusi* in elderly human immunodeficiency virus–negative patients from Vigo, Spain. *Clin Infect Dis*. 2002;34:918-921.
120. Bethony J, Chen J, Lin S, et al. Emerging patterns of hookworm infection: Influence of aging on the intensity of *Necator* infection in Hainan Province, People's Republic of China. *Clin Infect Dis*. 2002;35:1336-1344.
121. Van de Beek D, de Gans J, Spanjaard L, et al. Clinical features and prognostic factors in adults with bacterial meningitis. *N Engl J Med*. 2004;351:1849-1859.
122. Kastenbauer S, Pfister HW. Pneumococcal meningitis in adults: Spectrum of complications and prognostic factors in a series of 87 cases. *Brain*. 2003;126:1015-1025.
123. Choi C. Bacterial meningitis. *Clin Geriatr Med*. 1992;8:889-901.
124. Behrman RE, Meyers BR, Mendelson MH, et al. Central nervous system infections in the elderly. *Arch Intern Med*. 1989;149: 1596-1599.
125. Gorse GJ, Thrupp LD, Nudleman KL, et al. Bacterial meningitis in the elderly. *Arch Intern Med*. 1984;144:1603-1607.
126. Choi C. Bacterial meningitis in aging adults. *Clin Infect Dis*. 2001;33:1380-1385.
127. Nash D, Mostashari F, Fine A, et al. The outbreak of West Nile virus infection in the New York City area in 1999. *N Engl J Med*. 2001;344:1807-1814.
128. Watson JT, Pertel PE, Jones RC, et al. Clinical characteristics and functional outcomes of West Nile fever. *Ann Intern Med*. 2004;141:360-365.
129. Peterson LR, Marfin AA. West Nile virus: A primer for the clinician. *Ann Intern Med*. 2002;137:173-179.
130. Gottfried K, Quinn R, Jones T. Clinical description and follow-up investigation of human West Nile virus cases. *South Med J*. 2005;98:603-606.
131. Bhangoo S, Chua R, Hammond C, et al. Focal neurological injury caused by West Nile virus infection may occur independent of patient age and premorbid health. *J Neurol Sci*. 2005; 234:93-98.
132. Gavet F, Tournadre A, Soubrier M, et al. Septic arthritis in patients aged 80 and older: A comparison with younger adults. *J Am Geriatr Soc*. 2005;53:1210-1213.
133. McGuire NM, Kauffman CA. Septic arthritis in the elderly. *J Am Geriatr Soc*. 1985;33:170-174.
134. Gomolin IH, Lester P, Pollack S. Older is colder: observations on body temperature among nursing home subjects. *J Am Med Dir Assoc*. 2007;8:335-337.
135. Fox RH, MacGibbon R, Davies L, et al. Problem of the old and the cold. *BMJ*. 1973;1:21-24.
136. McAlpine CH, Martin BJ, Lennox IM, et al. Pyrexia in infection in the elderly. *Age Ageing*. 1986;15:230-234.
137. Marco CA, Schoenfeld CN, Hansen KN, et al. Fever in geriatric emergency patients: Clinical features associated with serious illness. *Ann Emerg Med*. 1995;26:18-24.
138. Norman DC, Wong MB, Yoshikawa TT. Fever of unknown origin in older persons. *Infect Dis Clin Am*. 2007;21:937-945.
139. Tal S, Guller V, Gurevich A. Fever of unknown origin in older adults. *Clin Geriatr Med*. 2007;23:649-668.
140. Stalam M, Kaye D. Antibiotic agents in the elderly. *Infect Dis Clin N Am*. 2004;18:533-549.
141. Herring AR, Williamson JC. Principles of antimicrobial use in older adults. *Clin Geriatr Med*. 2007;23:481-497.
142. Monette J, Miller MA, Monnette M, et al. Effect of an educational intervention on optimizing antibiotic prescribing in long-term care facilities. *J Am Geriatr Soc*. 2007;55:1231-1235.
143. O'Fallon E, Harper J, Shaw S, et al. Antibiotic and infection tracking in Minnesota long-term care facilities. *J Am Geriatr Soc*. 2007;55:1243-1247.
144. Schwartz D, Abiad H, DeMarais PL, et al. An educational intervention to improve antimicrobial use in a hospital-based long-term care facility. *J Am Geriatr Soc*. 2007;55:1236-1242.
145. Centers for Disease Control and Prevention. Resistance of *Streptococcus pneumoniae* to fluoroquinolones—United States 1995-1999. *MMWR Morb Mortal Wkly Rep*. 2001;50:800-804.
146. Yokota S, Sato K, Kuwahara O, et al. Fluoroquinolone-resistant *Streptococcus pneumoniae* strains occur frequently in elderly

patients in Japan. *Antimicrob Agents Chemother.* 2002;46:3311-3315.

147. Mamdani M, McNeely D, Evans G, et al. Impact of a fluoroquinolone restriction policy in an elderly population. *Am J Med.* 2007;120:893-900.

148. Marcus EL, Clarfield AM, Moses AE. Ethical issues relating to the use of antimicrobial therapy in older adults. *Clin Infect Dis.* 2001;33:1697-1705.

149. Leder, K, Weller PF, Wilson ME. Travel vaccines and elderly persons: Review of vaccines available in the United States. *Clin Infect Dis.* 2001;33:1553-1566.

150. Genton B, D'Acremont V, Furrer HJ, et al. Hepatitis A vaccines and the elderly. *Travel Med Infect Dis.* 2006;4:303-312.

151. Barnett ED. Yellow fever: epidemiology and prevention. *Clin Infect Dis.* 2007;44:850-856.

152. Khromova AY, Eidex RB, Weld LH, et al. The Yellow Fever Vaccine Safety Working Group. Yellow fever vaccine: An updated assessment of advanced age as a risk factor for serious adverse events. *Vaccine.* 2005;23:3256-3263.

153. Ceddia T, Natellis C, Zigrino AG. Antibody response to rabies vaccine prepared in tissue culture of human diploid cells and inactivated, evaluated in different classes of age. *Ann Sclavo.* 1982;24:491-495.

154. Mastroeni I, Vescia N, Pompa MG, et al. Immune response of the elderly to rabies vaccine. *Vaccine.* 1994;12:518-520.

155. Harpaz R, Ortega-Sanchez IR, Seward JF, Advisory Committee on Immunization Practices (ACIP) Centers for Disease Control and Prevention (CDC). Prevention of herpes zoster: Recommendations of the Advisory Committee on Immunization Practices (ACIP). *MMWR Recomm Rep.* 2008;57:1-30.

Infections in Asplenic Patients

LARRY I. LUTWICK

This member hath propritie by itself sometimes, to hinder a man's running. . . . They say that the splene may be taken out of the body by way of incision, and yet the creature lives nevertheless.

Plinius Secundus

Pliny, living in the malarious Mediterranean basin, could indeed have observed impaired athletic performances due to large *Plasmodium*-affected spleens.[1] His words, moreover, reflect the difficulties in understanding splenic function, which lasted for more than 25 centuries. The Grecian theory of bodily humors had deemed the spleen's black bile to be a source of melancholia, producing the concept of *venting one's spleen*. An association with laughter, putatively a therapeutic process, led to the prophetic idea that the spleen expurgated unclean material from both blood and spirit. Overall, however, the prevailing opinion relegated this organ to a nonessential role, wherein it was able to be removed without adverse effects.

Interest in splenic absence as a risk for serious infection was not truly aroused until King and Schumacker's 1952 seminal report of life-threatening infection in splenectomized infants.[2] The relationship between an absent or a hypofunctioning organ and severe infection, termed postsplenectomy sepsis (PSS) or overwhelming postsplenectomy infection (OPSI), is now well documented by illnesses evolving from good health to death within a day. Such septic deaths, almost entirely caused by certain encapsulated bacteria, may occur 600 times more frequently than in eusplenic persons,[3] influenced by factors including age at and cause of spleen removal.

Causes of Surgical Splenectomy

With an enlightened approach toward preserving splenic tissue, newer indications for spleen removal have resulted in a more conservative attitude toward resection. As examples, salvage procedures are being performed in traumatic splenic injury, and splenectomy is avoided in Hodgkin's disease. The maneuver, however, remains significant in the management of patients with hereditary hemolytic anemias, spherocytosis in particular.

Nonsurgical Equivalents of Splenectomy

CONGENITAL ASPLENIA

Asplenia, rarely, can be congenital rather than acquired. In infants, it is usually linked with serious organ malformations (Ivemark's syndrome). Isolated congenital asplenia, however, can be diagnosed even in the sixth or seventh decade of life, when the patient presents with life-threatening sepsis.[4] As such, congenital asplenia, which can be a genetically dominant trait, may be first recognized at autopsy in an individual who has succumbed to fulminant infection. The combination of Howell-Jolly bodies (see later) and thrombocytosis in the blood of an individual without a palpable spleen or an abdominal scar suggests the diagnosis of congenital asplenia. Classical PSS-like disease has also been very rarely reported in persons with seemingly normal spleens.

FUNCTIONAL HYPOSPLENISM

Although mostly related to splenectomy, PSS may occur with an anatomically present, albeit poorly performing organ.[5] Functional hyposplenism can be associated with a mélange of disorders (Table 315-1). Common mechanisms responsible for splenic dysfunction are repeated infarction, infiltration, intrasplenic blood flow redistribution, and antigen-antibody complex blockade.

Hyposplenism may be partially reversible, as exemplified by improved splenic function in celiac disease using a gluten-free diet[8] and in immune complex disease treated with plasma exchange.[9] Interestingly, transient splenic dysfunction can result from pneumococcemia,[10,11] perhaps contributing to PSS in hyposplenic persons.

Splenic Function and Its Assessment

As man's largest lymphoid organ, encamped in the midst of the blood's antigenic superhighway, the spleen has a bevy of immunologic functions, which include the production of opsonizing antibody and the efficient clearance of encapsulated bacteria. Increased amounts of specific antibody are needed in asplenia for the remaining reticuloendothelial system, particularly the liver, to effectively clear intravascular opsonized microorganisms.[12] Splenic absence or dysfunction is not well compensated for, however, with virulent pathogens, especially pneumococci.[13]

Mechanistically, circulating IgM memory B cells prominently decrease postsplenectomy.[14] These cells have a very significant role in the production of both natural and specific IgM antibodies vital to the early control of infection due to encapsulated bacteria. IgM memory cells are also diminished in hyposplenic disorders such as celiac disease[15] and inflammatory bowel disease.[16] Of note, anti-tumor necrosis factor can improve splenic function in Crohn's disease with parallel increases in this cell pool.[17]

IgM memory B cells originate in the splenic marginal zone B (MZB), found at the junction between red pulp and white pulp. Cells in the MZB have a low threshold for activation and a high expression of complement receptors to rapidly respond to T-cell–independent polysaccharide antigens such as those in bacterial capsules, facilitating both the innate and adaptive immune systems. Macrophages in the MZB express a lectin (referred to as SIGN-R1 in the mouse) that mediates the uptake of pneumococcal polysaccharides[18] and appears to be involved in protecting mice against pneumococcemia.[19]

The spleen also appears to have anti-inflammatory functions. An out-of-control production of proinflammatory cytokines contributes a deleterious role in sepsis. The central nervous system can dampen this *cytokine storm* through the efferent vagus nerve. Mediated through the spleen via a nicotinic acetylcholine receptor, the effect is absent in asplenic mice.[20] The spleen seems to play a role in dampening the febrile response as well.[21]

The architecture of the spleen functions as the blood's sieve, removing blood cells, microorganisms, and immune complexes. Addition-

TABLE 315-1	Conditions That May Be Associated with Functional Hyposplenism

Autoimmune Disorders

APECED*
Biliary cirrhosis
Chronic active hepatitis
Graves' disease
Hashimoto's thyroiditis
Mixed connective tissue disease
Rheumatoid arthritis
Sjögren's syndrome
Systemic lupus erythematosus
Vasculitis

Hematologic Diseases

Essential thrombocythemia
Fanconi syndrome
Hemophilia
Sickle cell hemoglobinopathies
  SS
  SC
  S-β thalassemia

Neoplasia

Breast carcinoma
Chronic myelogenous leukemia
Hemangiosarcoma of the spleen
Non-Hodgkin's lymphoma
Sézary syndrome

Infiltrative Diseases

Amyloidosis
Sarcoidosis

Liver/Intestinal Disorders

Celiac disease
Collagenous colitis
Crohn's disease†
Dermatitis herpetiformis
Intestinal lymphangiectasis
Portal hypertension
Tropical sprue
Ulcerative colitis
Whipple's disease

Miscellaneous

Alcoholism
Age
  Elderly (>70)‡
  Neonates/premature infants
Bone marrow transplantation
Chronic graft vs. host reaction
Hypopituitarism
Parenteral nutrition, chronic
Primary pulmonary hypertension
Splenic irradiation
  External
  Thoratrast
Thrombosis of splenic vessels
Wandering spleen with autoinfarction

*APECED, autoimmune polyendocrinopathy-candidiasis-ectodermal dystrophy.
†The degree of hyposplenism appears to be less in Crohn's disease than ulcerative colitis.[6]
‡Although splenic function is somewhat reduced with old age, it is usually not in the hyposplenic range.[7]

ally, after passing through the splenic microvasculature, red blood cells (RBCs) that contain inclusions may return to the circulation after undergoing remodeling (pitting). As such, finding Howell-Jolly bodies (nuclear remnants) and pocked RBCs in the peripheral blood reflect decreased remodeling and clearance, indicators of splenic dysfunction. Pocks are actually hemoglobin-containing vacuoles, found primarily in the older RBCs, that are removed by the normal spleen.[22]

The presence of Howell-Jolly bodies (Fig. 315-1A), a simple screening test for asplenia, is relatively insensitive in the hyposplenic patient without significant impairment of function.[23] An increased pocked RBC count is a more sensitive indicator of splenic dysfunction,[24] visualized using interference phase microscopy (see Fig. 315-1B). In eusplenic persons, less than 2% of red cells are pocked, whereas hyposplenic persons can demonstrate greater than 12% and asplenic persons as high as 50%.[25] As the pocked cell count increases, increasing

numbers of Howell-Jolly bodies can be seen, correlating well with the pock count.[23] An absent spleen is assessable by a variety of radiologic techniques and a technetium 99m sulfur colloid scan may detect hypofunction but can be discordant with other tests.

Clinical Characteristics of Postsplenectomy Sepsis

FREQUENCY

Factors contributing to difficulties in estimating PSS frequency[26,27] include a variable disease definition, differences in duration of follow-up, and considerations of age at and cause of splenectomy. Styrt assessed reports for the risk of fatal PSS to factor out milder, nonclassical infections.[26] In children, an incidence of one fatal case per approximately 350 patient-years of follow-up was found, or (assuming a 50% case fatality) one case per 175 patient-years. Postsplenectomy sepsis frequency is more variable after spleen removal in the adult. Overall, Styrt concluded that the risk is lower than after childhood splenectomy,[26] estimating an overall risk of one fatal case in 800 to 1000 patient-years, or one case in 400 to 500 patient-years.

The risk can also be stratified by splenectomy cause as seen in Table 315-2.[1,3,26,28] It is lowest related to trauma and idiopathic thrombocytopenic purpura (ITP), intermediate with spherocytosis, portal hypertension, and Hodgkin's disease, and the highest risk with thalas-

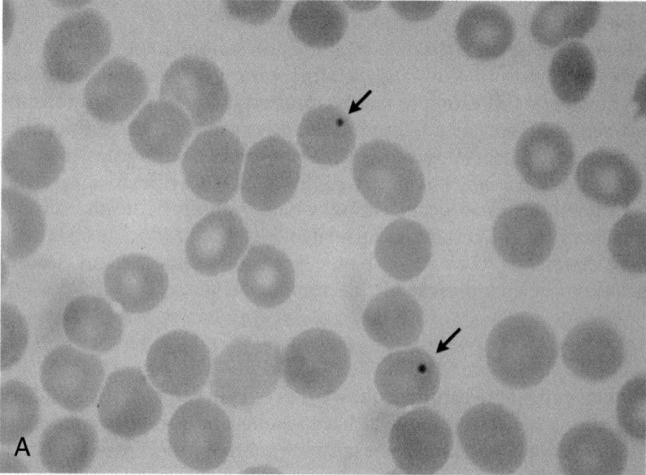

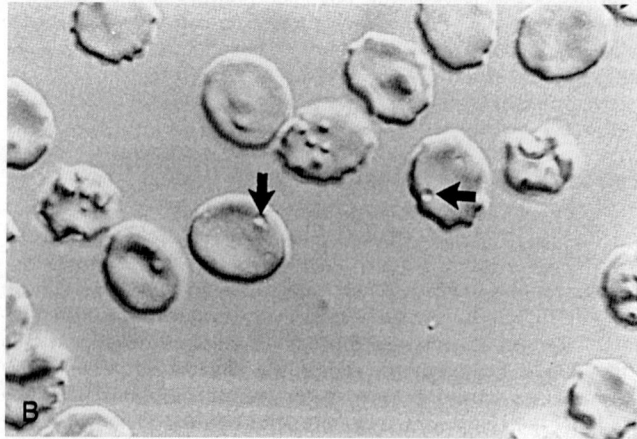

Figure 315-1 **A,** Photomicrograph of Howell-Jolly bodies in the circulating erythrocytes of a patient with a surgical splenectomy. **B,** An interference microscopy photomicrograph of pocked (intraerythrocytic vesicle) red cells. (**A,** *Courtesy of Dr. Carol Luhrs, Veterans Affairs New York Harbor Health System, Brooklyn Campus;* **B,** *Courtesy of Dr. George Buchanan, University of Texas.*)

TABLE 315-2	The Risk of Postsplenectomy Sepsis Related to Splenectomy Cause*† (Cases/100 Patient-Years)		
	Risk	*N*	*Range*
Low Attack Rate			
Incidental surgical	1.17	2521	1.0-2.4
Idiopathic thrombocytopenic purpura (ITP)	2.03	2728	1.5-3.3
Trauma	2.07	6612	1.5-2.4
Intermediate Attack Rate			
Spherocytosis	3.15	4816	2.4-3.6
Hodgkin's disease	6.15	2507	4.1-11.6
Portal hypertension	6.72	610	4.1-8.6
High Attack Rate			
Thalassemia	11.6	852	7.0-24.8
Autoimmune lymphoproliferative syndrome	31.3[22]	16	

*From references 1, 3, 26, and 28; all are reviews and the cases may have overlapped between them.

†In these reviews, how many of the cases are prototypical PSS as compared with bacteremias and other serious infections is unclear.

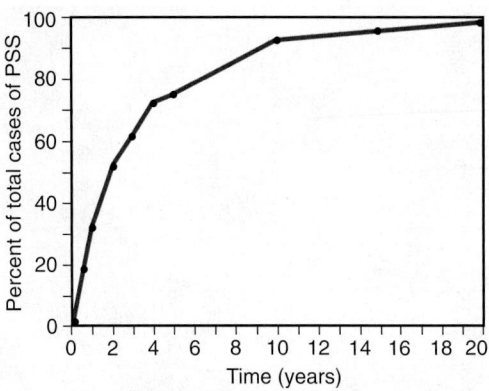

Figure 315-3 **The interval from splenectomy to postsplenectomy sepsis.** Of the total (N = 288), 3.1% occurred more than 20 years after splenectomy. *(Derived from data from Holdsworth RJ, Irving AD, Cuschieri A. Postsplenectomy sepsis and its mortality rate: Actual versus perceived risks. Br J Surg. 1991;78:1031-1038.)*

semia. Autoimmune lymphoproliferative syndrome (ALPS), a disorder with defective lymphocyte apoptosis that can require splenectomy for hypersplenism, also has a high potential for PSS.[29] In 5491 patient-years of follow-up after splenectomy for hereditary spherocytosis, risks of one case per 365 patient-years and one fatal case every 910 patient-years were found.[30] Coexisting hepatic disease, if Kupffer cell phagocytic function is depressed, may add to the risk of PSS. The percentage of cases of PSS linked to different causes of asplenia are illustrated in Figure 315-2. Repeated PSS may occur after splenectomy with reports of the risk of a second episode 6-fold higher than the first and for a third, 14-fold higher.[31] Overall, about 6% of total PSS cases occur in hyposplenic hosts.[27] In one cause of hyposplenism, pneumococcal sepsis in celiac disease occurred 3.9 times more frequently than that of the general population.[32]

Singer, comparing the frequency of PSS in his 1973 and 2001 reports, suggested that an overall 18% decrease in the risk of PSS had occurred.[1] A report regarding asplenic children in Toronto, moreover, showed that when the period between 1958 and 1970 was compared

with the period between 1971 and 1995, a 47% decrease in bacteremia with encapsulated organisms had occurred.[33] These studies affirm a significant role of prophylactic antimicrobials and immunization in PSS prevention.

TIMING RELATED TO SPLENECTOMY

PSS risk is highest in the first few years after spleen removal. The infection, however, has appeared many years later, with intervals in excess of four decades.[34] Styrt found 9 of 46 cases falling within the first year, followed by four to five new cases in each year from second to the seventh postsplenectomy year.[26] In a more extensive review of 288 PSS cases, 32% of cases occurred within the first year and 52% within the second (Fig. 315-3).[27] In general, the younger the person is at the time of splenectomy, the shorter the interval to PSS.

TYPICAL PRESENTATION

PSS has a short prodrome with low-grade fever, chills, pharyngitis, muscle aches, and often vomiting or diarrhea, or both. If enough detail were reported, true rigors might have been present for 1 to 2 days prior to clinical deterioration.[26] In the setting of known asplenia or a dysfunctional splenic state, any febrile illness with or without gastrointestinal or other focal symptoms must be suspected to be PSS. Usually, no clinically demonstrable site of infection is found in adult PSS. In children younger than 5 years old, however, focal infections, particularly meningitis, are more prominent.[27]

Overt deterioration is abrupt and progressive, measured in hours rather than days, with a picture that continues to remain disturbingly unchanged. An asplenic individual may walk into a health care facility complaining of fever and diarrhea only to be in shock within a few hours. Cardiovascular collapse often with disseminated intravascular coagulopathy (DIC), seizures, and coma accompanies this rapid downhill course. Tissue damage can be compounded by the development of purpura fulminans,[35] in which hypotension and endovascular injury contribute to extremity gangrene and the possibility of one, or often multiple, amputations. Thrombotic microangiopathy (thrombotic thrombocytopenic purpura/hemolytic uremic syndrome) can also occur[36] and may have been underdiagnosed in the past.

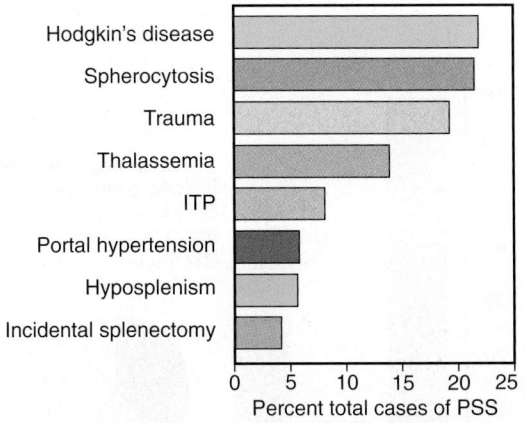

Figure 315-2 **Underlying cause of splenic deficiency in 688 episodes of postsplenectomy sepsis.** *(Derived from Hansen K, Singer DB. Asplenic-hyposplenic overwhelming sepsis: Postsplenectomy sepsis revisited. Pediatr Dev Pathol. 2001;4:105-121; Singer DB. Postsplenectomy sepsis. In: Rosenberg HS, Bolande RP, eds. Perspectives in Pediatric Pathology. Vol 1. Chicago: Year Book Medical; 1973:285-311; Styrt B. Infection associated with asplenia: Risks, mechanisms, and prevention. Am J Med. 1990;88[5N]:33N-42N; and Holdsworth RJ, Irving AD, Cuschieri A. Postsplenectomy sepsis and its mortality rate: Actual versus perceived risks. Br J Surg. 1991;78:1031-1038.)*

DIAGNOSIS

Early consideration of PSS is vital to facilitate an aggressive, immediate intervention. A high index of clinical suspicion must be maintained for febrile presentations in the asplenic patient or one with a chronic disease that can produce a dysfunctional spleen. The diag-

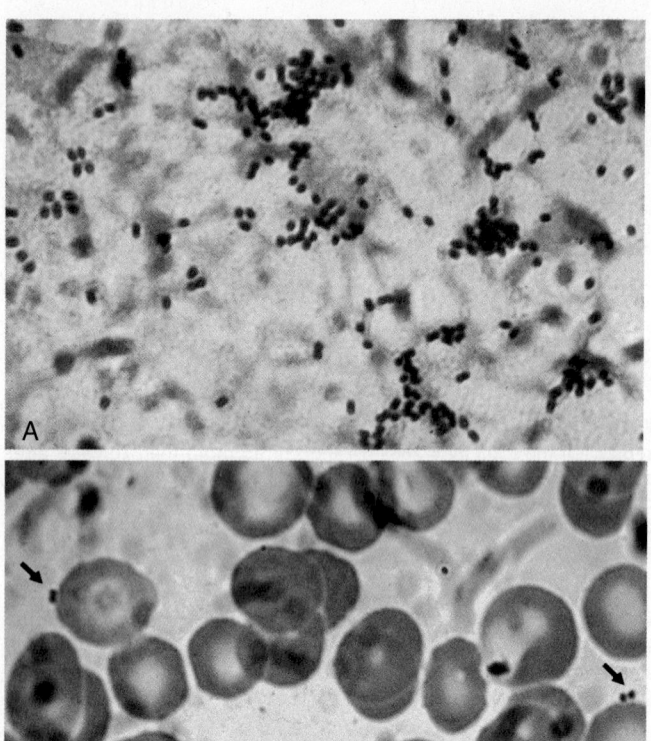

Figure 315-4 **A,** The Gram stain of a buffy coat smear from a patient with rapidly fatal pneumococcal postsplenectomy sepsis, 7 years after a staging laparotomy for Hodgkin's disease, showing many gram-positive diplococci. **B,** A more magnified Wright stain of a peripheral blood smear from the same patient, showing extracellular diplococci. *(From Lynch AM, Kapila R. Overwhelming postsplenectomy infection. Infect Dis Clin North Am. 1996;10:693-707. Used with permission of the publisher.)*

nostic workup should never delay use of empirical antimicrobial therapy.

An extremely high degree of bacteremia, greatly contributing to morbidity and mortality, allows a diagnosis to be made quickly. Bacteria can often be visualized on a Gram or Wright stain of the peripheral blood buffy coat (Fig. 315-4A) and may be seen on a peripheral blood smear (see Fig. 315-4B). This latter finding reflects greater than $10^6/mL$, as much as 4 logs or greater than that of a usual bacteremia.[37] Because of this, blood cultures are often positive within 6 to 12 hours. Petechial or purpuric lesions should be aspirated for Gram stain and culture, and a CSF examination may be needed, particularly in children. Examination of the peripheral blood for malaria or babesiosis may be necessary, guided by the patient's history. Furthermore, Howell-Jolly bodies or other evidence of hyposplenism should be sought in all septic patients, especially in an individual with a possibility of hyposplenism.

MORTALITY

PSS is particularly problematic because of its high mortality rates, classically in the range of 50% to 70% despite appropriate antimicrobial therapy and intensive medical support.[26,27] The dramatic nature of this illness is further underscored by the short time between the initial

symptoms and death, with 68% of the mortality within 24 hours and 80% within 48 hours. A substantial decrease in mortality associated with bacteremia involving encapsulated organisms has been reported when an earlier asplenic cohort (1958-1970) was compared with a more recent one (1971-1995).[33] This suggests that early diagnosis and aggressive treatment are effective in lowering the case fatality rate of PSS.

It is important to be aware that, unlike incidence, PSS case fatality rate is independent of the indication for spleen removal. This is likely to be the case, as well, in hyposplenia-associated PSS. A lower mortality (31.8%) has been observed in a small number of *Haemophilus influenzae* cases as compared to pneumococcal PSS.[27] In total, however, mortality from pneumococcal cases does not differ from those of non-pneumococcal etiology.

◼ Microbiology of Postsplenectomy Sepsis

STREPTOCOCCUS PNEUMONIAE (PNEUMOCOCCUS)

The pneumococcus is singularly the most important organism in PSS, involved in 50% to 90% of cases.[26,27] In a review of 349 PSS cases, *Streptococcus pneumoniae* was causative in 66% of episodes in which a bacterium could be identified (Fig. 315-5).[27] Although common in all age groups, the percentage of pneumococcal PSS cases increases with age. A predominant polysaccharide serotype is not found, and the distribution of serotypes involved in PSS does not differ from that in other invasive pneumococcal infections.

Antimicrobial resistance in *S. pneumoniae* is increasingly prevalent. In some areas, a significant percentage of pneumococci demonstrate penicillin resistance, either relative or absolute. Such isolates can be resistant to the extended-spectrum cephalosporins, such as ceftriaxone, as well. Penicillin-resistant pneumococci (PRP), as well as the increase in quinolone resistance, require consideration in the empirical therapy of PSS.

HAEMOPHILUS INFLUENZAE

Type b *H. influenzae* (Hib) is the second most common organism in PSS.[26,27] Most Hib-associated PSS cases have occurred in children younger than 15 years, 86% in one review,[27] with a frequency about 10 times lower than that of the pneumococcus. Neither nontypable nor non-b capsular strains (a, c-f) are significant PSS pathogens. Use

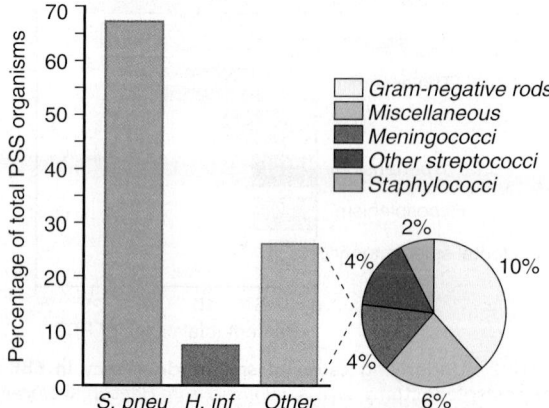

Figure 315-5 **The microbiology of postsplenectomy sepsis based on 298 culture-positive episodes including those due to the meningococcus.** Of the total, 51 (14.6%) additional episodes did not have a reported organism. Data are not stratified by age or cause of splenectomy. *(Derived from Holdsworth RJ, Irving AD, Cuschieri A. Postsplenectomy sepsis and its mortality rate: Actual versus perceived risks. Br J Surg. 1991;78:1031-1038.)*

of the conjugated Hib vaccine has dramatically decreased the incidence of invasive Hib disease. The consequences of this protection should be a falloff in PSS cases due to Hib. Some Hib-associated PSS may be related to more virulent isolates possessing multiple copies of the capsulation locus and this has been reported in an adult case of Hib PSS.[38] β-Lactamase production by many *H. influenzae* strains needs accounting for choosing empirical therapy.

OTHER BACTERIAL ORGANISMS

Neisseria meningitidis, the meningococcus, is often cited as the third most common cause of PSS. Although invasive meningococcal disease occurs in the asplenic[39,40] and it was reported in King and Schumacker's original series,[2] meningococcemia is neither less frequent nor milder in eusplenics than in this cohort.[41] Data in asplenic mice further support the lack of this association.[41] Some other encapsulated organisms such as Group A and B streptococci, the yeast *Cryptococcus neoformans* and the hyperviscous *Klebsiella pneumoniae* strains also are not significant causes of infection in the asplenic/hyposplenic cohort.

Capnocytophaga canimorsus and *C. cynodegmi,* zoonotic gram-negative rods formerly classified as CDC group DF-2 and DF-2-like, respectively, are part of canine and feline oral flora. Typically, both species are transmitted from dog contact, usually a bite. Both species can infect healthy persons and infections tend to be mild. Of reported severe cases, almost all due to *C. canimorsus,* 80% have predisposing conditions, primarily asplenia and hyposplenism.[42,43] An illness with gram-negative bacilli in the buffy coat or peripheral blood smear or an eschar at the bite site,[44] manifesting 1 to 7 days after the bite, suggests *Capnocytophaga* spp., as the cause. β-Lactamase activity can be seen in 30% of strains.

Severe salmonellosis is associated with the hyposplenism of chronic reticuloendothelial blockage in bartonellosis, and the infection is prominent in children with sickle cell anemia–associated splenic dysfunction. Nonetheless, *Salmonella enterica* subtypes do not play a large role in PSS. Most cases are associated with illnesses where defects in cell-mediated immunity from either the disease or its treatment predispose to salmonellosis.

A wide compendium of other bacteria has been anecdotally linked to PSS. Of note, *Streptococcus suis* has caused PSS in those with swine exposure[45] and 22 of the 26 reported bacteremias due to *Bordetella holmesii* occurred in asplenics or hyposplenics.[46] Of note, at least in a murine model, splenectomy may induce higher resistance to listeriosis.[47]

Relationship of Splenectomy to Other Infections

POSTOPERATIVE PERIOD

Early postoperative infections after splenectomy are related to the usual suspects in pulmonary, urinary, and superficial or deep operative sites. In trauma patients requiring splenectomy, both focal infections and bacteremias are more common in individuals with additional nonsplenic injuries.[48] The microbiology of these infections is primarily staphylococci and enteric gram-negative bacilli, not the characteristic PSS organisms. Whether splenectomy is an independent risk factor for postoperative infection remains ill defined. The risk may be higher but without a parallel increase in mortality.[49,50]

INTRAERYTHROCYTIC PARASITEMIAS (BABESIOSIS AND MALARIA)

In babesiosis, most severe infections occur in the asplenic host.[51] It is these individuals who have higher-grade parasitemias, develop significant hemolysis, and even with specific treatment can relapse. Babesiosis in eusplenic persons is, by and large, mild or subclinical, not requiring therapy.

Splenectomy allows adaptation of human malaria to primates, and the spontaneous resolution (*crisis*) of malaria is spleen-mediated in some nonhuman species. Whether malaria in humans is clinically affected by removal of the spleen, however, is less well established. In partially malaria-immune asplenic individuals, the course of *Plasmodium falciparum* infection was not altered in a Thai study,[52] but illness was more frequent and more severe in a report from Malawi.[53] The human spleen does play a pivotal role in malarial parasite clearance, removing intraerythrocytic parasites without red cell destruction (pitting). These pitted cells can be detected in the circulation by the presence of ring-associated erythrocyte surface antigen (RESA),[54] not found in malarious asplenic.[55] Since pitting does not occur in the *Plasmodium*-infected asplenic patient, parasite removal is delayed, so higher levels of parasitemia are noted, but this does not necessarily reflect resistance to the antimalarial used.[55] It is quite important for the asplenic/hyposplenic cohort to avoid both malaria and babesiosis by vector avoidance techniques and, with malaria, appropriate oral prophylaxis use.

EHRLICHIOSIS (ANAPLASMOSIS)

Human granulocytic ehrlichiosis, caused by *Anaplasma phagocytophilum,* has been reported to be recurrent, prolonged, or more severe, or some combination of the three, in asplenic persons.[56] Ehrlichiosis should be added to the list of severe infections in asplenic or hyposplenic persons if this is confirmed.

HEMOTROPIC BACTERIAL INFECTIONS

Bartonella bacilliformis is a gram-negative rod endemic in the western Peruvian Andes. During acute human infection (Oroyo fever), bacilli are found adherent to RBCs and a severe hemolytic anemia occurs. Asplenia seemed to be a factor in prolonged bacteremia without hemolysis in a splenectomized Peruvian with *B. bacilliformis* infection.[57] A 1979 report described an asplenic American patient without travel who had an uncultivatable organism adhering to most of his RBCs,[58] but additional cases have not surfaced.

INFECTION WITH THE HUMAN IMMUNODEFICIENCY VIRUS

There is no evidence of either a higher risk of PSS in human immunodeficiency virus (HIV)-infected asplenic patients or any relationship of risk to CD4 cell levels. After removal of the spleen, absolute CD4 and CD8 lymphocyte levels rise in both HIV-infected and noninfected individuals.[59] The CD4/CD8 ratio does not change and becomes more important in therapeutic decision-making processes for the splenectomized HIV-infected person.

Therapeutic Strategies

IMMEDIATE SELF-TREATMENT

Because of the potential for fulminant PSS, self-administration of an antimicrobial agent at the first sign of a suspicious illness in the asplenic or hyposplenic person is commonly advised, despite the absence of any controlled studies. Never a substitute for immediate medical evaluation, the procedure should be instituted especially if the delivery of medical care is not immediate. Treatment indications include any undifferentiated rigor or a febrile illness with prostration.

Choices, based on drug allergy and local antimicrobial resistance, include a quinolone, amoxicillin/clavulanic acid, trimethoprim/sulfamethoxazole (SXT), or a newer macrolide. Amoxicillin/clavulanic acid has activity against β-lactamase–producing *H. influenzae* and *Capnocytophaga* but not against PRP, and neither SXT nor the macrolides have consistent PRP activity. A quinolone with PRP activity (such as levofloxacin or moxifloxacin) could be used in high-risk individuals although pneumococci resistant to these antimicrobials also exist.

THERAPEUTIC INTERVENTIONS

If a patient suspected to have PSS is seen in a physician's office, an antimicrobial such as ceftriaxone should be given parenterally prior to hospital transfer, whether or not blood cultures can be obtained. Empirical antimicrobial options for suspected PSS that can be given on hospital arrival are shown in Table 315-3. Potential adjuvant immunologic interventions are also shown in this table.

Prevention Strategies

PROPHYLACTIC ANTIMICROBIALS

After splenectomy, pediatric patients are often given oral penicillin V prophylaxis for the first few years. In children with sickle hemoglobin-opathies, this practice has produced an 84% reduction in pneumococcal bacteremia.[68] The degree of protection in the asplenic child against PSS is not as well quantified and failures of prophylaxis are reported. In a 1986 review before the widespread emergence of PRP, 14 reports of prophylaxis failure were cited with none of the isolates being penicillin resistant.[69] In another 1986 study of 248 person-years in 88 children

with sickle cell anemia receiving both oral penicillin and pneumococcal vaccination, 8 episodes (3 fatal) of pneumococcal sepsis occurred, primarily due to penicillin therapy nonadherence.[70]

Prophylaxis has been discontinued in children older than 5 years with sickle cell anemia after pneumococcal vaccination and at least 2 years of treatment. No statistically significant increase in the incidence of pneumococcal events was found compared with those still receiving penicillin.[71] PRP strains were isolated equally in placebo and antimicrobial-treated breakthrough patients. A similar approach may be taken in the asplenic child who has not had PSS, although lifelong prophylaxis has been suggested,[72] more so in those with other underlying immune defects. A previous episode of PSS can be an indication for lifelong prophylaxis in both children and adults.

Little information is available on the utility of this modality in older asplenic persons. Because of the lower incidence of PSS in adults, the possibility of adverse effects from therapy, the selection of resistant strains, adherence issues, and the psychosocial burden of lifelong therapy, long-term prophylaxis in adults without a past episode of PSS is not generally recommended.[26] The role of antibiotic prophylaxis in hyposplenic patients without S-hemoglobinopathies remains unknown.

VACCINATION

Immunization against pneumococci using the 23-valent unconjugated capsular pneumococcal polysaccharide vaccine (PPV23) is uniformly recommended for both asplenic and hyposplenic hosts. The specific antibody responses (particularly IgM) to immunization in this cohort can be delayed and the magnitudes are often lower than in normal individuals.[73] Wide variation in response from patient to patient and to different vaccine capsular types is seen.

In elective splenectomy, PPV23 has been given at least 2 weeks before the procedure to optimize the antibody response.[72] After emergent spleen removal, immunization may be administered at hospital discharge or 2 weeks postoperatively, whichever is first. It is unclear if the timing of vaccination has an effect on efficacy, but it is reasonable to allow recovery from perioperative catabolism before immunization. Use is also often delayed for at least 3 months or more after chemotherapy or therapeutic irradiation.[72] If chemotherapy is given before splenectomy, however, functional humoral immunity may be restored as soon as 24 days after chemotherapy.[74]

How protective PPV23 is in the asplenic host remains inadequately defined, and anecdotal reports of failures related to vaccine-associated and non-vaccine–associated strains exist. Some efficacy in hyposplenic and asplenic patients, however, has been demonstrated.[75,76] Reimmunization in this cohort is reasonable even though PPV23 contains only T-cell–independent type 2 antigens that do not evoke immunologic memory. Indeed, PPV23 can induce hyporesponsiveness to a subsequent dose.[77] Because specific antibody levels can decrease more rapidly in the asplenic patient,[78] revaccination as often as every 2 to 3 years has been suggested.[79] The Centers for Disease Control and Prevention (CDC) adult immunization schedule, however, still recommends only a one-time revaccination after 5 years.[80] Local adverse reactions to repeat vaccination with PPV23 can occur, significantly correlated with prebooster antibody titer. In general, however, a third or even fourth PPV23 dose in adults has no increased risk of adverse reactions than initial doses.[81,82]

The more recently licensed heptavalent pneumococcal vaccine (PCV7) contains polysaccharides conjugated to a protein carrier. Conjugation allows the antigens to be T-cell dependent, not only inducing a protective antibody response but also priming the immune system for boosting.[83] This effect occurs even in children younger than 2 years old, where PPV23 is not immunogenic, in individuals with a genetic predisposition not to respond to polysaccharides, and in the elderly.[84] Since U.S. licensure of PCV7, an overall decline in invasive pneumococcal disease has occurred. Reductions, most prominent in children younger than 2 years old, were also noted in non-PCV7–immunized adults.[85] Breakthrough disease due to non-PCV7 serotypes have been

TABLE 315-3	Postsplenectomy Sepsis Therapeutic Considerations	
Consideration	*Treatment Options*
Empirical PSS Antimicrobial Treatment*	
Gram stain evidence of *Streptococcus pneumoniae* or no organism seen.	Vancomycin plus ceftriaxone or moxifloxacin
Gram stain evidence of a gram-negative bacillus or diplococcus or no organism is seen.	Based on circumstances, if a gram-negative bacillus resistant to ceftriaxone is suspected, cefepime ± gentamicin may be used ± vancomycin.
Potential Immunologic Interventions	
Corticosteroids	Despite the common use of physiologic doses of corticosteroids, it remains unclear how useful the therapy is.[60]
Intravenous human immunoglobulin	In asplenic animals, immunoglobulin decreased mortality from infection.[61,62]
Granulocyte-macrophage colony-stimulating factor (GM-CSF)	GM-CSF increased macrophage bactericidal activity in eusplenic and asplenic mice and treated animals had improved survival after pneumococcal challenge.[63]
Recombinant human activated protein C	This modality has been anecdotally used in pneumococcal PSS with survival[64] and in other septic events but has a high risk of bleeding.[65]
Interleukin-18 (IL-18)	IL-18 pretreatment in splenectomized mice protected against pneumococcal sepsis.[66] Natural IgM, stimulated by IL-18 in vivo was useful postexposure.[66]
Vagus nerve stimulation	In hyposplenic patients, it may be possible to modulate cytokine production via the cholinergic anti-inflammatory pathway.[67]

*Adult dosages: ceftriaxone: 2-4 g IV every 24 hours; vancomycin: 1 g IV every 12 hours; cefepime 2 g IV every 8-12 hours; moxifloxacin 400 mg IV every 24 hours, equivalent doses of other fluoroquinolones can be used. These regimens may need modification in renal or hepatic disease. Many patients with IgE-mediated penicillin allergy can tolerate cephalosporins but they ought to be given with caution or an alternative sought. Higher doses of vancomycin may be needed if meningitis is present. Modifications of the regimen chosen should be made when culture and sensitivity data is available.

TABLE 315-4	Shortcomings of Current Pneumococcal Vaccines

Protection is capsular serotype-specific
A limited number of serotypes can be contained in any vaccine
 • especially in conjugated vaccines
Unconjugated polysaccharides
 • produce no immunological memory
 • are nonimmunogenic in children < 2 years of age
 • 5%-10% of adults are genetically predisposed to fail to respond
 • can produce hyporesponsiveness to subsequent doses

The capsular serotypes in PCV7 are 4, 6B, 9V, 14, 18C, and 23F. PPV23 serotypes not in PCV7 include 1, 2, 3, 5, 7F, 8, 10A, 11A, 12F, 15B, 20, 22F, and 33F.

TABLE 315-5	Educational Issues for the Asplenic or Hyposplenic Host

Persons without a functioning spleen are more susceptible to certain infections.
The infection can progress very rapidly and be life-threatening.
The risk of the infection is lifelong but highest in the first year or two after the surgery.
All physicians tending to the patient should be informed of the condition, no matter how long after the splenectomy.
Both vaccination and antimicrobial agents may be used for prevention.

increasingly reported, notably serotype 19a[86] which is also not contained in PPV23.

In children with sickle cell anemia[87] and in Hodgkin's disease patients,[88] two doses of PCV7 followed by PPV23 produces higher levels of type-specific antibody for serotypes contained in both vaccines than PPV23 alone. The additional serotypes in PPV23 increase the coverage in adults from the 50% of isolates (80% in children) for PCV7.[87] Conjugate vaccine, additionally, can produce a more functional immunoglobulin by eliciting an antibody with heightened target avidity.[89] This effect may be related to a shift in IgG subtypes from IgG_2 to IgG_1, the latter with increased opsonic activity, facilitating opsonophagocytosis. How well this conjugate vaccine will perform in asplenic and hyposplenic individuals is not yet defined, but use in conjunction with PPV23 for asplenic persons has been suggested[72] and PCV7 is safe after previous PPV23 use, as well as more immunogenic than repeat PPV23.[90] In a rat model,[91] a conjugate vaccine could overcome splenic dependency of the antibody response to polysaccharides. Additionally, PCV7 was immunogenic in asplenics who developed PSS despite PPV23 use, seemingly due to a genetically regulated failure to respond to unconjugated polysaccharide antigens.[92] Expanding the number of conjugates in a single vaccine to improve serotype coverage, importantly, is limited by the carrier protein levels above which the immune response may be inhibited. The various shortcomings of current pneumococcal vaccines (Table 315-4) may be able to be circumvented by the use of virulence proteins, common to all serotypes, as antigens.[93]

Conjugated Hib polysaccharide vaccination is often given to those asplenic and hyposplenic persons not immunized in childhood. In splenectomized children and adults, the vaccine is immunogenic but antibody titers may not reach the level reached in eusplenic persons.[94] No recommendations have been made for boosters.[72,80] Booster doses are reasonable in the asplenic, however, because of lower peak titers, the need for higher levels of opsonins in this cohort,[12] and some evidence suggesting Hib infections may occur even in vaccinated normal children, in part due to the production of low avidity antibody.[95]

Quadrivalent polysaccharide meningococcal vaccines (types A, C, Y, and W135)[96] are immunogenic in the asplenic individual but less so in those treated with chemotherapy and radiotherapy.[97] Both nonconjugated and conjugated products are available, but in the asplenic, the conjugated vaccine is preferable for use.[96] A lack of an increased risk and absence of type B in the vaccine suggest that this immunization may not be necessary in the asplenic host. The CDC, however, recommends immunization in asplenic adults[80] and children,[96] with consideration of booster use.[96]

Influenza vaccine should be given yearly to the asplenic/hyposplenic cohort. In addition, it is important to note that asplenia and hyposplenia have never been contraindications to routine immunizations including live, attenuated vaccines.[72]

PATIENT AND FAMILY EDUCATION

A low level of knowledge about PSS risk exists. In one study, only 16% of asplenic persons were aware of any health precautions; this increased to 40% after prompting.[98] Issues to impart to the patient and family are listed in Table 315-5 and should be delivered in both an oral and written form. Because the half-life of knowledge is short, repeated emphasis during follow-up is vital.[99] The patient should wear a medical alert and carry a card documenting asplenia or hyposplenism, immunization, prophylactic antimicrobials, and an emergency plan. The use of a splenectomy registry has been proposed to further PSS education and prevention.[100]

SPLEEN-SPARING TREATMENTS

The risk of PSS has focused attention on alternatives to total spleen removal. Splenic preservation after traumatic rupture has been successful using conservative management, splenic repair, or partial splenectomy,[101] and it may be accomplished in greater than 90% of transcapsular splenic injuries.[102] Some return of splenic function after splenectomy for traumatic rupture has suggested that splenosis (growth of peritoneal implants of splenic tissue) could explain a lower PSS risk after trauma. Surgeons may autotransplant splenic tissue during splenectomy to augment splenosis. Fatal pneumococcal PSS has, however, occurred with as much as 92 g of splenosis, suggesting that splenic blood supply alterations may also play a role in PSS risk.[103] Supporting these limitations, in rabbits undergoing the procedure, not only did the transplant shrink in size and the parenchyma and vasculature degenerate over 6 months but also the clearance of pneumococci was no better than in asplenic animals.[104]

Partial removal of the spleen can be used in children with thalassemia[105] or hereditary hemolytic anemias such as spherocytosis.[106] Although regrowth may require total splenectomy, the delay is likely to be beneficial in young children. Splenic function is greater after partial splenectomy or splenic repair than after autotransplantation.[107]

REFERENCES

1. Hansen K, Singer DB. Asplenic-hyposplenic overwhelming sepsis: Postsplenectomy sepsis revisited. *Pediatr Dev Pathol.* 2001;4:105-121.
2. King H, Schumacker HB. Splenic studies. I. Susceptibility to infection after splenectomy performed in infancy. *Ann Surg.* 1952;136:239-242.
3. Singer DB. Postsplenectomy sepsis. In: Rosenberg HS, Bolande RP, eds. *Perspectives in Pediatric Pathology.* Vol 1. Chicago: Year Book Medical; 1973:285-311.
4. Gilbert B, Menetrey C, Belin V, et al. Familial isolated congenital asplenia. A rare, frequently hereditary dominant condition, often detected too late as a cause of overwhelming pneumococcal sepsis. Report of a case and review of 31 others. *Eur J Pediatr.* 2002;161:368-372.
5. Basem MW, Corazza GR. Hyposplenism: A comprehensive review. Part I: Basic concepts and causes. *Hematology.* 2007;12:1-13.
6. Muller AF, Cornford E, Toghill PJ. Splenic function in inflammatory bowel disease: Assessment by differential interference microscopy and splenic ultrasound. *Q J Med.* 1993;86:333-340.
7. Ravaglia G, Forti P, Biagi F, et al. Splenic function in old age. *Gerontology.* 1998;44: 91-94.
8. Corazza GR, Frisoni M, Vaira D, et al. Effect of gluten-free diet on splenic hypofunction of adult coeliac disease. *Gut.* 1983;24: 228-230.
9. Lockwood CM, Worlledge S, Nicholas A, et al. Reversal of impaired splenic function in patients with nephritis or vasculitis (or both) by plasma exchange. *N Engl J Med.* 1979;300:524-530.
10. Boughton BJ, Simpson A, Chandler S. Functional hyposplenism during pneumococcal septicaemia. *Lancet.* 1983;1:121-122.
11. Pelly MD, Huo Z, Henderson DC, et al. Severe pneumococcal disease and temporary splenic dysfunction. *Postgrad Med J.* 1997;73:173-174.
12. Hosea SW, Brown EJ, Hamburger MI, et al. Opsonic requirements for intravascular clearance after splenectomy. *N Engl J Med.* 1981;304:245-250.
13. Brown EJ, Hosea SW, Frank MM. The role of the spleen in experimental pneumococcal bacteremia. *J Clin Invest.* 1981;67:975-982.

14. Kruetzmann S, Rosado MM, Weber H, et al. Human immunoglobulin M memory B cells controlling *Streptococcus pneumoniae* infections are generated in the spleen. *J Exp Med.* 2003; 197:939-945.

15. Di Sabatino A, Rosado MM, Miele L, et al. Impairment of splenic IgM-memory but not switched-memory B cells in a patient with celiac disease and splenic atrophy. *J Allergy Clin Immunol.* 2007;120:1461-1463.

16. Di Sabatino A, Rosado MM, Ciccocioppo R, et al. Depletion of immunoglobulin M memory cells is associated with splenic hypofunction in inflammatory bowel disease. *Am J Gastroenterol.* 2005;100:1788-1795.

17. Di Sabatino A, Rosado MM, Cazzola P, et al. Splenic function and IgM-memory cells in Crohn's disease patients treated with infliximab. *Inflamm Bowel Dis.* 2008;14:591-596.

18. Kang Y-S, Kim JY, Bruening SA, et al. The C-type lectin SIGN-R1 mediates uptake of the capsular polysaccharide of *Streptococcus pneumoniae* in the marginal zone of the mouse spleen. *Proc Natl Acad Sci USA.* 2004;101:215-220.

19. Lanoue A, Clatworthy MR, Smith P, et al. SIGN-R1 contributes to protection against lethal pneumococcal infections in mice. *J Exp Med.* 2004;200:1383-1393.

20. Huston JM, Ochani M, Rosas-Ballina M, et al. Splenectomy inactivates the cholinergic anti-inflammatory pathway during lethal endotoxemia and polymicrobial sepsis. *J Exp Med.* 2006; 203:1623-1628.

21. Felder C, Blatteis CM. The role of the spleen in the febrile response induced by endotoxin in guinea pigs. *J Thermal Biol.* 2006;31:220-228.

22. Willekens FL, Roerdinkholder-Stoelwinder B, Groenen-Dopp YA, et al. Hemoglobin loss from erythrocytes in vivo results from spleen-facilitated vesiculation. *Blood.* 2003;101: 747-751.

23. Corazza GR, Ginaldi L, Zoli G, et al. Howell-Jolly body counting as a measure of splenic function: A reassessment. *Clin Lab Haematol.* 1990;12:269-275.

24. Buchanan GR, Holtkamp CA, Horton JA. Formation and disappearance of pocked erythrocytes: Studies in human subjects and laboratory animals. *Am J Hematol.* 1987;25:243-251.

25. Muller AF, Toghill PJ. Hyposplenism in gastrointestinal disease. *Gut.* 1995;36:165-167.

26. Styrt B. Infection associated with asplenia: Risks, mechanisms, and prevention. *Am J Med.* 1990;88:33N-42N.

27. Holdsworth RJ, Irving AD, Cuschieri A. Postsplenectomy sepsis and its mortality rate: Actual versus perceived risks. *Br J Surg.* 1991;78:1031-1038.

28. Bisharat N, Omari H, Lavi I, Raz R. Risk of infection and death among post-splenectomy patients. *J Infect.* 2001;43:182-186.

29. Straus SE, Sneller M, Lenardo MJ, et al. An inherited disorder of lymphocyte apoptosis: The autoimmune lymphoproliferative syndrome. *Ann Intern Med.* 1999;130:551-560.

30. Schilling RF. Estimating the risk for sepsis after splenectomy in hereditary spherocytosis. *Ann Intern Med.* 1995;122:187-188.

31. Kyaw MH, Holmes EM, Toolis F, et al. Evaluation of severe infection and survival after splenectomy. *Am J Med.* 2006; 119:e1-e7.

32. Ludvigsson JF, Olén O, Bell M, et al. Coeliac disease and risk of sepsis. *Gut.* 2008;57:1074.

33. Jugenburg M, Haddock G, Freedman MH, et al. The morbidity and mortality of pediatric splenectomy: Does prophylaxis make a difference? *J Pediatr Surg.* 1999;34:1064-1067.

34. Evans DI. Postsplenectomy sepsis 10 years or more after operation. *J Clin Pathol.* 1985;38:309-311.

35. Childers BJ, Cobanov B. Acute infectious purpura fulminans: A 15-year review of 28 consecutive cases. *Am Surg.* 2003;69: 86-90.

36. von Eyben FE, Szpirt W. Pneumococcal sepsis with hemolytic-uremic syndrome in the adult. *Nephron.* 1985;40:501-502.

37. Lynch AM, Kapila R. Overwhelming postsplenectomy infection. *Infect Dis Clin North Am.* 1996;10:693-707.

38. Cerquetti M, Cardines R, Giufrè M, et al. Detection of six copies of the capsulation b locus in a *Haemophilus influenzae* type b strain isolated from a splenectomized patient with fulminant septic shock. *J Clin Microbiol.* 2006;44:640-642.

39. Shah A, Lettieri CJ. Fulminant meningococcal sepsis in a woman with previously unknown hyposplenism. *Medscape J Med.* 2008; 10:36.

40. Condon RJ, Riley TV, Kelly H. Invasive meningococcal infection after splenectomy. *BMJ.* 1994;308:792-793.

41. Loggie BW, Hinchey EJ. Does splenectomy predispose to meningococcal sepsis? An experimental study and clinical review. *J Pediatr Surg.* 1986;21:326-330.

42. Zumla A, Lipscomb G, Corbett M, et al. Dysgonic fermenter—type 2: A zoonosis. Report of two cases and review. *Q J Med.* 1988;68:741-752.

43. Khawari AA, Myers JW, Ferguson DA Jr, et al. Sepsis and meningitis due to *Capnocytophaga cynodegmi* after splenectomy. *Clin Infect Dis.* 2005;40:1709-1710.

44. Kalb R, Kaplan MH, Tenebaum MJ, et al. Cutaneous infection at dog bite wounds associated with fulminant DF-2 septicemia. *Am J Med.* 1985;78:687-690.

45. Kopič J, Tomič Paradžik M, Pandak N. *Streptococcus suis* infection as a cause of severe illness: 2 cases from Croatia. *Scand J Infect Dis.* 2002;34:683-709.

46. Shepard CW, Daneshvar MI, Kaiser RM, et al. Bordetella holmesii bacteremia: A newly recognized entity among asplenic patients. *Clin Infect Dis.* 2004;38:799-804.

47. Kuranaga N, Kinoshita M, Kawabatta T, et al. A defective Th1 response of the spleen in the initial phase may explain why splenectomy helps prevent a Listeria infection. *Clin Exp Immunol.* 2005;140:11-21.

48. Malangoni MA, Dillon LD, Klamer TW, et al. Factors influencing the risk of early and late serious infection in adults after splenectomy for trauma. *Surgery.* 1984;96:775-783.

49. Weitz J, Jaques DP, Brennan M, et al. Association of splenectomy with postoperative complications in patients with proximal gastric and gastroesophageal junction cancer. *Ann Surg Oncol.* 2004;11:682-689.

50. Wiseman J, Brown CVR, Weng J, et al. Splenectomy for trauma increases the rate of early postoperative infection. *Am Surgeon.* 2006;72:947-950.

51. Krause PJ, Gewurz BE, Hill D, et al. Persistent and relapsing babesiosis in immunocompromised patients. *Clin Infect Dis.* 2008;46:370-376.

52. Looareesuwan S, Suntharasamai P, Webster HK, et al. Malaria in splenectomized patients: Report of four cases and review. *Clin Infect Dis.* 1993;16:361-366.

53. Bach O, Baier M, Pullwitt A, et al. Falciparum malaria after splenectomy: A prospective controlled study of 33 previously splenectomized Malawian adults. *Trans Roy Soc Trop Med Hyg.* 2005;99:861-867.

54. Angus BJ, Chotivanich K, Udomsangpetch R, et al. In vivo removal of malaria parasites from red blood cells without their destruction in acute falciparum malaria. *Blood.* 1997;90:2037-2040.

55. Chotivanich K, Udomsangpetch R, McGready R, et al. Central role of the spleen in malaria parasite clearance. *J Infect Dis.* 2002; 185:1538-1541.

56. Rabinstein A, Tikhomirov V, Kaluta A, et al: Recurrent and prolonged fever in asplenic patients with human granulocytic ehrlichiosis. *Q J Med.* 2000;93:198-201.

57. Henríquez C, Hinojosa JC, Ventosilla P, et al. Report of an unusual case of persistent bacteremia by *Bartonella bacilliformis* in a splenectomized patient. *Am J Trop Med Hyg.* 2004;71: 53-55.

58. Archer GL, Coleman PH, Cole RM, et al. Human infection from an unidentified erythrocyte-associated bacterium. *N Engl J Med.* 1979;301:897-900.

59. Domingo P, Fuster M, Muñiz-Diaz E, et al. Spurious postsplenectomy CD4 and CD8 lymphocytosis in HIV-infected patients. *AIDS.* 1996;10:106-107.

60. Sprung CL, Annane D, Keh D, et al. Hydrocortisone therapy for patients with septic shock. *N Engl J Med.* 2008;358:111-124.

61. Offenbartl K, Christensen P, Gullstrand P, et al. Treatment of pneumococcal postsplenectomy sepsis in the rat with human γ-globulin. *J Surg Res.* 1986;40:198-201.

62. Camel JE, Kim KS, Tchejeyan GH, et al. Efficacy of passive immunotherapy in experimental postsplenectomy sepsis due to *Haemophilus influenzae* type B. *J Pediatr Surg.* 1993;28:1441-1445.

63. Hebert JC, O'Reilly M. Granulocyte-macrophage colony-stimulating factor (GM-CSF) enhances pulmonary defenses against pneumococcal infections after splenectomy. *J Trauma.* 1996;41: 663-666.

64. Schumann C, Triantafilou K, Kamenz J, et al. Septic shock caused by *Streptococcus pneumoniae* in a post-splenectomy patient successfully treated with recombinant human activated protein C. *Scand J Infect Dis.* 2006;38:139-142.

65. Vincent JL, Nadel S, Kutsogiannis DJ, et al. Drotrecogin alfa (activated) in patients with severe sepsis presenting with purpura fulminans, meningitis, or meningococcal disease: A retrospective analysis of patients enrolled in recent clinical studies. *Crit Care.* 2005;9:R331-R343.

66. Kuritsugu N, Kinoshita M, Kawabata T, et al. Interleukin-18 protects splenectomized mice from lethal *Streptococcus pneumoniae* sepsis independent of interferon-γ by inducing IgM production. *J Infect Dis.* 2006;194:993-1002.

67. Huston JM, Gallowitsch-Puerta M, Ochani M, et al. Transcutaneous vagus nerve stimulation reduces serum high mobility group box 1 levels and improves survival in murine sepsis. *Crit Care Med.* 2007;35:2762-2768.

68. Gaston MH, Verter JI, Woods G, et al. Prophylaxis with oral penicillin in children with sickle cell anemia: A randomized trial. *N Engl J Med.* 1986;314:1593-1599.

69. Zarrabi MH, Rosner F. Rarity of failure of penicillin prophylaxis to prevent postsplenectomy sepsis. *Arch Intern Med.* 1986;146:1207-1208.

70. Buchanan GR, Smith SJ. Pneumococcal septicemia despite pneumococcal vaccine and prescription of penicillin prophylaxis in children with sickle cell anemia. *Am J Dis Child.* 1986; 140:428-432.

71. Falletta JM, Woods GM, Verter JI, et al. Discontinuing penicillin prophylaxis in children with sickle cell anemia. *J Pediatr.* 1995;127:685-690.

72. Davies JM, Barnes R, Milligan D. Update of guidelines for the prevention and treatment of infection in patients with an absent or dysfunctional spleen. *Clin Med.* 2002;2:440-443.

73. Molrine DC, Silber GR, Samra Y, et al. Normal IgG and impaired IgM responses to polysaccharide vaccines in asplenic patients. *J Infect Dis.* 1999;179:513-517.

74. Zandvoort A, Ludewijk ME, Klok PA, et al. After chemotherapy, functional humoral response capacity is restored before complete restoration of lymphoid compartment. *Clin Exp Immunol.* 2003;131:8-16.

75. Ammann AJ, Addiego J, Wara DW, et al. Polyvalent pneumococcal-polysaccharide immunization of patients with sickle-cell anemia and patients with splenectomy. *N Engl J Med.* 1977;297:897-900.

76. Foss Abrahamsen A, Hoiby EA, Hannisdol E, et al. Systemic pneumococcal disease after staging for Hodgkin's disease 1969-1980 without pneumococcal vaccine protection: A follow-up study 1994. *Eur J Haematol.* 1997;58:73-77.

77. Törling J, Hedlund J, Konradsen HB, et al. Revaccination with the 23-valent pneumococcal polysaccharide vaccine in middle-aged and elderly persons previously treated for pneumonia. *Vaccine.* 2003;22:96-103.

78. Giebink GS, Le CT, Cosio FG, et al. Serum antibody responses of high-risk children and adults to vaccination with capsular polysaccharide of *Streptococcus pneumoniae.* *Rev Infect Dis.* 1981;3(Suppl):168-178.

79. Rutherford EJ, Livengood J, Higginbotham M, et al. Efficacy and safety of pneumococcal revaccination after splenectomy for trauma. *J Trauma.* 1995;39:448-452.

80. Centers for Disease Control and Prevention. Recommended adult immunization schedule—United States, 2009. *MMWR Morbid Mortal Wkly Rep.* 2009;57:Q1-Q4.

81. Walker FJ, Singleton RJ, Bulkow LR, et al. Reactions after 3 or more doses of pneumococcal polysaccharide vaccine in adults in Alaska. *Clin Infect Dis.* 2005;40:1730-1735.

82. Jackson LA, Nelson JC, Whitney CG, et al. Assessment of the safety of a third dose of pneumococcal polysaccharide in the Vaccine Safety Database population. *Vaccine.* 2006;24: 151-156.

83. Centers for Disease Control and Prevention. Preventing pneumococcal disease among infants and young children: Recommendations of the Advisory Committee on Immunization Practices (ACIP). *MMWR Morbid Mortal Wkly Rep.* 2000;49:1-35.

84. de Roux A, Schmöele-Thomas B, Siber G, et al. Comparison of pneumococcal conjugate polysaccharide and free polysaccharide vaccines in elderly adults: Conjugate vaccine elicits improved antibacterial immune responses and immunological memory. *Clin Infect Dis.* 2008;46:1015-1023.

85. Whitney CG, Farley MM, Hadler J, et al. Decline in invasive pneumococcal disease after the introduction of protein-polysaccharide conjugate vaccine. *N Engl J Med.* 2003;348:1737-1746.

86. Singleton RJ, Hennessy T, Bulkow LR, et al. Invasive pneumococcal disease caused by nonvaccine serotypes among Alaskan native children with high levels of 7-valent pneumococcal conjugate vaccine coverage. *JAMA.* 2007;297:1784-1792.

87. Vernacchio L, Neufeld EJ, MacDonald K, et al. Combined schedule of 7-valent pneumococcal conjugate vaccine followed by 23-valent pneumococcal vaccine in children and young adults with sickle cell anemia. *J Pediatr.* 1998;133:275-278.

88. Chan CY, Molrine DC, George S, et al. Pneumococcal conjugate vaccine primes for antibody responses to polysaccharide pneumococcal vaccine after Hodgkin's disease. *J Infect Dis.* 1996;173:256-258.

89. Vidarsson G, Sigurdardottir ST, Gudnason T, et al. Isotypes and opsonophagocytosis of pneumococcus type 6B antibodies elicited in infants and adults by an experimental pneumococcus type 6B-tetanus toxoid vaccine. *Infect Immun.* 1998;66:2866-2870.

90. Smets F, Bourgois A, Vermylen C, et al. Randomised revaccination with pneumococcal polysaccharide or conjugate vaccine in asplenic children previously vaccinated with polysaccharide vaccine. *Vaccine.* 2007;25:5278-5282.

91. Breukels MA, Zandvoort A, van den Dobbelsteen GP, et al. Pneumococcal conjugate vaccines overcome splenic dependency of antibody response to pneumococcal polysaccharides. *Infect Immun.* 2001;69:7583-7587.

92. Musher DM, Ceasar H, Kojic EM, et al. Administration of protein-conjugate pneumococcal vaccine to patients who have invasive disease after splenectomy despite their having received 23-valent pneumococcal polysaccharide vaccine. *J Infect Dis.* 2005;191:1063-1067.

93. Ogunniyi AD, Grabowicz M, Briles DE, et al. Development of a vaccine against invasive pneumococcal disease based on combinations of virulence proteins of *Streptococcus pneumoniae. Infect Immun.* 2007;75:350-357.

94. Cimaz R, Mensi C, D'Angelo E, et al. Safety and immunogenicity of a conjugate vaccine against *Haemophilus influenzae* type b in splenectomized and nonsplenectomized patients with Cooley anemia. *J Infect Dis.* 2001;183:1819-1821.

95. Lee YC, Kelly DF, Yu LM, et al. *Haemophilus influenzae* vaccine failure in children is associated with inadequate production of high-quality antibody. *Clin Infect Dis.* 2008;46:186-192.

96. Centers for Disease Control and Prevention. Recommended immunization schedule for persons aged 0-18 years—United States, 2009. *MMWR Morbid Mortal Wkly Rep.* 2009;57:Q1-Q4.

97. Ruben FL, Hankins WA, Zeigler Z, et al. Antibody responses to meningococcal polysaccharide vaccine in adults without a spleen. *Am J Med.* 1984;76:115-121.

98. White KS, Covington D, Churchill P, et al. Patient awareness of health precautions after splenectomy. *Am J Infect Control.* 1991;19:36-41.

99. Corbett SM, Rebuck JA, Rogers FB, et al. Time lapse of comorbidities influence patient knowledge and pursuit of medical care after traumatic splenectomy. *J Trauma.* 2007;62: 397-403.

100. Woolley I, Jones P, Spelman D, et al. Cost-effectiveness of a post-splenectomy registry for prevention of sepsis in the asplenic. *Aust N Z J Public Health*. 2006;30:558-561.

101. Cooper MJ, Williamson RCN. Splenectomy: Indications, hazards and alternatives. *Br J Surg*. 1984;71:173-180.

102. Rozinov VM, Salel'ev SB, Keshishyan RA, et al. Organ-sparing treatment for closed spleen injuries in children. *Clin Orthoped*. 1995;320:34-39.

103. Rice HM, James PD. Ectopic splenic tissue failed to prevent fatal pneumococcal septicaemia after splenectomy for trauma. *Lancet*. 1980;1:565-566.

104. Tang WH, Wu FL, Huang MK, et al. Splenic tissue autotransplantation in rabbits: No restoration of host defense. *Langenbecks Arch Surg*. 2003;387:379-385.

105. Tracey ET, Rice HE. Partial splenectomy for hereditary spherocytosis. *Pediatr Clin N Am*. 2008;55:503-519.

106. Sheikha AK, Salih ZT, Kasnazan KH, et al. Prevention of overwhelming postsplenectomy infection in thalassemia patients by partial rather than total splenectomy. *Can J Surg*. 2007;50:382-386.

107. Traub A, Giebink GS, Smith C, et al. Splenic reticuloendothelial function after splenectomy, spleen repair, and spleen autotransplantation. *N Engl J Med*. 1987;317:1559-1564.

316

Infections in Injection Drug Users

DONALD P. LEVINE | PATRICIA D. BROWN

According to a 2006 report by the United Nations Office on Drugs and Crimes, 200 million people worldwide used illicit drugs at least once in the preceding year. The 2007 National Survey on Drug Use and Health found an estimated 19.9 million Americans aged 12 or older were current illicit drug users. This estimate represents 8% of the population aged 12 years or older. In the United States, 106,000 individuals older than 12 years used heroin for the first time.[1] Injection drug users (IDUs) have higher rates of bacterial, viral, and fungal infection than the general population, and infection is undoubtedly the major reason for contact between the illicit drug user and the health care system. The social circumstances of many addicts, including living in shelters or crowded conditions, increases the risk of pulmonary tuberculosis, including multidrug-resistant infections, and the reluctance of IDUs to seek medical attention and their failure to adhere to treatment regimens are responsible for the further spread of infection. Malnutrition contributes to altered host defenses, making infection more likely. Poor hygiene that frequently accompanies the drug use habit may exacerbate the risk of infection due to commensal organisms. In addition, IDUs have a higher rate of nasal and skin colonization with potential pathogens than do nonusers. Frequent injection into heavily colonized sites, such as the groin region, likely increases the risk of infection with enteric flora. Among addicts in San Francisco, 22.8% were found to have nasal colonization with *Staphylococcus aureus*, 12% of which were community-acquired *S. aureus* (CA-MRSA).[2] Indeed, the major risk factor among illicit drug users for colonization with *S. aureus* was ever injecting drugs and, among those who are colonized, ever using was associated with colonization by MRSA. The fact that addicts have frequent hospitalizations and exposure to antibiotics secondary to complications of injection drug use leads to an increased risk of MRSA colonization and infection.

Certain practices that are unique to IDUs, such as crushing capsules or tablets in the mouth before injection of the drug, may be responsible for infection caused by oral flora. Some addicts lick their needles to make the injection easier, a practice that doubles the risk of cellulitis or abscess caused by oral streptococci or anaerobes.[3] The use of "speedball" (a mixture of heroin and cocaine) or the practice of "booting" (repeatedly withdrawing small amounts of blood into the injection equipment before administering the complete contents) have also been associated with an increased risk of infection. Speedball use leads to tissue necrosis, with the formation of abscesses, and injection using poor technique or sclerosing substances causes a loss of usable veins, which may lead the addict to resort to "skin popping" or injection directly into the skin or muscle, leading to an increase in the odds of wound botulism.

Although early studies failed to detect pathogenic bacteria contaminating the illicit drugs, recent evidence demonstrating a connection between the use of black tar heroin and severe *Clostridium* infection indicates that certain substances or practices enhance the growth of particular organisms and account for infections that are unique to the drug-using population. Alternatively, failure to adequately cleanse the injection paraphernalia and sharing of equipment are also responsible for transmission of infection. The close contact among addicts may also be responsible for outbreaks of severe infections in certain locales. An outbreak of infection caused by *Clostridium novyi* in 2000 was associated with severe infection and a high mortality rate and appeared to be secondary to close contact in the IDU social network and use of shared substances and needles.[4] Between 1999 and 2001 there was a marked increase in cases caused by group A *Streptococcus*, and the number increased by 15% during 2002. Infection was caused by M nontypeable strains in 38%. A marked increase in needle and syringe sharing that took place in the late 1990s may have been responsible.[4]

Ultimately, infection drives a need for care in both the outpatient and inpatient environment. In the British health care system, IDUs infected with the human immunodeficiency virus (HIV) are less likely than others to use outpatient services but are more likely to have frequent and prolonged hospitalizations.[5] Substance abuse treatment programs can have a major impact on the utilization of health care services. The mortality rate among IDUs who are not enrolled in formal substance treatment programs is three times higher than that for those in treatment programs, mostly secondary to the high incidence of infection, although trauma also plays a role. The type of program also makes a difference. Addicts who continue to inject but who are enrolled in needle exchange programs are six times more likely to have injection-related infection than those enrolled in methadone maintenance programs.[5] In addition, the frequency of infection increases with the number of injections per day from a rate of 1.8% for drug users who do not inject, 3.5% for those with single daily injections, 6.1% for those who inject twice daily, to 11.4% for those with three or more injections per day.[5] Infection in IDUs is not just a problem for persons in that population but in many cases may spread to other members of the community. Examples of infections that can spread beyond the group of drug injectors include HIV, hepatitis B and C, and resistant organisms such as MRSA. As noted earlier, opiate maintenance programs have been demonstrated to significantly reduce the infection rate among drug users and can play a major role in reducing the spread of infection to nonusers.[6] Programs that include counseling and psychosocial services as well as medical care to methadone maintenance programs can decrease drug use, and secondarily the spread of infection.

An effort to decrease infections in IDUs requires multiple strategies. Education programs designed to teach addicts safe injecting techniques can prevent local disease as well as the spread of infection to others. Needle exchange programs have reduced the incidence of abscesses but are not available in many locales. In addition, making methadone or other opiate substitution programs more accessible can have the overall effect of improving the health status of addicts while decreasing their use of illegal substances and participating in illegal activity. When successful, these programs prevent the spread of HIV and other blood-borne pathogens as well as skin abscesses and cellulitis. The infections associated with injection drug use are frequently the consequence of the illegal status of street drugs. Heroin reduction programs, safer injecting facilities, and opiate substitution programs can reduce the incidence of a number of infections among addicted individuals.[6,7]

Host Defenses

Although it has been recognized for more than a century that opioid abuse is associated with an increased risk of infectious complications, a clear understanding of the effects of opioids on the immune system is still lacking. Studies have examined the effects of in vivo opioid exposure on the function of cells of the immune system isolated from drug users, the effect of in vitro exposure to opioids on immune cells isolated from healthy nonaddicts, and the effects of in vivo and in vitro exposure to opioids in animal models. The results of studies performed after the beginning of the HIV epidemic but before the availability of a serologic test may be confounded by the effects of immunodeficiency caused by unrecognized HIV infection. Previously, it was thought that immunologic dysfunction played a relatively minor role in the pathogenesis of infection in IDUs, compared with that of the repeated parenteral introduction or injection of nonsterile material and lifestyle factors associated with injection drug use. However, there is growing evidence of a direct effect of opioids on immune system function. These effects have been reviewed and summarized.[8-10]

Opiates have been demonstrated to reduce chemotaxis, phagocytosis, and the production of cytokines and chemokines. Both heroin and morphine (a major metabolite of heroin) have been shown to decrease natural killer cell activity and decrease lymphocyte proliferation in response to phytohemagglutinin and other mitogens. In addition to their direct effects on cells of the immune system (which have been demonstrated to have opiate receptors), opiates affect the immune system indirectly through the neuroendocrine system (mainly via the hypothalamic-pituitary-adrenal axis). Immunosuppression mediated through effects on the autonomic nervous system is also suggested. In spite of the depressed cell-mediated immunity demonstrated in IDUs, opportunistic infections characteristic of T-cell deficiency were rarely reported before the HIV epidemic. In the lung, heroin appears to reduce the activity of inducible nitric oxide synthase, which may increase susceptibility to pulmonary infections.[11,12]

Prolonged methadone maintenance has been shown to reverse some of the immunosuppressive effects of heroin.[13-15] Buprenorphine, which is increasingly used as substitution therapy, also appears to allow a reversal of the immunosuppressive effects associated with heroin addiction.[15]

Serum levels of immunoglobulin M and, to a lesser extent, immunoglobulin G are frequently elevated in IDUs, whereas serum immunoglobulin A levels are usually normal. Increased immunoglobulin levels tend to normalize after prolonged opiate withdrawal. Elevated immunoglobulin concentrations are accompanied by a high frequency of autoantibodies, such as rheumatoid factor, as well as those directed against various microorganisms. The latter phenomenon often manifests as a biologic false-positive Venereal Disease Research Laboratory (VDRL) test result, which may create diagnostic confusion in IDUs who are at high risk for acquiring sexually transmitted infections (STIs). Hypergammaglobulinemia resulting from polyclonal B-cell activation may be the result of recurrent immunologic stimulation by injected foreign antigens as well as associated chronic liver disease and chronic infections with other pathogens.

It has been shown that morphine may depress the monocyte functions essential for antiviral defense.[16] These alterations could contribute to the high efficiency of transmission of certain viral pathogens in IDUs, including hepatitis B virus (HBV), hepatitis C virus (HCV), and HIV. In vitro, morphine has been shown to enhance HIV infection of human mononuclear cells through the downregulation of β-chemokine production and the upregulation of CCR5 receptor expression.[17]

Skin and Soft Tissue Infections

Skin and soft tissue infections are the most common reason for IDUs to be admitted to hospital. Such infections also account for a substantial proportion of emergency department encounters in urban medical centers. In response, San Francisco General Hospital established the ISIS clinic (Integrated Soft-Tissue Infection Clinic), an outpatient facility at which patients can receive care for lesions that would otherwise be treated in the emergency department. Over a 3-year period, 6156 patients were seen for a total of 12,012 visits.[18] Fifty-eight percent of the patients were IDUs. Evidence exists that skin and soft tissue infections are increasing in this population. Among IDUs in England, between 1997 and 2004 there was a 566% increase in the number of patients admitted for abscesses of the trunk or groin and a 469% increase in patients with cellulitis of the trunk or groin.[19]

The distribution of soft tissue lesions is as varied as the sites used for injection and reflects both the duration of drug use and local practices among drug users. Typically, IDUs go through a progression of injection sites, starting with the upper extremity in the antecubital fossa, followed after approximately 2 years by the forearm. After about 4 years of use, they switch to injecting into the veins of the hand, and, approximately 6 years after first injecting, the veins of the neck, feet, and leg. By the 10th year of drug use they resort to the groin and peripheral digits.[20] The groin becomes a favored site after other injection sites have been exhausted, although in some cases femoral injection is preferred for convenience and ease of use or as a means of insuring immediate blood levels of the drug rather than facing the risk of the reduced euphoric effect associated with "skin popping," that is, either intended or accidental injection of drugs into the skin and subcutaneous tissues.[20]

After repeated injections into a site, frequently without benefit of sterile technique, local ischemia or necrosis develops and the tissues become susceptible to infection. In addition, the substances injected frequently contain materials added as diluents that commonly cause norepinephrine release and vasospasm or local damage to the vascular intima. This leads to thrombosis and further compromise of the soft tissues. Cocaine use may be associated with vascular thrombus at sites distant from injections and may cause muscle and skin infections even after inhalational use.[21,22] Opiates also have immunosuppressive properties that may predispose to infection.[23] HIV infection is now recognized as an important risk factor for skin abscesses. Women are at greater risk, presumably because of the difficulty they have accessing veins and the consequent injury to skin and subcutaneous tissues.[24]

Abscesses are the most common form of soft tissue infection, followed closely by cellulitis and skin ulcers.[25] The location of lesions is as varied as are injection sites. In one study, infections of the arm (50%) were more common than lesions of the leg (22.7%) or buttocks (19.8%). Abscesses confined to the deltoid region accounted for 14.1% of cases.[25] Although abscesses occur with injection of heroin as a single drug, they are also found frequently in addicts who inject a mixture of heroine and cocaine, known as "speedball," and are more likely in IDUs with a long history of drug use and skin popping.[26] Booting is also an independent risk factor for abscess formation.[26] Additional risk factors for abscesses are female gender (odds ratio [OR] 1.7, $P = .002$), recent incarceration (OR 1.7, $P = .001$), involvement in sex trade (OR 1.4, $P = .030$), frequent cocaine use (OR 1.5, $P = .002$), and being seropositive for HIV (OR 1.5, $P = .003$).[27]

Abscesses may spread to adjacent tissues, frequently with disastrous consequences. Mediastinitis may result from the extension of a cervical abscess, whereas lesions in the carotid triangle can erode into the carotid arteries, resulting in massive hemorrhage. Thrombosis of the internal jugular vein has been reported as a complication of a deep neck abscess, as has acute vocal cord paralysis.[28,29] This can lead to acute, severe airway obstruction and may necessitate immediate tracheostomy. Local venous thrombosis or extension to the retroperitoneal space may result from abscess in the femoral triangle.

S. aureus is the most common pathogen, followed by streptococci, either as the sole pathogen or in combination with other organisms. Even in patients with negative nares cultures, *S. aureus* was isolated from 66.4% of infection site cultures, 77% of which were MRSA.[30] Methamphetamine was found to be a risk factor for MRSA infection in IDUs presenting to emergency departments in Georgia. Unsterile injection practices did not appear to be a risk factor, as only 12.5% of patients injected the drug compared with 62.5% who either smoked or inhaled. The most significant risk factor among methamphetamine users was having a skin infection within the previous 3 months (adjusted OR 7.92). The authors noted that methamphetamine use causes formication, a sensation of something crawling on the skin. This sensation prompts the user to pick at the skin, which can lead to skin breakdown and subsequently serves as a focus for infection.[31] Among the staphylococci, MRSA have become the predominant strain, particularly CA-MRSA. Disease caused by CA-MRSA is most often a single lesion in an extremity, although multiple furuncles are also seen. Recurrences are common.[32] Coagulase-negative staphylococci and α-hemolytic streptococci are also seen. Among the latter, *Streptococcus* of the anginosus (*milleri*) group is most important, especially in addicts in Scotland, who inject tablets of buprenorphine and temazepam after crushing them between their teeth.[33,34] Other oral flora have been reported, in particular *Eikenella corrodens*, which in some centers has become the third most common pathogen. IDUs who lick their needles or contaminate their drugs with saliva are particularly prone to this infection. The pneumococcus is also occasionally found in this setting. Gram-negative bacilli are found with variable frequency. In the past, anaerobes were found infrequently, particularly in upper extremity infection. In a recent study, isolates from 39% of IDUs contained both aerobes and anaerobes, compared with only 27% in nonusers. In addition, anaerobes, either alone or as part of a mixed flora, were detected more frequently in drug users than in nonusers (44% vs. 35%).[35]

The diagnosis of abscesses in an IDU can be difficult, especially if surrounding cellulitis and induration are found. Bedside ultrasound has been used in an emergency department setting with a high degree of accuracy. These machines are portable, have the advantage of being available while the patient is in the department, can be completed in less than 1 minute, and are comfortable for the patient. In one large study in an emergency department, abscesses were found in 37% of addicts who were tested. There were only five false-positive studies, two of which were determined to be hematomas rather than abscesses. The sensitivity of ultrasound was 98%, compared with only 86% for clinical examination alone. The specificity was 85%, giving a positive predictive value of 93% and a negative predictive value of 97%. An unanticipated but important additional benefit of using ultrasound is that pseudoaneurysms that otherwise might have been misidentified as abscesses were also detected, thus avoiding a dangerous attempted incision and drainage.[36]

The first decision in the management of patients with soft tissue infections is whether the patient should be admitted to hospital. This can be a difficult decision, but it depends on the severity of the illness. Eron and colleagues recommend an approach in which patients are assigned to one of four classes.[37] Class 1 patients have no signs of systemic toxicity and have no uncontrolled comorbid conditions. These patients usually respond to topical or oral therapy. Class 2 patients either have evidence of systemic illness, but without any unstable, comorbid conditions, or are systemically well, but have one or more comorbid conditions that may complicate the outcome. Class 3 patients are toxic or are not toxic but have unstable comorbid conditions that may interfere with the response to therapy. Class 4 patients have the sepsis syndrome or a serious, life-threatening infection, such as necrotizing fasciitis. Predictors of severe infection are hypotension, tachycardia, temperature lower than 35°C or higher than 40°C, confusion, or a depressed level of consciousness. Patients with two or more of these findings have a blunted response to antibiotics and poor outcome. In terms of the decision whether to admit the patient to hospital, class 1 patients most likely will do well if managed as outpatients. Class 2 patients may benefit from a period of observation; those who respond quickly can be treated as outpatients, but others will require hospital admission. Patients in class 3 and 4 should be treated as inpatients.

The selection of antibiotic therapy is the next decision. Class 1 patients usually respond to oral antibiotics, as do some in class 2. Initial therapy with parenteral agents with rapid switch to oral agents may be preferable for class 2 patients. Patients with more serious illness should be treated with parenteral therapy, at least until they respond satisfactorily. Data from randomized trials to guide the duration of therapy are insufficient. In most cases 1 to 2 weeks of treatment are adequate, but infection may recur in up to 20%, thus prevention of future infections cannot be ignored.[37]

Regardless of antibiotic use, incision and drainage remain the mainstay of the treatment of abscesses in IDUs. In some reports, patients who received ineffective antibiotics based on culture data responded well to drainage alone. Others have demonstrated that the outcome is still better if patients receive appropriate therapy based on the antibiotic susceptibility of the isolated pathogens, especially if treatment is initiated within the first 48 hours.[38] Some data indicate that drainage alone may be sufficient to eliminate minor abscesses. Cultures of infected material are helpful to determine the infecting pathogen and

to ensure appropriate antibiotic selection. Whether antibiotics actually play in role in the outcome is controversial. Numerous patients have responded well to drainage alone. In some cases, patients admitted for abscess had shorter lengths of hospital stay than those with cellulitis or infected skin ulcers. Infection in the deltoid region is a consequence of skin-popping and subsequent necrosis of the underlying fascia. IDUs with abscesses of the deltoid were far more likely to receive surgical care than those with other lesions, no doubt a reflection of the fact that abscess drainage is often a major component of abscess treatment. However, cellulitis is an independent risk factor for hospitalization, along with elevated heart rate, increased white blood cell count, and fever. Forty percent of patients seeking care who were admitted to hospital with abscesses were more likely to require hospital admission (72%) compared with those who had cellulitis (51%).

Cleansing the skin with alcohol before injection protects against abscess and offers a potential intervention to reduce disease and hospital admissions.[26] Original optimism that needle exchange programs might reduce the incidence has not been realized. Widespread access to sterile needles and syringes through high-volume needle exchanges and medically supervised safer injection facilities did not prove to be effective in preventing high rates of abscesses among IDUs. In one study in Vancouver, despite such a program, 21.5% of IDUs had an abscess in the previous 6 months.[27] Either complete cessation from injecting or scrupulous attention to sterile technique is probably the only effective measure to eliminate abscesses in this population.

Synergy between streptococcal infection and cocaine-induced tissue ischemia may lead to large necrotic ulcerations and extensive tissue loss.[33] Alternatively, skin ulcerations may result from necrosis induced by the illicit substance injected.

Cellulitis may be extensive and can lead to overwhelming sepsis and death.[39,40] The diagnosis is seldom obscure, and most patients present with signs and symptoms referable to the involved site; however, blood cultures should be obtained, because it is difficult to predict bacteremia.[41] In contrast, the diagnosis of an abscess can be difficult. Patients typically have single lesions. The signs and symptoms are similar to patients with cellulitis alone. Indeed, most patients will also have an area of adjacent cellulitis. Fewer than half the patients are febrile. Erythema, pain, and tenderness of the affected site are common, but fluctuance is absent in approximately 25%.[42] Deep abscesses may be particularly difficult to detect.[43] Computed tomography (CT) is useful for locating cervical abscesses[44] and is probably effective for detecting abscesses in the groin and femoral region. Magnetic resonance imaging (MRI) is also useful, particularly in infection of the extremities.[45] Ultrasonography has been reported to be useful but is of variable accuracy, particularly when diagnosing lesions in the groin.

Antibiotic therapy is directed at the organisms recovered from the blood or purulent material. In uncomplicated cellulitides, cultures are seldom helpful. In such cases, therapy is empirical and is based on the pathogens most commonly encountered in that geographic location. Prolonged antibiotic treatment is frequently required.[46] Early surgical drainage of abscesses is essential, and, because of the tendency of these lesions to spread to adjacent or even distant regions, multiple drainage procedures may be required.[47] Deep infections of the hand are far more common in IDUs than in nonusers, and they mandate a unique approach. The microbiology of such infections varies, depending on the injected substances. Patients who primarily inject cocaine have a high frequency of mixed anaerobic infection,[42] whereas heroin users are more likely to harbor streptococci and staphylococci.[48] In either case, surgical débridement is far more likely to be required in IDUs than in nonusers.[48] Some caution is indicated before incising a lesion in the vicinity of blood vessels, because a mycotic pseudoaneurysm can easily be misdiagnosed as an abscess. Inadvertent entry into such a lesion can have disastrous consequences.

Skin ulcers are extremely common in IDUs. They are found at every conceivable site but are particularly common below the knee, close to the ankle.[49] They arise from tissue damage caused by repeated nonsterile injection into the same site with associated thrombosis and infection. Skin ulcers may persist for years and are a frequent reason for hospitalization. Typically they have ragged edges and seropurulent drainage. Patients complain of severe pain, and it is often the pain, rather than the ulcer itself, that brings the patient to medical attention. The microbiology of these lesions is similar to that of other soft tissue infections in addicts, although they more frequently contain more than one organism. *S. aureus* and β-hemolytic streptococci remain the most common isolates, with gram-negative bacilli—most often *Klebsiella*, *Pseudomonas*, *Escherichia coli*, and *Proteus*—playing an important role. They present particularly difficult management problems when ulcers involve the hands and feet and may ultimately lead to loss of function.

Treatment of skin ulcers requires administration of systemic antibiotics and prolonged local wound care, including gentle washing, wet-to-dry dressings, and application of topical antibacterial creams. Elevation of the leg to reduce edema is an important component of the therapy and also plays a role in pain management.[50] Generally, parenteral antibiotics are continued until the wound is covered by granulation tissue. Very large lesions may require skin grafting or muscle flaps, but these are only effective after all necrotic tissue has been removed and the wound is clean and granulating. An important adjuvant treatment is the application of compression dressings, such as Unna boots, which, when properly applied, serve to reduce the edema as well as to promote wound healing.[51] With time, most skin ulcers heal completely, leaving circular, punched-out scars. The most important complication is contiguous osteomyelitis, which may be difficult to diagnose because frequently radiologic evidence indicates periosteal reaction in bones immediately beneath large ulcers. When there is still a question of osteomyelitis, a triple-phase bone scan may be helpful. Ultimately a diagnosis of osteomyelitis may be impossible without a bone biopsy, which may be difficult to obtain without traversing infected superficial tissues. In such cases, prolonged parenteral antibiotic therapy directed at the organism cultured from the ulcer and careful radiographic follow-up may be the best approach. Recurrent and chronic infections are occasionally complicated by renal amyloidosis.

Necrotizing fasciitis, without or with myositis, is the single infection in IDUs that is most likely to need immediate and appropriate treatment; however, the clinical picture is subtle and rarely elicits the emergency response required. At San Francisco General Hospital, 1% of IDUs in need of incision and drainage for soft tissue infection were found to have necrotizing infection requiring extensive débridement. The classic findings of high fever, bullae, crepitance, and skin necrosis are usually absent initially, and the impression may be that of mild cellulitis.[48] In some cases, the true nature of the disease may be so subtle as to be missed during a procedure to débride an abscess or cellulitis. Alternatively, infection may spread after apparently effective incision and drainage.[52] The major indication of the true nature of the infection is the fact that signs and symptoms, such as pain and hemodynamic instability, are disproportionate to the apparent extent of the local process.[48] However, this can be misleading because the clinical presentation may be no different from routine cellulitis with no more than erythema of the involved area, providing no clue to the serious underlying pathology.[53] Also, because addicts are frequently viewed as drug-seeking complainers, what appears to be excessive complaint for minor disease may be interpreted as narcotic-seeking behavior, further delaying recognition of the need for aggressive and rapid action. Thus, a high index of suspicion is required so as not to miss the diagnosis. Additional clues to the serious nature of the problem are hemodynamic instability, local anesthesia, rapid progression of inflammation, or the presence of blue or hemorrhagic bullae. When present, crepitance is an important clue. Finally, a slow response to appropriate antibiotic treatment suggests a deeper underlying problem. An MRI or CT scan may be a useful diagnostic tool. Characteristic findings include asymmetrical fascial thickening and fat stranding, followed by gas tracking along fascial planes. Abscesses may also be seen.[54] CT scans may be misleading because both false-positive and false-negative results have been reported and contrast enhancement contributes no additional information. The only definitive test is surgical exploration,

which is both diagnostic and therapeutic. The finding of necrosis is characteristic, however, it may be necessary to explore more than one area. A negative biopsy result from one location does not preclude the diagnosis in adjacent tissues.[55]

As with most addict-related infections, gram-positive organisms are usually found. However, β-hemolytic streptococci predominate in approximately 50% of cases, followed by *S. aureus*, α-hemolytic streptococci, and coagulase-negative staphylococci. Gram-negative organisms are infrequent and are usually represented by enteric pathogens, especially *E. coli*, *Klebsiella*, *Proteus mirabilis*, *Pseudomonas*, and *Enterobacter*. Anaerobes are recovered in 12% of cases; yeasts (*Candida*) are uncommon. Polymicrobial infection is common.[56]

Management of necrotizing fasciitis by antibiotics alone leads to progression of the infection in 75% of patients. Parenteral antibiotics and aggressive surgery coupled with reexploration at 24 hours and as often as necessary afterward to ensure complete removal of all necrotic tissue offer the best prognosis. In a recent study, IDUs required an average of 3.4 débridements for necrotizing fasciitis.[56] Aggressive nutritional support and early coverage of the soft tissue defect have been shown to improve the outcome,[57] which for addicts, who tend to be young and relatively healthy, is the best of any patient group with this disease. Even with aggressive treatment, the mortality rate is high, ranging from 10% to 23%, and amputation is required in up to 10%.[56]

Recently, IDUs in Scotland and England were treated for a syndrome that included abscess, fasciitis, or myositis. The mortality rate for the aggregate was 45%. Preliminary evidence suggests the infection was due to *C. novyi*. At autopsy evidence of a diffuse toxic process with pleural effusions, soft tissue edema, or necrosis was found.[58]

Pyomyositis, a less serious infection involving the musculature, occurs frequently in IDUs. Direct inoculation of bacteria into the musculature has been implicated. Hematogenous spread also occurs, occasionally as a complication of endocarditis.[59] Most patients who have pyomyositis present with pain and swelling of the affected area. Lesions have been reported in the deltoid, psoas, biceps, gastrocnemius, gluteal, and quadriceps muscles. Ultrasound, CT, or MRI reveals the underlying defect within the muscle. *S. aureus* is the most common pathogen; viridans streptococci, aerobic gram-negative bacilli, and mixed infection with anaerobes have also been reported. Patients respond well to drainage and antibiotic therapy. A rare but related condition, uterine pyomyoma, has also been reported. The cause appears to be hematogenous dissemination to an infarcted leiomyoma.[60]

Just as needle exchange programs reduce HIV infection among IDUs, combining those services with a wound and abscess clinic may substantially reduce the cost of care (to as low as $5.00 per patient) and the number of visits to emergency departments. Widespread implementation of such clinics could have a major impact on the management of skin and soft tissue infections among IDUs.[61]

Bone and Joint Infections

Skeletal infections are common in IDUs, most occurring via hematogenous seeding by bacteria or fungi.[62] Target sites for infection are determined by the blood supply and predominantly affect the axial skeleton. The original source of these infections may be inapparent, or the infections may represent metastatic complications of endocarditis. IDU has been identified as a risk factor for osteoarticular infection in patients with endocarditis.[63] In addition, bone and joint infections frequently result from contiguous spread from adjacent, often neglected, areas of infection in skin and soft tissues. IDUs with hematogenous infection often have multiple sites involved simultaneously, and blood cultures frequently are negative at the time of presentation. IDUs with HIV infection do not appear to be at increased risk for osteoarticular infections, and when these infections do occur, they are most frequently caused by the usual bacterial pathogens, not opportunistic pathogens.[64,65]

IDUs with skeletal infection tend to be young and otherwise healthy. Clinical findings include constitutional manifestations as well as local signs and symptoms depending on the site involved. Patients with osteomyelitis often have a paucity of findings, presenting with local pain and tenderness only. Lack of signs and symptoms frequently results in delay in diagnosis. Fever is absent in one third of patients.[62] Similarly, signs of sepsis and leukocytosis and radiologic signs may be absent in patients with osteomyelitis.

Pyogenic infections predominate, with almost 90% being bacterial in origin, although virtually any organism can cause skeletal infections. The predominant pathogens isolated are *S. aureus* and group A and group G streptococci. Although less common, gram-negative bacilli, particularly *Pseudomonas aeruginosa*, are well known, as are polymicrobial infections. IDUs who lick their needles or the skin surface before injection may develop osteomyelitis or septic arthritis with *E. corrodens* ("needle licker's osteomyelitis").[66] *Candida* species have been increasingly recognized as a possible etiology of skeletal infections in IDUs, particularly spondylodiscitis and vertebral osteomyelitis.[67] A characteristic form of systemic candidiasis has been reported among IDUs who inject heroin that includes folliculitis, usually of the scalp and beard; endophthalmitis; and bone and joint lesions, most often costochondritis. Lastly, *Mycobacterium tuberculosis* should always be considered among the possible etiologies of skeletal infection in IDUs, particularly vertebral osteomyelitis. Skeletal infections caused by mycobacteria, including those caused by atypical species, are often associated with involvement of the lungs, adrenals, or pelvic organs.

Joint infections usually involve the extremities, most commonly affecting the knee. The incidence of left-sided involvement exceeds that of right-sided knee arthritis, possibly because of the tendency of right-handed IDUs to inject into the left groin veins; this suggests a relation between site of injection and infection.[62] IDUs are particularly susceptible to vertebral osteomyelitis. The lumbosacral spine is the most common site of infection, and a higher incidence of cervical spine involvement is seen in IDUs than in non-IDUs with vertebral osteomyelitis.[68] IDUs with vertebral osteomyelitis present with symptoms of a shorter duration than do other patients with infection of the spine.[68] Primary sternal osteomyelitis, often associated with an antecedent history of blunt trauma to the sternum, is reported in IDUs. This group is also prone to septic arthritis in unusual sites, such as the sternoclavicular and costochondral joints and the pubic symphysis. Other sites frequently involved include wrist, shoulder, hip, and sacroiliac joints. Vertebral osteomyelitis may extend into the subdural or epidural spaces and may cause formation of an abscess, with consequent cord compression and paraplegia. In addition, lumbosacral vertebral osteomyelitis may be associated with psoas abscess.

Because of the wide spectrum of organisms that may be involved, diagnostic needle aspiration for smear and culture is necessary in all cases. Even when blood cultures are positive, invasive diagnostic steps are advised, because skeletal and bloodstream infection may represent two separate processes and infections may be polymicrobial. Frequent arthrocentesis, arthroscopic or open drainage, and débridement of nonviable bone are also advised if clinically indicated. Antibiotic therapy is required for 4 to 6 weeks, the selection of drug being based on the identity of the responsible microorganisms and susceptibility data. Increasingly, oral antimicrobials with high bioavailability and good bone penetration are utilized for at least a portion of the therapeutic course.[69] Overall, with early diagnosis, the immediate prognosis of bone and joint infection in IDUs is excellent, but long-term follow-up data are lacking.[62] Many IDUs present late in the clinical course, and delays in diagnosis and institution of therapy are accompanied by a high likelihood of chronic osteomyelitis and late relapse of disease. Also contributing to this late but frequent complication is the problem of noncompliance. IDUs tend to leave the hospital against medical advice when confronted with prolonged inpatient IV antibiotic therapy, and many physicians are reluctant to consider outpatient parenteral antibiotic therapy in patients who are active IDUs. A tendency for medical personnel to underappreciate and undertreat the pain associated with skeletal infection may also lead to patients leaving the hospital before therapy can be completed.

A musculoskeletal syndrome, characterized by fever, arthralgia, myalgia (especially of paraspinal muscles), and periarticular tissue swelling thought to represent hypersensitivity to heroin contaminants was reported over 3 decades ago, but subsequent case reports have not appeared.[70]

Infective Endocarditis

Infective endocarditis (IE) is a common cause of bacteremia in IDUs. In the Detroit Medical Center, 74 of 180 addicts with bacteremia had endocarditis.[41] In a community teaching hospital in Ohio, between 1980 and 1990, 16% of endocarditis cases were related to injection drug use.[71] In another hospital emergency department, IE was diagnosed in 15% of febrile addicts.[72] Men are affected more often than women (5.4:1 in the Detroit Medical Center, 2:1 in Chicago). Men with IE are also older than women and have significantly longer histories of drug use (10.2 vs. 7.1 years). Recurrent endocarditis is also more common in IDUs, and the median interval between episodes is far shorter in addicts than in nonaddicts.[73] *S. aureus* remains the most common pathogen, affecting the tricuspid or pulmonary valve in approximately 90% of cases. Cocaine use and HIV infection are additional risk factors.[24,74]

S. aureus remains the commonest pathogen, with methicillin-resistant strains becoming more prevalent. Coagulase-negative staphylococci are now an uncommon cause of endocarditis in IDUs. Streptococci, particularly groups A, B, and G, are the second most common cause.[41,75] These two organisms account for up to 75% of cases.[41] *Enterococcus* played a major role in the past, but its prevalence is decreasing.[41,75] Gram-negative organisms are infrequent causes, although intermittent epidemics of *P. aeruginosa* endocarditis occurred in Detroit and Chicago,[41,69,76,77] and *Serratia marcescens* was responsible for a sustained epidemic in the Oakland, California, area.[78,79] Fungi, especially *Candida parapsilosis* and *Candida tropicalis*, account for approximately 4% of cases,[80] and several cases of IE caused by *Aspergillus* were recently reported.[81] Two of three patients were HIV-infected. Duration of symptoms ranged from 2 weeks to 1 month before detection. Blood cultures were negative, but there were large vegetations and peripheral embolization. *Aspergillus* frequently contaminates illicit drugs, but whether the inoculum associated with injection is sufficient to cause endocarditis is unclear. That two of three patients were HIV-positive is of interest and may indicate that altered immune status played a role. Polymicrobial endocarditis is being observed with increasing frequency among drug users. Usually only a few organisms are involved, but rarely there may be numerous pathogens. In such cases, standard laboratory techniques may be inadequate to isolate and identify the full microbial spectrum, placing a burden on the clinician to suspect polymicrobial endocarditis caused by salivary contamination of needles or injection sites whenever uncommon oropharyngeal organisms are cultured from the blood.[82] Among the fastidious organisms, most cases are caused by *Eikenella*; however, there are reports of endocarditis caused by anaerobes such as *Fusobacterium* spp. and *Clostridium*. In addition, numerous reports describe endocarditis in IDUs caused by a variety of organisms that are frequently considered nonpathogens. These infections may be related to altered host immunity resulting from HIV infection[83] or to unusual practices among addicts, such as licking needles before use or "cleaning" the injection site with saliva.

The pathophysiology of endocarditis in addicts is poorly understood. The organism is most often part of the patient's own flora,[41,84] although injection paraphernalia have been implicated in the case of *P. aeruginosa* endocarditis. Environmental contamination was also considered in the initial outbreak of *Serratia* endocarditis in California when it was learned that years earlier *Serratia* had been sprayed into the air to study wind currents. However, these strains were not the same ones that caused disease, and the regional predilection for this infection remains a mystery. It is also unclear why certain valves are affected in IDUs with endocarditis. It is known that, unlike native valve endocarditis in nonaddicts, the affected cardiac valve is almost always previously normal.[41,76,85] In an autopsy study of addicts who died from endocarditis, Dressler and Roberts reported that 81% of the valves were normal, including all right-side valves.[85] Early reports of endocarditis in addicts noted a predominance of tricuspid valve involvement. Left-side involvement predominates in some recent studies, and multiple valves are frequently involved.[75,86] Pulmonary involvement remains rare. Nevertheless, tricuspid valve involvement is seen almost exclusively in IDUs.

Clearly no single hypothesis explains the prevalence of right-sided involvement in IDUs. Potential explanations include damage to right-side endothelium by repeated exposure to injected particulate matter; vasospasm caused by injected diluents or illicit drugs, particularly cocaine; or drug-induced thrombus formation and subsequent bacterial aggregation. The fact that endocarditis caused by *Enterococcus* and *Serratia* is primarily a left-sided phenomenon suggests that other mechanisms must be important. Mitral valve prolapse has been proposed to explain the predilection for mitral valve endocarditis in female IDUs, but studies showing equal numbers of men and women with mitral involvement make this explanation unlikely. Specific surface properties of the common infecting pathogens, especially *S. aureus*, might favor attachment to extracellular matrix proteins that may have greater expression on right-side valves. *S. aureus* is also phagocytosed by endothelial cells, where it is protected from host defenses. This may activate the clotting system, leading to vegetation formation. The production of coagulase by *S. aureus* may further promote clotting and vegetation formation. Cytokines produced after phagocytosis may enhance immune-complex deposition that leads to valvulitis, thereby creating a lesion that is susceptible to vegetation formation and bacterial seeding. Finally, endothelial differences between the right and left sides of the heart might contribute to the predilection for tricuspid valve involvement. Additional hypotheses invoke an association between large, directly injected bacterial inocula and immune abnormalities that may contribute to sustained bacteremia and valvulitis.[87] Which, if any, of these mechanisms proves to be responsible for the preponderance of right-sided involvement depends on future studies. Whatever the reason, *S. aureus* predominantly affects the tricuspid valve but may also involve the mitral or aortic valves. *S. marcescens*, *Streptococcus pyogenes*, and enterococci affect left-side valves almost exclusively.[78,88,89]

HIV infection plays a significant role in the pathophysiology of endocarditis in IDUs. HIV-infected addicts are significantly more likely to develop endocarditis than addicts who are not infected with HIV, and those with the lowest CD4 lymphocyte counts are the most likely.[74] In contrast, alcohol consumption confers protection against endocarditis, perhaps by inducing an inhibitory effect on platelet function.[90]

Unlike nonaddicts, who generally present with symptoms of longer than 2 weeks' duration,[91] most addicts with IE present within the first week of illness with signs indicative of severe, acute infection.[41,75,92] Typically, they have acute onset of fever, chills, and dyspnea. Chest pain, often pleuritic in nature, occurs in up to half the cases and is due to septic pulmonary emboli.[41,75] Cough is frequently present; it may be nonproductive or associated with blood-streaked sputum. Radiologic evidence of pneumonia is detected in 23% and congestive heart failure in 13%.[75] Pneumothorax, occasionally bilateral, is a complication of septic pulmonary embolism.[93] Involvement of other organ systems is similar to that observed in endocarditis in nonaddicts. Initially, central nervous system (CNS) involvement may be confused with toxic effects of illicit drugs, but the diagnosis usually becomes rapidly apparent when blood cultures become positive.

The overall severity of the clinical picture depends on the valve or valves involved and whether there is any associated damage to the heart itself, such as valve ring abscess or valve rupture, or metastatic infection involving other organs. Osler's nodes and Janeway lesions are rare in addicts. Splenomegaly occurs in only 10% to 15%, and heart murmurs are found with variable frequency. When the infection is confined to the tricuspid valve, the presence of murmurs varies from 35% to 72%.[41]

Because of the high-grade bacteremia and acute nature of endocarditis in addicts, every organ is affected to some degree. Complications involving the heart, although infrequent, may be life threatening. When cardiac problems dominate the picture, which is most likely with mitral or aortic valve infections, the prognosis is poor, especially if congestive heart failure develops. As noted earlier, recurrent IE is common in addicts. Most patients survive the first episode, but with such severely damaged valves that dysfunction occurs in almost 70%. Previous valve damage predisposes to subsequent episodes, which frequently are fatal. Additional cardiac lesions include left-ventricular abscesses, which are multifocal and are found in conjunction with clusters of bacteria in intramural arteries, and myocardial infarction. Valve ring abscesses and, rarely, focal, acute interstitial myocarditis are also found.[85,94] Cardiac abscesses may also lead to further serious complications, such as a pseudoaneurysm of the heart, which can be demonstrated by MRI and color Doppler ultrasound.[95] As with nonaddicts, left-sided infection predisposes to systemic emboli and acute pericarditis. Certain organisms, especially *Serratia* and *Candida*, are notable for their tendency to induce large, systemic emboli. Their isolation in a patient with endocarditis should alert the clinician to the probability of left-sided infection and the likelihood of a serious embolic event. CNS complications of endocarditis are similar to those in non-IDUs and include mycotic aneurysms, brain abscess, stroke, meningitis, and epidural abscess. Splenic abscesses are seen, especially with *S. aureus* infection, and should be assessed before cardiac surgery to avoid valve replacement in a patient likely to remain bacteremic from a noncardiac source. Drug users are more likely than nonusers to develop bone and joint infection, particularly vertebral osteomyelitis, secondary to endocarditis.[96]

The diagnosis of endocarditis in IDUs is often easily made on the basis of the characteristic clinical picture. The modified Duke criteria effectively classify IDUs with either definite or possible endocarditis and can be utilized in difficult cases, particularly when difficult therapeutic decisions must be made.[97] Those with definite IE frequently have no obvious focus of infection and are more likely to have vascular phenomena and multiple opacities on chest radiographs.[98] However, in the emergency department setting, the absence of signs specific for endocarditis and the limited information available make the diagnosis particularly difficult.[99] At the time of the initial presentation, there are no differences in age, sex, maximum temperature, or leukocyte count between addicts with and without endocarditis. Those with endocarditis account for only 13% of addicts admitted for infection, and only positive echocardiogram findings, pulmonary or systemic emboli, and bacteremia distinguish patients with endocarditis from those without.[72]

Rothman and colleagues further modified the Duke criteria in an effort to improve diagnostic accuracy in an urban emergency department.[100] Major criteria are the same as the Duke criteria, although an echocardiogram performed upon arrival at the hospital is added and only data available in the first 24 hours are used. Minor criteria are unchanged. The definition of definite endocarditis is the same as in the Duke system; possible endocarditis requires either one major and two minor or four minor criteria. The diagnosis is rejected if these criteria are not met. The results were almost identical to published results using the standard Duke criteria, but the investigators were able to make admission and therapeutic decisions much earlier than was otherwise possible. The same investigators also evaluated the contribution to diagnosis of transthoracic echocardiography (TTE) in the emergency department. Adding TTE proved diagnostic for nearly 70% of patients who failed to meet major culture criteria.[101] In another attempt to arrive at earlier diagnosis, investigators utilized polymerase chain reaction to detect universal 16S ribosomal RNA. They found a sensitivity and specificity of only 86.7% and 86.9%, respectively, but accurately identified all eight patients with blood culture–positive endocarditis.[102] If validated, this method may provide an additional diagnostic tool for the emergency department clinician.

The most sensitive indicator of endocarditis in IDUs is a blood culture, which is positive in 80% to 100% of cases. However, because many addicts take oral antibiotics before admission, initial cultures may be negative. Subsequent blood cultures will reveal the pathogen.[103] Even after several days of appropriate parenteral therapy, blood cultures are still likely to be positive.[104,105] Because culture-negative IE is rare in IDUs, negative blood cultures suggest an alternative diagnosis.

Additional blood studies are not of particular benefit in diagnosing endocarditis. Anemia is common in IDUs as a result of the continual blood loss associated with the act of injecting. Elevated white blood cell (WBC) count, usually with a left-shift, is also common, although neutropenia and thrombocytopenia are occasionally found. Hyponatremia in the range of 125 to 133 mEq/L is found in approximately 40% of cases immediately after admission and predicts prolonged fever and greater morbidity.[41] The etiology is unclear, and the abnormality corrects immediately after fluid administration. Additional laboratory abnormalities reflect the high-grade bacteremia associated with endocarditis and routinely normalize soon after bacteremia clears. The cerebrospinal fluid (CSF) is abnormal in many cases, with increased WBC and protein in patients showing no overt CNS symptoms or signs.[106] The echocardiogram has a relatively high sensitivity (approximately 90%), and false-positive results are unusual.[72] The TTE is at least equivalent to the transesophageal echocardiogram (TEE) for detecting right-sided lesions. In cases with a high pretest probability, they are equivalent. Hence, a TTE might be performed first, and, if negative, a TEE may be ordered. Alternatively, TEE might be reserved for patients thought to have left-sided involvement or those with perivalvular lesions, such as valve ring abscess or perforation or a vestigial eustachian valve.[107] It is important to recognize that a negative TEE does not rule out endocarditis.

Addicts with IE who are stable and only moderately ill can be observed safely without antibiotic therapy while the results of blood cultures are awaited. Transient fever and bacteremia occur in this population, and because bacteremia is the most sensitive indicator of endocarditis, a commitment to therapy before the nature of the septic condition is documented can lead to unnecessary and prolonged hospitalization for administration of antibiotics. Even when the patient is acutely ill, several blood cultures should be obtained before antibiotic therapy is initiated. The initial empirical regimen is based in part on knowledge of the organisms most likely to cause endocarditis in that geographic location. In most settings, coverage is directed against *S. aureus*. Where MRSA is prevalent, vancomycin is the preferred agent. Where methicillin-resistant organisms are rare, nafcillin or a similar β-lactamase–resistant penicillin is preferred. When vancomycin is used, both fever and bacteremia are considerably prolonged, compared with treatment with nafcillin.[104]

Trimethoprim-sulfamethoxazole may be an alternative for both methicillin-sensitive *S. aureus* and MRSA soft tissue infections, but its efficacy in treating endocarditis is questionable.[108] Traditionally, endocarditis in IDUs was treated with 4- to 6-week courses of parenteral antibiotics. However, some patients with uncomplicated right-sided endocarditis may be successfully treated for 2 weeks with nafcillin plus an aminoglycoside[109] or even cloxacillin alone.[110] When quinolones are used, therapy may consist entirely of oral medication.[111] The addition of an aminoglycoside to an initial empirical regimen to provide coverage against a gram-negative pathogen is controversial. The standard aminoglycoside dose used with an antistaphylococcal penicillin is likely to have little effect against the most worrisome gram-negative organisms, particularly *Pseudomonas*. Reyes and colleagues noted that an aminoglycoside dose of 8 mg/kg/day in divided doses was required to achieve acceptable antipseudomonal activity.[112,113] Using a high-dose aminoglycoside and a synergistic β-lactam antibiotic, the outcome in *Pseudomonas* endocarditis is much more favorable than with any other initial regimen.[114] Quinolones also have utility against *Pseudomonas*, but the data are insufficient to permit a recommendation for their use.[115]

Combined therapy with penicillin (or vancomycin) plus an aminoglycoside is standard against enterococcal endocarditis, but the prevalence of resistant strains makes such a selection less reliable without first screening for susceptibility. Frequently, gentamicin-resistant enterococci are susceptible to streptomycin, and synergy can be obtained with use of the latter.[116]

Fungal endocarditis is usually treated with amphotericin B plus surgery. Currently, the need for surgery in all patients is being questioned. Recent information suggests the outcome in patients treated with medical management alone may be similar to that for those having valve replacement surgery. In either case, many clinicians prefer to prescribe long-term suppression with oral fluconazole following the initial treatment phase.[80] The role of newer triazoles and echinocandins in treating endocarditis has yet to be studied.

In most cases of IE in IDUs, the survival rate is good using antibiotics alone, despite complications and prolonged fever.[117] Septic emboli frequently occur after the initiation of therapy but do not affect the prognosis and are not necessarily an indication for removal or replacement of the infected valve.[41,117] The relationship between vegetation size, as determined by echocardiography, and the likelihood of an embolus is controversial. However, vegetations larger than 2 cm are associated with a 33% mortality rate, compared with 1.3% for patients with vegetations smaller than 2 cm ($P < .001$).[117] Hence, some clinicians consider large vegetations as an indication for surgery. In general, the indications for surgery and the final result are the same in IDUs with endocarditis as in the general population. Although surgery carries substantial risk, the mortality rate in patients who fail medical management approaches 100%, so surgical treatment is indicated and clearly improves survival.[118] The patient's HIV-1 status is a significant prognostic indicator. The CD4 cell count drops after cardiopulmonary bypass, which may lead to an acceleration of the progress toward the acquired immunodeficiency syndrome (AIDS).[119] Addicts with HIV-1 infection whose IE is poorly controlled at the time of cardiac surgery and those with advanced AIDS also have a poor prognosis.[120] The major problem after cardiac surgery for endocarditis in IDUs is their propensity to continue illicit drug use. In one study, only 4 of 57 addicts remained drug free, and the 10-year survival rate was only 10%.[120] Hence, some investigators advocate excision of the tricuspid valve or repair of the left-side valves rather than replacement for IDUs needing surgical intervention.[121] Prognosis is not affected by the duration of symptoms before initiation of therapy, antibiotic use before admission, right-sided heart failure, pulmonary embolism, or results of the following laboratory tests: leukocyte count, hemoglobin, and serum creatinine.[117]

Noncardiac Vascular Infections

As arm and leg veins become thrombosed, sclerosed, and unusable, femoral, axillary, and neck vessels are increasingly selected for injection. Vessels used frequently for injection become injured or infected, leading to the formation of hematomas, thrombosis, septic thrombophlebitis, mycotic aneurysm, or traumatic arteriovenous fistula.[122,123] The predominant pathogens are gram-positive cocci, usually *S. aureus*, although gram-negative pathogens, particularly *P. aeruginosa*, are not infrequently found. Findings with septic thrombophlebitis include local pain, swelling, and fever together with bacteremia and sepsis. Local signs of infection may be masked when deep vessels are involved. Infection or sclerosis of proximal large veins is frequently complicated by venous stasis and supervening thrombosis. Septic pulmonary embolization follows and closely resembles right-sided bacterial endocarditis.[41] The management of septic thrombophlebitis, which most frequently involves the femoral veins, remains controversial. Parenteral antimicrobial therapy is standard, but the value of anticoagulant use has not been established. Furthermore, hemorrhagic complications from unrecognized coexistent femoral and cerebral mycotic aneurysms may occur. Difficulty performing venography in IDUs precludes controlled studies evaluating efficacy and complications of anticoagulant use. Some experienced clinicians believe the risks of short-term anticoagulation are outweighed by the risk of major pulmonary emboli.

A major vascular complication in IDUs is the formation of mycotic aneurysms, most frequently involving femoral and, less commonly, neck vessels. True aneurysms, involving all three layers of the arterial wall, are rare. In the IDU, frequent direct trauma to peripheral vessels produces damage to the vessel wall and an initial sterile perivascular hematoma. Injection of chemical agents in illicit drugs also causes tissue necrosis. The vascular wall usually becomes infected by contiguous spread from adjacent subcutaneous abscesses or areas of cellulitis. Infection causes liquefaction of the central portion of the hematoma in communication with the arterial or, less commonly, the venous wall, forming a secondary (false) pseudoaneurysm.[123,124] The common femoral artery is the most frequent location, followed by the deep femoral and superficial femoral arteries. Because most IDUs are right handed, left-sided groin infections and aneurysms are more common. Primary mycotic aneurysms in which the damaged vessel wall is infected secondary to unrelated bacteremia are rare and are more likely to involve cerebral vessels as a complication of endocarditis. Pathogenesis includes septic embolization from valvular vegetations to the vasa vasorum of smaller vessels, such as the middle or posterior cerebral and visceral intra-abdominal arteries, which are more frequently involved than the aorta.

Clinical manifestations of a mycotic aneurysm include a painful, often enlarging, tender, and frequently pulsatile mass, accompanied by variable constitutional symptoms. Distal extremity ischemia and nerve compression are often present, and detection of a bruit or thrill over the mass strongly supports the diagnosis. Often addicts report "hitting the pinky," indicating unintended arterial injection. Bleeding from an injection site may be evidence of an aneurysm. Because drug abusers usually present with cellulitis and accompanying edema and induration, the pulsatile mass may be masked, obscuring the aneurysm. When rupture of the aneurysm occurs, it is usually preceded by severe pain that may be misdiagnosed as thrombophlebitis or soft tissue abscess. In contrast to an aneurysm in the lower limb, distal ischemia in the upper extremity (hand) from induced arterial spasm occurs commonly.

Anemia, leukocytosis, and an elevated sedimentation rate, although frequently present, are of limited diagnostic value. A high index of suspicion together with angiographic confirmation is essential, because misdiagnosis is common and cellulitis, abscess, or infected hematoma may mimic or mask an aneurysm (Fig. 316-1).

Ultrasonography, although useful, may fail to differentiate an abscess from an aneurysm. In one study, ultrasound had a false-negative rate of 54%.[125] CT, especially with injected contrast material, is extremely useful and delineates the pathology in the adjacent soft tissues. Color Doppler sonography may confirm the diagnosis, especially in the extremities, but may not define the vascular anatomy clearly.[126] Thus, angiography remains the definitive diagnostic procedure, not only for delineating the lesion but also for planning the approach to surgery, and digital subtraction angiography may replace traditional arteriography in diagnosing femoral and other peripheral aneurysms.[127] Magnetic resonance angiography (MRA) may prove to be helpful in the diagnosis of mycotic aneurysms. Needle aspiration, incision, and drainage should be avoided in inguinal masses that have not been investigated, even if nonpulsatile, because of the risk of uncontrolled bleeding from an unrecognized mycotic aneurysm.

Successful management of a mycotic aneurysm requires early diagnosis before rupture occurs. Surgical treatment should not be delayed, because rupture is frequent. It consists of proximal and distal ligation of the aneurysm, followed by excision of all necrotic and infected material, including the infected vessel. Vascular reconstruction as a delayed procedure is recommended only in patients who develop ischemia after excision of the aneurysm, and then only when a graft can be positioned through an uninfected tissue plane.

Because *S. aureus* is the most common pathogen, initial empirical antibiotic therapy should include a β-lactamase–resistant penicillin such as nafcillin. When MRSA is prominent, vancomycin should be started. An aminoglycoside is added initially if there is suspicion or evidence of gram-negative bacilli on Gram staining of sanguinopurulent drainage. Subsequent cultures obtained from blood and local

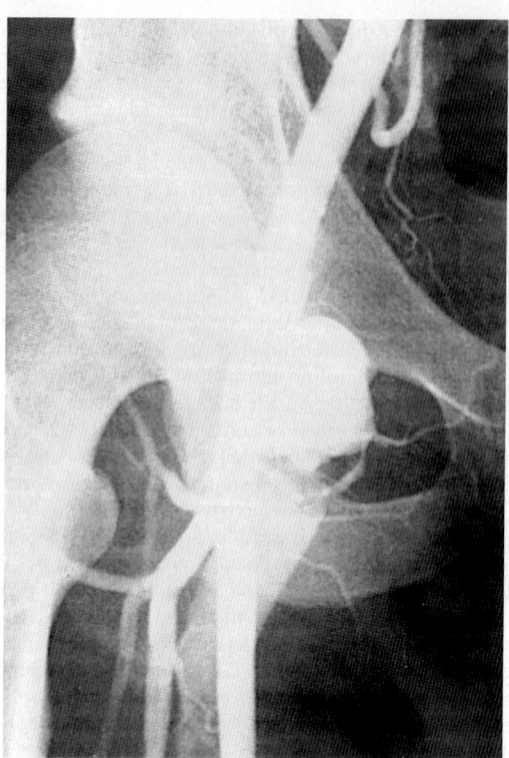

Figure 316-1 Arteriogram demonstrating a mycotic aneurysm of the right common iliac artery in an injection drug user.

exudate influence antibiotic selection. Recommended therapy is intravenous and lasts for 4 to 6 weeks.

Pulmonary Infections

Pulmonary manifestations are extremely common in IDUs. The lung is the target of numerous infectious and noninfectious insults. The latter include bronchospasm, airflow obstruction, diffusion impairment, emphysema, and pulmonary hypertension in heroin users.[128] Pulmonary hypertension and alveolar hemorrhage are associated with the injection of cocaine.[128] Heroin overdose may be associated with unilateral or bilateral pulmonary edema as a consequence of capillary-alveolar leak and may be accompanied by fever and leukocytosis; however, this complication of heroin overdose has been reported much less frequently in recent series.[129] Granulomatous lesions occur in reaction to particles of cotton (used to filter the drug before injection) and fillers (mainly from injection of crushed pills). Starch can cause mild transient pulmonary granuloma formation, whereas cotton fibers and talc (used as a filler) can cause permanent intravascular and perivascular granulomas in pulmonary arteries and arterioles.[130] The resultant baseline abnormalities of chest radiographic films and blood gases may cause diagnostic confusion in febrile IDUs. IDUs have a 10-fold increased risk of pneumonia compared with that for nondrug users.[131] Among patients with HIV infection on antiretroviral therapy, bacterial pneumonia was more common in those who were IDUs.[132] The incidence of pneumonia is increased in IDUs for a number of reasons, including impaired clearance of secretions, aspiration, increased exposure, decreased immune function, and the higher prevalence of HIV infection. In a series of pulmonary complications of injection drug use, septic pulmonary emboli were the most common complication, followed by community-acquired pneumonia and *M. tuberculosis* infection.[133]

Most pulmonary infections are community-acquired episodes of pneumonia caused by common respiratory pathogens. In one series of febrile IDUs, pneumonia was the most common cause of fever[134]; in a second series, pneumonia was second only to cellulitis as a cause of fever in IDUs.[135] Bacterial pneumonia must be distinguished from septic emboli originating from right-sided endocarditis or more distal thrombophlebitis and resultant pulmonary infarcts. Septic emboli result in multiple round or wedge-shaped lesions that may cavitate (Fig 316-2). Pleural involvement is common in both conditions and results in chest pain, pleural effusion, or empyema. Recurrent pulmonary emboli may also result in pulmonary hypertension. The usual pathogens in bacterial pneumonia include *Streptococcus pneumoniae* and oral anaerobes by the bronchogenic route, and *S. aureus* or, less commonly, *P. aeruginosa* by the hematogenous route. One study of the etiology of community-acquired pneumonia in an urban public hospital emphasized the importance of aspiration pneumonia in this patient population, particularly among patients with pneumonia necessitating admission to the intensive care unit.[136] Injection drug use has been identified as a risk factor for bacteremia in patients with community-acquired pneumococcal pneumonia.[137] A high incidence of bacterial pneumonia caused by *Haemophilus influenzae* has been described in IDUs with concomitant HIV infection.[138-141] However, in a more recent series of HIV patients with community-acquired bacterial pneumonia, the majority of whom were IDUs, *S. pneumoniae* was much more common than *H. influenzae*.[142] Lung abscesses may arise from aspiration pneumonia, necrotizing pneumonitis, or septic emboli. Opportunistic pulmonary infections, especially *Pneumocystis jirovecii* pneumonia, must also be considered in febrile IDUs.

Pulmonary tuberculosis (TB) is a major problem in both HIV-infected and non–HIV-infected drug users. Homelessness and nonadherence to medication regimens further complicate the problem. The risk of TB is still substantial in HIV-positive individuals taking antiretroviral therapy.[143] Among IDUs in New York City during the resurgence of TB in the 1990s, risk factors for active TB included HIV

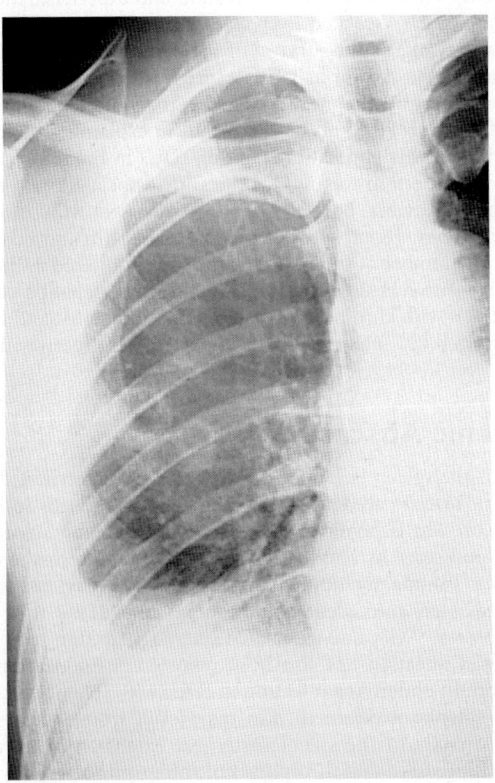

Figure 316-2 Anteroposterior radiograph of chest demonstrating pleural effusion and multiple cavitating nodular infarcts resulting from septic emboli in a patient with tricuspid endocarditis.

infection, receipt of less than 6 months of isoniazid for treatment of latent TB, CD4 count less than 200, and a positive result on the tuberculin skin test (TST).[144] TB in IDUs with AIDS is more frequently extrapulmonary, and patients present with less cavitary pulmonary disease and fewer acid-fast bacillus–positive organisms in sputum than those in other TB patients. Coughing induced by the use of marijuana or crack cocaine may increase the transmission of TB. HIV-negative IDUs should receive therapy for treatment of latent TB infection with isoniazid for 9 months if the TST is 10 mm or larger. IDUs with HIV infection should receive treatment for latent TB infection as recommended for other HIV-infected persons—that is, if the TST is 5 mm or larger or if the patient is a close contact of persons who have active TB, regardless of skin test results or previous courses of therapy for latent infection.[145] The recommended duration of treatment for latent TB infection in HIV-infected patients is 9 months, 2 months if the combination of rifampin and pyrazinamide is utilized. The latter combination is no longer recommended because of hepatotoxicity. Some experts also recommend that TST-negative and anergic HIV-infected persons from risk groups (such as IDUs) or geographic areas with a high prevalence of *M. tuberculosis* infection receive treatment for latent TB infection, but the efficacy of this approach has not been proved. The use of a two-step TST increases the proportion of IDUs diagnosed with latent TB infection.[146] Interferon-γ release assays have a moderate concordance with TST results in current and former IDUs and may increase the chances of diagnosis because the individual does not need to return for a skin test reading.[147,148] The potential risk of isoniazid-induced hepatotoxicity in IDUs, who have a higher frequency of background hepatitis and who may also be abusing other hepatotoxic agents such as alcohol and cocaine, is a concern. However, a study of isoniazid therapy in an IDU population with an HCV seroprevalence of 95% found that the risks of hepatotoxicity and isoniazid discontinuation were similar to those reported for populations with a lower prevalence of HCV.[149] Monetary incentives have been shown to be highly effective in increasing the return rates for TST reading and promoting adherence to a program of directly observed preventive therapy in IDUs.[150,151]

The febrile IDU with pulmonary infiltrates constitutes an enormous diagnostic challenge given the wide differential diagnosis, which includes noninfectious causes. Accordingly, initial treatment often involves multiple therapeutic agents to cover several pathogens, and empirical coverage for TB may be needed in critically ill patients.

Hepatitis

Hepatitis has long been recognized as a complication of injection drug use. A significant number of HCV-infected IDUs also screen positive for problem alcohol use despite demonstrating knowledge of the dangers.[152] The combination of alcohol plus HBV or HCV infection results in more severe liver disease than either alone and is associated with more rapid acceleration to cirrhosis. Heroin itself is not known to be hepatotoxic, but cocaine can cause severe liver injury. Buprenorphine, which is used as a substitution drug in the treatment of opiate addiction, has been reported to cause hepatitis, both when diverted and injected and when used sublingually.[153,154] Knowledge regarding risks and transmission of viral hepatitis among IDUs has been shown to be significantly lower than knowledge regarding risks and transmission of HIV.[61] Needle exchange programs have been shown to be less effective at preventing the transmission of HCV and HBV than HIV.[155,156] Needle exchange programs decrease the sharing of needles, but IDUs may still share other injection paraphernalia that can facilitate HCV and HBV transmission.[157] The validity of self-reported serostatus of hepatitis A, B, and C and HBV vaccination status by IDUs is poor.[158,159]

IDUs currently account for 16% of cases of acute HBV in the United States.[160] It has been thought that most acquire infection within the first few years of beginning injection drug use, although a recent study of IDUs younger than 30 years of age found that 22% had serologic evidence of vaccine-mediated immunity and 56% had no HBV markers, suggesting that vaccine prevention programs targeted to younger IDUs could still prevent a significant number of infections.[161] Clinically apparent HBV infection is uncommon, and many IDUs end up with a serologic pattern indicative of naturally acquired immunity. In the United States 60% to 80% of IDUs have serum antibody against hepatitis B surface antigen (HBsAg); however, only 5% to 10% become chronic carriers.[162,163] Spontaneous reactivation of chronic HBV infection has been described in IDUs, but the diagnosis may be difficult because the clinical presentation is indistinguishable from that of acute hepatitis, anti-HBV core immunoglobulin M may increase during a reactivation, and information on the patient's previous serologic status usually is unknown.[164,165] HIV-infected persons with HBV infection are more likely to become chronic carriers.[166] In addition, a high prevalence of occult HBV infection has been reported in IDUs with HIV infection.[167] The Centers for Disease Control and Prevention Advisory Committee on Immunization Practices has recommended HBV vaccination for IDUs since 1991, yet current vaccine coverage rates are low.[159,168] Although there is a tendency toward a decreased antibody response to immunization in HIV-positive and HIV-negative IDUs, there is not convincing evidence of decreased protection from infection, and all susceptible IDUs should be offered vaccination.[169] The incorporation of HBV vaccination into needle exchange programs may be cost-effective and improve coverage rates.[170] IDUs with isolated anti-HBV core antibody have been shown to have strong resistance to reinfection and do not need vaccination.[171] Guidelines for the treatment of chronic HBV infection are available, but they do not specifically address the issue of treatment of active IDUs, in contrast to guidelines for the treatment of HCV.[172,173]

Hepatitis delta virus (HDV) is a defective RNA virus that can replicate and cause hepatitis only in the presence of active HBV infection. HDV may be acquired along with HBV as a primary coinfection or as a superinfection in persons who are carriers of HBV. Because of the interdependent nature of the two viruses, immunity to HBV provides protection against HDV. In some areas where HBV is prevalent, HDV is also seen with relatively high frequency. In nonendemic areas, such as the United States, HDV infection is confined almost exclusively to particular high-risk groups, such as IDUs.[174,175] It had been previously reported that the incidence of HDV in IDUs who are HBsAg carriers approaches 50%,[176] but current data regarding the seroprevalence of HDV among IDUs in the United States are lacking. The association of injection drug use with HBV and HDV was clarified in a study comparing the transmission and carriage of each agent in two populations known to be at risk, IDUs and men who have sex with men.[177] Among 372 IDUs, 52.4% had evidence of current or past HBV infection; of these, 8.7% were chronic carriers of HBV. Among the chronic carriers, 70.6% were also chronic carriers of HDV. In contrast, only 27.4% of the men who have sex with men had serologic evidence of HBV infection (current or remote), of whom 7.9% were chronic carriers. Only a third of these chronic HBV carriers had evidence of HDV infection—a significant difference from the IDUs, demonstrating that injection drug use is a much more efficient means of transmission of HDV infection than is sexual contact.

Superinfection of HDV on previous HBV infection is the most common pattern of dual infection. Simultaneous acquisition of both viruses is more common among IDUs and is more likely to result in fulminant infection.[175] Outbreaks of HBV and HDV coinfection continue to be reported among IDUs in the United States.[178] IDUs who experience coinfection frequently have a biphasic illness.[177] The initial phase of the disease is caused by HDV, and the second by HBV.[179] The closer the proximity of the biphasic peaks, the greater is the risk of a fatal outcome. IDUs who survive such an illness usually have a complete recovery and clear both viruses.[180] Prevention of HDV can be accomplished by vaccination of IDUs against HBV.

Injection drug use is a major risk factor for HCV infection. IDUs accounted for 54% of cases of acute HCV infection in 2006.[160] The seroprevalence of anti-HCV antibody among IDUs in four U.S. cities decreased between 1994 and 2004 from 65% to 35%.[181] However, IDUs remain an important reservoir of HCV infection in the general popula-

tion and injection drug use is the primary mode of HCV transmission in the United States. Maternal drug use, independent of HIV coinfection, has been identified as a major risk factor for perinatal transmission of HCV.[182] Studies of HCV seroconversion among young IDUs have identified sharing of needles and drug preparation equipment, pooling money with another IDU to purchase drugs, requiring assistance to inject, and injecting more than once daily as independent risk factors for the acquisition of HCV.[183-185] Although injection drug use is more efficient at transmitting HCV infection than sexual activity, exchanging sex for money and having a sexual partner who uses injection drugs were also risk factors for seroconversion. Even if syringes are not shared, the sharing of equipment used to prepare drugs for injection such as cookers and cotton filters is a risk factor for the transmission of HCV.[186] Studies from the mid 1980s and 1990s showed that HCV infection was acquired after a very brief interval of IDU; more recent work, however, has demonstrated that this is no longer the case.[181] The average time to seroconversion among HCV-negative IDUs in Seattle was 3.4 years, certainly long enough to justify the allocation of resources to try and reduce risky injection practices.[185] There may be other benefits to reducing risky injection practices, beyond the reduction of infection with blood-borne viral infections. IDUs without HCV infection who were enrolled in an HCV risk reduction program had a lower risk of bacterial infections than those in other IDU cohorts.[187] It has been shown that IDUs who successfully cleared HCV infection in the past are less likely to develop persistent HCV viremia, despite continued exposure, and this appears to correlate with T-cell responses to HCV.[188-190]

Chronic HCV infection occurs in 60% to 80% of IDUs.[162] Current guidelines for the treatment of HCV state that the treatment of active IDUs must be considered on a case by case basis.[173] Response rates to treatment are comparable to those reported in non-IDUs, even with ongoing drug use, especially in multidisciplinary programs that incorporate treatment for addiction and directly observed therapy.[191-193] Despite a willingness to be treated, low uptake of HCV treatment among IDUs is reported.[191,194] HIV-HCV coinfected patients are less likely to clear HCV viremia after infection and experience more rapid progression to HCV-related liver disease. In addition, HCV coinfection negatively affects the survival of patients with HIV.[195]

IDUs are also at risk for hepatitis A virus (HAV) infection. Although parenteral transmission of HAV has been reported in IDUs, other lifestyle factors are likely more important in explaining the increased risk of HAV in this population. Among IDUs in Baltimore, evidence of past HAV infection was not significantly associated with high-risk drug-using behaviors but rather was associated with low annual income.[196] A more recent study of IDUs in Alaska did find a correlation between the number of times an individual had injected in the past 30 days and positive HAV serostatus.[197] Fulminant hepatitis caused by HAV in IDUs with chronic liver disease caused by HBV and HCV has been reported.[198,199] Nonimmune IDUs should receive the HAV vaccine.

Splenic Abscess

Abscess of the spleen is a major complication of injection drug use. The splenic arteries are end arteries; any occlusion leads to ischemia or infarction. The ischemic or infarcted areas are highly susceptible to infection and serve as a nidus for abscess formation in the event of bacteremia. Trauma, including blunt trauma, also may lead to splenic injury and is an antecedent condition in some IDUs who develop splenic abscess.[200] Cocaine-associated splenic infarction with secondary bacterial infection has also been reported.[201] Endocarditis is the most common underlying infection in IDUs with splenic abscess,[200,202] although splenic involvement also may result from spread of local infection directly to the splenic artery or extension of an adjacent process with erosion and thrombosis of the splenic artery.[203]

Splenic lesions may be multiple and small or solitary, occasionally becoming large.[200,202,203] Lesions within the spleen are most often found in the upper pole (53.1%). Lower-pole lesions (21.9%) and midspleen lesions (15.6%) are found less often.[203] Staphylococci and streptococci are the organisms most often implicated; however, gram-negative bacilli and anaerobes are isolated in approximately 25% and 5% of cases, respectively.[203] IDUs who lick their needles are susceptible to splenic abscesses caused by mouth anaerobes, in particular *Fusobacterium* spp.[204] *M. tuberculosis* has been reported as a cause of splenic abscess in IDUs who are infected with HIV.[205] Bacteremia is common in patients with splenic abscess, and usually the same organism is cultured from the blood and from the splenic cavity. However, IDUs have a tendency to have multiple infected sites that contain different organisms. Therefore, isolation of an organism from the blood is not assurance that the same organism will be found in the spleen.[202]

The signs and symptoms of splenic abscess may be vague or overshadowed by underlying endocarditis. Almost all patients have fever and some degree of abdominal pain or discomfort.[200,202,203] Pleuritic chest pain is common.[200,202,203] Left shoulder pain has also been described. Abdominal tenderness, which is frequently confined to the left upper quadrant, is found in approximately 50% of patients.[200,202,203] Splenomegaly may be present, but a splenic rub is unusual.[200] Abnormalities within the thorax are detected in two thirds of cases, including left lower lobe lung infiltrate and pleural effusion. The differential diagnosis includes subphrenic abscess, pulmonary empyema, perinephric abscess, and bland splenic infarct. The possibility of splenic abscess must always be excluded in IDUs with infective endocarditis who fail to clear their bacteremia or remain persistently febrile despite negative blood cultures. There are no characteristic laboratory abnormalities, although an extremely high leukocyte count has been correlated with a poor prognosis.[203] The chest radiograph may reveal an elevated hemidiaphragm, infiltrate, or a pleural effusion; however, abdominal radiography is seldom useful. The most reliable diagnostic tests are ultrasound and CT of the abdomen,[200] which also define the extent and location of the lesions and hence are useful postoperatively to exclude any residual collections or intra-abdominal abscesses.

Traditionally, splenectomy has been recommended for the treatment of splenic abscess; although randomized controlled trials are not possible, a recent case series suggests that splenectomy may still be associated with better outcomes.[206] Removal of the spleen may be difficult if it adheres to adjacent structures; removal or partial resection of these organs may be required.[200,202-204] Laparoscopic splenectomy for splenic abscess has been reported.[207] Successful percutaneous drainage of splenic abscess utilizing either ultrasound or CT guidance has increasingly been reported and should be considered, especially in cases with a solitary lesion.[208,209]

The complications of splenic abscess include spontaneous rupture, which can be so subtle in some cases that the patient has no signs of generalized peritonitis or purulence in the abdominal cavity.[200] Other manifestations include recurrent bacteremia and intestinal obstruction.[203] Although associated with significant morbidity and mortality, splenic abscess detected early and treated promptly has a good prognosis.

Central Nervous System Infections

IDUs may present with a variety of CNS manifestations that may or may not be infectious in origin. The differential diagnosis is extensive and frequently difficult. Complications related to the injection of illicit drugs include coma caused by overdose or intoxication, postanoxic encephalopathy, delirium, and acute confusion states. Seizures, cerebral edema, and dementia may result from noninfectious as well as infectious causes. Hemorrhage and infarction may be secondary to infection or compromise of the neurovascular system. Parkinsonism is most often the result of drug effects but has been reported in infection.[210] The etiology of these disorders may be obscure, necessitating a thorough workup to exclude an infectious cause. Infections of the CNS may be local or secondary to an infectious process elsewhere. When infection is the primary problem, focal findings and fever are usually

present. When present, focal findings suggest the possibility of a mass lesion requiring immediate surgical intervention. Therefore, an IDU with neurologic findings requires a differential diagnosis that includes both infectious and noninfectious causes and an effort to differentiate between a local process and a complication of a distant primary infection.

CNS manifestations are more common in IDUs than in nonusers and are found in 45% to 58% of addicts with endocarditis.[211] In one study of IDUs with left-sided IE, CNS complications were found in 52% of patients with mitral valve infection but in only 28% of those with aortic valve disease.[106] Other investigators found a greater incidence in aortic valve disease, especially when *S. aureus* was involved and the patients had congestive heart failure.[212] Endocarditis, particularly when caused by *S. aureus* or *S. pneumoniae*,[213] is the most common cause of CNS disease in IDUs, and it also accounts for the most serious complications, including brain abscess, meningitis, encephalopathy, and hemorrhage from ruptured mycotic aneurysms.[41,214] Mycotic aneurysms may manifest as a progressive focal neurologic deficit resulting from expansion of the aneurysm or as an acute subarachnoid or intracerebral hemorrhage.[215] Before rupture, patients may complain of severe localized headache. This should prompt immediate evaluation. CT adequately identifies mycotic aneurysms in most cases and may also be used to demonstrate brain abscess. MRA may be more effective, and, in one study, when combined with MRI, had a sensitivity of 86% and a specificity of 100% for aneurysms greater than 3 mm in diameter.[216] If a strong suspicion remains, a negative study should be followed by four-vessel cerebral angiography, which remains the definitive test. Even with a negative test result, if symptoms persist, repeated angiography might reveal lesions that were not detected previously.

The management of cerebral mycotic aneurysms remains undefined. In some cases, lesions resolve completely, or decrease in size, with antibiotic treatment alone. In other cases, the lesion may enlarge, or new aneurysms may appear. Surgery is important for control of ruptured aneurysms of peripheral arteries or when an intracranial location or masslike lesion occurs. Some researchers recommend serial angiograms to assess the progress of aneurysms; others call for aggressive surgical management, especially if the lesion is accessible. When the patient's condition precludes surgery, an endovascular procedure to embolize the lesion may be advised.[217] The presence of multiple aneurysms might make a surgical approach impossible. In some of these cases, patients do well with antimicrobial treatment, but each case must be treated individually.[218]

Focal abnormalities also result from septic emboli (which frequently result in transient focal neurologic deficits) and multiple cerebral abscesses. These lesions tend to resolve in 1 to 2 weeks with appropriate antibiotic therapy.[41] IDUs also commonly develop a diffuse encephalopathy that may be due to bacteremia or injected toxins.

Localized CNS infection in this population is confined primarily to brain abscess and subdural empyema. Pyogenic bacteria usually cause brain abscess; *Nocardia* has also been reported. Fungi, including *Aspergillus* spp., *Chaetomium strumarium*, and mucormycosis, have also been reported. Mucormycosis in IDUs is rarely associated with HIV infection and manifests as focal cerebritis or abscess, in contrast to the more extensive aggressive process observed in immunocompromised hosts. There may be a predilection for multifocal involvement and, in particular, involvement of the basal ganglia, with this region being affected far more often in addicts than in nonaddicts.[219] Cerebral mucormycosis is not caused by spread from sinuses. It appears the organism is either a contaminant in the illicit drugs or enters the bloodstream from an infected injection site, finding its way to areas of the brain predisposed by earlier drug-induced injury. The patient usually presents with signs and symptoms of a mass lesion. The differential diagnosis of such lesions includes toxoplasmosis, lymphoma, TB, and cryptococcosis. Isolated involvement of the basal ganglia is uncommon in toxoplasmosis and lymphoma. Radiologic contrast enhancement may or may not be seen in patients with mucormycosis and therefore lends little to the diagnosis. Biopsy of the lesion is required to establish the diagnosis; failure to do so is associated with a very high mortality rate.[219] Remarkably, the outcome of this disease is very good, with survival in most cases after prolonged amphotericin B therapy and excision of as much of the infected tissue as possible.[210,220,221]

The clinical signs and symptoms of brain abscesses in IDUs are the same as in nonaddicts and depend on the location of the lesion within the brain. They usually result from infected cerebral emboli in patients with mitral or aortic valve endocarditis.[41,92,106,214] Rarely, emboli travel through or originate in the pulmonary circulation. Alternatively, pathogens may seed the brain after an inadvertent injection into the arterial system during an attempted jugular vein injection. Tuberculous brain abscesses may also be seen, particularly in IDUs who are coinfected with HIV. The lesions are typically solitary, multiloculated, and contrast enhancing. They must be distinguished from those due to *Toxoplasma*, which usually causes multiple lesions that are not multiloculated, and lymphoma, which can be necrotic with multiple loculations but is more often located near an ependymal surface.[222] IDUs with HIV infection who have characteristic lesions may be treated empirically for toxoplasmosis, but failure to respond within 2 weeks should prompt a biopsy, which will lead to the correct diagnosis. Subdural empyema is also seen in IDUs and may be secondary to direct extension from a local infectious process or complicated bacteremia.

Meningitis in IDUs is most often secondary to endocarditis[214] and is usually due to *S. aureus* or *S. pneumoniae*.[211] However, abnormal CSF is common in patients with CNS complications of endocarditis. Findings in patients with meningitis include purulent CSF with a neutrophilic pleocytosis and elevated proteins, with normal or decreased glucose. A hemorrhagic CSF may also be found. A pattern consistent with aseptic meningitis is seen in 25% of cases; normal CSF is seen in only 30%.[211] Positive CSF cultures are seen in the minority of patients, most of whom have *S. aureus* infection and purulent CSF.

A spinal epidural abscess should be considered in any addict presenting with spinal ache or back pain, especially if focal neurologic signs are present. On occasion blunt trauma may predispose an area of the spine to infection following an episode of transient bacteremia.[223] Patients tend to have a prolonged symptomatic course, often as long as several months. Typically disease progresses from focal vertebral pain to root pain, neurologic deficits (motor or sensory), and, finally, paralysis. Fever is frequently absent. The thoracic or lumbar spine is most often involved, although cervical spine lesions are also seen. *S. aureus* is the most common cause, but other grampositive and gram-negative organisms have been reported, occasionally in combination with other organisms. *M. tuberculosis* also causes spinal epidural abscess, and it too may be found in combination with other organisms,[224] making careful definition of the microbial etiology imperative. The pathophysiology is usually direct spread to the epidural space from adjacent disk or vertebral body infection or hematogenous dissemination from a distant focus of infection. In most cases immediate drainage relieves symptoms; although once a chronic condition ensues there may be nothing but granulation tissue, requiring multiple-level laminectomy to relieve pressure on the spinal cord.

Intramedullary spinal cord abscess has been reported in an IDU with symptoms resembling those of an epidural abscess. Myelography demonstrated cord enlargement that was confirmed to be a result of intramedullary pus. The infection was caused by *Pseudomonas cepacia* but failed to respond to antibiotic therapy to which the organism was susceptible in vitro.[225]

Toxin-mediated diseases, specifically wound botulism and tetanus, are being seen with increasing frequency among IDUs and must be considered in addicts who have neurologic symptoms. Epidemics of both tetanus and wound botulism have occurred in California,[226,227] and cases are likely to be found elsewhere. The patient with tetanus is likely to be a long-time user who has poor venous access and multiple skin lesions caused by failed attempts at intravenous injections or by skin-popping (intentional injection into the subcutaneous tissues). These lesions become colonized by multiple pathogens, including *Clostridium* spp. In the proper anaerobic environment, toxin is generated and produces disease.[228] Among the patients from California who had tetanus, 89% were Hispanic Americans, which may be explained by a study finding that only 58% of Mexican-Americans had protective levels of antibody to tetanus toxoid, compared with 73% of non-Hispanic whites.[226] Wound botulism in IDUs was first described in New York City in 1982. Subsequently, sporadic cases were reported from different locations. Since 1990, a dramatic increase in the number of wound botulism cases has occurred in California.[228] With rare exceptions, patients were IDUs who injected black tar heroin, a black, gummy form of the drug synthesized in Mexico and distributed widely throughout the western United States. Skin-popping of black tar heroin was the major risk factor for acquisition of wound botulism. The greatest risk was seen among heavy users, but disease also occurred in occasional subcutaneous or intramuscular injection users. Most likely the drug was contaminated during the dilution process, when substances were added to the heroin to increase the amount of the product and thereby increase the seller's profits. Wound botulism results from colonization of wounds by *Clostridium botulinum* with subsequent toxin production. Initially patients experience blurred vision or diplopia, dysarthria and dysphagia, followed by descending muscle weakness and respiratory failure. The symptoms are similar to those of botulism in nonaddicts except that gastrointestinal symptoms are absent. Also, unlike nonaddicts, who usually have a dietary history to suggest the diagnosis, in IDUs the organism can usually be recovered from wound cultures. Frequently, fever results from the associated wound infection. Serum assays for botulism toxin are rarely positive; administration of antitoxin, which is helpful only if given within the first 24 hours, must be done on the basis of a high index of suspicion, rather than after culture identification.[227, 228]

Drug users were once the most common population in the United States to develop tetanus; now they account for only 40% of cases.[226] As noted previously, skin-popping plays a major role, providing the lesions with an environment conducive to toxin production. Skin-popping probably also accounts for the higher mortality rate in addicts than in nonaddicts. One proposed reason is that, because of the number and severity of skin lesions in addicts, there is greater opportunity for large amounts of toxin to be produced. In addition, an addict presenting with the typical symptoms of tetanus may be thought to be manifesting the effects of illicit drug toxicity, overdose, or drug withdrawal.[229] In view of the risk for tetanus associated with injection drug use, it is worthwhile to consider giving a tetanus booster to any addict who is being treated for any other condition unless the patient has been immunized recently.

▣ Ocular Manifestations

Endophthalmitis is a common and serious complication of injection drug use.[230] Both fungal endophthalmitis and bacterial endophthalmitis are hematogenous in origin and frequently manifest as complications of infective endocarditis. *Candida* is the most common fungal cause, and endophthalmitis may also occur as part of a disseminated syndrome involving eyes, bone, and skin in heroin users. Fungal endophthalmitis has been reported after injection of crack cocaine dissolved in lemon juice (a practice that may be increasing due to the lower cost and easy availability of crack cocaine) and after injection of diverted sublingual buprenorphine.[231,232] Symptoms of endophthalmitis include blurred vision, pain, and decreased visual acuity. White, cotton-like exudative lesions are found in the choroid and retina with vitreous haziness. Diagnosis requires a high index of suspicion, and because blood cultures are usually negative at the time of ocular symptoms, definitive diagnosis often involves vitreous sampling. The antifungal agent that has been used most extensively for the treatment of *Candida* chorioretinitis is amphotericin B. Successes have been reported with fluconazole and voriconazole.[233] Very limited experience is reported with the use of the echinocandins, despite the increasing use of these agents for the treatment of candidemia. If extension into the vitreous humor has occurred (i.e., endophthalmitis), then intravitreal amphotericin B with or without pars plana vitrectomy is frequently recommended (see Chapter 112).[230,234]

Aspergillus spp. are the second most common cause of fungal endophthalmitis in IDUs. As with *Candida*, the pathogenesis reflects mycotic contamination of drug paraphernalia or of the heroin injected, rather than host immunosuppression. Physical findings and treatment are similar to those of *Candida* infection.

Bacterial endophthalmitis is less common, and the presentation is often acute with rapid progression of symptoms. Inflammation usually is present in the anterior and posterior chambers. In addition to pain, redness, and lid swelling, flame-shaped hemorrhages and cotton-wool spots may be present. *S. aureus* is the organism most frequently isolated. A rapidly destructive form of endophthalmitis has been reported for *Bacillus cereus*, which has been cultured from heroin and drug paraphernalia.[235] Bacterial endophthalmitis is treated primarily with intravitreal antimicrobials with or without vitrectomy, although the role of systemic antibiotics continues to be debated (see Chapter 112). In both mycotic and bacterial endophthalmitis, early diagnosis and intervention increase the chance of a favorable outcome. Whereas bacterial endophthalmitis is rare, ocular peripheral emboli are frequent complications of infective endocarditis in the IDU. These include subconjunctival hemorrhages and retinal emboli (Roth's spots), which manifest as petechiae, retinal hemorrhage, and ischemia.

Acquired Immunodeficiency Syndrome

Early in the AIDS epidemic, injection drug use was identified as being associated with a high risk of contracting the disease. In the United States, the incidence of HIV infection among IDUs has steadily decreased; IDUs now account for 21% of infections in females and 16% of infections in males.[236] Sexual contact with IDUs still accounts for a significant number of cases among persons whose primary risk is heterosexual contact. In the United States, HIV infection associated with injection drug use disproportionally affects racial and ethnic minorities, particularly minority women and children.[237] Globally, of the estimated 13 million persons who inject illicit drugs, 10 million live in developing or transitional countries; injection drug use accounts for 10% of new infections globally, but 30% of new infections outside of sub-Saharan Africa are attributed to IDU.[238] A transition from an epidemic concentrated almost exclusively in IDUs to a generalized epidemic among heterosexuals has been described in several countries in Southeast Asia and eastern Europe. Needle exchange programs have been shown to be an effective means of reducing the incidence of new HIV infections. In addition to sterile injection equipment, these programs serve as a point of entry into substance abuse treatment and provide other health and preventive care services. Participation in needle exchange programs has been shown to reduce emergency department utilization among IDUs and promote entry into formal drug treatment programs.[239,240] In many states, needles and syringes are available for sale without prescription in retail pharmacies. It has been shown that in cities in which needle distribution or exchange is illegal, IDUs are more likely to obtain injection equipment from unsafe sources and engage in risky injection behaviors.[241] The existence of supervised injection facilities, where IDUs can inject their drugs under the supervision of health care professionals, has been shown to reduce public injecting, syringe sharing, and drug overdose and increase access to addiction treatment.[242,243] Despite the fact that no scientific evidence supports the contention that safe injection programs lead to an increase in injection drug use, these programs remain controversial. Substitution therapy for opioid addiction appears to reduce injection-related HIV risk behaviors but has less effect on risky sexual behaviors.[244,245]

In the era before the availability of highly active antiretroviral therapy (HAART), cohort studies failed to demonstrate any difference in the rate of progression to AIDS among IDUs, men who have sex with men, and heterosexuals.[246] The availability of HAART has increased the disease-free survival of HIV-infected IDUs but not to as great an extent as that for non-IDUs.[247] A number of different factors are likely contributing to the fact that, as a group, IDUs have not achieved the full benefits of HAART. Injection drug use is an independent predictor for delay in initiation of care after the diagnosis of HIV infection.[248] In care, IDUs are less likely to receive a prescription for HIV medications. Lack of response to HAART among IDUs can be related to poorer adherence to medication regimens. In patients with a sustained virologic response to HAART, injection drug use has been shown to be a predictor of a suboptimal immunologic (CD4 cell) response[249] and immunologic failure after initial response.[250] Despite these observations, in a recently published population-based cohort study of more than 3000 patients (of whom almost one third were IDUs), injection drug use was not associated with decreased survival among HIV-positive patients who initiated HAART.[251]

The medical management of HIV-infected IDUs must incorporate the diagnosis and treatment of substance abuse. Substitution therapy can facilitate social stability and support adherence to HAART. The drug interactions between HAART and methadone and buprenorphine have been recently reviewed and summarized.[252]

Other Sexually Transmitted Diseases

A major contributing factor to the prevalence of STIs is unsafe sexual practices associated with the use of illicit drugs.[253] Among almost 3000 active IDUs in Baltimore, 60% reported a history of an STI; 24.1% were HIV seropositive.[254] A more recent study of young IDUs in Baltimore found that the prevalence of chlamydia, gonorrhea, and trichomonas were similar to that in the general population despite the fact that 68% of subjects had two or more sex partners in the past 3 months and less than half consistently used condoms.[255] This same study reported a high prevalence of bacterial vaginosis among young female IDUs. The prevalence of human papillomavirus infection was found to be high among young IDUs in Baltimore and was significantly higher in women than in men.[256] Alcohol use and alcohol intoxication are associated with an increase in risky sexual behavior among IDUs.[257] Interestingly, the use of alcohol among drug users appears to be more strongly associated with risky sexual behavior than with risky injection practices.[258] In a large cohort of female IDUs in Vancouver, condoms were rarely used with regular partners but were more likely to be used with casual partners and paying partners.[259] More than half of the women in the cohort reported more than 100 lifetime sexual partners. In a study of young male IDUs, less than 20% used condoms consistently with heterosexual partners, and condom use was identical among males with multiple partners and those in monogamous relationships.[260] Female sex workers who are IDUs have a higher prevalence of STIs and are more likely to engage in risky sexual behaviors and have unsafe sex with clients than sex workers who do not inject drugs.[261] Male IDUs who have sex with men, especially those who engage in commercial sex work, are much more likely to report risky sexual behavior.[262,263] It has been observed that reducing risky sexual behavior among IDUs is much more difficult than reducing risky injection behavior.

Risk factors for syphilis among IDUs include recent initiation of injection drug use, injecting with other people, and injecting in public places.[264] The diagnosis and treatment of syphilis in IDUs may be complicated by the high rate of biologic false-positive, nonspecific serologic screening test results. In contrast to the poor reliability of self-reported hepatitis serostatus, self reports of syphilis infection history by IDUs were found to have good reliability.[265]

Given the importance of STIs as cofactors in the sexual transmission of HIV, reducing the prevalence of STIs in IDUs is an additional strategy to diminish the spread of HIV among IDUs and from them to their non–drug-using sexual contacts.

REFERENCES

1. Services, D.O.H.A.H., S.A.a.M.H.S. Administration, and O.o.A. Studies, Results from the 2007 National Survey on Drug Use and Health: National Findings in ⟨http://oas.samhsa.gov/nsduh/2k7nsduh/2k7Results.pdf⟩. 2007, Department of Health and Human Services Substance Abuse and Mental Health Services Administration Office of Applied Studies.
2. Charlebois ED, et al. Population-based community prevalence of methicillin-resistant *Staphylococcus aureus* in the urban poor of San Francisco. *Clin Infect Dis.* 2002;34:425-433.
3. Gordon RJ, Lowy FD. Bacterial infections in drug users. *N Engl J Med.* 2005;353:1945-1954.
4. Efstratiou A, et al. Increasing incidence of group A streptococcal infections amongst injecting drug users in England and Wales. *J Med Microbiol.* 2003;52:525-526.
5. Stein MD, Anderson B. Injection frequency mediates health service use among persons with a history of drug injection. *Drug Alcohol Depend.* 2003;7:159-168.
6. Bassetti S, Battegay M. *Staphylococcus aureus* infections in injection drug users: risk factors and prevention strategies. *Infection.* 2004;32:163-169.
7. Hankins C, Palmer D, Singh R. Unintended subcutaneous and intramuscular injection by drug users. *CMAJ.* 2000;163:1425-1426.
8. Alonzo NC, Bayer BM. Opioids, immunology, and host defenses of intravenous drug abusers. *Infect Dis Clin North Am.* 2002;16:553-569.
9. Friedman H, Newton C, Klein TW. Microbial infections, immunomodulation, and drugs of abuse. *Clin Microbiol Rev.* 2003;16:209-219.
10. Vallejo R, de Leon-Casasola O, Benyamin R. Opioid therapy and immunosuppression: a review. *Am J Ther.* 2004;11:354-365.
11. Lanier RK, et al. Self-administration of heroin produces alterations in the expression of inducible nitric oxide synthase. *Drug Alcohol Depend.* 2002;66:225-233.
12. Lysle DT, How T. Heroin modulates the expression of inducible nitric oxide synthase. *Immunopharmacology.* 2000;46:181-192.
13. Brown SM, et al. Immunologic dysfunction in heroin addicts. *Arch Intern Med.* 1974;134:1001-1006.
14. Novick DM, et al. Natural killer cell activity and lymphocyte subsets in parenteral heroin abusers and long-term methadone maintenance patients. *J Pharmacol Exp Ther.* 1989; 250:606-610.
15. Sacerdote P, et al. Buprenorphine and methadone maintenance treatment of heroin addicts preserves immune function. *Brain Behav Immun.* 2008;22:606-613.
16. Stoll-Keller F, et al. Effects of morphine on purified human blood monocytes. Modifications of properties involved in antiviral defences. *Int J Immunopharmacol.* 1997;19:95-100.
17. Guo CJ, et al. Morphine enhances HIV infection of human blood mononuclear phagocytes through modulation of beta-chemokines and CCR5 receptor. *J Investig Med.* 2002;50: 435-442.
18. Young DM, et al. An epidemic of methicillin-resistant *Staphylococcus aureus* soft tissue infections among medically underserved patients. *Arch Surg.* 2004;139:947-951; discussion 951-953.
19. Irish C, et al. Skin and soft tissue infections and vascular disease among drug users, England. *Emerg Infect Dis.* 2007;13:1510-1511.
20. Maliphant J, Scott J. Use of the femoral vein ("groin injecting") by a sample of needle exchange clients in Bristol, UK. *Harm Reduct J.* 2005;2:6.
21. Zamora-Quezada JC, et al. Muscle and skin infarction after free-basing cocaine (crack). *Ann Intern Med.* 1988;108: 564-566.
22. Cregler LL, Mark H. Medical complications of cocaine abuse. *N Engl J Med.* 1986;315:1495-1500.
23. Risdahl JM, et al. Opiates and infection. *J Neuroimmunol.* 1998;83:4-18.
24. Spijkerman IJ, et al. Human immunodeficiency virus infection and other risk factors for skin abscesses and endocarditis among injection drug users. *J Clin Epidemiol.* 1996;49: 1149-1154.
25. Takahashi TA, et al. Type and location of injection drug use-related soft tissue infections predict hospitalization. *J Urban Health.* 2003;80:127-136.
26. Murphy EL, et al. Risk factors for skin and soft-tissue abscesses among injection drug users: a case-control study. *Clin Infect Dis.* 2001;33:35-40.
27. Lloyd-Smith E, et al. Prevalence and correlates of abscesses among a cohort of injection drug users. *Harm Reduct J.* 2005;2:24.
28. Tom MB, Rice DH. Presentation and management of neck abscess: a retrospective analysis. *Laryngoscope.* 1988;98:877-880.
29. Hillstrom RP, Cohn AM, McCarroll KA. Vocal cord paralysis resulting from neck injections in the intravenous drug use population. *Laryngoscope.* 1990;100:503-506.
30. Frazee BW, et al. High prevalence of methicillin-resistant *Staphylococcus aureus* in emergency department skin and soft tissue infections. *Ann Emerg Med.* 2005;45:311-320.
31. Cohen AL, et al. Methamphetamine use and methicillin-resistant *Staphylococcus aureus* skin infections. *Emerg Infect Dis.* 2007;13:1707-1713.
32. Stryjewski ME, Chambers HF. Skin and soft-tissue infections caused by community-acquired methicillin-resistant *Staphylococcus aureus. Clin Infect Dis.* 2008;46(Suppl):S368-S377.
33. Hoeger PH, Haupt G, Hoelzle E. Acute multifocal skin necrosis: synergism between invasive streptococcal infection and cocaine-induced tissue ischaemia? *Acta Derm Venereol.* 1996;76:239-241.
34. Hemingway DM, et al. *Streptococcus milleri* and complex groin abscesses in intravenous drug abusers. *Scott Med J.* 1992;37: 116-117.
35. Talan DA, Summanen PH, Finegold SM. Ampicillin/sulbactam and cefoxitin in the treatment of cutaneous and other soft-tissue abscesses in patients with or without histories of injection drug abuse. *Clin Infect Dis.* 2000;31:464-471.
36. Squire BT, Fox JC, Anderson C. ABSCESS: applied bedside sonography for convenient evaluation of superficial soft tissue infections. *Acad Emerg Med.* 2005;12:601-606.
37. Eron LJ, et al. Managing skin and soft tissue infections: expert panel recommendations on key decision points. *J Antimicrob Chemother.* 2003;52(Suppl 1):i3-i17.
38. Madaras-Kelly KJ, et al. Efficacy of oral beta-lactam versus non-beta-lactam treatment of uncomplicated cellulitis. *Am J Med.* 2008;121:419-425.
39. Whittiker DM. A fatal case of toxic shock associated with group A streptococcal cellulitis. *J Am Board Fam Pract.* 1992;5: 523-526.
40. Organ CH Jr. Surgical procedures upon the drug addict. *Surg Gynecol Obstet.* 1972;134:947-952.
41. Levine DP, Crane LR, Zervos MJ. Bacteremia in narcotic addicts at the Detroit Medical Center. II. Infectious endocarditis: a prospective comparative study. *Rev Infect Dis.* 1986;8:374-396.
42. Bergstein JM, et al. Soft tissue abscesses associated with parenteral drug abuse: presentation, microbiology, and treatment. *Am Surg.* 1995;61:1105-1108.
43. Henriksen BM, et al. Soft tissue infections from drug abuse. A clinical and microbiological review of 145 cases. *Acta Orthop Scand.* 1994;65:625-628.
44. Alcantara AL, Tucker RB, McCarroll KA. Radiologic study of injection drug use complications. *Infect Dis Clin North Am.* 2002;16:713-743, ix-x.
45. Towers JD. The use of intravenous contrast in MRI of extremity infection. *Semin Ultrasound CT MR.* 1997;18:269-275.
46. Schnall SB, Holtom PD, Lilley JC. Abscesses secondary to parenteral abuse of drugs. A study of demographic and bacteriological characteristics. *J Bone Joint Surg Am.* 1994;76:1526-1530.
47. Wallace JR, Lucas CE, Ledgerwood AM. Social, economic, and surgical anatomy of a drug-related abscess. *Am Surg.* 1986;52:398-401.
48. Simmen HP, et al. Soft tissue infections of the upper extremities with special consideration of abscesses in parenteral drug abusers. A prospective study. *J Hand Surg Br.* 1995;20: 797-800.
49. Pieper B. A retrospective analysis of venous ulcer healing in current and former users of injected drugs. *J Wound Ostomy Continence Nurs.* 1996;23:291-296.
50. Pieper B, Rossi R, Templin T. Pain associated with venous ulcers in injecting drug users. *Ostomy Wound Manage.* 1998;44:54-58, 60-67.
51. Dow G, Browne A, Sibbald RG. Infection in chronic wounds: controversies in diagnosis and treatment. *Ostomy Wound Manage.* 1999;45:23-27, 29-40; quiz 41-42.
52. Gonzalez MH, et al. Necrotizing fasciitis of the upper extremity. *J Hand Surg Am.* 1996;21:689-692.
53. Callahan TE, Schecter WP, Horn JK. Necrotizing soft tissue infection masquerading as cutaneous abcess following illicit drug injection. *Arch Surg.* 1998;133:812-817; discussion 817-819.
54. Wysoki MG, et al. Necrotizing fasciitis: CT characteristics. *Radiology.* 1997;203:859-863.
55. Falasca GF, Reginato AJ. The spectrum of myositis and rhabdomyolysis associated with bacterial infection. *J Rheumatol.* 1994;21:1932-1937.
56. Chen JL, Fullerton KE, Flynn NM. Necrotizing fasciitis associated with injection drug use. *Clin Infect Dis.* 2001;33:6-15.
57. Sudarsky LA, et al. Improved results from a standardized approach in treating patients with necrotizing fasciitis. *Ann Surg.* 1987;206:661-665.
58. Soft tissue infections among injection drug users—San Francisco, California, 1996-2000. *MMWR Morb Mortal Wkly Rep.* 2001;50:381-384.
59. Lo TS, Mooers MG, Wright LJ. Pyomyositis complicating acute bacterial endocarditis in an intravenous drug user. *N Engl J Med.* 2000;342:1614-1615.
60. Prahlow JA, Cappellari JO, Washburn SA. Uterine pyomyoma as a complication of pregnancy in an intravenous drug user. *South Med J.* 1996;89:892-895.
61. Grau LE, et al. Expanding harm reduction services through a wound and abscess clinic. *Am J Public Health.* 2002;92:1915-1917.
62. Chandrasekar PH, Narula AP. Bone and joint infections in intravenous drug abusers. *Rev Infect Dis.* 1986;8:904-911.
63. Lamas C, Boia M, Eykyn SJ. Osteoarticular infections complicating infective endocarditis: a study of 30 cases between 1969 and 2002 in a tertiary referral centre. *Scand J Infect Dis.* 2006;38: 433-440.
64. Munoz-Fernandez S, et al. Osteoarticular infection in intravenous drug abusers: influence of HIV infection and differences with non drug abusers. *Ann Rheum Dis.* 1993;52:570-574.
65. Zalavras CG, et al. Microbiology of osteomyelitis in patients infected with the human immunodeficiency virus. *Clin Orthop Relat Res.* 2005;439:97-100.
66. Swisher LA, Roberts JR, Glynn MJ. Needle licker's osteomyelitis. *Am J Emerg Med.* 1994;12:343-346.
67. Miller DJ, Mejicano GC. Vertebral osteomyelitis due to *Candida* species: case report and literature review. *Clin Infect Dis.* 2001;33:523-530.
68. Sapico FL, Montgomerie JZ. Vertebral osteomyelitis in intravenous drug abusers: report of three cases and review of the literature. *Rev Infect Dis.* 1980;2:196-206.
69. Kak V, Chandrasekar PH. Bone and joint infections in injection drug users. *Infect Dis Clin North Am.* 2002;16:681-695.
70. Pastan RS, Silverman SL, Goldenberg DL. A musculoskeletal syndrome in intravenous heroin users: association with brown heroin. *Ann Intern Med.* 1977;87:22-29.
71. Watanakunakorn C, Burkert T. Infective endocarditis at a large community teaching hospital, 1980-1990. A review of 210 episodes. *Medicine (Baltimore).* 1993;72:90-102.
72. Weisse AB, et al. The febrile parenteral drug user: a prospective study in 121 patients. *Am J Med.* 1993;94: 274-280.
73. Baddour LM, Twelve-year review of recurrent native-valve infective endocarditis: a disease of the modern antibiotic era. *Rev Infect Dis.* 1988;10:1163-1170.
74. Manoff SB, et al. Human immunodeficiency virus infection and infective endocarditis among injecting drug users. *Epidemiology.* 1996;7:566-570.
75. Mathew J, et al. Clinical features, site of involvement, bacteriologic findings, and outcome of infective endocarditis in intravenous drug users. *Arch Intern Med.* 1995;155:1641-1648.
76. Reyes MP, Palutke WA, Wylin RF, et al. *Pseudomonas* endocarditis in the Detroit Medical Center, 1969-1972. *Medicine (Baltimore).* 1973;52:173-194.
77. Shekar R, et al. Outbreak of endocarditis caused by *Pseudomonas aeruginosa* serotype O11 among pentazocine and tripelennamine abusers in Chicago. *J Infect Dis.* 1985;151:203-208.
78. Mills J, Drew D. *Serratia marcescens* endocarditis: a regional illness associated with intravenous drug abuse. *Ann Intern Med.* 1976;84:29-35.
79. Cooper R, Mills J. *Serratia* endocarditis. A follow-up report. *Arch Intern Med.* 1980;140:199-202.
80. Pierrotti LC, Baddour LM. Fungal endocarditis, 1995-2000. *Chest.* 2002;122:302-310.
81. Petrosillo N, et al. Endocarditis caused by *Aspergillus* species in injection drug users. *Clin Infect Dis.* 2001;33:E97-E99.
82. Adler AG, et al. Seven-pathogen tricuspid endocarditis in an intravenous drug abuser. Pitfalls in laboratory diagnosis. *Chest.* 1991;99:490-491.
83. Szabo S, Lieberman JP, Lue YA. Unusual pathogens in narcotic-associated endocarditis. *Rev Infect Dis.* 1990;12:412-415.
84. Tuazon CU, Sheagren JN. Staphlococcal endocarditis in parenteral drug abusers: source of the organism. *Ann Intern Med.* 1975;82:788-790.
85. Dressler FA, Roberts WC. Infective endocarditis in opiate addicts: analysis of 80 cases studied at necropsy. *Am J Cardiol.* 1989;63:1240-1257.
86. Graves MK, Soto L. Left-sided endocarditis in parenteral drug abusers: recent experience at a large community hospital. *South Med J.* 1992;85:378-380.
87. Frontera JA, Gradon JD. Right-side endocarditis in injection drug users: review of proposed mechanisms of pathogenesis. *Clin Infect Dis.* 2000;30:374-379.
88. El-Khatib MR, Wilson FM, Lerner AM. Characteristics of bacterial endocarditis in heroin addicts in Detroit. *Am J Med Sci.* 1976;271:197-201.
89. Crane LR, et al. Bacteremia in narcotic addicts at the Detroit Medical Center. I. Microbiology, epidemiology, risk factors, and empiric therapy. *Rev Infect Dis.* 1986;8:364-373.
90. Wilson LE, et al. Prospective study of infective endocarditis among injection drug users. *J Infect Dis.* 2002;185: 1761-1766.
91. Stimmel B, Donoso E, Dack S. Comparison of infective endocarditis in drug addicts and nondrug users. *Am J Cardiol.* 1973;32:924-929.
92. Chambers HF, Korzeniowski OM, Sande MA. *Staphylococcus aureus* endocarditis: clinical manifestations in addicts and nonaddicts. *Medicine (Baltimore).* 1983;62:170-177.
93. Corzo JE, et al. Pneumothorax secondary to septic pulmonary emboli in tricuspid endocarditis. *Thorax.* 1992;47:1080-1081.
94. Dressler FA, Roberts WC. Modes of death and types of cardiac diseases in opiate addicts: analysis of 168 necropsy cases. *Am J Cardiol.* 1989;64:909-920.
95. Roberts JH, et al. Myocardial abscess resulting in a pseudoaneurysm: case report. *Cardiovasc Intervent Radiol.* 1991;14: 307-310.

96. Sapico FL, Liquete JA, Sarma RJ. Bone and joint infections in patients with infective endocarditis: review of a 4-year experience. *Clin Infect Dis.* 1996;22:783-787.
97. Li JS, et al. Proposed modifications to the Duke criteria for the diagnosis of infective endocarditis. *Clin Infect Dis.* 2000;30: 633-638.
98. Palepu A, et al. Factors other than the Duke criteria associated with infective endocarditis among injection drug users. *Clin Invest Med.* 2002;25:118-125.
99. Young GP, et al. Inability to validate a predictive score for infective endocarditis in intravenous drug users. *J Emerg Med.* 1993;11:1-7.
100. Rothman RE, Walker T, Weiss JL, et al. *Diagnostic importance of transthoracic echocardiography (TTE) in febrile intravenous drug users (IDUs) at risk for infective endocarditis (IE): Is there a role for ultrasound in the emergency department (ED)?* Poster #66. In 7th International Symposium on Modern Concepts in Endocarditis and Cardiovascular Infections. 2003. Chamonix Mont Blanc, France.
101. Rothman RE Walker T, Majumdar M, et al. *Criteria for the diagnosis of infective endocarditis (IE) in febrile intravenous drug users: A new gold standard for the acute care setting,* Abstract #38. In 7th International Symposium on Modern Concepts in Endocarditis and Cardiovascular Infections. 2003. Chamonix Mont Blanc, France.
102. Rothman RE, et al. Detection of bacteremia in emergency department patients at risk for infective endocarditis using universal 16S rRNA primers in a decontaminated polymerase chain reaction assay. *J Infect Dis.* 2002;186:1677-1681.
103. Pazin GJ, Saul S, Thompson ME. Blood culture positivity: suppression by outpatient antibiotic therapy in patients with bacterial endocarditis. *Arch Intern Med.* 1982;142:263-268.
104. Levine DP, Fromm BS, Reddy BR. Slow response to vancomycin or vancomycin plus rifampin in methicillin-resistant *Staphylococcus aureus* endocarditis. *Ann Intern Med.* 1991;115: 674-680.
105. Korzeniowski O, Sande MA. Combination antimicrobial therapy for *Staphylococcus aureus* endocarditis in patients addicted to parenteral drugs and in nonaddicts: A prospective study. *Ann Intern Med.* 1982;97:496-503.
106. Pruitt AA, et al. Neurologic complications of bacterial endocarditis. *Medicine (Baltimore).* 1978;57:329-343.
107. Brown PD, Levine DP. Infective endocarditis in the injection drug user. *Infect Dis Clin North Am.* 2002;16:645-665, viii-ix.
108. Markowitz N, Quinn EL, Saravolatz LD. Trimethoprim-sulfamethoxazole compared with vancomycin for the treatment of *Staphylococcus aureus* infection. *Ann Intern Med.* 1992;117: 390-398.
109. Chambers HF, Miller RT, Newman MD. Right-sided *Staphylococcus aureus* endocarditis in intravenous drug abusers: two-week combination therapy. *Ann Intern Med.* 1988;109:619-624.
110. Ribera E, et al. Effectiveness of cloxacillin with and without gentamicin in short-term therapy for right-sided *Staphylococcus aureus* endocarditis. A randomized, controlled trial. *Ann Intern Med.* 1996;125:969-974.
111. Heldman AW, et al. Oral antibiotic treatment of right-sided staphylococcal endocarditis in injection drug users: prospective randomized comparison with parenteral therapy. *Am J Med.* 1996;101:68-76.
112. Reyes MP, Brown WJ, Lerner AM. Treatment of patients with *Pseudomonas* endocarditis with high dose aminoglycoside and carbenicillin therapy. *Medicine (Baltimore).* 1978;57:57-67.
113. Reyes MP, et al. Synergy between carbenicillin and an aminoglycoside (gentamicin or tobramycin) against *Pseudomonas aeruginosa* isolated from patients with endocarditis and sensitivity of isolates to normal human serum. *J Infect Dis.* 1979;140: 192-202.
114. Wieland M, et al. Left-sided endocarditis due to *Pseudomonas aeruginosa*. A report of 10 cases and review of the literature. *Medicine (Baltimore).* 1986;65:180-189.
115. Daikos GL, et al. Long-term oral ciprofloxacin: experience in the treatment of incurable infective endocarditis. *Am J Med.* 1988;84:786-790.
116. Libertin CR, McKinley KM. Gentamicin-resistant enterococcal endocarditis: the need for routine screening for high-level resistance to aminoglycosides. *South Med J.* 1990;83:458-460.
117. Hecht SR, Berger M. Right-sided endocarditis in intravenous drug users. Prognostic features in 102 episodes. *Ann Intern Med.* 1992;117:560-566.
118. Mathew J, et al. Results of surgical treatment for infective endocarditis in intravenous drug users. *Chest.* 1995;108: 73-77.
119. Lemma M, et al. Cardiac surgery in HIV-positive intravenous drug addicts: influence of cardiopulmonary bypass on the progression to AIDS. *Thorac Cardiovasc Surg.* 1992;40: 279-282.
120. Frater RW. Surgical management of endocarditis in drug addicts and long-term results. *J Card Surg.* 1990;5:63-67.
121. Monsuez JJ, et al. Recurrent infective endocarditis one year after mitral repair in a woman addicted to drugs. *J Thorac Cardiovasc Surg.* 1997;114:864-866.
122. Benitez PR, Newell MA. Vascular trauma in drug abuse: patterns of injury. *Ann Vasc Surg.* 1986;1:175-181.
123. Yeager RA, et al. Vascular complications related to drug abuse. *J Trauma.* 1987;27:305-308.
124. Reddy DJ, et al. Infected femoral artery false aneurysms in drug addicts: evolution of selective vascular reconstruction. *J Vasc Surg.* 1986;3:718-724.
125. McIlroy MA, et al. Infected false aneurysms of the femoral artery in intravenous drug addicts. *Rev Infect Dis.* 1989;11: 578-585.
126. Tsao JW, et al. Presentation, diagnosis, and management of arterial mycotic pseudoaneurysms in injection drug users. *Ann Vasc Surg.* 2002;16:652-662.
127. Shetty PC, et al. Mycotic aneurysms in intravenous drug abusers: the utility of intravenous digital subtraction angiography. *Radiology.* 1985;155:319-321.
128. Wolff AJ, O'Donnell AE. Pulmonary effects of illicit drug use. *Clin Chest Med.* 2004;25:203-216.
129. Sporer KA, Dorn E. Heroin-related noncardiogenic pulmonary edema: a case series. *Chest.* 2001;120:1628-1632.
130. Pare JA, et al. Pulmonary "mainline" granulomatosis: talcosis of intravenous methadone abuse. *Medicine (Baltimore).* 1979;58:229-239.
131. Hind CR. Pulmonary complications of intravenous drug misuse. 2. Infective and HIV related complications. *Thorax.* 1990;45:957-961.
132. Le Moing V, et al. Incidence and risk factors of bacterial pneumonia requiring hospitalization in HIV-infected patients started on a protease inhibitor-containing regimen. *HIV Med.* 2006;7:261-267.
133. O'Donnell AE, Pappas LS. Pulmonary complications of intravenous drug abuse. Experience at an inner-city hospital. *Chest.* 1988;94:251-253.
134. Marantz PR, et al. Inability to predict diagnosis in febrile intravenous drug abusers. *Ann Intern Med.* 1987;106: 823-828.
135. Samet JH, et al. Hospitalization decision in febrile intravenous drug users. *Am J Med.* 1990;89:53-57.
136. Park DR, et al. The etiology of community-acquired pneumonia at an urban public hospital: influence of human immunodeficiency virus infection and initial severity of illness. *J Infect Dis.* 2001;184:268-277.
137. Jover F, et al. A comparative study of bacteremic and non-bacteremic pneumococcal pneumonia. *Eur J Intern Med.* 2008;19:15-21.
138. Casadevall A, et al. *Haemophilus influenzae* type b bacteremia in adults with AIDS and at risk for AIDS. *Am J Med.* 1992;92:587-590.
139. Polsky B, et al. Bacterial pneumonia in patients with the acquired immunodeficiency syndrome. *Ann Intern Med.* 1986;104:38-41.
140. Schlamm HT, Yancovitz SR. *Haemophilus influenzae* pneumonia in young adults with AIDS, ARC, or risk of AIDS. *Am J Med.* 1989;86:11-14.
141. Witt DJ, Craven DE, McCabe WR. Bacterial infections in adult patients with the acquired immune deficiency syndrome (AIDS) and AIDS-related complex. *Am J Med.* 1987;82:900-906.
142. Madeddu G, et al. Bacterial community acquired pneumonia in HIV-infected inpatients in the highly active antiretroviral therapy era. *Infection.* 2008;36:231-236.
143. Girardi E, et al. Incidence of tuberculosis among HIV-infected patients receiving highly active antiretroviral therapy in Europe and North America. *Clin Infect Dis.* 2005;41:1772-1782.
144. Scholten JN, et al. Effectiveness of isoniazid treatment for latent tuberculosis infection among human immunodeficiency virus (HIV)-infected and HIV-uninfected injection drug users in methadone programs. *Clin Infect Dis.* 2003;37:1686-1692.
145. Masur H, Kaplan JE, Holmes KK. Guidelines for preventing opportunistic infections among HIV-infected persons—2002. Recommendations of the U.S. Public Health Service and the Infectious Diseases Society of America. *Ann Intern Med.* 2002;137:435-478.
146. Swaminathan S, et al. Two-step tuberculin skin testing in drug users. *J Addict Dis.* 2007;26:71-79.
147. Dewan PK, et al. Feasibility, acceptability, and cost of tuberculosis testing by whole-blood interferon-gamma assay. *BMC Infect Dis.* 2006;6:47.
148. Shah SS, et al. Agreement between Mantoux skin testing and QuantiFERON-TB assay using dual mycobacterial antigens in current and former injection drug users. *Med Sci Monit.* 2006;12:MT11-MT16.
149. Sadaphal P, et al. Isoniazid preventive therapy, hepatitis C virus infection, and hepatotoxicity among injection drug users infected with *Mycobacterium tuberculosis*. *Clin Infect Dis.* 2001;33:1687-1691.
150. Malotte CK, Hollingshead JR, Rhodes F. Monetary versus nonmonetary incentives for TB skin test reading among drug users. *Am J Prev Med.* 1999;16:182-188.
151. Lorvick J, et al. Incentives and accessibility: a pilot study to promote adherence to TB prophylaxis in a high-risk community. *J Urban Health.* 1999;76:461-467.
152. Campbell JV, et al. High prevalence of alcohol use among hepatitis C virus antibody positive injection drug users in three US cities. *Drug Alcohol Depend.* 2006;81:259-265.
153. Berson A, et al. Hepatitis after intravenous buprenorphine misuse in heroin addicts. *J Hepatol.* 2001;34:346-350.
154. Herve S, et al. Acute hepatitis due to buprenorphine administration. *Eur J Gastroenterol Hepatol.* 2004;16:1033-1037.
155. Hagan H, et al. Syringe exchange and risk of infection with hepatitis B and C viruses. *Am J Epidemiol.* 1999;149: 203-213.
156. Mansson AS, et al. Continued transmission of hepatitis B and C viruses, but no transmission of human immunodeficiency virus among intravenous drug users participating in a syringe/needle exchange program. *Scand J Infect Dis.* 2000;32:253-258.
157. Dubois-Arber F, Balthasasr H, Huissoud T, et al. Trends in drug consumption and risk of transmission of HIV and hepatitis C virus among injecting drug users in Switzerland, 1993-2006. *Euro Surveill.* 2008;13:pii:18881.
158. Schlicting EG, et al. Validity of injecting drug users' self report of hepatitis A, B, C *Clin Lab Sci.* 2003;16:99-106.
159. Kuo I, et al. Poor validity of self-reported hepatitis B virus infection and vaccination status among young drug users. *Clin Infect Dis.* 2004;38:587-590.
160. Wasley A, Grytdal S, Gallagher K. Surveillance for acute viral hepatitis—United States, 2006. *MMWR Surveill Summ.* 2008; 57:1-24.
161. Lum PJ, et al. Hepatitis B virus infection and immunization status in a new generation of injection drug users in San Francisco. *J Viral Hepat.* 2008;15:229-236.
162. Lemberg BD, Shaw-Stiffel TA. Hepatic disease in injection drug users. *Infect Dis Clin North Am.* 2002;16:667-679.
163. Murrill CS, et al. Age-specific seroprevalence of HIV, hepatitis B virus, and hepatitis C virus infection among injection drug users admitted to drug treatment in 6 US cities. *Am J Public Health.* 2002;92:385-387.
164. Davis GL, Hoofnagle JH. Reactivation of chronic type B hepatitis presenting as acute viral hepatitis. *Ann Intern Med.* 1985;102:762-765.
165. Davis GL, Hoofnagle JH, Waggoner JG. Spontaneous reactivation of chronic hepatitis B virus infection. *Gastroenterology.* 1984;86:230-235.
166. Thio CL. Hepatitis B in the human immunodeficiency virus-infected patient: epidemiology, natural history, and treatment. *Semin Liver Dis.* 2003;23:125-136.
167. Torbenson M, et al. High prevalence of occult hepatitis B in Baltimore injection drug users. *Hepatology.* 2004;39:51-57.
168. Carey J, et al. Knowledge of hepatitis among active drug injectors at a syringe exchange program. *J Subst Abuse Treat.* 2005;29:47-53.
169. Baral S, et al. Vaccine immunogenicity in injecting drug users: a systematic review. *Lancet Infect Dis.* 2007;7: 667-674.
170. Hu Y, et al. Economic evaluation of delivering hepatitis B vaccine to injection drug users. *Am J Prev Med.* 2008;35: 25-32.
171. Quaglio G, et al. Isolated presence of antibody to hepatitis B core antigen in injection drug users: do they need to be vaccinated? *Clin Infect Dis.* 2001;32:E143-E144.
172. Hoofnagle JH, et al. Management of hepatitis B: summary of a clinical research workshop. *Hepatology.* 2007;45: 1056-1075.
173. Strader DB, et al. Diagnosis, management, and treatment of hepatitis C. *Hepatology.* 2004;39:1147-1171.
174. De Cock KM, et al. Delta hepatitis in the Los Angeles area: a report of 126 cases. *Ann Intern Med.* 1986;105:108-114.
175. Lettau LA, et al. Outbreak of severe hepatitis due to delta and hepatitis B viruses in parenteral drug abusers and their contacts. *N Engl J Med.* 1987;317:1256-1262.
176. Ponzetto A, et al. Hepatitis B markers in United States drug addicts with special emphasis on the delta hepatitis virus. *Hepatology.* 1984;4:1111-1115.
177. Smith HM, et al. Hepatitis B and delta virus infection among "at risk" populations in south east London. *J Epidemiol Community Health.* 1992;46:144-147.
178. Bialek SR, et al. Risk factors for hepatitis B in an outbreak of hepatitis B and D among injection drug users. *J Urban Health.* 2005;82:468-478.
179. Shattock AG, et al. Epidemic hepatitis B with delta-antigenaemia among Dublin drug-abusers. *Ir J Med Sci.* 1982;151: 334-338.
180. Bonino F, Smedile A. Delta agent (type D) hepatitis. *Semin Liver Dis.* 1986;6:28-33.
181. Amon JJ, et al. Prevalence of hepatitis C virus infection among injection drug users in the United States, 1994-2004. *Clin Infect Dis.* 2008;46:1852-1858.
182. Resti M, et al. Maternal drug use is a preeminent risk factor for mother-to-child hepatitis C virus transmission: results from a multicenter study of 1372 mother-infant pairs. *J Infect Dis.* 2002;185:567-572.
183. Miller CL, et al. Opportunities for prevention: hepatitis C prevalence and incidence in a cohort of young injection drug users. *Hepatology.* 2002;36:737-742.
184. Hahn JA, et al. Hepatitis C virus seroconversion among young injection drug users: relationships and risks. *J Infect Dis.* 2002;186:1558-1564.
185. Hagan H, Thiede H, Des Jarlais DC. Hepatitis C virus infection among injection drug users: survival analysis of time to seroconversion. *Epidemiology.* 2004;15:543-549.
186. Thorpe L, et al. The multiperson use of non-syringe injection equipment and risk of hepatitis c infection in a cohort of young adult injection drug users, Chicago 1997-1999. *Ann Epidemiol.* 2000;10:472-473.

187. Phillips KT, Anderson BJ, Stein MD. Predictors of bacterial infections among HCV-negative injection drug users in Rhode Island. *Am J Drug Alcohol Abuse.* 2008;34:203-210.

188. Grebely J, et al. Hepatitis C virus reinfection in injection drug users. *Hepatology.* 2006;44:1139-1145.

189. Mehta SH, et al. Protection against persistence of hepatitis C. *Lancet.* 2002;359:1478-1483.

190. Mizukoshi E, et al. Hepatitis C virus (HCV)-specific immune responses of long-term injection drug users frequently exposed to HCV. *J Infect Dis.* 2008;198:203-212.

191. Grebely J, et al. Current approaches to HCV infection in current and former injection drug users. *J Addict Dis.* 2008; 27:25-35.

192. Grebely J, et al. Treatment uptake and outcomes among current and former injection drug users receiving directly observed therapy within a multidisciplinary group model for the treatment of hepatitis C virus infection. *Int J Drug Policy.* 2007;18:437-443.

193. Seal KH, et al. Hepatitis C treatment candidacy and outcomes among 4318 US veterans with chronic hepatitis C virus infection: does a history of injection drug use matter? *J Clin Gastroenterol.* 2007;41:199-205.

194. Mehta SH, et al. Limited uptake of hepatitis C treatment among injection drug users. *J Community Health.* 2008;33: 126-133.

195. Anderson KB, Guest JL, Rimland D. Hepatitis C virus coinfection increases mortality in HIV-infected patients in the highly active antiretroviral therapy era: data from the HIV Atlanta VA Cohort Study. *Clin Infect Dis.* 2004;39:1507-1513.

196. Villano SA, et al. Hepatitis A among homosexual men and injection drug users: more evidence for vaccination. *Clin Infect Dis.* 1997;25:726-728.

197. Wells R, et al. Hepatitis A prevalence among injection drug users. *Clin Lab Sci.* 2006;19:12-17.

198. Vento S, et al. Fulminant hepatitis associated with hepatitis A virus superinfection in patients with chronic hepatitis C. *N Engl J Med.* 1998;338:286-290.

199. Keeffe EB. Is hepatitis A more severe in patients with chronic hepatitis B and other chronic liver diseases? *Am J Gastroenterol.* 1995;90:201-205.

200. Nallathambi MN, et al. Pyogenic splenic abscess in intravenous drug addiction. *Am Surg.* 1987;53:342-346.

201. Dettmeyer R, Schlamann M, Madea B. Cocaine-associated abscesses with lethal sepsis after splenic infarction in an 17-year-old woman. *Forensic Sci Int.* 2004;140:21-23.

202. Fry DE, Richardson JD, Flint LM. Occult splenic abscess: an unrecognized complication of heroin abuse. *Surgery.* 1978;84:650-654.

203. Chun CH, et al. Splenic abscess. *Medicine (Baltimore).* 1980;59:50-65.

204. Sastre J, et al. Splenic abscess due to *Fusobacterium necrophorum. Rev Infect Dis.* 1991;13:1249-1250.

205. Soriano V, et al. Multifocal splenic abscesses caused by *Mycobacterium tuberculosis* in HIV-infected drug users. *AIDS.* 1991;5:901-902.

206. Tung CC, Chen FC, Lo CJ. Splenic abscess: an easily overlooked disease? *Am Surg.* 2006;72:322-325.

207. Carbonell AM, et al. Laparoscopic splenectomy for splenic abscess. *Surg Laparosc Endosc Percutan Tech.* 2004;14: 289-291.

208. Kang M, et al. Image guided percutaneous splenic interventions. *Eur J Radiol.* 2007;64:140-146.

209. Zerem E, Bergsland J. Ultrasound guided percutaneous treatment for splenic abscesses: The significance in treatment of critically ill patients. *World J Gastroenterol.* 2006;12:7341-7345.

210. Adler CH, Stern MB, Brooks ML. Parkinsonism secondary to bilateral striatal fungal abscesses. *Mov Disord.* 1989;4:333-337.

211. Tunkel AR, Pradhan SK. Central nervous system infections in injection drug users. *Infect Dis Clin North Am.* 2002;16:589-605.

212. Garvey GJ, Neu HC. Infective endocarditis—an evolving disease. A review of endocarditis at the Columbia-Presbyterian Medical Center, 1968-1973. *Medicine (Baltimore).* 1978;57:105-127.

213. Roberts WC, Buchbinder NA. Right-sided valvular infective endocarditis. A clinicopathologic study of twelve necropsy patients. *Am J Med.* 1972;53:7-19.

214. Lerner PI. Neurologic complications of infective endocarditis. *Med Clin North Am.* 1985;69:385-398.

215. Gilroy J, Andaya L, Thomas VJ. Intracranial mycotic aneurysms and subacute bacterial endocarditis in heroin addiction. *Neurology.* 1973;23:1193-1198.

216. Ross JS, et al. Intracranial aneurysms: evaluation by MR angiography. *AJNR Am J Neuroradiol.* 1990;11:449-455.

217. Turtz AR, Yocom SS. Contemporary Approaches to the Management of Neurosurgical Complications of Infective Endocarditis. *Curr Infect Dis Rep.* 2001;3:337-346.

218. Frazee JG, Cahan LD, Winter J. Bacterial intracranial aneurysms. *J Neurosurg.* 1980;53:633-641.

219. Abbott SP, et al. Fatal cerebral mycoses caused by the ascomycete *Chaetomium strumarium. J Clin Microbiol.* 1995;33: 2692-2698.

220. Hopkins RJ, et al. Cerebral mucormycosis associated with intravenous drug use: three case reports and review. *Clin Infect Dis.* 1994;19:1133-1137.

221. Blazquez R, et al. Nonsurgical cure of isolated cerebral mucormycosis in an intravenous drug user. *Eur J Clin Microbiol Infect Dis.* 1996;15:598-599.

222. Farrar DJ, et al. Tuberculous brain abscess in a patient with HIV infection: case report and review. *Am J Med.* 1997;102: 297-301.

223. Nussbaum ES, et al. Spinal epidural abscess: a report of 40 cases and review. *Surg Neurol.* 1992;38:225-231.

224. Fraimow HS, et al. *Salmonella* meningitis and infection with HIV. *AIDS.* 1990;4:1271-1273.

225. Koppel BS, et al. Epidural spinal infection in intravenous drug abusers. *Arch Neurol.* 1988;45:1331-1337.

226. Centers for Disease Control and Prevention. Tetanus among injecting-drug users—California, 1997. *JAMA.* 1998; 279:987.

227. Centers for Disease Control and Prevention. Wound botulism—California, 1995. *JAMA.* 1996;275:95-96.

228. Passaro DJ, et al. Wound botulism associated with black tar heroin among injecting drug users. *JAMA.* 1998;279:859-863.

229. Redmond J, Stritch M, Blaney P. Severe tetanus in a narcotic addict. *Ir Med J.* 1984;77:325-326.

230. Kim RW, Juzych MS, Eliott D. Ocular manifestations of injection drug use. *Infect Dis Clin North Am.* 2002;16:607-622.

231. Aboltins CA, Allen P, Daffy JR. Fungal endophthalmitis in intravenous drug users injecting buprenorphine contaminated with oral *Candida* species. *Med J Aust.* 2005;182:427.

232. Albini TA, et al. Lemon juice and *Candida* endophthalmitis in crack-cocaine misuse. *Br J Ophthalmol.* 2007;91:702-703.

233. Hariprasad SM, et al. Voriconazole in the treatment of fungal eye infections: a review of current literature. *Br J Ophthalmol.* 2008;92:871-878.

234. Narendran N, et al. Five-year retrospective review of guideline-based management of fungal endophthalmitis. *Acta Ophthalmol.* 2008;86:525-532.

235. Young EJ, et al. Panophthalmitis due to *Bacillus cereus. Arch Intern Med.* 1980;140:559-560.

236. Trends in HIV/AIDS diagnoses—33 states, 2001-2004. *MMWR Morb Mortal Wkly Rep.* 2005;54:1149-1153.

237. Santibanez SS, et al. Update and overview of practical epidemiologic aspects of HIV/AIDS among injection drug users in the United States. *J Urban Health.* 2006;83:86-100.

238. Joint United Nations Programme on HIV/AIDS (UNAIDS) (UNAIDS), J.U.N.P.o.H.A., *2008 Report on the global AIDS epidemic.* <http://www.unaids.org/en/KnowledgeCentre/HIVData/GlobalReport/2008/2008/Globalreport.asp> Accessed: 12/18/2008

239. Cohn JA. HIV-1 infection in injection drug users. *Infect Dis Clin North Am.* 2002;16:745-770.

240. Pollack HA, et al. The impact of needle exchange-based health services on emergency department use. *J Gen Intern Med.* 2002;17:341-348.

241. Neaigus A, et al. Greater drug injecting risk for HIV, HBV, and HCV infection in a city where syringe exchange and pharmacy syringe distribution are illegal. *J Urban Health.* 2008;85: 309-322.

242. Kerr T, et al. The role of safer injection facilities in the response to HIV/AIDS among injection drug users. *Curr HIV/AIDS Rep.* 2007;4:158-164.

243. Kerr T, Montaner J, Wood E. Supervised injecting facilities: time for scale-up? *Lancet.* 2008;372:354-355.

244. Gowing L, et al. Substitution treatment of injecting opioid users for prevention of HIV infection. *Cochrane Database Syst Rev* 2008:CD004145.

245. Sullivan LE, et al. Buprenorphine/naloxone treatment in primary care is associated with decreased human immunodeficiency virus risk behaviors. *J Subst Abuse Treat.* 2008; 35:87-92.

246. Pezzotti P, et al. Direct comparison of time to AIDS and infectious disease death between HIV seroconverter injection drug users in Italy and the United States: results from the ALIVE and ISS studies. AIDS Link to Intravenous Experiences. Italian Seroconversion Study. *J Acquir Immune Defic Syndr Hum Retrovirol.* 1999;20:275-282.

247. Poundstone KE, Chaisson RE, Moore RD. Differences in HIV disease progression by injection drug use and by sex in the era of highly active antiretroviral therapy. *Aids.* 2001;15:1115-1123.

248. Torian LV, et al. Risk factors for delayed initiation of medical care after diagnosis of human immunodeficiency virus. *Arch Intern Med.* 2008;168:1181-1187.

249. Gutierrez F, et al. Patients' characteristics and clinical implications of suboptimal CD4 T-cell gains after 1 year of successful antiretroviral therapy. *Curr HIV Res.* 2008;6:100-107.

250. Dragsted UB, et al. Predictors of immunological failure after initial response to highly active antiretroviral therapy in HIV-1-infected adults: a EuroSIDA study. *J Infect Dis.* 2004; 190:148-155.

251. Wood E, et al. Highly active antiretroviral therapy and survival in HIV-infected injection drug users. *JAMA.* 2008; 300:550-554.

252. Bruce RD, Altice FL. Case series on the safe use of buprenorphine/naloxone in individuals with acute hepatitis C infection and abnormal hepatic liver transaminases. *Am J Drug Alcohol Abuse.* 2007;33:869-874.

253. Kanno MB, Zenilman J. Sexually transmitted diseases in injection drug users. *Infect Dis Clin North Am.* 2002;16:771-780.

254. Nelson KE, et al. Sexually transmitted diseases in a population of intravenous drug users: association with seropositivity to the human immunodeficiency virus (HIV). *J Infect Dis.* 1991;164:457-463.

255. Plitt SS, et al. Prevalence and correlates of *Chlamydia trachomatis, Neisseria gonorrhoeae, Trichomonas vaginalis* infections, and bacterial vaginosis among a cohort of young injection drug users in Baltimore, Maryland. *Sex Transm Dis.* 2005;32:446-453.

256. Plitt SS, et al. Human papillomavirus seroprevalence among young male and female drug users. *Sex Transm Dis.* 2007;34:676-680.

257. Arasteh K, Des Jarlais DC, Perlis TE. Alcohol and HIV sexual risk behaviors among injection drug users. *Drug Alcohol Depend.* 2008;95:54-61.

258. Rees V, et al. Association of alcohol consumption with HIV sex- and drug-risk behaviors among drug users. *J Subst Abuse Treat.* 2001;21:129-134.

259. Tyndall MW, et al. Risky sexual behaviours among injection drugs users with high HIV prevalence: implications for STD control. *Sex Transm Infect.* 2002;78(suppl 1):i170-i175.

260. Kapadia F, et al. Correlates of consistent condom use with main partners by partnership patterns among young adult male injection drug users from five US cities. *Drug Alcohol Depend.* 2007;91(Suppl 1):S56-S63.

261. Strathdee SA, et al. Correlates of injection drug use among female sex workers in two Mexico-U.S. border cities. *Drug Alcohol Depend.* 2008;92:132-140.

262. Bacon O, et al. Commercial sex work and risk of HIV infection among young drug-injecting men who have sex with men in San Francisco. *Sex Transm Dis.* 2006;33:228-234.

263. Deiss RG, et al. High-risk sexual and drug using behaviors among male injection drug users who have sex with men in two Mexico-US border cities. *Sex Transm Dis.* 2008;35:243-249.

264. Lopez-Zetina J, et al. Predictors of syphilis seroreactivity and prevalence of HIV among street recruited injection drug users in Los Angeles County, 1994-6. *Sex Transm Infect.* 2000;76: 462-469.

265. Fisher DG, et al. Reliability, sensitivity and specificity of self-report of HIV test results. *AIDS Care.* 2007;19:692-696.

317

Surgical Site Infections and Antimicrobial Prophylaxis

THOMAS R. TALBOT

In 1862, Louis Pasteur's ingenious experiments into the nature of putrefaction were officially endorsed by the Paris Academy of Science. The endorsement signaled an end to the long-held belief that the exposure of organic material to air brought about the spontaneous generation of microorganisms, and the concepts of *sepsis* and *asepsis* became firmly established. A mere 3 years later, Joseph Lister demonstrated the incredible implications of antisepsis in his practice of orthopedic surgery. For the first time in recorded history, major surgical procedures could be performed with a reasonable expectation of primary wound healing and recovery. Essential enhancements for preventing and controlling wound sepsis were provided by the antibiotic revolution of the 1940s, ushering in the highly technical, highly invasive, and highly successful era of modern surgery. As noted by McDermott and Rogers,[1] the great achievements of the antibiotic era may be related, in the long run, to its essential role in supporting the advancements of modern surgery. Indeed, surgery as we know it today would be impossible in an environment in which infection was likely or, once established, untreatable.

Despite the fundamental role of antisepsis and antibiotics in the development of modern surgery, implementation of these discoveries in the practice of surgery has not occurred without opposition. As late as 1880, for example, William Halstead was ordered from the operating theater when he challenged a senior surgeon's disregard for antiseptic techniques. The early use of antibiotics for prophylaxis in surgical procedures was also questioned as respected academicians freely voiced their disapproval of antibiotic prophylaxis in clean surgical procedures.[2] For a number of years, the value of prophylactic antibiotics in preventing infections of the surgical wound remained in doubt. A consensus in favor of their use did not emerge until two concepts of perioperative prophylaxis and infection were established. First, investigators in Cincinnati and Boston demonstrated that, despite the use of standard aseptic techniques, *Staphylococcus aureus* could be regularly isolated from the operative field.[3-5] It became apparent that aseptic technique could decrease but not eliminate bacterial contamination of the surgical field. Therefore, it appeared plausible that perioperative antibiotics could supplement aseptic techniques in containing the inevitable contamination of the operative wound.

The second major finding involved the timing of the administration of the prophylactic antibiotic. As early as 1946, Howes had noted a correlation between the amelioration of infection and the interval between the contamination of the wounds and the administration of antibiotics.[6] Several years later, Miles and colleagues[7] and Burke,[8] working with a guinea pig model of wound infection, demonstrated the remarkable brevity of the "window" of prophylactic efficacy. They noted that antibiotics given shortly before or at the time of bacterial inoculation of the subcutaneous tissue of the guinea pig produced a notable diminution in the size of the subsequent wound induration compared with lesions in animals not receiving antibiotic prophylaxis (Fig. 317-1). By delaying the administration of antibiotics by only 3 or 4 hours, resulting lesions were identical in size to those of animals receiving no antibiotic prophylaxis whatsoever. Thus "failures" of antimicrobial prophylaxis that had been noted in earlier clinical studies were related to the fact that administration of preoperative antibiotics had been inappropriately timed.[9-11] While these observations have been challenging to reproduce in vitro,[12] the experience of current practice has evolved to mandate that, whenever possible, surgical antimicrobial prophylaxis should be administered so as to ensure adequate tissue levels of antimicrobials from the time of the initial surgical incision until closure. The efficacy of prophylactic antibiotics has now been verified for most major surgical procedures with a wide variety of antimicrobials when care has been given to provide adequate serum and tissue levels of antibiotics during the surgical procedure. Perioperative antibiotics and aseptic techniques have become routine aspects of care in most major surgical procedures.

Despite efforts to prevent surgical site infections (SSIs), these outcomes are not uncommon. While an exact determination of the burden of SSIs in the United States has not been performed, analysis of data from the National Center for Health Statistics[13] and the National Healthcare Safety Network (NHSN)[14] suggests that between 250,000 and 1 million SSIs complicate the approximately 26.6 million inpatient surgical procedures performed annually in the United States. The impact of SSIs in the United States alone has been estimated to be 3.7 million excess hospital days and $1.6 billion in excess costs.[15] A patient who develops an SSI while hospitalized has a greater than 60% greater risk of being admitted to the intensive care unit, is 15 times more likely to be readmitted to the hospital within 30 days after discharge, and incurs an attributable extra hospital stay of 6.5 days, leading to a direct cost of an additional $3000 per infection.[16] SSIs due to methicillin-resistant *S. aureus* (MRSA) in particular have also been shown to have a higher mortality than those due to methicillin-sensitive strains of the organism.[17]

New technological advances (e.g., the introduction of minimally invasive procedures) and the emergence of antibiotic-resistant organisms (e.g., community-acquired MRSA [CA-MRSA]) have led to additional challenges in the prevention and identification of SSIs. In addition, through the advent of programs centered around adherence to basic key principles of surgical care and antimicrobial prophylaxis, such as the Centers for Medicare & Medicaid Services' (CMS) Surgical Care Improvement Project (SCIP),[18] the prevention of SSI has moved to the forefront of surgical quality improvement and pay-for-performance programs, highlighting unresolved issues regarding antimicrobial prophylaxis (e.g. drug dosing in obese patients, the specific timing of antibiotic administration, and the role of anti-MRSA prophylaxis). Now, nearly 150 years since the discoveries of Pasteur and Lister, much remains to be learned about the pathophysiology, prevention, and surveillance of SSIs.

Principles of Prevention and Control

DETERMINANTS AND PATHOPHYSIOLOGY

Whether a wound infection occurs after surgery depends on a complex interaction between the following: (1) patient-related factors (e.g., host immunity, nutritional status, the presence or absence of diabetes); (2) procedure-related factors (e.g., implantation of foreign bodies, degree of trauma to the host tissues); (3) microbial factors (tissue adherence and invasion); and (4) perioperative antimicrobial prophylaxis.

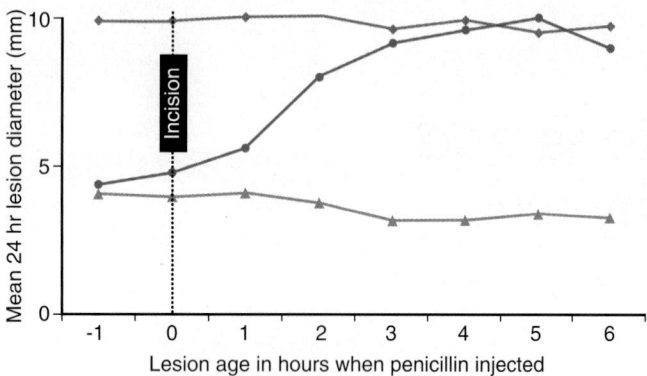

Figure 317-1   Importance of the timing of antimicrobial administration. Relationship between the timing of antimicrobial administration and the effectiveness of prophylaxis as shown by the size of wound infection in a guinea pig model.[8] Lesion sizes were measured as mean diameter (mm) of induration developing 24 hours after intradermal inoculation of *Staphylococcus aureus* (SA). *Red line* indicates animals injected with live SA who received placebo; *blue line* indicates animals injected with live SA who received penicillin; *green line* indicates animals injected with killed SA.

Species and Sources of Wound Bacteria

Bacterial contamination of the surgical wound is inevitable. State-of-the-art aseptic technique has been associated with a dramatic drop in, but not the elimination of, this phenomenon. Even under laminar flow operating room environments, bacteria can be isolated from wound surfaces at the close of the surgical procedure.[19] The importance of the microbial load in determining whether or not a wound becomes infected has been appreciated for decades and is relevant even in the era of the routine administration of antimicrobial prophylaxis for most major surgical procedures (Fig. 317-2).[20] Historically, surgeons and hospital epidemiologists have stratified operations on the basis of the expected quantity of bacteria introduced into the operative site during surgery (Table 317-1). Although the magnitude of bacterial inoculation into the wound still has some predictive value regarding the risk of developing a wound infection, patient- and procedure-related risk factors also contribute greatly to this risk (Table 317-2).[21] Acknowledging the role such factors play in the pathogenesis of SSIs, newer predic-

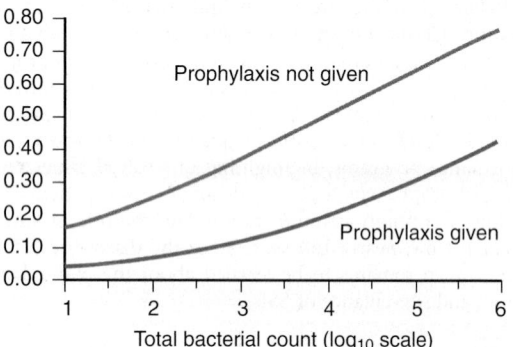

Figure 317-2   Wound infection and febrile morbidity. Plot of the probability of wound infection, febrile morbidity, or both according to total bacterial counts at the operative site in patients undergoing abdominal hysterectomy. The administration of antimicrobial prophylaxis reduces the likelihood of infection or fever for a given level of bacterial contamination of the wound. Stated another way, the administration of prophylaxis increases the magnitude of the bacterial inoculum needed to produce infection. (*From Houang ET, Ahmet Z. Intraoperative wound contamination during abdominal hysterectomy. J Hosp Infect. 1991;19:181-189. Copyright 1991, with permission from The Hospital Infection Society.*)

TABLE 317-1	Classification of Operative Wounds by Level of Bacterial Contamination

Class I/Clean Wound

An uninfected operative wound in which no inflammation is encountered and the respiratory, alimentary, genital, or uninfected urinary tract is not entered. In addition, clean wounds are primarily closed and, if necessary, drained with closed drainage. Operative incisional wounds that follow nonpenetrating (blunt) trauma should be included in this category if they meet the criteria.

Class II/Clean-Contaminated Wound

An operative wound in which the respiratory, alimentary, genital, or urinary tracts are entered under controlled conditions and without unusual contamination. Specifically, operations involving the biliary tract, appendix, vagina, and oropharynx are included in this category, provided no evidence of infection or major break in technique is encountered.

Class III/Contaminated Wound

Open, fresh, accidental wounds. In addition, operations with major breaks in sterile technique (e.g., open cardiac massage) or gross spillage from the gastrointestinal tract, and incisions in which acute, nonpurulent inflammation is encountered are included in this category.

Class IV/Dirty-Infected Wound

Old traumatic wounds with retained devitalized tissue and those that involve existing clinical infection or perforated viscera. This definition suggests that the organisms causing postoperative infection were present in the operative field before the operation.

Adapted from Mangram AJ, Horan TC, Pearson ML, et al. Guideline for prevention of surgical site infection, 1999. Hospital Infection Control Practices Advisory Committee. *Infect Control Hosp Epidemiol.* 1999; 20:250-278; quiz 279-280.

tive indices to determine the infection risk for a particular surgical site incorporate not only these measures of bacterial inoculation but also assessments of patient comorbidities and procedural characteristics that afford an increased risk for infection (see Risk Factors).

Numerous species have been described as wound pathogens, and the origin of the inoculum is not established with certainty for most infections. The patient's endogenous skin flora, with gram-positive organisms, in general, and staphylococcal species, in particular, are the predominant cause of incisional infections of clean surgical procedures (Table 317-3).[22] Over the past decade, the microbiology of SSIs appears to be evolving due to the emergence of various multidrug-resistant pathogens, particularly CA-MRSA, as suggested by a report from a large network of community hospitals that noted a doubling in the prevalence of MRSA SSIs from 2000 to 2005 (see Table 317-3).[23] *S. aureus* colonization of the patient's nares is a major risk factor for

TABLE 317-2	Selected Patient and Procedural Characteristics Associated with Increased Risk for Surgical Site Infection

Patient Factors	*Procedural Factors*
Diabetes mellitus/perioperative hyperglycemia	Shaving of site the night prior to procedure
Concurrent tobacco use	Use of razor for hair removal
Remote infection at time of surgery	Improper preoperative skin preparation
Obesity	
Malnutrition	Improper antimicrobial prophylaxis (wrong drug, wrong dose, wrong time of administration)
Low preoperative serum albumin	
Concurrent steroid use	
Prolonged preoperative stay*	Failure to timely redose antibiotics in prolonged procedures
Prior site irradiation	
Colonization with *S. aureus*	Inadequate OR ventilation
	Increased OR traffic
	Poor surgical technique (poor hemostasis, tissue trauma)
	Break in sterile technique and asepsis
	Perioperative hypothermia, hypoxia
	Improper use of flash sterilization of instruments

*Likely a surrogate marker for severity of underlying illness and comorbidities OR, operating room.

Adapted from Mangram AJ, Horan TC, Pearson ML, et al. Guideline for prevention of surgical site infection, 1999. Hospital Infection Control Practices Advisory Committee. *Infect Control Hosp Epidemiol.* 1999;20:250-78; quiz 279-80.

TABLE 317-3	Major Pathogens in Surgical Site Infections		
	NHSN (2007)	DICON Community Hospitals (2005)	
Pathogen	Percent of Infections*	Percent of Infections†	Prevalence Rate per 100 Procedures
Staphylococcus aureus	30	33	0.37
MRSA	N/A	17	0.20
MSSA	N/A	15	0.17
Coagulase-negative staphylococci	14	11	0.13
Enterococcus sp.	11	8	0.09
Escherichia coli	10	6	0.06
Pseudomonas aeruginosa	6	4	0.05
Enterobacter spp.	4		
Streptococcus spp.		3	0.04
Klebsiella sp.	4	4	0.04
Fungi (*Candida* spp.)	2	3	0.03
Anaerobes (*Bacteroides fragilis,* gram-positive anaerobes)		3	0.03
Acinetobacter spp.	1		
Other	19		

*From a total of 7025 isolates, as reported by the National Healthcare Safety Network (NHSN), January 2006 to October 2007.[22]

†From a total of 1,010 surgical site infections among 89,302 procedures performed during 2005 at 26 community-based hospitals within the Duke Infection Control Outreach Network (DICON).[23]

N/A, not available.

developing a *S. aureus* SSI, a particular concern in selected populations such as diabetic individuals and recipients of hemodialysis, who have *S. aureus* colonization rates in excess of 50%. A study of elective cardiothoracic, general, oncologic, gynecologic, and neurologic surgical procedures found a more than 4-fold increased odds of *S. aureus* SSI in colonized patients when compared with non-colonized persons.[24] *S. aureus* and *S. epidermidis* wound infections can also occur in clusters, sometimes with a particular surgeon or nurse implicated in their spread. Unusual and hard-to-culture species, including nontuberculous mycobacteria, *Nocardia* spp., *Legionella* spp., *Mycoplasma hominis*, and *Propionibacterium acnes*, have occasionally caused surgical site infections as well.

Modern methods of antisepsis can reduce but not eliminate the skin-associated bacteria of surgical patients. This limitation derives, in part, from the localization of up to 20% of skin-associated bacteria in skin appendages such as hair follicles and sebaceous glands (Fig. 317-3).[25] Because these sites are beneath the skin's surface, bacteria residing there are not eliminated by topical antisepsis. Transection of these skin structures by surgical incision may carry the patient's resident bacteria deep into the wound and set the stage for subsequent infection.

For contaminated procedures, wound pathogens frequently are among the bacterial species that comprise the normal flora of the viscus entered during the surgical procedure. Enteric gram-negative pathogens and anaerobic bacteria (e.g. *Bacteroides fragilis*) are common pathogens of wounds after colonic procedures, and polymicrobial infections are common in this setting. Infection by a particular species, however, does not correlate directly with its quantitative presence among the normal flora, but by the particular virulence attributes of bacteria.

Although numerous sources of bacterial contamination of surgical wounds have been described, it is virtually impossible to identify with certainty the source(s) and route(s) of contamination. The direct inoculation of a patient's endogenous flora at the time of surgery is believed to be the most common mechanism; however, others undoubtedly occur. Transmission from contaminated surgical instruments or surgical material, hematogenous seeding from preexisting infection of a nonwound site, and contamination from either the skin, mucous membranes, or clothing of operating room staff, or a combination of them, have all been implicated as potential sources of microbial contamination. Outbreaks of group A streptococcal wound infection have been traced to the anal or vaginal carriage of this organism by operating room personnel,[26,27] and epidemiologic investigation of these outbreaks indicated that airborne contamination of the operative field had occurred. Infections, including *Candida albicans* osteomyelitis and diskitis after lumbar laminectomy, have been traced to the use of artificial fingernails worn by surgical staff.[28] Organisms harbored between the artificial and natural fingernails are shielded from standard hand hygiene, leading to potential surgical field contamination. Many hospitals now ban the use of artificial or long natural fingernails in any health care workers with direct patient care responsibilities.

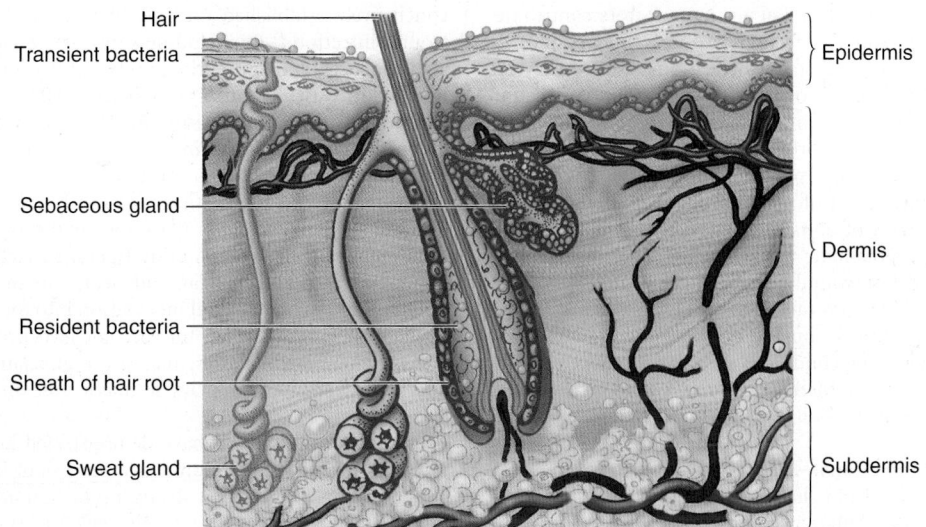

Figure 317-3 Diagram of the skin. Schematic diagram of the skin demonstrating the location of the transient bacteria on the skin surface, which are easily removed, and the deep resident bacteria, which cannot be destroyed by skin antiseptics. *(From Postlethwaite RW. Principles of operative surgery: Antisepsis, technique, sutures, and drains. In: Sabiston DC, ed. Davis-Christopher Textbook of Surgery. 12th ed. Philadelphia: WB Saunders; 1981:322.)*

The relative importance of hematogenous seeding (i.e., *inside to out*) of the surgical wound is somewhat unclear. Evidence of this route of seeding of the surgical wound site has been mainly noted with procedures involving implantation of prosthetic devices[23]; however, the report of SSIs related to the use of extrinsically-contaminated propofol provides strong epidemiologic support for this concept in other procedures.[29] In addition, although it is generally accepted that prosthetic valves and hips are at risk for an indefinite period of time for hematogenous seeding and infection post-operatively, it is difficult to ascertain with certainty whether a late postoperative infection results from intraoperative bacterial seeding of the prosthetic device followed by prolonged dormancy or from a true postoperative hematogenous event. In a randomized, prospective, controlled study of antibiotic prophylaxis in total hip replacement, Carlsson and co-workers demonstrated that deep wound infections that developed over 2.5 years after surgery were more likely to have occurred among placebo versus cloxacillin recipients (13.7% vs. 3.3%, respectively; $P < .05$).[30] These data strongly suggest that bacteria inoculated into wounds at the time of surgery may lie dormant for years, rendering differentiation of the precise source of late wound infection virtually impossible. If late hematogenous seeding of a surgical wound with or without prosthetic material can occur, it is reasonable to assume that wounds are even more vulnerable to seeding and secondary infection during the immediate postoperative period. During this time, surgical incisions are hyperemic from the trauma of the surgery and endothelialization of intravascular prosthetic materials has not yet had time to occur. Moreover, the regular use of indwelling intravascular catheters probably increases the risk of bacteremia. However, information with which to judge the relative contribution of intraoperative versus postoperative hematogenous seeding of the surgical incision is unavailable.

Virulence Factors of Major Wound Pathogens

Clean Wound Infections. The requirement for large inocula in the early models of *S. aureus* soft tissue infection gave the misleading impression that cooperative interaction between bacteria may be required to establish a wound infection.[7,8] Later models involving foreign bodies have demonstrated median infective dose (ID_{50}) values of less than 100 colony-forming units (CFU) with polytetrafluoroethylene (PTFE) tissue cages,[31] 10 CFU with PTFE vascular grafts,[32] and as low as 1 CFU with dextran microbeads.[33] These data demonstrate the pathogenic potential of a single bacterium to produce wound infection, provided that it is inoculated into a suitable niche.

Determinants of *S. aureus* virulence have been studied for decades and include a wide variety of enzymes and toxins with diverse effects on the host. Which of the staphylococcal virulence factors contribute to the development of a wound infection is poorly understood. *S. aureus* and the coagulase-negative staphylococci bind to a variety of biologic molecules, including fibronectin, fibrinogen, vitronectin, collagen, laminin, and platelet thrombospondin.[34-36] Blood clots and the subendothelium are rich in fibronectin, and adherence to such sites may be the first step in the pathogenesis of a clean surgical wound infection. Administration of a recombinant fragment of the fibronectin-binding domains of *S. aureus* has been shown to inhibit abscess formation and to potentiate the benefit of cefazolin prophylaxis in a guinea pig model of wound infection.[37] Once in the wound, several staphylococcal exoenzymes can damage host tissues, including hyaluronidase, lipase, proteases, nucleases, and four membrane-damaging toxins.[38] Under some conditions, protein A competes with phagocytic cells for F_c receptors, thereby reducing antibody-mediated opsonization.[39] Coagulase may also interfere with phagocytosis.

Contaminated Wound Infections. The role of coliforms and anaerobes in abdominal sepsis has been elucidated in a model that involves inserting a gelatin capsule containing a standardized inoculum of pooled cecal contents into the peritoneal cavities of rats.[40,41] Acute peritonitis and septicemia from coliforms caused rapid death in 37% of the animals, and all of the survivors developed abscesses with anaerobes as the predominant organisms. The capsular polysaccharide of

Bacteroides fragilis promotes abscess formation and may reduce phagocytosis. In experimental models, immunization against capsular polysaccharide can protect against abscess formation after inoculation with *B. fragilis* by a T-cell-dependent mechanism, except in the presence of foreign material.[42] Also, *B. fragilis* produces a variety of tissue-damaging enzymes, including fibrinolysin, chondroitin sulfatase, collagenase, and hyaluronidase.

Wound Microenvironment and Operative Effects on Immunity

Much of our understanding of the pathophysiology of wound infection and the nature of the surgical wound derives from investigational models. Early investigations suggesting that the efficacy of antibiotics in preventing wound infection is limited to only a few hours after the moment of bacterial inoculation suggested that the wound microenvironment is not static.[6,7] It is likely that rapid changes are occurring among microbial factors, such as a shift from exponential to stationary-phase growth with an accompanying decrease in bacterial susceptibility to antibiotics and possibly the expression of different microbial virulence factors. Wound-related changes must also occur, such as gradually diminishing tissue perfusion and antibiotic delivery related to increased tissue oncotic pressure brought about by the effect of inflammatory mediators on vascular permeability.

Multiple host defense mechanisms are involved in the response to bacteria inoculated at the surgical site. Neutrophils are probably the most important effector cells, and the most common wound pathogens are highly susceptible to killing by reactive oxygen intermediates. Opsonization by antibodies and complement facilitate phagocytosis. An additional host defense mechanism against abscess formation by *S. aureus* has been described by Dye and Kapral.[43] Abscess homogenates are bactericidal for staphylococci, and this activity is mediated by 2-monoglycerides and unsaturated free fatty acids. Most strains of *S. aureus* produce fatty-acid metabolizing enzyme (FAME), which inactivates the bactericidal lipids. Strains deficient in this enzyme are eliminated rapidly from intraperitoneal abscesses in mice, whereas strains producing FAME are capable of prolonged survival in vivo. Phospholipase A_2, found in inflammatory exudates, has been noted to have potent antistaphylococcal activity.[44] T-cell-dependent immune mechanisms have been shown to be important in protection against *B. fragilis* infection,[42] but their importance with regard to other common wound pathogens is not as well established.

Foreign Material and Operative Trauma to Tissue. Investigations of *S. aureus* infection in the skin of human volunteers by Elek and Conen conclusively established the role of foreign material in potentiating wound infection.[45] By including suture material with the intradermal staphylococcal inoculum, the number of organisms required to establish a skin pustule could be reduced 10,000-fold relative to lesions without sutures (i.e., a fall from 5×10^6 organisms to 3×10^2 organisms in the inoculum). These investigators further suggested that "other circumstances may lead to the unhindered growth of small inocula, including heavily traumatized tissues, burns, or devitalized tissues distal to the ligated vessels. This may be the explanation of the traditional surgical view that untidy operative techniques predispose to infection."[45] Because in clean and clean-contaminated surgical procedures, quantitative bacterial inoculation into the wound is small, tissue devitalization at a gross or microscopic level provides a niche wherein a small bacterial inoculum may grow in relative isolation from the host's defenses, which plays a major role in the pathogenesis of infection.

Investigational models have demonstrated how technical variables of the surgical procedure influence the risk of infection. Some suture materials appear to have a stronger adjuvant effect on infection than others.[46] Whether the use of the electrosurgical knife, which can damage host tissues via the transfer of heat, is an adjuvant for infection is controversial.[47,48] In an in vitro system, thermally killed fibroblasts activate the alternative complement pathway, leading ultimately to impaired neutrophilic activity against bacteria.[49]

Effect of Operative Procedures on Systemic and Local Immunity. Operative procedures produce systemic and local changes in the immune defense mechanisms of the host. Neutrophil function and serum opsonizing capacity become impaired. The microbicidal activity of neutrophils obtained postoperatively from patients undergoing abdominal hysterectomy is 25% less than that of neutrophils harvested from the same patients preoperatively, and it takes 9 days to return to normal.[50] The depletion of opsonizing factors within the abscess milieu also may contribute to decreased neutrophilic bactericidal function.[51]

Major surgical procedures compromise the host defenses in other ways. Surface levels of HLA-DR antigens on the circulating monocytes of patients are reduced following major surgery.[52] However, it has been shown that defects in T-cell proliferation and cytokine secretion after major surgery involve an inability of T cells to respond to T-cell receptor- and CD28 coreceptor-mediated signals rather than problems with antigen presentation by monocytes-macrophages.[53] Perioperative hypothermia brought on by anesthetic-induced impairment of thermoregulation and exposure to the low ambient temperatures of the operating room may accompany major surgery. In the setting of perioperative hypothermia, neutrophils have reduced chemotaxis, impaired ingestion of staphylococci, and diminished superoxide production.[54] Hypothermia can also trigger vasoconstriction and lead to low tissue oxygen tension, which is itself a risk factor for SSI.[55] Because of these risks, interventions aimed at reducing perioperative normothermia and hypoxia have been examined to prevent SSIs (see Prevention).

Perioperative blood transfusion has been associated with an increased rate of postoperative infections, including wound infection, with donated white blood cell (WBC)-induced immunosuppression implicated as the culprit.[56] Decreases in cell-mediated immunity and increases in cytokine levels (interleukin [IL]-2 receptor, IL-6) have been demonstrated in mice and humans following transfusion.[57] However, clinical trials comparing the receipt of standard whole or buffy-coat-depleted blood products (which, despite the moniker, still retain some donor WBCs) to WBC-depleted products, or the administration of allogenic versus autologous blood have failed to provide a consensus answer to transfusion's role in the development of postoperative infections.[58] Studies describing this potential transfusion effect have been criticized for using nonstandardized outcome definitions, failing to account for known risk factors for postoperative infection, and using only univariate analyses.[58] Blood transfusion may simply serve as a marker for unidentified patient comorbidities, and more rigorously designed studies are needed before general conclusions regarding the role of blood transfusion in wound infection can be determined.

In cardiac surgery, the patient may be exposed to hypothermia, cardiopulmonary bypass, and relative arterial hypotension throughout much of the procedure. Exposure of blood to cardiopulmonary bypass depletes serum complement, causes systemic release of pro-inflammatory cytokines, and adversely affects neutrophilic function.[59-61] Furthermore, protein denaturation and chylomicron aggregation may contribute to small vessel occlusion and tissue hypoxia as well as overwhelm the capacity of the reticuloendothelial system to clear infectious agents from the blood.[62] This raises the possibility that post-bypass patients may be predisposed to develop infections via hematogenous bacterial seeding as a result of reduced reticuloendothelial clearance.

The release of cytokines at the wound site may have a protective effect against infection. Pretreatment of tissue cages with tumor necrosis factor, either administered directly or generated in vivo by exposure to staphylococcal cell wall components, inhibited abscess formation by an inoculum of *S. aureus* that under normal circumstances would have produced infection 100% of the time.[63] Also, the use of fibrinolytic agents prevents abscess formation in investigational models.[64] This is consistent with the hypothesis that the adherence of bacteria to fibrinous exudates is an essential step in the pathogenesis of a wound infection.

RISK FACTORS FOR SURGICAL SITE INFECTION

Patient Factors

Various host factors have been associated with an increased risk of SSI (see Table 317-2), including underlying comorbid illnesses (e.g., diabetes mellitus),[65] malnutrition,[66] obesity,[67] history of irradiation at the site of the procedure,[68] and use of immunosuppressants.[69] Tobacco use may lead to SSI, due to nicotine's effects of vasoconstriction and inhibition of wound healing.[70] As noted earlier, colonization with *S. aureus* can also increase one's risk for developing staphylococcal SSI.

While diabetes mellitus has often been noted as a risk for SSI, acute fluctuations in glucose control may also be important. In a prospective study of 1000 cardiothoracic surgery patients, hyperglycemia (serum glucose > 200 mg/dL) in the 48 hours postprocedure was associated with a 102% increase in the risk for wound infection.[71] Risk also increased incrementally with further elevations in glucose; however, the degree of long-term glucose control (as measured by glycosylated hemoglobin levels at time of surgery) did not impact infection risk. As a result of this and similar studies, intensive glucose control during the perioperative period among cardiac surgical patients is now considered a basic SSI prevention practice.[18]

Increasing age in adults has often been noted as a risk factor for SSI; however, questions often arise as to whether age serves simply as a marker for underlying illness or whether immunosenescence associated with increased age leads to an increased risk of infection. In contrast, a recent study of greater than 72,000 surgical patients found that, after adjustment for hospital type, procedure type and duration, wound class, and American Society of Anesthesiologists (ASA) score, the risk of SSI decreased with advancing age (decrease of 1.1%/year as patient age increased).[72]

Procedural Factors

Attributes of the surgical procedure itself can lead to an increased risk for SSI. Breaks in sterile technique during the procedure, failure or incomplete preparation of the skin with antiseptic cleansers, improper ventilation of the operative suite, and use of flash (i.e., emergent/immediate) sterilization of surgical instruments[73] can all contribute to the development of SSIs. The rate of contamination of sterile instrument trays correlates with the duration such trays are left exposed and uncovered.[74] Increased traffic in the operating room (OR) may lead to increased bacterial shedding and airborne contamination. A study of nearly 3,000 surgical procedures noted a four fold increase in SSI frequency between surgical cases with 0 to 8 people entering the OR during the case and those with more than 17 people in the room.[75] While this finding was not significant in a multivariate analysis, it seems prudent that OR traffic be minimized as a part of good surgical practice. The method of hair removal is important, as shaving with a razor (vs. use of clippers or no hair removal at all) leaves small microabrasions around the operative site that may harbor bacteria. Finally, failure to appropriately administer prophylactic antibiotics (correct drug, correct dose, correct timing prior to incision) is a major factor in the development of SSI (see discussion later in this chapter).

Assessment of Patient Risk

Many risk factors for infection are interrelated, hence a patient with one risk factor is also likely to have others. Methods to ascertain an individual's overall risk for the development of an SSI have been devised to account for the multiple factors involved in the pathogenesis of wound infections. Developed and tested on more than 58,000 patients during the Centers for Disease Control and Prevention Study on the Efficacy of Nosocomial Infection Control (SENIC), one such index takes into account the traditional assessment of the level of wound contamination together with three patient- and procedure-related risk factors (Table 317-4).[76] Undergoing an operation involving the abdomen, having a procedure lasting longer than 2 hours, and the presence of three or more discharge diagnoses (as a surrogate for identifying the complicated patient) were all independent risk factors for a wound infection. Their inclusion with the traditional wound

TABLE 317-4	Indices to Assess Individual Risk of Developing Surgical Site Infection[14,21,76]	
Index		**Scoring**
SENIC (Study of the Efficacy of Nosocomial Infection Control)		
Operative time > 2 hours		1 point
Abdominal procedure		1 point
Contaminated or dirty procedure		1 point
≥ 3 discharge diagnoses		1 point
NNIS (National Nosocomial Infection Surveillance system)		
ASA score of 3, 4, or 5		1 point
Contaminated or dirty procedure		1 point
Length of procedure > T hours (75th percentile duration of specific procedure)		1 point
Use of laparoscope*		Minus 1 point

*Use of laparoscope reduces surgical site infection rates in all patients (regardless of other risk factors) undergoing cholecystectomy and colon surgery, and in those without other risk factors (NNIS score = 0) undergoing gastric surgery or appendectomy. This scoring criterion should, therefore, be applied to those select subgroups when assessing infection risk.

ASA, American Society of Anesthesiologists.

classification system predicted the risk of wound infection about twice as well as the wound classification system alone.

This model has been modified further, resulting in the National Nosocomial Infection Surveillance system (NNIS) risk index (see Table 317-4), which includes the three following variables: (1) a patient with an ASA preoperative assessment score of 3, 4, or 5; (2) an operation classified as contaminated or dirty-infected; and (3) an operation lasting longer than T hours, where T refers to the 75th percentile duration for the specific procedure.[77-79] Use of a laparoscope has been found to reduce the rates of SSIs in selected surgical populations (all patients undergoing laparoscopic cholecystectomy and colonic surgery regardless of risk and those with no risk factors for infection [NNIS score of 0] undergoing laparoscopic appendectomy or gastric surgery). Laparoscope use has therefore been added to the NNIS index for these patient subgroups.[14] Risk assessment using such indices has allowed detailed stratified descriptions of procedure-specific SSI rates to be generated over the past decade (Table 317-5).[14] Even with the improvement in risk assessment afforded by these indices, critics have noted that for some procedures, such as cesarean section and various neurosurgical procedures, the NNIS index may not adequately stratify risk.[80] Therefore, further modification of risk assessment tools for SSI will need to occur in order to accurately stratify postsurgical infection risk, particularly in the new era of public reporting and inter-facility comparison of infection rates.

Prevention

While an admirable goal, the increasingly noted perception that all SSIs are preventable is unrealistic and incorrect, given the presence of many risk factors noted above that are largely unalterable (such as patient comorbid diseases and obesity). That said, the goal should be to eliminate all potentially preventable infections through the use of evidenced-based processes. Stemming from the concepts of wound infection pathogenesis and the risk factors noted earlier, a number of such interventions have been put into practice over the past century to reduce the risk of SSI. These interventions can be grouped into two major categories (Table 317-6). The first line of defense involves measures that reduce bacterial inoculation into the wound site. These include familiar rituals such as the application of antiseptics to the skin of the patient, the washing and gloving of the surgeon's hands, the use of sterile drapes, strict adherence to sterile technique, airflow control, and the use of sterile gowns, caps, and masks by operating room personnel.

Efforts to reduce patient colonization with staphylococci may also be of benefit. A randomized, placebo-controlled trial found that mupirocin applied to the nares of patients undergoing elective car-

diothoracic, neurosurgical, oncologic, gynecologic, and general surgical procedures beginning on the day prior to surgery and continued for up to 5 consecutive days resulted in a reduction in *S. aureus* nosocomial infections from 7.7% to 4.0% in those with preoperative nasal carriage of *S. aureus*. However, the rates of nosocomial and, specifically, SSIs in all patients, regardless of *S. aureus* carriage status, were not reduced with the use of mupirocin.[24] Preoperative showering with a solution containing chlorhexidine suppresses bacterial colonization of the skin; however, a meta-analysis of six trials encompassing more than 10,000 patients did not find a significant impact of chlorhexidine showering on SSI rates.[81] Such findings may be due to the removal of the chlorhexidine during or soon after showering, which may minimize chlorhexidine's beneficial quality of prolonged bacterial killing.

For preoperative hair removal, methods that do not create microabrasions, such as clippers or depilatories, are preferred.[82] This recommendation is supported by a large randomized trial of 1,013 patients in which SSIs occurred in 3.2% of patients following hair removal with

TABLE 317-5	Surgical Site Infection Rates, by Selected Operative Procedure and NNIS Risk Index Category, January 1992 to June 2004*				
	Infection Rates† (No. of Procedures) for NNIS Risk Index =				
Operative Procedure Category	**M (−1)‡**	**0**	**1**	**2**	**3**
Cardiac		0.70	1.5	2.21	
CABG–chest only		0	2.19	3.72	
CABG–chest and donor site		1.25	3.39	5.43	9.76
Thoracic surgery		0.42	0.99	2.47	
Appendectomy (open)		1.31	2.55	4.85	
Appendectomy (laparoscopic)§		0.67			
Gastric surgery (open)		2.58	4.69	8.34	
Gastric surgery (laparoscopic)§		0.68			
Cholecystectomy	0.45	0.68	1.78	3.27	5.68
Colon surgery	3.98		5.66	8.54	11.25
Small bowel surgery		4.97	7.11	8.63	11.60
Laparotomy		1.71	3.08	4.71	7.19
Prostatectomy		0.81	2.05		
Genitourinary other than prostatectomy/nephrectomy		0.36	0.85	2.92	
Head and neck surgery		2.27	5.30	12.50	
Herniorrhaphy		0.81	2.14	4.53	
Mastectomy		1.74	2.20	3.42	
Craniotomy		0.91	1.72	2.40	
Ventricular shunt		4.42	5.36		
Cesarean section		2.71	4.14	7.53	
Abdominal hysterectomy		1.36	2.32	5.17	
Vaginal hysterectomy		1.31			
Limb amputation		3.50			
Open reduction of fracture		0.79	1.41	2.81	4.97
Organ transplant		4.63		13.71	26.0
Hip prosthesis		0.86	1.65	2.52	
Knee prosthesis		0.88	1.28	2.26	
Laminectomy		0.88	1.35	2.46	
Spinal fusion		1.04	2.64	6.35	
Vascular surgery		0.90	1.72	4.34	

*As reported by the National Nosocomial Infections Surveillance System.[14] Surgical site infection rates for adjacent risk index groupings that were not significantly different are grouped together.

†Per 100 operations.

‡For cholecystectomy and colon operations, 1 point is subtracted from the NNIS risk score if a laparoscope is used. When no risk factors are present and a laparoscope is used, the score is designated "M" or −1.

§Use if laparoscope was found only to reduce the rate of surgical site infection (SSI) in those with NNIS risk index of 0; Rates of SSI for laparoscopic appendectomy and gastric surgery in patients with NNIS risk index of 1 or greater are similar to that found with open procedure.

CABG, coronary artery bypass graft.

TABLE 317-6	Interventional Maneuvers of Proven or Theoretical Benefit in Diminishing the Risk of Surgical Wound Infection

Maneuvers to Diminish Inoculation of Bacteria into Wound

Preoperative Factors

- Avoid preoperative antibiotic use (excluding surgical prophylaxis)
- Minimize preoperative hospitalization
- Treat remote sites of infection
- Avoid shaving or razor use at operative site
- Delay hair removal at operative site until time of surgery and remove hair (*only* if necessary) with electric clippers or depilatories
- Ensure timely administration (including appropriate dose) of prophylactic antibiotics
- Consider elimination of *Staphylococcus aureus* nasal carriage via decolonization techniques

Intraoperative and Postoperative Factors

- Carefully prepare patient's skin with povidone-iodine or chlorhexidine-containing solution
- Rigorously adhere to routine aseptic techniques
- Isolate clean from contaminated surgical fields (e.g., reglove and change instruments used to harvest saphenous vein before working in intrathoracic field)
- Maintain high flow of filtered air
- Consider laminar flow environment
- Redose prophylactic antibiotics in prolonged procedures
- Minimize operative personnel traffic
- Minimize flash sterilization of surgical instruments
- Minimize use of drains
- Bring drains, if used, through a separate stab wound

Maneuvers to Improve Host Containment of Contaminating Bacteria

Preoperative Factors

- Resolve malnutrition or obesity
- Discontinue cigarette smoking
- Maximize diabetes control

Intraoperative and Postoperative Factors

- Minimize dead space, devitalized tissue, and hematomas
- Consider use of supplemental oxygen therapy
- Maintain perioperative normothermia
- Maintain adequate hydration and nutrition
- Identify and minimize hyperglycemia (through 48 hours post-procedure)

clippers the morning of surgery versus 10.0% in those who underwent day-of-surgery shaving with a razor.[83] Although some recommendations advocate no preoperative hair removal,[21] there is minimal evidence to support an increased risk of wound infection with hair removal by clippers or depilatories on the morning of surgery as compared with no hair removal.[82] Infection at sites remote from the operative field is a host risk factor for postoperative infection that is potentially correctable prior to surgery.[84] Drains and intravascular devices should be removed as quickly as possible to avoid the risk of direct and hematogenous seeding of the operative site.

The second major class of prevention measures is directed toward improving host containment and elimination of bacteria that have circumvented the front line of defense and have been inoculated into the wound. Most authorities have emphasized that the single most important factor in preventing wound infection is surgical technique. Gentle handling of wound tissues, avoidance of dead space, devitalized tissues, and hematomas, and careful approximation of tissue planes are believed to be critical in maintaining an infection-free incision. Good surgical technique, along with minimizing hypothermia and the use of vasoconstrictive medications help to improve tissue perfusion and oxygenation, thereby improving the delivery and function of neutrophils. Prophylaxis with antimicrobial therapy is another essential component of SSI prevention which is highlighted in detail later in this chapter.

In colorectal surgery, active measures to maintain normothermia during surgery have been associated with a reduction in SSIs compared to patients allowed to experience routine mild perioperative hypothermia.[85] The role of hypoxia prevention, however, is somewhat unclear. In colorectal patients, administration of supplemental oxygen (fraction of inspired oxygen [F_{IO_2}] 80%) resulted in significantly lower SSI rates

(5.2% vs. 11.2% in those receiving 30% F_{IO_2}).[86] A second randomized, double-blind trial of patients undergoing major intra-abdominal surgical procedures randomized to receive either 80% or 35% F_{IO_2} intraoperatively, however, found that the incidence of infection was significantly *higher* in those patients who received the higher oxygen concentration (25.0% in the 80% F_{IO_2} group vs. 11.3% in the 35% F_{IO_2} group).[87] A third study, again in colorectal surgical patients, noted reduction in SSI risk with 80% F_{IO_2} (14.9% vs. 24.4% in the group receiving 30% F_{IO_2}).[88] Pooling the data from these three studies results in relative reduction in SSI of 24% when 80% F_{IO_2} is used.[89] Although this does not reach statistical significance, these data, when coupled with the pathophysiologic rationale for preventing hypoxia of the wound bed, suggest that use of supplemental oxygen may be beneficial.

Intensive glucose control via continuous insulin infusion (CII) targeted to maintain glucose levels less than 200 mg/dL during the perioperative period (lasting through the second post-operative day) has been shown to reduce SSI in cardiac surgery patients.[90] When compared in a study of more than 2,400 diabetic patients, intensive glucose control with CII led to a reduction in the incidence of deep wound infection in diabetic cardiac surgery patients from 2.0% to 0.8% ($P = .01$).[91] Although only studied in cardiac surgical patients, the pathophysiologic effects of hyperglycemia on wound healing and immune function should not differ for other patients. Thus, it is my opinion that the benefit of strict glucose control to prevent SSIs should translate to other surgical procedures. Avoiding malnourishment also may reduce the risk of postoperative infection.[92] Conversely, investigations of mechanisms to directly modify the host immune system (administration of granulocyte-macrophage colony stimulating factor,[93] exclusive use of autologous blood transfusions,[56] or administration of histamine type 2 [H_2] receptor antagonist),[94] are either too preliminary or too inconclusive to provide guidelines for clinical practice.

PERIOPERATIVE ANTIMICROBIAL PROPHYLAXIS

The in vivo interaction between inoculated bacteria and prophylactically administered antibiotic is one of the most important determinants of the fate of the wound. For example, without antibiotic prophylaxis the reported risk of developing a *S. aureus* SSI after cardiac surgery is 21% to 44%,[95,96] an incidence that approximates the frequency of skin/nares colonization with *S. aureus*. Over the past 20 years, the efficacy of antibiotic prophylaxis in clean surgery has been clearly established. The guiding principle of systemic antibiotic prophylaxis is the belief that antibiotics in the host tissues can augment natural immune defense mechanisms and help to kill bacteria that are inoculated into the wound. The rationale for the administration of oral antibiotics in colonic surgery differs in that, although some agents exhibit systemic absorption and penetrate into host tissues (e.g., erythromycin and metronidazole, but not neomycin), the primary goal in this setting is a reduction in potential pathogens among the normal gut flora at the time of surgery. Oral prophylaxis is generally combined with mechanical preparation of the bowel to reduce colonic flora.

Every effort should be made to ensure that adequate antibiotic levels are maintained above the minimum inhibitory concentration (MIC) of the pathogens of concern throughout the surgical procedure (Fig. 317-4). Although prolonged surgical procedures are associated with a higher infection rate, it is not clear whether this increased risk is inevitable or primarily attributable to the greater likelihood of there being low or undetectable tissue concentrations of antibiotics during long procedures. In cardiothoracic procedures in particular, the use of cardiopulmonary bypass can dramatically reduce serum vancomycin levels as a result of alterations in drug clearance and volume of distribution, potentially placing the wound at increased risk for infection.[97] In contrast, cephalosporin levels tend to fall at a slower rate during bypass periods. Understanding the pharmacokinetics of the various antimicrobials used in perioperative prophylaxis is therefore vital to ensure adequate antibiotic levels at the surgical wound site during the entire procedure.

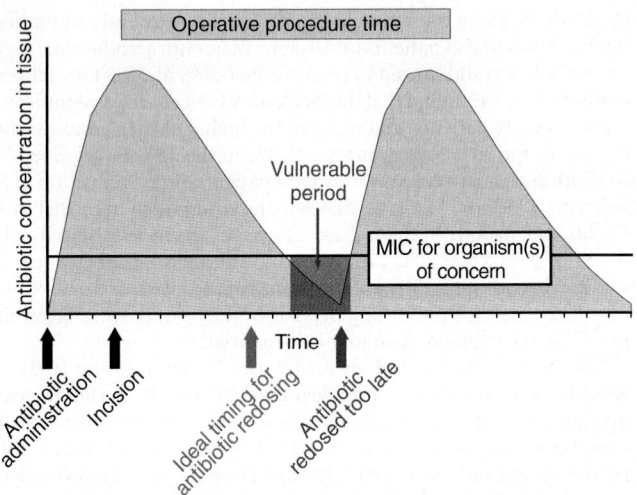

Figure 317-4 Tissue antibiotic concentration over time. Dynamics of tissue antibiotic concentration during the course of a surgical procedure. After an initial dose of antibiotic (noted on the far left of the x axis), tissue concentrations reach their peak rapidly, with a subsequent decline over time. As illustrated, the goal of antibiotic prophylaxis is to have tissue concentrations above the minimum inhibitory concentration (MIC) for the specific pathogens of concern at the time of the incision and throughout the procedure. Antibiotics should be redosed in prolonged procedures to prevent a period with tissue levels below the MIC (*blue arrow*). Failure to redose antibiotics appropriately (*red arrow*) may result in a period during which the wound is vulnerable.

The efficacy of perioperative prophylaxis in preventing SSI after many surgical procedures is unquestioned. Not only have the benefits of early antibiotic administration been duplicated by numerous investigators using different animal models, different pathogens, and different antibiotics, literally hundreds of clinical trials have verified the efficacy of perioperative antibiotics. Nevertheless, issues regarding the optimal choice, frequency, and duration of perioperative antibiotic prophylaxis remain.

Antimicrobial Prophylaxis: Drug Selection and Dosing

The CDC recommends that antibiotic prophylaxis be used for all clean-contaminated procedures and certain clean procedures (i.e., those in which intravascular prosthetic material or a prosthetic joint will be inserted and those in which an incisional or organ/space SSI would pose catastrophic risk).[21] Dirty or contaminated procedures usually do not require specific antimicrobial prophylaxis because patients undergoing these procedures are already on targeted antimicrobial therapy for established infections; however, if the treatment regimen does not adequately cover all pathogens of concern, consideration should be given to providing additional prophylaxis (i.e., in a procedure with a high incidence of MRSA SSI, additional prophylaxis with vancomycin may be warranted if the treatment regimen does not include coverage against MRSA). The use of antibiotic prophylaxis for all clean procedures, however, is less clear. For some clean, minimally-invasive procedures with low risk for SSI, the benefit of prophylaxis may be outweighed by the potential risks of antimicrobial therapy. In addition, adequately powered randomized clinical trials of antibiotic prophylaxis in such procedures are limited, because of the need for very large sample sizes to demonstrate a significant reduction in SSI.[98]

The keys in selecting an appropriate prophylactic antibiotic regimen include coverage against the expected endogenous flora at the surgical site (Table 317-7), consideration of patient allergies and antimicrobial costs, knowledge of the ecology of local nosocomial wound pathogens, consideration of antibiotic penetration into the specific surgical site tissue, and assurance of appropriate antibiotic dosing and delivery. Based on prospective studies of antibiotic prophylaxis, prophylactic

regimens have been recommended for a wide variety of surgical procedures (Table 317-8),[99-103] and many acceptable combinations of antibiotic prophylaxis have been used. Although only some regimens have been tested in controlled clinical trials, others with similar antimicrobial coverage and tissue penetration should provide similar protection, provided dosing guidelines are followed.

Based on their antibacterial spectrum and low incidence of allergy and side effects, the cephalosporins have traditionally been the drugs of choice for the vast majority of operative procedures. Even in clean-contaminated procedures such as hysterectomy and cholecystectomy, in which cephalosporins with improved in vitro activity against anaerobic bacteria are often advocated, most clinical studies indicate that cefazolin is equivalent in its prophylactic efficacy. For procedures in which anaerobic coverage is also justified (e.g., distal gastrointestinal tract, major head and neck, biliary, and gynecologic procedures) addition of metronidazole or use of second-generation cephalosporins with anaerobic activity (e.g., cefoxitin) are appropriate selections for prophylaxis.[21]

It should not be presumed that cephalosporins will remain the prophylactic agents of choice. Various classes of antibiotics have been shown to differ appreciably in activity against bacteria in the stationary phase of growth, postantibiotic effect, diffusibility into devitalized tissue or fibrin clots, resistance to enzymatic degradation, activity within abscesses, and penetration of and activity within neutrophils that may have ingested but be unable to kill wound bacteria. Each of these variables may affect the efficacy of an agent used for prophylaxis, and it is likely that preferred prophylactic regimens will change over time in response to an improved understanding of the pathophysiology of infection and to antimicrobial resistance among wound pathogens.

In particular, the emergence of CA-MRSA as a cause of SSI has clouded the issue of appropriate antimicrobial prophylaxis.[104] Current recommendations suggest consideration of using vancomycin as empiric therapy for treatment and prophylaxis of presumptive staphylococcal infection when the local rates of MRSA are high; however, the exact threshold at which vancomycin use should occur has not been clearly defined. Routine administration of vancomycin for surgical

TABLE 317-7	Typical Microbiologic Flora at Surgical Sites for Various Operative Procedures
Operation	*Likely Pathogens**
Placement of all grafts, prostheses, or implants	*Staphylococcus aureus,* CoNS
Cardiac	*S. aureus,* CoNS
Neurosurgery	*S. aureus,* CoNS
Breast	*S. aureus,* CoNS, streptococci
Ophthalmic	*S. aureus,* CoNS, streptococci, GNR
Orthopedic	*S. aureus,* CoNS, streptococci, GNR
Noncardiac thoracic	*S. aureus,* CoNS, *Streptococcus pneumoniae,* GNR
Vascular	*S. aureus,* CoNS
Appendectomy	GNR, anaerobes
Biliary tract	GNR, anaerobes
Colorectal	GNR, anaerobes
Gastroduodenal	GNR, streptococci, oropharyngeal anaerobes
Head and neck (with incision through oropharyngeal mucosa)	*S. aureus,* streptococci, oropharyngeal anaerobes
Obstetric and gynecologic	GNR, enterococci, group B streptococci, anaerobes
Urologic	GNR

*Staphylococci will be associated with surgical site infections following all types of operations.

CoNS, coagulase-negative staphylococci; GNR, gram-negative rods/bacilli.

Adapted from Mangram AJ, Horan TC, Pearson ML, et al. Guideline for prevention of surgical site infection, 1999. Hospital Infection Control Practices Advisory Committee. *Infect Control Hosp Epidemiol* 1999; 20:250-78; quiz 279-80.

TABLE 317-8	Summary of Antibiotic Prophylaxis Recommendations for the Most Commonly Performed Surgical Procedures
Procedure	**Antibiotic**
Cardiac (Prosthetic valve surgery, CABG, other open heart procedure, pacemaker and automated defibrillator placement)	Cefazolin 1-2 g Cefuroxime 1.5 g Vancomycin† 1 g
Colon	**Oral:** After appropriate diet and catharsis: Neomycin sulfate 1 g + erythromycin base 1 g orally at 1 PM, 2 PM, and 11 PM before 8 AM operation Neomycin sulfate 2 g + metronidazole 2 g 7 PM and 11 PM the day before 8 AM operation **IV:** Cefoxitin 1-2 g Ampicillin/sulbactam 3 g Ertapenem 1 g Cefazolin 1-2 g + metronidazole 500 mg Cefuroxime 1.5 g + metronidazole 500 mg
Total knee/hip arthroplasty	Cefazolin 1-2 g Cefuroxime 1.5 g Vancomycin† 1 g (If tourniquet used, drug should be infused prior to inflation).
Hysterectomy	Cefazolin 1-2 g Cefoxitin 1-2 g Cefuroxime 1.5 g Ampicillin/sulbactam 3 g
Vascular	Cefazolin 1-2 g Cefuroxime 1.5 g Vancomycin† 1 g
Neurosurgical (e.g. craniotomy, CSF shunt placement)	Cefazolin 1 g Vancomycin† 1 g
Timing of dose	Infusion started within 60 min (between 60-120 min if vancomycin or fluoroquinolone used) before incision. Redosing should occur in prolonged procedures. Recommended redosing intervals: Cefazolin—between 3-5 h after first dose, Cefuroxime—between 3-4 h after first dose Cefoxitin—between 2-3 h after first dose Metronidazole—between 6-8 h after first dose Vancomycin—between 6-12 h after first dose
Duration of prophylaxis	For most procedures, a single dose of prophylaxis is necessary. At most, duration should be 24 hr or less. Duration for cardiac procedures should be 48 hr or less.

Adapted from recommendations from the Surgical Care Improvement Project,[99] The Medical Letter (2006),[103] The Sanford Guide (2008),[100] the American Society of Health System Pharmacists (1999),[101] and the Surgical Infection Society (1993).[102] Antibiotics are recommended for IV dosing unless otherwise noted.

†Vancomycin use should be discouraged for routine prophylaxis unless patient is allergic to β-lactam antibiotics or the procedure involves implantation of prosthetic materials or devices at institutions with a high rate of infections caused by methicillin-resistant *Staphylococcus aureus* or methicillin-resistant coagulase negative staphylococci. In procedures in which gram-negative pathogens are likely (e.g., vascular surgery involving groin incisions, lower extremity vascular procedures, hysterectomy, or abdominal procedures), another agent with gram-negative activity should be used with vancomycin.

CABG, coronary artery bypass graft; CSF, cerebrospinal fluid.

prophylaxis has been a controversial proposal. A randomized trial of 855 cardiac surgical patients comparing routine use of vancomycin versus cefazolin for prophylaxis noted that, while the rate of MRSA SSI was higher in the cefazolin group, those who received vancomycin had a higher rate of methicillin-sensitive *S. aureus* SSI. Thus, there was no significant difference in overall SSI rates between the two groups.[105] An interrupted time series analysis of more than 6,000 cardiac surgery patients, however, found that in coronary artery bypass graft (CABG) patients, following a switch from cefazolin to vancomycin, the monthly

SSI rates decreased by 2.1 per 100 procedures, primarily due to a decrease in SSI due to vancomycin-sensitive pathogens (e.g., MRSA).[106] This decline was significant when compared to rates in patients undergoing valve replacement who had received routine prophylaxis with vancomycin during the entire study period, suggesting that other infection prevention interventions performed during the study period in both populations may not explain the reduction in the CABG patients.[106]

Practical limitations that may affect the use of vancomycin in surgery include its narrow spectrum of antimicrobial activity and the need for a slow rate of infusion. Furthermore, the growing prevalence of vancomycin-resistant enterococci and the emergence of vancomycin-resistant *S. aureus* (VRSA) raise concerns about potential adverse effects on the antimicrobial susceptibility of nosocomial pathogens induced by the selective pressure of surgical antibiotic prophylaxis.[107] Thus, as the prevalence of CA-MRSA increases, its role as a key agent of postsurgical infections will become more substantial, and use of vancomycin for routine surgical prophylaxis will have to be balanced against concerns for its inappropriate use.

A risk-based approach in which persons with specific risk factors for MRSA (e.g. history of recurrent furunculosis, prior MRSA infection, history of dialysis or recent health care exposure) may help limit vancomycin use to those at higher risk of developing MRSA SSI. The Society of Thoracic Surgeons recommends use of vancomycin with cefazolin in persons with a known history of MRSA colonization, those undergoing placement of a prosthetic valve or vascular graft, and those "susceptible to colonization" (e.g. hospitalized longer than 3 days, transfer from an inpatient facility, or on antibiotics at time of procedure).[108] CA-MRSA complicates these recommendations, however, because healthy patients with few of these traditional comorbidities and risk factors may be at increased risk of MRSA colonization and subsequent infection. Screening of patients for nasal carriage of MRSA prior to surgery followed by adaptation of prophylactic regimens to include anti-MRSA coverage in carriers (+/− decolonization) may be a reasonable strategy to address the growing issue of MRSA SSI.[109] Patients undergoing elective surgical procedures could be screened during the initial pre-operative evaluation, but clarifications of other issues related to screening (i.e., need for a second screening test to identify intermittent MRSA carriers, type of screening test to be utilized, and cost-effectiveness of screening in the pre-surgical population) must be determined.

For colorectal procedures, the following three approaches to antimicrobial prophylaxis have generally been used: (1) use of oral (often non-absorbable) agents; (2) use of IV agents, and (3) combination therapy using both types of agents.[99] Many surgeons use combination therapy, with the rationale to decrease intraluminal flora as well to provide adequate subcutaneous tissue concentrations. A meta-analysis of 13 studies examining the use of combination oral and IV prophylaxis versus IV prophylaxis alone in colorectal surgery noted a significant 49% risk reduction for SSI with the use of combination therapy.[110] Thus, it seems prudent to use both oral and IV agents for prophylaxis in colorectal surgical cases.

The use of higher doses of antibiotic is probably needed for obese patients. Following administration of a 1 g dose of cefazolin, tissue and serum concentrations of the antibiotic were significantly decreased in morbidly obese patients when compared to non-obese controls.[111] A higher (2 g) dose of cefazolin did provide tissue levels greater than the MIC for the most likely infecting pathogens. Another study of obese patients given 2 g doses of cefazolin, however, found therapeutic tissue levels of the drug in only 48% of persons with a body mass index (BMI) between 40 and 49, 29% in those with a BMI between 50 and 59, and 10% in those with a BMI 60 or higher, leading the authors to propose using continuous cefazolin administration in the morbidly obese patient to improve tissue concentrations.[112]

Antimicrobial Prophylaxis: Timing of Administration
Except in elective colonic surgical procedures in which oral antibiotics must be administered several hours before the procedure, the initial

dose of systemic antibiotics must be administered in a timely fashion so that antibiotic levels in the tissue at the time of the incision are adequate. Administration too early before or after the time of incision will result in suboptimal tissue levels and potentially increased risk of postoperative wound infection. Guidelines and studies vary somewhat on the exact timing, ranging from 2 hours to no more than 30 minutes before incision. The SCIP quality improvement project defines appropriately timed antibiotic prophylaxis as delivery of the antibiotic within 1 hour prior to incision, with the exception that vancomycin and the fluoroquinolones should be given within 2 hours prior to incision because of the need for a longer infusion time. This definition has become widely used as a metric that indicates delivery of standard, high-quality surgical care.[18]

Several large-scale studies have examined the relationship between the timing of delivery of antibiotic prophylaxis and the risk of SSI. The seminal study by Classen and colleagues noted that the risk of SSI was reduced when antibiotics were administered within 2 hours prior to incision (Fig. 317-5A).[11] More recently, the Trial to Reduce Antimicrobial Prophylaxis Errors (TRAPE) examined the association between SSI and timing of prophylaxis in cardiac, orthopaedic, and hysterectomy patients.[113] The TRAPE investigators found that SSI risk was lowest in those patients who received prophylaxis within 30 minutes (if given cephalosporins) or within 1 hour (if given vancomycin or a fluoroquinolone) prior to incision (Fig. 317-5B). Post-incision administration was associated with a significantly increased risk for SSI. These results have also been reproduced in a study of 1,922 patients undergoing total hip arthroplasty in which the rate of SSI was lowest in those who received antibiotics 1 to 30 minutes before incision.[114]

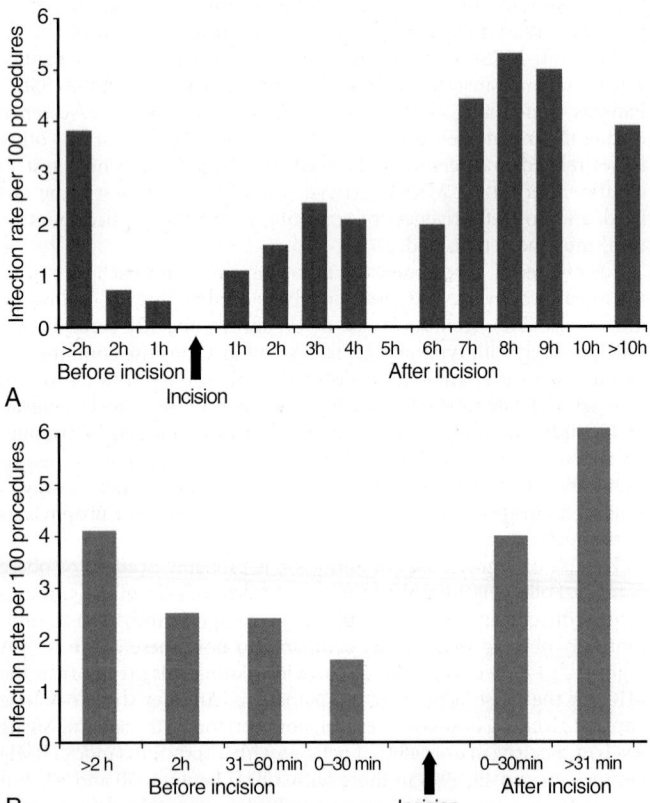

Figure 317-5 **Timing of administration and infection rate.** Relationship between timing of administration of prophylactic antibiotics and surgical site infection rate from two large studies. **A,** Data from 2,847 elective surgical patients (Classen 1992);[11] **B,** Data from 3,656 cardiac, orthopaedic and gynecologic surgical patients (Trial to Reduce Antimicrobial Prophylaxis Errors 2008).[113]

There also may be a threshold where, even though penetration into tissue for many drugs occurs in minutes, administration of antibiotic right before the incision may not provide enough time for tissue concentrations of the drug to reach the desired level at the time of incision. Weber and colleagues noted a twofold increased odds of SSI when cefuroxime prophylaxis was delivered less than 30 minutes before incision, as opposed to between 30 and 59 minutes pre-incision.[115] Curiously, when examined with more granularity, the risk was higher in those who received the antibiotic between 15 and 29 minutes versus those who received a dose between 0 and 14 minutes pre-incision. A study of vancomycin use in cardiac surgery patients found that prophylaxis was most effective when given between 16 and 60 minutes before incision (relative risk [RR] = 7.8 compared to receipt between 15 and 0 minutes pre-incision).[116] This may be explained by the need for an hour-long infusion of vancomycin to prevent infusion-related side effects, suggesting that a small proportion of the dose had been infused at the time of the incision. What is curious, however, is that those given a dose between 16 and 60 minutes pre-incision may not have had complete infusion of the drug dose (but perhaps enough to allow for adequate tissue penetration). The TRAPE study, however, did not note such an increase in risk if antibiotics were given "too close" to the incision. Thus, while the window of appropriate timing of surgical prophylaxis is narrowing, more investigation is needed into such nuances of the delivery of surgical prophylaxis.

Administration of prophylaxis in patients undergoing cesarean section has traditionally been held until after umbilical cord clamping to address concerns about delivery of drug to the neonate, which may mask signs of developing neonatal sepsis. Such a strategy, however, does not provide the mother with desired tissue concentrations of antibiotics at the time of incision. Two randomized trials have now shown that administration of prophylactic antibiotics prior to incision does not result in an increase in adverse neonatal outcomes (e.g., neonatal sepsis, sepsis workups, and admissions to the intensive care unit), indicating that provision of antibiotic prophylaxis in the hour before incision is acceptable.[117,118] For orthopedic procedures in which a tourniquet is used, full infusion of the drug should occur prior to tourniquet inflation.[99]

As critical as providing an appropriately timed initial dose of antibiotic is ensuring that tissue concentrations remain well above the MIC values of common pathogens during the entire procedure. To achieve this goal, antibiotics should also be re-administered during long surgical procedures,[119] as introduction of bacteria into the surgical wound occurs not only at the time of incision but continuously throughout the surgical procedure. In prolonged procedures or with antibiotics with short half-lives, patients may be inadequately protected if redosing is not routinely provided.[120]

Historically, it has proven to be more difficult to administer pre- and intraoperative antimicrobial prophylaxis at the optimal times than might be supposed. An analysis in 2001 of Medicare patients undergoing major surgical procedures for which antibiotic prophylaxis is recommended found that only 55.7% received an antibiotic within 1 hour prior to incision, while only 40.7% had prophylaxis discontinued at 24 hours after surgery.[18] Quality standards for antimicrobial prophylaxis in surgery recommend incorporating the administration of perioperative antimicrobial prophylaxis into the routine procedures executed within the operating room by either the anesthesiologist or the circulating nurse.[119] Some groups have also used the now-commonplace "time-out" prior to incision or computer-generated dosing reminders to ensure appropriate delivery of antibiotic prophylaxis.[121,122]

Antimicrobial Prophylaxis: Duration
In the early years of surgical prophylaxis, prolonged courses (7-10 days) of antibiotics seemed routine.[123] Over time, the benefit of prolonged courses of antimicrobials has been appropriately questioned, particularly due to pathophysiologic changes at the area of incision (i.e., coagulative necrosis, induced hemostasis via cautery of blood vessels) that likely limit the ability of antibiotics to reach the wound bed during the early postoperative period.[123]

A few studies have noted a benefit with prolonged prophylaxis in select subpopulations of patients, including those undergoing cesarean section,[124] major joint repair,[125] vascular surgery,[126] and colorectal surgery.[127] However, many more studies comparing short-course versus long-course prophylaxis have reflected no increase in infection rates among the short-course recipients. A systematic review of 28 randomized trials of single versus multiple doses of antimicrobial prophylaxis found no advantage of prolonged duration of prophylaxis in preventing SSI in a wide array of surgical procedures.[128] Prolonged antibiotic prophylaxis (>48 hours post-incision) has been significantly associated with an increased risk of acquiring an antibiotic-resistant pathogen.[129] A commonly espoused rationale for prolonging the duration of surgical prophylaxis following incision closure includes a desire to "cover" the wound while surgical drains remain in place or to "protect" against infection of central venous catheters (CVCs). However, a study in the United Kingdom found that prolonged prophylaxis until the patient's CVC was removed (vs. 3 doses of cefuroxime perioperatively) did not lead to a reduction in CVC colonization, a surrogate for CVC infection.[130]

The effectiveness of surgical prophylaxis is minimized after incision closure. Most guidelines for surgical prophylaxis recommend discontinuation of prophylactic antibiotics within 24 hours, a metric that also is part of the SCIP program and a marker of appropriate surgical care for an increasing number of quality and regulatory programs. For cardiac surgery, experts recommend continuing prophylaxis for 48 hours, based on concerns that more data are needed before uniformly recommending a shorter duration in this population.[131] Prompt discontinuation of prophylaxis does not impact the risk of developing SSI (as is the case with timely administration of antibiotics), but failure to do so contributes to unnecessary antimicrobial use and the subsequent problems related to such overuse.

Novel Methods of Antibiotic Prophylaxis

Newer methods for delivery of antimicrobial prophylaxis have expanded the available armamentarium for the prevention of SSIs. First introduced in 1939,[132] antibiotic-impregnated cement placed directly into the operative wound (as a local antimicrobial *brachytherapy*) is increasingly being used as a method of antibiotic prophylaxis and treatment, particularly in procedures involving the replacement of infected prosthetic joints. Brachytherapy uses powdered antibiotic mixed with a cement polymer (such as polymerized polymethylmethacrylate) to form a compound that may be directly applied onto prosthetic material or manufactured into beads (usually 3 to 10 mm in diameter) that are placed into the wound. Candidate antibiotics for use as brachytherapy must be available as a pharmaceutical-grade powder, must be heat stable (because of the exothermic reaction induced with polymerization), and must have an appropriate microbiologic spectrum of activity for the predominant pathogens at the operative site.[132] The aminoglycosides and vancomycin are the compounds most commonly used for brachytherapy; oxacillin and cefazolin have comparable elution characteristics but are less frequently used because of concerns regarding β-lactam allergy.

The majority of antibiotic elution occurs in the first days after implantation, but elution from impregnated cement has been detected years following surgery.[132,133] The use of antibiotic-impregnated cement (in conjunction with systemic prophylaxis) was significantly associated with a reduction in SSIs in studies from several large clinical registries in Europe.[134] Concerns remain, however, regarding routine use of this mode of prophylaxis because of possible adverse effects, such as allergic reactions.[135] Systemic absorption of antibiotic brachytherapy is also a concern because potentially high boluses of antibiotic may lead to toxicity. In one series of 14 subjects, 1 patient developed permanent and 2 others temporary high-frequency hearing loss following implantation of gentamicin-impregnated beads.[136] Renal failure attributed to impregnated cement, while rare, has also been reported.[137] Further studies into the systemic absorption, efficacy, and adverse effects of these brachytherapeutic compounds appear warranted.

Side Effects of Prophylaxis

Adverse effects of prophylaxis for the patient include allergic reactions ranging in severity from minor skin rashes to anaphylaxis. *Clostridium difficile*–associated diarrhea (CDAD) has been noted with several prophylactic agents, and in one study the rate of CDAD was 14.9 cases per 1000 in surgical patients who received antibiotic prophylaxis as their sole antibiotic exposure.[138,139] Another notable side effect is profound hypotension and flushing associated with vancomycin prophylaxis (the red-man syndrome), usually associated with rapid infusions of the antibiotic.[140]

The use of prophylactic antibiotics has consequences for the institution as well as the individual patient. Antibiotic use, and specifically prophylactic use, has been shown to have a critical role in the selection of antibiotic-resistant bacteria to become the dominant colonizing flora as well as nosocomial pathogens of hospitalized patients.[141] At least two mechanisms for this process have been documented. First, the antibiotic-resistant flora may be endemic within the institution and transferred to the patient during the course of hospitalization.[142] Second, a small population of antibiotic-resistant bacteria that are part of the patient's endogenous flora at the time of hospitalization may emerge under the selective pressure of perioperative prophylaxis to become the dominant flora.[143] The increasing prevalence of MRSA and resistant gram-negative bacteria has profound implications for a continued or expanded role of prophylactic antibiotics in surgery. In view of the improvement in overall surgical wound infection rates over recent decades, the consensus is that prophylactic antibiotics are clearly worth this potential side effect.

Resistance to Perioperative Antibiotics

The success of prophylaxis in clean surgery correlates directly with the susceptibility of bacteria to the antibiotic in vitro, with some failures of prophylaxis attributable to bacterial resistance.[144] Because cephalosporins have become the mainstay of prophylaxis, the increasing prevalence of cephalosporin-resistant pathogens has important implications for prophylaxis. Some *S. aureus* SSIs are caused by strains reported by the clinical laboratory to be cephalosporin susceptible, but that produce the type A variant of staphylococcal β-lactamase and can degrade less stable cephalosporins such as cefazolin relatively rapidly.[145] Studies involving a guinea pig model of wound infection and isogeneic strains of *S. aureus* that differ only in the presence or absence of the gene encoding type A staphylococcal β-lactamase have shown that, when cefazolin is administered as prophylaxis, the number of CFU required to establish infection 50% of the time (ID_{50}) is significantly smaller for the β-lactamase-producing isolate than for the non-β-lactamase-producing isolate.[146] A subpopulation of *S. aureus* belonging to phage group 94/96 and characterized by borderline susceptibility to oxacillin, the presence of a unique 17.2-kb plasmid, and the production of large quantities of type A staphylococcal β-lactamase has been associated with deep wound infections among surgical patients receiving cefazolin as perioperative prophylaxis.[147] β-Lactamase-mediated degradation of cephalosporins in vivo appears to enable a bacterium to survive beyond the time of its initial lodgment in antibiotic-containing tissues, ultimately contributing to the development of a wound infection.[145]

In addition, over recent years several multiple antibiotic-resistant bacteria have become important pathogens in the post-surgical patient, including strains of *Enterococcus faecium* resistant to vancomycin, ampicillin, gentamicin or a combination of the three; *S. aureus* resistant to β-lactams and the quinolones; and *Escherichia coli* and *Klebsiella* isolates that are resistant to cefotaxime and ceftazidime.[148,149] The arrival of VRSA[107] portends an ominous change in the complexity of the ecology of nosocomial infections.

Cost-Benefit of Prophylaxis

Prophylactic antibiotics add some cost to the routine care of surgical patients. In major surgical centers, the perioperative use of antibiotics may represent a large portion of the pharmacy's expenditures for antibiotics, and surgeons may be encouraged to reduce or eliminate antibiotics given for prophylaxis in certain settings. For example, in carotid endarterectomy and cholecystectomy, infections develop only infrequently, are seldom life threatening, and may cost more to prevent than to treat. However, it seems inappropriate to evaluate antibiotic use on the basis of cost alone. When prophylaxis or a particular form of prophylaxis offers a clear advantage to the patient, the health care system should advocate the better treatment without consideration of its cost. Moreover, an analysis of the cost of prophylactic antibiotics can be complicated. Not only the cost of the antibiotic per se but the cost of preparing, transporting, and administering multiple doses of antibiotic must be included. Perhaps of more importance, the cost in terms of mortality, morbidity, and resources of managing wound infections that develop when using inadequate prophylaxis must be considered.[150]

SURGICAL SITE INFECTION SURVEILLANCE

A key component in the prevention of SSIs is the establishment of a surveillance infrastructure to regularly detect and monitor rates of procedure-specific infections, to define the changing ecology of resistant pathogens that cause surgical infections, and to provide accurate analysis of the pervading antimicrobial sensitivity patterns in each specific institution to allow for tailoring of prophylactic regimens. Adequate surveillance for postsurgical infections with comparisons of infection rates to national benchmarks also allows for continued evaluation and assessment of the quality of an individual hospital's prevention strategies. In order to allow such comparisons, such surveillance must utilize standardized infection definitions, such as those used by the CDC's National Healthcare Safety Network (Table 317-9). Studies of risk factors for SSI as well as evaluations of interventions to reduce post-surgical infections use a wide array of outcome definitions, such as purulence at the incision site with a positive wound culture or attending physician diagnosis of wound infection. Thus, care must be taken when assessing the literature and comparing the results of different studies, as the outcome of interest may vary considerably.[151] The presence of purulence within a surgical incision generally serves as initial evidence of a SSI, but culture results of surgical wounds or exudates should not be used solely as a guide to the presence or absence of infection. Surveillance systems should also utilize the input of representatives with surgical, infectious diseases, and hospital epidemiology expertise in the analysis and evaluation of data.

In health care settings associated with a high volume of surgical procedures, surgical wound isolates should be maintained, if possible, for several weeks after isolation. Clusters or outbreaks of SSIs caused by a common pathogen are usually identified retrospectively, and the availability of infecting pathogens for pulsed-field gel electrophoresis or another means of molecular typing may be instrumental in identifying and eliminating the cause of the outbreak.

Highlighted by the landmark SENIC project, maintaining and publicizing surgeon-specific infection rates may be used to indirectly decrease SSI rates.[152] Such data may identify unsuspected problems among the surgical staff or may encourage individual surgeons to rigorously adhere to standards of perioperative aseptic techniques. If such a program is used, it is vital that any analysis include an assessment of procedure-specific infection rates. Wide differences in infection rates exist among surgical procedures, even among those procedures within the same surgical subspecialty and category of bacterial contamination. For example, in vascular surgery, infection rates after carotid endarterectomy are exceedingly low (< 0.1%). In contrast, bypass grafting in the femoral-popliteal area may be associated with

an infection rate of 2% to 3% despite the fact that both procedures are clean and may be performed by the same vascular surgeons. Other important variables such as the incidence of underlying patient risk factors must also be considered when comparing infection rates among surgeons.

Surveillance systems for postsurgical infections will face growing challenges in the future, such as the migration of surgical procedures to the outpatient arena and the growing push to decrease lengths of hospital stay with earlier discharge postsurgery. Sands and colleagues noted that 84% of SSIs occurred following hospital discharge and would, therefore, have been missed with traditional hospital-based surveillance.[153] Methods to improve detection of surgical site infections that arise post-discharge, including direct examination of wounds during follow-up visits, patient and practitioner surveys, and computerized queries of outpatient diagnostic codes and antibiotic prescriptions, have met with limited success and concerns regarding costs and the ability to generalize results.[142,154,155] Any method of postdischarge surveillance must address these concerns and accommodate the unique attributes of each specific hospital and patient population.

TABLE 317-9	National Healthcare Safety Network (NHSN) Definitions for Surgical Site Infections
Infection Type	**Definition**
Soft Tissue Infection	
Superficial	Infections involving only skin and subcutaneous tissue of the incision occurring within 30 days after the procedure with one or more of the following: • Purulent drainage from the incision; • Positive culture from superficial incision; • Pain or tenderness, swelling, erythema, or heat at surgical wound that has been deliberately opened by a surgeon; *or* • Diagnosis by a surgeon or attending physician.
Deep	Infections involving deep soft tissue (fascia/muscle layers) occurring within 30 days (or up to 1 yr if implant* is placed during surgery) after the procedure with one of the following: • Purulent drainage from deep incision but not from organ space; • Spontaneous dehiscence or deliberate opening by a surgeon with a positive incision culture *or*, if not cultured, has the presence of fever or local pain; • Abscess involving a deep incision found by direct exam, radiologic exam or during reoperation; *or* • Diagnosis by a surgeon or attending physician.
Organ/Space	Infections that involve any part of the body opened or manipulated during the operative procedure, excluding skin incision/fascia/muscle layers, within 30 days after procedure (or up to 1 year if implant is placed) with one of the following: • Purulent drainage from a drain that is placed through a stab wound into the organ/space; • Positive culture growth of a specimen of tissue or fluid aseptically obtained during operation or aspiration; • Evidence of infection during surgical procedure or by radiologic or histopathologic examination; *or* • Diagnosis by a surgeon or attending physician.

*Implant defined as a nonhuman-derived object, material, or tissue (e.g., prosthetic heart valve, nonhuman vascular graft, or hip prosthesis) that is permanently placed in a patient during an operative procedure.

REFERENCES

1. McDermott W, Rogers DE. Social ramifications of control of microbial disease. *Johns Hopkins Med J.* 1982;151:302-312.
2. Finland M. Antibacterial agents: Uses and abuses in treatment and prophylaxis. *R I Med J.* 1960;43:499-504 passim.
3. Culbertson WR, Altemeier WA, Gonzalez LL, et al. Studies on the epidemiology of postoperative infection of clean operative wounds. *Ann Surg.* 1961;154:599-610.
4. Howe CW, Marston AT. A study on sources of postoperative staphylococcal infection. *Surg Gynecol Obstet.* 1962;115:266-275.
5. Burke JF. Identification of the sources of Staphylococci contaminating the surgical wound during operation. *Ann Surg.* 1963;158:898-904.
6. Howes EL. Prevention of wound infection by the injection of nontoxic antibacterial substances. *Ann Surg.* 1946;124:268-276.

7. Miles AA, Miles EM, Burke J. The value and duration of defence reactions of the skin to the primary lodgement of bacteria. *Br J Exp Pathol.* 1957;38:79-96.
8. Burke JF. The effective period of preventive antibiotic action in experimental incisions and dermal lesions. *Surgery.* 1961;50: 161-168.
9. Sanchez-Ubeda R, Fernand E, Rousselot LM. Complication rate in general surgical cases; The value of penicillin and streptomycin as postoperative prophylaxis; a study of 511 cases. *N Engl J Med.* 1958;259:1045-1050.
10. Johnstone FR. An assessment of prophylactic antibiotics in general surgery. *Surg Gynecol Obstet.* 1963;116:1-10.
11. Classen DC, Evans RS, Pestotnik SL, et al. The timing of prophylactic administration of antibiotics and the risk of surgical-wound infection. *N Engl J Med.* 1992;326:281-286.
12. Warren MD, Kernodle DS, Kaiser AB. Correlation of in-vitro parameters of antimicrobial activity with prophylactic efficacy in an intradermal model of Staphylococcus aureus infection. *J Antimicrob Chemother.* 1991;28:731-740.
13. National Center for Health Statistics. National Hospital Discharge Survey: 2005 Annual Summary with Detailed Diagnosis and Procedure Data. Available at http://www.cdc.gov/nchs/data/series/sr_13/sr13_165.pdf. Accessed on August 15, 2008.
14. National Nosocomial Infections Surveillance (NNIS) System Report, data summary from January 1992 through June 2004, issued October 2004. *Am J Infect Control.* 2004;32:470-485.
15. Martone WJ, Nichols RL. Recognition, prevention, surveillance, and management of surgical site infections: Introduction to the problem and symposium overview. *Clin Infect Dis.* 2001; 33(suppl 2):S67-S68.
16. Kirkland KB, Briggs JP, Trivette SL, et al. The impact of surgical-site infections in the 1990s: Attributable mortality, excess length of hospitalization, and extra costs. *Infect Control Hosp Epidemiol.* 1999;20:725-730.
17. Engemann JJ, Carmeli Y, Cosgrove SE, et al. Adverse clinical and economic outcomes attributable to methicillin resistance among patients with Staphylococcus aureus surgical site infection. *Clin Infect Dis.* 2003;36:592-598.
18. Bratzler DW, Hunt DR. The surgical infection prevention and surgical care improvement projects: National initiatives to improve outcomes for patients having surgery. *Clin Infect Dis.* 2006;43:322-330.
19. Aglietti P, Salvati EA, Wilson PD Jr, et al. Effect of a surgical horizontal unidirectional filtered air flow unit on wound bacterial contamination and wound healing. *Clin Orthop Relat Res.* 1974:99-104.
20. Houang ET, Ahmet Z. Intraoperative wound contamination during abdominal hysterectomy. *J Hosp Infect.* 1991;19:181-189.
21. Mangram AJ, Horan TC, Pearson ML, et al. Guideline for prevention of surgical site infection, 1999. Hospital Infection Control Practices Advisory Committee. *Infect Control Hosp Epidemiol.* 1999;20:250-278; quiz 279-280.
22. Hidron AI, Edwards JR, Patel J, et al. NHSN annual update: antimicrobial-resistant pathogens associated with healthcare-associated infections: annual summary of data reported to the National Healthcare Safety Network at the Centers for Disease Control and Prevention, 2006-2007. *Infect Control Hosp Epidemiol.* 2008;29:996-1011.
23. Anderson DJ, Sexton DJ, Kanafani ZA, et al. Severe surgical site infection in community hospitals: Epidemiology, key procedures, and the changing prevalence of methicillin-resistant Staphylococcus aureus. *Infect Control Hosp Epidemiol.* 2007; 28:1047-1053.
24. Perl TM, Cullen JJ, Wenzel RP, et al. Intranasal mupirocin to prevent postoperative Staphylococcus aureus infections. *N Engl J Med.* 2002;346:1871-1877.
25. Postlethwaite RW. Principles of operative surgery: Antisepsis, technique, sutures, and drains. In: Sabiston DC, ed. *Davis-Christopher Textbook of Surgery.* Philadelphia: WB Saunders; 1981:322.
26. Schaffner W, Lefkowitz LB Jr, Goodman JS, et al. Hospital outbreak of infections with Group A streptococci traced to an asymptomatic anal carrier. *N Engl J Med.* 1969;280:1224-1225.
27. Stamm WE, Feeley JC, Facklam RR. Wound infections due to group A streptococcus traced to a vaginal carrier. *J Infect Dis.* 1978;138:287-292.
28. Parry MF, Grant B, Yukna M, et al. Candida osteomyelitis and diskitis after spinal surgery: An outbreak that implicates artificial nail use. *Clin Infect Dis.* 2001;32:352-357.
29. Bennett SN, McNeil MM, Bland LA, et al. Postoperative infections traced to contamination of an intravenous anesthetic, propofol. *N Engl J Med.* 1995;333:147-154.
30. Carlsson AK, Lidgren L, Lindberg L. Prophylactic antibiotics against early and late deep infections after total hip replacements. *Acta Orthop Scand.* 1977;48:405-410.
31. Zimmerli W, Waldvogel FA, Vaudaux P, et al. Pathogenesis of foreign body infection: Description and characteristics of an animal model. *J Infect Dis.* 1982;146:487-497.
32. Arbeit RD, Dunn RM. Expression of capsular polysaccharide during experimental focal infection with Staphylococcus aureus. *J Infect Dis.* 1987;156:947-952.
33. Kaiser AB, Kernodle DS, Parker RA. Low-inoculum model of surgical wound infection. *J Infect Dis.* 1992;166:393-399.
34. Patti JM, Jonsson H, Guss B, et al. Molecular characterization and expression of a gene encoding a Staphylococcus aureus collagen adhesin. *J Biol Chem.* 1992;267:4766-7472.
35. Paulsson M, Ljungh A, Wadstrom T. Rapid identification of fibronectin, vitronectin, laminin, and collagen cell surface binding proteins on coagulase-negative staphylococci by particle agglutination assays. *J Clin Microbiol.* 1992;30:2006-2012.
36. Froman G, Switalski LM, Speziale P, et al. Isolation and characterization of a fibronectin receptor from Staphylococcus aureus. *J Biol Chem.* 1987;262:6564-6571.
37. Menzies BE, Kourteva Y, Kaiser AB, et al. Inhibition of staphylococcal wound infection and potentiation of antibiotic prophylaxis by a recombinant fragment of the fibronectin-binding protein of Staphylococcus aureus. *J Infect Dis.* 2002;185:937-943.
38. Rogolsky M. Nonenteric toxins of Staphylococcus aureus. *Microbiol Rev.* 1979;43:320-360.
39. Dossett JH, Kronvall G, Williams RC Jr, et al. Antiphagocytic effects of staphylococcal protein A. *J Immunol.* 1969;103:1405-1410.
40. Weinstein WM, Onderdonk AB, Bartlett JG, et al. Experimental intra-abdominal abscesses in rats: Development of an experimental model. *Infect Immun.* 1974;10:1250-1255.
41. Onderdonk AB, Bartlett JG, Louie T, et al. Microbial synergy in experimental intra-abdominal abscess. *Infect Immun.* 1976;13: 22-26.
42. Onderdonk AB, Markham RB, Zaleznik DF, et al. Evidence for T cell-dependent immunity to Bacteroides fragilis in an intraabdominal abscess model. *J Clin Invest.* 1982;69:9-16.
43. Dye ES, Kapral FA. Partial characterization of a bactericidal system in staphylococcal abscesses. *Infect Immun.* 1980;30:198-203.
44. Weinrauch Y, Elsbach P, Madsen LM, et al. The potent anti-*Staphylococcus aureus* activity of a sterile rabbit inflammatory fluid is due to a 14-kD phospholipase A2. *J Clin Invest.* 1996;97:250-257.
45. Elek SD, Conen PE. The virulence of Staphylococcus pyogenes for man: A study of the problems of wound infection. *Br J Exp Pathol.* 1958;38:573-586.
46. McGeehan D, Hunt D, Chaudhuri A, et al. An experimental study of the relationship between synergistic wound sepsis and suture materials. *Br J Surg.* 1980;67:636-638.
47. Soballe PW, Nimbkar NV, Hayward I, et al. Electric cautery lowers the contamination threshold for infection of laparotomies. *Am J Surg.* 1998;175:263-266.
48. Kumagai SG, Rosales RF, Hunter GC, et al. Effects of electrocautery on midline laparotomy wound infection. *Am J Surg.* 1991;162:620-622; discussion 622-623.
49. Yamada Y, Hefter K, Burke JF, et al. An in vitro model of the wound microenvironment: Local phagocytic cell abnormalities associated with in situ complement activation. *J Infect Dis.* 1987;155:998-1004.
50. El-Maallem H, Fletcher J. Effects of surgery on neutrophil granulocyte function. *Infect Immun.* 1981;32:38-41.
51. Bamberger DM, Herndon BL. Bactericidal capacity of neutrophils in rabbits with experimental acute and chronic abscesses. *J Infect Dis.* 1990;162:186-192.
52. Cheadle WG, Hershman MJ, Wellhausen SR, et al. HLA-DR antigen expression on peripheral blood monocytes correlates with surgical infection. *Am J Surg.* 1991;161:639-645.
53. Hensler T, Hecker H, Heeg K, et al. Distinct mechanisms of immunosuppression as a consequence of major surgery. *Infect Immun.* 1997;65:2283-2291.
54. Clardy CW, Edwards KM, Gay JC. Increased susceptibility to infection in hypothermic children: Possible role of acquired neutrophil dysfunction. *Pediatr Infect Dis.* 1985;4:379-782.
55. Hopf HW, Hunt TK, West JM, et al. Wound tissue oxygen tension predicts the risk of wound infection in surgical patients. *Arch Surg.* 1997;132:997-1004; discussion 1005.
56. Vamvakas EC, Moore SB. Blood transfusion and postoperative septic complications. *Transfusion.* 1994;34:714-727.
57. Jensen LS, Hokland M, Nielsen HJ. A randomized controlled study of the effect of bedside leucocyte depletion on the immunosuppressive effect of whole blood transfusion in patients undergoing elective colorectal surgery. *Br J Surg.* 1996;83: 973-977.
58. Vamvakas EC. Transfusion-associated cancer recurrence and postoperative infection: Meta-analysis of randomized, controlled clinical trials. *Transfusion.* 1996;36:175-186.
59. Tarnok A, Schneider P. Pediatric cardiac surgery with cardiopulmonary bypass: Pathways contributing to transient systemic immune suppression. *Shock.* 2001;16(suppl 1):24-32.
60. Silva J Jr, Hoeksema H, Fekety FR Jr. Transient defects in phagocytic functions during cardiopulmonary bypass. *J Thorac Cardiovasc Surg.* 1974;67:175-183.
61. Parker DJ, Cantrell JW, Karp RB, et al. Changes in serum complement and immunoglobulins following cardiopulmonary bypass. *Surgery.* 1972;71:824-827.
62. Subramanian VA, Gay WA Jr, Dineen PA. Effect of cardiopulmonary bypass on in vivo clearance of live Klebsiella aerogens. *Surg Forum.* 1977;28:255-257.
63. Vaudaux P, Grau GE, Huggler E, et al. Contribution of tumor necrosis factor to host defense against staphylococci in a guinea pig model of foreign body infections. *J Infect Dis.* 1992;166: 58-64.
64. Rotstein OD, Kao J. Prevention of intra-abdominal abscesses by fibrinolysis using recombinant tissue plasminogen activator. *J Infect Dis.* 1988;158:766-772.
65. Talbot TR. Diabetes mellitus and cardiothoracic surgical site infections. *Am J Infect Control.* 2005;33:353-359.
66. Gibbs J, Cull W, Henderson W, et al. Preoperative serum albumin level as a predictor of operative mortality and morbidity: Results from the National VA Surgical Risk Study. *Arch Surg.* 1999;134:36-42.
67. Bamgbade OA, Rutter TW, Nafiu OO, et al. Postoperative complications in obese and nonobese patients. *World J Surg.* 2007;31:556-560; discussion 561.
68. Konishi T, Watanabe T, Kishimoto J, et al. Elective colon and rectal surgery differ in risk factors for wound infection: Results of prospective surveillance. *Ann Surg.* 2006;244:758-763.
69. Busti AJ, Hooper JS, Amaya CJ, et al. Effects of perioperative antiinflammatory and immunomodulating therapy on surgical wound healing. *Pharmacotherapy.* 2005;25:1566-1591.
70. Myles PS, Iacono GA, Hunt JO, et al. Risk of respiratory complications and wound infection in patients undergoing ambulatory surgery: Smokers versus nonsmokers. *Anesthesiology.* 2002; 97:842-847.
71. Latham R, Lancaster AD, Covington JF, et al. The association of diabetes and glucose control with surgical-site infections among cardiothoracic surgery patients. *Infect Control Hosp Epidemiol.* 2001;22:607-612.
72. Kaye KS, Schmit K, Pieper C, et al. The effect of increasing age on the risk of surgical site infection. *J Infect Dis.* 2005;191: 1056-1062.
73. Carlo A. The new era of flash sterilization. *AORN J.* 2007;86:58-68; quiz 69-72.
74. Dalstrom DJ, Venkatarayappa I, Manternach AL, et al. Time-dependent contamination of opened sterile operating-room trays. *J Bone Joint Surg Am.* 2008;90:1022-1025.
75. Pryor F, Messmer PR. The effect of traffic patterns in the OR on surgical site infections. *AORN J.* 1998;68:649-660.
76. Haley RW, Culver DH, Morgan WM, et al. Identifying patients at high risk of surgical wound infection. A simple multivariate index of patient susceptibility and wound contamination. *Am J Epidemiol.* 1985;121:206-215.
77. Culver DH, Horan TC, Gaynes RP, et al. Surgical wound infection rates by wound class, operative procedure, and patient risk index. National Nosocomial Infections Surveillance System. *Am J Med.* 1991;91:152S-157S.
78. Emori TG, Culver DH, Horan TC, et al. National nosocomial infections surveillance system (NNIS): Description of surveillance methods. *Am J Infect Control.* 1991;19:19-35.
79. Owens WD, Felts JA, Spitznagel EL Jr. ASA physical status classifications: A study of consistency of ratings. *Anesthesiology.* 1978;49:239-243.
80. Gaynes RP. Surgical-site infections and the NNIS SSI Risk Index: Room for improvement. *Infect Control Hosp Epidemiol.* 2000;21:184-185.
81. Webster J, Osborne S. Preoperative bathing or showering with skin antiseptics to prevent surgical site infection. Cochrane Database Syst Rev 2006(2):CD004985.
82. Kjonniksen I, Andersen BM, Sondenaa VG, et al. Preoperative hair removal—a systematic literature review. *AORN J.* 2002;75: 928-938, 940.
83. Alexander JW, Fischer JE, Boyajian M, et al. The influence of hair-removal methods on wound infections. *Arch Surg.* 1983;118:347-352.
84. Valentine RJ, Weigelt JA, Dryer D, et al. Effect of remote infections on clean wound infection rates. *Am J Infect Control.* 1986;14:64-67.
85. Kurz A, Sessler DI, Lenhardt R. Perioperative normothermia to reduce the incidence of surgical-wound infection and shorten hospitalization. Study of Wound Infection and Temperature Group. *N Engl J Med.* 1996;334:1209-1215.
86. Greif R, Akca O, Horn EP, et al. Supplemental perioperative oxygen to reduce the incidence of surgical-wound infection. Outcomes Research Group. *N Engl J Med.* 2000;342:161-167.
87. Pryor KO, Fahey TJ 3rd, Lien CA, et al. Surgical site infection and the routine use of perioperative hyperoxia in a general surgical population: A randomized controlled trial. *JAMA.* 2004;291:79-87.
88. Belda FJ, Aguilera L, Garcia de la Asuncion J, et al. Supplemental perioperative oxygen and the risk of surgical wound infection: A randomized controlled trial. *JAMA.* 2005;294:2035-2042.
89. Dellinger EP. Increasing inspired oxygen to decrease surgical site infection: Time to shift the quality improvement research paradigm. *JAMA.* 2005;294:2091-2092.
90. Zerr KJ, Furnary AP, Grunkemeier GL, et al. Glucose control lowers the risk of wound infection in diabetics after open heart operations. *Ann Thorac Surg.* 1997;63:356-361.
91. Furnary AP, Zerr KJ, Grunkemeier GL, et al. Continuous intravenous insulin infusion reduces the incidence of deep sternal wound infection in diabetic patients after cardiac surgical procedures. *Ann Thorac Surg.* 1999;67:352-360; discussion 360-362.
92. Klein JD, Hey LA, Yu CS, et al. Perioperative nutrition and postoperative complications in patients undergoing spinal surgery. *Spine.* 1996;21:2676-2682.
93. Meropol NJ, Wood DE, Nemunaitis J, et al. Randomized, placebo-controlled, multicenter trial of granulocyte-macrophage colony-stimulating factor as infection prophylaxis in oncologic surgery. Leukine Surgical Prophylaxis Research Group. *J Clin Oncol.* 1998;16:1167-1173.
94. Moesgaard F, Jensen LS, Christiansen PM, et al. The effect of ranitidine on postoperative infectious complications following emergency colorectal surgery: A randomized, placebo-controlled, double-blind trial. *Inflamm Res.* 1998;47:12-17.

95. Fong IW, Baker CB, McKee DC. The value of prophylactic antibiotics in aorta-coronary bypass operations: A double-blind randomized trial. *J Thorac Cardiovasc Surg.* 1979;78:908-913.

96. Austin TW, Coles JC, Burnett R, et al. Aortocoronary bypass procedures and sternotomy infections: A study of antistaphylococcal prophylaxis. *Can J Surg.* 1980;23:483-485.

97. Ortega GM, Marti-Bonmati E, Guevara SJ, et al. Alteration of vancomycin pharmacokinetics during cardiopulmonary bypass in patients undergoing cardiac surgery. *Am J Health Syst Pharm.* 2003;60:260-265.

98. Sanchez-Manuel FJ, Lozano-Garcia J, Seco-Gil JL. Antibiotic prophylaxis for hernia repair. *Cochrane Database Syst Rev* 2007(3):CD003769.

99. Bratzler DW, Houck PM. Antimicrobial prophylaxis for surgery: An advisory statement from the National Surgical Infection Prevention Project. *Clin Infect Dis.* 2004;38:1706-1715.

100. Gilbert DN, Moellering RC Jr, Eliopoulos GM, et al. *The Sanford Guide to Antimicrobial Therapy.* Sperryville, VA: Antimicrobial Therapy Inc.; 2008.

101. ASHP Therapeutic Guidelines on Antimicrobial Prophylaxis in Surgery. American Society of Health-System Pharmacists. *Am J Health Syst Pharm.* 1999;56:1839-1888.

102. Page CP, Bohnen JM, Fletcher JR, et al. Antimicrobial prophylaxis for surgical wounds. Guidelines for clinical care. *Arch Surg.* 1993;128:79-88.

103. Antimicrobial prophylaxis for surgery. *Treat Guidel Med Lett.* 2006;4:83-88.

104. Kourbatova EV, Halvosa JS, King MD, et al. Emergence of community-associated methicillin-resistant Staphylococcus aureus USA 300 clone as a cause of health care-associated infections among patients with prosthetic joint infections. *Am J Infect Control.* 2005;33:385-391.

105. Finkelstein R, Rabino G, Mashiah T, et al. Vancomycin versus cefazolin prophylaxis for cardiac surgery in the setting of a high prevalence of methicillin-resistant staphylococcal infections. *J Thorac Cardiovasc Surg.* 2002;123:326-332.

106. Garey KW, Lai D, Dao-Tran TK, et al. Interrupted time series analysis of vancomycin compared to cefuroxime for surgical prophylaxis in patients undergoing cardiac surgery. *Antimicrob Agents Chemother.* 2008;52:446-451.

107. Chang S, Sievert DM, Hageman JC, et al. Infection with vancomycin-resistant Staphylococcus aureus containing the vanA resistance gene. *N Engl J Med.* 2003;348:1342-1347.

108. Engelman R, Shahian D, Shemin R, et al. The Society of Thoracic Surgeons practice guideline series: Antibiotic prophylaxis in cardiac surgery, part II: Antibiotic choice. *Ann Thorac Surg.* 2007;83:1569-1576.

109. Jog S, Cunningham R, Cooper S, et al. Impact of preoperative screening for meticillin-resistant Staphylococcus aureus by real-time polymerase chain reaction in patients undergoing cardiac surgery. *J Hosp Infect.* 2008;69:124-130.

110. Lewis RT. Oral versus systemic antibiotic prophylaxis in elective colon surgery: A randomized study and meta-analysis send a message from the 1990s. *Can J Surg.* 2002;45:173-180.

111. Forse RA, Karam B, MacLean LD, et al. Antibiotic prophylaxis for surgery in morbidly obese patients. *Surgery.* 1989;106:750-756; discussion 756-775.

112. Edmiston CE, Krepel C, Kelly H, et al. Perioperative antibiotic prophylaxis in the gastric bypass patient: Do we achieve therapeutic levels? *Surgery.* 2004;136:738-747.

113. Steinberg JP, Braun BI, Hellinger WC, et al. Timing of antimicrobial prophylaxis and the risk of surgical site infections: Results from the Trial to Reduce Antimicrobial Prophylaxis Errors (TRAPE). *Arch Surg.* (in press). 2009.

114. van Kasteren ME, Mannien J, Ott A, et al. Antibiotic prophylaxis and the risk of surgical site infections following total hip arthroplasty: Timely administration is the most important factor. *Clin Infect Dis.* 2007;44:921-927.

115. Weber WP, Marti WR, Zwahlen M, et al. The timing of surgical antimicrobial prophylaxis. *Ann Surg.* 2008;247:918-926.

116. Garey KW, Dao T, Chen H, et al. Timing of vancomycin prophylaxis for cardiac surgery patients and the risk of surgical site infections. *J Antimicrob Chemother.* 2006;58:645-650.

117. Thigpen BD, Hood WA, Chauhan S, et al. Timing of prophylactic antibiotic administration in the uninfected laboring gravida: A randomized clinical trial. *Am J Obstet Gynecol.* 2005;192:1864-1868; discussion 1868-1871.

118. Sullivan SA, Smith T, Chang E, et al. Administration of cefazolin prior to skin incision is superior to cefazolin at cord clamping in preventing postcesarean infectious morbidity: A randomized, controlled trial. *Am J Obstet Gynecol.* 2007;196:455 e1-e5.

119. Dellinger EP, Gross PA, Barrett TL, et al. Quality standard for antimicrobial prophylaxis in surgical procedures. The Infectious Diseases Society of America. *Infect Control Hosp Epidemiol.* 1994;15:182-188.

120. Platt R, Munoz A, Stella J, et al. Antibiotic prophylaxis for cardiovascular surgery. Efficacy with coronary artery bypass. *Ann Intern Med.* 1984;101:770-774.

121. Rosenberg AD, Wambold D, Kraemer L, et al. Ensuring appropriate timing of antimicrobial prophylaxis. *J Bone Joint Surg Am.* 2008;90:226-232.

122. St Jacques P, Sanders N, Patel N, et al. Improving timely surgical antibiotic prophylaxis redosing administration using computerized record prompts. *Surg Infect (Larchmt).* 2005;6:215-221.

123. Nichols RL, Condon RE, Barie PS. Antibiotic prophylaxis in surgery—2005 and beyond. *Surg Infect (Larchmt).* 2005;6:349-361.

124. Elliott JP, Freeman RK, Dorchester W. Short versus long course of prophylactic antibiotics. *Am J Obstet Gynecol.* 1982;143:740-744.

125. Gatell JM, Garcia S, Lozano L, et al. Perioperative cefamandole prophylaxis against infections. *J Bone Joint Surg Am.* 1987;69:1189-1193.

126. Hall JC, Christiansen KJ, Goodman M, et al. Duration of antimicrobial prophylaxis in vascular surgery. *Am J Surg.* 1998;175:87-90.

127. Fujita S, Saito N, Yamada T, et al. Randomized, multicenter trial of antibiotic prophylaxis in elective colorectal surgery: Single dose vs 3 doses of a second-generation cephalosporin without metronidazole and oral antibiotics. *Arch Surg.* 2007;142:657-661.

128. McDonald M, Grabsch E, Marshall C, et al. Single- versus multiple-dose antimicrobial prophylaxis for major surgery: A systematic review. *Aust N Z J Surg.* 1998;68:388-396.

129. Harbarth S, Samore MH, Lichtenberg D, et al. Prolonged antibiotic prophylaxis after cardiovascular surgery and its effect on surgical site infections and antimicrobial resistance. *Circulation.* 2000;101:2916-2921.

130. Sandoe JA, Kumar B, Stoddart B, et al. Effect of extended perioperative antibiotic prophylaxis on intravascular catheter colonization and infection in cardiothoracic surgery patients. *J Antimicrob Chemother.* 2003;52:877-879.

131. Edwards FH, Engelman RM, Houck P, et al. The Society of Thoracic Surgeons practice guideline series: Antibiotic prophylaxis in cardiac surgery, Part I: Duration. *Ann Thorac Surg.* 2006;81:397-404.

132. Wininger DA, Fass RJ. Antibiotic-impregnated cement and beads for orthopedic infections. *Antimicrob Agents Chemother.* 1996;40:2675-2679.

133. Goodell JA, Flick AB, Hebert JC, et al. Preparation and release characteristics of tobramycin-impregnated polymethylmethacrylate beads. *Am J Hosp Pharm.* 1986;43:1454-1461.

134. Bourne RB. Prophylactic use of antibiotic bone cement: An emerging standard—in the affirmative. *J Arthroplasty.* 2004;19:69-72.

135. Hanssen AD. Prophylactic use of antibiotic bone cement: An emerging standard—in opposition. *J Arthroplasty.* 2004;19:73-77.

136. Haydon RC, Blaha JD, Mancinelli C, et al. Audiometric thresholds in osteomyelitis patients treated with gentamicin-impregnated methylmethacrylate beads (Septopal). *Clin Orthop Relat Res.* 1993:43-46.

137. Patrick BN, Rivey MP, Allington DR. Acute renal failure associated with vancomycin- and tobramycin-laden cement in total hip arthroplasty. *Ann Pharmacother.* 2006;40:2037-2042.

138. Wren SM, Ahmed N, Jamal A, et al. Preoperative oral antibiotics in colorectal surgery increase the rate of Clostridium difficile colitis. *Arch Surg.* 2005;140:752-756.

139. Carignan A, Allard C, Pepin J, et al. Risk of Clostridium difficile infection after perioperative antibacterial prophylaxis before and during an outbreak of infection due to a hypervirulent strain. *Clin Infect Dis.* 2008;46:1838-1843.

140. Dajee H, Laks H, Miller J, et al. Profound hypotension from rapid vancomycin administration during cardiac operation. *J Thorac Cardiovasc Surg.* 1984;87:145-146.

141. Roberts NJ Jr, Douglas RG Jr. Gentamicin use and Pseudomonas and Serratia resistance: Effect of a surgical prophylaxis regimen. *Antimicrob Agents Chemother.* 1978;13:214-220.

142. Archer GL, Armstrong BC. Alteration of staphylococcal flora in cardiac surgery patients receiving antibiotic prophylaxis. *J Infect Dis.* 1983;147:642-649.

143. Kernodle DS, Barg NL, Kaiser AB. Low-level colonization of hospitalized patients with methicillin-resistant coagulase-negative staphylococci and emergence of the organisms during surgical antimicrobial prophylaxis. *Antimicrob Agents Chemother.* 1988;32:202-208.

144. Kaiser AB, Clayson KR, Mulherin JL Jr, et al. Antibiotic prophylaxis in vascular surgery. *Ann Surg.* 1978;188:283-289.

145. Kernodle DS, Classen DC, Burke JP, et al. Failure of cephalosporins to prevent Staphylococcus aureus surgical wound infections. *JAMA.* 1990;263:961-966.

146. Kernodle DS, Voladri RK, Kaiser AB. Beta-lactamase production diminishes the prophylactic efficacy of ampicillin and cefazolin in a guinea pig model of Staphylococcus aureus wound infection. *J Infect Dis.* 1998;177:701-706.

147. Kernodle DS, Classen DC, Stratton CW, et al. Association of borderline oxacillin-susceptible strains of Staphylococcus aureus with surgical wound infections. *J Clin Microbiol.* 1998;36:219-222.

148. Archibald L, Phillips L, Monnet D, et al. Antimicrobial resistance in isolates from inpatients and outpatients in the United States: Increasing importance of the intensive care unit. *Clin Infect Dis.* 1997;24:211-215.

149. Neu HC. Emergence and mechanisms of bacterial resistance in surgical infections. *Am J Surg.* 1995;169:13S-20S.

150. Roach AC, Kernodle DS, Kaiser AB. Selecting cost-effective antimicrobial prophylaxis in surgery: Are we getting what we pay for? *DICP.* 1990;24:183-185.

151. Lee JT. Nomenclature nightmare. *Surg Infect (Larchmt).* 2003;4:293-296.

152. Haley RW, Culver DH, White JW, et al. The efficacy of infection surveillance and control programs in preventing nosocomial infections in US hospitals. *Am J Epidemiol.* 1985;121:182-205.

153. Sands K, Vineyard G, Platt R. Surgical site infections occurring after hospital discharge. *J Infect Dis.* 1996;173:963-970.

154. Kent P, McDonald M, Harris O, et al. Post-discharge surgical wound infection surveillance in a provincial hospital: Follow-up rates, validity of data and review of the literature. *ANZ J Surg.* 2001;71:583-589.

155. Mitchell DH. Post-discharge surgical wound surveillance. *ANZ J Surg.* 2001;71:563.

318

Burns

CLINTON K. MURRAY*

Injuries secondary to severe burns rank among the most serious forms of trauma, resulting in anatomic, physiologic, endocrinologic, and immunologic stresses, especially when burns involve more than 20% of the total body surface area (TBSA). In 2006, U.S. municipal fire departments responded to an estimated 1.6 million fires, with 3,245 nonfirefighter fatalities.[1] Approximately 75% of deaths occur at the scene, primarily because of inhalation of soot or absorption of carboxyhemoglobin in the blood.[2,3] Annually, 500,000 burn injuries receive medical treatment and approximately 40,000 require hospitalization, of which 60% are admitted to specialized burn centers.[3,4] Improvements in the care of patients who suffer burns, especially initial burn shock resuscitation, has resulted in remarkably improved survival rates.[5,6] In the early 1970s, there were approximately 15,000 deaths/year secondary to burns, in contrast to 3,250 today. In addition, a 30% TBSA burn was associated with a 50% survival rate in the 1970s whereas patients with an 80% TBSA burn now have a 50% survival rate.[4,7]

The metabolic stress associated with burn injuries has recently been reviewed but many issues remain unclear.[8,9] A review of the immunologic alterations associated with burns is beyond the scope of this chapter; however, the innate and adaptive immunologic alterations associated with burn injuries are numerous and can persist for weeks to months.[6,10-25] The National Institute of General Medicine Sciences and the National Institutes of Health have established a multicenter study of the genomic and proteomic response to severe burns that should enhance our knowledge in this area.[26]

The primary insult from a burn is the wound itself, which has three characteristic areas of involvement.[11] The first associated burn wound area is the zone of coagulation nearest the heat source and includes dead tissue forming the burn eschar. Adjacent to the necrotic tissue in the coagulation zone is the second area, known as the zone of stasis, which is viable but at risk of ischemia because of perfusion defects. The zone of hyperemia is the third area, which consists of relatively normal skin with increased blood flow and vasodilatation, and minimal cellular injury. Overall, the primary concern of burn wound injuries is the burn wound eschar, with its avascular nature preventing immune cells and systemically administered antibiotics from being delivered.[27] At the same time, homeostasis is attempted through various vascular alterations, including contraction, retraction, and coagulation.

There are several mechanisms resulting in burn injuries in addition to thermal burns that cause cellular damage based on duration and temperature of exposure. Chemical burns can involve reducing agents such as hydrochloric acid, oxidizing agents such as sodium hypochlorite, and corrosive agents such as phenol, all with varying modes of action resulting in burns. Other burn mechanisms include scalding, which is more common in children, contact with hot objects, electrical injuries, and radiation. Burn units also manage certain skin disorders such as Stevens-Johnson syndrome.

*The opinions or assertions contained herein are the private views of the author and are not to be construed as official or reflecting the views of the U.S. Department of the Army, the U.S. Department of Defense, or the federal government. The author is an employee of the U.S. government and this work was performed as part of official duties. All material in this chapter is in the public domain, with the exception of any borrowed figures or tables.

Epidemiology

The American Burn Association (ABA) maintains a national burn repository that provides a 10-year rolling review of ongoing data collected from 73 hospitals from 33 states and the District of Columbia.[28] For the period of 1998 to 2007, almost 70% of patients were men. The mean age was 35 years, with 12% of patients younger than 5 years and 14% age 60 years or older. The total burn size was less than 10% TBSA in 69% of cases, with a mortality of 0.7%. Increasing TBSA was associated with increased mortality—40% to 49.9% TBSA had a 25% mortality, 70% to 79.9% TBSA had a 58% mortality, and more than 90% TBSA experienced a 81% mortality. The overall mortality rate was 5%, mostly occurring 2 and 3 weeks after injury; however, mortality was 8% for fire or flame injuries, the most common cause of burn. Inhalation injury increased the likelihood of death by 15 times. For survivors, the average length of hospitalization was slightly more than 1 day/TBSA (%) burned. Overall, predictors of mortality remain extremes of age, percentage of TBSA, presence of full-thickness burns, and inhalation injury, with some data supporting gender-dependent diffferences.[29-34]

Improvements in the morbidity and mortality associated with burns have been attributed to advances in burn shock resuscitation, airway management and ventilatory strategies, nutritional support, burn wound care, and infection control practices.[5,35-39] If patients survive the initial burn and resuscitative phase, infections are a leading cause of mortality (75% of cases).[36,40-44] Six of the top ten complications in the 10-year rolling review of those suffering fire or flame injury (13,666 complications) were infectious: 4.6% of patients had pneumonia; 2.7%, septicemia; 2.6%, cellulitis or traumatic injury; 2.5%, respiratory failure; 2.2%, wound infection; 2.0%, other infection; 1.5%, renal failure; 1.4%, line infection; 1.2%, acute respiratory distress syndrome; and 1.0%, arrhythmia. Older patients with burns had more urinary tract infections. Scalds and burn injuries involving contact with a hot object had higher rates of wound infections and cellulitis. The number of patients suffering from pneumonia increased with mechanical ventilation longer than 4 days.

Infection preceded multiorgan dysfunction by a median of 4 days, with increasing mortality based on severity of sepsis and an odds ratio (OR) of mortality of 12.5 for septic shock versus uncomplicated sepsis.[40] Primary sites of infections are the bloodstream, lungs, wound, and urinary tract, with either lung or wound being the most common, depending on the diagnostic definitions used.[40,45-48] Pneumonias appear to occur more frequently when there is a concomitant inhalation injury.[49-52] Infected patients tend to be older, female, and intubated, with higher percentage TBSA burn, longer length of stay, more central venous and arterial catheters, and more operations.[45] Outcomes appear worse with polymicrobial infections.[53] Nosocomial infection rates have been reported from 77 to 90 infections/100 patients or an incident density of 32 to 48 infections/1000 patient days.[46] Catheter-associated bloodstream infections have been reported at 34/1000 central line days and ventilator-associated pneumonias at 26/1000 ventilator days.[48] The National Healthcare Safety Network has indicated that burn units have the highest rates in comparison to other units for urinary catheter–associated urinary tract infections, ventilator-associated pneumonias, and central line–associated bloodstream infections.[54] Endocarditis occurs in approximately 0.4% of burn unit admissions and in 9% of patients with persistent bacteremia.[55]

The organisms responsible for infections in patients who suffer severe burns may be endogenous or exogenous and include bacteria, fungus, and viruses which can change over time in the individual patient. Severe burns cause a mechanical disruption of the skin, allowing microbes to penetrate deeper tissues.[56] At the time of the burn, the normal skin structure is replaced by a moist, protein-rich, avascular eschar that is an ideal environment for microorganisms. Typically, the burn surface is sterile immediately following thermal injury, but after 48 hours the wound is colonized with skin pathogens that typically reside in sweat glands and hair follicles before the burn.[57-59] After 5 to 7 days, wounds become colonized with yeast and/or gram-positive and gram-negative bacteria from the host's normal gastrointestinal and upper respiratory tracts, or from the hospital environment and health care workers' hands.[57-67] The most commonly recovered pathogens depend on the site of culture and reflect a hospital's nosocomial pathogens.[57,68] Although *Streptococcus pyogenes* was the most frequently recovered pathogen historically, this has been replaced with *Staphylococcus aureus* and gram-negative pathogens, such as *Pseudomonas aeruginosa*, *Klebsiella pneumoniae*, and *Acinetobacter baumannii*, with higher resistance profiles as patients stay in the hospital longer.[68-72] Becoming infected with increasingly resistant pathogens is likely more reflective of cross-contamination rather than acquisition of new resistance mechanisms by the patient's endogenous bacteria.[73] In addition, within a hospital, isolates from the burn unit are often more resistant than those in other ICUs or wards.[74] Although anaerobic bacteria are noted in numerous wound studies, anaerobic bacteria do not appear to be associated with systemic infections such as bacteremia.[75]

Numerous fungal agents are associated with burn injuries, including *Aspergillus, Candida,* and agents of mucormycosis (zygomycosis), hyalohyphomycosis, and phaeohyphomycosis, but *Aspergillus* is associated with increased mortality.[76-78] Fungal infections typically involve the skin or lungs and occur in older patients with greater percentage of TBSA and stays in the hospital longer than 14 to 28 days.[78,79] A single-site study has shown that the presence of fungal wound infection increases mortality by an OR of 8.2, equivalent to raising the TBSA burn by 33%.[77] The mortality associated with fungal wound colonization was 27% compared with 76% for fungal wound infections.

The role of viral infections has not been clearly elucidated in patients with burns but likely includes reactivation, primary infection, or exogenous reinfection of cytomegalovirus (CMV), herpes simplex virus, or varicella-zoster virus.[11] Varicella-zoster virus in children has been associated with pulmonary disease.[80] Herpes simplex virus typically occurs in healing or recently healed partial-thickness burns and occasionally around the margins of skin graft donor sites 2 to 6 weeks following thermal injury.[11,27] Although CMV has been associated with patients who suffer severe burn, the clinical impact is unclear.[81,82]

Diagnosis

The traditional parameters used to detect infection, including temperature, white blood cell (WBC) count, respiratory status, and heart rate, are not sensitive or specific enough to be used in the same fashion in burn patients because of the metabolic perturbations associated with burns. Extremes or changes in temperature, WBC count, percentage of neutrophils, and inflammatory biochemical markers, including C-reactive protein, procalcitonin, and numerous cytokines, are not adequate in predicting ongoing infections.[24,25,83-85] With these limitations in mind, the ABA recently released criteria for sepsis that could be used as a trigger for the concern of ongoing infection; however, there are limited controlled studies for these recommendations, especially in adults (Table 318-1).[86]

Pneumonia is defined by a clinical syndrome consisting of two or more of the following: a new or persistent infiltrate, consolidation, or cavitation on chest x-ray (CXR), sepsis (as defined in Table 318-1) and a recent change in sputum or purulence in the sputum.[86,87] The diagnosis is confirmed if a patient meets the clinical syndrome with microbiologic confirmation, probable if a patient meets the clinical syndrome without microbiologic confirmation, and possible with an abnormal

TABLE 318-1	American Burn Association Sepsis Criteria*

I. Temperature: >39° or <36.5°C

II. Progressive tachycardia
- Adults: >110 beats/min
- Children: >2 SD above age-specific norms (85% age-adjusted heart rate)

III. Progressive tachypnea
- Adults: >25 breaths/min if not ventilated or minute ventilation >12 L/min if ventilated
- Children: >2 SD above age-specific norms (85% age-adjusted respiratory rate)

IV. Thrombocytopenia (only applicable >3 days post–initial resuscitation)
- Adults: <100,000/μL
- Children: >2 SD below age-specific norms

V. Hyperglycemia (only applicable to patients without a prior history of diabetes)
- Untreated plasma glucose >200 mg/dL
or
- Insulin resistance (>7 units of insulin/hr IV drip or >25% increase in insulin requirement over 24 hr)

VI. Inability to continue enteral feedings longer than 24 hr
- Abdominal distention
or
- Residual twice the feeding rate for adults or >150 mL/hr in children
or
- Uncontrolled diarrhea (>2,500 mL/day for adults or >400 mL/day for children)

*Sepsis is of concern if three or more of these six triggers are seen.
SD, standard deviation.
Adapted from Greenhalgh DG, Saffle JR, Holmes JH, et al. American Burn Association consensus conference to define sepsis and infection in burns. *J Burn Care Res.* 2007;28:776-790.

CXR with low or moderate clinical suspicions but microbiologic confirmation. Microbiologic criteria include tracheal aspirate with 10^5 organisms or more, bronchoalveolar lavage with 10^4 organisms or more, or protected bronchial brush with 10^3 organisms or more. Similar to other critically ill patients, these evaluations are not always routinely performed. Purulent tracheobronchitis, defined as fever and increased sputum without CXR findings or purulent discharge coating the trachea during bronchoscopy, is encountered in burn patients. There is evidence that the presence of tracheobronchitis is associated with prolonged durations of mechanical ventilation and that antibiotic therapy may mitigate this effect.[88]

Bloodstream infections are diagnosed using the standard analysis of pathogen, clinical syndrome, and number of positive cultures.[86] The needed quantity of blood or type of bottles at the time of culturing is not clear, and whether the recently published recommendations for fever in the critically ill apply to a burn population has yet to be defined.[75,89] Although patients can develop bacteremia after burn wound manipulation in the early postburn period, the clinical relevance of this bacteremia is uncertain.

Criteria for diagnosis of wound infections have been described by the ABA (Table 318-2) and others.[6,86,90] Changes of the eschar appearance to include development of a dark brown, black, or violaceous discoloration or edema at the wound margin are of concern for ongoing infection. Culturing the skin through swabs or biopsies are of limited clinical usefulness because they do not always correlate with each other, are associated with sampling bias, and are not always associated with ongoing bacteremia.[91-94] Although the definitive diagnosis of wound infection is probably histopathologic diagnosis with invasion of bacteria into viable tissue or blood vessels, the expertise and rapid turn-around is lacking in most centers. *Pseudomonas aeruginosa* can colonize the wound resulting in a yellow-green exudates but invasive infection should only be considered when there are purple-black and punched-out areas of the wound.[95] *Candida* infections can appear as small papules of purulence whereas *Aspergillus* appears as gray-brown plaques that can be removed out of the wound. Histology is used in some specialized burn centers using predefined criteria; however, this

TABLE 318-2	Diagnosis of Burn Wound Infection (American Burn Association Guidelines)
Syndrome	*Clinical and Pathologic Criteria (Burn Sepsis Guidelines)*
Wound colonization	Bacteria on wound surface at low concentration ($<10^5$ bacteria/g tissue); no invasive infection
Wound infection	Bacteria in the wound and wound eschar at high concentration ($>10^5$ bacteria/g tissue); no invasive infection
Invasive infection	Pathogens in burn wound at a sufficient concentration ($>10^5$ bacteria/g tissue [frequently]), depth, and surface area to cause suppurative separation of eschar or graft loss, invasion of adjacent unburned tissue, or sepsis syndrome (see Table 318-1)
Cellulitis	Bacteria present in wound and/or wound eschar at high concentrations ($>10^5$ bacteria/g tissue) with surrounding tissue revealing erythema (but this alone does not require therapy), induration, warmth, and/or tenderness
Necrotizing infection, fasciitis	Aggressive, invasive infection with involvement below the skin resulting in tissue necrosis

NOTES:
1. Quantitative biopsy can assist in identifying pathogen and antimicrobial resistance profiles but its ability to confirm a diagnosis is limited.
2. Quantitative swabs are unreliable but might assist in pathogen identification and antimicrobial resistance profiles.
3. Tissue histology can be used but limited expertise exists.
4. Clinical parameters of wound infection: pain, erythema, color change; unexpected changes in wound appearance and depth; systematic changes; premature separation of burn eschar.

Adapted from Greenhalgh DG, Saffle JR, Holmes JH, et al. American Burn Association consensus conference to define sepsis and infection in burns. *J Burn Care Res.* 2007;28:776-790.

is time-consuming, many facilities lack the expertise, and correlation between culture results and systemic infections is lacking.[27,96] Histology for fungal diagnosis must be augmented with culture because of inaccuracies of histology, presence of mixed cultures, and providing definitive identification of fungi to assist in antifungal selection.[78]

Treatment

Therapy of infections in patients with burns is focused on the site of infection and offending pathogen. Empirical therapy should rely on a burn unit's own specific antibiogram because resistance profiles in burn units might not be reflective of other units or wards in the same hospital.[74] Some burn units rely on individual patients' quantitative wound cultures on admission and use routine periodic screening of the skin to predict infecting pathogens. The usefulness of this method is unclear with sampling and technique bias.[58,96-100] Empirical therapeutic choices should focus on pathogens with notable mortality, such as *Klebsiella pneumoniae*, instead of pathogens with increased antimicrobial resistance but less virulence, such as *Acinetobacter baumannii*.[69,71] The pharmacokinetics of antimicrobial agents in patients who suffer burns may be dramatically altered and the use of serum creati-

nine concentrations to predict creatinine clearance using standard equations is questionable.[101,102] Vancomycin is noted to have a higher clearance rate, even after the initial burn shock period, because patients remain in a hypermetabolic period with increased cardiac output.[103] Variability has also been noted for aminoglycosides, carbapenems, and cephalosporins.[104-107] Close monitoring of drug levels and more accurate measurement of renal function might improve clinical outcomes.

Alternative routes of drug delivery have been considered to improve outcomes. Although antibiotic aerosol as adjunctive treatment of pneumonia has been assessed in general intensive care unit (ICU) patients, no clear benefit or harm has been shown in burn patients.[108,109] Historically, subeschar clysis was used in deep burns when early excision was not the standard of care, and is still used in areas where early surgical interventions and adequate support are not available. Methods include introduction of antimicrobial agents or other antimicrobials, such as povidone-iodine plus Neosporin (polymyxin B, neomycin, gramicidin).[110,111]

Therapy of fungal infections is dependent on identifying the genus and species as well as site of infection. One burn unit has reported a larger number of *Aspergillus terreus* infections, limiting the use of amphotericin B as empirical therapy for molds.[78] The role of empirical or preemptive therapy when a fungus is recovered from the skin but is not yet invasive is intriguing, especially in patients with 30% to 60% TBSA burned, because they may benefit the most from early therapy to prevent invasive infection and subsequent excess morbidity and mortality.[77]

Although surgical management is regarded as care of the wound, it can also treat and prevent infections.[56] The impact of early excision, typically within 5 days of burn, appears to be associated with an improved mortality rate compared with standard therapy only in patients without inhalation injury, but its impact on sepsis is unclear.[112-114] Coverage of the burn area is fundamental to burn care and includes autografts (cadaveric skin), xenografts (typically porcine skin), and synthetic coverage, as well as allografts.[115] Coverage provides a wound barrier and prevents evaporative losses, but the new coverage can develop infections, as can donor sites in cases of allografts.

Topical therapies are used to prevent and treat the development of infection and include mafenide acetate, silver sulfadiazine, silver nitrate, and silver dressings (Table 318-3).[116,117] These agents have various adverse event profiles, clinical application characteristics, and antimicrobial activity. It is unclear whether the limited fungal coverage of these agents results in increased fungal infections.[77]

Prevention

Infection control is fundamental to decreasing infectious complications associated with burns. Bacterial propagation involves hospital equipment such as mattresses, patient care with hydrotherapy, and movement of patients and equipment between the general ICU and burn unit.[62,65,73,118] Other studies have shown aerosolization of bacteria during wound dressing changes.[119] Burn units should be designed to

TABLE 318-3	Application of Topical Agents				
Agent	*Penetration*	*Spectrum*	*Side Effects*	*Comments*
Mafenide acetate (Sulfamylon)	Penetrates eschar	Gram-positive and gram-negative bacteria	Painful on application; metabolic acidosis	Twice daily or alternative with silver sulfadiazine
Silver sulfadiazine (Silvadene, Thermazene, Falmazine)	Poor eschar penetration	Gram-positive and gram-negative bacteria; *Candida* spp.	Leukopenia	Can treat through leukopenia
Silver nitrate	Poor eschar penetration	Gram-positive and gram-negative bacteria	Discolors wound bed; electrolyte changes, including hyponatremia, hypocalcemia, hypokalemia, hypomagnesemia	Apply in thick layers with mesh gauze frequently to keep moist; stains environment black; change dressing twice daily
Silver dressing (Acticoat, Silverlon)	Limited eschar penetration	Gram-positive and gram-negative bacteria; *Candida* spp.*	Discolors wound	

*Data are limited.

minimize transmission through dedicated burn space, no common treatment rooms, centralized dedicated operating rooms and facilities, and individual patient rooms with anterooms or individual doors. In addition, aggressive standard infection control procedures for resistant pathogens are recommended.[6,58,66]

Central catheter–related sepsis appears to be associated with the number of lines placed and total number of central line days, but not the site (upper or lower body) of insertion.[120] Distancing the insertion site from the burned area can decrease infections, but it is unclear whether guidewire exchange is comparable to insertion at a new site.[121,122] Changing lines every 3 days has been associated with fewer infections than changes every 4 days in one study.[123]

The use of perioperative antibiotics at the time of débridement or dressing changes has been shown to modify rates of bacteremia but not necessarily clinical or graft outcome and is of questionable usefulness, especially in patients with a TBSA lower than 40% to 60%.[93,124] Prophylactic antibiotics in children have been associated with a higher secondary infection rate.[125]

Selective decontamination of the digestive tract has been associated with a reduced mortality and lower rates of pneumonia but this is not routinely performed.[126] In addition, early enteral feeding may blunt the hypermetabolic response and decrease intestinal permeability, thus preserving the intestinal barrier and potentially affecting enterogenic infections.[127-131] Each unit of blood transfused in patients with burn injuries is associated with increased mortality and infectious complications, even after controlling for severity of disease.[132] Hyperbaric oxygen therapy has been evaluated, with mixed results.[133-135]

Conclusions

Patients who suffer burn injuries are subjected to the most physiologic stresses. Because infections are the highest cause of mortality after surviving the initial early postburn period, efforts are required to mitigate excessive death rates through adequate preventive measures and enhanced vigilance for infections and appropriate therapy. Burn units are ideal for outbreaks of multidrug-resistant pathogens, which can affect other patients and the entire health care facility if adequate infection control measures are not in place. The management of burned patients requires a multidisciplinary approach, including infectious disease physicians.

REFERENCES

1. Karter MJ Jr. Fire Loss in the United States 2007. Available at: http://www.nfpa.org/assets/files/PDF/OS.fireloss.pdf.
2. Gerling I, Meissner C, Reiter A, et al. Death from thermal effects and burns. *Forensic Sci Int.* 2001;115:33-41.
3. American Burn Association. Burn Incidence and Treatment in the US: 2007 Fact Sheet. Available at: http://www.ameriburn.org/resources_factsheet.php.
4. Latenser BA, Miller SF, Bessey PQ, et al. National Burn Repository 2006: A ten-year review. *J Burn Care Res.* 2007;28:635-658.
5. Pham TN, Cancio LC, Gibran NS. American Burn Association practice guidelines burn shock resuscitation. *J Burn Care Res.* 2008;29:257-266.
6. Mayhall CG. The epidemiology of burn wound infections: Then and now. *Clin Infect Dis.* 2003;37:543-550.
7. Holmes JH, Heimbach DM. Burns. In Brunicardi FC, ed. *Schwartz's Principles of Surgery.* New York: McGraw Hill; 2005:189-223.
8. Wolf SE. Nutrition and metabolism in burns: State of the science, 2007. *J Burn Care Res.* 2007;28:572-576.
9. Atiyeh BS, Gunn SW, Dibo SA. Metabolic implications of severe burn injuries and their management: A systematic review of the literature. *World J Surg.* 2008;32:1857-1859.
10. Shankar R, Melstrom KA Jr, Gamelli RL. Inflammation and sepsis: Past, present, and the future. *J Burn Care Res.* 2007;28:566-571.
11. Church D, Elsayed S, Reid O, et al. Burn wound infections. *Clin Microbiol Rev.* 2006;19:403-434.
12. Padfield KE, Zhang Q, Gopalan S, et al. Local and distant burn injury alter immuno-inflammatory gene expression in skeletal muscle. *J Trauma.* 2006;61:280-292.
13. Cohen MJ, Carroll C, He LK, et al. Severity of burn injury and sepsis determines the cytokine responses of bone marrow progenitor-derived macrophages. *J Trauma.* 2007;62:858-867.
14. Venet F, Tissot S, Debard AL, et al. Decreased monocyte human leukocyte antigen-DR expression after severe burn injury: Correlation with severity and secondary septic shock. *Crit Care Med.* 2007;35:1910-1917.
15. Schneider DF, Glenn CH, Faunce DE. Innate lymphocyte subsets and their immunoregulatory roles in burn injury and sepsis. *J Burn Care Res.* 2007;28:365-379.
16. Miller AC, Rashid RM, Elamin EM. The "T" in trauma: The helper T-cell response and the role of immunomodulation in trauma and burn patients. *J Trauma.* 2007;63:1407-1417.
17. Cairns BA, Barnes CM, Mlot S, et al. Toll-like receptor 2 and 4 ligation results in complex altered cytokine profiles early and late after burn injury. *J Trauma.* 2008;64:1069-1077.
18. Cairns B, Maile R, Barnes CM, et al. Increased Toll-like receptor 4 expression on T cells may be a mechanism for enhanced T cell response late after burn injury. *J Trauma.* 2006;61:293-298.
19. Barber RC, Chang LY, Arnoldo BD, et al. Innate immunity SNPs are associated with risk for severe sepsis after burn injury. *Clin Med Res.* 2006;4:250-255.
20. Summer GJ, Romero-Sandoval EA, Bogen O, et al. Proinflammatory cytokines mediating burn-injury pain. *Pain.* 2008;135:98-107.
21. Wang K, Wang DC, Feng YQ, et al. Changes in cytokine levels and CD4+/CD8+ T cells ratio in draining lymph node of burn wound. *J Burn Care Res.* 2007;28:747-753.
22. Suber F, Carroll MC, Moore FD Jr. Innate response to self-antigen significantly exacerbates burn wound depth. *Proc Natl Acad Sci U S A.* 2007;104:3973-3977.
23. Bhat S, Milner S. Antimicrobial peptides in burns and wounds. *Curr Protein Pept Sci.* 2007;8:506-520.
24. Dehne MG, Sablotzki A, Hoffmann A, et al. Alterations of acute phase reaction and cytokine production in patients following severe burn injury. *Burns.* 2002;28:535-542.
25. Jeschke MG, Barrow RE, Herndon DN. Extended hypermetabolic response of the liver in severely burned pediatric patients. *Arch Surg.* 2004;139:641-647.
26. Klein MB, Silver G, Gamelli RL, et al. Inflammation and the host response to injury: An overview of the multicenter study of the genomic and proteomic response to burn injury. *J Burn Care Res.* 2006;27:448-451.
27. Pruitt BA Jr, McManus AT, Kim SH, et al. Burn wound infections: Current status. *World J Surg.* 1998;22:135-145.
28. American Burn Association. National Burn repository: 2007 Report. Available at: http://www.ameriburn.org/2007NBRAnnualReport.pdf.
29. Lumenta DB, Hautier A, Desouches C, et al. Mortality and morbidity among elderly people with burns—evaluation of data on admission. *Burns.* 2008;34:965-974.
30. Cancio LC, Galvez E Jr, Turner CE, et al. Base deficit and alveolar-arterial gradient during resuscitation contribute independently but modestly to the prediction of mortality after burn injury. *J Burn Care Res.* 2006;27:289-296.
31. Tobiasen J, Hiebert JM, Edlich RF. The abbreviated burn severity index. *Ann Emerg Med.* 1982;11:260-262.
32. Ryan CM, Schoenfeld DA, Thorpe WP, et al. Objective estimates of the probability of death from burn injuries. *N Engl J Med.* 1998;338:362-366.
33. Moreau AR, Westfall PH, Cancio LC, et al. Development and validation of an age-risk score for mortality predication after thermal injury. *J Trauma.* 2005;58:967-972.
34. O'Keefe GE, Hunt JL, Purdue GF. An evaluation of risk factors for mortality after burn trauma and the identification of gender-dependent differences in outcomes. *J Am Coll Surg.* 2001;192:153-160.
35. Ipaktchi K, Arbabi S. Advances in burn critical care. *Crit Care Med.* 2006;34(Suppl):S239-S244.
36. Benmeir P, Sagi A, Greber B, et al. An analysis of mortality in patients with burns covering 40/cent BSA or more: a retrospective review covering 24 years (1964-88). *Burns.* 1991;17:402-405.
37. Bang RL, Sharma PN, Sanyal SC, et al. Septicaemia after burn injury: A comparative study. *Burns.* 2002;28:746-751.
38. Atiyeh BS, Gunn SW, Hayek SN. State of the art in burn treatment. *World J Surg.* 2005;29:131-148.
39. Merrell SW, Saffle JR, Larson CM, et al. The declining incidence of fatal sepsis following thermal injury. *J Trauma.* 1989;29:1362-1366.
40. Fitzwater J, Purdue GF, Hunt JL, et al. The risk factors and time course of sepsis and organ dysfunction after burn trauma. *J Trauma.* 2003;54:959-966.
41. Singh D, Singh A, Sharma AK, et al. Burn mortality in Chandigarh zone: 25 years' autopsy experience from a tertiary care hospital of India. *Burns.* 1998;24:150-156.
42. Kumar V, Mohanty MK, Kanth S. Fatal burns in Manipal area: A 10-year study. *J Forensic Leg Med.* 2007;14:3-6.
43. Pereira CT, Barrow RE, Sterns AM, et al. Age-dependent differences in survival after severe burns: A unicentric review of 1,674 patients and 179 autopsies over 15 years. *J Am Coll Surg.* 2006;202:536-548.
44. Sharma BR, Harish D, Singh VP, et al. Septicemia as a cause of death in burns: An autopsy study. *Burns.* 2006;32:545-549.
45. Appelgren P, Bjornhagen V, Bragderyd K, et al. A prospective study of infections in burn patients. *Burns.* 2002;28:39-46.
46. Wurtz R, Karajovic M, Dacumos E, et al. Nosocomial infections in a burn intensive care unit. *Burns.* 1995;21:181-184.
47. Soares de Macedo JL, Santos JB. Nosocomial infections in a Brazilian burn unit. *Burns.* 2006;32:477-481.
48. Santucci SG, Gobara S, Santos CR, et al. Infections in a burn intensive care unit: Experience of seven years. *J Hosp Infect.* 2003;53:6-13.
49. Rue LW 3rd, Cioffi WG, Mason AD Jr, et al. The risk of pneumonia in thermally injured patients requiring ventilatory support. *J Burn Care Rehabil.* 1995;16(Pt 1):262-268.
50. Herndon DN, Thompson PB, Traber DL. Pulmonary injury in burned patients. *Crit Care Clin.* 1985;1:79-96.
51. Edelman DA, Khan N, Kempf K, et al. Pneumonia after inhalation injury. *J Burn Care Res.* 2007;28:241-246.
52. de La Cal MA, Cerda E, Garcia-Hierro P, et al. Pneumonia in patients with severe burns: A classification according to the concept of the carrier state. *Chest.* 2001;119:1160-1165.
53. Still JM Jr, Belcher K, Law EJ. Experience with polymicrobial sepsis in a regional burn unit. *Burns.* 1993;19:434-436.
54. Edwards JR, Peterson KD, Andrus ML, et al. National Healthcare Safety Network (NHSN) Report, data summary for 2006, issued June 2007. *Am J Infect Control.* 2007;35:290-301.
55. Regules JA, Glasser JS, Wolf SE, et al. Endocarditis in burn patients: Clinical and diagnostic considerations. *Burns.* 2007;34:610-616.
56. Barret JP, Herndon DN. Effects of burn wound excision on bacterial colonization and invasion. *Plast Reconstr Surg.* 2003;111:744-750.
57. Erol S, Altoparlak U, Akcay MN, et al. Changes of microbial flora and wound colonization in burned patients. *Burns.* 2004;30:357-361.
58. Sharma BR. Infection in patients with severe burns: Causes and prevention thereof. *Infect Dis Clin North Am.* 2007;21:745-759.
59. de Macedo JL, Santos JB. Bacterial and fungal colonization of burn wounds. *Mem Inst Oswaldo Cruz.* 2005;100:535-539.
60. Magnotti LJ, Deitch EA. Burns, bacterial translocation, gut barrier function, and failure. *J Burn Care Rehabil.* 2005;26:383-391.
61. Gosain A, Gamelli RL. Role of the gastrointestinal tract in burn sepsis. *J Burn Care Rehabil.* 2005;26:85-91.
62. Bayat A, Shaaban H, Dodgson A, et al. Implications for Burns Unit design following outbreak of multi-resistant Acinetobacter infection in ICU and Burns Unit. *Burns.* 2003;29:303-306.
63. Manson WL, Pernot PC, Fidler V, et al. Colonization of burns and the duration of hospital stay of severely burned patients. *J Hosp Infect.* 1992;22:55-63.
64. Mayhall CG, Polk RE, Haynes BW. Infections in burned patients. *Infect Control.* 1983;4:454-459.
65. Sherertz RJ, Sullivan ML. An outbreak of infections with Acinetobacter calcoaceticus in burn patients: Contamination of patients' mattresses. *J Infect Dis.* 1985;151:252-258.
66. Weber J, McManus A. Infection control in burn patients. *Burns.* 2004;30:A16-A24.
67. Fleming RY, Zeigler ST, Walton MA, et al. Influence of burn size on the incidence of contamination of burn wounds by fecal organisms. *J Burn Care Rehabil.* 1991;12:510-515.
68. Agnihotri N, Gupta V, Joshi RM. Aerobic bacterial isolates from burn wound infections and their antibiograms—a five-year study. *Burns.* 2004;30:241-243.
69. Albrecht MC, Griffith ME, Murray CK, et al. Impact of Acinetobacter infection on the mortality of burn patients. *J Am Coll Surg.* 2006;203:546-550.
70. Altoparlak U, Erol S, Akcay MN, et al. The time-related changes of antimicrobial resistance patterns and predominant bacterial

profiles of burn wounds and body flora of burned patients. *Burns.* 2004;30:660-664.

71. Ressner RA, Murray CK, Griffith ME, et al. Outcomes of bacteremia in burn patients involved in combat operations overseas. *J Am Coll Surg.* 2008;206:439-444.

72. Oncul O, Yuksel F, Altunay H, et al. The evaluation of nosocomial infection during 1-year-period in the burn unit of a training hospital in Istanbul, Turkey. *Burns.* 2002;28:738-744.

73. Ferreira AC, Gobara S, Costa SE, et al. Emergence of resistance in Pseudomonas aeruginosa and Acinetobacter species after the use of antimicrobials for burned patients. *Infect Control Hosp Epidemiol.* 2004;25:868-872.

74. Yildirim S, Nursal TZ, Tarim A, et al. Bacteriological profile and antibiotic resistance: Comparison of findings in a burn intensive care unit, other intensive care units, and the hospital services unit of a single center. *J Burn Care Rehabil.* 2005;26:488-492.

75. Regules JA, Carlson MD, Wolf SE, et al. Analysis of anaerobic blood cultures in burned patients. *Burns.* 2007;33:561-564.

76. Ballard J, Edelman L, Saffle J, et al. Positive fungal cultures in burn patients: A multicenter review. *J Burn Care Res.* 2008;29: 213-221.

77. Horvath EE, Murray CK, Vaughan GM, et al. Fungal wound infection (not colonization) is independently associated with mortality in burn patients. *Ann Surg.* 2007;245:978-985.

78. Schofield CM, Murray CK, Horvath EE, et al. Correlation of culture with histopathology in fungal burn wound colonization and infection. *Burns.* 2007;33:341-346.

79. Murray CK, Loo FL, Hospenthal DR, et al. Incidence of systemic fungal infection and related mortality following severe burns. *Burns.* 2008;34:1108-1112.

80. Sheridan RL, Weber JM, Pasternak MM, et al. A 15-year experience with varicella infections in a pediatric burn unit. *Burns.* 1999;25:353-356.

81. Hamprecht K, Pfau M, Schaller HE, et al. Human cytomegalovirus infection of a severe-burn patient: Evidence for productive self-limited viral replication in blood and lung. *J Clin Microbiol.* 2005;43:2534-2536.

82. Rennekampff HO, Hamprecht K. Cytomegalovirus infection in burns: A review. *J Med Microbiol.* 2006;55(Pt 5):483-487.

83. Murray CK, Hoffmaster RM, Schmit DR, et al. Evaluation of white blood cell count, neutrophil percentage, and elevated temperature as predictors of bloodstream infection in burn patients. *Arch Surg.* 2007;142:639-642.

84. Lavrentieva A, Kontakiotis T, Lazaridis L, et al. Inflammatory markers in patients with severe burn injury. What is the best indicator of sepsis? *Burns.* 2007;33:189-194.

85. Bargues L, Chancerelle Y, Catineau J, et al. Evaluation of serum procalcitonin concentration in the ICU following severe burn. *Burns.* 2007;33:860-864.

86. Greenhalgh DG, Saffle JR, Holmes JH, et al. American Burn Association consensus conference to define sepsis and infection in burns. *J Burn Care Res.* 2007; 28:776-790.

87. Still J, Newton T, Friedman B, et al. Experience with pneumonia in acutely burned patients requiring ventilator support. *Am Surg.* 2000;66:206-209.

88. Nseir S, Di Pompeo C, Pronnier P, et al. Nosocomial tracheobronchitis in mechanically ventilated patients: Incidence, aetiology and outcome. *Eur Respir J.* 2002;20:1483-1489.

89. O'Grady NP, Barie PS, Bartlett JG, et al. Guidelines for evaluation of new fever in critically ill adult patients: 2008 update from the American College of Critical Care Medicine and the Infectious Diseases Society of America. *Crit Care Med.* 2008;36: 1330-1349.

90. Horan TC, Andrus M, Dudeck MA. CDC/NHSN surveillance definition of health care-associated infection and criteria for specific types of infections in the actue care setting. *Am J Infect Control.* 2008;36:309-332.

91. Sjoberg T, Mzezewa S, Jonsson K, et al. Comparison of surface swab cultures and quantitative tissue biopsy cultures to predict sepsis in burn patients: A prospective study. *J Burn Care Rehabil.* 2003;24:365-370.

92. Uppal SK, Ram S, Kwatra B, et al. Comparative evaluation of surface swab and quantitative full-thickness wound biopsy culture in burn patients. *Burns.* 2007;33:460-463.

93. Steer JA, Hill GB, Wilson AP. The effect of burn wound surgery and teicoplanin on the bactericidal activity of polymorphonuclear leucocytes against Staphylococcus aureus. *J Antimicrob Chemother.* 1995;36:851-855.

94. Danilla S, Andrades P, Gomez ME, et al. Concordance between qualitative and quantitative cultures in burned patients. Analysis of 2886 cultures. *Burns.* 2005;31:967-971.

95. McManus AT, Mason AD Jr, McManus WF, et al. Twenty-five year review of Pseudomonas aeruginosa bacteremia in a burn center. *Eur J Clin Microbiol.* 1985;4:219-223.

96. McManus AT, Kim SH, McManus WF, et al. Comparison of quantitative microbiology and histopathology in divided burn-wound biopsy specimens. *Arch Surg.* 1987;122:74-76.

97. Ramzy PI, Herndon DN, Wolf SE, et al. Comparison of wound culture and bronchial lavage in the severely burned child: Implications for antimicrobial therapy. *Arch Surg.* 1998;133:1275-1280.

98. Steer JA, Papini RP, Wilson AP, et al. Quantitative microbiology in the management of burn patients. II. Relationship between bacterial counts obtained by burn wound biopsy culture and surface alginate swab culture, with clinical outcome following burn surgery and change of dressings. *Burns.* 1996;22:177-181.

99. Steer JA, Papini RP, Wilson AP, et al. Quantitative microbiology in the management of burn patients. I. Correlation between quantitative and qualitative burn wound biopsy culture and surface alginate swab culture. *Burns.* 1996;22:173-176.

100. Miller PL, Matthey FC. A cost-benefit analysis of initial burn cultures in the management of acute burns. *J Burn Care Rehabil.* 2000;21:300-303.

101. Conil JM, Georges B, Fourcade O, et al. Assessment of renal function in clinical practice at the bedside of burn patients. *Br J Clin Pharmacol.* 2007;63:583-594.

102. Boucher BA, Kuhl DA, Hickerson WL. Pharmacokinetics of systemically administered antibiotics in patients with thermal injury. *Clin Infect Dis.* 1992;14:458-463.

103. Rybak MJ, Albrecht LM, Berman JR, et al. Vancomycin pharmacokinetics in burn patients and intravenous drug abusers. *Antimicrob Agents Chemother.* 1990;34:792-795.

104. Bracco D, Landry C, Dubois MJ, et al. Pharmacokinetic variability of extended interval tobramycin in burn patients. *Burns.* 2008;34:791-796.

105. Dailly E, Kergueris MF, Pannier M, et al. Population pharmacokinetics of imipenem in burn patients. *Fundam Clin Pharmacol.* 2003;17:645-650.

106. Conil JM, Georges B, Lavit M, et al. Pharmacokinetics of ceftazidime and cefepime in burn patients: The importance of age and creatinine clearance. *Int J Clin Pharmacol Ther.* 2007;45: 529-538.

107. Hoey LL, Tschida SJ, Rotschafer JC, et al. Wide variation in single, daily-dose aminoglycoside pharmacokinetics in patients with burn injuries. *J Burn Care Rehabil.* 1997;18:116-124.

108. Michalopoulos A, Fotakis D, Virtzili S, et al. Aerosolized colistin as adjunctive treatment of ventilator-associated pneumonia due to multidrug-resistant Gram-negative bacteria: A prospective study. *Respir Med.* 2008;102:407-412.

109. Ioannidou E, Siempos II, Falagas ME. Administration of antimicrobials via the respiratory tract for the treatment of patients with nosocomial pneumonia: A meta-analysis. *J Antimicrob Chemother.* 2007;60:1216-1226.

110. Sinha R, Sharma N, Agarwal RK. Subeschar clysis in deep burns. *Burns.* 2003;29:854-856.

111. McManus WF, Goodwin CW Jr, Pruitt BA Jr. Subeschar treatment of burn-wound infection. *Arch Surg.* 1983;118:291-294.

112. Ong YS, Samuel M, Song C. Meta-analysis of early excision of burns. *Burns.* 2006;32:145-150.

113. Herndon DN, Barrow RE, Rutan RL, et al. A comparison of conservative versus early excision. Therapies in severely burned patients. *Ann Surg.* 1989;209:547-552.

114. Subrahmanyam M. Early tangential excision and skin grafting of moderate burns is superior to honey dressing: A prospective randomised trial. *Burns.* 1999;25:729-731.

115. Atiyeh BS, Hayek SN, Gunn SW. New technologies for burn wound closure and healing—review of the literature. *Burns.* 2005;31:944-956.

116. Mooney EK, Lippitt C, Friedman J. Silver dressings. *Plast Reconstr Surg.* 2006;117:666-669.

117. Brown TP, Cancio LC, McManus AT, et al. Survival benefit conferred by topical antimicrobial preparations in burn patients: A historical perspective. *J Trauma.* 2004;56:863-866.

118. Simor AE, Lee M, Vearncombe M, et al. An outbreak due to multiresistant Acinetobacter baumannii in a burn unit: Risk factors for acquisition and management. *Infect Control Hosp Epidemiol.* 2002;23:261-267.

119. Dansby W, Purdue G, Hunt J, et al. Aerosolization of methicillin-resistant Staphylococcus aureus during an epidemic in a burn intensive care unit. *J Burn Care Res.* 2008;29:331-337.

120. Still JM, Law E, Thiruvaiyaru D, et al. Central line-related sepsis in acute burn patients. *Am Surg.* 1998;64:165-170.

121. Ramos GE, Bolgiani AN, Patino O, et al. Catheter infection risk related to the distance between insertion site and burned area. *J Burn Care Rehabil.* 2002;23:266-271.

122. O'Mara MS, Reed NL, Palmieri TL, et al. Central venous catheter infections in burn patients with scheduled catheter exchange and replacement. *J Surg Res.* 2007;142:341-350.

123. King B, Schulman CI, Pepe A, et al. Timing of central venous catheter exchange and frequency of bacteremia in burn patients. *J Burn Care Res.* 2007;28:859-860.

124. Piel P, Scarnati S, Goldfarb IW, et al. Antibiotic prophylaxis in patients undergoing burn wound excision. *J Burn Care Rehabil.* 1985;6:422-424.

125. Ergun O, Celik A, Ergun G, et al. Prophylactic antibiotic use in pediatric burn units. *Eur J Pediatr Surg.* 2004;14:422-426.

126. de La Cal MA, Cerda E, Garcia-Hierro P, et al. Survival benefit in critically ill burned patients receiving selective decontamination of the digestive tract: a randomized, placebo-controlled, double-blind trial. *Ann Surg.* 2005;241:424-430.

127. Peng YZ, Yuan ZQ, Xiao GX. Effects of early enteral feeding on the prevention of enterogenic infection in severely burned patients. *Burns.* 2001;27:145-149.

128. Wasiak J, Cleland H, Jeffery R. Early versus late enteral nutritional support in adults with burn injury: A systematic review. *J Hum Nutr Diet.* 2007;20:75-83.

129. Chen Z, Wang S, Yu B, et al. A comparison study between early enteral nutrition and parenteral nutrition in severe burn patients. *Burns.* 2007;33:708-712.

130. Kowal-Vern A, McGill V, Gamelli RL. Ischemic necrotic bowel disease in thermal injury. *Arch Surg.* 1997;132:440-443.

131. Peck MD, Kessler M, Cairns BA, et al. Early enteral nutrition does not decrease hypermetabolism associated with burn injury. *J Trauma.* 2004;57:1143-1148.

132. Palmieri TL, Caruso DM, Foster KN, et al. Effect of blood transfusion on outcome after major burn injury: A multicenter study. *Crit Care Med.* 2006;34:1602-1607.

133. Brannen AL, Still J, Haynes M, et al. A randomized prospective trial of hyperbaric oxygen in a referral burn center population. *Am Surg.* 1997;63:205-208.

134. Villanueva E, Bennett MH, Wasiak J, et al. Hyperbaric oxygen therapy for thermal burns. *Cochrane Database Syst Rev.* 2004; (3):CD004727.

135. Wasiak J, Bennett M, Cleland HJ. Hyperbaric oxygen as adjuvant therapy in the management of burns: Can evidence guide clinical practice? *Burns.* 2006;32:650-652.

319

Bites

ELLIE J. C. GOLDSTEIN

Bite wounds are common injuries that are often mistakenly considered innocuous by both patients and physicians. Most data on the incidence of infection, bacteriology, and the value of various medical and surgical methods of treatment come from small studies or anecdotal case reports that are further biased by the types of patients who elect to seek medical attention. Bite wounds consist of lacerations, evulsions, punctures, and scratches. Although 80% of patients never seek and do not need medical care, awareness of the magnitude of the infectious complications from bites is growing. The bacteria associated with bite infections may come from the environment, from the victim's skin flora, or most frequently, from the "normal" flora of the biter (Table 319-1).

The reader is referred to Chapter 163 for details on management of bites that carry a risk of rabies.

Animal Bites

In 2008 the Humane Society of the United States estimated that 74.8 million dogs and 88.3 million cats were kept as pets with about one-third of households owning dogs and cats.[1] Previously, it was estimated that one of every two Americans will be bitten in their lifetime, usually by a dog. Bites occur in 4.7 million Americans yearly[2] and account for 800,000 medical visits, including approximately 1% of all emergency department visits.[3] Most dog bites (85%) are provoked attacks by either the victim's own pet or a dog known to the victim and occur during the warm weather months.[4] Bite wounds that require attention are often those to the extremities, especially the dominant hand. Facial bites are more frequent in children younger than 10 years and lead to 5 to 10 deaths per year, often because of exsanguination.[5] Larger dogs can exert more than 450 lb/in.[2] of pressure with their jaws, which can lead to extensive crush injury.

Patients who present within 8 hours after injury are usually concerned with crush injury, care of disfiguring wounds, or the need for rabies or tetanus therapy.[4] These wounds are frequently contaminated with multiple strains of aerobic and anaerobic bacteria, similar to the spectrum found in documented bite infections. Between 2% and 30% of "treated" wounds will become infected and may require hospitalization.[6-10] Patients presenting longer than 8 hours after injury usually have established infection.[4,6,8,9,11] Infection is usually manifested by localized cellulitis, pain at the site of injury, and a purulent discharge, often gray and malodorous.[12] Temperature greater than 37.2° C, regional adenopathy, and lymphangitis occur in less than 10% of patients. Puncture wounds may become infected more frequently than evulsions and lead to abscess formation. Wounds close to bones or joints may penetrate these structures and cause septic arthritis, osteomyelitis, tenosynovitis, or local abscesses in any potential anatomic space. Osteomyelitis is a frequent and severe complication of bite wounds and should always be considered in the presence of pain in a joint or limited range of motion.

Rarely, sepsis, endocarditis, meningitis, or brain abscesses may develop after a bite injury. Fatal infection caused by *Capnocytophaga canimorsus* (formerly designated DF-2) in association with asplenia or liver disease has been noted.[13-15] This organism may be difficult to isolate and identify and may require up to 14 days of incubation to grow on blood culture. *C. canimorsus* has the potential capacity to escape the host immune system by both passive and active mechanisms.[16] It is generally susceptible to penicillin, cephalosporins, and fluoroquinolones but variably resistant to aztreonam and aminoglycosides (Table 319-2).[17]

Women who have undergone radical or modified radical mastectomy, patients with edema of an extremity due to any cause, patients with lupus erythematosus, especially if taking corticosteroids, and compromised hosts (e.g., patients with acute leukemia) may be prone to more severe infections, including sepsis, from the usual isolates that cause only limited cellulitis in immunocompetent patients.

Dog bite wound infections are considered to be predominantly related to the dog's oral flora.[4,7,11,12,18-20] Although most attention has focused on *Pasteurella multocida*, the spectrum of organisms associated with bite wound infections is much greater. Holst and colleagues[21] noted the following distribution of 159 *P. multocida* strains isolated over a period of 3 years from human infections, mostly from bite wounds: *P. multocida* (60%), which was the isolate in all bacteremia cases; *P. multocida* subsp. *septica* (13%), which has a greater prevalence in cats than in dogs and may have a preferential affinity for the central nervous system; *P. canis* biotype 1 (18%), which was isolated exclusively from dog bite infections; *P. stomatis* (6%); and *P. dagmatis* (3%), which may cause systemic infections. A study[12] of 107 dog and cat bite wounds showed that 75% of cat bites grew *Pasteurella* spp. on culturing (*P. multocida* subsp. *multocida*, 54%), as did 50% of dog bites (*P. canis*, 26%; *P. multocida* subsp. *multocida*, 12%). Other common isolates include streptococci (50%), *Staphylococcus aureus* (20% to 40%), and anaerobes (70%). Table 319-1 lists common bite pathogens. *Staphylococcus intermedius* is coagulase positive, is often mistaken for *S. aureus,* and is fourfold more common in canine flora[22,23] but possesses β-galactosidase activity, which differentiates it from *S. aureus*. It may masquerade as MRSA owing to false-positive rapid penicillin binding protein 2a latex tests[24] although an increasing number (~30%) of isolates may be resistant to oxacillin. MRSA has been cultured from a variety of companion animals including cats and has been documented to be transmitted from a healthy pet cat to humans, and the human strains and feline strains are indistinguishable.[25,26] Although not yet reported as isolated from animal bite wounds, MRSA should be considered as a potential causitive secondary invader agent, especially in patients with known risk factors for MRSA carriage. *C. canimorsus*[15] (DF-2) is difficult to grow on most routine solid media but can grow on chocolate agar and heart infusion agar with 5% rabbit blood when incubated in CO_2 and a variety of liquid media, including BACTEC aerobic medium.[14] This species can be differentiated from other *Capnocytophaga* spp. by the presence of positive oxidase and catalase reactions.[15] "DF-2–like" strains have been classified as *Capnocytophaga cynodegmi*. M5 has been classified as *Neisseria weaveri*[27] and has been associated with dog bites. EF-4 a is now called *Neisseria animaloris*, and EF-4b is *Neisseria zoodegmatis*. *Haemophilus felis*, which may be identical to *Aggregatibacter (Haemophilus) paraphrophilus,* requires factor V and CO_2 for growth, and is common in cat nasopharyngeal flora.[28] *Bergeyella (Weeksella) zoohelcum* has been associated with bite cellulitis, sepsis, and meningitis.[29] Other new aerobic species include *Neisseria canis* from a cat bite,[30] *Flavobacterium* IIb-like isolates from a pig bite,[31] *Actinobacillus lignieresii* and *Actinobacillus equi*-like bacterium from horse bites,[32] and NO1, a nonoxidative gram-negative rod[33] different from *Acinetobacter* spp. Orf virus infection has been transmitted by a sheep bite.[34] Anaerobes are isolated in up to 70% of animal bite wounds, always in mixed culture.[4,9,11] Approximately 50% to 60% of cat and dog bite wounds contain *Bacteroides tectum, Pre-*

TABLE 319-1	Common Bacterial Isolates from Dog and Cat Bite Wounds

Acinetobacter spp.
Aggregatibacter (Actinobacillus) actinomycetemcomitans
Aggregatibacter (Haemophilus) aphrophilus
Bacteroides tectus
Burgeyella (Weeksella) zoohelcum
Capnocytophaga canimorsus
Capnocytophaga cynodegmi
Corynebacterium minutissimum
Eikenella corrodens
Enterococcus spp.
Finegoldia magna
Fusobacterium nucleatum
Fusobacterium russii
Leifsonia (Corynebacterium) aquaticum
Leptotrichia buccalis
Micrococcus luteus
Moraxella spp.
Neisseria canis
Neisseria weaveri
Pasteurella multocida subsp. *multocida*
Pasteurella multocida subsp. *septica*
Pasteurella dagmatis
Pasteurella canis
Pasteurella stomatis
Peptostreptococci
Porphyromonas asaccharolytica
Porphyromonas gulae (gingivalis)
Porphyromonas canoris
Prevotella bivia
Prevotella heparinolytica
Prevotella melaninogenica
Prevotella intermedia
Prevotella zoogleoformans
Staphylococcus aureus
Staphylococcus intermedius
Staphylococcus epidermidis
Streptococci, α-hemolytic, β-hemolytic
Veillonella parvula

votella heparinolytica, Prevotella zoogleoformans, Prevotella bivia, Porphyromonas gingivalis, Porphyromonas canoris, fusobacteria, and peptostreptococci.[35-38] *Fusobacterium canifelinum* is an intrinsically fluoroquinolone-resistant species isolated from dog and cat bites.[39]

Gram stains of bite wounds are specific but nonsensitive indicators of bacterial growth. When compared, little difference was noted in the types of bacteria isolated from noninfected wounds seen early and infected wounds seen later.[4] All moderate to severe dog bite wounds, except those not clinically infected and more than 1 day old, should be considered contaminated with potential pathogens.

Wounds inflicted by cats are frequently scratches or tiny punctures located on the extremities and are likely to become infected.[40] *P. multocida* has been isolated from 50% to 70% of healthy cats and is a frequent pathogen in cat-associated wounds.[12,21,40] *Erysipelothrix rhusiopathiae* has been isolated from cat bite wounds.[12] Punctures over or near a joint, especially on the hands, should be treated aggressively with antibiotics and elevation because of a high incidence of osteomyelitis and septic arthritis. Cougar, tiger, and other feline bites also yield *P. multocida*.[32] Tularemia has likewise been transmitted by cat bites.[41] People are also bitten by a variety of other animals, including unusual domestic pets, farm animals, wild animals, aquatic animals, and laboratory animals.[3,42-45] Monkey bites cause more swelling and infection than do many other animal bites.[46] Old World monkeys may transmit potentially lethal subtype B virus (herpesvirus simiae; see Chapter 142).[47] Case reports of bear, caiman, and kinkajou bites with unusual isolates have been reported.[48-50] The bacteriology of most of these wounds is based on single case reports.

MANAGEMENT OF ANIMAL BITES

Table 319-3 notes the elements for treatment of animal bite wounds. The most problematic elements of the management of wounds seen early include the following:

1. The use of "prophylactic" antibiotics in wounds that are seen early but as yet are uninfected. Because 85% of such wounds harbor potential pathogens and one cannot reliably predict which wounds will become infected, selected wounds should be treated with oral therapy for 3 to 5 days (see Table 319-2). Recommendations about patient selection vary.[51]
2. The decision to suture the wound. Facial wounds are usually sutured after copious irrigation and the use of antibiotics in all but the most trivial wounds. No prospective studies are available to determine whether the risk of infection is increased. It is the author's experience and recommendation that other wounds need not be primarily closed, but after irrigation and débridement they can be approximated and be closed by delayed primary or secondary intention.

TABLE 319-2	Antimicrobial Susceptibilities of Bacteria Frequently Isolated from Animal Bite Wounds*					
	Percentages of Isolates Susceptible					
	*Staphylococcus aureus***	*Eikenella corrodens*	Anaerobes	*Pasteurella multocida*	*Capnocytophaga canimorsus*	*Staphylococcus intermedius*
Penicillin	10	99	50/95†	95	95	30
Dicloxacillin	99	5	50‡§	30	NS	70
Amoxicillin/clavulanic acid	100	100	100‡§	100	95	70
Cephalexin	100	20	40‡§	30	NS	95
Cefuroxime	100	70	40‡§	90	NS	NS
Cefoxitin	100	95	100‡§	95	95	NS
Erythromycin	100	20	40‡§	20	95	95
Tetracycline	95	85	60‡§	90	95	NS
TMP-SMX	100	95	0‡§	95	V	NS
Ciprofloxacin	100	100	40‡§	95	100	100
Levofloxacin	100	100	60‡§	100	100	100
Moxifloxacin	100	100	85‡§	100	100	100
Azithromycin	100	80	70‡§	100	100	NS
Clarithromycin	100	60	70‡§	70	100	NS
Clindamycin	100	0	100‡§	0	95	95

*Data are compiled from various studies.
**MRSA has been rarely reported in bite wounds but is an increasing possibility. In animal bites, *S. intermedius* may be mistakenly identified as MRSA.[24]
†Percentage of human bite isolates/percentage of animal bite isolates.
‡*Fusobacterium canifelinum* are intrinsically resistant, while human *Fusobacterium nucleatum* are susceptible.
§Some peptostreptococci are resistant.
NS, not studied; TMP-SMX, trimethoprim-sulfamethoxazole; V, variable.

TABLE 319-3	Management of Bite Wounds

History

Animal bite: Ascertain the type of animal, whether the bite was provoked or unprovoked, and the situation/environment in which the bite occurred. If the species can be rabid, locate the animal for 10 days' observation or sacrifice.

Patient: Obtain information on antimicrobial allergies, current medications, splenectomy, mastectomy, liver disease, and immunosuppression.

Physical Examination

Record a diagram of the wound with the location, type, and depth of injury; range of motion; possibility of joint penetration; presence of edema or crush injury; nerve and tendon function; signs of infection; and odor of exudate.

Culture

Infected wounds should be cultured and a Gram stain performed. Anaerobic cultures should be obtained in the presence of abscesses, sepsis, serious cellulitis, devitalized tissue, or foul odor of the exudate. Small tears and infected punctures should be cultured with a minitipped (nasopharyngeal) swab.

Irrigation

Copious amounts of normal saline should be used for irrigation. Puncture wounds should be irrigated with a "high-pressure jet" from a 20-mL syringe and an 18-gauge needle or catheter tip.

Débridement

Devitalized or necrotic tissue should be cautiously débrided. Debris and foreign bodies should be removed.

Radiographs

Radiographs should be obtained if fracture or bone penetration is possible to provide a baseline for future osteomyelitis.

Wound Closure

Wound closure may be necessary for selected, fresh, uninfected wounds, especially facial wounds, but primary wound closure is not usually indicated. Wound edges should be approximated with adhesive strips in selected cases.

Antimicrobial Therapy

Prophylaxis: Consider prophylaxis (1) for moderate to severe injury less than 8 hours old, especially if edema or crush injury is present, (2) if bone or joint penetration is possible, (3) for hand wounds, (4) for immunocompromised patients (including those with mastectomy, liver disease, or steroid therapy), (5) if the wound is adjacent to prosthetic joint, and (6) if the wound is in the genital area. Coverage should include *Pasteurella multocida, Staphylococcus aureus,* and anaerobes (see Table 319-2).

Treatment: Cover *P. multocida, S. aureus,* and anaerobes (see Table 319-2). Use oral medication if the patient is seen early after a bite and only mild to moderate signs of infection are present. The following can be considered for cat or dog bites in adults:

- First choice: Amoxicillin/clavulanic acid, 875/125 mg bid or 500/125 mg tid with food.
- Penicillin allergy: No alternative treatment for animal bites has been established for penicillin-allergic patients. The following regimens can be considered for adults:
    ○ Clindamycin 300 mg PO qid plus either levofloxacin 500 mg PO daily or trimethoprim-sulfamethoxazole two double-strength tablets PO bid.
    ○ Doxycycline 100 mg PO bid.
    ○ Moxifloxacin 400 mg PO daily.
    ○ In the highly penicillin-allergic pregnant patient, macrolides have been used, but the wounds must be watche carefully.

On emergency department discharge, a single starting dose of parenteral antibiotic, such as ertapenem 1 g, may be useful in selected cases. If hospitalization or closely monitored outpatient follow-up is required, intravenous agents should be used. Current choices include ampicillin/sulbactam and cefoxitin. The rising incidence of community-acquired *S. aureus* isolates that are methicillin resistant and therefore resistant to the drugs recommended here emphasizes the importance of susceptibility-testing any *S. aureus* isolates.

Hospitalization

Indications include fever, sepsis, spread of cellulitis, significant edema or crush injury, loss of function, a compromised host, patient noncompliance.

Immunizations

Give tetanus booster (Td, tetanus and diphtheria toxoids for adults) if original three-dose series has been given but none in the past 5 years. Adults who have not received acellular pertussis vaccine (Tdap), should be given this instead of Td. Give a primary series and tetanus immune globulin if the patient was never immunized (see Chapter 320).

Rabies vaccine (on days 0, 3, 7, 14, and 28) with hyperimmune globulin may be required, depending on the type of animal, ability to observe the animal, and locality (see Chapter 163).

Elevation

Elevation may be required if any edema is present. Lack of elevation is a common cause of therapeutic failure.

Immobilization

Immobilize the extremity, especially hands, with a splint.

Follow-up

Follow-up should occur at 24 and perhaps 48 hours for outpatients.

Reporting

Reporting the incident to a local health department may be required.

bid, two times a day; PO, orally; qid, four times a day; tid, three times a day.

The most common causes of therapeutic failure are the following:

1. Failure to stress the importance of, or noncompliance of the patient, in elevating an edematous wound. If the wound is on the hands, slings must be recommended because compliance is unlikely unless passively accomplished.
2. Selection of the incorrect antimicrobial agent (see Table 319-2). Most fastidious animal pathogens are susceptible to penicillin/amoxicillin. Because of resistance of certain bacteria, including *P. multocida,* first-generation cephalosporins, dicloxacillin, and erythromycin should be avoided or used cautiously. In vitro data suggest that some fluoroquinolones (ciprofloxacin, levofloxacin, and moxifloxacin), sulfamethoxazole-trimethoprim, and sec-ond-generation oral cephalosporins (cefuroxime) are active against many bite isolates.[52-58]
3. Failure to recognize joint penetration. Pain, diminished range of motion, local edema, and proximity of the puncture wound to a joint should alert one to the possibility of septic arthritis.

Venomous Snake Bites

Venomous snakes, usually vipers (rattlesnakes, copperheads, cottonmouths, or water moccasins), bite approximately 8000 people in the United States yearly, of which five or six result in death, usually of children or the elderly, who receive either no or delayed antivenom.[59]

The majority of bites occur in the southwestern United States between April and September and are to the extremities of males between 17 and 27 years old.[59] Envenomation can cause extensive tissue destruction and devitalization that predisposes to infection from the snake's normal oral flora. Sparse data exist on the incidence and bacteriology of snakebite infections. In rattlesnakes, the oral flora appears to be fecal in nature because the live prey usually defecates in the snake's mouth coincident with ingestion. Common oral isolates include *Pseudomonas aeruginosa, Proteus* spp., coagulase-negative staphylococci, and *Clostridium* spp.[60,61] Other potential pathogens isolated from rattlesnakes' mouths include *Bacteroides fragilis* and *Salmonella arizonae* (*Salmonella* groups IIIa and IIIb). *Crotalus* rattlesnake venom has innate broad activity against aerobic gram-positive and gram-negative bacteria but not against anaerobes.[62,63] The role of empirical antimicrobial therapy for noninfected wounds is not well defined. Specific therapy based on culturing of infected wounds should be instituted.

Lip Wounds and Paronychia

Wounds of the lip and paronychia and infections of the structure surrounding the nail account for most self-inflicted bite wounds that come to medical attention. Paronychia is more frequent in children who suck their fingers and results from direct inoculation of the oral flora into the fingers. Brook[64] took cultures from 33 children with paronychia. Aerobes and anaerobes were each found in pure culture in 27% of cases, whereas mixed infection was found in 46% of cases. The most frequent aerobic organisms isolated were viridans streptococci, group A streptococci, *S. aureus, Haemophilus parainfluenzae, Klebsiella pneumoniae*, and *Eikenella corrodens*. The most frequently isolated anaerobic bacteria were *Bacteroides* spp., *Fusobacterium* spp., and gram-positive cocci. Therapy should include drainage, appropriate antibiotics, and avoidance of further bacterial contamination.

Human Bites

Human bites have higher complication and infection rates than do animal bites. Occlusional human bites may affect any part of the body but most often involve the distal phalanx of the long or index fingers of the dominant hand. About 10% to 20% of wounds are "love nips" to the breasts and genital areas.[18,65,66] Bites to the hand are more serious and more frequently become infected than do bites to other areas.[67] Bites may also be caused by or be harbingers of child abuse.[68]

Important prognostic factors for the development of infection include the extent of tissue damage, the depth of the wound and which compartments are entered, and the pathogenicity of the inoculated oral bacteria.[69-72] The typical patient is a 27-year-old man who is assaulted by a 28-year-old man; first infectious symptoms occur approximately 22 hours postinjury, but patients do not seek medical care until approximately 36 hours later.[72] Viridans streptococci, especially *S. anginosus*, are the most common wound isolates. *S. aureus* infection occurred in 30% to 40% of wounds and was usually present in patients who had attempted self-débridement and presented 3 to 4 days after injury. As yet, MRSA has been rarely reported from human bite wounds. Although *H. influenzae* was occasionally isolated, other *Haemophilus* spp. including *H. parainfluenzae, Aggregatibacter (H.) aphrophilus*, and *Aggregatibacter (H.) paraphrophilus*, and some penicillin-resistant gram-negative rods, such as *Klebsiella* spp., and *Enterobacter cloacae*, were occasionally isolated. *Prevotella* spp., *Peptostreptococcus* spp., and *Fusobacterium nucleatum* were also frequent isolates.[59,72] Up to 45% of the anaerobic gram-negative bacilli isolated from human bite wounds may be penicillin resistant and β-lactamase positive.[54,73] *Candida* spp. were found in 8% of patients in one study although their pathogenicity was not determined.[72]

MANAGEMENT OF HUMAN BITES

A Gram stain and aerobic and anaerobic cultures should be obtained for all infected wounds before any therapy is given. Wounds should be copiously irrigated, surgically débrided, and diagrammed or photographed (or both). Immobilization of the affected area, including splinting if necessary, and elevation should be instituted. Empirical antimicrobial therapy should be based on the Gram stain (specific but not sensitive) or knowledge of the susceptibility of the oral flora. Patients who present early with uninfected wounds should also be given antimicrobial therapy of shorter duration and may be considered for outpatient management. Amoxicillin/clavulanic acid or penicillin plus a penicillinase-resistant penicillin or cephalosporin should be used. First-generation cephalosporins are not as effective as monotherapy because of resistance of some anaerobic bacteria and *E. corrodens*. The role of MRSA in bite wounds remains to be defined. The role of the newer fluoroquinolones with anaerobic activity has not been clinically evaluated. Many patients (32% in one study[72]) require hospitalization. Baseline radiographs should be taken of wounds close to the bone to compare for osteomyelitis later. Most physicians advise against primary closure, even for uninfected human bite wounds, especially those on the hands. Facial wounds may present a special situation because of the possibility of scarring and disfigurement, and many investigators recommend primary closure. Approximation of the wound margins or delayed primary closure (3 to 5 days) is often possible even in infected cases.

Clenched-fist Injuries

Clenched-fist injuries are traumatic lacerations that occur when one person strikes another in the mouth with a clenched fist. These injuries are most common over the third and fourth metacarpophalangeal joints of the dominant hand, but they may also occur over the proximal interphalangeal joints. These lacerations are often only 12 to 14 mm long but, despite their innocuous appearance, frequently lead to serious complications because of the proximity of the skin over the knuckles to the joint capsule and the potential spread of infection into subcutaneous, subfascial, subtendinous, subaponeurotic, and web spaces.

Typically, patients sustain a clenched-fist injury and attempt to cleanse it or, more often, ignore it until 36 hours postinjury, when they awaken with a painful, throbbing, and swollen hand. The swelling usually spreads proximally but not distally and results in decreased range of motion. A purulent discharge is often present. Lymphangitis, adenopathy, fever, or other signs of systemic infection are infrequent.

The bacteriology of clenched-fist injuries is similar to that of human bites and usually consists of the normal oral flora.[8,69,74] Viridans streptococci, especially *S. anginosus*, are the most frequent isolates, but *S. aureus* may be present in 20% to 40% of cases. Anaerobic bacteria can be recovered in more than 55% of clenched-fist injuries, including *Prevotella* spp., *F. nucleatum*, and peptostreptococci (including *Finegoldia magna*). *E. corrodens* is an often overlooked but especially important pathogen in clenched-fist injury infections.[74-77] It has a prevalence rate of 59% in human gingival plaque[66] and may be isolated in 25% of clenched-fist injuries.[75] It can act synergistically with viridans streptococci and is a common cause of osteomyelitis. Although *E. corrodens* is susceptible to penicillin, it is resistant to penicillinase-resistant penicillins, clindamycin, and metronidazole and is variably resistant to cephalosporins.[54-58]

Management should include examination by an experienced hand surgeon to evaluate nerve and muscular function and the extent of injury to tendons, bones, and joints. Débridement and copious irrigation are often required. Elevation and immobilization with a plaster splint from the fingers to the elbow are essential and should be continued until marked improvement is noted. Aerobic and anaerobic cultures and radiographic films (to check for fracture and osteomyelitis) should be obtained. Many authors suggest the use of tetanus toxoid or both toxoid and antitoxin when indicated. Secondary débridement to remove necrotic bone and tissue or to drain abscesses may be advisable.

Empirical antimicrobial therapy is often intravenous and should include either cefoxitin or ampicillin/sulbactam or a carbapenem (imipenem, ertapenem, meropenem or doripenam) until culture results are known. Failure of first-generation cephalosporins and penicillinase-resistant penicillins, when used alone, has been reported and is often due to *E. corrodens*.[75-80] If resistant gram-negative rods are isolated, therapy should be altered according to the results of culture. What role β-lactamase-positive *Prevotella* and *Porphyromonas* spp. will have in the selection of antimicrobial therapy remains to be determined.

REFERENCES

1. The Humane Society of the United States. American Pet Products Manufacturers Association (APPMA) 2007-2008 National Pet Owners Survey. ⟨http://www.americanpetproducts.org/pubs_survey.asp⟩; Accessed 3/31/09.
2. Sacks JJ, Kresnow M, Houston B. Dog bites: how big a problem? *Inj Prev*. 1996;2:52-54.
3. Weiss HB, Friedman DJ, Cohen JH. Incidence of dog bite injuries treated in emergency departments. *JAMA*. 1998;279:51-53.
4. Goldstein EJC, Citron DM, Finegold SM. Dog bite wounds and infection: a prospective clinical study. *Ann Emerg Med*. 1980;9:508-512.
5. Lockwood R. Dog-bite-related fatalities—United States, 1995-1996. *MMWR Morb Mortal Wkly Rep*. 1997;46:463-467.
6. Brakenbury PH, Muwanga C. A comparative double blind study of amoxycillin/clavulanate vs placebo in the prevention of infection after animal bites. *Arch Emerg Med*. 1989;6:251-256.
7. Feder HM, Shanley JD, Barbera JA. Review of 59 patients hospitalized with animal bites. *Pediatr Infect Dis J*. 1987;6:24-28.
8. Goldstein EJC. Bite wounds and infection. *Clin Infect Dis*. 1992;14:633-640.
9. Goldstein EJC, Citron DM, Nesbit C, et al. Prevalence and characterization of anaerobic bacteria from 50 patients with infected dog and cat bite wounds. In: Ely A, Bennett K, eds. *Anaerobic Pathogens*. Sheffield, England: Sheffield Academic; 1997: 177-185.
10. Zook EG, Miller M, Van Beek AL, et al. Successful treatment protocol of canine fang injuries. *J Trauma*. 1980;20:243-247.
11. Brook I. Microbiology of human and animal bite wounds in children. *Pediatr Infect Dis J*. 1987;6:29-32.
12. Talan DA, Citron DM, Abrahamian FM, et al. Bacteriologic analysis of infected dog and cat bites. Emergency Medicine Animal Bite Infection Study Group. *N Engl J Med*. 1999;340:85-92.
13. Gallen IW, Ispahani P. Fulminant *Capnocytophaga canimorsus* (DF-2) septicaemia. *Lancet*. 1991;337:308.
14. Hicklin H, Verghese A, Alvarez S. Dysgonic fermenter 2 septicemia. *Rev Infect Dis*. 1987;9:884-890.
15. Brenner DJ, Hollis DG, Fanning GR, et al. *Capnocytophaga canimorsus* sp. nov. (formerly CDC group DF2), a cause of septicemia following dog bite, and *C. cynodegmi* sp. nov., a cause of localized wound infection following dog bite. *J Clin Microbiol*. 1989;27: 231-235.
16. Shin H, Mally M, Kuhn M, et al. Escape from immune surveillance by *Capnocytophaga canimorsus*. *Clin Infect Dis*. 2007; 195:375-386.
17. Verghese A, Hamati F, Berk S, et al. Susceptibility of dysgonic fermenter 2 to antimicrobial agents in vitro. *Antimicrob Agents Chemother*. 1988;32:78-80.
18. Goldstein EJC, Citron DM, Finegold SM. Role of anaerobic bacteria in bite wound infections. *Rev Infect Dis*. 1984;6(Suppl 1):S177-S183.
19. Stucker FJ, Shaw GY, Boyd S, et al. Management of animal and human bites in the head and neck. *Arch Otolaryngol Head Neck Surg*. 1990;116:789-793.
20. Brook I. Human and animal bite infections. *J Fam Pract*. 1989;28: 713-718.
21. Holst E, Rollof J, Larsson L, et al. Characterization and distribution of *Pasteurella* species recovered from human infections. *J Clin Microbiol*. 1992;30:2984-2987.
22. Talan DA, Staatz D, Staatz A, et al. *Staphylococcus intermedius* in canine gingiva and canine inflicted human wound infections: laboratory characterization of a newly recognized zoonotic pathogen. *J Clin Microbiol*. 1989;27:78-81.
23. Talan DA, Goldstein EJC, Staatz D, et al. *Staphylococcus intermedius*: clinical presentation of a new human dog bite pathogen. *Ann Emerg Med*. 1989;18:410-413.
24. Pottumurthy S, Schapiro JM, Prentoce JL, et al. Clinical isolates of *Staphylococcus intermedius* masquerading as methicillin-resistant *Staphylococcus aureus*. *J Clin Microbiol*. 2004;42:5881-5884.
25. Leonard FC, Markey BK. Methicillin-resistant *Staphylococcus aureus* in animals: a review. *Vet J*. 2008;175:27-36.
26. Singh A, Tuschak C, Hormansdorfer S. Methicillin-resistant *Staphylococcus aureus* in a family and its pet cat. *New Engl J Med*. 2008;358:1200-1201.
27 Andersen BM, Steigerwalt AG, O'Conner SP, et al. *Neisseria weaveri* sp. nov., formerly CDC group M-5, a gram-negative bacterium associated with dog bite wounds. *J Clin Microbiol*. 1993;31:2456-2466.
28. Inzana TJ, Johnson JL, Shell L, et al. Isolation and characterization of a newly identified *Haemophilus* species from cats: *Haemophilus felis*. *J Clin Microbiol*. 1992;30:2108-2112.
29. Holmes B, Steigerwalt AG, Weaver RE, et al. *Weeksella zoohelcum* sp. nov. (formerly group IIj) from human clinical specimens. *Syst Appl Microbiol*. 1986;8:191-196.
30. Guibourdenche M, Lamber T, Riou JY. Isolation of *Neisseria canis* in mixed culture from a patient after a cat bite. *J Clin Microbiol*. 1989;27:1673-1674.
31. Goldstein EJC, Citron DM, Merkin TE, et al. Recovery of an unusual *Flavobacterium* IIb-like isolate from a hand infection following pig bite. *J Clin Microbiol*. 1990;28:1709-1781.
32. Peel NM, Hornridge KA, Luppino M, et al. *Actinobacillus* spp. and related bacteria in infected wounds of humans bitten by horses and sheep. *J Clin Microbiol*. 1991;29:2535-2538.
33. Hollis DG, Moss CW, Daneshaver MI, et al. Characterization of Centers for Disease Control group NO1, a fastidious, nonoxidative, gram negative organism associated with dog and cat bites. *J Clin Microbiol*. 1993;31:746-748.
34. Green G, Schnurr D, Knoll D, et al. Orf virus infection in humans—New York, Illinois, California, and Tenessee, 2004-2005. *MMWR Morb Mortal Wkly Rep*. 2006;55:65-68.
35. Citron DM, Gerardo SH, Claros MC, et al. Frequency of isolation of *Porphyromonas* species from infected dog and cat bite wounds in humans and their characterization by biochemical tests and arbitrarily primed-polymerase chain reaction fingerprinting. *Clin Infect Dis*. 1996;23(Suppl 1):S78-S82.
36. Alexander CJ, Citron DM, Gerardo SH, et al. Characterization of saccharolytic *Bacteroides* and *Prevotella* isolates from infected dog and cat bite wounds in humans. *J Clin Microbiol*. 1997;35: 406-411.
37. Hudspeth MK, Gerardo SH, Citron DM, et al. Growth characteristics and a novel method of identification (the WEE-TAB system) of *Porphyromonas* species isolated from infected dog and cat bite wounds in humans. *J Clin Microbiol*. 1997;35: 2450-2453.
38. Love DN, Cato EP, Johnson JL, et al. Deoxyribonucleic acid hybridization among strains of fusobacteria isolated from soft tissue infections of cats: comparison with the human and animal type strains from oral and other sites. *Int J Syst Bacteriol*. 1987; 37:23-26.
39. Conrads G, Citron DM, Goldstein EJC. Genetic determinant of intrinsic quinolone resistance in *Fusobacterium canifelinum*. *Antimicrob Agents Chemother*. 2005;49:434-437.
40. Lucas GL, Bartlett DH. *Pasteurella multocida* infection in the hand. *Plast Reconstr Surg*. 1981;67:49-53.
41. Capellan J, Fong IW. Tularemia from a cat bite: case report and review. *Clin Infect Dis*. 1993;16:472-475.
42. Ordog GJ, Balasubramianium S, Wasserberger J. Rat bites: fifty cases. *Ann Emerg Med*. 1985;14:126-130.
43. Paisley JW, Lauer BA. Severe facial injuries to infants due to unprovoked attacks by pet ferrets. *JAMA*. 1988;259:2005-2006.
44. Barnham M. Pig bite injuries and infection: report of seven human cases. *Epidemiol Infect*. 1988;101:641-645.
45. Flandry F, Lisecki EJ, Domingue GJ, et al. Initial antibiotic therapy for alligator bites. *South Med J*. 1989;82:262-266.
46. Goldstein EJC, Pryor EP III, Citron DM. Simian bites and bacterial infection. *Clin Infect Dis*. 1995;20:1551-1552.
47. Holmes GP, Chapman LE, Stewart J, et al. Guidelines for the prevention and treatment of B virus infections in exposed persons. *Clin Infect Dis*. 1995;20:421-439.
48. Kunimoto D, Rennie R, Citron DM, et al. Bacteriology of a bear bite wound infection and review. *J Clin Microbiol*. 2004;42: 3374-3376.
49. Hertner G. Caiman bite. *Wilderness Env Med*. 2006;17:267-270.
50. Lawson PA, Malnick H, Collins MD, et al. Description of *Kingella potus* sp. nov., an organism isolated from a wound caused by an animal bite. *J Clin Microbiol*. 2005;3526-3529.
51. Medeiros I, Saconato H. Antibiotic prophylaxis for mamilian bites. Cochrane Database Syst Rev 2001;2:CD001738.
52. Goldstein EJC, Citron DM, Richwald GA. Lack of in vitro efficacy of oral forms of certain cephalosporins, erythromycin and oxacillin against *Pasteurella multocida*. *Antimicrob Agents Chemother*. 1988;32:213-215.
53. Gaillot O, Guilbert L, Maruejouls C, et al. In vitro susceptibility to thirteen of *Pasteurella* spp. and related bacteria isolated from humans. *J Antimicrob Chemother*. 1995;36:878-880.
54. Goldstein EJC, Citron DM, Hudspeth M, et al. In vitro activity of Bay 12-8039, a new 8-methoxy-quinolone, compared to the activities of 11 other oral antimicrobial agents against 390 aerobic and anaerobic bacteria isolated from human and animal bite wounds in skin and soft tissue infections in humans. *Antimicrob Agents Chemother*. 1997;41:1552-1557.
55. Goldstein EJC, Citron DM, Merriam CV, et al. In vitro activities of the des-fluoro [6]-quinolone, BMS 284756, against aerobic and anaerobic pathogens isolated from skin and soft tissue animal and human bite wound infections. *Antimicrob Agents Chemother*. 2002;46:866-870.
56. Goldstein EJC, Citron DM, Merriam CV, et al. In vitro activity of GAR-936 against aerobic and anaerobic animal and human bite pathogens. *Antimicrob Agents Chemother*. 2000;44: 2747-2751.
57. Goldstein EJC, Citron DM, Merriam CV, et al. Comparative in vitro activity of ertapenem and 11 other antimicrobial agents against aerobic and anaerobic pathogens isolated from skin and soft tissue animal and human bite wound infections. *J Antimicrob Chemother* 2001;48:641-651.
58. Goldstein EJC, Citron DM, Gerardo SH, et al. Activities of HMR 3004 (RU 64004) and HMR 3647 (RU 6647) compared to those of erythromycin, azithromycin, clarithromycin, roxithromycin and eight other antimicrobial agents against unusual aerobic and anaerobic human and animal bite pathogens isolated from skin and soft tissue. *Antimicrob Agents Chemother*. 1998;42:1127-1132.
59. Gold B, Dart RC, Barish RA. Bites of venomous snakes. *N Engl J Med*. 2002;347:347-356.
60. Russell FE. Clinical aspects of snake venom poisoning in North America. *Toxicon*. 1969;7:33-37.
61. Goldstein EJC, Citron DM, Gonzalez H, et al. Bacteriology of rattlesnake venom and implications for therapy. *J Infect Dis*. 1979;140:818-821.
62. Williams FE, Freeman M, Kennedy E. The bacterial flora of the mouths of Australian venomous snakes in captivity. *Med J Aust*. 1934;2:190-193.
63. Talan D, Citron DM, Overturf GD, et al. Antibacterial activity of crotalid venoms against oral snake flora and other clinical bacteria. *J Infect Dis*. 1991;164:195-198.
64. Brook I. Bacteriology study of paronychia in children. *Am J Surg*. 1981;141:703.
65. Al Fallouji M. Traumatic love bites. *Br J Surg*. 1990;77: 100-101.
66. Wolf JS, Gomez R, McAninch JW. Human bites to the penis. *J Urol*. 1992;147:2065-2067.
67. Mann RJ, Hoffeld TA, Farmer CB. Human bites of the hand: Twenty years of experience. *J Hand Surg*. 1977;2:97-104.
68. Sperber ND. Bite marks, oral and facial injuries: harbingers of severe child abuse? *Pediatrician*. 1989;16:207-211.
69. Goldstein EJC, Citron DM, Wield B, et al. Bacteriology of human and animal bite wounds. *J Clin Microbiol*. 1978;8: 667-672.
70. Chuinard RG, D'Ambrosia RD. Human bite infections of the hand. *J Bone Joint Surg Am*. 1977;59:416-418.
71. Zubowicz VN, Gravier M. Management of early human bites of the hand: a prospective randomized study. *Plastic Reconstr Surg*. 1991;88:111-114.
72. Talan DA, Abrahamian FM, Moran GJ, et al. Clinical presentation and bacteriologic analysis of infected human bites presenting to emergency departments. *Clin Infect Dis*. 2003;37:1481-1489.
73. Brook I. Microbiology of human and animal bite wounds in children. *Pediatr Infect Dis*. 1987;6:29-32.
74. Merriam CV, Fernandez HT, Citron DM et al. Bacteriology of human bite wound infections. *Anaerobe* 2003;9:83-86.
75. Goldstein EJC, Miller TA, Citron DM, et al. Infections following clenched-fist injury: a new perspective. *J Hand Surg*. 1978;3: 455-457.
76. Goldstein EJC, Barone M, Miller TA. *Eikenella corrodens* in hand infections. *J Hand Surg*. 1983;8:563-567.
77. McDonald I. *Eikenella corrodens* infections of the hand. *Hand*. 1979;11:224-227.
78. Goldstein EJC, Tarenzi LA, Agyare EO, et al. Prevalence of *Eikenella corrodens* in dental plaque. *J Clin Microbiol*. 1983;17: 636-639.
79. Goldstein EJC, Sutter VL, Finegold SM. Susceptibility of *Eikenella corrodens* to ten cephalosporins. *Antimicrob Agents Chemother*. 1978;14:639-641.
80. Goldstein EJC, Gombert ME, Agyare EO. Susceptibility of *Eikenella corrodens* to newer beta-lactam antibiotics. *Antimicrob Agents Chemother*. 1980;18:832-833.

320

Immunization

WALTER A. ORENSTEIN | LARRY K. PICKERING | ALISON MAWLE |
ALAN R. HINMAN | MELINDA WHARTON

The two most effective means of preventing disease, disability, and death from infectious diseases have been sanitation and immunization. Both these approaches antedated understanding of the germ theory of disease. Artificial induction of immunity began centuries ago with variolation, the practice of inoculating fluid from smallpox lesions into the skin of susceptible persons. Although this technique usually produced mild illness without complications, spread of disease did occur, with occasional complications. In 1796, Jenner demonstrated that milkmaids who had contracted cowpox (vaccinia) were immune to smallpox. He inoculated the vesicular fluid from cowpox lesions into the skin of susceptible individuals and induced protection against smallpox, thus beginning the era of immunization.

Immunization is the act of artificially inducing immunity or providing protection from disease; it can be active or passive. Active immunization consists of inducing the body to develop defenses against disease. This is usually accomplished by the administration of vaccines or toxoids that stimulate the body's immune system to produce antibodies or cell-mediated immunity, or both, which protects against the infectious agent.[1] Passive immunization consists of providing temporary protection through the administration of exogenously produced antibody. Two situations in which passive immunization commonly occurs are through the transplacental transfer of antibodies to the fetus, which may provide protection against certain diseases for the first 3 to 6 months of life, and the injection of immunoglobulins for specific preventive purposes. A more detailed description of the immune mechanisms involved follows.

Immunizing agents include vaccines, toxoids, and antibody-containing preparations from human or animal donors. Some important definitions follow.

1. Vaccine: a suspension of attenuated live or killed microorganisms (bacteria, viruses, or rickettsiae), or fractions thereof, administered to induce immunity and thereby prevent infectious disease
2. Toxoid: a modified bacterial toxin that has been rendered nontoxic but retains the ability to stimulate the formation of antitoxin
3. Immunoglobulin: a sterile solution for intramuscular administration containing antibody from human blood. It contains 15% to 18% protein obtained by cold ethanol fractionation of large pools of blood plasma. It is primarily indicated for routine protection of certain immunodeficient persons and for passive immunization against measles and hepatitis A. Immune globulin intravenous (IGIV), a specialized preparation allowing intravenous administration, is indicated primarily for replacement therapy in immunoglobulin G (IgG) deficiency, treatment of Kawasaki disease, and idiopathic thrombocytopenic purpura.
4. Specific immunoglobulin: special preparations obtained from donor pools preselected for high antibody content against a specific disease, for example, hepatitis B immune globulin (HBIG), varicella-zoster immune globulin (VZIG), rabies immune globulin (RIG), and tetanus immune globulin (TIG)

The constituents of immunizing agents include the following:

1. Suspending fluid: This frequently is as simple as sterile water or saline, but it may be a complex fluid containing small amounts of proteins or other constituents derived from the medium or biologic system in which the immunizing agent is produced (serum proteins, egg antigens, cell culture–derived antigens).
2. Preservatives, stabilizers, antibiotics: These components of vaccines are used (1) to inhibit or prevent bacterial growth in viral culture or the final product or (2) to stabilize the antigen. They include materials such as mercurials (thimerosal), gelatin, and specific antibiotics. Allergic reactions may occur if the recipient is sensitive to any of these additives. A review of the mercury content of vaccines indicated some children had received quantities of ethyl mercury from thimerosal in excess of some federal guidelines for methyl mercury. As a precautionary measure, it was recommended that thimerosal be removed from the immunization schedule to the extent feasible.[2] In the United States, thimerosal, as a preservative, has been removed from almost all vaccines routinely recommended for children during the first 7 years of life, although some of these vaccines may still contain trace amounts (http://www.fda.gov/cber/vaccine/thimerosal.htm). Some vaccines for children contain other preservatives or do not need a preservative because they are packaged as single doses. Some vaccines, particularly those used in adults, may still contain thimerosal as a preservative, such as some influenza vaccine (25 µg per 0.5-mL dose) and combined adult-type tetanus and diphtheria toxoids (Td). Influenza vaccine, which is routinely recommended for children 6 months to 18 years of age, may contain about 12.5 to 25 µg of mercury as a preservative per dose (0.25 mL for children 6 to 35 months of age and 0.5 mL for older children).
3. Adjuvants: An aluminum salt is used in some vaccines to enhance the immune response to vaccines containing inactivated microorganisms or their products (e.g., toxoids and hepatitis B vaccine). Vaccines with such adjuvants should usually be injected deeply into muscle masses because subcutaneous or intracutaneous administration can cause local irritation, inflammation, granuloma formation, or necrosis.[3] Oil-in-water adjuvants are used in some vaccines licensed outside the United States and have been documented to have markedly enhanced immunogenicity for some vaccines such as inactivated influenza H5N1 vaccines.[4]

Immunologic Basis of Vaccination

Two major approaches to active immunization have been employed: the use of live (generally attenuated) infectious agents or the use of inactivated, or detoxified, agents or their extracts. For many diseases (including influenza, poliomyelitis, typhoid, and measles), both approaches have been employed. Live attenuated vaccines are believed to induce an immunologic response more similar to that resulting from natural infection than do killed vaccines. Inactivated or killed vaccines can consist of inactivated whole organisms (e.g., Japanese encephalitis), detoxified exotoxin (e.g., diphtheria and tetanus toxoids), soluble capsular material either alone (e.g., pneumococcal polysaccharide) or covalently linked to carrier proteins (e.g., *Haemophilus influenzae* type b conjugate vaccines), chemically purified components of the organism (e.g., acellular pertussis, inactivated influenza vaccines), or recombinant proteins (human papillomavirus [HPV], hepatitis B virus [HBV]).

DETERMINANTS OF IMMUNOGENICITY

The immune system is complex, and antigen composition and presentation are critical for stimulation of the desired immune response. Immunogenicity is determined not only by the chemical and physical states of the antigen but also by the genetic characteristics of the responding individual, the physiologic condition of the individual (e.g., age, nutrition, gender, pregnancy status, stress, infections, immune status), and the manner in which the antigen is presented (route of administration, dose or doses and timing of doses, and presence of adjuvants).[5,6]

LIVE VERSUS KILLED OR SUBUNIT VACCINES

Because the organisms in live vaccines multiply in the recipient, antigen production generally increases logarithmically until checked by the onset of the immune response it is intended to induce. The live attenuated viruses (e.g., measles, mumps, and rubella) generally are believed to confer lifelong protection in those who respond. By contrast, killed vaccines generally do not induce permanent immunity with one dose, making repeated vaccination and subsequent boosters necessary to develop and maintain high levels of antibody (e.g., diphtheria, tetanus, rabies, typhoid). Exceptions to this general rule may include hepatitis B vaccine, for which long-term immunologic memory has been demonstrated for at least 10 years after vaccination, and inactivated polio vaccine (IPV), for which the duration of immunity is unknown. Although the amount of antigen initially introduced is greater with inactivated vaccines, multiplication of organisms in the host results in a cumulatively greater antigenic input with live vaccines.

Most vaccines comprise protein antigens, which generate a T-cell–dependent immune response with induction of immunologic memory, booster effects on repeat administration, and good immunogenicity in all age groups. However, purified bacterial capsular polysaccharide vaccines induce a T-cell–independent immune response, which does not lead to immune memory and cannot be boosted with repeated injections.[7] Polysaccharide vaccines have poor immunogenicity in infants and young children. Covalent linkage of the polysaccharide to a carrier protein converts it from a T-cell–independent to a T-cell–dependent antigen (e.g. Hib, pneumococcal vaccine), which produces a good immune response in these important populations.

DOSE

The amount of antigen is important. The presentation of an insufficient amount may result in an absence of immune responsiveness. There is usually a dose-response curve relationship between antigen dose and peak response obtained beyond a threshold; however, responsiveness may reach a plateau, failing to increase beyond a certain level despite increasing doses of vaccine.

ADJUVANTS

The immune response to some inactivated vaccines or toxoids can be enhanced by the addition of adjuvants, such as aluminum salts. They are particularly useful with inactivated products, such as diphtheria and tetanus toxoids, and acellular pertussis vaccines (DTaP) and hepatitis B vaccine. The mechanism of enhancement of antigenicity by adjuvants is not well defined; however, it is increasingly clear that they activate the innate immune system through pathogen-associated molecular patterns (PAMPs). Although aluminum salts are currently the only licensed adjuvants for use in humans in the United States, other adjuvants based on oil-in-water emulsion of squalene or monophosphoryl lipid A have shown promising results.[8]

ROUTE OF ADMINISTRATION

The route of administration can determine the nature of the immune response to a vaccine or toxoid. Intramuscular and subcutaneous delivery results in a predominantly IgG response. Oral or nasal vaccination is more likely to result in production of local IgA compared with intramuscular injection, although systemic IgG also is induced. The immunogenicity of some vaccines is reduced when not given by the recommended route. For example, administration of hepatitis B vaccine subcutaneously into the fatty tissue of the buttock was associated with substantially lower seroconversion rates than injection intramuscularly into the deltoid muscle.[9]

Most vaccines are administered either intramuscularly or subcutaneously. However, there is increasing interest in the intradermal route, particularly with the potential of reducing the amount of antigen per dose, thereby decreasing strains on production capacity and potentially vaccine cost.[10]

AGE

The immune response to a vaccine varies with age. Although children and young adults usually respond well to all vaccines, differences in response capability exist during early infancy and old age. The presence of high levels of passively acquired maternal antibody in the first few months of life impairs the initial immune response to some killed vaccines (e.g., hepatitis A vaccine,[11] diphtheria toxoid) and many live vaccines (e.g., measles). Prematurely born infants of low birth weight should be immunized at the usual chronologic age in most cases. Infants with birth weights less than 2000 g may require modification of the timing of hepatitis B immunoprophylaxis depending on maternal hepatitis B surface antigen (HBsAg) status. Some studies suggest a reduced immune response in very low birth weight infants (less than 1500 g) immunized by the usual schedule; however, antibody concentrations achieved are usually protective. In elderly people, the response to antigenic stimulation may be diminished (e.g., influenza, hepatitis B vaccines).

◼ Components of the Immune Response

The immune response is traditionally divided into two components: the innate immune response, which is rapid, nonspecific and serves as an immediate first line of defense against an infection; and the adaptive immune response, which develops over a matter of days, is specific for the foreign antigen, and results in long-term immune memory. The latter protects the host against subsequent challenge with the same or immunologically similar pathogens and is the underlying principle of vaccination. The innate immune response is mediated by natural killer (NK) cells, which recognize and kill virally infected cells; by complement, which is activated by components of bacterial cell walls; and by phagocytes, including macrophages and dendritic cells (DCs), which ingest microorganisms and foreign particulates.[12] The adaptive immune response relies on antigen-presenting cells (APCs), such as DCs, for activation, and is mediated by T and B lymphocytes. T cells can be divided into CD4 (helper) and CD8 (cytotoxic) cells and are responsible for cell-mediated immune responses. CD4 helper T cells can be further subdivided into Th1 cells, which predominantly lead to cell-mediated responses, and Th2 cells, which predominantly lead to humoral responses. B cells produce antibody specific for the immunizing agent and require CD4 T-cell help. Interactions between APCs, helper T cells, and B cells involve class II major histocompatibility antigens (MHCs), whereas interactions between cytotoxic T cells and their target involve MHC class I antigens.[13] Soluble mediators or cytokines are secreted by all cell types and serve as activation and differentiation factors for the different cell lineages. These include interleukins, interferons, and others.[14] A further class of CD4 T cell (Treg) plays an essential role in the regulation of the adaptive immune response.[15]

It has become increasingly clear that the innate immune response is able to respond differently to different types of pathogens and that these differential responses help determine the nature of the subsequent adaptive response.[16] Pattern recognition receptors (PRRs) encoded in the germline recognize PAMPs such as toll-like receptors (TLRs), NOD-like receptors (NLRs), and others, all of which contribute to immune activation by inducing proinflammatory cytokines, which in turn modulate the adaptive immune response. As alluded to earlier, this has significant implications for adjuvant development.[17,18]

Mobilization of the Adaptive Immune Response

Upon exposure to an infectious organism or a vaccine, the innate immune system is mobilized through APC recognition of PAMPs that are present either in the organism or in the adjuvant. Activated APCs (macrophages and DCs) secrete proinflammatory cytokines and chemokines, which recruit other leukocytes to the site of infection. When activated, DCs migrate to the draining lymph nodes, where they interact with T cells through the MHC-peptide complex.[19] Once the organism or antigen is internalized, it is killed and broken down into peptides. These peptides are transported to the cell surface through membrane trafficking and bind to MHC class I or class II molecules. MHC class I molecules are able to bind peptides that are 8 to 10 amino acids in length, whereas MHC class II molecules are more permissive, binding peptides of 13 amino acids and greater.[20]

The first step in the induction of a T-cell–dependent antibody response is the activation of naïve CD4 helper T cells by presentation of an antigen by phagocytes or dendritic cells. The T-cell receptor recognizes the MHC-peptide complex, and this recognition triggers the secretion of cytokines, which stimulate the maturation of naïve helper T cells. In the presence of interleukin-12 (IL-12), Th1 cells will differentiate, and these in turn will secrete IL-2 and interferon-γ. In the presence of IL-4, Th2 will differentiate and secrete IL-4 and IL-5. These two cytokines are essential for the differentiation and maturation of B cells into antibody-secreting plasma cells.

Naïve B cells recognize a specific antigenic epitope on native antigen through the immunoglobulin receptor on their surface but are unable to differentiate into antibody-secreting cells without T-cell help. A given B cell can only be activated by a T cell responding to the same antigen. A helper T cell will recognize the MHC class II complex on the surface of the B cell and deliver a signal for B-cell differentiation. This leads to B-cell proliferation and maturation in a clonal manner. Class switching (from IgM to IgG and IgA) and affinity maturation take place, and antigen-specific plasma cells develop. However, not all B cells become plasma cells. Some mature into memory B cells, which are long-lived, and form the basis of the rapid secondary response on the next encounter with the pathogen.[21] Although the mechanism of maintenance of these cells is not clear, the ability to mount a strong secondary response after many years argues for a homeostatic mechanism that regulates these cells. The antibodies formed after vaccination express a variety of antigen-binding specificities (i.e., recognize different structures on a complex multideterminant antigen), reflecting the sum of the large number of individual clonal B-cell responses that make up an antibody response.

Antibodies mediate protection through a variety of mechanisms. They may inactivate soluble toxic protein products of bacteria (antitoxins), facilitate intracellular digestion of bacteria by phagocytes (opsonization), interact with components of serum complement to damage the bacterial membrane with resultant bacteriolysis (lysins), prevent infectious virus from infecting cells (neutralizing antibodies), or interact with components of the bacterial surface to prevent adhesion to mucosal surfaces (antiadhesins). Antibodies cannot readily reach intracellular sites of infection, the sites of viral and some bacterial replication. However, antibodies are effective against many viral diseases by interacting with virus before initial intracellular penetration occurs, and by preventing locally replicating virus from disseminating from the site of entry to an important target organ, as in the spread of poliovirus from the gut to the central nervous system or rabies from a puncture wound to peripheral neural tissue.

Virally infected cells can be killed by cytotoxic CD8 T cells. As the virus replicates in a cell, viral proteins are processed and presented on the cell surface as an MHC class I–peptide complex, which is then recognized by cytotoxic T cells. Cells infected with intracellular bacteria such as *Mycobacterium leprae* are recognized and killed in the same way.

Unanticipated Responses

Independent of antibody production, the stimulation of the immune system by vaccination may, on occasion, elicit a hypersensitivity response. Killed measles vaccine, in use in the United States between 1963 and 1967, induced incomplete humoral immunity and cell-mediated hypersensitivity, resulting in the development of a syndrome of atypical measles in some children on subsequent challenge.[22] In addition, some antibodies produced may not be protective but "block" the reaction of protective antibodies with antigens, inhibiting the body's defenses. Some vaccines may induce immunologic tolerance that results in blunting of the immune response on subsequent exposure to the antigen (e.g., meningococcal polysaccharide vaccine).[23] Concerns have been raised that immunizations might induce chronic allergic or autoimmune disorders. However, careful reviews of both the possible biologic mechanisms and epidemiologic evidence have generally failed to confirm vaccines as causes of these disorders.[24] Concerns have also been raised that the number of antigens today in the vaccine schedule might overwhelm an infant's immune system, leading to chronic diseases and predisposing to serious other infections. As a result of the removal of whole-cell pertussis vaccine and smallpox vaccine from the current immunization schedule, the number of immunogenic proteins and polysaccharides a child is exposed to today is actually smaller than in the past. Estimates suggest that an infant is capable of responding to 10,000 vaccines simultaneously.[25] The Institute of Medicine concluded that available evidence favored rejection of a causal relationship between vaccines and increased risk for infections and type 1 diabetes. The evidence was insufficient to accept or reject a causal relationship between vaccines and allergic disorders, particularly asthma.[26] A subsequent epidemiologic study failed to show an association between vaccines and asthma.[27]

Temporal Course of the Immune Response

On first exposure to a vaccine, a primary response is induced, and a protective immune response will develop in about 2 weeks. Circulating antibodies do not usually appear for 7 to 10 days, and the immunoglobulin class of the response changes over this period of time. Early-appearing antibodies are usually IgM class and of low affinity; late-appearing antibodies are usually IgG and display a high affinity. IgM antibodies may fix complement, making lysis and phagocytosis possible. As the titer of IgG rises during the second week (or later) after immunogenic stimulation, the IgM titer falls. IgG antibodies are produced in large amounts and function in the neutralization, precipitation, and fixation of complement. The antibody titer frequently reaches a peak in about 2 to 6 weeks and then falls gradually. The switch from IgM synthesis to predominantly IgG synthesis in B cells is mediated by T-cell help. Uncommonly, individuals may not respond to a vaccine, experiencing a primary vaccine failure. This may be due to a genetic inability to respond to vaccine, but other factors are involved. For example, almost all children who do not respond immunologically to the first dose of measles, mumps, rubella (MMR) vaccine will acquire measles immunity after a second dose.[28]

After a second exposure to the same antigen, a heightened humoral or cell-mediated response, an anamnestic response, is observed. These secondary responses occur sooner than the primary response, usually within 4 to 5 days, and depend on a marked proliferation of antibody-producing cells or effector T cells. The secondary response depends on immunologic memory after the first exposure mediated by both T and B cells. Infection with measles or varicella vaccine strains has been shown to evoke a cell-mediated as well as humoral response.

Many pathogens replicate at mucosal surfaces before host invasion and may induce secretory IgA along the respiratory and gastrointestinal mucous membranes and at other localized sites (e.g., polio, rubella, influenza). IgA antibodies are efficient at virus neutralization (e.g., polio), fix complement through the alternative pathway (e.g., cholera), prevent adsorption of organisms to the intestinal wall (e.g., *Escherichia coli*, cholera), and can lyse gram-negative bacteria (with the aid of both complement and lysozyme).[29] Current parenteral, especially inactivated, vaccines rarely induce high levels of secretory IgA antibodies.

Measurement of the Immune Response

Response to vaccines is often gauged by measuring the appearance and concentration of specific antibodies in the serum.[30] For some viral vaccines, such as those for measles, rubella, and hepatitis B, the presence of circulating antibodies correlates with clinical protection. Although this has served as a dependable indicator of immunity, seroconversion measures only the humoral parameter of the immune response. Secondary vaccine failure occurs when an individual who had previously had an adequate immune response loses measurable antibodies over time. This waning immunity can be attributed to a loss of long-lived memory B or T cells, in the absence of repeated exposure to the pathogen. Evaluating persistence of antibody has been used to determine duration of vaccine-induced immunity. However, the absence of measurable antibody may not mean that the individual is unprotected. Although a fall in titer takes place for some vaccines over time (e.g., measles, rubella, hepatitis B), on revaccination or challenge, a rapid secondary response is observed in IgG antibodies with little or no detectable IgM response, suggesting persistent protection. With some vaccines and toxoids, the mere presence of antibodies is not sufficient to ensure clinical protection, but rather a minimal circulating level of antibody is required (e.g., 0.01 IU/mL of tetanus antitoxin). Functional antibody is important in assessing immunity to bacterial polysaccharide vaccines. Opsonophagocytic activity (OPA) is considered the assay of choice for monitoring vaccine response[31] because the vaccines also induce nonfunctional antibodies that are detected in standard enzyme immunosorbent assay (EIA), although the EIA can be used as a proxy. Some immune responses may not in themselves confer immunity but may be sufficiently associated with protection that they remain useful proxy measures of protective immunity (e.g., vibriocidal serum antibodies in cholera). The measurement of cell-mediated immunity, which would be helpful in assessing the degree of ongoing protection in many circumstances, is usually limited to research laboratories and to only a few vaccines.

Vaccine Development

Most vaccines in use today have been developed by conventional techniques.[32] For live attenuated viral vaccines, organisms are repeatedly passaged in various tissue culture cell lines to reduce virulent properties while maintaining immunogenicity. Inactivated vaccines usually have been developed by growing microorganisms, followed by concentration, purification, and inactivation, not necessarily in that order. Component vaccines usually are derived from chemical separation of the needed component from the parent organism.

Future vaccines are likely to be derived from new methods of biotechnology—especially recombinant techniques. Currently available hepatitis B vaccines were developed by cloning the HBsAg gene into yeast, leading to synthesis of HBsAg within the yeast cell. Other new approaches for producing vaccines include live vectors, in which one or more genes encoding critical determinants of immunity from pathogenic microorganisms are inserted into the genome of the vector. These vectors may include viruses such as poxviruses (vaccinia or canarypox) or bacteria such as salmonella or bacillus Calmette-Guérin (BCG). Other newer techniques include microencapsulation of critical antigens in polymers that can lead to sustained release or pulse release over prolonged periods, mimicking the effect of multiple injections of an antigen over a several-month interval. New technologies also include use of nucleic acids, which encode critical antigens. Injection of the DNA leads to production of antigen without risk for producing whole infectious organisms. Live attenuated influenza vaccine was developed using genetic reassortment of the genes encoding two of the surface glycoproteins from wild virus isolates with six other genes contributed from a cold-adapted, temperature-sensitive influenza strain. Similar techniques were used to develop bovine rotavirus vaccines.[33]

GENERAL PRINCIPLES OF IMMUNIZATION

The introduction and widespread use of vaccines has resulted in global eradication of smallpox, elimination of poliomyelitis caused by wild viruses in the United States, and dramatic reductions in the incidence rates of other diseases (Table 320-1). Measles and rubella are no longer considered endemic in the United States.[34,35] Diphtheria and rubella have been greatly reduced in developed countries (more than 90%) and, if global vaccination efforts can be sustained, may eventually be eliminated from many countries. The World Health Assembly had established a goal to eradicate polio from the world by the end of 2000.[36] Although that goal was not achieved, by the end of 2008, only four countries in the world had never interrupted wild poliovirus transmission, although several others in Africa had been reinfected[37] (http://www.polioeradication.org). The last case of polio due to wild virus in the Western Hemisphere was in 1991, and both the European and Western Pacific Regions of the World Health Organization have been certified free of poliomyelitis.[38-40] Global use of hepatitis B vaccine in infants will potentially have an impact comparable to that of other vaccines in childhood. *Haemophilus influenzae* type b vaccines have only recently come into widespread use, but disease incidence has been markedly reduced in many developed countries.[41-43]

TABLE 320-1	Representative 20th-Century Morbidity Cases in 2007 and Change					
Disease	*20th-Century Annual Morbidity*	*2007*	*Decrease (%)*	*Healthy People 2010 Goal**	*Coverage 2007 (%)*
Diphtheria	21,053	0	100	4 doses, ≥90%	85
Measles	530,217	43	99.9	1 dose, ≥90%	93
Mumps	162,344	800	99.5	1 dose, ≥90%	93
Pertussis	200,752	10,452	94.8	4 doses, ≥90%	85
Polio (paralytic)	16,316	0	100	3 doses, ≥90%	92
Rubella	47,745	12	99.9	1 dose, ≥90%	93
Congenital rubella syndrome	152	0	99.3	1 dose, ≥90%	—
Smallpox	29,005	0	100	—	—
Tetanus	580	28	95.2	4 doses, ≥90%	85
Haemophilus influenzae type b and unknown (<5 yr)	20,000	202	99	3 doses, ≥90%	94

*Includes 19- through 35-month-old children. (See Centers for Disease Control and Prevention. National, state, and local area vaccination coverage among children aged 19-35 months—United States, 2007. *MMWR Morb Mortal Wkly Rep*. 2008;57:961-966.)

Adapted from Centers for Disease Control and Prevention. Notice to readers: Final 2007 reports of nationally notifiable infections disease. *MMWR Morb Mortal Wkly Rep*. 2008; 57:901,903-913.

Pneumococcal conjugate vaccines have had a marked impact on invasive pneumococcal disease in countries where they have been used widely in children.[44] Decreases in disease were observed not only in children but also in adults, who presumably are not being exposed to infectious children because the latter have been vaccinated.

Modern vaccines are very safe and effective; however, they are not completely so. Each vaccine is associated with some adverse effects, which may range from very mild to life threatening, and each vaccine falls short of 100% effectiveness. Consequently, some persons who have received a full course of vaccine or toxoid may acquire disease on exposure. The effectiveness of vaccines recommended for universal use in children is well defined, with most vaccines protecting 80% to more than 90% to 95% of recipients following a primary series. Acellular pertussis vaccines range in efficacy from 71% to 89% in most studies.[45-47] Varicella vaccine is 95% or more effective against severe varicella but is less effective against varicella of any severity.[48-49] In 2006, reductions of 95% or more from baseline 20th-century morbidity have been reported in the United States for smallpox, diphtheria, tetanus, polio, measles, mumps, and rubella. Similar reductions, based on historical estimates, have been achieved for congenital rubella syndrome and *H. influenzae* type b invasive disease.[50] Table 320-1 shows the impact has been maintained through 2007.

Although the high efficacy of each of these vaccines is readily apparent, there has been substantial controversy over reported adverse events temporally associated with vaccination. Because of these controversies, the Institute of Medicine (IOM) reviewed available information during the early 1990s regarding 9 of the 12 vaccines universally recommended for children and the serious adverse effects that have been reported in association with them.[51-55] For most events, the available evidence was insufficient to make a causal evaluation. However, evidence related to several events was sufficient to (1) support rejection of vaccine playing a causal role, (2) support vaccine playing a causal role, or (3) more definitively establish that vaccine has a causal role.[54] The evidence favored rejection of a causal relationship between combined diphtheria and tetanus toxoids (DT) and encephalopathy and between conjugate Hib vaccines and early-onset Hib disease. Specifically, for vaccines in use in the United States today, the IOM concluded that the evidence favored a causal relationship between RA27/3 rubella vaccine and chronic arthritis and established a causal relationship between MMR and thrombocytopenia, between rubella vaccine and acute arthritis, between DT and brachial neuritis and Guillain-Barré syndrome (GBS), and between a variety of vaccines and anaphylaxis. The Advisory Committee on Immunization Practices (ACIP) of the Centers for Disease Control and Prevention (CDC) subsequently reviewed the IOM findings along with new data available regarding GBS. Most of the IOM conclusions were accepted. However, data reported subsequent to the IOM evaluation from population-based studies of GBS and vaccines as well as information from a Finnish study do not support a causal relationship between oral polio vaccine, diphtheria and tetanus toxoids and pertussis vaccine (DTP), or tetanus toxoid and GBS.[54,56] Likewise, more recent studies have found no evidence of increased risk for new onset of chronic arthropathies among women vaccinated with RA27/3 vaccine, arguing against RA27/3 rubella vaccine as a cause of chronic arthropathy.[57-59]

More recently, the IOM had been asked to review the relationship between a variety of disorders and vaccines[54,55] (http://www.iom.edu/imsafety). They concluded that evidence did not support a relationship between MMR or thimerosal and autism, between multiple immunizations and heterologous infections, between multiple immunizations and type 1 diabetes, or between hepatitis B vaccine and incident or relapsed multiple sclerosis. The relationship of vaccines to autism has been particularly controversial, primarily among members of the lay public. However, there is a strong scientific database that has been accumulated that does not support any role of vaccines in autism.[60]

In the development of vaccines, the initial studies are typically conducted in animal models to demonstrate protection (or at least production of antibodies) and relative safety, and then limited numbers of doses are administered to humans to demonstrate antibody production and safety (phase I). After this stage, clinical trials in humans are typically carried out in a limited number of individuals to select optimal vaccine schedules and to demonstrate further safety (phase II). Larger trials are carried out to demonstrate efficacy (phase III). Because of their limited size, these field trials can only be expected to detect adverse events that occur relatively frequently (1 per 1000 doses or higher). After clinical trials, licensure may be sought. In the United States, vaccine production is strictly regulated by the Center for Biologics Evaluation and Research of the Food and Drug Administration. Only after a vaccine is found to be safe and effective is it licensed for use. Postmarketing surveillance (phase IV) is necessary to detect rare adverse events associated with vaccination and to monitor safety of vaccination practices such as simultaneous immunization.

Although there is no direct evidence of risk to the fetus when pregnant, women are given routinely recommended vaccines. Most live virus vaccines induce viremia, which at least theoretically could result in infection of the fetus, so live virus vaccines are not generally administered to pregnant women except in unusual circumstances.

The decision to use a vaccine involves assessment of the risks of disease, the benefits of vaccination, and the risks associated with vaccination. The relative balance of risks and benefits may change over time; consequently, continuing assessment of vaccines is essential. Recommendations for vaccine use are developed by several different bodies: the ACIP develops recommendations for vaccines for children adolescents and adults in the civilian population. These recommendations are available at http://www.cdc.gov/vaccines/recs/acip/default.htm. The Committee on Infectious Diseases of the American Academy of Pediatrics (the "Red Book" committee) develops recommendations for vaccine use in infants, children, and adolescents.[61] Since 1995, the ACIP, the American Academy of Pediatrics, and the American Academy of Family Physicians have collaborated to issue a harmonized childhood immunization schedule, which is updated annually.[62] The ACIP also issues annually an adult immunization schedule in two parts: (1) recommendations based on age group, and (2) recommendations based on underlying medical condition, which can be found at http://www.cdc.gov/vaccines/recs/schedules/adult-schedule.htm. The Adult Immunization Schedule for 2009 has also been approved by the American Academy of Family Physicians, the American College of Obstetricians and Gynecologists, and the American College of Physicians.

Currently Available Immunizing Agents

Tables 320-2 and 320-3 list currently licensed immunizing agents and immunoglobulins. This section presents brief information about most immunizing agents, primary indications for use, relative efficacy, number and spacing of doses required, known adverse effects, and precautions and contraindications for use. Package inserts and specific references and recommendations should be consulted for more detailed information. In addition to these licensed products, several other vaccines are under development and may soon become available.

VACCINES

Anthrax Vaccine

Anthrax vaccine is prepared from microaerophilic cultures of an avirulent nonencapsulated strain of *Bacillus anthracis*. The vaccine is a cell-free filtrate that contains a mixture of components, including protective antigen (the antigen that is thought to confer immunity) as well as other bacterial products. Because of concerns about potential use of *B. anthracis* as a biological warfare agent, vaccination of members of the U.S. Armed Forces was begun in 1998. Following the intentional release of anthrax in the United States in 2001, anthrax vaccine was recommended for civilians at risk for repeated exposure to *B. anthracis* spores, including laboratory personnel handling environmental specimens and performing confirmatory testing for *B. anthracis* in selected

TABLE 320-2	Currently Available Vaccines and Toxoids and Year Licensed*	
Product		**Year Licensed**
Anthrax vaccine adsorbed		1970
Bacille Calmette-Guérin vaccine		1950
Diphtheria and tetanus toxoids and acellular pertussis vaccine		1991
Diphtheria and tetanus toxoids adsorbed (pediatric use, DT)		1949
Diphtheria and tetanus toxoids and acellular pertussis vaccine absorbed, *Haemophilus* B conjugate vaccine, and inactivated polio vaccine combined		2008
Diphtheria and tetanus toxoids and acellular pertussis vaccine absorbed, plus *Haemophilus* B conjugate vaccine		1996
Diphtheria and tetanus toxoids and acellular pertussis vaccine absorbed and inactivated polio vaccine combined		2008
Diphtheria and tetanus toxoids and acellular pertussis adsorbed, hepatitis B (recombinant), and inactivated poliovirus vaccine combined		2002
Haemophilus influenzae type B conjugate vaccine		1987
Hepatitis A vaccine		1995
Hepatitis A inactivated and hepatitis B (recombinant) vaccine		2001
Hepatitis B recombinant vaccine		1987
Hepatitis B recombinant vaccine and *Haemophilus influenzae* type B conjugate vaccine		1996
Influenza virus vaccine (inactivated)		1945
Influenza virus vaccine, live, intranasal		2003
Japanese encephalitis vaccine		2009
Lyme disease vaccine		1998
Measles virus vaccine, live, attenuated		1963
Measles, mumps, rubella, varicella		2005
Measles, mumps, and rubella virus vaccine, live		1971
Meningococcal polysaccharide vaccine, groups A, C, Y, W135 combined		1981
Meningococcal polysaccharide (serogroups A, L, Y and W135) conjugated to diphtheria toxoid		2005
Mumps virus vaccine, live		1967
Pneumococcal conjugate vaccine (7 valent)		2000
Pneumococcal polysaccharide vaccine (23 valent)		1983
Poliomyelitis vaccine (inactivated, enhanced potency)		1987
Rabies vaccine (human diploid)		1980
Rotavirus vaccine		2006
Rubella virus vaccine, live		1969
Smallpox vaccine		1903
Tetanus and diphtheria toxoids, adsorbed (adult use, Td)		1955
Tetanus toxoid		1933
Tetanus toxoid adsorbed		1949
Tetanus toxoid, reduced diphtheria toxoid and acellular pertussis vaccine, absorbed		2005
Typhoid vaccine (polysaccharide)		1994
Typhoid vaccine (oral)		1990
Varicella vaccine		1995
Yellow fever vaccine		1953
Zoster vaccine		2006

*As of May 2009.

laboratories and workers making repeated entries into sites known to be contaminated with *B. anthracis* spores. Anthrax vaccine was also used after exposure, in conjunction with antimicrobial prophylaxis, under an investigational protocol.[63] Other groups for whom the vaccine is recommended include persons working with production quantities of *B. anthracis* cultures or in activities with a high potential for aerosol production and selected other workers at high risk for exposure to *B. anthracis* spores.[64] Efficacy has been demonstrated in protection against cutaneous disease. Data on clinical efficacy against inhaled anthrax in humans are limited, but available human and animal data are consistent with protection.[65] The vaccine induces antibodies in 90% or more of adults who received the currently recommended primary course of five intramuscular injections given at time zero, 4 weeks, 6 months, 12 months, and 18 months followed by

annual boosters.[64,66] A controlled study of a vaccine similar to the currently available vaccine demonstrated protective efficacy against cutaneous disease of 92.5% among mill workers.[67] Experience suggests that two doses of vaccine confer some protection.[68] Mild local reactions at the site of injection occur in about 30% of recipients. More severe local reactions occur infrequently (<4%) and systemic reactions are rare (0.2%). Surveillance for adverse events in the military program revealed no pattern of serious adverse events.[69,70] Adverse events, including injection site reaction incidence and duration, were less often seen after intramuscular injection compared with subcutaneous injection.[66] Vaccines containing only recombinant protective antigen are under active development and may be less reactogenic than the current vaccine.[71,72]

Bacille Calmette-Guérin Vaccine
BCG vaccine contains living Calmette-Guérin bacillus, an attenuated strain of *Mycobacterium bovis*. In many countries, BCG is widely used in infants and young children to prevent disseminated tuberculosis infection. In the United States, use of the vaccine is recommended only in special circumstances because the general risk for infection is low and because BCG vaccination results in conversion of the tuberculin skin test, thereby removing one of the most important indicators of tuberculosis infection (tuberculin conversion). Although BCG is widely used throughout the world, there has been much controversy regarding its efficacy. Studies suggest that the vaccine is effective, particularly for preventing complications of disseminated tuberculosis in young children.[73-75] In the United States, use of BCG should be considered for individuals, such as infants, whose skin test results are negative and who have prolonged, close contact with patients with active tuberculosis who are untreated, are ineffectively treated, or have antibiotic-resistant infection. BCG may also be considered for health care workers in areas in which multidrug-resistant *Mycobacterium tuberculosis* infection has become a significant problem.[76]

A single dose of vaccine is administered intradermally or by the percutaneous route. Known adverse effects include regional adenitis, disseminated BCG infection, and osteitis caused by the BCG organism. Adenitis occurs in about 1% to 10% of vaccinees, whereas disseminated infections and osteitis are apparently quite rare (about 1 case per 1 million vaccinees). Hypertrophic scars at the injection site occur in up to one third of vaccinated persons, and keloids occur in 2% to 4%. Immunocompromised individuals should not receive the vaccine because of increased risk for disseminated BCG infection.[76]

Cholera Vaccine
A killed whole-cell cholera vaccine was available in the United States from the 1940s until 2001.[77] The vaccine's efficacy was 50% or less,

TABLE 320-3	Immune Globulin Preparations Made from Human Plasma*		
Name	**Abbreviation**	**Route of Administration**	**Year Licensed**
Immune globulin	IG	Intramuscular	1943
Hepatitis B immune globulin	HBIG	Intramuscular	1977
Rabies immune globulin	RIG	Intramuscular	1974
Tetanus immune globulin	TIG	Intramuscular	1957
Varicella-zoster immune globulin	VZIG†	Intramuscular	1980
Immune globulin intravenous	IGIV	Intravenous	1981
Cytomegalovirus immune globulin intravenous	CMV IGIV	Intravenous	1990
Botulism intravenous immune globulin	Baby BIG	Intravenous	2003
Vaccinia immune globulin intravenous	VIG-IGIV	Intravenous	2005
Immune globulin subcutaneous	IG-SQ	Subcutaneous	2006

*Antitoxin preparations from animal sera other than humans are available for botulism and diphtheria.
†Available as the investigational product VariZIG.

and protection was short-lived. The vaccine required booster doses every 6 months. Killed whole-cell vaccines are still available in some countries, and improved killed vaccines are being developed, some of which include the B subunit of cholera toxin.[78] Live cholera vaccine, containing engineered strains of *Vibrio cholerae,* is available in some countries. Additional live attenuated cholera vaccines are under development.

Diphtheria Toxoid

Diphtheria toxoid is a purified preparation of inactivated diphtheria toxin. It is highly effective in inducing antibodies that will prevent disease, although they may not prevent acquisition or carriage of the organism. The toxoid is available in adsorbed form, combined with tetanus toxoid (adult formulation Td and pediatric formulation DT) or with tetanus toxoid and acellular pertussis vaccine (DTaP, childhood formulation, or Tdap, adult formulation). Single-antigen diphtheria toxoid is not distributed in the United States. Two dosage formulations are generally available, one for use up to the seventh year of life, and one for use in older children and adults. The adult formulation has a lower concentration of diphtheria toxoid (≤ 2.5 Lf) than the pediatric formulation (6.7 to 25 Lf), because local reactions are thought to relate to both age and dosage. With all formulations, levels of antitoxin considered protective are induced in excess of 90% of recipients who complete the schedule.[45,79,80]

Immunization against diphtheria is recommended for all residents in the United States. For children younger than 7 years of age with no contraindications to pertussis immunization, DTaP is recommended, and the primary series is three doses administered 4 to 8 weeks apart followed by a fourth dose 6 to 12 months later and a booster dose at school entry (4 through 6 years of age). For infants with contraindications to pertussis vaccine, DT is administered in the same schedule as DTaP (see "Pertussis Vaccine" and Fig. 320-1). The primary immunizing series of DT (for children 1 to 6 years of age) or Td (for older children and adults) consists of at least two doses administered 4 to 8 weeks apart followed by a third dose 6 to 12 months later. There is no need to restart a series if the schedule is interrupted; the next dose in the series should be given. Booster doses of Td should be given every 10 years. All persons 10 through 64 years of age should have one dose of Tdap, which can serve as one of the recommended booster doses for diphtheria and tetanus. Known adverse effects include local reactions and mild or moderate systemic reactions such as fever; anaphylaxis occurs rarely. Brachial neuritis appears to be a rare consequence of immunization and is most likely due to tetanus antigen.[52] The only contraindications are in individuals who have previously had neurologic or severe hypersensitivity reactions after diphtheria or tetanus toxoids or, if combined with pertussis, have had previous similar adverse events to those antigens.

Haemophilus influenzae Type b Vaccine

Conjugated vaccines to prevent *H. influenzae* type b (Hib) invasive disease were first licensed at the end of 1987 and have replaced the earlier polysaccharide vaccines because they elicit substantially higher antibody titers and are effective in young infants.[81] The polysaccharide in these vaccines is covalently linked to protein carriers converting them from T-cell–independent antigens to T-cell–dependent antigens. There are two available conjugate vaccines, licensed for use in infants.[82] Carrier proteins include a *Neisseria meningitidis* outer membrane protein complex (PRP-OMP) and tetanus toxoid (PRP-T). PRP-OMP has been demonstrated to be 95% effective in a clinical trial in infants. PRP-T has been licensed for use in infants because it elicits comparable antibody responses to other conjugate vaccines that have been shown to be highly effective.

PRP-OMP behaves differently from PRP-T, inducing high levels of antibody after a single dose. A second dose 2 months later increases those levels; less benefit appears to be derived from a third dose. The basic series for PRP-OMP is two doses given 2 months apart beginning at 2 months of age followed by a reinforcing dose at 12 through 15 months of age.[81] In contrast, PRP-T does not induce substantial

antibody levels until dose 2, and high levels of protection are achieved only after three doses 2 months apart. The basic series for PRP-T starts at 2 months of age with three doses 2 months apart followed by a booster dose at 12 through 15 months of age.[81] Although use of a single conjugate vaccine for the primary series has been recommended, several studies suggest that mixed sequences of Hib conjugate vaccines induce an adequate immune response.[83-85] Thus, for infants younger than 6 months of age, three doses of any licensed Hib vaccine administered at 2-month intervals should confer protection; a fourth dose is given at 12 through 15 months. For infants starting immunization between 7 and 11 months, two doses of any of the Hib vaccines licensed for infants should be given 2 months apart followed by a reinforcing dose at 12 through 15 months provided that at least 2 months have elapsed since the second dose. Any of the conjugates can be used for the booster dose.[81]

Children beginning immunization between 12 and 14 months of age can receive two doses of any conjugate, with the second dose given after age 15 months, at least 2 months after dose 1. Children who are initially immunized at 15 months of age need only one dose of any of the conjugate vaccines. A combination vaccine, DTaP-IPV/Hib, is licensed for any of the recommended first four doses during the first 2 years of life (http://www.fda.gov/cber/products/pentacel.htm). Decreased immune responses to the Hib component when it is combined with some acellular pertussis vaccines have slowed approval for some combinations for infant indications.[86]

Based on the epidemiology of invasive *H. influenzae* type b infection in the United States, vaccination is not routinely recommended beyond the fifth year of life, except for specific risk groups. Although vaccine is not indicated for children who had documented invasive *H. influenzae* type b infection at 2 years of age or older, it is indicated for younger children because of their inadequate antibody response after natural infection.

The vaccines appear to be quite safe. Local reactions at the injection site and fever have been noted in less than 4% of vaccinees. They can be administered simultaneously with MMR, DTaP, PCV7, rotavirus vaccine, and IPV with no increased risk for adverse reactions or compromise in efficacy of any of the vaccines. The vaccines should not be administered if there is a history of anaphylaxis to the specific vaccine or to other vaccine components. Although a slight increase in risk for invasive *H. influenzae* type b disease was observed shortly after receipt of the original unconjugated polysaccharide vaccine, available data show no such association with conjugate vaccines.

Hepatitis A Vaccine

There are two inactivated single antigen hepatitis A vaccines available in the United States, HAVRIX from GlaxoSmithKline Biologicals and VAQTA from Merck & Company. More than 97% of persons 2 years of age and older acquire antibody titers considered protective after a single dose of either vaccine. More than 85% of children and adults acquire protective levels within 15 days of a dose of HAVRIX. An efficacy trial of HAVRIX using doses of 360 ELISA units 1 month apart in children 1 to 16 years of age demonstrated a 94% efficacy against hepatitis A.[87] Efficacy of one 25-unit dose of VAQTA in children 2 to 16 years of age was 100%.[88]

The vaccine is recommended for use among populations known to be at increased risk for infection, including persons traveling to hepatitis A–endemic areas; children in communities with high rates of hepatitis A; men who have sex with men; illegal drug users; and persons who work with hepatitis A virus–infected primates or who do research with the virus; and recipients of clotting factors. Persons with chronic liver disease may be at increased risk for fulminant hepatitis A and should be vaccinated as well.[89] Nonetheless, most cases of hepatitis A occur among persons who are not among these risk groups, but instead are acquired as part of community-wide outbreaks. Preventing hepatitis A at the community level requires widespread vaccination of children and adults.[90] In 1999, the ACIP recommended that children living in states, counties, or communities with reported annual rates of hepatitis A of 20 per 100,000 or higher between 1987

Recommended Immunization Schedule for Persons Aged 0 through 6 Years, United States, 2009

Vaccine ▼ Age ▶	Birth	1 Month	2 Months	4 Months	6 Months	12 Months	15 Months	18 Months	19–23 Months	2–3 Years	4–6 Years
Hepatitis B[1]	HepB	HepB		see footnote 1		HepB					
Rotavirus[2]			RV	RV	RV[2]						
Diphtheria, Tetanus, Pertussis[3]			DTaP	DTaP	DTaP	see footnote 3	DTaP				DTaP
Haemophilus influenzae type b[4]			HiB	HiB	Hib[4]	Hib					
Pneumococcal[5]			PCV	PCV	PCV	PCV				PPSV	
Inactivated Poliovirus			IPV	IPV		IPV					IPV
Influenza[6]						Influenza (Yearly)					
Measles, Mumps, Rubella[7]						MMR			see footnote 7		MMR
Varicella[8]						Varicella			see footnote 8		Varicella
Hepatitis A[9]						HepA (2 doses)				HepA Series	
Meningococcal[10]										MCV	

☐ Range of recommended ages for vaccination   ☐ Certain high-risk groups

This schedule indicates the recommended ages for routine administration of currently licensed childhood vaccines, as of December 1, 2008, for children aged 0–6 years. Any dose not administered at the recommended age should be administered at a subsequent visit, when indicated and feasible. Licensed combination vaccines may be used whenever any component of the combination is indicated and other components are not contraindicated and if approved by the Food and Drug Administration for that dose of the series. Providers should consult the relevant Advisory Committee on Immunization Practices statement for detailed recommendations, including high-risk conditions: http://www.cdc.gov/vaccines/pubs/acip-list.htm. Clinically significant adverse events that follow immunization should be reported to the Vaccine Adverse Event Reporting System (VAERS). Guidance about how to obtain and complete a VAERS form is available at http://vaers.hhs.gov or by telephone 800-822-7967.

1. **Hepatitis B vaccine (HepB).** *(Minimum age: birth)*
   At birth:
   - Administer monovalent HepB to all newborns before hospital discharge.
   - If mother is hepatitis B surface antigen (HBsAg)-positive, administer HepB and 0.5 mL of hepatitis B immune globulin (HBIG) within 12 hours of birth.
   - If mother's HGsAg status is unknown, administer HepB within 12 hours of birth. Determine mother's HBsAg status as soon as possible and, if HBsAg-positive, administer HBIG (no later that age 1 week).
   After the birth dose:
   - The HepB series should be completed with either monovalent HepB or a combination vaccine containing HepB. The second dose should be administered at age 1 or 2 months. The final dose should be administered no earlier than age 24 weeks.
   - Infants born to HBsAg-positive mothers should be tested for HBsAG and antibody to HBsAg (anti-HBs) after completion of at least 3 doses of the HepB series, at age 9 through 18 months (generally at the next well-child visit).
   4-month dose:
   - Administration of 4 doses of HepB to infants is permissible when combination vaccines containing HepB are administered after the birth dose.
2. **Rotavirus vaccine (RV).** *(Minimum age: 6 weeks)*
   - Administer the first dose at age 6 through 14 weeks (maximum age: 14 weeks 6 days). Vaccination should not be initiated for infants aged 15 weeks or older (i.e., 15 weeks 0 days or older).
   - Administer the final dose in the series by age 8 months 0 days.
   - If Rotarix® is administered at ages 2 and 4 months, a dose at 6 months is not indicated.
3. **Diphtheria and tetanus toxoids and acellular pertussis vaccine (DTaP).** *(Minimum age: 6 weeks)*
   - The fourth dose may be administered as early as age 12 months, provided at least 6 months have elapsed since the third dose.
   - Administer the final dose in the series at age 4 through 6 years.
4. ***Haemophilus influenzae* type b conjugate vaccine (Hib).** *(Minimum age: 6 weeks)*
   - If PRP-OMP (PedvaxHIB® or Comvax® [HepB-Hib]) is administered at ages 2 and 4 months, a dose at age 6 months is not indicated.
   - TriHiBit® (DTaP/Hib) should not be used for doses at ages 2, 4, or 6 months but can be used as the final dose in children aged 12 months or older.
5. **Pneumococcal vaccine.** *(Minimum age 6 weeks for pneumococcal conjugate vaccine [PCV]; 2 years for pneumococcal polysaccharide vaccine [PPSV])*
   - PCV is recommended for all children aged younger than 5 years. Administer 1 dose of PCV to all healthy children aged 24 through 59 months who are not completely vaccinated for their age.
   - Administer PPSV to children aged 2 years or older with certain underlying medical conditions (see *MMWR* 2000; 49[No. RR-9]), including a cochlear implant.
6. **Influenza vaccine.** *(Minimum age: 6 months for trivalent inactivated influenza vaccine [TIV]; 2 years for live, attenuated influenza vaccine [LAIV])*
   - Administer annually to children aged 6 months through 18 years.
   - For healthy nonpregnant persons (i.e., those who do not have underlying medical conditions that predispose them to influenza complications) aged 2 through 49 years, either LAIV or TIV may be used.
   - Children receiving TIV should receive 0.25 mL if aged 6 through 35 months or 0.5 mL if aged 3 years or older.
   - Administer 2 doses (separated by at least 4 weeks) to children aged younger than 9 years who are receiving influenza vaccine for the first time or who were vaccinated for the first time during the previous influenza season but only received 1 dose.
7. **Measles, mumps, and rubella vaccine (MMR).** *(Minimum age: 12 months)*
   - Administer the second dose at age 4 through 6 years. However, the second dose may be administered before age 4, provided at least 28 days have elapsed since the first dose.
8. **Varicella vaccine.** *(Minimum age: 12 months)*
   - Administer the second dose at age 4 through 6 years. However, the second dose may be administered before age 4, provided at least 3 months have elapsed since the first dose.
   - For children aged 12 months through 12 years the minimum interval between doses is 3 months. However, if the second dose was administered at least 28 days after the first dose, it can be accepted as valid.
9. **Hepatitis A vaccine (HepA).** *(Minimum age 12 months)*
   - Administer to all children aged 1 year (i.e., aged 12 through 23 months). Administer 2 doses at least 6 months apart.
   - Children not fully vaccinated by age 2 years can be vaccinated at subsequent visits.
   - HepA also is recommended for children older than 1 year who live in areas where vaccination programs target older children or who are at increased risk of infection. See *MMWR* 2006; 55(No. RR-7).
10. **Meningococcal vaccine.** *(Minimum age: 2 years for meningococcal conjugate vaccine [MCV] and for meningococcal polysaccharide vaccine [MPSV])*
    - Administer MCV to children aged 2 through 10 with terminal complement component deficiency, anatomic or functional asplenia, and certain other high-risk groups. See *MMWR* 2005; 54(No. RR-7).

Figure 320-1 **Recommended immunization schedule for persons aged 0 through 6 years, United States, 2009.** *(From Centers for Disease Control and Prevention: http://www.cdc.gov/vaccines/recs/schedules/child-schedule.htm#printable.)*

and 1997 be routinely vaccinated beginning at 2 years of age or older. In 2006, the ACIP recommended all children in their second year of life be vaccinated.[91] HAVRIX is recommended in a two-dose schedule with doses separated by 6 to 12 months. The dose for children 1 through 18 years of age is 720 ELISA units, and for adults, it is 1440 ELISA units. Two doses of 25 units of VAQTA 6 through 18 months apart are recommended for persons 1 through 18 years, and two doses of 50 units 6 months apart are recommended for persons 19 years of age or older. Hepatitis A vaccine is not licensed for use in children younger than 12 months of age. The vaccine is poorly immunogenic in infants born to women who are seropositive for hepatitis A.[11,92] Simultaneous administration with immune globulin may decrease immunogenicity slightly but should not cause any decrease in protection.[93] The ACIP recommends hepatitis A vaccine for international travelers to countries with high or intermediate hepatitis A endemicity. Although immune globulin may be used, vaccine alone is preferred.[91] For persons 12 months to 40 years of age, vaccine alone may be given for postexposure prophylaxis. For persons older than 40 years, those with immune deficiency, and those with liver disease, immune globulin is preferred.

No serious adverse events have been attributed to either hepatitis A vaccine. The most frequent side effects are local reactions. The only contraindication is for persons sensitive to vaccine components.[91]

Hepatitis B Vaccine

Hepatitis B vaccine consists of purified inactivated HBsAg particles obtained either from the plasma of chronic carriers or from yeast through recombinant DNA technology. In the United States, plasma-derived vaccines have been replaced by recombinant vaccines, although the former are still available abroad. There are two single antigen hepatitis B vaccines available in the United States—Recombivax HB (Merck & Company) and Engerix-B (GlaxoSmithKline Biologicals), and each is available as a combination product: with *Haemophilus influenzae* b conjugate vaccine (Comvax; Merck & Company), hepatitis A vaccine (Twinrix; GlaxoSmithKline Biologicals), or DTaP and inactivated polio vaccine (Pediarix; GlaxoSmithKline Biologicals). Because recommended doses vary by age, the package insert should be consulted for the proper dose of each product. When initially licensed, use of vaccine was targeted to individuals at high risk for exposure to hepatitis B, including certain categories of health care workers (those with risk for exposure to blood or blood products), hemodialysis patients, recipients of certain blood products, men who have sex with men, certain institutionalized individuals, parenteral drug abusers, and household or sexual contacts of chronic carriers of HBsAg. Vaccine continues to be indicated for these groups, and federal regulations now mandate that the vaccine be made available at no charge to all health care and public safety workers who anticipate exposure to human blood or body fluids during work.[94] Failure of vaccination targeted only to high-risk groups to have substantial impact on disease incidence, along with the appreciation that hepatitis B affects larger groups in the general population (such as heterosexuals with multiple partners), has led to the development of population-based control strategies.[95,96]

Currently, hepatitis B vaccine is recommended for all infants in the United States. Acceptable schedules include (1) doses at birth, 1 through 2 months, and 6 through 18 months of age, or (2) doses at 1 to 2 months, 4 months, and 6 through 18 months, but it is preferred that the hepatitis B vaccine series be initiated at birth. When using combination vaccines, a four-dose schedule including a birth dose of single antigen hepatitis B vaccine is acceptable. It is anticipated that those immunized as infants will still be protected when they become adolescents and young adults, the greatest risk period in the United States.[95] To protect infants at highest risk for the development of chronic hepatitis B infection, all pregnant women should be routinely screened for HBsAg, preferably during an early prenatal visit. The vaccine should be administered within 12 hours of birth along with hepatitis B immune globulin to infants born of HBsAg-positive mothers. The immunizing course consists of three doses given intramuscularly at birth, 1 month, and 6 months of age.[96]

For adolescents and adults, the usual schedule is doses at 0, 1, and 6 months.[97] All adolescents who have not previously been vaccinated should receive three doses of vaccine. The second and third doses should be administered 1 to 2 months and 4 to 6 months, respectively, after the first dose. An alternate two-dose regimen of one licensed hepatitis B vaccine (Recombivax; Merck & Company) is available for routine vaccination of adolescents with doses at 0 and 4 to 6 months. A good time to begin adolescent immunization is at 11 to 12 years of age when other immunizations are also recommended.[98]

The vaccine should be administered intramuscularly to infants in the anterolateral thigh with a 1-inch 23-gauge needle and to children and adults in the deltoid region. For deltoid vaccination, a 5/8-inch, 25-gauge needle may be used in children up to 10 years of age, and a 1-inch, 23-gauge needle should be used in older children and adults. Gluteal administration is associated with poorer antibody responses.[9] A series of three intramuscular doses produces a protective antibody response (antibody to HbsAg greater than 10 mIU/mL) in more than 95% of infants and children, more than 90% of adults younger than 40 years of age, and 75% to 90% of adults older than 40 years of age. Host factors such as smoking and obesity contribute to decreased immunogenicity of the primary vaccine series, but age is the major determinant of vaccine response. Vaccine immunogenicity may also be lower in immunocompromised patients. Follow-up for up to 12 years has shown the virtual absence of clinically significant infections in persons who initially achieved a protective antibody titer.[99] Most persons who lose detectable antibody appear to retain immunologic memory against significant infections. A small study that followed Alaskan children, vaccinated at birth, suggested almost half of cases lacked anamnestic responses following a booster dose 15 years later.[100] However, none of the children had been infected, as measured by the presence of core antibody. Thus, there is no indication at this time for booster doses of vaccine after immunization of immunocompetent children or adults. Additional experience will be necessary to know whether there will be any need for booster doses in the second decade after immunization.

Adverse effects associated with hepatitis B vaccine have been few; they consist primarily of local reactions and low-grade fever. Serious reactions have been rare and, aside from anaphylaxis, have not convincingly been established to be caused by vaccination. Some reports suggest that hepatitis B vaccine may rarely cause alopecia. The condition has been reported primarily in adults and has been reversible in most cases.[101] A number of case reports have linked hepatitis B vaccine to demyelinating syndromes, including multiple sclerosis.[102,103] However, data available do not support a causal relationship. The IOM's Immunization Safety Review Committee reviewed available data and concluded that the evidence did not support a relationship between hepatitis B vaccination in adults and multiple sclerosis; the evidence was inadequate to accept or reject a causal relationship with other demyelinating conditions.[26]

Recombinant hepatitis B vaccine is contraindicated in persons with hypersensitivity to yeast. It is not effective in eliminating the carrier state, but there is no known risk for vaccinating individuals who are carriers or who are already immune.[96]

Human Papillomavirus Vaccines

Two major HPV vaccines have been developed containing L1 capsid proteins, which self-assemble into viral-like particles that are similar in conformation to the structures associated with the natural virus.[104] Both are produced using recombinant techniques, which incorporate the gene expressing L1 into *Saccharomyces cerevisiae* or baculovirus-infected insect cells. As of May 2009, only one of the vaccines was licensed in the United States: a quadrivalent preparation, containing types 16 and 18, which cause about 70% of cervical cancers worldwide, and types 6 and 11, which cause about 90% of genital warts.[105] The vaccine is produced in yeast and contains an aluminum hydroxide adjuvant. Efficacy was demonstrated in preventing cervical intraepithelial neoplasia (CIN) or adenocarcinoma in situ (AIS) in women. A combined analysis of four studies evaluating high-grade lesions (CIN

2/3 or AIS) associated with types 16 and 18 reported an efficacy of 100% with a lower bound of the 95% confidence limit of 92.9%. Effectiveness against genital warts related to any of the four types was 98.9% (95% confidence interval [CI], 93.7% to 100%). The duration of protection is unclear. However, preliminary data suggest that protection against vaccine-related CIN or external genital lesions was more than 95% three years after vaccination. Studies are pending regarding efficacy in males, and future discussions will involve whether vaccines should be recommended for this population as well, both to protect them individually and to decrease transmission of the virus and provide herd immunity. In clinical trials, the occurrence of systemic adverse events was similar between vaccine and placebo recipients.

Local reactions were more common in vaccine recipients. After licensure, concerns were raised about serious adverse events, temporally related to HPV vaccine, but the occurrence of these events appears to be compatible with expected incidence. The vaccine is recommended in a schedule of three doses at 0, 2, and 6 months, for all females 9 to 26 years of age. The usual age for starting vaccination is 11 to 12 years.

A second vaccine, produced using baculovirus, contains types 16 and 18, and is not yet licensed in the United States. This bivalent vaccine contains the proprietary adjuvant ASO4, which is composed of aluminum hydroxide and 3-deacylated monophosphoryl lipid A.[104] Early studies of the vaccine have shown it is at least 96% effective against persistent infection, with continued protection for more than 3 years. The vaccine has been used in a three-dose schedule at 0, 1, and 6 months of age.

Influenza Virus Vaccines—Inactivated

Trivalent influenza virus vaccine (TIV) is composed of inactivated disrupted ("split") influenza viruses or purified surface antigens. Because of the frequent antigenic changes in influenza viruses, the antigenic content of influenza virus vaccines is changed annually to reflect the influenza A and B virus strains in circulation. Persons for whom influenza vaccine is recommended should be vaccinated annually. The efficacy of the vaccine in protecting against influenza is directly related to the degree of concordance between the virus strains included in the vaccine and the strains that are circulating in the community. When periodic major changes in antigenic structure of circulating influenza viruses occur, vaccine that contains antigens representative of prior viruses has decreased or shown no effectiveness. Influenza vaccine has been estimated to be 70% to 90% effective in preventing influenza in healthy adults younger than 65 years of age. Efficacy appears to be lower in elderly persons. A meta-analysis of 20 cohort studies estimated effectiveness rates of 56%, 53%, 50%, and 68% for preventing respiratory illness, pneumonia, hospitalization, and death, respectively.[106] In nursing home settings, efficacy has often been substantially lower, on the order of 30% to 40%. However, prevention of complications of influenza in such settings has been considerably higher, averaging from about 50% to 60% in preventing hospitalization or pneumonia to 80% in preventing death.[107] Efficacy data among young children are limited. Estimates vary from 22% to 91%, with most studies documenting protection of 56% or more.[108] In comparative studies, younger children tend to have lower rates of protection than older children. In one study that followed a small number of children, efficacy was 66% among 6- to 24-month-old children in year 1, but no efficacy was demonstrated in year 2 when attack rates among placebo recipients were low.[109]

Influenza immunization strategy in the United States is directed at reducing the complications and mortality associated with influenza.[110] Because these occur primarily in chronically ill and elderly persons, these groups are advised most strongly to receive vaccine. Specifically, annual immunization is recommended for all persons 65 years of age or older; residents of nursing homes and other chronic care facilities with chronic medical conditions regardless of age; persons with chronic cardiovascular or pulmonary disorders, including children with asthma; persons requiring regular medical follow-up or those

hospitalized in the preceding year with chronic metabolic disease (including diabetes mellitus), renal dysfunction, hemoglobinopathies, or immunosuppression; and children and teenagers on long-term aspirin therapy. Women who will be pregnant during the influenza season (usually December through March) should be vaccinated. Because a high proportion of persons aged 50 through 64 years have high-risk medical conditions, and because age-based recommendations tend to be better followed than risk-based recommendations, annual vaccination is recommended for all persons 50 through 64 years of age. Physicians and other personnel caring for high-risk persons should be vaccinated to reduce the chances that such patients will be exposed to influenza. Similar recommendations apply to employees in nursing homes, those who provide home care, and household members of persons with high-risk conditions. Many of the persons in need of influenza vaccine are hospitalized frequently and should be vaccinated on discharge if hospitalized during autumn.[110] Starting in 2002, the ACIP encouraged annual vaccination of children 6 through 23 months of age, when feasible, because of data documenting an increased risk for hospitalization in this age group compared with older children. In October 2003, the ACIP voted to recommend influenza vaccination annually for all children 6 through 23 months of age and for all contacts of children younger than 2 years of age.[110]

In 2008, The ACIP recommended that no later than the 2009-2010 influenza vaccination season, all children 6 months through 18 years of age be vaccinated annually.[111] This should provide individual benefits to those who are vaccinated but also has the potential to reduce community transmission of the virus and provide indirect benefit to others. A child 6 months through 8 years of age, being vaccinated for the first time, should receive two doses of vaccine with an interval of at least 4 weeks between them; children in that age group who have previously received two doses require only a single dose in subsequent years. Children who received only a single dose when they were initially vaccinated against influenza require two doses the subsequent season and one dose annually thereafter. Influenza seasons can peak anywhere from November to May, although most occur in January or later, February being the most common month. Thus, although October and November have been the traditional months for influenza vaccination, vaccination through February and even March will provide benefit during most influenza seasons. As of 2009, about 83% of the U.S. population is recommended for vaccination, including all children 6 months through 18 years of age, household contacts and out of home caregivers of children younger than 5 years of age, all adults older than 50 years, persons with underlying chronic conditions that place them at high risk for complications from influenza, pregnant women, household contacts of high-risk persons, and health care workers. However, the ACIP has a permissive recommendation allowing anyone without contraindications, who wants to prevent influenza, to be vaccinated. Adverse events associated with current influenza vaccines are infrequent. Three to 5% of recipients report local tenderness or low-grade fever. During the swine influenza immunization program of 1976, an elevated incidence rate of GBS was noted in recipients of the swine flu vaccine.[112] The risk for GBS after influenza vaccine during six subsequent seasons that were studied was not significantly elevated compared with expected rates. However, studies during the 1992-1993 and 1993-1994 influenza seasons suggest that influenza vaccines may have been associated with GBS at an attributable risk of about 1 case per 1 million doses in those years.[113] No cases of GBS within 6 weeks of vaccination were detected in persons 18 to 44 years of age despite administration of about 4 million doses of vaccine over the two influenza seasons studied.[113] The overall risk for GBS in these studies was about one tenth the risk of GBS after swine flu vaccine. If GBS is ever caused by current influenza vaccines, it is rare. In contrast, the risk for hospitalization from influenza disease and its complications is orders of magnitude higher in most populations for whom vaccine is recommended. Given the substantial benefits of influenza vaccine among the targeted populations, the risk for GBS, if any, is exceeded by the benefits. Persons with an immediate hypersensitivity reaction to a prior dose or those with anaphylactic hypersensitivity to eggs, in which vaccine viruses are grown, should be vaccinated only after careful assessment that the benefits are likely to outweigh the risks.[111] Protocols have been developed for vaccinating such patients.[114] Concerns have been raised regarding vaccination of human immunodeficiency virus (HIV)–infected individuals. Persons with severe immunocompromise do not respond well, and some studies have shown a transient increase in HIV-1 in the plasma in the 2 to 4 weeks after vaccination, which has not been associated with clinical deterioration. On the other hand, the risk for influenza-associated deaths is higher in HIV-infected persons than in the general population. Therefore, influenza vaccine should be considered for HIV-infected persons.[111] The IOM reviewed the relationship between influenza vaccine and neurologic disorders. They concluded that the evidence favored acceptance of a causal relationship between GBS and the 1976 influenza vaccine, although the evidence was insufficient to accept or reject a causal relationship for subsequent years. The IOM concluded that the evidence favored rejection of a relationship between influenza vaccine and exacerbation of multiple sclerosis. Although the evidence was insufficient with regard to incident cases of multiple sclerosis, the committee concluded that given the evidence that influenza vaccine does not cause exacerbation of multiple sclerosis, vaccine was unlikely to cause new cases.[115] In 2009, a novel influenza A (H1N1) virus was reported to infect people throughout the world. For current status of the epidemiology, detection, antiviral drugs, and prevention including immunization and recommendations for travel and care of ill people see www.cdc.gov/H1N1flu/index.htm.[165]

Live Attenuated Influenza Vaccine

In 2003, the U.S. Food and Drug Administration (FDA) licensed a live attenuated influenza reassortant vaccine (LAIV) to be administered intranasally. Each viral strain in the trivalent vaccine consists of six internal genes from a cold-adapted, temperature-sensitive, attenuated mutant.[111,116,117] The hemagglutinin and neuraminidase are derived from circulating wild strains. The cold adaptation is supportive of growth of the vaccine viruses in the upper airways, and temperature sensitivity decreases their growth in the lower airways. The vaccine is trivalent with reassortants for each of the major circulating influenza viruses: A (H3N2), A (H1N1), and B.

In a study of healthy children, vaccine was 87% effective after two doses in those 60 to 71 months of age in year 1, with a good match between vaccine and circulating wild virus, and 87% in 60- to 84-month-old children in year 2, when vaccine and circulating strains substantially diverged. In addition, vaccine reduced influenza-associated febrile otitis media by 30%. A small challenge study among healthy adults, 18 to 41 years of age, was associated with 85% efficacy. An effectiveness study among adults during a year in which the circulating virus was not well matched to the vaccine strains still demonstrated a 19% reduction in severe febrile illnesses of any etiology and a 24% reduction in febrile respiratory illnesses.

Side effects in adults that have been significantly higher than among placebo recipients include coryza or nasal congestion, headache, and sore throat. Among children, coryza, headache, fever, and myalgias were more common among vaccinees than placebo recipients. Abdominal pain and occasional vomiting were also seen more frequently in vaccinees. Young children (12 to 59 months of age), who were vaccinated, had an unexplained but statistically significant increase in asthma or reactive airways disease over placebo recipients that was not seen in older age groups. No serious adverse events were observed. Shedding of vaccine virus from the nasopharynx is common, especially for young children. A study in a Finnish daycare center detected shedding of at least one strain in 80% of children with a mean duration of 7.6 days. However, transmission to unvaccinated contacts was rare (0.6% to 2.4%).

Comparative studies of LAIV and TIV in young children suggest that LAIV may provide better efficacy than TIV with both well-matched A/H1N1 strains and not well-matched A/H3N2 strains, but not for influenza B.[118] Nevertheless, the attack rates for laboratory-confirmed influenza among TIV recipients were still low, implying that TIV still provided substantial protection. In contrast, in adults there appears to be no advantage of LAIV over TIV.[119]

Vaccine is recommended for persons 2 through 49 years of age who do not have medical conditions that put them at high risk for complications from influenza.[111] This includes all persons 2 through 18 years of age who require annual influenza vaccination and other age-eligible persons who have contacts with persons with high-risk medical conditions. With the exception of contact with severely immunocompromised individuals (e.g., stem cell transplant recipients), there is no preference between LAIV and TIV. TIV is preferred for persons who come in close contact with severely immunocompromised individuals, although LAIV is not contraindicated. Children younger than 9 years old require two doses separated by at least 4 weeks unless they have received two doses of any influenza vaccine previously.[111]

Japanese Encephalitis

Japanese encephalitis (JE) vaccine is grown in mouse brains and inactivated and purified in at least a five-step process; it is no longer being produced.[120] No myelin basic protein has been detected in the vaccine. The vaccine has proved 91% effective in a large-scale trial in Thailand.[121] The vaccine is indicated for some persons traveling to or residing in endemic or epidemic areas, particularly those spending 30 or more days in high-risk areas (especially rural areas) in Asia during transmission season.[122] Persons traveling to such areas for shorter periods may warrant vaccine under special circumstances. The primary immunization schedule for persons 4 years of age or older consists of three 1-mL doses administered subcutaneously on days 0, 7, and 30. An abbreviated schedule with the third dose at 14 days may be used if time constraints do not permit the full schedule. The dose is 0.5 mL for children 1 to 3 years of age given by the same schedule. The remaining stockpile of this vaccine is being restricted for use in children from 1 through 16 years of age. A new, inactivated Vero cell–derived JE vaccine (IXIARO) has been licensed by the FDA in the United States for use in adult travelers 18 years of age and older. The vaccine was licensed in the United States based on a noninferiority immunogenicity study comparing neutralizing antibodies elicited by the new vaccine with the previously available JE vaccine. Fewer vaccine-associated hypersensitivity or neurologic adverse events are expected to occur compared with the previously used vaccine.

Measles Vaccine

Measles vaccine is a live attenuated virus vaccine recommended for use in all children 12 months of age and older who do not have contraindications.[123] When administered to a child 12 through 15 months of age or older, efficacy is greater than 95%. Only a single dose is needed to provide long-lasting, probably lifelong, immunity in those who respond to the vaccine. However, evidence suggests that measles transmission can be sustained among the 2% to 5% of vaccinated persons who fail to seroconvert after an initial dose of vaccine. Therefore, beginning in 1989, a two-dose schedule was recommended in the United States. The first dose should be administered at 12 through 15 months of age. Lower levels of maternal antibody from today's vaccinated mothers allow higher rates of seroconversion at 12 months than in the past when most maternal antibody came from mothers with naturally acquired disease.[124]

The second dose should be administered at 1 month or more after the first dose, typically at entry to school (4 to 6 years of age). Both doses should routinely be given as combined MMR vaccine or MMR and varicella (MMRV).[123] Recent data suggest that MMRV, because it is associated with a higher risk for fever than the separate administration of MMR and varicella, may also cause an increased risk for febrile seizures after dose 1 of the two-dose series.[125]

All college entrants who have not received two doses of MMR vaccine on or after their first birthday should receive them.[123] If necessary, the two doses can be given separated by 1 month. Immunization is recommended for all individuals not known to be immune. Because individuals born before 1957 are likely to have been infected naturally, they are usually considered immune. Other acceptable evidence of measles immunity is documentation of adequate vaccination, laboratory evidence of immunity to measles, or documentation of prior physician-diagnosed measles. Similar recommendations apply to health care workers. Health care facilities should consider recommending a dose of MMR to unvaccinated workers born before 1957 who do not have a history of physician-diagnosed measles or laboratory evidence of immunity to both measles and rubella.[126,127]

Because measles is much more prevalent outside the United States, adequate vaccination is recommended for all travelers born after 1956. Such persons should receive a second dose if they have not previously been vaccinated and lack other evidence of measles immunity.[123]

Untoward reactions associated with measles vaccine include fever of 39.4° C or greater in 5% of recipients and transient rashes in about 5% of vaccinees. Fever and rash generally begin 7 to 12 days after vaccination and last 1 to 2 days. Because measles vaccine causes fever, it can be associated with febrile convulsions.[128] Children with prior personal histories of convulsions or histories of convulsions in the immediate family may be at increased risk for febrile convulsions following MMR vaccination.[129] Antipyretics may prevent febrile seizures after MMR vaccination if administered before onset of fever and continued for 5 to 7 days. However, fever is difficult to anticipate, making the use of antipyretics impractical in most situations. Aspirin should not be used to prevent or control fever because of its association with Reye syndrome. Anaphylaxis and thrombocytopenic purpura also appear to be caused rarely by MMR.[52] Encephalopathy with onset about 10 days after vaccination has been reported in vaccine recipients, with a frequency of about 1 in 2 million vaccinations, although a causal role for measles vaccine has not been established.[130] The available evidence favors rejection of a causal role for MMR in autism.[55,131]

Measles vaccine is contraindicated for pregnant women and in persons who are immunocompromised because of either congenital or acquired disorders (e.g., leukemia or immunosuppressive drugs), with the exception of people infected with HIV. Because measles may cause severe disease in HIV-infected persons, asymptomatic and mildly symptomatic HIV-infected persons may be vaccinated if measles vaccination is otherwise indicated. However, vaccination is contraindicated for people who are severely immunocompromised. Persons with a history of anaphylactic reactions to eggs may be vaccinated and observed for at least 20 minutes because most persons with such histories do not have serious reactions to vaccine. Skin testing of persons with such histories is no longer recommended because such tests appear not to predict severe reactions.[123]

Meningococcal Vaccines

Two meningococcal vaccines are available in the United States.[132] A vaccine containing purified meningococcal capsular polysaccharides of groups A, C, Y, and W135 only, which may be given to persons greater than 2 years of age (MPSV4), and a vaccine consisting of each of the four polysaccharides, each conjugated to diphtheria toxoid (MCV4), which may be given to persons 2 through 55 years of age. The antibody responses to each of the four polysaccharides included in each of the quadrivalent vaccines are serogroup-specific and independent. Meningococcal vaccines are routinely indicated for control of outbreaks of serogroup C meningococcal disease and for use among certain high-risk groups such as persons with terminal complement component deficiencies, those with anatomic or functional asplenia, and laboratory personnel who routinely are exposed to *N. meningitidis* in solutions that may be aerosolized. MCV4 is preferred over MPSV4 for persons eligible for both vaccines. MCV4 is routinely recommended as a single dose for all adolescents beginning at 11 through 12 years of age. College freshmen, especially those living in dormitories, should receive a dose if not previously vaccinated. Children 2 through 10 years of age with high-risk conditions should also receive MCV4, but the vaccine is not routinely recommended for other children in this age group.[133]

Military recruits, who previously had high rates of meningococcal disease, are also routinely vaccinated with MCV4. Vaccine may be of

benefit to travelers to countries with endemic or hyperendemic disease who are expected to have prolonged contact with the local population. Frequent epidemics, generally between December and June, occur in the "meningitis belt" of sub-Saharan Africa (which stretches from Senegal to Ethiopia).[134] A single intramuscular injection of MPSV4 induces protection in 85% or more of school-aged recipients and adults against types C and A. The vaccine is immunogenic in 2- to 5-year-old children. MCV4 induces equivalent immune responses to MPSV4. For children first vaccinated before 4 years of age with MPSV4, revaccination should be considered after 3 years if they remain at high risk. The vaccines are not effective for children younger than 2 years of age with the exception of group A for MPSV4. Short-term protection may be achieved against this group in children as young as 3 months of age. When vaccinating 3- through 18-month-old children, two doses 3 months apart are recommended. Adverse effects associated with meningococcal polysaccharide vaccine are mild and consist primarily of pain and redness at the injection site. More than 40% of recipients have reported local reactions in some studies, but in others, reactions have been much more infrequent.[135,136] Up to 2% of children experience fever. There are no known contraindications to the use of this vaccine.

Conjugation of meningococcal polysaccharide to protein results in a vaccine that is immunogenic in infants and young children, by induction of T-cell–dependent responses, and induces immunologic memory to meningococcal polysaccharide.[23,136,137] Conjugate vaccines also reduce carriage and induce herd immunity.[138] Meningococcal type C conjugate vaccines also appear to be able to overcome immunologic hyporesponsiveness induced by meningococcal polysaccharide vaccine in young children and in adults.[139,140] In the United Kingdom, use of meningococcal C conjugate vaccines among infants, children, and adolescents since November 1999 has resulted in dramatic reductions in serogroup C disease without evidence of serotype replacement.[138,141,142] Infants received a three-dose primary series at 2, 3, and 4 months of age, and catch-up immunization for children through age 17 years was implemented with two (5- through 11-month-olds) or one (12 months through 17 years) dose of vaccine. Among adolescents, the effectiveness of the vaccine was 97% (95% CI, 77% to 99%), and in toddlers 92% (95% CI, 65% to 98%).[141] Effectiveness was also high among infants who had received at least two doses of vaccine, at 89% (95% CI, 58% to 97%).[141] Surveillance of adverse events in the United Kingdom has demonstrated that the vaccine is well tolerated; anaphylactic reactions were reported at a rate of 1 in 500,000 doses distributed.[138] MCV4 is administered as a single dose.[132] Boosters are not recommended at this time. Reports of adverse events suggest that MCV4 may be associated with an increased risk for GBS. The risk, if real, is very low, estimated at about 1.25 cases per 1 million doses distributed to persons 11 to 19 years of age.[143]

Systemic reactions to MCV4 are similar to the incidence after MPSV4 with the exception of low-grade fever, which may occur slightly more often with MCV4. Local reactions are also more common after MCV4.[132]

Mumps Vaccine

Mumps vaccine is a live attenuated virus vaccine that is recommended for use in all children 12 months of age or older who do not have contraindications. Mumps vaccine is routinely administered as MMR or MMRV at 12 through 15 months of age.[123] When administered on or after the first birthday, 90% or more of recipients can be expected to acquire protective antibodies. Although protection had been thought to be lifelong, investigations following a resurgence of mumps in 2006 suggested some persons may lose immunity over time.[144] A second dose is recommended with MMR or MMRV, usually at 4 through 6 years of age.[123] As with measles, most persons born before 1957 are likely to have been infected naturally by mumps virus and can generally be considered immune; otherwise, individuals should be considered susceptible unless they have documentation of having received live mumps vaccine on or after their first birthday, laboratory evidence of mumps immunity, or documentation of physician-diagnosed mumps disease.[123] For health care workers, acceptable evidence of immunity consists of two doses of mumps-containing vaccines.[145] Contraindications to mumps vaccine are pregnancy and an immunocompromised state (see "Measles Vaccine"). Persons with a history of anaphylactic reactions to eggs may be vaccinated. Adverse events associated with mumps vaccine are very few. Parotitis and orchitis have been reported rarely. Thrombocytopenic purpura and anaphylaxis appear to be caused rarely by MMR.[52] Aseptic meningitis has been associated with the Urabe and Leningrad-Zagreb strains of mumps vaccine, strains not available in the United States.[146,147] The Jeryl Lynn strain used in U.S. vaccines has not been proved to cause aseptic meningitis.[52]

Pertussis Vaccine

Acellular pertussis vaccines are made from purified components of the organism *Bordetella pertussis* and detoxified pertussis toxin (PT); whole-cell pertussis vaccines, made from suspensions of killed whole *B. pertussis,* are no longer available in the United States, although they continue to be widely used internationally.[45] Acellular pertussis vaccines currently available in the United States contain pertussis toxoid and filamentous hemagglutinin (FHA). In addition, they may contain pertactin (69-kDa protein) or fimbriae and pertactin.[46] Pertussis vaccines are combined with diphtheria and tetanus toxoids as DTaP (acellular pertussis vaccines for children) or TdaP (for adolescents and adults). The primary immunizing course for children consists of three doses of DTaP administered intramuscularly at 4- to 8-week intervals typically given at 2, 4, and 6 months of age. A fourth dose is given about 6 to 12 months later (15 through 18 months of age) and a fifth dose at 4 through 6 years of age. Acellular pertussis vaccines are preferred over whole-cell pertussis vaccines because the efficacy of acellular vaccines is comparable to whole-cell vaccines and because the incidence of adverse events after acellular vaccines is significantly lower than after whole-cell vaccines. As of May 2009, three acellular vaccines for children were available in the United States: Tripedia (Sanofi Pasteur, Inc.), which contains PT and FHA; Infanrix (GlaxoSmith-Kline Pharmaceuticals), which contains PT, FHA, and pertactin; and DAPTACEL (Sanofi Pasteur, Inc.), which contains PT, FHA, pertactin, and fimbriae types 2 and 3. Efficacy in preventing classic pertussis, consisting of 21 or more days of paroxysmal cough, has ranged from 71% to 89% for three doses.[46] This is considerably higher than the efficacy found for one of the old U.S. whole-cell vaccines after three doses in clinical trials in Europe (36% to 48%).[148,149] However, in comparative trials, most acellular vaccines have had slightly lower efficacy than whole-cell vaccines.

Symptoms and signs of local reactions occur about one tenth to one half as frequently after acellular vaccines compared with whole-cell vaccines. For example, the incidence of erythema by the third evening after any of the first three doses of acellular vaccines for children ranged from 26.3% to 39.2% in one large comparative trial, compared with 72.7% in those who received the whole-cell vaccine. In that study, the incidence of fever (greater than 39.4°C) after acellular vaccines was 3.3% to 5.2%, compared with 15.9% after receipt of whole-cell vaccine.[46,150] More serious adverse events such as seizures and hypotonic hyporesponsive episodes also appear to occur less frequently after acellular vaccines than after whole-cell vaccines.[151,152] The lower incidence of fever associated with acellular vaccines would be expected to decrease febrile seizures, especially after the fourth dose.

Contraindications to DTaP vaccines include an immediate anaphylactic reaction or encephalopathy within the 7 days after a prior dose. The following events are considered precautions: (1) temperature greater than or equal to 40.5°C within 48 hours of a prior dose without other identifiable cause, (2) collapse or shocklike state (hypotonic hyporesponsive episode) within 48 hours, (3) persistent inconsolable crying lasting 3 hours or more within 48 hours, and (4) convulsions with or without fever occurring within 3 days. Although under most circumstances such children will not be vaccinated, the physician may elect to continue pertussis vaccination if the benefits are judged to outweigh the risks, such as when there is a pertussis outbreak in the community. Children with evolving neurologic disorders should have

immunization deferred until the situation is clarified. Once stable, they can receive pertussis vaccine. Decisions about vaccinating children with underlying neurologic disease should be made no later than the first birthday. If pertussis vaccine is not used, the pediatric preparation of DT is indicated.[45]

Children with a personal or family history of convulsions appear to be at higher risk for seizures after pertussis vaccination than the general population. However, the benefits of vaccination outweigh the risks. Children with stable seizure disorders or with family histories of seizures may be vaccinated. Use of acetaminophen, 15 mg/kg, at the time of vaccination, and subsequently every 4 hours for 24 hours, and then as needed reduces the risk for fever after pertussis vaccination and may decrease the likelihood of postvaccination seizures.

Extensive swelling of the thigh or entire upper arm following the fourth or fifth doses of the DTaP series has been reported. The frequency appears to be 2% to 3%, and the pathogenesis is unclear. It is unknown whether children who experience entire limb swelling after a fourth dose of DTaP are at increased risk for this reaction after the fifth dose. Because of the benefits of the preschool booster and because the swelling reactions appear to be self-limited, a history of extensive swelling after the fourth dose is not a contraindication for receipt of the fifth dose of the DTaP series.[45]

DTaP is available in four combination formulations: with inactivated polio and hepatitis B vaccines (Pediarix; GlaxoSmithKline Pharmaceuticals), with inactivated polio and Hib vaccines (Pentacel, Sanofi Pasteur) with inactivated polio (KINRIX, GlaxoSmithKline Pharmaceuticals), and with Hib (TriHIB, Sanofi Pasteur). Combinations of acellular vaccines with Hib have generally resulted in diminished antibody response to the Hib component when administered to infants.[86] However, the immune response to Hib in persons who receive Pentacel is considered adequate. KINRIX is licensed only for dose 5 of DTaP, which is usually administered at the same time as dose 4 of inactivated polio vaccine at 4 to 6 years of age. TriHIBit is licensed for the fourth dose at 15 through 18 months after 3 doses of DTaP and a primary series of any Hib vaccine. Data are insufficient to document the safety, immunogenicity, and efficacy of using DTaP vaccines from different manufacturers in a mixed sequence. For this reason, whenever feasible, the same brand of DTaP should be used for all doses in the vaccination series. However, if the type of vaccine previously administered is unknown or is not available, any of the available licensed DTaP vaccines can be used to complete the vaccination series.

Concerns about the safety of whole-cell pertussis vaccines have led to decreased vaccine coverage in some countries. In the United Kingdom, pertussis vaccine uptake declined markedly in the period 1974 to 1978. The result was a major epidemic of pertussis in the years 1977 to 1979, with a second epidemic in 1982. This experience and similar ones in Japan and other countries illustrate the necessity for maintaining protection against pertussis.[153]

Studies of pertussis epidemiology suggest that adults may play an important role in sustaining transmission.[154-161] In a prospective study of persons 10 to 14 years of age with cough illness, laboratory testing for pertussis was positive in 13%, for an estimated annual incidence of pertussis of 507 cases per 100,000 person-years.[158] Pertussis in adolescents and adults may account for increases in pertussis among infants too young to be protected by vaccination.[161] Studies suggest acellular vaccines are safe and immunogenic in adults.[162]

During 2005, two acellular pertussis-containing vaccines were licensed. Both vaccines are combined with tetanus toxoid and reduced quantities of diphtheria toxoid (Tdap).[80,163] ADACEL (Sanofi Pasteur) contains detoxified pertussis toxin (PT), filamentous hemagglutinin, pertactin, and fimbriae types 2 and 3, similar to the pertussis components of DAPTACEL, the childhood preparation. The pertussis components of BOOSTRIX (GlaxoSmithKline) consist of PT, pertactin, and filamentous hemagglutinin. Both vaccines contain aluminum adjuvants. The vaccines were licensed on the basis of inducing antibody responses to pertussis antigens similar in magnitude to the responses associated with early childhood vaccination, although efficacy was also demonstrated in adults with a vaccine similar to BOOS-

TRIX.[164] The childhood vaccines were proved effective in preventing pertussis.

BOOSTRIX is licensed for administration to persons 10 through 64 years of age, whereas ADACEL is licensed for persons 11 through 64 years of age. TdaP is indicated routinely as a booster for adolescents at 11 to 12 years of age in place of the previously recommended tetanus and diphtheria toxoids for adult use (Td). In addition, all persons beyond 12 years of age but younger than 65 years should receive a single dose of Tdap, which can replace any of the decennial boosters of Td. Tdap is not indicated for primary immunization. However, it can be used for any one of the doses in the primary series of Td for unimmunized adolescents and adults. Because of concerns that TdaP might result in Arthus reactions in persons who recently received tetanus- and diphtheria-containing vaccines, it was originally recommended that a 5-year minimum interval between DTaP and Tdap or between Td and Tdap be observed. However, data from several studies suggest intervals less than 2 years are acceptable. Health care workers should also be vaccinated. TdaP is especially indicated for adults who will be caring for young infants because such children are susceptible to pertussis before active immunity can be induced by DTaP. Data are not available on the safety of administering Tdap to pregnant women. Ideally, such women should be vaccinated before becoming pregnant or immediately in the postpartum period. Some experts have recommended vaccination in late pregnancy as a way of reducing infant pertussis through both decreasing the risk for transmission of disease to the infant from the mother and through transfer of maternal antibodies against pertussis across the placenta.[165] This may be especially important for women who may be at increased risk for pertussis, such as adolescents, health care workers, and women employed in institutions in which there is a pertussis outbreak ongoing. The frequencies of both local and systemic reactions after Tdap are similar to those after Td.

Plague Vaccine

Plague vaccine is no longer available in the United States. Killed whole-cell vaccines and live attenuated vaccines are used elsewhere in the world, and new subunit and mucosal vaccines are under development.[166]

Pneumococcal Polysaccharide Vaccine

Pneumococcal polysaccharide vaccine was initially licensed as a purified preparation of 14 different serotypes of pneumococcal capsular polysaccharide in 1979. Since 1983, vaccine containing 23 types has replaced the earlier version. The types included in the current vaccine and immunologically related types are responsible for about 85% to 90% of all bacteremic pneumococcal disease in the United States. Demonstrable antibody rises to the serotypes contained in the vaccine are noted in 80% to 95% or more of healthy recipients. The vaccine has been highly effective in reducing pneumococcal disease among South African gold miners (a group at particularly high risk) and among military recruits.[167-169] In populations at high risk for pneumococcal infections, such as elderly persons and patients with high-risk medical conditions, the vaccine has generally been found to be effective against pneumococcal bacteremia but not against nonbacteremic pneumococcal pneumonia. Studies of patients with isolates from normally sterile body fluids have generally reported efficacies of 50% to 80% overall, with lower efficacy in persons who have compromised immune systems.[170-173] A study of Navaho adults did not demonstrate efficacy against invasive pneumococcal disease in this high-risk population.[174] Vaccine is primarily recommended for adults at high risk for complications from respiratory tract infections, particularly those with cardiovascular and chronic pulmonary disease, adults and children 2 years of age or older at high risk for pneumococcal disease (e.g., splenic dysfunction or anatomic asplenia, Hodgkin's disease, multiple myeloma, chronic liver disease, including cirrhosis, alcoholism, renal failure, cerebrospinal fluid leaks, cochlear implant recipients, and immunocompromised state), and otherwise healthy elderly persons (≥65 years of age).[175]

Polysaccharide vaccines are not effective in children younger than 2 years of age. Children who have completed the pneumococcal conjugate vaccine series before age 2 years and who are in these high-risk groups should receive one dose of pneumococcal polysaccharide vaccine at age 2 years.[176]

A single dose is administered by intramuscular injection. Revaccination is recommended for persons 65 years of age or older who received an initial vaccination before age 65 years, if at least 5 years has elapsed since that dose. Revaccination is also recommended for persons younger than 65 years with anatomic or functional asplenia or those who are immunocompromised, including patients with chronic renal failure and nephrotic syndrome. For such patients who are older than 10 years of age, revaccination should take place 5 years or more after the first dose. For younger patients, revaccination should be considered 3 years after the first dose.[176]

In some studies, mild reactions such as erythema and mild pain at the site of injection occurred in about half of recipients. Anaphylactic reactions have rarely been reported. Revaccination at intervals of 4 years may be associated with an increased risk for local reactions after vaccination, but these reactions tend to be self-limited and would not be a contraindication.[177] No contraindications are known, although its safety in pregnant women has not been evaluated.[172] Although transient increases in plasma HIV levels have been documented after vaccination in some studies, these have not been demonstrated to be of clinical significance. Conversely, risk for pneumococcal disease is increased in HIV-infected persons, and therefore they should be vaccinated as soon as possible after diagnosis to optimize immune response to the vaccine.[178]

Pneumococcal Conjugate Vaccine

Pneumococcal conjugate vaccines in which pneumococcal capsular polysaccharide is covalently linked to protein carriers have been developed, and a seven-valent conjugate vaccine (Prevnar; Wyeth Lederle Vaccines, PCV7) was licensed for use in infants and young children in 2000. The seven polysaccharide types included in the licensed vaccine account for 80% of invasive infections in children younger than age 6 years in the United States.[176] In a prelicensure efficacy trial in northern California, the efficacy of the conjugate vaccine was 97% against invasive disease caused by serotypes in the vaccine.[179] The vaccine was also effective in prevention of pneumonia, with the greatest impact in the first year of life, with a 32% reduction,[180] and in prevention of acute otitis media caused by serotypes of pneumococcus included in the vaccine.[179] Efficacy against invasive pneumococcal disease has been demonstrated in Native American children, a population at increased risk for disease.[181]

Pneumococcal conjugate vaccine is administered as a four-dose series, with doses at 2, 4, and 6 months of age, followed by a booster dose at 12 through 15 months of age.[176] The vaccine is recommended for all children younger than 2 years of age, as well as children aged 24 through 59 months. Children 24 through 59 months who have not completed the recommended schedule should receive one dose.[182] Children with underlying conditions who have received three doses of PCV7 should receive an additional dose. Such children who have received fewer than three doses should be vaccinated with two doses of PCV7, separated by 8 weeks.

High-risk conditions include sickle cell disease, congenital or acquired asplenia, HIV infection, congenital immunodeficiencies, renal failure and nephrotic syndrome, diseases associated with immunosuppressive therapy or radiation therapy, chronic cardiac or pulmonary disease, diabetes mellitus, cerebrospinal fluid leaks, or cochlear implants.[175,176] Other children aged 24 through 59 months may also be at increased risk for pneumococcal disease, including those aged 24 through 35 months, children of Alaska Native or American Indian descent, children of African American descent, and children who attend group daycare; use of the pneumococcal conjugate vaccine should be considered in these groups.

The primary series of the pneumococcal conjugate vaccine, administered simultaneously with other recommended childhood vaccines, is associated with an increased incidence of fever 100.4° F or higher within 48 hours of vaccination.[176]

Widespread use of the conjugate vaccine has resulted in dramatic decreases in disease incidence among young children, for whom the vaccine is recommended. In addition, decreases in disease incidence have also been observed among adults, which may be due to decreased transmission of pneumococci from children to adults.[183-184] Surveillance to date has revealed some evidence of serotype replacement, but in most studies, such replacement has been far outweighed by the reduction in disease caused by serotypes in the vaccine.[183]

Other pneumococcal conjugate vaccines containing additional pneumococcal serotypes are under development and may be licensed in the future. Use of pneumococcal conjugate vaccines in adults, either alone or in conjunction with pneumococcal polysaccharide vaccine, remains under investigation.

Polio Vaccine

Although two types of polio vaccine are available in the world to control polio, live attenuated oral polio vaccine (OPV) and IPV, which is administered by injection, only IPV is available in the United States. The schedule consists of four doses of IPV at 2 months, 4 months, 6 through 18 months, and 4 to 6 years.[185] IPV is available as a single vaccine or in combination with DTaP and hepatitis B vaccines (Pediarix; GlaxoSmithKline), DTaP and Hib vaccines (Pentacel; Sanofi Pasteur), or DTaP alone (Kinrix; GlaxoSmithKline). Although Pediarix can be used for the first three doses of IPV at 2, 4, and 6 months, single IPV is needed for the fourth dose. Pentacel can be used for any of the first three doses of IPV. Separate IPV would be needed at age 4 through 6 years. There is no need to restart a series if the primary immunization schedule is interrupted; the next dose in the series should be given.[3] Prior doses of OPV should be counted when considering whether there is a need for further polio immunization.

The decision to move to an all-IPV schedule in the United States was based on concerns that OPV could rarely cause paralytic polio, with the greatest risk after the first dose (overall risk 1 in every 750,000 first doses), and the fact that IPV given to a high proportion of people in developed countries like Sweden had eliminated disease without risk for serious side effects. In 1988, the World Health Assembly endorsed a goal to eradicate polio from the world. The major vaccine used in the worldwide eradication effort is OPV. Advantages include ease of use, better induction of intestinal immunity to prevent wild polio virus spread than IPV, spread of vaccine virus to unvaccinated contacts, and lower cost than IPV. Extensive efforts in the Americas, including mass campaigns with OPV twice a year targeted to all children younger than 5 years regardless of prior immunization status, have led to the elimination of polio in the Western Hemisphere. The last known case of polio due to wild poliovirus in the Americas had onset in Peru in 1991, and the Western Hemisphere was certified free of polio in 1994.[40] Since 1988, almost all countries with endemic polio have conducted National Immunization Days, and even with greatly improved surveillance, cases of polio have decreased from an estimated 350,000 in 1988 to about 1700 cases in 2008. By the end of 2008, only four countries had never interrupted wild poliovirus transmission, although some countries in Africa had been reinfected after being polio free.[37]

Polio vaccine is not routinely recommended for persons 18 years of age or older in the United States because the risk from wild virus is low. However, if vaccine is needed, such as for persons traveling to polio-endemic areas, previously unvaccinated adults should receive two doses of IPV at intervals of 4 to 8 weeks and a third dose 6 to 12 months after the second. Adults who have had a primary series of OPV or IPV and who are at increased risk for exposure to poliovirus may receive an additional dose of IPV.

Rabies Vaccine

Rabies vaccine is an inactivated virus vaccine prepared either in human diploid cell culture (HDCV) or in purified chick embryo cell culture (PCEC).[186] Rabies vaccination is recommended in two situations: as a routine in individuals likely to be exposed to rabies (e.g., veterinarians, forest rangers) and after exposure to animals known or suspected to be rabid. The primary pre-exposure immunizing course is three doses

of rabies vaccine given intramuscularly at 0, 7 days, and 21 to 28 days. The three-dose course results in formation of protective levels of antibodies in virtually 100% of vaccinees. HDCV is immunogenic when administered intradermally, but the manufacturer discontinued distribution of the only preparation approved for pre-exposure vaccination by the intradermal route in March 2001. Serologic testing every 2 years is recommended to ensure that high-risk vaccinees maintain protective levels of antibody. Those whose titer falls to less than the recommended level should receive a booster. Alternatively, boosters may be administered every 2 years without serologic testing for those at high risk for exposure. In the postexposure setting, four doses of rabies vaccine are given intramuscularly in a relatively short period (on days 0, 3, 7, and 14) to previously unimmunized persons. Previously fully vaccinated persons who are exposed to rabies should receive intramuscular doses of rabies vaccine on days 0 and 3. In all postexposure settings for previously unimmunized persons, rabies vaccine should always be used in conjunction with rabies immune globulin (see "Rabies Immune Globulin"). Rabies vaccine should be administered by intramuscular injection into the deltoid muscle for adults and children or the anterolateral thigh of infants; there have been reports of possible vaccine failure following gluteal administration.[187,188] Corticosteroids, other immunosuppressive agents, antimalarial drugs, and immunosuppressive illnesses can interfere with the immune response to rabies vaccine. Adverse events associated with current rabies vaccines include local reactions in 30% to 74% of recipients and systemic reactions, including headache, nausea, myalgia, abdominal pain, and dizziness, in 5% to 40% of recipients. As many as 6% of persons may develop an immune complex–like reaction 2 to 21 days after boosters, with generalized urticaria, sometimes accompanied by arthralgia, arthritis, angioedema, nausea, vomiting, fever, and malaise. There have been rare reports of transient neurologic reactions in association with the current vaccine; however, a causal relationship has not been demonstrated. There are no known contraindications to rabies vaccination in persons at risk or exposed[186] (see Chapter 163).

Rotavirus Vaccines

There are two licensed rotavirus vaccines in the United States: RotaTeq (RV5) (Merck Vaccine Division) and Rotarix (RV1) (GlaxoSmithKline Pharmaceuticals).[189] V5 was developed by reassortment of a parent bovine rotavirus strain (WC3) with human strains, which donate either outer capsid proteins (G proteins) or attachment proteins (P proteins) to the WC3 strain. The resultant vaccine contains five separate viruses expressing human G1, G2, G3, G4, and P1A(8). The G proteins in the vaccine cover about 90% of the wild rotavirus strains detected in the United States from 1996 to 2005. Many of the other strains have the P1A(8) attachment protein. After a three-dose series, the efficacy against any G1 to G4 virus–associated gastroenteritis was 74% and against severe gastroenteritis was 98%. RV5 reduced emergency room visits in an 11-country analysis by 94% and hospitalization by 96%. Of interest, the vaccine was effective against G9 wild-type rotaviruses. The incidence of intussusception among almost 35,000 vaccinated infants during the 42 days after any dose was not different from the incidence among 35,000 placebo recipients. There was no difference in incidence of fever between infants receiving vaccine or placebo. However, there were slightly higher rates of vomiting after dose 1 (6.7% vaccinees vs. 5.4% placebo) and diarrhea after dose 1 (10.4% vaccines vs. 9.1% placebo) and dose 2 (8.6% vaccinees vs. 6.4% placebo). RV5 is recommended routinely in three doses, administered usually at 2, 4, and 6 months of age. The minimum age for dose 1 is 6 weeks, and the maximum age is 14 weeks and 6 days. The minimum interval between doses is 4 weeks, and no doses should be administered after the infant reaches 8 months of age. Preliminary data from population surveillance systems suggest that RV5 not only induces individual protection but may also provide community protection through herd immunity.[190]

RV1 is an attenuated vaccine, derived from a wild human rotavirus [G1P1A(8)].[189] In a large Latin American trial, the efficacy against severe rotavirus infection following two doses of vaccine was 85% up to year 1 and 81% up to age 2 years. In a European trial, efficacy was higher, 87% against any rotavirus infection and 96% against severe disease. Concerns have been raised about whether RV1 will provide protection against disease caused by G2 wild rotaviruses. Although the number of cases of G2 disease was limited in both the European and Latin American trials, efficacy tended to be positive, although there were wide confidence intervals. There were no significant differences in rates of intussusception among vaccine or placebo recipients in a trial including 63,000 infants. Other adverse events were generally similar in vaccine and placebo recipients, with the exception of grade 3 (interfered with normal everyday activity) cough or runny nose, which was slightly higher in vaccinees (3.6% vaccinees vs. 3.2% placebo recipients). RV1 is recommended in a two-dose schedule, usually at 2 and 4 months of age. Minimum ages, minimum intervals, and maximum ages are the same as for RV5. There is no preference for one vaccine over another. Use of the same vaccine for all doses is recommended. When this is not feasible or when the type of vaccine used for prior doses is unknown, a total of three doses should be administered.

Rubella Vaccine

Rubella vaccine contains live attenuated rubella virus grown in human diploid cells (RA27/3).[123] Other substrates, such as duck embryo cells or rabbit kidney cells, have also been used for rubella vaccines, but these vaccines are no longer available in the United States. When administered to a person on or after the first birthday, 95% or more of recipients can be expected to become immune. Immunity after a single dose is long lasting and appears likely to be lifelong. Boosters are not necessary, although many persons will receive a second dose as part of the two-dose MMR schedule to prevent measles. Rubella vaccine is recommended for all individuals on or after the first birthday, except those who have documentation of having received live rubella vaccine and those who have laboratory documentation of immunity to rubella. Most persons born before 1957 can be considered immune. It is particularly important to ensure that women of childbearing age are immune to rubella. Rubella vaccine virus is known to be able to cross the placenta and infect fetal tissue. Nonetheless, there have been no instances of congenital rubella syndrome in the offspring of 226 susceptible women who received RA27/3 rubella vaccine within 3 months of conception and who carried their pregnancies to term.[191] This indicates that the risk for congenital rubella syndrome from vaccine virus is so small as to be negligible. The ACIP has stated that rubella vaccination during pregnancy should not ordinarily be a reason to consider termination of pregnancy. Notwithstanding the fact that no observable risk has been associated with rubella vaccine administered during pregnancy, rubella vaccine should not knowingly be administered to a pregnant woman. A reasonable approach is to ask women whether they are pregnant or may become pregnant within the next 3 months, exclude those who answer affirmatively, and vaccinate the others, after explaining the theoretical risk to them.[123]

Known adverse events associated with rubella vaccine include low-grade fever and rash in 5% to 10% of recipients and joint pains with or without objective manifestations of arthritis. The latter occur with increasing frequency in older individuals; about 25% of susceptible adult females may have transient arthralgia after rubella vaccination.[192,193] Acute arthritis is seen in about 10% of susceptible women. The risk for arthritis after rubella vaccine is substantially lower than the risk after natural rubella. The IOM reviewed the adverse consequences of rubella vaccination and concluded that the vaccine was an established cause of acute arthritis and that the evidence was consistent with a causal role of vaccine in rare cases of chronic arthritis.[51] However, more recent studies have found no evidence of increased risk for new onset of chronic arthropathies among women vaccinated with RA27/3 vaccine.[57-59] With regard to other illnesses temporally related to rubella vaccine, the IOM concluded that the evidence was insufficient to implicate rubella vaccine as a cause of thrombocytopenic purpura, radiculoneuritis, and other neuropathies. Thrombocytopenic purpura has been associated with MMR vaccine.[52]

Previous experience with programs involving serologic screening and subsequent vaccination of susceptible individuals has demonstrated a low success rate in delivering vaccinations to identified susceptible persons (typically on the order of 30% to 50%). Because of the importance of ensuring that adult women are immune to rubella and because reactions appear to occur only in susceptible individuals, it is recommended that women be vaccinated without serologic testing unless it can be ensured that they can be successfully contacted and recalled for vaccination if serologic testing indicates they are susceptible. Contraindications to rubella vaccination are pregnancy and an immunocompromised state (see "Measles Vaccine").[123]

Smallpox Vaccine

Effective use of smallpox vaccine eradicated smallpox as a naturally occurring disease in 1977.[194] The vaccine is a live unattenuated preparation of vaccinia virus that induces protection against smallpox virus in 95% or more of recipients. Two licensed preparations are available: Dryvax, an animal lymph vaccine last produced by Wyeth in 1978, and ACAM 2000 (Acambis Inc.), produced in Vero cells.[195]

Routine use of smallpox vaccine among the civilian population in the United States was discontinued in 1971 and by the military in 1990. In May 1983, Wyeth Laboratories, Inc., the only active licensed producer in the United States, discontinued general distribution of smallpox vaccine, making it no longer available for general civilian use. With concerns that smallpox could become an agent for bioterrorism, selected lots of smallpox vaccine were tested and, on October 25, 2002, were licensed; ACAM 2000 was licensed in 2007. Smallpox vaccine was recommended for members of public health and health care response teams[196] and for selected military personnel; it continues to be available as an investigational new drug for individuals working with vaccinia or other orthopoxviruses. Smallpox vaccine is administered intradermally by the multiple puncture technique using a presterilized bifurcated needle. With the bifurcated needle held perpendicular to the skin, punctures are made rapidly, with sufficient pressure that a trace of blood appears after 15 to 20 seconds.

Previously recognized adverse events associated with smallpox vaccine include disseminated vaccinia, eczema vaccinatum, vaccinia necrosum (progressive vaccinia), and encephalitis.[197-199] The risk for transmission of vaccinia virus from the inoculation site can be reduced by keeping the vaccine site covered with gauze and a layer of clothing and by good hand hygiene. For persons involved in patient care, addition of a semipermeable dressing is recommended.[198] In the current pre-event vaccination program, smallpox vaccine is contraindicated for persons with a history or presence of eczema, atopic dermatitis, or other dermatologic conditions; who have conditions associated with immunosuppression; who are pregnant or breastfeeding; or who have a serious allergy to any component of the vaccine. Following reports of ischemic cardiac events in recent vaccinees, persons with known underlying heart disease or three or more known major cardiac risk factors were also excluded from the pre-event vaccination program,[199] although no causal relationship has been established between receipt of the vaccine and ischemic cardiac disease.

Inflammatory cardiac disease (myocarditis, pericarditis, or myopericarditis) was recognized in 2003 among recipients of smallpox vaccine in both military and civilian programs.[200] Although myocarditis had been previously reported in Europe and Australia following administration of other vaccinia strains, it was not previously recognized as an adverse event following the New York City Board of Health (NYCBOH) strain, the strain used for production of smallpox vaccine in the United States. The clinical spectrum of illness ranges from mildly symptomatic to heart failure, and the natural history remains unknown; it is unclear if all patients recover completely, or if some persons with subclinical myocarditis may later develop dilated cardiomyopathy, as is thought to occur with some patients who have other types of myocarditis. Histopathologic data are limited, but in one patient who underwent endomyocardial biopsy, an eosinophilic infiltrate without presence of vaccinia virus was found. Onset is typically 7 to 19 days after vaccination; the frequency appears to be about 1 in 10,000 vaccinees.[200]

Other vaccinia strains, such as modified vaccinia Ankara, which only undergoes limited replication in humans, are under active study as vaccine strains that might be associated with a lower incidence of adverse events or might be safe to use in populations in which current smallpox vaccines are contraindicated (e.g., immunocompromised persons).[194]

Tetanus Toxoid

Tetanus toxoid, a purified preparation of inactivated tetanus toxin, is one of the most effective immunizing agents known. The preferred preparation is adsorbed (alum-precipitated) because it is more immunogenic than the fluid preparation. Tetanus toxoid is recommended for use in all residents of the United States for whom contraindications do not exist.[79] It should always be used in combination either with diphtheria toxoid alone or with diphtheria toxoid and pertussis vaccine to ensure protection against both diseases. A primary course of two doses administered 4 to 8 weeks apart, with a third dose given 6 to 12 months later, induces protective antibodies in more than 95% of recipients and is recommended for all unvaccinated older children (see Table 320-4) and adults. Following primary immunization, booster doses with adult formulation tetanus and diphtheria toxoids (Td) are recommended every 10 years. A one-time dose of Tdap may be substituted for one of the recommended Td boosters. When tetanus toxoid is given to children younger than 7 years of age as DTaP, five doses are given beginning at 2 months of age. For unvaccinated children in the first year of life, for whom pertussis vaccine is contraindicated, pediatric DT should be substituted for DTaP. For unvaccinated children in the second year of life for whom pertussis vaccine is contraindicated, two doses of DT should be administered 4 to 8 weeks apart, with a third dose 6 to 12 months later (see "Pertussis Vaccine"). Common adverse effects include local reactions and fever. In some individuals who have received multiple doses of tetanus toxoid, Arthus-like reactions have been described.[201] Tetanus toxoid has been suggested as a rare cause of brachial plexus neuropathy. The IOM concluded that tetanus toxoid causes brachial neuritis in the 1 month after immunization at a rate of 0.5 to 1 case per 100,000 toxoid recipients.[52] Tetanus toxoid has also been implicated as a cause of GBS. The most convincing evidence comes from a case report of one individual who acquired GBS three times with successive administrations of toxoid.[202] However, population-based studies in both children and adults have revealed an incidence of GBS within expected limits and do not support a causal role. If tetanus toxoid causes GBS, it does so very rarely.[203] The only contraindication is in individuals who previously had neurologic or severe hypersensitivity reactions after tetanus toxoid. Table 320-4 summarizes the ACIP recommended approach to use of tetanus toxoid and tetanus immune globulin for postexposure prophylaxis of tetanus.

TABLE 320-4	Summary Guide to Tetanus Prophylaxis in Routine Wound Management: United States*			
History of Adsorbed Tetanus Toxoid (Doses)	Clean, Minor Wounds		All Other Wounds†	
	Td‡	TIG	Td‡	TIG
Unknown or less than three	Yes	No	Yes	Yes
Three§	No‖	No	No¶	No

*Important details are in the text.
†Such as, but not limited to, wounds contaminated with dirt, feces, soil, saliva, and so on; puncture wounds; avulsions; and wounds resulting from missiles, crushing, burns, and frostbite.
‡For children younger than 7 years, DTaP or DTP (DT if pertussis vaccine is contraindicated) is preferred to tetanus toxoid alone. For persons 7 years and older, Td is preferred to tetanus toxoid alone.
§If only three doses of fluid toxoid have been received, a fourth dose of toxoid, preferably an absorbed toxoid, should be given.
‖Yes, if more than 10 years since last dose.
¶Yes, if more than 5 years since last dose. (More frequent boosters are not needed and can accentuate side effects.)

Typhoid Vaccine

Two preparations of typhoid vaccine are available in the United States: an oral live attenuated strain of *Salmonella typhi* (Ty21a) and a Vi capsular polysaccharide vaccine (ViCPS). The two vaccines provide between 50% and 80% protection after a primary series.[204] Typhoid vaccines are indicated for travelers who will have prolonged exposure to contaminated food and drinks in developing countries, those with prolonged exposure to typhoid carriers, and laboratory workers who work with *S. typhi*.

The oral vaccine comes as an enteric-coated capsule that should be taken on alternate days with cool liquid about 1 hour before a meal. The four recommended doses should be refrigerated until needed. Data are not available to make recommendations about the need for boosters with the oral vaccine, although the manufacturer recommends a new complete series every 5 years. The ViCPS is recommended as a single 0.5-mL dose. Boosters are recommended every 2 years. The Ty21a vaccine is not recommended for children younger than 6 years. The ViCPS is recommended for persons 2 years of age or older. The Ty21a and the ViCPS vaccines cause fever and headache in fewer than 6% of recipients. Other adverse reactions to the oral preparation are rare and consist of abdominal discomfort, nausea, and vomiting. Local reactions to the ViCPS have been reported in 7% of recipients. The oral vaccine should not be given to persons who are immunocompromised, including those with HIV infection. Ty21a should not be given to a person taking the antimalarial mefloquine or antibiotics, especially sulfonamides, unless at least 24 hours has elapsed since the last dose.

Varicella Vaccine

Two forms of varicella vaccine are available in the United States: a stand-alone product (VARIVAX; Merck & Co.) and a combined vaccine with MMR (MMRV, Pro Quad; Merck & Co.).[48] Both use the Oka strain. The titer in MMRV (minimum of 3.99 $\log_{10}$ PFU per dose is higher than the stand-alone vaccine, which is about 3.13 $\log_{10}$ PFU per dose). Live attenuated varicella vaccine (Oka strain) was licensed in the United States in 1995. The vaccine has generally been found to be highly effective against severe varicella (95% to 100%) and less effective against mild disease (70% to 90% in most studies).[205-210] Most vaccinees who acquire varicella tend to have mild illness with fewer than 50 lesions compared with 250 to 500 lesions in unvaccinated persons with disease. Immunity appears to be long lasting. However, breakthrough disease in the 10 years following a single dose was 7.3% in one study.[211] Most of the breakthroughs occurred in the first 5 years. In contrast, only 2.2% of children who received two doses had varicella. Given the benefits of two doses in reducing vaccine failure, a two-dose schedule is now recommended.[48] The vaccine is recommended routinely for all children at 12 through 15 months of age with a second dose usually at 4 through 6 years of age as varicella vaccine or MMRV. Vaccine also can be given to any susceptible older child or adult. Persons 13 years of age and older should receive two doses 4 to 8 weeks apart. Vaccination is recommended for susceptible persons aged 13 years or older who (1) live or work in settings where varicella transmission is likely or can occur, such as schools, child care centers, institutional settings, colleges, prisons, and the military; (2) are nonpregnant women of childbearing age; (3) live in households with children; or (4) are international travelers. Because adults are at higher risk for complications from varicella than are children, vaccination of all susceptible adolescents and adults is desirable. Persons with a reliable history of varicella can be considered immune. Although a negative or uncertain history of varicella in young children is predictive of susceptibility, most young adults with such histories are immune. In some settings, serologic screening of persons with negative or unknown prior histories of varicella is cost-effective.[212] However, recalling and vaccinating identified susceptible persons may be difficult, making vaccination using history as the determinant of need more attractive. Vaccination has also been demonstrated to be effective for outbreak control.[213,214]

The most common adverse events are local reactions and rash. In children, about 3% acquire a varicella-like rash at the injection site with a median of two lesions, and 4% acquire a generalized rash with a median of five lesions. For adults, 3% and 1% acquire localized rashes after doses 1 and 2, respectively, whereas 6% and 1% acquire more generalized rashes.[48] Transmission of vaccine virus has been reported rarely and only from persons with rash. There is no evidence that vaccination increases the risk for zoster. In fact, zoster incidence after vaccination appears lower than would be expected after natural infection. Vaccine is contraindicated in persons with anaphylactic hypersensitivity to vaccine components, including neomycin and gelatin, and in most persons with deficiencies of cell-mediated immunity.[48] Available data on the safety and efficacy of varicella vaccine in HIV-infected children who were not severely immunocompromised suggests that varicella vaccine is immunogenic and that the vaccine safety profile is acceptable.[215] HIV-infected children who are asymptomatic and not immunosuppressed should receive two doses of varicella vaccine with the first dose at 12 through 15 months of age or older and with a 3-month interval between doses.[48,216] Previously, children with acute lymphoblastic leukemia in remission could qualify for vaccine under an investigational new drug protocol, but the protocol has been terminated. Pregnant women should not be vaccinated, and women should be warned not to become pregnant for 1 month after vaccination.[48]

Varicella vaccine is more thermolabile than other vaccines. It must be stored frozen at an average temperature of −15°C or less.

Yellow Fever Vaccine

Yellow fever vaccine is a live attenuated virus preparation that is highly effective in inducing protection in recipients.[217] It is indicated for use in travelers going to yellow fever–endemic areas and may be required for entry into some countries. Only a single dose of vaccine is required; it is administered by subcutaneous inoculation. Boosters are recommended every 10 years, although their need has not been conclusively established. Local and mild systemic reactions occur in 2% to 5% of recipients 5 to 10 days after vaccination; more severe reactions, primarily encephalitis and encephalopathy, are rare. Children younger than 4 months of age appear to be at highest risk for severe neurotropic reactions, and vaccine is contraindicated in this age group. Other contraindications include anaphylactic hypersensitivity to eggs and immunocompromised states. If possible, vaccination of infants should be delayed until 9 months of age. Pregnancy is not considered an absolute contraindication; however, it is recommended that administration of the vaccine be postponed until after completion of pregnancy, if possible. A severe adverse event, vaccine-associated viscerotropic disease, has been identified in persons receiving their first dose of vaccine, particularly older adults. This event is characterized by multiorgan failure. Clinical manifestations have included fever, hypotension, respiratory failure, liver disease, renal failure, thrombocytopenia, and other manifestations. The estimated incidence in the United States is 1 in 400,000 doses distributed.[217]

Zoster Vaccine

Zoster vaccine is designed to boost immunity to varicella-zoster virus in persons previously infected with the virus to either prevent shingles by inhibiting the reactivation of virus from dorsal nerve ganglia or to lower the health burden of shingles, should it occur.[218] The vaccine is a lyophilized preparation of the Oka-Merck strain and differs from varicella vaccine in potency. The minimum potency of zoster vaccine ($4.29 \log_{10}$ PFU per dose) is about 14-fold greater than varicella vaccine and is similar in potency to the varicella component of MMRV ($3.993 \log_{10}$ PFU per dose).[48,213] In a trial of vaccine in adults 60 years or older and a history of prior varicella, a single dose of vaccine was 51% effective in decreasing the incidence of zoster, 61% effective in reducing the overall burden of illness from shingles, and 67% effective in reducing the incidence of postherpetic neuralgia (PHN) in the vaccinated cohort. Of persons who actually developed zoster, PHN was reduced by 39% in vaccinees compared with placebo recipients who had shingles. Effectiveness in preventing zoster tended to decrease with increasing age with the highest efficacy among 60- to 69-year-olds. For persons 80 years and older, the efficacy rate was positive, but the

95% CI overlapped zero, indicating that efficacy was not statistically significant.

Injection site reactions are more common in vaccinees than placebo recipients (48.3% vs. 16.6%). Most resolved within 4 days. Varicella-like rashes at the injection site were reported in 0.1% of vaccinees compared with 0.04% of placebo recipients. The rate of serious adverse events was 1.9% in vaccine recipients compared with 1.3% in placebo recipients, a difference that was significant. However, no particular clinical pattern was noted to implicate vaccine in causing specific adverse events. Zoster vaccine is indicated for the routine vaccination of persons 60 years and older without contraindications. Persons with a prior history of zoster can be vaccinated. The vaccine is contraindicated in persons with allergy to vaccine components and primary or acquired immune deficiency.

IMMUNOGLOBULIN PREPARATIONS

Passive immunization can be provided by preformed antibodies in several types of products used to treat people with primary and less frequently secondary immune deficiency and to either prevent or less frequently to treat certain infectious diseases. The choice is made in part by the types of products available, the type of antibody desired, route of administration, and condition or diseases being treated. Products used include (1) immune globulin administered by the intramuscular route; (2) specific or hyperimmune immune globulin preparations administered by the intramuscular (IM) route; (3) IGIV; (4) specific (hyperimmune) immune globulin administered by the IV route; (5) antibodies of animal origin; (6) monoclonal antibodies; and (7) immune globulin subcutaneous (human), which has been approved for treatment of patients with primary immune deficiency states (see Table 320-3). Indications for administration of immune globulin preparations other than those relevant to infectious diseases are not included in this chapter.

Intramuscular Immune Globulin

Intramuscular immune globulin is prepared from pooled human adult plasma by an alcohol-fractionation procedure (see Chapter 6). Immune globulin consists primarily of IgG and trace amounts of IgA and IgM, is sterile, and is not known to transmit any infectious agents, including hepatotropic viruses and HIV. Immune globulin is a concentrated protein solution containing specific antibodies reflective of the infectious disease exposure and immunization experience of people from whom the plasma was obtained to prepare the immune globulin. More than 1000 and up to 60,000 donors per lot are used to include immune globulin from people with a broad spectrum of antibodies. Individual donors are screened for markers of a variety of viruses to minimize potential transmission of infection. Immune globulin is licensed and recommended for administration deep into a large muscle mass such as the gluteal region or into the anterior thigh of a child. Intravenous use of human immune globulin is contraindicated.

Indications for Use of Intramuscular Immune Globulin. The three indications for use of immune globulin are replacement therapy for antibody deficiency disorders and for prophylaxis against hepatitis A and measles viruses.[34,91,123,219]

Replacement Therapy for Antibody Deficiency Disorders. For most patients, intramuscular immune globulin has been replaced by IGIV or subcutaneously administered immune globulin because use of IGIV results in higher total plasma immune globulin concentrations, and higher titers of specific antibodies can be achieved with minimal discomfort.

Hepatitis A Prophylaxis. In persons aged 12 months through 40 years, hepatitis A immunization is preferred over immune globulin for postexposure prophylaxis (PEP) against hepatitis A virus infections and for protection of persons traveling to areas where hepatitis A is endemic.[219] For persons younger than 12 months of age or older than 40 years of age, immunocompromised persons of all ages, and patients with chronic liver disease, immune globulin is preferred over hepatitis A immunization. Immune globulin is effective in preventing hepatitis A when administered within 14 days of exposure (a dose of 0.02 mL/kg) or when given before exposure in somewhat larger quantities (dose of 0.02 mL/kg for trips of 1 to 2 months, 0.06 mL/kg every 5 months for longer trips).

Measles Prophylaxis. Immunization against measles is the optimal method for achieving protection against measles. Immune globulin administered to exposed, measles-susceptible people will prevent or modify measles if administered within 6 days of exposure (a dose of 0.25 mL/kg for immunocompetent people, 0.5 mL/kg for immunocompromised hosts, up to a maximum of 15 mL).[34,123]

Specific Intramuscular Immune Globulin Preparations. The term *hyperimmune globulin* is used to refer to a group of products known as specific immune globulins. These products differ from other preparations in selection of donors who have been immunized or given booster immunizations, and often in the number of donors from whom plasma is included in the product pool. Donors known to have high titers of the desired antibody are selected. Specific immune globulin preparations are prepared by the same procedure as used for other immune globulin preparations. Products in this category include HBIG, RIG, TIG, and investigational VZIG.

Hepatitis B Immune Globulin. HBIG is prepared from plasma preselected for high titer of antibody to HBsAg. In the United States, HBIG has an anti-HBsAg titer of more than 1:100,000 by radioimmunoassay.[96,99] HBIG is recommended for use in postexposure settings for susceptible individuals who have been exposed to known hepatitis B virus–infected sexual partners or to blood containing HBsAg by the percutaneous or mucous membrane route. The dose is 0.06 mL/kg given immediately for both sexual contacts and people exposed percutaneously. The hepatitis B vaccine series should be started simultaneously in those who previously have not been vaccinated. Alternatively, a second dose of HBIG may be given 1 month later for persons for whom hepatitis B vaccine is not indicated. All pregnant women should be tested for circulating HBsAg. HBIG is recommended for infants born to HBsAg-positive women. A dose of 0.5 mL should be given as soon as possible after birth but within 12 hours of delivery in conjunction with a dose of hepatitis B vaccine. Additional doses of vaccine are indicated at 1 month and 6 months of age. The only known adverse effect is local discomfort at the site of injection. There are no known precautions or contraindications.[96,97]

Rabies Immune Globulin. RIG is a hyperimmune globulin prepared from humans who have been immunized against rabies and have very high titers of antibodies to rabies.[186] RIG is designed for management of people who have been exposed to rabid animals. RIG always should be used in conjunction with rabies vaccine in previously unvaccinated people. However, if more than 8 days has elapsed since the first dose of rabies vaccine, RIG is unnecessary because an active antibody response to the vaccine presumably has begun. Experience indicates that administration of a full course of HDCV or PCEC vaccine with RIG is 100% effective in preventing development of rabies after exposure to known rabid animals. As much as possible of the 20-IU/kg dose should be infiltrated into and around the wound. Any remaining RIG should be administered intramuscularly at a different site from vaccine. Adverse effects include minor local discomfort. There are no known contraindications.[186]

Tetanus Immune Globulin. TIG is a hyperimmune globulin indicated for management of tetanus-prone wounds in people who have no prior history of tetanus immunization.[79,80,163] The standard dose is 250 units intramuscularly, although some experts recommend doses as high as 500 units. Local reactions are rare, and there are no known contraindications. If used, TIG should be administered simultaneously with, but at a different site from, combined tetanus-diphtheria toxoids. Primary immunization against tetanus and diphtheria should then be completed using the routine schedule. Table 320-4 summarizes the ACIP-recommended approach to postexposure prophylaxis of tetanus.[79] TIG in large doses (3000 to 6000 units) also is recommended

with wound cleaning and débridement, antibiotics, and supportive care in the treatment of tetanus.

Varicella-Zoster Immune Globulin. VZIG is a purified human immune globulin preparation made from plasma containing high titers of varicella-zoster antibodies.[48] The VZIG product in use in the United States is VariZIG, available under Investigational New Drug protocol, and can be requested by calling the 24-hour telephone number of FFF Enterprises (800-843-7477). The decision to administer VariZIG depends on these factors: (1) the likelihood that the exposed person has no evidence of immunity to varicella, (2) the probability that a given exposure to varicella or zoster will result in infection; and (3) the likelihood that complications of varicella will develop if the person is infected. VariZIG administration includes newborns whose mothers acquire varicella within 5 days before to 48 hours after delivery. VariZIG should be administered within 96 hours of exposure, but ideally as soon after exposure as possible. VariZIG is given intramuscularly at the recommended dose of 125 units per 10 kg of body weight up to 625 units (i.e., five vials). The product may not prevent infection; however, if infection occurs, it is usually subclinical or mild. Any person to whom VariZIG is administered to prevent varicella subsequently should receive age-appropriate varicella vaccine, provided the vaccine is not contraindicated. Varicella vaccine should be delayed until 5 months after VariZIG administration to ensure optimal response. Varicella vaccine is not needed if the patient develops varicella after VariZIG administration. Local reactions are rare, and there are no known contraindications.[48] Episodes of inadvertent administration of varicella vaccine to pregnant women in whom VZIG was indicated continue to occur despite recognition of the problem of product confusion and should be reported (http://www.merckpregnancyregistries.com). Providers and others involved in administering this product should take steps to ensure that product confusion does not occur.

Immune Globulin Intravenous

IGIV is made from pool plasma of adults using methods designed to prepare a product for intravenous use. The number of donors ranges from 15,000 to 60,000. IGIV consists of greater than 95% immune globulin and trace amounts of IgA and IgM. The FDA specifics that all IGIV preparations must have a minimum concentration of antibodies to measles virus, *Corynebacterium diphtheriae*, poliovirus, and hepatitis B virus. Antibody concentrations against other pathogens vary widely among products. Not all IGIV products have been approved or studied for all FDA-approved indications.

Indications for Use of Immune Globulin Intravenous

IGIV initially was formulated for IV use in patients with primary immunodeficiencies; enabling them to receive enough immune globulin at regular intervals for protection against certain infections. Administration of IGIV results in an immediate rise in both total IgG and titers of specific antibodies. IGIV is approved by the FDA for six conditions: (1) primary immunodeficiency status, (2) Kawasaki disease, (3) immune-mediated thrombocytopenia, (4) pediatric HIV infection, (5) secondary immunodeficiency in chronic lymphocytic leukemia, and (6) prevention of graft-versus-host disease and infection in hematopoietic cell transplantation in adults. IGIV products also are used for many other conditions, although demonstrated efficacy from controlled trials is not available in all cases.

Specific Immune Globulins for Intravenous Use

There are three specific plasma-derived immune globulin products for intravenous administration for prophylaxis or therapy of infectious diseases: cytomegalovirus (CMV) IGIV, botulism IGIV (for infant botulism), and vaccinia immune globulin. An intramuscular humanized mouse monoclonal antibody preparation used to prevent respiratory syncytial virus (RSV) is available (see later).

CMV IGIV has been developed and is indicated for prophylaxis of disease in seronegative organ transplant recipients. Use of CMV IGIV for prophylaxis of CMV disease varies among transplantation centers. Risk factors for development of CMV among transplant recipients include type of organ, immunosuppressive therapy, and the donor-recipient CMV status. CMV-negative transplant recipients who receive an organ from a CMV-positive donor are at the highest risk for CMV disease and generally receive some form of CMV prophylaxis.

Botulism IGIV for human use (Baby-BIG) is a human-derived anti-toxin licensed by the FDA for treatment of infant botulism caused by *Clostridium botulinum* type A or type B. Baby-BIG is made and distributed by the California Department of Public Health (24-hour telephone number; 510-231-7600; http://www.infantbotulism.org). Baby-BIG has been shown to decrease significantly the number of days on mechanical ventilation, days of intensive care unit stays, and overall hospital stay.[220] An equine-derived antitoxin is available for use in adults with botulism but is *not* used in infants.

Vaccinia Immune Globulin

Vaccinia immune globulin (VIG), an intramuscular preparation, is a hyperimmune globulin prepared for treatment of certain complications of vaccinia vaccination. VIG is indicated for treatment of severe cases of inadvertent inoculation, eczema vaccinatum, severe generalized vaccinia, and progressive vaccinia. VIG use should be considered in patients with severe ocular complications other than isolated keratitis. VIG is not recommended for treatment of postvaccinial encephalitis or encephalomyelitis; myopericarditis following smallpox vaccination; mild cases of generalized vaccinia; erythema multiforme; or isolated vaccinia keratitis. A preparation of VIG suitable for IV use (VIG-IGIV) has been approved by the FDA. All preparations of VIG are currently available only under Investigational New Drug protocols through the CDC (http://www.bt.cdc.gov/agent/smallpox) and the U.S. Department of Defense.[197]

Respiratory Syncytial Virus Immune Globulin and Palivizumab

One product is licensed in the United States for administration to infants and children at high risk for severe disease due to RSV; groups at high risk include infants and children younger than 24 months with chronic lung disease or a history of premature birth (≤35 weeks' gestation). RSV-IGIV, a hyperimmune globulin formulated for IV administration, is no longer produced in the United States.[221] Palivizumab is a humanized monoclonal antibody against the F protein of RSV and is produced by recombinant DNA technology. The recommended dosage is 15 mg/kg administered intramuscularly monthly throughout the RSV season. Palivizumab has been demonstrated to be effective in reducing the risk for RSV hospitalization.[222] No significant adverse events have been associated with palivizumab, and there is no interference with the immune response to live virus vaccines. The American Academy of Pediatrics has recommended that because of the high cost of these interventions, their use be limited to those infants and children at highest risk for severe RSV disease. The American Academy of Pediatrics recommendations for use in premature infants are based on gestational age and chronologic age at the start of the RSV season.[223-225]

Adverse Reactions to Immune Globulin Preparations

The most common adverse effects of intramuscularly administered immune globulin include local pain at the injection site and, less commonly, flushing, headache, chills, and nausea. Serious systemic events are rare. Anaphylactic reactions have been reported after repeated administration to IgA-deficient people.[226] Other than prior anaphylactic reactions, there are no known contraindications to use of the product. Immune globulin inhibits response to certain live virus vaccines (e.g., measles and rubella vaccines) for between 3 and 9 months, depending on the dose administered.[227]

Adverse events after intravenous administration of immune globulin are common and include minor systemic reactions, pyrogenic reactions (high fever and systemic symptoms), vasomotor or cardiovascular manifestations (change in blood pressure and heart rate), and infrequent but serious reactions (aseptic meningitis, acute renal failure, hypersensitivity reactions, and anaphylaxis). Severe reactions to IGIV

occur infrequently, but mild adverse events have been associated with up to 20% of infusions. The Adverse Reactions sections of package inserts of specific products provide details.

Simultaneous administration of immune globulin with hepatitis A vaccine may result in a decrease of the ultimate titer of hepatitis A antibody achieved but does not influence seroconversion and presumed protection.[91]

Hepatitis C has been transmitted by IGIV in both Europe and the United States and by an intravenous Rh immune globulin preparation in Ireland.[228-230] Hepatitis C virus RNA has been detected by polymerase chain reaction in various immune globulin preparations,[231] but the significance of this finding is unclear; disease has not been associated with products other than those noted previously. In response to these findings, manufacturing procedures have been modified to add new viral inactivation steps.[232]

IMMUNE GLOBULIN SUBCUTANEOUS

Subcutaneous administration of immune globulin using battery-driven pumps has been shown to be safe and effective in adults and children with primary immunodeficiencies. Smaller doses, administered more frequently (i.e., weekly), result in more even serum IgG concentrations over time. Systemic reactions are less frequent than with intravenous therapy, and some parents or patients can be taught to infuse at home. The most common adverse effects of subcutaneous administration of immune globulin are injection-site reactions, including local swelling, redness, itching, soreness, induration, and local heat. There is only one product licensed in the United States for subcutaneous use. There are no data on administration of IgG by the subcutaneous route for conditions requiring high-dose immune globulin therapy.

Rh Immune Globulin

Rh immune globulin is a hyperimmune globulin prepared for use in Rh-negative women who have just delivered Rh-positive infants or have had a miscarriage or abortion of an Rh-positive fetus. When administered within 24 hours of the time of delivery or abortion, it is highly effective in preventing sensitization of the mother to Rh-positive red blood cells that might be present in a future pregnancy. Appropriate administration of Rh immune globulin has reduced the occurrence of Rh hemolytic disease of the newborn in the United States to very low levels. Further reductions will require more careful attention to the administration of the product after abortion or delivery in all women for whom it is indicated. There are essentially no adverse effects associated with the product, and there are no known contraindications.[233]

Use of Vaccines

ROUTINE

Children

The recommended schedule for administration of vaccines to infants, children, and adolescents are shown in Figures 320-1 and 320-2.[62] Catch-up schedules for children 4 months through 6 years of age and 7 years through 18 years of age and adolescents are shown in Table 320-5. All children and adolescents are recommended to receive all vaccines listed in the table unless medical contraindications exist.[62] Five doses of DTaP and four doses of polio-containing vaccines are recommended. The fifth dose of DTaP and the fourth dose of polio vaccine are recommended at 4 through 6 years of age.[62] Tdap boosters should be administered at 11 through 12 years of age, and Td boosters every 10 years thereafter.[80,163] A single dose of combined measles, mumps, and rubella vaccine at 12 through 15 months of age or older provides long-lasting, probably lifelong, immunity in more than 95% of recipients. The second dose of MMR at 4 through 6 years of age should provide immunity to most children not protected by the first dose.[34,123] There is no contraindication to giving DTaP, MMR, Hib,

Recommended Immunization Schedule for Persons Aged 7 through 18 Years, United States, 2009

Vaccine ▼ Age ▶	7–10 Years	11–12 Years	13–18 Years
Tetanus, Diphtheria, Pertussis[1]	see footnote 1	Tdap	Tdap
Human Papillomavirus[2]	see footnote 2	HPV (3 doses)	HPV Series
Meningococcal[3]	MCV	MCV	MCV
Influenza[4]	Influenza (Yearly)		
Pneumococcal[5]	PPSV		
Hepatitis A[6]	HepA Series		
Hepatitis B[7]	HepB Series		
Inactivated Poliovirus[8]	IPV Series		
Measles, Mumps, Rubella[9]	MMR Series		
Varicella[10]	Varicella Series		

☐ Range of recommended ages for vaccination ☐ Catch-up immunization ☐ Certain high-risk groups

This schedule indicates the recommended ages for routine administration of currently licensed childhood vaccines, as of December 1, 2008, for children aged 7 through 18 years. Any dose not administered at the recommended age should be administered at a subsequent visit, when indicated and feasible. Licensed combination vaccines may be used whenever any component of the combination is indicated and other components are not contraindicated and if approved by the Food and Drug Administration for that dose of the series. Providers should consult the relevant Advisory Committee on Immunization Practices statement for detailed recommendations, including high-risk conditions: http://www.cdc.gov/vaccines/pubs/acip-list.htm. Clinically significant adverse events that follow immunization should be reported to the Vaccine Adverse Event Reporting System (VAERS). Guidance about how to obtain and complete a VAERS form is available at http://vaers.hhs.gov or by telephone 800-822-7967.

1. **Tetanus and diphtheria toxoids and acellular pertussis vaccine (Tdap).** *(Minimum age: 10 years for BOOSTRIX® and 11 Years for ADACEL®)*
   - Administer at age 11 or 12 years for those who have completed the recommended childhood DTP/DTaP vaccination series and have not received a tetanus and diphtheria toxoid (Td) booster dose.
   - Persons aged 13 through 18 years who have not received Tdap should receive a dose.
   - A 5-year interval from the last Td dose is encouraged when Tdap is used as a booster dose; however, a shorter interval may be used if pertussis immunity is needed.
2. **Human papillomavirus vaccine (HPV).** *(Minimum age: 9 years)*
   - Administer the first dose to females at age 11 or 12 years
   - Administer the second dose 2 months after the first dose and the third dose 6 months after the first dose (at least 24 weeks after the first dose).
   - Administer the series to females at age 13 through 18 years if not previously vaccinated.
3. **Meningococcal conjugate** *vaccine (MCV).*
   - Administer at age 11 or 12 years, or at age 13 through 18 years if not previously vaccinated.
   - Administer to previously unvaccinated college freshmen living in a dormitory.
   - MCV is recommended for children aged 2 through 10 years with terminal complement component deficiency, anatomic or functional asplenia, and certain other groups at high-risk. See *MMWR* 2005; 54(No. RR-7).
   - Persons who received MPSV 5 or more years previously and remain at increased risk for meningococcal disease should be revaccinated with MCV.
4. **Influenza vaccine.**
   - Administer annually to children aged 6 months through 18 years.
   - For healthy nonpregnant persons (i.e., those who do not have underlying medical conditions that predispose them to influenza complications) aged 2 through 49 years, either LAIV or TIV may be used.
   - Administer 2 doses (separated by at least 4 weeks) to children aged younger than 9 years who are receiving influenza vaccine for the first time or who were vaccinated for the first time during the previous influenza season but only received 1 dose.

5. **Pneumococcal polysaccharide vaccine (PPSV).**
   - Administer to children with certain underlying medical conditions (see *MMWR* 1997; 46[No. RR-8]), including a cochlear implant. A single revaccination should be administered to children with functional or anatomic asplenia or other immunocompromising condition after 5 years.
6. **Hepatitis A vaccine (HepA).**
   - Administer 2 doses at least 6 months apart.
   - HepA is recommended for children older than 1 year who live in areas where vaccination programs target older children or who are at increased risk of infection. See *MMWR* 2006; 55(No. RR-7).
7. **Hepatitis B vaccine (HepB).**
   - Administer the 3-dose series to those not previously vaccinated.
   - A 2-dose series (separated by at least 4 months) of adult formulation Recombivax HB® is licensed for children aged 11 through 15 years.
8. **Inactivated poliovirus vaccine (IPV).**
   - For children who received an all-IPV or all-oral poliovirus (OPV) series, a fourth dose is not necessary if the third dose was administered at age 4 years or older.
   - If both OPV and IPB were administered as part of a series, a total of 4 doses should be administered, regardless of the child's current age.
9. **Measles, mumps, and rubella vaccine (MMR).**
   - If not previously vaccinated, administer 2 doses or the second dose for those who have received only 1 dose, with at least 28 days between doses.
10. **Varicella vaccine.**
   - For persons aged 7 through 18 years without evidence of immunity (see *MMWR* 2007; 56[No.RR-4]), administer 2 doses if not previously vaccinated or the second dose if they have received only 1 dose.
   - For persons aged 7 through 12 years, the minimum interval between doses is 3 months. However, if the second dose was administered at least 28 days after the first dose, it can be accepted as valid.
   - For persons aged 13 years and older, the minimum interval between doses is 28 days.

Figure 320-2 **Recommended immunization schedule for persons aged 7 through 18 years, United States, 2009.** *(From Centers for Disease Control and Prevention: http://www.cdc.gov/vaccines/.)*

TABLE 320-5	Catch-Up Immunization Schedule for Persons Aged 4 Months Through 6 Years Who Start Late or Who Are More than 1 Month Behind—United States, 2009				

		Minimum Interval Between Doses			
Vaccine	Minimum Age for Dose 1	Dose 1 to Dose 2	Dose 2 to Dose 3	Dose 3 to Dose 4	Dose 4 to Dose 5
Catch-Up Schedule for Persons Aged 4 Months through 6 Years					
Hepatitis B[1]	Birth	4 wk	8 wk (and at least 16 wk after first dose)		
Rotavirus[2]	6 wk	4 wk	4 wk[2]		
Diphtheria, tetanus, pertussis[3]	6 wk	4 wk	4 wk	6 mo	6 mo[3]
Haemophilus influenzae type b[4]	6 wk	4 wk, if first dose administered at younger than age 12 mo 8 wk (as final dose), if first dose administered at age 12-14 mo No further doses needed if first dose administered at age 15 mo or older	4 wk,[4] if current age is younger than 12 mo 8 wk (as final dose),[4] if current age is 12 mo or older and second dose administered at younger than age 15 mo No further doses needed, if previous dose administered at age 15 mo or older	8 wk (as final dose); this dose only necessary for children aged 12 mo through 59 mo who received 3 doses before age 12 mo	
Pneumococcal[5]	6 wk	4 wk, if first dose administered at younger than age 12 mo 8 wk (as final dose for healthy children), if first dose administered at age 12 or older or current age 24-59 mo No further doses needed, for healthy children if first dose administered at age 24 mo or older	4 wk, if current age is younger than 12 mo 8 wk (as final dose for healthy children), if current age is 12 mo or older No further doses needed for healthy children if previous dose administered at age 24 mo or older	8 wk (as final dose); this dose only necessary for children aged 12-59 mo who received 3 doses before age 12 mo or for high-risk children who received 3 doses at any age	
Inactivated poliovirus[6]	6 wk	4 wk	4 wk	4 wk[6]	

1. Hepatitis B vaccine (HepB).
   - Administer the 3-dose series to those not previously vaccinated.
   - A 2-dose series (separated by at least 4 months) of adult formulation of Recombivax HB® is licensed for children aged 11 through 15 years.
2. Rotavirus vaccine (RV)
   - The maximum age for the first dose is 14 weeks, 6 days. Vaccination should not be initiated for infants aged 15 weeks or older (i.e., 15 weeks, 0 days or older).
   - Administer the final dose in the series by age 8 months, 0 days.
   - If Rotarix® was administered for the first and second doses, a third dose is not indicated.
3. Diphtheria and tetanus toxoids and acellular pertussis vaccine (DTaP).
   - The fifth dose is not necessary if the fourth dose was administered at age 4 years or older.
4. Haemophilus influenzae type b conjugate vaccine (Hib)
   - Hib vaccine is not generally recommended for persons aged 5 years or older. No efficacy data are available on which to base a recommendation concerning use of Hib vaccine for older children and adults. However, studies suggest good immunogenicity in persons who have sickle cell disease, leukemia, or HIV infection, or those who have had a splenectomy; administering 1 dose of Hib vaccine to these persons is not contraindicated.
   - If the first 2 doses were PRP-OMP (PedvaxHIB® or Comvax®), and administered at age 11 months or younger, the third (and final) dose should be administered at age 12 through 15 months and at least 8 weeks after the second dose.
   - If the first dose was administered at age 7 through 11 months, administer 2 doses separated by 4 weeks and a final dose at age 12 through 15 months.
5. Pneumococcal vaccine
   - Administer 1 dose of pneumococcal conjugate vaccine (PCV) to all healthy children aged 24 through 59 months who have not received at least 1 dose of PCV on or after age 12 months.
   - For children aged 24 through 59 months with underlying medical conditions, administer 1 dose of PCV if 3 doses were received previously.
   - Administer pneumococcal polysaccharide vaccine (PPSV) to children aged 2 years or older with certain underlying medical conditions (see MMWR Morb Mortal Wkly Rep. 2000;49(RR-9), including a cochlear implant, at least 8 weeks after the last dose of PCV.
6. Inactivated poliovirus vaccine (IPV)
   - For children who received an all-IPV, or all-oral poliovirus (OPV) series, a fourth dose is not necessary if the third dose was administered at age 4 years or older.
   - If both OPV and IPV were administered as part of a series, a total of 4 doses should be administered, regardless of the child's current age.

hepatitis B, polio, pneumococcal conjugate, rotavirus, hepatitis A, influenza, and varicella vaccines at the same time as any of the other vaccines. Although all potential simultaneous administration schemes have not been evaluated, experience to date suggests that simultaneous administration of most vaccines does not increase reaction rates nor interfere with the immune responses.[1,2,234,235] Stress for infants, as measured by serum cortisol, does not increase when a second injection is given simultaneously with the first.[235a,235b] Hib should be given in two doses (PRP-OMP) or three doses (HbOC, PRP-T) in the first year of life followed by a reinforcing dose at 12 through 15 months of age.[62] Hepatitis B vaccine should be initiated at birth, and the three-dose series should be completed by 18 months of age; hepatitis B vaccine can be given simultaneously with all other childhood vaccines.[96] Combination vaccines containing hepatitis B are not licensed for use before 6 weeks of age. Pneumococcal conjugate vaccine should be administered in a four-dose series with the first three doses administered at 2, 4, and 6 months of age, and the fourth dose at 12 through 15 months. Children should receive varicella vaccine routinely at 12

through 18 months of age.[48] Annual influenza vaccine is recommended for children 5 through 18 years.[111] Children younger than 8 years of age receiving influenza vaccine for the first time should have two doses separated by at least 4 weeks. Children 6 through 35 months of age should receive half doses (0.25 mL). There are two rotavirus vaccine preparations. Bovine rotavirus vaccine should be given as a three-dose series at 2, 4, and 6 months of age, and human attenuated rotavirus vaccine should be administered in a two-dose series at 2 and 4 months of age. For both vaccines, the first dose should be given at 6 through 14 weeks (maximum, 14 weeks, 6 days) of age. Vaccination should not be initiated for infants 15 weeks, 0 days or older. The final dose in the series should be given by 8 months, 0 days of age. All children should receive two doses of varicella vaccine, the first at 12 through 18 months of age and the second at 4 through 6 years of age. Hepatitis A vaccine should be given as a two-dose series, with the first dose given at 12 through 23 months of age and the second at least 6 months later. The minimum age for the first dose is 6 months of age.

| TABLE 320-5 | Catch-Up Immunization Schedule for Persons Aged 7 Through 18 Years Who Start Late or Who Are More than 1 Month Behind— United States, 2009—cont'd |

Vaccine	Minimum Age for Dose 1	Minimum Interval Between Doses			
		Dose 1 to Dose 2	Dose 2 to Dose 3	Dose 3 to Dose 4	Dose 4 to Dose 5
Measles, mumps, rubella[7]	12 mo	4 wk			
Varicella[8]	12 mo	3 mo			
Hepatitis A[9]	12 mo	6 mo			
Catch-Up Schedule for Persons Aged 7 through 18 Years					
Tetanus, diphtheria/ tetanus, diphtheria, pertussis[10]	7 yr[10]	4 wk	4 wk, if current age is younger than 12 mo 6 mo, if current age is 12 mo or older	6 mo, if first dose administered at younger than age 12 mo	
Human papillomavirus[11]	9 yr	Routine dosing intervals are recommended[11]			
Hepatitis A[9]	12 mo	6 mo			
Hepatitis B[1]	Birth	4 wk	8 wk (and at least 16 wk after first dose)		
Inactivated poliovirus[6]	6 wk	4 wk	4 wk	4 wk[6]	
Measles, mumps, rubella[7]	12 mo	4 wk			
Varicella[8]	12 mo	3 mo, if the person is younger than age 13 yr 4 wk, if the person is aged 13 yr or older			

7. Measles, mumps, and rubella vaccine (MMR)
   - Administer the second dose at age 4 through 6 years. However, the second dose may be administered before age 4 years, provided at least 28 days have elapsed since the first dose.
   - If not previously vaccinated, administer 2 doses with at least 28 days between doses.
8. Varicella vaccine
   - Administer the second dose at age 4 through 6 years. However, the second dose may be administered before age 4, provided at least 3 months have elapsed since the first dose.
   - For persons 12 months through 12 years, the minimum interval between doses is 3 months. However, if the second dose was administered at least 28 days after the first dose, it can be accepted as valid.
   - For persons aged 13 years and older, the minimum interval between doses is 28 days.
9. Hepatitis A vaccine (HepA)
   - HepA is recommended for children older than 1 year who live in areas where vaccination programs target older children or who are at increased risk of infection. See *MMWR* 2006;55(RR-7).
10. Tetanus and diphtheria toxoids vaccine (Td) and tetanus and diphtheria toxoids and acellular pertussis vaccine (Tdap)
    - Doses of DTaP are counted as part of the Td/Tdap series.
    - Tdap should be substituted for a single dose of Td in the catch-up series or as a booster for children aged 10 through 18 years; use Td for other doses.
11. Human papillomavirus vaccine (HPV)
    - Administer the series to females at age 13 through 18 years if not previously vaccinated.
    - Use recommended routine dosing intervals for series catch-up (i.e., the second and third doses should be administered at 2 and 6 months after the first dose). However, the minimum interval between the first and second doses is 4 weeks. The minimum interval between the second and third doses is 12 weeks, and the third dose should be given at least 24 weeks after the first dose.

From Centers for Disease Control and Prevention: http://www.cdc.gov/vaccines.

Adolescents

An adolescent preventive medicine visit has been established at 11 through 12 years of age.[62] This is the appropriate time to administer the following vaccines: (1) a booster dose of Tdap for adolescents who completed the recommended childhood DTP/DTaP vaccination series and have not received a Td booster dose, (2) HPV vaccine to females 11 though 18 years of age if not previously immunized (the vaccine is licensed for females 9 through 26 years of age), (3) MCV4 at 11 through 18 years of age, if not previously immunized, (4) influenza vaccine annually through 18 years of age, (5) a second dose of MMR if not previously received, (6) a dose of varicella vaccine if the patient is susceptible, (7) the three-dose hepatitis B vaccination series should be administered if not previously received, and (8) polio immunization history should be reviewed. Other immunizations, including pneumococcal, and hepatitis A should be given, if indicated.

Adults

Routine immunizations for adults have received increasing attention in recent years with recognition of the large burden of vaccine-preventable diseases in this age group. Two adult immunization schedules have been published each year since 2002. One focuses on vaccines needed by five age groups and the second on vaccines needed for adults based on eight medical and other indications (Figs. 320-3 and 320-4). All adults should be immune to diphtheria and tetanus and if not previously immunized should be given a primary immunizing course (three doses of Td administered at time zero, 4 to 8 weeks, and 6 to 12 months) with boosters administered every 10 years thereafter.[80,236] A one-time dose of Tdap for adults 19 through 64 years of age should

replace one of the Td booster doses. HPV vaccine is recommended for all females 11 through 26 years of age who have not completed the immunization series. A complete series consists of three doses. The second dose should be given 2 months after the first dose, and the third dose should be given 6 months after the first dose. A quadrivalent HPV vaccine is licensed by the FDA, and a bivalent vaccine is under consideration. FDA is considering HPV vaccination for females 27 through 46 years of age and adolescent males. All adults without evidence of immunity to varicella should receive two doses of single-antigen varicella vaccine if not previously vaccinated or the second dose if they have received only one dose, unless they have a medical contraindication. Special consideration should be given to those who (1) have close contact with people at high risk for severe disease (e.g., health care personnel and family contacts of persons with immunocompromising conditions), or (2) are at high risk for exposure or transmission (e.g., teachers, child care employees, residents and staff members of institutional settings and including correctional institutions, college students, military personnel, adolescents and adults living in households with children, nonpregnant women of childbearing age, and international travelers). Evidence of immunity to varicella in adults includes any of the following[48]: (1) documentation of two doses of varicella vaccine at least 4 weeks apart; (2) born in the United States before 1980 (although for health care personnel and pregnant women, birth before 1980 should not be considered evidence of immunity); (3) history of varicella based on diagnosis or verification of varicella by a health care provider (for a patient reporting a history of or presenting with an atypical case, a mild case, or both, health care providers should seek either an epidemiologic link with a typical varicella case or to a labo-

Recommended Adult Immunization Schedule, by Vaccine and Age Group, 2009

Vaccine ▼ Age Group ▶	19–26 years	27–49 years	50–59 years	60–64 years	≥ 65 years
Tetanus, diphtheria, pertussis (Td/Tdap)[1,*]	Substitute 1-time dose of Tdap for Td booster; then boost with Td every 10 yrs				Td booster every 10 years
Human papillomavirus (HPV)[2]	3 doses (females)				
Varicella[3]	2 doses				
Zoster[4]				1 dose	
Measles, mumps, rubella (MMR)[5,*]	1 or 2 doses		1 dose		
Influenza[6,*]			1 dose annually		
Pneumococcal (polysaccharide)[7,8]	1 or 2 doses				1 dose
Hepatitis A[9,*]	2 doses				
Hepatitis B[10,*]	3 doses				
Meningococcal[11,*]	1 or more doses				

* Covered by the Vaccine Injury Compensation Program.

For all persons in this category who meet the age requirements and who lack evidence of immunity (e.g., lack documentation of vaccination or have no evidence of prior infection)

Recommended if some other risk factor is present (e.g., on the basis of medical, occupational, lifestyle, or other indications)

No recommendation

Figure 320-3 Recommended adult immunization schedule, by vaccine and age group. *(From Centers for Disease Control and Prevention: http://www.cdc.gov/vaccines/.)*

ratory-confirmed case or evidence of laboratory confirmation, if it was performed at the time of acute disease); (4) history of herpes zoster based on health care provider diagnosis or verification of herpes zoster by a health care provider; or (5) laboratory evidence of immunity or laboratory confirmation of disease. A single dose of zoster vaccine is

recommended for adults 60 years of age and older regardless of whether they report a prior episode of herpes zoster.[218] People with chronic medical conditions may be vaccinated unless their condition constitutes a contraindication. All adults should be immune to measles, mumps, and rubella. For practical purposes, people born before 1957

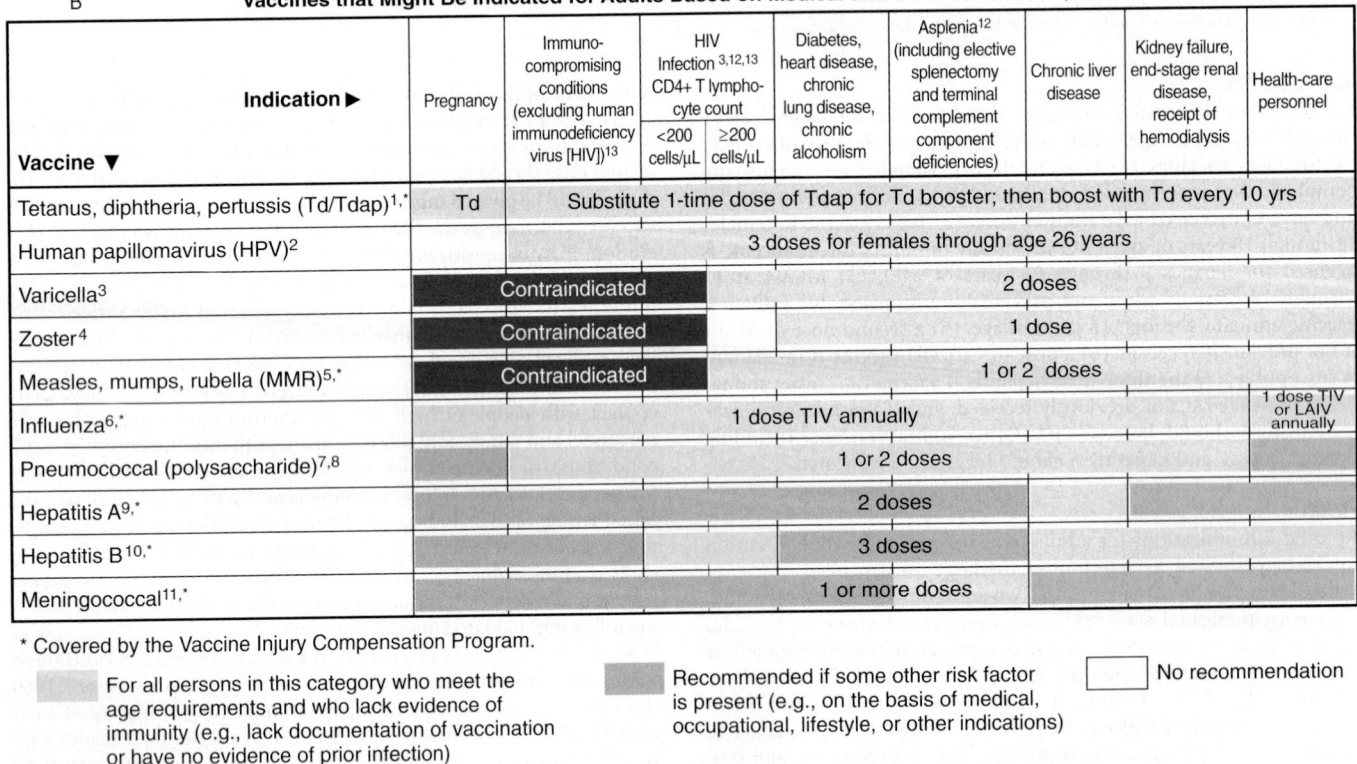

B

Vaccines that Might Be Indicated for Adults Based on Medical and Other Indications, 2009

Indication ▶ Vaccine ▼	Pregnancy	Immuno-compromising conditions (excluding human immunodeficiency virus [HIV])[13]	HIV Infection [3,12,13] CD4+ T lymphocyte count <200 cells/μL	HIV Infection [3,12,13] CD4+ T lymphocyte count ≥200 cells/μL	Diabetes, heart disease, chronic lung disease, chronic alcoholism	Asplenia[12] (including elective splenectomy and terminal complement component deficiencies)	Chronic liver disease	Kidney failure, end-stage renal disease, receipt of hemodialysis	Health-care personnel
Tetanus, diphtheria, pertussis (Td/Tdap)[1,*]	Td	Substitute 1-time dose of Tdap for Td booster; then boost with Td every 10 yrs							
Human papillomavirus (HPV)[2]		3 doses for females through age 26 years							
Varicella[3]	Contraindicated			2 doses					
Zoster[4]	Contraindicated			1 dose					
Measles, mumps, rubella (MMR)[5,*]	Contraindicated			1 or 2 doses					
Influenza[6,*]	1 dose TIV annually								1 dose TIV or LAIV annually
Pneumococcal (polysaccharide)[7,8]	1 or 2 doses								
Hepatitis A[9,*]	2 doses								
Hepatitis B[10,*]	3 doses								
Meningococcal[11,*]	1 or more doses								

* Covered by the Vaccine Injury Compensation Program.

For all persons in this category who meet the age requirements and who lack evidence of immunity (e.g., lack documentation of vaccination or have no evidence of prior infection)

Recommended if some other risk factor is present (e.g., on the basis of medical, occupational, lifestyle, or other indications)

No recommendation

Figure 320-4 Vaccines that might be indicated for adults based on medical and other indications. *(From Centers for Disease Control and Prevention: http://www.cdc.gov/vaccines/.)*

generally can be considered immune to these three diseases. All other adults should receive one or more doses of MMR unless they have a medical contraindication, documentation of one or more doses after the first birthday, have had physician-diagnosed measles or laboratory evidence of immunity. One dose of MMR vaccine is recommended for women whose rubella vaccination history is unreliable or who lack laboratory evidence of immunity. For women of childbearing age, regardless of birth year, rubella immunity should be determined, and women should be counseled regarding congenital rubella syndrome. Women who do not have evidence of immunity should receive MMR upon completion or termination of pregnancy and before discharge from the health care facility. Adults born before 1957 generally are considered immune to mumps. Adults born during or after 1957 should receive one dose of MMR unless they have a medical contraindication, history of mumps based on health care provider diagnosis, or laboratory evidence of immunity. Influenza vaccine is recommended for routine annual administration to adults 50 years of age and older and to adults at any age who have specified medical indications, for health care professionals, caregivers of children younger than 5 years of age, residents of nursing homes and other long-term care and assisted living facilities, people likely to transmit influenza to people at high risk, and anyone who wants to decrease their risk for getting influenza. Healthy, nonpregnant adults younger than 50 years without high-risk medical conditions who are not contacts of severely immunocompromised people in special care units can receive either intranasally administered live attenuated influenza vaccine (FluMist; MedImmune, Gaithersburg, Md) or inactivated vaccine. Other people should receive the inactivated vaccine.[111] Pneumococcal polysaccharide vaccine is recommended for administration to elderly patients and those with specific medical or other indications.[172] Hepatitis B vaccine is recommended for people with specific medical, occupational, and behavioral indications as a three-dose series at 0, 1, and 6 months. If the combined hepatitis A and hepatitis B vaccine (Twinrix) is used, three doses are administered at 0, 1, and 6 months; alternatively, a four-dose schedule, administered on days 0, 7, and 21 to 30 followed by a booster dose at month 12 may be used.[91,96,97] For adult patients receiving hemodialysis or with other immunocompromising conditions, 1 dose of 40 µg/mL (Recombivax HB) administered on a three-dose schedule or two doses of 20 µg/mL (Engerix-B) administered simultaneously on a four-dose schedule at 0, 1, 2, and 6 months can be used.[237] Hepatitis A vaccine is given to adults with behavioral, occupational, and other indications. Single-antigen vaccine formulations should be administered in a two-dose schedule at either 0 and 6 to 12 months (HAVRIX) or 0 and 6 to 18 months (VAQTA).[91] If the combined hepatitis A and hepatitis B vaccine (Twinrix) is used, administer three doses at 0, 1, and 6 months; alternatively, a four-dose schedule, administered on days 0, 7, and 21 to 30, followed by a booster dose at month 12, may be used. Meningococcal vaccine is given to adults with medical and other indications.[132] Meningococcal conjugate (MCV4) vaccine is preferred for adults with any of the preceding indications who are 55 years of age or younger, although meningococcal polysaccharide vaccine (MPSV4) is an acceptable alternative. Revaccination with MCV4 after 5 years might be indicated for adults previously vaccinated with MPSV4.

SPECIAL CIRCUMSTANCES

Travel

People travel internationally for business, tourism, and education and to visit relatives and friends (see Chapter 329). The two major categories of immunizations to consider for international travelers are status of the routinely recommended immunizations and the need for specific immunizations. Specific travel immunizations should be based on evidence of benefit and risks and on expert opinion when few or no data are available. Immunizations for international travel may be grouped into two categories: *required* (those that may be required to cross international borders) and *recommended* (those recommended according to risk for infection in the area of travel.) Country-specific

immunization is available for all countries (http://www.cdc.gov/travel and http://www.who.int/ith/en). The International Health Regulations allow countries to impose requirements for yellow fever vaccine as a condition for admission. Consequently, travelers should be aware of whether this vaccine is required for entry into the country of their destination. Other vaccines commonly considered for travelers include measles vaccine, polio vaccine, and boosters for tetanus and diphtheria. In addition, travelers to specified areas may wish to consider plague, typhoid, rabies, Japanese encephalitis, yellow fever, hepatitis A, hepatitis B, and meningococcal vaccines. Information on vaccines recommended for travel is summarized regularly in *Health Information for International Travel* (http://www.cdc.gov/travel/contentYellow-Book.aspx). Information on specific regions and diseases is available from the CDC Fax Information Service at 888-232-3299.

Occupational Exposure

A complete set of recommendations for vaccination for most occupational groups has not been developed. Specific recommendations are available for health care professionals.[126,127,236] Federal regulations require that health care and public safety workers who anticipate exposure to human blood or blood-derived body fluids are offered hepatitis B vaccination free of charge.[94,237] Transmission of rubella in medical facilities can occur to or from health care professionals. Consequently, it is important that all health care professionals who might transmit rubella to pregnant patients be immune to rubella. Documentation of a single dose of a rubella-containing vaccine on or after the first birthday or serologic evidence of immunity is acceptable. Health care professionals are at greater risk from measles than the general public. All health care professionals should be immune, defined as documentation of receipt of two doses of live measles vaccine on or after the first birthday, at least 1 month apart, health care professional–diagnosed measles, or serologic evidence of immunity. Although most people born before 1957 have been considered to be immune to measles, about 4% of cases in health care professionals in the past were in people born before this date. Therefore, a second dose of measles is recommended for adults who work in a health care setting. Mumps transmission in health settings has been reported, and mumps immunity can be ensured at the same time as measles and rubella by use of MMR.[123,145] A second dose of MMR is recommended for adults who work in a health care setting. Because health care professionals caring for patients with chronic diseases may transmit influenza to their patients, all health care professionals should be vaccinated against influenza annually.[111] Health care professionals also should be immune to varicella.[48] Those without evidence of immunity to varicella should receive two doses of single-antigen vaccine if not vaccinated previously, or the second dose if they have received only one dose, unless medically contraindicated.

Pregnancy

Because of lack of efficacy and safety studies of vaccines in pregnant women, recommendations for vaccine use in pregnancy are based on disease burden and severity for mothers and infants, studies from other countries, and expert opinion. The only vaccines recommended in the United States for pregnant women are adult-type tetanus and reduced diphtheria (Td) and inactivated trivalent influenza vaccines. Transfer of maternal antibodies to tetanus toxin is an important means of preventing neonatal tetanus. If a pregnant woman has not received a Td vaccination within the past 10 years, Td should be administered during the second or third trimester.[79] If the woman received the last Td vaccination less than 10 years previously, Tdap should be administered during the immediate postpartum period.[165] The postpartum Tdap should be administered before discharge from the hospital or birthing center or, if not possible, as soon as feasible thereafter. A dose of Tdap is not only recommended for those postpartum women but also for close contacts of infants less than 12 months of age, and all health care personnel with direct patient contact if they have not previously received Tdap. An interval for Tdap administration as short as 2 years from the last Td is suggested; shorter intervals can be used. Td can be deferred during pregnancy and Tdap substituted in the immediate postpartum period, or Tdap can be administered instead of Td to a pregnant woman after an informed discussion with the woman.

Inactivated TIV should be administered to all women who will be pregnant during the influenza season, regardless of trimester. Influenza immunization of women during pregnancy not only protects the pregnant woman but also appears to protect infants younger than 6 months of age.[111,238] Infants younger than 6 months cannot be immunized or receive antiviral prophylaxis because no products are licensed for this age group. LAIV is not licensed for use in pregnant women and should not be administered. However, pregnant women do not need to avoid contact with people immunized with LAIV. In general, live virus vaccines are contraindicated in pregnancy, with the exception of yellow fever virus vaccine, which may be administered if the risk for exposure to the disease during international travel is great. If indicated, some inactivated vaccines, such as hepatitis B, MCV4 (preferred, but MPS4 is acceptable), hepatitis A, and PPSV23, can be administered to pregnant women with medical or exposure conditions that put them at risk for certain vaccine-preventable infectious diseases. ACIP recommendations for pregnant women can be found at http://www.cdc.gov/vaccines/recs/schedules/adult-schedule.htm.

Immunocompromised States

Immunocompromised people (from primary or secondary immune deficiency conditions) particularly are susceptible to many infections, may be more susceptible to adverse effects from live virus vaccines,[51,52] and may respond poorly to inactivated vaccines. Consequently, in general, live virus vaccines are not administered to immunocompromised people, although inactivated vaccines are safe and are indicated.[1] Varicella vaccine is contraindicated in people with most deficiencies of cell-mediated immunity but can be safely given to people with deficiencies of humoral immunity. Recommendations for vaccination of people with specific immunocompromising conditions have been summarized (e.g., recipients of transplants of hematopoietic stem cells[239] or solid organs.)[240-242] and are provided on the recommended adult immunization schedule. The efficacy of inactivated vaccines in immunocompromised people may be less than that in healthy patients, although inactivated vaccines are safe and indicated for many patients.[243-245] In addition, household contacts of patients with immunocompromised conditions should be immunized appropriately, including annual influenza vaccine, to reduce risk for exposure of immunocompromised people.

Human Immunodeficiency Virus

Live attenuated vaccines generally are contraindicated in immunocompromised people, including people with symptomatic HIV infection. Limited studies in HIV-infected people generally have failed to show an increased risk for adverse events from live or inactivated vaccines. Exceptions include BCG given to patients with AIDS and measles-containing vaccine in patients with severe immunodeficiency.[245-247] Known susceptible HIV-infected adults who are asymptomatic should receive live attenuated MMR and varicella vaccines if CD4 and T-lymphocyte counts are above 15% and are greater than 200 cells/μL. Because of reports of severe measles disease, including death, in symptomatic HIV-infected children and adults, MMR vaccine should be considered with caution for symptomatic HIV-infected people.[123,248] MMR and varicella vaccines are contraindicated in people with severe immunodeficiency. Recommendations from the CDC, National Institutes of Health (NIH), and Infectious Diseases Society of America (IDSA) for administration of vaccines for adults are listed in Figure 320-5.[248a] Although transient increases of HIV in the blood of patients have been documented in the month after receipt of both pneumococcal and influenza vaccines, their clinical significance is unknown. Adults with HIV infection who meet the age requirements and lack evidence of immunity (lack documentation of immunization or have no evidence of prior infection) should be immunized with Td/Tdap, influenza (annually), PPSV23, MMR, varicella, and HepB. Women younger than 27 years of age should receive HPV. If specific risk factors are present, hepatitis A and MCV4 (MPSV4 if 55 years of age or older) should be considered. Although a protective immune

---

Immunization Schedule for Adults Infected with Human Immunodeficiency Virus (HIV)*

Vaccine ▼ Age Group ▶	19–49 years	50–64 years	≥ 65 years
Influenza[†]	1 dose annually		
Pneumococcal (polysaccharide)	1 dose		
Hepatitis B[†]	3 doses (0, 1–2, 4–6 mos)		
Tetanus, diphtheria, pertussis (Td/Tdap)[†]	Substitute 1-time dose of Tdap booster; then boost with Td every 10 yrs		1 dose Td booster every 10 yrs
Human papillomavirus (HPV)[†]			
Measles, mumps, rubella (MMR)[†]	Do not administer to severely immunosuppressed persons		
Varicella[†]	Do not administer to severely immunosuppressed persons		
Hepatitis A[†]	2 doses		
Meningococcal[†]	1 or more doses		

For all persons in this category who meet the age requirements and who lack evidence of immunity (e.g., lack documentation of vaccination or have no evidence of prior infection)

Recommended if some other risk factor is present (e.g., on the basis of medical, occupational, lifestyle, or other indications)

* Modified from the Advisory Committee on Immunization Practices (ACIP) Adult Immunization Schedule. For detailed information on immunization against influenza, pneumococcal disease, hepatitis B, human papillomavirus, varicella, and hepatitis A, see disease-specific sections in the text and Table 1 in reference 248a. For information on immunization against tetanus, diphtheria, pertussis, measles, mumps, rubella, and meningococcal disease, refer to recommendations of the ACIP (www.cdc.gov/vaccines/pubs/ACIP-list.htm).

† Covered by the Vaccine Injury Compensation Program.

Figure 320-5 Immunization schedule for adults infected with HIV. (Adapted from Kaplan JE, Benson C, Holmes KK, et al. Guidelines for prevention and treatment of opportunistic infections in HIV-infected adults and adolescents. MMWR Morb Mort Wkly Rep. 2009;58(RR04):1-98.)

response to vaccines and toxoids cannot be ensured in these patients, some protection may be provided. Publications from CDC, NIH, and IDSA entitled *Prevention and Treatment of Opportunistic Infections in Adults with HIV* are available (http://aidsinfo.nih.gov/Guidelines/GuidelineDetail.aspx?GuidelineID=14).

Postexposure Immunization

For certain diseases, administration of an immune globulin product soon after exposure can prevent or attenuate expression of disease.[249] Passive prophylaxis using various immune globulin preparations has been discussed previously. People who have received a complete course of immunization against tetanus are in general well protected against development of tetanus, particularly if a booster dose has been administered within 10 years. More problematic is the situation with individuals who cannot recall their immune status or who have not been immunized. Table 320-4 shows the ACIP recommended approach to postexposure prophylaxis of tetanus. In addition to passive prophylaxis, there is evidence that administration of measles vaccine within 6 days after exposure may prevent manifestations of the illness.[250] If the exposure did not result in infection, the vaccination should provide protection against future exposure. Varicella vaccine prevents varicella in exposed persons if administered within 3 to 5 days of exposure.[48,251,252]

OTHER CONSIDERATIONS

Storage and Handling of Vaccines

Inattention to vaccine handling and storage conditions can contribute to vaccine failure.[1,253] Live virus vaccines, including MMR, MMRV, varicella, yellow fever, live attenuated influenza, rotavirus, and OPV vaccines, are sensitive to increased temperature (heat sensitive). Inactivated vaccines may tolerate limited exposure to elevated temperatures but are damaged rapidly by freezing (cold sensitive). Exposure of inactivated vaccines to freezing temperature ($0.0°$ C [$32°$ F] or colder is the most common storage error.) Examples of cold-sensitive vaccines include diphtheria and tetanus toxoids and acellular pertussis (DTaP) and tetanus toxoid, reduced diphtheria toxoid, and acellular pertussis (Tdap) vaccines; IPV vaccine; Hib vaccine; pneumococcal polysaccharide and conjugate vaccines; hepatitis A and hepatitis B vaccines; inactivated influenza vaccine; and meningococcal polysaccharide and conjugate vaccines. Some vaccines must be protected from light. Physical appearance is not an appropriate basis for determining whether a vaccine has lost its potency because of inappropriate storage or handling. All personnel responsible for handling vaccines in an office or clinic setting should be familiar with standard procedures designed to minimize risk for vaccine failure. Recommendations for handling and storage of selected biologics are summarized in several areas, including the package insert for each product; in a publication entitled *Vaccine Management* available from the CDC (Centers for Disease Control and Prevention. *Vaccine Management: Recommendations for Handling and Storage of Selected Biologicals*. Atlanta, GA: US Department of Health and Human Services. Public Health Service. 2007; http://www.cdc.gov/vaccines/recs/storage/default.htm). This information is also available in a web-based toolkit (http://www2a.cdc.gov/vaccines/ed/shtoolkit/). The most current information about recommended vaccine storage conditions and handling instructions can be obtained directly from manufacturers, and their telephone numbers are listed in product labels (package inserts) and in the *Physician's Desk Reference*, which is published yearly.

Assessing the Need for Immunization

Immunization traditionally has been viewed as the task of the pediatrician and general practitioner caring for children, but with licensure of new vaccines (Tdap, MCV4, HPV, zoster) and expansion of vaccine recommendations (MMR, MMRV), physicians who care for adolescents and adults need to become aware of current recommendations. Health care providers should assess the immunization status of their patients at first contact and, depending on immunization status and

age, at selected contacts thereafter. In general, people should be viewed as susceptible unless they can prove immunity through documentation of having received vaccine, laboratory evidence of immunity, or for some diseases, documentation of physician-diagnosed disease.

A high proportion of elderly adults in the United States have never been immunized against tetanus or diphtheria. This is reflected in the fact that 36% of all cases of tetanus in the United States in the period 1998 to 2000 have occurred in people older than the age of 60 years.[254] Internists and other physicians caring for adults, especially elderly patients, should be particularly attuned to the need for administering tetanus and diphtheria toxoids to these individuals. Similarly, studies repeatedly demonstrate that less than 70% of people 65 years of age or older receive influenza immunization in a given year or have ever received pneumococcal vaccine.[255] It is vital that internists and family practitioners remind themselves and their patients of the need for annual influenza immunization of people with medical indications, people 50 years of age and older, household contacts or care providers of children 0 through 59 months of age, contacts of immunocompromised people, health care providers, and anyone who wants to be protected from influenza.

Substantial progress has been made in implementing hepatitis B vaccination programs for children and adolescents. Progress also has been made in immunizing adults with risk factors for HBV infection.

Immunization Records

In 2002, the National Vaccine Advisory Committee (NVAC) revised immunization standards that included the recommendations that immunization of patients be documented through use of immunization records that are accurate, complete, and easily accessible. The standards also recommend use of tracking systems to provide reminder-recall notices when immunizations are due or overdue. In children, Immunization Information Systems (IIS) address record-keeping needs and tracking functions and have additional capabilities (http://www.cdc.gov/vaccines/programs/iis/default.htm). Every individual should have an immunization record that is up to date and that contains information about each dose of vaccine received, including the date.[1] Patients should be asked to bring this record with them to all health care visits, and the record should be reviewed to ensure that it is current. Official immunization record cards should be used; they are available through local or state health departments. The National Childhood Vaccine Injury Act requires that all providers of vaccines covered by the program (i.e., listed on the vaccine injury table) record on the patient's permanent medical record the date, manufacturer, and lot number of each dose of vaccine administered and the name of the person giving the vaccine.[256] It is prudent to record the same information for other vaccines as well.

Every physician should ensure that the immunization record of each patient is maintained in a permanent, confidential manner that can be reviewed and updated easily whether the record is in hard copy or electronic health record format. The format of all records should facilitate identification and recall of patients in need of immunization.

Parent and Patient Education

All patients (or their parents or guardians) should be informed of the benefits and risks associated with vaccination.[253] The discussion should be conducted in language that is comprehensible to the recipient (or parent or guardian), and ample opportunity for questions and discussion should be given. Vaccine Information Statements (VIS) have been developed for all vaccines routinely recommended for children and adults and are available in several languages. The National Childhood Vaccine Injury Act requires physicians administering vaccines covered by the Vaccine Injury Compensation Program, whether purchased with private or public funds, to provide the relevant VIS at the time of each immunization. In addition, the Public Health Service has developed forms that explain the benefits as well as the risks of vaccination with other vaccines. Interested health care providers can receive

PART IV Special Problems

copies of these forms through local health departments or from the Internet (http://www.cdc.gov/vaccines/pubs/vis/default.htm).

Simultaneous Administration and Intervals between Immunizations

Vaccines can be given safely and effectively at the same time.[1] In general, inactivated vaccines can be administered simultaneously at separate sites, and field observations indicate that simultaneous administration of the most widely used live virus vaccines has not resulted in impaired antibody responses or increased rates of adverse reactions.[234] When vaccines are administered simultaneously, they should be given in separate limbs. When this is not feasible, they should be separated by at least 1 to 2 inches. However, simultaneous administration of immune globulin and MMR vaccines should be avoided because this may result in interference with antibody responses. With those vaccines, immune globulin should not be given for at least 2 weeks after vaccination. People receiving high doses of immune globulin or other blood products may have impaired responses to vaccines for as long as 11 months, depending on the dose received.[1,227] People who received standard doses of immune globulin for hepatitis A prophylaxis should wait to receive live vaccines until 3 months after immune globulin, whereas children treated for Kawasaki disease with IGIV in a dose of 2 g/kg should be vaccinated until 11 months after the dose. Similar recommendations apply to varicella vaccine. Immune globulin does not appear to interfere with the response to yellow fever or rotavirus vaccines.[257] In general, the antigenic mass of inactivated vaccines is so great that immune globulin will not interfere with the antibody response.

With live vaccines, there is the theoretical possibility of interference in the development of antibody responses when live vaccines are administered at intervals of 3 to 14 days. If more than one live vaccine is needed, the vaccines should be administered simultaneously or at intervals of about 1 month between different vaccines.[1] In general, there are no restrictions on intervals between doses of different inactivated vaccines or between different inactivated and live vaccines. The only exceptions are cholera and yellow fever vaccines, which should ideally be administered at least 3 weeks apart to achieve maximal immune responses to both vaccines.

Combination Vaccines

The routine immunization schedule has become increasingly complex over the years as more vaccines have been added. Currently, all male children should be protected against 15 diseases and all female children against 16 diseases. This can require as many as 22 injections of various vaccines by 18 months of age and an additional 9 injections excluding influenza vaccines by 18 years, a major challenge for any health care delivery system. This does not include influenza vaccine, which requires two injections for children younger than 9 years when they are first vaccinated and then one injection annually through age 18 years. Combination vaccines can provide equivalent protection with substantially fewer doses.[235,258-264] Vaccines combining antigens against multiple diseases have been a part of the routine immunization schedule for years.

For children and adolescents, many combination vaccines are available for use (Table 320-6). Combination vaccines may be used instead of their equivalent component vaccines when any component is indicated for the patient's age and other components are not contraindicated as licensed by the FDA. Combination vaccines represent an opportunity to reduce the number of injections. Table 320-6 shows combination vaccines licensed for use in the United States and recommendations for administration. Table 320-6 does not include MMR, DTaP, Tdap, and IPV, for which single antigen products are not available in the United States.

For adults, combination hepatitis A and hepatitis B vaccine (Twinrix) is available as a three- or four-dose regimen. This vaccine can be administered at 0, 1, and 6 months or alternatively at days 7 and 21 to 30 followed by a booster dose at month 12.

Interrupted Schedules

Immunologic memory induced by vaccines is usually long term. Therefore, when doses in a schedule of doses are missed, there is no need to restart the series. Instead, continue from where the schedule left off.

Reporting of Disease and Adverse Events

Public health officials at state health departments and the CDC collaborate in determining which diseases should be nationally notifiable. A disease may be added to the list as new pathogens emerge or may be deleted as the incidence decreases. Reporting of national notifiable diseases to the CDC by states is voluntary. Reporting is mandated by legislation or regulation by individual states. The list of reportable diseases (http://www.cdc.gov/ncphi/disss/nndss/phs/infdis2009.htm) includes many diseases preventable by vaccination. Health care providers should ensure that each suspected case of vaccine-preventable

TABLE 320-6	FDA-Licensed Combination Vaccines*			
			FDA Licensure	
Vaccine†	**Trade Name (Year Licensed)**	**Age Group**	**Recommendations**	
Hib-HepB	Comvax (1996)	6 wk through 71 mo	Three dose schedule given at 2, 4, and 12 through 15 mo of age	
DTaP/Hib	TriHIBit (1996)	15 through 18 mo of age	Fourth dose of Hib and DTaP series	
Hep A-HepB	Twinrix (2001)	≥18 yr	Three doses on a 0, 1, and 6 mo schedule	
DTaP-HepB-IPV	Pediarix (2002)	6 wk through 6 yr	Three dose series at 2, 4 and 6 mo of age	
MMRV	ProQuad (2005)	12 mo through 12 yr	Two doses 28 days apart on or after the first birthday	
DTaP-IPV	KINRIX (2008)	4-6 yr	Booster for fifth dose DTaP and fourth dose IPV	
DTaP-IPV/Hib	Pentacel (2008)	6 wk through 4 yr	Four dose series at 2, 4, 6, and 15-18 mo of age	

*Excludes MMR, DTaP, Tdap, and IPV, for which single antigen products are not available in the United States.
†Dash (-) indicates that products are supplied in their final form by the manufacturer and do not require mixing or reconstitution by user; slash (/) indicates that products are mixed or reconstituted by user.

DTaP, diphtheria and tetanus toxoids and acellular pertussis vaccine; HepA, hepatitis A vaccine; HepB, hepatitis B vaccine; IPV/Hib, Trivalent inactivated polio vaccine and Haemophilus influenzae type b vaccine; MMRV, measles-mumps-rubella and varicella vaccine.

Adapted with permission from American Academy of Pediatrics. Active immunization. In: Pickering LK, Baker CJ, Kimberlin DW, Long SS, eds. *Red Book: 2009 Report of the Committee on Infectious Diseases*, 28th ed. Elk Grove Village, IL: American Academy of Pediatrics, 2009:1-55.

Adapted from CDC. Notice to readers. FDA approval for infants of a *Haemophilus influenzae* type b conjugate and hepatitis B (recombinant) combined vaccine. *MMWR Morb Mortal Wkly Rep.* 1997;46:107-109; CDC. FDA approval of a *Haemophilus* b conjugate vaccine combined by reconstitution with an acellular pertussis vaccine. *MMWR Morb Mortal Wkly Rep.* 1996;45:993-995; CDC. Notice to Readers: FDA Approval for a Combined Hepatitis A and B Vaccine. *MMWR Morb Mortal Wkly Rep.* 2001;50:806-807; CDC. Notice to readers. FDA Licensure of Diphtheria and Tetanus Toxoids and Acellular Pertussis Adsorbed, Hepatitis B (Recombinant), and Poliovirus Vaccine Combined, (PEDIARIX™) for Use in Infants. *MMWR Morb Mortal Wkly Rep.* 2003;52:203-204; CDC. Notice to readers. Licensure of a Combined Live Attenuated Measles, Mumps, Rubella, and Varicella Vaccine. *MMWR Morb Mortal Wkly Rep.* 2005;54:1212-1214; CDC. Licensure of a Diphtheria and Tetanus Toxoids and Acellular Pertussis Adsorbed and Inactivated Poliovirus Vaccine and Guidance for Use as a Booster Dose. *MMWR Morb Mortal Wkly Rep.* 2008;57:1078-1079; and CDC. Licensure of a Diphtheria and Tetanus Toxoids and Acellular Pertussis Adsorbed, Inactivated Poliovirus, and Haemophilus b Conjugate Vaccine and Guidance for Use in Infants and Children. *MMWR Morb Mortal Wkly Rep.* 2008;57:1079-1080.

disease is reported promptly to the local or state health department. Similarly, serious adverse events after immunization should be reported to the Vaccine Adverse Events Reporting System (VAERS). Forms for VAERS can be obtained by calling 800-822-7967 or downloading from the website (http://vaers.hhs.gov). The National Childhood Vaccine Injury Act requires providers to report specified adverse events if they occur within a designated timeframe following immunization.[256,265] However, all serious events temporally related to vaccination should be reported regardless of whether they are thought to be caused by the vaccine. Only through accurate reporting and follow-up of both disease and adverse vaccine effects can the changing balance of the benefits and risks of vaccination be properly assessed.

Compensation for Vaccine Injuries

The National Childhood Vaccine Injury Act of 1986 established a no-fault compensation program for persons injured by vaccines.[256] The covered vaccines, adverse events, and time intervals for which people are eligible for compensation in the absence of other known causes for the events can be found at http://www.hrsa.gov/vaccinecompensation/. All people with alleged injuries from covered vaccines must file first under the compensation program. Those who meet the criteria of the table (and other legal requirements) are entitled to compensation without proving that vaccine caused the injury. People alleging a condition not included in the table or who otherwise do not meet criteria in the table must prove that the vaccine was the cause. People may accept decisions of the program or reject those decisions and go to the tort system. If compensation decisions are accepted, manufacturers and vaccine administrators are protected from litigation.[256,256a] More

TABLE 320-8	Standards for Adult Immunization Practices

Make Vaccinations Available.
1. Adult vaccination services are readily available.
2. Barriers to receiving vaccines are identified and minimized.
3. Patient "out-of-pocket" vaccination costs are minimized.
Assess Patients' Vaccination Status.
4. Health care professionals routinely review the vaccination status of patients.
5. Health care professionals assess for valid contraindications.
Communicate Effectively with Patients.
6. Patients are educated about risks and benefits of vaccination in easy-to-understand language.
Administer and Document Vaccinations Properly.
7. Written vaccination protocols are available at all locations where vaccines are administered.
8. Persons who administer vaccines are properly trained.
9. Health care professionals recommend simultaneous administration of indicated vaccine doses.
10. Vaccination records for patients are accurate and easily accessible.
11. All personnel who have contact with patients are appropriately vaccinated.
Implement Strategies to Improve Vaccination Rates.
12. Systems are developed and used to remind patients and health care professionals when vaccinations are due and to recall patients who are overdue.
13. Standing orders for vaccinations are employed.
14. Regular assessments of vaccination coverage levels are conducted in a provider's practice.
Partner with the Community.
15. Patient-oriented and community-based approaches are used to reach target populations.

From Poland GH, Shefer AM, McCauley M, et al. Standards for Adult Immunization Practices. *Am J Prev Med.* 2003;25:144-150. Reprinted with permission from the American Journal of Preventive Medicine.

TABLE 320-7	Standards for Child and Adolescent Immunization Practices

Availability of Vaccines
1. Vaccination services are readily available.
2. Vaccinations are coordinated with other health care services and provided in a medical home when possible.
3. Barriers to vaccination are identified and minimized.
4. Patient costs are minimized.
Assessment of Vaccination Status
5. Health care professionals review the vaccination and health status of patients at every encounter to determine which vaccines are indicated.
6. Health care professionals assess for and follow only medically accepted contraindications.
Effective Communication about Vaccine Benefits and Risks
7. Parents/guardians and patients are educated about the benefits and risks of vaccination in a culturally appropriate manner and in easy-to-understand language.
Proper Storage and Administration of Vaccines and Documentation of Vaccinations
8. Health care professionals follow appropriate procedures for vaccine storage and handling.
9. Up-to-date, written vaccination protocols are accessible at all locations where vaccines are administered.
10. Persons who administer vaccines and staff members who manage or support vaccine administration are knowledgeable and receive ongoing education.
11. Health care professionals simultaneously administer as many indicated vaccine doses as possible.
12. Vaccination records for patients are accurate, complete, and easily accessible.
13. Health care professionals report adverse events following vaccination promptly and accurately to the Vaccine Adverse Event Reporting System (VAERS) and are aware of a separate program, the National Vaccine Injury Compensation Program (VICP).
14. All personnel who have contact with patients are appropriately vaccinated.
Implementation of Strategies to Improve Vaccination Coverage
15. Systems are used to remind parents, guardians, patients, and health care professionals when vaccinations are due and to recall those who are overdue.
16. Office- or clinic-based patient record reviews and vaccination coverage assessments are performed annually.
17. Health care professionals practice community-based approaches.

From National Vaccine Advisory Committee. Standards for Child and Adolescent Immunization Practices. *Pediatrics.* 2003;112:958-963. Used with permission of the American Academy of Pediatrics.

information on the compensation program can be obtained by calling 800-338-2382 or through the Division of Vaccine Injury Compensation's home page (http://www.hrsa.gov/vaccinecompensation/).

Standards for Immunization Practices

To improve the quality of immunization delivery, standards for child and adolescent immunization practices, as well as standards for adult immunization practices, have been developed by the National Vaccine Advisory Committee (Tables 320-7 and 320-8).[266-268] These standards seek to minimize missed opportunities for immunization, ensure that appropriate contraindications are observed, and ensure that prospective vaccinees or their parents are adequately educated about vaccine risks and benefits. In addition, the standards include other measures to enhance the safe and effective use of vaccines.

Some of the more critical standards include providing vaccines in all health care settings; minimizing prevaccination requirements such as full physician evaluation when those services are not readily obtainable; screening for contraindications including, at a minimum, observation of the child, soliciting illness history from the parents, and verbally asking questions about contraindications; use of simultaneous immunization except when, in the judgment of the provider, nonsimultaneous vaccination will not compromise the immunization status of the patient; providing valid information on vaccine benefits and risks; and regular audits of patient records to determine the vaccination levels of the patients in each provider's practice. Valid contraindications can be viewed at http://www.cdc.gov/vaccines/recs/vac-admin/contraindications.htm.

The IDSA has established 46 guidelines that combine relevant aspects of both the pediatric and adult standards.[253]

Methods to Improve Immunization Coverage

The Task Force on Community Preventive Services has carefully reviewed the literature to determine effective interventions to improve immunization coverage for children, adolescents, and adults.[269] Provider-based interventions have been some of the most successful.[270,271] Two of the most important include assessment of immunization levels in a given practice with provision of information back to the provider and use of reminder-recall systems.[270-272]

Studies have shown that providers (as well as parents) tend to overestimate the level of coverage in their patients (or children), and formal review of records can be useful in making practitioners aware of the need to continue to pay attention.[269-271] Bushnell asked physicians and nurses from both public and private sectors in Massachusetts to estimate immunization coverage of their patient populations. Estimates ranged from 85% to 100%. Record reviews documented a median coverage of 61% (range, 19% to 93%).[272] Giving this information back to providers has been shown to lead to improvements in coverage.[273]

Reminder systems entail providing reminders to patients and parents or providers that an individual is due for an immunization. Recall systems notify individuals that they are past due for an immunization. Both patient and provider reminder-recall systems have been extensively studied and demonstrated effective.[271] The ACIP, American Academy of Pediatrics, and American Academy of Family Physicians have recommended "the regular use of R-R (reminder-recall) systems by public and private health-care providers in settings that have not achieved high documented levels of age-appropriate vaccinations."[274]

Immunization Information Systems (IIS), sometimes called immunization registries, can automate assessment, reminder and recall, and a number of other activities, such as assisting the practitioner in deciding whether a vaccine is needed, consolidating multiple records into a single complete record for a given individual, generating immunization records, and generating immunization coverage information for reports such as those called for in managed care settings by the Health Plan Employer Data Information System.[275] Registries are increasingly being developed and used throughout the United States, and there is a Healthy People 2010 objective to "increase to 95% the number of children enrolled in a fully functional population-based immunization registry (birth through age 5 years)."[270] As of December 31, 2007, 71% of children younger than 6 years in the United States were included in IIS, as were 64% of adolescents 11 to 18 years of age and 20% of adults (>18 years of age). Most public health authorities believe that a nationwide network of community-state population-based registries capable of exchanging information while maintaining privacy and confidentiality is essential to maintain the improvements in vaccine coverage that have been achieved.

Sources of Information

Lists of websites that provide comprehensive information on immunization are available from a number of sources.[253,276]

REFERENCES

1. General Recommendations on Immunization. Recommendations of the Advisory Committee on Immunization Practices (ACIP) and the American Academy of Family Physicians (AAFP). *MMWR Morb Mortal Wkly Rep*. 2010 (in press).
2. Thimerosal in vaccines: a joint statement of the American Academy of Pediatrics and the Public Health Service. *MMWR Morb Mortal Wkly Rep*. 1999;48:563-565.
3. Atkinson WL, Kroger AL, Pickering LS. General immunization practices. In: Plotkin SA, Orenstein WA, Offit PA, eds. *Vaccines*. 5th ed. Philadelphia: Elsevier; 2008:83-110.
4. Levie K, Leroux-Roels I, Hoppenbrouwers K, et al. An adjuvanted, low-dose, pandemic influenza A (H5N1) vaccine candidate is safe, immunogenic, and induces cross-reactive immune responses in healthy adults. *J Infect Dis*. 2008;198:642-649.
5. Claman HN. The biology of the immune response. *JAMA*. 1992;268:2790-2796.
6. Poland GA, Ovsyannikova IG, Jacobson RM. Vaccine immunogenetics: bedside to bench to population. *Vaccine*. 2008;26:6183-6188.
7. Fagarasan S, Honjo T. T-Independent immune response: new aspects of B cell biology. *Science*. 2000;290:89-92.
8. Vogel FR, Hem SL. Immunologic Adjuvants. In: Plotkin SA, Orenstein WA, Offit PA, eds. *Vaccines*. 5th ed. Philadelphia: Elsevier; 2008:59-71.
9. Shaw FE Jr, Guess HA, Roets JM, et al. Effect of anatomic injection site, age and smoking on the immune response to hepatitis B vaccination. *Vaccine*. 1989;7:425-430.
10. Nicolas JF, Guy B. Intradermal, epidermal and transcutaneous vaccination: from immunology to clinical practice. *Expert Rev Vaccines*. 2008;7:1201-1214.
11. Lieberman JM, Marcy SM, Partridge S, et al. Evaluation of hepatitis A vaccine in infants: Effect of maternal antibodies on the antibody response. *Infectious Diseases Society of America 36th Annual Meeting*. Denver, CO, 1998.
12. Ezekowitz RAB, Hoffmann JA, eds. *Innate Immunity*. Totowa, NJ: Humana Press; 2003.
13. Krogsgaard M, Davis MM. How T cells "see" antigen. *Nat Immunol*. 2005;6:239-245.
14. Kotb M, Calandra T. *Cytokines and Chemokines in Infectious Diseases Handbook*. Totowa, NJ: Humana Press; 2003.
15. O'Garra A, Vieira P. Regulatory T cells and mechanisms of immune system control. *Nat Med*. 2004;10:801-805.
16. Pulendran B, Ahmed R. Translating innate immunity into immunological memory: implications for vaccine development. *Cell*. 2006;124:849-863.
17. Pulendran B, Palucka K, Banchereau J. Sensing pathogens and tuning immune responses. *Science*. 2001;293:253-256.
18. Petrilli V, Dostert C, Muruve DA, et al. The inflammasome: a danger sensing complex triggering innate immunity. *Curr Opin Immunol*. 2007;19:615-622.
19. Siegrist CA. Vaccine immunology. In: Plotkin SA, Orenstein WA, Offit PA, eds. *Vaccines*. 5th ed. Philadelphia: Elsevier; 2008:18-36.
20. Sercarz EE, Maverakis E. MHC-guided processing: binding of large antigen fragments. *Nat Rev Immunol*. 2003;3:621-629.
21. McHeyzer-Williams LJ, McHeyzer-Williams MG. Antigen-specific memory B cell development. *Annu Rev Immunol*. 2005;23:487-513.
22. Fulginiti VA, Eller JJ, Downie AW, et al. Altered reactivity to measles virus. Atypical measles in children previously immunized with inactivated measles virus vaccines. *JAMA*. 1967;202:1075-1080.
23. MacDonald NE, Halperin SA, Law BJ, et al. Induction of immunologic memory by conjugated vs plain meningococcal C polysaccharide vaccine in toddlers: a randomized controlled trial. *JAMA*. 1998;280:1685-1689.
24. Offit PA, Hackett CJ. Addressing parents' concerns: do vaccines cause allergic or autoimmune diseases? *Pediatrics*. 2003;111:653-659.
25. Offit PA, Quarles J, Gerber MA, et al. Addressing parents' concerns: do multiple vaccines overwhelm or weaken the infant's immune system? *Pediatrics*. 2002;109:124-129.
26. *Immunization Safety Review: Multiple Immunizations and Immune Dysfunction*. Washington, DC: Institute of Medicine; 2002.
27. DeStefano F, Gu D, Kramarz P, et al. Childhood vaccinations and risk of asthma. *Pediatr Infect Dis J*. 2002;21:498-504.
28. Watson JC, Pearson JA, Markowitz LE, et al. An evaluation of measles revaccination among school-entry-aged children. *Pediatrics*. 1996;97:613-618.
29. Eriksson K, Holmgren J. Recent advances in mucosal vaccines and adjuvants. *Curr Opin Immunol*. 2002;14:666-672.
30. Milgrom F, Abeyounis CJ, Kano K. *Principles of Immunological Diagnosis in Medicine*. Philadelphia: Lea & Febiger; 1981.
31. Romero-Steiner S, Libutti D, Pais LB, et al. Standardization of an opsonophagocytic assay for the measurement of functional antibody activity against Streptococcus pneumoniae using differentiated HL-60 cells. *Clin Diagn Lab Immunol*. 1997;4:415-422.
32. Ellis RW. Technologies for making new vaccines. In: Plotkin SA, Orenstein WA, Offit PA, eds. *Vaccines*. 5th ed. Philadelphia: Elsevier; 2008:1335-1356.
33. Dennehy PH. Rotavirus vaccines: an overview. *Clin Microbiol Rev*. 2008;21:198-208.
34. Measles—United States, 1999. *MMWR Morb Mortal Wkly Rep*. 2000;49:557-560.
35. Reef SE, Cochi SL. The evidence for the elimination of rubella and congenital rubella syndrome in the United States: a public health achievement. *Clin Infect Dis*. 2006;43(Suppl 3):S123-S125.
36. Recommendations of the International Task Force for Disease Eradication. *MMWR Recomm Rep*. 1993;42:1-38.
37. Progress toward interruption of wild poliovirus transmission—worldwide—2008. *MMWR Morb Mortal Wkly Rep*. 2009;58:308-312.
38. Certification of poliomyelitis eradication—European Region, June 2002. *MMWR Morb Mortal Wkly Rep*. 2002;51:572-574.
39. Certification of poliomyelitis eradication—Western Pacific Region, October 2000. *MMWR Morb Mortal Wkly Rep*. 2001;50:1-3.
40. Certification of poliomyelitis eradication—the Americas, 1994. *MMWR Morb Mortal Wkly Rep*. 1994;43:720-722.
41. Peltola H, Kilpi T, Anttila M. Rapid disappearance of *Haemophilus influenzae* type b meningitis after routine childhood immunisation with conjugate vaccines. *Lancet*. 1992;340:592-594.
42. Progress toward eliminating *Haemophilus influenzae* type b disease among infants and children—United States, 1987-1997. *MMWR Morb Mortal Wkly Rep*. 1998;47:993-998.
43. Progress toward introduction of *Haemophilus influenzae* type b vaccine in low-income countries—worldwide, 2004-2007. *MMWR Morb Mortal Wkly Rep*. 2008;57:148-151.
44. Invasive pneumococcal disease in children 5 years after conjugate vaccine introduction—eight states, 1998-2005. *MMWR Morb Mortal Wkly Rep*. 2008;57:144-148.
45. Pertussis vaccination: use of acellular pertussis vaccines among infants and young children. Recommendations of the Advisory Committee on Immunization Practices (ACIP). *MMWR Recomm Rep*. 1997;46:1-25.
46. Edwards KM, Decker MD. Pertussis vaccines. In: Plotkin SA, Orenstein WA, Offit PA, eds. *Vaccines*. Philadelphia: Elsevier; 2008:467-518.
47. Use of diphtheria toxoid-tetanus toxoid-acellular pertussis vaccine as a five-dose series. Supplemental recommendations of the Advisory Committee on Immunization Practices (ACIP). *MMWR Recomm Rep*. 2000;49:1-8.
48. Marin M, Guris D, Chaves SS, et al. Prevention of varicella: recommendations of the Advisory Committee on Immunization Practices (ACIP). *MMWR Recomm Rep*. 2007;56:1-40.
49. Izurieta HS, Strebel PM, Blake PA. Postlicensure effectiveness of varicella vaccine during an outbreak in a child care center. *JAMA*. 1997;278:1495-1499.
50. Roush SW, Murphy TV. Historical comparisons of morbidity and mortality for vaccine-preventable diseases in the United States. *JAMA*. 2007;298:2155-2163.
51. Howson CP, Howe CJ, Fineberg HV. *Adverse Effects of Pertussis and Rubella Vaccines*. Washington, DC: Institute of Medicine. 1991.
52. Stratton KR, Howe CJ, Johnston RB Jr. Adverse events associated with childhood vaccines other than pertussis and rubella. Summary of a report from the Institute of Medicine. *JAMA*. 1994;271:1602-1605.
53. Howson CP, Fineberg HV. Adverse events following pertussis and rubella vaccines. Summary of a report of the Institute of Medicine. *JAMA*. 1992;267:392-396.
54. Chen RT, Davis RL, Sheedy KM. Safety of immunizations. In: Plotkin SA, Orenstein WA, eds. *Vaccines*. 4th ed. Philadelphia: WB Saunders; 2004:1557-1581.
55. *Immunization Safety Review: Vaccines and Autism*: Immunization Safety Review Committee, Board on Health Promotion, Institute of Medicine. 2004.
56. Rantala H, Cherry JD, Shields WD, et al. Epidemiology of Guillain-Barre syndrome in children: relationship of oral polio vaccine administration to occurrence. *J Pediatr*. 1994;124:220-223.
57. Slater PE, Ben-Zvi T, Fogel A, et al. Absence of an association between rubella vaccination and arthritis in underimmune postpartum women. *Vaccine*. 1995;13:1529-1532.
58. Frenkel LM, Nielsen K, Garakian A, et al. A search for persistent rubella virus infection in persons with chronic symptoms after rubella and rubella immunization and in patients with juvenile rheumatoid arthritis. *Clin Infect Dis*. 1996;22:287-294.
59. Ray P, Black S, Shinefield H, et al. Risk of chronic arthropathy among women after rubella vaccination. Vaccine Safety Datalink Team. *JAMA*. 1997;278:551-556.
60. Gerber JS, Offit PA. Vaccines and autism: A tale of shifting hypotheses. *Clin Infect Dis* 2009.
61. *Report of the Committee on Infectious Diseases*. Elk Grove Village, IL: American Academy of Pediatrics. 2009.
62. Recommended schedules for persons 0 through 18 years immunization schedule—United States. Centers for Disease Control

and Prevention. *MMWR Morb Mortal Wkly Rep.* 2009;57: Q1-Q4.
63. Use of anthrax vaccine in response to terrorism: supplemental recommendations of the Advisory Committee on Immunization Practices. *MMWR Morb Mortal Wkly Rep.* 2002;51:1024-1026.
64. Use of anthrax vaccine in the United States. Recommendations of the Advisory Committee on Immunization Practices (ACIP). Centers for Disease Control and Prevention. *MMWR Morb Mortal Wkly Rep* 2009 (in press).
65. Friedlander AM, Pittman PR, Parker GW. Anthrax vaccine: evidence for safety and efficacy against inhalational anthrax. *JAMA.* 1999;282:2104-2106.
66. Marano N, Plikaytis BD, Martin SW, et al. Effects of a reduced dose schedule and intramuscular administration of anthrax vaccine adsorbed on immunogenicity and safety at 7 months: a randomized trial. *JAMA.* 2008;300:1532-1543.
67. Brachman PS, Gold H, Plotkin SA, et al. Field evaluation of a human anthrax vaccine. *Am J Public Health Nations Health.* 1962;52:632-645.
68. Abramowicz M. Anthrax vaccine. *Med Lett Drugs Ther.* 1998; 40:52-53.
69. Sever JL, Brenner AI, Gale AD, et al. Safety of anthrax vaccine: a review by the Anthrax Vaccine Expert Committee (AVEC) of adverse events reported to the Vaccine Adverse Event Reporting System (VAERS). *Pharmacoepidemiol Drug Saf.* 2002;11:189-202.
70. Lange JL, Lesikar SE, Rubertone MV, et al. Comprehensive systematic surveillance for adverse effects of anthrax vaccine adsorbed, US Armed Forces, 1998-2000. *Vaccine.* 2003;21:1620-1628.
71. Leppla SH, Robbins JB, Schneerson R, et al. Development of an improved vaccine for anthrax. *J Clin Invest.* 2002;110:141-144.
72. Campbell JD, Clement KH, Wasserman SS, et al. Safety, reactogenicity and immunogenicity of a recombinant protective antigen anthrax vaccine given to healthy adults. *Hum Vaccin.* 2007;3:205-211.
73. Snider DE Jr, Rieder HL, Combs D, et al. Tuberculosis in children. *Pediatr Infect Dis J.* 1988;7:271-278.
74. Rodrigues LC, Diwan VK, Wheeler JG. Protective effect of BCG against tuberculous meningitis and miliary tuberculosis: a meta-analysis. *Int J Epidemiol.* 1993;22:1154-1158.
75. Colditz GA, Brewer TF, Berkey CS, et al. Efficacy of BCG vaccine in the prevention of tuberculosis. Meta-analysis of the published literature. *JAMA.* 1994;271:698-702.
76. The role of BCG vaccine in the prevention and control of tuberculosis in the United States. A joint statement by the Advisory Council for the Elimination of Tuberculosis and the Advisory Committee on Immunization Practices. *MMWR Recomm Rep.* 1996;45:1-18.
77. Cholera vaccine. *MMWR Morb Mortal Wkly Rep.* 1988;37:617-618, 23-4.
78. Tacket CO, Sack DA. Cholera vaccines. In: Plotkin SA, Orenstein WA, Offit PA, eds. *Vaccines.* 5th ed. Philadelphia: Elsevier; 2008:127-138.
79. Diphtheria, tetanus, and pertussis: recommendations for vaccine use and other preventive measures. Recommendations of the Immunization Practices Advisory committee (ACIP). *MMWR Recomm Rep.* 1991;40:1-28.
80. Kretsinger K, Broder KR, Cortese MM, et al. Preventing tetanus, diphtheria, and pertussis among adults: Use of tetanus toxoid, reduced diphtheria toxoid and acellular pertussis vaccine. Recommendations of the Advisory Committee on Immunization Practices (ACIP) and recommendation of ACIP, supported by the Healthcare Infection Control Practices Advisory Committee (HICPAC), for use of Tdap among health-care personnel. *MMWR Recomm Rep.* 2006;55:1-37.
81. Haemophilus b conjugate vaccines for prevention of *Haemophilus influenzae* type b disease among infants and children two months of age and older. Recommendations of the immunization practices advisory committee (ACIP). *MMWR Recomm Rep.* 1991;40:1-7.
82. Recommendations for use of Haemophilus b conjugate vaccines and a combined diphtheria, tetanus, pertussis, and Haemophilus b vaccine. Recommendations of the advisory Committee on Immunization Practices (ACIP). *MMWR Recomm Rep.* 1993;42: 1-15.
83. Anderson EL, Decker MD, Englund JA, et al. Interchangeability of conjugated *Haemophilus influenzae* type b vaccines in infants. *JAMA.* 1995;273:849-853.
84. Greenberg DP, Lieberman JM, Marcy SM, et al. Enhanced antibody responses in infants given different sequences of heterogeneous *Haemophilus influenzae* type b conjugate vaccines. *J Pediatr.* 1995;126:206-211.
85. Bewley KM, Schwab JG, Ballanco GA, et al. Interchangeability of *Haemophilus influenzae* type b vaccines in the primary series: evaluation of a two-dose mixed regimen. *Pediatrics.* 1996;98:898-904.
86. Unlicensed use of combination of *Haemophilus influenzae* type b conjugate vaccine and diphtheria and tetanus toxoid and acellular pertussis vaccine for infants. Centers for Disease Control and Prevention. *MMWR Morb Mortal Wkly Rep.* 1998;47:787.
87. Innis BL, Snitbhan R, Kunasol P, et al. Protection against hepatitis A by an inactivated vaccine. *JAMA.* 1994;271:1328-1334.
88. Werzberger A, Mensch B, Kuter B, et al. A controlled trial of a formalin-inactivated hepatitis A vaccine in healthy children. *N Engl J Med.* 1992;327:453-457.
89. Prevention of hepatitis A through active or passive immunization: Recommendations of the Advisory Committee on Immunization Practices (ACIP). *MMWR Recomm Rep.* 1996;45:1-30.
90. Bell BP, Shapiro CN, Alter MJ, et al. The diverse patterns of hepatitis A epidemiology in the United States-implications for vaccination strategies. *J Infect Dis.* 1998;178:1579-1584.
91. Fiore AE, Wasley A, Bell BP. Prevention of hepatitis A through active or passive immunization: recommendations of the Advisory Committee on Immunization Practices (ACIP). *MMWR Recomm Rep.* 2006;55:1-23.
92. Shapiro CN, Letson GW, Kuehn D, et al. Effect of maternal antibody on immunogenicity of hepatitis A vaccine in infants. *35th Interscience Conference on Antimicrobial Agents and Chemotherapy.* San Francisco, 1995.
93. Green MS, Cohen D, Lerman Y, et al. Depression of the immune response to an inactivated hepatitis A vaccine administered concomitantly with immune globulin. *J Infect Dis.* 1993;168:740-743.
94. U.S. Department of Labor, Occupational Safety and Health Administration. 29 CFR Part 1910, 1030. Occupational exposure to bloodborne pathogens: final rule. *Federal Register.* 1991; 56:64004-64182.
95. Hepatitis B virus: a comprehensive strategy for eliminating transmission in the United States through universal childhood vaccination. Recommendations of the Immunization Practices Advisory Committee (ACIP). *MMWR Recomm Rep.* 1991;40:1-25.
96. Mast EE, Margolis HS, Fiore AE, et al. A comprehensive immunization strategy to eliminate transmission of hepatitis B virus infection in the United States: recommendations of the Advisory Committee on Immunization Practices (ACIP). Part 1: immunization of infants, children, and adolescents. *MMWR Recomm Rep.* 2005;54:1-31.
97. Mast EE, Weinbaum CM, Fiore AE, et al. A comprehensive immunization strategy to eliminate transmission of hepatitis B virus infection in the United States: recommendations of the Advisory Committee on Immunization Practices (ACIP). Part II: immunization of adults. *MMWR Recomm Rep.* 2006;55:1-33; quiz, CE1-4.
98. Immunization of adolescents. Recommendations of the Advisory Committee on Immunization Practices, the American Academy of Pediatrics, the American Academy of Family Physicians, and the American Medical Association. *MMWR Recomm Rep.* 1996;45:1-16.
99. Mast E, Ward S. Hepatitis B vaccines. In: Plotkin SA, Orenstein WA, Offit PA, eds. *Vaccines.* 5th ed. Philadelphia: Elsevier; 2008: 205-242.
100. Hammitt LL, Hennessy TW, Fiore AE, et al. Hepatitis B immunity in children vaccinated with recombinant hepatitis B vaccine beginning at birth: a follow-up study at 15 years. *Vaccine.* 2007; 25:6958-6964.
101. Wise RP, Kiminyo KP, Salive ME. Hair loss after routine immunizations. *JAMA.* 1997;278:1176-1178.
102. Pirmohamed M, Winstanley P. Hepatitis B vaccine and neurotoxicity. *Postgrad Med J.* 1997;73:462-463.
103. DeStefano F, Verstraeten T, Jackson LA, et al. Vaccinations and risk of central nervous system demyelinating diseases in adults. *Arch Neurol.* 2003;60:504-509.
104. Schiller JT, Frazer IH, Lowy DR. Human papillomavirus vaccines In: Plotkin SA, Orenstein WA, Offit PA, eds. *Vaccines.* 5th ed. Philadelphia: Elsevier; 2008:243-257.
105. Markowitz LE, Dunne EF, Saraiya M, et al. Quadrivalent Human Papillomavirus Vaccine: Recommendations of the Advisory Committee on Immunization Practices (ACIP). *MMWR Recomm Rep.* 2007;56:1-24.
106. Gross PA, Hermogenes AW, Sacks HS, et al. The efficacy of influenza vaccine in elderly persons. A meta-analysis and review of the literature. *Ann Intern Med.* 1995;123:518-527.
107. Patriarca PA, Arden NH, Koplan JP, et al. Prevention and control of type A influenza infections in nursing homes. Benefits and costs of four approaches using vaccination and amantadine. *Ann Intern Med.* 1987;107:732-740.
108. Bridges CB, Katz JM, Levandowski RA, et al. Inactivated influenza vaccines. In: Plotkin SA, Orenstein WA, Offit PA, eds. *Vaccines.* 5th ed. Philadelphia: Elsevier; 2008:259-290.
109. Hoberman A, Greenberg DP, Paradise JL, et al. Effectiveness of inactivated influenza vaccine in preventing acute otitis media in young children: a randomized controlled trial. *JAMA.* 2003;290: 1608-1616.
110. Bridges CB, Harper SA, Fukuda K, et al. Prevention and control of influenza. Recommendations of the Advisory Committee on Immunization Practices (ACIP). *MMWR Recomm Rep.* 2003;52: 1-34; quiz CE1-4.
111. Prevention and control of influenza: recommendations of the Advisory Committee on Immunization Practices (ACIP). Centers for Disease Control and Prevention. *MMWR Morb Mortal Wkly Rep* 2009 (in press).
112. Schonberger LB, Bregman DJ, Sullivan-Bolyai JZ, et al. Guillain-Barre syndrome following vaccination in the National Influenza Immunization Program, United States, 1976-1977. *Am J Epidemiol.* 1979;110:105-123.
113. Lasky T, Terracciano GJ, Magder L, et al. The Guillain-Barre syndrome and the 1992-1993 and 1993-1994 influenza vaccines. *N Engl J Med.* 1998;339:1797-1802.
114. Murphy KR, Strunk RC. Safe administration of influenza vaccine in asthmatic children hypersensitive to egg proteins. *J Pediatr.* 1985;106:931-933.
115. *Immunization Safety Review: Influenza vaccine and neurological complications*: Institute of Medicine. 2003.
116. Harper SA, Fukuda K, Cox NJ, et al. Using live, attenuated influenza vaccine for prevention and control of influenza: supplemental recommendations of the Advisory Committee on Immunization Practices (ACIP). *MMWR Recomm Rep.* 2003;52: 1-8.
117. Belshe RB, Walker R, Stoddard JJ, et al. Influenza vaccine-live. In: Plotkin SA, Orenstein WA, Offit PA, eds. *Vaccines.* 5th ed. Philadelphia: Elsevier; 2008:291-309.
118. Belshe RB, Edwards KM, Vesikari T, et al. Live attenuated versus inactivated influenza vaccine in infants and young children. *N Engl J Med.* 2007;356:685-696.
119. Ohmit SE, Victor JC, Teich ER, et al. Prevention of symptomatic seasonal influenza in 2005-2006 by inactivated and live attenuated vaccines. *J Infect Dis.* 2008;198:312-317.
120. Halstead SB, Jacobson J. Japanese encephalitis vaccines. In: Plotkin SA, Orenstein WA, Offit PA, eds. 5th ed. *Vaccines.* Phildelphia: Elsevier; 2008:311-352.
121. Hoke CH, Nisalak A, Sangawhipa N, et al. Protection against Japanese encephalitis by inactivated vaccines. *N Engl J Med.* 1988;319:608-614.
122. Inactivated Japanese encephalitis virus vaccine. Recommendations of the Advisory Committee on Immunization Practices (ACIP). *MMWR Recomm Rep.* 1993;42:1-15.
123. Watson JC, Hadler SC, Dykewicz CA, et al. Measles, mumps, and rubella—vaccine use and strategies for elimination of measles, rubella, and congenital rubella syndrome and control of mumps: recommendations of the Advisory Committee on Immunization Practices (ACIP). *MMWR Recomm Rep.* 1998;47: 1-57.
124. Pabst HF, Spady DW, Marusyk RG, et al. Reduced measles immunity in infants in a well-vaccinated population. *Pediatr Infect Dis J.* 1992;11:525-529.
125. Update: recommendations from the Advisory Committee on Immunization Practices (ACIP) regarding administration of combination MMRV vaccine. *MMWR Morb Mortal Wkly Rep.* 2008;57:258-260.
126. Immunization of health-care workers: recommendations of the Advisory Committee on Immunization Practices (ACIP) and the Hospital Infection Control Practices Advisory Committee (HICPAC). *MMWR Recomm Rep.* 1997;46:1-42.
127. Weber DJ, Rutala WA. Vaccines for health care workers. In: Plotkin SA, Orenstein WA, Offit PA, eds. *Vaccines.* 5th ed. Philadelphia: Elsevier; 2008:1453-1478.
128. *Adverse events following immunization.* Atlanta: Centers for Disease Control and Prevention; 1989.
129. Griffin MR, Ray WA, Mortimer EA, et al. Risk of seizures after measles-mumps-rubella immunization. *Pediatrics.* 1991;88:881-885.
130. Measles and Mumps Vaccine: *In Adverse Events Associated With Childhood Vaccines: Evidence Bearing on Causality.* Washington, DC: Institute of Medicine; 1994.
131. Hornig M, Briese T, Buie T, et al. Lack of association between measles, virus vaccine and autism with enteropathy: a case-control study. *PLoS ONE* 2008;3:e3140.
132. Bilukha OO, Rosenstein N. Prevention and control of meningococcal disease. Recommendations of the Advisory Committee on Immunization Practices (ACIP). *MMWR Recomm Rep.* 2005;54:1-21.
133. Notice to readers: recommendation from the Advisory Committee on Immunization Practices (ACIP) for use of quadrivalent meningococcal conjugate vaccine (MCV4) in children aged 2-10 years at increased risk for invasive meningococcal disease. *MMWR Morb Mortal Wkly Rep.* 2007;56:1265-1266.
134. Riedo FX, Plikaytis BD, Broome CV. Epidemiology and prevention of meningococcal disease. *Pediatr Infect Dis J.* 1995;14: 643-657.
135. Scheifele DW, Bjornson G, Boraston S. Local adverse effects of meningococcal vaccine. *CMAJ.* 1994;150:14-15.
136. Lepow ML, Beeler J, Randolph M, et al. Reactogenicity and immunogenicity of a quadrivalent combined meningococcal polysaccharide vaccine in children. *J Infect Dis.* 1986;154:1033-1036.
137. Richmond P, Borrow R, Miller E, et al. Meningococcal serogroup C conjugate vaccine is immunogenic in infancy and primes for memory. *J Infect Dis.* 1999;179:1569-1572.
138. Miller E, Salisbury D, Ramsay M. Planning, registration, and implementation of an immunisation campaign against meningococcal serogroup C disease in the UK: a success story. *Vaccine.* 2001;20(Suppl 1):S58-S67.
139. Richmond P, Kaczmarski E, Borrow R, et al. Meningococcal C polysaccharide vaccine induces immunologic hyporesponsiveness in adults that is overcome by meningococcal C conjugate vaccine. *J Infect Dis.* 2000;181:761-764.
140. Borrow R, Goldblatt D, Andrews N, et al. Influence of prior meningococcal C polysaccharide vaccination on the response and generation of memory after meningococcal C conjugate vaccination in young children. *J Infect Dis.* 2001;184:377-380.
141. Balmer P, Borrow R, Miller E. Impact of meningococcal C conjugate vaccine in the UK. *J Med Microbiol.* 2002;51:717-722.

142. Ramsay ME, Andrews N, Kaczmarski EB, et al. Efficacy of meningococcal serogroup C conjugate vaccine in teenagers and toddlers in England. *Lancet.* 2001;357:195-196.
143. Centers for Disease Control and Prevention. Update: Guillain-Barré Syndrome among recipients of Menactra meningococcal conjugate vaccine - United States, June 2005-September 2006. *MMWR Morb Mortal Wkly Rep.* 2006;55:1120-1124.
144. Dayan GH, Quinlisk MP, Parker AA, et al. Recent resurgence of mumps in the United States. *N Engl J Med.* 2008;358:1580-1589.
145. Notice to readers: updated recommendations of the Advisory Committee on Immunization Practices (ACIP) for the control and elimination of mumps. *MMWR Morb Mortal Wkly Rep.* 2006;55:629-630.
146. Miller E, Goldacre M, Pugh S, et al. Risk of aseptic meningitis after measles, mumps, and rubella vaccine in UK children. *Lancet.* 1993;341:979-982.
147. da Silveira CM, Kmetzsch CI, Mohrdieck R, et al. The risk of aseptic meningitis associated with the Leningrad-Zagreb mumps vaccine strain following mass vaccination with measles-mumps-rubella vaccine, Rio Grande do Sul, Brazil, 1997. *Int J Epidemiol.* 2002;31:978-982.
148. Gustafsson L, Hallander HO, Olin P, et al. A controlled trial of a two-component acellular, a five-component acellular, and a whole-cell pertussis vaccine. *N Engl J Med.* 1996;334:349-355.
149. Greco D, Salmaso S, Mastrantonio P, et al. A controlled trial of two acellular vaccines and one whole-cell vaccine against pertussis. Progetto Pertosse Working Group. *N Engl J Med.* 1996;334:341-348.
150. Decker MD, Edwards KM, Steinhoff MC, et al. Comparison of 13 acellular pertussis vaccines: adverse reactions. *Pediatrics.* 1995;96:557-566.
151. Heijbel H, Rasmussen F, Olin P. Safety evaluation of one whole-cell and three acellular pertussis vaccines in Stockholm trial II. *Dev Biol Stand.* 1997;89:99-100.
152. Heijbel H, Ciofi degli Atti M, Harzer E, et al. Hypotonic hyporesponsive episodes in eight pertussis vaccine studies. *Dev Biol Stand.* 1997;89:101-103.
153. Gangarosa EJ, Galazka AM, Wolfe CR, et al. Impact of anti-vaccine movements on pertussis control: the untold story. *Lancet.* 1998;351:356-361.
154. Deen JL, Mink CA, Cherry JD, et al. Household contact study of *Bordetella* pertussis infections. *Clin Infect Dis.* 1995;21:1211-1219.
155. Izurieta HS, Kenyon TA, Strebel PM, et al. Risk factors for pertussis in young infants during an outbreak in Chicago in 1993. *Clin Infect Dis.* 1996;22:503-507.
156. Mink CM, Cherry JD, Christenson P, et al. A search for *Bordetella* pertussis infection in university students. *Clin Infect Dis.* 1992;14:464-471.
157. Wright SW, Edwards KM, Decker MD, et al. Pertussis infection in adults with persistent cough. *JAMA.* 1995;273:1044-1046.
158. Nennig ME, Shinefield HR, Edwards KM, et al. Prevalence and incidence of adult pertussis in an urban population. *JAMA.* 1996;275:1672-1674.
159. Edwards KM, Decker MD, Graham BS, et al. Adult immunization with acellular pertussis vaccine. *JAMA.* 1993;269:53-56.
160. Strebel P, Nordin J, Edwards K, et al. Population-based incidence of pertussis among adolescents and adults, Minnesota, 1995-1996. *J Infect Dis.* 2001;183:1353-1359.
161. Tanaka M, Vitek CR, Pascual FB, et al. Trends in pertussis among infants in the United States, 1980-1999. *JAMA.* 2003;290:2968-2975.
162. Keitel WA, Muenz LR, Decker MD, et al. A randomized clinical trial of acellular pertussis vaccines in healthy adults: dose-response comparisons of 5 vaccines and implications for booster immunization. *J Infect Dis.* 1999;180:397-403.
163. Broder KR, Cortese MM, Iskander JK, et al. Preventing tetanus, diphtheria, and pertussis among adolescents: use of tetanus toxoid, reduced diphtheria toxoid and acellular pertussis vaccines recommendations of the Advisory Committee on Immunization Practices (ACIP). *MMWR Recomm Rep.* 2006;55:1-34.
164. Ward JI, Cherry JD, Chang SJ, et al. Efficacy of an acellular pertussis vaccine among adolescents and adults. *N Engl J Med.* 2005;353:1555-1563.
165. Murphy TV, Slade BA, Broder KR, et al. Prevention of pertussis, tetanus, and diphtheria among pregnant and postpartum women and their infants recommendations of the Advisory Committee on Immunization Practices (ACIP). *MMWR Recomm Rep.* 2008;57:1-51.
166. Williamson ED, Simpson AJ, Titball RW. Plauge vaccines. In: Plotkin SA, Orenstein WA, Offit PA, eds. *Vaccines.* 5th ed. Philadelphia: Elsevier; 2008:519-529.
167. MacLeod CM, Hodges RG, Heidelberger M, et al. Prevention of pneumococcal pneumonia by immunization with specific capsular polysaccharides. *J Exp Med.* 1945;82:445-465.
168. Smit P, Oberholzer D, Hayden-Smith S, et al. Protective efficacy of pneumococcal polysaccharide vaccines. *JAMA.* 1977;238:2613-2616.
169. Austrian R, Douglas RM, Schiffman G, et al. Prevention of pneumococcal pneumonia by vaccination. *Trans Assoc Am Physicians.* 1976;89:184-194.
170. Shapiro ED, Berg AT, Austrian R, et al. The protective efficacy of polyvalent pneumococcal polysaccharide vaccine. *N Engl J Med.* 1991;325:1453-1460.
171. Butler JC, Breiman RF, Campbell JF, et al. Pneumococcal polysaccharide vaccine efficacy. An evaluation of current recommendations. *JAMA.* 1993;270:1826-1831.
172. Prevention of pneumococcal disease: recommendations of the Advisory Committee on Immunization Practices (ACIP). *MMWR Recomm Rep.* 1997;46:1-24.
173. Jackson LA, Neuzil KM, Yu O, et al. Effectiveness of pneumococcal polysaccharide vaccine in older adults. *N Engl J Med.* 2003;348:1747-1755.
174. Benin AL, O'Brien KL, Watt JP, et al. Effectiveness of the 23-valent polysaccharide vaccine against invasive pneumococcal disease in Navajo adults. *J Infect Dis.* 2003;188:81-89.
175. Pneumococcal vaccination for cochlear implant candidates and recipients: updated recommendations of the Advisory Committee on Immunization Practices. *MMWR Morb Mortal Wkly Rep.* 2003;52:739-740.
176. Preventing pneumococcal disease among infants and young children. Recommendations of the Advisory Committee on Immunization Practices (ACIP). *MMWR Recomm Rep.* 2000;49:1-35.
177. Jackson LA, Benson P, Sneller VP, et al. Safety of revaccination with pneumococcal polysaccharide vaccine. *JAMA.* 1999;281:243-248.
178. Dworkin MS, Ward JW, Hanson DL, et al. Pneumococcal disease among human immunodeficiency virus-infected persons: incidence, risk factors, and impact of vaccination. *Clin Infect Dis.* 2001;32:794-800.
179. Black S, Shinefield H, Fireman B, et al. Efficacy, safety and immunogenicity of heptavalent pneumococcal conjugate vaccine in children. Northern California Kaiser Permanente Vaccine Study Center Group. *Pediatr Infect Dis J.* 2000;19:187-195.
180. Black SB, Shinefield HR, Ling S, et al. Effectiveness of heptavalent pneumococcal conjugate vaccine in children younger than five years of age for prevention of pneumonia. *Pediatr Infect Dis J.* 2002;21:810-815.
181. O'Brien KL, Moulton LH, Reid R, et al. Efficacy and safety of seven-valent conjugate pneumococcal vaccine in American Indian children: group randomised trial. *Lancet.* 2003;362:355-361.
182. Updated recommendation from the Advisory Committee on Immunization Practices (ACIP) for use of 7-valent pneumococcal conjugate vaccine (PCV7) in children aged 24-59 months who are not completely vaccinated. *MMWR Morb Mortal Wkly Rep.* 2008;57:343-344.
183. Hsu HE, Shutt KA, Moore MR, et al. Effect of pneumococcal conjugate vaccine on pneumococcal meningitis. *N Engl J Med.* 2009;360:244-256.
184. Whitney CG, Farley MM, Hadler J, et al. Decline in invasive pneumococcal disease after the introduction of protein-polysaccharide conjugate vaccine. *N Engl J Med.* 2003;348:1737-1746.
185. Recommendations of the Advisory Committee on Immunization Practices: revised recommendations for routine poliomyelitis vaccination. *MMWR Morb Mortal Wkly Rep.* 1999;48:590.
186. Manning SE, Rupprecht CE, Fishbein D, et al. Human rabies prevention—United States, 2008: recommendations of the Advisory Committee on Immunization Practices. *MMWR Recomm Rep.* 2008;57:1-28.
187. Shill M, Baynes RD, Miller SD. Fatal rabies encephalitis despite appropriate post-exposure prophylaxis. A case report. *N Engl J Med.* 1987;316:1257-1258.
188. Human rabies despite treatment with rabies immune globulin and human diploid cell rabies vaccine—Thailand. *MMWR Morb Mortal Wkly Rep.* 1987;36:759-760, 65.
189. Cortese MM, Parashar UD. Prevention of rotavirus gastroenteritis among infants and children: recommendations of the Advisory Committee on Immunization Practices (ACIP). *MMWR Recomm Rep.* 2009;58:1-25.
190. Clark HF, Lawley D, Mallette LA, et al. Decline in cases of rotavirus gastroenteritis presenting to The Children's Hospital of Philadelphia after introduction of a pentavalent rotavirus vaccine. *Clin Vaccine Immunol.* 2009;16:382-386.
191. Rubella vaccination during pregnancy–United States, 1971-1988. *MMWR Morb Mortal Wkly Rep.* 1989;38:289-293.
192. Freestone DS, Prydie J, Smith SG, et al. Vaccination of adults with Wistar RA 27/3 rubella vaccine. *J Hyg (Lond).* 1971;69:471-477.
193. Polk BF, Modlin JF, White JA, et al. A controlled comparison of joint reactions among women receiving one of two rubella vaccines. *Am J Epidemiol.* 1982;115:19-25.
194. Henderson DA, Borio LL, Grabenstein JD. Smallpox and vaccinia. In: Plotkin SA, Orenstein WA, Offit PA, eds. *Vaccines.* 5th ed. Philadelphia: Elsevier; 2008:773-803.
195. Weltzin R, Liu J, Pugachev KV, et al. Clonal vaccinia virus grown in cell culture as a new smallpox vaccine. *Nat Med.* 2003;9:1125-1130.
196. Wharton M, Strikas RA, Harpaz R, et al. Recommendations for using smallpox vaccine in a pre-event vaccination program. Supplemental recommendations of the Advisory Committee on Immunization Practices (ACIP) and the Healthcare Infection Control Practices Advisory Committee (HICPAC). *MMWR Recomm Rep.* 2003;52:1-16.
197. Cono J, Casey CG, Bell DM. Smallpox vaccination and adverse reactions. Guidance for clinicians. *MMWR Recomm Rep.* 2003;52:1-28.
198. Talbot TR, Ziel E, Doersam JK, et al. Risk of vaccinia transfer to the hands of vaccinated persons after smallpox immunization. *Clin Infect Dis.* 2004;38:536-541.
199. Supplemental recommendations on adverse events following smallpox vaccine in the pre-event vaccination program: recommendations of the Advisory Committee on Immunization Practices. *MMWR Morb Mortal Wkly Rep.* 2003;52:282-284.
200. Halsell JS, Riddle JR, Atwood JE, et al. Myopericarditis following smallpox vaccination among vaccinia-naive US military personnel. *JAMA.* 2003;289:3283-3289.
201. Relyveld EH, Henocq E, Bizzini B. Studies on untoward reactions to diphtheria and tetanus toxoids. *Dev Biol Stand.* 1979;43:33-37.
202. Pollard JD, Selby G. Relapsing neuropathy due to tetanus toxoid. Report of a case. *J Neurol Sci.* 1978;37:113-125.
203. Update: vaccine side effects, adverse reactions, contraindications, and precautions. Recommendations of the Advisory Committee on Immunization Practices (ACIP). *MMWR Recomm Rep.* 1996;45:1-35.
204. Typhoid immunization. Recommendations of the Immunization Practices Advisory Committee (ACIP). *MMWR Recomm Rep.* 1990;39:1-5.
205. Kuter BJ, Weibel RE, Guess HA, et al. Oka/Merck varicella vaccine in healthy children: final report of a 2-year efficacy study and 7-year follow-up studies. *Vaccine.* 1991;9:643-647.
206. White CJ, Kuter BJ, Ngai A, et al. Modified cases of chickenpox after varicella vaccination: correlation of protection with antibody response. *Pediatr Infect Dis J.* 1992;11:19-23.
207. Watson BM, Piercy SA, Plotkin SA, et al. Modified chickenpox in children immunized with the Oka/Merck varicella vaccine. *Pediatrics.* 1993;91:17-22.
208. Bernstein HH, Rothstein EP, Watson BM, et al. Clinical survey of natural varicella compared with breakthrough varicella after immunization with live attenuated Oka/Merck varicella vaccine. *Pediatrics.* 1993;92:833-837.
209. Vazquez M, LaRussa PS, Gershon AA, et al. Effectiveness over time of varicella vaccine. *JAMA.* 2004;291:851-855.
210. Vessey SJ, Chan CY, Kuter BJ, et al. Childhood vaccination against varicella: persistence of antibody, duration of protection, and vaccine efficacy. *J Pediatr.* 2001;139:297-304.
211. Kuter B, Matthews H, Shinefield H, et al. Ten year follow-up of healthy children who received one or two injections of varicella vaccine. *Pediatr Infect Dis J.* 2004;23:132-137.
212. Lieu TA, Finkler LJ, Sorel ME, et al. Cost-effectiveness of varicella serotesting versus presumptive vaccination of school-age children and adolescents. *Pediatrics.* 1995;95:632-638.
213. Watson B, Seward J, Yang A, et al. Postexposure effectiveness of varicella vaccine. *Pediatrics.* 2000;105:84-88.
214. Hall S, Galil K, Watson B, et al. The use of school-based vaccination clinics to control varicella outbreaks in two schools. *Pediatrics.* 2000;105:e17.
215. Levin MJ, Gershon AA, Weinberg A, et al. Immunization of HIV-infected children with varicella vaccine. *J Pediatr.* 2001;139:305-310.
216. Kaplan JE, Masur H, Holmes KK. Guidelines for preventing opportunistic infections among HIV-infected persons—2002. Recommendations of the U.S. Public Health Service and the Infectious Diseases Society of America. *MMWR Recomm Rep.* 2002;51:1-52.
217. Cetron MS, Marfin AA, Julian KG, et al. Yellow fever vaccine. Recommendations of the Advisory Committee on Immunization Practices (ACIP), 2002. *MMWR Recomm Rep.* 2002;51:1-11; quiz, CE1-4.
218. Harpaz R, Ortega-Sanchez IR, Seward JF. Prevention of herpes zoster: recommendations of the Advisory Committee on Immunization Practices (ACIP). *MMWR Recomm Rep.* 2008;57:1-30; quiz, CE2-4.
219. Update: Prevention of hepatitis A after exposure to hepatitis A virus and in international travelers. Updated recommendations of the Advisory Committee on Immunization Practices (ACIP). *MMWR Morb Mortal Wkly Rep.* 2007;56:1080-1084.
220. Arnon SS, Schechter R, Maslanka SE, et al. Human botulism immune globulin for the treatment of infant botulism. *N Engl J Med.* 2006;354(5):462-471.
221. Meissner HC, Long SS. Revised indications for the use of palivizumab and respiratory syncytial virus immune globulin intravenous for the prevention of respiratory syncytial virus infections. *Pediatrics.* 2003;112:1447-1452.
222. Reduction of respiratory syncytial virus hospitalization among premature infants and infants with bronchopulmonary dysplasia using respiratory syncytial virus immune globulin prophylaxis. The PREVENT Study Group. *Pediatrics.* 1997;99:93-99.
223. Simoes EA, Sondheimer HM, Top FH Jr, et al. Respiratory syncytial virus immune globulin for prophylaxis against respiratory syncytial virus disease in infants and children with congenital heart disease. The Cardiac Study Group. *J Pediatr.* 1998;133:492-499.
224. Palivizumab, a humanized respiratory syncytial virus monoclonal antibody, reduces hospitalization from respiratory syncytial virus infection in high-risk infants. The IMpact-RSV Study Group. *Pediatrics.* 1998;102:531-537.
225. American Academy of Pediatrics. Respiratory syncytial virus. In: Pickering LK, Baker CJ, Kimberlin DW, Long SS, eds. *Red Book 2009: Report of the Committee on Infectious Diseases,* 28th ed. Elk Grove Village, IL: American Academy of Pediatrics; 2009:560-569.
226. Ellis EF, Henney CS. Adverse reactions following administration of human gamma globulin. *J Allergy.* 1969;43:45-54.

227. Siber GR, Werner BG, Halsey NA, et al. Interference of immune globulin with measles and rubella immunization. *J Pediatr.* 1993;122:204-211.
228. Outbreak of hepatitis C associated with intravenous immunoglobulin administration—United States, October 1993-June 1994. *MMWR Morb Mortal Wkly Rep.* 1994;43:505-509.
229. Hepatitis C virus and intravenous anti-D immunoglobulin. *Commun Dis Rep CDR Wkly.* 1995;5:111.
230. Schiff RI. Transmission of viral infections through intravenous immune globulin. *N Engl J Med.* 1994;331:1649-1650.
231. Yu MY, Mason BL, Tankersley DL. Detection and characterization of hepatitis C virus RNA in immune globulins. *Transfusion.* 1994;34:596-602.
232. Khabbaz RF, Chamberland M. From prions to parasites: issues and concerns in blood safety. In: Scheld WM, Craig WA, Hughes JM, eds. *Emerging Infections 2.* Washington, DC: ASM Press; 1998:295-309.
233. *Selective Rho (D) immune globulin (RHIG).* Chicago: American College of Obstetricians and Gynecologists (ACOG); 1981.
234. King GE, Hadler SC. Simultaneous administration of childhood vaccines: an important public health policy that is safe and efficacious. *Pediatr Infect Dis J.* 1994;13:394-407.
235. Combination vaccines for childhood immunization. *MMWR Recomm Rep.* 1999;48:1-14.
235a. Ramsay DS, Lewis M. Developmental change in infant cortisol and behavioral response to inoculation. *Child Dev* 1999;65:1491-1502.
235b. Lewis M, Ramsay DS, Suomi SJ. Validating current immunization practice with young infants. *Pediatrics* 1992;90:771-773.
236. Recommended adult immunization schedule—United States, 2009. *MMWR Morb Mortal Wkly Rep.* 2009;57:Q1-Q4.
237. Centers for Disease Control and Prevention. A comprehensive immunization strategy to eliminate transmission of hepatitis B virus in the United States. Recommendations of the Advisory Committee on Immunization Practices. Part II: Immunization of Adults. *MMWR Morbid Mortal Wkly Rep.*
238. Zaman K, Roy E, Arifeen SE, et al. Effectiveness of maternal influenza immunization in mothers and infants. *N Engl J Med.* 2008;359:1555-1564.
239. Recommendations of the Advisory Committee on Immunization Practices (ACIP): use of vaccines and immune globulins for persons with altered immunocompetence. *MMWR Recomm Rep.* 1993;42:1-18.
240. Avery RK, Ljungman P. Prophylactic measures in the solid-organ recipient before transplantation. *Clin Infect Dis.* 2001;33(Suppl 1):S15-S21.
241. Stark K, Gunther M, Schonfeld C, et al. Immunisations in solid-organ transplant recipients. *Lancet.* 2002;359:957-965.
242. Duchini A, Goss JA, Karpen S, et al. Vaccinations for adult solid-organ transplant recipients: current recommendations and protocols. *Clin Microbiol Rev.* 2003;16:357-364.
243. Pirofski LA, Casadevall A. Use of licensed vaccines for active immunization of the immunocompromised host. *Clin Microbiol Rev.* 1998;11:1-26.
244. Ljungman P. Vaccination in the immunocompromised host. In: Plotkin SA, Orenstein WA, Offit PA, eds. *Vaccines.* 5th ed. Philadelphia: Elsevier; 2008:1403-1416.

245. Moss WJ, Halsey NA. Vaccination of human immunodeficiency virus-infected persons. In: Plotkin SA, Orenstein WA, Offit PA, eds. *Vaccines.* 5th ed. Philadelphia: Elsevier; 2008:1417-1430.
246. Ninane J, Grymonprez A, Burtonboy G, et al. Disseminated BCG in HIV infection. *Arch Dis Child.* 1988;63:1268-1269.
247. Disseminated *Mycobacterium bovis* infection from BCG vaccination of a patient with acquired immunodeficiency syndrome. *MMWR Morb Mortal Wkly Rep.* 1985;34:227-228.
248. Measles pneumonitis following measles-mumps-rubella vaccination of a patient with HIV infection, 1993. *MMWR Morb Mortal Wkly Rep.* 1996;45:603-606.
248a. Kaplan SE, Benson C, Holmes KK, et al. Guidelines for prevention and treatment of opportunistic infections in HIV-infected adults and adolescents. Recommendations from CDC, the National Institutes of Health, and the HIV Medicine Association of the Infectious Diseases Society of America. *MMWR Morb Mort Wkly Rep.* 2009;58(RR04):1-198.
249. Siber GR, Snydman DR. Use of immune globulins in the prevention and treatment of infections. *Curr Clin Top Infect Dis.* 1992;12:208-256.
250. Ruuskanen O, Salmi TT, Halonen P. Measles vaccination after exposure to natural measles. *J Pediatr.* 1978;93:43-46.
251. Asano Y, Hirose S, Iwayama S, et al. Protective effect of immediate inoculation of a live varicella vaccine in household contacts in relation to the viral dose and interval between exposure and vaccination. *Biken J.* 1982;25:43-45.
252. Salzman MB, Garcia C. Postexposure varicella vaccination in siblings of children with active varicella. *Pediatr Infect Dis J.* 1998;17:256-257.
253. Pickering LK, Baker CJ, Freed GL, et al. Immunization Programs for Infants, Children, Adolescents, and Adults; Clinical Practice Guidelines by the Infectious Diseases Society of America (IDSA). *Clin Infect Dis.* 2009 (in press).
254. Pascual FB, McGinley EL, Zanardi LR, et al. Tetanus surveillance—United States, 1998-2000. *MMWR Surveill Summ.* 2003;52:1-8.
255. Centers for Disease Control and Prevention. *Early Release of Selected Estimates Based on Data from the 2002 National Health Interview Survey* 2004.
256. Evans G, Levine EM, Saindon EH. Legal issues. In: Plotkin SA, Orenstein WA, Offit PA, eds. *Vaccines.* 5th ed. Philadelphia: Elsevier; 2008:1651-1676.
256a. Stewart AM. When vaccine injury claims go to court. *N Engl J Med.* 2009;360:2498-2500.
257. Kaplan JE, Nelson DB, Schonberger LB, et al. The effect of immune globulin on the response to trivalent oral poliovirus and yellow fever vaccinations. *Bull World Health Organ.* 1984;62:585-590.
258. FDA approval for a combined hepatitis A and B vaccine. *MMWR Morb Mortal Wkly Rep.* 2001;50:806-807.
259. FDA approval for infants of a *Haemophilus influenzae* type b conjugate and hepatitis B (recombinant) combined vaccine. *MMWR Morb Mortal Wkly Rep.* 1997;46:107-109.
260. FDA approval of a Haemophilus b conjugate vaccine combined by reconstitution with an acellular pertussis vaccine. *MMWR Morb Mortal Wkly Rep.* 1996;45:993-995.

261. FDA licensure of diphtheria and tetanus toxoids and acellular pertussis adsorbed, hepatitis B (recombinant), and poliovirus vaccine combined, (PEDIARIX) for use in infants. *MMWR Morb Mortal Wkly Rep.* 2003;52:203-204.
262. Notice to readers: licensure of a combined live attenuated measles, mumps, rubella, and varicella vaccine. Centers for Disease Control and Prevention. *MMWR Morb Mortal Wkly Rep.* 2005;54:1212-1214.
263. Licensure of a diphtheria and tetanus toxoids and acellular pertussis adsorbed and inactivated poliovirus vaccine and guidance for use as a booster dose. *MMWR Morb Mortal Wkly Rep.* 2008;57:1078-1079.
264. Licensure of a diphtheria and tetanus toxoids and acellular pertussis adsorbed, inactivated poliovirus, and Haemophilus B conjugate vaccine and guidance for use in infants and children. *MMWR Morb Mortal Wkly Rep.* 2008;57:1079-1080.
265. National Childhood Vaccine Injury Act: requirements for permanent vaccination records and for reporting of selected events after vaccination. *MMWR Morb Mortal Wkly Rep.* 1988;37:197-200.
266. Standards for child and adolescent immunization practices. National Vaccine Advisory Committee. *Pediatrics.* 2003;112:958-963.
267. Poland GA, Shefer AM, McCauley M, et al. Standards for adult immunization practices. *Am J Prev Med.* 2003;25:144-150.
268. The measles epidemic. The problems, barriers, and recommendations. The National Vaccine Advisory Committee. *JAMA.* 1991;266:1547-1552.
269. Recommendations regarding interventions to improve vaccination coverage in children, adolescents, and adults. Task Force on Community Preventive Services. *Am J Prev Med.* 2000;18(Suppl 1):92-96.
270. Orenstein WA, Rodewald LE, Hinman AR, et al. Immunization in the United States. In: Plotkin SA, Orenstein WA, Offit PA, eds. *Vaccines.* 5th ed. Philadelphia: Elsevier; 2008:1479-1510.
271. Shefer A, Briss P, Rodewald L, et al. Improving immunization coverage rates: an evidence-based review of the literature. *Epidemiol Rev.* 1999;21:96-142.
272. Bushnell CJ. The ABC's of practice-based immunization assessments. Paper presented at 28th National Immunization Conference; 1994; Washington, DC.
273. Dini EF, Chaney M, Moolenaar RL, et al. Information as intervention: how Georgia used vaccination coverage data to double public sector vaccination coverage in seven years. *J Public Health Manag Pract.* 1996;2:45-49.
274. Recommendations of the Advisory Committee on Immunization Practices, the American Academy of Pediatrics, and the American Academy of Family Physicians: use of reminder and recall by vaccination providers to increase vaccination rates. *MMWR Morb Mortal Wkly Rep.* 1998;47:715-717.
275. Linkins RW, Feikema SM. Immunization registries: the cornerstone of childhood immunization in the 21st century. *Pediatr Ann.* 1998;27:349-354.
276. Wexler DL, Anderson TA, eds. Websites that contain information about immunization. In: Plotkin SA, Orenstein WA, Offit PA, eds. *Vaccines.* 5th ed. Philadelphia: Elsevier; 2008.

321

Bioterrorism: An Overview

LUCIANA BORIO | NOREEN A. HYNES | DONALD A. HENDERSON

Concerns about the possible use of microbes by bioterrorists have increased significantly over the past decade.[1,2] The havoc that could be generated by such an attack was illustrated in 2001 when a small number of letters laced with *Bacillus anthracis* spores were disseminated via the U.S. postal system.[3] Although only 22 persons became ill and five geographic areas were actually affected, fear and apprehension extended across the country and around the world.[4-6]

There is general consensus (among those who are most knowledgeable about bioterrorism and the potential use of biotechnology for subversive goals) that the release of one or more biological agents is inevitable.[7,8] The release and subsequent spread of a contagious agent, such as smallpox virus, could prove catastrophic if measures for control were not promptly and effectively applied. Equally serious would be a large-scale release of a highly lethal but non-transmissible agent, such as anthrax or botulinum toxin. The possible use of genetically modified agents offers yet another dimension to the threat. It is clear that the world, including the United States, is ill prepared to deal with serious microbial challenges, whatever their source.[9,10] Complacency about present capabilities to deal with these problems, such as has characterized the public health and the medical communities, is no longer an acceptable policy.

Use of Biological Weapons before the 21st Century

USE BEFORE THE 20TH CENTURY

Attempts to deliberately induce infectious diseases among enemy forces dates back to the Roman era when Roman armies used the bodies of animals and humans to contaminate water supplies.[11] The effectiveness of these efforts is not clear. Given the problems of sanitation in earlier times and the natural prevalence of waterborne infections, a further degradation of water quality probably contributed only marginally to general morbidity and it is doubtful that such efforts altered significantly the course of history. An often cited exception was the plague of Caffensistera, also known as Caffa or Kaffa, in the 14th century, which was said to have resulted from cadavers being slung from trebuchets into the city by its Mongol besiegers who had carried plague with them from Asia.[12] The Genoese defenders fled and, coincident with their flight, the Black Death began to spread across Europe, killing perhaps one-third of the population.[12] However, the explanation for the Kaffa episode as the instigator of the Black Death ignores the fact that plague-transmitting fleas leave cadavers soon after death in order to parasitize living hosts. The corpses were, thus, unlikely to have been bearing competent vectors.[13] A more likely explanation is that infection occurred as the result of the natural spread of disease through urban and sylvatic rodent populations.

Smallpox, at least in the Americas, was seen to be a particularly useful weapon soon after its inadvertent introduction by Cortez in 1520. Native American communities experienced case-fatality rates of 70% or more after virus introduction. The French, Spanish, English, and, later, the Americans are cited as having deliberately initiated outbreaks, sometimes using fomites, such as blankets, to transmit infection.[14] A particularly well-documented episode occurred in 1763 during the French and Indian Wars in which British officers took blankets from patients in the Smallpox Hospital and gave them to the Indians "to convey the Smallpox to the Indians."[15]

During the years of the American Revolution, there were a number of reports of civilians afflicted with smallpox being sent or transported by British army officers to infect Revolutionary troops and citizens.[16] Smallpox posed a more serious threat to the Americans because British and Hessian soldiers had grown up in more densely populated Europe, where most smallpox cases occurred in children. Those who survived to adulthood were fully protected against a second attack.

The first deliberate attempts on the part of British forces to spread smallpox during the American Revolutionary War were reported during the 1775-1776 siege of Boston, and later reports emanated from Quebec, Virginia, and New Hampshire. How many such outbreaks were deliberately induced is not known. With the advent of war and the movement of people and armies, smallpox could and did spread widely by natural means. Although smallpox played an important role during the Revolutionary War period, it is thought to be unlikely that its use as a weapon contributed significantly to deciding the conflict.

USE DURING THE 20TH CENTURY

The potential use of other pathogens as biological weapons had to await the development of modern microbiology when specific agents could be identified, grown, and produced in quantity. In the early part of the 20th century biological weapons were developed by states as part of their warfare armamentarium. However, with later evolution of the biological and microbiological sciences, the state's infrastructure was no longer essential for the production and dissemination of bioweapons, thus adding the words bioterrorism and biocrime to our vocabulary.

State-Sponsored Biological Weapons Programs

World War I Activities. The advent of World War I provided the stimulus for the development of "special" weapons systems, but most efforts were directed to the development and application of chemical weapons. However, German scientists did work with two agents intended for use in animals: *Bacillus anthracis* (for anthrax) and *Burkholderia mallei* (for glanders). German saboteurs, working in Allied countries, including the United States, endeavored to infect horses, mules, and sheep, primarily to impact transport and cavalry operations.[17] Attempts to spread cholera in Italy and plague in Russia were alleged but are probably not credible. In brief, biological weapons in World War I were, at most, a minor nuisance.

The horrors of chemical warfare effects during World War I precipitated international efforts to develop a treaty that would prohibit the future use of chemicals as offensive weapons. It was decided to extend this to biological weapons as well. Thus, in 1925, a unique treaty was agreed upon that, for the first time in history, banned an entire class of weapons.[13] The "1925 Geneva Protocol for the Prohibition of the Use in War of Asphyxiating, Poisonous or Other Gases and of Bacteriological Methods of Warfare" was eventually signed by 108 nations. It did not, however, proscribe basic research, production, or possession of biological weapons. Many countries ratified the protocol while stipulating that they had the right to retaliate should they be attacked. No provision was made for verification. Following World War I, a number of the signatories began biological weapons programs, including Belgium, Canada, France, Great Britain, Italy, Japan, the Netherlands, Poland, and the Soviet Union. The United States was not a signatory to the treaty until 1972, but it did not begin its own biological weapons program until 1942.[13]

PART IV Special Problems

World War II Activities. Biological weapons are known to have been used during World War II only by Japan and possibly by the Soviet Union and the Polish Resistance, although consequential research and development programs were conducted by the United States, Germany, and the United Kingdom. The Japanese biological weapons program was a vast enterprise. It consisted of a major center in Pingfan, Manchuria (termed Unit 731) with more than 3000 scientists plus smaller units at a number of other sites in China. Another center (Unit 100) worked primarily with animal and plant diseases including glanders, sheep and cattle plague, and red rust and mosaic plant diseases. More than 10,000 prisoners died as a result of experimental infections or execution following experimentation.[13,18] At least 11 cities in China were attacked using, variously, anthrax, cholera, shigella, salmonella, and plague organisms to contaminate food and water supplies. Fleas were infected with the plague bacillus and released by aircraft over cities. Data regarding the success of the efforts to infect civilian populations is sketchy. Large outbreaks of cholera and plague are known to have occurred, but it is believed that transmission in any given area was not long sustained.

Except for the Japanese initiative, whose impact is difficult to gauge, biological weapons played no significant role in World War II. Information about the possible use of biological weapons by the Soviet Union was provided by Alibek, who believes that tularemia was used at Stalingrad in 1942 against German panzers and Q fever in 1943 among German troops on leave in the Crimea.[19] Germany undertook a number of experimental studies of a variety of agents and was thought, at the time, to be preparing to use organisms as biological weapons. In consequence, Britain and the United States also undertook a variety of studies of different agents and, with Britain, prepared to utilize anthrax in cattle feed or bombs should retaliatory measures be decided upon. No actions, however, were ever taken.

Immediate Post–World War II Biological Weapons Program Development. The extent and sophistication of the Japanese program came to be known after the war when Japanese scientists were offered amnesty from war crimes prosecution for the information provided. This information served as an impetus to the expansion of biological weapons programs in a number of countries, including the United States, United Kingdom, Australia, France, and Canada. These programs grew and developed from 1945 until the Biological and Toxin Weapons Convention[20] came into effect in 1972.

In the United States, the principal biological weapons research site was located at Fort Detrick, Maryland; a production facility was constructed at Pine Bluff, Arkansas.[13] Studies conducted were wide-ranging. Seven human disease organisms were weaponized and stockpiled: *B. anthracis* (anthrax), botulinum toxin, *Francisella tularensis* (tularemia), *Brucella suis* (brucellosis), *Coxiella burnetii* (Q fever), staphylococcal enterotoxin B (food poisoning), and Venezuelan equine encephalitis. Countermeasures were developed, including vaccines and antibiotics, and technical advances were made that permitted large-scale fermentation and storage of agents. Studies of animal responses were conducted at Fort Detrick, in atolls in the Pacific, and at desert sites in the United States. Experiments using simulant organisms in aerosols were conducted in a number of cities to gain information about the survival time of organisms and patterns of dispersal.[21]

The Cold War Era. As time passed, there was increasing international concern regarding the population risks posed by biological weapons and concern that the 1925 Geneva Protocol was not sufficiently explicit about what could and could not be done. Moreover, the Protocol lacked verification procedures. Accordingly, in 1969, draft proposals for a new protocol were submitted to the Committee on Disarmament of the United Nations. Meanwhile, President Nixon terminated the U.S. offensive biological weapons program by Executive Orders in 1969 and 1970. A Biological Weapons Convention[20] was eventually agreed upon in 1972 and went into effect in 1975. The agreement reached by the 103 co-signing nations was "never to develop, produce, stockpile or otherwise acquire or retain microbial or other biological agents or toxins, whatever their origin or method of production, of types and in quantities that have no justification for prophylactic, protective or other peaceful purpose; and weapons, equipment or means of delivery designed to use such agents or toxins for hostile purposes or in armed conflict."[17]

During the 27 years that elapsed between the end of World War II and the signing of the Biological Weapons Convention, the United States was engaged in conflicts in Korea and Vietnam. During this period, there were a number of allegations, primarily by Communist bloc countries, that the United States was guilty of having used one or more agents against their adversaries. There were other allegations that biological agents had been used by those engaged in the Middle East conflict.[17] No convincing evidence of such actions was ever produced.

In the late 1980s and early 1990s serious new concerns arose regarding the bioweapons capability of the Soviet Union. Through defectors, it was learned that the Soviet bioweapons program was an enterprise far more extensive and sophisticated than any had imagined at the end of the Cold War.[19] Following the signing of the 1972 Biological Weapons Convention, the Soviet Union had decided to invest heavily in a greatly expanded program. By the 1990s, its complement of some 60,000 staff working on biological weapons research equaled or exceeded that which worked in its nuclear weapons program. One of the larger and more sophisticated of the facilities, called VECTOR, is located in Koltsovo, Novosibirsk. Through the early 1990s, VECTOR was a 4000-person, 30-building complex with high biological security facilities for laboratories and for isolation of human cases. It was at VECTOR that, during the 1980s, the technical problems were solved for the large-scale production of smallpox virus intended for use as an offensive weapon. With the dissolution of the Soviet Union, more than half of the scientific staff has left VECTOR, as has staff from other bioweapons laboratories, because of diminished government funding. Many have been recruited to laboratories in other parts of the world. The VECTOR laboratory and the Centers for Disease Control and Prevention (CDC), in Atlanta, are the only two repositories now designated by the World Health Organization (WHO) for smallpox virus. Both continue to do research on smallpox, albeit under the sanction of a specially constituted WHO committee. VECTOR has also continued work on other biological agents of concern such as Ebola, Marburg, and other hemorrhagic fever viruses.

Another facility of concern was the Soviet Union's principal production center for smallpox virus located near Moscow, at Sergiev Posad. It was able to produce upwards of 20 tons of smallpox virus annually, primarily for use in intercontinental ballistic missiles (ICBMs). The laboratory is still intact and is still a top secret facility operated by the Ministry of Defense of the Russian Federation.[22]

At the End of the 20th Century. Near the close of the last century, the U.S. Departments of State and Defense identified seven countries with confirmed (Iran, Iraq, Libya, North Korea, and Syria) or suspected (Cuba, Sudan) biological weapons programs.[23-25] Five years following the Gulf War of 1990, Iraq was discovered to have had a startlingly large biological weapons program. The discovery followed the defection and revelations by Hussein Kamal, Saddam Hussein's son-in-law, who had responsibility for the Iraqi program. Thereafter, Iraq documented, in a report to the United Nations, that it had produced, filled, and deployed bombs, rockets, and aircraft with spray tanks containing *Bacillus anthracis* and botulinum toxin.[26,27] Notably, since the onset of the Iraq War in 2003, no biological weapons have been found in Iraq.

Non–State-Sponsored Development and Use of Biological Weapons

Non–state-sponsored use of biological weapons can either be bioterrorism, committed by terrorists in support of a specific ideology and often directed at a large number of persons, or biocrimes, directed at one or a few people. There was low-level biological weapon use throughout most of the 20th century. Among 881 non–state-sponsored bioweapons casualties, 751 (85%) resulted from one incident of bioterrorism and 130 (15%) from biocrimes; all 10 fatal cases were among victims of biocrimes.[2] Some bioterrorism was directed at animals rather than humans or failed to have its intended effect in people.[28]

Then, in September 1984, members of the Rajneeshee religious cult deliberately contaminated contents of salad bars along a stretch of an Oregon interstate highway with *Salmonella typhimurium* (now *Salmonella enterica* subsp. *enterica* serovar Typhimurium), causing 751 persons to become ill; 45 persons were hospitalized. There were no deaths.[29] Additionally, a particularly disturbing event occurred in 1995 in Japan when a little-known apocalyptic religious cult, Aum Shinrikyo, released the nerve gas sarin in the Tokyo subway. The cult was later discovered to have had plans for biological terrorism,[30] and, in fact, it undertook on several occasions to spray an aerosol of anthrax organisms throughout metropolitan Tokyo. Fortunately, there were no casualties, as the cult mistakenly used a greatly attenuated anthrax vaccine strain rather than a naturally occurring virulent strain. In addition, members of this group traveled to Zaire in 1992 to try to obtain samples of Ebola virus for weapons development.[31]

The Changing Perspective Regarding the Threat from Biological Weapons

Serious concerns about the potential use of the so-called "weapons of mass destruction" arose in the context of the Cold War and focused originally on nuclear weapons and the potential of these to result in the ultimate scenario of a "nuclear winter."[32] Chemical weapons remained on the agenda of concerns given their extensive use during World War I. Concern about biological weapons waned even more significantly in the 1970s, coincident with President Nixon's initiative in 1969 to terminate the U.S. offensive biological weapons program and the subsequent endorsement by many countries of the 1972 Convention on the Prohibition, Production, and Stockpiling of Bacteriological (Biological) and Toxin Weapons and on their Destruction (usually referred to as the Biological Weapons Convention, BWC, or the Biological and Toxin Weapons Convention, BTWC).[20] The Convention called for the destruction of all stocks of biological weapons and the cessation of research on their use as offensive agents.

Among those in national policy circles, and the public health and medical communities, three points of view predominated until about 1995 that served to discourage consideration of biological weapons as more than a theoretical possibility:

1. That biological weapons had been deployed so rarely that precedent would suggest they would not be used.
2. That their use is so morally repugnant that no nation state or organized group would deign to use them.
3. That it is technologically so difficult to produce organisms in quantity and to disperse them that the science is beyond the reach of any but the most sophisticated laboratories.

Each of these arguments has been shown to be invalid. We now know that there are nations and dissident groups who have both the motivation and access to skills to cultivate successfully some of the most dangerous pathogens and to deploy them as agents in acts of terrorism or war. This was borne out in the anthrax attacks of late 2001 during which a yet to be definitely identified person or group (despite claims to the contrary by the U.S. Federal Bureau of Investigation) for yet undefined reasons sent letters containing anthrax spores to various media and political figures. The aerosolization of the spores both in high-speed processing machines and upon opening of the letters led to 22 cases of anthrax (11 inhalational, 11 cutaneous) with a case fatality rate of 54% among those with inhalational disease.[3] Methods for transforming biological agents into weapons are known, and the requirements for space and sophisticated equipment to produce them are modest.

It is clear that preventing the proliferation and use of biological weapons or countering them will be extremely difficult. Detection or interdiction of those intending to use biological weapons is next to impossible. Thus, the first evidence of intent to use such weapons will very likely be the appearance of sick people in hospital emergency rooms. The rapidity with which those front-line health care workers and others, such as infectious disease specialists and laboratory scientists, can reach a proper diagnosis and the speed with which preventative and/or therapeutic measures are applied could well spell the difference between thousands and, perhaps, tens of thousands of casualties. Indeed, the survival of the health care staff caring for the patients may be at stake. A challenge, however, is that few have ever seen patients with diseases caused by those agents most likely to be employed—as, for example, smallpox, plague, or anthrax.

Assessing Which Biological Organisms Are of Greatest Concern

ASSESSING THE THREAT AND RISK OF A BIOLOGICAL WEAPONS ATTACK

In theory, hundreds if not thousands of infectious agents and toxins could conceivably be employed as biological weapons, but few possess characteristics of virulence or contagiousness that would seriously disrupt normal community life or threaten the continuity of government. Indeed, each year, countless naturally transmitted infectious disease outbreaks occur throughout the world, some carried in water or food, some transmitted by the respiratory route, and some by vectors. Most of these outbreaks are small although some, such as influenza, can be regional or global, leading to significant morbidity and mortality burden. However, at least in the industrialized countries, the existing infrastructure of medical and public health staff is able to cope with most of these without undue difficulty. Contagious diseases have not seriously tested the U.S. health care system or significantly disrupted civilian life in most industrialized countries since the 1918 influenza pandemic.[33] Conversely, non-communicable diseases have had significant impacts. For example, the anthrax letter attacks for 2001, despite low morbidity and mortality, had a profound impact upon the U.S. population.[5,34] The attacks also highlighted gaps in the public health infrastructure in the United States and beyond.[35-37]

It is clear that certain agents if used as biological weapons could result in public health catastrophes and that special measures need to be taken to prevent their occurrence or, at least, to deal with them. Determining how to focus limited resources is a key to preparedness and response efforts. Two critical elements are used to assess and to estimate which biological organisms are of greatest concern: threat assessment and risk assessment.

Threat assessment is traditionally carried out by the intelligence community and is focused on three areas. These critical areas include the probability of an attack, given identified near-term threats; an evaluation of an adversary's capability to acquire, produce, and disseminate an agent; and an assessment of vulnerabilities that increase the likelihood of a successful attack.[38-40]

Risk assessment, either qualitative or quantitative, falls within the purview of science, medicine, and public health. An assessment includes four components: hazard identification, dose-response assessment, exposure assessment, and risk characterization, all leading to the estimated incidence of illness or other adverse outcomes from a particular biological agent.[39,40] A risk assessment seeks to answer critical questions needed for policy decision makers on how to focus finite resources and to guide those responsible for communicating the results of the assessment and related decisions to the population.

In the past, different governments and agencies compiled lists of organisms that represented potential biological weapons threats, but few had given appropriate consideration as to which were of sufficient concern to civilian populations to warrant special preparedness measures. Until 1998, no review of this sort had been undertaken by U.S. federal authorities. It was clear that there was a need to identify agents of the highest priority, to develop a basic strategy for containing outbreaks caused by these agents, and to get agreement on the best methods for treatment of patients. Accordingly, in 1998, a broadly representative, informal Working Group on Civilian Biodefense was convened at the Johns Hopkins Center for Civilian Biodefense Studies to examine these issues. Included in the group were federal experts from the CDC, the Food and Drug Administration (FDA), the Army Medical Research Institute of Infectious Diseases (USAMRIID) at Fort Detrick, state and local health officials, clinicians, and scientists with special expertise and knowledge of the most serious bioweapons agents.

It was decided by the group that the agents of special concern should be those that, under epidemic circumstance, could threaten the functioning of civil government. Many factors had to be weighed with respect to each candidate biological agent, including the magnitude of disease morbidity and mortality, contagiousness, number of organisms needed to infect, availability of therapeutic or preventive measures, difficulties in diagnosis, feasibility of organisms being obtained and grown in quantity, stability of the organisms in the environment, and the likely response of a population to an epidemic of an historically feared disease such as plague or smallpox. Eventually, five agents and a diagnostic group were identified as being those of special concern, warranting the development of special preparatory measures to respond to an attack. The diseases were smallpox, anthrax, plague, botulinum toxin poisoning, and tularemia and the "viral hemorrhagic fevers" (such as Ebola, Marburg, and Lassa fever). None of these are known clinically to more than a very few medical or public health staff in the United States and, until the Working Group had met, there had been no consensus on their preventive or therapeutic measures. Special reviews of each of these agents were undertaken and published in the *Journal of the American Medical Association* (JAMA).[41-46] These were later updated and, with additional papers dealing with the U.S. anthrax outbreak, published by JAMA in 2002 under the title, *Bioterrorism: Guidelines for Medical and Public Health Management*.[47]

Some months after the Working Group had met and decided on this list, a meeting was convened by the CDC at which the same consensus was reached as to the agents of greatest concern. These are now commonly referred to as Category A agents. A lower priority group was identified and labeled as Category B agents. A Category C list was compiled that included emerging pathogens (Table 321-1).

OBTAINING AND PRODUCING BIOLOGICAL WEAPONS

Some have assumed that because the likely pathogens to be used as biological weapons are comparatively rare it would be difficult for a prospective terrorist to acquire the organisms. This is not the case. The Russian Federation is one of several possible sources of organisms, including some that have been genetically engineered. All the organisms of greatest concern were subjects of study in the former Soviet biological weapons program. Most of the laboratories are still in operation, and many scientists, like those at the smallpox laboratory in Novosibirsk, continue work on organisms that could be used as biological weapons. Many that were employed by the program were among the Soviet Union's best scientists, but half or more have left the laboratories for work elsewhere, some having gone to countries now suspected of having their own bioweapons programs. Whether they have carried specimens with them is unknown.

There are other sources for strains of the Category A agents. Cases of plague, anthrax, tularemia, and botulism occur regularly in many countries of the world, including the United States. After processing such specimens, it was customary, until recently, for microbiologists to preserve the isolates in freezers for possible future reference. Thus, there are a great many laboratories around the world that have such isolates in their possession. On request, laboratories often would send strains of organisms to other laboratories and, as of December 2001, some 46 laboratories outside the United States advertised the availability of anthrax isolates on their Web sites. However, since the anthrax letter attacks of 2001, certain selected microbial agents and toxins are closely regulated under the oversight of the CDC and the Animal and Plant Health Inspection Service. These government programs regulate the possession, use, and transfer of these agents and require registration of all U.S. laboratories that handle these agents.[48]

GROWING AND "WEAPONIZING" THE AGENTS

In contrast to the challenges of acquiring functional nuclear weapons, production of biological weapons is simpler and less expensive. For many of the Category A agents, production is reasonably straightforward, especially for those with expertise. Those without access to such expertise now can obtain it from the Internet as well as through academic courses, including sophisticated methods that could be used for genetic engineering of pathogens. Existing or new biomedical production facilities or industries could be converted to the production of microorganisms for bioweapons owing to the dual-use nature of manufacturing equipment and supplies. Notably, comparatively little space is required, and for most agents, comparatively small quantities need to be aerosolized to produce large numbers of casualties. In 1999, Defense Threat Reduction Agency (DTRA) undertook project BACCHUS (Biotechnology Activity Characterization by Unconventional Signatures) to assess whether production of biological weapons would lead to signatures that would allow detection. The project found it would be relatively simple for a terrorist to assemble such a facility without being detected. This finding is supported by noting that a small team of scientists without prior training in biological weapons development built a clandestine laboratory in Nevada and produced

TABLE 321-1	CDC Bioterrorism Agents and Disease Categories		
Category	*A*	*B*	*C*
Priority	*1*	*2*	*3*
Characteristics	Easily disseminated or spread person-to-person Highly lethal Serious public health effects May cause great panic and social disruption	Moderately easy to disseminate Moderate morbidity Less lethal than category A agents Requires fewer special public health preparations	Includes emerging infectious diseases Potential for wide dissemination in the future could result in high morbidity, lethality, and major public health effects
Disease (agent)	Anthrax (*Bacillus anthracis*) Botulism (*Clostridium botulinum* toxin) Plague (*Yersinia pestis*) Smallpox (*Variola*) Tularemia (*Francisella tularensis*) Hemorrhagic fever viruses	Brucellosis (*Brucella* species) Epsilon toxin of *Clostridium perfringens* Food safety threats (e.g., *Salmonella*) Glanders (*Burkholderia mallei*) Melioidosis (*Burkholderia pseudomallei*) Psittacosis (*Chlamydia psittaci*) Q fever (*Coxiella burnetii*) Ricin toxin from *Ricinus communis* (castor beans) Staphylococcal enterotoxin B Typhus fever (*Rickettsia prowazekii*) Viral encephalitis (e.g., Venezuelan equine encephalitis) Water safety threats (e.g., *Vibrio cholerae*)	Emerging infectious disease threats such as Nipah virus and Hantavirus

simulated anthrax with materials purchased on the open market, mostly from a local hardware store, with a budget of less than $1.5 million.[49]

Various methods might be used for dispersing biological weapons, the most common being contamination of food or water supplies and aerosol dispersion. There is general consensus that aerosols pose the most serious threat to the civilian population. Organisms dispersed by other means could cause disease outbreaks, but they would be much less likely to cause epidemic disease on a scale great enough to threaten the integrity of civil government. Each of the Category A agents could be disseminated in a fine particle aerosol in the range of 1 to 5 microns. Such particles are inhaled and penetrate deeply into the lung. Larger sized particles, in contrast, are trapped in the upper airways and usually do not succeed at initiating infection. An aerosol of this size is invisible to the naked eye and behaves much like smoke in that it is able to penetrate most interior air spaces. With an appropriate coating of most organisms, aerosolized particles can remain suspended and viable for many hours to days. In the Sverdlovsk anthrax outbreak, humans became ill who were as far as 4 km from the point of release; animals that were 50 km away also developed anthrax.[50]

Generating an aerosol is comparatively straightforward with any of a number of off-the-shelf devices such as paint sprayers, fogging machines that disseminate insecticides, purse-size perfume atomizers, and hand-held drug delivery devices such as used by asthma patients. Even small releases of an agent would, almost certainly, result in serious public concern as was witnessed during the anthrax release in the United States in 2001. Repeated releases in different parts of the country could be devastating, especially if the public health response were seen as deficient. A large-scale release, of itself, could be as devastating as a nuclear weapon. An Office of Technology Assessment report estimated that if 100 kg of anthrax spores was released upwind of Washington, D.C. by means of a crop-duster aircraft, between 130,000 and 3 million deaths would result.[51]

With respect to other methods of dispersion, some cities have expressed special concerns about water reservoirs being contaminated and have invested in costly preventive measures. However, most Category A agents cannot be disseminated by water. For those that can, the quantities needed to contaminate a reservoir sufficient to infect the consumer would be prodigious. This reflects the facts that of the water distributed from reservoirs, only a small proportion is actually consumed and normal water treatment itself destroys many organisms. Contamination of food, likewise, is viewed with concern by some, primarily because of the threat posed by botulinum toxin. A successful attack, however, faces several barriers, including difficulties in producing the toxin in quantity and at a level of purity that would not cause the food to be unpalatable, and the identification of a food of proper chemical constituents that would enable the toxin to survive. Because botulinum toxin acts rapidly and has distinctive clinical symptoms, cases, in any event, would be likely to be diagnosed quickly and the contaminated products removed from commerce. One scenario has suggested the possibility of contaminating raw milk in a tanker truck, thereby potentially permitting a large number of persons to be poisoned over a short period of time and before much of the milk could be withdrawn.[52] Given the number of barriers to overcome in executing so complex an attack, it is difficult to recommend this as a priority concern.

◾ Pathogens of Greatest Concern

Most agencies that have developed lists of agents that might be used as biological weapons customarily identify a substantial number of possibilities but agree that only a handful of agents share the characteristics of being reasonably simple to prepare and disperse, and of being able to inflict sufficiently severe disease to paralyze a city, perhaps even a nation. In 1994, Vorobjev, a Soviet bioweapons expert, presented to a working group of the U.S. National Academy of Sciences the conclusions of Soviet experts as to the agents most likely to be used as bioweapons.[53] Smallpox headed the list and was followed closely by

anthrax and plague. A Russian defector later reported that the Soviet Union had regularly stockpiled 30 metric tons of dried anthrax spores and 20 tons each of smallpox, plague, and tularemia—all of which had been modified for use as weapons.[19] What effect the release of one of these agents might have is not certain and relies mainly on imperfect mathematical models. None has so far been deployed effectively as a biological weapon in significant quantities, and thus no real-world events exist that provide the basis for suggesting likely scenarios.

SMALLPOX AS A BIOLOGICAL WEAPON

Smallpox spreads from person to person in a continuing chain of infection. Among those who have never been vaccinated, 30% die of the disease. Although specific antiviral therapies are being developed,[54] none is currently licensed for this indication.

Many have forgotten how concerned countries of the world were about smallpox. For example, until 1972, the United States mandated smallpox vaccination for all children at school entry despite the fact that no cases had occurred in the country since 1949. In the United Kingdom, through the 1970s, four standby hospitals were maintained, to be opened only if cases of smallpox were imported. In Germany, two state-of-the-art smallpox isolation hospitals were constructed in the 1960s. Tourists everywhere carried yellow vaccination books attesting to the fact that they had been successfully vaccinated within the preceding 3 years. Until 1980, essentially all countries conducted routine vaccination programs of some sort whether or not they had endemic disease.[1]

Two importations of smallpox into Europe during the 1970s illustrate the nature of the threat posed. The potential for smallpox as an aerosolized agent was illustrated in an outbreak in Germany in 1970.[55] That year, a German electrician returning from Pakistan became desperately ill with high fever and diarrhea. On January 11, he was admitted to a local hospital and isolated in a private room because it was feared he might have typhoid fever. He had contact with only two nurses during his stay. On January 14, he developed a rash and 2 days later, the diagnosis of smallpox was confirmed. After diagnosis, the patient was immediately transported to a special isolation hospital; more than 100,000 area residents were promptly vaccinated; and hospital patients and staff were vaccinated and quarantined. The patient had had a cough, a symptom seldom seen with smallpox. Coughing produces a small-particle aerosol much as one could expect were smallpox to be used as a terrorist weapon. Subsequently, 19 cases occurred in the hospital, including three in other rooms on the patient's floor of the hospital, seven on the floor above, and nine on the third floor. One of those afflicted was a visitor who had spent less than 15 minutes in the hospital and had only briefly opened a corridor door, easily 30 feet from the patient's room, to ask for directions. The outbreak illustrated the potential for smallpox virus in aerosol form to spread over a great distance and to infect at very low doses.

An outbreak in Yugoslavia in February 1972 was instructive in demonstrating the havoc created even by a small number of cases.[56] Yugoslavia's last previous case of smallpox had occurred 45 years before, in 1927. Nevertheless, Yugoslavia, like most countries, had continued a routine vaccination program to protect itself should an importation occur. In 1972, a pilgrim returning from the Middle East became ill with an undiagnosed febrile disease. Friends and relatives visited from a number of different areas and 2 weeks later, 11 of them developed high fever and rash. None of the physicians who saw the patients diagnosed the cases as smallpox. Few had ever seen a case.

One of the eleven who acquired smallpox was a 30-year-old teacher who quickly became critically ill with the hemorrhagic form of the disease. This form of smallpox is not readily diagnosed even by experts. He was treated first at a local clinic, but as he became increasingly ill, he was transferred to a large city hospital and, eventually, to a critical care unit because he was bleeding profusely and in shock. He died without a definitive diagnosis. Four weeks elapsed after the first patient became ill before cases were correctly diagnosed. By then, 150 persons were ill. Among them were 38 who were infected by the young teacher in the hospital. The cases occurred in widely separated areas of the country, and by the time of diagnosis, they had already begun to expose yet another generation.

Each of the neighboring countries closed its borders to all traffic. Government health authorities saw no alternative but to launch a nation-wide vaccination campaign. Mass vaccination clinics were held, and check points along roads were established where vaccination certificates were examined. Twenty million persons were vaccinated. Hotels and residential apartments were taken over, cordoned off by the military, and all known contacts of cases forcibly moved into these centers under military guard. Some 10,000 persons spent 2 weeks or more under such surveillance. The outbreak stopped 9 weeks after the first patient became ill—175 patients had developed smallpox and 35 had died—in a generally well-vaccinated population. It was, in fact, a small outbreak.

What might happen if smallpox were to be released today in a modern city? Because routine vaccination stopped more 30 years ago, there are large numbers who have never been vaccinated. For others, vaccine immunity has been waning for more than 30 years. It is likely that no more than 25% of the population in the United States or most other countries have significant residual protective immunity.[57] Suppose that some modest quantity of virus were to be released as an aerosol. The event would probably go unnoticed until the first patients developed fever and rash some 7 to 10 days later. With patients being treated in different clinics and by those who almost certainly had never before seen a smallpox case, several days might elapse before the first cases would be diagnosed and an alert sounded.

Even if no more than 100 persons had actually been infected, dealing even with that number would be a challenge. All would have to be isolated, and as soon as smallpox was suspected, many others with fever and rash would be identified as possible cases and would also have to be screened and isolated until the diagnosis was certain. Most hospitals have no more than a handful of rooms that can ensure airborne isolation precautions, and few communities have developed plans to accommodate large numbers of contagious patients. Couple this with the problems posed by the occurrence of one or two severe hemorrhagic cases, which typically have very short incubation periods, are highly contagious, and would have already been admitted to hospitals before smallpox was suspected. They would have been cared for by a large number of unprotected emergency room and intensive care health care workers.

Predictably, there would be an immediate clamor for vaccination such as occurred in the cited outbreaks in Germany and Yugoslavia. The United States now has a large stock of vaccine, but most countries have little or none. How widely should the vaccine be distributed? Comparatively few doses might be needed if vaccine were limited strictly to close contacts of confirmed cases. However, the realities of dealing with even a modest-sized epidemic coupled with severe public anxiety would almost certainly preclude a cautious, measured vaccination effort. In most countries, such reserves of vaccine as may be present would rapidly disappear. There is, at the moment, only a limited manufacturing capacity to produce additional vaccine in only a small number of countries.

ANTHRAX AS A BIOLOGICAL WEAPON

Anthrax was a principal weapon in the arsenal of the former Soviet Union and is known to have been produced as a weapon by Iraq and the Aum Shinrikyo religious cult. The organism is reasonably readily available, easy to produce in large quantity, and extremely stable in its spore form. See Chapter 325 for a complete discussion of anthrax as an agent of bioterrorism.

■ Preparing for an Attack

The challenges of bioterrorism are uniquely different from those associated with dealing with an explosion or the release of a chemical agent. The worst effects of the latter, even when involving many casualties,

are quickly apparent; efforts for stabilization and recovery can begin immediately; and the toll of injuries and deaths can soon be ascertained. For biological attacks, outbreak identification signaling that an attack may have occurred would not be likely until a number of days had passed; the magnitude of the attack might not be certain for a week or more; and with smallpox, the implicit threat of further cases would cause many to live in fear that they or their families might be the next victims.[4,5,34,58] The realities of dealing with a comparatively straightforward release of a modest quantity of either smallpox or anthrax are staggering, let alone the problems that would be faced were genetically modified organisms to be used.

In the United States, health services have begun to take steps to deal with the possibility of outbreaks of disease following biological attacks that may be contagious and have high rates of morbidity and mortality. In the near term, public health systems must be prepared to promptly detect and diagnose, to characterize epidemiologically, and to respond appropriately to epidemic disease. There is a need at international, national, and local levels for a greater capacity for surveillance; a far better network of laboratories with expedient laboratory capacity; a larger cadre of trained epidemiologists, clinicians, and researchers; and better communication and coordination among those responsible for the response at the different levels. In addition to continued robust support for basic research, applied to a better understanding of pathogenesis and immunity, there is a special need to improve the organization, funding, and undertaking of research and development programs for improved therapeutic agents.

The task of anticipating the public response so as to minimize needless anxiety and encourage prosocial behavior is especially important but very difficult. There is little practical experience upon which to build, extrapolation from historical data (for example, the influenza pandemic of 1918) is problematic as many societal changes have occurred since, and surveys are inherently limited in predicting future behavior. Most importantly, the public's behavior will be influenced by the government's response and communication efforts, and these, too, are difficult to predict.

■ Response to Bioterrorism—Medical and Public Health Emergency Preparedness

It is clear that preventing the proliferation and use of biological weapons or countering them will be extremely difficult. Recipes for making biological weapons have been available on the Internet, and even groups with modest finances and basic training in biology and engineering could develop an effective weapon[59] at minimal cost. Detection or interdiction of those intending to use biological weapons is next to impossible. Thus, the first evidence of intent to use such weapons will very likely be the appearance of cases in hospital emergency rooms and physician offices. The rapidity with which these providers, both clinicians and laboratory scientists, can reach a proper diagnosis and the speed with which preventative and therapeutic measures are applied could well spell the difference between thousands, and perhaps tens of thousands, of casualties. Indeed, the survival of the health care staff caring for the patients may be at stake. However, few providers have ever seen patients with diseases caused by those agents most likely to be employed—as, for example, smallpox, plague, or anthrax.

Successful preparedness and response require political will, leadership, and transparency to all stakeholders, adequate resources (both funding and personnel), and competent personnel.[60] From the clinician's perspective, preparing to optimally respond to a bioterrorism event includes appropriate training, exercises to "harden" these training efforts, and enhanced horizontal and vertical communication between the medicine–public health interface and local, state, and federal governments.

BEFORE 9/11/2001

Most physicians and public health practitioners viewed the threat of biological weapons as negligible as recently as 1997. In most schools of medicine and schools of public health, biological and chemical weapons were regarded as being morally repugnant and not subjects that should be discussed, even from the standpoint of the threats they posed.

The terrorist events in Tokyo, Oklahoma City, and New York in the 1990s; revelations about the Soviet bioweapons program; and the discovery of Iraq's considerable investment in biological weapons created the impetus for the U.S. Congress to take more definitive steps to strengthen the country's national preparedness. As noted earlier, Congress, in 1996, passed the Defense against Weapons of Mass Destruction act. Responsibility for this activity was assigned to the Department of Defense; little money or responsibility was provided for the Department of Health and Human Services (DHHS).

Following the urging of the late Nobel laureate Joshua Lederberg, JAMA devoted its special August 6, 1997, issue to bioterrorism. The following month, the sitting Infectious Disease Society of America President, John Bartlett, convened the first symposium on biological weapons at the Society's annual meeting. With interest in the subject growing, the first National Symposium on the Medical and Public Health Response to Bioterrorism was held in Washington, D.C., in February 1998. It was convened by the Johns Hopkins Center for Civilian Biodefense Strategies and DHHS; 12 other organizations co-sponsored the event.

In May 1998, President Clinton requested that Congress provide $133 million in funds to DHHS for fiscal year 1999 in support of a new program of public health preparedness. The Assistant Secretary of Health, Dr. Margaret Hamburg, formerly Commissioner of Health for the City of New York, was given responsibility for developing a strategic plan. Most of the funds were allocated to CDC. Of the funds provided, $51 million was earmarked for the development of an emergency stockpile of antibiotics (the National Pharmaceutical Stockpile, or NPS), primarily for anthrax, and for smallpox vaccine. The balance, $82 million, provided for the initial steps to rebuild the long-neglected public health infrastructure at federal, state, and local levels. Some of these funds were used in 1999 to create a laboratory network, under the direction of CDC, to provide laboratory surge capacity, emergency assistance and support to state and local public health laboratories initially for the identification of biological threat agents and then expanded to include chemical threats. Subsequently, veterinary, military, government food testing, military, and some international laboratories were added to the network.

FOLLOWING 9/11/2001

Following the anthrax letter attacks in fall 2001, the inadequacy of the United States to respond to a sizable bioterrorism attack became evident. Preparedness and response gaps were identified in both medical and public health arenas and at all levels of government. Widespread actions were taken to address the identified gaps in preparedness to respond.

Since the 2001 terrorist attacks on the United States through fiscal year (FY) 2008, the Federal government has spent or allocated over $40 billion to 11 cabinet-level departments, $27.5 billion (69%) of which has been to DHHS (Table 321-2).[61,62] This allotment does not include the $5.6 billion placed in a special reserve fund created in October 2003 at the Department of Homeland Security for the purchase of medical countermeasures over a 10-year period by DHHS, as outlined in the Project BioShield Act of 2004.

In October 2007, the White House released Homeland Security Presidential Directive-21 (HSPD-21) establishing a "National Strategy for Public Health and Medical Preparedness." HSPD-21 was created to specifically address preparedness for catastrophic health events, defined as "any natural or manmade incident, including terrorism, that results in a number of ill or injured persons sufficient to over- whelm the capabilities of immediate local and regional emergency response and health care systems."[63]

PROVIDER AND HEALTH CARE SYSTEM PREPAREDNESS

The early detection of a potential bioterrorism event is key to minimizing morbidity and mortality. Clinically suspect cases require prompt laboratory confirmation, which is an essential step for any emergency response. Following an attack that employs any one of the Category A agents, the majority of patients would be severely, acutely ill and would be expected soon to be referred to emergency rooms with early consultation by infectious disease specialists. Thus, through a variety of educational approaches and training programs, emphasis has been placed on assuring that emergency room staff and the infectious disease specialists, in particular, are knowledgeable of the agents of greatest concern; know of the importance of prompt reporting to public health officials; and have access to laboratories that are prepared to provide rapid disease diagnosis.

Clinician Preparedness

Since 2001 most clinical professional societies have provided bioterrorism training opportunities through publications in peer-reviewed journals, on-line training modules, or symposia at professional meetings. The American Board of Internal Medicine includes questions on the diagnosis and management of patients with infections due to biological threat agents on its certifying examination in internal medicine as well as its subspecialty examination in infectious diseases. The American Association of Medical Colleges issued a 2003 report on bioterrorism training in medical school curricula and recommended integration of appropriate training in both the basic and clinical sciences. The report identified six medical schools with innovative training in bioterrorism and recommended that medical schools also train students in preparedness and response efforts. No follow-up report has been issued to reflect training changes that have been made. Also in 2003, DHHS began providing funds for bioterrorism training and curriculum development, first through the Health Resources and Services Administration (HRSA) and then from the Office of the Assistant Secretary for Preparedness and Response (ASPR). Over a 5-year period ending in FY2007, $126 million was spent on this effort.

The difficulties of sharing health care providers licensed in one state but not another was highlighted following the events of September 2001. In response, a mandated federal system of guidelines and standards was created to register, certify, and allow deployment of medical professionals across state jurisdictions in the event of a large-scale national emergency. The state-based system, called the Emergency System for Advance Registration of Volunteer Health Professionals (ESAR-VHP) is implemented at the state level with federal assistance, initially from HRSA and since December 2006 from ASPR.

In the event of a large bioterrorist incident requiring supplementation of clinical response efforts, both the National Disaster Medical System (NDMS) and the Medical Reserve Corps (MRC) can be activated. NDMS, a system coordinated by DHHS, acts to temporarily supplement state and local medical care needs following a disaster of any kind. NDMS can provide personnel, supplies, equipment at the site or at definitive care sites in unaffected areas, and needed patient care movement. Disaster Medical Assistance Teams (DMATs) are local units activated for 2-week deployments with sufficient supplies and equipment to be self-sustaining for 72 hours before resupply is needed. In the event of a national disaster, DMATs may be moved from their local area at which time they are made federal employees with medical credentials recognized in all states and protected under the Federal Tort Claims Act against any malpractice claim. Pre-disaster employment is protected under the Uniformed Services Employment and Reemployment Rights Act (USERRA). MRC was created in 2002 as community-based and locally organized groups of health care volunteers who donate their time and expertise to prepare for and respond to supplement existing emergency medical and public health resources

TABLE 321-2	Department of Health and Human Services (DHHS) Bioterrorism-Related Budget Breakdown (in $ Millions [M]), Fiscal Years (FY) 2001-2008*							
DHHS Office or Agency	FY2001	FY2002	FY2003	FY2004	FY2005	FY2006	FY2007	FY2008
Office of the Secretary (OS)								
Office of Public Health and Emergency Preparedness (OPHEP)†	63	49	42	41	41	41		
Office of the Assistant Secretary for Preparedness and Response (ASPR)‡							8	10
Operations							14	17
Preparedness and Emergency Operations							47	46
National Disaster Medical System (NDMS)§							474	423
Hospital Preparedness Grants‖							21	0
Training and Curriculum Development¶							104	102
Advanced Research and Development (for Medical Countermeasures)#							16	21
Project BioShield Management							9	9
International Early Warning Surveillance							3	4
Media/Public Information Campaign								
Subtotal ASPR							693	632
Metropolitan Medical Response System (MMRS)**	(17)‖‖	22	50	0	0	0	0	0
Healthcare Provider Credentialing System							0	0
Medical Reserve Corps	0	3	10	10	10	10	10	10
Revitalization/Transformation of the Commissioned Corps of the U.S. Public Health Service	0	0	0	3	3	4	10	4
Subtotal, OS	80	74	102	54	54	54	716	646
Food and Drug Administration (FDA)								
Food Safety and Defense††	1	98	97	116	150	158	172	171
Medical Countermeasures (MCM): Vaccines, Drugs, Diagnostics	6	46	53	53	57	57	57	56
Physical Security	2	13	7	7	7	7	7	7
Subtotal FDA	9	157	157	176	214	222	235	237
Health Resources and Services Administration (HRSA)								
Bioterrorism Hospital Preparedness‖	0	135	514	515	487	474	0	0
Bioterrorism Training and Curriculum Development¶	0	0	28	28	28	21	0	0
Smallpox Vaccination Compensation Program	0	0	42	0	0	0	0	0
Subtotal HRSA	0	135	584	543	515	494	0	0

*From DHHS Budget in Brief for FY2003, FY2004, FY2005, FY2006, FY2007, FY2008. Available at: http://www.hhs.gov/budget/docbudget.htm except where specifically noted.

†OPHEP was formed in FY2002 from a merger of the Office of Emergency Preparedness and the Office of Public Health Preparedness. The two offices combined included $63M in FY2001. These figures include $30M for "advanced research" in FY2001, $5M in FY2002, and $5M in FY2003. No information is available in the budget regarding research in subsequent years.

‡OPHEP ceased to exist on Dec. 19, 2006, when *The Pandemic and All-Hazards Preparedness Act* (Public Law 109-417) was enacted and created the ASPR. Functions previously carried out by OPHEP were transferred to ASPR.

§NDMS was originally part of the Office of Emergency Preparedness (OEP) and part of DHHS. It merged with the Office of Public Health Preparedness to become OPHEP. Certain functions of OEP, including NDMS and the Metropolitan Medical Response System (MMRS) were transferred to the Department of Homeland Security pursuant to the *Homeland Security Act of 2002*. NDMS and MMRS returned to DHHS with the enactment of P.L. 109-417, *The Pandemic and All-Hazards Preparedness Act*.

‖This is a continuation of the "Bioterrorism Hospital Preparedness" program previously under the auspices of the Health Resources and Services Administration. The program was transferred to ASPR in FY2007.

¶This is a continuation of the "Bioterrorism Training and Curriculum Development" program previously under the auspices of the Human Resources and Services Administration. The program was transferred to ASPR in FY2007.

#This was in the NIH budget in FY2006 and was transferred to the ASPR pursuant to P.L. 109-417, *The Pandemic and All-Hazards Preparedness Act*. Funds for late-stage development of medical countermeasures targeted for acquisition by DHHS for use during large-scale public health emergencies.

when needed. There are over 300 MRC units in the United States. Units have been active, for example, in providing services following hurricanes in 2004 and 2005. The Office of the U.S. Surgeon General acts as a clearinghouse for information and best practices in establishing and maintaining MRC units. Liability protection for individual MRC practitioners is determined by each state.

Emergency Use Authorization

During a public health catastrophic event, new drugs, vaccines, biologics, or diagnostics may be needed before they have completed their regulatory pathway to approval (drugs), licensure (vaccines and biologics), or clearance (diagnostics) by FDA. Although individual physicians may engage in off-label use of an approved or licensed product, investigational products require a detailed informed consent. In a catastrophic public health emergency, this requirement could lead to delayed care with possible heightened morbidity and mortality. Under Public Law (P.L.) 108-276, the Project BioShield Act of 2004, the DHHS Secretary can, after designation of a public health emergency, authorize the use of such medical countermeasures under the Emergency Use Authorization (EUA). This statute requires that informed consent be obtained but it no longer must be written. Additionally,

adverse effects must be tracked, to the extent possible in the emergency.[64]

Laboratory Preparedness

A network of national, reference, and sentinel laboratories define the Laboratory Response Network (LRN), which was established by DHHS at CDC in 1999 in accordance with Presidential Decision Directive 39 of 1999, which outlined national anti-terrorism policies and assigned specific missions to federal departments and agencies.

LRN includes the Laboratory Network for Biological Terrorism (NBT) in collaboration with the Association of Public Health Laboratories and the Federal Bureau of Investigation. The NBT defines a tiered system of laboratories for the identification and verification of biological agents. Approximately 25,000 sentinel laboratories (SLs), composed of hospital and commercial diagnostic laboratories, form the base of the network providing routine diagnostic services and ruling out the presence of biological threat agents in Biosafety Level (BSL) 1 and 2 environments. The American Society of Microbiology works closely with CDC and SLs to provide needed threat-agent rule-out protocols and training to laboratorians. SLs refer questionable samples to the second tier of approximately 100 reference laboratories

TABLE 321-2	Department of Health and Human Services (DHHS) Bioterrorism-Related Budget Breakdown (in $ millions [M]), Fiscal Years (FY) 2001-2008*—cont'd							
DHHS Office or Agency	FY2001	FY2002	FY2003	FY2004	FY2005	FY2006	FY2007	FY2008
Centers for Disease Control and Prevention (CDC)[‡‡]								
CDC Physical Security and Facilities	3	46	20	0	0	0	0	0
Upgrading State and Local Capacity	67	940	939	918	919	823	767	746
Biosurveillance Initiative	0	0	0	22	79	133[§§]	71	53
Upgrading CDC Capacity	22	143	159	151	141	137	123	121
Anthrax Research	18	18	18	18	17	14	8	0
Strategic National Stockpile[‖‖]	51	645	398	0	467	524	496	522
Supplemental Appropriations (smallpox vaccine)	0	512	100	0	0	0	0	0
Independent Studies	11	2	2	0	0	0	0	0
Other (Planning, Deterrence)	10	19	0	0	0	0	0	0
Subtotal CDC	182	2,324	1,634	1,110	1,623	1,631	1,465	1,442
National Institutes of Health (NIH)								
Research	53	198	687	1,629	1,548	1,604	1,624	1,633
Advanced Development Fund (non-add)[#]	0	0	0	0	0	54	0	0
Extramural Laboratory Construction	0	0	373	0	149	30	14	0
Intramural Physical Security and Facilities	0	92	370	0	0	0	0	0
rPA Anthrax Vaccine Intermediate Development–Manufacturing Scale-up[¶¶]	0	0	123	117	0	0	0	0
Modified Vaccinia Ankara (MVA) Smallpox Vaccine Intermediate Development–Manufacturing Scale-up[¶¶]	0	0	0	75	45	0	0	0
National Science Advisory Board for Biosecurity (NSABB)[##]	0	0	0	1	1	1	1	1
Subtotal NIH	53	290	1,553	1,822	1,743	1,689	1,639	1,634
Agency for Healthcare Research and Quality (AHRQ)	0	0	5	0	0	0	0	0
Total DHHS bioterrorism expenditures	324	2,980	4,035	3,704	4,148	4,090	4,055	3,956

**MMRS was originally part of the Office of Emergency Preparedness (OEP) and part of DHHS. It merged with the Office of Public Health Preparedness to become OPHEP. Certain functions of OEP, including MMRS and the National Disaster Medical System (NDMS) were transferred to the Department of Homeland Security pursuant to the *Homeland Security Act of 2002*. NDMS and MMRS returned to DHHS with the enactment of P.L. 109-417, *The Pandemic and All-Hazards Preparedness Act*.

[††]Multiple areas funded including but not limited to increasing regulatory personnel for threat-agent medical countermeasures, food biosurveillance, crisis/incident management, the Food Emergency Response Network.

[‡‡]Details of CDC bioterrorism spending is from CDC Budget Request Summaries for FY2006 and FY2008 and the CDC Detail Table for FY2007. All available at: http://www.cdc.gov/FMO/FMOFYBUDGET.HTM.

[§§]Includes $55M transferred from the Department of Defense.

[‖‖]Congress first appropriated $51M to CDC in FY1999 to create a stockpile of drugs, vaccines, biologics, and medical equipment and supplies needed to respond to large-scale public health emergencies, including biological, chemical, and nuclear or radiological attacks. In FY2006 and FY2007, $11M and $50M were added for the purchase of portable hospital units called Federal Medical Shelters to assist in response to mass casualty events. Initially the cache was named the National Pharmaceutical Stockpile. Renamed the Strategic National Stockpile (SNS) in the *Homeland Security Act of 2002*, the stockpile and its budget were transferred to the Department of Homeland Security under that Act but remained operationally in the hands of CDC. The SNS was returned to DHHS/CDC with the enactment, on Dec. 19, 2006, of P.L. 109-417, *The Pandemic and All-Hazards Preparedness Act*.

[¶¶]Following the attacks in fall 2001, NIH created an accelerated program for recombinant protective antigen (rPA) anthrax vaccine and Modified Vaccinia Ankara (MVA) smallpox vaccine with the plan to incentivize the accelerated development of these vaccines through large-scale manufacturing scale-up. This activity is outside the usual scope of NIH research and was undertaken owing to exigent circumstances. *The Project BioShield Act* of 2004 did not provide funds for this stage of development. However, with the enactment of P.L. 109-417, *The Pandemic and All-Hazards Preparedness Act*, these activities are carried out by ASPR.

[##]Costs are estimates based upon the estimates found in the 2004 charter for the NSABB. Available at: http://www.biosecurityboard.gov/SIGNED%20NSABB%20Charter.pdf. NIH provides the personnel to support the advisory board. Funding has traditionally come from the subordinate OPHEP and then ASPR offices.

(RLs) that function at up to the BSL-3 level for further identification and investigation. Final confirmation of a threat agent is done at national laboratories (NLs) capable of functioning at the BSL-4 level, if needed. These highest tier laboratories have capabilities to conduct specialized strain characterization and bioforensics and are found at CDC, the U.S. Army Medical Research Institute of Infectious Diseases (USAMRIID), and the Naval Medical Research Laboratory. Notably, by the end of 2007 six state public health laboratories and the District of Columbia lacked sufficient capabilities to test for biological threat agents.[9]

Hospital Preparedness

Efforts to improve hospital preparedness have also been undertaken. In 2003, although most urban hospitals in the United States had engaged in basic bioterrorism planning activities and 80% had written plans, few were deemed adequate. Fewer than 50% exercised their emergency response plans, and only 17% had 10 or more ventilators to support critically ill patients.[65] Beginning in FY2002 HRSA began funding the Bioterrorism Hospital Preparedness Cooperative Agreements Program with the program continuing as the Hospital Preparedness Grants Program under the ASPR beginning in FY2007. Between FY2002 and FY008 DHHS provided $3.022 billion for these efforts, or approximately $400 to $500 million per year. However, these seemingly large amounts provide only an average of $100,000 per

hospital per year despite estimates that at least $200,000 per year is needed after an initial one-time cost of $1 million per hospital.[66] By 2005, only one third of hospitals had the adequate surge capacity to support the infectious disease standard of 500 cases per million population,[67] rapidly consult with infection control experts, or prioritize the distribution of drugs and vaccines to health care workers; only two states had sufficient plans, incentives, or provisions to encourage health care workers to continue to come to work during such an event.[68] The results of a 2007 hospital emergency survey conducted by the Association for Practitioners in Infection Control and Epidemiology (APIC) demonstrated improvements, with 76% of hospitals reported as having an appropriate surge capacity plan and 53% a written plan for bringing needed providers into care sites. However, only 43% had plans to offer incentives to providers to continue or come back to work during such an emergency.[9]

Public Health System Preparedness

Although an astute clinician or laboratorian is anticipated to be the person who might first send out the clarion call that a possible bioterrorist event is under way, there is a desire to detect the event before patients present to emergency departments or doctors' offices. However a bioterrorist event is first identified—by the clinician, laboratory or public health surveillance—the response will require constant real-time communication and collaboration between these elements at all levels—local, state, and federal. Therefore, the importance of the establishment of a strong health care–public health partnership before such an event occurs cannot be overemphasized.

The importance of upgrading state and local public health capacity to respond to a bioterrorist event was beginning to be addressed even before late 2001. However, only in the aftermath of the terrorist attacks of that year did funding to improve overall public health capacity increase significantly. In the period FY2002 to FY2008, $6.052 billion was provided to upgrade public health departments. At the end of August 2002, only 28 states had completed bioterrorism response plans, public health surveillance systems continued to be suboptimally funded with untimely reporting, and the public health work force continued to erode.[69] Surveillance, monitoring, and outbreak alerting systems at the state level were known to be suboptimal or nonexistent in many states.

Pathogen Detection

In early 2002 legislation was introduced, but not enacted, to create a nationwide health tracking system. However, a multi-component interagency Biosurveillance Initiative (BI) was created and funded beginning in FY2004 to fill the gap in surveillance and early warning of a potential terrorist attack or infectious disease outbreak. The BI has three integrated elements.

The first BI component is BioSense, a multi-state data sharing program using existing health databases in near-real-time to identify possible bioterrorist events or epidemics using an experimental approach called syndromic surveillance.[70-73] The program monitors the number of cases with various general types of symptoms such as diarrhea, fever, and rash or febrile respiratory infection by tracking clinics, emergency rooms, or 911 calls. The belief is that the early nonspecific symptoms of several Category A agents may not serve to alert the busy clinician that an unusual cluster of cases is occurring. Although intuitively attractive, it remains to be determined whether this or any other surveillance system can be satisfactorily sustained, and at what cost, in the absence of regularly occurring and valid alarms that test the system.[74]

It would seem probable that, long before BioSense detected a sufficient number of cases that exceeded some threshold, emergency room physicians would already be raising an alarm based on only a few cases. It should not require many cases to alert even the minimally suspicious clinician: for example, three or four very sick patients with a pustular rash (possible smallpox), or a few previously healthy people with pneumonia and hemoptysis (possible pneumonic plague); or a few otherwise healthy people with fever, difficulty breathing, a widened mediastinum on chest radiography, and a rapid downhill course (inhalational anthrax). Sensitized staff in the nation's 2000 emergency rooms and assured lines of communication between them and infectious disease and public health specialists would seem to offer a better alarm system than large volumes of crude data collected by the BioSense system ostensibly created to provide situational awareness.[74]

Expansion of quarantine stations at U.S. ports of entry is the second BI element and specifically aims to improve monitoring of travelers, important foodstuffs, and research materials.

The third component is expansion of the LRN to include food safety and animal diagnostic laboratories, as early warning of an attack may be noted by contamination of the food supply or new or unusual animal diseases that could be transmitted to humans. By the end of 2007, 12 states did not have an electronic disease surveillance and reporting system that could interact with the national system at CDC.[9]

In a separate but related activity funded by the Department of Homeland Security, the LRN and the Environmental Protection Agency (EPA) participate in the BioWatch Program. The goals of the program are to provide early warning of a biological attack, thereby minimizing casualties in an affected area; to assist in establishing forensic evidence to aid law enforcement in identifying perpetrators; and to determine a preliminary spatial distribution of biological contamination, including what populations have been exposed. Daily col-

lection and testing is performed on up to 50 air sampling filters per city. The system uses existing EPA air sampling sites around the country; the filters are tested for CDC Category A agents by participants of the LRN using polymerase chain reaction. The intent is to detect and commence a response to a biological agent attack within 36 hours of release. The program, which has invested over $400 million to date in creating and operating this piggybacked system, is not without its critics. Proper sample handling and reporting have been recurring issues.[75] The current atmospheric samplers use an old sampling method and cannot preserve live organisms, and the system is costly to operate. Beginning in late 2008 this program is being evaluated by the National Academies of Science. The occurrence of one or two false alarms accompanied by the frenzy and publicity of response that would follow could seriously damage the credibility of government leadership. Illustrative of the problem was an event in October 2003 when two air monitors in Houston, Texas, detected the presence of tularemia on 2 consecutive days. Area hospitals and infectious disease specialists were warned about the possibility that a release had taken place, but authorities refrained from taking further action such as distributing antibiotics. Three to five cases of tularemia occur in Texas every year,[76] and officials rapidly discounted the possibility of bioterrorism.[77]

PUBLIC HEALTH RESPONSE

Key to the response to a bioterrorist event is advanced planning across the spectrum of anticipated response elements. As part of the preparation, exercises and drills can provide insights into areas of needed improvement and provide communication opportunities among medical, public health, emergency response, law enforcement, and military personnel who otherwise would not normally communicate. During 2007 all 50 U.S. states and the District of Columbia conducted emergency preparedness drills.[9]

Identification that a biological weapon has been released demands an immediate response by public health authorities. Most important is the need to determine as soon as possible when and where a release may have taken place so that all who were or might have been exposed can be dealt with. An epidemiological investigation should trace patients' movements so as to determine, along with other patients, a common time and site of exposure. A useful tool for determining time of release has been described by Sartwell.[78] It consists of plotting cases by time on a log scale on one axis, and the cumulative percentage of cases, likewise on a log scale, on the other axis. The intercept of the line through the points provides a remarkably accurate time of release for a common source exposure.

If the disease is contagious (e.g., smallpox; plague; Ebola, Marburg, or Lassa virus), the patient will need to be isolated and close contacts identified. If smallpox, all persons who have been in contact with the patient *since the onset of fever* should be vaccinated and placed under daily surveillance for the detection of symptoms. If the case is plague, prophylaxis of all close contacts with a suitable antibiotic[46] and daily surveillance for symptoms is recommended. If it is one of the contagious hemorrhagic fever viruses, there should be surveillance of contacts with immediate isolation if symptoms develop.[42]

The major challenge to public health officials is that of instituting necessary measures to avoid panic in the face of an epidemic of a traditionally feared disease. Reviews of past epidemics indicate that the most essential factor is effective leadership and competent, frequent, and open communication with the public, the press, professionals, and others concerned with dealing with the epidemic. This is an area that is too often neglected. The 2001 anthrax outbreak in the United States illustrated well the problems resulting from inadequate lines of communication.[79] Health departments at all levels were overwhelmed by requests for information from the public, health professionals, and especially the media. None had experienced an epidemic threat such as this, and none were prepared. Frequent, authoritative, up-to-date reports through the media to the public proved absolutely vital, but it took time before a pattern for these became established. The need for communication between and among professionals was clear, and this is now being addressed in part by the national Health Alert Network, which is financed by federal preparedness funds. It was also apparent that command centers were required to coordinate and direct operations and to facilitate the flow of information, but these took time to become established and to begin to function well. Sophisticated centers are now in place in the Secretary's Office at DHHS, CDC, and in many states and cities; they are now staffed on a continuous basis. Information and education materials have been prepared with respect to Category A diseases and are available throughout the health system. Of importance is the fact that at federal, state and local levels, exercises are being conducted to test response systems to determine how well they are functioning.

A second factor in muting the likelihood of panic is to do all possible to keep the normal day-to-day activities of citizens and the city as minimally disrupted as possible. Public officials at all levels have often been prone to want to invoke quarantine measures, whether to close airports or other parts of the transportation network or to forbid entry or departure from cities or other large areas. This was the case in all countries that reported cases of SARS in 2003. Experience has shown that quarantine measures are seldom effective and, in fact, often lead to more serious problems as many seek to flee an area or deny the presence of cases in family or friends, thus precluding appropriate containment measures.[80]

The Strategic National Stockpile (SNS) is an important part of the response armamentarium following a bioterrorist attack. Formerly known as the National Pharmaceutical Stockpile, or NPS, it was renamed when it was transferred from CDC to the newly created Department of Homeland Security in FY2003 and transferred back to DHHS in FY2005. It is currently under the oversight of the ASPR and operated by the CDC. The SNS contains antibiotics, antitoxins, vaccines, life-support medications, and medical supplies that can be used to supplement state and local resources during a large-scale public health emergency. Within 12 hours of a request, a Push-Package containing an initial supplemental cache of medical countermeasures and supplies can be at the targeted destination. These packages have been pre-positioned in strategically located secure warehouses to facilitate prompt delivery. If additional support is needed, a vendor-managed inventory is called upon to deliver ongoing needed medical countermeasures and supplies. Current annual operating costs for the SNS are about $500 million per year. However, by the end of 2007 10 states did not have adequate plans to distribute SNS resources upon delivery.[9]

Research and Development to Meet Preparedness and Response Needs

Research specifically directed at problems posed by the development and application of biological weapons was, until very recently, primarily conducted by the Department of Defense, principally, USAMRIID in Frederick, Maryland. Under the provisions of the 1972 Biological Weapons Convention, the research related basically to defensive measures against validated threat agents.[20] As concerns about the potential use of biological agents have mounted and preparedness programs have begun to be elaborated, it has become abundantly clear that many facets of a public health and medical response could be better handled if there were a better understanding of disease pathogenesis and immune response, and if there were available more appropriate technologies for detection, diagnosis, treatment, prevention, and environmental mitigation. Some of these items represent immediate-term needs, such as that of producing a contemporary, second-generation smallpox vaccine grown in tissue cell culture; others require a longer term vision and are dependent on basic science initiatives to broaden the understanding of health and disease. The importance of a major research effort was reinforced by the sudden emergence of SARS in spring 2003 and the extraordinary impact it had on Asian countries and the city of Toronto, Canada. To deal with SARS, there is an urgent

need for diagnostics, sensitive detection devices, a vaccine, and antiviral agents. As has become clear, the challenge of a new, naturally emergent microbial agent was remarkably congruent with that related to national security against a biological weapons attack, whether utilizing known agents or genetic mutants.

After the September 11 attack on the United States, one of the most urgent challenges was to prepare to deal with the two agents that had received the most attention during the course of the Soviet biological weapons program and which presumably could have been acquired or developed by any of a number of countries—smallpox and anthrax. Only 15 million doses of smallpox vaccine remained in storage from the 1970s, when smallpox had been virtually eradicated and vaccination had stopped. This amount was woefully insufficient to cope with epidemic smallpox should the virus be released. The old vaccine had been a crude preparation produced on the skin of calves and would not meet the standards of a contemporary vaccine. Moreover, there were no remaining vaccine production facilities anywhere in the world. It was estimated then that 5 to 8 years would be required, following traditional vaccine development protocols, to develop, produce, and license a new vaccine, grown, as are contemporary vaccines, in tissue cell culture. In the autumn of 2001 DHHS set the goal of securing, as soon as possible, sufficient vaccine for every American. In less than 18 months, the vaccine had been produced and tested for antigenicity, and was ready for use as an investigational new drug in the event of an emergency. While under IND it was delivered to the SNS for use under EUA, if needed, before licensure, which was granted by the FDA on September 1, 2007. Furthermore, the anthrax letter attacks highlighted the limitations of the existing six-dose anthrax vaccine produced by early 20th century technology. Prior to the attacks the Institute of Medicine had recommended the development of a new vaccine as both pre-exposure vaccine and post-exposure treatment in combination with antibiotics.[81] These experiences demonstrated the need to be prepared to act quickly and, as necessary, to develop and quickly procure vaccines, antitoxins, or antimicrobial agents, and to be able to make these available for field use.

The pathway from discovery through development, production, and final FDA approval is expensive as well as time consuming with a single product price tag estimated to be between $800 million and $1.2 billion.[82] Important in this process is encouraging discovery and development. The National Institutes of Health (NIH), primarily the National Institute of Allergy and Infectious Diseases (NIAID), received $9.4 billion from FY2002 to FY2008 to fund needed research into biological threat agents and support the construction of needed extramural research laboratories. Additionally, in the immediate post-9/11 period NIH/NIAID provided $360 million for late-stage development of recombinant protective antigen anthrax and modified vaccinia Ankara smallpox vaccines. The former effort has been less successful than the latter in terms of final product delivery.[83]

In an effort to encourage the private sector to develop and manufacture needed security medical countermeasures, a special reserve fund of $5.6 billion was created and appropriated to DHS in October 2003. The use of this fund by DHHS for the acquisition of vaccines, biologics, drugs, and diagnostics against security threat agents was authorized under P.L. 108-276, the Project BioShield Act of 2004.[84] Although Project BioShield had some success, the incentives were too meager for large pharmaceutical companies. In addition, the so-called "valley of death" between the stage of development funded by NIH research and scaling-up for product manufacturing and licensure, left many in the private sector loathe to enter into development of these products.[85] In an attempt to remedy the funding gap between advanced product stages and the regulatory finish-line, the Biomedical Advanced Research and Development Authority (BARDA) was created by Public Law No. 109-417, the Pandemic and All Hazards Preparedness Act enacted on December 19, 2006. Under BARDA contracts to purchase needed products can be delayed until products are more developed. However, given the research and development price tag for a single product, with 60% to 80% of a company's costs in the scale-up and manufacturing phase, it is unclear whether the current funding is adequate to provide the needed incentive to engage industry. Advanced development funds for BARDA in FY2007 and FY2008 are a little more than $100 million per year.

Efforts to accelerate the development and production of a second-generation recombinant anthrax vaccine have not been as successful[86] although progress in the development of an attenuated, non-replicating smallpox vaccine, which is anticipated to induce fewer adverse reactions, is ongoing.[83]

The Two-Edged Sword of Modern Biology

The rapidly accruing knowledge base of modern biology is making it possible to understand such factors as mechanisms for immune system or host restriction evasion. Further, it is now possible to synthesize and manipulate genomes. Examples of microbial manipulations of greatest concern include the transfer of antibiotic resistance, modification of the antigenic properties, modification of the stability in the environment, and the transfer of pathogenic properties.[87,88] What once were the tools of exploration for only the most sophisticated laboratories are now increasingly present in laboratories around the world and even in high school laboratories. For those interested in bioterrorism, a new world is opening.

Several scientists have reported in the open literature on the development of an antibiotic-resistant strain of anthrax[19,89,90] Apart from research dealing directly with biological agents, unexpected and unintended results are possible working with other microbes as happened with researchers at the John Curtin School in Australia.[91] They added a single gene to the mousepox virus and found, to their surprise, that it shut down the immunological response even of vaccinated mice, which are normally fully protected. The question of whether the addition of this gene to smallpox, a closely related virus, would shut down the immune defenses of humans cannot be definitively answered. Some believe it might, whereas others do not, owing to redundancies in the human immune system. Certainly, the potential of many more experiments to have unintended consequences, some of which could be catastrophic, must be anticipated.

How to deal with the problems of access to known biological pathogens of concern and how to ensure control, or at least responsible stewardship, of laboratory work is a vexing question yet to be answered. The problem is that the more extensive and restrictive the controls, the more difficult it will be to undertake studies that are needed to produce better vaccines, drugs, and other products. To know precisely which gene of an organism causes damage and how it acts may permit a highly targeted vaccine or drug but, at the same time, it identifies a gene that if inserted into another organism could produce a devastating effect.

Appropriate restrictions on work in laboratories will undoubtedly be required as never before but determining what these should be, balancing security and the needs of freedom for inquiry, will not be easy. Two acts have been passed by Congress and both are problematic in various ways—the Patriot Act (enacted in 2001[92] and reauthorized in 2006,[93] when it repealed the sunset date for, thus making permanent, most of its provisions with a few exceptions) and the Public Health Security and Bioterrorism Preparedness and Response Act (2002).[88,94] The first act criminalizes possession of biological agents unless justified by a prophylactic, protective, bona fide research or other peaceful purpose and prohibits the possession, transport, and receipt of selected agents by convicted felons; foreign nationals from terrorism-sponsoring nations; individuals dishonorably discharged from the Armed Services; and users of controlled substances. The second act requires that the Secretary of DHHS maintain a list of selected agents; requires research facilities possessing selected agents to register their possession to the CDC; requires background checks of those in possession of selected agents to ensure that they are not convicted felons, etc.; and requires the establishment of safeguard and security measures to prevent access to such agents and toxins for use in domestic or international terrorism or for any other criminal purpose.

The direct and indirect costs and complexity of physical facilities and procedures that limit access are consequential. For example, both NIH and CDC have undergone costly major infrastructure modifications to their respective campuses to enhance security and strengthen procedures to limit access to potentially dangerous pathogens. Furthermore, security enhancements and requirements to limit access to potentially dangerous pathogens have led some laboratories to abandon or forego studies on these microbial threat agents simply because the requirements related to undertaking such research are deemed as onerous. The costs of registering and policing compliance are likewise substantial. More salient is the question of what efficacy these procedures may have in deterrence, recognizing that few other nations have implemented measures that are, in any way, comparable.

Discussions are taking place in the United States and international forums with hopes that some rational and effective systems can be agreed upon that will act to lessen the likelihood of biological agents being developed and used for sinister purposes, but their impact is questionable. In 2003, the U.S. National Academies of Sciences' Committee on Research Standards and Practices to Prevent the Destructive Application of Biotechnology issued a report (colloquially known as the Fink report) on ways to balance national security and scientific openness. In response to this report, the National Science Advisory Board for Biosecurity (NSABB) was created to "provide advice to federal departments and agencies on ways to minimize the possibility that knowledge and technologies emanating from vitally important biological research will be misused to threaten public health or national security."[95] While NSABB has not made definitive recommendations, they have offered suggestions about how to best communicate the relative importance of why dual-use research is being conducted. The Committee recommended that a system of responsible oversight, consisting of voluntary self-governance by the scientific community and an expansion of existing regulatory processes, be developed for scientific experimentation in the life sciences in order to hinder their unintentional development as weapons.[96] It will be difficult at best to achieve reasonable goals, but the need is real and urgent.

REFERENCES

1. O'Toole T, Inglesby TV, Henderson DA. Why understanding biological weapons matters to medical and public health professionals. In: O'Toole T, Inglesby TV, Henderson DA, eds. *Bioterrorism: Guidelines for Medical and Public Health Management.* Chicago: AMA Press; 2002:1-7.
2. Carus WS, Center for Counterproliferation Research. *Bioterrorism and biocrimes: The illicit use of biological agents since 1900.* Washington, D.C.: Center for Counterproliferation Research, National Defense University; Feb. 2001 rev.
3. Inglesby TV, O'Toole T, Henderson DA, et al. Anthrax as a biological weapon: Updated recommendations for management. In: O'Toole T, Inglesby TV, Henderson DA, eds. *Bioterrorism: Guidelines for Medical and Public Health Management.* Chicago: AMA Press; 2002:63-97.
4. Austin PC, Mamdani MM, Chan BT, et al. Anxiety-related visits to Ontario physicians following September 11, 2001. *Can J Psychiatry.* 2003;48:416-419.
5. Allegra PC, Cochrane D, Dunn E, et al. Emergency department visits for concern regarding anthrax—New Jersey, 2001. *MMWR Morb Mortal Wkly Rep.* 2005;54(Suppl):163-167.
6. Baldauf S. Pakistan, other allies grapple with anthrax scares. *Christian Science Monitor,* November 5, 2001.
7. Fauci AS. Infectious diseases: Considerations for the 21st century. *Clin Infect Dis.* 2001;32:675-685.
8. Preparing for the Inevitable: Bioterrorism and Emerging Infectious Diseases. Biosecurity Conference. June 9, 2005. Available at: <http://ihcrp.georgetown.edu/lifescienceandsociety/pdfs/biosecurityconferencetranscript.pdf>; Accessed 04/02/09.
9. Levi J, Vinter S, Segal LM, Trust for America's Health. *Ready or not? Protecting the public's health from diseases, disasters, and bioterrorism.* Washington, D.C.: Trust for America's Health; 2007.
10. Gershon RR, Qureshi KA, Sepkowitz KA, et al. Clinicians' knowledge, attitudes, and concerns regarding bioterrorism after a brief educational program. *J Occup Environ Med.* 2004;46:77-83.
11. Gould R, Connell ND. The public health effects of biological weapons. In: Levy BS, Sidel VW, eds. *War and Public Health.* New York: Oxford Press; 1997:98-116.
12. Derbes VJ. Demussis and the great plague of 1348: a forgotten episode of biological warfare. *JAMA.* 1966;196:59-62.
13. Christopher GW, Cieslak TJ, Pavlin JA, et al. Biological warfare: a historical perspective. *JAMA.* 1997;278:412-417.
14. Hopkins DR. *The Greatest Killer: Smallpox in History.* Chicago: Univ. of Chicago Press; 2002.
15. Volwiler AT. William Trent's Journal at Fort Pitt. *Mississippi Valley Hist Rev.* 1763;11:390-413.
16. Fenn EA. *Pax Americana.* New York: Hill and Wang; 2001.
17. Eitzen EM, Takafuji ET. Historical overview of biological warfare. In: Siddel FR, Takafuji ET, Franz DR, eds. *Medical Aspects of Chemical and Biological Warfare.* Washington, D.C.: Office of the Surgeon General; 1997:415-423.

18. Williams P, Wallace D. *Unit 731*. New York: The Free Press, Macmillan; 1989.
19. Alibek K. *Biohazard*. New York: Random House; 1999.
20. *Convention on the Prohibition of the Development, Production, and Stockpiling of Bacteriological (Biological) and Toxin Weapons and on Their Destruction (1972)*. Washington, D.C.: U.S. Government Printing Office; 1972.
21. Page WF, Young HA, Crawford HM, Institute of Medicine Advisory Panel for the Study of Long-Term Health Effects of Participation in Project SHAD. *Long-term Health Effects of Participation in Project SHAD (Shipboard Hazard and Defense)*. Washington, D.C.: National Academies Press; 2007.
22. Guillemin J. *Biological Weapons: From the Invention of State-Sponsored Programs to Contemporary Bioterrorism*. New York: Columbia University Press; 2005.
23. U.S. Department of State. Patterns of Global Terrorism Report. 1996. Available at: <http://www.state.gov/www/global/terrorism/1996Report/1996index.html>; Accessed 04/02/09.
24. U.S. Arms Control and Disarmament Agency. Adherence to and Compliance With Arms Control Agreements. 1996. <http://dosfan.lib.uic.edu/acda/reports/annual/comp.htm>; Accessed 04/02/09.
25. Cohen W. *Proliferation: Threat and Response*. U.S. Government; 1997. Available at: <http://www.ciaonet.org/book/cohen02/index.html>; Accessed 04/02/09.
26. Ekeus R. Iraq's biological weapons programme: UNSCOM's experience. Memorandum report to the United Nations Security Council. New York; November 20, 1996.
27. Zilinskas RA. Iraq's biological weapons: the past as future? *JAMA*. 1997;278:418-424.
28. Lax AJ. *Toxin: The Cunning of Bacterial Poisons*. New York: Oxford University Press; 2005.
29. Torok TJ, Tauxe RV, Wise RP, et al. A large community outbreak of salmonellosis caused by intentional contamination of restaurant salad bars. *JAMA*. 1997;278:389-395.
30. Daplan E, Marchell A. *The Cult at the End of the World*. New York: Crown; 1996.
31. *Global Proliferation of Weapons of Mass Destruction: Hearings before the Permanent Subcommittee on Investigations of the Committee on Governmental Affairs, United States Senate, One Hundred Fourth Congress, first-second session*. Washington, D.C.: U.S. Government Printing Office; 1996.
32. Ehrlich PR, Harte J, Harwell MA, et al. Long-term biological consequences of nuclear war. *Science*. 1983;222:1293-1300.
33. Schoenbaum SC. The impact of pandemic influenza, with special reference to 1918. *International Congress Series*. 2001;1219:43-51.
34. Begley S, Isikoff M. War on terror: anxious about anthrax. *Newsweek* 2001;138:28-35.
35. Anderson A, Eisold JF. Anthrax attack at the United States Capitol: front line thoughts. *AAOHN J*. 2002;50:170-173.
36. Miro S, Kaufman SG. Anthrax in New Jersey: a health education experience in bioterrorism response and preparedness. *Health Promot Pract*. 2005;6:430-436.
37. Venkatesh S, Memish ZA. Bioterrorism—a new challenge for public health. *Int J Antimicrob Agents*. 2003;21:200-206.
38. Rosenswieg P, Kochem A. *Risk assessment and risk management: Necessary tools for homeland security. Backgrounder No 1889*. Washington, D.C.: Center for Legal and Judicial Studies, Heritage Foundation. Available at: <http://www.heritage.org/research/homelandsecurity/bg1889.cfm>; Accessed 04/02/09.
39. National Research Council (U.S.), Committee on the Institutional Means for Assessment of Risks to Public Health. *Risk Assessment in the Federal Government: Managing the Process*. Washington, D.C.: National Academy Press; 1983.
40. Stern PC, Fineberg HV, National Research Council (U.S.), Committee on Risk Characterization. *Understanding Risk: Informing Decisions in a Democratic Society*. Washington, D.C.: National Academy Press; 1996.
41. Arnon SS, Schechter R, Inglesby TV, et al. Botulinum toxin as a biological weapon: medical and public health management. *JAMA*. 2001;285:1059-1069.
42. Borio L, Inglesby TV, Peters CJ, et al. Hemorrhagic fever viruses as biological weapons: medical and public health management. *JAMA*. 2002;287:2391-2405.
43. Dennis DT, Inglesby TV, Henderson DA, et al. Tularemia as a biological weapon: medical and public health management. *JAMA*. 2001;285:2763-2773.
44. Henderson DA, Inglesby TV, Bartlett JG, et al. Smallpox as a biological weapon: medical and public health management. *JAMA*. 1999;281:2127-2137.
45. Inglesby TV, Henderson DA, Bartlett JG, et al. Anthrax as a biological weapon: medical and public health management. *JAMA*. 1999;281:1735-1745.
46. Inglesby TV, Dennis DT, Henderson DA, et al. Plague as a biological weapon: medical and public health management. *JAMA*. 2000;283:2281-2291.
47. *Bioterrorism: Guidelines for Medical and Public Health Management*. Chicago: American Medical Association; 2002.
48. Centers for Disease Control and Prevention. The Select Agent Program. Available at: <http://www.selectagents.gov/>; Accessed 04/02/09.
49. MacKenzie D. Trail of terror. *New Scientist*. Issue 2314; October 27, 2001.
50. Meselson M, Guillemin V, Hugh-Jones M, et al. The Sverdlovsk anthrax outbreak of 1979. *Science*. 1994;266:1202-1208.
51. Office of Technology Assessment, U.S. Congress. *Proliferation of Weapons of Mass Destruction. Publication OTA-ISC-559*. Washington, D.C.: U.S. Government Printing Office; 1993.
52. Wein LM, Liu Y. Analyzing a bioterror attack on the food supply: the case of botulinum toxin in milk. *Proc Natl Acad Sci U S A*. 2005;102:9984-9989.
53. Vorobjev AA, Cherkassky BL, Stepanov AV, et al. "Criterion rating" as a measure of probable use of bioagents as biological weapons. Presented to Working Group on Biological Weapons Control of the Committee on International Security and Arms Control. Washington, D.C.: National Academy of Sciences; April 1994.
54. Quenelle DC, Prichard MN, Keith KA, et al. Synergistic efficacy of the combination of ST-246 with CMX001 against orthopoxviruses. *Antimicrob Agents Chemother*. 2007;51:4118-4124.
55. Wehrle PF, Posch J, Richter KH, et al. An airborne outbreak of smallpox in a German hospital and its significance with respect to other recent outbreaks in Europe. *Bull World Health Organ*. 1970;43:669-679.
56. Fenner F, Henderson DA, Arita I, et al. *Smallpox and Its Eradication*. Geneva: World Health Organization; 1988.
57. Cohen J. Bioterrorism—Smallpox vaccinations: how much protection remains? *Science*. 2001;294:985.
58. van Furth AM, Zaaijer HL. Meningococcal disease in the Netherlands: media hype, but not an epidemic. *Ned Tijdschr Geneeskd*. 2001;145:1716-1718.
59. Roberts B. New challenges and new policy priorities for the 1990s. In: *Biologic Weapons: Weapons of the Future*. Washington, D.C.: Center for Strategic and International Studies; 1993.
60. Hynes NA. BioShield, BARDA, and HHS. Presented at Center for Biosecurity of UPMC. Baltimore, Maryland; January 2008.
61. Center for Arms Control and Non-Proliferation, Biological and Chemical Weapons Program. Federal Funding for Biological Weapons Prevention and Defense, Fiscal Years 2001 to 2008. Available at: <http://www.armscontrolcenter.org/resources/fy2008_bw_budget.pdf>; Accessed 04/02/09.
62. U.S. Department of Health and Human Services, Budget in Brief, Fiscal Year 2009. Available at: <http://www.hhs.gov/budget/09budget/2009BudgetInBrief.pdf>; Accessed 04/02/09.
63. *Homeland Security Presidential Directive/HSPD-21 [news release]*. Washington, DC: The White House; October 18, 2007. Available at: <http://www.whitehouse.gov/news/releases/2007/10/20071018-10.html>; Accessed 04/02/09.
64. Nightingale SL, Prasher JM, Simonson S. Emergency Use Authorization (EUA) to enable use of needed products in civilian and military emergencies, United States. *Emerg Infect Dis*. 2007;13:1046-1051.
65. *Hospital Preparedness: Most Urban Hospitals Have Emergency Plans but Lack Certain Capacities for Bioterrorism Response—Report to Congressional Committees*. Washington, D.C.: U.S. General Accounting Office; 2003.
66. Toner E, Waldhorn R, Maldin B, et al. Hospital preparedness for pandemic influenza. *Biosecur Bioterror*. 2006;4:207-217.
67. U.S. Department of Health and Human Services, Agency for Healthcare Research and Quality. Optimizing Surge Capacity: Regional Efforts in Bioterrorism Readiness. Bioterrorism and Health System Preparedness, Issue Brief No. 4. <http://www.ahrq.gov/news/ulp/btbriefs/btbrief4.htm>; Accessed 04/02/09.
68. Hearne SA, Segal LM, Earls MJ, et al. Trust for America's Health. *Ready or Not? Protecting the Public's Health from Diseases, Disasters, and Bioterrorism*. Washington, D.C.: Trust for America's Health; 2005.
69. *Public Health Preparedness: Progress and Challenges since September 11th, 2001—A Progress Report*. Washington, D.C.: Trust for America's Health; 2002.
70. Lazarus R, Kleinmann K, Dashevsky I, et al. Use of automated ambulatory-care encounter records for detection of acute illness clusters, including potential bioterrorism events. *Emerg Infect Dis*. 2002;8:753-760.
71. Lewis MD, Pavlin JA, Mansfield JL, et al. Disease outbreak detection system using syndromic data in the greater Washington, D.C. area. *Am J Prev Med*. 2002;23:180-186.
72. Lombardo J, Burkom H, Elbert E, et al. A systems overview of the electronic surveillance system for the early notification of community-based epidemics (ESSENCE II). *J Urban Health* 2003;80(Suppl 1):i32-i42.
73. Mostashari F, Fine A, Das D, et al. Use of ambulance dispatch data as an early warning system for communitywide influenzalike illness, New York City. *J Urban Health*. 2003;80(2 Suppl 1):i43-i49.
74. Reingold A. If syndromic surveillance is the answer, what is the question? *Biosecur Bioterror*. 2003;1:77-81.
75. Department of Homeland Security, Office of Inspector General. DHS' Management of BioWatch Program. No. OIG-07-22; January 2007. Available at: <http://www.dhs.gov/xoig/assets/mgmtrpts/OIG_07-22_Jan07.pdf>; Accessed 04/02/09.
76. Chang MH, Glynn MK, Groseclose SL. Endemic, notifiable bioterrorism-related diseases, United States, 1992-1999. *Emerg Infect Dis*. 2003;9:556-564.
77. Berger E. Suspicious bacteria detected: security monitors spot germ; terrorism discounted. Houston Chronicle Medical Writer. October 10, 2003.
78. Sartwell P. The distribution of incubation periods of infectious diseases. *Am J Hyg*. 1950;51:310-318.
79. Gursky E, Inglesby TV, O'Toole T. Anthrax 2001: observations on the medical and public health response. *Biosecur Bioterror*. 2003;1:97-110.
80. Barbera J, Macintyre A, Gostin L, et al. Large-scale quarantine following biological terrorism in the United States. *JAMA*. 2002;286:2711-2717.
81. Institute of Medicine (U.S.), Committee to Assess the Safety and Efficacy of the Anthrax Vaccine. *The Anthrax Vaccine: Is It Safe? Does It Work?* Washington, D.C.: National Academy Press; 2002.
82. DiMasi JA, Hansen RW, Grabowski HG, et al. Research and development costs for new drugs by therapeutic category: a study of the U.S. pharmaceutical industry. *Pharmacoeconomics*. 1995;7:152-169.
83. U.S. Department of Health and Human Services. Chemical, Biological, Radiological, and Nuclear (CBRN) Funding Activities. Available at: <http://www.hhs.gov/aspr/barda/procurement/cbrnactivities.html>; Accessed 04/02/09.
84. Gottron F. CRS Report for Congress. Project BioShield: Purposes and Authorities. Available at: <http://ftp.fas.org/sgp/crs/terror/RS21507.pdf>; Accessed 04/02/09.
85. *Crossing the Valley of Death: Bringing Promising Medical Countermeasures to BioShield. Hearing before the Subcommittee on Bioterrorism and Public Health Preparedness of the Committee on Health, Education, Labor, and Pensions, U.S. Senate, 109th Congress, 1st Session. June 9, 2005*. Washington, D.C.: U.S. Government Printing Office; 2005.
86. Miller JD. U.S. cancels anthrax vaccine contract. *The Scientist*. December 21, 2006.
87. National Research Council (U.S.), Committee on Research Standards and Practices to Prevent the Destructive Application of Biotechnology. *Biotechnology Research in an Age of Terrorism*. Washington, D.C.: National Academies Press; 2004.
88. Kwik G, Fitzgerald J, Inglesby TV, et al. Biosecurity: responsible stewardship of bioscience in an age of catastrophic terrorism. *Biosecur Bioterror*. 2003;1:27-35.
89. Pomerantsev AP, Mockov YV, et al. Expression of cereolysine AB genes in *Bacillus anthracis* vaccine strain ensure protection against experimental hemolytic anthrax infection. *Vaccine*. 1997;15:1846-1850.
90. Athamna A, Athamna M, Abu-Rashed N, et al. Selection of *Bacillus anthracis* isolates resistant to antibiotics. *J Antimicrob Chemother*. 2004;54:424-428.
91. Jackson RJ, Ramsay AJ, Christensen CD, et al. Expression of mouse interleukin-4 by a recombinant ectromelia virus suppresses cytolytic lymphocyte responses and overcomes genetic resistance to mouse pox. *J Virol*. 2001;75:8353-8355.
92. 107th Congress. Uniting and Strengthening America by Providing Appropriate Tools Required to Intercept and Obstruct Terrorism (USA PATRIOT Act) Act of 2001. Public Law 107-56; 2001.
93. 109th Congress. USA PATRIOT Improvement and Reauthorization Act of 2005. Public Law 109-177 2006.
94. 107th Congress. Public Health Security and Bioterrorism Preparedness and Response Act of 2002. Public Law 107-188; 2002.
95. *The National Science Advisory Board for Biosecurity*. Available at: <http://www.biosecurityboard.gov>; Accessed 04/02/09.
96. Committee on Research Standards and Practices to Prevent the Destructive Application of Biotechnology NRC. *Biotechnology Research in an Age of Terrorism: Confronting the Dual Use Dilemma*. Washington, D.C.: National Academies Press; 2003.

322

Plague as a Bioterrorism Weapon

LUCIANA BORIO | NOREEN A. HYNES

Yersinia pestis, the etiologic agent of plague, has caused pandemics and been responsible for more social and economic devastation than armed conflict.[1] Between the 6th and 20th centuries CE, three great plague pandemics resulted in over 200 million deaths. The first pandemic originated in Central Africa and spread throughout the Mediterranean basin, affecting the Byzantine Empire during the reign of Justinian I in the 6th century. It resulted in the loss of approximately 25% of the population of southern Europe and contributed to the demise of the Roman Empire. The second pandemic, infamously known as the Black Death, reportedly decimated between 30% and 40% of the populations of major European cities between 1347 and 1351. Epidemic cycles continued to occur until the end of the 17th century. The third, or "modern" pandemic, arose in China in the late 19th century and spread throughout the world until the mid-20th century. In India alone, 12.5 million people died,[2] and by 1899 pandemic plague had reached San Francisco. Today, zoonotic foci of plague exist on every major continent except Australia,[1] and the disease continues to sicken several thousand people per year, mostly in Africa.[3] However, the relatively late introduction of *Y. pestis* in the United States at the turn of the 20th century has resulted in many fewer genetically and phenotypically diverse strains compared with other parts of the world where the pathogen has been present since antiquity.[4]

History of *Yersinia Pestis* Use as a Biological Weapon

The first recorded use of *Y. pestis* in warfare occurred in 1346, during the siege of the Crimean Sea port city of Caffensistera, also known as Caffa or Kaffa (now Feodosiya, Ukraine) on the Black Sea.[5] The port city served as a gateway to the Silk Road trade route and was thus an important military target. The invading Mongols slung bodies of bubonic plague victims over the city walls using trebuchets while fighting Genoese sailors.[5] It is unclear the extent to which this warfare tactic contributed to the subsequent plague epidemic in this port city. However, the plague epidemic led the Genoese sailors to flee to Italy, likely in plague- and rat-infested ships, entering several Italian ports, possibly causing the second great pandemic (Black Death). The same technique was used by the Russians in 1710, while besieging Swedish forces in Reval, Estonia.[6]

In World War II, the Japanese Military Unit 731 (a secret biowarfare research unit) and a predecessor facility used several pathogens, including *Y. pestis*, to infect prisoners of war in Ping Fan and Beiyinhe, Manchuria, respectively.[7,8] This Japanese wartime effort is believed to have resulted in the deaths of approximately 3000 prisoners. The Japanese also repeatedly released plague in the civilian population in Chekiang Province, China, during that time period. The weapons effort was led by Major (subsequently General) Shiro Ishii, a physician, who developed a mechanism for dropping plague-infected human fleas (*Pulex irritans*) that had been placed inside clay bombs from airplanes. Eighty percent of the fleas were shown to survive this method of delivery, in contrast to bacteria-filled aerial bombs, which were ineffective owing to harsh pressure and temperature effects of explosions on the bacteria.[9,10]

During the Cold War era, both the United States and the Soviet Union had active offensive biological weapons programs. Prior to the abandonment of its program in 1969, the United States produced no plague for use as a weapon, deeming difficult to grow virulent organism in large batches.[11] In 1989, Vladmir Pasechnik, a Soviet biologist who had directed the Institute for Ultrapure Biological Preparations in Leningrad, defected to Britain.[11,12] He revealed that the Soviets had succeeded in preparing *Y. pestis* as an aerosolizable powder, genetically engineering it to be resistant to several antibiotics. The Soviets had the capacity to load this "superplague" into bombs, rocket warheads, and artillery shells, as well as strategic intercontinental ballistic missiles. The Soviets may have produced up to 1500 metric tons of this formulation yearly and undertook field tests with it. According to Sergei Popov, another former Soviet bioweapons scientist who defected to Britain in 1992, the Soviets also engineered *Y. pestis* to produce diphtheria toxin.[13,14] The resulting organism was highly virulent in laboratory animals.

Y. pestis has not only been envisioned for use in warfare, but potentially for terrorist and criminal purposes. In 1995, a white supremacist and microbiologist, Larry Wayne Harris, succeeded in purchasing vials of lyophilized *Y. pestis* from the American Type Culture Collection via a fraudulent request.[15] Although his intended use of the organism was never determined, Harris served an 18-month probation for illegal acquisition of the *Y. pestis*.[16] The episode caused alarm and in 1996 prompted Congress to pass the first of several regulations governing the acquisition, use, and transfer of biological agents that could be developed as bioweapons.[17-19]

Yersinia Pestis as a Potential Bioweapon Today

Y. pestis is one of ten agents deemed by the U.S. Army Research Medical Research Institute of Infectious Diseases to be most suitable for development as a bioweapon.[20] *Y. pestis* is also one of six agents deemed by the Centers for Disease Control and Prevention (CDC) to be of highest concern, the so-called Category A biological threat agents.[21] After conducting threat assessments, the Department of Homeland Security has determined that *Y. pestis* poses a "material threat" to U.S. national security.[22]

Today, several factors characterize *Y. pestis* as a potential bioterrorist weapon:[23] *Y. pestis* is available from microbial pathogen and strain collections in a number of different countries; it may be produced in large quantity and disseminated as an aerosol; and the disease is contagious and, if untreated, is associated with a high fatality rate. The impact of modern biotechnology in enhancing bacterial virulence cannot be underestimated—antimicrobial resistant strains have been developed, as have factor 1 (F1)–deficient strains that retain virulence[24,25] but evade F1 antigen–based immunity and certain diagnostic tests. (F1 is an anti-phagocytic capsular glycoprotein expressed by *Y. pestis*.)

The public's perception and historical familiarity with the disease is such that even a small or potential outbreak could possibly result in generalized panic in the community.[26] Although advances in living conditions, medicine, and public health make naturally occurring plague pandemics highly improbable, an intentional plague outbreak could have serious consequences. Civil unrest characterized the plague outbreak in Surat, India, in 1994,[26] and provides an indication of the perception of plague in a modern society. The small outbreak, which led to only 52 deaths, resulted in mass exodus of up to one-half million people from the city and consequent serious economic loss.

Characteristics of a Deliberate Attack Using Plague

CLINICAL CHARACTERISTICS

The deliberate use of *Y. pestis* as a biowarfare or bioterrorism weapon is unlikely to be declared by the perpetrators at the time of the attack. Even in places where a biodetection system such as BioWatch (see Chapter 321) is in place, the identification of a deliberate aerosol release would likely coincide with or be later than the initial clinical cases presenting in the acute care setting.[27] Therefore, a high index of suspicion is required, first by the astute clinician and hospital laboratorian who are likely to be the first to assess infected, ill persons, and then by the state or local public health professional to whom the suspect case is reported. The clinical spectrum of disease among initial cases presenting following an attack may be different from that seen among reported endemic cases with a preponderance of pneumonic rather than bubonic cases, respectively. In the United States, 381 cases of plague occurred between 1970 and 2001,[28] bubonic infection accounting for the vast majority secondary to local inoculation from an animal bite or scratch. Primary pneumonic plague is rare and most likely acquired by inhalation of infectious respiratory droplets from infected animals, such as domestic cats.[29]

Aerosol release of *Y. pestis* would be odorless, colorless, and likely to be unnoticed until the first victims fell ill 1 to 7 days after exposure. However, individuals nearest to the aerosol release site may receive the highest dose of organisms.[23] In such a case, the natural history of the disease might be altered by a very short incubation period and overwhelming septicemia without classic pneumonia.

The appearance of more than one patient during a brief period presenting with fever; cough productive of mucopurulent sputum that is watery, bloody, and containing gram-negative rods; hemoptysis; chest pain; and evidence of bronchopneumonia (without widened mediastinum) on chest radiography should alert the provider to the possibility of pneumonic plague.[30] The last outbreak of pneumonic plague that resulted in person-to-person transmission in the United States occurred in 1924-25 in Los Angeles.[1] Thus, a pneumonic plague case suggests that a bioterrorist attack may have taken place.

Aerosol dissemination of *Y. pestis* would lead to an outbreak of predominantly pneumonic plague, with a different epidemiologic pattern from a naturally occurring outbreak. The likely size of an epidemic after an aerosol attack is not possible to predict given the many variables involved, including the amount of agent used, environmental conditions, methods of aerosolization, and population density at the epicenter. Transmission of plague via respiratory droplets or aerosols requires an infectious dose of as little as 100-500 organisms.[1] In experimentally infected rhesus macaques, the LD_{50} is approximately 20,000 inhaled bacteria.[31] In 1970, the World Health Organization (WHO) assessed that, in a worst-case scenario, 50 kg of *Y. pestis* released as an aerosol over a city of 5 million people could result in 150,000 cases of pneumonic plague, leading to 80,000-100,000 hospitalizations and 36,000 deaths.[32] That report estimated that plague bacilli would remain viable as an aerosol for 1 hour and cover an area extending up to 10 km from the point of release.

Unlike *Y. pestis*, the other two bacterial species of *Yersinia* pathogenic for humans, *Y. enterocolitica* and *Y. pseudotuberculosis*, are almost exclusively transmitted by the fecal-oral route and affect the gastrointestinal tract. On the basis of studies examining environmental persistence to *Y. pestis* noted above, it may be possible to disseminate *Y. pestis* via the water or food supply, but the effects are unknown. Animal reservoirs of *Y. pestis* (e.g., rats, ground squirrels, prairie dogs, and field mice) occasionally acquire the infection by ingesting contaminated animal tissues.[33] Humans rarely acquire the infection via the oral route, but oropharyngeal infection with and without lower gastrointestinal symptoms has been reported in the Middle East after ingestion of infected raw camel meat.[34,35] Additionally, *Y. pestis* remains viable in refrigerated or frozen, experimentally contaminated, raw ground pork.[36] It has been reported that *Y. pestis* cultures were used by the Japanese army during World War II to contaminate food supplies of Chinese cities.[10,37-39] Plague following ingestion of contaminated food has been reported to occur naturally among such groups who have eaten killed raw meat from infected animals.[40,41] Infection by the oral route, whether due to a naturally occurring or deliberate exposure, is likely to produce exudative pharyngitis with or without lower gastrointestinal symptoms and/or septicemia with or without the classic bubo of bubonic plague.[42] In such a case the initial red flag is likely to be raised by the laboratory identification of gram-negative bipolar staining rods on blood culture.

Unprotected close contacts of persons with pneumonic or bubonic plague have previously been shown to have culturable organisms in the oropharynx.[43] It is unknown what percentage of such patients would proceed to develop symptomatic illness requiring treatment.

PUBLIC HEALTH CHARACTERISTICS

The public health agency receiving the report of a case of suspected plague will investigate a subsequent laboratory-confirmed case as a potential deliberate event. An outbreak, whether large or small, will be treated as a deliberate bioterrorism or biowarfare event until proved otherwise. A public health differential diagnosis is applied upon further investigation of the event and includes a naturally occurring event in an endemic area or re-emerging area for infection, a laboratory accident, and an intentional attack. Furthermore, animal plague cases in species not usually associated with endemic infection would increase suspicion for a deliberate event. The initial epidemic curve would suggest a point source epidemic, and if identification is delayed, secondary cases would follow pneumonic plague cases. In the case of an aerosol release, the epidemic curve would be steep with hundreds or more cases identified in a short period of time, far in excess of the annual number of U.S. cases reported annually from endemic areas.

Plague Medical Countermeasures

DIAGNOSTIC TESTS

In the case of pneumonic plague, stain and culture of bronchial washings or expectorated sputum may yield a putative diagnosis.[44] The organisms may also be identified by stain and culture of blood or aspirates of tissue (such as a bubo or a lymph node). Gram stain reveals plump, gram-negative rods, 1 to 2 $\mu m \times 0.5$ μm. In liquid media, these appear mostly as single cells, pairs, or short chains. Although the Gram stain may reveal a bipolar staining (or "safety-pin" shape) that is characteristic (but not diagnostic) of *Y. pestis* (and other *Yersinia* spp.), the Romanovsky-type Wright-Giemsa or Wayson stains are generally preferred as they are more likely to demonstrate this characteristic.

Y. pestis grows best at ambient temperatures (22 to 28°C) and atmosphere, and slower at 35 to 37°C and 5% CO_2. Plates should be held for 5 days (or 7 days in the event of the patient having been exposed to antimicrobials). Since the organism's growth rate is slower than that of most other bacteria, its presence may be masked by co-incubating organisms that replicate faster. On agar plates, colonies are small (1 to 2 mm) and gray-white to opaque. Under magnification or longer incubation, they may develop a "fried egg" appearance and are slightly raised. There is minimal or no hemolysis on sheep red blood agar, and colonies do not ferment lactose on selective agar such as MacConkey or eosin methylene blue. In broth, *Y. pestis* grows in clumps. *Y. pestis* is oxidase, urease, and indole negative, catalase positive, and alkaline-slant/acid-butt on triple sugar iron agar. *Y. pestis* is relatively inert biochemically, and has been misidentified as non–*Y. pestis* (e.g., *Shigella*, H_2S-negative *Salmonella*, *Acinetobacter*, and *Y. pseudotuberculosis*) in automated identification systems.[45]

A tiered laboratory approach, the Laboratory Response Network, is used for the identification of *Y. pestis* and other biological threat agents (see Chapter 321). The American Society of Microbiology, in coordination with CDC and the Association of Public Health Laboratories (APHL), has developed protocols to assist the first-tier, Sentinel Level,

Clinical Microbiology Laboratories with information to rule out microorganisms that might be suspected as agents of bioterrorism.[44] Sentinel laboratories should consult with the state public health laboratory prior to or concurrent with testing if *Y. pestis* is suspected by the physician, and should immediately notify the local and state public health department and laboratory if *Y. pestis* cannot be ruled out for confirmation. The state public health department will notify the appropriate law enforcement officials as appropriate.

Confirmatory laboratories, generally at the major county or state health department level, and other reference laboratories, use a variety of additional tests to identify and confirm the presence of *Y. pestis* infection. These include direct fluorescent antibody test to detect the F1 envelope antigen, polymerase chain reaction, antigen-capture ELISA, and serologic tests (passive hemagglutination or ELISA). Passive hemagglutination antibody detection in acute- or convalescent-phase plasma, showing a four-fold increase in titer or a single titer ≥1:16 specific to F1 antigen of *Y. pestis*, would meet presumptive criteria for plague infection.[46] This test is of retrospective value only because it takes days for hemagglutination antibodies to form after disease onset.[47]

A number of rapid diagnostic tests have been described, and some are under development. An F1 antigen-capture ELISA and immunogold chromatography dipstick were found to be highly specific but sensitive only if specimens were bubo aspirates.[48] A point-of-care rapid, hand-held dipstick test using monoclonal antibodies to detect F1 antigen has shown promise in preliminary field studies in Madagascar.[49] The test allows for a presumptive diagnosis at the patient's bedside within 15 minutes, but an unused test has a shelf-life of only 21 days, making commercial off-the-shelf availability unlikely until the test's shelf life can be extended.

In the event of a bioterrorist attack, determination of antimicrobial susceptibility of the organisms is essential given the possibility that a naturally occurring or an engineered strain resistant to multiple antibiotics might have been employed. Until such results are obtained, the choice of antibiotics will have to take this possibility into account.

ANTIMICROBIAL AGENTS

Postexposure Prophylaxis

For asymptomatic persons known to have been exposed to an aerosol of *Y. pestis*, as well as for those who have had close contact (within 6 feet) of the coughing, ill person, antimicrobial prophylaxis for 7 days is recommended.[23]

A consensus statement developed by the Working Group on Civilian Biodefense in 2000 recommends a 7-day course of antimicrobial prophylaxis for asymptomatic people with a common-source exposure to an aerosol of *Y. pestis*, or with household, health care, or close (i.e., <2 m) contact with a patient suspected of having pneumonic plague[23] (Table 322-1). Of note, mice infected with F1 negative strain of *Y. pestis* have been shown to have a diminished response to prophylaxis with doxycycline,[50] but no data support this finding in humans. Persons presumed to have been exposed or who have had close contact with an infected person should also be placed under surveillance for the development of symptoms. Those who have symptoms consistent with pneumonic plague, such as fever or cough, should receive treatment.

Treatment

In the setting of an outbreak, treatment should not be delayed to await laboratory confirmation. Pneumonic plague is rapidly progressive, and antimicrobial therapy is effective only when administered early in the course of disease.[31]

The Working Group on Civilian Biodefense offered consensus recommendations,[23] based on existing limited evidence,[51-53] for the treatment of plague following a bioterrorist event (see Table 322-1). Historically, streptomycin has been the drug of choice in the treatment of plague.[1] However, it requires parenteral administration and is available only in limited supply. Only tetracyclines and streptomycin are licensed by the FDA to be used in the treatment of plague. A number

TABLE 322-1	Working Group on Civilian Biodefense Recommendations for Treatment of Adult Patients with Pneumonic Plague*	
Contained Casualty Setting		
Preferred Choices		
Streptomycin	1 g IM twice daily	
Gentamicin	5 mg/kg IM or IV once daily or 2 mg/kg loading dose followed by 1.7 mg/kg IM or IV 3 times daily	
Alternative Choices		
Doxycyline‡	100 mg IV twice daily or 200 mg IV once daily	
Ciprofloxacin†	400 mg IV twice daily	
Chloramphenicol	25 mg/kg IV 4 times daily	
Mass Casualty Setting or Postexposure Prophylaxis		
Preferred Choices		
Doxycycline‡	100 mg orally twice daily	
Ciprofloxacin†	500 mg orally twice daily	
Alternative Choices		
Chloramphenicol	25 mg/kg orally 4 times daily	

*Only streptomycin and drugs of the tetracycline class are approved by FDA for treatment of plague. Duration of therapy (parenteral or oral) should be 10 days; oral therapy may be substituted when the patient's condition improves. Duration of postexposure prophylaxis should be 7 days.
†Other fluoroquinolones may be substituted.
‡Tetracycline may be substituted for doxycycline.
IM, intramuscularly; IV, intravenously.
Adapted from Inglesby TV, Dennis DT, Henderson DA, et al. Plague as a biological weapon: Medical and public health management. Working Group on Civilian Biodefense. *JAMA.* 2000;283:2281-2290. With permission from the American Medical Association.

of other antimicrobials are thought to be useful but have not been licensed by the FDA owing to lack of adequate published human trials. Fluoroquinolones are effective in mice with experimentally induced pneumonic plague.[53-55] Chloramphenicol is considered the drug of choice in the setting of meningitis, because it crosses the blood-brain barrier, but no clinical trials are available. Although sulfonamides have been used, WHO found sulfadiazine to be ineffective against pneumonic plague.[56]

An additional consideration in the event of a bioterrorist attack is the potential use of multidrug-resistant strains of *Y. pestis*. Although resistance is infrequent in naturally occurring outbreaks,[1] a multidrug-resistant (plasmid-mediated) outbreak occurred in Madagascar.[57,58] Russian scientists have reportedly engineered a multidrug-resistant strain of *Y. pestis*,[14] and there is one Russian manuscript reporting a quinolone-resistant strain.[59] If *Y. pestis* is used as an agent of bioterrorism, there should be an initial high index of suspicion of antimicrobial resistance, susceptibility testing performed rapidly, and responses to treatment closely monitored. Treatment (and prophylaxis) might have to be altered accordingly.

Special Considerations

Only antimicrobials of the tetracycline class (including doxycycline, minocycline, and demeclocycline) and streptomycin are currently approved by the U.S. Food and Drug Administration (FDA) to treat infections caused by *Y. pestis*. Several antimicrobials (e.g., ciprofloxacin, gentamicin, and doxycycline) are included in the U.S. Government's Strategic National Stockpile (SNS), have been recommended by the Working Group on Civilian Biodefense,[23] and could be deployed in response to an intentional release of *Y. pestis*. Gentamicin, for example, has been used with success in naturally occurring outbreaks.[60] However, neither ciprofloxacin nor gentamicin is currently FDA approved for the management of plague. The paucity of FDA-approved antimicrobials to prevent or treat plague poses a logistical challenge in responding to a bioterrorist attack. If gentamicin and ciprofloxacin are federally supplied from the SNS for the treatment of plague, they would need to be used under an Emergency Use Authorization (EUA) or an Investigational New Drug (IND) application (see Chapter 321).

In preparation, CDC has submitted both IND and pre-EUA applications to the FDA for the use of gentamicin for the treatment of plague and for ciprofloxacin for plague prophylaxis and treatment.[61] The existence of an IND should help expedite the issuance of the EUA should it be needed. The successful distribution of prophylactic antibiotics in a mass casualty situation is resource intensive and requires extensive pre-event planning.[62] Individual physicians may decide to use ciprofloxacin or gentamicin, both approved for other purposes, for the off-label use for the prevention or treatment of plague. The "off-label" use of locally available antimicrobials would be subject to provider discretion and would not require an IND or EUA.

Vaccines

The short incubation period of pneumonic plague obviates the need for a plague vaccine for postexposure treatment in this setting. Rather, its use would be pre-exposure immunization for laboratorians and military personnel or for those in the post-event setting who might be at risk for recurring reexposure.

Despite over 100 years of research, a safe and effective vaccine against the pneumonic form of plague has been elusive.[63] However, there has been a degree of success in development of vaccines that are efficacious against bubonic plague, the most common form of naturally occurring plague, including postexposure efficacy as demonstrated by Haffkine.[64] However, the efficacy of these initial heat-killed whole-cell broth vaccines and then formalin-killed whole-cell vaccines against bubonic plague was empiric and without the benefit of modern clinical trials.

There is currently no licensed plague vaccine in the United States. A killed whole-cell (KWC) vaccine was first produced in the United States in 1946 (Army Vaccine), and subsequent improvements yielded plague vaccine United States Pharmacopoeia (USP), a formalin-killed preparation using the virulent 195/P strain of *Y. pestis*.[65] This latter vaccine was licensed for use in the United States until 1999. It was commonly used among U.S. military forces deployed to plague endemic areas such as Vietnam to protect against bubonic plague but was not efficacious against pneumonic plague. It required a series of injections, up to 10% of recipients experienced an adverse effect,[66] and it did not appear to be protective against pneumonic plague either in humans[67,68] or in experimentally infected animals.[69] The Commonwealth Serum Laboratories (CSL Australia) currently produces a KWC vaccine that is licensed for clinical use in Australia.

Live-attenuated vaccines have been developed and used in the former U.S.S.R. and former French colonies,[66] but their safety and efficacy have never been established in controlled, randomized clinical trials.[70] In mice, a live-attenuated vaccine composed of the EV76 strain proved protective against an inhalation challenge with *Y. pestis* but resulted in 1% fatality.[69]

The development of subunit vaccines using one or a combination of virulence factors, such as the F1 capsular protein or low calcium response virulence (LcrV) protein, has been the focus of recent efforts because they have been shown to protect mice against an aerosol challenge.[66] A vaccine in which the F1 antigen is the sole protective immunogen would, of course, not be effective in infections caused by F1-deficient *Y. pestis*.[25] Two recombinant vaccines are in clinical development. A recombinant rF1 and rV antigen candidate vaccine produced in *Escherichia coli*, named rYP, originally developed by the U.K. Ministry of Defence, is currently undergoing phase II trials,[71] as is an rF1V vaccine candidate, originally identified and developed at the Army Medical Research Institute of Infectious Diseases (USAMRIID) in conjunction with the DynPort Vaccine Company.[72]

Biologics

An alternative to antimicrobial therapy would be desired in the event that a strain was found to be resistant to available antibiotics and also for persons with allergies to all plague bactericidal antibiotics. In the 1940s it was demonstrated that serum from a convalescent plague patient would provide passively transferred immunity to mice.[73] Furthermore, passive administration of antibodies that target the F1 or LcrV proteins of *Y. pestis* can protect animals against plague.[74] Neutralizing monoclonal antibodies raised against the V antigen,[74] as well as passive transfer of F1+V immune serum,[75] seem to protect mice against infection with *Y. pestis*.

However, the utility of passive immunization might be limited by the relatively short period of protection afforded and also because concomitant administration of vaccine and passive antibody, in a mouse model, impairs the development of protective antibody responses.[76] The combined utility of antimicrobials with monoclonal or polyclonal anti-plague antibodies is unknown.

Preparedness and Response

Preparedness activities in anticipation of and response activities following an identified plague attack involve clinicians, health care and public health delivery systems, governmental authorities, and the public. A key element to an optimal response is coordinated pre-event planning across the spectrum of anticipated response elements based upon their roles. The use of drills and exercises as well as tabletop exercises may help highlight areas of needed improvement for increased response effectiveness.

ROLE OF HEALTH CARE PROVIDERS

It is important for clinicians to alert laboratory personnel processing specimens of patients with suspected or confirmed *Y. pestis* infections so that appropriate measures to avoid laboratory-acquired infection may be undertaken.[77] Additionally, all plague cases are reportable by physicians or laboratories to the local/state public health authorities, who in turn report cases to CDC.[78] Most clinicians have never diagnosed or treated a patient with plague. Therefore, continuing education is a key element in preparedness for providers. Professional societies and hospitals as well as local, state, and federal government agencies provide opportunities for continuing education in the clinical diagnosis and treatment of biological threat agents, including plague.

HOSPITAL INFECTION CONTROL MEASURES

CDC and the Association of Practitioners of Infection Control (APIC) have formulated a bioterrorism planning template for health care facilities, including pathogen-specific actions to be taken during an event.[79] The management of patients with pneumonic, bubonic, and septicemic plague, postexposure prophylaxis of health care workers, and environmental controls are the same for intentional and naturally occurring infections and are discussed above and in Chapter 16.

ROLE OF THE PUBLIC HEALTH SYSTEM

Although the astute clinician or laboratorian is anticipated to be the person who first suspects that a plague bioterrorist event is under way, the response to such an event will require constant real-time communication and collaboration between these elements at all levels—local, state, and federal. Therefore, the importance of the establishment of a strong health care–public health partnership before such an event occurs cannot be overemphasized.

Local/state health departments receiving a report of a case or outbreak of plague or suspected plague would report it to CDC.[79] Under the new International Health Regulations of 2005, in force beginning in July 2007, an outbreak of plague would likely be reportable as a "public health event of international importance" by the designated National Focal Point at the Department of Health and Human Services (DHHS).[80]

The federal government likely will play a role in the response to a plague attack or other bioterrorist event (see Chapter 321). DHHS and its subordinate operating divisions and agencies, including the Office of the Assistant Secretary for Preparedness and Response (ASPR), serve as the medical and public health interface with state and local governments preparing for and responding to medical and public health consequences of a bioterrorism event. The Office of Preparedness and Emergency Operations (OPEO), a section within ASPR, develops operational plans and training exercises to ensure the preparedness of DHHS, the Federal Government, and the public to respond to domestic and international public health and medical threats and emergencies. OPEO is the lead for federal interagency planning and response activities required to fulfill DHHS responsibilities under the National Response Framework's Emergency Support Function No. 8[81,82] and Homeland Security Presidential Directive No. 10.[83] OPEO maintains a regional planning and response coordination capability and operates the National Disaster Medical Systems (NDMS).

ASPR oversees the Public Health Emergency Medical Countermeasure Enterprise among DHHS agencies. This entity has multiple functions related to the availability, stockpiling, and storage of medical countermeasures and equipment needed to supplement local resources in a public health emergency. The Strategic National Stockpile, operated by the CDC Office of Terrorism Preparedness and Emergency Response, includes large caches of antibiotics for treatment of biological agents, including plague, as well as respirators that may be needed to supplement local resources. DHHS agencies including CDC, the Health Resources and Services Administration, FDA, and the Substance Abuse and Mental Health Administration all have preparedness roles that provide requested assistance to local area providers, hospitals, public health departments, and the public.

A "detect to treat" surveillance system, the BioWatch Program, is run under the auspices of the Department of Homeland Security in collaboration with DHHS and its subordinate agency, CDC, and the Environmental Protection Agency (EPA).[27] BioWatch uses a series of pathogen detectors co-located with EPA air quality monitors to collect and analyze airborne particles. The objective of this yet unproven system is to decrease morbidity and mortality through the early identification of a pathogen release with subsequent early treatment. EPA maintains the sampling component and sensors, and CDC coordinates the laboratory testing through the existing system of state and local public health laboratories, which constitute a major portion of the CDC-sponsored Laboratory Response Network (LRN).[84] The LRN is a consortium of academic, private, and public health laboratories that follow consensus protocols to rule out and identify plague and other microorganisms deemed to be possible agents in bioterrorism (see Chapter 321). To date, there is no published evidence about the sensitivity, specificity, or efficacy of BioWatch to detect a release of *Y. pestis*. The BioWatch system is currently being evaluated by the Institute of Medicine of the National Academies.

Postevent Recovery and Environmental Mitigation

PREVENTING OCCUPATIONAL EXPOSURE

A covert attack involving aerosolized plague is unlikely to involve emergency responders soon after the release, as the first evidence that an attack has occurred would likely be diagnosis of the ill people days after the actual release upon presentation to clinicians, including emergency medical technicians. These providers would be at risk for infection from these index cases. However, if emergency responders are expected to enter a likely contaminated area, as would occur if authorities received notification regarding an aerosol dissemination device, disease preventive measures are warranted. In addition to antimicrobial prophylaxis as describe above, field workers who may be occupationally exposed should don personal protective equipment (PPE) prior to entering a known contaminated area. According to CDC, a minimum of Biosafety Level 3 PPE (i.e., Tyvek outer clothing, gloves, booties, and positive-pressure HEPA-filtered respirators) should be used for field work posing possible infective exposure. Further, all PPE must be decontaminated or disposed of as biohazardous waste.[61]

The same infection control precautions as described for health care workers should be applied to morticians, forensic personnel, and veterinarians involved in the postmortem care of plague patients.[85] As for laboratory workers, comprehensive recommendations on biosafety practices have been published.[86]

ENVIRONMENTAL PERSISTENCE

Persistence of viable *Y. pestis* outside the host species is dependent on several factors including exposure to ultraviolet (UV) radiation spectrum in sunlight, relative humidity, temperature, desiccation, and the environmental setting and surface. A WHO report estimated that a plague aerosol would be nonviable after 1 hour owing to environmental factors such as sunlight and heat.[32] In experiments using heart brain infusion broth diluent, an avirulent form of aerosolized *Y. pestis* demonstrated linear decay kinetics at ambient temperature and relative humidity up to 50%, with a three-log decay over 90 minutes. Furthermore, there was a dramatic decrease in viability at higher relative humidity.[87] Decay kinetics are more rapid at a given relative humidity in the presence of higher temperatures and in the presence of UV light. In aggregate, these experimental data suggest that the bacterium would persist for only a short period after a release. However, there are reports suggesting that plague bacilli may survive in the soil for a prolonged period of time, risking establishment in the environment if permissive conditions exist, such as rodent reservoirs and efficient flea vectors, in the area of dissemination.[88]

Experimental evidence suggests that high levels of contamination in sewage would be decreased but not removed by standard treatment processes.[89] However, the effect of subsequent UV exposure on treated effluent discharged into rivers, streams, or lakes may decrease viable organisms further. Notably, viable but non-culturable organisms could persist for approximately 2 weeks in well and tap water.[90] The ability of drinking of contaminated water to cause gastrointestinal or septicemic plague is unknown.

Surveillance of human disease and a limited environmental assessment following the release of *Y. pestis* are needed to evaluate unlikely risk to humans from exposure to infected animals, infectious fleas, or contaminated surfaces, soils, and water supplies. If the outbreak is found to spread in animal populations or to new regions, further control and prevention measures will need to be undertaken.

REFERENCES

1. Perry RD, Fetherston JD. *Yersinia pestis*—etiologic agent of plague. *Clin Microbiol Rev.* 1997;10:35-66.
2. Titball RW, Leary SE. Plague. *Br Med Bull.* 1998;54:625-633.
3. World Health Organization. Human plague in 2002 and 2003. *Wkly Epidemiol Rec.* 2004;79:301-306.
4. Anisimov AP, Lindler LE, Pier GB. Intraspecific diversity of *Yersinia pestis*. *Clin Microbiol Rev.* 2004;17:434-464.
5. Derbes VJ. De Mussis and the great plague of 1348: a forgotten episode of bacteriological warfare. *JAMA.* 1966;196:59-62.
6. Hughes L. *Peter the Great: A Biography.* New Haven: Yale University Press; 2002.
7. Block SM. The growing threat of biological weapons. *American Scientist* January-February 2001. Available at: <http://www.americanscientist.org/issues/feature/2001/1/the-growing-threat-of-biological-weapons>; Accessed 04/04/09.

8. Harris SH. *Factories of Death: Japanese Biological Warfare, 1932-45, and the American Cover-up.* New York: Routledge; 1994.
9. Williams P, Wallace D. *Unit 731: Japan's Secret Biological Warfare in World War II.* 1st American ed. New York: Free Press; 1989.
10. Barenblatt D. *A Plague upon Humanity: The Secret Genocide of Axis Japan's Germ Warfare Operation.* New York: HarperCollins; 2004.
11. Miller J, Engelberg S, Broad WJ. *Germs: Biological Weapons and America's Secret War.* 1st Touchstone ed. New York: Simon & Schuster; 2002.
12. Mangold T, Goldberg J. *Plague Wars.* 1st U.S. ed. New York: St. Martin's Press; 2000.
13. ANSER Institute for Homeland Defense. Interview with Serguei Popov. November 17, 2000. Available at: <http://homelanddefense.org/journal/Search.aspx?s=popov>; Accessed 04/04/09.

14. Alibek K, Handelman S. *Biohazard.* New York: Random House; 1999.
15. Tucker JB. *Toxic Terror.* Cambridge, MA: MIT Press; 2000.
16. Carus WS. National Defense University. Working Paper: Bioterrorism and Biocrimes: The Illicit Use of Biological Weapons Since 1900. February 2001. Available at: <http://oai.dtic.mil/oai/oai?verb=getRecord&metadataPrefix=html&identifier=ADA402108>; Accessed 04/04/09.
17. National Agriculture and Food Defense Act of 2007. Available at: <http://www.fas.org/biosecurity/resource/legislation/s1804.html>; Accessed 04/04/09.
18. Public Health Security and Bioterrorism Preparedness Response Act of 2002. Available at: <http://www.fda.gov/oc/bioterrorism/PL107-188.html>; Accessed 04/04/09.
19. U.S. Patriot Act of 2001, Title II, "Enhancing Controls on Dangerous Biological Agents and Toxins." Available at: <http://

fl1.findlaw.com/news.findlaw.com/cnn/docs/terrorism/hr3162. pdf>; Accessed 04/02/08.

20. Franz DR, Jahrling PB, Friedlander AM, et al. Clinical recognition and management of patients exposed to biological warfare agents. *JAMA*. 1997;278:399-411.

21. Rotz LD, Khan AS, Lillibridge SR, et al. Public health assessment of potential biological terrorism agents. *Emerg Infect Dis*. 2002;8:225-230.

22. DHHS Office of the Assistant Secretary for Preparedness and Response. HHS Public Health Emergency Medical Countermeasures Enterprise Implementation Plan For Chemical, Biological, Radiological and Nuclear Threats. Notice. *Federal Register*. 2007;72:20117-20128.

23. Inglesby TV, Dennis DT, Henderson DA, et al. Plague as a biological weapon: medical and public health management. *JAMA*. 2000;283:2281-2290.

24. Worsham PL, Stein MP, Welkos SL. Construction of defined F1 negative mutants of virulent *Yersinia pestis*. *Contrib Microbiol Immunol*. 1995;13:325-328.

25. Davis KJ, Fritz DL, Pitt ML, et al. Pathology of experimental pneumonic plague produced by fraction 1-positive and fraction 1-negative *Yersinia pestis* in African green monkeys. *Arch Pathol Lab Med*. 1996;120:156-163.

26. Ramalingaswami V. Psychosocial effects of the 1994 plague outbreak in Surat, India. *Mil Med*. 2001;166:29-30.

27. Shea DA, Lister SA. The BioWatch Program: Detection of Bioterrorism, Congressional Research Service Report No. RL 32152; November 19, 2003. Available at: <http://www.fas.org/sgp/crs/terror/RL32152.html#_1_3>; Accessed 04/04/09.

28. Centers for Disease Control and Prevention. Summary of notifiable diseases—United States, 2001. *MMWR Morb Mortal Wkly Rep*. 2003;50:1-108.

29. Centers for Disease Control and Prevention. Prevention of plague: Recommendations of the Advisory Committee on Immunization Practices (ACIP). *MMWR Recomm Rep*. 1996;45:1-15.

30. Recognition of illness associated with the intentional release of a biologic agent. *MMWR Morb Mortal Wkly Rep*. 2001;50:893-897.

31. Meyer KF. Pneumonic plague. *Bacteriol Rev*. 1961;25:249-261.

32. World Health Organization. Health aspects of chemical and biological weapons: Report of a WHO Group of Consultants. Geneva; 1970.

33. Butler T, Dennis DT. *Yersinia* species, including plague. In: Mandell GL, Bennett JE, Dolin R, eds. *Mandell, Douglas, and Bennett's Principles and Practice of Infectious Diseases*. 6th ed. Philadelphia: Elsevier Churchill Livingstone; 2005.

34. Arbaji A, Kharabsheh S, Al-Azab S, et al. A 12-case outbreak of pharyngeal plague following the consumption of camel meat, in north-eastern Jordan. *Ann Trop Med Parasitol*. 2005;99:789-793.

35. Christie AB, Chen TH, Elberg SS. Plague in camels and goats: their role in human epidemics. *J Infect Dis*. 1980;141:724-726.

36. Sommers CH, Niemira BA. Effect of temperature on the radiation resistance of *Yersinia pestis* suspended in raw ground pork. *J Food Safety*. 2007;27:317-325.

37. Burrows WD, Renner SE. Biological warfare agents as threats to potable water. *Environ Health Perspect*. 1999;107:975-984.

38. Eitzen E, U.S. Army Medical Research Institute of Infectious Diseases. *Medical Management of Biological Casualties: Handbook*. 3rd ed. Frederick, MD: U.S. Army Medical Research Institute of Infectious Diseases, Fort Detrick; 1998.

39. McGovern T, Friedlander A. Plague. In: Sidell F, Takafuji E, Franz D, eds. *Textbook of Military Medicine. Part I*. Falls Church, VA: Office of the Surgeon General, United States Army; 1997:479-502.

40. Bin Saeed AA, Al-Hamdan NA, Fontaine RE. Plague from eating raw camel liver. *Emerg Infect Dis*. 2005;11:1456-1457.

41. von Reyn CF, Barnes AM, Weber NS, et al. Bubonic plague from exposure to a rabbit: a documented case, and a review of rabbit-associated plague cases in the United States. *Am J Epidemiol*. 1976;104:81-87.

42. Hull HF, Montes JM, Mann JM. Plague masquerading as gastrointestinal illness. *West J Med*. 1986;145:485-487.

43. Marshall JD Jr, Quy DV, Gibson FL. Asymptomatic pharyngeal plague infection in Vietnam. *Am J Trop Med Hyg*. 1967;16:175-177.

44. American Society for Microbiology. Sentinel Laboratory Guidelines for Suspected Agents of Bioterrorism: *Yersinia pestis*. August 15, 2005. Available at: <http://www.asm.org/ASM/files/LeftMarginHeaderList/DOWNLOADFILENAME/000000000524/Ypestis81505.pdf>; Accessed 04/04/09.

45. Wilmoth BA, Chu MC, Quan TJ. Identification of *Yersinia pestis* by BBL Crystal Enteric/Nonfermenter Identification System. *J Clin Microbiol*. 1996;34:2829-2830.

46. Butler T. Yersinia infections: centennial of the discovery of the plague bacillus. *Clin Infect Dis*. 1994;19:655-661.

47. Butler T. *Yersinia* species (including plague). In: Mandell GL, Douglas RG, Bennett JE, Dolin R, eds. *Mandell, Douglas, and Bennett's Principles and Practice of Infectious Diseases*. 5th ed. Philadelphia: Churchill Livingstone; 2000:2406-2411.

48. Chanteau S, Rahalison L, Ratsitorahina M, et al. Early diagnosis of bubonic plague using F1 antigen capture ELISA assay and rapid immunogold dipstick. *Int J Med Microbiol*. 2000;290:279-283.

49. Chanteau S, Rahalison L, Ralafiarisoa L, et al. Development and testing of a rapid diagnostic test for bubonic and pneumonic plague. *Lancet*. 2003;361:211-216.

50. Samokhodkina ED, Ryzhko IV, Shcherbaniuk AI, et al. [Doxycycline in the prevention of experimental plague induced by plague microbe variants.] *Antibiot Khimioter*. 1992;37:26-28.

51. Byrne WR, Welkos SL, Pitt ML, et al. Antibiotic treatment of experimental pneumonic plague in mice. *Antimicrob Agents Chemother*. 1998;42:675-681.

52. Smith MD, Vinh DX, Nguyen TT, et al. *In vitro* antimicrobial susceptibilities of strains of *Yersinia pestis*. *Antimicrob Agents Chemother*. 1995;39:2153-2154.

53. Bonacorsi SP, Scavizzi MR, Guiyoule A, et al. Assessment of a fluoroquinolone, three beta-lactams, two aminoglycosides, and a cycline in treatment of murine *Yersinia pestis* infection. *Antimicrob Agents Chemother*. 1994;38:481-486.

54. Russell P, Eley SM, Bell DL, et al. Doxycycline or ciprofloxacin prophylaxis and therapy against experimental *Yersinia pestis* infection in mice. *J Antimicrob Chemother*. 1996;37:769-774.

55. Russell P, Eley SM, Green M, et al. Efficacy of doxycycline and ciprofloxacin against experimental *Yersinia pestis* infection. *J Antimicrob Chemother*. 1998;41:301-305.

56. World Health Organization. *Expert Committee on Plague: Third Report*. Geneva: WHO; 1970.

57. Galimand M, Guiyoule A, Gerbaud G, et al. Multidrug resistance in *Yersinia pestis* mediated by a transferable plasmid. *N Engl J Med*. 1997;337:677-680.

58. Rasoamanana B, Coulanges P, Michel P, et al. [Sensitivity of *Yersinia pestis* to antibiotics: 277 strains isolated in Madagascar between 1926 and 1989.] *Arch Inst Pasteur Madagascar*. 1989;56:37-53.

59. Ryzhko IV, Shcherbaniuk AI, Samokhodkina ED, et al. [Virulence of rifampicin and quinolone resistant mutants of strains of plague microbe with Fra+ and Fra- phenotypes.] *Antibiot Khimioter*. 1994;39:32-36.

60. Mwengee W, Butler T, Mgema S, et al. Treatment of plague with gentamicin or doxycycline in a randomized clinical trial in Tanzania. *Clin Infect Dis*. 2006;42:614-621.

61. Centers for Disease Control and Prevention. Plague training module. Available at: <http://www.bt.cdc.gov/agent/plague/trainingmodule/index.asp>; Accessed 04/04/09.

62. Blank S, Moskin LC, Zucker JR. An ounce of prevention is a ton of work: mass antibiotic prophylaxis for anthrax, New York City, 2001. *Emerg Infect Dis*. 2003;9:615-622.

63. Titball RW, Williamson ED. *Yersinia pestis* (plague) vaccines. *Expert Opin Biol Ther*. 2004;4:965-973.

64. Haffkine WM. Discourse on preventive inoculation. *Lancet*. 1899;156:1694-1699.

65. Williams JE, Altieri PL, Berman S, et al. Potency of killed plague vaccines prepared from avirulent *Yersinia pestis*. *Bull World Health Organ*. 1980;58:753-756.

66. Titball RW, Williamson ED. Vaccination against bubonic and pneumonic plague. *Vaccine*. 2001;19:4175-4184.

67. Meyer KF. Effectiveness of live or killed plague vaccines in man. *Bull World Health Organ*. 1970;42:653-666.

68. Cohen RJ, Stockard JL. Pneumonic plague in an untreated plague-vaccinated individual. *JAMA*. 1967;202:365-366.

69. Russell P, Eley SM, Hibbs SE, et al. A comparison of Plague vaccine, USP and EV76 vaccine induced protection against *Yersinia pestis* in a murine model. *Vaccine*. 1995;13:1551-1556.

70. Jefferson T, Demicheli V, Pratt M. Vaccines for preventing plague. *Cochrane Database Syst Rev*. 2000: CD000976.

71. PharmAthene. Available at: <http://www.pharmathene.com/pdf/Fact%20Sheet%20-%20Investor.pdf>; Accessed 04/04/09.

72. CSC'S DynPort Vaccine Company to Continue Plague Vaccine Development. June 5, 2008. Available at: <http://www.csc.com/mms/dvc/en/ne/pr/articleDetail.jsp?id=12925>; Accessed 04/04/09.

73. Jawetz E, Meyer KF. Studies on plague immunity in experimental animals. 2. Some factors of the immunity mechanism in bubonic plague. *J Immunol*. 1944;49:15-30.

74. Hill J, Leary SE, Griffin KF, et al. Regions of *Yersinia pestis* V antigen that contribute to protection against plague identified by passive and active immunization. *Infect Immun*. 1997;65:4476-4482.

75. Green M, Rogers D, Russell P, et al. The SCID/Beige mouse as a model to investigate protection against *Yersinia pestis*. *FEMS Immunol Med Microbiol*. 1999;23:107-113.

76. Eyles JE, Butcher WA, Titball RW, et al. Concomitant administration of *Yersinia pestis* specific monoclonal antibodies with plague vaccine has a detrimental effect on vaccine mediated immunity. *Vaccine*. 2007;25:7301-7306.

77. Burmeister R. Laboratory-acquired pneumonic plague. *Ann Intern Med*. 1962;56:789-800.

78. Centers for Disease Control and Prevention. Nationally Notifiable Infectious Diseases: United States 2008. Available at: <http://www.cdc.gov/ncphi/disss/nndss/PHS/infdis2008.htm>; Accessed 04/04/09.

79. English JF. Overview of bioterrorism readiness plan: a template for health care facilities. *Am J Infect Control*. 1999;27:468-469.

80. World Health Organization. World Health Assembly 58. WHA58.3 Revision of the International Health Regulations. 2005. Available at: <http://www.who.int/ipcs/publications/wha/ihr_resolution.pdf>; Accessed 04/04/09.

81. U.S. Dept. of Homeland Security. *National Response Framework*. Washington, DC: U.S. Dept. of Homeland Security; 2008.

82. Department of Homeland Security. National Response Plan Emergency Support Function #8—Public Health and Medical Services Annex. Available at: <http://www.fema.gov/pdf/emergency/nrf/nrf-esf-08.pdf>; Accessed 04/04/09.

83. Homeland Security Presidential Directive–10: Biodefense for the 21st Century. April 28, 2004. Available at: <http://www.dhs.gov/xabout/laws/editorial_0607.shtm>; Accessed 04/04/09.

84. Centers for Disease Control and Prevention. Laboratory Response Network: Partners in Preparedness. Available at: <http://www.bt.cdc.gov/lrn/pdf/lrnhistory.pdf>; Accessed 04/04/09.

85. U.S. Department of Labor. Occupational Safety & Health Administration. Plague controls. <http://www.osha.gov/SLTC/plague/controls.html>; Accessed 04/04/09.

86. Centers for Disease Control and Prevention, National Institutes of Health. *Biosafety in Microbiological and Biomedical Laboratories*. 4th ed. Atlanta, GA: U.S. Government Printing Office; 1999.

87. Won WD, Ross H. Effect of diluent and relative humidity on apparent viability of airborne *Pasteurella pestis*. *Appl Microbiol*. 1966;14:742-745.

88. Foley JE, Zipser J, Chomel B, et al. Modeling plague persistence in host-vector communities in California. *J Wildl Dis*. 2007;43:408-424.

89. Filipkowska Z. Sanitary and bacteriological aspects of sewage treatment. *Acta Microbiol Pol*. 2003;52(Suppl):57-66.

90. Mitscherlich E, Marth EH. *Microbial Survival in the Environment: Bacteria and Rickettsiae Important in Human and Animal Health*. Berlin. New York: Springer-Verlag; 1984.

Francisella tularensis (Tularemia) as an Agent of Bioterrorism

LISA S. HODGES | ROBERT L. PENN

*F*rancisella tularensis has become a national and global public health issue because of its potential use in biological warfare by organized military or independent terrorist groups. It was weaponized by freeze drying a bacteria-laden slurry that was then milled into a fine powder for aerosolized attack and incorporated into the biological warfare program of the United States during the 1950s to 1960s.[1] The potential impact of this organism is demonstrated by a report from the Centers for Disease Control and Prevention: If 100,000 people were exposed to a "tularemic cloud," 82,500 cases (82.5% attack rate) with 6188 deaths (6.2% death rate) would be expected. The medical costs of tularemia from this bioterrorist attack would range from $456 million to $561.8 million.[2]

History and Potential Use

The Centers for Disease Control and Prevention has classified *F. tularensis* as a category A bioterrorism agent, one most likely to be used as a weapon due to its ease of dissemination, potential to cause disease and death, impact on public health, and overall social disruption.[3] Table 323-1 lists the specific features of *F. tularensis* and the disease of tularemia that render this organism particularly useful as an agent of bioterrorism. Features that render it a less desirable weapon than other category A agents are its lack of a stable spore phase and its difficulty in handling without infecting those who process and disperse the pathogen.[4] The potential for *F. tularensis* to cause natural outbreaks has been well archived in the medical literature (see Chapter 227). Furthermore, *F. tularensis* is a well-described hazardous material for laboratory workers.

The highly infectious nature of this organism in concert with its ability to cause significant morbidity and mortality make *F. tularensis* an attractive biological agent. Japanese Germ Warfare Units recognized this potential as early as 1932 and began experiments on their prisoners with various forms of tularemia.[5] In 1955, U.S. military and civilian volunteers entered a steel chamber termed "The Eight Ball" at the U.S. Army Medical Research Institute of Infectious Diseases at Fort Detrick, MD, where they inhaled aerosolized *F. tularensis* organisms. The test allowed military researchers to study vaccine and antibiotic efficacy as well as the aerosolization parameters.[6] After the disposal of bioweapons stockpiles during the early 1970s, defensive research has continued in the areas of immunology, genomics, and vaccinology.

Characteristics of a Deliberate Attack Using Tularemia

The clinical manifestations of a deliberate attack using *F. tularensis* depend on the site of inoculation, the infecting dose, and virulence of the selected strain. The 2001 Tularemia Consensus Statement developed by The Working Group on Civilian Biodefense concluded that aerosolization would be the most likely method for dispersing *F. tularensis,* as inhalation of bacilli would affect the largest number of people and cause the most devastating manifestations of disease.[7] Children are theorized to be more vulnerable than adults to an aerosolized agent because of their higher respiratory rate, more permeable skin, and higher skin-to-mass ratio.[8]

After an aerosol release and an incubation period of 3 to 5 days, patients may present with the acute onset of fever (38°C to 40°C), malaise, headache, rigors, coryza, and sore throat. The subsequent clinical syndrome depends on the immune status of the host, the inhaled inoculum, and the subspecies of the released agent. In past outbreaks, *F. tularensis* subspecies *tularensis* (type A), found in North America, has been responsible for more serious disease than *F. tularensis* subspecies *holarctica* (type B), found in Europe, Asia, and North America. After inhalation, one of two acute presentations of tularemia is most likely to be seen: either typhoidal or pneumonic disease. Much of the experience with pneumonic tularemia in the United States is derived from the result of naturally occurring inhalational disease on Martha's Vineyard.[9] Primary pneumonic tularemia results from direct inoculation of the lung parenchyma with inhaled organisms. The typical initial manifestations on Martha's Vineyard have been some combination of fever, malaise, headache, sore throat, myalgias, anorexia and prostration, but the initial chest radiograph is often unremarkable.[9] Later symptoms generally include fever, cough, and retrosternal and pleuritic chest pain. Dermatologic manifestations in association with pneumonic tularemia are well described, particularly erythema nodosum (see Chapter 227). In the absence of treatment, fevers become hectic, respiratory findings become more prominent, and the chest radiograph becomes abnormal.[9] Chest radiography usually demonstrates peribronchial cuffing or lobar consolidation and may reveal an exudative pleural effusion and hilar lymphadenopathy. Less common manifestations include nodular or rounded infiltrates. Adenopathy has been more frequent in European cases believed to have been acquired by inhalation.[10] Pleural effusions accompanying pneumonic tularemia are common and may be detected as early as 3 days after the onset of symptoms. Effusions are characteristically exudative, appearing turbid with elevated protein and with a lymphocytic leukocytosis.[11]

Findings in nonhuman primates reveal a sequence of pathologic changes after inhalation of a virulent strain of *F. tularensis*. Initially there is acute bronchiolitis that rapidly spreads to the peribronchial tissues and alveolar septa, accompanied by tracheobronchial lymphadenopathy. Areas of inflammation are diffuse, evolving to consolidation, granuloma formation, and eventually chronic interstitial fibrosis.[12] Similarly, biopsy and autopsy specimens of human lungs from patients with tularemia pneumonia reveal an intense inflammatory edema that accompanies regions of necrotizing bronchiolitis and bronchopneumonia. Necrotic exudates are often found along the bronchial tree and along the interlobular septa. The involvement of vessels causes narrowing of their lumina, and complete occlusion by thrombosis is often found.[13,14] Humans exposed to low-dose aerosols of virulent strains may potentially become ill from dissemination to other organs without significant radiographic evidence of pulmonary disease. However, inhalation of a large number of *F. tularensis*, as could occur in a bioterrorism event, could cause a rapidly fatal pneumonia with or without extensive involvement of other organs. Thus, the degree of pulmonary involvement is multifactoral, determined by the dose and route of inoculation, virulence of the infecting strain, disease duration, and damage to small and medium-sized blood vessels.

A significant number of patients progress to frank respiratory failure, requiring mechanical ventilation; they may also develop the systemic inflammatory response syndrome. Recognizing this pneu-

<table>
<tr><td>TABLE 323-1</td><td colspan="2">**Characteristics of *Francisella tularensis* and Tularemia That Render the Organism a Suitable Bioterrorism Agent**</td></tr>
<tr><td>*Characteristic*</td><td colspan="2">*Comments*</td></tr>
</table>

Characteristic	Comments
Virulence	Low inhalation inocula: 10 organisms required to cause pneumonic tularemia Potential to infect all ages Populace highly susceptible to infection
Diversity of infectious sources	Water, animal hides, infected meat, aerosolized feces or animal matter, insect vectors
Pathogenicity	Substantial morbidity and mortality in untreated disease Increased pediatric susceptibility due to increased respiratory rate, higher skin/mass ratio, more permeable skin, and less fluid reserve[8]
Stability	Organisms and by-products stable in various environments
Assembly and distribution	Large quantities easily manufactured with potential for silent release into air or water supply
Diagnosis and public response	Difficult diagnosis in certain areas as disease is rarely seen Rapid pediatric diagnosis difficult because of inability of young children to describe symptomatology Public panic may overwhelm health and law enforcement agencies
Epidemiologic investigations	Identification of exposure site difficult if affected patients are far from site of release Potential to infect laboratory and autopsy workers

monic syndrome as tularemia is challenging because of the difficulty in distinguishing it from a plethora of other acute infections, including community-acquired pneumonia, *Legionella pneumonia*, psittacosis, Q fever, pneumonic plague, inhalation anthrax, and, more recently, severe acute respiratory syndrome. Characteristics that may help distinguish among some of these etiologies are presented in Table 323-2. The case-fatality rate of untreated severe pneumonic tularemia has approached 60%.

The second likely presentation of disease after inhalation is typhoidal tularemia. This presentation is marked by fever, a relative bradycardia, prostration, and signs of sepsis with no skin or lymph node manifestations of infection (see Chapter 227). Hematogenous dissemination of the organism is the rule, but blood cultures are often negative. This is due in part to intracellular sequestration of organisms and their fastidious culture characteristics. Secondary pneumonia and pleural effusion may result from hematogenous seeding of the lung where areas of focal necrosis can progress to bronchopneumonia, or become discrete nodules that may caseate. In some instances, a heavy pulmonary dispersion creates diffuse miliary foci mimicking those of miliary tuberculosis.[15] Patients with this clinical presentation are difficult to distinguish from those with primary pneumonic tularemia. In patients not gravely ill with typhoidal tularemia, fever can persist for months, causing significant debilitation. Involvement of the mouth or pharynx has been reported in as many as 35% of cases of typhoidal disease including pharyngitis, ulcerative tonsillitis, and pharyngeal abscess.[16] The typhoidal form has been complicated by rhabdomyolysis, renal dysfunction, osteomyelitis, endocarditis, meningitis, and hepatitis.[17,18] Renal dysfunction is common and, in severe cases, may progress to oliguria and acute renal failure. Acute renal failure is frequently an important contributing factor in fatal cases of typhoidal tularemia. Gastrointestinal symptoms mimicking enteric fever may be present. Many patients with typhoidal tularemia also develop erythema multiforme or erythema nodosum, further confusing the clinical picture. Historically, case-fatality rates of 35% to 60% have been observed in patients with untreated typhoidal tularemia[19]; however, the reported U.S. case-fatality rate is less than 2%, illustrating the importance of prompt recognition and institution of appropriate antimicrobial agents.[20]

It should be emphasized that not all patients inhaling aerosolized *F. tularensis* present with typhoidal or pneumonic tularemia. Airborne exposure can result in presentations of oculoglandular, ulceroglandular, glandular, or pharyngeal disease (see Chapter 227). It is also important to recognize that patients exposed to low-dose aerosols of virulent

<table>
<tr><td>TABLE 323-2</td><td colspan="6">**Comparison among Community-Acquired Pneumonias and Tularemia Pneumonia**</td></tr>
<tr><td>*Parameter*</td><td>*Tularemia*</td><td>*Pneumococcal Pneumonia*</td><td>*Common Atypical Pneumonias**</td><td>*Influenza Viral Pneumonia*</td><td>*Q Fever*</td><td>*SARS*</td></tr>
<tr><td>Incubation period</td><td>3-5 days after experimental aerosol exposure[†]</td><td>Often several days after onset of upper respiratory symptoms</td><td>*Legionella pneumophila*, 2-10 days
Mycoplasma pneumoniae, 14-21 days
Chlamydia pneumoniae, 21 days</td><td>Progression of typical influenza illness to include signs and symptoms of pneumonia</td><td>20 days</td><td>2-10 days</td></tr>
<tr><td>Underlying illness</td><td>No</td><td>Yes</td><td>Yes or no</td><td>Yes or no</td><td>No</td><td>No</td></tr>
<tr><td>Previous animal or insect exposures</td><td>Common
None if act of bioterrorism</td><td>No</td><td>No</td><td>No</td><td>Common
None if act of bioterrorism</td><td>No</td></tr>
<tr><td>Chest radiograph</td><td>Peribronchial cuffing
Alveolar consolidation
Parapneumonic effusion
Hilar lymphadenopathy</td><td>Alveolar consolidation
Parapneumonic effusion</td><td>Interstitial infiltrates
Patchy alveolar consolidation with predominant changes in lower lobes and perihilar regions</td><td>Bilateral infiltrates without consolidation</td><td>Alveolar consolidation
Reticulonodular infiltrates
Parapneumonic effusion
Atelectasis
Hilar lymphadenopathy
Multiple rounded opacities in cat-associated illness</td><td>Early: focal or patchy reticulonodular interstitial infiltrates
Late: alveolar consolidation</td></tr>
<tr><td>Diagnosis</td><td>Sputum GS, DFA
Enriched media culture
Serology
Fluid/tissue PCR</td><td>Sputum GS
Blood cultures
Urinary antigen</td><td>Serology
Urinary antigens
Culture of respiratory specimens (*Legionella*)</td><td>Rapid antigen assay
Viral culture
PCR</td><td>Serology (IFA)
Tissue PCR</td><td>Exclusion of other diagnoses
Exposure history
Serology
SARS-CoV RNA by RT-PCR</td></tr>
<tr><td>Person-to-person spread</td><td>No</td><td>No</td><td>Possible</td><td>Yes</td><td>No</td><td>Yes</td></tr>
</table>

*Pneumonias caused by *Legionella*, *Mycoplasma*, and *Chlamydia*.
[†]Dennis DT, Inglesby TV, Henderson DA, et al. Tularemia as a biological weapon. *JAMA*. 2001;285:2763-2773.
DFA, direct fluorescent antibody stain; GS, Gram stain; IFA, immunofluorescent antibody assay; PCR, polymerase chain reaction assay; RT-PCR, real-time polymerase chain reaction assay; SARS, severe acute respiratory syndrome; SARS-CoV RNA, SARS-coronavirus ribonucleic acid.

strains may present with disseminated disease in the absence of pneumonia. During a 1966 outbreak of aerosolized *F. tularensis* subspecies *holarctica* in Sweden, conjunctival involvement was noted in 26% of cases, skin ulcers in 12%, and pharyngeal and anterior cervical node involvement in 31%.[21] Although pharyngitis can occur after inhalation, this presentation is more commonly associated with ingestion, and several clustered cases of tularemic pharyngitis suggest a contaminated water or food source.

Clustered severe respiratory or typhoidal illness in previously healthy individuals of any age suggests inhalation tularemia, especially when patients develop pleural effusions and tracheobronchial or hilar lymphadenopathy. Knowledge of the current local epidemiology of tularemia is helpful when evaluating new cases for possible bioterrorist implications.[22] Previous outbreaks have occurred in settings with appropriate epidemiologic exposures[22]; an urban outbreak of tularemia lacking in animal, insect, and water or farming exposures suggests a possible bioterrorist attack. Reporting cases of tularemia to state health departments and to national databases is of utmost importance.

Diagnosis

Diagnosis of tularemia requires a high index of suspicion and most often is made on clinical grounds supported by results of microbial cultures and serologic studies (see Chapter 227). Serologic tests are preferred to cultures for routine diagnosis of endemic tularemia. However, antibodies usually are not measurable before week 2 of the illness, rendering serologic studies impractical for rapid diagnosis after an intentional release.

Highly specific and sensitive polymerase chain reaction (PCR) and real-time PCR assays have been developed for use on various human specimens, including blood products.[23-30] Sjöstedt and colleagues[25] demonstrated the advantage of PCR testing over testing with conventional cultures in the examination of human tularemic skin lesions; 73% of lesions were PCR positive for *F. tularensis* compared with only 25% using growth in culture. PCR has many advantages over culture-based methods, including rapidity of diagnosis, accuracy, reproducibility, and reduced biohazard risk. In addition, PCR-based assays may permit the rapid detection of antibiotic resistance genes or other genetic modifications in weaponized *F. tularensis* strains. Current research is focusing on the rapid transport of field specimens for PCR testing, and the development of field-stable PCR and other techniques for the simultaneous detection of multiple potential bioterrorism agents.[1,26,29-31] PCR assays have been used most often on swabs of an ulcer for the diagnosis of ulceroglandular tularemia, and the sensitivity of PCR when applied to other clinical specimens and disease presentations is not known. Antigen detection assays, PCR, enzyme-linked immunosorbent assays, immunoblotting, and electrophoresis are available in research and reference laboratories.[7] Novel genetic, proteomic, and immunologic approaches to rapid diagnosis are being explored; however, their clinical relevance is uncertain at this time (see Chapter 227).[31-34a] In the event of a bioterrorist attack, the emergency department is the most likely site where patients will initially present, highlighting the need for translating advances in rapid diagnostics to the bedside for use during acute care.

When entertaining a diagnosis of tularemia, the physician should alert the microbiology laboratory to allow for implementation of specialized diagnostic and safety procedures. Appropriate specimens depend on the clinical manifestations and may include blood cultures; swabs from skin, conjunctiva, and pharyngeal lesions; respiratory secretions from bronchoalveolar lavage washings, endotracheal aspirates, and expectorated sputum; lymph node aspirates; and tissue biopsy specimens. Biohazard level 2 recommendations should be followed in the laboratories processing clinical specimens. The organism is a known laboratory hazard owing to its highly virulent nature and should not be manipulated in the microbiology laboratory on an open bench.[35-37]

Smears may reveal faintly staining, tiny, intracellular and extracellular gram-negative coccobacilli that exhibit fastidious culture characteristics (see Chapter 227). Cysteine-enriched media should be used, but the organism may not grow well in broth even when enriched. Growth of the organism is slow, and it exhibits interesting temperature variation. Poor growth at 28°C can distinguish *F. tularensis* subspecies *tularensis* from other, less virulent subspecies as well as from *Yersinia pestis*, another small gram-negative coccobacillus that also grows well at 28°C. Additionally, *F. tularensis* does not exhibit the bipolar Gram stain appearance typical of *Y. pestis*. Differentiating *F. tularensis* from *Y. pestis* is critical because both are potential agents of bioterrorism and may cause clinical pneumonia after inhalation.

Visualization of the organism in clinical specimens can also be done by using direct fluorescent antibody and immunohistochemical staining techniques, but these tests are performed only at specialized laboratories in the National Public Health Network. During a possible biological attack, these laboratories should be contacted and the specimens shipped to them to use their specialized technology for urgent diagnosis (see Chapter 227). Clinicians should contact their hospital infection control practitioner or state health department to obtain information on submission of specimens and reporting of possible infection.[7] The Office of Health and Safety web page of the Centers for Disease Control and Prevention (www.cdc.gov/od/ohs/biosfty/biosfty.htm) and the American Society of Microbiology biodefense resources web page (http://www.asm.org/policy/index.asp?bid=520) can provide useful after-hours information on specimen testing and shipping.

Antimicrobial Agents for Treatment and Prophylaxis

Recommendations for therapy of tularemia in the context of a bioterrorism event presented in the Working Group consensus report[7] are summarized in Tables 323-3 and 323-4. Before determining a treatment strategy, case clusters should be evaluated for mass casualty potential, wherein large numbers of potentially infected people prohibit individual medical management, as would be possible in a contained casualty situation. Hence the recommended regimens differ for the two circumstances. Formulating optimal strategies for antibiotic use requires understanding the intracellular nature of *F. tularensis*. Treatment failures are highest with bacteriostatic drugs such as tetracycline, doxycycline, and chloramphenicol, especially for central nervous system infections.[38] Relapse is theorized to result in part from sequestration of organisms within host macrophages and other cells. Treatment using bacteriostatic drugs should be continued for a longer duration than the traditional 10-day course recommended for the bactericidal drugs (see Table 323-3). When treating individuals with ciprofloxacin, doxycycline, or chloramphenicol, intravenous regimens can be changed to oral regimens after substantial clinical improvement is noted. Note that in mass casualty situations, a minimum of 14 days is recommended for all regimens; this is due to the exclusive use of oral agents beginning from the initiation of therapy (see Table 323-4). The bacteriostatic regimens are not recommended for immunosuppressed patients because of the higher rates of treatment failure generally observed with these agents.[7] Furthermore, giving the entire minimum of 10 days of therapy parenterally should be considered for immunocompromised patients. Although quinolones and tetracyclines have been associated with adverse consequences in children and immature laboratory animals, short courses of these agents in children have not been detrimental in prospective studies.[39] When considering the use of these agents for tularemia in a specific setting, the risks in children should be weighed in proportion to the potential benefits.

There are few scientific data concerning postexposure prophylaxis for tularemia, a term generally meant to include therapy initiated during the incubation period of infection. Only a handful of studies used "prophylaxis" dosing of antimicrobials before an actual challenge with *F. tularensis*.[40] The 2001 Working Group on Civilian Biodefense

TABLE 323-3	Recommendations for Therapy of Contained Casualties after Intentional Release of *Francisella tularensis*

Adults

Serious Disease

Streptomycin 1 g IM q12h for 10 days

Gentamicin 5 mg/kg IM or IV qd for 10 days

Alternatives for Less Serious Disease

Streptomycin or gentamicin in doses listed above

Ciprofloxacin 400 mg IV bid for 10 days

Doxycycline 100 mg IV bid for 14-21 days

Chloramphenicol 15 mg/kg IV qid for 14-21 days

Children

Serious Disease

Streptomycin 15 mg/kg IM q12h for 10 days, not to exceed 2 g/day

Gentamicin 2.5 mg/kg IM or IV q8h for 10 days

Alternatives for Less Serious Disease

Streptomycin or gentamicin in doses listed above

Ciprofloxacin 15 mg/kg IV q12h for 10 days, not to exceed 1 g/day

Doxycycline 100 mg IV q12h for 14-21 days if weight ≥45 kg; 2.2 mg/kg IV q12h if weight <45 kg

Chloramphenicol 15 mg/kg IV q6h for 14-21 days

Pregnancy

Serious Disease

Gentamicin 5 mg/kg IM or IV qd for 10 days

Streptomycin 1 g IM q12h for 10 days

Alternatives for Less Serious Disease

Gentamicin or streptomycin in doses listed above

Ciprofloxacin 400 mg IV q12h for 10 days

Doxycycline 100 mg IV q12h for 14-21 days

Immunosuppressed Persons

Minimum of 10 days of treatment (see text)

Gentamicin 5 mg/kg/day IM or IV in divided doses

Streptomycin 1 g IM q12h

Choices are listed in our order of preference for use. Gentamicin may be more readily available than streptomycin. Initial intravenous therapy with doxycycline, ciprofloxacin, or chloramphenicol may be changed to oral dosing after patients are clinically improved.

Adapted from Dennis DT, Inglesby TV, Henderson DA, et al. Tularemia as a biological weapon: medical and public health management. *JAMA*. 2001;285:2763-2773.

recommendation for postexposure prophylaxis with 14 days of ciprofloxacin or doxycycline (see Table 323-4) is primarily based on two publications.[40,41] Patients offered prophylaxis need to be warned about potential side effects of these antimicrobials, most commonly gastrointestinal upset and rash.

Subsequent to intentional release of a biological agent, public health services will attempt to ensure the dissemination of accurate information to communities, but the media and the Internet may serve as potential sources of inflammatory material, thereby aggravating public

TABLE 323-4	Recommendations for Therapy of Mass Casualties and for Postexposure Prophylaxis after Intentional Release of *Francisella tularensis*

Adults

Ciprofloxacin 500 mg PO bid for 14 days

Doxycycline 100 mg PO bid for 14 days

Children

Ciprofloxacin 15 mg/kg PO bid for 14 days, not to exceed 1 g/day

Doxycycline 100 mg PO bid for 14 days if weight ≥45 kg; 2.2 mg/kg PO bid if weight <45 kg

Pregnancy

Ciprofloxacin 500 mg PO bid for 14 days

Doxycycline 100 mg PO bid for 14 days

Choices listed in our order of preference for use.

Adapted from Dennis DT, Inglesby TV, Henderson DA, et al. Tularemia as a biological weapon: medical and public health management. *JAMA*. 2001;285:2763-2773.

insecurity and leading to hoarding of antimicrobial agents, as was observed after the 2001 U.S. anthrax attacks. This behavior should be proactively discouraged by infectious diseases experts so that it does not contribute to the potential development of antimicrobial resistance.

Potential Use of Vaccines during the Postexposure Period

Attempts to manufacture a vaccine against *F. tularensis* have been ongoing worldwide since the 1930s. The completion of the genome sequence of *F. tularensis* subspecies *tularensis* Schu S4 has allowed new approaches to vaccine development through genetic and proteomic analyses. A pivotal issue is determining the safest and most effective route of exposure that will elicit protective immunity against an aerosol challenge. The live vaccine strain of *F. tularensis* developed in the 1950s is no longer available for use (see Chapter 227). Currently, vaccination cannot be recommended for postexposure use, and a vaccine available for general use in the population is not forthcoming. Thus, antimicrobial agents are likely to remain the mainstay of management in the near future.

Hospital Infection Control Measures

Special isolation in the hospital setting for persons with tularemia is not necessary because the organism is not transmitted person-to-person.

Microbiology laboratory workers and autopsy personnel are the most likely individuals to encounter *F. tularensis* organisms in the hospital setting. Guidelines for the safe handling of *F. tularensis* are available.[35-37] A critical component to prevent nosocomial transmission is notification of at-risk personnel about suspected cases or positive cultures, thereby facilitating appropriate use of personal protective measures and biosafety cabinets.

Once organisms suspected of being *F. tularensis* are isolated from clinical specimens, additional procedures that may produce droplets (centrifuging, grinding, vigorous shaking, growing cultures in volume) should be conducted under biosafety level 3 procedures.[35,36] Other members of the health care team, such as the medical examiner or coroner, also should be alerted to suspected cases of tularemia because certain procedures (e.g., sawing of bone) may aerosolize infected tissues. In fact, infection resulting from inoculation during an autopsy has been documented.[42] The responsibility to notify laboratory and pathology services rests solely with members of the primary health care team and cannot be overemphasized.

Shapiro and Schwartz[43] detailed the unnecessary exposure of 11 laboratory workers and 2 autopsy personnel to *F. tularensis* when the primary team failed to notify these services of their suspicions. Although tularemia was not transmitted to any of the workers, undue risk was assumed; 13 workers required prophylaxis with doxycycline, and the diagnosis was delayed.[43] This exposure occurred at a large teaching hospital in Boston where laboratory guidelines regarding isolation of potential biological agents were already in place, but their integration into the routine workup of clinical specimens had not been accomplished.[43] Their report illustrated the potential pitfalls of implementing local bioterrorism guidelines even with the heightened awareness stemming from the events of September 11, 2001.

Identification of *F. tularensis* in the microbiology laboratory is complex, and even experienced laboratory personnel can make mistakes when identifying the organism (see Chapter 227). The bacteria can be confused with other gram-negative bacilli, including *Haemophilus* species. Automated systems may incorrectly identify the organism (see Chapter 227). Confusion with *Legionella* may occur when *F. tularensis* grows on buffered charcoal yeast extract agar. If the laboratory is not notified in advance of the clinical suspicion of tularemia, procedures for any of these organisms may be carried out on an open bench with unnecessary risk to laboratory personnel.

Environmental Surveillance and Decontamination

Biothreat air monitors in Houston, TX, reported a false-positive detection signal for airborne *F. tularensis* in 2003.[44] In response to this event, DNA extracts of soil samples from the Houston area were studied using PCR amplification and several unique species of *Francisella*-like organisms were identified.[44] The natural reservoirs for these diverse species remain largely unknown. Further characterization of environmental *Francisella* and the development of high-resolution DNA-based strain typing systems will provide a basis for improved environmental surveillance and bioforensic analyses.[34a]

Because *F. tularensis* can cause disease in various mammals and rodents, public health officials should stay abreast of zoonotic epidemics because they may parallel disease in humans, especially if a common water source is used as a vehicle for intentional release. Veterinarians may be the first to observe an increase in the incidence of tularemia, and observation of the rates of animal disease and open dialogue with animal experts may prove to be an important surveillance tactic. During a possible epizoonosis, public education regarding methods of transmission via insect vectors should be emphasized.

The Working Group expects aerosolized *F. tularensis* to undergo desiccation, solar radiation, and oxidation, limiting secondary dispersal.[7] Body surfaces and clothes of individuals exposed should be washed with soapy water. Water contamination can be eradicated through standard chlorination, but chlorinating natural water reservoirs is complicated. Identified infected natural water sources must be contained to prevent public and animal use. Inanimate surfaces contaminated with *F. tularensis*, as in laboratory accidents, can be cleaned with a 10% bleach solution. Following up the bleach with a 70%

alcohol solution can reduce the harmful effects of bleach on countertop material without impairing decontamination. Soapy water can clean less concentrated areas of contamination in the laboratory.[7] Standard sterilizing autoclave cycles will eliminate *F. tularensis* from contaminated objects before disposal.

Other Resources

We have listed in Table 323-5 some sites with useful information on tularemia. These sites are likely to remain active or have links routed to other functioning websites.

TABLE 323-5	Useful Bioterrorism Websites with Information on Tularemia	
Source	*Address*	*Comments*
Centers for Disease Control and Prevention	http://www.bt.cdc.gov/ Agent/Agentlist.asp	Fact sheets and articles
	http://www.bt.cdc.gov/ LabIssues/index.asp	Testing, identification, biosafety, shipping, training, Laboratory Response Network description
Center for Biosecurity of the University of Pittsburgh Medical Center	http://www. upmc-biosecurity. org	Fact sheets, articles, consensus statements
St. Louis University School of Public Health	http://www. bioterrorism.slu.edu/ tularemia.htm	Fact sheets

Adapted from Ferguson NE, Steele L, Crawford CY, et al. Bioterrorism web site resources for infectious disease clinicians and epidemiologists. *Clin Infect Dis.* 2003;36:1458-1473.

REFERENCES

1. Franz DR, Jahrling PB, Friedlander AM, et al. Clinical recognition and management of patients exposed to biological warfare agents. *JAMA.* 1997;278:399-411.
2. Kaufmann AF, Meltzer MI, Schmid GP. The economic impact of a bioterrorist attack: are prevention and postattack intervention programs justifiable? *Emerg Infect Dis.* 1997;3:83-94.
3. Centers for Disease Control and Prevention. Biological and chemical terrorism: strategic plan for preparedness and response. Recommendations of the CDC Strategic Planning Workgroup. *MMWR Recomm Rep.* 2000;49:1-14.
4. Cunha BA. Anthrax, tularemia, plague, ebola or smallpox as agents of bioterrorism: recognition in the emergency room. *Clin Microbiol Infect.* 2002;8:489-503.
5. Harris S. Japanese biological warfare research on humans: a case study of microbiology and ethics. *Ann N Y Acad Sci.* 1992; 666:21-52.
6. Christopher GW, Cieslak TJ, Pavlin JA, et al. Biological warfare. A historical perspective. *JAMA.* 1997;278:412-417.
7. Dennis DT, Inglesby TV, Henderson DA, et al. Tularemia as a biological weapon: medical and public health management. *JAMA.* 2001;285:2763-2773.
8. Patt HA, Feigin RD. Diagnosis and management of suspected cases of bioterrorism: a pediatric perspective. *Pediatrics.* 2002;109:685-692.
9. Matyas BT, Nieder HS, Telford SR, 3rd. Pneumonic tularemia on Martha's Vineyard: clinical, epidemiologic, and ecological characteristics. *Ann N Y Acad Sci.* 2007;1105:351-377.
10. Ketai L, Tchoyoson Lim CC. Radiology of biological weapons—old and the new? *Semin Roentgenol.* 2007;42:49-59.
11. Hodges L, Penn RL. Tularemia and bioterrorism. In: Fong IW, Alibek K, eds. *Bioterrorism and Infectious Agents: A New Dilemma for the 21st Century.* New York, NY: Springer Science+Business Media; 2005:71-98.
12. White JD, Rooney JR, Prickett PA, et al. Pathogenesis of experimental respiratory tularemia in monkeys. *J Infect Dis.* 1964; 114:277-283.
13. Case records of the Massachusetts General Hospital. Weekly clinicopathological exercises. Case 14-2000. A 60-year-old farm worker with bilateral pneumonia. *N Engl J Med.* 2000;342:1430-1438.
14. Permar HH, Maclahlan WWG. Tularemia pneumonia. *Ann Intern Med.* 1931;5:687-698.
15. Foshay L. Tularemia: a summary of certain aspects of the disease including methods for early diagnosis and the results of serum treatment in 600 patients. *Medicine (Baltimore).* 1940;19:1-83.
16. Dienst FT Jr. Tularemia: a perusal of three hundred thirty-nine cases. *J La State Med Soc.* 1963;115:114-124.
17. Penn RL, Kinasewitz GT. Factors associated with a poor outcome in tularemia. *Arch Intern Med.* 1987;147:265-268.
18. Rodgers BL, Duffield RP, Taylor T, et al. Tularemic meningitis. *Pediatr Infect Dis J.* 1998;17:439-441.
19. Tularemia. In: Chin J, Ascher MS, eds. *Control of Communicable Diseases Manual.* 17th ed. Washington, DC: American Public Health Association; 2000:532-535.
20. Evans ME, Gregory DW, Schaffner W, et al. Tularemia: a 30-year experience with 88 cases. *Medicine (Baltimore).* 1985;64:251-269.
21. Dahlstrand S, Ringertz O, Zetterberg B. Airborne tularemia in Sweden. *Scand J Infect Dis.* 1971;3:7-16.
22. Chang MH, Glynn MK, Groseclose SL. Endemic, notifiable bioterrorism-related diseases, United States, 1992-1999. *Emerg Infect Dis.* 2003;9:556-564.
23. Fulop M, Leslie D, Titball R. A rapid, highly sensitive method for the detection of *Francisella tularensis* in clinical samples using the polymerase chain reaction. *Am J Trop Med Hyg.* 1996;54:364-366.
24. Grunow R, Splettstoesser W, McDonald S, et al. Detection of *Francisella tularensis* in biological specimens using a capture enzyme-linked immunosorbent assay, an immunochromatographic handheld assay, and a PCR. *Clin Diagn Lab Immunol.* 2000;7:86-90.
25. Sjöstedt A, Eriksson U, Berglund L, et al. Detection of *Francisella tularensis* in ulcers of patients with tularemia by PCR. *J Clin Microbiol.* 1997;35:1045-1048.
26. Skottman T, Piiparinen H, Hyytiäinen H, et al. Simultaneous real-time PCR detection of *Bacillus anthracis*, *Francisella tularensis* and *Yersinia pestis*. *Eur J Clin Microbiol Infect Dis.* 2007;26:207-211.
27. Tomaso H, Scholz HC, Neubauer H, et al. Real-time PCR using hybridization probes for the rapid and specific identification of *Francisella tularensis* subspecies *tularensis*. *Mol Cell Probes.* 2007;21:12-16.
28. Tomioka K, Peredelchuk M, Zhu X, et al. A multiplex polymerase chain reaction microarray assay to detect bioterror pathogens in blood. *J Mol Diagn.* 2005;7:486-494.
29. Wilson WJ, Erler AM, Nasarabadi SL, et al. A multiplexed PCR-coupled liquid bead array for the simultaneous detection of four biothreat agents. *Mol Cell Probes.* 2005;19:137-144.
30. Yang S, Rothman RE, Hardick J, et al. Rapid polymerase chain reaction-based screening assay for bacterial biothreat agents. *Acad Emerg Med.* 2008;15:388-392.
31. Huelseweh B, Ehricht R, Marschall HJ. A simple and rapid protein array based method for the simultaneous detection of biowarfare agents. *Proteomics.* 2006;6:2972-2981.
32. Andersson H, Hartmanova B, Bäck E, et al. Transcriptional profiling of the peripheral blood response during tularemia. *Genes Immun.* 2006;7:503-513.
33. Eliasson H, Olcen P, Sjöstedt A, et al. Kinetics of the immune response associated with tularemia: comparison of an enzyme-linked immunosorbent assay, a tube agglutination test, and a novel whole-blood lymphocyte stimulation test. *Clin Vaccine Immunol.* 2008;15:1238-1243.
34. Tärnvik A, Chu MC. New approaches to diagnosis and therapy of tularemia. *Ann N Y Acad Sci.* 2007;1105:378-404.
34a. Taitt CR, Malanoski AP, Lin B, et al. Discrimination between biothreat agents and "near neighbor" species using a resequencing array. *FEMS Immunol Med Microbiol.* 2008;54:356-364.
35. Lindquist D, Chu MC, Probert WS. *Francisella* and *Brucella*. In: Murray PR, Baron EJ, Jorgensen JH, et al., eds. Manual of Clinical Microbiology. 9th ed. Vol. 1. Washington, DC: American Society for Microbiology Press; 2007:815-834.
36. Robinson-Dunn B. The microbiology laboratory's role in response to bioterrorism. *Arch Pathol Lab Med.* 2002;126:291-294.
37. Sewell DL. Laboratory safety practices associated with potential agents of biocrime or bioterrorism. *J Clin Microbiol.* 2003;41:2801-2809.
38. Enderlin G, Morales L, Jacobs RF, et al. Streptomycin and alternative agents for the treatment of tularemia: review of the literature. *Clin Infect Dis.* 1994;19:42-47.
39. American Academy of Pediatrics. Antimicrobial agents and related therapy. In: Pickering LK, Baker CJ, Long SS, et al., eds. *Red Book: 2006 Report of the Committee on Infectious Diseases.* Elk Grove Village, IL: American Academy of Pediatrics; 2006:735-737.
40. Russell P, Eley SM, Fulop MJ, et al. The efficacy of ciprofloxacin and doxycycline against experimental tularaemia. *J Antimicrob Chemother.* 1998;41:461-465.
41. Sawyer WD, Dangerfield HG, Hogge AL, et al. Antibiotic prophylaxis and therapy of airborne tularemia. *Bacteriol Rev.* 1966;30:542-550.
42. Weilbacher JO, Moss ES. Tularemia following injury while performing post-mortem examination of a human case. *J Lab Clin Med.* 1938;24:34-38.
43. Shapiro DS, Schwartz DR. Exposure of laboratory workers to *Francisella tularensis* despite a bioterrorism procedure. *J Clin Microbiol.* 2002;40:2278-2281.
44. Barns SM, Grow CC, Okinaka RT, et al. Detection of diverse new *Francisella*-like bacteria in environmental samples. *Appl Environ Microbiol.* 2005;71:5494-5500.

324

Smallpox as an Agent of Bioterrorism

LISA D. ROTZ | JOANNE CONO | INGER K. DAMON

Over the past several years, general concerns over bioterrorism and biologic warfare involving smallpox have greatly increased. These are neither novel concepts nor newly identified threats. The history of smallpox as a weapon is given in Chapter 322.

After the official World Health Organization (WHO) declaration of smallpox eradication in 1980, laboratories worldwide were asked to voluntarily destroy or consolidate their stores of variola virus in one of two WHO Collaborating Centers (Centers for Disease Control and Prevention [CDC], Atlanta, Georgia, and the State Research Center of Virology and Biotechnology, Koltsovo, Novosibirsk Region, Russia).[1] All legitimate research with infectious variola virus is now conducted under biosafety level 4 (BSL-4) containment conditions within these two institutions only, using a WHO-approved research agenda.

Concerns about bioterrorism using the smallpox virus (variola) remain, with the belief that illegitimate stores of the virus may exist outside the two WHO collaborating centers (as nondestroyed products of the former Soviet biologic warfare program or as laboratory specimens not surrendered to the WHO repositories) and could be used in a malevolent manner.[2,3] It is for this reason that medical, research, and public health authorities must remain familiar with the clinical, epidemiologic, and scientific characteristics of this disease.

Smallpox Epidemiology Relative to Bioterrorism

There is no known environmental source or animal reservoir for the variola virus; therefore, a single case of confirmed smallpox would constitute an epidemic and raise great concern for bioterrorism. In addition, variola virus does not persist or reactivate in individuals who have recovered from the disease. Because legitimate research with infectious variola virus is carried out in only two laboratories by routinely vaccinated researchers under high-containment BSL-4 conditions, it is unlikely that an outbreak would be the result of an accidental infection or release from these facilities.

Examples of previously cited criteria used to identify biologic agents for further development in weapons programs include (1) high lethality or toxicity, (2) no medical countermeasures for prevention or treatment, (3) environmental stability and ease of large-scale production, (4) infectious via aerosol, and (5) high infectivity (low infectious dose), person-to-person transmissibility, or both.[2] Variola major has many of these attributes. The true infectious dose is not known, but it is thought to be low. The overall mortality rate for smallpox is about 30% (but can increase to almost 100% with the rare hemorrhagic and flat-type forms of the disease).[3,4] Human-to-human transmission of variola virus normally occurs by inhalation of large, virus-containing airborne droplets of saliva, although infection can result from contact with contaminated bedding or clothing or direct inoculation of virus into the skin. Even with a potentially low infectious dose, transmission usually requires prolonged, close contact (face to face). However, airborne transmission over greater distances has been infrequently reported.[5]

After a bioterrorism release of smallpox, the epidemiologic characteristics of transmission would be expected to be similar to those seen historically. Household contacts were at highest risk for secondary transmission from a smallpox-infected individual because of the usual need for more prolonged, close contact to transmit the disease effectively. Therefore identification, vaccination, and surveillance of this group would be among the highest priorities after diagnosis of smallpox in an individual or group of individuals after intentional release of the agent.

During the smallpox era, the overall average secondary attack rate was 58.4% in previously nonvaccinated close household contacts and 3.8% in previously vaccinated household contacts.[4] Because of the general lack of natural or vaccine-induced immunity in today's population, it is difficult to predict the exact attack rates that would result from person-to-person transmission after intentional release of the smallpox virus. Medical personnel caring for or evaluating potential smallpox cases after a smallpox virus release should be vaccinated as soon as possible because smallpox vaccine given before exposure or up to 3 days after exposure may prevent the disease or greatly lessen its severity.[3,6]

The usual incubation period for smallpox is 10 to 14 days (range, 7 to 17 days). Individuals are not infectious during this asymptomatic period. At the end of the incubation period, they develop a febrile prodrome that lasts 1 to 5 days and is characterized by myalgia, backache, headache, and occasionally nausea, vomiting, and delirium. Oral lesions appear in the mouth about 24 hours before the onset of the visible rash. These oral lesions quickly break down and shed large amounts of virus into the oral secretions. It is at this point that a person becomes infectious to others. Patients are most infectious during the first week of rash, with the infectiousness dropping dramatically as the oral and skin lesions heal and form scabs.[3]

Pathogenesis and Clinical Presentation

Natural infection by variola normally occurs through inhalation of saliva droplets from infected individuals. The index case (first person infected) releases infectious viral particles from sloughing oropharyngeal lesions during the first week of the rash.[7] Smallpox virus released from secretions of oropharyngeal lesions is contained mainly in large respiratory droplet particles.[8] Although smallpox scabs may contain viable virus for a long time,[9] the virus is contained in large fragments of inspissated (thickened, dried) material, accounting for the low transmissibility associated with scabs.

Typically, the smallpox virus initially infects the respiratory tract of a susceptible individual. When smallpox was endemic, modern tools for understanding disease pathogenesis and host response were not available. Therefore, descriptions of smallpox disease pathogenesis are derived from studies of systemic orthopoxvirus infections in other species and from clinical and laboratory observations of human disease. One study[4] concluded that antigen-presenting macrophages in the respiratory tract or skin are infected by the third day after viral transmission. These virally infected macrophages enter the lymphatic system and travel to the regional lymph nodes. The virus then multiplies in the draining lymph nodes and enters the bloodstream, largely cell-associated, by the fourth day after infection, subsequently seeding and replicating in reticuloendothelial organs. These initial phases of infection are typically asymptomatic and occur during the incubation period.

Symptoms present around the time of the secondary viremia. At this time, 10 to 14 days after infection (range, 7 to 17 days), patients present with the prodromal symptoms, followed in 1 to 5 days by disseminated rash lesions. Activated macrophages and lymphocytes are thought to produce inflammatory cytokines and interferons, which mediate the immune response and stimulate natural killer cell activity to destroy infected cells. In immunocompetent individuals, antigen-presenting cells trigger cytotoxic T-cell clonal expansion to destroy infected cells and prevent infectious virus release. The humoral immune response also plays a role in recovery from poxvirus infection and in protection against reinfection. For example, neutralizing antibodies directed against viral outer membrane antigens function to neutralize the infectivity of virions. Neutralizing antibodies are detectable by the sixth day of the rash[10] and are long-lived. Both the activity of cytotoxic T cells and the antibody titer increase over time.

The three major clinical forms of smallpox include the ordinary, flat, and hemorrhagic types. An early, vigorous immunocompetent cellular immune response inhibits viral multiplication, although the virus generally breaks through the host's immune response and produces characteristic skin lesions with a discrete distribution (ordinary smallpox). In contrast, a late, deficient cellular immune response is believed to lead to a rare manifestation of the disease termed *flat-type smallpox*. Flat-type smallpox is characterized by intense toxemia and delayed skin lesion appearance with slow evolution. The skin lesions are usually flat and soft, and sections of the skin may slough. Most of the flat-type smallpox cases are fatal. In patients with a highly compromised immune response, there is extensive multiplication of the virus in the spleen and bone marrow, producing a rare condition known as *hemorrhagic smallpox*. This rare type of smallpox is associated with petechiae in the skin and bleeding from the conjunctiva and mucous membranes. Severe toxemia results, followed by early death, often before the characteristic lesions of smallpox rash develop. Hemorrhagic-type smallpox is more common in pregnant women than in other adults. The underlying reasons for toxemia and other severe systemic effects that can be associated with smallpox are still unclear.

The prodrome is sometimes accompanied by an erythematous rash or, rarely, a petechial rash in pale-skinned subjects. Three to four days after the onset of the prodromal symptoms, the characteristic rash of ordinary-type smallpox appears, first on the buccal and pharyngeal mucosa, the face, the forearms, and the hands. The rash spreads downward, and within a day or so the trunk and lower limbs are involved, with the back more involved than the abdomen. Ultimately, the distribution of the variola rash is centrifugal: it is most profuse on the face and is more abundant on the forearms than the upper arms and on the lower legs than the thighs (Figs. 324-1 and 324-2). Prominences and surfaces exposed to irritation are involved more heavily by the rash

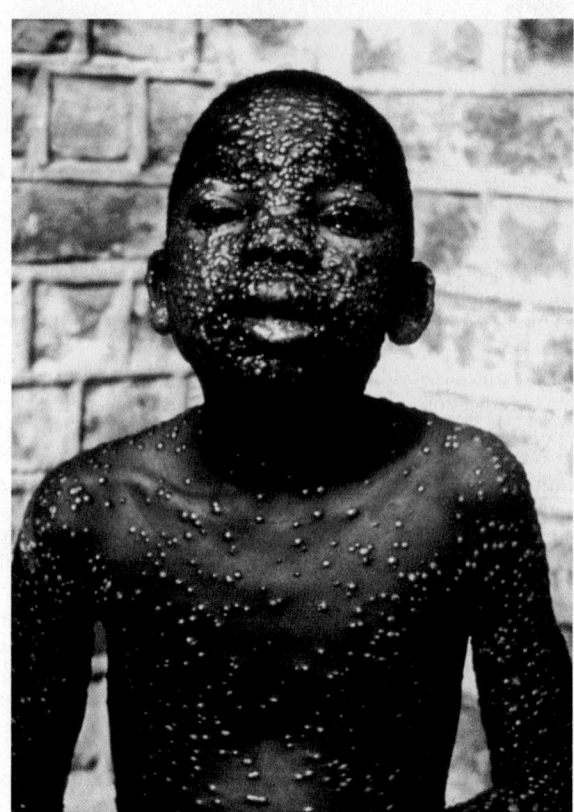

Figure 324-2 **African child displaying the typical centrifugal rash distribution of smallpox on his face, chest, and arms.** *(From the U.S. Centers for Disease Control and Prevention [CDC] Public Health Image Library [PHIL] at http://phil.cdc.gov/phil/default.asp. Image ID 3268. Photograph taken in 1970.)*

than the protected surfaces, flexures, and depressions, which are usually somewhat spared. In contrast to chickenpox, which is the disease most often confused with the early rash stage of smallpox, all lesions on any one part of the body are at the same stage of development (see Chapter 133). Furthermore, the distribution of the chickenpox rash is centripetal (with a predominance of lesions on the trunk and relative sparing of face and distal limbs), and abdominal involvement is equivalent to back involvement.

The lesions of the smallpox rash begin as circular macules (small, discolored skin patches). The macules form firm papules and then vesicles (usually multiloculated), which soon become opaque and pustular. The vesicles are typically raised and well circumscribed, deep, and firm to the touch (Fig. 324-3). Approximately 8 to 9 days after the onset of the rash, the pustules become pitlike and dimpled; around day 14 the pustules dry up and become crusted. The rash of chickenpox, in contrast, develops as uniloculated vesicles that do not umbilicate, and the vesicles may have irregular borders. By the end of the third week of smallpox infection, most of the lesion crusts separate, with those on the palms and soles separating last.

Sequelae often follow recovery. The most common are pockmarks, which may occur all over the body but are usually most prominent on the face owing to the large number of sebaceous glands affected by the lesions. Rarely, blindness occurs as a result of keratitis or corneal ulcerations. Recovery results in prolonged immunity to reinfection. Variola virus does not persist in the body after recovery.

Diagnosis

The CDC has developed several resources that can be used to assist clinicians in evaluating acute, generalized vesicular or pustular rash illnesses with regard to their likelihood of being smallpox in a nonout-

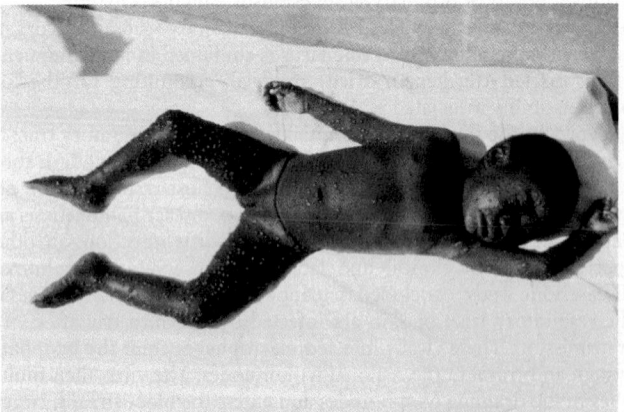

Figure 324-1 **Distribution of smallpox lesions on the body of a child during the fifth day of infection.** Note the greater numbers of discrete lesions on the face and extremities compared with the trunk. *(From the U.S. Centers for Disease Control and Prevention [CDC] Public Health Image Library [PHIL] at http://phil.cdc.gov/phil/default.asp. Image ID 3262. Photograph taken in 1972 by Dr. Paul B. Dean, CDC.)*

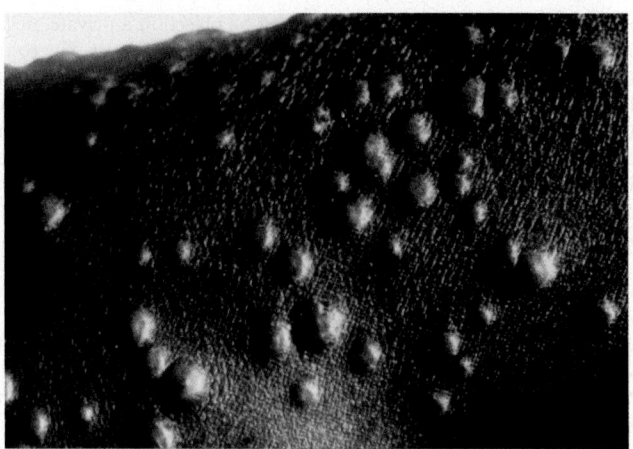

Figure 324-3 **Close-up view of smallpox pustules that are round, smooth, firm, and all at the same stage of development.** *(Originally from the World Health Organization Diagnosis of Smallpox Slide Series. Image downloaded from the U.S. Centers for Disease Control and Prevention [CDC] Public Health Image Library [PHIL] at http://phil.cdc. gov/phil/default.asp. Image ID 2009. Photograph taken in 1969.)*

break setting. These tools can be found on the CDC website (http://emergency.cdc.gov/agent/smallpox/diagnosis/#diagnosis) and include an interactive online version of the clinical evaluation algorithm. Because the positive predictive value of smallpox-specific diagnostics decreases considerably in the absence of existing disease, these tests should be performed on patients only when the clinical illness is compatible with a high risk for smallpox. Public health authorities should be immediately notified about patients with suspected smallpox to assist with the assessment and help expedite testing for smallpox through the national Laboratory Response Network (LRN), if indicated.

Historically, smallpox was diagnosed through clinical observation and laboratory diagnostics. Laboratory methods used during the eradication campaign included electron microscopy, agarose gel diffusion, culture on chick chorioallantoic membrane, growth characteristics on scarified rabbit skin, and growth on HeLa cells. These methods would still provide robust information to differentiate variola from other orthopoxviruses, but for a variety of reasons most are no longer used. Modern nucleic acid methods are more widely used today.

SPECIMEN COLLECTION

Virus can be easily recovered from active skin lesions. Appropriate specimens to collect for smallpox diagnostic testing are the lesion roof, base scrapings from unroofed lesions, tonsillar swabs, whole blood and serum, and lesion punch biopsies. Details of diagnostic specimen collection procedures can be found on the Internet (http://emergency.cdc. gov/agent/smallpox/response-plan/files/guide-d.pdf). Specimen collection for suspected smallpox cases should be done by vaccine-protected individuals using appropriate airborne infection isolation (AII; formerly "airborne precautions") and the prescribed personal protective measures, or by individuals using AII and the prescribed personal protective measures with no contraindications to vaccination who can be immediately vaccinated if the diagnosis of smallpox is confirmed.

NUCLEIC ACID TESTING

Through previous work and efforts by the U.S. smallpox research agenda, a variety of nucleic acid testing methodologies targeting poxviruses have been published and reviewed[11] or are in use at U.S. Public Health laboratories and other member laboratories of the LRN. The LRN, founded in 1999, is a national network of local, state, and federal public health, hospital-based, veterinary, agriculture, food, and envi-

ronmental testing laboratories that provide laboratory diagnostic capacity to respond to biologic and chemical terrorism and other public health emergencies. Several international laboratories are also members of the network.

Among tests described in the literature that allow both identification and quantification of the agent[12-19] are the standard polymerase chain reaction (PCR) assays, which generically amplify a segment of orthopoxvirus nucleic acid and allow speciation (e.g., variola, monkeypox, vaccinia) on the basis of fragment sizes after restriction endonuclease digestion; multiplex assays that permit simultaneous analysis of orthopoxvirus species in one reaction tube; and real-time PCR assays.

ELECTRON MICROSCOPY

Electron microscopic (EM) visualization of negatively stained poxvirus virions was a valuable technique for confirming poxvirus infections during the smallpox eradication campaign. Historically, skilled practitioners of negative-stain transmission EM successfully detected orthopoxvirus particles in approximately 95% of clinical specimens from patients with variola infections and in approximately 75% from patients with vaccinia infections.[20] In the event of a deliberate release of smallpox virus and subsequent human disease, or for generalized vaccinia infections resulting from vaccination, negatively stained preparations derived from lesions or scab material would again provide a valuable method for assisting in poxvirus diagnosis and ruling out other causes of rash illness. However, EM visualization of virions compatible with orthopoxvirus by itself does not constitute proof of a smallpox infection because variola, vaccinia, monkeypox, and molluscum viruses, for example, are morphologically indistinguishable by that method. Negative-stain EM, however, is valuable for discerning morphologic structures in primary clinical specimens compatible with other infectious agents, in the differential diagnosis of suspected smallpox that includes the herpesviruses (varicella, herpes simplex viruses 1 and 2 [HSV-1, HSV-2][21]; see Chapter 133).

HISTOPATHOLOGY AND IMMUNOHISTOCHEMISTRY

The presence of cytoplasmic inclusions is characteristic of poxvirus infections but cannot be used to specifically identify variola in a biopsy specimen. There are two types of inclusion bodies: A-type and B-type. B-type inclusion bodies (Guarnieri bodies) are the sites of viral replication and are found in those infected by all species of poxvirus. A-type inclusion bodies are produced by certain poxviruses in the genus Orthopoxvirus (cowpox virus [Downie body]); the ectromelia virus (Marchal body); and the raccoon, vole, and skunk poxviruses. They are also produced in the genus Avipoxvirus (fowlpox virus [Borrel body]).

Poxvirus inclusion bodies can be presumptively identified in hematoxylin and eosin (H&E)–stained specimens using light microscopy. In the early smallpox lesions in the skin and mucous membranes, B-type inclusion bodies are readily observed in H&E-stained sections as faintly basophilic bodies lying in the cytoplasm, usually close to the nucleus. In more advanced lesions, suitably stained sections showed faintly basophilic granular inclusions occupying a large part of the cytoplasm of infected cells. They are particularly evident in epithelial cells at the base of vesicles or pustules. (May-Grünwald Giemsa stain may also be used; here the basophilic inclusions appear magenta red.) Histopathologic staining of tissues provides another mechanism for evaluating if orthopoxvirus is present in the tissue. Again, these methods are not specific for variola.[22,23]

CELL CULTURE

Orthopoxviruses can be grown in a variety of established cell culture lines, including Vero, BS-C-1, CV-1, LLCMK-2 monkey kidney cells, human embryonic lung fibroblast cells, HeLa cells, chick embryo fibroblast cells, and MRC-5 human diploid fibroblast cells. Characteristic growth and the cytopathic effect in any of these cell lines do not identify which orthopoxvirus is present. Methods for growing and discriminating the morphology of orthopoxviruses on the chorioallantoic membrane of 12-day-old chick embryos have been described.[20,24] At this time, attempts to isolate variola virus by cell culture should be conducted only in an approved BSL-4 laboratory by appropriately trained and vaccinated personnel.

Pre-Event and Post-Event Exposure Preparedness

As previously stated, the world's population is largely not vaccinated against smallpox and therefore highly susceptible to infection should smallpox be intentionally released as a bioterrorism agent. It is imperative, therefore, that preparations for a medical and public health response to a smallpox outbreak be in place before such an outbreak occurs. Smallpox response planning involves many national and international health and emergency response agencies. In the United States, the Department of Health and Human Services (DHHS) and the CDC are the lead department and agency for the public health response to an outbreak. The CDC has prepared several guidance and planning documents to assist state and local public health and medical authorities to identify and plan essential local response measures (see http://www.bt.cdc.gov/planning/index.asp and http://www.bt.cdc.gov/agent/smallpox/prep/).

Education of medical and public health staff about the clinical presentation of smallpox and the control measures necessary to contain an outbreak, including vaccination strategies, is essential for responding to an outbreak of smallpox. Clinical evaluation and the collection of clinical laboratory specimens are covered elsewhere in this section (rash illness and laboratory algorithms). In addition, smallpox vaccination and training of identified public health and medical smallpox response teams was undertaken to enhance federal, state, and local rapid response capabilities to contain a smallpox outbreak.[25]

Surveillance and containment (SC) is the mainstay of smallpox outbreak control. Also called *ring vaccination* and *search and containment*, this strategy targets vaccination of close contacts of patients with smallpox and close monitoring to initiate isolation if symptoms of the disease occur. This ensures more rapid administration of vaccine to those who are at the greatest risk of contracting the disease. It thus represents the best chance for preventing further smallpox transmission. By vaccinating persons at highest risk of smallpox, this strategy can also help minimize the risk of adverse events in persons least likely to be exposed to a case of smallpox. Adverse events associated with smallpox vaccine are described in Chapter 133. Patients must first be identified and isolated and their close contacts (face-to-face or household contacts) identified and vaccinated; optimally, this occurs within 3 days of exposure to prevent or at least significantly lessen the severity of smallpox symptoms in most of the people.[26] Vaccination 4 to 7 days after exposure likely offers some protection from disease or at least modifies the severity of the disease.[27,28] Household family members of contacts to individuals with smallpox are also vaccinated to provide protection should the household member still develop smallpox. During the eradication campaign, when outbreaks sometimes still occurred despite 80% vaccination coverage of the population, this vaccination strategy was highly effective for stopping chains of disease transmission.[29] Large-scale voluntary vaccination may also be offered to unaffected populations (who have a low risk of vaccine complications) to augment SC activities (by decreasing the overall population susceptibility); however, SC activities should continue because they are the mainstay for outbreak control.

Infection Control Measures

Person-to-person spread of smallpox virus occurs largely through droplet transmission within 6 feet of the patient, although contact and airborne transmission have been documented.[5] Because airborne transmission is possible, it is imperative that all persons caring for smallpox patients maintain AII, in addition to standard and contact precautions. AII requires that the patient be placed in a private, negative–air-pressure room, with 6 to 12 air exchanges per hour. The room is monitored for negative pressure. There must also be appropriate discharge of air to the outdoors, or the air must be subjected to high-efficiency filtration before being recirculated to other parts of the facility. When AII is not available or the number of patients exceeds the number of rooms, patients with smallpox may be housed in another wing or facility that does not share untreated airflow with other areas.

Under AII, only essential personnel enter the room, and they wear fitted N95 (or higher-degree) respirators at all times. Other personnel protective equipment, such as gowns, gloves, and eye protection, is worn, and it is removed and discarded before leaving the areas. Patients with smallpox should be moved from the room only when necessary. When it must be done, the patient should wear a mask to limit the potential spread of droplet particles.[30]

During the smallpox era, inadequate infection control practices sometimes led to increased transmission in hospitals.[5,31] A review of importations into Europe during 1950 to 1971 concluded that more than 50% of the cases were associated with hospitals, with health care workers constituting approximately 20% of the cases.[31] A review of European smallpox outbreaks showed that the communicability of smallpox decreased by approximately one half when hospital-based transmission was excluded.[32] Therefore, it is advisable that all persons caring for patients with smallpox have a current vaccination against smallpox and maintain AII precautions to ensure that there is no accidental breech of protocol. Isolation of infected patients and vaccination with close monitoring of the patients' contacts at greatest risk for infection have been demonstrated to effectively interrupt transmission of smallpox.[4,33]

Public Health Issues and Preparedness Efforts

An outbreak of smallpox is a public health emergency, and all suspected cases of smallpox should be immediately reported to local public health officials. Local and state health authorities can provide medical personnel with guidance regarding the evaluation and infection control precautions to initiate. They can help expedite testing for varicella, HSV, and smallpox, if appropriate. Through their partnership with the CDC and participation in the LRN, several local and all state pubic health laboratories possess or have access to diagnostic resources for smallpox and other potential bioterrorism agents, as well as diagnostics for varicella, vaccinia, and other herpesviruses. In addition, CDC consultation and technical assistance is available 24 hours a day and can be initiated through the CDC Director's Emergency Operation Center at 770-488-7100.

Smallpox preparedness activities and response planning have been ongoing at the federal, state, and local levels since 1999. State and local authorities are working to enhance their preparedness for smallpox by identifying, training, and vaccinating smallpox response team personnel to be immediately available to initiate control measures in the event of a smallpox outbreak. In addition, response planning efforts for the initiation of control measures and rapid establishment of vaccination clinics in response to a smallpox outbreak are ongoing. Public health laboratory diagnostics, bioterrorism surveillance and epidemiologic capacity, and emergency communication capabilities have also been enhanced.[34]

At the federal level, major efforts have focused on (1) increasing smallpox education and outreach to the medical, public health, and general public communities; (2) developing rapid diagnostic tests that use modern genetic methods and increasing national diagnostic capacity through the LRN; (3) supporting national smallpox responder vaccination with the assistance of state and local public health organizations; (4) developing a comprehensive smallpox vaccine adverse events monitoring and investigation program to support safe vaccination efforts for pre-event responder preparedness; and (5) increasing the national stores of smallpox vaccine to an amount adequate for vaccinating the entire U.S. population if needed.

This last effort has included the initiation of research studies to evaluate the immunizing effectiveness of diluted formulations of several smallpox vaccines. Comparison of humoral and cellular responses of volunteers vaccinated with 1:10 diluted vaccine demonstrated little difference from those vaccinated with undiluted vaccine.[35] Vaccine "take" (demonstration of the expected skin reaction at the site 6 to 8 days after vaccination) rates, classically used as a sign of successful vaccination and protection, were similar in those vaccinated with a 1:5 dilution.[36] Diluted formulations of smallpox vaccine could be used under an investigative new drug (IND) protocol or an Emergency Use Authorization (http://www.fda.gov/oc/guidance/emergencyuse.html) should it ever be needed in an emergency.

In addition, a new, clonally derived, cell culture–grown vaccinia vaccine was licensed by the U.S. Food and Drug Administration in August, 2007.[37] ACAM2000 (Acambis, Inc., Cambridge, Mass) is derived from the vaccine previously used in the United States (New York City Board of Health strain) and licensed as Dryvax by Wyeth Laboratories.[38] Dryvax was originally prepared using calf skin production methods. Because of the adverse events associated with the original vaccine and its clonal derivatives,[39-41] additional efforts are being made to develop more attenuated vaccines. Recent National Institutes of Health–sponsored efforts have focused on the vaccinia strain MVA.[42,43] It is hoped that these efforts will yield a vaccine that retains its effectiveness but is safer for immunosuppressed individuals, including those with acquired immunodeficiency syndrome, who are at risk for the more severe adverse events associated with vaccinia[44] (see Chapter 133). Other, more fundamental research has focused on potential subunit vaccines, using envelope and membrane proteins.[45]

Additional information regarding smallpox, public health and medical actions that should be initiated in response to a smallpox outbreak, and current smallpox preparedness activities and response planning efforts can be found on the Internet (http://emergency.cdc.gov/agent/smallpox/).

REFERENCES

1. World Health Organization. *The Global Eradication of Smallpox: Final Report of the Global Commission for the Certification of Smallpox Eradication. History of International Public Health.* Geneva: World Health Organization; 1980:4.
2. Kortepeter MG, Parker GW. Potential biological weapons threats. *Emerging Infect Dis.* 1999;5:523-527.
3. Henderson DA, Inglesby TV, Bartlett JG, et al. Smallpox as a biological weapon: medical and public health management. Working Group on Civilian Biodefense. *JAMA.* 1999;281:2127-2137.
4. Fenner F, Henderson DA, Arita I, et al. *Smallpox and Its Eradication.* Geneva: World Health Organization; 1988:31-38, 121-168, 200, 1341-1343.
5. Gelfand HM, Posch J. The recent outbreak of smallpox in Meschede, West Germany. *Am J Epidemiol.* 1971;93:234-237.
6. Centers for Disease Control and Prevention. Vaccinia (smallpox) vaccine: recommendations of the Advisory Committee on Immunization Practices (ACIP), 2001. *MMWR Morb Mortal Wkly Rep.* 2001;50(RR-10):1-25.
7. Sarkar JK, Mitra AC, Mukherjee MK, et al. Virus excretion in smallpox: 2. Excretion in the throats of household contacts. *Bull WHO.* 1973;48:523-527.
8. Downie AW, Meiklejohn M, St Vincent L, et al. The recovery of smallpox virus from patients and their environment in a smallpox hospital. *Bull WHO.* 1965;33:615-622.
9. Rao AR. *Infected Inanimate Objects (Fomites) and Their Role in Transmission of Smallpox.* Geneva: World Health Organization; 1972:72.40.
10. Downie AW, McCarthy K. The antibody response in man following infection with viruses of the pox group: III. Antibody response in smallpox. *J Hyg (Lond).* 1958;56:479-487.
11. Damon I, Esposito JJ. Poxviruses that infect humans. In: Murray P, Baron E, Jorgenson J, et al., eds. *Manual of Clinical Microbiology.* Washington DC: ASM Press; 2003:1583-1592.
12. Meyer H, Ropp SL, Esposito JJ. Diagnostic virology protocols. In: Warnes A, Stephenson J, eds. *Methods in Molecular Biology.* Totowa, NJ: Humana Press; 1998:199-211.
13. Meyer H, Ropp SL, Esposito JJ. Gene for A-type inclusion body protein is useful for a polymerase chain reaction assay to differentiate orthopoxviruses. *J Virol Methods.* 1997;64:217-221.
14. Ropp SL, Jin Q, Knight JC, et al. PCR strategy for identification and differentiation of small pox and other orthopoxviruses. *J Clin Microbiol.* 1995;33:2069-2076.
15. Loparev VN, Massung RF, Esposito JJ, et al. Detection and differentiation of Old World orthopoxviruses: restriction fragment length polymorphism of the crmB gene region. *J Clin Microbiol.* 2001;39:94-100.
16. Dhar AD, Werchniak AE, Li Y, et al. Tanapox infection in a college student. *N Engl J Med.* 2004;350:361-366.
17. Lapa S, Mikheev M, Shchelkunov S, et al. Species-level identification of orthopoxviruses with an oligonucleotide microchip. *J Clin Microbiol.* 2002;40:753-757.
18. Ibrahim M, Kulesh D, Saleh S, et al. Real-time PCR assay to detect smallpox virus. *J Clin Microbiol.* 2003;8:3385-3839.
19. Espy MJ, Cockerill FR III, Meyer RF, et al. Detection of smallpox virus DNA by LightCycler PCR. *J Clin Microbiol.* 2002;40:1985-1988.
20. Nakano J. Poxviruses. In: Lennette E, Schmidt N, eds. *Diagnostic Procedures for Viral, Rickettsial and Chlamydial Infections.* 5th ed. Washington, DC: American Public Health Association; 1979:257-308.
21. Long GW, Nobel J Jr, Murphy FA, et al. Experience with electron microscopy in the differential diagnosis of smallpox. *Appl Microbiol.* 1970;20:497-504.
22. Reed KD, Melski JW, Graham MB, et al. The detection of monkeypox in humans in the Western Hemisphere. *N Engl J Med.* 2004;350:342-350.
23. Guarner J, Johnson B, Paddock C, et al. Monkeypox transmission and pathogens in prairie dogs. *Emerg Infect Dis.* 2004;3:426-431.
24. World Health Organization. *Guide to the Laboratory Diagnosis of Smallpox for Smallpox Eradication Programmes. WHO Technical Report Series.* Geneva: World Health Organization; 1960:1-47.
25. Wharton M, Strikas RA, Harpaz R, et al. Recommendations for using smallpox vaccine in a pre-event vaccination program: supplemental recommendations of the Advisory Committee on Immunization Practices (ACIP) and the Healthcare Infection Control Practices Advisory Committee (HICPAC). *MMWR Recomm Rep.* 2003;52:1-16.
26. Massoudi MS, Barker L, Schwartz B. Effectiveness of postexposure vaccination for the prevention of smallpox: Results of a Delphi analysis. *J Infect Dis.* 2003;188:973-976.
27. Mack TM, Thomas DB, Ali A, et al. Epidemiology of smallpox in West Pakistan: I. Acquired immunity and the distribution of disease. *Am J Epidemiol.* 1972;95:157-168.
28. Rao AR, Jacob ES, Kamalakshi S, et al. Epidemiological studies in smallpox: a study of intrafamilial transmission in a series of 254 infected families. *Indian J Med Res.* 1968;56:1826-1854.
29. Fenner F, Henderson DA, Arita I, et al. *Smallpox and Its Eradication.* Geneva: World Health Organization; 1988:481, 484, 494.
30. Garner JS, Simmons BP. Guideline for isolation precautions in hospitals. *Infect Control.* 1983;4(suppl):245-325.
31. Mack TM. Smallpox in Europe, 1950-1971. *J Infect Dis.* 1972;125:161-169.
32. Gani R, Leach S. Transmission potential of smallpox in contemporary populations. *Nature.* 2001;414:748-751.
33. Foege WH, Millar JD, Henderson DA. Smallpox eradication in West and Central Africa. *Bull WHO.* 1975;52:209-222.
34. LeDuc JW, Damon I, Relman DA, et al. Smallpox research activities: U.S. interagency collaboration, 2001. *Emerg Infect Dis.* 2002;8:743-745.
35. Frey SE, Newman FK, Cruz J, et al. Dose-related effects of smallpox vaccine. *N Engl J Med.* 2002;346:1275-1280.
36. Frey SE, Couch RB, Tacket CO, et al. Clinical responses to undiluted and diluted smallpox vaccine. *N Engl J Med.* 2002;346:1265-1274.
37. U.S. Food and Drug Administration. Product approval information. Available at: <http://www.fda.gov/cber/products/acam2000.htm>.
38. Greenberg RN, Kennedy JS. ACAM2000: A newly licensed cell culture-based live vaccinia smallpox vaccine. *Expert Opin Investig Drugs.* 2008;17:555-564.
39. Neff JM, Lane JM, Pert JH, et al. Complications of smallpox vaccination: I. National survey in the United States, 1963. *N Engl J Med.* 1967;276:125-132.
40. Lane JM, Ruben FL, Neff JM, et al. Complications of smallpox vaccination, 1968. *N Engl J Med.* 1969;281:1201-1208.
41. Lane JM, Ruben FL, Neff JM, et al. Complications of smallpox vaccination, 1968: results of ten statewide surveys. *J Infect Dis.* 1970;122:303-309.
42. Meyer H, Sutter G, Mayr A. Mapping of deletions in the genome of the highly attenuated vaccinia virus MVA and their influence on virulence. *J Gen Virol.* 1991;72(Pt 5):1031-1038.
43. National Institute of Allergy and Infectious Diseases. NIAID Biodefense Research Agenda for CDC Category A Agents—Progress Report. Bethesda, MD: NIAID; 2003.
44. Redfield RR, Wright DC, James WD, et al. Disseminated vaccinia in a military recruit with human immunodeficiency virus (HIV) disease. *N Engl J Med.* 1987;316:673-676.
45. Hooper JW, Custer DM, Thompson E. Four-gene-combination DNA vaccine protects mice against a lethal vaccinia virus challenge and elicits appropriate antibody responses in nonhuman primates. *Virology.* 2003;306:181-195.

325

Anthrax as an Agent of Bioterrorism

GREGORY J. MARTIN | ARTHUR M. FRIEDLANDER

When bioterrorism became reality in the autumn of 2001, the focus of the world shifted from a vision of passenger jets flying into the World Trade Center to that of *Bacillus anthracis*, a bacterium associated with what had become a relatively obscure disease of the developing world. With a few grams of anthrax spores dispersed in letters, the recognition that the threat of bioterrorism had been ignored for too long prompted a dramatic increase in research, training, public health preparedness, countermeasures, and response infrastructure. The general level of understanding of all the agents of bioterrorism was raised not only in the medical community but also among first responders, legislators, and the general public.

Anthrax remains the agent of greatest concern for future use as a bioterrorist's weapon. With naturally occurring cases not uncommon in much of the world, *B. anthracis* is readily accessible to terrorists; easy to grow in even a rudimentary laboratory; and, in the spore form, stable, easily stored, and portable in small quantities that can wreak havoc when dispersed.

Although physicians had an understanding of natural anthrax infections prior to 2001, the realization that there are unique considerations in a bioterrorist attack prompted the development of this bioterrorism section. The reader is referred to Chapter 208 for a review of the microbiology, clinical features, and treatment of anthrax infections. This chapter focuses on aspects of anthrax when used as an agent of bioterrorism.

History of *Bacillus anthracis* as a Bioterrorist Agent

The history of anthrax being spread intentionally to infect others is relatively recent (in comparison to that of plague and smallpox), extending only as far back as World War I when Germans were reported to have shipped infected horses and cattle with *B. anthracis* to be used by the Allies.[1] A more bizarre story is that of Finnish independence activist Baron Otto Karl von Rosen, who was apprehended by Norwegian police in 1917 with 19 sugar cubes, each with an embedded glass capillary tube supposedly filled with anthrax. Apparently, the plan was to infect reindeer and horses used to haul British arms through Norway. The sugar cubes would be fed to the animals, whose teeth would break the glass tubes inside, thereby lacerating their gums and allowing oropharyngeal or gastrointestinal anthrax to ensue. A British and Norwegian team successfully isolated viable anthrax from the one remaining vial 80 years later.[2]

During World War II, both the Axis and Allies had biologic warfare programs that involved anthrax, including the British, whose spore bomb experiments on the Scottish Gruinard Island rendered areas of the island heavily contaminated for decades.[3] The Japanese carried out extensive research on biological weapons. They used anthrax-infected animals to spread the disease in Russia and intentionally infected Chinese residents of Manchuria and China by various means, including an unsuccessful attempt to infect children with anthrax-laden chocolate.[4]

Beginning in the 1940s, the United States maintained an offensive biowarfare program that performed numerous studies on anthrax weaponization and defense that remain the basis of much of our understanding of bioterrorism today. The offensive program at Fort Detrick, Maryland, was disestablished by President Nixon in 1969 and replaced by the U.S. Army Medical Research Institute of Infectious Diseases, which has been focused on biodefense for more than 40 years.

The Soviet Union maintained an active anthrax program well into the 1990s. The widely studied accidental release of anthrax spores in 1979 from a Soviet military microbiology facility in Sverdlovsk, Russia, was responsible for approximately 70 human cases of inhalational anthrax.[5,6] It remains the largest outbreak of inhalational anthrax known.

During the rein of Saddam Hussein, Iraq was known to have an active biological warfare program, and 16 other nations were suspected of having biowarfare programs, but it is unknown which may have been be working with anthrax.[7] At the close of the first Gulf War, Iraqi authorities admitted to having produced 8500 L of anthrax and placed 6500 L into munitions but denied ever having used them.[8,9]

Far more widely known is the use of the U.S. Postal Service in 2001 to mail anthrax spore-laden letters in which 22 people developed anthrax, 11 with inhalational and 11 with cutaneous infections. There were five deaths among the inhalation cases. An astute infectious diseases physician first considered the diagnosis when a Florida man was noted to have gram-positive rods in his cerebrospinal fluid. Subsequent letters were sent to recipients in New York City and Washington, DC, including media outlets and offices in the U.S. Capitol of Senators Daschle and Leahy.

The epidemiology of the 2001 anthrax cases completely changed our understanding of the dispersal of anthrax spores. The ease with which spores were released from sealed envelopes during mail handling was a startling development that was not recognized until hospitalization of postal employees with inhalational anthrax occurred in those never suspected to have been exposed. Approximately 10,000 Americans subsequently received anthrax postexposure prophylaxis (PEP) with antibiotics because of possible exposure. The extensive cross-contamination of mail that led to additional cases geographically distant from the source was a completely unpredicted finding.[10,11] Finally, the substantial reaerosolization of spores from surfaces was not anticipated from studies performed decades previously and contributed to the $100 million spent on anthrax remediation (decontamination) in the United States, with $23 million spent at the U.S. Capitol complex alone.[12-14]

The anthrax events of 2001 fueled a massive investment by the U.S. government in broad areas of research on the agents of bioterrorism. Since these events, new rapid, sensitive, and specific diagnostics tests have become available and are dispersed regionally as part of the Laboratory Response Network's system of labs with varying biosafety levels (BSLs): sentinel (BSL-2), reference (BSL-3), and national (BSL-4) laboratories. Extensive bioterrorism educational efforts were made with physicians, nurses, infection control practitioners, and first responders. The intensive search for the source of the anthrax spores drove rapid improvements in microbial forensics, and the decontamination efforts in postal facilities, the U.S. Capitol, and multiple media outlets advanced the science behind environmental remediation.[13,15,16] The anthrax events, occurring soon after the terrorist attacks of September 11, 2001, provoked a sense of urgency in both legislators and the scientific and medical communities that has led to considerable improvements in countermeasures such as antibiotics, therapeutic antibodies, and vaccines. Project Bioshield was created in 2004 to provide the Strategic National Stockpile funds to maintain a supply of antibiotics and other therapeutics, vaccines, and diagnostics in the event of a national emergency. Furthermore, Bioshield not only provides funding for phase III clinical trials to obtain approval by the Food and Drug Administration (FDA) but also gives the option of using supplies that may not have been fully approved by the FDA if the Centers for Disease Control and Prevention (CDC) declares an emergency.[17]

Dissemination of Anthrax as a Bioterrorist Agent

History has already presented a number of methods in which anthrax can be weaponized. Anthrax has proven itself to be a versatile agent for a terrorist to utilize. Spores can be dispersed or sprayed as a powder or liquid, or animals can be infected and released with the intent to spread infection among others. Anthrax can be delivered by an aerosol in bombs, sprayed from a plane or backpack sprayer, or sent in the mail. It is generally believed that an intentional release of anthrax would most likely be associated with aerosols and subsequent inhalational infections. Although contamination of human food or water could cause gastrointestinal anthrax, evidence from experimental animals suggests that it is not an efficient route and requires very high doses of spores to lead to infection.[18] Anthrax is also an efficient agent; the 2 g of spores that were in the letter sent to Senator Daschle in 2001 were estimated to contain more than 10 million human LD_{50} (lethal dose for 50% of individuals) doses.[12]

In a report to the U.S. Congress, it was estimated that 100 kg of anthrax spores released from a plane over Washington, DC, would kill 1 to 3 million people under ideal meteorological conditions.[19] Other studies indicate there could be 50% fatalities as far as 160 km downwind from an aerosol spore release.[20]

A 1999 Canadian study that investigated the effect of aerial spraying of *Bacillus thuringiensis* for control of gypsy moths in British Columbia was indicative of why anthrax is considered such a high-threat agent. *B. thuringiensis* is a spore-forming Bacillus closely related to *B. anthracis* but a nonpathogen in animals. A plane sprayed a slurry of spores at a droplet size of 110 to 130 μm and samples were taken from the environment, inside homes, and from nasal swabs of asthmatic children. Thirty minutes after release, spore concentrations were highest in the outdoor environment (mean, 739 spores/m³ of air), but 5 or 6 hours later spore concentration inside homes exceeded outdoor concentrations (mean, 245 spores/m³). A significant amount of small droplet aerosolization occurred with droplets of 2 to 7 μm formed in sufficient quantities to penetrate houses, yielding positive nasal swabs in 76%. (Droplets <5 μm can reach the alveoli). If this had been *B. anthracis*, some estimates are that potentially 15% of the population sprayed may have been exposed to a lethal dose of anthrax.[21] Furthermore, the spray formulations and equipment used are readily available to the public through agricultural supply stores, and these formulations do not clog spray nozzles.[22]

Determinations of the number of inhaled spores per hour raise questions about the infective dose (ID) and lethal dose (LD) of anthrax spores. Obviously, controlled studies cannot be performed on humans and therefore we must rely on extrapolation of data from estimates of known inhalational cases and from studies in nonhuman primates. Even this is difficult because different animals have markedly different sensitivities to anthrax spores: Some are very sensitive and others quite resistant.[23,24] Despite the uncertainty inherent in extrapolation, the LD_{50} for humans is generally considered to range from approximately 4000 to 12,000 to 55,000 spores based on studies in nonhuman primates.[23,25-27] Data from nonhuman primates suggest that inhaled doses of 1000 to 5500 spores results in mortalities from 10% to 25%.[6] The determination of the LD_1 (or ID_1) is even more difficult to ascertain and it may be significantly lower,[25] but there are no data on this point. From a public health perspective, even an LD_1 or LD_{10} release may be significant because a city of 1 million would suffer tens of thousands of cases of anthrax.[21]

Studies from mill workers in the 1950s and 1960s revealed that many employees were inhaling hundreds of anthrax spores less than 5 μm

on a daily basis and yet inhalational anthrax was extraordinarily rare.[28-30] Furthermore, 15% of workers developed measurable anti-anthrax antibodies, demonstrating some degree of exposure by an unknown route, suggesting some degree of innate immunity in avoiding clinically evident infections.[31] Even in the absence of measurable antibodies, exposures in the U.S. Capitol appear to have been associated with evidence of a cellular immune response in a few cases.[32] What may be a "safe" number of spores for a healthy 20-year-old may be a lethal dose for an immunocompromised individual. Historically, some individuals with inhalational anthrax had evidence of preexisting pulmonary disease and some were welders.[33,34]

Outbreak Characteristics after Use of Anthrax as a Bioterrorist Agent

A terrorist considering using anthrax may contemplate which route to deliver spores to reach his objective. Although spores could be introduced into food supplies or water, the cutaneous, oropharyngeal and gastrointestinal disease that would result is far less dramatic, and far less fatal, than inhalational anthrax.[12] Knowledge of the number of spores needed to infect humans via ingestion is not available. It is generally understood that significantly more are needed than via inhalation, and experiments in nonhuman primates suggest it is very difficult to infect by the oral route.[18] In addition, the majority of ingestions are not associated with full-blown gastrointestinal anthrax, which is frequently fatal, but, rather, with gastroenteritis, a far less dramatic presentation than inhalational anthrax.[35]

An aerosol release, whether from an envelope, a sprayer on the ground, or on a larger scale from a plane, is considered the most likely terrorist scenario. Studies done in Canada with envelopes containing *Bacillus globigii* spores demonstrated how spores spread like a gas in an office after opening an envelope containing 1 g of spores (Fig. 325-1). The estimates were that with 10 minutes of exposure, hundreds to thousands of times a human LD_{50} would be inhaled by those in the room.[36,37]

Individual *B. anthracis* spores are 1.5 to 3 μm in size; in nature they are most likely clustered together to form aggregates that are 10 to 100 μm in diameter or greater. As Figure 325-2 demonstrates, particles larger than 5 μm typically cannot reach the terminal bronchioles and alveoli; they are captured in the respiratory tract mucous, removed by the mucociliary elevator to the mouth, and swallowed.[38] This is likely why inhalational anthrax has been uncommon in natural settings but was somewhat more common in factories where wool, hair, or hides were dried and manipulated by machinery, resulting in particle sizes of 1 to 5 μm. When spores are grown and engineered in a laboratory with the intent of preventing clumping by coating with silica or other substances, they may not cluster at all or may form small spore aggre-

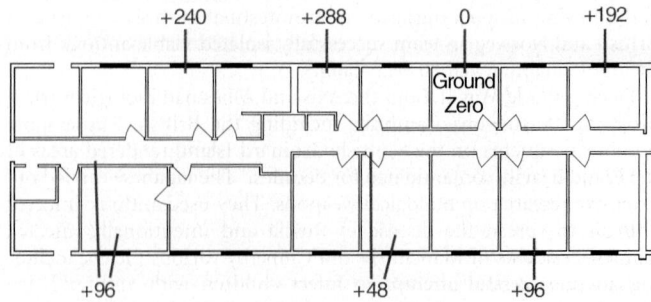

Figure 325-1 **Spores released in an office spread very rapidly through doors and in hallways.** Time in seconds for peak spore deposition at a site after release of spores from an envelope at "Ground Zero." *(From Kournikakis B, Ho J. Objective assessment of the hazard from anthrax terrorist attacks in an office environment. Presented at the Anthrax Incident Management Workshop, Medicine Hat, Alberta, Canada. April 30, 2002.)*

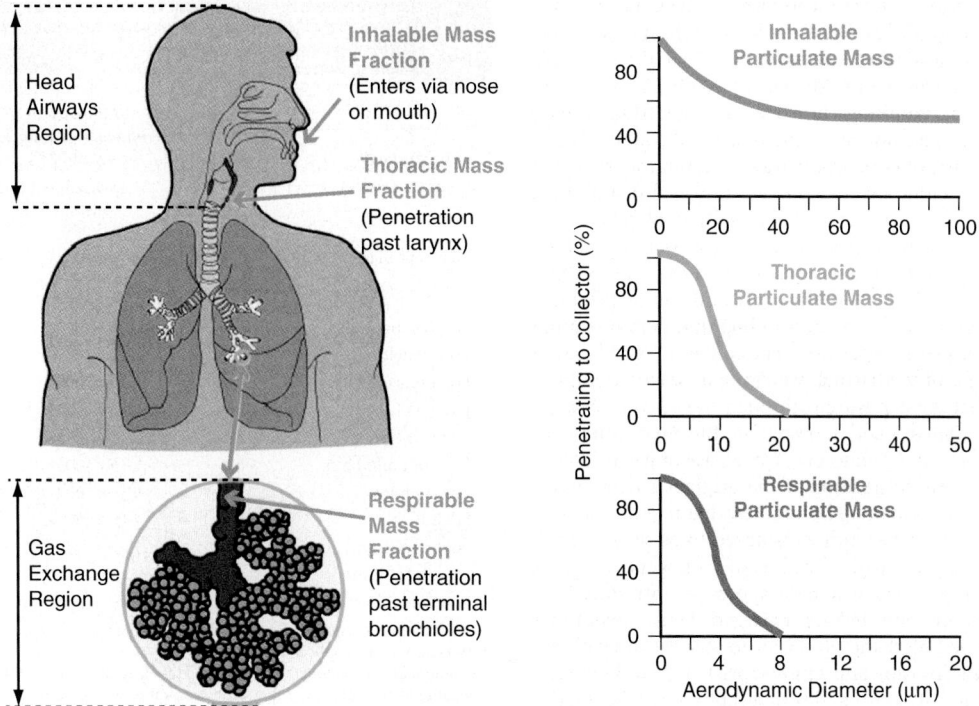

Figure 325-2   Deposition of anthrax spores in the human respiratory tract is dependent on the size of spore aggregates. Individual spores are 1 to 1.5 µm but form aggregates 10 to 100 µm or larger that are deposited in the upper airways and cleared; weaponized spores may not cluster and are efficiently delivered to the alveoli, where they may lead to inhalational anthrax. *(Adapted from Hoover MD. Uncertainty and probability distribution analyses for anthrax dispersion and human exposure. Paper presented at the Anthrax Incident Management Workshop, Medicine Hat, Alberta, Canada. April 30, 2002.)*

gates that may be efficiently delivered to the alveoli. It can be assumed that a sophisticated terrorist utilizing anthrax spores would ensure:

1. Engineering of spores to neutralize electrostatic charges, thereby reducing clusters and maintaining spores in small respirable aggregates less than 5 µm
2. Use of high concentrations of spores to overcome any degree of innate immunity
3. Selection of a strain demonstrating antimicrobial resistance
4. Genetic modifications to decrease protection from vaccination or increase toxin production

When anthrax spores pass the terminal bronchioles into the alveoli, they are rapidly scavenged by alveolar phagocytic cells and move through the lymphatics to the tracheobronchial and then mediastinal lymph nodes. Some spores rapidly transform to the vegetative state within the macrophages, whereas others are thought to remain quiescent potentially for months.

The incubation period in natural inhalational anthrax is generally considered to be 2 to 10 days, but with large inocula it may be as short as 1 day. In the 2001 cases for which the date of exposure was known, the incubation period was 4 to 6 days.[39] There is some controversy regarding how long the incubation can potentially be and whether small spore inocula may be associated with extended incubation periods.[11,30,34] The often cited last case of anthrax in Sverdlovsk occurred 43 days after the release of spores, but those closest to the release had a median incubation of 10 days and those farthest away of 21 days.[5] However, these data are of dubious value because critical details are not available and patients may have received antibiotics, which are known to extend the incubation period. The case of the 94-year-old woman in Connecticut who developed anthrax in 2001, presumably related to the terrorism cases that year, occurred 35 days after the last letter was mailed and 56 days after the first, suggesting she may have inhaled a small dose. However, the possibility of exposure resulting from a different unrecognized intentional release of spores cannot be

excluded.[11] In a series of 58 nonhuman primates, the time to death after exposure to spores varied from 2 to 9 days (Arthur M. Friedlander, unpublished observations). However, there are reports of three animals with possible times to death of 7, 14, and 98 days after exposure.[6,25] Animals sacrificed 42 days after inhalation had a large number of spores in the lungs, and even after 100 days small numbers of viable anthrax spores remained.[26]

The pathophysiology of anthrax infections and anthrax toxins are more thoroughly discussed in Chapter 208.

The ability to detect an aerosol release of anthrax spores soon after their release or to diagnose the first case of anthrax has improved significantly in the past decade. In a large spore release over a city, every day earlier that the exposure is recognized will result in earlier initiation of PEP and thousands of fewer deaths and millions of dollars in saved resources.[40,41] Even with an extensive system of detection in place, it is likely that the first evidence of anthrax bioterrorism, as in 2001, will be a critically ill patient discovered to have *B. anthracis* in a blood culture. Also as in 2001, it can be expected that some patients will present with cutaneous disease (because aerosolized spores deposited on the body can be introduced into the skin) and others with inhalational disease or meningitis. If an extensive outbreak is recognized, local medical resources will be severely taxed attempting to initiate PEP, evaluating those potentially developing symptoms, and caring for those already confirmed infected and potentially critically ill.

Although there are numerous rapid assays in development, there is currently no rapid method approved to diagnose anthrax early in disease. The early symptoms of inhalational anthrax are nonspecific and similar to those of influenza. It will be important to rapidly determine who has inhalational anthrax (IA), influenza or influenza-like illness (ILI), or community-acquired pneumonia (CAP) so that appropriate therapy can be initiated.[42-44] Kuehnert and associates combined data from patients presenting with each of these diagnoses and developed a scoring system.[44] They found that compared with patients who had ILI, patients who had IA were more likely to have tachycardia, high hematocrit, low albumin, and low sodium levels and were less likely to have myalgias, headache, sore throat, and nasal symptoms. Compared with patients who had CAP, patients with IA were more likely to have nausea or vomiting, tachycardia, high transaminase levels, low sodium levels, and normal white blood cell counts (Tables 325-1 and 325-2).[44] The use of rapid influenza and respiratory syncytial virus diagnostics in the clinic or emergency room is also indicated. Patients with fever and spore exposure should also have blood cultures obtained because all 7 patients with IA in 2001 who were not taking antibiotics had positive blood cultures. Kyriacou and co-workers compared 47 IA cases with 376 CAP or ILI cases and found the most accurate predictor of anthrax was a chest radiograph demonstrating mediastinal widening or pleural effusion.[45] The epidemiological as well as diagnostic significance of mediastinal widening needs to be emphasized in recognizing that the exposure is through the aerosol route. It has been erroneously stated[46] and repeated in the literature[47] that mediastinal widening was reported to occur in a case of gastrointestinal anthrax. However, a careful reading of the original article reveals no mention of mediastinal widening but, rather, that pneumonia was present on chest x-ray, which the authors believed to be secondary to bacteremia.[48] This is consistent with our ideas of pathogenesis in that the lymph nodes draining the site where the spores are introduced are those anticipated to become infected and enlarged. Thus, mediastinal widening on x-ray should alert the physician to suspect inhalational anthrax from an aerosol exposure and a bioterrorist event until proved otherwise. The evolution of computed tomography scans in inhalational anthrax is demonstrated in U.S. cases from 2001 in Figure 325-3.[49] The Center for Infectious Disease Research and Policy developed a helpful clinical pathway to guide clinicians assessing the probability of anthrax exposure and evaluating patients with possible inhalational anthrax (Fig. 325-4; Table 325-3).[50]

Anthrax Countermeasures

DIAGNOSTICS

Laboratory specimens for patients suspected to have any form of anthrax should be obtained as described in Chapter 208.

TABLE 325-1	Sign and Symptoms of Patients Presenting with Inhalation Anthrax, Influenza or Influenza-like Illness, and Community-Acquired Pneumonia		
Sign or Symptom	Inhalation Anthrax (n = 11), %	Influenza or Influenza-like Illness (n = 684), %	Community-Acquired Pneumonia (n = 650), %
Tachycardia	82	14 (p = .0001)	49 (p = .04)
Sore throat	18	76 (p = .0001)	25 (p = 1.0)
Nasal symptoms	27	81 (p = .0002)	34 (p = .76)
Headache	45	86 (p = .002)	38 (p = .76)
Myalgias	64	91 (p = .01)	41 (p = .21)
Fever >37.8°C	73	57 (p = .37; with flu p < .05)	53 (p = .23)
Cough	91	89 (p = 1.0)	79 (p = .47)
Fatigue	100	98 (p = 1.0)	NA
Abdominal pain	27	NA	21 (p = .71)
Diarrhea	9	NA	20 (p = .70)
Nausea or vomiting	82	NA	35 (p = .002)
Chest pain	64	NA	31 (p = .04; if pneumococcal bacteremia p > .05)
Dyspnea	82	NA	80 (p = 1.0)
Chills	82	NA	59 (p = .21)

NA, not applicable.
Modified from Kuehnert M, Doyle T, Hill H, et al. Clinical features that discriminate inhalational anthrax from other acute respiratory illnesses. *Clin Infect Dis* 2003;36:328-336.

TABLE 325-2	Laboratory Findings in Patients Presenting with Inhalation Anthrax, Influenza or Influenza-like Illness, and Community-Acquired Pneumonia		
Lab Parameter	Inhalation Anthrax (n = 8-11), %	Influenza or Influenza-like Illness (n = 630-687), %	Community-Acquired Pneumonia (n = 185-645)
Leukocytosis	27	7 (p = .04; without confirmed flu, p > .05)	61 (p = .03)
Neutrophilia	72	43 (p = .06; without confirmed flu, p < .05)	78 (p = .71)
High hematocrit	36	6 (p = .004)	NA
Low platelets	22	4 (p = .05)	NA
High bilirubin	38	6 (p = .009)	NA
High AST	89	18 (p < .0001)	29 (p = .0004)
High ALT	89	32 (p = .0008)	29 (p = .0005)
Low albumin level	67	2 (p < .0001)	NA
Low sodium	80	9 (p < .0001)	35 (p = .0005)
High BUN	50	4 (p < .0002)	23 (p = .10)
High creatinine	0	1 (p = 1.0)	NA
Low potassium	10	2 (p = .21)	NA
Low calcium	100	44 (p = .002)	74 (p = .21)

ALT, alanine aminotransferase; AST, aspartate aminotransferase; BUN, blood urea nitrogen; NA, not applicable.
Modified from Kuehnert M, Doyle T, Hill H, et al. Clinical features that discriminate inhalational anthrax from other acute respiratory illnesses. *Clin Infect Dis* 2003;36:328-336.

It is important to notify the laboratory that anthrax is in the differential diagnosis because the typical clinical laboratory may discard gram-positive rods as probable contaminants or not work them up beyond *Bacillus* sp. Furthermore, if *B. anthracis* is isolated, it should be handled in at least a BSL-2 lab (i.e., under a hood) because secondary cases have occurred among laboratory workers.

The frequency of encountering other *Bacillus* species has been part of the problem in developing sensitive and specific rapid tests for anthrax from both environmental and clinical sources. When Dahlgren and co-workers reported on *B. anthracis* aerosols in goat hair mills, they noted the difficulty in finding the organism because it was obscured by other spore-forming bacteria in a ratio of 115:1 to 700:1.[29] Recently developed, more specific polymerase chain reaction assays have become available that should aid in rapid diagnosis and minimize the number of false-positive samples.[51]

The role of nasal swabs in the "diagnosis" of anthrax must also be clarified. In the 2001 outbreak, patients considered nasal swabs as a determination of whether they had been exposed or not. The reality is that although a positive nasal culture for anthrax clearly indicates an exposure, a negative culture does not rule out an exposure. In Senator Daschle's suite in the Hart Building of the U.S. Capitol, all 13 staff members in the room where the spore-laden letter was opened had heavy growth on blood agar plates from their nasal swabs. Many of these individuals had a separate swab from each nostril, and in at least two cases one nostril yielded heavy growth and the other nostril yielded no *B. anthracis* growth (Gregory J. Martin, personal observation). Nasal swabs essentially use the nose to sample whether the individual has filtered anthrax spores in the recently (nasally) inhaled air. They are therefore helpful as a public health tool in determining the zone of exposure. Demonstrating that one individual in a space has a positive nasal swab requires that everyone in that space receive PEP regardless of the negative nasal swabs for the others. The optimal timing of obtaining nasal swabs after exposure has not been determined, but clearly the sooner the better, and it is likely that the yield 24 hours later (after showering, etc.) is much lower. Thus, obtaining nasal swabs more than 24 hours after exposure should be discouraged. All 28 positive cultures in the U.S. Capitol were obtained within hours of exposure; the remaining 6000 cultures done during the subsequent days

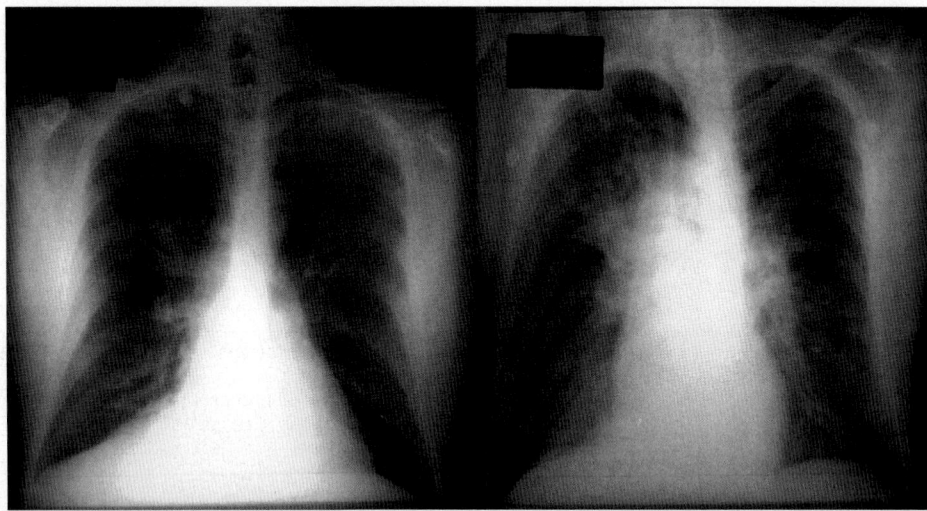

10/21/01 0300 (intital ER visit)   10/22/01 0530 (hospital admit)

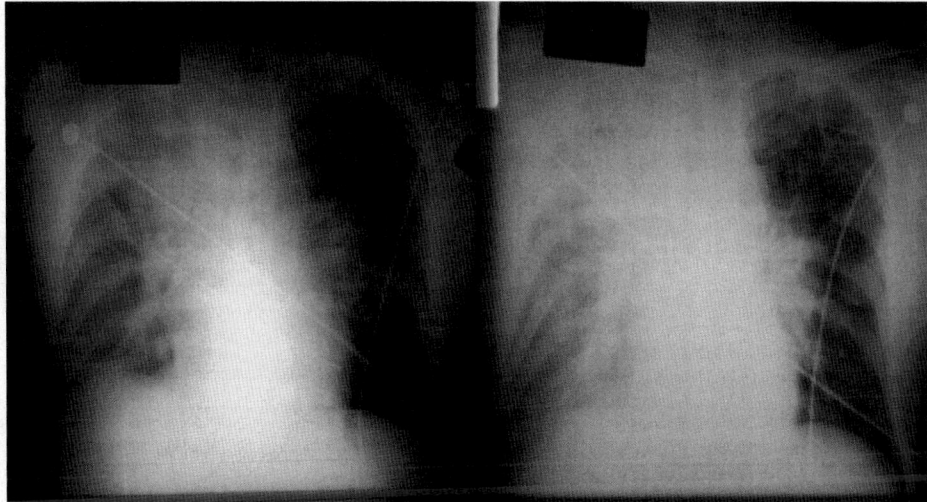

10/22/01 0900   10/22/01 1100 (shortly before death)

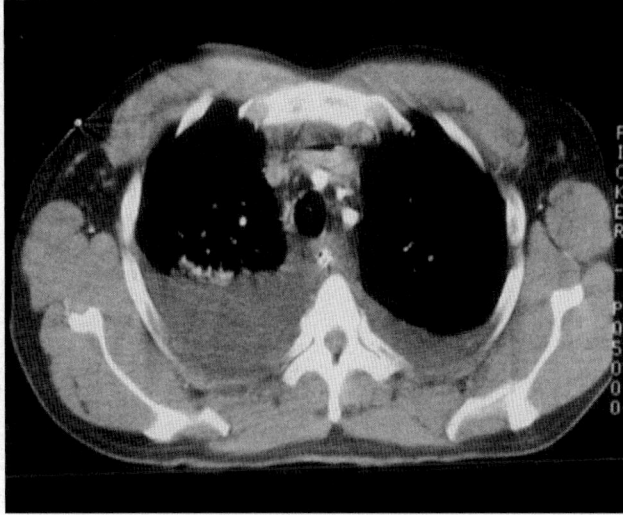

10/22/01 (shortly before death)

Figure 325-3   Chest radiographs and computed tomography scan from a 47-year-old postal worker who had been ill for 5 days when he presented to the hospital with inhalational anthrax. Note progressive bilateral perihilar and infrahilar infiltrates, widened mediastinum, and rapid evolution. Computed tomography scan demonstrates mediastinitis and large right and smaller left pleural effusions. (*Adapted from Borio L, Frank D, Mani V, et al. Death due to bioterrorism-related inhalational anthrax. JAMA. 2001;286:2554-2559.*)

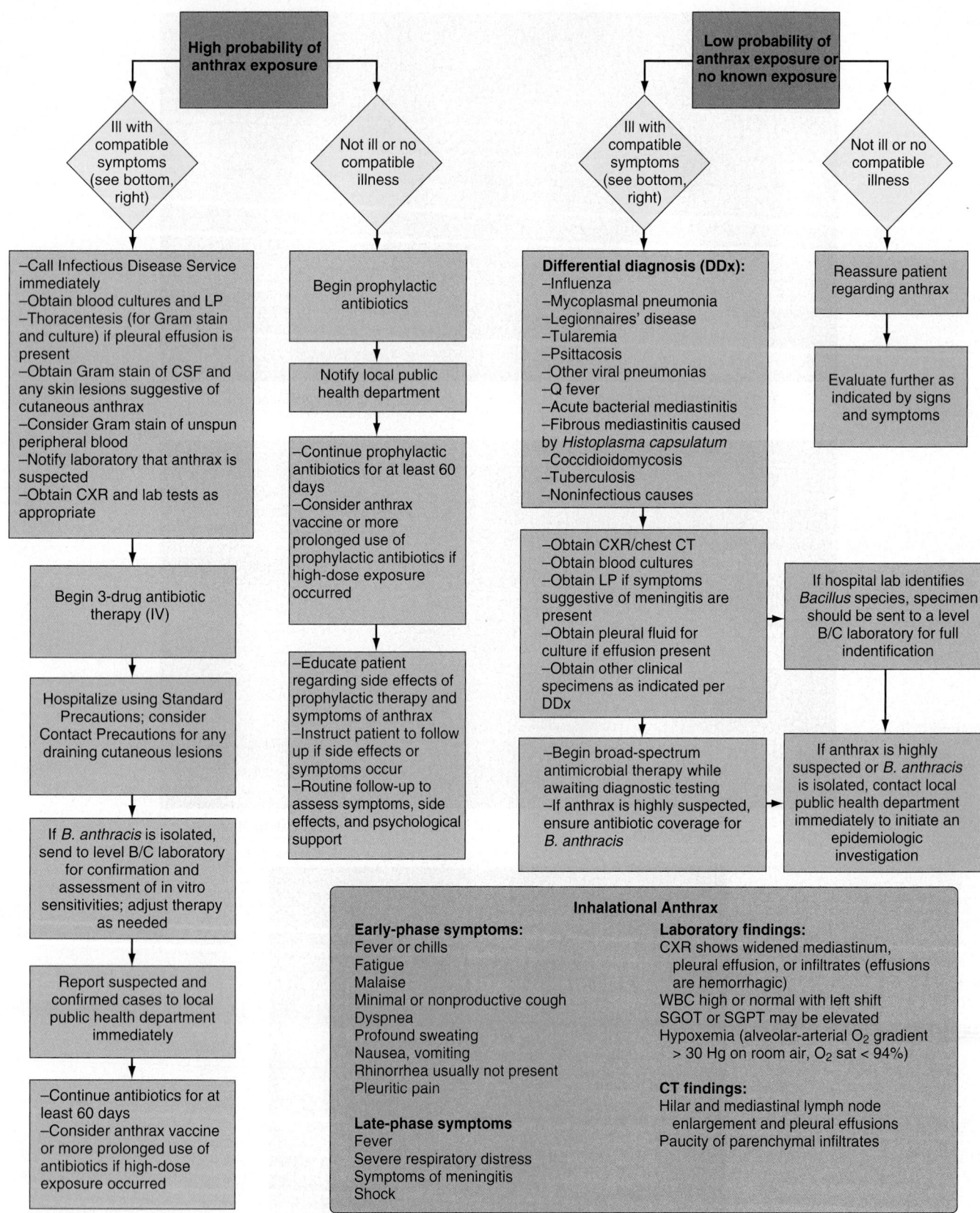

Figure 325-4 Clinical pathway: anthrax inhalational exposure. (*From the Center for Infectious Disease Research and Policy. Available at www. cidrap.umn.edu.*)

TABLE 325-3	Assessing the Probability of Anthrax Exposure

High Probability

During a known anthrax event

Persons exposed to an airspace where a suspicious material may have been aerosolized (e.g., near a suspicious powder-containing letter during opening)

Persons who shared an airspace likely to be the source of an inhalational anthrax case (e.g., being exposed to a shared ventilation system)

Persons who may have been exposed to an item contaminated with *Bacillus anthracis* (e.g., an envelope or other vehicle) along the transit path of the item (e.g., a postal sorting facility in which an envelope containing *B. anthracis* was processed)

*In situations in which anthrax has not previously been identified**

Persons who opened a suspicious letter or package that was found to contain a white powder suspected to be a source of *B. anthracis*

Persons exposed to an airspace where suspicious material may have been aerosolized (e.g., near a suspicious powder-containing letter during opening)

Sudden appearance of multiple patients with acute onset of characteristic illness (suggests common source exposure such as would be seen with a bioterrorist attack)

Low Probability

No history of exposure to an item (e.g., an envelope or other vehicle) or powder confirmed or suspected to harbor *B. anthracis* spores

No history of exposure to an airspace where a suspicious material could have been aerosolized (e.g., being present at the time a powder-containing letter was opened)

No history of exposure to an airspace likely to have been the source for a confirmed case of inhalational anthrax

*In situations in which anthrax exposure is suspected but no prior cases of anthrax have been confirmed, a risk assessment should be conducted by local public health and law enforcement officials. If the probability of anthrax exposure is considered high on the basis of the risk assessment, prophylactic antimicrobial therapy should be initiated for asymptomatic exposed persons while the suspect material is being tested for *B. anthracis*. Any persons who have symptoms compatible with anthrax should be treated with appropriate antibiotics until anthrax can be confirmed or ruled out.

From the Center for Infectious Disease Research and Policy (www.cidrap.umn.edu).

were negative despite environmental samples demonstrating varying levels of contamination from multiple other U.S. Capitol sites. Repeat nasal swabs of all the culture-positive individuals in the Capitol 1 week after exposure were negative (Gregory J. Martin, personal observation). In evaluation of future exposures, efforts to determine if an individual was exposed might also include culturing pharyngeal washings because a study of wool mill workers revealed that addition of such cultures doubled the number of individuals with positive cultures compared to culturing only nasal swabs.[11] Gram stain of cutaneous or oral lesions, pleural fluid, cerebrospinal fluid, or even buffy coats of blood may be positive for gram-positive rods indicative (in the right setting) of anthrax, and culture will confirm the diagnosis. Nasal swab, pharyngeal washes, and stool samples should be cultured for anthrax, but gram staining of these samples is not helpful.

In the 2001 outbreak, there were no serologic tests readily available for anthrax. In the aftermath, numerous serologic assays have been in development, and a rapid enzyme-linked immunosorbent assay (QuickELISA Anthrax-PA kit, Immunetics, Boston, MA) that measures total antibody to protective antigen (PA) has been FDA approved. This assay can be used on serum to diagnose all types of anthrax or demonstrate seroconversion after immunization. Retrospectively, it was positive in 100% of both cutaneous and inhalation cases from 2001. Unfortunately, it only becomes positive after approximately 1 week of symptoms. This was demonstrated in the 2006 inhalational anthrax case.[52,53] Numerous other assays are in the development stages, including assays for anti-lactoferrin antibodies.[54] Further research on new rapid diagnostic tests yielding results in a few hours, based on detection of toxin proteins[55,56] and capsule in the serum,[57] are in development and anticipated to be licensed in the near future.

Clinicians seriously considering anthrax in the differential diagnosis should consult the CDC website, http://emergency.cdc.gov/agent/anthrax/lab-testing/inhalationspecimens.asp, to ensure they are obtaining all the appropriate specimens and preparing and shipping them correctly.

ANTIBIOTICS

The role of antibiotics in preventing the development of anthrax after exposure to inhaled spores has been well documented in animal studies since the 1940s and in humans after the 2001 anthrax attacks. Antibiotic PEP and therapy are the most important countermeasures currently available for bioterrorism-associated anthrax. Chapter 208 reviews the use of antibiotics for treatment of all stages of anthrax, whereas this discussion focuses on PEP and newer agents approaching approval for anthrax.

Current recommendations for PEP are for initiation of 60 days of antibiotic prophylaxis with appropriate drugs as dictated by public health authorities and summarized in Table 325-4.[58] In the event of a release of anthrax spores, the determination of which antibiotic should be used will obviously be guided by the sensitivity profile of the *B. anthracis* isolated. Although ciprofloxacin 500 mg or doxycycline 100 mg administered orally twice daily have been recommended by the CDC as first-line agents to be used as PEP, it is relatively easy to develop resistant strains of anthrax through serial passages in low concentrations of antibiotics and a terrorist may develop and utilize a highly resistant strain.[59] Furthermore, in an unrecognized outbreak of inhalation disease many patients may be treated for community-acquired pneumonia with third-generation cephalosporins, to which even most natural occurring strains of *B. anthracis* are resistant.[60,61]

Initiation of antibiotics as soon as possible after (or before) exposure ensures the presence of antibiotics as spores germinate. Ungerminated

TABLE 325-4	Centers for Disease Control and Prevention Recommendations for Postexposure Prophylaxis after Exposure to *Bacillus anthracis* Spores	
Patient	*Recommended Initial Antibiotic*	*Duration*
Adults (including immunocompromised)	Ciprofloxacin, 500 mg orally twice daily *or* Levofloxacin, 500 mg orally once daily *or* Doxycycline, 100 mg orally twice daily	60 days
Pregnant or breast-feeding women	Ciprofloxacin, 500 mg orally twice daily *or* Levofloxacin, 500 mg orally once daily *or* Doxycycline, 100 mg orally twice daily (Amoxicillin 500 mg orally three times daily may be substituted if anthrax isolate has been determined to be a penicillin-sensitive strain)*	60 days
Children (including immunocompromised)	Ciprofloxacin, 10-15 mg/kg orally twice daily, not to exceed 500 mg twice daily *or* Levofloxacin, 16 mg/kg orally twice daily, not to exceed 250 mg twice daily *or* Doxycycline >8 years and >45 kg: 100 mg orally twice daily >8 years and <45 kg: 2.2 mg/kg orally twice daily <8 years: 2.2 mg/kg orally twice daily not to exceed 100 mg twice daily If anthrax isolate is penicillin sensitive amoxicillin may be substituted* <20 kg: 80 mg/kg orally divided three times daily >20 kg: 500 mg orally three times daily	60 days

*Although amoxicillin is not FDA approved for postexposure prophylaxis, it may be used in children and pregnant women if the anthrax strain is susceptible to avoid potential effects of quinolones and tetracyclines in these groups.

From Centers for Disease Control and Prevention. Update: investigation of bioterrorism-related anthrax and interim guidelines for exposure management and antimicrobial therapy. *MMWR Morb Mortal Wkly Rep.* 2001;50:889-893.

spores, while sequestered in the lung or macrophages, do not appear to be affected by antibiotics, which are only active on germinated spores or vegetative bacilli. The question of how long antibiotics should be maintained remains uncertain. A competing-risks model to determine the optimal duration of PEP suggests that this is dependent on the size of the inhaled inocula, with small exposures requiring shorter courses and large exposures requiring 4 months or more.[62]

The concern about prolonged PEP is that adherence to a 60-day course of antibiotics is quite poor. In the 2001 anthrax attacks, the overall adherence with 60 days of antibiotics was only 44%. Adverse events were common, seen in 57% during the first 60 days of PEP and occurred nearly equally with either ciprofloxacin or doxycycline. These data are somewhat deceptive in that many of the approximately 10,000 individuals placed on PEP did not perceive themselves to have been at high risk and so were less likely to continue PEP if they were experiencing even a mild adverse event. Conversely, those who enrolled in the investigational new drug (IND) application, involving the use of anthrax vaccine and prolonged antibiotics, actually had the best compliance.[63] This was reported to be a surrogate marker of individuals' perceived risk of exposure but also reflects the recommendations of clinicians who strongly advised those who had been most highly exposed in Senate offices to maintain strict adherence with PEP as well as enroll in the IND vaccine protocol (Gregory J. Martin, personal observation).

A number of new drugs are being tested for their efficacy in the prophylaxis and treatment of anthrax. Oritavancin, a novel lipoglycopeptide in late development for skin and soft tissue infections, was very effective in the mouse model for pre- and postexposure use. In addition, development of resistance to oritavancin in the laboratory has been much more difficult than with current drugs used for anthrax.[64] Cethromycin, a novel ketolide in development for pneumonia and sinusitis, has also demonstrated promise for *B. anthracis* infection. It can be administered orally once daily, and it showed efficacy equal to that of ciprofloxacin in the mouse model.[65]

VACCINES

Current CDC guidelines are for 60 days of PEP with either doxycycline or ciprofloxacin and initiation of anthrax immunization (given as an IND under protocol). Anthrax vaccine adsorbed (AVA or Biothrax), the currently approved vaccine in the United States, is only approved for use in preventing anthrax preexposure. The recommendation to add postexposure anthrax immunization to antibiotic PEP is due to the concern that retained spores may still be present at the end of 60 days and could germinate and lead to inhalational anthrax after discontinuance of antibiotics. Even after heavy spore exposures, animals taking antibiotics do not usually develop a significant humoral immune response. By initiating anthrax immunization, antibodies develop while the individual is protected by antibiotics. After the 60-day course of antibiotics is completed, there should be an adequate immune response provided by immunization to protect against remaining spores that might germinate and cause anthrax.

For PEP, AVA/Biothrax given as part of a CDC IND with only the initial three doses at 0, 2, and 4 weeks results in excellent antibody responses in nearly 100% of recipients. Although the FDA approved eliminating the week 2 dose in the preexposure regimen it is maintained in the postexposure IND regimen. The pre- and postexposure schedules are outlined in Table 325-5.

TABLE 325-5	Comparison of Anthrax Vaccine for Preexposure and Postexposure Use			
Clinical Setting	No. of Doses	Schedule	FDA-Licensed	IND Required*
Preexposure	5	Weeks 0, 4 Months 6, 12, 18	Yes	No
Postexposure	3	Weeks 0, 2, 4	No	Yes

*IND, investigational new drug. An IND is required by the FDA in the postexposure setting for this vaccine for two reasons: (1) the vaccine was approved for preexposure use but not for postexposure use; and (2) a total of three doses of vaccine over 1 month is recommended for postexposure vaccination, unlike the six-dose vaccine schedule given for preexposure vaccination as part of the FDA licensure.

Animal studies have demonstrated this and have even raised the prospect of shorter courses of antibiotics for those who are immunized. In rhesus macaques given approximately 1600 LD_{50} of inhaled spores and begun on PEP with oral ciprofloxacin for 14 days, 44% survived, whereas 100% of those administered three doses of anthrax vaccine in conjunction with the same course of 14 days of ciprofloxacin survived.[66]

Review of anthrax vaccines currently available and in development is presented in Chapter 208.

IMMUNOTHERAPY

The role of anthrax hyperimmune sera in the treatment of anthrax in the preantibiotic era is well documented[67] and discussed in Chapter 208. Its modern counterpart, anthrax immunoglobulin (AIG), was used in conjunction with antibiotics in the U.S. inhalation case in 2006,[68] and the role of immunotherapy in potential future bioterrorist attacks has not been defined but is almost certain. Through Project Bioshield, the U.S. government has purchased large amounts of both AIG and anti-PA monoclonal antibody for the Strategic National Stockpile, although these products are in still in the final stages of approval by the FDA.[69,70]

The protective effect of immune therapy in animals has been dramatic, and with the prospect of a highly antibiotic-resistant strain of anthrax being utilized by a terrorist, it may become necessary for both PEP and therapy of established disease.[71]

INFECTION CONTROL

Fortunately, *B. anthracis* has not been demonstrated to spread in household or health care settings from individuals who are infected with anthrax, with the exception of two cases associated with direct contact with cutaneous lesions.[72] Inhalational anthrax is not an airspace disease and is usually not associated with sputum production; when it is, sputa usually do not contain *B. anthracis*. Furthermore, vegetative anthrax bacteria, unlike the spores, are not hardy in the environment.

Anthrax-infected patients may be managed in a standard hospital room with standard universal precautions. Cutaneous lesions should be covered and dressings from lesions, chest tube drainage, blood, etc. should be considered potentially infectious and incinerated or autoclaved. Hand washing with soap and water, 2% chlorhexidine, or chlorine-containing towels decreased spores of other *Bacillus* sp. in testing, but the use of waterless ethyl alcohol-containing hand sanitizers was not effective in removing or destroying spores.[73]

The main concern for health care workers, especially in emergency rooms, is from exposed individuals who have not been decontaminated and may pass spores from clothing, skin, or hair to those caring for them. Similarly, hazardous materials and remediation teams may inadvertently carry spores outside the contaminated areas and expose other individuals. These teams often wear personal protective equipment (PPE) in buildings with HVAC shut down, so they are prone to heat-associated injuries and emergency room visits. Potentially exposed individuals should be decontaminated outside the emergency room if possible by individuals wearing PPE. Patients' clothes should be removed and bagged, they should shower, and skin and hair should be washed thoroughly with soap and water and thoroughly rinsed. Surfaces they contact (ambulances, benches, etc.) should be wiped down with a solution of 1:10 household bleach. PEP prophylaxis should be considered for those who have cared for these individuals.

Inadvertent contamination of laboratory workers can also occur as *B. anthracis* sporulates on blood agar plates, and if not handled carefully under BSL-2 or higher conditions, it could cause secondary infections.

REMEDIATION (DECONTAMINATION)

One of the more controversial topics regarding bioterrorist-associated use of anthrax is the method and cost associated with making spore-contaminated areas safe. Clearly, this is an additional advantage to the

TABLE 325-6	Recommended Steps in the Remediation of Sites Contaminated with Anthrax Spores

1. Perform a site assessment to include environmental sampling to assess contamination
2. Isolate contaminated areas
3. Remove any critical items, artifacts, antiques, etc
4. Source reduction if ongoing contamination
5. Remediate contaminated areas and contaminated articles removed from areas
6. Perform post remediation environmental sampling
7. Perform repeat remediation of persistently contaminated areas, consider using a different remediation method
8. Safely dispose of all contaminated waste

Adapted from Canter D. Remediating sites with anthrax contamination: building on experience. In: *AWMA/EPA Indoor Air Quality Problems and Engineering Solutions Specialty Conference and Exhibition*. Research Triangle Park, N.C.; 2003.

terrorist of using an agent that has the demonstrated persistence of the anthrax spore. During the massive cleanup effort in the wake of the 2001 attacks, there has been increased understanding of decontamination of spores that has continued during the remainder of the decade.

The Environmental Protection Agency has outlined eight steps in the remediation process of contaminated sites that are presented in Table 325-6.[15]

Fortunately, one of the least expensive and most commonly available compounds used to destroy anthrax spores is household bleach, and many of the high-tech remediation methods use chloride in some manner. Bleach, chlorine dioxide, ethylene oxide, hydrogen peroxide, peroxyacetic acid, methyl bromide, paraformaldehyde, and vaporized hydrogen peroxide were all used to some degree in the federal decontamination process in 2001 and 2002.[74] As might be expected, one

agent is not suitable for all applications. Chlorine dioxide gas and liquid were used extensively in the U.S. Capitol's Hart Senate Office Building but were not found to be very effective for porous surfaces such as carpeting, chairs, and fabric surfaces, which were subsequently decontaminated with other agents.

In the event of widespread contamination of individuals and households where the public will be expected to be performing much of the decontamination efforts, it is likely that household bleach in 1:10 dilution will be recommended because it is readily available. Contaminated individuals should be advised to remove clothing and place it in a bag either before entering their home or immediately after entering (to minimize spores coming off clothes into the home). They should shower using soap and water and shampoo their hair. Clothes can be decontaminated by washing in hot water with bleach and machine drying. Dry cleaning will also destroy spores.

How extensively remediation must be performed remains controversial. Because it is well-known from studies of wool mill workers and nonhuman primates that the innate immune system can eradicate an as yet undefined number of spores preventing the development of inhalational anthrax, must every spore be removed from every surface? There may be an acceptable level of contamination that will allow for a more timely and cost-effective remediation effort after a citywide exposure without serious compromise to the public health of the community.[24] Potentially coupling immunization with more modest remediation efforts may make reoccupation of buildings safer.[75,76] These are likely to remain contentious issues for the foreseeable future.

Disclaimer: The opinions and assertions herein are those of the authors and should not be construed as official or representing the views of the Department of the Navy, the Department of the Army, the Department of Defense, or the U.S. government.

REFERENCES

1. Stockholm International Peace Research Institute. The rise of CB weapons. In: *The Problem of Chemical and Biological Warfare*. New York: Humanities Press; 1971.
2. Redmond C, Pearce M, Manchee R, et al. Deadly relic of the Great War. *Nature*. 1998;393:747-748.
3. Manchee R, Broster M, Stagg A, et al. Formaldehyde solution effectively inactivates spores of *Bacillus anthracis* on the Scottish island of Gruinard. *Appl Environ Microbiol*. 1994;60:4167-4171.
4. Harris S. Japanese biological warfare research on humans: a case study of microbiology and ethics. *Ann N Y Acad Sci*. 1992; 666:21-52.
5. Meselson M, Guillemin J, Hugh-Jones M, et al. The Sverdlovsk anthrax outbreak of 1979. *Science*. 1994;266:1202.
6. Abramova F, Grinberg L, Yamplskaya O, et al. Pathology of inhalational anthrax in 42 cases from the Sverdlovsk outbreak of 1979. *Proc Natl Acad Sci USA*. 1993;90:2291-2294.
7. Cole L. The specter of biological weapons. *Sci Am*. 1996; 275:60-66.
8. Zilinskas R. Iraq's biological weapons: the past as future? *JAMA*. 1997;278:418-424.
9. Stone R. Peering into the shadows: Iraq's bioweapons program. *Science*. 2002;297:1110-1112.
10. Fennelly K, Davidow A, Miller S, et al. Airborne infection with *Bacillus anthracis*—from mills to mail. *Emerg Inf Dis*. 2004; 10:996-1001.
11. Barakat L, Quentzel H, Jernigan J, et al. Fatal inhalational anthrax in a 94-year-old Connecticut woman. *JAMA*. 2002;287:863-868.
12. Bartlett J, Inglesby T Jr, Borio L. Management of anthrax. *Clin Infect Dis*. 2002;35:851-858.
13. Stuart A, Wilkening D. Degradation of BIOLOGICAL weapons agents in the environment: implications for terrorism response. *Environ Sci Technol*. 2005;39:2736-2743.
14. Weis C, Intrepido A, Miller A, et al. Secondary aerosolization of viable *Bacillus anthracis* spores in a contaminated US Senate office. *JAMA*. 2002;288:2853-2858.
15. Canter D. Remediating sites with anthrax contamination: building on experience. In: *AWMA/EPA Indoor Air Quality Problems and Engineering Solutions Specialty Conference and Exhibition*. Research Triangle Park, NC; 2003.
16. Spotts Whitney E, Beatty M, Taylor T, et al. Inactivation of *Bacillus anthracis* spores. *Emerg Infect Dis*. 2003;9:623-627.
17. Gottron F. *CRS Report for Congress: Project Bioshield*. Washington, DC: Library of Congress; 2003.
18. Lincoln R, Hodges D, Klein F, et al. Role of the lymphatics in the pathogenesis of anthrax. *J Infect Dis*. 1965;115:481-486.
19. U.S. Congress. *Proliferation of Weapons of Mass Destruction: Assessing the Risks*. Washington, DC: Office of Technology Assessment; 1993.

20. Cieslak T, Eitzen E. Clinical and epidemiologic principles of anthrax. *Emerg Inf Dis*. 1999;5:552-555.
21. Hartley D, Peters C. Aerosols from insect control measures show dangers of bioterrorism. *Biosec Bioterror*. 2003;1:221-222.
22. Levin D, Valadares de Amorim G. Potential for aerosol dissemination of biological weapons: lessons from biological control of insects. *Biosec Bioterror*. 2003;1:37-42.
23. Coleman M, Thran B, Morse S, et al. Inhalation anthrax: dose response and risk analysis. *Biosec Bioterror*. 2008;6:147-159.
24. Lincoln R, Walker J, Klein F, et al. Value of field data for extrapolation in anthrax. *Fed Proc*. 1967;26:1558-1562.
25. Peters C, Hartley D. Anthrax inhalation and lethal human infection. *Lancet*. 2002;359:710-711.
26. Henderson D, Peacock S, Belton F. Observations on the prophylaxis of experimental pulmonary anthrax in the monkey. *J Hyg*. 1956;54:28-36.
27. Friedlander A, Welkos S, Pitt M. Postexposure prophylaxis against experimental inhalation anthrax. *J Infect Dis*. 1993; 167:1239-1242.
28. Carr E, Rew R. Recovery of *Bacillus anthracis* from the nose and throat of apparently healthy workers. *J Infect Dis*. 1957;100: 169-171.
29. Dahlgren C, Buchanan L, Decker H, et al. *Bacillus anthracis* aerosols in goat hair processing mills. *Am J Hyg*. 1960;72.
30. Glassman H. Discussion—industrial inhalation anthrax. *Bacteriol Rev*. 1966;30:657-659.
31. Norman P, Ray J, Brachman P, et al. Serological testing for anthrax antibodies in workers in a goat hair processing mill. *Am J Hyg*. 1960;72:32-37.
32. Doolan DL, Freilich DA, Brice GT, et al. The U.S. capitol bioterrorism anthrax exposures: clinical epidemiological and immunological characteristics. *J Infect Dis*. 2007;195:174-184.
33. Brachman P. Inhalation anthrax. *Ann N Y Acad Sci*. 1980; 353:83-93.
34. Brachman P, Kaufmann A, Dalldorf F. Industrial inhalation anthrax. *Bacteriol Rev*. 1966;30:646-657.
35. Sirisanthana T, Brown A. Anthrax of the gastrointestinal tract. *Emerg Infect Dis*. 2002;8:649-651.
36. Kournikakis B, Armour S, Boulet C, et al. *Risk Assessment of Anthrax Threat Letters*. Technical report No. DRES TR-2001-048. Ralston, Alberta, Canada: Defence Research Establishment Suffield; 2001.
37. Kournikakis B, Ho J. Objective assessment of the hazard from anthrax terrorist attacks in an office environment. Paper presented at the Anthrax Incident Management Workshop, Medicine Hat, Alberta, Canada. April 30, 2002.
38. Hoover M. Uncertainty and probability distribution analyses for anthrax dispersion and human exposure. Paper presented at the

Anthrax Incident Management Workshop, Medicine Hat, Alberta, Canada. April 30, 2002.
39. Jernigan J, Stephens D, Ashford D, et al. Bioterrorism-related inhalational anthrax: the first 10 cases reported in the United States. *Emerg Infect Dis*. 2001;7:933-943.
40. Buckeridge D, Owens D, Switzer P, et al. Evaluating detection of an inhalational anthrax outbreak. *Emerg Infect Dis*. 2006;12: 1942-1949.
41. Wein L, Craft D, Kaplan E. Emergency response to an anthrax attack. *Proc Natl Acad Sci USA*. 2003;100:4346-4351.
42. Centers for Disease Control and Prevention. Notice to readers: considerations for distinguishing influenza-like illness from inhalational anthrax. *MMWR Morb Mortal Wkly Rep*. 2001;50: 984-986.
43. Fine A, Wong J, Fraser H, et al. Is it influenza or anthrax? A decision analytic approach to the treatment of patients with influenza-like illnesses. *Ann Emerg Med*. 2004;43:318-328.
44. Kuehnert M, Doyle T, Hill H, et al. Clinical features that discriminate inhalational anthrax from other acute respiratory illnesses. *Clin Infect Dis*. 2003;36:328.
45. Kyriacou D, Stein A, Yarnold P, et al. Clinical predictors of bioterrorism-related inhalational anthrax. *Lancet*. 2004;364: 449-452.
46. Dixon T, Meselson M, Guillemin J, et al. Anthrax. *N Engl J Med*. 1999;341:815-826.
47. Beatty M, Ashford D, Griffin P, et al. Gastrointestinal anthrax. *Arch Intern Med*. 2003;163:2527-2531.
48. Paulet R, Caussin C, Coudray J, et al. Forme viscerale de charbon humain importée d'Afrique. *Presse Med*. 1994;23:477-478.
49. Wood B, DeFranco B, Ripple M, et al. Inhalational anthrax: radiologic and pathologic findings in two cases. *Am J Roentgenol*. 2003;181:1071-1078.
50. Regents of the University of Minnesota. Clinical pathway: Anthrax inhalational exposure. Available at <www.cidrap.umn.edu/cidrap/files/17/anthrax-clinical-pathway.pdf>, 2002. Accessed August 14, 2008.
51. Volokhov D, Pomerantsev A, Kivovich V, et al. Identification of *Bacillus anthracis* by multiprobe microarray hybridization. *Diag Micro Infect Dis*. 2004;49:163-171.
52. Centers for Disease Control and Prevention. Inhalation anthrax associated with dried animal hides—Pennsylvania and New York City, 2006. *MMWR Morb Mortal Wkly Rep*. 2006;55:280-282.
53. Quinn C, Dull P, Semenova V, et al. Immune responses to *Bacillus anthracis* protective antigen in patients with bioterrorism-related cutaneous or inhalation anthrax. *J Infect Dis*. 2004; 190:1228-1236.
54. Selinsky CL, Whitlow VD, Smith LR, et al. Qualification and performance characteristics of a quantitative enzyme-linked

immunosorbent assay for human IgG antibodies to anthrax lethal factor antigen. *Biologicals.* 2006;35:123-129.

55. Mabry R, Brasky K, Geiger R, et al. Detection of anthrax toxin in the serum of animals infected with *Bacillus anthracis* by using engineered immunoassays. *Clin Vaccine Immunol.* 2006;16: 671-677.

56. Boyer A, Quinn C, Woolfitt A, et al. Detection and quantification of anthrax lethal factor in serum by mass spectrometry. *Anal Chem.* 2007;79:8463-8470.

57. Kozel TR, Murphy W, Brandt S, et al. mAbs to *Bacillus anthracis* capsular antigen for immunoprotection in anthrax and detection of antigenemia. *Proc Natl Acad Sci USA.* 2004;101:5042-5047.

58. Centers for Disease Control and Prevention. Update: investigation of bioterrorism-related anthrax and interim guidelines for exposure management and antimicrobial therapy. *MMWR Morb Mortal Wkly Rep.* 2001;50:889-893.

59. Brook I, Elliott T, Pryor H II, et al. In vitro resistance of *Bacillus anthracis* Sterne to doxycycline, macrolides and quinolones. *Int J Antimicrob Agents.* 2001;18:559-562.

60. Cavallo J, Ramisse F, Girardet M, et al. Antibiotic susceptibilities of 96 isolates of *Bacillus anthracis* isolated in France between 1994 and 2000. *Antimicrob Agents Chemother.* 2002;46:2307-2309.

61. Turnbull P, Sirianni N, LeBron C. MICs of selected antibiotics for *Bacillus anthracis, Bacillus cereus, Bacillus thuringiensis,* and *Bacillus mycoides* from a range of clinical and environmental sources as determined by the Etest. *J Clin Microbiol.* 2004; 42:3626-3634.

62. Brookmeyer R, Johnson E, Bollinger R. Modeling the optimum duration of antibiotic prophylaxis in an anthrax outbreak. *Proc Natl Acad Sci USA.* 2003;100:10129-10132.

63. Shepard C, Soriano Gabarro M, Zell E, et al. Antimicrobial post-exposure prophylaxis for anthrax: adverse events and adherence. *Emerg Infect Dis.* 2002;8:1124-1132.

64. Heine H, Bassett J, Miller L, et al. Efficacy of oritavancin in a murine model of *Bacillus anthracis* spore inhalation anthrax. *Antimicrob Agents Chemother.* 2008;52:3350-3357.

65. AdisDataInformation. Cethromycin. *Drugs Res Dev.* 2007; 8:95-102.

66. Vietri N, Purcell B, Lawler J, et al. Short-course postexposure antibiotic prophylaxis combined with vaccination protects against experimental inhalational anthrax. *Proc Natl Acad Sci USA.* 2006;102:7813-7816.

67. Regan J. The advantage of serum therapy as shown by comparison of various methods of treatment of anthrax. *Am J Med Sci.* 1921;162:406-423.

68. Walsh J, Pesik N, Quinn C, et al. A case of naturally acquired inhalation anthrax: clinical care and analyses of anti-protective antigen immunoglobulin G and lethal factor. *Clin Infect Dis.* 2007;44:968-971.

69. Mohamed N, Clagett M, Li J. A high-affinity monoclonal antibody to anthrax protective antigen passively protects rabbits before and after aerosolized *Bacillus anthracis* spore challenge. *Infect Immun.* 2005;73:795-802.

70. Subramanian G, Cronin P, Poley G, et al. A phase 1 study of PAmAb, a fully human monoclonal antibody against *Bacillus anthracis* protective antigen, in healthy volunteers. *Clin Infect Dis.* 2005;41:1220.

71. Vitale L, Blanset D, Lowy I, et al. Prophylaxis and therapy of inhalational anthrax by a novel monoclonal antibody to protective antigen that mimics vaccine-induced immunity. *Infect Immun.* 2006;74:5840-5847.

72. Friedlander A. Anthrax: clinical features, pathogenesis, and potential biological warfare threat. *Curr Clin Top Infect Dis.* 2000;20:335-349.

73. Weber D, Sickbert-Bennett E, Gergen M, et al. Efficacy of selected hand hygiene agents used to remove *Bacillus atrophaeus* (a surrogate of *Bacillus anthracis*) from contaminated hands. *JAMA.* 2003;289:1274-1277.

74. Environmental Protection Agency. Anthrax spore decontamination using chlorine dioxide. Available at <www.epa.gov/pesticides/factsheets/chemicals/chlorinedioxidefactsheet.htm>; 2007. Accessed March 13, 2008.

75. Baccam P, Boechler M. Public health response to an anthrax attack: an evaluation of vaccination policy options. *Biosecur Bioterror.* 2007;5:26-34.

76. Schmitt B, Dobrez D, Parada JP, et al. Responding to a small-scale bioterrorist anthrax attack: cost-effectiveness analysis comparing preattack vaccination with postattack antibiotic treatment and vaccination. *Arch Intern Med.* 2007;167:655-662.

326

Botulinum Toxin as a Biological Weapon

PAVANI REDDY | THOMAS P. BLECK

The clostridial neurotoxins are among the most potent lethal substances present in the world, with median lethal doses (LD_{50}) for humans in the nanogram per kilogram range. These toxins are closely related proteins, synthesized as a single polypeptide chain, and then nicked to produce a heavy chain and a light chain connected by disulfide bonds. The seven botulinum toxins are encoded on the bacterial chromosome, and tetanospasmin, the tetanus neurotoxin, is encoded on a plasmid. Only three of the botulinum toxins (A, B, E) commonly cause human disease. Both types of clostridial neurotoxin are relatively simple to produce. *Clostridium botulinum* has been considered a high enough probability for use in bioterrorism that it has been targeted by a blue ribbon panel for special research emphasis. The botulinum toxins exert their effects at the neuromuscular junction and at muscarinic peripheral autonomic synapses; thus, their major manifestations are neuromuscular weakness and autonomic dysfunction. The predominant effect of tetanospasmin is on the central nervous system (CNS), where it produces failure of inhibition leading to hypertonia and spasms. The two conditions are discussed in detail in Chapter 245 (*Clostridium botulinum*) and Chapter 244 (*Clostridium tetani*).

Tetanospasmin is not a useful weapon candidate because of widespread immunity due to vaccination, although at least one group attempted to do so.[1] The botulinum toxins have proven a more interesting target for weapon development because the public health strategy for botulism has been to prevent exposure rather than immunization.

Although tetanus has been known since antiquity, botulism first emerged during the late eighteenth century as a consequence of changes in production methods for sausages.[2] The first clear clinical description of botulism emerged from epidemics of *wurstvergiftung* (sausage poisoning) near Stuttgart in 1812.

Rumors of the intentional use of botulinum toxin date back to the turn of the twentieth century.[3] The first known development of botulinum toxin as a bioweapon occurred in Manchuria during the 1930s under the auspices of Unit 731, the Japanese biological warfare research unit. During World War II, the United States developed methods for large-scale production of botulinum toxin. Scientists working in this program did not discuss the subject of their work by name but, rather, referred to it as agent X.[4] The United States also produced large quantities of botulinum toxoid for use as a vaccine.[5] Because of the fear that they would be exposed to botulinum toxin during the Normandy invasion, Allied troops involved in the invasion may have been immunized with this toxoid; debate persists about the historical record.[4,6] It appears likely that the Germans were dissuaded from using biological weapons in this war because of concern that the Allies would retaliate in kind. Other countries have also experimented with techniques to weaponize botulinum toxin, including the former Soviet Union.[5]

Iraq conducted one of the largest known military botulinum toxin programs, producing approximately 19,000 liters of concentrated toxin, more than half of which had been loaded into weapons systems.[7] The Iraqi military also deployed several other biological weapons systems before the first Gulf War (1990 to 1991). The seed culture for the Iraqi program was purchased legally from an American microbiological supply house. In preparation for potential exposure to this toxin, about 8000 American service personnel were vaccinated in 1991.[4]

The Aum Shinrikyo cult in Japan, best known for its attacks on civilians using the nerve agent sarin,[8] attempted to use botulinum toxin as a weapon on at least three occasions during the early 1990s.[9] Although these attempts were not successful, perhaps in part because of the reticence of some cult members to carry out their orders, the ease with which cult members were able to produce the toxin demonstrates the potential for small groups to use this substance as a bioterror weapon. At least some of their cultures of *C. botulinum* were grown from spores obtained from local soil, highlighting the ubiquitous nature of the organism and our inability to eliminate this threat by controlling the commercial supply of microorganisms.

Botulinum Toxin as a Weapon

Natural poisoning with botulinum toxin is almost always a consequence of ingesting preformed toxin produced by the growth of *C. botulinum* in improperly prepared or stored food. The exceptions (e.g., infant botulism, wound botulism) are described in Chapter 245. A bioterrorist attack with this toxin could cause intoxication via ingestion or an aerosol. One method by which botulinum toxin could be employed as a weapon would be the contamination of food with the toxin. The signs and symptoms of the victims of such an attack would be indistinguishable from a natural outbreak of botulism, except that epidemiologic investigation might reveal that the common food ingested was not typically associated with botulism, or that different foods in the same area were all contaminated. Introduction of toxin into milk trucks or other large, closed food or beverage transports would produce sporadic cases. In such a circumstance, individual clinicians would be unlikely to recognize an attack early in its development. Automated systems for the collection of epidemiologic data are required for this purpose.[10]

The premonitory gastrointestinal symptoms of nausea, vomiting, diarrhea, and abdominal cramping in patients with natural gastrointestinal botulism are probably not a consequence of botulinum toxin, which by itself would cause constipation. Smith argued that these effects were due to other bacterial products.[11] As a consequence, an outbreak of botulism cases without these other gastrointestinal symptoms should raise the suspicion of a toxin attack. Toxin would be detectable in serum, and in stool as well, if the gastrointestinal tract were the route of entry.

Predicting the consequences of dissemination into the environment is more problematic, as there are no data regarding the stability of the toxin in water or sunlight. One Centers for Disease Control and Prevention (CDC) expert estimated that an aerosol release of toxin could affect 10% of people within 500 meters.[5] Once in the atmosphere, the decay rate of the toxin is estimated at 1% to 4% per minute. Modeling an aerosol exposure suggests that substantial inactivation may take up to 2 days.[5] This would be accelerated by extremes of temperature and humidity. Aerosol exposure to the toxin would not result in substantial recovery of toxin in stool, but it would still be detectable in serum and potentially in respiratory secretions.

The effects of inhaling botulinum toxin by humans have been reported only following the accidental exposure of three German laboratory workers after they performed autopsies on animals that had been subjected to a type A botulinum aerosol.[12] They presumably inhaled a small amount of toxin wafted into the air from the fur of the animals. They exhibited no symptoms for the first two days after their exposure but on the third day began to have difficulty swallowing and experienced coryza without fever. A description of *mental numbness* is difficult to interpret, as the toxin would not be expected to affect the CNS. On the fourth day, they noted generalized weakness and difficulty with extraocular movements, and they were found to have modest pupillary dilation and slight rotary nystagmus, along with dysarthria and gait disturbance. They received antitoxin on the fourth and fifth days. Their symptoms apparently stopped progressing after the antitoxin was administered, and they had improved sufficiently to be discharged from the hospital within two weeks.

Primate experiments designed to study the efficacy of treatments for inhaled toxin revealed that doses of 5 to 10 median lethal dose (LD_{50}) caused death within 2 to 4 days in animals that were neither immunized nor treated with antitoxin.[13] The authors reported the development of signs of intoxication about 12 to 18 hours prior to death, beginning with diffuse weakness and then followed by ptosis and neck weakness.

Current approaches to the diagnosis of botulism and the detection of botulinum toxin would be of limited value during an attack. The diagnosis can be confirmed most rapidly with electromyography. Assays for toxin in serum, stool, and respiratory secretions requires an in vivo mouse assay. The increasing concern about bioterrorism in recent years has resulted in several new rapid detection methods, some of which are potentially applicable to both environmental and patient samples.[14,15,16]

Management

The management of individual cases of botulism is discussed in Chapter 245. In the event of a bioterrorist attack, several logistic issues would become problematic. Based on the limited information available, a large-scale attack (either food-borne or by aerosol) would probably not begin to produce symptomatic victims for more than a day. In one large common-source food-borne outbreak, the initial neurologic symptoms arose 24 to 108 hours after exposure.[17] Thus, recognition of the attack, and hence the potential magnitude of the problem, would initially be difficult. Although vaccination as a strategy to limit disease is important for a contagious disease such as smallpox, it would not be useful in the acute setting for the following reasons: (1) there is no risk of person-to-person transmission and (2) a vaccination series takes about 12 weeks. Thus, vaccination is useful only for those in whom a predictable exposure is anticipated. The current investigational pentavalent vaccine (types A to E) is, thus, reserved for laboratory workers and the military.

The cornerstones of botulism management are airway protection, mechanical ventilation, antitoxin administration, and supportive therapy. In the event of deliberate aerosolized release of botulinum toxin, some protection may be achieved by covering the mouth and nose with a scarf or handkerchief.[5] Individuals with botulism are usually observed for problems with airway protection, such as difficulty handling secretions, and are monitored for ventilatory difficulties by measuring vital capacity, the negative inspiratory pressure, and the respiratory rate. Endotracheal intubation is performed when either problem threatens the patient's safety. For a large attack with many casualties, measurements of ventilatory function would not be practical, and decisions regarding intubation would have to be based on the observation of difficulty with secretions or tachypnea. These observations would be facilitated by having the victims concentrated in a large open area.

The Strategic National Stockpile "push packs" contain laryngoscopes, endotracheal tubes, and Ambu bags, along with a limited number of mechanical ventilators. More information is available on the Internet (http://www.bt.cdc.gov/stockpile/index.asp). However, this equipment would not arrive until up to 24 hours after requested by the state governor, so the state health departments are responsible for organizing strategies for the first day. Because the number of intubated patients requiring ventilation may easily exceed the number of available ventilators, it might become necessary to recruit healthy civilians to perform bag ventilation on these patients. Such a process was highly successful in saving lives in Scandinavia during the poliomyelitis epidemics of the 1950s.[18]

The supply of antitoxins is small, reflecting the low incidence of the natural disease. With a large-scale attack, the available antitoxin would be quickly exhausted. Thus, airway protection and ventilation would remain the only viable options. To minimize additional exposures, exposed skin and clothing should be washed with soap and water while contaminated surfaces should be cleaned with 0.1% hypochlorite bleach solution if they cannot be avoided for the hours to days required for natural degradation.[5]

Updated resources are provided by the Infectious Disease Society of America on its website (http://www.cidrap.umn.edu/idsa/bt/botulism/resources/botreslist.html).

REFERENCES

1. Williams P, Wallace D. *Unit 731: Japan's secret biological warfare in World War II.* New York: Free Press; 989:27-28.
2. Dickson EC. Botulism: A clinical and experimental study. *Rockefeller Inst Med Res Monogr.* 1918;8:1-117.
3. CDC video. The history of bioterrorism. 1999; (available at: http://www.bt.cdc.gov/training/historyofbt/index.asp).
4. Middlebrook JL, Franz DR. Botulinum toxins. In: Sidell FR, Takafuji ET, Franz DR, eds. *Medical Aspects of Chemical and Biological Warfare.* Washington, DC: Office of the Surgeon General; 1997; (available at: https://ccc.apgea.army.mil).
5. Arnon SS, Schechter R, Inglesby TV, et al. Botulinum toxin as a biological weapon: Medical and public health management. *JAMA.* 2001;285:1059-1070.
6. Williams P, Wallace D. *Unit 731. Japan's secret biological warfare in World War II.* New York: Free Press; 1989:124.
7. Zilinskas RA. Iraq's biological weapons: The past as future? *JAMA.* 1997;278:418-424.
8. Kortepeter MG, Cieslak TJ, Eitzen EM. Bioterrorism. *J Environ Health.* 2001;63:21-24.
9. Lifton RJ. *Destroying the World to Save It.* New York: Henry Holt; 2000:39, 186-39, 188.
10. M'ikantha NM, Southwell B, Lautenbach E. Automated laboratory reporting of infectious diseases in a climate of bioterrorism. *Emerg Infect Dis.* 2003;9:1053-1057.
11. Smith LDS. *Botulism: The Organism, Its Toxins, the Disease.* Springfield, Ill.: Charles C Thomas; 1977.
12. Holzer VE. Botulismus durch inhalation. *Med Klin.* 1962;57:1735-1738.
13. Franz DR, Pitt LM, Clayton MA, et al. Efficacy of prophylactic and therapeutic administration of antitoxin for inhalation botulism. In: Das Gupta BR, ed. *Botulinum and Tetanus Neurotoxins: Neurotransmission and Biomedical Aspects.* New York: Plenum; 1993:473-476.
14. Peruski AH, Johnson LH III, Peruski LF Jr. Rapid and sensitive detection of biological warfare agents using time-resolved fluorescence assays. *J Immunol Methods.* 2002;263:35-41.
15. Liu W, Montana V, Chapman ER, et al. Botulinum toxin type B micro-mechanosensor. *Proc Natl Acad Sci U S A.* 2003;100:13621-13625.
16. Ahn-Yoon S, DeCory TR, Durst RA. Ganglioside-liposome immunoassay for the detection of botulinum toxin. *Anal Bioanal Chem.* 2004;378:68-75.
17. Terranova W, Breman JG, Locey RP, et al. Botulism type B: Epidemiologic aspects of an extensive outbreak. *Am J Epidemiol.* 1978;108:150-156.
18. Wackers GL. Modern anaesthesiological principles for bulbar polio: Manual IPPR in the 1952 polio-epidemic in Copenhagen. *Acta Anaesthesiol Scand.* 1994;38:420-431.

327

Viral Hemorrhagic Fevers as Agents of Bioterrorism

C. J. PETERS

Viral Hemorrhagic Fevers as Bioterrorist Agents

The viral hemorrhagic fevers (VHFs) are important considerations in bioterrorism (BT) preparedness (Table 327-1). BT may take many forms, ranging from hoaxes to mass casualties. Even small attacks may be disruptive, produce fear, and have a severe economic impact. The 2001 anthrax attacks interrupted activities we regard as constants of ordinary life and commerce, such as mail service; caused a hiatus in legislative function; induced fear and uncertainty in the population of the northeastern United States; and cost billions of dollars even though there were only 22 cases and 5 fatalities (see Chapter 325). VHFs lend themselves to a public disruption attack because of their reputation from popular literature and the dramatic clinical syndrome produced.[1]

This chapter mainly addresses the issue of mass casualty attacks and shows that some of the VHFs have the potential for large area coverage with many thousands of infected humans. Biological weapons were brought to a mature state by both the United States (the program was stopped and weapons destroyed in 1968) and the Soviet Union.[2-4] Fortunately, these weapons have never been used in a situation in which their full potential could be seen, although there are examples of abortive attempts.[5] Nevertheless, each step of the process was tested and found to be feasible for inducing human disease, and the overall process was tested at a practical level with experimental animals after open air exposure.[6]

The most dangerous format in which these agents could be dispersed is via small particle aerosols (1 to 5 μm in diameter), which are carried invisibly on wind currents and penetrate ventilated buildings. They are deposited in the fine airways of the lung and establish an infection. An aerosol chemical or biological attack is at the whim of meteorologic conditions, and the effects of biological weapons are delayed by their incubation period. These points may be seen as disadvantages in their tactical use, but the ability for stealthy, standoff delivery, and time for the perpetrators to escape may be useful for terrorists.[1] For this type of attack, one needs agents that are stable and infectious in the aerosol form and have a high case-to-infection ratio. VHFs meet these criteria.[7] Their experimental properties resemble those of that archetypical biological warfare virus Venezuelan equine encephalitis or of influenza.[6,8]

Among the aerosol agents some are judged to be more dangerous than others, but certainly anthrax and smallpox are at the top of most lists.[6] Comparison of anthrax spores to VHFs is instructive for understanding their relative likelihood of use and impact. Anthrax is widely available in nature, and most of the VHFs are as well, with the notable exception of the filoviruses. Anthrax is readily grown in commonly available culture media, sporulates when the cultures reach saturation, and is easily concentrated and purified in ordinary centrifuges. The VHFs are often propagated in cell culture, but titers fall short of the ideal for production of weapons of mass destruction. A state-sponsored program could make VHF production a practical enterprise through the use of fermentation technology and simple partial purification of the viruses by precipitation, filtration, or continuous-flow ultracentrifugation modeled on some commercial vaccine production methods. The isolated terrorist would probably rely on animal propagation of the agents to obtain high-titer starting material. Several of the viruses replicate exceedingly well in rodents or lambs, and, indeed, the Soviet program is said to have used guinea pigs to produce Marburg virus weapons.

Anthrax spores are highly stable in aerosol and on storage, but the VHFs are of lesser aerosol stability and require ultracold storage if kept for more than a few days in the liquid state. A state-sponsored program could reliably enhance aerosol stability problems by the appropriate additives, and by production of dried material that maintains bulk infectivity for much longer periods. This, of course, involves a period of experimentation and measurement of aerosol stability. An example of the stabilization principle is seen in Table 327-2, in which addition of glycerin to the Marburg virus diluted in saliva results in a marked increase in aerosol stability.[9] A simpler approach would involve proceeding with liquids and performing the attack relatively soon after preparing the virus suspension, but this imposes logistic constraints on the attacker.

Smallpox presents a different set of contrasts. It is extremely stable and infectious in aerosol form, and it is readily propagated. It is unobtainable from nature and is by international agreement confined to two laboratories, although clandestine stocks probably exist (see Chapter 324). In marked distinction to all the major biological warfare (BW) agents, smallpox is a natural human pathogen that is readily transmissible between patients and can be expected to cause large numbers of cases in multiple generations of transmission until limited by vaccination or other active means of control. The VHFs, in contrast, are all caused by zoonotic viruses and are expected to be of limited risk only to close family contacts and medical personnel. Because of the infectivity of smallpox for humans, it is likely that a smallpox attack would result in severe limitation of movement of humans in the country attacked and certainly to other countries. There is a similar corollary for Rift Valley fever (RVF) virus; it is an important domestic animal pathogen and use of that virus would result in an immediate cessation of movement of sheep and cattle in the country and a block on exported U.S. materials from these animals. Unlike the other VHFs, RVF has the ability to spread beyond its initial targets, mediated by mosquito vectors that are present in the United States.[10] It is unknown whether this can occur by interhuman transmission via arthropods or if it would require a substrate of viremic domestic animals.

In summary, then, the stability and infectivity of most of the VHFs is sufficient (or could be made so) to produce large numbers of casualties.[6] Terrorists, using VHF, as with plague and tularemia, would most likely require some prior knowledge of the stabilizers and manufacturing process to produce mass casualties.

Control of Bioterrorism from VHFs

Most of the VHFs are widely available in the environment by sampling their natural reservoir or through patients and virology laboratories in areas of the world in which they are endemic. Hence, the select agent restrictions in the United States will have little impact on preventing their use by any terrorist capable of turning them into significant weapons. Filoviruses are the exception because their reservoir is uncertain, and they are present in relatively few laboratories. Their genome could be synthesized in segments and reconstituted through reverse genetics, but this is a project that would require a sophisticated molecular virology laboratory.[11]

<table>
<tr><td colspan="3">TABLE 327-1   **Viral Hemorrhagic Fevers**</td></tr>
</table>

Family/Genus	Disease (Virus)	Chapter
Arenaviridae		167
	Lassa fever	
	Bolivian HF (Machupo virus)	
	Argentine HF (Junin virus)	
	Other South American HF	
Bunyaviridae		166
Phlebovirus	Rift Valley fever	
Nairovirus	Crimean Congo HF	
Hantavirus	HF with renal syndrome, HFRS (Hantaan and others)	
	Hantavirus pulmonary syndrome, HPS (Sin Nombre, Andes, and others)	
Filoviridae	Marburg HF	154
	Ebola HF	
Flaviviridae	Yellow fever	153
	Dengue HF	
	Tick-borne flavivirus HF (Kyasanur Forest, Omsk, and Al Alkhurma)	153

HF, hemorrhagic fever; HFRS, HF with renal syndrome; HPS, hantavirus pulmonary syndrome.

Any biological weapon requires a large amount of agent to disperse, and this currently limits the utility of Crimean Congo hemorrhagic fever (CCHF) virus and hantaviruses. These practical constraints could be overcome by an applied research program.

The methods for stabilizing the viruses in aerosol could be developed by trial and error or could be brought about by knowledgeable persons, particularly the scientists who previously worked in the Soviet programs, that have undergone the same downsizing as in their nuclear arena. The production of bioweapons is an industrial process that requires two sets of skills. The expertise to propagate the agents is available through microbiologists, and the development of the 1- to 5-μm powders that can be disseminated to infect large numbers of targets efficiently via aerosol clouds in buildings or open air situations, resides in pharmaceutical, cosmetic, insecticide, and other industries.[6,8] The equipment needed for production of bioweapons has multiple industrial uses and has no unique signature, so the prospects for controlling these weapons is far less likely than for nuclear devices.[12] The failed efforts of the Japanese Aum Shinrikyo sect are often cited as an example of how even a well-financed nonstate group cannot produce these weapons. This should not be comforting because of the naiveté of the sect's persons who headed the microbiological and dissemination efforts.[13]

▣ What Are VHFs and How Can We Respond Medically?

The VHFs comprise several viruses from different taxons in four virus families (see Table 327-1). These viruses share a number of properties (small RNA genome, lipid envelope, acid sensitivity, zoonotic natural cycle, aerosol infectivity), but they differ in others (replication strategy,

<table>
<tr><td colspan="2">TABLE 327-2   **Aerosol Stability of Some Viruses**</td></tr>
</table>

Virus	Stability (%/min)
Vaccinia	0.3
Influenza	1.9
Venezuelan equine encephalitis	3.0
Marburg (saliva)	11.5
Marburg (+10% glycerin)	1.5

Data are from Belanov Y, Muntyanov VP, Kryuk VD, et al. Retention of Marburg virus infecting capability on contaminated surfaces and in aerosol particles. *Vopr Virusol.* 1996;41:32-34.

morphogenesis, natural cycle, pathogenesis). One of the remarkable findings is that they are all aerosol-infectious with the exception of the dengue viruses, which cause dengue hemorrhagic fever (DHF) by a different mechanism, which involves secondary infections leading to enhanced pathogenesis. Thus, DHF is not a bioterrorism threat by virtue of the lack of aerosol infectiousness of the viruses and the need for sequential infections to produce the syndrome. The aerosol infectious properties of the VHF agents include both the viruses thought to be transmitted to humans in nature by aerosols and those that are primarily spread by mosquitoes or ticks (Table 327-3).

The pathogenesis varies among the various diseases with direct viral damage, disseminated intravascular coagulation (DIC), hepatic damage, vascular damage, and cytokine release being implicated to varying degrees. Fatal cases usually have extensive lymphoid depletion, except for the hantavirus diseases, in which immunopathology is an important mechanism.

Diagnosis of these infections, when they occur naturally, relies on an index of suspicion for travelers to the endemic areas within an incubation period (see Table 327-3). Of course, the absence of a travel history in a confirmed case is equally compelling evidence of a bioterrorism event. High throughput molecular techniques for detection are under development.[14]

The clinical course varies among the VHFs (Table 327-4),[15,16] but a typical patient might experience a prodrome of fever, myalgia, and malaise that typically lasts 3 to 4 days. The next events include worsening of these symptoms with prostration, evidence of capillary leak (nondependent edema, effusions), hemorrhage, and central nervous system depression. Hemorrhage occurs in most cases with some of the VHFs (e.g., South American hemorrhagic fevers) or in less than half in others (e.g., Lassa fever) and seems to require thrombocytopenia plus capillary damage. Patients with shock, florid hemorrhage, and extensive central nervous system damage have a poor prognosis.

Physical findings early in the course may be suggestive. Some patients have somewhat low blood pressure and postural hypotension. Conjunctival injection is common except in hantavirus pulmonary syndrome (HPS). Evidence of petechial hemorrhage should be sought carefully in good light. Later, more obvious signs and symptoms supervene.

Clinical laboratory findings vary by disease. Hemoconcentration is often found and may be extreme, particularly with the hantavirus diseases. All of the patients have thrombocytopenia except those with Lassa fever. Leukopenia is common with most of the VHFs and is particularly constant with South American HF. However, those with Lassa fever may have low, normal, or elevated white blood cell counts, and hantavirus infections result in normal to elevated and even leukemoid counts. Clotting studies are usually modestly abnormal, including the activated partial thromboplastin time and the prothrombin time, but no specific patterns are known to be diagnostic. Evidence of DIC is regularly found in CCHF, filovirus infections, severe RVF, and the early phase of HF with renal syndrome (HFRS) but is rare with arenavirus HF. Aspartate aminotransferase may be elevated, as may the serum amylase. With the exception of HFRS and some RVF cases, renal function reflects the circulatory status. Proteinuria is common, presumably reflecting the capillary leak.

Specific laboratory diagnosis during the acute phase relies on detection of RNA by reverse transcription–polymerase chain reaction, finding viral proteins by an enzyme-linked immunosorbent assay (ELISA), or virus isolation in the biosafety level 4 (BSL4) laboratory. As patients improve, markers of acute infection disappear and immunoglobin M (IgM) antibodies can be detected. Hantaviruses are exceptional in that they have antibodies present in serum at the time of onset of disease that can be readily detected in an IgM capture ELISA. Most of these tests are not readily available in the United States outside the Center for Disease Control and Prevention (CDC) and the U.S. Army Medical Research Institute of Infectious Diseases.

The differential diagnosis is most difficult with rickettsial disease, leptospirosis, and relapsing fever. Malaria, typhoid, shigellosis, sepsis, and other conditions may be confused with illnesses caused by VHF.

TABLE 327-3	Some Characteristics of the VHFs				

Virus	Disease	Geography	Incubation (days)	Vector/Reservoir	Human Infection
Arenaviridae					
Junin	Argentine HF	Argentine pampas	7-14	Chronic infection of small field rodent, *Calomys musculinus*.	Mainly agricultural workers. Major transmission in fall season. Aerosol transmission to humans. Interhuman transmission rare.
Machupo	Bolivian HF	Bolivia, Beni Province	—	Chronic infection of small field rodent, *Calomys callosus*.	Rural residents and farmers; rodent can invade towns with urban disease. Aerosol transmission to humans. Interhuman transmission not usual but occurs.
Guanarito	Venezuelan HF	Venezuela, Portuguesa state	—	Chronic infection of field rodent *Zygodontomys brevicauda*.	Rural residents in cleared area in Venezuela with small farms.
Sabia	?	Rural area near Sao Paulo, Brazil	—	Presumably chronic infection of unidentified rodents.	Single infection observed in nature: little information on potential. Two laboratory infections, one treated with ribavirin.
Lassa	Lassa fever	West Africa	5-16	Chronic infection of rodents of the genus *Mastomys*.	The reservoir rodent is very common in Africa, and the disease is a major cause of severe febrile illness in West Africa. Spread to humans occurs by aerosols and by capturing the rodent for consumption, as well as person-to-person transmission. Lassa fever is the most commonly exported HF.
Bunyaviridae					
Rift Valley fever	RVF	Sub-Saharan Africa	2-5	Vertical infection of flood-water *Aedes* mosquitoes maintains the virus. Epidemics occur during heavy rainfall with horizontal transmission by many mosquito species between domestic animals, particularly sheep and cattle.	Humans acquire by mosquito bite; contact with blood of infected sheep, cattle, or goats; and aerosols generated from infected domestic animal blood. No interhuman transmission observed.
Crimean Congo HF	Crimean Congo HF	Africa, Middle East, Balkans, southern Soviet Union, western China	3-12	Tick–mammal–tick infection. Vertical infection occurs in ticks. Hyalomma ticks are thought to be the natural reservoir, but other genera may become infected and transmit.	Tick bite; squashing ticks; and exposure to aerosols or fomites from slaughtered cattle and sheep. (Domestic animals do not have evidence of illness but may become infected when transported to market or when held in pens for slaughter.) Numerous nosocomial epidemics.
Hantaan, Seoul, Puumala, and others	HFRS	Worldwide, depending on rodent reservoir	9-35	Horizontal infection in a single rodent species typical of the virus. Viruses associated with HFRS have been obtained only from rodents of the family Muridae, subfamilies Murinae or Arvicolinae.	Aerosols, mainly from freshly shed urine of infected rodents. Some infections are acquired from secondary aerosols or droplets from previously shed rodent excreta and secreta or from rodent bites. Rural disease. Interhuman transmission never documented.
Sin Nombre, Bayou, Andes, and others	HPS	Americas	7-28	As for hantaviruses causing HFRS. All viruses associated with HPS have come from Muridae (subfamily Sigmodontinae) rodents.	As for hantaviruses causing HFRS. Entering unused, closed buildings may be a particular risk. Interhuman transmission observed with Andes virus; mechanisms unknown.
Filoviridae					
Marburg, Ebola	Marburg HF, Ebola HF	Africa, Philippines	3-16	Unknown.	Infection of index case occurs from unknown source. Infected nonhuman primates sometimes provide link to humans. Later spread among humans by close contact with another infected person or hospitalization.
Flaviviridae					
Yellow fever	Yellow fever	Africa, South America	3-6	Mosquito–monkey–mosquito maintenance with occasional human infection when unvaccinated humans enter forest. Formerly large epidemics among humans with *Aedes aegypti* as mosquito vector.	Mosquito infection of humans entering forests and encountering infected sylvatic vector. Emergence of epidemics into African savannas using specific *Aedes* mosquito vectors. In cities or villages, interhuman transmission by *A. aegypti*. Fully developed cases are no longer viremic, and direct interhuman transmission not believed to be a problem.
Dengue (types 1-4)	DHF/DSS	Tropics and subtropics worldwide	3-15	Maintained by *A. aegypti*–human–*A. aegypti* transmission with frequent geographic transport of viruses by travelers.	DHF/DSS occurs in areas where multiple dengue viruses are being transmitted. With the increased worldwide distribution of *A. aegypti* and movement of dengue viruses by travelers, this zone is enlarging. DSS first noted in Southeast Asia but is now common in the Americas and the Caribbean.
Kyasanur Forest disease	KFD	Limited area of Mysore State, India	3-8	Tick–vertebrate–tick.	Most infections occur from tick bite acquired in rural areas of the endemic zone. Monkey die-offs may accompany increased virus activity.
Omsk HF	OHF	Western Siberia	3-8	Poorly understood cycle involving ticks, voles, muskrats, and possibly waterborne transmission.	Few cases in recent years.
Al Khumrah	—	Middle East? Africa?	—	Unknown.	Discovered in Saudi Arabia but may have been introduced with imported livestock. Transmitted to humans working in livestock-related occupations by unknown route.

DHF, Dengue HF; DSS, Dengue shock syndrome; HF, hemorrhagic fever; HFRS, HF with renal syndrome; HPS, hantavirus pulmonary syndrome; KFD, Kyasanur Forest disease; OHF, Omsk HF; RVF, Rift Valley fever.

TABLE 327-4	Some Clinical Features of VHFs		
Disease	**Clinical Features**	**Therapeutic Synopsis**
South American HF	Most cases have hemorrhage. Neurologic symptoms such as dysarthria and tremor usual.	Treatment with intravenous ribavirin is likely to be beneficial. Safe, effective vaccine for Argentine HF but available only in Argentina.
Lassa fever	Prostration and shock but hemorrhage and neurologic signs much less common than South American HF.	Treatment with intravenous ribavirin shown to be beneficial. Deafness is common in convalesence.
Rift Valley fever	Incidence of HF low among total infections. May be associated with DIC and hepatitis. Infected may develop retinal vasculitis or encephalitis.	Ribavirin useful in animal models but human evidence is not impressive, perhaps owing to rapid course. Inactivated and live-attenuated vaccines are safe and effective but are not generally available.
Crimean Congo HF	Typical HF with florid hemorrhage. DIC common. Nosocomial infections common.	Ribavirin used with anecdotal success. No acceptable vaccine.
HFRS	Febrile prodrome followed by shock and renal failure. Hemoconcentration can be marked.	Supportive care, dialysis. Ribavirin may be useful adjunct. Vaccines available in Korea and China but do not meet U.S. manufacturing standards.
HPS	Similar to HFRS but acute pulmonary edema rather than renal failure.	ICU management of pulmonary edema and shock. Ribavirin not helpful.
Marburg or Ebola HF	Most severe of the HF. Marked weight loss and prostration. Maculopapular rash common. Hepatitis, uveitis, orchitis, arthralgia reported during convalescence.	Supportive care. In Ebola-infected monkeys, tissue factor inhibitors and activated protein C helpful. Investigational Ebola vaccine in Phase I studies.
Yellow fever	Severe HF with jaundice common.	Excellent vaccine.
Dengue HF	Not a BT threat but enters into differential diagnosis. Rare cause of primary HF. An important cause of HF in Asia and Latin America after infection with multiple dengue viruses, particularly in children.	Responds well to supportive care. Vaccines under development.
Tick-borne flavivirus HF	Biphasic illness with fever, thrombocytopenia, and hemorrhage during first phase and often a second phase with neurologic signs.	No therapy or vaccine.

BT, bioterrorism; DIC, disseminated intravascular coagulation; HF, hemorrhagic fever; HFRS, HF with renal syndrome; HPS, hantavirus pulmonary syndrome; ICU, intensive care unit.

The general principles of therapy are similar for all the HFs: rapid atraumatic hospitalization, intensive care unit admission if available, careful maintenance of fluid balance to avoid overhydration in the face of fragile systemic and pulmonary capillary beds and myocardial compromise, management of the bleeding diathesis according to the usual principles, and the specific therapy appropriate to each disease (see Table 327-4). Ribavirin should be given intravenously to all arenavirus infections (not an approved use) and should be considered for infections by *Bunyaviridae*,[17] particularly CCHF.

The issue of secondary spread is important, but there is no simple answer. Occasional secondary cases occur with most of the VHFs, and rarely there are miniepidemics. We know that long chains of transmission occur only with filoviruses and then only in settings with virtually no use of masks, gowns, or gloves. These viruses are highly infectious by aerosol spread in the laboratory, but spread between patients via this route is uncommon. Presumably, this is related to the small amount of virus in external secretions and a low output of aerosols by the patient.[18] The VHFs most commonly associated with nosocomial disease are CCHF and Ebola, and spread is usually associated with extensive exposure to blood in a setting of poor hospital hygiene.[19] Careful barrier nursing as recommended by the CDC limits or stops hospital transmission.[15]

As new viruses are isolated, new significant pathogens will be added to this list. There are new arenaviruses and a new filovirus that are not included now because of their limited distribution and limited knowledge of their properties.

REFERENCES

1. Danzig R. *Catastrophic Bioterrorism—What Is to Be Done?* Washington, DC: Center for Technology and National Security Policy at the National Defense University; 2003.
2. Alibek K, Handelman S. *Biohazard.* 1st ed. New York City: Random House; 1999.
3. Miller J, Engelberg S, Broad W. *Germs: Biological Weapons and America's Secret War.* 1st ed. New York: Simon and Schuster; 2001.
4. Harris R, Paxman J. *A Higher Form of Killing.* New York: Hill and Wang; 1982.
5. Christopher GW, Cieslak TJ, Pavlin JA, et al. Biological warfare: a historical perspective. In: Knobler SL, Mahmoud AAF, Pray LA, eds. *Biological Threats and Terrorism.* Washington, DC: National Academy Press; 1997:412-417.
6. Peters CJ, Spertzel R, Patrick W. Aerosol technology and biological weapons. In: Knobler SL, Mahmoud AAF, Pray LA, eds. *Biological Threats.* Washington, DC: National Academy Press; 2002:66-77.
7. Sinclair R, Boone SA, Greenberg D. Persistence of category A select agents in the environment. *Appl Environ Microbiol.* 2008;74(3):555-563.
8. Peters CJ. Are hemorrhagic fever viruses practical agents for biological terrorism? In: Scheld WM, Craig WA, Hughes JM, eds. *Emerging Infections.* vol 4. Washington: ASM Press; 2000:203-211.
9. Belanov Y, Muntyanov VP, Kryuk VD, et al. Retention of Marburg virus infecting capability on contaminated surfaces and in aerosol particles. *Vopr Virusol.* 1996;41:32-34.
10. Gargan TP, Clark GG, Dohm DJ, et al. Vector potential of selected North American mosquito species for Rift Valley fever virus. *Am J Trop Med Hyg.* 1988;38:440-446.
11. Volchkov VE, Volchkova VA, Muhlberger E, et al. Recovery of infectious Ebola virus from complementary DNA: RNA editing of the GP gene and viral cytotoxicity. *Science.* 2001;291:1965-1969.
12. Kadlec RP, Zelicoff AP, Vrtis AM. Biological weapons control: prospects and implications for the future. In: Lederberfg J, ed. *Biological Weapons: Limiting the Threat.* Cambridge, MA: MIT Press; 1999:95-111.
13. Smithson AE, Levy LA. *Ataxia: The Chemical and Biological Terrorism Threat and the U.S. Response.* Washington, DC: Henry L. Stimson Center; 2000.
14. Towner JS, Sealy TK, Ksiazek TG, et al. High-throughput molecular detection of hemorrhagic fever virus threats with applications for outbreak settings. *J Infect Dis.* 2007;196(Suppl 2):S205-S212.
15. Borio L, Inglesby T, Peters CJ, et al. Hemorrhagic fever viruses as biological weapons. *JAMA.* 2002;287:2391-2405.
16. Peters CJ, Zaki SR. Overview of viral hemorrhagic fevers. In: Guerrant RL, ed. *Essentials of Tropical Infectious Diseases.* Philadelphia: WB Saunders; 2000:552-559.
17. Enria D, Peters CJ. Other viruses and emerging viruses of concern. In: Boucher CAB, ed. *Practical Guidelines in Antiviral Therapy.* Amsterdam: Elsevier; 2002:279-301.
18. Peters CJ, Jahrling PB, Khan AS. Patients infected with high-hazard viruses: scientific basis for infection control. *Arch Virol.* 1996;11(Suppl):141-168.
19. Dowell SF, Mukunu R, Ksiazek TG, et al. Transmission of Ebola hemorrhagic fever: a study of risk factors in family members, Kikwit, Democratic Republic of the Congo, 1995; Commission de Lutte contre les Epidemies a Kikwit. *J Infect Dis.* 1999;179(Suppl 1):S87-S91.

328

Zoonoses

CAMILLE NELSON KOTTON | ARNOLD N. WEINBERG

Zoonoses are a complex group of diseases caused by a remarkable diversity of pathogenic microorganisms with varied life cycles and modes of spread that ordinarily reside and cause illness in the nonhuman animal world.[1] As rapid transportation and varied forms of commerce bring people closer in our "global village," as climate and other geophysical changes result in unpredictable distributions of arthropod vectors for pathogen carriage and transmission, as migration of individuals and groups results in urbanization with crowding and/or sylvatic encroachment of susceptible individuals, we can predict that zoonotic diseases will appear and reappear at unpredictable locations and times. In addition to their natural occurrence, many of these microorganisms are prime candidates for biological weapons.[2] Response to this potential threat, as well as to the awareness of naturally occurring zoonotic diseases, has stimulated renewed resolve to develop rapid diagnostic tests and protective vaccines and coordinate efforts by the World Health Organization and the Centers for Disease Control and Prevention to upgrade public health communications nationally and globally.[3]

Efforts to identify and monitor emerging zoonotic and other infectious diseases and their distribution in specific geographic regions have revealed important information regarding the maldistribution of the surveillance, research, and funding devoted to emerging infectious diseases. A recent report found that over a 64-year span, zoonoses account for 60% of emerging infectious diseases, the majority of which (72%) originate in wildlife and are primarily identified in resource-limited areas of the world.[4] The influence of geoclimatic change and spread of infectious diseases, especially focusing on zoonoses and vectors, was the subject of a robust report of a 2007 conference sponsored by the Institute of Medicine. Influences such as rainfall extremes, temperature changes at various latitudes and elevations, and examples of the interplay of these conditions on the spread of infectious diseases were thoughtfully presented. Clearly, alterations in ocean and terrestrial temperatures, increasing acidity of the seas, expansion of the ranges of competent vectors and pathogens, and socioeconomic fluctuations are all occurring; the consensus of the conference was strongly in support of these observations, but urged the need for specific studies and hard data to support further conclusions.[5]

The Conundrum: Defining a Zoonotic Disease

Criteria used to define a zoonotic infection vary and depend on how strictly the definition includes a vertebrate intermediate, other than humans, in the natural cycle of infection. For the purposes of this chapter, we define zoonotic diseases as those caused by pathogens naturally maintained or residing in living animals and not recognized as predictably adapted to humans or responsible for interhuman transmission on a regular basis. Zoonoses can cause illness in their natural hosts and are capable of infecting humans via contact (tularemia, anthrax, orf), animal bites (rabies, *Capnocytophaga*), ingestion (giardiasis, *Escherichia coli* O157 H7, vibriosis, salmonellosis, listeriosis), inhalation (tularemia, psittacosis), and arthropod intermediates (yellow fever, chikungunya) (with many more examples listed in Table 328-1). Some microbes, such as *Francisella tularensis,* can spread to humans or to other animals via all five of these routes of transmission. Inadvertently, zoonoses can be spread from one infected person to another, through blood or stem cell transfusions (e.g., dengue fever,

babesiosis)[6,7] or organ and tissue transplantations (e.g., lymphocytic choriomeningitis virus, rabies, Chagas disease).[6,8,9] Zoonoses, especially viral pathogens, have presented a significant stumbling block for xenotransplantation and the use of animal organs, cells, and contact through hemoperfusion (e.g., pig liver or spleen), but are not addressed here.[2] Ordinarily excluded from the group of zoonotic diseases are environmental microbes, such as *Burkholderia pseudomallei* and *Legionella* spp. Likewise, fungi are not considered except to acknowledge that bats have spread *Histoplasma capsulatum* and birds have been responsible for cases of *Cryptococcus neoformans* in humans. Reverse zoonoses are human illnesses that may cause illnesses in animals, such as hepatitis viruses, *Staphylococcus aureus*, tuberculosis, and *Streptococcus* infections.

In this chapter, malaria has been excluded because it exclusively cycles between mosquitoes and humans without the necessity of residence in nonhuman animals. Babesiosis, a disease caused by an animal protozoan, is included because transmission occurs from vertebrate nonhuman hosts via infected *Ixodes* ticks. Most arthropod-borne zoonoses (e.g., Lyme borreliosis, tularemia, Rocky Mountain spotted fever) have cycles that include an animal intermediate, although transovarial and transtadial (from the egg to the adult stage) life cycles can sometimes lead to direct transmission from ticks to humans without a nonhuman animal phase. Ingestion of *Vibrio* species with raw shellfish or of *Salmonella, E. coli, Yersinia pseudotuberculosis,* or *Cryptosporidium* in water or contaminated vegetable crops, represent diseases acquired from both nonvertebrate and vertebrate animals. Any rigid definition needs to be qualified by newly recognized or evolving exceptions, common or rare. *Plasmodium knowlesi*, a malarial pathogen in monkeys, has recently been identified as the causative agent of human malaria in Malaysia.[10] Many influenza viruses have mutated from their natural residence in nonhuman hosts to become fully adapted to humans, subsequently defined as anthroponotic pathogens (i.e., spread exclusively among humans). Influenza A subtype H5N1 or avian flu currently remains classified as a zoonotic illness and perhaps will not evolve to an anthroponotic disease. The coronavirus responsible for severe acute respiratory syndrome is a perplexing example of how cautious we must be in defining infectious agents. Originating in bats, this virus spread to humans either directly or through intermediate animals like the masked civet in crowded markets in Guangdong Province, Republic of China. After entering the human plane, the virus and disease spread rapidly among people, primarily by inhalation. Thus, severe acute respiratory syndrome, originating as a zoonotic illness, rapidly evolved into an anthroponotic disease; its current status in humans is uncertain based on current research and clinical data.

Influence on Individuals and Economies

The diversity of the zoonoses, their global distribution in mundane and exotic niches, the glamorous or complex names given to some (e.g., Kyasanur Forest disease), and the increasing enthusiasm that people have for travel and outdoor adventure all contribute to the aura and complexity surrounding this group of diseases. Domestic and laboratory animal contacts and diverse household pets,[11,12] including exotic imports,[13] have economic and emotional implications. It should be apparent that animal infections that can be transmitted to humans

TABLE 328-1	Diseases Acquired Directly or Indirectly from Animals or from Arthropod Vectors							
		Mode of Spread				Epidemiology		
Pathogen	Disease	Contact/Bite	Ingestion	Respiratory	Arthropod Vector	Public	Occupational	Environmental
VIRAL								
Alphavirus	Chikungunya				×			×
Alphavirus	**Eastern equine encephalitis**				×	×	×	×
Alphavirus	Mayaro virus disease				×			×
Alphavirus	Oropouche virus				×			×
Alphavirus	Ross River polyarthritis				×			×
Alphavirus	Semliki Forest				×			×
Alphavirus	**Venezuelan equine encephalitis**			×	×	×	×	×
Arenavirus	Lassa fever	×					×	×
Arenavirus	**Lymphocytic choriomeningitis**	×		×		×	×	×
Bat paramyxovirus	Hendra respiratory syndrome	×		×			×	×
Bat paramyxovirus	Nipah encephalitis	×	×	×			×	×
Bunyavirus	**California encephalitis**				×	×	×	×
Flavivirus	Eastern Hemisphere tick-borne encephalitis		×		×			×
Flavivirus	Japanese encephalitis				×			×
Flavivirus	Kyasanur Forest disease				×			×
Flavivirus	Murray Valley encephalitis				×			×
Flavivirus	Omsk hemorrhagic fever	×		×	×		×	×
Flavivirus	**Powassan virus encephalitis**		×		×	×	×	×
Flavivirus	**St. Louis encephalitis**				×	×	×	
Flavivirus	**West Nile virus**				×	×		×
Flavivirus	Yellow fever				×			×
Flavivirus spp.	**Dengue fever**				×	×		×
Hantavirus spp.	Hemorrhagic fever renal syndrome	×	×	×			×	×
Hantavirus spp. (New World)	**Hantavirus pulmonary syndrome**	×		×			×	×
Herpesvirus simiae	B virus	×				×	×	
Orbivirus	**Colorado tick fever**				×		×	×
Orthopox	Tanapox	×				×		×
Orthopoxvirus	**Monkeypox**	×				×	×	×
Parapoxvirus	**Contagious ecthyma (Orf)**	×					×	
Parapoxvirus	**Milker's nodule**	×					×	
Phlebovirus	Rift Valley fever	×	×	×	×			×
Prion	**Variant Creutzfeldt-Jakob encephalitis**		×			×		
Rhabdovirus	**Rabies**	×				×	×	×
BACTERIAL								
Anaplasma phagocytophilum	**Anaplasmosis**				×	×		×
Bacillus anthracis	**Anthrax**	×	×	×		×	×	×
Bartonella henselae	**Cat-scratch disease, bacillary angiomatosis**	×			×	×	×	×
Bartonella quintana	**Trench fever**	×			×	×		
Borrelia spp.	**Relapsing fever**				×	×	×	
Borrelia burgdorferi	**Lyme borreliosis**				×	×	×	×
Brucella spp.	**Brucellosis**	×	×	×		×	×	×
Burkholderia mallei	**Glanders**	×	×	×			×	
Campylobacter jejuni	**Campylobacteriosis**		×			×	×	
Capnocytophaga canimorsus	**Septicemia-canine bite associated**	×						×
Chlamydia psittaci	**Psittacosis, ornithosis**			×		×	×	
Coxiella burnetii	**Q fever**		×		×	×	×	×
Edwardsiella tarda	*Edwardsiella* infection		×			×	×	×
Ehrlichia chaffeensis	**Ehrlichiosis, monocytic**				×	×		
Erysipelothrix rhusiopathiae	**Erysipeloid**	×					×	×
Escherichia coli O157-H7, other serotypes	**Enterohemorrhagic gastroenteritis**	×	×			×	×	

TABLE 328-1	Diseases Acquired Directly or Indirectly from Animals or from Arthropod Vectors—cont'd							
		Mode of Spread				**Epidemiology**		
Pathogen	Disease	Contact/Bite	Ingestion	Respiratory	Arthropod Vector	Public	Occupational	Environmental
Francisella tularensis	**Tularemia**	X	X	X	X	X	X	X
Leptospira interrogans spp.	**Leptospirosis**	X	X			X	X	X
Listeria monocytogenes	Listeriosis		X			X	X	
Mycobacterium bovis	Tuberculosis		X			X	X	
Orientia tsutsugamushi	Scrub typhus				X		X	X
Pasteurella multocida	**Pasteurellosis**	X		X		X		X
Plesiomonas shigelloides	*Plesiomonas* gastroenteritis	X	X			X	X	
Rhodococcus equi	*Rhodococcus* pneumonia			X		X		
Rickettsia akari	Rickettsialpox				X	X		
Rickettsia rickettsii	**Rocky Mountain spotted fever**	X			X	X	X	X
Rickettsia spp.	Eastern Hemisphere spotted fevers				X	X		X
Rickettsia typhi	**Murine typhus**				X	X	X	X
Salmonella enteritidis	**Salmonellosis**		X			X	X	X
Spirillum minor	Rat-bite fever (Sodoku)	X				X	X	X
Streptobacillus moniliformis	**Rat-bite fever (Haverill fever)**	X	X			X	X	
Streptococcus iniae	**Streptococcal cellulitis**	X				X	X	
Vibrio cholerae	Cholera		X			X	X	X
Vibrio parahaemolyticus	Gastroenteritis		X			X	X	X
Vibrio vulnificus, other vibrios	**Skin gangrene sepsis-saltwater associated**	X	X			X	X	X
Yersinia enterocolitica	Yersiniosis		X			X	X	X
Yersinia pestis	**Plague**	X	X	X	X	X	X	X
Yersinia pseudotuberculosis	**Yersiniosis**		X			X	X	X
PARASITIC								
Angiostrongylus spp.	Angiostrongyliasis		X			X		
Babesia microti	**Babesiosis**				X		X	X
Clonorchis sinensis	Clonorchiasis		X					X
Cryptosporidia spp.	**Cryptosporidiosis**		X			X	X	X
Cyclospora cayetanensis	Cyclosporiasis		X			X		X
Diphyllobothrium latum	Fish tapeworm		X			X		
Dirofilaria immitis	**Dirofilariasis**				X			X
Echinococcus granulosus	Echinococcosis		X				X	
Fasciola hepatica	Fascioliasis		X				X	X
Giardia lamblia	**Giardiasis**		X			X	X	X
Leishmania donovani	Visceral leishmaniasis (kala-azar)				X			X
Leishmania mexicana	Cutaneous leishmaniasis				X			X
Leishmania spp.	Cutaneous leishmaniasis				X			X
Microsporidia spp.	**Chronic microsporidial diarrhea**		X				X	X
Paragonimus westermani	Paragonimiasis		X				X	X
Parastrongylus cantonensis	Angiostrongyliasis	X	X					X
Plasmodium knowlesi	Monkey malaria				X			X
Taenia solium	**Cysticercosis**		X			X		
Toxocara canis, cati	**Toxocariasis**	X	X			X		X
Toxoplasma gondii	**Toxoplasmosis**		X			X		
Trichinella spiralis	**Trichinosis**		X			X		
Trypanosoma brucei	African trypanosomiasis				X			X
Trypanosoma cruzi	Chagas' disease				X			X

Table includes selected common or interesting pathogens and is not comprehensive of all zoonoses. Bold type indicates acquired in North America, although the disease may have a wider distribution. Mode of spread includes contact (direct contact, including bites, scratches, or water), ingestion, respiratory, arthropod vector (e.g., mosquito, tick, flea, mite). Epidemiology includes public, people with pets or living in urban areas; occupational exposures, farmers, livestock and animal processing workers, fishers and others in aquatic environments, health care (both veterinary and human) and laboratory personnel; and environmental exposures, i.e., travelers, those who live in indigenous areas or those involved in outdoor recreational activities.

can have a significant impact on everyone, including physicians and veterinarians as well as local and national economies.

The long-term economic impact of animal husbandry and human disease reached a new dimension with the emergence in the United Kingdom in 1986 of the prion disease bovine spongiform encephalopathy (mad cow disease). Farmers fought to preserve their herds, the beef-eating public became increasingly upset as human cases of variant Creutzfeldt-Jakob disease were discovered and political turmoil intensified as other European countries recognized the disease in native or imported cattle. The slaughter of millions of head of cattle ensued, with restriction of beef imports and exports and to date more than 200 human deaths, predominantly in the United Kingdom. The efforts of basic scientists and epidemiologists and the involvement of the World Health Organization have resulted in considerable clarification of the etiology of the disease and its probable initiation in cattle fed protein supplements containing ruminant nervous system tissues. Confidence in food safety and movement of cattle continues to be a great concern. Latency of prion diseases in both animals and humans has not eliminated the economic or health impacts after more than two decades. Influenza A subtype H5N1 or avian flu emergence represents the most profound new threat to global health and disease. Widespread epizootics (zoonotic epidemics) in poultry have led to culling of flocks, compromising protein nutrition, and precipitating economic hardships in developing countries, as well as creating anxiety that successful adaptation and subsequent human-to-human spread could result in an influenza pandemic. As a result of these experiences, the World Health Organization has assumed a greater responsibility for surveillance, protocol development, and laboratory investigations, an indication of the globalization of concern, organization, and action in approaching emerging and resurging infectious diseases.[14]

Pets may harbor significant zoonotic pathogens. A pet guinea pig transmitted subclinical lymphocytic choriomeningitis virus to an organ donor from whom four organ transplant recipients were subsequently infected, three fatally.[8] Reptile contact accounts for an estimated 6% of human Salmonella infections in the United States. Turtles commonly carry Salmonella with fecal carriage rates as high as 90%; in 2007, an outbreak of 103 cases of Salmonella paratyphi B var. Java was found to be linked to exposure to small turtles (even though turtles with carapaces smaller than 4 inches had been banned in 1975 due to the high risk of Salmonella carriage).[15] In a survey of survivors of human plague (due to Yersinia pestis), dog ownership, especially sleeping in the same bed as a pet dog, were significantly associated with risk of infection.[16] A humanitarian shipment of 24 dogs and cats from Iraq to the United States (later distributed to 16 states), brought to reunite servicemen returning to the United States with animals they had adopted in Iraq, resulted in the transport of a dog who later died of rabies, later typed to be a rabies virus variant associated with dogs in the Middle East (the other animals were immediately vaccinated and placed under a 6-month quarantine).[17]

Importance of Zoonoses in Contemporary Infectious Disease

Perusal of Tables 328-1 and 328-2 reinforces both the global significance of animal-associated infectious agents as well as the large proportion that are indigenous to North America in wild and domestic animal reservoirs. In absolute numbers, zoonotic pathogens are common, and illness in humans constitutes a significant worldwide impact on morbidity and mortality. Without reviewing historical reports on epidemic bubonic plague, typhus, or woolsorter's disease, numerous contemporary examples illustrate the real and potential impact of zoonotic diseases in urban and rural settings. The criminal anthrax spore mail delivery incident of September 2001 is an example of the infectious potential of zoonotic microorganisms. The severity of illnesses, the fear factor, and the expense involved in surveillance and clean up of the environment reflect the complexity of dealing with a bioterrorist act.[18] Predicting the extent of spread through the animal and arthropod vector planes and subsequent human infection is difficult. The pandemic potential of avian flu has been appreciated, if

TABLE 328-2 Selected Zoonotic Diseases Transmitted Via Contact with Animals or Animal Products

Animal	Anthrax	Bartonellosis	Brucellosis	Campylobacterosis	Capnocytophaga sepsis	Cryptosporidiosis	Erysipiloid	Escherichia coli O157:H7 gastroenteritis	Giardiasis	Hantaviral pneumonia	Lymphocytic choriomeningitis	Leptospirosis	Listeriosis	Mycobacteria spp.	Ornithosis/Psittacosis	Pasteurellosis	Plague	Q fever	Rabies	Rat-bite fever	Salmonellosis	Toxoplasmosis	Tularemia	Vibriosis	Yersiniosis other than plague
Aquatic mammal							×		×												×	×			
Birds				×			×						×		×						×				
Cat	×	×		×		×		×				×				×	×	×	×		×	×	×		
Cattle	×		×	×		×		×				×	×	×				×			×	×			×
Dog	×		×	×	×	×		×				×				×			×		×				×
Fish/shellfish							×							×							×			×	
Goats/sheep	×		×	×		×			×			×						×			×	×		×	×
Horse	×							×													×				×
Rabbit/hare								×				×				×					×		×		
Reptiles, amphibians																					×				
Rodent		×								×	×						×			×	×		×		
Subhuman primate				×					×			×	×	×							×				×
Swine	×		×	×			×	×				×	×	×				×			×				×
Wildlife/bats	×					×		×	×	×		×	×			×	×	×	×		×	×	×		

In addition, animals (especially pet cats and dogs) can serve as carriers for vector-borne diseases, such as babesiosis, ehrlichiosis/anaplasmosis, Lyme disease, plague, and tularemia.

influenza A subtype H5N1 converts from a zoonotic to anthroponotic virus. The histories of Lyme borreliosis, Rocky Mountain spotted fever, chikungunya, and West Nile virus all portray the major impact of zoonoses, based on the numbers of cases and extension of geographic ranges.

CONTINENTAL UNITED STATES

Before 1991, the average yearly number of endemic and imported zoonotic infections (excluding salmonellosis) was approximately 2400 cases.[19] By 2007, the number expanded to approximately 40,000, associated with the addition of Lyme borreliosis, cryptosporidiosis, and *E. coli* O157:H7 to the list of reportable diseases.[20] This increase reflects increased awareness of these diseases, as well as the influences of expanded vector capacity, movements of animal and hosts, proximity of people to rural outdoors, and contamination of food sources. Regrowth of forests in the northeastern United State has resulted in ballooning populations of white-tailed deer, white-footed mice, and *Ixodes scapularis* ticks. The agents of Lyme disease and ehrlichiosis/anaplasmosis have been identified in and around cities, including an urban park on the edge of New York City.[21] Babesiosis, a rare protozoan zoonotic disease primarily afflicting elderly and splenectomized individuals, is being reported more frequently in young, healthy people. *Babesia microti* is transmitted naturally via the feeding of *Ixodes* ticks that may simultaneously transmit Lyme borreliosis or ehrlichiosis/anaplasmosis; concomitant triple infections have been described.[22] Cryptosporidiosis, responsible for sporadic and epidemic gastroenteritis, is being reported with increasing frequency in waterborne epidemics[23] as well as in patients ill with acquired immunodeficiency syndrome.[24,25] This chlorine-resistant protozoan is spread during contact with recreational water sources, as seen in Utah in 2007 where an outbreak of more than 1900 cases occurred, many with direct exposure to recreational water venues or to ill contacts.[23] *Cryptosporidium* is commonly transmitted through ingestion of contaminated food or water supplies; there are also many examples of transmission due to direct animal contacts.[26] Importation of a few subclinically infected rabid raccoons from Florida to stock hunting camps in West Virginia in 1978 initiated a rapidly spreading rabies epizootic, primarily into contiguous Middle Atlantic states,[27] followed by invasion of New York and New England. Other terrestrial wild animals, especially skunks, were infected and the epizootic spread to a wide variety of domestic animals, such as unvaccinated cats and pet rabbits. Isolation, containment, and sacrifice of companion pets and the threat posed to individuals added an emotional burden to the monetary drain placed on public health resources.

Hantaviruses have been documented, by serologic and virologic methods, to occur in the United States in a variety of New World rodents.[28] No clinical human disease had been recognized, although globally hemorrhagic fever with renal syndrome (e.g., Korean hemorrhagic fever) and nephropathia epidemica (milder Scandinavian nephropathy) are familiar illnesses caused by members of the Bunyaviridae family. The dramatic appearance of acute respiratory distress syndrome that afflicts primarily outdoor-oriented young adults and that carries significant mortality was first described in newspapers and in *Morbidity Mortality Weekly Report* in 1993 in the Four Corners area of four southwestern states.[29] This virulent respiratory disease, caused by a number of previously unidentified Hantaviruses, has now been identified throughout the United States and in Central and South America in a variety of rodent reservoirs.[30] The epidemiology of this new respiratory syndrome appears to be inhalation of virus in dried excreta or via contact. Using satellite imagery and mammalian sampling after the El Niño Southern Oscillation event, researchers were able to predict environmental conditions that supported vector growth, potentially identifying areas of high-risk hantaviral transmission and refugia (disease persistence).[31]

Two illnesses that illustrate the impact of zoonotic diseases on animals and humans appeared in the United States in the past decade. Neither had ever been identified in the Western Hemisphere before

the clinical diseases surfaced. West Nile viral encephalitis was diagnosed in the summer of 1999 in Queens, New York, in a number of elderly patients. Rapid collaboration among clinicians, epidemiologists, veterinary pathologists, and virologists isolated the causal agent that was transmitted from birds to people via *Culex* and other mosquitoes.[32] Although uncertain how the virus arrived in the States, it has now spread from the East Coast in recent years and is responsible for morbidity and mortality in people, birds, horses, and other animals in a relentless march westward to California and southward into Mexico.[33]

Monkeypox arrived in a shipment of exotic pets from West Africa in the spring of 2003. A virus that is carried by small mammals in forested areas of central and West Africa, monkeypox is responsible for sporadic and epidemic disease in subhuman primates and people. A Gambian giant pouched rat and several other small mammals at a pet distribution center in Illinois infected prairie dogs later sold as pets in a number of Midwestern states. The prairie dogs, in turn, infected approximately 80 people.[34] A ban on the sale of prairie dogs as pets and on the importation of African rodents is now in place and Public Health officials are alert to the potential for spread of monkeypox in the wild animal plane, in caged animals, and in humans. During the investigation of the first reported case of prairie dog-to-human tularemia transmission in Texas in 2002, it was noted that more than a thousand additional animals were shipped to Europe and Asia.[13] These examples illustrate the unexpected emergence of zoonotic diseases in new areas, carried in obvious or obscure vehicles from distant regions. A vigilant medical and veterinary community, sensible quarantine procedures, and a reliable public health infrastructure with sophisticated research laboratories are vital for the rapid identification of new pathogens occurring naturally or as acts of bioterrorism.[2]

GLOBAL EXPERIENCES

Our responsibility for patients' well-being often includes travel advice. The distribution of zoonotic diseases and their modes of spread often dictate the choice of protective immunizations, medications, and specific instructions about food and drink. In practical terms, many problems result from failed communication or incomplete advice. For example, in Boston and some other cities in the United States, more cases of Eastern Hemisphere spotted fever (e.g., South African tick bite fever) are seen in a decade than of indigenous Rocky Mountain spotted fever. Analysis of most of these cases reveals that no precautionary measures were discussed by the physician during the pretravel visit even though the patient's itinerary included a walking safari in an endemic region. The incubation period may influence the time of appearance of an emerging zoonotic infection, often after travel is completed and the patient is home.

Movement of large numbers of susceptible young soldiers to areas of the world endemic for contagious diseases, including infectious zoonoses, has always been a concern. Hemorrhagic fever emerged as an acute clinical problem among United Nations troops in the Korean conflict, as well as for practicing physicians in the West dealing with returning soldiers. The editor of *Reviews of Infectious Diseases* demonstrated his prescience by inviting experts to prepare a monograph supplement in the autumn of 1990 on the subject of infectious disease problems related to the Persian Gulf area.[35] A wide circulation of this supplement reached infectious disease specialists just as the Desert Storm conflict erupted. The major zoonoses endemic in the region were reviewed thoughtfully. In the aftermath of that brief conflict, rare reports of animal-associated diseases, such as Q fever that had become clinically active after a period of latency, appeared in the literature. Conflicts have continued to erupt in other regions of the globe, including Iraq and Afghanistan. Responsible reporting in the medical and military literature has been timely in bringing regional zoonoses to the attention of physicians and should be a continuing responsibility of the armed forces medical profession, the World Health Organization, and the Centers for Disease Control and Prevention.[36] Hundreds of cases of visceral and cutaneous leishmaniasis in U.S. military personnel stationed in Iraq, Kuwait, and Afghanistan have been described, as well as cases of brucellosis and Q fever in Iraq.[37]

The resurgence of dengue fever as a global health problem is another illustration of the unpredictability of arbovirus dissemination and the many factors influencing local outbreaks and epidemics.[38] In the Western Hemisphere, the epidemic of dengue fever clearly relates to failure of mosquito control, urbanization and population growth, and lack of proper water storage and waste removal procedures. Competent mosquitoes, including *Aedes aegypti* and *Aedes albopictus*, have spread dengue virus throughout the Caribbean and Central and South America. The southernmost indigenous case of dengue fever was recently documented in South America, likely due to the spread of the principal dengue vector, *Aedes aegypti*, southward to latitude 35° S near Buenos Aires (out of the torrid zone and well into the southern temperate zone, with a northern latitude corresponding to the Carolinas).[39] The presence of competent arthropod vectors in the southern United States increases the likelihood of dengue outbreaks locally (autochthonous spread), not just among tourists returning from vacationing in endemic areas.[40] Dengue is just one of more than 150 arboviruses worldwide known to cause human disease. Some of these viruses, like the agent of yellow fever, infect animal species where they persist as reservoirs with potential human spread. Selected examples are included in the tables. New arboviruses will emerge as threats to human health as remote forested regions are "developed" and extremes of rain, temperature, and climate are magnified.[5]

At a time when people seek adventure in the outdoors, when travel time around the globe is shorter than the incubation period of many zoonotic diseases, and when immunocompromised patients crowd foreign travel experiences into periods of wellness, our efforts must be assiduous in providing advance warning and in investigating new clinical symptoms in returning travelers. A useful text that covers geographic distribution of infections is available,[41] and the CDC provides excellent health information for international travelers via the *CDC Health Information for International Travel*[42] (available at http://wwwn.cdc.gov/travel/contentYellowBook.aspx).

Distribution of Zoonotic Pathogens in Nature

The emergence of newly recognized zoonoses and the spread of established animal diseases to new regions of the globe signal the need for urgent study of the interrelatedness of the many contributing factors. Zoonotic spread frequently involves some or all of the topics included in Table 328-3. The spread of West Nile virus in the United States serves as an excellent example of the confluence of all these factors, including geoclimatic conditions, with excessive rainfall leading to areas of standing water and increased vector capacity; human influence on ecosystems with urban crowding and suburban sprawl optimizing factors leading to disease transmission; migration patterns of birds resulting in transcontinental spread; mammalian and avian hosts encouraging spread to other animals, including horses; arthropod reservoirs and vectors, with overwintering mosquito populations apparently providing transovarial viral persistence; and global trade and travel, by which the virus was purportedly introduced into the United States. Individually or collectively, these factors affect commerce, economic development, human and animal health and behavior, clandestine activities, and urban and wild regional development as well as focusing on the significant concern for the effects of geoclimatic changes on the health of planet earth.

GEOCLIMATIC CONDITIONS AND GLOBAL WARMING

Numerous examples illustrate the influence of temperature, moisture, and soil conditions on the distribution of zoonotic agents and diseases. Tropical diseases imply that an environment is extant that supports the growth and transmission of infectious agents requiring high tem-

TABLE 328-3	Factors Associated with the Distribution and Potential Emergence of Zoonotic Pathogens in Nature
Geoclimatic conditions and global warming	
Temperature extremes: terrestrial and water	
Rainfall patterns, floods, standing water	
Soil characteristics	
Human influence on ecosystems	
Migration patterns of animals and birds	
Mammalian, avian, and aquatic hosts as reservoirs	
Arthropod reservoirs and vectors	
Effects of global trade	
Food	
Live animals and birds	
Inert conveyors (e.g., used tires, contaminated ballast water)	

peratures and abundant rainfall in which arthropod vectors thrive and appropriate animal hosts exist. Global temperature extremes are an example of a geoclimatic issue that is changing zoonotic disease distribution.[43] Arthropod vectors such as mosquitoes and ticks, enhanced or suppressed growth and distribution of plants, and animal migrations are intimately tied to changes in ambient temperature. Researchers in Sweden found that the increase in tick-borne encephalitis incidence since the mid-1980s was related to the increase in milder winters and early arrival of spring.[44] There were more than 200 cases of chikungunya infection in Italy during the summer of 2007, encouraged by the concentration of competent vectors (i.e., *Aedes albopictus*) at the time index human cases arrived, likely from the Indian Ocean. Subsequent indigenous cases have been reported, suggesting that chikungunya may have gained a foothold in southern Europe, although the ability of the virus to "winter over" in mosquitos or in animal hosts remains to be discovered.[45] The presence of *Anopheles* mosquitoes and the increasing number of cases of malaria at higher elevations support scientists who argue that climate change is already occurring.[46] A Kenyan study compared forested with deforested highland regions with respect to microclimates and sporogonic development of *Plasmodium falciparum* parasites in *Anopheles gambiae* mosquitoes.[47] Sporozoites appeared earlier, and vectorial capacity was estimated to be 78% higher in the deforested highland site, significantly increasing the risk of malaria in these regions. Researchers in East Africa found an association between rainfall and unusually high maximum temperatures and the number of inpatient malaria cases 3 to 4 months later, which allowed for the development of a malaria epidemic prediction model.[48]

Bacillus anthracis spores and vegetative growth of organisms are strongly influenced by ambient temperatures in "incubator" areas where plant decay adds warmth and moisture in the presence of a supportive alkaline soil containing adequate calcium salts.[49] The halophilic and nonhalophilic vibrios of the Northern Hemisphere winter in estuarine mud and appear in significant numbers only as water temperatures warm to approximately 20° C. Cases of gastroenteritis, necrotizing cellulitis, and septicemia due to *Vibrio* species are being diagnosed in individuals exposed to New England, Alaskan, and Danish coastal sea waters, regions traditionally considered too cold to support the growth of these organisms.[50,51]

HUMAN INFLUENCE ON ECOSYSTEMS

The ability of humans to exert significant influence on wind velocity, rainfall, temperature extremes, and soil conditions pales when compared with the natural forces operating around the globe. There are numerous small- and large-scale examples in irrigation practices, waste distribution, water purification, agricultural technologies, insecticide use, and incursions into areas of virgin vegetation, however, that illustrate the profound effects of human activities on the establishment and spread of zoonoses.[52]

Dramatic examples can be found in epidemics after pollution of water supplies, the most contemporary being the massive outbreak of cryptosporidial gastroenteritis after torrential rains and flooding that affected more than 400,000 Milwaukee, Wisconsin, residents.[26] Water-borne cryptosporidiosis remains a major threat, especially among immunocompromised individuals.[53] The first of many microbiologically documented *Giardia* epidemics, reported in 1993, spread from wild beavers through fecally contaminated water supplied to residents of several towns in western Canada.[54] We are not protecting our water systems adequately to kill and remove selected zoonotic pathogens that encyst and therefore are resistant to purification methods.

Recreational swimming holes can be contaminated by *Leptospira* spp. brought downstream from neighboring farms[55]; the largest outbreak of leptospirosis in the United States was in Illinois in 1998 during a triathlon after heavy rains.[56] Airplanes can facilitate the inadvertent transport of potentially infectious arthropod vectors of zoonoses in the wheel bays of intercontinental and transcontinental flights.[57] Indiscriminate use of insecticides has influenced avian populations instrumental in the control of various disease-carrying arthropod vectors. Perhaps the most devastating influence affecting the distribution of zoonotic pathogens occurs when virgin forests are cleared or are invaded by new roads and new towns in the name of economic development. It has been theorized that many undiscovered potentially pathogenic viruses and bacteria reside in animal hosts that are inaccessible to humans in remote ecosystems until such areas are developed and susceptible people begin moving to and fro. An example often quoted is the recognition of the viral disease Oropouche several years after a new road was built connecting Belem with Brasilia in Brazil.[58]

As human communities expand and encroach on shrinking wildlife habitats, more zoonoses (and reverse zoonoses) will be exchanged bidirectionally. In a prospective study of bacterial transmission among humans, nonhuman primates, and livestock in western Uganda, humans living near certain forest areas harbored *E. coli* bacteria that were approximately 75% more similar to bacteria from primates in those areas than to bacteria from primates in nearby undisturbed forests. Genetic similarity between human, primate, and livestock bacteria increased approximately threefold as anthropogenic disturbance within forest regions increased from moderate to high. Bacteria harbored by humans and livestock were approximately twice as similar to those of red-tailed guenons, which habitually enter human settlements to raid crops, than to bacteria of other primate species. Conservation efforts and awareness may guide interventions that reduce zoonotic disease transmission and emergence in selected regions.[59]

MIGRATION PATTERNS OF ANIMALS AND BIRDS

Tularemia appeared in Vermont for the first time in the late 1960s, brought there by infected muskrats migrating via a water route from Canada and New York State.[60] Cases of Rocky Mountain spotted fever appear in new and unexpected places, such as a small park surrounded by concrete and asphalt in Bronx, New York.[61] Did a dog bring the rickettsiae in dog ticks acquired from a visit to eastern Long Island? Did a hawk carry an infected rabbit from an endemic area? Can *Rickettsia rickettsii* be transported by migrating birds carrying infected arthropods? In nature, when considering the potential for emergence of zoonoses, no haven is safe. Even in a verdant park in New York City, ticks have been discovered carrying *Borrelia burgdorferi* and *Anaplasma* (*Ehrlichia*) *phagocytophila*, probably transported by roaming white-footed mice.[21] The questions are many; the answers are few. Observations of zoonotic disease spread confirms the influence of animal reservoir movements, the necessity of cohosts for long-term survival of some pathogens (e.g., *B. burgdorferi*),[62] and the importance of overwintering sedentary birds as well as migratory patterns for persistence and dissemination of selected zoonoses (e.g., West Nile virus). The presence of favorable conditions for growth, survival, and multiplication of ticks, biting flies, and mosquitoes, important vectors of many zoonotic pathogens (see Table 328-1), illustrates the potential for widespread movements of microorganisms carried by these vectors to new geographic regions. An acute respiratory illness in horses and

caretakers in Queensland, Australia, and an outbreak of severe encephalitis in pig farmers in Malaysia was first reported in 1994 and 1998, respectively; two closely related atypical paramyxoviruses, named Hendra and Nipah, were isolated and both viruses were found associated with pteropid bats (fruit-eating flying foxes) that probably serve as reservoirs and spread virus to horses and pigs.[63,64] The unprecedented encroachment of long-distance flying pteropid bats into cultivated fruit orchards (where piggeries were located) may have precipitated these novel outbreaks. The bat encroachment was likely due to a reduction in flowering and fruiting forest trees due to slash-and-burn deforestation and subsequent severe haze that blanketed much of Southeast Asia in the months directly preceding the Nipah virus disease outbreak, exacerbated by a drought driven by the severe 1997 to 1998 El Niño Southern Oscillation event.[65]

MAMMALIAN, AVIAN, AND AQUATIC HOSTS AS RESERVOIRS

Zoonotic spread is influenced by human and animal susceptibility factors, including genetic characteristics and immunity, both innate and acquired. Interactions with domestic animals can be a major factor. Vaccination of dogs in developed countries has all but eliminated rabies acquired from these pets, but in the developing world, rabies is frequently related to dog bites.[27] When domestic animals are allowed to stray or become feral, they can acquire many zoonotic infections, including tularemia, plague, and rabies.[66] Household pets can carry infected arthropod vectors into homes or to other geographic areas. The penchant of raccoons for suburban areas clearly facilitated the spread of rabies to domestic animals in the Middle Atlantic and New England states, primarily to cats, but also to dogs, cattle, horses, and even to pet rabbits.[67] The Hantavirus pulmonary syndrome, first described in the southwestern United States, emerged clinically when an abundance of food led to increased numbers of rodents living in proximity to susceptible humans.[29] Migrating and overwintering sedentary birds provide a reservoir for arboviruses, including West Nile virus, and aquatic mammals are sources of multiplication and dissemination of *Giardia lamblia*[54] and *F. tularensis*.[60] Petting farms and open zoos have been associated with a plethora of pathogens, with a predominance of those causing gastrointestinal disease, ranging from *E. coli* O157:H7 to *Salmonella*, *Shigella*, *Cryptosporidium*, monkeypox, and sealpox[68]; tuberculosis can be transmitted as both a zoonosis and reverse zoonosis between humans and elephants in such settings.[69]

ARTHROPOD RESERVOIRS AND VECTORS

Vectorial capacity, the summation of many factors that contribute to the ability of a pathogen to perpetuate in an arthropod host, is often enhanced by actions that increase survival and multiplication of the arthropod and vertebrate host intermediates.[70] Although incompletely understood, it appears that the spread of Lyme borreliosis to the majority of the lower 48 states resulted from a population explosion of white-tailed deer and white-footed mice, which allowed overwintering of the pathogen and enhanced distribution of the dependent *Ixodes* ticks. A provocative report linking eastern United States oak forests to a chain reaction involving gypsy moth activity, white-footed mouse density, acorn production, and white-tailed deer presence illustrates the delicate balance that can eventuate in the distribution and prevalence of Lyme disease.[71] The appearance in the southeastern United States of a mosquito vector from Asia, the Asian tiger mosquito *Aedes albopictus*, corresponded to the commercial stockpiling of used tire casings imported into the Houston, Texas, area in the early 1980s.[40,72] Subsequent spread via tires from the United States to the Veneto region of Italy was noted,[73] completing a tricontinental passage, emphasizing the major impact of global trade and transport on zoonotic vectors. This mosquito, a competent laboratory vector for more than 20 arboviruses, has now been identified in the majority of the United States, including Hawaii.[40] In a surveillance effort initiated in

Polk County, Florida, 14 strains of eastern equine encephalitis virus have been isolated from these mosquitoes.[74] *F. tularensis* can be maintained in *Dermacentor* ticks through transovarial passage, and thus the tick is an important reservoir in nature, capable of disseminating the pathogen to small mammals and people.[75]

GLOBAL TRADE: FOOD, LIVE ANIMALS AND BIRDS, INERT CONVEYORS

Numerous examples of international spread of zoonotic diseases have been mentioned or discussed in this chapter. Bovine spongiform encephalitis clearly resulted from widespread use of animal carcasses as protein supplements; several hundred cases of variant Creutzfeldt-Jakob encephalopathy occurred in the United Kingdom and elsewhere. Fresh berries from Central and South America have precipitated epidemics of cyclosporiasis elsewhere. Many of the most common foodborne pathogens are associated with animal sources, including *Campylobacter*, *Listeria*, *Salmonella*, *Shigella*, Shiga-toxin–producing *E. coli* O157, *Vibrio*, *Yersinia*, and *Cryptosporidium*. Three of the top four causes of gastroenteritis (nontyphoidal *Salmonella*, *Campylobacter*, and Shiga-toxin producing *E. coli* have animal reservoirs.[76] Increases in multiple factors, including the expanded global food chain, the consumption of mass processed fresh produce, and eating in restaurants all augment our risk of food-borne zoonotic illness. To reduce the incidence of such infections, concerted efforts are needed throughout the food supply chain, from farm to processing plant to kitchen or restaurant. Investigation of a national outbreak in the United States of *E. coli* O157:H7 in 2006 due to bagged spinach from California found that isolates from feral swine, cattle, surface water, sediment, and soil at one ranch all matched the outbreak strain, suggesting that the feral swine may have been the initial source of the outbreak.[77]

Transport of live animals and birds may establish zoonoses in new locales. The recent introduction of monkeypox virus in exotic animals from West Africa (see previously) and the spread of West Nile virus via bird movements in North America are good examples. Transportation of raccoons from Florida to Virginia and North Carolina for hunting purposes in the 1970s and 1980s may have contributed to an epizootic of raccoon rabies in the middle Atlantic states.[78] Imported psittacosis has resulted in important and rigid quarantine measures for the parrot family and other bird species. Additional examples of zoonoses that can be transported in live animals include influenza H5N1, *Leishmania*, and echinococcosis.[79]

Inert conveyers may also transport zoonoses, as seen with the transport of old tires (see previously), resulting in the tricontinental spread of the Asian tiger mosquito *Aedes albopictus*. A recent case of inhalation anthrax in a drum maker who carried goatskins into the United States emphasizes the need for appropriate education and importation controls.[80] Ballast water in ships has transported toxigenic *Vibrio* species and other pathogens as well as phytoplankton and other species that may alter ecosystems elsewhere. It is abundantly clear that with enhanced global trade and movements of many commodities among nations that the specter of disseminating zoonotic pathogens is a very real concern that requires thoughtful and vigorous control measures.[2]

Diagnostic Approach to Zoonoses

Few areas of our specialty demand the precision in extracting details of a travel, occupation, or exposure history than that which is required when we confront a patient ill with a perplexing febrile illness who has been roughing it in the United States or abroad or who has had an animal, animal product, or arthropod encounter. The possibility of a zoonotic infection can surface quickly from even a superficial history or features of the physical examination, or both. The following should be assessed for potential zoonotic risk factors: residence and travel history, occupation (e.g., abattoir worker, veterinarian, farmer), ingestion of potentially contaminated food and water, outside interests (e.g., hunting, trapping, other outdoor activities), or the presence of a characteristic skin lesion (e.g., erythema migrans of Lyme borreliosis, peripheral petechial lesions of Rocky Mountain spotted fever, *tache noire* of Eastern Hemisphere spotted fever). Knowledge of the local epidemiology of characteristic illnesses, such as St. Louis encephalitis in Texas and eastern equine encephalitis in New Jersey, may alert a physician to similar diagnoses in other patients.

There are hundreds of well-described zoonotic diseases, of which close to 100 are included in Table 328-1. By using Tables 328-1 through 328-3 as cross-referencing guides, an individual's at-risk activities or animal contacts can help narrow the etiologic possibilities. Potential modes of spread can be evaluated through careful attention to historical details. Geographic considerations and clinical data can then help in selecting possible etiologic diagnoses. The epidemic of Q fever that occurred after a group of poker players were exposed to a parturient cat in urban Halifax, Nova Scotia, in winter, attests to the potential usefulness of Table 328-2 in identifying diseases specific to selected animal species that should be considered.[81] The multiplicity of possible etiologies for a cluster of patients, for example, with an acute respiratory disease, allows greater precision in diagnosis by having a reference to animal reservoirs characteristic of specific pathogens.[82]

Laboratory studies, including appropriate cultures, paired serologic specimens, molecular diagnostic assays, chemistries selected to evaluate target organ involvement, and evaluation for specific parasites can help to confirm a suspected diagnosis. Rapid nonculture-based diagnostic tests are in use or are being developed to identify selected zoonoses, including enzyme-linked immunosorbent assay methodology, fluorescent antibody staining, polymerase chain reaction (both qualitative and quantitative), and DNA/RNA probes.[2,83] In addition, the Internet allows for better surveillance, tracking, and communication regarding certain zoonoses. Rapid diagnostics blossomed as a field with the recent increased concern for bioterrorism, where rapid and efficient tests are essential for effective defense. In acute circumstances, empirical therapy guided by the available data should be instituted before confirming a specific diagnosis, such as with tularemia. Most of the sophisticated studies to unravel the identity of a zoonotic infectious disease, however, ultimately rely on a detailed and accurate history from which specific tests and effective therapy can emerge.

REFERENCES

1. Waltner-Toews D. Caught in the causal web: analytical problems in the epidemiology of zoonoses. *Acta Vet Scand Suppl.* 1988;84:296-298.
2. Burroughs T, Knobler S, Lederberg J, eds. *The Emergence of Zoonotic Diseases: Understanding the Impact on Animal and Human Health.* Washington, DC: Institute of Medicine, National Academy Press; 2002:1-123.
3. Centers for Disease Control and Prevention (CDC). Terrorism preparedness in state health departments—United States, 2001-2003. *MMWR Morb Mortal Wkly Rep.* 2003;52:1051-1053.
4. Jones KE, Patel NG, Levy MA, et al. Global trends in emerging infectious diseases. *Nature.* 2008;451:990-993.
5. Relman DA, Hamburg MA, Choffnes ER, et al. *Global Climate Change and Extreme Weather Events: Understanding the Contributions to Infectious Disease Emergence: Workshop Summary.* Washington, DC: National Academy Press; 2008.
6. Kotton CN. Zoonoses in solid-organ and hematopoietic stem cell transplant recipients. *Clin Infect Dis.* 2007;44:857-866.
7. Tambyah PA, Koay ES, Poon ML, et al. Dengue hemorrhagic fever transmitted by blood transfusion. *N Engl J Med.* 2008;359:1526-1527.
8. Fischer SA, Graham MB, Kuehnert MJ, et al. Transmission of lymphocytic choriomeningitis virus by organ transplantation. *N Engl J Med.* 2006;354:2235-2249.
9. Srinivasan A, Burton EC, Kuehnert MJ, et al. Transmission of rabies virus from an organ donor to four transplant recipients. *N Engl J Med.* 2005;352:1103-1111.
10. Kantele A, Marti H, Felger I, et al. Monkey malaria in a European traveler returning from Malaysia. *Emerg Infect Dis.* 2008;14:1434-1436.
11. Fox JG, Lipman NS. Infections transmitted by large and small laboratory animals. *Infect Dis Clin.* 1991;5:131-163.
12. Goldstein EJC. Household pets and human infections. *Infect Dis Clin North Am.* 1991;5:117-130.
13. Avashia SB, Petersen JM, Lindley CM, et al. First reported prairie dog-to-human tularemia transmission, Texas, 2002. *Emerg Infect Dis.* 2004;10:483-486.
14. Meslin FX. Global aspects of emerging and potential zoonoses: a WHO perspective. *Emerg Infect Dis.* 1997;3:223-228.
15. Multistate outbreak of human *Salmonella* infections associated with exposure to turtles—United States, 2007-2008. *MMWR Morb Mortal Wkly Rep.* 2008;57:69-72.
16. Gould LH, Pape J, Ettestad P, et al. Dog-associated risk factors for human plague. *Zoonoses Public Health.* 2008;55:448-454.
17. Rabies in a dog imported from Iraq—New Jersey, June 2008. *MMWR Morb Mortal Wkly Rep.* 2008;57:1076-1078.

18. Jernigan DB, Raghunathan PL, Bell BP, et al. Investigation of bioterrorism-related anthrax, United States, 2001: epidemiologic findings. *Emerg Infect Dis.* 2002;8:1019-1028.
19. Summary of notifiable diseases, United States-1991. *MMWR Morb Mortal Wkly Rep.* 1991;40:1-63.
20. McNabb SJ, Jajosky RA, Hall-Baker PA, et al. Summary of notifiable diseases—United States, 2006. *MMWR Morb Mortal Wkly Rep.* 2008;55:1-92.
21. Daniels TJ, Falco RC, Schwartz I, et al. Deer ticks (*Ixodes scapularis*) and the agents of Lyme disease and human granulocytic ehrlichiosis in a New York City park. *Emerg Infect Dis.* 1997;3:353-355.
22. Krause PJ, McKay K, Thompson CA, et al. Disease-specific diagnosis of coinfecting tickborne zoonoses: babesiosis, human granulocytic ehrlichiosis, and Lyme disease. *Clin Infect Dis.* 2002;34:1184-1191.
23. Communitywide cryptosporidiosis outbreak—Utah, 2007. *MMWR Morb Mortal Wkly Rep.* 2008;57:989-993.
24. Vannier E, Gewurz BE, Krause PJ. Human babesiosis. *Infect Dis Clin North Am.* 2008;22:469-488, viii-ix.
25. Karp CL, Auwaerter PG. Coinfection with HIV and tropical infectious diseases. II. Helminthic, fungal, bacterial, and viral pathogens. *Clin Infect Dis.* 2007;45:1214-1220.
26. Guerrant RL. Cryptosporidiosis: an emerging, highly infectious threat. *Emerg Infect Dis.* 1997;3:51-57.
27. Fishbein DB. Rabies. *Infect Dis Clin North Am.* 1991;5:53-71.
28. Tsai TF, Bauer SP, Sasso DR, et al. Serological and virulogical evidence of a Hantaan virus-related enzootic in the United States. *Infect Dis.* 1985;152:126-136.
29. Update: Hantavirus infection—United States, 1993. *MMWR Morb Mortal Wkly Rep.* 1993;42:517-519.
30. Mertz GJ, Hjelle B, Crowley M, et al. Diagnosis and treatment of new world Hantavirus infections. *Curr Opin Infect Dis.* 2006;196:437-442.
31. Glass GE, Yates TL, Fine JB, et al. Satellite imagery characterizes local animal reservoir populations of Sin Nombre virus in the southwestern United States. *Proc Natl Acad Sci U S A.* 2002;99:16817-16822.
32. Nash D, Mostashari F, Fine A, et al. The outbreak of West Nile virus infection in the New York City area in 1999. *N Engl J Med.* 2001;344:1807-1814.
33. West Nile virus update—United States, January 1-August 19, 2008. *MMWR Morb Mortal Wkly Rep.* 2008;57:899-900.
34. Reed KD, Melski JW, Graham MB, et al. The detection of monkeypox in humans in the Western Hemisphere. *N Engl J Med.* 2004;350:342-350.
35. Oldfield EC, Wallace MR, Hyams KC, et al. Endemic infectious diseases of the Middle East. *Rev Infect Dis.* 1991;13(Suppl 3):S119-217.
36. Deresinski S. Health hazards in Somalia. *Infect Dis Alert.* 1993;12:69-72.
37. Nguyen DR. Illness in a redeployed soldier. *Mil Med.* 2007;172:541-543.
38. Gould EA, Solomon T. Pathogenic flaviviruses. *Lancet.* 2008;371:500-509.
39. Natiello M, Ritacco V, Morales MA, et al. Indigenous dengue fever, Buenos Aires, Argentina. *Emerg Infect Dis.* 2008;14:1498-1499.

40. Charrel RN, de Lamballerie X, Raoult D. Chikungunya outbreaks—the globalization of vectorborne diseases. *N Engl J Med.* 2007;356:769-771.
41. Wilson ME. *A World Guide to Infections: Disease, Distribution, Diagnosis.* New York: Oxford University Press; 1991.
42. Centers for Disease Control and Prevention. *Health Information for International Travel 2008: The Yellow Book.* Atlanta, GA: US Department of Health and Human Services, Public Health Service, 2007. Available at <http://wwwn.cdc.gov/travel/content/yellowbook/home-2008.aspx>. Accessed June 18, 2009. See also <http://www.cdc.gov/travel/desinations/list.aspx>. Accessed June 18, 2009.
43. Colwell R, Epstein P, Gubler D, et al. Global climate change and infectious diseases. *Emerg Infect Dis.* 1998;4:451-452.
44. Lindgren E, Gustafson R. Tick-borne encephalitis in Sweden and climate change. *Lancet.* 2001;358:16-18.
45. Angelini P, Macini P, Finarelli AC, et al. Chikungunya epidemic outbreak in Emilia-Romagna (Italy) during summer 2007. *Parassitologia.* 2008;50:97-98.
46. Epstein RP, Diaz HF, Elias S, et al. Biological and physical signs of climate change: focus on mosquito-borne disease. *Bull Am Meteorol Soc.* 1998;78:409-417.
47. Afrane YA, Little TJ, Lawson BW, et al. Deforestation and vectorial capacity of *Anopheles gambiae* Giles mosquitoes in malaria transmission, Kenya. *Emerg Infect Dis.* 2008;14:1533-1538.
48. Githeko AK, Ndegwa W. Predicting malaria epidemics in the Kenyan highlands using climate data: a tool for decision makers. *Global Change and Human Health.* 2001;2:54-63.
49. Van Ness GB. Ecology of anthrax. *Science.* 1971;172:1303-1307.
50. Kontoyiannis DP, Calia KE, Basgoz N, et al. Primary septicemia caused by *Vibrio cholerae* non-O1 acquired on Cape Cod, Massachusetts. *Clin Infect Dis.* 1995;21:1330-1333.
51. McLaughlin JB, DePaola A, Bopp CA, et al. Outbreak of *Vibrio parahaemolyticus* gastroenteritis associated with Alaskan oysters. *N Engl J Med.* 2005;353:1463-1470.
52. Wilson ME, Levins R, Speilman A, eds. Diseases in evolution: global changes and emergence of infectious diseases. *Ann N Y Acad Sci.* 1994;740:1-461.
53. Tzipori S, Widmer G. A hundred-year retrospective on cryptosporidiosis. *Trends Parasitol.* 2008;24:184-189.
54. Isaac-Renton JL, Cordeiro C, Sarafis K, et al. Characterization of *Giardia duodenalis* isolates from a waterborne outbreak. *J Infect Dis.* 1993;167:431-440.
55. Jackson LA, Kaufmann AF, Adams WG, et al. Outbreak of leptospirosis associated with swimming. *Pediatr Infect Dis J.* 1993;12:48-54.
56. Morgan J, Bornstein SL, Karpati AM, et al. Outbreak of leptospirosis among triathlon participants and community residents in Springfield, Illinois, 1998. *Clin Infect Dis.* 2002;34:1593-1599.
57. Russell RC. Survival of insects in the wheel bays of a Boeing 747 aircraft on flights between tropical and temperate airports. *Bull World Health Organ.* 1987;65:659-662.
58. Momen H. Emerging infectious diseases—Brazil. *Emerg Infect Dis.* 1998;4:1-3.
59. Goldberg TL, Gillespie TR, Rwego IB, et al. Forest fragmentation as cause of bacterial transmission among nonhuman primates, humans, and livestock, Uganda. *Emerg Infect Dis.* 2008;14:1375-1382.

60. Young LS, Bicknell DS, Archer BG, et al. Tularemia epidemic: Vermont 1968. *N Engl J Med.* 1969;280:1253-1260.
61. Salgo MP, Telzak BE, Currie B, et al. A focus of Rocky Mountain spotted fever within New York City. *N Engl J Med.* 1988;318:1345-1348.
62. Steere AC. Lyme disease. *N Engl J Med.* 1989;321:586-596.
63. Field H, Young P, Yob JM, et al. The natural history of Hendra and Nipah viruses. *Microbes Infect.* 2001;3:307-314.
64. Lam SK, Chu KB. Nipah virus encephalitis outbreak in Malaysia. *Clin Infect Dis.* 2002;34(Suppl 2):548-551.
65. Chua KB, Chua BH, Wang CW. Anthropogenic deforestation, El Nino and the emergence of Nipah virus in Malaysia. *Malays J Pathol.* 2002;24:15-21.
66. Capellan J, Fong IW. Tularemia from a cat bite: case report and review of feline-associated tularemia. *Clin Infect Dis.* 1993;16:472-475.
67. Extension of the raccoon rabies epizootic—United States, 1992. *MMWR Morb Mortal Wkly Rep.* 1992;41:661-664.
68. Stirling J, Griffith M, Dooley JS, et al. Zoonoses associated with petting farms and open zoos. *Vector Borne Zoonotic Dis.* 2008;8:85-92.
69. Payeur JB, Jarnagin JL, Marquardt JG, Whipple DL. Mycobacterial isolations in captive elephants in the United States. *Ann N Y Acad Sci.* 2002;969:256-258.
70. Telford SR 3rd, Pollack RJ, Spielman A. Emerging vector-borne infections. *Infect Dis Clin North Am.* 1991;5:7-18.
71. Jones CO, Ostfeld RS, Richard MP, et al. Chain reactions linking acorns to gypsy moth outbreaks and Lyme disease risk. *Science.* 1998;279:1023-1026.
72. Kennedy D. A tiger tale. *Science.* 2002;297:1445.
73. Dalla Pozza GL, Romi R, Severini C. Source and spread of *Aedes albopictus* in the Veneto region of Italy. *J Am Mosq Control Assoc.* 1994;10:589-592.
74. Mitchell O, Niebylski ML, Smith GC, et al. Isolation of eastern equine encephalitis virus from *Aedes albopictus* in Florida. *Science.* 1992;257:526-527.
75. Parker RR, Spencer RR. Hereditary transmission of tularemia infection by the wood tick, *Dermacentor andersoni*, Stiles. *Public Health Rep.* 1926;41:1341-1355.
76. DuPont HL. The growing threat of foodborne bacterial enteropathogens of animal origin. *Clin Infect Dis.* 2007;45:1353-1361.
77. Jay MT, Cooley M, Carychao D, et al. *Escherichia coli* O157:H7 in feral swine near spinach fields and cattle, central California coast. *Emerg Infect Dis.* 2007;13:1908-1911.
78. Jenkins SR, Winkler WG. Descriptive epidemiology from an epizootic of raccoon rabies in the Middle Atlantic states, 1982-1983. *Am J Epidemiol.* 1987;126:429-437.
79. Fevre EM, Bronsvoort BM, Hamilton KA, Cleaveland S. Animal movements and the spread of infectious diseases. *Trends Microbiol.* 2006;14:125-131.
80. Inhalation anthrax associated with dried animal hides—Pennsylvania and New York City, 2006. *MMWR Morb Mortal Wkly Rep.* 2006;55:280-282.
81. Langley JM, Marrie TJ, Covert A, et al. Poker players' pneumonia: an urban outbreak of Q fever following exposure to a parturient cat. *N Engl J Med.* 1988;319:354-356.
82. Weinberg AN. Respiratory infections transmitted from animals. *Infect Dis Clin North Am.* 1991;5:649-661.
83. Relman DA. Detection and identification of previously unrecognized microbial pathogens. *Emerg Infect Dis.* 1998;4:382-389.

329

Protection of Travelers

DAVID O. FREEDMAN

The pretravel management of the international traveler should be based on risk management principles. Prevention strategies and medical interventions need to be individualized according to both the itinerary and factors that are dependent on the traveler. A structured approach to patient interaction (Table 329-1) is the most efficient way to cover the necessary educational and preventive interventions. As many of these measures will be initiated only much later at the traveler's destination, clearly printed instructions in lay language are advisable. The worldwide epidemiology of travel-related diseases is constantly changing. A body of knowledge in travel medicine has been published, and online and print resources (Table 329-2) should be consulted frequently[1,2] to keep current.

Epidemiology of Travel-Related Illness

Globally, approximately 100 million people travel from industrialized to developing countries each year. Of note, travel to Africa, which presents a particularly high risk for a number of infectious diseases, is undertaken each year by many fewer (800,000) U.S. residents than European residents. Much of the most widely quoted travel-related health data is older than a decade and may not all be applicable at present.[3] Two recent analyses have provided much needed new data on the profiles of travel-related illness determined by destination of travel.[4,5] Depending on destination, 22% to 64% of travelers report some illness; most of these problems are mild, self-limited illnesses such as diarrhea, respiratory infections, and skin disorders.[3] Rates are significantly higher in summer. Approximately 8% of travelers consult a physician either during or after a trip, but less than 1% require hospitalization. Infectious diseases account for up to 10% of the morbidity during travel but only 1% of the deaths, with malaria being the most common disease. Causes of death vary according to population studied. At destinations that attract seniors, cardiovascular events predominate, whereas in developing countries motor vehicle accidents and drowning prevail.

Immunization

The choice of vaccines for an individual traveler is based on risk of exposure to vaccine-preventable diseases on the chosen itinerary, the severity of disease if acquired, and any risks presented by the vaccine itself. Travelers differ in their tolerance of risk. Requests for immunization against diseases that are actually of negligible risk to the traveler but have the potential for poor outcome if acquired are often difficult for the physician to refuse, because sporadic travel-related cases do occur each year. For the vaccine-preventable diseases, the monthly incidence for non-immune travelers to developing countries is most significant for symptomatic hepatitis A (HA) at .03% per month overall and is still considerable for perceived low-risk destinations such as Mexico.[6] The risk of symptomatic hepatitis B (HB) is most significant for long-stay travelers and expatriates at .25% per month. Enteric fever (typhoid and paratyphoid) has a risk of .03% per month on the Indian subcontinent and is 10 times lower in Africa and parts of Latin America.[5,7] Risk of yellow fever (YF) may be as high as .1% per month of travel to an area with current epidemic transmission, but the risk varies greatly between destinations encompassed by the endemic area map.[8] The risk of meningococcal meningitis, rabies, cholera, polio, measles, varicella, and Japanese encephalitis in travelers is not known but is thought to be small (<.0001%) even for travel to highly endemic areas.

Table 329-3 provides data on dosing, administration, need for boosters, and possible accelerated regimens for vaccines administered in the travel medicine setting. Details on vaccine composition, mechanism of action, use for routine adult and childhood primary vaccination, and adverse reactions can be found in Chapter 320. The following discussion focuses on indications for each vaccine in the context of travel.

UPDATE OF ROUTINE IMMUNIZATIONS

Because of the increased prevalence of many infections in the developing world, routine adult immunizations need to be current.[9] Tetanus/diphtheria/acellular pertussis boosters should usually be given if more than 10 years have elapsed since the last tetanus/diphtheria vaccination, but travelers to remote areas where tetanus toxoid (which would be indicated in cases of dirty trauma) will be inaccessible, should get boosters at 5-year intervals. Persons born in the United States before 1957 or born anytime in the developing world are considered immune to measles. Other adult travelers should have received at least two doses of live measles containing vaccine during their life unless a history of measles infection can be documented. Although persons born before 1957 in the United States are presumed to be immune, one dose of MMR or one dose each of single-antigen mumps vaccine and single-antigen measles vaccine should be considered for such persons without other evidence of immunity who are traveling for purposes of health care or humanitarian work that has the potential to put them in close contact with persons who are ill. Unvaccinated persons who have the accepted routine indications for influenza or pneumococcal vaccines (see Chapter 320) should receive these during the pretravel consultation. Varicella is primarily a disease of adolescents and young adults in tropical, nonindustrialized countries. Two doses of varicella vaccine spaced by at least 4 weeks should be considered for adult travelers without evidence of varicella immunity. Adults born before 1980 in the United States are considered immune.

VACCINES TO CONSIDER FOR ALL DESTINATIONS IN THE DEVELOPING WORLD

Hepatitis A

HA vaccine is indicated for every non-immune traveler to countries or areas with moderate to high risk of infection (Fig. 329-1), which includes essentially everyone traveling outside the United States, Canada, Japan, Australia, New Zealand, Scandinavian countries, and developed countries in Europe. A single dose of hepatitis A vaccine given any time before travel provides adequate protection. The Centers for Disease Control and Prevention (CDC) recommends ancillary concomitant immune globulin for travelers older than 40 years of age who are planning to depart in 2 weeks or less,[9] but this recommendation has not been widely adopted in practice. Individuals born in the developing world are generally immune to HA. Persons with a history of hepatitis or who previously lived in an endemic country for a prolonged period may benefit from prevaccination serum antibody testing.

Hepatitis B

Travelers born in the United States after 1992 already have received a HB vaccine series. Pretravel HB vaccination is indicated for all nonvac-

TABLE 329-1	A Structured Approach to the Pretravel Office Visit with a Traveler to the Developing World

Perform Risk Assessment

The following must always be ascertained to determine appropriate preventive medical recommendations. Preprinted medical record forms may be used to record these.

Exact itinerary, including regions within each country to be visited
Dates of travel to assess risk of seasonal diseases
Age
Past vaccination history
Underlying illness(es)
Current medications
Pregnancy status
Allergies
Purpose of trip
Risk exposures—blood, body fluids, adventure or extensive outdoor exposures
Urban versus rural travel
Type of accomodations
Level of aversion to risk
Financial limitations that may necessitate prioritization of interventions

Administer Immunizations

Administer routine vaccinations that are not up to date.
Administer indicated travel vaccines.
Provide to patient legally mandated Vaccine Information Statements from the Centers for Disease Control and Prevention (http://www.cdc.gov/vaccines/pubs/vis/).
Provide printed checklist to patient listing vaccines administered.
Record in the clinic record vaccines administered, lot number, and date. Document vaccines offered to but declined by patient, as well as nonrecommended vaccines administered at the patient's request.

Provide Malaria Prevention (if Indicated)

Determine whether malaria risk exists for the destination country. If yes:
  Does the patient's itinerary within that country put him or her at risk? If yes:
    Recommend malaria chemoprophylaxis. Several equally effective drugs of choice may be indicated. Ascertain which is best suited to the individual patient and itinerary.
Educate on personal protection against arthropods.

Educate on Traveler's Diarrhea

Recommend food and water precautions.
Prescribe and educate on standby therapy with a quinolone antibiotic or azithromycin and advise on use of loperamide and oral hydration if needed.

Teach Essential Preventive Behaviors

Most travel-related health problems, including vaccine-preventable diseases, can be avoided through simple behaviors initiated by the traveler.
Educate on appropriate strategies in the following categories (some topics are not applicable to all destinations): blood-borne and sexually transmitted diseases, safety and crime avoidance, injury prevention, swimming safety, rabies, skin/wound care, tuberculosis, packing for healthy travel, obtaining health care abroad.

Discuss Other Applicable Heath Issues

Advise and prescribe for altitude illness, motion sickness, or jet-leg.
Discuss prevention of specific travel-related infections that are of some risk to the traveler and have a possible preventive strategy not included in strategies above.
Discuss any minimal-risk conditions (e.g., hemorrhagic fevers) that are a frequent cause of patient anxiety.

TABLE 329-2	In-depth Information Resources for Travel Medicine

Authoritative Websites Updated Constantly with Epidemiologic and Outbreak Information

Centers for Disease Control and Prevention (CDC) Travelers Health
www.cdc.gov/travel
World Health Organization (WHO) Travelers Health
www.who.int/ith
Health Canada. Committee to Advise on Tropical Medicine And Travel (CATMAT)
http://www.phac-aspc.gc.ca/tmp-pmv/catmat-ccmtmv/index-eng.php
WHO Disease Outbreak News
http://www.who.int/csr/don/en/
WHO Weekly Epidemiological Record
www.who.int/wer
CDC Morbidity and Mortality Weekly Report
www.cdc.gov/mmwr
WHO Disease by Disease Health Topics
www.who.int/health_topics/en/
In-Depth References on Specialized Topics
Centers for Disease Control and Prevention. Health Information for International Travel 2010. (The "CDC Yellow Book"). U.S. Public Health Service. Atlanta. Order from www.phf.org. Full text and hard copy order information at http://wwwn.cdc.gov/travel/contentYellowBook.aspx
World Health Organization. International Travel and Health 2009. (WHO "Green" Book). Published annually. Available from authorized WHO book agents. Full text online at www.who.int/ith
Keystone JS, Kozarsky P, Freedman DO, et al, eds. Travel Medicine. 2nd ed. St. Louis: Mosby 2008. (ISBN: 9780323034531)
Plotkin SA, Orenstein WA, Offit P. Vaccines. 5th ed. Philadelphia: WB Saunders; 2008. (ISBN:9781416036111)
Schlagenhauf-Lawlor P. Travelers' Malaria. 2nd ed. Hamilton, Ontario, Canada: BC Decker; 2008. (ISBN 9781550093360)
Auerbach PS. Wilderness Medicine. 5th ed. St. Louis: Mosby; 2007. (ISBN 9780323032285)

istering all three primary doses necessary for high assurance of protection in the frequent circumstance in which the traveler is leaving in a very short time and is at risk of HB exposure.[10]

Combination Hepatitis A and Hepatitis B Vaccine

The combined HA and HB vaccine provides convenience for travelers with an overlap of indications for use of the individual vaccines. The accelerated 3-week schedule (see Table 329-3) was licensed in the United States in 2007.[11]

Typhoid

Typhoid vaccine is indicated for all travelers to the Indian subcontinent and considered for those traveling to other endemic areas under all but the most deluxe and protected of conditions. Risk increases with trip duration, lodging and/or eating with local residents, and extent of travel off the usual tourist itineraries. In risk areas, food and water precautions should still be followed rigorously, as typhoid vaccines are only from 53% to 72% protective[12] and a large oral inoculum may overwhelm even an optimal antibody response. The recent increase in quinolone-resistant *Salmonella typhi* in Asia has decreased the threshold for typhoid vaccination, because infection, once acquired, requires in-patient parenteral therapy with ceftriaxone or a carbapenem.[13] Current typhoid vaccines do not protect against *Salmonella paratyphi*, which is emerging in many areas.[13] Adherence to the oral vaccine regimen may be as low as 70%.[14]

Influenza

Influenza is transmitted year round in the tropics. Increasing data show that influenza may be the most common vaccine-preventable illness in travelers.[15-17] An increased risk of influenza has been reported among cruise ship passengers.[18] All travelers to destinations with current influenza virus circulation, not just those with the usual risk factors, should strongly consider influenza vaccination.[19] No proven benefit has been demonstrated to revaccinating persons before summer travel who were already vaccinated the previous fall.

cinated travelers with standard indications, such as health care workers, and all longer-stay travelers who will be visiting or residing in high- or moderate-risk areas (see Fig. 329-1). Transmission via routes such as sexual contact, blood transfusions, contaminated medical equipment, body piercing, tattooing, acupuncture, and sharing of cooking and bathroom facilities is difficult to control or predict in the context of travel. Vaccination is usually advocated for short-term travelers, especially younger travelers and those anticipating close contact with local populations, even if they have no specific risk factors. Adventure travelers (accident prone), backpackers, and those with underlying medical conditions are more likely to require contact with the medical system. Business and other regular travelers who fly internationally on multiple but short trips have a cumulative risk that increases with time, and such individuals should receive the HB vaccine. Accelerated and hyperaccelerated schedules (see Table 329-3) are used widely in practice and are approved in many countries. These are helpful in admin-

TABLE 329-3	Travel-Related Vaccines of Adults				
Disease	*Vaccine*	*Primary Course*	*Route*	*Further Boosters*
Vaccines to Consider for All Destinations				
Hepatitis A	Killed virus	0, 6-18 mo*	IM	None
Hepatitis B	Recombinant viral antigen	0, 1, 6 mo	IM	None
		A: 0, 1, 2, and 12 mo	IM	None
		A: 0, 1, 3 wk and 12 mo†	IM	
Hepatitis A/B	Combination of monovalent preparations	0, 1, 6 mo	IM	None
		A: 0, 1, 3 wk and 12 mo	IM	None
Typhoid	Capsular Vi polysaccharide	Single dose	IM	2-3 yr
	Live attenuated Ty21a bacteria	0, 2, 4, 6 days	Oral	5 yr
Influenza	Inactivated viral	Single dose	IM	Annual
	Live attenuated virus	Single dose	Nasal	Annual
Varicella	Live attenuated virus	0, 4-8 wk	SC	None
Vaccines for Selected Destinations				
Yellow fever	Live attenuated 17D virus	Single dose	SC	10 yr
Meningococcus	Quadrivalent conjugated polysaccharide (A, C, Y, W135)	Single dose	IM	>10 yr
Rabies	Inactivated cell culture viral	0, 7, 21-28 days	IM‡	None routinely but two doses after each exposure
Japanese encephalitis (Vero cell)	Inactivated viral	0, 28 days	IM	Unknown at present
Polio§	Inactivated viral	Single dose if adequate childhood series	SC; IM acceptable	None
Cholera	Killed bacteria + recombinant B toxin subunit¶	0, 1 wk	Oral	2 yr for cholera; 3 mo for ETEC
Tick-borne encephalitis**	Inactivated viral	0, 1-3 mo, 9-12 mo	IM	3 yr

*Second dose may be delayed up to 8 years without diminished efficacy.
†Regimen not approved by the U.S. Food and Drug Administration for monovalent HB vaccine but approved for combination Hep A/B vaccine containing the same quantity of HB antigen.
‡Intradermal rabies pre-exposure vaccine is no longer produced, and the intramuscular 1.0-mL vials are not licensed for intradermal use in a 0.1-mL dose.
§Oral polio vaccine is no longer produced in the United States.
‖Not available in the United States but available in Canada and most European countries. No cholera vaccine of any kind is currently available in the United States.
¶Also licensed in some countries for traveler's diarrhea due to enterotoxigenic *Escherichia coli*.
**Not available in United States but available in endemic areas and in Canada and the United Kingdom by special release.
A, accelerated regimen to be used for imminent departures; ETEC, enterotoxigenic *E. coli;* IM, intramuscular; SC, subcutaneous.

VACCINES TO CONSIDER ONLY FOR CERTAIN DESTINATIONS

Yellow Fever

The primary indication for YF vaccination is to prevent infection in individuals at risk. However, YF is currently the only vaccine that falls under the International Health Regulations that may necessitate vaccination purely for regulatory reasons.[20] Neither YF vaccine nor any other vaccine is currently required for readmission to the United States. In general, all healthy adult travelers to areas with a risk of yellow fever transmission (see Fig. 329-1) should be vaccinated. This endemic area may be restricted to only a portion of a country. Because of rare but serious vaccine-associated adverse side effects (see Chapter 320), persons who are not at any risk of exposure should not be vaccinated.[21] Urban YF rarely occurs in South America, but a number of urban areas are considered to have potential risk. Short-term travel that is restricted to very large urban areas in the endemic zone of South America carries negligible, if any, risk, but the situation may change rapidly. It is prudent to vaccinate persons who have anything less than a definite, fixed itinerary and who will travel anywhere close to regions with risk of transmission.

A number of African countries (Angola, Benin, Burkina Faso, Burundi, Cameroon, Central African Republic, Congo, Côte d'Ivoire, Democratic Republic of Congo, Gabon, Ghana, Liberia, Mali, Niger, Rwanda, São Tomé, Sierra Leone, Togo) and one in South America (French Guiana) require proof of YF vaccination from all arriving travelers. Other countries, both within and outside the risk zone, have submitted more complex requirements to the World Health Organization. They may require an official vaccination certificate only for individuals arriving directly from or via (may include a brief transit

stop) a country in the YF endemic zone but not from arriving travelers from other countries. These YF-free countries usually have the conditions and vectors to initiate a YF transmission cycle, and the purpose of the vaccine requirement is to prevent entry of viremic travelers. Current country-by-country YF entry requirements are at www.who.int/ith. The requirement often applies even if the arriving traveler has not visited an area within a country of departure that is endemic for YF.

A special permit, obtainable in the United States from state health departments, is required to legally stamp an international certificate of vaccination as an authorized YF vaccine center. The International Health Regulations enable clinicians who decide that YF vaccine is contraindicated on medical grounds to provide the traveler with a letter stating the reasons for that opinion, which can be presented to immigration authorities upon arrival at the destination. Acceptance of such "waiver letters" is at the complete discretion of the destination country.[20] On arrival, the receiving country may also quarantine the traveler for up to 6 days or request that the traveler be placed under surveillance.

No specific format exists for written documentation of medical contraindication. Letters of waiver are most appropriate for individuals needing a certificate purely for regulatory reasons. Waiver letters should be given with great reluctance for those with medical contraindications to vaccination (see Chapter 320) who plan to visit an endemic area. The variable risk within the endemic regions of the world needs to be considered (in consultation with an expert, if necessary), and cancellation of travel should be recommended strongly if the risk is more than negligible. A YF certificate becomes valid for entry 10 days after it is stamped and dated. Although officially valid for 10 years, the true duration of immunity from YF vaccination is probably

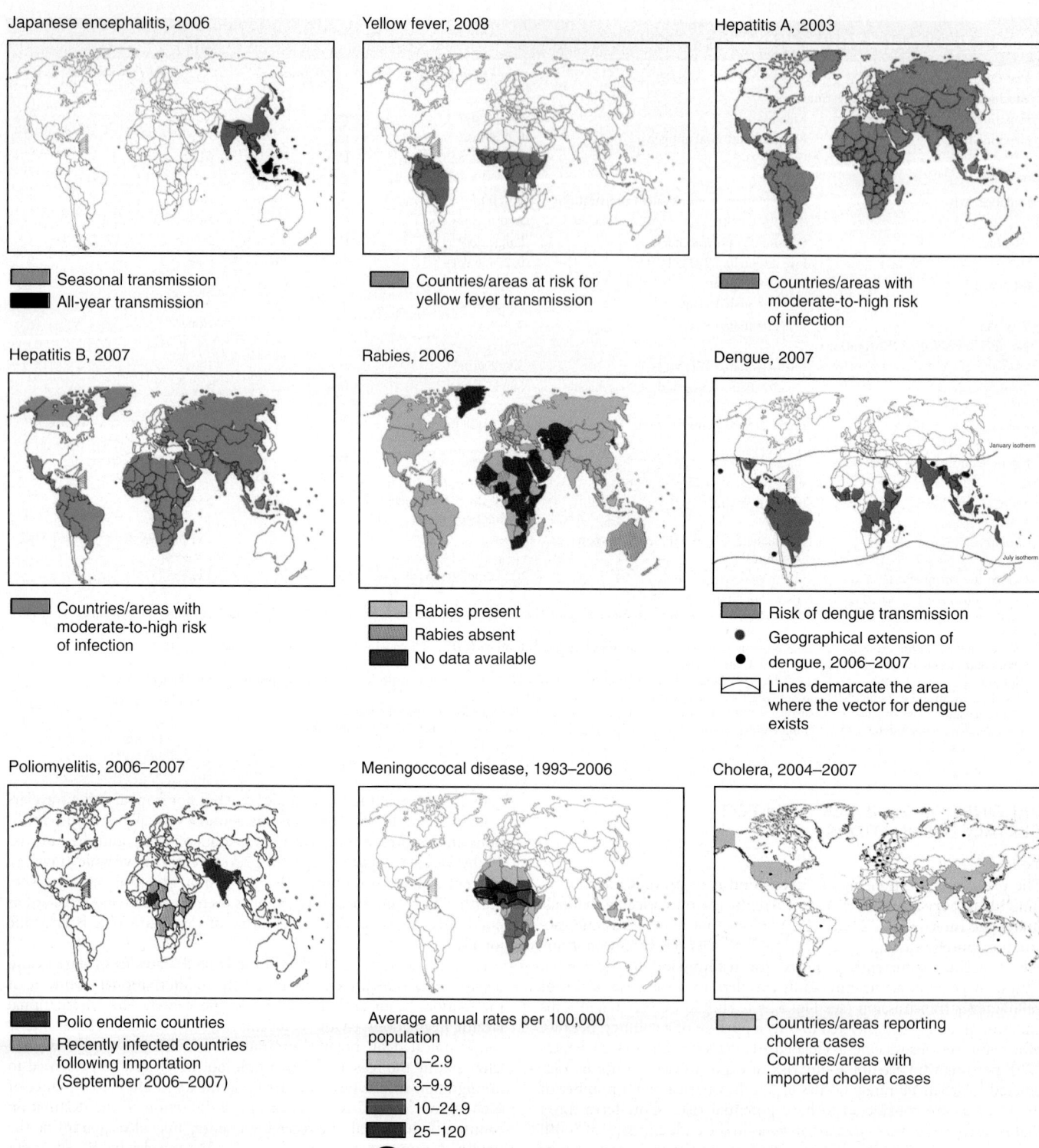

Japanese encephalitis, 2006
- Seasonal transmission
- All-year transmission

Yellow fever, 2008
- Countries/areas at risk for yellow fever transmission

Hepatitis A, 2003
- Countries/areas with moderate-to-high risk of infection

Hepatitis B, 2007
- Countries/areas with moderate-to-high risk of infection

Rabies, 2006
- Rabies present
- Rabies absent
- No data available

Dengue, 2007
- Risk of dengue transmission
- Geographical extension of dengue, 2006–2007
- Lines demarcate the area where the vector for dengue exists

Poliomyelitis, 2006–2007
- Polio endemic countries
- Recently infected countries following importation (September 2006–2007)

Meningoccocal disease, 1993–2006
Average annual rates per 100,000 population
- 0–2.9
- 3–9.9
- 10–24.9
- 25–120
- Meningitis belt

Cholera, 2004–2007
- Countries/areas reporting cholera cases
- Countries/areas with imported cholera cases

Figure 329-1 **Worldwide distribution of important travel-related diseases.** *(Reprinted with permission of the World Health Organization <http://www.who.int/ith/maps/en/>.)*

much longer and may exceed 30 years. A few countries may enforce YF regulations on individuals who have been in endemic areas as much as 30 days previously even though the International Health Regulations recognize only up to a 6-day requirement.

Meningococcus
Meningococcal vaccine is recommended for travelers to Africa's sub-Saharan "meningitis belt" (see Fig. 329-1) during the dry season from December through June, especially if prolonged contact with the local populace is likely. Out-of-season epidemics have recently begun to occur in Ethiopia, Somalia, and Tanzania, indicating possible changes in epidemiologic trends perhaps due to climate changes.[22,23] Muslims undertaking Hajj and Umrah pilgrimages in Saudi Arabia are at a higher risk of meningococcal disease, and proof of vaccination with quadrivalent vaccine within the past 3 years is required to obtain pilgrimage visas.[24]

Rabies

A pre-exposure rabies series is indicated for long-stay travel to endemic areas of Latin America, Asia, or Africa (see Fig. 329-1), where the rabies threat is constant and where access to adequate postexposure rabies immune globulin and vaccine is likely to be limited. Countries with the highest risk of rabies include the Indian subcontinent, Thailand, Vietnam, and most sub-Saharan African countries. For short-term travel, risk groups for whom immunization should be considered include adventure travelers, bikers, hikers, cave explorers, or business travelers who travel for short but frequent trips and plan to go running outdoors on these trips. Regardless of vaccination status, travelers should be instructed to cleanse well with soapy water any bite or animal scratch involving broken skin immediately and to seek postexposure treatment for rabies (see Chapter 163).

Japanese Encephalitis

Japanese encephalitis (JE) is endemic to many rural farming areas of Southeast Asia and the Indian subcontinent (see Fig. 329-1). Sporadic cases with severe sequelae continue to occur in travelers. In temperate regions, the transmission season is from April through November. In tropical or subtropical regions of Oceania and Southeast Asia, transmission may occur year round. Vaccination is recommended for (1) long-stay travel to an endemic rural area; (2) expatriation to anywhere in an endemic country; (3) short-term travel to endemic rural areas with extensive unprotected outdoor exposure, such as with adventure travel; or (4) short-term travel in the face of a current local epidemic.[25] A new, inactivated vero cell JE vaccine with an excellent safety profile replaced the older more toxic mouse brain JE vaccine in 2009 and is FDA-approved for sale in the United States.[26,27]

Polio

Because of eradication efforts, poliomyelitis remains in only a few countries, but complete control remains elusive (see Fig. 329-1). Adults traveling to countries that are currently polio endemic (updated information at www.polioeradication.org) and who have previously completed a primary vaccine series should receive a one-time single dose of inactivated polio vaccine as a booster if the last dose or booster dose was administered at least 10 years previously.

Cholera

Cholera vaccination is no longer required by any country, and the risk to typical travelers is insignificant.[28] However, medical and aid workers staying for short periods in disaster areas or refugee camps may consider cholera vaccine. The parenteral inactivated vaccine is no longer available in the United States and has been officially disowned by World Health Organization. A highly effective oral killed whole cell–B subunit vaccine[28] is available widely outside the United States. This vaccine also has about 50% efficacy against enterotoxigenic *Escherichia coli* and a 7% to 23% efficacy against all traveler's diarrhea (TD) and has this indication in some countries (see Fig. 329-1).

Tick-Borne Encephalitis

Tick-borne encephalitis (TBE) is an emerging, important, and serious flavivirus central nervous system infection in endemic areas. Distribution is highly focal in a range that extends in a swath from Germany through Scandinavia and the Baltic to Siberia and Vladivostok in the east. Risk to travelers is low unless extensive outdoor activities are planned in forested regions in endemic areas.[29] Immunization against TBE is recommended for adventure travel, extensive outdoor exposure, or camping in the forests of the endemic countries between April and October. Tick precautions are also recommended. The vaccine is available in most endemic countries and by special release in Canada and the United Kingdom.[30]

SPACING AND INTERACTIONS OF TRAVEL-RELATED VACCINES

All currently indicated immunizations can and should be given at the same time and in any combination. If two live viral antigens are not administered on the same day, they must be spaced by a month. However, YF vaccine can be given at any interval with respect to single-antigen measles vaccine. Live oral vaccines (typhoid, polio) can be administered at any interval with respect to any live virus vaccine. Minimum intervals between vaccine doses must be respected, although 4 or fewer days before the next interval are acceptable.[31] Regimens that involve 1-week intervals (rabies, JE, accelerated hepatitis) are exceptions. There is not a maximum interval between doses of a primary vaccine series; interrupted series (except oral typhoid and rabies) need not be restarted but can be resumed beginning with the dose that is overdue. Anaphylactic egg allergy precludes administration of YF, influenza, and measles/mumps/rubella (MMR) vaccines. No current vaccine contains penicillin. Baseline purified protein derivative (PPD) skin tests, often done in the pretravel setting, can be given on the day that live viral vaccines are administered or else must be done more than 4 weeks later. Antibacterial drugs should not be given within 24 hours of a dose of live oral typhoid or oral cholera vaccine. Concomitant mefloquine may interfere with oral typhoid vaccine.

Malaria Chemoprophylaxis

An average of 1500 imported cases of malaria are reported annually in the United States. Estimates of risk in travelers not taking chemoprophylaxis vary widely by destination but range from 3.4% per month in West Africa to one tenth that on the Indian subcontinent and a further 10-fold reduction in South America.[5,32] The majority of cases of imported malaria in the United States and Europe occur in noncitizen immigrants visiting friends and relatives abroad.[33] Malaria chemoprophylactic drugs are underutilized by these ethnic minority travelers. Eighty percent of all imported falciparum malaria originates in Africa.

Risk of travelers' malaria may not be the same as the risk for those in local populations. Travelers often operate in a more protected environment. Transmission, and in particular high transmission, is quite focal even within the shaded areas in Figure 329-2. In addition to the precise locations within the country or countries to be visited, the risk of travelers' malaria depends on the length of the trip, the season, whether the traveler adheres to precautions concerning mosquitoes, and whether the traveler spends the evening and nighttime hours where significant exposure to the vector may occur. Restriction of nighttime activities to air-conditioned hotels or other locations where there are few mosquitoes reduces the risk. With the exception of sub-Saharan Africa and certain cities in India, travel restricted to capital cities and other urban areas (as is typical of business travel) is associated with no risk or an insignificant risk of contracting malaria, despite the risk in areas nearby. The lifetime range of flight of an *Anopheles* mosquito is 1 km. Daytime side trips to malarious areas present no risk. At the same time, exposure to mosquitoes for even a few hours in an area with a high risk of transmission may result in infection. The decision regarding whether to prescribe chemoprophylaxis should also take into account the possibility of deviation from the preset itinerary brought to the pretravel consultation, as well as the traveler's personal tolerance for what may be an epidemiologically insignificant level of risk for the specific trip.

Resources describing current country-specific malaria microepidemiology should be accessible immediately to those prescribing malaria prophylaxis (see Table 329-1). Dosing and pharmaceutical properties of antimalarial drugs are described in Chapters 44 and 275. Drug resistance patterns that affect the choice of an antimalarial drug for chemoprophylaxis are shown in Figure 329-2. In the limited number of countries where it is still effective, chloroquine, 500 mg salt (300 mg base) per week beginning the week before the first exposure to malaria and continuing for 4 weeks after the last exposure, is still the drug of choice, however atovaquone/proguanil may still be used by short-stay travelers who prefer the shorter duration of that regimen.

For all other areas of the world, three drugs are equally effective, and the choice depends on both traveler and itinerary factors. Atovaquone/proguanil (250/100 mg) is a well-tolerated, once-a-day drug that should be started 1 day before arrival in the malarious area (may not

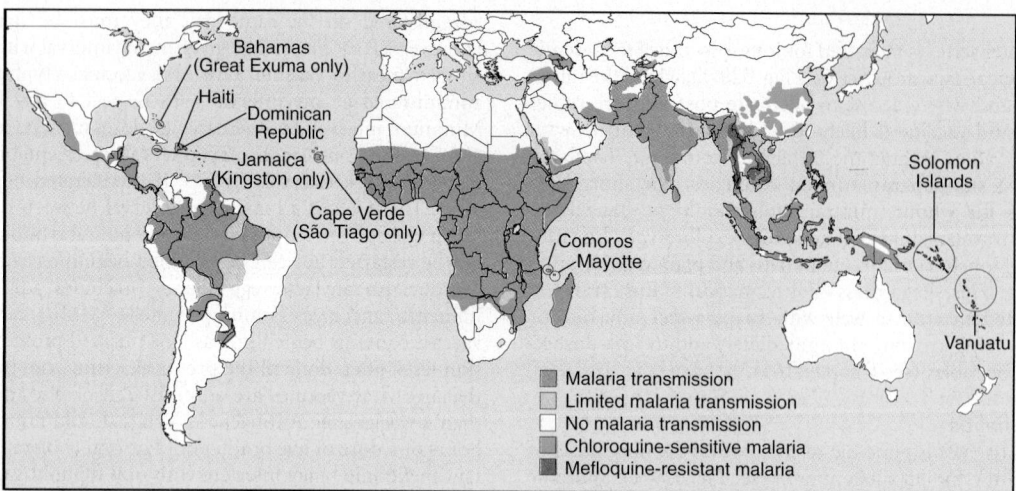

Figure 329-2 Shading indicates areas where malaria is endemic, and stippling indicates drug sensitivity patterns that affect choice of prophylactic agent. *(Reprinted with permission from Freedman DO. Clinical practice. Malaria prevention in short-term travelers. N Engl J Med. 2008;359:603-612.)*

coincide with first overseas destination) and continued for 7 days after the last exposure. The short period of postexposure use makes it convenient for the many travelers on typical 1- to 3-week itineraries. High cost and daily dosing make it difficult to use for extended periods. Weekly mefloquine (250 mg) is given 2 and preferably 3 weeks before the first exposure to malaria and continued for 4 weeks thereafter. Weekly dosing and a long track record of efficacy make this drug the most effective for long-stay travelers. If contraindications to mefloquine exist for long-stay travelers, daily doxycycline (100 mg) beginning 1 day before exposure can be used; unlike atovaquone/proguanil, it must be continued for 4 weeks after exposure. Generic doxycycline is by far the cheapest of the antimalarials, so it is attractive to both short- and long-stay budget travelers. For travelers to chloroquine-sensitive areas who are unable to tolerate chloroquine, any of the three latter drugs are effective. Approximately 5% of individuals who take either mefloquine or doxycycline discontinue therapy because of side effects.[34] Chemoprophylaxis may be started well before departure (3 to 4 weeks for mefloquine) in those concerned about possible intolerance to any drug. Mefloquine has been associated with neuro-psychiatric side effects[35] in some and should not be prescribed for persons with active depression or a recent history of depression, generalized anxiety disorder, psychosis, schizophrenia, or other major psychiatric disorder. It should be used with caution in patients with a previous history of depression. If prodromal psychiatric symptoms occur during use, the drug should be discontinued and an alternative medication substituted. Doxycycline is an esophageal and gastric irritant. It needs to be taken with a full glass of water on a full stomach, and the user should not go to sleep or lie down for 30 minutes after ingestion. Female travelers may get vaginal candidiasis and should carry self-therapy for candidiasis when prescribed doxycycline. The rare traveler intolerant of all of the three drugs may consider daily primaquine after consultation with a malaria expert and after G6PD testing.

Travelers should be reminded in writing to continue antimalarial drugs for the appropriate period after the last possible exposure, that malaria can still occur despite chemoprophylaxis, and that a malaria smear or malaria rapid card test is mandatory for any febrile illness occurring within 3 months after travel. Unless primaquine itself is used for primary prophylaxis during the trip, none of the primary prophylactic drugs discussed earlier is effective against the dormant hepatic hypnozoites of *Plasmodium vivax* or *Plasmodium ovale,* which may cause delayed relapses of malaria. Presumptive antirelapse therapy refers to a regimen at the end of the exposure period to kill residual hypnozoites of these two species. Per CDC guidelines, primaquine

30 mg base per day for 14 days, after checking G6PD levels, is indicated only for those with prolonged and extensive exposure to *P. vivax* or *P. ovale.* This effectively excludes most short-term travelers. Malaria chemoprophylaxis recommendations are likely to change periodically. Physicians may check the CDC or World Health Organization travel websites (see Table 329-2).

In destinations with mainly *P. vivax*, the CDC now recommends that primaquine can be considered as one of the first-line choices for primary malaria prophylaxis, as it has the added benefit of eliminating dormant hypnozoites and preventing later relapses with the use of a single drug regimen. Chloroquine-resistant *P. vivax* occurs only in areas in which the other drugs are already indicated for prophylaxis because of the concomitant presence of resistant *Plasmodium falciparum.*

For stays in areas with very low transmission rates of malaria, some physicians, notably in Europe, may advise that only a standby drug be carried, which should be taken in the event that symptoms suggestive of malaria occur and that there is no access to a physician or facility that can perform a competent malaria smear within 6 to 12 hours. This strategy is especially attractive for long-stay travelers. In areas with chloroquine-resistant *P. falciparum,* atovaquone/proguanil, four 250/100 tablets orally as a single daily dose for 3 consecutive days, or artemether/lumefantrine, four 20/120 mg tablets twice a day for 3 consecutive days, are recommended. In areas without chloroquine-resistant *P. falciparum,* chloroquine is the drug of choice. Prevention of malaria in travelers residing in malarious areas for 6 months or more presents complex problems that have been reviewed elsewhere.[36]

Dengue

An estimated 100 million cases of dengue fever (DF) and 250,000 cases of dengue hemorrhagic fever (DHF) occur annually (see Chapter 153). The past 20 years have seen a dramatic geographic expansion of epidemic DF and DHF (see Fig. 329-1). Dengue accounts for up to 2% of all illness in returned travelers who visit GeoSentinel clinics, and dengue is the most common systemic febrile illness in returned travelers from every region except sub-Saharan Africa, where malaria still predominates. Prospective seroconversion studies have estimated the attack rate of DF in travelers to the tropics to be 2.9% in Dutch travelers who spent 1 month in Asia; the seroconversion rate was 6.7% among Israelis who traveled for an average of 5 months. DF in returned travelers demonstrates seasonality in many parts of the world, with region-specific peaks for Southeast Asia (June, September), South Central Asia (October), South America (March), and the Caribbean

(August, October).[37] Several dengue vaccine candidates are in advanced clinical trials. DF is transmitted by day-biting *Aedes* mosquitoes, reinforcing the need to instruct travelers to the tropics in the need for both day and night use of repellents.

Traveler's Diarrhea

TD is the most common affliction of travelers to developing countries. Classic TD is defined as three or more unformed stools per day combined with one clinical sign, such as abdominal cramps, fever, nausea, or vomiting. The incidence varies from about 8% for travel to highly developed countries to about 20% in southern Europe, Israel, Japan, South Africa, and some Caribbean islands. In most developing countries, the risk is 20% to 66% in the first 2 weeks abroad and then somewhat less thereafter. The most frequent cause of TD is enterotoxigenic *E. coli* and in some locations enteroaggregative *E. coli*. *Salmonella*, *Shigella*, and *Campylobacter* each account for about 5% to 15%, and in Asia noncholera vibrios are significant. Protozoa account for less than 5%, and in adults, rarely, norovirus or rotavirus may be detected. Norovirus outbreaks may occur aboard cruise ships. About 30% of diarrheal episodes remain unexplained in routine clinical practice but apparently are of bacterial origin, because they appear to respond to antibacterials. Enteroaggregative *E. coli*, which is not routinely sought, may account for many of these cases. The mean duration of TD, even if untreated, is 4 days. A number of limited studies indicate that the incidence of postinfective irritable bowel syndrome at 6 months after an acute episode of TD may range from 4% to14%. The true incidence of this syndrome has not been determined, and ancillary contributing factors and possible preemptive interventions are still being investigated.[38]

Antibiotic prophylaxis for TD with a quinolone or with rifamixin has been demonstrated to be effective in many settings. Most guidelines do not recommend prophylaxis for the typical traveler because of potential adverse drug effects while away from medical care and because effective rapid onset therapy is available for diarrhea should it occur.[39] However, chemoprophylaxis can be considered for travelers with advanced human immunodeficiency virus (HIV) infection, for those who have an underlying chronic medical problem that makes them more prone to adverse consequences from diarrhea, and for travelers on a vital mission for a short period (less than 1 week) who cannot tolerate even a day of disability. Antibiotic prophylaxis should be carried out with a quinolone once per day or with rifamixin if travel is to an *E. coli*–predominant area; prophylaxis should only be used for trips of 2 weeks or less.

The risk of TD can be reduced but not eliminated by educating the traveler to avoid dietary indiscretions. Nevertheless, increasing evidence suggests surprisingly small differences in the incidence of TD in individuals who self-report meticulous rather than adventurous eating habits.[40-44] All travelers to the developing world should be thoroughly educated in self-therapy for diarrheal disease and carry the appropriate agents while traveling. Eighty percent of patients respond to a regimen of loperamide and an antibiotic within 24 hours. A single dose of a self-administered quinolone is usually sufficient, but patients should be instructed to complete 3 days of therapy with 500 mg of levofloxacin each day or 500 mg of ciprofloxacin twice daily should the TD not resolve within 24 hours. Because of a significant increase in quinolone-resistant *Campylobacter* in Southeast Asia, India, and Nepal, travelers to those destinations should self-treat with azithromycin, 500 mg per day for 3 days, or a single dose of 1000 mg.[45] Instructions on when to seek medical care should be given. Rifamixin can be used for TD caused by *E. coli* in adults and can be carried to *E. coli*-predominant areas but is not recommended when the patient has fever or blood in the stool.

Key Preventive Behaviors

Most travel-related health problems, including many infectious diseases, can be significantly reduced through appropriate behavior by the traveler.

PERSONAL PROTECTION AGAINST ARTHROPODS

Antimalarial chemoprophylactic drugs are less than 100% effective. Protection against arthropods will help prevent dengue (see Fig. 329-1), leishmaniasis, filariasis, and a number of important arboviral diseases. Travelers should be instructed to clothe themselves to reduce as much exposed skin as practicable and to apply a repellent containing DEET (concentration 30% to 35%) to all exposed, nonsensitive areas of the body every 4 to 6 hours.[46,47] More frequent application is required for agents containing lower concentrations of DEET. Agents containing 20% or higher concentrations of picaridin (KBR 3023) are similar to those containing DEET at the same concentration with regard to activity against *Anopheles* mosquitoes. Travelers should sleep under a permethrin-impregnated bed net in malarious areas unless they are in a sealed air-conditioned environment. When risk factors are especially high, travelers should treat outer clothing with permethrin. Although anopheline mosquitoes are night biters, *Aedes* spp. and culicine mosquitoes are usually day biters, so vigilance at all times of day is necessary.

PROTECTION AGAINST FOODBORNE DISEASE

Travelers to developing countries should be diligent in washing their hands frequently; avoiding food from dubious eating places, markets, and roadside vendors; avoiding buffets where there are no food covers or fly controls; avoiding high-risk food such as shellfish, reef fish (ciguatera risk), undercooked meats and poultry, dairy products, unpeeled fruits, cold sauces, and salads; avoiding both tap water and drinks or ice made from tap water; and using sealed bottled water or chemically treated, filtered, or boiled water for drinking and brushing their teeth.

SEX

Education on the incidence of HIV and sexually transmitted diseases among professional sex workers abroad, on the usage of condoms, and on the failure rate of condoms (3% to 5% breakage/slippage) should be given regardless of the apparent circumstances of the traveler. Unprotected sex even with fellow travelers is considered high risk. Travel is a disinhibiting experience in itself, and alcohol consumption tends to increase during travel. Between 19% and 26% of all travelers report a new sexual contact during their last trip abroad.[48,49] Condom use during casual travel sex is uniformly below 25% even in those who had received pretravel counseling. Discussion of emergency contraception strategies for female travelers is sometimes appropriate.

PROTECTION AGAINST BLOOD-BORNE DISEASE

Blood, blood products, syringes, and contaminated medical or dental instruments are a risk following accidents or trauma. Travelers should consider carrying an infusion set, needles, and a suture kit for high-risk areas. If possible, they should defer medical treatment and travel to a facility where safety can be ensured. Tattooing, acupuncture, and body piercing carry similar risks. Health care workers and others at risk in high HIV prevalence areas without sophisticated medical infrastructure may consider carrying a 1- to 2-week supply of Combivir (zidovudine/3TC), and Kaletra (lopinavir/ritonovir) to begin immediate twice daily postexposure prophylaxis, with the understanding that this is only an initial measure to allow time for travel to an adequate medical facility able to provide sophisticated testing and counseling.

PROTECTION AGAINST SKIN DISEASES[50]

Infected mosquito bites are common. Practicing good hand hygiene in dirty environments and covering open wounds are preventive measures that all travelers should take. Scabies and lice infestations can be prevented by carrying out good personal hygiene. In Africa, all clothes dried outdoors should be ironed to avoid cutaneous myiasis due to the tumbu fly. Hats and sunscreen are mandatory in the tropics. Sunscreen should always be applied to skin before, and not after, an application of N,N-diethyl-meta-toluamide (DEET).

PROTECTION AGAINST PATHOGENS DUE TO SWIMMING AND WATER EXPOSURE

Travelers should be instructed to avoid recreational (swimming, rafting, wading) or other exposure to fresh water in areas that are endemic for schistosomiasis. Hikers, bikers, and adventure travelers should consider prophylaxis with 200 mg of doxycycline once per week because of the significant risk of leptospirosis that exists in fresh water throughout the developing world. Walking barefoot in tropical areas predisposes to hookworm, *Strongyloides* infection, cutaneous larva migrans, and tungiasis.

PREVENTION OF TUBERCULOSIS

A predeparture baseline tuberculin skin test with annual retesting is indicated for long-stay travelers to developing countries.[51] Aggressive treatment of skin-test converters will prevent cases of active tuberculosis later. Travelers should avoid crowded public transportation or crowded public places and distance themselves immediately from anyone with a chronic or heavy cough. Expatriates should screen domestic help for tuberculosis.

◼ Noninfectious Travel Problems

MEDICAL KIT AND MEDICAL CARE ABROAD

Travelers should carry a compact medical kit. In addition to items mentioned elsewhere in the chapter, simple first-aid supplies like bandages, gauze, antiseptic, antibiotic ointment, and splinter forceps will allow early self-treatment of minor wounds before infection ensues. A thermometer to document elevations in temperature should be carried along with antipyretics. Antifungal creams, cough and cold remedies, antacids, hydrocortisone cream, and blister pads should be considered. The contact details of hometown medical providers should be recorded and accessible at all times. Long-stay travelers should plug themselves into the local expatriate medical infrastructure immediately after arrival so as to be able to seek competent care rapidly for any ensuing illness early in its course. Adequate medical and evacuation insurance should be arranged. A copy of a recent electrocardiogram should be carried by all cardiac patients on a portable USB drive or be accessible by Internet.

AIRLINE-RELATED MORBIDITY

A causal relationship between travel-related immobility and deep venous thrombosis/pulmonary embolism in otherwise healthy travelers has become established. Risk of pulmonary embolus is essentially absent on flights lasting less than 6 hours, rising to 5 per million on flights longer than 10 hours. Risk of a deep venous thrombosis, most often asymptomatic, is approximately 1:5000 for flights longer than 4 hours, but the data do not separate out those with risk factors.[52] Those with previously covert coagulopathies may manifest for the first time during travel. Those with clear, known risk factors are at highest risk. These include a personal or family history of deep venous thrombosis or pulmonary embolism; a personal or family history of a known blood clotting disorder predisposing to thrombosis (thrombophilia); major surgery, significant trauma, or prolonged immobilization (includes limb casts) in the previous 6 weeks; malignancy; late pregnancy; estrogen therapy, including oral contraceptives; age older than 50 years; severe obesity; and being very tall or very short. All travelers should avoid dehydration, avoid alcohol, and exercise the legs regularly in flight. Prophylactic subcutaneous low-molecular-weight heparin just before departure and again 24 hours later for those with thrombophilia or previous thrombotic events is often used in practice, although no definitive studies showing benefit from this practice have been published. Aspirin therapy is of no proven benefit in this setting. Jet lag occurs after crossing three or more time zones, and zolpidem taken for a few nights at bedtime at the destination is effective.[53] Those prone to motion sickness should sit in the center of airplanes, boats, or other conveyance and visually fix on distant objects. Meclizine or scopolamine is of benefit. Most in-flight medical emergencies are related to underlying illnesses and are difficult to predict at the time of the pretravel consultation. To avoid decompression sickness, established waiting periods for flying after diving have been determined.[54]

Altitude

Whether ascending by car or airplane, acute mountain sickness occurs in at least 25% of people who ascend rapidly to 2500 m or more and in most people who go quickly to 3000 m or more. Gradual ascent over days is rarely practiced by modern travelers. For prevention of altitude illness, acetazolamide, 125 to 250 mg twice a day beginning the morning of the day before ascent and continuing through the day after ascent, is effective. If symptoms of mountain sickness, such as nausea, vomiting, anorexia, light-headedness, fatigue, or insomnia, persist beyond the day after ascent, travelers may continue to take one tablet each evening.[55] Severe complications, such as pulmonary or cerebral edema, occur uncommonly under 3500 m and are best treated by oxygen and immediate descent. Those traveling above 3500 m for longer than a brief transit of a few hours should consult an expert.

◼ Traveling Adults with Special Needs

IMMUNOCOMPROMISED TRAVELERS AND THOSE INFECTED WITH THE HUMAN IMMUNODEFICIENCY VIRUS

Immunocompromised travelers are at risk for a complication or exacerbation of the underlying disease in a medically unfamiliar or underserved destination. Potential travelers need to understand the risks of the trip in the context of their personal situation. Precautions for immunocompromised travelers against malaria (including chemoprophylaxis), food- and water-borne diseases, and vector-borne diseases generally do not differ from those for healthy travelers. Live vaccines (YF, varicella, measles, oral typhoid, oral polio) should be avoided by those who are truly immunocompromised, even if the result is deferral of the trip. Other vaccines, although safe, likely will have suboptimal efficacy in compromised hosts, and the implications of this need to be discussed with the traveler.

HIV-infected individuals with adequate immune function (CD4 counts in the 350/mm^3 or higher range) as well as travelers using less than 20 mg prednisone daily for greater than 2 weeks are not at risk of infection and can be immunized as normal. Those on short courses (<2 weeks) of high-dose steroids and steroid inhalers and those who have received intra-articular steroids can be treated as normal hosts. However, asymptomatic HIV-infected individuals, even those with adequate immune function, should be given a waiver letter if the only reason for YF vaccination is to fulfill regulatory requirements. In those discontinuing truly immunosuppressive drugs, a 1-month waiting period before administration of live vaccines is advisable. Individuals with hematologic malignancies in remission should wait 3 months after their last chemotherapy before receiving live virus vaccines. Individuals with low-grade immune defects, such as chronic renal, hepatic or endocrine disease, should be counseled regarding increased risks of various infections, but no changes in pretravel immunizations are generally indicated. Functionally hyposplenic individuals should be vaccinated against pneumococci, meningococci, *Haemophilus influenzae* type B, and influenza, if they have not been already. The elderly may have suboptimal responses to many travel-related vaccines.

THE PREGNANT TRAVELER

Pregnancy presents several complex issues for travel, especially with regard to many commonly used travel medications. Determination of direct maternal-fetal–related contraindications to travel should be handled by the obstetrician. Travel is best undertaken in the second trimester. In general, pregnant travelers should not be given live vaccines. YF vaccine should be given only when the risk of contracting the disease is substantial and travel cannot be discouraged by the physician. Even killed vaccines are best delayed until the second trimester, if possible. Hepatitis A and B, tetanus, and meningococcal vaccines can be given without reservation. Other killed vaccines such as rabies, JE, typhoid, *H. influenzae* B, and pneumococcus should be given on a case-by-case basis when risk is high. In general, pregnant women should not travel to a malarious area unless the travel is absolutely necessary. Chloroquine is safe if travel is to one of the few countries where it is still the drug of choice. For other countries, mefloquine is recommended and likely safe, but extensive data on its safe use during pregnancy, especially during the first trimester, do not exist. Doxycycline, atovaquone/proguanil, and primaquine should not be used during pregnancy. Azithromycin is the treatment of choice for TD in pregnancy. Skiing, scuba diving, water skiing, and high altitude travel are not advisable during pregnancy. No vaccine affects the safety of breast-feeding. Mefloquine and chloroquine are safe during breast-feeding. Insufficient data are available for the use of doxycycline, atovaquone/proguanil, or primaquine. Twenty percent DEET used sparingly is safe in pregnancy.

REFERENCES

1. Freedman DO. Sources of travel medicine information. In: Keystone J, Kozarsky P, Freedman DO, eds. *Travel Medicine*. 2nd ed. St. Louis: Mosby Elsevier; 2008:29-34.
2. Kozarsky PE. Body of knowledge for the practice of travel medicine—2006. *J Travel Med*. 2006;13:251-254.
3. Steffen R, deBernardis C, Banos A. Travel epidemiology—A global perspective. *Int J Antimicrob Agents*. 2003;21:89-95.
4. Freedman DO, Weld LH, Kozarsky PE, et al. Spectrum of disease and relation to place of exposure among ill returned travelers. *N Engl J Med*. 2006;354:119-130.
5. Steffen R, Amitirigala I, Mutsch M. Health risks among travelers—need for regular updates. *J Travel Med*. 2008;15:145-146.
6. Mutsch M, Spicher VM, Gut C, et al. Hepatitis A virus infections in travelers, 1988-2004. *Clin Infect Dis*. 2006;42:490-497.
7. Steffen R, Banos A, deBernardis C. Vaccination priorities. *Int J Antimicrob Agents*. 2003;21:175-180.
8. Monath TP, Cetron MS. Prevention of yellow fever in persons traveling to the tropics. *Clin Infect Dis*. 2002;34:1369-1378.
9. Recommendations and Guidelines. Adult immunization schedule—United States. Updated annually. <http://www.cdc.gov/vaccines/recs/schedules/adult-schedule.htm>.
10. Marchou B, Excler JL, Bourderioux C, et al. A 3-week hepatitis B vaccination schedule provides rapid and persistent protective immunity: A multicenter, randomized trial comparing accelerated and classic vaccination schedules. *J Infect Dis*. 1995;172:258-260.
11. Connor BA, Blatter MM, Beran J, et al. Rapid and sustained immune response against hepatitis A and B achieved with combined vaccine using an accelerated administration schedule. *J Travel Med*. 2007;14:9-15.
12. Typhoid vaccines: WHO position paper. *Wkly Epidemiol Rec*. 2008;83:49-59
13. Connor BA, Schwartz E. Typhoid and paratyphoid fever in travellers. *Lancet Infect Dis*. 2005;5:623-628.
14. Stubi CL, Landry PR, Petignat C, et al. Compliance to live oral Ty21a typhoid vaccine, and its effect on viability. *J Travel Med*. 2000;7:133-137.
15. Leder K, Sundararajan V, Weld L, et al. Respiratory tract infections in travelers: A review of the GeoSentinel surveillance network. *Clin Infect Dis*. 2003;36:399-406.
16. Mutsch M, Tavernini M, Marx A, et al. Influenza virus infection in travelers to tropical and subtropical countries. *Clin Infect Dis*. 2005;40:1282-1287.
17. Marti F, Steffen R, Mutsch M. Influenza vaccine: a travelers' vaccine? *Expert Rev Vaccines*. 2008;7:679-687.
18. Miller JM, Tam TW, Maloney S, et al. Cruise ships: High-risk passengers and the global spread of new influenza viruses. *Clin Infect Dis*. 2000;31:433-438.
19. Prevention and control of influenza: recommendations of the Advisory Committee on Immunization Practices (ACIP), 2008. *MMWR Recomm Rep*. 2008;57(Aug 8(RR-7)):1-60.

20. Wilder-Smith A, Hill DR, Freedman DO. The revised International Health Regulations (2005): impact on yellow fever vaccination in clinical practice. *Am J Trop Med Hyg*. 2008;78:359-360.
21. Lindsey NP, Schroeder BA, Miller ER, et al. Adverse event reports following yellow fever vaccination. *Vaccine*. 2008;26:6077-6082.
22. Wilder-Smith A. Meningococcal vaccine in travelers. *Curr Opin Infect Dis*. 2007;20:454-460.
23. Meningococcal disease, Ethiopia. *Wkly Epidemiol Rec*. 2000;75:273.
24. Memish ZA. Meningococcal disease and travel. *Clin Infect Dis*. 2002;34:84-90.
25. Shlim DR, Solomon T. Japanese encephalitis vaccine for travelers: Exploring the limits of risk. *Clin Infect Dis*. 2002;35:183-188.
26. Tauber E, Kollaritsch H, Korinek M, et al. Safety and immunogenicity of a Vero-cell–derived, inactivated Japanese encephalitis vaccine: a non-inferiority, phase III, randomised controlled trial. *Lancet*. 2007;370:1847-1853.
27. Tauber E, Kollaritsch H, von Sonnenburg F, et al. Randomized, double-blind, placebo-controlled phase 3 trial of the safety and tolerability of IC51, an inactivated Japanese encephalitis vaccine. *J Infect Dis*. 2008;198:493-499.
28. Hill DR, Ford L, Lalloo DG. Oral cholera vaccines: use in clinical practice. *Lancet Infect Dis*. 2006;6:361-373.
29. Zent O, Bröker M. Tick-borne encephalitis vaccines: past and present. *Expert Rev Vaccines*. 2005;4:747-755.
30. Kaiser R. Tick-borne encephalitis. *Infect Dis Clin North Am*. 2008;22:561.
31. Kroger AT, Atkinson WL, Marcuse EK, et al. General recommendations on immunization: recommendations of the Advisory Committee on Immunization Practices (ACIP). *MMWR Recomm Rep*. 2006;55(Dec 1(RR-15)):1-48.
32. Leder K, Black J, O'Brien D, et al. Malaria in travelers: a review of the GeoSentinel surveillance network. *Clin Infect Dis*. 2004;39:1104-1112.
33. Leder K, Tong S, Weld L, et al. Illness in travelers visiting friends and relatives: a review of the GeoSentinel Surveillance Network. *Clin Infect Dis*. 2006;43:1185-1193.
34. Freedman DO. Clinical practice. Malaria prevention in short-term travelers. *N Engl J Med*. 2008;359:603-612.
35. Chen LH, Wilson ME, Schlagenhauf P. Controversies and misconceptions in malaria chemoprophylaxis for travelers. *JAMA*. 2007;297:2251-2263.
36. Chen LH, Wilson ME, Schlagenhauf P. Prevention of malaria in long-term travelers. *JAMA*. 2006;296:2234-2244.
37. Schwartz E, Weld LH, Wilder-Smith A, et al. Seasonality, annual trends, and characteristics of dengue among ill returned travelers, 1997-2006. *Emerg Infect Dis*. 2008;14:1081-1088.
38. DuPont AW. Postinfectious irritable bowel syndrome. *Clin Infect Dis*. 2008;46:594-599.

39. Hill DR, Ericsson CD, Pearson RD, et al. The practice of travel medicine: guidelines by the Infectious Diseases Society of America. *Clin Infect Dis*. 2006;43:1499-1539.
40. Hoge CW, Shlim DR, Echeverria P, et al. Epidemiology of diarrhea among expatriate residents living in a highly endemic environment. *JAMA*. 1996;275:533-538.
41. Steffen R, Tornieporth N, Clemens SA, et al. Epidemiology of travelers' diarrhea: details of a global survey. *J Travel Med*. 2004;11:231-237.
42. Shlim DR, Hoge CW, Rajah R, et al. Persistent high risk of diarrhea among foreigners in Nepal during the first 2 years of residence. *Clin Infect Dis*. 1999;29:613-616.
43. Steffen R, Collard F, Tornieporth N, et al. Epidemiology, etiology, and impact of traveler's diarrhea in Jamaica. *JAMA*. 1999;281:811-817.
44. von Sonnenburg F, Tornieporth N, Waiyaki P, et al. Risk and aetiology of diarrhoea at various tourist destinations. *Lancet*. 2000;356:133-134.
45. Tribble DR, Sanders JW, Pang LW, et al. Traveler's diarrhea in Thailand: randomized, double-blind trial comparing single-dose and 3-day azithromycin-based regimens with a 3-day levofloxacin regimen. *Clin Infect Dis*. 2007;44:338-346.
46. Fradin MS. Mosquitoes and mosquito repellents: A clinician's guide. *Ann Intern Med*. 1998;128:931-940.
47. Fradin MS, Day JF. Comparative efficacy of insect repellents against mosquito bites. *N Engl J Med*. 2002;347:13-18.
48. Cabada MM, Echevarria JI, Seas CR, et al. Sexual behavior of international travelers visiting Peru. *Sex Transm Dis*. 2002;29:510-513.
49. Mulhall BP. Sex and travel: Studies of sexual behaviour, disease and health promotion in international travellers—A global review. *Int J STD AIDS*. 1996;7:455-465.
50. Lederman E, Weld LH, Elyazar IRF, et al. Dermatologic conditions of the ill returned traveler: an analysis from the GeoSentinel Surveillance Network. *Int J Infect Dis*. 2008;12:593-602.
51. Cobelens FG, van Deutekom H, Draayer-Jansen IW, et al. Association of tuberculin sensitivity in Dutch adults with history of travel to areas of with a high incidence of tuberculosis. *Clin Infect Dis*. 2001;33:300-304.
52. WHO Research into Global Hazards of Travel (WRIGHT) project on air travel and venous thromboembolism. <http://www.who.int/cardiovascular_diseases/wright_project/en/>
53. Suhner A, Schlagenhauf P, Hofer I, et al. Effectiveness and tolerability of melatonin and zolpidem for the alleviation of jet lag. *Aviat Space Environ Med*. 2001;72:638-646.
54. Freiberger JJ, Denoble PJ, Pieper CF, et al. The relative risk of decompression sickness during and after air travel following diving. *Aviat Space Environ Med*. 2002;73:980-984.
55. Hackett PH, Roach RC. High-altitude illness. *N Engl J Med*. 2001;345:107-114.

330

Infections in Returning Travelers

DAVID O. FREEDMAN

Of the approximately 80 million people who travel from industrialized to developing countries each year, 22% to 64% of travelers report some illness.[1-3] The approach to the patient requires knowledge of world geography, the epidemiology of disease patterns in 230 or so countries, and the clinical presentation of a wide spectrum of disorders.[4] Most illnesses are mild, most are self-limited, and many are noninfectious. Up to 10% of travelers may consult a physician during or after a trip and approximately 1 in 100,000 travelers will die.

The ill travelers that do come to the attention of infectious diseases clinicians are generally either the most seriously ill or are suspected of harboring infectious agents not familiar in their home country. Based on 17,353 ill-returned travelers seen by the GeoSentinel Surveillance Network at 31 different clinical sites on 6 continents, in patients presenting to infectious or tropical diseases specialists after travel to the developing world, specific travel destinations are associated with the probability of the diagnosis of certain diseases.[5] Diagnostic approaches and empiric therapies can be guided by these destination-specific differences. Important region-specific disease occurrence data indicate that febrile illness is most important from Africa and Southeast Asia; malaria is one of the top three diagnoses from every region, yet over the past decade dengue has become the most common febrile illness from every region outside of sub-Saharan Africa; in sub-Saharan Africa, rickettsial disease is second only to malaria as a cause of fever; respiratory disease is most important in Southeast Asia; and acute diarrhea is disproportionately from South Central Asia. When individual diagnoses are collected into syndrome groups and examined for all regions together, 226 of every 1000 ill-returned travelers have a systemic febrile illness, 222 have acute diarrhea, 170 have a dermatologic disorder, 113 have chronic diarrhea, and 77 have a respiratory disorder.

Travelers who become ill during, or any time up to several months after, a foreign trip will frequently associate that illness with a possible travel-specific etiology. This may be the case, but often it is not. Routine things are common, and common things are common whether actually acquired during travel or at sometime after the trip. Thus fever, sore throat, and cervical adenopathy in a college student who returned 2 weeks earlier from a developing country is still more likely to be streptococcal pharyngitis or infectious mononucleosis than diphtheria. Presented with an ill patient with a history of travel, the physician must maintain discipline in making two separate lists of differential diagnoses, the first with the travel history factored in and the second considering the same presenting symptoms and signs as if in any other patient. The approach and workup must then proceed in parallel, with appropriate priority given to the most urgent or the most treatable diagnoses at the top of each list.

In this chapter, travelers are considered to be those returning from short visits to developing countries, and the term does not include immigrants, refugees, and very long-term residents arriving from those countries. Constellations of exposures and clinical presentations highly suggestive of particular diagnoses in returned travelers are shown in Table 330-1. Highly exotic endemic diseases very rarely, if ever, acquired by travelers are not discussed. The focus is on the identification of infectious causes of the presenting illness, on travel-associated risk factors, and on manifestations of those diseases that are particular to travelers. Detailed discussions of pathophysiology, spectrum of clinical manifestations, and therapy of each infectious agent are found in the disease-specific chapters of this book. Fever, traveler's diarrhea, and skin problems are the most common presenting illnesses in returned travelers. Eosinophilia is less common but is a frequent source of referral to the infectious diseases specialist. Each is discussed in turn.

Fever

EPIDEMIOLOGY

Fever occurs in 2% to 3%[1-3] of European or American travelers to the developing world. The proportion of ill-returned travelers who present to specialists with a febrile illness is 28%, with variation by region of travel: Americas (18%); South-Central Asia (includes India) (27%); Southeast Asia (33%); and sub-Saharan Africa (41%).

Several large case series from busy tropical disease units indicate malaria to be the cause of the fever in 27% to 42%.[6-8] The other most common tropical etiologies specific to returning travelers are dengue, rickettsial disease, typhoid fever, and enteric pathogens. Less common but important considerations are leptospirosis, chikungunya, acute schistosomiasis, and amebic liver abscess. All of these diseases have widespread distribution in the tropics and need to be considered initially in all febrile travelers. Some may be ruled out quickly based on a detailed travel and exposure history and consultation with relevant information sources on disease distribution. Upper and lower respiratory tract infection, including streptococcal pharyngitis and influenza, as well as urinary tract infections, are cosmopolitan, nontropical febrile etiologies that are remarkably common in travelers and should always be considered. In every series from sophisticated referral centers, up to 22% to 25% of those presenting with fever have self-limited illnesses that never have an etiologic diagnosis made.[8] These are mostly viral syndromes caused by one of hundreds of viral agents that exist outside of developed countries for which diagnostic tests may not be available anywhere. In many cases, the time and expense of a large panel of viral isolation and serologic assays is not warranted outside the research setting. Fever due to deep venous thrombosis or pulmonary embolism may be related to travel, especially in those with preexisting conditions or underlying coagulopathy. Thromboembolic disease always needs to be considered from the outset, but is not discussed further here.[9]

HISTORY

A good patient history is always important in clinical medicine, but nowhere is it as important as in the returning traveler. The cumulative list of infectious agents in 230 separate countries is daunting. A day-by-day travel itinerary, knowledge of risk factors and exposures for the common travel diseases, knowledge of usual incubation periods of those diseases, and knowledge of or access to the known geographic distribution of possible infectious diseases, will lead to an appropriately focused workup.[10,11] Much time, expense, and patient discomfort due to sometimes invasive diagnostic tests can be avoided when diagnoses that are not epidemiologically or chronologically possible are eliminated based on the patient history.

The fever pattern and clinical findings by themselves are often nonspecific and overlap greatly between many of the most common tropical infectious diseases. The history should include the key elements detailed in the following sections.

TABLE 330-1	Constellations of Exposures and Clinical Presentations Suggestive of Particular Diagnoses in Returned Travelers*	

Exposure Scenario	Distinctive Findings	Diagnosis
Any exposure in any area with documented malaria transmission	Fever with or without any other finding	Malaria
Most tropical countries	Fever and altered mental status	Malaria, meningococcal meningitis, rabies, West Nile virus
Budget travel to India, Nepal, Pakistan, or Bangladesh	Insidious-onset, high, unremitting fever, toxic patient, paucity of physical findings	Enteric fever due to *Salmonella typhi* or *Salmonella paratyphi*
Freshwater recreational exposure in Africa	Fever, eosinophilia, hepatomegaly, negative malaria smear	Acute schistosomiasis (Katayama fever)
Bitten by *Aedes aegypti* in Central America, Southeast Asia, or the South Pacific	Fever, headache, myalgia, diffuse macular rash, mild to moderate thrombocytopenia	Dengue
Bitten by *A. aegypti* or *Aedes albopictus* in India, Malaysia, Singapore, or an island in the Indian Ocean	Fever, headache, myalgia, diffuse macular rash, arthralgia, tenosynovitis often followed by chronic polyarthritis after the fever resolves	Chikungunya fever
Hunting or visiting game reserves in southern Africa	Fever, eschar, diffuse petechial rash	African tick typhus due to *Rickettsia africae*
Travel to Southeast Asia	Fever, eschar, diffuse petechial rash	Scrub typhus due to *Orientia tsutsugamushi*
Hiking, biking, swimming, rafting with exposure to fresh surface water	Fever, myalgia, conjunctival suffusion, mild to severe jaundice, variable rash	Leptospirosis
Summertime cruise to Alaska, elderly traveler	Influenza-like illness	Influenza A or B
Outdoor exposure anywhere in the Americas	Large, single furuncular lesion anywhere on body, with sense of movement inside	Myiasis due to *Dermatobia hominis* (botfly)
Clothing washed or dried out of doors in Africa	Multiple furuncular lesions around clothing contact points with skin	Myiasis due to *Cordylobia anthropophaga* (tumbu fly)
New sexual partner during travel	Fever, rash, mononucleosis-like illness	Acute human immunodeficiency virus infection
Travel to any developing country	Coryza, conjunctivitis, Koplik spots, rash	Measles
Longer visit to humid areas of Africa, the Americas or Southeast Asia	Asymptomatic eosinophilia or with periodic cough or wheezing	Strongyloidiasis
Sandfly bite in either New or Old World tropical area	Painless skin ulcer with clean, moist base in exposed area	Cutaneous leishmaniasis
Resort hotel in southern Europe, ± exposure to whirlpool spas	Pneumonia	Legionnaires' disease
Explored a cave in the Americas	Fever, cough, retrosternal chest pain, hilar adenopathy	Histoplasmosis
Ingestion of unpasteurized goat cheese	Chronic fever, fatigue	*Brucella melitensis*
Long trip to West/Central Africa	Afebrile, intensely pruritic, evanescent truncal maculopapular rash	Onchocerciasis
Long trip to West/Central Africa	Migratory localized angioedema or swellings over large joints, eosinophilia	Loiasis
Safari to game parks of East Africa	Fever, nongenital chancre, fine macular rash	East African trypanosomiasis
Travel to Australia	Fever, fatigue, polyarthritis	Ross River virus
Farming areas of India and Southeast Asia	Fever, altered mental status, paralysis	Japanese encephalitis
Forested areas of central and eastern Europe and across Russia	Fever, altered mental status, paralysis	Tick-borne encephalitis
Rodent exposure in West Africa	Fever, sore throat, jaundice, hemorrhagic manifestations	Lassa fever
Ingestion of sushi, ceviche, or raw freshwater fish	Migratory nodules in truncal areas with overlying erythema or mild hemorrhage	Gnathostomiasis
Returning Hajj pilgrim or family contact	Fever, meningitis	Meningococcal meningitis
Ingestion of snails, fish, or shellfish in Asia	Eosinophilic meningitis	Angiostrongyliasis, gnathostomiasis
Summertime exposure to rodent droppings in Scandinavia	Fever with decreased renal function	Puumala virus
Ingestion of undercooked meat of any animal in any country	Fever, facial edema, myositis, increased creatine phosphokinase, massive eosinophilia, normal erythrocyte sedimentation rate	Trichinosis
Unvaccinated, returning from sub-Saharan Africa or forested areas of Amazonia	Fever, jaundice, proteinuria, hemorrhage	Yellow fever
Exposure to farm animals	Pneumonia, mild hepatitis	Q fever
Possible tick exposure almost anywhere	Fever, headache, rash, conjunctival injection, hepatosplenomegaly	Tick-borne relapsing fever
Poor hygienic conditions with possible body louse exposure in Ethiopia or Sudan	Fever, headache, rash, conjunctival injection, hepatosplenomegaly	Louse-borne relapsing fever

*The table includes illnesses of travelers (listed first) as well as less common diseases with presentations that should suggest the possibility of the appropriate diagnosis. Many diseases have a spectrum of presentation and the table describes the most common presentations of these diseases. Many diseases have a spectrum of geographic origins and the table describes the most common exposures seen in daily practice.

Detailed Travel Itinerary

This should include every locale visited in every country visited, including transit stops. Some individuals are frequent travelers, so all travel for at least the previous 6 months must be considered initially. If the diagnosis remains elusive, a more remote travel history, especially that involving malarious areas, may be sought. The exact date of arrival back in the home country is often crucial to ascertain the last possible exposure date to an exotic pathogen. These details are most efficiently ascertained using a waiting room questionnaire. For example, it is insufficient to know simply that the patient visited Peru. Some parts of Peru are malarious and others are not, only some have risk of yellow fever, high-altitude destinations have little risk of vector-borne disease, and there is no risk of strongyloidiasis along the desert coastal strip.

Chronology of Travel and Illness

This should include the exact dates spent in each locale with respect to the onset of illness. Knowledge of typical incubation periods (Table 330-2) of possible infectious etiologies is a key tool in narrowing the differential diagnosis. Many agents are simply not biologically possible outside their usual incubation period. Arboviral diseases such as dengue uniformly have short incubation periods. Onset of illness more than 2 weeks after last possible exposure effectively rules out this class of viral illness. None of the known hemorrhagic fever viruses has a possible incubation longer than 21 days. Long-incubation infections like schistosomiasis cannot present less than several weeks after first possible exposure. Some diseases such as malaria or enteric fever have more variable incubation periods but nevertheless have a typical incubation period during which time the majority of the patients present. A number of diseases, especially those that are arthropod borne, have a strict seasonality whereby transmission stops during either cold or dry weather. Examples would include malaria in nontropical countries such as Korea, Tajikistan, or northern China, as well as Lyme borreliosis or tick-borne encephalitis, all of which completely cease transmission during winter months. Recent GeoSentinel surveillance data indicate that dengue cases in travelers show marked region-specific peaks for Southeast Asia (June, September), South-Central Asia (October), South America (March), and the Caribbean (August, October).[12]

Exposures

This should include a detailed dietary history. Budget travel and associated high-risk eating habits predispose to a variety of common enteric pathogens. A history of specific foods associated with known pathogens should also be elicited. This includes unpasteurized dairy products (*Brucella*, *Campylobacter*, *Salmonella*, tuberculosis), shellfish (vibrios, enteric viruses, viral hepatitis), uncooked beef such as carpaccio and steak tartare (*Toxoplasma*, *Campylobacter*, *Escherichia coli*

O157-H7), undercooked fish such as sushi and ceviche (vibrios, *Anisakis*, *Gnathostoma*), and undercooked pork or game meat (trichinosis). Exposure to fresh water or surface water in recreational or other settings may be associated with schistosomiasis[13,14] or leptospirosis.[15] A history of exposure to mosquitoes and flies is generally unhelpful, but history of tick bite (rickettsiae, relapsing fever, tick-borne encephalitis) or tsetse fly bite should be sought in the right setting. Exposures to new sexual partners,[16,17] needles, or blood should be ascertained. Rodent exposure is associated with Lassa fever, hantavirus infection, and rat-bite fever. A history of contact with other sick people is especially important in the post-travel setting. Travelers usually move in groups or with families or companions, all of whom will likely have shared the same exposures.

Immunization History

This should include exact dates of the last dose of each vaccine received and in some instances whether an adequate primary series was completed in the first place. Most vaccines, with the notable exception of typhoid vaccines, are very highly efficacious. Thus, hepatitis A or B, yellow fever, measles, or diphtheria are unlikely diagnoses in those with a substantiated history of adequate and current immunization.

Antimalarial Intake

If malaria is a possibility, a complete pill-by-pill history of ingestion of antimalarial drugs, including the name and dose of all drugs taken for prophylaxis or treatment, must be obtained. Patients often misunderstand the dosing or timing instructions given at the pretravel visit, or they may have been prescribed an inappropriate drug for their destination. Patients may have been treated with appropriate or inappropriate drugs en route for febrile illnesses. Some very efficacious drugs are not available in the United States and an international pharmacopeia such as Martindale's may need to be consulted by those unfamiliar with these drugs. A history of appropriate prophylaxis diminishes the possibility of malaria but does not eliminate the need for a malaria thick film, which may be preceded by a malaria rapid card test for any patient legitimately exposed to malaria.

Other Medications Ingested

Travelers who fall ill during the travel often self-treat with antibiotics or see a local physician and are prescribed a broad-spectrum antibiotic. Again, an international pharmacopeia may need to be consulted. Recent ingestion of a 1-week course of a quinolone, tetracycline, or cephalosporin antibiotic may alter the course of the illness or even affect the possibility of certain diagnoses. In particular, malaria may be suppressed by azithromycin, doxycycline, quinolones, or clindamycin.

PHYSICAL EXAMINATION

Common tropical infections often present as undifferentiated fever without focal findings. However, when a focal finding such as arthritis, meningitis, or pneumonia is present, the differential diagnosis can often be narrowed. Unfortunately, physical findings such as jaundice, hepatomegaly, splenomegaly, and lymphadenopathy occur at least a portion of the time in many of the most common travel-related infections and so are not specific enough to greatly narrow the differential diagnosis.[18] Most imported febrile rash illnesses engender the same differential diagnosis as for nontravelers. However, arbovirus infections, typhoid, rickettsial illness, leptospirosis, measles, early stages of viral hemorrhagic fevers, relapsing fever, and acute African trypanosomiasis should always be kept in mind.

CONSIDERATIONS FOR THE COMMON TRAVEL-RELATED FEBRILE ILLNESSES

Malaria

Fever in a traveler returning from a malarious area is an emergency and the instinctive performance of an immediate malaria smear will

TABLE 330-2	Incubation Periods of Common Travel-Related Infections*		
Short Incubation (<10 Days)	**Medium Incubation (10-21 Days)**	**Long Incubation (>21 Days)**
Malaria	Malaria	Malaria
Arboviruses including dengue, yellow fever, Japanese encephalitis	Flaviviruses—tick-borne encephalitis and Japanese encephalitis	Schistosomiasis
Hemorrhagic fevers—Lassa, Ebola, South American arenaviruses	Hemorrhagic fevers—Lassa, Ebola, Crimean-Congo hemorrhagic fever	Tuberculosis
Respiratory viruses including severe acute respiratory syndrome (SARS)	Acute HIV infection	Acute HIV infection
		Viral hepatitis
		Filariasis
		Rickettsia—Q fever
		Secondary syphilis
Typhoid and paratyphoid	Typhoid and paratyphoid	Epstein-Barr virus including mononucleosis
Bacterial enteritis	*Giardia*	Amebic liver disease
Rickettsia—spotted fever group: Rocky Mountain spotted fever, African tick typhus, Mediterranean spotted fever, scrub typhus, Q fever	*Rickettsia*—flea-borne, louse-borne, and scrub typhus, Q fever, spotted fevers (rare)	Leishmaniasis
		Brucella
		Bartonellosis (chronic)
	Cytomegalovirus	Babesiosis
	Toxoplasma	Rabies
	Amebic dysentery	African trypanosomiasis (chronic)
Bacterial pneumonia including *Legionella*	Histoplasmosis	Cytomegalovirus
Relapsing fever	*Brucella*	
Amebic dysentery	Leptospirosis	
Meningococcemia	Babesiosis	
Brucella (rarely)	Rabies	
Leptospirosis	African trypanosomiasis (acute), East African	
Fascioliasis	Hepatitis A (rarely)	
Rabies (rarely)	Measles	
African trypanosomiasis (acute), East African (rarely)		

*Diseases that commonly have variable incubation periods are shown more than once. However, most diseases may rarely have an atypical incubation period, and this is not shown here.

HIV, human immunodeficiency virus.

prevent unnecessary deaths. Malaria rapid diagnostic card tests may hasten the diagnosis, but a negative test does not rule out malaria and must always.be followed by a blood film.[19] Malaria due to *Plasmodium falciparum* is easily treatable if diagnosed early, but even with optimum treatment has a mortality rate of 20% or more if treatment is begun only after end-organ complications arise. Smears need to be repeated at least every 12 to 24 hours a minimum of three times to rule out malaria. Rapid deterioration can occur over a period of hours. Unreliable smear-negative patients with a high index of suspicion for *P. falciparum* malaria may need to be admitted for inpatient observation.

Because malaria is overwhelmingly an African disease, with about 80% of all *P. falciparum* imported into developed countries originating there,[20,21] suspicion of malaria is especially acute for Africa returnees. Beyond this, trends in the geographic origin of imported malaria cases do not always correlate well with regional transmission patterns because absolute numbers of cases from particular geographic areas may also mirror the intensity of travel to the affected region. Ethnic minority travelers returning home to visit friends and relatives in malarious areas have the highest risk of infection. Resources describing current country-specific malaria microepidemiology should be immediately accessible to those assessing tropical fevers.[11] In general, malaria is a rural disease, but the cities of Africa and India are exceptions.

P. falciparum malaria in nonimmune travelers most commonly has an incubation period of 9 to 14 days and 90% of cases occur within 1 month of last exposure. Non–*P. falciparum* malaria is only rarely life threatening but can present much later after arrival. Incubation periods are prolonged in those taking inadequate or incomplete chemoprophylaxis. Relapses of disease due to *Plasmodium vivax* or *Plasmodium ovale* may occur many months after travel in those whose initial attack was clinically silent because of suppressive chemoprophylaxis, but in whom terminal prophylaxis with primaquine was not used (see Chapter 275).

The presenting signs and symptoms of imported malaria remain sufficiently protean so as to mimic a number of common tropical or nontropical conditions.[22-24] No constellation of symptoms or signs differentiates *P. falciparum* from non–*P. falciparum* malaria. Classic periodic malarial fever is not a usual manifestation of imported malaria, although when fever does occur in discrete, repeated 48- or 72-hour cycles, the diagnosis is almost certain. The simian malaria parasite *Plasmodium knowlesi*, which is now known to commonly infect humans in Malaysia and Indonesia, uniquely has a periodicity of 24 hours. The exact geographic range of this species is not yet clear. Infected patients have high parasitemias (>1%) with a plasmodium that is morphologically almost identical to *Plasmodium malariae*. *P. malariae* typically has a parasitemia of less than 1%. Fever is absent at the exact time of the initial medical assessment in up to 40% of patients with malaria. Respiratory or gastrointestinal symptoms may be predominant. The presence of rash, lymphadenopathy, or leukocytosis indicates another diagnosis. Anemia is uncommon in travelers who present in the early days of their malarial illness. Thrombocytopenia occurs in over 50% and is a reliable if nonspecific indicator of malarial etiology when present.

Many other serious infections are present in malarious areas. The search for malaria should not hamper the simultaneous workup for other pathogens in smear-negative patients. Similarly, semi-immune residents of endemic areas may be mildly parasitemic on a chronic basis with little ill effect, so a positive malaria smear in these patients should not hamper a search for any other clinically suspected infections.

Dengue

Dengue, transmitted by the day-biting *Aedes aegypti* mosquito, is an important travel-related problem most notably in heavily visited areas of Southeast Asia, the South Pacific, and Central America and the Caribbean.[12,25] Travelers to Thailand seem particularly prone to infection,[26] and dengue is relatively uncommon in Africa. In contrast to many other tropical fevers, it is predominantly an urban infection so that it can even affect upscale business travelers in urban centers. The incubation period is usually 2 to 7 days after the mosquito bite, so many travelers initially become ill while still overseas. The clinical spectrum ranges widely from asymptomatic through a range of clinical manifestations up to the severe myalgia and arthralgia of "breakbone fever" (see Chapter 153). Malaria, other arbovirus diseases including chikungunya fever, leptospirosis, rickettsial disease, measles, or typhoid may present similar initial findings. However, in cases where one of several associated rashes manifests (Fig. 330-1A), dengue becomes more likely than the other possibilities.

A positive tourniquet test is found in up to 50% of patients with classic dengue and in almost all patients with dengue hemorrhagic fever, but it is a nonspecific finding that may also be present in leptospirosis. The test is performed by inflating a blood pressure cuff halfway between systolic and diastolic for 5 minutes and upon release counting the number of petechiae in a 2.5 × 2.5-cm patch below the cuff. Greater than 20 petechiae is considered positive.

Serologic confirmation most often must be sent to a reference laboratory. Immunoglobulin M (IgM) is not elevated until 5 or more days after illness onset, but most patients initially present earlier than this. If an IgM drawn more than 5 days into illness is negative, a third visit to test for fourfold elevations of IgG is required. Because most patients will be better by the time results of any confirmatory tests would be available and because treatment is supportive, many clinicians do not seek laboratory confirmation. Virus isolation from blood is possible only during the first 5 days of illness but is not routinely available. Polymerase chain reaction testing during the viremic phase is increasingly available. A postviral fatigue lasting up to 6 months may occur. Patients need to be reminded that another visit to a dengue-endemic area could result in infection with another serotype, with risk of ensuing dengue hemorrhagic fever.

Chikungunya Fever

Although chikungunya fever, a mosquito-borne alphavirus (chikungunya virus [CHIKV]) infection, was first isolated in the early 1950s when it caused epidemics in East Africa and is endemic in tropical Africa and Asia, it has been unknown to most clinicians in the Americas and Europe for the past 2 decades. Chikungunya fever has reappeared as a paradigm of an emerging infectious disease that was globalized on a wide scale with highly viremic travelers acting as efficient vectors. CHIKV emerged in 2004 in East Africa, spread to adjacent West Indian Ocean islands, causing an outbreak of unprecedented magnitude in 2005-2006, and with a jump to India affected millions of people before continuing its expansion into eastern Asia. Since 2006, CHIKV infection has been identified in more than 2000 U.S. and European travelers after return home from the epidemic areas. An outbreak affecting local populations in Italy in August 2007 demonstrated the reality of introduced transmission of significant pathogenic agents by receptive vectors such *Aedes* spp. mosquitoes, which are indigenous to much of Europe. The acute illness resembles dengue but with more prominent joint symptoms. Patients have fever, arthralgia, and sometimes acute arthritis. Rash, which occurs in about 50% of cases, may resemble that seen in dengue and is pruritic and macular or maculopapular. Although acute symptoms usually subside within a week, disabling joint symptoms may persist for months.

Typhoid and Paratyphoid Fever

Typhoid fever is often the most nondescript of the relatively common causes of travel-related fever.[27-29] The incubation period is most often a week but can be as long as 3 weeks. Risk is at least 10 times higher on the Indian subcontinent than anywhere else, but risk exists throughout the tropics in the setting of poor sanitation. In contrast to malaria, dengue, or rickettsial infection, onset is insidious and abnormal physical findings usually absent. Abdominal discomfort and constipation are common, but diarrhea is frequent enough so as to not rule out the diagnosis. Patients often look and feel particularly unwell, with severe prostration and high, unremitting fever. Leukopenia and

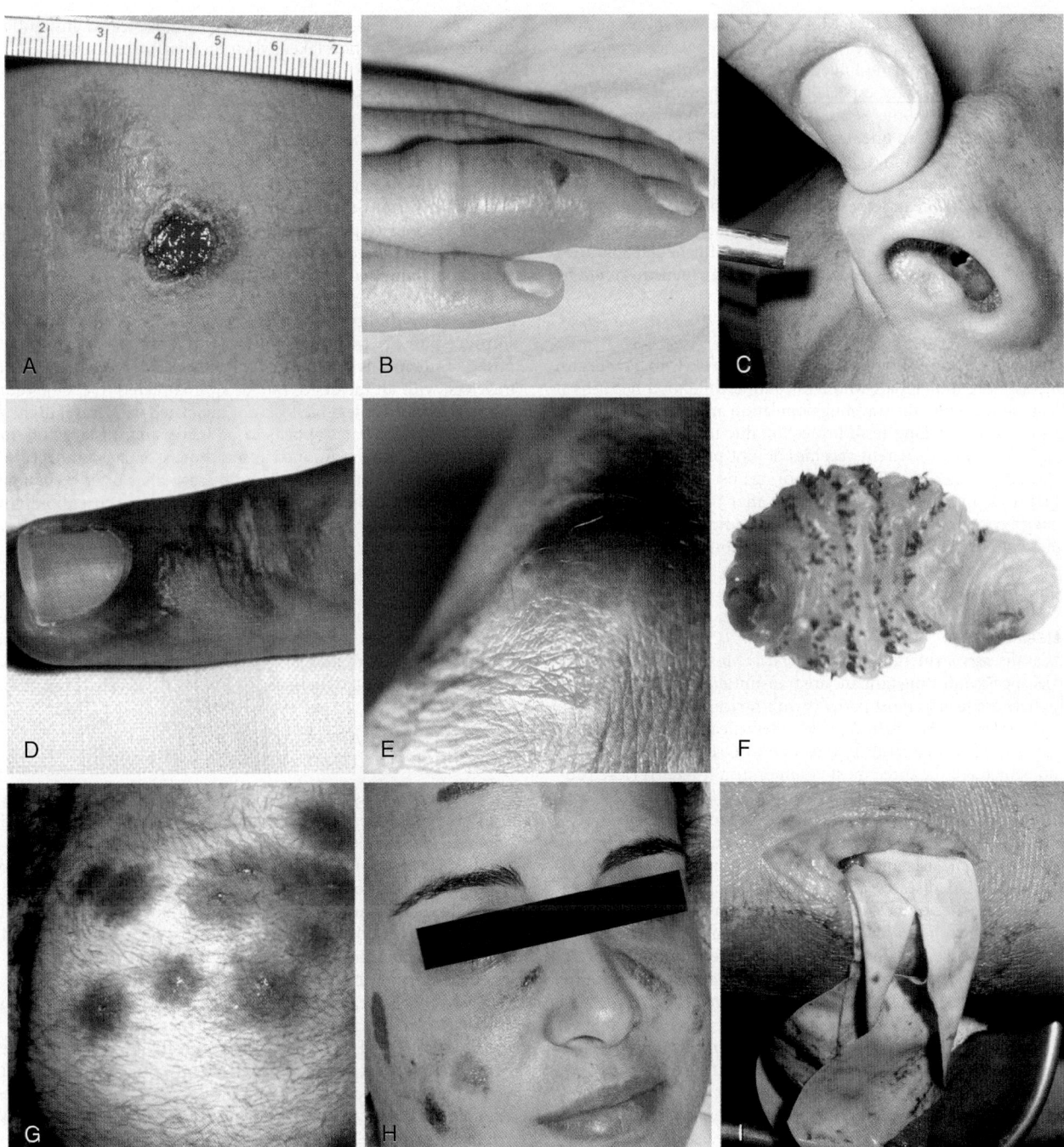

Figure 330-1   Some common diseases of travelers with pathologic effects localized to circumscribed areas of the skin and underlying tissue.
A, Painless ulcer with a clean base in a traveler to Peru with New World cutaneous leishmaniasis due to *Leishmania braziliensis*. **B,** More nodular and inflammatory lesions with crusting but only slight ulceration in a traveler to Afghanistan, which is more characteristic of Old World cutaneous leishmaniasis due to *Leishmania major*. **C,** Painless nasal perforation, which is often the earliest manifestation of mucocutaneous leishmaniasis due to metastatic spread of *L. braziliensis* from an earlier cutaneous lesion. **D,** Cutaneous larva migrans or creeping eruption due to the canine hookworm *Ancylostoma caninum*. **E,** Furuncular myiasis due to *Dermatobia hominis* (botfly). Patients often report a sense of movement inside; note tiny hole for the respiratory spicule of the botfly. **F,** *D. hominis* larva after migration to surface when the respiratory spicule was blocked with petroleum jelly. **G,** Characteristic multilesion presentation of African furuncular myiasis due to *Cordylobia anthropophaga* (tumbu fly). **H,** Phytophotodermatitis in a traveler to Ecuador after application of a lime juice–containing mixture by a shaman during a native ceremony; the same effect is seen when common tropical cocktails are spilled on sun-exposed areas. Pigmented lesions may take weeks to resolve. **I,** Tropical pyomyositis in a traveler to the Amazon. Pyomyositis due to deep staphylococcal infection is common in moist, warm climates and is characterized by brown pus as the muscle fibers dissolve. Initial lesions are characterized by exquisitely painful, localized erythematous areas overlying the affected muscle. (*Images reprinted with permission of the Instituto de Medicina Tropical Alexander von Humboldt, Universidad Peruana Cayetano Heredia, Lima, Peru; and the Gorgas Memorial Institute, University of Alabama, Birmingham, Ala.*)

thrombocytopenia often occur. Blood cultures are not always positive but bone marrow cultures increase the yield. Serologic assays, including agglutination and enzyme-linked immunosorbent assay (ELISA), have overall poor sensitivity, especially early in the course, and some lack of specificity in some settings, and enjoy poor reputations. However, when present, an unequivocal high titer in a previously naive traveler provides a more rapid diagnosis than will blood cultures. Up-to-date vaccination against typhoid provides only partial protection against *Salmonella typhi* and does not protect at all against *Salmonella paratyphi*.[30] Because of resistance, fluoroquinolones are no longer an option for empiric treatment in the Indian subcontinent and Southeast Asia, and third-generation cephalosporins or a carbapenem should be used.[27]

Viral Hepatitis

Incidence rates for travel-related viral hepatitis are likely to have begun a decline as more individuals who had routine childhood hepatitis B vaccine are moving into the traveling population and as more high-risk travelers are receiving long-term protection due to pretravel hepatitis A and B vaccination.[31] Current vaccines do not protect against hepatitis E, which is enterically acquired,[32] or against hepatitis C, which, like hepatitis B, may be acquired overseas after blood transfusion or contact with contaminated syringes, medical equipment, or tattoo and body-piercing implements. Viral hepatitis is a long-incubation infection so that acquisition may not always be readily linked by the patient or the physician to the travel.

Rickettsial Disease

Rickettsial disease is emerging in travelers.[5,33] Most of the long list of rickettsial species infecting humans are transmitted by ticks, mites, and fleas. Eschars are seen in most patients with African tick typhus due to *Rickettsia africae* (see Fig. 330-2F),[34] Mediterranean spotted fever due to *Rickettsia conori*, and scrub typhus due to *Orientia tsutsugamushi* infection, which are the three most common travel-related rickettsioses. In a group of 940 travelers to South Africa, 4% of all travelers and 27% of all travelers with flulike symptoms had infection with *R. africae*.[35] *R. africae* is the second most common cause of fever in travelers to Africa after malaria and is most prevalent in South Africa itself. Although rickettsial diseases are present in most countries of the world, individual species have restricted geographic distributions (see Chapter 186), which helps in the diagnostic formulation. High fever, headache, leukopenia, and thrombocytopenia are common. Rickettsiae infect endothelial cells and often cause widespread vasculitic-looking lesions (see Fig. 330-2F). Severe infections may present with disseminated intravascular coagulation and mimic a viral hemorrhagic fever. Because African tick-bite fever and scrub typhus both occur in malarious areas, a thick film is indicated even in febrile patients with pathognomonic skin lesions. Because response to tetracyclines is uniformly prompt and dramatic and the results of serologic tests slow to return, clinical suspicion and clinical diagnosis are usually relied upon. The diagnosis should be reconsidered in those who do not respond within 48 hours of initiation of doxycycline or tetracycline.

Leptospirosis

Leptospirosis is thought of as an occupational disease and a disease of urban slum dwellers with rodent exposure. In recent years, large leptospirosis outbreaks in adventure travelers and adventure racers such as whitewater rafters, triathletes, and participants in the 2000 Borneo Eco-Challenge race have occurred.[15] Doxycycline prophylaxis is now recommended for both civilians and military personnel who will hike, bike, swim, or raft in tropical environments.[15] The protean clinical manifestations, which include fever, headache, proximal lower extremity myalgia, and abdominal wall pain, are impossible to distinguish clinically from dengue but may also mimic a number of other common tropical infections. Conjunctival suffusion and jaundice occur in a subset and are more common than in the other undifferentiated febrile diseases, although both may occur in relapsing fever. A reliable, rapid IgM dipstick test for leptospirosis is widely available and used. Recog-

nition of possible leptospirosis affects therapy because antibiotic treatment is generally undertaken when the diagnosis is suspected.[36]

Respiratory Illness

Travelers spend long periods in confined spaces and tend to meet many different people during the course of their trip. Acute respiratory infections occur in 10% to 20% of all travelers, with rates as high as 1261 per 100,000 travelers for a 1-month stay in a developing country. For all ill-returning travelers seen at GeoSentinel Surveillance Network sites, 7.8% had respiratory infection diagnosed, with almost half of these being lower respiratory tract infections such as pneumonia or atypical pneumonia.[37]

Respiratory diseases are second only to gastrointestinal infections as a cause of morbidity in travelers. In outbreaks of infections on cruise ships, respiratory tract infections constitute the most common diagnosis.[38] Influenza is the most common vaccine-preventable disease of travelers, with an incidence rate of approximately 1%. One fourth or more of all cases of legionellosis are associated with travel in the previous 2 weeks, and rates appear to be increasing. Risk factors include stays at large air-conditioned resort hotels or spas and cruise ship travel.[39,40] Acute histoplasmosis can be seen after brief excursions into caves anywhere in the Americas, and travel-related coccidioidomycosis is reported.[41] Tuberculosis is a clear risk in those who spend longer periods in very high-risk countries and especially those who are doing medical or aid work.[42,43] Pulmonary infiltrates and symptoms may be seen during the migratory phases of helminthiases such as schistosomiasis, strongyloidosis, hookworm infestation, and ascariasis. Hemorrhagic pneumonitis may be seen with leptospirosis. Q fever should be sought in those with animal exposure. Workup should be guided by clinical and radiologic findings.

INITIAL OFFICE APPROACH TO THE FEBRILE PATIENT

The first priority is assessment for dangerous or immediately life-threatening disease, such as when hemorrhagic manifestations are apparent. If the patient has the appropriate exposures for a viral hemorrhagic fever, he or she needs to be immediately isolated and public health authorities contacted. None of the isolatable hemorrhagic fever viruses have incubation periods exceeding 3 weeks. Arenavirus infection, whether from West Africa (Lassa virus) or South America (Junin, Machupo, Guanarito viruses), should be treated with ribavirin. Most also recommend treating Crimean-Congo hemorrhagic fever with ribavirin.[44] Other rare hemorrhagic fevers of travelers such as Rift Valley fever, yellow fever, dengue hemorrhagic fever, and Ebola hemorrhagic fever need to be supported with the best possible intensive care.[45] Meningococcemia and rickettsial infection present with purpuric lesions, and bacterial sepsis and severe malaria are serious but treatable causes of hemorrhage due to disseminated intravascular coagulation. Any febrile patient with altered sensorium or any other evidence of end-organ damage consistent with malaria and in whom *P. falciparum* malaria is a possibility should receive empiric therapy for malaria regardless of the result of a blood film. The smear is often negative in advanced disease because of sequestration of parasites in capillary beds.

In the patient who is not severely ill but who has an undifferentiated fever without any localizing symptoms or signs, three blood films, if epidemiologically indicated, are the first priority. At the same time, other mandatory diagnostic tests in the workup of every tropical fever include blood cultures (for enteric fever), complete blood count with differential and platelets, liver function tests, urinalysis, and a chest radiograph. The blood film may also diagnose bartonellosis, acute trypanosomiasis, and relapsing fever. Leukopenia militates away from common bacterial infections and toward dengue, typhoid, brucellosis, rickettsial disease, or acute human immunodeficiency virus (HIV) infection. Thrombocytopenia is indicative of malaria, dengue, or brucellosis. Eosinophilia may indicate early migratory stages of a number of helminths (see later). Liver function test results will be consistently abnormal in viral hepatitis or toxin damage and variably abnormal in leptospirosis, rickettsial disease (including Q fever), relapsing fever, yellow fever, amebic abscess, brucellosis, typhoid, hemorrhagic fever, and dengue. An indirect benefit of chest radiography is the finding of an elevated right hemidiaphragm in many cases of amebic liver abscess.

The second wave of diagnostic testing is driven by any abnormalities that emerge from initial test results. In the absence of enlightening abnormalities, additional serologies may need to be sent based on travel itinerary, incubation periods, and known exposures, as discussed previously. HIV infection and its complications, syphilis, and tuberculosis should be sought at this stage if there is any suggestive exposure at all. After ruling out potentially serious as well as potentially treatable infections by history, physical examination, and routine laboratory work, and especially if patient financial resources are limiting, the clinician must then decide whether to wait 48 to 72 hours before serology and sophisticated diagnostic studies are pursued. Because up to 25% of all febrile illnesses in returning travelers are self-limited viral syndromes, a patient who was highly febrile and quite toxic looking at initial assessment is quite often perfectly well 48 hours later with no intervention. Reasonable clinical and local laboratory experience and confidence are required for this approach, but from the patient standpoint it is the most desirable course. At a minimum, acute serum should be stored for possible later use. If the patient is stable, has no laboratory abnormalities and no clinical evidence of end-organ damage, and has a reliable companion, he or she may be followed as an outpatient during the clinical evolution and the appropriate workup pursued according to any ensuing clinical findings.

Oral ciprofloxacin is sometimes given as empiric therapy for the slightest chance of typhoid fever because of the ease of treatment and the difficulty making the diagnosis. However, quinolone-resistant typhoid and paratyphoid fever is now predominant in the Indian subcontinent and Southeast Asia, where much of the travel-related enteric fever originates. Thus, in this situation, if clinical suspicion is high, the patient may need to be admitted for parenteral therapy. Empiric therapy for malaria without a positive blood film is appropriate only if clinical evidence of cerebral dysfunction or any other end-organ damage consistent with malaria is present. Otherwise, examination of these patients and of serial blood smears over several days by someone with appropriate experience will always lead to the parasitologic diagnosis of malaria, when present.[46] Such expertise is rarely so far away as to compromise patient care. In addition to potential drug toxicities, empiric treatment will necessarily eliminate any possibility of making a species diagnosis if the patient, in fact, does have malaria. After empiric treatment the clinician is then probably obligated to a course of primaquine, a potentially toxic drug, to cover the possibility that the antecedent infection was due to relapsing (*P. vivax* or *P. ovale*) malaria.

Febrile patients who present initially with focal symptoms or signs should have a more directed workup that takes into consideration appropriate disease distribution, incubation period, and possible exposures. Altered mental status or other central nervous system deficits are present as nonspecific sequelae of many systemic infections. However, appropriate itinerary, exposure, and incubation periods for the following less common infections should be sought: Japanese encephalitis, rabies, West Nile virus, tickborne encephalitis, African trypanosomiasis, angiostrongyliasis, gnathostomiasis, and, in recent Hajj pilgrims to Mecca, meningococci.[47]

Diarrhea in Travelers

ACUTE TRAVELER'S DIARRHEA

Diarrhea is by far the most common cause of illness during travel, affecting up to 60% of travelers to some high-risk destinations. South Asia is by far the highest-risk region for traveler's diarrhea (TD).[48] The most frequent cause of TD is enterotoxigenic *E. coli* (6% to 70%). Other types of *E. coli* (especially enteroaggregative *E. coli*),[49] *Salmonella*, *Shigella*, and *Campylobacter* each account for about 5% to 15%.

Vibrio parahaemolyticus is related to shellfish ingestion and is seen almost exclusively in Asia. Protozoa account for less than 5% and in adults, rarely, norovirus or rotavirus may be detected.[50-52] However, norovirus outbreaks aboard cruise ships are apparently increasing.[53] About 30% of diarrheal episodes remain unexplained but many are likely due to enteroaggregative *E. coli*, which is not usually cultured for because these episodes respond to antibacterial drugs.

Bacterial diarrhea generally manifests as the abrupt onset of uncomfortable, crampy diarrhea.[54,55] Fever, nausea, or vomiting, if present, further increase the likelihood of a bacterial etiology. In contrast, protozoal diarrhea (most often due to *Giardia lamblia* or *Entamoeba histolytica*) begins gradually, with loose stools occurring in distinct episodes and gradually becoming more disabling over 1 to 2 weeks. In protozoal diarrhea, medical care usually is not sought immediately because of the low-grade nature of the symptoms. Because most TD is bacterial, many travelers are instructed to self-treat with quinolone antibiotics and are told to seek medical assistance if diarrhea does not resolve after 3 to 5 days of treatment.[56]

Classic TD is defined as three or more unformed stools per day, although a syndrome of nonclassic TD with fewer stools but with accompanying symptoms is defined by some. Travelers may vary in their own definition of what is an abnormal bowel pattern and this needs to be established with the patient in a quantitative way at the outset. Returned travelers with acute diarrhea of a few days' duration who have not yet had a course of quinolone antibiotic can be prescribed an empiric course without any workup or stool culture. Toxic patients with bloody diarrhea should have a wet prep of stool and an immediate sigmoidoscopic examination to look for amebic trophozoites. Nonresponders at 36 to 48 hours should then have stool sent for performance of bacterial culture, ova and parasite (O&P) testing, acid-fast bacilli testing (to detect *Cryptosporidium* and *Cyclospora*), *Giardia* ELISA or immunofluorescence assay, *Entamoeba* ELISA, and *Clostridium difficile* toxin assay. *Vibrio* cultures usually require a special request. Quinolone-resistant *Campylobacter* is increasing worldwide and is the rule in Southeast Asia, so an empiric course of azithromycin can be given while awaiting culture if the patient is still moderately ill.[57] Rifaximin has recently been approved for TD due to *E. coli*.[58] Because of the difficulty of giardiasis diagnosis, an empiric course of tinidazole is often given in practice to those with subacute symptoms and a negative workup. Reiter's syndrome is an occasional sequela of enteritis due to *Shigella* or *Campylobacter*.

PERSISTENT DIARRHEA IN THE TRAVELER

Two percent of those with TD go on to develop chronic diarrhea lasting a month or more. These patients can be extremely frustrating to deal with because diagnosis is most often elusive despite extensive diagnostic testing.[59] Clearly, some undiscovered enteric pathogens remain. A number of limited studies indicate that the incidence of postinfective irritable bowel syndrome at 6 months after an acute episode of TD may range from 4% to 14%. The true incidence of this syndrome is not clear and ancillary contributing factors and possible preemptive interventions are still being investigated.[60] Appropriate studies, in addition to those already listed, include HIV serology, 5-hydroxyindoleacetic acid (5-HIAA) levels, thyroid function tests, serum calcium, testing for malabsorption, and upper and lower endoscopy with all aspirates and biopsies examined carefully for parasitic etiologies. *G. lamblia*, *Strongyloides stercoralis*, *Cryptosporidium parvum*, and *Cyclospora cayetanensis* are occasional etiologies of persistent diarrhea and may be discovered only after invasive workup. Serology for *S. stercoralis*, *Schistosoma mansoni*, or *E. histolytica* is indicated where exposure to these agents may have occurred. Intestinal biopsy almost always yields nonspecific findings, although cases of tropical or nontropical sprue are occasionally discovered or an initial diagnosis of inflammatory bowel disease made. In many patients, the etiology of the frequently found nonspecific villus blunting is unclear. This syndrome has often been called *tropical enteropathy* or *postinfective tropical malabsorption*[61] and is thought to be the residual damage caused by an initial bacterial or other insult. A temporary luminal disaccharidase deficiency may occur. Diarrhea may persist for months before resolving. In the absence of definitive diagnosis in patients with chronic TD, symptomatic treatment with loperamide is indicated. Elimination diets with restriction of lactose, fructose, gluten, and fat are sometimes of benefit. Those with preexisting irritable bowel syndrome may have it unmasked by travel and frequently have exacerbations during or after travel. Tegaserod, alosetron, antispasmodics, or other appropriate medication for their underlying disease may be needed.[62]

Skin Problems

Eruptions accompanying febrile illness have been discussed in the preceding sections and some are illustrated in Figure 330-2. Some common primary dermatologic infections are illustrated in Figure 330-1. The proportion of ill-returned travelers that present to infectious and tropical diseases specialists that have a dermatologic problem is 18%, with variation by region of travel. The most common skin-related diagnoses are cutaneous larva migrans (9.8% of all skin diagnoses), insect bites including superinfected bites (15%), skin abscess (7.7%), and allergic reaction (5.5%). Dengue (3.4%), leishmaniasis (3.3%), myiasis (2.7%) and spotted-fever–group rickettsial diseases (1.5%) are other important reasons for presentation. Arthropod-related skin diseases accounted for 31% of all skin diagnoses.[63,64] Ulcerative lesions of travelers include leishmaniasis, mycobacterial disease, deep mycoses, and, rarely, anthrax. Rickettsial diseases frequently include black eschars at the site of the arthropod bite. Loiasis,[65] gnathostomiasis,[66] and cysticercosis present as painless subcutaneous nodules. Arthropod bites and infestations such as scabies, fleas, lice, and mites present similarly as in nontropical environments. Onchocerciasis presents as an intensely pruritic, evanescent papular rash.[67,68] Varicella, measles, or other childhood exanthems occur in nonimmune travelers and should not be forgotten in the quest for exotic diagnoses. Seabather's eruption (sometimes called *sea-lice*) is a pruritic papular rash notable for being distributed only on skin covered by the patient's bathing suit.[69] Larval sea anemones become trapped by the fabric while the patient is swimming. The indurated erythematous chancre of *Trypanosoma rhodesiense* infection (see Chapter 278) should not be overlooked.[70] Arboviral eruptions usually present as acute febrile illnesses and not as predominant rash illnesses. HIV and STDs need always be considered as a cause of exanthems and ulcerative lesions.

Eosinophilia

In addition to parasitic causes, peripheral blood eosinophilia may be associated with a variety of dermatologic, immunologic, inflammatory, neoplastic, and idiopathic etiologies. Returning travelers and long-term residents of tropical countries are as prone to nonparasitic causes of eosinophilia as is the general population, and these must be considered when obtaining a history and initiating a diagnostic workup in a returned traveler. Schistosomiasis and strongyloidiasis are the most common parasitic causes of significant eosinophilia in returning travelers and serology should be sent on every traveler with potential exposure to either.[71,72]

Eosinophilia is a reaction to a tissue-invasive helminth, with its intensity being proportional to the degree of tissue invasion. During the initial larval migration phase after a new infection with a specific parasite (e.g., hookworm), there may be an intense eosinophilia (up to 5000/mm³). Weeks or months later, when the mature adults reside in the intestine with only minimal tissue contact, eosinophilia will be mild or absent. Although eosinophilia is not seen in protozoan infection, local eosinophilic infiltrates exceptionally occur in areas of the intestinal tract penetrated by *E. histolytica*, *G. lamblia*, or *Isospora belli*.

Although most laboratory reports express the eosinophil count as a percentage of the total white blood cell count, this practice can make it difficult to follow serial determinations in an individual patient. The

TABLE 330-3	Parasitic Causes of Eosinophilia	
Widespread Geographic Distribution	*Limited Geographic Distribution*
Ascariasis (migratory phase)	Clonorchiasis[†]
Hookworm[†]	Paragonimiasis[†]
Strongyloidiasis*[‡]	Fascioliasis[†]
Tropical pulmonary eosinophilia*	Angiostrongyliasis
Lymphatic filariasis	Opisthorchiasis[†]
Schistosomiasis	Onchocerciasis, loiasis, and other
Toxocariasis*	nonlymphatic filariases
Cysticercosis (*Taenia solium*)	Gnathostomiasis
Echinococcosis (cyst rupture)	Capillariasis
Trichinosis*	Trichostrongyliasis
Trichuriasis	
Aberrant helminthiasis from animals	

*Most frequent parasitic causes of massive eosinophilia (>5000/mm³).
[†]Moderate to marked during larval migration in early infection; most often absent or very mild during chronic infection.
[‡]Absent in disseminated infection in compromised hosts.

absolute eosinophil count can be calculated easily and ranges from 0 to 350/mm³ (mean, 120/mm³). Because the list of helminths inducing eosinophilia (Table 330-3) is extensive, and because many of the parasitologic and serologic techniques required for specific diagnosis are laborious and expensive, a well-obtained epidemiologic history is needed to narrow the differential diagnosis down to a manageable size. Some helpful physical findings are dermatitis (onchocerciasis, cutaneous larva migrans, larva currens); migratory swellings (loiasis, gnathostomiasis), wheezing or cough (*Strongyloides*, hookworm, *Ascaris*, or *Schistosoma* larvae in the lung), hemoptysis (*Paragonimus*), hepatomegaly (*Toxocara*, *Echinococcus*); lymphedema (filariasis); facial edema, myositis (trichinosis); subcutaneous mass (cysticercosis); meningeal signs (angiostrongyliasis, gnathostomiasis); abdominal tenderness (angiostrongyliasis, anisakiasis, fascioliasis).

The examination of stools for O&P is the first step and, unfortunately, this crucial diagnostic procedure is dependent on the expertise of the individual laboratory. A concentration technique should be used and at least three separate stools examined. Eggs are produced only by mature adult worms so stool examinations will be negative during the initial larval migratory phase of intestinal helminths for up to 6 weeks after exposure. *Strongyloides* eggs hatch while still in the intestine and Baermann concentration or agar plate cultures are indicated if suspicion is high. Because most anthelmintic drugs only work on adult worms and not immature larvae, empiric therapy of a traveler with eosinophilia soon after return is of no benefit.

The following ancillary procedures are indicated when epidemiologically appropriate[73] or when dictated by specific symptoms: day and night blood concentrations (filariasis); skin snips (onchocerciasis); rectal snips or scrapings (schistosomiasis); urine concentration (schistosomiasis); duodenal aspirate (strongyloidiasis); sputum for O&P (migrating larvae, *Strongyloides*, *Paragonimus*); and biopsy of any abnormal lesions. Serology is available for many of the common helminthic infections, but is hampered by lack of standardization and broad cross-reactivity among many helminth species. Nevertheless, an unequivocally elevated parasite-specific serum IgG level can be extremely helpful when positive in the setting of a previously naive traveler with a history of exposure to only one or a few specific parasites. Schistosomiasis and strongyloidiasis are the two most common causes of parasitic eosinophilia. Stool and more invasive examination is often negative and diagnosis often depends on positive serology.

The detection of one parasitic infection does not preclude the presence of another. All individuals should complete the diagnostic workup that is clinically and epidemiologically indicated. Similarly, all treated patients should be followed up to be certain that both infection and eosinophilia have resolved. An anomalous exacerbation of the eosinophilia may occur for 2 to 3 weeks after treatment as parasites die and release their antigens. Eosinophilia may not totally resolve for 6 months or more after adequate treatment of the inciting helminth, but no response whatsoever for a month or more after treatment may be a sign of inadequate response to treatment.

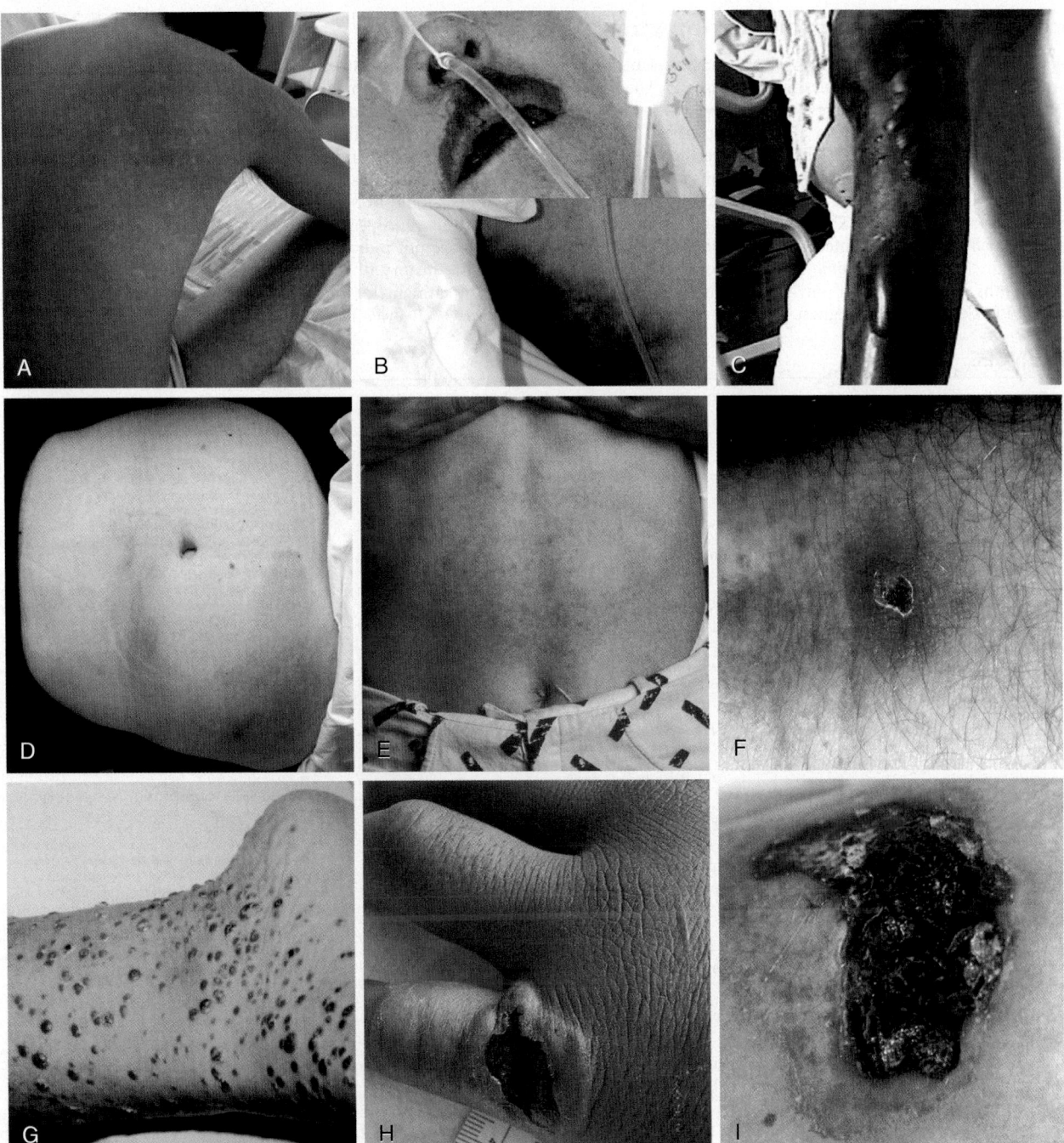

Figure 330-2   Cutaneous manifestations of some common systemic or widely disseminated diseases. A, Generalized macular rash of dengue; rash usually appears after 4 or 5 days but an earlier, faint, flushlike rash may be present as well. **B,** Viral hemorrhagic fever due to yellow fever infection; typical signs of viral hemorrhagic fevers include bleeding from orifices and intravenous sites as well as diffuse petechiae or ecchymoses, especially over pressure points. **C,** Sepsis due to *Vibrio vulnificus* infection after ingestion of contaminated shellfish; hemorrhagic bullae are seen in sepsis, envenomation, and autoimmune disease but not with viral hemorrhagic fevers. **D,** Migratory lesions of infection with *Gnathostoma spinigerum* after ingestion of uncooked freshwater fish; larvae often leave a mildly hemorrhagic track. **E,** Faint, papular, highly pruritic dermatitis due to *Onchocerca volvulus* infection after travel to Sierra Leone; travelers who may not present for a year or more after travel are usually lightly infected and have no ocular manifestation. **F,** Typical eschar of African tick typhus due to *Rickettsia africae*; widely disseminated petechial vasculitic lesions are often present as well. **G,** Verruga peruana due to chronic infection with *Bartonella bacilliformis*, present only if the patient is not treated for and survives the acute bacteremic phase. **H,** Painless lesions of cutaneous anthrax; surrounding edema is characteristic and the base quickly evolves to become totally black and necrotic. **I,** Spider bite due to *Loxosceles laeta*; unlike anthrax, spider bites are painful and usually have very irregular borders without significant edema. *(Images reprinted with permission of the Instituto de Medicina Tropical Alexander von Humboldt, Universidad Peruana Cayetano Heredia, Lima, Peru; and the Gorgas Memorial Institute, University of Alabama, Birmingham, Ala.)*

Screening for Asymptomatic Infection

Completely asymptomatic returned travelers may present with a request to be checked for possible tropical disease. The limited number of available cost-effectiveness studies have yet to show significant benefit to this approach on a population basis.[74-76] Neither a clinic visit nor any nondirected laboratory screening of returned very short-term travelers is indicated. Exceptions are those with known discrete high-risk exposure events in situations conducive to transmission of specific agents. This would include testing for HIV and other sexually transmitted infections, a purified protein derivative (PPD) skin test, or *Schistosoma* serology. For those who have spent 6 months or more under any conditions in a developing country, a PPD skin test is the highest priority even without a specific exposure. For those living under harsher conditions, any abnormalities found on a complete physical examination, including a dermatologic assessment, that would lead to specific laboratory testing should be sought first. For general screening, stool for O&P and an eosinophil count are used by most. Serology for schistosomiasis, filarial infection, and strongyloidiasis is often performed but should be strictly limited to those with extended travel to a known endemic area for each pathogen tested for. Those with new sexual partners should be screened for HIV and sexually transmitted infections at an appropriate interval after last potential exposure. Malaria smears are not indicated in asymptomatic travelers, even those with a remote history of malaria exposure during the travel, but primaquine treatment for those at risk of later relapse of disease due to *P. vivax* or *P. ovale* is.

REFERENCES

1. Steffen R, deBernardis C, Banos A. Travel epidemiology—A global perspective. *Int J Antimicrob Agents.* 2003;21:89-95.
2. Steffen R, Rickenbach M, Wilhelm U, et al. Health problems after travel to developing countries. *J Infect Dis.* 1987;156:84-91.
3. Hill DR. Health problems in a large cohort of Americans traveling to developing countries. *J Travel Med.* 2000;7:259-266.
4. Ryan ET, Wilson ME, Kain KC. Illness after international travel. *N Engl J Med.* 2002;347:505-516.
5. Freedman DO, Weld LH, Kozarsky PE, et al. GeoSentinel Surveillance Network. Spectrum of disease and relation to place of exposure among ill returned travelers. *N Engl J Med.* 2006; 354:119-130.
6. Doherty JF, Grant AD, Bryceson AD. Fever as the presenting complaint of travellers returning from the tropics. *QJM.* 1995;88:277-281.
7. O'Brien D, Tobin S, Brown GV, et al. Fever in returned travelers: review of hospital admissions for a 3-year period. *Clin Infect Dis.* 2001;33:603-609.
8. Wilson ME, Weld LH, Boggild A, et al. GeoSentinel Surveillance Network. Fever in returned travelers: results from the GeoSentinel Surveillance Network. *Clin Infect Dis.* 2007;44:1560-1568.
9. World Health Organization. WHO Research into Global Hazards of Travel (WRIGHT) Project on Air Travel and Venous Thromboembolism. Available at: <http://www.who.int/cardiovascular_diseases/wright_project/en/>.
10. D'Acremont V, Ambresin AE, Burnand B, et al. Practice guidelines for evaluation of fever in returning travelers and migrants. *J Travel Med.* 2003;10(suppl 2):S25-S52.
11. Keystone JS. GIDEON computer program for diagnosing and teaching geographic medicine. *J Travel Med.* 1999;6:152-154.
12. Schwartz E, Weld LH, Wilder-Smith A, et al. GeoSentinel Surveillance Network. Seasonality, annual trends, and characteristics of dengue among ill returned travelers, 1997-2006. *Emerg Infect Dis.* 2008;14:1081-1088.
13. Cetron MS, Chitsulo L, Sullivan JJ, et al. Schistosomiasis in Lake Malawi. *Lancet.* 1996;348:1274-1278.
14. Nicolls DJ, Weld LH, Schwartz E, et al. GeoSentinel Surveillance Network. Characteristics of schistosomiasis in travelers reported to the GeoSentinel Surveillance Network 1997-2008. *Am J Trop Med Hyg.* 2008;79:729-734.
15. Sejvar J, Bancroft E, Winthrop K, et al. Leptospirosis in "Eco-Challenge" athletes, Malaysian Borneo, 2000. *Emerg Infect Dis.* 2003;9:702-707.
16. Cabada MM, Echevarria JI, Seas CR, et al. Sexual behavior of international travelers visiting Peru. *Sex Transm Dis.* 2002;29:510-513.
17. Mulhall BP. Sex and travel: studies of sexual behaviour, disease and health promotion in international travellers—a global review. *Int J STD AIDS.* 1996;7:455-465.
18. Felton JM, Bryceson AD. Fever in the returning traveller. *Br J Hosp Med.* 1996;55:705-711.
19. Farcas GA, Zhong KJ, Lovegrove FE, et al. Evaluation of the Binax NOW ICT test versus polymerase chain reaction and microscopy for the detection of malaria in returned travelers. *Am J Trop Med Hyg.* 2003;69:589-592.
20. Mali S, Steele S, Slutsker L, et al. Malaria surveillance—United States, 2006. *MMWR Surveill Summ* 2008;57(SS-5):24-39.
21. Leder K, Black J, O'Brien D, et al. Malaria in travelers: a review of the GeoSentinel surveillance network. *Clin Infect Dis.* 2004;39:1104-1112.
22. Dorsey G, Gandhi M, Oyugi JH, et al. Difficulties in the prevention, diagnosis, and treatment of imported malaria. *Arch Intern Med.* 2000;160:2505-2510.
23. Svenson JE, MacLean JD, Gyorkos TW, et al. Imported malaria: clinical presentation and examination of symptomatic travelers. *Arch Intern Med.* 1995;155:861-868.
24. D'Acremont V, Landry P, Mueller I, et al. Clinical and laboratory predictors of imported malaria in an outpatient setting: an aid to medical decision making in returning travelers with fever. *Am J Trop Med Hyg.* 2002;66:481-486.
25. Lindback H, Lindback J, Tegnell A, et al. Dengue fever in travelers to the tropics, 1998 and 1999. *Emerg Infect Dis.* 2003;9:438-442.

26. Schwartz E, Moskovitz A, Potasman I, et al. Changing epidemiology of dengue fever in travelers to Thailand. *Eur J Clin Microbiol Infect Dis.* 2000;19:784-786.
27. Connor BA, Schwartz E. Typhoid and paratyphoid fever in travellers. *Lancet Infect Dis.* 2005;5:623-628.
28. Steinberg EB, Bishop R, Haber P, et al. Typhoid fever in travelers: who should be targeted for prevention? *Clin Infect Dis.* 2004;39:186-191.
29. Crump JA, Luby SP, Mintz ED. The global burden of typhoid fever. *Bull World Health Organ.* 2004;82:346-353.
30. Schwartz E, Shlim DR, Eaton M, et al. The effect of oral and parenteral typhoid vaccination on the rate of infection with *Salmonella typhi* and *Salmonella paratyphi* A among foreigners in Nepal. *Arch Intern Med.* 1990;150:349-351.
31. Mutsch M, Spicher VM, Gut C, et al. Hepatitis A virus infections in travelers, 1988-2004. *Clin Infect Dis.* 2006;42:490-497.
32. Piper-Jenks N, Horowitz HW, Schwartz E. Risk of hepatitis E infection to travelers. *J Travel Med.* 2000;7:194-199.
33. Cazorla C, Socolovschi C, Jensenius M, et al. Tick-borne diseases: tick-borne spotted fever rickettsioses in Africa. *Infect Dis Clin North Am.* 2008;22:531-544.
34. Raoult D, Fournier PE, Fenollar F, et al. *Rickettsia africae*, a tick-borne pathogen in travelers to sub-Saharan Africa. *N Engl J Med.* 2001;344:1504-1510.
35. Jensenius M, Fournier PE, Vene S, et al. African tick bite fever in travelers to rural sub-Equatorial Africa. *Clin Infect Dis.* 2003;36:1411-1417.
36. Yersin C, Bovet P, Smits HL, et al. Field evaluation of a one-step dipstick assay for the diagnosis of human leptospirosis in the Seychelles. *Trop Med Int Health.* 1999;4:38-45.
37. Leder K, Sundararajan V, Weld L, et al. Respiratory tract infections in travelers: a review of the GeoSentinel surveillance network. *Clin Infect Dis.* 2003;36:399-406.
38. Miller JM, Tam TW, Maloney S, et al. Cruise ships: high-risk passengers and the global spread of new influenza viruses. *Clin Infect Dis.* 2000;31:433-438.
39. Ricketts KD, McNaught B, Joseph CA; European Working Group for *Legionella* Infections. Travel-associated legionnaires' disease in Europe: 2004. *Eurosurveillance.* 2006;11:107-110.
40. Centers for Disease Control and Prevention (CDC). Surveillance for travel-associated legionnaires disease—United States, 2005-2006. *MMWR Morb Mortal Wkly Rep.* 2007;56:1261-1263.
41. Panackal AA, Hajjeh RA, Cetron MS, et al. Fungal infections among returning travelers. *Clin Infect Dis.* 2002;35:1088-1095.
42. Cobelens FG, van Deutekom H, Draayer-Jansen IW, et al. Association of tuberculin sensitivity in Dutch adults with history of travel to areas of with a high incidence of tuberculosis. *Clin Infect Dis.* 2001;33:300-304.
43. Updated guidelines on tuberculosis and air travel. *Wkly Epidemiol Rec.* 2008;83:209-213.
44. Ergonul O. Treatment of Crimean-Congo hemorrhagic fever. *Antiviral Res.* 2008;78:125-131.
45. Peters CJ. Emerging infections: ebola and other filoviruses. *West J Med.* 1996;164:36-38.
46. Svenson JE, Gyorkos TW, MacLean JD. Diagnosis of malaria in the febrile traveler. *Am J Trop Med Hyg.* 1995;53:518-521.
47. Memish ZA. Meningococcal disease and travel. *Clin Infect Dis.* 2002;34:84-90.
48. Greenwood Z, Black J, Weld L, et al. GeoSentinel Surveillance Network. Gastrointestinal infection among international travelers globally. *J Travel Med.* 2008;15:221-228.
49. Adachi JA, Jiang ZD, Mathewson JJ, et al. Enteroaggregative *Escherichia coli* as a major etiologic agent in traveler's diarrhea in 3 regions of the world. *Clin Infect Dis.* 2001;32:1706-1709.
50. von Sonnenburg F, Tornieporth N, Waiyaki P, et al. Risk and aetiology of diarrhoea at various tourist destinations. *Lancet.* 2000;356:133-134.
51. Steffen R, Collard F, Tornieporth N, et al. Epidemiology, etiology, and impact of traveler's diarrhea in Jamaica. *JAMA.* 1999;281:811-817.
52. Paredes P, Campbell-Forrester S, Mathewson JJ, et al. Etiology of travelers' diarrhea on a Caribbean island. *J Travel Med.* 2000;7:15-18.

53. Centers for Disease Control and Prevention. Outbreaks of gastroenteritis associated with noroviruses on cruise ships—United States, 2002. *MMWR Morb Mortal Wkly Rep.* 2002;51:1112-1115.
54. Farthing MJ. Travellers' diarrhoea. *Gut.* 1994;35:1-4.
55. Shlim DR, Hoge CW, Rajah R, et al. Persistent high risk of diarrhea among foreigners in Nepal during the first 2 years of residence. *Clin Infect Dis.* 1999;29:613-616.
56. Adachi JA, Ostrosky-Zeichner L, DuPont HL, et al. Empirical antimicrobial therapy for traveler's diarrhea. *Clin Infect Dis.* 2000;31:1079-1083.
57. Tribble DR, Sanders JW, Pang LW, et al. Traveler's diarrhea in Thailand: randomized, double-blind trial comparing single-dose and 3-day azithromycin-based regimens with a 3-day levofloxacin regimen. *Clin Infect Dis.* 2007;44:338-346.
58. DuPont HL, Jiang ZD, Ericsson CD, et al. Rifaximin versus ciprofloxacin for the treatment of traveler's diarrhea: a randomized, double-blind clinical trial. *Clin Infect Dis.* 2001;33:1807-1815.
59. Cook GC. Persisting diarrhoea and malabsorption. *Gut.* 1994;35:582-586.
60. DuPont AW. Postinfectious irritable bowel syndrome. *Clin Infect Dis.* 2008;46:594-599.
61. Veitch AM, Kelly P, Zulu IS, et al. Tropical enteropathy: a T-cell–mediated crypt hyperplastic enteropathy. *Eur J Gastroenterol Hepatol.* 2001;13:1175-1181.
62. Talley NJ, Spiller R. Irritable bowel syndrome: a little understood organic bowel disease? *Lancet.* 2002;360:555-564.
63. Caumes E, Carriere J, Guermonprez G, et al. Dermatoses associated with travel to tropical countries: a prospective study of the diagnosis and management of 269 patients presenting to a tropical disease unit. *Clin Infect Dis.* 1995;20:542-548.
64. Lederman ER, Weld LH, Elyazar IR, et al. Dermatologic conditions of the ill returned traveler: an analysis from the GeoSentinel Surveillance Network. *Int J Infect Dis.* 2008;12:593-602.
65. Klion AD, Massougbodji A, Sadeler BC, et al. Loiasis in endemic and nonendemic populations: immunologically mediated differences in clinical presentation. *J Infect Dis.* 1991;163:1318-1325.
66. Moore DA, McCroddan J, Dekumyoy P, et al. Gnathostomiasis: an emerging imported disease. *Emerg Infect Dis.* 2003;9:647-650.
67. McCarthy JS, Ottesen EA, Nutman TB. Onchocerciasis in endemic and nonendemic populations: differences in clinical presentation and immunologic findings. *J Infect Dis.* 1994;170:736-741.
68. Lipner EM, Law MA, Barnett E, et al. GeoSentinel Surveillance Network. Filariasis in travelers presenting to the GeoSentinel Surveillance Network. *PLoS Negl Trop Dis.* 2007;1:e88.
69. Freudenthal AR, Joseph PR. Seabather's eruption. *N Engl J Med.* 1993;331:542-544.
70. McGovern TW, Williams W, Fitzpatrick JE, et al. Cutaneous manifestations of African trypanosomiasis. *Arch Dermatol.* 1995;131:1178-1182.
71. Schulte C, Krebs B, Jelinek T, et al. Diagnostic significance of blood eosinophilia in returning travelers. *Clin Infect Dis.* 2002;34:407-411.
72. Whitty CJ, Mabey DC, Armstrong M, et al. Presentation and outcome of 1107 cases of schistosomiasis from Africa diagnosed in a non-endemic country. *Trans R Soc Trop Med Hyg.* 2000;94:531-534.
73. Whetham J, Day JN, Armstrong M, et al. Investigation of tropical eosinophilia: assessing a strategy based on geographical area. *J Infect.* 2003;46:180-185.
74. Carroll B, Dow C, Snashall D, et al. Post-tropical screening: how useful is it? *BMJ.* 1993;307:541.
75. MacLean JD, Libman M. Screening returning travelers. *Infect Dis Clin North Am.* 1998;12:431-443.
76. Whitty CJ, Carroll B, Armstrong M, et al. Utility of history, examination and laboratory tests in screening those returning to Europe from the tropics for parasitic infection. *Trop Med Int Health.* 2000;5:818-823.

Note: Page numbers followed by f or t indicate figures or tables, respectively.

A

Abacavir, 706t-709t, 1834f, 1835t, 1836
  dosage of, 740t-741t
  drug interactions with, 742t-761t
  formulations of, 717t
  for HIV-infected children, 1820t-1821t
  hypersensitivity reaction to, 269, 1733-1734, 1836
  resistance to, 1836
Abacavir-lamivudine, 717t
Abacavir-lamivudine-zidovudine, 717t
Abdomen
  anatomy of, 1012f, 1013-1030
  doughy, in tuberculous peritonitis, 3157
  infections within. See Intra-abdominal infections; Peritonitis.
Abdominal abscess, in liver transplant recipients, 3843
Abdominal actinomycosis, 1400t-1401t, 1404, 3212-3214, 3213f
Abdominal angiostrongyliasis, 3618t, 3620-3621
Abdominal cramps
  with diarrhea, 1414-1415
  without diarrhea, 1415
Abdominal pain
  and/or diarrhea with eosinophilia, syndrome of, 1407-1409, 1407t
  in Campylobacter infection, 2797
  in peritonitis, 1020
Abdominal tenderness, in peritonitis, 1020
Abdominal wall rigidity, in peritonitis, 1020
Abiotrophia, 2670t, 2673
Abiotrophia defectiva, 2673
  prosthetic valve endocarditis from, 1121-1122
ABO blood group
  cholera and, 51t
  in disease susceptibility, 52-53
  malaria and, 50, 50t, 3443
Abortion
  in brucellosis, 2923
  medical, toxic shock syndrome after, 1514
  pelvic infection after, 1513-1514
  septic, from Campylobacter jejuni, 2797
Abscess
  abdominal, in liver transplant recipients, 3843
  brain. See Brain abscess.
  Brodie's, 1465
  cutaneous. See also Skin infections.
    in chromoblastomycosis, 3278-3279, 3279f
    gonococcal, 2761
  epidural, 1281-1283, 1283f, 1460-1461, 1461f, 3886
  in glanders, 2877, 2877f
  in injection drug users, 3876, 3884-3886
  injection site, 1309
  internal, in melioidosis, 2872, 2874f-2875f
  intracranial
    from Blastomyces dermatitidis, 3326, 3326f
    hyperbaric oxygen therapy for, 628
  intraperitoneal, 1030-1032
    bacterial findings in, 1030
    diagnosis of, 1030-1031, 1031f
    etiology of, 1030
    treatment of, 1031-1032
  liver. See Liver abscess.
  lung, 925-929, 926t, 927f. See also Lung abscess.
  muscle, 1319
  myocardial, in endocarditis, 1074
  orbital. See Orbital abscess/cellulitis.
  pancreatic, 1046t, 1047
  paraspinal, 3155-3156, 3337-3338, 3338f
  pelvic, 1515-1516
  periapical, 858
  pericolonic, 3085, 3086f
  perihepatic, 1011, 1030

Abscess (Continued)
  perinephric, 976-979, 977f
  periodontal, 860, 3085
  peritonsillar
    gram-negative anaerobe rods in, 3115
    from pharyngitis, 820
  prostatic, 1523-1524, 1524f, 2872-2873, 2875f
  psoas, 1319, 2874f
  renal, 976-979, 976f-977f
  self-induced, 1309
  specimens from, 235t-236t, 243
  splenic
    in endocarditis, 1074-1075
    in injection drug users, 3884-3885
    in melioidosis, 1055-1057, 2874f-2875f
    microbiology of, 1055, 1056t
  subcutaneous, 1300, 1309-1310
  subperiosteal, 1572-1573, 1572f-1573f
    in suppurative thrombophlebitis, 1097
  subphrenic, 1030
  tuboovarian, 1518
Absidia, 3257, 3258f, 3258t
Absorption, drug, 297
Absorption rate constant, 297
Abuse
  alcohol
    cirrhosis from, 1013-1014, 2165-2166
    hepatitis from, 1588
    pulmonary host defense and, 894
  sexual, of children, HIV infection in, 1828
  substance. See also Injection drug users.
    chronic pneumonia and, 932-933
ABVD regimen, for Hodgkin's disease, 1776
Acanthamoeba, 3427-3436
  characteristics of, 3427, 3428f-3429f, 3430t
  disseminated disease from, 3434
  encephalitis from, 3427-3436. See also Amebic encephalitis, granulomatous.
  keratitis from, 1550, 3427-3436. See also Amebic keratitis.
  meningitis from, chronic, 1240
Accessory gene regulator, in Staphylococcus aureus pathogenesis, 2547-2548, 2548f
  ecologic and epidemiologic implication of, 2549
  role of, 2549
Acedapsone, for leprosy, 546
Acellular pertussis vaccine, 2961
Acetaminophen, antipyretic activity of, 774
Acetazolamide, for altitude sickness, 4016
Achromobacter, 3016t-3017t, 3021-3022
Achromobacter xylosoxidans, 3021-3022
Acid-fast staining, 244, 244t
  of Mycobacterium tuberculosis, 3130-3131, 3130t
Acidification of urine, during methenamine therapy, 518
Acinetobacter, 2881-2885
  antibiotic resistance to, 2883
  bacteremia from, 2883
  carbapenems for, 342t
  characteristics of, 2881, 2882t
  clinical manifestations of, 2882-2883
  community-acquired, 2882
  epidemiology of, 2881-2882
  genitourinary, 2883
  intracranial, 2883
  laboratory detection of, 240t-242t
  microbiology of, 2881
  miscellaneous, 2883
  nomenclature for, 2881, 2882t
  pathogenesis of, 2882
  respiratory, 2882-2883
  soft tissue, 2883
  treatment of, 2883-2884

Acinetobacter baumannii
  bloodstream infections from, 3700
  multidrug resistant, polymyxins for, 469
  resistance of, mechanisms of, 290t
Acinetobacter calcoaceticus, 2881
Acinetobacter calcoaceticus–Acinetobacter baumannii complex, 2881
Acne vulgaris. See also Propionibacterium acnes.
  topical antibacterials for, 526-527, 528t
Acquired immunodeficiency syndrome. See AIDS entries; Human immunodeficiency virus infection.
Acremonium, mycetoma from, 3281, 3282t, 3283f
Acridine orange stain, 244, 244t
Acrodermatitis chronica atrophicans, 801, 3076
Actinobacillus, 3015-3017, 3016t
Actinomucor, 3257, 3258t
Actinomyces. See also Actinomycosis.
  appendicitis from, 3212-3213
  endocarditis from, 3211-3215
  laboratory detection of, 240t-242t
  meningitis from, 1240
  in oral cavity, 855-856, 856t
  osteomyelitis from, 3211, 3211f
  pericarditis from, 3211-3215
  subcutaneous abscess from, 1309
Actinomyces meyeri, 3215
Actinomycetes, aerobic
  epidemiology of, 254
  identification of, 254
  laboratory tests for, 253-254
  specimens containing
    collection and transport of, 253
    direct detection of, 253
    processing and planting of, 253-254
  susceptibility testing of, 254
Actinomycetoma, 3214, 3281, 3284
Actinomycosis, 3209-3219
  abdominal, 1400t-1401t, 1404, 3212-3214, 3213f
  central nervous system disease in, 3214
  clinical manifestations of, 3210-3211, 3210f-3212f
  diagnosis of, 3215-3216, 3216f
  disseminated, 3215
  epidemiology of, 3209
  etiologic agents in, 3209
  of gallbladder, 3213-3214
  hepatic, 3213, 3213f
  mediastinal, 3211-3212
  musculoskeletal, 3214-3215
  oral-cervicofacial, 3210-3211, 3210f-3211f
  pathology and pathogenesis of, 3209-3210
  pelvic, 3214, 3214f
  perianal /perirectal, 3213
  pleuropulmonary, 918
  thoracic, 3211, 3212f
  treatment of, 3216-3217, 3217t
  urogenital, 3213
Acute respiratory distress syndrome (ARDS)
  methylprednisolone for, 619
  severe. See Severe acute respiratory syndrome (SARS).
Acute-phase proteins, 770, 771t
Acute-phase response, 990-992. See also Inflammatory response, initial.
  anti-infective, 990-991
  anti-inflammatory, 991
  febrile response and, 770-771, 770t-771t
  innate immunity and, 37, 41-44, 42t-43t
  metabolic, 991
  procoagulant, 991, 992f
  thermoregulatory, 992
Acyclovir, 566t-567t, 568-571, 706t-709t
  activity spectrum of, 568, 568t
  for acute retinal necrosis, 1567

Acyclovir *(Continued)*
  clinical studies of, 570-571
  for cytomegalovirus, 571
  dosage of, 738t-739t
  drug interactions with, 569, 742t-761t
  formulations of, 717t
  for herpes B virus, 2025
  for herpes simplex virus, 570-571, 1956, 1957t, 1958
  for herpes simplex virus esophagitis, 1355t
  for herpetic anterior uveitis, 1567
  for lymphoproliferative disease, 2004
  mechanism of action of, 568
  pharmacokinetics of, 569, 569t
  prophylactic
    for cancer-related infections, 3800t, 3802
    in transplant recipients, 3815
  resistance to, 568-569
  structure of, 568f
  toxicity of, 569-570
  for varicella-zoster virus, 571, 1966-1967
Adalimumab, leprosy and, 3174
Adefovir, 566t-567t, 572-573, 706t-709t
  clinical studies of, 573
  dosage of, 738t-739t
  formulations of, 717t
  for hepatitis B infection, chronic, 1598-1599, 1601t, 2076, 2076t
  in renal insufficiency, 572, 572t
  structure of, 572f
Adenitis, mesenteric. *See* Mesenteric lymphadenitis.
Adenoidectomy, for otitis media, 835
Adenopathy, preauricular, 1531
Adenosine deaminase
  deficiency of, 167-168, 169t-170t
  in tuberculous pleural effusion, 921
Adenoviruses, 2027-2033
  bronchiolitis from, 886t
  central nervous system infections from, 2030
  classification of, 2027, 2028t
  clinical syndromes associated with, 2029-2030, 2029f
  conjunctivitis from, 1531
  croup from, 825-826, 826f
  description of, 2027, 2028f
  detection of, 259t-260t, 2031, 2031f
  encephalitis from, 1251t-1252t
  epidemiology of, 2028-2029
  gastrointestinal infections from, 2029-2030
  genitourinary tract infections from, 2030
  in hematopoietic stem cell transplant recipients, 2030, 3830
  in HIV infection, 2031
  host interactions with, 2027-2028
  keratitis from, 1547
  latency of, 2028
  MHC class I downregulation by, 134
  myocarditis from, 1153
  ocular disease from, 2029
  pharyngitis from, 818
  prevention of, 2032
  receptors for, 2027
  in solid organ transplant recipients, 2030-2031
  transmission of, 2029
  treatment of, 2031-2032
  type 14, 204-205
  urinary tract infection from, 964
  vaccine for, 2032
  as vectors for gene therapy and vaccination, 2032
  as vectors for HIV vaccines, 1889, 1891-1892
Adenylate cyclase toxin, 28t, 30
  of *Bordetella pertussis*, 30, 2955
Adherence, 15-25
  antibody inhibition of, 15
  of *Bacillus*, 2728
  biofilms in, 22-23, 23t
  in diarrhea, 1341-1342
  in endocarditis, 1144
  of *Entamoeba histolytica*, 3413-3414
  mechanisms of, 18-21
  P fimbriae in, 16f, 20-21, 20f
  of *Staphylococcus epidermidis*, 2580-2581
  of *Streptococcus agalactiae* (group B), 2657
  in urinary tract infection, 962

Adhesins
  bacterial, 1341-1342
    role of, 2568-2569
  of *Bordetella pertussis*, 2955
  of *Campylobacter jejuni*, 2795-2796
  of Enterobacteriaceae organisms, 2818-2819
  Gal/GalNAc, 19-20, 19f
  of group A *Streptococcus*, 2594
  HIV gp120/160, 18-19, 18f
  identification of, 15, 16t
  microbial synergy and, 21
  of *Moraxella catarrhalis*, 2771-2772, 2772t
  receptors for
    identification of, 15-16, 16t
    interactions between, 17-18, 17f, 17t
  of *Staphylococcus aureus*, 2550-2551, 2551f, 2551t
  as therapeutic targets, 21-22, 21t
  of uropathogenic *Escherichia coli*, 16f, 20-21, 20f, 959-960, 959t
  of vesicular stomatitis, 16f
Adolescents
  HIV infection in, 1639, 1809-1810, 1819, 1827-1828
  immunization schedule for, 3939
  pertussis resurgence in, 2957, 2957f
  tuberculosis in, 3139, 3139f-3140f
ADP-ribosylating toxins, 28t
Adrenal infections, from *Paracoccidioides brasiliensis*, 3360
Adrenal insufficiency
  in sepsis, 998
  in septic shock, 1001
  in subacute progressive disseminated histoplasmosis, 3313
Adrenergic agents, as nasal decongestants, 811
Adrenocorticotropic hormone, innate immunity and, 45
Adult Pertussis Trial (APERT), 2961
Adult T-cell leukemia/lymphoma, 2313f-2314f, 2315-2316
Aedes aegypti
  chikungunya from, 207
  dengue from, 207, 207f. *See also* Dengue fever.
  distribution of, 2136, 2136f
  infection from, 4022
Aedes albopictus, chikungunya from, 207
Aedes flavicollis, hemorrhagic fever with renal syndrome from, 2290
Aedes mcintoshi, Rift Valley fever from, 2289-2290
Aerobactin, 2820
Aerobic actinomycetes
  epidemiology of, 254
  identification of, 254
  laboratory tests for, 253-254
  specimens containing
    collection and transport of, 253
    direct detection of, 253
    processing and planting of, 253-254
  susceptibility testing of, 254
Aerobic infections, from gram-negative bacilli
  classification of, 3017t
  meningitis from, 1193, 1218
Aerodigestive tract, gram-negative anaerobic rod infections of, 3115-3117
Aeromonas, 3016t-3017t, 3017-3019
Aeromonas caviae, 3018
Aeromonas hydrophila, 3018
  cellulitis from, 1296
  myonecrosis from, 1319
Aerosol release
  of anthrax spores, 3995
  of *Bacillus*, 3984-3985
  of biological weapons, 3955
  of *Francisella tularensis*, 3971
  of smallpox, 3995
  of viral agents, 3995, 3996t
  of *Yersinia pestis*, 3966
Africa, sub-Saharan
  HIV infection in, 1620-1622, 1621f
  HIV-infected children in, 1810
African histoplasmosis, 3314
African horse sickness virus, 2098
African tick fever, 3450, 3653-3654, 3653t
African tick typhus, from *Rickettsia africae*, 4024

African trypanosomiasis, 3489-3494
  clinical course of, 3491
  diagnosis of, 3490f, 3491-3492
  epidemiology of, 3490-3491, 3490t
  etiology of, 3489
  versus malaria, 3450
  melarsoprol for, 656
  pathology and pathogenesis of, 3489-3490
  prevention of, 3493
  treatment of, 3492-3493, 3492t
Agammaglobulinemia, 72
  Bruton's, 72
  enteroviral meningoencephalitis in, 1205, 1215, 2359-2360
  pneumococcal infection and, 2628
  X-linked, 72, 169t-170t, 171
Agar dilution tests, 249
Age. *See also* Children; Elderly; Infants; Neonates.
  antimicrobial agents and, 268-269
  chronic pneumonia and, 931
  gastrointestinal infections and, 1336
  HAV incidence rate and, 2374, 2374f
  tuberculosis and, 3133, 3139
  vaccines and, 3918
Agent, 186-187
  host versus, 185-188
Agglutination assay, 65, 248, 249t
  latex
    in bacterial meningitis, 1208
    in rotavirus infection, 2111
  microscopic, in leptospirosis, 3063
  particle, in HIV infection, 1669, 1669f
  in toxoplasmosis, 3509-3510
Agglutinins, cold
  in *Mycoplasma pneumoniae*, 2484-2486
  Raynaud phenomenon and, 2485
Aggregatibacter, 240t-242t, 2917-2918, 2917t, 3015-3017, 3016t-3017t
Aggregatibacter actinomycetemcomitans, 3015-3017
Aggregatibacter aphrophilus, 2917-2918, 2917t
Aggregatibacter israelii, 3015
Aggregatibacter paraphrophilus, 2917-2918, 2917t
Agr regulation, in *Staphylococcus aureus* pathogenesis, 2547-2548, 2548f
Agranulocytosis, congenital, 172
AIDS (acquired immunodeficiency syndrome). *See also* Human immunodeficiency virus infection.
  in children, 1644-1645, 1645f
  demography of, 1640-1641, 1641t
  geographic distribution of, 1641-1642, 1642f
  mortality in, 1644
  trends in, 1640, 1641f
AIDS dementia, 1746-1749
  brain biopsy in, 1747-1748
  clinical presentation in, 1746-1747, 1747t
  histologic analysis in, 1747-1748
  imaging studies in, 1747, 1748f
  laboratory findings in, 1747
  pathogenesis of, 1748, 1748t
  treatment of, 1748-1749, 1749t
AIDS surveillance case definition, 1635-1636, 1636t-1637t
AIDS-indicator diseases, 1643-1644
Airborne precautions, transmission-based, 3674-3675, 3674t-3675t
Airborne transmission, 188
Air-conditioning cooling towers, *Legionella pneumophila*–contaminated, 2979
Airline-related morbidity, in travelers, 4016
Airport malaria, 3445
Airway
  colonization of, prevention of, 3723
  obstruction of, in epiglottitis, 853
  pathology of, in chronic obstructive pulmonary disease, 877
  in pulmonary host defense, 891, 893t
Airway surface liquid, 891
Ajellomyces dermatitidis, 3319
Albaconazole, 559
  for *Scedosporium prolificans*, 3366
Albendazole, 706t-709t
  for ascariasis, 3579-3580
  for cysticercosis, 3613
  dosage of, 645
  for echinococcosis, 3614

Albendazole *(Continued)*
  for enterobiasis, 3584
  for giardiasis, 3531, 3531t
  for hookworm, 3581
  for intestinal parasitic infections, 632t-635t,
    644-646
  for liver flukes, 3601
  for microsporidiosis, 3401t, 3402
  resistance to, 645
  for strongyloidiasis, 3583
  for trichinellosis, 3588
  for trichuriasis, 3580-3581
Albumin, in nutritional assessment, 151, 152t
Alcaligenes, 3016t, 3021-3022
Alcohol(s), disinfection with, 521, 522t, 3681-3682
Alcohol abuse
  cirrhosis from, 1013-1014, 2165-2166
  hepatitis from, 1588
  pulmonary host defense and, 894
Alemtuzumab, 3812
Algae, toxic
  disease from, 3569-3571
  sites and types of, 3569, 3570f
Alginate, in *Pseudomonas aeruginosa* spread, 2847
Alimentary tract
  microflora of, 3784-3786
  mucosal barrier injury to, 3785-3786, 3785f
Alitretinoin gel, for Kaposi's sarcoma, 1767
Allergic bronchopulmonary aspergillosis
  clinical manifestations of, 3245-3246
  in cystic fibrosis, 951, 3246, 3246t
  pathogenesis of, 3245
Allergic croup, 825. *See also* Croup.
Allergic fungal sinusitis, 3245-3246, 3248, 3248f,
    3368, 3368f
Allergy
  to erythromycin, 431
  Helicobacter pylori infection and, 2806t, 2807-2808
  to penicillin, 350. *See also* Beta-lactam antibiotics,
    allergy to.
    CDC recommendations for, 3047t
    syphilis treatment and, 3050
Allograft, aortic, 1117
Alphaviruses, 2117-2125, 2118t, 4000t-4001t
  arthritis from, 1450
  clinical manifestations of, 2122-2123
  description of, 2117-2118, 2119f
  diagnosis of, 2123-2124
  encephalitis-causing, 2118-2120, 2122-2123
  epidemiology of, 2118-2121
  epizootic spread of, 2120, 2120f
  fever from, 2120-2121, 2123
  historical background on, 2117
  infections from, 4022
  New World, 2117
  Old World, 2117
  pathogenesis of, 2121-2122, 2122f
  polyarthritis from, 2120-2121, 2123
  rash from, 2120-2121, 2123
  treatment and prevention of diseases caused by,
    2124
Alternative and complementary therapy, 669-676,
    670t. *See also specific therapy.*
Alternative hypothesis, in clinical trials, 691
Altitude, effect of, on travelers, 4016
Alveolar cysts, 3608t, 3614-3615
Alveolar hemorrhage, diffuse, in transplant
    recipients, 3823
Amanita, poisoning from, 1417t, 1418
Amantadine, 566t-567t, 573-576
  activity spectrum of, 573
  clinical studies of, 575-576
  dosage of, 738t-739t
  drug interactions with, 575, 742t-761t
  formulations of, 717t
  for influenza, 2277-2278, 2277t, 2284
  mechanism of action of, 573
  pharmacokinetics of, 574, 574t-575t
  resistance to, 573-574, 2278
  structure of, 573f
  toxicity of, 575
Ambler classification of beta-lactamases, 282t, 311t
Amblyomma americanum, 3649, 3650f, 3652
Ambulatory care, in emergency preparedness,
    229-230

AMD-070, for HIV infection, 21-22
AMD-3100, for HIV infection, 21-22
Amdinocillin, 706t-709t, 718t-719t
Amebae, *Legionella pneumophila* interaction with,
    2970, 2970f
Amebiasis. *See Entamoeba histolytica.*
Amebic colitis, 3418, 3419f, 3422t
Amebic dysentery, 1391-1392, 3411
  clinical manifestations of, 3418, 3419f
  diagnosis of, 1393
Amebic encephalitis, granulomatous
  clinical manifestations of, 3432
  epidemiology of, 3430-3431
  etiology of, 3427, 3430t
  laboratory diagnosis of, 3433
  pathology and pathogenesis of, 3431
  treatment of, 3434
Amebic infections
  from *Acanthamoeba*, 3427-3436. *See also*
    Acanthamoeba.
  from *Balamuthia*, 3427-3436
  from *Entamoeba histolytica*, 3411-3425. *See also*
    Entamoeba histolytica.
  from free-living amebas, 3427-3436
  from *Naegleria*, 3427-3436
  from *Sappinia diploidea*, 3427-3436. *See also*
    Sappinia diploidea.
Amebic keratitis, 1550, 3427-3436
  clinical manifestations of, 1550, 1550f, 3432,
    3432f
  epidemiology of, 3431
  etiology of, 3427, 3430t
  laboratory diagnosis of, 3433
  pathology and pathogenesis of, 3431
  prevention of, 3435
  treatment of, 1551, 3434
Amebic liver abscess, 918, 921, 3412, 3416-3417,
    3417f
  clinical manifestations of, 1037, 3418, 3420f
  diagnosis of, 1037-1038
  epidemiology/etiology of, 1035
  microbiology of, 1036
  pathogenesis of and pathophysiology of, 1035
  treatment of, 632t-635t, 1038, 3422, 3422t
Amebic lung abscess, 925
Amebic meningitis, 1193, 1207, 1210-1211, 1220
Amebic meningoencephalitis, 3427-3436
  clinical manifestations of, 3432
  epidemiology of, 3429-3430
  etiology of, 3427, 3430t
  laboratory diagnosis of, 3432
  pathology and pathogenesis of, 3431
  prevention of, 3435
  treatment of, 632t-635t, 3433-3434
American cutaneous leishmaniasis, 3464t, 3469-3471,
    3470f
American mucosal leishmaniasis, 3464t, 3471f,
    3472-3473, 3476
American trypanosomiasis, 3481-3488
  acute, 3484-3485, 3484f
  chronic, 3484-3486, 3484f-3485f
  clinical course of, 3483-3484
  diagnosis of, 3485-3486
  epidemiology of, 3482-3484
  etiology of, 3481, 3482f
  in HIV infection, 1860t-1870t
  in immunocompromised hosts, 3484-3485
  myocarditis in, 1156
  pathology of, 3481-3482, 3482f
  prevention of, 3487
  transfusion-related, 3748
  transmission of, 3481, 3482f, 3483
  treatment of, 3486-3487
Amikacin, 359, 360f, 360t-361t, 706t-709t
  for actinomycetoma, 3284
  for brain abscess, 1274t
  dosage of, 724t-725t
    in children, 378t
    multiple daily
      loading dose in, 374, 374t
      in renal insufficiency, 374
    once-daily, 376, 377t
  for endophthalmitis, 1557
  for febrile neutropenia, 3804t
  formulations of, 715t

Amikacin *(Continued)*
  for meningitis, 1213t
  for *Mycobacterium abscessus* pulmonary disease,
    3193t, 3194
  for *Mycobacterium avium* complex disease, 3184t
  for nocardiosis, 3204-3205, 3204t
  for nontuberculous mycobacterial infections, 543
  for nosocomial pneumonia, 3718t
  for tuberculosis, 541
Aminoalcohols, 639-641
Aminocandin, 561
Aminoglycosides, 359-384
  administration of, 367
  adverse reactions to, 368-372, 368t
  antimicrobial activity of
    in animal models, 365-366
    combination therapy and, 365, 365t-366t
    dosing regimen and, 366
    mechanisms of, 362
    microbiology of, 363-364
    postantibiotic effect in, 364
    structure and, 359, 361f
    synergy in, 364-365, 365t
    time course of, 364
    in vitro, 363-365
  beta-lactam antibiotics with, 273
  biologic activity of, 359-361
  in bone cement, 379
  chemical characteristics of, 361
  cochlear toxicity from, 371-372
  distribution of, 367
  dosage of, 374-379, 724t-725t
    in children, 378, 378t
    in cystic fibrosis, 378-379
    in endocarditis, 379
    individualized, 375-376
    multiple daily, 374-376
      in dialysis, 375, 375t
      loading dose in, 374, 374t
      maintenance dose in, 375, 375t
      renal function and, 375, 375t
    once-daily, 376-378
      regimens for, 376-377, 377t-378t
      serum level monitoring with, 378
  drug interactions with, 361, 742t-761t
  for *Enterococcus*, 2647-2648
  enzymatic inactivation of, 362
  excretion of, 367
  formulations of, 715t
  indications for, 373-374
    empirical, 373, 373t
    prophylactic, 374
    specific, 373-374, 373t
  metabolism of, 367
  names and sources of, 359, 360t
  nephrotoxicity of, 368-371, 368f, 369t-370t
  neuromuscular blockade after, 372
  for nontuberculous mycobacterial infections, 543
  ototoxicity of, 371-372
  for parasitic infections, 641
  penicillins with, 273
  for peritonitis, 1022t, 1025, 1029t
    during continuous ambulatory peritoneal
      dialysis, 379
    experimental models of, 366-367
  pharmacokinetics of, 367-368
  pharmacology of, 367-368, 724t-725t
  for *Pseudomonas aeruginosa* bacteremia, 2850
  renal handling of, 368f
  resistance to, 362-363
    acquired, 362-363
    adaptive, 362
    clinical epidemiology of, 363
    in enterococci, 363
    enzymatic, 284-285, 285t
    intrinsic, 362
    prevention of, 366
    ribosomal binding site alteration in, 287
  structure of, 359, 360f, 361t
  vestibular toxicity from, 372
Aminopenicillins, 317-318, 318f
  indications for, 315
  susceptibility to, 311
4-Aminoquinolines, 631-636
8-Aminoquinolines, 636-639

Aminosalicylic acid, 706t-709t
  dosage of, 734t-735t
  drug interactions with, 742t-761t
  formulations of, 717t
Amithiozone, for tuberculosis, 542
Ammonium compounds, disinfection with, 3684
Amnesic shellfish poisoning, 1416-1417, 1417t, 3570,
    3570t
Amodiaquine
  for malaria, 631
  resistance to, 3445
Amoxicillin, 318, 318f, 706t-709t
  allergy to, 351
  for anthrax, 2721
  for Chlamydia trachomatis infections, 2455
  dosage of, 316t, 718t-719t
  formulations of, 715t
  for group A streptococcal pharyngitis, 819-820
  for Helicobacter pylori infection, 2809t
  indications for, 315
  for leptospirosis, 3064t
  for lower urinary tract infection, 973
  for Lyme disease, 3079t
  for lymphadenitis, 1330
  for lymphangitis, 1331-1332
  for otitis media, 834
    prophylactic, 834-835
  prophylactic, 316
  for sinusitis, 845t
  for streptococcal pharyngitis, 2598t
  susceptibility to, 311t-312t
  for syphilis, 3047t, 3049-3050
  for typhoid fever, 2899
Amoxicillin-clavulanate, 319t, 320, 706t-709t
  for bite wounds, 3913t
  for cellulitis, 1297-1298
  dosage of, 718t-719t
  for febrile neutropenia, 3804t
  formulations of, 715t
  for lung abscess, 927
  for melioidosis, 2876
  prophylactic, for cancer-related infections, 3800t
  for sinusitis, 844-845, 845t
AmpC beta-lactamase, 283
AmpC cephalosporinase, 329
Amphoric breath sounds, in tuberculosis, 3143
Amphotericin B, 549-553, 706t-709t
  activity spectrum of, 549
  for Blastomyces dermatitidis infection, 3330
  for brain abscess, 1273t-1274t, 1275
  for Candida esophagitis, 1355t
  for candidiasis, 3235
  for Coccidioides infection, 3340-3341
  for cryptococcal meningitis, 3298
    in HIV infection, 1746
  dosage of, 736t-737t
  drug interactions with, 742t-761t
  for febrile neutropenia, 3804t
  plus flucytosine, 554
  formulations of, 549-553, 717t
  for fungal arthritis, 1451-1452
  for Fusarium infection, 3370
  for histoplasmosis, 3315-3316
  inhaled, 553
  for leishmaniasis, 632t-635t
  lipid complex, 552-553, 706t-709t, 717t
  lipid-associated, 552-553
    for aspergillosis, 3251, 3251t
  liposomal, 552-553, 706t-709t
    for cutaneous leishmaniasis, 3476
    formulations of, 717t
    for leishmaniasis, 632t-635t
    for mucosal leishmaniasis, 3476
    for post-kala-azar dermal leishmaniasis, 3474
    for visceral leishmaniasis, 3473
  mechanism of action of, 549, 551f
  for mucormycosis, 1275, 3265-3266
  for Paracoccidioides brasiliensis infection, 3361
  for parasitic infections, 641
  for Penicillium marneffei infection, 3372
  for peritonitis, 1029t
  for prosthetic valve endocarditis, 1121t
  resistance of, 549
  for Scedosporium prolificans infection, 3366
  structure of, 550f-551f
  for suppurative thrombophlebitis, 1098

Amphotericin B cholesteryl sulfate complex,
    706t-709t, 717t
Amphotericin B colloidal dispersion, 552-553
Amphotericin B deoxycholate, 549-552
  administration of, 552
  adverse reactions to, 552
  for aspergillosis, 3251, 3251t
  dosage of, 552
  for leishmaniasis, 632t-635t
  for mucormycosis, 3265
  nephrotoxicity of, 550-551
  pharmacology of, 549-550
  for post-kala-azar dermal leishmaniasis, 3474
  for visceral leishmaniasis, 3474
Ampicillin, 318, 318f
  allergy to, 351
  for brain abscess, 1274t
  dosage of, 316t, 718t-719t
  for endocarditis, 1089-1090
  for Enterococcus infection, 2647-2648
  for Enterococcus endocarditis, 1120t
  formulations of, 715t
  for leptospirosis, 3064t
  for meningitis, 1213t
  for osteomyelitis, 1459t
  for peritonitis, 1024-1025, 1029t
  for pneumococcal pneumonia, 2636
  in pregnancy, 270
  prophylactic, 316
  rash from, in infectious mononucleosis,
    1993-1994, 1994f
  for Streptococcus agalactiae (group B) infection,
    2662t
  susceptibility to, 311t-312t
  for typhoid fever, 2899
  for Yersinia pseudotuberculosis infection, 2951
Ampicillin sodium, 706t-709t
Ampicillin trihydrate, 706t-709t
Ampicillin-probenecid, 706t-709t
Ampicillin-sulbactam, 321, 706t-709t
  for acute pyelonephritis, 972
  for cellulitis, 1297
  dosage of, 718t-719t
  for Enterococcus endocarditis, 1120t
  for epiglottitis, 853
  formulations of, 715t
  for HACEK endocarditis, 1121t
  for nosocomial pneumonia, 3718t
  for peritonitis, 1029t
  prophylactic, for surgical procedures, 3899t
Amplicon contamination, 247
Amprenavir, 1841
Amyloid, 2425
Amyloid A, serum, in febrile response, 771
Amyloid plaques
  in Gerstmann-Straussler-Scheinker syndrome,
    2428
  in variant Creutzfeldt-Jakob disease, 2430
Amyotrophic lateral sclerosis, in HIV infection,
    1758-1759
Anaerobes
  definition of, 3083
  in normal flora, 3083-3084, 3084t
  in pulmonary cystic fibrosis, 950-951
  virulence factors associated with, 3087, 3087t
Anaerobic bacterial infections, 3083-3089
  bacteremia in, 3086-3087
  of bone, 3086
  of central nervous system, 3086, 3086f
  clinical manifestations of, 3084-3085, 3084t, 3085f
  diagnosis of, 3088
  endocarditis from, 1084-1085
  etiology of, 3084
  from gram-negative cocci
    description of, 3121-3122
    microbiology of, 3121
  from gram-positive cocci, 3121-3128
    antimicrobial susceptibility of, 3122, 3123t,
      3127t
    clinical isolates in, 3122, 3125-3126
    commensal microbiota in, 3125
    description of, 3121-3122
    identification, 3122
    microbiology of, 3121, 3126
    taxonomy in, 3121, 3122t, 3125-3126
    treatment of, 3122, 3123t, 3126-3127, 3127t

Anaerobic bacterial infections (Continued)
  intra-abdominal, 3085, 3086f
  of joints, 3086
  Meleney's gangrene from, 3084, 3085f
  meningitis from, 1193
  metronidazole for, 422t, 424
  of mouth, head, and neck, 3084-3085
  pathogenesis of, 3087-3088, 3087t
  of pelvis, 3085-3086
  pleuropulmonary, 3085-3087
  of skin, 3086
  of soft tissue, 3086
  treatment of, 3088-3089, 3088t
Anaerobic myonecrosis
  streptococcal, 1318
  synergistic nonclostridial, 1318
Anaerococcus lactolyticus, 3123t
Anaerococcus murdochii, 3123t
Anaerococcus prevotii, 3123t
Anaerococcus tetradius, 3123t
Anaerococcus vaginalis, 3123t
Anal. See also Anogenital entries; Perianal entries.
Anal cancer
  clinical management of, 1775
  HIV-related, 1774
  human papillomavirus in, 1773-1774
Anal neoplasia, HIV-related, 1773-1774
Analytic studies, 182, 182t
Anaphylactoid reactions, to vancomycin, 454
Anaphylatoxin, 83
Anaphylatoxin inactivator, 78t, 81t
Anaphylaxis. See also Hypersensitivity reactions.
  to penicillin, 347
  to rifamycins, 404
Anaplasma, 2531. See also Anaplasmosis.
  bacteriology of, 2495, 2496t
  clinical findings in, 2496, 2498t
  diagnosis of, 2496
  epidemiology of, 2495-2496
  genetics of, 2495
  historical perspective on, 2495, 2497t
  medical and veterinary disease caused by, 2532t
  pathophysiology of, 2495
  taxonomy of, 2531
  treatment of, 2496
  ultrastructure of, 2531-2532
Anaplasma marginale, 2531-2532, 2532t
Anaplasma phagocytophilum, 2531-2532, 2532t
  human granulocytotropic anaplasmosis from,
    2533-2534
  laboratory detection of, 240t-242t
  transmission of, 2533
Anaplasma platys, 2531-2532, 2532t
Anaplasmosis, 803
  human granulocytotropic, 3657t
    diagnosis of, 2535-2536, 2536f
    epidemiology and epizootiology of, 2533
    pathogenesis and pathology of, 2533-2534
    prevention of, 2536
    versus Rocky Mountain spotted fever, 2535t
    signs and symptoms of, 2534t, 2535
    treatment of, 2536
  tick-borne, 3656, 3657t
  transfusion-related, 3748
Ancylostoma, 632t-635t
Ancylostoma braziliense, 3619
Ancylostoma caninum, 3619
  eosinophilic gastroenteritis from, 3621
Ancylostoma duodenale, 632t-635t, 3578t, 3581-3582
Anemia
  in African trypanosomiasis, 3490
  aplastic, from chloramphenicol, 396
  hemolytic
    from chloramphenicol, 397
    from cytomegalovirus, 1975
    in infectious mononucleosis, 1994
    from nitrofurantoin, 517
  in HIV infection, 1720
  iron deficiency, from hookworm, 3581
  from linezolid, 473
  in malaria, 3441, 3449
  megaloblastic, from Diphyllobothrium latum, 3609
  in parvovirus B19 infection
    persistent, 2090
    transient, 2090
  in visceral leishmaniasis, 3468

Aneurysm
    coronary artery, in Kawasaki syndrome,
        3663-3664
    mycotic, 1099-1103. *See also* Mycotic aneurysms.
    Rasmussen's, 3142-3143
Angina
    Ludwig's, 862t, 863, 863f
        mediastinitis from, 1173
    Vincent's, 859-860, 861t, 3085, 3115
Angioedema, hereditary, C1 inhibitor deficiency in,
    91-92
Angiogenesis inhibitors, for Kaposi's sarcoma,
    1767-1768
Angiography, magnetic resonance
    in myocarditis, 1158
    in suppurative intracranial thrombophlebitis,
        1285, 1285f
Angiomatosis, bacillary. *See* Bacillary angiomatosis.
Angioplasty, percutaneous transluminal coronary,
    bloodstream infection after, 1136-1137,
    1136t
Angiostrongyliasis, abdominal, 3618t, 3620-3621
Angiostrongylus cantonensis, 3619
    meningitis from, 1193-1194, 1207, 1211,
        1220-1222, 3619-3620
        chronic, 1240
    treatment of, 632t-635t
Angiostrongylus costaricensis, 3620-3621
    abdominal pain and/or diarrhea with eosinophilia
        from, 1407t, 1408
    treatment of, 632t-635t
Angular cheilitis, in HIV infection, 1714, 1714f
Anidulafungin, 560, 706t-709t
    for aspergillosis, 3251t, 3252
    dosage of, 736t-737t
    drug interactions with, 742t-761t
    formulations of, 717t
    structure of, 550f-551f, 559
Animal(s). *See also* Zoonoses.
    as hosts for Lyme disease, 3071-3072
    respiratory syncytial virus in, 2208
Animal bites, 3911-3913, 3912t
    to head and neck, 862t, 868
    management of, 3912-3913, 3912t-3913t
    Pasteurella infection from, 2939, 2941-2942
Animal models
    for HIV vaccines, 1889-1890
    of pharmacodynamics, 301
Anisakiasis, 632t-635t, 3618-3619
    abdominal pain and/or diarrhea with eosinophilia
        from, 1407t, 1408
Anisakis, life cycle of, 3618
Anncaliia, 3391, 3392t. *See also* Microsporidia.
Anogenital neoplasia, HIV-related, 1772-1775
    clinical implications of, 1774, 1774t
    histopathology of, 1773
    human papillomavirus in, 1772
    treatment recommendations for, 1774-1775
Anogenital warts. *See* Condylomata acuminata.
Antacids, quinolone interactions with, 494
Anthrax, 2715-2725. *See also* Bacillus anthracis.
    as biological weapon, 3956, 3983-3992
        aerosol release of, 3995
        countermeasures for, 3986-3991
        diagnosis of, 3986-3989
        dissemination of, 3984
        exposure to, assessment of, 3989t
        history of, 3983-3984
        immunotherapy for, 3990-3991
        incubation period for, 3985
        infection control for, 3990
        infective dose (ID) of, 3984
        lethal dose (LD) of, 3984
        outbreak characteristics of, 3984-3986,
            3984f-3985f, 3986t, 3987f-3988f, 3989t
        post-exposure prophylaxis for, 3989t, 3990
        signs and symptoms of, 3985-3986, 3986t
        site remediation (decontamination) for,
            3990-3991, 3991t
        vaccines for, 3990, 3990t
    cerebral edema in, 2723
    clinical manifestations of, 2717-2721
    cutaneous
        chancriform lesion of, 1293-1294, 1294f, 1294t
        clinical manifestations of, 2717-2718, 2718f
        treatment of, 2721-2722

Anthrax *(Continued)*
    diagnosis of, 2717-2721, 2719t
    epidemiology of, 2716-2717, 2717f
    gastrointestinal
        clinical manifestations of, 2720
        treatment of, 2721t, 2722-2723
    immunotherapy for, 2723, 3990
    inhalation of, 3984
        clinical pathway in, 3988f
        incubation period after, 3985
    inhalational (pulmonary)
        clinical manifestations of, 2718-2720
        treatment of, 2721t, 2722-2723
    intestinal, 1400t-1401t, 1403, 2720
    laboratory specimen collection and transport in,
        2719t
    meningitis from, 2720-2723
    oropharyngeal, 2720
    pleural effusion in, 2723
    quinolones for, 500
    treatment of, 2721-2724, 2721t-2722t
    vaccines for, 2723-2724, 3921-3922, 3922t, 3990,
        3990t
Anthropophilic dermatophytosis, 3346-3347,
    3346t
Antibiotics. *See* Antimicrobial agents.
Antibody(ies), 59-75. *See also* B cells;
        Immunoglobulin *entries.*
    affinity of, 60
    allotypes of, 59
    antigen binding with, 60
    antigen-specific, 69
    anti-idiotypic, 70
    autoreactive
        origin of, 71
        rheumatoid, 72
    avidity of, 60
    blocking function of, 62
    cellular cytotoxicity dependence on, 63
    cleavage fragments of, 60, 60f-61f
    in complement activation, 62
    effector functions mediated by, 62
    in encephalitis, 1249-1250
        HSV-specific, 1249
    functional, measurement of, 64-66
    heavy chains of, 59
    idiotypes of, 59
    isotypes of, 59-62, 60t
    laboratory measurement of, 64-66, 64f
    light chains of, 60
    monoclonal, 64
        therapeutic uses of, 74
        for transplant immunosuppression, infections
            and, 3811, 3811t
    natural, in immunity, 45
    neutralizing function of, 62
    in opsonization, 62-63
    pathology mediated by, 70-72
    polyclonal, for transplant immunosuppression,
            infections and, 3811, 3811t
    primary response of, 63, 63f
    production of
        B cell maturation and, 66-70
        downregulation of, 70
        kinetics of, 63-64, 63f
    secondary response of, 63, 63f
    structure of, 59-63, 60f
    therapeutic uses of, 73-74
    in urinary tract infection, 962-963
Anticoagulants
    for sepsis, 1004
    for suppurative intracranial thrombophlebitis,
        1285-1286
Anticytokine therapy, infection risk associated with,
    620
Antifungal agents, 549-563. *See also specific agent.*
    amphotericin B–based. *See* Amphotericin B.
    for aspergillosis, 3250-3252, 3251t
    azole. *See* Azoles.
    in combination, 274
    dosage of, 736t-737t
    echinocandin. *See* Echinocandins.
    formulations of, 717t
    mechanisms of action of, 551f
    mucorales resistance of, 3264-3265
    for mucormycosis, 3265-3266

Antifungal agents *(Continued)*
    pharmacology of, 736t-737t
    prophylactic
        for cancer-related infections, 3800t, 3801
        in transplant recipients, 3816
    structures of, 550f-551f
    for vulvovaginal candidiasis, 1501
Antigen(s)
    antibody binding with, 60
    B cells activated by, 69
    epitopes of, 60
    measurement of, assays for, 64f, 66
    T cell–independent, 69-70
Antigen processing
    by CD1, 137, 137f
    mechanisms of, 133-137
    by MHC class I molecules, 133-135, 135f
    by MHC class II molecules, 135-136, 136f
    transporter associated with, 134
Antigen testing, 245-246, 246t, 258, 264
    in bacterial meningitis, 1208
    in pneumonia, 898
    in rhinoviral infections, 2395
Antigen-binding sites, generation of, 66-67, 67f, 67t
Antigenicity, 186
Antigen-presenting cells, 139
    antigen-specific, B cells as, 69
    B7 ligands of, 69
    pattern recognition receptors of, 69
    T cells and, interface between, 132
Anti-HBc
    detection of, 2066
    isolated presence of, 2074
Anti-HBs, development of, 2066
Antihelmintics
    for cysticercosis, 3612-3613
    for echinococcosis, 3614
    for tapeworms, 3611
Antiherpesvirus agents, 576f
Antihistamines
    for otitis media with effusion, 834
    for rhinorrhea, 811
Anti-inflammatory drugs
    for bacterial meningitis, 1220-1221
    for cystic fibrosis, 951
    nonsteroidal
        antipyretic activity of, 774-775
        quinolone interactions with, 494
        for reactive arthritis, 1492
    for sepsis, 1003-1004
Anti-inflammatory response, acute, 991
Antimicrobial agents. *See also specific agent.*
    adverse reactions to, 268
    age and, 268-269
    clinical trials for, 687-698
        analysis of results of, 694-695, 695f
        end points in, 693-694
        examination of conclusions in, 695-697, 696t
        goals of, 688-690
        inclusion and exclusion criteria in, 690
        practice and research observations in,
            687-688
        randomization, blinding, and stratification in,
            690-691
        research study designs in, 688, 688t
        sample size, hypothesis testing, and error in,
            691-692
        selection of control regimen in, 692
        sources of bias in, 692-693
    colitis associated with, 1375-1387. *See also*
        Pseudomembranous colitis.
    concentration of, 705
    dosing of, 275-276, 705, 718t-719t
    drug interactions with, 742t-761t
    efficacy of, 276
    in elderly, 3861-3862
    generic names of, 706t-709t
    genetic abnormalities and, 269-270
    inappropriate use of, 213, 677-678
    interactions between
        antagonistic, 274-275
        synergistic, 273-274
    for intraventricular use, 1234, 1234t
    in liver disease, 271
    metabolic disorders and, 269
    novel, 511-513

Antimicrobial agents (Continued)
 oral rinses containing, 869
 organism identification for, 267
 organism susceptibility to, 267-268
 pharmacodynamics of, 300-306
 pharmacokinetics of, 297. See also
  Pharmacokinetics.
 pharmacology of, tables of, 705
 in pregnancy, 270
 prophylactic, 189-190. See also Chemoprophylaxis.
  for bite wounds, 3912, 3913t
  for cancer-related infections, 3799-3801, 3800t
  for catheter-related infections, 3709
   of urinary tract, 3731
    at catheter removal or replacement, 3732
  in complement deficiency, 95
  for neutrophil defects, 117
  for surgical site infections
   cost-benefit analysis of, 3901-3902
   drug selection and dosing in, 3898-3899,
    3898t-3899t
   duration of, 3900-3901
   novel methods of, 3901
   preoperative, 3897-3902, 3898f
   resistance to, 3901
   side effects of, 3901
   timing of administration of, 3891, 3892f,
    3899-3900, 3900f
  in transplant recipients, 3815, 3815t
  for traveler's diarrhea, 4015
 in renal insufficiency, 270-271
  dosage adjustment for, 705
 resistance to, 212-214, 213f
  antimicrobial stewardship programs and,
   681-682
  auxotrophs in, 289
  cell wall precursor target alterations in, 288,
   288t
  control of, 292, 292f
  DNA integration elements in, 281, 281f
  efflux promotion in, 286-287
  enzymatic alterations in, 281-286
  formulary decisions and, 682
  mechanisms of, 281-291, 282t, 290t
  membrane permeability in, 286
  molecular mechanisms of, 279-295, 280f
  multidrug, mechanisms of, 291-292, 291f
  plasmids in, 279
  prevention of, 273
  ribosomal binding site alteration in, 287-288
  surveillance for, 182
  target enzyme alteration in, 288-289
  target overproduction in, 289
  target site alterations in, 287-289
  target site protection in, 289
  transposable genetic elements in, 279-281, 280f
  vancomycin-intermediate Staphylococcus aureus
   and, 289-290
 rotation of, 682
 site of infection and, 271-272
 susceptibility testing of. See Susceptibility testing.
 teratogenicity of, 270
 therapy with
  administration route in, 275
  agent selection in, 267-272
  combination, 272-274
   adverse effects of, 275
   antagonism from, 274-275
   cost of, 275
   decreased toxicity with, 273
   disadvantages of, 274-275
   against fungal pathogens, 274
   indications for, 272-274
   for polymicrobial infections, 273
   synergism with, 273-274
   in vitro results of, 272, 272f
  heterogeneity in, 682
  host factors in, 268-272
  nosocomial infections and, 3670
  outpatient parenteral, 699-703
   future of, 702-703
   infections amenable to, 699-700, 700t
   modes of delivery of, 699, 700t
   patient monitoring in, 702
   patient selection for, 701-702, 701t-702t

Antimicrobial agents (Continued)
  suitability of, 700-701, 701t
   technology of, 701
  philosophy of, 677-678
  principles of, 267-278
  response monitoring in, 276
  stewardship over. See Antimicrobial
   stewardship.
  topical. See Topical antibacterial therapy.
  trade names of, 710t-714t
 Antimicrobial lock prophylaxis, for catheter-related
  infections, 3709
 Antimicrobial peptides and proteins, 37, 39t
 Antimicrobial stewardship, 677-685
  antibiotic rotation in, 682
  computer-assisted, 680
  educational programs in, 678
  focus of, 677
  formulary decisions in, 678-679, 682
  future of, 683-684
  multidisciplinary approaches to, 680
  outcomes of, 680-681, 680t
  prior-approval programs in, 679
  program design and implementation for, 682-683,
   683t
  prospective audit and feedback programs in,
   679-680
  resistance prevention with, 681-682
  strategies for, 678-680, 678f, 678t
 Antimicrobial-coated catheters, 3709-3710, 3731
 Antimonials
  for cutaneous leishmaniasis, 3475
  for mucosal leishmaniasis, 3476
  for parasitic infections, 641-642
  for visceral leishmaniasis, 3473-3474
 Antimotility agents
  for Clostridium difficile–associated colitis, 1383
  for cryptosporidiosis, 3554
 Antimycobacterial agents, 533-548
  dosage of, 734t-735t
  formulations of, 717t
  for leprosy, 544-546
  for nontuberculous mycobacterial infections,
   542-544
  pharmacology of, 734t-735t
  for tuberculosis. See Antituberculous agents.
 Antimyosin antibody imaging, in myocarditis, 1158
 Antiparasitic agents, 631-668, 632t-635t
  for cryptosporidiosis, 3554
 Antipseudomonal beta-lactam, for Pseudomonas
  aeruginosa bacteremia, 2849-2850
 Antipyretics, 773-776
  benefits versus risks of, 775-776
  diagnostic considerations in, 775
  endogenous, 771-772, 772f
  indications for, 776
  physical, 774-775
 Antiretroviral Pregnancy Registry, 3765-3766, 3765t
 Antiretroviral therapy, 1833-1853. See also specific
  agent.
  agents for, 1833-1844
  for AIDS dementia, 1748-1749, 1749t
  changing regimens in, 1848
  for cryptosporidiosis, in HIV infection, 3554
  dosage of, 740t-741t
  effects of, on hepatitis C infection, 2176-2177
  entry inhibitors in, 1842-1843, 1843f, 1843t
  formulations of, 717t
  future directions in, 1849
  hepatotoxicity of, 1741
  highly active
   for anal cancer, 1774
   for cervical cancer, 1773
   and chemotherapy, for HIV-related non-
    Hodgkin's lymphoma, 1769-1770
   for CNS lymphoma, 1772
   for esophagitis, 1356
   for HIV infection, 1784
    during breast-feeding, 1787
    with cryptococcosis, 3294
    with HBV coinfection, 1602
    natural history effects of, 1710-1711,
     1710f-1711f
   for HIV-related non-Hodgkin's lymphoma,
    1769

Antiretroviral therapy (Continued)
  for Hodgkin's disease, 1776
  for HPV infection, 1798
  for Kaposi's sarcoma, 1768
  progressive multifocal leukoencephalopathy
   and, 2052-2055
  for HIV infection, 210
  in children
   clinical trials of, 1821
   combination, complications of, 1816-1817
   failure of, evidence for, 1824t
   guidelines for, 1819-1821, 1820t-1823t
   management issues in, 1801-1802
   metabolic complications of, 1801
   pharmacokinetics and adverse events in, 1801
  in pregnancy, 1788, 1790t, 1792t-1793t
   discontinuation of, 1794
   in intrapartum period, 1795
   for perinatal transmission prophylaxis,
    1810-1811, 1811t
   potential mechanisms of, 1788-1789
   recommended guidelines on, 1789
   teratogenicity of, 1795
  response to, 1800-1801
  HIV replication cycle targets in, 1833, 1834f
  HIV transmission effect of, 1646, 1786
  immune reconstitution syndrome in, 1849
  initiation of, 1844-1847, 1845f
  integrase strand transfer inhibitors in, 1843f,
   1843t, 1844
  interrupting therapy with, 1846-1847
  laboratory testing during, 1847-1848, 1847t
  neurotoxicity of, 1757t
  non-nucleoside reverse transcriptase inhibitors in,
   1837, 1837f, 1837t
  nucleoside and nucleotide reverse transcriptase
   inhibitors in, 1833, 1834f, 1835t
  penetration-effectiveness scores of, 1749t
  pharmacodynamics of, 305
  pharmacology of, 740t-741t
  pneumonia risk and, 1727-1728
  for postexposure prophylaxis, 1848-1849
   adverse effects of, 3764-3765
   follow-up in, 3766-3767
   indications for, 3766
   nonoccupational, 1849, 3766
   occupational, 1848-1849, 3761-3767,
    3764t-3765t
   in pregnancy, 3765-3766, 3765t
   rationale for, 3762-3763
   regimen for, 3755t, 3763-3764
   resources on, 3765t
   in "source unknown" exposures, 3766
   timing and duration of, 3766
  for pre-exposure prophylaxis, 1652
  protease inhibitors in, 1838-1839, 1839f,
   1840t
  resistance to, testing for, 1848
  resources available for, 1630f-1631f, 1631
  with rifabutin, 539t
  with rifampin, 535-536, 537t
 Antiseptics, 3677
 Antithymocyte globulin
  in hematopoietic stem cell transplant recipients,
   3821
  for transplant immunosuppression, infections and,
   3811-3812, 3811t
 Antituberculous agents, 3144-3145. See also
  Tuberculosis, treatment of; specific agent.
  first-line, 533-539
  in hepatic or renal failure, 534t
  novel, 542
  second-line, 540-542
  selection of regimen for, 3145, 3145t
  standard regimens for, 3145-3146
 Anti–tumor necrosis factor therapy, infection risk
  associated with, 620
 Antivenin, 73
 Antiviral agents, 565-610. See also Antiretroviral
  therapy; specific agent.
  for acute viral hepatitis, 1589
  administration of, 566
  for avian influenza, 2280
  combinations of, 566
  for cytomegalovirus infection, 1976-1979

Antiviral agents (Continued)
 cross-resistance to, 1978, 1978f
 dosage of, 566, 566t-567t, 738t-739t
 for enteroviruses, 2341-2342
 formulations of, 717t
 for hepatitis B infection, chronic
  choice of, 1601-1602, 1601t
  optimal use of, 1600, 1600t
  recommendations for, 1600-1602, 1601t
 for hepatitis C infection
  chronic
   candidates for, 1609-1610, 1609t
   efficacy of, 1606-1607, 1606t
   registrations trials of, 1607-1608, 1607t
   tailored, 1608
  small molecule, 2174-2175, 2175f
 host immune response and, 565
 for infectious mononucleosis, 2003
 for influenza, 2277, 2277t, 2284
 interferon alfa with, 615
 investigational, 598-600, 599f
 for lymphoproliferative disease, 2004
 mechanisms of action of, 565
 for orthopoxvirus infection, 1930
 pharmacology of, 738t-739t
 prophylactic, for cancer-related infections, 3800t,
  3802
 resistance to, 565-566
 susceptibility testing for, 261-262
 targeted development of, 1913
 topical, 566
 viral kinetics after initiation of, 1596
Aorta
 mycotic aneurysm of, 1101. See also Mycotic
  aneurysms.
 tuberculosis of, 3159
Aortic allograft, 1117
Aortic valve, endocarditis of, 1067-1068
Aphthous ulcers
 esophageal, 1355, 1355t
 in HIV infection, 1712, 1712f
 in Marshall's syndrome, 1327
 oral, 866
 of vagina, 1482
Aplastic anemia, from chloramphenicol, 396
Aplastic crisis, transient, from parvovirus B19, 2090
Apnea
 in bronchiolitis, 888
 in respiratory syncytial virus infection, 2215
Apodemus agrarius, hemorrhagic fever with renal
  syndrome from, 2290
Apophysomyces, 3257, 3258t
Apoptosis
 in bacterial meningitis, 1203
 complement in, 84
 of neutrophils, 108
 virus, 1913, 1913f
Appendectomy, open versus laparoscopic,
  1060-1061
Appendicitis, 1059-1062
 actinomycotic, 3212-3213
 computed tomography in, 1060, 1060f
 versus mesenteric lymphadenitis, 1406
 pain in, 1060, 1060t
 with perforation, 1017
 versus primary peritonitis, 1014
 recurrent, 1061
 retrocecal, 1324
 treatment of, 1060-1061
Appendix, 1059
 gangrenous, 1059
 normal, in appendectomy, 1060
Arbekacin, 359, 360f, 360t-361t
Arboviruses
 detection of, 259t-260t
 encephalitis from, 1246t, 1255-1258
  incidence of, 1246-1247, 1247f
  pathogenesis of, 1256
 serologic tests for, 261
Arcanobacterium, 2699-2701
 pharyngitis from, 2596
Arcanobacterium bernardiae, 2701
Arcanobacterium haemolyticum, 2700, 2700f
 pharyngitis from, 816
Arcanobacterium pyogenes, 2700-2701

Arenaviruses, 2295-2301, 4000t-4001t
 characteristics of, 2295, 3997t
 clinical manifestations of, 2298-2299
 detection of, 259t-260t
 diagnosis of, 2299-2300
 epidemiology/epizootiology of, 2295-2297, 2296t
 pathogenesis of, 2297-2298
 prevention of, 2300
 treatment of, 2300
Argentine hemorrhagic fevers. See South American
  hemorrhagic fevers.
Argyll Robertson pupil, in ocular syphilis, 3042
Arizona, mycotic aneurysms from, 1102
Arm, mycetoma of, 3282f. See also Mycetoma.
Arrhythmias
 in leptospirosis, 3062
 in myocarditis, 1157
Arsenicals, for African trypanosomiasis, 3492-3493
Arteether, for malaria, 642-643
Artemether, 706t-709t
 for malaria, 642-643
Artemether-lumefantrine, 639-641
 for malaria, 4014
Artemisinins
 for malaria, 642-644, 669, 671f, 3452t, 3453-3454
  mechanism of action of, 3447
 neurotoxicity of, 643
 resistance to, 3445-3447
 for schistosomiasis, 3596t, 3599-3600
Arterial monitoring lines, infections of, 3706-3707,
  3707t. See also Catheter-related infections.
Arteritis
 coronary, in Kawasaki syndrome, 3663
 temporal (giant cell), fever of unknown origin in,
  787
Artesunate, 706t-709t
 for malaria, 632t-635t, 642-643
Arthralgia
 in HIV infection, 1759
 in Mycoplasma pneumoniae infection, 2484
Arthritis, 1443-1456
 bacterial
  approach to patient with, 1447-1448
  causes of, 1448t
  differential diagnosis of, 1448
  gonococcal, 1446-1447, 1447f
  nongonococcal, 1443-1446, 1444t-1446t,
   1445f-1446f
  predisposing factors for, 1443, 1444t
  treatment of, 1447-1449, 1448t
 from Blastomyces dermatitidis, 1451, 3326
 from Brucella, 2923
 from Candida, 1451, 3233
 chronic infectious, 1450-1453
 from Coccidioides immitis, 1451
 from Coccidioides posadasii, 1451
 from Cryptococcus neoformans, 1451
 daptomycin for, 464
 in elderly, 3861
 fungal, 1450-1452
 gonococcal, 1444t, 1446-1447
  clinical features of, 1447, 1447f
  pathogenesis of, 1447
  quinolones for, 496
 from Haemophilus influenzae, 1444, 1444t
 from Haemophilus influenzae type b, 2914
 from Histoplasma capsulatum, 1451
 Lyme, 3076, 3079-3080, 3079f
 mycobacterial, 1452-1453, 1452f
 from Mycobacterium leprae, 1453
 from Mycobacterium marinum, 1453
 from Mycobacterium tuberculosis, 1452, 1452f,
  3156
 nongonococcal, 1443-1446
  clinical features of, 1445-1446, 1445f, 1446f
  microbiology of, 1444-1445, 1444t-1445t
  pathophysiology of, 1443-1444
  radiographic features of, 1446, 1446f
 from Pantoea agglomerans, 1444-1445, 1445t
 from Pasteurella, 2940
 of prosthetic joints, quinolones for, 500
 from Pseudomonas aeruginosa, 1444, 1444t
 in rat-bite fever, 2965-2966
 reactive, 1448. See also Reiter's syndrome.
  urethritis and, 1491-1492

Arthritis (Continued)
 in rheumatic fever, 2613-2614
 rheumatoid
  versus bacterial arthritis, 1448
  juvenile, fever of unknown origin in, 787
 in rubella, 2128
 from Scedosporium prolificans, 3366, 3366f
 septic, 1450t, 1453
 sexually reactive, from Chlamydia trachomatis,
  1491-1492, 2453
 from Sporothrix schenckii, 1451
 from Staphylococcus aureus, 1443-1444,
  1444t-1445t, 2574
 from Streptobacillus moniliformis, 1444-1445,
  1445t
 from Streptococcus, 2614
 from Streptococcus agalactiae (group B), 2660
 from Streptococcus group C and group G,
  2675-2676
 from Streptococcus pneumoniae, 1444, 1444t
 from Streptococcus pyogenes, 1444, 1444t
 viral, 1449-1450, 1449f
Arthritis-dermatitis syndrome, gonococcal,
  2762-2763
Arthrobacter, 2701
Arthrocentesis, for inflammatory arthritis, 1448
Arthroconidia, inhalation of, coccidioidomycosis
  from, 3334-3335. See also Coccidioides.
Arthropathy
 from Histoplasma capsulatum, 3317
 from parvovirus B19, 2090
 from quinolones, 503
Arthropods
 in travelers, personal protection against,
  4015
 as zoonotic reservoirs and vectors, 4005-4006
Arthrospores, 3347
Ascariasis, 3577-3580, 3578t
 abdominal pain and/or diarrhea with eosinophilia
  from, 1407t, 1408
 clinical manifestations of, 3578-3579
 diagnosis of, 3579
 epidemiology of, 3577-3578
 life cycle in, 3577, 3578f-3579f
 treatment of, 632t-635t, 3579-3580
Aschoff nodule, in rheumatic fever, 2612
Ascites, in peritonitis, 1013-1015
Asia, HIV infection in, 1622-1623, 1623f-1624f
Aspergilloma, 3245-3246
Aspergillosis
 allergic bronchopulmonary
  clinical manifestations of, 3245-3246
  in cystic fibrosis, 951, 3246, 3246t
  pathogenesis of, 3245
 bone, 3249, 3249f
 in cancer patients, 3796t, 3798-3799
 caspofungin for, 560
 cerebral, 3248-3249, 3249f
 clinical presentation in, 3245-3249
 cutaneous, 3249, 3249f
 diagnosis of, 3249-3250
 disseminated, 3248
 endocarditis in, 3249
 epidemiology of, 3244, 3244t
 in hematopoietic stem cell transplant recipients,
  3831-3832
 in HIV infection, 1860t-1870t, 1878
 invasive, 3247-3248
 keratitis in, 3247
 onychomycosis in, 3247
 otomycosis in, 3247
 pericarditis in, 3249
 prevention of, 3252-3253
 pulmonary
  chronic necrotizing, 942f
  in HIV infection, 1732
  in lung transplant recipients, 3842
  manifestations of, 3247, 3247f-3248f
  pathogenesis of, 3244, 3245f
 saprophytic colonization by, 3246-3247
 sinusitis in, 3245-3246, 3248, 3248f
 superficial, 3246-3247
 tracheobronchitis in, 3247-3248
 treatment of, 3250-3252, 3251t
 voriconazole for, 558

Aspergillus, 3241-3255. *See also* Aspergillosis.
  brain abscess from, 1266, 1266t, 1269, 1271-1272,
    3248-3249, 3249f
    treatment of, 1275
  characteristics of, 3241-3243, 3242t
  in chronic granulomatous disease, 174, 174f
  culture of, 3249-3250
  endocarditis from, 1085
  endophthalmitis from, 1555-1556
  epidemiology of, 3244
  immune response to, 3244-3245
  microscopic features of, 3241, 3242f-3243f, 3242t
  mycotic aneurysms from, 1102
  pathogenicity of, 3244-3245
  susceptibility testing for, 3250
  toxins of, 3245
Aspergillus calidoustus, 3243
Aspergillus flavus, 3242-3243, 3242f, 3242t
Aspergillus fumigatus
  characteristics of, 3241-3242, 3242f, 3242t
  in cystic fibrosis, 951
  in transplant recipients, 3846
Aspergillus fumigatus species complex, 3242-3243
Aspergillus nidulans, 3243
Aspergillus niger, 3242t, 3243, 3243f
Aspergillus terreus, 3242t, 3243, 3243f
Aspiration
  of amebic liver abscess, 3422
  of brain abscess, 1271, 1275
  in bronchiolitis, 888
  chronic pneumonia and, 933
  of liver abscess, 1038-1039, 1038f
  of lung abscess, 928
  of peritoneal cavity, 1021
  in respiratory syncytial virus infection, 2215
  of subglottic secretions, 3723
  of vitreous, 1556, 1556f
Aspiration pneumonia, 903
  lung abscess from, 925
Aspirin
  antipyretic activity of, 774
  for Kawasaki syndrome, 3665-3666
  for rheumatic fever, 2616t
Asplenia
  antimicrobial prophylactic therapy in, 3870-3871,
    3870t
  babesiosis in, 3869
  Bartonella bacilliformis in, 3869
  congenital, 3865
  diagnosis of, 3865-3866, 3866f
  ehrlichiosis in, 3869
  HIV infection in, 3869
  immunizations in, 3870-3871, 3871t
  infections in, 3865-3873
  malaria in, 3869
  surgical, 3865. *See also* Splenectomy.
Assistant Secretary for Preparedness and Response
  (ASPR), 3968-3969
Asthma
  from *Chlamydophila pneumoniae*, 2471-2472,
    2471t
  in *Helicobacter pylori* infection, 2806t,
    2807-2808
  human metapneumovirus and, 2224-2225
  in *Mycoplasma pneumoniae* infection, 2483
  from rhinoviruses, 2392, 2394
  vaccines and, 3919
Astroviruses, 2407-2408, 2408f, 2408t
  gastroenteritis from, 1363
Ataxia-telangiectasia, 169t-170t, 171
Atazanavir, 706t-709t, 1839f, 1840t, 1841-1842
  dosage of, 740t-741t
  for HIV-infected children, 1820t-1821t, 1823t
Atelectasis, in spinal cord injury patients, 3853
Atherosclerosis, from *Chlamydophila pneumoniae*,
  2472-2473
Athlete's foot, 3348
Atopodium, 3126
Atovaquone, 706t-709t
  for *Pneumocystis jirovecii* pneumonia, 1860t-1870t,
    1872, 3382
  prophylactic, 1858t-1859t, 1874, 3386, 3800t
    in children, 1824-1825
  for *Toxoplasma* encephalitis, 1750-1751
  for toxoplasmosis, in HIV infection, 3518t

Atovaquone-azithromycin
  for babesiosis, 3544, 3544t
  for brain abscess, 1274t
Atovaquone-proguanil, 706t-709t
  for malaria, 632t-635t, 644, 3451, 3452t,
    4013-4014
    prophylactic, 3455t, 3456
  mechanism of action of, 3447
  resistance to, 3445, 3447
Atrioventricular block, in Lyme disease, 3075, 3075t,
  3079t
Attack rate, secondary, 186
Attributable risk/fraction, 181, 181f
Auditory canal infection, external. *See* Otitis externa.
Auramine-rhodamine stain, 244, 244t
Australian bat lyssavirus, 2249, 2250t
Autism
  measles, mumps, rubella (MMR) vaccine and,
    2234
  vaccines and, 3921
Autoclave, gravity displacement, 3686
Autoimmune disease, Epstein-Barr virus and, 1999
Autoimmune regulator (AIRE), 141
Autolysin, 2627, 2629t
Autonomic dysfunction, in sepsis, 998
Autophagy, in host defense, 41
Auxotrophs, in antimicrobial resistance, 289-290
AVA/Biothrax vaccine, for anthrax, 3990, 3990t
Avian influenza, 203-204, 203t, 204f, 2270-2271,
  2280
Axillary bubo, in bubonic plague, 2946, 2946f
Axillary lymphadenitis, 1324
Azalides
  dosage of, 726t-727t
  formulations of, 716t
Azaspiracid shellfish poisoning, 3570, 3570t
Azithromycin, 434-438, 706t-709t
  adverse reactions to, 435-436
  antimicrobial activity of, 429t, 434-435
  for bacillary dysentery, 2908-2909, 2909t
  for brain abscess, 1274t
  for cat-scratch disease, 3005
  for chancroid, 2917
  chemistry of, 434, 434f
  for *Chlamydia trachomatis* infections, 2455
  for *Chlamydophila* atherosclerosis, 2473
  for *Chlamydophila* respiratory infection, 2471,
    2471t
  for cholera, 2782-2783, 2782t
  for donovanosis, 3013
  dosage of, 726t-727t
  drug interactions with, 431t, 742t-761t
  formulations of, 716t
  for Legionnaires' disease, 2978t
  for lymphadenitis, 1330
  mechanism of action of, 434
  for *Mycobacterium avium* complex disease,
    3184t-3186t
  for *Neisseria gonorrhoeae* infection, 2765
  for nontuberculous mycobacterial infections, 543
  for nosocomial pneumonia, 3718t
  for parasitic infections, 655
  pharmacology of, 435
  preparations of, 434
  for Q fever pneumonia, 2514
  resistance to, mechanism of, 434
  for scrub typhus, 2530
  for sinusitis, 845t
  for streptococcal pharyngitis, 2598t
  for *Toxoplasma* encephalitis, 1750-1751
  for toxoplasmosis, in HIV infection, 3518t
  for traveler's diarrhea prophylaxis, 4015
  for urethritis, 1490-1491, 1491t
  uses of, 432t-433t, 436-438
Azlocillin, 318, 319f, 706t-709t
  dosage of, 718t-719t
  formulations of, 715t
Azoles, 554-559
  for cryptococcal meningitis, 3298-3299
  drug-drug interactions of, 556t
  mechanism of action of, 551f, 554-555
Azotemia. *See also* Nephrotoxicity.
  from amphotericin B, 550-551
Aztreonam, 706t-709t
  for acute pyelonephritis, 972

Aztreonam (*Continued*)
  antibacterial activity of, 343, 344t
  for brain abscess, 1274t
  dosage of, 344, 722t
  drug interactions with, 742t-761t
  formulations of, 716t
  half-life of, 344
  for meningitis, 1213t
  for peritonitis, 1025, 1029t
  for *Pseudomonas aeruginosa* bacteremia, 2849-2850
  for septic bursitis, 1450t
  structure of, 343, 343f

B

B cell follicles, 143, 143f
B cell lymphoma, chronic hepatitis C infection with,
  1611
B cells
  antibody production by, 65-70
  antigen-activated, 69
  assay of, 171t, 172
  autoreactive antibody production by, 71
  autoreactive clonal deletion in, 67
  congenital defects in, 169t-170t, 171-172
  coreceptor complex of, 68
  development of, stages of, 67f
  DNA rearrangement in, 66-67, 67f, 67t
  in HIV infection, 1697
  in lymph nodes, 142, 144
  in primary immune response, 63, 63f
  in sepsis, 998
  signals for
    antigen-mediated, 67-68, 68f
    second, 68-69, 68f
  in spleen, 143-144, 143f
  T cell activation by, 69, 70f
  T cell interactions with, 68-69, 68f
  T cell–independent antigens and, 69-70
  in vaccine immune response, 3919
B1 cells, 70
Babesia, 3539-3541. *See also* Babesiosis.
Babesia bigemina, 3539
Babesia bovis, 3539
Babesia divergens, 3539, 3543, 3656, 3658t
Babesia duncani, 3539, 3544
Babesia microti, 3539-3540, 3656-3657, 3658f, 3658t
  classification of, 3540
  clinical manifestations of, 3542
  epidemiology of, 3541
  treatment of, 3543-3544, 3544t
Babesiosis, 3539-3545, 3656-3657, 3658f, 3658t, 4003
  in asplenia, 3869
  clinical features of, 3542-3543
  diagnosis of, 3543
  epidemiology of
    in Europe, 3541-3542
    in rest of world, 3542
    in U.S., 3541
  pathogenesis of, 3543
  pathogen-host interactions in, 3539-3541
    tick events in, 3539-3540
    vertebrate host events in, 3540, 3540f
  prevention of, 3544
  transfusion-related, 3544, 3748
  transmission of, 3539
  treatment of, 632t-635t, 3543-3544, 3544t
Bacampicillin, 706t-709t, 715t, 718t-719t
Bacillary angiomatosis
  from *Bartonella*, 2997-2999, 2997f-2998f
  in HIV infection, 1302-1303, 1716-1717
  treatment of, 3005
Bacillary dysentery, 1389-1391, 1390f, 2905-2910. *See
  also Shigella.*
  communicability of, 2905-2906, 2906t
  complications of, 2909
  control of, 2909-2910
  cyclic patterns of, 2907
  diagnosis of, 2908
  epidemiology of, 2907-2908
  immunity to, 2909-2910
  incidence of, 2907
  laboratory findings in, 2908
  pathogenesis of, 2905-2907, 2906t
  transmission of, 2907-2908

Bacillary dysentery (Continued)
  treatment of, 2908-2909, 2909t
  vaccines for, 2909
Bacillary peliosis, 2999, 3005
Bacille Calmette-Guérin (BCG) vaccine, 3151, 3922,
    3922t
  in HIV-infected children, 1826
  in leprosy prevention, 3174
  mycobacterial exposure to, 3138
Bacillus, 2727-2731
  adherence of, 2728
  central nervous system infections from, 2729
  commercial uses of, 2728
  contamination by, 2727-2728
  endocarditis from, 1081t, 1083-1084, 1093
  epidemiology of, 2727
  eye infections from, 2729
  food poisoning from, 2728-2729
  gram-negative aerobic
    classification of, 3017t
    meningitis from, 1193, 1218
  infection prophylaxis for, 2730
  microbiology of, 2727
  muscle infections from, 2729-2730
  pseudoinfection from, 2727-2728
  respiratory infections from, 2729
  skin infections, 2729-2730
  soft tissue infections from, 2729-2730
  systemic infections from, 2729, 2729t
  treatment of, 2730
Bacillus anthracis, 2715-2725, 2727. See also Anthrax.
  antibiotic minimum inhibitory concentrations for,
    2722t
  as biological weapon, 3951-3952
  culture of, 2718, 2719t
  infection control of, 3990
  laboratory detection of, 240t-242t
  microbiology of, 2715-2716, 2716f
  spores of, 3984-3985, 3984f-3985f
  toxins of, 30
  virulence factors of, 5t
Bacillus cereus, 2727, 2729t
  foodborne disease from, 1413-1415, 1414t-1415t,
    1418, 2728
  laboratory confirmation of, 1422
Bacillus circulans, 2729t
Bacillus globigii, spores of, 3984, 3984f
Bacillus licheniformis, 2728, 2729t
  food poisoning from, 2728
Bacillus megaterium, 2729t
Bacillus pumilus, 2729t
Bacillus sphaericus, 2729t
Bacillus subtilis, 2728, 2729t
  food poisoning from, 2729
Bacillus thuringiensis, 2728
  aerial spraying of, 3984
Bacitracin, 527-528, 706t-709t, 742t-761t
Bacterascites, in peritonitis, 1013-1014
Bacteremia, 1303-1304. See also Septicemia.
  from Acinetobacter, 2883
  from Aeromonas hydrophila, 3018
  in anaerobic infections, 3086-3087
  in bacterial meningitis, 1196-1197
  from Bartonella, 2996-2997
  in burn patients, 3906
  from Campylobacter jejuni, 2796-2797
  in cancer patients, 3796-3798, 3796f-3797f, 3797t
  catheter-related, 3788
  from Clostridium, 3107-3108
  from coagulase-negative Staphylococcus, 2581-2585
  definition of, 987, 988t
  device-associated, 1128. See also Catheter-related
    infections.
    differential diagnosis of, 3700-3701, 3700t
    microbiology of, 3700, 3700t
    pathogenesis of, 3707-3710
    prevention of, 3707-3710
    risk factors for, 3699, 3699t
  in elderly, 3859-3860
  from Enterococcus, 2646
  from Erysipelothrix rhusiopathiae, 2733-2734
  from gram-negative anaerobic rods, 3114
  from Haemophilus influenzae, 1304
    nontypeable, 2913-2914
    type b, 2914

Bacteremia (Continued)
  from Helicobacter cinaedi, 1304
  in immunocompromised hosts, 3788
  from Kingella, 2775
  from Listeria monocytogenes, 2709
  versus malaria, 3450
  from Moraxella catarrhalis, 2773
  mucosal barrier injury related to, 3785f
  from Neisseria gonorrhoeae, 1304, 2762-2763
  from Neisseria meningitidis, 1304
  neonatal, from Escherichia coli, 2822
  from Ochrobactrum anthropi, 3024
  from Pseudomonas aeruginosa, 1303-1304,
    2848-2850, 2849f
  quinolones for, 501
  from Salmonella, 2896, 2899
  from Salmonella typhi, 1304
  in solid organ transplant recipients, 3844
  in spinal cord injury patients, 3855
  from Staphylococcus aureus, 1303
    community-onset, 2568
    daptomycin for, 464
  from Streptococcus agalactiae (group B), 2660
    postpartum, 2659
  from Streptococcus anginosus group, 2683
  from Streptococcus group C and group G,
    2676-2677
  from Streptococcus viridans group, 2670-2671
  in subcutaneous abscess, 1300
  transient, in endocarditis, 1069-1070, 1070t
  as trigger for severe sepsis, 996
  vancomycin for, 455-456
Bacteria. See also Microbial flora; specific bacterium.
  antigen tests for, 245-246, 246t
  biochemical tests for, 247-248, 247t
  classification of, 248t, 2539
  cultivatable, from oral cavity, 856t
  culture media for, 244-245, 245t
  detection methods for, 240t-242t, 243-247
  evolution of, 2540
  extracellular, 140
  gram-negative, current and previous names of,
    3016t
  gram-positive, vancomycin-resistant, 452
  host defense avoidance by, 110-118
  identification methods for, 247-249
  ingested, 104-105, 105f
    intracellular disposition of, 105-108
  intracellular, 139-140
  microscopic stains for, 244, 244t
  molecular tests for, 246t, 248-249
  as new causes for old diseases, 2540
  nonpyogenic, regional lymphadenitis from,
    1325-1327
  nucleic acid–based tests for, 246-247, 246t
  pyogenic, regional lymphadenitis from, 1323
  serologic tests for, 248, 249t
  specimen collection and transport for, 234,
    235t-236t
  specimen guidelines and initial processing for,
    236-243
  in surgical site infections
    species and sources of, 3892-3894, 3892f-3893f,
      3892t-3893t
    virulence factors of, 3894
  taxonomic changes for, 233, 234t
  therapeutic uses of, 2540-2541
Bacterial infections. See also specific infection.
  in acute bronchitis, 873, 874t
  anaerobic. See Anaerobic bacterial infections.
  arthritis from. See Arthritis, bacterial.
  blood culture for, 236-238, 237t
  cellular immune response to, 139-140
  conjunctivitis from. See Conjunctivitis, bacterial.
  in COPD exacerbations, 879-880
  disease mechanisms in, 2539, 2540t
  endocarditis from, 1084-1085. See also
    Endocarditis.
  after hematopoietic stem cell transplantation,
    3827-3828
  keratitis from, 1541-1544
  in liver transplant recipients, 3842
  meningitis from. See Meningitis, bacterial.
  pneumonia from. See Pneumonia, bacterial.
  polymorphism and, 2539

Bacterial infections (Continued)
  systemic, cutaneous involvement in, 1303-1305
  tick-borne, 3650-3656
  time course in, 2539, 2540t
  transfusion-related, 3746-3748, 3747f, 3747t
  in transplant recipients, 3812t
  vaginosis from. See Vaginosis, bacterial.
  variation in, 2539
  zoonotic, 4000t-4001t
Bacterial overgrowth, of small bowel, 1367-1368
  rifamycins for, 413
  in tropical sprue, 1429-1430
Bacterial rDNA polymerase chain reaction, in
    microorganism identification, 1115-1116
Bacterial translocation, in peritonitis, 1014
Bactericide, 3677
Bacteriologic statistics, 267
Bacteriuria. See also Urinary tract infections.
  in adult, 965
  asymptomatic, 970, 974
  catheter-associated
    asymptomatic, 3725
      screening and treatment of, 3733
    complications of, 3725-3726
    definition of, 3725
    incidence and prevalence of, 3725
    prevention of, 3728-3732
    risk factors for, 3725
    treatment of, 3733
      choice of antibiotic in, 3733
      duration of antibiotic in, 3733
      urine culture and catheter replacement
        before, 3733
  in children, 964-965, 965f
  definition of, 957
  in elderly, 965-966, 3857
  epidemiology of, 964-966
  in pregnancy, 975-976
  pyuria in, 967, 973-974
  recurring, methenamine for, 519
  significant, diagnosis of, 3727-3728
  in spinal cord injury patients, 3855
  true, 968
Bacteroides
  brain abscess from, 1265, 1266t
  in colon, 3112
  in female urogenital tract, 3113
  immunomodulatory effects of, 3112-3113
  microbiology of, 3111, 3112f, 3112t
  in oropharynx, 3113
  resistance of, mechanisms of, 290t
  suppurative thrombophlebitis from, 1098
Bacteroides fragilis
  abscesses from, 3116
  antibiotic sensitivities of, 3117t
  cardiovascular infections from, 3116
  early colonization by, 3112
  enteritis from, 3116
  enterotoxins of, 32
  peritonitis from, 1017-1018
  resistance of, to clindamycin, 440-441
  treatment of, 342t, 442-443
Bacteroides thetaiotaomicron, 3112-3113
BAD-1 protein
  antibody to, 3322
  in Blastomyces dermatitidis, 3321
Balamuthia, 3427-3436
Balamuthia mandrillaris, 3427-3436. See also
    Granulomatous amebic encephalitis.
  characteristics of, 3427, 3428f-3429f, 3430f
  epidemiology of, 3431
  meningitis from, 632t-635t
Balanitis, from Candida, 3229
Balanoposthitis, 1482
Balantidiasis, 632t-635t, 3565-3566
Balantidium coli, 3565-3566, 3566f
  dysentery from, 1392
  life cycle of, 3565
Balofloxacin, 706t-709t
Banna virus, 2102
Barbiturates, for intracranial hypertension, 1187, 1221
Bare lymphocyte syndrome, 133
Barotrauma, from hyperbaric oxygen therapy, 626
Barrett's esophagus, in Helicobacter pylori infection,
    2806t, 2807

Bartonella, 2995-3009
   antimicrobial susceptibility testing for, 3004
   background on, 2995
   classification of, 2995, 2996t
   clinical manifestations of, 2995-3002
   culture of, 3003-3004
   direct examination of, 3003
   diseases due to, 803
   epidemiology of, 2995
   in HIV infection, 1858t-1871t, 1881, 3002
   identification of, 3004, 3004f
   laboratory diagnosis of, 240t-242t, 3003-3005
   pathogenesis of, 3002-3003
   polymerase chain reaction assay for, 3004
   prevention of, 3005-3006
   serologic testing of, 3004-3005
   specimen collection and handling of, 3003
   treatment of, 3005-3006
Bartonella bacilliformis, 2995
   in asplenia, 3869
   clinical manifestations of, 2995-2996, 2996f
   epidemiology of, 2995
   pathogenesis of, 3002
   treatment of, 3005
Bartonella clarridgeiae
   cat-scratch disease from, 2999
   epidemiology of, 2995
Bartonella elizabethae
   bacteremia and endocarditis from, 2997
   epidemiology of, 2995
Bartonella henselae, 803
   bacillary angiomatosis/peliosis from, 2997-2999,
      2997f-2998f
   bacteremia and endocarditis from, 2996-2997
   cat-scratch disease from, 1326, 2999-3002. *See also*
      Cat-scratch disease.
   epidemiology of, 2995
   in HIV infection, 3002
   identification of, 3004, 3004f
   Parinaud's syndrome from, 1565
   pathogenesis of, 3002
   treatment of, 3005
Bartonella koehlerae, epidemiology of, 2995
Bartonella quintana, 803
   bacillary angiomatosis/peliosis from, 2997-2999,
      2997f-2998f
   bacteremia and endocarditis from, 2996-2997
   epidemiology of, 2995
   in HIV infection, 3002
   treatment of, 3005
Bartonellosis (Oroya fever), 1400t-1401t, 1403,
   2995-2996, 2996f, 3005
Basidiobolomycosis, 3267
Basidiobolus, 3258t
Basilar skull fracture, meningitis from, 1209, 1223
Bats, rabies in, 2251
Battery-driven, computer-operated pumps, for
      outpatient parenteral antimicrobial therapy, 701
Baylisascariasis, 632t-635t, 3618
Bed rest, for acute viral hepatitis, 1588-1589
Beef tapeworms, 3608t, 3609f, 3610
Behçet's syndrome, meningitis in, 1241
Bejel, 3056-3057
Bell's palsy, 580, 1948
Belmont Report, on ethical principles and guidelines,
   687-688
Benzathine penicillin. *See* Penicillin G.
Benzimidazoles, 644-649
Benznidazole, 658
   for American trypanosomiasis, 3486
Benzodiazepines, for tetanus, 3094, 3094t
Benzoyl benzoate, for scabies, 3636t
Benztropine, for tetanus, 3094t
Bergeyella, 3016t-3017t, 3028
Beta-lactam antibiotics
   allergy to, 347-354
      classification of
         by clinical manifestations, 348, 349t
         Gell and Coombs, 347, 348f-349f, 348t
         by time of onset, 347-348, 348t
      desensitization in, 351, 352t
      diagnosis of, 350-351
      risk factors for, 349-350
      semisynthetic penicillins and, 351
   aminoglycosides with, 273

Beta-lactam antibiotics (*Continued*)
   with beta-lactamase inhibitor, 319, 319t
   cross-reactivity among, 352-353
   desensitization to, 351, 352t
   dosage of, 722t
   for *Enterococcus*, 2647-2648
   for gram-negative anaerobic rod infections, 3117
   immunochemistry of, 348-349, 349f
   for nontuberculous mycobacterial infections,
      544
   for osteomyelitis, 1459
   for peritonitis, 1025
   pharmacology of, 722t
   resistance to, 281
      beta-lactamase in, 284
      efflux promotion in, 287
      mechanisms of, 284t, 310-311
      by *Neisseria gonorrhoeae*, 2755-2756
      by *Staphylococcus aureus*, 2558-2560, 2559f
      target enzyme alteration in, 288
   semisynthetic, allergy to, 351
   for *Staphylococcus aureus* infection, 2562
   structure of, 349f
   for tuberculosis, 542
Beta-lactamase
   AmpC, 283
   in anaerobic antibiotic resistance, 284
   in antimicrobial resistance, 281-286
   in beta-lactam antibiotic resistance, 284, 284t
   classification of, 281-282, 282t-283t, 310, 311t
   CTX-M–derived, 283
   extended-spectrum, 283-284, 283f
   OXA–derived, 283
   production of, detection of, 250
   SHV–derived, 283, 283f
   TEM-derived, 283, 283f
Beta-lactamase inhibitors, 319-321, 319t
Beta-lactam/beta-lactamase inhibitor combination,
   274
   for anaerobic infections, 3088-3089, 3088t
   for peritonitis, 1022t
Bias, in clinical trials, 688, 692-693
Bifidobacteria, 161, 162t-163t, 3126. *See also*
   Probiotics.
Bile, *Campylobacter jejuni* colonization in, 2795
Bilharzial dysentery, 1392
Biliary disease
   in cryptosporidiosis, 3554
   in HIV infection, 1738-1739
Biliary tract infections, 1039-1042
   clinical presentation in, 1040
   from *Clostridium*, 3108
   diagnosis of, 1040
   imaging of, 1040-1041, 1041f
   microbiology of, 1041, 1041t
   pathogenesis of, 1039-1040, 1039f
   pyogenic liver abscess in, 1035-1036
   quinolones for, 497
   treatment of, 1041-1042
Bioavailability, 297
Biochemical tests, for bacterial infections, 247-248,
   247t
Biofilm(s), 855
   microbial, 22-23, 23t
   Pseudomonas aeruginosa, quorum sensing and,
      2846-2847
   Staphylococcus aureus, 2549-2550
   Staphylococcus epidermidis, 2580-2581, 2581f
Biologic gradient, 186
Biologic response modifiers. *See* Immunomodulators.
Biological weapons. *See* Bioterrorism.
Biological Weapons Convention, 3952
Biopsy
   brain. *See* Brain biopsy.
   CT-guided, in fever of unknown origin, 785
   duodenal, in Whipple's disease, 1438, 1438f
   endomyocardial, in myocarditis, 1157-1158
   intestinal
      in cryptosporidiosis, 3550, 3550f
      in Whipple's disease, 1438, 1438f
   liver
      in acute viral hepatitis, 1580
      in hepatitis A infection, 2379
      in hepatitis C infection, 2169, 2169t
   lung. *See* Lung biopsy.

Biopsy (*Continued*)
   renal, in BK virus-associated nephropathy, 2056,
      2056f
Biosynthetic valve prosthesis, 1116-1117. *See also*
   Prosthetic heart valve.
Bioterrorism, 3951-3963
   agents of, inactivation of, 3689-3690
   anthrax in, 3956, 3983-3992. *See also* Anthrax.
   biological weapons in
      before 20th century, 3951
      during 20th century, 3951-3953
      during Cold War era, 3952
      at end of 20th century, 3952
      during immediate post–World War II era, 3952
      non–state-sponsored development of,
         3952-3953
      obtaining and producing, 3954
      pathogens of greatest concern as, 3955-3956
      state-sponsored programs of, 3951-3952
      during World War I, 3951
      during World War II, 3952
   botulinum toxin in, 3100, 3993-3994
   CDC pathogens and disease categories in, 3954t
   challenges of, 3956
   emergency preparedness for, 221-231. *See also*
      Emergency preparedness.
   modern, two-edged sword of, 3962
   pathogens in, growing and "weaponizing,"
      3954-3955
   preparation for attack of, 3956
      research and development in, 3961-3962
   response to
      clinician preparedness in, 3957-3958
      emergency use authorization in, 3958
      hospital preparedness in, 3959
      laboratory preparedness in, 3958-3959
      medical and public health emergency
         preparedness in, 3956-3961
         before 9/11/2001, 3957
         following 9/11/2001, 3957, 3958t-3959t
      pathogen detection in, 3960
      provider and health care system in, 3957-3960
      public health response in, 3960-3961
      public health system preparedness in,
         3959-3960
      research and development to meet, 3961-3962
   risk of, assessment of, 3953
   smallpox in, 3951, 3955-3956. *See also* Smallpox.
   threat from
      assessment of, 3953
      changing perspective regarding, 3953
   tularemia in, 2927, 3975, 3975t. *See also*
      Tularemia.
   viral hemorrhagic fever in, 3995-3998. *See also*
      Viral hemorrhagic fevers.
   Yersinia pestis in, 2943. *See also* Plague.
Biotherapy
   for HIV-related non-Hodgkin's lymphoma, 1770
   for plague, 3968
Biothreat air monitors, for tularemia, 3975
Biotransformation, 299
Bird exposure, psittacosis after, 2463-2465
Bird influenza, 203-204, 203t, 204f, 2270-2271, 2280
Bird mites, 3645
Bites, 3911-3915
   animal, 3911-3913, 3912t
      to head and neck, 862t, 868
      management of, 3912-3913, 3912t-3913t
      Pasteurella infection from, 2939, 2941-2942
   human, 3914
      to head and neck, 862t, 868
      management of, 3914
   mosquito, 4015-4016
   snake, venomous, 1297, 1297t, 3913-3914
Bithionol, 706t-709t
   for liver flukes, 3602
   for parasitic infections, 649
BK virus
   hemorrhagic cystitis from, 2056
   history of, 2051
   nephropathy from, 2055-2056
      clinical manifestations of, 2055-2056
      diagnosis of, 2056, 2056f
      epidemiology of, 2055
      pathogenesis of, 2055

BK virus *(Continued)*
    prognosis for, 2056
    in solid organ transplant recipients, 3848
    treatment of, 2056
    receptor for, 2052
    ureteral stenosis from, 2056
Black Death, 2945, 2945f. *See also* Plague.
Black piedra, 3355
Bladder
    antiadherence mechanism of, 962
    dysfunction of, in HIV infection, 1525
    flushing mechanism of, 962
    infection in, localization of, 969
    irrigation of, urinary tract infection prevention
        with, 3732
Blanket therapy, hypothermia, antipyretic effects of,
    774-775
Blastocystis hominis, 3566-3567, 3566f
Blastocytosis, 3567
Blastomyces dermatitidis, 3319-3332
    antigen detection assay for, 3328-3329
    arthritis from, 1451, 3326
    brain abscess from, 1266
    central nervous system infections from, 3326,
        3326f
    characteristics of, 3319, 3320f
    in children, 3327
    clinical manifestations of, 3322t-3323t, 3322-3327,
        3323f
    culture of, 3328
    cytology of, 3327-3328
    diagnosis of, 3327-3329, 3328f
    epidemiology of, 3319-3320, 3320f
    genitourinary infections from, 3326
    history of, 3319
    in HIV infection, 3327
    immune response to, 3320-3322
    in immunocompromised hosts, 3327
    lymphocyte transformation assay for, 3329
    molecular identification of, 3328
    mycelial form of, 3319
    osteomyelitis from, 3325-3326, 3326f
    pathogenesis and pathology of, 3320
    in pregnancy, 3327
    pulmonary infections from, 3320
        acute, 3322, 3324f
        chest radiography in, 943f-944f
        chronic/recurrent, 3323-3327, 3324f-3325f
        in HIV infection, 1732
    serology of, 3328
    serotypes of, 3319
    skin lesions from, 3325, 3325f-3326f
    in solid organ transplant recipients, 3327
    staining of, 3328, 3328f
    subcutaneous nodules from, 3325
    treatment of, 3329-3330
        chemotherapy in, 3329-3330, 3329t
        surgery in, 3330
    yeast form of, 3319, 3320f
Blastomycosis
    of eyelid, 1569, 1570f
    meningitis in, 1239
    South American, gastrointestinal manifestations
        of, 1395
Blastoschizomyces capitatus, 3371
Bleb-related endophthalmitis, 1553-1554
Bleomycin
    for HIV-related non-Hodgkin's lymphoma,
        1769
    pulmonary disease from, chest radiography in,
        937f
Blepharitis
    from herpes simplex virus, 1569, 1952
    marginal, 1569, 1570f
Blepharoconjunctivitis, 1536, 1569
Blindness. *See also* Visual loss.
    in leprosy, 3171
    river. *See* Onchocerciasis.
Blisters, in staphylococcal scalded skin syndrome,
    2553, 2554f
Blood
    clinical-biochemical examination of, in prosthetic
        valve endocarditis, 1116
    microscopic examination of
        for parasites, 262, 263t

Blood *(Continued)*
    specimen collection and transport guidelines
        for, 235t-236t
Blood culture
    for bacterial and fungal infections, 236-238, 237t
    incubation period for, 237-238
    in pneumococcal pneumonia, 2632, 2632t
    in pneumonia, 900
    in shunt infections, 1233
    skin antisepsis for, 237
    specimen collection and transport guidelines for,
        235t-236t
    for viral infections, 257t
Blood groups. *See also specific blood group.*
    in disease susceptibility, 52-53
Blood transfusions. *See* Transfusions.
Blood-borne disease, in travelers, protection against,
    4015
Blood-borne pathogen standard, OSHA, 3688-3690
Blood-brain barrier, in bacterial meningitis,
    1200-1201
Bloodstream infections. *See also* Vascular infections.
    central line-associated, 3697
        from *Acinetobacter baumannii,* 3700
        prevention of, 3709-3710
    definition of, 2567-2568
    after invasive nonsurgical cardiologic procedures,
        1136-1137, 1136t
    in solid organ transplant recipients, 3844
    from *Staphylococcus aureus,* 2567-2568
        community-onset, 2568
        management of, 2568
        nosocomial, 2568
    viral, 1914f, 1915
BMS-806, for HIV infection, 21
Bocavirus, 2093
Boceprevir, 598, 599f, 706t-709t
Body fluids
    discoloration of, from rifamycins, 407
    laboratory processing of, 238
    specimen collection and transport guidelines for,
        235t-236t
Body mass index, classification of, 152t
Body temperature. *See* Temperature.
Boerhaave syndrome, 1173
Boils, 1292-1293
    from *Staphylococcus aureus,* 2566
Bolivian hemorrhagic fever. *See* South American
    hemorrhagic fevers.
Bombesin, antipyretic activity of, 772
Bone
    avascular necrosis of, in HIV infection, 1715
    lesions of, in adult T-cell leukemia/lymphoma,
        2312, 2313f
Bone cement, aminoglycoside-impregnated, 379
Bone infections. *See also* Osteomyelitis.
    from *Actinomyces,* 3214
    anaerobic, 3086
    from *Cryptococcus neoformans,* 3293t, 3296
    of implant, rifamycins for, 409-410
    in injection drug users, 3878-3879
    from *Pasteurella,* 2940
    from *Pseudomonas aeruginosa,* 2852
    quinolones for, 499-500
Bone marrow
    aspiration of, in African trypanosomiasis, 3492
    chloramphenicol effects on, 396
    specimen collection and transport guidelines for,
        235t-236t
Bone marrow transplantation. *See also*
    Hematopoietic stem cell transplantation.
    granulocyte-macrophage colony-stimulating factor
        after, 614
    herpes simplex virus infection in, 1954, 1954f
    intravenous immune globulin after, 617-618
    for neutrophil defects, 118
    toxoplasmosis in, 3504
Bone scintigraphy, in prosthetic joint infections,
    1470-1471
Bordetella ansorpii, 2955
Bordetella avium, 2955
Bordetella bronchiseptica, 2955
Bordetella hinzii, 2955
Bordetella holmesii, 2955
Bordetella parapertussis, 2955

Bordetella pertussis. See also Pertussis.
    carrier state for, 2958
    culture of, 2958-2959
    description of, 2955
    direct fluorescent antibody test for, 2959
    evolution of, 7
    history of, 2955
    laboratory detection of, 240t-242t
    molecular diagnosis of, 2959
    serologic tests for, 2959
    toxins of, 30-31, 2955-2956
    transmission of, chemoprophylaxis against,
        2961-2962
    virulence determinants for, 2955
    virulence regulatory systems for, 8t
Bordetella trematum, 2955
Boric acid
    for bacterial meningitis, 1504
    for vulvovaginal candidiasis, 1502
Bornholm disease, 2356-2357
Borrel body, 3979
Borrelia
    laboratory detection of, 240t-242t
    pathogenic species of, 3071
    relapsing fever from, 3067-3069. *See also* Relapsing
        fever.
Borrelia afzelii, 3071, 3650
Borrelia burgdorferi, 801, 3071, 3649-3650, 3650f. *See
    also* Lyme disease.
    antibody titers to, 3077, 3077f
    coinfection with, 3077
    dissemination of, 3073
    electron micrographs of, 3072f
    genome of, 3071
    meningitis from, 1193, 1206, 1210, 1210f, 1212t,
        1219-1220
    myocarditis from, 1156
    outer surface proteins of, 3071, 3073
    transmission of
        transplacental, 3076
        vectors in, 3071-3072
Borrelia garinii, 3071, 3650
Borrelia lonestari, 3649, 3650f
Borrelioses, spirochetal, 3650-3653, 3651t-3652t
Botryomycosis, 3281
Botulinum toxin, 31, 3097
    as biological weapon, 3100, 3993-3994
    immunity to, 3100-3101
    release mechanism of, 3098, 3098f
    synthesis of, 3098
    therapeutic uses of, 34, 3099
    transport of, 3098
Botulism, 3097-3102. *See also Clostridium botulinum.*
    adult, 3097
    clinical manifestations of, 3098-3099, 3099t
    diagnosis of, 3099-3100, 3100f
    epidemiology of, 3097
    foodborne, 1416, 1419, 3097-3098
    history of, 3097
    infant, 3097, 3099
    pathogenesis of, 3098, 3098f
    prevention of, 3100-3101
    treatment of, 1423, 3100
    wound, 3097, 3099
        in injection drug users, 3886
Botulism intravenous immune globulin, 3922t, 3936
Boutonneuse fever, 2504, 3653-3654, 3653t
Bovine papular stomatitis virus, 1933
Bovine prion disease, 2432, 4002
Bowenoid papulosis, 2040, 2040f
Bowen's disease, 2040
BPI, in neutrophil bactericidal activity, 109
Brachiola, 3391. *See also* Microsporidia.
Brachytherapy, antibiotic, 3901
Bradykinin, in pharyngitis, 815
Brain abscess, 1265-1278
    from *Actinomyces,* 3214
    anaerobic, 3086, 3086f
    from *Aspergillus,* 1266, 1266t, 1269, 1271-1272,
        3248-3249, 3249f
    bacterial
        etiology of, 1265-1266, 1266t
        treatment of, 1273-1275, 1273t-1274t
    from *Bacteroides,* 1265, 1266t
    from *Blastomyces dermatitidis,* 1266

Brain abscess *(Continued)*
  from *Candida,* 1266, 1266t, 1275
  clinical manifestations of, 1184, 1269-1270, 1269t
  computed tomography in, 1270-1271, 1270f
  from *Cryptococcus neoformans,* 1266, 1266t
  diagnosis of, 1270-1272, 1270f-1271f
  from *Enterobacteria,* 1265, 1266t
  epidemiology of, 1265-1267
  etiology of, 1265-1267, 1266t
  fungal, 1266, 1266t, 1275
  from *Haemophilus influenzae,* 1265-1266, 1266t
  from head trauma, 1267
  helminthic, 1266-1267
  host defense mechanisms in, 1268-1269
  initiation of infection in, 1267-1268
  in injection drug users, 3885-3886
  from *Listeria monocytogenes,* 1265-1266, 2710
  magnetic resonance imaging in, 1270-1271, 1271f
  microbiology of, 1266t
  mortality from, 1265
  from *Mycobacterium tuberculosis,* 1266
  natural history of, 1268
  neurologic sequelae in, 1265
  from *Nocardia,* 1266, 1266t, 3201, 3202f
  pathogenesis of, 1267
  in phaeohyphomycosis, 3367-3368, 3367f-3368f
  predisposing conditions for, 1266t, 1272t
  from *Prevotella,* 1265, 1266t
  from *Proteus,* 1265
  protozoal, 1266-1267
  from *Pseudallescheria boydii,* 1266, 3365
  from *Pseudomonas aeruginosa,* 1267-1268
  from *Salmonella,* 1266
  from *Scedosporium,* 1266, 1266t
  signs and symptoms of, 1237
  single-photon emission computed tomography in, 1272
  from *Staphylococcus,* 1265, 1266t, 1267-1269
  from *Streptococcus,* 1265-1268, 1266t
  from *Toxoplasma gondii,* 1266-1267, 1266t
  treatment of, 1273-1275
    antimicrobial, 1273-1275, 1273t
      recommended dosages of, 1274t
    initial approach to, 1272-1273, 1272t-1273t
    surgical, 1275
Brain biopsy
  in AIDS dementia, 1747-1748
  in central nervous system lymphoma, 1751
  in central nervous system mass lesions, 1754
  in cytomegalovirus encephalitis, 1754
  in progressive multifocal leukoencephalopathy, 1753, 2053
  in *Toxoplasma* encephalitis, 1750
  in toxoplasmosis, 3513
Brain herniation, after lumbar puncture, 1184
Brain stem encephalitis, from *Listeria monocytogenes,* 2710, 2711f
Brainerd's diarrhea, 1366
Brazilian purpuric fever, 2916
Brazilian spotted fever, 3653-3654, 3653t
Breast cancer, in HIV-infected women, 1796
Breast implant infections, from coagulase-negative *Staphylococcus,* 2585
Breast milk
  antimicrobial agents in, 270
  HCV transmission via, 2171-2172
  HIV transmission via, 1653, 1787, 1811-1812
  protective effects of, 1339
    against giardiasis, 3529
    against rotaviruses, 2110
Breastfeeding, HAART during, 1787
Brevibacillus brevis, 2729t
Brevibacillus laterosporus, 2729t
Brevibacterium, 2701
Brevibacterium casei, 2701
Brill-Zinsser disease, 2522-2523
Brivudin, 578f, 598
Brodie's abscess, 1465
Bronchial cleft cyst, infected, 862t, 867
Bronchiectasis, from *Pseudomonas aeruginosa,* 2851
Bronchiolitis, 885-890
  from adenoviruses, 886t
  from bocavirus, 886t
  clinical manifestations of, 887-888
  complications of, 888

Bronchiolitis *(Continued)*
  definition of, 885
  diagnosis of, 888
  from enteroviruses, 885
  epidemiology of, 886
  etiology of, 885, 886t
  from human metapneumovirus, 885, 886t
  from influenza viruses, 886t
  from non-SARS coronaviruses, 885, 886t
  from parainfluenza viruses, 885, 886t
  pathophysiology of, 886-887, 887f
  from respiratory syncytial virus, 885, 886t, 2209
  from rhinoviruses, 885, 886t
  treatment of, 888-889
Bronchiolitis obliterans organizing pneumonia (BOOP), 936f
Bronchitis
  acute, 873-876
    clinical presentation in, 874
    diagnosis of, 874-875
    microbial etiology of, 873, 874t
    pathogenesis of, 873-874
    treatment of, 875
  chronic
    in chronic obstructive pulmonary disease, 877-878
    quinolones for, 498
  exacerbation of
    from rhinoviruses, 2393
    from *Streptococcus pneumoniae,* 2631
  trimethoprim-sulfamethoxazole for, 481
Bronchoalveolar lavage
  laboratory processing after, 239
  in pneumonia
    acute, 899
    chronic, 934-938
    non-bronchoscopic, 899
    nosocomial, 3720
    from *Pneumocystis,* 1729, 3383
Bronchodilators
  for bronchiolitis, 889
  for chronic obstructive pulmonary disease, 880t
  for cystic fibrosis, 951
Bronchopleural fistula
  empyema in, 922-923
  tuberculous, 3155
Bronchopneumonia, 935t-936t
Bronchopulmonary aspergillosis, allergic
  clinical manifestations of, 3245-3246
  in cystic fibrosis, 951, 3246, 3246t
  pathogenesis of, 3245
Bronchoscopy
  in chronic pneumonia, 942
  for lung abscess drainage, 928
  in *Pneumocystis* pneumonia, 3383
  in pneumonia, 899, 937-938
  in tuberculosis, 3143-3144
Broth dilution tests, 249, 268
Brucella, 2921-2925
  characteristics of, 2921
  immunity to, 2922
  laboratory detection of, 240t-242t, 2923-2924
  pathogenesis of, 2922
  vaccine for, 2924
Brucella suis, as biological weapon, 3952
Brucellosis, 2921-2925
  clinical manifestations of, 2922
  complications of, 2922-2923
  diagnosis of, 2923-2924
  enteric fever from, 1400t-1401t, 1403
  epidemiology of, 2921-2922, 2922f
  history of, 2921
  meningitis in, 1240
  prevention of, 2924
  rifamycins for, 412
  treatment of, 2924
  uveitis in, 1566
Brudzinski's sign, in bacterial meningitis, 1205
Brugia, 654
Brugia malayi
  filariasis from, 3590, 3590t. *See also* Filariasis, lymphatic.
  tropical pulmonary eosinophilia from, 3592
Brugia timori, 3590, 3590t. *See also* Filariasis, lymphatic.

Bruton's agammaglobulinemia, 72
Buboes
  in bubonic plague, 2945-2946
    axillary, 2946, 2946f
    femoral and inguinal, 1326-1327, 2946, 2946f
  in sexually transmitted disease, inguinal, 1326
Bubonic plague, 2945-2946, 2946f, 3639t. *See also* Plague.
  inguinal lymphadenitis in, 1326-1327
  treatment of, 1330
Buccal space, infections of, 863. *See also* Odontogenic infections.
Budd-Chiari syndrome, hepatitis in, 1588
Budesonide, for croup, 2198
Bulbar paralytic poliomyelitis, 2346-2347
Bullae, 792, 1303
  hemorrhagic, from *Vibrio vulnificus,* 2788-2789, 2789f
Bullous erysipelas, 1294
Bullous impetigo, 799, 1291, 2554, 2554f
Bullous lesions, with sepsis, 792, 796
Bull's eye lesions, 794
Bunyaviridae, 2289-2293, 2290t, 3997t
Burkholderia ambifaria, 2861
Burkholderia anthina, 2861
Burkholderia cepacia, 2861-2868
  clinical manifestations of, 2865, 2865f
  in cystic fibrosis, 949-950, 2864-2865, 2865f
  device-associated infections from, 3697, 3700
  epidemiology of, 2863-2864
  microbiology, taxonomy, and identification of, 2861
  pathogenesis of, 2861-2863, 2862f
  prevention and control of, 2866
  treatment of, 2866
    carbapenems in, 342t
    rifamycins in, 411
  virulence factors of, 2861-2863
Burkholderia cepacia complex, 240t-242t
Burkholderia dolosa, 2861
Burkholderia mallei, 2877-2878, 2877f
  as biological weapon, 3951
Burkholderia multivorans, 2861, 2865-2866
Burkholderia pseudomallei, 2869-2877. *See also* Melioidosis.
  culture of, 2875
  etiology of, 2869
  history of, 2869
  laboratory detection of, 240t-242t
  pathogenesis of, 2870-2871
  reactivation of, 2873-2875
  transmission of, 2870, 2870f
Burkholderia pyrrocinia, 2861
Burkholderia stabilis, 2861
Burkholderia ubonensis, 2861
Burkholderia vietnamiensis, 2861
Burkitt's lymphoma, from Epstein-Barr virus, 1989, 1996t, 1997
Burn infections, 3905-3909. *See also* Wound infections.
  criteria for, 3906-3907, 3907t
  diagnosis of, 3906-3907, 3906t-3907t
  epidemiology of, 3905-3906
  mechanisms of, 3905
  prevention of, 3907-3908
    topical antibacterials in, 525-526, 528t
  from *Pseudomonas aeruginosa,* 2837-2838, 2854
  suppurative thrombophlebitis and, 1097
  treatment of, 3906t, 3907
Bursitis
  olecranon, from *Pseudallescheria boydii,* 3365, 3366f
  septic, 1453
    from *Staphylococcus aureus,* 2574
    treatment of, 1450t, 1453
Buschke-Lowenstein tumors, 2040
Bush-Jacoby-Medeiros classification of beta-lactamases, 283t
Butoconazole nitrate, 706t-709t

C

C1
  in complement activation, 78
  regulation of, 81, 81t

C1 inhibitor, 81t
  deficiency of, in hereditary angioedema, 91-92
  purified, 91-92
  replacement of, in endotoxic shock, 93
C1-esterase, in severe sepsis, 994
C1q, 78t
  deficiency of, 88, 169t-170t
    in systemic lupus erythematosus, 86-88
C1qR, 81t, 82
C1r, 78t
  in complement activation, 78-79
  deficiency of, 169t-170t
C1s, 78t
  in complement activation, 78-79
  deficiency of, 169t-170t
C2, 78t
  deficiency of, 88, 169t-170t
    in systemic lupus erythematosus, 86
C3, 78t
  activation of, 79, 80f
  in adaptive immune response, 83-84
  in complement cascade, 77-78
  deficiency of, 89, 169t-170t
    in endotoxic shock, 93
C3 convertase
  in alternate pathway activation, 79-80, 79f-80f
  in classic pathway activation, 78-79, 79f-80f
  regulation of, 81-82, 81t
C3a/C4aR, 81t
C3b, 79-80
  as opsonin, 62
C4, 78t
  deficiency of
    in endotoxic shock, 93
    in systemic lupus erythematosus, 86
C4a
  in complement activation, 79
  deficiency of, 88, 169t-170t
C4b, 78t
  deficiency of, 88, 169t-170t
C4b BP, 81t
C5, 78t
  deficiency of, 89-91, 169t-170t
  monoclonal antibody to, 93
  in sepsis, 93-94
C5a, in severe sepsis, 994
C5aR, 81t, 82
C5b-7 complex, 82
C6, 78t
  deficiency of, 89-91, 169t-170t
C7, 78t
  deficiency of, 89-91, 169t-170t
C8, 78t
  deficiency of, 89-91, 169t-170t
C9, 78t, 82
  deficiency of, 89-91, 169t-170t
Caffeine, quinolone interactions with, 494
CagA gene, in *Helicobacter pylori* infection,
    2803-2805
CagA protein, in *Helicobacter pylori* infection,
    2803-2805
Calcium plus vitamin D, for osteoporosis, 1801
Calculi
  biliary. *See* Cholecystitis.
  urinary, 963, 964f
Caliciviruses, 2399-2405. *See also* Noroviruses.
California encephalitis group, meningitis from, 1190
California Encephalitis Project (CEP), 1243
California encephalitis virus, 1258
  characteristics of, 2290t
  clinical manifestations of, 2291
  diagnosis of, 2292
  epidemiology of, 2289-2291
  geographic distribution of, 1246-1247, 1247f,
    2289-2290
  prevention and treatment of, 2292
  transmission of, 2290
cAMP factor, in coryneform bacteria, 2696
Campylobacter
  diarrhea from, 206
  enteritis from, 1391
  in HIV infection, 1860t-1870t, 1880
  infections from, 2798
  laboratory detection of, 240t-242t
Campylobacter coli, 1391, 2794, 2794t, 2798

Campylobacter fetus
  clinical manifestations of, 2797-2798, 2797t
  enteric fever–like syndrome from, 1400t-1401t,
    1402
  etiology of, 2793, 2794t
  pathogenesis of, 2796, 2796f
  prognosis for, 2799
Campylobacter hyointestinalis, 2794, 2794t, 2798
Campylobacter insulaenigrae, 2798
Campylobacter jejuni, 1391, 2793-2802
  biochemical characteristics of, 2804t
  clinical manifestations of, 2796-2798, 2797t
  diagnosis of
    bacteriologic studies in, 2798
    fecal examination in, 2798, 2798f
  epidemiology of, 2794-2795
  etiology of, 2793-2794, 2794f, 2794t
  foodborne disease from, 1414t, 1415
  gastric acid and, 1337
  immunity to, 2796
  pathogenesis of, 2795-2796, 2796f
  prognosis for, 2799
  quinolone resistance in, 502
  treatment of, 2798-2799
Campylobacter lari, 2794t
Campylobacter sputorum, 2798
Campylobacter upsaliensis, 2794, 2794t, 2798
Canaliculitis, 1570-1571
Cancer. *See also* Tumor(s); *specific types.*
  antibody deficiencies in, 73
  chemoprophylaxis for, toxins in, 33-34
  HIV-related, 1765-1779. *See also* Anogenital
    neoplasia; Kaposi's sarcoma; Lymphoma.
    in women, 1796
  infections in, 3793-3807. *See also* Febrile
    neutropenia.
    bacterial, antibiotic resistance to, 3796-3798,
      3796f-3797f
    central venous access–related, 3795, 3797t
    chemoprophylaxis for, 3799-3801, 3800t
      antibacterial, 3799-3801, 3800t
      antifungal, 3800t, 3801
      antiviral, 3800t, 3802
      colony-stimulating factors in, 3800t, 3802
      immunoglobulins in, 3800t, 3802
      against *Pneumocystis jirovecii,* 3800t,
        3801-3802
      toxins from, 33-34
      against tuberculosis, 3800t, 3802
    clinical approach to, 3793, 3794t
    complications of, 3795t, 3797f
    epidemiology of, 3793-3795, 3794t-3796t
    etiology of, 3796-3799
    fungal, 3793, 3796t, 3798-3799
    viral, 3799
  tuberculosis in, 3144
  from viral infections, 1916-1917
Candida, 3225-3240. *See also* Candidiasis.
  arthritis from, 1451, 3233
  balanitis from, 1482, 3229
  brain abscess from, 1266, 1266t, 1275
  conjunctivitis from, 1536-1537, 1537f
  costochondritis from, 3233
  cystitis from, 3233
  ecology of, 3225
  endocarditis from, 1071, 1085, 3232, 3236
  endophthalmitis from, 1555-1556, 1555f, 1565,
    3234, 3234f
  esophagitis from, 1353-1354, 1354f, 3227-3228,
    3228f
    treatment of, 1355-1357, 1355t, 3237
  folliculitis from, 1292, 3229, 3229f
  forms of, 3225
  of gastrointestinal tract, 3227
  genital lesions in, 1482
  granuloma from, 3231, 3231f
  historical perspective on, 3225
  keratitis from, 1549
  meningitis from, 1239, 3231-3232
  mycotic aneurysms from, 1102
  myocarditis from, 3232
  myositis from, 3233
  osteomyelitis from, 3233, 3233f
  peritonitis from, 1017-1018
  pneumonia from, 3232

Candida (Continued)
  route of entry of, 3226-3227
  suppurative thrombophlebitis from, 1098
  urinary tract infections from, 3726-3727,
    3733-3734
  vaginitis from. *See* Vaginitis/vulvovaginitis, from
    Candida.
  virulence factors in, 3227
Candida albicans, 3225
Candida dubliniensis, 3225
Candida glabrata, 1500, 3225
Candida guilliermondii, 3225
Candida krusei, 3225
Candida lusitaniae, 3225
Candida parapsilosis, 3225, 3733-3734
  device-associated infections from, 3697
Candida pseudotropicalis, 3225
Candida tropicalis, 1500, 3225
Candidemia, 3234-3235
  treatment of
    in neutropenic patients, 3236
    in non-neutropenic patients, 3236
Candidiasis
  anidulafungin for, 560
  in cancer patients, 3796t, 3798-3799
  cardiac, 3232, 3236
  of central nervous system, 1239, 3231-3232, 3236
  clinical manifestations of, 3227-3235
  cutaneous, 3228-3231
    in diaper area, 3230, 3230f
    disseminated, 801-802, 1304-1305, 3229-3230,
      3230f
    of fingers and toes, 3228, 3229f
    generalized, 3228, 3229f
    in intertriginous region, 3230
    of nails, 3230, 3230f
    in perianal area, 3230, 3231f
  disseminated, 3234-3235
    premortem diagnosis of, 3235
    skin lesions in, 801-802, 1304-1305, 3229-3230,
      3230f
    vulvovaginal, in HIV infection, 1796-1797
  epidemiology of, 3225
  esophageal
    as AIDS indicator, 1643
    in HIV infection, 1737
  of gallbladder, 3233, 3237
  gastrointestinal, 1395
    nonesophageal, 3228
  in hematopoietic stem cell transplant recipients,
    3831
  in HIV infection, 1858t-1871t, 1877
    oral, 1714-1715, 1714f
    prophylaxis against, 1858t-1859t, 1871t
    treatment of, 1860t-1870t
    vulvovaginal, 1796-1797
  of liver, 3233, 3234f
  miscellaneous, 3235, 3238
  mucocutaneous
    chronic, 3230-3231, 3231f, 3238
    treatment of, 3237-3238
  of mucus membranes, 3227-3228, 3227f-3229f
  ocular, 3234, 3234f, 3238
  oral (thrush), 3227, 3227f
    in HIV infection, 1714-1715, 1714f
    treatment of, 3237
  oropharyngeal, posaconazole prophylaxis in, 559
  pathology and pathogenesis of, 3226-3227
  perianal, 3230, 3231f
  of peritoneum, 3233, 3237
  predisposing factors to, 3226
  of respiratory tract, 3232
  of spleen, 3233, 3234f
  after transplantation, 3816
  treatment of, 3235-3238
    caspofungin in, 559-560
    echinocandins in, 3236
    fluconazole in, 557
    flucytosine in, 3236
    general comments in, 3235
    micafungin in, 560-561
    polyenes in, 3235
    systemic, 3235-3236
    triazoles in, 3235-3236
  of urinary tract, 3232-3233, 3237, 3733-3734

Candidiasis *(Continued)*
  of vasculature, 3234
  vulvovaginal. *See* Vaginitis/vulvovaginitis, from
      Candida.
Candiduria, 3233
  eradication of, 3237
  postcatheterization, 3237
Canine spaces, infections of, 863. *See also*
      Odontogenic infections.
Capillaria philippinensis, 3621
  abdominal pain and/or diarrhea with eosinophilia
      from, 1407t, 1408
Capillariasis, 632t-635t, 648, 3618t, 3621
Capnocytophaga, 2991-2994
  animal-associated infections from, 2992, 2992t
  diagnosis and laboratory identification of,
      2992-2993, 2992f
  epidemiology of, 2992
  human oral-associated infections from, 2991-2992,
      2992t
  pathogenesis of, 2991-2992
  prevention of, 2993
  taxonomy of, 2991
  treatment of, 2993
Capnocytophaga canimorsus, 2991-2992, 3020-3021
  fatal infection with, 3911
  rash from, 801
Capnocytophaga cynodegmi, 2991-2992
Capnocytophaga gingivalis, 2991
Capnocytophaga granulosa, 2991
Capnocytophaga ochracea, 2991
  blepharoconjunctivitis from, 1569
Capnocytophaga sputigena, 2991
Capreomycin, 706t-709t
  dosage of, 734t-735t
  drug interactions with, 742t-761t
  formulations of, 717t
  for tuberculosis, 541
Capsid-binding agents, for rhinovirus infections,
      2396-2397
Capsules, of enterobacteriaceae, 2816, 2820
Carbapenemases, 284
Carbapenems. *See also* Beta-lactam antibiotics.
  adverse reactions to, 343
  antibacterial activity of, 341-342, 342t
  chemistry of, 341, 342f
  clinical use of, 343
  cross-reactivity with, 353
  for gram-negative anaerobic rod infections,
      3117
  mechanism of action of, 341
  pharmacology of, 342
  resistance to, 341
  structure of, 349f
Carbenicillin, 318, 319f
  dosage of, 718t-719t
  formulations of, 715t
Carbenicillin indanyl sodium, 706t-709t
  dosage of, 718t-719t
  formulations of, 715t
Carbohydrate, group A, in rheumatic valvulitis,
      2612
Carbol-fuchsin, 706t-709t
Carboxypenicillins, 311, 318, 319f
Carboxypeptidase N, 78t, 81t
Carbuncles, 1292-1293
  from *Staphylococcus aureus,* 2566
Cardiac catheterization, bloodstream infection after,
      1136-1137, 1136t
Cardiac conditions, endocarditis and, 1144t,
      1145-1146, 1146t
Cardiac output, in peritonitis, 1020
Cardiac rhythm management device infections,
      1127-1131
  clinical manifestations of, 1128
  from coagulase-negative *Staphylococcus,* 2583
  complications of, 1129
  diagnosis of, 1128-1129
  echocardiography in, 1129
  epidemiology of, 1127
  management of, 1129, 1130f
  microbiology of, 1127-1128, 1128f
  pathogenesis of, 1127
  prevention of, 1129-1131
  risk factors for, 1127, 1128t

Cardiac surgery
  endocarditis prophylaxis during, 1148-1149
  hypothermia during, 3895
Cardiac suture line infection, 1140
Cardiac vegetations, in endocarditis, 1073-1074
Cardiobacterium, 3016t-3017t, 3019
Cardiobacterium hominis, endocarditis from, 3019
  prosthetic valve, 1121t, 1123
Cardiobacterium valvarum, endocarditis from,
      prosthetic valve, 1121t, 1123
Cardiologic procedures, invasive nonsurgical,
      bloodstream infection after, 1136-1137, 1136t
Cardiomyopathy
  dilated
      as end stage of viral myocarditis, 1158
      from enteroviruses, 2358
  in HIV infection, 1720
Cardiothoracic surgery, mediastinitis secondary to,
      1173-1175, 1175t
Cardiovascular device infections, 1127-1142, 1128t.
      See also specific device types, e.g., Cardiac rhythm
      management device infections.
Cardiovascular disease
  from cytomegalovirus, 1982-1983
  in HIV-infected children, 1816
  odontogenic infections associated with, 865
Cardiovascular system
  gram-negative anaerobic rod infections of, 3116
  syphilis of, 3043
Cardioverter-defibrillator, implantable, infection of,
      1127-1131, 1128f, 1128t, 1130f. *See also* Cardiac
      rhythm management device infections.
Carditis. *See also* Endocarditis; Myocarditis;
      Pericarditis.
  in Kawasaki syndrome, 3663
  in rheumatic fever, 2613-2614
Caribbean, HIV infection in, 1623-1624, 1624f
Caries. *See* Dental caries.
Carotid artery erosion, in odontogenic infections,
      864-865
Carotid patch, dacron, infection of, 1139-1140
Case series studies, 183
Case-control studies, 183-184
Case-fatality rate, 186
Caspofungin, 559-560, 706t-709t
  for aspergillosis, 3251t, 3252
  for *Candida* esophagitis, 1355t, 1356-1357
  for *Coccidioides,* 3342
  dosage of, 736t-737t
  drug interactions with, 742t-761t
  for febrile neutropenia, 3804t
  formulations of, 717t
  structure of, 550f-551f, 559
Castleman's disease, multicentric, from human
      herpesvirus 8, 2020-2021, 2021f
Cat bites, 3912, 3912t
  Pasteurella infection from, 2939, 2941-2942
Cataract surgery, advances in, 1553
CATCH 22, 169t-170t
Catheter(s)
  antibiotic-impregnated, for cerebrospinal fluid
      shunts, 1235
  antimicrobial-coated, 3709-3710, 3731
  bacteremia from, 3788
  bacteriuria from. *See* Bacteriuria,
      catheter-associated.
  hub and lumen of, contamination of, 3698
  indwelling, alternatives to, 3729-3730
  infusate in, contamination of, 3697
  insertion and maintenance of, techniques for,
      3730
  insertion site of, contamination of, 3698
  long-term, infectious complications associated
      with, 3704t, 3705t
  peripherally inserted central
      for intermediate and long-term access, 3705
      for outpatient parenteral antimicrobial therapy,
          701
  pulmonary artery, infections of, 3706
  removal or replacement of, antimicrobial
      prophylaxis at, 3732
  routine changes of, 3732
  specimen collection and transport guidelines for,
      235t-236t
  urinary, in elderly, 3858

Catheter hub-infusion tubing, contamination of,
      3698
Catheterization
  cardiac, bloodstream infection after, 1136-1137,
      1136t
  condom, 3729-3730
  intermittent, 3730
  suprapubic, 3730
  unnecessary, reduction of, 3729
  for urine collection, 968
Catheter-related infections, 3697-3715
  in arterial lines, transducers, and transducer
      domes, 3706-3707, 3707t
  in cancer patients, 3793-3807. *See also* Cancer,
      infections in.
  chemoprophylaxis for, 3799-3801, 3800t
  from *Candida,* 3233
  in central venous access
      in cancer patients, 3795, 3797t
      long-term issues in, 3698, 3705t
      short-term issues in, 3698, 3704t
  epidemiology of, 3698-3700
  from hub and lumen contamination, 3698
  in immunocompromised hosts, 3788-3789
  from infusate contamination, 3697
  from insertion site contamination, 3698
  from nontuberculous mycobacteria, 3196
  from *Ochrobactrum anthropi,* 3024
  pathogenesis of, 3697-3698, 3698f
  in peripheral intravenous cannulization, 3697
  prevention of, 3707-3710
      antimicrobial catheters in, 3709-3710
      antimicrobial lock prophylaxis in, 3709
      antimicrobial prophylaxis in, 3709
      after catheter insertion, 3708-3709
      at catheter insertion, 3707-3708
      before catheter insertion, 3707
      other issues in, 3710
      rifamycin for, 410
      topical antibacterials in, 524
  in pulmonary artery catheterization, 3706
  risk factors for, 3698-3700
  from *Staphylococcus aureus,* 2567-2568
  in total parenteral nutrition, 3698, 3704t
  of urinary tract, 3725-3737. *See also* Urinary tract
      infections, catheter-associated.
Cat-scratch disease, 2999-3002, 3639t
  computed tomography in, 3000-3001, 3000f
  diagnosis of, 3001-3002
  differential diagnosis of, 3002
  encephalopathy in, 3001
  epidemiology of, 2995
  inflammatory response in, 3002-3003
  lymphadenitis/lymphadenopathy in, 1326, 2999,
      2999f-3000f
  musculoskeletal manifestations of, 2999-3000
  neuroretinitis in, 3001, 3001f, 3005
  papilledema in, 3001, 3001f
  papule or pustule in, 2999, 2999f
  Parinaud's oculoglandular syndrome in, 3000,
      3000f
  skin lesions in, 803
  treatment of, 1330, 3005
  "typical," 2999, 2999f-3000f
  uveitis in, 1565, 1566f
Cavernous sinus thrombophlebitis, 1571-1573
Cavernous sinus thrombosis, septic, 865, 865f,
      1283-1286, 1284f
Cavitation, pulmonary, 934, 935t-936t
CCL3 gene, in HIV susceptibility, 51-52
CCR2 gene, in HIV susceptibility, 51-52, 51t
CCR5
  defect in, 43-44
  HIV nonprogression and, 1692
  as HIV receptor, 1687, 1688f
  in HIV replication, 18, 18f, 2324-2325
  in HIV susceptibility, 51-52, 51t, 54-55
CCR5 antagonist, maraviroc as, 1843-1844
CD1, 136-137
  antigen processing and loading by, 137, 137f
  antigens presented by, 137
  host defenses and, 140
  isoforms of, 137
  structure of, 136-137, 136f
CD2, in disease susceptibility, 52

CD4
  in anal cancer, 1774
  antigen presentation to, 133
  apoptosis of, 1695-1696
  count of
    in antiretroviral therapy, 1845, 1847
    HIV prognosis and, 1708-1709, 1708f, 1708t
    in HIV staging, 1706, 1706t
    in HIV-infected children, 1813t-1814t, 1817
    opportunistic infections and, 1709, 1709f
    Pneumocystis jirovecii pneumonia and, 1727
    pneumonia and, 895
  in cryptococcosis, 3292
  in cryptosporidiosis, 3550-3551
  decreased production of, 1696
  depletion of, 1695-1696
  in disseminated *Mycobacterium avium* complex
    disease, 3177
  in hepatitis B infection, 1595, 2066-2067
  in hepatitis C infection, 2164
  in herpes simplex virus infection, 1946-1947
  in HIV infection, 1691-1692, 1695-1696,
    1796-1797
    pregnancy and, 1788, 1794-1795
  as HIV receptor, 1687, 1688f
  lymphocyte turnover and, 1696
  in microsporidiosis, 3395
  in non-Hodgkin's lymphoma, 1769-1770
  overview of, 129-131
  redistribution of, 1696
  resting, as HIV reservoir, 1693
  soluble, for HIV infection, 21
  subsets of, 168-171
  thymic selection of, 141-142
  in toxoplasmosis, 3499
  in tuberculosis response, 3136
  in tularemia, 2931
  in vivo responses to infection of, 130-131
  in Whipple's disease, 1436
CD4 lymphopenia, idiopathic, 176-177, 1642
CD4 receptor binding, 1842-1843
  in HIV replication, 18, 18f, 2325
CD8
  antigen presentation to, 132-133
  in cryptococcosis, 3292
  in hepatitis B infection, 1595, 2067
  in hepatitis C infection, 2164
  in herpes simplex virus infection, 1945-1947
  in HIV infection, 1696-1697
    cytotoxic, 1690-1691, 1690t
    noncytolytic antiviral activity of, 1691
  in microsporidiosis, 3395
  overview of, 131
  thymic selection of, 141-142
  in toxoplasmosis, 3499
  in tularemia, 2931
  in viral infections, 139
  in Whipple's disease, 1436
CD18, deficiency of, in leukocyte adhesion
    deficiency, 172
CD19, 68
CD21, 68
CD28, 71
CD28 receptor, activation of, 69
CD36, in *Plasmodium falciparum* malaria, 3440-3441
CD40, 132
CD40L, 132
CD59, 81t, 82
  deficiency of, 92-93
CD81, 68
Cefaclor, 706t-709t
  dosage of, 720t-722t
  formulations of, 715t
  structure of, 324f
  uses of, 334
Cefadroxil, 706t-709t
  for cellulitis, 1297-1298
  dosage of, 720t-722t
  formulations of, 715t
  structure of, 324f
  uses of, 333-334
Cefamandole, 706t-709t
  dosage of, 720t-722t
  formulations of, 715t
Cefapirin. *See* Cephapirin.

Cefazolin, 706t-709t
  for cellulitis, 1297-1298
  dosage of, 720t-722t
  for endocarditis, 1089, 1093
  formulations of, 715t
  for osteomyelitis, 1459t
  for peritonitis, 1029t
  prophylactic
    for postoperative mediastinitis, 1178
    for surgical procedures, 3899t
    for *Staphylococcus aureus* endocarditis,
      2571t
  structure of, 324f
  uses of, 333-334
Cefdinir, 706t-709t
  dosage of, 720t-722t
  formulations of, 715t
  for sinusitis, 844-845, 845t
  structure of, 325f
  uses of, 334-335
Cefditoren
  dosage of, 720t-722t
  drug interactions with, 742t-761t
  structure of, 325f
  uses of, 334-335
Cefditoren pivoxil, 706t-709t, 715t
Cefepime, 706t-709t
  for acute pyelonephritis, 972
  for brain abscess, 1274t
  dosage of, 720t-722t
  for febrile neutropenia, 3804t
  formulations of, 715t
  for meningitis, 1213t
  for osteomyelitis, 1459t
  for peritonitis, 1029t
  for *Pseudomonas aeruginosa* bacteremia,
    2849-2850
  for septic bursitis, 1450t
  structure of, 325f
  uses of, 335-336
Cefeptine, for nosocomial pneumonia, 3718t
Cefixime, 706t-709t
  dosage of, 720t-722t
  for febrile neutropenia, 3804t
  formulations of, 715t
  for gonococcal arthritis, 1449
  for *Neisseria gonorrhoeae* infection, 2764, 2764t,
    2766
  for sinusitis, 845t
  structure of, 325f
  for typhoid fever, 2898-2899, 2898t
  for urethritis, 1491, 1491t
  uses of, 334-335
Cefmetazole, 706t-709t
  dosage of, 720t-722t
  formulations of, 715t
Cefonicid, 706t-709t
  dosage of, 720t-722t
  formulations of, 715t
Cefoperazone, 706t-709t
  dosage of, 720t-722t
  formulations of, 715t
Cefoperazone-sulbactam, 706t-709t
Ceforanide, 706t-709t
Cefotaxime, 706t-709t
  for brain abscess, 1273t-1274t, 1274
  dosage of, 720t-722t
  for epiglottitis, 853
  formulations of, 715t
  for *Haemophilus influenzae* type b, 2915
  for meningitis, 1213t
  for peritonitis, 1029t
  structure of, 325f
  for typhoid fever, 2898-2899, 2898t
  uses of, 334-335
Cefotetan, 706t-709t
  dosage of, 720t-722t
  formulations of, 715t
  for *Neisseria gonorrhoeae* infection, 2765t
  for peritonitis, 1022t, 1024
  structure of, 324f
  uses of, 334
Cefoxitin, 706t-709t
  dosage of, 720t-722t
  formulations of, 715t

Cefoxitin (*Continued*)
  for *Mycobacterium abscessus* pulmonary disease,
    3193t, 3194
  for peritonitis, 1022t, 1024
  prophylactic, for surgical procedures, 3899t
  structure of, 324f
  uses of, 334
Cefpirome, 706t-709t
  structure of, 325f
  uses of, 335-336
Cefpodoxime, 706t-709t
  dosage of, 720t-722t
  formulations of, 715t
  for *Neisseria gonorrhoeae* infection, 2764
  for sinusitis, 844-845, 845t
  structure of, 325f
  uses of, 334-335
Cefprozil, 706t-709t
  dosage of, 720t-722t
  formulations of, 715t
  for sinusitis, 845t
  structure of, 324f
  uses of, 334
Cefsulodin, 706t-709t
  dosage of, 720t-722t
  formulations of, 715t
Ceftaroline
  structure of, 325f
  uses of, 336
Ceftazidime, 706t-709t
  for acute pyelonephritis, 972
  for brain abscess, 1273t-1274t, 1274
  dosage of, 720t-722t
  for endophthalmitis, 1557
  for febrile neutropenia, 3804t
  formulations of, 715t
  for melioidosis, 2876, 2876t
  for meningitis, 1213t
  for osteomyelitis, 1459t
  for peritonitis, 1029t
  for *Pseudomonas aeruginosa* bacteremia, 2849-2850
  for *Pseudomonas aeruginosa* burn wound sepsis,
    2854
  for *Pseudomonas aeruginosa* meningitis, 2852
  for septic bursitis, 1450t
  structure of, 325f
  uses of, 334-335
Ceftibuten, 706t-709t
  dosage of, 720t-722t
  formulations of, 715t
  structure of, 325f
  uses of, 334-335
Ceftizoxime, 706t-709t
  dosage of, 720t-722t
  formulations of, 715t
  for peritonitis, 1024
Ceftizoxime-alapivoxil, 706t-709t
Ceftobiprole, 706t-709t
  dosage of, 720t-722t
  formulations of, 715t
  structure of, 325f
  uses of, 336
Ceftriaxone, 706t-709t
  for brain abscess, 1273t-1274t, 1274
  for chancroid, 2917
  dosage of, 720t-722t
  for endocarditis, 1089-1090
  for *Enterococcus* endocarditis, 1120t
  for epiglottitis, 853
  for febrile neutropenia, 3804t
  formulations of, 715t
  for gonococcal arthritis, 1449
  for HACEK endocarditis, 1121t
  for *Haemophilus influenzae* type b infection, 2915
  for leptospirosis, 3064t
  for Lyme disease, 3079t
  for lymphangitis, 1331-1332
  for meningitis, 1213t
  for meningococcal infection, 2746t
  for *Neisseria gonorrhoeae* infection, 2764,
    2764t-2765t, 2766
  for *Neisseria meningitidis* nasal carriage, 2747-2748
  for neurosyphilis, in HIV infection, 1746
  for non-HACEK endocarditis, 1121t
  for nosocomial pneumonia, 3718t

Ceftriaxone (*Continued*)
for osteomyelitis, 1459t
outpatient parenteral delivery of, 700
for pneumococcal pneumonia, 2636
for septic bursitis, 1450t
for *Staphylococcus aureus* osteomyelitis, 2574
for streptococcal endocarditis, 2669-2670, 2670t
for streptococcal meningitis, 2636
for *Streptococcus* endocarditis, 1119t
structure of, 325f
for syphilis, 3047t, 3049-3050
for typhoid fever, 2898-2899, 2898t
for urethritis, 1491, 1491t
uses of, 334-335
for Whipple disease, 1439-1440, 1440t
Cefuroxime
dosage of, 720t-722t
formulations of, 715t
for Lyme disease, 3079t
for pancreatic infections, 1050
prophylactic, for surgical procedures, 3899t
structure of, 324f
uses of, 334
Cefuroxime axetil, 706t-709t
Cefuroxime sodium, 706t-709t
Cell surface determinants, in *Staphylococcus aureus* pathogenesis, 2549-2553, 2550f
Cell wall antigens, meningococcal, 2738
Cellulitis, 1295-1298. *See also* Soft tissue infections.
from *Acinetobacter,* 2883
from *Aeromonas hydrophila,* 1296
anaerobic
clostridial, 1305-1307, 1306t
nonclostridial, 1304, 1306t
anatomic variants of, 1296
from *Cryptococcus neoformans,* 1296-1297, 3295, 3295f
cuff, 1515
from *Erysipelothrix rhusiopathiae,* 1296, 2733, 2734f
gangrenous, 1298-1300, 1299f, 1303
differential diagnosis of, 1300, 1301t
in immunocompromised hosts, 1299-1300
from *Haemophilus influenzae,* 1296
from *Haemophilus influenzae* type b, 2914
in injection drug users, 3877
orbital. *See* Orbital abscess/cellulitis.
from *Pasteurella multocida,* 1296
preseptal, 1571-1574, 1571f-1573f
processes distinguished from, 1297, 1297t
quinolones for, 500
recurrent (pseudoerysipelas), 1295-1296
from *Staphylococcus aureus,* 2567, 2567f
from *Streptococcus pyogenes* (group A), 1295, 2602
perianal, 2606
synergistic necrotizing, 1306t, 1309, 1318
from *Vibrio alginolyticus,* 1296-1297
from *Vibrio parahaemolyticus,* 1296-1297
from *Vibrio vulnificus,* 1296
Cell-virus interactions, 1909-1913, 1910f, 1910t
Cement, antibiotic-impregnated, 3901
Centers for Disease Control and Prevention, 3028
anthrax postexposure prophylaxis recommendations of, 3989, 3989t
bioterrorism agent disease categories of, 3954t
group EF-4, 3016t-3017t, 3021
group NO-1, 3028
group O-1, O-2, O-3, 3028
group WO-1, 3028
group WO-2, 3028
HIV transmission prevention approach of, 1785
listeriosis prophylaxis recommendations of, 1425, 1425t
Central Asia, HIV infection in, 1620
Central line-associated bloodstream infections (CLABSIs), 3697
from *Acinetobacter baumannii,* 3700
prevention of, 3709-3710
Central nervous system
prion diseases of, 2423-2438. *See also* Prion disease.
in systemic response to infection, 990
Central nervous system infections, 1183-1188. *See also specific site and type.*
from *Actinomyces,* 3214

Central nervous system infections (*Continued*)
from adenoviruses, 2030
in African trypanosomiasis, 3490
anaerobic, 3086, 3086f
from *Bacillus* spp., 2729
from *Blastomyces dermatitidis,* 3326, 3326f
from *Campylobacter fetus,* 2798
from *Candida,* 1239, 3231-3232, 3236
from *Capnocytophaga,* 2991
clinical manifestations of, 1183-1184
from *Cryptococcus neoformans,* 3293t, 3294-3295, 3295f
microscopic examination of, 3296, 3296f-3297f
treatment of, 3298-3300
from cytomegalovirus, 1976
in elderly, 3861
encephalitis in, 1183-1184. *See also* Encephalitis.
endocarditis in, 1074
focal lesions in, 1184
from gram-negative anaerobic rod, 3115
from herpes simplex virus, 1950, 1952, 1957t
in histoplasmosis, 3313
in injection drug users, 3885-3886
from *Listeria monocytogenes,* 2709-2710
lumbar puncture in, 1184-1186, 1185t
management of, 1187-1188
adjunctive therapy in, 1187-1188
antimicrobial therapy in, 1187
outpatient parenteral, 699, 700t
surgical, 1187
meningitis in, 1183. *See also* Meningitis.
from microsporidia, 3397
neuroimaging studies in, 1186-1187
from nontuberculous mycobacteria, 3196
from *Pasteurella,* 2940
from *Pseudallescheria boydii,* 3365
from *Pseudomonas aeruginosa,* 2852
in solid organ transplant recipients, 3846, 3846t
from *Streptococcus anginosus* group, 2683
syphilis in, 3040-3041. *See also* Neurosyphilis.
from *Toxoplasma gondii,* 3501. *See also* Encephalitis, from *Toxoplasma gondii,* in HIV infection.
tuberculous, 3153-3154, 3153f
Whipple's disease in, 1437
Central nervous system lymphoma, HIV-related, 1771-1772
EBV DNA in, 2002
treatment of, 1772
Central nervous system mass lesions, in HIV infection, 1749-1754, 1755f
brain biopsy for, 1754
Central venous catheter infections. *See also* Catheter-related infections.
in cancer patients, 3795, 3797t
long-term issues in, 3698, 3705t
short-term issues in, 3698, 3704t
Cephalexin, 706t-709t
for bullous impetigo, 1291
dosage of, 720t-722t
formulations of, 715t
for lymphangitis, 1331-1332
for pyogenic lymphadenitis, 1330
structure of, 324f
uses of, 333-334
Cephalic tetanus, 3093, 3093f
Cephalosporinase, AmpC, 329
Cephalosporins, 323-339
activity spectrum of, 326, 327t-328t
for acute pyelonephritis, 972
adverse reactions to, 331-333, 333t
Aggregatibacter actinomycetemcomitans susceptibility to, 3016-3017
for bacillary dysentery, 2908-2909, 2909t
for brain abscess, 1273t-1274t, 1274
chemistry of, 323-324, 324f
classification of, 324-325, 326t
cross-reactivity of, 331, 352-353
distribution of, 330-331, 330t
dosage of, 333, 333t, 720t-722t
in renal disease, 331, 332t
drug interactions with, 742t-761t
for *Enterococcus* infection, 2649
first-generation
chemistry of, 323, 324f
dosage of, 333t

Cephalosporins (*Continued*)
uses of, 333-334
formulations of, 715t
fourth-generation
chemistry of, 323, 325f
dosage of, 333t
uses of, 335-336
mechanism of action of, 325-326
for meningococcal infection, 2745, 2746t
MRSA-active
chemistry of, 324, 325f
dosage of, 333t
uses of, 336
with MTT side chain, adverse reactions to, 331-332
for peritonitis, 1022t, 1024, 1029t
pharmacology of, 329-331, 330t, 720t-722t
in pregnancy, 333
pseudomembranous colitis from, 1378
resistance to
mechanisms of, 326-329
by *Streptococcus pneumoniae,* 2634
second-generation
chemistry of, 323, 324f
dosage of, 333t
uses of, 334
structure of, 349f
third-generation
chemistry of, 323, 325f
dosage of, 333t
uses of, 334-335
uses of, 333-336
Cephalothin, 706t-709t
dosage of, 720t-722t
for endocarditis, 1088-1089
formulations of, 715t
structure of, 324f
uses of, 333-334
Cephapirin, 706t-709t
dosage of, 720t-722t
formulations of, 715t
Cephradine, 706t-709t
dosage of, 720t-722t
formulations of, 715t
Cerebellar ataxia, in varicella, 1964-1965
Cerebral aspergillosis, 3248-3249, 3249f
Cerebral blood flow, in bacterial meningitis, 1202-1203
Cerebral cryptoccomas, 3294-3295, 3295f
Cerebral edema. *See also* Intracranial hypertension.
from anthrax, 2723
in bacterial meningitis, 1201-1202
Cerebral embolus, in endocarditis, 1074
Cerebral function, in sepsis, 997
Cerebral malaria, 3440f, 3441, 3449
Cerebral mucormycosis, 1266
in injection drug users, 3885-3886
Cerebrospinal fluid
appearance of, 1184-1185
collection of, 1184
drug penetration of, 1187
in HIV infection, 1747
laboratory processing of, 238
vancomycin in, 453
Cerebrospinal fluid analysis
in African trypanosomiasis, 3492
in AIDS dementia, 1747
cell count in, 1185
in central nervous system infections, 1184-1186, 1185t
in central nervous system lymphoma, 1751
culture in, in shunt infections, 1233
in encephalitis, 1249
in immunocompromised patients, 1245
glucose concentration in, 1185, 1185t
gram stain in, 1186
India ink smear in, 1186
in meningitis, 1185, 1185t
aseptic, 1950
bacterial, 1208-1209, 1208t
chronic, 1238
viral, 1207-1208
in meningococcal infection, 2744-2745
in neurosyphilis, 3041, 3041t
opening pressure in, 1184-1185

Cerebrospinal fluid analysis (Continued)
  polymerase chain reaction in, 1186
  in prion diseases, 2432-2433
  in progressive multifocal leukoencephalopathy, 1752, 2053
  protein concentration in, 1185-1186, 1185t
  in shunt infections, 1233
  in toxoplasmosis, 3512
  in tuberculous meningitis, 3153
Cerebrospinal fluid hypoglycorrhachia, 1185
Cerebrospinal fluid pleocytosis, 1185
Cerebrospinal fluid shunt infections, 1231-1236
  clinical features of, 1232-1233
  from coagulase-negative Staphylococcus, 2584
  diagnosis of, 1233
  epidemiology of, 1231
  etiology of, 1231, 1232t
  pathogenesis of, 1232
  prevention of, 1235
  risk factors for, 1231, 1232t
  shunt reimplantation after, 1235
  shunt removal in, 1234-1235
  timing of, 1232
  treatment of, 1233-1235, 1234t
Cervical cancer
  as AIDS indicator, 1643-1644
  clinical management of, 1774
  HIV-related, 1773, 1797-1798
  pathogenesis of, human papillomaviruses in, 2037
  screening for, 2045, 2045t
Cervical cytomegalovirus infection, in pregnancy, 1983-1984, 1984t
Cervical intraepithelial neoplasia
  HIV-related, 1772-1773, 1796-1798
  human papillomavirus in, 1773, 2041
Cervical lymphadenitis, 862t, 867, 1323-1324. See also Lymphadenitis/lymphadenopathy.
  in Kawasaki syndrome, 3663
  tuberculous, 1325
Cervical spinal cord tumors, 3660t
Cervicitis, 1505-1506, 1506f, 1506t
  from Chlamydia trachomatis, 2453
  gonococcal, 2759-2763, 2760f
  from herpes simplex virus, 1949, 1949f
  mucopurulent, in HIV-infection women, 1797
Cervicofacial actinomycosis, 3210-3211, 3211f
Cervicofacial lymphadenitis, in Mycobacterium avium complex, 3182
Cervicovaginal shedding, in HIV infection, 1784, 1796
Cervix, normal, 1497, 1497f
Cesarean section
  antibiotic prophylaxis for, 3900
  elective, HIV transmission prevention by, 1786
  endomyometritis after, 1511-1513, 1512f
Cestodes. See Tapeworms.
Cethromycin, 706t-709t
  dosage of, 726t-727t
  drug interactions with, 742t-761t
CFRT gene, 947
CFRT protein, 947-948
CH$_{50}$ test, in complement deficiency, 94
Chagas' disease, 3481-3488. See also Trypanosomiasis, American.
Chagoma, 3481, 3482f
Chain of infection, 185
Chalazion, 1569
Chancre
  in African trypanosomiasis, 3489
  in syphilis, 1477, 1477f, 1480-1481, 3038-3039, 3039f
Chanciform lesions, 1293-1294, 1294f, 1294t
Chancroid, 1477, 1478f, 1481, 2916-2917
  inguinal adenopathy in, 1326
Chandipura virus, 2246
Changuinola virus, 2098
Chapare arenavirus, 2296t. See also South American hemorrhagic fevers.
Chaperones, 9
Chédiak-Higashi syndrome, 169t-170t, 172
  Staphylococcus aureus infection in, 2563
Chemical agents
  HAV A resistance to, 2368
  rhinovirus inactivation by, 2391
Chemical disinfectants, 3681-3684

Chemical sterilants, 3677, 3680t
Chemical tick repellents, for tularemia prophylaxis, 2935-2936
Chemical warfare, during World War I, 3951
Chemoattractants, in neutrophil migration, 104
Chemokine(s). See also specific chemokine.
  CC, 43-44
  CD8 cell production of, 131
  in cryptosporidiosis, 3550
  CXC, 43-44
  HIV infection and, 2331
  in innate immunity, 41-44, 42t
  in Legionnaires' disease, 2971
  in neutrophil migration, 104
  in Pseudomonas aeruginosa resistance, 2838-2839
Chemokine receptors, in infection susceptibility, 51-52, 54
Chemoprophylaxis, 189-190
  against Bordetella pertussis, 2961-2962
  for cancer-related infections, 3799-3801, 3800t
    antibacterial, 3799-3801, 3800t
    antifungal, 3800t, 3801
    antiviral, 3800t, 3802
    colony-stimulating factors in, 3800t, 3802
    immunoglobulins in, 3800t, 3802
    against Pneumocystis jirovecii, 3800t, 3801-3802
    against tuberculosis, 3800t, 3802
  for Legionnaires' disease, 2979
  for malaria, in travelers, 4013-4014
  for Neisseria meningitidis nasal carriage, 2747-2748
Chemotaxis, defective, 112-114, 113f
Chemotherapy
  for adult T-cell leukemia/lymphoma, 2316
  cytotoxic, chronic hepatitis B and, 1602-1603, 2079
  granulocyte-macrophage colony-stimulating factor after, 614
  in hematopoietic stem cell transplant recipients, 3821
  for HIV-related non-Hodgkin's lymphoma
    HAART and, 1769-1770
    infusional, 1770
  influence of, on tuberculous spread, 3134-3135
  for Kaposi's sarcoma
    intralesional, 1767
    systemic, 1767
  mucosal barrier injury from, 3785-3786, 3785f
  posaconazole prophylaxis during, 558-559
  pseudomembranous colitis associated with, 1378
Chest pain, in pericarditis, 1163
Chest percussion, for cystic fibrosis, 951
Chest radiography. See Radiography, chest.
Chest tube, for pleural effusion/empyema, 922
Chickenpox. See Varicella.
Chiggers, 3643, 3645f, 3646t
Chikungunya fever, 207, 1450
  in travelers, 4022
Chikungunya virus, 2117-2125, 2118t. See also Alphaviruses.
  encephalitis from, 1251t-1252t
  isolation of, 207
  rash from, 802
  uveitis from, 1566
Childcare centers
  diarrhea in, 1365
  HAV outbreaks in, 2375-2376
  pertussis in, 2962
Children. See also Infants; Neonates.
  aminoglycosides in, 378, 378t
  antimicrobial therapy in, 269
  bacillary dysentery in, 2908-2909, 2909t
  bacterial meningitis in, 1206, 1213t
  bacteriuria in, 964-965, 965f
  Blastomyces dermatitidis in, 3327
  chloramphenicol in, 396
  cryptosporidiosis in, 3552
    malnutrition and, 3552
  diarrhea in
    from Cryptosporidium, 3552
    mortality from, 1335
    zinc for, 670t, 672-673
  endocarditis prophylaxis for, 1149
  enterovirus infections in, 2339-2340
  febrile seizure in, 774-775
  fever of unknown origin in, 779-781, 783

Children (Continued)
  hepatitis A in, vaccination against, 2381-2382, 2382t
  Histoplasma capsulatum in, 3312
  HIV exposure in
    accidental, 1828
    without infection, 1812
  HIV infection in, 1644-1645, 1645f, 1809-1832
    from accidental exposure, 1828
    antiretroviral therapy for
      clinical trials of, 1821
      combination, complications of, 1816-1817
      failure of, evidence for, 1824t
      guidelines for, 1819-1821, 1820t-1823t
    cardiovascular disease in, 1816
    central nervous system complications in, 1815-1816
    classification of, 1813, 1813t-1814t
    clinical manifestations of, 1812-1817
    counseling in, 1827
    culture in, 1818
    daily life management in, 1828
    developmental abnormalities in, 1813-1814
    diagnostic tests in, 1817-1819
    disclosure of, 1826-1827
    encephalopathy in, 1815-1816
    epidemiology of, 1809-1812
    global overview of, 1809-1810
    growth abnormalities in, 1813-1814
    hematologic disorders in, 1816
    immune reconstitution inflammatory syndrome in, 1817
    immunizations in, 1825, 1826f-1827f
    informed consent in, 1819
    intravenous immune globulin in, 1825
    laboratory findings in, 1813t, 1817
    lymphocytic interstitial pneumonitis in, 1815, 1815f
    natural history of, 1812-1813, 1812f
    neoplastic disease in, 1816
    nutritional abnormalities in, 1813-1814
    opportunistic infections in, 1814-1815, 1815f
      prophylaxis against, 1821-1825
    oral manifestations of, 1816
    p24 antigen assay in, 1818
    perinatal transmission of, 1810-1812, 1811t. See also Human immunodeficiency virus infection, transmission of, perinatal.
    Pneumocystis jirovecii pneumonia in, 1814, 1815f
      prophylaxis against, 1821-1825
    polymerase chain reaction assay in, 1817-1818
    rapid tests in, 1818
    renal disease in, 1816
    RNA assay in, 1818
    serologic tests in, 1818
    stroke in, 1816
    treatment of, 1819-1826
    in United States, 1809-1810, 1810f
    websites on, 1824t
  immunizations in, 189
    schedule for, 3924f, 3936-3938, 3937f, 3938t-3939t
  influenza vaccine in, 3926-3927
  Kawasaki syndrome in, 3663-3666, 3664f, 3664t
  Legionnaires' disease in, 2973
  Neisseria gonorrhoeae infection in, 2763, 2766
  nitrofurantoin in, 517
  pertussis in, 2958
  pleural effusion/empyema drainage in, 923
  primary peritonitis in, 1013
  quinolones in, 503
  recurrent respiratory papillomatosis in. See Papillomatosis, recurrent respiratory.
  respiratory syncytial virus in, 2211-2213, 2212f, 2213t-2214t
  respiratory tract infections in, from Haemophilus influenzae, nontypeable, 2913
  sexual abuse/assault of, HIV infection in, 1828
  temperature in, 768
  tuberculosis in, 3139-3140, 3149
  urinary tract infection in
    imaging of, 981, 981f-982f
    natural history of, 969
    symptoms of, 966

China, HIV-infected children in, 1810
Chinese restaurant syndrome, 1417
Chlamydia
    comparative aspects of, 2439-2442, 2440t
    conjunctivitis from, 1533-1534
    elementary body of, 2439, 2443
    genital infection from, quinolones for, 496
    genome of, 2440
    inclusions in, 2439-2440, 2440f
    life cycle of, 2439, 2440f, 2443-2444, 2444f
    natural history of, 2441
    reticulate body of, 2439, 2440f, 2443-2444
Chlamydia pneumoniae. See Chlamydophila pneumoniae.
Chlamydia psittaci. See Chlamydophila psittaci.
Chlamydia trachomatis, 2443-2461
    antigen detection for, 2447-2448
    antigenic composition of, 2445
    biovars of, 2439
    cervicitis from, 2453
    characteristics of, 2439-2442, 2440f, 2440t
    clinical manifestations of, 2449-2456, 2450f, 2452t
    conjunctivitis from, 1533
        inclusion
            in adults, 2450-2451, 2452t
            in neonates, 2455-2456
        in neonates, 1535-1536
    ectopic pregnancy from, 2454
    endometritis from, 2454
    epidemiology of, 2443, 2444f
    epididymitis from, 1524, 2451-2452, 2452t
    in female urethra, 1490
    genitourinary tract infections from, 2451, 2452t
        female, 2453, 2455
        treatment of, 2455
    genome of, 2445
    immunity to, 2446-2447
    inclusions in, 2439-2440, 2440f
    infertility from, 2454
    isolation of, 2447
    keratitis from, 1544-1545
    laboratory diagnosis of, 240t-242t, 243, 2447-2449, 2448t
    life cycle of, 2439, 2440f, 2443-2444, 2444f
    lymphogranuloma venereum from, 1477-1478, 1480-1481, 2449-2450
        treatment of, 2450
    Neisseria gonorrhoeae coinfection with, 2765
    nongonococcal urethritis from, 1488-1489. *See also* Urethritis, nongonococcal.
    nucleic acid amplification tests for, 2448
    nucleic acid hybridization assay for, 2447-2448
    ocular trachoma from, 2446, 2449, 2449t
    otitis media from, 833
    pathogenesis of, 2445-2446
    pelvic inflammatory disease from, 2454-2455
    perinatal infections in, 2455-2456
    persistence of, 2444
    pneumonia from, 2455
        in infants, 2456, 2456f
    in pregnancy, 2454-2455
    prevention of, 2456-2457, 2457t
    proctitis and proctocolitis from, 2452-2453, 2452t
    prostatitis from, 2451-2452, 2452t
    reinfection with, 2446
    rifamycins for, 411
    salpingitis from, 2454
    screening for, 2457, 2457t
    serologic tests for, 2448-2449
    serovars of, 2445
    sexually reactive arthritis from, 1491-1492, 2453
    urethritis from, 2451, 2452t, 2453-2454
    vaccine for, 2446-2447
Chlamydophila pecorum, 2439-2442, 2440t
Chlamydophila pneumoniae, 2467-2475
    asthma in, 2471-2472, 2471t
    atherosclerosis in, 2472-2473
    characteristics of, 2439-2442, 2440t
    chronic disease in, 2471-2474
    in chronic obstructive pulmonary disease, 879
    clinical manifestations of, 2470
    conjunctivitis from, 1533
    epidemiology of, 2470, 2470t
    history of, 2467
    laboratory testing for, 240t-242t, 2468-2469

Chlamydophila pneumoniae (Continued)
    antigen detection in, 2468-2469
    cell culture in, 2468, 2469f
    nucleic acid amplification techniques in, 2469
    serologic tests in, 2469
    life cycle of, 2467, 2468f
    long-term, 2467-2468
    microbiology of, 2467-2468
    multiple sclerosis in, 2473-2474
    Mycoplasma pneumoniae coinfection with, 2470
    pharyngitis from, 817
    prevalence of, 2439
    respiratory, 2470-2474
    Streptococcus pneumoniae coinfection with, 2470
    treatment of, 2470-2474, 2471t
Chlamydophila psittaci, 240t-242t, 2463-2465
    characteristics of, 2439-2442, 2440t
    endocarditis from, 1086, 1094
Chloramphenicol, 394-398, 706t-709t
    assay for, 396
    for *Bartonella bacilliformis* infection, 3005
    for brain abscess, 1274t
    in children, 269, 396
    dosage of, 726t-727t
    drug interactions with, 397, 397t, 742t-761t
    for endocarditis, 1093
    for *Enterococcus*, 2651
    for epidemic typhus, 2523
    formulations of, 716t
    gray baby syndrome from, 397
    hematologic effects of, 396-397
    indications for, 397-398
    in liver disease, 396
    mechanism of action of, 394-395
    for melioidosis, 2876
    for meningitis, 1213t
    minimal inhibitory concentrations of, 395, 395t
    for murine typhus, 2527
    optic neuritis from, 397
    for peritonitis, 1023
    pharmacology of, 395-396, 395f
    for plague, 2948
    for pneumonic plague, 3967t
    preparations of, 394
    in renal failure, 396
    resistance to, chloramphenicol acetyltransferase in, 285
    for Rocky Mountain spotted fever, 2503
    for scrub typhus, 2530
    for spotted fever rickettsia, 2505
    Staphylococcus aureus resistance to, 2559t
    structure of, 394, 394f
    toxicity of, 396-397
    for tularemia, 2935, 3974t
    for typhoid fever, 2899
    in vitro activity of, 395, 395t
Chloramphenicol acetyltransferase, 285
Chloramphenicol palmitate, 706t-709t
Chloramphenicol sodium succinate, 706t-709t
Chlorhexidine
    for amebic keratitis, 3434
    disinfection with, 521-522, 522t
    prophylactic
        for dental caries prophylaxis, 869
        for ventilator-assisted pneumonia, 3723
Chlorine, disinfection with, 3682
Chloroguanide, for malaria, 650
Chloroquine
    drug interactions with, 742t-761t
    for malaria, 631-636, 632t-635t, 3451, 3452t, 4013
        in nonfalciparum disease, 3454
        for prophylaxis, 3455, 3455t
    mechanism of action of, 3446-3447
    resistance to, 635, 3445-3447
Chloroquine hydrochloride, 706t-709t
Chloroquine phosphate, 706t-709t
Chloroquine-resistant *Plasmodium falciparum*, 211-212
    halofantrine for, 632t-635t, 639
    mechanism of action of, 3447
    mortality trends and, 3437, 3438f
Chloroquine-resistant *Plasmodium vivax*, 632t-635t
Chlorpheniramine, for cough, 875
Cholangiography, magnetic resonance, 1040-1041
Cholangiopathy, AIDS, 1041, 1738-1739

Cholangitis
    clinical presentation in, 1040
    diagnosis of, 1040
    in liver transplant recipients, 3843
    microbiology of, 1041, 1041t
    pathogenesis of, 1040
    pyogenic liver abscess in, 1035-1036
    treatment of, 1042
Cholecystitis
    acalculous, 1040
        in HIV infection, 1738
    from *Candida*, 3237
    clinical presentation in, 1040
    diagnosis of, 1040
    imaging of, 1040-1041, 1041f
    microbiology of, 1041, 1041t
    pathogenesis of, 1039-1040, 1039f
    treatment of, 1041-1042
Cholelithiasis
    in HIV infection, 1738
    in spinal cord injury patients, 3855
Cholera, 2777-2785. *See also Vibrio cholerae.*
    clinical manifestations of, 2780-2781, 2781f, 2781t
        in children, 2781
    diarrhea in, 1363
    epidemiology of, 2778-2780, 2779t
    laboratory abnormalities in, 2780-2781
    modern era of, 2777
    pandemic of, 2777
    pathophysiology of, 2778, 2778t
    prevention of, 2783
    reported cases of, 2777, 2778f
    seasonality in, 2779-2780, 2780f
    transmission of
        host factors in, 2780
        risk factors in, 2779
        via contaminated food and water, 2779
    treatment of, 2781-2783, 2782f
        antibiotics in, 2782-2783, 2782t
        fluid therapy in, 2781, 2782t
        quinolones in, 496
    vaccines for, 1346, 2783, 3922-3923
        in travelers, 4011t, 4013
Cholera toxin, 31-32
Cholera-like syndrome, diarrhea in, 1363
Cholescintigraphy, radionuclide, 1040
Cholestatic hepatitis, from erythromycin, 431
Cholestatic hepatitis E infection, 2416-2417
Cholesterol-binding cytolysins, pore-forming toxins of, 33
Chorea, in rheumatic fever, 2613-2614
Chorioamnionitis, 1511-1514
    from oral *Capnocytophaga*, 2991
Chorioretinitis
    from herpes simplex virus, 1952
    toxoplasmic
        in AIDS patient, 3501, 3505, 3505f
        in immunocompetent patient, 3502
Choroid, 1561
Chromobacterium, 3016t-3017t, 3019-3020
Chromobacterium violaceum, 3016t, 3020, 3020f
Chromoblastomycosis, 3277-3280
    clinical manifestations of, 3277-3278, 3278f
    from dark-walled fungi, 3367-3369, 3367t
    diagnosis of, 3278-3279, 3279f
    epidemiology of, 3277
    etiologic agents in, 3277
    pathology and pathogenesis of, 3277, 3278f
    treatment of, 3279
Chronic fatigue syndrome, 1897-1904
    clinical manifestations of, 1900
    consensus definition of, 1897, 1898t
    epidemiology of, 1897-1898
    history of, 1897
    laboratory findings in, 1900
    management of, 1900-1901
    pathogenesis of, 1898-1900
    proposed infectious causes of, 1897, 1898t
Chronic obstructive pulmonary disease, 877-883
    airway pathology in, 877
    antimicrobial agents for, 880-881, 881t
        prophylactic, 880
    chronic bronchitis in, 877-878
    chronic pulmonary histoplasmosis and, 3311
    clinical presentation in, 877-878

Chronic obstructive pulmonary disease *(Continued)*
  definition of, 877
  exacerbations of, 878-880
    from *Haemophilus influenzae,* nontypeable,
      2912-2913
    infections and, 878-879
    from influenza, 2276
    microbiology of, 879-880
    treatment of, 880-881, 881t
  Moraxella catarrhalis in, 2771-2773, 2773f
  pneumonia and, 895
  prevalence of, 877
  risk factors for, 877
  stable
    atypical bacteria in, 879
    bacteria in, 878
    viruses in, 878-879
    treatment of, 880-881, 880t-881t
Chryseobacterium, 3016t-3017t, 3022-3023
Ciclopirox, 706t-709t
Cidofovir, 566t-567t, 576-578, 706t-709t
  activity spectrum of, 568t, 576
  clinical studies of, 577-578
  for condylomata acuminata, 2044
  in cytomegalovirus infection, 1978
  dosage of, 738t-739t
  drug interactions with, 742t-761t
  formulations of, 717t
  for orthopoxvirus infection, 1930
  outpatient parenteral delivery of, 700, 701t
  structure of, 576f
Ciguatera fish poisoning, 1417, 1417t, 1423, 3569
Ciguatoxin, 1417
Ciliary body, 1561
Ciliary dysentery, 1392
Ciliary neurotropic factor, in febrile response, 769
Cinoxacin, 706t-709t
  dosage of, 732t-733t
  formulations of, 716t
Ciprofloxacin
  for acute pyelonephritis, 972-973
  for anthrax, 1294t, 2721t, 3989t
  antimicrobial activity of, 491t-492t
  for brain abscess, 1274t
  for *Campylobacter* infections, 2799
  for cellulitis, 1297-1298
  for chancroid, 2917
  for *Chlamydophila* respiratory infection, 2471t
  for cholera, 2782t
  for cyclosporiasis, 3562-3563
  dosage of, 493t, 732t-733t
  for *Enterococcus,* 2651
  for febrile neutropenia, 3804t
  formulations of, 716t
  for gonococcal arthritis, 1449
  for HACEK endocarditis, 1121t
  for *Isospora belli* infection, 3563
  for Legionnaires' disease, 2978t
  for lower urinary tract infection, 973
  for meningitis, 1213t
  for meningococcal infection, 2746t
  for nosocomial pneumonia, 3718t
  for osteomyelitis, 1459t
  for pancreatic infections, 1050
  for parasitic infections, 660
  for peritonitis, 1022t, 1025, 1029t
  pharmacology of, 492t
  for pneumonic plague, 3967t
  prophylactic
    for bacterial infections in cancer patients, 3800t
    after intentional release of *Francisella tularensis,*
      3974t
    for primary peritonitis, 1016
    for traveler's diarrhea, 4015
  for *Pseudomonas aeruginosa* osteomyelitis, 2852
  resistance to, mechanisms of, 489
  for septic bursitis, 1450t
  for spotted fever, 2505
  structure of, 487, 488f
  for tularemia, 2935, 3974t
  for typhoid fever, 2898t, 2898t
Ciprofloxacin hydrochloride, 706t-709t
Ciprofloxacin lactate, 706t-709t
Circulation, in sepsis, 998-999
Circumcision, HIV transmission and, 1625-1626

Cirrhosis
  alcoholic, 2165-2166
  in hepatitis C infection, 2165-2166
  peritonitis in, 1013-1014
Citrobacter, 342t, 2828
Citrobacter freundii, 2828
  device-associated, 3700
Citrobacter koseri, 2828
Clam digger's itch, 3622
Clarithromycin, 434-438, 706t-709t
  adverse reactions to, 435-436
  antimicrobial activity of, 429t, 434-435
  chemistry of, 434, 434f
  for *Chlamydophila* respiratory infection, 2471,
    2471t
  dosage of, 726t-727t
  drug interactions with, 431t, 436, 742t-761t
  formulations of, 716t
  for *Helicobacter pylori* infection, 2809t
  for Legionnaires' disease, 2978t
  mechanism of action of, 434
  for *Mycobacterium abscessus* pulmonary disease,
    3193t, 3194
  for *Mycobacterium avium* complex disease,
    3184t-3186t
  for nontuberculous mycobacterial infections,
    542-543
  pharmacology of, 435
  preparations of, 434
  resistance to, mechanism of, 434
  for sinusitis, 845t
  for streptococcal pharyngitis, 2598t
  for toxoplasmosis, in HIV infection, 3518t
  uses of, 432t-433t, 436-438
Class II transactivator protein (CIITA), 133
Clavicle, osteomyelitis of, 1463-1464
Clavulanate, 320, 320f
Clean wound infections, 3892t, 3894
  prevention of, 522-523
Clean-catch method of urine collection, 968
Cleaning, 3677
Clearance
  distribution, 298-299
  nonrenal, 300
  renal, 300
  total body, 300
Clenched-fist injuries, 3914-3915
Clethrionomys glareolus, hemorrhagic fever with renal
    syndrome from, 2290
Clevudine, 598-599, 599f
  for chronic hepatitis B, 1600
Clindamycin
  for actinomycosis, 3217t
  adverse reactions to, 442, 3516-3517
  antimicrobial activity of, 440-441, 441t
  for babesiosis, 3543, 3544t
  for bacterial meningitis, 1504
  for bite wounds, 3913t
  for brain abscess, 1274t
  chemistry of, 440, 440f
  for desquamative inflammatory vaginitis, 1505
  dosage of, 726t-727t
  drug interactions with, 442, 742t-761t
  formulations of, 716t
  for gram-negative anaerobic rod infections, 3117
  for lung abscess, 927
  for lymphadenitis, 1330
  mechanism of action of, 440
  for *Neisseria gonorrhoeae* infection, 2765t
  for parasitic infections, 649
  for peritonitis, 1023-1024
  pharmacology of, 441-442
  for *Pneumocystis* pneumonia, 3382
  resistance to, mechanisms of, 440
  for streptococcal pharyngitis, 2598t
  for suppurative thrombophlebitis, 1098-1099
  topical, 443
  for *Toxoplasma* encephalitis, 1750-1751
  for toxoplasmosis
    in HIV infection, 3518t
    ocular, 3520
  uses of, 442-443
Clindamycin hydrochloride, 706t-709t
Clindamycin palmitate hydrochloride, 706t-709t
Clindamycin phosphate, 706t-709t

Clindamycin-benzoyl peroxide gel, for acne vulgaris,
    527, 528t
Clindamycin-primaquine, for *Pneumocystis jirovecii*
    pneumonia, 1860t-1870t, 1872
Clindamycin-quinine, for babesiosis, 3544, 3544t
Clinical trials, 185, 687-698
  bias in, 688, 692-693
  binding in, 690-691
  conclusions of, 695-697, 696t
  control regimen selection in, 692
  end points in, 693-694
  error types in, 691-692
  exclusion criteria in, 690
  goals of, 688-690
  hypothesis testing in, 691-692
  inclusion criteria in, 690
  interpretation of, 688, 688t
  observations in, 687-688
  randomization in, 690-691
  results of, 694-695, 695f
  sample size in, 691-692
  stratification in, 690-691
  study designs in, 688, 688t
Clinician preparedness, for bioterrorist attack,
    3957-3958
Clioquinol, 706t-709t
Clofazimine, 706t-709t
  dosage of, 734t-735t
  drug interactions with, 742t-761t
  formulations of, 717t
  for leprosy, 545, 3172
  for leprosy reversal reactions, 3173
  for nontuberculous mycobacterial infections, 544
Clones, in multilocus sequencing, 2546
Clonorchis sinensis, 3596f, 3597f, 3600-3602, 3601f
Clostridium
  abdominal infections from, 3108
  antibiotic-associated colitis from, 3104-3106
  bacteremia from, 3107-3108
  biliary tract infections from, 3108
  characteristics of, 3103-3104, 3104t
  classification of, 3103
  female genitourinary tract infections from, 3108
  Gram stain characteristics of, 3105f
  historical perspective on, 3103
  myonecrosis from. *See* Gas gangrene.
  neurotoxins of, 31
  pleuropulmonary infections from, 3108
  spores of, 3104
  toxins of, 3103
Clostridium botulinum, 3097-3102. *See also* Botulism.
  characteristics of, 3097
  foodborne disease from, 1414t-1415t, 1416, 1419
  laboratory detection of, 240t-242t
  spores of, 3097
  toxins of, 31, 3097. *See also* Botulinum toxin.
  virulence factors of, 5t
Clostridium difficile
  age effects on, 1336
  antibiotic-associated colitis from, 1375-1387,
    3104-3106, 3106f. *See also* Pseudomembra-
    nous colitis, from *Clostridium difficile.*
  in cancer patients, 3798
  carbapenems for, 342t
  culture for, 1381
  detection of, 240t-242t, 242
  diarrhea from, 206, 1335
    antibiotic prophylaxis and, 3901
  epidemic strains of, 1379
  foodborne disease from, 1413
  in HIV infection, 1880
  laboratory detection of, 1381, 1381t
  microbiology of, 1376-1377
  reservoirs of, 1378-1379
  rifamycins for, 412
  toxins of, 32, 1340t, 1341, 1376
    assay for, 1344
    detection of, 1377f, 1380-1381
Clostridium novyi, 3105f
Clostridium perfringens, 3105f
  abdominal infections from, 3108
  biliary tract infections from, 3108
  carbapenems for, 342t
  foodborne disease from, 1414-1415, 1414t, 1418,
    3107

Clostridium perfringens (Continued)
gas gangrene from, 1316-1317, 3106-3107
laboratory confirmation of, 1422
peritonitis from, 1013, 1017-1018
pleuropulmonary infections from, 3108
toxins of, 1340t, 1341, 3106, 3106t
Clostridium ramosum, 3105f
Clostridium septicum, 3107-3108, 3108f
gas gangrene from, 1317
Clostridium tetani, 3091-3096. *See also* Tetanus.
characteristics of, 3091
culturing of, 3093
gram stain of, 3092f
laboratory detection of, 240t-242t
passive immunization against, 73
toxins of, 31
virulence factors of, 5t
Clotrimazole, 706t-709t, 717t
Clotting factors, in sepsis, 998-999
Cloxacillin, 317, 317f, 706t-709t
dosage of, 316t, 718t-719t
formulations of, 715t
Clubbing, in endocarditis, 1076
Clumping factor (Clf) protein, in prosthetic valve
infections, 1113-1114
Clusterin, 78t
Clutton's joints, in congenital syphilis, 3044
Coagulation
disseminated intravascular, in sepsis, 998-999
inflammation-activated, 991, 992f
Coagulopathy, in severe sepsis, 994
Co-artemether, 639-641
for malaria, 4014
Cobalamin, 153
deficiency of, in HIV/AIDS, 155
Coccidioides, 3333-3344
clinical manifestations of, 3335-3338
culture of, 3339
diagnosis of, 3339-3340
epidemiology of, 3333-3334, 3334f
extrapulmonary dissemination of, 3337-3338,
3338f, 3341
histopathology of, 3335
history of, 3333
host defenses against, 3335
meningitis from, 1238-1239, 3338, 3341
mycelial (saprobic) growth of, 3333
mycology of, 3333
pathogenesis of, 3334-3335
prevention of, 3342
pulmonary infections from
cavitary, 3336, 3337f-3338f, 3341
chronic fibrocavitary, 939f, 3336, 3341
diffuse, 3341
early, 3335-3336, 3336f, 3341
in HIV infection, 1732
nodular, 3336, 3336f
serology of, 3339
skin tests for, 3340
spherule (parasitic) growth of, 3333, 3334f
treatment of, 3340-3342
vaccine for, 3342
Coccidioides immitis, 3333
arthritis from, 1451
mycotic aneurysms from, 1102
Coccidioides posadasii, 3333
arthritis from, 1451
Coccidioidomycosis, in HIV infection, 1858t-1871t,
1878
Coccidiosis, diarrhea in, 1396
Cochlea, aminoglycoside-induced injury to,
371-372
Coenurosis, 3615
Cognitive/motor disorder, HIV-1–associated
major. *See* AIDS dementia.
minor, 1746
Cohort studies, 184
Colanic acid, 2816
Cold agglutinins
in *Mycoplasma pneumoniae*, 2484-2486
Raynaud phenomenon and, 2485
Colds. *See* Common cold.
Colistimethate, 706t-709t
dosage of, 728t-729t
formulations of, 716t

Colistin
for cystic fibrosis, 952
for nosocomial pneumonia, 3718t
for *Pseudomonas aeruginosa* infection, 2856
Colitis. *See also* Enterocolitis.
amebic, 3418, 3419f, 3422t. *See also Entamoeba
histolytica.*
antibiotic-associated, 1375-1387. *See also*
Pseudomembranous colitis.
from *Clostridium*, 3104-3106
cytomegalovirus, in HIV infection, 1976
pseudomembranous. *See* Pseudomembranous
colitis.
Collagen shields, antibiotic administration through,
for keratitis, 1543
Collectins, in *Pseudomonas aeruginosa* resistance,
2838
Colon
abnormalities of
in HIV infection, 1741-1742
in tropical sprue, 1432
abscess of, 3085, 3086f
bacterial colonization of, 3112
enlarged, in American trypanosomiasis, 3484,
3485f, 3487
resection of, for diverticulitis, 1064
Colonization factors, of enterotoxigenic *Escherichia
coli*, 2822
Colonoscopy, for *Entamoeba histolytica* infection,
3421
Colony-stimulating factor(s), 611-615
granulocyte. *See* Granulocyte colony-stimulating
factor.
granulocyte-macrophage. *See* Granulocyte-
macrophage colony-stimulating
factor.
for Kaposi's sarcoma, 1767
macrophage, 614-615
for neutropenia, in cancer, 3806
prophylactic, for cancer-related infections, 3800t,
3802
Colorado tick fever virus, 2101-2102
encephalitis from, 1259
meningitis from, 1190
Colorectal surgery, maintenance of normothermia
during, 3897
Colposcopy, in human papillomaviruses, 2041
Coltiviruses, 2101-2102
tick-borne, 3659-3660
Comamonas, 3016t-3017t, 3023
Comamonas acidovorans, 3023
Comamonas testosteroni, 3023
Common cold, 809-813. *See also* Respiratory tract
infections.
attack rate in, 809
clinical manifestations of, 810, 2393, 2394f
complications of, 811, 2393-2394
cough in, 810, 812
diagnosis of, 2395
differential diagnosis of, 810-811
duration of, 2393
echinacea for, 670t, 673-674, 812
epidemiology of, 809-810
etiology of, 809, 810t
immunity in, 810
laboratory findings in, 811
nasal congestion in, 810-811
pathogenesis of, 810, 2392
pharyngitis in, 810-812
prevention of, 812
protection against, 2392-2393
rhinorrhea in, 810-811
from rhinoviruses, 2389-2398. *See also*
Rhinoviruses/rhinovirus infection.
seasonal incidence of, 809, 2391
sneezing in, 811
transmission of, 809-810, 2391
treatment of, 811-812, 811t, 2395-2397
vitamin C for, 153
zinc for, 153, 670t, 673, 812
Communication plan, for emergency preparedness,
221, 223f
Community intervention trials, 185
Community support, for emergency preparedness,
221-222

Community-acquired infections
from *Acinetobacter*, 2882
from *Corynebacterium*, 2695, 2696t
versus health care–associated methicillin-resistant
Staphylococcus aureus infection, 2559-2560
from *Legionella pneumophila*, 2973-2974
from methicillin-resistant *Staphylococcus aureus*,
799, 2558
pneumonia in. *See* Pneumonia,
community-acquired.
from *Staphylococcus aureus*, 2568
Complement, 77-98
activation of, 77-81, 79f
by alternate pathway, 79-80, 79f-80f
antibodies in, 62
in bacterial meningitis, 1196
by classic pathway, 78-79, 79f-80f
by mannose-binding lectin pathway, 79, 79f
overview of, 77-78
properdin-directed model of, 80
regulation of, 81-82, 81t
in severe sepsis, 994
by *Streptococcus pneumoniae*, 2627
tickover model of, 79-80, 80f
in adaptive immune response, 83-84
in apoptosis, 84
assay of, 171t
catabolism of, 77
deficiency of, 85-93, 87t
in alternate pathway, 89, 89t, 169t-170t
in bacterial infections, 88
in classic pathway, 86-88, 169t-170t
congenital, 169t-170t, 176
evaluation of, 94-95
incidence of, 85-86, 86f
late, 89-91
in mannose-binding lectin pathway, 88-89
in meningococcal disease, 86, 86f, 89-90, 89t
molecular basis of, 86, 88
in pneumococcal infection, 2629
in systemic lupus erythematosus, 86-88
treatment of, 95
distribution of, 77
in febrile response, 771, 771t
functions mediated by, 83-84
in immune complexes, 84
in infectious diseases, 93-94
in inflammation, 83
microbial interactions with, 84-85
in microorganism elimination, 83
plasma proteins of, 77, 78t
in preterm infants, 77
in *Pseudomonas aeruginosa* resistance, 2838
regulatory proteins of, 81t
deficiencies of, 91-93
in renal disorders, 94
in rheumatologic disorders, 94
in self–non-self distinction, 82
synthesis of, 77
in systemic lupus erythematosus, 94
Complement cascade, 77-81, 79f
Complement fixation assays, 65
Complement proteins, 77, 78t, 83. *See also specific
protein, e.g.,* C1.
Complement receptors, 82-83
Complementary and alternative medicine, 669-676,
670t. *See also specific therapy.*
Computed tomography
in acute pyelonephritis, 978, 978f-979f
in anthrax, 3987f
in appendicitis, 1060, 1060f
in bacterial meningitis, 1209, 1209f, 1212
in biliary tract infections, 1040
in brain abscess, 1270-1271, 1270f, 3086, 3086f
in cat-scratch disease, 3000-3001, 3000f
in central nervous system infections, 1186-1187
in cranial subdural empyema, 1280
in cryptococcal meningoencephalitis, 3298
in disseminated *Mycobacterium avium* complex
disease, 3182f
in diverticulitis, 1064
in fever of unknown origin, 785
high resolution
in chronic pneumonia, 934, 935t-936t
in paracoccidioidomycosis, 3359, 3359f

Computed tomography *(Continued)*
    in *Pneumocystis* pneumonia, 3382-3383, 3383f
    in intraperitoneal abscess, 1031, 1031f
    in intrarenal abscess, 977, 977f
    before lumbar puncture, 1184
    in mediastinal fibrosis, 3310f
    in mediastinitis, 1176-1177, 1176f
    in osteomyelitis, 1457-1458, 1458f
    in perinephric abscess, 977, 977f
    in pleural effusion, 919, 920f
    in pneumonia, 903-904
    in prosthetic vascular graft infection, 1133-1134,
        1134t
    in pulmonary aspergillosis, 3247, 3248f, 3250
    in pulmonary *Mycobacterium avium* complex
        disease, 3180, 3180f-3181f
    in pyomyositis, 1315-1316
    in rabies, 2254, 2254f
    in septic arthritis, 1446, 1446f
    single-photon emission, in brain abscess, 1272
    in sinopulmonary mucormycosis, 3260-3261, 3261f
    in sinusitis, 844
    in splenic abscess, 1056
    in subperiosteal abscess, 1573, 1573f
    in suppurative intracranial thrombophlebitis, 1285
    in toxoplasmosis, 3510-3512, 3511f
    in tuberculous meningitis, 3153, 3153f
Computer-assisted antimicrobial stewardship, 680
Concentration, steady-state, 300
Concentration-dependent killing agents, 301-302,
    301f
Condom(s)
    in HIV infection prevention, 1650-1651
        in women, 1651, 1784-1785, 1800
    HIV transmission and, 1626, 1626f
    in HPV infection prevention, 2045
    in *Neisseria gonorrhoeae* infection prevention, 2767
Condom catheterization, 3729-3730
Condylomata acuminata, 1478, 1478f, 1481. *See also*
    Human papillomaviruses.
    antiviral agents for, 566t-567t
    clinical manifestations of, 2039-2040, 2039f-2040f
    diagnosis of, 2041-2042
    green tea extract for, 670t, 674, 674f
    incidence and prevalence of, 2036
    oral, 2041, 2044
    penile, 2040, 2040f
    transmission of, 2036
    treatment of, 2042-2044
    vulvar, 2039f, 2040
Condylomata lata, 1477, 1477f, 3039-3040
Congenital heart disease
    closure devices for, infectious complications of,
        1140
    respiratory syncytial virus infection and, 2214
Congenital infections
    from *Toxoplasma gondii*, 3506-3508. *See also*
        Toxoplasma gondii/toxoplasmosis.
        diagnosis of, 3516, 3517f
        serologic screening and prophylaxis for,
            3521-3522, 3521t
        treatment of, 3520
    from *Treponema pallidum*, 3043-3044, 3043t. *See*
        also Syphilis.
        diagnosis of, 3048
        treatment of, 3047t
Conidiobolomycosis, 3267
Conidiobolus, 3258t
Conjunctiva, *Rhinosporidium seeberi* infection of,
    1536-1537, 1537f
Conjunctival injection and discharge, in keratitis,
    1540
Conjunctivitis, 1529-1538. *See also* Keratitis;
    Keratoconjunctivitis; Ocular infections.
    acute hemorrhagic, 1532, 1532f, 2360-2361
    adenoviral, 1531
    anatomy in, 1529
    bacterial, 1534-1535
        acute (mucopurulent), 1534-1535
        chronic, 1535
        hyperacute (purulent), 1535
        pathogenesis of, 1534
    from *Candida*, 1536-1537, 1537f
    from *Chlamydophila (Chlamydia) pneumoniae*,
        1533

Conjunctivitis *(Continued)*
    from *Chlamydia trachomatis*, 1533
        in neonates, 1535-1536
    chlamydial, 1533-1534
    clinical presentation in, 1529-1531
    in epidemic keratoconjunctivitis, 1531-1532
    fungal, 1536-1537, 1537f
    gonococcal, 2761
        in neonates, 1536, 2763
        treatment of, 2764t
    granulomatous, in Parinaud's oculoglandular
        syndrome, 3000, 3000f
    from *Haemophilus influenzae*, nontypeable, 2914
    herpes simplex, 1532, 1952
        in neonates, 1536
    herpes zoster, 1532
    inclusion
        adult, 1534
        from *Chlamydia trachomatis*
            in adults, 2450-2451, 2452t
            in neonates, 2455-2456
    in Kawasaki syndrome, 3663, 3664f
    laboratory evaluation of, 1531
    from *Leishmania*, 1536
    in lymphogranuloma venereum, 1534
    from microsporidia, 1536
    neonatal, 1535-1536
    parasitic, 1536
    Parinaud's oculoglandular, 1536
    in pharyngoconjunctival fever, 1531
    in reactive arthritis, 1492
    from silver nitrate, 1535-1536
    from *Streptococcus pneumoniae*, 2633
    vaccinia, 1532-1533, 1533t
    varicella, 1532
    variola (smallpox), 1532
    viral, 1531-1533, 1532f, 1533t
Conjunctivochalasis, 1530
Constitutional disease, in HIV infection, 1713
Contact lens
    antibiotic administration through, for keratitis,
        1543
    keratitis associated with, 1539-1540
Contact precaution, transmission-based, 3674t-
    3675t, 3675-3676
Continuous-source disease outbreaks, 195, 195f
Contraceptives. *See also* Condom(s); Intrauterine
    devices.
    for HIV-infected women, 1800, 1800t
    oral, HIV transmission and, 1647, 1800, 1800t
Control regimen, selection of, in clinical trials,
    692
Cooling, external, for fever, 774-776
Corinub poisoning, 1417-1418, 1417t
Cornea
    anatomy of, 1539
    edema of, 1541
    inflammation of. *See* Keratitis;
        Keratoconjunctivitis.
    neovascularization of, 1541
Corneal anesthesia, in herpes zoster keratitis, 1546
Corneal infiltrate, 1540
Corneal transplants, Creutzfeldt-Jakob disease
    associated with, 2431
Coronary arteritis, in Kawasaki syndrome, 3663
Coronary artery aneurysm, in Kawasaki syndrome,
    3663-3664
Coronary artery bypass grafting, mediastinitis in,
    1173-1175
Coronary artery stent infection, 1137
Coronary vasoconstriction, from antipyretic drugs,
    775
Coronaviruses, 2187-2194
    colds from, clinical features of, 2191, 2191t
    description of, 2188-2189, 2188f-2189f
    detection of, 259t-260t
    disinfection/sterilization and, 3689
    gastrointestinal, 2187
        clinical manifestations of, 2191-2192
        laboratory diagnosis of, 2192
    history of, 2187
    non-SARS, bronchiolitis from, 885, 886t
    phylogeny of, 2187, 2188f
    respiratory, 2187, 2188f
        clinical manifestations of, 2191, 2191t

Coronaviruses *(Continued)*
    epidemiology of, 2189
    laboratory diagnosis of, 2192
    multiple sclerosis and, 2192
    pathogenesis of, 2190-2191
    SARS and, 2187. *See also* Severe acute
        respiratory syndrome (SARS).
    vaccines for, 2192
Correctional facilities
    HIV infection in, 1639
    tuberculosis in, spread of, 3135
Corticosteroids. *See also* specific agent.
    for amebic keratitis, 3434
    for anthrax meningitis, 2723
    antipyretic activity of, 772, 774
    for bronchiolitis, 889
    for chronic obstructive pulmonary disease, 880t
    for chronic pneumonia, 942
    critical illness–related insufficiency of, 998
    for croup, 2198
    as immunomodulators, 618-619
    for infectious mononucleosis, 2003
    for Kawasaki syndrome, 3665
    for meningitis, 1212-1214
    for neutropenia, in cancer, 3806
    for otitis media with effusion, 834
    for *Pneumocystis jirovecii* pneumonia, in HIV
        infection, 1860t-1870t, 1872-1873
    for septic shock, 1003
    strongyloidiasis and, 3582
    topical, for keratitis, 1544
    for toxoplasmic encephalitis, 3518-3519
    for transplant immunosuppression, infections and,
        3810-3811
    for tuberculosis, 3147-3148
    for tuberculous meningitis, 3154
    for tuberculous pericarditis, 1164-1165, 3155
Corticotropin, antipyretic activity of, 772
Corticotropin-releasing hormone, antipyretic activity
    of, 772
CORYNE database, of coryform bacteria, 2695-2696
Corynebacterium, 2695-2701, 2696t
    biochemical testing of, 2695-2696
    CAMP test for, 2696
    community-acquired infections from, 2695, 2696t
    lipophilic, 2698-2699
    medically relevant, 2695, 2697t
    microbiology of, 2695-2696
    miscellaneous, 2701
    nonlipophilic
        fermentative, 2696-2698
        nonfermentative, 2698
    nosocomial infections from, 2695, 2696t
    susceptibility testing for, 2696
    taxonomy of, 2695, 2697t
Corynebacterium accolens, 2699
Corynebacterium afermentans subsp. *afermentans*,
    2698
Corynebacterium afermentans subsp. *lipophilum*, 2699
Corynebacterium amycolatum, 2698
Corynebacterium argentoratense, 2698
Corynebacterium auris, 2698
Corynebacterium bovis, 2699
Corynebacterium confusum, 2698
Corynebacterium diphtheriae, 2687-2693. *See also*
    Diphtheria.
    biovars of, 2687
    description of, 2687-2688
    exotoxin production by, 2687-2688
    history of, 2687
    laboratory detection of, 240t-242t
    membranous ulcers from, 1298
    pharyngitis from, 816-817
    reservoirs of, 2688
    toxins of, 30-31
    virulence factors of, 5t
Corynebacterium glucuronolyticum, 2698
Corynebacterium jeikeium, 2698-2699
Corynebacterium kroppenstedtii, 2699
Corynebacterium kutscheri, 2699
Corynebacterium lipophiloflavum, 2699
Corynebacterium macginleyi, 2699
Corynebacterium matruchotii, 2698
Corynebacterium minutissimun, 2697
Corynebacterium propinquum, 2698

Corynebacterium pseudodiphtheriticum, 2698
Corynebacterium pseudotuberculosis, 2696-2697
    lymphadenitis from, 1325
Corynebacterium resistens, 2699
Corynebacterium riegelii, 2698
Corynebacterium striatum, 2697
Corynebacterium tuberculostearicum, 2699
Corynebacterium ulcerans, 2696-2697
Corynebacterium urealyticum, 2698-2699
    urinary tract infection from, 964
Corynebacterium ureicelerivorans, 2699
Corynebacterium xerosis, 2697
Coryneform bacteria, 2695-2701, 2696t. *See also*
        Corynebacterium entries.
    miscellaneous, 2701
Coslistimethate, 469-470
Coslistin, 469-470
Costochondritis, from *Candida,* 3233
Cotrimoxazole. *See* Trimethoprim-sulfamethoxazole.
Cotton-ball vititis, 1555-1556
Cough
    in acute bronchitis, 874-875
    in chronic obstructive pulmonary disease, 878
    in common cold, 810, 812
    in croup, 826-827
    from *Mycoplasma pneumoniae,* 2482
    paroxysmal, in pertussis, 2958
    in tuberculosis, 3141-3143
Cowpox, 1929-1930
Coxiella burnetii, 2512f, 3654-3655
    as biological weapon, 3952
    endocarditis from, 1086, 2515-2516, 2515f. *See
        also* Q fever.
        treatment of, 1094, 2515-2516, 2515f
    hepatitis from, 2516
    laboratory detection of, 240t-242t
    pneumonia from, 2512-2515, 2513f-2514f
Coxsackie B virus–adenovirus receptor, 2027
Coxsackievirus(es)
    acute hemorrhagic conjunctivitis from, 2360-2361
    characteristics of, 2337
    communicability period of, 2341
    diabetes mellitus and, 2361-2362
    dilated cardiomyopathy from, 2358
    encephalitis from
        in immunocompromised hosts, 2359-2360
        nonpoliovirus, 2354
    epidemiology of, 2339-2341, 2340t
    exanthems from, 2354-2355
    gastrointestinal disorders from, 2361
    hand-foot-and-mouth disease from, 2355
    herpangina from, 2355-2356
    host range of, 2338t
    immune response to, 2339
    incidence of, 2340-2341
    incubation period of, 2341
    laboratory diagnosis of, 2341
    meningitis from, 2353-2354
        in immunocompromised hosts, 2359-2360
    molecular biology of, 2337-2338, 2338t
    mutation of, 2339
    myocarditis from, 1153, 1155, 1155f
    myopericarditis from, 2357-2358
    myositis from, 2356-2357
    in neonates, 2358-2359
    paralysis from, nonpoliovirus, 2354
    pathogenesis of, 2338-2339
    pericarditis from, 1161
    pleurodynia from, 1320, 2356-2357
    prevention of, 2341-2342
    receptors for, 2337, 2338t
    respiratory infections from, 2355-2356
    transmission of, 2340
    treatment of, 2341-2342
Coxsackievirus B3, cardiovirulence of, 1155
CPAF (chlamydial protease-like activity factor), 2446
C-polysaccharide, 2623-2624
CR1 (CD35), 81t, 83
CR2 (CD21), 81t, 83
CR3 (CD11b/CD18), 81t, 83
CR4 (CD11c/CD18), 81t, 83
Crackles, in tuberculosis, 3143
Cranberry products
    for catheter-associated urinary tract infections,
        3732

Cranberry products *(Continued)*
    for urinary tract infection prophylaxis, 22,
        669-671, 670t, 671f, 971
Cranial. *See also* Intracranial *entries.*
Cranial nerve palsy, in encephalitis, 1246
Cranial subdural empyema, 1279, 1281f-1282f
Craniotomy
    for brain abscess, 1275
    for subdural empyema, 1280
CRASPs (complement regulator–acquiring surface
        proteins), 84
C-reactive protein
    in bacterial meningitis, 1209
    in febrile response, 770-771
Creatine kinase MB isoenzyme, in myocarditis, 1157
Creatinine, urinary excretion of, in nutritional
        assessment, 151, 152t
Creeping eruption, 3618t, 3619
Creutzfeldt-Jakob disease
    diagnosis of, 2431t, 2432-2434, 2433f
    genetic, 2424f, 2428-2429
    genetic susceptibility to, 51t, 52, 55
    iatrogenic, 2431-2432
    magnetic resonance imaging in, 2433-2434, 2433f
    prions of, decontamination and, 3689
    sporadic, 2427-2428, 2431t
    transfusion-related, 3748
    variant, 2429-2431, 2431t
Crimean-Congo hemorrhagic fever, 2289-2292,
        2290t
Critical illness
    antimicrobial combination therapy in, 273
    corticosteroid insufficiency in, 998
    nutritional support in, 154-155
    polyneuropathy and myopathy in, in sepsis, 998
Cross-sectional surveys, 184
Crotamiton, for scabies, 3636t
Croup, 825-829
    allergic, 825
    assessment of, Westley clinical score in, 828
    versus bacterial epiglottitis, 827
    versus bacterial tracheitis, 827-828
    classification of, 828, 828t
    clinical manifestations of, 827, 2197
    diagnosis of, 827-828
    differential diagnosis of, 827-828
    epidemiology of, 826
    versus epiglottitis, 851
    etiology of, 825-826, 826f
    versus foreign body aspiration, 828
    history of, 825
    hospital admissions for, 825, 2196-2197
    incidence of, 825
    from influenza, 2276
    membranous or true, 825
    outcome of, 828
    pathophysiology of, 826, 826f
    radiographic findings in, 827, 827f
    recurrent, 825, 827
    spasmodic, 825, 827
    treatment of, 828, 828t, 2198
Cryoglobulinemia, HCV-related, 2168
Cryotherapy
    for condylomata acuminata, 2043
    for cutaneous warts, 2042
    for Kaposi's sarcoma, 1767
Cryptoccomas, cerebral, 3294-3295, 3295f
Cryptococcosis, in HIV infection, 1718, 1718f, 3290,
        3294, 3296
    treatment of, 3299
Cryptococcus, taxonomy of, 3287-3288
Cryptococcus albidus, 3287-3288
Cryptococcus laurentii, 3287-3288
Cryptococcus neoformans, 3287-3303
    arthritis from, 1451
    of bone and joints, 3293t, 3296
    brain abscess from, 1266, 1266t
    capsule of, 3291
    cellulitis from, 1296-1297, 3295, 3295f
    of central nervous system, 3293t, 3294-3295, 3295f
        microscopic examination of, 3296, 3296f-3297f
        treatment of, 3298-3300
    clinical manifestations of, 3293-3296, 3293t
    cultures of, 3297
    ecology of, 3289

Cryptococcus neoformans (Continued)
    endocarditis from, 1085-1086, 1094
    epidemiology of, 3289-3290, 3289t
    of eye, 3293t, 3296
    genetics of, 3287
    high-temperature growth of, 3291
    history of, 3287
    HIV coinfection with, 3290, 3294, 3296
        treatment of, 3299
    host responses to, 3292
    identification of, 3288-3289
    immune reconstitution inflammatory syndrome
        and, 3296
    incidence of, 3289-3290
    laboratory diagnosis of, 3296-3298
    life cycle of, 3287
    of lung, 3293-3294, 3293t, 3294f
        chest radiograph of, 3298
        microscopic examination of, 3296, 3297f
    melanin production in, 3291
    meningitis from, 1238
        fluconazole for, 557
        in HIV infection, 1746, 1877
            prophylaxis against, 1858t-1859t, 1871t
            treatment of, 1860t-1870t
        microscopic examination of, 3296, 3296f-3297f
        in transplant recipients, 3846
        treatment of, 3298-3300
    pathogenesis of, 3290-3293
    peritonitis from, 3296
    phospholipase B gene of, 3291-3292
    pneumonia from, in HIV infection, 1731
    prevention of, 3300
    prognosis for, 3300
    of prostate, 3293t, 3295-3296
    radiography in, 3298
    of rare body sites, 3293t, 3296
    serologic tests for, 3297-3298
    serotypes of
        A, D, and AD, 3289
        B and C, 3289
    of skin, 3293t, 3295, 3295f
    strains of, 3291
    taxonomic classification of, 3287-3288
    transmission of, 3290
    treatment of, 3298-3300
        strategies in, 3298-3300
        in vitro drug analysis in, 3298
    ulcers from, 3295, 3295f
    virulence factors of, 3291
Cryptococcus neoformans var. *gattii,* 3287, 3289
    taxonomic classification of, 3287-3288
Cryptococcus neoformans var. *grubii,* 3287-3289
Cryptococcus neoformans var. *neoformans,* 3287-3289
Cryptosporidiosis, 3547-3560, 4003
    clinical manifestations of, 3551-3553
    in developing countries, childhood diarrhea and,
        3552
    diagnosis of, 3553-3554, 3553f
    diarrhea in, 1363-1364
    epidemiology of, 3547-3550
    in HIV infection, 1860t-1870t, 1880, 3553-3554
        treatment of, 3554-3555
    host response to, 3551
    immunity to, 3551
    in immunocompetent host, 3552
    infectious dose in, 3549
    macrolides for, 438
    malnutrition and, 3552
    management of, 3554-3555
    parasites in, 3547, 3548f
    pathology and pathogenesis of, 3550-3551, 3550f
    prevention of, 3555-3556
    pulmonary, in HIV infection, 1733
    transmission of, 3547, 3548f
        person-to-person, 3549
        secondary, 3549
        sexual, 3549
    treatment of, 632t-635t
    as waterborne disease, 4004-4005
Cryptosporidium, 3547-3560
    characteristics of, 3547
    diarrhea from, 1396
        in children, 3552
    infectious dose of, 3549

Cryptosporidium (Continued)
  life cycle of, 3547, 3548f
  oocysts of, 3549
Cryptosporidium andersoni, 3547
Cryptosporidium baylei, 3547
Cryptosporidium felis, 3547
Cryptosporidium hominis, 3547
Cryptosporidium meleagridis, 3547
Cryptosporidium muris, 3547
Cryptosporidium parvum, 3547, 3549-3550
  disinfection/sterilization and, 3688
  rifamycins for, 412
Cryptosporidium suis, 3547
Crystalloids, for sepsis, 1002
CTX-M–derived beta-lactamase, 283
Cuff cellulitis, 1515
Culiseta inornata, Jamestown Canyon virus infection from, 2292
Culture. *See also specific pathogen.*
  blood. *See* Blood culture.
  cerebrospinal fluid, in shunt infections, 1233
  for fungi, 255
  in liver abscess, 1037
  media for, for bacteria, fungi, and parasites, 244-245, 245t
  for microbacteria, 250-251
  operative, in prosthetic joint infections, 1471, 1471t
  for parasites, 264
  in sepsis, 1000-1001
  sputum
    in acute pneumonia, 897-898
    in pneumococcal pneumonia, 2632, 2632f, 2632t
  throat, in streptococcal pharyngitis, 819
  urine, 967-969, 968f
  for viruses, 258, 259t-260t
Cunninghamella, 3257, 3258t
Cupriavidus, 3016t, 3025-3026
CURB and CURB-65 scoring systems for pneumonia, 909
Curvularia geniculata, mycetoma from, 3281, 3282t, 3283f
Cutaneous. *See also* Skin *entries.*
Cutaneous abscess. *See also* Skin infections.
  in chromoblastomycosis, 3278-3279, 3279f
  gonococcal, 2761
Cutaneous larva migrans, 3618t, 3619
  treatment of, 632t-635t, 647, 654
Cutaneous leishmaniasis. *See* Leishmaniasis, cutaneous.
CXCR4
  as HIV receptor, 1687, 1688f
  in HIV replication, 18, 18f, 2325
Cyanobacteria, exposure syndromes from, 3570-3571, 3570t
Cyclacillin, 706t-709t
  dosage of, 718t-719t
  formulations of, 715t
Cyclitis, 1561
Cyclooxygenase variants, antipyretic drug affinities for, 774
Cyclophilin A, in HIV replication, 2325
Cyclophosphamide, for HIV-related non-Hodgkin's lymphoma, 1769
Cycloserine, 706t-709t
  dosage of, 734t-735t
  drug interactions with, 742t-761t
  formulations of, 717t
  for tuberculosis, 541-542
Cyclospora, 3561-3563
  diarrhea from, 1396
  foodborne disease from, 1419
  in HIV infection, 1880
  life cycle of, 3561
Cyclospora cayetanensis, 3561
  diarrhea from, 205
  transmission of, 3561
Cyclosporiasis
  clinical manifestations of, 3562
  diagnosis of, 3562, 3562f
  epidemiology of, 3561-3562
  treatment of, 632t-635t, 3562-3563
Cyclosporine
  for myocarditis, 1160

Cyclosporine *(Continued)*
  for transplant immunosuppression, infections and, 3811
Cyst(s)
  alveolar, 3608t, 3614-3615
  embryologic, infected, 862t, 867
  epidermal, infected, 1303
  hydatid, 3608t, 3613-3615, 3613f-3614f
Cyst wall protein, of *Giardia lamblia*, 3527
Cysteine proteinases, in *Entamoeba histolytica*, 3415
Cystic fibrosis, 947-955
  allergic bronchopulmonary aspergillosis in, 3246, 3246t
  aminoglycosides in, 378-379
  anaerobes in, 950-951
  Burkholderia cepacia complex in, 949-950, 2864-2865, 2865f
  clinical manifestations of, 947
  fungi in, 951
  genetic susceptibility to, 52, 55
  macrolides in, 438
  Mycobacterium avium complex in, 3180
  nontuberculous mycobacteria in, 950
  pathogenesis of, 947-948
  Pseudomonas aeruginosa in, 949
    alginate and, 2847
  pulmonary infections in
    microbiology of, 948-951
    treatment of, 951-952
  quinolones in, 499
  Staphylococcus aureus in, 948-949
  viruses in, 951
Cystic fibrosis transmembrane regulator, 52, 55
  in *Pseudomonas aeruginosa*, 2840, 2841f
Cystic hygroma, infected, 862t, 867
Cysticercosis, 632t-635t, 1321, 3611-3613, 3612f
Cysticidal agents, for echinococcosis, 3614
Cystitis. *See also* Urinary tract infections.
  from *Acinetobacter*, 2883
  from *Candida*, 3233
  definition of, 957
  in elderly, 3858
  hemorrhagic
    from adenoviruses, 2030
    BKV-induced, 2056
    in transplant recipients, 3822
  quinolones for, 495
  uncomplicated, nitrofurantoin for, 516
Cystourethrography, voiding, in urinary tract infection, 981, 981f-982f
Cytochrome P-450 3A4 isoenzyme system
  capsular, of *Staphylococcus aureus*, 2544t
  quinupristin-dalfopristin inhibition of, 461
Cytochrome P-450 system, 299-300
Cytokines. *See also specific cytokine.*
  in bacterial meningitis subarachnoid space inflammation, 1199
  CD4 cell production of, 129-130
  CD8 cell production of, 131
  in cryptosporidiosis, 3550
  dendritic cell production of, 139
  in hepatitis C infection, 2166
  in HIV infection, 1699
  as immunomodulators, 611, 612t
  in infection susceptibility, 54
  in innate immunity, 41-43, 42t
  intracellular staining of, 145, 145f
  in Legionnaires' disease, 2971
  in peritonitis, 1014, 1019-1020
  protective effect of, postsurgical, 3895
  in *Pseudomonas aeruginosa* resistance, 2838-2839
  pyrogenic
    in febrile response, 769-770, 770f, 772
    receptors for, shedding of, 772
  in sepsis, 1001
  in severe sepsis, 993-994
  in streptococcal toxic shock syndrome, 2604
  in tuberculosis response, 3136
  in urinary tract infection, 961
Cytolethal distending toxin, of *Salmonella typhi*, 30
Cytolysins, cholesterol-binding, pore-forming toxins of, 33

Cytomegalovirus/cytomegalovirus infection, 1938t-1940t, 1971-1987
  antiviral therapy for, 1976-1979
    acyclovir in, 571
    cidofovir in, 1978
    cross-resistance to, 1978, 1978f
    foscarnet in, 1977-1978
    ganciclovir in, 1976-1977
      resistance to, 1977, 1977f
    maribavir in, 1978-1979
    valganciclovir in, 1977
  in cancer patients, 3799
  cardiovascular diseases and, 1982-1983
  cell types infected by, 1972
  complications of, 1974-1975, 1974f
  congenital, 1983
  cultivation of, 1973
  description of, 1971-1972
  detection of, 259t-260t
  encephalitis from, 1254
  esophageal, in HIV infection, 1737-1738
  esophagitis from, 1354, 1355t, 1356
  gastric, in HIV infection, 1738
  genome of, 1971
  Guillain-Barré syndrome from, 1974-1975
  in hematopoietic stem cell transplant recipients, 3826, 3828-3829, 3828t-3829t
  hemolytic anemia from, 1975
  hepatitis from, 1587, 1593, 1974
  in HIV infection, 1710-1711, 1710f, 1875-1877, 1975-1976, 1975f
    colitis from, 1976
    diarrhea from, 1976
    encephalopathy from, 1750f, 1753-1754
    enterocolitis from, 1742
    oral ulcers from, 1715
    pelvic inflammatory disease from, 1797
    pneumonitis from, 1732
    polyradiculopathy from, 1758, 1976
    proctitis from, 1742
    retinitis from, 1719, 1975
      HAART and, 1721
      treatment of, 1975-1976
  infectious mononucleosis from, 1973-1974, 2002-2003
  interstitial pneumonia from, 1974, 1974f
  laboratory diagnosis of, 1972-1973
  latency of, 1972
  meningoencephalitis from, 1975
  MHC class I downregulation by, 134
  myocarditis from, 1156, 1975
  nosocomial, 3775-3777
  in pregnancy, 1983-1984, 1984t
  prevention of, 584, 1979-1980
  rash from, 1975
  retinitis from, 1563, 1975-1976, 1975f
    treatment of, 1976
      antiviral agents in, 566t-567t
      cidofovir in, 577
      fomivirsen in, 580
      foscarnet in, 582
      ganciclovir/valganciclovir in, 584
  serologic tests for, 261
  skin eruptions from, 1975
  in solid organ transplant recipients, 3847
  thrombocytopenia from, 1975
  in transplant recipients, 1980-1982, 3746, 3813-3814, 3816
    from donor organ, 1980
    drug resistance in, 1982
    drug resistance to, 1982
    immunosuppressive therapy and, 1980
    from kidney transplantation, 1981-1982
    from liver transplantation, 1981
    monitoring for, 3813
    prevention of, 3815
    from stem cell transplantation, 1980-1981
Cytomegalovirus DNA, 1972-1973
Cytomegalovirus intravenous immune globulin, 618, 3922t, 3935-3936
  in hematopoietic stem cell transplant recipients, 3833
Cytometry, flow, 144, 145f
Cytoplasmic pathogens, 140

D

Dacron carotid patch, infection of, 1139-1140
Dacryoadenitis, 1569
Dacryocystis, 1571
Dalbavancin, 706t-709t, 728t-729t
Dallas criteria for myocarditis, 1154-1155, 1158
Dapsone, 651, 706t-709t
    adverse reactions to, 545
    for brain abscess, 1274t
    dosage of, 730t
    drug interactions with, 742t-761t
    formulations of, 716t
    for leprosy, 544-545, 3172
    for *Pneumocystis* pneumonia, 3382
        in HIV infection, 1860t-1870t, 1872
    for *Pneumocystis* prophylaxis, 3386, 3800t
        in children, 1824-1825
        in HIV infection, 1858t-1859t, 1873-1874
    for toxoplasmosis, in HIV infection, 3518, 3518t
Dapsone-pyrimethamine, for *Pneumocystis*
        pneumonia prophylaxis, 1858t-1859t,
        1873-1874
Dapsone-trimethoprim, 480
Daptomycin, 462-465, 706t-709t
    administration of, 463
    adverse reactions to, 463-464
    antimicrobial activity of, 462
    for cellulitis, 1297-1298
    clinical uses of, 464-465
    distribution and elimination of, 463
    dosage of, 463, 728t-729t
    drug interactions with, 463-464, 742t-761t
    for endocarditis, 464, 1091
    for enterococcal infections, 464-465, 2649-2650
    formulations of, 716t
    mechanism of action of, 462
    minimal inhibitory concentration susceptibility
        for, 460t
    for MRSA joint infections, 1449
    for osteoarticular infections, 464
    for osteomyelitis, 1459-1460, 1459t
    pharmacodynamics of, 463
    pharmacokinetics of, 463
    resistance to, 291, 291t, 462-463
    for skin infections, 464
    for soft tissue infections, 464
    for *Staphylococcus aureus* bacteremia, 464
    Staphylococcus aureus resistance to, 2559t,
        2560-2561
    surfactant binding to, 271-272
Darkfield examination, for syphilis, 3044, 3045f
Dark-walled fungi, 3367-3369, 3367t, 3374t. See also
        Phaehyphomycosis.
Darmbrand, 1394
Darunavir, 706t-709t, 1839f, 1840t, 1842
    dosage of, 740t-741t
    drug interactions with, 742t-761t
    formulations of, 717t
    for HIV-infected children, 1820t-1821t, 1823t
Daycare centers. See Childcare centers.
Deamidating toxins, 28t
Débridement
    for gingivitis, 869
    for mediastinitis, 1178
    for osteomyelitis, 1460
    for streptococcal toxic shock syndrome, 869, 2605
Decay-accelerating factor (CD55), 81t
Decolonization, in *Staphylococcus aureus* carriers,
        2565
Decongestants
    for common cold, 811
    for otitis media with effusion, 834
    for sinusitis, 846
Decontamination, 3677
    environmental, for Legionnaires' disease
        outbreaks, 2975
    gut
        after liver transplantation, 3816
        selective, for pancreatic infections, 1048, 1049t
    for methicillin-resistant *Staphylococcus aureus*,
        2563, 2564t
    after terrorist-associated anthrax contamination,
        3990-3991, 3991t
    after terrorist-associated tularemia contamination,
        3975

Dectin-1, in innate immunity, 138
Decubitus ulcers, 1300
    in elderly, 3859
    in spinal cord injury patients, 3854
Deep fascial space infections, 859f, 860-864, 863f. See
        also Odontogenic infections.
Deep vein thrombosis, air travel-related, 4016
Deer fly fever. See Tularemia.
Deer tick, 3071, 3072f
DEET
    arthropod protection with, 4015
    skin disease protection with, 4015-4016
Defensins, in neutrophil bactericidal activity, 109
Degranulation, of neutrophils, 107-108
Dehydration, in bronchiolitis, 887-888
Dehydroemetine, 706t-709t
    for parasitic infections, 650
Delavirdine, 706t-709t, 1837f, 1837t, 1838
    dosage of, 740t-741t
    drug interactions with, 742t-761t
    formulations of, 717t
Delivery
    cesarean
        antibiotic prophylaxis for, 3900
        elective, HIV transmission prevention by,
            1786
        endomyometritis after, 1511-1513, 1512f
    HIV testing at, 1678
    premature, in acute pyelonephritis, 975
Demeclocycline, 387t, 706t-709t
    dosage of, 724t
    formulations of, 715t
Dementia, AIDS. See AIDS dementia.
Demodex mites, 3645
Dendritic cells
    in antimicrobial defense, 139
    in HIV infection, 1698
    infection of, 139
    in lymph nodes, 142
Dengue fever, 206-207, 207f, 4004
    Aedes aegypti in, 207, 207f
    clinical features of, 2144-2145
    versus enteric fever, 1400t-1401t, 1404
    epidemiology of, 2135-2136
    historical perspective on, 2133
    versus malaria, 3450
    in neonates, 2145
    pathogenesis of, 2142-2143
    in travelers, 4014-4015, 4022
    treatment of, 2150
Dengue hemorrhagic fever
    clinical features of, 2142f, 2144-2145
    epidemiology of, 2135-2136
    pathogenesis of, 2142-2143, 2142f
    in travelers, 4014-4015
    treatment of, 2150
Dengue shock syndrome, 2143, 2145
Dental caries
    mechanisms preventing, 857
    prevention of, 861t
    from *Streptococcus mutans*, 855-857, 856t
    from *Streptococcus sobrinus*, 856-857
    treatment of, 869
Dental infections. See Odontogenic infections.
Dental plaque
    accumulation of, prevention of, 861t
    anaerobes in, 3085
    microorganisms residing in, 855, 856f
Dental procedures
    endocarditis prophylaxis during, 1144t, 1145,
        1146t, 1148, 1148t
    injury prevention during, 3759
Dental pulp, infections of, 858
Dentoalveolar infections, 858-859, 861t. See also
        Odontogenic infections.
Deoxyguanosine, 568f
2-Deoxystreptamine, 359, 360f
Department of Health and Human Services
        (DHHS) bioterrorism-related budget,
        3958t-3959t
Dependoviruses, 2093
Depression, in brucellosis, 2923
Dermabacter hominis, 2701
Dermacentor andersoni, 2101
Dermacentor variabilis, 3655, 3655f

Dermatitis. See also Skin infections.
    from *Pseudomonas aeruginosa*, 2854
    schistosomal, 3597, 3618t, 3622
    seborrheic
        in HIV infection, 1717-1718, 1717f
        from *Malassezia*, 3354
Dermatitis syndrome, from HTLV, 2315
Dermatobia hominis, myiasis from, 3637, 4023f
Dermatophyte(s)
    antibody production by, 3345
    characteristics of, 3345
    classification and taxonomy of, 3345, 3346t
    immune response to, 3347
    species of, 3345-3347
Dermatophyte mycetoma, 3281
Dermatophytosis, 3345-3355. See also Tinea *entries*.
    age and, 3347
    anthropophilic, 3346-3347, 3346t
    clinical features of, 3347-3351
    deep, 3350-3351, 3351f
    epidemiology of, 3345-3347, 3346t
    of face, 3349, 3349f
    of foot, 3348, 3352, 3352t
    geophilic, 3346, 3346t
    of groin, 3348
    of hand, 3349
    "id" reactions in, 3351
    laboratory diagnosis of, 3351
    of nails, 3350, 3352
    pathogenesis of, 3347
    of scalp, 3346t, 3349-3350, 3350f, 3352t
    treatment of, 3351-3352, 3352t
    zoophilic, 3345, 3346t
Dermonecrotic toxin, of *Bordetella pertussis*, 31,
        2955-2956
Descriptive studies, 182, 182t
Desert rheumatism, 3335
Desethylchloroquine, 635-636
Developing countries
    diarrhea in
        childhood, from *Cryptosporidium*, 3552
        zinc for, 670t, 672-673
    HIV transmission in, 1624-1628
    poliomyelitis in, 2349-2350
    travel to
        immunizations for, 4009-4010, 4012f
        pretravel office visit for, 4010t
    tuberculosis in, 3133, 3133t
Developmental abnormalities, in HIV-infected
        children, 1813-1814
Dexamethasone
    for bacterial meningitis, 619
    for bronchiolitis, 889
    for central nervous system lymphoma, 1751
    for croup, 828, 828t, 2198
    for *Haemophilus influenzae* type b meningitis,
        2915
    for HIV-related non-Hodgkin's lymphoma, 1769
    for meningitis, 1212-1214, 1220
    for tuberculous meningitis, 618-619
    for typhoid fever, 2899
Diabetes mellitus
    antimicrobial therapy and, 269
    cellulitis in, 1297
    after congenital rubella, 2129
    foot ulcers in, 1300-1302, 1461-1462, 1462t
    insulin-dependent, enteroviruses and, 2361-2362
    juvenile, mumps and, 2204
    osteomyelitis in, 1461-1463, 1462f, 1462t
    urinary tract infections in, 966, 970
Diagnostic procedures, endocarditis prophylaxis
        during, 1144t, 1146t, 1148
Dialysis. See also Hemodialysis; Peritoneal dialysis.
    catheter-related infections in, 1028. See also
        Catheter-related infections.
        antibacterial prophylaxis for, 524-525
        from coagulase-negative *Staphylococcus*, 2584
    quinolone dosage in, 493-494, 493t
    for streptococcal toxic shock syndrome, 2605
Diaper rash, from *Candida*, 3230, 3230f
Diarrhea, 205-206. See also Gastroenteritis.
    abdominal cramps with, 1414-1415
    from *Aeromonas*, 3018
    and/or abdominal pain with eosinophilia,
        syndrome of, 1407-1409, 1407t

Diarrhea *(Continued)*
  antibiotic-associated, 1379. *See also* Pseudomem-
      branous colitis.
  from *Bacillus*, 2728
  bacterial adherence in, 1341-1342
  bacterial overgrowth in, 1367-1368
  Brainerd's, 1366
  from *Campylobacter jejuni*, 206, 2796
  in children
      from *Cryptosporidium*, 3552
      mortality from, 1335
      zinc for, 670t, 672-673
  from *Chromobacterium violaceum*, 3019-3020
  from *Clostridium difficile*, 206
      antibiotic prophylaxis and, 3901
  in coccidiosis, 1396
  from *Cryptosporidium*, 3550
      in children, 3552
      in immunocompetent host, 3552
  from *Cyclospora cayetanensis*, 205
  from cytomegalovirus, 1976
  in daycare centers, 1365
  from *Dysgonomonas capnocytophagoides*, 3020
  in elderly, 3860
  from *Entamoeba histolytica*, 3418. *See also*
      Entamoeba histolytica.
  from enteroinvasive *Escherichia coli*, 1391
  from enteropathogenic *Escherichia coli*, 1395
  epidemic, in newborn nurseries, 1359-1360, 1360t
  from *Escherichia coli*, 205-206, 1339-1340, 1339t,
      2821t
  in foodborne disease
      abdominal cramps and, 1414-1415
      nonbloody, 1415
      persistent, 1416
      without fever, 1415-1416
  from *Giardia lamblia*, 3530, 3530t
  from giardiasis, 1396
  global pattern of, 206
  after hematopoietic stem cell transplantation, 3823
  in HIV infection, 1364-1365, 1364t
  in hospitals, 1365
  idiopathic, chronic, 1366
  infantile, epidemic, 1359-1360, 1360t
  infectious
      diagnosis of, 1344-1346, 1345f
      oral rehydration therapy for, 1347
  in institutions, 1365
  in long-term care facilities, 1365
  malnutrition and, 1335
  in military campaigns, role of, 1335
  noninflammatory
      acute, 1363-1364, 1367
      chronic, 1367
  from noroviruses, 205
  outbreaks of, 205
  from *Plesiomonas shigelloides*, 3021
  probiotics for, 670t, 674-675
  from rotaviruses, 206
      clinical manifestations of, 2107
      diagnosis of, 1361, 2106f, 2111
      pathogenesis of, 2107-2108
      seasonality of, 2109, 2110f
      treatment of, 2111-2112
      weanling, 1361
  from *Salmonella*, 205-206
  in travelers, 1365-1367, 4015, 4025-4026
      acute, 4025
      amebic, 3416-3417, 3417f
      definition of, 4025
      etiology of, 1366, 1366t
      persistent, 4025-4026
      prevention of, 1367
      treatment of, 1367
  in tropical sprue, 1431
  from *Vibrio cholerae*, 205
  weanling, 1360-1362
  in winter vomiting disease, 1362
Diarrhetic shellfish poisoning, 3569-3570, 3570t
Diarylquinoline-TMC207, for tuberculosis, 542
Diazepam, for tetanus, 3094, 3094t
Dibekacin, 359, 360f, 360t-361t
Dicloxacillin, 317, 317f, 706t-709t
  for bullous impetigo, 1291
  for cellulitis, 1297-1298

Dicloxacillin *(Continued)*
  dosage of, 316t, 718t-719t
  formulations of, 715t
  for lymphangitis, 1331-1332
  for pyogenic lymphadenitis, 1330
Didanosine, 706t-709t, 1834f, 1835, 1835t
  dosage of, 740t-741t
  drug interactions with, 742t-761t
  formulations of, 717t
  for HIV-infected children, 1820t-1821t
  pancreatitis from, 1741
Dientamebiasis, 632t-635t
Dietary history, of traveler, 4021
Diethylcarbamazine, 659, 706t-709t
  for angiostrongyliasis, 3621
  for filariasis, 3591
  for loiasis, 3592
Differential fluorescence induction, 11
DiGeorge syndrome, 169t-170t, 171
Digital necrosis, in sickle cell disease with
      Mycoplasma pneumoniae infection, 2483f, 2484
Dihydrofolate reductase inhibitors, 650
Dihydropteroate synthetase inhibitors, 651
Diloxanide, for *Entamoeba histolytica* infection,
      3422t
Diloxanide furoate, 649, 706t-709t
Diphtheria. *See also Corynebacterium diphtheriae*.
  clinical manifestations of, 2690-2691
  cutaneous, 1298, 2691
  diagnosis of, 2691
  differential diagnosis of, 2691
  epidemiology of, 2688-2689, 2688f
  versus epiglottitis, 851
  immunization recommendations for, 2692-2693
  incidence of
      in Russia and Baltic States, 2688, 2688f
      in United States, 2688, 2688f
  invasive, 2691
  pathogenesis of, 2689, 2689f
  prevention of, 2692-2693
  respiratory, 2690-2691, 2690f
  treatment of, 2691-2692
      antibiotics in, 2692
      diphtheria antitoxin in, 2691-2692
      supportive care in, 2692
Diphtheria antitoxin (DAT), 1298, 2691-2692
Diphtheria toxin, 30-31
Diphtheria toxoid, 3922t, 3923
Diphtheria-pertussis-tetanus (DPT) vaccine, 2689,
      2692-2693, 2960-2961, 3094t, 3095, 3922t, 3923
Diphtheria-tetanus-accellular pertussis (DTaP)
      vaccine, 3922t, 3923, 3924f, 3929-3930
      recommended schedule for, 3924f
Diphyllobothrium, 3610
Diphyllobothrium caninum, 632t-635t
Diphyllobothrium latum, 632t-635t, 3608-3609,
      3608t, 3609f
Dipylidium caninum, 3610
Direct fluorescent antibody test
  for *Bordetella pertussis*, 2959
  for *Legionella pneumophila*, 2977, 2977t
  for rabies, 2254
  stains for, 244, 244t
Direct transmission, 187
Dirithromycin, 706t-709t
  dosage of, 726t-727t
  drug interactions with, 742t-761t
  formulations of, 716t
Dirofilaria immitis, 3621
Dirofilaria repens, 3594
Dirofilariasis, 3621
Disaster Medical Assistance Teams (DMATs),
      activation of, 3957-3958
Disc space infection, 1460-1461, 1461f
Disease prevention and control, 188-190. *See also*
      Infection control.
  assessment of, 188-189
  levels of, 188
  primary, 189-190
  secondary, 190
  tertiary, 190
Disease surveillance. *See* Surveillance.
Disinfectants, 3677
  chemical, 3681-3684
  high-level, 3677, 3680t

Disinfectants *(Continued)*
  intermediate-level, 3677
  low-level, 3677
Disinfection
  with alcohols, 521, 522t, 3681-3682
  of bioterrorism agents, 3689-3690
  with chlorhexidine, 521-522, 522t
  with chlorine and chlorine compounds, 3682
  current issues in, 3690-3692
  definition of, 3677
  with glutaraldehyde, 3680t, 3682-3683
  of health care equipment, 3681-3684
  in hospitals, 3681-3684
  with hydrogen peroxide, 3680t, 3683
  with iodophors, 521, 522t, 3683
  methods of, 3678t-3679t
  of noncritical items, 3678t-3679t, 3681, 3690
  with ortho-phthalaldehyde, 3680t, 3683-3684
  OSHA blood-borne pathogen standard and,
      3688-3690
  with peracetic acid, 3680t, 3684
  with peracetic acid/hydrogen peroxide, 3680t,
      3684
  with phenolics, 3684
  with povidone-iodine, 521, 522t
  with quaternary ammonium compounds, 3684
  rational approach to, 3677-3681
  of semicritical items, 3678t-3679t, 3680-3681,
      3690
  of skin, 521-522
  with trilosan, 522, 522t
Disposable gown, 3673, 3674t
Distribution, drug, 297-300, 298f
Distribution clearance, 298-299
Disulfiram effect, of metronidazole, 423
Diverticulitis, 1063-1064
  actinomycotic, 3212-3213
  definition of, 1063
DMSA scan, in acute pyelonephritis, 981, 982f
DNA, 1115
  bacterial
      persistence of, 1115-1116
      in synovial fluid, 1446
DNA gyrase, in quinolone resistance, 289, 487, 489
DNA integration elements, in antimicrobial
      resistance, 281, 281f
DNA microarrays, 11
DNA polymerase chain reaction assay. *See*
      Polymerase chain reaction assay.
DNA rearrangement, in B cells, 66-67, 67f, 67t
DNA-binding protein(s)
  activated agrA as, 2548
  in *Staphylococcus aureus* pathogenesis, 2548-2549,
      2548f
Dobra virus, 2291
Docosanol, 566t-567t, 578
Dogs
  bites of, 3911-3912, 3912t
  Pasteurella infection from, 2939, 2941-2942
  rabies in, 2250-2251, 2255
Domoic acid, in marine foods, 3570
Donovan bodies, 3012-3013, 3012f
Donovanosis, 1476-1477, 1478f, 1480, 1480f,
      3011-3013
  clinical manifestations of, 3011-3012, 3012f
  diagnosis of, 3012-3013, 3012f
  epidemiology of, 3011
  geographic distribution of, 3011
  pathogen in, 3011
  treatment of, 3013
Dopamine, for septic shock, 1003
Doripenem, 706t-709t
  antibacterial activity of, 342t
  chemistry of, 341, 342f
  clinical use of, 343
  dosage of, 722t
  drug interactions with, 742t-761t
  formulations of, 716t
  for nosocomial pneumonia, 3718t
  pharmacology of, 342
  for *Pseudomonas aeruginosa*, 2856
  recommended dose of, 343
  for septic bursitis, 1450t
Down syndrome, *Staphylococcus aureus* infection in,
      2563

Downie body, 3979
Doxorubicin, for HIV-related non-Hodgkin's
    lymphoma, 1769
Doxycycline, 387t
    for actinomycetoma, 3284
    for actinomycosis, 3217t
    for anthrax, 1294t, 2721t, 3989t
    for bacillary angiomatosis/peliosis, 3005
    for bite wounds, 3913t
    for brucellosis, 2924
    for cellulitis, 1297-1298
    for Chlamydia trachomatis infections, 2455
    for Chlamydophila respiratory infection, 2471,
        2471t
    for cholera, 2782, 2782t
    for donovanosis, 3013
    dosage of, 724t
    for ehrlichiosis, 2536
    for epidemic typhus, 2523
    food interactions with, 393t
    formulations of, 715t
    for Francisella tularensis prophylaxis, 3974t
    for gingivitis, 861t, 869
    indications for, 392-394, 393t
    for Legionnaires' disease, 2978t
    for leptospirosis, 3064, 3064t
    for Lyme disease, 3079t
    for malaria, 4013-4014
        prophylactic, 3455t, 3456
    mechanism of action of, 3447
    for meningitis, 1213t
    for murine typhus, 2527
    for Mycoplasma pneumoniae infections, 2487
    for Neisseria gonorrhoeae infection, 2765-2766,
        2765t
    for neuroretinitis, 3005
    for nontuberculous mycobacterial infections, 544
    for onchocerciasis, 3593
    for parasitic infections, 661
    pharmacology of, 387-390, 390t
    for plague, 2948
        prophylactic, 2949
    for pneumonic plague, 3967t
    for psittacosis, 2465
    for Q fever pneumonia, 2514
    for Rickettsia infections, 2496
    for rickettsialpox, 2509
    for Rocky Mountain spotted fever, 2503
    for scrub typhus, 2530
    side effects of, 391t
    for spotted fever, 2505
    for syphilis, 3047t, 3049-3050
    for toxoplasmosis, in HIV infection, 3518
    for tularemia, 3974t
    for urethritis, 1490-1491, 1491t
Doxycycline calcium, 706t-709t
Doxycycline hyclate, 706t-709t
Doxycycline monohyclate, 706t-709t
Doxycycline-hydrochloroquine, for Whipple disease,
    1440, 1440t
Dr hemagglutinin family, uropathogenic, 960
Dracunculiasis, 3589, 3589f
    treatment of, 632t-635t, 648
Dracunculus medinensis, 3589, 3589f
Drainage
    of amebic liver abscess, 3422
    of brain abscess, 1275
    gastrointestinal, for peritonitis, 1026
    of liver abscess, 1038-1039, 1038f
    of lung abscess, 928
    of pleural effusion, 922-923
Drainage bag, antimicrobials in, for catheter-
    associated urinary tract infections, 3732
Droplet precautions, transmission-based, 3674t-
    3675t, 3675
Drotrecogin alfa (activated), 706t-709t
Drug(s). See also specific drug or drug group.
    abuse of. See also Injection drug users.
        chronic pneumonia and, 932-933
    antimicrobial. See Antimicrobial agents.
    antiviral. See Antiviral agents.
    pharmacodynamics of, 300-306. See also
        Pharmacodynamics.
    pharmacokinetics of, 297. See also
        Pharmacokinetics.

Drug fever, 787
Duck hepatitis virus (DHV), 2059
Duct tape occlusion, for cutaneous warts, 2042
Duffy antigen negativity, malaria and, 3443-3444
Duffy blood group, in malaria susceptibility, 50,
    50t
Duke criteria, in endocarditis diagnosis, 1116,
    3880
Duodenal biopsy, in Whipple's disease, 1438, 1438f
Duodenal ulceration, in Helicobacter pylori infection,
    2806-2807, 2806t
Dura mater grafts, Creutzfeldt-Jakob disease
    associated with, 2431
Dust mites, 3643
Dwarf tapeworms, 3608t, 3609-3610, 3609f
Dysentery. See also Diarrhea; Gastroenteritis.
    acute, 1389-1393
    amebic, 1391-1392, 3411. See also Entamoeba
        histolytica.
        clinical manifestations of, 3418, 3419f
        diagnosis of, 1393
    bacillary. See Bacillary dysentery.
    bilharzial, 1392
    ciliary, 1392
    diagnosis of, 1389, 1390f, 1393-1394
    differential diagnosis of, 1390t
    epidemiology of, 1389
    from Escherichia coli, 1390-1391, 1390t
    fecal leukocytes in, 1389, 1390f
    history of, 1389
    ipecac bark for, 3411
    spirillar or spirochetal, 1393
    treatment of, 1393-1394
    in trichuriasis, 3580
Dysgonomonas, 3016t-3017t, 3020-3021
Dysgonomonas capnocytophagoides, 3020-3021
Dysphagia, in HIV infection, 1737
Dystrophin-glycoprotein complex, in enteroviral
    myocarditis, 1156
Dysuria
    acute onset of, 968-969, 968f
    herpes simplex virus infection and, 1949
    treatment of, 971
    trichomoniasis and, 1490
Dysuria syndrome, 973-974

E

E test, 250
Ear
    barotrauma to, from hyperbaric oxygen therapy,
        626
    infections of. See Otitis.
    specimen collection and transport guidelines for,
        235t-236t
East African trypanosomiasis, 3489-3494. See also
    African trypanosomiasis.
Eastern equine encephalitis, 1246t, 1257-1258,
    2117-2125, 2118t. See also Alphaviruses.
    geographic distribution of, 1246-1247, 1247f
Eastern Europe, HIV infection in, 1620
Ebola virus
    characteristics of, 2259, 2260f
    clinical manifestations of, 2262
    diagnosis of, 2262
    epidemiology of, 2259-2262, 2261f
    pathology and pathogenesis of, 2262
    prevention and treatment of, 2262-2263
    Reston subtype of, 2260
    transmission of, 2260-2262
    Zaire, Sudan, and Cote d'Ivoire subtypes of,
        2259-2260
Ecchymoses, subcutaneous, in meningococcal sepsis,
    2741-2743, 2742f
Echinacea, for common cold, 670t, 673-674, 812
Echinocandins, 559-561
    for Blastomyces dermatitidis, 3330
    for candidiasis, 3236
    investigational, 561
    mechanism of action of, 551f, 559
    structure of, 550f-551f, 559
Echinococcosis, 632t-635t, 3608t, 3613-3615,
    3613f-3614f
Echinococcus granulosus, 632t-635t
Echinococcus multilocularis, 632t-635t

Echocardiography
    in cardiac rhythm management device infections,
        1129
    in endocarditis, 1077, 1079-1080
    in Kawasaki syndrome, 3666
    in myocarditis, 1157
    in pericarditis, 1163
    in prosthetic valve endocarditis, 1116
Echoviruses
    acute hemorrhagic conjunctivitis from, 2360-2361
    characteristics of, 2337
    communicability period of, 2341
    diabetes mellitus and, 2361-2362
    dilated cardiomyopathy from, 2358
    encephalitis from
        in immunocompromised hosts, 2359-2360
        nonpoliovirus, 2354
    epidemiology of, 2339-2341, 2340t
    exanthems from, 2354-2355
    gastrointestinal disorders from, 2361
    hand-foot-and-mouth disease from, 2355
    herpangina from, 2355-2356
    host range of, 2338t
    immune response to, 2339
    incidence of, 2340-2341
    incubation period of, 2341
    laboratory diagnosis of, 2341
    meningitis from, 1241, 2353-2354
        in immunocompromised hosts, 2359-2360
    molecular biology of, 2337-2338, 2338t
    mutation of, 2339
    myopericarditis from, 2357-2358
    myositis from, 2356-2357
    in neonates, 2358-2359
    paralysis from, nonpoliovirus, 2354
    pathogenesis of, 2338-2339
    pleurodynia from, 2356-2357
    prevention of, 2341-2342
    receptors for, 2337, 2338t
    respiratory infections from, 2355-2356
    transmission of, 2340
    treatment of, 2341-2342
Econazole, 706t-709t, 717t
Ecosystem disruption, zoonoses and, 4004-4005
Ecthyma, 1293
Ecthyma gangrenosum, 798-799, 1303
    in Pseudomonas aeruginosa bacteremia, 2849, 2849f
    in sepsis, 1000
Ectoparasites. See also specific parasite.
    common, 3626t
    taxonomy of, 3625, 3626t
Ectoparasitic diseases, 3625-3627
    clinical manifestations of, 3626t
    epidemiology of, 3625
    mechanisms of, 3625
    selected, 3627t
Ectopic pregnancy, from Chlamydia trachomatis,
    2454
Eculizumab, 93
Eczema vaccinatum, 803
Edema
    cerebral. See also Intracranial hypertension.
        from anthrax, 2723
        in bacterial meningitis, 1201-1202
    conjunctival, 1530
    corneal, 1541
    lip, in Kawasaki syndrome, 3663, 3664f
    periorbital, from sinusitis, 846
    in poststreptococcal glomerulonephritis, 2619
    pulmonary, in malaria, 3441-3442
Edema factor, of Bacillus anthracis, 30, 2715
Education
    on antimicrobial stewardship, 678
    on emergency preparedness, 227
    on nosocomial infections, 3670
    parent and patient, on immunization, 3943-3944
Edwardsiella tarda, 2829
Efavirenz, 706t-709t, 1837f, 1837t, 1838
    dosage of, 740t-741t
    drug interactions with, 742t-761t
    formulations of, 717t
    for HIV postexposure prophylaxis, 3755t, 3764
    for HIV-infected children, 1820t-1821t
    resistance to, 1838
    toxicity of, 1838

Efavirenz-emtricitabine-tenofovir, 717t
Efflux pumps
    in antimicrobial resistance, 286-287
    in cephalosporin resistance, 329
    in multidrug resistance, 291, 291f
    in quinolone resistance, 490
Eflornithine, 649-650
    for African trypanosomiasis, 3492
Eggerthella, 3126
Ehrlichia, 2531
    bacteriology of, 2495, 2496t
    epidemiology of, 2495-2496
    genetics of, 2495
    historical perspective on, 2495, 2497t
    medical and veterinary disease caused by,
        2532t
    taxonomy of, 2531
    ultrastructure of, 2531-2532
Ehrlichia canis, 2531-2532, 2532t
Ehrlichia chaffeensis, 2531-2532, 2532t, 3656f
    laboratory detection of, 240t-242t
Ehrlichia ewingii, 2531-2532, 2532t, 2535
    laboratory detection of, 240t-242t
Ehrlichia muris, 2531-2532, 2532t, 2535
Ehrlichia ruminantium, 2531-2532, 2532t
Ehrlichiosis, 803
    in asplenia, 3869
    clinical findings in, 2496, 2498t
    diagnosis of, 2496
    versus enteric fever, 1400t-1401t, 1404
    human granulocytotropic, 3657t
    human monocytotropic, 3657t
        clinical manifestations of, 2534-2536
        course of, 2534
        diagnosis of, 2534-2535
        differential diagnosis of, 2535, 2535t
        epidemiology of, 2532-2533
        etiology of, 2531-2532, 2532f
        pathogenesis and pathology of, 2533
        prevention of, 2536
        versus Rocky Mountain spotted fever,
            2535t
        signs and symptoms of, 2534, 2534t
        treatment of, 2536
    pathophysiology of, 2495
    rifamycins for, 412
    tick-borne, 3656, 3656f, 3657t
    transfusion-related, 3748
    treatment of, 2496
Eikenella, 240t-242t, 3016t-3017t, 3023-3024
Eikenella corrodens, 3023-3024
Elderly, 3857-3864
    antimicrobial therapy in, 269, 3861-3862
    bacteremia in, 3859-3860
    bacterial meningitis in, 1206
    bacteriuria in, 965-966, 3857
    central nervous system infections in, 3861
    community-acquired pneumonia in, 905
    diarrhea in, 3860
    endocarditis in, 3860
    fever of unknown origin in, 781, 781t, 3861
    hypersensitivity reactions in, 269
    immunity in, 44-45
    immunizations in, 3862
    influenza vaccine in, 3926
    malnutrition in, 156-157, 156t
    meningitis in, 3861
    parainfluenza virus infection in, 2197
    physiologic changes in, 269
    pneumonia in, 894-895, 3858-3859
    pressure sores in, 3859
    respiratory syncytial virus infection in, 2212-2213,
        2213t
    septic arthritis in, 3861
    skin infections in, 3859
    temperature in, 766, 768
    tuberculosis in, 3140, 3859
        progressive lower lobe, 3142
    urinary tract infections in, 966-967, 970,
        3857-3858
    West Nile virus infection in, 3861
Electrocardiography
    in mumps virus, 2203
    in myocarditis, 1157
    in pericarditis, 1163

Electroencephalography
    in Creutzfeldt-Jakob disease, 2434
    in encephalitis, 1250
Electrolyte therapy
    for Campylobacter infections, 2798-2799
    for peritonitis, 1026
Electron microscopy
    of hepatitis C virus, 2158f
    of rotavirus, 2106f, 2111
    of smallpox virions, 3979
Electrophoresis
    pulse field gel, 180, 249
        in Staphylococcus aureus diagnosis, 2546
    serum protein, for monoclonal gammopathies, 64,
        64f
Electrophysiological studies, bloodstream infection
    after, 1136-1137, 1136t
Elimination, drug, 300
Elizabethkingia, 3016t, 3022-3023
Elizabethkingia meningoseptica, 3016t, 3022-3023,
    3023f
Embolus (embolism)
    in endocarditis, 1074, 1077
        cerebral, 1074
        pulmonary, 1075
        from Staphylococcus aureus, 2569, 2570f
    pulmonary. See Pulmonary embolism.
Embryologic cyst, infected, 862t, 867
Emergency preparedness, 221-231
    ambulatory care in, 229-230
    communication plan for, 221, 223f
    education in, 227
    emergency department issues in, 229-230
    general plans for, 221-223, 222f-223f
    health care worker surveillance and exposure
        management in, 227
    infection control in, 223-225
        detection and diagnosis for, 223-224, 224t
        policies, procedures, and administrative
            controls for, 224-225, 225t
        syndromic surveillance for, 223
    infrastructural, 228-229, 228f, 228t
    isolation technique in, 225-226, 225t, 226f
    media management in, 230
    patient and community support for, 221-222
    patient flow in, 222-223
    patient transport in, 229, 229f
    personal protective equipment in, 225-226
    respiratory isolation precautions in, 225,
        226f
    screening procedures in, 227-228, 228f
    surge capacity in, 222-223
    team approach to, 222
    visitors in, 229
Emergency use authorization, in bioterrorist attack,
    3958
Emerging diseases. See Infectious disease, emerging
    and reemerging.
Emetine, for parasitic infections, 650
Emphysema
    in chronic obstructive pulmonary disease, 877
    in HIV infection, 1733
    in tuberculosis, 3155
Emphysematous pyelonephritis, 973, 973f, 976-977,
    979-980
Empirical therapy, 689
    antifungal, 3805
    anti-inflammatory, for fever of unknown origin,
        785-786
    failure of, proposed definition of, 3804-3805,
        3805t
    for febrile neutropenia, 3804t
    limitations and risks of, 786
    for tuberculous meningitis, 1241
Empyema, 917-924
    in bronchopleural fistula, 922-923
    clinical manifestations of, 919
    from Haemophilus influenzae type b, 2914
    imaging of, 919-920, 919f-920f
    laboratory findings in, 920-921, 920t
    microbiology of, 917-919
    pathophysiology of, 917
    in pneumococcal pneumonia, 2633
    subdural, 1279, 1281f-1282f
    treatment of, 921-923, 921t

Emtricitabine, 599, 706t-709t, 1834f, 1835t, 1836
    dosage of, 740t-741t
    formulations of, 717t
    for HIV postexposure prophylaxis, 3755t, 3764
    for HIV-infected children, 1820t-1821t
    resistance to, 1836
    structure of, 578f
Emtricitabine-tenofovir, 717t
ENA-78, in pleural effusion, 917
Encephalitis. See also Meningoencephalitis.
    acute, 1183
    from alphaviruses, 2117-2125, 2118t. See also
        Alphaviruses.
    amebic
        granulomatous. See Granulomatous amebic
            encephalitis.
        nongranulomatous, 3427, 3430t
    antibody testing in, HSV-specific, 1249
    from arboviruses, 1246t, 1255-1258
        incidence of, 1246-1247, 1247f
        pathogenesis of, 1256
    California, 1258, 2289-2292, 2290t
    cerebrospinal fluid profile in, 1249
    chronic, 1183-1184
    clinical approach to, 1243-1250, 1244f, 1244t,
        1248f
    clinical features of, 1183-1184, 1245-1247, 1247f
    from Colorado tick fever virus, 1259
    from cytomegalovirus, 1254
        in HIV infection, 1750f, 1753-1754
    definition of, 1243
    diagnosis of, 1247-1250
    Eastern equine, 1246t, 1257-1258, 2117-2125,
        2118t
    geographic distribution of, 1246-1247, 1247f
    electroencephalography in, 1250
    from enteroviruses, 1259
        in immunocompromised hosts, 2359-2360
        nonpoliovirus, 2354
    from Epstein-Barr virus, 1254-1255, 1994-1995
    equine, 2117-2125, 2118t
    etiologic agents of, 1246t
    European, 2138t
    Far Eastern, 2138t
    from flaviviruses, 2141f, 2143-2144, 2150-2152,
        2151f
    from Hendra virus, 2242
    from herpes simplex virus, 1250-1253, 1952
        antiviral agents for, 566t-567t, 571
        magnetic resonance imaging in, 1247-1248,
            1248f
    from herpesvirus B, 1255
    from human herpesvirus 6, 1255, 2012-2013
    Japanese, 1258-1259. See also Japanese
        encephalitis.
    Kyasanur Forest, 2152-2153
    from Listeria monocytogenes, 2710
    management of, 1250
    from measles virus, 1260, 2231
    from mumps virus, 2203
    Murray Valley, 2152
    neuroimaging in, 1247-1249, 1248f
    from Nipah virus, 1251t-1252t, 2238-2241. See
        also Nipah virus, encephalitis from.
    from nonpoliovirus enteroviruses, 1259
    nonviral causes of, 1183
    from parvovirus B19 infection, 2091
    in poliomyelitis, 2347
    from poliovirus, 1259
    polymerase chain reaction analysis in, 1249-1250
    Powassan, 2148
    from rabies virus, 1259-1260
    Rocio, 2152
    in rubella, 2129
    St. Louis, 1257. See also St. Louis encephalitis.
    Siberian, 2138t
    signs and symptoms of, 1237. See also Central
        nervous system infections.
    subacute sclerosing, from measles virus, 2230
    tick-borne. See Tick-borne encephalitis.
    from Toxoplasma gondii, in HIV infection,
        1270-1271, 1749-1751, 1750f, 3501
        incidence of, 3498
        treatment of, 3518-3519
    from varicella-zoster virus, 1253-1254, 1965

Encephalitis (Continued)
  vector-borne, 1255-1258. See also Tick-borne
      encephalitis.
  Venezuelan equine, 1258
  viral, 1183, 1243-1263
      etiologies of, 1250-1260, 1251t-1252t
  West Nile, 1256-1257. See also West Nile
      encephalitis.
  Western equine, 1258
Encephalitozoon, 3391, 3392t. See also Microsporidia.
  in HIV infection, 3399
Encephalomyelitis
  acute disseminated, 1243-1250, 1244f, 1244t, 1246t
      from rabies vaccine, 2255
  in melioidosis, 2872-2873, 2875f
  postvaccination, 1925
Encephalopathy, 1243. See also
      Leukoencephalopathy, progressive multifocal.
  in cat-scratch disease, 3001
  hepatic, rifamycins for, 413
  HIV-1. See AIDS dementia.
  in HIV-infected children, 1815-1816
  JC virus-associated, 2053
  Lyme, 3076
  postvaccination, in infants, 1925
  transmissible spongiform, genetic agents in,
      259t-260t
Endarteritis, obliterative, in syphilis, 3038, 3038f
Endemic infections, versus epidemics, 193
Endobronchial tuberculosis, 3142
Endocarditis, 1067-1112. See also Myocarditis;
      Pericarditis.
  from Actinomyces, 3211-3215
  from Aggregatibacter actinomycetemcomitans,
      3015-3016
  from anaerobic bacilli, 1093
  from anaerobic bacteria, 1084-1085
  from Aspergillus, 1085, 3249
  from Bacillus, 1081t, 1083-1084, 1093
  from Bartonella, 2996-2997
  from Brucella, 2923
  from Candida, 1071, 1085, 3232, 3236
  cardiac conditions and, 1144t, 1145-1146, 1146t
  from cardiac rhythm management device
      infection, 1128
  from Cardiobacterium hominis, 3019
  central nervous system in, 1074
  from Chlamydia, 1094
  from Chlamydophila psittaci, 1086
  clinical manifestations of, 1075-1077, 1076t
  from Coxiella burnetii, 1086, 2515-2516, 2515f
      treatment of, 1094, 2515-2516, 2515f
  culture-negative, 1086, 1094
  dental/diagnostic/therapeutic procedures causing
      bacteremia and, 1144t, 1145, 1146t, 1148,
      1148t
  diagnosis of
      criteria in, 1080, 1080t-1081t
      tests in, 1078-1080
  in drug addicts, 1077
      etiology of, 1085
      management of, 2570, 2571t
  in elderly, 3860
  from Enterobacteriaceae, 1092-1093
  from Enterococcus, 1070-1073, 1070t, 2646
      treatment of, 2648, 2648f
  epidemiology of, 1067-1068
  from Erysipelothrix rhusiopathiae, 2733-2734
  etiologic agents in, 1081-1086, 1081t
  experimental, 1147
  eye in, 1075, 1075f
  fever in, 1076
  fever of unknown origin in, 787
  from fungi, 1085-1086, 1093-1094
  from gram-negative bacilli, 1081t, 1083-1084
  from gram-negative bacteria, 1084
  from gram-positive bacilli, 1084
  from HACEK organisms, 3015-3016
  from Haemophilus, 2918
  health care-associated, 1067
  heart in, 1073-1074
  hemodynamic factors in, 1069
  from Histoplasma capsulatum, 3313, 3317
  immunopathologic factors in, 1073
  in injection drug users, 1077, 3879-3881

Endocarditis (Continued)
  central nervous system manifestations of, 3885
  etiology of, 1085
      HIV and, 3880-3881
      right-sided, 2570, 2571t, 3880
  kidney in, 1074
  from Kingella, 2775
  laboratory findings in, 1077-1080
  from Listeria monocytogenes, 2710
  lung in, 1075
  meningococcal, 1093
  myalgia in, 1320
  mycotic aneurysms in, 1074. See also Mycotic
      aneurysms.
  from Neisseria gonorrhoeae, 1093, 2763
  nonbacterial thrombotic, 1069, 1115-1116
  Osler's nodes in, 799, 1076
  from Pasteurella, 2940
  pathogenesis of, 1068-1073, 1069f
  pathologic changes in, 1073-1075
      cardiac manifestations of, 1073-1074
      cutaneous manifestations of, 1075, 1075f
      mycotic aneurysms as, 1074
      neurologic manifestations of, 1074
      ocular manifestations of, 1075, 1075f
      pulmonary manifestations of, 1074-1075
      renal manifestations of, 1074
      splenic manifestations of, 1074-1075
  pathophysiology of, 1068-1073
  pneumococcal, 1093
  polymicrobial, 1086
  portals of entry in, elimination of, 1143-1144
  predisposing conditions for, correction of, 1143
  prevention of, 1143-1151
      antibiotics in, 1144-1145
      bacterial adherence inhibition in, 1144
      during cardiac surgery, 1148-1149
      chemoprophylaxis in
          for children, 1149
          cost-benefit and cost-effectiveness analyses of,
              1147-1148
          duration of, 1149
          efficacy of, 1146-1147
          evolution of, 1148
          procedural considerations for, 1148-1149
          timing of, 1149
      during diagnostic procedures, 1149
      elimination of portals of entry in, 1143-1144
      immunization in, 1144
      during invasive procedures involving infected
          sites, 1149
      medicolegal liability issues in, 1149
      pathogenetic considerations in, 1143, 1144t
      potential interventions for, 1143-1145
      predisposing conditions and, 1143
      recommendations for, 1148-1149, 1148t
  procedures causing, 1144t, 1145, 1146t, 1148,
      1148t
  prosthetic valve, 1113-1126
      clinical presentation of, 1114-1115
      community-acquired, 1113
      diagnosis of, 1115-1116
          Duke criteria in, 1116
      early-onset, 1114, 1122t, 1123
      epidemiology of, 1113
      health care-associated, 1113
      incidence of, 1113
      inflammatory processes in, 1116
      late-onset, 1114, 1122t, 1123
      microorganisms in, 1115-1116, 1115t
      mortality in
          factors associated with, 1116, 1117t
          in-hospital, 1123
      outcome of, 1123-1124
          after medical versus combined medical-
              surgical therapy, 1123-1124
      pathogenesis of, 1113-1114
      pathology of, 1114
      prevention of, 1148-1149, 1148t
      treatment of, 1116-1123, 1117t
          AHA recommended regimens for, 1118-1123
          combined medical-surgical approach in,
              1116-1117, 1117t
          medical approach in, 1117-1118, 1118t-1122t
          vancomycin/gentamicin in, 456

Endocarditis (Continued)
  from Pseudomonas, 1092-1093
  from Pseudomonas aeruginosa, 2854-2855
  rheumatoid factor in, 1073
  risk for, 1145-1146
      dental/diagnostic/therapeutic procedures and,
          1144t, 1145, 1146t
      preexisting cardiac conditions and, 1144t,
          1145-1146, 1146t
      rate of infection and, 1144t
  skin lesions in, 799, 1075, 1075f, 1304
  from Spirillum minus, 1086
  spleen in, 1074-1075
  from Staphylococcus, 1081t, 1082-1083, 1091-1092
  from Staphylococcus aureus, 1071-1073, 2568-2570
      bacterial adhesins in, 2568-2569
      clinical features of, 2569-2570, 2570f
      diagnosis of, 2570
      epidemiology of, 2568
      host defense in, 2569
      management of, 2570, 2571t
      neurologic complications of, 2569-2570
      pathogenesis of, 2568-2569
      platelets in, 2569
      prosthetic valve, 1113-1115, 1115t
      rifamycins for, 409
      vascular complications of, 2569, 2570f
  from Staphylococcus epidermidis, 409, 1120-1121,
      2582-2583
  from Streptococcus, 1070-1073, 1070t, 1081-1082,
      1081t
      penicillin-resistant, 1089-1090
      penicillin-sensitive, 1088-1089
      treatment of, 1088-1094
  from Streptococcus agalactiae (group B), 2660
  from Streptococcus anginosus group, 2683
  from Streptococcus gordonii, 1071
  from Streptococcus group C and G, 2676
  from Streptococcus mutans, 1070, 1070t
  from Streptococcus pneumoniae, 2633
  from Streptococcus sanguis, 1070-1071, 1070t
  from Streptococcus viridans group, 2668-2670,
      2670t
  transient bacteremia in, 1069-1070, 1070t
  treatment of, 1086-1095
      aminoglycosides in, 379
      antimicrobial, 1088-1094
          monitoring of, 1087-1088
      daptomycin in, 464
      outpatient parenteral antimicrobials in, 699,
          700t
      principles in, 1087
      quinolones in, 501
      surgical, 1094-1095
      teicoplanin in, 459
      vancomycin in, 455-456
          prophylactic, 453
  from Tropheryma whipplei, 1086
  in Whipple's disease, 1437
Endocytosis
  receptor-mediated, 1911, 1911f
  by Salmonella, 2892, 2892f
Endometritis
  from Chlamydia trachomatis, 2454
  postpartum, 1511-1513, 1512f
Endomyocardial biopsy, in myocarditis, 1157-1158
Endomyometritis, postpartum, 1511-1513, 1512f
Endophthalmitis, 1553-1559. See also Ocular
      infections.
  acute postcataract, 1553, 1554f
  anatomic aspects of, 1553, 1554f
  from Aspergillus, 1555-1556
  from Bacillus, 2729
  bacterial
      endogenous, 1554-1555
      treatment of, 1557
      visual outcome after, 1558
  bleb-related, 1553-1554
  from Candida, 1555-1556, 1555f, 1565, 3234,
      3234f
  chronic pseudophakic, 1555, 1557
  classification of, 1553-1556, 1554t
  from coagulase-negative Staphylococcus, 1553,
      2584
  diagnosis of, 1556-1557, 1556f

Endophthalmitis (Continued)
 fungal, 1555-1556, 1555f
  treatment of, 1557-1558
  visual outcome after, 1558
 in injection drug users, 3886-3887
 from Klebsiella pneumoniae, 1554-1555
 pathogenesis of, 1553
 post-traumatic, 1554
 from Propionibacterium acnes, 1555, 1558, 1565
 from Pseudomonas aeruginosa, 2853
 from Sporothrix schenckii, 3272
 from Staphylococcus epidermidis, 1553
 treatment of, 1557-1558
  vancomycin in, 457
 visual outcome after, 1558
Endophthalmitis Vitrectomy Study (EVS), 1557
Endoscopic sinus surgery, 846
Endoscopy
 in Candida esophagitis, 1353, 1354f
 in Clostridium difficile–associated colitis, 1381
 in Helicobacter pylori infection, 2808, 2808t
 in Whipple's disease, 1437f, 1438
Endothelial activation or injury, in severe sepsis,
  993
Endotoxemia, as trigger for severe sepsis, 996-997
Endotoxic shock, complement in, 93
Endotoxin, 2816
Endotracheal aspirate, in nosocomial pneumonia,
  3719-3720
Endotracheal suctioning, blind, in pneumonia, 899
Endotracheal tube
 bacterial colonization of, prevention strategies in,
  3721-3723
 silver-coated, 3723
Endovascular infections, from Pseudomonas
  aeruginosa, 2854-2855
Enfuvirtide, 706t-709t, 1843, 1843f, 1843t
 dosage of, 740t-741t
 formulations of, 717t
 for HIV infection, 22
 for HIV-infected children, 1820t-1821t
Enoxacin, 706t-709t
 dosage of, 732t-733t
 formulations of, 716t
Entamoeba, 3411-3425
Entamoeba chattoni, 3411
Entamoeba dispar, 1035, 3411
 dysentery from, 1392
Entamoeba gingivalis, 3411
Entamoeba hartmannii, 3411
Entamoeba histolytica, 3411-3425
 activated mast cells in, 3416
 adherence of, 3413-3414
 antigen testing for, 3421
 cell biology of, 3412-3413, 3413f
 cell-mediated response to, 3416, 3417f
 clinical manifestations of, 3417-3418
  in amebic diarrhea, 3418
  in amebic dysentery or colitis, 3418, 3419f
  in amebic liver abscess, 3418, 3420f
  in asymptomatic intraluminal disease,
   3417-3418
  in metastatic disease, 3418
 colonoscopy and biopsy in, 3421
 complement interactions with, 85
 culture of, 3421
 cysteine proteinases in, 3415
 cytolysis of, 3414
 diagnosis of, 3420-3422, 3420t
  versus enteric fever, 1400t-1401t, 1404
 epidemiology of, 3416-3417, 3417f
 Gal/GalNAc adherence lectin of, 19-20, 19f
 genome structure in, 3413
 genotypes of, 3411-3412
 gut bacteria effect on, 3415
 immunity to
  acquired, 3416
  innate, 3415-3416, 3415f
 intestinal epithelial cells in, 3416
 life cycle of, 3412, 3412f
 lysis of, complement-mediated, 3416
 macrophages in, 3415, 3415f
 metabolism of, 3412
 metastatic, 3418
 mucosal IgA response to, 3416, 3416f

Entamoeba histolytica (Continued)
 natural killer cells in, 3416
 neutrophils in, 3415
 pathogenesis of, 3413-3415, 3413f
 phagocytosis of, 3414
 polymerase chain reaction testing for, 3421
 prevention of, 3422
 receptors of, 3415
 mRNA expression in, 3413
 serologic tests for, 3421-3422
 stool ova and parasite examination in, 3420-3421
 in travelers, 3416-3417, 3417f
 treatment of, 632t-635t, 650, 3422, 3422t
Entamoeba histolytica DNA, 3413
Entamoeba moshkovskii, 3411
Entamoeba polecki, 3411
Entamoeba suis, 3411
Entecavir, 578-579, 706t-709t
 clinical studies of, 579
 dosage of, 738t-739t
 drug interactions with, 578, 742t-761t
 formulations of, 717t
 for hepatitis B infection, chronic, 1599, 1601t,
  2076, 2076t
 structure of, 578f
Enteral immunonutrition, 155, 155f
Enteral nutrition, 154-155, 155f
Enteric fever. See Typhoid fever.
Enteric fever–like syndromes, 1402-1403
Enteric pathogens
 attachment of, 1341-1342
 in HIV infection, 1860t-1870t, 1880
 host, 1336-1337
 invasiveness of, 1342
Enteritis. See also Diarrhea; Dysentery;
  Gastroenteritis.
 from Campylobacter, 1391, 2796
 from gram-negative anaerobic rods, 3116
 necrotizing, 1394
 parasitic, 1395-1396
 regional, abdominal pain and/or diarrhea with
  eosinophilia from, 1407t, 1409
 from trichinosis, 1392
Enterobacter, 2827
 brain abscess from, 1265, 1266t
 carbapenems for, 342t
 suppurative thrombophlebitis from, 1097-1098
Enterobacter aerogenes, 2827
Enterobacter cloacae, 2827
Enterobacter sakazakii, 2827
Enterobacteriaceae, 2815-2833, 2816t
 adhesins of, 2818-2819
 capsules of, 2816, 2820
 endocarditis from, 1092-1093
 epidemiology of, 2815
 fimbriae of, 2817-2819, 2818f
 flagellae of, 2816-2817, 2818f
 inner membrane of, 2815
 iron acquisition by, 2820
 lipopolysaccharide of, 2816, 2820
 meningitis from, 1212t
 outer membrane of, 2816
 peptidoglycan cell wall of, 2816
 periplasmic space of, 2815-2816
 pili of, 2818-2819
 plasmids of, 2820
 secretion systems of, 2819-2820
 structure and surface antigenic features of,
  2815-2818, 2817f-2818f
 surface polysaccharides of, 2816
 toxins of, 2819-2820
 urinary tract infections from, 3726-3727
 virulence factors of, 2818
Enterobacterial common antigen, 2816
Enterobactin, 2820
Enterobiasis, 632t-635t, 3578t, 3579f-3580f,
  3583-3584
Enterococcus, 2643-2653
 aminoglycoside resistance in, 363
 antimicrobial susceptibility of, 2647-2651, 2648f,
  2649t
 bacteremia from, 2646
 colonization by, 2643
 drug-resistant, mechanisms of, 290t
 endocarditis from, 1070-1073, 1070t, 2646

Enterococcus (Continued)
 prosthetic valve, 1120t, 1122-1123
  treatment of, 2648, 2648f
 epidemiology of, 2645-2646
 genomics of, 2645
 historical perspective on, 2643
 intra-abdominal infections from, 2647
 meningitis from, 2646-2647, 2651
 microbiology of, 2643, 2644f, 2644t-2645t
 neonatal infections from, 2647
 pelvic infections from, 2647
 phenotypic characteristics of, 2644t
 skin and soft tissue infections from, 2647
 taxonomy of, 2643, 2645t
 treatment of, 2647-2651, 2648f, 2649t
  with beta-lactam antibiotics and
   aminoglycosides, 2647-2648
  with daptomycin, 464-465, 2649-2650
  with glycopeptides and lipoglycopeptides, 2649
  with linezolid, 2650
  with quinupristin-dalfopristin, 2650-2651
  with rifamycins, 410
  with tigecycline, 2650
 urinary tract infections from, 2646, 2651
 vancomycin-dependent, 450-451
 vancomycin-resistant, 450-451
  detection of, 242
  epidemiology of, 2645-2646
  linezolid for, 473
  metronidazole and, 423-425
  in spinal cord injury patients, 3855
  treatment of, 2648f
 virulence of, 2643-2644
Enterococcus faecalis
 endocarditis from, prosthetic valve, 1122-1123
 genomics of, 2645
 microbiology of, 2644f, 2645
 quinupristin-dalfopristin-resistant, 460
 suppurative thrombophlebitis from, 1098
 vancomycin-resistant, 2648f
 virulence of, 2644-2645
Enterococcus faecium
 in cancer patients, 3796-3798
 vancomycin-resistant, 461, 2648f
Enterocolitis
 in HIV infection, 1741-1742, 1742t
 inflammatory, differential diagnosis of, 1390t
 necrotizing, in neonates, 1393-1394
 neutropenic (typhlitis), 1064-1065
 from Salmonella, 1392
Enterocytozoonidae. See also Microsporidia.
 in HIV infection, 3398-3399
Enterotoxin(s), 31-32. See also Toxin(s).
 of Bacteroides fragilis, 32
 of Clostridium difficile, 32
 epidemic infantile diarrhea from, 1359-1360,
  1360t
 of Escherichia coli, 2822-2823. See also Escherichia
  coli, enterotoxigenic.
  heat-labile, 32
  heat-stable, 32
 in gastrointestinal infections, 1340-1341, 1340t
 staphylococcal, 2543, 2556
 of Vibrio cholerae, 31-32
Enterovirus 71, 2362
Enteroviruses
 acute hemorrhagic conjunctivitis from, 2360-2361
 bronchiolitis from, 885
 characteristics of, 2337
 classification of, 2337, 2338t
 communicability period of, 2341
 croup from, 825-826, 826f
 detection of, 259t-260t
 diabetes mellitus and, 2361-2362
 dilated cardiomyopathy from, 2358
 encephalitis from, 1246t, 1259
  in immunocompromised hosts, 2359-2360
  nonpoliovirus, 1259, 2354
  poliovirus, 1259
 epidemiology of, 2339-2341, 2340t
 exanthems from, 2354-2355
 gastrointestinal disorders from, 2361
 hand-foot-and-mouth disease from, 2355
 herpangina from, 2355-2356
 host range of, 2338t

Enteroviruses *(Continued)*
  immune response to, 2339
  incidence of, 2340-2341
  incubation period of, 2341
  laboratory diagnosis of, 2341
  meningitis from, 1189, 1204-1205, 1207, 1220,
      2353-2354
    in immunocompromised hosts, 2359-2360
  meningoencephalitis agammaglobulinemia from,
      1205, 1215, 2359-2360
  molecular biology of, 2337-2338, 2338t
  mutation of, 2339
  myocarditis from, 1153, 1155-1156
  myopericarditis from, 2357-2358
  myositis from, 2356-2357
  in neonates, 2358-2359
  paralysis from, nonpoliovirus, 2354
  pathogenesis of, 2338-2339
  pharyngitis from, 817-818
  pleurodynia from, 2356-2357
  prevention of, 2341-2342
  receptors for, 2337, 2338t
  respiratory infections from, 2355-2356
  transmission of, 2340
  treatment of, 2341-2342
Entomophthoramycosis, 3266-3267
  agents of, taxonomic organization of, 3258t
  diagnosis of, 3267
  differential diagnosis of, 3267
  therapy and prevention of, 3267
Entry inhibitors, 1842-1843, 1843f, 1843t
Envelope protein human immunodeficiency virus
      vaccines, 1888, 1890-1891
Envenomation, 1297, 1297t, 3913-3914
Environmental cultures, of *Legionella,* 2980
Environmental decontamination, for Legionnaires'
      disease outbreaks, 2975
Environmental factors, in gastrointestinal infections,
      1336, 1336t
Environmental Protection Agency (EPA),
      bioterrorism and, 3969
Environmental stimuli, in virulence regulation,
      7, 8t
Enzyme(s)
  in antimicrobial resistance, 281-286
  of gram-negative anaerobic rods, 3114
  in quinolone resistance, 490
  of *Staphylococcus aureus,* 2544t, 2553
Enzyme immunoassays
  for *Bartonella,* 3005
  for *Coccidioides,* 3340
  for hepatitis C, 2168-2171
  in HIV-infected children, 1818
  for *Mycoplasma pneumoniae,* 2486
  for noroviruses, 2403
Enzyme-linked immunosorbent assay, 64-65, 64f
  for *Bacillus anthracis,* 3989
  for *Bordetella pertussis,* 2959
  for *Cryptosporidium,* 3553-3554
  for *Entamoeba histolytica,* 3421
  for histoplasmosis, 3314
  for HIV infection
    alternative, 1669-1670
    history of, 1663
    saliva for, 1670
    standard, 1668-1669, 1669f
    urine for, 1670
  for Lyme disease, 3077-3079, 3077f
  for toxoplasmosis, 3509-3510
  for *Yersinia pestis,* 2947-2948
Enzyme-linked immunospot assay, 65-66, 144-145,
      145f
  for ocular syphilis, 1567
  for tuberculosis, 3138
Eosinophil(s), 118-119
  circulating, 119
  development of, 118-119
  granules in, 118-119, 118f
  migration of, 119
Eosinophilia
  abdominal pain and/or diarrhea with, syndrome
      of, 1407-1409, 1407t
  in helminthic infections, 3574
  myalgia with, 1320-1321
  pleural fluid, 920

Eosinophilia *(Continued)*
  pulmonary, tropical, 3592
  in schistosomiasis, 3598
  in strongyloidiasis, 3582
  in travelers, 4026t, 4026t
Eosinophilic folliculitis
  in HIV infection, 1717-1718, 1718f
  pustular, 1292
Eosinophilic gastroenteritis, 3618t, 3621
  abdominal pain and/or diarrhea with eosinophilia
      from, 1407t, 1409
Eosinophilic meningitis, 3618t, 3619-3620
Eosinophilic pneumonia, 908-909
Eperezolid, 472f, 473
Epidemic(s). *See also specific infection.*
  definition of, 193
  emergency preparedness for. *See* Emergency
      preparedness.
  versus endemic infection, 193
Epidemic curves, 194, 195f
Epidemic infantile diarrhea, 1359-1360, 1360t
Epidemic keratoconjunctivitis, 1531-1532
  from adenoviruses, 2029
  differential diagnosis of, 1547
  treatment of, 1548
Epidemic typhus, 2521-2524, 2522f, 2522t-2523t
Epidemiologic studies
  analytic, 182, 182t
  case definition in, 180
  descriptive, 182, 182t
  design considerations in, 181-182
  experimental, 185
  incidence in, 180
  infection versus disease in, 179-180, 185
  methods in, 179-182
  observational, 182-185
  population at risk in, 179-180
  prevalence in, 180
  risk in, 180-181, 181f
  statistics in, 180-181
  types of, 182-185, 182t
Epidemiologist, hospital, 3671
Epidemiology
  agent factors in, 186-187
  of disease outbreaks, 193-197. *See also* Infectious
      disease, outbreaks of.
  disease prevention and control in, 188-190
    assessment of, 188-189
    levels of, 188
    primary, 189-190
    secondary, 190
    tertiary, 190
  goals of, 179
  hospital programs for, 3667-3672, 3670t
  host factors in, 187, 187t
  host-agent relationship in, 185-188
  principles of, 179-191
  transmission routes in, 187-188
Epidermal cyst, infected, 1303
Epidermodysplasia verruciformis, from human
      papillomaviruses, 2039, 2044
Epidermophyton floccosum, 3345-3346
Epididymis, anatomy of, 1521, 1522f
Epididymitis, 1524-1525
  from *Blastomyces dermatitidis,* 3326
  from *Chlamydia trachomatis,* 2451-2452, 2452t
  follow-up in, 1525
  gonococcal, 2759, 2766
  in HIV infection, 1525-1526
  nonspecific bacterial, 1524
  sexually transmitted, 1524-1525
  tuberculous, 1524
Epididymo-orchitis, from mumps virus, 2203
Epidural abscess, 1281-1283, 1283f, 1460-1461, 1461f
  in injection drug users, 3886
Epigallocatechin gallate, 674, 674f
Epiglottitis, 851-854, 852f, 852t
  in adults, 851
  bacterial, 827
  differential diagnosis of, 851
  from *Haemophilus influenzae* type b, 2914
  immunity in, 853
  in immunocompromised hosts, 851-852
  treatment of, 852-853
Epinephrine, nebulized, for croup, 828, 828t

Episiotomy infections, 1513
Epithelial cells
  intestinal, in *Entamoeba histolytica* infection, 3416
  in *Pseudomonas aeruginosa* resistance, 2840, 2841f
Epithelial defect, in keratitis, 1540
Epitope, 60
Epitope spreading, 71
Epitrochlear lymphadenitis, 1324
Epstein-Barr virus/Epstein-Barr virus infection,
      1938t-1940t, 1989-2010
  antibodies to, 2000, 2000t
  autoimmune disease and, 1999
  Burkitt's lymphoma from, 1989, 1996t, 1997
  chronic active, 1995-1996
  chronic fatigue syndrome from, 1897
  in chronic obstructive pulmonary disease, 879
  clinical manifestations of, 1993-1999
  CNS lymphoma from, 1771-1772
  complement interactions with, 85
  detection of, 259t-260t, 2000
  encephalitis from, 1254-1255
  epidemiology of, 1991-1993
  in hematopoietic stem cell transplant recipients,
      3830
  hemophagocytic lymphohistiocytosis from, 1996
  hepatitis from, 1587, 1593
  heterophile antibodies in, 1992, 1999-2000, 1999t
  histopathology of, 1992-1993
  history of, 1989
  in HIV infection, 1877
  Hodgkin's lymphoma from, 1996t, 1997, 1998f,
      2004
  host immune response to, 1992
  infectious mononucleosis from, 1993-1995, 1993t.
      See also Infectious mononucleosis.
  laboratory diagnosis of, 1999-2001
  latency of, 1990-1991, 1990t
  life cycle of, 1990, 1990t
  lymphocytosis in, 1992, 1999, 1999t
  lymphomatoid granulomatosis from, 1998
  lymphoproliferative disease from, 1990t,
      1996-1997, 1996t
    posttransplant, 1996-1997, 1997f, 2001-2002
    treatment of, 2003-2004
    X-linked, 1995
  lytic infections from, 1991
  malignant diseases associated with, 1996-1999,
      1996t
    latency of, 1990t, 1991
    treatment of, 2004
  meningitis from, 1201-1202
  multiple sclerosis and, 1999
  nasal NK and T-cell lymphoma from, 1998
  nasopharyngeal carcinoma from, 1996t,
      1997-1998, 1998f, 2001, 2001f-2002f, 2004
  nosocomial, 3777-3778
  oncogenicity of, 1916, 1940
  oral hairy leukoplakia from, 1996, 2004-2005
  pathogenesis of, 1992-1993
  pharyngitis from, 817
  physical properties of, 1989
  prevention of, 2005
  primary effusion lymphoma from, 1998-1999
  serologic tests for, 261
  serum antibody prevalence of, 1991
  shedding of, 1990, 1990t
  in solid organ transplant recipients, 3848-3849
  transmission of, 1991-1992
  treatment of, 2003-2005
    antiviral agents in, 571
  vaccine for, 2005
  viral load in, 2001
Equine encephalitis, 2117-2125, 2118t. *See also*
      Alphaviruses.
Equivalence trials, 688t, 689. *See also* Clinical trials.
Erm genes, 460
Erosio interdigitalis blastomycetica, 3228, 3229f
Error types, in clinical trials, 691-692
Ertapenem, 706t-709t
  for acute pyelonephritis, 972
  chemistry of, 341, 342f
  clinical use of, 343
  dosage of, 722t
  drug interactions with, 742t-761t
  formulations of, 716t

Ertapenem (Continued)
  pharmacology of, 342
  prophylactic, for surgical procedures, 3899t
Erwinia, 2829
Erysipelas, 1294-1295, 1295f
  from *Staphylococcus aureus*, 2567
  from *Streptococcus pyogenes*, 2601, 2601f
Erysipeloid of Rosenbach, 2733, 2734f
Erysipelothrix rhusiopathiae, 2601, 2733-2735, 2734f
  bite infections from, 3912
  cellulitis from, 1296
  laboratory detection of, 240t-242t
Erythema, 792. *See also* Rash.
  diffuse, 795
Erythema infectiosum, from parvovirus B19,
    2089-2090, 2090f
Erythema marginatum, 795
  in rheumatic fever, 2613-2614, 2615f
Erythema migrans
  in Lyme disease, 3074, 3074f, 3075t
    treatment of, 3079, 3079t
  in tick-borne infections, 3650-3651, 3651f
Erythema multiforme, 794
  from herpes simplex virus, 1948
Erythema multiforme major. *See* Stevens-Johnson
    syndrome.
Erythema necroticans, in leprosy, 3171, 3171f
Erythema nodosum
  in leprosy, 546, 3169-3171, 3171f, 3173
  in *Yersinia enterocolitica* infection, 2951
Erythrasma, 526, 1300
Erythrocyte sedimentation rate, in endocarditis,
    1077
Erythroderma, in sepsis, 1000
Erythroid cells, parvovirus B19 susceptibility of,
    2088
Erythromycin, 427-434, 706t-709t
  for actinomycosis, 3217t
  adverse reactions to, 431
  anti-inflammatory effects of, 430
  antimicrobial activity of, 428-430, 429t
  for bacillary angiomatosis/peliosis, 3005
  for *Campylobacter* infections, 2799
  for cellulitis, 1298
  chemistry of, 427, 428f
  for *Chlamydophila* respiratory infection, 2471,
    2471t
  for cutaneous diphtheria, 1298
  for diphtheria, 2692
  distribution of, 430
  for donovanosis, 3013
  drug interactions with, 431-432, 431t, 742t-761t
  for erysipelas, 1295
  for erythrasma, 1300
  for Legionnaires' disease, 2978t
  for louse-borne relapsing fever, 3068-3069
  for Lyme disease, 3079t
  for lymphadenitis, 1330
  mechanism of action of, 427
  for *Mycoplasma pneumoniae*, 2487
  for *Neisseria gonorrhoeae* infection, 2765
  for perinatal chlamydial infections, 2456
  for pertussis, 2960
  pharmacology of, 430-431, 430t
  preparations of, 427
  prokinetic effects of, 430
  for Q fever pneumonia, 2514
  resistance to
    enzymes in, 285
    mechanisms of, 427-428
  serum levels of, 430, 430t
  for tick-borne relapsing fever, 3068-3069
  for urethritis, 1490-1491
  uses of, 432-434, 432t-433t
Erythromycin base, 427, 428f
  for chancroid, 2917
  dosage of, 726t-727t
  formulations of, 716t
Erythromycin estolate, 706t-709t, 716t, 726t-727t
Erythromycin ethyl succinate, 706t-709t
  dosage of, 726t-727t
  formulations of, 716t
Erythromycin gluceptate, 706t-709t
  dosage of, 726t-727t
  formulations of, 716t

Erythromycin lactobionate, 706t-709t
  dosage of, 726t-727t
  formulations of, 716t
Erythromycin stearate, 706t-709t
  dosage of, 726t-727t
  formulations of, 716t
Erythroplasia of Queyrat, 2040
Eschar
  in rickettsialpox, 2509, 2509f
  in scrub typhus, 2529
Escherichia albertii, 2826, 2828
Escherichia blattae, 2826
Escherichia coli, 2820-2826
  clonal analysis of, 7
  dacryocystitis from, 1571
  diarrhea from, 205-206
  diarrheogenic
    pathogenic mechanisms of, 1339-1340, 1339t
    summary of, 2821t
  diffusely adherent, 2821t, 2824f, 2826
  disinfection/sterilization and, 3688
  enteroaggregative, 2821t, 2824f, 2825-2826
    chronic enteritides from, 1395
  enterohemorrhagic, 2821t, 2824-2825, 2825f
    detection of, 242
    virulence factors of, 5t
  enteroinvasive, 2821t, 2826
    diarrhea from, 1391
    dysentery from, 1390-1391, 1390t
    virulence factors of, 5t
  enteropathogenic, 2821t, 2823-2824, 2823f-2824f
    attaching and effacing effect of, 2823, 2823f
    breastfeeding protection against, 2824
    chronic diarrhea from, 1395
    epidemic infantile diarrhea from, 1359-1360,
      1360t
    pseudopod formation by, 9, 9f
  enterotoxigenic, 1340-1341, 1340t, 2821t,
      2822-2823
    cholera-like syndrome from, 1363
    travelers diarrhea from, 1366, 1366t
    travelers' diarrhea from, 2823
    virulence factors of, 5t
    weanling diarrhea from, 1361
  enterotoxins of, 2822-2823
    heat-labile, 32
    heat-stable, 32
  extraintestinal
    pathogenic, 2821-2822
    virulence factors of, 5t
  fecal examination for, 1344
  foodborne disease from, 1414t, 1415-1416,
      1418-1419
  hemolysins of, 2819
  inner membrane of, 2815
  invasive
    dysentery from, 2905, 2906f
    laboratory findings in, 2908
    mucosal invasion by, 2906
  invasiveness of, 1342
  laboratory diagnosis of, 240t-242t, 1422
  meningitis from, 1211t
  multidrug resistance AcrAB-TolC efflux pump in,
      291, 291f
  peritonitis from, 1013-1014
  quinolone resistance in, 489, 502
  Shiga toxin–producing, 2821t, 2824-2825, 2825f
  Shigella-like, 2905
  toxins of, 1340t, 1341
  urinary tract infections from, 3726-3727
  uropathogenic, 958-961, 964, 2821
    adhesins of, 16f, 20-21, 20f, 959-960, 959t
    P fimbriae of, 16f, 20-21, 20f, 959-960
    type 1 fimbriae of, 960
    type 3 fimbriae of, 960
    virulence characteristics of, 960
    virulence regulatory systems for, 8t
Escherichia coli O157:H7, 180
Escherichia fergusonii, 2826
Escherichia vulneris, 2826
ESKAPE pathogens, 511
Esophageal candidiasis, as AIDS indicator, 1643
Esophageal disease
  in *Helicobacter pylori* infection, 2806t, 2807
  in HIV infection, 1737-1738

Esophagitis, 1353-1358
  from *Candida*, 1353-1354, 1354f, 3227-3228, 3228f
    treatment of, 1355-1357, 1355t, 3237
  clinical manifestations of, 1353
  from cytomegalovirus, 1354
  etiology of, 1353-1355, 1354f, 1354t
  from herpes simplex virus, 1354-1355, 1355f,
      1952-1953
  in HIV infection, 1737
  treatment of, 1355-1357
    general considerations in, 1355-1356, 1355t
    in HIV infection, 1356-1357, 1356t
Esophagography, in *Candida* esophagitis, 1353-1354,
      1354f
Esophagus
  aphthous ulceration of, 1355, 1355t
  Barrett's, in *Helicobacter pylori* infection, 2806t,
      2807
  enlarged, in American trypanosomiasis, 3484,
      3485f, 3487
  perforation of, mediastinitis secondary to, 1173,
      1175t
Espundia, 3471f, 3472-3473
Estrogen
  deficiency of
    urinary tract infection and, 958
    vaginitis from, 1506
  innate immunity and, 45
  for urinary tract infection prophylaxis, 975
  vulvovaginal candidiasis and, 1500
Ethambutol, 706t-709t
  adverse reactions to, 538
  for brain abscess, 1274t
  dosage of, 734t-735t
  formulations of, 717t
  for *Mycobacterium avium* complex disease,
      3184t-3186t
  for *Mycobacterium kansasii* pulmonary disease
      from, 3193, 3193t
  for nontuberculous mycobacterial infections,
      543
  for tuberculosis, 534t, 537t, 538, 3144-3145, 3145t,
      3149
Ethionamide, 706t-709t
  dosage of, 734t-735t
  drug interactions with, 742t-761t
  formulations of, 717t
  for leprosy, 546
  for tuberculosis, 542
Ethmoid sinus, anatomy and physiology of, 839
Ethnicity
  chronic pneumonia and, 931
  HAV incidence rate by, 2374-2375, 2374f
  HIV infection and, 1781
  Neisseria gonorrhoeae infection and, 2758, 2758t
  tuberculosis and, 3132-3133
Ethylene oxide, sterilization with, 3685t, 3686-3687
Ethylenediamine-SQ109, for tuberculosis, 542
Etoposide, for Kaposi's sarcoma, 1767
Etravirine, 706t-709t, 1837f, 1837t, 1838
  dosage of, 740t-741t
  drug interactions with, 742t-761t
  formulations of, 717t
  for HIV-infected children, 1820t-1821t
  resistance to, 1838
Eubacterium, 3126
Eugonic fermenter-4 bacteria, 3021
Eumycetoma, 3281, 3282t, 3283f
  treatment of, 3284-3285
European encephalitis, 2138t
Eustachian tube, rhinoviral infection affecting, 2393
Evernimicin, 728t-729t
Ewingella americana, 2829
Exanthem(s), 792, 797. *See also* Rash.
  in acute HIV infection, 1716
  from enteroviruses, 2354-2355
  vesicular stomatitis with. *See* Hand-foot-and-
      mouth disease.
Exanthem subitum, from human herpesvirus 6,
      2012, 2012f
Exclusion criteria, in clinical trials, 690
Exercise, for chronic fatigue syndrome, 1901
Exfoliative toxins, of *Staphylococcus aureus*,
      2553-2554
Exoenzymes, of *Pseudomonas aeruginosa*, 2845

Exophiala (Wangiella) jeanselmei, 3371
Exotoxin(s). *See also* Toxin(s).
   Corynebacterium diphtheriae, 2687-2688
   Pseudomonas, 30
   streptococcal, 33, 2604
Exotoxin A, of *Pseudomonas aeruginosa,* 2844-2845
Experimental studies, 185
   clinical trials as, 185
   community intervention trials as, 185
Explanatory trials, 689. *See also* Clinical trials.
External auditory canal infection. *See* Otitis externa.
Extracutaneous sporotrichosis, 3271-3272,
      3272f-3273f. *See also* Sporotrichosis.
   multifocal, 3272-3273, 3273f
EYAV virus, 2102
Eye. *See also* Ocular *entries.*
   candidemic seeding of, 1555, 1555f
   in host defense, 41
   pain in, in keratitis, 1540
   pink, 1531-1533, 1532f, 1533t
   protection for, 3673, 3674t
   red, differential diagnosis of, 1537
Eyelid
   anatomy of, 1569, 1570f
   infections of, 1569, 1570f

F

Fab fragment, 60, 60f-61f
Face, dermatophytosis of, 3349, 3349f
Face mask, isolation, 3673, 3674t
Facial infections. *See* Orofacial infections.
Facial palsy, in Lyme disease, 3074-3075, 3075t
Factitial disease, 1309
Factitious fever, 787-788
Factor H, 78t, 81t, 82
   deficiency of, 92, 169t-170t
Factor I, 78t, 81t
   deficiency of, 169t-170t
Famciclovir, 566t-567t, 579-580, 706t-709t
   clinical studies of, 580
   dosage of, 738t-739t
   formulations of, 717t
   for herpes simplex virus esophagitis, 1355t
   for herpes simplex virus infection, 1956, 1957t
   prophylactic, for cancer-related infections, 3802
   in renal insufficiency, 579, 579t
   for varicella-zoster virus, 1967
Familial insomnia, fatal, 2428-2429
Familial Mediterranean fever, 1297, 1297t
Far Eastern encephalitis, 2138t
Fascial spaces
   anatomy of, 858, 859f
   deep, infections of, 859f, 860-864, 863f. *See also*
      Odontogenic infections.
Fasciitis, necrotizing. *See* Necrotizing fasciitis.
Fasciola hepatica, 3596t, 3597f, 3600-3602, 3601f
Fascioliasis, 648-650
Fasciolopsis buski, 3596t, 3602
Fat, dietary, in tropical sprue, 1430-1431
Fatigue
   chronic, 1897-1904, 1898t. *See also* Chronic
      fatigue syndrome.
   postinfection, 1898
   after Q fever, 2516-2517
Fatty acids, 154
   omega-3, 154
Favus, 3347, 3350
Fc receptors, 60, 60f, 63, 63t
Fc region of antibodies, 60, 60f-61f
FcγR, in opsonization, 63
FcγRIIB, 68
FcgRIII receptor, in disease susceptibility, 52
Febrile neutropenia, 782, 782t. *See also* Cancer,
      infections in; Neutropenia.
   in cancer patients, treatment of, 3802-3806
      with abdominal symptoms, 3805-3806
      for catheter-related infection, 3805
      colony-stimulating factors in, 3806
      empirical antibacterial, 3804-3805, 3805t
      empirical or preemptive antifungal, 3805
      granulocyte transfusions in, 3806
      in high-risk patient, 3803-3804, 3804t
      in low-risk patient, 3802-3803, 3803t
      with pulmonary infiltrates, 3805

Febrile neutropenia *(Continued)*
   steroids in, 3806
   caspofungin for, 560
   origin of, 3787-3788, 3787f
   Pseudomonas aeruginosa in, 2855-2856
   quinolones for, 501
   vancomycin for, 457
   voriconazole for, 558
Febrile response. *See also* Fever.
   acute-phase response and, 770-771, 770t-771t
   definition of, 765
   endogenous antipyretics in, 771-772, 772f
   endogenous pyrogens in, 769-770, 770f, 772
   evolutionary perspective on, 772-773, 772f
   exogenous pyrogens in, 769
   model for, 770f
Febrile seizure, 774-775
Fecal examination
   in *Campylobacter* infections, 2798, 2798f
   in *Cryptosporidium* infections, 3553-3554,
      3553f
   in *Entamoeba histolytica* infection, 3420-3421
Fecal flora, metronidazole effects on, 423
Fecal pH, 1344
Femoral buboes, in bubonic plague, 2946, 2946f
Fermenters, glucose, 3015-3021, 3016t-3017t
Ferripyochelin, 2844
Fertility. *See* Infertility.
Fetus
   maternal HIV infection impact on, 1788
   monitoring of, in HIV-infected mother,
      1794-1795
   parvovirus B19 infection in, 2091
   rubella vaccine effects on, 2131
   rubella virus effects on, 2129, 2129t
Fever. *See also* Febrile *entries; specific fever.*
   from alphaviruses, 2120-2121, 2123
   beneficial effects of, 772-773
   dermatologic conditions associated with, 797
   in elderly, 3861
   in endocarditis, 1076, 1114-1115
   evaluation of, thermometry in, 765-768, 767f
   hemorrhagic. *See* Hemorrhagic fever.
   historical perspective on, 765
   in HIV infection, 1713
   from influenza, 2274
   in leprosy, 546
   patterns in, 783, 784f
   periodic, 788
      with aphthous ulcers, pharyngitis, and adenitis,
         1327
      of unknown origin, 788
   postoperative, 781
   postpartum, of undetermined origin, 1513
   rat-bite, 2965-2968, 2966t. *See also* Rat-bite
      fever.
   relapsing. *See* Relapsing fever.
   rheumatic, 2611-2622. *See also* Rheumatic
      fever.
   risk-benefit considerations for, 772-773
   in spinal cord injury patients, 3851-3852
   terminology of, 765, 779, 783
   in transplant recipients, 3816-3817
   travel-related, 4019-4025
      considerations for, 4021-4024
      initial approach to, 4024-4025
      skin eruptions accompanying, 4026, 4027f
   treatment of, 773-776. *See also* Antipyretics.
   of unknown origin, 779-789
      in children, 779-781, 783
      classical, 779-781, 780f, 780t
      clinical evaluation of, 782-786, 783t
      comprehensive history in, 783
      definitions of, 779, 780t
      in disseminated granulomatoses, 786
      drug-induced, 787
      in elderly, 781, 781t, 3861
      in endocarditis, 787
      factitious, 787-788
      fever patterns in, 783, 784f
      fever verification in, 783
      health care-associated, 780t, 781-782
      HIV infection-related, 782, 783t
      imaging studies in, 785
      immune-deficient, 780t, 782

Fever *(Continued)*
   in infants, 779-781, 783
   infections responsible for, 779, 780t
   in intensive care unit patients, 781-782
   invasive diagnostic procedures in, 785
   laboratory tests in, 784-785
   in lymphoma, 786
   neutropenic, 782, 782t. *See also* Febrile
      neutropenia.
   periodic, 788
   physical findings in, 783-784, 785t
   in polymyalgia rheumatica, 787
   in postoperative patients, 781
   prognosis for, 786
   in returning travelers, 781, 781t
   selected causes of, 786-788
   in Still's disease, 787
   in stroke patients, 782
   in temporal arteritis, 787
   therapeutic trials in, 785-786
   in thromboembolic disease, 786-787
   treatment of, 786
      limitations and risks of, 786
   verification of, 783
F(ab′₂) fragment of antibodies, 60, 61f
Fibrin, in peritoneal cavity, 1018
Fibrinolytic therapy, for pleural effusion/empyema,
      922
Fibromyalgia, 1901
Fibrosing mediastinitis, tuberculous, 3158
Fibrosis
   cystic. *See* Cystic fibrosis.
   hepatitis C–related, 2166
      noninvasive markers of, 2169-2170
   mediastinal, from *Histoplasma capsulatum,* 3310,
      3310f, 3316
   pulmonary, diffuse, 935t-936t, 938
Fifth disease. *See* Erythema infectiosum.
Filariasis, 2495, 3589-3592, 3590t
   in lymphadenitis, 1327
   in lymphangitis, 1331
   lymphatic, 3590-3592
      clinical features of, 3590-3591, 3591f
      diagnosis of, 3591
      epidemiology of, 3590
      parasites in, 3590
      pathogenesis of, 3591
      prevention, control, and eradication of,
         3591-3592
      treatment of, 3591
   treatment of, 632t-635t
Filgrastim, 611-612
Filoviruses, 2259-2263
   characteristics of, 2259, 2260f, 3997t
   clinical manifestations of, 2262
   detection of, 259t-260t
   diagnosis of, 2262
   epidemiology of, 2259-2262, 2261f
   pathology and pathogenesis of, 2262
   prevention and treatment of, 2262-2263
   rash from, 802
   transmission of, 2260-2262
FimA gene, 1071
Fimbriae
   in bacterial meningitis, 1195
   of enterobacteriaceae, 2817-2819, 2818f
   of gram-negative anaerobic rods, 3113
   of uropathogenic *Escherichia coli*
      P, 16f, 20-21, 20f, 959-960
      type 1, 960
      type 3, 960
Finegoldia magna, 3123t
Finger(s)
   Candida infection between, 3228, 3229f
   herpes simplex virus infection of, 1951-1952
First-pass effect, 297
Fish, poisonous, 1416-1417, 1417t, 1419-1420, 3569,
      3570t
Fish oils, 154
Fish tapeworms, 3608-3609, 3608t, 3609f
Fistula
   bronchopleural
      empyema in, 922-923
      tuberculous, 3155
   pharyngocutaneous, postradiation, 868

Fite staining, of *Mycobacterium leprae*, 3169, 3169f-3170f
Fitz-Hugh–Curtis syndrome
  Neisseria gonorrhoeae infection in, 2761
  in peritonitis, 1014
Flagellae
  of *Campylobacter jejuni*, 2795-2796
  of Enterobacteriaceae organisms, 2816-2817, 2818f
  of *Pseudomonas aeruginosa*, 2842-2843
Flash sterilization, 3686
Flaviviruses, 2133-2156, 4000t-4001t
  characteristics of, 2135, 3997t
  clinical features of, 2144-2148
  encephalitis from, 2141f, 2143-2144, 2150-2152, 2151t
  epidemiology of, 2135-2141
  geographic distribution of, 2134f
  historical perspective on, 2133-2135
  laboratory diagnosis of, 2148-2149
  less common, 2152-2153, 2152t
  pathogenesis of, 2141-2144
  prevention of, 2149-2152
  rash from, 802
  treatment of, 2149-2152
Flavobacterium, 3016t, 3024
Fleas
  infectious diseases from, 3639, 3639t
  plague from, 2944-2945, 2945f
  sand, tungiasis from, 3639-3641, 3639t, 3640f
Flies
  myiasis from, 3637-3639, 3638t
  sand, in leishmaniasis transmission, 3464-3465, 3465f
  tsetse, in African trypanosomiasis transmission, 3489
Flomoxef, 706t-709t
Flow cytometry, 144, 145f
Flucloxacillin, 317, 317f, 706t-709t
  dosage of, 316t, 718t-719t
  formulations of, 715t
  for *Staphylococcus aureus* endocarditis, 2571t
  for *Staphylococcus aureus* osteomyelitis, 2574
Fluconazole, 555-557, 706t-709t
  for *Blastomyces dermatitidis* infection, 3329t, 3330
  for brain abscess, 1274t
  for *Candida* esophagitis, 1355t, 1356-1357
  for candiduria, 3237
  for *Coccidioides* infection, 3340-3341
  for cryptococcal meningitis, 3298-3299
    in HIV infection, 1746, 3299
  for cutaneous leishmaniasis, 3475
  for dermatophytosis, 3352
  dosage of, 736t-737t
  drug interactions with, 556t, 742t-761t
  for febrile neutropenia, 3804t
  formulations of, 717t
  for fungal arthritis, 1451-1452
  for fungal endophthalmitis, 1557-1558
  for mucosal candidiasis, 1797
  for peritonitis, 1029t
  prophylactic
    for cancer-related infections, 3800t
    in transplant recipients, 3816
  for prosthetic valve endocarditis, 1121t
  for sporotrichosis, 3274
  structure of, 550f-551f
  for suppurative thrombophlebitis, 1098
  for vulvovaginal candidiasis, 1501
Flucytosine, 553-554, 706t-709t
  for brain abscess, 1274t
  for candidiasis, 3236
  for cryptococcal meningitis, 3298
    in HIV infection, 1746
  dosage of, 736t-737t
  formulations of, 717t
  mechanism of action of, 551f
  for prosthetic valve endocarditis, 1121t
Fludrocortisone, for sepsis, 619
Fluid balance, gastrointestinal, 1343, 1343f
Fluid overload, in poststreptococcal glomerulonephritis, 2619
Fluid therapy
  for *Campylobacter* infections, 2798-2799
  for cholera, 2781, 2782t
  for CNS infections, 1187-1188

Fluid therapy *(Continued)*
  for cryptosporidiosis, 3554
  for infectious diarrhea, 1347
  for peritonitis, 1026
  for sepsis, 1002-1003
  for streptococcal toxic shock syndrome, 2605
  in urinary tract infection, 970
Flukes, 3574t, 3595-3605
  abdominal pain and/or diarrhea with eosinophilia from, 1407t, 1409
  foodborne disease from, 3603
  intestinal, 3596t, 3602
  life cycle of, 3597f
  liver, 1407t, 1409, 3596t, 3597f, 3600-3602, 3601f
  lung, 3596t, 3602-3603
  treatment of, 632t-635t
Fluorescence-activated cell sorting (FACS) analysis, 168
Fluorescence-linked immunosorbent assay (FLISA), 64-65
Fluorescent antibody test
  direct
    for *Bordetella pertussis*, 2959
    for *Legionella pneumophila*, 2977, 2977t
    for rabies, 2254
    stains for, 244, 244t
  indirect
    for ehrlichiosis, 2534-2535
    for *Toxoplasma gondii*, 3509
Fluorescent stains, 244, 244t
  for microbacteria, 251
Fluorescent treponemal antibody absorption test
  for neurosphylitic meningitis, 1210
  for syphilis, 3045-3046
Fluoride, for dental caries prophylaxis, 869
5-Fluorocytosine
  for endocarditis, 1093-1094
  structure of, 550f-551f
  for suppurative thrombophlebitis, 1098
Fluorodeoxyglucose positron emission tomography, in prosthetic joint infections, 1470-1471
Fluorometric assays, for chronic granulomatous disease, 115-116
Fluoroquinolones. *See* Quinolones.
5-Fluorouracil, for condylomata acuminata, 2044
Flying squirrels, typhus borne by, 2522
Folate, 153
  deficiency of, in tropical sprue, 1431
  trimethoprim effects on, 479
  for tropical sprue, 1432
Folate antagonists
  formulations of, 716t
  for parasitic infections, 650-651
Folinic acid
  for *Isospora belli* infection, 3563
  for *Toxoplasma* encephalitis, 1750-1751
  for toxoplasmosis
    in HIV infection, 3516, 3518, 3518t
    in pregnant patient, 3520
Follicle mites, 3645
Follicles, conjunctival, 1530
Folliculitis, 1292
  from *Candida*, 1292, 3229, 3229f
  eosinophilic
    in HIV infection, 1717-1718, 1718f
    pustular, 1292
  hot tub, 798, 2854
  from *Malassezia*, 3354
  from *Pseudomonas aeruginosa*, 1292
  from *Staphylococcus aureus*, 2566
Fomivirsen, 566t-567t, 580
Food(s)
  biological weapon dispersal via, 3955
  drug interactions of
    with metronidazole, 421t, 423
    with tetracycline, 392, 393t
  selection, preparation, and storage of, in infection prevention, 1424
Foodborne disease, 1413-1427
  abdominal cramps and diarrhea in
    within 6 to 48 hours, 1415
    within 8 to 16 hours, 1414-1415
    within 16 to 72 hours, 1415
  abdominal cramps without diarrhea in, 1415
  from *Amanita*, 1417t, 1418

Foodborne disease *(Continued)*
  from *Bacillus cereus*, 1413-1415, 1414t-1415t, 1418
  from *Bacillus* spp., 2728-2729
  from *Campylobacter jejuni*, 1414t, 1415
  clinical features of, 1413-1418
  from *Clostridium botulinum*, 1414t-1415t, 1416, 1419, 3097-3098
  from *Clostridium difficile*, 1413
  from *Clostridium perfringens*, 1414-1415, 1414t, 1418, 3107
  from *Corinub*, 1417-1418, 1417t
  from *Cyclospora*, 1419
  diarrhea in
    abdominal cramps and, 1414-1415
    persistent, 1416
    vomiting and, 1415
    without fever, 1415-1416
  epidemiology of, 1418-1421, 1419t-1420t
  from *Escherichia coli*, 1414t, 1415-1416, 1418-1419
  etiology of, 1419t
  from fish, 1416-1417, 1417t, 1419-1420
  food in, 1418-1420, 1419t
  food-specific attack rates of, 1420-1421, 1420t
  geographic location of, 1419t, 1420
  from *Gyromitra*, 1417t, 1418
  from heavy metals, 1419
  from hepatitis A, 2372, 2376
  incidence of
    from 1996-2007, 1413, 1414f
    associated with different pathogens, 1413, 1414t
    of known cause reported to CDC, 1413, 1414t
  laboratory diagnosis of, 1421-1423, 1421t
  from *Listeria monocytogenes*, 1413, 1414t, 1415, 1418-1419
  nausea and vomiting in, 1413-1414, 1416
    with diarrhea and paralysis, 1416
  from noroviruses, 1414t, 1415, 1419, 2401
  outbreaks of, 194
  paresthesia in, 1416-1418
  pathogenesis of, 1413-1418
  population changes in, 1420
  postinfection syndromes in, 1416
  prevention of, 1424-1425, 1425t
  from *Salmonella*, 1414t, 1415, 1418-1419, 2889-2891, 2889f, 2900
  seasonality of, 1419t, 1420
  from shellfish, 1416-1417, 1417t
  from *Shigella*, 1414t, 1415, 1419
  spectrum of, 1413
  from *Staphylococcus aureus*, 2556
  from *Staphylococcus epidermidis*, 1413
  surveillance of, 182-183, 1424
  systemic illness in, 1416
  toxins in
    bacterial, 1413-1416, 1415t
    nonbacterial, 1416-1418, 1417t
  in travelers, 4021
    protection against, 4015
  treatment of, 1423-1424, 1423t
  from *Trichinella*, 1414t, 1416, 1419
  from *Vibrio cholerae*, 1413, 1414t, 1415, 1419
  from *Vibrio parahaemolyticus*, 1414t, 1415
  from *Vibrio vulnificus*, 1416
  vomiting and nonbloody diarrhea in, 1415
  from *Yersinia enterocolitica*, 1414t, 1415, 1419
Food-handling errors, 1424-1425
FoodNet, 182-183
Foot
  athlete's, 3348
  chromoblastomycosis of, 3277, 3278f
  dermatophytosis of, 3348, 3352, 3352t
  insensitive, in leprosy, 3174
  mycetoma of, 3282f. *See also* Mycetoma.
  osteomyelitis of, 1461-1462
  ulceration of, in diabetic patient, 1300-1302, 1461-1462, 1462t
Foramen of Winslow, 1011, 1012f
Foreign bodies
  and antimicrobial activity, 272
  aspiration of, versus croup, 828
  infection from, rifamycin prophylaxis for, 410
  in surgical site infections, 3894

Formaldehyde, in urine, factors affecting, 518
Formulary decisions, in antimicrobial stewardship,
    678-679, 682
Fosamprenavir, 706t-709t, 1839f, 1840t, 1841
    dosage of, 740t-741t
    drug interactions with, 742t-761t
    formulations of, 717t
    for HIV-infected children, 1820t-1821t, 1823t
Foscarnet, 566t-567t, 580-582, 706t-709t
    activity spectrum of, 580-581
    clinical studies of, 582
    for cytomegalovirus encephalitis, 1754
    for cytomegalovirus esophagitis, 1355t, 1356
    for cytomegalovirus infection, 1977-1978
        in hematopoietic stem cell transplant recipients,
            3828, 3829t
    dosage of, 738t-739t
    drug interactions with, 581, 742t-761t
    formulations of, 717t
    for herpes simplex virus esophagitis, 1355t
    for herpes simplex virus infection, 1957t
    mechanism of action of, 581
    pharmacokinetics of, 581, 581t
    for progressive outer retinal necrosis, 1567
    resistance to, 581
    structure of, 576f
    toxicity of, 581-582
Fosfomycin, 706t-709t
    dosage of, 732t-733t
    formulations of, 716t
Fournier's gangrene, 627, 1308
Fracture
    basilar skull, meningitis from, 1209, 1223
    contaminated open, osteomyelitis after, 1460
Francisella holarctica, 2927, 2928t
Francisella novicida, 2927, 2928t
Francisella pathogenicity island (FPI) genes,
    2928-2929
Francisella philomiragia, 2928t, 2929
Francisella tularensis, 2927-2937, 3655-3656. See also
    Tularemia.
    as biological weapon, 2927, 3952, 3971-3975
    description of, 2927-2929
    differentiation of, 2928
    genomic and proteomic analyses of, 2928-2929
    growth characteristics of, 2928
    laboratory detection of, 240t-242t
    subspecies of, 2927, 2928t
Frequency, urinary, 968-969, 968f, 973-974
Friedlander's disease, 2826
Frontal sinus, anatomy and physiology of, 839
Fumagillin, 651
    for microsporidiosis, 3401t, 3402-3403
Fungal infections. See also specific infection.
    antifungal agents for, 549-563. See also Antifungal
        agents.
    blood culture for, 236-238, 237t
    brain abscess from, 1266, 1266t, 1275
    in cancer patients, 3793, 3796t, 3798-3799
    conjunctivitis from, 1536-1537, 1537f
    diagnosis of, 3222-3223, 3223f-3224f, 3224t
    endemic, 1302
    endocarditis from, 1085-1086, 1093-1094
        prosthetic valve, 1121t, 1123
    endophthalmitis from, 1555-1556, 1555f
        treatment of, 1557-1558
        visual outcome after, 1558
    epidemiology of, 3223-3224
    granulocyte-macrophage colony-stimulating factor
        for, 614
    after hematopoietic stem cell transplantation,
        3830
    in HIV infection, fluconazole prophylaxis for, 557
    interferon-gamma for, 616
    keratitis from, 1548-1550, 1549f
    in liver transplant recipients, 3842
    of nails. See Onychomycosis.
    opportunistic, 3370
    in pancreatitis, 1052
    pneumonia from, 892t
    rifamycins for, 412
    sinusitis from, 841-842, 842t
        allergic, 3245-3246, 3248, 3248f, 3368, 3368f
    systemic, cutaneous involvement in, 1303-1305
    in transplant recipients, 3812t

Fungemia, skin lesions in, 1304-1305
Fungi, 3221-3224. See also specific fungus.
    antigen tests for, 245-246, 246t
    appearance of, 3223f-3224f, 3224t
    culture media for, 244-245, 245t
    in cystic fibrosis, 951
    dark-walled, 3367-3369, 3367t, 3374t
    epidemiology of, 256
    identification of, 256
    isolation of, significance of, 256
    laboratory tests for, 236-243, 254-257, 255t
    microscopic stains for, 244, 244t
    nucleic acid–based tests for, 246-247, 246t
    pathogenic, features of, 3221-3222, 3222t
    relationship of microsporidia to, 3394
    safety issues for, 254-255
    serologic tests for, 256-257, 3222-3223
    in sinusitis, 841-842, 842t
    specimens containing
        collection and transport, and processing of, 255
        direct detection of, 255-256
    spores of, 3221-3222
    susceptibility testing of, 256
    taxonomy of, 3221
    terminology for, 254, 255t
    yeast-like
        appearance of, 3223f-3224f, 3224t
        features of, 3221-3222
Fungicide, 3677
Furazolidone, 706t-709t
    for cholera, 2782t
    drug interactions with, 742t-761t
    for giardiasis, 3531, 3531t
    for microsporidiosis, 3402
    for parasitic infections, 651-652
Furuncles (boils), 1292-1293
    from Staphylococcus aureus, 2566
Fusarium, 3369-3370, 3369f-3370f, 3374t
    keratitis from, 1549
Fusidic acid, 355-357, 528t, 530
    adverse reactions to, 356, 530
    antimicrobial activity of, 355, 356t
    dosage of, 355, 356t, 728t-729t
    drug interactions with, 356
    formulations of, 716t
    mechanism of action of, 355
    pharmacology of, 355-356, 356t
    resistance to, 355
    Staphylococcus aureus resistance to, 2559t
    structure of, 355
    uses of, 356
Fusobacterium
    antibiotic sensitivities of, 3117t
    microbiology of, 3112, 3112f, 3112t
Fusobacterium necrophorum, virulence factors
    associated with, 3087-3088, 3087t
Fusobacterium nucleatum
    dental caries from, 856, 856t
    virulence factors associated with, 3087-3088, 3087t

G
Galactomannan assay, in chronic pneumonia,
    934-937
α-Galactosyl ceramide, CD1-presented, 137
Gal/GalNac adherence lectin of Entamoeba
    histolytica, 19-20, 19f, 3413-3414
Gallbladder
    actinomycosis of, 3213-3214
    fungus balls in, 3233
GALT, as HIV reservoir, 1693-1694
Ganciclovir, 566t-567t, 582-585, 706t-709t
    activity spectrum of, 568t, 582
    clinical studies of, 584-585
    for cytomegalovirus, 1976-1977
        in hematopoietic stem cell transplant recipients,
            3828, 3829t
        prophylactic, 1979-1980
        resistance to, 1977, 1977f
    for cytomegalovirus colitis, 1976
    for cytomegalovirus encephalitis, 1754
    for cytomegalovirus esophagitis, 1355t
    for cytomegalovirus retinitis, 1975-1976
        sustained-release, 1976
    dosage of, 738t-739t

Ganciclovir (Continued)
    drug interactions with, 583-584, 742t-761t
    formulations of, 717t
    for herpes B virus, 2025
    for lymphoproliferative disease, 2004
    mechanism of action of, 582
    pharmacokinetics of, 583, 583t
    for progressive outer retinal necrosis, 1567
    prophylactic, in transplant recipients, 3815
    resistance to, 583
    structure of, 568f
    toxicity of, 584
    in transplant recipients, 1981
Gangosa, 3056, 3056f
Gangrene
    differential diagnosis of, 1301t
    Fournier's, 1308
    gas. See Gas gangrene.
    infectious, 1298-1300
    Meleney's, 3084, 3085f
    progressive bacterial synergistic, 1299, 1299f, 1301t
    pulmonary, 926
    streptococcal, 1299, 1301t, 2602
    symmetric peripheral, 797-798
    treatment of, 1300
    vascular, infected, 1319
Gangrenous stomatitis, 861t, 866
Gardnerella, 3028-3029
Gardnerella vaginalis, 3028-3029
    bacterial vaginosis from, 1503
    culture for, 1503
Garenoxacin, 706t-709t
    dosage of, 732t-733t
    formulations of, 716t
    structure of, 487
Gas gangrene, 1316-1318, 3106-3107
    clinical findings in, 1317, 1317f
    differential diagnosis of, 1306t, 1318
    after episiotomy, 1513
    etiologic agents in, 1318
    hyperbaric oxygen therapy for, 626-627
    laboratory findings in, 1317
    treatment of, 1318
Gastric acid
    age and, 268
    in gastrointestinal colonization prevention, 1337
Gastric carcinoma, in Helicobacter pylori infection,
    2806t, 2807
Gastric disorders, in HIV infection, 1738
Gastric lymphoma, in Helicobacter pylori infection,
    2806t, 2807
Gastric ulceration, in Helicobacter pylori infection,
    2806t, 2807
Gastritis, in HIV infection, 1738
Gastroduodenal ulcers, in HIV infection, 1738
Gastroenteritis. See also Diarrhea; Dysentery;
    Enteritis.
    from adenoviruses, 2029-2030
    from astroviruses, 2407-2408, 2408t
    from caliciviruses, 2399-2405
    eosinophilic, 3618t, 3621
        abdominal pain and/or diarrhea with
            eosinophilia from, 1407t, 1409
    febrile, from Listeria monocytogenes, 2711
    from nontyphoidal Salmonella, 2894-2895
    from picobirnaviruses, 2408
    quinolones for, 496
    in reactive arthritis, 1492
    from rotaviruses, 1361. See also Rotaviruses,
        diarrhea from.
    viral, 1362-1363, 1362t
Gastroesophageal reflux disease
    in Helicobacter pylori infection, 2806t, 2807
    in HIV infection, 1737
Gastrointestinal tract
    cephalosporin effects on, 332
    disorders of
        from penicillin, 314
        probiotics for, 670t, 674-675
        from rifamycins, 405
        in tropical sprue, 1431-1432
    drainage of, for peritonitis, 1026
    flora of, 1336-1339, 1336t
    fluid balance in, 1343, 1343f
    in host defense, 40, 1336-1339, 1336t

Gastrointestinal tract *(Continued)*
immunity of, 1338-1339
injury to, in sepsis, 999-1000
microbiology of, 3112
motility of, 1337
nitrofurantoin effects on, 517
in peritonitis, 1020
in plague, 2947
specimens from, 242
in syphilis, 3041
Gastrointestinal tract infections. *See also specific infection and pathogen.*
from adenoviruses, 2029-2030
age in, 1336
from *Candida*, 3227
nonesophageal, 3228
control of, 1346-1347
from coronaviruses, 2187, 2191-2192
from cytomegalovirus, 1976
cytotoxins in, 1340t, 1341
diagnosis of, 1344-1346, 1345f
enteric microflora in, 1337-1338
enterotoxins in, 1340-1341, 1340t
from enteroviruses, 2361
epidemiologic and environmental factors in, 1336, 1336t
gastric acidity in, 1337
genotype in, 1336-1337
in histoplasmosis, 3312-3313
host factors in, 1336-1339, 1336t
host species in, 1336-1337
human milk protection in, 1339
immunity in, 1338-1339
in immunocompromised hosts, 3786, 3786f, 3789
intestinal motility in, 1337
microbial factors in, 1339-1343, 1339t
from microsporidia, 3395-3397, 3396f, 3401-3402
from mucormycosis agents, 3262
neurotoxins in, 1340, 1340t
occurrence of, 1335
pathogen attachment in, 1341-1342
pathogen invasiveness in, 1342
personal hygiene in, 1337, 1337t
physical barriers in, 1337
physiologic derangements in, 1343-1344, 1343t
prevention of, 1346-1347
scope of, 1335
serum protective factors in, 1339
in solid organ transplant recipients, 3845-3846
treatment of, 1346-1347
trimethoprim-sulfamethoxazole for, 481
tropical sprue from, 1429
tuberculous, 3157
in HIV infection, 3157
types of, 1343-1344, 1343t
virulence factors in, 1342-1343
water-related, 1336, 1336t
Gatifloxacin, 706t-709t
antimicrobial activity of, 491t-492t
for *Chlamydophila* respiratory infection, 2471t
dosage of, 493t
pharmacology of, 492t
structure of, 487, 488f
Gaucher's disease, 1464
Gell and Coombs classification of hypersensitivity reactions, 70-72, 347, 348t
Gemella morbillorum, 2667-2668, 2668t
Gemifloxacin, 706t-709t
antimicrobial activity of, 491t-492t
dosage of, 493t, 732t-733t
formulations of, 716t
for nosocomial pneumonia, 3718t
pharmacology of, 492t
structure of, 487, 488f
Gender. *See also* Women.
body temperature and, 766, 768
chronic pneumonia and, 931
HIV infection and, 1627-1628, 1640-1641, 1641t
Gene(s). *See also specific gene.*
resistance, 52-55
susceptibility, 49-50, 50t-51t
Gene therapy
for cystic fibrosis, 952
for neutrophil defects, 118
vectors for, adenoviruses as, 2032

Genetics, 49-58
of hepatitis, 52
of HIV/AIDS, 51-52, 51t, 1664f, 2324f, 2326-2327, 2327t
variation in, 2332
of infectious disease, 50-52
applications of, 55
evolutionary aspects of, 55
magnitude of, 49-50, 50t
of malaria, 50, 50t, 3442-3444
of mycobacterial diseases, 50-51, 51t
of toxoplasmosis, 3500
of tuberculosis, 49, 50t, 3140
Genital lesions, 1475-1484
clinical manifestations of, 1475-1479
duration of, 1478-1479
epidemiology of, 1479, 1479t
etiology of, 1475, 1476t
history of presentation in, 1475
in HIV infection, 1479
HIV transmission and, 1624-1625, 1646
laboratory tests in, 1479-1481, 1480f
location of, 1475-1476
lymphadenopathy in, 1476
morphology of, 1476-1478, 1476f-1479f
nonvenereal, 1476t, 1482
treatment of, 1481
venereal, 1475, 1476t. *See also* Sexually transmitted diseases.
Genital specimens, 235t-236t, 242-243
Genital tuberculosis
female, 3157
male, 3156-3157
Genital ulcers
in chancroid, 2917
in HIV infection, 1798-1799
Genital warts. *See* Condylomata acuminata.
Genitourinary prosthesis infections, from coagulase-negative *Staphylococcus*, 2585
Genitourinary tract
female, gram-negative anaerobic rods in, 3113
in host defense, 40-41
Genitourinary tract infections. *See also* Urinary tract infections.
from *Actinomyces*, 3213
from adenoviruses, 2030
anaerobic, 3085-3086
from *Blastomyces dermatitidis*, 3326
from *Chlamydia trachomatis*, 2451, 2452t
female, 2453, 2455
treatment of, 2455
female
from *Chlamydia trachomatis*, 2453, 2455
from *Clostridium*, 3108
gram-negative anaerobic rod, 3116-3117
from HIV, 1784
from *Streptococcus agalactiae* (group B), 2660
male, 1521-1527. *See also* Epididymitis; Orchitis; Prostatitis.
anatomic aspects of, 1521, 1522f
in HIV infection, 1525-1526
host defenses in, 1521
from microsporidia, 3397
from *Mycoplasma* species, 2491-2492, 2492f, 2492t
tuberculous, 3156, 3156t
in HIV infection, 3157
Genomic hybridization, comparative, 11
Genomic islands. *See* Pathogenicity islands.
Genomic sequencing, for enteroviruses, 2341
Gentamicin, 359, 360f, 360t-361t, 706t-709t
for actinomycetoma, 3284
for acute pyelonephritis, 972
for bacillary angiomatosis/peliosis, 3005
for brain abscess, 1274t
for brucellosis, 2924
for donovanosis, 3013
dosage of, 724t-725t
in children, 378t
multiple daily
loading dose in, 374, 374t
in renal insufficiency, 374
once-daily, 376, 377t
for endocarditis, 1068-1069, 1088-1089, 1091
for *Enterococcus* endocarditis, 1120t
formulations of, 715t

Gentamicin *(Continued)*
intraventricular, 1234, 1234t
for meningitis, 1213t
for *Neisseria gonorrhoeae* infection, 2765t
for non-HACEK endocarditis, 1121t
for nosocomial pneumonia, 3718t
for osteomyelitis, 1459t
for peritonitis, 1029t
for plague, 2948
for pneumonic plague, 3967t
for prosthetic valve endocarditis, 1122t
resistance to
in enterococci, 363
high-level, 273
for *Staphylococcus aureus* endocarditis, 2571t
Staphylococcus aureus resistance to, 2559t
for *Staphylococcus* endocarditis, 1118t
for *Streptococcus agalactiae* (group B) infection, 2662t
for *Streptococcus* endocarditis, 1119t, 1122
for suppurative thrombophlebitis, 1098
for tularemia, 2935, 3974t
for viridans streptococcal endocarditis, 2670, 2670t
Gentian violet, 706t-709t
Geographic clustering, 195
Geophilic dermatophytosis, 3346, 3346t
German measles. *See* Rubella.
Germicide, 3677
Gerstmann-Sträussler-Scheinker syndrome, 2428
Gianotti-Crosti syndrome, from hepatitis B, 2072
Giant cell (temporal) arteritis, fever of unknown origin in, 787
Giardia agilis, 3527, 3528t
Giardia duodenalis, 3527
Giardia intestinalis, 3527
Giardia lamblia, 3527-3534, 3528t. *See also* Giardiasis.
acquisition of, 3528
cyst stage of, 3527, 3528f
description of, 3527-3528
life cycle of, 3527, 3528f
transmission of, 3528
trophozoite stage of, 3527, 3528f
waterborne disease from, 1418, 1418t
Giardia microti, 3527, 3528t
Giardia muris, 3527, 3528t
Giardiasis
clinical manifestations of, 3530, 3530t
diagnosis of, 3530-3531
diarrhea from, 1367, 1396
epidemiology of, 3528-3529
immune response to, 3529
pathogenesis of, 3529-3530
predisposition to, 3529
in pregnancy, 3532
prevention of, 3532
susceptibility to, 3529
treatment of, 632t-635t, 3531-3532, 3531t
Giemsa stain, 244, 244t
for African trypanosomes, 3490f, 3491-3492
for malaria, 3446f, 3448
GILT, in MHC class I antigen processing, 135-136
Gingivitis, 859-860. *See also* Odontogenic infections; Periodontal disease/periodontitis.
acute necrotizing ulcerative, 859-860, 861t, 3085, 3115
clinical manifestations of, 859-860
gonococcal, 2761
from herpes simplex virus, 1948, 1948f
in HIV infection, 1715
treatment of, 861t, 869
Glanders, 2877-2878, 2877f
Glands of Zeis, 1569
Glandular tularemia, 2932f, 2933
Glasgow Coma Scale, brain abscess and, 1265
Global Fund to Fight AIDS, Tuberculosis and Malaria, 1630
Global Outbreak Alert and Response Network (GOARN), 214
Global Public Health Intelligence Network (GPHIN), 214
Global trade, zoonoses and, 4005-4006
Global warming, zoonoses and, 4004

Glomerulonephritis. *See also* Nephritis.
  in endocarditis, 1074
  membranoproliferative, type II, factor H
    deficiency in, 92
  from parvovirus B19 infection, 2091
  poststreptococcal, 2617-2620, 2675
    diagnosis of, 2619
    epidemiology of, 2618, 2618t
    etiology and pathogenesis of, 2612t, 2617-2618
    history of, 2617
    manifestations of, 2619
    pathology of, 2618
    prevention of, 2619-2620
    prognosis in, 2620
    treatment of, 2619
Gloves, in standard precautions, 3673-3674
Glucocorticoids. *See* Corticosteroids.
Glucose
  in cerebrospinal fluid, 1185, 1185t
  metabolism of, quinolone interactions with, 494
  perioperative, reduced surgical site infections with,
    3897
  screening for, in HIV-infected pregnant patient,
    1795
  in sepsis, 998
Glucose control, in sepsis, 1005
Glucose fermenters, 3015-3021, 3016t-3017t
Glucose nonfermenters (weak fermenters),
    3016t-3017t, 3021-3029
Glucose-6-phosphate dehydrogenase, 116
  deficiency of
    antimicrobial therapy and, 269
    primaquine and, 637
    tafenoquine and, 638
    malaria and, 50, 50t, 53, 3443
Glucosylating toxins, 28t
Glutamate, in bacterial meningitis, 1204
Glutaraldehyde, disinfection with, 3680t, 3682-3683
Glycerol, for intracranial pressure reduction, 1221
Glycolipids, CD1-presented, 137
Glycopeptides, 449-459. *See also* Teicoplanin;
    Vancomycin.
  for *Enterococcus*, 2649
  Staphylococcus aureus resistance to, 2559t, 2560
Glycosphingolipases, urinary tract, 959-960
Glycylcyclines, 386-387
Gnathostomiasis, 632t-635t, 654, 3620
Gomori methenamine silver stain
  for *Blastomyces dermatitidis*, 3328, 3328f
  for *Paracoccidioides brasiliensis*, 3361, 3361f
Gonococcal infections, 2753-2770. *See also Neisseria
    gonorrhoeae.*
  arthritis in, 1444t, 1446-1447
  arthritis-dermatitis syndrome in, 2762
  bacteremia in, 1304, 2762-2763
  cervicitis in, 2759-2763, 2760f
  in children, 2763, 2766
  Chlamydia trachomatis coinfection with, 2765
  clinical manifestations of, 2759-2763
  complement interactions with, 85
  complications of, 2759
  conjunctival, 2761
    in neonates, 1536, 2763
    treatment of, 2764t
  cutaneous abscess in, 2761
  diagnosis of, 2763-2764
    cultures in, 2763
    DNA probe tests in, 2764
    gram-stained smears in, 2764
    nucleic acid amplification tests in, 2763
  disseminated, 2762-2763, 2762f, 2764t, 2766
  endocarditis in, 1093, 2763
  endocervical, 2759-2763, 2760f
  epidemiology of, 2756-2759
  epididymal, 2759, 2766
  epididymitis in, 1524
  Fitz-Hugh–Curtis syndrome in, 2761
  genital
    in men, 2759, 2759f-2760f
    in women, 2759-2763, 2760f
  gingival, 2761
  incidence of, 2756-2758, 2756f-2757f
  keratitis in, 1542
  in men who have sex with men, 2756-2758, 2757f
  in neonates, 2763

Gonococcal infections *(Continued)*
    conjunctival, 2763
    rectal, 2763
  pathology of, 2756, 2756f
  pelvic inflammatory disease in, 2761, 2765-2766,
    2765t
  peritonitis in, 1018
  pharyngeal, 2760, 2764t
  pharyngitis in, 817
  in pregnancy, 2761-2762
  prevention and control of, 2766-2767
    condoms and microbicides in, 2767
    public health strategies in, 2766-2767
    systemic antibiotics in, 2767
    vaccine development in, 2767
  proctitis in, 1393
  quinolone resistance in, 502
  race/ethnicity and, 2758, 2758t
  rectal, 2760
    in neonates, 2763
    treatment of, 2764t
  skin lesions in, 798
  transmission of, 2758
  treatment of, 2764-2766
    azithromycin in, 2765
    carbapenems in, 342t
    cefixime in, 2764, 2764t, 2766
    cefotetan in, 2765t
    cefpodoxime in, 2764
    ceftriaxone in, 2764, 2764t-2765t, 2766
    with chlamydial coinfection, 2765
    clindamycin in, 2765t
    doxycycline in, 2765-2766, 2765t
    erythromycin in, 2765
    fluoroquinolones in, 2764-2765
    gentamicin in, 2765t
    initial single-dose, 2764-2765, 2764t
    levofloxacin in, 2753, 2766
    metronidazole in, 2765, 2765t
    ofloxacin in, 2753
    quinolones in, 495-496
    sex partner management in, 2766
    spectinomycin in, 2765
    trimethoprim-sulfamethoxazole in, 481
  uncomplicated, 2759, 2759f-2760f
    follow-up of patients with, 2766
    treatment of, 2764-2765, 2764t
  urethral, 2759, 2759f-2760f
    in men, 2759, 2759f-2760f
  urethral exudate in, 1486, 1486f
  urethritis in, 1487-1489, 1487f, 1487t, 2759,
    2759f-2760f
    purulent discharge from, 1487-1488, 1487f
    quinolones for, 496
Gonococcemia, skin lesions of, 1304
Gonorrhea. *See* Gonococcal infections; *Neisseria
    gonorrhoeae.*
Gordonia bronchialis, 2703-2704
Gordonia rubripertinctus, 2703-2704
Gown, isolation, 3673, 3674t
Gp91*phox*, 107
  defective, 114-115, 114t
Gp120/160 adhesin, HIV, 18-19, 18f
Gradenigo's syndrome, 1282
Graft infections, vascular
  from coagulase-negative *Staphylococcus*, 2583
  prosthetic, 1132-1135
Graft-versus-host disease
  after hematopoietic stem cell transplantation,
    3821-3822, 3826
  posaconazole prophylaxis in, 558-559
Grain itch mite, 3645-3646, 3646f
Grains. *See also* Granules.
  in actinomycetoma, 3282t, 3284f
  in eumycetoma, 3282t, 3283f
  in mycetoma, 3281-3284, 3282t
Gram stain, 244, 244t, 267
  in bacterial meningitis, 1208
  in brain abscess, 1271
  of cerebrospinal fluid, 1186
  in *Neisseria gonorrhoeae* infection, 2756f, 2764
  in pneumococcal pneumonia, 2632, 2632f,
    2632t
  of sputum, in acute pneumonia, 896, 897f-898f
  of vaginal flora, 1498

Gram-negative anaerobic cocci infections
  description of, 3121-3122
  microbiology of, 3121
Gram-negative anaerobic rod(s)
  bacteremia from, 3114
  capsular polysaccharides in, 3113
  endotoxic lipopolysaccharides in, 3113
  enteritis from, 3116
  enzymes of, 3114
  history of, 3111
  host immune response to, 3114
  medically important, 3112t
  metabolic end products of, 3114
  microbiology of, 3111-3112, 3112f
  opportunism of, 3113
  in oropharynx, 3113
  otitis media from, 3115
  overview of, 3111
  peritonitis from, 3116
  pili and fimbriae of, 3113
  symbiosis and mutualism of, 3112-3115
  toxins of, 3114
  in urogenital tract, 3113
Gram-negative anaerobic rod infections, 3114
  aerodigestive, 3115-3117
  cardiovascular, 3116
  central nervous system, 3115
  intra-abdominal, 3116
  oropharyngeal, 3115
  salivary gland, 3116
  skeletal, 3114-3115
  skin, 3115
  soft tissue, 3115
  thoracic, 3116
  treatment of, 3117-3118
    antibiotic therapy in, 3117-3118, 3117t
    surgical, 3117
  urogenital tract, 3116-3117
Gram-negative bacilli infections
  endocarditis from, 1081t, 1083-1084
  multidrug resistant, polymyxins for, 469
  nosocomial pneumonia from, 3717
Gram-negative bacterial infections, endocarditis
  from, 1084
Gram-positive anaerobic cocci infections, 3121-3128
  antimicrobial susceptibility of, 3122, 3123t
  clinical isolates in, 3122, 3125-3126
  commensal microbiota in, 3125
  description of, 3121-3122
  identification, 3122
  microbiology of, 3121, 3126
  taxonomy in, 3121, 3122t, 3125-3126
  treatment of, 3122, 3123t, 3126-3127, 3127t
Gram-positive bacilli infections, endocarditis from,
  1084
Gram-positive bacterial infections
  anaerobic, 3125-3128
    clinical isolates in, 3125-3126
    commensal microbiota in, 3125
    microbiological aspects of, 3126
    taxonomy in, 3125-3126
    treatment of, 3126-3127, 3127t
  quinolone resistance in, 489-490
Granule cell neuronopathy, JC virus–associated, 2053
Granules. *See also* Grains.
  eosinophilic, 118-119, 118f
  neutrophilic
    deficiency of, 116-117
    primary (azurophilic), 100, 100t
    specific (secondary), 100, 100t
      deficiency of, 117
Granulicatella, 2670t, 2673
Granulicatella adiacens, endocarditis from, prosthetic
  valve, 1119t, 1121
Granulocyte(s). *See also* Eosinophil(s); Neutrophil(s).
  maturation of, 100
  transfusion of
    for neutropenia, in cancer, 3806
    for neutrophil defects, 117
Granulocyte colony-stimulating factor, 611-614
  adverse effects of, 613-614
  for community-acquired pneumonia, 613
  for diabetic foot infection, 613
  dosage of, 613
  endogenous, 611

Granulocyte colony-stimulating factor *(Continued)*
  formulations of, 611-612
  after hematopoietic stem cell transplantation, 613
  for Kaposi's sarcoma, 1767
  for neutropenia, 612
    acquired, 111
    in cancer, 3806
    in children, 612
    in HIV infection, 612
  for sepsis, 613
  for septicemic melioidosis, 2877
Granulocyte-macrophage colony-stimulating factor, 614
  adverse effects of, 614
  dosage of, 614
  formulations of, 614
  for Kaposi's sarcoma, 1767
  for neutropenia, 111
  uses of, 614
Granulocytopenia
  in immunocompromised host, 3781, 3782t, 3789, 3789f
  leukocyte transfusion for, 117
Granuloma
  actinomycotic, 3214
  from *Candida*, 3231, 3231f
  conjunctival, 1530
  from *Histoplasma capsulatum*, 3308, 3308f
  Majocchi's, in dermatophytosis, 3351
  in *Paracoccidioides brasiliensis* infection, 3359
  in schistosomiasis, 3596-3597
  swimming pool, 1331
  in tuberculous pericarditis, 1162-1163, 1163f
Granuloma inguinale. *See* Donovanosis.
Granulomatosis
  disseminated, fever in, 786
  lymphomatoid, from Epstein-Barr virus, 1998
  Wegener's, 943f
Granulomatous amebic encephalitis
  clinical manifestations of, 3432
  epidemiology of, 3430-3431
  etiology of, 3427, 3430t
  laboratory diagnosis of, 3433
  pathology and pathogenesis of, 3431
  treatment of, 3434
Granulomatous conjunctivitis, in Parinaud's oculoglandular syndrome, 3000, 3000f
Granulomatous disease
  chronic, 114-116, 114t, 169t-170t, 173-175
    from *Chromobacterium violaceum*, 3019-3020
    diagnosis of, 115-116
    infections in, 174, 174f
    interferon-gamma for, 616
    lymphadenitis in, 1325
    management of, 116
    nicotinamide adenine dinucleotide phosphate oxidase in, 173-174, 173f
    X-linked, 174
  disseminated, fever in, 786
Granulomatous lymphadenitis/lymphadenopathy, from nondiphtheria *Corynebacterium*, 1325
Granulomatous lymphangitis, chronic, 1331
Granulomatous prostatitis, 1523
Granulomatous uveitis, 1561, 1562f
Gravity displacement autoclave, 3686
Gray baby syndrome, from chloramphenicol, 397
Green nail syndrome, 2856
Green tea extract, for genital warts, 670t, 674, 674f
Griseofulvin, 706t-709t
  for dermatophytosis, 3352
  dosage of, 736t-737t
  drug interactions with, 742t-761t
  formulations of, 717t
Groin, dermatophytosis of, 3348
Growth abnormalities, in HIV-infected children, 1813-1814
Growth factors, for cancer-related infections, 3800t
Guanarito virus, 2296t. *See also* South American hemorrhagic fevers.
Guanosine, 593f
Guarnieri bodies, 3979
Guillain-Barré syndrome
  from *Campylobacter jejuni*, 1416, 2797
  from cytomegalovirus, 1974-1975
  differential diagnosis of, 3660t

Guillain-Barré syndrome *(Continued)*
  after influenza, 2276
  after influenza vaccine, 2280
  poliomyelitis versus, 2347
Gumma, in syphilis, 3043
Gut decontamination
  after liver transplantation, 3816
  selective, for pancreatic infections, 1048, 1049t
Gynecologic examination, in vaginitis/vulvovaginitis, 1497-1498, 1497f-1498f, 1497t
Gynecologic infections. *See also* Genitourinary tract infections; Sexually transmitted diseases.
  in HIV infection, 1796-1799
Gynecologic surgery, surgical site infection after, 1514-1516, 1514t, 1515f
Gyromitra poisoning, 1417t, 1418

H
H2-M3, 141
HAART. *See* Highly active antiretroviral therapy (HAART).
HACEK bacteria, 3015-3017
  endocarditis from, prosthetic valve, 1113
    treatment of, 1121t, 1123
  Haemophilus in, 2918
Haemophilus, 2911-2919, 2917t
Haemophilus aphrophilus. See Aggregatibacter aphrophilus.
Haemophilus ducreyi, 2916-2918, 2917t
  genital lesions in, 1479-1480, 1479t, 1480f
  laboratory detection of, 240t-242t, 243
Haemophilus haemolyticus, 2911, 2917-2918, 2917t
Haemophilus influenzae, 2911-2916
  adhesins of, 2912, 2912t
  arthritis from, 1444, 1444t
  bacteremia from, 1304
  biofilms of, 2912
  brain abscess from, 1265-1266, 1266t
  cellulitis from, 1296
    preseptal, 1572
  clinical manifestations of, 2913-2914
  dacryocystitis from, 1571
  description of, 2911
  diagnosis of, 2914-2915
  epidemiology of, 2911-2912
  epiglottitis from, 851, 853
  in HIV infection, 1878-1879
  host-agent interactions in, 187
  immunity to, 2912-2913
  laboratory detection of, 240t-242t
  meningitis from
    epidemiology and etiology of, 1190t-1191t, 1191-1192
    prevention of, 1222-1223
    treatment of, 1211t-1212t, 1215-1216
  nontypeable, 2912t
    bacteremia from, 2913-2914
    community-acquired pneumonia from, 2913
    conjunctivitis from, 2914
    COPD exacerbations from, 2912-2913
    diagnosis of, 2914-2915
    immunity to, 2912-2913
    invasive infections from, 2913-2914
    neonatal sepsis from, 2913
    otitis media from, 2912-2913
    pediatric respiratory tract infections from, 2913
    postpartum sepsis from, 2913
    sinusitis from, 2913
    treatment of, 2915
  otitis media from, 833
  pneumonia from, in HIV infection, 1730-1731
  postsplenectomy sepsis from, 3868-3869
  quinolones for, 498
  respiratory tract colonization by, 2911-2912
  treatment of, 2915-2916
    carbapenems in, 342t
    rifamycins in, 411
  type b, 2912t
    bacteremia from, 2914
    cellulitis from, 2914
    chemoprophylaxis for, 2915
    diagnosis of, 2915
    empyema from, 2914
    epiglottitis from, 2914

Haemophilus influenzae (Continued)
  immunity to, 2913
  invasive infections from, 2912
  meningitis from, 2914
  pneumonia from, 2914
  septic arthritis from, 2914
  treatment of, 2915-2916
  vaccines for, 2913, 2915-2916, 2916t, 3922t, 3923, 3924f
  VκA2 gene deficiency in, 73
Haemophilus influenzae biogroup aegyptius, 2916
Haemophilus parahaemolyticus, 2917-2918, 2917t
Haemophilus parainfluenzae, 2917-2918, 2917t
Haemophilus paraphrophilus. See Aggregatibacter paraphrophilus.
Hafnia alvei, 2826, 2828
Hair, specimen collection and transport guidelines for, 235t-236t
Hallucinations, from voriconazole, 558
Halo sign, 3201
Halofantrine, 706t-709t
  drug interactions with, 742t-761t
  for malaria, 639
Hamman's sign, 1176
Hand, dermatophytosis of, 3349
Hand hygiene, 3673
Hand-foot-and-mouth disease, from enteroviruses, 817-818, 2355
Hand-rub, alcohol-based, 3673
Hansen's disease. *See* Leprosy.
Hantaviruses, 2290-2291, 4003
  detection of, 259t-260t
  hantavirus pulmonary syndrome from, 2290t, 2292
  hemorrhagic fever with renal syndrome from, 2290t, 2291-2292
  rash from, 802
Haptenization, by penicillin, 348-349, 349f
Hartmann procedure, for diverticulitis, 1064
Hawaii virus, 2400-2402, 2401f
Haycockema perplexum, 3588-3589
Hazard Analysis Critical Control Point (HACCP) program, in infection prevention, 1424
HBx, 2063
  in hepatocellular carcinoma, 2067-2068
Head and neck. *See also* Neck.
  bites to, 862t, 868
  infections of, 855. *See also* Orofacial infections.
    anaerobic, 3084-3085, 3084t, 3085f
    mediastinitis secondary to, 1173, 1175t
    miscellaneous, 867-868
      from *Streptococcus anginosus* group, 2683
    suppurative, antimicrobial regimens for, 862t
  radiation therapy to, complications of, 868
Head trauma, brain abscess from, 1267
Headache
  from brain abscess, 1269, 1269t
  after lumbar puncture, 1184
Health care equipment, disinfection of, 3681-3684
Health care providers
  HAV transmission in, 2376
  HCV transmission in, 2171
  health of, nosocomial infections and, 3670
  HIV exposure in, 1648-1649, 1652-1653, 3753-3770. *See also* Human immunodeficiency virus infection, occupational.
  HIV-infected, management of, 3761
  pertussis immunization for, 2961
  role of, in plague terrorist event, 3968
  standard precautions for, 3673-3674, 3674t
  surveillance and exposure management of, emergency preparedness for, 227
  tuberculosis in, 932
Health care–associated infections. *See also* Nosocomial infections.
  versus community acquired methicillin-resistant *Staphylococcus aureus*, 2559-2560
  endocarditis as, 1067
  fever of unknown origin in, 780t, 781-782
  hematologic, from *Staphylococcus aureus*, 2568
  hospital epidemiology programs for, 3667-3672, 3670t
  of skin/soft tissue, from nontuberculous mycobacteria, 3195

Hearing loss
  from aminoglycosides, 371-372
  from erythromycin, 431
Heart disease
  congenital
    closure devices for, infectious complications of,
      1140
    respiratory syncytial virus infection and, 2214
  in endocarditis, 1073-1074
Heart failure
  in American trypanosomiasis, 3484, 3484f
  in rheumatic fever, 2614
Heart murmurs, in endocarditis, 1076
Heart rate, temperature and, 768
Heart transplant recipients
  endocarditis prophylaxis in, 1149
  infections in, 3841-3842, 3841t
  mediastinitis in, 1174
  survival data for, 3839, 3840f, 3840t
  toxoplasmosis in, 3503
Heart valve. See also specific valve.
  isolated infection of, 1437
  prosthetic
    choice of, 1116-1117
    infections of, endocarditis in, 1113-1126. See
      also Endocarditis, prosthetic valve.
  replacement of, in endocarditis, 1094-1095
Heart valve surgery
  contraindications to, 1116, 1117t
  indications for, 1116, 1117t
Heart-lung transplant recipients
  infections in, 3841t, 3842
  survival data for, 3839, 3840t
Heart-reactive antibodies, in rheumatic fever, 2612
Heat shock protein 60, aphthous ulcers and, 866
Heat stroke, 765
Heavy metal poisoning, 1419, 1422, 1424
Heck's disease, 2041
Helicobacter cinaedi, 2793, 2798
  bacteremia from, 1304
Helicobacter felis, 2804t
Helicobacter fennelliae, 2793, 2798
Helicobacter heilmannii, 2810
Helicobacter mustelae, 2804t
Helicobacter pylori, 2803-2813
  acute acquisition of, 2805
  allergic disorders in, 2806t, 2807-2808
  asthma in, 2806t, 2807-2808
  in cancer patients, 3798
  clinical consequences associated with, 2803, 2804t,
    2805-2807, 2806f, 2806t
  colonization of
    persistent, 2805-2806, 2806f
    prevalence of, 2804-2805, 2804f
  detection of, 240t-242t, 242
  diagnosis of, 2808-2809, 2808t
  disinfection/sterilization and, 3688
  duodenal ulceration in, 2806-2807, 2806t
  epidemiology of, 2804-2805, 2804f
  esophageal disease in, 2806t, 2807
  gastric carcinoma in, 2806t, 2807
  gastric lymphoma in, 2806t, 2807
  gastric ulceration in, 2806t, 2807
  genetic susceptibility to, 49, 50t
  in HIV infection, 1738
  idiopathic thrombocytopenic purpura in, 2806t,
    2808
  macrolides for, 437
  metabolic disorders in, 2808
  microbiology of, 2803-2804, 2804t
  pathology and pathogenesis of, 2803
  treatment of, 2809-2810
    indications for, 2809
    quinolones in, 497
    rifamycins in, 411
    therapies in, 2809-2810, 2809t
  Vibrio cholerae coinfection with, 2780
Helium/oxygen therapy, for croup, 828
HELLP syndrome, hepatitis in, 1588
Helminthic infections, 3573-3575, 3617-3623. See
    also specific infection.
  biology of, 3573
  brain abscess from, 1266-1267
  clinical syndromes associated with, 3618t
  diagnosis of, 3574-3575, 3574t

Helminthic infections (Continued)
  epidemiology of, 3573
  host-parasite relationship in, 3573-3574
  meningitis from
    adjunctive therapy for, 1221-1222
    antimicrobial therapy for, 1220
    clinical features of, 1207
    diagnosis of, 1210-1211
    epidemiology and etiology of, 1193-1194
  pathogenesis of, 3573-3574
  prevention of, 3575
  treatment of, 3575
Hemagglutinin, 15, 17, 17f
Hematochromatosis, in mucormycosis, 3259
Hematogenous dissemination, brain abscess from,
  1267
Hematogenous osteomyelitis, 1462. See also
  Osteomyelitis.
Hematologic disorders, in HIV-infected children,
  1816
Hematologic toxicity
  of linezolid, 473
  of rifamycins, 405
Hematopoietic stem cell transplantation, 3821-3837.
    See also Bone marrow transplantation.
  adenoviruses in, 2030
  autologous versus allogeneic, 3821
  chemotherapy in, 3821
  cytomegalovirus in, 1980-1981
    late-onset, 1981
  diarrhea after, 3823
  graft-versus-host disease after, 3821-3822, 3826
  granulocyte colony-stimulating factor after, 613
  hemorrhagic cystitis after, 3822
  hepatitis after, 3822-3823
  HLA matching in, 3822
  immune globulin after, 3833
  immune system reconstitution after, 3832-3833,
    3833t
  immunization after, 3832-3833, 3833t
  infections after, 3824-3826, 3824t, 3825f
    bacterial, 3827-3828
    fungal, 3831-3832
    infection control measures for, 3827
    natural history of, 3827-3832
    parasitic, 3832
    prevention of, 3822
    risk periods for, 3824-3826, 3824t, 3825f
    sequence of events in, 3782, 3783t
    viral, 3828-3831
  micafungin prophylaxis in, 561
  mortality rate in, 3802
  myeloablative, 3824-3826, 3824t, 3825f
  nonmyeloablative, 3822, 3826-3827
  osteomyelitis after, 3824
  pneumonia syndromes after, 3823
  radiation therapy in, total body, 3821-3822
  rash after, 3823
  techniques of, 3821-3822
  toxoplasmosis in, 3504
  veno-occlusive disease after, 3822
Hematuria
  in endocarditis, 1077
  in urinary tract infection, 967
Hemodialysis. See also Dialysis; Peritoneal dialysis.
  aminoglycoside dosing in, 375, 375t
  osteomyelitis in, 1464
Hemofiltration, continuous arteriovenous,
    aminoglycoside dosing in, 375, 375t
Hemoglobin C, malaria and, 50, 3442-3443
Hemoglobin E, malaria and, 3442-3443
Hemoglobin F, malaria and, 3443
Hemoglobin gene
  in thalassemia susceptibility, 53
  variants of, 53
Hemoglobin S, malaria and, 53, 3442-3443
Hemoglobinuria, in malaria, 3449
Hemolysins
  of Escherichia coli, 2819
  of Pseudomonas aeruginosa, 2844-2845
  of Staphylococcus aureus, 2553
  streptococcal, 2594
Hemolysis
  from primaquine, 637
  pyelonephritis and, 961

Hemolytic anemia
  from chloramphenicol, 397
  from cytomegalovirus, 1975
  in infectious mononucleosis, 1994
  from nitrofurantoin, 517
Hemolytic uremic syndrome
  from enterohemorrhagic Escherichia coli,
    2824-2825
  factor H deficiency in, 92
Hemoperfusion, for streptococcal toxic shock
  syndrome, 2605
Hemophagocytic lymphohistiocytosis, from
  Epstein-Barr virus, 1996
Hemophagocytic syndrome, from parvovirus B19,
  2091
Hemoptysis, in tuberculosis, 3142-3143
Hemorrhage
  diffuse alveolar, in transplant recipients, 3823
  local, after lumbar puncture, 1184
  pulmonary, in leptospirosis, 3062
  in rubella, 2128-2129
  splinter, in endocarditis, 1076
Hemorrhagic bullae, from Vibrio vulnificus,
  2788-2789, 2789f
Hemorrhagic conjunctivitis, acute, 1532, 1532f,
  2360-2361
Hemorrhagic cystitis
  from adenoviruses, 2030
  from BK virus, 2056
  in transplant recipients, 3822
Hemorrhagic fever
  Crimean-Congo, 2289-2292, 2290t
  dengue
    clinical features of, 2142f, 2144-2145
    epidemiology of, 2135-2136
    pathogenesis of, 2142-2143, 2142f
    in travelers, 4014-4015
    treatment of, 2150
  filovirus, 2259-2263. See also Filoviruses.
  Omsk, 2153
  with renal syndrome, 595, 2290t, 2291-2292
  South American, 2295-2301. See also South
    American hemorrhagic fevers.
  viral. See Viral hemorrhagic fevers.
Hemorrhagic telangiectasia, hereditary, brain abscess
  from, 1267
Henderson-Paterson bodies, in molluscum
  contagiosum, 1934
Hendra virus, 208-209
  clinical features of, 2241-2242
  detection of, 259t-260t
  diagnostic tests for, 2242
  emergence of, 2237
  encephalitis from, 1251t-1252t
  epidemiology of, 2241
  outbreaks of, 2238t
  pathology of, 2242
  structure and molecular biology of, 2237
  treatment of, 2242
Henipaviruses. See also Hendra virus; Nipah virus.
  classification of, 2237, 2238f
  emergence of, 2242
  genomes of, 2237
HEPA filters, in hematopoietic stem cell transplant
  recipients, 3831
HEPA-filtered mobile isolation device, 229, 229f
Hepatic. See also Liver entries.
Hepatic actinomycosis, 3213, 3213f
Hepatic encephalopathy, rifamycins for, 413
Hepatic fibrosis, hepatitis C–related, 2166,
  2169-2170
Hepatic tuberculosis, 3153
Hepatitis
  acute viral, 1577-1592
    asymptomatic, 1579
    background on, 1577-1581, 1578t
    characteristics of, 1577, 1578t
    clinical features of, 1579
    differential diagnosis of, 1587-1588, 1587t
    disease spectrum of, 1579-1580
    epidemiology of, 1577-1578, 1578f-1579f, 1578t
    fulminant, 1580
    from HAV, 1581-1582. See also Hepatitis A virus.
    from HBV, 1582-1584. See also Hepatitis B virus.
    from HCV, 1584-1585. See also Hepatitis C virus.

Hepatitis (*Continued*)
  from HDV, 1584. *See also* Hepatitis D virus.
  from HEV, 1585-1586. *See also* Hepatitis E virus.
  from HGV, 1586. *See also* Hepatitis G virus.
  historical perspective on, 1577
  management of, 1588-1590
  physical findings in, 1580
  prevention of, 1590, 1590t
  autoimmune, 1588
  cholestatic, 2377-2378
    fibrosing, 1579-1580
    from HAV, 1579
  chronic, 1593-1617
    histologic classification of, 1594t
    milk thistle for, 674, 674f
  from *Coxiella burnetii*, 2516
  from cytomegalovirus, 1593, 1974
  in duck, 2059
  versus enteric fever, 1400t-1401t, 1404
  fulminant, 1580
    from HBV, 2070
    from HSV, 1587
    management of, 1589-1590
  genetic susceptibility to, 52
  from herpes simplex virus, 1953
  histopathology of, 1580
  in HIV infection, 1881-1882
    HAART and, 1721
  versus infectious mononucleosis, 2003
  ischemic, 1588
  from isoniazid, 534, 3146, 3150
  in neonates, from enteroviruses, 2359
  non–A to E, 1578
    transfusion-related, 3746
  nosocomial, 3739-3742, 3740t
    blood-borne transmission of, 3739-3742
    fecal-oral transmission of, 3739
  from parvovirus B19 infection, 2091
  pathogenesis of, 1586-1587
  relapsing/biphasic, 1579
  from rifampin, 535
  schistosomiasis coinfection in, 3599
  serologic tests for, 261
  syphilitic, 3041
  in transplant recipients, 3822-3823, 3845-3846
  in travelers, 4024
  in woodchuck, 2059
Hepatitis A vaccine, 1590, 3922t, 3923-3925
  active immunization with, 2380-2381
  in children, 2381-2382, 2382t
  for chronic hepatitis B infection, 2079
  inactive, 2380-2381
    recommended doses and schedules for, 2382t
  live attenuated, 2381
  passive immunization in, 2379-2380
  in persons at increased risk, 2382-2383
  postexposure, 2380t, 2381-2383
  for travelers, 4009, 4011t
Hepatitis A virus, 1581-1582, 2367-2387
  antigenic composition of, 2369, 2369f
  biology of, 2369-2371
  cell culture of, 2369-2371
  characteristics of, 1577, 1578t, 1581-1582
  classification of, 2367-2371
  detection of, 259t-260t
  diversity of, 2369
  genetics of, 1581-1582
  genome of, 2368-2369, 2369f
  host range for, 2371
  neutralization sites for, 2369
  pathogenesis of, 1586
  physiochemical and biologic properties of, 2367-2371
  proteins of, 2368-2369, 2369f
  purification of, 2367
  replication of, site of, 2376-2377
  resistance of, to physical and chemical agents, 2368
  structure of, 2367, 2368f
Hepatitis A virus infection
  in childcare centers, schools, and institutions, 2375-2376
  in children, routine vaccination against, 2381-2382, 2382t

Hepatitis A virus infection (*Continued*)
  cholestatic, 1579
  in chronic liver disease, vaccination against, 2383
  clinical features of, 1579, 1581-1582, 1582t, 2377-2378, 2378t
  complications of, 2377-2378, 2378t
  epidemiology of, 1577-1578, 1578f, 1578t, 1581, 1581f, 2371-2376, 2371f
    in United States, 2373-2374, 2373f-2374f
  fulminant, 1580
  future directions in, 2383
  in health care settings, 2376
  historical perspective on, 1577, 2367
  in HIV infection, 1858t-1859t
  immunity to, 2379
  incidence of
    by age, 2374-2375, 2374f
    by race and ethnicity, 2374-2375, 2374f
    by region, 2374-2375, 2375f
  incubation period for, 2376
  in injection drug users, 2376, 3884
    vaccination against, 2382
  in international travelers, 2376
    vaccination against, 2383, 4009, 4011t
  laboratory diagnosis of, 2378-2379
  in men who have sex with men, 2376
    vaccination against, 2382
  outbreaks of, vaccination during, 2383
  pathogenesis of, 2376-2377
  potential sources of, 2375, 2375f
  in pregnancy, 2377
  in prevaccine era, 2373-2374, 2373f-2374f
  prevention of, 1590, 1590t, 2379-2381
    disease control strategies in, 2381-2383, 2382t
    intramuscular immune globulin for, 3934-3935
    postexposure, 2380t, 2381
    preexposure, 2381, 2382t
    recommendations for, 2381-2383
  relapse of, 1579
  risk factors for, 1581, 1581t, 2375, 2375f
  in specific groups and settings, 2375-2376
  symptoms of, 2377
  time course of, 1582, 1582f
  transfusion-related, 2372, 2376
    vaccination against, 2383
  transmission of
    blood-borne, 2372
    foodborne, 2372, 2376
    modes of, 2371-2376
    nosocomial, 3739, 3740t
    person-to-person, 2372
    transfusion-related, 3746
    vertical, 2372
    waterborne, 2372, 2376
  treatment of, 1589, 2383
  in vaccine era, 2374
  worldwide disease patterns of, 2372-2373, 2372f-2373f
Hepatitis A/hepatitis B vaccine, for travelers, 4010, 4011t
Hepatitis B core antigen (HBcAg), 2059
Hepatitis B DNA, 1583-1584, 1593-1594, 2059, 2060f
  treatment-related suppression of, 1596-1600, 1600t
Hepatitis B early antigen, 1583-1584, 2061-2062
  negative, 1594-1595, 2071
  reactive, 1594
Hepatitis B immune globulin, 1590, 3922t, 3935
Hepatitis B surface antigen, 1583, 2059, 2061-2062
  structure of, 2059, 2060f
Hepatitis B surface antigen escape mutants, 2081
Hepatitis B vaccine, 1583, 1590, 3922t, 3925
  active immunization in, 2080
  for contacts of HVB-infected persons, 2079
  dose regimen in, 2080, 2080t
  efficacy of, 2081
  epidemiologic studies of, 180
  indications for, 2080
  postexposure, 2079-2080
  for prenatal transmission prophylaxis, 2080-2081
  response durability of, 2081
Hepatitis B virus, 1582-1584, 2059-2086
  antibody to, 1583
  attachment of, 2059-2061
  biology of, 2059

Hepatitis B virus (*Continued*)
  characteristics of, 1577, 1578t
  classification of, 2059
  detection of, 259t-260t
  entry of, 2059-2061
  genetic susceptibility to, 49, 50t
  genetics of, 1582
  genome of, 2059, 2060f
  HBx and, 2063
  life cycle of, 2059-2061, 2061f
  morphogenesis and assembly of, 2063-2064
  pathogenesis of, 1586
  precore or HBe-negative mutants of, 2071
  replication of, 1593, 1594t, 2063, 2064f
    measures of, 2074
  structure of, 2059, 2060f
  transcription of, 2062
  translation of, 2062-2063, 2063f
  variants of, 1594, 1594t
Hepatitis B virus infection
  acute
    clinical manifestations of, 2069
    diagnosis of, 2073, 2073t
    incidence of, 2068, 2068f
    laboratory findings in, 2069-2070
    pathogenesis of, 2066, 2066f
    prognosis for, 2069
    treatment of, 2074
  arthritis in, 1450
  in cancer patients, 3799
  chronic, 1593-1603
    clinical features of, 1595, 2070
    definition of, 2070
    diagnosis of, 2073-2074, 2073t
    distinctions between patients in
      based on epidemiologic considerations, 1594, 1594t
      based on HBV replication, 1593, 1594t
      based on viral variants, 1594, 1594t
    laboratory testing for, 2070
    after liver transplantation, 1602, 2078
    natural history of, 1595, 2070-2071
    pathogenesis of, 2066-2067, 2066f
    pathophysiology of, 1595
    precore or HBe-negative mutants in, 2071
    in pregnancy, 1602
    prognosis for, 2071-2072
    treatment of, 1595-1600, 2074
      adefovir in, 572, 1598-1599, 1601t, 2076, 2076t
      antiviral agents in, 566t-567t, 573, 1596
        choice of, 1601-1602, 1601t
        optimal use of, 1600, 1600t
      clevudine in, 1600
      combination therapy in, 2078
      in cytotoxic chemotherapy recipients, 1602-1603, 2079
      entecavir in, 1599, 1601t, 2076, 2076t
      famciclovir in, 580
      HIV coinfection and, 1602
      immune-complex disease and, 1602
      interferon-alfa in, 588-589, 1596-1597, 1601t, 2074-2075
      issues in, 2079
      lamivudine in, 590, 1597-1598, 1601t, 2075-2076, 2076t
      patient selection for, 2074, 2075t
      in pregnancy, 1602
      recommendations for, 1600-1602, 1601t
      in special populations, 1602-1603, 2078-2079
      telbivudine in, 1600, 1601t, 2076-2077, 2076t
      tenofovir in, 1600, 1601t, 2077
      viral resistance in, 2077-2078
  clinical features of, 1579, 2069-2072
  diagnosis of, 2073-2074, 2073t
  epidemiology of, 1577-1578, 1578f, 1578t, 1582-1583, 1582t, 1583f, 2067-2069, 2068f, 2068t
  extrahepatic manifestations of, 2072
  fulminant, 1580
  global prevalence of, 2067-2068, 2068f, 2068t
  hepatitis C coinfection with, 2073
    cirrhosis and, 2165-2166
  hepatocellular carcinoma in, 2067-2068
  hepatotropism of, 2059-2061

Hepatitis B virus infection (Continued)
  historical perspective on, 1577, 2059
  HIV coinfection with, 2072
    prophylaxis against, 1858t-1859t
    treatment of, 1860t-1870t, 2078-2079
  in injection drug users, 3883-3884
  past, diagnosis of, 2073, 2073t
  pathogenesis of, 2066-2067
  postexposure prophylaxis for, 2079-2080
  post-transplant reactivation of, 2072-2073, 2078
  prevention of, 1590, 2079-2081
  prognosis for, 2069-2072
  risk factors for, 1583, 1583f
  serologic markers of, 1583
  transmission of, 1583, 1583f, 2069, 2069t
    nosocomial, 3739-3741, 3740t
    transfusion-related, 3745
  in transplant recipients, 3823, 3845
  treatment of, 1589, 2074-2078
    entecavir in, 579
    ganciclovir in, 585
    interferon-alfa for, 615
    telbivudine in, 596
    tenofovir in, 596
Hepatitis B virus polymerase protein, 2062-2063, 2063f
Hepatitis C RNA
  direct detection of, 2168
  nontranslated, 2157
Hepatitis C virus, 1584-1585, 2157-2185
  antibody to, 1584-1585
  characteristics of, 1577, 1578t
  classification of, 2157
  detection of, 259t-260t
  genetic diversity of, 2160-2161
  genome of, 2157-2160, 2158f-2159f
  genotypes of, 2161, 2161f-2162f
    determination of, 2168
    and response to therapy, 1607-1609
  geographic distribution of, 2161, 2162f
  nonstructural proteins of, 2159-2160
  NS2 proteins of, 2159
  p7 proteins of, 2159
  pathogenesis of, 1587
  polyprotein of, 2157, 2158f
  quasispecies variation of, 2160-2161
  replication of, 2160
    in animal models, 2162-2163
    autonomous, 2161-2162, 2163f
    in cell cultures, 2162, 2163f
    experimental models of, 2161-2163
    suppression of, 2175
  structural proteins of, 2157-2159, 2159f
  tropism of, 2161
  vaccine for, 2175
  virion properties of, 2157, 2158f
Hepatitis C virus infection
  acute
    with chronic hepatitis C, 1610
    clinical manifestations of, 2167
    treatment of, 2174
  antiretroviral therapy effects on, 2176-2177
  arthritis in, 1449-1450
  cancer from, 1916-1917
  in cancer patients, 3799
  chronic, 1585, 1603-1611
    with acute hepatitis C, 1610
    with B-cell lymphoma, 1611
    clinical features of, 1605-1606
    with HIV coinfection, 1606, 1610-1611
    with immune-complex disease, 1611
    after liver transplantation, 1610
    natural history of, 1604-1605
    pathophysiology of, 1604-1605
    progression of, 1605
    treatment of, 1606-1609, 1606t-1607t
      amantadine in, 576
      antiviral agents in, 566t-567t
      candidates for, 1595-1600, 1609t
      clinical benefits of, 1609
      future therapies in, 1611
      interferon-alfa in, 1606
      peginterferon-alfa in, 1606-1607, 1606t-1607t
      response to, 1608
      ribavirin in, 595

Hepatitis C virus infection (Continued)
    ribavirin/peginterferon-alfa in, 1607-1608, 1607t
      side effects of, 1607
      in special populations, 1610-1611
      tailored therapy in, 1608
  cirrhosis in, 2165-2166
  clinical manifestations of, 1584-1585, 2167-2168
  diagnosis of, 2168-2169
  direct detection of, 2168
  disease progression in, 2165-2167, 2165f, 2166f
  epidemiology of, 1577-1578, 1578t, 1579f, 1584, 2170-2172
  extrahepatic manifestations of, 2168
  fulminant, 1580, 2167
  hepatic fibrosis in, 2166
    noninvasive markers of, 2169-2170
  hepatitis B coinfection with, 2073
    cirrhosis and, 2165-2166
  hepatocellular carcinoma in, 2166-2167
  historical perspective on, 1577
  HIV coinfection with, 1606, 1610-1611, 2176-2177
    diagnosis of, 2177
    epidemiology of, 2176
    and impact on course of HCV infection, 2176
    and impact on course of HIV infection, 2176
    natural history of, 2176-2177
    pathogenesis of, 2177
    serologic tests for, 2177
    treatment of, 1860t-1870t, 2177
  immunity to
    cellular, 2164
    humoral, 2163-2164
  incidence of, 2170
  in injection drug users, 3884
  laboratory assessment of, 2168-2170
  liver biopsy in, 2169, 2169t
  natural history of, 2163-2167, 2165f
  nosocomial, 2171
  pathogenesis of, 2163-2167
  pretreatment evaluation of, 2169
  prevalence of, 2170
  prevention of, 2175-2176
    post-exposure, 2176
    pre-exposure, 2175
  retreatment of, 2174
  serology of, 2168
  tests for, clinical application of, 2168-2169
  transmission of, 2170-2172
    biologic basis of, 2170
    cofactors in, 2172
    maternal-infant, 2171-2172
    nosocomial, 2171, 3740t, 3741-3742
    percutaneous, 2170-2171
    sexual, 2171
    transfusion-related, 3745-3746
  in transplant recipients, 3823, 3845
  treatment of, 1589, 2172-2175
    adverse reactions to, 2174
    efficacy of and response indicators in, 2173-2174, 2173f
    histologic and clinical responses to, 2172
    interferon-alfa in, 589, 615, 2172-2173
    peginterferon-alfa in, 2173
    ribavirin/interferon-alfa in, 2173, 2173f
    small molecule antivirals in, 2174-2175, 2175f
    virologic responses to, 2172, 2172f
  viral persistence in, 2163-2165, 2163f
    mechanisms of, 2164-2165
Hepatitis D antigen, 1584, 2065, 2065f
Hepatitis D RNA, 2065
Hepatitis D virus, 1584, 2065-2066
  antibody to, 1584
  characteristics of, 1577, 1578t
  detection of, 259t-260t
  genetics of, 1584
  genome of, 2065
  geographic distribution of, 1584
  pathogenesis of, 1586
  replication of, 2065-2066, 2065f
  structure of, 2065, 2065f
Hepatitis D virus infection
  chronic, 1603
    treatment of, 1603
  clinical manifestations of, 1584, 2072

Hepatitis D virus infection (Continued)
  epidemiology of, 2069
  hepatitis B coinfection with, 1584
  in injection drug users, 3884
  pathogenesis of, 2067
  transmission of
    nosocomial, 3740t, 3742
    transfusion-related, 3745
  treatment of, 1589, 2079
Hepatitis E virus, 2411-2421
  antigenic composition of, 2413
  characteristics of, 1577, 1578t, 2411-2415
  classification of, 2412
  detection of, 259t-260t
  genetics of, 1585, 2412-2413, 2413f
  genome of, 2411, 2412f
  geographic distribution of, 2412-2413, 2413f
  host range of, 2415
  incubation period for, 2415
  replication of, 2415-2416, 2416f
  structure of, 2411-2412, 2412f
  vaccine for, 1590, 2419
Hepatitis E virus infection
  in animals, 2415
  cholestatic, 2416-2417
  clinical manifestations of, 1585-1586, 2417
  complications of, 2417
  epidemics of, 1585, 1585t
  epidemiology of, 2413-2414, 2414f
  fulminant, 1580, 2416-2417
  historical perspective on, 2411
  immune response to, 2416-2417, 2417f
  immunity to, 2419
  laboratory diagnosis of, 2417-2419
  molecular tests for, 2419
  pathogenesis of, 2415-2417
  pathology of, 2416
  in pregnancy, 1585, 2416-2417
  prevention of, 2419
  serologic tests for, 2418-2419, 2418f
  time course of, 1586, 1586f
  transmission of, 1585, 2414-2415
    nosocomial, 3739, 3740t
    transfusion-related, 3746
  in transplant recipients, 3846
  treatment of, 2419
Hepatitis F virus, 1578
Hepatitis G virus, 259t-260t, 1578, 1586
Hepatocellular carcinoma
  clinical manifestations of, 2167
  HBx in, 2067-2068
  hepatitis B-related, 1593-1594, 2067
    prognosis for, 2071-2072
  hepatitis C-related, 1605, 2166-2167
  surveillance of, 2079
Hepatomegaly
  in schistosomiasis, 3598
  in Still's disease, 787
Hepatorenal failure, foodborne disease and, 1417t, 1418
Hepatosplenic candidiasis, 3233, 3234f, 3237
Hepatotoxicity
  of pyrazinamide, 537
  of quinolones, 504
  of rifamycins, 405
  of telithromycin, 439
Hepatotropism, of hepatitis B, 2059-2061
Herbal medicine, 669-676, 670t
  hepatitis from, 1588
Hereditary factors, in innate immunity, 37-38, 38f
Hereditary hemorrhagic telangiectasia, brain abscess from, 1267
Herniation, brain, after lumbar puncture, 1184
Heroin
  abuse of. See Injection drug users.
  immune effects of, 3876
Herpangina, from enteroviruses, 817-818, 2355-2356
Herpes B virus, 1938t-1940t, 2023-2025
  characteristics of, 2023
  clinical manifestations of, 2023
  diagnosis of, 2023-2025
  encephalitis from, 1246t, 1255
  epidemiology of, 2023
  history of, 2023
  pathogenesis of, 2023, 2024f

Herpes B virus (*Continued*)
  postexposure prophylaxis for, 2024-2025, 2024t
  prevention of, 2025
  treatment of, 2025
Herpes gladiatorum, 1952
Herpes labialis, 566t-567t, 570-571
  recurrent, 1948
Herpes simplex virus, 1943-1962
  acyclovir-resistant, 568-569
  of central nervous system, 1950, 1952, 1957t
  conjunctivitis from, 1532
    in neonates, 566t-567t, 1536
  counseling for, 1958
  description of, 1943-1944
  detection of, 259t-260t
  diagnosis of, 1956
  disseminated, 1950
  encephalitis from, 1250-1253, 1952
    antiviral agents for, 566t-567t, 571
    magnetic resonance imaging in, 1247-1248,
      1248f
  epidemiology of, 1944, 1945t
  esophagitis from, 1354-1355, 1355f, 1952-1953
    treatment of, 1355t, 1356
  of eye, 1952, 1952f
  of finger (whitlow), 1951-1952
  genital, 1948-1950, 1949f
    antiviral agents for, 566t-567t, 570
    complications of, 1950-1951
    extragenital lesions in, 1950
    inguinal adenopathy in, 1326
    lesions in, 1476-1481, 1476f-1477f
    in pregnancy, 1955
    superinfection in, 1950-1951
    treatment of, 1957t
  in hematopoietic stem cell transplant recipients,
    3828
  hepatitis from, 1587, 1953
  in HIV infection, 1875, 1953-1954, 1953t
    oral ulcers from, 1715
    prophylaxis against, 1858t-1859t, 1871t
    skin lesions from, 1716, 1716f
    treatment of, 1860t-1870t
  in immunocompromised hosts, 1954, 1954f, 1957t
  incidence of, 1944
  inguinal adenopathy from, 1326
  keratitis from, 1545, 1547, 1547t
  latency of, 1943-1944
  meningitis from, 1189-1190, 1201-1202,
    1207-1208, 1950
  MHC class I downregulation by, 134
  mucocutaneous, 1954, 1954f
    foscarnet for, 582
    in immunocompromised hosts, 566t-567t, 571,
      577
    recurrent, 1951
    treatment of, 1956, 1957t
  myelitis from, 1950
  in neonates, 1954
  nosocomial, 3771-3772
  orofacial, 1948, 1948f
  orolabial, 566t-567t, 570-571, 1948
  pathogenesis of, 1945-1947, 1946f-1947f
  pharyngitis from, 818
  pneumonitis from, 1953
  in pregnancy, 1954-1955, 1955t
    clinical course of, 1955
    prevention of, 1955-1956
  prevention of, 1958
  reactivation of
    frequency of, 1946, 1947f, 1951
    treatment for, 1957t
  replication of, 1943, 1945
  sacral radiculopathy from, 1950
  in solid organ transplant recipients, 3847
  spectrum of diseases caused by, 1947-1948
  transmission of, 1944-1945
  in transplant recipients, 1954, 1954f
  treatment of
    acyclovir in, 570-571
    antiviral agents in, 566t-567t, 1956-1958, 1957t
    docosanol in, 578
    famciclovir in, 580
    idoxuridine in, 585
    interferon-alfa in, 589

Herpes simplex virus (*Continued*)
    trifluridine in, 596
  type 1, 1938t-1940t, 1943
    antibodies to, 1944
    complement interactions with, 85
    latency-associated transcription of, 1944
    seroprevalence of, 1945t, 1956
  type 2, 1938t-1940t, 1943
    acquisition of, cofactors for risk of, 1944
    antibodies to, 1944
    latency-associated transcription of, 1944
    screening for, 1956
    seroprevalence of, 1945t, 1956
    uveitis from, 1562-1563, 1567
    visceral, 1952-1953, 1957t
Herpes simplex virus DNA, 1943
Herpes zoster. *See also* Varicella-zoster virus.
  chronic, 1966
  clinical manifestations of, 1965-1966, 1965f
  conjunctivitis from, 1532
  diagnosis of, 1966
  epidemiology of, 1964
  historical perspective on, 1963
  in HIV infection, 1858t-1859t, 1875
    HAART and, 1721
    prophylaxis against, 1858t-1859t, 1871t
    retinitis from, 1719-1720
    skin lesions from, 1716, 1716f
    treatment of, 1860t-1870t
  keratitis from, 1546-1547, 1548t
  meningitis from, 1189-1190
  pathogenesis of, 1964
  treatment of, 1966-1967
  vaccine for, 1967-1968
Herpes zoster ophthalmicus, 1546, 1965
Herpesvirus(es)/herpesvirus infection(s), 1937-1942.
    See also Human herpesvirus *entries.*
  alpha, 1937
  beta, 1937
  classification of, 1937
  clinical manifestations of, 1939, 1939t-1940t
  diagnosis of, 1940, 1941f
  drug-resistant, 1941
  epidemiology of, 1939
  gamma, 1937
  genome of, 1937, 1938t
  immunity in, 1939-1940
  in immunocompromised hosts, 1939, 1939t
  latency of, 1937-1938
  meningitis from, 1189-1190, 1205
  nosocomial, 3771-3780
  oncogenicity of, 1940
  pathogenesis of, 1938
  prevention of, 1941
  rash from, 802
  reactivation of, 1938
  replication of, 1937
  structure of, 1937, 1938f
  transfusion-related, 3746
  treatment of, 1940-1941
Herpetic whitlow, 1951-1952
Herpetiform exanthems, from enteroviruses, 2355
Heterophile antibodies, in Epstein-Barr virus, 1992,
    1999-2000, 1999t
Heterophyes heterophyes, 3596t, 3602
Hexaplex assay, 260
Hidradenitis suppurativa, 1303
  from *Staphylococcus aureus*, 2566
High endothelial venules (HEVs), in lymph nodes,
    142
Highly active antiretroviral therapy (HAART). *See
    also* Antiretroviral therapy.
  for anal cancer, 1774
  for cervical cancer, 1773
  and chemotherapy, for HIV-related non-Hodg-
    kin's lymphoma, 1769-1770
  for CNS lymphoma, 1772
  for esophagitis, 1356
  for HIV infection, 1784
    during breast-feeding, 1787
    with cryptococcosis, 3294
    with HBV coinfection, 1602
    natural history effects of, 1710-1711,
      1710f-1711f
  for HIV-related non-Hodgkin's lymphoma, 1769

Highly active antiretroviral therapy (HAART)
    (*Continued*)
  for Hodgkin's disease, 1776
  for HPV infection, 1798
  for Kaposi's sarcoma, 1768
  for microsporidiosis, 3401, 3401t
  progressive multifocal leukoencephalopathy and,
    2052-2055
  for toxoplasmosis, 3505
High-mobility group box (HMGB)-1, in severe
    sepsis, 993
Histamine fish poisoning, 1416-1417, 1417t,
    1419-1420, 1422
Histiocytic necrotizing lymphadenitis, 1327-1329
Histiocytosis, sinus, with lymphadenopathy, 1329
Histologic activity index, in liver biopsy, 2169, 2169t
Histoplasma capsulatum (histoplasmosis), 3305-3318
  African, 3314
  arthritis from, 1451
  arthropathy from, 3317
  in children, 3312
  clinical manifestations of, 3309t
  culture of, 3314
  diagnosis of, 3314-3315, 3315f
  ecology of, 3305
  endocarditis from, 3313, 3317
  epidemiology of, 3305, 3306f
  gastrointestinal manifestations of, 1395
  granulomas from, 3308, 3308f
  history of, 3305
  in HIV infection, 1718, 1718f, 1858t-1871t, 1878,
    3311-3312, 3312f, 3317
  in immunocompromised hosts, 3312, 3317
  laryngeal infections from, 823
  mediastinal granuloma and fibrosis from, 3310,
    3310f, 3316
  mediastinitis from, 1179
  meningitis from, 1239, 3313, 3317
  mycelial phase of, 3305-3306, 3306f
  mycology of, 3305-3307, 3306f-3307f
  ocular infections from, 3313-3314, 3317
  pathogenesis of, 3307-3308, 3308f
  pericarditis from, 3317
  in pregnancy, 3317
  presumed ocular histoplasmosis syndrome from,
    1566
  prevention of, 3317
    in HIV infection, 3317
    in immunocompromised hosts, 3317
  progressive disseminated, 3311-3313
    acute, 3312, 3312f, 3316
    chronic, 3313, 3313f, 3316-3317
    subacute, 3312-3313, 3316-3317
  pulmonary infections from, 3308-3310
    acute primary, 3308-3310, 3309f, 3315-3316
    acute reinfection, 3310
    cavitary, 3310-3311, 3310f, 3316
    chronic, 3310-3311, 3310f
    chronic fibrocavitary, 938f
    in HIV infection, 1732
  serology of, 3314-3315
  skin test for, 3315
  staining of, 3315, 3315f
  travel-related, 4024
  treatment of, 3315-3317
  vaccine for, 3317
  yeast phase of, 3306, 3307f
Histoplasma capsulatum var. *duboisii*, 3314
Histoplasmoma, 3310, 3313, 3316
HIV. *See* Human immunodeficiency virus.
HLA (human leukocyte antigen)
  alleles of, 141
  in hepatitis B susceptibility, 52
  HIV nonprogression and, 1692
  in HIV susceptibility, 51, 55
  in infection susceptibility, 50, 53-54
  in malaria susceptibility, 50, 55
  matching of, in hematopoietic stem cell
    transplantation, 3822
  rheumatic fever and, 2612
HLA-A, 141
HLA-B27
  in HIV nonprogression, 51
  in reactive arthritis, 1491-1492
HLA-B35, in HIV susceptibility, 51

HLA-B53, in malaria resistance, 50, 53, 55
HLA-B57, in HIV nonprogression, 51
HLA-B*5701
    abacavir hypersensitivity reaction and, 269
    screening for, during antiretroviral therapy, 1847
HLA-DM, in MHC class I antigen processing,
        135-136
HLA-DQ
    in hepatitis C resistance, 51t
    in toxoplasmosis susceptibility, 3500
HLA-DR, following surgery, 3895
HLA-DR2, in leprosy susceptibility, 51t, 53
HLA-DR13, in malaria resistance, 50
HLA-DRB1
    in hepatitis B susceptibility, 51t, 52-53
    in Lyme arthritis, 3076
HLA-E, 141
HLA-G, 141
HN protein, of parainfluenza viruses, 2195
Hoarseness, in croup, 826
Hodgkin's disease
    from Epstein-Barr virus, 1996t, 1997, 1998f, 2004
    from HIV infection, 1775-1776
Hollow fiber model system, 300-301
Home parenteral therapy, for actinomycosis, 3216
Home testing, for HIV infection, 1680
Homeland Security Presidential Directive-21
        (HSPD-21), 3957
Homeless shelters, tuberculosis spread in, 3135
Hookworms, 632t-635t, 3578t, 3579f-3580f,
        3580-3581
    cutaneous larva migrans from, 3618t, 3619
    eosinophilic gastroenteritis from, 3618t, 3621
Hordeolum, 1569
Hormones, immunity and, 45
Hospital(s)
    accreditation of, in infection control, 3671-3672
    disinfection in, 3681-3684. See also Disinfection.
        rational approach to, 3677-3681, 3678t-3679t
    emergency preparedness of. See Emergency
        preparedness.
    infection control in, 3667-3672, 3670t
        in plague terrorist event, 3968
        in tularemia terrorist event, 3974
    infections acquired in. See Health care–associated
        infections; Nosocomial infections.
    sterilization in, 3684-3688. See also Sterilization.
        rational approach to, 3677-3681, 3678t-3679t
    tuberculosis in, 3135
Hospital epidemiologist, 3671
Hospital epidemiology programs, 3667-3672, 3670t
Hospital waste, 3690-3692
    disposal of, 3691t
Hospital-acquired pneumonia, 3717. See also
        Pneumonia, nosocomial.
Host, 187, 187t
    agent versus, 185-188
    genetics of
        approaches to, 49-50
        in disease susceptibility, 49-50, 50t
        variations in, 49
Host defenses, 988-992
    acute phase, 990-992. See also Acute-phase
        response.
    autophagy in, 41
    cutaneous, 38-40
    enteric, 1336-1339, 1336t
    eye in, 41
    genitourinary tract in, 40-41
    innate, 37-47, 38t. See also Immunity, innate.
    intestinal tract in, 40
    local, 988-989, 989f, 990t
    of male lower urogenital tract, 1521
    mechanism of, at surgical site, 3894
    metabolic, 44
    mucous membranes in, 40
    neutrophil-dependent, defects in, 110-118, 111t
    pathologic, 992-995
    phagocytosis in, 41
    pulmonary, 891-893, 893t
        impairment of, 893-894
    respiratory tract in, 40
    in sepsis, augmentation of, 1005
    subversion of, 10
    systemic, 989-990, 990t

Host factors, in antimicrobial therapy, 268-272
Host-agent relationship, 185-188
Host-virus interactions, 1913-1918, 1914f-1915f,
        1914t
Hot tub folliculitis, 798, 2854
Hourglass sign, in croup, 827, 827f
House-mouse mites, 3643, 3646t
Howell-Jolly bodies, in asplenia, 3866, 3866f
Human bites, 3914
    to head and neck, 862t, 868
    management of, 3914
Human bocavirus, 202, 2093
    bronchiolitis from, 886f
    croup from, 825-826, 826f
Human dependoviruses, 2093
Human granulocytotropic anaplasmosis. See
        Anaplasmosis, human granulocytotropic.
Human growth hormone, cadaver-derived,
        Creutzfeldt-Jakob disease associated with, 2431
Human herpesvirus 4. See Epstein-Barr virus/
        Epstein-Barr virus infection.
Human herpesvirus 6, 1938t-1940t, 2011-2014
    characteristics of, 2011
    clinical manifestations of, 2011-2013, 2012f, 2012t
    congenital, 2013
    detection of, 259t-260t
    diagnosis of, 2013-2014
    encephalitis from, 1255, 2012-2013
    epidemiology of, 2011, 2012f
    exanthem subitum from, 2012, 2012f
    in hematopoietic stem cell transplant recipients,
        3830
    history of, 2011
    in HIV infection, 1860t-1870t, 1877
    in immunocompromised hosts, 2013-2014
    infantile fever from, 2011-2012, 2012f
    infectious mononucleosis from, 2013, 2013f
    multiple sclerosis from, 2013
    nosocomial, 3778
    pathogenesis of, 2011
    rash from, 802
    seizures from, 2011-2012
    treatment of, 2014
Human herpesvirus 7, 1938t-1940t, 2014-2015
    clinical manifestations of, 2014-2015
    detection of, 259t-260t
    diagnosis of, 2015
    epidemiology of, 2012f, 2014
    history of, 2014
    nosocomial, 3778
    pathogenesis of, 2014
    rash from, 802
    treatment of, 2015
Human herpesvirus 8, 2017-2022
    biology of, 2017-2018
    classification of, 2017
    clinical manifestations of, 2018-2021
    detection of, 259t-260t
    epidemiology of, 2018
    history of, 2017
    in HIV infection, 1860t-1870t, 1881
    Kaposi's sarcoma from, 1765-1766, 2018-2020,
        2019f-2020f. See also Kaposi's sarcoma.
    MHC class I downregulation by, 134
    multicentric Castleman's disease from, 2020-2021,
        2021f
    nosocomial, 3778
    oncogenicity of, 1940
    pathogenesis of, 2018
    prevention of, 2021
    primary effusion lymphoma from, 2020, 2020f
    primary infection syndrome for, 2018
    in solid organ transplant recipients, 3848
    targeting of, 1768
    transfusion-related, 3746
    transmission of, 1766
    treatment of, 2021
Human immunodeficiency virus, 2323-2335
    accessory/regulatory genes of, 2329-2330
    chemokines and, 2331
    classification of, 2323-2324
    complement interactions with, 85
    co-receptor usage by, 1848
    detection of, 259t-260t
    emergence of, 209-210

Human immunodeficiency virus (Continued)
    entry into cell of, 1687, 1688f
    envelope glycoproteins in, 2328-2329
    Gag proteins in, 2327-2328, 2327t
    genetics of, 51-52, 51t, 1664f, 2324f, 2326-2327,
        2327t
        variation in, 2332
    genome of, 2324f
    genotypes of, 1786
    gp120/160 adhesin of, 18-19, 18f
    immune response to, 1667-1668, 1668f
    integrase in, 2328
    life cycle of, 2324-2327, 2324f, 2327f
    long terminal repeats in, 2331, 2331f
    in menstrual blood, 1784
    Nef protein in, 2330
    oncogenicity of, 2332-2333
    origin of, 2323-2324
    Pol protein in, 2328
    protease in, 2328
    receptors for, 1687, 1688f, 2331
    replication cycle of, antiretroviral therapy targeted
        to, 1833, 1834f
    reservoirs for, 1693-1694
    Rev protein in, 2330
    reverse transcriptase in, 2328
    RNA viral load in, 1800-1801
    structural proteins of, 2326f, 2327-2331, 2327t
    structure of, 2326-2327, 2326f
    subtype O, 1678
    Tat protein in, 2329
    tropism of, 2331
    type 2, 1650
        HIV transmission and, 1625
        in sub-Saharan Africa, 1622
        transfusion-related, 3745
    variability of, 2332
    Vif protein in, 2330
    viral enzymes in, 2328
    viral load of, 2331-2332
    virus-cell fusion in, 2329, 2329f
    Vpr protein in, 2330
    Vpu protein in, 2330
    Western blot assay for, 65
Human immunodeficiency virus entry inhibitors, as
        therapeutic targets, 21-22, 21t
Human immunodeficiency virus infection, 176-177
    acute (primary), 1642
        exanthem of, 1716
        HIV testing in, 1675, 1679
        versus infectious mononucleosis, 2003
    acute retroviral syndrome in, 817, 1711-1713,
        1712f, 1712t
    AIDS case definition in, 1635-1636, 1636t-1637t
    AIDS trends in, 1640, 1641f
    AIDS-indicator diseases in, 1643-1644
    American trypanosomiasis in, 3485
    amyotrophic lateral sclerosis in, 1758-1759
    anogenital neoplasia in, 1772-1775
        clinical implications of, 1774, 1774t
        histopathology of, 1773
        human papillomavirus in, 1772
        treatment recommendations for, 1774-1775
    aphthous ulcer in, 1712, 1712f
    in Asia, 1622-1623, 1623f-1624f
    aspergillosis in, 1860t-1870t, 1878
    in asplenia, 3869
    B cell response in, 1697
    bacillary angiomatosis in, 1302-1303, 1716-1717
    Bartonella in, 1858t-1871t, 1881, 3002
    biliary tract disorders in, 1738-1739
    Blastomyces dermatitidis in, 3327
    Campylobacter in, 1860t-1870t, 1880
    Campylobacter jejuni in, 2796
    cancer in, 1765-1779, 2332-2333. See also specific
        neoplasm.
    candidiasis in, 1858t-1871t, 1877
        esophageal, 1737
        oral, 1714-1715, 1714f
        prophylaxis against, 1858t-1859t, 1871t
        treatment of, 1860t-1870t
        vulvovaginal, 1796-1797
    cardiac manifestations of, 1720
    CD4 cell response in, 1691-1692, 1695-1696
    CD8 cell response in, 1690-1691, 1690t, 1696-1697

Human immunodeficiency virus infection
    (*Continued*)
    central nervous system lymphoma in, 1771-1772
        EBV DNA in, 2002
        treatment of, 1772
    central nervous system mass lesions in, 1749-1754,
        1755f
    cerebrospinal fluid in, 1747
    cervical cancer in, 1773, 1797-1798
    cervical intraepithelial neoplasia in, 1772-1773,
        1796-1798
    Chagas disease in, 1860t-1870t
    in children, 1644-1645, 1645f, 1809-1832. *See also*
        Children, HIV infection in.
    cholangiopathy in, 1041, 1738-1739
    classification of, 1705-1706, 1706t-1707t
    clinical manifestations of, 1642-1644, 1705-1725
        antiretroviral therapy impact on, 1710-1711,
            1710f-1711f
    Clostridium difficile in, 1880
    coccidioidomycosis in, 1858t-1871t, 1878
    colonic disorders in, 1741-1742
    constitutional disease in, 1713
    counseling for, 1653-1654
    cryptococcal meningitis in, 1877
        prophylaxis against, 1858t-1859t, 1871t
        treatment of, 1860t-1870t
    cryptococcosis in, 1718, 1718f, 3290, 3294, 3296
        treatment of, 3299
    cryptosporidiosis in, 1880, 3553-3554
        treatment of, 1860t-1870t, 3554-3555
    cutaneous manifestations of, 1716-1718
    Cyclospora in, 1880
    cytokine dysregulation in, 1699
    cytomegalovirus in, 1710-1711, 1710f, 1875-1877,
        1975-1976, 1975f
        colitis from, 1976
        diarrhea from, 1976
        encephalitis from, 1750f, 1753-1754
        oral ulcers from, 1715
        pelvic inflammatory disease from, 1797
        polyradiculopathy from, 1758, 1976
        retinitis from, 1719, 1975
            HAART and, 1721
            treatment of, 1975-1976
    dementia in. *See* AIDS dementia.
    demography of, 1640-1641, 1641t
    dendritic cell response in, 1698
    diagnosis of, 1642, 1663-1686. *See also* Human
        immunodeficiency virus infection, testing for.
        algorithms for, 1675, 1676f
        alternative strategies for, 1677
        antibody testing in, 1653-1654
        background/perspective on, 1663-1665,
            1664f-1665f
        confirmatory assays in, 1666f, 1672-1677,
            1673f-1674f
        distribution issues in, 1681
        enzyme-linked immunosorbent assays in
            alternative, 1669-1670
            history of, 1663
            saliva for, 1670
            standard, 1668-1669, 1669f
            urine for, 1670
        FDA-approved assays in, 1666, 1667t
        in HIV-1/2 dual infections, 1677-1678
        immunofluorescence assay in, 1673-1674
        laboratory methods in, 1667-1677
        in non-B subtypes, 1678
        nonserologic assays in, 1671-1672
        nucleic acid testing in, 1664, 1671-1672, 1671f
        particle agglutination assays in, 1669, 1669f
        perinatal, 1678-1679, 1818-1819
        point-of-care (home) testing in, 1680
        positive predictive value in, 1665-1666, 1666f,
            1667t, 1671
        in pregnancy, 1678
        quantitative immunocapture and sensitive/less
            sensitive assays in, 1670
        radioimmunoprecipitaiton assay in, 1674-1675
        rapid tests in, 1669-1670
        recommendations for, 1675-1677, 1676f
        regulatory issues in, 1681
        screening assays in, 1668-1672, 1669f
        serologic assays in, 260-261

Human immunodeficiency virus infection
    (*Continued*)
        for antibody detection, 1668-1670, 1669f
        for p24 antigen detection, 1663, 1670-1671
        terminology in, 1665-1666, 1666t
        test performance characteristics in, 1665-1666,
            1666f, 1666t-1667t
        virologic techniques in, 1675
        Western blot in, 1672-1673, 1673f-1674f
        window period in, 1667, 1668f
    diarrhea in, 1364-1365, 1364t
    diffuse infiltrative lymphocytosis syndrome–
        associated neuropathy in, 1758
    dissemination of, 1687-1688, 1689f
    distal sensory polyneuropathy in, 1756
    early phases of, viral proteins required for, 2326f
    in eastern Europe and Central Asia, 1620
    encephalitis in, 1251t-1252t
    endocrine disorders in, 1713-1714
    enteric pathogens in, 1860t-1870t, 1880
    enterocolitis in, 1741-1742, 1742t
    eosinophilic folliculitis in, 1717-1718, 1718f
    epidemic of
        global responses to, 1630-1631, 1630f-1631f
        impact of, 1627f, 1629-1630
        outside United States, 1649-1650
        serologic monitoring of, 1637-1640
    epidemiology of, 179, 1635-1661
    epiglottitis in, 851
    Epstein-Barr virus in, 1877
    esophageal disorders in, 1737-1738
    esophageal ulceration in, 1355
    esophagitis in, 1353-1357, 1356t, 1737
    exposure categories in, 1640
    factitious, 1680
    fever of unknown origin in, 782, 783t
    fungal infections in, fluconazole prophylaxis for,
        557
    gastric disorders in, 1738
    genetic susceptibility to, 51-52, 51t
    genital lesions in, 1479
    genitourinary tract infections in, 1525-1526, 1784
    geographic distribution of, 1641-1642, 1642f
    gingivitis in, 1715
    global impact of, 209-210
    global perspectives on, 1619-1633, 1620f, 1620t
    granulocyte-macrophage colony-stimulating factor
        for, 614
    Haemophilus influenzae in, 1878-1879
    hematologic manifestations of, 1720
    hepatic disorders in, 1739-1741, 1739t
    hepatitis A in, 1858t-1859t
    hepatitis B in, 1739, 2072
        prophylaxis against, 1858t-1859t
        treatment of, 1602, 1860t-1870t, 2078-2079
    hepatitis C in, 1606, 1610-1611, 1740, 2176-2177
        diagnosis of, 2177
        epidemiology of, 2176
        and impact on course of HCV infection, 2176
        and impact on course of HIV infection, 2176
        natural history of, 2176-2177
        pathogenesis of, 2177
        serologic tests for, 2177
        treatment of, 1860t-1870t, 2177
    hepatitis in, 1881-1882
        HAART and, 1721
    herpes simplex virus in, 1875, 1953-1954, 1953t
        oral ulcers from, 1715
        prophylaxis against, 1858t-1859t, 1871t
        skin lesions from, 1716, 1716f
        treatment of, 1860t-1870t
    herpes zoster in, 1858t-1859t, 1875, 1966
        HAART and, 1721
        prophylaxis against, 1858t-1859t, 1871t
        retinitis from, 1719-1720
        skin lesions from, 1716, 1716f
        treatment of, 1860t-1870t
    Histoplasma capsulatum in, 3311-3312, 3312f
        prophylaxis against, 3317
    histoplasmosis in, 1718, 1718f, 1858t-1871t, 1878
    historical background on, 1705, 2323
    Hodgkin's disease in, 1775-1776
    human herpesvirus 6 in, 1860t-1870t, 1877
    human herpesvirus 8 in, 1860t-1870t, 1881
    human papillomavirus in, 1858t-1870t

Human immunodeficiency virus infection
    (*Continued*)
    human T-cell lymphotrophic virus and, 2315-2316
    hyperbaric oxygen therapy in, 628
    immune dysfunction from, 1694-1698
    immune reconstitution syndrome in, 1720-1721.
        See also Immune reconstitution syndrome.
    immune response to, 1688-1692, 1887
        cellular, 1690-1692, 1690t, 1887
        humoral, 1688-1690, 1887
    immunology of, 1687-1703
    incidence of, 1636-1637
    inflammatory demyelinating polyneuropathy in,
        1755-1756
    influenza A and B in, 1858t-1859t
    influenza vaccine in, 3926-3927
    in injection drug users, 1620, 1621f, 1625, 1638,
        1781-1782, 3887
        pneumonia risk and, 1728
        transmission of, 1625, 1647, 1652
        tuberculosis with, 3883
    intravenous immune globulin in, 617
    Isospora in, 1858t-1871t, 1880
    Kaposi's sarcoma in, 1329, 1765-1768, 1881,
        2332-2333. *See also* Kaposi's sarcoma.
        oral lesions from, 1715
        skin lesions from, 1717, 1717f
        in women, 1796-1797
    in Latin America and the Caribbean, 1623-1624,
        1624f
    leiomyosarcoma in, 1775
    leishmaniasis in, 1860t-1871t
    leprosy in, 3174
    liver disease in, 1739-1741, 1739t
    long-term nonprogressors in, 1692-1693, 1692t,
        1707-1708
    lymphadenitis in, 1329-1330
    lymphadenopathy in, persistent generalized, 1713
    lymphoma in, 1768-1772, 2333. *See also*
        Non-Hodgkin's lymphoma, in HIV infection.
        central nervous system, 1751, 1752f
        gastrointestinal, 1738
        hepatic, 1741
        Hodgkin's, 1775-1776
        pulmonary, 1733
    malaria in, 1858t-1870t
    malnutrition in, 155-156, 156t
    measles vaccine in, 2234
    measles virus in, 2232
    in men who have sex with men, 1637-1638, 1640,
        1651
    meningitis in, 1190, 1745-1746
    metabolic disorders in, 1713-1714
    microsporidiosis in, 1858t-1871t, 1880, 3398-3399
    in Middle East and North Africa, 1622
    molluscum contagiosum skin lesions in, 1716,
        1717f
    monocyte-macrophage response in, 1698
    mononeuritis multiplex in, 1757
    mortality in, 1644
    musculoskeletal complications of, 1715
    musculoskeletal syndromes in, 1759-1761
    myalgia in, 1320
    mycobacterial disease in, disseminated nontuber-
        culous, 3196
    Mycobacterium avium complex in, 1710-1711,
        1710f, 1879-1880, 3177-3179, 3178f-3179f
        HAART and, 1721
        macrolides for, 437
        prophylaxis against, 1858t-1859t
        rifamycins for, 408
        treatment of, 1860t-1870t
    myelopathy in
        noncompressive, 1755
        vacuolar, 1754-1755
    myocarditis in, 1154
    myopathy in, 1759
    natural history of, 1706-1711, 1707f-1709f, 1708t
    natural killer cell response in, 1697-1698
    nephropathy from, 1719
    neurologic diseases in, 1745-1764, 1760t
        CD4 count and, 1760f
        temporal trends and aging in, 1761
    neuropathies in, 1755-1758
    neurosyphilis in, 1745-1746

Human immunodeficiency virus infection
  (Continued)
  neutralizing antibody responses to, 1887
  non-Hodgkin's lymphoma in, 1768-1771, 2333.
    See also Non-Hodgkin's lymphoma, in HIV
    infection.
  nonopportunistic infections in, 1857
  nosocomial, 3753-3770. See also Human
    immunodeficiency virus infection,
    occupational.
    from health care worker to patient, 3755-3757,
      3756t
    from patient to health care worker, 3753-3757,
      3754f, 3755t
    from patient to patient, 3757
    postexposure prophylaxis for, 3761-3767,
      3764t-3765t
    prevention of
      HIV testing in, 3761
      primary, 3757-3759
      secondary, 3761-3767, 3764t-3765t
  nucleoside neuropathy in, 1756-1757, 1757t
  occupational
    antiretroviral chemoprophylaxis for, 1848-1849,
      3761-3767, 3764t-3765t
    definition of, 3753-3754
    diagnosis of, 1679-1680
    follow-up for, 3766-3767
    initial management of, 3759-3760
    mechanisms of, 3753
    postexposure prophylaxis for, 3761-3767,
      3764t-3765t
    prevention of
      HIV testing in, 3761
      primary, 3757-3759
      secondary, 3761-3767, 3764t-3765t
    reported cases of, 3753, 3754f
    risk factors for, 3754-3755, 3755t
    transmission of, 1648-1649, 3753-3757, 3754f
  ocular complications of, 1719-1720
  opportunistic infections in, 1855-1886
    antiretroviral therapy impact on, 1710-1711,
      1710f-1711f, 1856
    drug interactions and, 1857
    management principles for, 1857-1858
    outpatient parenteral antimicrobial therapy for,
      700, 700t
    pathogens associated with, 1856-1857
    probability of, 1709, 1709f
    prophylaxis for, 1858t-1859t, 1871t
    prospective monitoring for, 1855-1856
    treatment of, 1858-1882, 1860t-1870t
  oral disease in, 1714-1715
  oral hairy leukoplakia in, 1715
  pancreatic disorders in, 1741
  pancreatitis in, 1045
  pathogenesis of, 2331-2332
    immune activation in, 1698-1699
  penicilliosis in, 1860t-1871t
  periodontitis in, 1715
  pharyngitis from, 817
  Pneumocystis pneumonia in, 1710-1711, 1710f,
    1729-1730, 1858-1874
    as AIDS indicator, 1643
    CD4+ counts in, 1727
    choroiditis from, 1720
    diagnosis of, 1870
    prophylaxis against, 1858t-1859t, 1871t, 1873
    treatment of, 1860t-1870t, 1872
  pneumonia in, 895
    antiretroviral therapy and, 1727-1728
    bacterial, 1730-1731, 1731f
    community-acquired, 906
    fungal, 1731-1732
    mycobacterial, 1731
    parasitic, 1732-1733
    from Pneumocystis jirovecii. See Human
      immunodeficiency virus infection,
      Pneumocystis pneumonia in.
    viral, 1732
  postexposure prophylaxis for. See Antiretroviral
    therapy, for postexposure prophylaxis.
  in pregnancy. See Pregnancy, HIV infection in.
  prevalence of, 1619, 1620f, 1636-1637
  prevention of, 1650-1653

Human immunodeficiency virus infection
  (Continued)
  in health care settings, 1652-1653
  in injection drug users, 1652
  perinatal, 1653
  sexual behavior modifications for, 1650-1652
  in transfusion settings, 1652
  in professional sex workers, 1638-1639, 4015
  progression of, 1642-1643, 1706-1711, 1707f-
    1709f, 1708t
  progressive multifocal leukoencephalopathy in,
    1752-1753, 1753f, 1860t-1870t, 1877, 2052
  progressive polyradiculopathy in, 1758
  pseudomembranous colitis in, 1378
  Pseudomonas aeruginosa in, 2856
  pulmonary manifestations of, 1727-1735
    diagnostic tests in, 1728-1729
    differential diagnosis of, 1727-1728, 1728t
    epidemiology of, 1727
    neoplastic, 1733-1734, 1733f
    noninfectious, 1733-1734, 1733f
    triage in, 1728
  pyomyositis in, 1313
  reactive arthritis in, 1492
  renal disease in, 1718-1719
  reporting of, 1664
  reservoirs of, 1693-1694
  respiratory bacterial infections in, 1860t-1870t
  respiratory syncytial virus infection in, 2215
  retinopathy from, 1719
  Rhodococcus equi in, 2702-2703
  Salmonella in, 1860t-1870t, 1880
    bacteremia from, 2899
    nontyphoidal, 2896
  scabies in, 1718, 1718f
  schistosomiasis coinfection in, 3599
  seborrheic dermatitis in, 1717-1718, 1717f
  seizures in, 1759-1760
  serologic monitoring of, 1637-1640
  Shigella in, 1860t-1870t, 1880
  small intestinal disorders in, 1741-1742
  spectrum of, 1642-1643
  spinal syndrome in, 1754-1755
  sporotrichosis in, 3273-3275, 3273f
  staging of, 1636, 1637t, 1705-1706, 1706t-1707t
  Streptococcus pneumoniae in, 1878-1879
  in sub-Saharan Africa, 1620-1622, 1621f
  subtype N, 1678
  surveillance case definition for, 1635-1636,
    1636t-1637t, 1705, 1706t
  syphilis coinfection with, 1639, 1860t-1870t,
    1880-1881, 3051
    treatment of, 3050
  T-cell depletion in, 2331-2332
  testing for. See also Human immunodeficiency
    virus infection, diagnosis of.
    in acute setting, 1675, 1679
    in blood donor screening, 1679
    counseling in, 1677
    as infection control procedure, 3761
    in occupational exposure, 1679-1680, 3760
    population proportion reporting, 1665, 1665f
    in tissue procurement for transplantation, 1679
    in vaccine studies, 1679
  toxoplasmosis in, 3504-3506, 3505f
    chorioretinitis from, 1720, 3501, 3504-3506,
      3505f
    encephalitis from, 1270-1271, 1874-1875
      incidence of, 3498
      prophylaxis against, 1858t-1859t
      treatment of, 3518-3519
    pulmonary, 1732-1733
  transmission of
    biology of, 2324
    by blood and other tissues, 1647-1648
    by casual contact, 1649
    demography/social context and, 1626-1627,
      1627f
    in developing world, 1624-1628
    gender and, 1627-1628
    heterosexual, 1638, 1640
    by injection drug users, 1625, 1647
    by insects, 1649
    male circumcision and, 1625-1626
    modes of, 1624-1625, 1645-1649

Human immunodeficiency virus infection
  (Continued)
  nosocomial, 1625
  occupational, 1648-1649, 3753-3757, 3754f
  patterns of, 1637-1640
  perinatal, 1625, 1785-1796, 1810-1812, 1811t
    antiretroviral therapy for, 1788
      discontinuation of, 1794
      in intrapartum period, 1795
      potential mechanisms of, 1788-1789
      recommended guidelines on, 1789
      teratogenicity of, 1795
    diagnosis of, 1818-1819
    and impact on pregnancy, 1787-1788
    postpartum follow-up in, 1795-1796
    pregnancy outcome after, 1788
    prevention of, 1653, 1810-1811, 1811t
    risk factors for, 1785-1787, 1785t
    timing of, 1785
  prevention of, 1628-1629, 1650-1653
  recipient partner susceptibility in, 1646-1647
  by saliva, 1649
  sexual behavior and, 1625-1626, 1626f,
    1645-1647
  sexually transmitted diseases and, 1624-1625,
    1647
  source partner infectiousness in, 1646
  stigma/discrimination and, 1628
  by transfusions, 1625, 1639-1640, 1647-1648,
    1652, 3745
  transplantation in, 3814
  in travelers, 4016
  treatment of
    adhesin-based therapies in, 21-22, 21t
    antiretroviral therapy in. See Antiretroviral
      therapy.
    cytokines in, 1699-1700
    hyperbaric oxygen therapy in, 628
    interferon-alfa in, 589
  trichomoniasis in, 3537
  tuberculosis in, 535-536, 536t, 1639, 1644, 1879,
    3132-3134
    extrapulmonary, 3151
    gastrointestinal, 3157
    genitourinary, 3157
    HAART and, 1721
    impact of, 1627f, 1629
    local epidemiology and, 1728
    miliary, 3153
    prophylaxis against, 1858t-1859t
    pulmonary, 3140, 3142, 3142t
    treatment of, 1860t-1870t, 3147-3148
  type 2
    detection of, 1677-1678
    plus HIV-1 infection, 1677-1678
  urologic manifestations of, 1525
  varicella-zoster virus in
    prophylaxis against, 1858t-1859t, 1871t
    treatment of, 1860t-1870t
  vector for, semen as, 1525-1526
  viral infections in, cutaneous, 1716, 1716f
  viral load in, prognosis and, 1708-1709, 1708f,
    1708t
  wasting in, 155-156, 156t, 1713-1714
  in western Europe, 1619-1620
  in women, 1781-1807
    antiretroviral therapy for
      management issues in, 1801-1802
      metabolic complications of, 1801
      pharmacokinetics and adverse events in, 1801
      response to, 1800-1801
    bacterial vaginosis in, 1796
    cervicovaginal shedding in, 1796
    clinical manifestations of, 1796-1802
    contraception and, 1800, 1800t
    donor insemination transmission of, 1782
    epidemiology of, 1640-1641, 1641t, 1781-1782
    female-to-female transmission of, 1782
    fertility issues in, 1799-1800
    of genital tract, 1784
    genital ulcer disease in, 1798-1799
    gynecologic infections in, 1796-1799
    heterosexual transmission of, 1783-1785
      efficiency of, 1783
      factors associated with, 1783-1784, 1783t

Human immunodeficiency virus infection
  (*Continued*)
    preventive strategies for, 1784-1785
  human papillomavirus infection in, 1797-1798
  Kaposi's sarcoma in, 1796-1797
  menstrual function in, 1799
  mucopurulent cervicitis in, 1797
  ovulation in, 1799
  pelvic inflammatory disease in, 1797
  perinatal transmission and. *See* Human
    immunodeficiency virus infection,
    transmission of, perinatal.
  progression of, 1800-1801
  proportion of, 1619, 1620f
  sex hormones in, 1799
  sexually transmitted disease prevention and,
    1800
  Trichomonas vaginitis in, 1797
  in United States, 1781-1782
  vulvovaginal candidiasis in, 1796-1797
  worldwide prevalence of, 1782
Human immunodeficiency virus RNA
  in acute retroviral syndrome, 1712
  in children, 1817
Human immunodeficiency virus vaccines,
    1887-1895, 3942-3943, 3942f
  adenovirus vectors for, 1889, 1891-1892
  animal models for, 1889-1890
  candidate, 1887-1889
  clinical trials of, 1890-1893
    phase I, 1890-1892
    phase II, 1890t, 1892
    phase IIB and III, 1890t, 1892-1893
  DNA, 1889, 1892
  envelope protein, 1888, 1890-1891
  HIV testing and, 1679
  internal or core protein, 1888
  live attenuated, 1888
  live vectors for, 1888-1889, 1891
  poxvirus vectors for, 1888-1889, 1891
  synthetic peptide, 1888, 1891
  whole killed, 1888
Human leukocyte antigen. *See* HLA *entries.*
Human metapneumovirus infection, 201-202,
    2223-2227
  in adults, 2225
  bronchiolitis from, 885, 886t
  characteristics of, 2223, 2224f
  in children, 2224-2225, 2224t, 2225f
  clinical manifestations of, 2224-2225, 2224t,
    2225f-2226f
  culture of, 2226, 2226f
  detection of, 259t-260t
  diagnosis of, 2225-2226, 2226f
  epidemiology of, 2223-2224
  genetics of, 202, 2223, 2224f
  in immunocompromised hosts, 2225, 2226f
  pathogenesis of, 2223
  treatment of, 2227
  vaccine for, 2227
Human papillomaviruses, 2035-2049
  in anal cancer, 1773-1774
  in anogenital neoplasia, 1772
  anogenital warts from. *See* Condylomata
    acuminata.
  cancer from, 1916
  in cervical cancer, 2037
  in cervical neoplasia, 1773
  clinical manifestations of, 2039-2041
  cutaneous warts from
    clinical manifestations of, 2039
    incidence and prevalence of, 2035-2036
    pathogenesis of, 2037, 2038f
    treatment of, 2042
  diagnosis of, 2041-2042
  disinfection/sterilization and, 3688
  epidemiology of, 2035-2037
  epidermodysplasia verruciformis from, 2039, 2044
  genital, 2036
  genome of, 2035
  in HIV infection, 1797-1798, 1858t-1870t
  immune response to, 2038
  incidence and prevalence of, 2035-2036
  interferon alfa for, 615
  oral lesions from, 2041, 2044

Human papillomaviruses (*Continued*)
  pathogenesis of, 2037-2039, 2038f
  prevention of, 2045-2046
  recurrent respiratory papillomatosis from. *See*
    Papillomatosis, recurrent respiratory.
  transmission of, 2036
  treatment of, 2042-2044
  types of, and disease associations, 2036t
  vaccine for, 2045, 3925-3926
  virology of, 2035, 2036t
Human parechovirus 1, 2342
  characteristics of, 2342
  classification of, 2337
  epidemiology of, 2342
  receptors for, 2338t, 2342
Human parvovirus 4, 2093
Human parvovirus B19. *See* Parvovirus B19.
Human T-cell lymphotrophic virus, 2303-2322
  adult T-cell leukemia/lymphoma from, 2313f-
    2314f, 2315-2316
    treatment of, 2316
  arthritis from, 1450
  asymptomatic, 2316
  biology of, 2305, 2306f
  clinical manifestations of, 2312-2316, 2312t
  demographic patterns of, 2308, 2309f
  detection of, 259t-260t, 2305-2307, 2307f
  discovery of, 2303, 2323-2324
  Env protein in, 2303-2304, 2304f, 2304t
  epidemiology of
    molecular, 2308-2310
    serologic, 2307-2308, 2308f-2309f
  Gag proteins in, 2303-2304, 2304f, 2304t
  genome of, 2303-2305, 2304f, 2304t, 2324f
  geographic distribution of, 2307-2308, 2308f
  HIV and, 2315-2316
  immune response to, 2311-2312
    cellular, 2312, 2312f
    humoral, 2311
  isolation of, 2305-2306
  myalgia from, 1320
  myelopathy from, 2314-2317
  Orf I/II proteins in, 2304f, 2304t, 2305
  Pol protein in, 2303-2304, 2304f, 2304t
  prevention of, 2317
  replication of, 2305, 2306f
  Rex proteins in, 2304f, 2304t, 2305
  structural and regulatory proteins of, 2303-2305,
    2304f, 2304t
  structure of, 2303-2305, 2304f, 2304t
  Tax proteins in, 2304-2305, 2304f, 2304t
  transfusion-related, 2311, 3745
  transmission of, 2305, 2306f, 2310-2311, 2310t
    mother-to-child, 2310-2311
    parenteral, 2311
    sexual, 2311
  treatment of, 2316-2317
  type I, 2308-2309, 2312-2314
  type II, 2309-2310, 2315-2316
  types III and IV, 2310
  vaccine for, 2317
Humidification, for croup, 828
Hutchinson's teeth, in congenital syphilis, 3044
Hyalomma, Crimean-Congo hemorrhagic fever
    from, 2290
Hybrid Capture CMV DNA assay, 1972-1973
Hybridization
  comparative genomic, 11
  subtractive, 11
Hydatid cysts, 3608t, 3613-3615, 3613f-3614f
Hydration. *See* Fluid therapy.
Hydrocephalus
  cerebrospinal fluid shunt for, 1231
  from coccidioidal meningitis, 3341
Hydrocortisone, for sepsis, 619, 1003
Hydrogen peroxide, disinfection with, 3680t, 3683
Hydrogen peroxide gas plasma, sterilization with,
    3685t, 3687
Hydrophobia, in furious rabies, 2253
Hydrops fetalis, from parvovirus B19 infection, 2091
Hydroxychloroquine, 636
  drug interactions with, 742t-761t
  for malaria, 632t-635t
  for Q fever endocarditis, 2515-2516
Hydroxychloroquine sulfate, 706t-709t

Hydroxyl radical, in neutrophil bactericidal activity,
    109
Hygiene
  in gastrointestinal infections, 1337, 1337t
  hand, 3673
  oral, 869
Hymenolepis diminuta, 3610
Hymenolepis nana, 632t-635t, 3608t, 3609-3610,
    3609f
Hyperbaric oxygen therapy, 625-629. *See also* Oxygen
    therapy.
  adverse effects of, 626, 626t
  for clostridial myonecrosis, 626-627
  contraindications to, 626
  equipment for, 625, 626f
  for Fournier's gangrene, 627
  for gas gangrene, 1318
  indications for, 625, 626t
  for mucormycosis, 628
  for necrotizing fasciitis, 627
  for osteomyelitis, 1460
  for peritonitis, 1026
  physiologic effects of, 625-626
  for refractory osteomyelitis, 627-628
Hyperbilirubinemia, in malaria, 3449
Hyperemia, conjunctival, 1530
Hypergammaglobulinemia, 72
Hyperimmunoglobulinema E, 113-114, 130,
    169t-170t, 176, 176f
  with impaired chemotaxis, 113-114
  Staphylococcus aureus infection in, 2563
Hyperimmunoglobulinema M, 72, 169t-170t, 171
Hyperleukocytosis, from granulocyte colony-
    stimulating factor, 614
Hyperparasitemia, in malaria, 3449
Hyperpyrexia, in malaria, 3449
Hypersensitivity pneumonitis, from *Mycobacterium
    avium* complex, 3183, 3186
Hypersensitivity reactions
  to abacavir, 269, 1733-1734, 1836
  cell-mediated (type IV), 347
  to cephalosporins, 331
  cytotoxic antibodies in (type II), 347
  in elderly, 269
  Gell and Coombs classification of, 70-72, 347, 348t
  idiopathic, 347
  immediate (type I), 347, 348f-349f, 348t
  immune complexes in (type III), 347
  to isoniazid, 534
  to penicillin, 313, 314f, 314t
  to rifampin, 535
  to rifamycins, 404
  to *Staphylococcus*, 1542
  to sulfonamides, 477
  to tetracycline, 390-392
  type I, 71
  type II, 71
  type III, 71-72
  type IV, 168, 171t
  to vaccines, 3919
Hypertension
  intracranial
    in bacterial meningitis, 1201-1202, 1221
    monitoring for
      in CNS infections, 1187
      in encephalitis, 1250
    in poststreptococcal glomerulonephritis, 2619
  pulmonary, in HIV infection, 1733
Hyperthermia, definition of, 765
Hyperventilation, for intracranial pressure reduction,
    1221
Hypochlorites, disinfection with, 3682
Hypochlorous acid, in neutrophil bactericidal
    activity, 109
Hypoesthesia, in leprosy, 3169
Hypogammaglobulinemia, 169t-170t
Hypoglycemia
  in malaria, 3441, 3449
  from quinolones, 504
Hypoglycorrhachia, cerebrospinal fluid, 1185
Hypogonadism, in HIV infection, 1713
Hypokalemia, from penicillin, 314
Hypotension
  postural, from ivermectin, 653
  sepsis-associated. *See* Septic shock.

Hypothalamic-pituitary-adrenal axis
  in chronic fatigue syndrome, 1899
  in sepsis, 997
Hypothalamus, in thermoregulation, 768-769, 768f
Hypothermia, during cardiac surgery, 3895
Hypothermia blanket therapy, antipyretic effects of, 774-775
Hypothesis testing, in clinical trials, 691-692
Hypovitaminosis E, 153
Hypoxia, cytopathic, in severe sepsis, 992-993
Hysterectomy
  cuff cellulitis after, 1515
  surgical site infection after, 1514-1516, 1514t, 1515f

I

IB4, for subarachnoid space inflammation, 1192
Ibuprofen, for cough, 875
Iclaprim, 482, 512, 706t-709t
"Id" reactions, in dermatophytosis, 3351
Idoxuridine, 576f, 585
Iliac artery, mycotic aneurysm of, 1101. See also Mycotic aneurysms.
Iliac lymphadenitis, 1324
Iliacus pyomyositis, 1319
Iliopsoas myositis, 1319
Imidazoles, 554
Imipenem
  for acute pyelonephritis, 972
  antibacterial activity of, 342t
  for brain abscess, 1274, 1274t
  chemistry of, 341, 342f
  clinical use of, 343
  dosage of, 722t
  drug interactions with, 742t-761t
  for febrile neutropenia, 3804t
  formulations of, 716t
  for melioidosis, 2876, 2876t
  for Mycobacterium abscessus pulmonary disease, 3193t, 3194
  for nosocomial pneumonia, 3718t
  for pancreatic infections, 1050
  pharmacology of, 342
  for Pseudomonas aeruginosa bacteremia, 2849-2850
  recommended dose of, 343
  for septic bursitis, 1450t
Imipenem-cilastatin, 706t-709t
  for Enterococcus endocarditis, 1120t
  for peritonitis, 1029t
Imiquimod, 566t-567t, 585-586, 585f, 620
  for condylomata acuminata, 2043
Immigrants, tuberculosis in, 3133, 3133t
Immune complex(es)
  complement in, 84
  in endocarditis, 1078
  measurement of, 66
Immune complex disease
  chronic hepatitis B in, 1602
  chronic hepatitis C in, 1611
Immune globulin(s), 3922t, 3934-3936. See also specific drug.
  adverse reactions to, 3936
  currently available, 3922t
  definition of, 3917
  for HAV, 2379-2380, 2380t, 2382t
  after hematopoietic stem cell transplantation, 3833
  in HIV-infected children, 1826
  intramuscular, 3934-3935
    for hepatitis A, 3934-3935
    indications for, 3934-3935
    for measles, 3935
    specific preparations of, 3935
  intravenous, 73-74, 3922t
    adverse effects of, 618
    for Clostridium difficile–associated colitis, 1383
    dosage of, 618
    for enteroviral meningitis, 1220
    in HIV-infected children, 1825
    for human metapneumovirus infection, 2227
    indications for, 3935
    for myocarditis, 1160
    for parvovirus B19 infection, 2092
    prophylactic, in transplant recipients, 3816
    specific preparations of, 3935-3936

Immune globulin(s) (Continued)
    for streptococcal toxic shock syndrome, 2605
    uses of, 617-618
  passive immunization with, 189
  prophylactic
    for cancer-related infections, 3800t, 3802
    for HAV, 1590, 1590t
  Rh, 3936
  specific, 3917
  subcutaneous, 3922t, 3936
Immune reconstitution syndrome, 619
  in antiretroviral therapy, 1849
  in cryptococcosis, 3296
  in HIV infection, 1720-1721
  in HIV-infected children, 1817
  Mycobacterium avium complex and, 3181, 3181f-3182f
  Pneumocystis pneumonia and, 3382
  in tuberculosis, 3148
Immune system
  in lymphoid tissues, 142-144, 142f-143f
  mucosal surfaces in, 144
  physical barriers in, 3783-3786, 3784f
  reconstitution of, after hematopoietic stem cell transplantation, 3832-3833, 3833t
  in sepsis, 1000
Immune-deficient fever of unknown origin, 780t, 782. See also Fever, of unknown origin.
Immunity
  adaptive, 37, 38t, 988, 990t. See also Inflammatory response, initial.
    complement in, 83-84
    innate immunity and, 138
    in viral infections, 1917
  aging and, 44-45
  capsular polysaccharides impact on, 3291
  cellular, 129-150. See also T cells.
    in immunocompromised hosts, 3781-3783, 3782t
    microbial pathogenesis and, 139-140
    type IV, 168, 171t
    in urinary tract infection, 957
    in viral infections, 1917
  commensal flora effects on, 45
  dysregulation of, 45
  hormones and, 45
  humoral. See also Antibody(ies); B cells; Immunoglobulin(s).
    in immunocompromised hosts, 3781-3783, 3782t
    in urinary tract infection, 962-963
    in viral infections, 1917-1918
  impaired, fever of unknown origin and, 782
  innate, 37-47, 38t, 137-140, 988, 990t
    adaptive immunity and, 138
    alterations in, 44-45
    chemokines in, 41-44, 42t
    cytokines in, 41-43, 42t
    dectin-1 in, 138
    hereditary factors in, 37-38, 38f
    initial inflammatory response and, 41-44, 42t-43t
    mannose receptor in, 138
    NODs in, 138
    pathogen interference with, 4, 10, 44
    physical barriers in, 38-41
    in Pseudomonas aeruginosa resistance, 2838-2839
    tissue tropisms in, 37-38
    Toll-like receptors in, 43, 138
    in urinary tract infection, 961
    in viral infections, 1917
  intestinal, 1338-1339
  natural antibodies in, 45
  nonspecific, 37, 38t
    alterations in, 44-45
  nutrition and, 44, 152-154
  oral mucosal, 857-858, 857f
  stress and, 45
  systemic and local, effect of operative procedures on, 3895
  tests of, 171t
  wound microenvironment effects on, 3894-3895

Immunization, 3917-3949. See also Vaccine(s).
  active, 189, 3917
  agents used for
    constituents of, 3917
    currently available, 3921-3936, 3922t
    definitions of, 3917
  in complement deficiency, 95
  coverage improvements for, 3945-3946
  documentation of, 3943
  in elderly, 3862
  in endocarditis prophylaxis, 1144
  after hematopoietic stem cell transplantation, 3832-3833, 3833t
  in HIV-infected children, 1825, 1826f-1827f
  information sources on, 3946
  intervals between, 3944
  need for, assessment of, 3943
  parent and patient education on, 3943-3944
  passive, 73, 189, 3917
  postexposure, 3943
  principles of, 3920-3921, 3920t
  recommended schedule for, 3921
    in adolescents, 3939
    in adults, 3939-3941, 3940f
    in children, 3924f, 3936-3938, 3937f, 3938t-3939t
  standards for, 3945, 3945t
  for travelers. See Travelers, immunizations for.
Immunochemistry, of smallpox, 3979
Immunocompromised hosts
  adenoviral infections in, 2030-2031
  American trypanosomiasis in, 3484-3485
  aspergillosis in, 3244, 3244t
  bacteremia in, 3788
  Blastomyces dermatitidis in, 3327
  catheter-related infections in, 3788-3789
  CNS toxoplasmosis in, 1270
  common pathogens in, 3782t
  concurrent illnesses in, 3787
  cryptosporidiosis in, 3552
  empyema in, 918
  enteroviral meningoencephalitis in, 2359-2360
  epiglottitis in, 851-852
  febrile neutropenia in, 3787-3788, 3787f. See also Febrile neutropenia.
  fever of unknown origin in, 782
  gastrointestinal tract infections in, 3786, 3786f, 3789
  granulocytopenia in, 3781, 3782t, 3789, 3789f
  herpes simplex virus infection in, 1954, 1954f, 1957t
  herpesviruses in, 1939, 1939t
  Histoplasma capsulatum in, 3312
    prophylaxis against, 3317
  human herpesvirus 6 infection in, 2013-2014
  human metapneumovirus infection in, 2225, 2226f
  immune defects in, 3781-3787, 3782t
    cellular, 3781-3783, 3782t
    humoral, 3781-3783, 3782t
  infections in
    fever and, origin of, 3787-3788, 3787f
    hosts defense deficiences and, 3781-3787, 3782t
    microbiologically defined, 3788
    principles of, 3781-3791
    sequence of events in, 3783t, 3789, 3789f
  influenza in, 2275
  leprosy in, 3174
  measles in, 2232
    prevention of, 2233
  mucosal barrier injury in, 3785-3786, 3785f
  mucositis in, 861t, 866-867, 866f
  myocarditis in, 1154
  nutritional deficiencies in, 3787
  opportunistic infections in, post-traumatic, 1302
  oral infections in, 3786, 3788
  organ dysfunction in, 3786-3787
  pneumonia in, 909
    chronic, 933
  Q fever in, 2516
  respiratory syncytial virus infection complications in, 2214-2215
  respiratory tract infections in, 3788
  rhinoviral infections in, 2394
  Rhodococcus equi infection in, 2703

Immunocompromised hosts *(Continued)*
    sepsis/systemic inflammatory response syndrome
        in, 3787-3788
    skin infections in, 3783-3784, 3788
    skin lesions in, 804-805, 804t
    stomatitis in, 866-867
    thrombocytopenia in, 3787
    toxoplasmosis in, 3502-3503
        diagnosis of, 3512-3513, 3514f
        serologic screening and prophylaxis for, 3521
        treatment of, 3518-3519, 3518t
    travel by, 4016
    trimethoprim-sulfamethoxazole in, for prophy-
        laxis, 482
    urinary tract infections in, 3789
    vaccines in, 3942
    varicella-zoster virus infection in, 1965
Immunodeficiency, 72-73, 167-178. *See also* Human
        immunodeficiency virus.
    acquired, 176-177
    in cancer, 73
    common variable, 72-73, 169t-170t, 172
    congenital, 169t-170t
    humoral, 73
    in immunocompromised hosts, 3781-3787,
        3782t
    index of suspicion for, 167, 168t-170t
    initial evaluation of, 167, 171t
    pathogens associated with, 167, 168t
    primary disorders of, intravenous immune
        globulin for, 617
    screening for, 167, 171t
    selective, 73
    severe combined, 73, 168, 169t-170t
Immunodiffusion test
    for *Blastomyces dermatitidis*, 3322
    for *Coccidioides*, 3340
Immunofluorescence assay, 65
    for *Babesia microti*, 3543
    for *Bartonella*, 3005
    for *Cryptosporidium*, 3553
    for flaviviruses, 2148
    in HIV infection, 1673-1674
    for human metapneumovirus, 2226
    for *Pneumocystis* pneumonia, 3383
Immunogenetics, 186
    of MHC molecules, 140-144, 141f
    of polysaccharides, 2738
Immunoglobulin(s), 59-75, 617-618. *See also*
        Antibody(ies).
    anthrax, 2723
    anti-*Cryptosporidium*, 3555
    classes of, 59-62, 60t
    in complement activation, 62
    defects of, 171
    in endocarditis, 1073
    in *Francisella tularensis*, 2934-2935
    in Kawasaki syndrome, 3665
    passive immunization with, 73
    preparations of, 3922t, 3934-3936. *See also*
        Immune globulin(s).
    structure of, 59-63, 60f
    total, quantification of, 64
Immunoglobulin A, 60t, 61
    blocking function of, 62
    in *Campylobacter jejuni*, 2796
    deficiency of, 72, 169t-170t
    measurement of, 64
    mucosal, 40
        in *Entamoeba histolytica* infection, 3416,
            3416f
    in opsonization, 62-63
    in Q fever endocarditis, 2515
    receptors for, 63
    in *Toxoplasma gondii* infection, 3499, 3510, 3516
Immunoglobulin A protease, in bacterial meningitis,
    1196
Immunoglobulin D, 62, 67
Immunoglobulin E, 60t, 62
    antibodies to, beta-lactam–specific, 347, 348f-349f
    excess of, 113-114, 130, 169t-170t, 176, 176f
        with impaired chemotaxis, 113-114
        Staphylococcus aureus infection in, 2563
    measurement of, 64
    in *Toxoplasma gondii* infection, 3499, 3510

Immunoglobulin G, 60t, 61
    in antibody-dependent cellular cytotoxicity, 63
    anti-*Toxoplasma*, 1271-1272, 3513
    in complement activation, 62
    deficiency of, in immunoglobulin A deficiency,
        72
    in *Helicobacter pylori* infection, 2808
    measurement of, 64
    as opsonin, 62
    in phagocytosis, 104-105
    receptors for, 63
    subclass deficiencies of, 73
    in *Toxoplasma gondii* infection, 3499, 3509, 3516
Immunoglobulin G avidity test, for toxoplasmosis,
    3509
Immunoglobulin G enzyme-linked immunosorbent
    assay, for toxoplasmosis, 3509
Immunoglobulin G immunoblot assay, for
    Bartonella, 3004-3005
Immunoglobulin M, 60-61, 60t
    anti-HAV, 2379
    in cytomegalovirus infection, 1974
    in dengue fever, 4022
    in diagnosis of infections, 63-64, 63f
    excess of, 72, 169t-170t, 171
    in *Helicobacter pylori* infection, 2808
    membrane, 67-68
    in opsonization, 62-63
    in Q fever, 2514-2515
    in *Toxoplasma gondii* infection, 3509, 3516
Immunoglobulin M enzyme-linked immunosorbent
    assay, for toxoplasmosis, 3509-3510
Immunohistochemistry, 65
    in Creutzfeldt-Jakob disease, 2434
Immunologic synapse, in T cell activation, 132
Immunologic techniques, 144-146, 145f-146f, 267
Immunomodulators, 611-623. *See also specific agent,*
        e.g., Colony-stimulating factor(s).
    classification of, 611
    cytokine, 611, 612t
    for *Mycobacterium avium* complex disease, 3185
    for viral infections, 565
Immunonutrition, enteral, 155, 155f
Immunoprophylaxis, 189
    for meningococcal infections, 2748-2749
Immunosuppression. *See also* Immunocompromised
        hosts.
    cytomegalovirus reactivation with, 1980
    for myocarditis, 1160
    pulmonary tuberculosis in, treatment of, 3149
    from rifamycins, 407
    in severe sepsis, 994
    in transplant recipients, infections and, 3810-3812,
        3811t
Immunotherapy
    adoptive, for lymphoproliferative disease, 2004
    for anthrax, 2723, 3990-3991
Impetigo, 1289-1291
    bullous, 799, 1291
        from *Staphylococcus aureus*, 2554, 2554f
    differential diagnosis of, 1289
    nonbullous, 1289, 2600
    from *Staphylococcus aureus*, 1289, 1291,
        2565-2566, 2566f
    streptococcal, 1289, 2600
    treatment of, 1291
Implant infections
    from coagulase-negative *Staphylococcus*, 2585
    outpatient parenteral antimicrobial therapy for,
        700, 700t
Implantable cardioverter-defibrillator, infection of,
    1127-1131, 1128f, 1128t, 1130f. *See also* Cardiac
        rhythm management device infections.
In vivo expression technology, 11
Incidence, 180
Inclusion bodies, 1912
    poxvirus, 3979
Inclusion body myositis, sporadic, in HIV infection,
    1759
Inclusion conjunctivitis
    adult, 1534
    from *Chlamydia trachomatis*
        in adults, 2450-2451, 2452t
        in neonates, 2455-2456
Inclusion criteria, in clinical trials, 690

Inclusions
    of *Chlamydia trachomatis*, 2439-2440, 2440f
    viral, 1912
Incubation period, 194
    definition of, 194
    for infectious disease, 194
    for travelers infections, 4021t
India, HIV-infected children in, 1810
India ink smear, of cerebrospinal fluid, 1186
Indinavir, 706t-709t, 1839f, 1840, 1840t
    dosage of, 740t-741t
    formulations of, 717t
    for HIV-infected children, 1820t-1821t, 1823t
Indium-111–tagged leukocyte scans, of
        intraperitoneal abscess, 1030-1031
Indomethacin, vasoconstrictor effects of, 775
Infants. *See also* Children; Neonates.
    agranulocytosis in, 111
    aminoglycosides in, 378, 378t
    bacterial meningitis in, 1206, 1213t
    botulism in, 3097, 3099
    Chlamydia trachomatis pneumonia in, 2456, 2456f
    epidemic diarrhea in, 1359-1360, 1360t
    fever in
        from human herpesvirus 6, 2011-2012, 2012f
        of unknown origin, 779-781, 783
    hypertrophic pyloric stenosis in, from erythromy-
        cin, 431
    malaria in, 3453
    pertussis immunization for, 2961
    pertussis in, 2958
    postvaccination encephalopathy in, 1925
    preterm
        complement in, 77
        fluconazole prophylaxis in, 557
        respiratory syncytial virus infection and, 2214
    Q fever in, 2516
    tuberculosis in, 3139
Infarction, splenic, in endocarditis, 1074-1075
Infection
    chain of, 185
    definition of, 3, 988t
    gradient of, 186
    host responses to, 988-992
        acute phase, 990-992. *See also* Acute-phase
            response.
        local, 988-989, 989f, 990t
        pathologic, 992-995. *See also* Sepsis.
        systemic, 989-990, 990t
Infection control. *See also* Disease prevention and
        control.
    in emergency preparedness, 223-225
        detection and diagnosis for, 223-224, 224t
        policies, procedures, and administrative
            controls for, 224-225, 225t
        syndromic surveillance for, 223
    after hematopoietic stem cell transplantation, 3827
    for HIV-related respiratory infections, 1728
    in hospitals, 3667-3672, 3670t. *See also* Nosoco-
        mial infections.
        accreditation in, 3671-3672
        functions of, 3669, 3670t
        organization of, 3671
    for respiratory syncytial virus, 2217, 2217t
    for urinary tract infections, 3728-3729
Infection-control committee, 3671
Infection-control professionals, 3671
Infectious disease
    in cancer patients, 3793-3807. *See also* Cancer,
        infections in.
    causes of death in, 199, 200f, 200t
    definition of, 3
    emerging and reemerging, 199-219, 802-805. *See*
        also specific infection.
        controlling threat of, 214-215, 215f
        emergency preparedness for. *See* Emergency
            preparedness.
        factors contributing to, 199, 201t
        morbidity and mortality in, 199-200, 200f
        newly identified microbes in, 199, 201t
        zoonotic origin of, 6
    genetics of, 50-52
        applications of, 55
        evolutionary aspects of, 55
        magnitude of, 49-50, 50t

Infectious disease (Continued)
    highly contagious, emergency preparedness for.
        See Emergency preparedness.
    after lumbar puncture, 1184
    outbreaks of
        consequences of, 197
        definitions of, 193
        epidemic curves in, 194, 195f
        epidemiology of, 194
        investigation of, 193-197
        key epidemiologic principles in, 194-195
        nosocomial, 3669-3670, 3670t
        observational studies in, 184-185
        response to, 196-197
            step-by-step approach to, 196, 196t
        surveillance of, 184, 193-194
    surveillance of. See Surveillance.
    susceptibility to
        genetic factors influencing, 199, 200t
        resistance genes in, 52-55
    travel-related, 4019-4028. See also Travelers.
Infectious mononucleosis
    clinical course in, 1995
    complications of, 1994-1995, 1994t
    from cytomegalovirus, 1973-1974, 2002-2003
    differential diagnosis of, 2002-2003
    versus enteric fever, 1400t-1401t, 1404
    epidemics of, 1992
    epidemiology of, 1991-1992
    from Epstein-Barr virus, 1993-1995, 1993t
    hemolytic anemia in, 1994
    heterophile antibodies in, 1992, 1999-2000, 1999t
    heterophile-negative, 2002
    historical perspective on, 1989
    from human herpesvirus 6, 2013, 2013f
    incidence of, 1991
    laboratory diagnosis of, 1999-2001, 1999t-2000t
    neurologic complications of, 1994-1995, 1994t
    neutropenia in, 1999
    pathogenesis of, 1992-1993
    pharyngitis in, 817
    public health impact of, 1992
    public health measures for, 2005
    signs of, 1993-1994, 1993t, 1994f
    splenic rupture in, 1994
    symptoms of, 1993, 1993t
    thrombocytopenia in, 1994, 1999
    treatment of, 2003
Infectious waste, 3690-3692
    disposal of, 3691t
Infectiousness, 186
Infective endocarditis. See Endocarditis.
Infectivity, 186
Inferior vena cava filter, infection of, 1139
Infertility
    from Chlamydia trachomatis, 2454
    in HIV infection, 1799-1800
    from pelvic inflammatory disease, 2761
Inflammasome, 10, 138
Inflammation
    complement in, 83
    local, 988-989, 989f
    neutrophils in, 101-108. See also Neutrophil(s),
        inflammatory response of.
    systemic, 989-990, 990t. See also Systemic
        inflammatory response syndrome (SIRS).
Inflammatory bowel disease, rifamycins for, 413
Inflammatory demyelinating polyneuropathy, in HIV
    infection, 1755-1756
Inflammatory enteritides, 1389-1398
    acute, 1389-1393. See also Dysentery.
    chronic, 1394-1396
Inflammatory response, initial. See also Acute-phase
        response.
    innate immunity and, 37, 41-44, 42t-43t
    metabolic changes in, 44
    Toll-like receptors in, 43
Infliximab, leprosy and, 3174
Influenza/influenza virus, 2265-2288
    antibody responses to, 2273-2274
    antigenic drift in, 2269
    antigenic shift in, 2269-2270, 2269f
    antigenic variation in, 2268
    avian, 203-204, 203t, 204f, 2270-2271
        treatment of, 2280

Influenza/influenza virus (Continued)
    bacterial pneumonia after, 21
    bronchiolitis from, 886t
    cellular pathogenesis of, 2271
    cellular responses to, 2274
    classification of, 2265, 2266t
    clinical findings in, 2274-2276
    complications of, 2275-2276
        nonpulmonary, 2276
        pulmonary, 2275-2276, 2275t
        treatment of, 2279-2280
    COPD exacerbation from, 2276
    croup from, 2276
    detection of, 259t-260t
    diagnosis of, 2276-2277
    encephalitis from, 1251t-1252t
    epidemic outbreaks of, 2267-2268, 2268f
    epidemiology of, 2265-2271
    Guillain-Barré syndrome after, 2276
    H5N1, 2270, 2280
    H7, 2270
    H9, 2270
    hemagglutinin adhesin of, 15, 17, 17f
    histopathology of, 2271-2272, 2272f-2273f
    historical background on, 2265
    in HIV infection, 1732, 1858t-1859t
    immune response to, 2273
    in immunocompromised hosts, 2275
    isolation of, 2276
    versus malaria, 3450
    morbidity and mortality of, 2265-2267, 2267f,
        2267t
    myalgia in, 1319-1320
    myositis from, 2276
    pandemic outbreaks of, 2268
    pathogenesis of, 2271-2274
    pathogenicity of, 2273
    pathophysiology of, 2272-2273
    pneumonia from, 2272-2273, 2272f, 2275, 2275t
    prevention of, 2280-2284
        chemoprophylaxis for, 2284
        immunoprophylaxis for. See Influenza vaccine.
    rapid tests for, 2276-2277
    versus respiratory syncytial virus infection, 2213,
        2213t-2214t
    Reye's syndrome after, 2276
    secondary bacterial pneumonia from, 2273, 2275,
        2275t
    shedding of, 2271, 2272f
    in solid organ transplant recipients, 3848
    structure of, 2265, 2266f
    swine, 2271
    toxic shock syndrome from, 2276
    travel-related, 4024
    treatment of
        amantadine/rimantadine in, 575-576,
            2277-2278, 2277t
        antiviral agents in, 566t-567t, 2277, 2277t
        oseltamivir in, 592
        peramivir in, 593
        zanamivir in, 598
        zanamivir/oseltamivir in, 2277t, 2278-2279
    type A, 2266t
        countries reporting, 203t
        outbreaks of, 203-204, 203t, 204f
        structure of, 2265, 2266f
        subtypes of, 2265, 2266t
    type B, 2266t
    type C, 2266t
    uncomplicated, 2274-2275
Influenza vaccine, 2280-2284
    in asplenia, 3871
    in children, 3926-3927
    comparison of, 2283
    in elderly, 3858, 3926
    in HIV infection, 3926-3927
    in HIV-infected children, 1825
    inactivated, 2280-2281, 3922t, 3926-3927
    live-attenuated (cold-adapted), 2281-2283, 2281f,
        3922t, 3927
    for pandemic outbreaks, 2283
    pneumonia and, 913
    recommendations for, 2283-2284, 2283t
    recommended schedule for, 3924f
    for travelers, 4010, 4011t

Influenza-like syndrome, from rifamycins, 407
Information resources
    for antiretroviral therapy, 1630f-1631f, 1631
    for travel medicine, 4010t
Informed consent, for HIV-infected children, 1819
Infrahyoid space infections, 864. See also
    Odontogenic infections.
Infusate, catheter, contamination of, 3697
Infusion center model, of outpatient parenteral
    antimicrobial delivery, 699, 700t
Infusion devices, for outpatient parenteral
    antimicrobial therapy, 701
Inguinal buboes, in bubonic plague, 2946, 2946f
Inguinal lymphadenitis
    in bubonic plague, 1326-1327
    in sexually transmitted disease, 1326
Inguinal lymphadenopathy
    in chancroid, 2917
    from Chlamydia trachomatis, 2449-2450
    in genital lesions, 1476
Inhibitory quotient, 305
Injection drug users, 3875-3890
    bone and joint infections in, 3878-3879
    central nervous system infections in, 3885-3886
    endocarditis in, 1077, 3879-3881
        central nervous system manifestations of,
            3885
        etiology of, 1085
        HIV and, 3880-3881
        right-sided, 2570, 2571t, 3880
    endophthalmitis in, 3886-3887
    hepatitis A infection in, 2376, 3884
        vaccination against, 2382
    hepatitis B infection in, 3883-3884
    hepatitis C infection in, 2171, 3884
    hepatitis D infection in, 3884
    HIV infection in, 1620, 1621f, 1625, 1638,
        1781-1782, 3887
        pneumonia risk and, 1728
        transmission of, 1625, 1647, 1652
        tuberculosis with, 3883
    host defenses in, 3875-3876
    mycotic aneurysms in, 3881-3882, 3882f, 3885
    ocular infections in, 3886-3887
    osteomyelitis in, 1464, 3878-3879
    pulmonary infections in, 3882-3883, 3883f
    pyomyositis in, 1313, 3878
    septic thrombophlebitis in, 3881
    sexually transmitted diseases in, 3887
    skin and soft tissue infections in, 3876-3878
    splenic abscess in, 3884-3885
    vascular infections in, noncardiac, 3881-3882
Injection site, abscess at, 1309
Injury prevention in HIV prophylaxis
    during procedures and surgery, 3758-3759
    during routine patient care, 3757-3758
Insertion sequences, in antimicrobial resistance,
    280-281
Insomnia, fatal familial, 2428-2429
Institutions
    HAV outbreaks in, 2375-2376
    tuberculosis spread in, 3135
Insulin infusion, perioperative, reduced surgical site
    infections with, 3897
Integrase strand transfer inhibitors, 1843f, 1843t,
    1844
Integrons, in antimicrobial resistance, 281, 281f
Integument, barrier function of, 3783-3784, 3784f
Intensive care unit patients
    fever of unknown origin in, 781-782
    streptococcal toxic shock syndrome in, 2605
Intention-to-treat population, in clinical trials, 694
Intercellular adhesion molecule-1, 103
    in malaria susceptibility, 50
    in Plasmodium falciparum malaria, 3440-3441
    of rhinoviruses, 2389
Intercellular adhesion molecule-1 receptor, blockade
    of, for rhinovirus infection, 2396
Intercellular adhesion molecule-2, 103
Intercellular adhesion molecule-3, 103
Interferon(s), 586-590, 615-616
    classification of, 586, 586t, 615
    clinical studies of, 588-590
    for condylomata acuminata, 2044
    drug interactions with, 588

Interferon(s) *(Continued)*
in febrile response, 769
interactions between, 587
mechanisms of action of, 586-587
for myocarditis, 1160
pharmacokinetics of, 587
plus ribavirin, for hepatitis C/HIV coinfection, 1740
toxicity of, 588
Interferon-alfa
adverse effects of, 615, 2174
for chronic hepatitis B virus, 588-589
drug interactions with, 742t-761t
for hepatitis B infection, chronic, 1596-1597, 1601t, 2074-2075
for hepatitis C infection, 589, 2172-2173
chronic, 1606
for herpes simplex virus infection, 589
in HIV infection, 589
for Kaposi's sarcoma, 1767
for papillomavirus, 589
pegylated, 587-588
for hepatitis B infection, chronic, 1597, 1601t, 2075, 2076t
for hepatitis C infection, 2173
chronic, 1606-1607, 1606t-1607t
for respiratory viruses, 589-590
for rhinovirus infection, 2395-2396
uses of, 615
Interferon-alfa-2a
dosage of, 738t-739t
formulations of, 717t
pegylated, 566t-567t, 706t-709t
formulations of, 717t
for hepatitis B virus, 588
plus ribavirin, 566t-567t
recombinant, 706t-709t
Interferon-alfa-2b, 566t-567t
dosage of, 738t-739t
formulations of, 717t
pegylated, 706t-709t
dosage of, 738t-739t
formulations of, 717t
plus ribavirin, formulations of, 717t
recombinant, 706t-709t
plus ribavirin, dosage of, 738t-739t
Interferon-alfacon-1, 706t-709t
dosage of, 738t-739t
Interferon-alfa/lamivudine, pegylated, for hepatitis B infection, chronic, 2078
Interferon-alfa-n3, 706t-709t
dosage of, 738t-739t
formulations of, 717t
Interferon-alfa/ribavirin
for hepatitis C infection, 2173, 2173f
pegylated, for hepatitis C infection, 2173
chronic, 1607-1608, 1607t
response of, 2173-2174, 2173f
Interferon-beta, 586, 586t
Interferon-gamma
in chronic granulomatous disease, 116
in *Entamoeba histolytica* infection, 3416, 3417f
expression of, in cryptosporidiosis, 3551
in infection susceptibility, 54
in MHC class I antigen processing, 134
in microsporidiosis, 3395
production of, by Th1 T cells, 129
in toxoplasmosis, 3499
in tuberculosis resistance, 51t
in tuberculous pleural effusion, 921
uses of, 616
Interferon-gamma receptor 1, deficiency of, 169t-170t, 175
Interferon-gamma receptor gene, mutations in, 49-51
Interferon-gamma signaling pathway, defects of, in disseminated *Mycobacterium avium* complex disease, 3179
Interleukin(s), in nasal secretions, in rhinoviral cold, 2392
Interleukin-1
for enhanced resistance to infection, 773
in febrile response, 769
in *Pseudomonas aeruginosa* resistance, 2838
uses of, 616

Interleukin-1 receptor–associated kinase-4 deficiency, 169t-170t
Interleukin-1β
in initial inflammatory response, 43
in streptococcal toxic shock syndrome, 2604
Interleukin-2
deficiency of, 169t-170t
for HIV infection, 1699-1700
uses of, 616-617
in Whipple's disease, 1436
Interleukin-6
in febrile response, 769
in initial inflammatory response, 43
in severe sepsis, 993
in Whipple's disease, 1436
Interleukin-7, for HIV infection, 1700
Interleukin-8, in pleural effusion, 917
Interleukin-10
antipyretic activity of, 772
in hepatitis B susceptibility, 52
induction of, by hyperbaric oxygen therapy, 626
in infection susceptibility, 54
in toxoplasmosis, 3499
uses of, 617
in Whipple's disease, 1436
Interleukin-12
in Legionnaires' disease, 2971
in microsporidiosis, 3395
production of, by Th1 T cells, 129
in toxoplasmosis, 3499
uses of, 617
Interleukin-12 p40, deficiency of, 169t-170t
Interleukin-12 receptor, deficiency of, 169t-170t, 175-176
Interleukin-18, in Legionnaires' disease, 2971
Internal mammary grafting, mediastinitis in, 1175
Interstitial nephritis
chronic, 957, 958f
from penicillin, 314
from quinolones, 503
tuberculous, 3156
Intertrigo, 3230, 3237-3238
Intestinal epithelium, *Salmonella* and, 2892-2893, 2892f
Intestinal flu, 1362-1363, 1362t
Intestinal flukes, 3596t, 3602
Intestinal immunity, 1338-1339
Intestinal intussusception, after rotavirus vaccine, 2112
Intestinal motility, 1337
Intestinal mucosa, T cells in, 144
Intestinal obstruction, in ascariasis, 3578-3579
Intestinal roundworms (nematodes), 3574t, 3577-3586, 3578f-3579f, 3578t
Intestinal transplant recipients
infections in, 3841t, 3843-3844
survival data for, 3839, 3840t
Intimate partner violence, HIV infection and, 1627-1628
Intra-abdominal infections, 1011. *See also* Peritonitis.
anaerobic, 3085, 3086f
bacteria causing, 1017
from *Candida*, 3233, 3234f, 3237
from *Clostridium*, 3108
death from, 1021
from *Enterococcus*, 2647
from gram-negative anaerobic rods, 3116
in liver transplant recipients, 3843
from *Pasteurella*, 2941
quinolones for, 497
in solid organ transplant recipients, 3845-3846
in spinal cord injury patients, 3855
from *Streptococcus anginosus* group, 2683
Intra-amniotic infection syndrome, 1511-1514
Intra-aortic balloon counterpulsation, catheter-related infection in, 1139, 1139t
Intracranial abscess
from *Blastomyces dermatitidis*, 3326, 3326f
epidural, 1281-1282
hyperbaric oxygen therapy for, 628
Intracranial hemorrhage, from tipranavir, 1842

Intracranial hypertension
in bacterial meningitis, 1201-1202, 1221
monitoring for
in CNS infections, 1187
in encephalitis, 1250
Intracranial mycotic aneurysms, 1101
Intracranial thrombophlebitis, suppurative, 1283-1286, 1285f-1286f
Intraluminal amebiasis, 3417-3418. *See also Entamoeba histolytica.*
Intramuscular immune globulin. *See* Immune globulin, intramuscular.
Intranuclear inclusions, in herpesviruses, 1940, 1941f
Intraocular inflammation, in keratitis, 1541
Intrapartum antibiotic prophylaxis, for *Streptococcus agalactiae* (group B) infection, 2662-2663, 2662t
Intraperitoneal abscess, 1030-1032
bacterial findings in, 1030
diagnosis of, 1030-1031, 1031f
etiology of, 1030
treatment of, 1031-1032
Intrathecal *T. pallidum* antibody (ITPA) index, calculation of, 3046
Intrauterine devices
for HIV-infected women, 1800
pelvic inflammatory disease and, from *Actinomycosis*, 3214, 3214f
Intravascular devices, percutaneous. *See* Percutaneous intravascular devices.
Intravenous drug users. *See* Injection drug users.
Intravenous immune globulin. *See* Immune globulin(s), intravenous.
Intravenous lines, infections of, 3697. *See also* Catheter-related infections.
Intussusception
from adenoviruses, 2030
intestinal, after rotavirus vaccine, 2112
Invasin-intimin family of proteins, 2819
Iodophors, disinfection with, 521, 522t, 3683
Iodoquinol, 652, 706t-709t
for balantidiasis, 3566
Ipecac bark, for dysentery, 3411
Ipratropium, for rhinorrhea, 811
Iridocyclitis, 1561
Iris, 1561
Iritis, 1561
Iron, 154
acquisition of
by enterobacteriaceae, 2820
by *Pseudomonas aeruginosa*, 2844
in urinary tract infection, 961
deficiency of, 154
serum, in initial inflammatory response, 44
in virulence regulation, 7
Iron deficiency anemia, from hookworm, 3581
Iron-binding proteins, 40
Irrigants, antimicrobial and antiseptic, for mediastinitis, 1178
Irritable bowel syndrome, rifamycins for, 413
Isavuconazole, 559
for aspergillosis, 3251-3252
Isepamicin, 706t-709t, 724t-725t
Isfahan virus, 2246
Isohemagglutinins, 172
Isolation device, HEPA-filtered mobile, 229, 229f
Isolation precautions, 188, 3673-3676
essential elements of, 3674t
standard, 3673-3674
gloves in, 3673-3674
hand hygiene in, 3673
transmission-based, 3674-3676
airborne, 3674-3675, 3675t
contact, 3675-3676, 3675t
droplet, 3675, 3675t
Isolation room, 228-229, 228f, 228t
Isolation technique, in emergency preparedness, 225-226, 225t, 226f
Isoniazid, 533-534, 706t-709t
adverse reactions to, 534-535
for brain abscess, 1274t
dosage of, 535, 734t-735t
drug interactions with, 534-535, 742t-761t
formulations of, 717t
hepatitis from, 3146, 3150
hepatotoxicity of, 269

Isoniazid (*Continued*)
  for *Mycobacterium kansaii* pulmonary disease from, 3193, 3193t
  for nontuberculous mycobacterial infections, 543-544
  for tuberculosis, 533-534, 534t, 537t, 3144-3145, 3145t, 3149
  for tuberculosis prophylaxis in cancer patients, 3800t
Isoniazid-pyrazinamide, for tuberculosis, 3146
Isoniazid-rifampin, for tuberculosis, 3146
Isospora, in HIV infection, 1858t-1871t, 1880
Isospora belli, 3563
Isosporiasis, 632t-635t, 3563
Isoxazolyn penicillins, 317, 317f
Itraconazole, 555, 706t-709t
  for aspergillosis, 3251, 3251t
  for *Blastomyces dermatitidis* infection, 3329-3330, 3329t
  for brain abscess, 1274t, 1275
  for *Candida* esophagitis, 1355t, 1356-1357
  for chromoblastomycosis, 3279
  for *Coccidioides* infection, 3340-3341
  for cryptococcal meningitis, 3299
  for cutaneous leishmaniasis, 3475
  for dermatophytosis, 3352
  dosage of, 736t-737t
  drug interactions with, 556t, 742t-761t
  for eumycetoma, 3284-3285
  formulations of, 717t
  for fungal arthritis, 1452
  for histoplasmosis, 3315-3317
    prophylactic, 3317
  for ocular microsporidiosis, 3402-3403
  for *Penicillium marneffei* infection, 3372
  for pityriasis (tinea) versicolor, 3354
  for sporotrichosis, 3274
    in HIV-infected patient, 3274-3275
  structure of, 550f-551f
Ivermectin, 652-655, 706t-709t
  for ascariasis, 3579-3580
  for cutaneous larva migrans, 654, 3619
  for enterobiasis, 3584
  for gnathostomiasis, 654, 3620
  hypotension from, 653
  for onchocerciasis, 652, 654, 3593
  for parasitic infections, 632t-635t, 652-655
  resistance to, 652
  for scabies, 3635, 3636t
  for strongyloidiasis, 654, 3583
Ixodes
  babesiosis from, 3539-3540. *See also* Babesiosis.
  life cycle of, 3539
  Lyme disease from, 3071-3072
Ixodes persulcatus, tick-borne encephalitis from, 2141
Ixodes ricinus, tick-borne encephalitis from, 2141

J

Jamestown Canyon virus, 2292
Janeway lesions, 799
  in endocarditis, 1075, 1075f
    from *Staphylococcus aureus*, 2569, 2570f
Japanese encephalitis, 1246t, 1258-1259
  clinical features of, 2145-2146
  epidemiology of, 2137-2139, 2138t, 2141f
  geographic distribution of, 2134f
  historical perspective on, 2133-2134
  magnetic resonance imaging in, 1249
  pathogenesis of, 2143-2144
  treatment of, 2150-2152
  vaccine for, 2150-2151, 2151t, 3922t, 3927
    for travelers, 4011t, 4013
Japanese spotted fever, 2504, 3653-3654, 3653t
Jarisch-Herxheimer reaction
  in relapsing fever treatment, 3069
  in syphilis treatment, 3050-3051
  in tick-borne infection treatment, 3652-3653
  in tularemia treatment, 2935
Jaundice, from hepatitis E infection, 2417
Jaw, osteomyelitis of, 862t, 865, 870
JC virus
  encephalitis from, 1251t-1252t
  encephalopathy from, 2053
  genomic map of, 2051, 2052f

JC virus (*Continued*)
  granule cell neuronopathy from, 2053
  history of, 2051
  meningitis from, 2053
  progressive multifocal leukoencephalopathy from, 2052-2055, 2053t
    clinical manifestations of, 2052-2053
    diagnosis of, 2053, 2054f-2055f
    epidemiology of, 2052
    pathogenesis of, 2052
    prognosis for, 2053-2054
    treatment of, 2054-2055
  receptor for, 2051-2052
Job's syndrome, 113-114, 130, 169t-170t, 176, 176f
  with impaired chemotaxis, 113-114
  Staphylococcus aureus infection in, 2563
Jock itch, 3348
Joint infections. *See also* Arthritis.
  anaerobic, 3086
  from *Coccidioides*, 3337-3338
  from *Cryptococcus neoformans*, 3293t, 3296
  in injection drug users, 3878-3879
  from *Pasteurella*, 2940
  prosthetic. *See* Prosthetic joint infections.
  from *Pseudomonas aeruginosa*, 2852
  quinolones for, 499-500
  from *Scedosporium prolificans*, 3366, 3366f
  from *Sporothrix schenckii*, 3271-3273, 3272f
Jones criteria for rheumatic fever, 2615, 2615t
Josamycin, 706t-709t, 726t-727t
Jugular suppurative thrombophlebitis (Lemierre disease), 862t, 864-865, 864f, 2700
Junction-associated proteins, viral, 1911
Junin virus, 2296t. *See also* South American hemorrhagic fevers.
Juvenile diabetes mellitus, mumps and, 2204
Juvenile rheumatoid arthritis, fever of unknown origin in, 787

K

Kala-azar, 3466-3468, 3466f
  antimonials for, 642
  skin lesions after, 3464t, 3468-3469, 3468f
    diagnosis of, 3469
    differential diagnosis of, 3469
    treatment of, 3474
Kanamycin, 359, 360f, 360t-361t, 706t-709t
  dosage of, 376, 377t, 724t-725t
  formulations of, 715t
  for tuberculosis, 541
Kaposi's sarcoma, 1765-1768
  clinical manifestations of, 1766, 2018-2020, 2019f-2020f
  cutaneous, 1766
  epidemiology of, 1765
  in HIV infection, 1329, 1881, 2332-2333
    gastric, 1738
    hepatic, 1741
    oral lesions from, 1715
    pulmonary, 1733, 1733f
    skin lesions from, 1717, 1717f
    in women, 1796-1797
  pathogenesis of, 1765-1766
  pre-HAART, 1765
  pulmonary, 1733, 1733f, 1766
  in solid organ transplant recipients, 3848
  treatment of, 1767-1768
    local therapy in, 1767
    recommendations for, 1768
    systemic therapy in, 1767-1768
  variants of, 2019
Kaposi's sarcoma–associated herpesvirus, 1765-1766, 1938t-1940t, 2017-2022. *See also* Human herpesvirus 8.
Katayama's fever, 3598. *See also* *Schistosoma*/schistosomiasis.
Kawasaki disease
  cardiac involvement in, 3663-3664
  versus cellulitis, 1297, 1297t
  clinical features of, 3663, 3664f, 3664t
  differential diagnosis of, 3664, 3664t
  epidemiology of, 3663
  etiology and pathogenesis of, 3665
  laboratory features of, 3664

Kawasaki disease (*Continued*)
  pathology of, 3665
  rash in, 3663, 3664f
  treatment of, 3665-3666
  in *Yersinia pseudotuberculosis* infection, 2951
Kell antigen system, 117
Kemerovo virus antigenic complex, 2098
Keratinocytes, oral, 857
Keratitis, 1539-1552
  from *Acanthamoeba*, 1550, 3427-3436. *See also* Amebic keratitis.
  adenoviral, 1547
  anatomic aspects of, 1539
  in aspergillosis, 3247
  from *Bacillus*, 2729
  bacterial, 1541-1544
    etiology of, 1541-1542
    geographic variation in, 1542
    gram-negative, 1542, 1542f
    gram-positive, 1542
    pathogenesis of, 1542
    treatment of, 1543-1544
  from *Candida*, 1549
  from *Chlamydia trachomatis*, 1544-1545
  conjunctival injection and discharge in, 1540
  contact lens–associated, 1539-1540
  etiology of, 1539-1540, 1540t
  fungal, 1548-1550, 1549f
  from *Fusarium*, 1549
  from herpes simplex virus, 1545, 1547, 1547t, 1562-1563, 1952, 1952f
  from herpes zoster, 1546-1547, 1548t
  interstitial, 1544-1545
  laboratory findings in, 1540-1541
  from microsporidia, 1550-1551
  from mycobacterial infection, 1542-1543
  neurotrophic, 1546
  in onchocerciasis, 1550-1551
  parasitic, 1550-1551
  from *Pseudomonas aeruginosa*, 2852-2853
  recurrent, 1545-1546
  risk factors for, 1539
  syphilitic, 1544-1545
  from trypanosomes, 1550-1551
  varicella-zoster, 1546-1547, 1548t
  viral, 1541, 1545-1548
Keratoconjunctivitis, 1530-1531. *See also* Conjunctivitis; Ocular infections.
  from *Candida guilliermondii*, 1536-1537, 1537f
  epidemic, 1531-1532
    from adenoviruses, 2029
    differential diagnosis of, 1547
    treatment of, 1548
Keratolysis, 1541
Kernig's sign, in bacterial meningitis, 1205
Ketoconazole, 555, 706t-709t
  for *Blastomyces dermatitidis* infection, 3329, 3329t
  for *Coccidioides*, 3340-3341
  for cutaneous leishmaniasis, 3476
  dosage of, 736t-737t
  drug interactions with, 742t-761t
  for eumycetoma, 3284-3285
  formulations of, 717t
  for *Paracoccidioides brasiliensis* infection, 3361
  for pityriasis (tinea) versicolor, 3354
  for sporotrichosis, 3274
  structure of, 550f-551f
Ketolides, 438-440. *See also* Telithromycin.
  dosage of, 726t-727t
  resistance to, ribosomal binding site alteration in, 287
KEX gene, of *Pneumocystis*, 3378
KI virus, 2051-2052
Kidney. *See also* Neph- and Renal *entries*.
  abscess of, 976-979, 976f-977f
  infection in
    barriers to, 41
    localization of, 969
  tuberculosis of, 3156, 3156t
Kidney transplant recipients
  adenoviral infections in, 2030-2031
  BK virus in, 2055-2056
  cytomegalovirus in, 1981-1982
  infections in, 3840-3841, 3841t
  survival data for, 3839, 3840t

Kidney transplant recipients (Continued)
  toxoplasmosis in, 3504
  urinary tract infection in, 966
Kikuchi's disease, 1327-1329
Kinases, transmembrane, in *Entamoeba histolytica*, 3412-3413, 3413f
Kingella, 2774-2775
  bacteremia from, 2775
  clinical manifestations of, 2775
  endocarditis from, 2775
  epidemiology of, 2774-2775
  history of, 2774
  laboratory diagnosis of, 240t-242t, 2775t
  microbiology of, 2774
  respiratory tract colonization by, 2774-2775
  skeletal, 2775
  treatment of, 2775
Kingella kingae
  history and microbiology of, 2774
  in respiratory tract, 2774-2775
  in skeletal system, 2775
Kinins, in nasal secretions, in rhinoviral cold, 2392
Kinyoun stain, 251
Kirby-Bauer disk diffusion method, 249-250
Klebsiella, 2826-2827
  suppurative thrombophlebitis from, 1097-1098
Klebsiella granulomatis, 2827. *See also* Donovanosis.
  biology of, 3011
  laboratory detection of, 240t-242t, 243
Klebsiella oxytoca, 2827
Klebsiella pneumoniae, 2826-2827
  endophthalmitis from, 1554-1555
  fish poisoning from, 1416-1417
  multidrug resistant, 2826-2827
  peritonitis from, 1013
  pneumonia from, 896, 897f-898f, 902f, 2826
  pyogenic liver abscess from, 1036-1037
  resistance of, mechanisms of, 290t
  urinary tract infection from, 2826
Klebsiella pneumoniae subsp. *ozaenae*, 2827
Klebsiella pneumoniae subsp. *rhinoscleromatis*, 2827, 2827f
Kluyvera, 2829
Knodell score, in liver biopsy, 2169, 2169t
Koch's postulate, pathogenicity and, 11
Koch's tuberculin, 3136-3137. *See also* Tuberculin skin test.
Koeppe nodules, 1561
Koplik spots, 797, 2231
Kuru, 2423, 2429-2430
Kyasanur Forest encephalitis, 2152-2153
Kytococcus schroeteri, prosthetic valve endocarditis from, 1123

L
Labetalol, for tetanus, 3094t
Laboratory Response Network (LRN), in bioterrorist attack, 3958-3959
Laboratory tests, 233-265
  for aerobic actinomycetes, 253-254
  for antimicrobial susceptibility. *See* Susceptibility testing.
  for bacteria, 236-249, 240t-242t
  for fungi, 236-243, 254-257, 255t
  metronidazole interference with, 423
  microbiologist/clinician responsibilities in, 233, 234t
  for mycobacteria, 240t-242t, 250-253, 252t
  for parasites, 262-264, 263t
  specimen collection and transport guidelines for, 234, 235t-236t
  specimen selection for, 234
  taxonomic changes and, 233, 234t
  for viruses, 257-262, 257t, 259t-260t
Lacazia loboi, 3372, 3372f, 3374t
Lacrimal system
  anatomy of, 1569, 1570f
  infections of, 1569-1571
    from *Actinomyces*, 3211
Lactate, in sepsis, 998
Lactate dehydrogenase
  in pleural effusion, 921
  in *Pneumocystis jirovecii* pneumonia, 1729

Lactobacillus, 161, 162t-164t, 3126. *See also* Probiotics.
  in oral cavity, 855, 856t
  in vaginal secretions, 1495, 1496f
Lactoferrin
  in neutrophil bactericidal activity, 109
  in oral mucosal immunity, 858
Lamivudine, 566t-567t, 590, 706t-709t, 1834f, 1835f, 1836
  clinical studies of, 590
  dosage of, 740t-741t
  drug interactions with, 742t-761t
  formulations of, 717t
  for hepatitis B infection
    chronic, 1597-1598, 1601t, 2075-2076, 2076t
    with HIV coinfection, 1602
  for HIV postexposure prophylaxis, 3755t, 3764
  for HIV-infected children, 1820t-1821t
  prophylactic, for cancer-related infections, 3800t, 3802
  resistance to, 590, 1836
  structure of, 572f
  toxicity of, 590
Laparoscopy, in fever of unknown origin, 785
Large intestine. *See* Colon.
Larva migrans
  cutaneous, 3618t, 3619
    treatment of, 632t-635t, 647, 654
  ocular, 3618
  visceral
    abdominal pain and/or diarrhea with eosinophilia from, 1407t, 1408
    from *Anisakis*, 3618, 3618t
    from *Baylisascaris procyonis*, 3618, 3618t
    versus enteric fever, 1400t-1401t, 1404
    from *Toxocara*, 3617-3618, 3618t
    treatment of, 632t-635t, 647
Laryngeal diphtheria, 2690-2691
Laryngeal infections, from *Histoplasma capsulatum*, 823
Laryngeal neuralgia, superior, 824
Laryngitis
  acute, 823-824, 824t
  tuberculous, 3159
Lassa fever, 2295-2301
  characteristics of, 2295
  clinical manifestations of, 2299
  diagnosis of, 2299-2300
  epidemiology/epizootiology of, 2296-2297, 2296t
  pathogenesis of, 2297-2298
  prevention of, 2300
  treatment of, 2300
Lateral pharyngeal (pharyngomaxillary) space
  infections of, 862t, 863-864
    mediastinitis from, 1173
  relation of, to cervical fascia, 858, 859f
Lateral sinus thrombosis, septic, 1283-1286
Latex agglutination test
  in bacterial meningitis, 1208
  in rotavirus infection, 2111
Latex tests, for *Coccidioides*, 3340
Latin America, HIV infection in, 1623-1624, 1624f
LDL receptor–related complement proteins, 83
Lebombo virus, 2098
Left ventricular assist device (LVAD), infection of, 1131-1132, 1131t
Leg, mycetoma of, 3282f. *See also* Mycetoma.
Legionella, 2985-2989, 2986t. *See also* Legionnaires' disease.
  clinical manifestations of, 2986-2987, 2987f-2988f
  description of, 2985
  diagnosis of, 2987
  ecology of, 2970
  versus enteric fever, 1400t-1401t, 1404
  environmental cultures for, 2980
  epidemiology of, 2985-2986
  laboratory detection of, 240t-242t
  prevention of, 2988
  treatment of, 2987-2988
  virulence factors of, 2973
Legionella bozemanii, 2985
  pneumonia from, in immunosuppressed patient, 2986-2987, 2988f
Legionella feeleii, 2985
Legionella longbeachae, 2971

Legionella maceachernii, 2985
Legionella micdadei, 2985-2987, 2987f
Legionella pneumophila, 2985. *See also* Legionnaires' disease.
  aerosolization of, 2974
    disinfection for, 2975
  in amoeba, 2970, 2970f
  cultures of, 2969-2970, 2970f, 2976-2977, 2977t
  ecology of, 2970, 2970f
  identification of, 2969
  in macrophage, 2971, 2972f
  pneumonia from, 908
  virulence factors of, 2972-2973
Legionellosis
  in hematopoietic stem cell transplant recipients, 3828
  rifamycins for, 411
Legionnaires' disease, 2969-2984
  affecting travelers, 2974
  causative agents in, 2969-2970, 2970f
  chemoprophylaxis for, 2979
  in children, 2973
  clinical presentation of, 2975-2976
  community-based, 2973-2974
  contagiousness of, 2973
  epidemiology of, 2973-2975
  extrapulmonary infections in, 2976
  history of, 2969
  incubation period for, 2973
  laboratory diagnosis of, 2976-2978, 2977t
  metastatic infections in, 2976
  mortality rates for, 2974
  nosocomial, 2973
  outbreaks of
    environmental decontamination for, 2975
    investigation of, 2975
  pathogenesis of, 2970-2973, 2972f
  patterns of, 2973-2974
  prevention of, 2979-2980
    engineering modifications and maintenance in, 2979-2980
  risk factors for, 2974
  transmission of, 2974-2975
  treatment of, 2978-2979, 2978t
    response to, 2979
Leifsonia aquatica, 2701
Leiomyosarcoma, HIV-related, 1775
Leishmania, 3463-3480
  classification of, 3464t, 3465
  conjunctivitis from, 1536
  keratitis from, 1550
  life cycle of, 3463, 3464f
  taxonomy of, 3464t, 3465
Leishmania amazonensis, 3471-3472
Leishmania braziliensis, 3471-3472
Leishmania donovani
  blepharoconjunctivitis from, 1569
  visceral leishmaniasis from, 3464t, 3466-3469
Leishmania guyanensis, 3470f, 3471-3472
Leishmania major
  cutaneous leishmaniasis from, 3471f, 3472
  defense against, T cells in, 129-130
Leishmania mexicana, 3470f, 3471
Leishmania panamensis, 3470f, 3471
Leishmania peruviana, 3470f, 3471
Leishmania tropica
  cutaneous leishmaniasis from, 3472
  leishmaniasis recidivans from, 3472
  viscerotropic leishmaniasis from, 3468
Leishmaniasis, 3463-3480
  antimonials for, 641-642
  cutaneous, 632t-635t, 3469-3472
    clinical manifestations of, 3472
    diagnosis of, 3472
    diffuse, 3464t, 3472, 3476
    epidemiology of, 3470-3471
    immune response to, 3471-3472
    New World (American), 3464t, 3469-3471, 3470f
    Old World, 3464t, 3470, 3471f
    pathogenesis of, 3471-3472
    treatment of, 3475-3476, 3475t
  diagnosis of, 3465
  disseminated, 3464t, 3472
  epidemiology of, 3463-3465, 3465f

Leishmaniasis (Continued)
  in HIV infection, 1860t-1871t
  interferon-gamma for, 616
  mucosal, 632t-635t, 3464t, 3471f, 3472-3473, 3476
  overview of, 3463-3466
  pathogenesis of, 3465, 3465f
  post–kala-azar dermal, 3464t, 3468-3469, 3468f
    diagnosis of, 3469
    differential diagnosis of, 3469
    treatment of, 3474
  prevention of, 3476-3477
  in travelers, 4023f
  treatment of, 632t-635t, 3465-3466, 3473-3476
  vaccine for, 3476-3477
  visceral, 632t-635t, 3464t, 3466-3469
    clinical manifestations of, 3467-3468
    epidemiology of, 3464t, 3466-3467
    in HIV infection, 3468
    late-stage (kala-azar), 3466-3468, 3466f
    natural history of, 3467
    pathogenesis of, 3467
    treatment of, 3473-3475
  viscerotropic, 3468
Leishmaniasis recidivans, 3464t, 3471f, 3472
Lemierre disease (jugular suppurative thrombophlebitis), 862t, 864-865, 864f, 2700
Lemierre's syndrome, from pharyngitis, 820
Lenograstim, 611-612
Lepromin reaction, 3170
Leprosy, 3165-3176. See also Mycobacterium leprae.
  borderline, 3168-3169
  chemotherapy-associated reactions in, 546
  classification of, 3167
  clinical manifestations of, 3168-3169
  complications of, 3171
  diagnosis of, 3169-3170, 3169f-3170f
  differential diagnosis of, 3169
  epidemiology of, 3165-3166
    global, 3165-3166
    in United States, 3166
  erythema nodosum leprosum in, 3169-3171, 3171f, 3173
  genetics of, 49-50, 50t, 3165-3167, 3166t
  history of, 3165
  in HIV infection, 3174
  hypoesthesia in, 3169
  in immunocompromised hosts, 3174
  immunology of, 3167
  lepromatous, 3167-3170, 3169f
  Lucio's phenomenon (erythema necroticans) in, 3171, 3171f
  multibacillary, 3167
  nerve damage in, 3167-3168, 3171
  paucibacillary, 3167, 3169, 3170f
  peripheral neuropathy in, 3168-3169
  prevention of, 3174
  rehabilitation in, 3174
  relapses in, 3173
  resistance testing in, 3173-3174
  reversal reactions in, 3169-3170, 3170f
    late, 3173
    treatment of, 3173
  supportive care in, 3174
  transmission of, 3165
  treatment of, 544-546, 3171-3173
    agents for, 3172
    interferon-gamma in, 616
    for reactions, 3173
    regimens for, 3172
    in relapse, 3173
    response to, 3172-3173
    rifamycins in, 408
  tuberculoid, 3167-3169
  uveitis in, 1566
Leptomeningitis, from Toxoplasma gondii, 3501
Leptospira/leptospirosis, 3059-3065
  biphasic nature of, 3061-3062, 3062f
  classification of, 3059, 3060f, 3060t
  clinical manifestations of, 3061-3062, 3061t, 3062f
  versus enteric fever, 1400t-1401t, 1403
  epidemiology of, 3059
  etiology of, 3059, 3060f
  hepatitis from, 1587
  history of, 3059

Leptospira/leptospirosis (Continued)
  laboratory diagnosis of, 240t-242t, 3062-3063, 3063f
  versus malaria, 3450
  microscopic agglutination test for, 3063
  pathogenesis of, 3059-3060
  prevention of, 3064, 3064t
  transmission of, 3059
  in travelers, 4024
  treatment of, 3063-3064, 3064t
  uveitis in, 1566
  vaccine for, 3064
  as waterborne disease, 4005
Leptospires
  indirect detection of, 3063
  isolation and identification of, 3063
  visualization of, 3059, 3060f, 3062-3063, 3063f
Lesser sac, 1011, 1012f
Lethal factor, of Bacillus anthracis, 30, 2715
Leuconostoc, 2644t, 2652
Leukemia
  acute myeloid, from granulocyte colony-stimulating factor, 613-614
  from chloramphenicol, 396-397
  T cell, adult, 2313f-2314f, 2315-2316
Leukocidin, of Pseudomonas aeruginosa, 2844
Leukocyte(s)
  in cerebrospinal fluid, 1185
    in bacterial meningitis, 1198
  in chronic pneumonia, 933-934
  fecal, in dysentery, 1389, 1390f
  in Pseudomonas aeruginosa resistance, 2839-2840
  in Q fever pneumonia, 2514
  in septic arthritis, 1445-1446, 1446t
  transfusion of, for granulocytopenia, 117
Leukocyte adhesion deficiency, 112, 172-173
  periodontal disease in, 167, 171f
  type 1, 112, 169t-170t, 172-173
  type 2, 112, 169t-170t, 173
  type 3, 112, 169t-170t
Leukocyte esterase test, in urinary tract infection, 967
Leukocyte function-associated antigen-1, 103
Leukocyte scans, indium-111–tagged, of intraperitoneal abscess, 1030-1031
Leukocytosis
  acute, 990-991
  in cellulitis, 1296
  in erysipelas, 1294-1295
  in liver abscess, 1037
  in mesenteric lymphadenitis, 1406
  in sepsis, 998
Leukoencephalopathy, progressive multifocal, 2052-2055, 2053t
  classic, 2052, 2053t
  clinical manifestations of, 2052-2053
  diagnosis of, 2053, 2054f-2055f
  epidemiology of, 2052
  in HIV infection, 1752-1753, 1753f, 1860t-1870t, 1877
  pathogenesis of, 2052
  prognosis for, 2053-2054
  in solid organ transplant recipients, 3848
  treatment of, 2054-2055
Leukoplakia, Candida, 3227, 3227f
Levamisole, for ascariasis, 655, 3579-3580
Levine's classification of beta-lactam allergy, 347-348, 348t
Levofloxacin, 706t-709t
  for anthrax, 3989t
  antimicrobial activity of, 491t-492t
  for Chlamydophila respiratory infection, 2471, 2471t
  for diabetic foot ulcer, 1462
  dosage of, 493t, 732t-733t
  formulations of, 716t
  for gonococcal arthritis, 1449
  for Helicobacter pylori infection, 2809t
  for Legionnaires' disease, 2978t
  for Neisseria gonorrhoeae infection, 2753, 2766
  for nosocomial pneumonia, 3718t
  for osteomyelitis, 1459t
  for peritonitis, 1022t, 1025
  pharmacology of, 492t

Levofloxacin (Continued)
  prophylactic
    for bacterial infections in cancer patients, 3800t
    for traveler's diarrhea, 4015
  for septic bursitis, 1450t
  for sinusitis, 844-845, 845t
  structure of, 487, 488f
  for urethritis, 1490
Levovirin, 599
Lice infestations, 3629-3632
  clinical manifestations of, 3629-3631
  control of, 2523
  diagnosis of, 3629, 3630f
  epidemiology of, 3629
  protection against, 3632, 4015-4016
  treatment of, 3631-3632, 3631t
  typhus borne by, 2521-2524, 2522f, 2522t
Lincomycin, 440-443, 706t-709t
  chemistry of, 440, 440f
  dosage of, 726t-727t
  formulations of, 716t
  mechanism of action of, 440
  resistance to, mechanisms of, 440
Lincosamides, 440-443. See also Clindamycin.
  dosage of, 726t-727t
  formulations of, 716t
  resistance to
    enzymes in, 285
    mechanisms of, 287t
    ribosomal binding site alteration in, 287
    Staphylococcus aureus resistance to, 2559t
Lindane, for scabies, 3636t
Linezolid, 471-474, 706t-709t
  adverse reactions to, 473
  antimicrobial activity of, 471, 472t
  for brain abscess, 1274-1275
  for cellulitis, 1297-1298
  chemistry of, 471, 472f
  for coagulase-negative staphylococcal infection, 473
  for diabetic foot ulcer, 1462
  dosage of, 728t-729t
  drug interactions with, 742t-761t
  for Enterococcus, 2650
  for Enterococcus endocarditis, 1120t
  formulations of, 716t
  mechanism of action of, 471
  for MRSA joint infections, 1449
  for nocardiosis, 3204t, 3205
  for nontuberculous mycobacterial infections, 544
  for nosocomial pneumonia, 3718t
  for osteomyelitis, 1459, 1459t
  pharmacology of, 471-472
  resistance to, 290-291, 291t, 473
  for Staphylococcus aureus, 472-473
  Staphylococcus aureus resistance to, 2559t, 2561
  for Staphylococcus endocarditis, 1118t
  for Streptococcus pneumoniae infection, 473
  for tuberculosis, 541
  uses of, 472-473, 472t
  for vancomycin-resistant enterococci, 473
Lip edema, in Kawasaki syndrome, 3663, 3664f
Lip wounds, 3914
Lipid A, 2816
Lipid(s)
  abnormalities of, in HIV infection, 1714
  mycobacterial, CD1-presented, 137, 140
  plasma, in sepsis, 998
Lipoglycopeptides
  for Enterococcus infection, 2649
  for Staphylococcus aureus infection, 2562-2563
  Staphylococcus aureus resistance to, 2559t
Lipo-oligosaccharides
  in Moraxella catarrhalis, 2772
  in Neisseria gonorrhoeae, 2755
Lipopeptides, 462-465. See also Daptomycin.
Lipopolysaccharides
  of Campylobacter jejuni, 2796
  endotoxic, of gram-negative anaerobic rods, 3113
  of enterobacteriaceae, 2816, 2820
  of Helicobacter pylori, 2805
  of Pseudomonas aeruginosa, 2835, 2836f, 2843
Lipoteichoic acids, of Staphylococcus aureus, 2551-2552
Lisofylline, 620

Listeria monocytogenes/listeriosis, 2707-2714
  bacteremia from, 2709
  brain abscess from, 1265-1266, 2710
  CNS infections from, 2709-2710
  complications of, 2711
  diagnosis of, 2711, 2712t
  encephalitis from, 2710
  endocarditis from, 2710
  epidemiology of, 2707-2708
  febrile gastroenteritis from, 2711
  focal infection from, 2710
  foodborne disease from, 1413, 1414t, 1415,
    1418-1419
  immunity to, 2709
  laboratory detection of, 240t-242t
  meningitis from, 1190t-1191t, 1192, 2709-2710,
    2710t
    treatment of, 1211t-1212t, 1217-1218
  microbiology of, 2707, 2708t
  in neonates, 2709
  pathogenesis of, 2708
  phagosome lysis by, 10
  in pregnancy, 2709
  prevention of, 2712-2713, 2712t
    CDC recommendations for, 1425, 1425t
  rhombencephalitis from, 2710, 2711f
  spinal cord infection from, 2710
  in transplant recipients, 3846
  treatment of, 2712
Liver. *See also* Hepatic; Hepato-; Hepatitis *entries.*
  enlarged
    in schistosomiasis, 3598
    in Still's disease, 787
  histology of, as indicator of disease, 2167
  nitrofurantoin effects on, 517
  in systemic response to infection, 990
Liver abscess, 1035-1039
  amebic, 918, 921, 3412, 3416-3417, 3417f
    clinical manifestations of, 1037, 3418, 3420f
    diagnosis of, 1037-1038
    epidemiology/etiology of, 1035
    microbiology of, 1036
    pathogenesis of and pathophysiology of, 1035
    treatment of, 632t-635t, 1038, 3422, 3422t
  clinical presentation in, 1037, 1037t
  diagnosis of, 1037-1038
  epidemiology/etiology of, 1035
  in liver transplant recipients, 3843
  microbiology of, 1036-1037, 1036t
  pathogenesis and pathophysiology of, 1035-1036,
    1036t
  pyogenic
    clinical presentation in, 1037, 1037t
    diagnosis of, 1037-1038
    epidemiology/etiology of, 1035
    from *Klebsiella pneumoniae*, 1036-1037
    microbiology of, 1036, 1036t
    pathogenesis and pathophysiology of,
      1035-1036, 1036t
    treatment of, 1038-1039, 1038f, 1039t
  staphylococcal, in chronic granulomatous disease,
    174, 174f
  treatment of, 1038-1039, 1038f, 1039t
Liver biopsy
  in acute viral hepatitis, 1580
  in hepatitis A infection, 2379
  in hepatitis C infection, 2169, 2169t
Liver disease
  antimicrobial agents in, 271
  chloramphenicol in, 396
  chronic, hepatitis A infection and, vaccination
    against, 2383
  HCV-related, in HIV infection, 2176
  in HIV infection, 1739-1741, 1739t
  quinolones in, 494
  tetracycline in, 389-390, 391t
  in tuberculosis, 3149
Liver enzymes, in hepatitis C infection, 2169
Liver failure
  acute
    definition of, 1580
    etiology of, 1580
  antituberculous agents in, 534t
  fulminant
    management of, 1589-1590

Liver failure *(Continued)*
    from viral hepatitis, 1580
  hyperacute, 1580
  in sepsis, 1000
  subacute, 1580
Liver flukes, 1407t, 1409, 3596t, 3597f, 3600-3602,
  3601f
Liver function tests, in infectious mononucleosis,
  2001
Liver transplant recipients
  abdominal infections in, 3843
  adenovirus infections in, 2030-2031
  cytomegalovirus infection in, 1981
  gut decontamination in, 3816
  hepatitis B in, 1602, 2072
  hepatitis C in, 1610
  infections in, 3810, 3810f, 3839, 3840f, 3841t,
    3842-3843
  survival data for, 3839, 3840t
  toxoplasmosis in, 3504
Ljungan virus, 2337. *See also* Parechoviruses.
Loa loa, 654, 3592
Lobar consolidation, 935t-936t
Lobectomy, for chronic pneumonia, 942
Lockjaw (trismus), from tetanus, 3092-3093, 3092f
Loiasis, 632t-635t, 3590t, 3592, 3592f
Lomefloxacin, 706t-709t
  dosage of, 732t-733t
  formulations of, 716t
Long bones, osteomyelitis of, 1458-1459
Long-term care facilities
  diarrhea in, 1365, 3860
  tuberculosis in, 3151
  urinary tract infections in
    incidence and prevalence of, 3725
    prevention of, 3728-3729
Lopinavir-ritonavir, 706t-709t, 1839f, 1840t, 1841
  dosage of, 740t-741t
  drug interactions with, 742t-761t
  formulations of, 717t
  for HIV postexposure prophylaxis, 3755t, 3764
  for HIV-infected children, 1820t-1821t, 1823t
Loracarbef, 706t-709t
  dosage of, 722t
  formulations of, 716t
  structure of, 324f
  uses of, 334
Lorazepam, for tetanus, 3094, 3094t
Louping ill virus, encephalitis from, 1251t-1252t
Louse-borne relapsing fever, 3067-3069
Lower respiratory tract specimens
  collection and transport guidelines for, 235t-236t
  laboratory processing of, 238-239
Lucio's phenomenon, in leprosy, 3171, 3171f
Ludwig's angina, 862t, 863, 863f
  mediastinitis from, 1173
Lumbar puncture, 1184-1186, 1185t. *See also*
  Cerebrospinal fluid.
  complications of, 1184
  neuroimaging studies before, 1184
Lumefantrine, 639-641, 706t-709t
  with artemether, 639-641
    for malaria, 4014
Lung. *See also* Pulmonary *entries;* Respiratory
  entries.
  barotrauma to, from hyperbaric oxygen therapy,
    626
  commensal bacteria in, 878
  effects of nitrofurantoin on, 517
  fungus ball of, 3245-3246
  Kaposi's sarcoma affecting, 1766
Lung abscess, 925-929
  amebic, 925
  classification of, 925
  clinical manifestations of, 926, 927f
  diagnosis of, 926-927, 927f
  differential diagnosis of, 926t, 927
  in melioidosis, 2872f-2873f
  microbiology of, 926, 926t
  pathophysiology of, 925
  prognosis in, 928
  treatment of, 927-928
Lung biopsy
  laboratory processing after, 239
  in *Pneumocystis jirovecii* pneumonia, 1729, 3383

Lung biopsy *(Continued)*
  in pneumonia, 899-900
  in Q fever pneumonia, 2514, 2514f
Lung cancer, in HIV infection, 1733
Lung consolidation, in melioidosis, 2871, 2873f
Lung flukes, 3596t, 3602-3603
Lung injury, acute, in sepsis, 999
Lung nodules, 935t-936t
  from *Coccidioides*, 3336, 3336f
  from *Nocardia*, 3201, 3202f
Lung transplant recipients
  infections in, 3810, 3810f, 3841t, 3842
  survival data for, 3839, 3840t
Lupus erythematosus
  complement deficiency in, 86-88
  complement in, 94
Lupus-like syndrome, from rifamycins, 407
Lyell's syndrome, in beta-lactam allergy, 347
Lyme disease, 3071-3081, 3650, 3651t-3652t
  acrodermatitis chronica atrophicans in, 3076
  animal hosts for, 3071-3072
  arthritis in, 3076, 3079-3080, 3079t
  cardiac involvement in, 3075, 3075t, 3079t
  causative agent in, 3071
  chronic, 3076
  clinical characteristics of, 3074-3076
  coinfection in, 3077
  congenital, 3076
  differential diagnosis of, 3079
  encephalopathy in, 3076
  epidemiology of, 3072-3073
  erythema migrans in, 3074, 3075t, 3079, 3079t
  interstitial keratitis in, 1545
  laboratory diagnosis of, 3077-3079, 3077f-3078f
  macrolides for, 437
  meningitis in, chronic, 1240
  neurologic abnormalities in, 3074-3075, 3075t,
    3079, 3079t
  ocular infections in, 3075, 3075t
  pathogenesis of, 3073-3074
  prevention of, 3080
  rash in, 801, 3651f
  stage 1 (localized infection), 3074, 3074f, 3075t
  stage 2 (disseminated infection), 3074-3075, 3074f,
    3075t
  stage 3 (persistent infection), 3074f, 3075t,
    3076
  tick-borne encephalitis versus, 2141
  treatment of, 3079-3080, 3079t
  uveitis in, 1565
  vectors of, 3071-3072
Lyme urine antigen test (LUAT), 3077
Lymph node, anatomy of, 142-143, 142f
Lymphadenitis/lymphadenopathy, 1323-1330
  acute, 1323
  axillary, 1324
  in cat-scratch disease, 1326, 2999, 2999f-3000f
  cervical, 862t, 867, 1323-1324
    in Kawasaki syndrome, 3663
    tuberculous, 1325
  chronic, 1323
  clinical features of, 1323
  deep neck space, 1324
  differential diagnosis of, 1327-1329, 1328t
  epitrochlear, 1324
  etiology of, 1327-1329, 1328t
  in filariasis, 1327, 3590f, 3591
  generalized, 1327, 1329-1330
  in genital lesions, 1476
  in glanders, 2877
  granulomatous, from nondiphtheria
    Corynebacterium, 1325
  in group A–associated streptococcal pharyngitis,
    816
  histiocytic necrotizing, 1327-1329
  in HIV infection
    generalized, 1329-1330
    persistent generalized, 1713
  from human T-cell lymphotrophic virus, 2315
  iliac, 1324
  inguinal
    in bubonic plague, 1326-1327
    in chancroid, 2917
    from *Chlamydia trachomatis*, 2449-2450
    filarial, 1327

Lymphadenitis/lymphadenopathy *(Continued)*
  in genital lesions, 1476
    in sexually transmitted disease, 1326
  in Kawasaki syndrome, 3663
  in Marshall's syndrome, 1327
  mediastinal, 1324, 1326, 3158
  mesenteric, 1405-1407
    clinical features of, 1405-1406, 1405t
    differential diagnosis of, 1406
    epidemiology of, 1406
    etiology and pathogenesis of, 1405
    treatment of, 1406-1407
    tuberculous, 3158
    in *Yersinia pseudotuberculosis* infection, 2951
  from *Mycobacterium,* 1325
  from *Mycobacterium avium* complex, 1325
    classification and microbiology of, 3179
    clinical presentation of, 3182, 3182f
    diagnosis of, 3183
    epidemiology of, 3177-3178
    host immunity to, 3179
    treatment of, 3186
  from *Mycobacterium avium-intracellulare,*
      1325
  nonpyogenic, 1325
    specific types of, 1325-1327
  from nontuberculous mycobacteria, 3194
  in oculoglandular (Parinaud's) syndrome,
      1326
  from *Paracoccidioides brasiliensis,* 3360
  pathogenesis and pathology of, 1323
  periauricular, 1326
  pyogenic, 1323
  recurrent, 1327
  regional, 1323
    nonpyogenic, 1325
      specific types of, 1325-1327
    pyogenic, 1323
  in Rosai-Dorfman disease, 1329
  from *Sporothrix schenckii,* 3271, 3272f, 3272t
  subpectoral, 1324
  suppurative, 1323-1324
    epitrochlear, 1324
    iliac, 1324
  tick-borne, 3653-3654, 3653t
  from *Toxoplasma gondii,* 1329
  in toxoplasmosis, 3500
  treatment of, 1330
  tuberculous, 3158, 3158f
  in tularemia, 2932-2933, 2932f
Lymphangioleiomyomatosis, chest radiography in,
    937f
Lymphangioma, infected, 862t, 867
Lymphangitis, 1330-1332
  acute, 1330-1331
  chronic granulomatous, 1331
  clinical features of, 1330-1331
  differential diagnosis of, 1331
  etiologic agents in, 1331, 1331t
  filarial, 1331
  pathogenesis and pathology of, 1330
  from *Streptococcus pyogenes,* 2606
  treatment of, 1331-1332
Lymphatic cutaneous metastases, versus cellulitis,
    1297, 1297t
Lymphedema, in deep dermatophytosis, 3350-3351,
    3351f
Lymphocytes
  B. *See* B cells.
  count of
    in immunodeficiency assessment, 168
    in nutritional assessment, 151, 152t
  pulmonary, 893
  T. *See* T cells.
Lymphocytic choriomeningitis virus, 2295-2301
  characteristics of, 2295
  clinical manifestations of, 2298-2299
  diagnosis of, 2299-2300
  encephalitis from, 1251t-1252t
  epidemiology/epizootiology of, 2295-2296,
      2296t
  meningitis from, 1190
  pathogenesis of, 2297-2298
  prevention of, 2300
  treatment of, 2300

Lymphocytic interstitial pneumonitis
  in HIV infection, 1733
  in HIV-infected children, 1815, 1815f
Lymphocytosis
  atypical, differential diagnosis of, 1999, 1999t
  diffuse infiltrative, neuropathy from, in HIV
      infection, 1758
  in Epstein-Barr virus infection, 1992, 1999, 1999t
Lymphogranuloma venereum, 1477-1478, 1480-1481
  from *Chlamydia trachomatis,* 2449-2450
  conjunctivitis in, 1534
  inguinal buboes in, 1326, 1329
Lymphohistiocytosis, hemophagocytic, from
    Epstein-Barr virus, 1996
Lymphoid anatomy, 142-144, 142f-143f
Lymphoid tissue, as HIV reservoir, 1693-1694
Lymphoma
  abdominal pain and/or diarrhea with eosinophilia
      from, 1407t, 1409
  B-cell, chronic hepatitis C coinfection with, 1611
  central nervous system, HIV-related, 1771-1772
    EBV DNA in, 2002
    treatment of, 1772
  fever of unknown origin in, 786
  gastric, in *Helicobacter pylori* infection, 2806t,
      2807
  in HIV infection, 1768-1772, 2333. *See also*
      Non-Hodgkin's lymphoma, in HIV infection.
    central nervous system, 1751, 1752f
    gastrointestinal, 1738
    hepatic, 1741
    Hodgkin's, 1775-1776
    pulmonary, 1733
  Hodgkin's. *See* Hodgkin's disease.
  primary effusion
    from Epstein-Barr virus, 1998-1999
    from human herpesvirus 8, 2020, 2020f
    pyothorax-associated, 1998-1999
  T cell, adult, 2313f-2314f, 2315-2316
Lymphomatoid granulomatosis, from Epstein-Barr
    virus, 1998
Lymphoproliferative disease
  from Epstein-Barr virus, 1990t, 1996-1997, 1996t
    posttransplant, 1996-1997, 1997f, 2001-2002
    treatment of, 2003-2004
  after transplantation, 1996-1997, 1997f,
      3848-3849
  X-linked, 73, 169t-170t, 171
    from Epstein-Barr virus, 1995
    hepatitis in, 1587
Lyngbya, exposure syndromes from, 3570-3571,
    3570f
Lysis, complement-mediated, of *Entamoeba
    histolytica,* 3416
Lysis-centrifugation system, for blood culture, 237,
    237t
Lysozyme
  in neutrophil bactericidal activity, 109
  in oral mucosal immunity, 858
Lyssavirus, 2249, 2250f, 2250t

M

M protein, in group A *Streptococcus,* 2593-2594
Machupo virus, 2296t. *See also* South American
    hemorrhagic fevers.
Macroevolutionary change, 279
Macrolides, 427-434. *See also* Azithromycin;
    Clarithromycin; Erythromycin.
  dosage of, 726t-727t
  formulations of, 716t
  for nontuberculous mycobacterial infections,
      542-543
  for parasitic infections, 655
  resistance to
    efflux promotion in, 287
    enzymes in, 285
    mechanisms of, 287t
    ribosomal binding site alteration in, 287
  Staphylococcus aureus resistance to, 2559t, 2561
  uses of, 432t-433t
Macronodular lesions, of disseminated candidiasis,
    3229-3230, 3230f
Macronutrients, supplementation of, in HIV/AIDS,
    156, 156t

Macrophage(s), 41
  in *Entamoeba histolytica,* 3415, 3415f
  in HIV infection, 1698
  in *Legionella pneumophila,* 2971, 2972f
  in *Salmonella,* 2893-2894
  in tuberculosis, 3136
  in Whipple's disease, 1436-1437
Macrophage colony-stimulating factor, 614-615
Macrophage migration inhibitory factor (MIF), in
    severe sepsis, 993
Macular degeneration, age-related, factor H
    deficiency in, 92
Macular lesions, 1303
Macules, 792
  in epidemic typhus, 2522
Maculopapular rash, 792-795, 793t, 1303. *See also*
    Rash.
  in CMV mononucleosis, 1975
Madurella, mycetoma from, 3281, 3282f, 3282t,
    3284-3285
Maduromycosis (madura foot), 3281
Mafenide acetate, 475-476, 706t-709t, 3907t
Magnetic resonance angiography
  in myocarditis, 1158
  in suppurative intracranial thrombophlebitis,
      1285, 1285f
Magnetic resonance cholangiography, 1040-1041
Magnetic resonance imaging
  in AIDS dementia, 1747, 1748f
  in brain abscess, 1270-1271, 1271f
  in central nervous system infections, 1186-1187,
      2710, 2711f
  in central nervous system lymphoma, 1751, 1752f
  in cranial subdural empyema, 1280, 1281f
  in Creutzfeldt-Jakob disease, 2433-2434, 2433f
  in cryptococcal meningoencephalitis, 3298
  in encephalitis, 1247-1249, 1248f
  in intraperitoneal abscess, 1031
  in myocarditis, 1158
  in neurocysticercosis, 3612, 3612f
  in Nipah virus encephalitis, 2240, 2240f
  in osteomyelitis, 1457-1458, 1458f, 1461, 1461f
  in pleural effusion, 919-920
  in progressive multifocal leukoencephalopathy,
      1752, 1753f, 2053, 2054f
  in prosthetic vascular graft infection, 1134, 1134t
  in pyomyositis, 1315-1316
  in rabies, 2254, 2254f
  in septic arthritis, 1446, 1446f
  in sinopulmonary mucormycosis, 3260-3261,
      3261f
  in spinal epidural abscess, 1282, 1283f
  in splenic abscess, 1056
  in suppurative intracranial thrombophlebitis,
      1285, 1285f-1286f
  in *Toxoplasma* encephalitis, 1749-1750, 1750f
  in toxoplasmosis, 3510-3512, 3511f
  in urinary tract infection, 980
  in West Nile encephalitis, 2147, 2147f
Maitotoxin, 1417
Majocchi's granuloma, in dermatophytosis, 3351
Major histocompatibility complex (MHC)
    molecules
  class I
    antigen processing by, 133-135, 135f
    cross priming by, 134-135
    structure of, 132-133, 133f
    in viral infections, 139
    viral intervention with, 134
  class Ib, 141
  class II
    antigen processing by, 135-136, 136f
    structure of, 133, 133f
  class III, 83
  defective, 169t-170t
  immunogenetics of, 140-144, 141f
Major histocompatibility complex (MHC) tetramer
    staining, 145-146, 146f
Major surface glycoprotein, of *Pneumocystis,*
    3377-3378
Major vault protein, in *Pseudomonas aeruginosa*
    resistance, 2840
Malabsorption
  from *Giardia lamblia,* 3530
  tropical, postinfectious. *See* Tropical sprue.

Malaria, 3437-3462
  ABO blood groups and, 3443
  airport, 3445
  anemia in, 3441, 3449
  in asplenia, 3869
  cerebral, 3440f, 3441, 3449
  chloroquine-resistant, 635
  clinical presentation in, 3447-3449
  diagnosis of, 3447-3449
    blood smears in, 3446f, 3448
    rapid tests in, 3448
    in severe disease, 3449, 3449t
  differential diagnosis of, 3449-3450, 3450t
  drug-resistant
    epidemiology of, 3444, 3445f
    geographic distribution of, 3445-3446, 3445f
    mortality trends and, 3437, 3438f
  Duffy antigen negativity and, 3443-3444
  emergence of, 211-212
  versus enteric fever, 1400t-1401t, 1403-1404, 3450
  epidemiology of, 3444-3445, 3445f
  general considerations in, 3438
  genetics of, 50, 50t, 3442-3444
  global efforts to control, 212
  glucose-6-phosphate dehydrogenase and, 50, 50t,
    53, 3443
  hemoglobin C and, 50, 3442-3443
  hemoglobin E and, 3442-3443
  hemoglobin F and, 3443
  hemoglobin S and, 53, 3442-3443
  hemoglobinuria in, 3449
  history in, 3447-3448
  in HIV infection, 1858t-1870t
  hyperbilirubinemia in, 3449
  hyperparasitemia in, 3449
  hyperpyrexia in, 3449
  hypoglycemia in, 3441, 3449
  immunology of, 3444, 3444f
  metabolic acidosis in, 3442
  mortality in, 3437, 3438f
  paroxysms in, 3438
  pathophysiology of, 3438-3442, 3439f-3440f
  physical examination in, 3447-3448
  placental, 3442
  from Plasmodium falciparum, 3438-3442,
    3439f-3440f
  from Plasmodium knowlesi, 3442
  from Plasmodium malariae, 3442
  from Plasmodium ovale, 3442
  from Plasmodium vivax, 3442
  in pregnancy, 3442, 3453
  prevention of, 3454-3456
    chemoprophylaxis for, 3455, 3455t
    mosquito repellent and avoidance measures for,
      3456
    risk assessment in, 3454-3455
  prostration in, 3449
  public health impact of, 3437, 3438f
  pulmonary edema in, 3441-3442
  rash in, 797
  renal insufficiency in, 3449
  respiratory distress in, 3441-3442, 3449
  severe
    criteria for, 3449, 3449t
    exchange transfusion in, 3454
    sepsis in, 3454
    treatment of, 3452t, 3453
  shock in, 3449
  Southeast Asian ovalocytosis and, 3443
  thalassemia and, 53, 3443
  transfusion-related, 3748
  transmission of, 3444
  in travelers, 4021-4022
    chemoprophylaxis for, 3455, 3455t, 4013-4014
    risk of, 4013, 4014f
    self-treatment of, 3453
  treatment of, 632t-635t, 3451-3454, 3452t
    artemisinins in, 669, 671f
    drug resistance in, 211-212
    exchange transfusion in, 3454
    general principles in, 3455-3456
    in infants, 3453
    macrolides in, 437-438
    mechanisms of action of, 3446-3447
    in nonfalciparum malaria, 3454

Malaria (Continued)
    in pregnancy, 3453
    resistance to, 3446-3447
    in severe disease, 3452t, 3453-3454
    in travelers, 3453, 4021
    in uncomplicated disease, 3451, 3452t
  vaccine for, 3456
  vomiting in, 3449
Malarone. See Atovaquone-proguanil.
Malassezia
  folliculitis from, 3354
  pityriasis (tinea) versicolor from, 3353-3354
  seborrheic dermatitis from, 3354
Malassezia furfur, 3371
  device-associated infections from, 3697
  in hematopoietic stem cell transplant recipients,
    3832
  suppurative thrombophlebitis from, 1098
Malathion, for scabies, 3636t
Malnutrition
  from ascariasis, 3578
  cryptosporidiosis and, 3552
  definition of, 151
  diagnosis of, 151, 152t
  diarrhea and, 1335
  in elderly, 156-157, 156t
  epidemiology of, 151
  in HIV/AIDS, 155-156, 156t
  in HIV-infected children, 1813-1814
  from hookworm, 3581
  in immunocompromised hosts, 3787
  pathogen virulence and, 157-158, 158f
  protein-energy, 151-152
Mammalian cells, pathogen recognition receptors on,
  2627
Management (strategy) trials, 689. See also Clinical
  trials.
Mandible
  actinomycosis of, 3211
  osteomyelitis of, 862t, 865, 870
Mannitol, for increased intracranial pressure,
  1202
Mannose receptor, in innate immunity, 138
Mannose-binding lectin
  complement activation by, 79, 79f
  deficiency of, 88-89
  in hepatitis B susceptibility, 52, 54
  in mycobacterial disease susceptibility, 51t, 54
  in phagocytosis, 104-105
Mannose-binding protein, 78t
  deficiency of, 88-89
Mannose-binding protein–associated serine protease
  2, deficiency of, 89
Mansonella, 654
Mansonella ozzardi, 3593
Mansonella perstans, 3593-3594
Mansonella streptocerca, 3594
Mansonellosis, 632t-635t, 3590t, 3593-3594
Maraviroc, 706t-709t, 1843-1844, 1843f, 1843t
  dosage of, 740t-741t
  drug interactions with, 742t-761t
  formulations of, 717t
  for HIV infection, 21-22
  for HIV-infected children, 1820t-1821t
Marburg virus
  characteristics of, 2259, 2260f
  clinical manifestations of, 2262
  diagnosis of, 2262
  ecology of, 2259, 2261f
  epidemiology of, 2259
  pathology and pathogenesis of, 2262
  prevention and treatment of, 2262-2263
  transmission of, 2260-2262
Marchal body, 3979
Maribavir, 599-600, 599f
  for cytomegalovirus infection, 1978-1979
Marshall's syndrome, 1327
Mask, isolation, 3673, 3674t
MASPs (MBP-associated serum proteases), 78t, 79
Mast cells, activated, in Entamoeba histolytica
  infection, 3416
Masticator spaces, infections of, 861-863. See also
  Odontogenic infections.
Mastitis, from Staphylococcus aureus, 2566
Mastoiditis, 835-836, 836f

Matrix metalloproteinases, in bacterial meningitis,
  1201
Maxilla, actinomycosis of, 3211, 3211f
Maxillary sinus, anatomy and physiology of, 839,
  840f
Maxillary sinusitis, 865
Maxillofacial trauma, 868
Maximal serum concentration, minimal inhibitory
  concentration relationship to, 302-303, 302f
Mayaro virus, 2117-2125, 2118t. See also
  Alphaviruses.
McBurney's point, in appendicitis, 1059
MDX-1303, for anthrax, 2723
Me Tri virus, encephalitis from, 1251t-1252t
Measles, 2229-2236
  in adults, 2233
  atypical, 2232
  characteristics of, 2229
  clinical manifestations of, 2231-2233, 2231f
  complications of, 2231-2232
  croup complicating, 826
  detection of, 259t-260t
  diagnosis of, 2233
  encephalitis from, 1260
  epidemiology of, 2229-2230
  German. See Rubella.
  immune response to, 2231
  in immunocompromised hosts, 2232
  Koplik's spots from, 2231
  modified, 2232
  pathogenesis of, 2230-2231
  in pregnancy, 2232
  prevention of, 2233-2234
    in immunocompromised hosts, 2233
    intramuscular immune globulin for, 3935
  rash from, 2231, 2231f
  subacute sclerosing panencephalitis from, 2230
  transmission of, 2230
  treatment of, 2234
  in tuberculosis, 2232
  vaccine for, 2233
    atypical measles after, 2232
Measles, mumps, rubella (MMR) vaccine, 2233,
  3922t, 3927-3928, 3932
  autism and, 2234
  in HIV-infected children, 1825
Measles, mumps, rubella, varicella (MMRV) vaccine,
  3922t, 3927, 3933
Measles immune globulin, 1826, 2233
Meatal care, enhanced, urinary tract infection
  prevention with, 3731-3732
Mebendazole, 706t-709t
  for angiostrongyliasis, 3621
  for ascariasis, 3579-3580
  for capillariasis, 3621
  drug interactions with, 742t-761t
  for echinococcosis, 3614
  for enterobiasis, 3584
  for hookworm, 3581
  for intestinal parasitic infections, 632t-635t,
    646-647
  for trichinellosis, 3588
  for trichuriasis, 3580-3581
MecA gene, in Staphylococcus, 2546, 2558
Mechanical débridement, for gingivitis, 869
Mechanical valve prosthesis, 1116-1117. See also
  Prosthetic heart valve.
Media management, in emergency preparedness, 230
Mediastinal actinomycosis, 3211-3212
Mediastinal fibrosis, from Histoplasma capsulatum,
  3310, 3310f, 3316
Mediastinal lymphadenitis, 1324
  tuberculous, 3158
Mediastinitis, 1173-1182
  acute, 1173-1179
  bacteriology of, 1175-1176, 1175t
  after cardiothoracic surgery, 1173-1175, 1175t
  causes of, 1174t
  chronic, 1179-1180, 1179t
  clinical manifestations of, 1176-1177
  complications of, 1178
  computed tomography in, 1176-1177, 1176f
  diagnosis of, 1176-1177, 1176f
  epidemiology of, 1173-1175
  after esophageal perforation, 1173, 1175t

Mediastinitis *(Continued)*
  fibrosing tuberculous, 3158
  from head and neck infections, 1173, 1175t
  in heart transplant recipients, 3841
  postoperative, antibiotic prophylaxis for, 1178
  prognosis for, 1179
  radiographic findings in, 1176, 1176f
  treatment of, 1177-1178
Mediastinum, anatomy of, 1173, 1174f
Medical and public health emergency preparedness
    for bioterrorist attack, 3956-3961
  before 9/11/2001, 3957
  following 9/11/2001, 3957, 3958t-3959t
Medical care abroad, for travelers, 4016
Medical countermeasures, in plague terrorist event,
    3966-3968
Medical kit, for travelers, 4016
Medical Reserve Corps (MRC), activation of,
    3957-3958
Medical waste, 3690-3692
  disposal of, 3691t
Medicolegal liability issues, in endocarditis
    prophylaxis, 1149
Mediterranean fever, familial, 1297, 1297t
Mediterranean spotted fever, 3653-3654, 3653t
  from *Rickettsia conori*, 4024
  rifamycins for, 411
Mefloquine, 706t-709t
  for malaria, 632t-635t, 655-656, 3451, 3452t,
    4013-4014
    for prophylaxis, 3455-3456, 3455t
  mechanism of action of, 3447
  neurotoxicity of, 656
  resistance to, 3445
Megaloblastic anemia, from *Diphyllobothrium latum*,
    3609
Meglumine antimonate, 706t-709t
  for parasitic infections, 632t-635t, 641-642
Meibomian glands, 1569, 1570f
Melanin, production of, in *Cryptococcus neoformans*,
    3291
α-Melanocyte–stimulating hormone, antipyretic
    activity of, 771-772
Melarsoprol, 656, 706t-709t
  for African trypanosomiasis, 3492-3493
Meleney's gangrene, 3084, 3085f
Melioidosis, 2869-2877
  chronic, 2871, 2873f
  clinical manifestations of, 2871-2875, 2876t
  cutaneous, 2872, 2874f
  encephalomyelitis in, 2872-2873, 2875f
  versus enteric fever, 1400t-1401t, 1403
  epidemiology of, 2869-2870
  etiology of, 2869
  history of, 2869
  internal abscesses in, 2872, 2874f-2875f
  laboratory diagnosis of, 2875
  lung consolidation in, 2871, 2873f
  natural history of, 2870, 2870f
  neurologic, 2872-2873, 2875f
  osteomyelitis in, 2872, 2874f
  pathogenesis of, 2870-2871
  pneumonia in, 2871, 2872f-2873f
  prevention of, 2877
  prostatic abscess in, 2872-2873, 2875f
  risk factors for, 2871, 2871t
  septicemia in, 2871, 2877
  treatment of, 2875-2877, 2876t
Membrane attack complex
  assembly of, 80-81
  regulation of, 82
Membrane cofactor protein (CD46), 81t
Membrane permeability, in antimicrobial resistance,
    286
Memory T cells, 131-132
Men who have sex with men (MSM)
  donovanosis in, 3011
  HAV outbreaks in, 2376
    vaccination against, 2382
  HCV prevalence among, 2171
  HIV infection in, 1637-1638, 1640, 1651
  methicillin-resistant *Staphylococcus aureus* in,
    481
  Neisseria gonorrhoeae infection in, 2756-2758,
    2757f

Menangle virus
  clinical features and diagnostic tests for,
    2242-2243
  emergence of, 2237
  epidemiology of, 2242
  outbreaks of, 2238t
  pathogenesis of, 2242
  rash in, 2242-2243
  structure and molecular biology of, 2237-2238
Mendelian susceptibility to mycobacterial disease,
    140
Meningitis. *See also* Meningoencephalitis.
  from *Acinetobacter*, 2883
  acute, 1183, 1189-1229
  from adenoviruses, 2030
  from aerobic gram-negative bacilli, 1193, 1218
  amebic, 1193, 1207, 1210-1211, 1220
  from *Angiostrongylus cantonensis*, 1193-1194, 1207,
    1211, 1220-1222, 3619-3620
  from anthrax, 2720-2723
  aseptic, 1189
    in HIV infection, 1745
    from parvovirus B19 infection, 2091
  bacterial
    adjunctive therapy for, 1220-1221
    anti-inflammatory agents for, 1220-1221
    antimicrobial therapy for, 1215-1219
    blood-brain-barrier alterations in, 1200-1201
    brain abscess from, 1268
    cerebral blood flow alterations in, 1202-1203
    cerebrospinal fluid examination in, 1208-1209,
      1208t
    clinical features of, 1205-1206, 1205t
    C-reactive protein in, 1209
    dexamethasone for, 619
    diagnosis of, 1208-1209, 1208t, 1209f
    in elderly, 1206
    epidemiology and etiology of, 1190-1193,
      1190t-1191t
    increased intracranial pressure in, 1201-1202,
      1221
    in infants and children, 1206, 1213t
    intravascular survival in, 1196
    meningeal invasion in, 1196-1197
    mucosal colonization and systemic invasion in,
      1195-1196
    in neonates, 1206, 1213t
    neuronal injury in, 1203-1204
    pathogenesis and pathophysiology of,
      1195-1204, 1195f, 1195t
    prevention of, 1222-1224
    procalcitonin in, 1209
    radiography in, 1209, 1209f
    subarachnoid space inflammation in,
      1199-1200, 1199t, 1220-1221
    subarachnoid space survival in, 1197-1199
    surgery for, 1221
  from basilar skull fracture, 1209, 1223
  from *Borrelia burgdorferi*, 1193, 1206, 1210, 1210f,
    1212t, 1219-1220
  from *Candida*, 1239, 3231-3232
  cerebrospinal fluid analysis in, 1185, 1185t
  chronic, 1183, 1237-1242
    from *Acanthamoeba*, 1240
    from *Actinomyces*, 3214
    in actinomycosis, 1240
    from *Angiostrongylus cantonensis*, 1240
    in Behçet's syndrome, 1241
    in blastomycosis, 1239
    blood tests in, 1238
    in brucellosis, 1240
    from *Candida*, 1239, 3231-3232
    cerebrospinal fluid analysis in, 1238
    from *Coccidioides*, 1238-1239
    from *Cryptococcus*, 1238
    differential diagnosis of, 1239t
    from echoviruses, 1241
    empirical therapy for, 1241
    from *Histoplasma*, 1239
    imaging in, 1238
    in Lyme borreliosis, 1240
    neoplastic, 1241
    in neurocysticercosis, 1240-1241
    from *Nocardia*, 1240
    past history in, 1237-1238

Meningitis *(Continued)*
    in phaeohyphomycosis, 1239
    physical signs of, 1237
    presentation of, 1237
    in sarcoidosis, 1241
    from *Scedosporium*, 1239
    in sporotrichosis, 1239
    syphilitic, 1240
    tuberculous, 1240
    in Vogt-Koyanagi-Harada syndrome, 1241
  clinical manifestations of, 1183, 1204-1207
  from *Coccidioides*, 3338, 3341
  from *Cryptococcus neoformans*, 1238
    fluconazole for, 557
    in HIV infection, 1746, 1877
      prophylaxis against, 1858t-1859t, 1871t
      treatment of, 1860t-1870t
    microscopic examination of, 3296, 3296f-3297f
    in transplant recipients, 3846
    treatment of, 3298-3300
  diagnosis of, 1207-1211
  differential diagnosis of, 1190t
  in elderly, 3861
  from *Elizabethkingia meningoseptica*, 3022-3023
  from enterobacteriaceae, 1212t
  from *Enterococcus*, 2646-2647, 2651
  from enteroviruses, 1189, 1204-1205, 1207, 1220,
    2353-2354
    in immunocompromised hosts, 2359-2360
  eosinophilic, 3618t, 3619-3620
  epidemiology and etiology of, 1189-1194
  from extraintestinal pathogenic *Escherichia coli*,
    2821
  from *Haemophilus influenzae*
    epidemiology and etiology of, 1190t-1191t,
      1191-1192
    prevention of, 1222-1223
    treatment of, 1211t-1212t, 1215-1216
    type b, 2914
  from herpes simplex virus, 1950
  from herpesviruses, 1189-1190, 1205
  from *Histoplasma capsulatum*, 3313, 3317
  in HIV infection, 1190, 1745-1746
  in injection drug users, 3886
  from JC virus, 2053
  in leptospirosis, 3061
  from *Listeria monocytogenes*, 1190t-1191t, 1192,
    2709-2710, 2710t
    treatment of, 1211t-1212t, 1217-1218
  meningococcal, 2737. *See also* Meningococcal
    infections.
  Mollaret's, 1950
  from mumps virus, 1189, 1205, 1205t, 1207
  from *Naegleria fowleri*, 632t-635t
  from *Neisseria meningitidis*, 2737, 2741. *See also*
    Meningococcal infections.
    clinical manifestations of, 1206
    epidemiology and etiology of, 1190t-1191t,
      1192
    prevention of, 1222-1224
    treatment of, 1211t-1212t, 1216
  neonatal, from *Escherichia coli*, 2822
  from *Pasteurella*, 2940
  pathogenesis and pathophysiology of, 1194-1204
  in plague, 2947
  prevention of, 1222-1224
    rifamycins for, 411
  protozoal and helminthic
    adjunctive therapy for, 1221-1222
    antimicrobial therapy for, 1220
    clinical features of, 1207
    diagnosis of, 1210-1211
    epidemiology and etiology of, 1193-1194
  from *Pseudallescheria boydii*, 3365
  from *Pseudomonas aeruginosa*, 2852
  shunt-related, 461
  spirochetal
    antimicrobial therapy for, 1219-1220
    clinical features of, 1206
    diagnosis of, 1209-1210
    epidemiology and etiology of, 1193
  from *Sporothrix schenckii*, 3272
  from *Staphylococcus aureus*, 1193, 1212t, 1218,
    2571
  from *Staphylococcus epidermidis*, 1193, 1212t

Meningitis *(Continued)*
  from *Streptococcus agalactiae,* 1190t-1191t,
    1192-1193, 1211t-1212t, 1218, 1223, 2661
  from *Streptococcus* group A, 1193
  from *Streptococcus* group C and group G, 2676
  from *Streptococcus pneumoniae,* 2631
    epidemiology and etiology of, 1190t-1191t, 1192
    prevention of, 1223-1224
    treatment of, 1211t-1212t, 1212-1214,
      1216-1217, 2636
  from *Streptococcus viridans* group, 2671
  subacute, 1183
  treatment of
    adjunctive, 1220-1222
    antimicrobial therapy in, 1211t-1213t,
      1215-1220
      empirical, 1211-1212, 1211t
    dexamethasone in, 1212-1214, 1220
    initial, 1211-1214, 1211f, 1211t
    quinolones in, 501-502
    vancomycin in, 456
  from *Treponema pallidum,* 1193, 1206, 1209-1210,
    1212t, 1219, 1745-1746
  tuberculous, 3153-3154, 3153f
    spinal, 3154
  viral
    adjunctive therapy for, 1220
    antimicrobial therapy for, 1215
    cerebrospinal fluid examination in, 1207-1208
    clinical features of, 1204-1205
    diagnosis of, 1207-1208
    epidemiology and etiology of, 1189-1194
    pathogenesis and pathophysiology of,
      1194-1195
Meningococcal infections. *See also Neisseria
    meningitidis.*
  capsular polysaccharides in, 2737-2738
  cell wall antigens in, 2738
  clinical manifestations of, 2741-2744, 2741f-2743f
  complement deficiency in, 86, 86f, 89-90, 89t
  endocarditis from, 1093
  epidemiology of, 2740-2741
  fulminant supraglottis, 2744
  immunoprophylaxis for, 2748-2749
  laboratory diagnosis of, 2744-2745
  treatment of, 2745-2749, 2746t
Meningococcal vaccine, 2748-2749, 3922t, 3928
  in asplenia, 3871
  recommendations for, 2749
  for travelers, 4011t, 4012
Meningococcemia
  chronic, 2744
  complement deficiency in, 2744
  fulminant, 996
  rash in, 798
    petechial, 2741-2743, 2741f-2742f
    rubella-like, 2737, 2743f
  skin lesions of, 1304
  without meningitis, 2741
Meningococcus
  antigenic structure of, 2737-2738
  respiratory infections with, 2744
  transmission of, 2739-2740
  urethritis from, 2744
Meningoencephalitis. *See also* Encephalitis;
    Meningitis.
  from adenoviruses, 2030
  amebic, 3427-3436
    clinical manifestations of, 3432
    epidemiology of, 3429-3430
    etiology of, 3427, 3430t
    laboratory diagnosis of, 3432
    pathology and pathogenesis of, 3431
    prevention of, 3435
    treatment of, 632t-635t, 3433-3434
  from *Campylobacter fetus,* 2798
  from *Coxiella burnetii,* 2516
  from cytomegalovirus, 1975
  enteroviral agammaglobulinemia in, 1205, 1215,
    2359-2360
  from mumps virus, 2203
  in West African trypanosomiasis, 3491
Menopause, in HIV-infected women, 1799
Menstrual blood, HIV in, 1784
Menstrual toxic shock syndrome, 2555

Menstruation, in HIV-infected women, 1799
Mephalan, mucositis risk with, 3785
Mercury, in vaccines, 3917
Merkel cell polyomavirus, 2051-2052
Meropenem, 706t-709t
  for acute pyelonephritis, 972
  antibacterial activity of, 342t
  for brain abscess, 1274, 1274t
  chemistry of, 341, 342f
  clinical use of, 343
  dosage of, 343, 722t
  drug interactions with, 742t-761t
  for febrile neutropenia, 3804t
  formulations of, 716t
  for melioidosis, 2876, 2876t
  for meningitis, 1213t
  for nosocomial pneumonia, 3718t
  for pancreatic infections, 1051
  pharmacology of, 342
  for *Pseudomonas aeruginosa* bacteremia, 2849-2850
  recommended dose of, 343
  for septic bursitis, 1450t
Mesenteric lymphadenitis, 1405-1407
  clinical features of, 1405-1406, 1405t
  differential diagnosis of, 1406
  epidemiology of, 1406
  etiology and pathogenesis of, 1405
  treatment of, 1406-1407
  tuberculous, 3158
  in *Yersinia pseudotuberculosis* infection, 2951
Metabolic acidosis, in malaria, 3442
Metabolic changes, in initial inflammatory response,
  44
Metabolic disorders
  antimicrobial agents and, 269
  in chronic hepatitis C infection, 2167
  from foscarnet, 581-582
  in *Helicobacter pylori* infection, 2808
  in HIV infection, 1713-1714
Metabolic end products, of gram-negative anaerobic
  rods, 3114
Metabolic response, acute, 991
Metabolism
  drug, 299
  in peritonitis, 1020
Metagonimus yokogawai, 3596t, 3602
Metalloprotease toxins, 28t
Metastatic infections, in Legionnaires' disease, 2976
Methacycline, 706t-709t
  dosage of, 724t
  formulations of, 715t
Methemoglobinemia, from primaquine, 637-638
Methenamine
  adverse effects of, 519
  for catheter-associated urinary tract infections,
    3731
  chemical structure of, 518, 518f
  clinical uses of, 518-519
  dosage of, 518
  drug interactions with, 742t-761t
  formulations of, 716t
  mechanism of action of, 518
  pharmacology of, 518
  for urinary tract infection, 971
Methenamine hippurate, 706t-709t, 732t-733t
Methenamine mandelate, 706t-709t, 732t-733t
Methicillin, 317, 317f
  dosage of, 718t-719t
  formulations of, 715t
  resistance to. *See also Staphylococcus aureus,*
    methicillin-resistant.
    target enzyme alteration in, 288-289
Methionine, for vacuolar myelopathy, 1755
Methotrexate, for HIV-related non-Hodgkin's
  lymphoma, 1769
Methylmethacrylate cement
  antimicrobial-impregnated, 1471-1472
  host responses to, 1470
  prosthetic joint infections and, 1469-1470
Methylprednisolone
  for acute respiratory distress syndrome, 619
  for histoplasmosis, 3316
  for Kawasaki syndrome, 3665
  for meningitis, 1212-1214
  for *Pneumocystis jirovecii* pneumonia, 618

Metrifonate, 656-657
  for schistosomiasis, 3596t, 3599-3600
Metronidazole, 419-426, 658, 706t-709t
  activity spectrum of, 419-420
  administration, 421, 422t
  adverse reactions to, 421-423
  for amebic liver abscess, 1038
  for anaerobic infections, 422t, 424
  for bacterial meningitis, 1504
  for balantidiasis, 3566
  for brain abscess, 1273-1274, 1273t-1274t
  for *Clostridium difficile*-associated colitis,
    1382-1383
  disulfiram effect of, 423
  dosage of, 420-421, 421t-422t, 726t-727t
  drug interactions with, 421t, 423, 742t-761t
  for *Entamoeba histolytica* infection, 3422t
  fecal floral effects of, 423
  food interactions with, 421t, 423
  formulations of, 716t
  for giardiasis, 3531, 3531t
  for gingivitis, 861t, 869
  for gram-negative anaerobic rod infections, 3118
  for *Helicobacter pylori* infection, 2809t
  indications for, 422t, 424
  laboratory test interference with, 423
  mechanism of action of, 419
  mutageneicity of, 422-423
  for *Neisseria gonorrhoeae* infection, 2765, 2765t
  for pancreatic infections, 1050-1051
  for parasitic infections, 422t, 424
  for peritonitis, 1022t, 1024
  pharmacokinetics of, 420-421, 421t
  in pregnancy, 422-423, 1500
  prophylaxis with, 422t, 424-425
  resistance to, 291, 291t, 420
  for suppurative thrombophlebitis, 1098-1099
  for tetanus, 3094t
  topical, 420-421
  for *Trichomonas vaginalis* infection, 1499
  for trichomoniasis, 3536-3537
    resistance to, 3537
  for urethritis, 1491
  vancomycin-resistant enterococci and, 423-425
Mezlocillin, 318, 319f, 706t-709t
  dosage of, 718t-719t
  formulations of, 715t
Micafungin, 560-561, 706t-709t
  for aspergillosis, 3251t, 3252
  dosage of, 736t-737t
  drug interactions with, 742t-761t
  formulations of, 717t
  structure of, 550f-551f, 559
Miconazole, 706t-709t
  dosage of, 736t-737t
  drug interactions with, 742t-761t
  formulations of, 717t
Microbacterium, 2701
Microbe-human relationships, diversity of, 3-4
Microbial adherence. *See* Adherence.
Microbial biofilms, 22-23, 23t. *See also* Biofilm(s).
Microbial factors, in gastrointestinal infections,
  1339-1343, 1339t
Microbial flora. *See also* Pathogens.
  of alimentary tract, 3784-3786
  anaerobes in, 3083-3084, 3084t
  complement interactions with, 84-85
  endogenous, 3
  in gastrointestinal infections, 1337-1338
  of gastrointestinal tract, 1336-1339, 1336t
  of oral cavity, 855, 856f
  in pancreatic infections, 1047
  primary versus opportunist, 3
  resident, on body surfaces, 3784f
  of skin, 3783, 3784f
  of vagina, 1498
Microbial surface components recognizing adhesive
    matrix molecules (MSCRAMMs), in prosthetic
    valve infections, 1113
Microbial synergy, adhesins and, 21
Microbicidal mechanisms, of neutrophils, 108-110
  impaired intracellular, 114-117, 114t
Microbicides
  in HIV infection prevention, 1800
  in *Neisseria gonorrhoeae* infection prevention, 2767

Microbiology laboratory, 233-265. *See also* Laboratory tests.
Microcirculatory dysfunction, in severe sepsis, 992-993
Microdilution tests, 249
Microevolutionary change, 279
β_2-Microglobulin, in peptide binding, 133
Microhemagglutination assay, for antibodies to *Treponema pallidum*, 65
Microimmunofluorescence, in psittacosis, 2464-2465
Micronutrients
  in immunity, 152-154
  supplementation of
    in elderly, 157, 157t
    in HIV/AIDS, 156
Microscopic agglutination test, for leptospirosis, 3063
Microscopy
  electron
    of hepatitis C virus, 2158f
    of rotavirus, 2106f, 2111
    of smallpox virions, 3979
  for parasites, 262-264, 263t
  specimen collection and transport guidelines for, 235t-236t
  stains for
    for bacteria, fungi, and parasites, 244, 244t
    for microbacteria, 251
  in urinary tract infection, 967, 967t
  for viruses, 258, 259t-260t
Microsporidia, 3391-3407
  characteristics of, 3391-3393
  conjunctivitis from, 1536
  germination of
    conditions promoting, 3391-3392
    polar tube in, 3391, 3393f
  keratitis from, 1550-1551
  life cycle of, 3393
  pathogenic, 3391, 3392t
  phylogeny of, 3393-3394
  polar tube of, 3391, 3393f
  relationship of fungi to, 3394
  sinusitis from, 3398
Microsporidia spore, structure of, 3391, 3392f
Microsporidiosis
  central nervous system, 3397
  clinical manifestations of, 3392t, 3398-3399
  cutaneous, 3398
  diagnosis of, 3399-3401, 3400t
  epidemiology of, 3394-3395
  gastrointestinal, 3395-3397, 3396f, 3401-3402
  genitourinary, 3397
  in HIV infection, 1858t-1871t, 1880, 3398-3399
  immunology of, 3395
  musculoskeletal, 3397-3398
  in non-AIDS patients, 3398
  ocular, 3397, 3397f, 3402-3403
  pathogenesis of, 3395-3398
  pathology of, 3395-3398
  prevention of, 3403
  pulmonary, in HIV infection, 1733
  respiratory, 3398
  treatment of, 632t-635t, 3401-3403, 3401t
Microsporum. See also Dermatophyte(s).
Microsporum audouinii, 3346-3347
Microsporum canis, 3345, 3350f
Microsporum gypseum, 3346
Microsporum nanum, 3345
Microsporum persicolor, 3345
Middle ear infection. *See* Otitis media.
Middle East, HIV infection in, 1622
Migration patterns, zoonoses and, 4005
Mikulicz cells, 2827, 2827f
Miliary tuberculosis, chest radiography in, 944f
Military service applicants, HIV infection in, 1639
Milk thistle, for chronic hepatitis, 674, 674f
Milker's nodes, 1933
Miltefosine, 657
  for leishmaniasis, 3474-3476
Minerals, trace, 153-154
  supplementation of, in elderly, 157, 157t
Minimal bactericidal concentration, 268
Minimal inhibitory concentration, 268, 300
  area under 24-hour serum concentration curve relationship to, 303-304, 303f

Minimal inhibitory concentration (Continued)
  of concentration-dependent killing agents, 301-302, 301f
  maximal serum concentration relationship to, 302-303, 302f
  pharmacodynamic relationships and, 301, 301f
  time above, 304
  of time-dependent (concentration-independent) killing agents, 302, 302f
Minimal inhibitory concentration test, 249
Minimal lethal concentration, 268
Minocycline, 387t, 706t-709t
  for actinomycosis, 3217t
  dosage of, 724t
  food interactions with, 393t
  formulations of, 715t
  for nocardiosis, 3204t, 3205
  for nontuberculous mycobacterial infections, 544
  pharmacology of, 387-390, 390t
  side effects of, 391t
  vertigo from, 392
Miscarriage, from parvovirus B19 infection, 2091
Mites and mite-transmitted diseases, 3643-3647
  diagnosis and management of, 3646t, 3647
  epidemiology of, 3643-3646
  prevention of, 3647
  taxonomy of, 3643, 3644t-3645t
Mitochondrial dysfunction
  from nucleoside and nucleotide reverse transcriptase inhibitors, 1833
  in severe sepsis, 992-993
Mitosome, of *Entamoeba histolytica*, 3412
Mitral valve, endocarditis of, 1067-1069
  from *Staphylococcus aureus*, 2569, 2570f
Mobiluncus, 3029, 3126
Mold infection
  in hematopoietic stem cell transplant recipients, 3832
  opportunistic, 3370
  posaconazole for, 559
Molds. *See also* Fungi.
  appearance of, 3222t, 3223f-3224f
  endophthalmitis due to, 1555-1556
  features of, 3221-3222
  terminology for, 254, 255t
Molecular mimicry
  in autoimmune reactions, 71
  in rheumatic fever, 2612
Molecular tests, for bacterial infections, 246t, 248-249
Molgramostim, 614
Mollaret's meningitis, 1950
Mollicutes, taxonomy and distribution of, 2477, 2479f
Molluscum contagiosum, 1478, 1478f, 1481, 1934-1935, 1934f
  versus condylomata acuminata, 2041
  in HIV infection, skin lesions from, 1716, 1717f
Monamine oxidase inhibition, by linezolid, 473
Monkey(s), arenavirus infection of, 2297-2298
Monkeypox, 209, 803-804, 1927-1929, 1929f, 4003
  clinical features of, 1928
  control of, 1929
  diagnosis of, 1928-1929
  encephalitis from, 1251t-1252t
  pathogenesis of, 1928
Monobactams, 343-344, 343f, 344t
  cross-reactivity with, 353
  structure of, 349f
Monochloramine, water treatment with, 2979
Monoclonal antibodies, 64
  therapeutic uses of, 74
  for transplant immunosuppression, infections and, 3811, 3811t
Monoclonal gammopathies, serum protein electrophoresis for, 64, 64f
Monocytes, 41
  in HIV infection, 1698
Mononeuritis multiplex, in HIV infection, 1757
Mononuclear cells, phagocyte and lymphocyte defects affecting, 175-177, 175f
Mononucleosis. *See* Infectious mononucleosis.
Monosodium glutamate (MSG) symptom complex, 1417

Monospot test, in infectious mononucleosis, 1999-2000
Moraxella, 2774
  identification of, laboratory procedures for, 2775t
  in oral cavity, 856t
Moraxella catarrhalis
  bacteremia from, 2773
  biochemistry of, 2774t
  clinical manifestations of, 2772-2773, 2772f-2773f
  COPD from, 2771-2773, 2773f
  epidemiology of, 2771
  growth characteristics of, 2774t
  history of, 2771
  microbiology of, 2771
  nosocomial, 2773
  otitis media from, 833, 2772, 2772f
  pathogenesis of, 2771-2772, 2772t
  pneumonia from, 2773
  respiratory tract colonization by, 2771
  sinusitis from, 2773
  treatment of, 2773
Morbilliform exanthems, from enteroviruses, 2354-2355
Morganella, carbapenems for, 342t
Morganella morganii, 2828-2829
Morphine, for tetanus, 3094t
Morrison's pouch, 1011-1012, 1012f
Mosquito(es)
  anopheline, in malaria transmission, 3444
  bites of, in travelers, 4015-4016
  repellent and avoidance measures for, 3456
  travel-associated exposure to, 4021
Mosquito-borne infections
  from *Aedes aegypti*, 4022. *See also* Dengue fever.
  from alphaviruses, 4022
  from Bunyavirdae, 2289-2293, 2290t
  from *Plasmodium. See* Malaria.
Motavizumab, for respiratory syncytial virus, 2218
Motility, intestinal, 1337
Mountain sickness, acute, in travelers, 4016
Mousepox virus, spread of, 1915, 1915f
Mouth. *See also* Oral *entries*.
  anaerobic infections of, 3084-3085, 3084t, 3085f
  diphtheria of, 2690, 2690f
  protection of, 3673, 3674t
Moxalactam, 706t-709t
  dosage of, 720t-722t
  formulations of, 715t
Moxifloxacin, 706t-709t
  antimicrobial activity of, 491t-492t
  for bite wounds, 3913t
  for brain abscess, 1274-1275
  for *Chlamydophila* respiratory infection, 2471, 2471t
  dosage of, 493t, 732t-733t
  for *Enterococcus*, 2651
  formulations of, 716t
  for Legionnaires' disease, 2978t
  for meningitis, 1213t
  for nosocomial pneumonia, 3718t
  for peritonitis, 1022t, 1025
  pharmacology of, 492t
  for sinusitis, 844-845, 845t
  structure of, 487, 488f
Mucociliary apparatus, dysfunction of, 840
Mucocutaneous candidiasis
  chronic, 3230-3231, 3231f, 3238
  treatment of, 3237-3238
Mucocutaneous herpes simplex virus infection, 1954, 1954f
  foscarnet for, 582
  in immunocompromised hosts, 566t-567t, 571, 577
  recurrent, 1951
  treatment of, 1956, 1957t
Mucopurulent cervicitis, in HIV infection, 1797
Mucor, 3257, 3258f, 3258t
Mucor indicus, 3262
Mucorales organisms
  blood vessel invasion by, 3260
  identification of, 3263-3264
  mycetoma formation by, 3262
  resistance of, to antifungal agents, 3264-3265

Mucormycosis
  agents of, taxonomic organization of, 3258t
  antifungal susceptibility of, 3264-3265
  cerebral, 1266
  clinical manifestations of, 3260-3263, 3260t
  cutaneous, 3262, 3263f
  diagnosis of, 3263-3265, 3264f
  disseminated, 3262-3263
  epidemiology of, 3257-3258, 3258f
  etiology of, 3257, 3258f
  gastrointestinal, 3262
  in hematopoietic stem cell transplant recipients,
      3832
  histopathologic features of, 3263, 3264f
  hyperbaric oxygen therapy for, 628
  less common presentations of, 3263
  pathogenesis of, 3258-3260, 3259f
  patterns of, by host population, 3260, 3260t
  prognosis for, 3266
  pulmonary, 3261-3262
  rhinocerebral, 1269, 3260-3261, 3260f-3261f
  sino-orbital, 3260, 3260f
  sinopulmonary, 3260-3261, 3261f
  soft tissue, 3262
  treatment of, 1275, 3265-3266
    adjunctive therapies in, 3266
    antifungal therapy in, 3265-3266
    surgical, 3266
Mucosa
  barrier injury to, in immunocompromised hosts,
      3785-3786, 3785f
  damaged, bacteremia related to, 3788
  immune tissues associated with, 144
  lesions of, from Paracoccidioides brasiliensis, 3360,
      3360f
  oral cavity, immunity of, 857-858, 857f
Mucosa-associated lymphoid tissue (MALT), oral,
    857-858
Mucosal leishmaniasis, 3464t, 3471f, 3472-3473, 3476
Mucositis, 3782t, 3785
  in immunocompromised hosts, 861t, 866-867,
      866f
Mucous membranes
  Candida infection of, 3227-3228, 3227f-3229f
  in host defense, 40
Multidrug resistance
  mechanisms of, 291-292, 291f
  in nosocomial pneumonia, 3717
    empirical antibiotic therapy for, 3720
  in tuberculosis, 533
    quinolones for, 500-501
    treatment of, 3146
Multifocal extracutaneous sporotrichosis, 3272-3273,
    3273f. See also Sporotrichosis.
Multilocus sequence typing, 249
  of Burkholderia cepacia, 2861
  of Staphylococcus aureus, 2546-2547
  of Staphylococcus epidermidis, 2580
Multinational Association for Supportive Care in
    Cancer (MASCC) study, 3802-3803, 3803t
Multiple sclerosis
  Chlamydophila pneumoniae and, 2473-2474
  coronaviruses and, 2192
  Epstein-Barr virus and, 1999
  from human herpesvirus 6, 2013
Multiple-locus variable-number tandem repeat
    analysis, of Francisella tularensis, 2927
Multiresistant bacteria, in spinal cord injury patients,
    3855
Multivitamin/mineral supplementation, in elderly,
    157, 157t
Mumps/mumps virus, 2201-2206
  characteristics of, 2201
  clinical manifestations of, 2202-2204, 2202t
  complications of, 2204
  detection of, 259t-260t
  diagnosis of, 2204-2205
  differential diagnosis of, 2205
  encephalitis from, 1251t-1252t
  epidemiology of, 2201-2202
  history of, 2201
  immunology of, 2204
  meningitis from, 1189, 1205, 1205t, 1207
  orchitis from, 1521
  parotitis from, 867

Mumps/mumps virus (Continued)
  pathogenesis of, 2202
  pathology of, 2202
  prevention of, 2205
  treatment of, 2205
  vaccine for, 2205, 3922t, 3928-3929. See also
      Measles, mumps, rubella (MMR) vaccine.
Mupirocin, 528t, 529-530, 706t-709t
  adverse effects of, 530
  antibacterial activity of, 529
  for impetigo, 1291
  pharmacokinetics of, 529
  prophylactic
    for catheter-related infections, 524-525
    for skin/soft tissue infections, 523
  for Staphylococcus aureus nasal carriage, 527, 530,
      1293
  structure of, 529
Murine typhus, 2525-2528, 3639t
Murmurs, in endocarditis, 1076
Murray Valley encephalitis, 1246t, 1251t-1252t, 2152
Muscle abscess, 1319
Muscle infections, from Bacillus spp., 2729-2730
Muscle proteolysis, in systemic infections, 1321
Muscle toxicity, from daptomycin, 463
Musculoskeletal infections
  from Actinomyces, 3214-3215
  in cat-scratch disease, 2999-3000
  from microsporidia, 3397-3398
  from nontuberculous mycobacteria, 3195-3196
Musculoskeletal syndromes, in HIV infection,
    1759-1761
Mushroom poisoning, 1417-1418, 1417t
  confirmation of, 1422
  treatment of, 1423-1424
Mutageneicity, of metronidazole, 422-423
Mutagenesis, signature-tagged, 10-11
Mutant prevention concentration, 300
Mutant selection window, 300
Myalgia, 1319-1320
  in endocarditis, 1320
  with eosinophilia, 1320-1321
  from influenza, 2274
  in influenza, 1319-1320
  from quinupristin-dalfopristin, 461
  in systemic infections, 1321
  in toxoplasmosis, 1320
Myasthenia gravis, exacerbation of, from
    telithromycin, 439
Mycelia sterila, 3222
Mycetoma, 3281-3285
  from Actinomyces, 3214-3215
  clinical manifestations of, 3282-3283, 3282f
  from Coccidioides, 3336, 3337f
  from dark-walled fungi, 3367-3369, 3367t
  diagnosis of, 3283-3284, 3283f-3284f
  epidemiology of, 3281
  etiologic agents of, 3281, 3282t
  from mucorales, 3262
  from Nocardia, 3200-3201, 3201f, 3281, 3282t,
      3283-3284, 3284f
  pathology and pathogenesis of, 3281-3282
  prevention of, 3285
  treatment of, 3284-3285
Mycobacteria
  classification of, 3178-3179
  epidemiology of, 253
  genetic susceptibility to, 50-51, 51t
  in hematopoietic stem cell transplant recipients,
      3827-3828
  identification of, 252
  isolation of, significance of, 252
  keratitis from, 1542-1543
  laboratory tests for, 240t-242t, 250-253, 252t
  mendelian susceptibility to, 140
  microbiology of, 3178-3179
  nontuberculous, 3191-3198. See also Mycobacte-
      rium avium complex.
    catheter-related infections from, 3196
    central nervous system infections from, 3196
    clinical syndromes associated with, 3192, 3192t
    culture of, 3196
    in cystic fibrosis, 950
    disseminated disease from, 3196
    environmental niches of, 3191-3192

Mycobacteria (Continued)
    geographic distribution of, 3192
    intermediately growing, 3191
    laboratory diagnosis of, 3196-3197
    lymphadenitis from, 3194
    musculoskeletal infections from, 3195-3196
    ocular infections from, 3196
    phagocyte and lymphocyte defects associated
        with, 175-177, 175f
    pulmonary disease from, 3192-3194,
        3192t-3193t
    quinolones for, 501
    rapidly growing, 3191, 3197
    rifamycins for, 408
    skin/soft tissue infections from, 3193t,
        3194-3195
    slowly growing, 3191, 3197
    strain comparison of, 3197
    susceptibility tests for, 544, 3197
    treatment of
      major drugs for, 542-543
      minor drugs for, 543-544
  quinolones for, 500-501
  safety issues for, 250
  specimens containing
    collection and transport of, 250-251
    direct detection of, 251
    processing and planting of, 251-252, 252t
    susceptibility testing of, 252-253
Mycobacterial interspersed repetitive unit analysis, of
    Mycobacterium tuberculosis, 3131-3132
Mycobacterium abscessus, 3191
  disseminated disease from, 3196
  pulmonary disease from, 3193t, 3194
  skin/soft tissue infections from, 3194
Mycobacterium avium complex, 252, 3177-3189. See
    also Mycobacteria, nontuberculous.
  atypical tuberculosis from, 938t
  clinical presentation of, 3179-3182
  cutaneous, 3184-3185
  in cystic fibrosis, 3180
  diagnosis of, 3182-3183
  disseminated
    classification and microbiology of, 3178-3179,
        3178f-3179f
    clinical presentation of, 3181-3182, 3181f-3182f
    diagnosis of, 3183
    epidemiology of, 3177
    host immunity to, 3179
    treatment of, 3186, 3186t
  epidemiology of, 3177-3178
  in HIV infection, 1710-1711, 1710f, 1879-1880,
      3177-3179, 3178f-3179f
    HAART and, 1721
    prophylaxis against, 1858t-1859t
    treatment of, 1860t-1870t
  in HIV-infected children, 1825
  host immunity to, 3179
  hypersensitivity pneumonitis from, 3183, 3186
  lymphadenitis in, 1325
    classification and microbiology of, 3179
    clinical presentation of, 3182, 3182f
    diagnosis of, 3183
    epidemiology of, 3177-3178
    host immunity to, 3179
    treatment of, 3186
  macrolid-resistant, 3185
  Mycobacterium avium in, 3177-3178
  prophylaxis for, 3187
  pulmonary
    classification and microbiology of, 3178
    clinical presentation of, 3179-3181, 3180f-3181f
    diagnosis of, 3182-3183
    epidemiology of, 3177
    host immunity to, 3179
    treatment of, 3185-3186, 3185t
  reservoir for, 3177
  rifamycins for, 408
  route of acquisition of, 3177
  treatment of, 3183-3185
    drug dosage in, 3184t-3186t, 3185
    drug interactions in, 3184-3185
    drug tolerability in, 3184, 3184t
    immunomodulatory, 3185
    principles in, 3183-3185

Mycobacterium avium complex *(Continued)*
  specific plans in, 3185-3186, 3185t
  surgical, 3186
  virulence of, 3178
Mycobacterium bovis, 3129
  in cancer patients, 3798
Mycobacterium chelonae, 3191
  disseminated disease from, 3196
  skin/soft tissue infections from, 3194
Mycobacterium fortuitum, 3191
  skin/soft tissue infections from, 3194
Mycobacterium genavense, 3191
Mycobacterium gordonae, 3191
Mycobacterium haemophilum, 3191
  skin/soft tissue infections from, 3195
Mycobacterium intracellulare, 3177-3178
Mycobacterium kansasii
  disseminated disease from, 3196
  in HIV infection, 1731
  pulmonary disease from, 3193, 3193t
Mycobacterium leprae, 50, 3165-3176. *See also*
    Leprosy.
  arthritis from, 1453
  defense against, T cells in, 130
  detection of, 3170
  Fite staining of, 3169, 3169f-3170f
  genome of, 3166-3167
  immune response to, 3167
  Lepromin reaction to, 3170
  microbiology of, 3166-3167
  nerve damage by, 3168, 3171
  reactions to, 3170-3171, 3170f-3171f
Mycobacterium leprae laminin-binding protein, 3168
Mycobacterium marinum, 3191
  arthritis from, 1453
  skin/soft tissue infections from, 3193t, 3194
Mycobacterium mucogenicum, 3191
Mycobacterium smegmatis, 3191
Mycobacterium tuberculosis, 3129-3163. *See also*
    Tuberculosis.
  acid-fast staining of, 3130-3131, 3130t
  arthritis from, 1452, 1452f, 3156
  brain abscess from, 1266
  cervical lymphadenitis from, 1325
  culturing of, 3130t, 3131
  defense against, T cells in, 129
  drug susceptibility testing of, 3130t, 3132
  drug-resistant, increased risk of infection from,
    3134, 3134t
  genotyping of, 3130t, 3131-3132
  global threat of, 210, 210f
  in hematopoietic stem cell transplant recipients,
    3827-3828
  laboratory detection of, 240t-242t
  latent, laboratory detection of, 252-253
  microbiology of, 3129-3132
  mycotic aneurysms from, 1102
  nucleic acid amplification of, 3130t, 3131
  osteomyelitis from, 1464-1465
  speciation of, 3130t, 3131
  susceptibility to infection from, 50-51
  tuberculin skin test for, 3136-3138
Mycobacterium tuberculosis complex, 252
Mycobacterium tuberculosis DNA, 3131-3132
Mycobacterium ulcerans, 3191
  skin/soft tissue infections from, 3195
Mycobacterium xenopi, 3191
Mycophenolate mofetil, for transplant
    immunosuppression, infections and, 3811
Mycoplasma, 2477-2480, 2491-2493
  animal, as human pathogens, 2478
  characteristics of, 2477, 2478t
  classification of, 2477, 2479f
  culture of, 2477, 2478f
  genital
    causing nongenital infection, 2478
    cultivation and detection of, 2491-2492, 2492f
    in men, 2491
    prevalence of, 2491, 2492t
    in women, 2491-2492
  pathogenesis of, 2477-2478
  susceptibility testing for, 2493
  uncommon, 2477-2478
Mycoplasma amphoriforme, 2477-2478
Mycoplasma argini, 2478

Mycoplasma fermentans, 2477-2478
  genital, 2491-2493, 2492t
Mycoplasma genitalium, 2491-2493, 2492f, 2492t
  detection of, 2492
  nongonococcal urethritis from, 1489, 2491, 2492t.
    See also Urethritis, nongonococcal.
Mycoplasma hominis, genital, 2491-2493, 2492t
Mycoplasma incognitus, 2477-2478
Mycoplasma penetrans, 2477-2478
  genital, 2491-2493, 2492t
Mycoplasma phocicerebrale, 2478
Mycoplasma pirum, 2477-2478
Mycoplasma pneumoniae/M. pneumoniae infection,
    2481-2489
  in cancer patients, 3798
  characteristics of, 2481
  Chlamydophila pneumoniae coinfection with, 2470
  in chronic obstructive pulmonary disease, 879
  clinical manifestation(s) of, 2482-2484
    cardiac, 2484
    dermatologic, 2483-2484, 2483f
    extrapulmonary, 2483
    musculoskeletal, 2484
    neurologic, 2484
    Raynaud phenomenon as, 2483f, 2484
    renal, 2484
    respiratory, 2482-2483, 2482f
  croup from, 825-826
  culture of, 2477, 2478f, 2485-2486
  diagnosis of, 2485-2486, 2486t
  versus enteric fever, 1400t-1401t, 1404
  epidemiology of, 2482
  history of, 2481
  immune response to, 2484-2485
  laboratory detection of, 240t-242t
  otitis media from, 833
  pathology and pathophysiology of, 2485
  pharyngitis from, 817
  pneumonia from, 2482-2483, 2482f
  prevention of, 2487
  risk factors for, 2484
  transmission of, 2482
  treatment of, 2486-2487
  vaccine for, 2487
Mycoplasma primatum, genital, 2491-2493, 2492t
Mycoplasma spermatophilum, genital, 2491-2493,
    2492t
Mycosis, gastrointestinal, 1395
Mycotic aneurysms, 1074, 1099-1103
  classification of, 1099t
  clinical manifestations of, 1100-1101
  in endocarditis, from *Staphylococcus aureus*, 2569
  epidemiology of, 1099
  etiologic agents in, 1101-1102
  in injection drug users, 3881-3882, 3882f, 3885
  intracranial, 1101
  laboratory findings in, 1101
  pathogenesis of, 1099-1100
  pathology of, 1100
  treatment of, 1102-1103
Myelitis, 1237. *See also* Encephalomyelitis.
  from herpes simplex virus, 1950
Myelodysplastic syndrome, from granulocyte
    colony-stimulating factor, 613-614
Myeloid differentiation primary response gene,
    169t-170t
Myelokathexis, 169t-170t
Myelopathy
  in HIV infection
    noncompressive, 1755
    vacuolar, 1754-1755
  from human T-cell lymphotrophic virus,
    2314-2317
Myeloperoxidase, deficiency of, 116-117, 169t-170t,
    173
Myeloradiculitis, 1237
Myiasis, 3637-3639, 3638f, 3638t, 4023f
Myocardial abscess, in endocarditis, 1074
Myocardial disease, in HIV infection, 1720
Myocarditis, 1153-1161. *See also* Endocarditis;
    Pericarditis.
  from adenoviruses, 1153, 2030
  from *Candida*, 3232
  clinical manifestations of, 1157
  from *Corynebacterium diphtheriae*, 2690

Myocarditis *(Continued)*
  from coxsackievirus B, 1153, 1155, 1155f
  from cytomegalovirus, 1975
  Dallas criteria for, 1154-1155
  diagnosis of, 1157-1159, 1159t
  from enteroviruses, 1153, 1155-1156
  etiology of, 1153-1154, 1154t
  fulminant, 1157, 1159
  in Kawasaki syndrome, 3663
  in neonates, from enteroviruses, 2359
  noninfectious causes of, 1159t
  nonviral causes of, 1154, 1154t
  from parvovirus B19 infection, 2091
  pathology and pathogenesis of, 1154-1156,
    1155f-1156f
  prevention of, 1160-1161
  from *Toxoplasma gondii*, 1156, 1156f
  in toxoplasmosis, 3501
    in immunocompetent patient, 3502
  treatment of, 1159-1160
  vaccine for, 1160-1161
  viral causes of, 1153-1154, 1154t
Myonecrosis
  from *Aeromonas hydrophila*, 1319
  anaerobic
    streptococcal, 1318
    synergistic nonclostridial, 1318
  clostridial. *See* Gas gangrene.
  after episiotomy, 1513
  from *Streptococcus pyogenes*, 2602-2603
Myopathy, critical illness, in sepsis, 998
Myopericarditis, from enteroviruses, 2357-2358
Myositis
  from adenoviruses, 2030
  from *Candida*, 3233
  classification of, 1314t
  clostridial. *See* Gas gangrene.
  cysticercus cellulosal, 1321
  from enteroviruses, 2356-2357
  iliopsoas, 1319
  from influenza, 2276
  nonclostridial (crepitant), 1318-1319
  nonpyogenic, 1314t, 1319-1320
  parasitic, 1320-1321
  pathogenesis of, 1316-1317
  psoas, 1319
  pyogenic, 1313-1316, 1314t, 1315f. *See also*
    Pyomyositis.
  streptococcal necrotizing, 1316
  from *Streptococcus pyogenes*, 2602-2603
  in toxoplasmosis, 3501
    in immunocompetent patient, 3502
Myringotomy, for otitis media, 835
Myroides, 3016t, 3024

N

Nadifloxacin, 706t-709t
Naegleria, 3427-3436
Naegleria fowleri
  characteristics of, 3427, 3428f, 3430t
  meningitis from, 632t-635t, 1193, 1212t,
    3427-3436. *See also* Amebic
    meningoencephalitis.
Nafcillin, 317, 317f, 706t-709t
  for brain abscess, 1274t
  for cellulitis, 1297-1298
  dosage of, 316t, 718t-719t
  for endocarditis, 1091
  formulations of, 715t
  for meningitis, 1213t
  for osteomyelitis, 1459t
  for staphylococcal scalded skin syndrome, 1291
  for *Staphylococcus aureus* endocarditis, 2571t
  for *Staphylococcus* endocarditis, 1118, 1118t
  for suppurative thrombophlebitis, 1098
Naftifine, 706t-709t
Nails
  fungal infections of. *See* Onychomycosis.
  specimen collection and transport guidelines for,
    235t-236t
Nalidixic acid, 706t-709t
  antimicrobial activity of, 491t-492t
  dosage of, 732t-733t
  drug interactions with, 742t-761t

Nalidixic acid *(Continued)*
  formulations of, 716t
  resistance to, mechanisms of, 489
  structure of, 487, 488f
Nalidixic acid–resistant nontyphoidal *Salmonella*, 2891, 2891f
Nanophyetiasis, 3622
Nanophyetus salmincola, 3622
Nasal cavity
  diphtheria of, 2690
  Neisseria meningitidis carriage in, 2739-2740
    chemoprophylaxis for, 2747-2748
  secretions in, 839
  Staphylococcus aureus carriage in, 2544
    eradication of, 527
    mupirocin for, 527, 530, 1293
    topical antibacterial therapy for, 527
Nasal congestion, in common cold, 810-811
Nasal NK and T-cell lymphoma, from Epstein-Barr virus infection, 1998
Nasal protection, 3673, 3674t
Nasal saline spray, for sinusitis, 846
Nasal secretion, rhinoviral shedding from, 2393
Nasal swabs
  anthrax diagnosis with, 3986-3989
  laboratory processing of, 239
Nasolabial ulcer, from *Coccidioides*, 3337, 3338f
Nasopharyngeal carcinoma, from Epstein-Barr virus infection, 1996t, 1997-1998, 1998f, 2001, 2001f-2002f, 2004
Nasopharynx, *Moraxella catarrhalis* colonization of, 2771
National Disaster Medical System (NDMS), 3957-3958
National Healthcare Safety Network (NHSN) definitions, of surgical site infections, 3902, 3902t
National Nosocomial Infection Surveillance System (NNIS) risk index, 3896, 3896t
Natural killer cells, 132
  in *Entamoeba histolytica* infection, 3416
  in hepatitis B infection, 2066
  in hepatitis C infection, 2164
  in HIV infection, 1697-1698
  in toxoplasmosis, 3499
Nausea and vomiting
  acute, 1362-1363, 1362t
  from *Bacillus*, 2728
  in foodborne disease, 1413-1414, 1416
    nonbloody diarrhea and, 1415
  in malaria, 3449
Necator americanus, 632t-635t, 3578t, 3581-3582
Neck. *See also* Head and neck.
  fascia of, relation of pharyngeal, retropharyngeal, and pretracheal spaces to, 858, 859f
Neck mass, in nasopharyngeal carcinoma, 2001, 2001f
Necrosis, in pancreatic infections, 1046, 1046f
Necrotizing enteritis, in adults, 1394
Necrotizing enterocolitis, in neonates, 1393-1394
Necrotizing fasciitis, 1306t, 1307-1309
  anatomic forms of, 1308
  clinical features of, 1307-1308
  after episiotomy, 1513
  hyperbaric oxygen therapy for, 627
  in injection drug users, 3878
  microbial etiologies of, 1308
  from *Staphylococcus aureus*, 2567
  streptococcal, 1316
  from *Streptococcus pyogenes*, 2602
  treatment of, 1308-1309
Necrotizing pneumonia, 925-926, 3085
Needle exchange programs, for HIV infection prophylaxis, 1652
Needle punctures, prevention of, 3757-3758
Negri bodies, in rabies, 2251, 2252f
Neisseria, 2773-2774
  biochemistry of, 2774t
  growth characteristics of, 2774t
Neisseria gonorrhoeae, 2753-2756. *See also* Gonococcal infections.
  bacteremia from, 1304, 2762-2763
  chromosomal mutations and transformation of, 2755-2756
  conjugative plasmids of, 2755

Neisseria gonorrhoeae (Continued)
  culture of, 2753, 2763
  description of, 2753
  DNA probe tests for, 2764
  epididymitis from, 1524
  in female urethra, 1490
  genetics of, 2755-2756
  gram-stained smears of, 2756f, 2764
  growth of, 2753
  laboratory detection of, 240t-242t, 243
  nucleic acid amplification tests for, 2763
  outer membrane of, 2754-2755, 2754f
  pili of, 2753-2754, 2754f
  resistance of, 290t, 2758-2759
  strain typing of, 2755
  surface structure of, 2753-2755, 2754f
Neisseria gonorrhoeae DNA, 2755
Neisseria meningitidis, 2737-2752. *See also* Meningococcal infections.
  antigenic structure of, 2737-2738
  bacteremia from, 1304
    without sepsis, 2741
  bactericidal antibody activity against, 2739
  capsular polysaccharides of, 2737-2738, 2738t
  carriers of, 2739-2740
    chemoprophylaxis for, 2747-2748
  cell wall antigens of, 2738
  clinical manifestations of, 2741-2744, 2741f-2743f
    community-acquired, 2741
  cross-reactivity of, 2739
  diagnosis of, 2744-2745
  epidemiology of, 2740-2741
  immunologic response to, 2739
  immunoprophylaxis for, 2748-2749
  laboratory detection of, 240t-242t
  meningitis from, 2737, 2741. *See also* Meningococcal infections.
    clinical manifestations of, 1206
    epidemiology and etiology of, 1190t-1191t, 1192
    prevention of, 1222-1224
    treatment of, 1211t-1212t, 1216
  meningococcemia from, 2744
  morphologic, cultural, and biochemical characteristics of, 2737-2740
  pathogenesis of, 2738-2739
  rash in, 2737, 2741-2743, 2741f-2743f
  respiratory infections from, 2744
  serotypes of, 2738
  skin lesions in, 798
  transmission of, 2739-2740
  treatment of, 2744-2745
    antibiotics in, 2745-2746, 2746t
    carbapenems in, 342t
    supportive care in, 2746-2747
Neisseria weaveri, 2773
Nelfinavir, 706t-709t, 1839f, 1840-1841, 1840t
  dosage of, 740t-741t
  formulations of, 717t
  for HIV-infected children, 1820t-1821t, 1823t
Nematodes. *See* Roundworms (nematodes).
Neomycin, 359, 360f, 360t-361t, 528, 706t-709t
  dosage of, 724t-725t
  formulations of, 715t
  prophylactic, for surgical procedures, 3899t
Neomycin-bacitracin-polymyxin spray, 528t
  prophylactic, for operative wound infections, 523
Neonates. *See also* Children; Infants.
  antimicrobial therapy in, 269
  bacterial meningitis in, 1206, 1213t
  Chlamydia trachomatis in, 2455-2456
    prevention and treatment of, 2456
  coagulase-negative *Staphylococcus* infection in, 2585-2586
  conjunctivitis in, 1535-1536
  dengue in, 2145
  diarrhea in, epidemic, 1359-1360, 1360t
  Elizabethkingia meningoseptica infection in, 3022-3023
  Enterococcus infections in, 2647
  enteroviral meningitis in, 1204-1205
  enteroviruses in, 2358-2359
  gray baby syndrome of, from chloramphenicol, 397
  hepatitis in, from enteroviruses, 2359
  herpes simplex virus infection in, 1954

Neonates *(Continued)*
  Listeria monocytogenes infection in, 2709
  myocarditis in, from enteroviruses, 2359
  necrotizing enterocolitis in, 1393-1394
  Neisseria gonorrhoeae infection in, 2763
    conjunctival, 2763
    rectal, 2763
  pneumonia in, from enteroviruses, 2359
  sepsis in
    from group C *Streptococcus*, 2676
    from *Haemophilus influenzae*, nontypeable, 2913
    Streptococcus agalactiae (group B) infection in, 2656
  tetanus in, 3093, 3093f
  toxoplasmosis in, 3506-3508
    diagnosis of, 3516, 3517f
    serologic screening and prophylaxis for, 3521-3522, 3521t
    treatment of, 3520
  varicella in, 1965
  vulvovaginitis in, 1495-1496
Neoplastic disease
  in HIV-infected children, 1816
  in meningitis, 1241
Neorickettsia, 2531-2532, 2532t
Neorickettsia risticii, 2531-2532, 2532t
Neorickettsia sennetsu, 2531-2532, 2532t
Neotestudina rosatii, mycetoma from, 3281, 3282t, 3283f
Nephritis. *See also* Glomerulonephritis; Pyelonephritis.
  interstitial
    chronic, 957, 958f
    from penicillin, 314
    from quinolones, 503
    tuberculous, 3156
  shunt, 1232-1233
  tuberculous interstitial, 3156
Nephropathy
  BKV-induced, 2055-2056
    clinical manifestations of, 2055-2056
    diagnosis of, 2056, 2056f
    epidemiology of, 2055
    pathogenesis of, 2055
    prognosis for, 2056
    treatment of, 2056
  from HIV infection, 1719
  reflux, 969
Nephrotic syndrome, from hepatitis B, 2072
Nephrotoxicity
  of acyclovir, 570
  of adefovir, 572
  of aminoglycosides, 368-371, 368f, 369t-370t
  of cidofovir, 577
  of foscarnet, 581
  of polymyxins, 470
  of teicoplanin, 459
  of tenofovir, 1837
  of vancomycin, 454
Netilmicin, 359, 360f, 360t-361t
  dosage of, 724t-725t
    once-daily, 376, 377t
  formulations of, 715t
Netilmicin sulfate, 706t-709t
Neuralgia, superior laryngeal, from laryngitis, 824
Neuramidase, 2627, 2629t
Neuritis, peripheral, from *Corynebacterium diphtheriae*, 2690
Neurocognitive disorder, HIV-1–associated. *See* AIDS dementia.
Neurocysticercosis, 3611-3612, 3612f
  meningitis in, 1240-1241
Neurodegeneration, in prion diseases, 2426
Neurodegenerative diseases, transmissible, 2423-2438. *See also* Prion disease.
Neurologic diseases, in HIV infection, 1745-1764, 1760t
  CD4 count and, 1760f
  temporal trends and aging in, 1761
Neurologic syndromes, in brucellosis, 2923
Neuromuscular blockade, after aminoglycosides, 372
Neuronal injury, in bacterial meningitis, 1203-1204
Neuronopathy, granule cell, JC virus–associated, 2053

Neuropathy. *See also* Polyneuropathy.
  from *Corynebacterium diphtheriae*, 2690
  in HIV infection, 1755-1758
  in leprosy, 3168-3169
  from linezolid, 473
  from nitrofurantoin, 517
  nucleoside, in HIV infection, 1756-1757, 1757t
  peripheral, from nitrofurantoin, 517
Neuroretinitis, in cat-scratch disease, 3001, 3001f, 3005
Neurosurgical instruments, contaminated, Creutzfeldt-Jakob disease associated with, 2431-2432
Neurosyphilis. *See also* Syphilis.
  acute, 3041-3042
  chronology of, 3049, 3050f
  classification of, 3041t
  clinical manifestations of, 3042t
  CSF examination in, 3041, 3041t
  in HIV infection, 1745-1746
  late, 3041-3043
  meningitis in, 1193, 1206, 1209-1210, 1212t, 1219, 1745-1746
  meningovascular, 3042
  parenchymatous, 3042
  tests for, 3046
  treatment of, 3043, 3049-3050
Neurotoxic shellfish poisoning, 1416-1417, 1417t, 3569, 3570t
Neurotoxicity
  of acyclovir, 569-570
  of amantadine, 575
  of ganciclovir, 584
  of HIV drugs, 1757t
  of isoniazid, 534
  of mefloquine, 656
  of polymyxins, 470
  of rimantadine, 575
Neurotoxins
  clostridial, 31
  in gastrointestinal infections, 1340, 1340t
Neurotrophic keratitis, 1546
Neurotrophic ulcers, in leprosy, 3174
Neutralizing gram-negative bacterial endotoxin, for sepsis, 1004
Neutrocytic ascites, in peritonitis, 1013-1014
Neutropenia, 111-112, 169t-170t, 172
  acquired, 111
  combination antimicrobial therapy in, 273
  cyclic, 111-112
  febrile. *See* Febrile neutropenia.
  fluconazole prophylaxis in, 557
  from ganciclovir, 584
  granulocyte colony-stimulating factor for, 612
    in cancer, 3806
    in children, 612
    in HIV infection, 612
  granulocyte-macrophage colony-stimulating factor for, 614
  hereditary, 111
  in HIV infection, 1720
  in infectious mononucleosis, 1999
  posaconazole prophylaxis in, 558-559
  prolonged, in mucormycosis, 3259
  Pseudomonas aeruginosa resistance in, 2839-2840
  sequence of events during, 3789, 3789f
  severe congenital, 111
  from vancomycin, 454
  in visceral leishmaniasis, 3468
Neutropenic enterocolitis, in transplant recipients, 3823
Neutropenic hosts, coagulase-negative *Staphylococcus* infection in, 2585
Neutrophil(s), 99-110
  apoptosis of, 108
  in Chédiak-Higashi syndrome, 113, 113f
  circulating, 101-102
  defects in
    antimicrobial prophylaxis for, 117
    bone marrow transplantation for, 118
    chemotactic, 112-114, 113f
    congenital, 169t-170t, 172-175
    gene therapy for, 118
    granulocyte transfusions for, 117
    host defense, 110-118, 111t

Neutrophil(s) *(Continued)*
    intracellular killing, 114-117, 114t
  degranulation of, 107-108
  in *Entamoeba histolytica* infection, 3415
  function of, evaluation of, 118, 118t
  half-life of, 108
  inflammatory response of, 101-108
    ingestion in, 104-105, 104f-105f
    phagosome disposition in, 105-108, 106f
    prologue in, 101-102
    recruitment in, 102-104, 102f
    resolution of, 108
  kinetics of, 101
  in leukocyte adhesion deficiency syndromes, 112
  mature, 100f-101f, 101
  microbial defenses against, 110
  microbicidal mechanisms of, 108-110
  migration of, 102-103, 102f
    tissue, 104
  morphology of, 99-101, 100f, 100t
  oxidative (respiratory) burst in, 105-107, 106f
    abnormal, 114-116
    in chronic granulomatous disease, 114-116, 114t
    in glucose-6-phosphate dehydrogenase, 116
  polymorphonuclear, 101
    in urethral specimen, 1485-1486
  priming of, 101-102
  structure of, 99-101, 100f, 100t
  surface receptors of, 101
Neutrophil-specific granule deficiency, 169t-170t, 173
Nevirapine, 706t-709t, 1837-1838, 1837f, 1837t
  dosage of, 740t-741t
  drug interactions with, 742t-761t
  formulations of, 717t
  for HIV-infected children, 1820t-1821t
  resistance to, 1838
New World (American) cutaneous leishmaniasis, 3464t, 3469-3471, 3470f
NF-κB essential modulator (NEMO), mutations in, 175
Ngari virus, 2293
Niacin poisoning, 1417
Niclosamide, 657, 706t-709t
  for tapeworms, 3611
Nicotinamide adenine dinucleotide phosphate oxidase, in chronic granulomatous disease, 173-174, 173f
Nifurtimox, 657, 706t-709t
  for American trypanosomiasis, 3486
Nikkomycin Z, 561
  for *Coccidioides* infection, 3342
Nikolsky's sign, 799-800, 2554
Nimodipine, for intracranial hypertension, 1202
Nipah virus, 209
  detection of, 259t-260t
  emergence of, 2237
  encephalitis from, 1251t-1252t, 2240-2241, 2240f
    clinical features of, 2240-2241, 2240f
    diagnostic tests for, 2241
    epidemiology of, 2238-2239
    incubation period for, 2240
    outbreaks of, 2238t
    pathology of, 2241
    prevention of, 2241
    relapsed or late-onset, 2240-2241
    treatment of, 2241
  isolates of, genetic differences among, 209
  reservoirs and intermediate hosts for, 2239-2240
  structure and molecular biology of, 2237, 2239f
Nitazoxanide, 657-658, 706t-709t
  for cryptosporidiosis, 3554-3555
  for cyclosporiasis, 3562-3563
  for giardiasis, 3531, 3531t
  for liver flukes, 3602
  for microsporidiosis, 3402
Nitric oxide
  in bacterial meningitis, 1203-1204
  in severe sepsis, 993
Nitrite, in urinary tract infection, 967
Nitroblue tetrazolium (NBT) slide test, for chronic granulomatous disease, 115
Nitrofurantoin, 515-517, 706t-709t
  adverse effects of, 517
  antimicrobial activity of, 515

Nitrofurantoin *(Continued)*
  chemical structure of, 515, 516f
  in children, 517
  clinical uses of, 516-517
  dosage of, 732t-733t
  drug interactions with, 742t-761t
  formulations of, 716t
  mechanism of action of, 515
  pharmacology of, 515-516
  in pregnancy, 517
  prophylactic, for urinary tract infections, 516-517, 975
  resistance to, 515
  for uncomplicated cystitis, 516
  for uncomplicated pyelonephritis, 516
  for urinary tract infections, 516
Nitroimidazoles, 658
Nitroimidazoles-PA-824, for tuberculosis, 542
NK lymphoma, nasal, from Epstein-Barr virus, 1998
National Disaster Medical System (NDMS), activation of, 3957-3958
Nocardia/nocardiosis, 3199-3207
  brain abscess from, 1266, 1266t, 3201, 3202f
  chest radiography in, 940f
  classification of, 3199
  clinical manifestations of, 3200-3201, 3201f-3202f
  clinical outcome of, 3206
  colonization by, 3201
  disseminated, 3201, 3202f
  DNA sequence analysis of, 3203
  ecology of, 3199
  epidemiology of, 3199
    clinical, 3200
  growth of, 3201-3202, 3203f
  in heart transplant recipients, 3842
  in hematopoietic stem cell transplant recipients, 3828
  laboratory diagnosis of, 240t-242t, 3201-3203, 3203f
  lung nodules from, 3201, 3202f
  meningitis from, 1193, 1240
  molecular identification of, 3203
  mycetoma from, 3200-3201, 3201f, 3281, 3282t, 3283-3284, 3284f
  pathogenesis of, 3199
  pathology of, 3199, 3200f, 3201, 3202f
  pneumonia from, in HIV infection, 1730-1731
  prognosis for, 3205-3206
  prophylaxis for, 3206
  pulmonary, 3199, 3200f, 3201, 3202f
  skin lesions from, 3200-3201, 3201f-3202f
  treatment of, 3203-3206, 3204t
    duration of, 3205-3206
    surgical, 3205
  virulence of, 3199-3200
Nocardia asteroides, 3199-3201
  sulfonamides for, 477
  in transplant recipients, 3846
Nocardia brasiliensis, 3199-3200
Nocardia farcinica, 3199-3200
Nocardia nova, 3199
Nodes
  milker's, 1933
  Osler's, in endocarditis, 799, 1076
Nodules, 792, 795
  Koeppe, 1561
  lung, 935t-936t
    from *Cryptococcus neoformans*, 3293-3294, 3294f
    from *Nocardia*, 3201, 3202f
  in molluscum contagiosum, 1934, 1934f
  subcutaneous, 795, 799, 1303
    from *Blastomyces dermatitidis*, 3325
  in rheumatic fever, 2613-2614
Noma, 862t, 866
Noma neonatorum, 2856
Non-HACEK bacteria, endocarditis from, prosthetic valve, 1121t, 1123
Non-Hodgkin's lymphoma, in HIV infection, 1768-1771, 2333
  clinical characteristics of, 1769
  epidemiology of, 1768
  oral lesions from, 1715
  pathogenesis of, 1768-1769
  prognosis for, 1769
  treatment of, 1769-1771

Non-Hodgkin's lymphoma, in HIV infection
    (Continued)
    biotherapy in, 1770
    HAART in, 1769
    HAART-chemothrapy in, 1769-1770
    infusional chemotherapy in, 1770
    pre-HAART, 1769
    recommendations in, 1771
    salvage therapy in, 1770-1771
Noninferiority trials, 689, 694-695, 695f. See also
    Clinical trials.
Noninvasive positive-pressure ventilation, for
    nosocomial pneumonia, 3722
Non–nucleoside reverse transcriptase inhibitors,
    1837, 1837f, 1837t
    for AIDS dementia, 1748
    for HIV-infected children, 1820t-1822t
    initial therapy with, 1846
    penetration-effectiveness scores of, 1749t
    pharmacokinetic interaction between oral
        contraceptives and, 1800, 1800t
    prophylactic, for perinatal HIV transmission,
        1790t, 1791, 1792t-1793t
Nonoxynol-9
    anti-HIV activity of, 1784
    for Chlamydia trachomatis prophylaxis,
        2456-2457
    in HIV infection prevention, 1651
    for Trichomonas vaginalis, 1499
Nonsteroidal anti-inflammatory drugs (NSAIDs)
    antipyretic activity of, 774-775
    quinolone interactions with, 494
    for reactive arthritis, 1492
Nontreponemal reaginic tests, for syphilis, 3045
Norfloxacin, 706t-709t
    antimicrobial activity of, 491t-492t
    for cholera, 2782t
    dosage of, 493t, 732t-733t
    formulations of, 716t
    pharmacology of, 492t
    prophylactic, for primary peritonitis, 1016
    structure of, 487, 488f
Normothermia, maintenance of, during colorectal
    surgery, 3897
Noroviruses/norovirus infection, 2399-2405
    characteristics of, 2399-2400, 2400f
    clinical manifestations of, 2402-2403, 2402f
    detection of, 259t-260t
    diagnosis of, 2403
    diarrhea from, 205
    disinfection/sterilization and, 3688-3689
    epidemiology of, 2400-2401
    foodborne disease from, 1414t, 1415, 1419
    gastroenteritis from, 1362
    history of, 2399
    immune response to, 2402
    laboratory confirmation of, 1421
    pathogenesis of, 2401-2402, 2401f
    treatment of, 2403
    vaccine for, 2403
North Africa, HIV infection in, 1622
Norwalk virus, 2399-2405, 2400f, 2402f. See also
    Noroviruses/norovirus infection.
Norwegian scabies, 3633, 3634f, 3635t
    in HIV infection, 1718, 1718f
Nose. See Nasal entries.
Nosema, 3391, 3392t. See also Microsporidia.
Nosocomial infections. See also Health care–
    associated infections.
    antimicrobial use and, 3670
    from Corynebacterium, 2695, 2696t
    from cytomegalovirus, 3775-3777
    education on, 3670
    employee health and, 3670
    environmental hygiene and, 3670-3671
    from Epstein-Barr virus, 3777-3778
    hematologic
        HCV-related, 2171
        outbreaks of, 194
        pneumonia as, 3717-3724. See also Pneumonia,
            nosocomial.
    from Staphylococcus aureus, 2568
    tuberculous
        control of, 3135
        spread of, 3135

Nosocomial infections (Continued)
    of urinary tract, 3725-3737. See also Urinary
        tract infections, nosocomial.
    from hepatitis, 3739-3742, 3740t
    from herpes simplex virus, 3771-3772
    from herpesviruses, 3771-3780
    from HIV, 3753-3770. See also Human immuno-
        deficiency virus infection, nosocomial.
    hospital epidemiology programs for, 3667-3672,
        3670t
        accreditation in, 3671-3672
        functions of, 3669, 3670t
        organization of, 3671
    from human herpesvirus 6 and herpesvirus 7, 3778
    from human herpesvirus 8, 3778
    from Legionella pneumophila, 2973, 2975
    from Moraxella catarrhalis, 2773
    new-product evaluation and, 3671
    outbreak investigation of, 3669-3670, 3670t
    policy development on, 3670
    quality improvement and, 3671-3672
    surveillance for, 3669
    from transfusions, 3742-3748, 3742t, 3743f-3744f,
        3747f, 3747t
    in transplant recipients, 3748, 3813
    from varicella-zoster virus, 3772-3775
Novobiocin sodium, 706t-709t
NS2 protein, 2159
NS3 protein, 2159-2160
NS3/4A protease, inhibition of, 2175
NS4A protein, 2160
NS5A protein, 2160
NS5B protein, 2160
Nuclear factor κB (NF-κB)
    in bacterial meningitis subarachnoid space
        inflammation, 1200
    in Pseudomonas aeruginosa resistance, 2840, 2841f
Nuclear imaging studies, in pneumonia, 904
Nucleic acid amplification tests
    of cerebrospinal fluid, 1186
    for Chlamydia trachomatis, 1486, 2448
    for genital lesions, 1481
    for microbacteria, 251
    for Mycobacterium tuberculosis, 3130t, 3131
    for Neisseria gonorrhoeae, 2763
    in pneumonia, 898
    for smallpox, 3979
    for Streptococcus anginosus group, 2681
Nucleic acid hybridization assay, for Chlamydia
    trachomatis, 2447-2448
Nucleic acid–based tests, 246-249, 246t, 258-260
    in HIV infection, 1664, 1671-1672, 1671f
    for parasites, 264
    for rhinoviruses, 2395
Nucleocapsid, 1907, 1909f
Nucleoside and nucleotide reverse transcriptase
    inhibitors, 1833, 1834f, 1835t
    for AIDS dementia, 1748
    for chronic hepatitis B infection, 2075
    dual therapy with, 1845-1846
    for HIV-infected children, 1820t-1822t
    neuropathy from, 1756-1757, 1757t
    neurotoxicity of, 1756-1757, 1757t
    penetration-effectiveness scores of, 1749t
    pharmacodynamics of, 305
    prophylactic, for perinatal HIV transmission,
        1790t, 1791, 1792t-1793t
    triple- and four-drug therapy with, 1846
Nucleotide oligomerization domain (NOD) proteins,
    988-989, 989f
Null hypothesis, in clinical trials, 691
Nursing home pneumonia, 905-906
Nursing homes. See Long-term care facilities.
Nutrition, 151-159. See also Malnutrition.
    assessment of, 151, 152t
    enteral, 154-155, 155f
    immunity and, 44, 152-154
    parenteral
        catheter-related infections during, 3698, 3704t
        contamination in, 3697
        total, 154
    status classification for, 152t
Nutritional support
    in acute viral hepatitis, 1589
    catheter-related infections during, 3698, 3704t

Nutritional support (Continued)
    in elderly, 156-157, 157t
    in HIV/AIDS, 155-156, 156t
    in pancreatic infections, 1048
    in sepsis, 1005
    in surgical and critically ill patients, 154-155
NXL103, 511-512
NXL104, 512
Nystatin, 706t-709t
    dosage of, 736t-737t
    formulations of, 717t
    liposomal, 706t-709t

O

O antigen, 2816
O blood group, in Helicobacter pylori infection
    susceptibility, 52
Oak leaf gall mite, 3645-3646, 3647f
Obesity, definition of, 151
Observation trials, 690. See also Clinical trials.
Observational studies, 182-185
    case series, 183
    case-control, 183-184
    cohort, 184
    cross-sectional survey, 184
    for disease surveillance, 182-183
    for outbreak investigations, 184-185
Obturator sign, 1059
Occupation, chronic pneumonia and, 931-932
Occupational exposure
    to HIV, 3753-3770. See also Human immunodefi-
        ciency virus infection, occupational.
    immunization for, 189, 3941
    to Yersinia pestis, prevention of, 3969
Occupational Safety and Health Administration
    (OSHA), blood-borne pathogen standard of,
        disinfection and, 3688-3690
Ochrobactrum, 3016t-3017t, 3024
Octreotide, for cryptosporidiosis, 3554
Ocular infections
    from adenoviruses, 2029
    from Bacillus spp., 2729
    from Candida albicans, 3234, 3234f, 3238
    from Capnocytophaga, 2991
    from Cryptococcus neoformans, 3293t, 3296
    in endocarditis, 1075, 1075f
    from herpes simplex virus, 1952, 1952f
    from Histoplasma capsulatum, 3313-3314, 3317
    in injection drug users, 3886-3887
    in Lyme disease, 3075, 3075t
    from microsporidia, 3397, 3397f, 3402-3403
    from nontuberculous mycobacteria, 3196
    from Pseudomonas aeruginosa, 2852-2853
    from Sporothrix schenckii, 3272
    syphilitic, 1563-1564
        Argyll Robertson pupil in, 3042
        treatment of, 1567, 3050
    from Toxocara, 1565, 3618
    from Toxoplasma gondii, 1565
        diagnosis of, 3513-3514
        in immunocompetent patient, 3506
        treatment of, 3519-3520
    tuberculous, 1564, 1564f
Ocular larva migrans, 3618
Ocular trachoma, from Chlamydia trachomatis, 2449,
    2449t
    pathogenesis of, 2446
    treatment of, 2449
Ocular vaccinia, 1546-1548
Oculoglandular syndrome. See Parinaud's syndrome.
Oculoglandular tularemia, 2933
Odds ratio, 180-181, 181f
Odontogenic infections, 858-868
    anatomic considerations in, 858, 858f-860f
    cardiovascular disease associated with, 865
    clinical manifestations of, 858-868, 860f
    complications of, 864-865
    deep fascial space, 859f, 860-864, 863f
    dentoalveolar, 858-859, 861t
    diagnosis of, 868-869
    gingival, 859-860
    host defenses against, 857-858, 857f
    imaging of, 868-869
    indigenous flora in, 855, 856t

Odontogenic infections (Continued)
microbiological investigation of, 868
microbiota associated with, 855
specificity of, 855-856, 856f
periodontal, 859-860
spread of, 858, 858f-860f
suppurative, 862t, 869-870
treatment of, 861t, 869-870
Odynophagia, in HIV infection, 1737
Oerskovia, 2701
Ofloxacin, 706t-709t
antimicrobial activity of, 491t-492t
for Chlamydia trachomatis infections, 2455
dosage of, 493t, 732t-733t
formulations of, 716t
for Neisseria gonorrhoeae infection, 2753
for Neisseria meningitidis carriage, 2747-2748
pharmacology of, 492t
structure of, 487, 488f
for typhoid fever, 2898, 2898t
for urethritis, 1490
Oklahoma tick fever, 2098
OKT3, for transplant immunosuppression, infections and, 3811-3812, 3811t
Old World cutaneous leishmaniasis, 3464t, 3470, 3471f
Olecranon bursitis, from Pseudallescheria boydii, 3365, 3366f
Oligella, 2775t, 3016t-3017t, 3024-3025
Oligella urethralis, 3024-3025
Olsenella, 3126
Omega-3 fatty acids, 154
Omsk hemorrhagic fever, 2153
Onchocerca lupi, 3594
Onchocerca volvulus, 3590
Onchocerciasis, 3590t, 3593
ivermectin for, 652, 654
keratitis in, 1550-1551
treatment of, 632t-635t
Oncogenicity, of herpesviruses, 1940
Oncolytic agent, reovirus as, 2097-2098
Onychomycosis, 3352t
in aspergillosis, 3247
from Candida, 3230, 3230f
from dermatophytes, 3350, 3352
from Scopulariopsis brevicaulis, 3353
from Scytalidium, 3353, 3353f
superficial white, 3353
O'nyong-nyong virus, 2117-2125, 2118t. See also Alphaviruses.
Oocysts
Cyclospora, 3562, 3562f
Isospora belli, 3563, 3564f
Sarcocystis, 3565, 3565f
Toxoplasma gondii, 3495, 3496f
Oophoritis, from mumps virus, 2203
Opa proteins, in Neisseria gonorrhoeae, 2754, 2754f
OPC-67683, for tuberculosis, 542
Operating room
infectious disease containment issues for, 229
injury prevention in, 3758-3759
Ophthalmia neonatorum, 1535-1536
Ophthalmicus, herpes zoster, 1546
Opiates/opioids
abuse of. See Injection drug users.
for cryptosporidiosis, 3554
immune effects of, 3875-3876
Opisthorchis felineus, 3596t, 3597f, 3600-3602, 3601f
Opisthorchis viverrini, 3596t, 3597f, 3600-3602, 3601f
Opportunism, of gram-negative anaerobic rods, 3113
Opportunistic infections
CD4 count in, 1709, 1709f
fungal, 3370
in HIV infection, 1855-1886
antiretroviral therapy impact on, 1856
in children, 1814-1815, 1815f
prophylaxis against, 1821-1825
drug interactions and, 1857
management principles for, 1857-1858
outpatient parenteral antimicrobial therapy for, 700, 700t
pathogens associated with, 1856-1857
pediatric, 1814-1815, 1815f
prophylaxis against, 1821-1825
prophylaxis for, 1858t-1859t, 1871t

Opportunistic infections (Continued)
prospective monitoring for, 1855-1856
treatment of, 1858-1882, 1860t-1870t
in women, 1796
post-traumatic, in immunocompromised patients, 1302
Opsonization
antibodies in, 62-63
of Streptococcus agalactiae (group B) infection, 2658
Opsonophagocytosis
complement-mediated, 83
in vaccine response monitoring, 3920
OPT-80, 512
Optic neuritis
from chloramphenicol, 397
from ethambutol, 538
Oral antiseptics, in prevention of ventilator-assisted pneumonia, 3723
Oral candidiasis (thrush), 3227, 3227f
in HIV infection, 1714, 1714f
treatment of, 3237
Oral cavity. See also Mouth.
flora of, 855, 856t
mucosa of
immunity and, 857-858, 857f
infections of, 866-867
Oral contraceptives, HIV transmission and, 1647, 1800, 1800t
Oral hairy leukoplakia
from Epstein-Barr virus, 1996, 2004-2005
in HIV infection, 1715
Oral hygiene, 869
Oral infections. See also Orofacial infections.
in HIV infection, 1714-1715
from human papillomaviruses, 2041, 2044
in immunocompromised hosts, 3786, 3788
Oral rehydration therapy
for infectious diarrhea, 1347
for rotavirus gastroenteritis, 2111
Oral temperature, 767, 767f
Oral ulcers
aphthous, 866
from cytomegalovirus in HIV infection, 1715
from herpes simplex virus in HIV infection, 1715
Oral warts, 2041, 2044
Orbital abscess/cellulitis, 1571, 1571f
clinical presentation of, 1572-1573, 1572f
epidemiology of, 1571-1572
etiology and bacteriology of, 1572
laboratory and radiologic studies of, 1573, 1573f
from sinusitis, 845f, 846
treatment of, 1573-1574
Orbital apex syndrome, 1573
Orbiviruses, 2098
Orchitis, 1525
bacterial (pyogenic), 1525
in HIV infection, 1525-1526
in melioidosis, 2875f
from mumps virus, 2203, 2205
viral, 1525
Orf virus, 1933
Organ failure
in sepsis, 999-1000, 999f
in toxic shock syndrome, 2604
Organ transplantation. See Solid organ transplant recipients.
Orientia tsutsugamushi, 2529-2530, 2529f, 2529t, 3643, 3645f, 3646t
Oritavancin, 706t-709t
dosage of, 728t-729t
for Enterococcus, 2649
Ornidazole, 658
Orofacial infections, 855-871
from Actinomyces, 3210-3211, 3210f-3211f
anatomic considerations in, 858, 858f-860f
from herpes simplex virus, 1948, 1948f
microbiologic considerations in, 855-856, 856f, 856t
nonodontogenic, 865-867, 866f
antimicrobial therapy for, 861t
odontogenic, 858-868. See also Odontogenic infections.
pathogenic mechanisms in, 856-857

Oropharyngeal colonization, reduction of, for endocarditis prophylaxis, 1143
Oropharyngeal infections
candidal, posaconazole prophylaxis in, 559
from gram-negative anaerobic rods, 3115
Oropharyngeal ulcer, in histoplasmosis, 3313, 3313f
Oropharynx, gram-negative anaerobic rods in, 3113
Oropouche virus, 2292
Oroya fever (bartonellosis), 1400t-1401t, 1403, 2995-2996, 2996f, 3005
Orthopedic. See also Bone entries.
Orthopedic prosthetic device infections, from coagulase-negative Staphylococcus, 2583-2584
Ortho-phthalaldehyde, disinfection with, 3680t, 3683-3684
Orthopoxvirus/orthopoxvirus infection, 803-804, 1923-1932
background on, 1923
cowpox as, 1929-1930
laboratory findings in, 1929-1930
monkeypox as, 1927-1929, 1929f
morphology and structure of, 1923, 1924f
pathogenesis of, 1923
treatment of, 1930
vaccinia (smallpox vaccine) as, 1924-1927, 1924f
variola (smallpox) as, 1924f, 1926-1927, 1927f
Orthoreoviruses, 2097-2098
Orungo virus, 2098
Oseltamivir, 566t-567t, 591-592, 706t-709t
for avian influenza, 2280
clinical studies of, 592
dosage of, 738t-739t
formulations of, 717t
for influenza, 2277t, 2278-2279, 2284
resistance to, 2279
structure of, 591f
Osler's nodes, in endocarditis, 799, 1076
Osler-Weber-Rendu syndrome, brain abscess from, 1267
Oslo study, of syphilis, 3038
Osteitis pubis, 1463
Osteoarticular tuberculosis, peripheral, 3156
Osteomyelitis, 1457-1467
from Aspergillus, 3249, 3249f
from Blastomyces dermatitidis, 3325-3326, 3326f
from Brucella, 2923
from Candida, 3233, 3233f
chronic, 1460
chronic contiguous, from Pseudomonas aeruginosa, 2851-2852
chronic recurrent multifocal, 1463
classification of, 1457, 1458t
of clavicle, 1463-1464
computed tomography in, 1457-1458, 1458f
after contaminated open fracture, 1460
from Coxiella burnetii, 2516
culture-negative, 1465
in diabetes mellitus, 1461-1463, 1462f, 1462t
diagnosis of, 1457-1458
experimental models of, 1457
of foot, from Pseudomonas aeruginosa, 2851
fungal, 1465
general principles of, 1457-1460, 1458f, 1459t
hematogenous, 1463
after hematopoietic stem cell transplantation, 3824
in hemodialysis patients, 1464
in injection drug users, 1464, 3878-3879
of jaw, 862t, 865, 870. See also Odontogenic infections.
of long bones, 1458-1459
magnetic resonance imaging in, 1457-1458, 1458f, 1461, 1461f
maxillary, from Actinomyces, 3211, 3211f
in melioidosis, 2872, 2874f
microbiology of, 1458-1459, 1459t
multifocal, chronic recurrent, 1463
from Mycobacterium tuberculosis, 1464-1465
from nontuberculous mycobacteria, 1465
from Pasteurella, 2940
in prosthetic joint infections, 1469
from Pseudomonas aeruginosa, 2851-2852
of pubis, 1516
refractory, hyperbaric oxygen therapy for, 627-628
of sacroiliac joint, 1464
in sickle cell disease, 1464

Osteomyelitis *(Continued)*
   in skeletal mycobacterial disease, 1464-1465
   in spinal cord injury patients, 3854-3855
   from *Sporothrix schenckii*, 3271, 3272f
   from *Staphylococcus aureus*, 1457-1459, 1461,
      1461f, 2572-2574
      clinical features of, 2572-2573
      diagnosis of, 2574
      epidemiology of, 2572, 2572t
      pathogenesis of, 2572, 2573f
      prosthetic joints in, 2573
      rifamycins for, 409-410
      treatment of, 2574
   from *Streptococcus agalactiae* (group B), 2660
   from *Streptococcus* group C and group G, 2676
   subcutaneous abscess in, 1309
   of symphysis pubis, 1463
   treatment of
      antimicrobial therapy in, 1459-1460, 1459t
         outpatient parenteral, 699-700, 700t
      daptomycin in, 464, 1459-1460, 1459t
      goal of, 1459
      hyperbaric oxygen therapy in, 1460
      quinolones in, 499
      surgical débridement in, 1460
      vancomycin in, 456-457
   tuberculous, 3156
   of vertebrae, 1460-1461, 1461f
Osteopenia, HIV infection and, 1715, 1801
Osteoporosis
   HIV infection and, 1801
   risk factors for, 1801
Otitis
   from *Pseudomonas aeruginosa*, 2853-2854
   syphilitic, treatment of, 3050
   tuberculous, 3159
Otitis externa, 831
   acute diffuse, 831
   chronic, 831
   malignant, 831
      hyperbaric oxygen therapy for, 628
Otitis media
   from *Actinomyces*, 3211
   bacterial, 832-833, 833t
   brain abscess from, 1266t, 1267, 1272t
   chemoprophylaxis for, 834-835
   from *Chlamydia trachomatis*, 833
   chronic suppurative, from *Pseudomonas
      aeruginosa*, 2853
   from common cold, 811
   course of, 833-834
   diagnosis of, 833-834
   with effusion, 832, 834
      from nontypeable *Haemophilus influenzae*, 2912
   epidemiology of, 832
   from gram-negative anaerobic rods, 3115
   from *Haemophilus influenzae*, nontypeable,
      2912-2913
   immunology of, 833
   macrolides for, 436
   malignant
      from *Pseudomonas aeruginosa*, 2853
      treatment of, 2853-2854
   mastoiditis from, 835-836, 836f
   microbiology of, 832-833, 833t
   from *Moraxella catarrhalis*, 2772, 2772f
   from *Mycoplasma pneumoniae*, 833
   pathogenesis of, 832
   prevention of, 834-835
   quinolones for, 499
   from respiratory syncytial virus, 2212
   from rhinoviruses, 2393
   from *Streptococcus pneumoniae*, 2625, 2629-2630
      treatment of, 2635
   suppurative, anaerobes in, 3085
   surgical management of, 835
   treatment of, 834
   trimethoprim-sulfamethoxazole for, 481
   uncommon forms of, 833
   vaccines for
      pneumococcal, 835, 835t
      respiratory virus, 835
   viral, 833
Otomycosis, in aspergillosis, 3247
Otosyphilis, 3041-3042

Ototoxicity
   of aminoglycosides, 371-372
   of erythromycin, 431
   of vancomycin, 454
Outbreak investigation, 193-197. *See also* Infectious
      disease, outbreaks of.
Outer surface proteins, of *Borrelia burgdorferi*, 3071,
   3073
Outpatient parenteral antimicrobial therapy (OPAT),
      699-703
   agent suitability in, 700-701, 701t
   future of, 702-703
   infections amenable to, 699-700, 700t
   modes of delivery of, 699, 700t
   patient monitoring in, 702
   patient selection for, 701-702, 701t-702t
   technology of, 701
Ovalocytosis, Southeast Asian, malaria and, 3443
Ovulation, in HIV-infected women, 1799
Oxacillin, 317, 317f, 706t-709t
   for brain abscess, 1274t
   dosage of, 316t, 718t-719t
   for endocarditis, 1091
   formulations of, 715t
   for meningitis, 1213t
   for osteomyelitis, 1459t
   for peritonitis, 1029t
   for *Staphylococcus* endocarditis, 1118, 1118t,
      2571t
   susceptibility to, 311t-312t
OXA–derived beta-lactamase, 283
Oxamniquine, 658, 706t-709t
   for schistosomiasis, 3596t, 3599-3600
Oxazolidinones, 471-474. *See also* Linezolid.
   resistance to, ribosomal binding site alteration in,
      288
Oxiconazole nitrate, 706t-709t
Oxidative (respiratory) burst
   abnormal, 114-116
   in chronic granulomatous disease, 114-116, 114t
   in glucose-6-phosphate dehydrogenase, 116
   in neutrophils, 105-107, 106f
Oxolinic acid, 706t-709t, 732t-733t
Oxygen metabolites, in neutrophil bactericidal
      activity, 109
Oxygen radicals, in bacterial meningitis, 1203
Oxygen therapy
   with helium, for croup, 828
   hyperbaric. *See* Hyperbaric oxygen therapy.
   supplemental, for bronchiolitis, 887-889
Oxygen toxicity, from hyperbaric oxygen therapy,
   626
Oxytetracycline, 387t, 706t-709t
   dosage of, 724t
   formulations of, 715t
Ozone, sterilization with, 3687

P

P antigen, on erythrocytes, 2088
P value, in statistical testing, 694-695
P7 protein, in hepatitis C virus, 2159
P22*phox*, 107
   defective, 114-115, 114t
P24 antigen
   in acute retroviral syndrome, 1712
   detection of, 1642, 1663, 1670-1671, 1818
   in HIV transmission, 1786
P40*phox*, 106-107
P47*phox*, 101-102, 106-107
   deficiency of, 114-116, 114t
P55 gene, of *Pneumocystis*, 3378
P67*phox*, 106-107
   deficiency of, 114-116, 114t
Pacemaker infection, 1127-1131, 1128f, 1128t, 1130f.
   See also Cardiac rhythm management device
      infections.
Paclitaxel, for Kaposi's sarcoma, 1767
Paeniibacillus alvei, 2729t
PAIR procedure, for echinococcosis, 3614
Palivizumab, 618, 706t-709t
   dosage of, 738t-739t
   formulations of, 717t
   for respiratory syncytial virus, 2217-2218
Palpation, fever detection by, 766

Palsy
   Bell's, 580, 1948
   cranial nerve, in encephalitis, 1246
   facial, in Lyme disease, 3074-3075, 3075t
PAMPs (pathogen-associated molecular patterns),
   41, 44
Panbronchiolitis, from *Pseudomonas aeruginosa*,
   2851
Pancreas transplant recipients, infections in, 3841t,
   3843
Pancreatic disorders, in HIV infection, 1741
Pancreatic infections, 1045-1053
   abscess in, 1046t, 1047
   in acute pancreatitis, 1045-1052
   definitions in, 1046-1047, 1046t
   diagnosis of, 1047
   enteral feeding for, 1048
   flora of, 1047
   management of, 1047-1048
   necrosis in, 1046, 1046t
   preemptive antibiotics for, 1048-1051, 1049t,
      1051t
   prevention of, 1048-1052
   pseudocyst in, 1046t, 1047
   selective gut decontamination for, 1048, 1049t
Pancreatitis
   acute, 1046t
      causes of, 1045, 1046t
         drug-induced, 1046t
      infection complicating, 1045-1052
      infectious causes of, 1045, 1046t
      severe, 1046t, 1047
   drug-induced, 1741
   fluid collection in, 1046t, 1047
   fungal infection in, 1052
   in HIV infection, 1045
   from mumps virus, 2203
   from probiotics, 164
PANDAS (poststreptococcal autoimmune
      neuropsychiatric disorders associated with
      streptococci), 2615
Pandemic. *See also specific infection.*
   of cholera, 2777
   definition of, 193
   emergency preparedness for. *See* Emergency
      preparedness.
   of influenza, 2268
   influenza vaccine for, 2283
Pantoea agglomerans, 2827
   arthritis from, 1444-1445, 1445t
Panton-Valentine toxins, of *Staphylococcus aureus*,
   2553, 2553f
Pap smear, 2045, 2045t
Papillae, conjunctival, 1530
Papillary necrosis, from infection, 957-958, 958f
Papilledema, in cat-scratch disease, 3001, 3001f
Papilloma, squamous cell, oral, 2041, 2044
Papillomatosis, recurrent respiratory
   clinical manifestations of, 2040-2041
   incidence and prevalence of, 2036
   transmission of, 2036
   treatment of, 2044
Papillomaviruses, 2035-2049. *See also* Human
      papillomaviruses.
   detection of, 259t-260t
   interferon-alpha for, 589
Papular stomatitis virus, bovine, 1933
Papules, 792
   in cat-scratch disease, 2999, 2999f
   in syphilis, 3039-3040
   waxy, in reactive arthritis, 1492
Papulopustular lesions, from *Blastomyces
      dermatitidis*, 3325, 3325f
Papulosis, bowenoid, 2040, 2040f
Para-aminosalicylic acid, for tuberculosis, 541
Paracoccidioides brasiliensis, 3357-3363
   adrenal infections from, 3360
   characteristics of, 3357, 3358f
   chronic adult form of, 3358
   clinical manifestations of, 3358-3359
   culture of, 3362
   differential diagnosis of, 3360
   ecology and epidemiology of, 3357-3358
   histopathology of, 3361, 3361f
   immune response to, 3358-3359

Paracoccidioides brasiliensis (Continued)
  juvenile form of, 3358
  laboratory diagnosis of, 3361-3362, 3361f
  lymphadenopathy from, 3360
  mucosal lesions from, 3360, 3360f
  pathogenesis of, 3358-3359
  pulmonary infections from, 3359, 3359f
  serology of, 3362
  skin test for, 3362
  treatment of, 3361
Paracolic gutter, 1011-1012, 1012f
Paragonimiasis, triclabendazole for, 649
Paragonimus westermani, 3596t, 3602-3603
Parainfluenza viruses, 2195-2199
  bronchiolitis from, 885, 886t
  classification of, 2195
  clinical manifestations of, 2197, 2197t
  croup from, 825-826, 826f, 2196-2197. *See also*
    Croup.
  detection of, 259t-260t
  diagnosis of, 2197
  epidemiology of, 2196-2197, 2197t
  in hematopoietic stem cell transplant recipients,
    3830
  history of, 2195
  immune response to, 2196, 2196f
  in immunocompromised hosts, 2197
  pathogenesis of, 2195-2196
  replication of, 2195
  treatment of, 2197-2198
  tropism of, 2195-2196
  vaccine for, 2198
Paralysis
  from enteroviruses, nonpoliovirus, 2354
  respiratory muscle, in poliomyelitis, 2347
  tick, 3660, 3660t
  in West Nile encephalitis, 2146-2147
Paralytic poliomyelitis
  bulbar, 2346-2347
  spinal, 2346
Paralytic (dumb) rabies, 2251-2253
Paralytic shellfish poisoning, 1416-1417, 1417t, 3569,
    3570t
Paramyxovirus(es), zoonotic, 2237-2244
  classification of, 2237, 2238f
  Hendra virus, 2241-2242
  Menangle virus, 2242-2243
  Nipah virus, 2238-2241
  structure and molecular biology of, 2237-2238
  virology of, 2237-2238
Paranasal sinuses. *See also* Sinusitis; *specific sinus.*
  anatomy and physiology of, 839, 840f
Parapharyngeal lymphadenitis, 1324
Paraplegia
  Pott's, 3156
  syphilitic (Erb's palsy), 3040-3041
Parapneumonic effusions, 900, 902f
Parapoxvirus, 1933-1934
Parasitemia, in babesiosis, 3542, 3544
Parasites
  antigen tests for, 245-246, 246t, 264
  classification of, 262, 262t
  culture for, 244-245, 245t, 264
  detection and identification of, 263
  laboratory tests for, 262-264, 263t
  microscopic stains for, 244, 244t
  microscopy for, 263-264
  nucleic acid–based tests for, 264
  serologic tests for, 264
  specimen collection and transport for, 262-263,
    263t
Parasitic infections. *See also* Ectoparasitic diseases;
    specific parasite.
  conjunctivitis from, 1536
  enteritis from, 1395-1396
  after hematopoietic stem cell transplantation,
    3832
  metronidazole for, 422t, 424
  transfusion-related, 3748
  treatment of, 631-668, 632t-635t. *See also*
    Antiparasitic agents.
  zoonotic, 4000t-4001t
Paraspinal abscess
  from *Coccidioides*, 3337-3338, 3338f
  in Pott's disease, 3155-3156

Paratyphoid fever
  quinolone-resistant, 4025
  from *Salmonella paratyphi,* 4022-4024
  in travelers, 4022-4024
Parechoviruses, 2342
  characteristics of, 2342
  classification of, 2337
  clinical manifestations of, 2362
  epidemiology of, 2342
  receptors for, 2338t, 2342
Parenteral antimicrobial therapy, outpatient. *See*
    Outpatient parenteral antimicrobial therapy
    (OPAT).
Parenteral nutrition. *See also* Nutritional support.
  catheter-related infections during, 3698, 3704t
  contamination in, 3697
  total, 154
PARESIS mnemonic, 3042
Paresthesia, in foodborne disease, 1416-1418
Parinaud's syndrome
  from *Bartonella henselae,* 1565
  in cat-scratch disease, 3000, 3000f
  conjunctivitis in, 1536
  lymphadenitis in, 1326
Parkinsonism, in encephalitis, 1245-1246
Paromomycin, 359, 360f, 360t-361t
  for cryptosporidiosis, 3555
  for cutaneous leishmaniasis, 3475
  for *Entamoeba histolytica* infection, 3422t
  for parasitic infections, 641
  for visceral leishmaniasis, 3474
Paromomycin sulfate, 706t-709t
Paromycin, 359, 360f, 360t-361t
Paronychia, 3914
  from *Candida,* 3230, 3230f, 3238
Parotid space, infections of, 863. *See also*
    Odontogenic infections.
Parotitis
  chronic bacterial, 867
  from mumps virus, 867, 2202, 2205
  suppurative, 861t, 867
Paroxysmal nocturnal hemoglobinuria, CD59
    deficiency in, 92-93
Paroxysms, in malaria, 3438
Particle agglutination assays, in HIV infection, 1669,
    1669f
Parvovirus(es)
  adeno-associated, 2093
  detection of, 259t-260t
  in hematopoietic stem cell transplant recipients,
    3831
Parvovirus 4, 2093
Parvovirus B19, 2087
  arthritis from, 1449, 1449f
  arthropathy from, 2090
  characteristics of, 2087-2088, 2088f
  clinical manifestations of, 2088t, 2089-2091, 2090f
  diagnosis of, 2092
  epidemiology of, 2089
  erythema infectiosum from, 2089-2090, 2090f
  fetal infection with, 2091
  immune response to, 2089f, 2091-2092
  pathogenesis of, 2088-2089, 2088f-2089f
  prevention of, 2092-2093
  pure red cell aplasia from, 2090-2091
  rash from, 795
  transfusion-related, 3746
  transient aplastic crisis from, 2090
  transmission of, 2089-2090
  treatment of, 2092
  vaccine for, 2092-2093
  virus-associated hemophagocytic syndrome from,
    2091
Passive immunization, 73
Pasteurella, 2939-2942
  from animal bites, 2939, 2941-2942
  bone and joint infections from, 2940
  central nervous system infections from, 2940
  clinical manifestations of, 2940-2941, 2941t
  description of, 2939, 2940f
  endocarditis from, 2940
  epidemiology of, 2939
  intra-abdominal infections from, 2941
  laboratory detection of, 240t-242t
  pathogenesis of, 2939-2940

Pasteurella (Continued)
  prevention of, 2941-2942
  respiratory tract infections from, 2940-2941
  septicemia from, 2940
  skin and soft tissue infections from, 2940
  treatment of, 2941-2942
Pasteurella canis, 2941t
Pasteurella dagmatis, 2941t
Pasteurella multocida, 2941t
  beta-lactamase–producing, 2941
  bite infections from, 868, 3911-3912
  cellulitis from, 1296
Pasteurella stomatis, 2941t
Pasteurization, 3684
Pathogenicity, 186
  evolution of, 7
  genomics of, 7
  Koch's postulate and, 11
  molecular perspective on, 1-13
  regulation of, 7-9, 8t
  virulence genes in, 5, 5t, 10-11
Pathogenicity islands, 7
  in *Staphylococcus aureus,* 2556-2558, 2557t
    mobilization of, 2557
    types and nomenclature of, 2557-2558
Pathogens. *See also specific pathogen.*
  attributes of, 4-6, 5t
  in bioterrorism. *See also* Bioterrorism.
    detection of, 3960
    of greatest concern, 3954t, 3955-3956
    growing and "weaponizing," 3954-3955
  cellular immune response to, 139-140
  clonal nature of, 6-7
  cytoplasmic, 140
  definition of, 3
  detection of, 11-12, 267
  emerging, 3688-3690. *See also* Infectious disease,
    emerging and reemerging.
  enteric
    attachment of, 1341-1342
    in HIV infection, 1860t-1870t, 1880
    host, 1336-1337
    invasiveness of, 1342
  host subversion mechanisms of, 10
  innate immunity interference by, 4, 10, 44
  as intracellular parasites, 9-10, 9f
  multiplication strategies of, 5
  phagosomal, 140
  primary versus opportunist, 3-4
  protection against, in travelers exposed to water,
    4016
  replication of, 10
  in surgical site infections, 3893t
  sources of, 3892, 3892f, 3892t
  species of, 3892-3893, 3893f, 3893t
  virulence factors of, 3894
Patient education, on immunization, 3943-3944
Patient transport, in emergency preparedness, 229,
    229f
Pattern recognition receptors, of antigen-presenting
    cells, 69
Pavlivizumab, 3936
Pazufloxacin, 706t-709t, 716t
PCV7 vaccine, for otitis media prophylaxis, 835,
    835t
Pediculicides, 3631-3632, 3631t
Pediculosis, 3629-3632. *See also* Lice infestations.
Pediococcus, 2678
Pefloxacin, 706t-709t
  antimicrobial activity of, 491t-492t
  dosage of, 493t, 732t-733t
  formulations of, 716t
  for pancreatic infections, 1051
  pharmacology of, 492t
  structure of, 487, 488f
Pegfilgrastim, 611-613
Peginterferon-alfa, 587-588
  for hepatitis B infection, chronic, 1597, 1601t,
    2075, 2076t
  for hepatitis C infection, 2173
    chronic, 1606-1607, 1606t-1607t
Peginterferon-alfa-2a, 566t-567t, 706t-709t
  formulations of, 717t
  for hepatitis B virus, 588
  plus ribavirin, 566t-567t

Peginterferon-alfa-2b, 706t-709t
  dosage of, 738t-739t
  formulations of, 717t
  plus ribavirin, formulations of, 717t
Peginterferon-alfa/lamivudine, for hepatitis B
    infection, chronic, 2078
Peginterferon-alfa/ribavirin, for hepatitis C infection,
    2173
  chronic, 1607-1608, 1607t
  response of, 2173-2174, 2173f
Peliosis, bacillary, 2999, 3005
Pellicle, acquired, 857
Pelvic abscess, 1515-1516
Pelvic infection(s), 1511-1519
  anaerobic, 3085-3086
  from *Enterococcus*, 2647
  episiotomy-related, 1513
  after gynecologic surgery, 1514-1516, 1514t, 1515f
  intrapartum, 1511-1514
  osteomyelitis pubis as, 1516
  postabortal, 1513-1514
  postpartum endometritis as, 1511-1513, 1512f
  postpartum fever of undetermined origin with,
    1513
Pelvic inflammatory disease, 1516-1518
  from *Actinomyces*, IUD-associated, 3214, 3214f
  from *Chlamydia trachomatis*, 2454-2455
  diagnosis of, 1517, 1517f
  in HIV infection, 1797
    cytomegalovirus and, 1797
  from *Neisseria gonorrhoeae*, 2761, 2765-2766,
    2765t
  quinolones for, 496
  risk factors for, 1516-1517
  sequelae of, 1518
  treatment of, 1514t, 1517-1518, 1518t
Pelvic pain, chronic
  chronic prostatitis with, 1522-1523
  in urethritis, 1490
Pelvic thrombophlebitis, septic, 1513
Penciclovir, 566t-567t, 579-580, 706t-709t
  activity spectrum of, 568t
  structure of, 568f
Penicillin(s), 309-322. *See also* Beta-lactam
    antibiotics.
  for actinomycosis, 3217t
  adverse reactions to, 313-314, 314f, 314t
  allergy to, 350. *See also* Beta-lactam antibiotics,
    allergy to.
    CDC recommendations for, 3047t
    syphilis treatment and, 3050
  aminoglycosides with, 273
  antimicrobial spectrum of, 315t
  antipseudomonal, 315-316
  for brain abscess, 1274t
  chemistry of, 309, 310f
  for chronic lymphangitis, 1332
  classification of, 311
  cross-reactivity with, 352-353
  dosage of, 316t, 718t-719t
    in renal disease, 312, 313t
  for endemic treponematoses, 3057
  for endocarditis, 1088-1090, 1093
  for erysipelas, 1295
  extended-spectrum, 315-316
  formulations of, 715t
  for group A streptococcal pharyngitis, 819, 820t
  haptenization by, 348-349, 349f
  immunochemistry of, 348-349, 349f
  for impetigo, 1291
  indications for, 314-316, 315t
  mechanism of action of, 309, 310f
  for meningococcal infection, 2745-2746, 2746t
  natural, 316
  for ocular syphilis, 1567
  for peritonitis, 1024-1025, 1029t
  pharmacology of, 312-313, 313t, 718t-719t
  for pneumococcal pneumonia, 2636
  for pneumonia, 910
  for poststreptococcal glomerulonephritis,
    2619-2620
  prophylactic, 316
  for rat-bite fever, 2966
  resistance to, 310-311
  semisynthetic, allergy to, 351

Penicillin(s) *(Continued)*
  Staphylococcus aureus resistance to, 2558, 2559t
  for streptococcal meningitis, 2636
  Streptococcus pneumoniae resistance to, 2633
  structure of, 349f
  susceptibility to, 311, 311t-312t
  tetracycline with, 392
Penicillin G, 316, 316f, 316t
  for brain abscess, 1273, 1273t
  for diphtheria, 2692
  dosage of, 316t, 718t-719t
  for endemic treponematoses, 3057
  for endocarditis, 1090
  for *Enterococcus* endocarditis, 1120t
  for erysipelas, 1295
  for *Erysipelothrix rhusiopathiae* infection,
    2733-2734
  formulations of, 715t
  for gas gangrene, 1318
  for gram-negative anaerobic rod infections, 3117
  indications for, 314-315
  for leptospirosis, 3064t
  for Lyme disease, 3079t
  for lymphadenitis, 1330
  for lymphangitis, 1331-1332
  for mediastinitis, 1177
  for meningitis, 1213t
  for meningococcal infection, 2746t
  for neurosyphilis, in HIV infection, 1746
  for osteomyelitis, 1459t
  for peritonitis, 1024-1025, 1029t
  plus phenoxymethyl penicillin, 706t-709t
  for plague, 2948-2949
  prophylactic, 316
  for *Staphylococcus aureus* osteomyelitis, 2574
  for streptococcal pharyngitis, 2598t
  for *Streptococcus agalactiae* (group B) infection,
    2662t
  for *Streptococcus anginosus* group infections, 2684
  for *Streptococcus* endocarditis, 1119t, 1122
  susceptibility to, 311, 311t-312t
  for syphilis, 3047t, 3049-3050
  for viridans streptococcal endocarditis, 2669, 2670t
  for viridans streptococcal meningitis, 2671
Penicillin G benzathine, 706t-709t
  dosage of, 718t-719t
  formulations of, 715t
  for rheumatic fever prophylaxis, 2617, 2617t
Penicillin G potassium, 706t-709t
Penicillin G procaine, 706t-709t
  dosage of, 718t-719t
  formulations of, 715t
Penicillin G sodium, 706t-709t
Penicillin V, 316f, 317
  for diphtheria, 2692
  dosage of, 316t
  for erysipelas, 1295
  for lymphadenitis, 1330
  for lymphangitis, 1331-1332
  prophylactic, 316
  for recurrent cellulitis, 1298
  for rheumatic fever prophylaxis, 2617, 2617t
  for streptococcal pharyngitis, 2598t
  susceptibility to, 311, 311t
Penicillin V potassium, 706t-709t
  dosage of, 718t-719t
  formulations of, 715t
Penicillinase, *Staphylococcus aureus* resistance to,
    2559t
Penicillinase-resistant penicillins, 317, 317f
  indications for, 315
Penicillin-binding protein, 309, 310f, 2558
Penicillin-clindamycin, for gas gangrene, 1318
Penicilliosis, in HIV infection, 1860t-1871t
Penicillium marneffei, 3371-3372, 3372f, 3374t
Penicilloyl polylysine (PPL) skin testing, in
    beta-lactam allergy, 350
Penicilloyl radioallergosorbent test, in beta-lactam
    allergy, 351
Penis, herpes simplex virus infection of, 1948-1949,
    1949f
Pentamidine
  drug interactions with, 742t-761t
  pancreatitis from, 1741
  for *Pneumocystis* pneumonia, 3385

Pentamidine *(Continued)*
    in HIV infection, 1860t-1870t, 1872
  for *Pneumocystis* prophylaxis, 3386, 3800t
    in HIV infection, 1858t-1859t, 1873-1874
Pentamidine isethionate, 658-659, 706t-709t
  for African trypanosomiasis, 3492
  for cutaneous leishmaniasis, 3476
  for visceral leishmaniasis, 3474
Pentoxifylline, 620
  for mucosal leishmaniasis, 3476
  for subarachnoid space inflammation, 1220-1221
Peptide binding
  by MHC class I, 132-133
  by MHC class II, 135-136
Peptide nucleic acid fluorescent in situ hybridization,
    in *Staphylococcus aureus* diagnosis, 2546
Peptidoglycan, 309, 2623-2624
  of *Neisseria gonorrhoeae*, 2755
  of *Staphylococcus aureus*, 2552-2553, 2553f
Peptidoglycan cell wall, of enterobacteriaceae, 2816
Peptidoglycan recognition protein (PGRP), in
    neutrophil bactericidal activity, 109
Peptococcus niger, 3121
Peptoniphilus anaerobius, 3123t
Peptoniphilus asaccharolyticus, 3123t
Peptoniphilus gorbachii, 3123t
Peptoniphilus harei, 3123t
Peptoniphilus micros, 3123t
Peptoniphilus olsenii, 3123t
Peptostreptococcus, 3121
  in oral cavity, 855-856, 856t
Peracetic acid
  disinfection with, 3680t, 3684
  with hydrogen peroxide, disinfection with, 3680t,
    3684
  sterilization with, 3685t, 3687-3688
Peramivir, 592-593
  clinical studies of, 593
  structure of, 591f
Percutaneous drainage, of splenic abscess, 1056
Percutaneous intravascular devices
  infections due to, 3697-3715. *See also* Catheter-
      related infections.
    from catheter hub and lumen contamination,
      3698
    diagnosis of, 3700-3702, 3700t
    epidemiology of, 3698-3700
    from infusate contamination, 3697
    from insertion site contamination, 3698
    microbiology of, 3700, 3700t
    pathogenesis of, 3697-3698, 3698f
    prevention of, 3707-3710
    risk factors for, 3699, 3699t
  specific. *See also* specific device.
    issues associated with, 3702-3707, 3704t-3705t,
      3707t
Percutaneous transluminal coronary angioplasty,
    bloodstream infection after, 1136-1137, 1136t
Perianal actinomycosis, 3213
Perianal candidiasis, 3230, 3231f
Perianal cellulitis, from *Streptococcus pyogenes*, 2606
Perianal herpetic lesions, 1949-1950
Periapical abscess, 858
Periarteriolar sheath, 143
Periauricular lymphadenopathy, 1326
Pericardial effusion, in HIV infection, 1720
Pericardial fluid, laboratory processing of, 238
Pericardial friction rub, in pericarditis, 1163
Pericardiocentesis, 3155
  in pericarditis, 1164
Pericardiotomy, in pericarditis, 1164
Pericarditis, 1161-1165. *See also* Endocarditis;
    Myocarditis.
  from *Actinomyces*, 3211-3215
  in aspergillosis, 3249
  bacterial, 1161-1163, 1161t
  clinical manifestations of, 1163
  constrictive, 1163-1165
  diagnosis of, 1163-1164, 1164t
  etiology of, 1161-1162, 1161t
  fungal, 1162
  from *Histoplasma capsulatum*, 3317
  noninfectious causes of, 1164t
  nonviral causes of, 1161-1162, 1161t
  pathology and pathogenesis of, 1162-1163, 1163f

Pericarditis *(Continued)*
   from *Staphylococcus aureus,* 2571
   from *Streptococcus pneumoniae,* 2633
   tamponade in, 1163
   treatment of, 1164-1165
   tuberculous, 1162-1165, 1163f, 3155
   viral causes of, 1161, 1161t
Pericolonic abscess, 3085, 3086f
Pericoronitis, 860. *See also* Odontogenic infections.
Perihepatic space, abscess in, 1011, 1030
Perimandibular actinomycosis, 3210-3211, 3211f
Perimandibular infections, anaerobic, 3085
Perinephric abscess, 976-979, 977f
Periodic fever, 788
   with aphthous ulcers, pharyngitis, and adenitis, 1327
   of unknown origin, 788
Periodic lateralizing epileptiform discharges
      (PLEDs), in encephalitis, 2291
Periodontal abscess, 860
   anaerobes in, 3085
Periodontal disease/periodontitis, 859-860. *See also*
      Gingivitis; Odontogenic infections.
   from *Aggregatibacter actinomycetemcomitans,* 3015
   from anaerobic infections, 3085
   clinical manifestations of, 860
   in HIV infection, 1715
   in leukocyte adhesion deficiency, 167, 171f
   microbiology of, 857
   treatment of, 869
      antimicrobial therapy in, 861t
Periorbital edema, from sinusitis, 846
Peripheral osteoarticular tuberculosis, 3156
Peripheral vascular stent infection, 1137-1138, 1137t
Peripherally inserted central catheter (PICC)
   for intermediate and long-term access, 3705
   for outpatient parenteral antimicrobial therapy, 701
Periplasmic space, of enterobacteriaceae, 2815-2816
Perirectal actinomycosis, 3213
Peritoneal cavity
   abscess in. *See* Intraperitoneal abscess.
   anatomy of, 1011-1012, 1012f
   intraperitoneal fluid and fibrin in, 1018
   needle aspiration of, 1021
Peritoneal dialysis. *See also* Dialysis; Hemodialysis.
   acute, 1029-1030
   catheter-related infections in, 1028. *See also*
      Catheter-related infections.
      from coagulase-negative *Staphylococcus,* 2584
   continuous ambulatory, 1027-1028
      aminoglycoside dosing in, 375, 375t
      peritonitis during, 1027-1028
      vancomycin in, 453
   long-term, 1027-1029
      peritonitis during, 1027-1030
      antimicrobial agents for, 1028-1029, 1029t
Peritoneal fluid, laboratory processing of, 238
Peritoneal membrane, 1013
Peritoneum, parietal, 1012
Peritonitis, 1013-1030
   aminoglycosides for
      during continuous ambulatory peritoneal
         dialysis, 379
      experimental models of, 366-367
   anaerobes in, 3085
   from *Candida,* 3233, 3237
   chemical, 1018
   from *Cryptococcus neoformans,* 3296
   dialysis-related, 1027-1030
      antimicrobial agents for, 1028-1029, 1029t
   fatal, 1018
   from gram-negative anaerobic rods, 3116
   in liver transplant recipients, 3843
   from *Pasteurella,* 2941
   primary, 1013-1016
      bacteriologic characteristics of, 1013-1014
      clinical manifestations of, 1014-1015
      diagnosis of, 1015
      etiology of, 1013
      laboratory findings in, 1015
      pathogenesis of, 1014
      prevention of, 1016
      prognosis for, 1015
      treatment of, 1016

Peritonitis *(Continued)*
   quinolones for, 497
   secondary, 1016-1027
      clinical manifestations of, 1020
      diagnosis of, 1020-1021
      differential diagnosis of, 1020-1021
      etiology of, 1016
      microbiologic characteristics of, 1016-1018
      pathogenesis of, 1018-1019
      pathophysiologic responses to, 1019-1020
         local, 1019-1020
         systemic, 1020
      physical findings in, 1020
      prevention of, 1027
      prognosis for, 1021
      treatment of, 1021-1027
         antimicrobial, 1021-1026, 1022t
            dosages of, 1029t
         blood and plasma transfusion in, 1026
         gastrointestinal drainage in, 1026
         hyperbaric oxygen therapy in, 1026
         pharmacodynamic considerations in, 1026
         respiratory support in, 1026-1027
         surgical, 1027
         water and electrolyte administration in, 1026
   spontaneous bacterial, 1013
      from *Streptococcus pneumoniae,* 2633
   tertiary, 1016
   tuberculous, 1014-1015, 3157
Peritonsillar abscess
   gram-negative anaerobe rods in, 3115
   from pharyngitis, 820
Periurethral region, bacterial adherence and
      colonization of, 962
Permethrin
   for lice control, 2523
   for scabies, 3635, 3636t
Peromyscus leucopus, Sin Nombre virus from, 2290
Peroxynitrite, in bacterial meningitis, 1204
Personal hygiene, in gastrointestinal infections, 1337, 1337t
Personal protective equipment, in emergency
      preparedness, 225-226
Person-to-person disease outbreaks, 194-195, 195f
   of cryptosporidiosis, 3549
   of hepatitis A, 2372
Pertussis, 2955-2964. *See also Bordetella pertussis.*
   in adults, 2958
   in adults and adolescents, issues concerning,
      2957-2958, 2957f
   chemoprophylaxis for, 2961-2962
   clinical manifestations of, 2958
   complications of, 2958
   diagnosis of, 2958-2959
   epidemiology of, 2956-2958, 2957f
   immunization against, 2960
      for health care workers, 2961
      for infants, 2961
      schedules for, 2961
   in infants, 2958
   pathogenesis of, 2955-2956, 2956f
   in prevaccine era, 2957
   prevention of, 2960-2962
   in schools and day care centers, 2962
   treatment of, 2959-2960
      antibiotics in, 2959-2960
      macrolides in, 437
      supportive care in, 2960
   in vaccine era, 2957
   WHO definition of, 2958
   in young children, 2958
Pertussis toxin, 30, 2955
Pertussis vaccines, 2960-2961, 3922t, 3929-3930. *See
      also* Diphtheria-pertussis-tetanus (DPT)
      vaccine.
   acellular, 2961
   for health care workers, 2961
   for infants, 2961
   schedules for, 2961
   whole-cell, 2960-2961
Petechiae, 792, 793t, 796-797. *See also* Rash.
   in endocarditis, 1075-1076, 1075f
   in meningococcemia, 2741-2743, 2741f-2742f
Petechial exanthems, from enteroviruses, 2355
Pfiesteria-associated syndrome, 3570t, 3571

pH
   and antimicrobial activity, 272
   fecal, 1344
   vaginal, 1497, 1498f
   in virulence regulation, 7
Phaeohyphomycosis, 3367-3369, 3367t, 3374t
   of brain, 3367-3368, 3367f-3368f
   cutaneous, 3369, 3369f
   meningitis in, 1239
   subcutaneous, 3367, 3367f, 3367t
Phaeoanellomyces werneckii, tinea nigra from,
      3354-3355
Phage-encoded virulence factors, 5, 5t
Phagocytes. *See also* Eosinophil(s); Neutrophil(s).
   assay of, 171t
   congenital defects in, 169t-170t, 172-175
      affecting mononuclear cells, 175-177, 175f
   function of, evaluation of, 118, 118t
   granulocytic, 99-127
   microbial defenses against, 110
   in pulmonary host defense, 891-892
   responses to, 110
   signaling defects in, 175, 175f
Phagocytosis, 104
   abnormal, 114
   of *Cryptococcus neoformans,* 3292
   of *Entamoeba histolytica,* 3414
   in host defense, 41
   immunoglobulin G in, 104-105
   mannose-binding lectin in, 104-105
Phagosomal pathogens, 140
Phagosome, pathogen lysis of, 10
Pharmacodynamics, 300-306
   abbreviations/definitions in, 298t
   animal models of, 301
   antimicrobial activity in, 300
   of antiretroviral agents, 305
   area under 24-hour serum concentration curve to
      minimal inhibitory concentration ratio in,
      303-304, 303f
   concentration-dependent killing agents in,
      301-302, 301f
   human trials of, 301, 301f
   indices of, 305-306
   maximal serum concentration to minimal
      inhibitory concentration ratio in, 302-303,
      302f
   pharmacokinetics and, interactions between, 298f
   postantibiotic effect in, 304-305
   study methodology for, 300-305
   time above minimal inhibitory concentration ratio
      in, 304
   time-dependent (concentration-independent)
      killing agents in, 302, 302f
   in vitro models of, 300-301
Pharmacokinetics, 297
   abbreviations/definitions in, 298t
   absorption in, 297
   biotransformation in, 299
   cytochrome P-450 system in, 299-300
   distribution in, 297-300, 298f
   elimination in, 300
   metabolism in, 299
   models for, 297
   pharmacodynamics and, interactions between,
      298f
Pharyngeal cleft cyst, infected, 862t, 867
Pharyngeal diphtheria, 2690, 2690f
Pharyngitis, 815-821
   acute lymphonodular, from coxsackievirus A10,
      2356
   from adenoviruses, 818
   from *Arcanobacterium,* 2596
   from *Arcanobacterium haemolyticum,* 816, 2700,
      2700f
   from *Chlamydophila pneumoniae,* 817
   clinical manifestations of, 816-818
   in common cold, 810-812
   complications of, 820
   from *Corynebacterium diphtheriae,* 816-817
   diagnosis of, 818-819, 818t
   from enteroviruses, 817-818
   epidemiology of, 815
   from Epstein-Barr virus, 817
   etiology of, 815, 816t

Pharyngitis (Continued)
  from Francisella tularensis, 2933
  from herpes simplex virus, 818, 1948
  from HIV infection, 817
  in Marshall's syndrome, 1327
  from Mycoplasma pneumoniae, 817
  from Neisseria gonorrhoeae, 817, 2760, 2764t
  pathogenesis of, 815-816
  in plague, 2947
  streptococcal
    group A–associated, 2595-2599
      clinical manifestations of, 816, 2595-2596
      complications of, 820
      diagnosis of, 818-819, 818t, 2596-2598
      epidemiology of, 815, 2595, 2595f
      etiology of, 815
      nonsuppurative complications of, 2596
      pathogenesis of, 815-816
      rapid antigen detection tests for,
        2597-2598
      suppurative complications of, 2596
      throat culture for, 2597
      treatment of, 819-820, 820t, 2598-2599, 2598t
    group C– and group G–associated, 816,
      2674-2675
    versus infectious mononucleosis, 2003
    rheumatic fever after, 2611
  from Yersinia enterocolitica, 2596, 2951
Pharyngoconjunctival fever
  from adenoviruses, 818, 2029
  conjunctivitis in, 1531
Pharyngocutaneous fistula, postradiation, 868
Pharyngomaxillary (lateral pharyngeal) space
  infections of, 863-864
    mediastinitis from, 1173
  relation of, to cervical fascia, 858, 859f
Phase I reactions, 299
Phase II reactions, 299
Phenazopyridine-sulfisoxazole, 706t-709t
Phenolics, disinfection with, 3684
Phenytoin, isoniazid interactions with, 534-535
Phlebitis, septic, lung abscess from, 925
Phlebotomus papatasi, Toscana virus infection from,
  2292-2293
PhoP/PhoQ regulatory system, of Salmonella,
  2893-2894
Phospholipase B gene, of Cryptococcus neoformans,
  3291-3292
Phospholipase C, of Pseudomonas aeruginosa,
  2844-2845
Photorhabdus asymbiotica, 2829
Photosensitivity reactions, to tetracycline, 390-392
Phototoxicity, of quinolones, 503
Phrenicocolic ligament, 1011, 1012f
Phthiriasis palpebrarum, 1569
Phycomycosis, gastrointestinal manifestations of,
  1395. See also Mucormycosis.
Physical agents
  HAV resistance to, 2368
  rhinoviruses inactivation by, 2391
Physical barriers, in innate immunity, 38-41
Phytophotodermatitis, 4023f
Pichia (Hansenula) anomala, 3371
Picobirnaviruses, 2408
Picornaviruses. See also Enteroviruses; Hepatitis A
  virus; Rhinoviruses/rhinovirus infection.
  adherence function of, 17f
  adhesin-based therapy for, 21t, 22
  classification of, 2389
Piedra
  black, 3355
  white, 3355
Piedraia hortae, black piedra from, 3355
Pig-bel, 1394
Pigmentation changes, from tetracycline, 390-392
Pigs, Toxoplasma gondii in, 3497
Pili
  of enterobacteriaceae, 2818-2819
  of gram-negative anaerobic rods, 3113
  of Neisseria gonorrhoeae, 9, 2753-2754, 2754f
  of Pseudomonas aeruginosa, 2842
Pink eye, 1531-1533, 1532f, 1533t
Pinta, from Treponema carateum, 3057
Pinworm, 3578t, 3579f-3580f, 3583-3584
Pipemidic acid, 706t-709t, 716t

Piperacillin, 318-319, 319f
  dosage of, 316t, 718t-719t
  formulations of, 715t
  indications for, 315-316
  for non-HACEK endocarditis, 1121t
  for peritonitis, 1029t
  susceptibility to, 311t-312t
Piperacillin sodium, 706t-709t
Piperacillin-tazobactam, 321, 706t-709t
  for acute pyelonephritis, 972
  dosage of, 718t-719t
  for febrile neutropenia, 3804t
  formulations of, 715t
  for nosocomial pneumonia, 3718t
  for Pseudomonas aeruginosa bacteremia,
    2849-2850
  for septic bursitis, 1450t
Piperazine, 659, 706t-709t, 742t-761t
Pityriasis (tinea) versicolor, 3353-3354
Pivmecillinam, 706t-709t, 715t
Placental malaria, 3442
Plague. See also Yersinia pestis.
  as biological weapon, 2943, 3965-3970
    characteristics of, 3966
    diagnostic tests for, 3966-3967
    health care providers' role in, 3968
    history of, 3965
    hospital infection control measures for, 3968
    medical countermeasures for, 3966-3968
    occupational exposure to, prevention of,
      3969
    post-event recovery from, 3969
    post-exposure prophylaxis for, 3967, 3967t
    potential for, 3965
    preparedness and response to, 3968-3969
    public health system's role in, 3968-3969
    transmission of, 3966
    treatment of, 3967
      biologics in, 3968
      special considerations in, 3967-3968
    vaccines for, 3968
  bubonic, 2945-2946, 3639t
    axillary bubo in, 2946, 2946f
    femoral and inguinal buboes in, 1326-1327,
      2946, 2946f
    treatment of, 1330
  chemoprophylaxis against, 2949
  clinical manifestations of, 2945-2947
  diagnosis of, 2947-2948
  versus enteric fever, 1400t-1401t, 1403
  epidemiology of, 2943-2945, 2945f
  gastrointestinal symptoms in, 2947
  history of, 2943, 2944f
  laboratory findings in, 2947, 2947f
  meningitis in, 2947
  pathogenesis of, 2945, 2945f
  pharyngitis in, 2947
  pneumonic, 2946-2947
    person-to-person transmission of, prevention
      of, 2947
    treatment of, 3967t
  prevention of, 2949
  reservoirs for, 2949
  septicemic, 2946
  transmission of, 2944, 2945f
  treatment of, 2948-2949
    antimicrobials in, 2948
    precaution protocols in, 2949
    supportive therapy in, 2948-2949
  vaccines for, 3930, 3968
  vector control for, 2949
Plant mites, 3645-3646, 3646f
Plaques, 792
Plasma transfusion
  for complement deficiencies, 95
  for peritonitis, 1026
  recipients of, vaccination against hepatitis A in,
    2383
Plasmid-encoded virulence factors, 5, 5t
Plasmids
  in antimicrobial resistance, 279
  of Campylobacter jejuni, 2795-2796
  conjugative, of Neisseria gonorrhoeae, 2755
  of enterobacteriaceae, 2820
  in quinolone resistance, 490

Plasmodium, 3437-3462
  antigenic variation in, 3444, 3444f
  characteristics of, 3437-3438, 3439f
  immune response to, 3444, 3444f
  life cycle of, 3437-3438, 3439f
Plasmodium falciparum, 211. See also Malaria.
  characteristics of, 3437-3438, 3439f
  chloroquine-resistant, 211-212
    halofantrine for, 632t-635t, 639
    mechanism of action of, 3447
    mortality trends and, 3437, 3438f
  drug-resistant, geographic distribution of,
    3445-3446, 3445f
  epidemiology of, 3444
  hemoglobin S protection against, 53
  immune response to, 50
  in nonimmune travelers, 4022
  pathogenesis of, 3438-3442, 3439f-3440f
Plasmodium falciparum erythrocyte membrane
  protein-1, 3439-3441
Plasmodium knowlesi, 211, 4022
  epidemiology of, 3444
  pathogenesis of, 3442
Plasmodium malariae, 211, 4022
  characteristics of, 3437-3438, 3439f
  epidemiology of, 3444
  pathogenesis of, 3442
  treatment of, 3454
Plasmodium ovale, 211
  characteristics of, 3437-3438, 3439f
  epidemiology of, 3444
  pathogenesis of, 3442
  treatment of, 3454
Plasmodium vivax, 211. See also Malaria.
  characteristics of, 3437-3438, 3439f
  chloroquine-resistant, 632t-635t
  Duffy blood group and, 50, 53
  epidemiology of, 3444
  pathogenesis of, 3442
  treatment of, 3454
Platelet(s), in Staphylococcus aureus endocarditis,
  2569
Platelet transfusions, bacterial infections from,
  3747-3748, 3747f
Platelet-endothelial cell adhesion molecule, 103
Pleconaril, 599f, 600
  for enteroviruses, 2341-2342
  for myocarditis, 1160
  for viral meningitis, 1215
Pleistophora, 3391, 3392t. See also Microsporidia.
Pleocytosis, cerebrospinal fluid, in CNS infections,
  1185
Plesiomonas, 3016t-3017t, 3021
Plesiomonas shigelloides, 2829, 3021
Pleural effusion, 917-924
  from anthrax, 2723
  clinical manifestations of, 919
  exudative versus transudative, 920, 920t
  imaging of, 919-920, 919f-920f
  laboratory findings in, 920-921, 920t
  microbiology of, 917-919
  in Mycoplasma pneumoniae, 2483
  pathophysiology of, 917
  in pneumonia, 900, 902f
  treatment of, 921-923, 921t
  tuberculous, 918, 921
Pleural fluid, laboratory processing of, 238
Pleural mesothelial cells, 917
Pleurisy, tuberculous, 3154-3155
Pleurodynia, from enteroviruses, 2356-2357
Pleurodynia syndromes, 1320
Pleuropulmonary infections
  anaerobic, 3085-3087
    from Clostridium, 3108
    from gram-negative anaerobic rods, 3116
Pneumatoceles
  in hyperimmunoglobulinema E, 176, 176f
  in Staphylococcus aureus pneumonia, 901-903,
    903f
Pneumococcal pneumonia, 2631-2633
  antibiotic susceptibility in, 910, 910t
  chest radiography in, 901-903, 901f-902f,
    2631
  clinical manifestations of, 2631
  community-acquired, 904

Pneumococcal pneumonia (*Continued*)
 complications of, 2633
 diagnostic microbiology of, 2632-2633, 2632f, 2632t
 in hematopoietic stem cell transplant recipients, 3827
 laboratory findings in, 2632
 predisposing factors for, 2631
 sputum in, 897, 897f
 treatment of, 910-912, 910t, 2635-2636
Pneumococcal surface adhesin A, 2627, 2629t
Pneumococcal surface protein A, 2627, 2629t
Pneumococcal vaccine, 2636-2638, 2637t, 2638f
 antibody levels after, 2637
 in asplenia, 3870, 3871t
 conjugate, 2637-2638, 2638f, 3922t, 3930-3931
 efficacy of, 2637
 in elderly, 3859
 in HIV-infected children, 1826
 for otitis media prophylaxis, 835, 835t
 pneumonia and, 913
 polysaccharide, 2637-2638, 3922t, 3930
 protection after, 2637, 2637t
 recommendations for, 2637-2638
 shortcomings of, 3871t
Pneumococcus. *See Streptococcus pneumoniae.*
Pneumocystis, 3377-3390
 antigens of, 3377-3378
 characteristics of, 3377-3378
 culture of, 3377, 3378f
 epidemiology of, 3378-3379
 extrapulmonary disease from, 3382
 genetics of, 3377
 histopathology of, 3380-3381, 3381f
 immune response to, 3379-3381, 3381f
 life cycle of, 3377, 3378f
 pneumonia from. *See Pneumocystis* pneumonia.
 serology of, 3383-3384
 staining of, 3383
 taxonomy of, 3377
 transmission of, 3379
Pneumocystis carinii. See Pneumocystis jirovecii.
Pneumocystis jirovecii, 3377
 detection of, 255
 pneumonia from. *See Pneumocystis* pneumonia.
 treatment of, 632t-635t
Pneumocystis pneumonia
 in cancer patients, chemoprophylaxis for, 3800t, 3801-3802
 clinical manifestations of, 3381-3382, 3382f
 corticosteroids for, 618
 course and prognosis in, 3384, 3384t
 diagnosis of, 3382-3384, 3382f
 epidemic form of, 3381
 epidemiology of, 3378-3379
 extrapulmonary manifestations of, 3382
 in hematopoietic stem cell transplant recipients, 3831
 in HIV infection, 1710-1711, 1710f, 1729-1734, 1858-1874
  as AIDS indicator, 1643
  CD4+ counts in, 1727
  choroiditis from, 1720
  diagnosis of, 1727, 1730, 1870
  prophylaxis against, 1727, 1858t-1859t, 1871t, 1873
  treatment of, 1860t-1870t, 1872
 in HIV-infected children, 1814, 1815f
  prophylaxis against, 1821-1825
 immune reconstitution inflammatory syndrome and, 3382
 pathology and pathogenesis of, 3379-3381, 3381f
 prevention of, 3386-3387
 primaquine for, 632t-635t, 636
 treatment of, 3382f, 3384-3386
 trimethoprim-sulfamethoxazole for, 481-482
Pneumolysin, 2626-2627, 2629t
Pneumonectomy, for chronic pneumonia, 942
Pneumonia. *See also* Pulmonary infections.
 acute
  clinical evaluation of, 894-904
  diagnostic tests in, 896
  etiology of, 891, 892t
  history in, 894-895, 895t
  pathogenesis of, 891-894

Pneumonia (*Continued*)
 physical examination in, 896
 predisposing factors in, 894-895
 treatment of, 909-913
  adjunctive, 912-913
  duration of, 912
  empirical, 910-912, 910t-911t
 versus acute bronchitis, 874
 from adenoviruses, 2029
 antigen detection in, 898
 aspiration, 903, 908
  bacterial, 908
  lung abscess from, 925
 atypical, 907-908, 2481-2489. *See also Mycoplasma pneumoniae.*
 bacterial
  as AIDS indicator, 1643
  chest radiography in, 901-903, 901f-903f
  in elderly, 905
  etiology of, 892t
  after influenza, 21
  from influenza, 2273, 2275, 2275t
 blind endotracheal suctioning in, 899
 blood culture in, 900
 bronchoalveolar lavage in, 899
 in burn patients, 3906
 from *Candida,* 3232
 chest radiography in, 901-904, 901f-903f
 from *Chlamydia pneumoniae,* 907. *See Chlamydophila pneumoniae.*
 from *Chlamydia trachomatis,* 907, 2455
  in infants, 2456, 2456f
 chronic, 931-945. *See also specific infections.*
  causes of, 931, 932t
  clinical features of, 933
  diagnosis of, 933-938
   chest radiography in, 934, 935t-936t
   initial laboratory studies in, 933-934
   invasive procedures in, 937-938
   in patients with radiographic evidence of diffuse infiltratration and fibrosis, 938
   in patients with radiographic evidence of localized infiltrates or cavitation, 934-937
  epidemiology of, 931-933
  noninfectious causes of, 931, 932t
  treatment of, 938-942
   antimicrobial agents in, 938-942
   bronchoscopy in, 942
   corticosteroids in, 942
   surgery in, 942
 community-acquired
  acute, 904-905
  in elderly, 905
  empirical treatment of, 910-912, 910t-911t
  granulocyte colony-stimulating factor for, 613
  from *Haemophilus influenzae,* nontypeable, 2913
  in HIV infection, 906
  macrolides for, 436
  quinolones for, 498
  severe, 906
  tetracycline for, 394
  versus tularemia pneumonia, 3971-3972, 3972t
 computed tomography in, 903-904
 COPD and, 895
 from *Coxiella burnetii,* 2512-2515, 2513f-2514f. *See also* Q fever.
  diagnosis of, 2514
  treatment of, 2514
 from *Cryptococcus neoformans,* 3293-3294, 3294f
 from cytomegalovirus, 1971, 1974, 1974f
 in elderly, 894-895, 3858-3859
 empyema in, 918
 eosinophilic, 908-909
 etiology of, environmental history and, 895, 895t
 fiberoptic bronchoscopy in, 899, 937-938
 from *Francisella tularensis,* 2933-2934, 2934f, 3971
  versus community-acquired pneumonia, 3971-3972, 3972t
 fungal, 892t
 from gram-negative bacilli, 905
 from *Haemophilus influenzae,* 897, 897f, 904
 from *Haemophilus influenzae* type b, 2914
 health care–associated, 895, 906-907
 in HIV infection, 895

Pneumonia (*Continued*)
 antiretroviral therapy and, 1727-1728
 bacterial, 1730-1731, 1731f
 community-acquired, 906
 fungal, 1731-1732
 mycobacterial, 1731
 parasitic, 1732-1733
 from *Pneumocystis jirovecii. See* Human immunodeficiency virus infection, *Pneumocystis* pneumonia in.
 viral, 1732
 hospitalization for, 909
 in immunocompromised hosts, 909
 in injection drug users, 3882-3883
 from *Klebsiella pneumoniae,* 896, 897f-898f, 902f, 2826
 from *Legionella,* 905, 908
 from *Legionella bozemanii,* in immunosuppressed patient, 2986-2987, 2988f
 lung biopsy in, 899-900
 in measles, 2231
 in melioidosis, 2871, 2872f-2873f
 from *Moraxella catarrhalis,* 905, 2773
 from mycobacteria, 897, 898f
 from *Mycoplasma pneumoniae,* 903, 907, 2482-2483, 2482f. *See also Mycoplasma pneumoniae.*
 necrotizing, 925-926, 3085
 in neonates, from enteroviruses, 2359
 nosocomial, 909, 3717-3724
  definition of, 3717
  diagnosis of, 3719-3720
  in elderly, 3858
  epidemiology of, 3717
  etiology of, 909, 3717, 3718t
  from *Legionella,* 2973
  pathogenesis of, 3717-3719, 3719f
  prevention of, 1005, 3721-3723, 3722t
   airway colonization in, 3723
   basic targets in, 3721
   endotracheal tube and bioflim issues in, 3721-3723
  risk factors for, 909
  treatment of, 3720-3721, 3720f
   antibiotic regimens in, 3718t, 3720-3721
   clinical nonresponders in, 3721
   limiting duration of therapy in, 3721
   quinolones in, 499
  ventilator-associated, 3717
 nuclear imaging studies in, 904
 nucleic acid amplification tests in, 898
 nursing home, 905-906
 from pertussis, 2958
 pleural effusion in, 900, 902f
 pneumococcal. *See* Pneumococcal pneumonia.
 from *Pneumocystis jirovecii. See Pneumocystis* pneumonia.
 prevention of, 913
 from *Pseudallescheria boydii,* 3365
 from *Pseudomonas aeruginosa,* 2847
  acute, 2850-2851
 pulmonary defense systems and, 891-893, 893t
 recurrent, 894
 from respiratory syncytial virus, 2210
 from *Rhodococcus equi,* 2702-2703
 risk factors for, 893-895, 895t
 scoring systems for, 906, 909
 serologic tests in, 900, 934-937
 in solid organ transplant recipients, 3841, 3841t, 3844
 in spinal cord injury patients, 3853-3854
 sputum examination in, 896-898, 897f-898f
 from *Staphylococcus aureus,* 897, 898f, 903f, 2553, 2553f
  community-acquired methicillin-resistant, 904-905
 from *Stenotrophomonas maltophilia,* 2864-2865, 2864f
 from *Streptococcus agalactiae* (group B), 2660
 from *Streptococcus* group C and group G, 2676
 from *Streptococcus pneumoniae. See* Pneumococcal pneumonia.
 from *Streptococcus pyogenes,* 2606
 from *Streptococcus viridans* group, 2672
 syndromes associated with, 904-909

Pneumonia (Continued)
  in transplant recipients, 3823
  urine antigen testing in, 901
  vancomycin for, 456
  ventilator-associated, 3717. See also Pneumonia, nosocomial.
  viral, 907
    chest radiography in, 903, 903f
    in elderly, 905
    etiology of, 892t
  vitamin A for, 670t, 671-672
  walking, 2482
Pneumonia severity index, 909
Pneumonic plague, 2946-2947. See also Plague.
  person-to-person transmission of, prevention of, 2947
  treatment of, 3967t
Pneumonitis
  from cytomegalovirus
    in hematopoietic stem cell transplant recipients, 3829
    in HIV infection, 1732
  from herpes simplex virus, 1953
  hypersensitivity, from Mycobacterium avium complex, 3183, 3186
  lymphocytic interstitial
    in HIV infection, 1733
    in HIV-infected children, 1815, 1815f
  trimethoprim-sulfamethoxazole for, 481
  in varicella, 1965
Pocket site infection, cardiac rhythm management device, 1128
Podofilox, for condylomata acuminata, 2043
Podophyllin, for condylomata acuminata, 2043
Point estimate, calculation of, in clinical trials, 694
Point-source disease outbreaks, 195, 195f
Polioencephalitis, 2347
Poliomyelitis
  abortive, 2346
  clinical manifestations of, 2346-2347, 2346f
  complications of, 2347
  in developing world, 2349-2350
  differential diagnosis of, 2347, 3660t
  encephalitis in, 2347
  eradication of, 2349-2350
  etiology of. See Polioviruses.
  genetic susceptibility to, 49, 50t
  historical perspective on, 2345
  laboratory diagnosis of, 2347
  nonparalytic, 2346
  paralytic
    bulbar, 2346-2347
    spinal, 2346
  pathogenesis of, 2346
  postpoliomyelitis syndrome after, 2348
  prognosis in, 2347
  risk factors for, 2347
  treatment of, 2347
  vaccine-associated, 2348-2350
Poliomyelitis vaccine, 2348
  in developing world, 2349
  inactivated, 2348, 3922t, 3924f, 3931
  live-attenuated, 2348
  monovalent oral, 2348
  poliomyelitis from, 2348-2349
  for travelers, 4011t, 4013
Polioviruses, 2345-2351. See also Enteroviruses.
  characteristics of, 2337, 2345
  clinical manifestations of. See Poliomyelitis.
  communicability period of, 2341
  encephalitis from, 1259
  epidemiology of, 2339-2341, 2340t
  history of, 2345
  host range of, 2338t
  immune response to, 2339
  incidence of, 2340-2341
  incubation period for, 2341, 2346
  laboratory diagnosis of, 2341, 2347
  molecular biology of, 2337-2338, 2338t
  mutation of, 2339
  pathogenesis of, 2338-2339, 2346
  prevention of, 2341-2342
  receptors for, 2337, 2338t
  risk factors for, 2347
  spread of, 1915-1916

Polioviruses (Continued)
  transmission of, 2340
  treatment of, 2341-2342
  tropism of, 1916
  vaccine for. See Poliomyelitis vaccine.
Polyarteritis nodosa, from hepatitis B, 2072
Polyarthritis
  from alphaviruses, 2120-2121, 2123
  from HTLV, 2315
  from mumps virus, 2203
  reactive, in Yersinia enterocolitica infection, 2951
Polyclonal antibodies, for transplant immunosuppression, infections and, 3811, 3811t
Polyenes, for candidiasis, 3235
Poly-gamma-DL-glutamic acid, Staphylococcus epidermidis production of, 2581
Polyhexamethylene biguanide, for amebic keratitis, 3434
Polymerase chain reaction assay, 247, 249
  in bacterial meningitis, 1208-1209
  for Bartonella, 3004
  in BK virus–associated nephropathy, 2056
  for Bordetella pertussis, 2959
  of cerebrospinal fluid
    in CNS infections, 1186
    in progressive multifocal leukoencephalopathy, 2053
  for Chlamydophila pneumoniae, 2469
  for Cryptosporidium parvum, 3554
  for Cyclospora, 3562
  for cytomegalovirus, 1972
  for ehrlichiosis, 2534
  for encephalitis, 1249-1250
  for Entamoeba histolytica, 3421
  for enteroviruses, 2341
  for flaviviruses, 2148
  for Francisella tularensis, 2934, 3973
  for herpesviruses, 1940
  for histoplasmosis, 3314
  in HIV-infected children, 1817-1818
  for human T-cell lymphotrophic virus, 2307
  for meningococcal infection, 2745
  in microorganism identification, 1115-1116
  multiplex real-time, for Staphylococcus aureus, 2546
  for Mycoplasma pneumoniae, 2486
  in myocarditis, 1159
  for neurosyphilis, 3046
  for Pneumocystis pneumonia, 3383
  for psittacosis, 2464-2465
  reverse transcriptase-. See Reverse transcriptase–polymerase chain reaction assay.
  in shunt infections, 1233
  for smallpox, 3979
  for Streptococcus agalactiae (group B), 2661
  for syphilis, 3048
  for Toxoplasma gondii, 1271, 3508
  for Tropheryma whipplei, 1438-1439
  for Trypansoma cruzi, 3486
  in tuberculous pleural effusion, 921
Polymicrobial bacterascites, in peritonitis, 1014
Polymorphic ventricular tachycardia, from erythromycin, 431
Polymorphisms, 299
  bacterial infections and, 2539
  in severe sepsis, 995
  single nucleotide, in human genome sequence, 49, 55
Polymorphonuclear neutrophils, 41, 101
  in urethral specimen, 1485-1486
Polymyalgia rheumatica, fever of unknown origin in, 787
Polymyositis
  in HIV infection, 1715
  from HTLV, 2315
Polymyxin B, 469-470, 528, 528t, 706t-709t
  dosage of, 728t-729t
  drug interactions with, 742t-761t
  for nosocomial pneumonia, 3718t
  resistance to, 290-291, 291t
Polymyxin E. See Colistin.
Polyneuropathy. See also Neuropathy.
  critical illness, in sepsis, 998
  distal sensory, in HIV infection, 1756

Polyneuropathy (Continued)
  inflammatory demyelinating, in HIV infection, 1755-1756
Polyomaviruses, 2051-2058. See also BK virus; JC virus.
  detection of, 259t-260t
  diseases associated with, 2052-2056, 2053t
  genomic map of, 2051, 2052f
  history of, 2051
  new human, 2052
  in solid organ transplant recipients, 3848
Polyphenon E
  for condylomata acuminata, 2043
  for genital warts, 670t, 674
Polyproteins, in hepatitis C virus, 2157, 2158f
Polyradiculitis, 1237
Polyradiculopathy, cytomegalovirus, in HIV infection, 1758, 1976
Polysaccharide(s), capsular
  of gram-negative anaerobic rods, 3113
  impact of, on host immunity, 3291
  of meningococcus, 2737-2738, 2738t
  of Staphylococcus aureus, 2544t
Polysaccharide antigen, cryptococcal, serologic tests for, 3297-3298
Polysaccharide capsule, in bacterial meningitis, 1196
Polyserositis, tuberculous, 3154
Polytetrafluoroethylene graft infection, in hemodialysis patients, 1135-1136, 1136t
Pontiac fever, 2969. See also Legionnaires' disease.
  clinical presentation of, 2976
  history of, 2969
  pathogenesis of, 2972
  patterns of, 2974
Population
  per-protocol, in clinical trials, 694
  at risk, 179-180
Pore-forming toxins, 33
PORF polyproteins, of hepatitis E virus, 2411, 2412f
Porins, in Neisseria gonorrhoeae, 2754-2755, 2754f
Pork tapeworms, 3608t, 3609f, 3610
Porphyria cutanea tarda, HCV-related, 2168
Porphyromonas
  antibiotic sensitivities of, 3117t
  dental caries from, 856, 856t
  microbiology of, 3111-3112, 3112t
Porphyromonas gingivalis, virulence factors associated with, 3087, 3087t
Portable steam sterilizers, 3686
Posaconazole, 558-559, 706t-709t
  for aspergillosis, 3251-3253, 3251t
  for Blastomyces dermatitidis infection, 3330
  for brain abscess, 1274t
  for chromoblastomycosis, 3279
  for Coccidioides infection, 3340-3341
  dosage of, 736t-737t
  drug interactions with, 556t, 742t-761t
  formulations of, 717t
  for mucormycosis, 3265-3266
  for Paracoccidioides brasiliensis infection, 3361
  prophylactic
    for cancer-related infections, 3800t
    in transplant recipients, 3816
  for Pseudallescheria boydii infection, 3365-3366
  structure of, 550f-551f
Positron emission tomography
  in fever of unknown origin, 785
  fluorodeoxyglucose, in prosthetic joint infections, 1470-1471
  in prosthetic vascular graft infection, 1134, 1134t
  in toxoplasmosis, 3510
Postantibiotic effect, 304-305
Postcataract endophthalmitis, acute, 1553, 1554f
Postgonococcal urethritis, 1489. See also Urethritis.
Postherpetic neuralgia, 1966
Postinfection syndromes, foodborne disease and, 1416
Postinfective tropical malabsorption, in travelers, 4025-4026
Post-Lyme disease syndrome, 3076
Postoperative infections. See Surgical site infections; Wound infections.
Postpartum bacteremia, from Streptococcus agalactiae, 2659
Postpartum endometritis, 1511-1513, 1512f

Postpartum fever of undetermined origin, 1513
Postpartum sepsis, from *Haemophilus influenzae*, nontypeable, 2913
Postpoliomyelitis syndrome, 2348
Post-Q fever fatigue syndrome, 2516-2517
Poststreptococcal autoimmune neuropsychiatric disorders associated with streptococci (PANDAS), 2615
Potassium iodide, saturated solution of, for sporotrichosis, 3274
Pott's disease, 1464, 3155-3156, 3155f
Pott's paraplegia, 3156
Poverty, HIV infection and, 1627
Povidone-iodine
  disinfection with, 521, 522t
  prophylactic, for catheter-related infections, 524-525
Powassan encephalitis, 1251t-1252t, 2148, 3658-3659, 3659t
Poxvirus(es)
  detection of, 259t-260t
  molluscum contagiosum as, 1934-1935, 1934f
  orthopoxvirus as, 1923-1932
  parapoxvirus as, 1933-1934
  yatapoxvirus as, 1935
Poxvirus inclusion bodies, 3979
Poxvirus vectors, for HIV vaccines, 1888-1889, 1891
Praziquantel, 706t-709t
  for cysticercosis, 3613
  for liver flukes, 3601
  for lung flukes, 3603
  for parasitic infections, 632t-635t, 659-660
  for schistosomiasis, 3596t, 3599-3600
  for tapeworms, 3611
Prealbumin, in nutritional assessment, 151, 152t
Preauricular adenopathy, 1531
Preauricular lymph node, in *Mycobacterium avium* complex lymphadenopathy, 3182, 3182f
Prebiotics, 161, 162t. *See also* Probiotics.
Prednisolone, for tuberculous meningitis, 618-619
Prednisone
  for aphthous esophageal ulceration, 1355t, 1356
  for cryptococcal meningitis, 3299-3300
  for histoplasmosis, 3316
  for Kawasaki syndrome, 3665
  for leprosy reversal reactions, 3173
  for Marshall's syndrome, 1327
  for myocarditis, 1160
  for ocular syphilis, 1567
  for *Pneumocystis jirovecii* pneumonia, 618
  for rheumatic fever, 2616t
  for tuberculous meningitis, 3154
  for tuberculous pericarditis, 1164-1165
  for varicella-zoster virus infection, 1967
Preemptive therapy, 689
Pregnancy
  acute fatty liver of, 1588
  antimicrobial agents in, 270
  arenavirus infection in, 2299
  bacterial vaginosis in, 1504
  bacteriuria in, 975-976
  Blastomyces dermatitidis in, 3327
  cephalosporins in, 333
  Chlamydia trachomatis in, 2454-2455
  cytomegalovirus infection in, 1983-1984, 1984t
  donovanosis in, 3011
  ectopic, from *Chlamydia trachomatis*, 2454
  giardiasis in, 3532
  hepatitis A infection in, 2377
  hepatitis B infection in, chronic, 1602
  hepatitis E infection in, 1585, 2416-2417
  herpes simplex virus infection in, 1954-1955, 1955t
    clinical course of, 1955
    prevention of, 1955-1956
  Histoplasma capsulatum in, 3317
  HIV infection in, 1678
    antiretroviral naivety and, 1791-1794
    fetal and maternal monitoring and, 1794-1795
    impact of, 1787-1788
    management of, 1789
      in antepartum period, 1789-1791, 1790t, 1792t-1793t
      in intrapartum period, 1795
    nutritional support in, 156

Pregnancy (*Continued*)
  outcome of, 1788
  transmission of, 1785-1796
    antiretroviral therapy for, 1788
      discontinuation of, 1794
      potential mechanisms of, 1788-1789
      recommended guidelines on, 1789
      teratogenicity of, 1795
    postpartum follow-up in, 1795-1796
    risk factors for, 1785-1787, 1785t
    timing of, 1785
  Listeria monocytogenes in, 2709
  malaria in, 3442, 3453
  measles virus in, 2232
  metronidazole in, 422-423
  Neisseria gonorrhoeae infection in, 2761-2762
  nitrofurantoin in, 517
  Q fever in, 2516
  quinolones in, 504
  rubella in, 2128
  Streptococcus agalactiae (group B) infection in, 2657
  tetracycline in, 389
  toxoplasmosis in, 3506, 3514-3516, 3515f, 3520
  travel during, 4017
  Trichomonas vaginalis infection in, 1500
  trichomoniasis in, 3537
  trimethoprim-sulfamethoxazole in, 482
  tuberculosis in, 3149, 3151
  urinary tract infection in, 975-976
  vaccines in, 3921, 3941
  vancomycin in, 455
Preoptic area, in thermoregulation, 768-769, 768f
Preseptal cellulitis, 1571-1574, 1571f-1573f
President's Emergency Plan for AIDS Relief, 1630
Pressor drugs, for sepsis, 1003
Pressure sores, 1300
  in elderly, 3859
  in spinal cord injury patients, 3854
Presumed ocular histoplasmosis syndrome (POHS), 1566, 3313-3314, 3317
Preterm infants
  complement in, 77
  fluconazole prophylaxis in, 557
  respiratory syncytial virus infection and, 2214
Pretracheal space
  infections of, 864
    mediastinitis from, 1173
  relation of, to cervical fascia, 858, 859f
Prevaccine era
  croup in, 826
  hepatitis A in, 2373-2374, 2373f-2374f
  pertussis in, 2957
Prevacuum sterilizer, high-speed, 3686
Prevalence, 180
Prevention. *See* Disease prevention and control.
Prevotella
  antibiotic sensitivities of, 3117t
  brain abscess from, 1265, 1266f
  microbiology of, 3111-3112, 3112f, 3112t
  virulence factors associated with, 3087t, 3088
Primaquine, 706t-709t
  drug interactions with, 742t-761t
  G6PD deficiency and, 637
  hemolysis from, 637
  for malaria, 636-638, 4014
    nonfalciparum, 3454
  oxidative stress from, 636
  for *Pneumocystis* pneumonia, 632t-635t, 636, 3382
  resistance to, 636
Prion(s), yeast, 2427
Prion disease, 2423-2438
  bovine, 2432, 4002
  chronic wasting disease as, 2432
  Creutzfeldt-Jakob disease as
    decontamination and, 3689
    genetic, 2424f, 2428-2429
    iatrogenic, 2431-2432
    sporadic, 2427-2428, 2431t
    variant, 2429-2431, 2431t
  fatal familial insomnia as, 2428-2429
  Gerstmann-Straussler-Scheinker syndrome as, 2428
  human, 2427-2432
  infectious prions in, 2424-2427, 2424t, 2426t

Prion disease (*Continued*)
  infectiously transmitted, 2429-2432
  kuru as, 2423, 2429
  laboratory diagnosis of, 2432-2434, 2433f
  long-duration, 2429
  molecular biology of, 2423-2427
  prion strains in, 2426, 2426t, 2427f
  in ruminants, 2432
  scrapie as, 2423, 2432
  transfusion-related, 3748
  treatment of, 2434-2435
Prion protein
  in infection susceptibility, 51t, 52, 55
  infectious, 2424-2427, 2424t
  normal, 2423-2424, 2424f, 2424t
PRNP gene
  in genetic Creutzfeldt-Jakob disease, 2424f, 2428
  in infection susceptibility, 51t, 52, 55
  polymorphisms in, 2429
PRO 140, for HIV infection, 21-22
PRO 542, for HIV infection, 21
Probenecid
  drug interactions with, 577
  pharmacokinetics of, 577
  for syphilis, 3047t, 3049-3050
Probiotics, 161-165
  adverse effects of, 164, 164t
  clinical studies of, 161-162, 162t-163t
  Cochrane reviews of, 161-162, 163t
  concerns about, 161, 162t
  future directions in, 164
  for gastrointestinal disease, 670t, 674-675
  with GRAS status, 161, 162t
  mechanisms of action of, 162-164
  for pancreatic infections, 1048
Procaine, 316t
Procalcitonin
  in bacterial meningitis, 1209
  in nosocomial pneumonia, 3720-3721
  in sepsis, 1001
Proctitis
  from *Chlamydia trachomatis*, 2452-2453, 2452t
  from herpes simplex virus, 1949-1950
  from *Neisseria gonorrhoeae*, 1393
Prodigiosin, 2827-2828
Progressive bacterial synergistic gangrene, 1299, 1299f, 1301t
  treatment of, 1300
Progressive outer retinal necrosis, 1563
  in HIV infection, 1860t-1870t
  treatment of, 1567
Progressive polyradiculopathy, in HIV infection, 1758
Proguanil, for malaria, 650
Project BioShield Act (2004), 3958
Properdin, 78t, 81t
  in complement activation, 80
  deficiency of, 89, 89t, 169t-170t
Prophylaxis
  definition of, in clinical trial, 688-689
  preemptive, 689
  secondary, 689
Propionibacterium, 3125-3126
Propionibacterium acnes, 526-527. *See also* Acne vulgaris.
  endophthalmitis from, 1555, 1565
    visual outcome after, 1558
Prostaglandin(s), in cryptosporidiosis, 3550
Prostaglandin E$_2$, in febrile response, 769
Prostate
  abscess of, 1523-1524, 1524f
    in melioidosis, 2872-2873, 2875f
  Cryptococcus neoformans infection of, 3293t, 3295-3296
Prostatic antibacterial factor, 1521
Prostatitis, 1521-1524
  acute bacterial, 1521-1522
  asymptomatic inflammatory, 1523
  from *Blastomyces dermatitidis*, 3326
  from *Chlamydia trachomatis*, 2451-2452, 2452t
  chronic
    with chronic pelvic pain syndrome, 1522-1523
    in urethritis, 1490
  chronic bacterial, 1522
  classification of, 1521-1524, 1522t

Prostatitis *(Continued)*
  granulomatous, 1523
  in HIV infection, 1525-1526
  host defenses against, 1521
  quinolones for, 495
Prosthetic heart valve
  choice of, 1116-1117
  infections of, endocarditis in, 1113-1126. *See also*
    Endocarditis, prosthetic valve.
Prosthetic joint infections, 1469-1474
  bacteriology of, 1469, 1470t
  clinical presentation in, 1470, 1470t
  diagnosis of, 1470-1471, 1471f, 1471t
  pathogenesis of, 1469-1470, 1470t
  prevention of, 1473
  quinolones for, 500
  from *Staphylococcus aureus*, 2573
  suppressive antibiotic therapy for, 1472-1473
  treatment of, 1471-1472
Prosthetic vascular graft infections, 1132-1135
  clinical manifestations of, 1133
  diagnosis of, 1133-1134, 1134t
  epidemiology of, 1132
  in hemodialysis patients, 1135-1136, 1136t
  management of, 1134-1135, 1134t-1135t
  microbiology of, 1133, 1133f
  pathogenesis of, 1132
  prevention of, 1135
  risk factors for, 1132-1133, 1133t
Prostitutes, HIV infection in, 1638-1639, 4015
Prostration, in malaria, 3449
Protease inhibitors, 1838-1839, 1839f, 1840t
  3C, for rhinovirus infections, 2397
  for AIDS dementia, 1748
  drug interactions with, 742t-761t
  for HIV-infected children, 1820t-1823t
  initial therapy with, 1846
  oral contraceptives and, pharmacokinetic
    interaction between, 1800, 1800t
  penetration-effectiveness scores of, 1749t
  pharmacodynamics of, 305
Proteases, of *Pseudomonas aeruginosa*, 2843-2844
Protective antigen, of *Bacillus anthracis*, 30,
  2715
Protein(s). *See also specific protein.*
  acute-phase, 770, 771t
  antimicrobial, 37, 39t
  in cerebrospinal fluid, 1185-1186, 1185t
  iron-binding, 40
  penicillin-binding, 2558
Protein binding, 299
  of antimicrobial agents, 271
Protein C, activated
  in acute-phase response, 991
  for severe sepsis, 1004
Protein synthesis inhibitors, *Staphylococcus aureus*
  resistance to, 2561
Protein-energy malnutrition, 151-152
Proteinuria
  in endocarditis, 1077
  in urinary tract infection, 967
Proteus, brain abscess from, 1265
Proteus mirabilis, 2828
Proteus vulgaris, 2828
Prothionamide, for leprosy, 546
Proton pump inhibitors, for *Helicobacter pylori*
  infection, 2809, 2809t
Prototheca, 3373, 3373f, 3374t
Protozoa, classification of, 3409-3410, 3409t
Protozoal infections, 3409-3410. *See also specific*
  infection.
  abdominal pain and/or diarrhea with eosinophilia
    from, 1407t, 1409
  brain abscess from, 1266-1267
  clinical syndromes caused by, 3410, 3410t
  diagnostic tests for, 3410, 3410t
  geographic distribution of, 3409t
  meningitis from
    adjunctive therapy for, 1221-1222
    antimicrobial therapy for, 1220
    clinical features of, 1207
    diagnosis of, 1210-1211
    epidemiology and etiology of, 1193-1194
  tick-borne, 3656-3657
  transmission of, 3409t

Protozoal infections *(Continued)*
  in transplant recipients, 3812t
  travelers diarrhea from, 1366
Providencia infection, carbapenems for, 342t
Providencia rettgeri, 2829
Providencia stuartii, 2828-2829
Provider and health care system response, to
  bioterrorist attack, 3957-3960
Provirus, 1912
Pruritus
  of cholestasis, rifamycins for, 412
  in enterobiasis, 3584
  in genital lesions, 1476
Pseudallescheria boydii, 3365-3366, 3366f, 3374t. *See*
  also Scedosporium apiospermum.
  brain abscess from, 1266
  mycetoma from, 3281-3282, 3282t, 3283f
Pseudoappendicitis, from *Campylobacter jejuni*, 2797
Pseudobuboes
  in donovanosis, 3011
  in granuloma inguinale, 1326
Pseudocowpox virus, 1933
Pseudocyst, pancreatic, 1046t, 1047
Pseudoerysipelas, 1295-1296
Pseudoinfection, from *Bacillus* spp., 2727-2728
Pseudolymphangitis, 1331
Pseudomembranous colitis
  from *Clostridium difficile*, 1375-1387
    clinical manifestations of, 1379
    diagnosis of, 1377f, 1380-1382, 1381t
    endoscopy in, 1381
    epidemic strains in, 1379
    epidemiology of, 1378-1379, 1378t
    factors contributing to, 1378
    inciting agents for, 1378, 1378t
    microbiology of, 1376-1377
    pathogenesis of, 1376-1377
    pathology of, 1379-1380, 1380f
    prevention of, 1384
    recurrent, 1383-1384
    reservoirs of, 1378-1379
    treatment of, 1382-1383, 1382t
  from erythromycin, 431
  historical overview of, 1375-1376, 1376f-1377f
  treatment of
    teicoplanin in, 458
    vancomycin in, 457
Pseudomonas, 3016t-3017t, 3025
  endocarditis from, 1092-1093
  exotoxins of, 30
  laboratory detection of, 240t-242t
  skin lesions from, 798-799
Pseudomonas aeruginosa, 2835-2860
  adherence of, 2842-2843
  anatomic and physiologic barriers to, 2837-2838
  antibiotic resistance to, 2856-2857
  antimicrobial combination therapy for, 274
  arthritis from, 1444, 1444t
  bacteremia from, 1303-1304, 2848-2850, 2849f
  biofilm formation by, quorum sensing and,
    2846-2847
  blepharoconjunctivitis from, 1569
  bloodstream dissemination of, 2847-2848
  bone and joint infections from, 2852
  brain abscess from, 1267-1268
  burn wound infections from, 2854
  central nervous system infections from, 2852
  chronic respiratory tract infections from, 2851
  clinical manifestations of, 2848-2857
  colonization by, 2837, 2842-2843
  community-acquired, 2836
  in cystic fibrosis, 949
  cystic fibrosis transmembrane regulator in, 2840,
    2841f
  ear infections from, 2853-2854
  endovascular infections from, 2854-2855
  entry of, 2842-2843
  epidemiology of, 2835-2837
  eye infections from, 2852-2853
  in febrile neutropenia, 2855-2856
  flagella of, 2842-2843
  folliculitis from, 1292
  history of, 2835
  in HIV infection, 2856
  iron acquisition by, 2844

Pseudomonas aeruginosa (Continued)
  keratitis from, 1542
  lipopolysaccharide of, 2835, 2836f, 2843
  lung disease from, 2847
  meningitis from, 1212t
  microbiology of, 2835
  morphology of, 2835, 2836f
  multidrug resistant, 2856-2857
    polymyxins for, 469
  nosocomial, 2835-2837
  pathogenesis of, 2837-2848
    bacterial factors in, 2841-2848, 2842t
    host factors in, 2837-2840, 2841f
  peritonitis from, 1016-1018
  pili of, 2842
  pneumonia from, 2847
    acute, 2850-2851
    in HIV infection, 1730-1731
  proteases of, 2843-2844
  quinolone resistance in, 489
  quorum sensing by, 2846-2847
  resistance to
    loss of, 2837-2838
    mechanisms of, 290t
  rifamycins for, 411
  secretion systems of, 2845
  sepsis from, skin lesions in, 798
  skin infections from, 2854
  soft tissue infections from, 2854
  structure of, 2835, 2836f
  tissue spread of, 2847
  toxin production by, 2844-2845
  typing of, 2837
  urinary tract infections from, 2854
  vaccines for, 2848, 2848t
  virulence factors of, 2841-2848, 2842t
  virulence of
    iron acquisition in, 2844
    pyocyanin in, 2845-2846
    quorum sensing and, 2846
    reactive oxygen species in, 2845-2846
Pseudomonas fluorescens, 3025
Pseudomonas luteola, 3025
Pseudomonas putida, device-associated infections
  from, 3697
Pseudomonas quinolone system, 2846
Pseudomonas stutzeri, 3025
Pseudophakic endophthalmitis, chronic, 1555, 1557
Pseudopod formation, by enteropathogenic
  Escherichia coli, 9, 9f
Pseudoterranova, 3618
Psittacosis, 1400t-1401t, 1404, 2463-2465
Psoas abscess, 1319
  in melioidosis, 2874f
Psoas sign, 1059
PTK 0796, 511
Puberty, delayed onset of, in HIV-infected children,
  1814
Pubis, osteomyelitis of, 1516
Public health emergencies of international concern
  (PHEIC), 214, 215f
Public health strategies
  for endemic treponematoses, 3058
  for infectious mononucleosis, 2005
  for *Neisseria gonorrhoeae*, 2766-2767
  for smallpox outbreak, 3980-3981
Public health system, bioterrorism and
  preparedness of, 3959-3960
  response of, 3960-3961
  role of, 3968-3969
Puerperal infection, from *Streptococcus* group C and
  group G, 2676
Pulmonary. *See also* Lung; Respiratory *entries.*
Pulmonary artery catheters, infections of, 3706. *See*
  also Catheter-related infections.
Pulmonary cavities, from *Coccidioides* infection,
  3336, 3337f-3338f, 3341
Pulmonary disease
  chronic obstructive. *See* Chronic obstructive
    pulmonary disease.
  drug-induced, 932-933
  in endocarditis, 1075
  from nontuberculous mycobacteria, 3192-3194,
    3192t-3193t
Pulmonary edema, in malaria, 3441-3442

Pulmonary embolism
  air travel–related, 4016
  in endocarditis, 1075
  pleural effusion and, 918-919, 921
  septic, in injection drug users, 3882-3883, 3883f
  in spinal cord injury patients, 3853-3854
Pulmonary eosinophilia, tropical, 3592
Pulmonary function testing, in chronic pneumonia,
      938
Pulmonary gangrene, 926
Pulmonary hemorrhage, in leptospirosis, 3062
Pulmonary host defenses, 891-893, 893t
  impairment of, 893-894
Pulmonary hypertension, in HIV infection, 1733
Pulmonary infections. See also Pneumonia;
      Respiratory tract infections; specific infection.
  in ascariasis, 3578
  in aspergillosis
    chronic necrotizing, chest radiography in, 942f
    manifestations of, 3247, 3247f-3248f
    pathogenesis of, 3244, 3245f
  from Blastomyces dermatitidis, 3320
    acute, 3322, 3324f
    chest radiography in, 3324f-3325f
    chronic/recurrent, 3323-3327, 3324f-3325f
    in HIV infection, 1732
  from Coccidioides
    cavitary, 3336, 3337f-3338f, 3341
    chronic fibrocavitary, 3336, 3341
    diffuse, 3341
    early, 3335-3336, 3336f, 3341
    nodular, 3336, 3336f
  from Cryptococcus neoformans, 3293-3294, 3293t,
      3294f
    chest radiograph of, 3298
    microscopic examination of, 3296, 3297f
  from Histoplasma capsulatum, 3308-3310
    acute primary, 3308-3310, 3309f, 3315-3316
    acute reinfection, 3310
    cavitary, 3310-3311, 3310f, 3316
    chronic, 3310-3311, 3310f
    chronic fibrocavitary, 3351f
    in HIV infection, 1732
  in injection drug users, 3882-3883, 3883f
  from mucormycosis agents, 3261-3262
  from Mycobacterium avium complex
    classification and microbiology of, 3178
    clinical presentation of, 3179-3181, 3180f-3181f
    diagnosis of, 3182-3183
    epidemiology of, 3177
    host immunity to, 3179
    treatment of, 3185-3186, 3185t
  in nocardiosis, 3199, 3200f, 3201, 3202f
  from Paracoccidioides brasiliensis, 3359, 3359f
  in pseudallescheriasis, 3365
  in sarcoidosis, 937f
  from Sporothrix schenckii, 3271-3272, 3273f
  from Staphylococcus aureus, 2571-2572
  in toxoplasmosis, 3501, 3505
Pulmonary infiltrates
  with eosinophilia, 908-909
  in febrile cancer patients, 3805
  localized, 934-937, 935t-936t
Pulmonary infiltration and fibrosis, diffuse,
      935t-936t, 938
Pulpitis, 858-859
Pulse field gel electrophoresis, 180, 249
  in Staphylococcus, 2546, 2580
Pulvinar sign, in Creutzfeldt-Jakob disease,
      2433-2434
Pupil, Argyll Robertson, in ocular syphilis, 3042
Purine nucleoside phosphorylase, deficiency of,
      167-168, 169t-170t
Purpura, 792, 793t, 796-797. See also Rash.
  thrombocytopenic
    idiopathic, in Helicobacter pylori infection, 2808
    thrombotic, in HIV infection, 1720
Purpuric fever, Brazilian, 2916
Pustular eosinophilic folliculitis, 1292
Pustular syphilids, 3039-3040
Pustules. See also Rash.
  in cat-scratch disease, 2999, 2999f
  in gonococcal arthritis, 1447, 1447f
  in melioidosis, 2872f
  in smallpox, 3978, 3979f

Puumala virus, 2291
Pyelonephritis. See also Urinary tract infections.
  from Acinetobacter, 2883
  acute
    antimicrobial agents for, 972-973, 983t
    definition of, 957
    imaging of, 978, 978f-980f, 981-983, 982f
    papillary necrosis in, 957-958, 958f
    pathology of, 957
    in pregnancy, 975
    premature delivery and, 975
  chronic
    definition of, 957
    pathology of, 957, 958f
  emphysematous, 973, 973f, 976-977, 979-980
  hemolysis role in, 961
  in kidney transplant recipients, 3840-3841
  renal function in, 967
  symptoms of, 966
  uncomplicated, nitrofurantoin for, 516
  xanthogranulomatous, 976-977, 980-981, 981f
Pyochelin, 2844
Pyocyanin, in Pseudomonas aeruginosa virulence,
      2845-2846
Pyoderma. See also specific type.
  primary, 1289-1300
    subcutaneous abscess in, 1309-1310
  quinolones for, 500
  from Streptococcus pyogenes, 2600, 2600f
  topical antibacterials for, 526
Pyogenic abscess
  hepatic
    clinical presentation in, 1037, 1037t
    diagnosis of, 1037-1038
    from epidemic Klebsiella pneumoniae infection,
        1036-1037
    epidemiology/etiology of, 1035
    microbiology of, 1036, 1036t
    pathogenesis and pathophysiology of,
        1035-1036, 1036t
    treatment of, 1038-1039, 1038f, 1039t
  intra-abdominal, versus enteric fever, 1400t-1401t,
      1404
Pyomyositis, 1313-1316
  clinical findings in, 1313-1314, 1315f
  diagnosis of, 1315-1316
  differential diagnosis of, 1315
  etiology of, 1314-1315
  in HIV infection, 1715
  iliacus, 1319
  in injection drug users, 3878
  pathogenesis of, 1313
  pyriformis, 1319
  from Staphylococcus aureus, 2574-2575
  streptococcal necrotizing, 1316
  treatment of, 1316
  tropical, 4023f
Pyonephrosis, 979, 980f
Pyothorax-associated lymphoma, 1998-1999
Pyoverdin, 2844
Pyrantel pamoate, 706t-709t
  for ascariasis, 3579-3580
  drug interactions with, 742t-761t
  for enterobiasis, 3584
  for parasitic infections, 660
  for trichuriasis, 3580-3581
Pyrazinamide, 706t-709t
  adverse reactions to, 537
  for brain abscess, 1274t
  dosage of, 734t-735t
  drug interactions with, 538
  formulations of, 717t
  for tuberculosis, 534t, 536-538, 537t, 3144-3145,
      3145t, 3149
Pyrethrin, for mite prophylaxis, 3647
Pyridoxine, 153
Pyriformis pyomyositis, 1319
Pyrimethamine, 706t-709t
  for brain abscess, 1274t
  for Isospora belli infection, 3563
  for parasitic infections, 632t-635t, 650-651
  prophylactic, in transplant recipients, 3816
  for Toxoplasma encephalitis, 1750-1751
  for toxoplasmosis, 3517
    congenital, 3520

Pyrimethamine (Continued)
  in HIV infection, 3518, 3518t
    ocular, 3519-3520
Pyrimethamine-sulfadiazine, for toxoplasmosis, 477
Pyrimethamine-sulfadoxine, 706t-709t
Pyrogenic exotoxins, 33
Pyrogens
  endogenous, 769-770, 770f, 772
  exogenous, 769
Pyroguanil, 706t-709t
Pyrrole-LL-3858, for tuberculosis, 542
Pyuria
  in bacteriuria, 967, 973-974
  from urethritis, 969
  in urinary tract infection, 3728

Q
Q fever, 2511-2519, 3654-3655
  clinical manifestations of, 2512-2517
  endocarditis in, 2511, 2512f, 2515-2516, 2515f
    treatment of, 2515-2516
  epidemiology of, 2511-2512
  fatigue syndrome after, 2516-2517
  febrile illness in, 2512
  hepatitis in, 1588, 2516
  in immunocompromised hosts, 2516
  in infants, 2516
  neurologic manifestations of, 2516
  osteomyelitis in, 2516
  pathogenesis of, 2512
  pneumonia in, 2512-2515, 2513f-2514f
    diagnosis of, 2514
    treatment of, 2514
  in pregnancy, 2516
  prevention of, 2517
  rifamycins for, 412
  transmission of, 2511
  vaccine for, 2517
QT interval prolongation
  from quinolones, 503-504
  from voriconazole, 558
Quadriplegia fever, 3851-3852
Quality improvement programs, infection control
      programs and, 3671-3672
Quantiferon-TB Gold test, 3138
Quantitative immunocapture assays, in HIV
      infection, 1670
Quarantine, 188
Quaternary ammonium compounds, disinfection
      with, 3684
Queensland tick typhus, 3653-3654, 3653t
Queyrat, erythroplasia of, 2040
Quinacrine, 706t-709t
  drug interactions with, 742t-761t
  for giardiasis, 3531, 3531t
  for parasitic infections, 660
Quinidine
  for malaria, 3452t, 3453-3454
  mechanism of action of, 3447
  for parasitic infections, 660
Quinine
  plus doxycycline, for malaria, 3451, 3452t
  drug interactions with, 742t-761t
  mechanism of action of, 3447
  for parasitic infections, 660
  resistance to, 3447
Quinine dihydrochloride, for malaria, 3452t, 3454
Quinine gluconate, for malaria, 632t-635t
Quinine sulfate, 706t-709t
  for malaria, 632t-635t
Quinolones, 487-510
  for acute pyelonephritis, 972-973
  adverse reactions to, 503-504, 540
  for anaerobic infections, 3089
  antimicrobial activity of, 490-491, 491t-492t
  for bacillary dysentery, 2908-2909, 2909t
  for bone and joint infections, 499-500
  in children, 269, 503
  in combination, 491
  distribution of, 493, 493t
  dosage of, 493-494, 493t, 732t-733t
  drug interactions with, 494, 742t-761t
  in elderly, 3861-3862
  elimination of, 493

Quinolones (Continued)
  for Enterococcus, 2651
  formulations of, 716t
  for gastrointestinal and abdominal infections, 496-497
  healing process of, on fractures, 1457
  for leprosy, 3172
  for lower urinary tract infection, 973
  mechanism of action of, 487-488
  for Mycoplasma pneumoniae, 2487
  for Neisseria gonorrhoeae infection, 2764-2765
  Neisseria gonorrhoeae resistance to, 2759
  for nontuberculous mycobacterial infections, 544
  for parasitic infections, 660
  for pelvic inflammatory disease, 1518
  for peritonitis, 1022t, 1025, 1029t
  pharmacology of, 491-494, 492t, 732t-733t
  for pneumonia, 910-912
  postantibiotic effect in, 491
  in pregnancy, 504
  prophylactic
    in transplant recipients, 3815
    for traveler's diarrhea, 4015
  for prostatitis, 495
  for psittacosis, 2465
  resistance to, 502-503
    efflux promotion in, 287
    mechanisms of, 489-490
    target enzyme alteration in, 289
    target site protection in, 289
  for respiratory tract infections, 497-499
  for sexually transmitted diseases, 495-496
  for skin and soft tissue infections, 500
  Staphylococcus aureus resistance to, 2559t, 2561-2562
  structure of, 487, 488f
  topical, for keratitis, 1543-1544
  for tuberculosis, 537t, 540-541, 3144
  for tularemia, 2935
  for typhoid fever, 2898, 2898t
  for urethritis, 1490
  for urinary tract infection, 495
  uses of, 495-502
Quinupristin-dalfopristin, 459-462, 706t-709t
  administration of, 461
  adverse reactions to, 461
  antimicrobial activity of, 460
  clinical uses of, 461-462
  distribution and elimination of, 461
  dosage of, 461, 728t-729t
  drug interactions with, 461
  for Enterococcus, 2650-2651
  for Enterococcus endocarditis, 1120t
  formulations of, 716t
  mechanism of action of, 459-460
  minimal inhibitory concentration susceptibility for, 460, 460t
  pharmacodynamics and pharmacokinetics of, 461
  resistance to, 460-461
  for Staphylococcus aureus infection, 2562
  Staphylococcus aureus resistance to, 2559t
Quorum sensing, 8
  by Pseudomonas aeruginosa, 2846-2847

R

Rabbit fever. See Tularemia.
Rabies, 2249-2258, 4003
  animal
    clinical manifestations of, 2253, 2253t
    epidemiology of, 2250-2251, 2251f
  clinical manifestations of, 2252-2253, 2252t
  detection of, 259t-260t
  diagnosis of, 2253-2255, 2254f
  differential diagnosis of, 2254-2255
  encephalitis from, 1246t, 1259-1260
  epidemiology of, 2249-2251, 2251f
  furious, 2251-2253, 2252f
  genome of, 2249, 2250t
  history of, 2249
  immune response to, 2252
  myocarditis from, 2252
  paralytic (dumb), 2251-2253
  pathology and pathogenesis of, 2251-2252, 2252f
  prevention of, 2255-2256

Rabies (Continued)
  postexposure, 2255-2256, 2256f
  preexposure, 2255
  replication of, 2249
  treatment of, 2256-2257
  virology of, 2249, 2250f, 2250t
Rabies immune globulin, 2255, 3922t, 3935
Rabies vaccine, 3922t, 3931
  acute disseminated encephalomyelitis from, 2255
  for animals, 2255
  for bite wounds, 3913t
  currently available, 2256
  postexposure, 2255-2256, 2256f
  preexposure, 2255
  for travelers, 4011t, 4013
Raccoons, rabies in, 2250-2251
Race
  chronic pneumonia and, 931
  HAV incidence rate by, 2374-2375, 2374f
  HIV infection and, 1637-1638, 1640-1641
  Neisseria gonorrhoeae infection and, 2758, 2758t
  tuberculosis and, 3132-3133
Racecadotril, for rotavirus gastroenteritis, 2111-2112
Racemose cysticercosis, 3612
Radiation therapy
  for CNS lymphoma, 1772
  to head and neck, complications of, 868
  for Kaposi's sarcoma, 1767
  mucosal barrier injury from, 3785-3786, 3785f
  total body, in hematopoietic stem cell transplant recipients, 3821-3822
Radiculopathy, sacral, from herpes simplex virus, 1950
Radioallergosorbent test, penicilloyl, in beta-lactam allergy, 351
Radiography
  in bacterial meningitis, 1209, 1209f
  chest
    in acute pneumonia, 901-904, 901f-903f
    in anthrax, 3987f
    in blastomycosis, 3323, 3324f-3325f
    in bleomycin-induced pulmonary disease, 937f
    in bronchiolitis obliterans organizing pneumonia (BOOP), 936f
    in chronic fibrocavitary pulmonary histoplasmosis, 938f
    in chronic necrotizing pulmonary aspergillosis, 942f
    in chronic pneumonia, 934, 935t-936t
    in coccidioidomycosis, 939f
    in croup, 827, 827f
    in histoplasmosis, 3309-3311, 3309f-3310f
    in HIV infection, 1728, 1729t
    in human metapneumovirus, 2225f
    in lung abscess, 926, 927f
    in lymphangioleiomyomatosis, 937f
    in mediastinitis, 1176, 1176f
    in miliary tuberculosis, 944f
    in Mycobacterium avium complex tuberculosis, 938f
    in nocardiosis, 940f
    in paracoccidioidomycosis, 3359, 3359f
    in pleural effusion, 919, 919f
    in pneumococcal pneumonia, 2631
    in Pneumocystis pneumonia, 3381-3382, 3382f
    in psittacosis, 2464
    in pulmonary aspergillosis, 3247, 3247f
    in pulmonary blastomycosis, 943f
    in pulmonary cryptococcosis, 3298
    in pulmonary Mycobacterium avium complex disease, 3180, 3180f
    in pulmonary sarcoidosis, 937f
    in Q fever pneumonia, 2513, 2513f
    in Rhodococcus equi pneumonia, 941f
    in sporotrichosis, 3271-3272, 3273f
    in tuberculosis, 940f, 3139f, 3141f-3142f, 3143
    in tularemia pneumonia, 2933-2934, 2934f
    in Wegener's granulomatosis, 943f
  in intraperitoneal abscess, 1030
  in prosthetic joint infections, 1470, 1471f
  in sinusitis, 844
Radioimmunoassay, 64-65
Radioimmunoprecipitation assay, in HIV infection, 1674-1675
Radionuclide cholescintigraphy, 1040

Radionuclide scanning, in fever of unknown origin, 785
Ralstonia, 3016t-3017t, 3025-3026
Ralstonia pickettii, 3026
Raltegravir, 706t-709t, 1843f, 1843t, 1844
  dosage of, 740t-741t
  drug interactions with, 742t-761t
  formulations of, 717t
  for HIV-infected children, 1820t-1821t
Ramoplanin, 512-513, 706t-709t
Randomization, in clinical trials, 690-691
Rapamycin, for transplant immunosuppression, infections and, 3811
Rapid antigen detection tests, for streptococcal pharyngitis, 819, 2597-2598
Rapid plasma reagin test, for syphilis, 3045
Rapid tests
  for HIV infection, 1669-1670, 1818
  for influenza, 2276-2277
  for malaria, 3448
  for syphilis, 3048
Rash, 791-807. See also Exanthem(s); Skin lesions.
  in acrodermatitis chronica atrophicans, 801
  in alphavirus infection, 2120-2121, 2123
  from ampicillin, in infectious mononucleosis, 1993-1994, 1994f
  in anaplasmosis, 803
  approach to patient with, 791-792, 793t
  in Arcanobacterium haemolyticum infection, 816, 2700, 2700f
  in bartonellosis, 803
  in beta-lactam allergy, 347
  in Borrelia burgdorferi infection, 801
  in candidiasis, 801-802
  in Capnocytophaga canimorsus infection, 801
  in Capnocytophaga infection, 2992
  in cat-scratch disease, 803
  in cytomegalovirus infection, 1975
  in dengue hemorrhagic fever, 2144
  in dermatophytosis, 3351
  diaper, from Candida, 3230, 3230f
  differential diagnosis of, 794t
  diffuse erythematous, 795
  in ecthyma gangrenosum, 798-799
  in eczema vaccinatum, 803
  in ehrlichiosis, 803
  in endocarditis, 799
  in epidemic typhus, 2522
  in erythema infectiosum, 2089-2090, 2090f
  in erythema marginatum, 795
  in erythema multiforme, 794
  febrile vesicular pustular, differential diagnosis of, 1927, 1928f
  in group A–associated streptococcal pharyngitis, 816
  after hematopoietic stem cell transplantation, 3823
  in herpesvirus infections, 802
  in hookworm, 3581
  in human herpesvirus 6 infection, 802
  in human herpesvirus 7 infection, 802
  in human parvovirus B19 infection, 795
  in Kawasaki syndrome, 3663, 3664f
  lesion characteristics of, 792-797, 793t
  in Lyme disease, 801
  maculopapular, 792-795, 793t
  in malaria, 797
  in measles, 2231, 2231f
  in Menangle virus infections, 2242-2243
  in meningococcemia, 798
    petechial, 2741-2743, 2741f-2742f
    rubella-like, 2737, 2743f
  in monkeypox, 803-804
  in murine typhus, 2526
  in Mycoplasma pneumoniae infection, 2483, 2483f
  in Neisseria gonorrhoeae infection, 798
  in Neisseria meningitidis infection, 798, 2741-2743, 2741f
  in orthopoxvirus infections, 803-804
  pathogenesis of, 792
  pathogens associated with, 793t, 796t, 797-802
  petechial, 793t, 796-797
  in Pseudomonas infections, 798-799
  purpuric, 793t, 796-797
  from quinolones, 503
  in rat-bite fever, 2965-2967

Rash (Continued)
  in rickettsial infections, 801
  in rickettsialpox, 2509
  from rifamycins, 406-407
  in Rocky Mountain spotted fever, 801, 2502,
      2502f, 3653-3654, 3654f
  in rubella, 2128
  rubelliform, in CMV mononucleosis, 1975
  in scarlet fever, 800, 2596
  in scrub typhus, 2529
  in sepsis, 797-798
  in smallpox, 803, 3978, 3978f-3979f
  in staphylococcal scalded skin syndrome, 799-800
  in staphylococcal toxic shock syndrome, 800, 800t
  in Staphylococcus aureus infections, 799-800
  in Stevens-Johnson syndrome, 792, 794-795
  in streptococcal infections, 800
  in streptococcal toxic shock syndrome, 800, 800t
  in Streptococcus pyogenes infections, 799-800
  in strongyloidiasis, 3582
  in syphilis, 795
  in tick-borne disease, 796-797, 803
  in toxic epidermal necrolysis, 792, 794-795
  in travelers, 4023f, 4026, 4027f
  in tularemia, 2934
  vesicobullous, 793t, 795-796
  in viral hemorrhagic fever, 802
  in West Nile virus infection, 792-794
Rasmussen's aneurysm, 3142-3143
Rat(s), plague from, 2944
Rat mites, 3645
Rat-bite fever, 2965-2968, 2966t
  clinical manifestations of, 2965-2966
  diagnosis of, 2966
  versus enteric fever, 1400t-1401t, 1403
  epidemiology of, 2965
  from Spirillum minus, 2966-2967, 2966t
  from Streptobacillus moniliformis, 2965, 2966t
  treatment of, 2966
Rattus norvegicus, Seoul virus infection from, 2291
Ravuconazole, 559, 706t-709t
  for aspergillosis, 3251-3252, 3251t
Raynaud phenomenon
  cold agglutinins and, 2485
  in Mycoplasma pneumoniae, 2483f, 2484
Reactive arthritis, 1448. See also Reiter's syndrome.
Reactive nitrogen species, in bacterial meningitis,
    1203-1204
Reactive oxygen species
  in bacterial meningitis, 1203-1204
  in Pseudomonas aeruginosa virulence, 2845-2846
Reactive polyarthritis, in Yersinia enterocolitica
    infection, 2951
Receptor-mediated endocytosis, 1911, 1911f
Recombinant immunoblot, for hepatitis C,
    2168-2169
Recreational spas, bacterial contamination of, 2980
Recreational water. See also Water entries.
  contaminated, Cryptosporidium in, 3549
Rectal temperature, 765-766
Rectum, Neisseria gonorrhoeae infection of, 2760
  in neonates, 2763
  treatment of, 2764t
Red blood cell transfusions, bacterial infections from,
    3747
Red cell aplasia, pure, from parvovirus B19,
    2090-2091
Red chicken mites, 3645, 3646f
Red eye, differential diagnosis of, 1537
Red man syndrome, from vancomycin, 454
Reduction-modifiable protein, in Neisseria
    gonorrhoeae, 2754-2755, 2754f
Reflux nephropathy, 969
Regramostim, 614
Reiter's syndrome
  versus bacterial arthritis, 1448
  from Chlamydia trachomatis, 2453
  in HIV infection, 1715
  urethritis in, 1491-1492
    clinical features of, 1492
    laboratory features of, 1492
    treatment of, 1492
Relapsing fever, 3067-3069
  clinical manifestations of, 3068, 3068t
  diagnosis of, 3068

Relapsing fever (Continued)
  versus enteric fever, 1400t-1401t, 1403
  epidemiology of, 3067
  etiology of, 3067
  louse-borne, 3067
  pathophysiology of, 3067-3068
  prevention of, 3069
  tick-borne, 3067, 3651t-3652t, 3652
  transmission of, 3067
  treatment of, 3068-3069
    Jarisch-Herxheimer reaction in, 3069
Relative risk, 180-181, 181f
Remediation, after terrorist-associated anthrax
    contamination, 3990-3991, 3991t
Renal. See also Kidney entries.
Renal biopsy, in BK virus-associated nephropathy,
    2056, 2056f
Renal clearance, 300
Renal disease
  complement in, 94
  in endocarditis, 1074
  end-stage, in tuberculosis, treatment of, 3149
  in HIV infection, 1718-1719
  in HIV-infected children, 1816
  from rifamycins, 406
Renal function, age and, 269
Renal insufficiency
  aminoglycosides in, 375-377, 375t, 378t
  antimicrobial agents in, 270-271
    dosage adjustment for, 705
  antituberculous agents in, 534t
  cephalosporins in, 331, 332t
  chloramphenicol in, 396
  in leptospirosis, 3061-3062
  in malaria, 3449
  in mumps, 2203
  quinolones in, 493-494, 493t
  in sepsis, 999
  tetracycline in, 389-390, 391t
  in urinary tract infection, 967
  vancomycin in, 453-454, 454t
  in visceral leishmaniasis, 3468
Renal scarring, vesicoureteral reflux and, 969
Renal scintigraphy, in urinary tract infection, 980,
    980f
Reolysin, 2097-2098
Reoviruses, 2097-2098
  apoptosis induced by, 1913, 1913f
Research study designs, types of, 688, 688t
Reservoirs
  for plague, 2949
  for zoonoses, 4002, 4002t, 4005-4006
Resiquimod, 585-586, 585f
Resistance island staphylococcal chromosome
    cassette mec, 2558
Respiratory burst. See Oxidative (respiratory) burst.
Respiratory distress
  acute
    methylprednisolone for, 619
    severe. See Severe acute respiratory syndrome
        (SARS).
  in malaria, 3441-3442, 3449
Respiratory isolation precautions, in emergency
    preparedness, 225, 226f
Respiratory muscle paralysis, in poliomyelitis, 2347
Respiratory papillomatosis, recurrent. See
    Papillomatosis, recurrent respiratory.
Respiratory support, for peritonitis, 1026-1027
Respiratory syncytial virus, 2207-2221
  in animals, 2208
  antigenic variation in, 2208-2209
  bronchiolitis from, 885, 886t
  characteristics of, 2207-2208, 2208f
  in chronic obstructive pulmonary disease, 878-879
  classification of, 2207
  clinical manifestations of, 2211-2213, 2212f,
      2213t-2214t
  complications of, 2213-2216
    acute, 2215
    in immunocompromised hosts, 2214-2215
    long-term, 2215-2216
    risk factors for, 2213-2215
  croup from, 825-826, 826f
  detection of, 259t-260t
  diagnosis of, 2216

Respiratory syncytial virus (Continued)
  epidemiology of, 2208-2209
  genome of, 2207, 2208f
  in hematopoietic stem cell transplant recipients,
      3830
  history of, 2207
  immune response to, 2210-2211, 2210f
  incidence and prevalence of, 2209
  infection control for, 2217, 2217t
  nosocomial, prevention of, 2217, 2217t
  in older children and adults, 2212-2213,
      2213t-2214t
  otitis media from, 2212
  pathogenesis of, 2209-2211
  pertussis coinfection with, 2958
  prevention of, 2217-2218, 2217t
  seasonal occurrence of, 2208
  in solid organ transplant recipients, 3847-3848
  treatment of, 2216-2217
    motavizumab in, 2218
    palivizumab in, 618, 2217-2218
    ribavirin in, 566t-567t, 595
  vaccine for, 2218
  in young children, 2211-2212, 2212f
Respiratory syncytial virus immune globulin, 3936
Respiratory tract
  deposition of Bacillus anthracis spores in,
      3984-3985, 3985f
  Haemophilus influenzae colonization of,
      2911-2912
  in host defense, 40
  Kingella colonization of, 2774-2775
  Moraxella catarrhalis colonization of, 2771
  in peritonitis, 1020
Respiratory tract infections. See also Pneumonia;
    Pulmonary infections; specific infection.
  from Acinetobacter, 2882-2883
  acute, 200-205
  from adenoviruses, 2028-2029
  from Bacillus spp., 2729
  bacterial, in HIV infection, 1860t-1870t
  from Candida, 3232
  from Chlamydophila pneumoniae, 2470-2474,
      2470t-2471t
  chronic, from Pseudomonas aeruginosa, 2851
  from coronaviruses, 2187, 2188f
    clinical manifestations of, 2191, 2191t
    epidemiology of, 2189
    laboratory diagnosis of, 2192
    multiple sclerosis and, 2192
    pathogenesis of, 2190-2191
    SARS and, 2187. See also Severe acute
        respiratory syndrome (SARS).
    vaccines for, 2192
  from Corynebacterium diphtheriae, 2690-2691,
      2690f
  from enteroviruses, 2355-2356
  in hematopoietic stem cell transplant recipients,
      3830
  from human bocavirus, 202
  from human metapneumovirus, 201-202
  in immunocompromised hosts, 3788
  from microsporidia, 3398
  from Moraxella catarrhalis, 2772-2773, 2773f
    nosocomial, 2773
  from Neisseria meningitidis, 2744
  nosocomial, 2773
  outbreaks of, 194
  outpatient parenteral antimicrobial therapy for,
      700, 700t
  from Pasteurella, 2940-2941
  quinolones for, 497-499
  from rhinoviruses in, 2394
  from Streptococcus group C and group G, 2676
  in travelers, 4024
  trimethoprim-sulfamethoxazole for, 481
  upper
    laryngitis in, 823-824, 824t
    from rhinoviruses, 2389-2398
  viral
    in COPD exacerbations, 879
    in solid organ transplant recipients, 3847-3848
Respiratory tract specimens
  collection and transport guidelines for, 235t-236t
  laboratory processing of, 238-239

Respiratory viruses
  detection of, 260
  treatment of
    interferon-alfa in, 589-590
    ribavirin in, 595
  vaccines for, for otitis media prophylaxis, 835
Respirovirus, 2195
Restriction fragment length polymorphism, 249
  of *Mycobacterium tuberculosis*, 3131-3132
Retamapulin, 528t, 530-531, 706t-709t
  adverse effects of, 531
  pharmacokinetics of, 530-531
  for pyoderma, 526
Reticular dysgenesis, 167-168, 169t-170t
Reticuloendothelial system, 41
Retina, peripheral, 1561
Retinal necrosis
  acute, 1563, 1563f
    acyclovir for, 1567
    in HIV infection, 1860t-1870t
  progressive outer, 1563, 1567
Retinitis, 1561. See also Chorioretinitis.
  from cytomegalovirus, 1563, 1975-1976, 1975f
    in HIV infection, 1719, 1975
      HAART and, 1721
      treatment of, 1975-1976
    treatment of, 1976
      antiviral agents in, 566t-567t
      cidofovir in, 577
      fomivirsen in, 580
      foscarnet in, 582
      ganciclovir/valganciclovir in, 584
    neurologic, in cat-scratch disease, 3001, 3001f,
      3005
Retinopathy, from HIV infection, 1719
Retroperitoneal space, 1012
Retropharyngeal space
  infections of, 862t, 864
    mediastinitis from, 1173
  lymphadenitis of, 1324
  relation of, to cervical fascia, 858, 859f
Retrovirology, 2323
Retroviruses
  human. See also Human immunodeficiency virus;
    Human T-cell lymphotrophic virus.
    diagnosis of, 1680-1681
    genomic organization of, 2324f
    origin of, 2323-2324
    structure of, 2326-2327, 2326f
    replication of, 2323
    survival advantage of, 2324
Revascularization, in prosthetic vascular graft
  infection, 1134-1135, 1134t-1135t
Reversal reactions, in leprosy, 3169-3170, 3170f
  late, 3173
  treatment of, 3173
Reverse transcriptase–polymerase chain reaction
  assay
  for croup, 825-827
  in HIV-infected children, 1818
  for human metapneumovirus, 2226
  for *Nocardia*, 3203
  for noroviruses, 2403
  for rabies, 2254
  for respiratory syncytial virus, 2216
  for respiratory viruses, 888
  for rhinoviruses, 2395
  for rotaviruses, 2111
Reverse transcription, in HIV replication, 2325
Reye's syndrome, after influenza, 2276
Rh immune globulin, 3936
Rhabdomyolysis
  acute, 1321
  statin-associated, in HIV infection, 1759
Rhabdoviruses, 2249-2258
  characteristics of, 2249, 2250t
  classification of, 2249, 2250t
Rhamnolipids, of *Pseudomonas aeruginosa*, 2845
Rheumatic fever, 2611-2622
  clinical manifestations of, 2613-2615, 2614f-2615f
  diagnosis of, 2615-2616, 2615t
  epidemiology of, 2613
  etiology and pathogenesis of, 2611-2612, 2612t
  history of, 2611
  pathology of, 2612

Rheumatic fever (*Continued*)
  prevention of, 2616-2617, 2617t
    versus endocarditis prophylaxis, 1149
  prognosis in, 2616
  treatment of, 2616, 2616t
Rheumatic heart disease, chronic, 2614, 2614f
Rheumatism, desert, 3335
Rheumatoid arthritis
  versus bacterial arthritis, 1448
  juvenile, fever of unknown origin in, 787
Rheumatoid factors, 72
  in endocarditis, 1073
Rheumatologic disorders, complement in, 94
Rhinocerebral mucormycosis, 1269, 3260-3261,
  3260f-3261f
Rhinoscleroma, from *Klebsiella pneumoniae* subsp.
  rhinoscleromatis, 2827, 2827f
Rhinorrhea, in common cold, 810-811
Rhinosinusitis. See also Sinusitis.
  chronic, 842
  pathogenesis of, 839-840
  viral, 2393. See also Common cold.
Rhinosporidium seeberi, 3372-3373, 3373f, 3374t
Rhinoviruses/rhinovirus infection, 2389-2398
  3C protease inhibitors for, 2397
  acid lability of, 2397
  antigen detection in, 2395
  asthma from, 2394
  bronchiolitis from, 885, 886t
  bronchitis exacerbation from, 2393
  capsid-binding agents for, 2396-2397
  characteristics of, 2390t
  classification of, 2389
  clinical manifestations of, 2393, 2394f
  colds from, 2191, 2191t. See also Common cold.
  complications of, 2393-2394
  croup from, 825-826, 826f
  detection of, 259t-260t
  diagnosis of, 2395
  epidemiology of, 2391
  genome of, 2389-2390
  geographic distribution of, 2391
  historical perspectives on, 2389
  in immunocompromised patients, 2394
  inactivation of, physical and chemical agents in,
    2391
  interferon-alfa for, 2395-2396
  isolation of, 2395, 2396f
    initial, 2389
  laboratory diagnosis of, 2395
  lower respiratory, 2394
  morphology and structure of, 2389-2390, 2390f
  nucleic acid detection in, 2395
  otitis media from, 2393
  pathogenesis of, 2392
  prevalence of, 2391
  prevention of, 2395-2397
  protection against, 2392-2393
  replication of, 2390
  seasonality of, 2391
  serologic assays for, 2395
  sinusitis from, 2393
  specificity of, 2391
  transmission of, 2391
  vaccines for, 2395
  virucidal therapy for, 2397
Rhizobium, 3016t-3017t, 3026
Rhizobium radiobacter, 3026
Rhizopus, 3257, 3258f, 3258t
Rhodococcus, 2702-2704
Rhodococcus equi, 2702-2703
  laboratory detection of, 240t-242t
  pneumonia from, 941f
    in HIV infection, 1731, 1731f
  rifamycins for, 411
Rhodococcus erythropolis, 2703-2704
Rhodococcus fascians, 2703-2704
Rhodococcus rhodochrous, 2703-2704
Rhombencephalitis, from *Listeria monocytogenes*,
  2710, 2711f
Ribavirin, 566t-567t, 593-595, 706t-709t
  activity spectrum of, 593-594
  adverse reactions to, 2174
  for arenaviruses, 2300
  clinical studies of, 595

Ribavirin (*Continued*)
  for Crimean-Congo hemorrhagic fever, 2292
  dosage of, 738t-739t
  drug interactions with, 594-595, 742t-761t
  formulations of, 717t
  for hemorrhagic fever with renal syndrome,
    2292
  for human metapneumovirus infection, 2227
  mechanism of action of, 594
  peginterferon alfa-2a plus, 566t-567t
  pharmacokinetics of, 594
  resistance to, 594
  for respiratory syncytial virus infection, 2216
  for Rift Valley fever, 2292
  structure of, 593f
  toxicity of, 594
Ribavirin–interferon alfa, for hepatitis C infection,
  2173, 2173f
Ribavirin–peginterferon alfa, for hepatitis C
  infection, 2173
  chronic, 1607-1608, 1607t
  response of, 2173-2174, 2173f
Ribosomal binding site alteration, in antimicrobial
  resistance, 287-288
Ribosomes, in *Staphylococcus aureus* resistance, 2561
Rickettsia/rickettsial infections
  bacteriology of, 2495, 2496t
  clinical findings in, 2496, 2498t
  criteria for, 2499
  diagnosis of, 2496
  versus enteric fever, 1400t-1401t, 1404
  epidemiology of, 2495-2496
  genetics of, 2495
  historical perspective on, 2495, 2497t
  pathophysiology of, 2495
  rash in, 801
  spotted fever group, 2499-2507, 3653-3654, 3653t,
    3654f
  in travelers, 4024
  treatment of, 2496
Rickettsia aeschlimanii, 2504-2505
Rickettsia africae, 2504, 4024
Rickettsia akari (rickettsialpox), 240t-242t,
  2509-2510, 2509f, 2509t, 3643, 3646t
Rickettsia australis, 2504
Rickettsia conorii, 2503-2504, 4024
Rickettsia felis, 2504-2505, 2525
Rickettsia heilongjiangensis, 2504
Rickettsia helvetica, 2504-2505
Rickettsia honei, 2504
Rickettsia massilae, 2504-2505
Rickettsia parkeri, 2504
Rickettsia prowazekii, 240t-242t, 2521-2524, 2522f,
  2522t-2523t
Rickettsia rickettsii, 2499. See also Rocky Mountain
  spotted fever.
  isolation of, 2503
  laboratory detection of, 240t-242t
  transmission of, 2500
Rickettsia sibirica, 2503-2504
Rickettsia slovaca, 2504-2505
Rickettsia typhi, 240t-242t, 2525-2528
Rifabutin, 706t-709t
  adverse reactions to, 539
  dosage of, 734t-735t
  drug interactions with, 404, 406t, 539-540, 539t
  formulations of, 717t
  for *Helicobacter pylori* infection, 2809t
  for leprosy, 546
  for *Mycobacterium avium* complex disease,
    3184t-3186t
  for *Mycobacterium kansasii* pulmonary disease
    from, 3193, 3193t
  for nontuberculous mycobacterial infections, 543
  structure of, 405f
  for tuberculosis, 539-540
    in HIV infection, 539t
Rifalazil, 413
Rifampin, 706t-709t. See also Rifamycins.
  adverse reactions to, 535
  antimicrobial activity of, 404t
  for *Bartonella bacilliformis* infection, 3005
  for brain abscess, 1274t
  for brucellosis, 2924
  for *Chlamydophila* respiratory infection, 2471t

Rifampin (Continued)
 dosage of, 734t-735t
 drug interactions with, 404, 406t, 535-536, 536t
 formulations of, 717t
 for Haemophilus influenzae type b prophylaxis, 2915
 for Legionnaires' disease, 2978t
 for leprosy, 545, 3172
 for meningitis, 1213t
 for meningococcal infection, 2746t
 for Mycobacterium avium complex disease, 3184t-3185t
 for Mycobacterium kansasii pulmonary disease from, 3193, 3193t
 for neuroretinitis, 3005
 for nontuberculous mycobacterial infections, 543
 for prosthetic joint infections, 1472
 for prosthetic valve endocarditis, 1122t
 for Q fever pneumonia, 2514
 for scrub typhus, 2530
 for Staphylococcus aureus endocarditis, 2571t
 Staphylococcus aureus resistance to, 2559t
 for Staphylococcus endocarditis, 1118t
 for streptococcal meningitis, 2636
 structure of, 405f
 for tuberculosis, 534t, 535-536, 537t, 3144-3145, 3145t, 3149
  alternatives to, 539-540
  in HIV infection, 535-536, 536t-537t
Rifamycins, 403-417
 adverse reactions to, 404-407
 antimicrobial activity of, 404t
 for brucellosis, 412
 for Burkholderia cepacia infection, 411
 for Chlamydia infection, 411
 for Chlamydophila infection, 411
 for Clostridium difficile infection, 412
 for Cryptosporidium parvum infection, 412
 drug interactions with, 404, 406t, 742t-761t
 for ehrlichiosis, 412
 for enterococcal infection, 410
 for foreign body infection prophylaxis, 410
 for fungal infections, 412
 for Haemophilus influenzae infection, 411
 for Helicobacter pylori infection, 411
 for hepatic encephalopathy, 413
 for inflammatory bowel disease, 413
 for irritable bowel syndrome, 413
 for legionellosis, 411
 mechanism of action of, 403
 for Mediterranean spotted fever, 411
 for meningitis prophylaxis, 411
 for nontuberculous mycobacterial infection, 408
 pharmacology of, 403-404
 for pruritus of cholestasis, 412
 for Pseudomonas aeruginosa infection, 411
 for Q fever, 412
 resistance to, mechanisms of, 403
 for Rhodococcus equi infection, 411
 for small intestinal bacterial overgrowth, 413
 for staphylococcal infection, 408-410
 for streptococcal infection, 410
 structure of, 405f
 for traveler's diarrhea, 412
 for tuberculosis, 407-408
 uses of, 407-413
Rifapentine, 706t-709t. See also Rifamycins.
 dosage of, 734t-735t
 formulations of, 717t
 for leprosy, 546
 structure of, 405f
 for tuberculosis, 407, 540, 3144
Rifaximin, 706t-709t. See also Rifamycins.
 for cryptosporidiosis, 3555
 formulations of, 716t
 structure of, 405f
Rift Valley fever virus, 2289-2292, 2290t
 encephalitis from, 1251t-1252t
Rimantadine, 566t-567t, 573-576, 706t-709t
 activity spectrum of, 573
 dosage of, 738t-739t
 drug interactions with, 575
 formulations of, 717t
 for influenza, 2277-2278, 2277t, 2284
 mechanism of action of, 573

Rimantadine (Continued)
 pharmacokinetics of, 574-575, 574t
 resistance to, 2278
 structure of, 573f
 toxicity of, 575
Ringworm, scalp. See Tinea capitis.
Risk, in epidemiologic studies, 180-181, 181f
Ritonavir, 706t-709t, 1839, 1839f, 1840t
 dosage of, 740t-741t
 drug interactions with, 742t-761t
 formulations of, 717t
 for HIV-infected children, 1820t-1821t, 1823t
Rituximab
 for HIV-related non-Hodgkin's lymphoma, 1770
 for lymphoproliferative disease, 2004
River blindness. See Onchocerciasis.
RNA
 splicing of, in HIV life cycle, 2326-2327, 2327f
 viral, replication of, 2390
rRNA gene, in microsporidia, 3392
16S rRNA gene, in cystic fibrosis patients, 950
RNA glycosidase toxins, 28t
RNA polymerase chain reaction assay. See Reverse transcriptase–polymerase chain reaction assay.
16S rRNA sequence analysis
 of Actinomyces, 3209
 of Nocardia, 3203
Rocio encephalitis, 1251t-1252t, 2152
Rocky Mountain spotted fever, 2499, 3653-3654, 3653t
 clinical manifestations of, 2501-2503, 2501t, 2502f
 diagnosis of, 2503
 versus ehrlichiosis and anaplasmosis, 2535t
 versus enteric fever, 1400t-1401t, 1404
 epidemiology of, 2499-2503, 2500f
 fulminant, 2502
 pathogen in, 2499
 pathogenesis of, 2501
 prevention of, 2503
 rash in, 801, 2502, 2502f, 3653-3654, 3654f
 treatment of, 2503
Rodents, arenavirus infection of, 2297-2298
Romaña's sign, in American trypanosomiasis, 3484, 3484f
Rosacea, topical antibacterials for, 526
Rosahn study, of syphilis, 3038
Rosai-Dorfman disease, lymphadenitis in, 1329
Rose spots
 in enteric fever, 1399-1401
 in typhoid fever, 1304, 2895, 2895f
Roseola infantum. See Exanthem subitum.
Roseoliform exanthems, from enteroviruses, 2355
Roseomonas, 3016t-3017t, 3026-3027
Roseomonas gilardii, 3026-3027
Rosetting, Plasmodium falciparum erythrocyte membrane protein-1 in, 3441
Rosoxacin, 706t-709t, 716t
Ross River virus, 2117-2125, 2118t. See also Alphaviruses.
Rotaviruses, 2105-2115
 deaths related to, 2109, 2109f
 detection of, 259t-260t
 diarrhea from, 206
  clinical manifestations of, 2107
  diagnosis of, 1361, 2106f, 2111
  pathogenesis of, 2107-2108
  seasonality of, 2109, 2110f
  treatment of, 2111-2112
  weanling, 1361
 epidemiology of, 2109-2110, 2109f-2110f
 historical perspective on, 2105
 immune response to, 2110-2111
 replication of, 2105-2107
 serologic classification of, 2108-2109
 structure of, 2105, 2106f
 vaccine for, 1361-1362, 2112, 3922t, 3931-3932
  in HIV-infected children, 1825
Roth spots, in endocarditis, 1075-1076, 1075f
Rothia dentocariosa, 2701
Rothia mucilaginosa, 2701
Roundworms (nematodes)
 intestinal, 3574t, 3577-3586, 3578f-3579f, 3578t
 tissue, 3574t, 3587-3594. See also Dracunculiasis; Filariasis; Trichinellosis.

Rovsing's sign, 1059
Roxithromycin, 706t-709t
 for Chlamydophila atherosclerosis, 2473
 dosage of, 726t-727t
 drug interactions with, 742t-761t
 formulations of, 716t
RpoB gene, in rifampin resistance, 403
RTX family toxins, 33
Rubella, 2127-2132
 arthritis from, 1449-1450
 clinical manifestations of, 2128-2129
 complications of, 2128-2129
 congenital, 2129, 2129t
 detection of, 259t-260t
 diagnosis of, 2129-2130
 encephalitis from, 1251t-1252t
 epidemiology of, 2127
 immunity to, maintenance of, 2127-2128
 pathogenesis of, 2128
 in pregnancy, 2128
 transmission of, 2127
 treatment of, 2130
 vaccine for, 2130-2131, 3922t, 3932. See also Measles, mumps, rubella (MMR) vaccine.
Rubelliform exanthems, from enteroviruses, 2354-2355
Rubelliform rash, in CMV mononucleosis, 1975
Rubeola virus. See Measles.
Rubulavirus, 2195, 2201. See also Mumps/mumps virus.
Rufloxacin, 706t-709t, 716t
Ruminants, prion disease in, 2432
Ruminococcus, 3123t
Runyoung mycobacterial groups, 252
Rural residence, HIV transmission and, 1626-1627, 1627f

S
S protein, 78t, 81t
Sabia virus, 2296t. See also South American hemorrhagic fevers.
Sabin-Feldman dye test, for toxoplasmosis, 3509
Saccharomyces boulardii, 161, 162t-164t. See also Probiotics.
Sacral radiculopathy, from herpes simplex virus, 1950
Sacroiliac joint, osteomyelitis of, 1464
Sacroiliitis
 from Brucella, 2923
 in reactive arthritis, 1492
Saddle nose, in congenital syphilis, 3044
St. Louis encephalitis, 1246t, 1257
 clinical features of, 2147
 epidemiology of, 2140, 2141f
 geographic distribution of, 1246-1247, 1247f
 historical perspective on, 2134
 meningitis from, 1190
 pathogenesis of, 2143-2144
 treatment of, 2150-2152
 vaccine for, 2151
Saksenaea, 3257, 3258t
Salicylic acid, for cutaneous warts, 2042
Saline, bladder irrigation with, for urinary tract infection prevention, 3732
Saliva
 HIV transmission by, 1649
 in oral mucosal immunity, 858
Saliva secretors, genetic determination of, 52
Salivaria, 3481
Salivary gland infections, 867
 from gram-negative anaerobic rods, 3116
Salmon River virus, 2102
Salmonella, 2887-2903
 bacteremia from, 2896
  in HIV infection, 2899
  treatment of, 2899
 brain abscess from, 1266
 classification of, 2887, 2888t
 clinical manifestations of, 2894-2896
 diarrhea from, 205-206
 endocytosis by, 2892, 2892f
 enteric fever from, 1399-1405, 2895-2896, 2895f.
  See also Typhoid fever.
 enterocolitis from, 1392

Salmonella (Continued)
epidemiology of, 2888-2891
extraintestinal complications of, 2896, 2897t, 2899
foodborne disease from, 1414t, 1415, 1418-1419, 2889-2891, 2889f, 2900
gastric acid and, 1337
genome of, 2887
history of, 2887
in HIV infection, 1860t-1870t, 1880
host cell entrance by, 9-10
host response to, 2894
innate immunity in, 2894
intestinal epithelium and, 2892-2893, 2892f
invasiveness of, 1342
laboratory detection of, 240t-242t, 1401-1402, 1422
macrophage response to, 2893-2894
meningitis from, 1218-1219
microbiology of, 2887-2888
multidrug-resistant, 1423
mycotic aneurysms from, 1101-1102
nontyphoidal
chronic carriage of, 2896, 2899-2900
epidemiology of, 2889-2891, 2889f-2891f
gastroenteritis from, 2894-2895
in HIV infection, 2896
multidrug-resistant, 2891, 2891f
nalidixic acid–resistant, 2891, 2891f
nosocomial, 2891
treatment of, 2899
pathogenesis of, 2892-2894
PhoP/PhoQ regulatory system of, 2893-2894
prevention of, 2900
schistosomiasis coinfection in, 3598-3599
secretory system of, 2892, 2894
SPI-1 translocated proteins of, 2892
taxonomy of, 2887, 2888t
vascular infections from, 2896
Salmonella bongori, 2887, 2888t
Salmonella choleraesuis, 1399, 1400t-1401t
Salmonella enterica, 2887, 2888t
Salmonella enterica serotype Typhi, 1399, 1400t-1401t
Salmonella paratyphi
enteric fever from, 2895-2896, 2895f. *See also*
Typhoid fever.
epidemiology of, 2888-2889, 2889f
paratyphoid fever from, 4022-4024. *See also*
Paratyphoid fever.
Salmonella paratyphi A, 1399, 1400t-1401t
Salmonella schottmuelleri, 1399, 1400t-1401t
Salmonella SopE, 10
Salmonella typhi
bacteremia from, 1304
enteric fever from, 2895-2896, 2895f. *See also*
Typhoid fever.
epidemiology of, 2888-2889, 2889f
gastrointestinal infection from, 1336
toxins of, 30
treatment of, 2898-2899, 2898t
typhoid from, 4022-4024. *See also* Typhoid fever.
vaccine for, 2896-2898
virulence of, 1342-1343
Salmonella typhimurium
defense against, T cells in, 129
evolution of, 7
gastrointestinal infection from, 1336-1338
virulence regulatory systems for, 8, 8t
Salpingitis
acute, 1517, 1517f
from *Chlamydia trachomatis,* 2454
Sand fleas, tungiasis from, 3639-3641, 3639t, 3640f
Sandflies, in leishmaniasis transmission, 3464-3465, 3465f
SAPHO syndrome, 1463
Sappinia diploidea, 3427-3436
characteristics of, 3427-3429, 3429f, 3430t
meningoencephalitis from, 3427-3436
Sappoviruses, 2399, 2401
Saquinavir, 706t-709t, 1839-1840, 1839f, 1840t
dosage of, 740t-741t
formulations of, 717t
for HIV-infected children, 1820t-1821t, 1823t
Sarcocystis, 3563-3565

Sarcocystosis, 3564-3565
muscular, 3565
Sarcoidosis
meningitis in, 1241
pulmonary, chest radiography in, 937f
Sarcoma, Kaposi's. *See* Kaposi's sarcoma.
Sarcoptes scabiei, 655, 3633-3636, 3634f. *See also*
Scabies.
Sargramostim, 614
Scabies, 3633-3636, 3634f, 3645
clinical manifestations of, 3633, 3634f
crusted (Norwegian), 3633, 3634f, 3635t
diagnosis of, 3633-3634
epidemiology of, 3633
genital lesions in, 1478, 1479f, 1481
in HIV infection, 1718, 1718f
prevention of, 3635
protection against, 4015-4016
sexually transmitted nodular, 3633, 3634f, 3635t
transmission of, 3633
treatment of, 3635, 3636t
Scalp
Bacillus infections of, 2729-2730
dermatophytosis of, 3346t, 3349-3350, 3350f, 3352t
Scalp ringworm. *See* Tinea capitis.
Scarlet fever
rash in, 800, 2596
staphylococcal, 800, 1291-1292
streptococcal, 2596
SCC*mec* resistance island, of methicillin-resistant
Staphylococcus aureus, 2558
Scedosporium, brain abscess from, 1266, 1266t
Scedosporium apiospermum
in cystic fibrosis, 951
meningitis from, 1239
Scedosporium prolificans, 3366, 3366f, 3374t
meningitis from, 1239
Schistosoma/schistosomiasis
abdominal pain and/or diarrhea with eosinophilia
from, 1407t, 1409
acute, 3598
characteristics of, 3595, 3596t, 3597f
chronic, 3598-3599
clinical syndromes of, 3597-3599
dermatitis in, 3597, 3618t, 3622
diagnosis of, 3599
dysentery from, 1392
versus enteric fever, 1400t-1401t, 1404
epidemiology of, 3595-3596, 3596t
etiology of, 3595, 3596t, 3597f
in hepatitis coinfection, 3599
in HIV coinfection, 3599
versus malaria, 3450
pathogenesis of, 3596-3597
prevention of, 3600
in *Salmonella* coinfection, 3598-3599
transmission of, 3595
treatment of, 632t-635t, 3596t, 3599-3600
Schistosoma mansoni, worm burden of, 52
Schools
HAV outbreaks in, 2375-2376
pertussis outbreaks in, 2962
Scleroma, respiratory (rhinoscleroma), from
Klebsiella pneumoniae subsp. *rhinoscleromatis,*
2827, 2827f
Sclerosing mediastinitis, 1179-1180, 1179t. *See also*
Mediastinitis.
Sclerotic body, of chromoblastomycosis, 3277, 3278f
Scopulariopsis brevicaulis, onychomycosis from, 3353
Scrapie, 2423, 2432
Scrofula, 1325, 3158, 3158f
Scrotum
swelling of, in epididymitis, 1524
ulcer of, in melioidosis, 2875f
Scrub typhus, 2495, 2529-2530, 2529f, 2529t, 3643, 3645f, 3646t
from *Orientia tsutsugamushi,* 4024
Scytalidium, 3353, 3353f
Scytalidium dimidiatum, 3353, 3353f
Scytalidium hyalinum, 3353
Sea lice, 4026
Sea-bather's eruption, 4026
Seadornaviruses, 2102

Seborrheic dermatitis
in HIV infection, 1717-1718, 1717f
from *Malassezia,* 3354
Secondary attack rate, 186
Secretion systems
of Enterobacteriaceae organisms, 2819-2820
of *Pseudomonas aeruginosa,* 2845
of *Salmonella,* 2892, 2894
for toxins, 29, 29t
Sedation, of ventilated patient, 3722-3723
Seizures
in CNS infections, 1185, 1187
in encephalitis, 1245-1246, 1250
toxoplasmic, 3519
febrile, 774-775
in HIV infection, 1759-1760
in human herpesvirus 6, 2011-2012
from penicillin, 314
Selectins, in neutrophil adhesion, 102
Selenium, 154
deficiency of, 154
in HIV/AIDS, 155
pathogen virulence and, 157-158, 158f
Self-administration model, of outpatient parenteral
antimicrobial delivery, 699, 700t
Self-limited febrile illness, in Q fever, 2512
Self–non-self distinction, complement in, 82
Semen, as vector for HIV infection, 1525-1526
Seminal vesicles, anatomy of, 1521, 1522f
Sendai virus, 2195
Sennetsu neorickettsiosis, 2536
Sensitivity, diagnostic, 179-180
Sensory polyneuropathy, distal, in HIV infection, 1756
Seoul virus, 2291
Sepsis, 987-1010. *See also* Septicemia.
acute lung injury in, 999
adrenal insufficiency in, 998
from *Arcanobacterium haemolyticum,* 2700
autonomic dysfunction in, 998
bacterial, antipyretic drugs during, 775-776
biomarker levels in, 1001
bullous lesions with, 792, 796
in burn patients, 3906, 3906t
from *Capnocytophaga,* 2991-2992
catheter-related, without suppurative thrombophlebitis, 1095-1096
cerebral function in, 997
circulation in, 998-999
clinical manifestations of, 997-1000
complement in, 93-94
continuum of, 999
corticosteroids for, 619
critical illness polyneuropathy and myopathy in, 998
cultures in, 1000-1001
cutaneous manifestations of, 1000
cytokine levels in, 1001
definitions of, 987, 988t, 992
diagnosis of, 1000-1001
diagnostic imaging in, 1001
differential diagnosis of, 1000
epidemiology of, 987-988
gastrointestinal tract injury in, 999-1000
glucose control in, 1005
granulocyte colony-stimulating factor for, 613
hepatic dysfunction in, 1000
host defenses in, augmentation of, 1005
hypothalamic-pituitary-adrenal axis in, 997
immune dysfunction in, 1000
in immunocompromised hosts, 3787-3788
intra-abdominal, imaging in, 1021
joint prosthesis. *See* Prosthetic joint infections.
versus malaria, 3450
meningococcal
petechial rash in, 2741-2743, 2741f-2742f
subcutaneous ecchymoses in, 2741-2743, 2742f
neonatal, enterococcal, 2647
nutritional support in, 1005
organ dysfunction in, 999-1000, 999f
pathogenesis of, 988-997
postsplenectomy, 3865-3873. *See also*
Splenectomy.
prognosis in, 1005

Sepsis *(Continued)*
  from *Pseudomonas aeruginosa*, 1303-1304, 2854
    skin lesions in, 798
  rash in, 797-798
  renal dysfunction in, 999
  secondary infections in, prevention of, 1005
  severe, 992-994
    antimicrobial therapy for, 1001-1003
    coagulopathy in, 994
    complement activation in, 994
    definition of, 987, 988t
    endothelial activation or injury in, 993
    gene polymorphisms in, 995
    immunosuppression in, 994
    mediators in, 993-994
    microbial triggers for, 995-997
    microcirculatory and mitochondrial dysfunction
      in, 992-993
    sites of infection in, 995, 995f
  treatment of, 1001-1003
    anticoagulants in, 1004
    anti-inflammatory, 619-620, 1003-1004
    antimicrobial therapy in, 1001, 1002t
    blood transfusion in, 1002-1003
    fluid resuscitation in, 1002-1003
    hydrocortisone in, 1003
    hyperbaric oxygen therapy in, 625
    intravenous immune globulin in, 618
    neutralizing gram-negative bacterial endotoxin
      and related molecules in, 1004
    pressor drugs in, 1003
    surgical drainage in, 1002
    vasopressin in, 1003
Septic abortion, from *Campylobacter jejuni*, 2797
Septic arthritis, 1450t, 1453
Septic bursitis, 1453
  from *Staphylococcus aureus*, 2574
  treatment of, 1450t, 1453
Septic shock
  adrenal insufficiency in, 1001
  cardiovascular impact of, 999
  continuum of, 994-995, 999
  definition of, 987, 988t
  streptococcal, viridans, 2669
Septicemia
  catheter-associated, 3700-3701, 3700t. *See also*
    Catheter-related infections.
  in leptospirosis, 3061
  in melioidosis, 2871, 2877
  from *Pasteurella*, 2940
  in *Yersinia enterocolitica* infection, 2951
Septicemic plague, 2946. *See also* Plague.
Seroincidence surveys, 184
Serologic tests, 247
  for arboviruses, 261
  for bacteria, 248, 249t
  in chronic meningitis, 1238
  for enteroviruses, 2341
  for fungi, 256-257, 3222-3223
  in HIV infection, 260-261
    for antibody detection, 1668-1670, 1669f
    for monitoring, 1637-1640
    for p24 antigen detection, 1663, 1670-1671
  for parasites, 264
  in pneumonia, 900, 934-937
  for viruses, 259t-260t, 260-261
Seroprevalence surveys, 184
Serratia, 2827-2828
Serratia marcescens, 2827-2828
  device-associated infections from, 3697
Serum bactericidal test, in prosthetic joint infections,
  1472
Serum opacity factor, of group A *Streptococcus*, 2594
Serum protective factors, in gastrointestinal
  infections, 1339
Serum sickness, from penicillin, 313
Setaria labiatopillosa, 3594
Severe acute respiratory syndrome (SARS), 202-203
  clinical manifestations of, 2191
  coronavirus (HCoV) in, 2187
    genome of, 2188, 2188f
  emergency preparedness for, 223-225. *See also*
    Emergency preparedness.
  epidemiology of, 2189-2190, 2190f
  identification of, 2187

Severe acute respiratory syndrome (SARS)
    (Continued)
  laboratory diagnosis of, 2192
  outbreaks of, 202
  pathogenicity of, 2190-2191
  prevention of, 2192
  pulmonary pathology of, 2191
  treatment of, 2192
Sex hormones, in HIV infection, 1799
Sexual abuse/assault, of children, HIV infection in,
  1828
Sexual behavior, HIV transmission and, 1625-1626,
  1626f, 1645-1647, 1650-1652
Sexual intercourse
  HCV transmission during, 2171
  unprotected, among travelers, 4015
  urinary tract infection and, 958, 962, 965
Sexual partners. *See also* Men who have sex with
    men (MSM).
  of men with nongonococcal urethritis, 1490
  Neisseria gonorrhoeae infection in, 2766
Sexually reactive arthritis, 1491-1492, 2453
Sexually transmitted diseases. *See also specific disease.*
  HIV transmission and, 1624-1625, 1647,
    1783-1784
    screening for, 1784
  inguinal lymphadenitis in, 1326
  in injection drug users, 3887
  outbreaks of, 194
  prevention of, in women, 1800
  in professional sex workers, 1638-1639, 4015
  public health strategies for, 2766-2767
  quinolones for, 495-496
  sex partner management of, 2766
  trimethoprim-sulfamethoxazole for, 481
Shell vial spin amplification (SVA) cultures, 258
Shellfish poisoning, 1416-1417, 1417t
  amnesic, 3570, 3570t
  azaspiracid, 3570, 3570t
  confirmation of, 1422
  diarrhetic, 3569-3570, 3570t
  neurotoxic, 1416-1417, 1417t, 3569, 3570t
  paralytic, 1416-1417, 1417t, 3569, 3570t
Shewanella, 3016t-3017t, 3027
Shiga toxin, 32, 2825
Shiga toxin–producing *Escherichia coli*, 2821t,
  2824-2825, 2825f
Shigella, 2905-2910
  anatomic localization of, 2906-2907
  diagnosis of, 2908
  dysentery from, 1389-1391, 1390f
  epidemiology of, 2907-2908
  foodborne disease from, 1414t, 1415, 1419
  gastric acid and, 1337
  in HIV infection, 1860t-1870t, 1880
  host cell entrance by, 9-10
  identification of, 2905
  infectivity of, 2905-2906, 2906t
  invasiveness of, 1342
  isolation of, 2905
  laboratory detection of, 240t-242t, 1422, 2908
  microbiology of, 2905
  mucosal invasion by, 2906
  pathogenesis of, 2905-2907, 2906t
  phagosome lysis by, 10
  reservoirs for, 2907-2908
  spread of, 2907-2908
  toxigenicity of, 2906
  treatment of, 2908-2909, 2909t
  virulence factors of, 5t
  virulence regulatory systems for, 8t
Shigella boydii, 1389
Shigella dysenteriae, 1389
  toxins of, 1340t, 1341
Shigella dysenteriae 1, 2907
Shigella flexneri, 1389, 2907
Shigella sonnei, 1389, 2907
Shigellosis
  pseudomembranous colitis from, 1389-1390, 1390f
  quinolones for, 496
Shingles. *See* Herpes zoster.
Shivering, 768
Shock
  in dengue shock syndrome, 2143, 2145
  endotoxic, complement in, 93

Shock *(Continued)*
  in malaria, 3449
  septic
    adrenal insufficiency in, 1001
    cardiovascular impact of, 999
    continuum of, 994-995, 999
    definition of, 987, 988t
    streptococcal, viridans, 2669
  in toxic shock syndrome, 2604. *See also* Toxic
    shock syndrome.
Short consensus repeats (SCRs), 82
Shunt infections. *See* Cerebrospinal fluid shunt
  infections.
Shunt meningitis, 461
Shunt nephritis, 1232-1233
SHV-derived beta-lactamase, 283, 283f
Sialic acid, 84
Siberian encephalitis, 2138t
Sickle cell disease
  Mycoplasma pneumoniae infection in, 2483f,
    2484
  osteomyelitis in, 1464
Sickle cell trait, bacteriuria and, 966
Siderophores, 2820
  Pseudomonas aeruginosa, 2844
Sifuvirtide, for HIV infection, 22
Signal transducer and activator of transcription 1
    (STAT1), mutations in, 169t-170t, 176
Silibinin, 674, 674f
Silver dressing, 3907t
Silver nitrate, 1535-1536, 3907t
Silver sulfadiazone, 475-476, 706t-709t, 3907t
Silymarin, 674, 674f
Simian herpesvirus. *See* Herpes B virus.
Simian immunodeficiency virus (SIV), 2323-2324
Sin Nombre virus, 2289-2290
Sindbis virus, 2117-2125, 2118t. *See also*
  Alphaviruses.
Single nucleotide polymorphisms (SNPs), in human
  genome sequence, 49, 55
Single-photon emission computed tomography, in
  brain abscess, 1272
Sinus(es), fungus ball of, 3246
Sinus histiocytosis, with lymphadenopathy, 1329
Sinus ostium, obstruction of, 839-840, 840t
Sinus thrombosis, septic cavernous, 865, 865f,
  1283-1286, 1284f
Sinusitis, 839-849
  anaerobes in, 3085
  bacterial, 841, 841t
  chronic, 842
    definition of, 842
    gram-negative anaerobe rods in, 3115
  clinical manifestations of, 843
  from common cold, 811
  community-acquired, 839, 841, 841t
  complications of, 846, 847f
  definition of, 839
  diagnosis of, 843-844, 843t
  diagnostic imaging in, 844
  endoscopic middle meatal culture versus sinus
    puncture in, 841, 841t
  epidemiology of, 842-843
  etiology of, 841, 841t
  fungal, 841-842, 842t
    allergic, 3245-3246, 3248, 3248f, 3368, 3368f
  from *Haemophilus influenzae*, nontypeable, 2913
  maxillary, 839, 865
  microbiology of, 840-842, 841t-842t
  from microsporidia, 3398
  from *Moraxella catarrhalis*, 2773
  nosocomial, 842, 842t
  pathogenesis of, 839-840, 840t
  prevention of, 846-847
  quinolones for, 499
  in rhinocerebral mucormycosis, 3260-3261, 3261f
  rhinoviral, 2393
  from streptococcus group C, 2676
  from *Streptococcus pneumoniae*, 2630-2631, 2635
  treatment of, 844-846
    adjunctive therapy in, 846
    antimicrobials in, 844-846, 845f, 845t-846t
    outpatient parenteral antimicrobial therapy in,
      700, 700t
  viral, 841, 2393. *See also* Common cold.

Sirolimus, for transplant immunosuppression, infections and, 3811
Sisomicin, 359, 360f, 360t-361t
Sitafloxacin, 706t-709t, 716t
Sixth disease. See Exanthem subitum.
Sjögren's syndrome, 867
Skeletal infections. See also Musculoskeletal infections.
    from gram-negative anaerobic rod, 3114-3115
    from Kingella, 2775
    from Mycobacterium tuberculosis, 3155-3156, 3155f
Skeletal specimens, 243
Skin. See also Cutaneous entries.
    barrier function of, 38-40, 3783-3784
    colonization of, reduction of, for endocarditis prophylaxis, 1143
    contamination of, at device insertion site, 3698
    disinfection of, 521-522
    microflora of, 3783, 3784f
    schematic diagram of, 3893, 3893f
    structure of, 522f
Skin infections. See also Dermatitis.
    anaerobic, 3086
    from Bacillus spp., 2729-2730
    from Candida. See Candidiasis, cutaneous.
    classification of, 1290t
    from Corynebacterium diphtheriae, 2691
    from Cryptococcus neoformans, 3293t, 3295, 3295f
    in elderly, 3859
    from Enterococcus, 2647
    from gram-negative anaerobic rod, 3115
    in immunocompromised hosts, 3783-3784, 3788
    in injection drug users, 3876-3878
    from microsporidia, 3398
    from mucormycosis agents, 3262, 3263f
    from Mycobacterium marinum, 1331
    from nontuberculous mycobacteria, 3193t, 3194-3195
    opportunistic, post-traumatic, in immunocompromised patients, 1302
    from Pasteurella, 2940
    PTK 0796 for, 511
    recurrent, prevention of, topical antibacterials in, 523, 528t
    secondary, 1300-1303
    self-induced, 1303
    in solid organ transplant recipients, 3844, 3844t
    from Sporothrix schenckii, 3271-3273, 3272f-3273f, 3272t
    from Staphylococcus aureus, 2565-2567, 2566f
        management of, 2567
    from Streptococcus agalactiae (group B), 2660-2661
    from Streptococcus group C and group G, 2675
    from Streptococcus pyogenes, 2600-2605
    in travelers, 4026, 4027f
        prevention of, 4015-4016
    treatment of
        daptomycin in, 464
        quinolones in, 500
        teicoplanin in, 459
        trimethoprim-sulfamethoxazole in, 481
        vancomycin in, 455
Skin lesions. See also Rash; specific lesion.
    in adult T-cell leukemia/lymphoma, 2312, 2313f
    from Blastomyces dermatitidis, 3325, 3325f-3326f
    in brucellosis, 2923
    characteristics of, 792-797, 793t
    in CMV mononucleosis, 1975
    from Coccidioides, 3337, 3338f
    in conjunctivitis, 1529

Skin lesions (Continued)
    in Mycoplasma pneumoniae infection, 2483-2484, 2483f
    in nocardiosis, 3200-3201, 3201f-3202f
    in post–kala-azar dermal leishmaniasis, 3468-3469, 3468f
    in Pseudomonas aeruginosa bacteremia, 2849, 2849f
    in sepsis, 1000
    in varicella, 1964
    in variola (smallpox), 1926, 1927f
Skin slit smears, for leprosy, 3169
Skin specimens, 235t-236t, 243
Skin temperature, 766
Skin tests
    in chronic pneumonia, 934
    for Coccidioides, 3340
    histoplasmin, 3315
    paracoccidioidin, 3362
Skin ulcers
    in chromoblastomycosis, 3277, 3278f
    from Cryptococcus neoformans, 3295, 3295f
    in injection drug users, 3877-3878
"Slapped cheek" disease. See Erythema infectiosum.
SLC11A1 gene, in tuberculosis susceptibility, 49, 51-52, 51t
Sleeping sickness, 3489-3494. See also Trypanosomiasis, African.
Slim disease, in HIV infection, 1714
Small bowel
    abnormalities of
        in HIV infection, 1741-1742
        in tropical sprue, 1431
    bacterial overgrowth of, 1367-1368
        rifamycins for, 413
        in tropical sprue, 1429-1430
Small bowel transplant recipients, infections in, 3841t, 3843-3844
Smallpox. See also Variola virus.
    as biological weapon, 3951, 3955-3956, 3977-3981
        aerosol release of, 3995
        epidemiology of, 3977
        infection control measures for, 3980
        pre- and post-event exposure preparedness for, 3980
        preparedness activities for, 3980-3981
        public health issues in, 3980-3981
    cell culture of, 3979-3980
    clinical presentation of, 3977-3978, 3978f-3979f
    conjunctivitis from, 1532
    diagnosis of, 3978-3980
    electron microscopy visualization of, 3979
    epidemiology of, relative to bioterrorism, 3977
    eradication of, 3977
    versus febrile vesicular pustular rash illnesses, 1927, 1928t
    flat-type, 3978
    hemorrhagic, 3978
    histopathology of, 3979
    immunochemistry of, 3979
    incubation period for, 3977
    nucleic acid testing for, 3979
    ordinary, 3978
    pathogenesis of, 3977-3978
    rash in, 803, 3978, 3978f-3979f
    specimen collection in, 3979
    transmission of, 3977
    vaccination against, 3977, 3980-3981
Smallpox vaccine, 803, 1924-1927, 1924f, 3922t, 3932-3933, 3977, 3980-3981
    complications of, 1925-1926
    immunity from, 1925
    recommendations for, 1926
Smoking
    chronic bronchitis and, 878
    chronic obstructive pulmonary disease and, 877
    in HIV infection, pneumonia risk and, 1728
Snake bites
    passive immunization against, 73
    venomous, 1297, 1297t, 3913-3914
SNARE complex, clostridial neurotoxins and, 31
Sneezing, in common cold, 811
Snow Mountain virus, 2399, 2400f
Snowshoe hare virus, encephalitis from, 1251t-1252t

Sodium stibogluconate, 706t-709t
    for parasitic infections, 632t-635t, 641-642
Sodoku, 2966-2967, 2966t
Soft tissue infections. See also Abscess; Cellulitis.
    from Acinetobacter, 2883
    from Aeromonas, 3018
    anaerobic, 3086
    from Arcanobacterium haemolyticum, 2700
    from Bacillus spp., 2729-2730
    from Enterococcus, 2647
    from gram-negative anaerobic rod, 3115
    in injection drug users, 3876-3878
    from mucormycosis agents, 3262
    from nontuberculous mycobacteria, 3193t, 3194-3195
    orofacial, 869-870
    from Pasteurella, 2940
    recurrent, prevention of, topical antibacterials in, 523, 528t
    in spinal cord injury patients, 3854
    from Staphylococcus aureus, 2565-2567, 2566f
    from Streptococcus agalactiae (group B), 2660-2661
    from Streptococcus group C and group G, 2675
    from Streptococcus pyogenes, 2600-2605
    treatment of
        daptomycin in, 464
        quinolones in, 500
        teicoplanin in, 459
        vancomycin in, 455
        trimethoprim-sulfamethoxazole for, 481
Soft tissue specimens, 243
Solid organ transplant recipients. See also under specific organ.
    adenoviruses in, 2030-2031
    blastomycosis in, 3327
    cytomegalovirus in, 1980, 3847
    Epstein-Barr virus in, 3848-3849
    herpes simplex virus in, 3847
    human herpesvirus 8 in, 3848
    infections in, 3839-3850
        abdominal, 3845-3846
        bloodstream, 3844
        central nervous system, 3846, 3846t
        chest, 3844-3845, 3848f
        gastrointestinal, 3845-3846
        sites and types of, 3844-3846
        skin and wound, 3844, 3844t
        timing of, 3839, 3840f
        by type of transplant, 3839-3844, 3841t
        urinary tract, 3844
        viral, 3846-3849
    Kaposi's sarcoma in, 3848
    polyomaviruses in, 3848
    post-transplant lymphoproliferative disorders in, 3848-3849
    respiratory viral infections in, 3847-3848
    survival data for, 3839, 3840f, 3840t
    varicella-zoster virus in, 3847
Sordarins, 561
Sore throat. See Pharyngitis.
South American blastomycosis, gastrointestinal manifestations of, 1395
South American hemorrhagic fevers, 2295-2301
    characteristics of, 2295
    clinical manifestations of, 2299
    diagnosis of, 2299-2300
    epidemiology/epizootiology of, 2296t, 2297
    pathogenesis of, 2297-2298
    prevention of, 2300
    treatment of, 2300
Southeast Asian ovalocytosis, malaria and, 3443
Southern tick-associated rash illness (STARI), 3071-3072, 3651f, 3651t-3652t, 3652
Soviet Bioweapons Program, 3952
SP-40,40, 78t
SPA-CLFS typing, of Staphylococcus aureus, 2547
Sparfloxacin, 706t-709t
    dosage of, 732t-733t
    formulations of, 716t
Sparganosis, 3608t, 3615
Spasm
    in croup, 825, 827
    in tetanus, 3092-3093, 3093f
SPATE (serine protease autotransporters of Enterobacteriaceae) family, 2819

Specificity, diagnostic, 179-180
Specimen collection and transport
    for aerobic actinomycetes, 253
    for fungi, 255
    guidelines for, 234, 235t-236t
    for mycobacteria, 250-251
    for parasites, 262-263, 263t
    for viruses, 257-258, 257t
Specimen selection, 234
Spectinomycin, 360f, 360t-361t, 706t-709t
    dosage of, 724t-725t
    drug interactions with, 742t-761t
    for Neisseria gonorrhoeae infection, 379, 2765
Sphenoid sinus, anatomy and physiology of, 839
Sphingobacterium, 3016t-3017t, 3027
Sphingomonas, 3016t-3017t, 3027-3028
Sphingomonas paucimobilis, 3028
SPI-1 translocated proteins, of Salmonella, 2892
Spinal cord abscess, in injection drug users, 3886
Spinal cord infection
    from Listeria monocytogenes, 2710
    from Toxoplasma gondii, in AIDS patient, 3505
Spinal cord injury patients
    abdominal infections in, 3855
    bacteremia in, 3855
    fever in, 3851-3852
    infections in, 3851-3856
        evaluation for, 3851-3852, 3852t
        predisposing factors for, 3851
    multiresistant bacteria in, 3855
    osteomyelitis in, 3854-3855
    pneumonia in, 3853-3854
    pressure sores in, 3854
    urinary tract infections in, 3852-3853
Spinal cord tumors, cervical, differential diagnosis of, 3660t
Spinal epidural abscess, 1281-1283, 1283f
    in injection drug users, 3886
Spinal meningitis, tuberculous, 3154
Spinal paralytic poliomyelitis, 2346
Spinal subdural empyema, 1279-1280
Spinal syndrome, in HIV infection, 1754-1755
Spinal tuberculosis, 3154
Spiramycin, 706t-709t
    for cryptosporidiosis, 3555
    dosage of, 726t-727t
    for toxoplasmosis, 655
        congenital, 3520
        in pregnant patient, 3520
Spirillar dysentery, 1393
Spirillum minus
    endocarditis from, 1086
    rat-bite fever from, 2966-2967, 2966t
Spirochetal borrelioses, 3650-3653, 3651t-3652t
Spirochetal dysentery, 1393
Spirochetal infections, meningitis from
    antimicrobial therapy for, 1219-1220
    clinical features of, 1206
    diagnosis of, 1209-1210
    epidemiology and etiology of, 1193
Spirochetemia, 3041
    direct examination of, 3044, 3045f
Spirometra mansonoides, 3608t
Spleen, 3865-3873
    anatomy of, 143-144, 143f
    congenital absence of, 3865
    enlarged, in endocarditis, 1074-1076
    evaluation of, 3865-3866, 3866f
    functions of, 3865-3866
    infarction of, in endocarditis, 1074-1075
    removal of. See Splenectomy.
    rupture of, in infectious mononucleosis, 1994
    in systemic response to infection, 990
    underfunctioning, causes of, 3865, 3866t
Splenectomy, 176-177. See also Asplenia.
    alternatives to, 3871
    causes of, 3865
    infections after, 3782-3783
    nonsurgical equivalents of, 3865, 3866t
    relationship to other infections, 3869
    sepsis after
        clinical characteristics of, 3866-3868, 3867f-3868f, 3867t
        education on, 3871, 3871t
        microbiology of, 3868-3869, 3868f

Splenectomy (Continued)
        prevention of, 3870-3871, 3871t
        treatment of, 3869-3870, 3870t
    for splenic abscess, 1056
Splenic abscess
    in endocarditis, 1074-1075
    in injection drug users, 3884-3885
    in melioidosis, 1055-1057, 2874f-2875f
    microbiology of, 1055, 1056t
Splinter hemorrhage, in endocarditis, 1076
Spondylitis
    from Brucella, 2923
    tuberculous, 3155-3156, 3155f
Spondylodiskitis, 1460-1461, 1461f
Spongiform encephalopathy, transmissible, genetic
        agents in, 259t-260t
Sponging, antipyretic effects of, 774-775
Sporicide, 3677
Sporothrix schenckii, 3271-3275
    arthritis from, 1451
    mycology of, 3271
    osteomyelitis from, 3271, 3272f
    syndromes caused by, 3271-3273
Sporotrichosis, 3271-3275
    clinical manifestations of, in HIV-infected patient, 3273-3274, 3273f
    clinical syndromes of, 3271-3273
    diagnosis of, 3274, 3274f
    differential diagnosis of, 3272t
    epidemiology of, 3271
    extracutaneous, 3271-3272, 3272f-3273f
        multifocal, 3272-3273, 3273f
    lymphocutaneous, 3271, 3272f
    meningitis in, 1239
    prognosis for, 3275
    treatment of, 3274-3275
        in HIV-infected patient, 3274-3275
Spotted fever, 2495, 2499-2507. See also Rickettsia/
        rickettsial infections.
    flea-borne, 3639t
    as group, 3653-3654, 3653t, 3654f
Sprue, tropical. See Tropical sprue.
Sputum
    in acute pneumonia, 896-898, 897f-898f
    in chronic pneumonia, 934-937
    laboratory processing of, 239
    Moraxella catarrhalis isolation from, 2771, 2773f
Sputum culture
    in acute pneumonia, 897-898
    in pneumococcal pneumonia, 2632, 2632f, 2632t
Squamous cell papilloma, oral, 2041, 2044
Squamous intraepithelial neoplasia
    anal, clinical management of, 1775
    cervical, 1772-1773, 1796-1798
        clinical management of, 1774
Squirrels, flying, typhus borne by, 2522
ST-246, for orthopoxvirus infection, 1930
Standard isolation precautions, 3673-3674
    gloves in, 3673-3674
    hand hygiene in, 3673
    in HIV prophylaxis, 3757
Stanford V regimen, for Hodgkin's disease, 1776
Staphylococcal chromosome cassette mec, resistance
        island, 2558
Staphylococcal scalded skin syndrome, 1291, 1292f,
        2553-2554, 2554f
    clinical aspects of, 2554
    generalized, 2554
    localized, 2554, 2554f
    molecular pathogenesis of, 2554
    rash in, 799-800
Staphylococcus
    coagulase-negative, 2579-2589. See also Staphylo-
        coccus epidermidis.
        antibiotic resistance to, 2579-2580
        bacteremia from, 2581-2585
        breast implant infection from, 2585
        cardiac device infection from, 2583
        catheter-related infection from, 2582, 2582f, 2584
        cerebrospinal fluid shunt infection from, 2584
        ecology of, 2579
        endocarditis from, 1120-1121, 2582-2583
        endophthalmitis from, 1553, 2584
        genitourinary prosthesis infection from, 2585

Staphylococcus (Continued)
        linezolid for, 473
        microbiology of, 2579
        miscellaneous device and implant infection
            from, 2585
        molecular epidemiology of, 2580
        neonates infected with, 2585-2586
        neutropenic hosts infected with, 2585
        non-epidermidis, 2586
        orthopedic prosthetic device infection from, 2583-2584
        surgical site infection from, 2584
        taxonomy of, 2580t
        transplant recipients infected with, 2585
        urinary tract infection from, 2585
        vancomycin-resistant, 452
        vascular graft infection from, 2583
        virulence factors of, 2580-2581, 2580t
    culture of, 2544-2545
    description of, 2543-2546, 2545t
    endocarditis from, 1081t, 1082-1083
        prosthetic valve, treatment of, 1118t, 1119
        treatment of, 1091-1092
    enterotoxins of, 2543
    habitat of, 2543-2544
    identification of, 2544-2545
    liver abscess from, in chronic granulomatous
        disease, 174, 174f
    treatment of
        clindamycin, 443
        fusidic acid for, 356
        linezolid in, 473
        rifamycins for, 408-410
    urinary tract infection from, 964
Staphylococcus aureus, 2543-2578
    adhesins of, 2550-2551, 2551f, 2551t
    antibiotic resistance of, 2558-2563, 2559t
        to beta-lactams, 2558-2560, 2559t
        burden of, 2563-2564
        to daptomycin, 2559t, 2560-2561
        drug efflux in, 2561
        to glycopeptides, 2559t, 2560
        to linezolid, 2561
        to penicillins, 2558, 2559t
        to protein synthesis inhibitors, 2561
        to quinolones, 2561-2562
        ribosome modification in, 2561
        to vancomycin, 288, 451, 1119, 2560
    arthritis from, 1443-1444, 1444t-1445t, 2574
    bacteremia from, 1303
        community-onset, 2568
    biofilm of, 2549-2550
    bloodstream infection from, 2567-2568
        community-onset, 2568
        health care-associated, 2568
        management of, 2568
        nosocomial, 2568
    brain abscess from, 1265, 1266t, 1267-1269
    capsule of, 2550
    carbuncles from, 2566
    carriage of, 2564-2565
        decolonization in, 2565
        nasal, 2544
            eradication of, 527
            mupirocin for, 527, 530, 1293
    cellulitis from, 2567, 2567f
    clinical aspects of, 2563-2565
    clinical spectrum of, 2563
    clinical syndromes of, 2565-2575
    colonization by, rifamycins for, 4
    in cystic fibrosis, 948-949
    description of, 2543-2546, 254?
    double-locus SPA-CLFS typin?
    endocarditis from, 1071-107?
        bacterial adhesins in, 256?
        clinical features of, 2569-
        diagnosis of, 2570
        epidemiology of, 2568
        host defense in, 2569
        management of, 257?
        neurologic compl?
        pathogenesis of?
        platelets in, 2?
        prosthetic ?
        rifamyci?

Staphylococcus aureus (Continued)
  vascular complications of, 2569, 2570f
  enterotoxins of, 2556
  enzymes of, 2553
  epidemiology of, 2563-2565
  erysipelas from, 2567
  fasciitis from, 2567
  folliculitis from, 2566
  foodborne disease from, 2556
  furuncles from, 2566
  fusidic acid resistance in, 355
  hemolysins of, 2553
  hidradenitis suppurativa from, 2566
  impetigo from, 1289, 1291, 2565-2566, 2566f
  laboratory detection of, 240t-242t
  linezolid for, 472-473
  lipoteichoic acids of, 2551-2552
  macrolide-resistant, 428-429, 429t
  mastitis from, 2566
  meningitis from, 1193, 1212t, 1218, 2571
  methicillin-resistant, 213, 2558-2560
    alternative treatments for, 2562-2563
    animal bite wounds and, 3911-3912
    burden of, 2563-2564
    carriage of, 2565
    carriers of, decolonization of, 2565
    community-associated, 799, 2558
    contact precautions for, 3675-3676
    mechanism of, 2560
    in men who have sex with men, 481
    molecular typing of, 2546
    postoperative mediastinitis from, 1175
    rifamycins for, 409
    SCC*mec* resistance island of, 2558
    in spinal cord injury patients, 3855
    surgical site infections from, 3892-3893, 3893t, 3898-3899
    vancomycin/gentamicin for, 455-456
  methicillin-susceptible
    evolution of, into methicillin-resistant *Staphylococcus aureus*, 2546-2547, 2547f
    postoperative mediastinitis from, 1175
  mobile genetic elements of, 2556-2558, 2557t
  molecular diagnosis of, 2546-2547
  molecular typing of, 2546
  morphology variants of, 2545-2546
  multilocus sequence typing of, 2546-2547
  mycotic aneurysms from, 1101-1102
  nasal carriage of, 2544
    eradication of, 527
    mupirocin for, 527, 530, 1293
  osteomyelitis from, 1457-1459, 1461, 1461f, 2572-2574
    clinical features of, 2572-2573
    diagnosis of, 2574
    epidemiology of, 2572, 2572t
    pathogenesis of, 2572, 2573f
    prosthetic joints in, 2573
    rifamycins for, 409-410
    treatment of, 2574
  otitis media from, 833
  pathogenesis of, 2547-2556
    accessory gene regulator in, 2547-2548, 2548f
      ecologic and epidemiologic implication of, 2549
      role of, 2549
    cell surface determinants in, 2549-2553, 2550f
    DNA-binding proteins and other regulators in, 2548-2549, 2548f
    extracellular factors involved in, 2544t
    pathogenicity (genomic) islands in, 2556-2558, 2557t
      mobilization of, 2557
      types and nomenclature of, 2557-2558
    potential regulatory factors and small RNAs in, 2548f, 2549
    regulatory systems in, 2547-2549
    two-component regulator in, 2547-2548
  peptidoglycan of, 2552-2553, 2553f
  pericarditis from, 2571
  peritonitis from, 1013, 1016
  in platelet activation, 1113-1114
  pneumonia from
    empyema in, 918
    in HIV infection, 1730-1731

Staphylococcus aureus (Continued)
  prevention of, 2563
  prospectives for, 2563
  prosthetic joint infections from, 2573
  pulmonary infections from, 2571-2572
  pulse field gel electrophoresis of, 2546
  pyomyositis from, 1314-1315, 2574-2575
  rash from, 799-800
  resistance of, mechanisms of, 290t
  risk factors for, 2563, 2564t
  scalded skin syndrome from, 2553-2554, 2554f.
    See also Staphylococcal scalded skin syndrome.
  septic bursitis from, 2574
  skin infections from, 2565-2567, 2566f
  small colony variants of, 2545-2546
  small RNA in pathogenesis of, 2549
  soft tissue infections from, 2565-2567, 2566f
  SPA typing of, 2547
  species in, 2543, 2545t
  superantigens of, 2554-2556
  suppurative thrombophlebitis from, 1097-1098
  surgical site infection from, 2566-2567
  teichoic acids of, 2551, 2552f
  toxic shock syndrome from, 2555-2556. *See also* Toxic shock syndrome, staphylococcal.
  toxins of, 1340t, 1341
    exfoliative, 2553-2554
    Panton-Valentine, 2553, 2553f
  treatment of
    alternative, 2562-2563
    beta-lactams in, 2562
    lipoglycopeptides in, 2562-2563
    quinupristin-dalfopristin in, 2562
    tigecycline in, 2562
  vancomycin-intermediate, 289-290, 1119
  virulence determinants of, 2547-2556
  virulence factors of, 5t
  virulence regulatory systems for, 8t
Staphylococcus capitis, 2543, 2545t
  endocarditis from, prosthetic valve, 1120
Staphylococcus epidermidis, 2543, 2545t
  adherence of, 2580-2581
  antibiotics produced by, 2581
  bacteremia from, 2581-2585
  biofilm formation in, 2580-2581, 2581f
  dispersal of, 2581
  endocarditis from, 2582-2583
    prosthetic valve, 1120
    rifamycins for, 409
  endophthalmitis from, 1553, 2584
  foodborne disease from, 1413
  infection from
    of breast implants, 2585
    of cardiac devices, 2583
    catheter-related, 2582, 2582f, 2584
    of cerebrospinal fluid shunt implant, 2584
    clinical syndromes of, 2581-2585
    of genitourinary prosthesis, 2585
    of orthopedic prosthetic devices, 2583-2584
    patient populations at risk for, 2585-2586
    of surgical site, 2584
    of urinary tract, 2585
    of vascular grafts, 2583
  keratitis from, 1542
  maturation of, 2581
  meningitis from, 1193, 1212t
  microbiology of, 2579, 2580t
  multilocus sequence typing of, 2580
  pathogenesis of, 2580-2581, 2580t, 2581f
  poly-gamma-DL-glutamic acid production by, 2581
  pulse field gel electrophoresis of, 2580
Staphylococcus haemolyticus, 2545t, 2586
Staphylococcus lugdunensis, 2545t, 2586
  endocarditis from, prosthetic valve, 1120
Staphylococcus saprophyticus, 2545t, 2586
Statin therapy
  anti-inflammatory effects of, 620
  pneumonia and, 912-913
  rhabdomyolysis from, in HIV infection, 1759
Statistics
  bacteriologic, 267
  in epidemiologic studies, 180-181

Stavudine, 706t-709t, 1834-1835, 1834f, 1835t
  dosage of, 740t-741t
  drug interactions with, 742t-761t
  formulations of, 717t
  for HIV-infected children, 1820t-1821t
Steam sterilization, 3685-3686, 3685t
Steeple sign, in croup, 827, 827f
Stem cell transplantation. *See* Hematopoietic stem cell transplantation.
Stenotrophomonas maltophilia, 2861-2868
  clinical manifestations of, 2864-2865, 2864f
  device-associated infections from, 3697
  epidemiology of, 2863-2864
  laboratory detection of, 240t-242t
  microbiology, taxonomy, and identification of, 2861
  pathogenesis of, 2861-2863
  pneumonia from, 2864-2865, 2864f
  prevention and control of, 2866
  resistance of, mechanisms of, 290t
  treatment of, 2865-2866
    ticarcillin-clavulanate in, 2865
    TMP-SMZ in, 2865
  virulence factors of, 2861-2863
Stent infection
  coronary artery, 1137
  peripheral vascular, 1137-1138, 1137t
Stercoraria, 3481
Sterilants, chemical, 3677, 3680t
Sterility assurance level (SAL), 3685
Sterilization. *See also* Disinfection.
  of bioterrorism agents, 3689-3690
  of critical items, 3678t-3679t, 3680, 3690
  current issues in, 3690-3692
  definition of, 3677
  ethylene oxide gas, 3685t, 3686-3687
  flash, 3686
  in hospitals, 3684-3688
  hydrogen peroxide gas plasma, 3685t, 3687
  methods of, 3678t-3679t
  ozone, 3687
  peracetic acid, 3685t, 3687-3688
  rational approach to, 3677-3681
  steam, 3685-3686, 3685t
  techniques of, 3685t
Sternoclavicular joint, septic arthritis of, from *Pseudomonas aeruginosa*, 2851
Steroids. *See* Corticosteroids.
Stevens-Johnson syndrome, 792, 794-795
  in beta-lactam allergy, 347
  in *Mycoplasma pneumoniae* infection, 2483, 2483f
Still's disease, fever of unknown origin in, 787
Stomatitis
  aphthous, 866
    variants of, 861t
  gangrenous, 861t, 866
  from herpes simplex virus, 1948, 1948f
  in immunocompromised hosts, 866-867
Stomatococcus, 2678
Stool specimens, 235t-236t, 242, 262
Strategic National Stockpile (SNS), bioterrorism and, 3961
Stratification, in clinical trials, 690-691
Straw itch mite, 3645-3646, 3646t
Strawberry tongue, 797
Streptidine, 359, 360f
Streptobacillus moniliformis
  arthritis from, 1444-1445, 1445t
  rat-bite fever from, 2965, 2966t
Streptococcal antibody test, in rheumatic fever, 2616
Streptococcus
  animal-isolated, 2592t
  beta-hemolytic, 2673-2674. *See also* Streptococcus group C; Streptococcus group G.
    clinical manifestations of, 2674-2677
    epidemiology of, 2674
    mesenteric lymphadenitis from, 1405
    microbiology of, 2673-2674
    treatment of, 2677-2678
  classification of, 2591-2592, 2591f, 2592t
  endocarditis from, 1070-1073, 1070t, 1088-1090
    prosthetic valve, 1113-1114
      treatment of, 1119t
    treatment of, 1088-1094

Streptococcus (Continued)
  gangrene from, 1299, 2602
  hemolytic, group A B-, postpartum endometritis
      from, 1512-1513
  human-isolated, 2592t
  keratitis from, 1542
  myonecrosis from, anaerobic, 1318
  nonsuppurative sequelae of, 2611-2622
  nutritionally variant (deficient), 2670t, 2673
  pyrogenic exotoxins of, 33
  rash from, 800
  rifamycins for, 410
Streptococcus agalactiae (group B), 2592t, 2655-2666
  adherence of, 2657
  arthritis from, 2660
  bacteremia from, 2660
  classification of, 2655
  clinical manifestations of, 2658-2661
      in adults, 2659-2661, 2659t
      in neonates, 2658-2659
      uncommon, 2661
  colonization with, factors influencing, 2656,
      2656t
  description of, 2655-2656
  diagnosis of, 2661
  endocarditis from, 2660
  epidemiology of, 2656-2657, 2656t
  genital tract infection from, in females, 2660
  historical perspective of, 2655
  host factors in, 2658
  identification of, 2655
  incidence of, 2656-2657
  inflammatory mediators in, 2658
  intrapartum antibiotic prophylaxis for, 2662-2663,
      2662t
  invasion of, 2657
  laboratory detection of, 240t-242t
  meningitis from, 1190t-1191t, 1192-1193,
      1211t-1212t, 1218, 1223, 2661
  morphologic characteristics of, 2655
  in neonates
      clinical manifestations of, 2658-2659
      transmission of, 2656
  osteomyelitis from, 2660
  pathogenetic mechanisms of, 2657-2658
  pneumonia from, 2660
  pregnancy-associated, 2657
  prevention of, 2662-2663, 2662t
  recurrent invasive, 2661
  reservoir for, 2656
  skin infections from, 2660-2661
  soft tissue infections from, 2660-2661
  treatment of, 2661-2662, 2662t
  typing of, 2655-2656
  vaccines for, 2663
  virulence of, 2657-2658
Streptococcus anginosus group, 2592t, 2667, 2668t,
    2681-2685
  bacteremia from, 2683
  bacteriologic characteristics of, 2681, 2682f,
      2682t
  brain abscess from, 1265-1268, 1266t
  empyema from, 917-918
  endocarditis from, 2683
  habitat of, 2681
  infection from
      abdominal, 2683
      central nervous system, 2683
      clinical manifestations of, 2683-2684
      head and neck, 2683
      miscellaneous, 2683-2684
      thoracic, 2683
      treatment of, 2683
  pathogenicity of, 2681-2683
  taxonomy in, 2681
Streptococcus bovis group, 2592t, 2644t, 2651-2652
Streptococcus canis, 2592t, 2674
Streptococcus dysgalactiae subsp. dysgalactiae, 2592t
Streptococcus dysgalactiae subsp. equisimilis, 2592t,
    2674
Streptococcus equi subsp. equi, 2592t
Streptococcus equi subsp. zooepidemicus, 2592t, 2674
Streptococcus gallolyticus, 2651
  endocarditis from, prosthetic valve, 1119t, 1121
Streptococcus gordonii, endocarditis from, 1071

Streptococcus group C, 2673-2674
  arthritis from, 2675
  bacteremia from, 2676-2677
  endocarditis from, 2676
  epidemiology of, 2674
  meningitis from, 2676
  microbiology of, 2674
  neonatal sepsis from, 2676
  osteomyelitis from, 2676
  pharyngitis from, 2675
  puerperal infection from, 2676
  respiratory tract infections from, 2676
  skin/soft tissue infections from, 2675
  treatment of, 2677
Streptococcus group G, 2673-2674
  arthritis from, 2675-2676
  bacteremia from, 2677
  endocarditis from, 2676
  epidemiology of, 2674
  meningitis from, 2676
  microbiology of, 2674
  osteomyelitis from, 2676
  pharyngitis from, 2675
  puerperal infection from, 2676
  respiratory tract infections from, 2676
  skin/soft tissue infections from, 2675
  treatment of, 2677-2678
Streptococcus iniae, 2592t, 2678
Streptococcus mitis, 2592t, 2667, 2668t
  dental caries from, 855, 856t
  in hematopoietic stem cell transplant recipients,
      3827
Streptococcus morbillorum, 2667-2668
Streptococcus mutans, 2592t, 2667, 2668t
  dental caries from, 855-857, 856t, 2669
  endocarditis from, 1070, 1070t
Streptococcus oralis, 856
Streptococcus pneumoniae, 2592t, 2623-2642
  adherence of, 2626
  anatomy and physiology of, 2623-2624, 2624f
  anticapsular antibody to, 2627-2628
  arthritis from, 1444, 1444t
  bronchitis exacerbation from, 2631
  capsule of, 2623-2624, 2624f
  Chlamydophila pneumoniae coinfection with, 2470
  clinical syndromes associated with, 2629-2633,
      2630f
  colonization by, 2626, 2628
  complement activation by, 2627
  conjunctivitis from, 2633
  endocarditis from, 2633
  epidemiology of, 2624-2625
  history of, 2623
  in HIV infection, 1730-1731, 1878-1879
  immunologic defenses against, 2627
  invasive, 2625-2626
  laboratory detection of, 240t-242t
  linezolid for, 473
  meningitis from, 2631
      epidemiology and etiology of, 1190t-1191t, 1192
      prevention of, 1223-1224
      treatment of, 1211t-1212t, 1212-1214,
          1216-1217, 2636
  microbiology of, 2623
  otitis media from, 832-833, 2625, 2629-2630, 2635
  pathogenetic mechanisms of, 2625-2627, 2629t
  pericarditis from, 2633
  peritonitis from, 1013, 1016, 2633
  phagocytosis of, avoidance of, 2626
  pneumonia from. See Pneumococcal pneumonia.
  postsplenectomy sepsis from, 3868
  predisposing factors for, 2628-2629, 2629t-2630t
  prevention of, 2636-2638, 2637t, 2638f
  resistance of, 306, 2633-2634, 2634t
      to cephalosporins, 2634
      to clindamycin, 441
      to macrolides, 428, 429t
      mechanisms of, 290t
      to penicillin, 2633
      prevalence of, 2634-2635, 2635t
      to quinolones, 502-503
      to vancomycin, 452
  serotypes of, 2624
  sinusitis from, 2630-2631, 2635
  splenic defenses against, 2628

Streptococcus pneumoniae (Continued)
  transformation in, 2624
  treatment of, 2635-2636
  vaccine for, 2636-2638, 2637f, 2638f. See also
      Pneumococcal vaccine.
  virulence factors of, 2626-2627, 2629t
Streptococcus porcinus, 2592t
Streptococcus pyogenes (group A), 2592t, 2593-2610
  arthritis from, 1444, 1444t
  bacteremia from, 2605-2606
  cellulitis from, 1295, 2602
      perianal, 2606
  description of, 2593-2595
  empyema from, 918
  erysipelas from, 2601, 2601f
  extracellular products of, 2594-2595
  genome sequence of, 2593
  history of, 2593
  impetigo from, 1289
  laboratory detection of, 240t-242t
  lymphangitis from, 2606
  M serotypes of
      glomerulonephritis from, 2612t, 2617-2618. See
          also Glomerulonephritis, poststreptococcal.
      rheumatic fever from, 2611-2612, 2612t
  meningitis from, 1193
  myonecrosis from, 2602-2603
  myositis from, 2602-2603
  necrotizing fasciitis from, 2602
  necrotizing myositis from, 1316
  otitis media from, 833
  pharyngitis from, 2595-2599. See also Pharyngitis,
      streptococcal, group A–associated.
  pneumonia from, 2606
  pyoderma from, 2600, 2600f
  rash from, 799-800
  resistance of
      to clindamycin, 441
      to macrolides, 428-429, 429t
  skin infections from, 2600-2605
  soft tissue infections from, 2600-2605
  somatic constituents of, 2593-2594, 2594f
  toxic shock syndrome from, 2603-2605, 2603f,
      2603t. See also Toxic shock syndrome,
      streptococcal.
  transmission of, 2595, 2595f
  virulence factors of, 5t
  vulvovaginitis from, 2606
Streptococcus salivarius, 2592t, 2667, 2668t
  in oral cavity, 855, 856t
Streptococcus sanguis, 2667, 2668t
  endocarditis from, 1070-1071, 1070t
      prosthetic valve, 1114, 1115t
  in oral cavity, 855-856, 856t
  in platelet activation, 1114
Streptococcus sobrinus, dental caries from, 856-857,
    2669
Streptococcus suis, 2592t
Streptococcus viridans group, 2667-2673
  antimicrobial susceptibility of, 2672-2673
  bacteremia from, 2670-2671
  biochemical characteristics of, 2667, 2668t
  classification of, 2667, 2668t
  clinical manifestations of, 2669-2672
  endocarditis from, 2668-2670, 2670t
      prosthetic valve, 1119t, 1121
  epidemiology of, 2668
  identification of, 2667-2668, 2668t
  meningitis from, 2671
  microbiology of, 2667
  pathogenicity of, 2668-2669
  pneumonia from, 2672
  tolerance of, 2672
  treatment of, 2669-2672
Streptogramins, 459-462. See also
    Quinupristin-dalfopristin.
  resistance to
      efflux promotion in, 287
      enzymes in, 285
      mechanisms of, 287t
      ribosomal binding site alteration in, 287
      Staphylococcus aureus, 2559t
Streptokinase, for pleural effusion/empyema, 922
Streptolysin O, 2594
Streptolysin S, 2594

Streptomycin, 359, 360f, 360t-361t
  for actinomycetoma, 3284
  adverse reactions to, 538
  for *Bartonella bacilliformis* infection, 3005
  for brucellosis, 2924
  for bubonic plague, 1330
  for donovanosis, 3013
  dosage of, 724t-725t, 734t-735t
    multiple daily, loading dose in, 374, 374t
    once-daily, 376, 377t
  for endocarditis, 1088-1089
  formulations of, 715t, 717t
  for *Mycobacterium avium* complex disease,
    3184t-3185t
  for plague, 2948
  for pneumonic plague, 3967t
  in pregnancy, 270
  for rat-bite fever, 2966
  resistance to
    in enterococci, 363
    high-level, 273
  for tuberculosis, 534t, 537t, 538-539, 3144
  for tularemia, 2935, 3974t
Streptomycin sulfate, 706t-709t
Stress
  immunity and, 45
  psychological, in immunocompromised hosts,
    3787
Stridor, in croup, 826-827
Stroke patients, fever of unknown origin in, 782
Stromal inflammation, in keratitis, 1546
Stromal melting, in keratitis, 1541
Stromal suppuration, in keratitis, 1541
Strongyloides stercoralis (strongyloidiasis), 3578t,
    3579f, 3582-3583
  abdominal pain and/or diarrhea with eosinophilia
    from, 1407, 1407t
  ivermectin for, 654
  pulmonary manifestations of, in HIV infection,
    1733
  treatment of, 632t-635t, 647
Strychnine poisoning, versus tetanus, 3093-3094
Stye, 1569
Subarachnoid space inflammation, in bacterial
    meningitis, 1199-1200, 1199t, 1220-1221
Subarachnoid space survival, in bacterial meningitis,
    1197-1199
Subcutaneous abscess, 1300, 1309-1310
Subcutaneous ecchymoses, in meningococcal sepsis,
    2741-2743, 2742f
Subcutaneous immune globulin, 3922t, 3936
Subcutaneous nodules, 795, 799, 1303
  from *Blastomyces dermatitidis*, 3325
  in rheumatic fever, 2613-2614
Subcutaneous tissue infections, 1305-1310
  clostridial, 1305-1307, 1306t
  in contiguous foci, 1309-1310
  differential diagnosis of, 1305, 1306t
  necrotizing, 1306t, 1307-1309
    synergistic, 1306t, 1309
  nonclostridial anaerobic, 1306t, 1307
  secondary, 1309
Subdural empyema, 1279, 1281f-1282f
Subglottic obstruction
  in croup, 826
  noninfectious sources of, 828
Subglottic secretions, continuous aspiration of, 3723
Subhepatic space, 1011, 1012f
Sublingual space, infections of, 863
Submandibular space, infections of, 863
Subpectoral lymphadenitis, 1324
Subperiosteal abscess, 1572-1573, 1572f-1573f
  in suppurative thrombophlebitis, 1097
Subphrenic space, 1011, 1012f
  abscess of, 1030
Substance abuse. *See also* Injection drug users.
  chronic pneumonia and, 932-933
Sudden infant death syndrome, pertussis vaccination
    and, 2959-2960
Sulbactam, 320-321, 320f
Sulfabenzamide-sulfacetamide-sulfathiazole,
    706t-709t
Sulfadiazine, 475, 476f, 706t-709t
  adverse reactions to, 477
  dosage of, 730t

Sulfadiazine *(Continued)*
  formulations of, 716t
  for *Neisseria meningitidis* carriage, 2747
  for *Paracoccidioides brasiliensis* infection, 3361
  for rheumatic fever prophylaxis, 2617, 2617t
  for *Toxoplasma* encephalitis, 1750-1751
  for toxoplasmosis
    congenital, 3520
    in HIV infection, 3518, 3518t
    ocular, 3519-3520
    in pregnant patient, 3520
Sulfadoxine, 651
  dosage of, 730t
  formulations of, 716t
Sulfadoxine-pyrimethamine
  drug interactions with, 742t-761t
  mechanism of action of, 3447
  resistance to, 3445, 3447
Sulfamethizole, 706t-709t
  dosage of, 730t
  formulations of, 716t
Sulfamethoxazole, 475, 476f, 706t-709t. *See also*
    Trimethoprim-sulfamethoxazole.
  dosage of, 730t
  formulations of, 716t
  for nontuberculous mycobacterial infections, 544
  Staphylococcus aureus resistance to, 2559t
Sulfanilamide, 706t-709t
Sulfisoxazole, 475, 476f, 706t-709t
  dosage of, 730t
  formulations of, 716t
  for otitis media prophylaxis, 834-835
Sulfisoxazole acetyl, 706t-709t
Sulfonamides, 475-478, 651
  adverse reactions to, 477, 636
  antimicrobial activity of, 476
  for brain abscess, 1273t-1274t, 1274-1275
  in children, 269
  clinical uses of, 477-478
  derivation of, 475-476
  distribution of, 476, 477t
  dosage of, 730t
  drug interactions with, 477, 742t-761t
  for gastrointestinal tract, 475
  long-acting, 475
  mechanisms of action of, 476
  medium-acting, 475
  for nocardiosis, 3203-3204
  for nontuberculous mycobacterial infections, 544
  for *Paracoccidioides brasiliensis* infection, 3361
  pharmacology of, 476-477, 477t, 730t
  in pregnancy, 270
  resistance to, 476
    target enzyme alteration in, 289
    target overproduction in, 289
  short-acting, 475
  structure of, 475, 476f
  topical, 475-476
  toxicity of, 477
  trimethoprim with, 274
Sulfoxone, for leprosy, 546
Sulfur, for scabies, 3636t
Sulfur granules, in actinomycosis, 3215, 3216f
Sulphones, 651
Superantigens
  bacterial toxins of, in Kawasaki syndrome, 3665
  of *Staphylococcus aureus*, 2544t, 2554-2556
Superinfection
  from erythromycin, 431
  in genital herpes, 1950-1951
  from tetracycline, 392
Superior sagittal sinus thrombosis, septic, 1283-1286,
    1285f
Superiority trials, 689, 694, 695f. *See also* Clinical
    trials.
Suppurative conditions. *See also* Sepsis.
Suppurative intracranial thrombophlebitis,
    1283-1286, 1285f-1286f
Suppurative lymphadenitis, 1323-1324
  epitrochlear, 1324
  iliac, 1324
Suppurative odontogenic infections, 862t, 869-870
Suppurative otitis media
  anaerobes in, 3085
  chronic, from *Pseudomonas aeruginosa*, 2853

Suppurative parotitis, 861t, 867
Suppurative streptococcal pharyngitis, group
    A–associated, 2596
Suppurative thrombophlebitis. *See*
    Thrombophlebitis, suppurative.
Suppurative thyroiditis, 862t, 868
Suprahyoid space infections, 863-864. *See also*
    Odontogenic infections.
Supramolecular activation complex, in T cell
    activation, 132
Suprapubic aspiration, for urine collection, 968
Suprapubic catheterization, 3730
Suramin, 706t-709t
  for African trypanosomiasis, 3492
  for parasitic infections, 632t-635t, 660-661
Surfactant
  daptomycin binding to, 271-272
  in *Pneumocystis*, 3381
  in pulmonary host defense, 891
Surgical drainage, for sepsis, 1002
Surgical gloves, 3758
Surgical patients, nutritional support in, 154-155
Surgical site infections, 3891-3904
  in clean wounds, 3892t, 3894
  from coagulase-negative *Staphylococcus*, 2584
  in contaminated wounds, 3892t, 3894
  control measures in, 3891-3896
  determinants of, 3891
  foreign material in, 3894
  after gynecologic surgery, 1514-1516, 1514t,
    1515f
  historical perspective of, 3891
  immunologic factors in, 3894-3895
  pathogens in, 3892-3893, 3893t
    sources of, 3892, 3892f, 3892t
    species of, 3892-3893, 3893f, 3893t
    virulence factors of, 3894
  pathophysiology of, 3891-3895, 3892f-3893f,
    3892t-3893t
  prevention of, 3896-3902, 3897t
    antimicrobial prophylaxis in
      cost-benefit analysis of, 3901-3902
      drug selection and dosing in, 3898-3899,
        3898t-3899t
      duration of, 3900-3901
      novel methods of, 3901
      preoperative, 3897-3902, 3898f
      resistance to, 3901
      side effects of, 3901
      timing of administration of, 3891, 3892f,
        3899-3900, 3900f
    cytokines in, 3895
    principles in, 3891-3896
    topical antibacterials in, 523-524
  risk factors for, 3895-3896
    assessment of, 3895-3896, 3896t
    patient, 3892, 3892t, 3895
    procedural, 3892, 3892t, 3895
  from *Staphylococcus aureus*, 2566-2567
  surveillance of, 3902, 3902t
  tissue trauma in, 3894
Surveillance
  active, 182-183
  for antimicrobial resistance, 182
  for nosocomial infections, 3669
  observational studies in, 182-183
  in outbreak detection, 184, 193-194
  passive, 182-183
  sentinel, 193
  syndromal, 182, 193
    in emergency preparedness, 223
Surveys
  cross-sectional, 184
  seroincidence, 184
  seroprevalence, 184
Susceptibility testing, 249-250, 267-268
  of aerobic actinomycetes, 254
  agar diffusion methods in, 249-250
  dilution methods in, 249
  of fungi, 256
  of mycobacteria, 252-253
  for nontuberculous mycobacteria, 3197
  specialized methods in, 250
  of viruses, 261-262
Suture needles, blunted, 3758

Sweet's syndrome, 797, 1529
  versus cellulitis, 1297, 1297t
Swimmer's ear, 831, 2853
Swimmer's itch, 3597, 3618t, 3622
Swimming, while traveling, protection against
    pathogens associated with, 4016
Swimming pool granuloma, 1331
Swine influenza, 2271
Sydenham's chorea, in rheumatic fever, 2614
Symmetric peripheral gangrene, 797-798
Symphysis pubis, osteomyelitis of, 1463
Synbiotics, 161, 162t. See also Probiotics.
Syncephalastrum, 3257, 3258t
Synctia, in parainfluenza virus infection, 2195-2196
Synergohymenotrop toxins, 2553
Synovial fluid
  laboratory evaluation of, in septic arthritis,
      1445-1446, 1446t
  laboratory processing of, 238
Syphilids, pustular, 3039-3040
Syphilis, 3035-3053. See also *Treponema pallidum*.
  atypical, 3044, 3049-3050
  cardiovascular, 3043
  causal agent of, 3036
  central nervous system in, 3040-3041. See also
      Neurosyphilis.
  chancre of, 1477, 1477f, 1480-1481, 3038-3039,
      3039f
  clinical manifestations of, 3038-3044
  condylomata lata in, 1477, 1477f, 3039-3040
  congenital, 3043-3044, 3043t
    diagnosis of, 3048
    treatment of, 3047t
  endemic, 3056-3057
  epidemiology of, 3036-3037, 3037f
  etiology of, 3036
  gastrointestinal, 1395, 3041
  gumma in, 3043
  hepatitis in, 3041
  historical aspects of, 3035-3036
  HIV coinfection with, 1639, 1860t-1870t,
      1880-1881, 3050-3051
  immunity to, 3051
  incubating, 3038
  in injection drug users, 3887
  keratitis in, 1544-1545
  laboratory diagnosis of, 3044-3048
  late, 3041-3043, 3041t-3042t
    benign, 3043
    treatment of, 3047t, 3049-3050
  latent, 3041
  meningitis in, 1240
    in HIV infection, 1745-1746
  mucous patches in, 3039-3040, 3040f
  nontreponemal reaginic tests for, 3045
  obliterative endarteritis in, 3038, 3038f
  ocular
    Argyll Robertson pupil in, 3042
    treatment of, 1567, 3050
    uveitis in, 1563-1564
  otitis in, 3050
  papules in, 3039-3040
  paraplegia in, 3040-3041
  pathogenesis of, 3037-3038
  pathologic characteristics of, 3038, 3038f
  persistent, 3050
  polymerase chain reaction assay for, 3048
  primary, 3038-3039, 3039f
  rapid tests for, 3048
  rash in, 795
  secondary (disseminated), 3039-3041, 3040f,
      3040t
  serologic tests for, 3044-3048, 3045t
    false-positive, 3046-3048, 3048t
  specific treponemal tests for, 3045-3046
  spirochetes in, 3041
    darkfield examination of, 3044, 3045f
  treatment of, 3047t, 3048-3051
    adequacy of, 3050
    follow-up and retreatment in, 3050
    Jarisch-Herxheimer reaction in, 3050-3051
    penicillin allergy and, 3050
  untreated, natural course of, 3038
Syringe pumps, for outpatient parenteral
    antimicrobial therapy, 701

Systemic inflammatory response syndrome (SIRS)
  in children, 987
  definition of, 987, 988t
  in immunocompromised hosts, 3787-3788

T

T cell leukemia/lymphoma
  adult, 2313f-2314f, 2315-2316
  nasal, from Epstein-Barr virus, 1998
T cell–independent antigens, 69-70
T cells. See also CD4; CD8.
  activation of, 132-137
    by B cells, 69, 70f
  antigen recognition by, 132-133
  antigen-presenting cells and, interface between,
      132
  assay of, 168, 171t
  in autoimmune reactions, 71
  B cell interactions with, 68-69, 68f
  in beta-lactam allergy, 347
  congenital defects in, 167-171, 169t-170t
  cytolytic, 131
  cytotoxic, in HIV infection, 1690-1691, 1690t
  depletion of, in HIV infection, 2331-2332
  in intestinal mucosa, 144
  in lymph nodes, 142, 144
  memory, 131-132
  natural killer, 132. See also Natural killer cells.
  peripheral, thymic selection and, 141
  in *Pseudomonas aeruginosa* resistance, 2839
  pulmonary, 893
  in sepsis, 998
  in spleen, 143-144, 143f
  subsets and phenotypic diversity of, 129-132
  Th1, 129
  Th2, 129-130
  Th17, 130
  thymic selection of, 141-142
  T-regulatory, 130
  in vaccine immune response, 3919
Tachyzoite, *Toxoplasma gondii*, 3495-3496, 3496f
Tacrolimus, for transplant immunosuppression,
    infections and, 3811
Taenia asiatica, 3610
Taenia multiceps, 3608t, 3615
Taenia saginata, 632t-635t, 3608t, 3609f, 3610
Taenia solium, 632t-635t, 3608t, 3609f, 3610
  cysticercosis from, 3611-3613, 3612f
Tafenoquine
  G6PD deficiency and, 638
  for malaria, 638-639
Tamm-Horsfall protein, 40, 961-962, 962f
Tamponade, in pericarditis, 1163
Tanapox virus, 1935
Tap water. See also Water *entries*.
  hypochlorite solutions in, 3682
Tapeworms, 3607-3616
  abdominal pain and/or diarrhea with eosinophilia
      from, 1407t, 1409
  anatomy of, 3607, 3609f
  beef, 3608t, 3609f, 3610
  diagnosis of, 3610-3611
  dwarf, 3608t, 3609-3610, 3609f
  fish, 3608-3609, 3608t, 3609f
  immune response to, 3608
  intestinal, 3574t
  invasive, 3611-3615
  larval, 3574t
  life cycle of, 3607-3608, 3608f-3609f
  pathogenecity of, 3608
  pork, 3608t, 3609f, 3610
  prevention of, 3615
  treatment of, 632t-635t, 3611
Taxonomy, bacterial, changes in, 233, 234t
Tazobactam, 321, 321f
Teichoic acids, 2623-2624
  of *Staphylococcus aureus*, 2551, 2552f
Teicoplanin, 457-459, 706t-709t
  adverse reactions to, 459
  antimicrobial activity of, 457-458
  clinical uses of, 459
  distribution of, 458
  dosage of, 458, 728t-729t
    in infants and children, 458

Teicoplanin (*Continued*)
  drug interactions with, 742t-761t
  for *Enterococcus* infections, 2649
  for febrile neutropenia, 3804t
  formulations of, 716t
  minimal inhibitory concentration susceptibility
      for, 460t
  peritoneal administration of, 458
  pharmacokinetics of, 458-459
  prophylactic, 459
  resistance to, 458
    cell wall precursor target alterations in, 288,
        288t
Telangiectasia, hereditary hemorrhagic, brain abscess
    from, 1267
Telaprevir, 599f, 600
  in NS3/4A protease inhibition, 2175
Telavancin, 706t-709t
  dosage of, 728t-729t
  for *Enterococcus* infections, 2649
Telbivudine, 595-596, 706t-709t
  clinical studies of, 596
  dosage of, 738t-739t
  formulations of, 717t
  for hepatitis B infection, chronic, 1600, 1601t,
      2076-2077, 2076t
  structure of, 572f
Telithromycin, 438-440, 706t-709t
  adverse reactions to, 439
  antimicrobial activity of, 429t, 439
  chemistry of, 438, 438f
  for *Chlamydophila* respiratory infection, 2471t
  dosage of, 726t-727t
  drug interactions with, 439, 742t-761t
  formulations of, 716t
  mechanism of action of, 438-439
  pharmacology of, 439
  preparations of, 438
  resistance to, 439
  uses of, 440
Temafloxacin, 504
TEM-derived beta-lactamase, 283, 283f
Temperature
  in children, 768
  core, 765
  diurnal variability in, 766, 768
  in elderly, 766, 768
  elevated. See Fever.
  gender and, 766, 768
  heart rate and, 768
  measurement of, 765-768
    anatomic variables in, 765-766
    physiologic variables in, 766-767
  mental health and, 766
  normal values for, 766-767, 767t
  oral, 767, 767f
  rectal, 765-766
  regulation of, 768-769, 768f
  right atrial, 766
  setpoint of, 769
  shell, 765
  skin, 766
  tympanic membrane, 766
  in virulence regulation, 8
Temporal (giant cell) arteritis, fever of unknown
    origin in, 787
Temporal clustering, 195
Tenofovir, 596, 706t-709t, 1834f, 1835t, 1836-1837
  dosage of, 740t-741t
  drug interactions with, 742t-761t
  formulations of, 717t
  for hepatitis B infection, chronic, 1600, 1601t,
      2077
  for HIV postexposure prophylaxis, 3755t, 3764
  for HIV-infected children, 1820t-1821t
  nephrotoxicity of, 1837
  resistance to, 1837
Tenosynovitis, from *Sporothrix schenckii*, 3271
  in HIV-infected patient, 3273-3274, 3273f
Teratogenicity
  of antimicrobial agents, 270
  of antiretroviral therapy, 1795
Terbinafine, 706t-709t
  for chromoblastomycosis, 3279
  for dermatophytosis, 3352

Terbinafine *(Continued)*
  dosage of, 736t-737t
  drug interactions with, 742t-761t
  for eumycetoma, 3284-3285
  formulations of, 717t
  for sporotrichosis, 3274
Terconazole, 706t-709t, 717t
Testis
  anatomy and physiology of, 1521, 1522f
  dysfunction of, in leprosy, 3171
  infection of. *See* Orchitis.
Tetanolysin, 3091
Tetanospasmin, 3091
Tetanus, 3091-3096. *See also Clostridium tetani.*
  cephalic, 3093, 3093f
  clinical manifestations of, 3092-3093
  diagnosis of, 3093-3094
  epidemiology of, 3091, 3092f
  generalized, 3092-3093, 3092f-3093f
  history of, 3091
  in injection drug users, 3886
  localized, 3093
  mortality rate in, 3091, 3092f, 3095
  neonatal, 3093, 3093f
  pathogenesis of, 3091-3092
  prophylaxis against, 3095. *See also* Diphtheria-
    pertussis-tetanus (DPT) vaccine; Tetanus
    immune globulin; Tetanus toxoid.
    for bite wounds, 3913t
    postexposure, 3943
  spasm in, 3092-3093, 3093f
  versus strychnine poisoning, 3093-3094
  treatment of, 3094-3095, 3094t
Tetanus immune globulin, 3092f, 3094-3095, 3922t,
  3935
  in HIV-infected children, 1826
Tetanus toxin, 31, 3091
Tetanus toxoid, 3095, 3922t, 3933
Tetanus-diphtheria (Td) toxoids, 2961, 3922t, 3923,
  3933
Tetanus–diphtheria–accelerated pertussis (TdaP)
  vaccine, 2961, 3095, 3922t, 3923, 3929-3930,
  3933
  during pregnancy, 2961
Tetracycline, 385-394, 706t-709t
  absorption of, 387-388, 390t
  for actinomycosis, 3217t
  activity spectrum of, 385-386, 388t
  for balantidiasis, 3566
  for brucellosis, 2924
  for *Campylobacter* infections, 2799
  in children, 269
  for *Chlamydophila* respiratory infection, 2471
  for cholera, 2782t
  classification of, 385
  for donovanosis, 3013
  dosage of, 724t
  drug interactions with, 392, 393t, 742t-761t
  for ehrlichiosis, 2536
  elimination of, 389
  for epidemic typhus, 2523
  food interactions with, 392, 393t
  formulations of, 387t, 715t
  gastrointestinal effects of, 392
  for *Helicobacter pylori* infection, 2809t
  hepatotoxicity of, 392
  history of, 385
  hypersensitivity reactions to, 390-392
  indications for, 392-394, 393t
  in liver disease, 389-390, 391t
  for louse-borne relapsing fever, 3068-3069
  mechanism of action of, 385-387
  minimal inhibitory concentrations of, 385-386,
    388t
  for *Mycoplasma pneumoniae* infection, 2487
  nephrotoxicity of, 392
  neurotoxicity of, 392
  for noninfectious conditions, 394
  for nontuberculous mycobacterial infections, 544
  for parasitic infections, 661
  penicillin with, 392
  for peritonitis, 1024
  pharmacology of, 387-390, 390t, 724t
  photosensitivity reactions to, 390-392
  pigmentation changes from, 390-392

Tetracycline *(Continued)*
  in pregnancy, 270, 389
  for psittacosis, 2465
  for Q fever, 2514
  for rat-bite fever, 2966
  in renal failure, 389-390, 391t
  resistance to
    efflux promotion in, 286, 386, 389t
    enzymes in, 285-286
    mechanisms of, 286t, 386-387, 388t-389t
    ribosomal binding site alteration in, 287, 386,
      389t
    Staphylococcus aureus, 2559t
    target site protection in, 289
  for Rocky Mountain spotted fever, 2503
  side effects of, 390-392, 391t
  structures of, 385, 386f
  superinfection from, 392
  for syphilis, 3047t
  teeth discoloration from, 392
  tissue distribution of, 388-389, 390t
  for tropical sprue, 1432
  for tularemia, 2935
  for urethritis, 1490
Tetramer staining, MHC, 145-146, 146f
Th1 immunity, to phagosomal pathogens, 140
Th1 T cells, 129
Th2 T cells, 129-130
Th17 T cells, 130
Thalassemia, malaria and, 53, 3443
Thalidomide
  for aphthous ulcers
    esophageal, 1355t, 1356
    oral, 866
  for erythema nodosum leprosum, 546, 3173
  as immunomodulator, 620
  for microsporidiosis, 3402
  for subarachnoid space inflammation, 1220-1221
Theophylline, quinolone interactions with, 494
Thermal injury, immunodeficiency in, 176-177
Thermogenesis, 768
  infection-regulated, 992
  nonshivering, 768
Thermometry, 765-768, 767f
Thermoregulation, 768-769, 768f
Thermotherapy, for cutaneous leishmaniasis, 3475
Thiabendazole, 706t-709t
  for angiostrongyliasis, 3621
  drug interactions with, 742t-761t
  for intestinal parasitic infections, 632t-635t,
    647-648
Thiacetazone, 706t-709t
  for leprosy, 545
Thiamphenicol, 394
Thienamycin, chemistry of, 341, 342f
Thimerosal, in vaccines, 3917
Thioester bond, in tickover model of complement
  activation, 79-80, 80f
Thoracentesis, for pleural effusion/empyema, 922
Thoracic actinomycosis, 3211, 3212f
Thoracic infections
  from gram-negative anaerobic rods, 3116
  from *Streptococcus anginosus* group, 2683
Thoracic surgery, video-assisted, for pleural effusion/
  empyema drainage, 923
Thoracoscopy, in pneumonia, 899-900
Thoracotomy, for chronic pneumonia, 942
Throat, sore. *See* Pharyngitis.
Throat culture, for streptococcal pharyngitis, 819,
  2597
Throat swabs, laboratory processing of, 238-239
Thrombocytopenia
  in cytomegalovirus infection, 1975
  in HIV infection, 1720
  in immunocompromised hosts, 3787
  in infectious mononucleosis, 1994, 1999
  from linezolid, 473
  from rifamycins, 405
  in sepsis, 998
  from teicoplanin, 459
Thrombocytopenic purpura
  idiopathic, in *Helicobacter pylori* infection, 2808
  thrombotic, in HIV infection, 1720
Thromboembolic disease, fever of unknown origin
  in, 786-787

Thrombophlebitis
  cavernous sinus, 1571-1573
  in injection drug users, 3881
  septic pelvic, 1513
  suppurative, 1095-1099
    in burn patients, 1097
    clinical manifestations of, 1096-1097
    epidemiology of, 1095-1096
    etiologic agents in, 1097-1098
    intracranial, 1283-1286, 1285f-1286f
    jugular, 862t, 864-865, 864f
    laboratory findings in, 1097
    pathogenesis of, 1096
    pathology of, 1096
    pelvic, 1097
    prevention of, 1099
    septic, 1095-1096
    from *Staphylococcus aureus,* 1097-1098
    subperiosteal abscess in, 1097
    superficial, 1096
    treatment of, 1098-1099
Thrombosis
  deep vein, air travel-related, 4016
  sinus, septic cavernous, 865, 865f, 1283-1286,
    1284f
Thrombotic thrombocytopenic purpura, in HIV
  infection, 1720
Thrush (oral candidiasis), 3227, 3227f
  in HIV infection, 1714, 1714f
  treatment of, 3237
ThyA gene, in *Staphylococcus,* 2545-2546
Thymic selection of T cells, 141-142
Thymidine analog mutations, in zidovudine
  resistance, 1834
Thymosin-alpha, 620
Thyroglossal duct cyst, infected, 862t, 867
Thyroiditis, suppurative, 862t, 868
TIBOLA (tick-borne lymphadenopathy), 2504-2505
Ticarcillin, 318, 319f, 706t-709t
  dosage of, 718t-719t
  formulations of, 715t
  indications for, 315-316
  susceptibility to, 311t-312t
Ticarcillin-clavulanate, 320, 706t-709t
  dosage of, 718t-719t
  formulations of, 715t
  for *Stenotrophomonas maltophilia* infection, 2865
Tick(s)
  argasid, 3649
  biology and ecology of, 3649, 3650f
  Ixodid, 3071, 3072f, 3649-3650, 3651f
Tick bite, in Rocky Mountain spotted fever,
  2499-2503
Tick fever, Oklahoma, 2098
Tick paralysis, 3660, 3660t
Tick repellents, prophylactic, for tularemia,
  2935-2936
Tick typhus, 2504
Tick-borne encephalitis
  clinical features of, 2147-2148
  epidemiology of, 2140-2141
  geographic distribution of, 2134f
  historical perspective on, 2134-2135
  immunization against, for travelers, 4011t, 4013
  subtypes of, 2138t
  treatment of, 2150-2152
  vaccine for, 2151
  viral etiology in, 1251t-1252t, 3657-3659, 3659t
Tick-borne infection(s), 3649-3662. *See also specific*
  infection.
  anaplasmosis as, 3656, 3657t
  babesiosis as, 3539-3545, 3656-3657, 3658f, 3658t
  bacterial, 3650-3656
  coltiviruses as, 3659-3660
  Crimean-Congo hemorrhagic fever as, 2289-2292,
    2290t
  ehrlichiosis as, 2531-2538, 3656, 3656f, 3657t
  epidemiology of, 3649-3650
  prevention and control of, 3661
  protozoal, 3656-3657
  Q fever as, 3654-3655
  rash in, 796-797, 803
  relapsing fever as, 3067
    treatment of, 3068-3069
  spirochetal borrelioses as, 3650-3653, 3651t-3652t

Tick-borne infection(s) (Continued)
  spotted fever group rickettsial, 3653-3654, 3653t, 3654f
  tick behavior and, 3649, 3650f
  transfusion-related, 3748
  tularemia as, 2927-2937, 3655-3656
  viral, 3657-3660
  viral encephalitides as, 3657-3659, 3659t
  viral hemorrhagic fevers as, 3659, 3659t
Tigecycline, 387t, 706t-709t
  activity spectrum of, 385-386, 388t
  for Chlamydophila respiratory infection, 2471t
  dosage of, 724t
  for Enterococcus infection, 2650
  formulations of, 715t
  for gram-negative anaerobic rod infections, 3117-3118
  indications for, 392-394, 393t
  for nontuberculous mycobacterial infections, 544
  for peritonitis, 1022t, 1026
  pharmacology of, 387-390, 390t
  resistance to, 291, 291t
  side effects of, 391t
  for Staphylococcus aureus infection, 2562
Time-dependent (concentration-independent) killing agents, 302, 302f
Tinea barbae, 3349
Tinea capitis, 3346t, 3349-3350, 3350f, 3352t
Tinea corporis, 3348, 3348f, 3352t
Tinea cruris, 3348
Tinea faciei, 3349, 3349f
Tinea imbricata, 3346, 3349, 3349f
Tinea incognito, 3347
Tinea manuum, 3349
Tinea nigra, 3354-3355
Tinea pedis, 3348, 3352, 3352t
Tinea versicolor, 3353-3354
Tinidazole, 658, 706t-709t
  for amebic liver abscess, 1038
  for bacterial meningitis, 1504
  dosage of, 726t-727t
  drug interactions with, 742t-761t
  for Entamoeba histolytica infection, 3422t
  formulations of, 717t
  for giardiasis, 3531, 3531t
  for Helicobacter pylori infection, 2809t
  in pregnancy, 1500
  for Trichomonas vaginalis infection, 1499
  for trichomoniasis, 3536-3537
  for urethritis, 1491
Tipranavir, 706t-709t, 1839f, 1840t, 1842
  dosage of, 740t-741t
  formulations of, 717t
  for HIV-infected children, 1820t-1821t, 1823t
Tissue roundworms (nematodes), 3574t
Tissue trauma, postsurgical, 3894
Tissue tropisms, in innate immunity, 37-38
Tissue-type plasminogen activator (t-PA), in bacterial meningitis, 1204
TMA/HPA assay, in HIV infection, 1671-1672, 1671f
Tobramycin, 359, 360f, 360t-361t
  for brain abscess, 1274t
  for cystic fibrosis, 952
  dosage of, 724t-725t
    in children, 378t
    multiple daily
      loading dose in, 374, 374t
      in renal insufficiency, 374
    once-daily, 376, 377t
  for endocarditis, 1093
  formulations of, 715t
  inhalation solution of, 706t-709t
  for meningitis, 1213t
  for non-HACEK endocarditis, 1121t
  for nosocomial pneumonia, 3718t
  for peritonitis, 1029t
  resistance to, in enterococci, 363
Tobramycin sulfate, 706t-709t
Toe(s)
  Candida infection between, 3228, 3229f
  osteomyelitis of, 1461-1462
Toe web infections, 2856
Tolevamer, for Clostridium difficile–associated colitis, 1383-1384

Toll-like receptor(s), 41, 42t
  activation of, in oral mucosa, 857
  in bacterial meningitis subarachnoid space inflammation, 1200
  cytokine cascade and, 42-43
  distribution of, 43, 43t
  genetic deficiency of, 43
  in initial inflammatory response, 43
  in innate immunity, 43, 138
  in Legionnaires' disease, 2971, 2974
  in phagocyte signaling, 175, 175f
  in Streptococcus agalactiae (group B) infection, 2658
Toll-like receptor 2, 54-55
Toll-like receptor 3, 169t-170t
Toll-like receptor 4, 54-55
Toll-like receptor 5, 54
Toll-like receptor pathway genes, 54-55
Tolnaftate, 706t-709t
TonB protein, 2820
Tonsillitis
  from Actinomyces, 3211
  from Corynebacterium diphtheriae, 2596, 2689, 2689f
Tooth (teeth). See also Dental entries.
  discoloration of, from tetracycline, 392
Topical antibacterial therapy, 521-532
  for acne vulgaris, 526-527
  advantages of, 521, 522t
  for burn infections, 3906t, 3907
  for erythrasma, 526
  general use of, 521-527
  for keratitis, 1543
  prophylactic
    for burn wound infections, 525-526
    for catheter-related infections, 524
    for clean wound infections, 522-523
    for dialysis catheter infections, 524-525
    for operative wound infections, 523-524
    for recurrent skin/soft tissue infections, 523
  for pyoderma, 526
  for rosacea, 526
  skin disinfection with, 521-522
  specific agents used in, 522t. See also specific agent.
  Staphylococcus aureus nasal carriage elimination with, 527
Topoisomerase IV, quinolone inhibition of, 289, 487, 489
Toronto virus, 2401
Toroviruses/torovirus infection, 2187, 2408
  clinical manifestations of, 2191-2192
  description of, 2189
  laboratory diagnosis of, 2192
  pathogenicity of, 2192
Torsades de pointes, from voriconazole, 558
Toscana virus, 2292-2293
  encephalitis from, 1251t-1252t
Tosufloxacin, 706t-709t
Tourniquet test, for dengue fever, 4022
Toxic algae
  disease from, 3569-3571
  sites and types of, 3569, 3570f
Toxic epidermal necrolysis, 792, 794-795
  in beta-lactam allergy, 347
Toxic shock syndrome, 2555-2556
  from influenza, 2276
  intravenous immune globulin for, 618
  after medical abortion, 1514
  menstrual, 2555
  nonmenstrual, 2555
  staphylococcal, 1292
    diagnosis of, 2555, 2556t
    menstrual, 2555
    nonmenstrual, 2555
    predisposing factors in, 2555
    rash in, 800, 800t
    treatment and prevention of, 2555-2556
  streptococcal, 2603-2605, 2603f
    case definition of, 2603t
    clinical manifestations of, 2604-2605
    cytokine induction of, 2604
    diagnosis of, 2555, 2556t
    exotoxins in, 2604
    factors in, 2603, 2603t
    pathogenesis of, 2603-2604

Toxic shock syndrome (Continued)
  rash in, 800, 800t
  risk of secondary cases of, 2606
  secondary, prophylaxis and, 2606
  treatment of, 2605
Toxic shock syndrome toxin, as trigger for severe sepsis, 997
Toxic shock syndrome toxin-1, 2554
Toxin(s), 27-35. See also Enterotoxin(s); Exotoxin(s).
  A-B, 27, 30
  adenylate cyclase, 28t, 30
  ADP-ribosylating, 28t
  attachment of, 29-30
  of Bacillus, 2728
  of Bacillus anthracis, 30
  of Bordetella pertussis, 30-31, 2955-2956
  botulinum, 3097
    as biological weapon, 3100
    immunity to, 3100-3101
    release mechanism of, 3098, 3098f
    synthesis of, 3098
    therapeutic uses of, 3099
    transport of, 3098
  cholera, 31-32
  ciguatera fish, 1416-1417, 1417t, 3569, 3570t
  classification of, 27, 28t
  of Clostridium, 3103
  of Clostridium botulinum, 31, 3097
  of Clostridium difficile, 32, 1340t, 1341, 1376
    assay for, 1344
    detection of, 1377f, 1380-1381
  of Clostridium perfringens, 1340t, 1341, 3106, 3106t
  of Clostridium tetani, 31
  of Cornebacterium diphtheriae, 30-31
  deamidating, 28t
  of Enterobacteriaceae organisms, 2819-2820
  entry of, 29-30
  of Escherichia coli, 1340t, 1341
  in foodborne disease
    bacterial, 1413-1416, 1415t
    nonbacterial, 1416-1418, 1417t
  in gastrointestinal infections, 1340-1341, 1340t
  glucosylating, 28t
  of gram-negative anaerobic rods, 3114
  metalloprotease, 28t
  pore-forming, 33
  of Pseudomonas aeruginosa, 2844-2845
  pyrogenic, 33
  regulation of, 27-29, 29t
  RNA glycosidase, 28t
  secretion of, 29, 29t
  shellfish, 1416-1417, 1417t, 3569-3570, 3570t
  Shiga and Shiga-like, 32
  of Shigella dysenteriae, 1340t, 1341
  of Staphylococcus aureus, 1340t, 1341
    exfoliative, 2553-2554
    Panton-Valentine, 2553, 2553f
  synergohymenotrop, 2553
  therapeutic uses of, 33-34
  toxic shock syndrome, 997
Toxocara, 632t-635t
Toxocara canis, 3617
Toxocara cati, 3617
Toxocariasis, 3617-3618, 3618t
  ocular, 1565, 3618
Toxoid. See also specific agent.
  currently available, 3922t
  definition of, 3917
Toxoplasma gondii/toxoplasmosis, 3495-3526
  in bone marrow transplant recipient, 3504
  brain abscess from, 1266-1267, 1266t
  central nervous system manifestations of, 1270, 3501
  chorioretinitis in, 3501
    in HIV infection, 1720, 3505, 3505f
  clinical manifestations of, 3502-3508
  congenital, 3506-3508
    diagnosis of, 3516, 3517t
    serologic screening and prophylaxis for, 3521-3522, 3521t
    treatment of, 3520
  diagnosis of, 3508-3516
    CSF abnormalities in, 3512
    histologic, 3508

Toxoplasma gondii/toxoplasmosis (*Continued*)
  in immunocompetent patient, 3512
  in immunodeficient patient, 3512-3513, 3514f
    polymerase chain reaction in, 3508
    radiologic, 3510-3512, 3511f
    serologic antibody tests in, 3508-3510
    specific clinical entities in, 3512
  encephalitis in, in HIV infection, 1270-1271, 1749-1751, 1750f, 1874-1875, 3501
    incidence of, 3498
    prophylaxis against, 1858t-1859t
    treatment of, 3518-3519
  epidemiology of, 3497-3498, 3497f
  etiology of, 3495-3497, 3496f
  genetic susceptibility to, 3500
  in heart transplant recipients, 3503, 3842, 3846
  in hematopoietic stem cell transplant recipients, 3504, 3832
  in HIV infection, 3504-3506, 3505f
    chorioretinitis in, 1720
    encephalitis in. See *Toxoplasma gondii*/ toxoplasmosis, encephalitis in.
    pulmonary, 1732-1733
  host cell entrance by, 9
  immune response to, 3498-3500
  in immunocompetent patient, 3502
    diagnosis of, 3512
    ocular, 3506
    treatment of, 3518
  in immunodeficient patient, 3502-3503
    diagnosis of, 3512-3513, 3514f
    serologic screening and prophylaxis for, 3521
    treatment of, 3518-3519, 3518t
  versus infectious mononucleosis, 2003
  isolation of, 3508
  in kidney transplant recipient, 3504
  life cycle of, 3497, 3497f
  in liver transplant recipient, 3504
  lymphadenitis from, 1329
  lymphadenitis in, 3500
  myalgia in, 1320
  myocarditis from, 1156, 1156f
  myocarditis in, 3501
  myositis in, 3501
  ocular, 1565
    diagnosis of, 3513-3514
    in immunocompetent patient, 3506
    treatment of, 3519-3520
  oocysts of, 3495, 3496f
  in organ transplant recipient, 3503, 3503t
  pathogenesis of, 3498-3500
  pathology of, 3500-3502, 3500f
  in pregnancy, 3506
    diagnosis of, 3514-3516, 3515f
    treatment of, 3520
  prevention of, 3521-3522
    general methods in, 3500f, 3521
    serologic screening and prophylaxis in, 3521-3522, 3521t
  pulmonary, 3501
    in HIV infection, 1732-1733, 3505
  tachyzoites of, 3495-3496, 3496f
  tissue cysts of, 3496-3497, 3496f
  transmission of, 3497, 3497f
  treatment of, 632t-635t, 3516-3520
    in congenital cases, 3520
    in immunocompetent patient, 3518
    in immunodeficient patient, 3518-3519, 3518t
    for ocular infections, 3519-3520
    in pregnancy, 3520
    sulfonamides in, 477
ToxR protein, 8
Trace minerals, 153-154
  supplementation of, in elderly, 157, 157t
Tracheal aspirates, laboratory processing of, 239
Tracheal cytotoxin, of *Bordetella pertussis*, 30
Tracheitis, bacterial, 827-828
Tracheobronchial diphtheria, 2690-2691
Tracheobronchitis
  in aspergillosis, 3247-3248
  in burn patients, 3906
  from *Mycoplasma pneumoniae*, 2482
  ventilator-associated, 3717-3719, 3723

Trachipleistophora, 3391, 3392t. See also Microsporidia.
  in HIV infection, 3399
Trachoma, 1533-1534
  keratitis in, 1544-1545
  macrolides for, 437
  ocular, from *Chlamydia trachomatis*, 2446, 2449, 2449t
Transducer/transducer dome, infections of, in hemodynamic monitoring, 3706-3707, 3707t
Transepithelial elimination, in chromoblastomycosis, 3277
Transesophageal echocardiography, in endocarditis, 1080
  prosthetic valve, 1116
Transferrin, in nutritional assessment, 151, 152t
Transfusions
  cost of, 3744
  Creutzfeldt-Jakob disease associated with, 2432
  granulocyte
    for neutropenia, in cancer, 3806
    for neutrophil defects, 117
  HAV-contaminated blood in, 2372, 2376
    vaccination for, 2383
  HCV-contaminated blood in, 2167, 2175
  HIV testing in, 1679
  HIV transmission through, 1625, 1639-1640, 1647-1648, 1652
  human T-cell lymphotrophic virus infection from, 2311
  infections from
    donor screening for, 3742, 3742t, 3743f-3744f
    nosocomial, 3742-3748, 3742t, 3743f-3744f, 3747f, 3747t
    in transplant recipients, 3813, 3813t
  for peritonitis, 1026
  plasma
    for complement deficiencies, 95
    for peritonitis, 1026
    recipients of, vaccination against hepatitis A in, 2383
  platelet, bacterial infections from, 3747-3748, 3747f
  red blood cell, bacterial infections from, 3747
  scope of, 3742-3744
  for sepsis, 1002-1003
Translocation, cytolysin-mediated, 33
Transmembrane kinases, in *Entamoeba histolytica*, 3412-3413, 3413f
Transmission, routes of, 187-188
Transmission-based isolation precautions, 3674-3676
  airborne, 3674-3675, 3675t
  contact, 3675-3676, 3675t
  droplet, 3675, 3675t
Transplantation. See also *under specific organ*.
  aspergillosis after, 3244, 3244t
  bone marrow. See Bone marrow transplantation.
  coagulase-negative *Staphylococcus* infection after, 2585
  cytomegalovirus after, 1980-1982. See also Cytomegalovirus/cytomegalovirus infection, in transplant recipients.
  fever after, approach to, 3816-3817
  hematopoietic stem cell. See Hematopoietic stem cell transplantation.
  hepatitis B after, 2072-2073
  HIV after, 1647-1648
  infections after, 3809-3819, 3813t
    fever and, 3816-3817
    host factors in, 3809
    immunosuppression and, 3810-3812, 3811t
    microbial agents causing, 3812-3813, 3812t-3813t
    monitoring for, 3814
    pathogen exposure prevention in, 3816, 3817t
    pretransplant evaluation for, 3813-3814, 3814t
    prevention of, 3815-3816, 3815t
    risk factors in, 3809, 3810t
    in stem cell transplants, 3821-3837. See also Hematopoietic stem cell transplantation.
    transmission of, 3748
    transplant type and, 3809-3810, 3810f
  leprosy after, 3174
  lymphoproliferative disease after, 1996-1997, 1997f, 2001-2002, 3848-3849

Transplantation (*Continued*)
  solid organ. See Solid organ transplant recipients.
  tissue procurement for, HIV testing in, 1679
  toxoplasmosis after, 3503, 3503t
Transporter associated with antigen processing (TAP), in MHC class I peptide transport, 134
Transposable genetic elements, in antimicrobial resistance, 279-281, 280f
Transposons, 10-11
  in antimicrobial resistance, 279-281, 280f
  conjugative, 280-281
  versus insertion sequences, 280-281
Transthoracic echocardiography, in endocarditis, 1079
Trauma
  brain abscess from, 1267
  clenched-fist, 3914-3915
  endophthalmitis after, 1554
  maxillofacial, 868
  miscellaneous infections secondary to, 1309
  opportunistic infections after, in immunocompromised patients, 1302
  tissue, postsurgical site, 3894
Travel itinerary, detailed, 4020
Travel medicine, information resources for, 4010t
Travelers
  acute mountain sickness in, 4016
  airline-related morbidity in, 4016
  altitude and, 4016
  arthropods in, personal protection against, 4015
  blood-borne disease in, protection against, 4015
  chikungunya fever in, 4022
  chronology of illness in, 4021, 4021t
  dengue in, 4014-4015, 4022
  to developing world
    immunizations for, 4009-4010, 4012f
    pretravel office visit for, 4010t
  diarrhea in, 1365-1367, 4015, 4025-4026
    acute, 4025
    amebic, 3416-3417, 3417f
    definition of, 4025
    from *Escherichia coli*, 2823
    etiology of, 1366, 1366t
    persistent, 4025-4026
    prevention of, 1367
    rifamycins for, 412
    treatment of, 1367
  eosinophilia in, 4026, 4026t
  fever in, 4019-4025
    considerations for, 4021-4024
    initial approach to, 4024-4025
    skin eruptions accompanying, 4026, 4027f
    of unknown origin, 781, 781t
  foodborne disease in, 4021
    protection against, 4015
  hepatitis A in, 2376
    vaccination against, 2383, 4009, 4011t
  HIV infection in, 4016
  immunization history in, 4021
  immunizations for, 189, 3941, 4009-4013, 4011t. See also *specific vaccine*.
    to all destinations in developing world, 4009-4010, 4012f
    to certain destinations, 4011-4013
    in elderly, 3862
    interactions among, 4013
    spacing of, 4013
    update of routine, 4009
  immunocompromised, 4016
  infections in, 4019-4028
    asymptomatic, screening for, 4028
    common, 4023f
    cutaneous manifestations of, 4026, 4027f
    epidemiology of, 4009, 4019
    exposure and clinical presentation of, 4019, 4020t
    incubation periods of, 4021t
    patient history for, 4019-4021, 4021t
    worldwide distribution of, 4012f
  Legionnaires' disease in, 2974
  leptospirosis in, 4024
  malaria in, 4021-4022
    chemoprophylaxis for, 3455, 3455t, 4013-4014
    risk of, 4013, 4014f
    self-treatment of, 3453

Travelers *(Continued)*
  medical care abroad for, 4016
  medical kit for, 4016
  medications ingested by, 4021
    antimalarial, 4021
  noninfectious problems in, 4016
  paratyphoid fever in, 4022-4024
  physical examination of, 4021
  pregnant, 4017
  protection of, 4009-4017
  rash in, 4023f, 4026, 4027f
  respiratory illness in, 4024
  rickettsial disease in, 4024
  sexually transmitted disease in, 4015
  skin disease in, prevention of, 4015-4016
  with special needs, 4016-4017
  swimming by, protection against pathogens due
    to, 4016
  tuberculosis in, 4024
    prevention of, 4016
  typhoid fever in, 4022-4024
  unprotected sex among, 4015
  viral hepatitis in, 4024
  water exposure of, protection against pathogens
    due to, 4016
T-regulatory T cells, 130
Trematodes. *See* Flukes; *Schistosoma*
  (schistosomiasis).
Trench fever, 2995-2997
Trench mouth (Vincent's angina), 859-860
  anaerobes in, 3085, 3115
  antimicrobial therapy for, 861t
Treponema carateum, 3055, 3057
Treponema pallidum, 3035. *See also* Syphilis.
  in central nervous system, 3041-3043. *See also*
    Neurosyphilis.
  isolation of, 3048
  laboratory detection of, 240t-242t, 243
  meningitis from, 1193, 1206, 1209-1210, 1212t,
    1219, 1745-1746
  uveitis from, 1564. *See also* Syphilis, ocular.
Treponema pallidum particle agglutination (TPPA)
  index, calculation of, 3046
Treponema pallidum subsp. *endemicum*, 3055-3057
Treponema pallidum subsp. *pertenue*, 3055-3056,
  3056f
Treponemal tests
  for endemic treponematoses, 3057
  specific, for syphilis, 3045-3046
Treponematoses, endemic, 3055-3058
  clinical manifestations of, 3055-3057, 3056f
  diagnosis of, 3057
  epidemiology of, 3055
  etiology of, 3055
  public health control of, 3058
  treatment of, 3057
Triazoles, 551f, 554-555
  for candidiasis, 3235-3236
  investigational, 559
Trichinella, 3587, 3588t
  foodborne disease from, 1414t, 1416, 1419
  larvae of, 3587, 3588f
  life cycle of, 3587
  transmission of, 3587
Trichinella britova, 3588t
Trichinella murrelli, 3588t
Trichinella nativa, 3588t
Trichinella nelsoni, 3588t
Trichinella pseudospiralis, 3588t
Trichinella spiralis
  abdominal pain and/or diarrhea with eosinophilia
    from, 1407t, 1408
  hosts and geographic distribution of, 3588t
Trichinellosis, 3587-3588
  clinical features of, 3588
  diagnosis of, 3588
  epidemiology of, 3587
  parasites in, 3587, 3588t
  pathology of, 3587, 3588f
  treatment and prevention of, 3588
  treatment of, 632t-635t
Trichinosis, 1320-1321
  versus enteric fever, 1400t-1401t, 1404
  enteritis from, 1392
  treatment of, 648

Trichloracetic acid, for condylomata acuminata,
  2043
Trichomonads, in urethral exudate, 1486
Trichomonas tenax, 3535
Trichomonas vaginalis, 1498-1500, 3535-3538
  diagnosis of, 1498-1499, 1499f
  etiology and pathogenesis of, 1498, 1498t
  nongonococcal urethritis from, 1489, 3535-3536.
    See also Urethritis, nongonococcal.
  in pregnancy, 1500
  treatment of, 1499-1500, 1499t
  vaginitis from, in HIV infection, 1797
Trichomoniasis, 3535-3538
  clinical features of, 3535-3536, 3536f, 3536t
  complications of, 3537
  diagnosis of, 3536
  dysuria in, 1490
  epidemiology of, 3535
  HIV associated with, 3537
  in pregnancy, 3537
  taxonomy in, 3535
  treatment of, 632t-635t, 3536-3537
Trichophyton, 3346t. *See also* Dermatophyte(s);
  Dermatophytosis.
Trichophyton concentricum, 3346, 3349, 3349f
Trichophyton erinacei, 3345, 3348f
Trichophyton interdigitale, 3346
Trichophyton mentagrophytes, 3345-3346, 3348
Trichophyton mentagrophytes quinckeanum, 3345
Trichophyton rubrum, 3346, 3348-3349, 3349f, 3351f
Trichophyton schoenleinii, 3347
Trichophyton tonsurans, 3346-3347
Trichophyton verrucosum, 3345
Trichophyton violaceum, 3346-3347
Trichosporon, 3370, 3374t
  white piedra from, 3355
Trichosporonosis, in hematopoietic stem cell
  transplant recipients, 3832
Trichostrongyliasis, 632t-635t
Trichuriasis, 632t-635t, 3578t, 3579f-3580f,
  3580-3581
Triclabendazole
  for liver flukes, 3602
  for parasitic infections, 648-649
Tricuspid valve, endocarditis of, 1077
  from *Staphylococcus aureus*, 2569, 2570f
Trifluorothymidine
  for orthopoxvirus infection, 1930
  structure of, 576f
Trifluridine, 566t-567t, 596, 706t-709t
  for ocular vaccinia, 1548
Trilosan, disinfection with, 522, 522t
Trimethoprim, 478-482, 706t-709t
  for acute pyelonephritis, 972
  antimicrobial activity of, 478-479
  derivation of, 478
  dosage of, 730t
  drug interactions with, 742t-761t
  formulations of, 716t
  for lower urinary tract infection, 973
  mechanism of action of, 478, 478f
  with other antimicrobial agents, 480
  pharmacology of, 479
  resistance to, 478-479
    target enzyme alteration in, 289
    target overproduction in, 289
  Staphylococcus aureus resistance to, 2559t
  structure of, 478, 478f
Trimethoprim-dapsone, 480
Trimethoprim-sulfamethoxazole, 706t-709t
  for actinomycetoma, 3284
  for acute pyelonephritis, 972
  antimicrobial activity of, 478
  for brain abscess, 1273t-1274t, 1274-1275
  for brucellosis, 2924
  for cholera, 2782t
  clinical uses of, 480-482
  for cyclosporiasis, 3562
  dosage of, 730t
  drug interactions with, 480, 480t
  for epiglottitis, 853
  formulations of, 716t
  for gastrointestinal infections, 481
  for *Isospora belli* infection, 3563
  for lower urinary tract infection, 973

Trimethoprim-sulfamethoxazole *(Continued)*
  for melioidosis, 2876
  for meningitis, 1213t
  for nocardiosis, 3204, 3204t, 3206
  for nontuberculous mycobacterial infections, 544
  for *Paracoccidioides brasiliensis* infection, 3361
  for peritonitis, 1029t
  for *Pneumocystis* pneumonia, 481-482
    in HIV infection, 1860t-1870t, 1872
  for *Pneumocystis* prophylaxis, 482, 632t-635t,
    3386-3387, 3800t
    in children, 1824-1825
    in HIV infection, 1858t-1859t, 1871t, 1873
  in pregnancy, 482
  prophylactic
    in immunocompromised patients, 482
    for nocardiosis, 3206
    for primary peritonitis, 1016
    in transplant recipients, 3815
    for urinary tract infection, 975
  resistance to, 479
  for respiratory tract infections, 481
  for sexually transmitted diseases, 481
  side effects of, 479-480
  for skin and soft tissue infections, 481
  for *Stenotrophomonas maltophilia* infection, 2865
  toxicity of, 479-480
  for toxoplasmosis
    in HIV infection, 3518, 3518t
    ocular, 3520
  for typhoid fever, 2899
  for urinary tract infections, 480-481
  for Whipple disease, 1439-1440, 1440t
Trimetrexate
  formulations of, 716t
  for *Pneumocystis* pneumonia, 3385
Trimetrexate glucuronate, 706t-709t
Triptans, for intracranial hypertension, 1202
Trismus (lockjaw), from tetanus, 3092-3093, 3092f
Trisulfapyrimidines, 706t-709t
  for nocardiosis, 3203-3204
Troleandomycin, 706t-709t
Tropheryma whipplei, 1435, 1436f. *See also* Whipple's
  disease.
  asymptomatic carriers of, 1437
  endocarditis from, 1086
  laboratory detection of, 240t-242t
  replication of, 1435-1436
Trophozoite, *Giardia lamblia*, 3527, 3528f
Tropical enteropathy, in travelers, 4025-4026
Tropical pulmonary eosinophilia, 3592
Tropical pyomyositis, 1313, 4023f
Tropical spastic paraparesis, from HTLV, 2314-2317
Tropical sprue, 1429-1433
  causes of, 1429-1431, 1431f
  clinical manifestations of, 1431
  diagnosis of, 1432
  epidemiology of, 1429
  histopathology of, 1432
  intestinal abnormalities in, 1431-1432
  treatment of, 1432
Tropinins, in myocarditis, 1157
Tropism
  of hepatitis C virus, 2161
  of viruses, 1916
Trovafloxacin, hepatotoxicity of, 504
Trypanosoma
  characteristics of, 3481
  classification of, 3481
  distribution of, 3481, 3482f
  keratitis from, 1550-1551
Trypanosoma brucei complex, 3489
Trypanosoma brucei gambiense
  distribution of, 3481, 3482f, 3490
  transmission of, 3489
  West African trypanosomiasis from, 3490, 3490t
Trypanosoma brucei rhodesiense
  detection of, 3490f, 3491-3492
  distribution of, 3481, 3482f, 3490-3491
  East African trypanosomiasis from, 3490-3491,
    3490t
  transmission of, 3489
Trypanosoma cruzi
  complement interactions with, 85
  distribution of, 3481, 3482f

Trypanosoma cruzi (Continued)
  in heart transplant recipients, 3842
  life cycle of, 3481, 3482f
  myocarditis from, 1154
  transmission of, 3481, 3482f
Trypanosomiasis
  African, 3489-3494
    clinical course of, 3491
    diagnosis of, 3490f, 3491-3492
    epidemiology of, 3490-3491, 3490t
    etiology of, 3489
    versus malaria, 3450
    melarsoprol for, 656
    pathology and pathogenesis of, 3489-3490
    prevention of, 3493
    treatment of, 3492-3493, 3492t
  American, 3481-3488
    acute, 3484-3485, 3484f
    chronic, 3484-3486, 3484f-3485f
    clinical course of, 3483-3484
    diagnosis of, 3485-3486
    epidemiology of, 3482-3484
    etiology of, 3481, 3482f
    in HIV infection, 1860t-1870t
    in immunocompromised hosts, 3484-3485
    myocarditis in, 1156
    pathology of, 3481-3482, 3482f
    prevention of, 3487
    transfusion-related, 3748
    transmission of, 3481, 3482f, 3483
    treatment of, 3486-3487
  East African, versus malaria, 3450
  treatment of, 632t-635t, 649-650
Tsetse flies, in African trypanosomiasis transmission, 3489
Tsukamurella paurometabola, 2703-2704
Tuberculin skin test, 3136-3138
  booster effect of, 3137
  in chronic pneumonia, 934
  dosage of, 3137
  false-negative/false-positive reaction to, 3137
  HIV infection and, 3137-3138
  interpretation of, 3137
  loss of reactivity of, 3137, 3138t
  positivity of, 3133
  targeted, 3137
  technical aspects of, 3137
  variant (delayed) reactivity of, 3137
Tuberculocide, 3677
Tuberculoid leprosy, 3167-3169
Tuberculoma, 3142, 3142f, 3154
Tuberculosis, 3129-3163. *See also Mycobacterium tuberculosis.*
  active
    clinical manifestations of, 3142t
    incidence of, 3133, 3133t
    progression to, 3135
    treatment of, 3150
  in adolescents, 3139, 3139f-3140f
  age distribution of, 3133
  age influence on, 3139
  aortic, 3159
  bronchopleural fistula in, 3155
  cancer in, 3144
  in cancer patients, chemoprophylaxis for, 3800t, 3802
  central nervous system, 3153-3154, 3153f
  chest radiography in, 940f
  in children, 3139-3140, 3149
  in correctional facilities, 3135
  cutaneous, 3158-3159
  in developing countries, 3133, 3133t
  diagnosis of, 3143-3144
    assays used in, 3130t
    at autopsy, 3144
    fiberoptic bronchoscopy in, 3143-3144
  drug-resistant, 3134, 3134t
    extensively, 533
    prevention of, 273
    treatment of, 3146
  in elderly, 3140, 3859
  emergence of, 210-211, 210f
  emphysema in, 3155
  epidemiology of, 3132-3135, 3132f
  epididymitis from, 1524

Tuberculosis (Continued)
  in ethnic/racial minorities, 3132-3133
  extrapulmonary, 3151-3159
    in AIDS patient, 3151
    treatment of, 3151
  fibrosing mediastinitis in, 3158
  gastrointestinal, 1395, 3157
    in HIV infection, 3157
  genetic factors in, 49, 50t, 3140
  genital
    female, 3157
    male, 3156-3157
  genitourinary, 3156, 3156t
    in HIV infection, 3157
  hematogenous spread of, 3140
  hepatic, 3153
  history of, 3129
  in HIV infection, 210, 210f, 1639, 1731, 1879, 3132-3134
    extrapulmonary, 3151
    gastrointestinal, 3157
    genitourinary, 3157
    HAART and, 1721
    impact of, 1627f, 1629
    local epidemiology and, 1728
    miliary, 3153
    prophylaxis against, 1858t-1859t
    pulmonary, 3140, 3142, 3142t
    treatment of, 1860t-1870t, 3147-3148
  in homeless shelters, 3135
  in hospitals, 3135
  in immigrants, 3133, 3133t
  immune reconstitution inflammatory syndrome in, 3148
  immunity to, 3135-3136
  in infancy, 3139
  intestinal, versus enteric fever, 1400t-1401t, 1403-1404
  laryngeal, 823
  laryngitis in, 3159
  latent
    newer assays for, 3138
    treatment of, 3149, 3149t
      drug regimens in, 3149-3150
      in HIV infection, 3150
      isoniazid hepatotoxicity risk in, 3150
      in patients with additional risk factors, 3150-3151
  lymphadenitis/lymphadenopathy in, 3158, 3158f
  measles virus in, 2232
  meningitis in, 618-619, 1240-1241
  microbiology of, 3130-3131
  in mid-adulthood, 3139-3140
  miliary, 3151
    chest radiography in, 944f
    cryptic, 3152
    hematologic abnormalities in, 3153
    in HIV infection, 3153
    pleurisy with effusion complicating, 3154-3155
    usual (acute), 3151-3152, 3152f, 3152t
  morbidity and mortality trends in, 3132-3134, 3132f, 3133t
  multidrug-resistant, 533
    quinolones for, 500-501
    treatment of, 3146
  nonreactive, 3152-3153
  nosocomial
    control of, 3135
    spread of, 3135
  ocular, 1564, 1564f
  otitis in, 3159
  pathogenesis of, 3138-3139
  pericarditis in, 1162-1165, 1163f, 3155
  peripheral osteoarticular, 3156
  peritonitis in, 3157
  from pleural effusion, 918, 921
  pleurisy in, 3154-3155
  primary infection in, 3138-3139
  pulmonary
    apical localization of, 3139
    in childhood, 3140
    chronic, 3139-3140
    corticosteroids for, 618-619
    diagnosis of, 3143-3144
    endobronchial, 3142

Tuberculosis (Continued)
  in HIV infection, 3140, 3142, 3142t. *See also* Tuberculosis, in HIV infection.
  in injection drug users, 3883
  intercurrent events in, 3140
  laboratory findings in, 3143
  lower lobe, 3142
  physical examination of, 3143
  pleurisy with effusion complicating, 3154
  postprimary, 3141, 3141f
  radiographic findings in, 3143
  symptoms of, 3142-3143
  quiescent, treatment of, 3150
  reinfection in, 3138-3139
    endogenous versus exogenous, 3139
  renal, 3156, 3156t
  reported cases of
    in immigrants, 3133, 3133t
    worldwide, 3133, 3133t
  resurgence of, 211
  re-treatment of, 3147
  risk of, 3134
  skeletal, 3155-3156, 3155f
  in small communities, 3133
  spinal, 3154
  spread of, 3134
    chemotherapy influence on, 3134-3135
    hematogenous, 3140
    institutional, 3135
  in transplant recipients, 3814
  travel-related, 4024
    prevention of, 4016
  treatment of, 3144-3151
    for active disease, 3150
    algorithm in, 3147, 3147f
    antituberculous drugs in, 3144-3145. *See also* Antituberculous agents; *specific agent.*
    corticosteroids in, 3147-3148
    course of, 3146-3147
    duration of, 3149
    duration of observation in, 3146-3147
    for extensively drug-resistant disease, 3146
    fixed-dose combination tablets in, 3146
    in HIV infection, 535-536, 536t, 3147-3148
    for latent disease, 3149, 3149t. *See also* Tuberculosis, latent, treatment of.
    for minimal disease, 3146
    for multidrug-resistant disease, 3146
    for quiescent disease, 3150
    selection of drug regimen in, 3145, 3145t
    special circumstances in, 3149
    standard drug regimens in, 3145-3146
    vaccination in, 3151
  tuberculin skin test for, 3136-3138. *See also* Tuberculin skin test.
  vaccine for, 3151
  in young adults, 3139, 3139f-3140f
Tuboovarian abscess, 1518
Tularemia, 2927-2937, 3655-3656
  as biological weapon, 2927, 3952, 3971-3975
    bioterrorism websites for, 3975, 3975t
    diagnosis of, 3973
    history of, 3971
    outbreak characteristics of, 3971-3973, 3972t
    in postexposure period
      environmental surveillance and decontamination for, 3975
      hospital isolation control measures for, 3974
      prophylaxis for, 3973-3974, 3974t
      vaccines for, 3974
    potential use of, 3971
    treatment of, 3973-3974, 3974t
  clinical classification of, 3655t
  clinical manifestations of, 2931-2934, 2932f, 2934f
  complications of, 2934
  diagnosis of, 2934-2935
  epidemiology of, 2929-2930, 2929f-2930f
  Francisella tularensis in, 2927. *See also Francisella tularensis.*
  glandular, 2932f, 2933
  history of, 2927
  incidence of, 2929-2930, 2930f
  incubation period for, 2931-2932
  oculoglandular, 2933
  outcome of, 2934

Tularemia (*Continued*)
  pathogenesis of, 2930-2931
  pharyngeal, 2933
  pneumonic, 2933-2934, 2934f, 3971
    versus community-acquired pneumonia,
      3971-3972, 3972t
  prevention of, 2935-2936
  skin rashes in, 2934
  tick vector of, 3655, 3655f
  transmission of, 2930
  treatment of, 2935
  typhoidal, 1400t-1401t, 1403, 2933, 3972
  ulceroglandular, 2932-2933, 2932f
  vaccine for, 2936
Tumor(s). *See also* Cancer.
  abdominal pain and/or diarrhea with eosinophilia
    from, 1407t, 1409
  Buschke-Lowenstein, 2040
  cervical spinal cord, 3660t
Tumor necrosis factor
  in hepatitis B susceptibility, 52
  in infection susceptibility, 54
  in leishmaniasis susceptibility, 52
Tumor necrosis factor-α
  in febrile response, 769
  in initial inflammatory response, 43
  for Kawasaki syndrome, 3665
  in Legionnaires' disease, 2971
  for meningococcal infection, 2746-2747
  in neutrophil apoptosis, 108
  in *Pseudomonas aeruginosa* resistance, 2838-2839
  in streptococcal toxic shock syndrome, 2604
  in *Streptococcus agalactiae* (group B) infection,
    2658
  in toxoplasmosis, 3499
Tungiasis, from sand fleas, 3639-3641, 3639t, 3640f
Turicella otitidis, 2701
Tuskegee study, of syphilis, 3036, 3038
24-hour serum concentration curve, area under,
    minimal inhibitory concentration relationship
    to, 303-304, 303f
Tympanic membrane temperature, 766
Tympanostomy tubes, for otitis media, 835
Typhlitis, 1064-1065
  in transplant recipients, 3823
Typhoid fever, 1399-1405, 2895-2896
  clinical features of, 1399-1402, 1400t-1401t
  diagnosis of, 1402, 2895-2896
  differential diagnosis of, 1400t-1401t,
    1402-1405
  versus enteric fever-like syndromes, 1402-1403
  epidemiology of, 1402, 2888-2889, 2889f
  history of, 2887
  intestinal hemorrhage in, 1392
  laboratory findings in, 1400t-1401t, 1401-1402
  versus malaria, 3450
  pathogenesis of, 1399
  physical findings in, 1399-1401, 1401t
  quinolone-resistant, 4025
  quinolones for, 496-497
  reporting system for, 2898
  rose spots in, 1304, 2895, 2895f
  from *Salmonella typhi,* 4022-4024
  symptoms of, 1399, 1401t
  versus systemic infections, 1403-1405
  in travelers, 4022-4024
  treatment of, 1405, 2898-2899, 2898t
Typhoid vaccine, 2896-2898, 3922t, 3933
  for travelers, 4010, 4011t
Typhoidal tularemia, 1400t-1401t, 1403, 2933,
    3972
Typhus
  African tick, 4024
  epidemic, 2521-2524, 2522f, 2522t-2523t
  murine, 2525-2528, 3639t
  recrudescent, 2522-2523
  scrub, 2495, 2529-2530, 2529f, 2529t, 3643, 3645f,
    3646t, 4024
  tick, 2504

U

Ulcerative gingivitis, acute necrotizing, 859-860,
    861t, 3085, 3115
Ulceroglandular tularemia, 2932-2933, 2932f

Ulcers
  actinomycotic, 3211
  aphthous
    esophageal, 1355, 1355t
    in HIV infection, 1712, 1712f
    in Marshall's syndrome, 1327
    oral, 866
    of vagina, 1482
  from *Blastomyces dermatitidis,* 3325, 3326f
  decubitus, 1300
    in elderly, 3859
    in spinal cord injury patients, 3854
  diabetic foot, 1300-1302, 1461-1462, 1462t
  duodenal, in *Helicobacter pylori* infection,
    2806-2807, 2806t
  gastric, in *Helicobacter pylori* infection, 2806t, 2807
  gastroduodenal, in HIV infection, 1738
  genital
    in chancroid, 2917
    in HIV infection, 1798-1799
  membranous, 1298
  nasolabial, from *Coccidioides,* 3337, 3338f
  neurotrophic, in leprosy, 3174
  oral
    aphthous, 866
    from cytomegalovirus in HIV infection, 1715
    from herpes simplex virus in HIV infection,
      1715
  oropharyngeal, in histoplasmosis, 3313, 3313f
  scrotal, in melioidosis, 2875f
  skin
    in chromoblastomycosis, 3277, 3278f
    from *Cryptococcus neoformans,* 3295, 3295f
    in injection drug users, 3877-3878
  in vulvovaginal candidiasis, 1500-1501, 1501f
Ultrasonography
  in acute pyelonephritis, 978, 979f-980f
  in cholecystitis, 1040, 1041f
  in intraperitoneal abscess, 1031
  in perinephric abscess, 977, 977f
  in pleural effusion, 919
  in prosthetic vascular graft infection, 1134, 1134t
  in pyomyositis, 1315
  in sinusitis, 844
  in splenic abscess, 1055-1056
Umbilical cord blood, in hematopoietic stem cell
    transplantation, 3821
UNC93B1 gene, in herpes encephalitis susceptibility,
    49-50
Undulant fever, 2922
Upper respiratory tract infection. *See also* Respiratory
    tract infections.
  laryngitis in, 823-824, 824t
  from rhinoviruses, 2389-2398
Upper respiratory tract specimens
  collection and transport guidelines for, 235t-236t
  laboratory processing of, 238-239
Urban residence, HIV transmission and, 1626-1627,
    1627f
Ureaplasma, 2477-2480
  characteristics of, 2477, 2478t
  classification of, 2477, 2479f
  susceptibility testing for, 2493
Ureaplasma urealyticum, 2491-2493, 2492t
  nongonococcal urethritis from, 1489, 2491, 2492t.
    See also Urethritis, nongonococcal.
Urease breath test, for *Helicobacter pylori* infection,
    2808-2809
Ureidopenicillins, 318-319, 319f
  indications for, 315-316
  susceptibility to, 311
Uremia
  in endocarditis, 1077
  in tuberculosis, 3149
Ureteral obstruction, urinary tract infection and, 963
Ureteral stenosis, BKV-induced, 2056
Urethra
  anatomic examination of, 1485
  female
    Chlamydia trachomatis in, 1490
    examination of, 1485
    Neisseria gonorrhoeae in, 1490
  specimen from, examination of, 1485-1487, 1486f,
    1486t
Urethral candidiasis, 3232

Urethral exudate, gonorrheal, 1486, 1486f
Urethral syndrome, 968-969, 1490
Urethritis, 1485-1494
  asymptomatic, 1489
  from *Chlamydia trachomatis,* 2451, 2452t,
    2453-2454
  clinical features of, 1492
  complications of, 1490
  gonococcal, 1487-1489, 1487f, 1487t, 2759,
    2759f-2760f
    purulent discharge from, 1487-1488, 1487f
    quinolones for, 496
  meningococcal, 2744
  nongonococcal, 1487-1489, 1487t, 1488f
    from *Chlamydia trachomatis,* 1488-1489
    etiology of, 1488-1489
    from *Mycoplasma genitalium,* 1489, 2491, 2492t
    reactive arthritis in, 1491-1492
    treatment of, 1490-1491, 1491t
      for sexual partners, 1490
    from *Trichomonas vaginalis,* 1489, 3535-3536
    from *Ureaplasma urealyticum,* 1489, 2491, 2492t
  noninfectious, 1487
  physical examination in, 1485
  postgonococcal, 1489
  pyuria from, 969
  recurrent, 1491
  treatment of, 1490-1491, 1491t
  urethral specimen examination in, 1485-1487,
    1486f, 1486t
  urethral syndrome from, 1490
Urgency, urinary, 968-969, 968f, 973-974
Urinalysis, in urinary tract infection, 967, 967t
Urinary calculi, 963, 964f
Urinary obstruction, urinary tract infection and,
    963-964, 964f
Urinary tract infections, 957-985. *See also*
    Bacteriuria; Cystitis; Genitourinary tract
    infections.
  ascending route of, 958
  bacterial adherence and colonization in, 962
  from *Candida,* 3232-3233, 3237, 3726-3727,
    3733-3734
  catheter-associated, 3725-3737
    epidemiology of, 3725-3727
    pathogenesis of, 3727
    prevention of, 3728-3732, 3729t
      alternatives to indwelling catheterization in,
        3729-3730
      antimicrobial prophylaxis in, 3731
        at catheter removal or replacement, 3732
      antimicrobial-coated catheters in, 3731
      antimicrobials in drainage bag in, 3732
      bladder irrigation in, 3732
      catheter insertion and maintenance in, 3730
      cranberry products in, 3732
      enhanced meatal care in, 3731-3732
      infection control programs in, 3728-3729
      reduction of unnecessary catheterization in,
        3729
      routine catheter change in, 3732
  in children
    imaging of, 981, 981f-982f
    natural history of, 969
    symptoms of, 966
  chronic, 957
  clinical manifestations of, 966-967
  from coagulase-negative *Staphylococcus,* 2585
  complicated, 957
  in diabetic women, 966, 970
  diagnosis of, 967-969
    culture in, 967-969, 968f
    presumptive, 967, 967t
    site localization in, 969
  in elderly, 966-967, 970, 3857-3858
  from *Enterococcus,* 2646, 2651
  epidemiology of, 964-966, 966t
  from *Escherichia coli,* 3726-3727
  from extraintestinal pathogenic *Escherichia coli,*
    2821-2822
  fungal, 975
  genetic risk factors for, 963
  hematogenous route of, 958
  in HIV infection, 1525
  host defense against, 961, 961t

Urinary tract infections *(Continued)*
  cellular immunity in, 963
  humoral immunity in, 962-963
  innate immunity in, 40-41, 961
  urine and bladder antibacterial activity in,
    961-962, 962f
  imaging of, 978-983, 978f-981f
  in immunocompromised hosts, 3789
  in kidney transplant recipients, 3840-3841
  from *Klebsiella pneumoniae*, 2826
  with low numbers of organisms, 968-969, 968f
  lower, 966
    antimicrobial agents for, 973, 983t
  lymphatic route of, 958
  microorganisms in, 958-961, 959t, 964
  natural history of, 969-970
  nosocomial, 3725-3737. *See also* Urinary tract
    infections, catheter-associated.
    asymptomatic, 3733
    complications of, 3725-3726
    diagnosis of, 3727-3728
    epidemiology of, 3725-3727
    fungal, 3733-3734
    incidence and prevalence of, 3725
    management of, 3733
    microbiology in, 3726-3727
    pathogenesis of, 3727
    prevention of, 3728-3732
      routine strategies in, 3728-3730, 3729t
      strategies for further investigation in, 3732
      strategies with little benefit in, 3731-3732
      strategies with possible benefit in, 3731
    risk factors for, 3725
    versus uncomplicated urinary tract infection,
      3725, 3726t
  pathogenesis of, 958-961
  pathology of, 957-958, 958f
  persistence of, 971-972
  in pregnancy, 975-976
  prevention of
    cranberry for, 22, 669-671, 670t, 671f
    long-term, 974-975
  from *Pseudomonas aeruginosa*, 2854
  rapid screening for, 239
  recurrent
    methenamine for, 518-519
    nitrofurantoin for, 516-517
  reinfection in, 957, 972, 974-975
  relapsing, 957, 966-967, 972, 974
  renal function in, 967
  risk factors for, 966t
  in solid organ transplant recipients tract, 3844
  in spinal cord injury patients, 3852-3853
  from *Streptococcus agalactiae* (group B), 2661
  structural abnormalities and, 963-964, 964f
  symptoms of, 966-967
  treatment of, 970-983
    analgesics in, 971
    antimicrobial agents in, 971-972
      concentrations of, 971
      dosage of, 732t-733t
      formulations of, 716t
      response to, 971-972
      by specific disorder, 972-975
    general considerations in, 970
    hydration in, 970
    nitrofurantoin in, 516
    quinolones for, 495
    summary of, 982f, 983, 983t
    surgical, 983
    trimethoprim-sulfamethoxazole in, 480-481
    urinary pH in, 970-971
  uncomplicated, versus nosocomial urinary tract
    infection, 3725, 3726t
  vesicoureteral reflux in, 964, 964f-965f
Urine
  acidification of, 970-971
    during methenamine therapy, 518
  antibacterial activity of, 40, 961-962, 962f
  collection methods for, 968
  culture of, 967-969, 968f
  examination of, in urinary tract infection, 967,
    967t
  formaldehyde concentrations in, factors affecting,
    518

Urine antigen testing
  for *Legionella pneumophila*, 2977
  in pneumonia, 901
Urine specimens
  collection and transport guidelines for, 235t-236t
  laboratory processing of, 239
Urogenital infections. *See* Genitourinary tract
  infections.
Urokinase, for pleural effusion/empyema, 922
Uromucoid, 961-962, 962f
Uropathogens, 958-961, 964
  in catheterized patients, 3727
  Escherichia coli. See Escherichia coli, uropathogenic.
Urosepsis, 957
Urovirulence, in bacteria, 958-961, 959t
Ushers, 9
Uterus, postpartum infection of, 1511-1513, 1512f
Uvea, 1561
Uveitis, 1561-1568
  in acute retinal necrosis, 1563, 1563f
  in brucellosis, 1566, 2923
  in cat-scratch disease, 1565, 1566f
  in chikungunya virus infection, 1566
  in chronic endophthalmitis, 1565
  classification of, 1562t
  in cytomegalovirus retinitis, 1563
  diagnosis of, 1566
  epidemiology of, 1561
  etiology of, 1561, 1562f
  granulomatous, 1561, 1562f
  from herpes simplex virus, 1562-1563, 1567
  from HTLV, 2315
  infectious etiologies of
    major, 1562-1565
    uncommon, 1565-1566
  in leprosy, 1566
  in leptospirosis, 1566
  in ocular Lyme disease, 1565
  in ocular syphilis, 1563-1564
  in ocular toxocariasis, 1565
  in ocular toxoplasmosis, 1565
  in ocular tuberculosis, 1564, 1564f
  pathophysiology of, 1561
  in presumed ocular histoplasmosis syndrome,
    1566
  in progressive outer retinal necrosis, 1563
  from rifamycins, 406
  treatment of, 1566-1567
  in West Nile virus infection, 1565
  in Whipple's disease, 1566

V
V factor, for *Haemophilus influenzae* growth, 2911
VacA gene, in *Helicobacter pylori*, 2804
VacA protein, in *Helicobacter pylori*, 2805
Vaccine(s), 3917-3949. *See also* Immunization;
  specific diseases or vaccine.
  adjuvants for, 3917-3918
  administration route for, 3918
  adverse effects of, 3921
  age and, 3918
  autism and, 3921
  combination, 3944, 3944t
  conjugate, 69, 70f
  constituents of, 3917
  currently available, 3921-3934, 3922t
  definition of, 3917
  development of, 3920-3921, 3920t
  dose of, 3918
  effectiveness of, 3921
  in HIV infection, 1887-1895, 3942-3943, 3942f.
    See also Human immunodeficiency virus
    vaccines.
  immune response to
    age and, 3918
    components of, 3918-3919
    measurement of, 3920
    mobilization of, 3919
    temporal course of, 3919-3920
    unanticipated, 3919
  immunization principles and, 3920-3921, 3920t
  in immunocompromised hosts, 3942
  immunogenicity determinants of, 3918
  immunologic basis of, 3917-3918

Vaccine(s) *(Continued)*
  impact of, 3920, 3920t
  injuries from, compensation for, 3945
  interrupted schedule for, 3944
  killed (inactivated), 3917-3918
  live attenuated, 3917-3918
  for myocarditis prophylaxis, 1160-1161
  for occupational exposure, 3941
  in pregnancy, 3921, 3941
  recommended schedule for, 3921
    in adolescents, 3939
    in adults, 3939-3941, 3940f
    in children, 3924f, 3936-3938, 3937f,
      3938t-3939t
  reporting of disease and adverse effects from,
    3944-3945
  simultaneous administration of, 3944
  storage and handling of, 3943
  for travelers. *See* Travelers, immunizations for.
  vectors for, adenoviruses as, 2032
Vaccine era
  hepatitis A infection in, 2374
  pertussis in, 2957
Vaccinia
  conjunctivitis from, 1532-1533, 1533t
  encephalitis from, 1251t-1252t
  generalized, 1925
  keratitis from, 1546-1548
  progressive, 1925
  as zoonosis, 1926
Vaccinia immune globulin, 1548, 3922t, 3936
Vaccinia vaccine. *See* Smallpox vaccine.
Vacuolar myelopathy, in HIV infection, 1754-1755
Vacuum-assisted closure (VAC) therapy, for
  mediastinitis, 1178
Vagina
  aphthous ulcers of, 1482
  flora of, assessment of, 1498
  infection in, barriers to, 41
Vaginal cuff cellulitis, after hysterectomy, 1515
Vaginal introitus, bacterial adherence and
  colonization of, 962
Vaginal secretions
  abnormal, 1495, 1496t
  examination of, 1497, 1497t, 1498f
  normal, 1495, 1496f, 1496t
  sampling of, 1497
Vaginitis/vulvovaginitis
  age and, 1495-1496
  bacterial, 243
  from *Candida*, 243, 1500-1502, 3228, 3229f
    clinical features of, 1500-1501, 1500t, 1501f
    complicated, 1502, 1502t
    diagnosis of, 1501, 1501f
    etiology and pathogenesis of, 1500
    in HIV infection, 1796-1797
    treatment of, 1501-1502, 1502t, 3238
    uncomplicated, 1501, 1502t
  desquamative inflammatory, 1504-1505, 1505f,
    1505t
  estrogen deficiency, 1506
  examination in, 1497-1498, 1497f-1498f, 1497t
  history in, 1495-1497, 1496t
  from *Streptococcus pyogenes*, 2606
  from *Trichomonas vaginalis*, 1498-1500,
    1498t-1499t, 1499f, 3536, 3536f
    in HIV infection, 1797
Vaginosis, bacterial, 1502-1504
  anaerobic, 3086
  diagnosis of, 1503-1504, 1503f-1504f, 1503t-1504t
  epidemiology of, 1503
  from *Gardnerella vaginalis*, 1503, 3028-3029
  in HIV infection, 1796
  pathophysiology of, 1503
  in pregnancy, 1504
  treatment of, 1504
Valacyclovir, 566t-567t, 568-571, 706t-709t
  activity spectrum of, 568
  clinical studies of, 570-571
  dosage of, 738t-739t
  drug interactions with, 569, 742t-761t
  formulations of, 717t
  for herpes B virus postexposure prophylaxis,
    2024-2025
  for herpes simplex virus, 570-571, 1956, 1957t

Valacyclovir *(Continued)*
  for herpes simplex virus esophagitis, 1355t
  mechanism of action of, 568
  pharmacokinetics of, 569, 570t
  prophylactic, for cancer-related infections, 3800t,
    3802
  resistance to, 568-569
  toxicity of, 569-570
  for varicella-zoster virus, 1967
Valganciclovir, 566t-567t, 582-585, 706t-709t
  activity spectrum of, 582
  clinical studies of, 584-585
  for cytomegalovirus, 1977
    in hematopoietic stem cell transplant recipients,
      3828
    prophylactic, 1979
  for cytomegalovirus encephalitis, 1754
  for cytomegalovirus esophagitis, 1355t
  dosage of, 738t-739t
  drug interactions with, 742t-761t
  formulations of, 717t
  pharmacokinetics of, 583, 583t
  prophylactic, in transplant recipients, 3815-3816
  toxicity of, 584
Valve, heart. *See* Heart valve.
Valvular regurgitation, in rheumatic fever,
    2615-2616
VanA gene cluster, 450-451, 458
VanB gene cluster, 450-451
Vancomycin, 449-457, 706t-709t
  administration of, 453
  adverse reactions to, 454-455
  antimicrobial activity of, 449
  for bacteremia, 455-456
  for brain abscess, 1273-1274, 1273t-1274t
  for cellulitis, 1297-1298
  clinical uses of, 455-457
  for *Clostridium difficile*–associated colitis,
    1382-1384
  distribution of, 452-453
  dosage of, 728t-729t
    in infants and children, 453
    monitoring of, 455
    in renal insufficiency, 453-454, 454t
  drug interactions with, 455, 742t-761t
  for endocarditis, 455-456, 1088-1090
    prosthetic valve, 1122t
  for *Enterococcus*, 2649
  for epiglottitis, 853
  excretion of, 453
  for febrile neutropenia, 457, 3804t
  formulations of, 716t
  intraventricular, 1234, 1234t
  mechanism of action of, 449
  for meningitis, 456, 1213t
  minimal inhibitory concentration susceptibility
    for, 460t
  for MRSA joint infections, 1449
  for nosocomial pneumonia, 3718t
  for osteomyelitis, 456-457, 1457, 1459t
  for peritonitis, 1029t
  pharmacodynamics and pharmacokinetics of,
    452-454
  for pneumonia, 456
  prophylactic, 457
    for endocarditis, 453
    for postoperative mediastinitis, 1178
    for surgical procedures, 3899t
  for pseudomembranous colitis, 457
  resistance to, 449-452
    cell wall precursor target alterations in, 288,
      288t
    by coagulase-negative *Staphylococcus*, 452
    by enterococci, 450-451
      detection of, 242
      epidemiology of, 2645-2646
      linezolid for, 473
      metronidazole and, 423-425
      in spinal cord injury patients, 3855
      treatment of, 2648f
    by gram-positive bacteria, 452
    by *Staphylococcus aureus*, 288, 451, 1119, 2560
    by *Streptococcus pneumoniae*, 452
  for septic bursitis, 1450t
  for skin and soft tissue infections, 455

Vancomycin *(Continued)*
  for *Staphylococcus* endocarditis, 1118t, 2571t
  for *Staphylococcus* osteomyelitis, 2574
  for *Streptococcus agalactiae* (group B) infection,
    2662t
  structure of, 449, 450f
  teicoplanin interaction with, 459
  for ventriculitis, 456
Vancomycin-intermediate *Staphylococcus aureus*,
    289-290
Vaporizers, for croup, 828
Variant-specific surface protein (VSP), of *Giardia
    lamblia*, 3527
Varicella. *See also* Varicella-zoster virus.
  clinical manifestations of, 1964-1965
  conjunctivitis from, 1532
  diagnosis of, 1966
  epidemiology of, 1963-1964
  historical perspective on, 1963
  in immunocompromised hosts, 1965
  pathogenesis of, 1964
  treatment of, 1966-1967
  vaccine for, 1967
Varicella vaccine, 3922t, 3933
  in HIV-infected children, 1825
  recommended schedule for, 3924f
  for travelers, 4011t
Varicella-zoster immune globulin, 1967, 3922t, 3935
  in HIV-infected children, 1826
  in prophylaxis, 3773
Varicella-zoster/varicella-zoster virus, 1938t-1940t,
    1963-1969. *See also* Herpes zoster.
  acyclovir-resistant, 569
  characteristics of, 1963
  clinical manifestations of, 1964-1966
  detection of, 259t-260t
  diagnosis of, 1966
  encephalitis from, 1253-1254
  epidemiology of, 1963-1964
  in hematopoietic stem cell transplant recipients,
    3829-3830
  historical perspective on, 1963
  in HIV infection
    prophylaxis against, 1858t-1859t, 1871t
    treatment of, 1860t-1870t
  in immunocompromised hosts, 1965
  keratitis from, 1546-1547, 1548t
  meningitis from, 1201-1202
  nosocomial, 3772-3775
  pathogenesis of, 1964
  prevention of, 1967-1968
  replication of, 1963
  in solid organ transplant recipients, 3847
  treatment of, 566t-567t, 571, 1966-1967
  vaccine for, 1941, 3922t, 3934
Variola virus, 1924f, 1926-1927, 1927f, 3977. *See
    also* Smallpox.
Vas deferens, anatomy of, 1521, 1522f
Vascular access site infection, in hemodialysis
    patients, 1135-1136, 1136f
Vascular closure device infection, percutaneous, 1138
Vascular gangrene, infected, 1319
Vascular graft infections
  from coagulase-negative *Staphylococcus*, 2583
  prosthetic, 1132-1135. *See also* Prosthetic vascular
    graft infections.
Vascular infections. *See also* Bloodstream infections.
  from *Candida*, 3234
  by mucorales, 3260
  noncardiac, in injection drug users, 3881-3882
  from *Salmonella*, 2896
Vasculitis
  abdominal pain and/or diarrhea with eosinophilia
    from, 1407t, 1409
  from parvovirus B19 infection, 2091
Vasoconstriction
  coronary, from antipyretic drugs, 775
  in septic shock, 994-995
Vasodilation, in septic shock, 994-995
Vasopressin
  antipyretic activity of, 771
  for sepsis, 1003
Vat genes, 461
VDRL test, cerebrospinal fluid, for neurosphylitic
    meningitis, 1210

VECTOR bioterrorism laboratory, 3952
Vector control, for plague, 2949
Vector-borne infections, 206-209. *See also specific
    infection.*
  outbreaks of, 194
  viral, 1255-1258
Vector-borne transmission, 188
Vecuronium, for tetanus, 3094t
Vehicle-borne transmission, 187-188
Veillonella, 3123t
  in oral cavity, 855, 856t
Velocardiofacial syndrome, 169t-170t
Vena cava filter, infection of, 1139
Venereal Disease Research Laboratory test, 3035
  for neurosyphilis, 3046
  for syphilis, 3045, 3045t
Venereal warts. *See* Condylomata acuminata.
Venezuelan equine encephalitis, 1246t, 1258,
    2117-2125, 2118t. *See also* Alphaviruses.
Venezuelan hemorrhagic fever. *See* South American
    hemorrhagic fevers.
Venomous snake bites, 1297, 1297t, 3913-3914
Veno-occlusive disease, after hematopoietic stem cell
    transplantation, 3822
Venous sinus thrombosis, suppurative intracranial,
    1283-1286, 1285f-1286f
Ventilation
  noninvasive positive-pressure, for nosocomial
    pneumonia, 3722
  weaning protocols for, 3722-3723
Ventilator-associated pneumonia, 3717. *See also*
    Pneumonia, nosocomial.
Ventilator-associated tracheobronchitis, 3717-3719,
    3723
Ventricular assist device, infection of, 1131-1132,
    1131t
Ventriculitis, vancomycin for, 456
Verrucae planae, 2035-2036, 2039
Verrucae plantaris, 2035-2036, 2039
Verrucae vulgaris, 2035-2036, 2039, 2042
Verruga peruana, 2995-2996, 2996f
Vertebral osteomyelitis, 1460-1461, 1461f
  from *Aspergillus*, 3249, 3249f
  in injection drug users, 3879
Vertigo, from minocycline, 392
Vesicles, 792, 1303
Vesicobullous eruptions, 793t, 795-796. *See also*
    Rash.
Vesicoureteral reflux
  imaging of, 981, 981f
  renal scarring and, 969
  urinary tract infection and, 964, 964f-965f
Vesicular rash, in rickettsialpox, 2509
Vesicular stomatitis virus, 2245-2247, 2246t
  adhesins of, 16f
  with exanthem. *See* Hand-foot-and-mouth
    disease.
Vesiculoviruses, 2245-2247, 2246t, 2249
Vestibular toxicity, from aminoglycosides, 372
Vestibulitis, vulvar, 1507-1508, 1507f
Vgb genes, 461
Viannia subgenus of *Leishmania*, 3463
Vibrio
  dysentery from, 1392
  halophilic, 2790
  laboratory detection of, 240t-242t
  nonhalophilic, 2790
Vibrio alginolyticus, 2789-2790
  cellulitis from, 1296-1297
Vibrio carchariae, 2790
Vibrio cholerae, 2777-2785. *See also* Cholera.
  O1, 2777
  O139, 2777
  diarrhea from, 205
  enterotoxins of, 31-32
  foodborne disease from, 1413, 1414t, 1415, 1419
  gastric acid and, 1337
  genomic sequence of, 2778
  identification of, 2777-2778
  isolation of, 2777-2778
  laboratory confirmation of, 1422
  life cycle of, 2778-2779, 2779f
  microbiology of, 2777-2778
  non-O1, 2790
  virulence factors of, 5t

Vibrio cholerae (Continued)
  virulence of, 1342-1343
  virulence regulatory systems for, 8, 8t
Vibrio cincinnatiensis, 2790
Vibrio damsela, 2790
Vibrio fluvialis, 2790
Vibrio hollisae, 2790
Vibrio metschnikovii, 2790
Vibrio mimicus, 2790
Vibrio parahaemolyticus, 2787-2788
  cellulitis from, 1296-1297
  dysentery from, 1392
  foodborne disease from, 1414t, 1415
  immune response to, 2788
Vibrio vulnificus, 2788-2789
  cellulitis from, 1296, 2789, 2789f
  foodborne disease from, 1416
  hemorrhagic bullae from, 2788-2789, 2789f
  virulence in, 2789
Vicriviroc, 706t-709t
  for HIV infection, 21-22
Vidarabine, 566t-567t, 596-597, 706t-709t
  dosage of, 738t-739t
  drug interactions with, 742t-761t
  for ocular vaccinia, 1548
  structure of, 576f
Video-assisted thoracic surgery, for pleural effusion/
    empyema drainage, 923
Vincent's angina (trench mouth), 859-860
  anaerobes in, 3085, 3115
  antimicrobial therapy for, 861t
Vincristine, for HIV-related non-Hodgkin's
    lymphoma, 1769
Vinorelbine, for Kaposi's sarcoma, 1767
Violence, intimate partner, HIV infection and,
    1627-1628
Viral attachment proteins, 1909-1910
Viral hemorrhagic fevers. *See also specific fever.*
  bioterrorism from, 3995, 3996t
    aerosol stability and, 3995, 3996t
    control of, 3995-3996
    medical response to, 3996-3998, 3997t-3998t
  characteristics of, 3996, 3997t
  clinical features of, 3996, 3998t
  laboratory diagnosis of, 3996
  rash in, 802
  secondary spread of, 3998
  tick-borne, 3659, 3659t
Viral inclusions, 1912
Viral infections. *See also specific infection.*
  in acute bronchitis, 873, 874t
  antiviral agents for. *See Antiviral agents.*
  cancer from, 1916-1917
  in cancer patients, 3799
  cellular immune response to, 139
  conjunctivitis from, 1531-1533, 1532f, 1533t
  in COPD exacerbations, 879
  in cutaneous HIV infection, 1716, 1716f
  encephalitis from, 1183, 1243-1263
    etiologies of, 1250-1260, 1251t-1252t
  gastroenteritis from, 1362-1363, 1362t
  in hematopoietic stem cell transplant recipients,
    3828-3831
  host responses to, 1917-1918
  immunomodulators for, 565
  meningitis from. *See Meningitis, viral.*
  myocarditis from, 1153-1154, 1154t
  pericarditis from, 1161, 1161t
  pneumonia from. *See Pneumonia, viral.*
  pulmonary host defense and, 894
  of respiratory tract
    in COPD exacerbations, 879
    in solid organ transplant recipients, 3847-3848
  rhinosinusitis from, 2393. *See also Common
    cold.*
  in solid organ transplant recipients, 3846-3849
  tick-borne, 3657-3660
  in transplant recipients, 3812t
  virucidal agents for, 565
  zoonotic, 4000t-4001t
Viral load monitoring, during antiretroviral therapy,
    1847-1848
Viral RNA, replication of, 2390
Viramidine, 599
Viremia, in viral meningitis, 1194

Viridans *Streptococcus* group. *See Streptococcus
    viridans* group.
Virions, 1907, 1908f
Virucidal agents, 565
Virucidal therapy, for rhinovirus infections, 2397
Virucide, 3677
Virulence, 186
  definition of, 3
  molecular perspective on, 1-13
  nutritional status and, 157-158, 158f
  regulation of, 7-9, 8t
  of viruses, determinants of, 1917
Virulence factors. *See also under specific pathogen.*
  definition of, 3
  of Enterobacteriaceae organisms, 2818
  in gastrointestinal infections, 1342-1343
  phage-encoded, 5, 5t
  plasmid-encoded, 5, 5t
Virulence genes, in pathogenicity, 5, 5t, 10-11
Virus(es), 1905-1921. *See also specific virus.*
  antibody neutralization of, 1917-1918
  antigen tests for, 245-246, 246t, 258
  assembly of, 1908-1909
  classification of, 257t, 1907, 1908t
  culture for, 258, 259t-260t
  enveloped, 1909, 1909f
  historical perspective on, 1907
  host entry by, 1914, 1914f
  interactions of
    with cell, 1909-1913, 1910f, 1910t
    with host, 1913-1918, 1914f-1915f, 1914t
  laboratory tests for, 257-262, 257t, 259t-260t
  microscopy for, 258, 259t-260t
  nucleic acid–based tests for, 246-247, 246t,
    258-260
  oncogenic, 1916-1917
  persistence of, 1916
  in pulmonary cystic fibrosis, 951
  receptor-mediated endocytosis of, 1911, 1911f
  receptors for, 1910-1911, 1910t
  replication of, 1909-1913, 1910t
    attachment in, 1909-1911, 1910f, 1910t
    cell killing in, 1913, 1913f
    cell penetration in, 1911, 1911f
    disassembly in, 1911
    drug targeting of, 1913
    genomic, 1911-1912
  serologic tests for, 259t-260t, 260-261
  specimen collection and transport for, 257-258,
    257t
  spread of, 1914-1916, 1914f-1915f
  structure of, 1907-1909, 1908f-1909f, 1908t
  symmetry of, 1908, 1908t
  tropism of, 1916
  virulence of, determinants of, 1917
Virus-associated hemophagocytic syndrome, from
    parvovirus B19, 2091
Visceral larva migrans
  abdominal pain and/or diarrhea with eosinophilia
    from, 1407t, 1408
  from *Anisakis*, 3618, 3618t
  from *Baylisascaris procyonis*, 3618, 3618t
  versus enteric fever, 1400t-1401t, 1404
  from *Toxocara*, 3617-3618, 3618t
  treatment of, 632t-635t, 647
Visceral leishmaniasis, 632t-635t, 3464t,
    3466-3469
  clinical manifestations of, 3467-3468
  epidemiology of, 3464t, 3466-3467
  in HIV infection, 3468
  late-stage (kala-azar), 3466-3468, 3466f
  natural history of, 3467
  pathogenesis of, 3467
  treatment of, 3473-3475
Viscerotropic disease, yellow fever vaccine–
    associated, 2149
Viscerotropic leishmaniasis, 3468
Visiting nurse model, of outpatient parenteral
    antimicrobial delivery, 699, 700t
Visitors, in emergency preparedness, 229
Visual disturbances, from voriconazole, 558
Visual loss
  after endophthalmitis, 1558
  from ethambutol, 538
  from linezolid, 473

Vitamin(s)
  fat-soluble, 152-153
  water-soluble, 153
Vitamin A, 152
  deficiency of, 152
    in HIV/AIDS, 155
    in pregnant HIV-infected women, 1786
  for measles, 2234
  for pneumonia, 670t, 671-672
  toxicity of, 152
Vitamin B_6 (pyridoxine), 153
Vitamin B_{12} (cobalamin), 153
  deficiency of, in HIV/AIDS, 155
Vitamin C, 153
  for colds, 153
  deficiency of, 153
Vitamin D, 152-153
  deficiency of, 152
Vitamin D receptor
  in hepatitis B susceptibility, 52, 55
  in tuberculosis resistance, 51t
Vitamin E, 153
  deficiency of, 153
  supplementation of, in elderly, 157
Vitamin K, in acute viral hepatitis, 1589
Vititis, cotton-ball, 1555-1556
Vitrectomy, 1556-1557, 1556f
Vitreous, aspiration of, 1556, 1556f
Vitreous washings, 1556
Vittaforma, 3391, 3392t. *See also* Microsporidia.
Vogt-Koyanagi-Harada syndrome, meningitis in,
    1241
Volume of distribution, 297
  total, 297-298
Volume of peripheral compartment, 298-299
Vomiting. *See* Nausea and vomiting.
Voriconazole, 557-558, 706t-709t
  for aspergillosis, 3250, 3251t
  for *Blastomyces dermatitidis*, 3330
  for brain abscess, 1274t, 1275
  for *Candida* esophagitis, 1355t, 1356-1357
  for *Coccidioides*, 3340-3341
  dosage of, 736t-737t
  drug interactions with, 556t, 742t-761t
  for febrile neutropenia, 3804t
  formulations of, 717t
  prophylactic, in transplant recipients, 3816
  for *Pseudallescheria boydii*, 3365-3366
  for *Scedosporium prolificans*, 3366
  structure of, 550f-551f
Vulva, herpes simplex virus infection of, 1948-1949,
    1949f
Vulvar vestibulitis, 1507-1508, 1507f
Vulvitis, 1507
Vulvovaginitis. *See* Vaginitis/vulvovaginitis.

W

Wak fermenters, 3016t-3017t, 3021-3029
Walking pneumonia, 2482
Warfarin, quinolone interactions with, 494
War-related injury, *Acinetobacter* in, 2883
Warts, 169t-170t. *See also* Human papillomaviruses.
  anogenital. *See* Condylomata acuminata.
  in chromoblastomycosis, 3277, 3278f
  common (verrucae vulgaris), 2035-2036, 2039,
    2042
  cutaneous
    clinical manifestations of, 2039
    incidence and prevalence of, 2035-2036
    pathogenesis of, 2037, 2038f
    treatment of, 2042
  imiquimod for, 620
  oral, 2041, 2044
  plane (verrucae planae), 2035-2036, 2039
  plantar (verrucae plantaris), 2035-2036, 2039
  vaginal, 2044
Wasting disease
  as AIDS indicator, 1643
  chronic, 2432
  in HIV infection, 155-156, 156t, 1713-1714
Water
  biological weapon dispersal via, 3955
  Chromobacterium violaceum-contaminated,
    3019-3020

Water (Continued)
  Cryptosporidium-contaminated, 3549
  Legionella-contaminated, 2975-2976
  tap, hypochlorite solutions in, 3682
Waterborne disease, 1418, 1418t
  cryptosporidiosis as, 4004-4005
  exposure to, while traveling, protection against pathogens due to, 4016
  hepatitis A as, 2372, 2376
  leptospirosis as, 4005
  monochloramine treatment of, 2979
  shigellosis as, 2907, 2909
Water-related infection, types of, 1336, 1336t
Weaning protocols, for ventilation, 3722-3723
Weanling diarrhea, 1360-1362
Weeksella, 3016t-3017t, 3028
Wegener's granulomatosis, 943f
Weight loss, in HIV/AIDS, 155-156, 156t
Weil-Felix test, in scrub typhus, 2530
Weil's disease, in leptospirosis, 3061
Well's syndrome, versus cellulitis, 1297, 1297t
West African trypanosomiasis, 3489-3494. See also Trypanosomiasis, African.
West Nile encephalitis, 1256-1257, 4003
  clinical features of, 2146-2147, 2146f-2147f
  epidemiology of, 2139-2140, 2139t, 2141f
  geographic distribution of, 1246-1247, 1247f, 2134f
  historical perspective on, 2134
  magnetic resonance imaging in, 1248-1249
  pathogenesis of, 2143-2144
  rash in, 792-794
  transmission of, 2140f
  vaccine for, 2151
West Nile virus infection, 207-208, 208f
  in elderly, 3861
  meningitis from, 1190
  transmission of, transfusion-related, 3746
  uveitis from, 1565
Western blot assay, 65
  for HIV infection, 1672-1673, 1673f-1674f
  for human T-cell lymphotrophic virus, 2306, 2307f
  for Lyme disease, 3077-3078, 3078f
Western equine encephalitis, 1258, 2117-2125, 2118t. See also Alphaviruses.
Western Europe
  HIV infection in, 1619-1620
  HIV-infected children in, 1810
Western immunoblotting assay, for syphilis, 3046
Westley clinical score, in croup assessment, 828
Wheezing
  in bronchiolitis, 888
  in chronic pneumonia, 933
  after respiratory syncytial virus infection, 2215
Whipple's disease, 1435-1441
  classic, 1437
  diagnosis of, 1438-1439, 1438f-1439f
  epidemiology of, 1435-1436
  etiology of, 1435
  laboratory tests for, 1439
  pathogenesis of, 1435-1436
  pathology of, 1436-1437, 1437f
  prognosis for, 1440
  signs and symptoms of, 1438t
  treatment of, 1439-1440, 1440t
  uveitis in, 1566
Whipworm, 3578t, 3580-3581
White blood cells. See Leukocyte(s).
White cell casts, in urinary tract infection, 967
White piedra, 3355
Whitfield's ointment, for Scytalidium, 3353
Whole-cell pertussis vaccine, 2960-2961
Widal test for typhoid fever, 1402, 2896
Wilson's disease, hepatitis in, 1588
WIN compounds, for picornaviruses, 21t, 22
Winter vomiting disease, 1362-1363, 1362t
Wisconsin protocol for rabies, 2256-2257
Wiskott-Aldrich syndrome, 169t-170t, 171
  Staphylococcus aureus infection in, 2563
Wolbachia, 2495
Women
  condoms for, 1651
  genital gonococcal infections in, 2759-2763, 2760f
  genital tuberculosis in, 3157

Women (Continued)
  genitourinary tract infections in. See Genitourinary tract infections, female.
  gynecologic surgery in, surgical site infection after, 1514-1516, 1514t, 1515f
  HIV infection in, 1781-1807. See also Human immunodeficiency virus infection, in women.
  mycoplasmal infections in, 2491-2492
  pelvic infections in, 1511-1519. See also Pelvic infection(s); Pelvic inflammatory disease.
    anaerobic, 3085-3086
  pregnant. See Pregnancy.
  urinary tract infection in, 958, 962, 965, 969-970
Woodchuck hepatitis virus (WHV), 2059
Woolsorter's disease, 2719
Wound botulism, 3097, 3099
Wound healing, hyperbaric oxygen therapy for, 625
Wound infections
  bacterial isolates from, 3912t
  from bites, 862t, 868
  from Capnocytophaga canimorsus, 3911
  clean, 3892t, 3894
    prevention of, 522-523
  contaminated, 3892t, 3894
    occupation-related, 1302
  from Erysipelothrix rhusiopathiae, 3912
  febrile morbidity and, 3892, 3892f
  in heart transplant recipients, 3841
  in kidney transplant recipients, 3841
  from Pasteurella multocida, 3911-3912
  pathogens in, 3893t
    virulence factors of, 3894
  postsurgical, 862t, 868. See also Surgical site infections.
  prevention of, topical antibacterials in, 522-523
  from Pseudomonas aeruginosa, loss of resistance to, 2837-2838
  risk of, interventional maneuvers diminishing, 3897t
  in solid organ transplant recipients, 3844, 3844t
  specimens in, 243
Wright-Giemsa stain, 244, 244t
WU virus, 2051-2052
Wuchereria bancrofti, 654
  filariasis from, 3590, 3590f, 3590t. See also Filariasis, lymphatic.
  life cycle of, 3590
  tropical pulmonary eosinophilia from, 3592

X
X factor, for Haemophilus influenzae growth, 2911
Xanthochromia, in centrifuged cerebrospinal fluid, 1184-1185
Xanthogranulomatous pyelonephritis, 976-977, 980-981, 981f
X-linked agammaglobulinemia, 72, 169t-170t, 171
X-linked chronic granulomatous disease, 174
X-linked immunodeficiency with hyperIgG syndrome, cryptosporidiosis in, 3551
X-linked lymphoproliferative disease, 73, 169t-170t, 171
  from Epstein-Barr virus, 1995
  hepatitis in, 1587

Y
Yaba monkey tumor virus, 1935
Yatapoxvirus, 1935
Yaws, from Treponema pallidum subsp. pertenue, 3055-3056, 3056f
Yeast. See also Fungi.
  appearance of, 3223f-3224f, 3224t
  terminology for, 254, 255t
Yeast infections, genital lesions in, 1482
Yeast prions, 2427
Yellow fever
  clinical features of, 2144
  epidemiology of, 2135-2136
  geographic distribution of, 2134f
  hepatitis from, 1587
  historical perspective on, 2133
  versus malaria, 3450
  pathogenesis of, 2141-2142
  treatment of, 2149-2150

Yellow fever (Continued)
  vaccine for, 2149, 3922t, 3934
    for travelers, 4011-4012, 4011t
Yersinia, 2943-2953
  appendicitis from, 1059
  virulence factors of, 5t
  virulence regulatory systems for, 8t
Yersinia enterocolitica, 2943
  clinical manifestations of, 1392-1393, 2950-2951
  complement interactions with, 85
  description of, 2949-2950
  diagnosis of, 2951
  enteric fever–like syndrome from, 1400t-1401t, 1402
  epidemiology of, 2950, 2950f
  erythema nodosum in, 2951
  foodborne disease from, 1414t, 1415, 1419
  history of, 2949
  laboratory diagnosis of, 240t-242t, 1422
  mesenteric lymphadenitis from, 1405-1406, 1405t
  pathogenesis of, 2950
  pharyngitis in, 2596, 2951
  prevention and treatment of, 2951-2952
  reactive polyarthritis in, 2951
  septicemia in, 2951
  transmission of, 3966
Yersinia frederksenii, 2952
Yersinia intermedia, 2952
Yersinia kristensenii, 2952
Yersinia pestis, 2943-2949. See also Plague.
  antimicrobial-resistant, 2948
  as biological weapon, 2943, 3965-3970, 3967t
    history of, 3965
    potential of, 3965
  classic biovars of, 2943
  culture of, 2943, 2947
  environmental persistence of, 3969
  evolution of, 7
  genomic studies of, 2943
  history of, 2943, 2944f
  laboratory detection of, 240t-242t
  virulence and transmission factors of, 2944t
Yersinia pseudotuberculosis, 2943
  clinical manifestations of, 2951
  description of, 2949-2950
  diagnosis of, 2951
  enteric fever–like syndrome from, 1400t-1401t, 1402
  epidemiology of, 2950
  history of, 2949
  mesenteric lymphadenitis from, 1405-1406, 1405t
  pathogenesis of, 2950
  prevention and treatment of, 2951
  transmission of, 3966
Yersinia YopH effector protein, 10
Yogurt, prophylactic, for vulvovaginal candidiasis, 1502

Z
Zanamivir, 566t-567t, 597-598, 706t-709t
  formulations of, 717t
  for influenza, 2277t, 2278-2279, 2284
  polymeric conjugates of, 590-591
  resistance to, 2279
  structure of, 591f
Zidovudine, 706t-709t, 1833-1834, 1834f, 1835t
  adverse effects of, 1833
  for AIDS dementia, 1748
  dosage of, 740t-741t
  drug interactions with, 742t-761t
  efficacy of, 1789
  formulations of, 717t
  for HIV-infected children, 1820t-1821t
  myopathy from, 1759
  prophylactic
    after HIV exposure, 3755t, 3764
    in intrapartum period, 1795
    for perinatal HIV transmission, 1786, 1788, 1790t, 1792t-1793t, 1810-1811, 1811t
  resistance to, 1834
Ziehl-Neelsen stain, 251
Zinc, 153
  for common cold, 153, 670t, 673, 812
  deficiency of, 153

Zinc *(Continued)*
    in HIV/AIDS, 155
    for diarrhea, in children, 670t, 672-673
    in initial inflammatory response, 44
    for rotavirus gastroenteritis, 2111
Zoonoses, 206-209, 3999-4007. *See also specific*
    infection and vector.
    animal reservoirs for, 4002, 4002t, 4005
    arthropod reservoirs and vectors for, 4005-4006
    classification of, 3999, 4000t-4001t
    defining criteria for, 3999
    diagnosis of, 4006

Zoonoses *(Continued)*
    distribution of pathogens in, factors influencing,
        4004-4006, 4004t
    epidemiology of, 4000t-4001t, 4002-4004
    etiology of, 4000t-4001t
    global experiences with, 4003-4004
    outbreaks of, 194
    from paramyxovirus, 2237-2244
        classification of, 2237, 2238f
        Hendra virus, 2241-2242
        Menangle virus, 2242-2243
        Nipah virus, 2238-2241

Zoonoses *(Continued)*
    structure and molecular biology of,
        2237-2238
    virology of, 2237-2238
    public health impact of, 3999-4002
    from retroviruses, 1680-1681
    transmission of, 4000t-4001t
    in United States, 4003
Zoophilic dermatophytosis, 3345, 3346t
Zoster sine herpete, 1189-1190